The MERCK Manual

TWENTIETH EDITION

1st Edition – 1899
2nd Edition – 1901
3rd Edition – 1905
4th Edition – 1911
5th Edition – 1923
6th Edition – 1934
7th Edition – 1940
8th Edition – 1950
9th Edition – 1956
10th Edition – 1961
11th Edition – 1966
12th Edition – 1972
13th Edition – 1977
14th Edition – 1982
15th Edition – 1987
16th Edition – 1992
17th Edition – 1999
18th Edition – 2006
19th Edition – 2011
20th Edition – 2018

FOREIGN LANGUAGE EDITIONS
of *The Merck Manual*

Arabic—Larike Publications Services, Cyprus
Chinese—People's Medical Publishing House, Beijing
Croatian—Placebo, Split
Czech—Egem, Prague
French—Editions de Médicine, Paris
German—Elsevier, Ltd., Munich
Greek—Broken Hill Publishers, Cyprus
Hungarian—Melania, Budapest
Italian—Springer-Verlag Italia Srl (Medicom), Milan
Japanese—Nikkei Business Publications, Tokyo
Korean—Shinil Publishing Co., Seoul
Polish—-Elsevier, Ltd., Wroclaw
Portuguese—Editora Guanabara Koogan Ltda., Rio de Janeiro
Romanian—Editura All Publishers, Bucharest
Russian—Remedium, Moscow
Spanish—PanAmericana, Madrid
Turkish—Yüce, Istanbul

OTHER MERCK BOOKS

THE MERCK INDEX (SOLD TO ROYAL SOCIETY OF CHEMISTRY IN 2012)
First Edition, 1889

THE MERCK VETERINARY MANUAL
First Edition, 1955

THE MERCK MANUAL OF GERIATRICS
First Edition, 1990

THE MERCK MANUAL OF MEDICAL INFORMATION—HOME EDITION
First Edition, 1997

THE MERCK MANUAL OF HEALTH & AGING
First Edition, 2004

THE MERCK/MERIAL MANUAL FOR PET HEALTH
First Edition, 2007

THE MERCK MANUAL OF PATIENT SYMPTOMS
First Edition, 2008

THE MERCK GO-TO HOME GUIDE FOR SYMPTOMS
First Edition, 2013

Merck books are published on a nonprofit basis as a service to the scientific community and the public.

The MERCK Manual

Of Diagnosis and Therapy

TWENTIETH EDITION

Robert S. Porter, MD, *Editor-in-Chief*
Justin L. Kaplan, MD, *Deputy Editor-in-Chief*
Richard B. Lynn, MD, and Madhavi T. Reddy, MD, *Senior Assistant Editors*

Published by
MERCK SHARP & DOHME CORP., A SUBSIDIARY OF MERCK & CO., INC.
Kenilworth, NJ
2018

Editorial and Production Staff

Library of Congress Catalog Card Number 1-31760
ISBN (13 digit) 978-0-911910-42-1
ISBN (10 digit) 0-911-910-42-5
ISSN 0076-6526

Printed in the USA.

Preface

As this 20th print edition of *The Merck Manual* becomes available, most medical reference sources, including *The Manual*, have become primarily digital products. Digital publishing allows for a wealth of features and functions that cannot be duplicated in print and can be updated with an immediacy unimagined by previous generations. However, many users still enjoy the tactile satisfaction provided by a print book. Also, there are still places in the world that have limited availability of the electronic connections many of us now take for granted.

Whatever the format, what is the role of a general medical reference work such as *The Merck Manual* when detailed subspecialty information is at one's fingertips electronically? With such a vast body of knowledge available, finding a good starting place can be difficult. *The Manual* has always intended to be the first stop on the road to understanding medicine for readers encountering a medical topic for the first time or for the first time in a long time. After digesting a *Merck Manual* topic, readers will be well prepared to understand and evaluate the wealth of more detailed information available elsewhere.

As it has for almost 120 years, *The Merck Manual* focuses on discussions of specific disorders, organized by organ system or medical specialty. In its structured introductions to medical disorders, *The Manual* provides health care practitioners and students with straightforward, practical explanations of "what to do" to diagnose and treat those conditions. We discuss when to suspect a disease, the proper sequence of evaluation, and the first-line options for treatment along with selected alternatives. In addition, we provide enough background information on etiology and pathophysiology to ensure comprehension of the management recommendations. Finally, most topics end with a bulleted list of Key Points, summing up that topic's most salient features.

The Manual continues to enhance its accessibility, particularly to accommodate readers accustomed to the more carefully structured, smaller bites of information typically presented digitally. Many larger blocks of text have been broken up into new topics, more subheaders have been added, and we have made more liberal use of bulleting and other indicators of text structure.

In the interest of brevity, *The Merck Manual* print versions have never before cited references to the medical literature. However, in response to reader demand, *The Manual* has begun providing select references to articles in the primary medical literature that provide background to and expansion of our content.

Although the printed *Merck Manual* has long since grown too big to be carried in a lab coat, it has returned to the pocket in the form of native apps that can be downloaded to mobile devices. The apps contain the entire contents of the print version along with a large amount of multimedia and interactive features—all of which also are provided on our website at www.merckmanuals.com. The apps and online versions both are available free of charge without registration or advertising. But whatever the platform, we will continue to strive to keep *The Merck Manual* as useful as ever.

We thank the numerous contributors who have worked diligently with us to craft this edition, and we hope you will find it worthy of continued and frequent use. As always, suggestions for improvements will be warmly welcomed and carefully considered.

Robert S. Porter, MD
Editor-in-Chief

Committed to Providing Medical Information: Merck and The Merck Manuals

In 1899, the American drug manufacturer Merck & Co. first published a small book titled *Merck's Manual of the Materia Medica*. It was meant as an aid to physicians and pharmacists, reminding doctors that "Memory is treacherous." Compact in size, easy to use, and comprehensive, *The Merck Manual* (as it was later known) became a favorite of those involved in medical care and others in need of a medical reference. Even Albert Schweitzer carried a copy to Africa in 1913, and Admiral Byrd carried a copy to the South Pole in 1929.

By the 1980s, the book had become the world's largest selling medical text and was translated into more than a dozen languages. While the name of the parent company has changed somewhat over the years, the book's name has remained constant, known officially as *The Merck Manual of Diagnosis and Therapy* but usually referred to as *The Merck Manual* and sometimes "The Merck."

In 1990, the editors of *The Merck Manual* introduced *The Merck Manual of Geriatrics*. This new book quickly became the best-selling textbook of geriatric medicine, providing specific and comprehensive information on the care of older people. The 3rd edition was published in five languages.

In 1997, *The Merck Manual of Medical Information—Home Edition* was published. In this revolutionary book, the editors translated the complex medical information in *The Merck Manual* into plain language, producing a book meant for all those people interested in medical care who did not have a medical degree. The book received critical acclaim and sold over 2 million copies. *The Second Home Edition* was released in 2003. Merck's commitment to providing comprehensive, understandable medical information to all people continued with *The Merck Manual Home Health Handbook*, published in 2009.

The Merck Manual of Health & Aging, published in 2004, continued Merck's commitment to education and geriatric care, providing information on aging and the care of older people in words understandable by the lay public.

In 2008, *The Merck Manual of Patient Symptoms* was introduced to complement *The Merck Manual* and was intended to help newcomers to clinical diagnosis approach patients who present with certain common symptoms. A consumer version, *The Merck Manual Go-To Home Guide for Symptoms,* was published in 2013.

As part of its commitment to ensuring that all who need and want medical information can get it, Merck provides the content of The Merck Manuals on the web for free (www.merckmanuals.com) and as free native apps for mobile devices. Non-English versions are available in nine languages online and four languages in the apps. Registration is not required, and use is unlimited. The web publications are continuously updated to ensure that the information is as up-to-date as possible.

Merck also is committed to meeting the animal-health information needs of veterinarians and veterinary students. *The Merck Veterinary Manual* was first published in 1955, and the 11th edition was released in 2016. It is the preeminent text in the field of veterinary medicine.

Merck & Co., Inc., is one of the world's largest pharmaceutical companies. Merck is committed to providing excellent medical information and, as part of that effort, continues to proudly provide all of The Merck Manuals as a service to the community.

Contents

Guide For Readers

The **Contents** (p. vii) shows the pages on which readers can find the Editors and the Editorial Board members, additional reviewers, and contributors, as well as titles of sections, appendixes, and the index. Thumb tabs with appropriate abbreviations and section numbers mark each section and the index.

Each **Section** begins with its own table of contents, listing chapters and topics in that section. Chapters are numbered serially from the beginning to the end of the book.

Most **Topics** begin with a **nutshell** of the key information about that topic, set in a different font to make it stand out. Most topics end with a bulleted list of **Key Points**. Also throughout the book are periodic **Pearls & Pitfalls**, those nuggets of information that bear calling out in a special way.

The **Index** is detailed and contains many cross-entries. In addition, readers will find many **cross-references** throughout the text to specific pages where additional or related information can be found.

Running heads carry the section number and title on left-hand pages and the chapter number and title on right-hand pages.

Abbreviations and symbols, used throughout the text as essential space savers, are listed on pages ix and x. Other abbreviations in the text are expanded at first mention in the chapter or topic.

Tables and figures are referenced in the index but are not listed in a separate table of contents. An insert of color plates contains photographs of many eye, ear, endocrine, skin, and gynecologic disorders as well as infectious diseases.

Laboratory values in the book are given in conventional units. In most cases, SI units follow in parentheses. Appendix II contains several tables listing normal laboratory values for many tests conducted on blood, plasma, serum, urine, CSF, and stool.

Drugs are designated in the text by generic (nonproprietary) names. In Appendix III, many of the drugs mentioned in the book are listed alphabetically, with each generic name followed by one or more trade names.

Important: The authors, reviewers, and editors of this book have made extensive efforts to ensure that treatments, drugs, and dosage regimens are accurate and conform to the standards accepted at the time of publication. However, constant changes in information resulting from continuing research and clinical experience, reasonable differences in opinions among authorities, unique aspects of individual clinical situations, and the possibility of human error in preparing such an extensive text require that the reader exercise individual judgment when making a clinical decision and, if necessary, consult and compare information from other sources. In particular, the reader is advised to check the product information provided by the manufacturer of a drug product before prescribing or administering it, especially if the drug is unfamiliar or is used infrequently.

Note: Readers can find more current information, additional photos and imaging studies, as well as numerous multimedia enhancements at www.merckmanuals.com. Visit the web site frequently for new enhancements and the latest information on clinical developments. The Manual also is available as a native app for mobile devices.

Abbreviations

The following abbreviations are used throughout the text; other abbreviations are expanded at first mention in the chapter or subchapter.

ABG	arterial blood gas
ACE	angiotensin converting enzyme
ACTH	adrenocorticotropic hormone
ADH	antidiuretic hormone
AIDS	acquired immunodeficiency syndrome
ALT	alanine transaminase (formerly SGPT)
AST	aspartate transaminase (formerly SGOT)
ATP	adenosine triphosphate
BCG	bacille Calmette-Guerin
bid	2 times a day (only in dosages)
BMR	basal metabolic rate
BP	blood pressure
BSA	body surface area
BUN	blood urea nitrogen
C	Celsius; centigrade
Ca	calcium
cAMP	cyclic adenosine monophosphate
CBC	complete blood count
cGy	centigray
Ci	curie
CK	creatine kinase
CK-MB	creatine kinase of muscle band
Cl	chloride; chlorine
cm	centimeter
CNS	central nervous system
CO_2	carbon dioxide
COPD	chronic obstructive pulmonary disease
CPR	cardiopulmonary resuscitation
CSF	cerebrospinal fluid
CT	computed tomography
cu	cubic
D & C	dilation and curettage
dL	deciliter (= 100 mL)
DNA	deoxyribonucleic acid
DTP	diphtheria-tetanus-pertussis (toxoids/vaccine)
D/W or D	dextrose
ECF	extracellular fluid
ECG	electrocardiogram, electrocardiography
EEG	electroencephalogram, electroencephalography
ENT	ear, nose, and throat
ERCP	endoscopic retrograde cholangiopancreatography
ESR	erythrocyte sedimentation rate
F	Fahrenheit
FDA	US Food and Drug Administration
ft	foot; feet (measure)
FUO	fever of unknown origin
g	gram
GFR	glomerular filtration rate
GI	gastrointestinal
G6PD	glucose-6-phosphate dehydrogenase
GU	genitourinary
Gy	gray
h	hour
Hb	hemoglobin
HCl	hydrochloric acid; hydrochloride
HCO_3	bicarbonate
Hct	hematocrit
Hg	mercury
HIV	human immunodeficiency virus
HLA	human leukocyte antigen
HMG-CoA	hydroxymethyl glutaryl coenzyme A
Hz	hertz (cycles/second)
ICF	intracellular fluid
ICU	intensive care unit
IgA, etc	immunoglobulin A, etc
IL-1, etc	interleukin-1, etc
IM	intramuscular(ly)
INR	international normalized ratio
IU	international unit
IV	intravenous(ly)
IVU	intravenous urography
K	potassium
kcal	kilocalorie (food calorie)
kg	kilogram
L	liter
lb	pound
LDH	lactic dehydrogenase
M	molar
m	meter
MAOI	monoamine oxidase inhibitor
MCH	mean corpuscular hemoglobin
MCHC	mean corpuscular hemoglobin concentration
mCi	millicurie
MCV	mean corpuscular volume

mEq milliequivalent
Mg magnesium
mg milligram
MI myocardial infarction
MIC minimum inhibitory concentration
min minute
mIU milli-international unit
mL milliliter
mm millimeter
mmol millimole
mo month
mOsm milliosmole
MRI magnetic resonance imaging
N nitrogen; normal (strength of solution)
Na sodium
NaCl sodium chloride
ng nanogram (= millimicrogram)
NGT nasogastric tube
nm nanometer (= millimicron)
nmol nanomole
npo nothing by mouth
NSAID nonsteroidal anti-inflammatorydrug
O_2 oxygen
OTC over-the-counter (pharmaceuticals)
oz ounce
P phosphorus
$PACO_2$ alveolar carbon dioxide partial pressure
$PaCO_2$ arterial carbon dioxide partial pressure
PAO_2 alveolar oxygen partial pressure
PaO_2 arterial oxygen partial pressure
PCO_2 carbon dioxide partial pressure (or tension)
PCR polymerase chain reaction
PET positron emission tomography
pg picogram (= micromicrogram)
pH hydrogen ion concentration
PMN polymorphonuclear leukocyte
po orally
PO_2 oxygen partial pressure (or tension)
PPD purified protein derivative (tubercullin)
ppm parts per million
prn as needed
PT prothrombin time
PTT partial thromboplastin time
q every (only in dosages)
qid 4 times a day (only in dosages)
RA rheumatoid arthritis
RBC red blood cell
RNA ribonucleic acid
SaO_2 arterial oxygen saturation
sc subcutaneous
sec second
SI International System of Units
SIDS sudden infant death syndrome
SLE systemic lupus erythematosus
sp species (when referring to the singular) [eg, *Clostridium* sp]
spp species (when referring to the plural) [eg, *Nocardia* and *Myocardia* spp]
sp gr specific gravity
sq square
SSRI selective serotonin reuptake inhibitor
TB tuberculosis
tid 3 times a day (only in dosages)
TNF tumor necrosis factor
TPN total parenteral nutrition
TSH thyroid-stimulating hormone
URI upper respiratory infection
UTI urinary tract infection
vs versus
WBC white blood cell
WHO World Health Organization
wk week
wt weight
yr year
μ micro-; micron
μCi microcurie
μg microgram
μL microliter
μm micrometer (= micron)
μmol micromole
μOsm micro-osmole
mμ millimicron

Editors

Editor-in-Chief

Deputy Editor-in-Chief

Senior Assistant Editors

Editorial Board

JAMES I. McMILLAN, MD
Associate Professor of Medicine, Nephrology Fellowship Program Director, Loma Linda University

DAVID F. MURCHISON, DDS, MMS
Clinical Professor, Department of Biological Sciences, The University of Texas at Dallas; Clinical Professor, Texas A&M University Baylor College of Dentistry

ROBERT J. RUBEN, MD
Distinguished University Professor, Departments of Otorhinolaryngology–Head & Neck Surgery and Pediatrics, Albert Einstein College of Medicine and Montefiore Medical Center

DAVID A. SPAIN, MD
The Ned and Carol Spieker Professor and Chief of Acute Care Surgery, Associate Chief of General Surgery, Department of Surgery, Stanford University

JERRY L. SPIVAK, MD
Professor of Medicine and Oncology and Director, Center for the Chronic Myeloproliferative Disorders, Johns Hopkins University School of Medicine

EVA M. VIVIAN, PharmD, MS
Professor, University of Wisconsin School of Pharmacy

MICHAEL R. WASSERMAN, MD
Chief Medical Officer, Rockport Healthcare Services, Los Angeles

DAVID S. WEINBERG, MD, MSc
Professor and Chair, Department of Medicine, and Audrey Weg Schaus and Geoffrey Alan Weg Chair in Medical Science, Fox Chase Cancer Center

Additional Reviewers

WILLIAM E. BRANT, MD
Professor Emeritus, Department of Radiology and Medical Imaging, University of Virginia

MICHAEL F. CELLUCCI, MD
Assistant Professor of Pediatrics, Sidney Kimmel Medical College at Thomas Jefferson University; Attending Physician, Diagnostic Referral Division/Solid Organ Transplantation, Nemours/AI duPont Hospital for Children

ROBERT B. COHEN, DMD
Clinical Associate Professor of Dentistry, Tufts University School of Dental Medicine

SIDNEY COHEN, MD
Professor of Medicine, Sidney Kimmel Medical College of Thomas Jefferson University; Co-Director, Gastrointestinal Motility Program, Jefferson University Hospitals

EUGENE P. FRENKEL, MD
Professor of Internal Medicine and Radiology, Patsy R. and Raymond D. Nasher Distinguished Chair in Cancer Research, Elaine Dewey Sammons Distinguished Chair in Cancer Research in honor of Eugene P. Frenkel, MD, A. Kenneth Pye Professorship in Cancer Research, The University of Texas Southwestern Medical Center at Dallas

J. CARLTON GARTNER, MD
Professor of Pediatrics, Sidney Kimmel Medical College at Thomas Jefferson University; Pediatrician-in-Chief, Nemours/AI duPont Hospital for Children

CHRISTOPHER P. RAAB, MD
Associate Professor of Pediatrics, Sidney Kimmel Medical College at Thomas Jefferson University; Attending Physician, Diagnostic Referral Division, Nemours/Alfred I. duPont Hospital for Children

MELVIN I. ROAT, MD
Clinical Associate Professor of Ophthalmology, Sidney Kimmel Medical College at Thomas Jefferson University; Cornea Service, Wills Eye Hospital

STEWART SHANKEL, MD
Emeritus Professor of Medicine, Loma Linda University

CATHERINE M. SOPRANO, MD
Clinical Assistant Professor of Pediatrics, Sidney Kimmel Medical College at Thomas Jefferson University; Attending Physician, Diagnostic Referral Division, Nemours/Alfred I. duPont Hospital for Children

Contributors

DENISE M. AARON, MD
Assistant Professor of Surgery, Section of Dermatology, Dartmouth-Hitchcock Medical Center; Staff Physician, Veterans Administration Medical Center, White River Junction
Benign Skin Tumors, Growths, and Vascular Lesions; Fungal Skin Infections

SIDDIQUE A. ABBASI, MD, MSc
Assistant Professor of Medicine, Warren Alpert Medical School of Brown University; Attending Cardiologist, Director of Heart Failure, and Director of Cardiac MRI, Providence VA Medical Center
Cardiac Tumors

BOLA ADAMOLEKUN, MD
Clinical Professor of Neurology, University of Tennessee Health Science Center
Seizure Disorders

CHRIS G. ADIGUN, MD
Board-Certified Dermatologist, Private Practice, Dermatology & Laser Center of Chapel Hill
Nail Disorders

MEHDI AFSHAR, MD
Clinical Fellow in Adult Cardiology, University of Toronto
Arteriosclerosis

THANIYYAH S. AHMAD, MD, MPH
Department of Cardiothoracic Surgery, University of North Carolina
Diseases of the Aorta and Its Branches

ROY D. ALTMAN, MD
Professor of Medicine, Division of Rheumatology and Immunology, David Geffen School of Medicine at UCLA
Paget Disease of Bone

GERALD L. ANDRIOLE, MD
Royce Distinguished Professor and Chief of Urologic Surgery, Barnes-Jewish Hospital, Washington University School of Medicine
Benign Prostate Disease

PARSWA ANSARI, MD
Assistant Professor and Program Director in Surgery, Hofstra Northwell–Lenox Hill Hospital, New York
Acute Abdomen and Surgical Gastroenterology; Anorectal Disorders; GI Bleeding

NOEL A. ARMENAKAS, MD
Clinical Professor of Urology, Weill Cornell Medical School; Attending Surgeon, New York Presbyterian Hospital and Lenox Hill Hospital
Genitourinary Tract Trauma

GUY P. ARMSTRONG, MD
Cardiologist, North Shore Hospital, Auckland; Cardiologist, Waitemata Cardiology, Auckland
Valvular Disorders

THOMAS ARNOLD, MD
Professor and Chairman, Department of Emergency Medicine, LSU Health Sciences Center–Shreveport
Bites and Stings

RAUL ARTAL, MD
Professor and Chair Emeritus, Department of Obstetrics/Gynecology and Women's Health, Saint Louis University School of Medicine
High-Risk Pregnancy

EVELYN ATTIA, MD
Professor of Psychiatry, Columbia University Medical Center, New York State Psychiatric Institute; Professor of Clinical Psychiatry, Weill Cornell Medical College, New York Presbyterian Hospital
Eating Disorders

JEANNE MARIE BAFFA, MD
Associate Professor of Pediatrics, Sidney Kimmel Medical College at Thomas Jefferson University; Program Director, Pediatric Cardiology Fellowship and Director of Echocardiography, Nemours/A.I. duPont Hospital for Children
Congenital Cardiovascular Anomalies

JAMES C. BAIRD, CPO (L)
Director of Education, Hanger Clinic
Limb Prosthetics

GEORGE L. BAKRIS, MD
Professor of Medicine and Director, ASH Comprehensive Hypertension Center, University of Chicago Medicine
Hypertension

RAGHAV BANSAL, MBBS
Assistant Professor, Ichan School of Medicine at Mount Sinai
Bezoars and Foreign Bodies; Pancreatitis

DAVID H. BARAD, MD, MS
Director of Assisted Reproductive Technology, Center for Human Reproduction
Approach to the Gynecologic Patient; Symptoms of Gynecologic Disorders

PEGGY P. BARCO, MS, BSW, OTR/L, SCDCM, CDRS
Assistant Professor of Occupational Therapy and Medicine, Washington University School of Medicine
The Older Driver

ROBERT A. BARISH, MD, MBA
Professor of Emergency Medicine and Vice Chancellor for Health Affairs, University of Illinois at Chicago
Bites and Stings

JENNIFER M. BARKER, MD
Associate Professor of Pediatrics, Division of Pediatric Endocrinology, Children's Hospital Colorado
Polyglandular Deficiency Syndromes

ROSEMARY BASSON, MD
Clinical Professor, Department of Psychiatry, University of British Columbia; Director, UBC Sexual Medicine Program
Sexual Dysfunction in Women

JAMES R. BERENSON, MD
President and Chief Medical Officer, Institute for Myeloma and Bone Cancer Research
Plasma Cell Disorders

JOHN L. BERK, MD
Associate Professor of Medicine and Assistant Director, Amyloidosis Center, Boston University Medical Center
Amyloidosis

BARBARA J. BERKMAN, DSW, PhD
Helen Rehr/Ruth Fitzdale Professor Emerita, Columbia University School of Social Work
Elder Abuse; Social Issues in the Elderly

CHESTON M. BERLIN, Jr., MD
University Professor of Pediatrics and Professor of Pharmacology, Penn State University College of Medicine
Principles of Drug Treatment in Children

RICHARD W. BESDINE, MD
Professor of Medicine, Greer Professor of Geriatric Medicine, and Director, Division of Geriatrics and Palliative Medicine and of the Center for Gerontology and Healthcare Research, Warren Alpert Medical School of Brown University
Approach to the Geriatric Patient; Aging and Quality of Life

RAJEEV BHATIA, MD
Associate Professor of Pediatrics, Northeast Ohio Medical University; Pediatric Pulmonologist, Akron Children's Hospital
Respiratory Disorders in Young Children

SCOTT W. BIEST, MD
Associate Professor of Obstetrics/Gynecology and Director of Minimally Invasive Gynecologic Surgery, Washington University School of Medicine
Uterine Fibroids

JOSEPH J. BIUNDO, MD
Clinical Professor of Medicine, Tulane Medical Center
Bursa, Muscle, and Tendon Disorders

DONALD W. BLACK, MD
Vice Chair for Education, Department of Psychiatry, University of Iowa, Roy J. and Lucille A. Carver College of Medicine
Idiopathic Environmental Intolerance

KAREN A. BLACKSTONE, MD
Assistant Professor of Medicine, Geriatrics and Palliative Care, George Washington University; Director, Palliative Care, Washington DC Veterans Administration Medical Center
The Dying Patient

MARCY B. BOLSTER, MD
Associate Professor of Medicine, Harvard Medical School; Director, Rheumatology Fellowship Training Program, Massachusetts General Hospital
Osteoporosis

JESSICA BON, MD, MS
Assistant Professor of Medicine, Division of Pulmonary, Allergy, and Critical Care Medicine, University of Pittsburgh School of Medicine
Pulmonary Rehabilitation

HERBERT L. BONKOVSKY, MD
Professor of Medicine and Chief, Liver Services and Laboratory for Liver and Metabolic Disorders, Wake Forest University School of Medicine
Porphyrias

CHARLES D. BORTLE, EdD
Director of Clinical Simulation, Office of Academic Affairs, Einstein Medical Center
Respiratory Arrest

ALFRED A. BOVE, MD, PhD
Professor (Emeritus) of Medicine, Lewis Katz School of Medicine, Temple University
Injury During Diving or Work in Compressed Air

THOMAS G. BOYCE, MD, MPH
Associate Professor of Pediatrics and Consultant in Pediatric Infectious Diseases and Immunology, Mayo Clinic College of Medicine
Gastroenteritis

SIMEON A. BOYADJIEV BOYD, MD
Professor of Pediatrics and Genetics, Section of Genetics, Department of Genetics, University of California, Davis
Congenital Craniofacial and Musculoskeletal Abnormalities

CHRISTOPHER J. BRADY, MD
Assistant Professor of Ophthalmology, Wilmer Eye Institute, Retina Division, Johns Hopkins University School of Medicine
Symptoms of Ophthalmologic Disorders

EVAN M. BRAUNSTEIN, MD, PhD
Assistant Professor of Medicine, Division of Hematology, Department of Medicine, Johns Hopkins School of Medicine
Anemias Caused by Deficient Erythropoiesis; Anemias Caused by Hemolysis; Approach to the Patient With Anemia

GEORGE R. BROWN, MD
Professor and Associate Chairman of Psychiatry, East Tennessee State University; Adjunct Professor of Psychiatry, University of North Texas
Sexuality, Gender Dysphoria, and Paraphilias

HAYWOOD L. BROWN, MD
F. Bayard Carter Professor of Obstetrics and Gynecology, Duke University Medical Center
Approach to the Pregnant Woman and Prenatal Care; Normal Labor and Delivery

CHRISTOPHER BRUNO, MD
Assistant Professor of Medicine, Division of infectious Diseases & HIV Medicine, Drexel University College of Medicine
Bacteria and Antibacterial Drugs

ERIKA F. BRUTSAERT, MD
Assistant Professor, Albert Einstein College of Medicine; Attending Physician, Montefiore Medical Center
Diabetes Mellitus and Disorders of Carbohydrate Metabolism

LARRY M. BUSH, MD
Affiliate Professor of Clinical Biomedical Sciences, Charles E. Schmidt College of Medicine, Florida Atlantic University; Affiliate Associate Professor of Medicine, University of Miami-Miller School of Medicine
Gram-Negative Bacilli; Gram-Positive Bacilli; Gram-Positive Cocci; Neisseriaceae; Spirochetes

JERROLD T. BUSHBERG, PhD, DABMP
Clinical Professor, Radiology and Radiation Oncology, and Director of Health Physics Program, School of Medicine, University of California, Davis
Radiation Exposure and Contamination

EDWARD R. CACHAY, MD, MAS
Professor of Clinical Medicine, Department of Medicine and Division of Infectious Diseases–Owen Clinic, University of California, San Diego
Human Immunodeficiency Virus Infection

ANDREW CALABRIA, MD
Assistant Professor of Pediatrics, Perelman School of Medicine at The University of Pennsylvania; Attending Physician, Division of Endocrinology & Diabetes, The Children's Hospital of Philadelphia
Endocrine Disorders in Children

DANIELLE CAMPAGNE, MD
Associate Clinical Professor, Department of Emergency Medicine, University of San Francisco–Fresno
Fractures, Dislocations, and Sprains

CAROLINE CARNEY, MD, MSc
Chief Medical Officer, Magellan Healthcare
Approach to the Patient With Mental Symptoms

DAVID B. CARR, MD
Alan A. and Edith L. Wolff Professor of Geriatric Medicine, Professor of Medicine and Neurology, and Clinical Director, Division of Geriatrics and Nutritional Science, Washington University School of Medicine
The Older Driver

MARY T. CASERTA, MD
Professor of Pediatrics, Division of Infectious Diseases, University of Rochester School of Medicine and Dentistry; Attending Physician, Golisano Children's Hospital, University of Rochester Medical Center
Enteroviruses; Infections in Neonates; Miscellaneous Viral Infections in Infants and Children; Pox Viruses

MICHAEL F. CELLUCCI, MD
Assistant Professor of Pediatrics, Sidney Kimmel Medical College at Thomas Jefferson University; Attending Physician, Diagnostic Referral Division/Solid Organ Transplantation, Nemours/A.I. duPont Hospital for Children
Dehydration and Fluid Therapy in Children

BRUCE A. CHABNER, MD
Director of Clinical Research, Massachusetts General Hospital Cancer Center; Professor of Medicine, Harvard Medical School
Overview of Cancer; Principles of Cancer Therapy

WALTER W. CHAN, MD, MPH
Assistant Professor of Medicine, Harvard Medical School; Director, Center for Gastrointestinal Motility, Division of Gastroenterology, Hepatology and Endoscopy, Brigham and Women's Hospital
Diagnostic and Therapeutic GI Procedures

IAN M. CHAPMAN, MBBS, PhD
Professor of Medicine, Discipline of Medicine, University of Adelaide, Royal Adelaide Hospital
Pituitary Disorders

LOIS CHOI-KAIN, MD
Assistant Professor of Psychiatry, Harvard Medical School; Medical and Program Director, Gunderson Residence of McLean Hospital; Director, McLean Borderline Personality Disorder Training Institute
Personality Disorders

ALFRED J. CIANFLOCCO, MD
Director, Primary Care Sports Medicine, Cleveland Clinic Sports Health; Department of Orthopaedic Surgery, Cleveland Clinic
Neck and Back Pain

JESSE M. CIVAN, MD
Assistant Professor and Medical Director, Liver Tumor Center, Thomas Jefferson University Hospital
Fibrosis and Cirrhosis

PAULA J. CLAYTON, MD
Professor Emeritus, University of Minnesota School of Medicine; American Foundation for Suicide Prevention
Suicidal Behavior and Self-Injury

ERIN G. CLIFTON, PhD
Department of Psychological Sciences, Case Western Reserve University
Domestic Violence and Rape

ELIZABETH L. COBBS, MD
Professor of Medicine, Geriatrics and Palliative Care, George Washington University; Chief, Geriatrics, Extended Care and Palliative Care, Washington DC Veterans Administration Medical Center
The Dying Patient

WILLIAM J. COCHRAN, MD
Associate, Department of Pediatric Gastroenterology and Nutrition, Geisinger Clinic, Danville, PA; Clinical Professor, Department of Pediatrics, Temple University School of Medicine
Congenital Gastrointestinal Anomalies; Gastrointestinal Disorders in Neonates and Infants

KATHRYN COLBY, MD, PhD
Louis Block Professor and Chair, Department of Ophthalmology & Visual Science, University of Chicago School of Medicine
Eye Trauma

RAFAEL ANTONIO CHING COMPANIONI, MD
Icahn School of Medicine at Mount Sinai, Elmhurst Hospital Center
Inflammatory Bowel Disease

DEBORAH M. CONSOLINI, MD
Assistant Professor of Pediatrics, Sidney Kimmel Medical College of Thomas Jefferson University; Chief, Division of Diagnostic Referral, Nemours/Alfred I. duPont Hospital for Children
Care of Newborns and Infants; Caring for Sick Children and Their Families; Health Supervision of the Well Child; Symptoms in Infants and Children

BAŞAK ÇORUH, MD
Assistant Professor, Division of Pulmonary, Critical Care, and Sleep Medicine, University of Washington
Bronchiectasis and Atelectasis

WILLIAM CORYELL, MD
George Winokur Professor of Psychiatry, Carver College of Medicine at University of Iowa
Mood Disorders

RICARDO A. CRUCIANI, MD, PhD
Chair and Professor, Department of Neurology, and Director, Center for Pain Palliative Medicine, Drexel University College of Medicine
Neurotransmission

JIMENA CUBILLOS, MD
Associate Professor of Clinical Urology and Pediatrics, University of Rochester School of Medicine and Dentistry
Congenital Renal and Genitourinary Anomalies

PATRICIA A. DALY, MD
Medical Director for Diabetes, Valley Health System; Visiting Assistant Professor of Clinical Medicine, University of Virginia
Multiple Endocrine Neoplasia Syndromes

DANIEL F. DANZL, MD
Professor and Chair, Department of Emergency Medicine, University of Louisville School of Medicine
Cold Injury

SHINJITA DAS, MD
Instructor in Dermatology, Harvard Medical School; Assistant in Dermatology, Massachusetts General Hospital
Pigmentation Disorders; Psoriasis and Scaling Diseases; Sweating Disorders

NORMAN L. DEAN, MD
Private Consultant, Internal/Pulmonary Medicine, Chapel Hill; Lifetime Fellow, American College of Physicians
Drowning

PETER J. DELVES, PhD
Professor of Immunology, Division of Infection & Immunity, Faculty of Medical Sciences, University College London
Allergic, Autoimmune, and Other Hypersensitivity Disorders; Biology of the Immune System

MARC A. De MOYA, MD
Chief, Division of Trauma, Critical Care, and Acute Care Surgery, Medical College of Wisconsin
Shock and Fluid Resuscitation

ARA DerMARDEROSIAN, PhD
Professor Emeritus of Biology and Pharmacognosy, University of the Sciences
Dietary Supplements

DEEPINDER K. DHALIWAL, MD, L.Ac
Professor, Department of Ophthalmology, University of Pittsburgh School of Medicine
Refractive Error

A. DAMIAN DHAR, MD, JD
Private Practice, North Atlanta Dermatology
Bacterial Skin Infections

MICHAEL C. DiMARINO, MD
Clinical Assistant Professor, Sidney Kimmel Medical College at Thomas Jefferson University
Diverticular Disease

JOEL E. DIMSDALE, MD
Professor Emeritus, Department of Psychiatry, University of California, San Diego
Somatic Symptom and Related Disorders

JAMES G. H. DINULOS, MD
Clinical Associate Professor of Surgery (Dermatology Section), Geisel School of Medicine at Dartmouth; Clinical Assistant Professor of Dermatology, University of Connecticut
Cornification Disorders; Parasitic Skin Infections; Viral Skin Diseases

KARL DOGHRAMJI, MD
Professor of Psychiatry, Neurology, and Medicine, and Medical Director, Jefferson Sleep Disorders Center, Thomas Jefferson University
Sleep and Wakefulness Disorders

JAMES D. DOUKETIS, MD
Professor, Divisions of General Internal Medicine, Hematology and Thromboembolism, Department of Medicine, McMaster University; Director, Vascular Medicine Research Program, St. Joseph's Healthcare Hamilton
Lymphatic Disorders; Peripheral Venous Disorders

ANTONETTE T. DULAY, MD
Attending Physician, Maternal-Fetal Medicine Section, Department of Obstetrics and Gynecology, Main Line Health System; Senior Physician, Axia Women's Health
Abnormalities of Pregnancy

JEFFREY S. DUNGAN, MD
Associate Professor, Clinical Genetics, Department of Obstetrics and Gynecology, Northwestern University Feinberg School of Medicine
Prenatal Genetic Counseling and Evaluation

DERRICK A. DUPRE, MD
Department of Neurosurgery, Allegheny General Hospital; Drexel University College of Medicine
Spinal Trauma; Traumatic Brain Injury

SOUMITRA R. EACHEMPATI, MD
Professor of Surgery, Professor of Medicine in Medical Ethics, and Director, Surgical Intensive Care Unit, Weill Cornell Medical College, New York Presbyterian Hospital
Approach to the Critically Ill Patient

JOSEPHINE ELIA, MD
Professor of Psychiatry and Human Behavior, Professor of Pediatrics, Sidney Kimmel Medical College of Thomas Jefferson University; Attending Physician, Nemours/A.I. duPont Hospital for Children
Mental Disorders in Children and Adolescents

B. MARK EVERS, MD
Professor and Vice-Chair of Surgery; Markey Cancer Foundation Endowed Chair; Director, Lucille P. Markey Cancer Center; Physician-in-Chief, Oncology Service Line UK Healthcare, University of Kentucky
Carcinoid Tumors

STEPHEN J. FALCHEK, MD
Director, Residency Program and formerly Division Chief of Pediatric Neurology, Nemours/A.I. duPont Hospital for Children; Instructor, Sidney Kimmel Medical College of Thomas Jefferson University
Congenital Neurologic Anomalies

MARK A. FARBER, MD
Professor of Surgery and Radiology, Division of Vascular Surgery, University of North Carolina; Program Director in Vascular Surgery; Director, University of North Carolina Aortic Network
Diseases of the Aorta and Its Branches

ABIMBOLA FARINDE, PhD, PharmD
Professor, Columbia Southern University, Orange Beach, AL
Pharmacodynamics

CHRISTOPHER M. FECAROTTA, MD
Attending Physician, Phoenix Children's Hospital
Eye Defects and Conditions in Children

NORAH C. FEENY, PhD
Professor, Department of Psychology, Case Western Reserve University
Domestic Violence and Rape

CAROLYN FEIN LEVY, MD
Assistant Professor, Hofstra Northwell School of Medicine
Histiocytic Syndromes

JAMES M. FERNANDEZ, MD, PhD
Clinical Assistant Professor of Medicine, Cleveland Clinic Lerner College of Medicine at Case Western Reserve University, Director, Allergy and Clinical Immunology, Louis Stokes VA Medical Center, Wade Park; Cleveland Clinic, Staff, Department of Allergy and Clinical Immunology
Immunodeficiency Disorders

BRADLEY D. FIGLER, MD
Assistant Professor of Urology, University of North Carolina
Genitourinary Tests and Procedures

T. ERNESTO FIGUEROA, MD
Professor of Urology and Pediatrics, Sidney Kimmel Medical College of Thomas Jefferson University; Chief, Division of Pediatric Urology, Nemours/A.I. duPont Nemours Hospital for Children
Incontinence in Children

DAVID N. FINEGOLD, MD
Professor of Human Genetics, Department of Human Genetics, Graduate School of Public Health, University of Pittsburgh
General Principles of Medical Genetics

MARVIN P. FRIED, MD
Professor and University Chairman, Department of Otorhinolaryngology-Head and Neck Surgery, Montefiore Medical Center, The University Hospital of Albert Einstein College of Medicine
Approach to the Patient With Nasal and Pharyngeal Symptoms; Nose and Paranasal Sinus Disorders

LARA A. FRIEL, MD, PhD
Associate Professor, Maternal-Fetal Medicine Division, Department of Obstetrics, Gynecology, and Reproductive Sciences, University of Texas Health Medical School at Houston, McGovern Medical School
Pregnancy Complicated by Disease

DMITRY GABRILOVICH, MD, PhD
Christopher M. Davis Professor in Cancer Research and Program Leader, Translational Tumor Immunology, The Wistar Institute; Professor, Department of Pathology and Laboratory Medicine, Perelman School of Medicine at the University of Pennsylvania
Tumor Immunology

PIERLUIGI GAMBETTI, MD
Professor of Pathology, Case Western Reserve University
Prion Diseases

JAMES A. GARRITY, MD
Whitney and Betty MacMillan Professor of Ophthalmology, Mayo Clinic College of Medicine
Eyelid and Lacrimal Disorders; Optic Nerve Disorders; Orbital Diseases

MARGERY GASS, MD
Board of Trustees, International Menopause Society
Menopause

DAVID M. GERSHENSON, MD
Professor and Chairman, Department of Gynecologic Oncology and Reproductive Medicine, The University of Texas MD Anderson Cancer Center
Gynecologic Tumors

ERIC B. GIBSON, MD
Associate Professor, Neonatal-Perinatal Medicine, Sidney Kimmel Medical College of Thomas Jefferson University; Attending Physician, Nemours/A.I. duPont Hospital for Children
Perinatal Problems

ELIAS A. GIRALDO, MD, MS
Professor of Neurology and Director, Neurology Residency Program, University of Central Florida College of Medicine
Stroke

MARK T. GLADWIN, MD
Jack D. Myers Professor and Chair, Department of Medicine, University of Pittsburgh School of Medicine; Director, Pittsburgh Heart, Lung, and Blood Vascular Medicine Institute
Pulmonary Hypertension

STEPHEN J. GLUCKMAN, MD
Professor of Medicine, Perelman School of Medicine at The University of Pennsylvania; Medical Director, Penn Global Medicine
Chronic Fatigue Syndrome

ANNE CAROL GOLDBERG, MD
Professor of Medicine, Division of Endocrinology, Metabolism and Lipid Research, Department of Medicine, Washington University School of Medicine
Lipid Disorders

MERCEDES E. GONZALEZ, MD
Clinical Assistant Professor of Dermatology, University of Miami Miller School of Medicine; Clinical Assistant Professor of Dermatology, Florida International University Herbert Wertheim College of Medicine; Medical Director, Pediatric Dermatology of Miami
Dermatitis

HECTOR A. GONZALEZ-USIGLI, MD
Professor of Neurology, HE UMAE Centro Médico Nacional de Occidente; Movement Disorders Clinic, Neurology at IMSS
Movement and Cerebellar Disorders

CARMEN E. GOTA, MD
Assistant Professor of Internal Medicine, Cleveland Clinic Lerner College of Medicine at Case Western Reserve University; Senior Staff, Department of Rheumatology, Orthopedic and Rheumatologic Institute, Center for Vasculitis Care and Research
Vasculitis

EVAN GRABER, DO
Clinical Assistant Professor of Pediatrics, Sidney Kimmel Medical College of Thomas Jefferson University; Pediatric Endocrinologist, Nemours/A.I. duPont Hospital for Children
Growth and Development

NORTON J. GREENBERGER, MD
Clinical Professor of Medicine, Harvard Medical School; Senior Physician, Brigham and Women's Hospital
Symptoms of GI Disorders

JOHN E. GREENLEE, MD
Professor and Executive Vice Chair, Department of Neurology, University of Utah School of Medicine
Brain Infections; Meningitis

JOHN J. GREGORY, Jr., MD
Assistant Professor of Pediatrics, Rutgers, New Jersey Medical School; Attending Physician, Goryeb Children's Hospital, Atlantic Health
Pediatric Cancers

JOHN H. GREIST, MD
Clinical Professor of Psychiatry, University of Wisconsin School of Medicine and Public Health; Distinguished Senior Scientist, Madison Institute of Medicine
Anxiety and Stressor-Related Disorders

ASHLEY B. GROSSMAN, MD
Emeritus Professor of Endocrinology, University of Oxford; Fellow, Green-Templeton College; Professor of Neuroendocrinology, Barts and the London School of Medicine; Consultant NET Endocrinologist, Royal Free Hospital, London
Adrenal Disorders

RAVINDU GUNATILAKE, MD
Director of Clinical Perinatal Medicine, Director of Obstetrical Research, Valley Perinatal Services
Drugs in Pregnancy

JENNIFER GURNEY, MD
Adjunct Assistant Professor, Uniformed Services of the Health Sciences
Care of the Surgical Patient

RULA A. HAJJ-ALI, MD
Associate Professor, Cleveland Clinic Lerner College of Medicine at Case Western Reserve University; Staff Physician, Center of Vasculitis Care and Research, Department of Rheumatic and Immunologic Disease, Cleveland Clinic
Autoimmune Rheumatic Disorders

JESSE B. HALL, MD
Professor Emeritus of Medicine and Anesthesia and Critical Care, University of Chicago School of Medicine
Respiratory Failure and Mechanical Ventilation

JOHN W. HALLETT, Jr., MD
Clinical Professor, Division of Vascular Surgery, Medical University of South Carolina
Peripheral Arterial Disorders

JAMES PETER ADAM HAMILTON, MD
Assistant Professor of Medicine, Division of Gastroenterology and Hepatology, Johns Hopkins University School of Medicine
Iron Overload

MARGARET R. HAMMERSCHLAG, MD
Professor of Pediatrics and Medicine and Director, Pediatric Infectious Disease Fellowship Program, State University of New York Downstate Medical Center
Chlamydia and Mycoplasmas

KEVIN C. HAZEN, PhD
Professor of Pathology and Director of Clinical Microbiology, Duke University Health System
Laboratory Diagnosis of Infectious Disease

L. AIMEE HECHANOVA, MD
Assistant Professor of Medicine, Loma Linda University; Attending Nephrologist, Loma Linda University Medical Center
Renal Replacement Therapy; Renal Transport Abnormalities

R. PHILLIPS HEINE, MD
Professor and Director, Division of Maternal-Fetal Medicine, Department of Obstetrics and Gynecology, Duke University Medical Center
Symptoms During Pregnancy

STEVEN K. HERRINE, MD
Professor of Medicine, Division of Gastroenterology and Hepatology, and Vice Dean for Academic Affairs, Sidney Kimmel Medical College at Thomas Jefferson University
Approach to the Patient With Liver Disease; Drugs and the Liver; Liver Masses and Granulomas

JEROME M. HERSHMAN, MD, MS
Distinguished Professor of Medicine Emeritus, David Geffen School of Medicine at UCLA; Director of the Endocrine Clinic, West Los Angeles VA Medical Center
Thyroid Disorders

MARTIN HERTL, MD, PhD
Jack Fraser Smith Professor of Surgery, Director of Solid Organ Transplantation, and Chief Surgical Officer, Rush University Medical Center
Transplantation

LYALL A. J. HIGGINSON, MD
Professor of Medicine, University of Ottawa; Clinical Cardiologist, Division of Cardiology, University of Ottawa Heart Institute
Symptoms of Cardiovascular Disorders

IRVIN H. HIRSCH, MD
Clinical Professor of Urology, Sidney Kimmel Medical College of Thomas Jefferson University
Male Reproductive Endocrinology and Related Disorders; Male Sexual Dysfunction

BRIAN D. HOIT, MD
Professor of Medicine and Physiology and Biophysics, Case Western Reserve University; Director of Echocardiography, Harrington HVI, University Hospitals Cleveland Medical Center
Pericarditis

JUEBIN HUANG, MD, PhD
Assistant Professor, Department of Neurology, Memory Impairment and Neurodegenerative Dementia (MIND) Center, University of Mississippi Medical Center
Delirium and Dementia; Function and Dysfunction of the Cerebral Lobes

WENDY W. HUANG, MD
Attending Physician, Phoenix Children's Hospital
Eye Defects and Conditions in Children

VICTOR F. HUCKELL, MD
Clinical Professor of Medicine, University of British Columbia; Staff Cardiologist, Vancouver General Hospital
Endocarditis

MICHAEL C. IANNUZZI, MD, MBA
Professor, Hofstra Northwell School of Medicine; Chair, Department of Medicine, Staten Island University Hospital
Sarcoidosis

HAKAN ILASLAN, MD
Associate Professor of Radiology, Cleveland Clinic Lerner College of Medicine at Case Western Reserve University; Staff Radiologist, Imaging Institute, Diagnostic Radiology
Principles of Radiologic Imaging; Tumors of Bones and Joints

TALHA H. IMAM, MD
Assistant Clinical Professor in Internal Medicine and Nephrology, University of Riverside School of Medicine; Attending Physician, Department of Nephrology, Kaiser Permanente
Urinary Tract Infections

HARRY S. JACOB, MD
George Clark Professor of Medicine and Laboratory Medicine (Emeritus), University of Minnesota Medical School; Founding Chief Medical Editor, *HemOnc Today*
Spleen Disorders

NAVIN JAIPAUL, MD, MHS
Associate Professor of Medicine, Loma Linda University School of Medicine; Chief of Nephrology, VA Loma Linda Healthcare System
Cystic Kidney Disease; Glomerular Disorders; Tubulointerstitial Diseases

LARRY E. JOHNSON, MD, PhD
Associate Professor of Geriatrics and Family and Preventive Medicine, University of Arkansas for Medical Sciences; Medical Director, Community Living Center, Central Arkansas Veterans Healthcare System
Mineral Deficiency and Toxicity; Vitamin Deficiency, Dependency, and Toxicity

BRIAN D. JOHNSTON
Director of Education, International Association of Resistance Trainers; Director of Education, Prescribed Exercise Clinics
Exercise

JAIME JORDAN, MD
Assistant Professor and Vice Chair, Acute Care College, David Geffen School of Medicine at UCLA; Associate Director, Residency Training Program, Department of Emergency Medicine, Harbor-UCLA Medical Center
Approach to the Trauma Patient

DOUGLAS E. JORENBY, PhD
Professor of Medicine, University of Wisconsin School of Medicine and Public Health; Director of Clinical Services, University of Wisconsin Center for Tobacco Research and Intervention
Tobacco Use

MICHAEL J. JOYCE, MD
Associate Clinical Professor of Orthopaedic Surgery, Cleveland Clinic Lerner School of Medicine at Case Western Reserve University
Tumors of Bones and Joints

JAMES O. JUDGE, MD
Associate Clinical Professor of Medicine, University of Connecticut School of Medicine; Senior Medical Director, Optum Complex Care Management
Gait Disorders in the Elderly

DANIEL B. KAPLAN, PhD
Assistant Professor, Adelphi University School of Social Work
Elder Abuse; Social Issues in the Elderly

KENNETH M. KAYE, MD
Associate Professor, Division of Infectious Diseases, Department of Medicine, Brigham and Women's Hospital, Harvard Medical School
Herpesviruses

JONETTE E. KERI, MD, PhD
Associate Professor of Dermatology and Cutaneous Surgery, University of Miami Miller School of Medicine; Chief, Dermatology Service, Miami VA Hospital
Acne and Related Disorders; Principles of Topical Dermatologic Therapy

BRADLEY W. KESSER, MD
Professor, Department of Otolaryngology - Head and Neck Surgery, University of Virginia School of Medicine
External Ear Disorders

LEILA M. KHAZAENI, MD
Associate Professor of Ophthalmology, Loma Linda University School of Medicine
Approach to the Ophthalmologic Patient; Cataract

JENNIFER F. KNUDTSON, MD
Assistant Professor, Reproductive Endocrinology and Infertility, Department of Obstetrics and Gynecology, University of Texas Health Science Center at San Antonio
Female Reproductive Endocrinology

APOSTOLOS KONTZIAS, MD
Assistant Professor of Medicine and Director, Autoinflammatory Clinic, Cleveland Clinic Foundation
Hereditary Periodic Fever Syndromes; Joint Disorders

MARY ANN KOSIR, MD
Professor of Surgery and Oncology, Wayne State University School of Medicine; Karmanos Cancer Institute
Breast Disorders

THOMAS KOSTEN, MD
JH Waggoner Chair and Professor of Psychiatry, Neuroscience, Pharmacology, Immunology and Pathology, Baylor College of Medicine/MD Anderson Cancer Center
Substance-Related Disorders

DANIELA KROSHINSKY, MD, MPH
Associate Professor of Dermatology, Harvard Medical School; Attending Physician and Director, Inpatient Dermatology, Massachusetts General Hospital
Pressure Ulcers

DAVID J. KUTER, MD, DPhil
Professor of Medicine, Harvard Medical School; Chief of Hematology, Massachusetts General Hospital
Bleeding Due to Abnormal Blood Vessels; Thrombocytopenia and Platelet Dysfunction

KARA C. LaMATTINA, MD
Assistant Professor of Ophthalmology, Boston University School of Medicine
Uveitis and Related Disorders

LEWIS LANDSBERG, MD
Irving S. Cutter Professor of Medicine and Dean Emeritus, Northwestern University Feinberg School of Medicine
Multiple Endocrine Neoplasia Syndromes

ALAN LANTZY, MD
Neonatologist, West Penn Hospital, Pittsburgh
Metabolic, Electrolyte, and Toxic Disorders in Neonates

CHRISTOPHER J. LaROSA, MD
Assistant Professor of Pediatrics, Perelman School of Medicine at The University of Pennsylvania; Attending Physician, Division of Pediatric Nephrology, Children's Hospital of Philadelphia
Congenital Renal Transport Abnormalities

JENNIFER LE, PharmD, MAS, BCPS-ID
Professor of Clinical Pharmacy and Director of Experiential Education in Los Angeles, Skaggs School of Pharmacy and Pharmaceutical Sciences, University of California San Diego
Pharmacokinetics

NOAH LECHTZIN, MD, MHS
Associate Professor of Medicine and Director, Adult Cystic Fibrosis Program, Johns Hopkins University School of Medicine
Approach to the Pulmonary Patient; Diagnostic and Therapeutic Pulmonary Procedures; Symptoms of Pulmonary Disorders

JOYCE S. LEE, MD, MAS
Assistant Professor, Division of Pulmonary Sciences and Critical Care Medicine, Department of Medicine, University of Colorado Denver
Interstitial Lung Diseases

JOSEPH R. LENTINO, MD, PhD
Chief, Infectious Disease Section and Professor of Medicine, Loyola University Medical Center
Anaerobic Bacteria

MICHAEL C. LEVIN, MD
Saskatchewan Multiple Sclerosis Clinical Research Chair and Professor of Neurology and Anatomy-Cell Biology, College of Medicine, University of Saskatchewan; Adjunct Professor of Neurology, University of Tennessee Health Science Center
Approach to the Neurologic Patient; Demyelinating Disorders; Neurologic Tests and Procedures; Symptoms of Neurologic Disorders

WENDY S. LEVINBOOK, MD
Private Practice, Hartford Dermatology Associates
Hair Disorders

ANDREA LEVINE, MD
Fellow, Division of Pulmonary, Allergy, and Critical Care Medicine, University of Pittsburgh Medical Center
Pulmonary Hypertension; Pulmonary Rehabilitation

MATTHEW E. LEVISON, MD
Former Professor, School of Public Health, Drexel University; Adjunct Professor and Former Chief, Division of Infectious Diseases, College of Medicine, Drexel University; Associate Editor, Bacterial Disease Moderator, ProMED-mail, International Society of Infectious Diseases
Arboviruses, Arenaviridae, and Filoviridae

SHARON LEVY, MD, MPH
Associate Professor of Pediatrics, Harvard Medical School; Director, Adolescent Substance Abuse Program, Boston Children's Hospital
Problems in Adolescents

JAMES L. LEWIS, III, MD
Attending Physician, Brookwood Baptist Health and Saint Vincent's Ascension Health, Birmingham
Acid-Base Regulation and Disorders; Electrolyte Disorders; Fluid Metabolism

PAUL L. LIEBERT, MD
Attending Physician, Orthopedic Surgery, Tomah Memorial Hospital, Tomah, WI
Sports Injury

JANE L. LIESVELD, MD
Professor, Department of Medicine, James P. Wilmot Cancer Institute, University of Rochester Medical Center
Eosinophilic Disorders; Myeloproliferative Disorders

RICHARD W. LIGHT, MD
Professor of Medicine, Vanderbilt University Medical Center
Mediastinal and Pleural Disorders

SUNNY A. LINNEBUR, PharmD, BCPS, BCGP
Professor of Clinical Pharmacy, University of Colorado Skaggs School of Pharmacy and Pharmaceutical Sciences
Drug Therapy in the Elderly

JEFFREY M. LIPTON, MD, PhD
Professor of Pediatrics and Molecular Medicine, Hofstra Northwell School of Medicine; Professor, The Center for Autoimmune and Musculoskeletal Disease, Feinstein Institute for Medical Research; Chief, Hematology/Oncology and Stem Cell Transplantation, Cohen Children's Medical Center of New York
Histiocytic Syndromes

JOHN LISSOWAY, MD
Department of Emergency Medicine, University of New Mexico; Department of Emergency Medicine, Presbyterian Hospital
Heat Illness

JAMES H. LIU, MD
Arthur H. Bill Professor and Chair, Departments of Obstetrics and Gynecology and Reproductive Biology, UH Cleveland Medical Center; Professor, Obstetrics and Gynecology, Case Western Reserve University School of Medicine
Endometriosis

ELLIOT M. LIVSTONE, MD
Emeritus Staff, Sarasota Memorial Hospital, Sarasota, FL
Tumors of the GI Tract

PHILLIP LOW, MD
Professor of Neurology, College of Medicine, Mayo Clinic; Consultant, Department of Neurology, Mayo Clinic
Autonomic Nervous System

ANDREW M. LUKS, MD
Professor, Division of Pulmonary, Critical Care, and Sleep Medicine, University of Washington
Altitude Diseases

LAWRENCE R. LUSTIG, MD
Howard W. Smith Professor and Chair, Department of Otolaryngology-Head & Neck Surgery, Columbia University Medical Center and New York Presbyterian Hospital
Hearing Loss; Inner Ear Disorders

KRISTLE LEE LYNCH, MD
Assistant Professor of Medicine, Perelman School of Medicine at The University of Pennsylvania
Esophageal and Swallowing Disorders

SHALINI S. LYNCH, PharmD
Associate Professor, Department of Clinical Pharmacy, University of California San Francisco School of Pharmacy
Concepts in Pharmacotherapy; Factors Affecting Response to Drugs

JOANNE LYNN, MD, MA, MS
Director, Center for Elder Care and Advanced Illness, Altarum Institute
The Dying Patient

JAMES MADSEN, MD, MPH
Adjunct Associate Professor of Preventive Medicine and Biometrics, Uniformed Services University of the Health Sciences; Chief, Consultant Branch, Chemical Casualty Care Division, US Army Medical Research Institute of Chemical Defense, Aberdeen Proving Ground South, MD
Mass Casualty Weapons

PAUL M. MAGGIO, MD, MBA
Associate Professor of Surgery, Associate Chief Medical Officer, and Co-Director, Critical Care Medicine, Stanford University Medical Center
Sepsis and Septic Shock

KENNETH MAIESE, MD
Member and Advisor, Biotechnology and Venture Capital Development, Office of Translational Alliances and Coordination, National Heart, Lung, and Blood Institute; Past Professor, Chair, and Chief of Service, Department of Neurology and Neurosciences, Rutgers University
Coma and Impaired Consciousness

ANNA MALKINA, MD
Assistant Clinical Professor of Medicine, Division of Nephrology, University of California, San Francisco
Chronic Kidney Disease

J. RYAN MARK, MD
Assistant Professor, Department of Urology, Sidney Kimmel Medical College at Thomas Jefferson University
Genitourinary Cancer

JOHN MARKMAN, MD
Director, Neuromedicine Pain Management, Director, Translational Pain Research and Associate Director, Department of Neurosurgery and Neurology, Neuromedicine Pain Management Center
Pain

MELISSA G. MARKO, PhD
Senior Clinical Scientist, Nestle Nutrition
Dietary Supplements

MARGARET C. McBRIDE, MD
Professor of Pediatrics, Northeast Ohio Medical University; Pediatric Neurologist, NeuroDevelopmental Science Center, Akron Children's Hospital
Neurocutaneous Syndromes; Neurologic Disorders in Children

DOUGLAS L. McGEE, DO
Chief Academic Officer and ACGME Designated Institutional Official, Einstein Healthcare Network
Clinical Decision Making

ROBERT S. McKELVIE, MD, PhD, MSc
Professor of Medicine, Western University; Cardiologist, Secondary Prevention and Heart Failure Programs, St. Joseph's Health Care
Sports and the Heart

JESSICA E. McLAUGHLIN, MD
Obstetrics and Gynecology, Division of Reproduction, Endocrinology, and Infertility, University of Texas Health and Science Center at San Antonio
Female Reproductive Endocrinology

JAMES I. McMILLAN, MD
Associate Professor of Medicine, Nephrology Fellowship Program Director, Loma Linda University
Acute Kidney Injury

S. GENE McNEELEY, MD
Clinical Professor, Michigan State University, College of Osteopathic Medicine; Center for Advanced Gynecology and Pelvic Health, Trinity Health
Benign Gynecologic Lesions; Pelvic Relaxation Syndromes

PAMELA J. McSHANE, MD
Assistant Professor of Medicine, Section of Pulmonary and Critical Care Medicine, University of Chicago
Respiratory Failure and Mechanical Ventilation

JAY MEHTA, MD
Assistant Professor of Pediatrics, Perelman School of Medicine at The University of Pennsylvania; Clinical Director, Division of Rheumatology, The Children's Hospital of Philadelphia
Juvenile Idiopathic Arthritis

NOSHIR R. MEHTA, DMD, MDS, MS
Professor, Department of Public Health and Community Service; Associate Dean for Global Relations; Senior Advisor, Craniofacial Pain and Sleep Center, Tufts University School of Dental Medicine
Temporomandibular Disorders

SONIA MEHTA, MD
Assistant Professor of Ophthalmology, Vitreoretinal Diseases and Surgery Service, Wills Eye Hospital, Sidney Kimmel Medical College at Thomas Jefferson University
Retinal Disorders

DANIEL R. MISHELL, Jr., MD (*DECEASED*)
Endowed Professor of Obstetrics and Gynecology, Keck School of Medicine, University of Southern California
Family Planning

L. BRENT MITCHELL, MD
Professor of Medicine, Department of Cardiac Services, Libin Cardiovascular Institute of Alberta, University of Calgary
Arrhythmias and Conduction Disorders

RICHARD T. MIYAMOTO, MD, MS
Arilla Spence DeVault Professor Emeritus and Past-Chairman, Department of Otolaryngology-Head and Neck Surgery, Indiana University School of Medicine
Middle Ear and Tympanic Membrane Disorders

JOEL L. MOAKE, MD
Professor Emeritus of Medicine, Baylor College of Medicine; Senior Research Scientist and Associate Director, J.W. Cox Laboratory for Biomedical Engineering, Rice University
Coagulation Disorders; Hemostasis; Thrombotic Disorders

PAUL K. MOHABIR, MD
Clinical Professor, Medicine - Pulmonary and Critical Care Medicine, Stanford University School of Medicine
Care of the Surgical Patient

JULIE S. MOLDENHAUER, MD
Associate Professor of Clinical Obstetrics and Gynecology in Surgery, Perelman School of Medicine at the University of Pennsylvania; Medical Director of the Garbose Family Special Delivery Unit and Attending High-Risk Obstetrician at the Center for Fetal Diagnosis and Treatment, The Children's Hospital of Philadelphia
Abnormalities and Complications of Labor and Delivery; Postpartum Care and Associated Disorders

STEPHANIE M. MOLESKI, MD
Assistant Professor of Medicine, Division of Gastroenterology and Hepatology, Sidney Kimmel Medical College at Thomas Jefferson University
Approach to the GI Patient; Irritable Bowel Syndrome

JOHN E. MORLEY, MB, BCh
Dammert Professor of Gerontology and Director, Division of Geriatric Medicine, Saint Louis University School of Medicine
Principles of Endocrinology; Undernutrition

ALEX MOROZ, MD
Associate Professor of Rehabilitation Medicine, Vice Chair of Education, and Residency Program Director, New York University School of Medicine
Rehabilitation

SHELDON R. MORRIS, MD, MPH
Associate Professor of Medicine, University of California San Diego
Sexually Transmitted Diseases

SAM P. MOST, MD
Chief, Division of Facial Plastic and Reconstructive Surgery, and Professor, Departments of Otolaryngology-Head & Neck Surgery (Plastic), Stanford University School of Medicine
Facial Trauma

DAVID F. MURCHISON, DDS, MMS
Clinical Professor, Department of Biological Sciences, The University of Texas at Dallas; Clinical Professor, Texas A & M University Baylor College of Dentistry
Dental Emergencies; Symptoms of Dental and Oral Disorders

DAVID G. MUTCH, MD
Ira C. and Judith Gall Professor of Obstetrics and Gynecology and Vice-Chair, Division of Gynecology, Washington University School of Medicine
Uterine Fibroids

SRI KAMESH NARASIMHAN, PhD
Assistant Professor, Sciences, University of Rochester
Pain

EDWARD A. NARDELL, MD
Professor of Medicine and Global Health and Social Medicine, Harvard Medical School; Associate Physician, Divisions of Global Health Equity and Pulmonary and Critical Care Medicine, Brigham & Women's Hospital
Mycobacteria

URSULA S. NAWAB, MD
Associate Medical Director, Newborn/Infant Intensive Care Unit and Attending Neonatologist, Division of Neonatology, Children's Hospital of Philadelphia
Perinatal Problems

GEORGE NEWMAN, MD, PhD
Chairman, Department of Neurosensory Sciences, Albert Einstein Medical Center
Neurologic Examination

LEE S. NEWMAN, MD, MA
Professor, Departments of Environmental and Occupational Health and Epidemiology, Colorado School of Public Health; Professor of Medicine, Division of Pulmonary Sciences and Critical Care Medicine, Colorado University Anschutz
Environmental Pulmonary Diseases

ALEXANDER S. NIVEN, MD
Adjunct Professor of Medicine, Uniformed Services University of the Health Sciences; Senior Associate Consultant, Division of Pulmonary and Critical Care Medicine, Mayo Clinic
Bronchiectasis and Atelectasis

STEVEN NOVELLA, MD
Assistant Professor of Neurology, Yale University School of Medicine
Complementary and Alternative Medicine

JAMES M. O'BRIEN, Jr., MD, MSc
System Vice President, Quality and Patient Safety, OhioHealth
Tests of Pulmonary Function

ROBERT E. O'CONNOR, MD, MPH
Professor and Chair of Emergency Medicine, University of Virginia School of Medicine
Cardiac Arrest and Cardiopulmonary Resuscitation

ADEDAMOLA A. OGUNNIYI, MD
Faculty, Department of Emergency Medicine, Harbor-UCLA Medical Center; Assistant Clinical Professor, David Geffen School of Medicine at UCLA
Motion Sickness

GERALD F. O'MALLEY, DO
Professor, Sidney Kimmel Medical College at Thomas Jefferson University; Director of Toxicology, Grand Strand Regional Medical Center, Myrtle Beach
Poisoning; Recreational Drugs and Intoxicants

RIKA O'MALLEY, MD
Attending Physician, Department of Emergency Medicine, Einstein Medical Center
Poisoning; Recreational Drugs and Intoxicants

NICHOLAS T. ORFANIDIS, MD
Clinical Assistant Professor of Medicine, Thomas Jefferson University Hospital
Alcoholic Liver Disease; Testing for Hepatic and Biliary Disorders; Vascular Disorders of the Liver

VICTOR E. ORTEGA, MD, PhD
Assistant Professor, Department of Internal Medicine, Section on Pulmonary, Critical Care, Allergy, and Immunologic Diseases, Center for Genomics and Personalized Medicine Research, Wake Forest School of Medicine
Asthma and Related Disorders

JAMES T. PACALA, MD, MS
Professor and Associate Head, Department of Family Medicine and Community Health, University of Minnesota Medical School
Prevention of Disease and Disability in the Elderly

ELIZABETH H. PAGE, MD
Assistant Clinical Professor of Dermatology, Harvard Medical School; Staff Physician, Lahey Hospital and Medical Center
Approach to the Dermatologic Patient; Reactions to Sunlight

ROY A. PATCHELL, MD
Chair of Neurology, Barrow Neurological Institute; Chair of Neurology, University of Arizona–Phoenix
Intracranial and Spinal Tumors

AVINASH S. PATIL, MD
Director, Center for Personalized Obstetric Medicine, Valley Perinatal Services, Phoenix
Drugs in Pregnancy

DAVID A. PAUL, MD
Professor of Pediatrics, Sidney Kimmel Medical College at Thomas Jefferson University; Chair, Department of Pediatrics, Christiana Care Health System
Perinatal Hematologic Disorders

RICHARD D. PEARSON, MD
Emeritus Professor of Medicine, University of Virginia School of Medicine
Approach to Parasitic Infections; Cestodes (Tapeworms); Extraintestinal Protozoa; Intestinal Protozoa and Microsporidia; Nematodes (Roundworms); Trematodes (Flukes)

ALICIA R. PEKARSKY, MD
Assistant Professor of Pediatrics, SUNY Upstate Medical University, McMahon/Ryan Child Advocacy Center
Child Maltreatment

EMILY J. PENNINGTON, MD
Pulmonologist, Wake Forest School of Medicine
Asthma and Related Disorders

DANIEL M. PERAZA, MD
Adjunct Assistant Professor of Surgery, Geisel School of Medicine at Dartmouth University
Bullous Diseases

FRANK PESSLER, MD, PhD
Helmholtz Centre for Infection Research, Braunschweig, Germany; Hannover Medical School, Hannover, Germany
Bone Disorders in Children; Connective Tissue Disorders in Children; Juvenile Idiopathic Arthritis

WILLIAM A. PETRI, Jr., MD, PhD
Wade Hampton Frost Professor of Medicine and Chief, Division of Infectious Diseases and International Health, University of Virginia School of Medicine
Rickettsiae and Related Organisms

KATHARINE A. PHILLIPS, MD
Professor of Psychiatry and Human Behavior, Warren Alpert Medical School of Brown University; Private Practice of Psychiatry, New York, NY
Obsessive-Compulsive and Related Disorders

JOANN V. PINKERTON, MD
Professor of Obstetrics and Gynecology and Division Director, Midlife Health Center, University of Virginia Health System; Executive Director, The North American Menopause Society
Menstrual Abnormalities

CAROL S. PORTLOCK, MD
Professor of Clinical Medicine, Weill Cornell University Medical College; Attending Physician, Lymphoma Service, Memorial Sloan-Kettering Cancer Center
Lymphomas

NINA N. POWELL-HAMILTON, MD
Clinical Assistant Professor of Pediatrics, Sidney Kimmel Medical College at Thomas Jefferson University; Medical Geneticist, Nemours/A.I. duPont Hospital for Children
Chromosome and Gene Anomalies

GLENN M. PREMINGER, MD
James F. Glenn Professor of Urology and Chief, Division of Urologic Surgery, Duke University Medical Center; Director, Duke Comprehensive Kidney Stone Center
Obstructive Uropathy; Urinary Calculi

CRAIG R. PRINGLE, BSc, PhD (*DECEASED*)
Professor Emeritus, School of Life Sciences, University of Warwick
Respiratory Viruses; Viruses

CHRISTOPHER P. RAAB, MD
Associate Professor of Pediatrics, Sidney Kimmel Medical College at Thomas Jefferson University; Attending Physician, Diagnostic Referral Division, Nemours/Alfred I. duPont Hospital for Children
Miscellaneous Disorders in Infants and Children

RONALD RABINOWITZ, MD
Professor of Urology and Pediatrics, University of Rochester Medical Center
Congenital Renal and Genitourinary Anomalies

PEDRO T. RAMIREZ, MD
Professor, Department of Gynecologic Oncology and Reproductive Medicine, David M. Gershenson Distinguished Professor in Ovarian Cancer Research, and Director of Minimally Invasive Surgical Research and Education, The University of Texas MD Anderson Cancer Center
Gynecologic Tumors

PATRICK M. REAGAN, MD
Senior Instructor, Department of Medicine, University of Rochester Medical Center
Eosinophilic Disorders; Myeloproliferative Disorders

ROBERT W. REBAR, MD
Professor and Chair, Department of Obstetrics and Gynecology, Western Michigan University Homer Stryker M.D. School of Medicine
Infertility

WINGFIELD E. REHMUS, MD, MPH
Clinical Assistant Professor of Pediatrics, Associate Member of Department of Dermatology, University of British Columbia; BC Children's Hospital, Division of Dermatology
Hypersensitivity and Inflammatory Disorders

BARBARA RESNICK, PhD, CRNP
Professor, OSAH, and Sonya Ziporkin Gershowitz Chair in Gerontology, University of Maryland School of Nursing
Provision of Care to the Elderly

SANJAY G. REVANKAR, MD
Professor of Medicine and Director, Infectious Disease Fellowship Program, Division of Infectious Diseases, Wayne State University School of Medicine
Fungi

DOUGLAS J. RHEE, MD
Chair, Department of Ophthalmology and Visual Sciences, UH Cleveland Medical Center; Visiting Professor of Ophthalmology, Case Western Reserve University School of Medicine; Director, Eye Institute, University Hospitals
Glaucoma

MELISSA M. RILEY, MD
Assistant Professor of Pediatrics, Children's Hospital of Pittsburgh; Associate Medical Director, NICU, and Medical Director, Neonatal Transport Services, UPMC Newborn Medicine Program
Perinatal Physiology

MELVIN I. ROAT, MD
Clinical Associate Professor of Ophthalmology, Sidney Kimmel Medical College at Thomas Jefferson University; Cornea Service, Wills Eye Hospital
Conjunctival and Scleral Disorders; Corneal Disorders

BERYL J. ROSENSTEIN, MD
Professor of Pediatrics, Johns Hopkins University School of Medicine
Cystic Fibrosis

LAURENCE Z. RUBENSTEIN, MD, MPH
Professor Emeritus of Geriatric Medicine, University of Oklahoma College of Medicine; Professor Emeritus of Medicine/Geriatrics at University of California, Los Angeles
Falls in the Elderly

MICHAEL RUBIN, MD
Professor of Clinical Neurology, Weill Cornell Medical College; Attending Neurologist and Director, Neuromuscular Service and EMG Laboratory, New York-Presbyterian/Weill Cornell Medical Center
Craniocervical Junction Abnormalities; Inherited Muscular Disorders; Neuro-ophthalmologic and Cranial Nerve Disorders; Peripheral Nervous System and Motor Unit Disorders; Spinal Cord Disorders

SEAN R. RUDNICK, MD
Assistant Professor, Department of Internal Medicine, Section on Gastroenterology, Wake Forest University School of Medicine
Porphyrias

ATENODORO R. RUIZ, Jr., MD
Consultant, Section of Gastroenterology, and Head, Colon Cancer Screening Task Force, The Medical City, Pasig City, Metro-Manila, Philippines
Malabsorption Syndromes

DANIEL P. RUNDE, MD
Clinical Assistant Professor of Emergency Medicine, Carver College of Medicine at University of Iowa
Electrical and Lightning Injuries

J. MARK RUSCIN, PharmD, BCPS
Professor and Chair, Department of Pharmacy Practice, Southern Illinois University Edwardsville School of Pharmacy
Drug Therapy in the Elderly

ANNA E. RUTHERFORD, MD, MPH
Assistant Professor of Medicine, Harvard Medical School; Clinical Director of Hepatology, Brigham and Women's Hospital
Hepatitis

LAWRENCE M. RYAN, MD
Professor of Medicine, Medical College of Wisconsin
Crystal-Induced Arthritides

CHARLES SABATINO, JD
Adjunct Professor, Georgetown University Law Center; Director, Commission on Law and Aging, American Bar Association
Medicolegal Issues

BIRENDRA P. SAH, MD
Assistant Professor, Pulmonary and Critical Care Medicine, and Medical ICU Director, Upstate Medical University
Sarcoidosis

GLORIA SALVO, MD
Rotating Research Resident, Department of Gynecologic Oncology and Reproductive Medicine, MD Anderson Cancer Center
Gynecologic Tumors

VAISHALI SANCHORAWALA, MD
Professor of Medicine, Director, Autologous Stem Cell Transplant Program, and Director, Amyloidosis Center, Boston Medical Center and University School of Medicine
Amyloidosis

LEE M. SANDERS, MD, MPH
Associate Professor of Pediatrics and Chief, General Division of Pediatrics, Stanford University School of Medicine
Inherited Disorders of Metabolism

CHRISTOPHER SANFORD, MD, MPH, DTM&H
Associate Professor, Family Medicine, Global Health, University of Washington
Medical Aspects of Travel

JEROME SANTORO, MD
Clinical Professor of Medicine, Sidney Kimmel Medical College at Thomas Jefferson University; Attending Physician, Lankenau Medical Center
Immunization

RAVINDRA SARODE, MD
Professor of Pathology, Director of Transfusion Medicine and Hemostasis, and Chief of Pathology and Medical Director of Clinical Laboratory Services, The University of Texas Southwestern Medical Center
Transfusion Medicine

CLARENCE T. SASAKI, MD
The Charles W. Ohse Professor of Surgery and Director, Yale Larynx Lab, Yale University School of Medicine
Laryngeal Disorders; Oral and Pharyngeal Disorders

BRADLEY A. SCHIFF, MD
Associate Professor, Department of Otorhinolaryngology-Head and Neck Surgery, Montefiore Medical Center, The University Hospital of Albert Einstein College of Medicine
Tumors of the Head and Neck

HANS P. SCHLECHT, MD, MMSc
Clinical Associate Professor of Medicine, Department of Medicine, Division of Infectious Diseases & HIV Medicine, Drexel University College of Medicine
Bacteria and Antibacterial Drugs

STEVEN SCHMITT, MD
Associate Professor of Medicine, Cleveland Clinic Lerner College of Medicine at Case Western Reserve University; Head, Section of Bone and Joint Infections, Department of Infectious Disease, Cleveland Clinic
Infections of Joints and Bones

S. CHARLES SCHULZ, MD
Professor Emeritus, University of Minnesota Medical School; Psychiatrist, Prairie Care Medical Group
Schizophrenia and Related Disorders

MARVIN I. SCHWARZ, MD
James C. Campbell Professor of Pulmonary Medicine, University of Colorado Denver
Diffuse Alveolar Hemorrhage and Pulmonary-Renal Syndrome

LAURA SECH, MD
Family Planning Fellow, Department of Obstetrics and Gynecology, Keck School of Medicine, University of Southern California
Family Planning

PENINA SEGALL-GUTIERREZ, MD, MSc
Adjunct Associate Professor of Family Medicine and Obstetrics and Gynecology, Keck School of Medicine, University of Southern California
Family Planning

SANJAY SETHI, MD
Professor and Chief, Pulmonary, Critical Care and Sleep Medicine, and Assistant Vice President for Health Sciences, University at Buffalo SUNY
Acute Bronchitis; Lung Abscess; Pneumonia

ANUJA P. SHAH, MD
Assistant Professor, David Geffen School of Medicine at UCLA; Los Angeles Biomedical Research Institute at Harbor-UCLA Medical Center
Approach to the Genitourinary Patient; Symptoms of Genitourinary Disorders

SANJIV J. SHAH, MD
Professor of Medicine, Division of Cardiology, Department of Medicine, Northwestern University Feinberg School of Medicine
Heart Failure

UDAYAN K. SHAH, MD
Professor, Sidney Kimmel Medical College at Thomas Jefferson University; Chief, Division of Otolaryngology, Nemours/A.I. duPont Hospital for Children
Some Ear, Nose, and Throat Disorders in Children

MICHAEL J. SHEA, MD
Professor of Internal Medicine, Michigan Medicine at the University of Michigan
Approach to the Cardiac Patient; Cardiovascular Tests and Procedures

PATRICK J. SHENOT, MD
Associate Professor and Deputy Chair, Department of Urology, Sidney Kimmel Medical College at Thomas Jefferson University
Penile and Scrotal Disorders; Voiding Disorders

DARYL SHORTER, MD
Staff Psychiatrist, Michael E. DeBakey VA Medical Center; Assistant Professor, Menninger Department of Psychiatry, Baylor College of Medicine
Substance-Related Disorders

ALI A. SIDDIQUI, MD
Professor of Medicine, Division of Gastroenterology, Sidney Kimmel Medical College at Thomas Jefferson University
Gallbladder and Bile Duct Disorders

STEPHEN D. SILBERSTEIN, MD
Professor of Neurology and Director, Headache Center, Sidney Kimmel Medical College at Thomas Jefferson University
Headache

EMILY SILVERSTEIN, MD
Research Project Manager, Department of Obstetrics and Gynecology, University of Southern California Keck School of Medicine
Family Planning

ADAM J. SINGER, MD
Professor and Vice Chair for Research, Department of Emergency Medicine, Stony Brook University School of Medicine
Lacerations

MICHAEL J. SMITH, MD, MSCE
Associate Professor of Pediatrics, Division of Pediatric Infectious Diseases, and Medical Director, Pediatric Antimicrobial Stewardship, Duke University Medical Center
Childhood Vaccination

DAPHNE E. SMITH-MARSH, PharmD, BC-ADM, CDE
Clinical Assistant Professor, Department of Pharmacy Practice, College of Pharmacy, University of Illinois at Chicago; Clinical Pharmacist, Mile Square Health Center, University of Illinois at Chicago
Adverse Drug Reactions

JACK D. SOBEL, MD
Dean and Distinguished Professor of Medicine, Wayne State University School of Medicine
Fungi

DAVID E. SOPER, MD
J. Marion Sims Professor, Department of Obstetrics and Gynecology, Medical University of South Carolina
Vaginitis, Cervicitis, and Pelvic Inflammatory Disease

DAVID SPIEGEL, MD
Jack, Samuel, and Lulu Willson Professor of Medicine, Associate Chair of Psychiatry and Behavioral Sciences, Director of the Center on Stress and Health, and Medical Director of the Center for Integrative Medicine, Stanford University School of Medicine
Dissociative Disorders

JERRY L. SPIVAK, MD
Professor of Medicine and Oncology and Director, Center for the Chronic Myeloproliferative Disorders, Johns Hopkins University School of Medicine
Leukemias

THOMAS D. STAMOS, MD
Chief, Clinical Cardiology and Associate Professor of Medicine, University of Illinois at Chicago
Cardiomyopathies

DAN J. STEIN, MD, PhD
Professor and Chair, Department of Psychiatry, University of Cape Town
Obsessive-Compulsive and Related Disorders

DAVID R. STEINBERG, MD
Associate Professor, Department of Orthopaedic Surgery, and Director, Hand and Upper Extremity Fellowship, Perelman School of Medicine at the University of Pennsylvania
Hand Disorders

MARVIN E. STEINBERG, MD
Professor Emeritus, Department of Orthopaedic Surgery, Perelman School of Medicine at the University of Pennsylvania
Osteonecrosis

LAUREN STRAZZULA, MD
Resident in Dermatology, Massachusetts General Hospital
Pressure Ulcers

KINGMAN P. STROHL, MD
Professor of Medicine, Case School of Medicine, Case Western Reserve University; Program Director, Case Fellowship in Sleep Medicine, UH Cleveland Medical Center
Sleep Apnea

STEPHEN BRIAN SULKES, MD
Professor of Pediatrics, Division of Developmental and Behavioral Pediatrics, University of Rochester Medical Center
Behavioral Concerns and Problems in Children; Learning and Developmental Disorders

ROSALYN SULYANTO, DMD, MS
Instructor in Developmental Biology, Harvard School of Dental Medicine and Boston Children's Hospital
Approach to the Dental Patient

WILLIAM D. SURKIS, MD
Clinical Associate Professor of Medicine, Sidney Kimmel Medical College at Thomas Jefferson University; Program Director, Internal Medicine Residency Program, Lankenau Medical Center
Immunization

GEETA K. SWAMY, MD
Associate Professor, Division of Maternal-Fetal Medicine, Department of Obstetrics and Gynecology, Duke University Medical Center
Symptoms During Pregnancy

VICTOR F. TAPSON, MD
Director, Venous Thromboembolism and Pulmonary Vascular Disease Research Program and Associate Director, Pulmonary and Critical Care Division, Cedars-Sinai Medical Center; Director, Clinical Research for the Women's Guild Lung Institute
Pulmonary Embolism

MARY TERRITO, MD
Emeritus Professor of Medicine, Division of Hematology and Oncology, David Geffen School of Medicine at UCLA
Leukopenias

GEORGE THANASSOULIS, MD, MSc
Associate Professor of Medicine, McGill University; Director, Preventive and Genomic Cardiology, McGill University Health Center
Arteriosclerosis

DAVID R. THOMAS, MD
Professor Emeritus, Saint Louis University School of Medicine
Nutritional Support

ELIZABETH CHABNER THOMPSON, MD, MPH
Founder, BFFL Co
Overview of Cancer; Principles of Cancer Therapy

DYLAN TIERNEY, MD, MPH
Instructor, Harvard Medical School; Associate Physician, Division of Global Health Equity, Brigham and Women's Hospital
Mycobacteria

AMAL N. TRIVEDI, MD, MPH
Associate Professor, Department of Health Services, Policy and Practice and Department of Medicine, Brown University
Financial Issues in Health Care; Funding Health Care for the Elderly

ANNE S. TSAO, MD
Associate Professor and Director, Mesothelioma Program; Director, Thoracic Chemo-Radiation Program, University of Texas M.D. Anderson Cancer Center
Tumors of the Lungs

DEBARA L. TUCCI, MD, MS, MBA
Professor, Head and Neck Surgery & Communication Sciences, Duke University Medical Center
Approach to the Patient With Ear Problems

ALLAN R. TUNKEL, MD, PhD
Professor of Medicine and Medical Services; Associate Dean for Medical Education, Warren Alpert Medical School of Brown University
Biology of Infectious Disease

JAMES T. UBERTALLI, DMD
Private Practice, Hingham, MA
Common Dental Disorders; Periodontal Disorders

NIMISH VAKIL, MD
Clinical Adjunct Professor, University of Wisconsin School of Medicine and Public Health
Gastritis and Peptic Ulcer Disease

PHILBERT YUAN VAN, MD
Assistant Professor of Surgery, Division of Trauma, Critical Care and Acute Care Surgery, Department of Surgery, Oregon Health and Science University
Abdominal Trauma

MARIA T. VAZQUEZ-PERTEJO, MD
Medical Director, Division of Pathology and Laboratory Medicine, JFK Medical Center; Integrated Regional Pathology Services
Gram-Negative Bacilli; Gram-Positive Bacilli; Gram-Positive Cocci; Neisseriaceae; Spirochetes

ALEXANDRA VILLA-FORTE, MD, MPH
Staff Physician, Center for Vasculitis Care and Research, Department of Rheumatic and Immunologic Diseases, Cleveland Clinic
Approach to the Patient With Joint Disease; Pain in and Around Joints

AARON E. WALFISH, MD
Clinical Assistant Professor, Mount Sinai Medical Center
Bezoars and Foreign Bodies; Inflammatory Bowel Disease

B. TIMOTHY WALSH, MD
Ruane Professor of Psychiatry, College of Physicians and Surgeons, Columbia University; Founding Director, Eating Disorders Research Unit, New York State Psychiatric Institute
Eating Disorders

JAMES WAYNE WARNICA, MD
Professor Emeritus of Cardiac Sciences and Medicine, The University of Calgary
Coronary Artery Disease

MICHAEL R. WASSERMAN, MD
Chief Medical Officer, Rockport Healthcare Services, Los Angeles
Nonspecific Symptoms

GEOFFREY A. WEINBERG, MD
Professor of Pediatrics, University of Rochester School of Medicine and Dentistry; Director, Clinical Pediatric Infectious Diseases and Pediatric HIV Program, Golisano Children's Hospital
Human Immunodeficiency Virus Infection in Infants and Children; Miscellaneous Bacterial Infections in Infants and Children

THOMAS G. WEISER, MD, MPH
Associate Professor, Department of Surgery, Section of Trauma & Critical Care, Stanford University School of Medicine
Thoracic Trauma

ERIC A. WEISS, MD
Professor of Surgery (Emergency Medicine), Stanford University Medical Center, Emeritus; Medical Director, Stanford University Fellowship in Wilderness Medicine
Heat Illness

GREGORY L. WELLS, MD
Staff Dermatologist, Ada West Dermatology, St. Luke's Boise Medical Center, and St. Alphonsus Regional Medical Center
Cancers of the Skin

KENDRICK ALAN WHITNEY, DPM
Associate Professor, Department of Biomechanics, Temple University School of Podiatric Medicine
Foot and Ankle Disorders

FRANK H. WIANS, Jr., PhD
Professor and Clinical Chemist, Department of Pathology, Texas Tech University Health Sciences Center El Paso
Normal Laboratory Values

JACK WILBERGER, MD
Professor of Neurosurgery, Drexel University College of Medicine; Jannetta Endowed Chair, Department of Neurosurgery, Allegheny General Hospital; DIO, Chairman Graduate Medical Education Committee, Allegheny Health Network Medical Education Consortium; Vice-President, Graduate Medical Education, Allegheny Health Network
Spinal Trauma; Traumatic Brain Injury

ROBERT A. WISE, MD
Professor of Medicine, Division of Pulmonary and Critical Care Medicine, Johns Hopkins University School of Medicine
Chronic Obstructive Pulmonary Disease and Related Disorders

STEVEN E. WOLF, MD
Golden Charity Guild Charles R. Baxter, MD Distinguished Chair in Burn Surgery; Professor and Vice-Chair for Research, Department of Surgery, University of Texas–Southwestern Medical Center
Burns

ADRIENNE YOUDIM, MD
Associate Professor of Medicine, David Geffen School of Medicine at UCLA; Associate Professor of Medicine, Cedars-Sinai Medical Center
Nutrition: General Considerations; Obesity and the Metabolic Syndrome

ZHIWEI ZHANG, MD
Associate Professor of Medicine, Loma Linda University; Attending Nephrologist, VA Loma Linda Healthcare System
Renovascular Disorders

Acknowledgments

Composition, design, indexing, and proofreading services were provided by S4Carlisle. Bridget Meyer and Brigitte Fenton provided production assistance, as did Kevin Farwell and Sandie Trevethan from Vasont. Most of the line illustrations are by Christopher C. Butts or Michael Reingold.

We thank the following people and institutions for allowing us to publish their photographs in the color plates:

© Springer Science+Business Media (**Plates 1–5, 19, 22, 26, 35, 38, 45, 57, 67, 68, 76, 81, 82, 92, 96, 97, and 99**); Image provided by Piet van Hasselt, MD (**Plate 6**); Image provided by Bechara Ghorayeb, MD (**Plate 7**); Image printed with permission of Science Photo Library (**Plates 8–18, 20, 24, 25, 28, 87, 91, and 94**); Image provided by Ralph C. Eagle, Jr., and Science Photo Library (**Plate 21**); Image provided by James Garrity, MD (**Plate 23**); Image provided by Thomas Habif, MD (**Plates 27, 29–33, 36, 37, 39–41, 42 [top], 43, 46–49, 51–54, and 59–63**); Image courtesy of Allen W. Mathies, MD, California Emergency Preparedness Office, Immunization Branch, via the Public Health Image Library of the Centers for Disease Control and Prevention (**Plate 34**); Image courtesy of Dennis D. Juranek, MD, via the Public Health Image Library of the Centers for Disease Control and Prevention (**Plate 42 [bottom]**); Image provided by Gregory L. Wells, MD (**Plate 44**); Image provided by Karen McKoy, MD (**Plate 50**); Image provided by Robert MacNeal, MD (**Plate 55**); Image courtesy of www.doctorfungus.com (**Plates 56 and 58**); By permission of the publisher. From Deitcher S. In *Atlas of Clinical Hematology*. Edited by JO Armitage. Philadelphia, Current Medicine, 2004 (**Plate 64**); By permission of the publisher. From Newman C. In *Atlas of Clinical Endocrinology: Neuroendocrinology and Pituitary Disease*. Edited by SG Korenman (series editor) and ME Molitch. Philadelphia, Current Medicine, 2000 (**Plate 65**); By permission of the publisher. From Biller B. In *Atlas of Clinical Endocrinology: Neuroendocrinology and Pituitary Disease*. Edited by SG Korenman (series editor) and ME Molitch. Philadelphia, Current Medicine, 2000 (**Plate 66**); By permission of the publisher. From Joe E, Soter N. In *Current Dermatologic Diagnosis and Treatment*, edited by I Freedberg, IM Freedberg, and MR Sanchez. Philadelphia, Current Medicine, 2001. (**Plate 69**); Images courtesy of the Public Health Image Library of the Centers for Disease Control and Prevention (**Plates 70, 83, 85, 86, and 89**); Image provided by David M. Martin, MD (**Plate 71**); Image provided by Jonathan Ship, MD (**Plate 72**); Image courtesy of Dr. S. E. Thompson and J. Pledger via the Public Health Image Library of the Centers for Disease Control and Prevention (**Plate 73**); Image courtesy of James Gathany via the Public Health Image Library of the Centers for Disease Control and Prevention (**Plate 74**); Image provided by Noel Armenakas, MD (**Plate 75**); Image courtesy of Susan Lindsley via the Public Health Image Library of the Centers for Disease Control and Prevention (**Plates 77–79**); Image courtesy of Joe Miller and Dr. Cornelio Arevalo via the Public Health Image Library of the Centers for Disease Control and Prevention (**Plate 80**); Image courtesy of Dr. Heinz F. Eichenwald, New York Hospital and Cornell Medical Center, via the Public Health Image Library of the Centers for Disease Control and Prevention (**Plate 84**); By permission of the publisher. From Kaufman R, Brown D. In *Atlas of Clinical Gynecology: Gynecologic Pathology*. Edited by M Stenchever (series editor) and B Goff. Philadelphia, Current Medicine, 1998 (**Plate 88**); By permission of the publisher. From Sobel JD. In *Atlas of Infectious Diseases: Fungal Infections*. Edited by GL Mandell and RD Diamond. Philadelphia, Current Medicine, 2000. Also from Sobel JD. In *Atlas of Infectious Diseases*. Edited by GL Mandell and MF Rein. Philadelphia, Current Medicine, 1996 (**Plate 90**); By permission of the publisher. From Scott I, Warman R, Murray T: *Atlas of Ophthalmology*. Edited by RK Parrish II and TG Murray. Philadelphia, Current Medicine, 2000 (**Plate 93**); Image provided by Thomas Arnold, MD (**Plate 95**); Image provided by Steven E. Wolf, MD (**Plates 98 and 100**).

SECTION 1

Nutritional Disorders

1 Nutrition: General Considerations

Nutrition is the science of food and its relationship to health. Nutrients are chemicals in foods that are used by the body for growth, maintenance, and energy.

Nutrients that cannot be synthesized by the body and thus must be derived from the diet are considered essential. They include

- Vitamins
- Minerals
- Some amino acids
- Some fatty acids

Nutrients that the body can synthesize from other compounds, although they may also be derived from the diet, are considered nonessential.

Macronutrients are required by the body in relatively large amounts; micronutrients are needed in minute amounts.

Lack of nutrients can result in undernutrition, which can lead to deficiency syndromes (eg, kwashiorkor, pellagra). Excess intake of macronutrients can lead to obesity (see p. 19) and related disorders; excess intake of micronutrients can be toxic. Also, the balance of various types of nutrients, such as how much unsaturated vs saturated fat is consumed, can influence the development of disorders.

Macronutrients

Macronutrients constitute the bulk of the diet and supply energy and many essential nutrients. Carbohydrates, proteins (including essential amino acids), fats (including essential fatty acids), macrominerals, and water are macronutrients. Carbohydrates, fats, and proteins are interchangeable as sources of energy; fats yield 9 kcal/g (37.8 kJ/g); proteins and carbohydrates yield 4 kcal/g (16.8 kJ/g).

Carbohydrates: Dietary carbohydrates are broken down into glucose and other monosaccharides. Carbohydrates increase blood glucose levels, supplying energy.

Simple carbohydrates are composed of small molecules, generally monosaccharides or disaccharides, which increase blood glucose levels rapidly.

Complex carbohydrates are composed of larger molecules, which are broken down into monosaccharides. Complex carbohydrates increase blood glucose levels more slowly but for a longer time.

Glucose and sucrose are simple carbohydrates; starches and fiber are complex carbohydrates.

The **glycemic index** measures how rapidly consumption of a carbohydrate increases plasma glucose levels. Values range from 1 (the slowest increase) to 100 (the fastest increase, equivalent to pure glucose—see Table 1–1). However, the actual rate of increase also depends on what foods are consumed with the carbohydrate.

Carbohydrates with a high glycemic index may increase plasma glucose to high levels rapidly. It is hypothesized that as a result, insulin levels increase, inducing hypoglycemia and hunger, which tends to lead to consumption of excess calories and weight gain. Carbohydrates with a low glycemic index increase plasma glucose levels slowly, resulting in lower postprandial insulin levels and less hunger, which probably makes consumption of excess calories less likely. These effects are predicted to result in a more favorable lipid profile and a decreased risk of obesity, diabetes mellitus, and complications of diabetes if present.

Table 1–1. GLYCEMIC INDEX OF SOME FOODS

CATEGORY	FOOD	INDEX*
Beans	Kidney	33
	Red lentils	27
	Soy	14
Bread	Pumpernickel	49
	White	69
	Whole wheat	72
Cereals	All bran	54
	Corn flakes	83
	Oatmeal	53
	Puffed rice	90
	Shredded wheat	70
Dairy	Milk, ice cream, yogurt	34–38
Fruit	Apple	38
	Banana	61
	Orange	43
	Orange juice	49
	Strawberries	32
Grains	Barley	22
	Brown rice	66
	White rice	72
Pasta	—	38
Potatoes	Instant mashed (white)	86
	Mashed (white)	72
	Sweet	50
Snacks	Corn chips	72
	Oatmeal cookies	57
	Potato chips	56
Sugar	Fructose	22
	Glucose	100
	Honey	91
	Refined sugar	64

*Values may vary.

Proteins: Dietary proteins are broken down into peptides and amino acids. Proteins are required for tissue maintenance, replacement, function, and growth. However, if the body is not getting enough calories from dietary sources or tissue stores (particularly of fat), protein may be used for energy.

As the body uses dietary protein for tissue production, there is a net gain of protein (positive nitrogen balance). During catabolic states (eg, starvation, infections, burns), more protein may be used (because body tissues are broken down) than is absorbed, resulting in a net loss of protein (negative nitrogen balance). Nitrogen balance is best determined by subtracting the amount of nitrogen excreted in urine and feces from the amount of nitrogen consumed.

Of the 20 amino acids, 9 are essential amino acids (EAAs); they cannot be synthesized and must be obtained from the diet. All people require 8 EAAs; infants also require histidine.

The weight-adjusted requirement for dietary protein correlates with growth rate, which decreases from infancy until adulthood. The daily dietary protein requirement decreases from 2.2 g/kg in

Table 1–2. ESSENTIAL AMINO ACID REQUIREMENTS IN MG/KG BODY WEIGHT

REQUIREMENT	INFANT (4–6 mo)	CHILD (10–12 yr)	ADULT
Histidine	29	—	—
Isoleucine	88	28	10
Leucine	150	44	14
Lysine	99	49	12
Methionine and cystine	72	24	13
Phenylalanine and tyrosine	120	24	14
Threonine	74	30	7
Tryptophan	19	4	3
Valine	93	28	13
Total essential amino acids (excluding histidine)	715	231	86

3-mo-old infants to 1.2 g/kg in 5-yr-old children and to 0.8 g/kg in adults. Protein requirements correspond to EAA requirements (see Table 1–2). Adults trying to increase muscle mass need very little extra protein beyond the requirements in the table.

The amino acid composition of protein varies widely. Biological value (BV) reflects the similarity in amino acid composition of protein to that of animal tissues; thus, BV indicates what percentage of a dietary protein provides EAAs for the body:

- A perfect match is egg protein, with a value of 100.
- Animal proteins in milk and meat have a high BV (~90).
- Proteins in cereal and vegetables have a lower BV (~40)
- Some derived proteins (eg, gelatin) have a BV of 0.

The extent to which dietary proteins supply each other's missing amino acids (complementarity) determines the overall BV of the diet. The recommended daily allowances (RDA) for protein assumes that the average mixed diet has a BV of 70.

Fats: Fats are broken down into fatty acids and glycerol. Fats are required for tissue growth and hormone production. Saturated fatty acids, common in animal fats, tend to be solid at room temperature. Except for palm and coconut oils, fats derived from plants tend to be liquid at room temperature; these fats contain high levels of monounsaturated fatty acids or polyunsaturated fatty acids (PUFAs).

Partial hydrogenation of unsaturated fatty acids (as occurs during food manufacturing) produces trans fatty acids, which are solid or semisolid at room temperature. In the US, the main dietary source of trans fatty acids is partially hydrogenated vegetable oils, used in manufacturing certain foods (eg, cookies, crackers, chips) to prolong shelf life. Trans fatty acids may elevate LDL cholesterol and lower HDL; they may also independently increase the risk of coronary artery disease.

Essential fatty acids (EFAs) are

- Linoleic acid, an omega-6 (n-6) fatty acid
- Linolenic acid, an omega-3 (n-3) fatty acid

Other omega-6 acids (eg, arachidonic acid) and other omega-3 fatty acids (eg, eicosapentaenoic acid, docosahexaenoic acid) are required by the body but can be synthesized from EFAs.

EFAs (see also p. 37) are needed for the formation of various eicosanoids (biologically active lipids), including prostaglandins, thromboxanes, prostacyclins, and leukotrienes. Consumption of omega-3 fatty acids may decrease the risk of coronary artery disease.

Requirements for EFAs vary by age. Adults require amounts of linoleic acid equal to at least 2% of total caloric needs and linolenic acid equal to at least 0.5%. Vegetable oils provide linoleic acid and linolenic acid. Oils made from safflower, sunflower, corn, soy, primrose, pumpkin, and wheat germ provide large amounts of linoleic acid. Marine fish oils and oils made from flaxseeds, pumpkin, soy, and canola provide large amounts of linolenic acid. Marine fish oils also provide some other omega-3 fatty acids in large amounts.

Macrominerals: Sodium, chloride, potassium, calcium, phosphate, and magnesium are required in relatively large amounts per day (see Tables 1–3, 1–4, and 2–2 on p. 9).

Table 1–3. MACROMINERALS

NUTRIENT	PRINCIPAL SOURCES	FUNCTIONS
Calcium	Milk and milk products, meat, fish, eggs, cereals, beans, fruits, vegetables	Bone and tooth formation, blood coagulation, nerve transmission, muscle contraction, myocardial conduction
Chloride	Many foods, mainly animal products but some vegetables; similar to sodium	Blood and intracellular acid-base balance, osmotic pressure, kidney function
Potassium	Many foods, including whole and skim milk, bananas, prunes, raisins, and meats	Muscle contraction, nerve transmission, intracellular acid-base balance, water retention
Magnesium	Green leaves, nuts, cereals, grains, seafood	Bone and tooth formation, nerve transmission, muscle contraction, enzyme activation
Sodium	Many foods, including beef, pork, sardines, cheese, green olives, corn bread, potato chips, and sauerkraut	Blood and intracellular acid-base balance, osmotic pressure, muscle contraction, nerve transmission, maintenance of cell membrane gradients
Phosphorus	Milk, cheese, meat, poultry, fish, cereals, nuts, legumes	Bone and tooth formation, blood and intracellular acid-base balance, energy production

Table 1–4. RECOMMENDED DIETARY REFERENCE INTAKES* FOR SOME MACRONUTRIENTS, FOOD AND NUTRITION BOARD, INSTITUTE OF MEDICINE OF THE NATIONAL ACADEMIES

CATEGORY	AGE OR TIME FRAME (yr)	PROTEIN (g/kg)	ENERGY (kcal/kg)	CALCIUM (mg/kg)	PHOSPHORUS (mg/kg)	MAGNESIUM (mg/kg)
Infants	0.0–0.5	2.2	108.3	66.7	50.0	6.7
	0.5–1.0	1.6	94.4	66.7	55.6	6.7
Children	1–3	1.2	100.0	61.5	61.5	6.2
	4–6	1.2	90.0	40.0	40.0	6.0
	7–10	1.0	71.4	28.6	28.6	6.1
Males	11–14	1.0	55.6	26.7	26.7	6.0
	15–18	0.9	45.5	18.2	18.2	6.1
	19–24	0.8	40.3	16.7	16.7	4.9
	25–50	0.8	36.7	10.1	10.1	4.4
	51+	0.8	29.9	10.4	10.4	4.5
Females	11–14	1.0	47.8	26.1	26.1	6.1
	15–18	0.8	40.0	21.8	21.8	5.5
	19–24	0.8	37.9	20.7	20.7	4.8
	25–50	0.8	34.9	12.7	12.7	4.4
	51+	0.8	29.2	12.3	12.3	4.3
Pregnant	—	0.9	4.6	18.5	18.5	4.9
Breastfeeding	1st yr	1.0	7.9	19.0	19.0	5.4

*These amounts, expressed as average daily intakes over time, are intended to provide for individual variations among most healthy people living in the US under usual environmental stresses.

Water: Water is considered a macronutrient because it is required in amounts of 1 mL/kcal (0.24 mL/kJ) of energy expended, or about 2500 mL/day. Needs vary with fever, physical activity, and changes in climate and humidity.

Micronutrients

Vitamins and minerals required in minute amounts (trace minerals) are micronutrients.

Water-soluble vitamins are vitamin C (ascorbic acid) and 8 members of the vitamin B complex: biotin, folate, niacin, pantothenic acid, riboflavin (vitamin B_2), thiamin (vitamin B_1), vitamin B_6 (pyridoxine), and vitamin B_{12} (cobalamin).

Fat-soluble vitamins are vitamins A (retinol), D (cholecalciferol and ergocalciferol), E (alpha-tocopherol), and K (phylloquinone and menaquinone).

Only vitamins A, E, and B_{12} are stored to any significant extent in the body; the other vitamins must be consumed regularly to maintain tissue health.

Essential trace minerals include chromium, copper, iodine, iron, manganese, molybdenum, selenium, and zinc. Except for chromium, each of these is incorporated into enzymes or hormones required in metabolism. Except for deficiencies of iron and zinc, micromineral deficiencies are uncommon in developed countries.

Other minerals (eg, aluminum, arsenic, boron, cobalt, fluoride, nickel, silicon, vanadium) have not been proved essential for people. Fluoride, although not essential, helps prevent tooth decay by forming a compound with calcium (calcium fluoride [CaF_2]), which stabilizes the mineral matrix in teeth.

All trace minerals are toxic at high levels, and some (arsenic, nickel, and chromium) may cause cancer.

Other Dietary Substances

The daily human diet typically contains as many as 100,000 chemicals (eg, coffee contains 1000). Of these, only 300 are nutrients, only some of which are essential. However, many nonnutrients in foods are useful. For example, food additives (eg, preservatives, emulsifiers, antioxidants, stabilizers) improve the production and stability of foods. Trace components (eg, spices, flavors, odors, colors, phytochemicals, many other natural products) improve appearance and taste.

Fiber: Fiber occurs in various forms (eg, cellulose, hemicellulose, pectin, gums). It increases GI motility, prevents constipation, and helps control diverticular disease. Fiber is thought to accelerate the elimination of cancer-causing substances produced by bacteria in the large intestine. Epidemiologic evidence suggests an association between colon cancer and low fiber intake and a beneficial effect of fiber in patients with functional bowel disorders, Crohn disease, obesity, or hemorrhoids. Soluble fiber (present in fruits, vegetables, oats, barley, and legumes) reduces the postprandial increase in blood glucose and insulin and can reduce cholesterol levels.

The typical Western diet is low in fiber (about 12 g/day) because of a high intake of highly refined wheat flour and a low intake of fruits and vegetables. Increasing fiber intake to about 30 g/day by consuming more vegetables, fruits, and high-fiber cereals and grains is generally recommended. However, very high fiber intake may reduce absorption of certain minerals.

NUTRITIONAL REQUIREMENTS

Good nutrition aims to achieve and maintain a desirable body composition and high potential for physical and mental work. Balancing energy intake with energy expenditure is necessary for a desirable body weight. Energy expenditure depends on age, sex, weight (see Table 1–4), and metabolic and physical activity. If energy intake exceeds expenditure, weight is gained. If energy intake is less than expenditure, weight is lost.

Daily dietary requirements for essential nutrients also depend on age, sex, weight, and metabolic and physical activity. Every 5 yr, the Food and Nutrition Board of the National Academy of Sciences/National Research Council and the US Department of Agriculture (USDA) issues the dietary reference intakes (DRIs) for protein, energy, and some vitamins and minerals (see Tables 1–4, 2–2 on p. 9, and 6–1 on p. 38). For vitamins and minerals about which less is known, safe and adequate daily dietary intakes are estimated.

Pregnant women and infants have special nutritional needs.

The USDA publishes MyPlate, which helps people develop a healthy eating style and make healthy food choices that suit their individual needs. The recommendations are individualized based on age, sex, and physical activity (see Table 1–5). The web site provides a tool (SuperTracker) that helps people plan, analyze, track, and manage their diet and physical activity.

Generally, the recommended intake decreases with aging because physical activity tends to decrease, resulting in less energy expended.

The the following general guidelines are emphasized:

- Increasing consumption of whole grains
- Increasing consumption of vegetables and fruits
- Substituting fat-free or low-fat milk products (or equivalents) for whole-fat milk products
- Reducing consumption of saturated fats
- Reducing or eliminating consumption of trans fatty acids
- Exercising regularly

Adequate fluid intake is also important.

Fats should constitute ≤ 28% of total calories, and saturated and trans fatty acids should constitute < 8%. Excess intake of saturated fats contributes to atherosclerosis. Substituting polyunsaturated fatty acids for saturated fats can decrease the risk of atherosclerosis.

Routine use of nutritional supplements is not necessary or beneficial; some supplements can be harmful. For example, excess vitamin A can lead to hypervitaminosis A, with headaches, osteoporosis, and rash.

NUTRITION IN CLINICAL MEDICINE

Nutritional deficiencies can often worsen health outcomes (whether a disorder is present or not), and some disorders (eg, malabsorption) can cause nutritional deficiencies. Also, many patients (eg, elderly patients during acute hospitalization) have unsuspected nutritional deficiencies that require treatment. Many medical centers have multidisciplinary nutrition support teams of physicians, nurses, dietitians, and pharmacists to help the clinician prevent, diagnose, and treat occult nutritional deficiencies.

Overnutrition may contribute to chronic disorders, such as cancer, hypertension, obesity, diabetes mellitus, and coronary artery disease. Dietary restrictions are necessary in many hereditary metabolic disorders (eg, galactosemia, phenylketonuria).

Evaluation of Nutritional Status

Indications for nutritional evaluation include the following:

- Undesirable body weight or body composition
- Suspicion of specific deficiencies or toxicities of essential nutrients
- In infants and children, insufficient growth or development

Nutritional status should be evaluated routinely as part of the clinical examination for

- Infants and children
- The elderly
- People taking several drugs
- People with psychiatric disorders
- People with systemic disorders that last longer than several days

Table 1–5. GENERAL RECOMMENDED DIETARY INTAKE[a] FOR 40-YR-OLDS WITH MODERATE PHYSICAL ACTIVITY[b]

FOOD GROUPS	AMOUNT/DAY	
	Men	Women
Grains[c]	7 oz	6 oz
Vegetables[d]	3.5 cups	2.5 cups
Fruits[e]	2 cups	1.5 cups
Dairy[f]	3 cups	3 cups
Protein[g]	6 oz	5 oz
Oils	6 tsp	5 tsp
Estimated daily intake[h]	2600 calories	2000 calories

[a]Actual needed intake varies based on height and weight and is determined most accurately be monitoring how body weight changes in response to changes in dietary intake. The amounts for men are based on a height of 5 ft 10 in and a weight of 150 lb. The amounts for women are based on a height of 5 ft 6 in and a weight of 130 lb.

[b]About 30 to 60 min of moderate or vigorous activity (eg, brisk walking, jogging, biking, aerobic exercise, yard work) daily.

[c]At least half should be whole grains. Generally, 1-ounce equivalents from the grains group = 1 slice of bread, 1 cup of ready-to-eat cereal, or 0.5 cup of cooked rice, cooked pasta, or cooked cereal.

[d]People should vary the vegetables they eat and include beans and peas, dark green vegetables (eg, broccoli, greens, lettuce, spinach), orange vegetables (eg, carrots, sweet potatoes, winter squash), starchy vegetables (eg, corn, potatoes), and other vegetables (eg, asparagus, cauliflower, mushrooms, tomatoes). Generally, 1 cup from the vegetable group = 1 cup of raw or cooked vegetables or vegetable juice or 2 cups of raw leafy greens.

[e]Generally, 1 cup from the fruit group = 1 cup of fruit or 0.5 cup of dried fruit.

[f]One cup from the dairy group = 1 cup of milk, yogurt, or soy milk (soy beverage), 1.5 ounces of natural cheese, or 2 ounces of processed cheese.

[g]The protein foods group includes meat, poultry, seafood, beans, peas, eggs, processed soy products, nuts, and seeds. Generally, 1-ounce equivalents from the protein foods group = 1 ounce of meat, poultry or fish; 0.25 cup of cooked beans; 1 egg; 1 tablespoon of peanut butter; or 0.5 ounce of nuts or seeds.

[h]These values are general estimates; daily caloric intake varies greatly from person to person.

NOTE: Individualized recommendations can be obtained by entering the relevant information at the USDA web site (www.myPlate.org) using the SuperTracker tool.

Table 1–6. EFFECTS OF SOME DRUGS ON APPETITE, FOOD ABSORPTION, AND METABOLISM

EFFECT	DRUGS
Increases appetite	Alcohol, antihistamines, corticosteroids, dronabinol, insulin, megestrol acetate, mirtazapine, many psychoactive drugs, sulfonylureas, thyroid hormone
Decreases appetite	Antibiotics, bulk agents (methylcellulose, guar gum), cyclophosphamide, digoxin, glucagon, indomethacin, morphine, fluoxetine
Decreases absorption of fats	Orlistat
Increases blood glucose levels	Octreotide, opioids, phenothiazines, phenytoin, probenecid, thiazide diuretics, corticosteroids, warfarin
Decreases blood glucose levels	ACE inhibitors, aspirin, barbiturates, beta-blockers, insulin, monoamine oxidase inhibitors (MAOIs), oral antihyperglycemic drugs, phenacetin, phenylbutazone, sulfonamides
Decreases blood lipid levels	Aspirin and *p*-aminosalicylic acid, L-asparaginase, chlortetracycline, colchicine, dextrans, glucagon, niacin, phenindione, statins, sulfinpyrazone, trifluperidol
Increases blood lipid levels	Adrenal corticosteroids, chlorpromazine, ethanol, growth hormone, oral contraceptives (estrogen-progestin type), thiouracil, vitamin D
Decreases protein metabolism	Chloramphenicol, tetracycline

Evaluating general nutritional status includes history, physical examination, and sometimes tests. If undernutrition is suspected, laboratory tests (eg, albumin levels) and skin tests for delayed hypersensitivity may be done. Body composition analysis (eg, skinfold measurements, bioelectrical impedance analysis) is used to estimate percentage of body fat and to evaluate obesity.

History includes questions about dietary intake, weight change, and risk factors for nutritional deficiencies and a focused review of systems (see Table 5–1 on p. 31). A dietitian can obtain a more detailed dietary history. It usually includes a list of foods eaten within the previous 24 h and a food questionnaire. A food diary may be used to record all foods eaten. The weighed ad libitum diet, in which the patient weighs and writes down all foods consumed, is the most accurate record.

A complete physical examination, including measurement of height and weight and distribution of body fat, should be done. Body mass index (BMI)—weight(kg)/height(m)^2, which adjusts weight for height (see Table 4–2 on p. 21), is more accurate than height and weight tables. There are standards for growth and weight gain in infants, children, and adolescents (see p. 2589).

Distribution of body fat is important. Disproportionate truncal obesity (ie, waist/hip ratio > 0.8) is associated with cardiovascular and cerebrovascular disorders, hypertension, and diabetes mellitus more often than fat located elsewhere. Measuring waist circumference in patients with a BMI of < 35 helps determine whether they have truncal obesity and helps predict risk of diabetes, hypertension, hypercholesterolemia, and cardiovascular disorders. Risk is increased if waist circumference is > 102 cm (> 40 in) in men or > 88 cm (> 35 in) in women.

NUTRIENT-DRUG INTERACTIONS

Nutrition can affect the body's response to drugs; conversely, drugs can affect the body's nutrition.

Foods can enhance, delay, or decrease drug absorption. Foods impair absorption of many antibiotics. They can alter metabolism of drugs; eg, high-protein diets can accelerate metabolism of certain drugs by stimulating cytochrome P-450. Eating grapefruit can inhibit cytochrome P-450 34A, slowing metabolism of some drugs (eg, amiodarone, carbamazepine, cyclosporine, certain calcium channel blockers). Diets that alter the bacterial flora may markedly affect the overall metabolism of certain drugs.

Some foods affect the body's response to drugs. For example, tyramine, a component of cheese and a potent vasoconstrictor, can cause hypertensive crisis in some patients who take monoamine oxidase inhibitors and eat cheese.

Nutritional deficiencies can affect drug absorption and metabolism. Severe energy and protein deficiencies reduce enzyme tissue concentrations and may impair the response to drugs by reducing absorption or protein binding and causing liver dysfunction. Changes in the GI tract can impair absorption and affect the response to a drug. Deficiency of calcium, magnesium, or zinc may impair drug metabolism. Vitamin C deficiency decreases activity of drug-metabolizing enzymes, especially in the elderly.

Many drugs affect appetite, food absorption, and tissue metabolism (see Table 1–6). Some drugs (eg, metoclopramide) increase GI motility, decreasing food absorption. Other drugs (eg, opioids, anticholinergics) decrease GI motility. Some drugs are better tolerated if taken with food.

Table 1–7. POSSIBLE EFFECTS OF DRUGS ON MINERAL METABOLISM

DRUGS	EFFECTS
Diuretics, especially thiazides, and corticosteroids	Can deplete body potassium*
Laxatives if used repeatedly	May deplete potassium*
Cortisol, desoxycorticosterone, and aldosterone†	Cause marked sodium and water retention, at least temporarily
Sulfonylureas and lithium	Impair uptake or release of iodine by the thyroid
Oral contraceptives	Lower blood zinc levels, increase copper levels
Certain antibiotics (eg, tetracyclines)	Reduce iron absorption

*Depletion of potassium increases susceptibility to digoxin-induced cardiac arrhythmias.
†Retention of sodium and water is much less with prednisone, prednisolone, and some other corticosteroid analogs.

Table 1–8. POSSIBLE EFFECTS OF DRUGS ON VITAMIN ABSORPTION OR METABOLISM

DRUGS	EFFECTS
Ethanol	Impairs thiamin utilization
Isoniazid	Interferes with niacin and pyridoxine metabolism
Ethanol and oral contraceptives	Inhibit folate absorption
Phenytoin, phenobarbital, primidone, or phenothiazines	In most patients, cause folate (folic acid) deficiency*, probably because hepatic microsomal drug-metabolizing enzymes are affected
Anticonvulsants	Can cause vitamin D deficiency
Aminosalicylic acid, slow-release potassium iodide, colchicine, trifluoperazine,metformin, ethanol, and oral contraceptives	Interfere with absorption of vitamin B_{12}
Oral contraceptives with a high progestin dose.	Can cause depression, probably because of metabolically induced tryptophan deficiency
Proton pump inhibitors	Can cause deficiencies of vitamin B_{12}, vitamin C, iron, calcium, and magnesium

*Folate supplements may make phenytoin less effective.

Certain drugs affect mineral metabolism (see Table 1–7). Certain antibiotics (eg, tetracyclines) reduce iron absorption, as can certain foods (eg, vegetables, tea, bran).

Certain drugs affect vitamin absorption or metabolism (see Table 1–8).

FOOD ADDITIVES AND CONTAMINANTS

Additives: Chemicals are often combined with foods to facilitate their processing and preservation or to enhance their desirability. Only amounts of additives shown to be safe by laboratory tests are permitted in commercially prepared foods.

Weighing the benefits of additives (eg, reduced waste, increased variety of available foods, protection against food-borne illness) against the risks is often complex. For example, nitrite, which is used in cured meats, inhibits the growth of *Clostridium botulinum* and improves flavor. However, nitrite converts to nitrosamines, which are carcinogens in animals. On the other hand, the amount of nitrite added to cured meat is small compared with the amount from naturally occurring food nitrates converted to nitrite by the salivary glands. Dietary vitamin C can reduce nitrite formation in the GI tract.

Rarely, some additives (eg, sulfites) cause food hypersensitivity (allergy) reactions. Most of these reactions are caused by ordinary foods.

Contaminants: Sometimes limited amounts of contaminants are allowed in foods because the contaminants cannot be completely eliminated without damaging the foods. Common contaminants are pesticides, heavy metals (lead, cadmium, mercury), nitrates (in green leafy vegetables), aflatoxins (in nuts and milk), growth-promoting hormones (in dairy products and meat), animal hairs and feces, and insect parts.

FDA-estimated safe levels are levels that have not caused illness or adverse effects in people. However, demonstrating a causal relationship between extremely low level exposures and adverse effects is difficult; long-term adverse effects, although unlikely, are still possible. Safe levels are often determined by consensus rather than by hard evidence.

2 Mineral Deficiency and Toxicity

Six **macrominerals** are required by people in gram amounts.

- Four cations: Sodium, potassium, calcium, and magnesium
- Two accompanying anions: Chloride and phosphorus

Daily requirements range from 0.3 to 2.0 g. Bone, muscle, heart, and brain function depend on these minerals.

Nine **trace minerals** (microminerals) are required by people in minute amounts (see Table 2–1):

- Chromium
- Copper
- Fluorine
- Iodine
- Iron
- Manganese
- Molybdenum
- Selenium
- Zinc

Dietary guidelines for trace minerals have been determined (see Table 2–2). All trace minerals are toxic at high levels; some minerals (arsenic, nickel, and chromium) may be carcinogens.

Mineral deficiencies (except for iodine, iron, and zinc) do not often develop spontaneously in adults on ordinary diets; infants are more vulnerable because their growth is rapid and intake varies. Trace mineral imbalances can result from hereditary disorders (eg, hemochromatosis, Wilson disease), kidney dialysis, parenteral nutrition, or restrictive diets prescribed for people with inborn errors of metabolism.

Table 2–1. TRACE MINERALS

NUTRIENT	PRINCIPAL SOURCES	FUNCTIONS	EFFECTS OF DEFICIENCY AND TOXICITY
Chromium	Liver, processed meats, whole-grain cereals, nuts	Promotion of glucose tolerance	**Deficiency:** Possibly impaired glucose tolerance
Copper	Organ meats, shellfish, nuts, dried legumes, dried fruits, whole-grain cereals, peas, cocoa, mushrooms, tomato products	Enzyme component, hematopoiesis, bone formation	**Deficiency:** Anemia in undernourished children, Menkes (kinky-hair) syndrome **Toxicity:** Wilson disease, copper poisoning
Fluorine	Seafood, tea, fluoridated water (sodium fluoride 1.0–2.0 ppm)	Bone and tooth formation	**Deficiency:** Predisposition to dental caries, possibly osteoporosis **Toxicity:** Fluorosis, mottling and pitting of permanent teeth, exostoses of spine
Iodine	Seafood, iodized salt, eggs, cheese, drinking water (content varies)	Thyroxine (T_4) and triiodothyronine (T_3) synthesis, development of fetus	**Deficiency:** Simple (colloid, endemic) goiter, cretinism, deaf-mutism, impaired fetal growth and brain development **Toxicity:** Hyperthyroidism or hypothyroidism
Iron	Many foods (except dairy products)—soybean flour, beef, kidney, liver, fish, poultry, beans, clams, molasses, enriched grains and cereals (bioavailability variable in plant sources)	Hemoglobin and myoglobin formation, cytochrome enzymes, iron-sulfur proteins	**Deficiency:** Anemia, pica, glossitis, angular cheilosis **Toxicity:** Hemochromatosis, cirrhosis, diabetes mellitus, skin pigmentation
Manganese	Whole-grain cereals, pineapple, nuts, tea, beans, tomato paste	Healthy bone structure Component of manganese-specific enzymes: glycosyltransferases, phosphoenolpyruvate carboxykinase, manganese-superoxide dismutase	**Deficiency:** Questionable **Toxicity:** Neurologic symptoms resembling those of parkinsonism or Wilson disease
Molybdenum	Milk, legumes, whole-grain breads and cereals, dark green vegetables	Component of coenzyme for sulfite oxidase, xanthine dehydrogenase, and one aldehyde oxidase	**Deficiency:** Tachycardia, headache, nausea, obtundation (sulfite toxicity)
Selenium	Meats, seafood, nuts, plant-based foods (selenium content varying with soil concentration)	Component of glutathione peroxidase and thyroid hormone iodinase	**Deficiency:** Keshan disease (viral cardiomyopathy), muscle weakness **Toxicity:** Hair loss, abnormal nails, nausea, dermatitis, peripheral neuropathy
Zinc	Meat, liver, oysters, seafood, fortified cereals, peanuts, whole grains (bioavailability variable in plant sources)	Enzyme component, skin integrity, wound healing, growth	**Deficiency:** Impaired growth and delayed sexual maturation, hypogonadism, hypogeusia **Toxicity:** RBC microcytosis, neutropenia, impaired immunity

CHROMIUM

Only 1 to 3% of biologically active trivalent chromium (Cr) is absorbed. Normal plasma levels are 0.05 to 0.50 µg/L (1.0 to 9.6 nmol/L).

Chromium potentiates insulin activity; however, it is not known whether chromium picolinate supplementation is beneficial in diabetes mellitus. Patients with diabetes should not take chromium supplements unless use is supervised by a diabetes specialist. Chromium supplements do not enhance muscle size or strength.

Chromium Deficiency

Four patients receiving long-term TPN developed possible chromium deficiency, with glucose intolerance, weight loss, ataxia, and peripheral neuropathy. Symptoms resolved in 3 who were given trivalent chromium 150 to 250 mg.

Chromium Toxicity

High doses of trivalent chromium given parenterally cause skin irritation, but lower doses given orally are not toxic. Exposure to hexavalent chromium (CrO_3) in the workplace may irritate the skin, lungs, and GI tract and may cause perforation of the nasal septum and lung carcinoma.

COPPER

Copper is a component of many body proteins; almost all of the body's copper is bound to copper proteins. Unbound (free) copper ions are toxic. Genetic mechanisms control the incorporation of copper into apoproteins and the processes that prevent toxic accumulation of copper in the body. Copper absorbed in excess of metabolic requirements is excreted through bile.

Copper deficiency may be acquired or inherited.

Table 2–2. GUIDELINES FOR DAILY INTAKE OF MINERALS

CATEGORY	AGE (YR) OR TIME FRAME	CHROMIUM (mcg)	COPPER (mcg)	FLUORIDE (mg)	IODINE (mcg)	IRON (mg)	MANGANESE (mg)	MOLYBDENUM (mcg)	SELENIUM (mcg)	ZINC (mg)
Recommended daily intake										
Infants	0.0–0.6	**0.2**	**200**	NR	**110**	**0.27**	**0.3**	**2**	**15**	**2**
	0.7–1.0	**5.5**	**220**	**0.01–0.5**	**130**	11	**0.6**	**3**	**20**	**3**
Children	1–3	**11**	340	**0.7**	90	7	1.2	17	20	3
	4–8	**15**	440	**1**	90	10	1.5	22	30	5
Males	9–13	**25**	700	**2**	120	8	1.9	34	40	8
	14–18	**35**	890	**3**	150	11	2.2	43	55	11
	19–30	**35**	900	**4**	150	8	2.3	45	55	11
	31–50	**35**	900	**4**	150	8	2.3	45	55	11
	51+	**30**	900	**4**	150	8	2.3	45	55	11
Females	9–13	**21**	700	**2**	120	8	1.6	34	40	8
	14–18	**24**	890	**3**	150	15	1.6	43	55	9
	19–30	**25**	900	**3**	150	18	1.8	45	55	8
	31–50	**25**	900	**3**	150	18	1.8	45	55	8
	51+	**20**	900	**3**	150	8	1.8	45	55	8
	Pregnant	**30**	1000	**3**	220	27	2.0	50	60	11
	Breastfeeding	45	1300	**3**	290	9	2.6	50	70	12
Upper limit (UL)										
Infants	< 1	ND	ND	0.7–0.9	ND	40	ND	ND	45–60	4–5
Children	1–8	ND	1000–3000	1.3–2.2	200–300	40	2–3	300–600	90–150	7–12
People	≥ 9	ND	5,000–10,000	10	600–1100	40–45	6–11	1100–2000	280–400	23–40

NOTE: **Recommended dietary allowances (RDAs)** are shown in regular type. RDAs are set to meet the needs of 97 to 98% of people in a group.

Adequate intakes (AIs) are shown in **bold** type. For healthy breastfed infants, AIs are the mean intake. For other groups, AIs are amounts believed to meet the needs of all people in the group, but because of lack of data, the percentage of people covered cannot be specified with confidence.

NR = not recommended; ND = not determinable because of lack of data, so sources of intake should be limited to foods.

Adapted from *Dietary Reference Intakes for Vitamin A, Vitamin K, Arsenic, Boron, Chromium, Copper, Iodine, Iron, Manganese, Molybdenum, Nickel, Silicon, Vanadium, and Zinc*, Food and Nutrition Board, Institute of Medicine. Washington, DC, National Academies Press, 2002, pp. 772–773. (See also U.S. Department of Agriculture.)

Copper toxicity may also be acquired or inherited (as Wilson disease).

Acquired Copper Deficiency

If the genetic mechanisms controlling copper metabolism are normal, dietary deficiency rarely causes clinically significant copper deficiency. Causes include

- Severe childhood protein deficiency
- Persistent infantile diarrhea (usually associated with a diet limited to milk)
- Severe malabsorption (as in sprue or cystic fibrosis)
- Gastric surgery (where vitamin B_{12} deficiency may also be present)
- Excessive zinc intake

Deficiency may cause neutropenia, impaired bone calcification, myelopathy, neuropathy, and hypochromic anemia not responsive to iron supplements.

Diagnosis of acquired copper deficiency is based on low serum levels of copper and ceruloplasmin, although these tests are not always reliable.

Treatment of acquired copper deficiency is directed at the cause, and copper 1.5 to 3 mg/day po (usually as copper sulfate) is given.

Inherited Copper Deficiency

(Menkes Syndrome)

Inherited copper deficiency occurs in male infants who inherit a mutant X-linked gene. Incidence is about 1 in 100,000 to 250,000 live births. Copper is deficient in the liver, serum, and essential copper proteins, including cytochrome-c oxidase, ceruloplasmin, and lysyl oxidase.

Symptoms and Signs

Symptoms of inherited copper deficiency are severe intellectual disability, vomiting, diarrhea, protein-losing enteropathy, hypopigmentation, bone changes, and arterial rupture; the hair is sparse, steely, or kinky.

Most affected children die by age 10 yr.

Diagnosis

- Serum copper and ceruloplasmin levels

Diagnosis of inherited copper deficiency is based on low copper and ceruloplasmin levels in serum. Because early diagnosis and treatment seem to result in a better prognosis, the disorder is ideally detected before age 2 wk. However, diagnostic accuracy of these tests is limited. Thus, other tests are being developed.

Treatment

- Copper histidine

Parenteral copper is usually given as copper histidine 250 mcg sc bid to age 1 yr, then 250 mcg sc once/day until age 3 yr; monitoring of kidney function is essential during treatment.

Despite early treatment, many children have abnormal neurodevelopment.

Acquired Copper Toxicity

Acquired copper toxicity can result from ingesting or absorbing excess copper (eg, from ingesting an acidic food or beverage that has had prolonged contact with a copper container). Self-limited gastroenteritis with nausea, vomiting, and diarrhea may occur.

More severe toxicity results from ingestion (usually with suicidal intent) of gram quantities of a copper salt (eg, copper sulfate) or from absorption of large amounts through the skin (eg, if compresses saturated with a solution of a copper salt are applied to large areas of burned skin). Hemolytic anemia and anuria can result and may be fatal.

Indian childhood cirrhosis, non-Indian childhood cirrhosis, and idiopathic copper toxicity are probably identical disorders in which excess copper causes cirrhosis. All appear to be caused by ingesting milk that has been boiled or stored in corroded copper or brass vessels. Studies suggest that idiopathic copper toxicity may develop only in infants with an unknown genetic defect.

Diagnosis of acquired copper toxicity usually requires liver biopsy, which may show Mallory hyalin bodies.

Treatment

- Chelation
- Supportive measures

For copper toxicity due to ingesting grams of copper, prompt gastric lavage is done. Copper toxicity that causes complications such as hemolytic anemia, anuria, or hepatotoxicity is also treated with chelation therapy with one of the following:

- Oral penicillamine 250 mg q 6 h to 750 mg q 12 h (1000 to 1500 mg/day in 2 to 4 doses)
- Dimercaprol 3 to 5 mg/kg IM q 4 h for 2 days, then q 4 to 6 h)

If used early, hemodialysis may be effective.

Occasionally, copper toxicity is fatal despite treatment.

Wilson Disease

(Inherited Copper Toxicity)

Wilson disease results in accumulation of copper in the liver and other organs. Hepatic or neurologic symptoms develop. Diagnosis is based on a low serum ceruloplasmin level, high urinary excretion of copper, and sometimes liver biopsy results. Treatment consists of a low-copper diet and drugs such as penicillamine or trientine.

Wilson disease is a disorder of copper metabolism that affects men and women; about 1 person in 30,000 has the disorder. Affected people are homozygous for the mutant recessive gene, located on chromosome 13. Heterozygous carriers, who constitute about 1.1% of the population, are asymptomatic.

Pathophysiology

The genetic defect in Wilson disease impairs copper transport. The impaired transport decreases copper secretion into the bile, thus causing the copper overload and resultant accumulation in the liver, which begins at birth. The impaired transport also interferes with incorporation of copper into the copper protein ceruloplasmin, thus decreasing serum levels of ceruloplasmin.

Hepatic fibrosis develops, ultimately causing cirrhosis. Copper diffuses out of the liver into the blood, then into other tissues. It is most destructive to the brain but also damages the kidneys and reproductive organs and causes hemolytic anemia. Some copper is deposited around the rim of the cornea and edge of the iris, causing Kayser-Fleischer rings. The rings appear to encircle the iris.

Symptoms and Signs

Symptoms of Wilson disease usually develop between ages 5 and 35 but can develop from age 2 to 72 yr.

In almost half of patients, particularly adolescents, the first symptom is

- Hepatitis—acute, chronic active, or fulminant

But hepatitis may develop at any time.

In about 40% of patients, particularly young adults, the first symptoms reflect

- CNS involvement

Motor deficits are common, including any combination of tremors, dystonia, dysarthria, dysphagia, chorea, drooling, and incoordination. Sometimes the CNS symptoms are cognitive or psychiatric abnormalities.

In 5 to 10% of patients, the first symptom is incidentally noted gold or greenish gold Kayser-Fleischer rings or crescents (due to copper deposits in the cornea), amenorrhea or repeated miscarriages, or hematuria.

Diagnosis

- Slit-lamp examination for Kayser-Fleischer rings
- Serum ceruloplasmin, sometimes serum copper, and 24-h urinary copper excretion
- Sometimes confirmation by penicillamine provocation test or liver biopsy

Wilson disease should be suspected in people < 40 with any of the following:

- An unexplained hepatic, neurologic, or psychiatric disorder
- An unexplained persistent elevation in hepatic transaminases
- A sibling, parent, or cousin with Wilson disease
- Fulminant hepatitis

If Wilson disease is suspected, slit-lamp examination for Kayser-Fleischer rings is required, and serum ceruloplasmin levels and 24-h urinary copper excretion are measured. Serum copper levels may be measured, but ceruloplasmin levels are usually sufficient. Transaminase levels are also often measured; high levels are consistent with the diagnosis.

Kayser-Fleischer rings: These rings plus typical motor neurologic abnormalities or a decrease in ceruloplasmin are nearly pathognomonic for Wilson disease. Rarely, these rings occur in other liver disorders (eg, biliary atresia, primary biliary cirrhosis), but ceruloplasmin levels should be unaffected.

Ceruloplasmin: Serum ceruloplasmin (normally 20 to 35 mg/dL) is usually low in Wilson disease but can be normal. It can also be low in heterozygous carriers and those with other liver disorders (eg, viral hepatitis, drug- or alcohol-induced liver disease). A low ceruloplasmin level in a patient with a

Kayser-Fleischer ring is diagnostic. Also, a level of < 5 mg/dL is highly suggestive regardless of clinical findings.

Serum copper: Serum copper levels are sometimes measured; they may be high, normal, or low.

Urinary copper excretion: In Wilson disease, 24-h urinary copper excretion (normally, ≤ 30 μg/day) is usually > 100 μg/day. If serum ceruloplasmin is low and urinary copper excretion is high, diagnosis is clear. If levels are equivocal, measuring urinary copper excretion after penicillamine is given (penicillamine provocation test) may confirm the diagnosis; this test is not usually done in adults because cutoff values are not well-established.

Liver biopsy: In unclear cases (eg, elevated transaminases, no Kayser-Fleischer rings, indeterminate values for ceruloplasmin and urinary copper), the diagnosis is made by doing a liver biopsy to measure hepatic copper concentration. However, false-negative results may occur because of a sampling error (due to large variations in copper concentrations in the liver) or fulminant hepatitis (causing necrosis that releases large amounts of copper).

Screening for Wilson disease: Because early treatment is most effective, screening is indicated for anyone who has a sibling, cousin, or parent with Wilson disease. Screening consists of a slit-lamp examination and measurement of transaminase levels, serum copper and ceruloplasmin, and 24-h urine copper excretion. If any results are abnormal, liver biopsy is done to measure hepatic copper concentration.

Infants should not be tested until after age 1 yr because ceruloplasmin levels are low during the first few months of life. Children < 6 yr with normal test results should be retested 5 to 10 yr later.

Genetic testing is under investigation.

Prognosis

Prognosis for patients with Wilson disease is usually good, unless disease is advanced before treatment begins.

Untreated Wilson disease is fatal, usually by age 30.

Treatment

- Penicillamine or trientine
- Low-copper diet
- For maintenance, lifelong low-dose penicillamine or trientine, or oral zinc

Continual, lifelong treatment of Wilson disease is mandatory regardless of whether symptoms are present. A low-copper diet (eg, avoiding beef liver, cashews, black-eyed peas, vegetable juice, shellfish, mushrooms, and cocoa) and use of penicillamine, trientine, and sometimes oral zinc can prevent copper from accumulating. Copper content in drinking water should be checked, and people should be advised not to take any vitamin or mineral supplements containing copper.

Penicillamine is the most commonly used chelating drug but has considerable toxicity (eg, fever, rash, neutropenia, thrombocytopenia, proteinuria). Cross-reactivity may occur in people with penicillin allergy. Patients > 5 yr are given oral doses of 62.5 mg q 6 h to 250 mg q 12 h (250 to 500 mg/day in 2 to 4 doses) and slowly increased to a maximum of 250 mg q 6 h to 750 mg q 12 h (1000 to 1500 mg/day in 2 to 4 doses). Younger children are given 10 mg/kg bid or 6.7 mg/kg tid (20 mg/kg/day) po. Pyridoxine 25 mg po once/day is given with penicillamine. Occasionally, use of penicillamine is associated with worsening neurologic symptoms.

Trientine hydrochloride, also a chelating drug, is an alternative treatment to penicillamine. Doses are 375 to 750 mg po bid or 250 to 500 mg po tid (750 to 1500 mg/day).

Zinc acetate 50 mg po tid can reduce intestinal copper absorption, thus preventing reaccumulation of copper in patients who cannot tolerate penicillamine or trientine or who have neurologic symptoms that do not respond to the other drugs. (CAUTION: *Penicillamine or trientine must not be taken at the same time as zinc because either drug can bind zinc, forming a compound with no therapeutic effect.*)

Poor long-term adherence to drug therapy is common. After 1 to 5 yr of therapy, lower dose maintenance drug therapy can be considered. Regular follow-up care with an expert in liver disease is recommended.

Liver transplantation may be lifesaving for patients who have Wilson disease and fulminant hepatic failure or severe hepatic insufficiency refractory to drugs.

KEY POINTS

- Wilson disease is a rare, autosomal recessive disorder in which copper accumulates in various organs.
- The disease manifests during childhood or adulthood, usually between ages 5 and 35.
- Suspect the disorder in people with a family history of the disorder or unexplained hepatic, neurologic, or psychiatric abnormalities (including elevated transaminase levels).
- Confirm the diagnosis primarily with a slit-lamp examination (for Kayser-Fleischer rings) and measurement of serum ceruloplasmin (which is low) and 24-h urinary copper excretion (which is high).
- Advise patients to follow a low copper diet, and treat them with penicillamine, trientine, or, if these drugs are intolerable or ineffective, oral zinc.

FLUORINE

Most of the body's fluorine (F) is contained in bones and teeth. Fluoride (the ionic form of fluorine) is widely distributed in nature. The main source of fluoride is fluoridated drinking water.

Fluorine Deficiency

Fluorine deficiency can lead to dental caries and possibly osteoporosis. Fluoridation of water that contains < 1 ppm (the ideal) reduces the incidence of dental caries. If a child's drinking water is not fluoridated, oral fluoride supplements can be prescribed.

Fluorine Toxicity

Excess fluorine can accumulate in teeth and bones, causing fluorosis. Drinking water containing > 10 ppm is a common cause. Permanent teeth that develop during high fluoride intake are most likely to be affected. Exposure must be much greater to affect deciduous teeth.

The **earliest signs** of fluorine toxicity are

- Chalky-white, irregularly distributed patches on the surface of the enamel

These patches become stained yellow or brown, producing a characteristic mottled appearance. Severe toxicity weakens the enamel, pitting its surface. Bony changes, including osteosclerosis, exostoses of the spine, and genu valgum, can develop but only in adults after prolonged high intake of fluoride.

No tests to diagnose toxicity are available.

Treatment of fluorine toxicity involves reducing fluoride intake; eg, in areas with high fluoride water levels, patients should not drink fluoridated water or take fluoride supplements. Children should always be told not to swallow fluoridated toothpastes.

IODINE

In the body, iodine (I) is involved primarily in the synthesis of 2 thyroid hormones, thyroxine (T_4) and triiodothyronine (T_3).

Iodine occurs in the environment and in the diet primarily as iodide. In adults, about 80% of the iodide absorbed is trapped by the thyroid gland. Most environmental iodine occurs in seawater as iodide; a small amount enters the atmosphere and, through rain, enters ground water and soil near the sea. Thus, people living far from the sea and at higher altitudes are at particular risk of iodine deficiency.

Fortifying table salt with iodide (typically 70 mcg/g) helps ensure adequate intake (150 mcg/day). Requirements are higher for pregnant (220 mcg/day) and lactating (290 mcg/day) women.

Iodine Deficiency

Iodine deficiency is rare in areas where iodized salt is used but common worldwide. Iodine deficiency develops when iodide intake is < 20 mcg/day.

Symptoms and Signs

In mild or moderate iodine deficiency, the thyroid gland, influenced by thyroid-stimulating hormone (TSH), hypertrophies to concentrate iodide in itself, resulting in colloid goiter. Usually, patients remain euthyroid; however, severe iodine deficiency in adults may cause hypothyroidism (endemic myxedema). It can decrease fertility and increase risk of stillbirth, spontaneous abortion, and prenatal and infant mortality.

Severe maternal iodine deficiency retards fetal growth and brain development, sometimes resulting in birth defects, and, in infants, causes cretinism, which may include intellectual disability, deaf-mutism, difficulty walking, short stature, and sometimes hypothyroidism.

Diagnosis

- Assessment of thyroid structure and function

Diagnosis of iodine deficiency in adults and children is usually based on thyroid function tests (see p. 1343), examination for goiter, and imaging tests identifying abnormalities in thyroid function and structure. All neonates should be screened for hypothyroidism by measuring the TSH level.

Treatment

- Iodide with or without levothyroxine

Infants with iodine deficiency are given levothyroxine 3 mcg/kg po once/day for a week plus iodide 50 to 90 mcg po once/day for several weeks to quickly restore a euthyroid state.

Children are treated with iodide 90 to 120 mcg once/day.

Adults are given iodide 150 mcg once/day. Iodine deficiency can also be treated by giving levothyroxine.

Serum TSH levels are monitored in all patients until the levels are normal (ie, < 5 μIU/mL).

Iodine Toxicity

Chronic toxicity may develop when intake is > 1.1 mg/day. Most people who ingest excess amounts of iodine remain euthyroid. Some people who ingest excess amounts of iodine, particularly those who were previously deficient, develop hyperthyroidism (Jod-Basedow phenomenon). Paradoxically, excess uptake of iodine by the thyroid may inhibit thyroid hormone synthesis (called Wolff-Chaikoff effect). Thus, iodine toxicity can eventually cause iodide goiter, hypothyroidism, or myxedema.

Very large amounts of iodide may cause a brassy taste in the mouth, increased salivation, GI irritation, and acneiform skin lesions. Patients frequently exposed to large amounts of radiographic contrast dyes or the drug amiodarone need to have their thyroid function monitored.

Diagnosis of iodine toxicity is usually based on results of thyroid function testing and imaging, which are correlated with clinical data. Iodine excretion may be more specific but is not usually measured.

Treatment of iodine toxicity consists of correcting thyroid abnormalities and, if intake is excessive, dietary modification.

IRON

Iron (Fe) is a component of hemoglobin, myoglobin, and many enzymes in the body. Heme iron, contained mainly in animal products, is absorbed much better than nonheme iron (eg, in plants and grains), which accounts for > 85% of iron in the average diet. However, absorption of nonheme iron is increased when it is consumed with animal protein and vitamin C.

Iron Deficiency

Iron deficiency is one of the most common mineral deficiencies in the world. It may result from the following:

- Inadequate iron intake, common in infants, adolescent girls, and pregnant women
- Malabsorption (eg, celiac disease)
- Chronic bleeding, including heavy menses and bleeding from GI lesions (eg, tumors)

Chronic bleeding due to colon cancer is a serious cause in middle-aged people and the elderly.

Iron deficiency and iron deficiency anemia are common among elite runners and triathlon athletes.[1]

When deficiency is advanced, microcytic anemia develops (see p. 1095).

In addition to anemia, iron deficiency may cause pica (a craving for nonfoods) and spoon nails and is associated with restless leg syndrome. Rarely, iron deficiency causes dysphagia due to postcricoid esophageal web.

Diagnosis of iron deficiency involves CBC, serum ferritin and iron levels, and possibly measurement of transferrin saturation (iron-binding capacity). In deficiency states, iron and ferritin levels tend to be low, and iron-binding capacity tends to be high.

Rarely, when the diagnosis of iron deficiency remains uncertain, examination of bone marrow for iron may be necessary.

Treatment of iron deficiency involves correcting the cause if possible (eg, treatment of a bleeding intestinal tumor). All people with moderate or severe iron deficiency and some people with mild deficiency require iron supplementation.

1. Coates A, Mountjoy M, Burr J: Incidence of iron deficiency and iron deficient anemia in elite runners and triathletes. *Clin J Sport Med* 1-6, 2016. doi: 10.1097/JSM.0000000000000390.

Iron Toxicity

Iron may accumulate in the body because of

- Iron therapy given in excessive amounts or for too long
- Repeated blood transfusions
- Chronic alcoholism
- Overdose of iron

Iron overload can also result from an inherited iron overload disease (hemochromatosis—see p. 1138), a potentially fatal but easily treatable genetic disorder in which too much iron is absorbed. Hemochromatosis affects > 1 million Americans.

An overdose of iron is toxic (see p. 3066), causing vomiting, diarrhea, and damage to the intestine and other organs.

Diagnosis of iron toxicity is similar to that for iron deficiency.

Treatment of iron toxicity often involves deferoxamine, which binds with iron and is excreted in urine.

MANGANESE

Manganese (Mn), necessary for healthy bone structure, is a component of several enzyme systems, including manganese-specific glycosyltransferases and phosphoenolpyruvate carboxykinase. Median intake is between 1.6 and 2.3 mg/day; absorption is 5 to 10%.

Manganese deficiency has not been conclusively documented, although one experimental case in a volunteer resulted in transient dermatitis, hypocholesterolemia, and increased alkaline phosphatase levels.

Manganese toxicity is usually limited to people who mine and refine ore; prolonged exposure causes neurologic symptoms resembling those of parkinsonism or Wilson disease.

MOLYBDENUM

Molybdenum (Mo) is a component of coenzymes necessary for the activity of xanthine oxidase, sulfite oxidase, and aldehyde oxidase.

Genetic and nutritional deficiencies of molybdenum have been reported but are rare. Genetic sulfite oxidase deficiency was described in 1967 in a child. It resulted from the inability to form the molybdenum coenzyme despite the presence of adequate molybdenum. The deficiency caused intellectual disability, seizures, opisthotonus, and lens dislocation.

Molybdenum deficiency resulting in sulfite toxicity occurred in a patient receiving long-term TPN. Symptoms were tachycardia, tachypnea, headache, nausea, vomiting, and coma. Laboratory tests showed high levels of sulfite and xanthine and low levels of sulfate and uric acid in the blood and urine. Ammonium molybdate 300 mcg/day IV caused dramatic recovery.

A case of molybdenum toxicity may have occurred in 1961; it caused goutlike symptoms and abnormalities of the GI tract, liver, and kidneys.

SELENIUM

Selenium (Se) is a part of the enzyme glutathione peroxidase, which metabolizes hydroperoxides formed from polyunsaturated fatty acids. Selenium is also a part of the enzymes that deiodinate thyroid hormones. Generally, selenium acts as an antioxidant that works with vitamin E.

Some epidemiologic studies associate low selenium levels with cancer. However, a recent study showed that selenium supplements did not prevent future colorectal adenomas in patients who had colorectal adenomas removed.[1]

Plasma levels of selenium vary from 8 to 25 mcg/dL, depending on selenium intake.

Diagnosis of selenium deficiency or toxicity is usually clinical; sometimes blood glutathione peroxidase is measured.

1. Thompson PA, Ashbeck EL, Roe DJ, et al: Selenium supplementation for prevention of colorectal adenomas and risk of associated type 2 diabetes. *J Natl Cancer Inst* 108(12), 2016. doi: 10.1093/jnci/djw152.

Selenium Deficiency

Selenium deficiency is rare, even in New Zealand and Finland, where selenium intake is 30 to 50 mcg/day, compared with 100 to 250 mcg/day in the US and Canada.

In certain areas of China, where intake averages 10 to 15 mcg/day, selenium deficiency predisposes patients to Keshan disease, an endemic viral cardiomyopathy affecting primarily children and young women. This cardiomyopathy can be prevented but not cured by sodium selenite supplements of 50 mcg/day po.

Patients receiving long-term TPN have developed selenium deficiency with muscle pain and tenderness that responded to a selenomethionine supplement.

In Siberian Russia and China, growing children with selenium deficiency may develop chronic osteoarthropathy (Kashin-Beck disease).

Selenium deficiency may contribute synergistically with iodine deficiency to the development of goiter and hypothyroidism.

Diagnosis of selenium deficiency is made clinically or sometimes by measuring glutathione peroxidase activity or plasma selenium, but neither of these tests is readily available.

Treatment of selenium deficiency consists of sodium selenite 100 mcg/day po.

Selenium Toxicity

At high doses (> 900 mcg/day), selenium causes toxicity.

Manifestations include hair loss, abnormal nails, dermatitis, peripheral neuropathy, nausea, diarrhea, fatigue, irritability, and a garlic odor of the breath.

Toxic levels of plasma selenium are not well defined.

Treatment of selenium toxicity involves reducing selenium consumption.

ZINC

Zinc (Zn) is contained mainly in bones, teeth, hair, skin, liver, muscle, leukocytes, and testes. Zinc is a component of several hundred enzymes, including many nicotinamide adenine dinucleotide (NADH) dehydrogenases, RNA and DNA polymerases, and DNA transcription factors as well as alkaline phosphatase, superoxide dismutase, and carbonic anhydrase.

A diet high in fiber and phytate (eg, in whole-grain bread) reduces zinc absorption.

Zinc Deficiency

Dietary deficiency is unlikely in healthy persons. Secondary zinc deficiency can develop in the following:

- Patients taking diuretics
- Patients with diabetes mellitus, sickle cell disease, chronic kidney disease, liver disease, chronic alcoholism, or malabsorption
- Patients with stressful conditions (eg, sepsis, burns, head injury)
- Elderly institutionalized and homebound patients (common)

Maternal zinc deficiency may cause fetal malformations and low birth weight.

Zinc deficiency in children causes impaired growth, impaired taste (hypogeusia), delayed sexual maturation, and hypogonadism. In children or adults, manifestations also include alopecia, impaired immunity, anorexia, dermatitis, night blindness, anemia, lethargy, and impaired wound healing.

Zinc deficiency should be suspected in undernourished patients with typical symptoms or signs. However, because many of the symptoms and signs are nonspecific, clinical diagnosis of mild zinc deficiency is difficult. Laboratory diagnosis is also difficult. Low albumin levels, common in zinc deficiency, make serum zinc levels difficult to interpret; diagnosis usually requires the combination of low levels of zinc in serum and increased urinary zinc excretion. If available, isotope studies can measure zinc status more accurately.

Treatment of zinc deficiency consists of elemental zinc 15 to 120 mg po once/day until symptoms and signs resolve.

Acrodermatitis enteropathica: Acrodermatitis enteropathica (a rare, once fatal autosomal recessive disorder) causes malabsorption of zinc. Psoriasiform dermatitis develops around the eyes, nose, and mouth; on the buttocks and perineum; and in an acral distribution. The disorder also causes hair loss, paronychia, impaired immunity, recurrent infection, impaired growth, and diarrhea. Symptoms and signs usually develop after infants are weaned from breast milk. In such cases, doctors suspect acrodermatitis enteropathica. If this diagnosis is correct, zinc sulfate 30 to 150 mg/day po usually results in complete remission.

Zinc Toxicity

The recommended upper limit in adults for zinc intake is 40 mg/day; the upper limit is lower for younger people. Toxicity is rare.

Ingesting doses of elemental zinc ranging from 100 to 150 mg/day for prolonged periods interferes with copper metabolism and causes low blood copper levels, RBC microcytosis, neutropenia, and impaired immunity; higher doses should be given only for short periods of time and the patient followed closely.

Ingesting larger amounts (200 to 800 mg/day), usually by consuming acidic food or drinking from a galvanized (zinc-coated) container, can cause anorexia, vomiting, and diarrhea. Chronic toxicity may result in copper deficiency and may cause nerve damage.

Metal fume fever, also called brass-founders' ague or zinc shakes, is caused by inhaling industrial zinc oxide fumes; it results in fever, dyspnea, nausea, fatigue, and myalgias. Symptom onset is usually 4 to 12 h after exposure. Symptoms usually resolve after 12 to 24 h in a zinc-free environment.

Diagnosis of zinc toxicity is usually based on the time course and a history of exposure.

Treatment of zinc toxicity consists of eliminating exposure to zinc; no antidotes are available.

3 Nutritional Support

Many undernourished patients need nutritional support, which aims to increase lean body mass. Oral feeding can be difficult for some patients with anorexia or with eating or absorption problems. Behavioral measures that sometimes enhance oral intake include the following:

- Encouraging patients to eat
- Heating or seasoning foods
- Providing favorite or strongly flavored foods
- Encouraging patients to eat small portions
- Scheduling around meals
- Assisting patients with feeding

If behavioral measures are ineffective, nutritional support—oral nutrition, enteral tube nutrition, or parenteral nutrition—is indicated, except sometimes for dying or severely demented patients.

Predicting Nutritional Requirements

Nutritional requirements are predicted so that interventions can be planned. Requirements can be estimated by formulas or measured by indirect calorimetry. Indirect calorimetry requires use of a metabolic cart (a closed rebreathing system that determines energy expenditure based on total CO_2 production), which requires special expertise and is not always available. Thus, total energy expenditure (TEE) and protein requirements usually are estimated.

Energy expenditure: TEE varies based on the patient's weight, activity level, and degree of metabolic stress (metabolic demands); TEE ranges from 25 kcal/kg/day for people who are sedentary and not under stress to about 40 kcal/kg/day for people who are critically ill. TEE equals the sum of

- Resting metabolic rate (RMR, or resting energy expenditure rate), which is normally about 70% of TEE
- Energy dissipated by metabolism of food (10% of TEE)
- Energy expended during physical activity (20% of TEE)

Undernutrition can decrease RMR up to 20%. Conditions that increase metabolic stress (eg, critical illness, infection, inflammation, trauma, surgery) can increase RMR but rarely by > 50%.

The Mifflin–St. Jeor equation estimates RMR more precisely and with fewer errors than the commonly used Harris-Benedict equation, usually providing results that are within 20% of those measured by indirect calorimetry. The Mifflin–St. Jeor equation estimates RMR as follows:

$$\textbf{Men}: kcal/day = (10 * weight[kg]) + (6.25 * height[cm]) - (5 * age[yr]) + 5$$

$$\textbf{Women}: kcal/day = (10 * weight[kg]) + (6.25 * height[cm]) - (5 * age[yr]) - 161$$

TEE can be estimated by adding about 10% (for sedentary people) to about 40% (for people who are critically ill) to RMR.

Protein requirements: For healthy people, protein requirements are estimated at 0.8 g/kg/day. However, for patients with metabolic stress or kidney failure and for elderly patients, requirements may be higher (see Table 3–1).

Table 3–1. ESTIMATED ADULT DAILY PROTEIN REQUIREMENT

CONDITION	REQUIREMENT (g/kg of ideal body wt/day)
Normal	0.8
Age > 70 yr	1.0
Kidney failure without dialysis (GFR < 25 mL/min/1.73 m^2)	0.6–0.75
Kidney failure with dialysis	1.2
Metabolic stress (eg, critical illness, trauma, burns, surgery)	1.5

Assessing Response to Nutritional Support

There is no gold standard to assess response. Clinicians commonly use indicators of lean body mass such as the following:

- Body mass index (BMI)
- Body composition analysis
- Body fat distribution (see pp. 21 and 31)

Nitrogen balance, response to skin antigens, muscle strength measurement, and indirect calorimetry can also be used.

Nitrogen balance, which reflects the balance between protein needs and supplies, is the difference between amount of nitrogen ingested and amount lost. A positive balance (ie, more ingested than lost) implies adequate intake. Precise measurement is impractical, but estimates help assess response to nutritional support:

- Nitrogen intake is estimated from protein intake: nitrogen (g) equals protein (g)/6.25.
- Estimated nitrogen losses consist of urinary nitrogen losses (estimated by measuring urea nitrogen content of an accurately obtained 24-h urine collection) plus stool losses (estimated at 1 g/day if stool is produced; negligible if stool is not produced) plus insensible and other unmeasured losses (estimated at 3 g).

Response to skin antigens, a measure of delayed hypersensitivity, often increases to normal as undernourished patients respond to nutritional support. However, other factors can affect response to skin antigens.

Muscle strength indirectly reflects increases in lean body mass. It can be measured quantitatively, by hand-grip dynamometry, or electrophysiologically (typically by stimulating the ulnar nerve with an electrode).

Levels of acute-phase reactant serum proteins (particularly short-lived proteins such as prealbumin [transthyretin], retinol-binding protein, and transferrin) sometimes correlate with improved nutritional status, but these levels correlate better with inflammatory conditions.

KEY POINTS

- Behavioral measures may avert the need for nutritional support.
- Predict the patient's energy requirements based on weight, sex, activity level, and degree of metabolic stress (eg, due to critical illness, trauma, burns, or recent surgery).
- Normal protein requirement is 0.8 mg/kg/day, but this amount is adjusted if age is > 70 or if the patient has kidney failure or metabolic stress.
- Assess the response to nutritional support by indicators of lean body mass and/or other indicators (eg, nitrogen balance, response to skin antigens, muscle strength measurement, indirect calorimetry).

ENTERAL TUBE NUTRITION

Enteral tube nutrition is indicated for patients who have a functioning GI tract but cannot ingest enough nutrients orally because they are unable or unwilling to take oral feedings. Compared with parenteral nutrition, enteral nutrition has the following advantages:

- Better preservation of the structure and function of the GI tract
- Lower cost
- Probably fewer complications, particularly infections

Specific indications for enteral nutrition include the following:

- Prolonged anorexia
- Severe protein-energy undernutrition
- Coma or depressed sensorium
- Liver failure
- Inability to take oral feedings due to head or neck trauma
- Critical illnesses (eg, burns) causing metabolic stress

Other indications may include bowel preparation for surgery in seriously ill or undernourished patients, closure of enterocutaneous fistulas, and small-bowel adaptation after massive intestinal resection or in disorders that may cause malabsorption (eg, Crohn disease).

Procedure: If tube feeding is needed for ≤ 4 to 6 wk, a small-caliber, soft nasogastric or nasoenteric (eg, nasoduodenal) tube made of silicone or polyurethane is usually used. If a nasal injury or deformity makes nasal placement difficult, an orogastric or other oroenteric tube can be placed.

Tube feeding for > 4 to 6 wk usually requires a gastrostomy or jejunostomy tube, placed endoscopically, surgically, or radiologically. Choice depends on physician capabilities and patient preference.

Jejunostomy tubes are useful for patients with contraindications to gastrostomy (eg, gastrectomy, bowel obstruction proximal to the jejunum). However, these tubes do not pose less risk of tracheobronchial aspiration than gastrostomy tubes, as is often thought. Jejunostomy tubes are easily dislodged and are usually used only for inpatients.

Feeding tubes are surgically placed if endoscopic and radiologic placement is unavailable, technically impossible, or unsafe (eg, because of overlying bowel). Open or laparoscopic techniques can be used.

Formulas: Liquid formulas commonly used include feeding modules and polymeric or other specialized formulas.

Feeding modules are commercially available products that contain a single nutrient, such as proteins, fats, or carbohydrates. Feeding modules may be used individually to treat a specific deficiency or combined with other formulas to completely satisfy nutritional requirements.

Polymeric formulas (including blenderized food and milk-based or lactose-free commercial formulas) are commercially available and generally provide a complete, balanced diet. For oral or tube feedings, they are usually preferred to feeding modules. In hospitalized patients, lactose-free formulas are the most commonly used polymeric formulas. However, milk-based formulas tend to taste better than lactose-free formulas. Patients with lactose intolerance may be able to tolerate milk-based formulas given slowly by continuous infusion.

Specialized formulas include hydrolyzed protein or sometimes amino acid formulas, which are used for patients who have difficulty digesting complex proteins. However, these formulas are expensive and usually unnecessary. Most patients with pancreatic insufficiency, if given enzymes, and most patients with malabsorption can digest complex proteins. Other specialized formulas (eg, calorie- and protein-dense formulas for patients whose fluids are restricted, fiber-enriched formulas for constipated patients) may be helpful.

Administration: Patients should be sitting upright at 30 to 45° during tube feeding and for 1 to 2 h afterward to minimize incidence of nosocomial aspiration pneumonia and to allow gravity to help propel the food.

Tube feedings are given in boluses several times a day or by continuous infusion. Bolus feeding is more physiologic and may be preferred for patients with diabetes. Continuous infusion is necessary if boluses cause nausea.

For bolus feeding, total daily volume is divided into 4 to 6 separate feedings, which are injected through the tube with a syringe or infused by gravity from an elevated bag. After feedings, the tube is flushed with water to prevent clogging.

Nasogastric or nasoduodenal tube feeding often causes diarrhea initially; thus, feedings are usually started with small amounts of dilute preparations and increased as tolerated. Most formulas contain 0.5, 1, or 2 kcal/mL. Formulas with higher caloric concentration (less water per calorie) may cause decreased gastric emptying and thus higher gastric residuals than when more dilute formulas with the same number of calories are used. Initially, a 1-kcal/mL commercially prepared solution may be given undiluted at 50 mL/h or, if patients have not been fed for a while, at 25 mL/h. Usually, these solutions do not supply enough water, particularly if vomiting, diarrhea, sweating, or fever has increased water loss. Extra water is supplied as boluses via the feeding tube or IV. After a few days, the rate or concentration can be increased as needed to meet caloric and water needs.

Jejunostomy tube feeding requires greater dilution and smaller volumes. Feeding usually begins at a concentration of ≤ 0.5 kcal/mL and a rate of 25 mL/h. After a few days, concentrations and volumes can be increased to eventually meet caloric and water needs. Usually, the maximum that can be tolerated is 0.8 kcal/mL at 125 mL/h, providing 2400 kcal/day.

Complications: Complications are common and can be serious (see Table 3–2).

KEY POINTS

- Consider enteral tube nutrition for patients who have a functioning GI tract but cannot ingest enough nutrients orally because they are unable or unwilling to take oral feedings.
- If tube feeding is expected to last > 4 to 6 wk, consider a gastrostomy or jejunostomy tube, placed endoscopically, surgically, or radiologically.

Table 3–2. COMPLICATIONS OF ENTERAL TUBE NUTRITION

PROBLEM	EFFECTS	COMMENTS
Tube-related		
Presence of tube	Damage to the nose, pharynx, or esophagus	The tube, particularly if large, can irritate tissues, causing them to erode.
	Sinusitis	Sinus ostia can become blocked.
Blockage of tube lumen	Inadequate feeding	Thick feedings or pills can block the lumen, particularly of small tubes. Sometimes blockages can be dissolved by instilling a solution of pancreatic enzymes or other commercial products.
Misplacement of a nasogastric tube intracranially	Brain trauma, infection	A tube may be misplaced intracranially if the cribriform plate is disrupted by severe facial trauma.
Misplacement of a nasogastric or orogastric tube in the tracheobronchial tree	Pneumonia	Responsive patients immediately cough and gag. Obtunded patients have few immediate symptoms. If misplacement is not recognized, feedings enter the lungs, causing pneumonia.
Dislodgement of a gastrostomy or jejunostomy tube	Peritonitis	After being dislodged, a tube may be replaced into the peritoneal cavity. If tubes were originally placed using invasive techniques, replacement is more difficult and more likely to cause complications.
Formula-related		
Intolerance of one of the formula's main nutrient components	Diarrhea, GI discomfort*, nausea, vomiting, mesenteric ischemia (occasionally)	Intolerance occurs in up to 20% of patients and 50% of critically ill patients and is more common with bolus feedings.
Osmotic diarrhea	Frequent, loose stools	Sorbitol, often contained in liquid drug preparations given through feeding tubes, can exacerbate diarrhea.
Nutrient imbalances	Electrolyte disturbances, hyperglycemia, volume overload, hyperosmolarity	Body weight and blood levels of electrolytes, glucose, Mg, and phosphate should be frequently monitored (daily during the first week).
Other		
Reflux of tube feedings or difficulty with oropharyngeal secretions	Aspiration	Aspiration may occur even though tubes are placed correctly and the head of the bed is elevated if patients have either of these problems.

*GI discomfort may have other causes, including reduced compliance of the stomach due to shrinkage caused by lack of feeding, distention due to volume of feeding, and decreased gastric emptying due to dysfunction of the pylorus.

- A polymeric formula is the most commonly used and usually the easiest formula to give.
- Keep patients sitting upright at 30 to 45° during tube feeding and for 1 to 2 h afterward to minimize incidence of nosocomial aspiration pneumonia and to allow gravity to help propel the food.
- Check patients periodically for complications of tube feedings (eg, tube-related, formula-related, aspiration).

TOTAL PARENTERAL NUTRITION

Parenteral nutrition is by definition given IV.

Partial parenteral nutrition supplies only part of daily nutritional requirements, supplementing oral intake. Many hospitalized patients are given dextrose or amino acid solutions by this method.

Total parenteral nutrition (TPN) supplies all daily nutritional requirements. TPN can be used in the hospital or at home. Because TPN solutions are concentrated and can cause thrombosis of peripheral veins, a central venous catheter is usually required.

Parenteral nutrition should not be used routinely in patients with an intact GI tract. Compared with enteral nutrition, it causes more complications, does not preserve GI tract structure and function as well, and is more expensive.

Indications: TPN may be the only feasible option for patients who do not have a functioning GI tract or who have disorders requiring complete bowel rest, such as the following:

- Some stages of ulcerative colitis
- Bowel obstruction
- Certain pediatric GI disorders (eg, congenital GI anomalies, prolonged diarrhea regardless of its cause)
- Short bowel syndrome due to surgery

Nutritional content: TPN requires water (30 to 40 mL/kg/day), energy (30 to 45 kcal/kg/day, depending on energy expenditure), amino acids (1.0 to 2.0 g/kg/day, depending on the degree of catabolism), essential fatty acids, vitamins, and minerals (see Table 3–3).

Children who need TPN may have different fluid requirements and need more energy (up to 120 kcal/kg/day) and amino acids (up to 2.5 or 3.5 g/kg/day).

Basic TPN solutions are prepared using sterile techniques, usually in liter batches according to standard formulas. Normally, 2 L/day of the standard solution is needed. Solutions may be modified based on laboratory results, underlying disorders, hypermetabolism, or other factors.

Most calories are supplied as carbohydrate. Typically, about 4 to 5 mg/kg/min of dextrose is given. Standard solutions contain up to about 25% dextrose, but the amount and concentration depend on other factors, such as metabolic needs and the proportion of caloric needs that are supplied by lipids.

Commercially available lipid emulsions are often added to supply essential fatty acids and triglycerides; 20 to 30% of total calories are usually supplied as lipids. However, withholding lipids and their calories may help obese patients mobilize endogenous fat stores, increasing insulin sensitivity.

Solutions: Many solutions are commonly used. Electrolytes can be added to meet the patient's needs.

Solutions vary depending on other disorders present and patient age, as for the following:

- For renal insufficiency not being treated with dialysis or for liver failure: Reduced protein content and a high percentage of essential amino acids
- For heart or kidney failure: Limited volume (liquid) intake
- For respiratory failure: A lipid emulsion that provides most of nonprotein calories to minimize CO_2 production by carbohydrate metabolism
- For neonates: Lower dextrose concentrations (17 to 18%)

Beginning TPN administration: Because the central venous catheter needs to remain in place for a long time, strict sterile technique must be used during insertion and maintenance. The TPN line should not be used for any other purpose. External tubing should be changed every 24 h with the first bag of the day. In-line filters have not been shown to decrease complications.

Table 3–3. BASIC ADULT DAILY REQUIREMENTS FOR TPN

NUTRIENT	AMOUNT
Water (/kg body wt/day)	30–40 mL
Energy* (/kg body wt/day)	
Medical patient	30 kcal
Postoperative patient	30–45 kcal
Hypercatabolic patient	45 kcal
Amino acids (/kg body wt/day)	
Medical patient	1.0 g
Postoperative patient	2.0 g
Hypercatabolic patient	3.0 g
Minerals	
Acetate/gluconate	90 mEq
Calcium	15 mEq
Chloride	130 mEq
Chromium	15 mcg
Copper	1.5 mg
Iodine	120 mcg
Magnesium	20 mEq
Manganese	2 mg
Phosphorus	300 mg
Potassium	100 mEq
Selenium	100 mcg
Sodium	100 mEq
Zinc	5 mg
Vitamins	
Ascorbic acid	100 mg
Biotin	60 mcg
Cobalamin	5 mcg
Folate (folic acid)	400 mcg
Niacin	40 mg
Pantothenic acid	15 mg
Pyridoxine	4 mg
Riboflavin	3.6 mg
Thiamin	3 mg
Vitamin A	4000 IU
Vitamin D	400 IU
Vitamin E	15 mg
Vitamin K	200 mcg

*Requirements for energy increase by 12% per 1° C of fever.

Dressings should be kept sterile and are usually changed every 48 h using strict sterile techniques.

If TPN is given outside the hospital, patients must be taught to recognize symptoms of infection, and qualified home nursing must be arranged.

The solution is started slowly at 50% of the calculated requirements, using 5% dextrose to make up the balance of fluid requirements. Energy and nitrogen should be given simultaneously. The amount of regular insulin given (added directly to the TPN solution) depends on the plasma glucose level; if the level is normal and the final solution contains 25% dextrose, the usual starting dose is 5 to 10 units of regular insulin/L of TPN fluid.

Monitoring: Progress should be followed on a flowchart. An interdisciplinary nutrition team, if available, should monitor patients. Weight, CBC, electrolytes, and BUN should be monitored often (eg, daily for inpatients). Plasma glucose should be monitored every 6 h until patients and glucose levels become stable. Fluid intake and output should be monitored continuously. When patients become stable, blood tests can be done much less often.

Liver function tests should be done. Plasma proteins (eg, serum albumin, possibly transthyretin or retinol-binding protein), prothrombin time, plasma and urine osmolality, and Ca, Mg, and phosphate should be measured twice/wk. Changes in transthyretin and retinol-binding protein reflect overall clinical status rather than nutritional status alone. If possible, blood tests should not be done during glucose infusion.

Full nutritional assessment (including BMI calculation and anthropometric measurements—see pp. 21 and 31) should be repeated at 2-wk intervals.

Complications: About 5 to 10% of patients have complications related to central venous access.

Catheter-related sepsis occurs in probably ≥ 50% of patients.

Glucose abnormalities (hyperglycemia or hypoglycemia) or liver dysfunction occurs in > 90% of patients.

Glucose abnormalities are common. Hyperglycemia can be avoided by monitoring plasma glucose often, adjusting the insulin dose in the TPN solution, and giving subcutaneous insulin as needed.

Hypoglycemia can be precipitated by suddenly stopping constant concentrated dextrose infusions. Treatment depends on the degree of hypoglycemia. Short-term hypoglycemia may be reversed with 50% dextrose IV; more prolonged hypoglycemia may require infusion of 5 or 10% dextrose for 24 h before resuming TPN via the central venous catheter.

Hepatic complications include liver dysfunction, painful hepatomegaly, and hyperammonemia. They can develop at any age but are most common among infants, particularly premature ones (whose liver is immature).

- **Liver dysfunction** may be transient, evidenced by increased transaminases, bilirubin, and alkaline phosphatase; it commonly occurs when TPN is started. Delayed or persistent elevations may result from excess amino acids. Pathogenesis is unknown, but cholestasis and inflammation may contribute. Progressive fibrosis occasionally develops. Reducing protein delivery may help.
- **Painful hepatomegaly** suggests fat accumulation; carbohydrate delivery should be reduced.
- **Hyperammonemia** can develop in infants, causing lethargy, twitching, and generalized seizures. Arginine supplementation at 0.5 to 1.0 mmol/kg/day can correct it.

If infants develop any hepatic complication, limiting amino acids to 1.0 g/kg/day may be necessary.

Abnormalities of serum electrolytes and minerals should be corrected by modifying subsequent infusions or, if correction is urgently required, by beginning appropriate peripheral vein infusions. Vitamin and mineral deficiencies are rare when solutions are given correctly. Elevated BUN may reflect dehydration, which can be corrected by giving free water as 5% dextrose via a peripheral vein.

Volume overload (suggested by > 1 kg/day weight gain) may occur when patients have high daily energy requirements and thus require large fluid volumes.

Metabolic bone disease, or bone demineralization (osteoporosis or osteomalacia), develops in some patients given TPN for > 3 mo. The mechanism is unknown. Advanced disease can cause severe periarticular, lower-extremity, and back pain.

Adverse reactions to lipid emulsions (eg, dyspnea, cutaneous allergic reactions, nausea, headache, back pain, sweating, dizziness) are uncommon but may occur early, particularly if lipids are given at > 1.0 kcal/kg/h. Temporary hyperlipidemia may occur, particularly in patients with kidney or liver failure; treatment is usually not required. Delayed adverse reactions to lipid emulsions include hepatomegaly, mild elevation of liver enzymes, splenomegaly, thrombocytopenia, leukopenia, and, especially in premature infants with respiratory distress syndrome, pulmonary function abnormalities. Temporarily or permanently slowing or stopping lipid emulsion infusion may prevent or minimize these adverse reactions.

Gallbladder complications include cholelithiasis, gallbladder sludge, and cholecystitis. These complications can be caused or worsened by prolonged gallbladder stasis. Stimulating contraction by providing about 20 to 30% of calories as fat and stopping glucose infusion several hours a day is helpful. Oral or enteral intake also helps. Treatment with metronidazole, ursodeoxycholic acid, phenobarbital, or cholecystokinin helps some patients with cholestasis.

KEY POINTS

- Consider parenteral nutrition for patients who do not have a functioning GI tract or who have disorders requiring complete bowel rest.
- Calculate requirements for water (30 to 40 mL/kg/day), energy (30 to 45 kcal/kg/day, depending on energy expenditure), amino acids (1.0 to 2.0 g/kg/day, depending on the degree of catabolism), essential fatty acids, vitamins, and minerals.
- Choose a solution based on patient age and organ function status; different solutions are required for neonates and for patients who have compromised heart, kidney, or lung function.
- Use a central venous catheter, with strict sterile technique for insertion and maintenance.
- Monitor patients closely for complications (eg, related to central venous access, glucose levels, electrolyte and mineral levels, hepatic or gallbladder effects, volume, or lipid emulsions).

NUTRITIONAL SUPPORT FOR DYING OR SEVERELY DEMENTED PATIENTS

Anorexia or loss of appetite is common among dying patients. Behavioral measures (eg, using flexible feeding schedules, feeding slowly, giving small portions or favorite or strongly flavored foods) can often increase oral intake. A small amount of a favorite alcoholic drink, given 30 min before meals, may also help. Certain antidepressants, megestrol acetate, and dronabinol may stimulate appetite. Metoclopramide enhances gastric emptying, but it may take 1 to 2 wk to reach peak effectiveness.

Advanced dementia eventually leads to inability to eat; sometimes affected patients are given tube feedings. However, there is no convincing evidence that tube feedings prolong life, provide comfort, improve function, or prevent complications (eg, aspiration, pressure ulcers).

Tube feedings and parenteral nutrition cause discomfort and are usually not indicated for patients who are dying or too demented to eat. Forgoing nutritional support may be difficult for family members to accept, but they should understand that patients are usually more comfortable eating and drinking as they choose. Sips of water and easy-to-swallow foods may be useful. Supportive care, including good oral hygiene (eg, brushing the teeth, moistening the oral cavity with swabs and ice chips as needed, applying lip salve), can physically and psychologically comfort the patients and the family members who provide the care.

Counseling may help family members who are dealing with anxieties about whether to use invasive nutritional support.

4 Obesity and the Metabolic Syndrome

OBESITY

Obesity is excess body weight, defined as a body mass index (BMI) of ≥ 30 kg/m². Complications include cardiovascular disorders (particularly in people with excess abdominal fat), diabetes mellitus, certain cancers, cholelithiasis, fatty liver, cirrhosis, osteoarthritis, reproductive disorders in men and women, psychologic disorders, and, for people with BMI ≥ 35, premature death. Diagnosis is based on body mass index. Treatment includes lifestyle modification (eg, in diet, physical activity, and behavior) and, for certain patients, drugs or bariatric (weight-loss) surgery.

See also Obesity in Adolescents on p. 2823.

Prevalence of obesity in the US is high in all age groups (see Table 4–1). Over 36.5% of adults are obese.[1]

Prevalence is highest among non-Hispanic blacks (48.1%), compared with Hispanics (42.5%), whites (34.5%), and Asians (11.7%).[1] Black and Mexican-American men in higher income groups are more likely to be obese than those in lower income groups. However, women in higher income groups, regardless of ethnic group, are less likely to be obese, and most obese adults are not in lower income groups.

In the US, obesity and its complications cause as many as 300,000 premature deaths each year, making it second only to cigarette smoking as a preventable cause of death.

1. CDC: Adult Obesity Facts. Accessed 10/11/16.

Etiology

Causes of obesity are probably multifactorial and include genetic predisposition. Ultimately, obesity results from a long-standing imbalance between energy intake and energy expenditure, including energy utilization for basic metabolic processes and energy expenditure from physical activity. However, many other factors appear to increase a person's predisposition to obesity, including endocrine disruptors (eg, bisphenol A [BPA]), gut microbiome, sleep/wake cycles, and environmental factors.

Genetic factors: Heritability of BMI is about 66%. Genetic factors may affect the many signaling molecules and receptors used by parts of the hypothalamus and GI tract to regulate food intake (see Sidebar 4–1). Genetic factors can be inherited or result from conditions in utero (called genetic imprinting). Rarely, obesity results from abnormal levels of peptides that

Sidebar 4–1. Pathways Regulating Food Intake

Preabsorptive and postabsorptive signals from the GI tract and changes in plasma nutrient levels provide short- and long-term feedback to regulate food intake:

- GI hormones (eg, glucagon-like peptide 1 [GLP-1], cholecystokinin [CCK], peptide YY [PYY]) reduce food intake.
- Ghrelin, secreted primarily by the stomach, increases food intake.
- Leptin, secreted from adipose tissue, informs the brain how much fat is stored. Leptin suppresses appetite in normal-weight people, but high leptin levels correlate with increased body fat. Leptin levels can decrease when weight is lost and then send a hunger signal to the brain.

The hypothalamus integrates various signals involved in the regulation of energy balance and then activates pathways that increase or decrease food intake:

- Neuropeptide Y (NPY), agouti-related peptide (ARP), alpha-melanocyte–stimulating hormone (alpha-MSH), cocaine- and amphetamine-related transcript (CART), orexin, and melanin-concentrating hormone (MCH) increase food intake.
- Corticotropic hormone (CRH) and urocortin decrease it.

Table 4–1. CHANGES IN PREVALENCE OF OBESITY ACCORDING TO NHANES

AGE GROUP	1976–1980	2003–2004	2007–2008	2009–2012	2013–2014*
2–5 yr	5%	13.9%	10.4%	12.1%	9.4%
6–11 yr	6.5%	18.8%	19.6%	18.0%	17.4%
12–19 yr	5%	17.4%	18.1%	18.4%	20.6%
20–74 yr	15%	32.9%	33.8%	35.7%	37.9%

*Data for 2013–2014 is from the CDC National Center for Health Statistics, derived from Health, United States, 2015, Table 53.
NHANES = National Health and Nutrition Examination Surveys.

regulate food intake (eg, leptin) or abnormalities in their receptors (eg, melanocortin-4 receptor).

Genetic factors also regulate energy expenditure, including BMR, diet-induced thermogenesis, and nonvoluntary activity–associated thermogenesis. Genetic factors may have a greater effect on the distribution of body fat, particularly abdominal fat (which increases the risk of metabolic syndrome—see p. 28), than on the amount of body fat.

Environmental factors: Weight is gained when caloric intake exceeds energy needs. Important determinants of energy intake include

- Portion sizes
- The energy density of the food

High-calorie foods (eg, processed foods), diets high in refined carbohydrates, and consumption of soft drinks, fruit juices, and alcohol promote weight gain. Diets high in fresh fruit and vegetables, fiber, complex carbohydrates, and lean proteins, with water as the main fluid consumed, minimize weight gain.

A sedentary lifestyle promotes weight gain.

Regulatory factors: Prenatal maternal obesity, prenatal maternal smoking, and intrauterine growth restriction can disturb weight regulation and contribute to weight gain during childhood and later. Obesity that persists beyond early childhood makes weight loss in later life more difficult.

The composition of the gut microbiome also appears to be an important factor; early use of antibiotics and other factors that alter the composition of the gut microbiome may promote weight gain and obesity later in life.[1]

About 15% of women permanently gain ≥ 20 lb with each pregnancy.

Insufficient sleep (usually considered < 6 to 8 h/night) can result in weight gain by changing the levels of satiety hormones that promote hunger.

Drugs, including corticosteroids, lithium, traditional antidepressants (tricyclics, tetracyclics, monoamine oxidase inhibitors [MAOIs]), benzodiazepines, anticonvulsants, thiazolidinediones (eg, rosiglitazone, pioglitazone), beta-blockers, and antipsychotic drugs, can cause weight gain.

Uncommonly, weight gain is caused by one of the following disorders:

- Brain damage caused by a tumor (especially a craniopharyngioma) or an infection (particularly those affecting the hypothalamus), which can stimulate consumption of excess calories
- Hyperinsulinism due to pancreatic tumors
- Hypercortisolism due to Cushing syndrome, which causes predominantly abdominal obesity
- Hypothyroidism (rarely a cause of substantial weight gain)

Eating disorders: At least 2 pathologic eating patterns may be associated with obesity:

- **Binge eating disorder** is consumption of large amounts of food quickly with a subjective sense of loss of control during the binge and distress after it (see p. 1755). This disorder does not include compensatory behaviors, such as vomiting. Binge eating disorder occurs in about 3.5% of women and 2% of men during their lifetime and in about 10 to 20% of people entering weight reduction programs. Obesity is usually severe, large amounts of weight are frequently gained or lost, and pronounced psychologic disturbances are present.
- **Night-eating syndrome** consists of morning anorexia, evening hyperphagia, and insomnia, with eating in the middle of the night. At least 25 to 50% of daily intake occurs after the evening meal. About 10% of people seeking treatment for severe obesity may have this disorder. Rarely, a similar disorder is induced by use of a hypnotic such as zolpidem.

Similar but less extreme patterns probably contribute to excess weight gain in more people. For example, eating after the evening meal contributes to excess weight gain in many people who do not have night-eating syndrome.

1. Ajslev TA, Andersen CS, Gamborg M, et al: Childhood overweight after establishment of the gut microbiota: The role of delivery mode, pre-pregnancy weight and early administration of antibiotics. *Int J Obes* 35(4):522–529, 2011. doi: 10.1038/ijo.2011.27.

Complications

Complications of obesity include the following:

- Metabolic syndrome
- Diabetes mellitus
- Cardiovascular disorders
- Liver disorders (nonalcoholic steatohepatitis [fatty liver], which may lead to cirrhosis)
- Gallbladder disease (cholelithiasis)
- Gastroesophageal reflux
- Obstructive sleep apnea
- Reproductive system disorders, including infertility, a low serum testosterone level in men, and polycystic ovary syndrome in women
- Many cancers (especially colon and breast cancers)
- Osteoarthritis
- Tendon and fascial disorders
- Skin disorders (eg, intertriginous infections)
- Social, economic, and psychologic problems

Insulin resistance, dyslipidemias, and hypertension (metabolic syndrome) can develop, often leading to diabetes mellitus and coronary artery disease. These complications are more likely in patients with fat that is concentrated abdominally, a high serum triglyceride level, a family history of type 2 diabetes mellitus or premature cardiovascular disease, or a combination of these risk factors.

Obstructive sleep apnea can result if excess fat in the neck compresses the airway during sleep. Breathing stops for moments, as often as hundreds of times a night. This disorder, often undiagnosed, can cause loud snoring and excessive daytime sleepiness and increases the risk of hypertension, cardiac arrhythmias, and metabolic syndrome.

Obesity may cause the obesity-hypoventilation syndrome (Pickwickian syndrome). Impaired breathing leads to hypercapnia, reduced sensitivity to carbon dioxide in stimulating respiration, hypoxia, cor pulmonale, and risk of premature death. This syndrome may occur alone or secondary to obstructive sleep apnea.

Skin disorders are common; increased sweat and skin secretions, trapped in thick folds of skin, are conducive to fungal and bacterial growth, making intertriginous infections especially common.

Being overweight probably predisposes to gout, deep venous thrombosis, and pulmonary embolism.

Obesity leads to social, economic, and psychologic problems as a result of prejudice, discrimination, poor body image, and low self-esteem. For example, people may be underemployed or unemployed.

Diagnosis

- BMI
- Waist circumference
- Sometimes body composition analysis

Table 4–2. BODY MASS INDEX

	NORMAL*	OVERWEIGHT	OBESE		EXTREMELY OBESE	
BMI†	**18.5–24**	**25–29**	**30–34**	**35–39**	**40–47**	**48–54**
Height (in)	**Body Weight (lb)**					
60–61	97–127	128–153	153–180	179–206	204–248	245–285
62–63	104–135	136–163	164–191	191–220	218–265	262–304
64–65	110–144	145–174	174–204	204–234	232–282	279–324
66–67	118–153	155–185	186–217	216–249	247–299	297–344
68–69	125–162	164–196	197–230	230–263	262–318	315–365
70–71	132–172	174–208	209–243	243–279	278–338	334–386
72–73	140–182	184–219	221–257	258–295	294–355	353–408
74–75	148–192	194–232	233–272	272–311	311–375	373–431
76	156–197	205–238	246–279	287–320	328–385	394–443

*BMIs less than those listed as normal are considered underweight.
†Calculations are done using metric units (kg, m), but the table is presented in inches and pounds for US readers.

In adults, BMI, defined as weight (kg) divided by the square of the height (m^2), is used to screen for overweight or obesity (see Table 4–2):

- Overweight = 25 to 29.9 kg/m^2
- Obesity = ≥ 30 kg/m^2

However, BMI is a crude screening tool and has limitations in many subpopulations. Some experts think that BMI cutoffs should vary based on ethnicity, sex, and age. For example, in certain nonwhite populations, complications of obesity develop at a much lower BMI than in whites.

In children and adolescents, overweight is defined as BMI at the ≥ 95th percentile, based on age- and sex-specific growth charts from the CDC at the CDC web site.

Asians, Japanese, and many aboriginal populations have a lower cut-off (23 kg/m^2) for overweight. In addition, BMI may be high in muscular athletes, who lack excess body fat, and may be normal or low in formerly overweight people who have lost muscle mass.

Waist circumference and the presence of metabolic syndrome appear to predict risk of metabolic and cardiovascular complications better than BMI does.

The waist circumference that increases risk of complications due to obesity varies by ethnic group and sex:

- White men: > 93 cm (> 36.6 in), particularly > 101 cm (> 39.8 in)
- White women: > 79 cm (> 31.1 in), particularly > 87 cm (> 34.2 in)
- Asian Indian men: > 78 cm (> 30.7 in), particularly > 90 cm (> 35.4 in)
- Asian Indian women: > 72 cm (> 28.3 in), particularly > 80 cm (> 31.5 in)

Body composition analysis: Body composition—the percentage of body fat and muscle—is also considered when obesity is diagnosed. Although probably unnecessary in routine clinical practice, body composition analysis can be helpful if clinicians question whether elevated BMI is due to muscle or excessive fat.

The percentage of body fat can be estimated by measuring skinfold thickness (usually over the triceps) or determining mid upper arm muscle area (see p. 31).

Bioelectrical impedance analysis (BIA) can estimate percentage of body fat simply and noninvasively. BIA estimates percentage of total body water directly; percentage of body fat is derived indirectly. BIA is most reliable in healthy people and in people with only a few chronic disorders that do not change the percentage of total body water (eg, moderate obesity, diabetes mellitus). Whether measuring BIA poses risks in people with implanted defibrillators is unclear.

Underwater (hydrostatic) weighing is the most accurate method for measuring percentage of body fat. Costly and time-consuming, it is used more often in research than in clinical care. To be weighed accurately while submerged, people must fully exhale beforehand.

Imaging procedures, including CT, MRI, and dual-energy x-ray absorptiometry (DXA), can also estimate the percentage and distribution of body fat but are usually used only for research.

Other testing: Obese patients should be screened for common comorbid disorders, such as obstructive sleep apnea, diabetes, dyslipidemia, hypertension, fatty liver, and depression. Screening tools can help; for example, for obstructive sleep apnea, clinicians can use an instrument such as the STOP-BANG questionnaire (see Table 239–4 on p. 2016) and often the apnea-hypopnea index (total number of apnea or hypopnea episodes occurring per hour of sleep). Obstructive sleep apnea is often underdiagnosed, and obesity increases the risk.

Prognosis

Untreated, obesity tends to progress. The probability and severity of complications are proportional to

- The absolute amount of fat
- The distribution of the fat
- Absolute muscle mass

After weight loss, most people return to their pretreatment weight within 5 yr, and accordingly, obesity requires a lifelong management program similar to that for any other chronic disorder.

Treatment

- Dietary management
- Physical activity
- Behavioral interventions

- Drugs (eg, phentermine, orlistat, lorcaserin, phentermine/topiramate, naltrexone/bupropion extended-release, liraglutide)
- Bariatric surgery

Weight loss of even 5 to 10% improves overall health, helps reduce risk of developing cardiovascular complications (eg, hypertension, dyslipidemia, insulin resistance) and helps lessen their severity, and may lessen the severity of other complications and comorbid disorders such as obstructive sleep apnea, fatty liver, infertility, and depression.

Support from health care practitioners, peers, and family members and various structured programs can help with weight loss and weight maintenance.

Diet: Balanced eating is important for weight loss and maintenance.

Strategies include

- Eating small meals and avoiding or carefully choosing snacks
- Substituting fresh fruits and vegetables and salads for refined carbohydrates and processed food
- Substituting water for soft drinks or juices
- Limiting alcohol consumption to moderate levels
- Including no- or low-fat dairy products, which are part of a healthy diet and help provide an adequate amount of vitamin D

Low-calorie, high-fiber diets that modestly restrict calories (by 600 kcal/day) and that incorporate lean protein appear to have the best long-term outcome. Foods with a low glycemic index (see Table 1–1 on p. 2) and marine fish oils or monounsaturated fats derived from plants (eg, olive oil) reduce the risk of cardiovascular disorders and diabetes.

Use of meal replacements can help with weight loss and maintenance; these products can be used regularly or intermittently.

Diets that are overly restrictive are unlikely to be maintained or to result in long-term weight loss. Diets that limit caloric intake to < 50% of basal energy expenditure (BEE), described as very low calorie diets, can have as few as 800 kcal/day. A very low calorie diet may be indicated for obese patients; however, such diets must be supervised by a physician, and after weight is lost, intake must be increased gradually to prevent patients from regaining weight.

Physical activity: Exercise increases energy expenditure, BMR, and diet-induced thermogenesis. Exercise also seems to regulate appetite to more closely match caloric needs. Other benefits associated with physical activity include

- Increased insulin sensitivity
- Improved lipid profile
- Lower BP
- Better aerobic fitness
- Improved psychologic well-being
- Decreased risk of breast and colon cancer
- Increased life expectancy

Exercise, including strengthening (resistance) exercises, increases muscle mass. Because muscle tissue burns more calories at rest than does fat tissue, increasing muscle mass produces lasting increases in BMR. Exercise that is interesting and enjoyable is more likely to be sustained. A combination of aerobic and resistance exercise is better than either alone. Guidelines suggest physical activity of 150 min/wk for health benefits and 300 to 360 min/wk for weight loss and maintenance. Developing a more physically active lifestyle can help with weight loss and maintenance.

Behavioral interventions: Clinicians can recommend various behavioral interventions to help patients lose weight. They include

- Support
- Self-monitoring
- Stress management
- Contingency management
- Problem solving
- Stimulus control

Support may come from a group, a buddy, or family members. Participation in a support group can improve adherence to lifestyle changes and thus increase weight loss. The more frequently people attend group meetings, the greater the support, motivation, and supervision they receive and the greater their accountability, resulting in greater weight loss.

Self-monitoring may include keeping a food log (including the number of calories in foods), weighing regularly, and observing and recording behavioral patterns. Other useful information to record includes time and location of food consumption, the presence or absence of other people, and mood. Clinicians can provide feedback about how patients may improve their eating habits.

Stress management involves teaching patients to identify stressful situations and to develop strategies to manage stress that do not involve eating (eg, going for a walk, meditating, deep breathing).

Contingency management involves providing tangible rewards for positive behaviors (eg, for increasing time spent walking or reducing consumption of certain foods). Rewards may be given by other people (eg, from members of a support group or a health care practitioner) or by the person (eg, purchase of new clothing or tickets to a concert). Verbal rewards (praise) may also be useful.

Problem solving involves identifying and planning ahead for situations that increase the risk of unhealthy eating (eg, travelling, going out to dinner) or that reduce the opportunity for physical activity (eg, driving across country).

Stimulus control involves identifying obstacles to healthy eating and an active lifestyle and developing strategies to overcome them. For example, people may avoid going by a fast-food restaurant or not keep sweets in the house. For a more active lifestyle, they may take up an active hobby (eg, gardening), enroll in scheduled group activities (eg, exercise classes, sports teams), walk more, make a habit of taking the stairs instead of elevators, and park at the far end of parking lots (resulting in a longer walk).

Internet resources, applications for mobile devices, and other technological devices may also help with adherence to lifestyle changes and weight loss. Applications can help patients set a weight-loss goal, monitor their progress, track food consumption, and record physical activity.

Drugs: Drugs (eg, orlistat, phentermine, phentermine/topiramate, lorcaserin) may be used if BMI is ≥ 30 or if BMI is ≥ 27 in patients who have complications (eg, hypertension, insulin resistance). Usually, drug treatment results in modest (5 to 10%) weight loss.

Orlistat inhibits intestinal lipase, decreasing fat absorption and improving blood glucose and lipids. Because orlistat is not absorbed, systemic effects are rare. Flatus, oily stools, and diarrhea are common but tend to resolve during the 2nd yr of treatment. A dose of 120 mg po tid should be taken with meals that include fat. A vitamin supplement should be taken at least 2 h before or after taking orlistat. Malabsorption and cholestasis are contraindications; irritable bowel syndrome and other GI disorders may make orlistat difficult to tolerate. Orlistat is available OTC.

Phentermine is a centrally acting appetite suppressant for short-term use (≤ 3 mo). Usual starting dose is 15 mg once/day, and dose may be increased to 30 mg once/day, 37.5 mg once/day, 15 mg bid, or 8 mg tid before meals. Common side effects include elevated BP and heart rate, insomnia, anxiety, and constipation. Phentermine should not be used in patients with preexisting cardiovascular disorders, poorly controlled hypertension, hyperthyroidism, or a history of drug abuse or addiction. Twice/day dosing may help control appetite better throughout the day.

The combination of **phentermine and topiramate** (used to treat seizures and migraines) is approved for long-term use. This combination drug results in weight loss for up to 2 yr. The starting dose of the extended-release form (phentermine 3.75 mg/topiramate 23 mg) should be increased to 7.5 mg/46 mg after 2 wk; then the dose can be gradually increased to a maximum of 15 mg/92 mg if needed to maintain weight loss. Because birth defects are a risk, the combination should be given to women of reproductive age only if they are using contraception and are tested monthly for pregnancy. Other potential adverse effects include sleep problems, cognitive impairment, and increased heart rate. Long-term cardiovascular effects are unknown, and postmarketing studies are ongoing.

Lorcaserin suppresses appetite via selective agonism of serotonin 2C (5-HT_{2C}) brain receptors. Unlike serotonergic drugs previously used for weight loss, lorcaserin selectively targets 5-HT_{2C} receptors in the hypothalamus, which, when targeted, result in hypophagia; it does not to stimulate the 5-HT_{2b} receptors on heart valves. In clinical studies, incidence of valvulopathy was not significantly increased in patients taking lorcaserin compared with those taking placebo. The usual and maximum dose of lorcaserin is 10 mg po q 12 h. The most common adverse effects in patients without diabetes are headache, nausea, dizziness, fatigue, dry mouth, and constipation; these effects are usually self-limited. Lorcaserin should not be used with serotonergic drugs, such as selective serotonin reuptake inhibitors (SSRIs), serotonin-norepinephrine reuptake inhibitors (SNRIs), or monoamine oxidase inhibitors (MAOIs), because serotonin syndrome is a risk.

Naltrexone/bupropion extended-release (ER) tablets can be used as a weight-loss adjunct. Naltrexone (used to aid in alcohol cessation) is an opioid antagonist and is thought to block negative feedback on satiety pathways in the brain. Bupropion (used to treat depression and aid in smoking cessation) can induce hypophagia by adrenergic and dopaminergic activity in the hypothalamus. The starting dose is a single tablet of naltrexone 8 mg/bupropion 90 mg; dose is titrated over 4 wk to the maximum dose of 2 tablets bid. The most common adverse effects include nausea, vomiting, headache, and increases in systolic and diastolic BP of 1 to 3 mm Hg. Contraindications to this drug include uncontrolled hypertension and a history of or risk factors for seizures because bupropion reduces the seizure threshold.

Liraglutide is a GLP-1 agonist used initially in the treatment of type 2 diabetes. Liraglutide augments glucose-mediated insulin release from the pancreas to induce glycemic control; liraglutide also stimulates satiety and reduces food intake. Studies have shown that liraglutide 3 mg daily results in a 12.2% weight loss after 56 wk. The initial dose is 0.6 mg once/day; the dose is increased 0.6 mg/wk to the maximum dose of 3 mg once/day. Liraglutide must be given by injection. Adverse effects include nausea and vomiting; liraglutide has warnings that include acute pancreatitis and risk of thyroid C-cell tumors.

Weight loss drugs should be stopped if patients do not have documented weight loss after 12 wk of treatment.

Most OTC weight-loss drugs are not recommended because they have not been shown to be effective. Examples of such drugs are brindleberry, L-carnitine, chitosan, pectin, grapeseed extract, horse chestnut, chromium picolinate, fucus vesiculosus, and ginkgo biloba. Some (eg, caffeine, ephedrine, guarana, phenylpropanolamine) have adverse effects that outweigh their advantages. Also, some of these drugs are adulterated or contain harmful substances banned by the FDA (eg, ephedra, bitter orange, sibutramine).

Surgery: Bariatric surgery is the most effective treatment for extremely obese patients.

Special Populations

Obesity is a particular concern in children and the elderly.

Children: For obese children, complications are more likely to develop because they are obese longer. More than 25% of children and adolescents are overweight or obese.

Risk factors for obesity in infants are low birth weight and maternal obesity, diabetes, and smoking.

After puberty, food intake increases; in boys, the extra calories are used to increase protein deposition, but in girls, fat storage is increased.

For obese children, psychologic complications (eg, poor self-esteem, social difficulties, depression) and musculoskeletal complications can develop early. Some musculoskeletal complications, such as slipped capital femoral epiphyses, occur only in children. Other early complications may include obstructive sleep apnea, insulin resistance, hyperlipidemia, and nonalcoholic steatohepatitis. Risk of cardiovascular, respiratory, metabolic, hepatic, and other obesity-related complications increases when these children become adults.

Risk of obesity persisting into adulthood depends partly on when obesity first develops:

- During infancy: Low risk
- Between 6 mo and 5 yr: 25%
- After 6 yr: > 50%
- During adolescence if a parent is obese: > 80%

In children, preventing further weight gain, rather than losing weight, is a reasonable goal. Diet should be modified, and physical activity increased. Increasing general activities and play is more likely to be effective than a structured exercise program. Participating in physical activities during childhood may promote a lifelong physically active lifestyle. Limiting sedentary activities (eg, watching TV, using the computer or handheld devices) can also help. Drugs and surgery are avoided but, if complications of obesity are life threatening, may be warranted.

Measures that control weight and prevent obesity in children may have the largest public health benefits. Such measures should be implemented in the family, schools, and primary care programs.

The elderly: In the US, the percentage of obese elderly people has been increasing.

With age, body fat increases and is redistributed to the abdomen, and muscle mass is lost, largely because of physical inactivity, but decreased androgens and growth hormone (which are anabolic) and inflammatory cytokines produced in obesity may also play a role.

Risk of complications depends on

- Body fat distribution (increasing with a predominantly abdominal distribution)
- Duration and severity of obesity
- Associated sarcopenia

Increased waist circumference, suggesting abdominal fat distribution, predicts morbidity (eg, hypertension, diabetes mellitus, coronary artery disease) and mortality risk better in the elderly than does BMI. With aging, fat tends to accumulate more in the waist.

For the elderly, physicians may recommend that caloric intake be reduced and physical activity be increased. However, if elderly patients wish to substantially reduce their caloric intake, their diet should be supervised by a physician. Physical activity also improves muscle strength, endurance, and overall well-being and reduces the risk of developing chronic disorders such as diabetes. Activity should include strengthening and endurance exercises.

Regardless of whether caloric restriction is considered necessary, nutrition should be optimized.

Weight-loss drugs are often not studied specifically in the elderly, and possible benefits may not outweigh the adverse effects. However, orlistat may be useful for obese elderly patients, particularly those with diabetes mellitus or hypertension. Surgery can be considered in healthy elderly patients with good functional status.

Prevention

Regular physical activity and healthy eating improve general fitness, can control weight, and help prevent obesity and diabetes mellitus. Even without weight loss, exercise decreases the risk of cardiovascular disorders. Dietary fiber decreases the risk of colon cancer and cardiovascular disorders.

Sufficient and good-quality sleep, management of stress, and moderation of alcohol intake are also important.

KEY POINTS

- Obesity increases the risk of many common health problems and causes up to 300,000 premature deaths each year in the US, making it second only to cigarette smoking as a preventable cause of death.
- Excess caloric intake and too little physical activity contribute the most to obesity, but genetic susceptibility and various disorders (including eating disorders) may also contribute.
- Screen patients using BMI and waist circumference and, when body composition analysis is indicated, by measuring skinfold thickness or using bioelectrical impedance analysis.
- Screen obese patients for common comorbid disorders, such as obstructive sleep apnea, diabetes, dyslipidemia, hypertension, fatty liver, and depression.
- Encourage patients to lose even 5 to 10% of body weight by changing their diet, increasing physical activity, and using behavioral interventions if possible.
- Try treating patients with orlistat, phentermine, phentermine/topiramate, lorcaserin, naltrexone/bupropion, or liraglutide if BMI is ≥ 30 or if BMI is ≥ 27 and they have complications (eg, hypertension, insulin resistance); however, for extreme obesity, surgery is most effective.
- Encourage all patients to exercise, to eat healthily, to get enough sleep, and to manage stress.

BARIATRIC SURGERY

Bariatric surgery is the surgical alteration of the stomach, intestine, or both to cause weight loss.

In the US, about 160,000 bariatric operations are done each year. Development of safer laparoscopic approaches has made this surgery more popular.

Indications

To qualify for bariatric surgery, patients should

- Have a body mass index (BMI) of > 40 kg/m^2 or a BMI > 35 kg/m^2 plus a serious complication (eg, diabetes, hypertension, obstructive sleep apnea, high-risk lipid profile)
- Have acceptable operative risk
- Be well-informed and motivated
- Have unsuccessfully tried all reasonable nonsurgical methods to lose weight and manage obesity-associated complications

Although studies have shown that surgery causes remission of diabetes in patients with a BMI of 30 to 35, long-term data are limited, and the use of bariatric surgery is controversial in patients with a lower BMI.

Contraindications include

- An uncontrolled psychiatric disorder such as major depression
- Current drug or alcohol abuse
- Cancer that is not in remission
- Another life-threatening disorder
- Inability to comply with nutritional requirements, including life-long vitamin replacement (when indicated)

Procedures

The most common procedures done in the US include

- Roux-en-Y gastric bypass (RYGB)
- Sleeve gastrectomy (SG)
- Adjustable gastric banding (AGB)

Most procedures are done laparoscopically, resulting in less pain and a shorter healing time than open surgery. Traditionally, bariatric surgery has been classified as restrictive and/or malabsorptive, referring to the presumptive mechanism of weight loss. However, other factors appear to contribute to weight loss; for example, RYGB (traditionally classified as malabsorptive) and SG (traditionally classified as restrictive) both result in metabolic or hormonal changes that favor satiety and weight loss and in other hormonal changes (eg, an increase in insulin release [incretin effect]) that appear to contribute to the rapid remission of diabetes. After RYGB (particularly) or SG, levels of GI hormones, such as glucagon-like peptide-1 (GLP-1) and peptide YY (PYY), are increased, possibly contributing to satiety, weight loss, and remission of diabetes. Increased insulin sensitivity is evident immediately postoperatively, before significant weight loss occurs, suggesting that neurohormonal factors are prominent in remission of diabetes. A change in gut microbiome may also contribute to changes in weight after RYGB.

Roux-en-Y gastric bypass surgery: RYGB is usually done laparoscopically. A small part of the proximal stomach is detached from the rest, creating a stomach pouch of < 30 mL (see Fig. 4–1). Also, food bypasses part of the stomach and small intestine, where it is normally absorbed, reducing the amount of food and calories absorbed. The pouch is connected to the proximal jejunum; the opening between them is narrow, limiting the rate of gastric emptying. The segment of small intestine connected to the bypassed stomach is attached to the distal small intestine. This arrangement allows bile acids and pancreatic enzymes to mix with GI contents, limiting malabsorption and nutritional deficiencies.

RYGB is particularly effective in treating diabetes; remission rates are up to 62% after 6 yr.

For many patients who have had RYGB, eating high-fat and high-sugar foods can cause dumping syndrome; symptoms can include light-headedness, diaphoresis, nausea, abdominal pain, and diarrhea. Dumping syndrome may inhibit the consumption of such foods by adverse conditioning.

Sleeve gastrectomy: In the past, SG was done only when patients are considered too high risk for procedures such as RYGB and biliopancreatic diversion (eg, patients with a BMI > 60), typically before one of these procedures or another similar procedure is done. However, because SG causes substantial and sustained weight loss, it is being used in the US as definitive treatment for severe obesity. Part of the stomach is removed, creating a tubular stomach passage. The procedure does not involve anatomic changes to the small intestine.

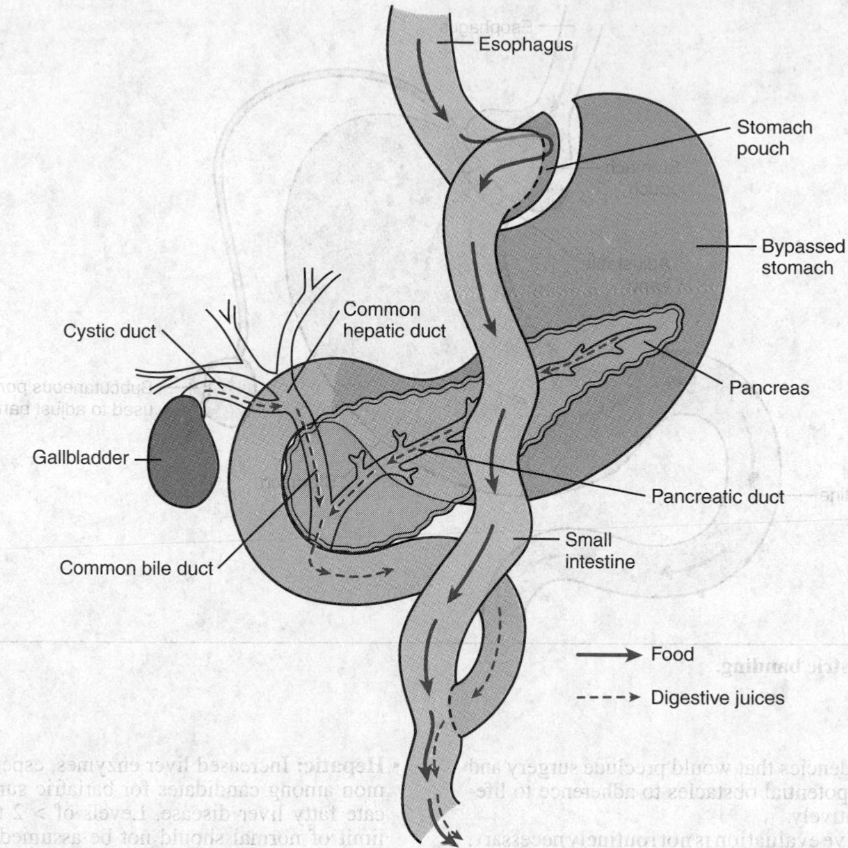

Fig. 4–1. Roux-en-Y gastric bypass surgery.

Mean excess weight loss tends to be higher than with that with AGB. Although SG is traditionally classified as a restrictive procedure, weight loss is probably also related to neurohormonal changes.

The most serious complication is gastric leak at the suture line; it occurs in 1 to 3% of patients.

Adjustable gastric banding: Use of AGB has dramatically decreased in the US. A band is placed around the upper part of the stomach to divide the stomach into a small upper pouch and a larger lower pouch (see Fig. 4–2). Typically, the band is adjusted 4 to 6 times by injecting saline into the band via a port that is placed subcutaneously. When saline is injected, the band expands, restricting the upper pouch of the stomach. As a result, the pouch can hold much less food, patients eat more slowly, and satiety occurs earlier. This procedure is usually done laparoscopically. Saline can be removed from the band if a complication occurs or if the band is overly restrictive.

Weight loss with the band varies and is related to the frequency of follow-up; more frequent follow-ups result in greater weight loss. Although postoperative morbidity and mortality are less than those with RYGB, long-term complications, including repeat operations, are more likely, possibly occurring in up to 15% of patients.

Biliopancreatic diversion with a duodenal switch: This procedure accounts for < 5% of bariatric procedures done in the US.

Part of the stomach is removed, causing restriction. The remaining part empties into the duodenum. The duodenum is cut and attached to the ileum, bypassing much of the small intestine, including the sphincter of Oddi (where bile acids and pancreatic enzymes enter); as a result, food absorption decreases. This procedure is technically demanding but can sometimes be done laparoscopically.

Malabsorption and nutritional deficiencies often develop.

Vertical banded gastroplasty: This procedure is no longer commonly done because complication rates are high and the resulting weight loss is insufficient. For this procedure, a stapler is used to divide the stomach into a small upper pouch and a larger lower pouch. A nonexpandable plastic band is placed around the opening where the upper pouch empties into the lower pouch.

Preoperative Evaluation

Preoperative evaluation consists of diagnosing and correcting comorbid conditions as much as possible, assessing readiness and ability to engage in lifestyle modification, and excluding contraindications to surgery. All patients should be evaluated by a dietician to review the postoperative diet and to assess their ability to make necessary lifestyle changes. All patients should also be evaluated by a psychologist or other qualified mental health care practitioner to identify any uncontrolled psychiatric

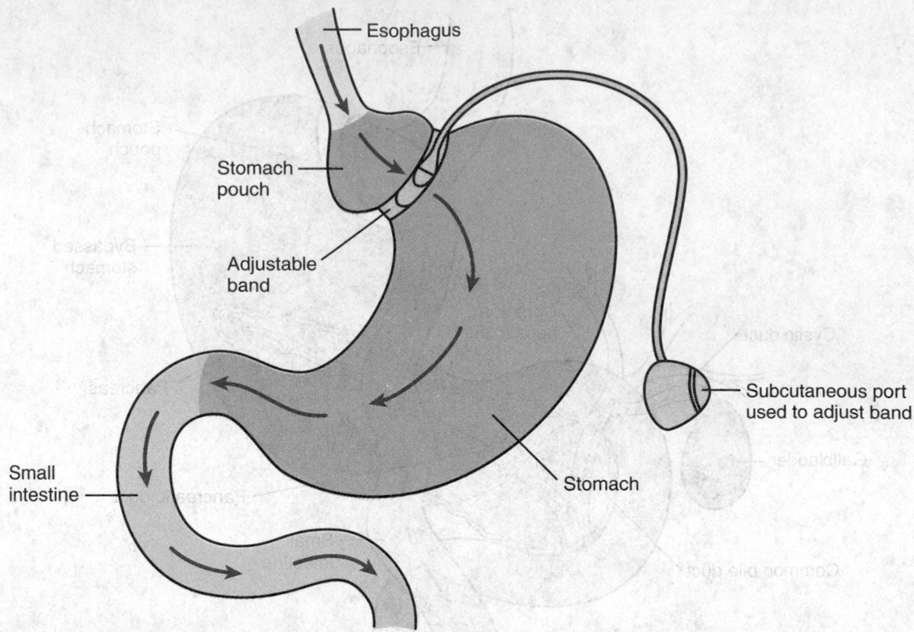

Fig. 4–2. Adjustable gastric banding.

disorder and any dependencies that would preclude surgery and to identify and discuss potential obstacles to adherence to lifestyle changes postoperatively.

Extensive preoperative evaluation is not routinely necessary, but preoperative testing may be necessary based on clinical findings, and measures to control certain conditions (eg, hypertension) or reduce risk may be taken.

- **Pulmonary:** Patients at risk of obstructive sleep apnea based on clinical suspicion should be screened with polysomnography, and if obstructive sleep apnea is present, patients should be treated with continuous positive airway pressure (CPAP). This diagnosis indicates risk of cardiovascular morbidity and premature death. Smoking increases risk of pulmonary complications, ulcers, and GI bleeding postoperatively. Smoking should be stopped ≥ 8 wk before surgery and indefinitely thereafter.
- **Cardiac:** Preoperative ECG is recommended, even for asymptomatic patients, to identify occult coronary artery disease. Even though obesity increases risk of pulmonary hypertension, echocardiography is not done routinely. Other cardiac testing is not done routinely; rather it is done based on the patient's risk factors for coronary artery disease, risk of surgery, and functional status. BP should be optimally controlled before surgery. During the perioperative period, risk of acute kidney disease is increased; thus, diuretics, ACE inhibitors, and angiotensin II receptor blockers (ARBs), if needed, should be used cautiously during this time.
- **GI:** An upper GI series or endoscopy is usually done preoperatively. To reduce the risk of marginal ulcers, clinicians may test for and treat *Helicobacter pylori* infection, although evidence for the necessity of such treatment preoperatively is inconsistent.
- **Hepatic:** Increased liver enzymes, especially ALT, are common among candidates for bariatric surgery and often indicate fatty liver disease. Levels of > 2 to 3 times the upper limit of normal should not be assumed to result from fatty liver and should prompt an investigation for other causes of abnormal liver enzyme levels. If prophylactic cholecystectomy is planned during bariatric surgery (to decrease risk of cholelithiasis), liver ultrasonography may be done.
- **Metabolic bone disease:** Obese patients are at risk of vitamin D deficiency and metabolic bone disease, sometimes with secondary hyperparathyroidism. Patients should be screened and treated for these disorders before surgery, particularly because vitamin D deficiency is common preoperatively and poor absorption develops postoperatively.
- **Diabetes:** Because poorly controlled diabetes increases the risk of adverse surgical outcomes, glycemic control should be optimized before surgery.
- **Nutrition:** Obese patients are at risk of nutritional deficiencies, which can be exacerbated postoperatively because food preferences and tolerance change, stomach acidity changes, and absorption from the small intestine is decreased. Routine measurement of vitamin D, vitamin B_{12}, folate, and iron levels is recommended. For certain patients, measuring levels of other nutrients, such as thiamin (vitamin B_1), may also be indicated.

Risks

Perioperative risks are lowest when bariatric surgery is done in an accredited center.

Complications include

- Gastric and/or anastomotic leaks (in 1 to 3%)
- Pulmonary complications (eg, ventilator dependence, pneumonia, pulmonary embolism)

- MI
- Wound infection
- Incisional hernia
- Small-bowel obstruction
- GI bleeding
- Ventral hernia
- Deep venous thrombosis

These complications can cause significant morbidity, prolong hospitalization, and increase costs. Tachycardia may be the only early sign of anastomotic leak.

Later problems may include prolonged nausea and vomiting secondary to small-bowel obstruction and anastomotic stenosis.

Nutritional deficiencies (eg, protein-energy undernutrition, vitamin B_{12} deficiency, iron deficiency) may result from inadequate intake, inadequate supplementation, or malabsorption. Malodorous flatulence, diarrhea, or both may develop, particularly after malabsorptive procedures. Calcium and vitamin D absorption may be impaired, causing deficiencies and sometimes hypocalcemia and secondary hyperparathyroidism. With prolonged vomiting, thiamin deficiency may occur.

Patients may have symptoms of reflux, especially after SG. During rapid weight loss, cholelithiasis (often symptomatic), gout, and nephrolithiasis may develop.

Incidence of psychologic disorders such as depression is increased in patients having bariatric surgery. A 2016 meta-analysis confirmed this increase in preoperative depression and reported a postoperative decrease in the prevalence and severity of depression.[1] One large study suggested that the risk of suicide in patients who had bariatric surgery was increased compared with that in controls (2.7 vs 1.2 per 10,000 person/yr; hazard ratio 1.71 [0.69 to 4.25]; P value = 0.25.[2] Incidence of alcohol use disorder also appears to be increased after bariatric surgery.[3]

Eating habits may be disordered. Adjusting to new eating habits can be difficult.

1. Dawes AJ, Maggard-Gibbons M, Maher AR, et al: Mental health conditions among patients seeking and undergoing bariatric surgery: A meta-analysis. *JAMA* 315(2):150–163, 2016. doi: 10.1001/jama.2015.18118.
2. Adams TD, Gress RE, Smith SC, et al: Long-term mortality after gastric bypass surgery. *N Engl J Med* 357:753–761, 2007.
3. Heinberg LJ, Ashton K, Coughlin J: Alcohol and bariatric surgery: review and suggested recommendations for assessment and management. *Surg Obes Relat Dis* 8(3):357–363, 2012. doi: 10.1016/j.soard.2012.01.016.

Prognosis

In hospitals accredited by the American Society of Bariatric Surgery as centers of excellence (COE), overall 30-day mortality is 0.2 to 0.3%. However, some data indicate that lower rates of serious complications are predicted more accurately by the number of procedures done in the hospital and by the surgeon than by COE status.

Mortality is higher with RYGB than laparoscopic AGB and higher with open procedures (2.1%) than laparoscopic procedures (0.2%). Factors that predict higher risk of mortality include a history of deep venous thrombosis or pulmonary embolism, obstructive sleep apnea, and poor functional status. Other factors such as severe obesity (BMI > 50), older age, and male sex have also been associated with higher risk, but the evidence is inconsistent.

Average excess weight loss depends on the procedure.

For **laparoscopic AGB,** weight loss is

- 45 to 72% at 3 to 6 yr
- 14 to 60% at 7 to 10 yr
- About 47% at 15 yr

Percentage of weight loss is related to the frequency of follow-ups and number of band adjustments. Patients with a lower BMI tend to lose more excess weight than those with a higher BMI.

For **SG,** weight loss is

- 33 to 58% at 2 yr
- 58 to 72% at 3 to 6 yr

Longer-term data are not available.

For **RYGB,** weight loss is

- 50 to 65% after 2 yr

Weight loss after RYGB is maintained for up to 10 yr.

Comorbid conditions that tend to abate or resolve after bariatric surgery include cardiovascular risk factors (eg, dyslipidemia, hypertension, diabetes), cardiovascular disorders, diabetes, obstructive sleep apnea, osteoarthritis, and depression. Diabetes is particularly likely to remit (eg, with RYGB, up to 62% of patients at 6 yr). All-cause mortality decreases by 25%, primarily because cardiovascular and cancer mortality is reduced.

Follow-up

Regular, long-term follow-up helps ensure adequate weight loss and prevent complications. After RYGB or SG, patients should be monitored every 4 to 12 wk during the period of rapid weight loss (usually about the first 6 mo after surgery), then every 6 to 12 mo thereafter. With laparoscopic AGB, results appear to be optimal when patients are monitored and the band is adjusted at least 6 times during the first year after surgery.

Weight and BP are checked, and eating habits are reviewed. Blood tests (usually CBC, electrolytes, glucose, BUN, creatinine, albumin, and protein and liver function tests) are done at regular intervals. Glycosylated Hb (HbA_{1c}) and fasting lipid levels should be monitored if they were abnormal before surgery. Depending on the type of procedure, vitamin and mineral levels, including calcium, vitamin D, vitamin B_{12}, folate, iron, and thiamin (vitamin B_1), may need to be monitored. Because secondary hyperparathyroidism is a risk, parathyroid hormone levels should also be monitored. Bone density should be measured after SG and RYGB.

Clinicians should check for any changes in response to antihypertensives, insulin, oral hypoglycemics, or lipid-lowering drugs during the period of rapid weight loss after surgery.

Patients should be regularly evaluated for gout, cholelithiasis, and nephrolithiasis, all of which can develop after bariatric surgery. Prophylactic ursodiol reduces risk of cholelithiasis and should be offered after bariatric surgery. Patients should also be regularly screened for depression and alcohol use, particularly if alcohol use was heavy preoperatively.

To minimize risk of hypoglycemia (due to increased insulin sensitivity after bariatric surgery) in patients with diabetes, clinicians should adjust the dose of insulin and decrease the dose of oral hypoglycemics (particularly sulfonylureas) or stop them after RYGB and SG.

KEY POINTS

- Consider weight loss surgery if patients are motivated, have not succeeded using nonsurgical treatments, and have a BMI of > 40 kg/m^2 or a BMI of > 35 kg/m^2 plus a serious complication (eg, diabetes, hypertension, obstructive sleep apnea, high-risk lipid profile).
- Weight loss surgery is contraindicated if patients have an uncontrolled psychiatric disorder (eg, major depression), drug or alcohol abuse, cancer that is not in remission, or another life-threatening disorder or if they cannot comply with nutritional requirements (including life-long vitamin replacement when indicated).
- The most common procedure is Roux-en-Y gastric bypass, followed by sleeve gastrectomy; use of adjustable gastric banding has decreased dramatically in the US.
- Monitor patients regularly after surgery for maintenance of weight loss, resolution of weight-related comorbid disorders, and complications of surgery (eg, nutritional deficiencies, metabolic bone disease, gout, cholelithiasis, nephrolithiasis, depression, alcohol abuse).

METABOLIC SYNDROME

(Insulin Resistance Syndrome; Syndrome X)

Metabolic syndrome is characterized by a large waist circumference (due to excess abdominal fat), hypertension, abnormal fasting plasma glucose or insulin resistance, and dyslipidemia. Causes, complications, diagnosis, and treatment are similar to those of obesity.

In developed countries, metabolic syndrome is a serious problem. It is very common; in the US, > 40% of people > 50 yr may have it. Children and adolescents can develop metabolic syndrome, but in these age groups, no definition is established.

Development of metabolic syndrome depends on distribution as well as amount of fat. Excess fat in the abdomen (called apple shape), particularly when it results in a high waist-to-hip ratio (reflecting a relatively low muscle-to-fat mass ratio), increases risk. The syndrome is less common among people who have excess subcutaneous fat around the hips (called pear shape) and a low waist-to-hip ratio (reflecting a higher muscle-to-fat mass ratio).

Excess abdominal fat leads to excess free fatty acids in the portal vein, increasing fat accumulation in the liver. Fat also accumulates in muscle cells. Insulin resistance develops, with hyperinsulinemia. Glucose metabolism is impaired, and dyslipidemias and hypertension develop. Serum uric acid levels are typically elevated (increasing risk of gout), and a prothrombotic state (with increased levels of fibrinogen and plasminogen activator inhibitor I) and an inflammatory state develop.

Risks of metabolic syndrome include

- Obstructive sleep apnea
- Nonalcoholic steatohepatitis
- Chronic kidney disease
- Polycystic ovary syndrome (for women)
- Low plasma testosterone, erectile dysfunction, or both (for men)

Diagnosis

- Waist circumference and BP
- Fasting plasma glucose and a lipid profile

Screening is important. A family history plus measurement of waist circumference and BP are part of routine care. If patients with a family history of type 2 diabetes mellitus, particularly those ≥ 40 yr, have a waist circumference greater than that recommended for race and sex, fasting plasma glucose and a lipid profile must be determined.

Metabolic syndrome has many different definitions, but it is most often diagnosed when ≥ 3 of the following are present (see Table 4–3):

- Excess abdominal fat
- A high fasting plasma glucose level
- Hypertension
- A high triglyceride level
- A low high-density lipoprotein (HDL) cholesterol level

Treatment

- Healthy diet and exercise
- Sometimes metformin
- Management of cardiovascular risk factors

Optimally, the management approach results in weight loss based on a healthy diet and regular physical activity, which includes a combination of aerobic activity and resistance training, reinforced with behavioral therapy. Metformin, an insulin sensitizer, or a thiazolidinedione (eg, rosiglitazone, pioglitazone) may be useful. Weight loss of ≈ 7% may be sufficient to reverse the syndrome, but if not, each feature of the syndrome should be managed to achieve recommended targets; available drug treatment is very effective.

Other cardiovascular risk factors (eg, smoking cessation) also need to be managed. Increased physical activity has cardiovascular benefits even if weight is not lost.

KEY POINTS

- Excess abdominal fat leads to abnormal fasting plasma glucose or insulinresistance, dyslipidemias, and hypertension.
- Metabolic syndrome is extremely common in developed countries (eg, prevalence of possibly > 40% in people > 50 yr).
- Determine waist circumference, BP, fasting plasma glucose, and lipid profile.
- Emphasize following a healthy diet and exercising, manage cardiovascular risk factors, and if these measures are not completely effective, consider use of metformin.

Table 4–3. CRITERIA OFTEN USED FOR DIAGNOSIS OF METABOLIC SYNDROME*

CRITERIA	VALUE
Waist circumference (cm [in])	≥ 102 (≥ 40) for men ≥ 88 (≥ 35) for women
Fasting glucose (mg/dL [mmol/L])	≥ 100 (≥ 5.6)
BP (mm Hg)	≥ 130/85
Triglycerides, fasting (mg/dL [mmol/L])	≥ 150 (≥ 1.7)
High-density lipoprotein (HDL) cholesterol (mg/dL [mmol/L])	< 40 (< 1.04) for men < 50 (< 1.29) for women

*At least 3 of the criteria must be present for the diagnosis.

5 Undernutrition

Undernutrition is a form of malnutrition. (Malnutrition also includes overnutrition—see p. 19). Undernutrition can result from inadequate ingestion of nutrients, malabsorption, impaired metabolism, loss of nutrients due to diarrhea, or increased nutritional requirements (as occurs in cancer or infection). Undernutrition progresses in stages; it may develop slowly when it is due to anorexia or very rapidly, as sometimes occurs when it is due to rapidly progressive cancer-related cachexia. First, nutrient levels in blood and tissues change, followed by intracellular changes in biochemical functions and structure. Ultimately, symptoms and signs appear. Diagnosis is by history, physical examination, body composition analysis, and sometimes laboratory tests (eg, albumin).

Risk Factors

Undernutrition is associated with many disorders and circumstances, including poverty and social deprivation.

Risk is also greater at certain times (ie, during infancy, early childhood, adolescence, pregnancy, breastfeeding, and old age).

Infancy and childhood: Infants and children are particularly susceptible to undernutrition because of their high demand for energy and essential nutrients. Because vitamin K does not readily cross the placenta, neonates may be deficient, so they are given a single injection of vitamin K within 1 h of birth to prevent hemorrhagic disease of the newborn (see p. 2785), a life-threatening disorder. Infants fed only breast milk, which is typically low in vitamin D, are given supplemental vitamin D; they can develop vitamin B_{12} deficiency if the mother is a vegan. Inadequately fed infants and children are at risk of protein-energy undernutrition (PEU—previously called protein-energy malnutrition) and deficiencies of iron, folate (folic acid), vitamins A and C, copper, and zinc.

During adolescence, nutritional requirements increase because the growth rate accelerates. Anorexia nervosa may affect adolescent girls in particular (see p. 1754).

Pregnancy and breastfeeding: Requirements for nutrients increase during pregnancy and breastfeeding. Aberrations of diet, including pica (consumption of nonnutritive substances, such as clay and charcoal), may occur during pregnancy. Anemia due to iron deficiency is common, as is anemia due to folate deficiency, especially among women who have taken oral contraceptives (see p. 2386). Vitamin D deficiency is common during late pregnancy, predisposing the child to decreased bone mass.

Old age: Aging—even when disease or dietary deficiency is absent—leads to sarcopenia (progressive loss of lean body mass), starting after age 40 and eventually amounting to a muscle loss of about 10 kg (22 lb) in men and 5 kg (11 lb) in women. Undernutrition contributes to sarcopenia, and sarcopenia accounts for many of the complications of undernutrition (eg, decreased nitrogen balance, increased susceptibility to infections).

Causes of sarcopenia include the following:

- Decreased physical activity
- Decreased food intake
- Increased levels of cytokines (particularly interleukin-6)
- Decreased levels of growth hormone and mechano growth factor (insulin-like growth factor-3)
- In men, decreasing androgen levels

Aging decreases basal metabolic rate (due mainly to decreased fat-free mass), total body weight, height, and skeletal mass; from about age 40 to age 65, mean body fat (as a percentage of body weight) increases to about 30% (from 20%) in men and to 40% (from 27%) in women.

From age 20 to 80, food intake decreases, especially in men. Anorexia due to aging itself has many causes, including

- Reduced adaptive relaxation of the stomach's fundus
- Increased release and activity of cholecystokinin (which produces satiation)
- Increased leptin (an anorectic hormone produced by fat cells)
- Diminished taste and smell, which can decrease eating pleasure but usually decrease food intake only slightly
- Depression (a common cause)
- Loneliness
- Inability to shop or prepare meals
- Dementia
- Some chronic disorders
- Use of certain drugs

Occasionally, anorexia nervosa (sometimes called anorexia tardive in the elderly), paranoia, or mania interferes with eating. Dental problems limit the ability to chew and subsequently to digest foods. Swallowing difficulties (eg, due to strokes, other neurologic disorders, esophageal candidiasis, or xerostomia) are common. Poverty or functional impairment limits access to nutrients.

The institutionalized elderly are at particular risk of PEU. They are often confused and may be unable to express hunger or preferences for foods. They may be physically unable to feed themselves. Chewing or swallowing may be very slow, making it tedious for another person to feed them enough food.

In the elderly, particularly the institutionalized elderly, inadequate intake and often decreased absorption or synthesis of vitamin D, increased demand for vitamin D, and inadequate exposure to sunshine contribute to vitamin D deficiency and osteomalacia.

Disorders and medical procedures: Diabetes, some chronic disorders that affect the GI tract, intestinal resection, and certain other GI surgical procedures tend to impair absorption of fat-soluble vitamins, vitamin B_{12}, calcium, and iron. Gluten enteropathy, pancreatic insufficiency, or other disorders can result in malabsorption. Decreased absorption possibly contributes to iron deficiency and osteoporosis.

Liver disorders impair storage of vitamins A and B_{12} and interfere with metabolism of protein and energy sources. Renal insufficiency predisposes to protein, iron, and vitamin D deficiencies.

Anorexia causes some patients with cancer or depression and many with AIDS to consume inadequate amounts of food.

Infections, trauma, hyperthyroidism, extensive burns, and prolonged fever increase metabolic demands. Any condition that increases cytokines may be accompanied by muscle loss, lipolysis, low albumin levels, and anorexia.

Vegetarian diets: Iron deficiency can occur in ovo-lacto vegetarians (although such a diet can be compatible with good health). Vegans may develop vitamin B_{12} deficiency unless they consume yeast extracts or Asian-style fermented foods. Their intake of calcium, iron, and zinc also tends to be low.

A fruit-only diet is not recommended because it is deficient in protein, sodium, and many micronutrients.

Fad diets: Some fad diets result in vitamin, mineral, and protein deficiencies; cardiac, renal, and metabolic disorders; and sometimes death. Very low calorie diets (< 400 kcal/day) cannot sustain health for long.

NESTLÉ NUTRITION SERVICES

Last name: ____ First name: ____ Sex: ____ Date: ____

Age: ____ Weight, kg: ____ Height, cm: ____ I.D. Number: ____

Complete the screen by filling in the boxes with the appropriate numbers.
Add the numbers for the screen. If score is 11 or less, continue with the assessment to gain a Malnutrition Indicator Score.

SCREENING

A Has food intake declined over the past 3 months due to loss of appetite, digestive problems, chewing or swallowing difficulties?
0 = severe loss of appetite
1 = moderate loss of appetite
2 = no loss of appetite ☐

B Weight loss during last months
0 = weight loss greater than 3 kg (6.6 lbs)
1 = does not know
2 = weight loss between 1 and 3 kg (2.2 and 6.6 lbs)
3 = no weight loss ☐

C Mobility
0 = bed or chair bound
1 = able to get out of bed/chair but does not go out
2 = goes out ☐

D Has suffered psychological stress or acute disease in the past 3 months
0 = yes 2 = no ☐

E Neuropsychological problems
0 = severe dementia or depression
1 = mild dementia
2 = no psychological problems ☐

F Body Mass Index (BMI) (weight in kg) / (height in m)^2
0 = BMI less than 19
1 = BMI19 to less than 21
2 = BMI 21 to less than 23
3 = BMI 23 or greater ☐

Screening Score (subtotal max. 14 points) ☐☐

12 points or greater	Normal—not at risk—no need to complete assessment
11 points or below	Possible malnutrition—continue assessment

ASSESSMENT

G Lives independently (not in a nursing home or hospital)
0 = no 1 = yes ☐

H Takes more than 3 prescription drugs per day
0 = yes 1 = no ☐

I Pressure sores or skin ulcers
0 = yes 1 = no ☐

J How many full meals does the patient eat daily?
0 = 1 meal
1 = 2 meals
2 = 3 meals ☐

K Selected consumption markers for protein intake
- At least one serving of dairy products (milk, cheese, yogurt) per day? yes ☐ no ☐
- Two or more servings of legumes or eggs per week? yes ☐ no ☐
- Meat, fish or poultry every day yes ☐ no ☐

0.0 = if 0 or 1 yes
0.5 = if 2 yes
1.0 = if 3 yes ☐.☐

L Consumes two or more servings of fruits or vegetables per day?
0 = no 1 = yes ☐

M How much fluid (water, juice, coffee, tea, milk. . .) is consumed per day?
0.0 = less than 3 cups
0.5 = 3 to 5 cups
1.0 = more than 5 cups ☐.☐

N Mode of feeding
0 = unable to eat without assistance
1 = self-fed with some difficulty
2 = self-fed without any problem ☐

O Self view of nutritional status
0 = views self as being malnourished
1 = is uncertain of nutritional state
2 = views self as having no nutritional problem ☐

P In comparison with other people of the same age, how do they consider their health status?
0.0 = not as good
0.5 = does not know
1.0 = as good
2.0 = better ☐.☐

Q Mid-arm circumference (MAC) in cm
0.0 = MAC less than 21
0.5 = MAC 21 to 22
1.0 = MAC 22 or greater ☐.☐

R Calf circumference (CC) in cm
0 = CC less than 31 1 = CC 31 or greater ☐

Assessment (max. 16 points) ☐☐.☐

Screening score ☐☐

Total Assessment (max. 30 points) ☐☐.☐

Malnutrition Indicator Score

17 to 23.5 points	at risk of malnutrition	☐
Less than 17 points	malnourished	☐

Fig. 5–1. Mini nutritional assessment. Guigoz Y and Garry PJ. Mini nutritional assessment. A practical assessment tool for grading the nutritional status of elderly patients. Facts and Research in Gerontology. Supplement 2:15–59, 1994. Rubenstein LZ, Jarker J, Guigoz Y, and Vellas B. Comprehensive geriatric assessment (CGA) and the MNA: An overview of the CGA, nutritional assessment and development of a shortened version of the MNA. In *Mini nutritional assessment (MNA): Research and practice in the elderly*. Vellas B, Garry PJ, and Guigoz Y, editors. Nestlé Nutrition Workshop Series. Clinical & Performance Programme, vol. 1, Karger, Bale, 1997. ® Société des Produits Nestlé S.A., Vevey, Switzerland, trademark owners. Reprinted with permission.

Drugs and nutritional supplements: Many drugs (eg, appetite suppressants, digoxin) decrease appetite; others impair nutrient absorption or metabolism. Some drugs (eg, stimulants) have catabolic effects. Certain drugs can impair absorption of many nutrients; eg, anticonvulsants can impair absorption of vitamins.

Alcohol or drug dependency: Patients with alcohol or drug dependency may neglect their nutritional needs. Absorption and metabolism of nutrients may also be impaired. IV drug addicts typically become undernourished, as do alcoholics who consume ≥ 1 quart of hard liquor/day. Alcoholism can cause deficiencies of magnesium, zinc, and certain vitamins, including thiamin.

Symptoms and Signs

Symptoms vary depending on the cause and type of undernutrition (eg, PEU, vitamin deficiency).

Evaluation

Diagnosis of undernutrition is based on results of medical and diet histories, physical examination, body composition analysis, and selected laboratory tests.

History: History should include questions about dietary intake (see Fig. 5–1), recent changes in weight, and risk factors for undernutrition, including drug and alcohol use. Unintentional loss of ≥ 10% of usual body weight during a 3-mo period indicates a high probability of undernutrition. Social history should include questions about whether money is available for food and whether the patient can shop and cook.

Review of systems should focus on symptoms of nutritional deficiencies (see Table 5–1). For example, impaired night vision may indicate vitamin A deficiency.

Physical examination: Physical examination should include

- Measurement of height and weight
- Inspection of body fat distribution
- Anthropometric measurements of lean body mass

Body mass index (BMI = weight[kg]/height[m]^2) adjusts weight for height (see Table 4–2 on p. 21). If weight is < 80% of what is predicted for the patient's height or if BMI is ≤ 18, undernutrition should be suspected. Although these findings are useful in diagnosing undernutrition and are acceptably sensitive, they lack specificity.

The **mid upper arm muscle area** estimates lean body mass. This area is derived from the triceps skinfold thickness (TSF) and mid upper arm circumference. Both are measured at the same site, with the patient's right arm in a relaxed position. The average mid upper arm circumference is about 34.1 cm for men and 31.9 cm for women.[1] The formula for calculating the mid upper arm muscle area in cm^2 is as follows:

$$\frac{[\text{midarm circumference (cm)} - (3.14 \times \text{TSF cm})]^2}{4\pi} - 10 \text{ (males) or } -6.5 \text{ (females)}$$

Table 5–1. SYMPTOMS AND SIGNS OF NUTRITIONAL DEFICIENCY

AREA/SYSTEM	SYMPTOM OR SIGN	DEFICIENCY
General appearance	Wasting	Energy
Skin	Rash	Many vitamins, zinc, essential fatty acids
	Rash in sun-exposed areas	Niacin (pellagra)
	Easy bruising	Vitamin C or vitamin K
Hair and nails	Thinning or loss of hair	Protein
	Premature whitening of hair	Selenium
	Spooning (upcurling) of nails	Iron
Eyes	Impaired night vision	Vitamin A
	Corneal keratomalacia (corneal drying and clouding)	Vitamin A
Mouth	Cheilosis and glossitis	Riboflavin, niacin, pyridoxine, iron
	Bleeding gums	Vitamin C, riboflavin
Extremities	Edema	Protein
Neurologic	Paresthesias or numbness in a stocking-glove distribution	Thiamin (beriberi)
	Tetany	Calcium, magnesium
	Cognitive and sensory deficits	Thiamin, niacin, pyridoxine, vitamin B_{12}
	Dementia	Thiamin, niacin, vitamin B_{12}
Musculoskeletal	Wasting of muscle	Protein
	Bone deformities (eg, bowlegs, knocked knees, curved spine)	Vitamin D, calcium
	Bone tenderness	Vitamin D
	Joint pain or swelling	Vitamin C
GI	Diarrhea	Protein, niacin, folate, vitamin B_{12}
	Diarrhea and dysgeusia	Zinc
	Dysphagia or odynophagia (due to Plummer-Vinson syndrome)	Iron
Endocrine	Thyromegaly	Iodine

Table 5–2. MID UPPER ARM MUSCLE AREA IN ADULTS

PERCENTAGE OF STANDARD (%)	MEN (cm^2)	WOMEN (cm^2)	MUSCLE MASS
100 ± 20*	54 ± 11	30 ± 7	Adequate
75	40	22	Marginal
60	32	18	Depleted
50	27	15	Wasted

*Mean mid upper arm muscle mass ± 1 standard deviation.
From the National Health and Nutrition Examination Surveys I and II.

This formula corrects the upper arm area for fat and bone. Average values for the mid upper arm muscle area are 54 ± 11 cm^2 for men and 30 ± 7 cm^2 for women. A value < 75% of this standard (depending on age) indicates depletion of lean body mass (see Table 5–2). This measurement may be affected by physical activity, genetic factors, and age-related muscle loss.

Physical examination should focus on signs of specific nutritional deficiencies. Signs of PEU (eg, edema, muscle wasting, skin changes) should be sought. Examination should also focus on signs of conditions that could predispose to nutritional deficiencies, such as dental problems. Mental status should be assessed, because depression and cognitive impairment can lead to weight loss.

The following assessment tools may be useful:

- The widely used Subjective Global Assessment (SGA) uses information from the patient history (eg, weight loss, change in intake, GI symptoms), physical examination findings (eg, loss of muscle and subcutaneous fat, edema, ascites), and the clinician's judgment of the patient's nutritional status.
- The Mini Nutritional Assessment (MNA) has been validated and is widely used, especially for elderly patients (see Fig. 5–1).
- The Simplified Nutrition Assessment Questionnaire (SNAQ), a simple, validated method of predicting future weight loss, may be used (see Fig. 5–2).

1. My appetite is
   a. very poor
   b. poor
   c. average
   d. good
   e. very good
2. When I eat
   a. I feel full after eating only a few mouthfuls
   b. I feel full after eating about a third of a meal
   c. I feel full after eating over half a meal
   d. I feel full after eating most of the meal
   e. I hardly ever feel full
3. Food tastes
   a. very bad
   b. bad
   c. average
   d. good
   e. very good
4. Normally, I eat
   a. < 1 meal a day
   b. 1 meal a day
   c. 2 meals a day
   d. 3 meals a day
   e. > 3 meals a day

Points are assigned for the patient's answers as follows: a = 1, b = 2, c = 3, d = 4, e = 5. The sum is the SNAQ score. A SNAQ score of ≤ 14 indicates high risk of at least 5% weight loss within 6 mo.

Adapted from Wilson MMG, et al: Appetite assessment: Simple appetite questionnaire predicts weight loss in community-dwelling adults and nursing home residents. *The American Journal of Clinical Nutrition* 82(5):1074-1081, 2005; used with permission.

Fig. 5–2. Simplified nutrition assessment questionnaire (SNAQ).

Testing: The extent of laboratory testing needed is unclear and may depend on the patient's circumstances. If the cause is obvious and correctable (eg, a wilderness survival situation), testing is probably of little benefit. Other patients may require more detailed evaluation.

Serum albumin measurement is the laboratory test most often used. Decreases in albumin and other proteins (eg, prealbumin [transthyretin], transferrin, retinol-binding protein) may indicate protein deficiency or PEU. As undernutrition progresses, albumin decreases slowly; prealbumin, transferrin, and retinol-binding protein decrease rapidly. Albumin measurement is inexpensive and predicts morbidity and mortality better than measurement of the other proteins. However, the correlation of albumin with morbidity and mortality may be related to nonnutritional as well as nutritional factors. Inflammation produces cytokines that cause albumin and other nutritional protein markers to extravasate, decreasing serum levels. Because prealbumin, transferrin, and retinol-binding protein decrease more rapidly during starvation than does albumin, their measurements are sometimes used to diagnose or assess the severity of acute starvation. However, whether they are more sensitive or specific than albumin is unclear.

Total lymphocyte count, which often decreases as undernutrition progresses, may be determined. Undernutrition causes a marked decline in CD4+ T lymphocytes, so this count may not be useful in patients who have AIDS.

Skin tests using antigens can detect impaired cell-mediated immunity in PEU and in some other disorders of undernutrition (see p. 1393).

Other laboratory tests, such as measuring vitamin and mineral levels, are used selectively to diagnose specific deficiencies.

1. McDowell MA, Fryar CD, Ogden CL, Flegal KM: Anthropometric reference data for children and adults: United States, 2003–2006. *Natl Health Stat Report* Oct 22(10):1–48, 2008.

PROTEIN-ENERGY UNDERNUTRITION

Protein-energy undernutrition (PEU), previously called protein-energy malnutrition, is an energy deficit due to deficiency of all macronutrients. It commonly includes deficiencies of many micronutrients. PEU can be sudden and total (starvation) or gradual. Severity ranges from subclinical deficiencies to obvious wasting (with edema, hair loss, and skin atrophy) to starvation. Multiple organ systems are often impaired. Diagnosis usually involves laboratory testing, including serum albumin. Treatment consists of correcting fluid and electrolyte deficits with IV solutions, then gradually replenishing nutrients, orally if possible.

In developed countries, PEU is common among the institutionalized elderly (although often not suspected) and among patients with disorders that decrease appetite or impair nutrient digestion, absorption, or metabolism. In developing countries, PEU affects children who do not consume enough calories or protein.

Classification and Etiology

PEU is graded as mild, moderate, or severe. Grade is determined by calculating weight as a percentage of expected weight for length or height using international standards (normal, 90 to 110%; mild PEU, 85 to 90%; moderate, 75 to 85%; severe, <75%).

PEU may be

- Primary: Caused by inadequate nutrient intake
- Secondary: Results from disorders or drugs that interfere with nutrient use

Primary PEU: Worldwide, primary PEU occurs mostly in children and the elderly who lack access to nutrients, although a common cause in the elderly is depression. PEU can also result from fasting or anorexia nervosa. Child or elder abuse may be a cause.

In children, chronic primary PEU has 2 common forms:

- Marasmus
- Kwashiorkor

The form depends on the balance of nonprotein and protein sources of energy. Starvation is an acute severe form of primary PEU.

Marasmus (also called the dry form of PEU) causes weight loss and depletion of fat and muscle. In developing countries, marasmus is the most common form of PEU in children.

Kwashiorkor (also called the wet, swollen, or edematous form) is a risk after premature abandonment of breastfeeding, which typically occurs when a younger sibling is born, displacing the older child from the breast. So children with kwashiorkor tend to be older than those with marasmus. Kwashiorkor may also result from an acute illness, often gastroenteritis or another infection (probably secondary to cytokine release), in a child who already has PEU. A diet that is more deficient in protein than energy may be more likely to cause kwashiorkor than marasmus. Less common than marasmus, kwashiorkor tends to be confined to specific parts of the world, such as rural Africa, the Caribbean, and the Pacific islands. In these areas, staple foods (eg, yams, cassavas, sweet potatoes, green bananas) are low in protein and high in carbohydrates. In kwashiorkor, cell membranes leak, causing extravasation of intravascular fluid and protein, resulting in peripheral edema.

In both marasmus and kwashiorkor, cell-mediated immunity is impaired, increasing susceptibility to infections. Bacterial infections (eg, pneumonia, gastroenteritis, otitis media, UTIs, sepsis) are common. Infections result in release of cytokines, which cause anorexia, worsen muscle wasting, and cause a marked decrease in serum albumin levels.

Starvation is a complete lack of nutrients. It occasionally occurs when food is available (as in fasting or anorexia nervosa) but usually occurs because food is unavailable (eg, during famine or wilderness exposure).

Secondary PEU: This type most commonly results from the following:

- **Disorders that affect GI function:** These disorders can interfere with digestion (eg, pancreatic insufficiency), absorption (eg, enteritis, enteropathy), or lymphatic transport of nutrients (eg, retroperitoneal fibrosis, Milroy disease).
- **Wasting disorders:** In wasting disorders (eg, AIDS, cancer, COPD) and renal failure, catabolism causes cytokine excess, resulting in undernutrition via anorexia and cachexia (wasting of muscle and fat). End-stage heart failure can cause cardiac cachexia, a severe form of undernutrition; mortality rate is particularly high. Factors contributing to cardiac cachexia may include passive hepatic congestion (causing anorexia), edema of the intestinal tract (impairing absorption), and, in advanced disease, increased O_2 requirement due to anaerobic metabolism. Wasting disorders can decrease appetite or impair metabolism of nutrients.

- **Conditions that increase metabolic demands:** These conditions include infections, hyperthyroidism, pheochromocytoma, other endocrine disorders, burns, trauma, surgery, and other critical illnesses.

Pathophysiology

The initial metabolic response is decreased metabolic rate. To supply energy, the body first breaks down adipose tissue. However, later, when these tissues are depleted, the body may use protein for energy, resulting in a negative nitrogen balance. Visceral organs and muscle are broken down and decrease in weight. Loss of organ weight is greatest in the liver and intestine, intermediate in the heart and kidneys, and least in the nervous system.

Symptoms and Signs

Symptoms of moderate PEU can be constitutional or involve specific organ systems. Apathy and irritability are common. The patient is weak, and work capacity decreases. Cognition and sometimes consciousness are impaired. Temporary lactose deficiency and achlorhydria develop. Diarrhea is common and can be aggravated by deficiency of intestinal disaccharidases, especially lactase. Gonadal tissues atrophy. PEU can cause amenorrhea in women and loss of libido in men and women.

Wasting of fat and muscle is common in all forms of PEU. In adult volunteers who fasted for 30 to 40 days, weight loss was marked (25% of initial weight). If starvation is more prolonged, weight loss may reach 50% in adults and possibly more in children.

In adults, cachexia is most obvious in areas where prominent fat depots normally exist. Muscles shrink and bones protrude. The skin becomes thin, dry, inelastic, pale, and cold. The hair is dry and falls out easily, becoming sparse. Wound healing is impaired. In elderly patients, risk of hip fractures and pressure (decubitus) ulcers increases.

With acute or chronic severe PEU, heart size and cardiac output decrease; pulse slows and BP falls. Respiratory rate and vital capacity decrease. Body temperature falls, sometimes contributing to death. Edema, anemia, jaundice, and petechiae can develop. Liver, kidney, or heart failure may occur.

Marasmus in infants causes hunger, weight loss, growth retardation, and wasting of subcutaneous fat and muscle. Ribs and facial bones appear prominent. Loose, thin skin hangs in folds.

Kwashiorkor is characterized by peripheral and periorbital edema due to the decrease in serum albumin. The abdomen protrudes because abdominal muscles are weakened, the intestine is distended, the liver enlarges, and ascites is present. The skin is dry, thin, and wrinkled; it can become hyperpigmented and fissured and later hypopigmented, friable, and atrophic. Skin in different areas of the body may be affected at different times. The hair can become thin, reddish brown, or gray. Scalp hair falls out easily, eventually becoming sparse, but eyelash hair may grow excessively. Alternating episodes of undernutrition and adequate nutrition may cause the hair to have a dramatic "striped flag" appearance. Affected children may be apathetic but become irritable when held.

Total starvation is fatal in 8 to 12 wk. Thus, certain symptoms of PEU do not have time to develop.

Diagnosis

- Diagnosis usually based on history
- To determine severity: Body mass index (BMI), serum albumin, total lymphocyte count, CD4+ count, serum transferrin
- To diagnose complications and consequences: CBC, electrolytes, BUN, glucose, calcium, magnesium, phosphate

Diagnosis of protein-energy undernutrition can be based on history when dietary intake is markedly inadequate. The cause of inadequate intake, particularly in children, needs to be identified. In children and adolescents, child abuse and anorexia nervosa should be considered.

Physical examination may include measurement of height and weight, inspection of body fat distribution, and anthropometric measurements of lean body mass. Body mass index (BMI = weight[kg]/height[m]^2) is calculated to determine severity. Findings can usually confirm the diagnosis.

Laboratory tests are required if dietary history does not clearly indicate inadequate caloric intake. Measurement of serum albumin, total lymphocyte count, CD4+ T lymphocytes, transferrin, and response to skin antigens may help determine the severity of PEU (see Table 5–3) or confirm the diagnosis in borderline cases. Many other test results may be abnormal: eg, decreased levels of hormones, vitamins, lipids, cholesterol, prealbumin, insulin-like growth factor-1, fibronectin, and retinol-binding protein. Urinary creatine and methylhistidine levels can be used to gauge the degree of muscle wasting. Because protein catabolism slows, urinary urea level also decreases. These findings rarely affect treatment.

Laboratory tests are required to identify causes of suspected secondary PEU. C-reactive protein or soluble interleukin-2 receptor should be measured when the cause of undernutrition is unclear; these measurements can help determine whether there is cytokine excess. Thyroid function tests may also be done.

Table 5–3. VALUES COMMONLY USED TO GRADE THE SEVERITY OF PROTEIN-ENERGY UNDERNUTRITION

MEASUREMENT	NORMAL	MILD UNDERNUTRITION	MODERATE UNDERNUTRITION	SEVERE UNDERNUTRITION
Normal weight (%)	90–110	85–90	75–85	< 75
BMI	19–24*	18–18.9	16–17.9	< 16
Serum albumin (g/dL)	3.5–5.0	3.1–3.4	2.4–3.0	< 2.4
Serum transferrin (mg/dL)	220–400	201–219	150–200	< 150
Total lymphocyte count (per μL)	2000–3500	1501–1999	800–1500	< 800
Delayed hypersensitivity index†	2	2	1	0

*In the elderly, BMI < 21 may increase mortality risk.

†Delayed hypersensitivity index uses a common antigen (eg, one derived from *Candida* sp or *Trichophyton* sp) to quantitate the amount of induration elicited by skin testing. Induration is graded: 0 = < 0.5 cm, 1 = 0.5–0.9 cm, 2 = ≥ 1.0 cm.

Other laboratory tests can detect associated abnormalities that may require treatment. Serum electrolytes, BUN, glucose, and possibly levels of calcium, magnesium, and phosphate should be measured. Levels of blood glucose, electrolytes (especially potassium, occasionally sodium), phosphate, calcium, and magnesium are usually low. BUN is often low unless renal failure is present. Metabolic acidosis may be present. CBC is usually obtained; normocytic anemia (usually due to protein deficiency) or microcytic anemia (due to simultaneous iron deficiency) is usually present.

Stool cultures should be obtained and checked for ova and parasites if diarrhea is severe or does not resolve with treatment. Sometimes urinalysis, urine culture, blood cultures, tuberculin testing, and a chest x-ray are used to diagnose occult infections because people with PEU may have a muted response to infections.

Prognosis

Children: In children, mortality varies from 5 to 40%. Mortality rates are lower in children with mild PEU and those given intensive care. Death in the first days of treatment is usually due to electrolyte deficits, sepsis, hypothermia, or heart failure. Impaired consciousness, jaundice, petechiae, hyponatremia, and persistent diarrhea are ominous signs. Resolution of apathy, edema, and anorexia is a favorable sign. Recovery is more rapid in kwashiorkor than in marasmus.

Long-term effects of PEU in children are not fully documented. Some children develop chronic malabsorption and pancreatic insufficiency. In very young children, mild intellectual disability may develop and persist until at least school age. Permanent cognitive impairment may occur, depending on the duration, severity, and age at onset of PEU.

Adults: In adults, PEU can result in morbidity and mortality (eg, progressive weight loss increases mortality rate for elderly patients in nursing homes). In elderly patients, PEU increases the risk of morbidity and mortality due to surgery, infections, or other disorders.

Except when organ failure occurs, treatment is uniformly successful.

Treatment

- Usually oral feeding
- Possibly avoidance of lactose (eg, if persistent diarrhea suggests lactose intolerance)
- Supportive care (eg, environmental changes, assistance with feeding, orexigenic drugs)
- For children, feeding delayed 24 to 48 h

Worldwide, the most important preventive strategy is to reduce poverty and improve nutritional education and public health measures.

Mild or moderate PEU, including brief starvation, can be treated by providing a balanced diet, preferably orally. Liquid oral food supplements (usually lactose-free) can be used when solid food cannot be adequately ingested. Diarrhea often complicates oral feeding because starvation makes the GI tract more likely to move bacteria into Peyer patches, facilitating infectious diarrhea. If diarrhea persists (suggesting lactose intolerance), yogurt-based rather than milk-based formulas are given because people with lactose intolerance can tolerate yogurt. Patients should also be given a multivitamin supplement.

Severe PEU or prolonged starvation requires treatment in a hospital with a controlled diet. The first priority is to correct fluid and electrolyte abnormalities (see p. 1298) and treat infections. (A recent study suggested that children may benefit from antibiotic prophylaxis.) The next priority is to supply macronutrients orally or, if necessary (eg, when swallowing is difficult), through a feeding tube, a nasogastric tube (usually), or a gastrostomy tube (enteral nutrition). Parenteral nutrition is indicated if malabsorption is severe (see p. 17).

Other treatments may be needed to correct specific deficiencies, which may become evident as weight increases. To avoid deficiencies, patients should take micronutrients at about twice the recommended daily allowance (RDA) until recovery is complete.

Children: Underlying disorders should be treated.

For children with diarrhea, feeding may be delayed 24 to 48 h to avoid making the diarrhea worse; during this interval, children require oral or IV rehydration. Feedings are given often (6 to 12 times/day) but, to avoid overwhelming the limited intestinal absorptive capacity, are limited to small amounts (< 100 mL). During the first week, milk-based formulas with supplements added are usually given in progressively increasing amounts; after a week, the full amounts of 175 kcal/kg and 4 g of protein/kg can be given. Twice the RDA of micronutrients should be given, using commercial multivitamin supplements. After 4 wk, the formula can be replaced with whole milk plus cod liver oil and solid foods, including eggs, fruit, meats, and yeast.

Energy distribution among macronutrients should be about 16% protein, 50% fat, and 34% carbohydrate. An example is a combination of powdered cow's skimmed milk (110 g), sucrose (100 g), vegetable oil (70 g), and water (900 mL). Many other formulas (eg, whole [full-fat] fresh milk plus corn oil and maltodextrin) can be used. Milk powders used in formulas are diluted with water.

Usually, supplements should be given with the formulas:

- Magnesium 0.4 mEq/kg/day IM is given for 7 days.
- B-complex vitamins at twice the RDA are given parenterally for the first 3 days, usually with vitamin A, phosphorus, zinc, manganese, copper, iodine, fluoride, molybdenum, and selenium.
- Because absorption of oral iron is poor in children with PEU, oral or IM iron supplementation may be necessary.

Parents are taught about nutritional requirements.

Adults: Underlying disorders should be treated. For example, if AIDS or cancer results in excess cytokine production, megestrol acetate or medroxyprogesterone may improve food intake. However, because these drugs dramatically decrease testosterone in men (possibly causing muscle loss), testosterone should be replaced. Because these drugs can cause adrenal insufficiency, they should be used only short-term (< 3 mo).

In patients with functional limitations, home delivery of meals and feeding assistance are key.

An orexigenic drug, such as the cannabis extract dronabinol, should be given to patients with anorexia when no cause is obvious or to patients at the end of life when anorexia impairs quality of life. An anabolic steroid (eg, testosterone enanthate, nandrolone) or growth hormone can benefit patients with cachexia due to renal failure and possibly elderly patients (eg, by increasing lean body mass or possibly by improving function).

Correction of PEU in adults generally resembles that in children; feedings are often limited to small amounts. However, for most adults, feeding does not need to be delayed. A commercial formula for oral feeding can be used. Daily nutrient supply should be given at a rate of 60 kcal/kg and 1.2 to 2 g of protein/kg. If liquid oral supplements are used with solid food, they should be given at least 1 h before meals so that the amount of food eaten at the meal is not reduced.

Treatment of institutionalized elderly patients with PEU requires multiple interventions:

- Environmental measures (eg, making the dining area more attractive)
- Feeding assistance
- Changes in diet (eg, use of food enhancers and caloric supplements between meals)
- Treatment of depression and other underlying disorders
- Use of orexigenic drugs, anabolic steroids, or both

The long-term use of gastrostomy tube feeding is essential for patients with severe dysphagia; its use in patients with dementia is controversial. Increasing evidence supports the avoidance of unpalatable therapeutic diets (eg, low salt, diabetic, low cholesterol) in institutionalized patients because these diets decrease food intake and may cause severe PEU.

Complications of treatment: Treatment of PEU can cause complications (refeeding syndrome), including fluid overload, electrolyte deficits, hyperglycemia, cardiac arrhythmias, and diarrhea. Diarrhea is usually mild and resolves; however, diarrhea in patients with severe PEU occasionally causes severe dehydration or death. Causes of diarrhea (eg, sorbitol used in elixir tube feedings, *Clostridium difficile* if the patient has received an antibiotic) may be correctable. Osmotic diarrhea due to excess calories is rare in adults and should be considered only when other causes have been excluded.

Because PEU can impair cardiac and renal function, overhydration can cause intravascular volume overload. Treatment decreases extracellular potassium and magnesium. Depletion of potassium or magnesium may cause arrhythmias. Carbohydrate metabolism that occurs during treatment stimulates insulin release, which drives phosphate into cells. Hypophosphatemia can cause muscle weakness, paresthesias, seizures, coma, and arrhythmias. Because phosphate levels can change rapidly during parenteral feeding, levels should be measured regularly.

During treatment, endogenous insulin may become ineffective, leading to hyperglycemia. Dehydration and hyperosmolarity can result. Fatal ventricular arrhythmias can develop, possibly caused by a prolonged QT interval.

KEY POINTS

- PEU can be primary (ie, caused by decreased intake of nutrients) or secondary to GI disorders, wasting disorders, or conditions that increase metabolic demand.
- In severe forms of PEU, body fat and eventually visceral tissue are lost, immunity is impaired, and organ function slows, sometimes resulting in multiple organ failure.
- To determine severity, measure body mass index (BMI), serum albumin, total lymphocyte count, CD4 count, and serum transferrin.
- To diagnose complications and consequences, measure CBC, electrolytes, BUN, glucose, calcium, magnesium, and phosphate.
- For mild PEU, recommend a balanced diet, sometimes avoiding foods that contain lactose.
- For severe PEU, hospitalize patients, give them a controlled diet, correct fluid and electrolyte abnormalities, and treat infections; common complications of treatment (refeeding syndrome) include fluid overload, electrolyte deficits, hyperglycemia, cardiac arrhythmias, and diarrhea.

CARNITINE DEFICIENCY

Carnitine deficiency results from inadequate intake of or inability to metabolize the amino acid carnitine. It can cause a heterogeneous group of disorders. Muscle metabolism is impaired, causing myopathy, hypoglycemia, or cardiomyopathy. Infants typically present with hypoglycemic, hypoketotic encephalopathy. Most often, treatment consists of dietary L-carnitine.

The amino acid carnitine is required for the transport of long-chain fatty acyl coenzyme A (CoA) esters into myocyte mitochondria, where they are oxidized for energy. Carnitine is obtained from foods, particularly animal-based foods, and via endogenous synthesis.

Causes of carnitine deficiency include the following:

- Inadequate intake (eg, due to fad diets, lack of access, or long-term TPN)
- Inability to metabolize carnitine due to enzyme deficiencies (eg, carnitine palmitoyltransferase deficiency, methylmalonicaciduria, propionicacidemia, isovalericacidemia)
- Decreased endogenous synthesis of carnitine due to a severe liver disorder
- Excess loss of carnitine due to diarrhea, diuresis, or hemodialysis
- A hereditary disorder in which carnitine leaks from renal tubules
- Increased requirements for carnitine when ketosis is present or demand for fat oxidation is high (eg, during a critical illness such as sepsis or major burns; after major surgery of the GI tract)
- Decreased muscle carnitine levels due to mitochondrial impairment (eg, due to use of zidovudine)
- Use of valproate

The deficiency may be generalized (systemic) or may affect mainly muscle (myopathic).

Symptoms

Symptoms and the age at which symptoms appear depend on the cause.

Carnitine deficiency may cause muscle necrosis, myoglobinuria, lipid-storage myopathy, hypoglycemia, fatty liver, and hyperammonemia with muscle aches, fatigue, confusion, and cardiomyopathy.

Diagnosis

- In neonates: Mass spectrometry
- In adults: Acylcarnitine levels

In neonates, carnitine palmitoyltransferase deficiency is diagnosed using mass spectrometry to screen blood. Prenatal diagnosis may be possible using amniotic villous cells.

In adults, the definitive diagnosis is based on acylcarnitine levels in serum, urine, and tissues (muscle and liver for systemic deficiency; muscle only for myopathic deficiency).

Treatment

- Avoidance of fasting and strenuous exercise
- Dietary interventions, based on cause

Carnitine deficiency due to inadequate dietary intake, increased requirements, excess losses, decreased synthesis, or (sometimes) enzyme deficiencies can be treated by giving L-carnitine 25 mg/kg po q 6 h.

All patients must avoid fasting and strenuous exercise. Consuming uncooked cornstarch at bedtime prevents early morning hypoglycemia.

Some patients require supplementation with medium-chain triglycerides and essential fatty acids (eg, linoleic acid, linolenic acid). Patients with a fatty acid oxidation disorder require a high-carbohydrate, low-fat diet.

ESSENTIAL FATTY ACID DEFICIENCY

Essential fatty acid (EFA) deficiency is rare, occurring most often in infants fed diets deficient in EFAs. Signs include scaly dermatitis, alopecia, thrombocytopenia, and, in children, intellectual disability. Diagnosis is clinical. Dietary replenishment of EFAs reverses the deficiency.

The EFAs linoleic and linolenic acid are substrates for the endogenous synthesis of other fatty acids that are needed for many physiologic processes, including maintaining the integrity of skin and cell membranes and synthesizing prostaglandins and leukotrienes. For example, eicosapentaenoic acid and docosahexaenoic acid, synthesized from EFAs, are important components of the brain and retina.

For EFA deficiency to develop, dietary intake must be very low. Even small amounts of EFAs can prevent EFA deficiency. Cow's milk has only about 25% of the linoleic acid in human milk, but when ingested in normal amounts, it has enough linoleic acid to prevent EFA deficiency. Total fat intake of people in many developing countries may be very low, but the fat is often vegetable based, with large amounts of linoleic acid and enough linolenic acid to prevent EFA deficiency.

Babies fed a formula low in linoleic acid, such as a skim-milk formula, can develop EFA deficiency. EFA deficiency used to result from long-term TPN if fat was not included. But now, most TPN solutions include fat emulsions to prevent EFA deficiency. In patients with fat malabsorption or increased metabolic needs (eg, because of surgery, multiple trauma, or burns), laboratory evidence of EFA deficiency may be present without clinical signs.

Dermatitis due to EFA deficiency is generalized and scaly; in infants, it can resemble congenital ichthyosis. The dermatitis increases water loss from the skin.

Diagnosis of fatty acid deficiency is usually clinical; however, laboratory assays are now available in large research centers.

Treatment of fatty acid deficiency consists of dietary EFAs, reversing the deficiency.

6 Vitamin Deficiency, Dependency, and Toxicity

Vitamins may be

- Fat soluble (vitamins A, D, E, and K)
- Water soluble (B vitamins and vitamin C)

The B vitamins include biotin, folate, niacin, pantothenic acid, riboflavin (B_2), thiamin (B_1), B_6 (eg, pyridoxine), and B_{12} (cobalamins).

For dietary requirements, sources, functions, effects of deficiencies and toxicities, blood levels, and usual therapeutic dosages for vitamins, see Tables 6–1 and 6–2.

Dietary requirements for vitamins (and other nutrients) are expressed as daily recommended intake (DRI). There are 3 types of DRI:

- **Recommended daily allowance (RDA):** RDAs are set to meet the needs of 97 to 98% of healthy people.
- **Adequate intake (AI):** When data to calculate an RDA are insufficient, AIs are based on observed or experimentally determined estimates of nutrient intake by healthy people.
- **Tolerable upper intake level (UL):** ULs are the largest amount of a nutrient that most adults can ingest daily without risk of adverse health effects.

In developed countries, **vitamin deficiencies** result mainly from the following:

- Poverty
- Food faddism
- Drugs (see p. 6 and Table 6–3)
- Alcoholism (see p. 3231)
- Prolonged and inadequately supplemented parenteral feeding
- Malabsorption

Mild vitamin deficiency is common among frail and institutionalized elderly people who have protein-energy undernutrition (see p. 33).

In developing countries, vitamin deficiencies can result from lack of access to nutrients.

Deficiencies of water-soluble vitamins (except vitamin B_{12}) may develop after weeks to months of undernutrition. Deficiencies of fat-soluble vitamins and of vitamin B_{12} take > 1 yr to develop because the body stores them in relatively large amounts. Intakes of vitamins sufficient to prevent classic vitamin deficiencies (such as scurvy or beriberi) may not be adequate for optimum health. This area remains one of controversy and active research.

Vitamin dependency results from a genetic defect involving metabolism of a vitamin. In some cases, vitamin doses as high as 1000 times the DRI improve function of the altered metabolic pathway.

Vitamin toxicity (hypervitaminosis) usually results from taking megadoses of vitamin A, D, C, B_6, or niacin.

Because many people eat irregularly, foods alone may provide suboptimal amounts of some vitamins. In these cases, the risk of certain cancers or other disorders may be increased. However, routine daily multivitamin supplements have not been proved to reduce cancer. Supplementation with vitamins does not appear to prevent cardiovascular disease,[1,2] or falls.[3-6]

1. Myung SK, Ju W, Cho B, et al: Efficacy of vitamin and antioxidant supplements in prevention of cardiovascular disease: systematic review and meta-analysis of randomized controlled trials. *BMJ* 346:f10, 2013.
2. Sesso HD, Christen WG, Bubes V, et al: Multivitamins in the prevention of cardiovascular disease in men: The Physicians' Health Study II randomized controlled trial. *JAMA*308(17):1751–1756, 2012.
3. Bischoff-Ferrari HA, Dawson-Hughes B, Orav EJ, et al: Monthly high-dose vitamin D treatment for the prevention of functional decline: A randomized clinical trial. *JAMA Intern Med* 176(2):175–183, 2016.
4. Cummings SR, Kiel DP, Black DM: Vitamin D supplementation and increased risk of falling: A cautionary tale of vitamin supplements retold. *JAMA Intern Med* 176(2):171–172, 2016.

Table 6–1. RECOMMENDED DAILY INTAKES FOR VITAMINS

AGE (yr)	FOLATE (mcg)	NIACIN (mg NE*)	RIBOFLAVIN (mg)	THIAMIN (mg)	VITAMIN A (mcg)	VITAMIN B_6 (mg)	VITAMIN B_{12} (mcg)	VITAMIN C (mg)	VITAMIN D (IU)†	VITAMIN E (mg)	VITAMIN K (mcg)
Infants											
0–6 mo	**65**	**2**	**0.3**	**0.2**	**400**	**0.1**	**0.4**	**40**	400	**4**	**2.0**
7–12 mo	**80**	**4**	**0.4**	**0.3**	**500**	**0.3**	**0.5**	**50**	400	**5**	**2.5**
Children											
1–3	150	6	0.5	0.5	300	0.5	0.9	15	**600**	6	**30**
4–8	200	8	0.6	0.6	400	0.6	1.2	25	**600**	7	**55**
Males											
9–13	300	12	0.9	0.9	600	1.0	1.8	45	**600**	11	**60**
14–18	400	16	1.3	1.2	900	1.3	2.4	75	**600**	15	**75**
19–70	400	16	1.3	1.2	900	1.3	2.4	90	**600**	15	**120**
> 70	400	16	1.3	1.2	900	1.7	2.4	90	**800‡**	15	**120**
Females											
9–13	300	12	0.9	0.9	600	1.0	1.8	45	**600**	11	**60**
14–18	400	14	1.0	1.0	700	1.2	2.4	65	**600**	15	**75**
19–70	400	14	1.1	1.1	700	1.3	2.4	75	**600**	15	**90**
≥ 70	400	14	1.1	1.1	700	1.5	2.4	75	**800‡**	15	**90**
Pregnant women											
19–50 yr	600	18	1.4	1.4	770	1.9	2.6	85	**600**	15	**90**
Breastfeeding women											
19–50 yr	500	17	1.6	1.4	1300	2.0	2.8	120	**600**	19	**90**
Upper limit (UL)§											
	1000	35	ND	ND	3000	100	ND	2000	4000	1000	ND

NOTE: **Recommended dietary allowances (RDAs)** are shown in regular type. RDAs are set to meet the needs of 97 to 98% of healthy people.

Adequate intakes (AIs) are shown in **bold** type. When data to calculate the RDA for a nutrient are insufficient, AIs are based on observed or experimentally determined estimates of nutrient intake by healthy people.

*1 niacin equivalent (NE) equals 1 mg niacin or 60 mg dietary tryptophan.

†200 IU of vitamin D equals 5 mcg cholecalciferol.

‡800 IU of vitamin D is recommended for people ≥ 70 yr.

§UL is the largest amount of a nutrient that most adults can ingest daily without risk of adverse effects. The more the UL is exceeded, the greater the risk of adverse effects.

ND = not determinable because of lack of data (sources of intake should be limited to foods); RAE = retinol activity equivalents (1 mcg RAE of preformed vitamin A= 3.33 IU).

Adapted from Dietary Reference Intakes, Food and Nutrition Board, Institute of Medicine. Washington, DC: National Academy Press.

5. Uusi-Rasi K, Patil R, Karinkanta S, Kannus P, et al: Exercise and vitamin D in fall prevention among older women: A randomized clinical trial. *JAMA Intern Med* 75(5):703–711, 2015.
6. LeBlanc ES, Chou R: Vitamin D and falls—Fitting new data with current guidelines. *JAMA Intern Med* 175(5):712–713, 2015.

BIOTIN AND PANTOTHENIC ACID

Biotin acts as a coenzyme for carboxylation reactions essential to fat and carbohydrate metabolism. Adequate intake for adults is 30 mcg/day.

Pantothenic acid is widely distributed in foods; it is an essential component of coenzyme A. Adults probably require about 5 mg/day. A beneficial role for pantothenic acid supplementation in lipid metabolism, RA, or athletic performance remains unproved.

Isolated deficiency of biotin or pantothenic acid virtually never occurs.

FOLATE

(Folic Acid)

Folate is now added to enriched grain foods in the US and Canada. Folate is also plentiful in various plant foods and meats, but its bioavailability is greater when it is in supplements or enriched foods than when it occurs naturally in food (see Table 6–2).

Folates are involved in RBC maturation and synthesis of purines and pyrimidines. They are required for development of the fetal nervous system. Absorption occurs in the duodenum and upper jejunum. Enterohepatic circulation of folate occurs.

Table 6–2. SOURCES, FUNCTIONS, AND EFFECTS OF VITAMINS

NUTRIENT	PRINCIPAL SOURCES	FUNCTIONS	EFFECTS OF DEFICIENCY AND TOXICITY
Folate (folic acid)	Raw green leafy vegetables, fruits, organ meats (eg, liver), enriched cereals and breads	Maturation of RBCs Synthesis of purines, pyrimidines, and methionine Development of fetal nervous system	**Deficiency:** Megaloblastic anemia, neural tube birth defects, confusion
Niacin (nicotinic acid, nicotinamide)	Liver, red meat, fish, poultry, legumes, whole-grain or enriched cereals and breads	Oxidation-reduction reactions Carbohydrate and cell metabolism	**Deficiency:** Pellagra (dermatitis, glossitis, GI and CNS dysfunction) **Toxicity:** Flushing
Riboflavin (vitamin B_2)	Milk, cheese, liver, meat, eggs, enriched cereal products	Many aspects of carbohydrate and protein metabolism Integrity of mucous membranes	**Deficiency:** Cheilosis, angular stomatitis, corneal vascularization
Thiamin (vitamin B_1)	Whole grains, meat (especially pork and liver), enriched cereal products, nuts, legumes, potatoes	Carbohydrate, fat, amino acid, glucose, and alcohol metabolism Central and peripheral nerve cell function Myocardial function	**Deficiency:** Beriberi (peripheral neuropathy, heart failure), Wernicke-Korsakoff syndrome
Vitamin A (retinol)	As preformed vitamin: fish liver oils, liver, egg yolks, butter, vitamin A–fortified dairy products As provitamin carotenoids: dark green and yellow vegetables, carrots, yellow and orange fruits	Formation of rhodopsin (a photoreceptor pigment in the retina) Integrity of epithelia Lysosome stability Glycoprotein synthesis	**Deficiency:** Night blindness, perifollicular hyperkeratosis, xerophthalmia, keratomalacia, increased morbidity and mortality in young children **Toxicity:** Headache, peeling of skin, hepatosplenomegaly, bone thickening, intracranial hypertension, papilledema, hypercalcemia
Vitamin B_6 group (pyridoxine, pyridoxal, pyridoxamine)	Organ meats (eg, liver), whole-grain cereals, fish, legumes	Many aspects of nitrogen metabolism (eg, transaminations, porphyrin and heme synthesis, tryptophan conversion to niacin) Nucleic acid biosynthesis Fatty acid, lipid, and amino acid metabolism	**Deficiency:** Seizures, anemia, neuropathies, seborrheic dermatitis **Toxicity:** Peripheral neuropathy
Vitamin B_{12} (cobalamins)	Meats (especially beef, pork, and organ meats [eg, liver]), poultry, eggs, fortified cereals, milk and milk products, clams, oysters, mackerel, salmon	Maturation of RBCs, neural function, DNA synthesis, myelin synthesis and repair	**Deficiency:** Megaloblastic anemia, neurologic deficits (confusion, paresthesias, ataxia)
Vitamin C (ascorbic acid)	Citrus fruits, tomatoes, potatoes, broccoli, strawberries, sweet peppers	Collagen formation Bone and blood vessel health Carnitine, hormone, and amino acid formation Wound healing	**Deficiency:** Scurvy (hemorrhages, loose teeth, gingivitis, bone defects)
Vitamin D (cholecalciferol, ergocalciferol)	Direct ultraviolet B irradiation of the skin (main source), fortified dairy products (main dietary source), fish liver oils, fatty fish, liver	Calcium and phosphate absorption Mineralization and repair of bone Tubular reabsorption of calcium Insulin and thyroid function, improvement of immune function, reduced risk of autoimmune disease	**Deficiency:** Rickets (sometimes with tetany), osteomalacia **Toxicity:** Hypercalcemia, anorexia, renal failure, metastatic calcifications
Vitamin E group (alpha-tocopherol, other tocopherols)	Vegetable oils, nuts	Intracellular antioxidant Scavenger of free radicals in biologic membranes	**Deficiency:** RBC hemolysis, neurologic deficits **Toxicity:** Tendency to bleed
Vitamin K group (phylloquinone, menaquinones)	Green leafy vegetables (especially collards, spinach, and salad greens), soy beans, vegetable oils Bacteria in the GI tract after neonatal period	Formation of prothrombin, other coagulation factors, and bone proteins	**Deficiency:** Bleeding due to deficiency of prothrombin and other factors, osteopenia

Table 6–3. POTENTIAL VITAMIN-DRUG INTERACTIONS

NUTRIENT	DRUG
Biotin	Antibiotics, anticonvulsants
Folate	Alcohol, 5-fluorouracil, metformin, methotrexate, oral contraceptives, anticonvulsants (eg, phenobarbital, phenytoin, primidone), sulfasalazine, triamterene, trimethoprim
Niacin	Alcohol, isoniazid
Riboflavin	Alcohol, barbiturates, phenothiazines, thiazide diuretics, tricyclic antidepressants
Thiamin	Alcohol; oral contraceptives; thiamin antagonists in coffee, tea, raw fish, and red cabbage
Vitamin A	Cholestyramine, mineral oil
Vitamin B_6	Alcohol, anticonvulsants, corticosteroids, cycloserine, hydralazine, isoniazid, levodopa, oral contraceptives, penicillamine
Vitamin B_{12}	Antacids, metformin, nitrous oxide (repeated exposure)
Vitamin C	Corticosteroids
Vitamin D	Antipsychotics, corticosteroids, mineral oil, anticonvulsants, rifampin
Vitamin E	Mineral oil, warfarin
Vitamin K	Antibiotics, anticonvulsants, mineral oil, rifampin, warfarin

Folate supplements do not protect against coronary artery disease or stroke (even though they lower homocysteine levels); current evidence does not support claims that folate supplementation increases or reduces the risk of various cancers.

The upper limit for folate intake is 1000 mcg; higher daily doses (up to 4 mg) are recommended for women who have had a baby with a neural tube defect. Folate is essentially nontoxic.

Women taking both oral contraceptives and anticonvulsants may need to take folate supplements to maintain birth control effectiveness.

Folate Deficiency

Folate deficiency is common. It may result from inadequate intake, malabsorption, or use of various drugs. Deficiency causes megaloblastic anemia (indistinguishable from that due to vitamin B_{12} deficiency). Maternal deficiency increases the risk of neural tube birth defects. Diagnosis requires laboratory testing to confirm. Measurement of neutrophil hypersegmentation is sensitive and readily available. Treatment with oral folate is usually successful.

Etiology

The most common causes of folate deficiency are

- Inadequate intake (usually in patients with undernutrition or alcoholism)
- Increased demand (eg, due to pregnancy or lactation)
- Impaired absorption (eg, in celiac disease or due to certain drugs)

Deficiency can also result from inadequate bioavailability and increased excretion (see Table 6–4).

Prolonged cooking destroys folate, predisposing to inadequate intake. Intake is sometimes barely adequate (eg, in alcoholics). Liver stores provide only a several-month supply.

Alcohol interferes with folate absorption, metabolism, renal excretion, and enterohepatic reabsorption and reduces healthy food intake. 5-Fluorouracil, metformin, methotrexate, phenobarbital, phenytoin, sulfasalazine, triamterene, and trimethoprim impair folate metabolism.

In the US and Canada, many dietary staples (eg, cereals, grain products) are routinely enriched with folate, tending to reduce risk of deficiency.

Symptoms and Signs

Folate deficiency may cause glossitis, diarrhea, depression, and confusion. Anemia may develop insidiously and, because of compensatory mechanisms, be more severe than symptoms suggest.

Folate deficiency during pregnancy increases the risk of fetal neural tube defects and perhaps other brain defects.

Diagnosis

- CBC and serum vitamin B_{12} and folate levels

CBC may indicate megaloblastic anemia indistinguishable from that of vitamin B_{12} deficiency.

If serum folate is < 3 mcg/L or ng/mL (< 7 nmol/L), deficiency is likely. Serum folate reflects folate status unless intake has recently increased or decreased. If intake has changed, erythrocyte (RBC) folate level better reflects tissue stores. A level of < 140 mcg/L or ng/mL (< 305 nmol/L) indicates inadequate status.

Also, an increase in the homocysteine level suggests tissue folate deficiency (but the level is also affected by vitamin B_{12} and vitamin B_6 levels, renal insufficiency, and genetic factors). A normal methylmalonic acid (MMA) level may differentiate folate deficiency from vitamin B_{12} deficiency because MMA levels rise in vitamin B_{12} deficiency but not in folate deficiency.

Treatment

- Supplemental oral folate

Folate 400 to 1000 mcg po once/day replenishes tissues and is usually successful even if deficiency has resulted from malabsorption. The normal requirement is 400 mcg/day. (CAUTION: *In patients with megaloblastic anemia, vitamin B_{12} deficiency must be ruled out before treating with folate. If vitamin B_{12} deficiency is present, folate supplementation can alleviate the anemia but does not reverse, and may even worsen, neurologic deficits.*)

Table 6–4. CAUSES OF FOLATE DEFICIENCY

CAUSE	SOURCE
Inadequate intake	Diet lacking raw green vegetables or enriched grains, chronic alcoholism, TPN
Impaired absorption	Celiac disease, sprue, other malabsorption syndromes, anticonvulsants, congenital or acquired folate malabsorption
Inadequate utilization	Folate antagonists (metformin, methotrexate, triamterene, trimethoprim), anticonvulsants, congenital or acquired enzyme deficiency, alcoholism
Increased demand	Pregnancy, lactation, infancy, increased metabolism
Increased excretion	Renal dialysis (peritoneal or hemodialysis)

For pregnant women, the recommended daily allowance (RDA) is 600 mcg/day. For women who have had a fetus or infant with a neural tube defect, the recommended dose is 4000 mcg/day, started 1 mo before conception (if possible) and continued until 3 mo after conception.

KEY POINTS

- Most commonly, folate deficiency results from reduced intake (eg, due to alcoholism), increased demand (eg, due to pregnancy), or impaired absorption (eg, due to drugs or malabsorption disorders).
- Prolonged cooking destroys folate, but many dietary staples are supplemented with folate.
- Deficiency causes megaloblastic anemia and sometimes glossitis, diarrhea, depression, and confusion.
- Measure serum folate and vitamin B_{12} levels in patients who have megaloblastic anemia.
- To treat deficiency, give patients supplemental folate 400 to 1000 mcg po once/day.

NIACIN

(Nicotinic Acid; Nicotinamide)

Niacin derivatives include nicotinamide adenine dinucleotide (NAD) and nicotinamide adenine dinucleotide phosphate (NADP), which are coenzymes in oxidation-reduction reactions. They are vital in cell metabolism.

Because dietary tryptophan can be metabolized to niacin, foods rich in tryptophan (eg, dairy products) can compensate for inadequate dietary niacin (see Table 6–2).

Niacin Deficiency

Dietary niacin deficiency (causing pellagra) is uncommon in developed countries. Clinical manifestations include the three Ds: localized pigmented rash (dermatitis); gastroenteritis (diarrhea); and widespread neurologic deficits, including cognitive decline (dementia). Diagnosis is usually clinical, and dietary supplementation (oral or, if needed, IM) is usually successful.

Etiology

Primary niacin deficiency results from extremely inadequate intake of both niacin and tryptophan, which usually occurs in areas where maize (Indian corn) constitutes a substantial part of the diet. Bound niacin, found in maize, is not assimilated in the GI tract unless it has been previously treated with alkali, as when tortillas are prepared. Corn protein is also deficient in tryptophan. The high incidence of pellagra in India among people who eat millet with a high leucine content has led to the hypothesis that amino acid imbalance may contribute to deficiency. Deficiencies of protein and many B vitamins commonly accompany primary niacin deficiency.

Secondary niacin deficiency may be due to diarrhea, cirrhosis, or alcoholism. Pellagra also may occur in carcinoid syndrome (tryptophan is diverted to form 5-hydroxytryptophan and serotonin) and in Hartnup disease (absorption of tryptophan by the intestine and kidneys is defective).

Symptoms and Signs

Pellagra is characterized by skin, mucous membrane, CNS, and GI symptoms. Advanced pellagra can cause a symmetric photosensitive rash, stomatitis, glossitis, diarrhea, and mental aberrations. Symptoms may appear alone or in combination.

Skin symptoms include several types of lesions, which are usually bilaterally symmetric. The distribution of lesions—at pressure points or sun-exposed skin—is more pathognomonic than the form of the lesions. Lesions can develop in a glove-like distribution on the hands (pellagrous glove) or in a boot-shaped distribution on the feet and legs (pellagrous boot). Sunlight causes Casal necklace and butterfly-shaped lesions on the face.

Mucous membrane symptoms affect primarily the mouth but may also affect the vagina and urethra. Glossitis and stomatitis characterize acute deficiency. As the deficiency progresses, the tongue and oral mucous membranes become reddened, followed by pain in the mouth, increased salivation, and edema of the tongue. Ulcerations may appear, especially under the tongue, on the mucosa of the lower lip, and opposite the molar teeth.

GI symptoms early in the deficiency include burning in the pharynx and esophagus and abdominal discomfort and distention. Constipation is common. Later, nausea, vomiting, and diarrhea may occur. Diarrhea is often bloody because of bowel hyperemia and ulceration.

CNS symptoms include psychosis, encephalopathy (characterized by impaired consciousness), and cognitive decline (dementia). Psychosis is characterized by memory impairment, disorientation, confusion, and confabulation; the predominant symptom may be excitement, depression, mania, delirium, or paranoia.

Diagnosis

- Clinical evaluation

Diagnosis of niacin deficiency is clinical and may be straightforward when skin and mouth lesions, diarrhea, delirium, and dementia occur simultaneously. More often, the presentation is not so specific. Differentiating the CNS changes from those in thiamin deficiency is difficult. A history of a diet lacking niacin and tryptophan may help establish the diagnosis. A favorable response to treatment with niacincan usually confirm it.

If available, laboratory testing can help confirm the diagnosis, particularly when the diagnosis is otherwise unclear. Urinary excretion of N^1-methylnicotinamide (NMN) is decreased; < 0.8 mg/day (< 5.8 mcmol/day) suggests a niacin deficiency.

Treatment

- Nicotinamide and other nutrients

Because multiple deficiencies are common, a balanced diet, including other B vitamins (particularly riboflavin and pyridoxine), is needed.

Nicotinamide is usually used to treat niacin deficiency, because nicotinamide, unlike nicotinic acid (the most common form of niacin), does not cause flushing, itching, burning, or tingling sensations. Nicotinamide is given in doses of 250 to 500 mg po daily.

KEY POINTS

- Niacin deficiency can cause pellagra, mainly in developing countries.
- Pellagra causes a photosensitivity rash, mucositis, GI disturbances, and neuropsychiatric dysfunction.
- Diagnose clinically if possible.
- Use nicotinamide to treat the deficiency; a favorable response can confirm the diagnosis.

Niacin Toxicity

Niacin (nicotinic acid) in large amounts is sometimes used to lower low-density lipoprotein (LDL) cholesterol and triglyceride levels and to increase high-density lipoprotein (HDL) cholesterol levels. Symptoms may include flushing and, rarely, hepatotoxicity.

Immediate- and sustained-release preparations of niacin (but not nicotinamide) may affect lipid levels. However, whether niacin reduces risk of coronary artery disease and stroke is unclear.

At intermediate doses (1000 mg/day), niacin has the following effects:

- Triglyceride levels decrease 15 to 20%.
- HDL cholesterol levels increase 15 to 30%.
- LDL cholesterol levels decrease < 10%.

Higher doses of niacin (3000 mg/day) reduce LDL cholesterol 15 to 20% but may cause jaundice, abdominal discomfort, blurred vision, worsening of hyperglycemia, and precipitation of preexisting gout. People with a liver disorder probably should not take high-dose niacin.

Flushing, which is prostaglandin-mediated, is more common with immediate-release preparations. It may be more intense after alcohol ingestion, aerobic activity, sun exposure, and consumption of spicy foods. Flushing is minimized if niacin is taken after meals or if aspirin (325 mg, which may work better than lower doses) is taken 30 to 45 min before niacin. The chance of severe flushing can be reduced by starting immediate-release niacin at a low dose (eg, 50 mg tid) and increasing it very slowly.

Hepatotoxicity may be more common with some sustained-release preparations. Some authorities recommend checking levels of uric acid, blood glucose, and plasma aminotransferases every 6 to 8 wk until the dose of niacin has been stabilized.

RIBOFLAVIN

(Vitamin B_2)

Riboflavin is involved in carbohydrate metabolism as an essential coenzyme in many oxidation-reduction reactions (see Table 6–2). Riboflavin is essentially nontoxic.

Riboflavin Deficiency

Riboflavin deficiency usually occurs with other B vitamin deficiencies. Symptoms and signs include sore throat, lesions of the lips and mucosa of the mouth, glossitis, conjunctivitis, seborrheic dermatitis, and normochromic-normocytic anemia. Diagnosis is usually clinical. Treatment consists of oral or, if needed, IM riboflavin.

Etiology

Primary riboflavin deficiency results from inadequate intake of the following:

- Fortified cereals
- Milk
- Other animal products

Secondary riboflavin deficiency is most commonly caused by the following:

- Chronic diarrhea
- Malabsorption syndromes
- Liver disorders
- Hemodialysis
- Peritoneal dialysis
- Long-term use of barbiturates
- Chronic alcoholism

Symptoms and Signs

The most common signs of riboflavin deficiency are pallor and maceration of the mucosa at the angles of the mouth (angular stomatitis) and vermilion surfaces of the lips (cheilosis), eventually replaced by superficial linear fissures. The fissures can become infected with *Candida albicans*, causing grayish white lesions (perlèche). The tongue may appear magenta.

Seborrheic dermatitis develops, usually affecting the nasolabial folds, ears, eyelids, and scrotum or labia majora. These areas become red, scaly, and greasy.

Rarely, neovascularization and keratitis of the cornea occur, causing lacrimation and photophobia.

Diagnosis

- Therapeutic trial
- Urinary excretion of riboflavin

The lesions characteristic of riboflavin deficiency are nonspecific. Riboflavin deficiency should be suspected if characteristic signs develop in a patient with other B vitamin deficiencies.

Diagnosis of riboflavin deficiency can be confirmed by a therapeutic trial or laboratory testing, usually by measuring urinary excretion of riboflavin.

Treatment

- Oral riboflavin and other water-soluble vitamins

Riboflavin 5 to 10 mg po once/day is given until recovery. Other water-soluble vitamins should also be given.

KEY POINTS

- Riboflavin deficiency causes various nonspecific skin and mucosal lesions, including maceration of mucosa at the angles of the mouth (angular stomatitis) and surfaces of the lips (cheilosis).
- Suspect riboflavin deficiency in patients with characteristic symptoms and other B vitamin deficiencies; confirm it with a therapeutic trial of riboflavin supplements or measurement of urinary excretion of riboflavin.
- Treat with supplement of riboflavin and other water-soluble vitamins.

THIAMIN

(Vitamin B_1; Thiamine)

Thiamin is widely available in the diet (see Table 6–2). Thiamin is involved in carbohydrate, fat, amino acid, glucose, and alcohol metabolism. Thiamin is essentially nontoxic.

Thiamin Deficiency

Thiamin deficiency (causing beriberi) is most common among people subsisting on white rice or highly refined carbohydrates in developing countries and among alcoholics. Symptoms include diffuse polyneuropathy, high-output heart failure, and Wernicke-Korsakoff syndrome. Thiamin is given to help diagnose and treat the deficiency.

Etiology

Primary thiamin deficiency is caused by

- Inadequate intake of thiamin

It is commonly due to a diet of highly refined carbohydrates (eg, polished rice, white flour, white sugar) in developing countries. It also develops when intake of other nutrients is inadequate, as may occur in young adults with severe anorexia; it often occurs with other B vitamin deficiencies.

Secondary thiamin deficiency is caused by

- Increased demand (eg, due to hyperthyroidism, pregnancy, lactation, strenuous exercise, or fever)
- Impaired absorption (eg, due to prolonged diarrhea)
- Impaired metabolism (eg, due to hepatic insufficiency)

In alcoholics, many mechanisms contribute to thiamin deficiency; they include decreased intake, impaired absorption and use, increased demand, and possibly an apoenzyme defect.

Pathophysiology

Thiamin deficiency causes degeneration of peripheral nerves, thalamus, mammillary bodies, and cerebellum. Cerebral blood flow is markedly reduced, and vascular resistance is increased.

The heart may become dilated; muscle fibers become swollen, fragmented, and vacuolized, with interstitial spaces dilated by fluid. Vasodilation occurs and can result in edema in the feet and legs. Arteriovenous shunting of blood increases. Eventually, high-output heart failure may occur.

Symptoms and Signs

Early symptoms are nonspecific: fatigue, irritability, poor memory, sleep disturbances, precordial pain, anorexia, and abdominal discomfort.

Different forms of beriberi cause different symptoms.

Dry beriberi refers to peripheral neurologic deficits due to thiamin deficiency. These deficits are bilateral and roughly symmetric, occurring in a stocking-glove distribution. They affect predominantly the lower extremities, beginning with paresthesias in the toes, burning in the feet (particularly severe at night), muscle cramps in the calves, pains in the legs, and plantar dysesthesias. Calf muscle tenderness, difficulty rising from a squatting position, and decreased vibratory sensation in the toes are early signs. Muscle wasting occurs. Continued deficiency worsens polyneuropathy, which can eventually affect the arms.

Wernicke-Korsakoff syndrome, which combines Wernicke encephalopathy (see p. 3248) and Korsakoff psychosis (see p. 3242), occurs in some alcoholics who do not consume foods fortified with thiamin. Wernicke encephalopathy consists of psychomotor slowing or apathy, nystagmus, ataxia, ophthalmoplegia, impaired consciousness, and, if untreated, coma and death. It probably results from severe acute deficiency superimposed on chronic deficiency. Korsakoff psychosis consists of mental confusion, dysphonia, and confabulation with impaired memory of recent events. It probably results from chronic deficiency and may develop after repeated episodes of Wernicke encephalopathy.

Cardiovascular (wet) beriberi is myocardial disease due to thiamin deficiency. The first effects are vasodilation, tachycardia, a wide pulse pressure, sweating, warm skin, and lactic acidosis. Later, heart failure develops, causing orthopnea and pulmonary and peripheral edema. Vasodilation can continue, sometimes resulting in shock.

Infantile beriberi occurs in infants (usually by age 3 to 4 wk) who are breastfed by thiamin-deficient mothers. Heart failure (which may occur suddenly), aphonia, and absent deep tendon reflexes are characteristic.

Because thiamin is necessary for glucose metabolism, glucose infusions may precipitate or worsen symptoms of deficiency in thiamin-deficient people.

Diagnosis

- Favorable response to thiamin

Diagnosis of thiamin deficiency is usually based on a favorable response to treatment with thiamin in a patient with symptoms or signs of deficiency. Similar bilateral lower extremity polyneuropathies due to other disorders (eg, diabetes, alcoholism, vitamin B_{12} deficiency, heavy metal poisoning) do not respond to thiamin. Single-nerve neuritides (mononeuropathies—eg, sciatica) and multiple mononeuropathies (mononeuritis multiplex) are unlikely to result from thiamin deficiency.

Electrolytes, including magnesium, should be measured to exclude other causes. For confirmation in equivocal cases, erythrocyte transketolase activity and 24-h urinary thiamin excretion may be measured.

Diagnosis of cardiovascular beriberi can be difficult if other disorders that cause heart failure are present. A therapeutic trial of thiamin can help.

Treatment

- Supplemental thiamin, with dose based on clinical manifestations

Ensuring that dietary supplies of thiamin are adequate is important regardless of symptoms.

Because IV glucose can worsen thiamin deficiency, alcoholics and others at risk of thiamin deficiency should receive IV thiamin 100 mg before receiving IV glucose solutions.

PEARLS & PITFALLS

- Give thiamin 100 mg IV before giving IV glucose to alcoholics and others at risk of thiamin deficiency.

The thiamin dose is

- For mild polyneuropathy: 10 to 20 mg po once/day for 2 wk
- For moderate or advanced neuropathy: 20 to 30 mg/day, continued for several weeks after symptoms disappear
- For edema and congestion due to cardiovascular beriberi: 100 mg IV once/day for several days

Heart failure is also treated.

For **Wernicke-Korsakoff syndrome,** thiamin 50 to 100 mg IM or IV bid must usually be given for several days, followed by 10 to 20 mg once/day until a therapeutic response is obtained. Anaphylactic reactions to IV thiamin are rare. Symptoms of ophthalmoplegia may resolve in a day; improvement in patients with Korsakoff psychosis may take 1 to 3 mo. Recovery from neurologic deficits is often incomplete in Wernicke-Korsakoff syndrome and in other forms of thiamin deficiency.

Because thiamin deficiency often occurs with other B vitamin deficiencies, multiple water-soluble vitamins are usually given for several weeks. Patients should continue to consume a nutritious diet, supplying 1 to 2 times the DRI of vitamins; all alcohol intake should stop.

KEY POINTS

- The risk of thiamin deficiency is increased in people who subsist on highly refined carbohydrates such as polished rice

and white flour (as occurs in developing countries) or who are alcoholics.
- Early findings can be nonspecific; peripheral neurologic deficits, high-output heart failure, and Wernicke-Korsakoff syndrome (mainly in alcoholics) may also develop.
- Diagnose based on clinical findings, including a favorable response to treatment with supplemental thiamin.

VITAMIN A

(Retinol)

Vitamin A is required for the formation of rhodopsin, a photoreceptor pigment in the retina (see Table 6–2). Vitamin A helps maintain epithelial tissues.

Normally, the liver stores 80 to 90% of the body's vitamin A. To use vitamin A, the body releases it into the circulation bound to prealbumin (transthyretin) and retinol-binding protein. Beta-carotene and other provitamin carotenoids, contained in green leafy and yellow vegetables and deep- or bright-colored fruits, are converted to vitamin A. Carotenoids are absorbed better from vegetables when they are cooked or homogenized and served with some fat (eg, oils).

Retinol activity equivalents (RAE) were developed because provitamin A carotenoids have less vitamin A activity than preformed vitamin A; 1 μg retinol = 3.33 IU.

Synthetic vitamin analogs (retinoids) are being used increasingly in dermatology. The possible protective role of beta-carotene, retinol, and retinoids against some epithelial cancers is under study. However, risk of certain cancers may be increased after beta-carotene supplementation.

Vitamin A Deficiency

Vitamin A deficiency can result from inadequate intake, fat malabsorption, or liver disorders. Deficiency impairs immunity and hematopoiesis and causes rashes and typical ocular effects (eg, xerophthalmia, night blindness). Diagnosis is based on typical ocular findings and low vitamin A levels. Treatment consists of vitamin A given orally or, if symptoms are severe or malabsorption is the cause, parenterally.

Etiology

Primary vitamin A deficiency is usually caused by

- Prolonged dietary deprivation

It is endemic in areas such as southern and eastern Asia, where rice, devoid of beta-carotene, is the staple food. Xerophthalmia due to primary deficiency is a common cause of blindness among young children in developing countries.

Secondary vitamin A deficiency may be due to

- Decreased bioavailability of provitamin A carotenoids
- Interference with absorption, storage, or transport of vitamin A

Interference with absorption or storage is likely in celiac disease, cystic fibrosis, pancreatic insufficiency, duodenal bypass, chronic diarrhea, bile duct obstruction, giardiasis, and cirrhosis. Vitamin A deficiency is common in prolonged protein-energy undernutrition not only because the diet is deficient but also because vitamin A storage and transport is defective.

Symptoms and Signs

Impaired dark adaptation of the eyes, which can lead to night blindness, is an early symptom of vitamin A deficiency. Xerophthalmia (which is nearly pathognomonic) results from keratinization of the eyes. It involves drying (xerosis) and thickening of the conjunctivae and corneas. Superficial foamy patches composed of epithelial debris and secretions on the exposed bulbar conjunctiva (Bitot spots) develop. In advanced deficiency, the cornea becomes hazy and can develop erosions, which can lead to its destruction (keratomalacia).

Keratinization of the skin and of the mucous membranes in the respiratory, GI, and urinary tracts can occur. Drying, scaling, and follicular thickening of the skin and respiratory infections can result.

Immunity is generally impaired.

The younger the patient, the more severe are the effects of vitamin A deficiency. Growth retardation and infections are common among children. Mortality rate can exceed 50% in children with severe vitamin A deficiency.

Diagnosis

- Serum retinol levels, clinical evaluation, and response to vitamin A

Ocular findings suggest vitamin A deficiency. Dark adaptation can be impaired in other disorders (eg, zinc deficiency, retinitis pigmentosa, severe refractive errors, cataracts, diabetic retinopathy). If dark adaptation is impaired, rod scotometry and electroretinography are done to determine whether vitamin A deficiency is the cause.

Serum levels of retinol are measured. Normal range is 28 to 86 mcg/dL (1 to 3 mcmol/L). However, levels decrease only after the deficiency is advanced because the liver contains large stores of vitamin A. Also, decreased levels may result from acute infection, which causes retinol-binding protein and transthyretin (also called prealbumin) levels to decrease transiently.

A therapeutic trial of vitamin A may help confirm the diagnosis.

Prevention

The diet should include dark green leafy vegetables, deep- or bright-colored fruits (eg, papayas, oranges), carrots, and yellow vegetables (eg, squash, pumpkin). Vitamin A–fortified milk and cereals, liver, egg yolks, and fish liver oils are helpful. Carotenoids are absorbed better when consumed with some dietary fat. If milk allergy is suspected in infants, they should be given adequate vitamin A in formula feedings.

In developing countries, prophylactic supplements of vitamin A palmitate in oil 200,000 IU (60,000 RAE) po every 6 mo are advised for all children between 1 and 5 yr of age; infants < 6 mo can be given a one-time dose of 50,000 IU (15,000 RAE), and those aged 6 to 12 mo can be given a one-time dose of 100,000 IU (30,000 RAE).

Treatment

- Vitamin A palmitate

Dietary deficiency of vitamin A is traditionally treated with vitamin A palmitate in oil 60,000 IU po once/day for 2 days, followed by 4500 IU po once/day. If vomiting or malabsorption is present or xerophthalmia is probable, a dose of 50,000 IU for infants < 6 mo, 100,000 IU for infants 6 to 12 mo, or 200,000 IU for children > 12 mo and adults should be given for 2 days, with a third dose at least 2 wk later. The same doses are recommended for infants and children with complicated measles.

Vitamin A deficiency is a risk factor for severe measles; treatment with vitamin A can shorten the duration of the disorder and may reduce the severity of symptoms and risk of death. The WHO recommends that all children with measles in developing countries should receive 2 doses of vitamin A, (100,000 IU for children < 12 mo and 200,000 IU for those > 12 mo) given 24 h apart (see also WHO: Measles Fact Sheet).

Infants born to HIV-positive mothers should receive 50,000 IU (15,000 RAE) within 48 h of birth. Prolonged daily administration of large doses, especially to infants, must be avoided because toxicity may result.

For pregnant or breastfeeding women, prophylactic or therapeutic doses should not exceed 10,000 IU (3000 RAE)/day to avoid possible damage to the fetus or infant.

KEY POINTS

- Vitamin A deficiency usually results from dietary deficiency, as occurs in areas where rice, devoid of beta-carotene, is the staple food, but it may result from disorders that interfere with the absorption, storage, or transport of vitamin A.
- Ocular findings include impaired night vision (early), conjunctival deposits, and keratomalacia.
- In children with severe deficiency, growth is slowed and risk of infection is increased.
- Diagnose based on ocular findings and serum retinol levels.
- Treat with vitamin A palmitate.

Vitamin A Toxicity

Vitamin A toxicity can be acute (usually due to accidental ingestion by children) or chronic. Both types usually cause headache and increased intracranial pressure. Acute toxicity causes nausea and vomiting. Chronic toxicity causes changes in skin, hair, and nails; abnormal liver test results; and, in a fetus, birth defects. Diagnosis is usually clinical. Unless birth defects are present, adjusting the dose almost always leads to complete recovery.

Acute vitamin A toxicity in children may result from taking large doses (> 300,000 IU [> 100,000 RAE]), usually accidentally. In adults, acute toxicity has occurred when arctic explorers ingested polar bear or seal livers, which contain several million units of vitamin A.

Chronic vitamin A toxicity in older children and adults usually develops after doses of > 100,000 IU (> 30,000 RAE)/day have been taken for months. Megavitamin therapy is a possible cause, as are massive daily doses (150,000 to 350,000 IU [50,000 to 120,000 RAE]) of vitamin A or its metabolites, which are sometimes given for nodular acne or other skin disorders. Adults who consume > 4500 IU (> 1500 RAE)/day of vitamin A may develop osteoporosis. Infants who are given excessive doses (18,000 to 60,000 IU [6,000 to 20,000 RAE]/day) of water-miscible vitamin A may develop toxicity within a few weeks. Birth defects occur in children of women receiving isotretinoin (which is related to vitamin A) for acne treatment during pregnancy.

Although carotene is converted to vitamin A in the body, excessive ingestion of carotene causes carotenemia, not vitamin A toxicity. Carotenemia is usually asymptomatic but may lead to carotenosis, in which the skin becomes yellow.

When taken as a supplement, beta-carotene has been associated with increased cancer risk; risk does not seem to increase when carotenoids are consumed in fruits and vegetables.

Symptoms and Signs

Although symptoms of vitamin A toxicity may vary, headache and rash usually develop during acute or chronic toxicity.

Acute toxicity causes increased intracranial pressure. Drowsiness, irritability, abdominal pain, nausea, and vomiting are common. Sometimes the skin subsequently peels.

Early symptoms of chronic toxicity are sparsely distributed, coarse hair; alopecia of the eyebrows; dry, rough skin; dry eyes; and cracked lips. Later, severe headache, pseudotumor cerebri, and generalized weakness develop. Cortical hyperostosis of bone and arthralgia may occur, especially in children. Fractures may occur easily, especially in the elderly. In children, toxicity can cause pruritus, anorexia, and failure to thrive. Hepatomegaly and splenomegaly may occur.

In carotenosis, the skin (but not the sclera) becomes deep yellow, especially on the palms and soles.

Diagnosis

- Clinical evaluation

Diagnosis of vitamin A toxicity is clinical. Blood vitamin levels correlate poorly with toxicity. However, if clinical diagnosis is equivocal, laboratory testing may help. In vitamin A toxicity, fasting serum retinol levels may increase from normal (28 to 86 mcg/dL [1 to 3 mcmol/L]) to > 100 mcg/dL (> 3.49 mcmol/L), sometimes to > 2000 mcg/dL (> 69.8 mcmol/L). Hypercalcemia is common.

Differentiating vitamin A toxicity from other disorders may be difficult. Carotenosis may also occur in severe hypothyroidism and anorexia nervosa, possibly because carotene is converted to vitamin A more slowly.

Prognosis

Complete recovery usually occurs if vitamin A ingestion stops. Symptoms and signs of chronic toxicity usually disappear within 1 to 4 wk. However, birth defects in the fetus of a mother who has taken megadoses of vitamin A are not reversible.

Treatment

- Vitamin A is stopped.

KEY POINTS

- Vitamin A toxicity can be caused by ingesting high doses of vitamin A—acutely (usually accidentally by children) or chronically (eg, as megavitamin therapy or treatment for skin disorders).
- Acute toxicity causes rash, abdominal pain, increased intracranial pressure, and vomiting.
- Chronic toxicity causes rash, increased intracranial pressure, sparse and coarse hair, dry and rough skin, and arthralgia; risk of fractures is increased, especially in the elderly.
- Diagnose based on clinical findings.
- When vitamin A is stopped, symptoms (except birth defects) usually resolve within 1 to 4 wk.

VITAMIN B_6

(Pyridoxine)

Vitamin B_6 includes a group of closely related compounds: pyridoxine, pyridoxal, and pyridoxamine. They are metabolized in the body to pyridoxal phosphate, which acts as a coenzyme in many important reactions in blood, CNS, and skin metabolism. Vitamin B_6 is important in heme and nucleic acid biosynthesis and in lipid, carbohydrate, and amino acid metabolism (see Table 6–2).

Vitamin B_6 Deficiency and Dependency

Because vitamin B6 is present in most foods, dietary deficiency is rare. Secondary deficiency may result from various conditions. Symptoms can include peripheral neuropathy, a pellagra-like syndrome, anemia, and seizures, which, particularly in infants, may not resolve when treated with anticonvulsants. Impaired metabolism (dependency) is rare; it causes various symptoms, including seizures, intellectual disability, and anemia. Diagnosis is usually clinical; no laboratory test readily assesses vitamin B6 status. Treatment consists of giving oral vitamin B6 and, when possible, treating the cause.

Etiology

Dietary vitamin B_6 deficiency, though rare, can develop because extensive processing can deplete foods of vitamin B_6.

Secondary vitamin B_6 deficiency most often results from

- Protein-energy undernutrition
- Malabsorption
- Alcoholism
- Use of pyridoxine-inactivating drugs (eg, anticonvulsants, isoniazid, cycloserine, hydralazine, corticosteroids, penicillamine)
- Excessive loss during hemodialysis

Rarely, secondary deficiency results from increased metabolic demand (eg, in hyperthyroidism).

Rare inborn errors of metabolism can affect pyridoxine metabolism.

Symptoms and Signs

Vitamin B_6 deficiency causes peripheral neuropathy and a pellagra-like syndrome, with seborrheic dermatitis, glossitis, and cheilosis, and, in adults, can cause depression, confusion, EEG abnormalities, and seizures.

Rarely, deficiency or dependency causes seizures in infants. Seizures, particularly in infants, may be refractory to treatment with anticonvulsants.

Normocytic, microcytic, or sideroblastic anemia can also develop.

Diagnosis

- Clinical evaluation

Vitamin B_6 deficiency should be considered in

- Any infant who has seizures
- Any patient who has seizures refractory to treatment with anticonvulsants
- Any patient with deficiencies of other B vitamins, particularly in patients with alcoholism or protein-energy undernutrition

Diagnosis of vitamin B_6 deficiency is usually clinical. There is no single accepted laboratory test of vitamin B_6 status; measurement of serum pyridoxal phosphate is most common.

PEARLS & PITFALLS

- If anticonvulsants do not stop seizures in infants, consider giving pyridoxine to treat possible vitamin B_6 deficiency.

Treatment

- Pyridoxine
- Elimination of risk factors when possible

For secondary vitamin B_6 deficiency, causes (eg, use of pyridoxine-inactivating drugs, malabsorption) should be corrected if possible.

Usually, pyridoxine 50 to 100 mg po once/day corrects the deficiency in adults. Most people taking isoniazid should also be given pyridoxine 30 to 50 mg po once/day. For deficiency due to increased metabolic demand, amounts larger than the DRI may be required. For most cases of inborn errors of metabolism, high doses of pyridoxine may be effective.

KEY POINTS

- Vitamin B_6 deficiency is usually caused by pyridoxine-inactivating drugs (eg, isoniazid), protein-energy undernutrition, malabsorption, alcoholism, or excessive loss.
- Deficiency can cause peripheral neuropathy, seborrheic dermatitis, glossitis, and cheilosis, and, in adults, depression, confusion, and seizures.
- Suspect and diagnose based on clinical findings.
- Correct secondary causes, or give supplemental pyridoxine.

Vitamin B_6 Toxicity

The ingestion of megadoses (> 500 mg/day) of pyridoxine (eg, taken to treat carpal tunnel syndrome or premenstrual syndrome although efficacy is unproved) may cause peripheral neuropathy with deficits in a stocking-glove distribution, including progressive sensory ataxia and severe impairment of position and vibration senses. Senses of touch, temperature, and pain are less affected. Motor and central nervous systems are usually intact.

Diagnosis of vitamin B_6 toxicity is clinical.

Treatment of vitamin B_6 toxicity is to stop taking vitamin B_6. Recovery is slow and, for some patients, incomplete.

VITAMIN B_{12}

(Cobalamins)

Cobalamin is a general term for compounds with biologic vitamin B_{12} activity. These compounds are involved in nucleic acid metabolism, methyl transfer, and myelin synthesis and repair. They are necessary for the formation of normal RBCs (see Table 6–2).

Food-bound vitamin B_{12} is released in the stomach's acid environment and is bound to R protein (haptocorrin). Pancreatic enzymes cleave this B_{12} complex (B_{12}-R protein) in the small intestine. After cleavage, intrinsic factor, secreted by parietal cells in the gastric mucosa, binds with vitamin B_{12}. Intrinsic factor is required for absorption of vitamin B_{12}, which takes place in the terminal ileum.

Vitamin B_{12} in plasma is bound to transcobalamins I and II. Transcobalamin II is responsible for delivering vitamin B_{12} to tissues. The liver stores large amounts of vitamin B_{12}. Enterohepatic reabsorption helps retain vitamin B_{12}. Liver vitamin B_{12} stores can normally sustain physiologic needs for 3 to 5 yr if B_{12} intake stops (eg, in people who become vegans) and for months to 1 yr if enterohepatic reabsorption capacity is absent.

Large amounts of vitamin B_{12} seem to be nontoxic but are not recommended for regular use (ie, as a general tonic).

Vitamin B_{12} Deficiency

Dietary vitamin B_{12} deficiency usually results from inadequate absorption, but deficiency can develop in vegans who do not take vitamin supplements. Deficiency causes megaloblastic anemia, damage to the white matter of the spinal cord and brain, and peripheral neuropathy. Diagnosis is usually made by measuring serum vitamin B_{12} levels. The Schilling test helps determine etiology. Treatment consists of oral or parenteral vitamin B_{12}. Folate (folic acid) should not be used instead of vitamin B_{12} because folate may alleviate the anemia but allow neurologic deficits to progress.

Etiology

Vitamin B_{12} deficiency can result from

- Inadequate intake
- Inadequate absorption
- Decreased utilization
- Use of certain drugs

Inadequate vitamin B_{12} intake is possible in vegans but is otherwise unlikely. Breastfed babies of vegan mothers may develop vitamin B_{12} deficiency by age 4 to 6 mo because in these babies, liver stores (which are normally extensive in other babies) are limited and their rapid growth rate results in high demand.

Inadequate vitamin B_{12} absorption is the most common cause of deficiency (see Table 6–5). In the elderly, inadequate absorption most commonly results from decreased acid secretion. In such cases, crystalline vitamin B_{12} (such as that available in vitamin supplements) can be absorbed, but food-bound vitamin B_{12} is not liberated and absorbed normally.

Inadequate absorption may occur in blind loop syndrome (with overgrowth of bacteria) or fish tapeworm infestation; in these cases, bacteria or parasites use ingested vitamin B_{12} so that less is available for absorption.

Vitamin B_{12} absorption may be inadequate if ileal absorptive sites are destroyed by inflammatory bowel disease or are surgically removed.

Table 6–5. CAUSES OF VITAMIN B_{12} DEFICIENCY

CAUSE	SOURCE
Inadequate diet	Vegan diet Breastfeeding of infants by vegan mothers Fad diets
Impaired absorption	Lack of intrinsic factor (due to autoimmune metaplastic atrophic gastritis, destruction of gastric mucosa, gastric surgery, or gastric bypass surgery) Intrinsic factor inhibition Decreased acid secretion Small-bowel disorders (eg, inflammatory bowel disease, celiac disease, cancer, biliary or pancreatic disorders) Competition for vitamin B_{12} (in fish tapeworm infestation or blind loop syndrome) AIDS
Inadequate utilization	Enzyme deficiencies Liver disorders Transport protein abnormality
Drugs	Antacids Metformin Nitrous oxide (repeated exposure)

Less common causes of inadequate vitamin B_{12} absorption include chronic pancreatitis, gastric or bariatric surgery, malabsorption syndromes, AIDS, use of certain drugs (eg, antacids, metformin), repeated exposure to nitrous oxide, and a genetic disorder causing malabsorption in the ileum (Imerslund-Graesbeck syndrome).

Less commonly, **decreased utilization of vitamin B_{12}** or **use of certain drugs** causes vitamin B_{12} deficiency (see Table 6–5).

Pernicious anemia is often used synonymously with vitamin B_{12} deficiency. However, pernicious anemia specifically refers to anemia resulting from vitamin B_{12} deficiency caused by an autoimmune metaplastic atrophic gastritis with loss of intrinsic factor. Patients with classic pernicious anemia, most commonly younger adults, are at increased risk of stomach and other GI cancers.

Symptoms and Signs

Anemia usually develops insidiously. It is often more severe than its symptoms indicate because its slow evolution allows physiologic adaptation.

Occasionally, splenomegaly and hepatomegaly occur. Various GI symptoms, including weight loss and poorly localized abdominal pain, may occur. Glossitis, usually described as burning of the tongue, is uncommon.

Neurologic symptoms develop independently from and often without hematologic abnormalities.

Subacute combined degeneration refers to degenerative changes in the nervous system due to vitamin B_{12} deficiency; they affect mostly brain and spinal cord white matter. Demyelinating or axonal peripheral neuropathies can occur.

In early stages, decreased position and vibratory sensation in the extremities is accompanied by mild to moderate weakness and hyporeflexia. In later stages, spasticity, extensor plantar responses, greater loss of position and vibratory sensation in the lower extremities, and ataxia emerge. These deficits may develop in a stocking-glove distribution. Tactile, pain, and temperature sensations are usually spared but may be difficult to assess in the elderly.

Some patients are also irritable and mildly depressed. Paranoia (megaloblastic madness), delirium, confusion, and, at times, postural hypotension may occur in advanced cases. The confusion may be difficult to differentiate from age-related dementias, such as Alzheimer disease.

Diagnosis

- CBC and vitamin B_{12} and folate levels
- Sometimes methylmalonic acid (MMA) levels or Schilling test

It is important to remember that severe neurologic disease may occur without anemia or macrocytosis.

Diagnosis of vitamin B_{12} deficiency is based on CBC and vitamin B_{12} and folate levels. CBC usually detects megaloblastic anemia. Tissue deficiency and macrocytic indexes may precede the development of anemia. A vitamin B_{12} level < 200 pg/mL (< 145 pmol/L) indicates vitamin B_{12} deficiency. The folate level is measured because vitamin B_{12} deficiency must be differentiated from folate deficiency as a cause of megaloblastic anemia; folate supplementation can mask vitamin B_{12} deficiency and may alleviate megaloblastic anemia but allow the neurologic deficits to progress or even accelerate.

When clinical judgment suggests vitamin B_{12} deficiency but the vitamin B_{12} level is low-normal (200 to 350 pg/mL [145 to 260 pmol/L]) or hematologic indexes are normal, other tests can be done. They include measuring the following:

- Serum MMA levels: An elevated MMA level supports vitamin B_{12} deficiency but may be due to renal failure. MMA levels can also be used to monitor the response to treatment. MMA levels remain normal in folate deficiency.

- Homocysteine levels: Levels may be elevated with either vitamin B_{12} or folate deficiency.
- Less commonly, holotranscobalamin II (transcobalamin II–B_{12} complex) content: When holotranscobalamin II is < 40 pg/mL (< 30 pmol/L), vitamin B_{12} is deficient.

After vitamin B_{12} deficiency is diagnosed, additional tests (eg, Schilling test) may be indicated for younger adults but usually not for the elderly. Unless dietary vitamin B_{12} is obviously inadequate, serum gastrin levels or autoantibodies to intrinsic factor may be measured; sensitivity and specificity of these tests may be poor.

Schilling test: The Schilling test is useful only if diagnosing intrinsic factor deficiency is important, as in classic pernicious anemia. This test is not necessary for most elderly patients. The Schilling test measures absorption of free radiolabeled vitamin B_{12}. Radiolabeled vitamin B_{12} is given orally, followed in 1 to 6 h by 1000 mcg (1 mg) of parenteral vitamin B_{12}, which reduces uptake of radiolabeled vitamin B_{12} by the liver. Absorbed radiolabeled vitamin B_{12} is excreted in urine, which is collected for 24 h. The amount excreted is measured, and the percentage of total radiolabeled vitamin B_{12} is determined. If absorption is normal, ≥ 9% of the dose given appears in the urine. Reduced urinary excretion (< 5% if kidney function is normal) indicates inadequate vitamin B_{12} absorption. Improved absorption with the subsequent addition of intrinsic factor to radiolabeled vitamin B_{12} confirms the diagnosis of pernicious anemia.

The test is often difficult to do or interpret because of incomplete urine collection or renal insufficiency. In addition, because the Schilling test does not measure absorption of protein-bound vitamin B_{12}, the test does not detect defective liberation of vitamin B_{12} from foods, which is common among the elderly. The Schilling test repletes vitamin B_{12} and can mask deficiency, so it should be done only after all other diagnostic tests and therapeutic trials.

If malabsorption is identified, the Schilling test can be repeated after a 2-wk trial of an oral antibiotic. If antibiotic therapy corrects malabsorption, the likely cause is intestinal overgrowth of bacteria (eg, blind-loop syndrome).

Treatment

- Supplemental vitamin B_{12}

Vitamin B_{12} 1000 to 2000 mcg po can be given once/day to patients who do not have severe deficiency or neurologic symptoms or signs. A nasal gel preparation of vitamin B_{12} is available at a higher price. Large oral doses can be absorbed by mass action, even when intrinsic factor is absent. If the MMA level (sometimes used to monitor treatment) does not decrease, patients may not be taking vitamin B_{12}.

For more severe deficiency, vitamin B_{12} 1 mg IM is usually given 1 to 4 times/wk for several weeks until hematologic abnormalities are corrected; then it is given once/mo.

Although hematologic abnormalities are usually corrected within 6 wk (reticulocyte count should improve within 1 wk), resolution of neurologic symptoms may take much longer. Neurologic symptoms that persist for months or years become irreversible. In most elderly people with vitamin B_{12} deficiency and dementia, cognition does not improve after treatment.

Vitamin B_{12} treatment must be continued for life unless the pathophysiologic mechanism for the deficiency is corrected.

Infants of vegan mothers should receive supplemental vitamin B_{12} from birth.

KEY POINTS

- Common causes of vitamin B_{12} deficiency include inadequate dietary amounts (eg, in vegans), impaired absorption, age-related decreased acid secretion, and autoimmune metaplastic atrophic gastritis (which causes pernicious anemia).
- The deficiency commonly causes megaloblastic anemia, loss of position and vibration sensation (which occurs early and progresses), and, when advanced, paranoia, delirium, and confusion.
- Do a CBC and measure vitamin B_{12} and folate levels.
- Do a Schilling test in young and middle-aged adults with vitamin B_{12} deficiency.
- Treat with supplemental vitamin B_{12}.

VITAMIN C

(Ascorbic Acid)

Vitamin C plays a role in collagen, carnitine, hormone, and amino acid formation. It is essential for wound healing and facilitates recovery from burns. Vitamin C is also an antioxidant, supports immune function, and facilitates the absorption of iron (see Table 6–2).

Vitamin C Deficiency

(Scurvy)

In developed countries, vitamin C deficiency can occur as part of general undernutrition, but severe deficiency (causing scurvy) is uncommon. Symptoms include fatigue, depression, and connective tissue defects (eg, gingivitis, petechiae, rash, internal bleeding, impaired wound healing). In infants and children, bone growth may be impaired. Diagnosis is usually clinical. Treatment consists of oral vitamin C.

Severe vitamin C deficiency results in scurvy, a disorder characterized by hemorrhagic manifestations and abnormal osteoid and dentin formation.

Etiology

In adults, primary vitamin C deficiency is usually due to

- Inadequate diet

The need for dietary vitamin C is increased by febrile illnesses, inflammatory disorders (particularly diarrheal disorders), achlorhydria, smoking, hyperthyroidism, iron deficiency, cold or heat stress, surgery, burns, and protein deficiency. Heat (eg, sterilization of formulas, cooking) can destroy some of the vitamin C in food.

Pathophysiology

When vitamin C is deficient, formation of intercellular cement substances in connective tissues, bones, and dentin is defective, resulting in weakened capillaries with subsequent hemorrhage and defects in bone and related structures.

Bone tissue formation becomes impaired, which, in children, causes bone lesions and poor bone growth. Fibrous tissue forms between the diaphysis and the epiphysis, and costochondral junctions enlarge. Densely calcified fragments of cartilage are embedded in the fibrous tissue. Subperiosteal hemorrhages, sometimes due to small fractures, may occur in children or adults.

Symptoms and Signs

In adults, symptoms of vitamin C deficiency develop after weeks to months of vitamin C depletion. Lassitude, weakness, irritability, weight loss, and vague myalgias and arthralgias may develop early.

Symptoms of scurvy (related to defects in connective tissues) develop after a few months of deficiency. Follicular hyperkeratosis, coiled hair, and perifollicular hemorrhages may develop. Gums may become swollen, purple, spongy, and friable; they bleed easily in severe deficiency. Eventually, teeth become loose and avulsed. Secondary infections may develop. Wounds heal poorly and tear easily, and spontaneous hemorrhages may occur, especially as ecchymoses in the skin of the lower limbs or as bulbar conjunctival hemorrhage.

Other symptoms and signs include femoral neuropathy due to hemorrhage into femoral sheaths (which may mimic deep venous thrombosis), lower extremity edema, and painful bleeding or effusions within joints.

In infants, symptoms include irritability, pain during movement, anorexia, and slowed growth. In infants and children, bone growth is impaired, and bleeding and anemia may occur.

Diagnosis

- Usually clinical (based on skin or gingival findings and risk factors)

Diagnosis of vitamin C deficiency is usually made clinically in a patient who has skin or gingival signs and is at risk of vitamin C deficiency. Laboratory confirmation may be available. CBC is done, often detecting anemia. Bleeding, coagulation, and prothrombin times are normal.

Skeletal x-rays can help diagnose childhood (but not adult) scurvy. Changes are most evident at the ends of long bones, particularly at the knee. Early changes resemble atrophy. Loss of trabeculae results in a ground-glass appearance. The cortex thins. A line of calcified, irregular cartilage (white line of Fraenkel) may be visible at the metaphysis. A zone of rarefaction or a linear fracture proximal and parallel to the white line may be visible as only a triangular defect at the bone's lateral margin but is specific. The epiphysis may be compressed. Healing subperiosteal hemorrhages may elevate and calcify the periosteum.

Laboratory diagnosis, which requires measuring blood ascorbic acid, is sometimes done at academic centers. Levels of < 0.6 mg/dL (< 34 mcmol/L) are considered marginal; levels of < 0.2 mg/dL (< 11 mcmol/L) indicate vitamin C deficiency. Measurement of ascorbic acid levels in the WBC-platelet layer of centrifuged blood is not widely available or standardized.

In adults, scurvy must be differentiated from arthritis, hemorrhagic disorders, gingivitis, and protein-energy undernutrition. Hyperkeratotic hair follicles with surrounding hyperemia or hemorrhage are almost pathognomonic. Bleeding gums, conjunctival hemorrhages, most petechiae, and ecchymoses are nonspecific.

Treatment

- Nutritious diet with supplemental ascorbic acid

For scurvy in adults, ascorbic acid 100 to 500 mg po tid is given for 1 to 2 wk, until signs disappear, and followed by a nutritious diet supplying 1 to 2 times the DRI.

In scurvy, therapeutic doses of ascorbic acid restore the functions of vitamin C in a few days. The symptoms and signs usually disappear over 1 to 2 wk. Chronic gingivitis with extensive subcutaneous hemorrhage persists longer.

Prevention

Vitamin C 75 mg po once/day for women and 90 mg po once/day for men prevents deficiency. Smokers should consume an additional 35 mg/day. Five servings of most fruits and vegetables (recommended daily) provide > 200 mg of vitamin C.

KEY POINTS

- The need for vitamin C is increased by fever, inflammation, diarrhea, smoking, hyperthyroidism, iron deficiency, cold or heat stress, surgery, burns, and protein deficiency.
- After weeks or months, the deficiency causes nonspecific symptoms (eg, weakness, lassitude, irritability, arthralgias, myalgias); later, connective tissue is affected, causing follicular hyperkeratosis, coiled hair, swollen and bleeding gums, loose teeth, poor wound healing, and spontaneous hemorrhages.
- In patients who have skin or gingival symptoms or risk factors for the deficiency, measure the ascorbic acid level.
- Treat with supplemental ascorbic acid and a nutritious diet.

Vitamin C Toxicity

The upper limit for vitamin C intake is 2000 mg/day.

Up to 10 g/day of vitamin C are sometimes taken for unproven health benefits, such as preventing or shortening the duration of viral infections or slowing or reversing the progression of cancer or atherosclerosis. Such doses may acidify the urine, cause nausea and diarrhea, interfere with the healthy antioxidant-prooxidant balance in the body, and, in patients with thalassemia or hemochromatosis, promote iron overload.

Intake of vitamin C below the upper limit does not have toxic effects in healthy adults.

VITAMIN D

Vitamin D has 2 main forms:

- D_2 (ergocalciferol)
- D_3 (cholecalciferol): The naturally occurring form and the form used for low-dose supplementation

Vitamin D_3 is synthesized in skin by exposure to direct sunlight (ultraviolet B radiation) and obtained in the diet chiefly in fish liver oils and salt water fish (see Table 6–2). In some developed countries, milk and other foods are fortified with vitamin D. Human breast milk is low in vitamin D, containing an average of only 10% of the amount in fortified cow's milk.

Vitamin D levels may decrease with age because skin synthesis declines. Sunscreen use and dark skin pigmentation also reduce skin synthesis of vitamin D.

Vitamin D is a prohormone with several active metabolites that act as hormones. Vitamin D is metabolized by the liver to 25(OH)D, which is then converted by the kidneys to $1,25(OH)_2D$ (1,25-dihydroxycholecalciferol, calcitriol, or active vitamin D hormone). 25(OH)D, the major circulating form, has some metabolic activity, but $1,25(OH)_2D$ is the most metabolically active. The conversion to $1,25(OH)_2D$ is regulated by its own concentration, parathyroid hormone (PTH), and serum concentrations of calcium and phosphate.

Vitamin D affects many organ systems (see Table 6–6), but mainly it increases calcium and phosphate absorption from the intestine and promotes normal bone formation and mineralization.

Vitamin D and related analogs may be used to treat psoriasis, hypoparathyroidism, and renal osteodystrophy. Vitamin D's usefulness in preventing leukemia and breast, prostate, and colon

Table 6–6. ACTIONS OF VITAMIN D AND ITS METABOLITES

ORGAN	ACTIONS
Bone	Promotes bone formation by maintaining appropriate calcium and phosphate concentrations
Immune system	Stimulates immunogenic and antitumor activity Decreases risk of autoimmune disorders
Intestine	Enhances calcium and phosphate transport (absorption)
Kidneys	Enhances calcium reabsorption by the tubules
Parathyroid glands	Inhibits parathyroid hormone secretion
Pancreas	Stimulates insulin production

cancers has not been proved, nor has its efficacy in preventing falls in the elderly.[1-3]

1. Cummings SR, Kiel DP, Black DM: Vitamin D supplementation and increased risk of falling: A cautionary tale of vitamin supplements retold. *JAMA Intern Med* 176(2):171–172, 2016.
2. Uusi-Rasi K, Patil R, Karinkanta S, Kannus P, et al: Exercise and vitamin D in fall prevention among older women: A randomized clinical trial. *JAMA Intern Med* 75(5):703–711, 2015.
3. LeBlanc ES, Chou R: Vitamin D and falls—Fitting new data with current guidelines. *JAMA Intern Med* 175(5):712–713, 2015.

Vitamin D Deficiency and Dependency

Inadequate exposure to sunlight predisposes to vitamin D deficiency. Deficiency impairs bone mineralization, causing rickets in children and osteomalacia in adults and possibly contributing to osteoporosis. Diagnosis involves measurement of serum 25(OH)D (D2 + D3). Treatment usually consists of oral vitamin D; calcium and phosphate are supplemented as needed. Prevention is often possible. Rarely, hereditary disorders cause impaired metabolism of vitamin D (dependency).

Vitamin D deficiency is common worldwide. It is a common cause of rickets and osteomalacia, but these disorders may also result from other conditions, such as chronic kidney disease, various renal tubular disorders, familial hypophosphatemic (vitamin D–resistant) rickets (see p. 2543), chronic metabolic acidosis, hyperparathyroidism, hypoparathyroidism, inadequate dietary calcium, and disorders or drugs that impair the mineralization of bone matrix.

Vitamin D deficiency causes hypocalcemia, which stimulates production of PTH, causing hyperparathyroidism. Hyperparathyroidism increases absorption, bone mobilization, and renal conservation of calcium but increases excretion of phosphate. As a result, the serum level of calcium may be normal, but because of hypophosphatemia, bone mineralization is impaired.

Etiology

Vitamin D deficiency may result from the following:

- Inadequate exposure to sunlight
- Inadequate intake of vitamin D
- Reduced absorption of vitamin D
- Abnormal metabolism of vitamin D
- Resistance to the effects of vitamin D

Inadequate exposure or intake: Inadequate direct sunlight exposure or sunscreen use and inadequate intake usually occur simultaneously to result in clinical deficiency. Susceptible people include

- The elderly (who are often undernourished and are not exposed to enough sunlight)
- Certain communities (eg, women and children who are confined to the home or who wear clothing that covers the entire body and face)

Inadequate vitamin D stores are common among the elderly, particularly those who are housebound, institutionalized, or hospitalized or who have had a hip fracture.

Recommended direct sunlight exposure is 5 to 15 min (suberythemal dose) to the arms and legs or to the face, arms, and hands, at least 3 times a week. However, many dermatologists do not recommend increased sunlight exposure because risk of skin cancer is increased.

Reduced absorption: Malabsorption can deprive the body of dietary vitamin D; only a small amount of 25(OH)D is recirculated enterohepatically.

Abnormal metabolism: Vitamin D deficiency may result from defects in the production of 25(OH)D or $1,25(OH)_2D$. People with chronic kidney disease commonly develop rickets or osteomalacia because renal production of $1,25\ (OH)_2D$ is decreased and phosphate levels are elevated. Hepatic dysfunction can also interfere with production of active vitamin D metabolites.

Type I hereditary vitamin D–dependent rickets is an autosomal recessive disorder characterized by absent or defective conversion of 25(OH)D to $1,25(OH)_2D$ in the kidneys. X-linked familial hypophosphatemia reduces vitamin D synthesis in the kidneys.

Many anticonvulsants and use of glucocorticoids increase the need for vitamin D supplementation.

Resistance to effects of vitamin D: Type II hereditary vitamin D–dependent rickets has several forms and is due to mutations in the $1,25(OH)_2D$ receptor. This receptor affects the metabolism of gut, kidney, bone, and other cells. In this disorder, $1,25(OH)_2D$ is abundant but ineffective because the receptor is not functional.

Symptoms and Signs

Vitamin D deficiency can cause muscle aches, muscle weakness, and bone pain at any age.

Vitamin D deficiency in a pregnant woman causes deficiency in the fetus. Occasionally, deficiency severe enough to cause maternal osteomalacia results in rickets with metaphyseal lesions in neonates.

In young infants, rickets causes softening of the entire skull (craniotabes). When palpated, the occiput and posterior parietal bones feel like a ping pong ball.

In older infants with rickets, sitting and crawling are delayed, as is fontanelle closure; there is bossing of the skull and costochondral thickening. Costochondral thickening can look like beadlike prominences along the lateral chest wall (rachitic rosary).

In children 1 to 4 yr, epiphyseal cartilage at the lower ends of the radius, ulna, tibia, and fibula enlarge; kyphoscoliosis develops, and walking is delayed.

In older children and adolescents, walking is painful; in extreme cases, deformities such as bowlegs and knock-knees develop. The pelvic bones may flatten, narrowing the birth canal in adolescent girls.

Tetany is caused by hypocalcemia and may accompany infantile or adult vitamin D deficiency. Tetany may cause paresthesias of the lips, tongue, and fingers; carpopedal and facial spasm; and, if very severe, seizures. Maternal deficiency can cause tetany in neonates.

Osteomalacia predisposes to fractures. In the elderly, hip fractures may result from only minimal trauma.

Diagnosis

- Levels of 25(OH)D ($D_2 + D_3$)

Vitamin D deficiency may be suspected based on any of the following:

- A history of inadequate sunlight exposure or dietary intake
- Symptoms and signs of rickets, osteomalacia, or neonatal tetany
- Characteristic bone changes seen on x-ray

X-rays of the radius and ulna plus serum levels of calcium, phosphate, alkaline phosphatase, PTH, and 25(OH)D are needed to differentiate vitamin D deficiency from other causes of bone demineralization.

Assessment of vitamin D status and serologic tests for syphilis can be considered for infants with craniotabes based on the history and physical examination, but most cases of craniotabes resolve spontaneously. Rickets can be distinguished from chondrodystrophy because the latter is characterized by a large head, short extremities, thick bones, and normal serum calcium, phosphate, and alkaline phosphatase levels.

Tetany due to infantile rickets may be clinically indistinguishable from seizures due to other causes. Blood tests and clinical history may help distinguish them.

X-rays: Bone changes, seen on x-rays, precede clinical signs. In rickets, changes are most evident at the lower ends of the radius and ulna. The diaphyseal ends lose their sharp, clear outline; they are cup-shaped and show a spotty or fringy rarefaction. Later, because the ends of the radius and ulna have become noncalcified and radiolucent, the distance between them and the metacarpal bones appears increased. The bone matrix elsewhere also becomes more radiolucent. Characteristic deformities result from the bones bending at the cartilage-shaft junction because the shaft is weak. As healing begins, a thin white line of calcification appears at the epiphysis, becoming denser and thicker as calcification proceeds. Later, the bone matrix becomes calcified and opacified at the subperiosteal level.

In adults, bone demineralization, particularly in the spine, pelvis, and lower extremities, can be seen on x-rays; the fibrous lamellae can also be seen, and incomplete ribbonlike areas of demineralization (pseudofractures, Looser lines, Milkman syndrome) appear in the cortex.

Laboratory tests: Because levels of serum 25(OH)D reflect body stores of vitamin D and correlate with symptoms and signs of vitamin D deficiency better than levels of other vitamin D metabolites, the best way to diagnose vitamin D deficiency is generally considered to be

- 25(OH)D ($D_2 + D_3$) levels

Target 25(OH)D levels are > 20 to 24 ng/mL (about 50 to 60 nmol/L) for maximal bone health; whether higher levels have other benefits remains uncertain, and higher absorption of calcium may increase risk of coronary artery disease.

If the diagnosis is unclear, serum levels of $1,25(OH)_2D$ and urinary calcium concentration can be measured. In severe deficiency, serum $1,25(OH)_2D$ is abnormally low, usually undetectable. Urinary calcium is low in all forms of the deficiency except those associated with acidosis.

In vitamin D deficiency, serum calcium may be low or, because of secondary hyperparathyroidism, may be normal. Serum phosphate usually decreases, and serum alkaline phosphatase usually increases. Serum PTH may be normal or elevated.

Type I hereditary vitamin D–dependent rickets results in normal serum 25(OH)D, low serum $1,25(OH)_2D$ and calcium, and normal or low serum phosphate.

Treatment

- Correction of calcium and phosphate deficiencies
- Supplemental vitamin D

Calcium deficiency (which is common) and phosphate deficiency should be corrected.

As long as calcium and phosphate intake is adequate, adults with osteomalacia and children with uncomplicated rickets can be cured by giving vitamin D_3 40 mcg 1600 IU po once/day. Serum 25(OH)D and $1,25(OH)_2D$ begin to increase within 1 or 2 days. Serum calcium and phosphate increase and serum alkaline phosphatase decreases within about 10 days. During the 3rd wk, enough calcium and phosphate are deposited in bones to be visible on x-rays. After about 1 mo, the dose can usually be reduced gradually to the usual maintenance level of 15 mcg (600 IU) once/day.

If tetany is present, vitamin D should be supplemented with IV calcium salts for up to 1 wk (see p. 1287).

Some elderly patients need vitamin D_3 25 to > 50 mcg (1000 to ≥ 2000 IU) daily to maintain a 25(OH)D level > 20 ng/mL (> 50 nmol/L); this dose is higher than the RDA for people < 70 yr (600 IU) or > 70 yr (800 IU). The current upper limit for vitamin D is 4000 IU/day. Higher doses of vitamin D_2 (eg, 25,000 to 50,000 IU every week or every month) are sometimes prescribed; because vitamin D_3 is more potent than vitamin D_2, it is now preferred.

Because rickets and osteomalacia due to defective production of vitamin D metabolites are vitamin D–resistant, they do not respond to the doses usually effective for rickets due to inadequate intake. Endocrinologic evaluation is required because treatment depends on the specific defect. When 25(OH)D production is defective, vitamin D_3 50 mcg (2000 IU) once/day increases serum levels and results in clinical improvement. Patients with kidney disorders often need $1,25(OH)_2D$ (calcitriol) supplementation.

Type I hereditary vitamin D–dependent rickets responds to $1,25(OH)_2D$ 1 to 2 mcg po once/day. Some patients with type II hereditary vitamin D–dependent rickets respond to very high doses (eg, 10 to 24 mcg/day) of $1,25(OH)_2D$; others require long-term infusions of calcium.

Prevention

Dietary counseling is particularly important in communities whose members are at risk of vitamin D deficiency. Fortifying unleavened chapati flour with vitamin D (125 mcg/kg) has been effective among Indian immigrants in Britain. The benefits of sunlight exposure for vitamin D status must be weighed against the increased skin damage and skin cancer risks.

All breastfed infants should be given supplemental vitamin D 10 mcg (400 IU) once/day from birth to 6 mo; at 6 mo, a more diversified diet is available. Any benefit of doses higher than the RDA is unproved.

KEY POINTS

- Vitamin D deficiency is common and results from inadequate exposure to sunlight and inadequate dietary intake (usually occurring together) and/or from chronic kidney disease.

- The deficiency can cause muscle aches and weakness, bone pain, and osteomalacia.
- Suspect vitamin D deficiency in patients who have little exposure to sunlight and a low dietary intake, typical symptoms and signs (eg, rickets, muscle aches, bone pain), or bone demineralization seen on x-rays.
- To confirm the diagnosis, measure the level of 25(OH)D ($D_2 + D_3$).
- To treat vitamin D deficiency, correct deficiencies of calcium and phosphate and give supplemental vitamin D.

Vitamin D Toxicity

Usually, vitamin D toxicity results from taking excessive amounts. In vitamin D toxicity, resorption of bone and intestinal absorption of calcium is increased, resulting in hypercalcemia. Marked hypercalcemia commonly causes symptoms. Diagnosis is typically based on elevated blood levels of 25(OH)D. Treatment consists of stopping vitamin D, restricting dietary calcium, restoring intravascular volume deficits, and, if toxicity is severe, giving corticosteroids or bisphosphonates.

Because synthesis of $1,25(OH)_2D$ (the most active metabolite of vitamin D) is tightly regulated, vitamin D toxicity usually occurs only if excessive doses (prescription or megavitamin) are taken. Vitamin D 1000 mcg (40,000 IU)/day causes toxicity within 1 to 4 mo in infants. In adults, taking 1250 mcg (50,000 IU)/day for several months can cause toxicity. Vitamin D toxicity can occur iatrogenically when hypoparathyroidism is treated too aggressively (see p. 1285).

Symptoms and Signs

The main symptoms of vitamin D toxicity result from hypercalcemia. Anorexia, nausea, and vomiting can develop, often followed by polyuria, polydipsia, weakness, nervousness, pruritus, and eventually renal failure. Proteinuria, urinary casts, azotemia, and metastatic calcifications (particularly in the kidneys) can develop.

Diagnosis

- Hypercalcemia plus risk factors or elevated serum 25(OH) D levels

A history of excessive vitamin D intake may be the only clue differentiating vitamin D toxicity from other causes of hypercalcemia. Elevated serum calcium levels of 12 to 16 mg/dL (3 to 4 mmol/L) are a constant finding when toxic symptoms occur. Serum 25(OH)D levels are usually elevated to > 150 ng/mL (> 375 nmol/L). Levels of $1,25(OH)_2D$, which need not be measured to confirm the diagnosis, may be normal.

Serum calcium should be measured often (weekly at first, then monthly) in all patients receiving large doses of vitamin D, particularly the potent $1,25(OH)_2D$.

Treatment

- IV hydration plus corticosteroids or bisphosphonates

After stopping vitamin D intake, hydration (with IV normal saline) and corticosteroids or bisphosphonates (which inhibit bone resorption) are used to reduce blood calcium levels.

Kidney damage or metastatic calcifications, if present, may be irreversible.

VITAMIN E

(Tocopherol)

Vitamin E is a group of compounds (including tocopherols and tocotrienols) that have similar biologic activities. The most biologically active is alpha-tocopherol, but beta-, gamma-, and delta-tocopherols, 4 tocotrienols, and several stereoisomers may also have important biologic activity. These compounds act as antioxidants, which prevent lipid peroxidation of polyunsaturated fatty acids in cellular membranes (see Table 6–2).

Plasma tocopherol levels vary with total plasma lipid levels. Normally, the plasma alpha-tocopherol level is 5 to 20 mcg/mL (11.6 to 46.4 mcmol/L).

High-dose vitamin E supplements do not protect against cardiovascular disorders; whether supplements can protect against tardive dyskinesia or increase or decrease the risk of prostate cancer is controversial. There is no convincing evidence that doses of up to 2000 IU/day slow the progression of Alzheimer disease.

Although the amount of vitamin E in many fortified foods and supplements is given in IU, current recommendations are to use mg.

Vitamin E Deficiency

Dietary vitamin E deficiency is common in developing countries; deficiency among adults in developed countries is uncommon and usually due to fat malabsorption. The main symptoms are hemolytic anemia and neurologic deficits. Diagnosis is based on measuring the ratio of plasma alpha-tocopherol to total plasma lipids; a low ratio suggests vitamin E deficiency. Treatment consists of oral vitamin E, given in high doses if there are neurologic deficits or if deficiency results from malabsorption.

Vitamin E deficiency causes fragility of RBCs and degeneration of neurons, particularly peripheral axons and posterior column neurons.

Etiology

In developing countries, the most common cause of vitamin E deficiency is

- Inadequate intake of vitamin E

In developed countries, the most common causes are

- Disorders that cause fat malabsorption, including abetalipoproteinemia (Bassen-Kornzweig syndrome, due to genetic absence of apolipoprotein B), chronic cholestatic hepatobiliary disease, pancreatitis, short bowel syndrome, and cystic fibrosis.

A rare genetic form of vitamin E deficiency without fat malabsorption results from defective liver metabolism.

Symptoms and Signs

The main symptoms of vitamin E deficiency are mild hemolytic anemia and nonspecific neurologic deficits. Abetalipoproteinemia results in progressive neuropathy and retinopathy in the first 2 decades of life.

Vitamin E deficiency may contribute to retinopathy of prematurity (also called retrolental fibroplasia) in premature infants and to some cases of intraventricular and subependymal hemorrhage in neonates. Affected premature neonates have muscle weakness.

In children, chronic cholestatic hepatobiliary disease or cystic fibrosis causes neurologic deficits, including spinocerebellar ataxia with loss of deep tendon reflexes, truncal and limb ataxia, loss of vibration and position senses, ophthalmoplegia, muscle weakness, ptosis, and dysarthria.

In adults with malabsorption, vitamin E deficiency very rarely causes spinocerebellar ataxia because adults have large vitamin E stores in adipose tissue.

Diagnosis

- Low alpha-tocopherol level or low ratio of serum alpha-tocopherol to serum lipids

Without a history of inadequate intake or a predisposing condition, vitamin E deficiency is unlikely. Confirmation usually requires measuring the vitamin level. Measuring RBC hemolysis in response to peroxide can suggest the diagnosis but is nonspecific. Hemolysis increases as vitamin E deficiency impairs RBC stability.

Measuring the serum alpha-tocopherol level is the most direct method of diagnosis. In adults, vitamin E deficiency is suggested if the alpha-tocopherol level is < 5 mcg/mL (< 11.6 mcmol/L). Because abnormal lipid levels can affect vitamin E status, a low ratio of serum alpha-tocopherol to lipids (< 0.8 mg/g total lipid) is the most accurate indicator in adults with hyperlipidemia.

In children and adults with abetalipoproteinemia, serum alpha-tocopherol levels are usually undetectable.

Treatment

- Supplemental alpha-tocopherol or mixed tocopherols (alpha-, beta-, and gamma-tocopherols)

If malabsorption causes clinically evident deficiency, alpha-tocopherol 15 to 25 mg/kg po once/day should be given. Or mixed tocopherols (200 to 400 IU) can be given. However, larger doses of alpha-tocopherol given by injection are required to treat neuropathy during its early stages or to overcome the defect of absorption and transport in abetalipoproteinemia.

Prevention

Although premature neonates may require supplementation, human milk and commercial formulas have enough vitamin E for full-term neonates.

KEY POINTS

- Vitamin E deficiency is usually caused by inadequate dietary intake in developing countries or by a disorder causing fat malabsorption in developed countries.
- The deficiency causes mainly mild hemolytic anemia and nonspecific neurologic deficits.
- In patients with inadequate intake or a predisposing condition plus compatible findings, measure the tocopherol level to confirm the diagnosis.
- Treat with supplemental tocopherol.

Vitamin E Toxicity

Many adults take relatively large amounts of vitamin E (alpha-tocopherol 400 to 800 mg/day) for months to years without any apparent harm. Occasionally, muscle weakness, fatigue, nausea, and diarrhea occur. The most significant risk is bleeding. However, bleeding is uncommon unless the dose is > 1000 mg/day or the patient takes oral coumarin or warfarin. Thus, the upper limit for adults aged ≥ 19 yr is 1000 mg for any form of alpha-tocopherol.

Analyses of previous studies report that high vitamin E intakes may increase the risk of hemorrhagic stroke and premature death.

VITAMIN K

Vitamin K_1 (phylloquinone) is dietary vitamin K. Dietary fat enhances its absorption. Infant formulas contain supplemental vitamin K.

Vitamin K_2 refers to a group of compounds (menaquinones) synthesized by bacteria in the intestinal tract; the amount synthesized does not satisfy the vitamin K requirement.

Vitamin K controls the formation of coagulation factors II (prothrombin), VII, IX, and X in the liver (see Table 6–2). Other coagulation factors dependent on vitamin K are protein C, protein S, and protein Z; proteins C and S are anticoagulants. Metabolic pathways conserve vitamin K. Once vitamin K has participated in formation of coagulation factors, the reaction product, vitamin K epoxide, is enzymatically converted to the active form, vitamin K hydroquinone.

The actions of vitamin K–dependent proteins require calcium. The vitamin K–dependent proteins, osteocalcin and matrix gamma-carboxy-glutamyl (Gla) protein, may have important roles in bone and other tissues. Forms of vitamin K are common therapy for osteoporosis in Japan and other countries.

Vitamin K Deficiency

Vitamin K deficiency results from extremely inadequate intake, fat malabsorption, or use of coumarin anticoagulants. Deficiency is particularly common among breastfed infants. It impairs clotting. Diagnosis is suspected based on routine coagulation study findings and confirmed by response to vitamin K. Treatment consists of vitamin K given orally or, when fat malabsorption is the cause or when risk of bleeding is high, parenterally.

Vitamin K deficiency decreases levels of prothrombin and other vitamin K–dependent coagulation factors, causing defective coagulation and, potentially, bleeding.

Worldwide, vitamin K deficiency causes infant morbidity and mortality.

Vitamin K deficiency causes hemorrhagic disease of the newborn, which usually occurs 1 to 7 days postpartum. In affected neonates, birth trauma can cause intracranial hemorrhage. A late form of this disease can occur in infants about 2 to 12 wk old, typically in infants who are breastfed and are not given vitamin K supplements. If the mother has taken phenytoin anticonvulsants, coumarin anticoagulants, or cephalosporin antibiotics, the risk of hemorrhagic disease is increased.

In **healthy adults,** dietary vitamin K deficiency is uncommon because vitamin K is widely distributed in green vegetables and the bacteria of the normal gut synthesize menaquinones.

Etiology

Neonates are prone to vitamin K deficiency because of the following:

- The placenta transmits lipids and vitamin K relatively poorly.
- The neonatal liver is immature with respect to prothrombin synthesis.
- Breast milk is low in vitamin K, containing about 2.5 mcg/L (cow's milk contains 5000 mcg/L).
- The neonatal gut is sterile during the first few days of life.

In **adults,** vitamin K deficiency can result from

- Fat malabsorption (eg, due to biliary obstruction, malabsorption disorders, cystic fibrosis, or resection of the small intestine)
- Use of coumarin anticoagulants

Coumarin anticoagulants interfere with the synthesis of vitamin–K dependent coagulation proteins (factors II, VII, IX, and X) in the liver. Certain antibiotics (particularly some cephalosporins and other broad-spectrum antibiotics), salicylates, megadoses of vitamin E, and hepatic insufficiency increase risk of bleeding in patients with vitamin K deficiency. Inadequate intake of vitamin K is unlikely to cause symptoms.

Symptoms and Signs

Bleeding is the usual manifestation. Easy bruisability and mucosal bleeding (especially epistaxis, GI hemorrhage, menorrhagia, and hematuria) can occur. Blood may ooze from puncture sites or incisions.

Hemorrhagic disease of the newborn and late hemorrhagic disease in infants may cause cutaneous, GI, intrathoracic, or, in the worst cases, intracranial bleeding. If obstructive jaundice develops, bleeding—if it occurs—usually begins after the 4th or 5th day. It may begin as a slow ooze from a surgical incision, the gums, the nose, or GI mucosa, or it may begin as massive bleeding into the GI tract.

Diagnosis

- Usually prolonged PT or elevated INR that decreases after phytonadione

Vitamin K deficiency or antagonism (due to coumarin anticoagulants) is suspected when abnormal bleeding occurs in a patient at risk. Blood coagulation studies can preliminarily confirm the diagnosis. PT is prolonged and INR is elevated, but PTT, thrombin time, platelet count, bleeding time, and levels of fibrinogen, fibrin-split products, and D-dimer are normal.

If phytonadione (USP generic name for vitamin K_1) 1 mg IV significantly decreases PT within 2 to 6 h, a liver disorder is not the likely cause, and the diagnosis of vitamin K deficiency is confirmed.

Some centers can detect vitamin K deficiency more directly by measuring the serum vitamin level. The serum level of vitamin K_1 ranges from 0.2 to 1.0 ng/mL in healthy people consuming adequate quantities of vitamin K_1 (50 to 150 mcg/day). Knowing vitamin K intake can help interpret serum levels; recent intake affects levels in serum but not in tissues.

More sensitive indicators of vitamin K status, such as PIVKA (protein induced in vitamin K absence or antagonism) and undercarboxylated osteocalcin, are under study.

Treatment

- Phytonadione

Whenever possible, phytonadione should be given po or sc. The usual adult dose is 1 to 20 mg. (Rarely, even when phytonadione is correctly diluted and given slowly, IV replacement can result in anaphylaxis or anaphylactoid reactions.) INR usually decreases within 6 to 12 h. The dose may be repeated in 6 to 8 h if INR has not decreased satisfactorily.

Phytonadione 1 to 10 mg po is indicated for nonemergency correction of a prolonged INR in patients taking anticoagulants. Correction usually occurs within 6 to 8 h. When only partial correction of INR is desirable (eg, when INR should remain slightly elevated because of a prosthetic heart valve), lower doses (eg, 1 to 2.5 mg) of phytonadione can be given.

In infants, bleeding due to vitamin K deficiency can be corrected by giving phytonadione 1 mg sc or IM once. The dose is repeated if INR remains elevated. Higher doses may be necessary if the mother has been taking oral anticoagulants.

Prevention

Phytonadione 0.5 to 1 mg IM (or 0.3 mg/kg for preterm infants) is recommended for all neonates within 6 h of birth to reduce the incidence of intracranial hemorrhage due to birth trauma and of classic hemorrhagic disease of the newborn (risk of increased bleeding 1 to 7 days after birth). It is also used prophylactically before surgery.

Some clinicians recommend that pregnant women taking anticonvulsants receive phytonadione 10 mg po once/day for the 1 mo or 20 mg po once/day for the 2 wk before delivery. The low vitamin K_1 content in breast milk can be increased by increasing maternal dietary intake of phylloquinone to 5 mg/day.

KEY POINTS

- Vitamin K deficiency causes infant morbidity and mortality worldwide.
- The deficiency causes bleeding (eg, easy bruisability, mucosal bleeding).
- Suspect the deficiency in at-risk patients with abnormal or excessive bleeding.
- Measure PT or INR before and after giving phytonadione; a decrease in prolonged PT or an elevated INR after phytonadione confirms the diagnosis.
- Treat with oral or sc phytonadione.

Vitamin K Toxicity

Vitamin K_1 (phylloquinone) is not toxic when consumed orally, even in large amounts. However, menadione (a synthetic, water-soluble vitamin K precursor) can cause toxicity and should not be used to treat vitamin K deficiency.

SECTION 2

Gastrointestinal Disorders

7 Approach to the GI Patient

GI symptoms and disorders are quite common. History and physical examination are often adequate to make a disposition in patients with minor complaints; in other cases, testing is necessary.

History

Using open-ended, interview-style questions, the physician identifies the location and quality of symptoms and any aggravating and alleviating factors.

Abdominal pain is a frequent GI complaint (see Acute Abdominal Pain on p. 83 and Chronic and Recurrent Abdominal Pain on p. 59). Determining the location of the pain can help with the diagnosis. For example, pain in the epigastrium may reflect problems in the pancreas, stomach, or small bowel. Pain in the right upper quadrant may reflect problems in the liver, gallbladder, and bile ducts such as cholecystitis or hepatitis. Pain in the right lower quadrant may indicate inflammation of the appendix, terminal ileum, or cecum, suggesting appendicitis, ileitis, or Crohn disease. Pain in the left lower quadrant may indicate diverticulitis or constipation. Pain in either the left or right lower quadrant may indicate colitis, ileitis, or ovarian (in women) etiologies.

Asking patients about radiation of pain may help clarify the diagnosis. For example, pain radiating to the shoulder may reflect cholecystis because the gallbladder may be irritating the diaphragm. Pain radiating to the back may reflect pancreatitis. Asking patients to describe the character of the pain (ie, sharp and constant, waves of dull pain) and the onset (sudden, such as resulting from a perforated viscus or ruptured ectopic pregnancy) can help differentiate causes.

Patients should be queried about changes in eating and elimination. Regarding eating, patients should be asked about difficulty swallowing (dysphagia), loss of appetite, and presence of nausea and vomiting. If patients are vomiting, they should be asked how often and for how long and whether they have noted blood or coffee-ground-like material suggestive of GI bleeding. Also, patients should be asked about the type and quantity of liquids they have tried to drink, if any, and whether they have been able to keep them down.

Regarding elimination, patients should be asked when their most recent bowel movement was, how frequently they have been having bowel movements, and whether this frequency represents a change from their typical frequency. It is more useful to ask for specific, quantitative information about bowel movements rather than simply asking whether they are constipated or have diarrhea because different people use these terms quite differently. Patients should also be asked to describe the color and consistency of the stool, including whether stool has appeared black or bloody (suggestive of GI bleeding), purulent, or mucoid. Patients who have noticed blood should be asked whether it was coating the stool, mixed with stool, or whether blood was passed without any stool.

A gynecologic history is important in women because gynecologic and obstetric disorders may manifest with GI symptoms.

Associated, nonspecific symptoms, such as fever or weight loss, must be assessed. Weight loss is an associated symptom that may indicate a more severe problem such as cancer, and the clinician should be prompted to do a more extensive evaluation.

Patients report symptoms differently depending on their personality, the impact of the illness on their life, and sociocultural influences. For example, nausea and vomiting may be minimized or reported indirectly by a severely depressed patient but presented with dramatic urgency by a histrionic one.

Important elements of the past medical history include presence of previously diagnosed GI disorders, previous abdominal surgery, and use of drugs and substances that might cause GI symptoms (eg, NSAIDs, alcohol).

Physical Examination

The physical examination might begin with inspection of the oropharynx to assess hydration, ulcers, or possible inflammation.

Inspection of the abdomen with the patient supine may show a convex appearance when bowel obstruction, ascites, or, rarely, a large mass is present. Auscultation to assess bowel sounds and determine presence of bruits should follow. Percussion elicits hyperresonance (tympany) in the presence of bowel obstruction and dullness with ascites and can determine the span of the liver. Palpation proceeds systematically, beginning gently to identify areas of tenderness and, if tolerated, palpating deeper to locate masses or organomegaly.

When the abdomen is tender, patients should be assessed for peritoneal signs such as guarding and rebound. Guarding is an involuntary contraction of the abdominal muscles that is slightly slower and more sustained than the rapid, voluntary flinch exhibited by sensitive or anxious patients. Rebound is a distinct flinch upon brisk withdrawal of the examiner's hand.

The inguinal area and all surgical scars should be palpated for hernias.

Digital rectal examination with testing for occult blood and (in women) pelvic examination complete the evaluation of the abdomen.

Testing

Patients with acute, nonspecific symptoms (eg, dyspepsia, nausea) and an unremarkable physical examination rarely require testing. Findings suggesting significant disease (alarm symptoms) should prompt further evaluation:

- Anorexia
- Anemia
- Blood in stool (gross or occult)
- Dysphagia
- Fever
- Hepatomegaly
- Pain that awakens patient
- Persistent nausea and vomiting
- Weight loss

Chronic or recurrent symptoms, even with an unremarkable examination, also warrant evaluation. See Ch. 9 on p. 78 for specific GI tests.

FUNCTIONAL GI ILLNESS

Often, no objectively measurable structural or physiologic abnormality for GI complaints is found, even after extensive evaluation. Such patients are said to have functional illness, which accounts for 30 to 50% of referrals to gastroenterologists. Functional illness may manifest with upper and/or lower GI symptoms. (See also Irritable Bowel Syndrome on p. 142.)

Functional GI disorders are disorders of the gut-brain interaction. Some evidence suggests that such patients have visceral hypersensitivity, a disturbance of nociception in which they experience discomfort caused by sensations (eg, luminal distention, peristalsis) that other people do not find distressing. Functional disorders are classified by symptoms related to a combination of not only visceral hypersensitivity but also motility disturbance, altered microbiota, mucosal and immune function, and CNS processing.[1]

In some patients, psychologic conditions such as anxiety (with or without aerophagia), conversion disorder, somatic symptom disorder, or illness anxiety disorder (previously called hypochondriasis) are associated with GI symptoms. Psychologic theories hold that some functional symptoms may satisfy certain psychologic needs. For example, some patients with chronic illness derive secondary benefits from being sick. For such patients, successful treatment of symptoms may lead to development of other symptoms.

Many referring physicians and GI specialists find functional GI complaints difficult to understand and treat, and uncertainty may lead to frustration and judgmental attitudes. An effective physician-patient interaction reduces health care–seeking behavior by the patient. Physicians should acknowledge the patient's symptoms and provide empathy. Physicians should avoid ordering repeated studies or multiple drug trials for insistent patients with inexplicable complaints because this may promote symptom anxiety and health care–seeking behavior.[2] When symptoms are not suggestive of serious illness, the physician should wait rather than embark on another diagnostic or therapeutic plan. In time, new information may direct evaluation and management. Functional complaints are sometimes present in patients with physiologic disease (eg, peptic ulcer, esophagitis); such symptoms may not remit even when a physiologic illness is addressed. In some patients, testing (eg, CT) may identify incidental abnormalities that are unrelated to the symptoms.

1. Drossman DA: Functional gastrointestinal disorders: History, pathophysiology, clinical features, and Rome IV. *Gastroenterology* 150:1262–1279, 2016. doi: http://dx.doi.org/10.1053/j.gastro.2016.02.032.
2. Drossman DA: 2012 David Sun Lecture: Helping your patient by helping yourself: How to improve the patient-physician relationship by optimizing communication skills. *Am J Gastroenterol* 108:521–528, 2013. doi: 10.1038/ajg.2013.56.

8 Symptoms of GI Disorders

Upper GI complaints include

- Chest pain
- Chronic and recurrent abdominal pain
- Dyspepsia
- Lump in the throat
- Halitosis
- Hiccups
- Nausea and vomiting
- Rumination

Some upper GI complaints represent functional illness (ie, no physiologic cause found after extensive evaluation).

Lower GI complaints include

- Constipation
- Diarrhea
- Gas and bloating
- Abdominal pain
- Rectal pain or bleeding

As with upper GI complaints, lower GI complaints result from physiologic illness or represent a functional disorder (ie, no radiologic, biochemical, or pathologic abnormalities are found even after extensive evaluation). The reasons for functional symptoms are not clear. Evidence suggests that patients with functional symptoms may have disturbances of motility, nociception, or both; ie, they perceive as uncomfortable certain sensations (eg, luminal distention, peristalsis) that other people do not find distressing.

No bodily function is more variable and subject to external influences than defecation. Bowel habits vary considerably from person to person and are affected by age, physiology, diet, and social and cultural influences. Some people have unwarranted preoccupation with bowel habits. In Western society, normal stool frequency ranges from 2 to 3/day to 2 to 3/wk. Changes in stool frequency, consistency, volume, or composition (ie, presence of blood, mucus, pus, or excess fatty material) may indicate disease.

CHRONIC AND RECURRENT ABDOMINAL PAIN

Chronic abdominal pain (CAP) persists for more than 3 mo either continuously or intermittently. Intermittent pain may be referred to as recurrent abdominal pain (RAP). Acute abdominal pain is discussed elsewhere. CAP occurs any time after 5 yr of age. Up to 10% of children require evaluation for RAP. About 2% of adults, predominantly women, have CAP (a much higher percentage of adults have some type of chronic GI symptoms, including nonulcer dyspepsia and various bowel disturbances).

Nearly all patients with CAP have had a prior medical evaluation that did not yield a diagnosis after history, physical, and basic testing.

Pathophysiology

Functional abdominal pain syndrome (FAPS) is pain that persists > 6 mo without evidence of physiologic disease, shows no relationship to physiologic events (eg, meals, defecation, menses), and interferes with daily functioning. FAPS is poorly understood but seems to involve altered nociception. Sensory neurons in the dorsal horn of the spinal cord may become abnormally excitable and hyperalgesic due to a combination of factors. Cognitive and psychologic factors (eg, depression, stress, culture, secondary gain, coping and support mechanisms) may cause efferent stimulation that amplifies pain signals, resulting in perception of pain with low-level inputs and persistence of pain long after the stimulus has ceased. Additionally, the pain itself may function as a stressor, perpetuating a positive feedback loop.

In addition, menopause increases GI symptoms in several disorders including irritable bowel syndrome, inflammatory bowel disease, endometriosis, and nonulcer dyspepsia.

Etiology

Perhaps 10% of patients have an occult physiologic illness (see Table 8–1); the remainder have a functional process. However, determining whether a particular abnormality (eg, adhesions, ovarian cyst, endometriosis) is the cause of CAP symptoms or an incidental finding can be difficult.

Evaluation

History: History of present illness should elicit pain location, quality, duration, timing and frequency of recurrence, and factors that worsen or relieve pain (particularly eating or moving bowels). A specific inquiry as to whether milk and milk products cause abdominal cramps, bloating, or distention is needed because lactose intolerance is common, especially among blacks.

Review of systems seeks concomitant GI symptoms such as gastroesophageal reflux, anorexia, bloating or "gas," nausea, vomiting, jaundice, melena, hematuria, hematemesis, weight loss, and mucus or blood in the stool. Bowel symptoms, such as diarrhea, constipation, and changes in stool consistency, color, or elimination pattern, are particularly important.

In adolescents, a diet history is important because ingestion of large amounts of cola beverages and fruit juices (which may contain significant quantities of fructose and sorbitol) can account for otherwise puzzling abdominal pain.

Past medical history should include nature and timing of any abdominal surgery and the results of previous tests that have been done and treatments that have been tried. A drug history should include details concerning prescription and illicit drug use as well as alcohol.

Family history of RAP, fevers, or both should be ascertained, as well as known diagnoses of sickle cell trait or disease, familial Mediterranean fever, and porphyria.

Physical examination: Review of vital signs should particularly note presence of fever or tachycardia.

General examination should seek presence of jaundice, skin rash, and peripheral edema.

Abdominal examination should note areas of tenderness, presence of peritoneal findings (eg, guarding, rigidity, rebound), and any masses or organomegaly. Rectal examination and (in women) pelvic examination to locate tenderness, masses, and blood are essential.

Red flags: The following findings are of particular concern:

- Fever
- Anorexia, weight loss
- Pain that awakens patient
- Blood in stool or urine
- Jaundice
- Edema
- Abdominal mass or organomegaly

Interpretation of findings: Clinical examination alone infrequently provides a firm diagnosis.

Determining whether CAP is physiologic or functional can be difficult. Although the presence of red flag findings indicates a high likelihood of a physiologic cause, their absence does not rule it out. Other hints are that physiologic causes usually cause pain that is well localized, especially to areas other than the periumbilical region. Pain that wakes the patient is usually physiologic. Some findings suggestive of specific disorders are listed in Table 8–1.

Functional CAP may result in pain similar to that of physiologic origin. However, there are no associated red flag findings, and psychosocial features are often prominent. A history of physical or sexual abuse or an unresolved loss (eg, divorce, miscarriage, death of a family member) may be a clue.

The Rome criteria for diagnosis of irritable bowel syndrome are the presence of abdominal pain or discomfort for at least 3 days/mo in the last 3 mo along with at least 2 of the following: (1) improvement with defecation; (2) onset (of each episode of discomfort) associated with a change in frequency of defecation; and (3) change in consistency of stool.

Testing: In general, simple tests (including urinalysis, CBC, liver tests, ESR, and lipase) should be done. Abnormalities in these tests, the presence of red flag findings, or specific clinical findings mandate further testing, even if previous assessments have been negative. Specific tests depend on the findings (see Table 8–1) but typically include ultrasonography for ovarian cancer in women > 50 yr, CT of the abdomen and pelvis with contrast, upper GI endoscopy or colonoscopy, and perhaps small-bowel x-rays or stool testing.

The benefits of testing patients with no red flag findings are unclear. Patients > 50 should probably have a colonoscopy; those ≤ 50 can be observed or have CT of the abdomen and pelvis with contrast if an imaging study is desired. Magnetic resonance cholangiopancreatography (MRCP), ERCP, and laparoscopy are rarely helpful in the absence of specific indications.

Between the initial evaluation and the follow-up visit, the patient (or family, if the patient is a child) should record any pain, including its nature, intensity, duration, and precipitating factors. Diet, defecation pattern, and any remedies tried (and the results obtained) should also be recorded. This record may reveal inappropriate behavior patterns and exaggerated responses to pain or otherwise suggest a diagnosis.

Treatment

Physiologic conditions are treated.

If the diagnosis of functional CAP is made, frequent examinations and tests should be avoided because they may focus on or magnify the physical complaints or imply that the physician lacks confidence in the diagnosis.

There are no modalities to cure functional CAP; however, many helpful measures are available. These measures rest on a foundation of a trusting, empathic relationship among the physician, patient, and family. Patients should be reassured that they are not in danger; specific concerns should be sought and addressed. The physician should explain the laboratory findings and the nature of the problem and describe how the pain is generated and how the patient perceives it (ie, that there is a constitutional tendency to feel pain at times of stress). It is important to avoid perpetuating the negative psychosocial consequences of chronic pain (eg, prolonged absences from school or work, withdrawal from social activities) and to promote independence, social participation, and self-reliance. These strategies help the patient control or tolerate the symptoms while participating fully in everyday activities.

Drugs such as aspirin, NSAIDs, H_2 receptor blockers, proton pump inhibitors, and tricyclic antidepressants can be effective. Opioids should be avoided because they invariably lead to dependency.

Cognitive methods (eg, relaxation training, biofeedback, hypnosis) may help by contributing to the patient's sense of well-being and control. Regular follow-up visits should be scheduled weekly, monthly, or bimonthly, depending on the patient's needs, and should continue until well after the problem has resolved. Psychiatric referral may be required if symptoms persist, especially if the patient is depressed or there are significant psychologic difficulties in the family.

Table 8–1. PHYSIOLOGIC CAUSES OF CHRONIC ABDOMINAL PAIN

CAUSE	SUGGESTIVE FINDINGS*	DIAGNOSTIC APPROACH
GU disorders		
Congenital abnormalities	Recurrent UTIs	IVU Ultrasonography
Endometriosis	Discomfort before or during menses	Laparoscopy
Ovarian cyst, ovarian cancer	Vague lower abdominal discomfort, bloating Sometimes a palpable pelvic mass	Pelvic ultrasonography Gynecologic consultation
Renal calculi	Fever, flank pain, dark or bloody urine	Urine culture IVU CT
Sequelae of acute PID	Pelvic discomfort History of acute PID	Pelvic examination Sometimes laparoscopy
GI disorders		
Celiac disease	In children, failure to thrive Abdominal bloating, diarrhea, and often steatorrhea Symptoms that worsen when gluten-containing products are ingested	Serologic markers Small-bowel biopsy
Chronic appendicitis	Several previous discrete episodes of RLQ pain	Abdominal CT Ultrasonography
Chronic cholecystitis	Recurrent colicky RUQ pain	Ultrasonography HIDA scan
Chronic hepatitis	Upper abdominal discomfort, malaise, anorexia Jaundice uncommon In about one-third of patients, a history of acute hepatitis	Liver tests Viral hepatitis titers
Chronic pancreatitis, pancreatic pseudocyst	Episodes of severe epigastric pain Sometimes malabsorption (eg, diarrhea, fatty stool) Usually a history of acute pancreatitis	Serum lipase levels (frequently not elevated) CT, MRCP
Colon cancer	Discomfort uncommon but possibly colicky discomfort if left colon is partially obstructed Often occult or visible blood in stool	Colonoscopy
Crohn disease	Episodic severe pain with fever, anorexia, weight loss, diarrhea Extraintestinal symptoms (joints, eyes, mouth, skin)	CT enterography or upper GI series with SBFT Colonoscopy and esophagogastroduodenoscopy with biopsies
Gastric cancer	Dyspepsia or mild pain Often occult blood in stool	Upper endoscopy
Granulomatous enterocolitis	Family history Recurrent infections in other sites (eg, lungs, lymph nodes)	ESR Barium enema CT enterography
Hiatus hernia with gastroesophageal reflux	Heartburn Sometimes cough and/or hoarseness Symptoms relieved by taking antacids Sometimes regurgitation of gastric contents into mouth	Barium swallow Endoscopy
Intestinal TB	Chronic nonspecific pain Sometimes palpable RLQ mass Fever, diarrhea, weight loss	Tuberculin test Endoscopy for biopsy CT with oral contrast
Lactose intolerance	Bloating and cramps after ingesting milk products	Hydrogen breath test Trial of elimination of lactose-containing foods
Pancreatic cancer	Severe upper abdominal pain that • Often radiates to the back • Occurs late in disease, when weight loss is often present May cause obstructive jaundice	CT MRCP or ERCP

Table continues on the following page.

Table 8–1. PHYSIOLOGIC CAUSES OF CHRONIC ABDOMINAL PAIN (*Continued*)

CAUSE	SUGGESTIVE FINDINGS*	DIAGNOSTIC APPROACH
Parasitic infestation (particularly giardiasis)	History of travel or exposure Cramps, flatulence, diarrhea	Stool examination for ova or parasites Stool enzyme immunoassay (for *Giardia*)
Peptic ulcer disease	Upper abdominal pain relieved by food and antacids May awaken patient at night	Endoscopy and biopsy for *Helicobacter pylori* *H. pylori* breath test Evaluation of NSAID use Stool examination for occult blood
Postoperative adhesive bands	Previous abdominal surgery Colicky discomfort accompanied by nausea and sometimes vomiting	Upper GI series, SBFT, or enteroclysis
Ulcerative colitis	Crampy pain with bloody diarrhea	Sigmoidoscopy Rectal biopsy Colonoscopy
Systemic disorders		
Abdominal epilepsy	Very rare Episodic pain No other GI symptoms	EEG
Familial angioneurotic edema	Family history Pain often with peripheral angioedema and fever	Serum complement level (C4) during attacks
Familial Mediterranean fever	Family history Fever and peritonitis often accompanying the bouts of pain Starting in childhood or adolescence	Genetic testing
Food allergy	Symptoms developing only after consuming certain foods (eg, seafood)	Elimination diet
Immunoglobulin A–associated vasculitis (formerly Henoch-Schönlein purpura)	Palpable purpuric rash Joint pains Occult blood in stool	Biopsy of skin lesions
Lead poisoning	Cognitive/behavioral abnormalities	Blood lead level
Migraine equivalent	Rare variant with epigastric pain and vomiting Mainly in children Usually family history of migraine	Clinical evaluation
Porphyria	Recurrent severe abdominal pain, vomiting Benign abdominal examination Sometimes neurologic symptoms (eg, muscle weakness, seizures, mental disturbance) In some types, skin lesions	Urine porphobilinogen and delta-aminolevulinic acid screening RBC deaminase assay
Sickle cell disease	Family history Severe episodes of abdominal pain lasting over a day Recurrent pain in nonabdominal sites	Sickle preparation Hb electrophoresis

*Findings are not always present and may be present in other disorders.

HIDA = hydroxyiminodiacetic acid; MRCP = magnetic resonance cholangiopancreatography; PID = pelvic inflammatory disease; RLQ = right lower quadrant; RUQ = right upper quadrant; SBFT = small-bowel follow-through.

Modified from Barbero GJ: Recurrent abdominal pain. *Pediatrics in Review* 4:30, 1982 and from Greenberger NJ: Sorting through nonsurgical causes of acute abdominal pain. *Journal of Critical Illness* 7:1602–1609, 1992.

School personnel should become involved for children who have CAP. Children can rest briefly in the nurse's office during the school day, with the expectation that they return to class after 15 to 30 min. The school nurse can be authorized to dispense a mild analgesic (eg, acetaminophen). The nurse can sometimes allow the child to call a parent, who should encourage the child to stay in school. However, once parents stop treating their child as special or ill, the symptoms may worsen before they abate.

KEY POINTS

- Most cases represent a functional process.
- Red flag findings indicate a physiologic cause and need for further assessment.
- Testing is guided by clinical features.
- Repeated testing after physiologic causes are ruled out is usually counterproductive.

DYSPEPSIA

Dyspepsia is a sensation of pain or discomfort in the upper abdomen; it often is recurrent. It may be described as indigestion, gassiness, early satiety, postprandial fullness, gnawing, or burning.

Etiology

There are several common causes of dyspepsia (see Table 8–2). Many patients have findings on testing (eg, duodenitis, pyloric dysfunction, motility disturbance, *Helicobacter pylori* gastritis, lactose deficiency, cholelithiasis) that correlate poorly with symptoms (ie, correction of the condition does not alleviate dyspepsia).

Nonulcer (functional) dyspepsia is defined as dyspeptic symptoms in a patient who has no abnormalities on physical examination and upper GI endoscopy.

Evaluation

History: History of present illness should elicit a clear description of the symptoms, including whether they are acute or chronic and recurrent. Other elements include timing and frequency of recurrence, any difficulty swallowing, and relationship of symptoms to eating or taking drugs. Factors that worsen symptoms (particularly exertion, certain foods, or alcohol) or relieve them (particularly eating or taking antacids) are noted.

Review of systems seeks concomitant GI symptoms such as anorexia, nausea, vomiting, hematemesis, weight loss, and bloody or black (melanotic) stools. Other symptoms include dyspnea and diaphoresis.

Past medical history should include known GI and cardiac diagnoses, cardiac risk factors (eg, hypertension, hypercholesterolemia), and the results of previous tests that have been done and treatments that have been tried. Drug history should include prescription and illicit drug use as well as alcohol.

Physical examination: Review of vital signs should note presence of tachycardia or irregular pulse.

General examination should note presence of pallor or diaphoresis, cachexia, or jaundice. Abdomen is palpated for tenderness, masses, and organomegaly. Rectal examination is done to detect gross or occult blood.

Red flags: The following findings are of particular concern:

- Acute episode with dyspnea, diaphoresis, or tachycardia
- Anorexia
- Nausea or vomiting
- Weight loss
- Blood in the stool
- Dysphagia or odynophagia
- Failure to respond to therapy with H_2 blockers or proton pump inhibitors (PPIs)

Interpretation of findings: Some findings are helpful (see Table 8–2).

A patient presenting with a single, acute episode of dyspepsia is of concern, particularly if symptoms are accompanied by dyspnea, diaphoresis, or tachycardia; such patients may have acute coronary ischemia. Chronic symptoms that occur with exertion and are relieved by rest may represent angina.

GI causes are most likely to manifest as chronic complaints. Symptoms are sometimes classified as ulcer-like, dysmotility-like, or reflux-like; these classifications suggest but do not confirm an

Table 8–2. SOME CAUSES OF DYSPEPSIA

CAUSE	SUGGESTIVE FINDINGS	DIAGNOSTIC APPROACH
Achalasia	Slowly progressive dysphagia Early satiety, nausea, vomiting, bloating, and symptoms that are worsened by food Sometimes nocturnal regurgitation of undigested food Chest discomfort	Barium swallow Esophageal manometry Endoscopy
Cancer (eg, esophageal, gastric)	Chronic, vague discomfort Later, dysphagia (esophageal) or early satiety (gastric) Weight loss	Upper endoscopy
Coronary ischemia	Symptoms described as gas or indigestion rather than chest pain by some patients May have exertional component Cardiac risk factors	ECG Serum cardiac markers Sometimes stress testing
Delayed gastric emptying (caused by diabetes, viral illness, or drugs)	Nausea, bloating, fullness	Scintigraphic test of gastric emptying
Drugs (eg, bisphosphonates, erythromycin and other macrolide antibiotics, estrogens, iron, NSAIDs, potassium)	Use apparent on history Symptoms coincident with use	Clinical evaluation
Esophageal spasm	Substernal chest pain with or without dysphagia for liquids and solids	Barium swallow Esophageal manometry
Gastroesophageal reflux disease	Heartburn Sometimes reflux of acid or stomach contents into mouth Symptoms sometimes triggered by lying down Relief with antacids	Clinical evaluation Sometimes endoscopy Sometimes 24-h pH testing
Peptic ulcer disease	Burning or gnawing pain relieved by food or antacids	Upper endoscopy

etiology. Ulcer-like symptoms consist of pain that is localized in the epigastrium, frequently occurs before meals, and is partially relieved by food, antacids, or H_2 blockers. Dysmotility-like symptoms consist of discomfort rather than pain, along with early satiety, postprandial fullness, nausea, vomiting, bloating, and symptoms that are worsened by food. Reflux-like symptoms consist of heartburn or acid regurgitation. However, symptoms often overlap.

Alternating constipation and diarrhea with dyspepsia suggests irritable bowel syndrome or excessive use of OTC laxatives or antidiarrheals.

Testing: Patients in whom symptoms suggest acute coronary ischemia, particularly those with risk factors, should be sent to the emergency department for urgent evaluation, including ECG and serum cardiac markers.

For patients with chronic, nonspecific symptoms, routine tests include CBC (to exclude anemia caused by GI blood loss) and routine blood chemistries. If results are abnormal, additional tests (eg, imaging studies, endoscopy) should be considered. Because of the risk of cancer, patients > 55 and those with new-onset red flag findings should undergo upper GI endoscopy. For patients < 55 with no red flag findings, some authorities recommend empiric therapy for 2 to 4 wk with antisecretory agents followed by endoscopy in treatment failures. Others recommend screening for *H. pylori* infection with a C_{14}-urea breath test or stool assay (see p. 118). However, caution is required in using *H. pylori* or any other nonspecific findings to explain symptoms.

Esophageal manometry and pH studies are indicated if reflux symptoms persist after upper GI endoscopy and a 2- to 4-wk trial with a PPI.

Treatment

Specific conditions are treated. Patients without identifiable conditions are observed over time and reassured. Symptoms are treated with PPIs, H_2 blockers, or a cytoprotective agent (see Table 8–3). Prokinetic drugs (eg, metoclopramide, erythromycin) given as a liquid suspension also may be tried in patients with dysmotility-like dyspepsia. However, there is no clear evidence that matching the drug class to the specific symptoms (eg, reflux vs dysmotility) makes a difference. Misoprostol and anticholinergics are not effective in functional dyspepsia. Drugs that alter sensory perception (eg, tricyclic antidepressants) may be helpful.

KEY POINTS

- Coronary ischemia is possible in a patient with acute "gas."
- Endoscopy is indicated for patients > 55 or with red flag findings.
- Empiric treatment with an acid blocker is reasonable for patients < 55 without red flag findings; patients who do not respond in 2 to 4 wk require further evaluation.

HICCUPS

(Hiccough; Singultus)

Hiccups are repeated involuntary spasms of the diaphragm followed by sudden closure of the glottis, which checks the inflow of air and causes the characteristic sound. Transient episodes are very common. Persistent (> 2 days) and intractable (> 1 mo) hiccups are uncommon but quite distressing.

Etiology

Hiccups follow irritation of afferent or efferent diaphragmatic nerves or of medullary centers that control the respiratory muscles, particularly the diaphragm. Hiccups are more common among men.

Cause is generally unknown, but transient hiccups are often caused by the following:

- Gastric distention
- Alcohol consumption
- Swallowing hot or irritating substances

Persistent and intractable hiccups have myriad causes (see Table 8–4).

Table 8–3. SOME ORAL DRUGS FOR DYSPEPSIA

DRUG	USUAL DOSE	COMMENTS
Proton pump inhibitors		
Dexlansoprazole	30 mg once/day	With long-term use, elevated gastrin levels, but no evidence that this finding causes dysplasia or cancer
Esomeprazole	40 mg once/day	May cause abdominal pain or diarrhea
Lansoprazole	30 mg once/day	
Omeprazole	20 mg once/day	
Pantoprazole	40 mg once/day	
Rabeprazole	20 mg once/day	
H_2 blockers		
Cimetidine	800 mg once/day	Doses reduced in elderly patients
Famotidine	40 mg once/day	With cimetidine and to a lesser extent with other drugs, minor antiandrogen effects and, less commonly, erectile dysfunction
Nizatidine	300 mg once/day	Delayed metabolism of drugs eliminated by cytochrome P-450 enzyme system (eg, phenytoin, warfarin, diazepam)
Ranitidine	300 mg once/day or 150 mg bid	May cause constipation or diarrhea
Cytoprotective agent		
Sucralfate	1 g po qid	Rarely constipation May bind to other drugs and interfere with absorption Cimetidine, ciprofloxacin, digoxin, norfloxacin, ofloxacin, and ranitidine avoided 2 h before or after taking sucralfate

Table 8–4. SOME CAUSES OF INTRACTABLE HICCUPS

CATEGORY	EXAMPLES
Esophageal	Gastroesophageal reflux disease Other esophageal disorders
Abdominal	Abdominal surgery Bowel diseases Gallbladder disease Hepatic metastases Hepatitis Pancreatitis Pregnancy
Thoracic	Diaphragmatic pleurisy Pericarditis Pneumonia Thoracic surgery
Other	Alcoholism Posterior fossa tumors or infarcts Uremia

Evaluation

History: History of present illness should note duration of hiccups, remedies tried, and relationship of onset to recent illness or surgery.

Review of systems seeks concomitant GI symptoms such as gastroesophageal reflux and swallowing difficulties; thoracic symptoms such as cough, fever, or chest pain; and any neurologic symptoms.

Past medical history should query known GI and neurologic disorders. A drug history should include details concerning alcohol use.

Physical examination: Examination is usually unrewarding but should seek signs of chronic disease (eg, cachexia). A full neurologic examination is important.

Red flags: The following is of particular concern:

- Neurologic symptoms or signs

Interpretation of findings: Few findings are specific. Hiccups after alcohol consumption or surgery may well be related to those events. Other possible causes (see Table 8–4) are both numerous and rarely a cause of hiccups.

Testing: No specific evaluation is required for acute hiccups if routine history and physical examination are unremarkable; abnormalities are pursued with appropriate testing.

Patients with hiccups of longer duration and no obvious cause should have testing, probably including serum electrolytes, BUN and creatinine, chest x-ray, and ECG. Upper GI endoscopy and perhaps esophageal pH monitoring should be considered. If these are unremarkable, brain MRI and chest CT may be done.

Treatment

Identified problems are treated (eg, proton pump inhibitors for gastroesophageal reflux disease, dilation for esophageal stricture).

For symptom relief, many simple measures can be tried, although none are more than slightly effective: $PaCO_2$ can be increased and diaphragmatic activity can be inhibited by a series of deep breath-holds or by breathing deeply in to and out of a paper bag. (CAUTION: *Plastic bags can cling to the nostrils and should not be used.*) Vagal stimulation by pharyngeal irritation (eg, swallowing dry bread, granulated sugar, or crushed ice; applying traction on the tongue; stimulating gagging) may work. Numerous other folk remedies exist.

Persistent hiccups are often recalcitrant to treatment. Many drugs have been used in anecdotal series. Baclofen, a gamma-aminobutyric acid agonist (5 mg po q 6 h increasing to 20 mg/dose), may be effective. Other drugs include chlorpromazine 10 to 50 mg po tid prn, metoclopramide 10 mg po bid to qid, and various anticonvulsants (eg, gabapentin). Additionally, an empiric trial of proton pump inhibitors may be given. For severe symptoms, chlorpromazine 25 to 50 mg IM or IV can be given. In intractable cases, the phrenic nerve may be blocked by small amounts of 0.5% procaine solution, with caution being taken to avoid respiratory depression and pneumothorax. Even bilateral phrenicotomy does not cure all cases.

KEY POINTS

- The cause is usually unknown.
- Rarely, a serious disorder is present.
- Evaluation is typically unrewarding but should be pursued for hiccups of long duration.
- Numerous remedies exist, none with clear superiority (or perhaps even effectiveness).

LUMP IN THROAT

(Globus Sensation)

Lump in the throat (globus sensation, globus hystericus) is the sensation of a lump or mass in the throat, unrelated to swallowing, when no mass is present. (See Neck Mass on p. 799 if a mass is present.)

Etiology

No specific etiology or physiologic mechanism has been established. Some studies suggest that elevated cricopharyngeal (upper esophageal sphincter) pressure or abnormal hypopharyngeal motility occur during the time of symptoms. The sensation may also result from gastroesophageal reflux disease (GERD) or from frequent swallowing and drying of the throat associated with anxiety or another emotional state. Although not associated with stress factors or a specific psychiatric disorder, globus sensation may be a symptom of certain mood states (eg, grief, pride); some patients may have a predisposition to this response.

Disorders that can be confused with globus sensation include cricopharyngeal (upper esophageal) webs, symptomatic diffuse esophageal spasm, GERD, skeletal muscle disorders (eg, myasthenia gravis, myotonia dystrophica, polymyositis), and mass lesions in the neck or mediastinum that cause esophageal compression.

Evaluation

The main goal is to distinguish globus sensation from true dysphagia, which suggests a structural or motor disorder of the pharynx or esophagus.

History: History of present illness should elicit a clear description of the symptom, particularly as to whether there is any pain with swallowing or difficulty swallowing (including sensation of food sticking). Timing of symptoms is important, particularly whether it occurs with eating or drinking or is independent of those activities; association with emotional events should be queried specifically.

Review of systems seeks weight loss (as evidence of a swallowing disorder) and symptoms of muscle weakness.

Past medical history should include known neurologic diagnoses, particularly those causing weakness.

Physical examination: The neck and floor of the mouth are palpated for masses. The oropharynx is inspected (including by direct laryngoscopy). Swallowing (of water and a solid food such as crackers) should be observed. Neurologic examination with particular attention to motor function is important.

Red flags: The following findings are of particular concern:

- Neck or throat pain
- Weight loss
- Abrupt onset after age 50
- Pain, choking, or difficulty with swallowing
- Regurgitation of food
- Muscle weakness
- Palpable or visible mass
- Progressive worsening of symptoms

Interpretation of findings: Symptoms unrelated to swallowing, with no pain or difficulty with swallowing, or sensation of food sticking in the throat in a patient with a normal examination imply globus sensation. Any red flag findings or abnormal findings on examination suggest a mechanical or motor disorder of swallowing. Chronic symptoms that occur during unresolved or pathologic grief and that may be relieved by crying suggest globus sensation.

Testing: Patients with findings typical of globus sensation need no testing. If the diagnosis is unclear or the clinician cannot adequately visualize the pharynx, testing as for dysphagia is done. Typical tests include plain or video esophagography, measurement of swallowing time, chest x-ray, and esophageal manometry.

Treatment

Treatment of lump in throat involves reassurance and sympathetic concern. No drug is of proven benefit. Underlying depression, anxiety, or other behavioral disturbances should be managed supportively, with psychiatric referral if necessary. At times, communicating to the patient the association between symptoms and mood state can be beneficial.

KEY POINTS

- Globus symptoms are unrelated to swallowing.
- Tests are not needed unless symptoms are related to swallowing, examination is abnormal, or there are red flag findings.

NAUSEA AND VOMITING

(Nausea and vomiting in infants and children is discussed on p. 2453.)

Nausea, the unpleasant feeling of needing to vomit, represents awareness of afferent stimuli (including increased parasympathetic tone) to the medullary vomiting center. Vomiting is the forceful expulsion of gastric contents caused by involuntary contraction of the abdominal musculature when the gastric fundus and lower esophageal sphincter are relaxed.

Vomiting should be distinguished from regurgitation, the spitting up of gastric contents without associated nausea or forceful abdominal muscular contractions. Patients with achalasia or rumination syndrome or a Zenker diverticulum may regurgitate undigested food without nausea.

Complications: Severe vomiting can lead to symptomatic dehydration and electrolyte abnormalities (typically a metabolic alkalosis with hypokalemia) or rarely to an esophageal tear, either partial (Mallory-Weiss) or complete (Boerhaave syndrome). Chronic vomiting can result in undernutrition, weight loss, and metabolic abnormalities.

Etiology

Nausea and vomiting occur in response to conditions that affect the vomiting center. Causes may originate in the GI tract or CNS or may result from a number of systemic conditions (see Table 8–5).

The **most common causes** of nausea and vomiting are the following:

- Gastroenteritis
- Drugs
- Toxins

Cyclic vomiting syndrome (CVS) is an uncommon disorder characterized by severe, discrete attacks of vomiting or sometimes only nausea that occur at varying intervals, with normal health between episodes and no demonstrable structural abnormalities. It is most common in childhood (mean age of onset 5 yr) and tends to remit with adulthood. CVS in adults is often due to chronic marijuana (cannabis) use.

Evaluation

History: History of present illness should elicit frequency and duration of vomiting; its relation to possible precipitants such as drug or toxin ingestion, head injury, and motion (eg, car, plane, boat, amusement rides); and whether vomitus contained bile (bitter, yellow-green) or blood (red or "coffee ground" material). Important associated symptoms include presence of abdominal pain and diarrhea; the last passage of stool and flatus; and presence of headache, vertigo, or both.

Review of systems seeks symptoms of causative disorders such as amenorrhea and breast swelling (pregnancy), polyuria and polydipsia (diabetes), and hematuria and flank pain (kidney stones).

Past medical history should ascertain known causes such as pregnancy, diabetes, migraine, hepatic or renal disease, cancer (including timing of any chemotherapy or radiation therapy), and previous abdominal surgery (which may cause bowel obstruction due to adhesions). All drugs and substances ingested recently should be ascertained; certain substances may not manifest toxicity until several days after ingestion (eg, acetaminophen, some mushrooms).

Family history of recurrent vomiting should be noted.

Physical examination: Vital signs should particularly note presence of fever and signs of hypovolemia (eg, tachycardia, hypotension, or both).

General examination should seek presence of jaundice and rash.

On abdominal examination, the clinician should look for distention and surgical scars; listen for presence and quality of bowel sounds (eg, normal, high-pitched); percuss for tympany; and palpate for tenderness, peritoneal findings (eg, guarding, rigidity, rebound), and any masses, organomegaly, or hernias. Rectal examination and (in women) pelvic examination to locate tenderness, masses, and blood are essential.

Neurologic examination should particularly note mental status, nystagmus, meningismus (eg, stiff neck, Kernig sign or Brudzinski sign), and ocular signs of increased intracranial pressure (eg, papilledema, absence of venous pulsations, 3rd cranial nerve palsy) or subarachnoid hemorrhage (retinal hemorrhage).

Red flags: The following findings are of particular concern:

- Signs of hypovolemia
- Headache, stiff neck, or mental status change
- Peritoneal signs
- Distended, tympanitic abdomen

Interpretation of findings: Many findings are suggestive of a cause or group of causes (see Table 8–5).

Table 8–5. SOME CAUSES OF NAUSEA AND VOMITING

CAUSE	SUGGESTIVE FINDINGS*	DIAGNOSTIC APPROACH
GI disorders		
Bowel obstruction	Obstipation, distention, tympany Often bilious vomiting, abdominal surgical scars, or hernia	Flat and upright abdominal x-rays
Gastroenteritis	Vomiting, diarrhea Benign abdominal examination	Clinical evaluation
Gastroparesis or ileus	Vomiting of partially digested food a few hours after ingestion Often in diabetics or after abdominal surgery	Flat and upright abdominal x-rays Succussion splash
Hepatitis	Mild to moderate nausea for many days, sometimes vomiting Jaundice, anorexia, malaise Sometimes slight tenderness over the liver	Serum aminotransferases, bilirubin, viral hepatitis titers
Perforated viscus or other acute abdomen (eg, appendicitis, cholecystitis, pancreatitis)	Significant abdominal pain Usually peritoneal signs	See p. 83
Toxic ingestion (numerous)	Usually apparent based on history	Varies with substance
CNS disorders		
Closed head injury	Apparent based on history	Head CT
CNS hemorrhage	Sudden-onset headache, mental status change Often meningeal signs	Head CT Lumbar puncture if CT is normal
CNS infection	Gradual-onset headache Often meningeal signs, mental status change Sometimes petechial rash* due to meningococcemia	Head CT Lumbar puncture
Increased intracranial pressure (eg, caused by hematoma or tumor)	Headache, mental status change Sometimes focal neurologic deficits	Head CT
Labyrinthitis	Vertigo, nystagmus, symptoms worsened by motion Sometimes tinnitus	See p. 792
Migraine	Headache sometimes preceded or accompanied by a neurologic aura or photophobia Often a history of recurrent similar attacks In patients with known migraine, possible development of other CNS disorders	Clinical evaluation Head CT and lumbar puncture considered if evaluation is unclear
Motion sickness	Apparent based on history	Clinical evaluation
Psychogenic disorders	Occurring with stress Eating food considered repulsive	Clinical evaluation
Systemic conditions		
Advanced cancer (independent of chemotherapy or bowel obstruction)	Apparent based on history	Clinical evaluation
Diabetic ketoacidosis	Polyuria, polydipsia Often significant dehydration With or without history of diabetes	Serum glucose, electrolytes, ketones
Drug adverse effect or toxicity	Apparent based on history	Varies with substance
Liver failure or renal failure	Often apparent based on history Often jaundice in advanced liver disease, uremic odor in renal failure	Laboratory tests of liver and renal function
Pregnancy	Often occurring in morning or triggered by food Benign examination (possibly dehydration)	Pregnancy test
Radiation exposure	Apparent based on history	Clinical evaluation
Severe pain (eg, due to a kidney stone)	Varies with cause	Clinical evaluation

*Sometimes forceful vomiting (caused by any disorder or condition) causes petechiae on the upper torso and face, which may resemble those of meningococcemia. Patients with meningococcemia are usually very ill, whereas those with petechiae caused by vomiting often appear otherwise quite well.

Vomiting occurring shortly after drug or toxin ingestion or exposure to motion in a patient with an unremarkable neurologic and abdominal examination can confidently be ascribed to those causes, as may vomiting in a woman with a known pregnancy and a benign examination. Acute vomiting accompanied by diarrhea in an otherwise healthy patient with a benign examination is highly likely to be infectious gastroenteritis; further assessment may be deferred.

Vomiting that occurs at the thought of food or that is not temporally related to eating suggests a psychogenic cause, as does personal or family history of functional nausea and vomiting. Patients should be questioned about the relationship between vomiting and stressful events because they may not recognize the association or even admit to feeling distress at those times.

Testing: All females of childbearing age should have a urine pregnancy test. Patients with severe vomiting, vomiting lasting over 1 day, or signs of dehydration on examination should have other laboratory tests (eg, electrolytes, BUN, creatinine, glucose, urinalysis, sometimes liver tests). Patients with red flag findings should have testing appropriate to the symptoms (see Table 8–5).

The assessment of chronic vomiting usually includes the previously listed laboratory tests plus upper GI endoscopy, small-bowel x-rays, and tests to assess gastric emptying and antral-duodenal motility.

Treatment

Specific conditions, including dehydration, are treated. Even without significant dehydration, IV fluid therapy (0.9% saline 1 L, or 20 mL/kg in children) often leads to reduction of symptoms. In adults, various antiemetics are effective (see Table 8–6). Choice of agent varies somewhat with the cause and severity of symptoms. Typical use is the following:

- Motion sickness: Antihistamines, scopolamine patches, or both
- Mild to moderate symptoms: Prochlorperazine or metoclopramide
- Severe or refractory vomiting and vomiting caused by chemotherapy: 5-HT_3 antagonists

Obviously, only parenteral agents should be used in actively vomiting patients.

For psychogenic vomiting, reassurance indicates awareness of the patient's discomfort and a desire to work toward relief of symptoms, regardless of cause. Comments such as "nothing is wrong" or "the problem is emotional" should be avoided. Brief symptomatic treatment with antiemetics can be tried. If long-term management is necessary, supportive, regular office visits may help resolve the underlying problem.

KEY POINTS

- Many episodes have an obvious cause and benign examination and require only symptomatic treatment.
- Be alert for signs of an acute abdomen or significant intracranial disorder.
- Always consider pregnancy in females of childbearing age.

Table 8–6. SOME DRUGS FOR VOMITING

DRUG	USUAL DOSE	COMMENTS
Antihistamines		
Dimenhydrinate	50 mg po q 4–6 h	Used to treat vomiting of labyrinthine etiology (eg, motion sickness, labyrinthitis)
Meclizine	25 mg po q 8 h	
5-HT_3 antagonists		
Dolasetron	12.5 mg IV at onset of nausea and vomiting	Used to treat severe or refractory vomiting, or vomiting caused by chemotherapy Possible adverse effects: Constipation, diarrhea, abdominal pain
Granisetron	1 mg po or IV tid	
Ondansetron	4–8 mg po or IV q 8 h	
Palonosetron	Prophylaxis: 0.25 mg IV as a single dose 30 min before chemotherapy	
Other drugs		
Aprepitant	125 mg po 1 h before chemotherapy on day 1, then 80 mg po daily in the morning on days 2 and 3 When used with ondansetron, 32 mg IV 30 min before chemotherapy on day 1 only When used with dexamethasone 12 mg po 30 min before chemotherapy on day 1 and 8 mg po daily in the morning on days 2, 3, and 4	Used with highly emetogenic chemotherapy regimens Possible adverse effects: Somnolence, fatigue, hiccups
Metoclopramide	5–20 mg po or IV tid to qid	Used to treat initial treatment of mild vomiting
Perphenazine	5–10 mg IM or 8–16 mg po daily in divided doses; maximum dose 24 mg/day	—
Prochlorperazine	5–10 mg IV or 25 mg per rectum	—
Scopolamine	1-mg patch worn for up to 72 h	Used to treat motion sickness Possible adverse effects: Diminished sweating, dry skin

RUMINATION

Rumination is the (usually involuntary) regurgitation of small amounts of food from the stomach (most often 15 to 30 min after eating) that are rechewed and, in most cases, again swallowed. Patients do not complain of nausea or abdominal pain.

Rumination is commonly observed in infants. The incidence in adults is unknown, because it is rarely reported by patients themselves.

Etiology

Patients with achalasia or a Zenker diverticulum may regurgitate undigested food without nausea. In the majority of patients who do not have these obstructive esophageal conditions, the pathophysiology is poorly understood. The reverse peristalsis in ruminants has not been reported in humans. The disorder is probably a learned, maladaptive habit and may be part of an eating disorder. The person learns to open the lower esophageal sphincter and propel gastric contents into the esophagus and throat by increasing gastric pressure via rhythmic contraction and relaxation of the diaphragm.

Symptoms and Signs

Nausea, pain, and dysphagia do not occur. During periods of stress, the patient may be less careful about concealing rumination. Seeing the act for the first time, others may refer the patient to a physician. Rarely, patients regurgitate and expel enough food to lose weight.

Diagnosis

- Clinical evaluation
- Sometimes endoscopy, esophageal motility studies, or both

Rumination is usually diagnosed through observation. A psychosocial history may disclose underlying emotional stress. Endoscopy or an upper GI series is necessary to exclude disorders causing mechanical obstruction or a Zenker diverticulum. Esophageal manometry and tests to assess gastric emptying and antral-duodenal motility may be used to identify a motility disturbance.

Treatment

- Behavioral techniques

Treatment of rumination is supportive. Drug therapy generally does not help. Motivated patients may respond to behavioral techniques (eg, relaxation, biofeedback, training in diaphragmatic breathing [using the diaphragm instead of chest muscles to breathe]). Psychiatric consultation may be helpful.

CONSTIPATION

Constipation is difficult or infrequent passage of stool, hardness of stool, or a feeling of incomplete evacuation.

Many people incorrectly believe that daily defecation is necessary and complain of constipation if stools occur less frequently. Others are concerned with the appearance (size, shape, color) or consistency of stools. Sometimes the major complaint is dissatisfaction with the act of defecation or the sense of incomplete evacuation after defecation. Constipation is blamed for many complaints (abdominal pain, nausea, fatigue, anorexia) that are actually symptoms of an underlying problem (eg, irritable bowel syndrome [IBS], depression). Patients should not expect all symptoms to be relieved by a daily bowel movement, and measures to aid bowel habits should be used judiciously.

Obsessive-compulsive patients often feel the need to rid the body daily of "unclean" wastes. Such patients often spend excessive time on the toilet or become chronic users of cathartics.

Etiology

Acute constipation suggests an organic cause, whereas chronic constipation may be organic or functional (see Table 8–7).

In many patients, constipation is associated with sluggish movement of stool through the colon. This delay may be due to drugs, organic conditions, or a disorder of defecatory function (ie, pelvic floor dysfunction), or a disorder that results from diet (see Table 8–8). Patients with disordered defecation do not generate adequate rectal propulsive forces, do not relax the puborectalis and the external anal sphincter during defecation, or both. In IBS, patients have symptoms (eg, abdominal discomfort and altered bowel habits) but generally normal colonic transit and anorectal functions. However, IBS-disordered defecation may coexist.

Excessive straining, perhaps secondary to pelvic floor dysfunction, may contribute to anorectal pathology (eg, hemorrhoids, anal fissures, and rectal prolapse) and possibly even to syncope. Fecal impaction, which may cause or develop from constipation, is also common among elderly patients, particularly with prolonged bed rest or decreased physical activity. It is also common after barium has been given by mouth or enema.

Evaluation

History: History of present illness should ascertain a lifetime history of the patient's stool frequency, consistency, need to strain or use perineal maneuvers (eg, pushing on the perineum, gluteal region, or recto-vaginal wall) during defecation, and satisfaction after defecation should be obtained, including frequency and duration of laxative or enema use. Some patients deny previous constipation but, when questioned specifically, admit to spending 15 to 20 min per bowel movement. The presence, amount, and duration of blood in the stool should also be elicited.

Review of systems should seek symptoms of causative disorders, including a change in caliber of the stool or blood in the stool (suggesting cancer). Systemic symptoms suggesting chronic diseases (eg, weight loss) should also be sought.

Past medical history should ask about known causes, including previous abdominal surgery and symptoms of metabolic (eg, hypothyroidism, diabetes mellitus) and neurologic (eg, Parkinson disease, multiple sclerosis, spinal cord injury) disorders. Prescription and nonprescription drug use should be assessed, with specific questioning about anticholinergic and opioid drugs.

Physical examination: A general examination is done to look for signs of systemic disease, including fever and cachexia. Abdominal masses should be sought by palpation. A rectal examination should be done not only for fissures, strictures, blood, or masses (including fecal impaction) but also to evaluate anal resting tone (the puborectalis "lift" when patients squeeze the anal sphincter), perineal descent during simulated evacuation, and rectal sensation. Patients with defecatory disorders may have increased anal resting tone (or anismus), reduced (ie, < 2 cm) or increased (ie, > 4 cm) perineal descent, and/or paradoxical contraction of the puborectalis during simulated evacuation.

Table 8–7. CAUSES OF CONSTIPATION

CAUSES	EXAMPLES
Acute constipation*	
Bowel obstruction	Volvulus, hernia, adhesions, fecal impaction
Adynamic ileus	Peritonitis, major acute illness (eg, sepsis), head or spinal trauma, bed rest
Drugs	Anticholinergics (eg, antihistamines, antipsychotics, antiparkinsonian drugs, antispasmodics), cations (iron, aluminum, Ca, barium, bismuth), opioids, Ca channel blockers, general anesthetics Constipation shortly after start of therapy with the drug
Chronic constipation*	
Colonic tumor	Adenocarcinoma of sigmoid colon
Metabolic disorders	Diabetes mellitus, hypothyroidism, hypocalcemia or hypercalcemia, pregnancy, uremia, porphyria
CNS disorders	Parkinson disease, multiple sclerosis, stroke, spinal cord lesions
Peripheral nervous system disorders	Hirschsprung disease, neurofibromatosis, autonomic neuropathy
Systemic disorders	Systemic sclerosis, amyloidosis, dermatomyositis, myotonic dystrophy
Functional disorders	Slow-transit constipation, irritable bowel syndrome, pelvic floor dysfunction (functional defecatory disorders)
Dietary factors	Low-fiber diet, sugar-restricted diet, chronic laxative abuse

*There is some overlap between acute and chronic causes of constipation. In particular, drugs are common causes of chronic constipation.

Red flags: Certain findings raise suspicion of a more serious etiology of chronic constipation:

- Distended, tympanitic abdomen
- Vomiting
- Blood in stool
- Weight loss
- Severe constipation of recent onset/worsening in elderly patients

Interpretation of findings: Certain symptoms (eg, a sense of anorectal blockage, prolonged or difficult defecation), particularly when associated with abnormal (ie, increased or reduced) perineal motion during simulated evacuation, suggest a defecatory disorder. A tense, distended, tympanitic abdomen, particularly when there is nausea and vomiting, suggests mechanical obstruction.

Patients with IBS typically have abdominal pain with disordered bowel habits. Chronic constipation with modest abdominal discomfort in a patient who has used laxatives for a long time suggests slow-transit constipation. Acute constipation coincident with the start of a constipating drug in patients without red flag findings suggests the drug is the cause. New-onset constipation that persists for weeks or occurs intermittently with increasing frequency or severity, in the absence of a known cause, suggests colonic tumor or other causes of partial obstruction. Excessive straining or prolonged or unsatisfactory defecation, with or without anal digitation, suggests a defecatory disorder. Patients with fecal impaction may have cramps and may pass watery mucus or fecal material around the impacted mass, mimicking diarrhea (paradoxic diarrhea).

Testing: Testing is guided by clinical presentation and the patient's diet history.

Constipation with a clear etiology (drugs, trauma, bed rest) may be treated symptomatically without further study. Patients with symptoms of bowel obstruction require flat and upright abdominal x-rays, possibly a water-soluble contrast enema to evaluate for colonic obstruction, and possibly a CT scan or barium x-ray of the small intestine (see p. 92). Most patients without a clear etiology should have colonoscopy and a laboratory evaluation (CBC, thyroid-stimulating hormone, fasting glucose, electrolytes, and calcium).

Further tests are usually reserved for patients with abnormal findings on the previously mentioned tests or who do not respond to symptomatic treatment. If the primary complaint is infrequent defecation, colonic transit times should be measured with radiopaque markers (Sitz markers) or scintigraphy. If the primary complaint is difficulty with defecation, anorectal manometry and rectal balloon expulsion should be assessed. In patients with chronic constipation, it is important to distinguish between slow-transit constipation (abnormal Sitz marker

Table 8–8. FOODS OFTEN AFFECTING GI FUNCTION

Foods likely to cause loose bowel movements and/or excessive gas
All caffeine-containing beverages especially coffee with chicory
Peaches, pears, cherries, apples
Fruit juices: Orange, cranberry, apple
Asparagus and cruciferous vegetables such as broccoli, cauliflower, cabbage, and Brussels sprouts
Bran cereal, whole wheat bread, high-fiber foods
Pastry, candy, chocolate, waffle syrup, doughnuts
Wine (> 3 glasses in susceptible people)
Milk and milk products (in lactose-sensitive people)
Foods likely to cause constipation or help control loose bowel movements
Rice, bread, potatoes, pasta
Meat, veal, poultry, fish
Cooked vegetables
Bananas

radiopaque study) and pelvic floor muscle dysfunction (markers retained only in distal colon).

Treatment

- Possibly discontinuation of causative drugs (some may be necessary)
- Increase in dietary fiber
- Possibly trial with a brief course of osmotic laxatives

Any identified conditions should be treated.

See Table 8–9 for a summary. Laxatives should be used judiciously. Some (eg, phosphate, bran, cellulose) bind drugs and interfere with absorption. Rapid fecal transit may rush some drugs and nutrients beyond their optimal absorptive locus. Contraindications to laxative and cathartic use include acute abdominal pain of unknown origin, inflammatory bowel disorders, intestinal obstruction, GI bleeding, and fecal impaction.

Diet and behavior: The diet should contain enough fiber (typically 15 to 20 g/day) to ensure adequate stool bulk. Vegetable fiber, which is largely indigestible and unabsorbable,

Table 8–9. AGENTS USED TO TREAT CONSTIPATION

AGENT	DOSAGE	SOME ADVERSE EFFECTS
Fiber*		
Bran	Up to 1 cup/day	Bloating, flatulence, iron and calcium malabsorption
Psyllium	Up to 10–15 g/day in divided doses of 2.5–7.5 g	Bloating, flatulence
Methylcellulose	Up to 6–9 g/day in divided doses of 0.45–3 g	Less bloating than with other fiber agents
Ca polycarbophil	2–6 tablets/day	Bloating, flatulence
Emollients		
Docusate Na	100 mg bid or tid	Ineffective for severe constipation
Glycerin	2–3 g suppository once/day	Rectal irritation
Mineral oil	15–45 mL po once/day	Lipid pneumonia, malabsorption of fat-soluble vitamins, dehydration, fecal incontinence
Osmotic agents		
Sorbitol	15–30 mL po of 70% solution once/day or bid 120 mL rectally of 25–30% solution	Transient abdominal cramps, flatulence
Lactulose	10–20 g (15–30 mL) once/day up to qid	Same as for sorbitol
Polyethylene glycol	17 g daily	Fecal incontinence (related to dosage)
Mg	$MgCl_2$ or Mg sulfate tablets 1–3 g qid Milk of Mg 30–60 mL/day Mg citrate 150–300 mL/day (up to 360 mL)	Magnesium toxicity, dehydration, abdominal cramps, fecal incontinence, diarrhea
Na phosphate	10 g po once as bowel preparation	Rare cases of acute renal failure
Stimulants		
Anthraquinones	Depends on brand used	Abdominal cramps, dehydration, melanosis coli, malabsorption, possible deleterious effects on intramural nerves
Bisacodyl	10-mg suppositories up to 3 times/wk 5–15 mg/day po	Fecal incontinence, hypokalemia, abdominal cramps, rectal burning with daily use of suppository form
Linaclotide	145–290 mcg po once/day at least 30 min before first meal	Abdominal pain, flatulence; contraindicated in children < 6 yr; avoided in children < 17 yr
Lubiprostone†	24 mcg po bid with food	Nausea, particularly on empty stomach
Enemas		
Mineral oil/olive oil retention	100–250 mL/day rectally	Fecal incontinence, mechanical trauma
Tap water	500 mL rectally	Mechanical trauma
Phosphate	60 mL rectally	Accumulated damage to rectal mucosa, hyperphosphatemia, mechanical trauma
Soapsuds	1500 mL rectally	Accumulated damage to rectal mucosa, mechanical trauma

*The dose of fiber supplements should be gradually increased over several weeks to the recommended dose.

†Lubiprostone is available by prescription only and is approved for long-term use.

Adapted from Romero Y, Evans JM, Fleming KC, Phillips SF: Constipation and fecal incontinence in the elderly population. *Mayo Clinic Proceedings* 71:81–92, 1996; by permission.

increases stool bulk. Certain components of fiber also absorb fluid, making stools softer and facilitating their passage. Fruits and vegetables are recommended sources, as are cereals containing bran. Fiber supplementation is particularly effective in treating normal-transit constipation but is not very effective for slow-transit constipation or defecatory disorders.

Behavioral changes may help. Patients should try to move their bowels at the same time daily, preferably 15 to 45 min after breakfast, because food ingestion stimulates colonic motility. Initial efforts at regular, unhurried bowel movements may be aided by glycerin suppositories.

Explanation is important, but it is difficult to convince obsessive-compulsive patients that their attitude toward defecation is abnormal. Physicians must explain that daily bowel movements are not essential, that the bowel must be given a chance to function, and that frequent use of laxatives or enemas (> once/3 days) denies the bowel that chance.

Types of laxatives: Bulking agents (eg, psyllium, calcium polycarbophil, methylcellulose) act slowly and gently and are the safest agents for promoting elimination. Proper use involves gradually increasing the dose—ideally taken tid or qid with sufficient liquid (eg, 500 mL/day of extra fluid) to prevent impaction—until a softer, bulkier stool results. Bloating may be reduced by gradually titrating the dose of dietary fiber to the recommended dose, or by switching to a synthetic fiber preparation such as methylcellulose.

Osmotic agents contain poorly absorbed polyvalent ions (eg, magnesium, phosphate, sulfate), polymers (eg, polyethylene glycol), or carbohydrates (eg, lactulose, sorbitol) that remain in the bowel, increasing intraluminal osmotic pressure and thereby drawing water into the intestine. The increased volume stimulates peristalsis. These agents usually work within 3 h.

In general, osmotic laxatives are reasonably safe even when used regularly. However, sodium phosphate should not be used for bowel cleansing because it may rarely cause acute renal failure even after a single use for bowel preparation. These events occurred primarily in elderly patients, those with preexisting renal disease, and those who were taking drugs that affect renal perfusion or function (eg, diuretics, ACE inhibitors, angiotensin II receptor blockers). Also, magnesium and phosphate are partially absorbed and may be detrimental in some conditions (eg, renal insufficiency). Sodium (in some preparations) may exacerbate heart failure. In large or frequent doses, these drugs may upset fluid and electrolyte balance. Another approach to cleansing the bowel for diagnostic tests or surgery or sometimes for chronic constipation uses large volumes of a balanced osmotic agent (eg, polyethylene glycol–electrolyte solution) given orally or via NGT.

Secretory or stimulant cathartics (eg, phenolphthalein, bisacodyl, anthraquinones, castor oil, anthraquinones) act by irritating the intestinal mucosa or by directly stimulating the submucosal and myenteric plexus. Although phenolphthalein was withdrawn from the US market after animal studies suggested the compound was carcinogenic, there is no epidemiologic evidence of this in humans. Bisacodyl is an effective rescue drug for chronic constipation. The anthraquinones senna, cascara sagrada, aloe, and rhubarb are common constituents of herbal and OTC laxatives. They pass unchanged to the colon where bacterial metabolism converts them to active forms.

Adverse effects include allergic reactions, electrolyte depletion, melanosis coli, and cathartic colon. Melanosis coli is a brownish black colorectal pigmentation of unknown composition. Cathartic colon refers to alterations in colonic anatomy observed on barium enema in patients with chronic stimulant laxative use. It is unclear whether cathartic colon, which has been attributed to destruction of myenteric plexus neurons by anthraquinones, is caused by currently available agents or other neurotoxic agents (eg, podophyllin), which are no longer available. There does not seem to be an increased risk of colon cancer with long-term anthraquinone use.

Enemas can be used, including tap water and commercially prepared hypertonic solutions.

Emollient agents (eg, docusate, mineral oil) act slowly to soften stools, making them easier to pass. However, they are not potent stimulators of defecation. Docusate is a surfactant, which allows water to enter the fecal mass to soften and increase its bulk.

Fecal impaction: Fecal impaction is treated initially with enemas of tap water followed by small enemas (100 mL) of commercially prepared hypertonic solutions. If these do not work, manual fragmentation and disimpaction of the mass is necessary. This procedure is painful, so perirectal and intrarectal application of local anesthetics (eg, lidocaine 5% ointment or dibucaine 1% ointment) is recommended. Some patients require sedation.

Geriatrics Essentials

Constipation is common among elderly people because of low-fiber diets, lack of exercise, coexisting medical conditions, and use of constipating drugs. Many elderly people have misconceptions about normal bowel habits and use laxatives regularly. Other changes that predispose the elderly to constipation include increased rectal compliance and impaired rectal sensation (such that larger rectal volumes are needed to elicit the desire to defecate).

KEY POINTS

- Drug causes are common (eg, chronic laxative abuse, use of anticholinergic or opioid drugs).
- Be wary of bowel obstruction when constipation is acute and severe.
- Symptomatic treatment is reasonable in the absence of red flag findings and after excluding pelvic floor dysfunction.

Dyschezia

(Disordered Evacuation; Dysfunction of Pelvic Floor or Anal Sphincters; Functional Defecatory Disorders; Dyssynergia)

Dyschezia is difficulty defecating. Patients sense the presence of stool and the need to defecate but are unable. It results from a lack of coordination of pelvic floor muscles and anal sphincters. Diagnosis requires anorectal testing. Treatment is difficult, but biofeedback may be of benefit.

Etiology

Normally, when a person tries to defecate, rectal pressure rises in coordination with relaxation of the external anal sphincter. This process may be affected by one or more dysfunctions (eg, impaired rectal contraction, excessive contraction of the abdominal wall, paradoxic anal contraction, failure of anal relaxation) of unclear etiology. Functional defecatory disorders may manifest at any age. In contrast, Hirschsprung disease, which is due to an absent recto-anal inhibitory reflex, is almost always diagnosed in infancy or childhood.

Symptoms and Signs

The patient may or may not sense that stool is present in the rectum. Despite prolonged straining, evacuation is tedious or impossible, frequently even for soft stool or enemas. Patients may complain of anal blockage and may digitally remove stool from their rectum or manually support their perineum or splint the vagina to evacuate. Actual stool frequency may or may not be decreased.

Diagnosis

Rectal and pelvic examinations may reveal hypertonia of the pelvic floor muscles and anal sphincters. With bearing down, patients may not demonstrate the expected anal relaxation and perineal descent. With excessive straining, the anterior rectal wall prolapses into the vagina in patients with impaired anal relaxation; thus rectoceles are usually a secondary rather than a primary disturbance. Long-standing dyschezia with chronic straining may cause a solitary rectal ulcer or varying degrees of rectal prolapse or excessive perineal descent or an enterocoele.

Anorectal manometry and rectal balloon expulsion, occasionally supplemented by defecatory or magnetic resonance proctography, are necessary to diagnose the condition.

Treatment

Because treatment with laxatives is unsatisfactory, it is important to assess anorectal functions in patients with refractory constipation. Biofeedback therapy can improve coordination between abdominal contraction and pelvic floor relaxation during defecation, thereby alleviating symptoms. However, pelvic floor retraining for defecatory disorders is highly specialized and available at select centers only. A collaborative approach (physiotherapists, dietitians, behavior therapists, gastroenterologists) is necessary.

DIARRHEA

Stool is 60 to 90% water. In Western society, stool amount is 100 to 200 g/day in healthy adults and 10 g/kg/day in infants, depending on the amount of unabsorbable dietary material (mainly carbohydrates). Diarrhea is defined as stool weight > 200 g/day. However, many people consider any increased stool fluidity to be diarrhea. Alternatively, many people who ingest fiber have bulkier but formed stools but do not consider themselves to have diarrhea.

Complications: Complications may result from diarrhca of any etiology. Fluid loss with consequent dehydration, electrolyte loss (sodium, potassium, magnesium, chloride), and even vascular collapse sometimes occur. Collapse can develop rapidly in patients who have severe diarrhea (eg, patients with cholera) or are very young, very old, or debilitated. Bicarbonate loss can cause metabolic acidosis. Hypokalemia can occur when patients have severe or chronic diarrhea or if the stool contains excess mucus. Hypomagnesemia after prolonged diarrhea can cause tetany.

Etiology

Normally, the small intestine and colon absorb 99% of fluid resulting from oral intake and GI tract secretions—a total fluid load of about 9 of 10 L daily. Thus, even small reductions (ie, 1%) in intestinal water absorption or increases in secretion can increase water content enough to cause diarrhea.

There are a number of causes of diarrhea (see Table 8–10). Several basic mechanisms are responsible for most clinically significant diarrheas: increased osmotic load, increased secretions, and decreased contact time/surface area. In many disorders,

Table 8–10. SOME CAUSES OF DIARRHEA*

TYPE	EXAMPLES
Acute	
Viral infection	Norovirus, rotavirus
Bacterial infection	*Salmonella,Campylobacter,* or *Shigella* sp; *Escherichia coli;Clostridium difficile*
Parasitic infection	*Giardia* sp, *Entamoeba histolytica,Cryptosporidia*sp
Food poisoning	Staphylococci, *Bacillus cereus,Clostridium perfringens*
Drugs	Laxatives, magnesium-containing antacids, caffeine, antineoplastic drugs, many antibiotics, colchicine, quinine/quinidine, prostaglandin analogs, excipients (eg, lactose) in elixirs
Chronic	
Drugs	See Acute
Functional	Irritable bowel syndrome
Dietary factors	See Table 8–11
Inflammatory bowel disease	Ulcerative colitis, Crohn disease
Surgery	Intestinal or gastric bypass or resection
Malabsorption syndromes	Celiac disease, pancreatic insufficiency Carbohydrate intolerance (particularly lactose intolerance)
Tumors	Colon carcinoma, lymphoma, villous adenoma of the colon
Endocrine tumors	Vipoma, gastrinoma, carcinoid, mastocytosis, medullary carcinoma of the thyroid
Endocrine	Hyperthyroidism Diabetes (multifactorial concurrent celiac disease, pancreatic insufficiency, autonomic neuropathy)

*Numerous causes exist. Some not mentioned may be likely causes in particular subgroups.

more than one mechanism is active. For example, diarrhea in inflammatory bowel disease results from mucosal inflammation, exudation into the lumen, and from multiple secretagogues and bacterial toxins that affect enterocyte function.

Osmotic load: Diarrhea occurs when unabsorbable, water-soluble solutes remain in the bowel and retain water. Such solutes include polyethylene glycol, magnesium salts (hydroxide and sulfate), and sodium phosphate, which are used as laxatives. Osmotic diarrhea occurs with sugar intolerance (eg, lactose intolerance caused by lactase deficiency). Ingesting large amounts of hexitols (eg, sorbitol, mannitol, xylitol) or high fructose corn syrups, which are used as sugar substitutes in candy, gum, and fruit juices, causes osmotic diarrhea because hexitols are poorly absorbed. Lactulose, which is used as a laxative, causes diarrhea by a similar mechanism. Overingesting certain foodstuffs (see Table 8–11) can cause osmotic diarrhea.

Increased secretions: Diarrhea occurs when the bowels secrete more electrolytes and water than they absorb. Causes of increased secretions include infections, unabsorbed fats, certain drugs, and various intrinsic and extrinsic secretagogues.

Infections (eg, gastroenteritis) are the most common causes of secretory diarrhea. Infections combined with food poisoning are the most common causes of acute diarrhea (< 4 days in duration). Most enterotoxins block sodium-potassium exchange, which is an important driving force for fluid absorption in the small bowel and colon.

Unabsorbed dietary fat and bile acids (as in malabsorption syndromes and after ileal resection) can stimulate colonic secretion and cause diarrhea.

Drugs may stimulate intestinal secretions directly (eg, quinidine, quinine, colchicine, anthraquinone cathartics, castor oil, prostaglandins) or indirectly by impairing fat absorption (eg, orlistat).

Various endocrine tumors produce secretagogues, including vipomas (vasoactive intestinal peptide), gastrinomas (gastrin), mastocytosis (histamine), medullary carcinoma of the thyroid (calcitonin and prostaglandins), and carcinoid tumors (histamine, serotonin, and polypeptides). Some of these mediators (eg, prostaglandins, serotonin, related compounds) also accelerate intestinal transit, colonic transit, or both.

Impaired absorption of bile salts, which can occur with several disorders, can cause diarrhea by stimulating water and electrolyte secretion. The stools have a green or orange color.

Reduced contact time/surface area: Rapid intestinal transit and diminished surface area impair fluid absorption and cause diarrhea. Common causes include small-bowel or large-bowel resection or bypass, gastric resection, and inflammatory bowel disease. Other causes include microscopic colitis (collagenous or lymphocytic colitis) and celiac disease.

Stimulation of intestinal smooth muscle by drugs (eg, magnesium-containing antacids, laxatives, cholinesterase inhibitors, SSRIs) or humoral agents (eg, prostaglandins, serotonin) also can speed transit.

Evaluation

History: History of present illness should determine duration and severity of diarrhea, circumstances of onset (including recent travel, food ingested, source of water), drug use (including any antibiotics within the previous 3 mo), abdominal pain or vomiting, frequency and timing of bowel movements, changes in stool characteristics (eg, presence of blood, pus, or mucus; changes in color or consistency; evidence of steatorrhea), associated changes in weight or appetite, and rectal urgency or tenesmus should be noted. Simultaneous occurrence of diarrhea in close contacts should be ascertained.

Review of systems should seek symptoms suggesting possible causes, including joint pains (inflammatory bowel disease, celiac disease); flushing (carcinoid, vipoma, mastocytosis); CAP (irritable bowel, inflammatory bowel disease, gastrinoma); and GI bleeding (ulcerative colitis, tumor).

Past medical history should identify known risk factors for diarrhea, including inflammatory bowel disease, irritable bowel syndrome, HIV infection, and previous GI surgical procedures (eg, intestinal or gastric bypass or resection, pancreatic resection). Family and social history should query about simultaneous occurrence of diarrhea in close contacts.

Physical examination: Fluid and hydration status should be evaluated. A full examination with attention to the abdomen and a digital rectal examination for sphincter competence and occult blood testing are important.

Red flags: Certain findings raise suspicion of an organic or more serious etiology of diarrhea:

- Blood or pus
- Fever
- Signs of dehydration
- Chronic diarrhea
- Weight loss

Interpretation of findings: Acute, watery diarrhea in an otherwise healthy person is likely to be of infectious etiology, particularly when travel, possibly tainted food, or an outbreak with a point-source is involved.

Acute bloody diarrhea with or without hemodynamic instability in an otherwise healthy person suggests an enteroinvasive infection. Diverticular bleeding and ischemic colitis also manifest with acute bloody diarrhea. Recurrent bouts of bloody diarrhea in a younger person suggest inflammatory bowel disease.

Table 8–11. DIETARY FACTORS THAT MAY WORSEN DIARRHEA

DIETARY FACTOR	SOURCE
Caffeine	Coffee, tea, cola, OTC headache remedies
Fructose (in quantities surpassing the gut's absorptive capacity)	Apple juice, pear juice, grapes, honey, dates, nuts, figs, soft drinks (especially fruit flavored), prunes
Hexitols, sorbitol, and mannitol	Sugar-free gum, mints, sweet cherries, prunes
Lactose	Milk, ice cream, frozen yogurt, yogurt, soft cheeses
Mg	Mg-containing antacids
Olestra	Certain fat-free potato chips or fat-free ice creams

Adapted from Bayless T: Chronic diarrhea. *Hospital Practice* Jan. 15, 1989, p. 131; used with permission.

In the absence of laxative use, **large-volume diarrhea** (eg, daily stool volume > 1 L/day) strongly suggests an endocrine cause in patients with normal GI anatomy. A history of oil droplets in stool, particularly if associated with weight loss, suggests malabsorption.

Diarrhea that consistently follows ingestion of certain foods (eg, fats) suggests food intolerance. Recent antibiotic use should raise suspicion for antibiotic-associated diarrhea, including *Clostridium difficile* colitis.

Diarrhea with green or orange stools suggests impaired absorption of bile salts.

The symptoms can help identify the affected part of the bowel. Generally, in small-bowel diseases, stools are voluminous and watery or fatty. In colonic diseases, stools are frequent, sometimes small in volume, and possibly accompanied by blood, mucus, pus, and abdominal discomfort. In irritable bowel syndrome (IBS), abdominal discomfort is relieved by defecation, associated with more loose or frequent stools, or both. However, these symptoms alone do not discriminate IBS from other diseases (eg, inflammatory bowel disease). Patients with IBS or rectal mucosal involvement often have marked urgency, tenesmus, and small, frequent stools (see p. 143).

Extra-abdominal findings that suggest an etiology include skin lesions or flushing (mastocytosis), thyroid nodules (medullary carcinoma of the thyroid), right-sided heart murmur (carcinoid), lymphadenopathy (lymphoma, AIDS), and arthritis (inflammatory bowel disease, celiac disease).

Testing: Acute diarrhea (< 4 days) typically does not require testing. Exceptions are patients with signs of dehydration, bloody stool, fever, severe pain, hypotension, or toxic features—particularly those who are very young or very old. These patients should have a CBC and measurement of electrolytes, BUN, and creatinine. Stool samples should be collected for microscopy, culture, fecal leukocyte testing, and, if antibiotics have been taken recently, *C. difficile* toxin assay.

Chronic diarrhea (> 4 wk) requires evaluation, as does a shorter (1 to 3 wk) bout of diarrhea in immunocompromised patients or those who appear significantly ill. Initial stool testing should include culture, fecal leukocytes (detected by smear or measurement of fecal lactoferrin), microscopic examination for ova and parasites, pH (bacterial fermentation of unabsorbed carbohydrate lowers stool pH < 6.0), fat (by Sudan stain), and electrolytes (sodium and potassium). If no standard pathogens are found, specific tests for *Giardia* antigen and *Aeromonas, Plesiomonas,* coccidia, and microsporidia should be requested. Sigmoidoscopy or colonoscopy with biopsies should follow to look for inflammatory causes. Chronic diarrhea develops in 10% of patients after an acute enteric infection (postinfectious irritable bowel syndrome).

If no diagnosis is apparent and Sudan stain is positive for fat, fecal fat excretion should be measured, followed by small-bowel enteroclysis or CT enterography (structural disease) and endoscopic small-bowel biopsy (mucosal disease). If evaluation still yields negative findings, assessment of pancreatic structure and function (see p. 156) should be considered for patients who have unexplained steatorrhea. Infrequently, capsule endoscopy may uncover lesions, predominantly Crohn disease or NSAID enteropathy, not identified by other modalities.

The stool osmotic gap, which is calculated 290 − 2 × (stool sodium + stool potassium), indicates whether diarrhea is secretory or osmotic. An osmotic gap < 50 mEq/L indicates secretory diarrhea; a larger gap suggests osmotic diarrhea. Patients with osmotic diarrhea may have covert magnesium laxative ingestion (detectable by stool magnesium levels) or carbohydrate malabsorption (diagnosed by hydrogen breath test, lactase assay, and dietary review).

Undiagnosed secretory diarrhea requires testing (eg, plasma gastrin, calcitonin, vasoactive intestinal peptide levels, histamine, urinary 5-hydroxyindole acetic acid [5-HIAA]) for endocrine-related causes. A review for symptoms and signs of thyroid disease and adrenal insufficiency should be done. Surreptitious laxative abuse must be considered; it can be ruled out by a fecal laxative assay.

Treatment

- Fluid and electrolytes for dehydration
- Possibly antidiarrheals for nonbloody diarrhea in patients without systemic toxicity

Severe diarrhea requires fluid and electrolyte replacement to correct dehydration, electrolyte imbalance, and acidosis. Parenteral fluids containing sodium chloride, potassium chloride, and glucose are generally required. Salts to counteract acidosis (sodium lactate, acetate, bicarbonate) may be indicated if serum bicarbonate is < 15 mEq/L. An oral glucose-electrolyte solution can be given if diarrhea is not severe and nausea and vomiting are minimal (see p. 2557). Oral and parenteral fluids are sometimes given simultaneously when water and electrolytes must be replaced in massive amounts (eg, in cholera).

Diarrhea is a symptom. When possible, the underlying disorder should be treated, but symptomatic treatment is often necessary. Diarrhea may be decreased by oral loperamide 2 to 4 mg tid or qid (preferably given 30 min before meals), diphenoxylate 2.5 to 5 mg (tablets or liquid) tid or qid, codeine phosphate 15 to 30 mg bid or tid, or paregoric (camphorated opium tincture) 5 to 10 mL once/day to qid.

Because antidiarrheals may exacerbate *C. difficile* colitis or increase the likelihood of hemolytic-uremic syndrome in *Shiga* toxin–producing *Escherichia coli* infection, they should not be used in bloody diarrhea of unknown cause. Their use should be restricted to patients with watery diarrhea and no signs of systemic toxicity. However, there is little evidence to justify previous concerns about prolonging excretion of possible bacterial pathogens with antidiarrheals.

Psyllium or methylcellulose compounds provide bulk. Although usually prescribed for constipation, bulking agents given in small doses decrease the fluidity of liquid stools. Kaolin, pectin, and activated attapulgite adsorb fluid. Osmotically active dietary substances (see Table 8–11) and stimulatory drugs should be avoided.

KEY POINTS

- In patients with acute diarrhea, stool examination (cultures, ova and parasites, *C. difficile* cytotoxin) is only necessary for those who have prolonged symptoms (ie, > 1 wk) or red flag findings.
- Be cautious when using antidiarrheals if *C. difficile* colitis, *Salmonella* infection, or shigellosis is possible.
- Postinfectious IBS develops in 10% of patients after acute infectious enteritis.

GAS-RELATED COMPLAINTS

The gut contains < 200 mL of gas, whereas daily gas expulsion averages 600 to 700 mL after consuming a standard diet plus 200 g of baked beans. About 75% of flatus is derived from colonic bacterial fermentation of ingested nutrients and endogenous glycoproteins. Gases include hydrogen (H_2), methane

(CH_4), and carbon dioxide (CO_2). Flatus odor correlates with hydrogen sulphide concentrations. Swallowed air (aerophagia) and diffusion from the blood into the lumen also contribute to intestinal gas. Gas diffuses between the lumen and the blood in a direction that depends on the difference in partial pressures. Thus, most nitrogen (N_2) in the lumen originates from the bloodstream, and most hydrogen in the bloodstream originates from the lumen.

Etiology

There are 3 main gas-related complaints: excessive belching, distention (bloating), and excessive flatus, each with a number of causes (see Table 8–12). Infants 2 to 4 mo of age with recurrent crying spells often appear to observers to be in pain, which in the past has been attributed to abdominal cramping or gas and termed colic. However, studies show no increase in H_2 production or in mouth-to-cecum transit times in colicky infants. Hence, the cause of infantile colic remains unclear.

Excessive belching: Belching (eructation) results from swallowed air or from gas generated by carbonated beverages. Aerophagia occurs normally in small amounts during eating and drinking, but some people unconsciously swallow air repeatedly while eating or smoking and at other times, especially when anxious or in an attempt to induce belching. Excessive salivation increases aerophagia and may be associated with various GI disorders (eg, gastroesophageal reflux disease), ill-fitting dentures, certain drugs, gum chewing, or nausea of any cause.

Most swallowed air is eructated. Only a small amount of swallowed air passes into the small bowel; the amount is apparently influenced by position. In an upright person, air is readily belched; in a supine person, air trapped above the stomach fluid tends to be propelled into the duodenum. Excessive eructation may also be voluntary; patients who belch after taking antacids may attribute the relief of symptoms to belching rather than to antacids and may intentionally belch to relieve distress.

Distention (bloating): Abdominal bloating may occur in isolation or along with other GI symptoms in patients with functional disorders (eg, aerophagia, nonulcer dyspepsia, gastroparesis, irritable bowel syndrome) or organic disorders (eg, ovarian cancer, colon cancer). Gastroparesis (and consequent bloating) also has many nonfunctional causes, the most important of which is autonomic visceral neuropathy due to diabetes; other causes include postviral infection, drugs with anticholinergic properties, and long-term opiate use. However, excessive intestinal gas is not clearly linked to these complaints. In most healthy people, 1 L/h of gas can be infused into the gut with minimal symptoms. It is likely that many symptoms are incorrectly attributed to "too much gas."

On the other hand, some patients with recurrent GI symptoms often cannot tolerate small quantities of gas: Retrograde colonic distention by balloon inflation or air instillation during colonoscopy often elicits severe discomfort in some patients (eg, those with irritable bowel syndrome) but minimal symptoms in others. Similarly, patients with eating disorders (eg, anorexia nervosa, bulimia) often misperceive and are particularly stressed by symptoms such as bloating. Thus, the basic abnormality in patients with gas-related symptoms may be a hypersensitive intestine. Altered motility may contribute further to symptoms.

Excessive flatus: There is great variability in the quantity and frequency of rectal gas passage. As with stool frequency, people who complain of flatulence often have a misconception of what is normal. The average number of gas passages is about 13 to 21/day.

Sidebar 8–1. Essay on Flatulence

(First printed in the 14th Edition of *The Merck Manual*)

Flatulence, which can cause great psychosocial distress, is unofficially described according to its salient characteristics:

1. The "slider" (crowded elevator type), which is released slowly and noiselessly, sometimes with devastating effect
2. The open sphincter, or "pooh" type, which is said to be of higher temperature and more aromatic
3. The staccato or drumbeat type, pleasantly passed in privacy
4. The "bark" type (described in a personal communication) is characterized by a sharp exclamatory eruption that effectively interrupts (and often concludes) conversation. Aromaticity is not a prominent feature.

Rarely, this usually distressing symptom has been turned to advantage, as with a Frenchman referred to as "Le Petomane," who became affluent as an effluent performer who played tunes with the gas from his rectum on the Moulin Rouge stage.

Objectively recording flatus frequency (using a diary kept by the patient) is a first step in evaluation.

Flatus is a metabolic by-product of intestinal bacteria; almost none originates from swallowed air or back-diffusion of gases (primarily nitrogen) from the bloodstream. Bacterial metabolism yields significant volumes of hydrogen, methane, and carbon dioxide.

Hydrogen is produced in large quantities in patients with malabsorption syndromes and after ingestion of certain fruits and vegetables containing indigestible carbohydrates (eg, baked beans), sugars (eg, fructose), or sugar alcohols (eg, sorbitol). In patients with disaccharidase deficiencies (most commonly lactase deficiency), large amounts of disaccharides pass into the colon and are fermented to hydrogen. Celiac disease, tropical sprue, pancreatic insufficiency, and other causes of carbohydrate malabsorption should also be considered in cases of excess colonic gas.

Methane is also produced by colonic bacterial metabolism of the same foods (eg, dietary fiber). However, about 10% of people have bacteria that produce methane but not hydrogen.

Carbon dioxide is also produced by bacterial metabolism and generated in the reaction of bicarbonate and hydrogen ions. Hydrogen ions may come from gastric hydrochloric acid or from fatty acids released during digestion of fats—the latter sometimes produces several hundred mEq of hydrogen ions. The acid products released by bacterial fermentation of unabsorbed carbohydrates in the colon may also react with bicarbonate to produce carbon dioxide. Although bloating may occasionally occur, the rapid diffusion of carbon dioxide into the blood generally prevents distention.

Diet accounts for much of the variation in flatus production among individuals, but poorly understood factors (eg, differences in colonic flora and motility) may also play a role.

Despite the flammable nature of the hydrogen and methane in flatulence, working near open flames is not hazardous. However, gas explosion, even with fatal outcome, has been reported during jejunal and colonic surgery and colonoscopy, when diathermy was used during procedures in patients with incomplete bowel cleaning.

Table 8–12. SOME CAUSES OF GAS-RELATED COMPLAINTS

CAUSE	SUGGESTIVE FINDINGS	DIAGNOSTIC APPROACH
Belching		
Aerophagia (swallowing air)	With or without awareness of swallowing air Sometimes in patients who smoke or chew gum excessively Sometimes in patients who have esophageal reflux or ill-fitting dentures	Clinical evaluation
Gas from carbonated beverages	Beverage consumption usually obvious based on history	Clinical evaluation
Voluntary	Patient usually admits when questioned	Clinical evaluation
Distention or bloating		
Aerophagia	See Belching	Clinical evaluation
Irritable bowel syndrome	Chronic, recurrent bloating or distention associated with a change in frequency of bowel movements or consistency of stool No red flag findings Typically beginning during the teens and 20s	Clinical evaluation Examination of stool Blood tests
Gastroparesis	Nausea, abdominal pain, sometimes vomiting Early satiety Sometimes in patients known to have a causative disorder	Upper endoscopy and/or nuclear scanning that evaluates stomach emptying
Eating disorders	Long-standing symptoms In patients who are thin but still very concerned about excess body weight, particularly young women	Clinical evaluation
Constipation if chronic	A long history of hard, infrequent bowel movements	Clinical evaluation
Non-GI disorders (eg, ovarian or colon cancer)	New, persistent bloating in middle-aged or older patients For colon cancer, sometimes blood in stool (blood may be visible or detected during a doctor's examination)	For ovarian cancer, pelvic ultrasonography For colon cancer, colonoscopy
Flatus		
Dietary substances, including beans, dairy products, vegetables, onions, celery, carrots, Brussels sprouts, fruits (eg, raisins, bananas, apricots, prune juice), and complex carbohydrates (eg, pretzels, bagels, wheat germ)	Symptoms that develop mainly after consuming food that can cause gas	Clinical evaluation Trial of elimination
Disaccharidase deficiency	Bloating, cramps, and diarrhea after consuming milk products	Breath tests
Celiac disease, tropical sprue	Symptoms of anemia, steatorrhea, loss of appetite, diarrhea For celiac disease, weakness, symptoms that often begin during childhood For tropical sprue, nausea, abdominal cramps, weight loss	Blood tests Biopsy of the small intestine
Pancreatic insufficiency	Diarrhea, steatorrhea Usually a known history of pancreatic disease	Abdominal CT Sometimes MRCP, endoscopic ultrasonography, or ERCP

MRCP = magnetic resonance cholangiopancreatography.

Evaluation

History: History of present illness in patients with belching should be directed at finding the cause of aerophagia, especially dietary causes.

In patients complaining of gas, bloating, or flatus, the relationship between symptoms and meals (both timing and type and amount of food), bowel movements, and exertion should be explored. Certain patients, particularly in the acute setting, may use the term "gas" to describe their symptoms of coronary ischemia. Changes in frequency and color and consistency of stool are sought. History of weight loss is noted.

Review of systems should seek symptoms of possible causes, including diarrhea and steatorrhea (malabsorption syndromes such as celiac sprue. tropical sprue, disaccharidase deficiency, and pancreatic insufficiency) and weight loss (cancer, chronic malabsorption).

Past medical history should review all components of the diet for possible causes (see Table 8–12).

Physical examination: The examination is generally normal, but in patients with bloating or flatus, signs of an underlying organic disorder should be sought on abdominal, rectal, and (for women) pelvic examination.

Red flags: The following findings are of concern:

- Weight loss
- Blood in stool (occult or gross)
- "Gas" sensation in chest

Interpretation of findings: Chronic, recurrent bloating or distention relieved by defecation and associated with change in frequency or consistency of stool but without red flag findings suggests irritable bowel syndrome.

Long-standing symptoms in an otherwise well young person who has not lost weight are unlikely to be caused by serious physiologic disease, although an eating disorder should be considered, particularly in young women. Bloating accompanied by diarrhea, weight loss, or both (or only after ingestion of certain foods) suggests a malabsorption syndrome.

Testing: Testing is not indicated for belching unless other symptoms suggest a particular disorder. Testing for carbohydrate intolerance (eg, lactose, fructose) with breath tests should be considered particularly when the history suggests significant consumption of these sugars. Testing for small-bowel bacterial overgrowth should also be considered, particularly in patients who also have diarrhea, weight loss, or both, preferably by aerobic and anaerobic culture of small-bowel aspirates obtained during upper GI endoscopy. Testing for bacterial overgrowth with hydrogen breath tests, generally glucose-hydrogen breath tests, is prone to false-positive (ie, with rapid transit) and false-negative (ie, when there are no hydrogen-producing bacteria) results. New, persistent bloating in middle-aged or older women (or those with an abnormal pelvic examination) should prompt pelvic ultrasonography to rule out ovarian cancer.

Treatment

Belching and bloating are difficult to relieve because they are usually caused by unconscious aerophagia or increased sensitivity to normal amounts of gas. Aerophagia may be reduced by eliminating gum and carbonated beverages, cognitive behavioral techniques to prevent air swallowing, and management of associated upper GI diseases (eg, peptic ulcer). Foods containing unabsorbable carbohydrates should be avoided. Even lactose-intolerant patients generally tolerate up to 1 glass of milk drunk in small amounts throughout the day. The mechanism of repeated belching should be explained and demonstrated. When aerophagia is troublesome, behavioral therapy to encourage open-mouth, diaphragmatic breathing and minimize swallowing may be effective.

Drugs provide little benefit. Results with simethicone, an agent that breaks up small gas bubbles, and various anticholinergics are poor. Some patients with dyspepsia and postprandial upper abdominal fullness benefit from antacids, a low dose of tricyclic antidepressants (eg, nortriptyline 10 to 50 mg po once/day), or both to reduce visceral hypersensitivity.

Complaints of excess flatus are treated with avoidance of triggering substances (see Table 8–12). Roughage (eg, bran, psyllium seed) may be added to the diet to try to increase colonic transit; however, in some patients, worsening of symptoms may result. Activated charcoal can sometimes help reduce gas and unpleasant odor; however, it stains clothing and the oral mucosa. Charcoal-lined undergarments are available. Probiotics may also reduce bloating and flatulence by modulating intestinal bacterial flora. Antibiotics are useful in patients with documented bacterial overgrowth.

Functional bloating, distention, and flatus may run an intermittent, chronic course that is only partially relieved by therapy. When appropriate, reassurance that these problems are not detrimental to health is important.

KEY POINTS

- Testing should be guided by the clinical features.
- Be wary of new-onset, persistent symptoms in older patients.

9 Diagnostic and Therapeutic GI Procedures

AMBULATORY PH MONITORING

Ambulatory 24-h esophageal pH monitoring with or without intraluminal impedance testing is currently the most common test for quantifying gastroesophageal reflux. The principal indications are

- To document excessive acid or nonacid reflux
- To correlate symptoms with reflux episodes
- To identify candidates for antireflux surgery
- To evaluate the effectiveness of medical or surgical treatments

Tests may use a transnasal continuous reflux-monitoring catheter or a wireless pH-monitoring device that is endoscopically attached to the distal esophagus.

Complications are very rare. Patients must have nothing by mouth (npo) after midnight but are free to eat as usual after the monitoring device is placed.

Catheter-based pH monitoring: A thin tube containing a pH probe is positioned 5 cm above the lower esophageal sphincter. The patient records symptoms, meals, and sleep for 24 h. Esophageal acid exposure is defined by the percentage of the total recording time that the pH is < 4.0. A value > 4.3% is considered abnormal if the patient has not been taking a proton pump inhibitor, and a value > 1.3% is abnormal if the patient has been taking a proton pump inhibitor for the duration of the test. Additional sensors along the more proximal regions of the pH probe allow identification of proximal reflux episodes.

A dual-channel esophageal and gastric pH probe has two separate pH sensors along the catheter; one sensor is placed 5 cm above the lower esophageal sphincter, and one sensor is placed in the stomach. The two sensors allow for simultaneous measurement of the pH level in the distal esophagus and in the stomach. This test is most useful for evaluating the efficacy and adequacy of acid-suppressing drugs.

The newer combined pH-impedance monitoring devices also do multichannel intraluminal impedance testing, which identifies reflux of any gastric contents into the esophagus regardless of pH level. In addition to acid reflux, this test helps detect weakly acidic reflux (pH between 4.0 and 7) and non-acidic reflux (pH > 7), which would be missed by conventional pH monitoring.

The correlation between patient-reported symptoms and reflux events can be assessed using the symptom index (SI) or symptom association probability (SAP). A significant SI value or SAP value suggests that the correlation between symptoms and reflux events is not due to chance. Excessive reflux and significant symptom-reflux correlation are positive predictors of a favorable outcome from antireflux surgery.

Wireless pH monitoring: Ambulatory esophageal pH monitoring can also be done using a wireless pH-sensing capsule that is attached to the distal esophagus. The device is endoscopically placed 5 cm above the lower esophageal sphincter and continuously monitors esophageal acid exposure (defined as pH < 4.0) for 48 h. Similar to the probe-based test, patients record symptoms, meals, and sleep for the duration of the test and excessive acid exposure and symptom-reflux correlation (SI or SAP) are identified. However, because the capsule is a pure pH sensor, only acid reflux is detected. The capsule usually falls off within a week of placement and is spontaneously passed in the stool. Because the capsule transmits data wirelessly while attached, it does not need to be retrieved.

ANOSCOPY AND SIGMOIDOSCOPY

Anoscopy and sigmoidoscopy are used to evaluate symptoms referable to the rectum or anus (eg, bright rectal bleeding, discharge, protrusions, pain). In addition, sigmoidoscopy also allows for biopsy of colonic tissues and application of intervention such as hemostasis or intraluminal stenting. There are no absolute contraindications, except contraindications for regular endoscopies should be considered. Patients with cardiac arrhythmias or recent myocardial ischemia should have the procedure postponed until the comorbid conditions improve; otherwise, patients will need cardiac monitoring. Per changes in American Heart Association guidelines, these procedures no longer require endocarditis prophylaxis.

The perianal area and distal rectum can be examined with a 7-cm anoscope, and the rectum and sigmoid can be examined with a rigid 25-cm or a flexible 60-cm instrument. Flexible sigmoidoscopy is much more comfortable for the patient and readily permits photography and biopsy of tissue. Considerable skill is required to pass a rigid sigmoidoscope beyond the recto-sigmoid junction (15 cm) without causing discomfort.

Sigmoidoscopy is done after giving an enema to empty the rectum. IV drugs are usually not needed. The patient is placed in the left lateral position. After external inspection and digital rectal examination, the lubricated instrument is gently inserted 3 to 4 cm past the anal sphincter. At this point, the obturator of the rigid sigmoidoscope is removed, and the instrument is inserted further under direct vision.

Anoscopy may be done without preparation. The anoscope is inserted its full length as described above for rigid sigmoidoscopy, usually with the patient in the left lateral position. Complications of anoscopy are exceedingly rare when the procedure is done properly.

ENDOSCOPY

Flexible endoscopes equipped with video cameras can be used to view the upper GI tract from pharynx to upper duodenum and the lower GI tract from anus to cecum (and, sometimes, terminal ileum). Several other diagnostic and therapeutic interventions also can be done endoscopically. The potential to combine diagnosis and therapy in one procedure gives endoscopy a significant advantage over studies that provide only imaging (eg, x-ray contrast studies, CT, MRI) and often outweighs endoscopy's higher cost and need for sedation.

Endoscopy generally requires IV sedation and, for upper endoscopy, topical anesthesia of the throat. Exceptions are anoscopy and sigmoidoscopy, which generally require no sedation. The overall complication rate of endoscopy is 0.1 to 0.2%; mortality is about 0.03%. Complications are usually drug related (eg, respiratory depression); procedural complications (eg, aspiration, perforation, significant bleeding) are less common.

Diagnostic GI endoscopy: Diagnostic procedures by conventional endoscopy include cell and tissue sample collection by brush or biopsy forceps. Several different types of endoscopes provide additional diagnostic and therapeutic functions. Ultrasound-equipped endoscopes can evaluate blood flow or provide imaging of mucosal, submucosal, or extraluminal lesions. Endoscopic ultrasound can provide information (eg, the depth and extent of lesions) that is not available via conventional endoscopy. Also, fine-needle aspiration of both intraluminal and extraluminal lesions can be done with endoscopic ultrasound guidance. Conventional endoscopes cannot visualize the vast majority of the small intestine. Push enteroscopy uses a longer endoscope that can be manually advanced into the distal duodenum or proximal jejunum.

Balloon-assisted enteroscopy provides additional assessment of the small intestine beyond push enteroscopy. It uses an endoscope with one or two inflatable balloons attached to an overtube fitted over the endoscope. When the endoscope is advanced to the farthest possible distance, the balloon is inflated and anchored to the intestinal mucosa. Pulling back of the inflated balloon pulls the small bowel over the overtube like a sleeve, thus shortening and straightening the small intestine and allowing further advancement of the endoscope. Balloon-assisted enteroscopy can be done in anterograde (caudad) or retrograde (cephalad) fashion, enabling examination of the entire small intestine.

Screening colonoscopy is recommended for patients at high risk of colon cancer and for everyone ≥ 50 yr. Colonoscopy should be done every 10 yr for patients with no risk factors or history of polyps. CT colonography (see p. 82) is an alternative to colonoscopy for screening for colonic tumors.

Therapeutic GI endoscopy: Therapeutic endoscopic procedures include

- Removal of foreign bodies
- Hemostasis by hemoclips placement, injection of drugs, thermal coagulation, laser photocoagulation, variceal banding, or sclerotherapy
- Debulking of tumors by laser or bipolar electrocoagulation
- Ablative therapy of premalignant lesions
- Dilation of webs or strictures
- Stent placement
- Reduction of volvulus or intussusception
- Decompression of acute or subacute colonic dilation
- Feeding tube placement

Contraindications to GI endoscopy: Absolute contraindications to endoscopy include

- Shock
- Acute MI
- Peritonitis
- Acute perforation
- Fulminant colitis

Relative contraindications include poor patient cooperation, coma (unless the patient is intubated), and cardiac arrhythmias or recent myocardial ischemia.

Patients taking anticoagulants or chronic NSAID therapy can safely undergo diagnostic endoscopy. However, if there is a possibility that biopsy or photocoagulation will be done, these drugs should be stopped for an appropriate interval before the procedure. Oral iron-containing drugs should be stopped 4 to 5 days before colonoscopy, because certain green vegetables interact with iron to form a sticky residue that is difficult to remove with a bowel preparation and interferes with visualization. The American Heart Association no longer recommends endocarditis prophylaxis for patients having routine GI endoscopy.

Preparation for GI endoscopy: Routine preparations for endoscopy include no solids for 6 to 8 h and no liquids for 4 h before the procedure. Additionally, colonoscopy requires cleansing of the colon. A variety of regimens may be used, but all typically include a full or clear liquid diet for 24 to 48 h and some type of laxative, with or without an enema. A common laxative preparation involves having the patient drink a high-volume (4 L) balanced electrolyte solution over a period of 3 to 4 h before the procedure. Patients who cannot tolerate this solution may be given magnesium citrate, sodium phosphate, polyethylene glycol, lactulose, or other laxatives. Enemas can be done with either sodium phosphate or tap water. Phosphate preparations should not be used in patients with renal insufficiency.

Video capsule endoscopy: In video capsule endoscopy (wireless video endoscopy), patients swallow a capsule containing a camera that transmits images to an external recorder. This noninvasive technology provides diagnostic imaging of the small bowel that is otherwise difficult to obtain by conventional endoscopies. This procedure is particularly useful in patients with occult GI bleeding and for detection of mucosal abnormalities. Capsule endoscopy is more difficult in the colon and is, therefore, not an adequate modality for colorectal cancer screening.

GASTRIC ANALYSIS

Gastric acid analysis is rarely done in current practice. When conducted, samples of stomach contents obtained via NGT are used to measure gastric acid output in a basal and stimulated state. This information may be useful in a patient who develops a recurrent ulcer after surgical vagotomy for peptic ulcer disease. In this case, a positive acid response to stimulation (sham feeding) indicates an incomplete vagotomy.

The test also is used to evaluate a patient with elevated serum gastrin levels. Hyperchlorhydria in the presence of elevated gastrin usually indicates Zollinger-Ellison syndrome. Hypochlorhydria in the presence of elevated gastrin indicates impairment of acid output, such as occurs in pernicious anemia, atrophic gastritis, and Ménétrier disease and after inhibition of gastric acid secretion by potent antisecretory drugs.

To do gastric analysis, an NGT is inserted and the gastric contents are aspirated and discarded. Gastric juice is then collected for 1 h, divided into four 15-min samples. These samples represent basal acid output.

Gastric analysis can also be done during catheter-based esophageal pH-monitoring. Complications are very rare.

LAPAROSCOPY

Diagnostic laparoscopy is a surgical procedure used to evaluate intra-abdominal or pelvic pathology (eg, tumor, endometriosis) in patients with acute or chronic abdominal pain and operability in patients with cancer. It also is used for lymphoma staging and liver biopsy.

Absolute contraindications to laparoscopy include

- A coagulation or bleeding disorder
- Poor patient cooperation
- Peritonitis
- Intestinal obstruction
- Infection of the abdominal wall

Relative contraindications include severe cardiac or pulmonary disease, large abdominal hernias, multiple abdominal operations, and tense ascites.

CBC, coagulation studies, and type and Rh testing are done before laparoscopy. X-rays of the chest and abdomen (kidneys, ureters, and bladder) are also taken. Laparoscopy is done with sterile technique in an operating room or a well-equipped endoscopy suite. The patient is given local anesthesia plus IV sedation and analgesia with an opioid and short-acting sedative (eg, midazolam, propofol).

The procedure involves insertion of a pneumoperitoneum needle into the peritoneal cavity and infusion of nitrous oxide to distend the abdomen. After the opening is enlarged, a peritoneoscope is inserted into the abdomen and the abdominal contents are examined. Surgical instruments for biopsy and other procedures are inserted through separate openings. When the procedure is completed, the nitrous oxide is expelled by the patient with a Valsalva maneuver and the cannula is removed. Complications can include bleeding, bacterial peritonitis, and perforation of a viscus.

MANOMETRY

Manometry is measurement of pressure within various parts of the GI tract. It is done by passing a catheter containing solid-state or liquid-filled pressure transducers through the mouth or anus into the lumen of the organ to be studied. Manometry typically is done to evaluate motility disorders in patients in whom structural lesions have been ruled out by other studies. Manometry is used in the esophagus, stomach and duodenum, sphincter of Oddi, and rectum. Aside from minor discomfort, complications are very rare. Patients must have nothing by mouth (npo) after midnight.

Anorectal manometry: In this test, a pressure transducer is placed in the anus to evaluate the anorectal sphincter mechanism and rectal sensation in patients with incontinence or constipation. It can help diagnose Hirschsprung disease and defecation disorders and provide biofeedback training for fecal incontinence. A barostat balloon is also inflated during the test to evaluate rectal sensation and accommodation. The balloon expulsion test, which is often done together with anorectal manometry, allows for objective assessment of evacuation function.

Barostat: This is a pressure-sensing device that is placed in the stomach to measure gastric accommodation. The device consists of a plastic balloon and an electronic controller that varies the amount of air in the balloon to maintain constant pressure. This device is used mainly in research studies assessing sensory threshold and altered visceral perception, particularly in functional GI disorders.

Esophageal manometry: This test is used to evaluate patients with dysphagia, heartburn, regurgitation, or chest pain. It measures the pressure in the upper and lower esophageal sphincters, determines the effectiveness and coordination of propulsive movements, and detects abnormal contractions. Manometry can be used to diagnose esophageal motility disorders such as achalasia, diffuse spasm, systemic sclerosis, and lower esophageal sphincter hypotension and hypertension. It also is used to evaluate esophageal function and anatomy such as hiatus hernia before certain therapeutic procedures (eg, antireflux surgery, pneumatic dilation for achalasia). Newer high-resolution manometry is often combined with impedance testing to simultaneously evaluate bolus transit through the esophagus during the test swallows.

Gastroduodenal manometry: In this test, transducers are placed in the gastric antrum, duodenum, and proximal jejunum. Pressure is monitored for 5 to 24 h in both fasting and fed states. This test is usually used in patients who have symptoms suggestive of dysmotility but have normal gastric emptying study results or who are unresponsive to therapy. It can help determine whether the patient's symptoms or dysmotility result from a muscular disorder (abnormal contraction amplitude but normal pattern) or nerve disorder (irregular contraction pattern but normal amplitude).

NASOGASTRIC OR INTESTINAL INTUBATION

Nasogastric or intestinal intubation is used to decompress the stomach. It is used to treat gastric atony, ileus, or obstruction; remove ingested toxins, give antidotes (eg, activated charcoal), or both; obtain a sample of gastric contents for analysis (volume, acid content, blood); and supply nutrients.

Contraindications to nasogastric intubation include

- Nasopharyngeal or esophageal obstruction
- Severe maxillofacial trauma
- Uncorrected coagulation abnormalities

Esophageal varices previously have been considered a contraindication, but evidence of adverse effects is lacking.

Several types of tubes are available. A Levin or Salem sump tube is used for gastric decompression or analysis and rarely for short-term feeding. A variety of long, thin, intestinal tubes are used for long-term enteral feeding.

For intubation, the patient sits upright or, if unable, lies in the left lateral decubitus position. A topical anesthetic sprayed in the nose and pharynx helps reduce discomfort. With the patient's head partially flexed, the lubricated tube is inserted through the nares and aimed back and then down to conform to the nasopharynx. As the tip reaches the posterior pharyngeal wall, the patient should sip water through a straw. Violent coughing with flow of air through the tube during respiration indicates that the tube is misplaced in the trachea. Aspiration of gastric juice verifies entry into the stomach. The position of larger tubes can be confirmed by instilling 20 to 30 mL of air and listening with the stethoscope under the left subcostal region for a rush of air.

Some smaller, more flexible intestinal feeding tubes require the use of stiffening wires or stylets. These tubes usually require fluoroscopic or endoscopic assistance for passage through the pylorus.

Complications are rare and include nasopharyngeal trauma with or without hemorrhage, pulmonary aspiration, traumatic esophageal or gastric hemorrhage or perforation, and (very rarely) intracranial or mediastinal penetration.

NUCLEAR GASTROINTESTINAL SCANS

Bleeding scans: Bleeding scans use ^{99m}Tc-labeled RBCs, or occasionally ^{99m}Tc-labeled colloid, to determine the origin of lower GI hemorrhage before surgery or angiography. Active bleeding sites are identified by focal areas of tracer that conform to bowel anatomy, increase with time, and move with peristalsis. Bleeding scans are useful mainly for colonic bleeding in patients with significant hemorrhage and an unprepared bowel, in whom endoscopic visualization is difficult.

Gastric emptying: Gastric emptying can be measured by having the patient ingest a radiolabeled meal (solid or liquid) and observing its passage out of the stomach with a gamma camera. Because this test cannot differentiate physical obstruction from gastroparesis, further diagnostic studies typically are done if emptying is delayed. The test also is useful in monitoring response to promotility drugs (eg, metoclopramide, erythromycin).

Meckel scans: A Meckel scan identifies ectopic gastric mucosa (as in a Meckel diverticulum) by using an injection of ^{99m}Tc pertechnetate, which is taken up by mucus-secreting cells of the gastric mucosa. Focal uptake outside of the stomach and in the small bowel indicates a Meckel diverticulum.

PARACENTESIS

Abdominal paracentesis is used to obtain ascitic fluid for testing. It also can be used to remove tense ascites causing respiratory difficulties or pain or as a treatment for chronic ascites.

Absolute contraindications to paracentesis include

- Severe, uncorrectable disorders of blood coagulation
- Intestinal obstruction
- An infected abdominal wall

Poor patient cooperation, surgical scarring over the puncture area, large intra-abdominal masses, and severe portal hypertension with abdominal collateral circulation are relative contraindications.

CBC, platelet count, and coagulation studies are done before the procedure. After emptying the bladder, the patient sits in bed with the head elevated 45 to 90°. In patients with obvious and marked ascites, a point is located at the midline between the umbilicus and the pubic bone and is cleaned with an antiseptic solution and alcohol. Two other possible sites for paracentesis are located about 5 cm superior and medial to the anterior superior iliac spine on either side. In patients with moderate ascites, precise location of ascitic fluid by abdominal ultrasound is indicated. Positioning the patient in a lateral decubitus position with the planned insertion site down also promotes the floating and migration of air-filled bowel loops up and away from the point of entry.

Under sterile technique, the area is anesthetized to the peritoneum with lidocaine 1%. For diagnostic paracentesis, an 18-gauge needle attached to a 50-mL syringe is inserted through the peritoneum (generally a popping sensation is noted). Fluid is gently aspirated and sent for cell count, protein or amylase content, cytology, or culture as needed. For therapeutic (large-volume) paracentesis, a 14-gauge cannula attached to a vacuum aspiration system is used to collect up to 8 L of ascitic fluid. Concurrent infusion of IV albumin is recommended during large-volume paracentesis to help avoid significant intravascular volume shift and postprocedural hypotension.

Hemorrhage is the most common complication of paracentesis. Occasionally, with tense ascites, prolonged leakage of ascitic fluid occurs through the needle site.

X-RAY AND OTHER IMAGING CONTRAST STUDIES OF THE GI TRACT

X-Ray Contrast Studies of the Abdomen

X-ray and other imaging contrast studies visualize the entire GI tract from pharynx to rectum and are most useful for detecting mass lesions and structural abnormalities (eg, tumors, strictures). Single-contrast studies fill the lumen with radiopaque material, outlining the structure. Better, more detailed images are obtained from double-contrast studies, in which a small amount of high-density barium coats the mucosal surface and gas distends the organ and enhances contrast. The gas is injected by the operator in double-contrast barium enema, whereas in other studies, intrinsic GI tract gas is adequate. In all cases, patients turn themselves to properly distribute the gas and barium. Fluoroscopy can monitor the progress of the contrast material. Either video or plain films can be taken for documentation, but video is particularly useful when assessing motor disorders (eg, cricopharyngeal spasm, achalasia).

The main contraindication to x-ray contrast studies is

- Suspected perforation

Perforation is a contraindication because free barium is highly irritating to the mediastinum and peritoneum; water-soluble contrast is less irritating and may be used if perforation is possible. Older patients may have difficulty turning themselves to properly distribute the barium and intraluminal gas.

Patients having upper GI x-ray contrast studies must have nothing by mouth (npo) after midnight. Patients having barium enema follow a clear liquid diet the day before, take an oral sodium phosphate laxative in the afternoon, and take a bisacodyl suppository in the evening. Other laxative regimens are effective.

Complications are rare. Perforation can occur if barium enema is done in a patient with toxic megacolon. Barium impaction may be prevented by postprocedure oral fluids and sometimes laxatives.

Barium enema: A barium enema can be done as a single- or double-contrast study. Single-contrast barium enemas are used for potential obstruction, diverticulitis, fistulas, and megacolon. Double-contrast studies are preferred for detection of tumors.

Enteroclysis: Enteroclysis (small-bowel enema) provides still better visualization of the small bowel but requires intubation of the duodenum with a flexible, balloon-tipped catheter. A barium suspension is injected, followed by a solution of methylcellulose, which functions as a double-contrast agent that enhances visualization of the small-bowel mucosa.

Small-bowel meal: A small-bowel meal is done by using fluoroscopy and provides a more detailed evaluation of the small bowel. Shortly before the examination, the patient is given metoclopramide 20 mg po to hasten transit of the contrast material.

Upper GI examination: An upper GI examination is best done as a biphasic study beginning with a double-contrast examination of the esophagus, stomach, and duodenum, followed by a single-contrast study using low-density barium. Glucagon 0.5 mg IV can facilitate the examination by causing gastric hypotonia.

CT Scanning of the Abdomen

CT scanning using oral and IV contrast allows excellent visualization of both the small bowel and colon as well as of other intra-abdominal structures.

CT colonography: CT colonography (virtual colonoscopy) generates 3D and 2D images of the colon by using MDCT and a combination of oral contrast and gas distention of the colon. Viewing the high-resolution 3D images somewhat simulates the appearance of optical endoscopy, hence the name. Optimal CT colonography technique requires careful cleansing and distention of the colon. Residual stool causes problems similar to those encountered with barium enema because it simulates polyps or masses. Three-dimensional endoluminal images are useful to confirm the presence of a lesion and to improve diagnostic confidence.

CT enterography: CT enterography provides optimal visualization of the small-bowel mucosa; it is preferably done by using a multidetector CT (MDCT) scanner. Patients are given a large volume (1350 mL) of 0.1% barium sulfate before imaging. For certain indications (eg, obscure GI bleeding, small-bowel tumors, chronic ischemia), a biphasic contrast-enhanced MDCT study is done.

CT enterography and CT colonoscopy have largely supplanted standard small-bowel series and barium enema examinations.

OTHER GI TESTING PROCEDURES

Breath tests: Breath tests typically involve ingestion of a substrate that is then metabolized by GI bacteria or digestive enzymes. The metabolites of the ingested substrate are then measured in the exhaled breath of the patient.

Various breath tests help diagnose conditions such as

- Helicobacter pylori infection: Urea breath test
- Carbohydrate intolerance: Hydrogen (H_2) breath test
- Bacterial overgrowth in the small intestine: ^{14}C-xylose breath test, H_2 breath test

Electrogastrography: Electrogastrography measures gastric electrical activity with adhesive cutaneous electrodes. This procedure is useful in patients with gastroparesis.

Wireless capsule motility: Wireless capsule motility involves an ingestible device that continuously measures the pressure and pH of the intraluminal environment as the device travels through the GI tract. It allows the measurement of transit time, pressure profile, and motility of the entire GI tract and individual regions (stomach, small intestine, colon). This procedure can help assess gastric emptying as well as small-bowel and colonic transit in patients presenting with symptoms suggestive of dysmotility.

10 Acute Abdomen and Surgical Gastroenterology

ACUTE ABDOMINAL PAIN

Abdominal pain is common and often inconsequential. Acute and severe abdominal pain, however, is almost always a symptom of intra-abdominal disease. It may be the sole indicator of the need for surgery and must be attended to swiftly: Gangrene and perforation of the gut can occur < 6 h from onset of symptoms in certain conditions (eg, interruption of the intestinal blood supply due to a strangulating obstruction or an arterial embolus). Abdominal pain is of particular concern in patients who are very young or very old and those who have HIV infection or are taking immunosuppressants (including corticosteroids).

Textbook descriptions of abdominal pain have limitations because people react to pain differently. Some, particularly elderly people, are stoic, whereas others exaggerate their symptoms. Infants, young children, and some elderly people may have difficulty localizing the pain.

The term *acute abdomen* refers to abdominal symptoms and signs of such severity or concern that disorders requiring surgery should be considered.

Pathophysiology

Visceral pain comes from the abdominal viscera, which are innervated by autonomic nerve fibers and respond mainly to the sensations of distention and muscular contraction—not to cutting, tearing, or local irritation. Visceral pain is typically vague, dull, and nauseating. It is poorly localized and tends to be referred to areas corresponding to the embryonic origin of the affected structure. Foregut structures (stomach, duodenum, liver, and pancreas) cause upper abdominal pain. Midgut structures (small bowel, proximal colon, and appendix) cause periumbilical pain. Hindgut structures (distal colon and GU tract) cause lower abdominal pain.

Somatic pain comes from the parietal peritoneum, which is innervated by somatic nerves, which respond to irritation from infectious, chemical, or other inflammatory processes. Somatic pain is sharp and well localized.

Referred pain is pain perceived distant from its source and results from convergence of nerve fibers at the spinal cord. Common examples of referred pain are scapular pain due to biliary colic, groin pain due to renal colic, and shoulder pain due to blood or infection irritating the diaphragm.

Peritonitis: Peritonitis is inflammation of the peritoneal cavity. The most serious cause is perforation of the GI tract (see p. 87), which causes immediate chemical inflammation followed shortly by infection from intestinal organisms. Peritonitis can also result from any abdominal condition that causes marked inflammation (eg, appendicitis, diverticulitis, strangulating intestinal obstruction, pancreatitis, pelvic inflammatory disease, mesenteric ischemia). Intraperitoneal blood from any source (eg, ruptured aneurysm, trauma, surgery, ectopic pregnancy) is irritating and results in peritonitis. Barium causes severe caking and peritonitis and should never be given to a patient with suspected GI tract perforation. However, water-soluble contrast agents can be safely used. Peritoneosystemic shunts, drains, and dialysis catheters in the peritoneal cavity predispose a patient to infectious peritonitis, as does ascitic fluid.

Rarely, **spontaneous bacterial peritonitis** occurs, in which the peritoneal cavity is infected by bloodborne bacteria. Spontaneous bacterial peritonitis occurs primarily in patients with cirrhosis and ascites.

Peritonitis causes fluid to shift into the peritoneal cavity and bowel, leading to severe dehydration and electrolyte disturbances. Adult respiratory distress syndrome can develop rapidly. Kidney failure, liver failure, and disseminated intravascular coagulation follow. The patient's face becomes drawn into the masklike appearance typical of hippocratic facies. Death occurs within days.

Etiology

Many intra-abdominal disorders cause abdominal pain (see Fig. 10–1); some are trivial but some are immediately life threatening, requiring rapid diagnosis and surgery. These include ruptured abdominal aortic aneurysm (AAA), perforated viscus, mesenteric ischemia, and ruptured ectopic pregnancy. Others (eg, intestinal obstruction, appendicitis, severe acute pancreatitis) are also serious and nearly as urgent. Several extra-abdominal disorders also cause abdominal pain (see Table 10–1).

Abdominal pain in neonates, infants, and young children has numerous causes not encountered in adults. These causes include necrotizing enterocolitis, meconium peritonitis, pyloric stenosis, volvulus of a gut with intestinal malrotation, imperforate anus, intussusception, and intestinal obstruction caused by atresia.

Evaluation

Evaluation of mild and severe pain follows the same process, although with severe abdominal pain, therapy sometimes proceeds simultaneously and involves early consultation with a surgeon. History and physical examination usually exclude all but a few possible causes, with final diagnosis confirmed by judicious use of laboratory and imaging tests. Life-threatening causes should always be ruled out before focusing on less serious diagnoses. In seriously ill patients with severe abdominal pain, the most important diagnostic measure may be expeditious surgical exploration. In mildly ill patients, watchful waiting and a diagnostic evaluation may be best.

History: A thorough history usually suggests the diagnosis (see Table 10–2). Of particular importance are pain location (see Fig. 10–1) and characteristics, history of similar symptoms, and associated symptoms. Concomitant symptoms such as heartburn, nausea, vomiting, diarrhea, constipation, jaundice, melena, hematuria, hematemesis, weight loss, and mucus or blood in the stool help direct subsequent evaluation. A drug history should include details concerning prescription and illicit drug use as well as alcohol. Many drugs cause GI upset. Prednisone or immunosuppressants may inhibit the inflammatory response to perforation or peritonitis and result in less pain, tenderness, or leukocytosis than might otherwise be expected. Anticoagulants can increase the chances of bleeding and hematoma formation. Alcohol predisposes to pancreatitis.

Known medical conditions and previous abdominal surgeries are important to ascertain. Women should be asked whether they are pregnant.

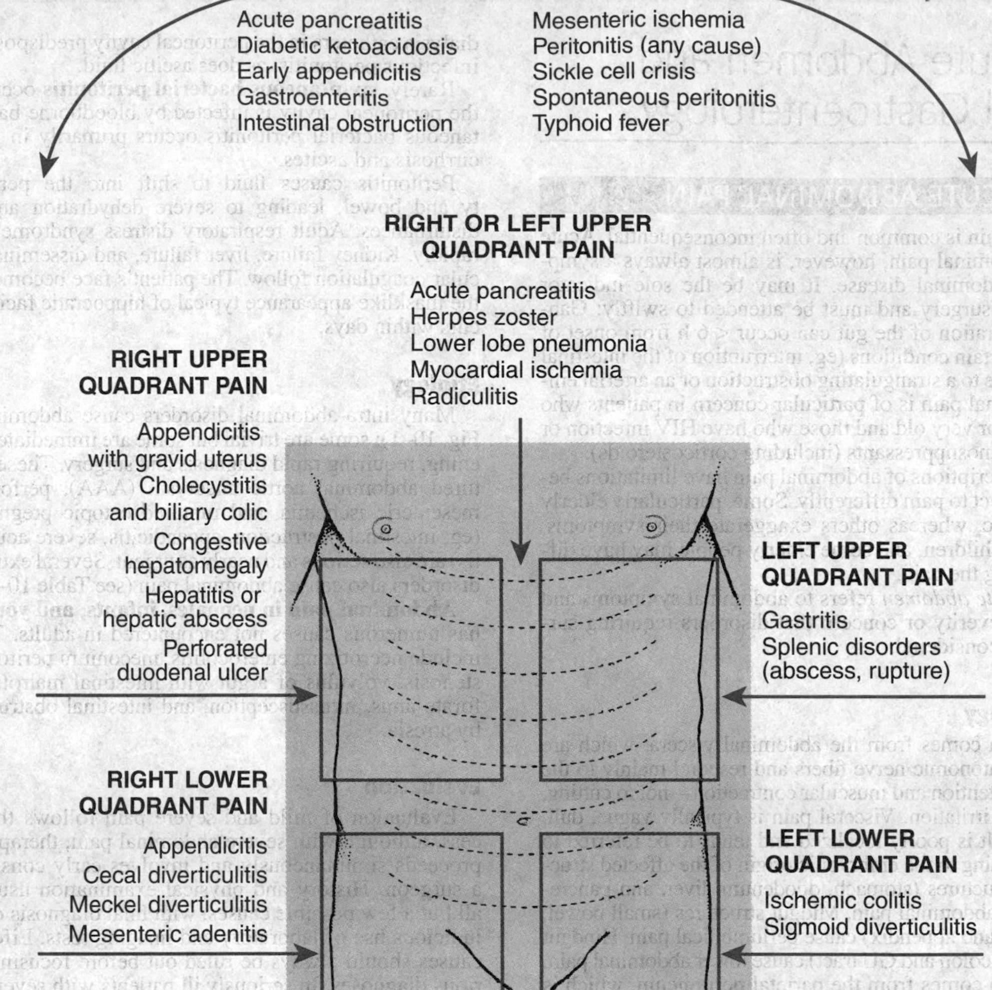
DIFFUSE ABDOMINAL PAIN
Acute pancreatitis
Diabetic ketoacidosis
Early appendicitis
Gastroenteritis
Intestinal obstruction
Mesenteric ischemia
Peritonitis (any cause)
Sickle cell crisis
Spontaneous peritonitis
Typhoid fever
RIGHT OR LEFT UPPER QUADRANT PAIN
Acute pancreatitis
Herpes zoster
Lower lobe pneumonia
Myocardial ischemia
Radiculitis
RIGHT UPPER QUADRANT PAIN
Appendicitis with gravid uterus
Cholecystitis and biliary colic
Congestive hepatomegaly
Hepatitis or hepatic abscess
Perforated duodenal ulcer
LEFT UPPER QUADRANT PAIN
Gastritis
Splenic disorders (abscess, rupture)
RIGHT LOWER QUADRANT PAIN
Appendicitis
Cecal diverticulitis
Meckel diverticulitis
Mesenteric adenitis
LEFT LOWER QUADRANT PAIN
Ischemic colitis
Sigmoid diverticulitis
RIGHT OR LEFT LOWER QUADRANT PAIN
Abdominal or psoas abscess
Abdominal wall hematoma
Cystitis
Endometriosis
Incarcerated or strangulated hernia
Inflammatory bowel disease
Mittelschmerz
Pelvic inflammatory disease
Renal stone
Ruptured abdominal aortic aneurysm
Ruptured ectopic pregnancy
Torsion of ovarian cyst or testis

Fig. 10–1. Location of abdominal pain and possible causes.

Table 10–1. EXTRA-ABDOMINAL CAUSES OF ABDOMINAL PAIN

Abdominal wall
Rectus muscle hematoma
GU
Testicular torsion
Infectious
Herpes zoster
Metabolic
Alcoholic ketoacidosis Corticosteroid insufficiency Diabetic ketoacidosis Hypercalcemia Porphyria Sickle cell disease
Thoracic
Costochondritis Myocardial infarction Pneumonia Pulmonary embolism Radiculitis
Toxic
Black widow spider bite Heavy metal poisoning Methanol poisoning Opioid withdrawal Scorpion sting

Physical examination: The general appearance is important. A happy, comfortable-appearing patient rarely has a serious problem, unlike one who is anxious, pale, diaphoretic, or in obvious pain. BP, pulse, state of consciousness, and other signs of peripheral perfusion must be evaluated. However, the focus of the examination is the abdomen, beginning with inspection and auscultation, followed by palpation and percussion. Rectal examination and pelvic examination (for women) to locate tenderness, masses, and blood are essential.

Palpation begins gently, away from the area of greatest pain, detecting areas of particular tenderness, as well as the presence of guarding, rigidity, and rebound (all suggesting peritoneal irritation) and any masses. Guarding is an involuntary contraction of the abdominal muscles that is slightly slower and more sustained than the rapid, voluntary flinch exhibited by sensitive or anxious patients. Rebound is a distinct flinch upon brisk withdrawal of the examiner's hand. The inguinal area and all surgical scars should be palpated for hernias.

Red flags: Certain findings raise suspicion of a more serious etiology:

- Severe pain
- Signs of shock (eg, tachycardia, hypotension, diaphoresis, confusion)
- Signs of peritonitis
- Abdominal distention

Interpretation of findings: Distention, especially when surgical scars, tympany to percussion, and high-pitched peristalsis or borborygmi in rushes are present, strongly suggests bowel obstruction.

Severe pain in a patient with a silent abdomen who is lying as still as possible suggests peritonitis; location of tenderness suggests etiology (eg, right upper quadrant suggests cholecystitis, right lower quadrant suggests appendicitis) but may not be diagnostic.

Table 10–2. HISTORY IN PATIENTS WITH ACUTE ABDOMINAL PAIN

QUESTION	POTENTIAL RESPONSES AND INDICATIONS
Where is the pain?	See Fig. 10–1
What is the pain like?	Acute waves of sharp constricting pain that "take the breath away" (renal or biliary colic) Waves of dull pain with vomiting (intestinal obstruction) Colicky pain that becomes steady (appendicitis, strangulating intestinal obstruction, mesenteric ischemia) Sharp, constant pain, worsened by movement (peritonitis) Tearing pain (dissecting aneurysm) Dull ache (appendicitis, diverticulitis, pyelonephritis)
Have you had it before?	Yes suggests recurrent problems such as ulcer disease, gallstone colic, diverticulitis, or mittelschmerz
Was the onset sudden?	Sudden: "Like a light switching on" (perforated ulcer, renal stone, ruptured ectopic pregnancy, ovarian torsion, testicular torsion, some ruptured aneurysms) Less sudden: Most other causes
How severe is the pain?	Severe pain (perforated viscus, kidney stone, peritonitis, pancreatitis) Pain out of proportion to physical findings (mesenteric ischemia)
Does the pain travel to any other part of the body?	Right scapula (gallbladder pain) Left shoulder region (ruptured spleen, pancreatitis) Pubis or vagina (renal pain) Back (ruptured aortic aneurysm, pancreatitis, sometimes perforated ulcer)
What relieves the pain?	Antacids (peptic ulcer disease) Lying as quietly as possible (peritonitis)
What other symptoms occur with the pain?	Vomiting precedes pain and is followed by diarrhea (gastroenteritis) Delayed vomiting, absent bowel movement and flatus (acute intestinal obstruction; the delay increases with a lower site of obstruction) Severe vomiting precedes intense epigastric, left chest, or shoulder pain (emetic perforation of the intra-abdominal esophagus)

Back pain with shock suggests ruptured AAA, particularly if there is a tender, pulsatile mass.

Shock and vaginal bleeding in a pregnant woman suggest ruptured ectopic pregnancy.

Ecchymoses of the costovertebral angles (Grey Turner sign) or around the umbilicus (Cullen sign) suggest hemorrhagic pancreatitis but are not very sensitive for this disorder.

History is often suggestive (see Table 10–2). Mild to moderate pain in the presence of active peristalsis of normal pitch suggests a nonsurgical disease (eg, gastroenteritis) but may also be the early manifestations of a more serious disorder. A patient who is writhing around trying to get comfortable is more likely to have an obstructive mechanism (eg, renal or biliary colic).

Previous abdominal surgery makes obstruction caused by adhesions more likely. Generalized atherosclerosis increases the possibility of MI, AAA, and mesenteric ischemia. HIV infection makes infectious causes more likely.

Testing: Tests are selected based on clinical suspicion.

- Urine pregnancy test for all women of childbearing age
- Selected imaging tests based on suspected diagnosis

Standard tests (eg, CBC, chemistries, urinalysis) are often done but are of little value due to poor specificity; patients with significant disease may have normal results. Abnormal results do not provide a specific diagnosis (the urinalysis in particular may show pyuria or hematuria in a wide variety of conditions), and they can also occur in the absence of significant disease. An exception is serum lipase, which strongly suggests a diagnosis of acute pancreatitis. A bedside urine pregnancy test should be done for all women of childbearing age because a negative result effectively excludes ruptured ectopic pregnancy.

An abdominal series, consisting of flat and upright abdominal x-rays and upright chest x-rays (left lateral recumbent abdomen and anteroposterior chest x-ray for patients unable to stand), should be done when perforation or obstruction is suspected. However, these plain x-rays are seldom diagnostic for other conditions and need not be otherwise automatically done. Ultrasound should be done for suspected biliary tract disease or ectopic pregnancy (transvaginal probe) and for suspected appendicitis in children. Ultrasound can also detect AAA but cannot reliably identify rupture. Noncontrast helical CT is the modality of choice for suspected renal stones. CT with oral and IV contrast is diagnostic in about 95% of patients with significant abdominal pain and has markedly lowered the negative laparotomy rate. However, advanced imaging must not be allowed to delay surgery in patients with definitive symptoms and signs.

Treatment

Some clinicians feel that providing pain relief before a diagnosis is made interferes with their ability to evaluate. However, moderate doses of IV analgesics (eg, fentanyl 50 to 100 mcg, morphine 4 to 6 mg) do not mask peritoneal signs and, by diminishing anxiety and discomfort, often make examination easier.

KEY POINTS

- Look for life-threatening causes first.
- Rule out pregnancy in women of childbearing age.
- Seek signs of peritonitis, shock, and obstruction.
- Blood tests are of minimal value.

ACUTE MESENTERIC ISCHEMIA

Acute mesenteric ischemia is interruption of intestinal blood flow by embolism, thrombosis, or a low-flow state. It leads to mediator release, inflammation, and ultimately infarction. Abdominal pain is out of proportion to physical findings. Early diagnosis is difficult, but angiography and exploratory laparotomy have the most sensitivity; other imaging modalities often become positive only late in the disease. Treatment is by embolectomy, revascularization of viable segments, or resection; sometimes vasodilator therapy is successful. Mortality is high.

Pathophysiology

The intestinal mucosa has a high metabolic rate and, accordingly, a high blood flow requirement (normally receiving 20 to 25% of cardiac output), making it very sensitive to the effects of decreased perfusion. Ischemia disrupts the mucosal barrier, allowing release of bacteria, toxins, and vasoactive mediators, which in turn leads to myocardial depression, systemic inflammatory response syndrome (see p. 569), multisystem organ failure, and death. Mediator release may occur even before complete infarction. Necrosis can occur as soon as 10 to 12 h after the onset of symptoms.

Etiology

Three major vessels serve the abdominal contents:

- Celiac trunk: Supplies the esophagus, stomach, proximal duodenum, liver, gallbladder, pancreas, and spleen
- Superior mesenteric artery (SMA): Supplies the distal duodenum, jejunum, ileum, and colon to the splenic flexure
- Inferior mesenteric artery (IMA): Supplies the descending colon, sigmoid colon, and rectum

Collateral vessels are abundant in the stomach, duodenum, and rectum; these areas rarely develop ischemia. The splenic flexure is a watershed between the SMA and IMA and is at particular risk of ischemia. Note that acute mesenteric ischemia is distinct from ischemic colitis, which involves only small vessels and causes mainly mucosal necrosis and bleeding.

Mesenteric blood flow may be disrupted on either the venous or arterial sides. In general, patients > 50 are at greatest risk and have the types of occlusions and risk factors shown in Table 10–3. However, many patients have no identifiable risk factors.

Symptoms and Signs

The early hallmark of mesenteric ischemia is severe pain but minimal physical findings. The abdomen remains soft, with little or no tenderness. Mild tachycardia may be present. Later, as necrosis develops, signs of peritonitis appear, with marked abdominal tenderness, guarding, rigidity, and no bowel sounds. The stool may be heme-positive (increasingly likely as ischemia progresses). The usual signs of shock develop and are frequently followed by death.

Sudden onset of pain suggests but is not diagnostic of an arterial embolism, whereas a more gradual onset is typical of venous thrombosis. Patients with a history of postprandial abdominal discomfort (which suggests intestinal angina) may have arterial thrombosis.

Diagnosis

- Clinical diagnosis more important than diagnostic tests
- Mesenteric angiography or CT angiography if diagnosis unclear

Table 10–3. CAUSES OF ACUTE MESENTERIC ISCHEMIA

OCCLUSION TYPE	RISK FACTORS
Arterial embolus (> 40%)	Coronary artery disease, heart failure, valvular heart disease, atrial fibrillation, history of arterial emboli
Arterial thrombosis (30%)	Generalized atherosclerosis
Venous thrombosis (15%)	Hypercoagulable states, inflammatory conditions (eg, pancreatitis, diverticulitis), trauma, heart failure, renal failure, portal hypertension, decompression sickness
Nonocclusive ischemia (15%)	Low-flow states (eg, heart failure, shock, cardiopulmonary bypass), splanchnic vasoconstriction (eg, vasopressors, cocaine)

Early diagnosis of mesenteric ischemia is particularly important because mortality increases significantly once intestinal infarction has occurred. Mesenteric ischemia must be considered in any patient > 50 with known risk factors or predisposing conditions who develops sudden, severe abdominal pain.

Patients with clear peritoneal signs should proceed directly to the operating room for both diagnosis and treatment. For others, selective mesenteric angiography or CT angiography is the diagnostic procedure of choice. Other imaging studies and serum markers can show abnormalities but lack sensitivity and specificity early in the course of the disease when diagnosis is most critical. Plain abdominal x-rays are useful mainly in ruling out other causes of pain (eg, perforated viscus), although portal venous gas or pneumatosis intestinalis may be seen late in the disease. These findings also appear on CT, which may also directly visualize vascular occlusion—more accurately on the venous side. Doppler ultrasonography can sometimes identify arterial occlusion, but sensitivity is low. MRI is very accurate in proximal vascular occlusion, less so in distal vascular occlusion. Serum markers (eg, creatine kinase, lactate) rise with necrosis but are nonspecific findings that are seen later.

Prognosis

If diagnosis and treatment take place before infarction occurs, mortality is low; after intestinal infarction, mortality approaches 70 to 90%. For this reason, clinical diagnosis of mesenteric ischemia should supersede diagnostic tests, which may delay treatment.

Treatment

- Surgical: Embolectomy, revascularization, with or without bowel resection
- Angiographic: Vasodilators or thrombolysis
- Long-term anticoagulation or antiplatelet therapy

If diagnosis is made during exploratory laparotomy, options are surgical embolectomy, revascularization, and resection. A "second look" laparotomy may be needed to reassess the viability of questionable areas of bowel. If diagnosis is made by angiography, infusion of the vasodilator papaverine through the angiography catheter may improve survival in both occlusive and nonocclusive ischemia. Papaverine is useful even when surgical intervention is planned and is sometimes given during and after surgical intervention as well. In addition, for arterial occlusion, thrombolysis or surgical embolectomy may be done. The development of peritoneal signs at any time during the evaluation suggests the need for immediate surgery. Mesenteric venous thrombosis without signs of peritonitis can be treated with papaverine followed by anticoagulation with heparin and then warfarin.

Patients with arterial embolism or venous thrombosis require long-term anticoagulation with warfarin. Patients with nonocclusive ischemia may be treated with antiplatelet therapy.

KEY POINTS

- Early diagnosis is critical because mortality increases significantly once intestinal infarction has occurred.
- Initially, pain is severe but physical findings are minimal.
- Surgical exploration is often the best diagnostic measure for patients with clear peritoneal findings.
- For other patients, mesenteric angiography or CT angiography is done.
- Treatment options include embolectomy, revascularization, and resection.

ACUTE PERFORATION OF THE GI TRACT

Any part of the GI tract may become perforated, releasing gastric or intestinal contents into the peritoneal space. Causes vary. Symptoms develop suddenly, with severe pain followed shortly by signs of shock. Diagnosis is usually made by the presence of free air in the abdomen on imaging studies. Treatment is with fluid resuscitation, antibiotics, and surgery. Mortality is high, varying with the underlying disorder and the patient's general health.

Etiology

Both blunt and penetrating trauma can result in perforation of any part of the GI tract (see Table 10–4). Swallowed foreign bodies, even sharp ones, rarely cause perforation unless they become impacted, causing ischemia and necrosis from local pressure (see p. 102). Foreign bodies inserted via the anus may perforate the rectum or sigmoid colon (see p. 104).

Symptoms and Signs

Esophageal, gastric, and duodenal perforation tends to manifest suddenly and catastrophically, with abrupt onset of acute abdomen with severe generalized abdominal pain, tenderness, and peritoneal signs. Pain may radiate to the shoulder.

Perforation at other GI sites often occurs in the setting of other painful, inflammatory conditions. Because such perforations are often small initially and frequently walled off by the omentum, pain often develops gradually and may be localized. Tenderness also is more focal. Such findings can make it difficult to distinguish perforation from worsening of the underlying disorder or lack of response to treatment.

In all types of perforation, nausea, vomiting, and anorexia are common. Bowel sounds are quiet to absent.

Table 10–4. SOME CAUSES OF GI TRACT PERFORATION

PERFORATION SITE	CAUSE	COMMENTS
All sites	Trauma	—
	Foreign bodies	—
Esophagus	Forceful vomiting	Termed Boerhaave syndrome
	Iatrogenic causes	Typically perforation with an esophagoscope, balloon dilator, or bougie
	Ingestion of corrosive material	—
Stomach or duodenum	Peptic ulcer disease	In about one-third of patients, no previous history of ulcer symptoms In about 20%, no free air visible on x-ray
	Ingestion of corrosive material	Typically stomach
Intestine	Strangulating obstruction	—
	Possibly acute appendicitis and Meckel diverticulitis	Free air rarely visible on x-rays
Colon	Obstruction	Typically perforates at cecum High risk: Colon ≥ 13 cm diameter, patients receiving prednisone or other immunosuppressants (symptoms and signs may be minimal in this group)
	Diverticulitis	—
	Inflammatory bowel disease (ulcerative colitis, Crohn disease)	—
	Toxic megacolon	—
	Sometimes spontaneous	
Gallbladder	Iatrogenic injury during cholecystectomy or liver biopsy	Usually the biliary tree or duodenum is injured
	Rarely, acute cholecystitis	Usually walled off by omentum

Diagnosis

- Abdominal series
- If nondiagnostic, abdominal CT

An abdominal series (supine and upright abdominal x-rays and chest x-rays) may be diagnostic, showing free air under the diaphragm in 50 to 75% of cases. As time passes, this sign becomes more common. A lateral chest x-ray is more sensitive for free air than a posteroanterior x-ray.

If the abdominal series is nondiagnostic, abdominal CT usually with oral and IV and/or rectal contrast may be helpful. Barium should not be used if perforation is suspected.

Treatment

- Surgery
- IV fluids and antibiotics

If a perforation is noted, immediate surgery is necessary because mortality caused by peritonitis increases rapidly the longer treatment is delayed. If an abscess or an inflammatory mass has formed, the procedure may be limited to drainage of the abscess.

An NGT is sometimes inserted before operation. Patients with signs of volume depletion should have urine output monitored with a catheter. Fluid status is maintained by adequate IV fluid and electrolyte replacement. IV antibiotics effective against intestinal flora should be given (eg, cefotetan 1 to 2 g bid, or amikacin 5 mg/kg tid plus clindamycin 600 to 900 mg qid).

KEY POINTS

- Pain is sudden and followed quickly by signs of peritonitis and shock.
- Imaging with plain x-rays and/or CT is done.
- Surgical repair is necessary in conjunction with IV fluid resuscitation and antibiotics.

APPENDICITIS

Appendicitis is acute inflammation of the vermiform appendix, typically resulting in abdominal pain, anorexia, and abdominal tenderness. Diagnosis is clinical, often supplemented by CT or ultrasonography. Treatment is surgical removal of the appendix.

In the US, acute appendicitis is the most common cause of acute abdominal pain requiring surgery. Over 5% of the population develops appendicitis at some point. It most commonly occurs in the teens and 20s but may occur at any age.

Other conditions affecting the appendix include carcinoids, cancer, villous adenomas, and diverticula. The appendix may also be affected by Crohn disease or ulcerative colitis with pancolitis (inflammatory bowel disease).

Etiology

Appendicitis is thought to result from obstruction of the appendiceal lumen, typically by lymphoid hyperplasia, but occasionally by a fecalith, foreign body, or even worms. The obstruction leads to distention, bacterial overgrowth, ischemia, and inflammation. If untreated, necrosis, gangrene, and perforation occur. If the perforation is contained by the omentum, an appendiceal abscess results.

Symptoms and Signs

The classic acute appendicitis symptoms are

- Epigastric or periumbilical pain followed by brief nausea, vomiting, and anorexia

After a few hours, the pain shifts to the right lower quadrant. Pain increases with cough and motion.

Classic signs of appendicitis are

- Right lower quadrant direct and rebound tenderness located at the McBurney point (junction of the middle and outer thirds of the line joining the umbilicus to the anterior superior spine)

Additional appendicitis signs are pain felt in the right lower quadrant with palpation of the left lower quadrant (Rovsing sign), an increase in pain caused by passive extension of the right hip joint that stretches the iliopsoas muscle (psoas sign), or pain caused by passive internal rotation of the flexed thigh (obturator sign). Low-grade fever (rectal temperature 37.7 to 38.3° C [100 to 101° F]) is common.

Unfortunately, these classic findings appear in < 50% of patients. Many variations of appendicitis symptoms and signs occur. Pain may not be localized, particularly in infants and children. Tenderness may be diffuse or, in rare instances, absent. Bowel movements are usually less frequent or absent; if diarrhea is a sign, a retrocecal appendix should be suspected. RBCs or WBCs may be present in the urine. Atypical symptoms are common among elderly patients and pregnant women; in particular, pain is less severe and local tenderness is less marked.

Diagnosis

- Clinical evaluation
- Abdominal CT if necessary
- Ultrasonography an option to CT

When classic appendicitis symptoms and signs are present, the appendicitis diagnosis is clinical. In such patients, delaying appendicitis surgery to do imaging tests only increases the likelihood of perforation and subsequent complications.

In patients with atypical or equivocal findings, imaging studies should be done without delay. Contrast-enhanced CT has reasonable accuracy in diagnosing appendicitis and can also reveal other causes of an acute abdomen. Graded compression ultrasonography can usually be done quickly and uses no radiation (of particular concern in children); however, it is occasionally limited by the presence of bowel gas and is less useful for recognizing nonappendiceal causes of pain.

Appendicitis remains primarily a clinical diagnosis. Selective and judicious use of radiographic studies may reduce the rate of negative laparotomy.

Laparoscopy can be used for diagnosis as well as definitive treatment of appendicitis; it may be especially helpful in women with lower abdominal pain of unclear etiology. Laboratory studies typically show leukocytosis (12,000 to 15,000/μL), but this finding is highly variable; a normal WBC count should not be used to exclude appendicitis.

Prognosis

Without surgery or antibiotics (eg, in a remote location or historically), the mortality rate for appendicitis is > 50%.

With early surgery, the mortality rate is < 1%, and convalescence is normally rapid and complete. With complications (rupture and development of an abscess or peritonitis) and/or advanced age, the prognosis is worse: Repeat operations and a long convalescence may follow.

Treatment

- Surgical removal of the appendix
- IV fluids and antibiotics

Treatment of acute appendicitis is open or laparoscopic appendectomy; because treatment delay increases mortality, a negative appendectomy rate of 15% is considered acceptable. The surgeon can usually remove the appendix even if perforated. Occasionally, the appendix is difficult to locate: In these cases, it usually lies behind the cecum or the ileum and mesentery of the right colon.

A contraindication to appendectomy is inflammatory bowel disease involving the cecum. However, in cases of terminal ileitis and a normal cecum, the appendix should be removed.

Appendectomy should be preceded by IV antibiotics. Third-generation cephalosporins are preferred. For nonperforated appendicitis, no further antibiotics are required. If the appendix is perforated, antibiotics should be continued until the patient's temperature and WBC count have normalized or continued for a fixed course, according to the surgeon's preference. If surgery is impossible, antibiotics—although not curative—markedly improve the survival rate.

When a large inflammatory mass is found involving the appendix, terminal ileum, and cecum, resection of the entire mass and ileocolostomy are preferable. In late cases in which a pericolic abscess has already formed, the abscess is drained either by an ultrasound-guided percutaneous catheter or by open operation (with appendectomy to follow at a later date).

KEY POINTS

- Patients with classic symptoms and signs should have laparotomy instead of imaging tests.
- Patients with nondiagnostic findings should have imaging with CT or, particularly for children, ultrasonography.
- Give a 3rd-generation cephalosporin preoperatively and, if the appendix has perforated, continue it postoperatively.

HERNIAS OF THE ABDOMINAL WALL

A hernia of the abdominal wall is a protrusion of the abdominal contents through an acquired or congenital area of weakness or defect in the wall. Many hernias are asymptomatic, but some become incarcerated or strangulated, causing pain and requiring immediate surgery. Diagnosis is clinical. Treatment is elective surgical repair.

Abdominal hernias are extremely common, particularly among males, necessitating about 700,000 operations each year in the US.

Classification of Abdominal Hernias

Abdominal hernias are classified as either abdominal wall or groin hernias. Strangulated hernias are ischemic from physical constriction of their blood supply. Strangulation can result in bowel infarction, perforation, and peritonitis.

Abdominal wall hernias: Abdominal wall hernias include

- Umbilical hernias
- Epigastric hernias
- Spigelian hernias
- Incisional (ventral) hernias

Umbilical hernias (protrusions through the umbilical ring) are mostly congenital, but some are acquired in adulthood secondary to obesity, ascites, pregnancy, or chronic peritoneal dialysis.

Epigastric hernias occur through the linea alba.

Spigelian hernias occur through defects in the transversus abdominis muscle lateral to the rectus sheath, usually below the level of the umbilicus.

Incisional hernias occur through an incision from previous abdominal surgery.

Groin hernias: Groin hernias include

- Inguinal hernias
- Femoral hernias

Inguinal hernias occur above the inguinal ligament. Indirect inguinal hernias traverse the internal inguinal ring into the inguinal canal, and direct inguinal hernias extend directly forward and do not pass through the inguinal canal.

Femoral hernias occur below the inguinal ligament and go into the femoral canal.

About 75% of all abdominal hernias are inguinal. Incisional hernias comprise another 10 to 15%. Femoral and unusual hernias account for the remaining 10 to 15%.

Sports hernias: A sports hernia is not a true hernia because there is no abdominal wall defect through which abdominal contents protrude. Instead, the disorder involves a tear of one or more muscles, tendons, or ligaments in the lower abdomen or groin, particularly where they attach to the pubic bone.

Symptoms and Signs

Most patients complain only of a visible bulge, which may cause vague discomfort or be asymptomatic. Most hernias, even large ones, can be manually reduced with persistent gentle pressure; placing the patient in the Trendelenburg position may help. An incarcerated hernia cannot be reduced and can be the cause of a bowel obstruction. A strangulated hernia causes steady, gradually increasing pain, typically with nausea and vomiting. The hernia itself is tender, and the overlying skin may be erythematous; peritonitis may develop depending on location, with diffuse tenderness, guarding, and rebound.

Diagnosis

- Clinical evaluation

The diagnosis of an abdominal hernia is clinical. Because the hernia may be apparent only when abdominal pressure is increased, the patient should be examined in a standing position. If no hernia is palpable, the patient should cough or perform a Valsalva maneuver as the examiner palpates the abdominal wall. Examination focuses on the umbilicus, the inguinal area (with a finger in the inguinal canal in males), the femoral triangle, and any incisions that are present.

Inguinal masses that resemble hernias may be the result of adenopathy (infectious or malignant), an ectopic testis, or lipoma. These masses are solid and are not reducible. A scrotal mass may be a varicocele, hydrocele, or testicular tumor. Ultrasound may be done if physical examination is equivocal.

Prognosis

Congenital umbilical hernias rarely strangulate and are not treated; most resolve spontaneously within several years. Very large defects may be repaired electively after age 2 yr. Umbilical hernias in adults cause cosmetic concerns and can be electively repaired; strangulation and incarceration are unusual but can happen and usually contain omentum rather than intestine.

Treatment

- Surgical repair

Groin hernias typically should be repaired electively because of the risk of strangulation, which results in higher morbidity (and possible mortality in elderly patients). Asymptomatic inguinal hernias in men can be observed; if symptoms develop, they can be repaired electively. Repair may be through a standard incision or laparoscopically.

An incarcerated or strangulated hernia of any kind requires urgent surgical repair.

ILEUS

(Paralytic Ileus; Adynamic Ileus; Paresis)

Ileus is a temporary arrest of intestinal peristalsis. It occurs most commonly after abdominal surgery, particularly when the intestines have been manipulated. Symptoms are nausea, vomiting, and vague abdominal discomfort. Diagnosis is based on x-ray findings and clinical impression. Treatment is supportive, with nasogastric suction and IV fluids.

Etiology

The most common cause of ileus is

- Abdominal surgery

Other causes include

- Intraperitoneal or retroperitoneal inflammation (eg, appendicitis, diverticulitis, perforated duodenal ulcer)
- Retroperitoneal or intra-abdominal hematomas (eg, from ruptured abdominal aortic aneurysm, blunt abdominal trauma)
- Metabolic disturbances (eg, hypokalemia)
- Drugs (eg, opioids, anticholinergics, sometimes calcium channel blockers)
- Sometimes renal or thoracic disease (eg, lower rib fractures, lower lobe pneumonias, MI)

Gastric and colonic motility disturbances after abdominal surgery are common. The small bowel is typically least affected, with motility and absorption returning to normal within hours after surgery. Stomach emptying is usually impaired for about 24 h or more. The colon is often most affected and may remain inactive for 48 to 72 h or more.

Symptoms and Signs

Symptoms and signs of ileus include abdominal distention, nausea, vomiting, and vague discomfort. Pain rarely has the classic colicky pattern present in mechanical obstruction. There may be obstipation or passage of slight amounts of watery stool. Auscultation reveals a silent abdomen or minimal peristalsis. The abdomen is not tender unless the underlying cause is inflammatory.

Diagnosis

- Clinical evaluation
- Sometimes x-rays

The most essential task is to distinguish ileus from intestinal obstruction. In both conditions, x-rays show gaseous distention of isolated segments of intestine. In postoperative ileus, however, gas may accumulate more in the colon than in the small bowel. Postoperative accumulation of gas in the small bowel often implies development of a complication (eg, obstruction, peritonitis). In other types of ileus, x-ray findings are similar to obstruction; differentiation can be difficult unless clinical features clearly favor one or the other. A contrast-enhanced CT may help differentiate between the two and suggest an underlying cause of the ileus.

Treatment

- NGT
- IV fluids

Treatment of ileus involves continuous nasogastric suction, npo status, IV fluids and electrolytes, a minimal amount of sedatives, and avoidance of opioids and anticholinergic drugs. Maintaining an adequate serum potassium level (> 4 mEq/L [> 4 mmol/L]) is especially important. Ileus persisting > 1 wk probably has a mechanical obstructive cause, and laparotomy should be considered.

Sometimes colonic ileus can be relieved by colonoscopic decompression; rarely, cecostomy is required. Colonoscopic decompression is helpful in treating pseudo-obstruction (Ogilvie syndrome), which consists of apparent obstruction at the splenic flexure, although no cause can be found by contrast enema or colonoscopy for the failure of gas and feces to pass this point. Some clinicians use IV neostigmine (which requires cardiac monitoring) to treat Ogilvie syndrome.

INTESTINAL OBSTRUCTION

Intestinal obstruction is significant mechanical impairment or complete arrest of the passage of contents through the intestine due to pathology that causes blockage of the bowel. Symptoms include cramping pain, vomiting, obstipation, and lack of flatus. Diagnosis is clinical, confirmed by abdominal x-rays. Treatment is fluid resuscitation, nasogastric suction, and, in most cases of complete obstruction, surgery.

Mechanical obstruction is divided into obstruction of the small bowel (including the duodenum) and obstruction of the large bowel. Obstruction may be partial or complete. About 85% of partial small-bowel obstructions resolve with nonoperative treatment, whereas about 85% of complete small-bowel obstructions require surgery.

Etiology

Overall, the most common causes of mechanical obstruction are adhesions, hernias, and tumors. Other general causes are diverticulitis, foreign bodies (including gallstones), volvulus (twisting of bowel on its mesentery), intussusception (telescoping of one segment of bowel into another), and fecal impaction. Specific segments of the intestine are affected differently (see Table 10–5).

Table 10–5. CAUSES OF INTESTINAL OBSTRUCTION

LOCATION	CAUSE
Colon	Tumors (usually in left colon), diverticulitis (usually in sigmoid), volvulus of sigmoid or cecum, fecal impaction, Hirschsprung disease, Crohn disease
Duodenum	
Adults	Cancer of the duodenum or cancer of the head of pancreas, ulcer disease
Neonates	Atresia, volvulus, bands, annular pancreas
Jejunum and ileum	
Adults	Hernias, adhesions (common), tumors, foreign body, Meckel diverticulum, Crohn disease (uncommon), *Ascaris* infestation, midgut volvulus, intussusception by tumor (rare)
Neonates	Meconium ileus, volvulus of a malrotated gut, atresia, intussusception

Pathophysiology

In simple mechanical obstruction, blockage occurs without vascular compromise. Ingested fluid and food, digestive secretions, and gas accumulate above the obstruction. The proximal bowel distends, and the distal segment collapses. The normal secretory and absorptive functions of the mucosa are depressed, and the bowel wall becomes edematous and congested. Severe intestinal distention is self-perpetuating and progressive, intensifying the peristaltic and secretory derangements and increasing the risks of dehydration and progression to strangulating obstruction.

Strangulating obstruction is obstruction with compromised blood flow; it occurs in nearly 25% of patients with small-bowel obstruction. It is usually associated with hernia, volvulus, and intussusception. Strangulating obstruction can progress to infarction and gangrene in as little as 6 h. Venous obstruction occurs first, followed by arterial occlusion, resulting in rapid ischemia of the bowel wall. The ischemic bowel becomes edematous and infarcts, leading to gangrene and perforation. In large-bowel obstruction, strangulation is rare (except with volvulus).

Perforation may occur in an ischemic segment (typically small bowel) or when marked dilation occurs. The risk is high if the cecum is dilated to a diameter ≥ 13 cm. Perforation of a tumor or a diverticulum may also occur at the obstruction site.

PEARLS & PITFALLS

- Strangulating obstruction can progress to infarction and gangrene in as little as 6 h.

Symptoms and Signs

Obstruction of the small bowel causes symptoms shortly after onset: abdominal cramps centered around the umbilicus or in the epigastrium, vomiting, and—in patients with complete obstruction—obstipation. Patients with partial obstruction may develop diarrhea. Severe, steady pain suggests that strangulation has occurred. In the absence of strangulation, the abdomen is not tender. Hyperactive, high-pitched peristalsis with rushes coinciding with cramps is typical. Sometimes, dilated loops of bowel are palpable. With infarction, the abdomen becomes tender and auscultation reveals a silent abdomen or minimal peristalsis. Shock and oliguria are serious signs that indicate either late simple obstruction or strangulation.

Obstruction of the large bowel usually causes milder symptoms that develop more gradually than those caused by small-bowel obstruction. Increasing constipation leads to obstipation and abdominal distention. Vomiting may occur (usually several hours after onset of other symptoms) but is not common. Lower abdominal cramps unproductive of feces occur. Physical examination typically shows a distended abdomen with loud borborygmi. There is no tenderness, and the rectum is usually empty. A mass corresponding to the site of an obstructing tumor may be palpable. Systemic symptoms are relatively mild, and fluid and electrolyte deficits are uncommon.

Volvulus often has an abrupt onset. Pain is continuous, sometimes with superimposed waves of colicky pain.

Diagnosis

- Abdominal series

Supine and upright abdominal x-rays should be taken and are usually adequate to diagnose obstruction. Although only laparotomy can definitively diagnose strangulation, careful serial clinical examination may provide early warning. Elevated WBCs and acidosis may indicate that strangulation has already occurred, but these signs may be absent if the venous outflow from the strangulated loop of bowel is decreased.

On plain x-rays, a ladderlike series of distended small-bowel loops is typical of small-bowel obstruction but may also occur with obstruction of the right colon. Fluid levels in the bowel can be seen in upright views. Similar, although perhaps less dramatic, x-ray findings and symptoms occur in ileus (paralysis of the intestine without obstruction); differentiation can be difficult. Distended loops and fluid levels may be absent with an obstruction of the proximal jejunum or with closed-loop strangulating obstructions (as may occur with volvulus). Infarcted bowel may produce a mass effect on x-ray. Gas in the bowel wall (pneumatosis intestinalis) indicates gangrene.

In large-bowel obstruction, abdominal x-ray shows distention of the colon proximal to the obstruction. In cecal volvulus, there may be a large gas bubble in the mid-abdomen or left upper quadrant. With both cecal and sigmoid volvulus, a contrast enema shows the site of obstruction by a typical "bird-beak" deformity at the site of the twist; the procedure may actually reduce a sigmoid volvulus. If contrast enema is not done, colonoscopy can be used to decompress a sigmoid volvulus but rarely works with a cecal volvulus.

Abdominal CT is being used more often in suspected small-bowel obstruction.

Treatment

- Nasogastric suction
- IV fluids
- IV antibiotics if bowel ischemia suspected

Patients with possible intestinal obstruction should be hospitalized. Treatment of acute intestinal obstruction must proceed simultaneously with diagnosis. A surgeon should always be involved.

Supportive care is similar for small- and large-bowel obstruction: nasogastric suction, IV fluids (0.9% saline or lactated Ringer's solution for intravascular volume repletion), and a urinary catheter to monitor fluid output. Electrolyte replacement should be guided by test results, but, in cases of repeated vomiting, serum sodium and potassium are likely to be depleted. If bowel ischemia or infarction is suspected, antibiotics should be given (eg, a 3rd-generation cephalosporin, such as cefotetan 2 g IV) before operative exploration.

Specific measures: Obstruction of the duodenum in adults is treated by resection or, if the lesion cannot be removed, palliative gastrojejunostomy (for treatment in children, see p. 2523).

Complete obstruction of the small bowel is preferentially treated with early laparotomy, although surgery can be delayed 2 or 3 h to improve fluid status and urine output in a very ill, dehydrated patient. The offending lesion is removed whenever possible. If a gallstone is the cause of obstruction, it is removed through an enterotomy, and cholecystectomy need not be done. Procedures to prevent recurrence should be done, including repair of hernias, removal of foreign bodies, and lysis of the offending adhesions. In some patients with early postoperative obstruction or repeated obstruction caused by adhesions, simple intubation with a long intestinal tube (many physicians consider a standard NGT to be equally effective), rather than surgery, may be attempted in the absence of peritoneal signs.

Disseminated intraperitoneal cancer obstructing the small bowel is a major cause of death in adult patients with GI tract cancer. Bypassing the obstruction, either surgically or with endoscopically placed stents, may palliate symptoms briefly.

Obstructing colon cancers can sometimes be treated by a single-stage resection and anastomosis, with or without a temporary colostomy or ileostomy. When this procedure is not possible, the tumor may be resected, and a colostomy or ileostomy is created; the stoma may possibly be closed at a later time. Occasionally, a diverting colostomy with delayed resection is required.

When diverticulitis causes obstruction, perforation is often present. Removal of the involved area may be very difficult but is indicated if perforation and general peritonitis are present. Resection and colostomy are done, and anastomosis is postponed.

Fecal impaction usually occurs in the rectum and can be removed digitally and with enemas. However, a fecal concretion alone or in a mixture (ie, with barium or antacids) that causes complete obstruction (usually in the sigmoid) requires laparotomy.

Treatment of cecal volvulus consists of resection and anastomosis of the involved segment or fixation of the cecum in its normal position by cecostomy in the frail patient. In sigmoid volvulus, an endoscope or a long rectal tube can often decompress the loop, and resection and anastomosis may be deferred for a few days. Without a resection, recurrence is almost inevitable.

KEY POINTS

- The most common causes of obstruction are adhesions, hernias, and tumors; a small-bowel obstruction in the absence of prior surgery or hernias is often caused by a tumor.
- Vomiting and third spacing of fluid cause volume depletion.
- Prolonged obstruction can cause bowel ischemia, infarction, and perforation.
- Use nasogastric suction and IV fluids prior to surgical repair.
- Consider a trial of nasogastric suction rather than immediate surgery for patients with recurrent obstruction due to adhesions.

INTRA-ABDOMINAL ABSCESSES

Abscesses can occur anywhere in the abdomen and retroperitoneum. They mainly occur after surgery, trauma, or

conditions involving abdominal infection and inflammation, particularly when peritonitis or perforation occurs. Symptoms are malaise, fever, and abdominal pain. Diagnosis is by CT. Treatment is with drainage, either surgical or percutaneous. Antibiotics are ancillary.

Etiology

Intra-abdominal abscesses are classified as intraperitoneal, retroperitoneal, or visceral (see Table 10–6). Many intra-abdominal abscesses develop after perforation of a hollow viscus or colonic cancer. Others develop by extension of infection or inflammation resulting from conditions such as appendicitis, diverticulitis, Crohn disease, pancreatitis, pelvic inflammatory disease, or indeed any condition causing generalized peritonitis. Abdominal surgery, particularly that involving the digestive or biliary tract, is another significant risk factor: The peritoneum may be contaminated during or after surgery from such events as anastomotic leaks. Traumatic abdominal injuries—particularly lacerations and hematomas of the liver, pancreas, spleen, and intestines—may develop abscesses, whether treated operatively or not.

The **infecting organisms** typically reflect normal bowel flora and are a complex mixture of anaerobic and aerobic bacteria. Most frequent isolates are aerobic gram-negative bacilli (eg, *Escherichia coli* and *Klebsiella*) and anaerobes (especially *Bacteroides fragilis*).

Symptoms and Signs

Abscesses may form within 1 wk of perforation or significant peritonitis, whereas postoperative abscesses may not occur until 2 to 3 wk after operation and, rarely, not for several months. Although manifestations vary, most abscesses cause fever and abdominal discomfort ranging from minimal to severe (usually near the abscess). Paralytic ileus, either generalized or localized, may develop. Nausea, anorexia, and weight loss are common.

Abscesses in the Douglas cul-de-sac, adjacent to the rectosigmoid junction, may cause diarrhea. Contiguity to the bladder may result in urinary urgency and frequency and, if caused by diverticulitis, may create a colovesical fistula.

Subphrenic abscesses may cause chest symptoms such as nonproductive cough, chest pain, dyspnea, and shoulder pain. Rales, rhonchi, or a friction rub may be audible. Dullness to percussion and decreased breath sounds are typical when basilar atelectasis, pneumonia, or pleural effusion occurs.

Generally, there is tenderness over the location of the abscess. Large abscesses may be palpable as a mass.

Complications: Undrained abscesses may extend to contiguous structures, erode into adjacent vessels (causing hemorrhage or thrombosis), rupture into the peritoneum or bowel, or form a cutaneous or genitourinary fistula. Subdiaphragmatic abscesses may extend into the thoracic cavity, causing an empyema, lung abscess, or pneumonia. An abscess in the lower abdomen may track down into the thigh or perirectal fossa. Splenic abscess is a rare cause of sustained bacteremia in endocarditis that persists despite appropriate antimicrobial therapy.

Diagnosis

- Abdominal CT
- Rarely radionuclide scanning

CT of the abdomen and pelvis with oral contrast is the preferred diagnostic modality for suspected abscess. Other imaging studies, if done, may show abnormalities; plain abdominal x-rays may reveal extraintestinal gas in the abscess, displacement of adjacent organs, a soft-tissue density representing the abscess, or loss of the psoas muscle shadow. Abscesses near the diaphragm may result in chest x-ray abnormalities such as ipsilateral pleural effusion, elevated or immobile hemidiaphragm, lower lobe infiltrates, and atelectasis.

Table 10–6. INTRA-ABDOMINAL ABSCESSES

LOCATION	ETIOLOGY	ORGANISMS
Intraperitoneal		
Subphrenic Right or left lower quadrant Interloop Paracolic Pelvic	Postoperative; perforation of hollow viscus, appendicitis, diverticulitis, or tumor; Crohn disease; pelvic inflammatory disease; generalized peritonitis of any etiology	Bowel flora, often polymicrobial
Retroperitoneal		
Pancreatic	Trauma, pancreatitis	Bowel flora, often polymicrobial
Perinephric	Spread of renal parenchymal abscess (complication of pyelonephritis or rarely hematogenous from a remote source)	Aerobic gram-negative bacilli
Visceral		
Hepatic	Trauma, ascending cholangitis, portal bacteremia	Aerobic gram-negative bacilli if origin is biliary, polymicrobial bowel flora, if portal bacteremia, possibly amebic infection (see p. 1644)
Splenic	Trauma, hematogenous, infarction (as in sickle cell disease and malaria)	Staphylococci, streptococci, anaerobes, aerobic gram-negative bacilli including *Salmonella, Candida* in immunocompromised patients

CBC and blood cultures should be done. Leukocytosis occurs in most patients, and anemia is common.

Occasionally, radionuclide scanning with indium^{111}-labeled leukocytes may be helpful in identifying intra-abdominal abscesses.

Prognosis

Intra-abdominal abscesses have a mortality rate of 10 to 40%. Outcome depends mainly on the patient's primary illness or injury and general medical condition rather than on the specific nature and location of the abscess.

Treatment

- IV antibiotics
- Drainage: Percutaneous or surgical

Almost all intra-abdominal abscesses require drainage, either by percutaneous catheters or surgery; exceptions include small (< 2 cm) pericolic or periappendiceal abscesses, or abscesses that are draining spontaneously to the skin or into the bowel. Drainage through catheters (placed with CT or ultrasound guidance) may be appropriate given the following conditions: Few abscess cavities are present; the drainage route does not traverse bowel or uncontaminated organs, pleura, or peritoneum; the source of contamination is controlled; and the pus is thin enough to pass through the catheter.

Antibiotics are not curative but may limit hematogenous spread and should be given before and after intervention. Therapy requires drugs active against bowel flora, such as a combination of an aminoglycoside (eg, gentamicin 1.5 mg/kg q 8 h) and metronidazole 500 mg q 8 h. Single-agent therapy with cefotetan 2 g q 12 h is also reasonable. Patients previously given antibiotics or those who have hospital-acquired infections should receive drugs active against resistant aerobic gram-negative bacilli (eg, *Pseudomonas*) and anaerobes.

Nutritional support is important, with the enteral route preferred. Parenteral nutrition should begin early if the enteral route is not feasible.

KEY POINTS

- Suspect abdominal abscess in patients with a previous causative event (eg, abdominal trauma, abdominal surgery) or condition (eg, Crohn disease, diverticulitis, pancreatitis) who develop abdominal pain and fever.
- Abscess may be the first manifestation of a cancer.
- Diagnosis is with abdominal CT.
- Treatment is percutaneous or surgical drainage; antibiotics are necessary but alone are not adequate treatment.

ISCHEMIC COLITIS

Ischemic colitis is a transient reduction in blood flow to the colon.

Necrosis may occur but is usually limited to the mucosa and submucosa, only occasionally causing full-thickness necrosis necessitating surgery. Ischemic colitis occurs mainly in older people (> 60) and is thought to be caused by small-vessel atherosclerosis. It can also be a complication of abdominal aortic aneurysm repair.

Symptoms of ischemic colitis are milder and of slower onset than those of acute mesenteric ischemia and consist of left lower quadrant pain followed by rectal bleeding.

Diagnosis

- CT or colonoscopy

Diagnosis of ischemic colitis is made by CT or colonoscopy. Angiography or magnetic resonance angiography is not indicated.

Treatment

- IV fluids, bowel rest, and antibiotics
- Rarely surgery

Treatment of ischemic colitis is supportive with IV fluids, bowel rest, and antibiotics.

Surgery is rarely required, unless ischemic colitis is a complication of a vascular procedure or there is full-thickness necrosis. About 5% of patients have a recurrence. Occasionally, strictures develop at the site of the ischemia several weeks later, necessitating surgical resection.

11 Anorectal Disorders

The **anal canal** begins at the anal verge and ends at the anorectal junction (pectinate line, mucocutaneous junction, dentate line), where there are 8 to 12 anal crypts and 5 to 8 papillae. The canal is lined with anoderm, a continuation of the external skin. The anal canal and adjacent skin are innervated by somatic sensory nerves and are highly susceptible to painful stimuli. Venous drainage from the anal canal occurs through the caval system, but the anorectal junction can drain into both the portal and caval systems. Lymphatics from the anal canal pass to the internal iliac nodes, the posterior vaginal wall, and the inguinal nodes. The venous and lymphatic distributions determine how malignant disease and infection spread.

The **rectum** is a continuation of the sigmoid colon beginning at the level of the 3rd sacral vertebra and continuing to the anorectal junction. The rectal lining consists of red, glistening glandular mucosa, which has an autonomic nerve supply and is relatively insensitive to pain. Venous drainage occurs through the portal system. Lymphatic return from the rectum occurs along the superior hemorrhoidal vascular pedicle to the inferior mesenteric and aortic nodes.

The **sphincteric ring** encircling the anal canal is composed of the internal sphincter, the central portion of the levators, and components of the external sphincter. Anteriorly, it is more vulnerable to trauma, which can result in incontinence. The puborectalis forms a muscular sling around the rectum for support and assistance in defecation.

History: History should include the details of bleeding, pain, protrusion, discharge, swelling, abnormal sensations, bowel movements, incontinence, stool characteristics, use of cathartics and enemas, and abdominal and urinary symptoms. All patients should be asked about anal intercourse and other possible causes of trauma and infection.

Physical examination: Examination should be done gently and with good lighting. It consists of external inspection, perianal and intrarectal digital palpation, abdominal examination, and rectovaginal bidigital palpation. Anoscopy and rigid or flexible sigmoidoscopy to 15 to 60 cm above the anal verge are often included (see p. 79). Inspection, palpation, and anoscopy and sigmoidoscopy are best done with the patient in the left lateral (Sims) position or inverted on a tilt table. In cases of painful anal lesions, topical (lidocaine 5% ointment), regional, or even general anesthesia may be required. If it can be tolerated, a cleansing phosphate enema may facilitate sigmoidoscopy. Biopsies, smears, and cultures may be taken, and imaging studies are done if indicated.

ANAL FISSURE

(Fissure in Ano; Anal Ulcer)

An anal fissure is an acute longitudinal tear or a chronic ovoid ulcer in the squamous epithelium of the anal canal. It causes severe pain, sometimes with bleeding, particularly with defecation. Diagnosis is by inspection. Treatment is local hygiene, stool softeners, topical measures, and sometimes botulinum toxin injection and/or a surgical procedure.

Anal fissures are believed to result from laceration by a hard or large stool or from frequent loose bowel movements. Trauma (eg, anal intercourse) is a rare cause. The fissure may cause internal sphincter spasm, decreasing blood supply and perpetuating the fissure.

Symptoms and Signs

Anal fissures usually lie in the posterior midline but may occur in the anterior midline. Those off the midline may have specific etiologies, particularly Crohn disease. An external skin tag (the sentinel pile) may be present at the lower end of the fissure, and an enlarged (hypertrophic) papilla may be present at the upper end.

Infants may develop acute fissures, but chronic fissures are rare. Chronic fissures must be differentiated from cancer, primary lesions of syphilis, TB, and ulceration caused by Crohn disease.

Fissures cause pain and bleeding. The pain typically occurs with or shortly after defecation, lasts for several hours, and subsides until the next bowel movement. Examination must be gentle but with adequate spreading of the buttocks to allow visualization.

Diagnosis

- Clinical evaluation

Diagnosis of anal fissure is made by inspection. Unless findings suggest a specific cause or the appearance and/or location is unusual, further studies are not required.

Treatment

- Stool softeners
- Protective ointments, sitz baths
- Nitroglycerin ointment, topical calcium channel blocker, or botulinum toxin type A injection

Fissures often respond to conservative measures that minimize trauma during defecation (eg, stool softeners, psyllium, fiber). Healing is aided by use of protective zinc oxide ointments or bland suppositories (eg, glycerin) that lubricate the lower rectum and soften stool. Topical anesthetics (eg, benzocaine, lidocaine) and warm (not hot) sitz baths for 10 or 15 min after each bowel movement and as needed give temporary relief.

Topical nitroglycerin 0.2% ointment, nifedipine cream 0.2%, 2% diltiazem gel, and injections of botulinum toxin type A into the internal sphincter relax the anal sphincter and decrease maximum anal resting pressure, allowing healing. When conservative measures fail, surgery (internal anal sphincterotomy or controlled anal dilation) is needed to interfere with the cycle of internal anal sphincter spasm.

ANORECTAL ABSCESS

An anorectal abscess is a localized collection of pus in the perirectal spaces. Abscesses usually originate in an anal crypt. Symptoms are pain and swelling. Diagnosis is primarily by examination and CT or pelvic MRI for deeper abscesses. Treatment is surgical drainage.

An abscess may be located in various spaces surrounding the rectum and may be superficial or deep. A **perianal abscess** is superficial and points to the skin. An **ischiorectal abscess** is deeper, extending across the sphincter into the ischiorectal space below the levator ani; it may penetrate to the contralateral side, forming a "horseshoe" abscess. An abscess above the levator ani (ie, supralevator abscess) is quite deep and may extend to the peritoneum or abdominal organs; this abscess often results from diverticulitis or pelvic inflammatory disease. Crohn disease (especially of the colon) sometimes causes anorectal abscess. A mixed infection usually occurs, with *Escherichia coli, Proteus vulgaris, Bacteroides,* streptococci, and staphylococci predominating.

Symptoms and Signs

Superficial abscesses can be very painful; perianal swelling, redness, and tenderness are characteristic. Fever is rare.

Deeper abscesses may be less painful but cause toxic symptoms (eg, fever, chills, malaise). There may be no perianal findings, but digital rectal examination may reveal a tender, fluctuant swelling of the rectal wall. High pelvirectal abscesses may cause lower abdominal pain and fever without rectal symptoms. Sometimes fever is the only symptom.

Diagnosis

- Clinical evaluation
- Sometimes examination under anesthesia or rarely CT

Patients who have a pointing cutaneous abscess, a normal digital rectal examination, and no signs of systemic illness do not require imaging. CT scan is useful when a deep abscess or Crohn disease are suspected. Higher (supralevator) abscesses require CT to determine the intra-abdominal source of the infection. Those with any findings suggestive of a deeper abscess or complex perianal Crohn disease should have an examination under anesthesia at the time of drainage.

Treatment

- Incision and drainage
- Antibiotics for high-risk patients

Prompt incision and adequate drainage are required and should not wait until the abscess points. Many abscesses can be drained as an in-office procedure; deeper abscesses may require drainage in the operating room. Febrile, neutropenic, or diabetic patients or those with marked cellulitis should also receive antibiotics (eg, ciprofloxacin 500 mg IV q 12 h and metronidazole 500 mg IV q 8 h, ampicillin/sulbactam 1.5 g IV q 8 h). Antibiotics are not indicated for healthy patients with superficial abscesses. Anorectal fistulas may develop after drainage.

KEY POINTS

- Anorectal abscesses may be superficial or deep.
- Superficial abscesses may be diagnosed clinically and drained in the office or emergency department.
- Deep abscesses often require imaging with CT scan and typically must be drained in the operating room.
- Immunocompromised patients and those with deep abscesses should receive antibiotics.

ANORECTAL FISTULA

(Fistula in Ano)

An anorectal fistula is a tubelike tract with one opening in the anal canal and the other usually in the perianal skin. Symptoms are discharge and sometimes pain. Diagnosis is by examination and sigmoidoscopy. Treatment often requires surgery.

Fistulas arise spontaneously or occur secondary to drainage of a perirectal abscess. Predisposing causes include Crohn disease and TB. Most fistulas originate in the anorectal crypts; others may result from diverticulitis, tumors, or trauma. Fistulas in infants are congenital and are more common among boys. **Rectovaginal fistulas** may be secondary to Crohn disease, obstetric injuries, radiation therapy, or cancer.

Symptoms and Signs

A history of recurrent abscess followed by intermittent or constant discharge is usual. Discharge material is purulent, serosanguineous, or both. Pain may be present if there is infection. On inspection, one or more secondary openings can be seen. A cordlike tract can often be palpated. A probe inserted into the tract can determine the depth and direction and often the primary opening.

Diagnosis

- Clinical evaluation
- Sigmoidoscopy

Diagnosis of anorectal fistula is by examination. Sigmoidoscopy should follow if there is suspicion of Crohn disease (see diagnosis of Crohn disease on p. 137).

Hidradenitis suppurativa, pilonidal sinus, dermal suppurative sinuses, and urethroperineal fistulas must be differentiated from cryptogenic fistulas.

Treatment

- Various surgical procedures
- Medical treatment if caused by Crohn disease

In the past, the only effective treatment was surgery, in which the primary opening and the entire tract are unroofed and converted into a "ditch." Partial division of the sphincters may be necessary. Some degree of incontinence may occur if a considerable portion of the sphincteric ring is divided. Alternatives to conventional surgery include advancement flaps, biologic plugs, and fibrin glue instillations into the fistulous tract. More recently, the ligation of intersphincteric fistula tract (LIFT) procedure, where the fistula tract is divided between the sphincter muscles, has gained acceptance as an alternative more likely to preserve continence.

If diarrhea or Crohn disease is present, fistulotomy is inadvisable because of delayed wound healing. For patients with Crohn disease, metronidazole, other appropriate antibiotics, and suppressive therapies can be given (see treatment of Crohn disease on p. 138). Infliximab is effective in closing anal fistulas caused by Crohn disease.

FECAL INCONTINENCE

Fecal incontinence is involuntary defecation.

Fecal incontinence can result from injuries or diseases of the spinal cord, congenital abnormalities, accidental injuries to the rectum and anus, procidentia, diabetes, severe dementia, fecal impaction, extensive inflammatory processes, tumors, obstetric injuries, and operations involving division or dilation of the anal sphincters.

Physical examination should evaluate gross sphincter function and perianal sensation and rule out fecal impaction. Anal sphincter endoscopic ultrasonography, pelvic and perineal MRIs, pelvic floor electromyography, and anorectal manometry are also useful.

Treatment

- Program of stool regulation
- Perineal exercises, sometimes with biofeedback
- Sometimes a surgical procedure

Treatment of fecal incontinence includes a bowel management program to develop a predictable pattern of defecation. The program includes intake of adequate fluid and sufficient dietary bulk. Sitting on a toilet or using another customary defecatory stimulant (eg, coffee) encourages defecation. A suppository (eg, glycerin, bisacodyl) or a phosphate enema may also be used. If a regular defecatory pattern does not develop, a low-residue diet and oral loperamide may reduce the frequency of defecation.

Simple perineal exercises, in which the patient repeatedly contracts the sphincters, perineal muscles, and buttocks, may strengthen these structures and contribute to continence, particularly in mild cases. Biofeedback (to train the patient to use the sphincters maximally and to better appreciate physiologic stimuli) should be considered before recommending surgery in well-motivated patients who can understand and follow instructions and who have an anal sphincter capable of recognizing the cue of rectal distention. About 70% of such patients respond to biofeedback.

A defect in the sphincter as assessed by endoscopic ultrasonography can be sutured directly. When there is insufficient residual sphincter for repair, particularly in patients < 50 yr of age, a gracilis muscle can be transposed. However, the positive results of these procedures typically do not last long. Some centers attach a pacemaker to the gracilis muscle, whereas others use an artificial sphincter; these or other experimental procedures are available in only a few centers in the US, as research protocols. Sacral nerve stimulation has shown promise in the treatment of fecal incontinence. Alternatively, a Thiersch wire or other material can be used to encircle the anus. When all else fails, a colostomy can be considered.

HEMORRHOIDS

(Piles)

Hemorrhoids are dilated veins of the hemorrhoidal plexus in the anal canal. Symptoms include irritation and bleeding. Thrombosed hemorrhoids are painful. Diagnosis is by inspection or anoscopy. Treatment is symptomatic or with rubber banding, injection sclerotherapy, or sometimes surgery.

Increased pressure in the veins of the anorectal area leads to hemorrhoids. This pressure may result from pregnancy, frequent heavy lifting, or repeated straining during defecation (eg, due to constipation). Hemorrhoids may be external or internal. In a few people, rectal varices result from increased blood pressure in the portal vein, and these are distinct from hemorrhoids.

External hemorrhoids are located below the dentate line and are covered by squamous epithelium.

Internal hemorrhoids are located above the dentate line and are lined by rectal mucosa. Hemorrhoids typically occur in the right anterior, right posterior, and left lateral zones. They occur in adults and children.

Symptoms and Signs

Hemorrhoids are often asymptomatic, or they may simply protrude. Pruritus ani is not commonly caused by hemorrhoids unless they are significantly prolapsed.

External hemorrhoids may become thrombosed, resulting in a painful, purplish swelling. Rarely, they ulcerate and cause minor bleeding. Cleansing the anal region may be difficult.

Internal hemorrhoids typically manifest with bleeding after defecation; blood is noted on toilet tissue and sometimes in the toilet bowl. Internal hemorrhoids may be uncomfortable but are not as painful as thrombosed external hemorrhoids. Internal hemorrhoids sometimes cause mucus discharge and a sensation of incomplete evacuation.

Strangulated hemorrhoids occur when protrusion and constriction occlude the blood supply. They cause pain that is occasionally followed by necrosis and ulceration.

Diagnosis

- Anoscopy
- Sometimes sigmoidoscopy or colonoscopy

Most painful hemorrhoids, thrombosed, ulcerated or not, are seen on inspection of the anus and rectum. Anoscopy is essential in evaluating painless or bleeding hemorrhoids. Rectal bleeding should be attributed to hemorrhoids only after more serious conditions are excluded (ie, by sigmoidoscopy or colonoscopy).

PEARLS & PITFALLS

- Rectal bleeding should be attributed to hemorrhoids only after more serious conditions are excluded.

Treatment

- Stool softeners, sitz baths
- Occasionally excision for thrombosed external hemorrhoids
- Injection sclerotherapy or rubber band ligation for internal hemorrhoids

Symptomatic treatment of hemorrhoids is usually all that is needed. It is accomplished with stool softeners (eg, docusate, psyllium), warm sitz baths (ie, sitting in a tub of tolerably hot water for 10 min) after each bowel movement and as needed, anesthetic ointments containing lidocaine, or witch hazel (hamamelis) compresses (which soothe by an unknown mechanism). Pain caused by a thrombosed external hemorrhoid can be treated with NSAIDs. Infrequently, simple excision of the external hemorrhoid is done, which may relieve pain rapidly; after infiltration with 1% lidocaine, the thrombosed portion of the hemorrhoid is excised, and the defect is closed with an absorbable suture.

Bleeding internal hemorrhoids can be treated by injection sclerotherapy with 5% phenol in vegetable oil or other sclerosing agents. Bleeding should cease at least temporarily.

Rubber band ligation is used for larger, prolapsing internal hemorrhoids or those that do not respond to conservative management. With mixed internal and external hemorrhoids, only the internal component should be rubber band ligated. The internal hemorrhoid is grasped and withdrawn through a stretched ½-cm diameter band, which is released to ligate the hemorrhoid, resulting in its necrosis and sloughing. Typically, one hemorrhoid is ligated every 2 wk; 3 to 6 treatments may be required. Sometimes, multiple hemorrhoids can be ligated at a single visit. External hemorrhoids should not be banded.

Infrared photocoagulation is useful for ablating nonprolapsing, bleeding internal hemorrhoids, hemorrhoids that cannot be rubber band ligated because of pain sensitivity, or hemorrhoids that are not cured with rubber band ligation.

Doppler-guided hemorrhoid artery ligation, in which a rectal ultrasound probe is used to identify vessels for suture ligation, is promising but requires further study to determine its overall utility. Laser destruction, cryotherapy, and various types of electrodestruction are of unproven efficacy.

Surgical hemorrhoidectomy is required for patients who do not respond to other forms of therapy. Significant postoperative pain is common, as are urinary retention and constipation. Stapled hemorrhoidopexy is an alternative procedure for circumferential hemorrhoids and causes less postoperative pain but has higher recurrence and complication rates than conventional surgical hemorrhoidectomy.

KEY POINTS

- External hemorrhoids may thrombose and become very painful but rarely bleed.
- Internal hemorrhoids often bleed but are not often painful.
- Stool softeners, topical treatments, and analgesics are usually adequate treatment for external hemorrhoids.
- Bleeding internal hemorrhoids may require injection sclerotherapy, rubber band ligation, or various other ablative methods.
- Surgery is a last resort.

LEVATOR SYNDROME

Episodic rectal pain caused by spasm of the levator ani muscle.

Proctalgia fugax (fleeting pain in the rectum) and **coccydynia** (pain in the coccygeal region) are variants of levator syndrome. Rectal spasm causes pain, typically unrelated to defecation, usually lasting < 20 min. The pain may be brief and intense or a vague ache high in the rectum. It may occur spontaneously or with sitting and can waken the patient from sleep. The pain may feel as if it would be relieved by the passage of gas or a bowel movement. In severe cases, the pain can persist for many hours and recur frequently. The patient may have undergone various rectal operations for these symptoms, with no benefit.

Diagnosis

- Clinical evaluation

Physical examination can exclude other painful rectal conditions (eg, thrombosed hemorrhoids, fissures, abscesses). Physical examination is often normal, although tenderness or tightness of the levator muscle, usually on the left, may be present. Occasional cases are caused by low back or prostate disorders. Other causes of pelvic pain (eg, cancer) must be ruled out. In most cases, a distinct cause of levator syndrome is not identified.

Treatment

- Analgesics, sitz baths
- Sometimes electrogalvanic stimulation

Treatment of levator syndrome consists of explanations to the patient of the benign nature of the condition. An acute episode may be relieved by the passage of gas or a bowel movement, by a sitz bath, or by a mild analgesic. When the symptoms are more intense, physical therapy may be effective. Skeletal muscle relaxants or anal sphincter massage under local or regional anesthesia can be tried, but the benefit is unclear.

PILONIDAL DISEASE

Pilonidal disease refers to an acute abscess or chronic draining sinus in the sacrococcygeal area.

Pilonidal disease usually occurs in young, hirsute, white males but can also occur in women. One or several midline or adjacent-to-the-midline pits or sinuses occur in the skin of the sacral region and may form a cavity, often containing hair. The lesion is usually asymptomatic; infected lesions are painful.

Treatment of an acute abscess is by incision and drainage. Usually, one or more chronic draining sinuses persist and must be extirpated by excision and primary closure or, preferably, by an open technique (eg, cystotomy, marsupialization). Antibiotics are typically not needed.

Larger cysts may require a rotation flap to close the defect.

PROCTITIS

Proctitis is inflammation of the rectal mucosa, which may result from infection, inflammatory bowel disease, or radiation. Symptoms are rectal discomfort and bleeding. Diagnosis is by sigmoidoscopy, usually with cultures and biopsy. Treatment depends on etiology.

Proctitis may be a manifestation of

- Sexually transmitted diseases (eg, *Neisseria gonorrhoeae, Chlamydia* sp)
- Certain enteric infections (eg, *Campylobacter, Shigella, Salmonella*—see p. 1577)
- Inflammatory bowel disease
- Radiation treatments

Proctitis associated with prior antibiotic use may be due to Clostridium difficile.

Sexually transmitted pathogens cause proctitis more commonly among men who have sex with men. Immunocompromised patients are at particular risk of infections with herpes simplex and cytomegalovirus.

Symptoms and Signs

Typically, patients report tenesmus (a strong feeling of need to defecate when stool is not present), rectal bleeding, or passage of mucus. Proctitis resulting from gonorrhea, herpes simplex, or cytomegalovirus may cause intense anorectal pain.

Diagnosis

- Proctoscopy or sigmoidoscopy
- Tests for sexually transmitted diseases and *C. difficile*

Diagnosis of proctitis requires proctoscopy or sigmoidoscopy, which may reveal an inflamed rectal mucosa. Small discrete ulcers and vesicles suggest herpes infection. Rectal swabs should be tested for *Neisseria gonorrhoeae and Chlamydia* sp (by culture or ligase chain reaction), enteric pathogens (by culture), and viral pathogens (by culture or immunoassay).

Serologic tests for syphilis and stool tests for *C. difficile* toxin are done. Sometimes mucosal biopsy is needed.

Colonoscopy may be valuable in some patients to rule out inflammatory bowel disease.

Treatment

- Various treatments depending on cause

Infective proctitis can be treated with antibiotics. Men who have sex with men who have nonspecific proctitis may be treated empirically with ceftriaxone 125 mg IM once (or ciprofloxacin 500 mg po bid for 7 days), plus doxycycline 100 mg po bid for 7 days. Antibiotic-associated proctitis is treated with metronidazole (250 mg po qid) or vancomycin (125 mg po qid) for 7 to 10 days.

Radiation proctitis is usually effectively treated with topical formalin carefully applied to the affected mucosa. Alternative treatments include topical corticosteroids as foam (hydrocortisone 90 mg) or enemas (hydrocortisone 100 mg or methylprednisolone 40 mg) bid for 3 wk, or mesalamine (4 g) enema at bedtime for 3 to 6 wk. Mesalamine suppositories 500 mg once/day or bid, mesalamine 800 mg po tid, or sulfasalazine 500 to 1000 mg po qid for ≥ 3 wk alone or in combination with topical therapy may also be effective. Patients unresponsive to these forms of therapy may benefit from a course of systemic corticosteroids. Various methods of coagulation have been tried, including argon plasma, lasers, electrocoagulation, and heater probes.

PRURITUS ANI

(Anal Itching)

The perianal skin tends to itch, which can result from numerous causes (see Table 11–1). This condition is also known as pruritus ani. Occasionally, the irritation is misinterpreted by the patient as pain, so other causes of perianal pain (eg, abscess or cancer) should be ruled out.

Etiology

Most anal itching is

- Idiopathic (the majority)
- Hygiene-related

Too little cleansing leaves irritating stool and sweat residue on the anal skin. Too much cleansing, often with sanitary wipes and strong soaps, can be drying or irritating or occasionally cause a contact hypersensitivity reaction. Large external hemorrhoids can make postdefecation cleansing difficult, and large internal hemorrhoids can cause mucus drainage or fecal soilage and consequent irritation.

Table 11–1. SOME CAUSES OF PRURITUS ANI

CAUSE	SUGGESTIVE FINDINGS	DIAGNOSTIC APPROACH
Anorectal disorders		
Inflammatory bowel disease (eg, Crohn disease)	Purulent discharge Pain in the rectum (sometimes) and/or abdomen (often) Sometimes draining fistula Sometimes diarrhea	Anoscopy, sigmoidoscopy, or colonoscopy
Hemorrhoids (internal or external)	With internal hemorrhoids, bleeding (a small amount of blood on toilet paper or in the toilet bowl) With external hemorrhoids, a painful, swollen lump on the anus	Clinical evaluation Usually anoscopy or sigmoidoscopy
Infections		
Bacterial infection (secondary to scratching)	Inflamed, excoriated area	Clinical evaluation
Candida	A rash around the anus	Clinical evaluation Sometimes examination of skin scrapings
Pinworms	Usually in children Sometimes present in several family members	Microscopic examination of transparent tape that was applied to the anal area to check for pinworm eggs (see diagnosis of pinworms on p. 1676)
Scabies	Intense itching, usually worse at night Possibly itching of other body areas Possibly pink, thin, slightly raised lines or bumps (burrows) on the affected areas	Clinical evaluation Examination of skin scrapings
Skin disorders		
Atopic dermatitis	An itchy, red, oozing, and crusty rash	Clinical evaluation
Perianal carcinoma (eg, Bowen disease, extramammary Paget disease)	Scaly or crusted lesion	Biopsy
Psoriasis	Typical psoriatic plaques Sometimes plaques on other areas of the skin	Clinical evaluation
Skin tags	Small flap of tissue on anus	Clinical evaluation
Drugs		
Antibiotics	Current or recent antibiotic use	Trial of elimination
Foods and dietary supplements		
Beer, caffeine, chocolate, hot peppers, milk products, nuts, tomato products, citrus fruits, spices, or vitamin C tablets	Symptoms only after ingestion of substance	Trial of elimination
Hygiene-related problems		
Excessive sweating	Excessive sweating described by the person, particularly with wearing of tight and/or synthetic clothing	Trial of measures to limit sweating (eg, wearing loose cotton underwear, changing underwear frequently)
Overly meticulous or aggressive cleansing of the anal area Poor cleansing	Inappropriate cleansing practices described by the patient	Trial of a change in cleansing practices
Skin irritants		
Local anesthetics, ointments, soaps, and sanitary wipes	Use of a possibly irritating or sensitizing substance described by the patient	Trial of elimination

Other distinct causes are rarely identified, but a variety of factors have been implicated (see Table 11–1).

In the very young and elderly, fecal and urinary incontinence predisposes to local irritation and secondary candidal infections.

Once itching occurs, resulting from any cause, an itch-scratch-itch cycle can begin, in which scratching begets more itching. Often, skin becomes excoriated and secondarily infected, causing yet more itching. Also, topical treatments for itching and infection may be sensitizing, causing further itching.

Evaluation

History: History of present illness should note whether the problem is acute or recurrent. The patient should be asked about topical agents applied to the anus, including wipes, ointments (even those used to treat itching), sprays, and soaps. Diet and drug profiles should be reviewed for causative agents (see Table 11–1), particularly acidic or spicy foods. A general sense of hygiene should be obtained by asking about frequency of showers and baths.

Review of systems should seek symptoms of causative disorders, including urinary or fecal incontinence (local irritation), anal pain or lump, blood on toilet paper (hemorrhoids), bloody diarrhea and abdominal cramps (inflammatory bowel disease), and skin plaques (psoriasis).

Past medical history should identify known conditions associated with pruritus ani, particularly prior anorectal surgery, hemorrhoids, and diabetes.

Physical examination: General examination should obtain a sense of overall hygiene and note any signs of anxiety or obsessive-compulsive behavior.

Physical examination focuses on the anal region, particularly looking for perianal skin changes, signs of fecal staining or soilage (suggesting inadequate hygiene), and hemorrhoids. External inspection should also note the integrity of the perianal skin, whether it appears dull or thickened (suggesting chronicity), and the presence of any cutaneous lesions, fistulas, excoriations, or signs of local infection. Sphincter tone is assessed by having the patient contract the sphincter during digital rectal examination. The patient should then be asked to bear down as if for a bowel movement, which may show prolapsing internal hemorrhoids. Anoscopy may be necessary to further evaluate the anorectum for hemorrhoids.

Dermatologic examination may reveal scabies burrows in the inter-digital webbing or scalp or signs of any other contributing systemic skin disease.

Red flags: The following findings are of particular concern:

- Draining fistula
- Bloody diarrhea
- Large external hemorrhoids
- Prolapsing internal hemorrhoids
- Perianal fecal soilage
- Dull or thickened perianal skin

Interpretation of findings: Hygiene issues, use of topical agents, and local disorders (eg, candidal infection, hemorrhoids) are usually apparent by history and examination.

In adults with acute itching without obvious cause, ingested substances should be considered; a trial of eliminating these substances from the diet may be useful. In children, pinworms should be suspected.

In adults with chronic itching and no apparent cause, overly aggressive anal hygiene may be involved.

Testing: For many patients, a trial of empiric, nonspecific therapy is appropriate unless particular findings are noted. For example, biopsy, culture, or both of visible lesions of uncertain etiology should be considered. If pinworms, which occur most often in school-aged children, are suspected, eggs can be detected by patting the perianal skinfolds with a strip of cellophane tape in the early morning; the tape is placed side down on a glass slide and viewed microscopically.

Treatment

Systemic causes and parasitic or fungal infections must be treated specifically.

Foods and topical agents suspected of causing pruritus ani should be eliminated.

General measures: Clothing should be kept loose, and bed clothing should be light. After bowel movements, the patient should clean the anal area with absorbent cotton or plain soft tissue moistened with water or a commercial perianal cleansing preparation for hemorrhoids; soaps and premoistened wipes should be avoided. Liberal, frequent dusting with nonmedicated talcum powder or cornstarch helps combat moisture. Hydrocortisone acetate 1% ointment, applied qid for a brief period (< 1 wk), may relieve symptoms. Sometimes, higher potency topical corticosteroids may be needed.

KEY POINTS

- Pinworms in children and hygiene-related issues in adults are common causes.
- Foods and detergents or soaps can cause anal itching.
- Practicing appropriate, nonirritating hygiene (ie, not too little but not too vigorous, avoiding strong soaps and chemicals) and decreasing local moisture can help alleviate symptoms.

RECTAL PROLAPSE AND PROCIDENTIA

Rectal prolapse is painless protrusion of the rectum through the anus. Procidentia is complete prolapse of the entire thickness of the rectum. Diagnosis is by inspection. Surgery is usually required in adults.

Transient, minor prolapse of just the rectal mucosa often occurs in otherwise normal infants. Mucosal prolapse in adults persists and may progressively worsen.

Procidentia is complete prolapse of the entire thickness of the rectum. The primary cause of procidentia is unclear. Most patients are women > 60.

Symptoms and Signs

The most prominent symptom of rectal prolapse and procidentia is protrusion. It may only occur while straining or while walking or standing. Rectal bleeding can occur, and incontinence is frequent. Pain is uncommon unless incarceration or significant prolapse occurs.

Diagnosis

- Clinical evaluation
- Sigmoidoscopy, colonoscopy, or barium enema

To determine the full extent of the prolapse, the clinician should examine the patient while the patient is standing or squatting and straining. Rectal procidentia can be distinguished from hemorrhoids by the presence of circumferential mucosal folds. Anal sphincter tone is usually diminished. Sigmoidoscopy, colonoscopy, or barium enema x-rays of the colon must be done to search for other disease. Primary neurologic disorders (eg, spinal cord tumors) must be ruled out.

Treatment

- Elimination of causes of straining
- For infants and children: Sometimes strapping buttocks together
- For adults: Sometimes surgery

In infants and children, conservative treatment is most satisfactory. Causes of straining should be eliminated. Firmly strapping the buttocks together with tape between bowel movements usually facilitates spontaneous resolution of the prolapse. For simple mucosal prolapse in adults, the excess mucosa can be excised. For procidentia, rectopexy, in which the rectum is mobilized and fixed to the sacrum, may be required. In patients who are very old or in poor health, a wire or synthetic plastic loop can encircle the sphincteric ring (Thiersch procedure). Other perineal operations (eg, Delorme or Altemeier procedure) can be considered.

SOLITARY RECTAL ULCER SYNDROME

Solitary rectal ulcer syndrome is a rare disorder that involves straining during defecation, a sense of incomplete evacuation, and sometimes passage of blood and mucus by rectum. It is probably caused by localized ischemic injury of the distal rectal mucosa. Diagnosis is clinical with confirmation by flexible sigmoidoscopy and biopsy. Treatment is a bowel regimen for mild cases, but surgery is sometimes needed if rectal prolapse is the cause.

Solitary rectal ulcer syndrome is caused by mucosal ischemia of the distal rectal mucosa resulting from trauma.

Causes include

- Rectal prolapse
- Paradoxical contraction of the puborectalis muscle
- Chronic constipation
- Attempts at manual disimpaction of hard stools

Symptoms and Signs

Affected patients have straining during defecation, a sense of incomplete evacuation or pelvic fullness, and sometimes passage of blood and mucus by rectum.

The syndrome is poorly named because associated lesions may be solitary or multiple and ulcerated or nonulcerated; they range from mucosal erythema to ulcers to small mass lesions. Lesions are typically located in the anterior rectal wall within 10 cm of the anal verge.

PEARLS & PITFALLS

- Solitary rectal ulcer syndrome is poorly named because associated lesions may be solitary or multiple and ulcerated or nonulcerated; they range from mucosal erythema to ulcers to small mass lesions.

Diagnosis

- Clinical evaluation
- Flexible sigmoidoscopy with biopsy

Diagnosis of solitary rectal ulcer syndrome is typically made by clinical history alone, but flexible sigmoidoscopy with biopsy is sometimes done for confirmation. Assessment for internal or full-thickness rectal prolapse should be done (see p. 100).

Histopathologic examination of the biopsy specimen shows a thickened mucosal layer with distortion of the crypt architecture and replacement of the lamina propria with smooth muscle and collagen, leading to hypertrophy and disorganization of the muscularis mucosa.

Treatment

- Bulk laxatives
- Sometimes surgery for rectal prolapse

Mild cases are treated with reassurance and establishment of a bowel regimen with bulk laxatives to relieve chronic constipation. If rectal prolapse is the cause, surgery may be needed (see treatment of rectal prolapse on p. 100).

12 Bezoars and Foreign Bodies

BEZOARS

A bezoar is a tightly packed collection of partially digested or undigested material that is unable to exit the stomach. Gastric bezoars are usually rare and can occur in all age groups. They often occur in patients with behavior disorder or abnormal gastric emptying and also after gastric surgery. Many bezoars are asymptomatic, but some cause symptoms. Some bezoars can be dissolved chemically, others removed endoscopically, and some require surgery.

Bezoars are classified according to their composition:

- Phytobezoars (vegetable—most common)
- Trichobezoars (hair)
- Pharmacobezoars (drugs; particularly common with sucralfate and aluminum hydroxide gel)
- Disopyrobezoars, a subset of phytobezoars (excessive intake of persimmon; occur most often in regions where the fruit is grown)
- Other (variety of other substances including tissue paper and polystyrene foam products such as cups)

Etiology

Trichobezoars, which can weigh several kilograms, most commonly occur in young females with psychiatric disorders who chew and swallow their own hair.

Phytobezoars are the most common form of bezoar. They often occur in adult patients as a postoperative complication after gastric bypass or partial gastrectomy, especially when partial gastrectomy is accompanied by vagotomy. Delayed gastric emptying due to diabetes mellitus or other systemic illness increases the risk of gastric bezoar formation. Other predisposing factors include hypochlorhydria, diminished antral motility, and incomplete mastication; these factors are more common among the elderly, who are thus at higher risk of bezoar formation.

Symptoms and Signs

Gastric bezoars are usually asymptomatic. When symptoms are present, the most common include postprandial fullness, abdominal pain, nausea, vomiting, anorexia, and weight loss.

Complications: Rarely, bezoars cause serious complications including

- Gastric outlet obstruction
- GI bleeding
- Small-bowel obstruction
- Peritonitis
- Intussusception

Diagnosis

- Endoscopy

Bezoars are detectable as a mass lesion on imaging studies (eg, x-ray, ultrasound, CT) that are often done to evaluate the patient's nonspecific upper GI symptoms. The findings may be mistaken for tumors.

Upper endoscopy is usually done to confirm the diagnosis. On endoscopy, bezoars have an unmistakable irregular surface and may range in color from yellow-green to gray-black. An endoscopic biopsy that yields hair or plant material is diagnostic.

Treatment

- Chemical dissolution
- Endoscopic removal
- Sometimes surgery

The optimal therapeutic intervention is controversial because randomized controlled trials comparing different options have not been done.

Chemical dissolution using agents such as cola and cellulase can be done for patients with mild symptoms. Cellulase dosage is 3 to 5 g dissolved in 300 to 500 mL of water; this is taken over the course of a day for 2 to 5 days. Metoclopramide 10 mg po is often given as an adjunct to promote gastric motility. Enzymatic digestion using papain is no longer recommended.

Endoscopic removal is indicated for patients who have bezoars that fail to dissolve, moderate to severe symptoms due to large bezoars, or both. If initial diagnosis is made by endoscopy, removal can be attempted at that time. Fragmentation with forceps, wire snare, jet spray, or even laser[1] may break up bezoars, allowing them to pass or be extracted.

Surgery is reserved for cases in which chemical dissolution and endoscopic intervention cannot be done or have failed or for patients with complications.

Persimmon fruit bezoars are usually hard and difficult to treat because persimmons contain the tannin shibuol, which polymerizes in the stomach.

1. Mao Y, Qiu H, Liu Q, et al: Endoscopic lithotripsy for gastric bezoars by Nd:YAG laser-ignited mini-explosive technique. *Lasers Med Sci* 29:1237–1240, 2014. doi: 10.1007/s10103-013-1512-1.

OVERVIEW OF FOREIGN BODIES IN THE GI TRACT

A variety of foreign bodies may enter the GI tract intentionally or accidentally. Many foreign bodies pass through the GI tract spontaneously, but some become impacted, causing symptoms and sometimes complications. The role of imaging in the management of foreign body ingestion is not standardized. Nearly all impacted objects can be removed endoscopically, but surgery is occasionally necessary. Timing of endoscopy varies depending on the type of foreign body ingested.

Foreign bodies in the GI tract may be

- Esophageal
- Gastric
- Intestinal
- Rectal

The majority of foreign body ingestions occur in children. Deliberate and recurrent foreign body ingestion is described more commonly among prison inmates and psychiatric patients. Denture wearers, the elderly, and inebriated people are prone to accidentally swallowing inadequately masticated food (particularly meat), which may become impacted in the esophagus. Smugglers who swallow drug-filled balloons, vials, or packages to escape detection (see p. 3229) may develop intestinal obstruction. The packaging may rupture, leading to drug overdose.

The **common complications** of foreign body ingestion include

- Ulceration
- Lacerations
- Perforation
- GI obstruction
- Fistula formation
- Bacteremia

1. ASGE Standards of Practice Committee, Ikenberry SO, Jue TL, Anderson MA, et al: Management of ingested foreign bodies and food impactions. *Gastrointest Endosc* 73:1085–1091, 2011. doi: 10.1016/j.gie.2010.11.010.

ESOPHAGEAL FOREIGN BODIES

Food and a variety of other swallowed objects can become impacted in the esophagus. Esophageal foreign bodies cause dysphagia and sometimes lead to perforation. Diagnosis is clinical, but imaging studies and endoscopy may be needed. Some objects pass spontaneously, but endoscopic removal is often required.

The esophagus is the most common site of foreign body impaction. Food impactions cause most esophageal foreign bodies. Large, smooth food pieces (eg, steak, hot dogs) are particularly easy to swallow inadvertently before being chewed sufficiently. Bones, particularly fish bones, may be swallowed if the meat in which they are embedded is not chewed sufficiently.

Infants and toddlers do not have fully mature oropharyngeal coordination and often inadvertently swallow small, round foods (eg, grapes, peanuts, candies), which may become impacted. In addition, infants and toddlers often swallow a wide variety of inedible objects (eg, coins, batteries), some of which become impacted in the esophagus. Impacted disc batteries are particularly worrisome because they may cause esophageal burns, perforation, or tracheoesophageal fistula.

Foreign bodies in the esophagus usually lodge in areas where physiologic or pathologic luminal narrowing exists. Luminal narrowing may be caused by webs, rings, strictures, benign and cancerous tumors, achalasia, and eosinophilic esophagitis.

Complications: The main complications of esophageal foreign bodies are

- Obstruction
- Perforation

Obstruction may be partial (eg, patient can swallow liquids or at least their oral secretions) or complete. Partial obstruction is less emergent unless it involves a sharp object embedded in the wall, which can lead to perforation. Complete obstruction is poorly tolerated clinically, and even a smooth object, if tightly impacted, may cause pressure necrosis and risk of perforation if allowed to remain in the esophagus for more than about 24 h.

Complications also depend on the nature of the object involved. Despite their small size, impacted disk or button batteries are objects of particular concern because liquefaction necrosis and perforation can occur rapidly.

Symptoms and Signs

The main presenting symptom is acute dysphagia. Patients with complete obstruction of the esophagus hypersalivate and are unable to swallow oral secretions. Other symptoms include retrosternal fullness, regurgitation, odynophagia, blood-stained saliva, and gagging and choking. Hyperventilation resulting from anxiety and discomfort often gives the appearance of respiratory distress, but actual dyspnea or auscultatory findings of stridor or wheezing strongly suggest the foreign body is in the airway rather than the esophagus.

Sometimes, foreign bodies scratch the esophagus but do not become lodged. In such cases, patients may report a foreign body sensation even though no foreign body is present.

Diagnosis

- Clinical evaluation
- Sometimes imaging studies
- Often endoscopic evaluation

Many patients give a clear history of ingestion; those with significant symptoms suggesting complete obstruction should have immediate therapeutic endoscopy. Patients with minimal symptoms who are able to swallow normally may not have an impacted foreign body and can be observed at home for resolution of symptoms. Other patients may require imaging studies.

Some patients, such as young children, mentally impaired adults, and those with psychiatric illness, may not be able to give an adequate history of ingestion. These patients may present with choking, refusal to eat, vomiting, drooling, wheezing, blood-stained saliva, or respiratory distress. Imaging studies also may be needed in these patients.

Some foreign bodies can be detected with plain x-rays (2 views preferred). These x-rays are best for detecting metallic foreign objects and steak bones as well as for detecting signs of perforation (eg, free air in the mediastinum or peritoneum). However, fish bones and even some chicken bones, wood, plastic, glass, and thin metal objects can be difficult to identify on plain x-rays. If there is any suspicion at all of a sharp or dangerous esophageal foreign body, imaging studies, such as CT, should be done to identify the foreign body. However, endoscopic evaluation is required in patients with suspected foreign body ingestions and ongoing symptoms despite negative imaging results. A contrast study typically should not be done because of the risk of aspiration and concern about the presence of residual contrast material making subsequent endoscopic retrieval more difficult.

Treatment

- Sometimes trial of observation and/or IV glucagon
- Often endoscopic removal

Some foreign bodies pass spontaneously into the stomach, after which they typically pass completely through the GI tract and are expelled. Patients without symptoms of high-grade obstruction and without ingestion of sharp objects or disk or button batteries typically can safely be observed for up to 24 h to await passage, which is indicated by relief of symptoms. Administration of glucagon 1 mg IV is a relatively safe and acceptable option that sometimes allows for spontaneous passage of a food bolus by relaxing the distal esophagus. Other methods, such as use of effervescent agents, meat tenderizer, and bougienage, are not recommended.

Foreign bodies that do not pass within 24 h[1] should be removed because delay increases the risk of complications, including perforation, and decreases the likelihood of successful removal.

Endoscopic removal is the treatment of choice. Removal is best achieved using a forceps, basket, or snare, preferably with an overtube placed in the esophagus or orotracheal intubation to prevent aspiration and protect the airway.

Emergent endoscopy is required for sharp-pointed objects, disk or button batteries, and any obstruction causing significant symptoms.

Follow-up care for the evaluation of structural and functional abnormalities is recommended for patients with esophageal food impaction.

1. ASGE Standards of Practice Committee, Ikenberry SO, Jue TL, Anderson MA, et al: Management of ingested foreign bodies and food impactions. *Gastrointest Endosc* 73:1085–1091, 2011. doi: 10.1016/j.gie.2010.11.010.

KEY POINTS

- The esophagus is the most common site of ingested foreign body impaction.
- The main presenting symptom is acute dysphagia; patients with complete obstruction of the esophagus hypersalivate and are unable to swallow oral secretions.
- Complete obstruction may cause pressure necrosis and increases the risk of perforation if present for more than about 24 h.
- Emergent endoscopy is required for sharp-pointed objects, disk or button batteries, and any obstruction causing significant symptoms.

GASTRIC AND INTESTINAL FOREIGN BODIES

A variety of swallowed objects can become lodged in the stomach or intestines. Some foreign bodies cause obstruction or perforation. Diagnosis is by x-ray. Some foreign bodies can be removed endoscopically.

Of the foreign bodies that reach the stomach, 80 to 90% pass spontaneously through the GI tract, 10 to 20% require nonoperative intervention, and ≤ 1% require surgery. Thus, conservative management is appropriate for most blunt objects in asymptomatic patients. However, objects > 6 cm in length or objects > 2.5 cm in diameter rarely pass through the stomach.[1]

Ingested drug packages (see Body Packing and Body Stuffing on p. 3229) are of great concern because of the risk of leakage and consequent drug overdose. Packages can also cause mechanical obstruction.

1. ASGE Standards of Practice Committee, Ikenberry SO, Jue TL, Anderson MA, et al: Management of ingested foreign bodies and food impactions. *Gastrointest Endosc* 73: 1085–1091, 2011. doi: 10.1016/j.gie.2010.11.010.

Symptoms and Signs

Foreign bodies that pass through the esophagus are asymptomatic unless perforation or obstruction occurs. Perforation of the stomach or intestines manifests with symptoms and signs of peritonitis such as abdominal pain, guarding, and rebound tenderness. Obstruction of the intestines causes abdominal pain and distention and vomiting.

Diagnosis

- Imaging studies

Abdominal x-rays may be done to identify the foreign object and are useful for following the progression of the object through the GI tract. Abdominal x-rays with chest x-rays are also important for identifying signs of perforation (eg, free air that is subdiaphragmatic, mediastinal, or subcutaneous). A hand-held metal detector can localize metallic foreign bodies and provide information comparable to that yielded by plain x-rays. If plain x-rays are negative, a CT scan may helpful.

Suspected body packers and stuffers are usually brought to medical attention by law enforcement officials. Plain x-rays can often confirm the presence of packets in the GI tract. If these x-rays are negative, a CT scan may be helpful.

Treatment

- Observation
- Sometimes endoscopic removal
- Rarely surgery

Management depends on several factors:

- Location of the object
- Nature of the object
- Symptoms and signs

Gastric foreign bodies: Sharp objects should be retrieved from the stomach because 15 to 35% will cause intestinal perforation. Small round objects (eg, coins) can simply be observed for a period of time that varies depending on the nature of the object. The patient's stools should be searched, and if the object does not appear, x-rays are taken at 48-h intervals and then at weekly intervals. The following objects should be removed endoscopically:

- Batteries that cause symptoms or signs of GI tract injury
- Cylindrical batteries and disk batteries that remain in the stomach for > 48 h *without* causing signs of GI injury
- Sharp-pointed objects in the stomach
- Objects > 2.5 cm diameter in the stomach
- Small, round objects (eg, coins) that remain in the stomach after 3 to 4 wk
- Any magnets within endoscopic reach

Intestinal foreign bodies: Most foreign objects that have passed into the small intestine usually traverse the GI tract without problem, even if they take weeks or months to do so. They tend to be held up just before the ileocecal valve or at any site of narrowing. Sometimes objects such as toothpicks remain within the GI tract for many years, only to turn up in a granuloma or abscess.

Single-balloon and double-balloon enteroscopy can be used to access the small bowel and may have a role in the treatment of small-bowel foreign body ingestions in some patients.

Surgical removal should be considered for short, blunt objects that are located in the small bowel, distal to the duodenum, but have not changed location for more than 1 wk and cannot be managed endoscopically.

Drug packages: Patients who have ingested drug packages and who present with symptoms and signs of drug toxicity should receive medical treatment immediately. Prompt surgical evaluation should be obtained when sympathomimetic toxicity, bowel obstruction, perforation, or drug leakage is suspected. Asymptomatic patients should be admitted to the hospital and closely monitored in an intensive care setting.

Endoscopic removal is not recommended for ingested drug packages because of the high risk of package perforation. Some clinicians advocate whole-body irrigation using oral polyethylene glycol solution as a cathartic to enhance passage of the material; others suggest surgical removal. The best practice is unclear.

KEY POINTS

- Foreign bodies that pass through the esophagus are asymptomatic unless perforation or obstruction occurs.
- Abdominal x-rays may identify the foreign object and are useful for following the progression through the GI tract.
- Management depends on the nature of the object, but sharp objects should be retrieved from the stomach.
- Impacted drug packages can cause serious or fatal toxicity; even asymptomatic patients require close monitoring.

RECTAL FOREIGN BODIES

Rectal foreign bodies are usually objects that have been inserted into the rectum but can be caused by swallowed objects. Sudden and excruciating pain during defecation can be caused by a foreign body penetrating the rectal wall. Diagnosis is by digital examination and sometimes x-ray. Removal of a rectal foreign body may be of high risk and should be done by a surgeon or gastroenterologist skilled in foreign body removal.

Gallstones, fecaliths, and swallowed foreign bodies (including toothpicks and chicken and fish bones) may lodge at the anorectal junction. Urinary calculi, vaginal pessaries, or surgical sponges or instruments may erode into the rectum. Foreign bodies, sometimes bizarre and/or related to sexual play, or drug packets inserted in an attempt to conceal them from law enforcement officials, may be introduced intentionally but become lodged unintentionally; occasionally perforation may occur during insertion. Some objects are caught in the rectal wall, and others are trapped just above the anal sphincter.

Symptoms and Signs

Sudden, excruciating pain during defecation should arouse suspicion of a penetrating foreign body, usually lodged at or just above the anorectal junction. The presence of frank blood indicates that a laceration or perforation has occurred. Other manifestations depend on the size and shape of the foreign body, its duration in situ, and the presence of infection or perforation.

Diagnosis

- Digital examination
- Sometimes imaging studies

Foreign bodies usually become lodged in the mid rectum, where they cannot negotiate the anterior angulation of the rectum. They may be felt on digital examination.

A plain x-ray of the abdomen is often helpful in identifying an object. An upright x-ray should also be done to evaluate for free air in the peritoneum due to perforation. CT may help identify radiolucent objects not seen on routine x-ray.

Treatment

- Manual extraction

Removal of a rectal foreign body may be of high risk and should be done by a surgeon or gastroenterologist skilled in foreign body removal. An anoscope, proctoscope, and/or speculum can facilitate direct visualization and removal of rectal foreign bodies.

If the foreign body can be palpated, inject a local anesthetic, dilate the anus with a rectal retractor, and attempt to grasp and remove the foreign body. Regional or general anesthesia is infrequently necessary.

If the object cannot be palpated or visualized, blind attempts to grasp and remove the foreign body should not be made. Peristalsis frequently moves the foreign body down to the mid rectum, and removal attempts can than be made.

Removal via a sigmoidoscope or proctoscope can be attempted but is not always successful. Sometimes sigmoidoscopy forces the foreign body proximally, further delaying its extraction. If attempts to remove the foreign body are unsuccessful, laparotomy with milking of the foreign body toward the anus or colotomy with extraction of the foreign body is rarely necessary. After extraction, sigmoidoscopy should be done to rule out significant rectal injury.

13 Diverticular Disease

Diverticula are saclike mucosal outpouchings that protrude from a tubular structure. True diverticula contain all layers of the parent structure. False or pseudodiverticula are mucosal projections through the muscular layer. Esophageal (see p. 112) and Meckel diverticula are true diverticula. Colonic diverticula are pseudodiverticula; they cause symptoms by trapping feces and becoming inflamed or infected, bleeding, or rupturing.

DIVERTICULOSIS

Diverticulosis is the presence of multiple diverticula in the colon, probably resulting from a lifelong low-fiber diet. Most diverticula are asymptomatic, but some become inflamed or bleed. Diagnosis is by colonoscopy or barium enema. Treatment varies depending on manifestation.

(See also the American College of Gastroenterology's practice guidelines on the diagnosis and management of diverticular disease of the colon in adults.)

Diverticula occur anywhere in the large bowel—usually in the sigmoid but rarely below the peritoneal reflection of the rectum. They vary in diameter from 3 mm to > 3 cm. Patients with diverticula usually have several of them. Diverticulosis is uncommon in people < 40 but becomes common rapidly thereafter; essentially every 90-yr-old person has many diverticula. Giant diverticula, which are rare, range in diameter from 3 to 15 cm and may be single.

Pathophysiology

Diverticula are probably caused by increased intraluminal pressure leading to mucosal extrusion through the weakest points of the muscular layer of the bowel—areas adjacent to intramural blood vessels. Diverticula are more common among people who eat a low-fiber diet; however, the mechanism is not clear. One theory is that increased intraluminal pressure is required to move low-bulk stool through the colon. Another theory is that low-stool bulk causes a smaller diameter colon, which by Laplace's law would have increased pressure.

The etiology of giant diverticula is unclear. One theory is that a valvelike abnormality exists at the base of the diverticulum, so bowel gas can enter but escapes less freely.

Symptoms and Signs

Most (70%) patients with diverticulosis are asymptomatic, 15 to 25% have symptomatic disease resulting from diverticulitis (inflammation of a diverticula), and 10 to 15% can have painless bleeding. The bleeding is probably caused by erosion of the adjacent vessel by local trauma from impacted feces in the diverticulum. Although most diverticula are distal, 75% of bleeding occurs from diverticula proximal to the splenic flexure. In 33% of patients (5% overall), bleeding is serious enough to require transfusion. Rarely, a patient may need surgery (colectomy or partial colectomy) for refractory bleeding.

Diagnosis

- Usually colonoscopy

Asymptomatic diverticula are usually found incidentally during colonoscopy, barium enema, or even CT of the abdomen. Diverticulosis is suspected when painless rectal bleeding develops, particularly in an elderly patient. Evaluation of rectal bleeding typically includes colonoscopy, which can be done electively after routine preparation unless there is significant ongoing bleeding. In such patients, a rapid preparation (5 to 10 L of polyethylene glycol solution delivered via NGT over 3 to 4 h) often allows adequate visualization. If colonoscopy cannot visualize the source and ongoing bleeding is sufficiently rapid (> 0.5 to 1 mL/min), angiography may localize the source. Some angiographers first do a radionuclide scan to focus the examination.

Treatment

- High-fiber diet
- Sometimes angiographic or endoscopic treatment of bleeding

Treatment of diverticulosis aims at reducing segmental spasm. A high-fiber diet helps and may be supplemented by psyllium seed preparations or bran. Low-fiber diets are contraindicated. The intuitive injunction to avoid seeds or other dietary material that might become impacted in a diverticulum has no established medical basis. Antispasmodics (eg, belladonna) are

PEARLS & PITFALLS

- Angiographic embolization can stop diverticular bleeding but causes bowel infarction in up to 20% of patients and is not recommended.

not of benefit and may cause adverse effects. Surgery is unwarranted for uncomplicated disease. Giant diverticula, however, may require surgery.

Diverticular bleeding stops spontaneously in 75% of patients. Treatment is often given during diagnostic procedures. If angiography was done for diagnosis, ongoing bleeding can be controlled in 70 to 90% of patients by intra-arterial injection of vasopressin. In some cases, bleeding recurs within a few days and requires surgery. Angiographic embolization effectively stops bleeding but leads to bowel infarction in up to 20% of patients and is not recommended. Colonoscopy allows heat or laser coagulation of vessels or injection of epinephrine. If these measures fail to stop bleeding, segmental resection or subtotal colectomy is indicated.

KEY POINTS

- Diverticulosis is the presence of multiple diverticula in the colon; diverticulitis is inflammation of a diverticulum.
- Diverticulosis is rare in people < 40 and becomes increasingly common with age, particularly among people who eat a low-fiber diet.
- Painless bleeding develops in 10 to 15% of patients, and painful inflammation (diverticulitis) develops in 15 to 25%.
- Treat asymptomatic patients with a high-fiber diet.
- Bleeding stops spontaneously in about 75% of patients; control the remainder during angiography with intra-arterial vasopressin or during colonoscopy with coagulation or epinephrine injection.

DIVERTICULITIS

Diverticulitis is inflammation of a diverticulum, which can result in phlegmon of the bowel wall, peritonitis, perforation, fistula, or abscess. The primary symptom is abdominal pain. Diagnosis is by CT. Treatment is with bowel rest, antibiotics (ciprofloxacin, or a 3rd-generation cephalosporin plus metronidazole), and occasionally surgery.

Diverticulitis occurs when a micro or macro perforation develops in a diverticulum, releasing intestinal bacteria. The resultant inflammation remains localized in about 75% of patients. The remaining 25% may develop abscess, free intraperitoneal perforation, bowel obstruction, or fistulas. The most common fistulas involve the bladder but may also involve the small bowel, uterus, vagina, abdominal wall, or even the thigh.

Diverticulitis is most serious in elderly patients, especially those taking prednisone or other drugs that increase the risk of infection. Nearly all serious diverticulitis occurs in the sigmoid.

Symptoms and Signs

Diverticulitis usually manifests with pain or tenderness in the left lower quadrant of the abdomen and fever. Peritoneal signs (eg, rebound or guarding) may be present, particularly with abscess or free perforation. Fistulas may manifest as pneumaturia, feculent vaginal discharge, or a cutaneous or myofascial infection of the abdominal wall, perineum, or upper leg. Patients with bowel obstruction have nausea, vomiting, and abdominal distention. Bleeding is uncommon.

Diagnosis

- Abdominal CT
- Colonoscopy after resolution

Clinical suspicion is high in patients with known diverticulosis. However, because other disorders (eg, appendicitis, colon or ovarian cancer) may cause similar symptoms, testing is required. Abdominal CT with oral and IV contrast is preferred, although findings in about 10% of patients cannot be distinguished from colon cancer. Colonoscopy, after resolution of the acute infection, is necessary for definitive diagnosis.

Treatment

- Varies with severity
- Liquid diet, oral antibiotics for mild disease
- IV antibiotics, npo for more severe disease
- CT-guided percutaneous drainage of abscess
- Sometimes surgery

A patient who is not very ill is treated at home with rest, a liquid diet, and oral antibiotics (eg, ciprofloxacin 500 mg bid amoxicillin/clavulanate 500 mg tid plus metronidazole 500 mg qid). Symptoms usually subside rapidly. Some recent data suggest some patients may recover from mild, acute, uncomplicated diverticulitis without antibiotic therapy. The patient gradually advances to a soft, low-fiber diet for 4 to 6 wk. The colon should be evaluated after 6 to 8 wk with a colonoscopy or barium enema. After 1 mo, a high-fiber diet is resumed.

Patients with more severe symptoms (eg, pain, fever, marked leukocytosis) should be hospitalized, as should patients taking prednisone (who are at higher risk of perforation and general peritonitis). Treatment is bed rest, npo, IV fluids, and IV antibiotics (eg, ceftazidime 1 g IV q 8 h plus metronidazole 500 mg IV q 6 to 8 h).

About 80% of patients can be treated successfully without surgery. An abscess may respond to percutaneous drainage (CT guided). If response is satisfactory, the patient remains hospitalized until symptoms are relieved and a soft diet is resumed. A colonoscopy or barium enema is done ≥ 4 wk after symptoms have resolved.

Surgery: Surgery is required immediately for patients with free perforation or general peritonitis and for patients with severe symptoms that do not respond to nonsurgical treatment within 48 h. Increasing pain, tenderness, and fever are other signs that surgery is needed. Surgery should also be considered in patients with any of the following: ≥ 3 previous attacks of mild diverticulitis (or one attack in a patient < 50); a persistent tender mass; clinical, endoscopic, or x-ray signs suggestive of cancer; and dysuria or pneumaturia associated with diverticulitis in men (or in women who have had a hysterectomy) because this symptom may presage fistula formation or perforation into the bladder.

The involved section of the colon is resected. The ends can be reanastomosed immediately in healthy patients without perforation, abscess, or significant inflammation. Other patients have a temporary colostomy with anastomosis carried out in a subsequent operation after inflammation resolves and their general condition improves.

KEY POINTS

- Diverticulosis is the presence of multiple diverticula in the colon; diverticulitis is inflammation of a diverticulum.
- Diverticulitis occurs when a diverticulum perforates, releasing intestinal bacteria.
- Inflammation remains localized in about 75% of patients; the remainder develop abscesses, free intraperitoneal perforation, bowel obstruction, or fistulas.
- Diagnose using abdominal CT with oral and IV contrast; do colonoscopy 6 to 8 wk after resolution to make definitive diagnosis.
- Management depends on severity but typically includes antibiotics and sometimes percutaneous or surgical drainage.

MECKEL DIVERTICULUM

Meckel diverticulum is a congenital sacculation of the distal ileum occurring in 2 to 3% of people. It is usually located within 100 cm of the ileocecal valve and often contains heterotopic gastric tissue, pancreatic tissue, or both. Symptoms are uncommon but include bleeding, bowel obstruction, and inflammation (diverticulitis). Diagnosis is difficult and often involves radionuclide scanning and barium studies. Treatment is surgical resection.

Pathophysiology

In early fetal life, the vitelline duct running from the terminal ileum to the umbilicus and yolk sac is normally obliterated by the 7th wk. If the portion connecting to the ileum fails to atrophy, a Meckel diverticulum results. This congenital diverticulum arises from the antimesenteric margin of the intestine and contains all layers of the normal bowel. About 50% of diverticula also contain heterotopic tissue of the stomach (and thus contain parietal cells that secrete HCl), pancreas, or both.

Only about 2% of people with Meckel diverticulum develop complications. Although diverticula are equally common among males and females, males are 2 to 3 times more likely to have complications. Complications include the following:

- Bleeding
- Obstruction
- Diverticulitis
- Tumors

Bleeding is more common among young children (< 5 yr) and occurs when acid secreted from ectopic gastric mucosa in the diverticulum ulcerates the adjacent ileum. Obstruction can occur at any age but is more common among older children and adults. In children, obstruction is most likely caused by intussusception of the diverticulum. Obstruction may also result from adhesions, volvulus, retained foreign bodies, tumors, or incarceration in a hernia (Littre hernia). Acute Meckel diverticulitis can occur at any age, but its incidence peaks in older children. Tumors, including carcinoids, are rare and occur mainly in adults.

Symptoms and Signs

In all ages, intestinal obstruction is manifested by cramping abdominal pain, nausea, and vomiting. Acute Meckel diverticulitis is characterized by abdominal pain and tenderness typically localized below or to the left of the umbilicus; it is often accompanied by vomiting and is similar to appendicitis except for location of pain.

Children may present with repeated episodes of painless, bright red rectal bleeding, which is usually not severe enough to cause shock. Adults may also bleed, typically resulting in melena rather than frank blood.

Diagnosis

- Based on symptoms
- Radionuclide scan for bleeding
- CT for pain

Diagnosis is difficult, and tests are chosen based on presenting symptoms. If rectal bleeding is suspected to originate from a Meckel diverticulum, a ^{99m}Tc pertechnetate scan may identify ectopic gastric mucosa and hence the diverticulum. Patients presenting with abdominal pain and focal tenderness should have CT with oral contrast. If vomiting and signs of obstruction are predominant, flat and upright x-rays of the abdomen are done. Sometimes diagnosis is made only during surgical exploration for presumed appendicitis; whenever a normal appendix is found, Meckel diverticulum should be suspected.

Treatment

- Surgery

Patients with intestinal obstruction caused by Meckel diverticulum require early surgery. For detailed treatment of intestinal obstruction, see p. 91.

A bleeding diverticulum with an indurated area in the adjacent ileum requires resection of this section of the bowel and the diverticulum. A bleeding diverticulum without ileal induration requires only resection of the diverticulum.

Meckel diverticulitis also requires resection. Small, asymptomatic diverticula encountered incidentally at laparotomy need not be removed.

KEY POINTS

- Meckel diverticulum is a common congenital sacculation of the distal ileum that occasionally bleeds, becomes inflamed, or causes obstruction.
- About half of diverticula contain heterotopic gastric tissue that secretes HCl, which can cause ulcers of the adjacent ileum.
- Patients may have pain similar to that of appendicitis, or painless bleeding.
- Select tests based on presenting symptoms.
- Remove symptomatic diverticula surgically; asymptomatic, incidentally discovered diverticula need not be removed.

DIVERTICULAR DISEASE OF THE STOMACH AND SMALL BOWEL

Diverticula rarely involve the stomach but occur in the duodenum in up to 25% of people. Most duodenal diverticula are solitary and occur in the second portion of the duodenum near the ampulla of Vater (periampullary). Jejunal diverticula occur in about 0.26% of patients and are more common among patients with disorders of intestinal motility. Meckel diverticulum occurs in the distal ileum.

Duodenal and jejunal diverticula are asymptomatic in > 90% of cases and are usually detected incidentally during radiologic or endoscopic investigation of the upper GI tract for an unrelated disease. Rarely, small-bowel diverticula bleed or become inflamed, causing pain and nausea. Some even perforate. For poorly understood reasons, patients with periampullary diverticula are at increased risk of gallstones and pancreatitis. Treatment is surgical resection; however, the clinician should be cautious of recommending surgery for patients with a diverticulum and vague GI symptoms (eg, dyspepsia).

14 Esophageal and Swallowing Disorders

(See also Esophageal Cancer on p. 164 and Esophageal Atresia on p. 2524.)

The swallowing apparatus consists of the pharynx, upper esophageal (cricopharyngeal) sphincter, the body of the esophagus, and the lower esophageal sphincter (LES). The upper third of the esophagus and the structures proximal to it are composed of skeletal muscle; the distal esophagus and LES are composed of smooth muscle. These components work as an integrated system that transports material from the mouth to the stomach and prevents its reflux into the esophagus. Physical obstruction or disorders that interfere with motor function (esophageal motility disorders) can affect the system.

The patient's history suggests the diagnosis almost 80% of the time. The only physical findings in esophageal disorders are cervical and supraclavicular lymphadenopathy caused by metastasis, swellings in the neck caused by large pharyngeal diverticula or thyromegaly, white plaques in the posterior oropharynx caused by *Candida* infection, and prolonged swallowing time (the time from the act of swallowing to the sound of the bolus of fluid and air entering the stomach—normally ≤ 12 sec—heard by auscultation with the stethoscope over the epigastrium). Watching the patient swallow may help diagnose aspiration or nasal regurgitation. Most esophageal disorders require specific tests for diagnosis.

Esophageal and swallowing disorders include the following:

- Achalasia
- Cricopharyngeal incoordination
- Dysphagia
- Dysphagia lusoria
- Eosinophilic esophagitis
- Esophageal diverticula
- Esophageal motility disorders
- Esophageal rupture
- Esophageal web
- Gastroesophageal reflux disease (GERD)
- Hiatus hernia
- Infectious esophageal disorders
- Lower esophageal ring
- Mallory-Weiss syndrome
- Obstructive disorders of the esophagus
- Symptomatic diffuse esophageal spasm

ACHALASIA

(Cardiospasm; Esophageal Aperistalsis; Megaesophagus)

Achalasia is a neurogenic esophageal motility disorder characterized by impaired esophageal peristalsis and a lack of LES relaxation during swallowing. Symptoms are slowly progressive dysphagia, usually to both liquids and solids, and regurgitation of undigested food. Evaluation typically includes manometry, barium swallow, and endoscopy. Treatments include dilation, chemical denervation, surgical myotomy, and peroral endoscopic myotomy.

(See also the American College of Gastroenterology's practice guidelines on the diagnosis and management of achalasia.)

Achalasia is thought to be caused by a loss of ganglion cells in the myenteric plexus of the esophagus, resulting in denervation of esophageal muscle. Etiology of the denervation is unknown, but viral and autoimmune causes are suspected, and certain tumors may cause achalasia either by direct obstruction or as a paraneoplastic process. Chagas disease, which causes destruction of autonomic ganglia, may result in achalasia.

Increased pressure at the LES causes obstruction with secondary dilation of the esophagus. Esophageal retention of undigested food and liquid is common.

Symptoms and Signs

Achalasia occurs at any age but usually begins between ages 20 and 60. Onset is insidious, and progression is gradual over months or years. Dysphagia for both solids and liquids is the major symptom. Nocturnal regurgitation of undigested food occurs in about 33% of patients and may cause cough and pulmonary aspiration. Chest pain is less common but may occur on swallowing or spontaneously. Mild to moderate weight loss occurs; when weight loss is pronounced, particularly in elderly patients whose symptoms of dysphagia developed rapidly, achalasia secondary to a tumor of the gastroesophageal junction should be considered.

Diagnosis

- Esophageal manometry
- Sometimes barium swallow

Esophageal manometry is the preferred diagnostic test for achalasia. This test shows incomplete relaxation of the LES with an integrated relaxation pressure ≥ 15, and 100% failed peristalsis.

Barium swallow is a complementary test that is often done during the initial phase of testing and that may show absence of progressive peristaltic contractions during swallowing. Typically, the esophagus is dilated, often enormously, but is narrowed and beaklike at the LES.

If esophagoscopy is done, there is esophageal dilation but no obstructing lesion, and a classic "pop" is often felt when the esophagoscope passes into the stomach. Rarely, these findings can result from a tumor; endoscopic ultrasonography with biopsies can be considered to rule out cancer.

Achalasia must be differentiated from a distal stenosing carcinoma and a peptic stricture, particularly in patients with systemic sclerosis, in whom esophageal manometry may also show aperistalsis. Systemic sclerosis is usually accompanied by a history of Raynaud phenomenon and symptoms of GERD due to low or absent LES pressure.

Achalasia due to cancer at the gastroesophageal junction can be diagnosed by CT of the chest and abdomen or by endoscopic ultrasound with biopsy.

Prognosis

Pulmonary aspiration and the presence of cancer are the determining prognostic factors. Nocturnal regurgitation and coughing suggest aspiration. Pulmonary complications secondary to aspiration are difficult to manage. Incidence of esophageal cancer in patients with achalasia may be increased; this point is controversial.

Treatment

- Balloon dilation or surgical myotomy of the LES
- Sometimes peroral endoscopic myotomy
- Sometimes botulinum toxin injection

No therapy restores peristalsis; treatment of achalasia is aimed at reducing the pressure at the LES.

Balloon dilation of the LES and surgical myotomy appear similarly effective. In 2016, a randomized, controlled trial involving achalasia patients found that at 5-yr follow-up pneumatic balloon dilation had comparable efficacy to laparoscopic Heller myotomy.[1] The most concerning complication of these procedures is esophageal perforation. Perforation rates vary by center, ranging from 0 to 14% for pneumatic balloon dilation and 0 to 4.6% for laparoscopic Heller myotomy.[2] Other current studies have shown peroral endoscopic myotomy to have a good short-term outcome.[3] Thus, choice between these three procedures depends on the operator and the particular type of achalasia.

In patients who are not candidates for these treatment options, chemical denervation of cholinergic nerves in the distal esophagus by direct endoscopic injection of botulinum toxin type A into the LES may be tried. Clinical improvement occurs in 70 to 80% of patients, but results may last only 6 mo to 1 yr.

Reducing pressure at the LES can increase the occurrence of GERD. The incidence varies depending on which type of treatment is done. On average, it is estimated that about 20% of patients have postprocedural GERD.

Drugs such as nitrates (eg, isosorbide dinitrate 5 to 10 mg sublingually before meals) or calcium channel blockers (eg, nifedipine 10 to 30 mg po 30 to 45 min before a meal) may be tried. These drugs are of limited effectiveness but may reduce LES pressure enough to prolong the time between dilations.

1. Moonen A, Annese V, Belmans A, et al: Long-term results of the European achalasia trial: A multicentre randomised controlled trial comparing pneumatic dilation versus laparoscopic Heller myotomy. *Gut* 65(5):732–739, 2016. doi: 10.1136/gutjnl-2015-310602.
2. Lynch KL, Pandolfino JE, Howden CW, et al: Major complications of pneumatic dilation and Heller myotomy for achalasia: Single-center experience and systematic review of the literature. *Am J Gastroenterol* 107(12):1817–1825, 2012. doi: 10.1038/ajg.2012.332.
3. Rentein DV, Fuchs K-H, Fockens P, et al: Peroral endoscopic myotomy for the treatment of achalasia: An international prospective multicenter study. *Gastroenterology* 145(2): 272–273, 2013. doi: 10.1053/j.gastro.2013.04.057

KEY POINTS

- A viral- or autoimmune-induced loss of ganglion cells in the myenteric plexus of the esophagus decreases esophageal peristalsis and impairs relaxation of the LES.
- Patients gradually develop dysphagia for both solids and liquids, and about one third regurgitate undigested food at night.
- Esophageal manometry is the preferred test for achalasia and shows an elevated integrated relaxation pressure in conjunction with 100% failed peristalsis.
- Barium swallow shows absence of progressive peristaltic contractions during swallowing and a markedly dilated esophagus with beaklike narrowing at the LES.
- No therapy restores peristalsis; treatment aims to reduce the pressure (and thus the obstruction) at the LES.
- Treatment is typically pneumatic balloon dilation or myotomy of the LES.

CRICOPHARYNGEAL INCOORDINATION

In cricopharyngeal incoordination, the cricopharyngeal muscle (the upper esophageal sphincter) is uncoordinated. It can cause a Zenker diverticulum. Repeated aspiration of material from the diverticulum can lead to chronic lung disease.

The condition can be treated by surgical section of the cricopharyngeal muscle.

DYSPHAGIA

Dysphagia is difficulty swallowing. The condition results from impeded transport of liquids, solids, or both from the pharynx to the stomach. Dysphagia should not be confused with globus sensation, a feeling of having a lump in the throat, which is unrelated to swallowing and occurs without impaired transport.

Complications: Dysphagia can lead to tracheal aspiration of ingested material, oral secretions, or both. Aspiration can cause acute pneumonia; recurrent aspiration may eventually lead to chronic lung disease. Prolonged dysphagia often leads to inadequate nutrition and weight loss.

Etiology

Dysphagia is classified as oropharyngeal or esophageal, depending on where it occurs.

Oropharyngeal dysphagia: Oropharyngeal dysphagia is difficulty emptying material from the oropharynx into the esophagus; it results from abnormal function proximal to the esophagus. Patients complain of difficulty initiating swallowing, nasal regurgitation, and tracheal aspiration followed by coughing.

Most often, oropharyngeal dysphagia occurs in patients with neurologic conditions or muscular disorders that affect skeletal muscles (see Table 14–1).

Esophageal dysphagia: Esophageal dysphagia is difficulty passing food down the esophagus. It results from either a motility disorder or a mechanical obstruction (see Table 14–2).

Evaluation

History: History of present illness begins with duration of symptoms and acuity of onset. Patients should describe what substances cause difficulty and where they feel the disturbance

Table 14–1. SOME CAUSES OF OROPHARYNGEAL DYSPHAGIA

MECHANISM	EXAMPLES
Neurologic	Stroke Parkinson disease Multiple sclerosis Some motor neuron disorders (amyotrophic lateral sclerosis, progressive bulbar palsy, pseudobulbar palsy) Bulbar poliomyelitis Giant cell arteritis
Muscular	Myasthenia gravis Dermatomyositis Muscular dystrophy Cricopharyngeal incoordination

Table 14–2. SOME CAUSES OF ESOPHAGEAL DYSPHAGIA

MECHANISM	EXAMPLES
Motility disorder	Achalasia Diffuse esophageal spasm Systemic sclerosis Eosinophilic esophagitis
Mechanical obstruction	Peptic stricture Esophageal cancer Lower esophageal rings Esophageal webs Radiation stricture Extrinsic compression (eg, caused by an enlarged left atrium, an aortic aneurysm, an aberrant subclavian artery [termed dysphagia lusoria], a substernal thyroid, a cervical bony exostosis, or a thoracic tumor) Caustic ingestion

is located. Specific concerns include whether patients have difficulty swallowing solids, liquids, or both; whether food comes out their nose; whether they drool or have food spill from their mouth; whether they have had food impaction; and whether they cough or choke while eating.

Review of symptoms should focus on symptoms suggestive of neuromuscular, GI, and connective tissue disorders and on the presence of complications. Important neuromuscular symptoms include weakness and easy fatigability, gait or balance disturbance, tremor, and difficulty speaking. Important GI symptoms include heartburn or other chest discomfort suggestive of reflux. Symptoms of connective tissue disorders include muscle and joint pain, Raynaud phenomenon, and skin changes (eg, rash, swelling, thickening).

Past medical history should ascertain known diseases that may cause dysphagia (see Tables 14–1 and 14–2).

Physical examination: Examination focuses on findings suggestive of neuromuscular, GI, and connective tissue disorders and on the presence of complications.

General examination should evaluate nutritional status (including body weight). A complete neurologic examination is essential, with attention to any resting tremor, the cranial nerves (note the gag reflex may normally be absent; this absence is thus not a good marker of swallowing dysfunction), and muscle strength. Patients who describe easy fatigability should be observed performing a repetitive action (eg, blinking, counting aloud) for a rapid decrement in performance. The patient's gait should be observed, and balance should be tested. Skin is examined for rash and thickening or texture changes, particularly on the fingertips. Muscles are inspected for wasting and fasciculations and are palpated for tenderness. The neck is evaluated for thyromegaly or other mass.

Red flags: Any dysphagia is of concern, but certain findings are more urgent:

- Symptoms of complete obstruction (eg, drooling, inability to swallow anything)
- Dysphagia resulting in weight loss
- New focal neurologic deficit, particularly any objective weakness

Interpretation of findings: Dysphagia that occurs in conjunction with an acute neurologic event is likely the result of that event; new dysphagia in a patient with a stable, long-standing neurologic disorder may have another etiology. Dysphagia for solids alone suggests mechanical obstruction; however, a problem with both solids and liquids is nonspecific. Drooling and spilling food from the mouth while eating or nasal regurgitation suggests an oropharyngeal disorder. Regurgitation of a small amount of food on lateral compression of the neck is virtually diagnostic of pharyngeal diverticulum.

Patients who complain of difficulty getting food to leave the mouth or of food sticking in the lower esophagus are usually correct about the condition's location; the sensation of dysphagia in the upper esophagus is less specific.

Many findings suggest specific disorders (see Table 14–3) but are of varying sensitivity and specificity and thus do not rule in or out a given cause; however, they can guide testing.

Table 14–3. SOME HELPFUL FINDINGS IN DYSPHAGIA

FINDING	POSSIBLE CAUSE
Tremor, ataxia, balance disturbance	Parkinson disease
Focal easy fatigability, particularly of facial muscles	Myasthenia gravis
Muscle fasciculation, wasting, weakness	Motor neuron disease, myopathy
Rapidly progressive, constant dysphagia, no neurologic findings	Esophageal obstruction, probably cancer
Food impaction	Eosinophilic esophagitis
GI reflux symptoms	Peptic stricture
Intermittent dysphagia	Lower esophageal ring or diffuse esophageal spasm
Slow progression (months to years) of dysphagia to solids and liquids, sometimes with nocturnal regurgitation	Achalasia
Neck mass, thyromegaly	Extrinsic compression
Dusky, erythematous rash, muscle tenderness	Dermatomyositis
Raynaud phenomenon, arthralgias, skin tightening/contractures of fingers	Systemic sclerosis
Cough, dyspnea, lung congestions	Pulmonary aspiration

Testing

- Upper endoscopy

Patients with dysphagia should always have upper endoscopy, which is extremely important to rule out cancer. During endoscopy, esophageal biopsies should also be done to look for eosinophilic esophagitis. A barium swallow (with a solid bolus, usually a marshmallow or tablet) can be done if the patient is unable to undergo an upper endoscopy. If the barium swallow is negative and the upper endoscopy is normal, esophageal motility studies should be done. Other tests for specific causes are done as suggested by findings.

Treatment

Treatment of dysphagia is directed at the specific cause. If complete obstruction occurs, emergent upper endoscopy is essential. If a stricture, ring, or web is found, careful endoscopic dilation is performed. Pending resolution, patients with oropharyngeal dysphagia may benefit from evaluation by a rehabilitation specialist. Sometimes patients benefit from changing head position while eating, retraining the swallowing muscles, doing exercises that improve the ability to accommodate a food bolus in the oral cavity, or doing strength and coordination exercises for the tongue. Patients with severe dysphagia and recurrent aspiration may require a gastrostomy tube.

Geriatrics Essentials

Chewing, swallowing, tasting, and communicating require intact, coordinated neuromuscular function in the mouth, face, and neck. Oral motor function in particular declines measurably with aging, even in healthy people. Decline in function may have many manifestations:

- Reduction in masticatory muscle strength and coordination is common, especially among patients with partial or complete dentures, and may lead to a tendency to swallow larger food particles, which can increase the risk of choking or aspiration.
- Drooping of the lower face and lips caused by decreased circumoral muscle tone and, in edentulous people, reduced bone support, is an aesthetic concern and can lead to drooling, spilling of food and liquids, and difficulty closing the lips while eating, sleeping, or resting. Sialorrhea (saliva leakage) is often the first symptom.
- Swallowing difficulties increase. It takes longer to move food from mouth to oropharynx, which increases the likelihood of aspiration.

After age-related changes, the most common causes of oral motor disorders are neuromuscular disorders (eg, cranial neuropathies caused by diabetes, stroke, Parkinson disease, amyotrophic lateral sclerosis, multiple sclerosis). Iatrogenic causes also contribute. Drugs (eg, anticholinergics, diuretics), radiation therapy to the head and neck, and chemotherapy can greatly impair saliva production. Hyposalivation is a major cause of delayed and impaired swallowing.

Oral motor dysfunction is best managed with a multidisciplinary approach. Coordinated referrals to specialists in prosthetic dentistry, rehabilitative medicine, speech pathology, otolaryngology, and gastroenterology may be needed.

KEY POINTS

- All patients complaining of esophageal dysphagia should undergo upper endoscopy to rule out cancer.
- If the upper endoscopy is normal, biopsies should be obtained to rule out eosinophilic esophagitis.
- Treatment of dysphagia is geared toward the cause.

DYSPHAGIA LUSORIA

Dysphagia lusoria is caused by compression of the esophagus from any of several congenital vascular abnormalities.

The vascular abnormality is usually an aberrant right subclavian artery arising from the left side of the aortic arch, a double aortic arch, or a right aortic arch with left ligamentum arteriosum. The dysphagia may develop in childhood or later in life as a result of arteriosclerotic changes in the aberrant vessel.

Barium swallow shows the extrinsic compression, but arteriography is necessary for absolute diagnosis.

Most patients require no treatment, but surgical repair is sometimes done.

EOSINOPHILIC ESOPHAGITIS

Eosinophilic esophagitis is a chronic immune-mediated disease of the esophagus resulting in eosinophil-predominant inflammation of the esophagus; it can cause reflux-like symptoms, dysphagia, and food impaction.

(See also the American College of Gastroenterology's Evidenced Based Approach to the Diagnosis and Management of Esophageal Eosinophilia and Eosinophilic Esophagitis [EoE].)

Eosinophilic esophagitis is an increasingly recognized disease that can begin at any time between infancy and young adulthood; it occasionally manifests in older adults. It is more common among males.

The cause is likely an immune response to dietary antigens in patients with genetic susceptibility; environmental allergens may also play a role. Untreated chronic esophageal inflammation ultimately can lead to esophageal narrowing and strictures.

Symptoms

Infants and children may present with food refusal, vomiting, and/or chest pain.

In adults, esophageal food impaction is sometimes the first manifestation, and most patients have dysphagia. Symptoms of GERD, such as heartburn, may occur.

Patients often also have manifestations of other atopic disorders (eg, asthma, eczema, allergic rhinitis).

Diagnosis

- Endoscopy with biopsy
- Sometimes a barium swallow

The diagnosis of eosinophilic esophagitis is often first considered when reflux symptoms fail to respond to acid-suppression therapy. It should also be considered in adults who present with esophageal food impaction or in adults who have noncardiac chest pain.

Diagnosis requires endoscopy with biopsy showing eosinophilic infiltration (> 15 eosinophils/high-powered field). Although visible abnormalities (eg, furrows, strictures, rings) may be apparent on endoscopy, the appearance can be normal, so biopsies are essential. Because GERD can also cause eosinophilic infiltrates, patients who have mainly reflux symptoms should probably have endoscopy only after failure of a 2-mo trial of a proton pump inhibitor.

A barium swallow may show a feline esophagus, ringed esophagus, narrow-caliber esophagus, or strictures.

Testing for food allergies is often done to identify possible triggers; alternatives include skin testing, radioallergosorbent testing (RAST), or trial of an elimination diet.

Treatment

- Topical corticosteroids
- Elimination diet
- Sometimes esophageal dilation

In adults, topical corticosteroids are often given to treat eosinophilic esophagitis. Patients may use a multi-dose inhaler of fluticasone (220 mcg) or budesonide (180 mcg) 30 min before breakfast and 30 min before dinner; they puff the drug into their mouth without inhaling and then swallow it. Budesonide (0.5 mg/2 mL mixed with a sugar substitute and swallowed 30 min before breakfast and 30 min before dinner) also can be mixed into a slurry and swallowed. They are given for 8 wk.

Dietary changes are also tried and are usually more effective in children than adults; food allergens identified by testing are eliminated from the diet or patients can follow a prespecified elimination diet (see Table 175–5 on p. 1386).

Patients who have significant strictures may need careful esophageal dilation using a balloon or esophageal dilator; multiple, careful, progressive dilations are done to help prevent esophageal tears or perforation.

ESOPHAGEAL DIVERTICULA

An esophageal diverticulum is an outpouching of mucosa through the muscular layer of the esophagus. It can be asymptomatic or cause dysphagia and regurgitation. Diagnosis is made by barium swallow; surgical repair is rarely required.

There are several types of esophageal diverticula, each of different origin.

- Zenker (pharyngeal) diverticula are posterior outpouchings of mucosa and submucosa through the cricopharyngeal muscle, probably resulting from an incoordination between pharyngeal propulsion and cricopharyngeal relaxation.
- Midesophageal (traction) diverticula are caused by traction from mediastinal inflammatory lesions or, secondarily, by esophageal motility disorders.
- Epiphrenic diverticula occur just above the diaphragm and usually accompany a motility disorder (achalasia, diffuse esophageal spasm).

Symptoms and Signs

A Zenker diverticulum fills with food that might be regurgitated when the patient bends or lies down. Aspiration pneumonitis may result if regurgitation is nocturnal. Rarely, the pouch becomes large, causing dysphagia and sometimes a palpable neck mass.

Traction and epiphrenic diverticula are rarely symptomatic, although their underlying cause may be.

Diagnosis

All diverticula are diagnosed by videotaped barium swallow.

Treatment

- Usually none
- Sometimes surgical resection

Specific treatment is usually not required, although resection is occasionally necessary for large or symptomatic diverticula. Diverticula associated with motility disorders require treatment of the primary disorder. For example, case reports suggest doing a cricopharyngeal myotomy when resecting a Zenker diverticulum.

ESOPHAGEAL MOTILITY DISORDERS

Esophageal motility disorders involve dysfunction of the esophagus that causes symptoms such as dysphagia, heartburn, and chest pain.

Primary esophageal causes of dysmotility include

- Achalasia
- Diffuse esophageal spasm
- Eosinophilic esophagitis

Esophageal motility also can be disturbed by systemic disorders such as

- Systemic sclerosis
- Chagas disease

Many generalized disorders of neuromuscular function (eg, myasthenia gravis, amyotrophic lateral sclerosis, stroke, Parkinson disease) can affect swallowing but are not typically classified as esophageal motility disorders.

Symptoms of esophageal motility disorders depend on the cause but typically include difficulty swallowing (dysphagia), chest pain, and/or heartburn.

Evaluation of esophageal motility disorders depends on the patient's presenting symptoms and may include upper GI endoscopy, barium swallow, esophageal manometry, and/or acid- and reflux-related tests.

ESOPHAGEAL RUPTURE

Esophageal rupture may be iatrogenic during endoscopic procedures or other instrumentation or may be spontaneous (Boerhaave syndrome). Patients are seriously ill, with symptoms of mediastinitis. Diagnosis is by esophagography with a water-soluble contrast agent. Immediate surgical repair and drainage are required.

Endoscopic procedures are the primary cause of esophageal rupture, but spontaneous rupture may occur, typically related to vomiting, retching, or swallowing a large food bolus. The most common site of rupture is the distal esophagus on the left side. Acid and other stomach contents cause a fulminant mediastinitis and shock. Pneumomediastinum is common.

Symptoms and Signs

Symptoms of esophageal rupture include chest and abdominal pain, fever, vomiting, hematemesis, and shock. Subcutaneous emphysema is palpable in about 30% of patients. Mediastinal crunch (Hamman sign), a crackling sound synchronous with the heartbeat, may be present.

Diagnosis

- Chest and abdominal x-rays
- Esophagography

Chest and abdominal x-rays showing mediastinal air, pleural effusion, or mediastinal widening suggest the diagnosis.

Diagnosis of esophageal rupture is confirmed by esophagography with a water-soluble contrast agent, which avoids potential mediastinal irritation from barium. CT of the thorax detects mediastinal air and fluid but does not localize the perforation well. Endoscopy may miss a small perforation.

Treatment

- Endoscopic stenting or surgical repair

Pending surgical repair or endoscopic stenting, patients should receive broad-spectrum antibiotics (eg, gentamicin plus metronidazole or piperacillin/tazobactam) and fluid resuscitation as needed for shock. Even with treatment, mortality is high.

ESOPHAGEAL WEB

(Plummer-Vinson Syndrome; Paterson-Kelly Syndrome; Sideropenic Dysphagia)

An esophageal web is a thin mucosal membrane that grows across the lumen and causes dysphagia.

Rarely, webs develop in patients with untreated severe iron deficiency anemia; they develop even more rarely in patients without anemia. Webs usually occur in the upper esophagus, causing dysphagia for solids. They are best diagnosed by barium swallow.

Webs resolve with treatment of the anemia but can be easily ruptured during esophagoscopy.

GASTROESOPHAGEAL REFLUX DISEASE

Incompetence of the LES allows reflux of gastric contents into the esophagus, causing burning pain. Prolonged reflux may lead to esophagitis, stricture, and rarely metaplasia or cancer. Diagnosis is clinical, sometimes with endoscopy, with or without acid testing. Treatment involves lifestyle modification, acid suppression using proton pump inhibitors, and sometimes surgical repair.

GERD is common, occurring in 10 to 20% of adults. It also occurs frequently in infants, typically beginning at birth (see p. 2582).

Etiology

The presence of reflux implies lower esophageal sphincter incompetence, which may result from a generalized loss of intrinsic sphincter tone or from recurrent inappropriate transient relaxations (ie, unrelated to swallowing). Transient LES relaxations are triggered by gastric distention or subthreshold pharyngeal stimulation.

Factors that contribute to the competence of the gastroesophageal junction include the angle of the cardioesophageal junction, the action of the diaphragm, and gravity (ie, an upright position). Factors that may contribute to reflux include weight gain, fatty foods, caffeinated or carbonated beverages, alcohol, tobacco smoking, and drugs. Drugs that lower LES pressure include anticholinergics, antihistamines, tricyclic antidepressants, calcium channel blockers, progesterone, and nitrates.

Complications: GERD may lead to esophagitis, peptic esophageal ulcer, esophageal stricture, Barrett esophagus, and esophageal adenocarcinoma. Factors that contribute to the development of esophagitis include the caustic nature of the refluxate, the inability to clear the refluxate from the esophagus, the volume of gastric contents, and local mucosal protective functions. Some patients, particularly infants, may aspirate the reflux material.

Symptoms and Signs

The most prominent symptom of GERD is heartburn, with or without regurgitation of gastric contents into the mouth. Infants present with vomiting, irritability, anorexia, and sometimes symptoms of chronic aspiration. Both adults and infants with chronic aspiration may have cough, hoarseness, or wheezing.

Esophagitis may cause odynophagia and even esophageal hemorrhage, which is usually occult but can be massive. Peptic strictures cause a gradually progressive dysphagia for solid foods. Peptic esophageal ulcers cause the same type of pain as gastric or duodenal ulcers, but the pain is usually localized to the xiphoid or high substernal region. Peptic esophageal ulcers heal slowly, tend to recur, and usually leave a stricture on healing.

Diagnosis

- Clinical diagnosis
- Endoscopy for patients not responding to empiric treatment
- 24-h pH testing for patients with typical symptoms but normal endoscopy

A detailed history points to the diagnosis. Patients with typical symptoms of GERD may be given a trial of acid-suppressing therapy. Patients who do not improve, or have long-standing symptoms or symptoms of complications, should undergo further testing.

Endoscopy, with cytologic washings and/or biopsy of abnormal areas, is the test of choice. Endoscopic biopsy is the only test that consistently detects the columnar mucosal changes of Barrett esophagus. Patients with unremarkable endoscopy findings who have typical symptoms despite treatment with proton pump inhibitors should undergo 24-h pH testing. Although barium swallow readily shows esophageal ulcers and peptic strictures, it is less useful for mild to moderate reflux; in addition, most patients with abnormalities require subsequent endoscopy.

Esophageal manometry is used to evaluate esophageal peristalsis before surgical treatment.

Treatment

- Head of bed elevated
- Coffee, alcohol, fats, and smoking avoided
- Proton pump inhibitors, H_2 blockers

Management of uncomplicated GERD consists of elevating the head of the bed about 15 cm (6 in) and avoiding the following:

- Eating within 2 to 3 h of bedtime
- Strong stimulants of acid secretion (eg, coffee, alcohol)
- Certain drugs (eg, anticholinergics)
- Specific foods (eg, fats, chocolate)
- Smoking

Weight loss is recommended for overweight patients and those who have gained weight recently.

Drug therapy is often with a proton pump inhibitor; all appear equally effective. For example, adults can be given omeprazole 20 mg, lansoprazole 30 mg, pantoprazole 40 mg, or esomeprazole 40 mg 30 min before breakfast. In some cases (eg, only partial response to once/day dosing), proton pump inhibitors may be given twice daily. Infants and children may be given these drugs at an appropriate lower single daily dose (ie, omeprazole 20 mg in children > 3 yr, 10 mg in children < 3 yr; lansoprazole 15 mg in children ≤ 30 kg, 30 mg in children > 30 kg). These drugs may be continued long-term, but the dose should be adjusted to the minimum required to prevent symptoms, including intermittent or as-needed dosing. H_2 blockers (eg, ranitidine 150 mg at bedtime) or promotility agents (eg, metoclopramide 10 mg po 30 min before meals and at bedtime) are less effective but may be added to a proton pump inhibitor regimen.

Antireflux surgery (usually fundoplication via laparoscopy) is done in patients with serious esophagitis, large hiatal hernias, hemorrhage, stricture, or ulcers. Esophageal strictures are managed by repeated endoscopic dilation.

Barrett esophagus may or may not regress with medical or surgical therapy. (See also the American College of Gastroenterology's updated guidelines for the diagnosis, surveillance, and therapy of Barrett's esophagus.) Because Barrett esophagus is a precursor to adenocarcinoma, endoscopic surveillance for malignant transformation is recommended every 3 to 5 yr in nondysplastic disease. The American College of Gastroenterology's 2015 guidelines recommend endoscopic ablative therapy for patients with confirmed low-grade dysplasia and without life-limiting comorbidity; however, endoscopic surveillance every 12 mo is an acceptable alternative. Patients with Barrett esophagus and confirmed high-grade dysplasia should be managed with endoscopic ablative therapy unless they have life-limiting comorbidity. Endoscopic ablative techniques for Barrett esophagus include mucosal resection, photodynamic therapy, cryotherapy, and laser ablation.

KEY POINTS

- LES incompetence and transient relaxations allow gastric contents to reflux into the esophagus and sometimes into the larynx or lungs.
- Complications include esophagitis, peptic esophageal ulcer, esophageal stricture, Barrett esophagus, and esophageal adenocarcinoma.
- The main symptom in adults is heartburn, and infants present with vomiting, irritability, anorexia, and sometimes symptoms of chronic aspiration; at any age, chronic aspiration may cause cough, hoarseness, or wheezing.
- Diagnose clinically; do endoscopy in patients not responding to empiric treatment and 24-h pH monitoring if endoscopy is normal in patients with typical symptoms.
- Treat with lifestyle changes (eg, head of bed elevation, weight loss, dietary trigger avoidance) and acid-suppressing therapy.
- Antireflux surgery can help patients with complications or a large amount of symptomatic nonacid reflux.

HIATUS HERNIA

Hiatus hernia is a protrusion of the stomach through the diaphragmatic hiatus. Most hernias are asymptomatic, but an increased incidence of acid reflux may lead to symptoms of GERD. Diagnosis is by barium swallow. Treatment is directed at symptoms of GERD if present.

Etiology

Etiology is usually unknown, but a hiatus hernia is thought to be acquired through stretching of the fascial attachments between the esophagus and diaphragm at the hiatus (the opening through which the esophagus traverses the diaphragm—see Fig. 14–1).

Pathophysiology

In a sliding hiatus hernia (the most common type), the gastroesophageal junction and a portion of the stomach are above the diaphragm. In a paraesophageal hiatus hernia, the gastroesophageal junction is in the normal location, but a portion of the stomach is adjacent to the esophagus in the diaphragmatic hiatus. Hernias may also occur through other parts of the diaphragm (see p. 2523).

A sliding hiatus hernia is common and is an incidental finding on x-ray in > 40% of the population; therefore, the relationship of hernia to symptoms is unclear. Although most patients with GERD have some degree of hiatus hernia, < 50% of patients with hiatus hernia have GERD.

Symptoms and Signs

Most patients with a sliding hiatus hernia are asymptomatic, but chest pain and other reflux symptoms can occur. A paraesophageal hiatus hernia is generally asymptomatic but, unlike a sliding hiatus hernia, may incarcerate and strangulate. Occult or massive GI hemorrhage may occur with either type.

Diagnosis

- Barium swallow
- Sometimes upper endoscopy

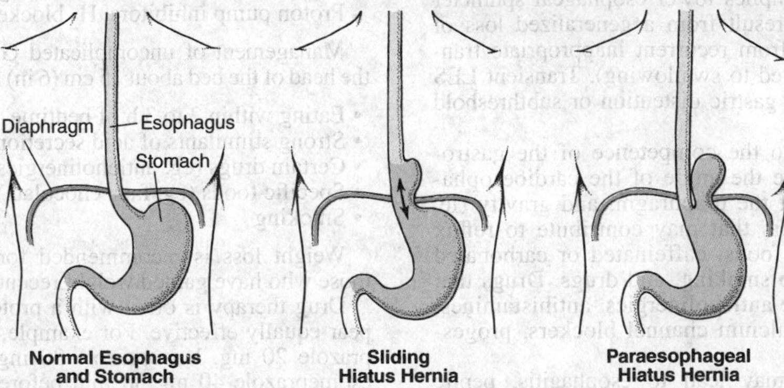

Fig. 14–1. Understanding hiatus hernia. A hiatus hernia is an abnormal bulging of a portion of the stomach through the diaphragm.

A large hiatus hernia is often discovered incidentally on chest x-ray. Smaller hernias are diagnosed with a barium swallow.

Hernias can also be seen with upper endoscopy.

Treatment

- Sometimes surgical repair
- Sometimes a proton pump inhibitor

An asymptomatic sliding hiatus hernia requires no specific therapy. Patients with accompanying GERD should be treated with a proton pump inhibitor.

A paraesophageal hernia should be reduced surgically because of the risk of strangulation.

INFECTIOUS ESOPHAGEAL DISORDERS

Esophageal infection occurs mainly in patients with impaired host defenses. Primary agents include *Candida albicans*, herpes simplex virus HSV, and cytomegalovirus (CMV). Symptoms are odynophagia and chest pain. Diagnosis is by endoscopic visualization and culture. Treatment is with antifungal or antiviral drugs.

Esophageal infection is rare in patients with normal host defenses. Primary esophageal defenses include saliva, esophageal motility, and cellular immunity. Thus, at-risk patients include those with AIDS, organ transplants, alcoholism, diabetes, undernutrition, cancer, and esophageal motility disorders. *Candida* infection may occur in any of these patients. HSV and CMV infections occur mainly in AIDS and transplant patients.

Candida esophagitis: Patients with *Candida* esophagitis usually complain of odynophagia and, less commonly, dysphagia. About two-thirds of patients have signs of oral thrush (thus its absence does not exclude esophageal involvement). Patients with odynophagia and typical thrush may be given empiric treatment, but if significant improvement does not occur in 5 to 7 days, endoscopic evaluation is required. Barium swallow is less accurate.

Treatment of *Candida* esophagitis is with fluconazole 200 to 400 mg po or IV once/day for 14 to 21 days. Alternatives include other azoles (eg, itraconazole, voriconazole, posaconazole) or echinocandins (eg, caspofungin, micafungin, anidulafungin). Topical therapy has no role.

HSV and CMV esophagitis: These infections are equally likely in transplant patients, but HSV occurs early after transplantation (reactivation) and CMV occurs 2 to 6 mo after. Among AIDS patients, CMV is much more common than HSV, and viral esophagitis occurs mainly when the CD4+ count is < 200/μL. Severe odynophagia results from either infection.

Endoscopy, with cytology or biopsy, is usually necessary for diagnosis. HSV is treated with IV acyclovir 5 mg/kg q 8 h for 7 days or valacyclovir 1 g po tid. CMV is treated with ganciclovir 5 mg/kg IV q 12 h for 14 to 21 days with maintenance at 5 mg/kg IV 5 days/wk for immunocompromised patients. Alternatives include foscarnet and cidofovir.

LOWER ESOPHAGEAL RING

(Schatzki Ring; B Ring)

A lower esophageal ring is a 2- to 4-mm mucosal stricture that causes a ringlike narrowing of the distal esophagus at the squamocolumnar junction that often causes dysphagia.

The etiology of lower esophageal rings is controversial; the leading theories are that they are congenital, or caused by acid reflux or pill-induced esophagitis.

These rings cause intermittent dysphagia for solids. Symptoms can begin at any age but usually do not begin until after age 25. The swallowing difficulty comes and goes and is especially aggravated by meat and dry bread. Symptoms usually occur only when the esophageal lumen is < 12 mm in diameter and never when it is > 20 mm.

Typically, evaluation of dysphagia begins with upper endoscopy, which should show a ring large enough to cause symptoms. If the distal esophagus is adequately distended, barium x-rays usually also show the ring.

Instructing the patient to chew food thoroughly is usually the only treatment required in wider rings, but narrow-lumen rings require dilation by endoscopy or bougienage. Surgical resection is rarely required.

MALLORY-WEISS SYNDROME

Mallory-Weiss syndrome is a nonpenetrating mucosal laceration of the distal esophagus and proximal stomach caused by vomiting, retching, or hiccuping.

Initially described in alcoholics, Mallory-Weiss syndrome can occur in any patient who vomits forcefully. It is the cause of about 5% of episodes of upper GI hemorrhage. The tear may also be accompanied by pain in the lower chest.

Diagnosis of Mallory-Weiss syndrome is suggested clinically by a typical history of hematemesis occurring after one or more episodes of non-bloody vomiting. In such cases, if the amount of bleeding is minimal and the patient is stable, testing may be deferred. Otherwise, if history is unclear or bleeding is ongoing, the patient should have standard evaluation for GI bleeding, typically with upper endoscopy and laboratory testing. Upper endoscopy can also be therapeutic because a clip can be placed over the tear to control bleeding.

Most episodes of bleeding stop spontaneously; severe bleeding occurs in about 10% of patients, who require significant intervention, such as transfusion or endoscopic hemostasis (by clip placement, injection of ethanol or epinephrine, or by electrocautery). Intra-arterial infusion of vasopressin or therapeutic embolization into the left gastric artery during angiography may also be used to control bleeding. Surgical repair is rarely required.

OBSTRUCTIVE DISORDERS OF THE ESOPHAGUS

(See also Benign Esophageal Tumors on p. 161 and Esophageal Cancer on p. 164.)

Most esophageal obstruction develops slowly and is incomplete when patients first seek care, typically for difficulty swallowing solids. However, sometimes complete esophageal obstruction develops suddenly because of an impacted esophageal foreign body or food bolus.

Obstruction may have intrinsic or extrinsic causes.

Intrinsic obstruction may be caused by

- Esophageal tumors (benign or malignant)
- Esophageal rings
- Esophageal webs
- Strictures caused by gastroesophageal reflux or, rarely, caustic ingestion

Extrinsic obstruction may be caused by compression resulting from

- An enlarged left atrium
- An aortic aneurysm
- An aberrant subclavian artery (termed dysphagia lusoria)
- A substernal thyroid gland
- Cervical bony exostosis
- A thoracic tumor

For evaluation of potential esophageal obstruction, see Dysphagia on p. 109.

SYMPTOMATIC DIFFUSE ESOPHAGEAL SPASM

(Spastic Pseudodiverticulosis; Rosary Bead or Corkscrew Esophagus)

Symptomatic diffuse esophageal spasm is part of a spectrum of motility disorders characterized variously by nonpropulsive contractions, hyperdynamic contractions, or elevated LES pressure. Symptoms are chest pain and sometimes dysphagia. Diagnosis is by barium swallow or manometry. Treatment is difficult but includes nitrates, calcium channel blockers, botulinum toxin injection, and antireflux therapy.

Abnormalities in esophageal motility correlate poorly with patient symptoms; similar abnormalities may cause different or no symptoms in different people. Furthermore, neither symptoms nor abnormal contractions are definitively associated with histopathologic abnormalities of the esophagus.

Symptoms and Signs

Diffuse esophageal spasm typically causes substernal chest pain with dysphagia for both liquids and solids. The pain may waken the patient from sleep. Very hot or cold liquids may aggravate the pain. Over many years, this disorder may evolve into achalasia.

Esophageal spasms can cause severe pain without dysphagia. This pain is often described as a substernal squeezing pain and may occur in association with exercise. Such pain may be indistinguishable from angina pectoris.

Diagnosis

- Barium swallow
- Esophageal manometry
- Possibly testing for coronary ischemia

Alternative diagnoses include coronary ischemia, which may need to be excluded by appropriate testing (eg, ECG, cardiac markers, stress testing—see Diagnosis of Acute Coronary Syndromes on p. 677). Definitive confirmation of an esophageal origin for symptoms is difficult.

Barium swallow may show poor progression of a bolus and disordered, simultaneous contractions or tertiary contractions. Severe spasms may mimic the radiographic appearance of diverticula but vary in size and position.

Esophageal manometry provides the most specific description of the spasms. At least 20% of test swallows must have a short distal latency (< 4.5 sec) to meet manometric criteria for diffuse esophageal spasm. However, spasms may not occur during testing.

Esophageal scintigraphy and provocative tests with drugs (eg, edrophonium chloride 10 mg IV) have not proved helpful.

Treatment

- Calcium channel blockers
- Botulinum toxin injection

Esophageal spasms are often difficult to treat, and controlled studies of treatment methods are lacking. Anticholinergics, tricyclic antidepressants, nitroglycerin, and long-acting nitrates have had limited success. Calcium channel blockers given orally (eg, verapamil 80 mg tid, nifedipine 10 mg tid) may be useful, as may injection of botulinum toxin type A into the LES.

Medical management is usually sufficient, but surgical myotomy along the full length of the esophagus has been tried in intractable cases.

15 Gastritis and Peptic Ulcer Disease

OVERVIEW OF ACID SECRETION

Acid is secreted by parietal cells in the proximal two thirds (body) of the stomach. Gastric acid aids digestion by creating the optimal pH for pepsin and gastric lipase and by stimulating pancreatic bicarbonate secretion. Acid secretion is initiated by food: the thought, smell, or taste of food effects vagal stimulation of the gastrin-secreting G cells located in the distal one third (antrum) of the stomach. The arrival of protein to the stomach further stimulates gastrin output. Circulating gastrin triggers the release of histamine from enterochromaffin-like cells in the body of the stomach. Histamine stimulates the parietal cells via their H_2 receptors. The parietal cells secrete acid, and the resulting drop in pH causes the antral D cells to release somatostatin, which inhibits gastrin release (negative feedback control).

Acid secretion is present at birth and reaches adult levels (on a weight basis) by age 2. There is a decline in acid output in elderly patients who develop chronic gastritis, but acid output is otherwise maintained throughout life.

Normally, the GI mucosa is protected by several distinct mechanisms:

- Mucosal production of mucus and HCO_3 creates a pH gradient from the gastric lumen (low pH) to the mucosa (neutral pH). The mucus serves as a barrier to the diffusion of acid and pepsin.
- Epithelial cells remove excess hydrogen ions (H^+) via membrane transport systems and have tight junctions, which prevent back diffusion of H^+ ions.
- Mucosal blood flow removes excess acid that has diffused across the epithelial layer.

Several growth factors (eg, epidermal growth factor, insulin-like growth factor I) and prostaglandins have been linked to mucosal repair and maintenance of mucosal integrity.

Factors that interfere with these mucosal defenses (particularly NSAIDs and *Helicobacter pylori* infection) predispose to gastritis and peptic ulcer disease.

NSAIDs promote mucosal inflammation and ulcer formation (sometimes with GI bleeding) both topically and systemically. By inhibiting prostaglandin production via blockage of the enzyme cyclooxygenase (COX), NSAIDs reduce gastric blood flow, reduce mucus and HCO_3 secretion, and decrease cell repair and replication. Also, because NSAIDs are weak acids and are nonionized at gastric pH, they diffuse freely across the mucus barrier into gastric epithelial cells, where H^+ ions are liberated, leading to cellular damage. Because gastric prostaglandin production involves the COX-1 isoform, NSAIDs that are selective COX-2 inhibitors have fewer adverse gastric effects than other NSAIDs.

OVERVIEW OF GASTRITIS

Gastritis is inflammation of the gastric mucosa caused by any of several conditions, including infection (*Helicobacter pylori*), drugs (NSAIDs, alcohol), stress, and autoimmune phenomena (atrophic gastritis). Many cases are asymptomatic, but dyspepsia and GI bleeding sometimes occur. Diagnosis is by endoscopy. Treatment is directed at the cause but often includes acid suppression and, for *Helicobacter pylori* infection, antibiotics.

Gastritis is classified as erosive gastritis or nonerosive gastritis based on the severity of mucosal injury. It is also classified according to the site of involvement (ie, cardia, body, antrum). Gastritis can be further classified histologically as acute or chronic based on the inflammatory cell type. No classification scheme matches perfectly with the pathophysiology; a large degree of overlap exists. Some forms of gastritis involve acid-peptic and H. pylori disease. Additionally, the term is often loosely applied to nonspecific (and often undiagnosed) abdominal discomfort and gastroenteritis.

Acute gastritis is characterized by PMN infiltration of the mucosa of the antrum and body.

Chronic gastritis implies some degree of atrophy (with loss of function of the mucosa) or metaplasia. It predominantly involves the antrum (with subsequent loss of G cells and decreased gastrin secretion) or the corpus (with loss of oxyntic glands, leading to reduced acid, pepsin, and intrinsic factor).

AUTOIMMUNE METAPLASTIC ATROPHIC GASTRITIS

Autoimmune metaplastic atrophic gastritis is an inherited autoimmune disease that attacks parietal cells, resulting in hypochlorhydria and decreased production of intrinsic factor. Consequences include atrophic gastritis, B_{12} malabsorption, and, frequently, pernicious anemia. Risk of gastric adenocarcinoma increases 3-fold. Diagnosis is by endoscopy. Treatment is with parenteral vitamin B_{12}.

Patients with autoimmune metaplastic atrophic gastritis (AMAG) have antibodies to parietal cells and their components (which include intrinsic factor and the proton pump H^+, K^+-ATPase). AMAG is inherited as an autosomal dominant trait. Some patients also develop Hashimoto thyroiditis and 50% have thyroid antibodies; conversely, parietal cell antibodies are found in 30% of patients with thyroiditis.

The lack of intrinsic factor leads to vitamin B_{12} deficiency that can result in a megaloblastic anemia (pernicious anemia) or neurologic symptoms (subacute combined degeneration).

Hypochlorhydria leads to G-cell hyperplasia and elevated serum gastrin levels (often > 1000 pg/mL). Elevated gastrin levels lead to enterochromaffin-like cell hyperplasia, which occasionally undergoes transformation to a carcinoid tumor.

In some patients, AMAG may be associated with chronic Helicobacter pylori infection, although the relationship is not clear. Gastrectomy and chronic acid suppression with proton pump inhibitors cause similar deficiencies of intrinsic factor secretion.

The areas of atrophic gastritis in the body and fundus may manifest as metaplasia. Patients with AMAG have a 3-fold increased relative risk of developing gastric adenocarcinoma.

Diagnosis of autoimmune metaplastic atrophic gastritis is made by endoscopic biopsy. Serum B_{12} levels should be obtained. Parietal cell antibodies can be detected but are not measured routinely. The issue of surveillance endoscopy for cancer screening is unsettled; follow-up examinations are unnecessary unless histologic abnormalities (eg, dysplasia) are present on initial biopsy or symptoms develop.

No treatment is needed other than parenteral replacement of vitamin B_{12}.

EROSIVE GASTRITIS

Erosive gastritis is gastric mucosal erosion caused by damage to mucosal defenses. It is typically acute, manifesting with bleeding, but may be subacute or chronic with few or no symptoms. Diagnosis is by endoscopy. Treatment is supportive, with removal of the inciting cause and initiation of acid-suppressant therapy. Certain ICU patients (eg, ventilator-bound, head trauma, burn, multisystem trauma) benefit from prophylaxis with acid suppressants.

Common causes of erosive gastritis include

- NSAIDs
- Alcohol
- Stress

Less common causes include

- Radiation
- Viral infection (eg, cytomegalovirus)
- Vascular injury
- Direct trauma (eg, NGTs)

Superficial erosions and punctate mucosal lesions occur. These may develop as soon as 12 h after the initial insult. Deep erosions, ulcers, and sometimes perforation may occur in severe or untreated cases. Lesions typically occur in the body, but the antrum may also be involved.

Acute stress gastritis, a form of erosive gastritis, occurs in about 5% of critically ill patients. The incidence increases with duration of ICU stay and length of time the patient is not receiving enteral feeding. Pathogenesis likely involves hypoperfusion of the GI mucosa, resulting in impaired mucosal defenses. Patients with head injury or burns may also have increased secretion of acid.

Symptoms and Signs

Patients with mild erosive gastritis are often asymptomatic, although some complain of dyspepsia, nausea, or vomiting. Often, the first sign is hematemesis, melena, or blood in the nasogastric aspirate, usually within 2 to 5 days of the inciting event. Bleeding is usually mild to moderate, although it can be massive if deep ulceration is present, particularly in acute stress gastritis.

Diagnosis

Acute and chronic erosive gastritis are diagnosed endoscopically.

Treatment

- For bleeding: Endoscopic hemostasis
- For acid suppression: A proton pump inhibitor or H_2 blocker

In severe gastritis, bleeding is managed with IV fluids and blood transfusion as needed. Endoscopic hemostasis should be attempted, with surgery (total gastrectomy) a fallback procedure. Angiography is unlikely to stop severe gastric bleeding because of the many collateral vessels supplying the stomach. Acid suppression should be started if the patient is not already receiving it.

For milder gastritis, removing the offending agent and using drugs to reduce gastric acidity (see p. 123) to limit further injury and promote healing may be all that is required.

Prevention

Prophylaxis with acid-suppressive drugs can reduce the incidence of acute stress gastritis. However, it mainly benefits certain high-risk ICU patients, including those with severe burns, CNS trauma, coagulopathy, sepsis, shock, multiple trauma, mechanical ventilation for > 48 h, hepatic or renal failure, multiorgan dysfunction, and history of peptic ulcer or GI bleeding.

Prophylaxis consists of IV H_2 blockers, proton pump inhibitors, or oral antacids to raise intragastric pH > 4.0. Repeated pH measurement and titration of therapy are not required. Early enteral feeding also can decrease the incidence of bleeding.

Acid suppression is not recommended for patients simply taking NSAIDs unless they have previously had an ulcer.

HELICOBACTER PYLORI INFECTION

Helicobacter pylori **is a common gastric pathogen that causes gastritis, peptic ulcer disease, gastric adenocarcinoma, and low-grade gastric lymphoma. Infection may be asymptomatic or result in varying degrees of dyspepsia. Diagnosis is by urea breath test, stool antigen test, and testing of endoscopic biopsy samples. Treatment is with a proton pump inhibitor plus two antibiotics.**

(See also the American College of Gastroenterology's guidelines for the management of *Helicobacter pylori* infection.)

H. pylori is a spiral-shaped, gram-negative organism that has adapted to thrive in acid. In developing countries, it commonly causes chronic infections and is usually acquired during childhood. In the US, infection is less common among children but increases with age: by age 60, about 50% of people are infected. Infection is most common among blacks, Hispanics, and Asians.

The organism has been cultured from stool, saliva, and dental plaque, which suggests oral-oral or fecal-oral transmission. Infections tend to cluster in families and in residents of custodial institutions. Nurses and gastroenterologists seem to be at high risk because bacteria can be transmitted by improperly disinfected endoscopes.

Pathophysiology

Effects of *H. pylori* infection vary depending on the location within the stomach.

Antral-predominant infection results in increased gastrin production, probably via local impairment of somatostatin release. Resultant hypersecretion of acid predisposes to prepyloric and duodenal ulcer.

Body-predominant infection leads to gastric atrophy and *decreased* acid production, possibly via increased local production of IL-1β. Patients with body-predominant infection are predisposed to gastric ulcer and adenocarcinoma.

Some patients have mixed infection of both antrum and body with varying clinical effects. Many patients with *H. pylori* infection have no noticeable clinical effects.

Ammonia produced by *H. pylori* enables the organism to survive in the acidic environment of the stomach and may erode the mucus barrier. Cytotoxins and mucolytic enzymes (eg, bacterial protease, lipase) produced by *H. pylori* may play a role in mucosal damage and subsequent ulcerogenesis.

Infected people are 3 to 6 times more likely to develop stomach cancer. *H. pylori* infection is associated with intestinal-type adenocarcinoma of the gastric body and antrum but not cancer of the gastric cardia. Other associated cancers include gastric lymphoma and mucosa-associated lymphoid tissue (MALT) lymphoma, a monoclonally restricted B-cell tumor.

Diagnosis

- Urea breath testing and stool antigen testing

Screening of asymptomatic patients is not warranted. Tests are done during evaluation for peptic ulcer and gastritis. Post-treatment testing is typically done to confirm eradication of the organism.

Noninvasive tests: Laboratory and office-based serologic assays for antibodies to *H. pylori* have a sensitivity and specificity of > 85% and previously were considered the noninvasive tests of choice for initial documentation of *H. pylori* infection. However, as the prevalence of infection has declined, the percentage of false-positive results with serologic assays has increased significantly, making these tests too unreliable in most countries and regions. As a result, urea breath testing and stool antigen testing are preferred for initial diagnosis. Qualitative assays remain positive for up to 3 yr after successful treatment and because quantitative antibody levels do not decline significantly for 6 to 12 mo after treatment, serologic assays are not usually used to assess cure.

Urea breath tests use an oral dose of ^{13}C- or ^{14}C-labeled urea. In an infected patient, the organism metabolizes the urea and liberates labeled CO_2, which is exhaled and can be quantified in breath samples taken 20 to 30 min after ingestion of the urea. Sensitivity and specificity are > 95%. Urea breath tests are well suited for confirming eradication of the organism after therapy. False-negative results are possible with recent antibiotic use or concomitant proton pump inhibitor therapy; therefore, follow-up testing should be delayed ≥ 4 wk after antibiotic therapy and 1 wk after proton pump inhibitor therapy. H_2 blockers do not affect the test.

Stool antigen assays seem to have a sensitivity and specificity near that of urea breath tests, particularly for initial diagnosis; an office-based stool test is under development.

Invasive tests: Endoscopy is used to obtain mucosal biopsy samples for a rapid urease test (RUT) or histologic staining. Bacterial culture is of limited use because of the fastidious nature of the organism. Endoscopy is not recommended solely for diagnosis of *H. pylori*; noninvasive tests are preferred unless endoscopy is indicated for other reasons.

The RUT, in which presence of bacterial urease in the biopsy sample causes a color change on a special medium, is the diagnostic method of choice on tissue samples. Histologic staining of biopsy samples should be done for patients with negative RUT results but suspicious clinical findings, recent antibiotic use, or treatment with proton pump inhibitors. RUT and histologic staining each have a sensitivity and specificity of > 90%.

Treatment

- Antibiotics (various regimens) plus a proton pump inhibitor
- For confirmation of cure, urea breath test, stool antigen assay, or upper endoscopy

Patients with complications (eg, ulcer, cancer) should have the organism eradicated. Eradication of *H. pylori* can even cure some cases of MALT lymphoma (but not other infection-related cancers). Treatment of asymptomatic infection has been controversial, but the recognition of the role of *H. pylori* in cancer has led to a recommendation for treatment. Vaccines, both preventive and therapeutic (ie, as an adjunct to treatment of infected patients), are under development.

H. pylori eradication requires multidrug therapy, typically antibiotics plus acid suppressants.[1] Proton pump inhibitors suppress *H. pylori,* and the increased gastric pH accompanying their use can enhance tissue concentration and efficacy of antimicrobials, creating a hostile environment for *H. pylori.*

Triple therapy is the most frequently prescribed regimen for *H. pylori* infection. The following drugs are given for 10 to 14 days:

- A proton pump inhibitor (lansoprazole 30 mg po bid, omeprazole 20 mg po bid, pantoprazole 40 mg po bid, rabeprazole 20 mg po bid, or esomeprazole 40 mg po once/day)
- Amoxicillin (1 g po bid) OR metronidazole 250 mg qid
- Clarithromycin (500 mg po bid)

However, in many regions of the world, the rate of clarithromycin resistance has been increasing and failure of triple therapy is increasingly likely. Thus, this regimen is not recommended for initial therapy unless ≥ 85% of local strains of *H. pylori* are known to be susceptible *or* the regimen is known to still be clinically effective in the local area.

For multidrug-resistance strains of *H. pylori*, triple therapy with rifabutin appears to be effective.[2]

Quadruple therapy is the best initial therapy in areas where the clarithromycin resistance rate is > 15%. In quadruple therapy, the following drugs are given for 10 to 14 days[3]:

- A proton pump inhibitor (lansoprazole 30 mg po bid, omeprazole 20 mg po bid, pantoprazole 40 mg po bid, rabeprazole 20 mg po bid, or esomeprazole 40 mg po once/day)
- Bismuth subsalicylate (524 mg po qid)
- Metronidazole 250 mg qid
- Tetracycline 500 mg qid

Infected patients with duodenal or gastric ulcer require continuation of the acid suppression for at least 4 wk. Eradication may be confirmed by a urea breath test, stool antigen test, or upper endoscopy done ≥ 4 wk after completion of therapy. Confirmation of eradication is reasonable in all treated patients but is mandatory in patients who have serious manifestations of *H. pylori* infection (eg, bleeding ulcer). Recurrent bleeding ulcer is likely if the infection is not eradicated.

Treatment is repeated if *H. pylori* is not eradicated. If two courses are unsuccessful, some authorities recommend endoscopy to obtain cultures for sensitivity testing.

1. Yang JC, Lin CJ, Wang HL, et al: High-dose dual therapy is superior to standard first-line or rescue therapy for *Helicobacter pylori* infection. *Clin Gastroenterol Hepatol* 13(5):895–905.e5, 2015. doi: 10.1016/j.cgh.2014.10.036.
2. Fiorini G, Zullo A, Vakil N, et al: Rifabutin triple therapy is effective in patients with multidrug-resistant strains of *Helicobacter pylori*. *J Clin Gastroenterol* 2016 Apr 30 [Epub ahead of print]. doi: 10.1097/MCG.0000000000000540.
3. Fallone CA, Chiba N, van Zanten SV, et al: The Toronto consensus for the treatment of *Helicobacter pylori* infection in adults. *Gastroenterology* 151(1):51–69, 2016. doi: 10.1053/j.gastro.2016.04.006.

KEY POINTS

- *H. pylori* is a gram-negative organism that is highly adapted to an acid environment and often infects the stomach; incidence of infection increases with age—by age 60, about 50% of people are infected.
- Infection predisposes to gastric, prepyloric, and duodenal ulcers and increases risk of gastric adenocarcinoma and lymphoma.
- Make initial diagnosis with a urea breath test or stool antigen assay; if endoscopy is being done for other reasons, analyze biopsy samples using a rapid urease test or histologic staining.
- Give treatment to eradicate the organism in patients with complications (eg, ulcer, cancer); a typical regimen includes a proton pump inhibitor plus two antibiotics (eg, clarithromycin plus either amoxicillin or metronidazole) or quadruple therapy in areas that have high resistance rates to clarithromycin.
- Confirm cure using a urea breath test, stool antigen test, or upper endoscopy.

NONEROSIVE GASTRITIS

Nonerosive gastritis refers to a variety of histologic abnormalities that are mainly the result of *Helicobacter pylori* infection. Most patients are asymptomatic. Diagnosis is by endoscopy. Treatment is eradication of *H. pylori* and sometimes acid suppression.

Pathology

Superficial gastritis: Lymphocytes and plasma cells mixed with neutrophils are the predominant infiltrating inflammatory cells. Inflammation is superficial and may involve the antrum, body, or both. It is usually not accompanied by atrophy or metaplasia. Prevalence increases with age.

Deep gastritis: Deep gastritis is more likely to be symptomatic (eg, vague dyspepsia). Mononuclear cells and neutrophils infiltrate the entire mucosa to the level of the muscularis, but exudate or crypt abscesses seldom result, as might be expected by such infiltration. Distribution may be patchy. Superficial gastritis may be present, as may partial gland atrophy and metaplasia.

Gastric atrophy: Atrophy of gastric glands may follow in gastritis, most often long-standing antral (sometimes referred to as type B) gastritis. Some patients with gastric atrophy have autoantibodies to parietal cells, usually in association with corpus (type A) gastritis and pernicious anemia.

Atrophy may occur without specific symptoms. Endoscopically, the mucosa may appear normal until atrophy is advanced, when submucosal vascularity may be visible. As atrophy becomes complete, secretion of acid and pepsin diminishes and intrinsic factor may be lost, resulting in vitamin B_{12} malabsorption.

Metaplasia: Two types of metaplasia are common in chronic nonerosive gastritis:

- Mucous gland
- Intestinal

Mucous gland metaplasia (pseudopyloric metaplasia) occurs in the setting of severe atrophy of the gastric glands, which are progressively replaced by mucous glands (antral mucosa), especially along the lesser curve. Gastric ulcers may be present (typically at the junction of antral and corpus mucosa), but whether they are the cause or consequence of these metaplastic changes is not clear.

Intestinal metaplasia typically begins in the antrum in response to chronic mucosal injury and may extend to the body. Gastric mucosa cells change to resemble intestinal mucosa—with goblet cells, endocrine (enterochromaffin or enterochromaffin-like) cells, and rudimentary villi—and may even assume functional (absorptive) characteristics.

Intestinal metaplasia is classified histologically as complete (most common) or incomplete. With complete metaplasia, gastric mucosa is completely transformed into small-bowel mucosa, both histologically and functionally, with the ability to absorb nutrients and secrete peptides. In incomplete metaplasia, the epithelium assumes a histologic appearance closer to that of the large intestine and frequently exhibits dysplasia. Intestinal metaplasia may lead to stomach cancer.

Symptoms and Signs

Most patients with *H. pylori*–associated gastritis are asymptomatic, although some have mild dyspepsia or other vague symptoms.

Diagnosis

- Endoscopy

Often, the condition is discovered during endoscopy done for other purposes. Testing of asymptomatic patients is not indicated. Once gastritis is identified, testing for *H. pylori* is appropriate.

Treatment

- Eradication of *H. pylori*
- Sometimes acid-suppressive drugs

Treatment of chronic nonerosive gastritis is *H. pylori* eradication. Treatment of asymptomatic patients is somewhat controversial given the high prevalence of *H. pylori*–associated superficial gastritis and the relatively low incidence of clinical sequelae (ie, peptic ulcer disease). However, *H. pylori* is a class 1 carcinogen; eradication removes the cancer risk.

In *H. pylori*–negative patients, treatment is directed at symptoms using acid-suppressive drugs (eg, H_2 blockers, proton pump inhibitors) or antacids.

PEPTIC ULCER DISEASE

A peptic ulcer is an erosion in a segment of the GI mucosa, typically in the stomach (gastric ulcer) or the first few centimeters of the duodenum (duodenal ulcer), that penetrates through the muscularis mucosae. Nearly all ulcers are caused by *Helicobacter pylori* infection or NSAID use. Symptoms typically include burning epigastric pain that is often relieved by food. Diagnosis is by endoscopy and testing for *Helicobacter pylori.* Treatment involves acid suppression, eradication of *H. pylori* (if present), and avoidance of NSAIDs.

Ulcers may range in size from several millimeters to several centimeters. Ulcers are delineated from erosions by the depth of penetration; erosions are more superficial and do not involve the muscularis mucosae. Ulcers can occur at any age, including infancy and childhood, but are most common among middle-aged adults.

Etiology

H. pylori and NSAIDs disrupt normal mucosal defense and repair, making the mucosa more susceptible to acid. *H. pylori* infection is present in 50 to 70% of patients with duodenal ulcers and in 30 to 50% of patients with gastric ulcers. If *H. pylori* is eradicated, only 10% of patients have recurrence of peptic ulcer disease, compared with 70% recurrence in patients treated with acid suppression alone. NSAIDs now account for > 50% of peptic ulcers.

Cigarette smoking is a risk factor for the development of ulcers and their complications. Also, smoking impairs ulcer healing and increases the incidence of recurrence. Risk correlates with the number of cigarettes smoked per day. Although alcohol is a strong promoter of acid secretion, no definitive data link moderate amounts of alcohol to the development or delayed healing of ulcers. Very few patients have hypersecretion of gastrin caused by a gastrinoma (Zollinger-Ellison syndrome).

A family history exists in 50 to 60% of children with duodenal ulcer.

Symptoms and Signs

Symptoms depend on ulcer location and patient age; many patients, particularly elderly patients, have few or no symptoms. Pain is most common, often localized to the epigastrium and relieved by food or antacids. The pain is described as burning or gnawing, or sometimes as a sensation of hunger. The course is usually chronic and recurrent. Only about half of patients present with the characteristic pattern of symptoms.

Gastric ulcer symptoms often do not follow a consistent pattern (eg, eating sometimes exacerbates rather than relieves pain). This is especially true for pyloric channel ulcers, which are often associated with symptoms of obstruction (eg, bloating, nausea, vomiting) caused by edema and scarring.

Duodenal ulcers tend to cause more consistent pain. Pain is absent when the patient awakens but appears in mid-morning and is relieved by food but recurs 2 to 3 h after a meal. Pain that awakens a patient at night is common and is highly suggestive of duodenal ulcer. In neonates, perforation and hemorrhage may be the first manifestation of duodenal ulcer. Hemorrhage may also be the first recognized sign in later infancy and early childhood, although repeated vomiting or evidence of abdominal pain may be a clue.

Diagnosis

- Endoscopy
- Sometimes serum gastrin levels

Diagnosis of peptic ulcer is suggested by patient history and confirmed by endoscopy. Empiric therapy is often begun without definitive diagnosis. However, endoscopy allows for biopsy or cytologic brushing of gastric and esophageal lesions to distinguish between simple ulceration and ulcerating stomach cancer. Stomach cancer may manifest with similar manifestations and must be excluded, especially in patients who are > 45, have lost weight, or report severe or refractory symptoms. The incidence of malignant duodenal ulcer is extremely low, so biopsies of duodenal lesions are generally not warranted. Endoscopy can also be used to definitively diagnose *H. pylori* infection, which should be sought when an ulcer is detected (see diagnosis of *H. pylori* infection on p. 118).

Gastrin-secreting cancer and gastrinoma should be considered when there are multiple ulcers, when ulcers develop in atypical locations (eg, postbulbar) or are refractory to treatment, or when the patient has prominent diarrhea or weight loss. Serum gastrin levels should be measured in these patients.

Complications

Hemorrhage: Mild to severe hemorrhage is the most common complication of peptic ulcer disease. Symptoms include hematemesis (vomiting of fresh blood or "coffee ground" material); passage of bloody stools (hematochezia) or black tarry stools (melena); and weakness, orthostasis, syncope, thirst, and sweating caused by blood loss.

Penetration (confined perforation): A peptic ulcer may penetrate the wall of the stomach. If adhesions prevent leakage into the peritoneal cavity, free penetration is avoided and confined perforation occurs. Still, the ulcer may penetrate into the duodenum and enter the adjacent confined space (lesser sac) or another organ (eg, pancreas, liver). Pain may be intense, persistent, referred to sites other than the abdomen (usually the back when caused by penetration of a posterior duodenal ulcer into the pancreas), and modified by body position. CT or MRI is usually needed to confirm the diagnosis. When therapy does not result in healing, surgery is required.

Free perforation: Ulcers that perforate into the peritoneal cavity unchecked by adhesions are usually located in the anterior wall of the duodenum or, less commonly, in the stomach. The patient presents with an acute abdomen. There is sudden, intense, continuous epigastric pain that spreads rapidly throughout the abdomen, often becoming prominent in the right lower quadrant and at times referred to one or both shoulders. The patient usually lies still because even deep breathing worsens the pain. Palpation of the abdomen is painful, rebound tenderness is prominent, abdominal muscles are rigid (boardlike), and bowel sounds are diminished or absent. Shock may ensue, heralded by increased pulse rate and decreased BP and urine output. Symptoms may be less striking in elderly or moribund patients and those receiving corticosteroids or immunosuppressants.

Diagnosis is confirmed if an x-ray or CT shows free air under the diaphragm or in the peritoneal cavity. Upright views of the chest and abdomen are preferred. The most sensitive view is the lateral x-ray of the chest. Severely ill patients may be unable to sit upright and should have a lateral decubitus x-ray of the abdomen. Failure to detect free air does not exclude the diagnosis.

Immediate surgery is required. The longer the delay, the poorer is the prognosis. IV antibiotics effective against intestinal flora (eg, cefotetan, or amikacin plus clindamycin) should be given. Usually, an NGT is inserted to do continuous nasogastric suction. In the rare cases when surgery cannot be done, prognosis is poor.

Gastric outlet obstruction: Obstruction may be caused by scarring, spasm, or inflammation from an ulcer. Symptoms include recurrent, large-volume vomiting, occurring more frequently at the end of the day and often as late as 6 h after the last meal. Loss of appetite with persistent bloating or fullness after eating also suggests gastric outlet obstruction. Prolonged vomiting may cause weight loss, dehydration, and alkalosis.

If the patient's history suggests obstruction, physical examination, gastric aspiration, or x-rays may provide evidence of retained gastric contents. A succussion splash heard > 6 h after a meal or aspiration of fluid or food residue > 200 mL after an overnight fast suggests gastric retention. If gastric aspiration shows marked retention, the stomach should be emptied and endoscopy done or x-rays taken to determine site, cause, and degree of obstruction.

Edema or spasm caused by an active pyloric channel ulcer is treated with gastric decompression by nasogastric suction and acid suppression (eg, IV H_2 blocker or IV proton pump inhibitor). Dehydration and electrolyte imbalances resulting from protracted vomiting or continued nasogastric suctioning should be vigorously sought and corrected. Prokinetic agents are not indicated. Generally, obstruction resolves within 2 to 5 days of treatment. Prolonged obstruction may result from peptic scarring and may respond to endoscopic pyloric balloon dilation. Surgery is necessary to relieve obstruction in selected cases.

Recurrence: Factors that affect recurrence of ulcer include failure to eradicate *H. pylori,* continued NSAID use, and smoking. Less commonly, a gastrinoma may be the cause. The 3-yr recurrence rate for gastric and duodenal ulcers is < 10% when *H. pylori* is successfully eradicated but is > 50% when it is not. Thus, a patient with recurrent disease should be tested for *H. pylori* and treated again if the tests are positive.

Although long-term treatment with H_2 blockers, proton pump inhibitors, or misoprostol reduces the risk of recurrence, their routine use for this purpose is not recommended. However, patients who require NSAIDs after having had a peptic ulcer are candidates for long-term therapy, as are those with a marginal ulcer or prior perforation or bleeding.

Stomach cancer: Patients with *H. pylori*–associated ulcers have a 3- to 6-fold increased risk of gastric cancer later in life. There is no increased risk of cancer with ulcers of other etiology.

Treatment

- Eradication of *H. pylori* (when present)
- Acid-suppressive drugs

Treatment of gastric and duodenal ulcers requires eradication of *H. pylori* when present (see also the Cochrane review abstract: Antibiotics for people with peptic ulcers caused by *Helicobacter pylori* infection) and a reduction of gastric acidity. For duodenal ulcers, it is particularly important to suppress nocturnal acid secretion.

Methods of decreasing acidity include a number of drugs, all of which are effective but which vary in cost, duration of therapy, and convenience of dosing. In addition, mucosal protective drugs (eg, sucralfate) and acid-reducing surgical procedures may be used. Drug therapy is discussed elsewhere (see p. 123).

Adjuncts: Smoking should be stopped, and alcohol consumption should be stopped or limited to small amounts of dilute alcohol. There is no evidence that changing the diet speeds ulcer healing or prevents recurrence. Thus, many physicians recommend eliminating only foods that cause distress.

Surgery: With current drug therapy, the number of patients requiring surgery has declined dramatically. Indications include perforation, obstruction, uncontrolled or recurrent bleeding, and, although rare, symptoms that do not respond to drug therapy.

Surgery consists of a procedure to reduce acid secretion, often combined with a procedure to ensure gastric drainage. The recommended operation for duodenal ulcer is highly selective, or parietal cell, vagotomy (which is limited to nerves at the gastric body and spares antral innervation, thereby obviating the need for a drainage procedure). This procedure has a very low mortality rate and avoids the morbidity associated with resection and traditional vagotomy. Other acid-reducing surgical procedures include antrectomy, hemigastrectomy, partial gastrectomy, and subtotal gastrectomy (ie, resection of 30 to 90% of the distal stomach). These are typically combined with truncal vagotomy. Patients who undergo a resective procedure or who have an obstruction require gastric drainage via a gastroduodenostomy (Billroth I) or gastrojejunostomy (Billroth II).

The incidence and type of postsurgical symptoms vary with the type of operation. After resective surgery, up to 30% of patients have significant symptoms, including weight loss, maldigestion, anemia, dumping syndrome, reactive hypoglycemia, bilious vomiting, mechanical problems, and ulcer recurrence.

Weight loss is common after subtotal gastrectomy; the patient may limit food intake because of early satiety (because the residual gastric pouch is small) or to prevent dumping syndrome and other postprandial syndromes. With a small gastric pouch, distention or discomfort may occur after a meal of even moderate size; patients should be encouraged to eat smaller and more frequent meals.

Maldigestion and steatorrhea caused by pancreaticobiliary bypass, especially with Billroth II anastomosis, may contribute to weight loss.

Anemia is common (usually from iron deficiency, but occasionally from vitamin B_{12} deficiency caused by loss of intrinsic factor or bacterial overgrowth) in the afferent limb, and osteomalacia may occur. IM vitamin B_{12} supplementation is recommended for all patients with total gastrectomy but may also be given to patients with subtotal gastrectomy if deficiency is suspected.

Dumping syndrome may follow gastric surgical procedures, particularly resections. Weakness, dizziness, sweating, nausea, vomiting, and palpitations occur soon after eating, especially hyperosmolar foods. This phenomenon is referred to as early dumping, the cause of which remains unclear but likely involves autonomic reflexes, intravascular volume contraction, and release of vasoactive peptides from the small intestine. Dietary modifications, with smaller, more frequent meals and decreased carbohydrate intake, usually help.

Reactive hypoglycemia or **late dumping** (another form of the syndrome) results from rapid emptying of carbohydrates from the gastric pouch. Early high peaks in blood glucose stimulate excess release of insulin, which leads to symptomatic hypoglycemia several hours after the meal. A high-protein, low-carbohydrate diet and adequate caloric intake (in frequent small feedings) are recommended.

Mechanical problems (including gastroparesis and bezoar formation) may occur secondary to a decrease in phase III gastric motor contractions, which are altered after antrectomy and vagotomy. Diarrhea is especially common after vagotomy, even without a resection (pyloroplasty).

Ulcer recurrence, according to older studies, occurs in 5 to 12% of patients after highly selective vagotomy and in 2 to 5% after resective surgery. Recurrent ulcers are diagnosed by endoscopy and generally respond to either proton pump inhibitors or H_2 blockers. For ulcers that continue to recur, the completeness of vagotomy should be tested by gastric analysis, *H. pylori* should be eliminated if present, and gastrinoma should be ruled out by serum gastrin studies.

KEY POINTS

- Peptic ulcers affect the stomach or duodenum and can occur at any age, including infancy and childhood.
- Most ulcers are caused by *H. pylori* infection or NSAID use; both factors disrupt normal mucosal defense and repair, making the mucosa more susceptible to acid.
- Burning pain is common; food may worsen gastric ulcer symptoms but relieve duodenal ulcer symptoms.
- Acute complications include GI bleeding and perforation; chronic complications include gastric outlet obstruction, recurrence, and, when *H. pylori* infection is the cause, stomach cancer.
- Diagnose with endoscopy and do tests for *H. pylori* infection.
- Give acid-suppressing drugs and therapy to eradicate *H. pylori*.

POSTGASTRECTOMY GASTRITIS

Postgastrectomy gastritis is gastric atrophy developing after partial or subtotal gastrectomy (except in cases of gastrinoma).

Metaplasia of the remaining corpus mucosa is common. The degree of gastritis is usually greatest at the lines of anastomosis. Several mechanisms are responsible:

- Bile reflux, which is common after such surgery, damages the gastric mucosa.
- Loss of antral gastrin decreases stimulation of parietal and peptic cells, causing atrophy.
- Vagotomy may result in a loss of vagal trophic action.

There are no specific symptoms of gastritis. Postgastrectomy gastritis often progresses to severe atrophy and achlorhydria. Production of intrinsic factor may cease with resultant vitamin B_{12} deficiency (which may be worsened by bacterial overgrowth in the afferent loop). The relative risk of gastric adenocarcinoma seems to increase 15 to 20 yr after partial gastrectomy; however, given the low absolute incidence of postgastrectomy cancer, routine endoscopic surveillance is probably not cost effective, but upper GI symptoms or anemia in such patients should prompt endoscopy.

UNCOMMON GASTRITIS SYNDROMES

Ménétrier disease: This rare idiopathic disorder affects adults aged 30 to 60 and is more common among men. It manifests as a significant thickening of the gastric folds of the gastric body but not the antrum. Gland atrophy and marked foveolar pit hyperplasia occur, often accompanied by mucous gland metaplasia and increased mucosal thickness with little inflammation. Hypoalbuminemia (the most consistent laboratory abnormality) caused by GI protein loss may be present (protein-losing gastropathy). As the disease progresses, the secretion of acid and pepsin decreases, causing hypochlorhydria.

Symptoms of Ménétrier disease are nonspecific and commonly include epigastric pain, nausea, weight loss, edema, and diarrhea. Differential diagnosis includes the following:

- Lymphoma, in which multiple gastric ulcers may occur
- MALT lymphoma, with extensive infiltration of monoclonal B lymphocytes
- Gastrinoma (Zollinger-Ellison syndrome) with associated gastric fold hypertrophy
- Cronkhite-Canada syndrome, a mucosal polypoid protein-losing syndrome associated with diarrhea

Diagnosis of Ménétrier disease is made by endoscopy with deep mucosal biopsy or full-thickness laparoscopic gastric biopsy.

Various treatments have been used, including anticholinergics, antisecretory drugs, and corticosteroids, but none have proved fully effective. Partial or complete gastric resection may be necessary in cases of severe hypoalbuminemia.

Eosinophilic gastritis: Extensive infiltration of the mucosa, submucosa, and muscle layers with eosinophils often occurs in the antrum. It is usually idiopathic but may result from nematode infestation. Symptoms of eosinophilic gastritis include nausea, vomiting, and early satiety.

Diagnosis of eosinophilic gastritis is by endoscopic biopsy of involved areas.

Corticosteroids can be successful in idiopathic cases; however, if pyloric obstruction develops, surgery may be required.

MALT lymphoma: This rare condition is characterized by massive lymphoid infiltration of the gastric mucosa, which can resemble Ménétrier disease.

Gastritis caused by systemic disorders: Sarcoidosis, TB, amyloidosis, and other granulomatous diseases can cause gastritis, which is seldom of primary importance.

Gastritis caused by physical agents: Radiation and ingestion of corrosives (especially acidic compounds) can cause gastritis. Exposure to > 6 Gy of whole-body radiation (see on p. 3093) causes marked deep gastritis, usually involving the antrum more than the corpus. Pyloric stenosis and perforation are possible complications of radiation-induced gastritis.

Infectious (septic) gastritis: Except for *Helicobacter pylori* infection, bacterial invasion of the stomach is rare and mainly occurs after ischemia, ingestion of corrosives, or exposure to radiation. On x-ray, gas outlines the mucosa. The condition can manifest as an acute surgical abdomen and has a very high mortality rate. Surgery is often necessary.

Debilitated or immunocompromised patients may develop viral or fungal gastritis with cytomegalovirus, *Candida,* histoplasmosis, or mucormycosis; these diagnoses should be considered in patients with exudative gastritis, esophagitis, or duodenitis.

DRUG TREATMENT OF GASTRIC ACIDITY

Drugs for decreasing acidity are used for peptic ulcer, gastroesophageal reflux disease (GERD), and many forms of gastritis. Some drugs are used in regimens for treating *Helicobacter pylori* infection. Drugs include

- Proton pump inhibitors
- H_2 blockers
- Antacids
- Prostaglandins

Proton pump inhibitors: These drugs are potent inhibitors of H^+, K^+-ATPase. This enzyme, located in the apical secretory membrane of the parietal cell, plays a key role in the secretion of H^+ (protons). These drugs can completely inhibit acid secretion and have a long duration of action. They promote ulcer healing and are also key components of *H. pylori* eradication regimens. Proton pump inhibitors have replaced H_2 blockers in most clinical situations because of greater rapidity of action and efficacy.

Proton pump inhibitors include esomeprazole, lansoprazole, and pantoprazole, all available orally and IV, and omeprazole and rabeprazole, available only orally in the US (see Table 15–1). Omeprazole, esomeprazole, and lansoprazole are available without a prescription in the US. For uncomplicated duodenal ulcers, omeprazole 20 mg po once/day or lansoprazole 30 mg po once/day is given for 4 wk. Complicated duodenal ulcers (ie, multiple ulcers, bleeding ulcers, those > 1.5 cm, or those occurring in patients with serious underlying illness) respond better to higher doses (omeprazole 40 mg once/day, lansoprazole 60 mg once/day or 30 mg bid). Gastric ulcers require treatment for 6 to 8 wk. Gastritis and GERD require 8 to 12 wk of therapy; GERD additionally often requires long-term maintenance.

Long-term proton pump inhibitor therapy produces elevated gastrin levels, which lead to enterochromaffin-like cell hyperplasia. However, there is no evidence of dysplasia or malignant transformation in patients receiving this treatment. Some may develop vitamin B_{12} malabsorption.

H_2 blockers: These drugs (cimetidine, ranitidine, famotidine, available IV and orally; and nizatidine available orally) are competitive inhibitors of histamine at the H_2 receptor,

Table 15–1. PROTON PUMP INHIBITORS

DRUG	MOST CONDITIONS*	GASTRIC ULCERS AND COMPLICATED DUODENAL ULCERS
Esomeprazole	40 mg once/day	40 mg bid
Lansoprazole	30 mg once/day (Pediatric doses: < 10 kg 7.5 mg once/day 10–20 kg 15 mg once/day ≥ 20 kg 30 mg once/day)†	30 mg bid
Omeprazole	20 mg once/day (Pediatric dose: 1 mg/kg/day in a single dose or divided bid)†	40 mg once/day
Pantoprazole	40 mg once/day	40 mg bid
Rabeprazole	20 mg once/day	20 mg bid

*Gastritis, gastroesophageal reflux disease, uncomplicated duodenal ulcers.
†Representative doses. Data are limited to the use of proton pump inhibitors in children.

thus suppressing gastrin-stimulated acid secretion and proportionately reducing gastric juice volume. Histamine-mediated pepsin secretion is also decreased. Nizatidine, famotidine, cimetidine, and ranitidine are available without a prescription in the US.

H_2 blockers are well absorbed from the GI tract, with onset of action 30 to 60 min after ingestion and peak effects at 1 to 2 h. IV administration produces a more rapid onset of action. Duration of action is proportional to dose and ranges from 6 to 20 h. Doses should often be reduced in elderly patients.

For duodenal ulcers, once daily oral administration of cimetidine 800 mg, ranitidine 300 mg, famotidine 40 mg, or nizatidine 300 mg given at bedtime or after dinner for 6 to 8 wk is effective. Gastric ulcers may respond to the same regimen continued for 8 to 12 wk, but because nocturnal acid secretion is less important, morning administration may be equally or more effective. Children ≥ 40 kg may receive adult doses. Below that weight, the oral dosage is ranitidine 2 mg/kg q 12 h and cimetidine 10 mg/kg q 12 h. For GERD, H_2 blockers are now mostly used for pain management. Gastritis heals with famotidine or ranitidine given bid for 8 to 12 wk.

Cimetidine has minor antiandrogen effects expressed as reversible gynecomastia and, less commonly, erectile dysfunction with prolonged use. Mental status changes, diarrhea, rash, drug fever, myalgias, thrombocytopenia, and sinus bradycardia and hypotension after rapid IV administration have been reported with all H_2 blockers, generally in < 1% of treated patients but more commonly in elderly patients.

Cimetidine and, to a lesser extent, other H_2 blockers interact with the P-450 microsomal enzyme system and may delay metabolism of other drugs eliminated through this system (eg, phenytoin, warfarin, theophylline, diazepam, lidocaine).

Antacids: These agents neutralize gastric acid and reduce pepsin activity (which diminishes as gastric pH rises to > 4.0). In addition, some antacids adsorb pepsin. Antacids may interfere with the absorption of other drugs (eg, tetracycline, digoxin, iron).

Antacids relieve symptoms, promote ulcer healing, and reduce recurrence. They are relatively inexpensive but must be taken 5 to 7 times/day. The optimal antacid regimen for ulcer healing seems to be 15 to 30 mL of liquid or 2 to 4 tablets 1 h and 3 h after each meal and at bedtime. The total daily dosage of antacids should provide 200 to 400 mEq neutralizing capacity. However, antacids have been superseded by acid-suppressive therapy in the treatment of peptic ulcer and are used only for short-term symptom relief.

In general, there are 2 types of antacids:

- Absorbable
- Nonabsorbable

Absorbable antacids (eg, sodium bicarbonate, calcium carbonate) provide rapid, complete neutralization but may cause alkalosis and should be used only briefly (1 or 2 days).

Nonabsorbable antacids (eg, aluminum or magnesium hydroxide) have fewer systemic adverse effects and are preferred.

Aluminum hydroxide is a relatively safe, commonly used antacid. With chronic use, phosphate depletion occasionally develops as a result of binding of phosphate by aluminum in the GI tract. The risk of phosphate depletion increases in alcoholics, undernourished patients, and patients with renal disease (including those receiving hemodialysis). Aluminum hydroxide causes constipation.

Magnesium hydroxide is a more effective antacid than aluminum but may cause diarrhea. To limit diarrhea, many proprietary antacids combine magnesium and aluminum antacids. Because small amounts of magnesium are absorbed, magnesium preparations should be used with caution in patients with renal disease.

Prostaglandins: Certain prostaglandins (especially misoprostol) inhibit acid secretion by decreasing the generation of cyclic AMP that is triggered by histamine stimulation of the parietal cell, and enhance mucosal defense. Synthetic prostaglandin derivatives are used predominantly to decrease the risk of NSAID-induced mucosal injury. Patients at high risk of NSAID-induced ulcers (ie, elderly patients, those with a history of ulcer or ulcer complication, those also taking corticosteroids) are candidates to take misoprostol 200 mcg po qid with food along with their NSAID. Common adverse effects of misoprostol are abdominal cramping and diarrhea, which occur in 30% of patients. Misoprostol is a powerful abortifacient and is absolutely contraindicated in women of childbearing age who are not using contraception.

Sucralfate: This drug is a sucrose-aluminum complex that dissociates in stomach acid and forms a physical barrier over an inflamed area, protecting it from acid, pepsin, and bile salts. It also inhibits pepsin-substrate interaction, stimulates mucosal prostaglandin production, and binds bile salts. It has no effect on acid output or gastrin secretion. Sucralfate seems to have trophic effects on the ulcerated mucosa, possibly by binding growth factors and concentrating them at an ulcer site. Systemic absorption of sucralfate is negligible. Constipation occurs in 3 to 5% of patients. Sucralfate may bind to other drugs and interfere with their absorption.

16 Gastroenteritis

(See also Food Allergy on p. 1384 and Mushroom Poisoning on p. 3062.)

Gastroenteritis is inflammation of the lining of the stomach and small and large intestines. Most cases are infectious, although gastroenteritis may occur after ingestion of drugs and chemical toxins (eg, metals, plant substances). Acquisition may be foodborne, waterborne, or via person-to-person spread. In the US, an estimated 1 in 6 people contracts foodborne illness each year. Symptoms include anorexia, nausea, vomiting, diarrhea, and abdominal discomfort. Diagnosis is clinical or by stool culture, although PCR and immunoassays are increasingly used. Treatment is symptomatic, although some parasitic and some bacterial infections require specific anti-infective therapy.

Gastroenteritis is usually uncomfortable but self-limited. Electrolyte and fluid loss is usually little more than an inconvenience to an otherwise healthy adult but can be grave for people who are very young (see p. 2554), elderly, or debilitated or who have serious concomitant illnesses. Worldwide, an estimated 1.5 million children die each year from infectious gastroenteritis; although high, this number represents one half to one quarter of previous mortality. Improvements in water sanitation in many parts of the world and the appropriate use of oral rehydration therapy for infants with diarrhea are likely responsible for this decrease.

Etiology

Infectious gastroenteritis may be caused by viruses, bacteria, or parasites. Many specific organisms are discussed further in the Infectious Diseases section.

Viruses: The viruses most commonly implicated are

- Rotavirus
- Norovirus

Viruses are the most common cause of gastroenteritis in the US. They infect enterocytes in the villous epithelium of the small bowel. The result is transudation of fluid and salts into the intestinal lumen; sometimes, malabsorption of carbohydrates worsens symptoms by causing osmotic diarrhea. Diarrhea is watery. Inflammatory diarrhea (dysentery), with fecal WBCs and RBCs or gross blood, is uncommon. Four categories of viruses cause most gastroenteritis: rotavirus and calicivirus (predominantly the norovirus [formerly Norwalk virus]) cause the majority of viral gastroenteritis, followed by astrovirus and enteric adenovirus.

Rotavirus is the most common cause of sporadic, severe, dehydrating diarrhea in young children (peak incidence, 3 to 15 mo). Rotavirus is highly contagious; most infections occur by the fecal-oral route. Adults may be infected after close contact with an infected infant. The illness in adults is generally mild. Incubation is 1 to 3 days. In temperate climates, most infections occur in the winter. Each year in the US, a wave of rotavirus illness begins in the Southwest in November and ends in the Northeast in March.

Norovirus most commonly infects older children and adults. Infections occur year-round, but 80% occur from November to April. Norovirus is the principal cause of sporadic viral gastroenteritis in adults and of epidemic viral gastroenteritis in all age groups; large waterborne and foodborne outbreaks occur. Person-to-person transmission also occurs because the virus is highly contagious. This virus causes most cases of gastroenteritis epidemics on cruise ships and in nursing homes. Incubation is 24 to 48 h.

Astrovirus can infect people of all ages but usually infects infants and young children. Infection is most common in winter. Transmission is by the fecal-oral route. Incubation is 3 to 4 days.

Adenoviruses are the 4th most common cause of childhood viral gastroenteritis. Infections occur year-round, with a slight increase in summer. Children < 2 yr are primarily affected. Transmission is by the fecal-oral route. Incubation is 3 to 10 days.

In immunocompromised patients, additional viruses (eg, cytomegalovirus, enterovirus) can cause gastroenteritis.

Bacteria: The bacteria most commonly implicated are

- *Salmonella*
- *Campylobacter*
- *Shigella*
- *Escherichia coli* (especially serotype O157:H7)
- *Clostridium difficile*

Bacterial gastroenteritis is less common than viral. Bacteria cause gastroenteritis by several mechanisms. Certain species (eg, *Vibrio cholerae,* enterotoxigenic strains of *E. coli*) adhere to intestinal mucosa without invading and produce enterotoxins. These toxins impair intestinal absorption and cause secretion of electrolytes and water by stimulating adenylate cyclase, resulting in watery diarrhea. *C. difficile* produces a similar toxin (see p. 1463).

Some bacteria (eg, *Staphylococcus aureus, Bacillus cereus, Clostridium perfringens*—see p. 1468) produce an exotoxin that is ingested in contaminated food. The exotoxin can cause gastroenteritis without bacterial infection. These toxins generally cause acute nausea, vomiting, and diarrhea within 12 h of ingestion of contaminated food. Symptoms abate within 36 h.

Other bacteria (eg, *Shigella, Salmonella, Campylobacter,* some *E. coli* subtypes—see p. 1468) invade the mucosa of the small bowel or colon and cause microscopic ulceration, bleeding, exudation of protein-rich fluid, and secretion of electrolytes and water. The invasive process and its results can occur whether or not the organism produces an enterotoxin. The resulting diarrhea contains WBCs and RBCs and sometimes gross blood.

Salmonella and *Campylobacter* are the most common bacterial causes of diarrheal illness in the US. Both infections are most frequently acquired through undercooked poultry; unpasteurized milk is also a possible source. *Campylobacter* is occasionally transmitted from dogs or cats with diarrhea. *Salmonella* can be transmitted by consuming undercooked eggs and by contact with reptiles, birds, or amphibians. Species of *Shigella* are the 3rd most common bacterial cause of diarrhea in the US and are usually transmitted person to person, although foodborne epidemics occur. *Shigella dysenteriae* type 1 (not present in the US) produces Shiga toxin, which can cause hemolytic-uremic syndrome (see p. 1204).

Several different subtypes of *E. coli* cause diarrhea. The epidemiology and clinical manifestations vary greatly depending on the subtype: (1) Enterohemorrhagic *E. coli* is the most clinically significant subtype in the US (see p. 1584). It produces Shiga toxin, which causes bloody diarrhea (hemorrhagic colitis). *E. coli* O157:H7 is the most common strain of this subtype in the US. Undercooked ground beef, unpasteurized milk and juice, and contaminated water are possible sources. Person-to-person transmission is common in the day care setting. Outbreaks associated with exposure to water in recreational settings (eg, pools, lakes, water parks) have also been reported. Hemolytic-uremic syndrome is a serious complication that develops in 2 to 7% of cases, most commonly among the young and old. (2) Enterotoxigenic *E. coli* produces two toxins (one similar to cholera toxin) that cause watery diarrhea. This subtype is the most common cause of traveler's diarrhea in people visiting the developing world. (3) Enteropathogenic *E. coli* causes watery diarrhea. Once a common cause of diarrhea outbreaks in nurseries, this subtype is now rare. (4) Enteroinvasive *E. coli* causes bloody or nonbloody diarrhea, primarily in the developing world. It is rare in the US.

In the past, *C. difficile* infection occurred almost exclusively in hospitalized patients receiving antibiotics. With the emergence of the hypervirulent NAP1 strain in the US in the late 2000s, many community-associated cases are now occurring.

Several other bacteria cause gastroenteritis, but most are uncommon in the US. *Yersinia enterocolitica* can cause gastroenteritis or a syndrome that mimics appendicitis. It is transmitted by undercooked pork, unpasteurized milk, or contaminated water. Several *Vibrio* species (eg, *V. parahaemolyticus*—see p. 1583) cause diarrhea after ingestion of undercooked seafood. *V. cholerae* (see p. 1582) sometimes causes severe dehydrating diarrhea in the developing world and is a particular concern after natural disasters or in refugee camps. *Listeria* causes food-borne gastroenteritis (see p. 1614). *Aeromonas* is acquired from swimming in or drinking contaminated fresh or brackish water. *Plesiomonas shigelloides* can cause diarrhea in patients who have eaten raw shellfish or traveled to tropical regions of the developing world.

Parasites: The parasites most commonly implicated are

- *Giardia*
- *Cryptosporidium*

Certain intestinal parasites, notably *Giardia intestinalis* (*lamblia*—see p. 1648), adhere to or invade the intestinal mucosa, causing nausea, vomiting, diarrhea, and general malaise. Giardiasis occurs in every region of the US and throughout the world. The infection can become chronic and cause a malabsorption syndrome. It is usually acquired via person-to-person transmission (often in day care centers) or from contaminated water.

Cryptosporidium parvum (see p. 1646) causes watery diarrhea sometimes accompanied by abdominal cramps, nausea, and vomiting. In healthy people, the illness is self-limited, lasting about 2 wk. In immunocompromised patients, illness may be severe, causing substantial electrolyte and fluid loss. *Cryptosporidium* is usually acquired through contaminated water. It is not easily killed by chlorine and is the most common cause of recreational waterborne illness in the US, accounting for about three-fourths of outbreaks.

Other parasites that can cause symptoms similar to those of cryptosporidiosis include *Cyclospora cayetanensis* and, in immunocompromised patients, *Cystoisospora (Isospora) belli*, and a collection of organisms referred to as microsporidia (eg, *Enterocytozoon bieneusi, Encephalitozoon intestinalis*). *Entamoeba histolytica* (amebiasis—see p. 1644) is a common cause of subacute bloody diarrhea in the developing world but is rare in the US.

Symptoms and Signs

The character and severity of symptoms vary. Generally, onset is sudden, with anorexia, nausea, vomiting, abdominal cramps, and diarrhea (with or without blood and mucus). Malaise, myalgias, and prostration may occur. The abdomen may be distended and mildly tender; in severe cases, muscle guarding may be present. Gas-distended intestinal loops may be palpable. Hyperactive bowel sounds (borborygmi) are present on auscultation even without diarrhea (an important differential feature from paralytic ileus, in which bowel sounds are absent or decreased). Persistent vomiting and diarrhea can result in intravascular fluid depletion with hypotension and tachycardia. In severe cases, shock, with vascular collapse and oliguric renal failure, occurs.

If vomiting is the main cause of fluid loss, metabolic alkalosis with hypochloremia can occur. If diarrhea is more prominent, acidosis is more likely. Both vomiting and diarrhea can cause hypokalemia. Hyponatremia may develop, particularly if hypotonic fluids are used in replacement therapy.

In viral infections, watery diarrhea is the most common symptom; stools rarely contain mucus or blood. Rotavirus gastroenteritis in infants and young children may last 5 to 7 days. Vomiting occurs in 90% of patients, and fever > 39° C (> 102.2° F) occurs in about 30%. Norovirus typically causes acute onset of vomiting, abdominal cramps, and diarrhea, with symptoms lasting only 1 to 2 days. In children, vomiting is more prominent than diarrhea, whereas in adults, diarrhea usually predominates. Patients may also experience fever, headache, and myalgias. The hallmark of adenovirus gastroenteritis is diarrhea lasting 1 to 2 wk. Affected infants and children may have mild vomiting that typically starts 1 to 2 days after the onset of diarrhea. Low-grade fever occurs in about 50% of patients. Astrovirus causes a syndrome similar to mild rotavirus infection.

Bacteria that cause invasive disease (eg, *Shigella, Salmonella*) are more likely to result in fever, prostration, and bloody diarrhea. *E. coli* O157:H7 infection usually begins with watery diarrhea for 1 to 2 days, followed by bloody diarrhea. Fever is absent or low grade. The spectrum of illness with *C. difficile* infection ranges from mild abdominal cramps and mucus-filled diarrhea to severe hemorrhagic colitis and shock. Bacteria that produce an enterotoxin (eg, *S. aureus, B. cereus, C. perfringens*) usually cause watery diarrhea.

Parasitic infections typically cause subacute or chronic diarrhea. Most cause nonbloody diarrhea; an exception is *E. histolytica,* which causes amebic dysentery. Fatigue and weight loss are common when diarrhea is persistent.

Diagnosis

- Clinical evaluation
- Stool testing in select cases

Other GI disorders that cause similar symptoms (eg, appendicitis, cholecystitis, ulcerative colitis) must be excluded (see p. 74). Findings suggestive of gastroenteritis include copious, watery diarrhea; ingestion of potentially contaminated food (particularly during a known outbreak), untreated surface water, or a known GI irritant; recent travel; or contact with certain animals or similarly ill people. *E. coli* O157:H7–induced diarrhea is notorious for appearing to be a hemorrhagic rather than an infectious process, manifesting as GI bleeding with little or no stool. Hemolytic-uremic syndrome (see p. 1204) may follow as evidenced by renal failure and hemolytic anemia. Recent oral antibiotic use (within 3 mo) must raise suspicion for *C. difficile* infection. However, about one-fourth of patients with community-associated *C. difficile* infection do not have a history of recent antibiotic use.

Stool testing: If a rectal examination shows occult blood or if watery diarrhea persists > 48 h, stool examination (fecal WBCs, ova, parasites) and culture are indicated. However, for the diagnosis of giardiasis or cryptosporidiosis, stool antigen detection using an enzyme immunoassay has a higher sensitivity. Rotavirus and enteric adenovirus infections can be diagnosed using commercially available rapid assays that detect viral antigen in the stool, but these assays are usually done only to document an outbreak. Norovirus can be detected by PCR in reference laboratories; this test is sometimes indicated to determine the cause of persistent diarrhea in an immunocompromised patient.

All patients with grossly bloody diarrhea should be tested for *E. coli* O157:H7, as should patients with nonbloody diarrhea during a known outbreak. Specific cultures must be requested because this organism is not detected on standard stool culture media. Alternatively, a rapid enzyme assay for the detection of Shiga toxin in stool can be done; a positive test indicates infection with *E. coli* O157:H7 or one of the other serotypes of enterohemorrhagic *E. coli*. (NOTE: *Shigella* species in the US do not produce Shiga toxin.) However, a rapid enzyme assay is not as sensitive as culture. PCR is used to detect Shiga toxin in some centers.

Adults with grossly bloody diarrhea should usually have sigmoidoscopy with cultures and biopsy. Appearance of the colonic mucosa may help diagnose amebic dysentery, shigellosis, and *E. coli* O157:H7 infection, although ulcerative colitis may cause similar lesions.

Patients with a history of recent antibiotic use or other risk factors for *C. difficile* infection (eg, inflammatory bowel disease, use of proton pump inhibitors) should have a stool assay for *C. difficile* toxin, but testing should also be done in patients with significant illness even when these risk factors are not present because about 25% of cases of *C. difficile* infection currently occur in people without identified risk factors. Historically, enzyme immunoassays for toxins A and B were used to diagnose *C. difficile* infection. However, nucleic acid amplification tests targeting one of the *C. difficile* toxin genes or their regulator have been shown to have higher sensitivity and are now the diagnostic tests of choice.

General tests: Serum electrolytes, BUN, and creatinine should be obtained to evaluate hydration and acid-base status in patients who appear seriously ill. CBC is nonspecific, although eosinophilia may indicate parasitic infection. Renal function tests and CBC should be done about a week after the start of symptoms in patients with *E. coli* O157:H7 to detect early-onset hemolytic-uremic syndrome.

Treatment

- Oral or IV rehydration
- Consideration of antidiarrheal agents if *C. difficile* or *E. coli* O157:H7 infection is not suspected
- Antibiotics only in select cases

Supportive treatment is all that is needed for most patients. Bed rest with convenient access to a toilet or bedpan is desirable. Oral glucose-electrolyte solutions, broth, or bouillon may prevent dehydration or treat mild dehydration. Even if vomiting, the patient should take frequent small sips of such fluids; vomiting may abate with volume replacement. For patients with *E. coli* O157:H7 infection, rehydration with isotonic IV fluids may attenuate the severity of any renal injury should hemolytic-uremic syndrome develop. Children may become dehydrated more quickly and should be given an appropriate rehydration solution (several are available commercially—see p. 2557). Carbonated beverages and sports drinks lack the correct ratio of glucose to Na and thus are not appropriate for children < 5 yr. If the child is breastfed, breastfeeding should continue. If vomiting is protracted or if severe dehydration is prominent, IV replacement of volume and electrolytes is necessary (see p. 576).

When the patient can tolerate fluids without vomiting and the appetite has begun to return, food may be gradually restarted. There is no demonstrated benefit from restriction to bland food (eg, cereal, gelatin, bananas, toast). Some patients have temporary lactose intolerance.

Antidiarrheal agents are safe for patients > 2 yr with watery diarrhea (as shown by heme-negative stool). However, antidiarrheals may cause deterioration of patients with *C. difficile* or *E. coli* O157:H7 infection and thus should not be given to any patient with recent antibiotic use or heme-positive stool, pending specific diagnosis. Effective antidiarrheals include loperamide 4 mg po initially, followed by 2 mg po for each subsequent episode of diarrhea (maximum of 6 doses/day or 16 mg/day), or diphenoxylate 2.5 to 5 mg tid or qid in tablet or liquid form. For children, loperamide is used. The dose for children 13 to 20 kg is 1 mg po tid; for children 20 to 30 kg, 2 mg po bid; and for children > 30 kg, up to age 12, 2 mg po tid. Adults and children ≥ 12 yr may receive 4 mg po after the first loose stool and then 2 mg after each subsequent loose stool, not to exceed 16 mg in any 24-h period.

If **vomiting** is severe and a surgical condition has been excluded, an antiemetic may be beneficial. Drugs useful in adults include prochlorperazine 5 to 10 mg IV tid or qid, or 25 mg per rectum bid and promethazine 12.5 to 25 mg IM tid or qid, or 25 to 50 mg per rectum qid. These drugs are usually avoided in children because of lack of demonstrated efficacy and the high incidence of dystonic reactions. Ondansetron is safe and effective in decreasing nausea and vomiting in children and in adults, including those with gastroenteritis, and is available as an standard tablet, oral disintegrating pill, or IV formulation. The dose for children ≥ 2 yr is 0.15 mg/kg po or IV tid, with a maximum single dose of 8 mg. The dose for adults is 4 or 8 mg po or IV tid.

Although probiotics appear to briefly shorten the duration of diarrhea, there is insufficient evidence that they affect major clinical outcomes (eg, decrease the need for IV hydration and/or hospitalization) to support their routine use in the treatment or prevention of infectious diarrhea.

Antimicrobials: Empiric antibiotics are generally not recommended except for certain cases of traveler's diarrhea or when suspicion of *Shigella* or *Campylobacter* infection is high (eg, contact with a known case). Otherwise, antibiotics should not be given until stool culture results are known, particularly in children, who have a higher rate of infection with *E. coli* O157:H7 (antibiotics increase the risk of hemolytic-uremic syndrome in patients infected with *E. coli* O157:H7).

In proven bacterial gastroenteritis, antibiotics are not always required. They do not help with *Salmonella* and prolong the duration of shedding in the stool. Exceptions include immunocompromised patients, neonates, and patients with *Salmonella* bacteremia. Antibiotics are also ineffective against toxic gastroenteritis (eg, *S. aureus, B. cereus, C. perfringens*). Indiscriminate use of antibiotics fosters the emergence of drug-resistant organisms. However, certain infections do require antibiotics (see Table 16–1).

Initial management of *C. difficile* colitis involves stopping the causative antibiotic if possible. Mild cases are treated with oral metronidazole. More severe cases should be treated with oral vancomycin. Unfortunately, recurrences are common with either regimen, occurring in about 20% of patients. A newer drug, fidaxomicin, may have a slightly lower relapse rate but is expensive. Many centers are using fecal microbial transplantation for patients with multiple recurrences of *C. difficile* colitis. This treatment has been shown to be safe and effective (see p. 1467).

For cryptosporidiosis, nitazoxanide may be helpful in immunocompetent patients. The dose is 100 mg po bid for children 1 to 3 yr, 200 mg po bid for children 4 to 11 yr, and 500 mg po bid for children ≥ 12 yr and adults.

Prevention

Two live-attenuated oral rotavirus vaccines are available that are safe and effective against the majority of strains responsible for disease. Rotavirus immunization is part of the recommended infant vaccination schedule (see Table 291–2 on p. 2462).

Prevention of infection is complicated by the frequency of asymptomatic infection and the ease with which many agents, particularly viruses, are transmitted from person to person. In general, proper procedures for handling and preparing food must be followed. Travelers must avoid potentially contaminated food and drink.

To prevent recreational waterborne infections, people should not swim if they have diarrhea. Infants and toddlers should have frequent diaper checks and should be changed in a bathroom and not near the water. Swimmers should avoid swallowing water when they swim.

Infants and other immunocompromised people are particularly predisposed to develop severe cases of salmonellosis and should not be exposed to reptiles, birds, or amphibians, which commonly carry *Salmonella*.

Breastfeeding affords some protection to neonates and infants. Caregivers should wash their hands thoroughly with soap and water after changing diapers, and diaper-changing areas should be disinfected with a freshly prepared solution of 1:64 household bleach (¼ cup diluted in 1 gallon of water). Children with diarrhea should be excluded from child care facilities for the duration of symptoms. Children infected with

Table 16–1. SELECTED ORAL ANTIBIOTICS FOR INFECTIOUS GASTROENTERITIS*

ORGANISM	ANTIBIOTIC	ADULT DOSAGE	PEDIATRIC DOSAGE
Vibrio cholerae	Ciprofloxacin	1 g once	NA
	Doxycycline[†]	300 mg single dose	6 mg/kg single dose
	TMP/SMX	1 DS tablet bid for 3 days	4–6 mg[‡]/kg bid for 5 days
Clostridium difficile	Metronidazole	250 mg qid or 500 mg tid for 10 days	7.5 mg/kg qid for 10–14 days
	Vancomycin	125–250 mg qid for 10 days	10 mg/kg qid for 10–14 days
	Fidaxomicin	200 mg bid for 10 days	NA
Shigella	Ciprofloxacin	500 mg bid for 5 days	NA
	TMP/SMX	1 DS tablet bid	4–6 mg[‡]/kg bid for 5 days
Giardia intestinalis (lamblia)	Metronidazole	250 mg tid for 5 days	10 mg/kg tid for 7–10 days (maximum 750 mg/day)
	Nitazoxanide	500 mg bid for 3 days	1–3 yr: 100 mg bid for 3 days 4–11 yr: 200 mg bid for 3 days ≥ 12 yr: 500 mg bid for 3 days
Entamoeba histolytica	Metronidazole[§]	750 mg tid for 5–10 days	12–16 mg/kg tid for 10 days (maximum 750 mg/day)
Campylobacter jejuni	Azithromycin	500 mg once/day for 3 days	10 mg/kg once/day for 3 days
	Ciprofloxacin	500 mg once/day for 5 days	NA

*Antibiotics are not indicated in most cases but may be used supportively with IV fluids to treat infections caused by specific organisms.
[†]This drug should not be given to children aged < 8 yr or to pregnant women.
[‡]Dose is based on trimethoprim component.
[§]Treatment should be followed by iodoquinol 10–13 mg/kg tid for 20 days or paromomycin 500 mg po tid for 7 days.
DS = double-strength; NA = not applicable; TMP/SMX = trimethoprim/sulfamethoxazole.

enterohemorrhagic *E. coli* or *Shigella* should also have two negative stool cultures before readmission to the facility.

TRAVELER'S DIARRHEA

(Turista)

Traveler's diarrhea is gastroenteritis that is usually caused by bacteria endemic to local water. Symptoms include vomiting and diarrhea. Diagnosis is mainly clinical. Treatment is with ciprofloxacin or azithromycin, loperamide, and replacement fluids.

(See also the Center for Disease Control and Prevention's health information for traveler's diarrhea.)

Etiology

Traveler's diarrhea may be caused by any of several bacteria, viruses, or, less commonly, parasites. However, enterotoxigenic *Escherichia coli* is most common. *E. coli* is common in the water supplies of areas that lack adequate purification. Infection is common among people traveling to developing countries. Norovirus infection has been a particular problem on some cruise ships.

Both food and water can be the source of infection. Travelers who avoid drinking local water may still become infected by brushing their teeth with an improperly rinsed toothbrush, drinking bottled drinks with ice made from local water, or eating food that is improperly handled or washed with local water. People taking drugs that decrease stomach acid (antacids, H_2 blockers, and proton pump inhibitors) are at risk of more severe illness.

Symptoms and Signs

Nausea, vomiting, hyperactive bowel sounds, abdominal cramps, and diarrhea begin 12 to 72 h after ingesting contaminated food or water. Severity is variable. Some people develop fever and myalgias. Most cases are mild and self-limited, although dehydration can occur, especially in warm climates.

Diagnosis

- Clinical evaluation

Specific diagnostic measures are usually not necessary. However, fever, severe abdominal pain, and bloody diarrhea suggest more serious disease and should prompt immediate evaluation.

Treatment

- Fluid replacement
- Sometimes antimotility drugs
- Antibiotics (eg, ciprofloxacin, azithromycin) for moderate to severe diarrhea

The mainstay of treatment is fluid replacement and an antimotility drug such as loperamide 4 mg po initially, followed by 2 mg po for each subsequent episode of diarrhea (maximum of 6 doses/day or 16 mg/day), or diphenoxylate 2.5 to 5 mg po tid or qid in tablet or liquid form. For drug treatment in children, see p. 127. Antimotility drugs are contraindicated in patients with fever or bloody stools and in children < 2 yr. Iodochlorhydroxyquin, which may be available in some developing countries, should not be used because it may cause neurologic damage.

Generally, antibiotics are not necessary for mild diarrhea. In patients with moderate to severe diarrhea (≥ 3 loose stools over 8 h), antibiotics are given, especially if vomiting, abdominal cramps, fever, or bloody stools are present. For adults, ciprofloxacin 500 mg po bid for 3 days or levofloxacin 500 mg po once/day for 3 days is recommended. Azithromycin 250 mg po once/day for 3 days or rifaximin 200 mg po tid for 3 days may also be used. For children, azithromycin 5 to 10 mg/kg po once/day for 3 days is preferred.

Prevention

Travelers should dine at restaurants with a reputation for safety and avoid foods and beverages from street vendors. They should consume only cooked foods that are still steaming hot, fruit that can be peeled, and carbonated beverages without ice served in sealed bottles (bottles of noncarbonated beverages can contain tap water added by unscrupulous vendors); uncooked vegetables (particularly including salsa left out on the table) should be avoided. Buffets and fast-food restaurants pose an increased risk.

Prophylactic antibiotics are effective in preventing diarrhea, but because of concerns about adverse effects and development of resistance, they should probably be reserved for immunocompromised patients.

DRUG-RELATED GASTROENTERITIS AND CHEMICAL-RELATED GASTROENTERITIS

Many drugs cause nausea, vomiting, and diarrhea as adverse effects. A detailed drug history must be obtained. In mild cases, cessation followed by reuse of the drug may establish a causal relationship. Commonly responsible drugs include antacids containing Mg, antibiotics, antihelminthics, cytotoxics (used in cancer therapy), colchicine, digoxin, heavy metals, laxatives, and radiation therapy. Use of antibiotics may lead to *Clostridium difficile*–induced diarrhea (see p. 1466).

Iatrogenic, accidental, or intentional heavy-metal poisoning frequently causes nausea, vomiting, abdominal pain, and diarrhea.

Laxative abuse, sometimes denied by patients, may lead to weakness, vomiting, diarrhea, electrolyte depletion, and metabolic disturbances.

Various plants and mushrooms cause a syndrome of gastroenteritis (see Mushroom Poisoning and Plant Poisoning on p. 3062).

17 GI Bleeding

GI bleeding can originate anywhere from the mouth to the anus and can be overt or occult. The manifestations depend on the location and rate of bleeding.

Hematemesis is vomiting of red blood and indicates upper GI bleeding, usually from a peptic ulcer, vascular lesion, or varix. Coffee-ground emesis is vomiting of dark brown, granular material that resembles coffee grounds. It results from upper GI bleeding that has slowed or stopped, with conversion of red Hb to brown hematin by gastric acid.

Hematochezia is the passage of gross blood from the rectum and usually indicates lower GI bleeding but may result from vigorous upper GI bleeding with rapid transit of blood through the intestines.

Melena is black, tarry stool and typically indicates upper GI bleeding, but bleeding from a source in the small bowel or right colon may also be the cause. About 100 to 200 mL of blood in the upper GI tract is required to cause melena, which may persist for several days after bleeding has ceased. Black stool that does not contain occult blood may result from ingestion of iron, bismuth, or various foods and should not be mistaken for melena.

Chronic occult bleeding can occur from anywhere in the GI tract and is detectable by chemical testing of a stool specimen. Acute, severe bleeding also can occur from anywhere in the GI tract. Patients may present with signs of shock. Patients with underlying ischemic heart disease may develop angina or MI because of coronary hypoperfusion.

GI bleeding may precipitate portosystemic encephalopathy or hepatorenal syndrome (kidney failure secondary to liver failure).

Etiology

There are many possible causes (see Table 17–1), which are divided into upper GI (above the ligament of Treitz), lower GI, and small bowel.

Bleeding of any cause is more likely, and potentially more severe, in patients with chronic liver disease (eg, caused by alcohol abuse or chronic hepatitis), in those with hereditary coagulation disorders, or in those taking certain drugs. Drugs associated with GI bleeding include anticoagulants (eg, heparin, warfarin), those affecting platelet function (eg, aspirin and certain other NSAIDs, clopidogrel, SSRIs), and those affecting mucosal defenses (eg, NSAIDs).

Evaluation

Stabilization with airway management, IV fluids, or transfusions is essential before and during diagnostic evaluation.

Table 17–1. COMMON CAUSES OF GI BLEEDING

Upper GI tract
Duodenal ulcer (20–30%)
Gastric or duodenal erosions (20–30%)
Varices (15–20%)
Gastric ulcer (10–20%)
Mallory-Weiss tear (5–10%)
Erosive esophagitis (5–10%)
Angioma (5–10%)
Arteriovenous malformations (< 5%)
Gastrointestinal stromal tumors
Lower GI tract (percentages vary with the age group sampled)
Anal fissures
Angiodysplasia (vascular ectasia)
Colitis: Radiation, ischemic, infectious
Colonic carcinoma
Colonic polyps
Diverticular disease
Inflammatory bowel disease: Ulcerative proctitis/colitis, Crohn disease
Internal hemorrhoids
Small-bowel lesions (rare)
Angiomas
Arteriovenous malformations
Meckel diverticulum
Tumors

History: History of present illness should attempt to ascertain quantity and frequency of blood passage. However, quantity can be difficult to assess because even small amounts (5 to 10 mL) of blood turn water in a toilet bowl an opaque red, and modest amounts of vomited blood appear huge to an anxious patient. However, most can distinguish between blood streaks, a few teaspoons, and clots.

Patients with hematemesis should be asked whether blood was passed with initial vomiting or only after an initial (or several) nonbloody emesis.

Patients with rectal bleeding should be asked whether pure blood was passed; whether it was mixed with stool, pus, or mucus; or whether blood simply coated the stool or toilet paper. Those with bloody diarrhea should be asked about travel or other possible exposure to GI pathogens.

Review of symptoms should include presence of abdominal discomfort, weight loss, easy bleeding or bruising, previous colonoscopy results, and symptoms of anemia (eg, weakness, easy fatigability, dizziness).

Past medical history should inquire about previous GI bleeding (diagnosed or undiagnosed); known inflammatory bowel disease, bleeding diatheses, and liver disease; and use of any drugs that increase the likelihood of bleeding or chronic liver disease (eg, alcohol).

Physical examination: General examination focuses on vital signs and other indicators of shock or hypovolemia (eg, tachycardia, tachypnea, pallor, diaphoresis, oliguria, confusion) and anemia (eg, pallor, diaphoresis). Patients with lesser degrees of bleeding may simply have mild tachycardia (heart rate > 100).

Orthostatic changes in pulse (a change of > 10 beats/min) or BP (a drop of ≥ 10 mm Hg) often develop after acute loss of ≥ 2 units of blood. However, orthostatic measurements are unwise in patients with severe bleeding (possibly causing syncope) and generally lack sensitivity and specificity as a measure of intravascular volume, especially in elderly patients.

External stigmata of bleeding disorders (eg, petechiae, ecchymoses) are sought, as are signs of chronic liver disease (eg, spider angiomas, ascites, palmar erythema) and portal hypertension (eg, splenomegaly, dilated abdominal wall veins).

A digital rectal examination is necessary to search for stool color, masses, and fissures. Anoscopy is done to diagnose hemorrhoids. Chemical testing of a stool specimen for occult blood completes the examination if gross blood is not present.

Red flags: Several findings suggest hypovolemia or hemorrhagic shock:

- Syncope
- Hypotension
- Pallor
- Diaphoresis
- Tachycardia

Interpretation of findings: The history and physical examination suggest a diagnosis in about 50% of patients, but findings are rarely diagnostic and confirmatory testing is required.

Epigastric abdominal discomfort relieved by food or antacids suggests peptic ulcer disease. However, many patients with bleeding ulcers have no history of pain. Weight loss and anorexia, with or without a change in stool, suggest a GI cancer. A history of cirrhosis or chronic hepatitis suggests esophageal varices. Dysphagia suggests esophageal cancer or stricture. Vomiting and retching before the onset of bleeding suggests a Mallory-Weiss tear of the esophagus, although about 50% of patients with Mallory-Weiss tears do not have this history.

A history of bleeding (eg, purpura, ecchymosis, hematuria) may indicate a bleeding diathesis (eg, hemophilia, hepatic failure). Bloody diarrhea, fever, and abdominal pain suggest ischemic colitis, inflammatory bowel disease (eg, ulcerative colitis, Crohn disease), or an infectious colitis (eg, *Shigella, Salmonella, Campylobacter,* amebiasis). Hematochezia suggests diverticulosis or angiodysplasia. Fresh blood only on toilet paper or the surface of formed stools suggests internal hemorrhoids or fissures, whereas blood mixed with the stool indicates a more proximal source. Occult blood in the stool may be the first sign of colon cancer or a polyp, particularly in patients > 45 yr.

Blood in the nose or trickling down the pharynx suggests the nasopharynx as the source. Spider angiomas, hepatosplenomegaly, or ascites is consistent with chronic liver disease and hence possible esophageal varices. Arteriovenous malformations, especially of the mucous membranes, suggest hereditary hemorrhagic telangiectasia (Rendu-Osler-Weber syndrome). Cutaneous nail bed and GI telangiectasia may indicate systemic sclerosis or mixed connective tissue disease.

Testing: Several tests are done to help confirm the suspected diagnosis.

- CBC, coagulation profile, and often other laboratory studies
- NGT for all but those with minimal rectal bleeding
- Upper endoscopy for suspected upper GI bleeding
- Colonoscopy for lower GI bleeding (unless clearly caused by hemorrhoids)

CBC should be obtained in patients with large-volume or occult blood loss. Patients with more significant bleeding also require coagulation studies (eg, platelet count, PT, PTT) and liver function tests (eg, bilirubin, alkaline phosphatase, albumin, AST, ALT). Type and cross-match are done if bleeding is ongoing. Hb and Hct may be repeated up to every 6 h in patients with severe bleeding. Additionally, one or more diagnostic procedures are typically required.

Nasogastric aspiration and lavage should be done in all patients with suspected upper GI bleeding (eg, hematemesis, coffee-ground emesis, melena, massive rectal bleeding). Bloody nasogastric aspirate indicates active upper GI bleeding, but about 10% of patients with upper GI bleeding have no blood in the nasogastric aspirate. Coffee-ground material indicates bleeding that is slow or stopped. If there is no sign of bleeding, and bile is returned, the NGT is removed; otherwise, it is left in place to monitor continuing or recurrent bleeding. Nonbloody, nonbilious return is considered a nondiagnostic aspirate.

Upper endoscopy (examination of the esophagus, stomach, and duodenum) should be done for upper GI bleeding. Because endoscopy may be therapeutic as well as diagnostic, it should be done rapidly for significant bleeding but may be deferred for 24 h if bleeding stops or is minimal. Upper GI barium x-rays have no role in acute bleeding, and the contrast used may obscure subsequent attempts at angiography. Angiography is useful in the diagnosis of upper GI bleeding and permits certain therapeutic maneuvers (eg, embolization, vasoconstrictor infusion).

Flexible sigmoidoscopy and anoscopy may be all that is required acutely for patients with symptoms typical of hemorrhoidal bleeding. All other patients with hematochezia should have colonoscopy, which can be done electively after routine preparation unless there is significant ongoing bleeding. In such patients, a rapid prep (5 to 6 L of polyethylene glycol solution delivered via NGT or by mouth over 3 to 4 h) often allows adequate visualization. If colonoscopy cannot visualize the source and ongoing bleeding is sufficiently rapid (> 0.5 to 1 mL/min), angiography may localize the source. Some angiographers first take a radionuclide scan to focus the examination, because angiography is less sensitive than the radionuclide scan.

Diagnosis of occult bleeding can be difficult, because heme-positive stools may result from bleeding anywhere in the

GI tract. Endoscopy is the preferred method, with symptoms determining whether the upper or lower GI tract is examined first. Double-contrast barium enema and sigmoidoscopy can be used for the lower tract when colonoscopy is unavailable or the patient refuses it.

If the results of upper endoscopy and colonoscopy are negative and occult blood persists in the stool, an upper GI series with small-bowel follow-through, CT enterography, small-bowel endoscopy (enteroscopy), capsule endoscopy (which uses a small pill-like camera that is swallowed), technetium-labeled colloid or RBC scan, and angiography should be considered. Capsule endoscopy is of limited value in an actively bleeding patient.

Treatment

- Secure airway if needed
- IV fluid resuscitation
- Blood transfusion if needed
- In some, angiographic or endoscopic hemostasis

(See also the American College of Gastroenterology's practice guidelines on management of the adult patient with acute lower GI bleeding and the practice guidelines on management of patients with ulcer bleeding.)

Hematemesis, hematochezia, or melena should be considered an emergency. Admission to an ICU, with consultation by both a gastroenterologist and a surgeon, is recommended for all patients with severe GI bleeding. General treatment is directed at maintenance of the airway and restoration of circulating volume. Hemostasis and other treatment depend on the cause of the bleeding.

Airway: A major cause of morbidity and mortality in patients with active upper GI bleeding is aspiration of blood with subsequent respiratory compromise. To prevent these problems, endotracheal intubation should be considered in patients who have inadequate gag reflexes or are obtunded or unconscious—particularly if they will be undergoing upper endoscopy.

Fluid resuscitation: Intravenous access should be obtained immediately. Short, large-bore (eg, 14- to 16-gauge) IV catheters in the antecubital veins are preferable to a central venous catheter unless a large (8.5 Fr) sheath is used. IV fluids are initiated immediately, as for any patient with hypovolemia or hemorrhagic shock (see p. 576). Healthy adults are given normal saline IV in 500- to 1000-mL aliquots until signs of hypovolemia remit—up to a maximum of 2 L (for children, 20 mL/kg, that may be repeated once).

Patients requiring further resuscitation should receive transfusion with packed RBCs. Transfusions continue until intravascular volume is restored and then are given as needed to replace ongoing blood loss. Transfusions in older patients or those with coronary artery disease may be stopped when Hct is stable at 30 unless the patient is symptomatic. Younger patients or those with chronic bleeding are usually not transfused unless Hct is < 23 or they have symptoms such as dyspnea or coronary ischemia.

Platelet count should be monitored closely; platelet transfusion may be required with severe bleeding. Patients who are taking antiplatelet drugs (eg, clopidogrel, aspirin) have platelet dysfunction, often resulting in increased bleeding. Platelet transfusion should be considered when patients taking these drugs have severe ongoing bleeding, although a residual circulating drug (particularly clopidogrel) may inactivate transfused platelets. Fresh frozen plasma should be transfused after every 4 units of packed RBCs.

Hemostasis: GI bleeding stops spontaneously in about 80% of patients. The remaining patients require some type of intervention. Specific therapy depends on the bleeding site. Early intervention to control bleeding is important to minimize mortality, particularly in elderly patients.

For **peptic ulcer,** ongoing bleeding or rebleeding is treated with endoscopic coagulation (with bipolar electrocoagulation, injection sclerotherapy, heater probes, clips, or laser). Nonbleeding vessels that are visible within an ulcer crater are also treated. If endoscopy does not stop the bleeding, angiographic embolization of the bleeding vessel may be attempted, or surgery is required to oversew the bleeding site. If the patient has been treated medically for peptic ulcer disease but has recurrent bleeding, surgeons do acid-reduction surgery (see p. 122) at the same time.

Active variceal bleeding can be treated with endoscopic banding, injection sclerotherapy, or a transjugular intrahepatic portosystemic shunting (TIPS) procedure.

Severe, ongoing **lower GI bleeding** caused by diverticula or angiomas can sometimes be controlled colonoscopically by clips, electrocautery, coagulation with a heater probe, or injection with dilute epinephrine. Polyps can be removed by snare or cautery. If these methods are ineffective or unfeasible, angiography with embolization or vasopressin infusion may be successful. However, because collateral blood flow to the bowel is limited, angiographic techniques have a significant risk of bowel ischemia or infarction unless super-selective catheterization techniques are used. In most series, the rate of ischemic complications is < 5%. Vasopressin infusion has about an 80% success rate for stopping bleeding, but bleeding recurs in about 50% of patients. Also, there is a risk of hypertension and coronary ischemia. Furthermore, angiography can be used to localize the source of bleeding more accurately.

Surgery may be done in patients with continued lower GI bleeding (requiring > 6 units transfusion), but localization of the bleeding site is very important. If the bleeding site cannot be localized, subtotal colectomy is recommended. Blind hemicolectomy (with no preoperative identification of the bleeding site) carries a much higher mortality risk than does directed segmental resection and may not remove the bleeding site; the rebleeding rate is 40%. However, assessment must be expeditious so that surgery is not unnecessarily delayed. In patients who have received > 10 units of packed RBCs, the mortality rate is about 30%.

Acute or chronic bleeding of internal hemorrhoids stops spontaneously in most cases. Patients with refractory bleeding are treated via anoscopy with rubber band ligation, injection, coagulation, or surgery.

Geriatrics Essentials

In the elderly, hemorrhoids and colorectal cancer are the most common causes of minor bleeding. Peptic ulcer, diverticular disease, and angiodysplasia are the most common causes of major bleeding. Variceal bleeding is less common than in younger patients.

Massive GI bleeding is tolerated poorly by elderly patients. Diagnosis must be made quickly, and treatment must be started sooner than in younger patients, who can better tolerate repeated episodes of bleeding.

KEY POINTS

- Rectal bleeding may result from upper or lower GI bleeding.
- Orthostatic changes in vital signs are unreliable markers for serious bleeding.
- About 80% of patients stop bleeding spontaneously; various endoscopic techniques are usually the first choice for the remainder.

VARICES

Varices are dilated veins in the distal esophagus or proximal stomach caused by elevated pressure in the portal venous system, typically from cirrhosis. They may bleed massively but cause no other symptoms. Diagnosis is by upper endoscopy. Treatment is primarily with endoscopic banding and IV octreotide. Sometimes a TIPS procedure is needed.

Portal hypertension results from a number of conditions, predominantly liver cirrhosis. If portal pressure remains higher than inferior vena caval pressure for a significant period, venous collaterals develop. The most dangerous collaterals occur in the distal esophagus and gastric fundus, causing engorged, serpentine submucosal vessels known as varices. These varices partially decompress portal hypertension but can rupture, causing massive GI bleeding. The trigger for variceal rupture is unknown, but bleeding almost never occurs unless the portal/systemic pressure gradient is > 12 mm Hg. Coagulopathies caused by liver disease may facilitate bleeding.

See also the American College of Gastroenterology's practice guidelines on variceal hemorrhage in cirrhosis.

PEARLS & PITFALLS

- NGT passage in a patient with varices has not been shown to trigger bleeding.

Symptoms and Signs

Patients typically present with sudden, painless, upper GI bleeding, often massive. Signs of shock may be present. Bleeding is usually from the distal esophagus, less often from the gastric fundus. Bleeding from gastric varices also may be acute but is more often subacute or chronic.

Bleeding into the GI tract may precipitate portal-systemic encephalopathy in patients with impaired hepatic function.

Diagnosis

- Endoscopy
- Evaluation for coagulopathy

Both esophageal and gastric varices are best diagnosed by endoscopy, which may also identify varices at high risk of bleeding (eg, those with red markings). Endoscopy is also critical to exclude other causes of acute bleeding (eg, peptic ulcer), even in patients known to have varices; perhaps as many as one third of patients with known varices who have upper GI bleeding have a nonvariceal source.

Because varices are typically associated with significant hepatic disease, evaluation for possible coagulopathy is important. Laboratory tests include CBC with platelets, PT, PTT, and liver function tests. Bleeding patients should have type and cross-match for 6 units of packed RBCs.

Prognosis

In about 40% of patients, variceal bleeding stops spontaneously. Previously, mortality was > 50%, but even with current management, mortality is at least 20% at 6 wk. Mortality depends primarily on severity of the associated liver disease rather than on the bleeding itself. Bleeding is often fatal in patients with severe hepatocellular impairment (eg, advanced cirrhosis), whereas patients with good hepatic reserve usually recover.

Surviving patients are at high risk of further variceal bleeding; typically, 50 to 75% have recurrence within 1 to 2 yr. Ongoing endoscopic or drug therapy significantly lowers this risk, but the overall effect on long-term mortality seems to be marginal, probably because of the underlying hepatic disease.

Treatment

- Fluid resuscitation
- Endoscopic banding (sclerotherapy second choice)
- IV octreotide
- Possibly a TIPS procedure

Fluid resuscitation, including transfusion as needed, is done to manage hypovolemia and hemorrhagic shock. Patients with coagulation abnormalities (eg, significantly elevated INR) can be treated with 1 to 2 units of fresh frozen plasma, but this should be given cautiously because giving large volumes of fluid to patients who are not hypovolemic may actually promote bleeding from varices. Patients with known cirrhosis with GI bleeding are at risk of bacterial infection and should receive antibiotic prophylaxis with norfloxacin or ceftriaxone.

Because varices are invariably diagnosed during endoscopy, primary treatment is endoscopic. Endoscopic banding of varices is preferred over injection sclerotherapy. At the same time, IV octreotide (a synthetic analog of somatostatin, which may also be used) should be given. Octreotide increases splanchnic vascular resistance by inhibiting the release of splanchnic vasodilator hormones (eg, glucagon, vasoactive intestinal peptide). The usual dose is a 50-μg IV bolus, followed by infusion of 50 μg/h. Octreotide is preferred over previously used agents such as vasopressin and terlipressin, because it has fewer adverse effects.

If bleeding continues or recurs despite these measures, emergency techniques to shunt blood from the portal system to the vena cava can lower portal pressure and diminish bleeding. A TIPS procedure is the emergency intervention of choice. TIPS is an invasive radiologic procedure in which a guidewire is passed from the vena cava through the liver parenchyma into the portal circulation. The resultant passage is dilated by a balloon catheter, and a metallic stent is inserted, creating a bypass between the portal and hepatic venous circulations. Stent size is crucial. If the stent is too large, portal-systemic encephalopathy results because of diversion of too much portal blood flow from the liver. If the stent is too small, it is more likely to occlude. Surgical portacaval shunts, such as the distal spleno-renal shunt, work by a similar mechanism but are more invasive and have a higher immediate mortality.

Mechanical compression of bleeding varices with a Sengstaken-Blakemore tube or one of its variants causes considerable morbidity and should not be used as primary management. However, such a tube may provide life-saving tamponade pending decompression with a TIPS or surgical procedure. The tube is a flexible NGT with one gastric balloon and one esophageal balloon. After insertion, the gastric balloon is inflated with a fixed volume of air, and traction is applied to the tube to pull the balloon snugly against the gastroesophageal junction. This balloon is often sufficient to control bleeding, but if not, the esophageal balloon is inflated to a pressure of 25 mm Hg. The procedure is quite uncomfortable and may result in esophageal perforation and aspiration; thus, endotracheal intubation and IV sedation are often recommended.

Liver transplantation can also decompress the portal system but is a practical option only for patients already on a transplant list.

Long-term medical therapy of portal hypertension (with β-blockers and nitrates) is discussed elsewhere (see p. 192). Treatment of portosystemic encephalopathy may be needed.

KEY POINTS

- Varices are the main but not the only cause of GI bleeding in patients with cirrhosis.
- The severity of the underlying liver disease is a major determinant of mortality of a bleeding episode.
- Endoscopy is done for diagnosis and treatment; banding or sclerotherapy can be used.
- Recurrence rate is 50 to 75% within 1 to 2 yr.

VASCULAR GI LESIONS

Several distinct congenital or acquired syndromes involve abnormal mucosal or submucosal blood vessels in the GI tract. These vessels may cause recurrent bleeding, which is rarely massive. Diagnosis is by endoscopy and sometimes angiography. Treatment is endoscopic hemostasis; occasionally, angiographic embolization or surgical resection may be needed.

Vascular ectasias (angiodysplasias, arteriovenous malformations) are dilated, tortuous vessels that typically develop in the cecum and ascending colon. They occur mainly in people > 60 and are the most common cause of lower GI bleeding in that age group. They are thought to be degenerative and do not occur in association with other vascular abnormalities. Most patients have 2 or 3 lesions, which are typically 0.5 to 1.0 cm, bright red, flat or slightly raised, and covered by very thin epithelium.

Vascular ectasias also occur in association with a number of systemic diseases (eg, renal failure, cirrhosis, CREST syndrome [calcinosis cutis, Raynaud phenomenon, esophageal dysmotility, sclerodactyly, telangiectasias]—see p. 266) and after radiation to the bowel.

Gastric antral vascular ectasia (watermelon stomach or GAVE) consists of large dilated veins running linearly along the stomach, creating a striped appearance suggestive of a watermelon. The condition occurs mainly in older women and is of unknown etiology.

Hereditary hemorrhagic telangiectasia (Rendu-Osler-Weber syndrome) is an autosomal dominant disorder that causes multiple vascular lesions in various parts of the body, including the entire GI tract. GI bleeding rarely occurs before age 40.

Dieulafoy lesion is an abnormally large artery that penetrates the gut wall, occasionally eroding through the mucosa and causing massive bleeding. It occurs mainly in the proximal stomach.

Arteriovenous malformations and **hemangiomas,** both congenital disorders of blood vessels, can occur in the GI tract but are rare.

Symptoms and Signs

Vascular lesions are painless. Patients often present with heme-positive stools or modest amounts of bright red blood from the rectum. Bleeding is often intermittent, sometimes with long periods between episodes. Patients with upper GI lesions may present with melena. Major bleeding is unusual.

Diagnosis

- Endoscopy

Vascular lesions are most commonly diagnosed endoscopically. If routine endoscopy is nondiagnostic, small-bowel endoscopy, capsule endoscopy, intraoperative endoscopy, or visceral angiography may be required. ^{99m}Tc-labeled RBC scans are less specific but may help localize the lesion enough to facilitate endoscopy or angiography.

Treatment

- Endoscopic coagulation

Endoscopic coagulation (with heater probe, laser, argon plasma, or bipolar electrocoagulation) is effective for many vascular lesions. Endoscopic clips may be applied to some lesions. Vascular ectasias often recur, although there is some evidence that oral estrogen-progesterone combinations may limit recurrence.

Mild recurrent bleeding can be treated simply with chronic iron therapy. More significant bleeding that is unresponsive to endoscopic measures may require angiographic embolization or surgical resection. However, rebleeding occurs in about 15 to 25% of surgically treated patients.

KEY POINTS

- A variety of inherited and acquired vascular abnormalities can cause mild to moderate GI bleeding (usually lower).
- Preferred treatment is endoscopy with coagulation of lesions.

18 Inflammatory Bowel Disease

Inflammatory bowel disease (IBD), which includes Crohn disease and ulcerative colitis (UC), is a relapsing and remitting condition characterized by chronic inflammation at various sites in the GI tract, which results in diarrhea and abdominal pain.

Inflammation results from a cell-mediated immune response in the GI mucosa. The precise etiology is unknown, but evidence suggests that the normal intestinal flora trigger an abnormal immune reaction in patients with a multifactorial genetic predisposition (perhaps involving abnormal epithelial barriers and mucosal immune defenses). No specific environmental, dietary, or infectious causes have been identified. The immune reaction involves the release of inflammatory mediators, including cytokines, interleukins, and TNF.

Although Crohn disease and UC are similar, they can be distinguished in most cases (see Table 18–1). About 10% of colitis cases are not initially distinguishable and are termed unclassified; if a surgical pathologic specimen cannot be classified, it is called indeterminate colitis. The term *colitis* applies only to inflammatory disease of the colon (eg, ulcerative, granulomatous, ischemic, radiation-induced, infectious). Spastic (mucous) colitis is a misnomer sometimes applied to a functional disorder, irritable bowel syndrome.

Table 18–1. DIFFERENTIATING CROHN DISEASE AND ULCERATIVE COLITIS

CROHN DISEASE	ULCERATIVE COLITIS
Small bowel is involved in 80% of cases.	Disease is confined to the colon.
Rectosigmoid is often spared; colonic involvement is usually right-sided.	Rectosigmoid is invariably involved; colonic involvement is usually left-sided.
Gross rectal bleeding is rare, except in 75–85% of cases of Crohn colitis.	Gross rectal bleeding is always present.
Fistula, mass, and abscess development is common.	Fistulas do not occur.
Perianal lesions are significant in 25–35% of cases.	Significant perianal lesions never occur.
On x-ray, bowel wall is affected asymmetrically and segmentally, with skip areas between diseased segments.	Bowel wall is affected symmetrically and uninterruptedly from rectum proximally.
Endoscopic appearance is patchy, with discrete ulcerations separated by segments of normal-appearing mucosa.	Inflammation is uniform and diffuse.
Microscopic inflammation and fissuring extend transmurally; lesions are often highly focal in distribution.	Inflammation is confined to mucosa except in severe cases.
Epithelioid (sarcoid-like) granulomas are detected in bowel wall or lymph nodes in 25–50% of cases (pathognomonic).	Typical epithelioid granulomas do not occur.

Epidemiology: Inflammatory bowel disease affects people of all ages but usually begins before age 30, with peak incidence from 14 to 24. IBD may have a second smaller peak between ages 50 and 70; however, this later peak may include some cases of ischemic colitis.

IBD is most common among people of Northern European and Anglo-Saxon origin and is 2 to 4 times more common among Ashkenazi Jews than non-Jewish whites from the same geographic location. The incidence is lower in central and southern Europe and lower still in South America, Asia, and Africa. However, the incidence is increasing among blacks and Latin Americans living in North America. Both sexes are equally affected. First-degree relatives of patients with IBD have a 4- to 20-fold increased risk; their absolute risk may be as high as 7%. Familial tendency is much higher in Crohn disease than in UC. Several gene mutations conferring a higher risk of Crohn disease (and some possibly related to UC) have been identified.

Cigarette smoking seems to contribute to development or exacerbation of Crohn disease but decreases risk of UC. Appendectomy done to treat appendicitis also appears to lower the risk of UC. NSAIDs may exacerbate IBD. Oral contraceptives may increase the risk of Crohn disease. Some data suggest that perinatal illness and the use of antibiotics in childhood may be associated with an increased risk of IBD.

For unclear reasons, people who have a higher socioeconomic status may have an increased risk of Crohn disease.

PEARLS & PITFALLS

- Cigarette smoking *decreases* the risk of ulcerative colitis.

Extraintestinal Manifestations

Crohn disease and UC both affect organs other than the intestines. Most extraintestinal manifestations are more common in UC and Crohn colitis than in Crohn disease limited to the small bowel. Extraintestinal manifestations of inflammatory bowel disease are categorized in 3 ways:

1. Disorders that usually parallel (ie, wax and wane with) IBD flare-ups: These disorders include peripheral arthritis, episcleritis, aphthous stomatitis, erythema nodosum, and pyoderma gangrenosum. Arthritis tends to involve large joints and be migratory and transient. One or more of these parallel disorders develops in more than one-third of patients hospitalized with IBD.

2. Disorders that are clearly associated with IBD but appear independently of IBD activity: These disorders include ankylosing spondylitis, sacroiliitis, uveitis, and primary sclerosing cholangitis. Ankylosing spondylitis occurs more commonly in IBD patients with the HLA-B27 antigen. Most patients with spinal or sacroiliac involvement have evidence of uveitis and vice versa. Primary sclerosing cholangitis, which is a risk factor for cancer of the biliary tract, is strongly associated with UC or Crohn colitis. Cholangitis may appear before or concurrently with the bowel disease or even 20 yr after colectomy. Liver disease (eg, fatty liver, autoimmune hepatitis, pericholangitis, cirrhosis) occurs in 3 to 5% of patients, although minor abnormalities in liver function tests are more common. Some of these conditions (eg, primary sclerosing cholangitis) may precede IBD by many years and, when diagnosed, should prompt an evaluation for IBD.

3. Disorders that are consequences of disrupted bowel physiology: These disorders occur mainly in severe Crohn disease of the small bowel. Malabsorption may result from extensive ileal resection and cause deficiencies of fat-soluble vitamins, vitamin B_{12}, or minerals, resulting in anemia, hypocalcemia, hypomagnesemia, clotting disorders, and bone demineralization. In children, malabsorption retards growth and development. Other disorders include kidney stones from excessive dietary oxalate absorption, hydroureter and hydronephrosis from ureteral compression by the intestinal inflammatory process, gallstones from impaired ileal reabsorption of bile salts, and amyloidosis secondary to long-standing inflammatory and suppurative disease.

Thromboembolic disease may occur as a result of multiple factors in all 3 categories.

Treatment

- Supportive care
- 5-Aminosalicylic acid
- Corticosteroids
- Immunomodulating drugs
- Biologic agents (anticytokine drugs)
- Sometimes antibiotics (eg, metronidazole, ciprofloxacin) and probiotics

Several classes of drugs are helpful for IBD. Details of their selection and use are discussed under each disorder.

Supportive care: Most patients and their families are interested in diet and stress management. Although there are anecdotal reports of clinical improvement on certain diets, including one with rigid carbohydrate restrictions, controlled trials have shown no consistent benefit. Stress management may be helpful.

DRUGS FOR INFLAMMATORY BOWEL DISEASE

Several classes of drugs are helpful for inflammatory bowel disease (IBD). Details of their selection and use are discussed under each disorder (see Crohn disease treatment on p. 138 and ulcerative colitis treatment on p. 139).

5-Aminosalicylic Acid (5-ASA, Mesalamine)

5-ASA blocks production of prostaglandins and leukotrienes and has other beneficial effects on the inflammatory cascade. Because 5-ASA is active only intraluminally and is rapidly absorbed by the proximal small bowel, it must be formulated for delayed absorption when given orally.

Sulfasalazine, the original agent in this class, delays absorption by complexing 5-ASA with a sulfa moiety, sulfapyridine. The complex is cleaved by bacterial flora in the lower ileum and colon, releasing the 5-ASA. The sulfa moiety, however, causes numerous adverse effects (eg, nausea, dyspepsia, headache), interferes with folate (folic acid) absorption, and occasionally causes serious adverse reactions (eg, hemolytic anemia or agranulocytosis and, rarely, hepatitis, pneumonitis, or myocarditis). Reversible decreases in sperm count and motility occur in up to 80% of men. If used, sulfasalazine should be given with food, initially in a low dosage (eg, 0.5 g po bid) and the dose and frequency gradually increased over several days to 1 to 1.5 g qid. Patients should take daily folate supplements (1 mg po) and have CBC and liver tests every 6 to 12 mo. Acute interstitial nephritis secondary to mesalamine occurs rarely; periodic monitoring of renal function is advisable because most cases are reversible if recognized early.

Drugs that complex 5-ASA with other vehicles seem almost equally effective but have fewer adverse effects. **Olsalazine** (a 5-ASA dimer) and **balsalazide** (5-ASA conjugated to an inactive compound) are cleaved by bacterial azoreductases (as is sulfasalazine). These drugs are activated mainly in the colon and are less effective for proximal small-bowel disease. Olsalazine dosage is 1000 mg po bid, and balsalazide is 2.25 g po tid. Olsalazine sometimes causes diarrhea, especially in patients with pancolitis. This problem is minimized by gradual escalation of dose and administration with meals.

Other formulations of 5-ASA use delayed-release and/or extended-release coatings. **Asacol HD**® (typical dose 1600 mg po tid) and **Delzicol**® (800 mg tid) are delayed-release forms of 5-ASA coated with an acrylic polymer whose pH solubility delays release of the drug until entry into the distal ileum and colon. **Pentasa**® (1 g po qid) is an extended-release 5-ASA encapsulated in ethylcellulose microgranules that release 35% of the drug in the small bowel. **Lialda**® (2400 to 4800 mg po once/day) and **Apriso**® (1500 mg po once/day) are combination delayed-release and extended-release formulations that may be given once/day; their less frequent dosing may improve adherence. All of these formulations of 5-ASA are therapeutically roughly equivalent.

5-ASA is also available as a suppository (500 or 1000 mg at bedtime or bid) or enema (4 g at bedtime or bid) for proctitis and left-sided colon disease. These rectal preparations are effective for both acute treatment and long-term maintenance in proctitis and left-sided colon disease and they have incremental benefit in combination with oral 5-ASA. Patients who cannot tolerate enemas due to rectal irritation should be given 5-ASA foam.

Corticosteroids

Corticosteroids are useful for acute flare-ups of most forms of IBD when 5-ASA compounds are inadequate. However, corticosteroids are not appropriate for maintenance.

IV hydrocortisone 300 mg/day or **methylprednisolone** 60 to 80 mg/day by continuous drip or in divided doses (eg, 30 to 40 mg IV bid) is used for severe disease; **oral prednisone** or **prednisolone** 40 to 60 mg once/day may be used for moderate disease. Treatment is continued until symptoms remit (usually 7 to 28 days) and then tapered by 5 to 10 mg weekly to 20 mg once/day. Treatment is then further tapered by 2.5 to 5 mg weekly depending upon clinical response, while instituting maintenance therapy with 5-ASA or immunomodulators. Adverse effects of short-term corticosteroids in high doses include hyperglycemia, hypertension, insomnia, hyperactivity, and acute psychotic episodes.

Hydrocortisone enemas or foam may be used for proctitis and left-sided colon disease; as an enema, 100 mg in 60 mL of isotonic solution is given once/day or bid. The enema should be retained in the bowel as long as possible; instillation at night, with the patient lying on the left side with hips elevated, may prolong retention and extend distribution. Treatment, if effective, should be continued daily for about 2 to 4 wk, then every other day for 1 to 2 wk, and then gradually discontinued over 1 to 2 wk.

Budesonide is a corticosteroid with a high (> 90%) first-pass liver metabolism; thus, oral administration may have a significant effect on GI tract disease but minimal adrenal suppression. Oral budesonide has fewer adverse effects than prednisolone but is not as rapidly effective and is typically used for less severe disease. Budesonide may be effective in maintaining remission for 3 to 6 mo but has not yet proved effective for long-term maintenance. The drug is approved for small-bowel Crohn disease, and an enteric-coated, delayed-release form is available for ulcerative colitis. Dosage is 9 mg once/day. It is also available outside the US as an enema.

All patients started on corticosteroids (including budesonide) should be given oral vitamin D 400 to 800 units/day and calcium 1200 mg/day.

Immunomodulating Drugs

The antimetabolites azathioprine, 6-mercaptopurine, and methotrexate are also used in combination therapy with biologic agents.

Azathioprine and 6-mercaptopurine: Azathioprine and its metabolite 6-mercaptopurine inhibit T-cell function and may induce T-cell apoptosis. They are effective long-term and may diminish corticosteroid requirements and maintain remission for years. These drugs often require 1 to 3 mo to produce clinical benefits, so corticosteroids cannot be completely withdrawn until at least the 2nd month. Dosage of azathioprine is usually 2.5 to 3.0 mg/kg po once/day and 6-mercaptopurine is 1 to 1.5 mg/kg po once/day but varies depending on individual metabolism.

The most common adverse effects are nausea, vomiting, and malaise. Signs of bone marrow suppression must be monitored with regular WBC count (biweekly for 1 mo, then every

1 to 2 mo). Pancreatitis or high fever occurs in about 3 to 5% of patients; either is an absolute contraindication to rechallenge. Hepatotoxicity is rarer and can be screened by blood tests every 6 to 12 mo. These drugs are associated with increased risk of lymphoma and nonmelanoma skin cancers.

Before starting these drugs, patients should have tests to measure the activity of thiopurine methyltransferase (TPMT), an enzyme that converts azathioprine and 6-mercaptopurine to their active metabolites 6-thioguanine (6-TG) and 6-methylmercaptopurine (6-MMP). Patients should also have genotype testing for known low-activity variants of this enzyme. After starting these drugs, it is useful to measure levels of 6-TG and 6-MMP to help ensure safe and effective drug dosages. Therapeutic efficacy correlates with 6-TG levels between 230 and 400 picomoles per 8×10^8 RBCs. Myelotoxicity can occur when 6-TG levels are > 400. Hepatotoxicity can occur when 6-MMP levels are > 5000 picomoles per 8×10^8 RBCs. The concentrations of metabolites are also useful in nonresponding patients to distinguish lack of adherence from resistance.

Methotrexate: Methotrexate 15 to 25 mg po or sc weekly is of benefit to many patients with corticosteroid-refractory or corticosteroid-dependent Crohn disease, even those who have not responded to azathioprine or 6-mercaptopurine.

Adverse effects include nausea, vomiting, and asymptomatic liver function test abnormalities. Folate 1 mg po once/day may diminish some of the adverse effects. Women taking methotrexate should be using at least one form of birth control. Additionally, women and perhaps men should stop methotrexate for at least 3 mo before trying to conceive. Monthly CBCs and liver function tests with albumin should be done for the first 3 mo of therapy then every 8 to 12 wk during therapy. Alcohol use, obesity, diabetes, and possibly psoriasis are risk factors for hepatotoxicity. Preferably, patients with these conditions should not be treated with methotrexate. Pretreatment liver biopsies are not recommended; liver biopsies are done if the results of 6 of 12 tests done in a 1-yr period show elevated levels of AST. Myelosuppression, pulmonary toxicity, and nephrotoxicity can also occur with methotrexate therapy.

Cyclosporine and tacrolimus: **Cyclosporine,** which blocks lymphocyte activation, may benefit patients with severe UC unresponsive to corticosteroids and who may otherwise require colectomy. Its only well-documented use in Crohn disease is for patients with refractory fistulas or pyoderma. Initial dose is 2 to 4 mg/kg IV in continuous infusion over 24 h; responders are converted to an oral dose of 6 to 8 mg/kg once/day with early introduction of azathioprine or 6-mercaptopurine. Long-term use (> 6 mo) is contraindicated by multiple adverse effects (eg, renal toxicity, seizures, opportunistic infections, hypertension, neuropathy). Generally, patients are not offered cyclosporine unless there is a reason to avoid the safer curative option of colectomy. If the drug is used, trough blood levels should be kept between 200 to 400 ng/mL and *Pneumocystis jirovecii* prophylaxis should be considered during the period of concomitant corticosteroid, cyclosporine, and antimetabolite treatment.

Tacrolimus, an immunosuppressant also used in transplant patients, seems as effective as cyclosporine and may be considered for use in patients with severe or refractory UC who do not require hospitalization.

Biologic Agents

Anti-TNF drugs: Infliximab, certolizumab, adalimumab, and golimumab are antibodies to tumor necrosis factor (TNF). Infliximab, certolizumab, and adalimumab are useful in Crohn disease, particularly in preventing or retarding postoperative recurrence. Infliximab, adalimumab, and golimumab are beneficial in UC for refractory or corticosteroid-dependent disease.

Infliximab is given as a single IV infusion of 5 mg/kg over 2 h. It is followed by repeat infusions at wk 2 and 6. Subsequently, it is given every 8 wk. To maintain remission in many if not most patients, the dose needs to be increased or the interval needs to be shortened within a year or so.

Adalimumab is given with an initial loading dose of 160 mg sc and then 80 mg sc at wk 2. After that dose, 40 mg sc is given every 2 wk. Patients who are intolerant or who have lost their initial response to infliximab may respond to adalimumab therapy.

Certolizumab is given as 400 mg sc q 2 wk for three doses and then q 4 wk for maintenance. Patients who are intolerant of or who have lost their initial response to infliximab may respond to certolizumab.

Monotherapy with anti-TNF agents is clearly effective for both induction and maintenance of remission, but some studies suggest better results when anti-TNF agents are initiated in combination with a thiopurine (eg, azathioprine) or methotrexate. Nevertheless, given the possible increase in adverse effects with combination therapy, treatment recommendations should be individualized. Corticosteroid tapering may begin after 2 wk. Adverse effects during infusion (infusion reaction) include immediate hypersensitivity reactions (eg, rash, itching, sometimes anaphylactoid reactions), fever, chills, headache, and nausea. Delayed hypersensitivity reactions have also occurred. Anti-TNF drugs given subcutaneously (eg, adalimumab) do not cause infusion reactions, although they may cause local erythema, pain, and itching (injection site reaction).

Several patients have died of sepsis after anti-TNF use, so these drugs are contraindicated when uncontrolled bacterial infection is present. Also, TB and hepatitis B reactivation has been attributed to anti-TNF drugs; therefore, screening for latent TB (with PPDs and/or interferon-gamma release assay and chest x-ray) and for hepatitis B is required before therapy.

Lymphoma, demyelinating disease, and liver and hematologic toxicity are other potential concerns with anti-TNF antibody treatment.

Other biologic agents: Several immunosuppressive interleukins and anti-interleukin antibodies also may decrease the inflammatory response and are being studied for Crohn disease.

Vedolizumab and **natalizumab** are antibodies to leukocyte adhesion molecules. Vedolizumab has been approved for moderate to severe UC and Crohn disease. Its effect is believed to be limited to the gut, making it safer than natalizumab, which is used only as a 2nd-line drug through a restricted-prescribing program for the most refractory cases of Crohn disease.

Other anticytokine, anti-integrin, and growth factors are under investigation, as is leukopheresis therapy to deplete activated immunocytes.

Antibiotics and Probiotics

Antibiotics: Antibiotics may be helpful in Crohn disease but are of limited use in UC, except in toxic colitis). Metronidazole 500 to 750 mg po tid for 4 to 8 wk may control mild Crohn disease and help heal fistulas. However, adverse effects (particularly neurotoxicity) often preclude completion of treatment. Ciprofloxacin 500 to 750 mg po bid may prove less toxic. Many experts recommend metronidazole and ciprofloxacin in combination. Rifaximin, a nonabsorbable antibiotic, at a dose of 200 mg po tid or 800 mg po bid may also be beneficial as treatment for active Crohn disease.

Probiotics: Various nonpathogenic microorganisms (eg, commensal *Escherichia coli, Lactobacillus* species, *Saccharomyces*) given daily serve as probiotics and may be effective in preventing pouchitis, but other therapeutic roles have yet to be clearly defined. Therapeutic infestation with the parasite *Trichuris suis* has been tried in an effort to stimulate T2-helper cell immunity and may decrease disease activity in UC.

CROHN DISEASE

(Regional Enteritis; Granulomatous Ileitis; Granulomatous Ileocolitis)

Crohn disease is a chronic transmural inflammatory bowel disease that usually affects the distal ileum and colon but may occur in any part of the GI tract. Symptoms include diarrhea and abdominal pain. Abscesses, internal and external fistulas, and bowel obstruction may arise. Extraintestinal symptoms, particularly arthritis, may occur. Diagnosis is by colonoscopy and imaging studies. Treatment is with 5-aminosalicylic acid, corticosteroids, immunomodulators, anticytokines, antibiotics, and often surgery.

(See also the American College of Gastroenterology's practice guidelines for management of Crohn's disease in adults.)

Pathophysiology

Crohn disease begins with crypt inflammation and abscesses, which progress to tiny focal aphthoid ulcers. These mucosal lesions may develop into deep longitudinal and transverse ulcers with intervening mucosal edema, creating a characteristic cobblestoned appearance to the bowel.

Transmural spread of inflammation leads to lymphedema and thickening of the bowel wall and mesentery. Mesenteric fat typically extends onto the serosal surface of the bowel. Mesenteric lymph nodes often enlarge. Extensive inflammation may result in hypertrophy of the muscularis mucosae, fibrosis, and stricture formation, which can lead to bowel obstruction.

Abscesses are common, and fistulas often penetrate into adjoining structures, including other loops of bowel, the bladder, or psoas muscle. Fistulas may even extend to the skin of the anterior abdomen or flanks. Independently of intra-abdominal disease activity, perianal fistulas and abscesses occur in 25 to 33% of cases; these complications are frequently the most troublesome aspects of Crohn disease.

Noncaseating granulomas can occur in lymph nodes, peritoneum, the liver, and all layers of the bowel wall. Although pathognomonic when present, granulomas are not detected in about half of patients with Crohn disease. The presence of granulomas does not seem to be related to the clinical course.

Segments of diseased bowel are sharply demarcated from adjacent normal bowel (called skip areas), hence the name regional enteritis.

- About 35% of Crohn disease cases involve the ileum alone (ileitis).
- About 45% involve the ileum and colon (ileocolitis), with a predilection for the right side of the colon.
- About 20% involve the colon alone (granulomatous colitis), most of which, unlike UC, spare the rectum.

Occasionally, the entire small bowel is involved (jejunoileitis). The stomach, duodenum, or esophagus is clinically involved only rarely, although microscopic evidence of disease is often detectable in the gastric antrum, especially in younger patients. In the absence of surgical intervention, the disease almost never extends into areas of small bowel that are not involved at first diagnosis.

Classification: The Vienna Classification and its recent Montreal modification categorize Crohn disease into 3 principal patterns: (1) primarily inflammatory, which after several years commonly evolves into (2) primarily stenotic or obstructing or (3) primarily penetrating or fistulizing.

These different clinical patterns dictate different therapeutic approaches. Some genetic studies suggest a molecular basis for this classification.

Complications: There is an increased risk of cancer in affected small-bowel segments. Patients with colonic involvement have a long-term risk of colorectal cancer equal to that of UC, given the same extent and duration of disease. Chronic malabsorption may cause nutritional deficiencies, particularly of vitamins D and B_{12}.

Toxic megacolon is a rare complication of colonic Crohn disease. It is a clinical syndrome of ileus accompanied by radiographic evidence of colonic dilation; many cases must be treated aggressively with surgical intervention.

Symptoms and Signs

The **most common initial manifestations** of Crohn disease are

- Chronic diarrhea with abdominal pain, fever, anorexia, and weight loss
- The abdomen is tender, and a mass or fullness may be palpable.

Gross rectal bleeding is unusual except in isolated colonic disease, which may manifest similarly to UC. Some patients present with an acute abdomen that simulates acute appendicitis or intestinal obstruction. About 33% of patients have perianal disease (especially fissures and fistulas), which is sometimes the most prominent or even initial complaint.

In children, extraintestinal manifestations frequently predominate over GI symptoms; arthritis, FUO, anemia, or growth retardation may be a presenting symptom, whereas abdominal pain or diarrhea may be absent.

With **recurrent disease,** symptoms vary. Pain is most common and occurs with both simple recurrence and abscess formation. Patients with severe flare-up or abscess are likely to have marked tenderness, guarding, rebound, and a general toxic appearance. Stenotic segments may cause bowel obstruction, with colicky pain, distention, obstipation, and vomiting. Adhesions from previous surgery may also cause bowel obstruction, which begins rapidly, without the prodrome of fever, pain, and malaise typical of obstruction due to a Crohn disease flare-up. An enterovesical fistula may produce air bubbles in the urine (pneumaturia). Draining cutaneous fistulas may occur. Free perforation into the peritoneal cavity is unusual.

Chronic disease causes a variety of systemic symptoms, including fever, weight loss, malnutrition, and other extraintestinal manifestations of IBD.

Diagnosis

- Barium x-rays of the stomach, small bowel, and colons
- Abdominal CT (conventional or CT enterography)
- Sometimes magnetic resonance (MR) enterography, upper endoscopy, colonoscopy, and/or video capsule endoscopy

Crohn disease should be suspected in a patient with inflammatory or obstructive symptoms or in a patient without prominent GI symptoms but with perianal fistulas or abscesses or with otherwise unexplained arthritis, erythema nodosum, fever, anemia, or (in a child) stunted growth. A family history of Crohn disease also increases the index of suspicion.

Similar symptoms and signs (eg, abdominal pain, diarrhea) may be caused by other GI disorders, particularly ulcerative colitis. Differentiation from UC may be an issue in the 20% of cases in which Crohn disease is confined to the colon. However, because treatment is similar, this distinction is critical only when surgery or experimental therapy is contemplated.

Patients presenting with an acute abdomen (either initially or during a relapse) should have flat and upright abdominal x-rays and an abdominal CT scan. These studies may show obstruction, abscesses or fistulas, and other possible causes of an acute abdomen (eg, appendicitis). Ultrasonography may better delineate gynecologic pathology in women with lower abdominal and pelvic pain.

If initial presentation is less acute, an upper GI series with small-bowel follow-through and spot films of the terminal ileum is preferred over conventional CT. However, newer techniques of CT or MR enterography, which combine high-resolution CT or MR imaging with large volumes of ingested contrast, are becoming the procedures of choice in some centers. These imaging studies are virtually diagnostic if they show characteristic strictures or fistulas with accompanying separation of bowel loops.

If findings are questionable, CT enteroclysis or video capsule enteroscopy may show superficial aphthous and linear ulcers. Barium enema x-ray may be used if symptoms seem predominantly colonic (eg, diarrhea) and may show reflux of barium into the terminal ileum with irregularity, nodularity, stiffness, wall thickening, and a narrowed lumen. Differential diagnoses in patients with similar x-ray findings include cancer of the cecum, ileal carcinoid, lymphoma, systemic vasculitis, radiation enteritis, ileocecal TB, and ameboma.

In atypical cases (eg, predominantly diarrhea, with minimal pain), evaluation is similar to suspected UC, with colonoscopy (including biopsy, sampling for enteric pathogens, and, when possible, visualization of the terminal ileum). Upper GI endoscopy may identify subtle gastroduodenal involvement even in the absence of upper GI symptoms.

Laboratory testing: Laboratory tests should be done to screen for anemia, hypoalbuminemia, and electrolyte abnormalities. Liver function tests should be done; elevated alkaline phosphatase and γ–glutamyl transpeptidase levels in patients with major colonic involvement suggest possible primary sclerosing cholangitis. Leukocytosis or increased levels of acute-phase reactants (eg, ESR, C-reactive protein) are nonspecific but may be used serially to monitor disease activity.

To detect nutritional deficiencies, levels of vitamin D and B_{12} should be checked every 1 to 2 yr. Additional laboratory measurements, such as levels of water-soluble vitamins (folic acid and niacin), fat-soluble vitamins (A, D, E, and K), and minerals (zinc, selenium, and copper) may be checked when deficiencies are suspected.

All patients with inflammatory bowel disease (IBD), whether male or female, young or old, should have their bone mineral density monitored, usually by dual-energy x-ray absorptiometry (DXA) scan.

Perinuclear antineutrophil cytoplasmic antibodies are present in 60 to 70% of patients with UC and in only 5 to 20% of patients with Crohn disease. Anti–*Saccharomyces cerevisiae* antibodies are relatively specific for Crohn disease. However, these tests do not reliably separate the 2 diseases and they are not recommended for routine diagnosis. Additional antibodies such as anti-OmpC and anti-CBir1 are now available, but the clinical value of these supplementary tests is uncertain; some studies suggest that high titers of these antibodies have adverse prognostic implications.

Prognosis

Established Crohn disease is rarely cured but is characterized by intermittent exacerbations and remissions. Some patients have severe disease with frequent, debilitating periods of pain. However, with judicious medical therapy and, where appropriate, surgical therapy, most patients function well and adapt successfully. Disease-related mortality is very low. GI cancer, including cancer of the colon and small bowel, is the leading cause of excess Crohn disease-related mortality. Thromboembolic complications (especially during active Crohn colitis) also may cause death. About 10% of people are disabled by Crohn disease and the complications it causes.

Treatment

- Loperamide or antispasmodics for symptom relief
- 5-Aminosalicylic acid (5-ASA) or antibiotics
- Other drugs depending on symptoms and severity
- Sometimes surgery

Details of specific drugs and dosages are discussed in Drugs for Inflammatory Bowel Disease on p. 135.

General management: Cramps and diarrhea may be relieved by oral administration of loperamide 2 to 4 mg or antispasmodic drugs up to 4 times/day (ideally before meals). Such symptomatic treatment is safe, except in cases of severe, acute Crohn colitis, which may progress to toxic colitis as in UC. Hydrophilic mucilloids (eg, methylcellulose or psyllium preparations) sometimes help prevent anal irritation by increasing stool firmness. Dietary roughage is to be avoided in stricturing disease or active colonic inflammation.

Mild to moderate disease: This category includes ambulatory patients who tolerate oral intake and have no signs of toxicity, tenderness, mass, or obstruction. 5-ASA (mesalamine) is commonly used as first-line treatment. Pentasa® is favored for small-bowel disease, and Asacol® HD is favored for distal ileal and colonic disease. However, the benefits of any 5-ASA drug for small-bowel Crohn disease are modest, and many experts advocate not using it in small-bowel Crohn disease.

Antibiotics are considered a first-line agent by some clinicians, or they may be reserved for patients not responding to 4 wk of 5-ASA; their use is strictly empiric. With any of these drugs, 8 to 16 wk of treatment may be required.

Responders should receive maintenance therapy.

Moderate to severe disease: Patients without fistulas or abscesses but with significant pain, tenderness, fever, or vomiting, or those who have not responded to treatment for mild disease, often have rapid relief of symptoms when given corticosteroids, either oral or parenteral. Oral prednisone or prednisolone may act more rapidly and reliably than oral budesonide, but budesonide has somewhat fewer adverse effects and is considered the corticosteroid of choice in many centers, especially in Europe.

Patients who do not respond rapidly to corticosteroids, or those whose doses cannot be tapered within a few weeks, must not be maintained on these drugs and require different therapy.

An antimetabolite (azathioprine, 6-mercaptopurine, or methotrexate), an anti-TNF agent (infliximab, adalimumab, or certolizumab pegol), or a combination of both, can be used as 2nd-line therapy after corticosteroids, and even as first-line therapy in preference to corticosteroids. These drugs, guided by measurements of drug and antibody levels, achieve clinical success in most cases. When these lines of treatment fail in patients for whom surgery is not feasible or appropriate, newer biologic drugs including anti-integrins (eg, natalizumab and vedolizumab) can be used. Furthermore, other biologic agents are emerging rapidly.

Obstruction is managed initially with nasogastric suction and IV fluids. Obstruction due to uncomplicated Crohn disease should resolve within a few days and therefore does not require either specific anti-inflammatory therapy or parenteral nutrition; absence of prompt response, however, indicates a complication or another etiology and requires immediate surgery.

Fulminant disease or abscess: Patients with toxic appearance, high fever, persistent vomiting, rebound, or a tender or palpable mass must be hospitalized for administration of IV fluids and antibiotics. Abscesses must be drained, either percutaneously or surgically. IV corticosteroids or biologic agents should be given only when infection has been ruled out or controlled. If there is no response to corticosteroids and antibiotics within 5 to 7 days, surgery is usually indicated.

Fistulas: Perianal fistulas are treated initially with metronidazole and ciprofloxacin. Patients who do not respond in 3 to 4 wk may receive an immunomodulator (eg, azathioprine, 6-mercaptopurine), with or without an induction regimen of infliximab or adalimumab for more rapid response. Anti-TNF therapy (infliximab or adalimumab) can also be used alone. Cyclosporine or tacrolimus are alternatives, but fistulas often relapse after treatment.

Severe refractory perianal fistulas may require temporary diverting colostomy but almost invariably recur after reconnection; hence, diversion is more appropriately considered a preparation for definitive surgery or at best an adjunct to infliximab or adalimumab rather than a primary treatment.

Maintenance therapy: Patients who require only 5-ASA or an antibiotic to achieve remission of Crohn disease can be maintained on that drug. Patients requiring acute treatment with corticosteroids or anti-TNF agents typically require azathioprine, 6-mercaptopurine, methotrexate, anti-TNF therapy, or combination therapy for maintenance. Many if not most patients brought into remission with an anti-TNF will require escalation of the dose or shortening of the treatment intervals within a year or two. Systemically active corticosteroids are neither safe nor effective for long-term maintenance, although budesonide has been shown to delay relapse with fewer adverse effects. Patients who respond to anti-TNF therapy for acute disease but who are not well maintained on antimetabolites may stay in remission with repeat doses of anti-TNF agents.

Monitoring during remission can be done by following symptoms and doing blood tests and does not require routine x-rays or colonoscopy (other than regular surveillance for dysplasia after 7 to 8 yr of disease).

Surgery: Even though about 70% of patients ultimately require an operation, surgery for Crohn disease is often done reluctantly. It is best reserved for recurrent intestinal obstruction or intractable fistulas or abscesses. Resection of the involved bowel may ameliorate symptoms but does not cure the disease, which is likely to recur even after resection of all clinically apparent lesions.

The recurrence rate, defined by endoscopic lesions at the anastomotic site, is

- > 70% at 1 yr
- > 85% at 3 yr

Defined by clinical symptoms, the recurrence rate is about

- 25 to 30% at 3 yr
- 40 to 50% at 5 yr

Ultimately, further surgery is required in nearly 50% of cases. However, recurrence rates seem to be reduced by early postoperative prophylaxis with 6-mercaptopurine or azathioprine, metronidazole, or infliximab. Moreover, when surgery is done for appropriate indications, almost all patients have improved quality of life.

Because smoking increases the risk of recurrence, especially in women, smoking cessation should be encouraged.

KEY POINTS

- Crohn disease affects the ileum and/or colon but spares the rectum (which is invariably affected in ulcerative colitis).
- Intermittent areas of diseased bowel are sharply demarcated from adjacent normal bowel (called skip areas).
- Symptoms primarily involve episodic diarrhea and abdominal pain; GI bleeding is rare.
- Complications include abdominal abscesses and enterocutaneous fistulas.
- Treat mild to moderate disease with 5-aminosalicylic acid and/or antibiotics (eg, metronidazole, ciprofloxacin, rifaximin).
- Treat severe disease with corticosteroids and sometimes immunomodulators (eg, azathioprine) or anti-TNF agents (eg, infliximab, adalimumab).
- About 70% of patients ultimately require an operation, typically for recurrent intestinal obstruction, intractable fistulas, or abscesses.

ULCERATIVE COLITIS

UC is a chronic inflammatory and ulcerative disease arising in the colonic mucosa, characterized most often by bloody diarrhea. Extraintestinal symptoms, particularly arthritis, may occur. Long-term risk of colon cancer is high. Diagnosis is by colonoscopy. Treatment is with 5-aminosalicylic acid, corticosteroids, immunomodulators, biologics, antibiotics, and occasionally surgery.

Pathophysiology

Ulcerative colitis usually begins in the rectum. It may remain localized to the rectum (ulcerative proctitis) or extend proximally, sometimes involving the entire colon. Rarely, it involves most of the large bowel at once.

The inflammation caused by UC affects the mucosa and submucosa, and there is a sharp border between normal and affected tissue. Only in severe disease is the muscularis involved. Early in the disease, the mucous membrane is erythematous, finely granular, and friable, with loss of the normal vascular pattern and often with scattered hemorrhagic areas. Large mucosal ulcers with copious purulent exudate characterize severe disease. Islands of relatively normal or hyperplastic inflammatory mucosa (pseudopolyps) project above areas of ulcerated mucosa. Fistulas and abscesses do not occur.

Toxic colitis: **Toxic colitis or fulminant colitis** occurs when transmural extension of ulceration results in localized ileus and peritonitis. Within hours to days, the colon loses muscular tone and begins to dilate.

The terms toxic megacolon and toxic dilation are discouraged because the toxic inflammatory state and its complications can occur without frank megacolon (defined as transverse colon > 6 cm diameter during an exacerbation).

Toxic colitis is a medical emergency that usually occurs spontaneously in the course of very severe colitis but is sometimes precipitated by opioid or anticholinergic antidiarrheal drugs. Colonic perforation may occur, which increases mortality significantly.

Symptoms and Signs

Bloody diarrhea of varied intensity and duration is interspersed with asymptomatic intervals. Usually an attack begins insidiously, with increased urgency to defecate, mild lower abdominal cramps, and blood and mucus in the stools. Some cases develop after an infection (eg, amebiasis, bacillary dysentery).

When ulceration is confined to the rectosigmoid, the stool may be normal or hard and dry, but rectal discharges of mucus loaded with RBCs and WBCs accompany or occur between bowel movements. Systemic symptoms are absent or mild. If ulceration extends proximally, stools become looser and the patient may have > 10 bowel movements per day, often with severe cramps and distressing rectal tenesmus, without respite at night. The stools may be watery or contain mucus and frequently consist almost entirely of blood and pus.

Toxic or fulminant colitis manifests initially with sudden violent diarrhea, fever to 40° C (104° F), abdominal pain, signs of peritonitis (eg, rebound tenderness), and profound toxemia.

Systemic symptoms and signs, more common with extensive UC, include malaise, fever, anemia, anorexia, and weight loss. Extraintestinal manifestations of IBD (particularly joint and skin complications) are most common when systemic symptoms are present.

Diagnosis

- Stool cultures and microscopy (to exclude infectious causes)
- Sigmoidoscopy with biopsy

Initial presentation: Diagnosis is suggested by typical symptoms and signs, particularly when accompanied by extraintestinal manifestations or a history of previous similar attacks. Ulcerative colitis should be distinguished from Crohn disease (see Table 18–1) but more importantly from other causes of acute colitis (eg, infection; in elderly patients, ischemia).

In all patients, stool cultures for enteric pathogens should be done, and *Entamoeba histolytica* should be excluded by examination of fresh stool specimens. When amebiasis is suspected because of epidemiologic or travel history, serologic titers and biopsies should be done. History of prior antibiotic use or recent hospitalization should prompt stool assay for *Clostridium difficile* toxin. Patients at risk should be tested for HIV, gonorrhea, herpesvirus, chlamydia, and amebiasis. Opportunistic infections (eg, cytomegalovirus, *Mycobacterium avium-intracellulare*) or Kaposi sarcoma must also be considered in immunosuppressed patients. In women using oral contraceptives, contraceptive-induced colitis is possible; it usually resolves spontaneously after hormone therapy is stopped.

Sigmoidoscopy should be done; it allows visual confirmation of colitis and permits direct sampling of stool or mucus for culture and microscopic evaluation, as well as biopsy of affected areas. Although visual inspection and biopsies may be nondiagnostic, because there is much overlap in appearance among different types of colitis, acute, self-limited, infectious colitis can usually be distinguished histologically from chronic idiopathic UC or Crohn colitis. Severe perianal disease, rectal sparing, absence of bleeding, and asymmetric or segmental involvement of the colon indicate Crohn disease rather than UC. Colonoscopy is usually unnecessary initially but should be done electively if inflammation has extended proximal to the reach of the sigmoidoscope.

Laboratory tests should be done to screen for anemia, hypoalbuminemia, and electrolyte abnormalities. Liver function tests should be done; elevated alkaline phosphatase and γ-glutamyl transpeptidase levels suggest possible primary sclerosing cholangitis. Perinuclear antineutrophil cytoplasmic antibodies are relatively specific (60 to 70%) for UC. Anti–*Saccharomyces cerevisiae* antibodies are relatively specific for Crohn disease. However, these tests do not reliably separate the 2 diseases and are not recommended for routine diagnosis. Other possible laboratory abnormalities include leukocytosis, thrombocytosis, and elevated acute-phase reactants (eg, ESR, C-reactive protein).

X-rays are not diagnostic but occasionally show abnormalities. Plain x-rays of the abdomen may show mucosal edema, loss of haustration, and absence of formed stool in the diseased bowel. Barium enema shows similar changes, albeit more clearly, and may also show ulcerations, but the enema should not be done during an acute presentation. A shortened, rigid colon with an atrophic or pseudopolypoid mucosa is often seen after several years of illness. X-ray findings of thumbprinting and segmental distribution are more suggestive of intestinal ischemia or possibly Crohn colitis rather than of UC.

Recurrent symptoms: Patients with known disease and a recurrence of typical symptoms should be examined, but extensive testing is not always required. Depending on duration and severity of symptoms, sigmoidoscopy or colonoscopy may be done and a CBC obtained. Cultures, ova and parasite examination, and *C. difficile* toxin assay should be done when there are atypical features to the relapse or when there is an exacerbation after prolonged remission, during a contagious outbreak, after antibiotic exposure, or whenever the clinician is suspicious.

Acute severe attacks: Patients require prompt hospitalization during severe flare-ups. Flat and upright abdominal x-rays should be taken; they may show megacolon or intraluminal gas accumulated over a long, continuous, paralyzed segment of colon—a result of lost muscle tone. Colonoscopy and barium enema should be avoided because of the risk of perforation, but a careful sigmoidoscopy is typically advisable to assess severity and rule out infection. CBC, platelet count, ESR, C-reactive protein, electrolytes, and albumin should be obtained; PT, PTT, and blood type and cross-match are also indicated in cases of severe bleeding.

The patient must be watched closely for progressive peritonitis or perforation. Percussion over the liver is important because loss of hepatic dullness may be the first clinical sign of free perforation, especially in a patient whose peritoneal signs are suppressed by high-dose corticosteroids. Abdominal x-rays are taken every 1 or 2 days to follow the course of colonic distention and to detect free or intramural air; CT is more sensitive in detecting extraluminal air or pericolic abscess.

Prognosis

Usually, UC is chronic with repeated exacerbations and remissions. In about 10% of patients, an initial attack becomes fulminant with massive hemorrhage, perforation, or sepsis and toxemia. Complete recovery after a single attack occurs in another 10%.

Patients with localized ulcerative proctitis have the best prognosis. Severe systemic manifestations, toxic complications, and malignant degeneration are unlikely, and late extension of the disease occurs in only about 20 to 30%. Surgery is rarely required, and life expectancy is normal. The symptoms, however, may prove stubborn and refractory. Moreover, because extensive UC may begin in the rectum and spread proximally, proctitis should not be considered localized until it has been observed for ≥ 6 mo. Localized disease that later extends is often more severe and more refractory to therapy.

Colon cancer: The risk of colon cancer is proportional to the duration of disease and amount of colon affected but not necessarily to the clinical severity of the attacks. Some studies suggest that sustained microscopic inflammation is a risk factor, and that use of 5-ASA to control inflammation is protective.

Cancer begins to appear by 7 yr from onset of illness in patients with extensive colitis and then develops in about 0.5 to 1% of patients each year thereafter. Thus, after 20 yr of disease, about 7% to 10% of patients will have developed cancer, and about 30% after 35 yr of disease. However, patients who have inflammatory bowel disease and primary sclerosing cholangitis are at a higher risk of cancer from the time of colitis diagnosis.

Regular colonoscopic surveillance, preferably during remission, is advised for patients with disease duration > 8 to 10 yr (except for those with isolated proctitis) or when there is concomitant primary sclerosing cholangitis, in which case surveillance colonoscopy should begin at the time of diagnosis. The most recent guidelines suggest doing *random* biopsies (taken every 10 cm throughout the colon) when using high-definition white-light colonoscopy but doing only *targeted* biopsies of visible lesions when using chromoendoscopy to detect dysplasia. Definite dysplasia of any grade within an area affected by colitis is liable to progress to more advanced neoplasia and even cancer. After complete removal of endoscopically resectable polypoid or nonpolypoid dysplastic lesions, colonoscopic surveillance is suggested rather than colectomy. Patients with dysplasia that is *not* visible endoscopically should probably be referred to a gastroenterologist with expertise in IBD surveillance using chromoendoscopy and/or high-definition colonoscopy to decide whether colectomy or continued colonoscopic surveillance should be done.

The optimal frequency of colonoscopic surveillance has not been established, but some authorities recommend every 2 yr during the 2nd decade of disease and annually thereafter.

Long-term survival after diagnosis of colitis-related cancer is about 50%, a figure comparable to that for colorectal cancer in the general population.

Treatment

- Dietary management and loperamide (except in acute severe attacks) for symptom relief
- 5-Aminosalicylic acid (5-ASA)
- Corticosteroids and other drugs depending on symptoms and severity
- Antimetabolites and biologic agents
- Sometimes surgery

Details of specific drugs and dosages are discussed in Drugs for Inflammatory Bowel Disease on p. 135.

General management: Avoiding raw fruits and vegetables limits trauma to the inflamed colonic mucosa and may lessen symptoms. A milk-free diet may help but need not be continued if no benefit is noted. Loperamide 2 mg po bid to qid is indicated for relatively mild diarrhea; higher oral doses (4 mg in the morning and 2 mg after each bowel movement) may be required for more intense diarrhea. Antidiarrheal drugs must be used with extreme caution in severe cases because they may precipitate toxic dilation. All patients with inflammatory bowel disease should be advised to take appropriate amounts of calcium and vitamin D.

Mild left-sided disease: Patients with proctitis, or colitis that does not extend proximally beyond the splenic flexure, are treated with 5-ASA (mesalamine) enemas once/day or bid depending on severity. Suppositories are effective for more distal disease and are usually preferred by patients. Corticosteroid and budesonide enemas are slightly less effective but should be used if 5-ASA is unsuccessful or not tolerated. Once remission is achieved, dosage is slowly tapered to maintenance levels. Oral 5-ASA drugs theoretically have some incremental benefit in lessening the probability of proximal spread of disease.

Moderate or extensive disease: Patients with inflammation proximal to the splenic flexure or left-sided disease unresponsive to topical agents should receive an oral 5-ASA formulation in addition to 5-ASA enemas. High-dose corticosteroids are added for more severe symptoms; after 1 to 2 wk, the daily dose is reduced by about 5 to 10 mg each wk. Immunomodulator therapy with azathioprine or 6-mercaptopurine can be used in patients who are refractory to maximal doses of 5-ASA and would otherwise need long-term corticosteroid therapy. Additionally, infliximab, adalimumab, and golimumab are beneficial in some patients and may be considered for those refractory to immunomodulator (thiopurine failure) or corticosteroid therapy as well as those who are corticosteroid-dependent. Moreover, a combination of immunomodulator and anti-TNF therapy is sometimes helpful. Finally, in some patients who fail to respond to corticosteroids, immunosuppressants, or anti-TNF drugs, a trial of vedolizumab can be considered.

Severe disease: Patients with > 10 bloody bowel movements per day, tachycardia, high fever, or severe abdominal pain require hospitalization to receive high-dose IV corticosteroids. 5-ASA may be continued. IV fluids and blood transfusion are given as needed for dehydration and anemia. The patient must be observed closely for the development of toxic colitis. Parenteral hyperalimentation is sometimes used for nutritional support but is of no value as primary therapy; patients who can tolerate food should eat.

Patients who do not respond within 3 to 7 days should be considered for IV cyclosporine or infliximab or else for surgery. Patients who do respond to a corticosteroid regimen are switched within a week or so to prednisone 60 mg po once/day, which may be gradually reduced at home based on clinical response. Patients who are started on IV cyclosporine and respond to therapy are switched to oral cyclosporine and concomitant azathioprine or 6-mercaptopurine. Oral cyclosporine is continued for about 3 to 4 mo, during which time corticosteroids are tapered and cyclosporine levels are closely monitored. Some clinicians recommend prophylaxis against *Pneumocystis jirovecii* pneumonia during the interval of overlapping treatment with corticosteroids, cyclosporine, and an antimetabolite.

Fulminant colitis: If fulminant or toxic colitis is suspected, the patient should

1. Stop all antidiarrheal drugs
2. Take nothing by mouth and have inserted a long intestinal tube attached to intermittent suction
3. Receive aggressive IV fluid and electrolyte therapy with 0.9% NaCl, and potassium chloride and blood as needed
4. Receive high-dose IV corticosteroids or cyclosporine
5. Receive antibiotics (eg, metronidazole 500 mg IV q 8 h and ciprofloxacin 500 mg IV q 12 h)

Having the patient roll over in bed from the supine to prone position every 2 to 3 h may help redistribute colonic gas and prevent progressive distention. Insertion of a soft rectal tube may also be helpful but must be done with extreme caution to avoid bowel perforation. Even if decompression of a dilated colon is achieved, the patient is not out of danger unless the underlying inflammatory process is controlled; otherwise, colectomy will still be necessary.

If intensive medical measures do not produce definite improvement within 24 to 48 h, immediate surgery is required or the patient may die of sepsis caused by bacterial translocation or even perforation.

Maintenance therapy: After effective treatment of a flare-up, corticosteroids are tapered based on clinical response and then stopped because they are ineffective as maintenance. Patients should remain on 5-ASA drugs—oral or rectal, depending on location of disease—indefinitely because stopping maintenance therapy often allows disease relapse. Dosage intervals for rectal preparations may be gradually lengthened to every 2nd or 3rd day. There is ample evidence that combination oral and rectal therapy is significantly more effective than either therapy alone.

Patients who cannot be withdrawn from corticosteroids should be given thiopurines (azathioprine or 6-mercaptopurine), anti-TNF drugs, or a combination. For more refractory cases, the anti-integrin vedolizumab can be used for both UC and Crohn disease. Also, infliximab, adalimumab, or golimumab are becoming more widely accepted as maintenance therapy for UC.

Surgery: Nearly one-third of patients with extensive UC ultimately require surgery. Total proctocolectomy is curative: Life expectancy is restored to normal, the disease does not recur (unlike Crohn disease), and the risk of colon cancer is significantly decreased. After total proctocolectomy with ileal pouch-anal anastomosis (IPAA), there remains a small risk of dysplasia or cancer in the rectal cuff anal transition zone and even in the ileal pouch. After proctocolectomy with ileostomy or IPAA, the quality of life is improved; however, new quality-of-life challenges are created.

Emergency colectomy is indicated for massive hemorrhage, fulminating toxic colitis, or perforation. Subtotal colectomy with ileostomy and rectosigmoid closure (Hartmann procedure) or mucous fistula is usually the procedure of choice because most critically ill patients cannot tolerate more extensive surgery. The rectosigmoid stump may be electively removed later or may be used for ileoanal anastomosis with a pouch. The intact rectal stump should not be allowed to remain indefinitely because of the risks of disease activation and malignant transformation.

Elective surgery is indicated for cancer, symptomatic strictures, growth retardation in children, or, most commonly, intractable chronic disease resulting in invalidism or corticosteroid dependence. Severe colitis-related extraintestinal manifestations (eg, pyoderma gangrenosum), now better controlled by intensive medical therapies,are only rarely indications for surgery.

The elective procedure of choice in patients with normal sphincter function is restorative proctocolectomy with ileoanal anastomosis. This procedure creates a pelvic reservoir or pouch from distal ileum, which is connected to the anus. The intact sphincter allows continence, typically with 4 to 9 bowel movements/day (including 1 or 2 at night).

Pouchitis is an inflammatory reaction occurring after restorative proctocolectomy with IPAA in about 50% of patients. The risk of pouchitis appears to be higher in patients with primary sclerosing cholangitis, in patients with preoperative extraintestinal manifestations, and possibly in patients with high preoperative serologic titers of perinuclear antineutrophilic antibodies and other inflammatory bowel disease biomarkers. Pouchitis is thought to be related to bacterial overgrowth and is treated with antibiotics (eg, quinolones). Probiotics may be protective. Most cases of pouchitis are readily controlled, but 5 to 10% prove refractory to all medical therapy and require conversion to a conventional (Brooke) ileostomy. For a minority of patients who are older, who have well-established families and lifestyles, who have poor sphincter tone or cannot tolerate frequent bowel movements, or who are simply unable or unwilling to face the consequences of frequent or chronic pouchitis, the Brooke ileostomy remains the procedure of choice.

In any event, the physical and emotional burdens imposed by any form of colon resection must be recognized, and care should be taken to see that the patient receives all the instructions and all the medical and psychologic support that is necessary before and after surgery.

KEY POINTS

- UC begins in the rectum and may extend proximally in a contiguous fashion without intervening patches of normal bowel.
- Symptoms are intermittent episodes of abdominal cramping and bloody diarrhea.
- Complications include fulminant colitis, which may lead to perforation; long-term, the risk of colon cancer is increased.
- Treat mild to moderate disease with 5-ASA per rectum and, for proximal disease, by mouth.
- Treat extensive disease with high-dose corticosteroids or immunomodulator therapy with azathioprine or 6-mercaptopurine.
- Treat fulminant disease with high-dose IV corticosteroids or cyclosporine and antibiotics (eg, metronidazole, ciprofloxacin); colectomy may be required.
- About one-third of patients with extensive UC ultimately require surgery.

19 Irritable Bowel Syndrome

(Spastic Colon)

Irritable bowel syndrome (IBS) is characterized by recurrent abdominal discomfort or pain that is accompanied by at least two of the following: relief by defecation, change in frequency of stool, or change in consistency of stool. The cause is unknown, and the pathophysiology is incompletely understood. Diagnosis is clinical. Treatment is symptomatic, consisting of dietary management and drugs, including anticholinergics and agents active at serotonin receptors.

Etiology

The cause of IBS is unknown. No anatomic cause can be found on laboratory tests, x-rays, and biopsies. Emotional factors, diet, drugs, or hormones may precipitate or aggravate GI symptoms. Historically, the disorder was often considered as purely psychosomatic. Although psychosocial factors are involved, IBS is better understood as a combination of psychosocial and physiologic factors.

Psychosocial factors: Psychologic distress is common among patients with IBS, especially in those who seek medical care. Some patients have anxiety disorders, depression, or a somatization disorder. Sleep disturbances also coexist. However, stress and emotional conflict do not always coincide with symptom onset and recurrence. Some patients with IBS seem to have a learned aberrant illness behavior (ie, they express emotional conflict as a GI complaint, usually abdominal pain). The physician evaluating patients with IBS, particularly those with refractory symptoms, should investigate for unresolved psychologic issues, including the possibility of sexual or physical abuse. Psychosocial factors also affect the outcome in IBS.

Physiologic factors: A variety of physiologic factors seem to be involved in IBS symptoms. These factors include altered motility, visceral hyperalgesia, and various genetic and environmental factors.

Visceral hyperalgesia refers to hypersensitivity to normal amounts of intraluminal distention and heightened perception of pain in the presence of normal quantities of intestinal gas; it may result from remodeling of neural pathways in the brain-gut axis. Some patients (perhaps 1 in 7) have reported their IBS symptoms began after an episode of acute gastroenteritis (termed postinfectious IBS). A subset of patients with IBS has autonomic dysfunctions. However, many patients have no demonstrable physiologic abnormalities, and, even in those that do, the abnormalities may not correlate with symptoms.

Constipation may be explained by slower colonic transit, and diarrhea may be explained by faster colonic transit. Some patients with constipation have fewer colonic high amplitude-propagated contractions, which propel colonic contents over several segments. Conversely, excess sigmoid motor activity may retard transit in functional constipation.

Postprandial abdominal discomfort may be attributed to an exaggerated gastro-colonic reflex (the colonic contractile response to a meal), the presence of colonic high amplitude-propagated contractions, increased intestinal sensitivity (visceral hyperalgesia), or a combination of these factors. Fat ingestion may increase intestinal permeability and exaggerate hypersensitivity. Ingestion of food high in fermentable oligosaccharides, disaccharides, monosaccharides, and polyols (collectively called FODMAPs) are poorly absorbed in the small intestine and may increase colonic motility and secretion.

Hormonal fluctuations affect bowel functions in women. Rectal sensitivity is increased during menses but not during other phases of the menstrual cycle. The effects of sex steroids on GI transit are subtle. The role of small-bowel bacterial overgrowth in IBS is controversial.

Symptoms and Signs

IBS tends to begin in adolescence and the 20s, causing bouts of symptoms that recur at irregular periods. Onset in late adult life is less common but not rare. Symptoms rarely rouse the sleeping patient. Symptoms are often triggered by food, particularly fats, or by stress.

Patients have abdominal discomfort, which varies considerably but is often located in the lower abdomen, steady or cramping in nature, and relieved by defecation. In addition, abdominal discomfort is temporally associated with alterations in stool frequency (increased in diarrhea-predominant IBS and decreased in constipation-predominant IBS) and consistency (ie, loose or lumpy and hard). Pain or discomfort related to defecation is likely to be of bowel origin; that associated with exercise, movement, urination, or menstruation usually has a different cause.

Although bowel patterns are relatively consistent in most patients, it is not unusual for patients to alternate between constipation and diarrhea. Patients may also have symptoms of abnormal stool passage (straining, urgency, or feeling of incomplete evacuation), pass mucus, or complain of bloating or abdominal distention. Many patients also have symptoms of dyspepsia. Extra-intestinal symptoms (eg, fatigue, fibromyalgia, sleep disturbances, chronic headaches) are common.

Diagnosis

- Clinical evaluation, based on Rome criteria
- Screening for organic causes with basic laboratory tests and sigmoidoscopy or colonoscopy
- Other tests for patients with red flag findings (rectal blood, weight loss, fever)

Diagnosis of IBS is based on characteristic bowel patterns, time and character of pain, and exclusion of other disease processes through physical examination and routine diagnostic tests.

Red flags: Diagnostic testing should be more intensive when the following red flags are present either at initial presentation or at any time after diagnosis:

- Older age
- Fever
- Weight loss
- Rectal bleeding
- Vomiting

Differential diagnosis: Because patients with IBS can develop organic conditions, testing for other conditions should also be considered in patients who develop alarm symptoms or markedly different symptoms during the course of IBS. Common illnesses that may be confused with IBS include

- Lactose intolerance
- Drug-induced diarrhea
- Postcholecystectomy syndrome
- Laxative abuse
- Parasitic diseases (eg, giardiasis)
- Eosinophilic gastritis or enteritis
- Microscopic colitis
- Small-bowel bacterial overgrowth
- Celiac disease
- Early inflammatory bowel disease

However, uninflamed colonic diverticula do not cause symptoms, and their presence should not be considered explanatory.

The bimodal age distribution of patients with inflammatory bowel disease makes it imperative to evaluate both younger and older patients. In patients > 60 with acute symptoms, ischemic colitis should be considered. Patients with constipation and no anatomic lesion should be evaluated for hypothyroidism and hyperparathyroidism. If the patient's symptoms suggest malabsorption, tropical sprue, celiac disease, and Whipple disease must be considered. Defecatory disorders should be considered as a cause of constipation in patients who report symptoms of difficult defecation.

Rare causes of diarrhea include hyperthyroidism, medullary cancer of the thyroid, or carcinoid syndrome, gastrinoma, and vipoma. However, secretory diarrhea caused by vasoactive intestinal peptide (VIP), calcitonin, or gastrin is typically accompanied by stool volumes > 1000 mL daily.

PEARLS & PITFALLS

- Uninflamed colonic diverticula do not cause symptoms, and their presence should not be considered explanatory.

History: Particular attention should be given to the character of the pain, bowel habits, familial interrelationships, and drug and dietary histories. Equally important are the patient's overall emotional state, interpretation of personal problems, and quality of life. The quality of the patient-physician interaction is key to diagnostic and therapeutic efficacy.

The **Rome criteria** are standardized symptom-based criteria for diagnosing IBS. The Rome criteria require the presence of abdominal pain for at least 1 day/wk in the last 3 mo along with ≥ 2 of the following:

- Pain that is related to defecation.
- Pain is associated with a change in frequency of defecation.
- Pain is associated with a change in consistency of stool.

Physical examination: Patients generally appear to be healthy. Palpation of the abdomen may reveal tenderness, particularly in the left lower quadrant, at times associated with a palpable, tender sigmoid. A digital rectal examination, including a test for occult blood, should be done on all patients. In women, a pelvic examination helps rule out ovarian tumors and cysts or endometriosis, which may mimic IBS.

Testing: The diagnosis of IBS can reasonably be made using the Rome criteria as long as patients have no red flag findings, such as rectal bleeding, weight loss, and fever, or other findings that might suggest another etiology. Many patients with IBS are overtested; however, CBC, biochemical profile (including liver tests), ESR, stool examination for ova and parasites (in patients with diarrhea predominance), thyroid-stimulating hormone and calcium for patients with constipation, and flexible sigmoidoscopy or colonoscopy should be done.

During flexible fiberoptic proctosigmoidoscopy, introduction of the instrument and air insufflation frequently trigger bowel spasm and pain. The mucosal and vascular patterns in IBS usually appear normal. Colonoscopy is preferred for patients > 50 with a change in bowel habits, particularly those with no previous IBS symptoms, to exclude colonic polyps and tumors. In patients with chronic diarrhea, particularly older women, mucosal biopsy can rule out possible microscopic colitis.

Additional studies (such as ultrasonography, CT, barium enema x-ray, upper GI esophagogastroduodenoscopy, and small-bowel x-rays) should be undertaken only when there are other objective abnormalities. Fecal fat excretion should be measured when there is a concern about steatorrhea. Testing for celiac disease and small-bowel x-rays are recommended when malabsorption is suspected. Testing for carbohydrate intolerance or small-bowel bacterial overgrowth should be considered in appropriate circumstances.

Intercurrent disease: Patients with IBS may subsequently develop additional GI disorders, and the clinician must not summarily dismiss their complaints. Changes in symptoms (eg, in the location, type, or intensity of pain; in bowel habits; in constipation and diarrhea) and new symptoms or complaints (eg, nocturnal diarrhea) may signal another disease process. Other symptoms that require investigation include fresh blood in the stool, weight loss, very severe abdominal pain or unusual abdominal distention, steatorrhea or noticeably foul-smelling stools, fever or chills, persistent vomiting, hematemesis, symptoms that wake the patient from sleep (eg, pain, the urge to defecate), and a steady progressive worsening of symptoms. Patients > 40 are more likely than younger patients to develop an intercurrent physiologic illness.

Treatment

- Support and understanding
- Normal diet, avoiding gas-producing and diarrhea-producing foods
- Increased fiber intake for constipation
- Drug therapy directed at the dominant symptoms

Therapy is directed at specific symptoms. An effective therapeutic relationship is essential for effectively managing IBS. Patients should be invited to express not only their symptoms but also their understanding of their symptoms and the reasons prompting a visit to the health care practitioner (eg, fear of serious disease). Patients should be educated about the disorder (eg, normal bowel physiology and the bowel's hypersensitivity to stress and food) and reassured, after appropriate tests, about the absence of a serious or life-threatening disease. Appropriate therapeutic goals (eg, expectations regarding the normal course or variability in symptoms, adverse effects of drugs, the appropriate and available working relationship between the physician and the patient) should be established.

Finally, patients can benefit by being actively involved in the management of their condition. When successful, this can enhance the patient's motivation to adhere to treatment, foster a more positive physician-patient relationship, and mobilize the coping resources of even the most chronically passive patients. Psychologic stress, anxiety, or mood disorders should be identified, evaluated, and treated. Regular physical activity helps relieve stress and assists in bowel function, particularly in patients with constipation.

Diet: In general, a normal diet can be followed. Meals should not be overly large, and eating should be slow and paced. Patients with abdominal distention and increased flatulence may benefit from reducing or eliminating beans, cabbage, and other foods containing fermentable carbohydrates. Reduced intake of sweeteners (eg, sorbitol, mannitol, fructose), which are constituents of natural and processed foods (eg, apple and grape juice, bananas, nuts, and raisins), may alleviate flatulence, bloating, and diarrhea. Patients with evidence of lactose intolerance should reduce their intake of milk and dairy products. A low-fat diet may reduce postprandial abdominal symptoms.

Dietary fiber supplements may soften stool and improve the ease of evacuation. A bland bulk-producing agent may be used (eg, raw bran, starting with 15 mL [1 tbsp] with each meal, supplemented with increased fluid intake). Alternatively, psyllium hydrophilic mucilloid with two glasses of water may be used. However, excessive use of fiber can lead to bloating and diarrhea, so fiber doses must be individualized. Occasionally, flatulence may be reduced by switching to a synthetic fiber preparation (eg, methylcellulose).

Drug therapy: (See also the American Gastroenterological Association's technical review and guideline on pharmacologic management of irritable bowel syndrome.)

Drug therapy is directed toward the dominant symptoms. Anticholinergic drugs (eg, hyoscyamine 0.125 mg po 30 to 60 min before meals) may be used for their antispasmodic effects.

In patients with constipation-predominant IBS (IBS-C), the chloride channel activator lubiprostone 8 mcg or 24 mcg po bid and the guanylate cyclase C agonist linaclotide 145 mcg or 290 mcg po once/day may be helpful. Polyethylene glycol laxatives have not been well-studied in IBS. However, they have been shown to be effective for use in chronic constipation and for bowel lavage before colonoscopy and are thus frequently used for IBS-C.

In patients with diarrhea-predominant IBS (IBS-D), oral diphenoxylate 2.5 to 5 mg or loperamide 2 to 4 mg may be given before meals. The dose of loperamide should be titrated upward to reduce diarrhea while avoiding constipation. Rifaximin is an antibiotic that has been shown to relieve symptoms of bloating and abdominal pain and to help decrease looseness of stools in patients with IBS-D. The recommended dose of rifaximin for IBS-D is 550 mg po tid for 14 days. Alosetron is a

5-hydroxytryptamine (serotonin) 3 (5HT3) receptor antagonist that may benefit women with severe IBS-D refractory to other drugs. Because alosetron has been associated with ischemic colitis, its use in the US is under a restricted prescribing program. Eluxadoline has mixed opioid receptor activity and is indicated for treatment of IBS-D.

For many patients, tricyclic antidepressants (TCAs) help relieve symptoms of diarrhea, abdominal pain, and bloating. These drugs are thought to reduce pain by down-regulating the activity of spinal cord and cortical afferent pathways arriving from the intestine. Secondary amine TCAs (eg, nortriptyline, desipramine) are often better tolerated than parent tertiary amines (eg, amitriptyline, imipramine, doxepin) because of fewer anticholinergic, sedating antihistaminic, and alpha-adrenergic adverse effects. Treatment should begin with a very low dose of a TCA (eg, desipramine 10 to 25 mg once/day at bedtime), increasing as necessary and tolerated up to about 100 to 150 mg once/day.

SSRIs are sometimes used in patients with anxiety or an affective disorder, but studies have not shown a significant benefit for patients with IBS and they may exacerbate diarrhea.

Preliminary data suggest that certain probiotics (eg, *Bifidobacterium infantis*) alleviate IBS symptoms, particularly bloating. The beneficial effects of probiotics are not generic to the entire species but specific to certain strains. Certain aromatic oils (carminatives) can relax smooth muscle and relieve pain caused by cramps in some patients. Peppermint oil is the most commonly used agent in this class.

Psychologic therapies: Cognitive-behavioral therapy, standard psychotherapy, and hypnotherapy may help some IBS patients.

KEY POINTS

- IBS is recurrent abdominal discomfort or pain accompanied by ≥ 2 of the following: relief by defecation, change in frequency of stool (diarrhea or constipation), or change in consistency of stool.
- Etiology is unclear but appears to involve both psychosocial and physiologic factors.
- Exclude more dangerous diseases by testing, particularly in patients with red flag findings, such as older age, fever, weight loss, rectal bleeding, or vomiting.
- Common illnesses that may be confused with IBS include lactose intolerance, drug-induced diarrhea, post-cholecystectomy diarrhea, laxative abuse, parasitic diseases, eosinophilic gastritis or enteritis, microscopic colitis, small-bowel bacterial overgrowth, celiac disease, and early inflammatory bowel disease.
- Typical testing includes CBC, biochemical profile (including liver tests), ESR, stool examination for ova and parasites (in patients with diarrhea predominance), thyroid-stimulating hormone and calcium (for patients with constipation), and flexible sigmoidoscopy or colonoscopy.
- A supportive, understanding, and therapeutic relationship is essential; direct drug therapy toward the dominant symptoms.

20 Malabsorption Syndromes

Malabsorption is inadequate assimilation of dietary substances due to defects in digestion, absorption, or transport.

Malabsorption can affect macronutrients (eg, proteins, carbohydrates, fats), micronutrients (eg, vitamins, minerals), or both, causing excessive fecal excretion, nutritional deficiencies, and GI symptoms. Malabsorption may be global, with impaired absorption of almost all nutrients, or partial (isolated), with malabsorption of only specific nutrients.

Pathophysiology

Digestion and absorption occur in three phases:

1. Intraluminal hydrolysis of fats, proteins, and carbohydrates by enzymes—bile salts enhance the solubilization of fat in this phase
2. Digestion by brush border enzymes and uptake of end-products
3. Lymphatic transport of nutrients

The term *malabsorption* is commonly used when any of these phases is impaired, but, strictly speaking, impairment of phase 1 is maldigestion rather than malabsorption.

Digestion of fats: Pancreatic enzymes (lipase and colipase) split long-chain triglycerides into fatty acids and monoglycerides, which combine with bile acids and phospholipids to form micelles that pass through jejunal enterocytes. Absorbed fatty acids are resynthesized and combined with protein, cholesterol, and phospholipid to form chylomicrons, which are transported by the lymphatic system. Medium-chain triglycerides are absorbed directly.

Unabsorbed fats trap fat-soluble vitamins (A, D, E, and K) and possibly some minerals, causing deficiency. Bacterial overgrowth results in deconjugation and dehydroxylation of bile salts, limiting the absorption of fats. Unabsorbed bile salts stimulate water secretion in the colon, causing diarrhea.

Digestion of carbohydrates: The pancreatic enzyme amylase and brush border enzymes on microvilli lyse carbohydrates and disaccharides into constituent monosaccharides. Colonic bacteria ferment unabsorbed carbohydrates into carbon dioxide, methane, hydrogen, and short-chain fatty acids (butyrate, propionate, acetate, and lactate). These fatty acids cause diarrhea. The gases cause abdominal distention and bloating.

Digestion of proteins: Gastric pepsin initiates digestion of proteins in the stomach (and also stimulates release of cholecystokinin that is critical to the secretion of pancreatic enzymes). Enterokinase, a brush border enzyme, activates trypsinogen into trypsin, which converts many pancreatic proteases into their active forms. Active pancreatic enzymes hydrolyze proteins into oligopeptides, which are absorbed directly or hydrolyzed into amino acids.

Etiology

Malabsorption has many causes (see Table 20–1). Some malabsorptive disorders (eg, celiac disease) impair the absorption of most nutrients, vitamins, and trace minerals (global malabsorption); others (eg, pernicious anemia) are more selective.

Pancreatic insufficiency causes malabsorption if > 90% of function is lost. Increased luminal acidity (eg, Zollinger-Ellison

Table 20–1. CAUSES OF MALABSORPTION

MECHANISM	CAUSE
Inadequate gastric mixing, rapid emptying, or both	Billroth II gastrectomy
	Gastrocolic fistula
	Gastroenterostomy
Insufficient digestive agents	Biliary obstruction and cholestasis
	Cirrhosis
	Chronic pancreatitis
	Cholestyramine-induced bile acid loss
	Cystic fibrosis
	Lactase deficiency
	Pancreatic cancer
	Pancreatic resection
	Sucrase-isomaltase deficiency
Abnormal milieu	Abnormal motility secondary to diabetes, scleroderma, hypothyroidism, or hyperthyroidism
	Bacterial overgrowth due to blind loops (deconjugation of bile salts), diverticula in the small intestine
	Zollinger-Ellison syndrome (low duodenal pH)
Acutely abnormal epithelium	Acute intestinal infections
	Alcohol
	Neomycin
Chronically abnormal epithelium	Amyloidosis
	Celiac disease
	Crohn disease
	Ischemia
	Radiation enteritis
	Tropical sprue
	Whipple disease
Short bowel	Intestinal resection (eg, for Crohn disease, volvulus, intussusception, or infarction)
	Jejunoileal bypass for obesity
Impaired transport	Abetalipoproteinemia
	Addison disease
	Blocked lacteals due to lymphoma or TB
	Intrinsic factor deficiency (as in pernicious anemia)
	Lymphangiectasia

syndrome) inhibits lipase and fat digestion. Cirrhosis and cholestasis reduce hepatic bile synthesis or delivery of bile salts to the duodenum, causing malabsorption. Other causes are discussed elsewhere in this chapter.

Acute bacterial, viral, and parasitic infections (see also Overview of Gastroenteritis on p. 124) may cause transient malabsorption, probably as a result of temporary, superficial damage to the villi and microvilli. Chronic bacterial infections of the small bowel are uncommon, apart from blind loops, systemic sclerosis, and diverticula. Intestinal bacteria may use up dietary vitamin B_{12} and other nutrients, perhaps interfere with enzyme systems, and cause mucosal injury.

Table 20–2. SYMPTOMS OF MALABSORPTION

SYMPTOM	MALABSORBED NUTRIENT
Anemia (hypochromic, microcytic)	Iron
Anemia (macrocytic)	Vitamin B_{12}, folate
Bleeding, bruising, petechiae	Vitamins K and C
Carpopedal spasm	Ca, Mg
Edema	Protein
Glossitis	Vitamins B_2 and B_{12}, folate, niacin, iron
Night blindness	Vitamin A
Pain in limbs, bones, pathologic fractures	Vitamins K and D, Mg, Ca
Peripheral neuropathy	Vitamins B_1, B_6, B_{12}

Symptoms and Signs

The effects of unabsorbed substances, especially in global malabsorption, include diarrhea, steatorrhea, abdominal bloating, and gas. Other symptoms result from nutritional deficiencies. Patients often lose weight despite adequate food intake.

Chronic diarrhea is the most common symptom and is what usually prompts evaluation of the patient. Steatorrhea—fatty stool, the hallmark of malabsorption—occurs when > 7 g/day of fat are excreted. Steatorrhea causes foul-smelling, pale, bulky, and greasy stools.

Severe vitamin and mineral deficiencies occur in advanced malabsorption; symptoms are related to the specific nutrient deficiency (see Table 20–2). Vitamin B_{12} deficiency may occur in blind loop syndrome or after extensive resection of the distal ileum or stomach. Iron deficiency may be the only symptom in a patient with mild malabsorption.

Amenorrhea may result from undernutrition and is an important manifestation of celiac disease in young women.

Diagnosis

- Diagnosis typically clinically apparent from a detailed patient history
- Blood tests to screen for consequences of malabsorption
- Stool fat testing to confirm malabsorption (if unclear)
- Cause diagnosed with endoscopy, contrast x-rays, or other tests based on findings

Malabsorption is suspected in a patient with chronic diarrhea, weight loss, and anemia. The etiology is sometimes obvious. For example, patients with malabsorption due to chronic pancreatitis usually have had prior bouts of acute pancreatitis. Patients with celiac disease can present with classic lifelong diarrhea exacerbated by gluten products and may have dermatitis herpetiformis. Patients with cirrhosis and pancreatic cancer can present with jaundice. Abdominal distention, excessive flatus, and watery diarrhea occurring 30 to 90 min after carbohydrate ingestion suggest deficiency of a disaccharidase enzyme, usually lactase. Previous extensive abdominal operations suggest short bowel syndrome.

If the history suggests a specific cause, testing should be directed to that condition (see Fig. 20–1). If no cause is readily apparent, blood tests can be used as screening tools (eg, CBC,

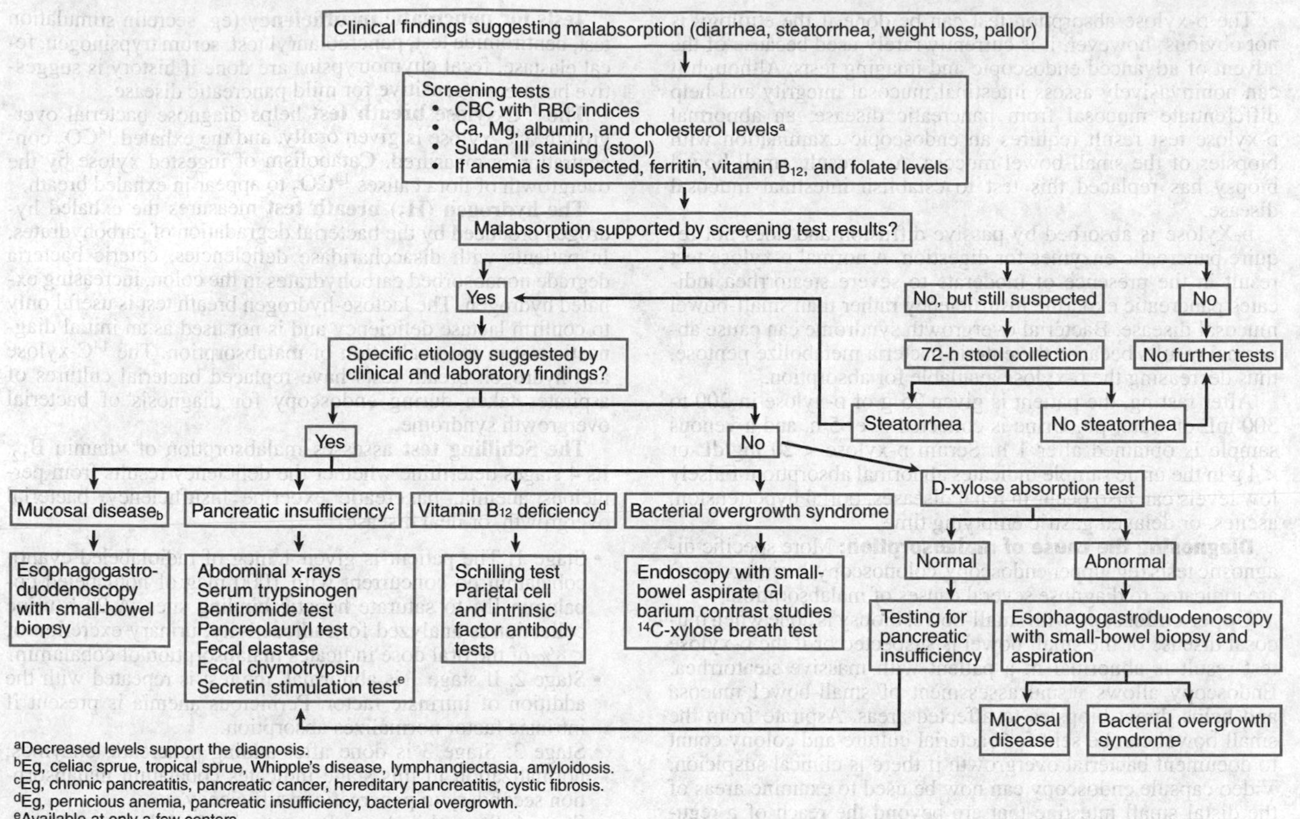

Fig. 20–1. Suggested evaluation for malabsorption.

RBC indices, ferritin, vitamin B_{12}, folate, calcium, albumin, cholesterol, PT). Test results may suggest a diagnosis and direct further investigation.

Macrocytic anemia should prompt measurement of serum folate and B_{12} levels. Folate deficiency is common in mucosal disorders involving the proximal small bowel (eg, celiac disease, tropical sprue, Whipple disease). Low B_{12} levels can occur in pernicious anemia, chronic pancreatitis, bacterial overgrowth, and terminal ileal disease. A combination of low B_{12} and high folate levels is suggestive of bacterial overgrowth, because intestinal bacteria use vitamin B_{12} and synthesize folate.

Microcytic anemia suggests iron deficiency, which may occur with celiac disease. Albumin is a general indicator of nutritional state. Low albumin can result from poor intake, decreased synthesis in cirrhosis, or protein wasting. Low serum carotene (a precursor of vitamin A) suggests malabsorption if intake is adequate.

Confirming malabsorption: Tests to confirm malabsorption are appropriate when symptoms are vague and the etiology is not apparent. Most tests for malabsorption assess fat malabsorption because it is relatively easy to measure. Confirmation of carbohydrate malabsorption is not helpful once steatorrhea is documented. Tests for protein malabsorption are rarely used because fecal nitrogen is difficult to measure.

Direct measurement of fecal fat from a 72-h stool collection is the gold standard test for establishing steatorrhea but unnecessary with gross steatorrhea of obvious cause. However, this test is available routinely in only a few centers. Stool is collected for a 3-day period during which the patient consumes ≥ 100 g fat/day. Total fat in the stool is measured. Fecal fat > 7 g/day is abnormal. Although severe fat malabsorption (fecal fat ≥ 40 g/day) suggests pancreatic insufficiency or small-bowel mucosal disease, this test cannot determine the specific cause of malabsorption. Because the test is messy, unpleasant, and time consuming, it is unacceptable to most patients and difficult to do.

Sudan III staining of a stool smear is a simple and direct, but nonquantitative, screening test for fecal fat. Acid steatocrit is a gravimetric assay done on a single stool sample; it has a reported high sensitivity and specificity (using 72-h collection as the standard). Near-infrared reflectance analysis (NIRA) simultaneously tests stool for fat, nitrogen, and carbohydrates and may become the preferred test in the future; this test is currently available in only a few centers.

Measurement of elastase and chymotrypsin in the stool can also help differentiate pancreatic and intestinal causes of malabsorption; both are decreased in pancreatic exocrine insufficiency, whereas both are normal in intestinal causes.

The D-xylose absorption test can be done if the etiology is not obvious; however, it is currently rarely used because of the advent of advanced endoscopic and imaging tests. Although it can noninvasively assess intestinal mucosal integrity and help differentiate mucosal from pancreatic disease, an abnormal D-xylose test result requires an endoscopic examination with biopsies of the small-bowel mucosa. As a result, small-bowel biopsy has replaced this test to establish intestinal mucosal disease.

D-Xylose is absorbed by passive diffusion and does not require pancreatic enzymes for digestion. A normal D-xylose test result in the presence of moderate to severe steatorrhea indicates pancreatic exocrine insufficiency rather than small-bowel mucosal disease. Bacterial overgrowth syndrome can cause abnormal results because the enteric bacteria metabolize pentose, thus decreasing the D-xylose available for absorption.

After fasting, the patient is given 25 g of D-xylose in 200 to 300 mL of water po. Urine is collected over 5 h, and a venous sample is obtained after 1 h. Serum D-xylose < 20 mg/dL or < 4 g in the urine sample indicates abnormal absorption. Falsely low levels can also occur in renal diseases, portal hypertension, ascites, or delayed gastric emptying time.

Diagnosing the cause of malabsorption: More specific diagnostic tests (eg, upper endoscopy, colonoscopy, barium x-rays) are indicated to diagnose several causes of malabsorption.

Upper endoscopy with small-bowel biopsy is done when mucosal disease of the small bowel is suspected or if the D-xylose test result is abnormal in a patient with massive steatorrhea. Endoscopy allows visual assessment of small-bowel mucosa and helps direct biopsies to affected areas. Aspirate from the small bowel can be sent for bacterial culture and colony count to document bacterial overgrowth if there is clinical suspicion. Video capsule endoscopy can now be used to examine areas of the distal small intestine that are beyond the reach of a regular endoscope. Histologic features on small-bowel biopsy (see Table 20–3) can establish the specific mucosal disease.

Small-bowel x-rays (eg, small-bowel follow-through, enteroclysis, CT enterography) can detect anatomic conditions that predispose to bacterial overgrowth. These include jejunal diverticula, fistulas, surgically created blind loops and anastomoses, ulcerations, and strictures. Abdominal flat plate x-rays may show pancreatic calcifications indicative of chronic pancreatitis. Barium contrast studies of the small bowel are neither sensitive nor specific but may show findings suggestive of mucosal disease (eg, dilated small-bowel loops, thinned or thickened mucosal folds, coarse fragmentation of the barium column). CT, magnetic resonance cholangiopancreatography (MRCP), and ERCP can establish the diagnosis of chronic pancreatitis.

Tests for pancreatic insufficiency (eg, secretin stimulation test, bentiromide test, pancreolauryl test, serum trypsinogen, fecal elastase, fecal chymotrypsin) are done if history is suggestive but are not sensitive for mild pancreatic disease.

The ^{14}C-xylose breath test helps diagnose bacterial overgrowth. ^{14}C-xylose is given orally, and the exhaled $^{14}CO_2$ concentration is measured. Catabolism of ingested xylose by the overgrowth of flora causes $^{14}CO_2$ to appear in exhaled breath.

The hydrogen (H_2) breath test measures the exhaled hydrogen produced by the bacterial degradation of carbohydrates. In patients with disaccharidase deficiencies, enteric bacteria degrade nonabsorbed carbohydrates in the colon, increasing exhaled hydrogen. The lactose-hydrogen breath test is useful only to confirm lactase deficiency and is not used as an initial diagnostic test in the evaluation of malabsorption. The ^{14}C-xylose and hydrogen breath tests have replaced bacterial cultures of aspirates taken during endoscopy for diagnosis of bacterial overgrowth syndrome.

The Schilling test assesses malabsorption of vitamin B_{12}. Its 4 stages determine whether the deficiency results from pernicious anemia, pancreatic exocrine insufficiency, bacterial overgrowth, or ileal disease.

- Stage 1: The patient is given 1 mcg of radiolabeled cyanocobalamin po concurrent with 1000 mcg of nonlabeled cobalamin IM to saturate hepatic binding sites. A 24-h urine collection is analyzed for radioactivity; urinary excretion of < 8% of the oral dose indicates malabsorption of cobalamin.
- Stage 2: If stage 1 is abnormal, the test is repeated with the addition of intrinsic factor. Pernicious anemia is present if intrinsic factor normalizes absorption.
- Stage 3: Stage 3 is done after adding pancreatic enzymes; normalization in this stage indicates cobalamin malabsorption secondary to pancreatic insufficiency.
- Stage 4: Stage 4 is done after antimicrobial therapy with anaerobic coverage; normalization after antibiotics suggests bacterial overgrowth.

Cobalamin deficiency secondary to ileal disease or ileal resection results in abnormalities in all stages.

Tests for less common causes of malabsorption include serum gastrin (Zollinger-Ellison syndrome), intrinsic factor and parietal cell antibodies (pernicious anemia), sweat chloride (cystic fibrosis), lipoprotein electrophoresis (abetalipoproteinemia), and serum cortisol (Addison disease).

To diagnose bile acid malabsorption, which may occur with diseases of the terminal ileum (eg, Crohn disease, extensive resection of terminal ileum), patients can be given a therapeutic trial of a bile acid binding resin (eg, cholestyramine).

Table 20–3. SMALL-BOWEL MUCOSAL HISTOLOGY IN CERTAIN MALABSORPTIVE DISORDERS

DISORDER	HISTOLOGIC CHARACTERISTICS
Normal	Fingerlike villi with a villous: crypt ratio of about 4:1; columnar epithelial cells with numerous regular microvilli (brush border); mild round cell infiltration in the lamina propria
Celiac disease (untreated)	Virtual absence of villi and elongated crypts; increased intraepithelial lymphocytes and round cells (especially plasma cells) in the lamina propria; cuboidal epithelial cells with scanty, irregular microvilli
Intestinal lymphangiectasia	Dilation and ectasia of the intramucosal lymphatics
Tropical sprue	Range from minimal changes in villous height and moderate epithelial cell damage to virtual absence of villi and elongated crypts with lymphocyte infiltration in the lamina propria
Whipple disease	Lamina propria densely infiltrated with periodic acid-Schiff–positive macrophages; villous structure possibly obliterated in severe lesions

Alternatively, the selenium homocholic acid taurine (SeHCAT) test can be done. In this test, ^{75}Se-labeled synthetic bile acid is given orally and, after 7 days, the retained bile acid is measured with a whole-body scan or gamma camera. If bile acid absorption is abnormal, retention is less than 5%.

BACTERIAL OVERGROWTH SYNDROME

Small-bowel bacterial overgrowth can result from alterations in intestinal anatomy or GI motility, or lack of gastric acid secretion. This condition can lead to vitamin deficiencies, fat malabsorption, and undernutrition. Diagnosis is by breath test or quantitative culture of intestinal fluid aspirate. Treatment is with oral antibiotics.

Under normal conditions, the proximal small bowel contains < 10^5 bacteria/mL, mainly gram-positive aerobic bacteria. This low bacterial count is maintained by normal peristalsis, normal gastric acid secretion, mucus, secretory IgA, and an intact ileocecal valve.

Etiology

Anatomic alterations of the stomach and/or small intestine promote stasis of intestinal contents, leading to bacterial overgrowth. Conditions that cause or require anatomic alterations include small-bowel diverticulosis, surgical blind loops, postgastrectomy states (especially in the afferent loop of a Billroth II), strictures, or partial obstruction. Intestinal motility disorders associated with diabetic neuropathy, systemic sclerosis, amyloidosis, hypothyroidism, and idiopathic intestinal pseudo-obstruction can also impair bacterial clearance. Achlorhydria and idiopathic changes in intestinal motility may cause bacterial overgrowth in elderly people.

Pathophysiology

The excess bacteria consume nutrients, including carbohydrates and vitamin B_{12}, leading to caloric deprivation and vitamin B_{12} deficiency. However, because the bacteria produce folate, this deficiency is rare. The bacteria deconjugate bile salts, causing failure of micelle formation and subsequent fat malabsorption. Severe bacterial overgrowth also damages the intestinal mucosa. Fat malabsorption and mucosal damage can cause diarrhea.

Symptoms and Signs

Many patients are asymptomatic and present with only weight loss or nutrient deficiencies. The most frequent symptoms are abdominal discomfort, diarrhea, bloating, and excess flatulence. Some patients have significant diarrhea or steatorrhea.

Diagnosis

- ^{14}C-xylose breath test or quantitative culture of intestinal aspirate
- Sometimes upper GI series with small-bowel follow-through

Some clinicians advocate response to empiric antibiotic therapy as a diagnostic test. However, because bacterial overgrowth can mimic other malabsorptive disorders (eg, Crohn disease) and adverse effects of the antibiotics can worsen symptoms, establishing a definitive etiology is preferred.

The standard for diagnosis of bacterial overgrowth syndrome is quantitative culture of intestinal fluid aspirate showing a bacterial count > 10^5/mL. This method, however, requires endoscopy. Breath tests, using substrates like glucose, lactulose, and xylose, are noninvasive and easy to do. The ^{14}C-xylose breath test (see p. 148) seems to perform better than the other breath tests.

If the anatomic alterations are not due to previous surgery, an upper GI series with small-bowel follow-through should be done to identify predisposing anatomic lesions.

Treatment

- Oral antibiotics (various)
- Dietary modification

Treatment of bacterial overgrowth syndrome is with 10 to 14 days of oral antibiotics that cover both aerobic and anaerobic enteric bacteria. Empiric regimens include use of one of the following: tetracycline 250 mg qid, amoxicillin/clavulanic acid 250 to 500 mg tid, cephalexin 250 mg qid, trimethoprim/sulfamethoxazole 160/800 mg bid, metronidazole 250 to 500 mg tid or qid, or rifaximin 400 to 550 mg bid. Antibiotic treatment can be cyclic, if symptoms tend to recur, and changed based on culture and sensitivity. Changing antibiotic treatment may be difficult, however, due to coexistence of multiple bacteria.

Because bacteria metabolize primarily carbohydrates in the intestinal lumen rather than fats, a diet high in fat and low in carbohydrates and fiber is beneficial.

Underlying conditions and nutritional deficiencies (eg, vitamin B_{12}) should be corrected.

KEY POINTS

- Anatomic alterations in stomach or intestines lead to GI stasis and thus bacterial overgrowth.
- Bacteria deconjugate bile salts, causing fat malabsorption.
- Diagnosis is made using the ^{14}C-xylose breath test and other breath tests or quantitative culture of intestinal aspirate.
- Oral antibiotics are used, and a high-fat, low-carbohydrate diet is followed.

CARBOHYDRATE INTOLERANCE

Carbohydrate intolerance is the inability to digest certain carbohydrates due to a lack of one or more intestinal enzymes. Symptoms include diarrhea, abdominal distention, and flatulence. Diagnosis is clinical and by a hydrogen (H_2) breath test. Treatment is removal of the causative disaccharide from the diet.

Pathophysiology

Disaccharides are normally split into monosaccharides by disaccharidases (eg, lactase, maltase, isomaltase, sucrase [invertase]) located in the brush border of small-bowel enterocytes. Undigested disaccharides cause an osmotic load that attracts water and electrolytes into the bowel, causing watery diarrhea. Bacterial fermentation of carbohydrates in the colon produces gases (hydrogen, carbon dioxide, and methane), resulting in excessive flatus, bloating and distention, and abdominal pain.

Etiology

Enzyme deficiencies can be

- Congenital (eg, rare deficiencies of lactase or sucrase-isomaltase)
- Acquired (primary)
- Secondary

Acquired lactase deficiency (primary adult hypolactasia) is the most common form of carbohydrate intolerance. Lactase levels are high in neonates, permitting digestion of milk; in most ethnic groups (80% of blacks and Hispanics, > 90% of Asians), the levels decrease in the post-weaning period rendering older children and adults unable to digest significant amounts of lactose. However, 80 to 85% of whites of Northwest European descent produce lactase throughout life and are thus able to digest milk and milk products. It is unclear why the normal state of > 75% of the world's population should be labeled a "deficiency."

Secondary lactase deficiency occurs in conditions that damage the small-bowel mucosa (eg, celiac disease, tropical sprue, acute intestinal infections [see Gastroenteritis on p. 124]). In infants, temporary secondary disaccharidase deficiency may complicate enteric infections or abdominal surgery. Recovery from the underlying disease is followed by an increase in activity of the enzyme.

Symptoms and Signs

Symptoms and signs of carbohydrate intolerance are similar in all disaccharidase deficiencies. A child who cannot tolerate lactose develops diarrhea after ingesting significant amounts of milk and may not gain weight. An affected adult may have watery diarrhea, bloating, excessive flatus, nausea, borborygmi, and abdominal cramps after ingesting lactose. The patient often recognizes early in life that dairy causes GI problems and avoids eating dairy products. Symptoms typically require ingestion of more than the equivalent of 250 to 375 mL (8 to 12 oz) of milk. Diarrhea may be severe enough to purge other nutrients before they can be absorbed. Symptoms may be similar to and can be confused with irritable bowel syndrome.

PEARLS & PITFALLS

- Most people with lactase deficiency can tolerate up to 250 to 375 mL of milk; symptoms that occur after consuming much smaller amounts may suggest another diagnosis.

Diagnosis

- Clinical diagnosis
- Hydrogen breath test for confirmation

Lactose intolerance can usually be diagnosed with a careful history supported by dietary challenge. Patients usually have a history of diarrhea and/or gas after ingestion of milk and dairy foods; other symptoms, such as rash, wheezing, or other anaphylactic symptoms (particularly in infants and children), suggest a cow's milk *allergy*. Milk allergy is rare in adults and also may cause vomiting and symptoms of esophageal reflux, which are not manifestations of carbohydrate intolerance. The diagnosis is also suggested if the stool from chronic or intermittent diarrhea is acidic (pH < 6) and can be confirmed by an H_2 breath test or a lactose tolerance test.

In the hydrogen breath test, 50 g of lactose is given orally and the hydrogen produced by bacterial metabolism of undigested lactose is measured with a breath meter at 2, 3, and 4 h postingestion. Most affected patients have an increase in expired hydrogen of > 20 ppm over baseline. Sensitivity and specificity are > 95%.

The lactose tolerance test is less sensitive, about 75%, although specificity is > 95%. Oral lactose (1.0 to 1.5 g/kg body weight) is given. Serum glucose is measured before ingestion and 60 and 120 min after. Lactose-intolerant patients develop diarrhea, abdominal bloating, and discomfort within 20 to 30 min, and their serum glucose levels do not rise to > 20 mg/dL (< 1.1 mmol/L) above baseline.

Treatment

- Dietary restriction

Carbohydrate malabsorption is readily controlled by avoiding dietary sugars that cannot be absorbed (ie, following a lactose-free diet in cases of lactase deficiency). However, because the degree of lactose malabsorption varies greatly, many patients can ingest up to 375 mL (18 g of lactose) of milk daily without symptoms. Yogurt is usually tolerated because it contains an appreciable amount of lactase produced by intrinsic *Lactobacilli*. Cheese contains lower amounts of lactose than milk and is often tolerated, depending on the amount ingested.

For symptomatic patients wishing to drink milk, lactose in milk can be predigested by the addition of a commercially prepared lactase, and pretreated milk is now available. Enzyme supplements should be an adjunct to, not a substitute for, dietary restriction. Lactose-intolerant patients must take calcium supplements (1200 to 1500 mg/day).

KEY POINTS

- Disaccharide deficiency (usually of lactase) can be acquired or, rarely, congenital.
- Undigested disaccharides, such as lactose, create an osmotic load that causes diarrhea.
- Intestinal bacteria metabolize some undigested disaccharides, producing gases that cause distention and flatus.
- Confirm clinical diagnosis by doing a hydrogen breath test.
- Dietary restriction is usually adequate treatment.

CELIAC DISEASE

(Gluten Enteropathy)

Celiac disease is an immunologically mediated disease in genetically susceptible people caused by intolerance to gluten, resulting in mucosal inflammation and villous atrophy, which causes malabsorption. Symptoms usually include diarrhea and abdominal discomfort. Diagnosis is by small-bowel biopsies showing characteristic though not specific pathologic changes of villous atrophy that resolve with a strict gluten-free diet.

(See also the ACG Clinical Guidelines: Diagnosis and Management of Celiac Disease.)

Etiology

Celiac disease is a hereditary disorder caused by sensitivity to the gliadin fraction of gluten, a protein found in wheat; similar proteins are present in rye and barley. In a genetically susceptible person, gluten-sensitive T cells are activated when gluten-derived peptide epitopes are presented. The inflammatory response causes characteristic mucosal villous atrophy in the small bowel.

Epidemiology: Celiac disease mainly affects people of northern European descent. Prevalence estimates based on serologic screens among blood donors (sometimes confirmed by biopsy) indicate the disorder may be present in about 1/150 in Europe, especially in Ireland and Italy, and perhaps 1/250 in some parts of the US. Current prevalence estimates in some regions are as high as 1/100.

The disease affects about 10 to 20% of 1st-degree relatives. Female:male ratio is 2:1. Onset is generally in childhood but may occur later.

Patients who have other diseases, such as lymphocytic colitis, Down syndrome, type 1 diabetes mellitus, and autoimmune (Hashimoto) thyroiditis, are at risk of developing celiac disease.

Symptoms and Signs

The clinical presentation varies; no typical presentation exists. Some patients are asymptomatic or have only signs of nutritional deficiency. Others have significant GI symptoms.

Celiac disease can manifest in infancy and childhood after introduction of cereals into the diet. The child has failure to thrive, apathy, anorexia, pallor, generalized hypotonia, abdominal distention, and muscle wasting. Stools are soft, bulky, clay-colored, and offensive. Older children may present with anemia or failure to grow normally.

In adults, lassitude, weakness, and anorexia are most common. Mild and intermittent diarrhea is sometimes the presenting symptom. Steatorrhea ranges from mild to severe (7 to 50 g of fat/day). Some patients have weight loss, rarely enough to become underweight. Anemia, glossitis, angular stomatitis, and aphthous ulcers are usually seen in these patients. Manifestations of vitamin D and calcium deficiencies (eg, osteomalacia, osteopenia, osteoporosis) are common. Both men and women may have reduced fertility; women may not have menstrual periods.

About 10% of patients have dermatitis herpetiformis, an intensely pruritic papulovesicular rash that is symmetrically distributed over the extensor areas of the elbows, knees, buttocks, shoulders, and scalp. This rash can be induced by a high-gluten diet.

Diagnosis

- Serologic markers
- Small-bowel biopsy

The diagnosis of celiac disease is suspected clinically and by laboratory abnormalities suggestive of malabsorption. Family incidence is a valuable clue. Celiac disease should be strongly considered in a patient with iron deficiency without obvious GI bleeding.

Confirmation requires a small-bowel biopsy from the second portion of the duodenum. Findings include lack or shortening of villi (villous atrophy), increased intraepithelial cells, and crypt hyperplasia. However, such findings can also occur in tropical sprue, severe intestinal bacterial overgrowth, eosinophilic enteritis, infectious enteritis (eg, giardiasis), and lymphoma.

Because biopsy lacks specificity, serologic markers can aid diagnosis. Anti-tissue transglutaminase antibody (tTG) and anti-endomysial antibody (EMA—an antibody against an intestinal connective tissue protein) have sensitivity and specificity > 90%. These markers can also be used to screen populations with high prevalence of celiac disease, including 1st-degree relatives of affected patients and patients with diseases that occur at a greater frequency in association with celiac disease. If either test is positive, the patient should have a diagnostic small-bowel biopsy. If both are negative, celiac disease is extremely unlikely. These antibodies decrease in titer in patients on a gluten-free diet and thus are useful in monitoring dietary adherence. All diagnostic serologic testing should be done with patients following a gluten-containing diet.

Other laboratory abnormalities often occur and should be sought. They include anemia (iron-deficiency anemia in children and folate-deficiency anemia in adults); low albumin, calcium, potassium, and sodium; and elevated alkaline phosphatase and PT.

Malabsorption tests are not specific for celiac disease. If done, common findings include steatorrhea of 10 to 40 g/day and abnormal results with D-xylose and (in severe ileal disease) positive Schilling tests.

PEARLS & PITFALLS

- Strongly consider celiac disease in patients with iron deficiency but no apparent GI bleeding.

Prognosis

Complications of celiac disease include refractory disease, collagenous sprue, and intestinal lymphomas. Intestinal lymphomas affect 6 to 8% of patients with celiac disease, usually manifesting after 20 to 40 yr of disease. The incidence of other GI cancers (eg, carcinoma of the esophagus or oropharynx, small-bowel adenocarcinoma) also increases. Adherence to a gluten-free diet can significantly reduce the risk of cancer. If people who have been doing well on a gluten-free diet for a long time once again develop symptoms of celiac disease, physicians usually do upper endoscopy with small bowel biopsy to check for signs of intestinal lymphoma.

Treatment

- Gluten-free diet
- Supplements to replace any serious deficiencies

Treatment of celiac disease is a gluten-free diet (avoiding foods containing wheat, rye, or barley). Gluten is so widely used (eg, in commercial soups, sauces, ice creams, and hot dogs) that a patient needs a detailed list of foods to avoid. Patients are encouraged to consult a dietitian and join a celiac support group. The response to a gluten-free diet is usually rapid, and symptoms resolve in 1 to 2 wk. Ingesting even small amounts of food containing gluten may prevent remission or induce relapse.

Small-bowel biopsy should be repeated after 3 to 4 mo of a gluten-free diet. If abnormalities persist, other causes of villous atrophy (eg, lymphoma) should be considered. Lessening of symptoms and improvement in small-bowel morphology are accompanied by a decrease in anti-tissue transglutaminase antibody and anti-endomysial antibody titers.

Supplementary vitamins, minerals, and hematinics may be given, depending on the deficiencies. Mild cases may not require supplementation, whereas severe cases may require comprehensive replacement. For adults, replacement includes ferrous sulfate 300 mg po once/day to tid, folate 5 to 10 mg po once/day, calcium supplements, and any standard multivitamin. Sometimes children (but rarely adults) who are seriously ill on initial diagnosis require bowel rest and TPN.

If a patient responds poorly to gluten withdrawal, either the diagnosis is incorrect or the disease has become refractory. Corticosteroids can control symptoms in refractory disease.

KEY POINTS

- Celiac disease involves an inflammatory response to gluten that causes villous atrophy and malabsorption.
- People of northern European heritage are most often affected.
- Suspect the diagnosis if the serologic markers anti-tissue transglutaminase antibody and anti-endomysial antibody are present and confirm the diagnosis with a small-bowel biopsy.
- Instruct the patient to follow a gluten-free diet and replace any vitamin or mineral deficiencies.

INTESTINAL LYMPHANGIECTASIA

(Idiopathic Hypoproteinemia)

Intestinal lymphangiectasia is a rare disorder characterized by obstruction or malformation of the intramucosal lymphatics of the small bowel. It primarily affects children and young adults. Symptoms include those of malabsorption, with edema and growth retardation. Diagnosis is by small-bowel biopsy. Treatment is usually supportive.

Malformation of the lymphatic system is congenital or acquired. Congenital cases usually manifest in children (typically diagnosed before age 3 yr) and less frequently in adolescents or young adults. Males and females are equally affected. In acquired cases, the defect may be secondary to retroperitoneal fibrosis, constrictive pericarditis, pancreatitis, neoplastic tumors, and infiltrative disorders that block the lymphatics.

Impaired lymphatic drainage leads to increased pressure and leakage of lymph into the intestinal lumen. Impairment of chylomicron and lipoprotein absorption results in malabsorption of fats and protein. Because carbohydrates are not absorbed through the lymphatic system, their uptake is not impaired.

Symptoms and Signs

Early manifestations of intestinal lymphangiectasia include massive and often asymmetric peripheral edema, intermittent diarrhea, nausea, vomiting, and abdominal pain. Some patients have mild to moderate steatorrhea. Chylous pleural effusions (chylothorax) and chylous ascites may be present. Growth is retarded if onset is in the first decade of life.

Diagnosis

- Endoscopic small-bowel biopsy
- Sometimes contrast lymphangiography

Diagnosis of intestinal lymphangiectasia usually requires endoscopic small-bowel biopsy, which shows marked dilation and ectasia of the mucosal and submucosal lymphatic vessels. Alternatively, contrast lymphangiography (injection of contrast material via the pedal lymphatics) can show abnormal intestinal lymphatics.

Laboratory abnormalities include lymphocytopenia and low levels of serum albumin, cholesterol, IgA, IgM, IgG, transferrin, and ceruloplasmin. Barium studies may show thickened, nodular mucosal folds that resemble stacked coins. D-Xylose absorption is normal. Intestinal protein loss can be shown by using chromium-51-labeled albumin.

Treatment

- Supportive care
- Sometimes surgical resection or repair

Abnormal lymphatics cannot be corrected. Supportive treatment of intestinal lymphangiectasia includes a low-fat (< 30 g/day), high-protein diet containing medium-chain triglyceride supplements. Supplemental calcium and fat-soluble vitamins are given. Intestinal resection or anastomosis of the abnormal lymphatics to the venous channels may be beneficial. Pleural effusions should be drained by thoracentesis.

SHORT BOWEL SYNDROME

Short bowel syndrome is malabsorption resulting from extensive resection of the small bowel (usually more than two thirds the length of the small intestine). Symptoms depend on the length and function of the remaining small bowel, but diarrhea can be severe, and nutritional deficiencies are common. Treatment is with small feedings, antidiarrheals, and sometimes TPN or intestinal transplantation.

Common reasons for extensive resection are Crohn disease, mesenteric infarction, radiation enteritis, cancer, volvulus, and congenital anomalies.

Because the jejunum is the primary digestive and absorptive site for most nutrients, jejunal resection leads to loss of absorptive area and significantly reduces nutrient absorption. In response, the ileum adapts by increasing the length and absorptive function of its villi, resulting in gradual improvement of nutrient absorption.

The ileum is the site of vitamin B_{12} and bile acid absorption. Severe diarrhea and bile acid malabsorption result when > 100 cm of the ileum is resected. Notably, there is no compensatory adaptation of the remaining jejunum (unlike that of the ileum in jejunal resection). Consequently, malabsorption of fat, fat-soluble vitamins, and vitamin B_{12} occurs. In addition, unabsorbed bile acids in the colon result in secretory diarrhea. Preservation of the colon can significantly reduce water and electrolyte losses. Resection of the terminal ileum and ileocecal valve can predispose to bacterial overgrowth.

Treatment

- TPN
- Eventual oral feeding if > 100 cm of jejunum remain
- Antidiarrheals, cholestyramine, proton pump inhibitors, vitamin supplements

In the immediate postoperative period, diarrhea is typically severe, with significant electrolyte losses. Patients typically require TPN and intensive monitoring of fluid and electrolytes (including calcium and magnesium). An oral iso-osmotic solution of sodium and glucose (similar to WHO oral rehydration formula—see p. 2557) is slowly introduced in the postoperative phase once the patient stabilizes and stool output is < 2 L/day.

Patients with extensive resection (< 100 cm of remaining jejunum) and those with excessive fluid and electrolyte losses require TPN for life.

Patients with > 100 cm of remaining jejunum can achieve adequate nutrition through oral feeding. Fat and protein in the diet are usually well tolerated, unlike carbohydrates, which contribute a significant osmotic load. Small feedings reduce the osmotic load. Ideally, 40% of calories should consist of fat.

Patients who have diarrhea after meals should take antidiarrheals (eg, loperamide) 1 h before eating. Cholestyramine 2 to 4 g taken with meals reduces diarrhea associated with bile acid malabsorption due to ileal resection. Monthly IM injections of vitamin B_{12} should be given to patients with a documented deficiency. Most patients should take supplemental vitamins, calcium, and magnesium.

Gastric acid hypersecretion can develop, which can deactivate pancreatic enzymes; thus, most patients are given H_2 blockers or proton pump inhibitors.

Small-bowel transplantation is advocated for patients who are not candidates for long-term TPN and in whom adaptation does not occur.

KEY POINTS

- Extensive resection or loss of small bowel can cause significant diarrhea and malabsorption.
- Patients with < 1 m of remaining jejunum require lifelong TPN; patients with > 1 m of remaining jejunum may survive on small feedings that are high in fat and protein and low in carbohydrate.
- Antidiarrheals, cholestyramine, proton pump inhibitors, and vitamin supplements are needed.

TROPICAL SPRUE

Tropical sprue is a rare acquired disease, probably of infectious etiology, characterized by malabsorption and megaloblastic anemia. Diagnosis is clinical and by small-bowel biopsy. Treatment is with tetracycline and folate for 6 mo.

Etiology

Tropical sprue occurs chiefly in the Caribbean, southern India, and Southeast Asia, affecting both natives and visitors. The illness is rare in visitors spending < 1 mo in areas where the disease is endemic. Although etiology is unclear, it is thought to result from chronic infection of the small bowel by toxigenic strains of coliform bacteria. Malabsorption of folate and vitamin B_{12} deficiency result in megaloblastic anemia. Tropical sprue has rarely been reported in the US, and the incidence worldwide has been decreasing in recent decades, perhaps because of increasing use of antibiotics for acute traveler's diarrhea.

Symptoms and Signs

Patients commonly have acute diarrhea with fever and malaise. A chronic phase of milder diarrhea, nausea, anorexia, abdominal cramps, and fatigue follows. Steatorrhea is common. Nutritional deficiencies, especially of folate and vitamin B_{12}, eventually develop after several months to years. The patient may also have weight loss, glossitis, stomatitis, and peripheral edema.

Diagnosis

- Endoscopy with small-bowel biopsy
- Blood tests to screen for consequences of malabsorption

Tropical sprue is suspected in people who live in or have visited areas where the disease is endemic and who have megaloblastic anemia and symptoms of malabsorption. The definitive test is upper GI endoscopy with small-bowel biopsy. Characteristic histologic changes (see Table 20–3) usually involve the entire small bowel and include blunting of the villi with infiltration of chronic inflammatory cells in the epithelium and lamina propria. Celiac disease and parasitic infection must be ruled out. Unlike in celiac disease, anti-tissue transglutaminase antibody (tTG) and anti-endomysial antibody (EMA) are negative in patients with tropical sprue.

Additional laboratory studies (eg, CBC; albumin; calcium; PT; iron, folate, and B_{12} levels) help evaluate nutritional status. Barium small-bowel follow-through may show segmentation of the barium, dilation of the lumen, and thickening of the mucosal folds. D-Xylose absorption is abnormal in > 90% of cases. However, these tests are not specific or essential for diagnosis of tropical sprue.

Treatment

- Long-term tetracycline

Treatment of tropical sprue is tetracycline 250 mg po qid for 1 or 2 mo, then bid for up to 6 mo, depending on disease severity and response to treatment. Doxycycline 100 mg po bid can be used instead of tetracycline. Folate 5 to 10 mg po once/day should be given for the first month along with vitamin B_{12} 1 mg IM weekly for several weeks. Megaloblastic anemia promptly abates, and the clinical response is dramatic. Other nutritional replacements are given as needed. Relapse may occur in 20%. Failure to respond after 4 wk of therapy suggests another condition.

WHIPPLE DISEASE

(Intestinal Lipodystrophy)

Whipple disease is a rare systemic illness caused by the bacterium *Tropheryma whipplei*. Main symptoms are arthritis, weight loss, abdominal pain, and diarrhea. Diagnosis is by small-bowel biopsy. Treatment is initially with ceftriaxone or penicillin followed by a minimum 1 yr of trimethoprim/sulfamethoxazole.

Whipple disease predominately affects white men aged 30 to 60. Although it affects many parts of the body (eg, heart, lung, brain, serous cavities, joints, eye, GI tract), the mucosa of the small bowel is almost always involved. Affected patients may have subtle defects of cell-mediated immunity that predispose to infection with *T. whipplei*. About 30% of patients have HLA-B27.

Symptoms and Signs

Clinical presentation varies depending on the organ systems affected. The four cardinal symptoms of Whipple disease are

- Arthralgia
- Diarrhea
- Abdominal pain
- Weight loss

Usually, the first symptoms are arthritis and fever. Intestinal symptoms (eg, watery diarrhea, steatorrhea, abdominal pain, anorexia, weight loss) usually manifest later, sometimes years after the initial complaint. Gross or occult intestinal bleeding may occur. Severe malabsorption may be present in patients diagnosed late in the clinical course. Other findings include increased skin pigmentation, anemia, lymphadenopathy, chronic cough, serositis, peripheral edema, and CNS symptoms.

Diagnosis

- Endoscopy with small-bowel biopsy

The diagnosis of Whipple disease may be missed in patients without prominent GI symptoms. Whipple disease should be suspected in middle-aged white men who have arthritis and abdominal pain, diarrhea, weight loss, or other symptoms of malabsorption. Such patients should have upper endoscopy with small-bowel biopsy; the intestinal lesions are specific and diagnostic. The most severe and consistent changes are in the proximal small bowel. Light microscopy shows periodic acid-Schiff–positive macrophages that distort the villus architecture. Gram-positive, acid fast–negative bacilli (*T. whipplei*) are seen in the lamina propria and in the macrophages. If *T. whipplei* are not seen but Whipple disease is still clinically suspected, PCR testing and immunohistochemistry should be done.

Whipple disease should be differentiated from intestinal infection with *Mycobacterium avium-intracellulare* (MAI), which has similar histologic findings. However, MAI stains positive with acid fast.

Treatment

- Antibiotics
- Late relapse a possibility

Untreated disease is progressive and fatal. Many antibiotics are curative (eg, trimethoprim/sulfamethoxazole, penicillin, cephalosporins). Treatment of Whipple disease is initiated with ceftriaxone (2 g IV daily) or penicillin G (1.5 to 6 million units IV q 6 h). This regimen is followed by a long-term course of trimethoprim/sulfamethoxazole (160/800 mg po bid for 1 yr) or a combination of doxycycline (100 mg po bid for 1 yr) and hydroxychloroquine (200 mg po tid for 1 yr). Sulfa-allergic patients may substitute oral penicillin VK or ampicillin. Prompt clinical improvement occurs, with fever and joint pains resolving in a few days. Intestinal symptoms usually abate within 1 to 4 wk.

To confirm response to treatment, PCR testing can be done on stool, saliva, or other tissue. However, other authorities recommend repeat biopsy after 1 yr with microscopy to document bacilli (not just macrophages, which may persist for years after successful treatment) in conjunction with PCR testing.

Relapses are common and may occur years later. If relapse is suspected, small-bowel biopsies or PCR testing should be done (regardless of affected organ systems) to determine presence of free bacilli.

KEY POINTS

- Infection by the bacteria *T. whipplei* affects many organs, including the GI tract.
- Small bowel mucosal involvement causes malabsorption.
- Suspect Whipple disease in middle-aged white men who have arthritis and abdominal pain, diarrhea, weight loss, or other symptoms of malabsorption.
- Endoscopic small-bowel biopsy is necessary.
- Long-term antibiotic treatment is necessary, and relapses are common.

21 Pancreatitis

Pancreatitis is classified as either acute or chronic.

Acute pancreatitis is inflammation that resolves both clinically and histologically.

Chronic pancreatitis is characterized by histologic changes that are irreversible and progressive and that result in considerable loss of exocrine and endocrine pancreatic function. Patients with chronic pancreatitis may have a flare-up of acute disease.

Pancreatitis can affect both the exocrine and endocrine functions of the pancreas. Pancreatic cells secrete bicarbonate and digestive enzymes into ducts that connect the pancreas to the duodenum at the ampulla of Vater (exocrine function). Pancreatic beta cells secrete insulindirectly into the bloodstream (endocrine function).

ACUTE PANCREATITIS

Acute pancreatitis is acute inflammation of the pancreas (and, sometimes, adjacent tissues). The most common triggers are gallstones and chronic heavy alcohol intake. The severity of acute pancreatitis is classified as mild, moderate, or severe based on the presence of local complications and transient or persistent organ failure. Diagnosis is based on clinical presentation and serum amylase and lipase levels. Treatment is supportive with IV fluids, analgesics, and nutritional support. Although overall mortality of acute pancreatitis is low, morbidity and mortality are significant in severe cases.

Acute pancreatitis is a common disorder and a major health-care concern.

Etiology

Gallstones and alcoholism account for ≥ 70% of acute pancreatitis cases. The remaining cases result from myriad causes (see Table 21–1).

Gallstones: Gallstones cause about 40% of cases of acute pancreatitis. The precise mechanism of gallstone pancreatitis is unknown but likely involves increased pressure in the pancreatic duct caused by obstruction at the ampulla secondary to a stone or edema caused by the passage of a stone. Ductal hypertension results in aberrant activation of digestive enzymes from acinar cells. The toxic effects of bile acid itself on acinar cells might also be a mechanism. Gallstone pancreatitis is rare in pregnancy and occurs most commonly in the 3rd trimester.

Alcohol: Alcohol causes about 30% of cases of acute pancreatitis. Alcohol-induced pancreatitis occurs only after many years of alcohol use. The risk of developing pancreatitis increases with increasing doses of alcohol (4 to 7 drinks/day in men and ≥ 3 drinks/day in women). Low or moderate levels of alcohol consumption are associated with progression from acute to chronic pancreatitis. Overt disease develops in only a few drinkers, suggesting additional triggers or cofactors are needed to precipitate pancreatitis.

Table 21–1. SOME CAUSES OF ACUTE PANCREATITIS

CAUSE	EXAMPLES
Drugs	ACE inhibitors, asparaginase, azathioprine, 2′,3′-dideoxyinosine, furosemide, 6-mercaptopurine, pentamidine, sulfa drugs, valproate
Infectious	Coxsackievirus B, cytomegalovirus, mumps
Inherited	Multiple known gene mutations, including a small percentage of cystic fibrosis patients
Mechanical/ structural	Gallstones, ERCP, trauma, pancreatic cancer or periampullary cancer, choledochal cyst, sphincter of Oddi stenosis, pancreas divisum
Metabolic	Hypertriglyceridemia, hypercalcemia (including hyperparathyroidism), estrogenuse associated with high lipid levels
Toxins	Alcohol, methanol
Other	Cigarette smoking, pregnancy, postrenal transplant, ischemia caused by hypotension or atheroembolism, tropical pancreatitis

Pancreatic acinar cells metabolize alcohol into toxic metabolites via both oxidative and nonoxidative pathways and exhibit effects that predispose the cells to autodigestive injury and predispose the pancreas to necrosis, inflammation, and cell death. These effects include increased enzyme content, destabilization of lysosomal and zymogen granules, sustained increase in calcium overload, and activation of pancreatic stellate cells. Another theory proposes that alcohol increases the propensity of formation of protein plugs within pancreatic ducts by altering the level of lithogenic proteins and increasing the viscosity of pancreatic secretions, causing obstruction, and, eventually, acinar atrophy.

Other causes: A number of genetic mutations predisposing to pancreatitis have been identified. An autosomal dominant mutation of the cationic trypsinogen gene causes pancreatitis in 80% of carriers; an obvious familial pattern is present. Other mutations have lesser penetrance and are not readily apparent clinically except through genetic testing. The gene that causes cystic fibrosis increases the risk of recurrent acute pancreatitis as well as chronic pancreatitis.

Acute pancreatitis is the most frequent serious complication that develops after endoscopic retrograde cholangiopancreatography (ERCP); frequency is 5 to 10% among patients undergoing ERCP.

Pathogenesis

Regardless of the etiology, the initial step in pathogenesis of acute pancreatitis is intra-acinar activation of pancreatic enzymes (including trypsin, phospholipase A_2, and elastase), leading to the autodigestive injury of the gland itself. The enzymes can damage tissue and activate the complement system and the inflammatory cascade, producing cytokines and causing inflammation and edema. This process causes necrosis in a few cases. Acute pancreatitis increases the risk of infection by compromising the gut barrier, leading to bacterial translocation from the gut lumen to the circulation.

Activated enzymes and cytokines that enter the peritoneal cavity cause a chemical burn and third spacing of fluid; those that enter the systemic circulation cause a systemic inflammatory response that can result in acute respiratory distress syndrome and acute kidney injury. The systemic effects are mainly the result of increased capillary permeability and decreased vascular tone, which result from the released cytokines and chemokines. Phospholipase A_2 is thought to injure alveolar membranes of the lungs.

In mild pancreatitis, inflammation is confined to the pancreas. Patients do not have organ failure or systemic or local complications. The mortality rate is < 5%.

In severe pancreatitis, there is persistent single or multiorgan failure (after about 48 h). Most patients have one or more local complications. The mortality rate is > 30%.

Complications

The types of complications of acute pancreatitis vary according to the timing after the onset of the disorder.

Acute pancreatitis appears to have 2 distinct phases:[1]

- An early phase (within 1 wk)
- A late phase (> 1 wk)

The **early phase** is related to the pathophysiology of the inflammatory cascade.

Patients with persistent systemic inflammatory response syndrome (SIRS) are at increased risk of multiorgan failure (eg, acute cardiovascular and/or respiratory failure, acute kidney injury), and shock in the early phase of acute pancreatitis. Mortality in the early phase of acute pancreatitis usually results from multiorgan failure.

The **late phase,** which develops in fewer than 20% of patients with acute pancreatitis, is characterized by persistence of systemic inflammation, local complications, or both. The local complications include

- Pseudocyst (risk of hemorrhage, rupture, or infection)
- Acute collections of necrotic material, called acute necrotic collections (risk of infection)
- Splenic vein thrombosis
- Pseudoaneurysm formation
- Pancreatic duct disruption leading to ascites
- Pleural effusion

Collections of enzyme-rich pancreatic fluid form in and around the pancreas. Most of these collections resolve spontaneously. In other patients, the collections form pseudocysts. A pseudocyst is a fluid collection usually outside the pancreas with minimal or no necrotic materials that persists for 4 to 6 wk. Pseudocysts have a fibrous capsule without an epithelial lining. Pseudocysts may hemorrhage, rupture, or become infected. Spontaneous resolution occurs in one third of patients with a pseudocyst.

Acute collections that occur in necrotizing pancreatitis have no definable wall and may contain both liquid and solid material. The necrosis can include the pancreatic parenchyma and/or the peripancreatic tissue. Walled-off necrosis is pancreatic necrosis that has liquefied after 5 to 6 wk. About one third of patients with pancreatic necrosis may become infected by gut bacteria, which has very high morbidity and mortality rates.

Mortality in the late phase of acute pancreatitis usually results from a combination of factors, including multiorgan failure, infection, or complications resulting from surgical and endoscopic intervention.

1. Banks PA, Bollen TL, Dervenis C, et al: Classification of acute pancreatitis 2012: Revision of the Atlanta

classification and definitions by international consensus. *Gut* 62:102–111, 2013. doi: 10.1136/gutjnl-2012-302779.

Symptoms and Signs

An acute attack causes steady, boring upper abdominal pain, typically severe enough to require large doses of parenteral opioids. The pain radiates through to the back in about 50% of patients. Pain usually develops suddenly in gallstone pancreatitis; in alcoholic pancreatitis, pain develops over a few days. The pain usually persists for several days. Sitting up and leaning forward may reduce pain, but coughing, vigorous movement, and deep breathing may accentuate it. Nausea and vomiting are common.

The patient appears acutely ill and sweaty. Pulse rate is usually 100 to 140 beats/min. Respiration is shallow and rapid. BP may be transiently high or low, with significant postural hypotension. Temperature may be normal or even subnormal at first but may increase to 37.7 to 38.3° C (100 to 101° F) within a few hours. Sensorium may be blunted to the point of semicoma. Scleral icterus is occasionally present because of obstruction of the bile duct by a gallstone or inflammation and swelling of the pancreatic head. The lungs may have limited diaphragmatic excursion and evidence of atelectasis.

Patients may have an ileus resulting in decreased bowel sounds and abdominal distention. Marked abdominal tenderness occurs, most often in the upper abdomen. Rarely, severe peritoneal irritation results in a rigid and boardlike abdomen. Pancreatic duct disruption may cause ascites (pancreatic ascites). The Grey Turner sign (ecchymoses of the flanks) and the Cullen sign (ecchymoses of the umbilical region) indicate extravasation of hemorrhagic exudate, occur in < 1% of cases, and portend a poor prognosis.

Infection in the pancreas or in an adjacent fluid collection should be suspected if the patient has a generally toxic appearance with fever and an elevated WBC count or if deterioration follows an initial period of stabilization. Patients with severe disease can manifest multiorgan failure (cardiovascular, renal, and respiratory).

Diagnosis

- Serum markers (amylase, lipase)
- Imaging studies

Pancreatitis is suspected whenever severe abdominal pain occurs, especially in a patient with significant alcohol use or known gallstones.

Diagnosis of acute pancreatitis is made by clinical suspicion and supported by lab and/or imaging findings. Amylase and lipase are done whenever pancreatitis is considered.

The diagnosis of acute pancreatitis is most often established by the presence of at least 2 of the following:

- Abdominal pain consistent with the disease
- Serum amylase and/or lipase > 3 times the upper limit of normal
- Characteristic findings on abdominal imaging

The **differential diagnosis** of the symptoms of acute pancreatitis includes

- Perforated gastric or duodenal ulcer
- Mesenteric infarction
- Strangulating intestinal obstruction
- Aortic aneurysm
- Biliary colic
- Appendicitis
- Diverticulitis
- Inferior wall MI
- Hematoma of the abdominal muscles or spleen

To exclude other causes of abdominal pain and to diagnose metabolic complications of acute pancreatitis, a broad range of tests is usually done at initial evaluation. These include laboratory and imaging tests.

Laboratory tests: Serum amylase and lipase concentrations increase on the first day of acute pancreatitis and return to normal in 3 to 7 days. Lipase is more specific for pancreatitis, but both enzymes may be increased in renal failure and various abdominal conditions (eg, perforated ulcer, mesenteric vascular occlusion, intestinal obstruction). Other causes of increased serum amylase include salivary gland dysfunction, macroamylasemia, and tumors that secrete amylase. Fractionation of total serum amylase into pancreatic type (p-type) isoamylase and salivary-type (s-type) isoamylase increases the accuracy of serum amylase. Both amylase and lipase levels may remain normal if destruction of acinar tissue during previous episodes precludes release of sufficient amounts of enzymes. The serum of patients with hypertriglyceridemia may contain a circulating inhibitor that must be diluted before an elevation in serum amylase can be detected.

Serum amylase levels may be chronically elevated in macroamylasemia where amylase is bound to a serum immunoglobulin to form a complex that is filtered slowly from the blood by the kidneys. Amylase:creatinine clearance ratio does not have sufficient sensitivity or specificity to diagnose pancreatitis. It is generally used to diagnose macroamylasemia when no pancreatitis exists.

A urine dipstick test for trypsinogen-2 has sensitivity and specificity of > 90% for acute pancreatitis.

The WBC count usually increases to 12,000 to 20,000/μL. Third-space fluid losses may increase the Hct to as high as 50 to 55% and elevate the BUN, indicating severe inflammation. Persistent elevations in BUN despite resuscitation raise suspicions of multiorgan failure. Hyperglycemia and hypocalcemia may occur. Patients may have abnormal liver function test results, including elevated serum bilirubin, due to a retained stone in the bile duct or compression of the bile duct by pancreatic edema. Patients with shock may have an anion gap metabolic acidosis or other electrolyte abnormalities. Magnesium levels are obtained to exclude hypomagnesemia as a cause of hypocalcemia.

Imaging studies: CT (with IV contrast) should be done early, but only when the diagnosis of acute pancreatitis is uncertain or to exclude other causes for the patient's symptoms. Also, once pancreatitis has been diagnosed, CT is generally done to identify the complications of acute pancreatitis such as necrosis, fluid collection, or pseudocysts. Necrotized pancreatic tissue does not enhance after IV contrast is given and may not appear on CT until 48 to 72 h after onset of acute pancreatitis. MRI without contrast is better than CT for detecting choledocholithiasis.

Abdominal ultrasonography should be done if gallstone pancreatitis is suspected (and another cause is not obvious) to detect gallstones or dilation of the common bile duct, which indicates biliary tract obstruction. Edema of the pancreas may be visible, but overlying gas frequently obscures the pancreas.

If done, plain x-rays of the abdomen may disclose calcifications within pancreatic ducts (evidence of prior inflammation and hence chronic pancreatitis), calcified gallstones, localized ileus of a segment of small intestine in the left upper quadrant or the center of the abdomen (a "sentinel loop"), or the colon cutoff sign (absence of air in left colonic flexure or descending colon) in more severe disease. However, the value of routine abdominal x-rays is controversial.

Chest x-rays should be done and may reveal atelectasis or a pleural effusion (usually left-sided or bilateral but rarely confined to the right pleural space), which are signs of severe disease.

The role of endoscopic ultrasonography is limited in acute pancreatitis. Endoscopic ultrasonography has a higher sensitivity than that of magnetic resonance cholangiopancreatography (MRCP) for detecting common bile duct stones, but MRCP has the advantage of being noninvasive.

ERCP to relieve bile duct obstruction should be done expeditiously in patients with gallstone pancreatitis who have increasing serum bilirubin and signs of sepsis.

Prognosis

The severity of acute pancreatitis is determined by the presence of organ failure, local and systemic complications, or a combination. Using patient-related risk factors to assess severity early in the course of disease can help identify patients at increased risk of developing organ dysfunction and other complications. These patients can then be given maximal supportive therapy at presentation to improve outcomes and decrease morbidity and mortality. For initial risk assessment, patient-related risk factors that predict a severe course include the following:

- Age ≥ 60 yr
- Comorbid health problems
- Obesity with body mass index > 30
- Long-term, heavy alcohol use
- Presence of SIRS
- Laboratory markers of hypovolemia (eg, elevated BUN, elevated Hct)
- Presence of pleural effusions and/or infiltrates on admission chest x-ray
- Altered mental status

Severity scoring systems require multiple measurements and may delay appropriate management. Some of these can be done at admission to assist in triage of patients, whereas others are not accurate until 48 to 72 h after presentation.

- Ranson criteria: This scoring system is cumbersome and takes 48 h to compute but has good negative predictive value.
- The APACHE II score: This system is complex and cumbersome to use but has good negative predictive value.
- SIRS score: This system is inexpensive, readily available, and can be applied at the bedside.
- Bedside index of severity in acute pancreatitis (BISAP) score: This score is simple and calculated during the first 24 h.
- Harmless acute pancreatitis score: This simple score is calculated within 30 min of admission.
- Organ failure–based scores: These scores do not directly measure the severity of acute pancreatitis.
- CT severity index (Balthazar score): This score is based on the degree of necrosis, inflammation, and the presence of fluid collections on CT.

The long-term risks after acute pancreatitis includes the risks of recurrent attacks and development of chronic pancreatitis. Risk factors include the severity and amount of pancreatic necrosis in the initial episode of acute pancreatitis as well as the etiology. Long-term, heavy alcohol use and cigarette smoking increase the risk of developing chronic pancreatitis.

Treatment

- Supportive measures
- For severe acute pancreatitis and complications, antibiotics and therapeutic interventions as needed

Treatment of acute pancreatitis is typically supportive. Patients who develop complications may require specific additional treatment. (See also the American College of Gastroenterology's guidelines for the management of acute pancreatitis.)

The basic treatment of acute pancreatitis includes

- Early fluid resuscitation
- Analgesia
- Nutritional support

Early aggressive IV fluid resuscitation improves pancreatic perfusion and helps prevent serious complications such as pancreatic necrosis. The 2013 American College of Gastroenterology (ACG) guidelines recommend that early aggressive hydration, defined as 250 to 500 mL/h of isotonic crystalloid solution (ideally lactated Ringer's solution), should be provided to all patients during the first 12 to 24 h unless cardiovascular, renal, or other related comorbid factors contraindicate doing so. Adequacy of fluid replacement can be assessed by reduction in Hct and BUN levels over the first 24 h, particularly if they were high at the onset. Other parameters include improvement in vital signs and maintenance of adequate urine output. The ACG guidelines also recommend that fluid requirements should be reassessed at frequent intervals in the first 6 h of admission and for the next 24 to 48 h. Patients undergoing volume resuscitation should undergo continuous pulse oximetry, receive supplemental oxygen as needed, and have their fluid intake and output strictly monitored.

Adequate pain relief requires use of parenteral opioids such as hydromorphone or fentanyl, which should be given in adequate doses. Antiemetic drugs should be given to relieve nausea and vomiting.

Studies have shown that providing enteral or parenteral nutrition to patients with acute pancreatitis results in a lower risk of death than if no supplemental nutrition is given. However, total parenteral nutrition should be avoided because infectious complications can result. Patients with mild pancreatitis can resume an oral diet as soon as their pain decreases and their overall clinical condition improves. Feeding with a low-residue, low-fat, soft diet can be initiated. A low-residue diet is designed to restrict stool volume and frequency by minimizing dietary fiber and foods that increase bowel activity. Early refeeding also seems to result in a shorter hospital stay.

Severe acute pancreatitis and complications: Treatment of severe acute pancreatitis and complications includes

- Usually ICU care
- Sometimes artificial nutritional support
- Antibiotics for extrapancreatic infections and infected necrosis
- Necrosectomy (removal of necrotic tissue) for infected necrosis
- ERCP for acute pancreatitis and concurrent acute cholangitis
- Drainage of pseudocysts

The management of patients with severe acute pancreatitis and its complications should be individualized using a multidisciplinary approach including therapeutic endoscopists, interventional radiologists, and a surgeon. Patients with severe acute pancreatitis should be monitored closely in the first 24 to 48 h in an ICU. Patients with worsening condition or widespread local complications requiring intervention should be transferred to centers of excellence focusing on pancreatic disease (if available).

Patients with severe acute pancreatitis may need artificial nutritional support, although the optimal starting time and duration of nutritional support are still unclear. ACG guidelines from 2013 recommend using enteral nutrition and only giving parenteral nutrition if the enteral route is not available, not tolerated, or not meeting caloric requirements. The enteral route is preferred because it

- Helps maintain the intestinal mucosal barrier
- Prevents the intestinal atrophy that can occur with prolonged bowel rest (and promotes translocation of bacteria that can seed pancreatic necrosis)
- Avoids the risk of infection of a central IV catheter
- Is less expensive

A nasojejunal feeding tube placed beyond the ligament of Treitz may help avoid stimulating the gastric phase of the digestive process; placement requires radiologic or endoscopic guidance. If a nasojejunal feeding tube cannot be placed, nasogastric feeding should be initiated. In both cases, patients should be placed in the upright position to decrease risk of aspiration. The ACG guidelines note that nasogastric and nasojejunal feeding appear comparable in their efficacy and safety.

According to the 2013 ACG guidelines, prophylactic antibiotics are not recommended in patients with acute pancreatitis, regardless of the type or disease severity. However, antibiotics should be started if patients develop an extrapancreatic infection (eg, cholangitis, pneumonia, bloodstream infection, UTI) or infected pancreatic necrosis.

Infection (pancreatic or extrapancreatic) should be suspected in patients who have signs of deterioration (eg, fever, increasing WBC count) or who fail to improve after 7 to 10 days of hospitalization. Most infections in pancreatic necrosis are caused by single bacterial species from the gut. The most common organisms are gram-negative bacteria; gram-positive bacteria and fungi are rare. In patients with infected necrosis, antibiotics known to penetrate pancreatic necrosis, such as carbapenems, fluoroquinolones, and metronidazole, are recommended.

For necrosectomy (removal of infected tissue), a minimally invasive approach is preferred over an open surgical approach and should be attempted initially. The 2013 ACG guidelines recommend that drainage of infected necrosis (radiologic, endoscopic, or surgical approach) should be delayed, preferably for > 4 wk in stable patients, to allow liquefication of the contents and the development of a fibrous wall around the necrosis (walled-off necrosis).

More than 80% of patients with gallstone pancreatitis pass the stone spontaneously and do not require ERCP. Patients with acute pancreatitis and concurrent acute cholangitis should undergo early ERCP. Patients with mild gallstone pancreatitis who spontaneously improve should undergo cholecystectomy before discharge to prevent recurrent attacks.

A pseudocyst that is expanding rapidly, infected, bleeding, or likely to rupture requires drainage. Whether drainage is percutaneous, surgical, or endoscopic ultrasound–guided cystogastrostomy depends on location of the pseudocyst and institutional expertise.

KEY POINTS

- There are many causes of acute pancreatitis, but the most common are gallstones and chronic, heavy alcohol intake.
- Inflammation is confined to the pancreas in mild cases, but, with increasing severity, a severe systemic inflammatory response may develop resulting in single or multiorgan failure.
- Once pancreatitis is diagnosed, assess risk using clinical criteria and sometimes scoring systems to triage appropriate patients to more intensive care and aggressive therapy and to help estimate prognosis.
- Treatment includes IV fluid resuscitation, pain control, and nutritional support.
- Complications, including pseudocyst and infected pancreatic necrosis, need to be identified and treated appropriately (eg, drainage of pseudocyst, necrosectomy).

CHRONIC PANCREATITIS

Chronic pancreatitis is persistent inflammation of the pancreas that results in permanent structural damage with fibrosis and ductal strictures, followed by a decline in exocrine and endocrine function. Drinking alcohol and smoking cigarettes are two of the major risk factors. Abdominal pain is the predominant symptom in most patients. Diagnosis is usually made by imaging studies and pancreatic function testing. Treatment mainly includes pain control and management of pancreatic insufficiency.

Chronic pancreatitis can be broadly classified into 3 forms:

- Chronic calcifying pancreatitis
- Chronic obstructive pancreatitis
- Chronic autoimmune pancreatitis

Chronic calcifying pancreatitis is the most common form and is characterized by calcification of the pancreatic parenchyma, formation of intraductal stones, or both.

Chronic obstructive pancreatitis results from partial or complete obstruction of the pancreatic duct.

Chronic autoimmune pancreatitis is a unique form that often responds to glucocorticoids.

Pathogenesis

The pathogenesis of chronic pancreatitis is not well understood.

The **stone and duct obstruction theory** proposes that disease is due to ductal obstruction caused by formation of protein-rich plugs as a result of protein–bicarbonate imbalance. These plugs may calcify and eventually form stones within the pancreatic ducts. If obstruction is chronic, persistent inflammation leads to fibrosis, pancreatic ductal distortion, strictures, and atrophy. After several years, progressive fibrosis and atrophy lead to loss of exocrine and endocrine function.

The **necrosis–fibrosis hypothesis** posits that repeated attacks of acute pancreatitis with necrosis are key to the pathogenesis of chronic pancreatitis. Over years, the healing process replaces the necrotic tissue with fibrotic tissue, leading to the development of chronic pancreatitis.

Neuronal sheath hypertrophy and perineural inflammation occur and may contribute to chronic pain.

Etiology

In the US, about 50% of cases of chronic pancreatitis result from alcoholism and are more common in men than women. Only a minority of alcoholics ultimately develop chronic pancreatitis, suggesting that there are other cofactors required to trigger overt disease. Cigarette smoking is an independent, dose-dependent risk factor for developing chronic pancreatitis.[1] Both alcohol abuse and smoking increase risk of disease progression, and their risks are likely additive. A large proportion of cases of chronic pancreatitis are idiopathic.

Table 21–2. CAUSES OF CHRONIC PANCREATITIS

CAUSES	EXAMPLES
Toxins	Alcohol
Genetic	Cationic trypsinogen gene (*PRSSI*) Serine peptidase inhibitor Kazal-type 1 (*SPINK1*) Cystic fibrosis transmembrane conductance regulator gene (*CFTR*) Other genetic disorders
Obstructive	Pancreatic duct stricture (traumatic, iatrogenic, anastomotic, or malignant) Mass effect due to a tumor Possibly pancreas divisum (congenital anomaly causing division of the pancreatic duct) Possibly sphincter of Oddi dysfunction
Autoimmune	Type 1, related to IgG4 disease, and type 2 autoimmune pancreatitis
Idiopathic	Tropical pancreatitis
Other	Cigarette smoking

Tropical pancreatitis is an idiopathic form of chronic pancreatitis that occurs in children and young adults in tropical regions such as India, Indonesia, and Nigeria. Tropical pancreatitis is characterized by an early age of onset, large ductal calculi, an accelerated course of the disease, and an increased risk of pancreatic cancer.

Less common causes of chronic pancreatitis include genetic disorders, systemic diseases, and ductal obstruction caused by stenosis, stones, or cancer (see Table 21-2).

1. Yadav D, Gawes RH, Brand RE, et al: Alcohol consumption, cigarette smoking, and the risk of recurrent acute and chronic pancreatitis. *Arch Intern Med* 169:1035–1045, 2009. doi: 10.1001/archinternmed.2009.125. Clarification and additional information. *Arch Intern Med* 171(7):710, 2011. doi:10.1001/archinternmed.2011.124.

Complications

When lipase and protease secretions are reduced to < 10% of normal, the patient develops malabsorption characterized by steatorrhea, the passing of greasy stools, or even oil droplets that float in water and are difficult to flush. In severe cases, undernutrition, weight loss, and malabsorption of fat-soluble vitamins (A, D, E, and K) may also occur.

Glucose intolerance may appear at any time, but overt diabetes mellitus usually occurs late in the course of chronic pancreatitis. Patients also are at risk of hypoglycemia because pancreatic alpha cells, which produce glucagon (a counter-regulatory hormone), are lost.

Other complications of chronic pancreatitis include

- Formation of pseudocysts
- Obstruction of the bile duct or duodenum
- Disruption of the pancreatic duct (resulting in ascites or pleural effusion)
- Thrombosis of the splenic vein (can cause gastric varices)
- Pseudoaneurysms of arteries near the pancreas or pseudocyst

Patients with chronic pancreatitis are at increased risk of pancreatic adenocarcinoma, and this risk seems to be greatest for patients with hereditary and tropical pancreatitis.

Symptoms and Signs

Abdominal pain and pancreatic insufficiency are the primary manifestations of chronic pancreatitis. Pain can occur during the early stages of chronic pancreatitis, before development of apparent structural abnormalities in the pancreas on imaging. Pain is often the dominant symptom in chronic pancreatitis and is present in most patients. Pain is usually postprandial, located in the epigastric area, and partially relieved by sitting up or leaning forward. The pain attacks are initially episodic but later tend to become continuous.

About 10 to 15% of patients have no pain and present with symptoms of malabsorption. Clinical manifestations of pancreatic insufficiency include flatulence, abdominal distention, steatorrhea, undernutrition, weight loss, and fatigue.

Diagnosis

- Imaging studies
- Pancreatic function tests

Diagnosis of chronic pancreatitis can be difficult because amylase and lipase levels are frequently normal secondary to significant loss of pancreatic function. Diagnosis relies on clinical assessment, imaging studies, and pancreatic function tests.

Patients with unexplained or sustained worsening of symptoms should be evaluated for cancer, particularly if assessment reveals a pancreatic duct stricture. Evaluation may include brushing of the strictures for cytology and measuring serum markers (eg, CA 19-9, carcinoembryonic antigen).

Imaging studies: In a patient with a typical history of alcohol abuse and recurrent episodes of acute pancreatitis, detection of pancreatic calcification on plain x-ray of the abdomen may be sufficient. However, such calcifications typically occur late in the disease and then are visible in only about 30% of patients. CT can also be used in patients with a history of alcohol abuse and in whom plain x-rays are not diagnostic.

In patients without a typical history but with symptoms suggesting chronic pancreatitis, abdominal CT is typically recommended to exclude pancreatic cancer as the cause of pain. Abdominal CT can be used to detect calcifications and other pancreatic abnormalities (eg, pseudocyst or dilated ducts) but still may be normal early in the disease.

MRI coupled with magnetic resonance cholangiopancreatography (MRCP) is now frequently used for diagnosis and can show masses in the pancreas as well as provide more optimal visualization of ductal changes consistent with chronic pancreatitis. Administration of IV secretin during MRCP increases sensitivity for detecting ductal abnormalities and also allows for functional assessment in patients with chronic pancreatitis. MRI is more accurate than CT and does not expose patients to radiation.

ERCP is invasive and rarely used for the diagnosis of chronic pancreatitis. ERCP findings could be normal in patients with early chronic pancreatitis. ERCP should be reserved for patients who may need therapeutic intervention.

Endoscopic ultrasonography is less invasive and enables detection of subtle abnormalities in the pancreatic parenchyma and in the pancreatic duct. This imaging modality has a high level of sensitivity and a low level of specificity.

Pancreatic function tests: The most common pancreatic function tests do not detect mild to moderate exocrine pancreatic insufficiency with adequate accuracy. Late in the disease, tests of pancreatic exocrine function more reliably become abnormal.

Pancreatic function tests are classified as

- Direct
- Indirect

Direct tests are done to monitor the actual secretion of pancreatic exocrine products (bicarbonate and enzymes), whereas indirect tests are done to measure the secondary effects resulting from the lack of pancreatic enzymes.

Direct pancreatic function tests are most useful in patients who have an earlier stage of chronic pancreatitis in whom imaging studies are not diagnostic. Direct tests involve infusion of the hormone cholecystokinin to measure the production of digestive enzymes or infusion of the hormone secretin to measure the production of bicarbonate. The duodenal secretions are collected using double-lumen gastroduodenal collection tubes or an endoscope. Direct tests are cumbersome, are time-consuming, and have not been well standardized. Direct pancreatic function tests have mostly been phased out of clinical practice and are done in only a few specialized centers.

Indirect pancreatic function tests are less accurate in diagnosing earlier stages of chronic pancreatitis. These tests involve blood or stool samples. The serum trypsinogen test is an inexpensive test and is available through commercial laboratories. Very low levels of serum trypsinogen (< 20 ng/mL) are highly specific for chronic pancreatitis. A 72-h test for stool fecal fat in patients who are following a high-fat diet is diagnostic for steatorrhea. This test is fairly reliable but cannot establish the cause of malabsorption. In other tests, fecal concentration of chymotrypsin and elastase may be decreased. The indirect tests are widely available, less invasive, inexpensive, and easier to do than the direct tests.

Treatment

- Pain control
- Pancreatic enzyme supplements
- Management of diabetes
- Management of other complications

The prognosis for chronic pancreatitis is variable and relatively poor.

Pain control: Pain control is the most challenging task in the management of patients with chronic pancreatitis. First, vigorous efforts and appropriate referrals to encourage smoking cessation and alcohol abstinence should be made for patients with chronic pancreatitis in an effort to slow the disease progression as early as possible. Second, treatable complications of chronic pancreatitis that can cause similar symptoms should be sought. Patients should consume a low-fat (< 25 g/day) diet to reduce secretion of pancreatic enzymes. Patients with chronic pancreatitis should be educated about healthy lifestyle practices, and this should be reinforced at each visit.

Pancreatic enzyme supplementation may reduce chronic pain by suppressing the release of cholecystokinin from the duodenum, thereby reducing the secretion of pancreatic enzymes. Enzyme therapy is more likely to be successful in patients with less advanced disease, in women, and in patients with idiopathic pancreatitis than in patients with alcoholic pancreatitis. Although enzyme therapy is often tried because of its safety and minimal adverse effects, it may not provide substantial benefit in improving pain.

Often these measures do not relieve pain, requiring increased amounts of opioids, which increases the risk of addiction. Adjunctive pain drugs, such as tricyclic antidepressants, gabapentin, pregabalin, and SSRIs, have been used alone or combined with opioids to manage chronic pain; results are variable. Drug treatment of pain in chronic pancreatitis is often unsatisfactory.

Other treatment modalities include endoscopic therapy, lithotripsy, celiac plexus nerve block, and surgery.

Endoscopic therapy is aimed at decompressing a pancreatic duct obstructed by stricture, stones, or both and may provide pain relief in carefully selected patients with appropriate ductal anatomy. If there is significant stricture at the papilla or distal pancreatic duct, ERCP with sphincterotomy, stent placement, or dilation may be effective. Pseudocysts can cause chronic pain. Some pseudocysts can be drained endoscopically.

Lithotripsy (extracorporeal shock wave lithotripsy or intraductal lithotripsy) is usually need to treat large or impacted pancreatic stones.

Percutaneous or endoscopic ultrasound-guided nerve blockade of the celiac plexus with a corticosteroid and long-acting anesthetic may provide short-term pain relief in some patients with chronic pancreatitis.

Surgical treatment may be effective for pain relief. Surgical options should be reserved for patients who have stopped using alcohol and who can manage diabetes that may be intensified by pancreatic resection. A variety of surgical options involve resection and/or decompression. The choice of surgical procedure depends on the anatomy of the pancreatic duct, consideration of local complications, the surgical history of the patient, and local expertise. For example, if the main pancreatic duct is dilated > 5 to 8 mm, a lateral pancreaticojejunostomy (Puestow procedure) or Partington-Rochelle modification of the Puestow procedure relieves pain in about 70 to 80% of patients. If the pancreatic duct is not dilated, a variation of the modified Puestow procedure called a V-plasty or Hamburg procedure can be done.

Other surgical approaches include a partial resection such as a distal pancreatectomy (for extensive disease at the tail of the pancreas), a Whipple procedure (for extensive disease at the head of the pancreas), a pylorus-sparing pancreaticoduodenectomy (similar to a Whipple procedure), or a total pancreatectomy with autotransplantation of islets. Overall, surgical drainage is more effective than endoscopic approaches in relieving obstruction and achieving pain relief.[1] A pancreatic pseudocyst can also be treated surgically, with decompression into a nearby structure to which it firmly adheres (eg, the stomach) or into a defunctionalized loop of jejunum (via a Roux-en-Y cystojejunostomy).

Pancreatic enzyme replacement: In patients with exocrine pancreatic insufficiency, malabsorption of fat is more severe than malabsorption of proteins and carbohydrates. Fat malabsorption also results in a deficit of fat-soluble vitamins (A, D, E, and K). Pancreatic enzyme replacement therapy (replacement of deficient hormones to treat pancreatic insufficiency) is used to treat steatorrhea. Various preparations are available, and a dose of up to 90,000 USP of lipase per meal and half that amount with snacks is needed for appropriate fat absorption. The treatment should be started at a low dose with subsequent titration based on clinical response. The preparations should be taken with meals. An H_2 blocker or proton pump inhibitor should be given to patients taking nonenteric–coated preparations to prevent acid breakdown of the enzymes.

Favorable clinical responses include weight gain, fewer bowel movements, elimination of oil droplet seepage, increases in levels of fat-soluble vitamins, and improved well-being. Clinical response can be documented by showing a decrease in stool fat after enzyme replacement therapy. If steatorrhea is particularly severe and refractory to these measures, medium-chain triglycerides can be provided as a source of fat because they are absorbed without pancreatic enzymes and other dietary fats should be reduced proportionally. Supplementation with fat-soluble vitamins A, D, and K should be given, including vitamin E, which may minimize inflammation.

Management of diabetes: The patient should be referred to an endocrine specialist for the management of diabetes. Insulin should be given cautiously because the coexisting deficiency of glucagon secretion by alpha cells means that the hypoglycemic effects of insulin are unopposed and prolonged hypoglycemia may occur. Oral hypoglycemic drugs rarely help treat diabetes caused by chronic pancreatitis.

1. Cahen DL, Gouma DJ, Nio Y, et al: Endoscopic versus surgical drainage of the pancreatic duct in chronic pancreatitis. *N Engl J Med* 356:676–684, 2007. doi: 10.1056/NEJMoa060610.

KEY POINTS

- Recurrent attacks of acute pancreatitis may cause chronic persistent inflammation, ductal damage, and ultimately fibrosis, leading to chronic pancreatitis.
- Patients have episodic abdominal pain, followed later in the disease by manifestations of malabsorption.
- Diagnosis is based on clinical presentation, imaging studies, and pancreatic function tests.
- Treatment of chronic pancreatitis principally includes pain control and management of complications, including pancreatic insufficiency.

22 Tumors of the GI Tract

ANORECTAL CANCER

Anorectal cancer accounts for an estimated 8080 cases and about 1080 deaths in the US annually.[1] The main symptom is bleeding with defecation. Diagnosis is by colonoscopy. Treatment options include excision and chemotherapy and radiation therapy.

The **most common anorectal cancer** is

- Adenocarcinoma

Squamous cell carcinoma (nonkeratinizing squamous cell or basaloid carcinoma) of the anorectum accounts for 3 to 5% of distal large-bowel cancers. Basal cell carcinoma, Bowen disease (intraepidermal squamous cell carcinoma), extramammary Paget disease, cloacogenic carcinoma, and malignant melanoma are less common. Other tumors include lymphoma and various sarcomas. Metastasis occurs along the lymphatics of the rectum and into the inguinal lymph nodes.

Risk factors for anorectal cancer include the following:

- Infection with human papillomavirus (HPV)
- Chronic fistulas
- Irradiated anal skin
- Leukoplakia
- Lymphogranuloma venereum
- Condyloma acuminatum

People having receptive anal intercourse are at increased risk. Patients with HPV infection may manifest dysplasia in slightly abnormal or normal-appearing anal epithelium (anal intraepithelial neoplasia—histologically graded I, II, or III). These changes are more common among HIV-infected patients (see Squamous cell cancer of the anus and vulva on p. 1644). Higher grades may progress to invasive carcinoma. It is unclear whether early recognition and eradication improve long-term outcome; hence, screening recommendations are unclear.

1. Siegel RL, Miller KD, Jemal A: Cancer statistics 2016. *CA Cancer J Clin* 66(1):7–30, 2016. doi: 10.3322/caac.21332.

Symptoms and Signs

Bleeding with defecation is the most common initial symptom of anorectal cancer. Some patients have pain, tenesmus, or a sensation of incomplete evacuation. A mass may be palpable on digital rectal examination.

Diagnosis

- Colonoscopy
- Sometimes biopsy

Whenever rectal bleeding occurs, even in patients with obvious hemorrhoids or known diverticular disease, coexisting cancer must be ruled out. Typically, colonoscopy is done, but skin biopsy by a dermatologist or surgeon might be needed for lesions near the squamocolumnar junction (Z line).

Staging by CT, MRI, or PET is advisable.

Treatment

- Combination chemotherapy and radiation therapy
- Sometimes surgical resection

Combination chemotherapy and radiation therapy result in a high rate of cure when used for anal squamous and cloacogenic tumors.

Abdominoperineal resection is indicated when radiation and chemotherapy do not result in complete regression of tumor and there are no metastases outside of the radiation field.

BENIGN ESOPHAGEAL TUMORS

There are many types of benign esophageal tumors, and many cause swallowing symptoms (see p. 109) and rarely ulceration or bleeding. Leiomyoma, the most common, may be multiple but usually has an excellent prognosis.

COLORECTAL CANCER

Colorectal cancer (CRC) is extremely common. Symptoms include blood in the stool and change in bowel habits. Screening is with fecal occult blood testing. Diagnosis is by colonoscopy. Treatment is surgical resection and chemotherapy for nodal involvement.

CRC accounts for an estimated 134,490 cases and 49,190 deaths in the US annually.[1] In Western countries, the colon and rectum account for more new cases of cancer per year than any anatomic site except the lung. Incidence begins to rise at age 40 and peaks at age 60 to 75. Overall, 70% of cases occur in the rectum and sigmoid, and 95% are adenocarcinomas. Colon cancer is more common among women; rectal cancer is more common among men. Synchronous cancers (more than one) occur in 5% of patients.

1. Siegel RL, Miller KD, Jemal A: Cancer statistics 2016. *CA Cancer J Clin* 66(1):7–30, 2016. doi: 10.3322/caac.21332.

Etiology

CRC most often occurs as transformation within adenomatous polyps. About 80% of cases are sporadic, and 20% have an inheritable component. Predisposing factors include chronic ulcerative colitis and Crohn colitis; the risk of cancer increases with the duration of these disorders.

Patients in populations with a high incidence of CRC eat low-fiber diets that are high in animal protein, fat, and refined carbohydrates. Carcinogens may be ingested in the diet but are more likely produced by bacterial action on dietary substances or biliary or intestinal secretions. The exact mechanism is unknown.

CRC spreads by direct extension through the bowel wall, hematogenous metastasis, regional lymph node metastasis, perineural spread, and intraluminal metastasis.

Symptoms and Signs

Colorectal adenocarcinoma grows slowly, and a long interval elapses before it is large enough to cause symptoms. Symptoms depend on lesion location, type, extent, and complications.

The right colon has a large caliber and a thin wall and its contents are liquid; thus, obstruction is a late event. Bleeding is usually occult. Fatigue and weakness caused by severe anemia may be the only complaints. Tumors sometimes grow large enough to be palpable through the abdominal wall before other symptoms appear.

The left colon has a smaller lumen, the feces are semisolid, and cancer tends to encircle the bowel, causing alternating constipation and increased stool frequency or diarrhea. Partial obstruction with colicky abdominal pain or complete obstruction may be the initial manifestation. The stool may be streaked or mixed with blood. Some patients present with symptoms of perforation, usually walled off (focal pain and tenderness), or rarely with diffuse peritonitis.

In rectal cancer, the most common initial symptom is bleeding with defecation. Whenever rectal bleeding occurs, even with obvious hemorrhoids or known diverticular disease, coexisting cancer must be ruled out. Tenesmus or a sensation of incomplete evacuation may be present. Pain is common with perirectal involvement.

Some patients first present with symptoms and signs of metastatic disease (eg, hepatomegaly, ascites, supraclavicular lymph node enlargement).

Diagnosis

- Colonoscopy

Screening tests

- Colonoscopy
- Fecal occult blood testing
- Sometimes flexible sigmoidoscopy
- Sometimes fecal DNA testing
- Sometimes CT colonography

For average-risk patients, screening for CRC should begin at age 50 yr and continue until age 75 yr. For adults aged 76 to 85, the decision whether to screen for CRC should be individualized, taking into consideration the patient's overall health and prior screening history.[2,3]

There are multiple options for CRC screening, including

- Colonoscopy every 10 yr
- Fecal occult blood test annually (fecal immunochemical tests [FIT] preferred)
- Flexible sigmoidoscopy every 5 yr (every 10 yr if combined with FIT)
- CT colonography every 5 yr
- Fecal DNA testing every 3 yr

The American College of Gastroenterology's guidelines recommend colonoscopy as the preferred screening test. Alternative CRC screening tests are available for patients who decline colonoscopy or for whom economic issues preclude screening with colonoscopy.[3] Patients with a positive family history (eg, 1st-degree relatives with early-onset CRC or advanced adenomatous polyps) should be screened more frequently starting at a younger age. Screening of patients with high-risk conditions (eg, ulcerative colitis) is discussed under the specific condition.

CT colonography (virtual colonoscopy) generates 3D and 2D images of the colon using multidetector row CT and a combination of oral contrast and gas distention of the colon. Viewing the high-resolution 3D images somewhat simulates the appearance of optical endoscopy, hence the name. It has some promise as a screening test for people who are unable or unwilling to undergo endoscopic colonoscopy but is less sensitive and highly interpreter dependent. It avoids the need for sedation but still requires thorough bowel preparation, and the gas distention may be uncomfortable. Additionally, unlike with optical colonoscopy, lesions cannot be biopsied during the diagnostic procedure.

Video capsule endoscopy of the colon has many technical problems and is not currently acceptable as a screening test.

Diagnostic tests

- Colonoscopic biopsy
- CT to evaluate extent of tumor growth and spread

Patients with positive fecal occult blood tests require colonoscopy, as do those with lesions seen during sigmoidoscopy or an imaging study. All lesions should be completely removed for histologic examination. If a lesion is sessile or not removable at colonoscopy, surgical excision should be strongly considered.

Barium enema x-ray, particularly a double-contrast study, can detect many lesions but is somewhat less accurate than colonoscopy and is not preferred as follow-up to a positive fecal occult blood test.

Once cancer is diagnosed, patients should have abdominal CT, chest x-ray, and routine laboratory tests to seek metastatic disease and anemia and to evaluate overall condition.

Elevated serum CEA levels are present in 70% of patients with CRC, but this test is not specific and therefore is not recommended for screening. However, if CEA is high preoperatively and low after removal of a colon tumor, monitoring CEA may help detect recurrence earlier. CA 199 and CA 125 are other tumor markers that may be similarly used.

2. US Preventive Services Task Force, Bibbins-Domingo K, Grossman DC, et al: Screening for colorectal cancer: US Preventive Services Task Force recommendation statement. *JAMA* 315(23):2564–2575, 2016. doi: 10.1001/jama.2016.5989.
3. Rex DK, Johnson DA, Anderson JC, et al: American College of Gastroenterology guidelines for colorectal cancer screening 2009 (corrected). *Am J Gastroenterol* 104:739–750, 2009. doi: 10.1038/ajg.2009.104.

Prognosis

Prognosis depends greatly on stage (see Table 22–1). The 10-yr survival rate for cancer limited to the mucosa approaches 90%; with extension through the bowel wall, 70 to 80%; with positive lymph nodes, 30 to 50%; and with metastatic disease, < 20%.

Treatment

- Surgical resection, sometimes combined with chemotherapy, radiation, or both

Surgery: Surgery for cure can be attempted in the 70% of patients presenting without metastatic disease. Attempt to cure consists of wide resection of the tumor and its regional lymphatic drainage with reanastomosis of bowel segments. If there is ≤ 5 cm of normal bowel present between the lesion and the anal verge, an abdominoperineal resection is done, with permanent colostomy.

Resection of a limited number (1 to 3) of liver metastases is recommended in select nondebilitated patients as a subsequent procedure. Criteria include patients whose primary tumor has been resected, whose liver metastases are in one hepatic lobe, and who have no extrahepatic metastases. Only a small number of patients with liver metastases meet these criteria, but 5-yr postoperative survival is 25%.

Adjuvant therapy: Chemotherapy (typically 5-fluorouracil and leucovorin) improves survival by 10 to 30% in colon cancer patients with positive lymph nodes. Rectal cancer patients with 1 to 4 positive lymph nodes benefit from combined radiation and chemotherapy; when > 4 positive lymph nodes are found, combined modalities are less effective. Preoperative radiation therapy and chemotherapy to improve the resectability rate of rectal cancer or decrease the incidence of lymph node metastasis are standard.

Follow-up: After curative surgical resection of CRC, surveillance colonoscopy should be done 1 yr after surgery or after the clearing preoperative colonoscopy.[4] A second surveillance colonoscopy should be done 3 yr after the 1-yr surveillance colonoscopy if no polyps or tumors are found. Thereafter, surveillance colonoscopy should be done every 5 yr. If the preoperative colonoscopy was incomplete because of an obstructing cancer, a completion colonoscopy should be done 3 to 6 mo after surgery to detect any synchronous cancers and to detect and resect any precancerous polyps.[4]

Additional screening for recurrence should include history, physical examination, and laboratory tests (eg, CBC, liver function tests) every 3 mo for 3 yr and then every 6 mo for 2 yr. Imaging studies (CT or MRI) are often recommended at 1-yr intervals but are of uncertain benefit for routine follow-up in the absence of abnormalities on examination or blood tests.

Palliation: When curative surgery is not possible or the patient is an unacceptable surgical risk, limited palliative surgery (eg, to relieve obstruction or resect a perforated area) may be indicated; median survival is 7 mo. Some obstructing tumors can be debulked by endoscopic laser treatment or electrocoagulation or held open by stents. Chemotherapy may shrink tumors and prolong life for several months.

Newer drugs used singly or in drug combinations include capecitabine (a 5-fluorouracil precursor), irinotecan, and oxaliplatin. Monoclonal antibodies such as bevacizumab, cetuximab, and panitumumab are also being used with some effectiveness. No regimen is clearly more effective for prolonging life in patients with metastatic CRC, although some have been shown to delay disease progression. Chemotherapy for advanced colon cancer should be managed by an experienced chemotherapist who has access to investigational drugs.

When metastases are confined to the liver, hepatic artery infusion with floxuridine or radioactive microspheres, given either intermittently in a radiology department or given continuously via an implantable sc pump or an external pump worn on the belt, may offer more benefit than systemic chemotherapy; however, these therapies are of uncertain benefit. When metastases are also extrahepatic, intrahepatic arterial chemotherapy offers no advantage over systemic chemotherapy.

4. Kahi CJ, Boland R, Dominitz JA, et al: Colonoscopy surveillance after colorectal cancer resection: Recommendations of the US multi-society task force on colorectal cancer. *Gastroenterology* 150:758–768, 2016. doi: 10.1053/j.gastro.2016.01.001.

Table 22–1. STAGING COLORECTAL CANCER*

STAGE	TUMOR (MAXIMUM PENETRATION)	REGIONAL LYMPH NODE METASTASIS	DISTANT METASTASIS
0	Tis	N0	M0
I	T1 or T2	N0	M0
II	T3	N0	M0
III	Any T or	Any N	M0
	T4	N0	M0
IV	Any T	Any N	M1

*TNM classification:

Tis = carcinoma in situ; T1 = submucosa; T2 = muscularis propria; T3 = penetrates all layers (for rectal cancer, includes perirectal tissue); T4 = adjacent organs or peritoneum.
N0 = none; N1 = 1–3 regional nodes; N2 = ≥ 4 regional nodes; N3 = apical or vascular trunk nodes.
M0 = none; M1 = present.

KEY POINTS

- CRC is the 2nd most common cancer in western countries, typically arising within an adenomatous polyp.
- Right-sided lesions usually manifest with bleeding and anemia; left-sided lesions usually manifest with obstructive symptoms (eg, change in stool frequency, colicky abdominal pain).
- Routine screening should begin at age 50 for patients with average risk; typical methods involve colonoscopy or fecal occult blood testing and/or flexible sigmoidoscopy.
- Serum CEA levels are often elevated but are not specific enough to be used for screening; however, after treatment, monitoring CEA levels may help detect recurrence.
- Treatment is with surgical resection, sometimes combined with chemotherapy and/or radiation; outcome varies widely depending on the stage of the disease.

ESOPHAGEAL CANCER

The most common malignant tumor in the proximal two thirds of the esophagus is squamous cell carcinoma; adenocarcinoma is the most common in the distal one-third. Symptoms are progressive dysphagia and weight loss. Diagnosis is by endoscopy, followed by CT and endoscopic ultrasound for staging. Treatment varies with stage and generally includes surgery with or without chemotherapy and radiation. Long-term survival is poor except for patients with local disease.

Esophageal cancer accounts for an estimated 16,910 cases and 15,690 deaths in the US annually.[1]

1. Siegel RL, Miller KD, Jemal A: Cancer statistics 2016. *CA Cancer J Clin* 66(1):7–30, 2016. doi: 10.3322/caac.21332.

Squamous cell carcinoma of the esophagus: About 8000 cases occur annually in the US. Squamous cell carcinoma is more common in parts of Asia and in South Africa. In the US, it is 4 to 5 times more common among blacks than whites, and 2 to 3 times more common among men than women.

The **primary risk factors for esophageal cancer** are

- Alcohol ingestion
- Tobacco use (in any form)

Other factors include achalasia, human papillomavirus, lye ingestion (resulting in stricture), sclerotherapy, Plummer-Vinson syndrome, irradiation of the esophagus, and esophageal webs. Genetic causes are unclear, but 50% of patients with tylosis (hyperkeratosis palmaris et plantaris), an autosomal dominant disorder, have esophageal cancer by age 45, and 95% have it by age 55.

Adenocarcinoma of the esophagus: Adenocarcinoma occurs in the distal esophagus. Its incidence is increasing; it accounts for 50% of esophageal carcinoma in whites. It is 4 times more common among whites than blacks. Alcohol is not an important risk factor, but smoking is contributory. Adenocarcinoma of the distal esophagus is difficult to distinguish from adenocarcinoma of the gastric cardia invading the distal esophagus.

Most adenocarcinomas arise in **Barrett esophagus,** which results from chronic gastroesophageal reflux disease and reflux esophagitis. In Barrett esophagus, a metaplastic, columnar, glandular, intestine-like mucosa with brush border and goblet cells replaces the normal stratified squamous epithelium of the distal esophagus during the healing phase of acute esophagitis when healing takes place in the continued presence of stomach acid. Obesity is associated with a 16-fold increased risk of esophageal adenocarcinoma, probably because obesity is a contributing factor to reflux.

Other malignant tumors of the esophagus: Less common malignant tumors include spindle cell carcinoma (a poorly differentiated variant of squamous cell carcinoma), verrucous carcinoma (a well-differentiated variant of squamous cell carcinoma), pseudosarcoma, mucoepidermoid carcinoma, adenosquamous carcinoma, cylindroma (adenoid cystic carcinoma), primary oat cell carcinoma, choriocarcinoma, carcinoid tumor, sarcoma, and primary malignant melanoma.

Metastatic cancer constitutes 3% of esophageal cancer. Melanoma and breast cancer are most likely to metastasize to the esophagus; others include cancers of the head and neck, lung, stomach, liver, kidney, prostate, testis, and bone. These tumors usually seed the loose connective tissue stroma around the esophagus, whereas primary esophageal cancers begin in the mucosa or submucosa.

Symptoms and Signs

Early-stage esophageal cancer tends to be asymptomatic. When the lumen of the esophagus becomes constricted to < 14 mm, dysphagia commonly occurs. The patient first has difficulty swallowing solid food, then semisolid food, and finally liquid food and saliva; this steady progression suggests a growing malignant process rather than a spasm, benign ring, or peptic stricture. Chest pain may be present, usually radiating to the back.

Weight loss, even when the patient maintains a good appetite, is almost universal. Compression of the recurrent laryngeal nerve may lead to vocal cord paralysis and hoarseness. Nerve compression elsewhere may cause spinal pain, hiccups, or paralysis of the diaphragm. Malignant pleural effusions or pulmonary metastasis may cause dyspnea. Intraluminal tumor involvement may cause odynophagia, vomiting, hematemesis, melena, iron deficiency anemia, aspiration, and cough. Fistulas between the esophagus and tracheobronchial tree may cause lung abscess and pneumonia. Other findings may include superior vena cava syndrome, malignant ascites, and bone pain.

Lymphatic spread to internal jugular, cervical, supraclavicular, mediastinal, and celiac nodes is common. The tumor usually metastasizes to lung and liver and occasionally to distant sites (eg, bone, heart, brain, adrenal glands, kidneys, peritoneum).

Diagnosis

- Endoscopy with biopsy
- Then CT and endoscopic ultrasonography

There are no screening tests. Patients suspected of having esophageal cancer should have endoscopy with cytology and biopsy. Although barium x-ray may show an obstructive lesion, endoscopy is required for biopsy and tissue diagnosis.

Patients in whom esophageal cancer is identified require CT of the chest and abdomen to determine extent of tumor spread. If CT results are negative for metastasis, endoscopic ultrasonography should be done to determine the depth of the tumor in the esophageal wall and regional lymph node involvement. Findings guide therapy and help determine prognosis.

Basic blood tests, including CBC, electrolytes, and liver function, should be done.

Prognosis

Prognosis depends greatly on stage, but overall is poor (5-yr survival: < 5%) because many patients present with advanced disease. Patients with cancer restricted to the mucosa have about an 80% survival rate, which drops to < 50% with submucosal involvement, 20% with extension to the muscularis propria, 7% with extension to adjacent structures, and < 3% with distant metastases.

Treatment

- Surgical resection, often combined with chemotherapy and radiation

Esophageal cancer treatment decisions depend on tumor staging, size, location, and the patient's wishes (many choose to forgo aggressive treatment).

General principles: Patients with stage 0, I, or IIa disease (see Table 22–2) respond well to surgical resection; preoperative chemotherapy and radiation provide additional benefit. Patients with stages IIb and III have poor survival with surgery alone; response and survival are enhanced by preoperative (neoadjuvant) use of radiation and chemotherapy to reduce tumor volume before surgery. Patients unable or unwilling to undergo surgery may receive some benefit from combined radiation and chemotherapy. Radiation or chemotherapy alone is of little benefit. Patients with stage IV disease require palliation and should not undergo surgery.

After treatment, patients are screened for recurrence by endoscopy and CT of the neck, chest, and abdomen at 6-mo intervals for 3 yr and annually thereafter.

Patients with Barrett esophagus require intense long-term treatment for gastroesophageal reflux disease and endoscopic surveillance for malignant transformation at 3- to 12-mo intervals depending on the degree of metaplasia.

Surgery: Superficial, early, noninvasive cancers may be treated with endoscopic mucosal resection (usually by gastroenterologists at tertiary care centers) if the superficial nature of the lesion has been confirmed by endoscopic ultrasound. However, in the large majority of cases, en bloc resection for cure requires removal of the entire tumor, proximal and distal margins of normal tissue, all potentially malignant lymph nodes, and a portion of the proximal stomach sufficient to contain the distal draining lymphatics. The procedure requires gastric pull-up with esophagogastric anastomosis, small-bowel interposition, or colonic interposition. Pyloroplasty (surgical widening of the pylorus) is required to ensure proper gastric drainage because esophagectomy necessarily results in bilateral vagotomy. This extensive surgery may be poorly tolerated by patients > 75 yr, particularly those with underlying cardiac or pulmonary disease (ejection fraction < 40%, or forced expiratory volume in 1 sec [FEV_1] < 1.5 L/min). Overall, operative mortality is about 5%.

Preoperative chemotherapy combined with radiation therapy can improve survival after surgical resection of thoracic esophageal cancer. Chemotherapy without radiation therapy followed by surgery may also be considered.[2,3]

Complications of surgery include anastomotic leaks, fistulas, and strictures; bilious gastroesophageal reflux; and dumping syndrome. The burning chest pain of bile reflux after distal esophagectomy can be more annoying than the original symptom of dysphagia and may require subsequent Roux-en-Y jejunostomy for bile diversion. An interposed segment of small bowel or colon in the chest has a tenuous blood supply, and torsion, ischemia, or gangrene of the interposed bowel may result.

External beam radiation therapy: Radiation is usually used in combination with chemotherapy for patients who are poor candidates for curative surgery, including those with advanced disease. Radiation is contraindicated in patients with tracheoesophageal fistula because tumor shrinkage enlarges the fistula. Similarly, patients with vascular encasement by tumor may experience massive hemorrhage with tumor shrinkage. During the early stages of radiation therapy, edema may worsen esophageal obstruction, dysphagia, and odynophagia. This problem may require esophageal dilation or preradiation placement of a percutaneous gastrostomy feeding tube. Other adverse effects of radiation therapy include nausea, vomiting, anorexia, fatigue, esophagitis, excess esophageal mucus production, xerostomia, stricture, radiation pneumonitis, radiation pericarditis, myocarditis, and myelitis (spinal cord inflammation).

Chemotherapy: Tumors are poorly responsive to chemotherapy alone. Response rates (defined as ≥ 50% reduction in all measurable areas of tumor) vary from 10 to 40%, but responses generally are incomplete (minor shrinkage of tumor) and temporary. No drug is notably more effective than another.

Most commonly, cisplatin and 5-fluorouracil are used in combination. However, several other drugs, including mitomycin, doxorubicin, vindesine, bleomycin, and methotrexate, also are active against squamous cell carcinoma.

Palliation: Palliation is directed at reducing esophageal obstruction sufficiently to allow oral intake. Suffering caused by esophageal obstruction can be significant, with salivation and recurrent aspiration. Options include manual dilation procedures (bougienage), orally inserted stents, radiation therapy,

Table 22–2. STAGING ESOPHAGEAL CANCER*

STAGE	TUMOR (MAXIMUM PENETRATION)	REGIONAL LYMPH NODE METASTASIS	DISTANT METASTASIS
0	Tis	N0	M0
I	T1	N0	M0
II	T2 or T3	N0	M0
III	T3 or T4	N1	M0
IV	Any T	Any N	M1

*TNM classification:

Tis = carcinoma in situ; T1 = lamina propria or submucosa; T2 = muscularis propria; T3 = adventitia; T4 = adjacent structures.
N0 = none; N1 = present.
M0 = none; M1 = present.

laser photocoagulation, and photodynamic therapy. In some cases, cervical esophagostomy with feeding jejunostomy is required.

Relief provided by esophageal dilation rarely lasts more than a few days. Flexible metal mesh stents are more effective at maintaining esophageal patency. Some plastic-coated models can also be used to occlude malignant tracheoesophageal fistulas, and some are available with a valve that prevents reflux when the stent must be placed near the lower esophageal sphincter.

Endoscopic laser therapy can palliate dysphagia by burning a central channel through the tumor and can be repeated if needed. Photodynamic therapy uses an injection of porfimer sodium, a hematoporphyrin derivative that is taken up by tissues and acts as a photosensitizer. When activated by a laser beam directed on the tumor, this substance releases cytotoxic oxygen singlets that destroy tumor cells. Patients receiving this treatment must avoid sun exposure for 6 wk after treatment because the skin is also sensitized to light.

Supportive care: Nutritional support by enteral supplementation enhances the tolerability and feasibility of all treatments. An endoscopically or surgically placed feeding tube provides a more distal route for feeding when the esophagus is obstructed.

Because many cases of esophageal cancer are fatal, end-of-life care should always aim to control symptoms, especially pain and inability to swallow secretions (see p. 3177). At some point, many patients need substantial doses of opioids. Patients should be advised to make end-of-life care decisions early in the course of disease and to record their wishes in an advance directive.

2. Sjoquist KM, Burmeister BH, Smithers BM, et al: Survival after neoadjuvant chemotherapy or chemoradiotherapy for resectable oesophageal carcinoma: An updated meta-analysis. *Lancet Oncol* 12(7):681–692, 2011. doi: 10.1016/S1470-2045(11)70142-5.
3. Kidane B, Coughlin S, Vogt K, Malthaner R: Preoperative chemotherapy for resectable thoracic esophageal cancer. *Cochrane Database Syst Rev* 9(5):CD001556. doi: 10.1002/14651858.CD001556.pub3.

KEY POINTS

- Alcohol, tobacco, and human papillomavirus infection are risk factors for squamous cell carcinoma; Barrett esophagus due to chronic reflux (often related to obesity) is a risk factor for adenocarcinoma.
- Early-stage cancer is typically asymptomatic; initial symptoms are usually progressive dysphagia, which results from significant encroachment on the lumen, and sometimes chest discomfort.
- Overall, survival is poor (5-yr survival: < 5%) because many patients present with advanced disease.
- Surgery for cure is extensive and often poorly tolerated by older patients and patients with comorbidities.
- Palliation may involve stenting or endoscopic laser therapy to reduce obstruction and allow oral intake.

FAMILIAL ADENOMATOUS POLYPOSIS

Familial adenomatous polyposis is a hereditary disorder causing numerous colonic polyps and resulting in colon carcinoma by age 40. Patients are usually asymptomatic but may have heme-positive stool. Diagnosis is by colonoscopy and genetic testing. Treatment is colectomy.

FAP is an autosomal dominant disease in which ≥ 100 adenomatous polyps carpet the colon and rectum. The disorder occurs in 1 in 8,000 to 14,000 people. Polyps are present in 50% of patients by age 15 yr, and 95% by age 35 yr. Cancer develops before age 40 in nearly all untreated patients.

Patients also can develop various extracolonic manifestations (previously termed Gardner syndrome), both benign and malignant. Benign manifestations include desmoid tumors, osteomas of the skull or mandible, sebaceous cysts, and adenomas in other parts of the GI tract. Patients are at increased risk of cancer in the duodenum (5 to 11%), pancreas (2%), thyroid (2%), brain (medulloblastoma in < 1%), and liver (hepatoblastoma in 0.7% of children < 5 yr).

Symptoms and Signs

Many patients are asymptomatic, but rectal bleeding, typically occult, occurs.

Diagnosis

- Colonoscopy
- Genetic testing of patient and 1st-degree relatives
- Offspring screened for hepatoblastoma

Diagnosis of FAP is made by finding > 100 polyps on colonoscopy. Diagnosed patients should have genetic testing to identify the specific mutation, which should then be sought in 1st-degree relatives. If genetic testing is unavailable, relatives should be screened with annual sigmoidoscopy beginning at age 12, reducing frequency with each decade. If no polyps are evident by age 50, screening frequency is then the same as for average-risk patients.

Children of parents with FAP should be screened for hepatoblastoma from birth to age 5 yr with annual serum alpha-fetoprotein levels and possibly liver ultrasound.

Treatment

- Colectomy
- Endoscopic surveillance of remainder of GI tract
- Perhaps coxibs

Colectomy should be done at the time of diagnosis. Total proctocolectomy, either with ileostomy or mucosal proctectomy and ileoanal pouch, eliminates the risk of colon and rectal cancer. If subtotal colectomy (removal of most of the colon, leaving the rectum) with ileorectal anastomosis is done, the rectal remnant must be inspected every 3 to 6 mo; new polyps must be excised or fulgurated. Coxibs may inhibit new polyp formation. If new ones appear too rapidly or prolifically to remove, excision of the rectum and permanent ileostomy are needed.

After colectomy, patients should have upper endoscopic surveillance at periodic intervals. The 2015 American College of Gastroenterology's guidelines for genetic testing and management of hereditary GI cancer syndromes recommend doing upper endoscopy including duodenoscopy starting at age 25 to 30 yr and repeating surveillance every 6 mo to 4 yr depending on the stage of duodenal polyposis. Annual screening of the thyroid with ultrasound also is recommended.

KEY POINTS

- FAP is an autosomal dominant disease in which ≥ 100 adenomatous polyps carpet the colon and rectum.
- Nearly all patients develop colon carcinoma by age 40, so total proctocolectomy is usually done at time of diagnosis.

- Patients have an increased risk of other cancers, particularly of the duodenum, and also the pancreas, thyroid, brain, and liver.
- After treatment, patients are screened regularly for other cancers and development of polyps in the upper GI tract.
- Children of parents with FAP should be screened for hepatoblastoma from birth to age 5 yr.

GASTROINTESTINAL STROMAL TUMORS

Gastrointestinal stromal tumors are tumors of the GI tract derived from mesenchymal precursor cells in the gut wall. They result from mutations of a growth factor receptor gene, *C-KIT*. Some are caused by previous radiation therapy to the abdomen for other tumors.

Tumors are slow growing, and malignant potential varies from minimal to significant. Most (60 to 70%) occur in the stomach, 20 to 25% in the small bowel, and a small number in the esophagus, colon, and rectum. Average age at presentation is 50 to 60.

Symptoms of gastrointestinal stromal tumors vary with location but include bleeding, dyspepsia, and obstruction.

Diagnosis of gastrointestinal stromal tumors is usually by endoscopy, with biopsy and endoscopic ultrasonography for staging.

Gastrointestinal stromal tumor treatment is surgical removal. The role of radiation and chemotherapy is unclear, but the tyrosine kinase inhibitor imatinib has been beneficial.

LYNCH SYNDROME

(Hereditary Nonpolyposis Colorectal Carcinoma [HNPCC])

Lynch syndrome is an autosomal dominant disorder responsible for 2 to 3% of cases of CRC. Symptoms, initial diagnosis, and treatment are similar to other forms of CRC. Lynch syndrome is suspected by history and is confirmed by genetic testing. Patients also require surveillance for other cancer, particularly endometrial and ovarian cancer.

Lynch syndrome is an autosomal dominant disorder in which patients with one of several known genetic mutations that impair DNA mismatch repair have a 70 to 80% lifetime risk of developing CRC. Compared to sporadic forms of colon cancer, Lynch syndrome occurs at a younger age (mid 40s), and the lesion is more likely to be proximal to the splenic flexure. The precursor lesion is usually a single colonic adenoma, unlike the multiple adenomas present in patients with FAP, the other main hereditary form of CRC.

However, similar to FAP, numerous extracolonic manifestations occur. Nonmalignant disorders include café-au-lait spots and sebaceous gland tumors. The low-grade skin cancer, keratoacanthoma, can occur. Other common associated cancers include endometrial tumors and ovarian tumors (39% risk of endometrial and 9% risk of ovarian by age 70). Patients also have an elevated risk of other cancers, including of the stomach, urinary tract, pancreas, biliary tree, small bowel, and brain.

Symptoms and Signs

Symptoms and signs of Lynch syndrome are similar to other forms of CRC, and diagnosis and management of the tumor itself are the same.

Diagnosis

- Detailed family history
- Clinical criteria followed by testing for microsatellite instability (MSI) or with immunohistochemistry (IHC)
- Genetic testing for confirmation

(See also the 2016 American Gastroenterological Association's guideline regarding diagnosis and management of Lynch syndrome.)

The specific diagnosis of Lynch syndrome is confirmed by genetic testing. However, deciding who to test is difficult because, unlike FAP, there is no typical clinical appearance. Thus, suspicion of Lynch syndrome requires a detailed family history, which should be obtained in all younger patients identified with CRC.

To meet the Amsterdam II criteria for Lynch syndrome, all three of the following historical elements must be present:

- Three or more relatives with CRC or a Lynch syndrome–associated cancer
- CRC involving at least two generations
- At least one case of CRC before age 50

Other prediction models (eg, the PREMM model) and other criteria (eg, the Bethesda criteria[1]) are used by some health care practitioners.

Patients meeting these criteria should have their tumor tissue tested either for MSI or with IHC to detect proteins responsible for DNA mismatch repair; however, most commercial and hospital pathology laboratories now routinely do this test on all colorectal adenocarcinoma specimens. The 2015 AGA guidelines recommend that tumors of all patients with CRC should be tested either with IHC or for MSI.[2] If MSI or IHC is positive, genetic testing for specific Lynch syndrome mutations is indicated.

Patients with Lynch syndrome should have a surveillance colonoscopy every 1 to 2 yr.[2] Patients with confirmed Lynch syndrome require ongoing screening for other cancers. For endometrial cancer, annual endometrial aspiration or transvaginal ultrasound is recommended. For ovarian cancer, options include annual transvaginal ultrasound and serum CA 125 levels. Prophylactic hysterectomy and oophorectomy are also options. Urinalysis may be used to screen for renal tumors.

First-degree relatives of patients with Lynch syndrome should have colonoscopy every 1 to 2 yr beginning in their 20s, and annually after age 40. Female 1st-degree relatives should be tested annually for endometrial and ovarian cancer. More distant blood relatives should have genetic testing; if results are negative, they should have colonoscopy at the frequency for average-risk patients.

1. Umar A, Boland CR, Terdiman JP, et al: Revised Bethesda guidelines for hereditary nonpolyposis colorectal cancer (Lynch syndrome) and microsatellite instability. *J Natl Cancer Inst* 96(4): 261–268, 2004.
2. Rubenstein JH, Enns R, Heidelbaugh J, et al: American Gastroenterological Association Institute guideline on the diagnosis and management of Lynch syndrome. *Gastroenterology* 149:777-782, 2015. doi: 10.1053/j.gastro.2015.07.036.

Treatment

- Surgical resection

The most common Lynch syndrome treatment is resection of the index lesion with frequent surveillance for another colon cancer and any associated tumors in other organs. Because most

Lynch syndrome tumors occur proximal to the splenic flexure, subtotal colectomy, leaving the rectosigmoid intact, has been suggested as an alternative. In either case, close follow-up is needed.

KEY POINTS

- Certain autosomal dominant mutations confer a 70 to 80% lifetime risk of developing CRC.
- Patients also have an increased risk of other cancers, particularly of the endometrium and ovary.
- Symptoms, initial diagnosis, and treatment are similar to other forms of CRC.
- Patients with certain familial risk factors should have their tumor tissue tested for microsatellite instability (MSI) or with immunohistochemistry (IHC); if positive, genetic testing is done.
- First-degree relatives should have colonoscopy every 1 to 2 yr beginning in their 20s, and annually after age 40; women should also be tested annually for endometrial and ovarian cancer.
- More distant relatives should have genetic testing.

PANCREATIC CANCER

Pancreatic cancer, primarily ductal adenocarcinoma, accounts for an estimated 53,000 cases and 41,800 deaths in the US annually.1 Symptoms include weight loss, abdominal pain, and jaundice. Diagnosis is by CT. Treatment is surgical resection and adjuvant chemotherapy and radiation therapy. Prognosis is poor because disease is often advanced at the time of diagnosis.

Most pancreatic cancers are exocrine tumors that develop from ductal and acinar cells. Pancreatic endocrine tumors are discussed elsewhere.

Adenocarcinomas of the exocrine pancreas arise from duct cells 9 times more often than from acinar cells; 80% occur in the head of the gland. Adenocarcinomas appear at the mean age of 55 yr and occur 1.5 to 2 times more often in men.

Prominent risk factors for pancreatic cancer include smoking, a history of chronic pancreatitis, obesity, and possibly long-standing diabetes mellitus (primarily in women). Heredity plays some role. Alcohol and caffeine consumption do not seem to be risk factors.

1. Siegel RL, Miller KD, Jemal A: Cancer statistics 2016. *CA Cancer J Clin* 66(1):7–30, 2016. doi: 10.3322/caac.21332.

Symptoms and Signs

Symptoms of pancreatic cancer occur late. By diagnosis, 90% of patients have locally advanced tumors that have involved retroperitoneal structures, spread to regional lymph nodes, or metastasized to the liver or lung.

Most patients have severe upper abdominal pain, which usually radiates to the back. The pain may be relieved by bending forward or assuming the fetal position. Weight loss is common. Adenocarcinomas of the head of the pancreas cause obstructive jaundice (often causing pruritus) in 80 to 90% of patients. Cancer in the body and tail may cause splenic vein obstruction, resulting in splenomegaly, gastric and esophageal varices, and GI hemorrhage.

The cancer causes diabetes in 25 to 50% of patients, leading to symptoms of glucose intolerance (eg, polyuria and polydipsia). Pancreatic cancer can also interfere with production of digestive enzymes by the pancreas (pancreatic exocrine insufficiency) in some patients and with the ability to break down food and absorb nutrients (malabsorption). This malabsorption causes bloating and gas and a watery, greasy, and/or foul-smelling diarrhea, leading to weight loss and vitamin deficiencies.

Diagnosis

- CT, endoscopic ultrasonography, or magnetic resonance cholangiopancreatography (MRCP)
- CA 19-9 antigen to follow (not for screening)

(See also the U.S. Preventive Services Task Force's summary of recommendations regarding screening for pancreatic cancer.)

The preferred tests are an abdominal helical CT, MRCP, or endoscopic ultrasonography. If these tests show apparent unresectable or metastatic disease, a percutaneous needle aspiration of an accessible lesion might be considered to obtain a tissue diagnosis. If CT shows a potentially resectable tumor or no tumor, MRCP or endoscopic ultrasound may be used to stage disease or detect small tumors not visible with CT. Patients with obstructive jaundice may have ERCP as the first diagnostic procedure.

Routine laboratory tests should be done. Elevation of alkaline phosphatase and bilirubin indicate bile duct obstruction or liver metastases. Pancreas-associated antigen CA 19-9 may be used to monitor patients diagnosed with pancreatic carcinoma and to screen those at high risk. However, this test is not sensitive or specific enough to be used for population screening. Elevated levels should drop with successful treatment; subsequent increases indicate progression. Amylase and lipase levels are usually normal.

Prognosis

Prognosis for pancreatic cancer varies with stage but overall is poor (5-yr survival: < 2%), because many patients have advanced disease at the time of diagnosis.

Treatment

- Whipple procedure
- Adjuvant chemotherapy and radiation therapy
- Symptom control

About 80 to 90% of cancers are considered surgically unresectable at time of diagnosis because of metastases or invasion of major blood vessels. Depending on location of the tumor, the procedure of choice for resection of the cancer is most commonly a Whipple procedure (pancreaticoduodenectomy). Adjuvant therapy with gemcitabine plus capecitabine is now recommended[2] and external beam radiation therapy is typically given, resulting in about 40% 2-yr and 25% 5-yr survival. This combination is also used for patients with localized but unresectable tumors and results in median survival of about 1 yr. Gemcitabine and capecitabine and perhaps other newer drugs (eg, irinotecan, paclitaxel, oxaliplatin, carboplatin) may be more effective than 5-FU–based chemotherapy, but no drug, singly or in combination, is clearly superior in prolonging survival. Patients with hepatic or distant metastases may be offered chemotherapy as part of an investigational program, but the outlook is dismal with or without such treatment and some patients may choose to forego it.

If an unresectable tumor is found at operation and gastroduodenal or bile duct obstruction is present or pending, a double gastric and biliary bypass operation is usually done to relieve obstruction. In patients with inoperable lesions and jaundice, endoscopic placement of a bile duct stent relieves jaundice. However, surgical bypass should be considered in patients with unresectable lesions if life expectancy is > 6 to 7 mo because of complications associated with stents.

Symptomatic treatment

- Analgesics, usually opioids
- Sometimes procedures to maintain biliary patency
- Sometimes pancreatic enzyme supplementation

Ultimately, most patients experience pain and die. Thus, symptomatic treatment is as important as controlling disease. Appropriate end-of-life care should be discussed (see p. 3175).

Patients with moderate to severe pain should receive an oral opioid in doses adequate to provide relief. Concern about addiction should not be a barrier to effective pain control. For chronic pain, long-acting preparations (eg, transdermal fentanyl, oxycodone, oxymorphone) are usually best. Percutaneous or operative splanchnic (celiac) block effectively controls pain in most patients. In cases of intolerable pain, opioids given sc or by IV, epidural, or intrathecal infusion provides additional relief.

If palliative surgery or endoscopic placement of a biliary stent fails to relieve pruritus secondary to obstructive jaundice, the patient can be managed with cholestyramine (4 g po once/day to qid).

Exocrine pancreatic insufficiency is treated with tablets of porcine pancreatic enzymes (pancrelipase). The patient should take enough to supply 16,000 to 20,000 lipase units before each meal or snack. If a meal is prolonged (as in a restaurant), some of the tablets should be taken during the meal. Optimal intraluminal pH for the enzymes is 8; thus, some clinicians give a proton pump inhibitor or H_2 blocker 2 times/day. Diabetes mellitus should be closely monitored and controlled.

2. Neoptolemos JP, Palmer DH, Ghaneh P, et al: Comparison of adjuvant gemcitabine and capecitabine with gemcitabine monotherapy in patients with resected pancreatic cancer (ESPAC-4): A multicentre, open-label, randomised, phase 3 trial. *Lancet* pii: S0140-6736(16)32409-6, 2017. doi: 10.1016/S0140-6736(16)32409-6.

KEY POINTS

- Pancreatic cancer is highly lethal, typically because it is diagnosed only at a late stage.
- Prominent risk factors include smoking and a history of chronic pancreatitis; alcohol use does not seem to be an independent risk factor.
- Diagnosis involves CT and/or magnetic resonance cholangiopancreatography (MRCP) or endoscopic ultrasound; amylase and lipase levels are usually normal, and the CA 19-9 antigen is not sensitive or specific enough to be used for population screening.
- About 80 to 90% of cancers are considered surgically unresectable at time of diagnosis because of metastases or invasion of major blood vessels.
- Do a Whipple procedure when surgery is feasible and also give adjuvant chemotherapy and radiation therapy.
- Control symptoms with adequate analgesia, gastric and/or biliary bypass to relieve symptoms of obstruction, and sometimes pancreatic enzyme supplements.

Cystadenocarcinoma

Cystadenocarcinoma is a rare adenomatous pancreatic cancer that arises as a malignant degeneration of a mucous cystadenoma and manifests as upper abdominal pain and a palpable abdominal mass.

Diagnosis of cystadenocarcinoma is made by abdominal CT or MRI, which typically shows a cystic mass containing debris; the mass may be misinterpreted as necrotic adenocarcinoma or pancreatic pseudocyst.

Unlike ductal adenocarcinoma, cystadenocarcinoma has a relatively good prognosis. Only 20% of patients have metastasis at the time of operation; complete excision of the tumor by distal or total pancreatectomy or by a Whipple procedure results in a 65% 5-yr survival.

Intraductal Papillary-Mucinous Tumor

Intraductal papillary-mucinous tumor is a rare cancer resulting in mucus hypersecretion and ductal obstruction. Histology may be benign, borderline, or malignant. Most (80%) tumors occur in women and in the tail of the pancreas (66%).

Symptoms of intraductal papillary-mucinous tumor consist of pain and recurrent bouts of pancreatitis.

Diagnosis of intraductal papillary-mucinous tumor is made by CT, sometimes along with endoscopic ultrasonography, magnetic resonance cholangiopancreatography, or ERCP.

Benign and malignant disease cannot be differentiated without surgical removal, which is the treatment of choice. With surgery, 5-yr survival is > 95% for benign or borderline cases, but 50 to 75% for malignant tumors.

PEUTZ-JEGHERS SYNDROME

Peutz-Jeghers syndrome is an autosomal dominant disease with multiple hamartomatous polyps in the stomach, small bowel, and colon along with distinctive pigmented skin lesions.

Patients are at a significantly increased risk of GI and non-GI cancers; possibly the genetic defect involves a tumor suppressor gene. GI cancers include those of the pancreas, small intestine, and colon. Non-GI cancers include those of the breast, lung, uterus, and ovaries.

The skin lesions are melanotic macules of the skin and mucous membranes, especially of the perioral region, lips and gums, hands, and feet (see Plate 1). All but the buccal lesions tend to fade by puberty. Polyps may bleed and often cause obstruction or intussusception.

Diagnosis of Peutz-Jeghers syndrome is suggested by the clinical picture. Genetic testing for STK11 mutation should be considered. First-degree relatives should be evaluated and have routine surveillance for cancers, but there is no firm consensus on specific tests and intervals.

Colonic polyps larger than 1 cm typically are removed.

POLYPS OF THE COLON AND RECTUM

An intestinal polyp is any mass of tissue that arises from the bowel wall and protrudes into the lumen. Most are asymptomatic except for minor bleeding, which is usually occult. The main concern is malignant transformation; most colon cancers arise in a previously benign adenomatous polyp. Diagnosis is by endoscopy. Treatment is endoscopic removal.

(See also the U.S. Multi-Society Task Force on Colorectal Cancer's guidelines for colonoscopy surveillance after screening and polypectomy.)

Polyps may be sessile or pedunculated and vary considerably in size. Incidence of polyps ranges from 7 to 50%; the higher figure includes very small polyps (usually hyperplastic polyps or adenomas) found at autopsy. Polyps, often multiple, occur most commonly in the rectum and sigmoid and decrease in frequency toward the cecum. Multiple polyps may represent FAP. About 25% of patients with cancer of the large bowel also have satellite adenomatous polyps.

Adenomatous (neoplastic) polyps are of greatest concern. Such lesions are classified histologically as tubular adenomas, tubulovillous adenomas (villoglandular polyps), or villous adenomas. The likelihood of cancer in an adenomatous polyp at the time of discovery is related to size, histologic type, and degree of dysplasia; a 1.5-cm tubular adenoma has a 2% risk of containing a cancer vs a 35% risk in 3-cm villous adenomas. Serrated adenomas, a somewhat more aggressive type of adenoma, may develop from hyperplastic polyps.

Nonadenomatous (nonneoplastic) polyps include hyperplastic polyps, hamartomas (see p. 169), juvenile polyps, pseudopolyps, lipomas, leiomyomas, and other rarer tumors. Juvenile polyps occur in children, typically outgrow their blood supply, and autoamputate some time during or after puberty. Treatment is required only for uncontrollable bleeding or intussusception. Inflammatory polyps and pseudopolyps occur in chronic ulcerative colitis and in Crohn disease of the colon. Multiple juvenile polyps (but not sporadic ones) convey an increased cancer risk. The specific number of polyps resulting in increased risk is not known.

Symptoms and Signs

Most polyps are asymptomatic. Rectal bleeding, usually occult and rarely massive, is the most frequent complaint. Cramps, abdominal pain, or obstruction may occur with a large lesion. Rectal polyps may be palpable by digital examination. Occasionally, a polyp on a long pedicle may prolapse through the anus. Large villous adenomas may rarely cause watery diarrhea that may result in hypokalemia.

Diagnosis

- Colonoscopy

Diagnosis of colonic polyps is usually made by colonoscopy. Barium enema, particularly double-contrast examination, is effective, but colonoscopy is preferred because polyps also may be removed during that procedure. Because rectal polyps are often multiple and may coexist with cancer, complete colonoscopy to the cecum is mandatory even if a distal lesion is found by flexible sigmoidoscopy.

Treatment

- Complete removal during colonoscopy
- Sometimes follow with surgical resection
- Follow-up surveillance colonoscopy

Polyps should be removed completely with a snare or electrosurgical biopsy forceps during total colonoscopy; complete excision is particularly important for large villous adenomas, which have a high potential for cancer. If colonoscopic removal is unsuccessful, laparotomy should be done. Tattooing the distal margin of the polyp with India ink helps the surgeon locate the polyp during laparotomy.

Subsequent treatment depends on the histology of the polyp. If dysplastic epithelium does not invade the muscularis mucosa, the line of resection in the polyp's stalk is clear, and the lesion is well differentiated, endoscopic excision and close endoscopic follow-up should suffice. Patients with deeper invasion, an unclear resection line, or a poorly differentiated lesion should have segmental resection of the colon. Because invasion through the muscularis mucosa provides access to lymphatics and increases the potential for lymph node metastasis, such patients should have further evaluation (as in colon cancer).

The scheduling of follow-up examinations after polypectomy is controversial and varies by the number, size, and type of polyps removed (see also American College of Gastroenterology's [ACG] guidelines for colonoscopy surveillance after polypectomy). For example, the 2012 ACG guidelines recommend a repeat total colonoscopy (or barium enema if total colonoscopy is impossible) 3 yr after removal of a tubular adenoma $\geq$ 10 mm or a villous adenoma of any size.

Prevention

Aspirin and COX-2 inhibitors may help prevent formation of new polyps in patients with polyps or colon cancer.[1]

1. Cook NR, Lee IM, Zhang SM, et al: Alternate-day, low-dose aspirin and cancer risk: Long-term observational follow-up of a randomized trial. *Ann Int Med* 159:77-85, 2013. doi: 10.7326/0003-4819-159-2-201307160-00002.

KEY POINTS

- Colonic polyps are common; the incidence ranges from 7 to 50% (depending on the diagnostic method used).
- The main concern is malignant transformation, which occurs at different rates depending on the size and type of polyp.
- The main symptom is bleeding, usually occult and rarely massive.
- Colonoscopy is the recommended diagnostic and therapeutic procedure.
- In patients with polyps, aspirin and COX-2 inhibitors may help prevent formation of new polyps.

SMALL-BOWEL TUMORS

Small-bowel tumors account for 1 to 5% of GI tumors. Small-bowel cancer accounts for an estimated 10,090 cases and about 1,330 deaths in the US annually.[1]

Benign tumors include leiomyomas, lipomas, neurofibromas, and fibromas. All may cause abdominal distention, pain, bleeding, diarrhea, and, if obstruction develops, vomiting. Polyps are not as common as in the colon.

Adenocarcinoma, a malignant tumor, is uncommon. Usually it arises in the duodenum or proximal jejunum and causes minimal symptoms. In patients with Crohn disease, the tumors tend to occur distally and in bypassed or inflamed loops of bowel; adenocarcinoma occurs more often in Crohn disease of the small bowel than in Crohn disease of the colon.

Primary malignant **lymphoma** arising in the ileum may cause a long, rigid segment. Small-bowel lymphomas arise often in long-standing untreated celiac disease.

Carcinoid tumors occur most often in the small bowel, particularly the ileum, and the appendix, and in these locations are often malignant. Multiple tumors occur in 50% of cases. Of those > 2 cm in diameter, 80% have metastasized locally or to the liver by the time of operation. About 30% of small-bowel carcinoids cause obstruction, pain, bleeding, or carcinoid syndrome. Treatment of carcinoid tumors is surgical resection; repeat operations may be required.

Kaposi sarcoma, first described as a disease of elderly Jewish and Italian men, occurs in an aggressive form in Africans, transplant recipients, and AIDS patients, who have GI tract involvement 40 to 60% of the time. Lesions may occur anywhere in the GI tract but usually in the stomach, small bowel, or distal colon. GI lesions usually are asymptomatic, but bleeding, diarrhea, protein-losing enteropathy, and intussusception may occur. Treatment of Kaposi sarcoma depends on the cell type and location and extent of the lesions.

1. Siegel RL, Miller KD, Jemal A: Cancer statistics 2016. *CA Cancer J Clin* 66(1):7–30, 2016. doi: 10.3322/caac.21332.

Diagnosis

- Enteroclysis
- Sometimes push endoscopy or capsule video endoscopy

Enteroclysis (sometimes CT enteroclysis) is probably the most common study for mass lesions of the small bowel. Push endoscopy of the small bowel with an enteroscope may be used to visualize and biopsy tumors. Video capsule endoscopy can help identify small-bowel lesions, particularly bleeding sites; a swallowed capsule transmits 2 images/sec to an external recorder. The original capsule is not useful in the stomach or colon because it tumbles in these larger organs; a colon capsule camera with better optics and illumination is under development for use in these larger-diameter organs.

Treatment

- Surgical resection

Treatment of small-bowel tumors is surgical resection. Electrocautery, thermal obliteration, or laser phototherapy at the time of enteroscopy or surgery may be an alternative to resection.

STOMACH CANCER

Etiology of stomach cancer is multifactorial, but *Helicobacter pylori* plays a significant role. Symptoms include early satiety, obstruction, and bleeding but tend to occur late in the disease. Diagnosis is by endoscopy, followed by CT and endoscopic ultrasonography for staging. Treatment is mainly surgery; chemotherapy may provide a temporary response. Long-term survival is poor except for patients with local disease.

Stomach cancer accounts for an estimated 26,370 cases and about 10,730 deaths in the US annually.[1] Gastric adenocarcinoma accounts for 95% of malignant tumors of the stomach; less common are localized gastric lymphomas and leiomyosarcomas. Stomach cancer is the 2nd most common cancer worldwide, but the incidence varies widely; incidence is extremely high in Japan, China, Chile, and Iceland. In the US, incidence has declined in recent decades to the 7th most common cause of death from cancer. In the US, it is most common among blacks, Hispanics, and American Indians. Its incidence increases with age; > 75% of patients are > 50 yr.

1. Siegel RL, Miller KD, Jemal A: Cancer statistics 2016. *CA Cancer J Clin* 66(1):7–30, 2016. doi: 10.3322/caac.21332.

Etiology

Helicobacter pylori infection is a risk factor for some stomach cancers.

Autoimmune atrophic gastritis and various genetic factors are also risk factors. Dietary factors are not proven causes; however, the WHO International Agency for Research on Cancer (IARC) has reported a positive association between consumption of processed meat and stomach cancer.[2] Smoking is a risk factor for stomach cancer, and people who smoke may have an impaired response to treatment.

Gastric polyps can be precursors of cancer. Inflammatory polyps may develop in patients taking NSAIDs, and fundic foveolar polyps are common among patients taking proton pump inhibitors. Adenomatous polyps, particularly multiple ones, although rare, are the most likely to develop cancer. Cancer is particularly likely if an adenomatous polyp is > 2 cm in diameter or has a villous histology. Because malignant transformation cannot be detected by inspection, all polyps seen at endoscopy should be removed. The incidence of stomach cancer is generally decreased in patients with duodenal ulcer.

2. Bouvard V, Loomis D, Guyton KZ, et al: Carcinogenicity of consumption of red and processed meat. *Lancet Oncol* 16(16):1599–1600, 2015. doi: 10.1016/S1470-2045(15)00444-1.

Pathophysiology

Gastric adenocarcinomas can be classified by gross appearance:

- Protruding: The tumor is polypoid or fungating.
- Penetrating: The tumor is ulcerated.
- Superficial spreading: The tumor spreads along the mucosa or infiltrates superficially within the wall of the stomach.
- Linitis plastica: The tumor infiltrates the stomach wall with an associated fibrous reaction that causes a rigid "leather bottle" stomach.
- Miscellaneous: The tumor shows characteristics of ≥ 2 of the other types; this classification is the largest.

Prognosis is better with protruding tumors than with spreading tumors because protruding tumors become symptomatic earlier.

Symptoms and Signs

Initial symptoms of stomach cancer are nonspecific, often consisting of dyspepsia suggestive of peptic ulcer. Patients and physicians alike tend to dismiss symptoms or treat the patient for acid disease. Later, early satiety (fullness after ingesting a small amount of food) may occur if the cancer obstructs the pyloric region or if the stomach becomes nondistensible secondary to linitis plastica. Dysphagia may result if cancer in the cardiac region of the stomach obstructs the esophageal outlet. Loss of weight or strength, usually resulting from dietary restriction, is common. Massive hematemesis or melena is uncommon, but secondary anemia may follow occult blood loss. Occasionally, the first symptoms are caused by metastasis (eg, jaundice, ascites, fractures).

Physical findings may be unremarkable or limited to heme-positive stools. Late in the course, abnormalities include an epigastric mass; umbilical, left supraclavicular, or left axillary lymph nodes; hepatomegaly; and an ovarian or rectal mass. Pulmonary, CNS, and bone lesions may occur.

Diagnosis

- Endoscopy with biopsy
- Then CT and endoscopic ultrasonography

Differential diagnosis of stomach cancer commonly includes peptic ulcer and its complications.

Patients suspected of having stomach cancer should have endoscopy with multiple biopsies and brush cytology. Occasionally, a biopsy limited to the mucosa misses tumor tissue in the submucosa. X-rays, particularly double-contrast barium studies, may show lesions but rarely obviate the need for subsequent endoscopy.

Patients in whom cancer is identified require CT of the chest and abdomen to determine extent of tumor spread. If CT is negative for metastasis, endoscopic ultrasonography should be done to determine the depth of the tumor and regional lymph node involvement. Findings guide therapy and help determine prognosis.

Basic blood tests, including CBC, electrolytes, and liver function tests, should be done to assess anemia, hydration, general condition, and possible liver metastases. CEA should be measured before and after surgery.

Screening: Screening with endoscopy is used in high-risk populations (eg, Japanese) but is not recommended in the US. Follow-up screening for recurrence in treated patients consists of endoscopy and CT of the chest, abdomen, and pelvis. If an elevated CEA level dropped after surgery, follow-up should include CEA levels; a rise signifies recurrence.

Prognosis

Prognosis depends greatly on stage but overall is poor (5-yr survival: < 5 to 15%) because most patients present with advanced disease. If the tumor is limited to the mucosa or submucosa, 5-yr survival may be as high as 80%. For tumors involving local lymph nodes, survival is 20 to 40%. More widespread disease is almost always fatal within 1 yr. Gastric lymphomas have a better prognosis.

Treatment

- Surgical resection, sometimes combined with chemotherapy, radiation, or both

Stomach cancer treatment decisions depend on tumor staging and the patient's wishes (some may choose to forgo aggressive treatment—see p. 3212).

Curative surgery involves removal of most or all of the stomach and adjacent lymph nodes and is reasonable in patients with disease limited to the stomach and perhaps the regional lymph nodes (< 50% of patients). Adjuvant chemotherapy or combined chemotherapy and radiation therapy after surgery may be beneficial if the tumor is resectable.

Resection of locally advanced regional disease results in a 10-mo median survival (vs 3 to 4 mo without resection).

Metastasis or extensive nodal involvement precludes curative surgery, and, at most, palliative procedures should be undertaken. However, the true extent of tumor spread often is not recognized until curative surgery is attempted. Palliative surgery typically consists of a gastroenterostomy to bypass a pyloric obstruction and should be done only if the patient's quality of life can be improved. In patients not undergoing surgery, combination chemotherapy regimens (5-fluorouracil, doxorubicin, mitomycin, cisplatin, or leucovorin in various combinations) may produce temporary response but little improvement in 5-yr survival. Radiation therapy is of limited benefit.

KEY POINTS

- *Helicobacter pylori* infection is a risk factor for some stomach cancers.
- Initial symptoms are nonspecific and often resemble those of peptic ulcer disease.
- Screening with endoscopy is used in high-risk populations (eg, Japanese) but is not recommended in the US.
- Overall, survival is poor (5-yr survival: 5 to 15%) because many patients present with advanced disease.
- Curative surgery, perhaps with combined chemotherapy and radiation therapy, is reasonable in patients with disease limited to the stomach and perhaps the regional lymph nodes.

OVERVIEW OF PANCREATIC ENDOCRINE TUMORS

Pancreatic endocrine tumors arise from islet and gastrin-producing cells and often produce many hormones. Although these tumors develop most often in the pancreas, they may appear in other organs, particularly the duodenum, jejunum, and lung.

These tumors have two general manifestations:

- Functioning
- Nonfunctioning

Nonfunctioning tumors may cause obstructive symptoms of the biliary tract or duodenum, bleeding into the GI tract, or abdominal masses.

Functioning tumors hypersecrete a particular hormone, causing various syndromes (see Table 22–3). These clinical syndromes can also occur in multiple endocrine neoplasia, in which tumors or hyperplasia affects two or more endocrine glands, usually the parathyroid, pituitary, thyroid, or adrenals.

Treatment

- Surgical resection

Treatment for functioning and nonfunctioning tumors is surgical resection. If metastases preclude curative surgery, various antihormone treatments (eg, octreotide, lanreotide) may be tried for functioning tumors. Because of tumor rarity, chemotherapy trials have not yet identified definitive treatment. Streptozotocin has selective activity against pancreatic islet cells and is commonly used, either alone or in combination with 5-fluorouracil or doxorubicin. Some centers use chlorozotocin and interferon.

Newer chemotherapeutic regimens that include temozolomide, either alone or in combination with other agents (eg, thalidomide, bevacizumab, everolimus, capecitabine), have shown good results in small clinical trials and are under active investigation in large prospective clinical trials.

GASTRINOMA

(Zollinger-Ellison Syndrome; Z-E Syndrome)

A gastrinoma is a gastrin-producing tumor usually located in the pancreas or the duodenal wall. Gastric acid hypersecretion and aggressive, refractory peptic ulceration result (Zollinger-Ellison syndrome). Diagnosis is by measuring serum gastrin levels. Treatment is proton pump inhibitors and surgical removal.

Gastrinomas are a type of pancreatic endocrine tumor that arises from islet cells but can also arise from the gastrin-producing cells in duodenum and, much less rarely, other sites in the body. Gastrinomas occur in the pancreas or duodenal wall 80 to 90% of the time. The remainder occur in the splenic hilum, mesentery, stomach, lymph node, or ovary. About 50% of patients have multiple tumors. Gastrinomas usually are small

Table 22–3. PANCREATIC ENDOCRINE TUMORS

TUMOR	HORMONE	TUMOR LOCATION	SYMPTOMS AND SIGNS
ACTHoma	ACTH	Pancreas	Cushing syndrome
Gastrinoma	Gastrin	Pancreas (60%) Duodenum (30%) Other (10%)	Abdominal pain, peptic ulcer, diarrhea
Glucagonoma	Glucagon	Pancreas	Glucose intolerance, rash, weight loss, anemia
GRFoma	Growth hormone releasing factor	Lung (54%) Pancreas (30%) Jejunum (7%) Other (13%)	Acromegaly
Insulinoma	Insulin	Pancreas	Fasting hypoglycemia
Somatostatinoma	Somatostatin	Pancreas (56%) Duodenum/jejunum (44%)	Glucose intolerance, diarrhea, gallstones
Vipoma	Vasoactive intestinal peptidase	Pancreas (90%) Other (10%)	Severe watery diarrhea, hypokalemia, flushing

(< 1 cm in diameter) and grow slowly. About 50% are malignant. About 40 to 60% of patients with gastrinoma have multiple endocrine neoplasia.

Symptoms and Signs

Zollinger-Ellison syndrome typically manifests as aggressive peptic ulcer disease, with ulcers occurring in atypical locations (up to 25% are located distal to the duodenal bulb). However, as many as 25% of patients do not have an ulcer at diagnosis. Typical ulcer symptoms and complications (eg, perforation, bleeding, obstruction) can occur. Diarrhea is the initial symptom in 25 to 40% of patients.

Diagnosis

- Serum gastrin level
- CT, scintigraphy, or PET to localize

Gastrinoma is suspected by history, particularly when symptoms are refractory to standard acid suppressant therapy.

The most reliable test is serum gastrin. All patients have levels > 150 pg/mL; markedly elevated levels of > 1000 pg/mL in a patient with compatible clinical features and gastric acid hypersecretion of > 15 mEq/h establish the diagnosis. However, moderate hypergastrinemia can occur with hypochlorhydric states (eg, pernicious anemia, chronic gastritis, use of proton pump inhibitors), in renal insufficiency with decreased clearance of gastrins, in massive intestinal resection, and in pheochromocytoma.

A secretin provocative test may be useful in patients with gastrin levels < 1000 pg/mL. An IV bolus of secretin 2 µg/kg is given with serial measurements of serum gastrin (10 and 1 min before, and 2, 5, 10, 15, 20, and 30 min after injection). The characteristic response in gastrinoma is an increase in gastrin levels, the opposite of what occurs in patients with antral G-cell hyperplasia or typical peptic ulcer disease. Patients also should be evaluated for Helicobacter pylori infection, which commonly results in peptic ulceration and moderate excess gastrin secretion.

Once the diagnosis of gastrinoma has been established, the tumor or tumors must be localized. The first test is abdominal CT or somatostatin receptor scintigraphy, which may identify the primary tumor and metastatic disease. PET or selective arteriography with magnification and subtraction is also helpful. If no signs of metastases are present and the primary is uncertain, endoscopic ultrasonography should be done. Selective arterial secretin injection is an alternative.

Prognosis

Five- and 10-yr survival is > 90% when an isolated tumor is removed surgically vs 43% at 5 yr and 25% at 10 yr with incomplete removal.

Treatment

- Acid suppression
- Surgical resection for localized disease
- Chemotherapy for metastatic disease

Acid suppression: Proton pump inhibitors are the drugs of choice (eg, omeprazole or esomeprazole 40 mg po bid). The dose may be decreased gradually once symptoms resolve and acid output declines. A maintenance dose is needed; patients need to take these drugs indefinitely unless they undergo surgery.

Octreotide injections, 100 to 500 mcg sc bid to tid, may also decrease gastric acid production and may be palliative in patients not responding well to proton pump inhibitors. A long-acting form of octreotide (20 to 30 mg IM once/mo) can be used.

Surgery: Surgical removal should be attempted in patients without apparent metastases. At surgery, duodenotomy and intraoperative endoscopic transillumination or ultrasonography help localize tumors. Surgical cure is possible in 20% of patients if the gastrinoma is not part of a multiple endocrine neoplasia syndrome.

Chemotherapy: In patients with metastatic disease, streptozocin in combination with 5-fluorouracil or doxorubicin is the preferred chemotherapy for islet cell tumors. It may reduce tumor mass (in 50 to 60%) and serum gastrin levels and is a useful adjunct to omeprazole. Newer chemotherapies under investigation for insulinoma include temozolomide-based regimens, everolimus, or sunitinib. Patients with metastatic disease are not cured by chemotherapy.

KEY POINTS

- Most gastrinomas manifest with peptic ulcer symptoms, but some patients present with diarrhea.
- About half of patients have multiple gastrinomas and about half have multiple endocrine neoplasia syndrome; half of gastrinomas are malignant.
- Serum gastrin levels are usually diagnostic, but patients with borderline elevated levels may need a secretin provocative test.
- Tumors can usually be localized with CT, somatostatin receptor scintigraphy, or PET.
- Acid secretion is suppressed with a proton pump inhibitor, sometimes also with octreotide, pending surgical removal.

GLUCAGONOMA

A glucagonoma is a pancreatic alpha-cell tumor that secretes glucagon, causing hyperglycemia and a characteristic rash. Diagnosis is by elevated glucagon levels and imaging studies. Tumor is localized with CT and endoscopic ultrasound. Treatment is surgical resection.

Glucagonomas are a type of pancreatic endocrine tumor that arises from the alpha cells of the pancreas. Glucagonomas are very rare but similar to other islet cell tumors in that the primary and metastatic lesions are slow-growing: 15-yr survival is common. Eighty percent of glucagonomas are malignant. The average age at symptom onset is 50 yr; 80% of patients are women. A few patients have multiple endocrine neoplasia type 1.

Symptoms and Signs

Because glucagonomas produce glucagon, the symptoms are the same as those of diabetes. Frequently, weight loss, normochromic anemia, hypoaminoacidemia, and hypolipidemia are present, but the most distinctive clinical feature is a chronic eruption involving the extremities, often associated with a smooth, shiny, vermilion tongue and cheilitis. The exfoliating, brownish red, erythematous lesion with superficial necrolysis is termed **necrolytic migratory erythema**.

Diagnosis

- Serum glucagon level
- CT and endoscopic ultrasonography to localize

Most patients with glucagonoma have glucagon levels > 1000 pg/mL (normal < 200). However, moderate elevations occur in renal insufficiency, acute pancreatitis, severe stress, and fasting. Correlation with symptoms is required.

Patients should have abdominal CT followed by endoscopic ultrasonography; MRI or PET may be used if CT is unrevealing.

Treatment

- Surgical resection for localized disease
- Chemotherapy for metastatic disease
- Octreotide to suppress glucagon production

Resection of the tumor alleviates all symptoms.

Unresectable, metastatic, or recurrent tumors are treated with combination streptozocin and doxorubicin, which may decrease levels of circulating immunoreactive glucagon, lessen symptoms, and improve response rates (50%) but are unlikely to improve survival. Newer chemotherapies under investigation for glucagonoma include temozolomide-based regimens, everolimus, or sunitinib.

Octreotide injections partially suppress glucagon production and relieve the erythema, but glucose tolerance may also decrease because octreotide decreases insulin secretion. Octreotide may quickly reverse anorexia and weight loss caused by the catabolic effect of glucagon excess. Patients who respond may be converted to a long-acting octreotide formulation given 20 to 30 mg IM once/mo. Patients using octreotide may also need to take supplemental pancreatic enzymes because octreotide suppresses pancreatic enzyme secretion.

Locally applied, oral, or parenteral zinc may cause the erythema to disappear, but resolution may occur after simple hydration or IV administration of amino or fatty acids, suggesting that the erythema is not solely caused by zinc deficiency.

INSULINOMA

An insulinoma is a rare pancreatic beta-cell tumor that hypersecretes insulin. The main symptom is fasting hypoglycemia. Diagnosis is by a 48- or 72-h fast with measurement of glucose and insulin levels, followed by endoscopic ultrasound. Treatment is surgery when possible. Drugs that block insulin secretion (eg, diazoxide, octreotide, calcium channel blockers, beta-blockers, phenytoin) are used for patients not responding to surgery.

Insulinomas are a type of pancreatic endocrine tumor that arises from islet cells. Of all insulinomas, 80% are single and may be curatively resected if identified. Only 10% of insulinomas are malignant. Insulinoma occurs in 1/250,000 at a median age of 50 yr, except in multiple endocrine neoplasia (MEN) type 1 (about 10% of insulinomas), when it occurs in the 20s. Insulinomas associated with MEN 1 are more likely to be multiple.

Surreptitious administration of exogenous insulin can cause episodic hypoglycemia mimicking insulinoma.

Symptoms and Signs

Hypoglycemia secondary to an insulinoma occurs during fasting. Symptoms of hypoglycemia due to insulinoma are insidious and may mimic various psychiatric and neurologic disorders. CNS disturbances include headache, confusion, visual disturbances, motor weakness, palsy, ataxia, marked personality changes, and possible progression to loss of consciousness, seizures, and coma.

Symptoms of sympathetic stimulation (faintness, weakness, tremulousness, palpitation, sweating, hunger, and nervousness) are often present.

Diagnosis

- Insulin level
- Sometimes C-peptide or proinsulin levels
- Endoscopic ultrasound

Plasma glucose should be measured during symptoms. If hypoglycemia is present (glucose < 40 mg/dL [2.78 mmol/L]), an insulin level should be measured on a simultaneous sample. Hyperinsulinemia of > 6 μU/mL (42 pmol/L) suggests an insulin-mediated cause, as does a serum insulin to plasma glucose ratio > 0.3 (μU/mL)/(mg/dL).

Insulin is secreted as proinsulin, consisting of an alpha chain and beta chain connected by a C peptide. Because pharmaceutical insulin consists only of the beta chain, surreptitious insulin administration can be detected by measuring C-peptide and proinsulin levels. In patients with insulinoma, 72C peptide is ≥ 0.2 nmol/L and proinsulin is ≥ 5 pmol/L. These levels are normal or low in patients with surreptitious insulin administration.

Because many patients have no symptoms (and hence no hypoglycemia) at the time of evaluation, diagnosis of insulinoma requires admission to the hospital for a 48- or 72-h fast. Nearly all (98%) patients with insulinoma develop symptoms within 48 h of fasting; 70 to 80% within 24 h. Hypoglycemia as the cause of the symptoms is established by the Whipple triad:

1. Symptoms occur during the fast.
2. Symptoms occur in the presence of hypoglycemia.
3. Ingestion of carbohydrates relieves the symptoms.

Hormone levels are obtained as described above when the patient is having symptoms.

If the Whipple triad is not observed after prolonged fasting and the plasma glucose after an overnight fast is > 50 mg/dL (> 2.78 mmol/L), a C-peptide suppression test can be done. During insulin infusion (0.1 U/kg/h), patients with insulinoma fail to suppress C peptide to normal levels (≤ 1.2 ng/ mL [≤ 0.40 nmol/L]).

Endoscopic ultrasonography has > 90% sensitivity and helps localize the tumor. PET also may be used. CT has not proved useful, and arteriography or selective portal and splenic vein catheterization is generally unnecessary.

Treatment

- Surgical resection
- Diazoxide or sometimes octreotide for hypoglycemia
- Chemotherapy

Overall surgical cure rates approach 90%. A small, single insulinoma at or near the surface of the pancreas can usually be enucleated surgically. If a single large or deep adenoma is within the pancreatic body or tail, if there are multiple lesions of the body or tail (or both), or if no insulinoma is found (an unusual circumstance), a distal, subtotal pancreatectomy is done. In < 1% of cases, the insulinoma is ectopically located in peripancreatic sites of the duodenal wall or periduodenal area and can be found only by diligent search during surgery. Pancreatoduodenectomy (Whipple procedure) is done for resectable malignant insulinomas of the proximal pancreas. Total pancreatectomy is done if a previous subtotal pancreatectomy proves inadequate.

If hypoglycemia continues, diazoxide starting at 1.5 mg/kg po bid with a natriuretic can be used. Doses can be increased up to 4 mg/kg. A somatostatin analog, octreotide (100 to 500 mcg sc bid to tid), is variably effective and should be considered for patients with continuing hypoglycemia refractory to diazoxide. Patients who respond may be converted to a long-acting octreotide formulation given as 20 to 30 mg IM once/mo. Patients using octreotide may also need to take supplemental pancreatic enzymes because octreotide suppresses pancreatic enzyme secretion. Other drugs that have modest and variable effect on insulin secretion include verapamil, diltiazem, and phenytoin.

If symptoms are not controlled, chemotherapy may be tried, but response is limited. Streptozotocin has a 30 to 40% response rate and, when combined with 5-fluorouracil, a 60% response rate lasting up to 2 yr. Other agents include doxorubicin, chlorozotocin, and interferon. Newer chemotherapies under investigation for insulinoma include temozolomide-based regimens, everolimus, or sunitinib.

KEY POINTS

- Only about 10% of insulinomas are malignant, but all cause fasting hypoglycemia.
- Glucose and insulin levels are measured during symptoms (either spontaneous or induced by fasting during hospitalization).
- Endoscopic ultrasonography has > 90% sensitivity for locating the tumor; PET also may be used, but CT is not useful.
- About 90% of insulinomas can be resected surgically.
- Control symptoms of hypoglycemia with diazoxide or sometimes octreotide.

VIPOMA

(Werner-Morrison Syndrome)

A vipoma is a non-beta pancreatic islet cell tumor secreting vasoactive intestinal peptide (VIP), resulting in a syndrome of watery diarrhea, hypokalemia, and achlorhydria (WDHA syndrome). Diagnosis is by serum VIP levels. Tumor is localized with CT and endoscopic ultrasound. Treatment is surgical resection.

Vipomas are a type of pancreatic endocrine tumor that arises from islet cells. Of these tumors, 50 to 75% are malignant, and some may be quite large (7 cm) at diagnosis. In about 6%, vipoma occurs as part of multiple endocrine neoplasia.

Symptoms and Signs

The major symptoms of vipoma are prolonged massive watery diarrhea (fasting stool volume > 750 to 1000 mL/day and nonfasting volumes of > 3000 mL/day) and symptoms of hypokalemia, acidosis, and dehydration. In half of patients, diarrhea is constant; in the rest, diarrhea severity varies over time. About 33% of patients have diarrhea < 1 yr before diagnosis, but 25% have diarrhea ≥ 5 yr before diagnosis.

Lethargy, muscular weakness, nausea, vomiting, and crampy abdominal pain occur frequently.

Flushing similar to that of carcinoid syndrome occurs in 20% of patients during attacks of diarrhea.

Diagnosis

- Confirmation of secretory diarrhea
- Serum VIP levels
- Endoscopic ultrasonography, PET, or scintigraphy can localize

Diagnosis of vipoma requires demonstration of secretory diarrhea (stool osmolality is close to plasma osmolality, and twice the sum of sodium and potassium concentration in the stool accounts for all measured stool osmolality). Other causes of secretory diarrhea and, in particular, laxative abuse must be excluded (see p. 73). In such patients, serum VIP levels should be measured (ideally during a bout of diarrhea). Markedly elevated levels establish the diagnosis, but mild elevations may occur with short bowel syndrome and inflammatory diseases. Patients with elevated VIP levels should have tumor localization studies, such as endoscopic ultrasonography, PET, and octreotide scintigraphy or arteriography to localize metastases.

Electrolytes and CBC should be measured. Hyperglycemia and impaired glucose tolerance occur in ≤ 50% of patients. Hypercalcemia occurs in 50% of patients.

Treatment

- Fluid and electrolyte replacement
- Octreotide
- Surgical resection for localized disease

Initially, fluids and electrolytes must be replaced. Bicarbonate must be given to replace fecal loss and avoid acidosis. Because fecal losses of water and electrolytes increase as rehydration is achieved, continual IV replacement may become difficult.

Octreotide usually controls diarrhea, but large doses may be needed. Responders may benefit from a long-acting octreotide formulation given 20 to 30 mg IM once/mo. Patients using octreotide may also need to take supplemental pancreatic enzymes because octreotide suppresses pancreatic enzyme secretion.

Tumor resection is curative in 50% of patients with a localized tumor. In patients with metastatic tumor, resection of all visible tumor may provide temporary relief of symptoms. The combination of streptozocin and doxorubicin may reduce diarrhea and tumor mass if objective response occurs (in 50 to 60%). Newer chemotherapies under investigation for vipoma include temozolomide-based regimens, everolimus, or sunitinib. Chemotherapy is not curative.

KEY POINTS

- More than half of vipomas are malignant.
- Copious watery diarrhea (often 1 to 3 L/day) is common, often resulting in electrolyte abnormalities and/or dehydration.
- Patients with confirmed watery diarrhea should have their serum VIP levels measured (ideally during a bout of diarrhea).
- Localize tumors with endoscopic ultrasonography, PET, or octreotide scintigraphy or arteriography.
- Remove tumors surgically when possible and suppress diarrhea with octreotide.

SECTION 3

Hepatic and Biliary Disorders

23 Approach to the Patient with Liver Disease

The liver is the most metabolically complex organ. Hepatocytes (liver parenchymal cells) perform the liver's metabolic functions:

- Formation and excretion of bile during bilirubin metabolism (see Sidebar 23–1)
- Regulation of carbohydrate homeostasis
- Lipid synthesis and secretion of plasma lipoproteins
- Control of cholesterol metabolism
- Formation of urea, serum albumin, clotting factors, enzymes, and numerous other proteins
- Metabolism or detoxification of drugs and other foreign substances

At the cellular level, portal triads consist of adjacent and parallel terminal branches of bile ducts, portal veins, and hepatic arteries that border the hepatocytes (see Fig. 23–1). Terminal branches of the hepatic veins are in the center of hepatic lobules. Because blood flows from the portal triads past the hepatocytes and drains via vein branches in the center of the lobule, the center of the lobule is the area most susceptible to ischemia.

Pathophysiology

Liver disorders can result from a wide variety of insults, including infections, drugs, toxins, ischemia, and autoimmune disorders. Occasionally, liver disorders occur postoperatively (see p. 194). Most liver disorders cause some degree of hepatocellular injury and necrosis, resulting in various abnormal laboratory test results and, sometimes, symptoms. Symptoms may be due to liver disease itself (eg, jaundice due to acute hepatitis) or to complications of liver disease (eg, acute GI bleeding due to cirrhosis and portal hypertension).

Despite necrosis, the liver can regenerate itself. Even extensive patchy necrosis can resolve completely (eg, in acute viral hepatitis). Incomplete regeneration and fibrosis, however, may result from injury that bridges entire lobules or from less pronounced but ongoing damage.

Sidebar 23–1. Overview of Bilirubin Metabolism

The breakdown of heme produces bilirubin (an insoluble waste product) and other bile pigments. Bilirubin must be made water soluble to be excreted. This transformation occurs in 5 steps: formation, plasma transport, liver uptake, conjugation, and biliary excretion.

Formation: About 250 to 350 mg of unconjugated bilirubin forms daily; 70 to 80% derives from the breakdown of degenerating RBCs, and 20 to 30% (early-labeled bilirubin) derives primarily from other heme proteins in the bone marrow and liver. Hb is degraded to iron and biliverdin, which is converted to bilirubin.

Plasma transport: Unconjugated (indirect-reacting) bilirubin is not water soluble and so is transported in the plasma bound to albumin. It cannot pass through the glomerular membrane into the urine. Albumin binding weakens under certain conditions (eg, acidosis), and some substances (eg, salicylates, certain antibiotics) compete for the binding sites.

Liver uptake: The liver takes up bilirubin rapidly but does not take up the attached serum albumin.

Conjugation: Unconjugated bilirubin in the liver is conjugated to form mainly bilirubin diglucuronide (conjugated [direct-reacting] bilirubin). This reaction, catalyzed by the microsomal enzyme glucuronyl transferase, renders the bilirubin water soluble.

Biliary excretion: Tiny canaliculi formed by adjacent hepatocytes progressively coalesce into ductules, interlobular bile ducts, and larger hepatic ducts. Outside the porta hepatis, the main hepatic duct joins the cystic duct from the gallbladder to form the common bile duct, which drains into the duodenum at the ampulla of Vater.

Conjugated bilirubin is secreted into the bile canaliculus with other bile constituents. In the intestine, bacteria metabolize bilirubin to form urobilinogen, much of which is further metabolized to stercobilins, which render the stool brown. In complete biliary obstruction, stools lose their normal color and become light gray (clay-colored stool). Some urobilinogen is reabsorbed, extracted by hepatocytes, and re-excreted in bile (enterohepatic circulation). A small amount is excreted in urine.

Because conjugated bilirubin is excreted in urine and unconjugated bilirubin is not, only conjugated hyperbilirubinemia (eg, due to hepatocellular or cholestatic jaundice) causes bilirubinuria.

Specific diseases preferentially affect certain hepatobiliary structures or functions (eg, acute viral hepatitis—see p. 222) is primarily manifested by damage to hepatocytes or hepatocellular injury; primary biliary cirrhosis, of biliary secretion; and cryptogenic cirrhosis, by liver fibrosis and resultant portal venous hypertension). The part of the hepatobiliary system affected determines the symptoms, signs, and laboratory abnormalities.

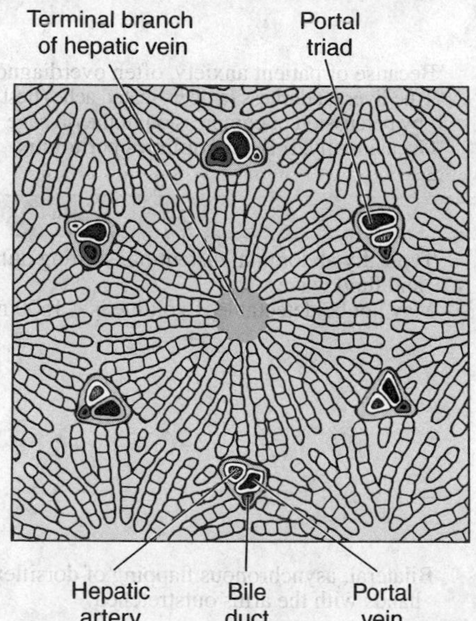

Fig. 23–1. Organization of the liver. The liver is organized into lobules around terminal branches of the hepatic vein. Between the lobules are portal triads. Each triad consists of branches of a bile duct, portal vein, and hepatic artery.

Some disorders (eg, severe alcoholic liver disease) affect multiple liver structures, resulting in a combination of patterns of symptoms, signs, and laboratory abnormalities.

The prognosis of serious complications is worse in older adults, who are less able to recover from severe physiologic stresses and to tolerate toxic accumulations.

EVALUATION OF THE PATIENT WITH A LIVER DISORDER

History: Various symptoms may develop, but few are specific for liver disorders:

- Common nonspecific symptoms include fatigue, anorexia, nausea, and, occasionally, vomiting, particularly in severe disorders.
- Loose, fatty stools (steatorrhea) can occur when cholestasis prevents sufficient bile from reaching the intestines. Patients with steatorrhea are at risk of deficiencies of fat-soluble vitamins (A, D, E, and K). Common clinical consequences may include osteoporosis and bleeding.
- Fever can develop in viral or alcoholic hepatitis.
- Jaundice, occurring in both hepatocellular dysfunction and cholestatic disorders, is the most specific symptom. It is often accompanied by dark urine and light-colored stools.
- Right upper quadrant pain due to liver disorders usually results from distention (eg, by passive venous congestion or tumor) or inflammation of the liver capsule.
- Erectile dysfunction and feminization develop; however, these symptoms may reflect the effects of alcohol more than liver disorders.

Family history, social history, and drug and substance use history should note risk factors for liver disorders (see Table 23–1).

Physical examination: Abnormalities detectable during a physical examination usually do not develop until late in the course of the disease. Some common findings suggest a cause (see Table 23–2).

Table 23–1. RISK FACTORS FOR LIVER DISORDERS

CATEGORY	RISK FACTORS
Acquired	Alcohol use Blood transfusions (particularly before 1992)* Body piercing* Drug (prescription and nonprescription) and herbal product use Exposure to other liver toxins Exposure to hepatitis* Needlesticks* Parenteral drug use* Shellfish ingestion* Tattoos*
Familial	Family history of disorders such as primary biliary cirrhosis, hemochromatosis, Wilson disease, or alpha-1-antitrypsin deficiency

*These factors increase risk of hepatitis in particular, as well as risk of liver disorders in general.

Testing: Testing for hepatic and biliary disorders, including blood tests, imaging, and sometimes liver biopsy, plays a prominent role in the diagnosis of liver disorders. Individual tests, particularly those of liver biochemistry and excretion, often have limited sensitivity and specificity. A combination of tests often best defines the cause and severity of disease.

THE ASYMPTOMATIC PATIENT WITH ABNORMAL LABORATORY TEST RESULTS

Because aminotransferases and alkaline phosphatase are included in commonly done laboratory test panels, abnormalities are often detected in patients without symptoms or signs of liver disease. In such patients, the physician should obtain a history of exposure to possible liver toxins, including alcohol, prescription and nonprescription drugs, herbal teas and remedies, and occupational or other chemical exposures.

Table 23–2. INTERPRETATION OF SOME PHYSICAL FINDINGS

FINDING	POSSIBLE CAUSES	COMMENTS
Hepatic abnormalities		
Hepatomegaly	Acute hepatitis Fatty liver Alcoholic liver disease Passive venous congestion Liver hemorrhage (into a cyst or the parenchyma) Metastatic cancer Biliary obstruction	—
Palpable lump	Cancer	—
Liver firmness, irregular shape, blunt edges, and few if any individual nodules	Cirrhosis	—
Tenderness	Acute hepatitis Passive congestion Liver hemorrhage Cancer	Because of patient anxiety, often overdiagnosed True liver tenderness (a deep-seated ache) best elicited by percussion or compression of the rib cage Occasionally, if severe, mimics peritonitis
Friction rubs or bruits (rare)	Tumor	—
Extrahepatic abnormalities		
Ascites	Portal hypertension Alcoholic hepatitis if chronic or severe Hepatic vein obstruction Peritoneal disorders Generalized fluid retention (eg, heart failure, nephrotic syndrome, hypoalbuminemia)	Typically abdominal distention, shifting dullness, and fluid wave May not be detectable if volume is < 1500 mL
Visibly dilated abdominal veins (caput medusae)	Portal hypertension Inferior vena cava obstruction	—
Splenomegaly	Portal hypertension Nonalcoholic cirrhosis Splenic disorders	—
Asterixis	Portosystemic encephalopathy Uremia Heart failure if severe	Bilateral, asynchronous flapping of dorsiflexed hands with the arms outstretched
Fetor hepaticus	Portosystemic encephalopathy or shunting	Sweet, pungent smell
Drowsiness and confusion	Portosystemic encephalopathy Drugs Brain or systemic disorders	Nonspecific
Wasted extremities plus protuberant abdomen with ascites (cirrhotic habitus)	Cirrhosis if advanced Cancers with peritoneal metastases if advanced	—

Table 23–2. INTERPRETATION OF SOME PHYSICAL FINDINGS (*Continued*)

FINDING	POSSIBLE CAUSES	COMMENTS
Extrahepatic abnormalities		
Male hypogonadism	Alcoholic cirrhosis Hemochromatosis Drugs Pituitary, genetic, systemic, and endocrine disorders	Testicular atrophy, erectile dysfunction, infertility, and loss of libido
In men, gynecomastia, loss of axillary or chest hair, and female pattern of pubic hair	Cirrhosis Alcohol abuse if chronic Drugs Endocrine disorders Chronic kidney disease	Gynecomastia differentiated from pseudogynecomastia (in overweight men) by examination
Gynecomastia plus testicular atrophy	Cirrhosis Alcohol abuse if chronic Anabolic steroid use Pituitary or endocrine disorders	—
Spider angiomas	Cirrhosis Feminization (in men) Pregnancy Undernutrition if severe Alcohol abuse if chronic (possibly)	After compression, peripherally directed blood flow (to the outside of the lesion) Possibly increased risk of severe cirrhosis and variceal hemorrhage as number of angiomas increases May occur as a normal variant (usually < 3)
Palmar erythema	Cirrhosis Feminization (in men) Hyperthyroidism Pregnancy RA Hematologic cancers Alcohol abuse if chronic (possibly)	Often most obvious on thenar and hypothenar eminences
In patients with cirrhosis, clubbing	Possibly advanced portosystemic shunting or biliary cirrhosis Lung disorders if chronic Cyanotic heart disease Infection (eg, infective endocarditis) if chronic Stroke Inflammatory bowel disease	—
Jaundice	Hyperbilirubinemia caused by conditions such as hepatic or biliary disorders, hemolysis, use of certain drugs, or inborn errors of metabolism	Visible when bilirubin level is > 2 to 2.5 mg/dL (> 34 to 43 μmol/L) Affects sclerae (unlike carotenemia)
Muddy skin pigmentation, excoriations caused by constant pruritus, and xanthelasmas or xanthomas (cutaneous lipid deposits)	Cholestasis (including primary biliary cirrhosis) if chronic	—
Parotid gland enlargement	Alcohol use if chronic (often present with alcoholic cirrhosis)	—
Slate gray or bronze skin	Hemochromatosis with deposition of iron and melanin	—
Dupuytren contracture	Alcoholic cirrhosis Alcohol use if chronic Cigarette use Complex regional pain syndrome Repetitive motion or vibration Diabetes Peyronie disease	—

Aminotransferases: Mild isolated elevations of ALT or AST (< 2 times normal) may require only repeat testing; they resolve in about one-third of cases. If abnormalities are present in other laboratory tests, are severe, or persist on subsequent testing, further evaluation is indicated as follows:

- Fatty liver should be considered; it can often be recognized clinically.
- Patients should be screened for hepatitis B and C.
- Patients > 40 should be screened for hemochromatosis.
- Patients < 30 should be screened for Wilson disease.
- Most patients, especially young or middle-aged women, should be screened for autoimmune disorders.
- Patients at risk should be screened for malaria and schistosomiasis.

If at this point the results are negative, screening for alpha-1 antitrypsin deficiency is indicated. If the entire evaluation reveals no cause, liver biopsy may be warranted.

Alkaline phosphatase: Isolated elevation of alkaline phosphatase levels in an asymptomatic patient requires confirmation of hepatic origin by showing elevation of 5´-nucleotidase or gamma-glutamyl transpeptidase. If hepatic origin is confirmed, liver imaging, usually with ultrasonography or magnetic resonance cholangiopancreatography, is indicated. If no structural abnormality is found on imaging, intrahepatic cholestasis is possible and may be suggested by a history of exposure to drugs or toxins. Infiltrative diseases and liver metastases (eg, due to colon cancer) should also be considered. In women, antimitochondrial antibody should be obtained to check for primary biliary cirrhosis. Persistent unexplained elevations or suspicion of intrahepatic cholestasis warrants consideration of liver biopsy.

ACUTE LIVER FAILURE

(Fulminant Liver Failure)

Acute liver failure is caused most often by drugs and hepatitis viruses. Cardinal manifestations are jaundice, coagulopathy, and encephalopathy. Diagnosis is clinical. Treatment is mainly supportive, sometimes with liver transplantation and/or specific therapies (eg, *N*-acetylcysteine for acetaminophen toxicity).

Liver failure can be classified in several ways, but no system is universally accepted (see Table 23–3).

Etiology

Overall, the **most common causes** of acute liver failure are

- Viruses
- Drugs and toxins

In developing countries, viral hepatitis is usually considered the most common cause; in developed countries, toxins are usually considered the most common cause.

Overall, the most common viral cause is hepatitis B; hepatitis C is not a common cause. Other possible viral causes include cytomegalovirus, Epstein-Barr virus, herpes simplex virus, human herpesvirus 6, parvovirus B19, varicella-zoster virus, hepatitis A virus (rarely), hepatitis E virus (especially if contracted during pregnancy), and viruses that cause hemorrhagic fever (see p. 1480).

The most common toxin is acetaminophen; toxicity is dose-related. Predisposing factors for acetaminophen-induced liver failure include preexisting liver disease, chronic alcohol use, and use of drugs that induce the cytochrome P-450 enzyme system (eg, anticonvulsants). Other toxins include amoxicillin/clavulanate, halothane, iron compounds, isoniazid, NSAIDs, some compounds in herbal products, and *Amanita phalloides* mushrooms (see p. 205). Some drug reactions are idiosyncratic.

Less common causes include

- Vascular disorders
- Metabolic disorders

Vascular causes include hepatic vein thrombosis (Budd-Chiari syndrome), ischemic hepatitis, portal vein thrombosis, and hepatic sinusoidal obstruction syndrome (also called hepatic veno-occlusive disease), which is sometimes drug- or toxin-induced. Metabolic causes include acute fatty liver of pregnancy, HELLP syndrome (hemolysis, elevated liver function tests, and low platelets), Reye syndrome, and Wilson disease. Other causes include autoimmune hepatitis, metastatic liver infiltration, heatstroke, and sepsis. The cause cannot be determined in up to 20% of cases.

Pathophysiology

In acute liver failure, multiple organ systems malfunction, often for unknown reasons and by unknown mechanisms. Affected systems include

- **Hepatic:** Hyperbilirubinemia is almost always present at presentation. The degree of hyperbilirubinemia is one indicator of the severity of liver failure. Coagulopathy due to impaired hepatic synthesis of coagulation factors is common. Hepatocellular necrosis, indicated by increased aminotransferase levels, is present.
- **Cardiovascular:** Peripheral vascular resistance and BP decrease, causing hyperdynamic circulation with increased heart rate and cardiac output.
- **Cerebral:** Portosystemic encephalopathy occurs, possibly secondary to increased ammonia production by nitrogenous substances in the gut. Cerebral edema is common among patients with severe encephalopathy secondary to acute liver failure; uncal herniation is possible and usually fatal.
- **Renal:** For unknown reasons, acute kidney injury occurs in up to 50% of patients. Because BUN level depends on hepatic synthetic function, the level may be misleadingly low; thus, the creatinine level better indicates kidney injury. As in hepatorenal syndrome, urine sodium and fractional sodium excretion decrease even when diuretics are not used and tubular injury is absent (as may occur when acetaminophen toxicity is the cause).
- **Immunologic:** Immune system defects develop; they include defective opsonization, deficient complement, and dysfunctional WBCs and killer cells. Bacterial translocation from the GI tract increases. Respiratory and urinary tract infections and sepsis are common; pathogens can be bacterial, viral, or fungal.

Table 23–3. CLASSIFICATION OF LIVER FAILURE*

SEVERITY	DESCRIPTION	COMMON FINDINGS
Acute (fulminant)	Portosystemic encephalopathy develops within • 2 wk after jaundice appears • 8 wk in a patient with no prior liver disease	Often cerebral edema
Subacute (subfulminant)	Encephalopathy develops within 6 mo but later than in acute liver failure.	Renal failure, portal hypertension (more common than in acute liver failure)
Chronic	Encephalopathy develops after 6 mo.	Often caused by cirrhosis

*No classification system is universally accepted.

- **Metabolic:** Metabolic and respiratory alkalosis may occur early. If shock develops, metabolic acidosis can supervene. Hypokalemia is common, in part because sympathetic tone is decreased and diuretics are used. Hypophosphatemia and hypomagnesemia can develop. Hypoglycemia may occur because hepatic glycogen is depleted and gluconeogenesis and insulin degradation are impaired.
- **Pulmonary:** Noncardiogenic pulmonary edema may develop.

Symptoms and Signs

Characteristic manifestations are altered mental status (usually part of portosystemic encephalopathy), bleeding, purpura, jaundice, and ascites. Other symptoms may be nonspecific (eg, malaise, anorexia) or result from the causative disorder. Fetor hepaticus (a musty or sweet breath odor) and motor dysfunction are common. Tachycardia, tachypnea, and hypotension may occur with or without sepsis. Signs of cerebral edema can include obtundation, coma, bradycardia, and hypertension. Patients with infection sometimes have localizing symptoms (eg, cough, dysuria), but these symptoms may be absent.

Diagnosis

- Prolongation of PT and/or clinical manifestations of encephalopathy in patients with hyperbilirubinemia and elevated aminotransferase levels
- To determine the cause: History of drug use, exposure to toxins, hepatitis virus serologic tests, autoimmune markers, and other tests based on clinical suspicion

Acute liver failure should be suspected if patients have acute jaundice, unexplained bleeding, or changes in mental status (possibly suggesting encephalopathy) or if patients with known liver disease quickly deteriorate in any way.

Laboratory tests to confirm the presence and severity of liver failure include liver enzyme and bilirubin levels and PT. Acute liver failure is usually considered confirmed if sensorium is altered or PT is prolonged by > 4 sec or if INR is > 1.5 in patients who have clinical and/or laboratory evidence of acute liver injury. Evidence of cirrhosis suggests that liver failure is chronic.

Patients with acute liver failure should be tested for complications. Tests usually done during the initial evaluation include CBC, serum electrolytes (including calcium, phosphate, and magnesium), renal function tests, and urinalysis. If acute liver failure is confirmed, ABGs, amylase and lipase, and blood type and screen should also be done. Plasma ammonia is sometimes recommended for diagnosing encephalopathy or monitoring its severity. If patients have hyperdynamic circulation and tachypnea, cultures (blood, urine, ascitic fluid) and chest x-ray should be done to rule out infection. If patients have impaired or worsening mental status, particularly those with coagulopathy, head CT should be done to rule out intracranial bleeding.

To determine the cause of acute liver failure, clinicians should take a complete history of toxins ingested, including prescription and OTC drugs, herbal products, and dietary supplements. Tests done routinely to determine the cause include

- Viral hepatitis serologic tests (eg, IgM antibody to hepatitis A virus [IgM anti-HAV], hepatitis B surface antigen [HBsAg], IgM antibody to hepatitis B core antigen [IgM anti-HBcAg], antibody to hepatitis C virus [anti-HCV])
- Autoimmune markers (eg, antinuclear antibodies [ANA], anti–smooth muscle antibodies, immunoglobulin levels)

Other testing is done based on findings and clinical suspicion, as for the following:

- Recent travel to developing countries: Tests for hepatitis A, B, D, and E
- Females of child-bearing age: Pregnancy testing
- Age < 40 and relatively normal aminotransferase levels: Ceruloplasmin level to check for Wilson disease
- Suspicion of a disorder with structural abnormalities (eg, Budd-Chiari syndrome, portal vein thrombosis, liver metastases): Ultrasonography and sometimes other imaging

Patients should be monitored closely for complications (eg, subtle changes in vital signs compatible with infection), and the threshold for testing should be low. For example, clinicians should not assume worsening mental status is due to encephalopathy; in such cases, head CT and often bedside glucose testing should be done. Routine laboratory testing (eg, daily PT, serum electrolytes, renal function tests, blood glucose, and ABGs) should be repeated frequently in most cases. However, testing may need to be more frequent (eg, blood glucose q 2 h in patients with severe encephalopathy).

Prognosis

Prediction of prognosis can be difficult. Important predictive variables include

- Degree of encephalopathy: Worse when encephalopathy is severe
- Patient age: Worse when age is < 10 or > 40 yr
- PT: Worse when PT is prolonged
- Cause of acute liver failure: Better with acetaminophen toxicity, hepatitis A, or hepatitis B than with idiosyncratic drug reactions or Wilson disease

Various scores (usually King's College criteria or Acute Physiologic Assessment and Chronic Health Evaluation II [APACHE II] score) can predict prognosis in populations of patients but are not highly accurate for individual patients.

Treatment

- Supportive measures
- *N*-Acetylcysteine for acetaminophen toxicity
- Sometimes liver transplantation

(See also the American Association for the Study of Liver Disease's practice guideline Management of Acute Liver Failure: Update 2011.)

Whenever possible, patients should be treated in an ICU at a center capable of liver transplantation. Patients should be transported as soon as possible because deterioration can be rapid and complications (eg, bleeding, aspiration, worsening shock) become more likely as liver failure progresses.

Intensive supportive therapy is the mainstay of treatment. Drugs that could worsen manifestations of acute liver failure (eg, hypotension, sedation) should be avoided or used in the lowest possible doses.

For **hypotension** and **acute kidney injury,** the goal of treatment is maximizing tissue perfusion. Treatment includes IV fluids and usually, until sepsis is excluded, empiric antibiotics. If hypotension is refractory to about 20 mL/kg of crystalloid solution, clinicians should consider measuring pulmonary capillary wedge pressure to guide fluid therapy. If hypotension persists despite adequate filling pressures, clinicians should consider using pressors (eg, dopamine, epinephrine, norepinephrine).

For **encephalopathy,** the head of the bed is elevated 30° to reduce risk of aspiration; intubation should be considered early.

When selecting drugs and drug doses, clinicians should aim to minimize sedation so that they can monitor the severity of encephalopathy. Propofol is the usual induction drug for intubation because it protects against intracranial hypertension and has a brief duration of action, allowing rapid recovery from sedation. Lactulose may be helpful for encephalopathy, but it is not given by mouth or nasogastric tube to patients who have altered mental status unless they are intubated; the dose is 50 mL q 1 to 2 h po until patients have ≥ 2 stools/day, or 300 mL in 1 L of saline can be given rectally. Measures are taken to avoid increasing intracranial pressure (ICP) and avoid decreasing cerebral perfusion pressure:

- To avoid sudden increases in ICP: Stimuli that could trigger a Valsalva maneuver are avoided (eg, lidocaine is given before endotracheal suctioning to prevent the gag reflex).
- To temporarily decrease cerebral blood flow: Mannitol (0.5 to 1 g/kg, repeated once or twice as needed) can be given to induce osmotic diuresis, and possibly brief hyperventilation can be used, particularly when herniation is suspected.
- To monitor ICP: It is not clear whether or when the risks of ICP monitoring (eg, infection, bleeding) outweigh the benefits of being able to detect cerebral edema early and being able to use ICP to guide fluid and pressor therapy; some experts recommend such monitoring if encephalopathy is severe. Goals of treatment are an ICP of < 20 mm Hg and a cerebral perfusion pressure of > 50 mm Hg.

Seizures are treated with phenytoin; benzodiazepines are avoided or used only in low doses because they cause sedation.

Infection is treated with antibacterial and/or antifungal drugs; treatment is started as soon as patients show any sign of infection (eg, fever; localizing signs; deterioration of hemodynamics, mental status, or renal function). Because signs of infection overlap with those of acute liver failure, infection is likely to be overtreated pending culture results.

Electrolyte deficiencies may require supplementation with sodium, potassium, phosphate, or magnesium.

Hypoglycemia is treated with continuous glucose infusion (eg, 10% dextrose), and blood glucose should be monitored frequently because encephalopathy can mask the symptoms of hypoglycemia.

Coagulopathy is treated with fresh frozen plasma if bleeding occurs, if an invasive procedure is planned, or possibly if coagulopathy is severe (eg, INR > 7). Fresh frozen plasma is otherwise avoided because it may result in volume overload and worsening of cerebral edema. Also, when it is used, clinicians cannot follow changes in PT, which are important because PT is an index of severity of acute liver failure and is thus sometimes a criterion for transplantation. Recombinant factor VII is sometimes used instead of or with fresh frozen plasma in patients with volume overload. Its role is evolving. H_2 blockers may help prevent GI bleeding.

Nutritional support may be necessary if patients cannot eat. Severe protein restriction is unnecessary; 60 g/day is recommended.

Acute acetaminophen overdose is treated with *N*-acetylcysteine. Because chronic acetaminophen toxicity can be difficult to diagnose, use of *N*-acetylcysteine should be considered if no cause for acute liver failure is evident. Whether *N*-acetylcysteine has a slight beneficial effect on patients with acute liver failure due to other conditions is under study.

Liver transplantation results in average 1-yr survival rates of about 80%. Transplantation is thus recommended if prognosis without transplantation is worse. However, prediction is difficult and scores, such as King's College criteria and the APACHE II score, are not sufficiently sensitive and specific to be used as the only criteria for transplantation; thus, they are used as adjuncts to clinical judgment (eg, based on risk factors).

KEY POINTS

- The most common causes of acute liver failure are viral hepatitis (in developing countries) and drugs and toxins (in developed countries).
- Acute liver failure is characterized by jaundice, coagulopathy, and encephalopathy.
- Confirm the diagnosis by finding prolongation of PT or clinical manifestations of encephalopathy in patients with hyperbilirubinemia and elevated aminotransferase levels.
- Determine the cause by assessing history of drug use and exposure to toxins and doing hepatitis virus serologic tests, autoimmune markers, and other tests based on clinical suspicion.
- Treat complications intensively, usually in an ICU.
- Consider *N*-acetylcysteine for acetaminophen-induced liver failure and liver transplantation for patients with poor prognostic factors (eg, age < 10 or > 40, severe encephalopathy, severe prolongation of PT, idiosyncratic drug reaction, Wilson disease).

ASCITES

Ascites is free fluid in the peritoneal cavity. The most common cause is portal hypertension. Symptoms usually result from abdominal distention. Diagnosis is based on physical examination and often ultrasonography or CT. Treatments include bed rest, dietary sodium restriction, diuretics, and therapeutic paracentesis. Ascitic fluid can become infected (spontaneous bacterial peritonitis), often with pain and fever. Diagnosis of infection involves analysis and culture of ascitic fluid. Infection is treated with antibiotics.

Etiology

Ascites can result from hepatic disorders, usually chronic but sometimes acute; conditions unrelated to the liver can also cause ascites.

Hepatic causes include the following:

- Portal hypertension (accounts for > 90% of hepatic cases), usually due to cirrhosis
- Chronic hepatitis
- Severe alcoholic hepatitis without cirrhosis
- Hepatic vein obstruction (eg, Budd-Chiari syndrome)

Portal vein thrombosis does not usually cause ascites unless hepatocellular damage is also present.

Nonhepatic causes include the following:

- Generalized fluid retention associated with systemic diseases (eg, heart failure, nephrotic syndrome, severe hypoalbuminemia, constrictive pericarditis)
- Peritoneal disorders (eg, carcinomatous or infectious peritonitis, biliary leak due to surgery or another medical procedure)
- Less common causes, such as renal dialysis, pancreatitis, SLE, and endocrine disorders (eg, myxedema)

Pathophysiology

Mechanisms are complex and incompletely understood. Factors include nitric oxide-induced splanchnic vasodilation, altered Starling forces in the portal vessels (low oncotic pressure due to hypoalbuminemia plus increased portal venous pressure), avid renal sodium retention (urinary sodium concentration is typically < 5 mEq/L), and possibly increased hepatic lymph formation.

Mechanisms that seem to contribute to renal sodium retention include activation of the renin-angiotensin-aldosterone system; increased sympathetic tone; intrarenal shunting of blood away from the cortex; increased formation of nitric oxide; and altered formation or metabolism of ADH, kinins, prostaglandins, and atrial natriuretic factor. Vasodilation in the splanchnic arterial circulation may be a trigger, but the specific roles and interrelationships of these abnormalities remain uncertain.

Symptoms and Signs

Small amounts of ascitic fluid cause no symptoms. Moderate amounts cause increased abdominal girth and weight gain. Massive amounts may cause nonspecific diffuse abdominal pressure, but actual pain is uncommon and suggests another cause of acute abdominal pain (see p. 83). If ascites results in elevation of the diaphragm, dyspnea may occur. Symptoms of spontaneous bacterial peritonitis (SBP) may include new abdominal discomfort and fever.

Signs include shifting dullness (detected by abdominal percussion) and a fluid wave. Volumes < 1500 mL may not cause physical findings. Massive ascites causes tautness of the abdominal wall and flattening of the umbilicus. In liver diseases or peritoneal disorders, ascites is usually isolated or disproportionate to peripheral edema; in systemic diseases (eg, heart failure), the reverse is usually true.

Diagnosis

- Ultrasonography or CT unless physical findings make diagnosis obvious
- Often tests of ascitic fluid

Diagnosis may be based on physical examination if there is a large amount of fluid, but imaging tests are more sensitive. Ultrasonography and CT reveal much smaller volumes of fluid (100 to 200 mL) than does physical examination. SBP is suspected if a patient with ascites also has abdominal pain, fever, or unexplained deterioration.

Diagnostic abdominal paracentesis should be done if any of the following occur:

- Ascites is newly diagnosed.
- Its cause is unknown.
- SBP is suspected.

About 50 to 100 mL of fluid is removed and analyzed for gross appearance, protein content, cell count and differential, cytology, culture, and, as clinically indicated, acid-fast stain, amylase, or both. In contrast to ascites due to inflammation or infection, ascites due to portal hypertension produces fluid that is clear and straw-colored, has a low protein concentration, a low PMN count (< 250 cells/μL), and, most reliably, a high serum-to-ascites albumin concentration gradient, which is the serum albumin concentration minus the ascitic albumin concentration. Gradients ≥ 1.1 g/dL are relatively specific for ascites due to portal hypertension. In ascitic fluid, turbidity and a PMN count of > 250 cells/μL indicate SBP, whereas bloody fluid can suggest a tumor or TB. The rare milky (chylous) ascites is most common with lymphoma or lymphatic duct occlusion.

Treatment

- Bed rest and dietary sodium restriction
- Sometimes spironolactone, possibly plus furosemide
- Sometimes therapeutic paracentesis

(See also the American Association for the Study of Liver Disease's practice guideline Management of Adult Patients with Ascites Due to Cirrhosis.)

Bed rest and dietary sodium restriction (2000 mg/day) are the first and least risky treatments for ascites due to portal hypertension. Diuretics should be used if rigid sodium restriction fails to initiate diuresis within a few days. Spironolactone is usually effective (in oral doses ranging from 50 mg once/day to 200 mg bid). A loop diuretic (eg, furosemide 20 to 160 mg po usually once/day or 20 to 80 mg po bid) should be added if spironolactone is insufficient. Because spironolactone can cause potassium retention and furosemide can cause potassium depletion, the combination of these drugs often provides optimal diuresis with a lower risk of potassium abnormalities. Fluid restriction is indicated only for treatment of hyponatremia (serum sodium < 120 mEq/L).

Changes in body weight and urinary sodium determinations reflect response to treatment. Weight loss of about 0.5 kg/day is optimal because the ascitic compartment cannot be mobilized much more rapidly. More aggressive diuresis depletes fluid from the intravascular compartment, especially when peripheral edema is absent; this depletion may cause renal failure or electrolyte imbalance (eg, hypokalemia) that may precipitate portosystemic encephalopathy. Inadequate dietary sodium restriction is the usual cause of persistent ascites.

Therapeutic paracentesis is an alternative. Removal of 4 L/day is safe; many clinicians infuse IV salt-poor albumin (about 40 g/paracentesis) at about the same time to prevent intravascular volume depletion. Even single total paracentesis may be safe. Therapeutic paracentesis shortens the hospital stay with relatively little risk of electrolyte imbalance or renal failure; nevertheless, patients require ongoing diuretics and tend to reaccumulate fluid more rapidly than those treated without paracentesis.

Techniques for the autologous infusion of ascitic fluid (eg, the LeVeen peritoneovenous shunt) often cause complications and are generally no longer used. Transjugular intrahepatic portosystemic shunting (TIPS) can lower portal pressure and successfully treat ascites resistant to other treatments, but TIPS is invasive and may cause complications, including portosystemic encephalopathy and worsening hepatocellular function.

(See also the American Association for the Study of Liver Disease's practice guideline The Role of Transjugular Intrahepatic Portosystemic Shunt (TIPS) in the Management of Portal Hypertension: Update 2009.)

KEY POINTS

- Ascites is free fluid in the abdominal cavity, usually caused by portal hypertension and sometimes by other hepatic or nonhepatic conditions.
- Moderate amounts of fluid can increase abdominal girth and cause weight gain, and massive amounts can cause abdominal distention, pressure, and dyspnea; signs may be absent if fluid accumulation is < 1500 mL.
- Unless the diagnosis is obvious, confirm the presence of ascites using ultrasonography or CT.
- If ascites is newly diagnosed, its cause is unknown, or SBP is suspected, do paracentesis and test ascitic fluid.
- Recommend bed rest and dietary sodium restriction, and if these measures are insufficiently effective, consider use of diuretics and therapeutic paracentesis.

CRIGLER-NAJJAR SYNDROME

This rare inherited disorder is caused by deficiency of the enzyme glucuronyl transferase.

Patients with autosomal recessive type I (complete) disease have severe hyperbilirubinemia. They usually die of kernicterus by age 1 yr but may survive into adulthood. Treatment may include phototherapy and liver transplantation.

Patients with autosomal dominant type II (partial) disease (which has variable penetrance) often have less severe hyperbilirubinemia (< 20 mg/dL [< 342 μmol/L]) and usually live into adulthood without neurologic damage. Phenobarbital 1.5 to 2 mg/kg po tid, which induces the partially deficient glucuronyl transferase, may be effective.

FATTY LIVER

(Hepatic Steatosis)

Fatty liver is excessive accumulation of lipid in hepatocytes, the most common liver response to injury.

Fatty liver develops for many reasons, involves many different biochemical mechanisms, and causes different types of liver damage. Clinically, it is most useful to distinguish fatty liver due to pregnancy or alcoholic liver disease from that occurring in the absence of pregnancy and alcoholism (nonalcoholic fatty liver disease [NAFLD]). NAFLD includes simple fatty infiltration (a benign condition) and nonalcoholic steatohepatitis, a less common but more important variant.

GILBERT SYNDROME

Gilbert syndrome is a presumably lifelong disorder in which the only significant abnormality is asymptomatic, mild, unconjugated hyperbilirubinemia. It can be mistaken for chronic hepatitis or other liver disorders.

Gilbert syndrome may affect as many as 5% of people. Although family members may be affected, a clear genetic pattern is difficult to establish.

Pathogenesis may involve complex defects in the liver's uptake of bilirubin. Glucuronyl transferase activity is low, though not as low as in Crigler-Najjar syndrome type II. In many patients, RBC destruction is also slightly accelerated, but this acceleration does not explain hyperbilirubinemia. Liver histology is normal.

Gilbert syndrome is most often detected in young adults serendipitously by finding an elevated bilirubin level, which usually fluctuates between 2 and 5 mg/dL (34 and 86 μmol/L) and tends to increase with fasting and other stresses.

Gilbert syndrome is differentiated from hepatitis by fractionation that shows predominantly unconjugated bilirubin, otherwise normal liver function test results, and absence of urinary bilirubin. It is differentiated from hemolysis by the absence of anemia and reticulocytosis.

Treatment is unnecessary. Patients should be reassured that they do not have liver disease.

INBORN METABOLIC DISORDERS CAUSING HYPERBILIRUBINEMIA

Hereditary or inborn metabolic disorders may cause unconjugated or conjugated hyperbilirubinemia.

- Unconjugated hyperbilirubinemia: Gilbert syndrome, Crigler-Najjar syndrome, and primary shunt hyperbilirubinemia
- Conjugated hyperbilirubinemia: Dubin-Johnson syndrome and Rotor syndrome

Primary Shunt Hyperbilirubinemia

This rare, familial, benign condition is characterized by overproduction of early-labeled bilirubin (bilirubin derived from ineffective erythropoiesis and nonhemoglobin heme rather than from normal RBC turnover).

Dubin-Johnson Syndrome and Rotor Syndrome

Dubin-Johnson syndrome and Rotor syndrome cause conjugated hyperbilirubinemia, but without cholestasis, causing no symptoms or sequelae other than jaundice. In contrast to unconjugated hyperbilirubinemia in Gilbert syndrome (which also causes no other symptoms), bilirubin may appear in the urine. Aminotransferase and alkaline phosphatase levels are usually normal. Treatment is unnecessary.

Dubin-Johnson syndrome: This rare autosomal recessive disorder involves impaired excretion of bilirubin glucuronides. It is usually diagnosed by liver biopsy; the liver is deeply pigmented as a result of an intracellular melanin-like substance but is otherwise histologically normal.

Rotor syndrome: This rare disorder is clinically similar to Dubin-Johnson syndrome, but the liver is not pigmented, and other subtle metabolic differences are present.

JAUNDICE

Jaundice is a yellowish discoloration of the skin and mucous membranes caused by hyperbilirubinemia. Jaundice becomes visible when the bilirubin level is about 2 to 3 mg/dL (34 to 51 μmol/L).

Pathophysiology

Most bilirubin is produced when Hb is broken down into unconjugated bilirubin (and other substances). Unconjugated bilirubin binds to albumin in the blood for transport to the liver, where it is taken up by hepatocytes and conjugated with glucuronic acid to make it water soluble. Conjugated bilirubin is excreted in bile into the duodenum. In the intestine, bacteria metabolize bilirubin to form urobilinogen. Some urobilinogen is eliminated in the feces, and some is reabsorbed, extracted by hepatocytes, reprocessed, and re-excreted in bile (enterohepatic circulation—see Sidebar 23–1 on p. 179).

Mechanisms of hyperbilirubinemia: Hyperbilirubinemia may involve predominantly unconjugated or conjugated bilirubin.

Unconjugated hyperbilirubinemia is most often caused by ≥ 1 of the following:

- Increased production
- Decreased hepatic uptake
- Decreased conjugation

Conjugated hyperbilirubinemia is most often caused by ≥ 1 of the following:

- Dysfunction of hepatocytes (hepatocellular dysfunction)
- Slowing of bile egress from the liver (intrahepatic cholestasis)
- Obstruction of extrahepatic bile flow (extrahepatic cholestasis)

Consequences: Outcome is determined primarily by the cause of jaundice and the presence and severity of hepatic dysfunction. Hepatic dysfunction can result in coagulopathy, encephalopathy, and portal hypertension (which can lead to GI bleeding).

Etiology

Although hyperbilirubinemia can be classified as predominantly unconjugated or conjugated, many hepatobiliary disorders cause both forms.

Many conditions (see Table 23–4), including use of certain drugs (see Table 23–5), can cause jaundice, but the most common causes overall are

- Inflammatory hepatitis (viral hepatitis, autoimmune hepatitis, toxic hepatic injury)
- Alcoholic liver disease
- Biliary obstruction

Evaluation

History: History of present illness should include onset and duration of jaundice. Hyperbilirubinemia can cause urine to darken before jaundice is visible. Therefore, the onset of dark urine indicates onset of hyperbilirubinemia more accurately than onset of jaundice. Important associated symptoms include fever, prodromal symptoms (eg, fever, malaise, myalgias) before jaundice, changes in stool color, pruritus, steatorrhea, and abdominal pain (including location, severity, duration, and radiation). Important symptoms suggesting severe disease include nausea and vomiting, weight loss, and possible symptoms of coagulopathy (eg, easy bruising or bleeding, tarry or bloody stools).

Review of systems should seek symptoms of possible causes, including weight loss and abdominal pain (cancer); joint pain and swelling (autoimmune or viral hepatitis, hemochromatosis, primary sclerosing cholangitis, sarcoidosis); and missed menses (pregnancy).

Past medical history should identify known causative disorders, such as hepatobiliary disease (eg, gallstones, hepatitis, cirrhosis); disorders that can cause hemolysis (eg, hemoglobinopathy, G6PD deficiency); and disorders associated with liver or biliary disease, including inflammatory bowel disease, infiltrative disorders (eg, amyloidosis, lymphoma, sarcoidosis, TB), and HIV infection or AIDS.

Table 23–4. MECHANISMS AND SOME CAUSES OF JAUNDICE IN ADULTS

MECHANISM	EXAMPLES	SUGGESTIVE FINDINGS*
Unconjugated hyperbilirubinemia		
Increased bilirubin production	Common: Hemolysis Less common: Resorption of large hematomas, ineffective erythropoiesis	Few or no clinical manifestations of hepatobiliary disease; sometimes anemia, ecchymoses Serum bilirubin level usually < 3.5 mg/dL (< 59 μmol/L), no bilirubin in urine, normal aminotransferase levels
Decreased hepatic bilirubin uptake	Common: Heart failure Less common: Drugs, fasting, portosystemic shunts	—
Decreased hepatic conjugation	Common: Gilbert syndrome Less common: Ethinyl estradiol, Crigler-Najjar syndrome, hyperthyroidism	—
Conjugated hyperbilirubinemia[†]		
Hepatocellular dysfunction	Common: Drugs, toxins, viral hepatitis Less common: Alcoholic liver disease, hemochromatosis, primary biliary cirrhosis, primary sclerosing cholangitis, steatohepatitis, Wilson disease	Aminotransferase levels usually > 500 U/L
Intrahepatic cholestasis	Common: Alcoholic liver disease, drugs, toxins, viral hepatitis Less common: Infiltrative disorders (eg, amyloidosis, lymphoma, sarcoidosis, TB), pregnancy, primary biliary cirrhosis, steatohepatitis	Gradual onset of jaundice, sometimes pruritus If severe, clay-colored stools, steatorrhea If long-standing, weight loss Alkaline phosphatase and GGT usually > 3 times normal Aminotransferase levels < 200 U/L
Extrahepatic cholestasis	Common: Common bile duct stone, pancreatic cancer Less common: Acute cholangitis, pancreatic pseudocyst, primary sclerosing cholangitis, common duct strictures caused by previous surgery, other tumors	Depending on cause, manifestations possibly similar to those of intrahepatic cholestasis or a more acute disorder (eg, abdominal pain or vomiting due to a common bile duct stone or acute pancreatitis) Alkaline phosphatase and GGT usually > 3 times normal Aminotransferase levels < 200 U/L
Other, less common mechanisms	Hereditary disorders (mainly Dubin-Johnson syndrome and Rotor syndrome)	Normal liver enzymes

*Symptoms and signs of the causative disorder may be present.
[†]Bilirubin is present in urine.
GGT = gamma-glutamyltransferase.

Table 23–5. SOME DRUGS AND TOXINS THAT CAN CAUSE JAUNDICE

MECHANISM	DRUGS OR TOXINS
Increased bilirubin production	Drugs that cause hemolysis (common among patients with G6PD deficiency), such as sulfa drugs and nitrofurantoin
Decreased hepatic uptake	Chloramphenicol, probenecid, rifampin
Decreased conjugation	Ethinyl estradiol
Hepatocellular dysfunction	Acetaminophen (high dose or overdose), amiodarone, isoniazid, NSAIDs, statins, many others, many drug combinations
	Amanita phalloides mushrooms, carbon tetrachloride, phosphorus
Intrahepatic cholestasis	Amoxicillin/clavulanate, anabolic steroids, chlorpromazine, pyrrolizidine alkaloids (eg, in herbal preparations), oral contraceptives, phenothiazines

Drug history should include questions about use of drugs or exposure to toxins known to affect the liver (see Table 23–5) and about vaccination against hepatitis.

Surgical history should include questions about previous surgery on the biliary tract (a potential cause of strictures).

Social history should include questions about risk factors for hepatitis (see Table 23–6), amount and duration of alcohol use, injection drug use, and sexual history.

Family history should include questions about recurrent, mild jaundice in family members and diagnosed hereditary liver disorders. The patient's history of recreational drug and alcohol use should be corroborated by friends or family members when possible.

Physical examination: Vital signs are reviewed for fever and signs of systemic toxicity (eg, hypotension, tachycardia).

General appearance is noted, particularly for cachexia and lethargy.

Head and neck examination includes inspection of the sclerae and tongue for icterus and the eyes for Kayser-Fleischer rings. Mild jaundice is best seen by examining the sclerae in natural light; it is usually detectable when serum bilirubin reaches 2 to 2.5 mg/dL (34 to 43 μmol/L). Breath odor should be noted (eg, for fetor hepaticus).

The abdomen is inspected for collateral vasculature, ascites, and surgical scars. The liver is palpated for hepatomegaly, masses, nodularity, and tenderness. The spleen is palpated for splenomegaly. The abdomen is examined for umbilical hernia, shifting dullness, fluid wave, masses, and tenderness. The rectum is examined for gross or occult blood.

Table 23–6. SOME RISK FACTORS FOR HEPATITIS

TYPE OF HEPATITIS	RISK FACTORS
A	Day care attendance or employment Residence or employment in a closed institution Travel to an endemic area Oral-anal sex Ingestion of raw shellfish
B	Injection drug use Hemodialysis Sharing of razor blades or toothbrushes Tattooing Body piercing Absence of vaccination in health care workers High-risk sexual activity Birth in areas of high endemicity
C	Blood transfusion before 1992 Injection drug use Hemodialysis Exposure during health care work or sexual activity Date of birth between 1945 and 1965

Men are checked for testicular atrophy and gynecomastia.

The upper extremities are examined for Dupuytren contractures.

Neurologic examination includes mental status assessment and evaluation for asterixis.

The skin is examined for jaundice, palmar erythema, needle tracks, vascular spiders, excoriations, xanthomas (consistent with primary biliary cirrhosis), paucity of axillary and pubic hair, hyperpigmentation, ecchymoses, petechiae, and purpura.

Red flags: The following findings are of particular concern:

- Marked abdominal pain and tenderness
- Altered mental status
- GI bleeding (occult or gross)
- Ecchymoses, petechiae, or purpura

Interpretation of findings: **Severity of illness** is indicated mainly by the degree (if any) of hepatic dysfunction. Ascending cholangitis is a concern because it requires emergency treatment.

Severe hepatic dysfunction is indicated by encephalopathy (eg, mental status change, asterixis) or coagulopathy (eg, easy bleeding, purpura, tarry or heme-positive stool), particularly in patients with signs of portal hypertension (eg, abdominal collateral vasculature, ascites, splenomegaly). Massive upper GI bleeding suggests variceal bleeding due to portal hypertension (and possibly coagulopathy).

Ascending cholangitis is suggested by fever and marked, continuous right upper quadrant abdominal pain; acute pancreatitis with biliary obstruction (eg, due to a common duct stone or pancreatic pseudocyst) may manifest similarly.

Cause of jaundice may be suggested by the following:

- Acute jaundice in the young and healthy suggests acute viral hepatitis, particularly when a viral prodrome, risk factors, or both are present; however, acetaminophen overdose is also common.
- Acute jaundice after acute drug or toxin exposure in healthy patients is likely to be due to that substance.
- A long history of heavy alcohol use suggests alcoholic liver disease, particularly when typical stigmata are present.
- A personal or family history of recurrent, mild jaundice without findings of hepatobiliary dysfunction suggests a hereditary disorder, usually Gilbert syndrome.
- Gradual onset of jaundice with pruritus, weight loss, and clay-colored stools suggests intrahepatic or extrahepatic cholestasis.
- Painless jaundice in elderly patients with weight loss and a mass but with minimal pruritus suggests biliary obstruction caused by cancer.

Other examination findings can also be helpful (see Table 23–7).

Testing: The following are done:

- Blood tests (bilirubin, aminotransferase, alkaline phosphatase)
- Usually imaging
- Sometimes biopsy or laparoscopy

Blood tests include measurement of total and direct bilirubin, aminotransferase, and alkaline phosphatase levels in all patients. Results help differentiate cholestasis from hepatocellular dysfunction (important because patients with cholestasis usually require imaging tests):

- Hepatocellular dysfunction: Marked aminotransferase elevation (> 500 U/L) and moderate alkaline phosphatase elevation (< 3 times normal)
- Cholestasis: Moderate aminotransferase elevation (< 200 U/L) and marked alkaline phosphatase elevation (> 3 times normal)
- Hyperbilirubinemia without hepatobiliary dysfunction: Mild hyperbilirubinemia (eg, < 3.5 mg/dL [< 59 μmol/L]) with normal aminotransferase and alkaline phosphatase levels

Table 23–7. FINDINGS SUGGESTING A CAUSE OF JAUNDICE

FINDING	POSSIBLE CAUSES
Risk factors	
Alcohol use (heavy)	Alcoholic liver disease, including alcoholic hepatitis and cirrhosis
GI cancer	Extrahepatic biliary obstruction
Hypercoagulable state	Hepatic vein thrombosis (Budd-Chiari syndrome)
Inflammatory bowel disease	Primary sclerosing cholangitis
Pregnancy	Intrahepatic cholestasis, steatohepatitis (acute fatty liver due to pregnancy)
Previous cholecystectomy	Biliary stricture Retained or recurrent common duct stone
Recent surgery	Ischemic hepatitis Benign postoperative intrahepatic cholestasis Lengthy cardiac bypass surgery
Symptoms	
Colicky right upper quadrant, right shoulder, or subscapular pain (current or previous)	Choledocholithiasis
Constant right upper quadrant pain	Acute alcoholic or viral hepatitis, acute cholangitis
Dark urine	Conjugated hyperbilirubinemia
Joint pain, swelling, or both	Hepatitis (autoimmune or viral) Hemochromatosis Primary sclerosing cholangitis Sarcoidosis
Nausea or vomiting before jaundice	Acute hepatitis Common bile duct obstruction by a stone (particularly if accompanied by abdominal pain or rigors)
Pruritus and clay-colored stools	Intrahepatic or extrahepatic cholestasis, possibly severe if stools are clay-colored
Viral prodrome (eg, fever, malaise, myalgias)	Acute viral hepatitis
Physical examination	
Abdominal collateral vasculature, ascites, and splenomegaly	Portal hypertension (eg, due to cirrhosis)
Cachexia in a patient with a hard, lumpy liver	Metastases (common) Cirrhosis (less often)
Diffuse lymphadenopathy in a patient with acute jaundice	Infectious mononucleosis
Diffuse lymphadenopathy in a patient with chronic jaundice	Lymphoma, leukemia
Dupuytren contractures, palmar erythema, paucity of axillary and pubic hair, and vascular spiders	Alcoholic liver disease
Gynecomastia and testicular atrophy	Alcoholic liver disease, anabolic steroid use
Hyperpigmentation	Hemochromatosis, primary biliary cirrhosis
Kayser-Fleischer rings	Wilson disease
Needle marks	Hepatitis B or C
Resolving hematoma	Extravasation of blood into tissues
Xanthomas	Primary biliary cirrhosis

Also, patients with hepatocellular dysfunction or cholestasis have dark urine due to bilirubinuria because conjugated bilirubin is excreted in urine; unconjugated bilirubin is not. Bilirubin fractionation also differentiates conjugated from unconjugated forms. When aminotransferase and alkaline phosphatase levels are normal, fractionation of bilirubin can help suggest causes, such as Gilbert syndrome or hemolysis (unconjugated) vs Dubin-Johnson syndrome or Rotor syndrome (conjugated).

Other blood tests are done based on clinical suspicion and initial test findings, as for the following:

- Signs of hepatic insufficiency (eg, encephalopathy, ascites, ecchymoses) or GI bleeding: Coagulation profile (PT/PTT)
- Hepatitis risk factors (see Table 23–6) or a hepatocellular mechanism suggested by blood test results: Hepatitis viral and autoimmune serologic tests
- Fever, abdominal pain, and tenderness: CBC and, if patients appear ill, blood cultures

Suspicion of hemolysis can be confirmed by a peripheral blood smear.

Imaging is done if pain suggests extrahepatic obstruction or cholangitis or if blood test results suggest cholestasis.

Abdominal ultrasonography is usually done first; usually, it is highly accurate in detecting extrahepatic obstruction. CT and MRI are alternatives. Ultrasonography is usually more accurate for gallstones, and CT is more accurate for pancreatic lesions. All these tests can detect abnormalities in the biliary tree and focal liver lesions but are less accurate in detecting diffuse hepatocellular disorders (eg, hepatitis, cirrhosis).

If ultrasonography shows extrahepatic cholestasis, other tests may be necessary to determine the cause; usually, magnetic resonance cholangiopancreatography (MRCP), endoscopic ultrasonography (EUS), or ERCP is used. ERCP is more invasive but allows treatment of some obstructive lesions (eg, stone removal, stenting of strictures).

Liver biopsy is not commonly required but can help diagnose certain disorders (eg, disorders causing intrahepatic cholestasis, some kinds of hepatitis, some infiltrative disorders, Dubin-Johnson syndrome, hemochromatosis, Wilson disease). Biopsy can also help when liver enzyme abnormalities are unexplained by other tests.

Laparoscopy (peritoneoscopy) allows direct inspection of the liver and gallbladder without the trauma of a full laparotomy. Unexplained cholestatic jaundice warrants laparoscopy occasionally and diagnostic laparotomy rarely.

Treatment

The cause and any complications are treated. Jaundice itself requires no treatment in adults (unlike in neonates—see p. 2725). Itching, if bothersome, may be relieved with cholestyramine 2 to 8 g po bid. However, cholestyramine is ineffective in patients with complete biliary obstruction.

Geriatrics Essentials

Symptoms may be attenuated or missed in the elderly; eg, abdominal pain may be mild or absent in acute viral hepatitis. A sleep disturbance or mild confusion resulting from portosystemic encephalopathy may be misattributed to dementia.

KEY POINTS

- Suspect acute viral hepatitis in patients, particularly young and healthy patients, who have acute jaundice, particularly with a viral prodrome.
- Suspect biliary obstruction due to cancer in elderly patients with painless jaundice, weight loss, an abdominal mass, and minimal pruritus.
- Suspect hepatocellular dysfunction if aminotransferase levels are > 500 U/L and alkaline phosphatase elevation is < 3 times normal.
- Suspect cholestasis if aminotransferase levels are < 200 U/L and alkaline phosphatase elevation is > 3 times normal.
- Hepatic dysfunction is significant if mental status is altered and coagulopathy is present.

NONALCOHOLIC STEATOHEPATITIS

Nonalcoholic steatohepatitis (NASH) is a syndrome that develops in patients who are not alcoholic; it causes liver damage that is histologically indistinguishable from alcoholic hepatitis. It develops most often in patients with at least one of the following risk factors: obesity, dyslipidemia, and glucose intolerance. Pathogenesis is poorly understood but seems to be linked to insulin resistance (eg, as in obesity or metabolic syndrome). Most patients are asymptomatic. Laboratory findings include elevations in aminotransferase levels. Biopsy is required to confirm the diagnosis. Treatment includes elimination of causes and risk factors.

(See also the American Gastroenterological Association's Medical Position Statement on nonalcoholic fatty liver disease [NAFLD] at www.gastro.org.)

NASH (sometimes called steatonecrosis) is diagnosed most often in patients between 40 yr and 60 yr but can occur in all age groups. Many affected patients have obesity, type 2 diabetes mellitus (or glucose intolerance), dyslipidemia, and/or metabolic syndrome.

Pathophysiology

Pathophysiology involves fat accumulation (steatosis), inflammation, and, variably, fibrosis. Steatosis results from hepatic triglyceride accumulation. Possible mechanisms for steatosis include reduced synthesis of very low density lipoprotein (VLDL) and increased hepatic triglyceride synthesis (possibly due to decreased oxidation of fatty acids or increased free fatty acids being delivered to the liver). Inflammation may result from lipid peroxidative damage to cell membranes. These changes can stimulate hepatic stellate cells, resulting in fibrosis. If advanced, NASH can cause cirrhosis and portal hypertension.

Symptoms and Signs

Most patients are asymptomatic. However, some have fatigue, malaise, or right upper quadrant abdominal discomfort. Hepatomegaly develops in about 75% of patients. Splenomegaly may develop if advanced hepatic fibrosis is present and is usually the first indication that portal hypertension has developed. Patients with cirrhosis due to NASH can be asymptomatic and may lack the usual signs of chronic liver disease.

Diagnosis

- History (presence of risk factors, absence of excessive alcohol intake)
- Serologic tests that rule out hepatitis B and C
- Liver biopsy

The diagnosis should be suspected in patients with risk factors such as obesity, type 2 diabetes mellitus, or dyslipidemia and in patients with unexplained laboratory abnormalities suggesting liver disease. The most common laboratory abnormalities are elevations in aminotransferase levels. Unlike in alcoholic liver disease, the ratio of AST/ALT in NASH is usually < 1. Alkaline phosphatase and gamma–glutamyl transpeptidase (GGT) occasionally increase. Hyperbilirubinemia, prolongation of PT, and hypoalbuminemia are uncommon.

For diagnosis, strong evidence (such as a history corroborated by friends and relatives) that alcohol intake is not excessive (eg, is < 20 g/day) is needed, and serologic tests should show absence of hepatitis B and C (ie, hepatitis B surface antigen and hepatitis C virus antibody should be negative). Liver biopsy reveals damage similar to that seen in alcoholic hepatitis, usually including large fat droplets (macrovesicular fatty infiltration). Indications for biopsy include unexplained signs of portal hypertension (eg, splenomegaly, cytopenia) and unexplained elevations in aminotransferase levels that persist for > 6 mo in a patient with diabetes, obesity, or dyslipidemia.

Liver imaging tests, including ultrasonography, CT, and particularly MRI, may identify hepatic steatosis. However, these tests cannot identify the inflammation typical of NASH and cannot differentiate NASH from other causes of hepatic steatosis.

Prognosis

Prognosis is hard to predict. Probably, most patients do not develop hepatic insufficiency or cirrhosis. However, some drugs (eg, cytotoxic drugs) and metabolic disorders are associated with acceleration of NASH. Prognosis is often good unless complications (eg, variceal hemorrhage) develop.

Treatment

- Elimination of causes and control of risk factors

The only widely accepted treatment goal is to eliminate potential causes and risk factors. Such a goal may include discontinuation of drugs or toxins, weight loss, and treatment for dyslipidemia or treatment for hyperglycemia. Preliminary evidence suggests that thiazolidinediones and vitamin E can help correct biochemical and histologic abnormalities in NASH. Many other treatments (eg, ursodeoxycholic acid, metronidazole, metformin, betaine, glucagon, glutamine infusion) have not been proved effective.

KEY POINTS

- NASH causes histologic liver damage similar to that in alcoholic hepatitis but occurs in patients who are not alcoholics and who often are obese or have type 2 diabetes mellitus or dyslipidemia.
- Symptoms are usually absent, but some patients have right upper quadrant discomfort, fatigue, and/or malaise.
- Signs of portal hypertension and cirrhosis can eventually occur and may be the first manifestations.
- Rule out alcoholism (based on corroborated history) and hepatitis B and C (with serologic tests) and do a liver biopsy.
- Eliminate causes and control risk factors when possible.

PORTAL HYPERTENSION

Portal hypertension is elevated pressure in the portal vein. It is caused most often by cirrhosis (in developed countries), schistosomiasis (in endemic areas), or hepatic vascular abnormalities. Consequences include esophageal varices and portosystemic encephalopathy. Diagnosis is based on clinical criteria, often in conjunction with imaging tests and endoscopy. Treatment involves prevention of GI bleeding with endoscopy, drugs, or both and sometimes with portacaval shunting or liver transplantation.

The portal vein, formed by the superior mesenteric and splenic veins, drains blood from the abdominal GI tract, spleen, and pancreas into the liver. Within reticuloendothelium-lined blood channels (sinusoids), blood from the terminal portal venules merges with hepatic arterial blood. Blood flows out of the sinusoids via the hepatic veins into the inferior vena cava.

Normal portal pressure is 5 to 10 mm Hg (7 to 14 cm H_2O), which exceeds inferior vena caval pressure by 4 to 5 mm Hg (portal venous gradient). Higher values are defined as portal hypertension.

Etiology

Portal hypertension results mainly from increased resistance to blood flow in the portal vein. A common cause of this resistance is disease within the liver; uncommon causes include blockage of the splenic or portal vein and impaired hepatic venous outflow (see Table 23–8). Increased flow volume is a rare cause, although it often contributes to portal hypertension in cirrhosis and in hematologic disorders that cause massive splenomegaly.

Pathophysiology

In cirrhosis, tissue fibrosis and regeneration increase resistance in the sinusoids and terminal portal venules. However, other potentially reversible factors contribute; they include contractility of sinusoidal lining cells, production of vasoactive substances

Table 23–8. MOST COMMON CAUSES OF PORTAL HYPERTENSION

MECHANISM OR LOCATION	CAUSE
Prehepatic	
Obstruction	Portal or splenic vein thrombosis
Increased portal flow (rare)	Arteriovenous fistula Massive splenomegaly caused by a primary hematologic disorder
Hepatic	
Presinusoidal	Idiopathic portal hypertension Other periportal disorders (eg, primary biliary cirrhosis, sarcoidosis, congenital hepatic fibrosis) Schistosomiasis
Sinusoidal	Cirrhosis (all etiologies)
Postsinusoidal	Hepatic sinusoidal obstruction syndrome (hepatic veno-occlusive disease)
Posthepatic	
Obstruction	Hepatic vein thrombosis (Budd-Chiari syndrome) Obstruction of the inferior vena cava
Resistance to right heart filling	Constrictive pericarditis Restrictive cardiomyopathy

(eg, endothelins, nitric oxide), various systemic mediators of arteriolar resistance, and possibly swelling of hepatocytes.

Over time, portal hypertension creates portosystemic venous collaterals. They may slightly decrease portal vein pressure but can cause complications. Engorged serpentine submucosal vessels (varices) in the distal esophagus and sometimes in the gastric fundus can rupture, causing sudden, catastrophic GI bleeding. Bleeding rarely occurs unless the portal pressure gradient is > 12 mm Hg. Gastric mucosal vascular congestion (portal hypertensive gastropathy) can cause acute or chronic bleeding independent of varices. Visible abdominal wall collaterals are common; veins radiating from the umbilicus (caput medusae) are much rarer and indicate extensive flow in the umbilical and periumbilical veins. Collaterals around the rectum can cause rectal varices that can bleed.

Portosystemic collaterals shunt blood away from the liver. Thus, less blood reaches the liver when portal flow increases (diminished hepatic reserve). In addition, toxic substances from the intestine are shunted directly to the systemic circulation, contributing to portosystemic encephalopathy (see below). Venous congestion within visceral organs due to portal hypertension contributes to ascites via altered Starling forces. Splenomegaly and hypersplenism (see p. 1196) commonly occur as a result of increased splenic vein pressure. Thrombocytopenia, leukopenia, and, less commonly, hemolytic anemia may result.

Portal hypertension is often associated with a hyperdynamic circulation. Mechanisms are complex and seem to involve altered sympathetic tone, production of nitric oxide and other endogenous vasodilators, and enhanced activity of humoral factors (eg, glucagon).

Symptoms and Signs

Portal hypertension is asymptomatic; symptoms and signs result from its complications. The most dangerous is acute variceal bleeding (see p. 132). Patients typically present with sudden painless upper GI bleeding, often massive. Bleeding from portal hypertensive gastropathy is often subacute or chronic. Ascites, splenomegaly, or portosystemic encephalopathy may be present.

Diagnosis

- Usually clinical evaluation

Portal hypertension is assumed to be present when a patient with chronic liver disease has collateral circulation, splenomegaly, ascites, or portosystemic encephalopathy. Proof requires measurement of the hepatic venous pressure gradient, which approximates portal pressure, by a transjugular catheter; however, this procedure is invasive and usually not done. Imaging may help when cirrhosis is suspected. Ultrasonography or CT often reveals dilated intra-abdominal collaterals, and Doppler ultrasonography can determine portal vein patency and flow.

Esophagogastric varices and portal hypertensive gastropathy are best diagnosed by endoscopy, which may also identify predictors of esophagogastric variceal bleeding (eg, red markings on a varix).

Prognosis

Mortality during acute variceal hemorrhage may exceed 50%. Prognosis is predicted by the degree of hepatic reserve and the degree of bleeding. For survivors, the bleeding risk within the next 1 to 2 yr is 50 to 75%. Ongoing endoscopic or drug therapy lowers the bleeding risk but decreases long-term mortality only marginally. For treatment of acute bleeding, see pp. 131 and 132.

Treatment

- Ongoing endoscopic therapy and surveillance
- Nonselective beta-blockers with or without isosorbide mononitrate
- Sometimes portal vein shunting

When possible, the underlying disorder is treated. Long-term treatment of esophagogastric varices that have bled is a series of endoscopic banding sessions to obliterate residual varices, then periodic surveillance endoscopy for recurrent varices.

Long-term drug therapy for varices that have bled involves nonselective beta-blockers; these drugs lower portal pressure primarily by diminishing portal flow, although the effects vary. They include propranolol (40 to 80 mg po bid), nadolol (40 to 160 mg po once/day), timolol (10 to 20 po bid), and carvedilol (6.25 to 12.5 mg po bid), with dosage titrated to decrease heart rate by about 25%. Adding isosorbide mononitrate 10 to 20 mg po bid may further reduce portal pressure. Combined long-term endoscopic and drug therapy may be slightly more effective than either alone.

Patients who do not adequately respond to either treatment should be considered for transjugular intrahepatic portosystemic shunting (TIPS) or, less frequently, a surgical portacaval shunt. In TIPS, the shunt is created by placing a stent between the portal and hepatic venous circulation within the liver. (See also the American Association for the Study of Liver Disease's practice guideline The Role of Transjugular Intrahepatic Portosystemic Shunt (TIPS) in the Management of Portal Hypertension: Update 2009.) Although TIPS may result in fewer immediate deaths than surgical shunting, particularly during acute bleeding, maintenance of patency may require repeat procedures because the stent may become stenosed or occluded over time. Long-term benefits are unknown. Liver transplantation may be indicated for some patients.

For patients with varices that have not yet bled, nonselective beta-blockers lower the risk of bleeding.

For bleeding due to portal hypertensive gastropathy, drugs can be used to decrease portal pressure. A shunt should be considered if drugs are ineffective, but results may be less successful than for esophageal variceal bleeding.

Because it rarely causes clinical problems, hypersplenism requires no specific treatment, and splenectomy should be avoided.

KEY POINTS

- Portal hypertension is caused most often by cirrhosis (in developed countries), schistosomiasis (in endemic areas), or hepatic vascular abnormalities.
- Complications can include acute variceal bleeding (with a high mortality rate), ascites, splenomegaly, and portosystemic encephalopathy.
- Diagnose portal hypertension based on clinical findings.
- To help prevent acute variceal bleeding, initiate periodic surveillance and endoscopic banding sessions.
- To help prevent rebleeding, treat with nonselective beta-blockers with or without isosorbide mononitrate, TIPS, or both.

PORTOSYSTEMIC ENCEPHALOPATHY

Portosystemic encephalopathy is a neuropsychiatric syndrome. It most often results from high gut protein or acute metabolic stress (eg, GI bleeding, infection, electrolyte abnormality) in a patient with portosystemic shunting. Symptoms are mainly neuropsychiatric (eg, confusion, asterixis, coma). Diagnosis is based on clinical findings. Treatment is usually correction of the acute cause, a diet that includes

vegetable protein as the primary protein source, oral lactulose, and nonabsorbable antibiotics such as rifaximin.

(See also the American College of Gastroenterology's practice guideline Hepatic Encephalopathy online at http://s3.gi.org.) Portosystemic encephalopathy better describes the pathophysiology than hepatic encephalopathy or hepatic coma, but all 3 terms are used interchangeably.

Etiology

Portosystemic encephalopathy may occur in fulminant hepatitis caused by viruses, drugs, or toxins, but it more commonly occurs in cirrhosis or other chronic disorders when extensive portosystemic collaterals have developed as a result of portal hypertension. Encephalopathy may also follow portosystemic anastomoses, such as surgically created anastomoses connecting the portal vein and vena cava (portacaval shunts, transjugular intrahepatic portosystemic shunting [TIPS]).

Precipitants: In patients with chronic liver disease, acute episodes of encephalopathy are usually precipitated by reversible causes. The most common are the following:

- Metabolic stress (eg, infection; electrolyte imbalance, especially hypokalemia; dehydration; use of diuretic drugs)
- Conditions that increase gut protein (eg, GI bleeding, high-protein diet)
- Nonspecific cerebral depressants (eg, alcohol, sedatives, analgesics)

Pathophysiology

In portosystemic shunting, absorbed products that would otherwise be detoxified by the liver enter the systemic circulation and reach the brain, causing toxicity, particularly to the cerebral cortex. The substances causing brain toxicity are not precisely known. Ammonia, a product of protein digestion, is an important cause, but other factors (eg, alterations in cerebral benzodiazepine receptors and neurotransmission by gamma–aminobutyric acid [GABA]) may also contribute. Aromatic amino acid levels in serum are usually high and branched-chain levels are low, but these levels probably do not cause encephalopathy.

Symptoms and Signs

Symptoms and signs of encephalopathy tend to develop in progressive stages (see Table 23–9).

Symptoms usually do not become apparent until brain function is moderately impaired. Constructional apraxia, in which patients cannot reproduce simple designs (eg, a star), develops early. Agitation and mania can develop but are uncommon. A characteristic flapping tremor (asterixis) is elicited when patients hold their arms outstretched with wrists dorsiflexed. Neurologic deficits are usually symmetric. Neurologic signs in coma usually reflect bilateral diffuse hemispheric dysfunction. Signs of brain stem dysfunction develop only in advanced coma, often during the hours or days before death. A musty, sweet breath odor (fetor hepaticus) can occur regardless of the stage of encephalopathy.

Diagnosis

- Clinical evaluation
- Often adjunctive testing with psychometric evaluation, ammonia level, EEG, or a combination
- Exclusion of other treatable disorders

Diagnosis is ultimately based on clinical findings, but testing may help:

- Psychometric testing may reveal subtle neuropsychiatric deficits, which can help confirm early encephalopathy.
- Ammonia levels are usually measured.
- An EEG usually shows diffuse slow-wave activity, even in mild cases, and may be sensitive but is not specific for early encephalopathy.

CSF examination is not routinely necessary; the only usual abnormality is mild protein elevation.

Other potentially reversible disorders that could cause similar manifestations (eg, infection, subdural hematoma, hypoglycemia, intoxication) should be ruled out. If portosystemic encephalopathy is confirmed, the precipitating cause should be sought.

Prognosis

In chronic liver disease, correction of the precipitating cause usually causes encephalopathy to regress without permanent neurologic sequelae. Some patients, especially those with portacaval shunts or TIPS, require continuous therapy, and irreversible extrapyramidal signs or spastic paraparesis rarely develops. Coma (stage 4 encephalopathy) associated with fulminant hepatitis is fatal in up to 80% of patients despite

Table 23–9. CLINICAL STAGES OF PORTOSYSTEMIC ENCEPHALOPATHY

STAGE	COGNITION AND BEHAVIOR	NEUROMUSCULAR FUNCTION
0 (subclinical)	Asymptomatic loss of cognitive abilities	None
1	Sleep disturbances Impaired concentration Depression, anxiety, or irritability	Monotone voice Tremor Poor handwriting Constructional apraxia
2	Drowsiness Disorientation Poor short-term memory Disinhibited behavior	Ataxia Dysarthria Asterixis Automatisms (eg, yawning, blinking, sucking)
3	Somnolence Confusion Amnesia Anger, paranoia, or other bizarre behavior	Nystagmus Muscular rigidity Hyperreflexia or hyporeflexia
4	Coma	Dilated pupils Oculocephalic or oculovestibular reflexes Decerebrate posturing

intensive therapy; the combination of advanced chronic liver failure and portosystemic encephalopathy is often fatal.

Treatment

- Treatment of the cause
- Bowel cleansing using oral lactulose or enemas
- A diet with vegetable as the primary protein source
- Oral nonabsorbable antibiotics such as rifaximin and neomycin

Treating the cause usually reverses mild cases. Eliminating toxic enteric products is the other goal and is accomplished using several methods. The bowels should be cleared using enemas or, more often, oral lactulose syrup, which can be tube-fed to comatose patients. This synthetic disaccharide is an osmotic cathartic. It also lowers colonic pH, decreasing fecal ammonia production. The initial dosage, 30 to 45 mL po tid, should be adjusted to produce 2 or 3 soft stools daily. Dietary protein should be about 1.0 mg/kg/day, primarily from vegetable sources. Oral nonabsorbable antibiotics such as rifaximin and neomycin are effective for hepatic encephalopathy. Rifaximin is usually preferred because neomycin is an aminoglycoside, which can precipitate ototoxicity or nephrotoxicity.

Sedation deepens encephalopathy and should be avoided whenever possible. For coma caused by fulminant hepatitis, meticulous supportive and nursing care coupled with prevention and treatment of complications increase the chance of survival. High-dose corticosteroids, exchange transfusion, and other complex procedures designed to remove circulating toxins generally do not improve outcome. Patients deteriorating because of fulminant hepatic failure may be saved by liver transplantation.

Other potential therapies, including levodopa, bromocriptine, flumazenil, sodium benzoate, infusions of branched-chain amino acids, keto-analogs of essential amino acids, and prostaglandins, have not proved effective. Complex plasma-filtering systems (artificial liver) show some promise but require more study.

KEY POINTS

- Portosystemic encephalopathy is a neuropsychiatric syndrome that occurs when portosystemic shunting allows absorbed products that are normally detoxified by the liver to reach the brain.
- Manifestations include cognitive and behavioral dysfunction (eg, confusion, obtundation, coma) and neuromuscular dysfunction (eg, flapping tremor, ataxia, hyperreflexia or hyporeflexia).
- Diagnose portosystemic encephalopathy based mainly on clinical findings, but usually measure the blood ammonia level, and if signs are subtle or absent, do neuropsychologic testing.
- Exclude other treatable disorders (eg, subdural hematoma, hypoglycemia, intoxication), and search for triggers of encephalopathy (eg, infection, GI bleeding, electrolyte abnormality).
- Treat the cause of encephalopathy and treat encephalopathy itself with bowel cleansing (using oral lactulose or enemas), restriction of dietary protein to vegetable sources, and oral rifaximin or neomycin.

SPONTANEOUS BACTERIAL PERITONITIS

Spontaneous bacterial peritonitis (SBP) is infection of ascitic fluid without an apparent source. Manifestations may include fever, malaise, and symptoms of ascites and worsening hepatic failure. Diagnosis is by examination of ascitic fluid. Treatment is with cefotaxime or another antibiotic.

SBP is particularly common in cirrhotic ascites. This infection can cause serious sequelae or death. The most common bacteria causing SBP are gram-negative *Escherichia coli* and *Klebsiella pneumoniae* and gram-positive *Streptococcus pneumoniae*; usually only a single organism is involved.

Symptoms and Signs

Patients have symptoms and signs of ascites. Discomfort is usually present; it typically is diffuse, constant, and mild to moderate in severity.

Signs of SBP may include fever, malaise, encephalopathy, worsening hepatic failure, and unexplained clinical deterioration. Peritoneal signs (eg, abdominal tenderness and rebound) are present but may be somewhat diminished by the presence of ascitic fluid.

Diagnosis

- Diagnostic paracentesis

Clinical diagnosis of SBP can be difficult; diagnosis requires a high index of suspicion and liberal use of diagnostic paracentesis, including culture. Transferring ascitic fluid to blood culture media before incubation increases the sensitivity of culture to almost 70%. PMN count of > 250 cells/μL is diagnostic of SBP. Blood cultures are also indicated. Because SBP usually results from a single organism, finding mixed flora on culture suggests a perforated abdominal viscus or contaminated specimen.

Treatment

- Cefotaxime or another antibiotic

If SBP is diagnosed, an antibiotic such as cefotaxime 2 g IV q 4 to 8 h (pending Gram stain and culture results) is given for at least 5 days and until ascitic fluid shows < 250 PMNs/μL. Antibiotics increase the chance of survival. Because SBP recurs within a year in up to 70% of patients, prophylactic antibiotics are indicated; quinolones (eg, norfloxacin 400 mg po once/day) are most widely used.

Antibiotic prophylaxis in ascitic patients with variceal hemorrhage decreases the risk of SBP.

POSTOPERATIVE LIVER DYSFUNCTION

Mild liver dysfunction sometimes occurs after major surgery even in the absence of preexisting liver disorders. This dysfunction usually results from hepatic ischemia or poorly understood effects of anesthesia. Patients with preexisting well-compensated liver disease (eg, cirrhosis with normal liver function) usually tolerate surgery well. However, surgery can increase the severity of some preexisting liver disorders; eg, laparotomy may precipitate acute liver failure in a patient with viral or alcoholic hepatitis.

Postoperative jaundice: Diagnosis of postoperative jaundice requires liver function tests. Timing of symptoms also aids in diagnosis.

Multifactorial mixed hyperbilirubinemia is the most common reason for postoperative jaundice. It is caused by increased formation of bilirubin and decreased hepatic clearance. This disorder most often occurs after major surgery or trauma requiring multiple transfusions. Hemolysis, sepsis, resorption of hematomas, and blood transfusions can increase the bilirubin load; simultaneously, hypoxemia, hepatic ischemia, and other poorly understood factors impair hepatic function. This condition is usually maximal within a few days of operation. Hepatic insufficiency is rare, and hyperbilirubinemia typically resolves slowly but completely. Liver laboratory tests can often differentiate multifactorial mixed hyperbilirubinemia from hepatitis. In multifactorial mixed hyperbilirubinemia, severe hyperbilirubinemia with mild aminotransferase and alkaline phosphatase elevations are common. In hepatitis, aminotransferase levels are usually very high.

Postoperative hepatitis: Ischemic postoperative "hepatitis" results from insufficient liver perfusion, not inflammation. The cause is transient perioperative hypotension or hypoxia. Typically, aminotransferase levels increase rapidly (often > 1000 units/L), but bilirubin is only mildly elevated. Ischemic hepatitis is usually maximal within a few days of the operation and resolves within a few days.

Halothane-related hepatitis can result from use of anesthetics containing halothane or related agents. It usually develops within 2 wk, is often preceded by fever, and is sometimes accompanied by a rash and eosinophilia.

True postoperative hepatitis is now rare. It used to result mainly from transmission of hepatitis C virus during blood transfusion.

Postoperative cholestasis: The most common cause of postoperative cholestasis is extrahepatic biliary obstruction due to intra-abdominal complications or drugs given postoperatively. Intrahepatic cholestasis occasionally develops after major surgery, especially after abdominal or cardiovascular procedures (benign postoperative intrahepatic cholestasis). The pathogenesis is unknown, but the condition usually resolves slowly and spontaneously. Occasionally, postoperative cholestasis results from acute acalculous cholecystitis or pancreatitis.

SYSTEMIC ABNORMALITIES IN LIVER DISEASE

Liver disease often causes systemic symptoms and abnormalities (see also Portosystemic Encephalopathy on p. 192.)

Circulatory Abnormalities

Hypotension in advanced liver failure may contribute to renal dysfunction. The pathogenesis of thc hyperdynamic circulation (increased cardiac output and heart rate) and hypotension that develop in advanced liver failure or cirrhosis is poorly understood. However, peripheral arterial vasodilation probably contributes to both. Factors that may contribute in cirrhosis may include altered sympathetic tone, production of nitric oxide and other endogenous vasodilators, and enhanced activity of humoral factors (eg, glucagon).

For specific disorders of hepatic circulation (eg, Budd-Chiari syndrome), see Ch. 31.

Endocrine Abnormalities

Glucose intolerance, hyperinsulinism, insulin resistance, and hyperglucagonemia are often present in patients with cirrhosis; the elevated insulin levels reflect decreased hepatic degradation rather than increased secretion, whereas the opposite is true for hyperglucagonemia. Abnormal thyroid function tests may reflect altered hepatic handling of thyroid hormones and changes in plasma binding proteins rather than thyroid abnormalities.

Sexual effects are common. Chronic liver disease commonly impairs menstruation and fertility. Males with cirrhosis, especially alcoholics, often have both hypogonadism (including testicular atrophy, erectile dysfunction, decreased spermatogenesis) and feminization (gynecomastia, female habitus). The biochemical basis is not fully understood. Gonadotropin reserve of the hypothalamic-pituitary axis is often blunted. Circulating testosterone levels are low, resulting mainly from decreased synthesis but also from increased peripheral conversion to estrogens. Levels of estrogens other than estradiol are usually increased, but the relationship between estrogens and feminization is complex. These changes are more prevalent in alcoholic liver disease than in cirrhosis of other etiologies, suggesting that alcohol, rather than liver disease, may be the cause. In fact, evidence indicates that alcohol itself is toxic to the testes.

Hematologic Abnormalities

Anemia is common among patients with liver disease. Contributing factors may include blood loss, folate (folic acid) deficiency, hemolysis, marrow suppression by alcohol, and a direct effect of chronic liver disease.

Leukopenia and **thrombocytopenia** often accompany splenomegaly in advanced portal hypertension.

Clotting and coagulation abnormalities are common and complex. Hepatocellular dysfunction and inadequate absorption of vitamin K may impair liver synthesis of clotting factors. An abnormal PT, depending on the severity of hepatocellular dysfunction, may respond to parenteral phytonadione (vitamin K_1) 5 to 10 mg once/day for 2 to 3 days. Thrombocytopenia, disseminated intravascular coagulation, and fibrinogen abnormalities also contribute to clotting disturbances in many patients.

Renal and Electrolyte Abnormalities

Renal and electrolyte abnormalities are common, especially among patients with ascites.

Hypokalemia may result from excess urinary potassium loss due to increased circulating aldosterone, renal retention of ammonium ion in exchange for K, secondary renal tubular acidosis, or diuretic therapy. Management consists of giving oral potassium chloride supplements and withholding K-wasting diuretics.

Hyponatremia is common even though the kidneys may avidly retain sodium (see p. 184); it usually occurs with advanced hepatocellular disease and is difficult to correct. Relative water overload is more often responsible than total body sodium depletion; potassium depletion may also contribute. Water restriction and potassium supplements may help; diuretics that increase free water clearance can be used in severe or refractory cases. Saline solution IV is indicated only if profound hyponatremia causes seizures or if total body sodium depletion is suspected; it should be avoided in patients with cirrhosis and fluid retention because it worsens ascites and only temporarily increases serum sodium levels.

Advanced liver failure can alter acid-base balance, usually causing metabolic alkalosis. BUN levels are often low because of impaired liver synthesis; GI bleeding causes elevations because of an increased enteric load rather than renal impairment. When GI bleeding elevates BUN, normal creatinine values tend to confirm normal kidney function.

Renal failure in liver disease may reflect

- Rare disorders that directly affect both the kidneys and the liver (eg, carbon tetrachloride toxicity)
- Circulatory failure with decreased renal perfusion, with or without frank acute tubular necrosis
- Functional renal failure, often called hepatorenal syndrome

Hepatorenal syndrome: This syndrome consists of progressive oliguria and azotemia in the absence of structural damage to the kidney; it usually occurs in patients with fulminant hepatitis or advanced cirrhosis with ascites. Its unknown pathogenesis probably involves extreme vasodilation of the splanchnic arterial circulation, leading to decreased central arterial volume. Neural or humoral reductions in renocortical blood flow follow, resulting in a diminished glomerular filtration rate. Low urinary sodium concentration and benign sediment usually distinguish it from tubular necrosis, but prerenal azotemia may be more difficult to distinguish; in equivocal cases, response to a volume load should be assessed.

Once established, renal failure due to untreated hepatorenal syndrome is usually rapidly progressive and fatal (type 1 hepatorenal syndrome), although some cases are less severe, with stable milder renal insufficiency (type 2).

Combination therapy with vasoconstrictors (typically, midodrine, octreotide, or terlipressin) and volume expanders (typically, albumin) can be effective.

Liver transplantation is another accepted treatment for type 1 hepatorenal syndrome; transjugular intrahepatic portosystemic shunting (TIPS) shows some promise, but more study is needed.

24 Testing for Hepatic and Biliary Disorders

Diagnosis of liver and biliary system disorders may include laboratory tests, imaging tests, and liver biopsy. Individual tests, particularly those of liver biochemistry and excretion, often have limited sensitivity and specificity. A combination of tests often best defines the cause and severity of disease. Useful algorithms (eg, Model of End-Stage Liver Disease [MELD], Child-Pugh score) have incorporated clinical and laboratory features to predict survival in patients with decompensated cirrhosis.

LABORATORY TESTS OF THE LIVER AND GALLBLADDER

(See also the American Gastroenterological Association Medical Position Statement and Technical Review on evaluation of liver chemistry tests at www.gastrojournal.org.)

Laboratory tests are generally effective for the following:

- Detecting hepatic dysfunction
- Assessing the severity of liver injury
- Monitoring the course of liver diseases and the response to treatment
- Refining the diagnosis

Many tests of liver biochemistry and excretory performance are called liver function tests. However, rather than assessing liver function, several of these tests measure liver enzymes that are released into the bloodstream (eg, release of aminotransferases from injured liver cells or of alkaline phosphatase due to cholestasis). Only certain tests actually assess liver function by evaluating hepatobiliary excretion (eg, bilirubin) or the liver's synthetic capability (eg, PT, usually reported as the INR; albumin).

The most useful laboratory tests to screen for liver disorders are serum aminotransferases (the most commonly used liver function tests), bilirubin, and alkaline phosphatase. Certain patterns of biochemical abnormalities help distinguish hepatocellular injury from impaired bile excretion (cholestasis—see Table 24–1). Tests that detect viral hepatitis, liver inflammation, or altered immunoregulation include hepatitis serologic tests and measurement of immunoglobulins, antibodies, and autoantibodies.

A few laboratory tests are diagnostic by themselves; they include the following:

- IgM antibody to hepatitis A virus (anti-HAV) for acute hepatitis A
- Hepatitis B surface antigen (HBsAg) for hepatitis B
- Antibody to hepatitis C virus (anti-HCV) and HCV-RNA for hepatitis C
- Antimitochondrial antibody for primary biliary cirrhosis
- Serum ceruloplasmin (reduced) and urinary copper (elevated) for Wilson disease
- Serum α_1-antitrypsin for α_1-antitrypsin deficiency
- α-Fetoprotein for hepatocellular carcinoma

Tests for Liver Injury

Aminotransferases: Alanine aminotransferase (ALT) and aspartate aminotransferase (AST) leak from damaged cells; thus, these enzymes are sensitive indicators of liver injury. Markedly high values (> 500 IU/L; normal, ≤ 40 IU/L), which indicate acute hepatocellular necrosis or injury, usually result from the following:

- Acute viral hepatitis
- Toxin- or drug-induced hepatitis
- Ischemic hepatitis or hepatic infarction

High levels continue usually for days or, in viral hepatitis, for weeks. The degree of elevation may not reflect the extent of liver injury. Serial measurements better reflect severity and prognosis than does a single measurement. A fall to normal indicates recovery unless accompanied by an increase in bilirubin and in PT or INR (which indicates fulminant liver failure). Fulminant liver failure results in fewer liver cells that can leak enzymes.

Aminotransferase levels may also be markedly high in the following:

- Acute exacerbation of autoimmune hepatitis
- Reactivation of chronic hepatitis B
- Acute Budd-Chiari syndrome
- Acute fatty liver of pregnancy
- Passage of a common duct stone

Modest elevations (300 to 500 IU/L) persist in chronic liver disorders (eg, chronic hepatitis, alcoholic hepatitis) and in biliary obstruction, except when passage of a common duct stone can transiently result in markedly high levels, sometimes into the thousands.

Mild increases (< 300 IU/L) are nonspecific and often present in disorders such as

- Cirrhosis secondary to viral hepatitis
- Nonalcoholic fatty liver disease (NAFLD)
- Cholestatic liver disorders
- Hepatocellular cancer

Aminotransferases can be normal in certain liver disorders, such as

- Hemochromatosis
- Methotrexate- or amiodarone-induced liver injury
- Chronic hepatitis C
- NAFLD

Table 24–1. COMMON PATTERNS OF LABORATORY TEST ABNORMALITIES

PATTERN	AMINOTRANSFERASE ELEVATIONS	ALKALINE PHOSPHATASE ELEVATIONS	PROLONGATION OF PT
Acute necrosis or injury	Marked	Often present but may be mild	Prolonged if hepatic function is severely impaired
Chronic hepatocellular disease	Mild to moderate	Often present but may be mild	Prolonged if hepatic function is severely impaired
Cholestasis	Often present but may be mild	Marked	Prolonged if chronic steatorrhea causes vitamin K malabsorption Can be corrected with parenteral (usually sc) vitamin K
Infiltration	Mild	Mild to moderate	Not usually prolonged
Liver failure	Depend on cause	Depend on cause	Prolonged but often only slightly if failure is chronic

Elevated ALT is somewhat specific for liver injury. Because AST is present in the heart, skeletal muscle, kidneys, and pancreas, elevated AST may reflect rhabdomyolysis or injury to one of these organs. In most liver disorders, the ratio of AST to ALT is < 1. However, in alcohol-related liver disease, the ratio is characteristically > 2 because pyridoxal-5'-phosphate is deficient in alcoholic patients; it is required for ALT synthesis but is less essential for AST synthesis. This deficiency also explains why elevations of ALT and AST are low (< 300 IU/L) in alcoholic patients.

Lactate dehydrogenase: LDH, commonly included in routine analysis, is present in many other tissues and is insensitive and nonspecific for hepatocellular injury. LDH is typically elevated in ischemic hepatitis and cancers that extensively infiltrate the liver.

Tests for Cholestasis

Bilirubin: Bilirubin, the pigment in bile, is produced from the breakdown of heme proteins, mostly from the heme moiety of hemoglobin in senescent RBCs. Unconjugated (free) bilirubin is insoluble in water and thus cannot be excreted in urine; most unconjugated bilirubin is bound to albumin in plasma. Bilirubin is conjugated in the liver with glucuronic acid to form the more water-soluble bilirubin diglucuronide. Conjugated bilirubin is then excreted through the biliary tract into the duodenum, where it is metabolized into urobilinogens (some of which are reabsorbed and resecreted into bile), then into orange-colored urobilins (most of which are eliminated in feces). These bile pigments give stool its typical color.

Hyperbilirubinemia results from one or more of the following:

- Increased bilirubin production
- Decreased liver uptake or conjugation
- Decreased biliary excretion

Normally, total bilirubin is mostly unconjugated, with values of < 1.2 mg/dL (< 20 μmol/L). Fractionation measures the proportion of bilirubin that is conjugated (ie, direct, so-called because it is measured directly, without the need for solvents). Fractionation is most helpful for evaluating neonatal jaundice and for evaluating elevated bilirubin when other liver test results are normal, suggesting that hepatobiliary dysfunction is not the cause.

Unconjugated hyperbilirubinemia (indirect bilirubin fraction > 85%) reflects increased bilirubin production (eg, in hemolysis) or defective liver uptake or conjugation (eg, in Gilbert syndrome). Such increases in unconjugated bilirubin are usually < 5 times normal (to < 6 mg/dL [< 100 μmol/L]) unless there is concurrent liver injury.

Conjugated hyperbilirubinemia (direct bilirubin fraction > 50%) results from decreased bile formation or excretion (cholestasis). When associated with other liver function test abnormalities, a high serum bilirubin indicates hepatocellular dysfunction. Serum bilirubin is somewhat insensitive for liver dysfunction. However, the development of severe hyperbilirubinemia in primary biliary cirrhosis, alcoholic hepatitis, and acute liver failure suggests a poor prognosis.

Bilirubinuria reflects the presence of conjugated bilirubin in urine; bilirubin spills into urine because blood levels are markedly elevated, indicating severe disease. Unconjugated bilirubin is water insoluble and bound to albumin and so cannot be excreted in urine. Bilirubinuria can be detected at the bedside with commercial urine test strips in acute viral hepatitis or other hepatobiliary disorders, even before jaundice appears. However, the diagnostic accuracy of such urine tests is limited. Results can be falsely negative when the urine specimen has been stored a long time, vitamin C has been ingested, or urine contains nitrates (eg, due to UTIs). Similarly, increases in urobilinogen are neither specific nor sensitive.

Alkaline phosphatase: Increased levels of this hepatocyte enzyme suggest cholestasis. Results may not be specific because alkaline phosphatase consists of several isoenzymes and has a widespread extrahepatic distribution (eg, in the placenta, the small intestine, WBCs, kidneys, and particularly bone).

Alkaline phosphatase levels increase to ≥ 4 times normal 1 to 2 days after onset of biliary obstruction, regardless of the site of obstruction. Levels may remain elevated for several days after the obstruction resolves because the half-life of alkaline phosphatase is about 7 days. Increases of up to 3 times normal occur in many liver disorders, including

- Hepatitis
- Cirrhosis
- Space-occupying lesions (eg, carcinoma)
- Infiltrative disorders (eg, amyloidosis, sarcoidosis, TB, metastases, abscesses)
- Syphilitic hepatitis (alkaline phosphatase may be disproportionately elevated compared with the modest changes in other liver tests)

Isolated elevations (ie, when other liver test results are normal) may accompany

- Focal liver lesions (eg, abscess, tumor)
- Partial or intermittent bile duct obstruction (eg, stone, stricture, cholangiocarcinoma)
- Syphilitic hepatitis
- Occasionally infiltrative disorders

Isolated elevations also occur in the absence of any apparent liver or biliary disorder, as in the following:

- Some cancers without apparent liver involvement (eg, bronchogenic carcinoma, Hodgkin lymphoma, renal cell carcinoma)
- After ingestion of fatty meals (because of an enzyme produced in the small intestine)
- Pregnancy (because of an enzyme produced in the placenta)
- Children and adolescents who are still growing (because of bone growth)
- Chronic renal failure (because of an enzyme produced in the intestine and bone)

Levels of γ-glutamyl transpeptidase or 5′-nucleotidase, which are more specific to the liver, can differentiate hepatic from extrahepatic sources of alkaline phosphatase better than fractionation of alkaline phosphatase, which is technically difficult. Also, in otherwise asymptomatic elderly people, an increase in alkaline phosphatase usually originates in bone (eg, in Paget disease) and does not require further investigation for liver injury.

5′-Nucleotidase: Increases in levels of this enzyme are as sensitive as alkaline phosphatase for detecting cholestasis and biliary obstruction but are more specific, almost always indicating hepatobiliary dysfunction. Because levels of alkaline phosphatase and 5′-nucleotidase do not always correlate, one can be normal while the other is increased.

γ-Glutamyl transpeptidase (GGT): Levels of this enzyme increase in hepatobiliary dysfunction, especially cholestasis, and correlate loosely with levels of alkaline phosphatase and 5′-nucleotidase. Levels do not increase because of bone lesions, during childhood, or during pregnancy. However, alcohol and certain drugs (eg, some anticonvulsants, warfarin) can induce hepatic microsomal (cytochrome P-450) enzymes, markedly increasing GGT and thus somewhat limiting its specificity.

Tests of Hepatic Synthetic Capacity

PT and INR: PT may be expressed in time (sec) or, preferably, as a ratio of the patient's measured PT to the laboratory's control value (INR—see p. 1132). The INR is more accurate than PT for monitoring anticoagulation. PT or INR is a valuable measure of the liver's ability to synthesize fibrinogen and vitamin K–dependent clotting factors: factors II (prothrombin), V, VII, and X. Changes can occur rapidly because some of the involved clotting factors have short biologic half-lives (eg, 6 h for factor VII). Abnormalities indicate severe hepatocellular dysfunction, an ominous sign in acute liver disorders. In chronic liver disorders, an increasing PT or INR indicates progression to liver failure. The PT or INR does not increase in mild hepatocellular dysfunction and is often normal in cirrhosis.

A prolonged PT and an abnormal INR can result from coagulation disorders such as a consumptive coagulopathy or vitamin K deficiency. Fat malabsorption, including cholestasis, can cause vitamin K deficiency. In chronic cholestasis, marked hepatocellular dysfunction can be ruled out if vitamin K replacement (10 mg sc) corrects PT by ≥ 30% within 24 h.

Serum proteins: Hepatocytes synthesize most serum proteins, including α- and β-globulins, albumin, and most clotting factors (but not factor VIII, produced by the vascular endothelium, or γ-globulin, produced by B cells). Hepatocytes also make proteins that aid in the diagnosis of specific disorders:

- α_1-Antitrypsin (absent in α_1-antitrypsin deficiency)
- Ceruloplasmin (reduced in Wilson disease)
- Transferrin (saturated with iron in hemochromatosis)
- Ferritin (greatly increased in hemochromatosis)

These proteins usually increase in response to damage (eg, inflammation) to various tissues, so that elevations may not specifically reflect liver disorders.

Serum albumin commonly decreases in chronic liver disorders because of an increase in volume of distribution (eg, due to ascites), a decrease in hepatic synthesis, or both. Values < 3 g/dL (< 30 g/L) suggest decreased synthesis, caused by one of the following:

- Advanced cirrhosis (the most common cause)
- Alcoholism
- Chronic inflammation
- Protein undernutrition

Hypoalbuminemia can also result from excessive loss of albumin from the kidneys (ie, nephrotic syndrome), gut (eg, due to protein-losing gastroenteropathies), or skin (eg, due to burns or exfoliative dermatitis).

Because albumin has a half-life of about 20 days, serum levels take weeks to increase or decrease.

Other Laboratory Tests

Ammonia: Nitrogen compounds that enter the colon (eg, ingested protein, secreted urea) are degraded by resident bacteria, liberating ammonia. The ammonia is then absorbed and transported via the portal vein to the liver. The healthy liver readily clears the ammonia from the portal vein and converts it to glutamine, which is metabolized by the kidneys into urea to be excreted. In patients with portosystemic shunting, the diseased liver does not clear ammonia, which then enters the systemic circulation, possibly contributing to portosystemic (hepatic) encephalopathy. Elevated ammonia levels occur in hepatic encephalopathy, but levels may be falsely low or high. In advanced liver disorders, the following may increase ammonia levels:

- High-protein meals
- GI bleeding
- Hypokalemia
- Metabolic alkalosis
- Certain drugs (eg, alcohol, barbiturates, diuretics, opioids, valproate)
- High-dose chemotherapy
- Parenteral nutrition
- Renal insufficiency
- Extreme muscle exertion and muscle wasting
- Salicylate intoxication
- Shock
- Ureterosigmoidostomy
- UTI with a urease-producing organism (eg, *Proteus mirabilis*)

Because the degree of elevation in the ammonia level correlates poorly with severity of hepatic encephalopathy, this level has limited usefulness in monitoring therapy.

Serum immunoglobulins: In chronic liver disorders, serum immunoglobulins often increase. However, elevations are not specific and are usually not helpful clinically. Levels increase slightly in acute hepatitis, moderately in chronic active hepatitis, and markedly in autoimmune hepatitis. The pattern of immunoglobulin elevation adds little information, although different immunoglobulins are usually very high in different disorders:

- IgM in primary biliary cirrhosis
- IgA in alcoholic liver disease
- IgG in autoimmune hepatitis

Antimitochondrial antibodies: These heterogeneous antibodies are positive, usually in high titers, in > 95% of patients with primary biliary cirrhosis. They are also occasionally present in the following:

- Autoimmune hepatitis
- Drug-induced hepatitis
- Other autoimmune disorders, such as connective tissue disorders, myasthenia gravis, autoimmune thyroiditis, Addison disease, and autoimmune hemolytic anemia

Antimitochondrial antibodies can help determine the cause of cholestasis because they are usually absent in extrahepatic biliary obstruction and primary sclerosing cholangitis.

Other antibodies: Other antibodies may help in diagnosis of the following:

- Autoimmune hepatitis: Smooth muscle antibodies against actin, antinuclear antibodies (ANA) that provide a homogeneous (diffuse) fluorescence, and antibodies to liver-kidney microsome type 1 (anti-LKM1) are often present.
- Primary biliary cirrhosis: Antimitochondrial antibody is key to the diagnosis.
- Primary sclerosing cholangitis: Perinuclear antineutrophil cytoplasmic antibodies (p-ANCA) can help raise the index of suspicion.

Isolated abnormalities of any of these antibodies are never diagnostic and do not elucidate pathogenesis.

α-Fetoprotein (AFP): AFP, a glycoprotein normally synthesized by the yolk sac in the embryo and then by the fetal liver, is elevated in neonates and hence the pregnant mother. AFP decreases rapidly during the first year of life, reaching adult values (normally, < 10 to 20 ng/mL or < 10 to 20 mg/L depending on the laboratory) by the age of 1 yr. An increase in AFP, no matter how small, should prompt consideration of primary hepatocellular carcinoma (HCC). Serum AFP generally correlates with tumor size, differentiation and metastatic involvement. Because small tumors may produce low levels of AFP, increasing values suggest the presence of HCC, especially when tumors are > 3 cm diameter. AFP also helps predict prognosis.

Mild AFP elevations also occur in acute and chronic hepatitis, probably reflecting liver regeneration; AFP can occasionally increase to 500 ng/mL in fulminant hepatitis. High AFP levels can occur in a few other disorders (eg, embryonic teratocarcinomas, hepatoblastomas in children, some hepatic metastases from GI tract cancers, some cholangiocarcinomas), but these circumstances are not common and usually can be differentiated based on clinical and histopathologic grounds.

Sensitivity, specificity, and peak levels of AFP in patients with HCC vary by population, reflecting differences in factors such as hepatitis prevalence and ethnicity. In areas with a relatively low prevalence of hepatitis (eg, North America, western Europe), AFP cutoff values of 20 ng/mL have a sensitivity of 39 to 64% and a specificity of 76 to 91%. However, not all HCCs produce AFP. Thus, AFP is not an ideal screening test but does have a role in detecting HCC. Levels exceeding normal (> 20 ng/mL), especially when increasing, strongly suggest HCC. In cirrhotic patients with a mass and a high value (eg, > 200 ng/mL), the predictive value is high. The combined use of AFP and ultrasonography currently provides the best surveillance.

IMAGING TESTS OF THE LIVER AND GALLBLADDER

Imaging is essential for accurately diagnosing biliary tract disorders and is important for detecting focal liver lesions (eg, abscess, tumor). It is limited in detecting and diagnosing diffuse hepatocellular disease (eg, hepatitis, cirrhosis).

Ultrasonography: Ultrasonography, traditionally done transabdominally and requiring a period of fasting, provides structural, but not functional, information. It is the least expensive, safest, and most sensitive technique for imaging the biliary system, especially the gallbladder. Ultrasonography is the procedure of choice for

- Screening for biliary tract abnormalities
- Evaluating the hepatobiliary tract in patients with right upper quadrant abdominal pain
- Differentiating intrahepatic from extrahepatic causes of jaundice
- Detecting liver masses

The kidneys, pancreas, and blood vessels are also often visible on hepatobiliary ultrasounds. Ultrasonography can measure spleen size and thus help diagnose splenomegaly, which suggests portal hypertension.

Use of endoscopic ultrasonography may further refine the approaches to hepatobiliary abnormalities.

Ultrasonography can be difficult in patients with intestinal gas or obesity and is operator-dependent. Endoscopic ultrasonography incorporates an ultrasound transducer into the tip of an endoscope and thus provides greater image resolution even when intestinal gas is present.

Gallstones cast intense echoes with distal acoustic shadowing that move with gravity. Transabdominal ultrasonography is extremely accurate (sensitivity > 95%) for gallstones > 2 mm in diameter. Endoscopic ultrasonography can detect stones as small as 0.5 mm (microlithiasis) in the gallbladder or biliary system. Transabdominal and endoscopic ultrasonography can also identify biliary sludge (a mixture of particulate material and bile) as low-level echoes that layer in the dependent portion of the gallbladder without acoustic shadowing.

Cholecystitis typically causes

- A thickened gallbladder wall (> 3 mm)
- Pericholecystic fluid
- An impacted stone in the gallbladder neck
- Tenderness when the gallbladder is palpated with the ultrasound probe (ultrasonographic Murphy sign)

Extrahepatic obstruction is indicated by dilated bile ducts. On transabdominal and endoscopic ultrasounds, bile ducts stand out as echo-free tubular structures. The diameter of the common duct is normally < 6 mm, increases slightly with age, and can reach 10 mm after cholecystectomy. Dilated ducts are virtually pathognomonic for extrahepatic obstruction in the appropriate clinical setting. Ultrasonography can miss early or intermittent obstruction that does not dilate the ducts. Transabdominal ultrasonography may not reveal the level or cause of biliary obstruction (eg, sensitivity for common duct stones is < 40%). Endoscopic ultrasonography has a better yield.

Focal liver lesions > 1 cm in diameter can usually be detected by transabdominal ultrasonography. In general, cysts are echo-free; solid lesions (eg, tumors, abscesses) tend to be echogenic. Carcinoma appears as a nonspecific solid mass. Ultrasonography has been used to screen for HCC in patients at high risk (eg, with chronic hepatitis B, cirrhosis, or hemochromatosis). Because ultrasonography can localize focal lesions, it can be used to guide aspiration and biopsy.

Diffuse disorders (eg, cirrhosis, sometimes fatty liver) can be detected with ultrasonography. Ultrasound elastography can measure liver stiffness as an index of hepatic fibrosis. In this procedure, the transducer emits a vibration that induces an elastic shear wave. The rate at which the wave is propagated through the liver is measured; liver stiffness speeds this propagation.

Doppler ultrasonography: This noninvasive method is used to assess direction of blood flow and patency of blood vessels around the liver, particularly the portal vein. Clinical uses include

- Detecting portal hypertension, (eg, indicated by significant collateral flow and the direction of flow)
- Assessing the patency of liver shunts (eg, surgical portocaval, percutaneous transhepatic)
- Evaluating portal vein patency before liver transplantation and detecting hepatic artery thrombosis after transplantation
- Detecting unusual vascular structures (eg, cavernous transformation of the portal vein)
- Assessing tumor vascularity before surgery

CT: CT is commonly used to identify hepatic masses, particularly small metastases, with an accuracy of about 80%. It is considered the most accurate imaging technique. CT with IV contrast is accurate for diagnosing cavernous hemangiomas of the liver as well as differentiating them from other abdominal masses. Neither obesity nor intestinal gas obscures CT images. CT can detect fatty liver and the increased hepatic density that occurs with iron overload. CT is less helpful than ultrasonography in identifying biliary obstruction but often provides the best assessment of the pancreas.

Cholescintigraphy: After patients fast, an IV technetium-labeled iminodiacetic compound (eg, hydroxy or diisopropyl iminodiacetic acid [HIDA or DISIDA]) is injected; these substances are taken up by the liver and excreted in bile, then enter the gallbladder.

In acute calculous cholecystitis, which is usually caused by impaction of a stone in the cystic duct, the gallbladder does not appear on a scintigraphic scan because the radionuclide cannot enter the gallbladder. Such nonvisualization is diagnostically quite accurate (except for false-positive results in some critically ill patients). However, cholescintigraphy is rarely needed clinically to diagnose acute cholecystitis.

If acalculous cholecystitis is suspected, the gallbladder is scanned before and after administration of cholecystokinin (used to initiate gallbladder contraction). The decrease in scintigraphic counts indicates the gallbladder ejection fraction. Reduced emptying, measured as the ejection fraction, suggests acalculous cholecystitis.

Cholescintigraphy also detects bile leaks (eg, after surgery or trauma) and anatomic abnormalities (eg, congenital choledochal cysts, choledochoenteric anastomoses). After cholecystectomy, cholescintigraphy can quantitate biliary flow; biliary flow helps identify sphincter of Oddi dysfunction.

Radionuclide liver scanning: Ultrasonography and CT have largely supplanted radionuclide scanning, which had been used to diagnose diffuse liver disorders and mass lesions of the liver. Radionuclide scanning shows the distribution of an injected radioactive tracer, usually technetium (^{99m}Tc sulfur colloid), which distributes uniformly within the normal liver. Space-occupying lesions > 4 cm, such as liver cysts, abscesses, metastases, and tumors, appear as defects. Diffuse liver disorders (eg, cirrhosis, hepatitis) decrease liver uptake of the tracer, with more appearing in the spleen and bone marrow. In hepatic vein obstruction (Budd-Chiari syndrome), liver uptake is decreased except in the caudate lobe because its drainage into the inferior vena cava is preserved.

Plain x-ray of the abdomen: Plain x-rays are not usually useful for diagnosis of hepatobiliary disorders. They are insensitive for gallstones unless the gallstones are calcified and large. Plain x-rays can detect a calcified (porcelain) gallbladder. Rarely, in gravely ill patients, x-rays show air in the biliary tree, which suggests emphysematous cholangitis.

MRI: MRI is used to image blood vessels (without using contrast), ducts, and hepatic tissues. Its clinical uses are still evolving. MRI is superior to CT and ultrasonography for diagnosing diffuse liver disorders (eg, fatty liver, hemochromatosis) and for clarifying some focal defects (eg, hemangiomas). MRI also shows blood flow and therefore complements Doppler ultrasonography and CT angiography in the diagnosis of vascular abnormalities and in vascular mapping before liver transplantation.

Magnetic resonance cholangiopancreatography (MRCP) is more sensitive than CT or ultrasonography in diagnosing common bile duct abnormalities, particularly stones. Its images of the biliary system and pancreatic ducts are comparable to those obtained with ERCP and percutaneous transhepatic cholangiography, which are more invasive. Thus, MRCP is a useful screening tool when biliary obstruction is suspected and before therapeutic ERCP (eg, for simultaneous imaging and stone removal) is done.

ERCP: ERCP combines endoscopy through the second portion of the duodenum with contrast imaging of the biliary and pancreatic ducts. The papilla of Vater is cannulated through an endoscope placed in the descending duodenum, and the pancreatic and biliary ducts are then injected with a contrast agent.

ERCP provides detailed images of much of the upper GI tract and the periampullary area, biliary tract, and pancreas. ERCP can also be used to obtain tissue for biopsy. ERCP is the best test for diagnosis of ampullary cancers. ERCP is as accurate as endoscopic ultrasonography for diagnosis of common duct stones. Because it is invasive, ERCP is used more for treatment (including simultaneous diagnosis and treatment) than for diagnosis alone. ERCP is the procedure of choice for treating biliary and pancreatic obstructing lesions, as for

- Removal of bile duct stones
- Stenting of strictures (inflammatory or malignant)
- Sphincterotomy (eg, for sphincter of Oddi dysfunction)

Morbidity from a diagnostic ERCP with only injection of contrast material is about 1%. Adding sphincterotomy raises morbidity to 4 to 9% (mainly due to pancreatitis and bleeding). ERCP with manometry to measure sphincter of Oddi pressure causes pancreatitis in up to 25% of patients.

Percutaneous transhepatic cholangiography (PTC): With fluoroscopic or ultrasound guidance, the liver is punctured with a needle, the peripheral intrahepatic bile duct system is cannulated above the common hepatic duct, and a contrast agent is injected.

PTC is highly accurate in diagnosing biliary disorders and can be therapeutic (eg, decompression of the biliary system, insertion of an endoprosthesis). However, ERCP is usually preferred because PTC causes more complications (eg, sepsis, bleeding, bile leaks).

Operative cholangiography: A contrast agent is directly injected during laparotomy to image the bile duct system.

Operative cholangiography is indicated when jaundice occurs and noninvasive procedures are equivocal, suggesting common duct stones. The procedure can be followed by common duct exploration for removal of biliary stones. Technical difficulties have limited its use, particularly during laparoscopic cholecystectomy.

LIVER BIOPSY

Liver biopsy provides histologic information about liver structure and evidence of liver injury (type and degree, any fibrosis); this information can be essential not only to diagnosis but also to staging, prognosis, and management. Although only a small core of tissue is obtained, it is usually representative, even for focal lesions.

Liver biopsy is usually done percutaneously at the bedside or with ultrasound guidance. Ultrasound guidance is preferred because its complication rate is slightly lower and it provides opportunity to visualize the liver and target focal lesions.

Indications: Generally, biopsy is indicated for suspected liver abnormalities that are not identified by less invasive methods or that require histopathology for staging (see Table 24–2). Biopsy is especially valuable for detecting TB or other granulomatous infiltrations and for clarifying graft problems (ischemic injury, rejection, biliary tract disorders, viral hepatitis) after liver transplantation. Serial biopsies, commonly done over years, may be necessary to monitor disease progression.

Gross examination and histopathology are often definitive. Cytology (fine-needle aspiration), frozen section, and culture may be useful for selected patients. Metal content (eg, copper in suspected Wilson disease, iron in hemochromatosis) can be measured in the biopsy specimen.

Limitations of liver biopsy include

- Sampling error
- Occasional errors or uncertainty in cases of cholestasis
- Need for a skilled histopathologist (some pathologists have little experience with needle specimens)

Contraindications: Absolute contraindications to liver biopsy include

- Patient's inability to remain still and to maintain brief expiration for the procedure
- Suspected vascular lesion (eg, hemangioma)
- Bleeding tendency (eg, INR > 1.2 despite receiving vitamin K, bleeding time > 10 min)
- Severe thrombocytopenia (< 50,000/mL)

Relative contraindications include profound anemia, peritonitis, marked ascites, high-grade biliary obstruction, and a subphrenic or right pleural infection or effusion. Nonetheless, percutaneous liver biopsy is sufficiently safe to be done on an outpatient basis. Mortality is 0.01%. Major complications (eg, intra-abdominal hemorrhage, bile peritonitis, lacerated liver) develop in about 2% of patients. Complications usually become evident within 3 to 4 h—the recommended period for monitoring patients.

Other routes: Transjugular venous biopsy of the liver is more invasive than the percutaneous route; it is reserved for patients with a severe coagulopathy. The procedure involves cannulating the right internal jugular vein and passing a catheter through the inferior vena cava into the hepatic vein. A fine needle is then advanced through the hepatic vein into the liver. Biopsy is successful in > 95% of patients. Complication rate is low; 0.2% bleed from puncture of the liver capsule.

Occasionally, liver biopsy is done during surgery (eg, laparoscopy); a larger, more targeted tissue sample can then be obtained.

Table 24–2. INDICATIONS FOR LIVER BIOPSY*

CONDITION	USE
Unexplained liver test abnormalities	Diagnosis
Alcoholic liver disease or nonalcoholic steatosis	Diagnosis and staging
Chronic hepatitis (viral or autoimmune)	Diagnosis and staging
Heavy metal storage disorders (eg, hemochromatosis, Wilson disease)	Diagnosis
Suspected rejection or another complication after liver transplantation	Diagnosis
Liver donor status	Evaluation
Hepatosplenomegaly of unknown cause	Diagnosis
Unexplained intrahepatic cholestasis (usually primary biliary cirrhosis or primary sclerosing cholangitis)	Diagnosis
Suspected cancer or unexplained focal lesions	Diagnosis
Unexplained systemic illness (eg, fever of unknown origin, inflammatory or granulomatous disorders)	Diagnosis (culture is done)
Use of hepatotoxic drugs (eg, methotrexate)	Monitoring

*Generally, biopsy is indicated for suspected liver abnormalities that are not identified by less invasive methods or that require histopathology for staging.

25 Alcoholic Liver Disease

(See also the 2010 American College of Gastroenterology's practice guidelines for alcoholic liver disease online at http://gi.org.)

Alcohol consumption is high in most Western countries. Among US adults, about 4.6% meet DSM-IV criteria for alcohol abuse and 3.8% for alcohol dependence. The male:female ratio is about 2:1. Disorders that occur in alcohol abusers, often in sequence, include

- Fatty liver (in > 90%)
- Alcoholic hepatitis (in 10 to 35%)
- Cirrhosis (in 10 to 20%)

Hepatocellular carcinoma may also develop in patients with cirrhosis, especially if iron accumulation coexists.

Risk Factors

The main risk factors for alcoholic liver disease are

- Quantity and duration of alcohol use (usually > 8 yr)
- Sex
- Genetic and metabolic traits
- Obesity

Quantity of alcohol: Among susceptible people, a linear correlation generally exists between the amount and duration of alcohol use and the development of liver disease.

Alcohol content is estimated to be the beverage volume (in mL) multiplied by its percentage of alcohol. For example, the alcohol content of 45 mL of an 80-proof (40% alcohol) beverage is 18 mL by volume. Each mL contains about 0.79 g of alcohol. Although values can vary, the percentage of alcohol averages 2 to 7% for most beers and 10 to 15% for most wines.

Thus, a 12-oz glass of beer contains between about 5 to 20 g of alcohol, and a 5-oz glass of wine contains between about 12 to 18 g, and a 1 1/2-oz shot of hard liquor contains about 14 g.

Risk of liver disease increases markedly for men who drink > 40 g, particularly > 80 g, of alcohol/day (eg, about 2 to 8 cans of beer, 3 to 6 shots of hard liquor, or 3 to 6 glasses of wine) for > 10 yr. For cirrhosis to develop, consumption must usually be > 80 g/day for > 10 yr. If consumption exceeds 230 g/day for 20 yr, risk of cirrhosis is about 50%. But only some chronic alcohol abusers develop liver disease. Thus, variations in alcohol intake do not fully explain variations in susceptibility, indicating that other factors are involved.

Sex: Women are more susceptible to alcoholic liver disease, even after adjustment for body size. Women require only 20 to 40 g of alcohol to be at risk—half of that for men. Risk in women may be increased because they have less alcohol dehydrogenase in their gastric mucosa; thus, more intact alcohol reaches the liver.

Genetic factors: Alcoholic liver disease often runs in families, suggesting genetic factors (eg, deficiency of cytoplasmic enzymes that eliminate alcohol).

Nutritional status: A diet high in unsaturated fat increases susceptibility, as does obesity.

Other factors: Other risk factors include iron accumulation in the liver (not necessarily related to iron intake) and concomitant hepatitis C.

Pathophysiology

Alcohol absorption and metabolism: Alcohol (ethanol) is readily absorbed from the stomach, but most is absorbed from the small intestine. Alcohol cannot be stored. A small amount is degraded in transit through the gastric mucosa, but most is catabolized in the liver, primarily by alcohol dehydrogenase (ADH) but also by cytochrome P-450 2E1 (CYP2E1) and the microsomal enzyme oxidation system (MEOS).

Metabolism via the ADH pathway involves the following:

- ADH, a cytoplasmic enzyme, oxidizes alcohol into acetaldehyde. Genetic polymorphisms in ADH account for some individual differences in blood alcohol levels after the same alcohol intake but not in susceptibility to alcoholic liver disease.
- Acetaldehyde dehydrogenase (ALDH), a mitochondrial enzyme, then oxidizes acetaldehyde into acetate. Chronic alcohol consumption enhances acetate formation. Asians, who have lower levels of ALDH, are more susceptible to toxic acetaldehyde effects (eg, flushing); the effects are similar to those of disulfiram, which inhibits ALDH.
- These oxidative reactions generate hydrogen, which converts nicotinamide-adenine dinucleotide (NAD) to its reduced form (NADH), increasing the redox potential (NADH/NAD) in the liver.
- The increased redox potential inhibits fatty acid oxidation and gluconeogenesis, promoting fat accumulation in the liver.

Chronic alcoholism induces the MEOS (mainly in endoplasmic reticulum), increasing its activity. The main enzyme involved is CYP2E1. When induced, the MEOS pathway can account for 20% of alcohol metabolism. This pathway generates harmful reactive O_2 species, increasing oxidative stress and formation of O_2-free radicals.

Hepatic fat accumulation: Fat (triglycerides) accumulates throughout the hepatocytes for the following reasons:

- Export of fat from the liver is decreased because hepatic fatty acid oxidation and lipoprotein production decrease.
- Input of fat is increased because the decrease in hepatic fat export increases peripheral lipolysis and triglyceride synthesis, resulting in hyperlipidemia.

Hepatic fat accumulation may predispose to subsequent oxidative damage.

Endotoxins in the gut: Alcohol changes gut permeability, increasing absorption of endotoxins released by bacteria in the gut. In response to the endotoxins (which the impaired liver can no longer detoxify), liver macrophages (Kupffer cells) release free radicals, increasing oxidative damage.

Oxidative damage: Oxidative stress is increased by

- Liver hypermetabolism, caused by alcohol consumption
- Free radical–induced lipid peroxidative damage
- Reduction in protective antioxidants (eg, glutathione, vitamins A and E), caused by alcohol-related undernutrition
- Binding of alcohol oxidation products, such as acetaldehyde, to liver cell proteins, forming neoantigens and resulting in inflammation
- Accumulation of neutrophils and other WBCs, which are attracted by lipid peroxidative damage and neoantigens
- Inflammatory cytokines secreted by WBCs

Accumulation of hepatic iron, if present, aggravates oxidative damage. Iron can accumulate in alcoholic liver disease through ingestion of iron-containing fortified wines; most often, the iron accumulation is modest. This condition must be differentiated from hereditary hemochromatosis.

Resultant inflammation, cell death, and fibrosis: A vicious circle of worsening inflammation occurs: Cell necrosis and apoptosis result in hepatocyte loss, and subsequent attempts at regeneration result in fibrosis. Stellate (Ito) cells, which line blood channels (sinusoids) in the liver, proliferate and transform into myofibroblasts, producing an excess of type I collagen and extracellular matrix. As a result, the sinusoids narrow, limiting blood flow. Fibrosis narrows the terminal hepatic venules, compromising hepatic perfusion and thus contributing to portal hypertension. Extensive fibrosis is associated with an attempt at regeneration, resulting in liver nodules. This process culminates in cirrhosis.

Pathology

Fatty liver, alcoholic hepatitis, and cirrhosis are often considered separate, progressive manifestations of alcoholic liver disease. However, their features often overlap.

Fatty liver (steatosis) is the initial and most common consequence of excessive alcohol consumption. Fatty liver is potentially reversible. Macrovesicular fat accumulates as large droplets of triglyceride and displaces the hepatocyte nucleus, most markedly in perivenular hepatocytes. The liver enlarges.

Alcoholic hepatitis (steatohepatitis) is a combination of fatty liver, diffuse liver inflammation, and liver necrosis (often focal)—all in various degrees of severity. The damaged hepatocytes are swollen with a granular cytoplasm (balloon degeneration) or contain fibrillar protein in the cytoplasm (Mallory or alcoholic hyaline bodies). Severely damaged hepatocytes become necrotic. Sinusoids and terminal hepatic venules are narrowed. Cirrhosis may also be present.

Alcoholic cirrhosis is advanced liver disease characterized by extensive fibrosis that disrupts the normal liver architecture. The amount of fat present varies. Alcoholic hepatitis may coexist. The feeble compensatory attempt at hepatic regeneration produces relatively small nodules (micronodular cirrhosis). As a result, the liver usually shrinks. In time, even with abstinence, fibrosis forms broad bands, separating liver tissue into large nodules (macronodular cirrhosis—see p. 208).

Symptoms and Signs

Symptoms usually become apparent in patients during their 30s or 40s; severe problems appear about a decade later.

Fatty liver is often asymptomatic. In one-third of patients, the liver is enlarged and smooth, but it is not usually tender.

Alcoholic hepatitis ranges from mild and reversible to life threatening. Most patients with moderate disease are undernourished and present with fatigue, fever, jaundice, right upper quadrant pain, tender hepatomegaly, and sometimes a hepatic bruit. About 40% deteriorate soon after hospitalization, with consequences ranging from mild (eg, increasing jaundice) to severe (eg, ascites, portosystemic encephalopathy, variceal bleeding, liver failure with hypoglycemia, coagulopathy). Other manifestations of cirrhosis may be present.

Cirrhosis, if compensated, may be asymptomatic. The liver is usually small; when the liver is enlarged, fatty liver or hepatoma should be considered. Symptoms range from those of alcoholic hepatitis to the complications of end-stage liver disease, such as portal hypertension (often with esophageal varices and upper GI bleeding, splenomegaly, ascites, and portosystemic encephalopathy). Portal hypertension may lead to intrapulmonary arteriovenous shunting with hypoxemia (hepatopulmonary syndrome), which may cause cyanosis and nail clubbing. Acute renal failure secondary to progressively decreasing renal blood flow (hepatorenal syndrome) may develop. Hepatocellular carcinoma develops in 10 to 15% of patients with alcoholic cirrhosis.

Chronic alcoholism, rather than liver disease, causes Dupuytren contracture of the palmar fascia, vascular spiders, myopathy, and peripheral neuropathy. In men, chronic alcoholism causes signs of hypogonadism and feminization (eg, smooth skin, lack of male-pattern baldness, gynecomastia, testicular atrophy, changes in pubic hair). Undernutrition may lead to multiple vitamin deficiencies (eg, of folate and thiamin), enlarged parotid glands, and white nails. In alcoholics, Wernicke encephalopathy and Korsakoff psychosis result mainly from thiamin deficiency. Pancreatitis is common. Hepatitis C occurs in > 25% of alcoholics; this combination markedly worsens the progression of liver disease.

Rarely, patients with fatty liver or cirrhosis present with Zieve syndrome (hyperlipidemia, hemolytic anemia, and jaundice).

Diagnosis

- Confirmed history of alcohol use
- Liver function tests and CBC
- Sometimes liver biopsy

Alcohol is suspected as the cause of liver disease in any patient who chronically consumes excess alcohol, particularly > 80 g/day. When the patient's alcohol consumption is in doubt, history should be confirmed by family members. Patients can be screened for alcoholism using the CAGE questionnaire (need to *C*ut down, *A*nnoyed by criticism, *G*uilty about drinking, and need for a morning *E*ye-opener). There is no specific test for alcoholic liver disease, but if the diagnosis is suspected, liver function tests (PT; serum bilirubin, aminotransferase, and albumin levels) and CBC are done to detect signs of liver injury and anemia.

Elevations of aminotransferases are moderate (< 300 IU/L) and do not reflect the extent of liver damage. The ratio of AST to ALT is ≥ 2. The basis for low ALT is a dietary deficiency of pyridoxal phosphate (vitamin B_6), which is needed for ALT to function. Its effect on AST is less pronounced. Serum gamma-glutamyl transpeptidase (GGT) increases, more because ethanol induces this enzyme than because patients have cholestasis or liver injury or use other drugs. Serum albumin may be low, usually reflecting undernutrition but occasionally reflecting otherwise obvious liver failure with deficient synthesis. Macrocytosis with an MCV > 100 fL reflects the direct effect of alcohol on bone marrow as well as macrocytic anemia resulting from folate deficiency, which is common among undernourished alcoholics. Indexes of the severity of liver disease are

- Serum bilirubin, which represents secretory function
- PT or INR, which reflects synthetic ability

Thrombocytopenia can result from the direct toxic effects of alcohol on bone marrow or from splenomegaly, which accompanies portal hypertension. Neutrophilic leukocytosis may result from alcoholic hepatitis, although coexisting infection (particularly pneumonia and spontaneous bacterial peritonitis) should also be suspected.

Imaging tests of the liver are not routinely needed for diagnosis. If done for other reasons, abdominal ultrasonography or CT may suggest fatty liver or show splenomegaly, evidence of portal hypertension, or ascites. Ultrasound elastography measures liver stiffness and thus detects advanced fibrosis. This valuable adjunct can obviate the need for liver biopsy to check for cirrhosis and help assess prognosis. Its exact role is under study.

If abnormalities suggest alcoholic liver disease, screening tests for other treatable forms of liver disease, especially viral hepatitis, should be done.

Because features of fatty liver, alcoholic hepatitis, and cirrhosis overlap, describing the precise findings is more useful than assigning patients to a specific category, which can only be determined by liver biopsy.

Not all experts agree on the indications for liver biopsy. Proposed indications include the following:

- Unclear clinical diagnosis (eg, equivocal clinical and laboratory findings, unexplained persistent elevations of aminotransferase levels)
- Clinical suspicion of > 1 cause of liver disease (eg, alcohol plus viral hepatitis)
- Desire for a precise prediction of prognosis

Liver biopsy confirms liver disease, helps identify excessive alcohol use as the likely cause, and establishes the stage of liver injury. If iron accumulation is observed, measurement of the iron content and genetic testing can eliminate hereditary hemochromatosis as the cause.

For stable patients with cirrhosis, alpha-fetoprotein measurement and liver ultrasonography should be done every 6 mo to screen for hepatocellular carcinoma.

Prognosis

Prognosis is determined by the degree of hepatic fibrosis and inflammation. Fatty liver and alcoholic hepatitis without fibrosis are reversible if alcohol is avoided. With abstinence, fatty liver may completely resolve within 6 wk. Fibrosis and cirrhosis are usually irreversible.

Certain biopsy findings (eg, neutrophils, perivenular fibrosis) indicate a worse prognosis. Proposed quantitative indexes to predict severity and mortality use primarily laboratory features of liver failure such as PT, creatinine (for hepatorenal syndrome), and bilirubin levels. The Maddrey discriminant function may be used; it is calculated from the formula:

$$4.6 \times (\text{PT} - \text{control PT}) + \text{serum bilirubin}$$

For this formula, bilirubin level is measured in mg/dL (converted from bilirubin in µmol/L by dividing by 17). A value of > 32 is associated with a high short-term mortality rate (eg, after 1 mo, 35% without encephalopathy and 45% with encephalopathy). Other indexes include the Model for End-Stage Liver Disease (MELD) score, Glasgow alcoholic hepatitis score, and

Lille model. For patients ≥ 12 yr, the MELD score is calculated using the following formula:

$$3.8\ [\text{Ln serum bilirubin (mg/dL)}] + 11.2\ [\text{Ln INR}] + 9.6\ [\text{Ln serum creatinine (mg/dL)}] + 6.4$$

Once cirrhosis and its complications (eg, ascites, bleeding) develop, the 5-yr survival rate is about 50%; survival is higher in patients who abstain and lower in patients who continue drinking. Coexisting iron accumulation or chronic hepatitis C increases risk of hepatocellular carcinoma.

Treatment

- Abstinence
- Supportive care
- Corticosteroids and enteral nutrition for severe alcoholic hepatitis
- Sometimes transplantation

Restricting alcohol intake: Abstinence is the mainstay of treatment; it prevents further damage from alcoholic liver disease and thus prolongs life. Because compliance is problematic, a compassionate team approach is essential. Behavioral and psychosocial interventions can help motivated patients; they include rehabilitation programs and support groups, brief interventions by primary care physicians, and therapies that explore and clarify the motivation to abstain (motivational enhancement therapy).

Drugs, if used, should only supplement other interventions. Opioid antagonists (naltrexone or nalmefene) and drugs that modulate gamma-aminobutyric acid receptors (baclofen or acamprosate) appear to have a short-term benefit by reducing the craving and withdrawal symptoms. Disulfiram inhibits aldehyde dehydrogenase, allowing acetaldehyde to accumulate; thus, drinking alcohol within 12 h of taking disulfiram causes flushing and has other unpleasant effects. However, disulfiram has not been shown to promote abstinence and consequently is recommended only for certain patients.

Supportive care: General management emphasizes supportive care. A nutritious diet and vitamin supplements (especially B vitamins) are important during the first few days of abstinence. Alcohol withdrawal requires use of benzodiazepines (eg, diazepam). In patients with advanced alcoholic liver disease, excessive sedation can precipitate portosystemic encephalopathy and thus must be avoided.

Severe acute alcoholic hepatitis commonly requires hospitalization, often in an ICU, to facilitate enteral feeding (which can help manage nutritional deficiencies) and to manage specific complications (eg, infection, bleeding from esophageal varices, specific nutritional deficiencies, Wernicke encephalopathy, Korsakoff psychosis, electrolyte abnormalities, portal hypertension, ascites, portosystemic encephalopathy—see elsewhere in THE MANUAL).

Specific treatment: Corticosteroids (eg, prednisolone 40 mg/day po for 4 wk, followed by tapered doses) improve outcome in patients who have severe acute alcoholic hepatitis and who do not have infection, GI bleeding, renal failure, or pancreatitis.

Other than corticosteroids and enteral feeding, few specific treatments are clearly established. Antioxidants (eg, *S*-adenosyl-L-methionine, phosphatidylcholine, metadoxine) show promise in ameliorating liver injury during early cirrhosis but require further study. Therapies directed at cytokines, particularly TNF-alpha, and aiming to reduce inflammation have had mixed results in small trials. Pentoxifylline, a phosphodiesterase inhibitor that inhibits TNF-alpha synthesis, had mixed results in clinical trials in patients with severe alcoholic hepatitis. When biologic agents that inhibit TNF-alpha (eg, infliximab, etanercept) are used, risk of infection outweighs benefit. Drugs given to decrease fibrosis (eg, colchicine, penicillamine) and drugs given to normalize the hypermetabolic state of the alcoholic liver (eg, propylthiouracil) have no proven benefit. Antioxidant remedies, such as silymarin (milk thistle) and vitamins A and E, are ineffective.

Liver transplantation can be considered if disease is severe. With transplantation, 5-yr survival rates are comparable to those for nonalcoholic liver disease—as high as 80% in patients without active liver disease and 50% in those with acute alcoholic hepatitis. Because up to 50% of patients resume drinking after transplantation, most programs require 6 mo of abstinence before transplantation is done; recent data suggest that earlier transplantation may offer a survival advantage, but currently, this approach is not standard of care.

KEY POINTS

- Risk of alcoholic liver disease increases markedly in men if they ingest > 40 g, particularly > 80 g, of alcohol/day (eg, about 2 to 8 cans of beer, about 3 to 6 glasses of wine or hard liquor) for > 10 yr; risk increases markedly in women if they ingest about half that amount.
- Screen patients using the CAGE questionnaire, and when in doubt about the patient's alcohol consumption, consider asking family members.
- To estimate prognosis, consider unfavorable histologic findings (eg, neutrophils, perivenular fibrosis) and use of a formula (eg, Maddrey discriminant function, Model for End-Stage Liver Disease [MELD] score).
- Emphasize abstinence, provide supportive care, and hospitalize and give corticosteroids to patients with severe acute alcoholic hepatitis.
- Consider transplantation for abstinent patients.

26 Drugs and the Liver

EFFECTS OF LIVER DISEASE ON DRUG METABOLISM

Liver disease may have complex effects on drug clearance, biotransformation, and pharmacokinetics. Pathogenetic factors include alterations in intestinal absorption, plasma protein binding, hepatic extraction ratio, liver blood flow, portal-systemic shunting, biliary excretion, enterohepatic circulation, and renal clearance. Sometimes alterations increase levels of bioavailable drug, causing normal drug doses to have toxic effects. However, levels and effects for an individual drug are unpredictable and do not correlate well with the type of liver injury, its severity, or liver function test results. Thus, no general rules are available for modifying drug dosage in patients with liver disease.

Clinical effects can vary independent of drug bioavailability, especially in chronic liver disease; eg, cerebral sensitivity to opioids and sedatives is often enhanced in patients with chronic liver disease. Thus, seemingly small doses of these drugs given to cirrhotic patients may precipitate encephalopathy. The mechanism of this effect probably involves alterations in cerebral drug receptors.

Adverse drug reactions do not appear to be more likely in patients with advanced liver disease; however, such patients may tolerate any hepatic adverse effects of drugs less well.

LIVER INJURY CAUSED BY DRUGS

Many drugs (eg, statins) commonly cause asymptomatic elevation of hepatic enzymes (ALT, AST, alkaline phosphatase). However, clinically significant liver injury (eg, with jaundice, abdominal pain, or pruritus) or impaired liver function—ie, resulting in deficient protein synthesis (eg, with prolonged PT or with hypoalbuminemia)—is rare.

The term *drug-induced liver injury* (DILI) may be used to mean clinically significant liver injury or all (including asymptomatic) liver injury. DILI includes injury caused by medicinal herbs, plants, and nutritional supplements as well as drugs.[1,2]

1. Chalasani N, Bonkovsky HL, Fontana R, et al: Features and outcomes of 899 patients with drug-induced liver injury: The DILIN prospective study. *Gastroenterology* 148(7):1340–1352, 2015.
2. Navarro VJ, Barnhart H, Bonkovsky HL, et al: Liver injury from herbals and dietary supplements in the U.S. Drug-Induced Liver Injury Network. *Hepatology* 60(4):1399–1408, 2014.

Pathophysiology

The pathophysiology of DILI varies depending on the drug (or other hepatotoxin) and, in many cases, is not entirely understood. Drug-induced injury mechanisms include covalent binding of the drug to cellular proteins resulting in immune injury, inhibition of cell metabolic pathways, blockage of cellular transport pumps, induction of apoptosis, and interference with mitochondrial function.

In general, the following are thought to increase risk of DILI:

- Age ≥ 18 yr
- Obesity
- Pregnancy
- Concomitant alcohol consumption
- Genetic polymorphisms (increasingly recognized)

Patterns of liver injury: DILI can be predictable (when injury usually occurs shortly after exposure and is dose-related) or unpredictable (when injury develops after a period of latency and has no relation to dose). Predictable DILI (commonly, acetaminophen poisoning) is a common cause of acute jaundice and acute liver failure in the US. Unpredictable DILI is a rare cause of severe liver disease. Subclinical DILI may be underreported.

Biochemically, 3 types of liver injury are generally noted (see Table 26–1):

- **Hepatocellular:** Hepatocellular hepatotoxicity generally manifests as malaise and right upper quadrant abdominal pain, associated with marked elevation in aminotransferase levels (ALT, AST, or both), which may be followed by hyperbilirubinemia in severe cases. Hyperbilirubinemia in this setting is known as hepatocellular jaundice and, according to Hy's law, is associated with mortality rates as high as 50%. If hepatocellular liver injury is accompanied by jaundice, impaired hepatic synthesis, and encephalopathy, chance of spontaneous recovery is low, and liver transplantation should be considered. This type of injury can result from drugs such as acetaminophen and isoniazid.

Table 26–1. POTENTIALLY HEPATOTOXIC DRUGS

FINDING	DRUG
Hepatocellular: Elevated ALT	Acarbose Acetaminophen Allopurinol Amiodarone ART drugs Bupropion Fluoxetine Germander Green tea extract Baclofen Isoniazid Kava Ketoconazole Lisinopril Losartan Methotrexate NSAIDs Omeprazole Paroxetine Pyrazinamide Rifampin Risperidone Sertraline Statins Tetracyclines Trazodone Trovafloxacin Valproate
Cholestatic: Elevated alkaline phosphatase and total bilirubin	Amoxicillin/clavulanate Anabolic steroids Chlorpromazine Clopidogrel Oral contraceptives Erythromycins Estrogens Irbesartan Mirtazapine Phenothiazines Terbinafine Tricyclic antidepressants
Mixed: Elevated alkaline phosphatase and ALT	Amitriptyline Azathioprine Captopril Carbamazepine Clindamycin Cyproheptadine Enalapril Nitrofurantoin Phenobarbital Phenytoin Sulfonamides Trazodone Trimethoprim/sulfamethoxazole Verapamil

ART = antiretroviral therapy.

- **Cholestatic:** Cholestatic hepatotoxicity is characterized by development of pruritus and jaundice accompanied by marked elevation of serum alkaline phosphatase levels. Usually, this type of injury is less serious than severe hepatocellular syndromes, but recovery may be protracted. Substances known to lead to this type of injury include amoxicillin/clavulanate and chlorpromazine. Rarely, cholestatic hepatotoxicity leads to chronic liver disease and vanishing bile duct syndrome (progressive destruction of intrahepatic bile ducts).

- **Mixed:** In these clinical syndromes, neither aminotransferase nor alkaline phosphatase elevations are clearly predominant. Symptoms may also be mixed. Drugs such as phenytoin can cause this type of injury.

Diagnosis

- Identification of characteristic patterns of laboratory abnormalities
- Exclusion of other causes

Presentation varies widely, ranging from absent or nonspecific symptoms (eg, malaise, nausea, anorexia) to jaundice, impaired hepatic synthesis, and encephalopathy. Early recognition of DILI improves prognosis.

Identification of a potential hepatotoxin and a pattern of liver test abnormalities that is characteristic of the substance (its signature) make the diagnosis likely.

Because there is no confirmatory diagnostic test, other causes of liver disease, especially viral, biliary, alcoholic, autoimmune, and metabolic causes, need to be excluded. Drug rechallenge, although it can strengthen evidence for the diagnosis, should be avoided. Suspected cases of DILI should be reported to MedWatch (the FDA's adverse drug reaction monitoring program).

PEARLS & PITFALLS

- Do not rechallenge with a drug suspected of causing liver injury.

Treatment

- Early drug withdrawal

Management emphasizes drug withdrawal, which, if done early, usually results in recovery. In severe cases, consultation with a specialist is indicated, especially if patients have hepatocellular jaundice and impaired liver function, because liver transplantation may be required. Antidotes for DILI are available for only a few hepatotoxins; such antidotes include *N*-acetylcysteine for acetaminophen toxicity and silymarin or penicillin for *Amanita phalloides* toxicity.

Prevention

Efforts to avoid DILI begin during the drug development process, although apparent safety in small preclinical trials does not ensure eventual safety of the drug after it is in widespread use. Postmarketing surveillance, now increasingly mandated by FDA, can call attention to potentially hepatotoxic drugs.

The National Institute of Diabetes and Digestive and Kidney Diseases (NIDDK) has established the LiverTox database to collect and analyze cases of severe liver injury caused by prescription drugs, OTC drugs, and alternative medicines, such as herbal products and dietary supplements. This is a searchable database that provides easily accessible and accurate information regarding known hepatotoxicity related to drugs and supplements.

Routine monitoring of liver enzymes has not been shown to decrease the incidence of hepatotoxicity. Use of pharmacogenomics may allow tailoring of drug use and avoidance of potential toxicities in susceptible patients.

KEY POINTS

- Drugs are much more likely to cause an asymptomatic abnormality in liver function than clinically evident liver damage or dysfunction.
- Risk factors for DILI include age ≥ 18 yr, obesity, pregnancy, concomitant alcohol consumption, and certain genetic polymorphisms.
- DILI can be predictable and dose-related or unpredictable and unrelated to dose.
- DILI can be hepatocellular, cholestatic (usually less serious than hepatocellular), or mixed.
- To confirm the diagnosis, exclude other causes of liver disease, especially viral, biliary, alcoholic, autoimmune, and metabolic disorders.
- Do not rechallenge patients with drugs suspected of causing DILI.

27 Fibrosis and Cirrhosis

HEPATIC FIBROSIS

Hepatic fibrosis is overly exuberant wound healing in which excessive connective tissue builds up in the liver. The extracellular matrix is overproduced, degraded deficiently, or both. The trigger is chronic injury, especially if there is an inflammatory component. Fibrosis itself causes no symptoms but can lead to portal hypertension (the scarring distorts blood flow through the liver) or cirrhosis (the scarring results in disruption of normal hepatic architecture and liver dysfunction). Diagnosis is based on liver biopsy. Treatment involves correcting the underlying condition when possible.

In hepatic fibrosis, excessive connective tissue accumulates in the liver; this tissue represents scarring in response to chronic, repeated liver cell injury. Commonly, fibrosis progresses, disrupting hepatic architecture and eventually function, as regenerating hepatocytes attempt to replace and repair damaged tissue. When such disruption is widespread, cirrhosis is diagnosed.

Various types of chronic liver injury can cause fibrosis (see Table 27–1). Self-limited, acute liver injury (eg, acute viral hepatitis A), even when fulminant, does not necessarily distort the scaffolding architecture and hence does not cause fibrosis, despite loss of hepatocytes. In its initial stages, hepatic fibrosis can regress if the cause is reversible (eg, with viral clearance). After months or years of chronic or repeated injury, fibrosis becomes permanent. Fibrosis develops even more rapidly in mechanical biliary obstruction.

Pathophysiology

Activation of the hepatic perivascular stellate cells (Ito cells, which store fat) initiates fibrosis. These and adjacent cells proliferate, becoming contractile cells termed myofibroblasts. These cells produce excessive amounts of abnormal matrix (consisting of collagen, other glycoproteins, and glycans) and

Table 27–1. DISORDERS AND DRUGS THAT CAN CAUSE HEPATIC FIBROSIS

Disorders with direct hepatic effects
Autoimmune hepatitis
Certain storage diseases and inborn errors of metabolism
• Alpha-1 antitrypsin deficiency
• Copper storage diseases (eg, Wilson disease)
• Fructosemia
• Galactosemia
• Glycogen storage diseases (especially types III, IV, VI, IX, and X)
• Iron-overload syndromes (hemochromatosis)
• Lipid abnormalities (eg, Gaucher disease)
• Peroxisomal disorders (eg, Zellweger syndrome)
• Tyrosinemia
Congenital hepatic fibrosis
Infections
• Bacterial (eg, brucellosis)
• Parasitic (eg, echinococcosis)
• Viral (eg, chronic hepatitis B or C*)
Nonalcoholic steatohepatitis (NASH)
Primary biliary cirrhosis
Primary sclerosing cholangitis
Disorders affecting hepatic blood flow
Budd-Chiari syndrome
Heart failure
Hepatic veno-occlusive disease†
Portal vein thrombosis
Drugs and chemicals
Alcohol*
Amiodarone
Chlorpromazine
Isoniazid
Methotrexate
Methyldopa
Oxyphenisatin
Tolbutamide
Mechanical obstruction
Scarring due to prior liver surgery
Bile duct strictures due to impacted gallstones

*Most common causes.
†Sometimes caused by pyrrolizidine alkaloids, present in herbal products such as bush teas.

matricellular proteins. Kupffer cells (resident macrophages), injured hepatocytes, platelets, and leukocytes aggregate. As a result, reactive O_2 species and inflammatory mediators (eg, platelet-derived growth factor, transforming growth factors, connective tissue growth factor) are released. Thus, stellate cell activation results in abnormal extracellular matrix, both in quantity and composition.

Myofibroblasts, stimulated by endothelin-1, contribute to increased portal vein resistance and increase the density of the abnormal matrix. Fibrous tracts join branches of afferent portal veins and efferent hepatic veins, bypassing the hepatocytes and limiting their blood supply. Hence, fibrosis contributes both to hepatocyte ischemia (causing hepatocellular dysfunction) and portal hypertension. The extent of the ischemia and portal hypertension determines how the liver is affected. For example, congenital hepatic fibrosis affects portal vein branches, largely sparing the parenchyma. The result is portal hypertension with sparing of hepatocellular function.

Symptoms and Signs

Hepatic fibrosis itself does not cause symptoms. Symptoms may result from the disorder causing fibrosis or, once fibrosis progresses to cirrhosis, from complications of portal hypertension. These symptoms include variceal bleeding, ascites, and portosystemic encephalopathy. Cirrhosis can result in hepatic insufficiency and potentially fatal liver failure.

Diagnosis

- Clinical evaluation
- Sometimes blood tests and/or noninvasive imaging tests
- Sometimes liver biopsy

Hepatic fibrosis is suspected if patients have known chronic liver disease (eg, chronic viral hepatitis C and hepatitis B, alcoholic liver disease) or if results of liver function tests are abnormal; in such cases, tests are done to check for fibrosis and, if fibrosis is present, to determine its severity (stage). Knowing the stage of fibrosis can guide medical decisions. For example, screening for hepatocellular carcinoma and for gastroesophageal varices is indicated if cirrhosis is confirmed, but it is generally not indicated for mild or moderate fibrosis. Also, if liver biopsy does not detect advanced fibrosis in patients with hepatitis C, many clinicians defer treatment with interferons because they anticipate that more effective, less toxic drugs will be available.

Tests used to stage fibrosis include noninvasive imaging tests, blood tests, liver biopsy, and newer tests that assess liver stiffness.

Noninvasive imaging tests include conventional ultrasonography, CT, and MRI and should include cross-sectional views. These tests can detect evidence of cirrhosis and portal hypertension, such as splenomegaly and varices. However, they are not sensitive for moderate or even advanced fibrosis if splenomegaly and varices are absent. Although fibrosis may appear as altered echogenicity on ultrasonography or heterogeneity of signal on CT, these findings are nonspecific and may indicate only liver parenchymal fat.

New technologies can increase the accuracy of ultrasonography and MRI for detecting fibrosis or early cirrhosis; they include ultrasound elastography, magnetic resonance elastography, and acoustic radiation force impulse imaging. For these tests, acoustic vibrations are applied to the abdomen with a probe. How rapidly these vibrations are transmitted through liver tissue is measured—an indication of how stiff (ie, fibrosed) the liver is. Ultrasound elastography and magnetic resonance elastography are gaining acceptance by insurance providers as documentation of hepatic fibrosis justifying treatment with costly new interferon-free drugs for viral hepatitis.

Liver biopsy remains the gold standard for diagnosing and staging hepatic fibrosis and for diagnosing the underlying liver disorder causing fibrosis. However, liver biopsy is invasive, resulting in a 10 to 20% risk of minor complications (eg, postprocedural pain) and a 0.5 to 1% risk of serious complications (eg, significant bleeding). Also, liver biopsy is limited by sampling error and imperfect interobserver agreement in interpretation of histologic findings. Thus, liver biopsy may not always be done.

Blood tests include commercially available panels that combine indirect markers (eg, serum bilirubin) and direct markers of hepatic function. Direct markers are substances involved in the pathogenesis of extracellular matrix deposition or cytokines that induce extracellular matrix deposition. These panels are best used to distinguish between 2 levels of fibrosis: absent to minimal vs moderate to severe; they do not accurately differentiate between degrees of moderate to severe fibrosis. Therefore, if fibrosis is suspected, one approach is to start with one of these panels and then do liver biopsy only if the panel indicates that fibrosis is moderate to severe.

Which tests are done may depend on the degree of clinical suspicion, based on clinical evaluation, including liver function test results. For example, noninvasive blood tests may be used to determine whether biopsy is indicated; in some of these cases, imaging tests may not be needed.

Treatment

- Treatment of cause

Because fibrosis represents a response to hepatic damage, primary treatment should focus on the cause (removing the basis of the liver injury). Such treatment may include eliminating hepatitis B virus or hepatitis C virus in chronic viral hepatitis, abstaining from alcohol in alcoholic liver disease, removing heavy metals such as iron in hemochromatosis or copper in Wilson disease, and decompressing bile ducts in biliary obstruction. Such treatments may stop the fibrosis from progressing and, in some patients, also reverse some of the fibrotic changes.

Treatments aimed at reversing the fibrosis are usually too toxic for long-term use (eg, corticosteroids, penicillamine) or have no proven efficacy (eg, colchicine). Other antifibrotic treatments are under study. Simultaneous use of multiple antifibrotic drugs may eventually prove most beneficial. Silymarin, present in milk thistle, is a popular alternative medicine used to treat hepatic fibrosis. It appears to be safe but to lack efficacy.

KEY POINTS

- Self-limited, acute liver injury (eg, due to acute viral hepatitis A), even when fulminant, tends not to cause fibrosis.
- The most common causes of hepatic fibrosis are hepatitis B and C and alcohol abuse.
- Fibrosis does not cause symptoms unless it progresses to cirrhosis.
- Liver biopsy, although imperfect, is the gold standard diagnostic test.
- Noninvasive testing, including ultrasound elastography and magnetic resonance elastography, is becoming increasingly important.
- Treat the cause of fibrosis.

CIRRHOSIS

Cirrhosis is a late stage of hepatic fibrosis that has resulted in widespread distortion of normal hepatic architecture. Cirrhosis is characterized by regenerative nodules surrounded by dense fibrotic tissue. Symptoms may not develop for years and are often nonspecific (eg, anorexia, fatigue, weight loss). Late manifestations include portal hypertension, ascites, and, when decompensation occurs, liver failure. Diagnosis often requires liver biopsy. Cirrhosis is usually considered irreversible. Treatment is supportive.

Cirrhosis is a leading cause of death worldwide. The causes of cirrhosis are the same as those of fibrosis (see Table 27–1). In developed countries, most cases result from chronic alcohol abuse or chronic hepatitis C. In parts of Asia and Africa, cirrhosis often results from chronic hepatitis B (see Table 29–2 on p. 224 for additional information on hepatitis B and C.) Cirrhosis of unknown etiology (cryptogenic cirrhosis) is becoming less common as many specific causes (eg, chronic hepatitis C, steatohepatitis) are identified. Injury to the bile ducts also can result in cirrhosis, as occurs in mechanical bile duct obstruction, primary biliary cirrhosis, and primary sclerosing cholangitis.

Pathophysiology

There are 2 primary ingredients:

- Hepatic fibrosis
- Regenerating liver cells

In response to injury and loss, growth regulators induce hepatocellular hyperplasia (producing regenerating nodules) and arterial growth (angiogenesis). Among the growth regulators are cytokines and hepatic growth factors (eg, epithelial growth factor, hepatocyte growth factor, transforming growth factor-α, tumor necrosis factor). Insulin, glucagon, and patterns of intrahepatic blood flow determine how and where nodules develop.

Angiogenesis produces new vessels within the fibrous sheath that surrounds nodules. These vessels connect the hepatic artery and portal vein to hepatic venules, restoring the intrahepatic circulatory pathways. Such interconnecting vessels provide relatively low-volume, high-pressure venous drainage that cannot accommodate as much blood volume as normal. As a result, portal vein pressure increases. Such distortions in blood flow contribute to portal hypertension, which increases because the regenerating nodules compress hepatic venules.

The progression rate from fibrosis to cirrhosis and the morphology of cirrhosis vary from person to person. Presumably, the reason for such variation is the extent of exposure to the injurious stimulus and the individual's response.

Complications: Portal hypertension is the most common serious complication of cirrhosis, and it, in turn, causes complications, including

- GI bleeding from esophageal, gastric, or rectal varices and portal hypertensive gastropathy
- Ascites
- Acute kidney injury (hepatorenal syndrome)
- Pulmonary hypertension (portopulmonary hypertension—see p. 506)

Ascites is a risk factor for spontaneous bacterial peritonitis. Portopulmonary hypertension can manifest with symptoms of heart failure. Complications of portal hypertension tend to cause significant morbidity and mortality.

Cirrhosis can cause other cardiovascular complications. Vasodilation, intrapulmonary right-to-left shunting, and ventilation/perfusion mismatch can result in hypoxia (hepatopulmonary syndrome).

Progressive loss of hepatic architecture impairs function, leading to hepatic insufficiency; it manifests as coagulopathy, acute kidney injury (hepatorenal syndrome), and hepatic encephalopathy. Hepatocytes secrete less bile, contributing to cholestasis and jaundice. Less bile in the intestine causes malabsorption of dietary fat (triglycerides) and fat-soluble vitamins. Malabsorption of vitamin D may contribute to osteoporosis. Undernutrition is common. It may result from anorexia with reduced food intake or, in patients with alcoholic liver disease, from malabsorption due to pancreatic insufficiency.

Blood disorders are common. Anemia usually results from hypersplenism, chronic GI bleeding, folate deficiency (particularly in patients with alcoholism), and hemolysis.

Cirrhosis results in decreased production of prothrombotic and antithrombotic factors. Hypersplenism and altered expression of thrombopoietin contribute to thrombocytopenia. Thrombocytopenia and decreased production of clotting factors can make clotting unpredictable, increasing risk of both bleeding and thromboembolic disease (even though INR is usually increased). Leukopenia is also common; it is mediated by hypersplenism and altered expression of erythropoietin and granulocyte-stimulating factors.

PEARLS & PITFALLS

- Consider thromboembolic complications in patients with cirrhosis, even if INR is elevated.

Hepatocellular carcinoma frequently complicates cirrhosis, particularly cirrhosis resulting from chronic hepatitis B or C, hemochromatosis, alcohol-related liver disease, alpha-1 antitrypsin deficiency, or glycogen storage disease.

Histopathology: Cirrhosis is characterized by regenerating nodules and fibrosis. Incompletely formed liver nodules, nodules without fibrosis (nodular regenerative hyperplasia), and congenital hepatic fibrosis (ie, widespread fibrosis without regenerating nodules) are not true cirrhosis.

Cirrhosis can be micronodular or macronodular. Micronodular cirrhosis is characterized by uniformly small nodules (< 3 mm in diameter) and thick regular bands of connective tissue. Typically, nodules lack lobular organization; terminal (central) hepatic venules and portal triads are distorted. With time, macronodular cirrhosis often develops. The nodules vary in size (3 mm to 5 cm in diameter) and have some relatively normal lobular organization of portal triads and terminal hepatic venules. Broad fibrous bands of varying thickness surround the large nodules. Collapse of the normal hepatic architecture is suggested by the concentration of portal triads within the fibrous scars. Mixed cirrhosis (incomplete septal cirrhosis) combines elements of micronodular and macronodular cirrhosis. Differentiation between these morphologic types of cirrhosis has limited clinical value.

Symptoms and Signs

Cirrhosis may be asymptomatic for years. One third of patients never develop symptoms. Often, the first symptoms are nonspecific; they include generalized fatigue (due to cytokine release), anorexia, malaise, and weight loss (see Table 27–2). The liver is typically palpable and firm, with a blunt edge, but is sometimes small and difficult to palpate. Nodules usually are not palpable.

Clinical signs that suggest a chronic liver disorder or chronic alcohol use but are not specific for cirrhosis include muscle wasting, palmar erythema, parotid gland enlargement, white nails, clubbing, Dupuytren contracture, spider angiomas (< 10 may be normal), gynecomastia, axillary hair loss, testicular atrophy, and peripheral neuropathy.

Once complications of cirrhosis develop, decompensation inexorably ensues.

Diagnosis

- Liver function tests, coagulation tests, CBC, and serologic tests for viral causes
- Sometimes biopsy (eg, when clinical and noninvasive tests are inconclusive or when biopsy results may change management)

Table 27–2. COMMON SYMPTOMS AND SIGNS DUE TO COMPLICATIONS OF CIRRHOSIS

SYMPTOM OR SIGN	POSSIBLE CAUSE
Abdominal distention	Ascites
Abdominal discomfort with fever or hepatic encephalopathy (infrequently with peritoneal signs)	Spontaneous bacterial peritonitis
Calf pain or swelling, symptoms of pulmonary embolism	Thromboembolism
Clubbing	Hepatopulmonary syndrome
Confusion, lethargy	Hepatic encephalopathy
Dyspnea, hypoxia	Hepatopulmonary syndrome Portopulmonary hypertension
Fatigue, pallor	Anemia due to bleeding, hypersplenism, undernutrition with deficiency of folate (or iron or vitamin B_{12}), chronic disease, or effects of alcohol (eg, bone marrow suppression)
Fluid overload, oliguria, symptoms of renal failure	Hepatorenal syndrome
Fragility fracture (due to a fall from standing height or less)	Osteoporosis
Symptoms of infection	Leukopenia
Jaundice	Cholestasis
Petechiae, purpura, bleeding	Thrombocytopenia caused by splenomegaly due to portal hypertension or the direct effects of alcohol on bone marrow Coagulopathy due to impaired liver synthetic function, vitamin K deficiency, or both
Pruritus, xanthelasmas	Cholestasis
Rectal bleeding	Rectal varices
Splenomegaly	Portal hypertension
Steatorrhea	Fat malabsorption
Upper GI bleeding	Esophageal varices Portal hypertensive gastropathy

- Sometimes ultrasound elastography or magnetic resonance elastography
- Identification of cause based on clinical evaluation, routine testing for common causes, and selective testing for less common causes

General approach: Cirrhosis is suspected in patients with manifestations of any of its complications, particularly portal hypertension or ascites. Early cirrhosis should be considered in patients with nonspecific symptoms or characteristic laboratory abnormalities detected incidentally during laboratory testing, particularly in patients who have a disorder or take a drug that might cause fibrosis.

Testing seeks to detect cirrhosis and any complications and to determine its cause.

Laboratory tests: Diagnostic testing begins with liver function tests, coagulation tests, CBC, and serologic tests for viral causes (eg, hepatitis B and C). Laboratory tests alone may increase suspicion for cirrhosis but cannot confirm or exclude it. Liver biopsy becomes necessary if a clear diagnosis would lead to better management and outcome.

Test results may be normal or may indicate nonspecific abnormalities due to complications of cirrhosis or alcoholism. ALT and AST levels are often modestly elevated. Alkaline phosphatase and γ-glutamyl transpeptidase (GGT) are often normal; elevated levels indicate cholestasis or biliary obstruction. Bilirubin is usually normal but increases when cirrhosis progresses, particularly in primary biliary cirrhosis (see p. 212). Decreased serum albumin and a prolonged PT directly reflect impaired hepatic synthesis—usually an end-stage event. Albumin can also be low when nutrition is poor. Serum globulin increases in cirrhosis and in most liver disorders with an inflammatory component.

Anemia is common and usually normocytic with a high RBC distribution width. Anemia is often multifactorial; contributing factors may include chronic GI bleeding (usually causing microcytic anemia), folate nutritional deficiency (causing macrocytic anemia, especially in alcohol abuse), hemolysis, and hypersplenism. CBC may also detect leukopenia, thrombocytopenia, or pancytopenia.

Diagnostic imaging: Conventional imaging tests are not highly sensitive or specific for the diagnosis of cirrhosis by themselves, but they can often detect its complications. Ultrasound elastography and magnetic resonance elastography are useful in detection of early cirrhosis when conventional imaging findings are equivocal and portal hypertension is not evident.

In advanced cirrhosis, ultrasonography shows a small, nodular liver. Ultrasonography also detects portal hypertension and ascites.

CT can detect a nodular texture, but it has no advantage over ultrasonography. Radionuclide liver scans using technetium-99m sulfur colloid may show irregular liver uptake and increased spleen and bone marrow uptake. MRI is more expensive than other imaging tests and has little advantage.

Identification of the cause: Determining the specific cause of cirrhosis requires key clinical information from the history and examination, as well as selective testing.

Alcohol is the likely cause in patients with a documented history of alcoholism and clinical findings such as gynecomastia, spider angiomas (telangiectasia), and testicular atrophy plus laboratory confirmation of liver damage (AST elevated more than ALT) and liver enzyme induction (a greatly increased GGT). Fever, tender hepatomegaly, and jaundice suggest the presence of alcoholic hepatitis.

Detecting hepatitis B surface antigen (HBsAg) and IgG antibodies to hepatitis B (IgG anti-HBc) confirms chronic hepatitis B. Identifying serum antibody to hepatitis C (anti-HCV) and HCV-RNA points to hepatitis C. Most clinicians also routinely test for the following:

- Autoimmune hepatitis: Suggested by a high antinuclear antibody titer (a low titer is nonspecific and does not always mandate further evaluation) and confirmed by hypergammaglobulinemia and the presence of other autoantibodies (eg, anti–smooth muscle or anti-liver/kidney microsomal type 1 antibodies)
- Hemochromatosis: Confirmed by increased serum Fe and transferrin saturation and possibly results of genetic testing
- Alpha-1 antitrypsin deficiency: Confirmed by a low serum alpha-1 antitrypsin level and genotyping

If these causes are not confirmed, other causes are sought:

- Presence of antimitochondrial antibodies (in 95%) suggests primary biliary cirrhosis.
- Strictures and dilations of the intrahepatic and extrahepatic bile ducts, seen on magnetic resonance cholangiopancreatography (MRCP), suggest primary sclerosing cholangitis.
- Decreased serum ceruloplasmin and characteristic copper test results suggest Wilson disease.
- The presence of obesity and a history of diabetes suggest NASH.

Liver biopsy: If clinical criteria and noninvasive testing are inconclusive, liver biopsy is usually done. For example, if well-compensated cirrhosis is suspected clinically and imaging findings are inconclusive, biopsy should be done to confirm the diagnosis. Sensitivity of liver biopsy approaches 100%. Nonalcoholic fatty liver disease (NAFLD) may be evident on ultrasound scans. However, NASH, often associated with obesity, diabetes, or the metabolic syndrome, requires liver biopsy for confirmation.

In obvious cases of cirrhosis with marked coagulopathy, portal hypertension, ascites, and liver failure, biopsy is not required unless results would change management. In patients with coagulopathy and thrombocytopenia, the transjugular approach to biopsy is safest. When this approach is used, pressures can be measured and thus the transsinusoidal pressure gradient can be calculated.

Monitoring: All patients with cirrhosis, regardless of cause, should be screened regularly for hepatocellular carcinoma (see p. 241). Currently, abdominal ultrasonography is recommended every 6 mo, and if abnormalities compatible with hepatocellular carcinoma are detected, contrast-enhanced MRI or triple-phase CT of the abdomen (contrast-enhanced CT with separate arterial and venous phase images) should be done. Contrast-enhanced ultrasonography appears promising as an alternative to CT or MRI but is still under study in the US.

Upper endoscopy to check for gastroesophageal varices should be done when the diagnosis is made and then every 2 to 3 yr. Positive findings may mandate treatment or more frequent endoscopic monitoring.

Prognosis

Prognosis is often unpredictable. It depends on factors such as etiology, severity, presence of complications, comorbid conditions, host factors, and effectiveness of therapy. Patients who continue to drink alcohol, even small amounts, have a very poor prognosis. The Child-Turcotte-Pugh scoring system uses clinical and laboratory information to stratify disease severity, surgical risk, and overall prognosis (see Tables 27–3 and 27–4).

Table 27–3. CHILD-TURCOTTE-PUGH SCORING SYSTEM

CLINICAL OR LABORATORY FACTOR	DEGREE OF ABNORMALITY	POINTS ASSIGNED*
Encephalopathy (grade[†])	None	1
	1–2	2
	3–4	3
Ascites	None	1
	Mild (or controlled by diuretics)	2
	At least moderate despite diuretic treatment	3
Albumin (g/dL)	> 3.5	1
	2.8–3.5	2
	< 2.8	3
Bilirubin (mg/dL)	< 2	1
	2–3	2
	> 3	3
PT (seconds prolonged)	< 4	1
	4–6	2
	> 6	3
or, instead of PT		
INR	< 1.7	1
	1.7–2.3	2
	> 2.3	3

*Risk (grade) is based on the total number of points:
Low (A): 5–6
Moderate (B): 7–9
High (C): 10–15

[†]Encephalopathy is graded based on symptoms:

1: Sleep disturbances; impaired concentration; depression, anxiety, or irritability
2: Drowsiness, disorientation, poor short-term memory, uninhibited behavior
3: Somnolence; confusion; amnesia; anger, paranoia, or other bizarre behavior
4: Coma

However, the Child-Turcotte-Pugh scoring system has limitations; for example, assessments of the severity of ascites and encephalopathy are subjective; interrater reliability of results is thus decreased. In contrast, the Model for End-Stage Liver Disease (MELD) score estimates the severity of end-stage liver disease, regardless of cause, based solely on objective results of laboratory tests: serum creatinine, serum total bilirubin, and INR. The MELD score is used to determine allocation of available organs to liver transplant candidates. Variations of the MELD score are sometimes used for other purposes (eg, to estimate risk of 90-day mortality in patients with alcoholic hepatitis, to predict risk of postoperative mortality in patients with cirrhosis). A variation that incorporates serum sodium (MELDNa) has been extensively studied but is not yet widely used clinically in the US.

Table 27–4. INTERPRETATION OF THE CHILD-TURCOTTE-PUGH SCORING SYSTEM

POINTS	RISK (GRADE)	SURVIVAL RATE (%)	
		1-yr	2-yr
5–6	Low (A)	100	85
7–9	Moderate (B)	80	60
10–15	High (C)	45	35

The MELD score should be calculated differently for patients who have hepatocellular carcinoma. For patients who are 12 to 17 yr old and who have a urea cycle disorder, organic acidemia, or hepatoblastoma, the MELD score is set at 30. Higher MELD scores predict higher risk.

For patients < 12 yr, the corresponding Pediatric End-Stage Liver Disease (PELD) score is calculated. Higher PELD scores predict higher risk.

Treatment

- Supportive care

In general, treatment is supportive and includes stopping injurious drugs, providing nutrition (including supplemental vitamins), and treating the underlying disorders and complications. Doses of drugs metabolized in the liver should be reduced. All alcohol and hepatotoxic substances must be avoided. Withdrawal symptoms during hospitalization should be anticipated in patients who have cirrhosis and have continued to abuse alcohol. Patients should be vaccinated against viral hepatitis A and B unless they are already immune.

Patients with varices need therapy to prevent bleeding. No evidence supports treating small esophageal varices. Medium and large esophageal varices should be treated prophylactically with nonselective beta-blockers or endoscopic banding (ligation). If gastric varices are not amenable to endoscopic banding and do not respond to nonselective beta-blockers, balloon-occluded retrograde transvenous obliteration or endoscopic cyanoacrylate injection may be used.

Transjugular intrahepatic portosystemic shunting (TIPS—see p. 132) should be considered if patients have complications of portal hypertension that are refractory to standard treatments, including ascites and recurrent variceal bleeding.

Liver transplantation is indicated for patients with end-stage liver disease or hepatocellular carcinoma. Risk of death without liver transplantation begins to exceed risks of transplantation (eg, perioperative complications, chronic immunosuppression) when the MELD score is more than about 15. Thus, if the score is ≥ 15 or if cirrhosis has decompensated clinically, patients should be referred to a transplantation center.

KEY POINTS

- Morbidity and mortality in cirrhosis usually result from its complications (eg, complications of portal hypertension, liver failure, hematologic problems).
- Do liver biopsy if a clear diagnosis would lead to better management and outcome.
- Evaluate all patients with cirrhosis for autoimmune hepatitis, hereditary hemochromatosis, and alpha-1 antitrypsin deficiency, as well as for the more common causes, alcoholic and viral hepatitis.
- Evaluate all patients periodically for gastroesophageal varices and hepatocellular carcinoma.
- Predict prognosis using the Child-Turcotte-Pugh and MELD scoring systems, and refer patients with a MELD score ≥ 15 to be evaluated for a liver transplant.
- Treat cirrhosis supportively, including using therapies to prevent bleeding.

PRIMARY BILIARY CIRRHOSIS

(Primary Biliary Cholangitis)

Primary biliary cirrhosis (PBC) is an autoimmune liver disorder characterized by the progressive destruction of intrahepatic bile ducts, leading to cholestasis, cirrhosis, and liver failure. Patients usually are asymptomatic at presentation but may experience fatigue or have symptoms of cholestasis (eg, pruritus, steatorrhea) or cirrhosis (eg, portal hypertension, ascites). Laboratory tests reveal cholestasis, increased IgM, and, characteristically, antimitochondrial antibodies in the serum. Liver biopsy may be necessary for diagnosis and staging. Treatment includes ursodeoxycholic acid, cholestyramine (for pruritus), supplementary fat-soluble vitamins, and, ultimately for advanced disease, liver transplantation.

Etiology

PBC is the most common liver disease associated with chronic cholestasis in adults. Most (95%) cases occur in women aged 35 to 70. PBC also clusters in families. A genetic predisposition, perhaps involving the X chromosome, probably contributes. There may be an inherited abnormality of immune regulation.

An autoimmune mechanism has been implicated; antibodies to antigens located on the inner mitochondrial membranes occur in > 95% of cases. These antimitochondrial antibodies (AMAs), the serologic hallmarks of PBC, are not cytotoxic and are not involved in bile duct damage.

PBC is associated with other autoimmune disorders, such as RA, systemic sclerosis, Sjögren syndrome, CREST syndrome, autoimmune thyroiditis, and renal tubular acidosis.

T cells attack the small bile ducts. CD4 and CD8 T lymphocytes directly target biliary epithelial cells. The trigger for the immunologic attack on bile ducts is unknown. Exposure to foreign antigens, such as an infectious (bacterial or viral) or toxic agent, may be the instigating event. These foreign antigens might be structurally similar to endogenous proteins (molecular mimicry); then the subsequent immunologic reaction would be autoimmune and self-perpetuating. Destruction and loss of bile ducts lead to impaired bile formation and secretion (cholestasis). Retained toxic materials such as bile acids then cause further damage, particularly to hepatocytes. Chronic cholestasis thus leads to liver cell inflammation and scarring in the periportal areas. Eventually, hepatic inflammation decreases as hepatic fibrosis progresses to cirrhosis.

Autoimmune cholangitis is sometimes considered to be a separate disorder. It is characterized by autoantibodies, such as antinuclear antibodies (ANAs), anti–smooth muscle antibodies, or both and has a clinical course and response to treatment that are similar to PBC. However, in autoimmune cholangitis, AMAs are absent.

Symptoms and Signs

About half of patients present without symptoms. Symptoms or signs may develop during any stage of the disease and may include fatigue or reflect cholestasis (and the resulting fat malabsorption, which may lead to vitamin deficiencies and osteoporosis), hepatocellular dysfunction, or cirrhosis.

Symptoms usually develop insidiously. Pruritus, fatigue, and dry mouth and eyes are the initial symptoms in > 50% of patients and can precede other symptoms by months or years. Other initial manifestations include right upper quadrant discomfort (10%); an enlarged, firm, nontender liver (25%); splenomegaly (15%); hyperpigmentation (25%); xanthelasmas (10%); and jaundice (10%). Eventually, all the features and complications of cirrhosis occur. Peripheral neuropathy and other autoimmune disorders associated with PBC may also develop.

Diagnosis

- Liver function tests
- Antimitochondrial antibodies
- Ultrasonography and often MRCP
- Liver biopsy

In asymptomatic patients, PBC is detected incidentally when liver function tests detect abnormalities, typically elevated levels of alkaline phosphatase and gamma-glutamyl transpeptidase (GGT). PBC is suspected in middle-aged women with classic symptoms (eg, unexplained pruritus, fatigue, right upper quadrant discomfort, jaundice) or laboratory results suggesting cholestatic liver disease: elevated alkaline phosphatase and GGT but minimally abnormal aminotransferases (ALT, AST). Serum bilirubin is usually normal in the early stages; elevation indicates disease progression and a worsening prognosis.

If PBC is suspected, liver function tests and tests to measure serum IgM (increased in PBC) and AMA should be done. Enzyme-linked immunosorbent assay (ELISA) tests are 95% sensitive and 98% specific for PBC; false-positive results can occur in autoimmune hepatitis (type 1). Other autoantibodies (eg, ANAs, anti–smooth muscle antibodies, rheumatoid factor) may be present. Extrahepatic biliary obstruction should be ruled out. Ultrasonography is often done first, but ultimately MRCP and sometimes ERCP are necessary. Unless life expectancy is short or there is a contraindication, liver biopsy is usually done. Liver biopsy confirms the diagnosis; it may detect pathognomonic bile duct lesions, even in early stages. As PBC progresses, it becomes morphologically indistinguishable from other forms of cirrhosis. Liver biopsy also helps stage PBC, which has 4 histologic stages:

- **Stage 1:** Inflammation, abnormal connective tissue, or both, confined to the portal areas
- **Stage 2:** Inflammation, fibrosis, or both, confined to the portal and periportal areas
- **Stage 3:** Bridging fibrosis
- **Stage 4:** Cirrhosis

Autoimmune cholangitis is diagnosed when AMAs are absent in a patient who otherwise would be diagnosed with PBC.

Prognosis

Usually, PBC progresses to terminal stages over 15 to 20 yr, although the rate of progression varies. PBC may not diminish quality of life for many years. Patients who present without symptoms tend to develop symptoms over 2 to 7 yr but may not do so for 10 to 15 yr. Once symptoms develop, median life expectancy is 10 yr. Predictors of rapid progression include the following:

- Rapid worsening of symptoms
- Advanced histologic changes
- Older patient age
- Presence of edema
- Presence of associated autoimmune disorders
- Abnormalities in bilirubin, albumin, PT, or INR

The prognosis is ominous when pruritus disappears, xanthomas shrink, jaundice develops, and serum cholesterol decreases.

Treatment

- Arresting or reversing liver damage
- Treating complications (chronic cholestasis and liver failure)
- Sometimes liver transplantation

All alcohol use and hepatotoxic drugs should be stopped. Ursodeoxycholic acid (15 mg/kg po once/day) decreases liver damage, prolongs survival, and delays the need for liver transplantation. About 20% of patients do not have biochemical improvement after ≥ 4 mo; they may have advanced disease and require liver transplantation in a few years. Other drugs proposed to decrease liver damage have not improved overall clinical outcomes or are controversial.

Pruritus may be controlled with cholestyramine 6 to 8 g po bid. This anionic-binding drug binds bile salts and thus may aggravate fat malabsorption. If cholestyramine is taken long-term, supplements of fat-soluble vitamins should be considered. Cholestyramine can decrease absorption of ursodeoxycholic acid, so these drugs should not be given simultaneously. Cholestyramine can also decrease absorption of various drugs; if patients take any drug that could be affected, they should be told not to take the drug within 3 h before or after taking cholestyramine.

Some patients with pruritus respond to ursodeoxycholic acid and ultraviolet light; others may warrant a trial of rifampin or an opioid antagonist, such as naltrexone.

Patients with fat malabsorption due to bile salt deficiency should be treated with vitamin A, D, E, and K supplements. For osteoporosis, weight-bearing exercises, bisphosphonates, or raloxifene may be needed in addition to calcium and vitamin D supplements. In later stages, portal hypertension or complications of cirrhosis require treatment.

Liver transplantation (see p. 1416) has excellent results. The general indication is decompensated liver disease (uncontrolled variceal bleeding, refractory ascites, intractable pruritus, and hepatic encephalopathy). Survival rates after liver transplantation are > 90% at 1 yr, > 80% at 5 yr, and > 65% at 10 yr. AMAs tend to persist after transplantation. PBC recurs in 15% of patients in the first few years and in > 30% by 10 yr. Recurrent PBC after liver transplantation appears to have a benign course. Cirrhosis rarely occurs.

KEY POINTS

- PBC is a chronic, progressive cholestatic liver disorder that is caused by an autoimmune attack on small bile ducts and that occurs almost exclusively in women aged 35 to 70.
- PBC typically progresses to a terminal stage over 15 to 20 yr.
- Suspect PBC if patients have unexplained elevated alkaline phosphatase and GGT but minimally abnormal aminotransferases, particularly if they have constitutional symptoms or manifestations of cholestasis (eg, pruritus, osteoporosis, vitamin D deficiency).
- Measure IgM and antimitochondrial antibodies, and do imaging (to rule out extrahepatic biliary obstruction) and liver biopsy.
- Stop use of hepatotoxins (including alcohol), and treat with ursodeoxycholic acid, which may delay the need for transplantation.
- Transplantation is indicated for decompensated liver disease (uncontrolled variceal bleeding, refractory ascites, intractable pruritus, hepatic encephalopathy).

28 Gallbladder and Bile Duct Disorders

The liver (see Fig. 28–1) produces about 500 to 600 mL of bile each day. Bile is isosmotic with plasma and consists primarily of water and electrolytes but also organic compounds: bile salts, phospholipids (mostly lecithin), cholesterol, bilirubin, and other endogenously produced or ingested compounds, such as proteins that regulate GI function and drugs or their metabolites. Bilirubin is a degradation product of heme compounds from worn-out RBCs and is the pigment that gives bile its yellow-green color.

Bile salts (bile acids) are the major organic component in bile. The liver uses active transport to secrete bile salts into the canaliculus, the cleft between adjacent hepatocytes. Canalicular transport is the rate-limiting step in bile formation. Once secreted, bile salts draw other bile components (particularly sodium and water) into the canaliculus by osmosis. Bile salts are also biologic detergents that enable the body to excrete cholesterol and potentially toxic compounds (eg, bilirubin, drug metabolites). The function of bile salts in the duodenum is to solubilize ingested fat and fat-soluble vitamins, facilitating their digestion and absorption. From the liver, bile flows from the intrahepatic collecting system into the right or left hepatic duct, then into the common hepatic duct.

During fasting, about 75% of the bile secreted passes from the common hepatic duct into the gallbladder via the cystic duct.

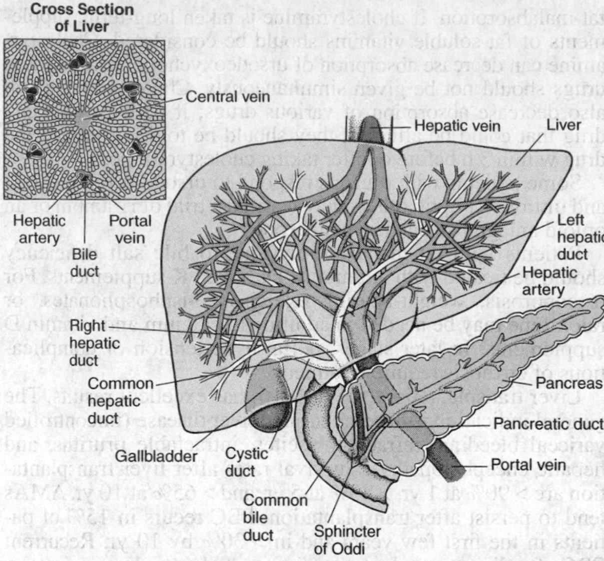

Fig. 28-1. View of the liver and gallbladder.

The rest flows directly into the common bile duct (formed by the junction of the common hepatic and cystic ducts) into the duodenum. During fasting, the gallbladder absorbs up to 90% of bile water, concentrating and storing bile.

Bile empties from the gallbladder into the common bile duct. The common bile duct joins with the pancreatic duct to form the ampulla of Vater, which empties into the duodenum. Before joining the pancreatic duct, the common bile duct tapers to a diameter of ≤ 0.6 cm.

The sphincter of Oddi, which surrounds both the pancreatic duct and the common bile duct, includes a sphincter for each duct. Bile does not normally flow retrograde into the pancreatic duct. These sphincters are highly sensitive to cholecystokinin and other gut hormones (eg, gastrin-releasing peptide) and to alterations in cholinergic tone (eg, by anticholinergic drugs).

Eating releases gut hormones and stimulates cholinergic nerves, causing the gallbladder to contract and the sphincter of Oddi to relax. As a result, the gallbladder empties 50 to 75% of its contents into the duodenum. Conversely, during fasting, an increase in sphincter tone facilitates gallbladder filling.

Bile salts are poorly absorbed by passive diffusion in the proximal small bowel; most intestinal bile salts reach the terminal ileum, which actively absorbs 90% into the portal venous circulation. Returned to the liver, bile salts are efficiently extracted, promptly modified (eg, conjugated if they arrive in the free form), and secreted back into bile. Bile salts circulate through this pathway from liver to gut to liver—the enterohepatic circulation—10 to 12 times/day.

Most disorders of the biliary tract result from gallstones, although acalculous biliary pain occurs in the absence of gallstones and postcholecystectomy syndrome occurs after the gallbladder itself has been removed. Gallstones in the gallbladder (cholelithiasis—see p. 218) are usually asymptomatic. Bile flow may be blocked by gallstones in the bile ducts (choledocholithiasis—see p. 217), triggering biliary colic or causing inflammation of the gallbladder (cholecystitis). Cholecystitis may be acute, developing over hours, or chronic, persisting for a long time.

Blockage of the bile ducts can also cause inflammation, usually with bacterial infection, of the bile ducts (acute cholangitis). Bile flow can be blocked or slowed (called cholestasis) by tumors or, in patients who have AIDS, by strictures caused by opportunistic infections (AIDS cholangiopathy—see below). Cholestasis can also lead to inflammation, fibrosis, and strictures of the bile ducts (called sclerosing cholangitis). Usually, the cause of sclerosing cholangitis is unknown (called primary sclerosing cholangitis).

ACALCULOUS BILIARY PAIN

Acalculous biliary pain is biliary colic without gallstones, resulting from structural or functional disorders; it is sometimes treated with laparoscopic cholecystectomy.

Biliary colic can occur in the absence of gallstones, particularly in young women. Acalculous biliary pain accounts for up to 15% of laparoscopic cholecystectomies. Common causes of such biliary pain include the following:

- Microscopic stones—not detected by routine abdominal ultrasonography
- Abnormal gallbladder emptying
- An overly sensitive biliary tract
- Sphincter of Oddi dysfunction
- Hypersensitivity of the adjacent duodenum
- Possibly gallstones that have spontaneously passed

Some patients eventually develop other functional GI disorders.

Diagnosis

- Unclear
- Usually ultrasonography and sometimes cholescintigraphy and/or ERCP

The best diagnostic approach remains unclear.

Acalculous biliary pain is suspected in patients with biliary colic when diagnostic imaging cannot detect gallstones. Imaging should include ultrasonography and, where available, endoscopic ultrasonography (for small stones < 1 cm).

Abnormal laboratory tests may reveal evidence of a biliary tract abnormality (eg, elevated alkaline phosphatase, bilirubin, ALT, or AST) or a pancreatic abnormality (eg, elevated lipase) during an episode of acute pain. Cholescintigraphy with cholecystokinin infusion measures gallbladder emptying (ejection fraction); potentially interfering drugs such as calcium channel blockers, opioids, and anticholinergics should not be used. ERCP with biliary manometry detects sphincter of Oddi dysfunction.

Treatment

- Unclear but sometimes laparoscopic cholecystectomy

Laparoscopic cholecystectomy improves outcomes for patients with microscopic stones and possibly abnormal gallbladder motility. The role of laparoscopic cholecystectomy or endoscopic sphincterotomy remains problematic. Drug therapies have no proven benefit.

AIDS CHOLANGIOPATHY

AIDS cholangiopathy is biliary obstruction secondary to biliary tract strictures caused by various opportunistic infections.

Before the advent of antiretroviral therapy, cholangiopathy occurred in 25% of patients with AIDS, especially in those with a low CD4 count (< 100/μL). The most common pathogen is *Cryptosporidium parvum*. Others include cytomegalovirus, microsporidia, and *Cyclospora* sp. Papillary stenosis or intrahepatic or extrahepatic sclerosing cholangitis develops in most patients. Over half have both.

Common symptoms include right upper quadrant and epigastric pain and diarrhea. A few patients have fever and jaundice. Severe pain usually indicates papillary stenosis. Milder pain suggests sclerosing cholangitis. The diarrhea reflects small-bowel infection, often cryptosporidiosis.

Diagnosis

- Usually ultrasonography and ERCP

Imaging usually begins with ultrasonography, which is noninvasive and very accurate (> 95%). However, ERCP is usually necessary. ERCP provides the diagnosis, enables clinicians to take a sample for small-bowel biopsy for identification of the causative organism, and provides a therapeutic opportunity to relieve strictures. CT and magnetic resonance cholangiopancreatography likely have supportive roles.

Abnormal liver function test results (especially a high alkaline phosphatase level) are consistent with cholestasis.

Treatment

- Endoscopic procedures

Endoscopic sphincterotomy, often done during ERCP, can markedly relieve pain, jaundice, and cholangitis in patients with papillary stenosis. Isolated or dominant strictures can be stented endoscopically. Antimicrobial therapy is given to treat the infection but alone does not reduce the biliary tract damage or relieve symptoms.

Because of its use in primary sclerosing cholangitis, ursodeoxycholic acid may have a role in treating intrahepatic ductal sclerosis and cholestasis.

ACUTE CHOLECYSTITIS

Acute cholecystitis is inflammation of the gallbladder that develops over hours, usually because a gallstone obstructs the cystic duct. Symptoms include right upper quadrant pain and tenderness, sometimes accompanied by fever, chills, nausea, and vomiting. Abdominal ultrasonography detects the gallstone and sometimes the associated inflammation. Treatment usually involves antibiotics and cholecystectomy.

Acute cholecystitis is the most common complication of cholelithiasis. Conversely, ≥ 95% of patients with acute cholecystitis have cholelithiasis. When a stone becomes impacted in the cystic duct and persistently obstructs it, acute inflammation results. Bile stasis triggers release of inflammatory enzymes (eg, phospholipase A, which converts lecithin to lysolecithin, which then may mediate inflammation).

The damaged mucosa secretes more fluid into the gallbladder lumen than it absorbs. The resulting distention further releases inflammatory mediators (eg, prostaglandins), worsening mucosal damage and causing ischemia, all of which perpetuate inflammation. Bacterial infection can supervene. The vicious circle of fluid secretion and inflammation, when unchecked, leads to necrosis and perforation.

If acute inflammation resolves then continues to recur, the gallbladder becomes fibrotic and contracted and does not concentrate bile or empty normally—features of chronic cholecystitis.

Acute acalculous cholecystitis: Acalculous cholecystitis is cholecystitis without stones. It accounts for 5 to 10% of cholecystectomies done for acute cholecystitis. Risk factors include the following:

- Critical illness (eg, major surgery, burns, sepsis, or trauma)
- Prolonged fasting or TPN (both predispose to bile stasis)
- Shock
- Immune deficiency
- Vasculitis (eg, SLE, polyarteritis nodosa)

The mechanism probably involves inflammatory mediators released because of ischemia, infection, or bile stasis. Sometimes an infecting organism can be identified (eg, *Salmonella* sp or cytomegalovirus in immunodeficient patients). In young children, acute acalculous cholecystitis tends to follow a febrile illness without an identifiable infecting organism.

Symptoms and Signs

Most patients have had prior attacks of biliary colic or acute cholecystitis. The pain of cholecystitis is similar in quality and location to biliary colic but lasts longer (ie, > 6 h) and is more severe. Vomiting is common, as is right subcostal tenderness. Within a few hours, the Murphy sign (deep inspiration exacerbates the pain during palpation of the right upper quadrant and halts inspiration) develops along with involuntary guarding of upper abdominal muscles on the right side. Fever, usually low grade, is common.

In the elderly, the first or only symptoms may be systemic and nonspecific (eg, anorexia, vomiting, malaise, weakness, fever). Sometimes fever does not develop.

Acute cholecystitis begins to subside in 2 to 3 days and resolves within 1 wk in 85% of patients even without treatment.

Complications: Without treatment, 10% of patients develop localized perforation, and 1% develop free perforation and peritonitis. Increasing abdominal pain, high fever, and rigors with rebound tenderness or ileus suggest empyema (pus) in the gallbladder, gangrene, or perforation. When acute cholecystitis is accompanied by jaundice or cholestasis, partial common duct obstruction is likely, usually due to stones or inflammation.

Other complications include the following:

- Mirizzi syndrome: Rarely, a gallstone becomes impacted in the cystic duct and compresses and obstructs the common bile duct, causing cholestasis.
- Gallstone pancreatitis: Gallstones pass from the gallbladder into the biliary tract and block the pancreatic duct.
- Cholecystoenteric fistula: Infrequently, a large stone erodes the gallbladder wall, creating a fistula into the small bowel (or elsewhere in the abdominal cavity); the stone may pass freely or obstruct the small bowel (gallstone ileus).

Acute acalculous cholecystitis: The symptoms are similar to those of acute cholecystitis with gallstones but may be difficult to identify because patients tend to be severely ill (eg, ICU setting) and may be unable to communicate clearly. Abdominal distention or unexplained fever may be the only clue. Untreated, the disease can rapidly progress to gallbladder gangrene and perforation, leading to sepsis, shock, and peritonitis; mortality approaches 65%.

PEARLS & PITFALLS

- Closely monitor patients at risk of acalculous cholecystitis (eg, critically ill, fasting, or immunocompromised patients) for subtle signs of the disorder (eg, abdominal distention, unexplained fever).

Diagnosis

- Ultrasonography
- Cholescintigraphy if ultrasonography results are equivocal or if acalculous cholecystitis is suspected

Acute cholecystitis is suspected based on symptoms and signs.

Transabdominal ultrasonography is the best test to detect gallstones. The test may also elicit local abdominal tenderness over the gallbladder (ultrasonographic Murphy sign). Pericholecystic fluid or thickening of the gallbladder wall indicates acute inflammation.

Cholescintigraphy is useful when results are equivocal; failure of the radionuclide to fill the gallbladder suggests an obstructed cystic duct (ie, an impacted stone). False-positive results may be due to the following:

- A critical illness
- Receiving TPN and no oral foods (because gallbladder stasis prevents filling)
- Severe liver disease (because the liver does not secrete the radionuclide)
- Previous sphincterotomy (which facilitates exit into the duodenum rather than the gallbladder)

Morphine provocation, which increases tone in the sphincter of Oddi and enhances filling, helps eliminate false-positive results.

Abdominal CT identifies complications such as gallbladder perforation or pancreatitis.

Laboratory tests are done but are not diagnostic. Leukocytosis with a left shift is common. In uncomplicated acute cholecystitis, liver function tests are normal or only slightly elevated. Mild cholestatic abnormalities (bilirubin up to 4 mg/dL and mildly elevated alkaline phosphatase) are common, probably indicating inflammatory mediators affecting the liver rather than mechanical obstruction. More marked increases, especially if lipase (amylase is less specific) is elevated > 2-fold, suggest bile duct obstruction. Passage of a stone through the biliary tract increases aminotransferases (ALT, AST).

Acute acalculous cholecystitis: Acute acalculous cholecystitis is suggested if a patient has no gallstones but has ultrasonographic Murphy sign or a thickened gallbladder wall and pericholecystic fluid. A distended gallbladder, biliary sludge, and a thickened gallbladder wall without pericholecystic fluid (due to low albumin or ascites) may result simply from a critical illness.

CT identifies extrabiliary abnormalities. Cholescintigraphy is more helpful; failure of a radionuclide to fill may indicate edematous cystic duct obstruction. Giving morphine helps eliminate a false-positive result due to gallbladder stasis.

Treatment

- Supportive care (hydration, analgesics, antibiotics)
- Cholecystectomy

Management includes hospital admission, IV fluids, and analgesics, such as an NSAID (ketorolac) or opioid. Nothing is given orally, and nasogastric suction is instituted if vomiting or an ileus is present. Parenteral antibiotics are usually initiated to treat possible infection, but evidence of benefit is lacking. Empiric coverage, directed at gram-negative enteric organisms, involves IV regimens such as ceftriaxone 2 g q 24 h plus metronidazole 500 mg q 8 h, piperacillin/tazobactam 4 g q 6 h, or ticarcillin/clavulanate 4 g q 6 h.

Cholecystectomy cures acute cholecystitis and relieves biliary pain. Early cholecystectomy is generally preferred, best done during the first 24 to 48 h in the following situations:

- The diagnosis is clear and patients are at low surgical risk.
- Patients are elderly or have diabetes and are thus at higher risk of infectious complications.
- Patients have empyema, gangrene, perforation, or acalculous cholecystitis.

Surgery may be delayed when patients have an underlying severe chronic disorder (eg, cardiopulmonary) that increases the surgical risks. In such patients, cholecystectomy is deferred until medical therapy stabilizes the comorbid disorders or until cholecystitis resolves. If cholecystitis resolves, cholecystectomy may be done ≥ 6 wk later. Delayed surgery carries the risk of recurrent biliary complications.

Percutaneous cholecystostomy is an alternative to cholecystectomy for patients at very high surgical risk, such as the elderly, those with acalculous cholecystitis, and those in an ICU because of burns, trauma, or respiratory failure.

KEY POINTS

- Most (≥ 95%) patients with acute cholecystitis have cholelithiasis.
- In the elderly, symptoms of cholecystitis may be nonspecific (eg, anorexia, vomiting, malaise, weakness), and fever may be absent.
- Although acute cholecystitis resolves spontaneously in 85% of patients, localized perforation or another complication develops in 10%.
- Do ultrasonography and, if results are equivocal, cholescintigraphy.
- Treat patients with IV fluids, antibiotics, and analgesics; do cholecystectomy when patients are stable.

CHRONIC CHOLECYSTITIS

Chronic cholecystitis is long-standing gallbladder inflammation almost always due to gallstones.

Chronic cholecystitis almost always results from gallstones and prior episodes of acute cholecystitis (even if mild). Damage ranges from a modest infiltrate of chronic inflammatory cells to a fibrotic, shrunken gallbladder. Extensive calcification due to fibrosis is called porcelain gallbladder.

Symptoms and Signs

Gallstones intermittently obstruct the cystic duct and so cause recurrent biliary colic. Such episodes of pain are not necessarily accompanied by overt gallbladder inflammation; the extent of inflammation does not correlate with the intensity or frequency of biliary colic. Upper abdominal tenderness may be present, but usually fever is not. Fever suggests acute cholecystitis. Once episodes begin, they are likely to recur.

Diagnosis

- Ultrasonography

Chronic cholecystitis is suspected in patients with recurrent biliary colic plus gallstones. Ultrasonography or another imaging test usually shows gallstones and sometimes a shrunken, fibrotic gallbladder. The diagnosis is made in patients with a history of recurrent biliary colic and ultrasonographic evidence of gallstones. Cholescintigraphy may show nonvisualization of the gallbladder but is less accurate.

Treatment

- Laparoscopic cholecystectomy

Laparoscopic cholecystectomy is indicated to prevent symptom recurrence and further biliary complications. This procedure is particularly appropriate for the porcelain gallbladder associated with gallbladder carcinoma.

CHOLEDOCHOLITHIASIS AND CHOLANGITIS

Choledocholithiasis is the presence of stones in bile ducts; the stones can form in the gallbladder or in the ducts themselves. These stones cause biliary colic, biliary obstruction, gallstone pancreatitis, or cholangitis (bile duct infection and inflammation). Cholangitis, in turn, can lead to strictures, stasis, and choledocholithiasis. Diagnosis usually requires visualization by magnetic resonance cholangiopancreatography or ERCP. Early endoscopic or surgical decompression is indicated.

Stones may be described as

- Primary stones (usually brown pigment stones), which form in the bile ducts
- Secondary stones (usually cholesterol), which form in the gallbladder but migrate to the bile ducts
- Residual stones, which are missed at the time of cholecystectomy (evident < 3 yr later)
- Recurrent stones, which develop in the ducts > 3 yr after surgery

In developed countries, > 85% of common duct stones are secondary; affected patients have additional stones located in the gallbladder. Up to 10% of patients with symptomatic gallstones also have associated common bile duct stones. After cholecystectomy, brown pigment stones may result from stasis (eg, due to a postoperative stricture) and the subsequent infection. The proportion of ductal stones that are pigmented increases with time after cholecystectomy.

Bile duct stones may pass into the duodenum asymptomatically. Biliary colic occurs when the ducts become partially obstructed. More complete obstruction causes duct dilation, jaundice, and, eventually, cholangitis (a bacterial infection). Stones that obstruct the ampulla of Vater can cause gallstone pancreatitis. Some patients (usually the elderly) present with biliary obstruction due to stones that have caused no symptoms previously.

In **acute cholangitis,** bile duct obstruction allows bacteria to ascend from the duodenum. Most (85%) cases result from common bile duct stones, but bile duct obstruction can result from tumors or other conditions (see Table 28–1). Common infecting organisms include gram-negative bacteria (eg, *Escherichia coli, Klebsiella* sp, *Enterobacter* sp); less common are gram-positive bacteria (eg, *Enterococcus* sp) and mixed anaerobes (eg, *Bacteroides* sp, *Clostridia* sp). Symptoms include abdominal pain, jaundice, and fever or chills (Charcot triad). The abdomen is tender, and often the liver is tender and enlarged (often containing abscesses). Confusion and hypotension predict about a 50% mortality rate and high morbidity.

Recurrent pyogenic cholangitis (Oriental cholangiohepatitis, hepatolithiasis) is characterized by intrahepatic brown pigment stone formation. This disorder occurs in Southeast Asia. It consists of sludge and bacterial debris in the bile ducts. Undernutrition and parasitic infestation (eg, *Clonorchis sinensis*, *Opisthorchis viverrini*) increase susceptibility. Parasitic infestation can cause obstructive jaundice with intrahepatic ductal inflammation, proximal stasis, stone formation, and cholangitis. Repeating cycles of obstruction, infection, and inflammation lead to bile duct strictures and biliary cirrhosis. The extrahepatic ducts tend to be dilated, but the intrahepatic ducts appear straight because of periductal fibrosis.

Table 28–1. CAUSES OF BILE DUCT OBSTRUCTION

Stones (common)
Duct trauma due to surgery (common)
Tumors
Scarring due to chronic pancreatitis
External compression by a cyst, a hernia of the common bile duct (choledochocele), or a pancreatic pseudocyst (rare)
Extrahepatic or intrahepatic strictures due to primary sclerosing cholangitis
AIDS-related cholangiopathy or cholangitis
Parasitic infestation with *Clonorchis sinensis* or *Opisthorchis viverrini*
Parasite migration of *Ascaris lumbricoides* into the common bile duct (rare)

In AIDS-related cholangiopathy or cholangitis, direct cholangiography may show abnormalities similar to those in primary sclerosing cholangitis or papillary stenosis (ie, multiple strictures and dilations involving the intrahepatic and extrahepatic bile ducts). Etiology is probably infection, most likely with cytomegalovirus, *Cryptosporidium* sp, or microsporidia.

Diagnosis

- Liver function tests
- Ultrasonography

Common duct stones should be suspected in patients with jaundice and biliary colic. Fever and leukocytosis further suggest acute cholangitis. Elevated levels of bilirubin and particularly alkaline phosphatase, ALT, and gamma-glutamyltransferase are consistent with extrahepatic obstruction, suggesting stones, particularly in patients with features of acute cholecystitis or cholangitis.

Ultrasonography may show stones in the gallbladder and occasionally in the common duct (less accurate). The common duct is dilated (> 6 mm in diameter if the gallbladder is intact; > 10 mm after a cholecystectomy). If the ducts are not dilated early in the presentation (eg, first day), stones have probably passed. If doubt exists, magnetic resonance cholangiopancreatography (MRCP) is highly accurate for retained stones. ERCP is done if MRCP is equivocal; it can be therapeutic as well as diagnostic. CT, though less accurate than ultrasonography, can detect liver abscesses.

For suspected acute cholangitis, CBC and blood cultures are essential. Leukocytosis is common, and aminotransferases may reach 1000 IU/L, suggesting acute hepatic necrosis, often due to microabscesses. Blood cultures guide antibiotic choice.

Treatment

- ERCP and sphincterotomy

If biliary obstruction is suspected, ERCP and sphincterotomy are necessary to remove the stones. Success rate exceeds 90%; up to 7% of patients have short-term complications (eg, bleeding, pancreatitis, infection). Long-term complications (eg, stone recurrence, fibrosis and subsequent duct stricture) are more common. Laparoscopic cholecystectomy, which is not as well-suited for operative cholangiography or common duct exploration, can be done electively after ERCP and sphincterotomy. Mortality and morbidity after open cholecystectomy with common duct exploration are higher. In patients at high risk of complications with cholecystectomy (eg, the elderly), sphincterotomy alone is an alternative.

Acute cholangitis is an emergency requiring aggressive supportive care and urgent removal of the stones, endoscopically or surgically. Antibiotics are given, similar to those used for acute alcalulous cholecystitis (see p. 216). An alternative regimen for very ill patients is imipenem and ciprofloxacin plus metronidazole to cover anaerobes.

For recurrent pyogenic cholangitis, management aims to provide supportive care (eg, broad-spectrum antibiotics), eradicate any parasites, and mechanically clear the ducts of stones and debris endoscopically (via ERCP) or surgically.

KEY POINTS

- In developed countries, > 85% of common duct stones form in the gallbladder and migrate to the bile ducts; most are cholesterol stones.
- Suspect common duct stones if patients have biliary colic, unexplained jaundice, and/or elevated alkaline phosphatase and gamma-glutamyltransferase levels.
- Do ultrasonography and, if inconclusive, MRCP.
- Do ERCP and sphincterotomy to remove a stone that causes obstruction.
- For acute cholangitis, remove stones as soon as possible and give antibiotics.

CHOLELITHIASIS

Cholelithiasis is the presence of one or more calculi (gallstones) in the gallbladder. In developed countries, about 10% of adults and 20% of people > 65 yr have gallstones. Gallstones tend to be asymptomatic. The most common symptom is biliary colic; gallstones do not cause dyspepsia or fatty food intolerance. More serious complications include cholecystitis; biliary tract obstruction (by stones in the bile ducts [choledocholithiasis]), sometimes with infection (cholangitis); and gallstone pancreatitis. Diagnosis is usually by ultrasonography. If cholelithiasis causes symptoms or complications, cholecystectomy is necessary.

Risk factors for gallstones include female sex, obesity, increased age, American Indian ethnicity, a Western diet, rapid weight loss, and a family history. Most disorders of the biliary tract result from gallstones.

Pathophysiology

Biliary sludge is often a precursor of gallstones. It consists of calcium bilirubinate (a polymer of bilirubin), cholesterol microcrystals, and mucin. Sludge develops during gallbladder stasis, as occurs during pregnancy or use of TPN. Most sludge is asymptomatic and disappears when the primary condition resolves. Alternatively, sludge can evolve into gallstones or migrate into the biliary tract, obstructing the ducts and leading to biliary colic, cholangitis, or pancreatitis.

There are several types of gallstones.

Cholesterol stones account for > 85% of gallstones in the Western world. For cholesterol gallstones to form, the following is required:

- Bile must be supersaturated with cholesterol. Normally, water-insoluble cholesterol is made water soluble by combining with bile salts and lecithin to form mixed micelles. Supersaturation of bile with cholesterol most commonly results from excessive cholesterol secretion (as occurs in obesity or diabetes) but may result from a decrease in bile salt secretion (eg, in cystic fibrosis because of bile salt malabsorption) or in lecithin secretion (eg, in a rare genetic disorder that causes a form of progressive intrahepatic familial cholestasis).
- The excess cholesterol must precipitate from solution as solid microcrystals. Such precipitation in the gallbladder is accelerated by mucin, a glycoprotein, or other proteins in bile.
- The microcrystals must aggregate and grow. This process is facilitated by the binding effect of mucin forming a scaffold and by retention of microcrystals in the gallbladder with impaired contractility due to excess cholesterol in bile.

Black pigment stones are small, hard gallstones composed of calcium (Ca) bilirubinate and inorganic Ca salts (eg, Ca carbonate, Ca phosphate). Factors that accelerate stone development include alcoholic liver disease, chronic hemolysis, and older age.

Brown pigment stones are soft and greasy, consisting of bilirubinate and fatty acids (Ca palmitate or stearate). They form during infection, inflammation, and parasitic infestation (eg, liver flukes in Asia).

Gallstones grow at about 1 to 2 mm/yr, taking 5 to 20 yr before becoming large enough to cause problems. Most gallstones form within the gallbladder, but brown pigment stones form in the ducts. Gallstones may migrate to the bile duct after cholecystectomy or, particularly in the case of brown pigment stones, develop behind strictures as a result of stasis and infection.

Symptoms and Signs

About 80% of people with gallstones are asymptomatic. The remainder have symptoms ranging from a characteristic type of pain (biliary colic) to cholecystitis to life-threatening cholangitis. Biliary colic is the most common symptom.

Stones occasionally traverse the cystic duct without causing symptoms. However, most gallstone migration leads to cystic duct obstruction, which, even if transient, causes biliary colic. Biliary colic characteristically begins in the right upper quadrant but may occur elsewhere in the abdomen. It is often poorly localized, particularly in diabetics and the elderly. The pain may radiate into the back or down the arm.

Episodes begin suddenly, become intense within 15 min to 1 h, remain at a steady intensity (not colicky) for up to 12 h (usually < 6 h), and then gradually disappear over 30 to 90 min, leaving a dull ache. The pain is usually severe enough to send patients to the emergency department for relief. Nausea and some vomiting are common, but fever and chills do not occur unless cholecystitis has developed. Mild right upper quadrant or epigastric tenderness may be present; peritoneal findings are absent. Between episodes, patients feel well.

Although biliary colic can follow a heavy meal, fatty food is not a specific precipitating factor. Nonspecific GI symptoms, such as gas, bloating, and nausea, have been inaccurately ascribed to gallbladder disease. These symptoms are common, having about equal prevalence in cholelithiasis, peptic ulcer disease, and functional GI disorders.

PEARLS & PITFALLS

- Fatty foods are not specific causes of biliary colic, and gas, bloating, and nausea are not specific symptoms of gallbladder disease.

Little correlation exists between the severity and frequency of biliary colic and pathologic changes in the gallbladder. Biliary colic can occur in the absence of cholecystitis. If colic lasts > 12 h, particularly if it is accompanied by vomiting or fever, acute cholecystitis or pancreatitis is likely.

Diagnosis

- Ultrasonography

Gallstones are suspected in patients with biliary colic. Abdominal ultrasonography is the imaging test of choice for detecting gallbladder stones; sensitivity and specificity are 95%. Ultrasonography also accurately detects sludge. CT, MRI, and oral cholecystography (rarely available now, although quite accurate) are alternatives. Endoscopic ultrasonography accurately detects small gallstones (< 3 mm) and may be needed if other tests are equivocal.

Laboratory tests usually are not helpful; typically, results are normal unless complications develop.

Asymptomatic gallstones and biliary sludge are often detected incidentally when imaging, usually ultrasonography, is done for other reasons. About 10 to 15% of gallstones are calcified and visible on plain x-rays.

Prognosis

Patients with asymptomatic gallstones become symptomatic at a rate of about 2%/yr. The symptom that develops most commonly is biliary colic rather than a major biliary complication. Once biliary symptoms begin, they are likely to recur; pain returns in 20 to 40% of patients/yr, and about 1 to 2% of patients/yr develop complications such as cholecystitis, choledocholithiasis, cholangitis, and gallstone pancreatitis.

Treatment

- For symptomatic stones: Laparoscopic cholecystectomy or sometimes stone dissolution using ursodeoxycholic acid
- For asymptomatic stones: Expectant management

Most asymptomatic patients decide that the discomfort, expense, and risk of elective surgery are not worth removing an organ that may never cause clinical illness. However, if symptoms occur, gallbladder removal (cholecystectomy) is indicated because pain is likely to recur and serious complications can develop.

Surgery: Surgery can be done with an open or a laparoscopic technique.

Open cholecystectomy, which involves a large abdominal incision and direct exploration, is safe and effective. Its overall mortality rate is about 0.1% when done electively during a period free of complications.

Laparoscopic cholecystectomy is the treatment of choice. Using video endoscopy and instrumentation through small abdominal incisions, the procedure is less invasive than open cholecystectomy. The result is a much shorter convalescence, decreased postoperative discomfort, improved cosmetic results, yet no increase in morbidity or mortality. Laparoscopic cholecystectomy is converted to an open procedure in 2 to 5% of patients, usually because biliary anatomy cannot be identified or a complication cannot be managed. Older age typically increases the risks of any type of surgery.

Cholecystectomy effectively prevents future biliary colic but is less effective for preventing atypical symptoms such as dyspepsia. Cholecystectomy does not result in nutritional problems or a need for dietary limitations. Some patients develop diarrhea, often because bile salt malabsorption in the ileum is unmasked. Prophylactic cholecystectomy is warranted in asymptomatic patients with cholelithiasis only if they have large gallstones (> 3 cm) or a calcified gallbladder (porcelain gallbladder); these conditions increase the risk of gallbladder carcinoma.

Stone dissolution: For patients who decline surgery or who are at high surgical risk (eg, because of concomitant medical disorders or advanced age), gallbladder stones can sometimes be dissolved by ingesting bile acids orally for many months. The best candidates for this treatment are those with small, radiolucent stones (more likely to be composed of cholesterol) in a functioning nonobstructed gallbladder (indicated by normal filling detected during cholescintigraphy or oral cholecystography or by absence of stones in the neck).

Ursodeoxycholic acid 4 to 5 mg/kg po bid or 3 mg/kg po tid (8 to 10 mg/kg/day) dissolves 80% of tiny stones < 0.5 cm in diameter within 6 mo. For larger stones (the majority), the success rate is much lower, even with higher doses of ursodeoxycholic acid. Further, after successful dissolution, stones recur in 50% within 5 yr. Most patients are thus not candidates and prefer laparoscopic cholecystectomy. However, ursodeoxycholic acid 300 mg po bid can help prevent stone formation in morbidly obese patients who are losing weight rapidly after bariatric surgery or while on a very low calorie diet.

Stone fragmentation (extracorporeal shock wave lithotripsy) to assist stone dissolution and clearance is now unavailable.

KEY POINTS

- In developed countries, about 10% of adults and 20% of people > 65 yr have gallstones, but 80% are asymptomatic.
- Abdominal ultrasonography is 95% sensitive and specific for detecting gallbladder stones.
- Once symptoms develop (usually biliary colic), pain returns in 20 to 40% of patients/yr.
- Treat most patients who have symptomatic gallstones with laparoscopic cholecystectomy.

POSTCHOLECYSTECTOMY SYNDROME

Postcholecystectomy syndrome is occurrence of abdominal symptoms after cholecystectomy.

Postcholecystectomy syndrome occurs in 5 to 40% of patients. It refers to presumed gallbladder symptoms that continue or that develop after cholecystectomy or to other symptoms that result from cholecystectomy. Removal of the gallbladder, the storage organ for bile, normally has few adverse effects on biliary tract function or pressures. In about 10%, biliary colic appears to result from functional or structural abnormalities of the sphincter of Oddi, resulting in altered biliary pressures or heightened sensitivity.

The most common symptoms are dyspepsia or otherwise nonspecific symptoms rather than true biliary colic. Papillary stenosis, which is rare, is fibrotic narrowing around the sphincter, perhaps caused by trauma and inflammation due to pancreatitis, instrumentation (eg, ERCP), or prior passage of a stone. Other causes include a retained bile duct stone, pancreatitis, and gastroesophageal reflux.

Diagnosis

- ERCP with biliary manometry or biliary nuclear scanning
- Exclusion of extrabiliary pain

Patients with postcholecystectomy pain should be evaluated as indicated for extrabiliary as well as biliary causes. If the pain suggests biliary colic, alkaline phosphatase, bilirubin,

ALT, amylase, and lipase should be measured, and ERCP with biliary manometry or biliary nuclear scanning should be done (see Laboratory Tests of the Liver and Gallbladder on p. 196 and Imaging Tests on p. 199). Elevated liver enzymes suggest sphincter of Oddi dysfunction; elevated amylase and lipase suggest dysfunction of the sphincter's pancreatic portion.

Dysfunction is best detected by biliary manometry done during ERCP, although ERCP has a 15 to 30% risk of inducing pancreatitis. Manometry shows increased pressure in the biliary tract when pain is reproduced. A slowed hepatic hilum-duodenal transit time on a scan also suggests sphincter of Oddi dysfunction. Diagnosis of papillary stenosis is based on a clear-cut history of recurrent episodes of biliary pain and abnormal liver (or pancreatic) enzyme tests.

Treatment

- Sometimes endoscopic sphincterotomy

Endoscopic sphincterotomy can relieve recurrent pain due to sphincter of Oddi dysfunction, particularly if due to papillary stenosis. ERCP and manometry have been used to treat postcholecystectomy pain; however, no current evidence indicates that this treatment is efficacious if patients have no objective abnormalities. These patients should be treated symptomatically.

PRIMARY SCLEROSING CHOLANGITIS

Primary sclerosing cholangitis (PSC) is patchy inflammation, fibrosis, and strictures of the bile ducts that has no known cause. However, 80% of patients have inflammatory bowel disease, most often ulcerative colitis. Other associated conditions include connective tissue disorders, autoimmune disorders, and immunodeficiency syndromes, sometimes complicated by opportunistic infections. Fatigue and pruritus develop insidiously and progressively. Diagnosis is by cholangiography (MRCP or ERCP). Liver transplantation is indicated for advanced disease.

PSC is the most common form of sclerosing cholangitis. Most (70%) patients with PSC are men. Mean age at diagnosis is 40 yr.

Etiology

Although the cause is unknown, PSC is associated with inflammatory bowel disease, which is present in 80% of patients. About 5% of patients with ulcerative colitis and about 1% with Crohn disease develop PSC. This association and the presence of several autoantibodies (eg, anti–smooth muscle and perinuclear antineutrophilic antibodies [pANCA]) suggest immune-mediated mechanisms. T cells appear to be involved in the destruction of the bile ducts, implying disordered cellular immunity. A genetic predisposition is suggested by a tendency for the disorder to develop in multiple family members and a higher frequency in people with HLAB8 and HLADR3, which are often correlated with autoimmune disorders. An unknown trigger (eg, bacterial infection, ischemic duct injury) probably causes PSC to develop in genetically predisposed people.

Symptoms and Signs

Onset is usually insidious, with progressive fatigue and then pruritus. Jaundice tends to develop later. About 10 to 15% of patients present with repeated episodes of right upper quadrant pain and fever, possibly due to ascending bacterial cholangitis. Steatorrhea and deficiencies of fat-soluble vitamins can develop. Persistent jaundice harbingers advanced disease. Symptomatic gallstones and choledocholithiasis tend to develop in about 75% of patients.

Some patients, asymptomatic until late in the course, first present with hepatosplenomegaly or cirrhosis. PSC tends to slowly and inexorably progress. The terminal phase involves decompensated cirrhosis, portal hypertension, ascites, and liver failure. The time from diagnosis to liver failure is about 12 yr.

Despite the association between PSC and inflammatory bowel disease, the two diseases tend to run separate courses. Ulcerative colitis may appear years before PSC and tends to have a milder course when associated with PSC. Similarly, total colectomy does not change the course of PSC.

The presence of both PSC and inflammatory bowel disease increases the risk of colorectal carcinoma, regardless of whether a liver transplantation has been done for PSC. Cholangiocarcinoma develops in 10 to 15% of patients.

Diagnosis

- MRCP

PSC is suspected in patients with unexplained abnormalities in liver function tests, particularly in those with inflammatory bowel disease. A cholestatic pattern is typical: elevated alkaline phosphatase and gamma-glutamyltransferase (GGT) rather than aminotransferases. Gamma globulin and IgM levels tend to be increased. Anti–smooth muscle antibodies and pANCA are usually positive. Antimitochondrial antibody, positive in primary biliary cirrhosis, is characteristically negative.

Imaging of the hepatobiliary system begins with ultrasonography to exclude extrahepatic biliary obstruction. Although ultrasonography or CT can show ductal dilation, diagnosis requires cholangiography to show multiple strictures and dilations in the intrahepatic and extrahepatic bile ducts. Cholangiography should begin with MRCP. ERCP is usually a 2nd choice because it is invasive. Liver biopsy is usually not required for diagnosis; when done, it shows bile duct proliferation, periductal fibrosis, inflammation, and loss of bile ducts. With disease progression, periductal fibrosis extends from the portal regions and eventually leads to secondary biliary cirrhosis.

Measurement of serum tumor markers and ERCP surveillance with brush cytology should be done regularly to check for cholangiocarcinoma.

Treatment

- Supportive care
- ERCP dilation for major (dominant) strictures
- Transplantation for recurrent bacterial cholangitis or complications of liver failure

Asymptomatic patients usually require only monitoring (eg, physical examination and liver function tests twice/yr). Ursodeoxycholic acid (eg, 5 mg/kg po tid, up to 15 mg/kg/day) reduces itching and improves biochemical markers but not survival. Chronic cholestasis and cirrhosis require supportive treatment. Episodes of bacterial cholangitis warrant antibiotics and therapeutic ERCP as needed. If a single stricture appears to be the major cause of obstruction (a dominant stricture, found in about 20% of patients), ERCP dilation (with brush cytology to check for tumors) and stenting can relieve symptoms.

Liver transplantation is the only treatment that improves life expectancy in patients with PSC and that offers a cure. Recurrent bacterial cholangitis or complications of end-stage liver disease (eg, intractable ascites, portosystemic encephalopathy, bleeding esophageal varices) are reasonable indications for liver transplantation.

KEY POINTS

- Most (80%) patients with PSC have inflammatory bowel disease, usually ulcerative colitis, and many have autoantibodies.
- Suspect PSC if patients, particularly those with inflammatory bowel disease, have an unexplained cholestatic pattern of abnormalities in liver function tests.
- Exclude extrahepatic biliary obstruction by ultrasonography, then do MRCP (or, as a second choice, ERCP).
- Monitor patients with periodic liver function testing, and treat symptoms and complications (eg, ERCP to dilate dominant strictures).
- Consider liver transplantation if recurrent cholangitis or complications of liver failure develop.

SCLEROSING CHOLANGITIS

Sclerosing cholangitis refers to chronic cholestatic syndromes characterized by patchy inflammation, fibrosis, and strictures of the intrahepatic and extrahepatic bile ducts. Progression obliterates the bile ducts and leads to cirrhosis, liver failure, and sometimes cholangiocarcinoma.

Sclerosing cholangitis may be primary (with no known cause) or secondary due to immune deficiencies (congenital in children, acquired in adults as AIDS cholangiopathy), often associated with superimposed infections (eg, cytomegalovirus, *Cryptosporidium*), histiocytosis X, or use of drugs (eg, intraarterial floxuridine). Both primary and secondary sclerosing cholangitis cause similar inflammatory and fibrosing lesions scarring the bile ducts. Other causes of bile duct strictures are choledocholithiasis, postoperative biliary stricture, ischemic bile duct injury (during liver transplantation), congenital biliary abnormalities, cholangiocarcinoma, and parasitic infestations.

Diagnosis of biliary strictures and dilations requires imaging techniques such as ultrasonography and cholangiography.

Treatment focuses on relieving biliary obstruction (eg, dilating and stenting strictures) and, when possible, eradicating responsible organisms or treating the cause (eg, HIV).

TUMORS OF THE GALLBLADDER AND BILE DUCTS

Gallbladder and bile duct tumors can cause extrahepatic biliary obstruction. Symptoms may be absent but often are constitutional or reflect biliary obstruction. Diagnosis is based on ultrasonography plus CT cholangiography or MRCP. Prognosis is grim. Mechanical bile drainage can often relieve pruritus, recurrent sepsis, and pain due to biliary obstruction.

Cholangiocarcinomas and other bile duct tumors are rare (1 to 2/100,000 people) but are usually malignant. Cholangiocarcinomas occur predominantly in the extrahepatic bile ducts: 60 to 70% in the perihilar region (Klatskin tumors), about 25% in the distal ducts, and the rest in the liver. Risk factors include primary sclerosing cholangitis, older age, infestation with liver flukes, and a choledochal cyst.

Gallbladder carcinoma is uncommon (2.5/100,000). It is more common among American Indians, patients with large gallstones (> 3 cm), and those with extensive gallbladder calcification due to chronic cholecystitis (porcelain gallbladder). Nearly all (70 to 90%) patients also have gallstones. Median survival is 3 mo. Cure is possible when cancer is found early (eg, incidentally at cholecystectomy).

Gallbladder polyps are usually asymptomatic benign mucosal projections that develop in the lumen of the gallbladder. Most are < 10 mm in diameter and composed of cholesterol ester and triglycerides; the presence of such polyps is called cholesterolosis. They are found in about 5% of people during ultrasonography. Other, much less common benign polyps include adenomas (causing adenomyomatosis) and inflammatory polyps. Small gallbladder polyps are incidental findings that do not require treatment.

Symptoms and Signs

Most patients with cholangiocarcinomas present with pruritus and painless obstructive jaundice, typically at age 50 to 70 yr. Early perihilar tumors may cause only vague abdominal pain, anorexia, and weight loss. Other features include fatigue, acholic stool, a palpable mass, hepatomegaly, or a distended gallbladder (Courvoisier sign, with distal cholangiocarcinoma). Pain may resemble that of biliary colic (reflecting biliary obstruction) or may be constant and progressive. Sepsis (secondary to acute cholangitis), although unusual, may be induced by ERCP.

Manifestations of gallbladder carcinoma may range from incidental findings at cholecystectomy done to relieve biliary pain to cholelithiasis to advanced disease with constant pain, weight loss, and an abdominal mass or obstructive jaundice.

Most gallbladder polyps cause no symptoms.

Diagnosis

- Ultrasonography (sometimes endoscopic), followed by CT cholangiography or MRCP
- Sometimes ERCP

Cholangiocarcinomas and gallbladder carcinomas are suspected when extrahepatic biliary obstruction is unexplained. Laboratory test results reflect the degree of cholestasis. In patients with primary sclerosing cholangitis, serum carcinoembryonic antigen (CEA) and cancer antigen (CA) levels 19-9 are measured periodically to check for cholangiocarcinoma.

Diagnosis is based on ultrasonography (or endoscopic ultrasonography), followed by CT cholangiography or MRCP (see p. 199). CT is sometimes done and may provide more information than ultrasonography, particularly for gallbladder carcinomas. When these methods are inconclusive, ERCP with percutaneous transhepatic cholangiography (PTC) becomes necessary. ERCP not only detects the tumor but also, with brushings, can provide a tissue diagnosis, sometimes making ultrasonography- or CT-guided needle biopsy unnecessary. Contrast-enhanced CT assists in staging.

Open laparotomy is necessary to determine disease extent, which guides treatment.

Treatment

- For cholangiocarcinomas, stenting (or another bypass procedure) or occasionally resection
- For gallbladder carcinoma, usually symptomatic treatment

For cholangiocarcinoma, stenting or surgically bypassing the obstruction relieves pruritus, jaundice, and perhaps fatigue.

Hilar cholangiocarcinomas with CT evidence of spread are stented via PTC or ERCP. Distal duct cholangiocarcinomas are stented endoscopically with ERCP. If cholangiocarcinoma appears localized, surgical exploration determines resectability by hilar resection or pancreaticoduodenectomy. However, successful resection is uncommon.

Liver transplantation is not indicated because of the high recurrence rate. Effectiveness of adjuvant chemotherapy and radiation therapy for cholangiocarcinomas is unproved as yet.

Many gallbladder carcinomas are treated symptomatically.

KEY POINTS

- Biliary tract cancer (usually cholangiocarcinoma or gallbladder carcinoma) is uncommon.
- Suspect cancer if patients have an unexplained extrahepatic biliary obstruction or abdominal mass.
- Diagnose cancers by imaging, beginning with ultrasonography, followed by CT cholangiography or MRCP.
- Treat cancers symptomatically (eg, by stenting or bypassing obstructions in cholangiocarcinoma); occasionally, resection is warranted.

29 Hepatitis

Hepatitis is an inflammation of the liver characterized by diffuse or patchy necrosis.

Hepatitis may be acute or chronic (usually defined as lasting > 6 mo). Most cases of acute viral hepatitis resolve spontaneously, but some progress to chronic hepatitis.

Common Causes

Common causes of hepatitis include

- Specific hepatitis viruses
- Alcohol
- Drugs (eg, isoniazid)

At least 5 specific viruses appear to be responsible. Other unidentified viruses probably also cause acute viral hepatitis.

Less Common Causes

Less common causes of hepatitis include other viral infections (eg, infectious mononucleosis, yellow fever, cytomegalovirus infection) and leptospirosis.

Parasitic infections (eg, schistosomiasis, malaria, amebiasis), pyogenic infections, and abscesses that affect the liver are not considered hepatitis. Liver involvement with TB and other granulomatous infiltrations is sometimes called granulomatous hepatitis, but the clinical, biochemical, and histologic features differ from those of diffuse hepatitis.

Various systemic infections and other illnesses may produce small focal areas of hepatic inflammation or necrosis. This nonspecific reactive hepatitis can cause minor liver function abnormalities but is usually asymptomatic.

Some types of infectious and noninfectious liver inflammation are summarized in Table 29–1.

OVERVIEW OF ACUTE VIRAL HEPATITIS

Acute viral hepatitis is diffuse liver inflammation caused by specific hepatotropic viruses that have diverse modes of transmission and epidemiologies. A nonspecific viral prodrome is followed by anorexia, nausea, and often fever or right upper quadrant pain. Jaundice often develops, typically as other symptoms begin to resolve. Most cases resolve spontaneously, but some progress to chronic hepatitis. Occasionally, acute viral hepatitis progresses to acute liver failure (indicating fulminant hepatitis). Diagnosis is by liver function tests and serologic tests to identify the virus. Good hygiene and universal precautions can prevent acute viral hepatitis. Depending on the specific virus, preexposure and postexposure prophylaxis may be possible using vaccines or serum globulins. Treatment is usually supportive.

Acute viral hepatitis is a common, worldwide disease that has different causes; each type shares clinical, biochemical, and morphologic features. Liver infections caused by nonhepatitis viruses (eg, Epstein-Barr virus, yellow fever virus, cytomegalovirus) generally are not termed acute viral hepatitis.

Table 29–1. SELECTED DISEASES OR ORGANISMS ASSOCIATED WITH LIVER INFLAMMATION

DISEASE OR ORGANISM	MANIFESTATIONS
Viruses	
Cytomegalovirus	**In neonates:** Hepatomegaly, jaundice, congenital defects **In adults:** Mononucleosis-like illness with hepatitis; may occur posttransfusion
Epstein-Barr	Infectious mononucleosis Clinical hepatitis with jaundice in 5–10%; subclinical liver involvement in 90–95% Acute hepatitis sometimes severe in young adults
Yellow fever	Jaundice, systemic toxicity, bleeding Liver necrosis with little inflammatory reaction
Other	Hepatic infection occasionally due to echovirus or coxsackievirus infections, varicella, herpes simplex, rubella, or rubeola
Bacteria	
Actinomycosis	Granulomatous reaction of liver with progressive necrotizing abscesses
Pyogenic abscess*	Serious infection acquired via portal pyemia, cholangitis, or hematogenous or direct spread; due to various organisms, especially gram-negative and anaerobic Illness and toxicity, yet only mild liver dysfunction
Tuberculosis	Hepatic involvement (common; usually subclinical) with granulomatous infiltration; jaundice (rare) Disproportionately increased alkaline phosphatase
Other	Minor focal hepatitis in numerous systemic infections (common; usually subclinical)

Table 29–1. SELECTED DISEASES OR ORGANISMS ASSOCIATED WITH LIVER INFLAMMATION (*Continued*)

DISEASE OR ORGANISM	MANIFESTATIONS
Fungi	
Histoplasmosis	Granulomas in liver and spleen (usually subclinical) that heal with calcification
Other	Granulomatous infiltration sometimes occurring in cryptococcosis, coccidioidomycosis, blastomycosis, or other infections
Protozoa	
Amebiasis*	Important disease, often without obvious dysentery Usually a large single abscess with liquefaction Systemic illness, tender hepatomegaly, surprisingly mild liver dysfunction
Malaria	A common cause of hepatosplenomegaly in endemic areas Jaundice absent or mild unless active hemolysis is present
Toxoplasmosis	Transplacental infection **In neonates:** Jaundice, CNS and other systemic manifestations
Visceral leishmaniasis	Infiltration of reticuloendothelial system by parasite, hepatosplenomegaly
Helminths	
Ascariasis	Biliary obstruction by adult worms, parenchymal granulomas caused by larvae
Clonorchiasis	Biliary tract infestation, cholangitis, stones, cholangiocarcinoma
Echinococcosis	One or more hydatid cysts, which usually have a calcified rim and may be large but which often are asymptomatic and do not disrupt liver function Can rupture into the peritoneum or biliary tract
Fascioliasis	**Acute:** Tender hepatomegaly, fever, eosinophilia **Chronic:** Biliary fibrosis, cholangitis
Schistosomiasis	Periportal granulomatous reaction to ova with progressive hepatosplenomegaly, pipestem fibrosis, portal hypertension, and varices Hepatocellular function preserved; not true cirrhosis
Toxocariasis	Visceral larva migrans syndrome Hepatomegaly with granulomas, eosinophilia
Spirochetes	
Leptospirosis	Acute fever, prostration, jaundice, bleeding, renal injury Liver necrosis (often mild despite severe jaundice)
Syphilis	**Congenital:** Neonatal hepatosplenomegaly, fibrosis **Acquired:** Variable hepatitis in secondary stage, gummas with irregular scarring in tertiary stage
Relapsing fever	*Borrelia* infection Systemic symptoms, hepatomegaly, sometimes jaundice
Unknown	
Idiopathic granulomatous hepatitis	Active chronic granulomatous inflammation not resulting from known causes (sarcoid variant?) May cause mainly systemic symptoms (eg, fever, malaise) and can occur when certain drugs are used
Sarcoidosis	Granulomatous infiltration (common, usually subclinical), jaundice (rare) Occasionally, progressive inflammation with scarring and portal hypertension
Ulcerative colitis, Crohn disease	Spectrum of hepatic disease, especially in ulcerative colitis; includes periportal inflammation (pericholangitis), sclerosing cholangitis, cholangiocarcinoma, and autoimmune hepatitis Poor correlation between hepatic function and activity of bowel disorder

*Differentiate from amebiasis with serologic tests for amebas and direct percutaneous abscess aspiration.

Etiology

At least 5 specific viruses appear to be responsible (see Table 29–2):

- Hepatitis A (HAV)
- Hepatitis B (HBV)
- Hepatitis C (HCV)
- Hepatitis D (HDV)
- Hepatitis E (HEV)

Other unidentified viruses probably also cause acute viral hepatitis.

Symptoms and Signs

Some manifestations of acute hepatitis are virus-specific (see discussions of individual hepatitis viruses), but in general, acute infection tends to develop in predictable phases:

- **Incubation period:** The virus multiplies and spreads without causing symptoms (see Table 29–2).
- **Prodromal (pre-icteric) phase:** Nonspecific symptoms occur; they include profound anorexia, malaise, nausea and vomiting, a newly developed distaste for cigarettes (in smokers), and often fever or right upper quadrant abdominal pain. Urticaria and arthralgias occasionally occur, especially in HBV infection.

Table 29–2. CHARACTERISTICS OF HEPATITIS VIRUSES

CHARACTERISTIC	HAV	HBV	HCV	HDV	HEV
Nucleic acid	RNA	DNA	RNA	*	RNA
Serologic diagnosis	IgM anti-HA	HBsAg	Anti-HCV	Anti-HDV	Anti-HEV
Major transmission	Fecal-oral	Blood	Blood	Needle	Water
Incubation period (days)	15–45	40–180	20–120	30–180	14–60
Epidemics	Yes	No	No	No	Yes
Chronicity	No	Yes	Yes	Yes	No
Liver cancer	No	Yes	Yes	Yes	No

*Incomplete RNA; requires presence of HBV for replication.

Anti-HCV = antibody to HCV; anti-HDV = antibody to HDV; anti-HEV = antibody to HEV; HBsAg = hepatitis B surface antigen; IgM anti-HAV = IgM antibody to HAV.

- **Icteric phase:** After 3 to 10 days, the urine darkens, followed by jaundice. Systemic symptoms often regress, and patients feel better despite worsening jaundice. The liver is usually enlarged and tender, but the edge of the liver remains soft and smooth. Mild splenomegaly occurs in 15 to 20% of patients. Jaundice usually peaks within 1 to 2 wk.
- **Recovery phase:** During this 2- to 4-wk period, jaundice fades.

Appetite usually returns after the first week of symptoms. Acute viral hepatitis usually resolves spontaneously 4 to 8 wk after symptom onset.

Anicteric hepatitis (hepatitis without jaundice) occurs more often than icteric hepatitis in patients with HCV infection and in children with HAV infection. It typically manifests as a minor flu-like illness.

Recrudescent hepatitis occurs in a few patients and is characterized by recurrent manifestations during the recovery phase.

Manifestations of cholestasis may develop during the icteric phase (called cholestatic hepatitis) but usually resolve. When they persist, they cause prolonged jaundice, elevated alkaline phosphatase, and pruritus, despite general regression of inflammation.

Diagnosis

- Liver function tests (AST and ALT elevated out of proportion to alkaline phosphatase, usually with hyperbilirubinemia)
- Viral serologic testing
- PT/INR measurement

Initial diagnosis of acute viral hepatitis: Acute hepatitis must first be differentiated from other disorders that cause similar symptoms. In the prodromal phase, hepatitis mimics various nonspecific viral illnesses and is difficult to diagnose. Anicteric patients suspected of having hepatitis based on risk factors are tested initially with nonspecific liver function tests, including aminotransferases, bilirubin, and alkaline phosphatase. Usually, acute hepatitis is suspected only during the icteric phase. Thus, acute hepatitis should be differentiated from other disorders causing jaundice (see Fig. 29–1 and p. 86).

Acute hepatitis can usually be differentiated from other causes of jaundice by

- Its marked elevations of AST and ALT (typically ≥ 400 IU/L)

ALT is typically higher than AST, but absolute levels correlate poorly with clinical severity. Values increase early in the prodromal phase, peak before jaundice is maximal, and fall slowly during the recovery phase. Urinary bilirubin usually precedes jaundice. Hyperbilirubinemia in acute viral hepatitis varies in severity, and fractionation has no clinical value. Alkaline phosphatase is usually only moderately elevated; marked elevation suggests extrahepatic cholestasis and prompts imaging tests (eg, ultrasonography).

Liver biopsy is usually not needed unless the diagnosis is uncertain.

If laboratory results suggest acute hepatitis, particularly if ALT and AST are > 1000 IU/L, PT/INR is measured.

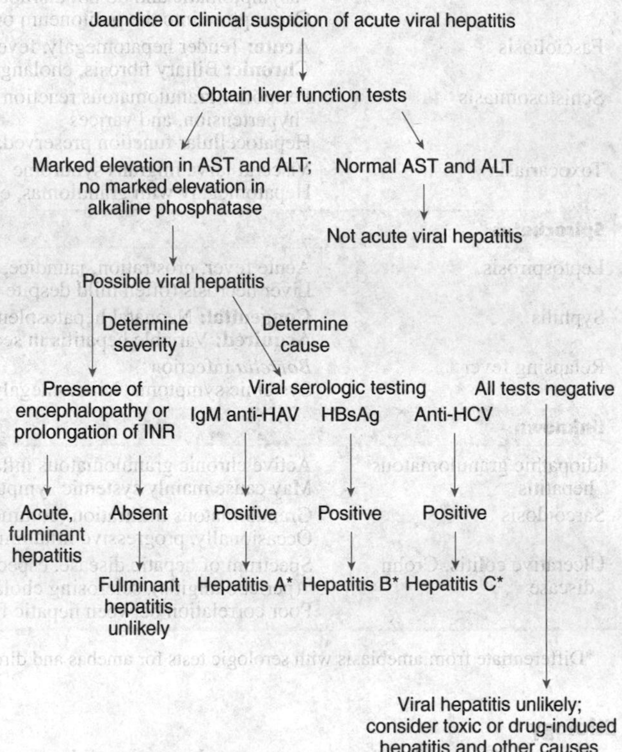

Fig. 29–1. Simplified diagnostic approach to possible acute viral hepatitis.

*Obtain additional laboratory studies for hepatitis A, hepatitis B, and hepatitis C.

Anti-HCV = antibody to HCV; HBsAg = hepatitis B surface antigen; IgM anti-HAV = IgM antibody to HAV.

Manifestations of portosystemic encephalopathy, bleeding diathesis, or prolongation of INR suggest acute liver failure, indicating fulminant hepatitis (see below).

If acute hepatitis is suspected, efforts are next directed toward identifying its cause. A history of exposure may provide the only clue of drug-induced or toxic hepatitis. The history should also elicit risk factors for viral hepatitis. Prodromal sore throat and diffuse adenopathy suggest infectious mononucleosis rather than viral hepatitis.

Alcoholic hepatitis is suggested by a history of drinking, more gradual onset of symptoms, and presence of vascular spiders or signs of chronic alcohol use or chronic liver disease (see p. 203); aminotransferase levels rarely exceed 300 IU/L, even in severe cases. Also, unlike in viral hepatitis, AST is typically higher than ALT, although this difference by itself does not reliably differentiate the two. In uncertain cases, liver biopsy usually distinguishes alcoholic from viral hepatitis.

Serology: In patients with findings suggesting acute viral hepatitis, the following studies are done to screen for HAV, HBV, and HCV:

- IgM antibody to HAV (IgM anti-HAV)
- Hepatitis B surface antigen (HBsAg)
- IgM antibody to hepatitis B core (IgM anti-HBc)
- Antibody to HCV (anti-HCV)

If any are positive, further serologic testing may be necessary to differentiate acute from past or chronic infection (see Tables 29–3, 29–4, and 29–6).

If serology suggests hepatitis B, testing for hepatitis B e antigen (HBeAg) and antibody to hepatitis B e antigen (anti-HBe) is usually done to help determine the prognosis and to guide antiviral therapy. If serologically confirmed HBV infection is severe, anti-HDV is measured.

If the patient has recently traveled to an endemic area, IgM antibody to HEV (IgM anti-HEV) should be measured if the test is available.

Biopsy: Biopsy is usually unnecessary but, if done, usually reveals similar histopathology regardless of the specific virus:

- Patchy cell dropout
- Acidophilic hepatocellular necrosis
- Mononuclear inflammatory infiltrate
- Histologic evidence of regeneration
- Preservation of the reticulin framework

HBV infection can occasionally be diagnosed based on the presence of ground-glass hepatocytes (caused by HBsAg-packed cytoplasm) and using special immunologic stains for the viral components. However, these findings are unusual in acute HBV infection and are much more common in chronic HBV infection.

HCV causation can sometimes be inferred from subtle morphologic clues.

Liver biopsy may help predict prognosis in acute hepatitis but is rarely done solely for this purpose. Complete histologic recovery occurs unless extensive necrosis bridges entire acini (bridging necrosis). Most patients with bridging necrosis recover fully. However, some cases progress to chronic hepatitis.

Treatment

- Supportive care

No treatments attenuate acute viral hepatitis. Alcohol should be avoided because it can increase liver damage. Restrictions on diet or activity, including commonly prescribed bed rest, have no scientific basis.

Most patients may safely return to work after jaundice resolves, even if AST or ALT levels are slightly elevated.

For cholestatic hepatitis, cholestyramine 8 g po once/day or bid can relieve itching.

Viral hepatitis should be reported to the local or state health department.

Prevention

Because treatments have limited efficacy, prevention of viral hepatitis is very important.

General measures: Good personal hygiene helps prevent transmission, particularly fecal-oral transmission, as occurs with HAV and HEV.

Blood and other body fluids (eg, saliva, semen) of patients with acute HBV and HCV infection and stool of patients with HAV infection are considered infectious. Barrier protection is recommended, but isolation of patients does little to prevent spread of HAV and is of no value in HBV or HCV infection.

Posttransfusion infection is minimized by avoiding unnecessary transfusions and screening all donors for HBsAg and anti-HCV. Screening has decreased the incidence of posttransfusion hepatitis, probably to about 1/100,000 units of blood component transfused.

Immunoprophylaxis: Immunoprophylaxis can involve active immunization using vaccines and passive immunization.

Vaccines for hepatitis A and hepatitis B are available in the US.

Routine vaccination for hepatitis A and B is recommended in the US for all children and adults at high risk.

A vaccine for hepatitis E is now available in China

Standard immune globulin prevents or decreases the severity of HAV infection and should be given to family members and close contacts of patients. Hepatitis B immune globulin (HBIG) probably does not prevent infection but prevents or attenuates clinical illness.

No product exists for immunoprophylaxis of HCV or HDV. However, prevention of HBV infection prevents HDV infection. The propensity of HCV for changing its genome hampers vaccine development.

KEY POINTS

- Transmission is the fecal-oral route for hepatitis A and parenterally or via blood for hepatitis B and C.
- Hepatitis B and C, unlike hepatitis A, predispose to chronic hepatitis and liver cancer.
- Patients with acute viral hepatitis may be anicteric or even asymptomatic.
- Do viral serologic testing (IgM anti-HAV, HBsAg, anti-HCV) if clinical findings are consistent with acute viral hepatitis and AST and ALT are elevated out of proportion to alkaline phosphatase.
- Treat patients supportively.
- Routine vaccination for hepatitis A and B is recommended in the US for all children and adults at high risk.

FULMINANT HEPATITIS

Fulminant hepatitis is a rare syndrome of massive necrosis of liver parenchyma and a decrease in liver size (acute yellow atrophy) that usually occurs after infection with certain hepatitis viruses, exposure to toxic agents, or drug-induced injury.

HBV is sometimes responsible for fulminant hepatitis, and up to 50% of cases of fulminant hepatitis B involve HDV coinfection. Fulminant hepatitis with HAV is rare but may be more likely in people with preexisting liver disorders. The role of HCV remains uncertain.

Patients rapidly deteriorate because portosystemic encephalopathy develops, progressing to coma and cerebral edema over a period of several days to several weeks. Coagulopathy commonly results from liver failure or disseminated intravascular coagulation, and functional renal failure (hepatorenal syndrome—see p. 195) may develop. Increasing PT or INR, portosystemic encephalopathy, and particularly renal failure are ominous.

Diagnosis

- Clinical evaluation
- Liver function tests
- PT/INR measurement

Fulminant hepatitis should be suspected if patients are acutely ill with new-onset jaundice, rapid changes in mental status, or unexplained bleeding or if patients with known liver disease rapidly deteriorate.

Laboratory tests to confirm the diagnosis of fulminant hepatitis include liver function tests and PT/INR.

Laboratory tests for acute HAV, HBV, and HCV, as well as some other viruses (eg, cytomegalovirus, Epstein-Barr virus, herpes simplex virus), are done to determine whether a virus is the cause.

Treatment

- Oral nucleoside or nucleotide analogs
- Liver transplantation

Meticulous nursing care and aggressive treatment of complications improve the outcome.

If fulminant hepatitis results from hepatitis B, treatment with oral nucleoside or nucleotide analogs can increase the likelihood of survival.

However, emergency liver transplantation provides the best hope for survival. Survival in adults is uncommon without transplantation; children tend to do better.

Patients who survive usually recover fully.

OVERVIEW OF CHRONIC HEPATITIS

Chronic hepatitis is hepatitis that lasts > 6 mo. Common causes include HBV and HCV, autoimmune liver disease (autoimmune hepatitis), steatohepatitis (nonalcoholic steatohepatitis or alcoholic hepatitis), and some drugs. Many patients have no history of acute hepatitis, and the first indication is discovery of asymptomatic aminotransferase elevations. Some patients present with cirrhosis or its complications (eg, portal hypertension). Biopsy is necessary to confirm the diagnosis and to grade and stage the disease. Treatment is directed toward complications and the underlying condition (eg, corticosteroids for autoimmune hepatitis, antiviral therapy for viral hepatitis). Liver transplantation is often indicated for decompensated cirrhosis.

Hepatitis lasting > 6 mo is generally defined as chronic, although this duration is arbitrary.

Etiology

Common causes: The most common causes are

- HBV
- HCV
- Nonalcoholic steatohepatitis (NASH)
- Alcoholic hepatitis
- Idiopathic (probably autoimmune)

HBV and HCV are frequent causes of chronic hepatitis; 5 to 10% of cases of HBV infection, with or without HDV coinfection, and about 75% of cases of HCV infection become chronic. Rates are higher for HBV infection in children (eg, up to 90% of infected neonates and 30 to 50% of young children). Although the mechanism of chronicity is uncertain, liver injury is mostly determined by the patient's immune reaction to the infection.

Rarely, HEV genotype 3 has been implicated in chronic hepatitis.

HAV does not cause chronic hepatitis.

Other causes of chronic hepatitis include NASH and alcoholic hepatitis. NASH develops most often in patients with at least one of the following risk factors:

- Obesity
- Dyslipidemia
- Glucose intolerance

Alcoholic hepatitis (a combination of fatty liver, diffuse liver inflammation, and liver necrosis) results from excess consumption.

Many cases are idiopathic. A high proportion of idiopathic cases have prominent features of immune-mediated hepatocellular injury (autoimmune hepatitis), including the following:

- The presence of serologic immune markers
- An association with histocompatibility haplotypes common in autoimmune disorders (eg, HLA-B1, HLA-B8, HLA-DR3, HLA-DR4)
- A predominance of T lymphocytes and plasma cells in liver histologic lesions
- Complex in vitro defects in cellular immunity and immunoregulatory functions
- An association with other autoimmune disorders (eg, RA, autoimmune hemolytic anemia, proliferative glomerulonephritis)
- A response to therapy with corticosteroids or immunosuppressants

Less common causes: Sometimes chronic hepatitis has features of both autoimmune hepatitis and another chronic liver disorder (eg, primary biliary cholangitis [formerly, primary biliary cirrhosis]). These conditions are called overlap syndromes.

Many drugs, including isoniazid, methyldopa, nitrofurantoin, and, rarely acetaminophen, can cause chronic hepatitis. The mechanism varies with the drug and may involve altered immune responses, cytotoxic intermediate metabolites, or genetically determined metabolic defects.

Less often, chronic hepatitis results from alpha-1 antitrypsin deficiency, celiac disease, a thyroid disorder, hereditary hemochromatosis, or Wilson disease.

Classification

Cases of chronic hepatitis were once classified histologically as chronic persistent, chronic lobular, or chronic active hepatitis. A more useful recent classification system specifies the following:

- Etiology
- Intensity of histologic inflammation and necrosis (grade)
- Degree of histologic fibrosis (stage)

Inflammation and necrosis are potentially reversible; fibrosis usually is not.

Symptoms and Signs

Clinical features of chronic hepatitis vary widely. About one third of cases develop after acute hepatitis, but most develop insidiously de novo.

Many patients are asymptomatic, especially in chronic HCV infection. However, malaise, anorexia, and fatigue are common, sometimes with low-grade fever and nonspecific upper abdominal discomfort. Jaundice is usually absent.

Often, particularly with HCV, the first findings are

- Signs of chronic liver disease (eg, splenomegaly, spider nevi, palmar erythema)
- Complications of cirrhosis (eg, portal hypertension, ascites, encephalopathy)

A few patients with chronic hepatitis develop manifestations of cholestasis (eg, jaundice, pruritus, pale stools, steatorrhea).

In autoimmune hepatitis, especially in young women, manifestations may involve virtually any body system and can include acne, amenorrhea, arthralgia, ulcerative colitis, pulmonary fibrosis, thyroiditis, nephritis, and hemolytic anemia.

Chronic HCV is occasionally associated with lichen planus, mucocutaneous vasculitis, glomerulonephritis, porphyria cutanea tarda, and, perhaps, non-Hodgkin B-cell lymphoma.

About 1% of patients develop symptomatic cryoglobulinemia with fatigue, myalgias, arthralgias, neuropathy, glomerulonephritis, and rashes (urticaria, purpura, leukocytoclastic vasculitis); asymptomatic cryoglobulinemia is more common.

Diagnosis

- Liver function test results compatible with hepatitis
- Viral serologic tests
- Possibly autoantibodies, immunoglobulins, alpha-1 antitrypsin level, and other tests
- Usually biopsy
- Serum albumin, platelet count, and PT/INR

(See also the American Association for the Study of Liver Disease's practice guideline Diagnosis, Management, and Treatment of Hepatitis C and the U.S. Preventive Services Task Force's clinical guideline Screening for Hepatitis C in Adults.)

The diagnosis is suspected in patients with any of the following:

- Suggestive symptoms and signs
- Incidentally noted elevations in aminotransferase levels
- Previously diagnosed acute hepatitis

In addition, to identify asymptomatic patients, the Centers for Disease Control and Prevention (CDC) recommends testing all people born between 1945 and 1965 once for hepatitis C.

Liver function tests: Liver function tests are needed if not previously done and include serum ALT, AST, alkaline phosphatase, and bilirubin.

Aminotransferase elevations are the most characteristic laboratory abnormalities. Although levels can vary, they are typically 100 to 500 IU/L. ALT is usually higher than AST. Aminotransferase levels can be normal during chronic hepatitis if the disease is quiescent, particularly with HCV.

Alkaline phosphatase is usually normal or only slightly elevated but is occasionally markedly high.

Bilirubin is usually normal unless the disease is severe or advanced.

However, abnormalities in these laboratory tests are not specific and can result from other disorders, such as alcoholic liver disease, recrudescent acute viral hepatitis, and primary biliary cirrhosis.

Other laboratory tests: If laboratory results are compatible with hepatitis, viral serologic tests are done to exclude HBV and HCV (see Tables 29–4 and 29–6). Unless these tests indicate viral etiology, further testing is required.

The next tests done include

- Autoantibodies (antinuclear antibody, anti–smooth muscle antibody, antimitochondrial antibody, liver-kidney microsomal antibody)
- Immunoglobulins
- Thyroid tests (thyroid-stimulating hormone)
- Tests for celiac disease (tissue transglutaminase antibody)
- Alpha-1 antitrypsin level
- Iron and ferritin levels and total iron-binding capacity

Children and young adults are screened for Wilson disease by measuring the ceruloplasmin level.

Marked elevations in serum immunoglobulins suggest chronic autoimmune hepatitis but are not conclusive.

Autoimmune hepatitis is normally diagnosed based on the presence of antinuclear (ANA), anti–smooth muscle (ASMA), or anti-liver/kidney microsomal type 1 (anti-LKM1) antibodies at titers of 1:80 (in adults) or 1:20 (in children). Antimitochondrial antibodies are occasionally present in patients with autoimmune hepatitis. (See also the American Association for the Study of Liver Disease's practice guideline Diagnosis and management of autoimmune hepatitis.)

Serum albumin, platelet count, and PT should be measured to determine severity; low serum albumin, a low platelet count, or prolonged PT may suggest cirrhosis and even portal hypertension.

Biopsy: Unlike in acute hepatitis, biopsy is necessary.

Mild cases may have only minor hepatocellular necrosis and inflammatory cell infiltration, usually in portal regions, with normal acinar architecture and little or no fibrosis. Such cases rarely develop into clinically important liver disease or cirrhosis.

In more severe cases, biopsy typically shows periportal necrosis with mononuclear cell infiltrates (piecemeal necrosis) accompanied by variable periportal fibrosis and bile duct proliferation. The acinar architecture may be distorted by zones of collapse and fibrosis, and frank cirrhosis sometimes coexists with signs of ongoing hepatitis.

Biopsy is also used to grade and stage the disease.

In most cases, the specific cause of chronic hepatitis cannot be discerned via biopsy alone, although cases caused by HBV can be distinguished by the presence of ground-glass hepatocytes and special stains for HBV components. Autoimmune cases usually have a more pronounced infiltration by lymphocytes and plasma cells. In patients with histologic but not serologic criteria for chronic autoimmune hepatitis, variant autoimmune hepatitis is diagnosed; many have overlap syndromes.

Screening for complications: If symptoms or signs of cryoglobulinemia develop during chronic hepatitis, particularly with HCV, cryoglobulin levels and rheumatoid factor should be measured; high levels of rheumatoid factor and low levels of complement suggest cryoglobulinemia.

Patients with chronic HBV infection should be screened every 6 mo for hepatocellular cancer with ultrasonography and serum alpha-fetoprotein measurement, although the cost-effectiveness of this practice is debated. (See also the Cochrane review abstract on alpha-fetoprotein and/or liver ultrasonography for liver cancer screening in patients with chronic hepatitis B.) Patients with chronic HCV infection should be similarly screened only if advanced fibrosis or cirrhosis is present.

Prognosis

Prognosis is highly variable.

Chronic hepatitis caused by a drug often regresses completely when the causative drug is withdrawn.

Without treatment, cases caused by HBV can resolve (uncommon), progress rapidly, or progress slowly to cirrhosis over decades. Resolution often begins with a transient increase in disease severity and results in seroconversion from hepatitis B e antigen (HBeAg) to antibody to hepatitis B e antigen (anti-HBe). Coinfection with HDV causes the most severe form of chronic HBV infection; without treatment, cirrhosis develops in up to 70% of patients.

Untreated chronic hepatitis due to HCV causes cirrhosis in 20 to 30% of patients, although development may take decades and varies because it is often related to a patient's other risk factors for chronic liver disease, including alcohol use and obesity.

Chronic autoimmune hepatitis usually responds to therapy but sometimes causes progressive fibrosis and eventual cirrhosis.

Chronic HBV infection increases the risk of hepatocellular cancer (see p. 241). The risk is also increased in chronic HCV infection, but only if cirrhosis or advanced fibrosis has developed.

Treatment

- Supportive care
- Treatment of cause (eg, corticosteroids for autoimmune hepatitis, antivirals for HBV and HCV infection)

There are specific antiviral treatments for chronic hepatitis B (eg, entecavir and tenofovir as first-line therapies; see Table 29–5) and antiviral treatments for chronic hepatitis C (eg, interferon-free regimens of direct-acting antivirals; see Table 29–6).

General treatment: Treatment goals for chronic hepatitis include treating the cause and managing complications (eg, ascites, encephalopathy) if cirrhosis and portal hypertension have developed.

Drugs that cause hepatitis should be stopped. Underlying disorders, such as Wilson disease, should be treated.

In chronic hepatitis due to HBV, prophylaxis (including immunoprophylaxis—see p. 225) for contacts of patients may be helpful. No vaccination is available for contacts of patients with HCV infection.

Corticosteroids and immunosuppressants should be avoided in chronic hepatitis B and C because these drugs enhance viral replication. If patients with chronic hepatitis B require treatment with corticosteroids, immunosuppressive therapies, or cytotoxic chemotherapy for other disorders, they should be treated with antiviral drugs at the same time to prevent a flare-up of acute hepatitis B or acute liver failure due to hepatitis B. A similar situation with hepatitis C being activated or causing acute liver failure has not been described.

NASH: (See also the American Association for the Study of Liver Disease's The diagnosis and management of non-alcoholic fatty liver disease at www.aasld.org.)

Treatment of NASH aims to

- Eliminate causes
- Control risk factors for NASH

It may involve recommending weight loss, treating hyperlipidemias and hyperglycemia, stopping drugs associated with NASH (eg, amiodarone, tamoxifen, methotrexate, corticosteroids such as prednisone or hydrocortisone, synthetic estrogens), and avoiding exposure to toxins (eg, pesticides).

Autoimmune hepatitis: (See also the American Association for the Study of Liver Disease's practice guideline Diagnosis and Management of Autoimmune Hepatitis at www.aasld.org.)

Corticosteroids, with or without azathioprine, prolong survival. Prednisone is usually started at 30 to 60 mg po once/day, then tapered to the lowest dose that maintains aminotransferases at normal or near-normal levels. To prevent long-term need for corticosteroid treatment, clinicians can transition to azathioprine 1 to 1.5 mg/kg po once/day or mycophenolate mofetil 1000 mg twice/day after corticosteroid induction is complete and then gradually taper the corticosteroid. Most patients require long-term, low-dose, corticosteroid-free maintenance treatment.

Liver transplantation may be required for decompensated cirrhosis.

KEY POINTS

- Chronic hepatitis is usually not preceded by acute hepatitis and is often asymptomatic.
- If liver function test results (eg, unexplained elevations in aminotransferase levels) are compatible with chronic hepatitis, do serologic tests for hepatitis B and C.
- If serologic results are negative, do tests (eg, autoantibodies, immunoglobulins, alpha-1 antitrypsin level) for other forms of hepatitis.
- Do a liver biopsy to confirm the diagnosis and assess the severity of chronic hepatitis.
- Consider entecavir and tenofovir as first-line therapies for chronic hepatitis B.
- Treat chronic hepatitis C of all genotypes with interferon-free regimens of direct-acting antivirals.
- Treat autoimmune hepatitis with corticosteroids and transition to maintenance treatment with azathioprine or mycophenolate mofetil.

HEPATITIS A, ACUTE

Hepatitis A is caused by an enterically transmitted RNA virus that, in older children and adults, causes typical symptoms of viral hepatitis, including anorexia, malaise, and jaundice. Young children may be asymptomatic. Fulminant hepatitis and death are rare. Chronic hepatitis does not occur. Diagnosis is by antibody testing. Treatment is supportive. Vaccination and previous infection are protective.

HAV is a single-stranded RNA picornavirus. It is the most common cause of acute viral hepatitis and is particularly common among children and young adults.

In some countries, > 75% of adults have been exposed to HAV. In the US, an estimated 3000 cases occur annually—a decrease from 25,000 to 35,000 annual cases before the hepatitis A vaccine became available in 1995 (see CDC Hepatitis A FAQs).

HAV spreads primarily by fecal-oral contact and thus may occur in areas of poor hygiene. Waterborne and food-borne epidemics occur, especially in developing countries. Eating contaminated raw shellfish is sometimes responsible. Sporadic cases are also common, usually as a result of person-to-person contact.

Fecal shedding of the virus occurs before symptoms develop and usually ceases a few days after symptoms begin; thus, infectivity often has already ceased when hepatitis becomes clinically evident. HAV has no known chronic carrier state and does not cause chronic hepatitis or cirrhosis.

Symptoms and Signs

In children < 6 yr, 70% of hepatitis A infections are asymptomatic, and in children with symptoms, jaundice is rare. In contrast, most older children and adults have typical manifestations of viral hepatitis, including anorexia, malaise, fever, nausea, and vomiting; jaundice occurs in over 70%. Manifestations typically resolve after about 2 mo, but in some patients, symptoms continue or recur for up to 6 mo.

Recovery from acute hepatitis A is usually complete. Fulminant hepatitis rarely occurs.

Diagnosis

- Serologic testing

In the initial diagnosis of acute hepatitis, viral hepatitis should be differentiated from other disorders causing jaundice. If acute viral hepatitis is suspected, the following tests are done to screen for HAV, HBV, and HCV:

- IgM antibody to HAV (IgM anti-HAV)
- Hepatitis B surface antigen (HBsAg)
- IgM antibody to hepatitis B core (IgM anti-HBc)
- Antibody to HCV (anti-HCV)

If the IgM anti-HAV test is positive, acute hepatitis A is diagnosed. The IgG antibody to HAV (IgG anti-HAV) test is done (see Table 29–3) to help distinguish acute from prior infection. A positive IgG anti-HAV test suggests prior HAV infection or acquired immunity. There is no further testing for hepatitis A.

HAV is present in serum only during acute infection and cannot be detected by clinically available tests.

IgM antibody typically develops early in the infection and peaks about 1 to 2 wk after the development of jaundice. It diminishes within several weeks, followed by the development of protective IgG antibody (IgG anti-HAV), which persists usually for life. Thus, IgM antibody is a marker of acute infection, whereas IgG anti-HAV indicates only previous exposure to HAV and immunity to recurrent infection.

Treatment

- Supportive care

No treatments attenuate acute viral hepatitis, including hepatitis A. Alcohol should be avoided because it can increase liver damage. Restrictions on diet or activity, including commonly prescribed bed rest, have no scientific basis.

Most patients may safely return to work after jaundice resolves, even if AST or ALT levels are slightly elevated.

For cholestatic hepatitis, cholestyramine 8 g po once/day or bid can relieve itching.

Table 29–3. HEPATITIS A SEROLOGY

MARKER	ACUTE HAV INFECTION	PRIOR HAV INFECTION*
IgM anti-HAV	+	–
IgG anti-HAV	–	+

*HAV does not cause chronic hepatitis.
HAV = hepatitis A virus; IgM anti-HAV = IgM antibody to HAV.

Viral hepatitis should be reported to the local or state health department.

Prevention

Good personal hygiene helps prevent fecal-oral transmission of hepatitis A. Barrier protection is recommended, but isolation of patients does little to prevent spread of HAV.

Spills and contaminated surfaces in the home of patients can be cleaned with dilute household bleach.

Vaccination: The hepatitis A vaccine is recommended for all children beginning at age 1 yr, with a 2nd dose 6 to 18 mo after the first (see p. Table 291–2 on p. 2462)

Preexposure HAV vaccination (see the CDC's Adult Immunization Schedule at www.cdc.gov) should be provided for

- Travelers to countries with high or intermediate HAV endemicity
- Diagnostic laboratory workers
- Men who have sex with men
- People who use injection or noninjection illicit drugs
- People with chronic liver disorders (including chronic hepatitis C) because they have an increased risk of developing fulminant hepatitis due to HAV
- People who receive clotting factor concentrates
- People who anticipate close contact with an international adoptee during the first 60 days after arrival from a country with high or intermediate HAV endemicity

Preexposure HAV prophylaxis can be considered for day-care center employees and for military personnel.

Several vaccines against HAV are available, each with different doses and schedules; they are safe, provide protection within about 4 wk, and provide prolonged protection (probably for > 20 yr).

Previously, travelers were advised to get the hepatitis A vaccine ≥ 2 wk before travel; those leaving in < 2 wk should also be given standard immune globulin. Current evidence suggests immune globulin is necessary only for older travelers and travelers with chronic liver disease or another chronic disorder.

Postexposure prophylaxis: Postexposure prophylaxis should be given to family members and close contacts of patients with hepatitis A.

For healthy, unvaccinated patients aged 1 to 40 yr, a single dose of hepatitis A vaccine is given.

For other patients, particularly those > 75 yr, those with chronic liver disease, and immunocompromised patients, standard immune globulin (formerly immune serum globulin) prevents or decreases the severity of hepatitis A. A dose 0.02 mL/kg IM is generally recommended, but some experts advise 0.06 mL/kg (3 to 5 mL for adults). It can be given up to 2 wk after exposure, but the earlier, the better.

KEY POINTS

- HAV is the most common cause of acute viral hepatitis; it is spread by the fecal-oral route.
- Children < 6 yr may be asymptomatic; older children and adults have anorexia, malaise, and jaundice.
- Fulminant hepatitis is rare, and chronic hepatitis, cirrhosis, and cancer do not occur.
- Treat supportively.
- Routine vaccination beginning at age 1 is recommended for all.
- Vaccinate people at risk (eg, travelers to endemic areas, laboratory workers), and provide postexposure prophylaxis with standard immune globulin or, for some, vaccination.

HEPATITIS B, ACUTE

Hepatitis B is caused by a DNA virus that is often parenterally transmitted. It causes typical symptoms of viral hepatitis, including anorexia, malaise, and jaundice. Fulminant hepatitis and death may occur. Chronic infection can lead to cirrhosis and/or hepatocellular carcinoma. Diagnosis is by serologic testing. Treatment is supportive. Vaccination is protective and postexposure use of hepatitis B immune globulin may prevent or attenuate clinical disease.

HBV is the most thoroughly characterized and complex hepatitis virus. The infective particle consists of a viral core plus an outer surface coat. The core contains circular double-stranded DNA and DNA polymerase, and it replicates within the nuclei of infected hepatocytes. A surface coat is added in the cytoplasm and, for unknown reasons, is produced in great excess.

HBV is the 2nd most common cause of acute viral hepatitis. Prior unrecognized infection is common but is much less widespread than that with HAV. In the US, about 3000 cases of acute hepatitis B infection are reported annually—a decrease from the 25,000 annual cases reported before use of hepatitis B vaccine became widespread. However, because many cases are not recognized or not reported, the Centers for Disease Control and Prevention (CDC) estimates that the actual number of new infections is close to 20,000 annually (see CDC Hepatitis B FAQs).

HBV, for unknown reasons, is sometimes associated with several primarily extrahepatic disorders, including polyarteritis nodosa, other connective tissue diseases, membranous glomerulonephritis, and essential mixed cryoglobulinemia. The pathogenic role of HBV in these disorders is unclear, but autoimmune mechanisms are suggested.

Transmission of hepatitis B: HBV is often transmitted parenterally, typically by contaminated blood or blood products. Routine screening of donor blood for hepatitis B surface antigen (HBsAg) has nearly eliminated the previously common posttransfusion transmission, but transmission through needles shared by drug users remains common. Risk of HBV is increased for patients in renal dialysis and oncology units and for hospital personnel in contact with blood.

Infants born to infected mothers have a 70 to 90% risk of acquiring hepatitis B during delivery (neonatal HBV infection—see p. 2630) unless they are treated with hepatitis B immune globulin (HBIG) and are vaccinated immediately after delivery. Earlier transplacental transmission can occur but is rare.

The virus may be spread through mucosal contact with other body fluids (eg, between sex partners, both heterosexual and homosexual; in closed institutions, such as mental health institutions and prisons), but infectivity is far lower than that of HAV, and the means of transmission is often unknown.

The role of insect bites in transmission is unclear. Many cases of acute hepatitis B occur sporadically without a known source.

Chronic HBV carriers provide a worldwide reservoir of infection. Prevalence varies widely according to several factors, including geography (eg, < 0.5% in North America and northern Europe, > 10% in some regions of the Far East and Africa).

Symptoms and Signs

Hepatitis B infection causes a wide spectrum of liver diseases, from a subclinical carrier state to severe hepatitis or acute liver failure (fulminant hepatitis), particularly in the elderly, in whom mortality can reach 10 to 15%.

Most patients have typical manifestations of viral hepatitis, including anorexia, malaise, fever, nausea, and vomiting, followed by jaundice. Symptoms persist from a few weeks up to 6 mo.

Five to 10% of all patients with HBV develop chronic hepatitis B or become inactive carriers. The younger the age when acute infection occurs, the higher the risk of developing chronic infection:

- For infants: 90%
- For children aged 1 to 5 yr: 25 to 50%
- Adults: About 5%

Cirrhosis can develop. Hepatocellular carcinoma can ultimately develop in chronic HBV infection, even without being preceded by cirrhosis.

Diagnosis

- Serologic testing

In the initial diagnosis of acute hepatitis, viral hepatitis should be differentiated from other disorders causing jaundice (see Fig. 29–1). If acute viral hepatitis is suspected, the following tests are done to screen for HAV, HBV, and HCV:

- IgM antibody to HAV (IgM anti-HAV)
- Hepatitis B surface antigen (HBsAg)
- IgM antibody to hepatitis B core (IgM anti-HBc)
- Antibody to HCV (anti-HCV)

If any of the hepatitis B tests are positive, further serologic testing may be necessary to differentiate acute from past or chronic infection (see Table 29–4). If serology suggests hepatitis B, testing for hepatitis B e antigen (HBeAg) and antibody to hepatitis B e antigen (anti-HBe) is usually done to help determine the prognosis and to guide antiviral therapy. If serologically confirmed HBV infection is severe, antibody to HDV (anti-HDV) is measured.

Hepatitis B has at least 3 distinct antigen-antibody systems that can be tested:

- HBsAg
- Hepatitis B core antigen (HBcAg)
- HBeAg

Table 29–4. HEPATITIS B SEROLOGY*

MARKER	ACUTE HBV INFECTION	CHRONIC HBV INFECTION	PRIOR HBV INFECTION†
HBsAg	+	+	–
Anti-HBs	–	–	+‡
IgM anti-HBc	+	–	–
IgG anti-HBc	–	+	±
HBeAg	±	±	–
Anti-HBe	–	±	±
HBV-DNA	+	+	–

*Antibody to HDV (anti-HDV) levels should be measured if serologic tests confirm HBV and infection is severe.

†Patients have had HBV infection and recovered.

‡Anti-HBs is also seen as the sole serologic marker after HBV vaccination.

Anti-HBc = antibody to hepatitis B core; anti-HBe = antibody to HBeAg; anti-HBs = antibody to HBsAg; HBeAg = hepatitis B e antigen; HBsAg = hepatitis B surface antigen; HBV = hepatits B virus.

HBsAg characteristically appears during the incubation period, usually 1 to 6 wk before clinical or biochemical illness develops, and implies infectivity of the blood. It disappears during convalescence. However, HBsAg is occasionally transient. The corresponding protective antibody (anti-HBs) appears weeks or months later, after clinical recovery, and usually persists for life; thus, its detection indicates past HBV infection and relative immunity. In 5 to 10% of patients, HBsAg persists and antibodies do not develop; these patients become asymptomatic carriers of the virus or develop chronic hepatitis.

HBcAg reflects the viral core. It is detectable in infected liver cells but not in serum except by special techniques. Antibody to HBcAg (anti-HBc) usually appears at the onset of clinical illness; thereafter, titers gradually diminish, usually over years or life. Its presence with anti-HBs indicates recovery from previous HBV infection. Anti-HBc is also present in chronic HBsAg carriers, who do not mount an anti-HBs response. In acute infection, anti-HBc is mainly of the IgM class, whereas in chronic infection, IgG anti-HBc predominates. IgM anti-HBc is a sensitive marker of acute HBV infection and occasionally is the only marker of recent infection, reflecting a window between disappearance of HBsAg and appearance of anti-HBs.

HBeAg is a protein derived from the viral core (not to be confused with HEV). Present only in HBsAg-positive serum, HBeAg tends to suggest more active viral replication and greater infectivity. In contrast, presence of the corresponding antibody (anti-HBe) suggests lower infectivity. Thus, e antigen markers are more helpful in prognosis than in diagnosis. Chronic liver disease develops more often among patients with HBeAg and less often among patients with anti-HBe.

HBV-DNA can be detected in the serum of patients with active HBV infection.

Other tests: Liver function tests are needed if not previously done; they include serum ALT, AST, alkaline phosphatase, and bilirubin.

Other tests should be done to evaluate disease severity; they include serum albumin, platelet count, and PT/INR.

Treatment

- Supportive care
- For fulminant hepatitis B, antiviral drugs and liver transplantation

No treatments attenuate acute viral hepatitis, including hepatitis B. Alcohol should be avoided because it can increase liver damage. Restrictions on diet or activity, including commonly prescribed bed rest, have no scientific basis.

If fulminant hepatitis occurs, treatment with oral nucleoside or nucleotide analogs can increase the likelihood of survival. However, emergency liver transplantation provides the best hope for survival. Survival in adults is uncommon without transplantation; children tend to do better.

Most patients may safely return to work after jaundice resolves, even if AST or ALT levels are slightly elevated.

For cholestatic hepatitis, cholestyramine 8 g po once/day or bid can relieve itching.

Viral hepatitis should be reported to the local or state health department.

Prevention

Patients should be advised to avoid high-risk behavior (eg, sharing needles to inject drugs, having multiple sex partners).

Blood and other body fluids (eg, saliva, semen) are considered infectious. Spills should be cleaned up using dilute bleach. Barrier protection is recommended, but isolation of patients is of no value.

Posttransfusion infection is minimized by avoiding unnecessary transfusions and screening all donors for HBsAg and anti-HCV. Screening has decreased the incidence of posttransfusion hepatitis, probably to about 1/100,000 units of blood component transfused.

Vaccination: Hepatitis B vaccination in endemic areas has dramatically reduced local prevalence.

Preexposure immunization has long been recommended for people at high risk. However, selective vaccination of high-risk groups in the US and other nonendemic areas has not substantially decreased the incidence of HBV infection; thus, vaccination is now recommended for all US residents < 18 beginning at birth (see Table 291–2 on p. 2462). Universal worldwide vaccination is desirable but is too expensive to be feasible.

Adults at high risk of HBV infection should be screened and vaccinated if they are not already immune or infected (see Adult Immunization Schedule at www.cdc.gov). These high-risk groups include

- Men who have sex with men
- People with a sexually transmitted disease
- People who have had > 1 sex partner during the previous 6 mo
- Health care and public safety workers potentially exposed to blood or other infectious body fluids
- People who have diabetes and are < 60 yr (or ≥ 60 yr if their risk of acquiring HBV is considered increased)
- People with end-stage renal disease, HIV, or chronic liver disease
- Household contacts and sex partners of people who are HBsAg-positive
- Clients and staff members of institutions and nonresidential day care facilities for people with developmental disabilities
- People in correctional facilities or facilities providing drug abuse treatment and prevention services
- International travelers to regions with high or intermediate HBV endemicity

Two recombinant vaccines are available; both are safe, even during pregnancy. Three IM deltoid injections are given: at baseline, at 1 mo, and at 6 mo. Children are given lower doses, and immunosuppressed patients and patients receiving hemodialysis are given higher doses.

After vaccination, levels of anti-HBs remain protective for 5 yr in 80 to 90% of immunocompetent recipients and for 10 yr in 60 to 80%. Booster doses of vaccine are recommended for patients receiving hemodialysis and immunosuppressed patients whose anti-HBs is < 10 mIU/mL.

Postexposure prophylaxis: Hepatitis B postexposure immunoprophylaxis combines vaccination with hepatitis B immune globulin (HBIG), a product with high titers of anti-HBs. HBIG probably does not prevent infection but prevents or attenuates clinical illness.

For infants born to HBsAg-positive mothers, an initial dose of vaccine plus 0.5 mL of HBIG is given IM in the thigh immediately after birth.

For anyone having sexual contact with an HBsAg-positive person or percutaneous or mucous membrane exposure to HBsAg-positive blood, 0.06 mL/kg of HBIG is given IM within days, along with vaccine.

Any previously vaccinated patient sustaining a percutaneous HBsAg-positive exposure is tested for anti-HBs; if titers are < 10 mIU/mL, a booster dose of vaccine is given.

KEY POINTS

- Hepatitis B is often transmitted by parenteral contact with contaminated blood but can result from mucosal contact with other body fluids.
- Infants born to mothers with hepatitis B have a 70 to 90% risk of acquiring infection during delivery unless the infants are treated with hepatitis B immune globulin (HBIG) and are vaccinated after delivery.
- Chronic infection develops in 5 to 10% of patients with acute hepatitis B and often leads to cirrhosis and/or hepatocellular carcinoma.
- Diagnose by testing for hepatitis B surface antigen and other serologic markers.
- Treat supportively.
- Routine vaccination beginning at birth is recommended for all.
- Postexposure prophylaxis consists of HBIG and vaccine; HBIG probably does not prevent infection but may prevent or attenuate clinical hepatitis.

HEPATITIS B, CHRONIC

Hepatitis B is a common cause of chronic hepatitis. Patients may be asymptomatic or have nonspecific manifestations such as fatigue and malaise. Without treatment, cirrhosis often develops; risk of hepatocellular carcinoma is increased. Antiviral drugs may help, but liver transplantation may become necessary.

Hepatitis lasting > 6 mo is generally defined as chronic hepatitis, although this duration is arbitrary.

Acute hepatitis B becomes chronic in about 5 to 10% of patients overall. However, the younger the age when acute infection occurs, the higher the risk of developing chronic infection:

- For infants: 90%
- For children aged 1 to 5 yr: 25 to 50%
- Adults: About 5%

The Centers for Disease Control and Prevention (CDC) estimates that 850,000 to 2.2 million people in the US and about 240 million people worldwide have chronic hepatitis B infection.

Without treatment, chronic hepatitis B can resolve (uncommon), progress rapidly, or progress slowly to cirrhosis over decades. Resolution often begins with a transient increase in disease severity and results in seroconversion from hepatitis B e antigen (HBeAg) to antibody to hepatitis B e antigen (anti-HBe). Coinfection with HDV causes the most severe form of chronic HBV infection; without treatment, cirrhosis develops in up to 70% of patients. Chronic HBV infection increases the risk of hepatocellular cancer.

Symptoms and Signs

Symptoms vary depending on the degree of underlying liver damage.

Many patients, particularly children, are asymptomatic. However, malaise, anorexia, and fatigue are common, sometimes with low-grade fever and nonspecific upper abdominal discomfort. Jaundice is usually absent.

Often, the first findings are

- Signs of chronic liver disease or portal hypertension (eg, splenomegaly, spider nevi, palmar erythema)
- Complications of cirrhosis (eg, portal hypertension, ascites, encephalopathy)

A few patients with chronic hepatitis develop manifestations of cholestasis (eg, jaundice, pruritus, pale stools, steatorrhea).

Extrahepatic manifestations may include polyarteritis nodosa and glomerular disease.

Diagnosis

- Serologic testing
- Liver biopsy

The diagnosis of chronic hepatitis B is suspected in patients with suggestive symptoms and signs, incidentally noted elevations in aminotransferase levels, or previously diagnosed acute hepatitis.

Diagnosis is confirmed by finding positive hepatitis B surface antigen (HBsAg) and IgG anti-HBc and negative IgM antibody to HBcAg (anti-HBc—see Table 29–4) and by measuring HBV DNA (quantitative HBV-DNA).

If chronic hepatitis B is confirmed, testing for hepatitis B e antigen (HBeAg) and antibody to hepatitis B e antigen (anti-HBe) is usually done to help determine the prognosis and to guide antiviral therapy. If serologically confirmed HBV infection is severe, antibody to HDV (anti-HDV) is measured.

Quantitative HBV-DNA tests are also used before and during treatment to assess response.

Biopsy is typically done to evaluate the extent of liver damage and to exclude other causes of liver disease. Liver biopsy is most useful in cases that do not meet clear-cut guidelines for treatment (see also the American Association for the Study of Liver Disease's practice guideline Diagnosis and Management of Autoimmune Hepatitis).

Other tests: Liver function tests are needed if not previously done; they include serum ALT, AST, alkaline phosphatase, and bilirubin.

Other tests should be done to evaluate disease severity; they include serum albumin, platelet count, and PT/INR.

Patients should also be tested for HIV and hepatitis C infection because transmission of these infections is similar.

If symptoms or signs of cryoglobulinemia develop during chronic hepatitis, cryoglobulin levels and rheumatoid factor should be measured; high levels of rheumatoid factor and low levels of complement suggest cryoglobulinemia.

Screening for complications: Patients with chronic HBV infection should be screened every 6 mo for hepatocellular cancer with ultrasonography and serum alpha-fetoprotein measurement, although the cost-effectiveness of this practice is debated. (See also the Cochrane review abstract on alpha-fetoprotein and/or liver ultrasonography for liver cancer screening in patients with chronic hepatitis B.)

Treatment

- Antiviral drugs
- Sometimes liver transplantation

(See also the American Association for the Study of Liver Disease's Practice Guidelines for the Treatment of Chronic Hepatitis B.)

Antiviral treatment is indicated for patients with

- Elevated aminotransferase levels
- Clinical or biopsy evidence of progressive disease
- Both of the above

The goal is to eliminate HBV-DNA.[1] Treatment can occasionally cause loss of hepatitis B e antigen (HBeAg), or, even more rarely, loss of hepatitis B surface antigen (HBsAg). However, the majority of patients treated for chronic hepatitis B must be treated indefinitely; thus, treatment may be very expensive.

Stopping treatment prematurely can lead to relapse, which may be severe. However, treatment may be stopped if one of the following occurs:

- HBeAg converts to antibody to HBeAg (anti-HBe).
- Tests for HBsAg become negative.

Drug resistance is also a concern.

Seven antiviral drugs—entecavir, adefovir, lamivudine, interferon alfa (INF-alpha), pegylated INF-alpha (peginterferon-alpha), telbivudine, and tenofovir—are available (see Table 29–5).

First-line treatment is usually with

- An oral antiviral drug, such as entecavir (a nucleoside analog) or tenofovir (a nucleotide analog)

Oral antiviral drugs have few adverse effects and can be given to patients with decompensated liver disease. Combination therapy has not proved superior to monotherapy, but studies continue to examine their comparative usefulness.

If HBsAg becomes undetectable and HBeAg seroconversion occurs in patients with HBeAg-positive chronic HBV infection, these patients may be able to stop antiviral drugs. Patients with HBeAg-negative chronic HBV infection almost always need to take antiviral drugs indefinitely to maintain viral suppression; they have already developed antibodies to HBeAg, and thus the only specific criterion for stopping HBV treatment would be HBsAg that becomes undetectable.

Entecavir has a high antiviral potency, and resistance to it is uncommon; it is considered a first-line treatment for HBV infection. Entecavir is effective against adefovir-resistant strains. Dosage is 0.5 mg po once/day; however, patients who have previously taken a nucleoside analog should take 1 mg po once/day. Dose reduction is required in patients with renal insufficiency. Serious adverse effects appear to be uncommon, although safety in pregnancy has not been established.

Tenofovir has replaced adefovir (an older nucleotide analog) as a first-line treatment. Tenofovir is the most potent oral antiviral for hepatitis B; resistance to it is minimal. It has few adverse effects. Dosage is 300 mg po once/day; dosing frequency may need to be reduced if creatinine clearance is reduced.

For **adefovir**, dosage is 10 mg po once/day.

Interferon alfa (IFN-alpha) can be used but is no longer considered first-line treatment. Dosage is 5 million IU sc once/day or 10 million IU sc 3 times/wk for 16 to 24 wk in patients with HBeAg-positive chronic HBV infection and for 12 to 24 mo in patients with HBeAg-negative chronic HBV infection. In about 40% of patients, this regimen eliminates HBV-DNA and causes seroconversion to anti-HBe; a successful response is usually presaged by a temporary increase in aminotransferase levels. The drug must be given by injection and is often poorly tolerated. The first 1 or 2 doses cause an influenza-like syndrome. Later, fatigue, malaise, depression, bone marrow suppression, and, rarely, bacterial infections or autoimmune disorders can occur.

Contraindications to INF-alpha include the following:

- Advanced cirrhosis: In patients with cirrhosis, IFN-alpha can precipitate decompensation of cirrhosis.
- Renal failure
- Immunosuppression
- Solid organ transplantation
- Cytopenia

In a few patients, treatment must be stopped because of intolerable adverse effects. The drug should be given cautiously or not at all to patients with ongoing substance abuse or a major psychiatric disorder.

Pegylated IFN-alpha can be used instead of IFN-alpha. Dosage is usually 180 mcg by injection once/wk for 48 wk. Adverse effects are similar to those of IFN-alpha but may be less severe.

Lamivudine (a nucleoside analog) is no longer considered first-line treatment for HBV infection because risk of resistance is higher and efficacy is lower than those of newer antiviral drugs. Dosage is 100 mg po once/day; it has few adverse effects.

Telbivudine is a newer nucleoside analog that has greater efficacy and potency than lamivudine but also has a high rate of resistance; it is not considered first-line treatment. Dosage is 600 mg po once/day.

Table 29–5. COMPARISON OF DRUGS COMMONLY USED TO TREAT CHRONIC VIRAL HEPATITIS B

EFFECT (% OF PATIENTS)	INF-ALPHA	PEG IFN-ALPHA	LAMIVUDINE	ADEFOVIR	ENTECAVIR	TELBIVUDINE	TENOFOVIR
Serum HBV-DNA becomes undetectable	37%	30–42%	44%	21%	61%	60%	76%
Seroconversion from HBeAg to anti-Hbe occurs	18%	29–36%	16–21%	12%	21–22%	22%	21%
ALT normalizes	23%	34–52%	41–75%	48%	68–81%	77%	68%
Histologic improvement occurs	NA	38%	49–56%	53%	72%	65%	74%
HBsAg becomes undetectable (at 1 yr)	8%	3%	< 1%	0%	2–3%	0%	3%
Resistance develops	None	None	At 1 yr: ~14–32% At 5 yr: ~60–70%	At 1 yr: 0% At 5 yr: 29%	At 1 yr: 0% At 6 yr: 1.2%	At 1 yr: 5% At 2 yr: 25%	After 6 yr: 0%

Anti-Hbe = antibody to HBeAg; HBeAg = hepatitis B e antigen; HBsAg = hepatitis B surface antigen; HBV = hepatitis B virus; INF-alpha = interferon alfa; PEG IFN-alpha = pegylated INF-alpha.

Adapted from Lok ASF, McMahon BJ: Chronic hepatitis B: Update 2009. American Association for the Study of Liver Diseases (AASLD) practice guidelines update. *Hepatology* 50:661–699, 2009 and Terrault NA, Bzowej NH, Chang KM, et al: AASLD guidelines for treatment of chronic hepatitis B. *Hepatology* 63:261–283, 2016.

Liver transplantation should be considered for end-stage liver disease caused by HBV. In patients with HBV infection, the long-term use of first-line oral antivirals and peritransplantation use of hepatitis B immune globulin (HBIG) has improved outcomes after liver transplantation. Survival is equal to or better than that after transplantation for other indications, and recurrences of hepatitis B are minimized.

1. Terrault NA, Bzowej NH, Chang KM, et al: AASLD guidelines for treatment of chronic hepatitis B. *Hepatology* 63: 261–283, 2016.

KEY POINTS

- Acute hepatitis B becomes chronic in about 5 to 10% of patients overall; risk is highest at a young age (90% for infants, 25 to 50% for children aged 1 to 5 yr, and about 5% for adults).
- The CDC estimates about 240 million people worldwide have chronic hepatitis B infection.
- Symptoms vary depending on the degree of underlying liver damage.
- Antiviral drugs can improve liver function test results and liver histology and delay progression to cirrhosis but may need to be taken indefinitely; drug resistance is a concern.
- Liver transplantation may be required in patients with decompensated cirrhosis due to hepatitis B.

HEPATITIS C, ACUTE

Hepatitis C is caused by an RNA virus that is often parenterally transmitted. It sometimes causes typical symptoms of viral hepatitis, including anorexia, malaise, and jaundice but may be asymptomatic. Fulminant hepatitis and death rarely occur. Chronic hepatitis develops in about 75% and can lead to cirrhosis and rarely hepatocellular carcinoma. Diagnosis is by serologic testing. Treatment is supportive. No vaccine is available.

In the US, about 2000 cases of acute hepatitis C infection are reported annually. However, because many cases are not recognized or not reported, the CDC estimates that the actual number of new infections is close to 30,000 annually (see CDC Hepatitis C FAQs).

HCV is a single-stranded RNA flavivirus that causes acute viral hepatitis and is a common cause of chronic viral hepatitis. Six major HCV subtypes exist with varying amino acid sequences (genotypes); these subtypes vary geographically and in virulence and response to therapy. HCV can also alter its amino acid pattern over time in an infected person, producing quasispecies.

HCV infection sometimes occurs simultaneously with specific systemic disorders, including the following:

- Essential mixed cryoglobulinemia
- Porphyria cutanea tarda (about 60 to 80% of porphyria patients have HCV infection, but only a few patients infected with HCV develop porphyria)
- Glomerulonephritis

The mechanisms are uncertain.

In addition, up to 20% of patients with alcoholic liver disease harbor HCV. The reasons for this high association are unclear because concomitant alcohol and drug use accounts for only a portion of cases. In these patients, HCV and alcohol act synergistically to worsen liver inflammation and fibrosis.

Transmission of hepatitis C: Infection is most commonly transmitted through blood, primarily when parenteral drug users share needles, but also through tattoos or body piercing.

Sexual transmission and vertical transmission from mother to infant are relatively rare.

Transmission through blood transfusion has become very rare since the advent of screening tests for donated blood.

Some sporadic cases occur in patients without apparent risk factors.

HCV prevalence varies with geography and other risk factors.

Symptoms and Signs

Hepatitis C may be asymptomatic during the acute infection. Its severity often fluctuates, sometimes with recrudescent hepatitis and roller-coaster aminotransferase levels for many years or even decades. Fulminant hepatitis is extremely rare.

HCV has the highest rate of chronicity (about 75%). The resultant chronic hepatitis C is usually asymptomatic or benign but progresses to cirrhosis in 20 to 30% of patients; cirrhosis often takes decades to appear. Hepatocellular carcinoma can result from HCV-induced cirrhosis but results only rarely from chronic infection without cirrhosis (unlike in hepatitis B).

Diagnosis

- Serologic testing

In the initial diagnosis of acute hepatitis, viral hepatitis should be differentiated from other disorders causing jaundice (see Fig. 29–1). If acute viral hepatitis is suspected, the following tests are done to screen for HAV, HBV, and HCV:

- IgM antibody to HAV (IgM anti-HAV)
- Hepatitis B surface antigen (HBsAg)
- IgM antibody to hepatitis B core (IgM anti-HBc)
- Antibody to HCV (anti-HCV)

If the anti-HCV test is positive, HCV-RNA is measured to distinguish active from past hepatitis C infection (see Table 29–6).

In hepatitis C, serum anti-HCV represents chronic, past, or acute infection; the antibody is not protective. In unclear cases, HCV-RNA is measured. Anti-HCV usually appears within 2 wk of acute infection but is sometimes delayed; however, HCV-RNA is positive sooner.

Other tests: Liver function tests are needed if not previously done; they include serum ALT, AST, alkaline phosphatase, and bilirubin.

Other tests should be done to evaluate disease severity; they include serum albumin, platelet count, and PT/INR.

Treatment

- Supportive care

Table 29–6. HEPATITIS C SEROLOGY

MARKER	ACUTE HCV INFECTION	CHRONIC HCV INFECTION	PRIOR HCV INFECTION*
Anti-HCV	+	+	+
HCV-RNA	+	+	–

*Patients have had HCV infection and spontaneously recovered or been successfully treated.

Anti-HCV = antibody to HCV; HCV = hepatitis C virus.

No treatments attenuate acute viral hepatitis, including hepatitis C.

There are a number of new, highly effective direct-acting antiviral drugs for chronic hepatitis C that may decrease the likelihood of developing chronic infection. However, the regimens are very expensive and have not been studied in acute infection; current recommendations are to follow patients for 6 mo to allow spontaneous clearance and then treat those who have persistent viremia (ie, chronic hepatitis C).

Alcohol should be avoided because it can increase liver damage. Restrictions on diet or activity, including commonly prescribed bed rest, have no scientific basis.

Most patients may safely return to work after jaundice resolves, even if AST or ALT levels are slightly elevated.

For cholestatic hepatitis, cholestyramine 8 g po once/day or bid can relieve itching.

Viral hepatitis should be reported to the local or state health department.

Prevention

Patients should be advised to avoid high-risk behavior (eg, sharing needles to inject drugs, getting tattoos and body piercings).

Blood and other body fluids (eg, saliva, semen) are considered infectious. Risk of infection after a single needlestick exposure is about 1.8%. Barrier protection is recommended, but isolation of patients is of no value in preventing acute hepatitis C.

Risk of transmission from HCV-infected medical personnel appears to be low, and there are no CDC recommendations to restrict health care workers with hepatitis C infection.

Posttransfusion infection is minimized by avoiding unnecessary transfusions and screening all donors for HBsAg and anti-HCV. Screening has decreased the incidence of posttransfusion hepatitis, probably to about 1/100,000 units of blood component transfused.

No product exists for immunoprophylaxis of HCV. The propensity of HCV for changing its genome hampers vaccine development.

KEY POINTS

- Hepatitis C is usually transmitted by parenteral contact with contaminated blood; transmission from mucosal contact with other body fluids and perinatal transmission from infected mothers are rare.
- About 75% of patients with acute hepatitis C develop chronic hepatitis C, which leads to cirrhosis in 20 to 30%; some patients with cirrhosis develop hepatocellular carcinoma.
- Diagnose by testing for antibody to HCV and other serologic markers.
- Treat supportively.
- There is no vaccine for hepatitis C.

HEPATITIS C, CHRONIC

Hepatitis C is a common cause of chronic hepatitis. It is often asymptomatic until manifestations of chronic liver disease occur. Treatment is with direct-acting antiviral drugs and other agents depending on genotype; permanent elimination of detectable viral RNA is possible.

Hepatitis lasting > 6 mo is generally defined as chronic hepatitis, although this duration is arbitrary.

There are 6 major genotypes of HCV, which vary in their response to treatment. Genotype 1 is more common than genotypes 2, 3, 4, 5, and 6; it accounts for 70 to 80% of cases of chronic hepatitis C in the US.

Acute hepatitis C becomes chronic in about 75% of patients. The Centers for Disease Control and Prevention (CDC) estimates that about 2.7 to 3.9 million people in the US have chronic hepatitis C infection. Worldwide 71 million people are estimated to have chronic hepatitis C. Chronic hepatitis C progresses to cirrhosis in 20 to 30% of patients; cirrhosis often takes decades to appear. Hepatocellular carcinoma can result from HCV-induced cirrhosis but results only rarely from chronic infection without cirrhosis (unlike in HBV infection).

Symptoms and Signs

Many patients are asymptomatic and do not have jaundice, although some have malaise, anorexia, fatigue, and nonspecific upper abdominal discomfort. Often, the first findings are signs of chronic liver disease (eg, splenomegaly, spider nevi, palmar erythema) or complications of cirrhosis (eg, portal hypertension, ascites, encephalopathy).

Chronic hepatitis C is occasionally associated with lichen planus, mucocutaneous vasculitis, glomerulonephritis, porphyria cutanea tarda, and, perhaps, non-Hodgkin B-cell lymphoma.

Diagnosis

- Serologic testing

The diagnosis of chronic hepatitis C is suspected in patients with suggestive symptoms and signs, incidentally noted elevations in aminotransferase levels, or previously diagnosed acute hepatitis.

Diagnosis is confirmed by finding positive anti-HCV and positive HCV-RNA ≥ 6 mo after initial infection (see Table 29–6).

Liver biopsy is useful for one or more of the following:

- Grading inflammatory activity
- Staging fibrosis or progression of disease (which can sometimes help determine which patients to treat and when)
- Excluding other causes of liver disease

However, the role of liver biopsy is evolving in hepatitis C, and biopsy is being supplanted by noninvasive imaging (eg, ultrasound elastography, magnetic resonance elastography) and serum markers of fibrosis, as well as scoring systems for fibrosis based on serologic markers.

HCV genotype is determined before treatment because genotype influences the course, duration, and success of treatment.

HCV-RNA detection and quantification is used to help diagnose hepatitis C and to evaluate treatment response during and after treatment. For most currently available quantitative HCV-RNA assays, the lower limit of detection is at least < 50 IU/mL. If a quantitative assay does not have that level of sensitivity, a qualitative assay can be used. Qualitative assays can detect very low levels of HCV-RNA, often as low as < 10 IU/mL, and provide results as positive or negative. Qualitative tests can be used to confirm a diagnosis of hepatitis C or a sustained virologic response (SVR), defined as no detectable HCV-RNA at 12 and 24 wk after completion of treatment, depending on the drug regimen used.

(See also the American Association for the Study of Liver Disease's practice guideline Diagnosis, Management, and Treatment of Hepatitis C [at www.hcvguidelines.org] and the U.S. Preventive Services Task Force's clinical guideline Screening for Hepatitis C in Adults [at www.uspreventiveservicestaskforce.org].)

Other tests: Liver function tests are needed if not previously done; they include serum ALT, AST, alkaline phosphatase, and bilirubin.

Other tests should be done to evaluate disease severity; they include serum albumin, platelet count, and PT/INR.

Patients should be tested for HIV and hepatitis B infection because transmission of these infections is similar.

If symptoms or signs of cryoglobulinemia develop during chronic hepatitis C, cryoglobulin levels and rheumatoid factor should be measured; high levels of rheumatoid factor and low levels of complement suggest cryoglobulinemia.

Screening for complications: Patients with chronic HCV infection and advanced fibrosis or cirrhosis should be screened every 6 mo for hepatocellular cancer with ultrasonography and serum alpha-fetoprotein measurement, although the cost-effectiveness of this practice is debated.

Prognosis

Prognosis depends on whether patients have an SVR (ie, no detectable HCV-RNA at 12 and 24 wk after completion of treatment, depending on the drug regimen used).

Patients who have an SVR have a > 99% chance of remaining HCV RNA–negative and are typically considered cured. Nearly 95% of patients with an SVR have improved histologic findings, including fibrosis and histologic activity index; in addition, risk of progression to cirrhosis, hepatic failure, and liver-related death is reduced. In patients who have cirrhosis and portal hypertension and who were treated with interferon-based regimens, an SVR has been shown to reduce portal pressures and significantly reduce risk of hepatic decompensation, liver-related death, all-cause mortality, and hepatocellular carcinoma.[1]

Achieving an SVR with interferon-based therapies is more likely when ≥ 1 of the following are present:

- Genotype other than genotype 1
- Low pretreatment viral loads
- Age < 40 yr
- Body weight < 75 kg
- No bridging fibrosis or cirrhosis
- Ethnicity other than African American
- No hepatic steatosis or insulin resistance

Likelihood of achieving an SVR with new interferon-free regimens seems to depend mostly on the following:

- Pretreatment viral load
- Degree of liver fibrosis
- Response to prior treatment

1. van der Meer AJ, Veldt BJ, Feld JJ, et al: Association between sustained virological response and all-cause mortality among patients with chronic hepatitis C and advanced hepatic fibrosis. *JAMA* 308(24):2584–2593, 2012.

Treatment

- Direct-acting antiviral drugs

Overview of HCV treatment: (See also the American Association for the Study of Liver Disease's [AASLD] practice guidelines Recommendations for Testing, Managing, and Treating Hepatitis C and the AASLD/Infectious Disease Society of America guidelines When and in Whom to Initiate HCV Therapy.)

For chronic hepatitis C, treatment is indicated if both of the following are present:

- Aminotransferase levels are elevated.
- Biopsy shows active inflammatory disease with evolving fibrosis.

The goal of treatment is permanent elimination of HCV-RNA (ie, SVR), which is associated with permanent normalization of aminotransferase and cessation of histologic progression. Treatment results are more favorable in patients with moderate fibrosis and a viral load of < 600,000 to 800,000 IU/mL than in patients with cirrhosis and a viral load of > 800,000 IU/mL.

Until late 2013, all genotypes were treated with pegylated IFN-alpha plus ribavirin. Now, most patients are treated with antiviral drugs (direct-acting antivirals [DAAs]) that affect specific HCV targets, such as proteases or polymerases (see below and p. 237).

DAAs used to treat HCV include

- Telaprevir and boceprevir: 1st-generation protease inhibitors with activity against HCV genotype 1
- Simeprevir: A 2nd-generation genotype 1–specific protease inhibitor
- Sofosbuvir: A polymerase inhibitor with activity against HCV genotypes 1 to 6
- Paritaprevir: A protease inhibitor
- Ledipasvir: A protease inhibitor
- Dasabuvir: A polymerase inhibitor
- Ombitasvir: An inhibitor of the viral nonstructural protein 5A (NS5A inhibitor)
- Daclatasvir: An NS5A inhibitor
- Elbasvir: An NS5A inhibitor
- Grazoprevir: A protease inhibitor
- Velpatasvir: An NS5A inhibitor used to treat all HCV genotypes

Telaprevir, boceprevir, and simeprevir were traditionally given with pegylated IFN and ribavirin, but interferon-based treatment regimens are no longer considered standard of care.

Sofosbuvir can be used without interferon; it can be given with ribavirin (for genotypes 1 to 6), simeprevir (for genotype 1), or daclatasvir (for genotypes 1 to 3) in all-oral regimens. Ledipasvir and sofosbuvir are available in a single pill to treat HCV genotypes 1, 4, and 6. Elbasvir/grazoprevir in a single pill is used to treat HCV genotypes 1 and 4.

Velpatasvir and sofosbuvir are available in a single pill to treat HCV genotypes 1 through 6.

The following 5-drug regimen is effective against genotypes 1 and 4:

- Paritaprevir/ritonavir/ombitasvir (in a single pill) given once/day
- Dasabuvir, given twice/day
- Ribavirin, given twice/day

Paritaprevir/ritonavir/ombitasvir plus dasabuvir is available in a single package.

Ritonavir increases levels of paritaprevir but has no direct antiviral activity. Ribavirin is often used with DAAs.

Because more and more DAAs are being developed, current recommendations for HCV treatment are evolving rapidly. Recommendations for testing, managing, and treating hepatitis C from the American Association for the Study of Liver Disease (AASLD) and the Infectious Diseases Society of America (IDSA), available online, are updated frequently.

Decompensated cirrhosis due to hepatitis C is the most common indication for liver transplantation in the US. HCV recurs almost universally in the graft, and both patient and graft survival are less favorable than when transplantation is done for other indications. Many DAAs and interferon-free regimens are being used in patients who have hepatitis C and have received a liver transplant. When DAAs are used, the SVR rate in patients who have had a liver transplant exceeds 95% whether they have cirrhosis or not.

HCV genotype 1: Genotype 1 is more resistant to treatment with dual therapy with pegylated IFN-alpha plus ribavirin than other genotypes. However, now with the use of IFN-free regimens of DAAs, the rate of SVR has increased from < 50% to up to 95%. Regimens include

- Simeprevir or daclatasvir plus sofosbuvir
- Ledipasvir/sofosbuvir
- Elbasvir/grazoprevir
- Velpatasvir/sofosbuvir
- The 5-drug regimen of paritaprevir/ritonavir/ombitasvir, dasabuvir, and ribavirin

Pegylated IFN alpha-2b 1.5 mcg/kg sc once/wk and **pegylated IFN alpha-2a** 180 mcg sc once/wk have comparable results. Adverse effects of pegylated IFN-alpha are similar to those of IFN-alpha but may be less severe; contraindications are also similar (see above). Interferons are no longer recommended as first-line treatment for hepatitis C.

For **ribavirin**, dosage is 500 to 600 mg po bid. Ribavirin is usually well-tolerated but commonly causes anemia due to hemolysis; dosage should be decreased if hemoglobin decreases to < 10 g/dL. Ribavirin is teratogenic in both men and women, requiring contraception during treatment and for 6 mo after treatment is completed. Patients who cannot tolerate ribavirin should still be given pegylated IFN-alpha, but not using ribavirin reduces the likelihood of successful treatment. Ribavirin monotherapy is of no value.

First-line treatments for HCV genotype 1 include

- Fixed-dose combination of ledipasvir 90 mg/sofosbuvir 400 mg po once/day for 8 to 24 wk depending on history of prior treatment, pretreatment viral load, and degree of liver fibrosis
- Fixed-dose combination of elbasvir 50 mg/grazoprevir 100 mg po once/day with or without ribavirin 500 to 600 mg po bid for 12 to 16 wk depending on history of prior treatment, degree of liver fibrosis, and, in patients with genotype 1a, the presence or absence of baseline NS5A resistance–associated variants to elbasvir
- Fixed-dose combination of paritaprevir 150 mg/ritonavir 100 mg/ombitasvir 25 mg once/day plus dasabuvir 250 mg po bid and ribavirin 500 to 600 mg po bid for 12 to 24 wk depending on degree of liver fibrosis
- Sofosbuvir 400 mg po once/day plus simeprevir 150 mg po once/day with or without ribavirin 500 to 600 mg po bid for 12 to 24 wk, depending of degree of liver fibrosis
- Sofosbuvir 400 mg po once/day plus daclatasvir 60 mg once/day with or without ribavirin 500 to 600 mg po bid for 12 to 24 wk, depending on degree of liver fibrosis and history of prior treatment
- Fixed-dose combination of sofosbuvir 400 mg/velpatasvir 100 mg once/day for 12 wk

Simeprevir can cause anemia and photosensitivity. All protease inhibitors have drug-drug interactions.

HCV genotypes 2, 3, 4, 5, and 6: For **genotype 2**, one of the following combinations is recommended:

- Sofosbuvir 400 mg po once/day plus daclatasvir 60 mg po once/day for 12 to 24 wk, depending on the degree of liver fibrosis
- Fixed-dose combination of sofosbuvir 400 mg/velpatasvir 100 mg once/day for 12 wk

For **genotype 3**, first-line treatments include

- Sofosbuvir 400 mg po once/day plus daclatasvir 60 mg po once/day with or without ribavirin 500 to 600 mg po bid for 12 to 24 wk depending on degree of liver fibrosis
- Fixed-dose combination of sofosbuvir 400 mg/velpatasvir 100 mg once/day for 12 wk

For **genotype 4,** first-line treatments include

- Ledipasvir 90 mg/sofosbuvir 400 mg po once/day for 12 wk
- Paritaprevir 150 mg/ritonavir 100 mg/ombitasvir 25 mg po once/day plus ribavirin 500 to 600 mg po bid for 12 wk
- Elbasvir 50 mg/grazoprevir 100 mg po once/day for 12 wk
- Sofosbuvir 400 mg/velpatasvir 100 mg once/day for 12 wk

For **genotypes 5 and 6,** first-line treatments include

- Ledipasvir 90 mg/sofosbuvir 400 mg po once/day for 12 wk
- Sofosbuvir 400 mg/velpatasvir 100 mg once/day for 12 wk

KEY POINTS

- Chronic hepatitis C infection develops in 75% of patients with acute infection and leads to cirrhosis in 20 to 30%; some patients with cirrhosis develop hepatocellular carcinoma.
- Diagnosis is confirmed by finding positive anti-HCV and positive HCV-RNA; then do biopsy and determine genotype.
- Treatment varies by genotype but includes use of one or more direct-acting antiviral drugs, sometimes with ribavirin.
- Pegylated IFN is no longer recommended for treatment of chronic hepatitis C
- New treatments can permanently eliminate HCV-RNA in many patients.

HEPATITIS D

Hepatitis D is caused by a defective RNA virus (delta agent) that can replicate only in the presence of hepatitis B virus. It occurs uncommonly as a coinfection with acute hepatitis B or as a superinfection in chronic hepatitis B.

Hepatitis D is usually transmitted by parenteral or mucosal contact with infected blood or body fluids. Infected hepatocytes contain delta particles coated with hepatitis B surface antigen (HBsAg).

Prevalence of HDV varies widely geographically, with endemic pockets in several countries. Parenteral drug users are at relatively high risk, but HDV, unlike HBV has not widely permeated the homosexual community.

Symptoms and Signs

Acute hepatitis D infection typically manifests as

- Unusually severe acute HBV infection (coinfection)
- An acute exacerbation in chronic HBV carriers (superinfection)
- A relatively aggressive course of chronic HBV infection

Diagnosis

- Serologic testing

In the initial diagnosis of acute hepatitis, viral hepatitis should be differentiated from other disorders causing jaundice (see Fig. 29–1). If acute viral hepatitis is suspected, the following tests are done to screen for HAV, HBV, and HCV:

- IgM antibody to HAV (IgM anti-HAV)
- Hepatitis B surface antigen (HBsAg)
- IgM antibody to hepatitis B core (IgM anti-HBc)
- Antibody to HCV (anti-HCV)

If serologic tests for hepatitis B confirm infection and clinical manifestations are severe, antibody to HDV (anti-HDV) levels should be measured. Anti-HDV implies active infection. It may not be detectable until weeks after the acute illness.

Treatment

- Supportive care

No treatments attenuate acute viral hepatitis, including hepatitis D. Alcohol should be avoided because it can increase liver damage. Restrictions on diet or activity, including commonly prescribed bed rest, have no scientific basis.

Most patients may safely return to work after jaundice resolves, even if AST or ALT levels are slightly elevated.

For cholestatic hepatitis, cholestyramine 8 g po once/day or bid can relieve itching.

The only drug approved for treatment of chronic hepatitis D is interferon-alfa, although pegylated IFN-alpha is likely equally effective. Treatment for 1 yr is recommended, although whether longer treatment courses are more effective has not been established.

Prevention

No product exists for immunoprophylaxis of hepatitis D (see p. 231). However, prevention of HBV infection prevents HDV infection.

KEY POINTS

- Hepatitis D occurs only with hepatitis B.
- Suspect hepatitis D particularly when cases of hepatitis B are severe or when symptoms of chronic hepatitis B are worsening.
- Treat and prevent infection as for hepatitis B.

HEPATITIS E

Hepatitis E is caused by an enterically transmitted RNA virus and causes typical symptoms of viral hepatitis, including anorexia, malaise, and jaundice. Fulminant hepatitis and death are rare, except during pregnancy. Diagnosis is by antibody testing. Treatment is supportive.

There are 4 genotypes of HEV. All can cause acute viral hepatitis.

Genotypes 1 and 2 usually cause waterborne outbreaks that are linked to fecal contamination of the water supply and fecal-oral person-to-person transmission. Outbreaks have occurred in China, India, Mexico, Pakistan, Peru, Russia, and central and northern Africa. These outbreaks have epidemiologic characteristics similar to hepatitis A virus epidemics. Sporadic cases also occur. No outbreaks have occurred in the US or in Western Europe. Most cases in the developed world occur in travelers returning from a developing country, but sporadic cases not associated with travel have been reported.

Genotypes 3 and 4 typically cause sporadic cases rather than outbreaks. Transmission is food-borne and can involve eating uncooked or undercooked meat; cases have been associated with consumption of pork, deer, and shellfish.

HEV was not originally thought to cause chronic hepatitis, cirrhosis, or chronic carrier state; however, reports document chronic genotype 3 hepatitis E exclusively in immunocompromised patients (including organ-transplant recipients, patients receiving cancer chemotherapy, and HIV-infected patients).

Symptoms and Signs

Typical manifestations of viral hepatitis occur: anorexia, malaise, nausea and vomiting, and fever, followed by jaundice. Hepatitis E may be severe, especially in pregnant women; in them, risk of fulminant hepatitis and death is increased.

Diagnosis

- IgM antibody test (when available)

In the initial diagnosis of acute hepatitis, viral hepatitis should be differentiated from other disorders causing jaundice (see Fig. 29–1). If acute viral hepatitis is suspected, the following tests are done to screen for HAV, HBV, and HCV:

- IgM antibody to HAV (IgM anti-HAV)
- Hepatitis B surface antigen (HBsAg)
- IgM antibody to hepatitis B core (IgM anti-HBc)
- Antibody to HCV (anti-HCV)

If tests for hepatitis A, B, and C are negative but the patient has typical manifestations of viral hepatitis and has recently traveled to an endemic area, IgM antibody to HEV (IgM anti-HEV) should be measured if the test is available.

Treatment

- Supportive care
- For chronic hepatitis E, possibly ribavirin

No treatments attenuate acute viral hepatitis, including hepatitis E.

Preliminary studies suggest antiviral efficacy for ribavirin in treatment of chronic hepatitis E.

Alcohol should be avoided because it can increase liver damage. Restrictions on diet or activity, including commonly prescribed bed rest, have no scientific basis.

Most patients may safely return to work after jaundice resolves, even if AST or ALT levels are slightly elevated.

For cholestatic hepatitis, cholestyramine 8 g po once/day or bid can relieve itching.

Viral hepatitis should be reported to the local or state health department.

Prevention

Good personal hygiene and standard universal precautions help prevent fecal-oral transmission of hepatitis E. Boiling water appears to reduce risk of infection. Because person-to-person transmission is rare, isolation of infected patients is not indicated.

A **vaccine for hepatitis E** is now available in China; it is not available in the US. The vaccine appears to have about 95% efficacy in preventing symptomatic infection in males and is safe. Efficacy in other groups, duration of protection, and efficacy in preventing asymptomatic infection are unknown.

KEY POINTS

- Transmission of hepatitis E is usually by the fecal-oral route.
- Most patients recover spontaneously, but pregnant women have an increased risk of fulminant hepatitis and death.
- Genotype 3 may cause chronic hepatitis in immunocompromised patients.
- Suspect hepatitis E in travelers to endemic regions; do IgM anti-HEV testing if available.
- Treat patients supportively; consider using ribavirin for chronic hepatitis E.
- A vaccine is available in China.

30 Liver Masses and Granulomas

HEPATIC CYSTS

Isolated cysts are commonly detected incidentally on abdominal ultrasonography or CT.[1] These cysts are usually asymptomatic and have no clinical significance. The rare congenital polycystic liver is commonly associated with polycystic disease of the kidneys and other organs. It causes progressive nodular hepatomegaly (sometimes massive) in adults. Nevertheless, hepatocellular function is remarkably well preserved, and portal hypertension rarely develops.

Other hepatic cysts include the following:

- Hydatid (echinococcal) cysts
- Caroli disease: This rare, autosomal recessive disorder is characterized by segmental cystic dilation of intrahepatic bile ducts; it often becomes symptomatic in adulthood, with stone formation, cholangitis, and sometimes cholangiocarcinoma.
- Cystadenoma: This rare disorder sometimes causes pain or anorexia and is evident on ultrasonography; treatment is cyst resection.
- Cystadenocarcinoma: This rare disorder is probably secondary to malignant transformation of a cystadenoma and is often multilobular; treatment is liver resection.
- Other true cystic tumors: These tumors are rare.

1. Marrero JA, Ahn J, Rajender Reddy K; American College of Gastroenterology. ACG clinical guideline: the diagnosis and management of focal liver lesions. *Am J Gastroenterol* 109(9):1328–1347, 2014. doi: 10.1038/ajg.2014.213.

HEPATIC GRANULOMAS

Hepatic granulomas have numerous causes and are usually asymptomatic. However, the underlying disorder may cause extrahepatic manifestations, hepatic inflammation, fibrosis, portal hypertension, or a combination. Diagnosis is based on liver biopsy, but biopsy is necessary only if a treatable underlying disorder (eg, infection) is suspected or if other liver disorders need to be ruled out. Treatment depends on the underlying disorder.

Hepatic granulomas, although sometimes insignificant, more often reflect clinically relevant disease. The term *granulomatous hepatitis* is often used to describe the condition, but the disorder is not true hepatitis, and the presence of granulomas does not imply hepatocellular inflammation.

Etiology

Hepatic granulomas have many causes (see Table 30–1); drugs and systemic disorders (often infections) are more common causes than primary liver disorders. Infections must be identified because they require specific treatments. TB and schistosomiasis are the most common infectious causes worldwide; fungal and viral causes are less common. Sarcoidosis is the most common noninfectious cause; the liver is involved in about two thirds of patients, and occasionally, clinical manifestations of sarcoidosis are predominantly hepatic.

Table 30–1. CAUSES OF HEPATIC GRANULOMAS

CAUSE	EXAMPLES
Drugs	Allopurinol, phenylbutazone, quinidine, sulfonamides
Infections, bacterial	Actinomycosis, brucellosis, cat-scratch fever, syphilis, TB*, other mycobacterial infections, tularemia, Q fever
Infections, fungal	Blastomycosis, cryptococcosis, histoplasmosis
Infections, parasitic	Schistosomiasis*, toxoplasmosis, visceral larva migrans
Infections, viral	Hepatitis C, cytomegalovirus infection
Liver disorders	Primary biliary cirrhosis
Systemic disorders	Hodgkin lymphoma, polymyalgia rheumatica, other connective tissue disorders, sarcoidosis*

*Most common causes.

Granulomas are much less common in primary liver disorders; primary biliary cirrhosis is the only important cause. Small granulomas occasionally occur in other liver disorders but are not clinically significant.

Idiopathic granulomatous hepatitis is a rare syndrome of hepatic granulomas with recurrent fever, myalgias, fatigue, and other systemic symptoms, which often occur intermittently for years. Some experts believe it is a variant of sarcoidosis.

Pathophysiology

A granuloma is a localized collection of chronic inflammatory cells with epithelioid cells and giant multinucleated cells. Caseation necrosis or foreign body tissue (eg, schistosome eggs) may be present. Most granulomas occur in the parenchyma, but in primary biliary cirrhosis, granulomas may occur in the hepatic triads.

Granuloma formation is incompletely understood. Granulomas may develop in response to poorly soluble exogenous or endogenous irritants. Immunologic mechanisms are involved.

Hepatic granulomas rarely affect hepatocellular function. However, when granulomas are part of a broader inflammatory reaction involving the liver (eg, drug reactions, infectious mononucleosis), hepatocellular dysfunction is present. Sometimes inflammation causes progressive hepatic fibrosis and portal hypertension, typically with schistosomiasis and occasionally with extensive sarcoidal infiltration.

Symptoms and Signs

Granulomas themselves are typically asymptomatic; even extensive infiltration usually causes only minor hepatomegaly and little or no jaundice. Symptoms, if they occur, reflect the underlying condition (eg, constitutional symptoms in infections, hepatosplenomegaly in schistosomiasis).

Diagnosis

- Liver function tests
- Imaging
- Biopsy

Hepatic granulomas are suspected in patients with

- Conditions that commonly cause granulomas
- Unexplained hepatic masses found during imaging tests
- Abnormalities detected by an imaging test that is done to evaluate asymptomatic elevations in liver enzymes, particularly alkaline phosphatase

When granulomas are suspected, liver function tests are usually done, but results are nonspecific and are rarely helpful in diagnosis. Alkaline phosphatase (and gamma-glutamyltransferase) is often mildly elevated but occasionally may be markedly elevated. Other test results may be normal or abnormal, reflecting additional hepatic damage (eg, widespread hepatic inflammation due to a drug reaction). Usually, imaging tests, such as ultrasonography, CT, or MRI, are not diagnostic; they may show calcification (if granulomas are long-standing) or filling defects, particularly with confluent lesions.

Diagnosis is based on liver biopsy. However, biopsy is usually indicated only to diagnose treatable causes (eg, infections) or to rule out nongranulomatous disorders (eg, chronic viral hepatitis). Biopsy sometimes detects evidence of the specific cause (eg, schistosome eggs, caseation of TB, fungal organisms). However, other tests (eg, cultures, skin tests, laboratory tests, imaging tests, other tissue specimens) are often needed.

In patients with constitutional or other symptoms suggesting infection (eg, FUO), specific measures are taken to increase the diagnostic sensitivity of biopsy for infections; eg, a portion of the fresh biopsy specimen is sent for culture, or special stains for acid-fast bacilli, fungi, and other organisms are used. Often, cause cannot be established.

Prognosis

Hepatic granulomas caused by drugs or infection regress completely after treatment. Sarcoid granulomas may disappear spontaneously or persist for years, usually without causing clinically important liver disease. Progressive fibrosis and portal hypertension (sarcoidal cirrhosis) rarely develop.

In schistosomiasis, progressive portal scarring (pipestem fibrosis) is typical; liver function is usually preserved, but marked splenomegaly and variceal hemorrhage can occur.

Treatment

- Treatment of cause

Treatment is directed at the underlying disorder. When the cause is unknown, treatment is usually withheld, and follow-up with periodic liver function tests is instituted. However, if symptoms of TB (eg, prolonged fever) and deteriorating health occur, empiric antituberculous therapy may be justified.

Corticosteroids may benefit patients with progressive hepatic sarcoidosis, although whether these drugs prevent hepatic fibrosis is unclear. However, corticosteroids are not indicated for most patients with sarcoidosis and are warranted only if TB and other infections can be excluded confidently.

KEY POINTS

- Hepatic granulomas can result from many drugs and systemic disorders; primary liver disorders are uncommon causes.
- TB and schistosomiasis are the most common infectious causes worldwide; sarcoidosis is the most common noninfectious cause.
- Symptoms and complications are due mainly to the underlying condition rather than the granulomas themselves.
- Treatment is directed at the cause.

BENIGN LIVER TUMORS

Benign liver tumors are relatively common. Most are asymptomatic, but some cause hepatomegaly, right upper quadrant discomfort, or intraperitoneal hemorrhage. Most are detected incidentally on ultrasound or other scans (see Imaging Tests of the Liver and Gallbladder on p. 199). Liver function tests are usually normal or only slightly abnormal. Diagnosis is usually possible with imaging tests but may require biopsy. Treatment is needed only in a few specific circumstances.

Hepatocellular adenoma: Hepatocellular adenoma is the most important benign tumor to recognize. It occurs primarily in women of childbearing age, particularly those taking oral contraceptives, possibly via estrogen's effects.[1]

Most adenomas are asymptomatic, but large ones may cause right upper quadrant discomfort. Rarely, adenomas manifest as peritonitis and shock due to rupture and intraperitoneal hemorrhage. Rarely, they become malignant.

Diagnosis is often suspected based on ultrasound or CT results, but biopsy is sometimes needed for confirmation.

Adenomas due to contraceptive use may regress if the contraceptive is stopped. If the adenoma does not regress or if it is subcapsular or > 5 cm, surgical resection is often recommended.

Focal nodular hyperplasia: This localized hamartoma may resemble macronodular cirrhosis histologically. Diagnosis is usually based on MRI or CT with contrast, but biopsy may be necessary for confirmation. Treatment is rarely needed.

Hemangiomas: Hemangiomas are usually small and asymptomatic; they occur in 1 to 5% of adults. Symptoms are more likely if they are > 4 cm; symptoms include discomfort, fullness, and, less often, anorexia, nausea, early satiety, and pain secondary to bleeding or thrombosis. These tumors often have a characteristic highly vascular appearance. Hemangiomas are found incidentally during ultrasonography, CT, or MRI. CT typically shows a well-demarcated, hypodense mass; when contrast is used, there is early peripheral enhancement, followed by later centrifugal enhancement. Treatment is usually not indicated. Resection can be considered if symptoms are troublesome or if a hemangioma is rapidly enlarging.

In infants, hemangiomas often regress spontaneously by age 2 yr. However, large hemangiomas occasionally cause arteriovenous shunting sufficient to cause heart failure and sometimes consumption coagulopathy. In these cases, treatment may include high-dose corticosteroids, sometimes diuretics and digoxin to improve heart function, interferon alfa (given sc), surgical removal, selective hepatic artery embolization, and, rarely, liver transplantation.

Other benign tumors: Lipomas (usually asymptomatic) and localized fibrous tumors (eg, fibromas) rarely occur in the liver.

Benign bile duct adenomas are rare, inconsequential, and usually detected incidentally. They are sometimes mistaken for metastatic cancer.

1. Marrero JA, Ahn J, Rajender Reddy K: American College of Gastroenterology. ACG clinical guideline: The diagnosis and management of focal liver lesions. *Am J Gastroenterol* 109(9):1328–1347, 2014. doi: 10.1038/ajg.2014.213.

HEPATOCELLULAR CARCINOMA

Hepatocellular carcinoma (hepatoma) usually occurs in patients with cirrhosis and is common in areas where infection with hepatitis B and C viruses is prevalent. Symptoms and signs are usually nonspecific. Diagnosis is based on alpha-fetoprotein (AFP) levels, imaging tests, and sometimes liver biopsy. Screening with periodic AFP measurement and ultrasonography is sometimes recommended for high-risk patients. Prognosis is poor when cancer is advanced, but for small tumors that are confined to the liver, ablative therapies are palliative and surgical resection or liver transplantation is sometimes curative.

Hepatocellular carcinoma is the most common type of primary liver cancer, with an estimated 23,000 new cases and about 14,000 deaths expected in 2012 in the US. However, it is more common outside the US, particularly in East Asia and sub-Saharan Africa where the incidence generally parallels geographic prevalence of chronic hepatitis B virus (HBV) infection.

Etiology

Hepatocellular carcinoma is usually a complication of cirrhosis.

The presence of HBV increases risk of hepatocellular carcinoma by > 100-fold among HBV carriers. Incorporation of HBV-DNA into the host's genome may initiate malignant transformation, even in the absence of chronic hepatitis or cirrhosis.

Other disorders that cause hepatocellular carcinoma include cirrhosis due to chronic hepatitis C virus (HCV) infection, hemochromatosis, and alcoholic cirrhosis. Patients with cirrhosis due to other conditions are also at increased risk.

Environmental carcinogens may play a role; eg, ingestion of food contaminated with fungal aflatoxins is believed to contribute to the high incidence of hepatocellular carcinoma in subtropical regions.

Symptoms and Signs

Most commonly, previously stable patients with cirrhosis present with abdominal pain, weight loss, right upper quadrant mass, and unexplained deterioration. Fever may occur. In a few patients, the first manifestation of hepatocellular carcinoma is bloody ascites, shock, or peritonitis, caused by hemorrhage of the tumor. Occasionally, a hepatic friction rub or bruit develops.

Occasionally, systemic metabolic complications, including hypoglycemia, erythrocytosis, hypercalcemia, and hyperlipidemia, occur. These complications may manifest clinically.

Diagnosis

- Alpha-fetoprotein (AFP) measurement
- Imaging (CT, ultrasonography, or MRI)

Clinicians suspect hepatocellular carcinoma if

- They feel an enlarged liver.
- Unexplained decompensation of chronic liver disease develops.
- An imaging test detects a mass in the right upper quadrant of the abdomen during an examination done for other reasons, especially if patients have cirrhosis.

However, screening programs enable clinicians to detect many hepatocellular carcinomas before symptoms develop.

Diagnosis is based on AFP measurement and an imaging test. In adults, AFP signifies dedifferentiation of hepatocytes, which most often indicates hepatocellular carcinoma; 40 to 65% of patients with the cancer have high AFP levels (> 400 μg/L). High levels are otherwise rare, except in teratocarcinoma of the testis, a much less common tumor. Lower values are less specific and can occur with hepatocellular regeneration (eg, in hepatitis). Other blood tests, such as AFP-L3 (an AFP isoform) and des-gamma–carboxyprothrombin, are being studied as markers to be used for early detection of hepatocellular carcinoma.

Depending on local preferences and capabilities, the first imaging test may be contrast-enhanced CT, ultrasonography, or MRI. Hepatic arteriography is occasionally helpful in equivocal cases and can be used to outline the vascular anatomy when ablation or surgery is planned.

If imaging shows characteristic findings and AFP is elevated, the diagnosis is clear. Liver biopsy, often guided by ultrasonography or CT, is sometimes indicated for definitive diagnosis.

Staging: If a hepatocellular carcinoma is diagnosed, evaluation usually includes chest CT without contrast, imaging of the portal vein (if not already done) by MRI or CT with contrast to exclude thrombosis, and sometimes bone scanning.

Various systems can be used to stage hepatocellular carcinoma; none is universally used. One system is the TNM system, based on the following (see Table 30–2).

- **T:** How many primary tumors, how big they are, and whether the cancer has spread to adjacent organs

Table 30–2. STAGING HEPATOCELLULAR CARCINOMA*

STAGE	DESIGNATION	DESCRIPTION
I	T1, N0, M0	Single tumor (any size) with no invasion of blood vessels
II	T2, N0, M0	Single tumor (any size) with invasion of blood vessels *or* Several tumors that are all < 5 cm
IIIA	T3a, N0, M0	Several tumors with at least one > 5 cm
IIIB	T3b, N0, M0	One or more tumors of any size with invasion of a major branch of the portal or hepatic vein
IIIC	T4, N0, M0	Tumor or tumors of any size with invasion of adjacent organs other than the gallbladder or with perforation of the visceral peritoneum
IVA	Any T, N1, M0	Tumor or tumors of any size with spread to nearby (regional) lymph nodes
IVB	Any T, Any N, M1	Tumor or tumors of any size with distant metastasis

*Adapted from the American Joint Committee on Cancer (AJCC): *AJCC Cancer Staging Manual,* ed. 7. New York, Springer, 2010.

- **N:** Whether the cancer has spread to nearby lymph nodes
- **M:** Whether the cancer has metastasized to other organs of the body

Numbers (0 to 4) are added after T, N, and M to indicate increasing severity.

Other scoring systems include the Okuda and the Barcelona-Clinic Liver Cancer staging systems. In addition to tumor size, local extension, and metastases, these systems incorporate information about the severity of liver disease.

The TNM system may predict prognosis better than other systems for patients who are having tumor resection (and possibly transplantation), whereas the Barcelona system may predict prognosis better for patients who are not having surgery.

Screening: An increasing number of hepatocellular carcinomas are being detected through screening programs. Screening patients with cirrhosis is reasonable, although this measure is controversial and has not been shown to reduce mortality. One common screening method is ultrasonography every 6 or 12 mo. Many experts advise screening patients with long-standing hepatitis B even when cirrhosis is absent.

Treatment

- Transplantation if tumors are small and few

Treatment of hepatocellular carcinoma depends on its stage.[1]

For single tumors < 5 cm or ≤ 3 tumors that are all ≤ 3 cm and that are limited to the liver, liver transplantation results in as good a prognosis as liver transplantation done for noncancerous disorders. Alternatively, surgical resection may be done; however, the cancer usually recurs.

Ablative treatments (eg, hepatic arterial chemoembolization, yttrium-90 microsphere embolization [selective internal radiation therapy, or SIRT], drug-eluting bead transarterial embolization, radiofrequency ablation) provide palliation and slow tumor growth; they are used when patients are awaiting liver transplantation.

If the tumor is large (> 5 cm), is multifocal, has invaded the portal vein, or is metastatic (ie, stage III or higher), prognosis is much less favorable (eg, 5-yr survival rates of about 5% or less). Radiation therapy is usually ineffective. Sorafenib appears to improve outcomes.

1. Bruix J, Reig M, Sherman M: Evidence-based diagnosis, staging, and treatment of patients with hepatocellular carcinoma. *Gastroenterology* 50(4):835–853, 2016. doi: 10.1053/j.gastro.2015.12.041.

Prevention

Use of vaccine against HBV eventually decreases the incidence, especially in endemic areas. Preventing the development of cirrhosis of any cause (eg, via treatment of chronic hepatitis C, early detection of hemochromatosis, or management of alcoholism) can also have a significant effect.

KEY POINTS

- Hepatocellular carcinoma is usually a complication of cirrhosis and is most common in parts of the world where hepatitis B is prevalent.
- Consider the diagnosis if physical examination or an imaging test detects an enlarged liver or if chronic liver disease worsens unexpectedly.
- Diagnose hepatocellular carcinoma based on the AFP level and liver imaging results, and stage it using chest CT without contrast, portal vein imaging, and sometimes bone scanning.
- Consider liver transplantation if tumors are small and few.
- Prevention involves use of the hepatitis B vaccine and management of disorders that can cause cirrhosis.

PRIMARY LIVER CANCER

Primary liver cancer is usually hepatocellular carcinoma. The first manifestations of liver cancer are usually nonspecific, delaying the diagnosis. Prognosis is usually poor.

Other Primary Liver Cancers

Other primary liver cancers are uncommon or rare. Diagnosis usually requires biopsy. Prognosis is typically poor.

Some cancers, if localized, can be resected. Resection or liver transplantation may prolong survival.

Fibrolamellar carcinoma: This distinct variant of hepatocellular carcinoma has a characteristic morphology of malignant hepatocytes enmeshed in lamellar fibrous tissue. It usually occurs in young adults and has no association with preexisting cirrhosis, HBV, HCV, or other known risk factors. Alpha-fetoprotein (AFP) levels are rarely elevated.

Prognosis is better than that for hepatocellular carcinoma, and many patients survive several years after tumor resection.

Cholangiocarcinoma: This tumor originates in the biliary epithelium. It is common in China, where underlying infestation with liver flukes is believed to contribute. Elsewhere, it is less common than hepatocellular carcinoma; histologically, the two may overlap. Primary sclerosing cholangitis greatly increases risk of cholangiocarcinoma.[1]

Hepatoblastoma: Although rare, hepatoblastoma is one of the most common primary liver cancers in infants, particularly those with a family history of familial adenomatous polyposis (see p. 166). It can also develop in children. Some patients with hepatoblastoma present with precocious puberty caused by ectopic gonadotropin production, but the cancer is usually detected because of deteriorating general health and a right upper quadrant mass. An elevated AFP level and abnormal imaging test results may help in the diagnosis.

Angiosarcoma: This rare cancer is associated with specific chemical carcinogens, including industrial vinyl chloride.

Cystadenocarcinoma: This rare disorder is probably secondary to malignant transformation of a cystadenoma and is often multilobular.

Treatment is liver resection.

1. Razumilava N, Gores GJ, Lindor KD: Cancer surveillance in patients with primary sclerosing cholangitis. *Hepatology* 54(5):1842–1852, 2011.

METASTATIC LIVER CANCER

Liver metastases are common in many types of cancer, especially those of the GI tract, breast, lung, and pancreas. The first symptoms of metastases are usually nonspecific (eg, weight loss, right upper quadrant discomfort); they are sometimes the first symptoms of the primary cancer. Liver metastases are suspected in patients with weight loss and hepatomegaly or with primary tumors likely to spread to the liver. Diagnosis is usually supported by an imaging test, most often ultrasonography, spiral CT with contrast, or MRI with contrast. Treatment usually involves palliative chemotherapy.

Metastatic liver cancer is more common than primary liver cancer and is sometimes the initial clinical manifestation of cancer originating in the GI tract, breast, lung, or pancreas.

Symptoms and Signs

Early liver metastases may be asymptomatic. Nonspecific symptoms of cancer (eg, weight loss, anorexia, fever) often develop first. The liver may be enlarged, hard, or tender; massive hepatomegaly with easily palpable nodules signifies advanced disease. Hepatic bruits and pleuritic-type pain with an overlying friction rub are uncommon but characteristic. Splenomegaly is occasionally present, especially when the primary cancer is pancreatic. Concomitant peritoneal tumor seeding may produce ascites, but jaundice is usually absent or mild initially unless a tumor causes biliary obstruction.

In the terminal stages, progressive jaundice and hepatic encephalopathy presage death.

Diagnosis

- CT with contrast or MRI with contrast
- Sometimes biopsy

Liver metastases are suspected in patients with weight loss and hepatomegaly or with primary tumors likely to spread to the liver. If metastases are suspected, liver function tests are often done, but results are usually not specific for the diagnosis. Alkaline phosphatase, gamma-glutamyl transpeptidase, and sometimes LDH typically increase earlier or to a greater degree than do other test results; aminotransferase levels vary. Imaging tests have good sensitivity and specificity. Ultrasonography is usually helpful, but CT with contrast or MRI with contrast is often more accurate.

Liver biopsy guided by imaging provides the definitive diagnosis and is done if other tests are equivocal or if histologic information (eg, cell type of the liver metastasis) may help determine the treatment plan.

Treatment

- Sometimes surgical resection
- Sometimes systemic chemotherapy; sometimes hepatic intra-arterial chemotherapy
- Occasionally, radiation therapy for palliation

Treatment depends on the extent of metastasis.

With solitary or very few metastases due to colorectal cancer, surgical resection may prolong survival.

Depending on characteristics of the primary tumor, systemic chemotherapy may shrink tumors and prolong life but is not curative; hepatic intra-arterial chemotherapy sometimes has the same effect but with fewer or milder systemic adverse effects.

Radiation therapy to the liver occasionally alleviates severe pain due to advanced metastases but does not prolong life. Extensive disease is fatal and is best managed by palliation for the patient and support for the family.

Hematologic Cancers and the Liver

The liver is commonly involved in advanced leukemia and related blood disorders. Liver biopsy is not needed. In hepatic lymphoma, especially Hodgkin lymphoma, the extent of liver involvement determines staging and treatment but may be difficult to assess. Hepatomegaly and abnormal liver function tests may reflect a systemic reaction to Hodgkin lymphoma rather than spread to the liver, and biopsy often shows nonspecific focal mononuclear infiltrates or granulomas of uncertain significance. Treatment is directed at the hematologic cancer.

31 Vascular Disorders of the Liver

The liver has a dual blood supply (see Fig. 31–1). The portal vein (which is rich in nutrients and relatively high in oxygen) provides two thirds of blood flow to the liver. The hepatic artery (which is oxygen-rich) supplies the rest. The hepatic veins drain the liver into the inferior vena cava. When portal vein blood flow increases, hepatic artery flow decreases and vice versa (the hepatic arterial buffer response). This dual, reciprocally compensatory blood supply provides some protection from hepatic ischemia in healthy people.

Despite its dual blood supply, the liver, a metabolically active organ, can be injured by

- Ischemia
- Insufficient venous drainage
- Specific vascular lesions

Ischemia results from reduced blood flow, reduced oxygen delivery, increased metabolic activity, or all 3. Diffuse ischemia can cause ischemic hepatitis; focal ischemia can cause hepatic infarction or ischemic cholangiopathy. Hepatic infarction results from hepatic artery disorders.

Insufficient venous drainage may result from focal or diffuse obstruction or from right-sided heart failure, as in congestive hepatopathy. Obstruction can occur in the intrahepatic or extrahepatic veins (Budd-Chiari syndrome) or in the intrahepatic terminal hepatic venules and hepatic sinusoids (veno-occlusive

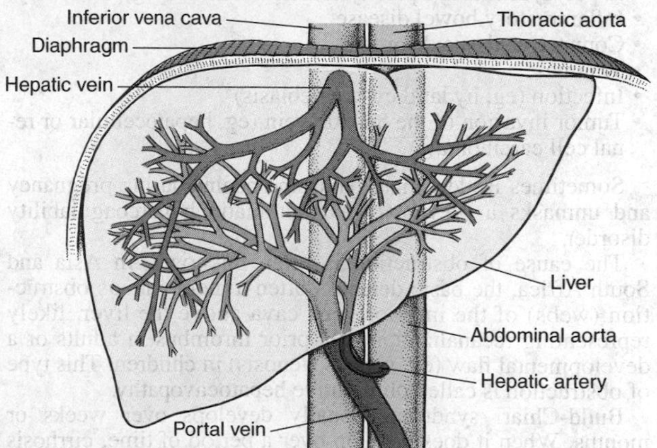

Fig. 31–1. Blood supply of the liver.

disease) but often occurs in both. Cirrhosis is the most common cause of diffuse intrahepatic venous outflow obstruction. Diffuse obstruction results in congestion of the sinusoids, hepatomegaly, portal hypertension, reduced portal blood flow, ascites, and splenomegaly. Manifestations of focal venous obstruction depend on the location.

Specific vascular lesions may occur in the hepatic artery, hepatic vein, or portal vein. The hepatic artery may be occluded. Uncommonly, aneurysms develop. In peliosis hepatis, blood-filled cystic spaces develop in the sinusoids (microvascular anastomoses between the portal and hepatic veins).

Hepatic vein disorders can result in focal or diffuse venous obstruction.

Nearly all portal vein disorders obstruct portal vein blood flow and cause portal hypertension. Obstruction can be

- Extrahepatic—portal vein thrombosis due to a hypercoagulable state, a vessel wall lesion (eg, pylephlebitis, omphalitis), an adjacent lesion (eg, pancreatitis, tumor), or congenital atresia of the portal vein
- Intrahepatic—eg, microvascular portal vein obstruction as occurs in schistosomiasis, primary biliary cirrhosis, sarcoidosis, and noncirrhotic portal hypertension

BUDD-CHIARI SYNDROME

Budd-Chiari syndrome is obstruction of hepatic venous outflow that originates anywhere from the small hepatic veins inside the liver to the inferior vena cava and right atrium. Manifestations range from no symptoms to fulminant liver failure. Diagnosis is based on ultrasonography. Treatment includes supportive medical therapy and measures to establish and maintain venous patency, such as thrombolysis, decompression with shunts, and long-term anticoagulation.

Etiology

In the Western world, the most common cause is a clot obstructing the hepatic veins and the adjacent inferior vena cava. Clots commonly result from the following:

- Thrombotic conditions (eg, protein C or S deficiency, antiphospholipid syndrome, antithrombin III deficiency, factor V Leiden mutation, pregnancy, oral contraceptive use)
- Hematologic disorders (eg, myeloproliferative disorders such as polycythemia and paroxysmal nocturnal hemoglobinopathy)
- Inflammatory bowel disease
- Connective tissue disorders
- Trauma
- Infection (eg, hydatid cyst, amebiasis)
- Tumor invasion of the hepatic vein (eg, hepatocellular or renal cell carcinoma)

Sometimes Budd-Chiari syndrome begins during pregnancy and unmasks a previously asymptomatic hypercoagulability disorder.

The cause of obstruction is often unknown. In Asia and South Africa, the basic defect is often a membranous obstruction (webs) of the inferior vena cava above the liver, likely representing recanalization of a prior thrombus in adults or a developmental flaw (eg, venous stenosis) in children. This type of obstruction is called obliterative hepatocavopathy.

Budd-Chiari syndrome usually develops over weeks or months. When it does develop over a period of time, cirrhosis and portal hypertension tend to develop.

Symptoms and Signs

Manifestations range from none (asymptomatic) to fulminant liver failure or cirrhosis. Symptoms vary depending on whether the obstruction occurs acutely or over time.

Acute obstruction (in about 20%) causes fatigue, right upper quadrant pain, nausea, vomiting, mild jaundice, tender hepatomegaly, and ascites. It typically occurs during pregnancy. Fulminant liver failure with encephalopathy is rare. Aminotransferase levels are quite high.

Chronic outflow obstruction (developing over weeks to months) may cause few or no symptoms until it progresses, or it may cause fatigue, abdominal pain, and hepatomegaly. Lower-extremity edema and ascites may result from venous obstruction, even in the absence of cirrhosis. Cirrhosis may develop, leading to variceal bleeding, massive ascites, splenomegaly, hepatopulmonary syndrome, or a combination. Complete obstruction of the inferior vena cava causes edema of the abdominal wall and legs plus visibly tortuous superficial abdominal veins from the pelvis to the costal margin.

Diagnosis

- Clinical evaluation and liver function tests
- Vascular imaging

Budd-Chiari syndrome is suspected in patients with hepatomegaly, ascites, liver failure, or cirrhosis when there is no obvious cause (eg, alcohol abuse, hepatitis) or when the cause is unexplained.

Liver function tests are usually abnormal; the pattern is variable and nonspecific. The presence of risk factors for thrombosis increase the consideration of this diagnosis.

Imaging usually begins with abdominal Doppler ultrasonography, which can show the direction of blood flow and the site of obstruction. Magnetic resonance angiography and CT are useful if ultrasonography is not diagnostic. Conventional angiography (venography with pressure measurements and arteriography) is necessary if therapeutic or surgical intervention is planned.

Liver biopsy is done occasionally to diagnose the acute stages and determine whether cirrhosis has developed.

Prognosis

Without treatment, most patients with complete venous obstruction die of liver failure within 3 yr. For patients with incomplete obstruction, the course varies.

Treatment

- Supportive care
- Restoration and maintenance of adequate venous outflow

Treatment varies according to onset (acute vs chronic) and severity (fulminant liver failure vs decompensated cirrhosis or stable/asymptomatic). The cornerstones of management are

- Giving supportive therapy directed at complications (eg, ascites, liver failure, esophageal varices
- Decompressing the congested liver (ie, maintaining venous outflow)
- Preventing propagation of the clot

Aggressive interventions (eg, thrombolysis, stents) are used when the disease is acute (eg, within 4 wk and in the absence of cirrhosis). Thrombolysis can dissolve acute clots, allowing recanalization and so relieving hepatic congestion. Radiologic procedures, such as angioplasty, stenting, and/or portosystemic shunts, can have a major role.

For caval webs or hepatic venous stenosis, decompression via percutaneous transluminal balloon angioplasty with intraluminal stents can maintain hepatic outflow. When dilation of a hepatic outflow narrowing is not technically feasible, transjugular intrahepatic portosystemic shunting (TIPS) and various surgical shunts can provide decompression by diverting blood flow into the systemic circulation. Portosystemic shunts are typically not used if hepatic encephalopathy is present; such shunts worsen liver function. Further, clots tend to form in shunts, especially if patients have a hematologic or thrombotic disorder.

Long-term anticoagulation is often necessary to prevent recurrence. Liver transplantation may be lifesaving in patients with fulminant disease or decompensated cirrhosis.

KEY POINTS

- The most common cause of Budd-Chiari syndrome (obstruction of hepatic venous outflow) is a clot blocking the hepatic veins and inferior vena cava.
- Consider the diagnosis if patients have typical findings (eg, hepatomegaly, ascites, liver failure, cirrhosis) that are unexplained or if they have abnormal liver function test results and risk factors for thrombosis.
- Confirm the diagnosis using Doppler ultrasonography or, if results are inconclusive, magnetic resonance angiography or CT.
- Restore venous outflow (eg, with thrombolysis, angioplasty, stents), and treat complications

CONGESTIVE HEPATOPATHY

(Passive Hepatic Congestion)

Congestive hepatopathy is diffuse venous congestion within the liver that results from right-sided heart failure (usually due to a cardiomyopathy, tricuspid regurgitation, mitral insufficiency, cor pulmonale, or constrictive pericarditis).

Moderate or severe right-sided heart failure increases central venous pressure, which is transmitted to the liver via the inferior vena cava and hepatic veins. Chronic congestion leads to atrophy of hepatocytes, distention of sinusoids, and centrizonal fibrosis, which, if severe, progresses to cirrhosis (cardiac cirrhosis). The basis for liver cell death is probably sinusoidal thrombosis that propagates to the central veins and branches of the portal vein, causing ischemia.

Most patients are asymptomatic. However, moderate congestion causes right upper quadrant discomfort (due to stretching of the liver capsule) and tender hepatomegaly. Severe congestion leads to massive hepatomegaly and jaundice. Ascites may result from the transmitted central venous hypertension; infrequently, splenomegaly results. With transmitted central venous hypertension, the hepatojugular reflex is present, unlike in hepatic congestion due to Budd-Chiari syndrome.

Diagnosis

- Clinical evaluation

Congestive hepatopathy is suspected in patients who have right-sided heart failure, jaundice, and tender hepatomegaly. Laboratory test results are modestly abnormal: unconjugated hyperbilirubinemia (total bilirubin < 3 mg/dL), elevated (usually < 2- to 3-fold) aminotransferases, and prolonged PT/INR. Ascitic fluid, if present, has a high albumin content (typically > 2.5 g/dL); in contrast, only 10% of patients with cirrhotic ascites have ascitic albumin levels that high.

Because the laboratory abnormalities are nonspecific, recognition of congestive hepatopathy is ultimately clinical. The liver disorder is more important as an index of the severity of heart failure than as a diagnosis by itself.

Treatment

- Targets underlying heart failure

Treatment is directed at the underlying heart failure.

HEPATIC ARTERY ANEURYSMS

Aneurysms of the hepatic artery are uncommon. They tend to be saccular and multiple. Causes include infection, arteriosclerosis, trauma, and vasculitis.

Untreated aneurysms may cause death by rupturing into the common bile duct (causing hemobilia), the peritoneum (causing peritonitis), or adjacent hollow viscera. Hemobilia may cause jaundice, upper GI bleeding, and abdominal pain in the right upper quadrant.

Diagnosis is suspected if typical symptoms occur or if imaging tests detect an aneurysm. Doppler ultrasonography, followed by contrast CT, is required for confirmation.

Treatment is embolization or surgical ligation.

HEPATIC ARTERY OCCLUSION

Causes of hepatic artery occlusion include thrombosis (eg, due to hypercoagulability disorders, severe arteriosclerosis, or vasculitis), emboli (eg, due to endocarditis, tumors, therapeutic embolization, or chemoembolization), iatrogenic causes (eg, ligation during surgery), vasculitis (via nonthrombotic mechanisms), structural arterial abnormalities (eg, hepatic artery aneurysm), eclampsia, cocaine use, and sickle cell crisis.

Usually, the result is an hepatic infarct. In patients with a liver transplant or preexisting portal vein thrombosis, hepatic artery thrombosis causes ischemic hepatitis. Because of the liver's dual blood supply, the liver is somewhat resistant to ischemic hepatitis and infarction.

Hepatic artery occlusion does not elicit symptoms unless hepatic infarction or ischemic hepatitis is present. Hepatic infarction may be asymptomatic or cause right upper quadrant pain, fever, nausea, vomiting, and jaundice. Leukocytosis and a high aminotransferase level are common.

Diagnosis

- Vascular imaging

Diagnosis of hepatic artery occlusion is confirmed by imaging with Doppler ultrasonography, usually followed by angiography. The choice between CT angiography, magnetic resonance angiography, and celiac arteriography largely depends on availability and expertise. CT may detect a wedge-shaped area of low attenuation.

Treatment

- Directed at the cause

Treatment is directed at the cause.

ISCHEMIC CHOLANGIOPATHY

Ischemic cholangiopathy is focal damage to the biliary tree due to disrupted flow from the hepatic artery via the peribiliary arterial plexus.

Common causes of ischemic cholangiopathy include

- Vascular injury during orthotopic liver transplantation or laparoscopic cholecystectomy
- Graft-rejection injury
- Chemoembolization
- Radiation therapy
- Thrombosis resulting from hypercoagulability disorders

Bile duct injury (ischemic necrosis) results, causing cholestatis, cholangitis, or biliary strictures (often multiple). Ischemic cholangiopathy most commonly occurs in people who have had a liver transplant.

Symptoms (eg, pruritus, dark urine, pale stools) and results of laboratory tests and imaging studies may indicate cholestasis.

Diagnosis

- Magnetic resonance cholangiopancreatography, ERCP, or both

The diagnosis is suspected when cholestasis is evident in patients at risk, particularly after liver transplantation. Ultrasonography is the first-line diagnostic imaging test for cholestasis, but most patients require magnetic resonance cholangiopancreatography, ERCP, or both to rule out other causes such as cholelithiasis or cholangiocarcinoma (see p. 199).

Treatment

- For rejection, antirejection therapy and possibly retransplantation
- For biliary strictures, balloon dilation and stenting

Treatment is directed at the cause. After liver transplantation, such treatment includes antirejection therapy and possible retransplantation. Biliary strictures warrant endoscopic balloon dilation and stenting.

ISCHEMIC HEPATITIS

(Acute Hepatic Infarction; Hypoxic Hepatitis; Shock Liver)

Ischemic hepatitis is diffuse liver damage due to an inadequate blood or oxygen supply.

Causes are most often systemic:

- Impaired hepatic perfusion (eg, due to heart failure or acute hypotension)
- Hypoxemia (eg, due to respiratory failure or carbon monoxide toxicity)
- Increased metabolic demand (eg, due to sepsis)

Focal lesions of the hepatic vasculature are less common causes. Ischemic hepatitis may develop when hepatic artery thrombosis occurs during liver transplantation or when thrombosis of the portal vein and hepatic artery develops in a patient with sickle cell crisis (thus compromising the dual blood supply to the liver). Centrizonal necrosis develops without liver inflammation (ie, not true hepatitis).

Symptoms may include nausea, vomiting, and tender hepatomegaly.

Diagnosis

- Clinical evaluation and liver function tests
- Doppler ultrasonography, MRI, or arteriography

Ischemic hepatitis is suspected in patients who have risk factors and laboratory abnormalities:

- Serum aminotransferase increases dramatically (eg, to 1000 to 3000 IU/L).
- LDH increases within hours of ischemia (unlike acute viral hepatitis).
- Serum bilirubin increases modestly, only to ≤ 4 times its normal level.
- PT/INR increases.

Diagnostic imaging helps define the cause: Doppler ultrasonography, MRI, or arteriography can identify an obstructed hepatic artery or portal vein thrombosis.

Treatment

- Hepatic reperfusion

Treatment is directed at the cause, aiming to restore hepatic perfusion, particularly by improving cardiac output and reversing any hemodynamic instability.

If perfusion is restored, aminotransferase decreases over 1 to 2 wk. In most cases, liver function is fully restored. Fulminant liver failure, although uncommon, can occur in patients with preexisting cirrhosis.

PELIOSIS HEPATIS

Peliosis hepatis is typically an asymptomatic disorder in which multiple blood-filled cystic spaces develop randomly in the liver.

Measuring a few millimeters to about 3 cm in diameter, the cysts of peliosis hepatis often lack a cell lining and are surrounded by hepatocytes. Some have an endothelial cell lining, accompanied by dilated hepatic sinusoids. The cause is probably damage to the sinusoidal lining cells. Peliosis hepatis is associated with use of hormones (eg, anabolic steroids, oral contraceptives, glucocorticoids), tamoxifen, vinyl chloride, vitamin A, and, particularly in kidney transplant recipients, azathioprine.

Peliosis hepatis is usually asymptomatic, but occasionally cysts rupture, resulting in hemorrhage and sometimes causing death. Some patients develop overt liver disease, characterized by jaundice, hepatomegaly, and liver failure.

Mild cases may be detected incidentally during imaging tests done because liver function test results are slightly abnormal or for other reasons. Ultrasonography or CT can detect cysts. Most cases are not treated.

PORTAL VEIN THROMBOSIS

Portal vein thrombosis causes portal hypertension and consequent GI bleeding from varices, usually in the lower esophagus or stomach. Diagnosis is based on ultrasonography. Treatment involves control of variceal bleeding (usually with endoscopic banding, IV octreotide, or both), prevention of recurrence using beta-blockers, and sometimes surgical shunts and thrombolysis for acute thrombosis.

Table 31–1. COMMON CAUSES OF PORTAL VEIN THROMBOSIS*

AGE GROUP	CAUSE	COMMENTS
Neonates	Umbilical stump infection or omphalitis (spread via the umbilical vein to the portal vein) Congenital portal vein abnormalities (less common)	Congenital abnormalities of the portal vein usually accompany congenital defects elsewhere.
Older children	Pylephlebitis	In acute appendicitis, infection enters the portal system; the vascular infection/inflammation then triggers thrombosis.
Adults	Surgery (eg, splenectomy) Hypercoagulable states (eg, myeloproliferative disorder, protein C or S deficiency, pregnancy) Cancer hepatocellular (eg, or pancreatic carcinoma, renal or adrenal cancers) Cirrhosis Trauma Possibly portal hypertension causing congestion and stasis	

*The cause is multifactorial in most cases and unknown in about one-third of cases.

Etiology

Common causes vary by age group (see Table 31–1).

Symptoms and Signs

Acute portal vein thrombosis is commonly asymptomatic unless associated with another event, such as pancreatitis (the cause), or another complication, such as mesenteric venous thrombosis. Most often, clinical features—splenomegaly (especially in children) and variceal hemorrhage—develop over a period of time secondary to portal hypertension. Ascites is uncommon (10%) in postsinusoidal portal hypertension. Ascites may be precipitated when cirrhosis is also present or when serum albumin (and thus oncotic pressure) deceases after high-volume fluid resuscitation for a major GI bleed.

Diagnosis

- Clinical evaluation and liver function tests
- Doppler ultrasonography

Portal vein thrombosis is suspected in patients with the following:

- Manifestations of portal hypertension without cirrhosis
- Mild abnormalities in liver function or enzymes plus risk factors such as neonatal umbilical infection, childhood appendicitis, or a hypercoagulability disorder

Doppler ultrasonography is usually diagnostic, showing diminished or absent portal vein flow and sometimes the thrombus. Difficult cases may require MRI or CT with contrast. Angiography may be required to guide shunt surgery.

Treatment

- For some acute cases, thrombolysis
- Long-term anticoagulation
- Management of portal hypertension and its complications

In acute cases, thrombolysis is sometimes successful, best reserved for recent occlusion, particularly in hypercoagulable states. Anticoagulation does not lyse clots but has some value for long-term prevention in hypercoagulable states despite the risk of variceal bleeding. In neonates and children, treatment is directed at the cause (eg, omphalitis, appendicitis). Otherwise, management is directed at the portal hypertension and its complications; treatment can include octreotide IV (a synthetic analog of somatostatin) and endoscopic banding to control variceal bleeding and nonselective beta-blockers to prevent rebleeding. These therapies have decreased the use of surgical shunts (eg, mesocaval, splenorenal), which can become occluded and have an operative mortality rate of 5 to 50%. Transjugular intrahepatic portosytemic shunting (TIPS) is not recommended. TIPS requires monitoring (including frequent angiography) to assess patency, may become blocked, and may not adequately decompress the liver.

KEY POINTS

- Causes of and risk factors for portal vein thrombosis include umbilical cord infection (in neonates), appendicitis (in children), and hypercoagulability states (in adults).
- Suspect portal vein thrombosis if patients have manifestations of portal hypertension in the absence of cirrhosis or if they have mild, nonspecific liver abnormalities plus risk factors.
- Confirm the diagnosis using Doppler ultrasonography or, if results are inconclusive, MRI or CT with contrast.
- Treat the cause of portal vein thrombosis and the complications of portal hypertension.

VENO-OCCLUSIVE DISEASE

(Sinusoidal Obstruction Syndrome)

Hepatic veno-occlusive disease is caused by endothelial injury, leading to nonthrombotic occlusion of the terminal hepatic venules and hepatic sinusoids, rather than of the hepatic veins or inferior vena cava (as in Budd-Chiari syndrome).

Venous congestion causes portal hypertension and ischemic necrosis (which leads to cirrhosis).

Common causes include

- Irradiation
- Graft-vs-host disease resulting from bone marrow or hematopoietic cell transplantation
- Pyrrolizidine alkaloids in crotalaria and senecio plants (eg, medicinal bush teas) and other herbs (eg, comfrey)
- Other hepatotoxins (eg, dimethylnitrosamine, aflatoxin, azathioprine, some anticancer drugs)

PEARLS & PITFALLS

- Ask patients who have cryptogenic liver abnormalities about use of herbal and natural products (including bush and herb teas) and anabolic steroids (which can cause peliosis hepatis).

Symptoms and Signs

Initial manifestations include sudden jaundice, ascites, and tender, smooth hepatomegaly. Onset is within the first 3 wk of transplantation in bone marrow or hematopoietic cell recipients, who either recover spontaneously within a few weeks (or sometimes, with mild cases, after an increase in immunosuppressant therapy) or die of fulminant liver failure. Other patients have recurrent ascites, portal hypertension, splenomegaly, and, eventually, cirrhosis.

Diagnosis

- Clinical evaluation and liver function tests
- Ultrasonography
- Sometimes invasive tests (eg, liver biopsy, measurement of portal-hepatic venous pressure gradient)

The diagnosis is suspected in patients with unexplained clinical or laboratory evidence of liver disease, particularly in those with known risk factors, such as bone marrow or hematopoietic cell transplantation.

Laboratory results are nonspecific: elevated aminotransferase and conjugated bilirubin levels. PT/INR becomes abnormal when disease is severe. Ultrasonography shows retrograde flow in the portal vein.

If the diagnosis is unclear, invasive tests become necessary—eg, liver biopsy or measurement of the portal-hepatic venous pressure gradient (a pressure gradient > 10 mm Hg suggests veno-occlusive disease). Measuring the pressure across the liver entails inserting a catheter percutaneously into a hepatic vein and then wedging it into the liver. This wedged pressure reflects portal vein pressure. (An exception is portal vein thrombosis; in this case, the pressure is normal despite portal hypertension.)

Treatment

- Supportive care
- Treatment of cause
- For progressive disease, TIPS or transplantation

Ursodeoxycholic acid helps prevent graft-vs-host disease in bone marrow or hematopoietic cell transplant recipients. Management includes withdrawing the causative agent (such as herbal teas) and providing supportive therapy.

Most patients have mild to moderate disease and do quite well. TIPS can be tried for relief of portal hypertension, but has not yet been shown to prolong survival, particularly when veno-occlusive disease is severe. In 25%, veno-occlusive disease is severe, accompanied by fulminant liver failure. Liver transplantation is a last resort.

Musculoskeletal and Connective Tissue Disorders

32 Approach to the Patient with Joint Disease

Some musculoskeletal disorders affect primarily the joints, causing arthritis. Others affect primarily the bones (eg, fractures, Paget disease of bone, tumors), muscles or other extra-articular soft tissues (eg, fibromyalgia), or periarticular soft tissues (eg, bursitis, tendinitis, sprain). Arthritis has myriad possible causes, including infection, autoimmune disorders, crystal-induced inflammation, and minimally inflammatory cartilage and bone disorders (eg, osteoarthritis). Arthritis may affect single joints (monarthritis) or multiple joints (polyarthritis) in a symmetric or asymmetric manner. Joints may suffer fractures or sprains (see elsewhere in The Manual).

History

The clinician should focus on systemic and extra-articular symptoms as well as joint symptoms. Many symptoms, including fever, chills, malaise, weight loss, Raynaud phenomenon, mucocutaneous symptoms (eg, rash, eye redness or pain, photosensitivity), and GI or cardiopulmonary symptoms, can be associated with various joint disorders.

Pain is the most common symptom of joint disorders. The history should address the character, location, severity, factors that aggravate or relieve pain, and time frame (new-onset or recurrent). The clinician must determine whether pain is worse when first moving a joint or after prolonged use and whether it is present upon waking or develops during the day. Usually, pain originating from superficial structures is better localized than pain originating from deeper structures. Pain originating in small distal joints tends to be better localized than pain originating in large proximal joints. Joint pain can be referred from extra-articular structures or from other joints. Arthritis often causes aching pain, whereas neuropathies often cause burning pain.

Stiffness refers to difficulty in moving a joint, but to patients, stiffness also may mean weakness, fatigue, or fixed limitation of motion. The clinician must separate the inability to move a joint from reluctance to move a joint because of pain. Characteristics of stiffness may suggest a cause, as in the following:

- Discomfort that occurs with motion when attempting to move a joint after a period of rest occurs in rheumatic disease.
- Stiffness is more severe and prolonged with increasing severity of joint inflammation.
- The theater sign (short-lived stiffness upon standing that necessitates walking slowly after sitting for several hours) is common in osteoarthritis.
- Morning stiffness in peripheral joints that lasts > 1 h can be an important early symptom of joint inflammation, such as in RA, psoriatic arthritis, or chronic viral arthritis (see Table 32–1).
- In the low back, morning stiffness that lasts > 1 h may reflect spondylitis.

Fatigue is a desire to rest that reflects exhaustion. It differs from weakness, inability to move, and reluctance to move because of pain with movement. Fatigue may reflect activity of a systemic inflammatory disorder.

Instability (buckling of a joint) suggests weakness of the ligaments or other structures that stabilize the joint, which are assessed by stress testing on physical examination. Buckling occurs most often in the knee and most often results from an internal joint derangement.

Physical Examination

Each involved joint should be inspected and palpated, and the range of motion should be estimated. With polyarticular disease, certain nonarticular signs (eg, fever, wasting, rash) may reflect systemic disorders.

The rest position of joints is noted, along with any erythema, swelling, deformity, and skin abrasions or punctures. Involved joints are compared with their uninvolved opposites or with those of the examiner.

Joints are gently palpated, noting the presence and location of tenderness, warmth, and swelling. Determining whether tenderness is present along the joint line or over tendon insertions or bursae is particularly important. Soft masses, bulges, or tissues that fill normal concavities or spaces (representing joint effusion or synovial proliferation) are noted. Palpation of swollen joints can sometimes differentiate among joint effusion, synovial thickening, and capsular or bony enlargement. Small joints (eg, acromioclavicular, tibiofibular, radioulnar) can be the source of pain that was initially believed to arise from a nearby major joint. Bony enlargement (often due to osteophytes) is noted.

Active range of motion (the maximum range through which the patient can move the joint) is assessed first; limitation may reflect weakness, pain, or stiffness as well as mechanical abnormalities. Then passive range of motion (the maximum range through which the examiner can move the joint) is assessed; passive limitation typically reflects mechanical abnormalities (eg, scarring, swelling, deformities) rather than weakness or pain. Active and passive movement of an inflamed joint (eg, due to infection or gout) may be very painful.

Inability to reproduce pain with motion or palpation of the joint suggests the possibility of referred pain.

Patterns of joint involvement should be noted. Symmetric involvement of multiple joints is common in systemic diseases (eg, RA); monarticular (involving one joint) or asymmetric oligoarticular (involving ≤ 4) joint involvement is more common in osteoarthritis and psoriatic arthritis. Small peripheral joints are commonly affected in RA, and the larger joints and spine are affected more in spondyloarthropathies. However, the full pattern of involvement may not be apparent in early disease.

Crepitus, a palpable or audible grinding produced by motion, is noted. It may be caused by roughened articular cartilage or by tendons; crepitus-causing motions should be determined and may suggest which structures are involved.

Specific features should be sought at each joint.

Elbow: Synovial swelling and thickening caused by joint disease occur in the lateral aspect between the radial head and olecranon, causing a bulge. Full 180° extension of the joint should be attempted. Although full extension is possible with nonarthritic or extra-articular problems such as tendinitis, its loss is an early change in arthritis. The area around the joint is examined for swellings. Rheumatoid nodules are firm, occurring especially along the extensor surface of the forearm. Tophi are sometimes visible under the skin as cream-colored aggregates and indicate gout. Swelling of the olecranon bursa occurs over the tip of the olecranon, is cystic, and does not limit joint motion; infection, trauma, gout, and RA are possible causes. Epitrochlear nodes occur above the medial epicondyle; they can result from inflammation in the hand but can also suggest sarcoidosis or lymphoma.

Shoulder: Because pain can be referred to areas around the shoulder, shoulder palpation should include the glenohumeral, acromioclavicular, and sternoclavicular joints, the coracoid process, clavicle, acromion process, subacromial bursa, biceps tendon, and greater and lesser tuberosities of the humerus, as well as the neck. Glenohumeral joint effusions may cause a bulge between the coracoid process and the humeral head. Possible causes include RA, osteoarthritis, septic arthritis, Milwaukee shoulder (see p. 276), and other arthropathies.

Limited motion, weakness, pain, and other disturbances of mobility caused by rotator cuff impairment can be quickly identified by having the patient attempt to abduct and raise both arms above the head and then to slowly lower them. Specific maneuvers against resistance can help determine which tendons are affected. Muscle atrophy and neurologic abnormalities should be sought.

Knee: At the knee, gross deformities such as swelling (eg, joint effusion, popliteal cysts), quadriceps muscle atrophy, and joint instability may be obvious when the patient stands and walks. With the patient supine, the examiner should palpate the knee, identifying the patella, femoral condyles, tibial tuberosity, tibial plateau, fibular head, medial and lateral joint lines, popliteal fossa, and quadriceps and patellar tendons. The medial and lateral joint lines correspond to locations of the medial and lateral menisci and can be located by palpation while slowly flexing and extending the knee. Tender extra-articular bursae such as the anserine bursa below the medial joint line should be differentiated from true intra-articular disturbances.

Detection of small knee effusions is often difficult and is best accomplished using the bulge sign. The knee is fully extended

Table 32–1. DISTINGUISHING INFLAMMATORY VS NONINFLAMMATORY JOINT DISEASE BY FEATURES

FEATURE	INFLAMMATORY	NONINFLAMMATORY
Systemic symptoms	Prominent, including fatigue	Unusual
Onset	Insidious Usually affecting multiple joints	Gradual 1 joint or a few joints
Morning stiffness	> 1 h	< 30 min
Worst time of day	Morning	As day progresses
Effect of activity on symptoms (joint pain and stiffness)	Lessen with activity Worse after periods of rest May also have pain with use	Worsen with activity Lessen with rest

and the leg slightly externally rotated while the patient is supine with muscles relaxed. The medial aspect of the knee is stroked to express any fluid away from this area. Placement of one hand on the suprapatellar pouch and gentle stroking or pressing on the lateral aspect of the knee can create a fluid wave or bulge, visible medially when an effusion is present. Larger effusions can be identified visually or by balloting the patella. Joint effusion can result from many joint diseases, including RA, osteoarthritis, gout, and trauma.

Full 180° extension of the knee is attempted to detect flexion contractures. The patella is tested for free, painless motion.

Hip: Examination begins with gait evaluation. A limp is common among patients with significant hip arthritis and may be caused by pain, leg shortening, flexion contracture, muscle weakness, or knee problems. Loss of internal rotation (an early change in hip osteoarthritis or any hip synovitis), flexion, extension, or abduction can usually be demonstrated. Placement of one hand on the patient's iliac crest detects pelvic movement that might be mistaken for hip movement. Flexion contracture can be identified by attempting leg extension with the opposite hip maximally flexed to stabilize the pelvis. Tenderness over the femoral greater trochanter suggests bursitis (which is extra-articular) rather than an intra-articular disorder. Pain with passive range of motion (assessed by internal and external rotation with the patient supine and the hip and knee flexed to 90°) suggests intra-articular origin. However, patients may have simultaneous intra-articular and extra-articular disorders.

Other: Hand examination is discussed elsewhere (see p. 287 and Pain in Multiple Joints on p. 332). Foot and ankle examination is discussed in on p. 277. Examination of the neck and back is discussed on p. 315.

Testing

Laboratory testing and imaging studies often provide less information than do the history and physical examination. Although some testing may be warranted in some patients, extensive testing is often not. Blood tests should be selected based on history and examination findings.

Blood tests: Some tests, although not specific, can be helpful in supporting the possibility of certain systemic rheumatic diseases, as for the following:

- Antinuclear antibodies (ANA) and anti–double-stranded DNA antibodies in SLE
- Rheumatoid factor and anti-cyclic citrullinated peptide (anti-CCP) antibodies in RA
- HLA-B27 in spondyloarthropathy (eg, with symptoms of inflammatory back pain and normal x-rays)
- Antineutrophil cytoplasmic antibodies (ANCA) in certain vasculitides (sometimes useful when systemic involvement is suspected)

Tests such as WBC count, ESR, and C-reactive protein may help determine the likelihood that arthritis is inflammatory due to infectious or other systemic disorders, but these tests are not highly specific or sensitive. For example, an elevated ESR or C-reactive protein level suggests articular inflammation or may be due to a large number of nonarticular inflammatory conditions (eg, infection, cancer). Also, such markers may not be elevated in all inflammatory disorders.

Imaging studies: Imaging studies are often unnecessary. Plain x-rays in particular reveal mainly bony abnormalities, and most joint disorders do not affect bone primarily. However, imaging may help in the initial evaluation of relatively localized, unexplained, persistent or severe joint and particularly spine abnormalities; it may reveal primary or metastatic tumors, osteomyelitis, bone infarctions, periarticular calcifications (as in calcific tendinitis), or other changes in deep structures that may escape physical examination. If chronic RA, gout, or osteoarthritis is suspected, erosions, cysts, and joint space narrowing with osteophytes may be visible. In pseudogout, Ca pyrophosphate deposition may be visible in intra-articular cartilage.

For musculoskeletal imaging, plain x-rays may be obtained first, but they are often less sensitive, particularly during early disease, than MRI, CT, or ultrasonography. MRI is the most accurate study for fractures not visible on plain x-rays, particularly in the hip and pelvis, and for soft tissues and internal derangements of the knee. CT is useful if MRI is contraindicated or unavailable. Ultrasonography, arthrography, and bone scanning may help in certain conditions, as can biopsy of bone, synovium, or other tissues.

Arthrocentesis: Arthrocentesis is the process of puncturing the joint with a needle to withdraw fluid. If there is an effusion and arthrocentesis is done correctly, fluid can typically be withdrawn. Examination of synovial fluid is the most accurate way to exclude infection, diagnose crystal-induced arthritis, and otherwise determine the cause of joint effusions. This procedure is indicated for all patients with acute or unexplained monarticular joint effusions and for patients with unexplained polyarticular effusions.

Arthrocentesis is done using strictly sterile technique. Infection or other rash over the site used to enter the joint is a contraindication. Preparations for collecting samples should be made before doing the procedure. Local anesthesia, with lidocaine or difluoroethane spray, is often used. Many joints are punctured on the extensor surface to avoid nerves, arteries, and veins, which are usually on the joint's flexor surface. A 20-gauge needle can be used for most larger joints. Smaller joints of the upper and lower extremities are probably easier to access using a 22- or 23-gauge needle. As much fluid as is possible should be removed. Specific anatomic landmarks are used (see Figs. 32–1, 32–2, and 32–3).

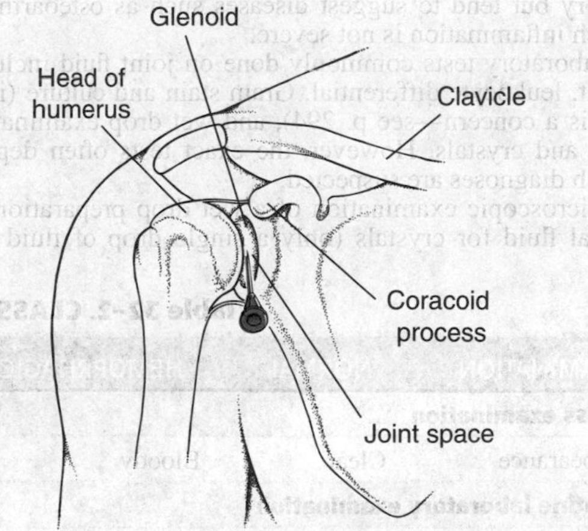

Fig. 32–1. Arthrocentesis of the shoulder. The glenohumeral joint is punctured while the patient sits with the arm at the side and the hand on the lap. The needle is inserted anteriorly, slightly inferior and lateral to the coracoid process, aiming posteriorly toward the glenoid fossa. A posterior approach is also possible.

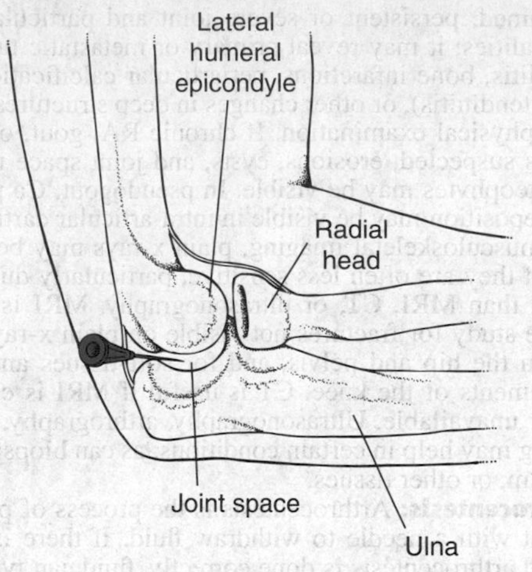

Fig. 32–2. Arthrocentesis of the elbow. The ulnohumeral joint is entered while the patient's elbow is flexed at 60° and the wrist is pronated. The needle enters the joint's lateral surface, between the lateral humeral epicondyle and the ulna.

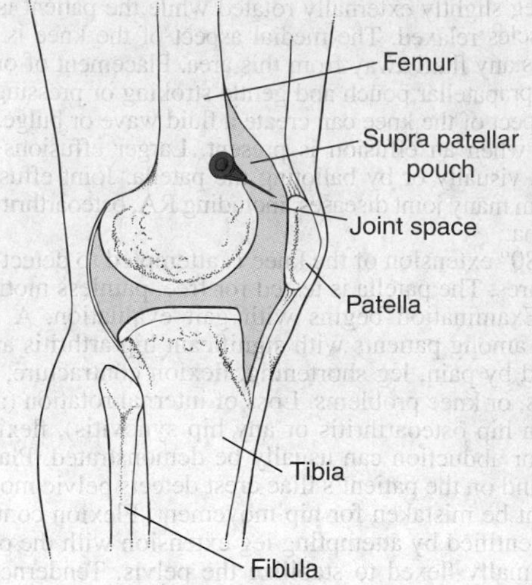

Fig. 32–3. Arthrocentesis of the knee. The knee and connecting suprapatellar pouch can be punctured while the patient is supine and the knee is extended. The needle, usually 20-gauge, can be inserted laterally, just under the cephalad edge of the patella. Alternatively, the needle can be inserted medially, under the cephalad half of the patella.

Metacarpophalangeal joints, metatarsophalangeal joints, and interphalangeal joints of the hands and feet are punctured similarly to each other, using a 22- or 23-gauge needle. The needle is inserted dorsally, to either side of the extensor tendon. Distraction (pulling) of the joint is sometimes useful to open the joint space and allow easier access.

Synovial fluid examination: At the bedside, gross characteristics of the fluid are assessed, such as its color and clarity.

Gross characteristics allow many effusions to be tentatively classified as noninflammatory, inflammatory, or infectious (see Table 32–2). Effusions can also be hemorrhagic. Each type of effusion suggests certain joint diseases (see Table 32–3). So-called noninflammatory effusions are actually mildly inflammatory but tend to suggest diseases such as osteoarthritis, in which inflammation is not severe.

Laboratory tests commonly done on joint fluid include cell count, leukocyte differential, Gram stain and culture (if infection is a concern—see p. 294), and wet drop examination for cells and crystals. However, the exact tests often depend on which diagnoses are suspected.

Microscopic examination of a wet drop preparation of synovial fluid for crystals (only a single drop of fluid from a joint is needed) using polarized light is essential for definitive diagnosis of gout, pseudogout, and other crystal-induced arthritides (see p. 272). A polarizer over the light source and another polarizer between the specimen and the examiner's eye allow visualization of crystals with a shiny white birefringence. Compensated polarized light is provided by inserting a first-order red plate, as is found in commercially available microscopes. The effects of a compensator can be reproduced by placing 2 strips of clear adhesive tape on a glass slide and placing this slide over the lower polarizer. Such a homemade system should be tested against a commercial polarizing microscope. The most common crystals seen are those diagnostic of gout (monosodium urate, negatively birefringent needle-shaped crystals) and pseudogout (Ca pyrophosphate, rhomboid- or rod-shaped crystals that are positively birefringent or not birefringent). If crystals appear atypical in a wet drop, several less common crystals (cholesterol, liquid lipid crystals, oxalate, cryoglobulins) or artifacts (eg, depot corticosteroid crystals) should be considered.

Table 32–2. CLASSIFICATION OF SYNOVIAL EFFUSIONS

EXAMINATION	NORMAL	HEMORRHAGIC	INFECTIOUS	INFLAMMATORY	NONINFLAMMATORY
Gross examination					
Appearance	Clear	Bloody	Turbid or purulent	Yellow, cloudy	Straw-colored, clear
Routine laboratory examination					
Culture	Negative	Negative	Often positive	Negative	Negative
PMN %*	< 25		Usually > 85	> 50	< 25
WBC count*	< 200/μL	Affected by amount of blood	5000–> 100,000/μL	1000–50,000/μL	200–1000/μL

*WBC count and PMN % in infectious arthritis are lower if the organism is less virulent (eg, in gonococcal, Lyme, tuberculous, or fungal arthritis) or partially treated. Some effusions in SLE and other connective tissue diseases are only equivocally inflammatory, with a WBC count of 500–2,000/μL. Noninfectious effusions rarely have up to 100,000 WBC/μL.

Table 32–3. DIFFERENTIAL DIAGNOSIS BASED ON SYNOVIAL FLUID CLASSIFICATION*†

TYPE OF EFFUSION	POSSIBLE CAUSES
Hemorrhagic	Anticoagulants Hemangioma Coagulopathy Neurogenic (neuropathic) arthropathy Pigmented villonodular synovitis Scurvy Thrombocytopenia Trauma with or without fracture Tumor
Infectious	Various organisms depending on patient characteristics (see Table 38–2 on p. 295)
Inflammatory	Acute crystal synovitis (gout and pseudogout) Ankylosing spondylitis Crohn disease Lyme disease Partially treated or less virulent bacterial infections Psoriatic arthritis Reactive arthritis (including what was previously called Reiter syndrome) RA Rheumatic fever SLE (mild inflammation) Synovial infarction (eg, caused by sickle cell disease) Ulcerative colitis
Noninflammatory	Amyloidosis Ehlers-Danlos syndrome Hypertrophic pulmonary osteoarthropathy Metabolic diseases causing osteoarthritis Neurogenic (neuropathic) arthropathy Osteoarthritis Osteochondritis dissecans Osteochondromatosis Osteonecrosis (including osteonecrosis caused by sickle cell disease) Progressive systemic sclerosis Rheumatic fever SLE Subsiding or early inflammation Trauma

*See Table 32–2 for classification. This differential diagnosis is only a partial listing.

†Some disorders span classifications (eg, neuropathic arthropathy can be hemorrhagic or noninflammatory; progressive systemic sclerosis can be inflammatory or noninflammatory).

Other synovial fluid findings that occasionally make or suggest a specific diagnosis include the following:

- Specific organisms (identifiable by Gram or acid-fast stain)
- Marrow spicules or fat globules (caused by fracture)
- Reiter cells (monocytes on Wright-stained smears that have phagocytized PMNs), which appear most often in reactive arthritis
- Amyloid fragments (identifiable by Congo red stain)
- Sickled RBCs (caused by sickle cell hemoglobinopathies)

33 Autoimmune Rheumatic Disorders

Autoimmune rheumatic disorders include diverse syndromes such as eosinophilic fasciitis, mixed connective tissue disease, polymyositis and dermatomyositis, relapsing polychondritis, Sjögren syndrome, SLE, and systemic sclerosis. RA and the spondyloarthropathies and their variants are also immune mediated. The triggers and precise pathophysiology remain unknown for all these disorders, although many aspects of pathogenesis are becoming clearer.

KEY POINTS

- Patients with most autoimmune rheumatic disorders are at increased risk of atherosclerosis.
- Patients who receive corticosteroids plus another immunosuppressive drug should usually receive prophylaxis for opportunistic infections such as *Pneumocystis jirovecii*.

EOSINOPHILIC FASCIITIS

Eosinophilic fasciitis (EF) is an uncommon disorder characterized by symmetric and painful inflammation, swelling, and induration of the arms and legs. Diagnosis is by biopsy of skin and fascia. Treatment is with corticosteroids.

The cause of EF is unknown. The disorder occurs mostly in middle-aged men but can occur in women and children.

Symptoms and Signs

The disease often begins after strenuous physical activity (eg, chopping wood). The initial features are pain, swelling, and inflammation of the skin and subcutaneous tissues, followed by induration, creating a characteristic orange-peel configuration most evident over the anterior surfaces of the extremities. The face and trunk are occasionally involved. Restriction of arm and leg movement usually develops insidiously. Contractures commonly evolve, secondary to induration and thickening of the fascia, but the process may also involve tendons, synovial membranes, and muscle. Typically, EF does not involve the fingers and toes (acral areas). Muscle strength is unimpaired, but myalgia and arthritis may occur. Carpal tunnel syndrome may also occur.

Fatigue and weight loss are common. Rarely, aplastic anemia, thrombocytopenia, and lymphoproliferative processes develop.

Diagnosis

- Biopsy

EF should be suspected in patients with typical symptoms. The cutaneous manifestations may suggest systemic sclerosis; however, patients with systemic sclerosis usually also have Raynaud phenomenon, acral involvement, telangiectasia, and visceral changes (eg, esophageal dysmotility). All of these are absent in EF.

Diagnosis is confirmed by biopsy, which should be deep enough to include fascia and adjacent muscle fibers. Characteristic findings are inflammation of the fascia, with or without eosinophils.

Blood tests are not diagnostic, but CBC shows eosinophilia (in early active disease), and serum protein electrophoresis shows polyclonal hypergammaglobulinemia. CBC should be done in all patients because the presence of eosinophilia helps in the diagnosis. Autoantibodies are usually absent. MRI, although not specific, can show thickened fascia, with the increased signal intensity in the superficial muscle fibers correlating with the inflammation.

Prognosis

Although the long-term outcome varies, EF is often self-limited after treatment.

Treatment

- Oral prednisone

Most patients respond rapidly to high doses of prednisone (40 to 60 mg po once/day followed by gradual reduction to 5 to 10 mg/day as soon as the fasciitis resolves). Continued low doses may be required for 2 to 5 yr. Some patients require longer courses and possibly other drugs (eg, hydroxychloroquine, methotrexate, azathioprine, rituximab, mycophenolate mofetil, cyclosporine). There are no controlled drug trials to guide therapy. NSAIDs and H_2 blockers (eg, cimetidine) also have been used to treat EF. Surgical release of contractions and the carpal tunnel may be necessary.

Monitoring with CBCs is advised because of the occasional hematologic complications. Prophylaxis for opportunistic infections, such as *Pneumocystis jirovecii,* should be added if combination immunosuppressive therapy is used.

KEY POINTS

- Patients develop symmetric and painful inflammation, swelling, and induration of the arms and legs in a characteristic orange-peel configuration.
- Although cutaneous manifestations may suggest systemic sclerosis, patients with EF usually do not have Raynaud phenomenon, acral involvement, telangiectasia, and visceral changes (eg, esophageal dysmotility).
- Confirm the diagnosis with a biopsy that includes fascia and adjacent muscle.
- Treat patients with prednisone, other immunosuppressants, or both.

MIXED CONNECTIVE TISSUE DISEASE

Mixed connective tissue disease (MCTD) is an uncommon, specifically defined overlap syndrome characterized by clinical features of SLE, systemic sclerosis, and polymyositis with very high titers of circulating antinuclear antibody to a ribonucleoprotein antigen. Hand swelling, Raynaud phenomenon, polyarthralgia, inflammatory myopathy, esophageal hypomotility, and pulmonary dysfunction are common. Diagnosis is by the combination of clinical features, antibodies to ribonucleoprotein, and absence of antibodies specific for other autoimmune diseases. Treatment varies with disease severity and organ involvement but usually includes corticosteroids and additional immunosuppressants.

MCTD occurs worldwide and in all races, with a peak incidence in the teens and 20s. About 80% of people who have this disease are women. The cause is unknown. In some patients, the disorder evolves into classic systemic sclerosis or SLE.

Symptoms and Signs

Raynaud phenomenon may precede other manifestations by years. Frequently, the first manifestations resemble early SLE, systemic sclerosis, polymyositis, or even RA. Many patients appear to have an undifferentiated connective tissue disease initially. The disease manifestations may progress and become widespread, and the clinical pattern changes over time.

Diffuse swelling of the hands is typical but not universal. Skin findings include lupus or dermatomyositis-like rashes. Diffuse systemic sclerosis-like skin changes and ischemic necrosis or ulceration of the fingertips may occasionally develop.

Almost all patients have polyarthralgias, and 75% have frank arthritis. Often the arthritis is nondeforming, but erosive changes and deformities similar to those in RA (eg, boutonnière and swan-neck deformities) may be present. Proximal muscle weakness with or without tenderness is common.

Renal involvement (most commonly membranous nephropathy) occurs in about 25% of patients and is typically mild; severe involvement, with morbidity or mortality, is atypical for MCTD. The lungs are affected in up to 75% of patients with MCTD. Interstitial lung disease is the most common lung manifestation; pulmonary hypertension is a major cause of death. Heart failure can occur. Sjögren syndrome may develop. A trigeminal sensory neuropathy may be the presenting feature and is considered the most frequent CNS manifestation.

Diagnosis

- Testing for antinuclear antibodies (ANA), antibodies to extractable nuclear antigen (antibodies to U1 ribonucleoprotein, or RNP), and Smith [Sm]) and anti-DNA antibodies
- Organ involvement determined as clinically indicated

MCTD should be suspected when additional overlapping features are present in patients appearing to have SLE, systemic sclerosis, or polymyositis.

Tests for ANA and antibody to U1 RNP antigen are done first. Almost all patients have high titers (often > 1:1000) of fluorescent ANA that produce a speckled pattern. Antibodies to U1 RNP are usually present at very high titers (> 1:100,000). Antibodies to the ribonuclease-resistant Sm component of extractable nuclear antigen (anti-Sm antibodies) and to double-stranded DNA (negative in MCTD by definition) are measured to exclude other disorders.

Rheumatoid factors are frequently present, and titers may be high. The ESR is frequently elevated.

Pulmonary hypertension should be detected as early as possible. Further evaluation depends on symptoms and signs; manifestations of myositis, renal involvement, or pulmonary involvement prompt tests of those organs (eg, CK, MRI, electromyogram, or muscle biopsy for diagnosis of myositis).

Prognosis

The overall 10-yr survival rate is 80%, but prognosis depends largely on which manifestations predominate. Patients with features of systemic sclerosis and polymyositis have a worse prognosis. Patients are at increased risk of atherosclerosis. Causes of death include pulmonary hypertension, renal failure, MI, colonic perforation, disseminated infection, and cerebral hemorrhage. Some patients have sustained remissions for many years without treatment.

Treatment

- NSAIDs or antimalarials for mild disease
- Corticosteroids for moderate to severe disease
- Sometimes other immunosuppressants

General management and initial drug therapy are tailored to the specific clinical problem and are similar to those of SLE or the dominant clinical phenotype. Most patients with moderate or severe disease respond to corticosteroids, particularly if treated early. Mild disease is often controlled by NSAIDs, antimalarials, or sometimes low-dose corticosteroids. Severe major organ involvement usually requires higher doses of corticosteroids (eg, prednisone 1 mg/kg po once/day) and additional immunosuppressants. If patients develop features of myositis or systemic sclerosis, treatment is as for those diseases.

All patients should be closely monitored for atherosclerosis. Patients on long-term corticosteroid therapy should receive osteoporosis prophylaxis. Prophylaxis for opportunistic infections, such as *Pneumocystis jirovecii,* should be added if combination immunosuppressive therapy is used.

KEY POINTS

- MCTD most often resembles SLE, systemic sclerosis, and/or polymyositis.
- Typically, ANA and antibodies to U1 RNP are present and anti-Sm and anti-DNA antibodies are absent.
- Anticipate pulmonary hypertension.
- Treat mild disease with NSAIDs or antimalarials and more severe disease with corticosteroids and sometimes other immunosuppressants.

POLYMYOSITIS AND DERMATOMYOSITIS

Polymyositis and dermatomyositis are uncommon systemic rheumatic disorders characterized by inflammatory and degenerative changes in the muscles (polymyositis) or in the skin and muscles (dermatomyositis). The most specific skin signs are Gottron papules over the knuckles and a periorbital heliotropic rash. Manifestations include symmetric weakness, some tenderness, and later atrophy, principally of the proximal limb girdle muscles. Complications can include visceral involvement and cancer. Diagnosis is by clinical findings and abnormalities on muscle tests, which may include muscle enzymes, MRI, electromyography, and muscle biopsy. Treatment is with corticosteroids, usually combined with immunosuppressants or IV immune globulin.

The female:male ratio is 2:1. These disorders may appear at any age but occur most commonly from age 40 to 60 or, in children, from age 5 to 15.

Etiology

The cause seems to be an autoimmune reaction to muscle tissue in genetically susceptible people. Familial clustering occurs, and HLA subtypes -DR3, -DR52, and -DR6 seem to be the genetic predisposition. Possible inciting events include viral myositis and underlying cancer. Picornavirus-like structures have been found in muscle cells, but their significance is not known, and viruses can trigger similar disorders in animals. The association of cancer with dermatomyositis (less so with polymyositis) suggests that a tumor may incite myositis as the result of an autoimmune reaction against a common antigen in muscle and tumor.

Pathophysiology

Pathologic changes in both disorders include cellular damage and atrophy, with variable degrees of inflammation. Muscles in the hands, feet, and face are affected less than other skeletal muscles. Involvement of muscles in the pharynx and upper esophagus and occasionally the heart can impair the functions of those organs. Inflammation may occur in joints and lungs, especially in patients with antisynthetase antibodies.

Dermatomyositis is characterized by immune complex deposition in the vessels and is considered a complement-mediated vasculopathy. In contrast, the main pathophysiologic abnormality in polymyositis is direct T cell-mediated muscle injury.

Classification

Myositis has been divided into several subtypes:

- Primary idiopathic polymyositis can occur at any age and does not involve the skin.

- Primary idiopathic dermatomyositis is similar to primary idiopathic polymyositis but also involves the skin.
- Polymyositis or dermatomyositis associated with cancer can occur at any age but is most common among older adults; the cancer can develop up to 2 yr before or after the myositis.
- Childhood dermatomyositis can be associated with systemic vasculitis.
- Polymyositis or dermatomyositis can occur with an associated disorder such as progressive systemic sclerosis, mixed connective tissue disease, RA, SLE, or sarcoidosis.

Inclusion body myositis is a separate disorder that has clinical manifestations similar to chronic idiopathic polymyositis; however, it develops at an older age, frequently involves distal muscles (eg, hand and foot muscles), has a longer duration, responds poorly to therapy, and has a different histologic appearance.

Symptoms and Signs

Onset of polymyositis may be acute (particularly in children) or insidious (particularly in adults). Polyarthralgias, Raynaud phenomenon, dysphagia, pulmonary symptoms, and constitutional complaints (notably fever, fatigue, and weight loss) may also occur.

Muscle weakness may progress over weeks to months. However, it takes destruction of 50% of muscle fibers to cause symptomatic weakness (ie, muscle weakness indicates advanced myositis). Patients may have difficulty raising their arms above their shoulders, climbing steps, or rising from a sitting position. Patients may become wheelchair-bound or bedridden because of weakness of pelvic and shoulder girdle muscles. The flexors of the neck may be severely affected, causing an inability to raise the head from the pillow. Involvement of pharyngeal and upper esophageal muscles may impair swallowing and predispose to aspiration. Muscles of the hands, feet, and face escape involvement. Limb contractures may eventually develop.

Joint manifestations include polyarthralgia or polyarthritis, often with swelling, effusions, and other characteristics of nondeforming arthritis, which occur in about 30% of patients. However, joint manifestations tend to be mild. They occur more often in a subset with Jo-1 or other antisynthetase antibodies.

Visceral involvement (except that of the pharynx and upper esophagus) is less common in polymyositis than in some other rheumatic disorders (eg, SLE, systemic sclerosis). Occasionally, and especially in patients with antisynthetase antibodies, interstitial pneumonitis (manifested by dyspnea and cough) is the most prominent manifestation. Cardiac arrhythmias, especially including conduction disturbances or ventricular dysfunction, can occur. GI symptoms, more common among children, are due to an associated vasculitis and may include hematemesis, melena, and ischemic bowel perforation.

Skin changes, which occur in dermatomyositis, tend to be dusky and erythematous. Periorbital edema with a purplish appearance (heliotrope rash) is relatively specific for dermatomyositis. Elsewhere, the rash may be slightly elevated and smooth or scaly; it may appear on the forehead, V of the neck and shoulders, chest and back, forearms and lower legs, elbows and knees, medial malleoli, and radiodorsal aspects of the proximal interphalangeal and metacarpophalangeal joints (Gottron papules—also a relatively specific finding). The base and sides of the fingernails may be hyperemic or thickened. Desquamating dermatitis with splitting of the skin may evolve over the radial aspects of the fingers. The primary skin lesions frequently fade completely but may be followed by secondary changes (eg, brownish pigmentation, atrophy, scarring, vitiligo). Rash on the scalp may appear psoriaform and be intensely pruritic. Subcutaneous calcification may occur, particularly in children.

Diagnosis

- Clinical criteria
- Muscle biopsy (definitive)

Polymyositis should be suspected in patients with proximal muscle weakness with or without muscle tenderness. Dermatomyositis should be suspected in patients with a heliotropic rash or Gottron papules, even without myositis, and in patients with symptoms of polymyositis and any skin findings compatible with dermatomyositis. Polymyositis and dermatomyositis share certain clinical findings with systemic sclerosis or, less frequently, with SLE or vasculitis. Establishing the diagnosis requires as many as possible of the following 5 criteria:

- Proximal muscle weakness
- Characteristic rash
- Elevated serum muscle enzymes (if CK is not elevated, aminotransferases or aldolase [which are less specific than CK])
- Characteristic electromyographic or MRI muscle abnormalities
- Muscle biopsy changes (the definitive test)

Muscle biopsy excludes some similar conditions such as inclusion body myositis and postviral rhabdomyolysis. Biopsy findings can be variable, but chronic inflammation and muscle degeneration and regeneration are typical. A definite diagnosis made by muscle biopsy is recommended before treatment of polymyositis to exclude other muscle disorders. To increase the sensitivity of the biopsy results, the biopsy sample should be obtained from a muscle that has one or more of the following characteristics:

- Weakness on clinical examination
- Inflammation identified on MRI
- Contralateral pair of a muscle shown to be abnormal on electromyography

Laboratory studies can increase or decrease suspicion for the disorder, assess its severity, identify overlaps, and help detect complications. Autoantibodies should be tested. ANA are positive in up to 80% of patients. Detailed testing of ANA, when present, is important in identifying other overlap syndromes, most often those with another autoimmune disorder. About 30% of patients have myositis-specific autoantibodies: antibodies to aminoacyl-tRNA synthetases (anti-synthetase antibodies), including anti–Jo-1; antibodies to signal recognition particle (SRP—anti-SRP antibodies); and antibodies to Mi-2, a nuclear helicase. The relationship between these autoantibodies and disease pathogenesis remains unclear, although antibody to Jo-1 is a significant marker for fibrosing alveolitis, pulmonary fibrosis, arthritis, and Raynaud phenomenon.

Periodic measurement of CK is helpful in monitoring treatment. However, in patients with widespread muscle atrophy, levels are occasionally normal despite chronic, active myositis. Muscle biopsy, MRI, or high CK levels can often differentiate a relapse of polymyositis from corticosteroid-induced myopathy. Aldolase is a less specific marker for muscle injury than CK.

Cancer screening is recommended by some authorities for patients ≥ 40 yr who have dermatomyositis or for patients ≥ 60 yr who have polymyositis because these patients often have unsuspected cancers. Screening should include a physical examination that includes breast, pelvis, and rectum (with occult blood testing); CBC; biochemical profile; mammogram; carcinoembryonic antigen; urinalysis; chest x-ray; and any other tests appropriate based on patient's age. Additional investigation should be based on history and physical examination findings. Some authorities recommend CT of the chest, abdomen, and pelvis. Younger patients without symptoms of cancer need not undergo screening.

Prognosis

Long remissions (even apparent recovery) occur in up to 50% of treated patients within 5 yr, more often in children. Relapse, however, may still occur at any time. Overall 5-yr survival rate is 75% and is higher in children. Death in adults is preceded by severe and progressive muscle weakness, dysphagia, undernutrition, aspiration pneumonia, or respiratory failure with superimposed pulmonary infection. Polymyositis tends to be more severe and resistant to treatment in patients with cardiac or pulmonary involvement. Death in children may be a result of bowel vasculitis. Cancer, if present, generally determines the overall prognosis.

Treatment

- Corticosteroids
- Sometimes immunosuppressants (eg, methotrexate, azathioprine, mycophenolate mofetil, rituximab, cyclosporine, IV immune globulin)

Physical activities should be modestly curtailed until the inflammation subsides. Corticosteroids are the drugs of choice initially. For acute disease, adults receive prednisone ≥ 40 to 60 mg po once/day. Serial measurements of CK provide the best early guide of therapeutic effectiveness, falling toward or reaching normal in most patients in 6 to 12 wk, followed by improved muscle strength. Once enzyme levels have returned to normal, prednisone can be gradually reduced. If muscle enzyme levels rise, the dose is increased. Patients who seem to recover can have treatment gradually withdrawn with close monitoring, but most adults require chronic maintenance with prednisone (up to 10 to 15 mg/day). Children require initial doses of prednisone of 30 to 60 mg/m^2 once/day. In children, it may be possible to stop prednisone after ≥ 1 yr of remission.

Occasionally, patients treated chronically with high-dose corticosteroids become increasingly weak because of a superimposed corticosteroid myopathy.

If a patient does not to respond to corticosteroids, depends on a high to moderate dose of corticosteroids, or develops a corticosteroid myopathy or another complication that necessitates stopping or decreasing prednisone, immunosuppressants (eg, methotrexate, azathioprine, mycophenolate mofetil, rituximab, cyclosporine, IV immune globulin) should be tried. Some clinicians combine prednisone with an immunosuppressant at the time treatment is initiated. Some patients have received only methotrexate (generally in higher doses than used for RA) for ≥ 5 yr. IV immune globulin can be effective in some patients refractory to drug treatment, but the prohibitive cost has discouraged comparative trials.

Myositis associated with cancer or inclusion body myositis usually is more refractory to corticosteroids. Cancer-associated myositis may remit if the tumor is removed.

People with an autoimmune disorder are at higher risk of atherosclerosis and should be closely monitored. Patients on long-term corticosteroid therapy should receive osteoporosis prophylaxis. Prophylaxis for opportunistic infections, such as *Pneumocystis jirovecii,* should be added if combination immunosuppressive therapy is used.

KEY POINTS

- Muscle weakness indicates advanced myositis.
- Heliotropic rash and Gottron papules are relatively specific for dermatomyositis.
- To establish the diagnosis, look for characteristic muscle weakness and rash, elevated CK level, and muscle changes on electromyography or MRI.
- If necessary, do a muscle biopsy to confirm the diagnosis.
- Screen patients ≥ 40 yr with dermatomyositis and patients ≥ 60 yr with polymyositis for cancer.
- Treat most patients with corticosteroids and sometimes other immunosuppressants.

RELAPSING POLYCHONDRITIS

Relapsing polychondritis is an episodic, inflammatory, and destructive disorder involving primarily cartilage of the ear and nose but also potentially affecting the eyes, tracheobronchial tree, heart valves, kidneys, joints, skin, and blood vessels. Diagnosis is by a combination of clinical, laboratory, imaging, and sometimes biopsy findings. Treatment usually requires prednisone and other immunosuppressants.

Relapsing polychondritis affects men and women equally; onset typically is in middle age. An association with RA, systemic vasculitis, SLE, and other connective tissue disorders suggests an autoimmune etiology.

Symptoms and Signs

Acute pain, erythema, and swelling most commonly affect the pinna cartilage. Nasal cartilage inflammation is the next most common manifestation, followed by arthritis that varies from arthralgias to symmetric or asymmetric nondeforming arthritis involving large and small joints, with a predilection for the costochondral joints and knees. The next most common manifestations, in decreasing order of frequency, are inflammation of the eye (eg, conjunctivitis, scleritis, iritis, keratitis, chorioretinitis); cartilaginous tissue of the larynx, trachea, or bronchi (causing hoarseness, cough, and tenderness over the laryngeal cartilage); internal ear; cardiovascular system (eg, aortic regurgitation, mitral regurgitation, pericarditis, myocarditis, aortic aneurysms, aortitis); kidney; and skin. Bouts of acute inflammation heal over weeks to months, with recurrences over several years.

Advanced disease can lead to destruction of supporting cartilage, causing floppy ears, saddle nose, pectus excavatum, and visual, auditory, and vestibular abnormalities. Tracheal narrowing can lead to dyspnea, pneumonia, or even tracheal collapse. Coexisting systemic vasculitis (leukocytoclastic vasculitis or polyarteritis nodosa), myelodysplastic syndrome, or cancer is possible.

Diagnosis

- Clinical criteria
- Sometimes biopsy

Diagnosis is established if the patient develops at least 3 of the following:

- Bilateral chondritis of the external ears
- Inflammatory polyarthritis
- Nasal chondritis
- Ocular inflammation
- Respiratory tract chondritis
- Auditory or vestibular dysfunction

Biopsy of involved cartilage, most often the pinna, is helpful if clinical diagnosis is not clear-cut.

Laboratory tests are done. They are not specific but may help exclude other disorders. Synovial fluid analysis reveals mild inflammatory changes that are nonspecific but help rule out an infectious process. Blood tests may show normocytic-normochromic anemia, leukocytosis, elevated ESR or γ-globulin levels, and occasionally positive rheumatoid factor, ANA, or, in up to 25% of patients, antineutrophil cytoplasmic antibodies (ANCA). Abnormal renal function may indicate an associated glomerulonephritis. A positive c-ANCA test (ANCA that are reactive mainly to proteinase-3) suggests granulomatosis with polyangiitis (previously Wegener granulomatosis), which can cause similar findings (see p. 351).

The upper and lower airways should be evaluated, including complete spirometric testing and chest CT, when the diagnosis is made.

Prognosis

Mortality rates have decreased with newer therapies. Survival is now 94% after 8 yr, with death typically resulting from collapse of laryngeal and tracheal structures or from cardiovascular complications such as large-vessel aneurysm, cardiac valvular insufficiency, or systemic vasculitis.

Treatment

- NSAIDs or dapsone for mild ear disease
- Corticosteroids
- Sometimes methotrexate or other immunosuppressants (eg, cyclosporine, cyclophosphamide, azathioprine, anti-TNF drugs)

Mild recurrent ear disease may respond to NSAIDs in anti-inflammatory doses, or dapsone (50 to 100 mg po once/day). However, most patients are treated with prednisone 30 to 60 mg po once/day, with tapering of the dose as soon as there is a clinical response. Some patients require chronic use. In such patients, methotrexate 7.5 to 20 mg po once/wk can reduce the requirement for corticosteroids. Very severe cases may require other immunosuppressants, such as cyclosporine, cyclophosphamide, anti-TNF drugs (eg, infliximab, etanercept), or azathioprine (see p. 310). None of these therapies has been tested in controlled trials or has been shown to decrease mortality. If tracheal narrowing causes stridor, a tracheostomy or stent may be needed.

More extensive tracheobronchial collapse may require tracheal reconstruction. Eye disease may sometimes be recalcitrant to treatment, especially when involving the sclera, and has a poor prognosis. All patients should be closely monitored for atherosclerosis given the risk of premature atherosclerosis in systemic vasculitides. Patients on long-term corticosteroid therapy should receive osteoporosis prophylaxis. Prophylaxis for opportunistic infections, such as *Pneumocystis jirovecii,* should be added if combination immunosuppressive therapy is used.

Endotracheal intubation can be technically difficult because of tracheal involvement and narrowing; also, intratracheal manipulation can lead to life-threatening postanesthetic deterioration by causing further glottal or subglottal inflammation. Thus, endotracheal intubation should be avoided whenever possible (eg, instead using local and regional anesthesia). When endotracheal intubation is unavoidable, preparations should be made for emergency cricothyrotomy.

KEY POINTS

- Consider relapsing polychondritis if patients develop inflammation of the pinna or nasal cartilage, particularly with symptoms and signs compatible with respiratory tract chondritis or unexplained arthritis, ocular inflammation, or auditory or vestibular dysfunction.
- Biopsy the affected cartilage if necessary to confirm the diagnosis.
- Treat mild disease with NSAIDs or dapsone.
- Treat more severe disease with corticosteroids and sometimes methotrexate or other immunosuppressants.
- Avoid endotracheal intubation or, if it is unavoidable, prepare for emergency cricothyrotomy.

SJÖGREN SYNDROME

Sjögren syndrome (SS) is a relatively common chronic, autoimmune, systemic, inflammatory disorder of unknown cause. It is characterized by dryness of the mouth, eyes, and other mucous membranes due to lymphocytic infiltration of the exocrine gland and secondary gland dysfunction. SS can affect various exocrine glands or other organs. Diagnosis is by specific criteria relating to eye, mouth, and salivary gland involvement, autoantibodies, and (occasionally) histopathology. Treatment is usually symptomatic.

SS occurs most frequently among middle-aged women. SS is classified as primary when there is no other associated disease. In about 30% of patients with autoimmune disorders such as RA, SLE, systemic sclerosis, mixed connective tissue disease, Hashimoto thyroiditis, primary biliary cirrhosis, or chronic autoimmune hepatitis, SS develops and, in such cases, is classified as secondary. Genetic associations have been found (eg, HLA-DR3 antigens in whites with primary SS).

Pathophysiology

Salivary, lacrimal, and other exocrine glands become infiltrated with CD4+ T cells and with some B cells. The T cells produce inflammatory cytokines (eg, IL-2, interferon-γ). Salivary duct cells also produce cytokines, eventually damaging the secretory ducts. Atrophy of the secretory epithelium of the lacrimal glands causes desiccation of the cornea and conjunctiva (keratoconjunctivitis sicca—see p. 927). Lymphocytic infiltration and intraductal cellular proliferation in the parotid gland cause luminal narrowing and in some cases formation of compact cellular structures termed myoepithelial islands; atrophy of the gland can result. Dryness and GI mucosal or submucosal atrophy and diffuse infiltration by plasma cells and lymphocytes may cause symptoms (eg, dysphagia).

Symptoms and Signs

Glandular manifestations: SS often affects the eyes or mouth initially and sometimes exclusively. Dry eyes can cause a sandy, gritty sensation. In advanced cases, the cornea is severely damaged, epithelial strands hang from the corneal surface (keratitis filiformis), and vision can be impaired. Diminished saliva (xerostomia) results in difficulty chewing and swallowing, secondary *Candida* infection, tooth decay, and calculi in the salivary ducts. Taste and smell may be diminished. Dryness may also develop in the skin and in mucous membranes of the nose, throat, larynx, bronchi, vulva, and vagina. Dryness of the respiratory tract may cause cough. Alopecia may occur. Parotid glands enlarge in 33% of patients and are usually firm, smooth, and mildly tender. Enlargement can be asymmetric, but highly disproportionate enlargement of one gland may indicate a tumor. Chronic salivary gland enlargement is rarely painful unless there is obstruction or infection.

Extraglandular manifestations: Joint disease in SS is typically nonerosive and nondeforming. Arthralgias occur in about 50% of patients. Arthritis occurs in about 33% of patients and is similar in distribution to RA but is not erosive.

Other common extraglandular manifestations include generalized lymphadenopathy, Raynaud phenomenon, parenchymal lung involvement (which is common but infrequently serious), and vasculitis. Vasculitis can occasionally affect the peripheral nerves (causing peripheral polyneuropathy or mononeuritis multiplex) or CNS or cause rashes (including purpura) and glomerulonephritis. Kidney involvement can cause renal tubular acidosis, impaired concentrating ability, kidney stones, or interstitial nephritis. Pseudolymphoma, malignant lymphoma, or Waldenström macroglobulinemia can develop; patients develop non-Hodgkin lymphoma at 40 times the normal rate. Chronic hepatobiliary disease and pancreatitis (exocrine pancreatic tissue is similar to that of salivary glands) may also occur.

Diagnosis

- Eye symptoms, oral symptoms, and eye and salivary gland testing
- Autoantibodies
- Sometimes salivary gland biopsy

SS should be suspected in patients with gritty or dry eyes or dry mouth, enlarged salivary glands, peripheral neuropathy, purpura, or unexplained renal tubular acidosis. Such patients should receive diagnostic tests that can include evaluation of the eyes and salivary glands and serologic tests. Different criteria have been proposed for classification of SS. The latest modifications to the American-European classification criteria for SS were proposed in 2002. These criteria were not developed for use in routine clinical practice, and not every patient who receives a clinical diagnosis of SS fulfills the proposed criteria (usually > 3 of 6 manifestations). The 6 manifestations are eye symptoms, oral symptoms, positive eye tests, salivary gland involvement, autoantibodies, and histopathology. The possibility of IgG4-associated disease (a newly recognized disease characterized by lymphoplasmacytic infiltration of various organs) should be considered if patients have submandibular gland enlargement, especially with a history of pancreatitis.

Eye symptoms are ≥ 3 mo of either dry eyes or use of tear substitutes ≥ 3 times/day; slit-lamp examination may also confirm dry eyes.

Oral symptoms are > 3 mo of daily dry mouth sensation, daily use of liquids to aid in swallowing, or swollen salivary glands.

Eye signs should be evaluated with the Schirmer test, which measures the quantity of tears secreted in 5 min after irritation from a filter paper strip placed under each lower eyelid. A young person normally moistens 15 mm of each paper strip. Most people with SS moisten < 5 mm, although about 15% of test results are false-positive and 15% are false-negative. Ocular staining with an eye drop of rose bengal or lissamine green solution is highly specific. Slit-lamp examination showing a fluorescein tear breakup in < 10 sec is also suggestive.

Salivary gland involvement can be confirmed by abnormally low saliva production (≤ 1.5 mL/15 min) as measured by salivary flow, sialography, or salivary scintiscanning, although these tests are used infrequently. Saliva production can be qualitatively evaluated by looking for normal pooling of saliva under the tongue. Alternatively, a tongue blade can be held against the buccal mucosa for 10 sec. If the tongue blade falls off immediately when released, salivary flow is considered normal. The more difficulty encountered removing the tongue blade, the more severe the dryness. In women, the lipstick sign, where lipstick adheres to the front teeth, may be a useful indicator of dry mouth. If a graduated container is available, the patient can expectorate once to empty the mouth and then expectorate all saliva into the container for several minutes. Normal production is 0.3 to 0.4 mL/min. Significant xerostomia is 0.1 mL/min.

Autoantibodies (serologic criteria) have limited sensitivity and specificity. They include antibodies to Ro (SS-A autoantibodies—see p. 262) or to nuclear antigens (termed La or SS-B autoantibodies), ANA, or an elevated level of antibodies against γ-globulin. Rheumatoid factor is present in > 70% of patients. ESR is elevated in 70%, 33% have anemia, and up to 25% have leukopenia.

Histopathology is assessed by biopsy of minor salivary glands in the buccal mucosa. Salivary gland biopsy is usually reserved for patients in whom the diagnosis cannot be established by autoantibody testing or when a major organ is involved. Histopathologic involvement is confirmed if labial minor salivary glands show multiple large foci of lymphocytes with atrophy of acinar tissue.

Most common causes of dry eyes and dry mouth (sicca symptoms) are aging and drugs, but when parotid enlargement occurs in addition to sicca symptoms, diseases such as hepatitis C, HIV, bulimia, and sarcoidosis should be differentiated from SS.

Prognosis

SS is chronic, and death may occasionally result from pulmonary infection and, rarely, from renal failure or lymphoma. Associated systemic autoimmune disorders may dictate prognosis.

Treatment

- Symptomatic treatment for sicca symptoms
- Avoidance of aggravating factors
- Occasionally oral corticosteroids, cyclophosphamide, or rituximab

SS should be initially managed by topical therapy of dry eyes and dry mouth. Other systemic manifestations of SS should be treated depending on the severity and the involved organ. Recognition of therapies for other conditions that can exacerbate dryness complaints is crucial. Hydroxychloroquine 200 to 400 mg po once/day is usually given to halt the progression of the disease and for the treatment of arthralgias.

Dry eyes should be treated with lubricating eye preparations (initially drops such as hypromellose or methylcellulose and an OTC ointment at bedtime). Other treatments include drainage (punctal) duct closure and topical cyclosporine. Skin and vaginal dryness can be treated with lubricants.

Mouth dryness may be avoided by sipping fluids throughout the day, chewing sugarless gum, and using a saliva substitute containing carboxymethylcellulose as a mouthwash. Drugs that decrease salivary secretion (eg, antihistamines, antidepressants, other anticholinergics) should be avoided. Fastidious oral hygiene and regular dental visits are essential. Stones must be promptly removed, preserving viable salivary tissue. The pain of suddenly enlarged salivary glands is generally best treated with warm compresses and analgesics. Pilocarpine 5 mg po tid to qid or cevimeline HCl 30 mg po tid can stimulate salivary production but should be avoided in patients with bronchospasm and closed-angle glaucoma.

Aggressive systemic treatment is occasionally indicated; it is usually reserved for patients with associated diseases (eg, severe vasculitis or visceral involvement). Corticosteroids (eg, prednisone 1 mg/kg po once/day), cyclophosphamide, or rituximab may be needed in severe disease, but there is concern regarding the increased baseline risk of lymphoma even without cytotoxic therapy.

KEY POINTS

- Suspect SS if patients have gritty or dry eyes or dry mouth, enlarged salivary glands, peripheral neuropathy, purpura, or unexplained renal tubular acidosis.
- Confirm the diagnosis usually by specific clinical criteria.
- Treat sicca symptoms symptomatically (eg, with topical lubricants) and avoid drying factors.
- If patients have severe disease (eg, severe vasculitis or visceral involvement), treat with corticosteroids, cyclophosphamide, or rituximab.

SYSTEMIC LUPUS ERYTHEMATOSUS

(Disseminated Lupus Erythematosus)

Systemic lupus erythematosus (SLE) is a chronic, multisystem, inflammatory disorder of autoimmune etiology, occurring predominantly in young women. Common manifestations may include arthralgias and arthritis, malar and other rashes, pleuritis or pericarditis, renal or CNS involvement, and hematologic cytopenias. Diagnosis requires clinical and serologic criteria. Treatment of severe, ongoing, active disease requires corticosteroids, often hydroxychloroquine, and sometimes immunosuppressants.

Of all cases, 70 to 90% occur in women (usually of child-bearing age). SLE is more common among blacks and Asians than whites. It can affect patients of any age, including neonates. Increased awareness of mild forms has resulted in a worldwide rise in reported cases. In some countries, the prevalence of SLE rivals that of RA. SLE may be precipitated by currently unknown environmental triggers that cause autoimmune reactions in genetically predisposed people. Some drugs (eg, hydralazine, procainamide, isoniazid) cause a reversible lupus-like syndrome.

Symptoms and Signs

Clinical findings vary greatly. SLE may develop abruptly with fever or insidiously over months or years with episodes of arthralgias and malaise. Vascular headaches, epilepsy, or psychoses may be initial findings. Manifestations referable to any organ system may appear. Periodic exacerbations (flares) may occur.

Joint manifestations: Joint symptoms, ranging from intermittent arthralgias to acute polyarthritis, occur in about 90% of patients and may precede other manifestations by years. Most lupus polyarthritis is nondestructive and nondeforming. However, in long-standing disease, deformities without bone erosions may develop (eg, the metacarpophalangeal and interphalangeal joints may rarely develop ulnar drift or swan-neck deformities without bony or cartilaginous erosions [Jaccoud arthritis]).

Skin and mucous membrane manifestations: Skin lesions include malar butterfly erythema (flat or raised) that generally spares the nasolabial folds. The absence of papules and pustules helps distinguish SLE from rosacea. A variety of other erythematous, firm, maculopapular lesions can occur elsewhere, including exposed areas of the face and neck, upper chest, and elbows. Skin blistering and ulceration are rare, although recurrent ulcers on mucous membranes (particularly the central portion of the hard palate near the junction of the hard and soft palate, the buccal and gum mucosa, and the anterior nasal septum) are common (sometimes called mucosal lupus); findings can sometimes mimic toxic epidermal necrolysis. Generalized or focal alopecia is common during active phases of SLE. Panniculitis can cause subcutaneous nodular lesions (sometimes called lupus panniculitis or profundus). Vasculitic skin lesions may include mottled erythema on the palms and fingers, periungual erythema, nailfold infarcts, urticaria, and palpable purpura. Petechiae may develop secondary to thrombocytopenia. Photosensitivity occurs in some patients. Lupus erythematosus tumidus is characterized by pink to violaceous urticarial nonscarring plaques and/or nodules, some annular, in a photo distribution. Chilblain lupus is characterized by tender, bright red to reddish blue nodules on the toes, fingers, nose, or ears that occur in cold weather. Some patients with SLE have features of lichen planus.

Cardiopulmonary manifestations: Cardiopulmonary symptoms commonly include recurrent pleurisy, with or without pleural effusion. Pneumonitis is rare, although minor impairments in pulmonary function are common. Severe alveolar hemorrhage occasionally occurs. Prognosis has traditionally been poor but seems to be improving, possibly because of better early and aggressive critical care. Other complications include pulmonary emboli, pulmonary hypertension, and shrinking lung syndrome. Cardiac complications include pericarditis (most commonly) and myocarditis. Serious, rare complications are coronary artery vasculitis, valvular involvement, and Libman-Sacks endocarditis. Accelerated atherosclerosis is an increasing cause of morbidity and mortality. Congenital heart block can develop in neonates.

Lymphoid tissue: Generalized adenopathy is common, particularly among children, young adults, and blacks; however, mediastinal adenopathy is not common. Splenomegaly occurs in 10% of patients.

Neurologic manifestations: Neurologic symptoms can result from involvement of any part of the central or peripheral nervous system or meninges. Mild cognitive impairment is common. There may also be headaches, personality changes, ischemic stroke, subarachnoid hemorrhage, seizures, psychoses, organic brain syndrome, aseptic meningitis, peripheral and cranial neuropathies, transverse myelitis, or cerebellar dysfunction.

Renal manifestations: Renal involvement can develop at any time and may be the only manifestation of SLE. It may be benign and asymptomatic or progressive and fatal. Renal lesions can range in severity from a focal, usually benign, glomerulitis to a diffuse, potentially fatal, membranoproliferative glomerulonephritis. Common manifestations include proteinuria (most often), an abnormal urinary sediment manifested by RBC casts and leukocytes, hypertension, and edema.

Obstetric manifestations: Obstetric manifestations include early and late fetal loss. In patients with antiphospholipid antibodies, the risk of recurrent miscarriages is increased. Pregnancy can be successful (see p. 2388), particularly after 6 to 12 mo of remission, but SLE flares are common during pregnancy. Pregnancy should be timed for when disease is in remission. During pregnancy, the patient should be monitored closely for any disease flare or thrombotic events by a multidisciplinary team that includes a rheumatologist, an obstetrician who specializes in high-risk pregnancies, and a hematologist.

Hematologic manifestations: Hematologic manifestations include anemia (autoimmune hemolytic), leukopenia (usually lymphopenia, with < 1500 cells/μL), and thrombocytopenia (sometimes life-threatening autoimmune thrombocytopenia). Recurrent arterial or venous thrombosis, thrombocytopenia, and a high probability of obstetric complications occur in patients with antiphospholipid antibodies. Thromboses probably account for many of the complications of SLE, including obstetric complications.

GI manifestations: GI manifestations can result from bowel vasculitis or impaired bowel motility. In addition, pancreatitis can result from SLE or perhaps from its treatment with high-dose corticosteroids or azathioprine. Manifestations may include abdominal pain resulting from serositis, nausea, vomiting, manifestations of bowel perforation, and pseudo-obstruction. SLE rarely causes parenchymal liver disease.

Diagnosis

- Clinical criteria
- Cytopenias
- Autoantibodies

SLE should be suspected in patients, particularly young women, with any of the symptoms and signs. However, early-stage SLE can mimic other connective (or nonconnective) tissue disorders, including RA if arthritic symptoms predominate. Mixed connective tissue disease (MCTD) can mimic SLE but also may involve features of systemic sclerosis, rheumatoid-like polyarthritis, and polymyositis. Infections (eg, bacterial endocarditis, histoplasmosis) can mimic SLE and may develop as a result of treatment-caused immunosuppression. Disorders such as sarcoidosis and paraneoplastic syndromes can also mimic SLE.

Laboratory testing differentiates SLE from other connective tissue disorders. Routine testing should include the following:

- ANA and anti–double-stranded (ds) DNA
- CBC
- Urinalysis
- Chemistry profile including renal and liver enzymes

Most clinicians rely on diagnostic criteria for SLE that were developed by the American Rheumatism Association. However, revised criteria proposed by the Systemic Lupus International Collaborating Clinics (SLICC), a consensus group of experts on SLE, are now favored. Classification as SLE by the SLICC criteria requires either of the following:

- At least 4 of 17 criteria, including at least 1 of the 11 clinical criteria and 1 of the 6 immunologic criteria (see Table 33–1)
- Biopsy-proven nephritis compatible with SLE plus ANA or anti-dsDNA antibodies

Fluorescent ANA: The fluorescent test for ANA is the best screen for SLE; positive ANA tests (usually in high titer: > 1:80) occur in > 98%. However, positive ANA tests can also occur in RA, other connective tissue disorders, cancers, and even in the general population. The false-positive rate varies from about 3% for ANA titers of 1:320 to about 30% for ANA titers of 1:40 among healthy controls. Drugs such as hydralazine, procainamide, and TNF-α antagonists can produce positive ANA results as well as a lupus-like syndrome; the ANA eventually becomes negative if the drug is stopped. Positive ANA should prompt more specific testing such as anti-dsDNA antibodies; high titers are highly specific for SLE but occur in only 25 to 30% of people with SLE.

Other ANA and anticytoplasmic antibodies: The ANA test is very sensitive, but it is not specific for SLE; thus, evidence of other autoantibodies is needed to establish the diagnosis. They include Ro (SSA), La (SSB), Smith (Sm), ribonucleoprotein (RNP), and dsDNA. Ro is predominantly cytoplasmic; anti-Ro antibodies are occasionally present in ANA-negative SLE patients presenting with chronic cutaneous lupus. Anti-Ro is the causal antibody for neonatal lupus and congenital heart block. Anti-Sm is highly specific for SLE but, like anti-dsDNA, is not sensitive. Anti-RNP occurs in patients with SLE, MCTD, and occasionally other systemic autoimmune disorders and systemic sclerosis.

Other blood tests: Leukopenia (usually lymphopenia) is common. Hemolytic anemia may occur. Thrombocytopenia in SLE may be difficult or impossible to differentiate from idiopathic thrombocytopenic purpura except that patients have other features of SLE. False-positive serologic tests for syphilis occur in 5 to 10% of SLE patients. These test results may be associated with the lupus anticoagulant and a prolonged PTT. Abnormal values in one or more of these assays suggest the presence of antiphospholipid antibodies (eg, anticardiolipin antibodies), which should then be measured directly by enzyme-linked immunosorbent assay (ELISA). Antiphospholipid antibodies are associated with arterial or venous thrombosis, thrombocytopenia, and, during pregnancy, spontaneous abortion or late fetal death but may be present in asymptomatic patients. A positive direct Coombs test in the absence of hemolytic anemia is one criterion for the diagnosis of lupus.

Other tests help monitor disease severity and determine the need for treatment. Serum complement levels (C3, C4) are often depressed in active disease and are usually lowest in patients with active nephritis. ESR is elevated frequently during active disease. C-reactive protein levels are not necessarily elevated.

Renal involvement: Screening for renal involvement begins with urinalysis. RBC and/or WBC casts suggest active nephritis. Urinalysis should be done at regular intervals, even for patients in apparent remission, because kidney disease may be asymptomatic. Renal biopsy is indicated when protein excretion is > 500 mg/day or if there is evidence of an active urinary sediment. Renal biopsy is helpful in evaluating the status of renal disease (ie, active inflammation vs postinflammatory scarring) and in guiding therapy. Patients with chronic renal insufficiency and mostly sclerotic glomeruli are not likely to benefit from aggressive immunosuppressive therapy.

Prognosis

The course is usually chronic, relapsing, and unpredictable. Remissions may last for years. If the initial acute phase is controlled, even if very severe (eg, with cerebral thrombosis or severe nephritis), the long-term prognosis is usually good. The 10-yr survival in most developed countries is > 95%. Improved prognosis is in part due to earlier diagnosis and more effective therapies. More severe disease requires more toxic therapies, which increase risk of mortality. Examples of such complications include infection from immunosuppression or

Table 33–1. SLICC CRITERIA FOR THE CLASSIFICATION OF SLE*

CRITERION	DEFINITION
Clinical criteria	
Acute cutaneous lupus	Lupus malar rash (malar discoid rash not counted), bullous lupus, toxic epidermal necrolysis variant of SLE, maculopapular lupus rash, photosensitive lupus rash (in the absence of dermatomyositis) *or* Subacute cutaneous lupus (nonindurated psoriaform and/or annular polycyclic lesions that resolve without scarring, sometimes with postinflammatory dyspigmentation or telangiectasias)
Chronic cutaneous lupus	Classic discoid rash, localized (above the neck) discoid rash, generalized (above and below the neck) discoid rash, hypertrophic (verrucous) lupus, lupus panniculitis (profundus), mucosal lupus, lupus erythematosus tumidus, chilblain lupus *or* Discoid lupus/lichen planus overlap
Nonscarring alopecia	Diffuse thinning or hair fragility with visible broken hairs (in the absence of other causes such as alopecia areata, drugs, iron deficiency, and androgenic alopecia)
Oral or nasal ulcers	Palate, buccal, and tongue ulcers *or* Nasal ulcers (in the absence of other causes, such as vasculitis, Behçet disease, infection [herpesvirus], inflammatory bowel disease, reactive arthritis, and acidic foods)
Joint disease	Synovitis involving ≥ 2 joints, characterized by swelling or effusion *or* Tenderness in ≥ 2 joints and at least 30 min of morning stiffness
Serositis	Typical pleurisy for > 1 day, pleural effusions, or pleural rub *or* Typical pericardial pain (pain with recumbency improved by sitting forward) for > 1 day, pericardial effusion, pericardial rub, or pericarditis by electrocardiography in the absence of other causes (eg, infection, uremia, Dressler syndrome)
Renal manifestations	Urine protein:creatinine ratio (or 24-h urine protein) representing 500 mg protein/24 h *or* RBC casts
Neurologic manifestations	Seizures, psychosis, multiple mononeuropathy (in the absence of other known causes such as primary vasculitis), myelitis, peripheral or cranial neuropathy (in the absence of other known causes such as primary vasculitis, infection, and diabetes mellitus) *or* Acute confusional state (in the absence of other causes, including toxic and metabolic causes, uremia, or drugs)
Hemolytic anemia	Hemolytic anemia
Leukopenia or lymphopenia	Leukopenia: < 4000/mm^3 at least once (in the absence of other known causes such as Felty syndrome, drugs, and portal hypertension) *or* Lymphopenia: < 1000/mm^3 at least once (in the absence of other known causes such as corticosteroids, drugs, and infections)
Thrombocytopenia	Thrombocytopenia (< 100,000/mm^3) at least once in the absence of other known causes such as drugs, portal hypertension, and thrombotic thrombocytopenic purpura
Immunologic criteria	
ANA	ANA level above laboratory reference range
Anti-dsDNA	Anti-dsDNA antibody level above laboratory range (or > 2-fold the reference range if tested by ELISA)
Anti-Sm	Presence of antibody to Sm nuclear antigen
Antiphospholipid	Antiphospholipid antibody positivity as determined by any of the following: • Positive test result for lupus anticoagulant • False-positive test result for rapid plasma reagin • Medium- or high-titer anticardiolipin antibody level (IgA, IgG, or IgM) • Positive test result for anti-β2-glycoprotein I (IgA, IgG, or IgM)
Low complement	Low C3, low C4 *or* Low CH50
Direct Coombs test	Direct Coombs test in the absence of hemolytic anemia

*Classification requires at least 4 of 17 criteria, including at least 1 clinical criterion and 1 immunologic criterion *or* biopsy-proven lupus nephritis.

ANA = antinuclear antibodies; Anti-dsDNA = anti–double-stranded DNA; ELISA = enzyme-linked immunosorbent assay; Sm = Smith; SLICC = Systemic Lupus International Collaborating Clinics.

osteoporosis from long-term corticosteroid use. Increased risk of coronary artery disease can contribute to premature death.

Treatment

- NSAIDs and often antimalarials for mild disease
- Corticosteroids and often immunosuppressants for severe disease

To simplify therapy, SLE should be classified as mild (eg, fever, arthritis, pleurisy, pericarditis, headache, rash) or severe (eg, hemolytic anemia, thrombocytopenic purpura, massive pleural and pericardial involvement, significant renal damage, acute vasculitis of the extremities or GI tract, florid CNS involvement).

Mild or remittent disease: Little or no therapy may be needed. Arthralgias are usually controlled with NSAIDs. Antimalarials help, particularly when joint and skin manifestations are prominent. Hydroxychloroquine 200 mg po once/day or bid reduces the frequency of SLE flares. Alternatives include chloroquine 250 mg po once/day and quinacrine 50 to 100 mg po once/day. Hydroxychloroquine can rarely cause retinal and skeletal or cardiac muscle toxicity. The eyes should be examined at 12-mo intervals.

Severe disease: Treatment includes induction therapy to control acute severe manifestations followed by maintenance therapy. Corticosteroids are first-line therapy. A combination of prednisone and immunosuppressants is recommended in active, serious CNS lupus, vasculitis especially affecting viscera or nerves, or active lupus nephritis. Methylprednisolone 1 g by slow (1-h) IV infusion on 3 successive days is often the initial treatment. Then, prednisone given in doses of 40 to 60 mg po once/day can be maintained, but the dose may vary according to the manifestation of SLE. Cyclophosphamide or mycophenolate mofetil (especially in African-Americans) is usually also used for induction therapy. In severe renal involvement, cyclophosphamide is usually given in intermittent IV pulses instead of daily oral doses; eg, about 500 mg to 1 g/m^2 IV (together with mesna and fluid loading to protect the bladder) monthly for 6 mo and then once q 3 mo for 18 mo (less frequently if there is renal or hematologic toxicity—see Table 33–2).

In CNS lupus or other critical crises, IgG 400 mg/kg IV once/day for 5 consecutive days may be useful for refractory thrombocytopenia. Patients with end-stage renal disease can undergo kidney transplantation, as an alternative to dialysis, with a successful outcome, especially if their disease has been in remission.

Table 33–2. PROTOCOL FOR CHEMOTHERAPY WITH CYCLOPHOSPHAMIDE AND IV MESNA

Use constant supervision regarding tolerance throughout entire procedure.

1. Using 50 mL of normal saline, mix ondansetron 10 mg and dexamethasone 10 mg and infuse over 10 to 30 min.
2. Using 250 mL of normal saline, mix in mesna 250–500 mg (used to bind acrolein, a metabolite of cyclophosphamide that is a bladder irritant) and infuse along with 500–1000 mL of normal saline before the infusion of cyclophosphamide.
3. Using 250 mL of normal saline, mix in cyclophosphamide 500–1000 mg/m^2 and infuse over 1 h.
4. Using 250 mL of normal saline, mix in mesna 250–500 mg and infuse second dose of mesna. Total dose of mesna should be equal to the total dose of cyclophosphamide used. Patient should be encouraged to drink plenty of fluids and to empty bladder every 2 h. Patient must take ondansetron 8 mg po the next morning.

Improvement of severe SLE often takes 4 to 12 wk. Thrombosis or embolism of cerebral, pulmonary, or placental vessels requires short-term treatment with heparin and longer treatment with warfarin, if the diagnosis of antiphospholipid syndrome is confirmed. The target INR is usually 3.

Maintenance therapy: For most patients, the risk of flares can be decreased without prolonged high-dose corticosteroids. Chronic disease should be treated with the lowest dose of corticosteroids and other drugs that control inflammation (eg, antimalarials, low-dose immunosuppressants) to maintain remission. Treatment should be guided by clinical features primarily, although anti-dsDNA antibody titers or serum complement levels may be followed. Other pertinent blood and urine tests may be used to assess specific organ involvement. Anti-dsDNA antibody titers or serum complement levels may not parallel nonrenal disease flares. If a patient needs long-term high-dose corticosteroids, alternative oral immunosuppressants such as azathioprine should be considered. Ca, vitamin D, and bisphosphonate therapy should be considered in patients taking corticosteroids long term.

Focal complications and coexisting medical conditions: All patients should be closely monitored for atherosclerosis. Long-term anticoagulation is vital in patients with antiphospholipid antibodies and recurrent thrombosis (see p. 757).

If a pregnant patient has antiphospholipid antibodies, thrombotic complications can be limited with corticosteroids (prednisone ≤ 30 mg po once/day), low-dose aspirin, or anticoagulation with heparin. Daily heparin given subcutaneously with or without one baby aspirin throughout the 2nd and 3rd trimesters may be the most successful prophylactic measure.

KEY POINTS

- Joint and skin manifestations are classic in SLE, but the disorder can affect various organ systems, such as the skin, heart and lungs, lymphoid tissue, kidneys, and GI, hematologic, reproductive, and nervous systems.
- Use the SLICC clinical and immunologic criteria to confirm the diagnosis when possible, or do a kidney biopsy.
- Among tests, use the highly sensitive ANA for screening, but use more specific autoantibodies (eg, anti-dsDNA, anti-Sm) for confirmation.
- Evaluate all patients for kidney involvement.
- Treat mild disease with an NSAID or an antimalarial such as chloroquine or hydroxychloroquine.
- Use corticosteroids for moderate or severe SLE and often an immunosuppressant for nephritis, CNS disease, and vasculitis or if corticosteroids are ineffective.
- Use corticosteroids at the lowest possible dose to maintain remission.

Variant Forms of Lupus

Discoid lupus erythematosus (DLE): DLE, also sometimes called chronic cutaneous lupus erythematosus, is a set of skin changes that can occur as part of lupus, with or without systemic involvement. Skin lesions begin as erythematous plaques and progress to atrophic scars (see Plate 2). They cluster in light-exposed areas of the skin, such as the face, scalp, and ears. Untreated, lesions extend and develop central atrophy and scarring. There may be widespread scarring alopecia. Mucous membrane involvement may be prominent, especially in the mouth. Sometimes lesions are hypertrophic and may mimic lichen planus (called hypertrophic or verrucous lupus).

Patients presenting with typical discoid lesions should be evaluated for SLE. Antibodies against dsDNA are almost invariably absent in DLE. Although it does not differentiate DLE from SLE, biopsy can rule out other disorders (eg, lymphoma or sarcoidosis). Biopsy should be done from the active margin of a skin lesion.

Early treatment can prevent permanent atrophy. Exposure to sunlight or ultraviolet light should be minimized (eg, using potent sunscreens when outdoors). Topical corticosteroid ointments (particularly for dry skin) or creams (less greasy than ointments) tid to qid (eg, triamcinolone acetonide 0.1 or 0.5%, fluocinolone 0.025 or 0.2%, flurandrenolide 0.05%, betamethasone valerate 0.1%, and, particularly betamethasone dipropionate 0.05%) usually cause involution of small lesions; they should not be used excessively or on the face (where they cause skin atrophy). Resistant lesions can be covered with plastic tape coated with flurandrenolide. Alternatively, intradermal injection with triamcinolone acetonide 0.1% suspension (< 0.1 mL per site) may resolve lesions, but secondary atrophy frequently follows. Antimalarials (eg, hydroxychloroquine 200 mg po once/day or bid) can help, including for facial lesions. In resistant cases, combinations (eg, hydroxychloroquine 200 mg/day plus quinacrine 50 to 100 mg po once/day) may be required for months to years.

Subacute cutaneous lupus erythematosus (SCLE): SCLE is a variant form of SLE in which skin involvement is prominent. Patients with SCLE develop extensive recurring rashes. Annular or papulosquamous lesions may develop on the face, arms, and trunk. Lesions are usually photosensitive and can develop hypopigmentation but rarely scar. Arthritis and fatigue are common in SCLE, but neurologic and renal manifestations are not. Patients may be ANA-positive or ANA-negative. Most have antibodies to Ro (SSA). Infants whose mothers have Ro antibodies may have congenital SCLE or congenital heart block. SCLE should be treated similarly to SLE.

SYSTEMIC SCLEROSIS

(Scleroderma)

Systemic sclerosis (SSc) is a rare chronic disease of unknown cause characterized by diffuse fibrosis, degenerative changes, and vascular abnormalities in the skin, joints, and internal organs (especially the esophagus, lower GI tract, lungs, heart, and kidneys). Common symptoms include Raynaud phenomenon, polyarthralgia, dysphagia, heartburn, and swelling and eventually skin tightening and contractures of the fingers. Lung, heart, and kidney involvement accounts for most deaths. Diagnosis is clinical, but laboratory tests help with confirmation. Specific treatment is difficult, and emphasis is often on treatment of complications.

SSc is about 4 times more common among women than men. It is most common among people aged 20 to 50 and is rare in children. SSc can develop as part of mixed connective tissue disease (MCTD).

Etiology

Immunologic mechanisms and heredity (certain HLA subtypes) play a role in etiology. SSc-like syndromes can result from exposure to vinyl chloride, bleomycin, pentazocine, epoxy and aromatic hydrocarbons, contaminated rapeseed oil, or L-tryptophan.

Pathophysiology

Pathophysiology involves vascular damage and activation of fibroblasts; collagen and other extracellular proteins in various tissues are overproduced.

In SSc, the skin develops more compact collagen fibers in the reticular dermis, epidermal thinning, loss of rete pegs, and atrophy of dermal appendages. T cells may accumulate, and extensive fibrosis in the dermal and subcutaneous layers develops. In the nail folds, capillary loops dilate and some microvascular loops are lost. In the extremities, chronic inflammation and fibrosis of the synovial membrane and surfaces and periarticular soft tissues occur.

Esophageal motility becomes impaired, and the lower esophageal sphincter becomes incompetent; gastroesophageal reflux and secondary strictures can develop. The intestinal muscularis mucosa degenerates, leading to pseudodiverticula in the colon and ileum. Interstitial and peribronchial fibrosis or intimal hyperplasia of small pulmonary arteries can develop; if long-standing, pulmonary hypertension can result. Diffuse myocardial fibrosis or cardiac conduction abnormalities occur. Intimal hyperplasia of interlobular and arcuate arteries can develop within the kidneys, causing renal ischemia and hypertension.

SSc varies in severity and progression, ranging from generalized skin thickening with rapidly progressive and often fatal visceral involvement (SSc with diffuse scleroderma) to isolated skin involvement (often just the fingers and face) and slow progression (often several decades) before visceral disease develops. The latter form is termed limited cutaneous scleroderma or CREST syndrome (calcinosis cutis, Raynaud phenomenon, esophageal dysmotility, sclerodactyly, telangiectasias). In addition, SSc can overlap with other autoimmune rheumatic disorders—eg, sclerodermatomyositis (tight skin and muscle weakness indistinguishable from polymyositis) and MCTD.

Symptoms and Signs

The most common initial symptoms and signs are Raynaud phenomenon and insidious swelling of the distal extremities with gradual thickening of the skin of the fingers. Polyarthralgia is also prominent. GI disturbances (eg, heartburn, dysphagia) or respiratory complaints (eg, dyspnea) are occasionally the first manifestations.

Skin and nail manifestations: Swelling of the skin is usually symmetric and progresses to induration. It may be confined to the fingers (sclerodactyly) and hands, or it may affect most or all of the body. The skin eventually becomes taut, shiny, and hypopigmented or hyperpigmented; the face becomes mask-like; and telangiectases may appear on the fingers, chest, face, lips, and tongue. Subcutaneous calcifications may develop, usually on the fingertips (pulps) and over bony eminences. Digital ulcers are common, especially on the fingertips, overlying the finger joints, or over calcinotic nodules. Abnormal capillary and microvascular loops in the nails can be seen with an ophthalmoscope or dissecting microscope.

Joint manifestations: Polyarthralgias or mild arthritis can be prominent. Flexion contractures may develop in the fingers, wrists, and elbows. Friction rubs may develop over the joints, tendon sheaths, and large bursae.

GI manifestations: Esophageal dysfunction is the most frequent visceral disturbance and occurs in most patients. Dysphagia (usually retrosternal) usually develops first. Acid reflux can cause heartburn and stricture. Barrett esophagus occurs in one third of patients and predisposes to complications (eg, stricture, adenocarcinoma). Hypomotility of the small bowel causes anaerobic bacterial overgrowth that can lead to malabsorption. Air may penetrate the damaged bowel wall and be visible on x-rays (pneumatosis intestinalis). Leakage of bowel contents into the peritoneal cavity can cause peritonitis. Distinctive wide-mouthed diverticula can develop in the colon. Biliary cirrhosis may develop in patients with CREST syndrome.

Cardiopulmonary manifestations: Lung involvement generally progresses indolently, with substantial individual variability, but is a common cause of death. Lung fibrosis can impair gas exchange, leading to exertional dyspnea and restrictive disease with eventual respiratory failure. Acute alveolitis (potentially responsive to therapy) can develop. Esophageal dysfunction can lead to aspiration pneumonia. Pulmonary hypertension may develop, as can heart failure, both of which are poor prognostic findings. Pericarditis with effusion or pleurisy can occur. Cardiac arrhythmias are common.

Renal manifestations: Severe, often sudden renal disease (renal crisis) may occur, most commonly in the first 4 to 5 yr and in patients with diffuse scleroderma. It is usually heralded by sudden, severe hypertension with features of thrombotic microangiopathic hemolytic anemia.

Diagnosis

- Clinical evaluation
- Usually ANA, Scl-70 (topoisomerase I), and anticentromere antibodies

SSc should be considered in patients with Raynaud phenomenon, typical musculoskeletal or skin manifestations, or unexplained dysphagia, malabsorption, pulmonary fibrosis, pulmonary hypertension, cardiomyopathies, or conduction disturbances. Diagnosis can be obvious in patients with combinations of classic manifestations, such as Raynaud phenomenon, dysphagia, and tight skin. However, in some patients, the diagnosis cannot be made clinically, and confirmatory laboratory tests can increase the probability of disease but do not rule it out.

Serum ANA and Scl-70 antibody should be obtained. ANA are present in ≥ 90%, often with an antinucleolar pattern. Antibody to centromeric protein (anticentromere antibody) occurs in the serum of a high proportion of patients with CREST syndrome and is detectable on the ANA. Scl-70 antigen is a DNA-binding protein sensitive to nucleases. Patients with diffuse scleroderma are more likely than those with CREST to have anti–Scl-70 antibodies. Rheumatoid factor also is positive in one third of patients.

If lung involvement is suspected, pulmonary function testing, chest CT, and echocardiography can begin to define its severity. Acute alveolitis is often detected by high-resolution chest CT.

Prognosis

The course depends on the type of SSc but is unpredictable. Typically, progression is slow. Overall 10-yr survival is about 65%. Most patients with diffuse skin disease eventually develop visceral complications, which are the usual causes of death. Prognosis is poor if cardiac, pulmonary, or renal manifestations are present early. Heart failure may be intractable. Ventricular ectopy, even if asymptomatic, increases the risk of sudden death. Acute renal insufficiency, if untreated, progresses rapidly and causes death within months. Patients with CREST syndrome may have disease that is limited and nonprogressive for long periods; visceral changes (eg, pulmonary hypertension caused by vascular disease of the lung, a peculiar form of biliary cirrhosis) eventually develop, but the course is often remarkably benign.

Treatment

- Treatment directed at symptoms and dysfunctional organs

No drug significantly influences the natural course of SSc overall, but various drugs are of value in treating specific symptoms or organ systems. NSAIDs can help arthritis but may cause GI problems. Corticosteroids may be helpful if there is overt myositis or MCTD but may predispose to renal crisis and thus are used only if necessary. Penicillamine, long used for treatment of skin thickening, has not shown clear efficacy in recent trials.

Various immunosuppressants, including methotrexate, azathioprine, mycophenolate mofetil, and cyclophosphamide, may help pulmonary alveolitis. Successful lung transplantation has been reported. Epoprostenol (prostacyclin) and bosentan may be helpful for pulmonary hypertension. Ca channel blockers, such as nifedipine 20 mg po tid or as an extended-release formulation, may help Raynaud phenomenon but may worsen gastric reflux. Bosentan, sildenafil, tadalafil, and vardenafil are other alternatives for severe Raynaud phenomenon. Patients should dress warmly, wear mittens, and keep their head warm. IV infusions of prostaglandin E1 (alprostadil) or epoprostenol or sympathetic blockers can be used for digital ischemia. Reflux esophagitis is relieved by frequent small feedings, high-dose proton pump inhibitors, and sleeping with the head of the bed elevated. Esophageal strictures may require periodic dilation; gastroesophageal reflux may possibly require gastroplasty. Tetracycline 500 mg po bid or another broad-spectrum antibiotic can suppress overgrowth of intestinal flora and may alleviate malabsorption symptoms. Physiotherapy may help preserve muscle strength but is ineffective in preventing joint contractures. No treatment affects calcinosis.

For acute renal crisis, prompt treatment with an ACE inhibitor can dramatically prolong survival. BP is usually, but not always, controlled. The mortality rate of renal crisis remains high. If end-stage renal disease develops, it may be reversible, but dialysis and transplantation may be necessary.

KEY POINTS

- Key pathologic changes include skin and joint changes, Raynaud phenomenon, and esophageal changes, but life-threatening effects may involve organs such as the lungs, heart, or kidneys.
- Consider the diagnosis if patients have Raynaud phenomenon, typical musculoskeletal or skin manifestations, or unexplained dysphagia, malabsorption, pulmonary fibrosis, pulmonary hypertension, cardiomyopathies, or conduction disturbances.
- Test for ANA, Scl-70 (topoisomerase I), and anticentromere antibodies.
- Because there is no clear disease-modifying therapy, direct treatment at the involved organs.

34 Bursa, Muscle, and Tendon Disorders

BURSITIS

Bursitis is acute or chronic inflammation of a bursa. The cause is usually unknown, but trauma, repetitive or acute, may contribute, as may infection and crystal-induced disease. Symptoms include pain (particularly with motion or pressure), swelling, and tenderness. Diagnosis is usually clinical; however, ultrasonography may be needed to evaluate deep bursae. Diagnosis of infection and crystal-induced disease requires analysis of bursal fluid. Treatment includes splinting, NSAIDs, sometimes corticosteroid injections, and treatment of the underlying cause.

Bursae are fluid-filled sac-like cavities or potential cavities that are located where friction occurs (eg, where tendons or muscles pass over bony prominences). Bursae minimize friction between moving parts and facilitate movement. Some communicate with joints.

Bursitis may occur in the shoulder (subacromial or subdeltoid bursitis), particularly in patients with rotator cuff tendinitis, which is usually the primary lesion in the shoulder. Other commonly affected bursae include olecranon (miner's or barfly's elbow), prepatellar (housemaid's knee), suprapatellar, retrocalcaneal, iliopectineal (iliopsoas), ischial (weaver's bottom), greater trochanteric, pes anserine, and first metatarsal head (bunion) bursae. Occasionally, bursitis causes inflammation in a communicating joint.

Etiology

Bursitis may be caused by the following:

- Injury
- Chronic overuse
- Inflammatory arthritis (eg, gout, RA, psoriatic arthritis, spondylitis)
- Acute or chronic infection (eg, pyogenic organisms, particularly *Staphylococcus aureus*)

Idiopathic and traumatic causes are by far the most common. Acute bursitis may follow unusual exercise or strain and usually causes bursal effusion. The olecranon and prepatellar bursae are the bursae most often involved when an infection is present.

Chronic bursitis may develop after previous attacks of bursitis or repeated trauma. The bursal wall is thickened, with proliferation of its synovial lining; bursal adhesions, villus formation, tags, and chalky deposits may develop.

Symptoms and Signs

Acute bursitis causes pain, particularly when the bursa is compressed or stretched during motion. Swelling, sometimes with other signs of inflammation, is common if the bursa is superficial (eg, prepatellar, olecranon). Swelling may be more prominent than pain in olecranon bursitis. Crystal- or bacterial-induced bursitis is usually accompanied by erythema, pitting edema, pain, and warmth in the area over the bursa.

Chronic bursitis may last for several months and may recur frequently. Bouts may last a few days to several weeks. If inflammation persists near a joint, the joint's range of motion may be limited. Prolonged limitation of motion may lead to muscle atrophy.

Diagnosis

- Clinical evaluation
- Ultrasonography or MRI for deep bursitis
- Aspiration for suspected infection, hemorrhage (due to trauma or anticoagulants), or crystal-induced bursitis

Superficial bursitis should be suspected in patients with swelling or signs of inflammation over bursae. Deep bursitis is suspected in patients with unexplained pain worsened by motion in a location compatible with bursitis. Usually, bursitis can be diagnosed clinically. Ultrasonography or MRI can help confirm the diagnosis when deep bursae are not readily accessible for inspection, palpation, or aspiration. These tests are done to confirm a suspected diagnosis or exclude other possibilities. These imaging techniques increase the accuracy of identifying the involved structures.

If bursal swelling is particularly painful, red, or warm or if the olecranon or prepatellar bursa is affected, infection and crystal-induced disease should be excluded by bursal aspiration. After a local anesthetic is injected, fluid is withdrawn from the bursa using sterile techniques; analysis includes cell count, Gram stain and culture, and microscopic search for crystals. Gram stain, although helpful, may not be specific, and WBC counts in infected bursae are usually lower than those in septic joints. Urate crystals are easily seen with polarized light microscopy, but the apatite crystals typical of calcific tendinitis appear only as shiny chunks that are not birefringent. X-rays should be taken if bursitis is persistent or if calcification is suspected.

Acute bursitis should be distinguished from hemorrhage into a bursa, which should be considered particularly when a patient taking warfarin develops acute bursitis. Hemorrhagic bursitis can cause similar manifestations because blood is inflammatory. Fluid in traumatic bursitis is usually serosanguinous. Cellulitis can cause signs of inflammation but does not normally cause bursal effusion; cellulitis overlying the bursa is a relative contraindication to bursal puncture through the cellulitis, but if septic bursitis is strongly suspected, aspiration must be done.

Treatment

- Rest
- High-dose NSAIDs
- Treatment of crystal-induced disease or infection
- Occasionally a corticosteroid injection

For crystal-induced disease, see p. 274. For infection, empiric antibiotics effective against *S. aureus* should be given initially (see treatment of staphylococcal infection on p. 1604). Subsequent choice of antibiotic is determined by results of Gram stain and culture. Infectious bursitis requires drainage or excision in addition to antibiotics.

Acute nonseptic bursitis is treated with temporary rest or immobilization and high-dose NSAIDs and sometimes with other analgesics. Voluntary movement should be increased as pain subsides. Pendulum exercises are helpful for the shoulder joint.

If oral drugs and rest are inadequate, aspiration and intrabursal injection of depot corticosteroids 0.5 to 1 mL (eg, triamcinolone acetonide 40 mg/mL) is the treatment of choice. About 1 mL of local anesthetic (eg, 2% lidocaine) can be injected before the corticosteroid injection. The same needle is used; it is kept in place and the syringes are changed. Dose and volume of the corticosteroid may vary according to the size of the bursa. Infrequently, a flare-up occurs within several hours of injection of a depot corticosteroid; the flare-up is probably a synovitis in reaction to crystals in the injection. It usually lasts ≤ 24 h and responds to cold compresses plus analgesics. Oral corticosteroids (eg, prednisone) can be used to treat the primary problem if a local injection is not feasible.

Chronic bursitis is treated the same as acute bursitis, except that splinting and rest are less likely to help, and range-of-motion exercises are especially important. Rarely, the bursa needs to be excised.

KEY POINTS

- The usual causes of bursitis are injury and overuse, but infection and crystal-induced disease are possible.
- Withdraw bursal fluid to diagnose bacterial or crystal-induced bursitis when the olecranon or prepatellar bursa is affected or when there is warmth, redness, tenderness, and pitting edema.
- If no infection is present, treat most cases with rest, high-dose NSAIDs, and sometimes intrabursal corticosteroid injection.

FIBROMYALGIA

(Fibromyositi; Fibrositis; Myofascial Pain Syndrome)

Fibromyalgia is a common nonarticular disorder of unknown cause characterized by generalized aching (sometimes severe); widespread tenderness of muscles, areas around tendon insertions, and adjacent soft tissues; muscle stiffness; fatigue; mental cloudiness; poor sleep; and a variety of other somatic symptoms. Diagnosis is clinical. Treatment includes exercise, local heat, stress management, drugs to improve sleep, and nonopioid analgesics.

In fibromyalgia, any fibromuscular tissues may be involved, especially those of the occiput, neck, shoulders, thorax, low back, and thighs. There is no specific histologic abnormality. Symptoms and signs of fibromyalgia are generalized, in contrast to localized soft-tissue pain and tenderness (myofascial pain syndrome), which is often related to overuse or microtrauma.

Fibromyalgia is common; it is about 7 times more common among women, usually young or middle-aged women, but can occur in men, children, and adolescents. Because of the sex difference, it is sometimes overlooked in men. It sometimes occurs in patients with other concomitant, unrelated systemic rheumatic disorders, thus complicating diagnosis and management.

Current evidence suggests fibromyalgia may be a centrally mediated disorder of pain sensitivity. The cause is unknown, but disruption of stage 4 sleep may contribute, as can emotional stress. Fibromyalgia may be precipitated by a viral or other systemic infection (eg, Lyme disease) or a traumatic event.

Symptoms and Signs

Stiffness and pain frequently begin gradually and diffusely and have an achy quality. Pain is widespread and may worsen with fatigue, muscle strain, or overuse.

Patients typically have a variety of somatic symptoms. Fatigue is common, as are cognitive disturbances such as difficulty concentrating and a general feeling of mental cloudiness. Many patients also have symptoms of irritable bowel syndrome, interstitial cystitis, or migraine or tension headaches. Paresthesias may be present, typically bilaterally.

Symptoms can be exacerbated by environmental or emotional stress, poor sleep, trauma, exposure to dampness or cold, or by a physician, family member, or friend who implies that the disorder is "all in the head."

Patients tend to be stressed, tense, anxious, fatigued, ambitious, and sometimes depressed. Patients may tend to be perfectionists.

Physical examination is unremarkable except that specific, discrete areas of muscle (tender points) often are tender when palpated. The tender areas are not swollen, red, or warm; such findings should suggest an alternative diagnosis.

Diagnosis

- Clinical criteria
- Usually testing and a detailed physical examination to exclude other disorders

Fibromyalgia is suspected in patients with the following:

- Generalized pain and tenderness, especially if disproportionate to physical findings
- Negative laboratory results despite widespread symptoms
- Fatigue as a predominant symptom

The diagnosis of fibromyalgia should be considered in people who have had widespread pain for at least 3 mo, particularly when accompanied by various somatic symptoms. Pain is considered widespread when patients have pain in the left and right side of the body, above and below the waist, and in the axial skeleton (cervical spine, anterior chest or thoracic spine, or low back).

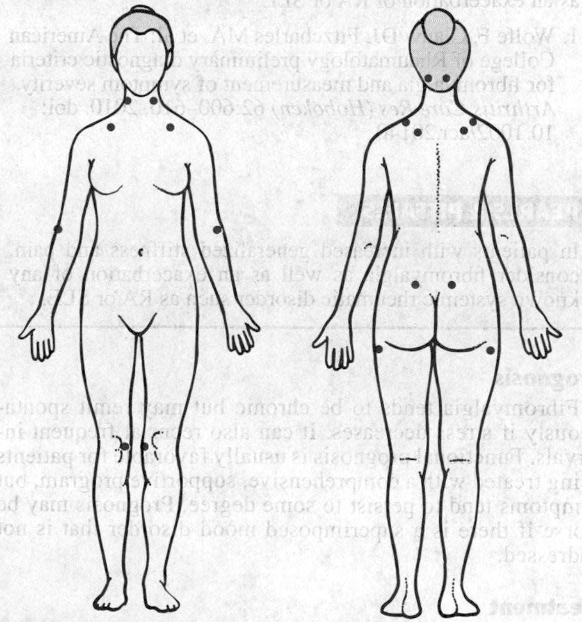

Fig. 34–1. Detecting tenderness in fibromyalgia. Current American College of Rheumatology diagnostic criteria no longer include the presence of tender points. However, patients do typically have widespread tenderness and this can be assessed systematically by palpation over 18 specific areas. Digital palpation should be done with a force of about 4 kg. A positive result requires that palpation be painful.

The diagnosis is based on clinical criteria from the American College of Rheumatology,[1] which include a combination of widespread pain and the presence of various other cognitive and somatic symptoms, such as those listed above, which are graded in severity. Previous criteria relied on the presence of tenderness at some of 18 specified tender points. This criterion was eliminated because nonspecialists sometimes have difficulty evaluating tenderness consistently, and because it was thought advantageous to have criteria that are entirely symptom-based. However, tenderness is quite common, and some specialists continue to assess it systematically (see Fig. 34–1).

Tests for other causes of patient symptoms should include ESR or C-reactive protein, CK, and probably tests for hypothyroidism and hepatitis C (which can cause fatigue and generalized myalgias). Other tests (eg, serologic testing for rheumatic disorders) are done only if indicated by findings on history and/or physical examination.

To avoid potential pitfalls, clinicians should consider the following:

- Fibromyalgia is often overlooked in men, children, and adolescents.
- Chronic fatigue syndrome (systemic exertion intolerance disease) can cause similar generalized myalgias and fatigue, and laboratory test results are typically normal.
- Polymyalgia rheumatica can cause generalized myalgias, particularly in older adults; it can be distinguished from fibromyalgia because it tends to affect proximal muscles selectively, is more symptomatic in the morning, and is accompanied by high ESR and C-reactive protein levels.
- In patients with systemic rheumatic disorders, diagnosing coexistent fibromyalgia may be more difficult, but it is quite common. For example, fibromyalgia may be misinterpreted as an exacerbation of RA or SLE.

1. Wolfe F, Clauw DJ, Fitzcharles MA, et al: The American College of Rheumatology preliminary diagnostic criteria for fibromyalgia and measurement of symptom severity. *Arthritis Care Res (Hoboken)* 62:600–610, 2010. doi: 10.1002/acr.20140.

PEARLS & PITFALLS

- In patients with increased generalized stiffness and pain, consider fibromyalgia as well as an exacerbation of any known systemic rheumatic disorder such as RA or SLE.

Prognosis

Fibromyalgia tends to be chronic but may remit spontaneously if stress decreases. It can also recur at frequent intervals. Functional prognosis is usually favorable for patients being treated with a comprehensive, supportive program, but symptoms tend to persist to some degree. Prognosis may be worse if there is a superimposed mood disorder that is not addressed.

Treatment

- Stretching and aerobic exercise, local heat, and massage
- Stress management
- Tricyclic antidepressants or cyclobenzaprine to improve sleep
- Nonopioid analgesics

Stretching exercises, aerobic exercises, sufficient sound sleep, local applications of heat, and gentle massage may provide relief. Overall stress management (eg, deep breathing exercises, meditation, psychologic support, counseling if necessary) is important.

Exercises to gently stretch the affected muscles should be done daily; stretches should be held for about 30 sec and repeated about 5 times. Aerobic exercise (eg, fast walking, swimming, exercise bicycling) can lessen symptoms.

Improving sleep is critical. Sedating drugs can be taken but only at night and only to improve sleep. Low-dose oral tricyclic antidepressants at bedtime (eg, amitriptyline 10 to 50 mg, trazodone 50 to 150 mg, doxepin 10 to 25 mg) or the pharmacologically similar cyclobenzaprine 10 to 30 mg may promote deeper sleep and decrease muscle pain. The lowest effective dose should be used. Drowsiness, dry mouth, and other adverse effects may make some or all of these drugs intolerable, particularly for the elderly.

Nonopioid analgesics (eg, tramadol, acetaminophen, NSAIDs) may help some patients. Opioids should be avoided. Pregabalin, duloxetine, and milnacipran are available for treatment of fibromyalgia, but should be used as adjuncts to exercise, measures to improve sleep, and stress management; they may help modestly to reduce pain.

Occasional injections of 0.5% bupivacaine or 1% lidocaine 1 to 5 mL are used to treat incapacitating areas of focal tenderness, but such injections should not be relied on as primary treatment because evidence does not support their regular use.

Drugs taken by the patient should be reviewed to identify those that may aggravate sleep problems. Such drugs should be avoided. Anxiety, depression, and especially bipolar disorder, if present, should be addressed.

KEY POINTS

- Fibromyalgia-related stiffness and pain can be exacerbated by environmental or emotional stress, poor sleep, trauma, exposure to dampness or cold, or by a physician, family member, or friend who implies that the disorder is "all in the head."
- Suspect fibromyalgia when generalized pain and tenderness and fatigue are unexplained or out of proportion to physical and laboratory findings.
- Do ESR or C-reactive protein, CK, and tests for hypothyroidism and hepatitis C, and consider chronic fatigue syndrome and polymyalgia rheumatica.
- Consider fibromyalgia in patients having apparent painful exacerbations of systemic rheumatic disorders such as RA or SLE but who have no clinical or laboratory evidence to confirm such exacerbations.
- Treat by emphasizing physical methods, stress management, and sleep improvement, and, when necessary for pain, by giving nonopioid analgesics.

TENDINITIS AND TENOSYNOVITIS

Tendinitis is inflammation of a tendon, often developing after degeneration (tendinopathy). Tenosynovitis is tendinitis with inflammation of the tendon sheath lining. Symptoms usually include pain with motion and tenderness with palpation. Chronic deterioration or inflammation of the tendon or tendon sheath can cause scars that restrict motion. Diagnosis is clinical, sometimes supplemented with imaging. Treatment includes rest, NSAIDs, and sometimes corticosteroid injections.

Tendinopathy usually results from repeated small tears or degenerative changes (sometimes with calcium deposits) that occur over years in the tendon.

Tendinitis and tenosynovitis most commonly affect tendons associated with the shoulder (rotator cuff), the tendon of the long head of the biceps muscle (bicipital tendon), flexor carpi radialis or ulnaris, flexor digitorumo, popliteus tendon, Achilles tendon (see p. 3107), and the abductor pollicis longus and extensor pollicis brevis, which share a common fibrous sheath (the resulting disorder is de Quervain syndrome—see p. 289).

Etiology

The cause of tendinitis is often unknown. It usually occurs in people who are middle-aged or older as the vascularity of tendons decreases; repetitive microtrauma may contribute. Repeated or extreme trauma (short of rupture), strain, and excessive or unaccustomed exercise probably also contribute. Some fluoroquinolone antibiotics may increase the risk of tendinopathy and tendon rupture.

Risk of tendinitis may be increased by certain systemic disorders—most commonly RA, systemic sclerosis, gout, reactive arthritis, and diabetes or, very rarely, amyloidosis or markedly elevated blood cholesterol levels. In younger adults, particularly women, disseminated gonococcal infection may cause acute migratory tenosynovitis.

Symptoms and Signs

Affected tendons are usually painful when actively moved or when natural motion is resisted. Occasionally, tendon sheaths become swollen and fluid accumulates, usually when patients have infection, RA, or gout. Swelling may be visible or only palpable. Along the tendon, palpation elicits localized tenderness of varying severity.

In systemic sclerosis, the tendon sheath may remain dry, but movement of the tendon in its sheath causes friction, which can be felt or heard with a stethoscope.

Diagnosis

- Clinical evaluation
- Sometimes imaging

Usually, the diagnosis can be based on symptoms and physical examination, including palpation or specific maneuvers to assess pain. MRI or ultrasonography may be done to confirm the diagnosis or rule out other disorders. MRI can detect tendon tears and inflammation (as can ultrasonography).

- **Rotator cuff tendinitis:** This disorder is the most common cause of shoulder pain. The rotator cuff is composed of four tendons, the supraspinatus, infraspinatus, subscapularis, and teres minor. The supraspinatus tendon is most frequently involved and the subscapularis is second. Active abduction in an arc of 40 to 120° and internal rotation cause pain (see p. 3103). Passive abduction causes less pain, but abduction against resistance can increase pain. Calcium deposits in the tendon just below the acromion are sometimes visible on x-ray. Ultrasonography or MRI may help with further evaluation and with treatment decisions.
- **Bicipital tendinitis:** Pain in the biceps tendon is aggravated by shoulder flexion or resisted supination of the forearm. Examiners can elicit tenderness proximally over the bicipital groove of the humerus by rolling (flipping) the bicipital tendon under their thumb.
- **Volar flexor tenosynovitis (digital flexor tendinitis):** This common musculoskeletal disorder is often overlooked (see p. 289). Pain occurs in the palm on the volar aspect of the thumb or other digits and may radiate distally. Palpation of the tendon and sheath elicits tenderness; swelling and sometimes a nodule are present. In later stages, the digit may lock when it is flexed, and forceful extension may cause a sudden release with a snap (trigger finger).
- **Gluteus medius tendinitis:** Patients with trochanteric bursitis almost always have gluteus medius tendinitis. In patients with trochanteric bursitis, palpation over the lateral prominence of the greater trochanter elicits tenderness. Patients often have a history of chronic pressure on the joint, trauma, a change in gait (eg, due to osteoarthritis, stroke, or leg-length discrepancy), or inflammation at this site (eg, in RA).

Treatment

- Rest or immobilization, heat or cold, followed by exercise
- High-dose NSAIDs
- Sometimes corticosteroid injection

Symptoms are relieved by rest or immobilization (splint or sling) of the tendon, application of heat (usually for chronic inflammation) or cold (usually for acute inflammation), and high-dose NSAIDs (see Table 39–3 on p. 307) for 7 to 10 days. Indomethacin or colchicine may be helpful if gout is the cause. After inflammation is controlled, exercises that gradually increase range of motion should be done several times a day, especially for the shoulder, which can develop contractures rapidly.

Injecting a sustained-release corticosteroid (eg, betamethasone 6 mg/mL, triamcinolone 40 mg/mL, methylprednisolone 20 to 40 mg/mL) in the tendon sheath may help; injection is usually indicated if pain is severe or if the problem has been chronic. Injection volume may range from 0.3 mL to 1 mL, depending on the site. An injection through the same needle of an equal or double volume of local anesthetic (eg, 1 to 2% lidocaine) confirms the diagnosis if pain is relieved immediately. Clinicians should be careful not to inject the tendon (which can be recognized by marked resistance to injection); doing so may weaken it, increasing risk of rupture. Patients are advised to rest the injected joint to reduce the slight risk of rupture. Infrequently, symptoms can worsen for up to 24 h after the injection.

PEARLS & PITFALLS

- Do not inject corticosteroids into a tendon; doing so will weaken it, increasing risk of rupture.

Repeat injections and symptomatic treatment may be required. Rarely, for persistent cases, particularly rotator cuff tendinitis, surgical exploration with removal of calcium deposits or tendon repair, followed by graded physical therapy, is needed. Occasionally, patients require surgery to release scars that limit function, remove part of a bone causing repetitive friction, or do tenosynovectomy to relieve chronic inflammation.

KEY POINTS

- Tendinitis and tenosynovitis, unlike tendinopathy (tendon degeneration), involve inflammation.
- Pain, tenderness, and swelling tend to be maximal along the tendon's course.
- Diagnose most cases by examination, including tendon-specific maneuvers, sometimes confirming the diagnosis with MRI or ultrasonography.
- Treat with rest, heat or cold, high-dose NSAIDs, and sometimes corticosteroid injection.

35 Crystal-Induced Arthritides

Arthritis can result from intra-articular deposition of crystals:

- Monosodium urate (MSU)
- Ca pyrophosphate dihydrate (CPPD)
- Basic Ca phosphate (apatite)
- Rarely, others such as Ca oxalate crystals

Diagnosis requires synovial fluid analysis. Polarized light microscopy is used to specifically identify most crystals; basic Ca phosphate (BCP) crystals are of ultramicroscopic size and require other methods. Crystals may be engulfed in WBCs or may be extracellular. The presence of crystals does not exclude the possibility of simultaneous infectious or other inflammatory forms of arthritis. Noninvasive identification of MSU and CPPD crystals is possible using ultrasonography, but currently few ultrasonographers have sufficient expertise to do this technique.

GOUT

Gout is precipitation of monosodium urate (MSU) crystals into tissue, usually in and around joints, most often causing recurrent acute or chronic arthritis. The initial attack of acute arthritis is usually monarticular and often involves the 1st metatarsophalangeal joint. Symptoms of gout include acute pain, tenderness, warmth, redness, and swelling. Diagnosis requires identification of crystals in synovial fluid. Treatment of acute attacks is with anti-inflammatory drugs. The frequency of attacks can be reduced by regular use of NSAIDs, colchicine, or both and by lowering the serum urate level with allopurinol, febuxostat, or uricosuric drugs.

Gout is more common among men than women. Usually, gout develops during middle age in men and after menopause in women. Gout is rare in younger people but is often more severe in people who develop the disorder before age 30. Gout often runs in families. Patients with the metabolic syndrome are at risk of gout.

Pathophysiology

The greater the degree and duration of hyperuricemia, the greater is the likelihood that gout will develop. Urate levels can be elevated because of

- Decreased excretion (most common)
- Increased production
- Increased purine intake

Why only some people with elevated serum uric acid (urate) levels develop gout is not known.

Decreased renal excretion is by far the most common cause of hyperuricemia. It may be hereditary and also occurs in patients receiving diuretics and in those with diseases that decrease GFR. Ethanol increases purine catabolism in the liver and increases the formation of lactic acid, which blocks urate secretion by the renal tubules, and ethanol may also stimulate liver urate synthesis. Lead poisoning and cyclosporine, usually in the higher doses given to transplant patients, damage renal tubules, leading to urate retention.

Increased production of urate may be caused by increased nucleoprotein turnover in hematologic conditions (eg, lymphoma, leukemia, hemolytic anemia) and in conditions with increased rates of cellular proliferation and cell death (eg, psoriasis, cytotoxic cancer therapy, radiation therapy). Increased urate production may also occur as a primary hereditary abnormality and in obesity, because urate production correlates with body surface area. In most cases, the cause of urate overproduction is unknown, but a few cases are attributable to enzyme abnormalities; deficiency of hypoxanthine-guanine phosphoribosyltransferase (complete deficiency is Lesch-Nyhan syndrome) is a possible cause, as is overactivity of phosphoribosylpyrophosphate synthetase.

Increased intake of purine-rich foods (eg, liver, kidney, anchovies, asparagus, consommé, herring, meat gravies and broths, mushrooms, mussels, sardines, sweetbreads) can contribute to hyperuricemia. Beer is particularly rich in guanosine, a purine nucleoside. However, a strict low-purine diet lowers serum urate by only about 1 mg/dL.

Urate precipitates as needle-shaped MSU crystals, which are deposited extracellularly in avascular tissues (eg, cartilage) or in relatively avascular tissues (eg, tendons, tendon sheaths, ligaments, walls of bursae) and skin around cooler distal joints and tissues (eg, ears). In severe, long-standing hyperuricemia, MSU crystals may be deposited in larger central joints and in the parenchyma of organs such as the kidney. At the acid pH of urine, urate precipitates readily as small platelike or diamond-shaped uric acid crystals that may aggregate to form gravel or stones, which may obstruct urine outflow. Tophi are MSU crystal aggregates that most often develop in joint and cutaneous tissue. They are usually encased in a fibrous matrix, which prevents them from causing acute inflammation.

Acute gouty arthritis may be triggered by trauma, medical stress (eg, pneumonia or other infection), surgery, use of thiazide diuretics or drugs with hypouricemic effects (eg, allopurinol, probenecid, nitroglycerin), or indulgence in purine-rich food or alcohol. Attacks are often precipitated by a sudden increase or, more commonly, a sudden decrease in serum urate levels. Why acute attacks follow some of these precipitating conditions is unknown. Tophi in and around joints can limit motion and cause deformities, called chronic tophaceous gouty arthritis. Chronic gout increases the risk of developing secondary osteoarthritis.

Symptoms and Signs

Acute gouty arthritis usually begins with sudden onset of pain (often nocturnal). The metatarsophalangeal joint of a great toe is most often involved (called podagra—see Plate 3), but the instep, ankle, knee, wrist, and elbow are also common sites. Rarely, the hip, shoulder, sacroiliac, sternoclavicular, or cervical spine joints are involved. The pain becomes progressively more severe, usually over a few hours, and is often excruciating. Swelling, warmth, redness, and exquisite tenderness may suggest infection. The overlying skin may become tense, warm, shiny, and red or purplish. Fever, tachycardia, chills, and malaise sometimes occur.

Course: The first few attacks usually affect only a single joint and last only a few days. Later attacks may affect several joints simultaneously or sequentially and persist up to 3 wk if untreated. Subsequent attacks develop after progressively shorter symptom-free intervals. Eventually, several attacks may occur each year.

Tophi: Tophi develop most often in patients with chronic gout, but they can rarely occur in patients who have never had acute gouty arthritis. They are usually firm yellow or white papules or nodules, single or multiple. They can develop in various locations, commonly the fingers, hands, feet, and around the olecranon or Achilles tendon. Tophi can also develop in the kidneys and other organs and under the skin on the ears. Patients with osteoarthritic Heberden nodes may develop tophi in the nodes. This development occurs most often in elderly women taking diuretics. Normally painless, tophi, especially in the olecranon bursae, can become acutely inflamed and painful, often after mild or inapparent injury. Tophi may even erupt through the skin, discharging chalky masses of urate crystals. Tophi may eventually cause deformities and secondary osteoarthritis.

Chronic gout: Chronic gouty arthritis can cause pain, deformity, and limited joint motion. Inflammation can be flaring in some joints while subsiding in others. About 20% of patients with gout develop urolithiasis with uric acid stones or Ca oxalate stones.

Complications include obstruction and infection, with secondary tubulointerstitial disease. Untreated progressive renal dysfunction, most often related to coexisting hypertension or, less often, some other cause of nephropathy, further impairs excretion of urate, accelerating crystal deposition in tissues.

Cardiovascular disease and the metabolic syndrome are common among patients with gout.

Diagnosis

- Clinical criteria
- Synovial fluid analysis

The diagnosis of gout should be suspected in patients with acute monoarticular or oligoarticular arthritis, particularly older adults or those with other risk factors. Podagra and recurrent instep inflammation are particularly suggestive. Previous attacks that began explosively and resolved spontaneously are also characteristic. Similar symptoms can result from the following:

- CPPD crystal deposition disease (however, CPPD generally occurs in larger joints, is not associated with tophi, and its clinical course is usually milder)
- Acute rheumatic fever with joint involvement and juvenile idiopathic arthritis (however, these disorders occur mostly in young people, who rarely get gout)
- RA (however, in RA, all affected joints flare, flares persist for longer, and flares in all joints subside together, whereas in gout, inflammation is usually flaring in some joints while subsiding in others)
- Acute fracture in patients unable to provide a history of injury
- Infectious arthritis (acute or chronic; differentiation requires synovial fluid analysis)
- Palindromic rheumatism
- Acute calcific periarthritis caused by BCP and Ca oxalate crystal deposition disease

Palindromic rheumatism is characterized by acute, recurrent attacks of inflammation in or near one or occasionally several joints with spontaneous resolution; pain and erythema can be as severe as in gout. Attacks subside spontaneously and completely in 1 to 3 days. Such attacks may herald the onset of RA, and rheumatoid factor tests can help in differentiation; they are positive in about 50% of patients (these tests are positive in 10% of gouty patients also).

Synovial fluid analysis: If acute gouty arthritis is suspected, arthrocentesis and synovial fluid analysis should be done at the initial presentation. A typical recurrence in a patient with known gout does not mandate arthrocentesis, but it should be done if there is any question of the diagnosis or if the patient's risk factors or any clinical characteristics suggest infectious arthritis.

Synovial fluid analysis can confirm the diagnosis by identifying needle-shaped, strongly negatively birefringent urate crystals that are free in the fluid or engulfed by phagocytes (see Table 35–1). Synovial fluid during attacks has inflammatory characteristics, usually 2,000 to 100,000 WBCs/μL, with > 80% polymorphonuclear WBCs. These findings overlap considerably with infectious arthritis, which must be excluded by Gram stain (which is insensitive) and culture.

Serum urate level: An elevated serum urate level supports the diagnosis of gout but is neither specific nor sensitive; at least 30% of patients have a normal serum urate level during an acute attack. However, the baseline serum urate level between attacks reflects the size of the extracellular miscible urate pool. The level should be measured on 2 or 3 occasions in patients with newly proven gout to establish a baseline; if elevated (> 7 mg/dL [> 0.41 mmol/L]), 24-h urinary urate excretion is sometimes measured. Normal 24-h excretion in people eating a regular diet is about 600 to 900 mg.

Quantification of urinary uric acid can indicate whether hyperuricemia results from impaired excretion or increased production and is useful if a uricosuric drug is used for urate-lowering therapy. However, urate excretion does not predict the patient's response to allopurinol or febuxostat. Patients with elevated urine excretion of urate are at increased risk of urolithiasis and uricosuric drugs are typically avoided.

Imaging: X-rays of the affected joint may be taken to look for bony tophi but are probably unnecessary if the diagnosis has been established by synovial fluid analysis. In CPPD,

Table 35–1. MICROSCOPIC EXAMINATION OF CRYSTALS IN JOINTS

CRYSTAL TYPE	BIREFRINGENCE	ELONGATION*	SHAPE	LENGTH (μm)
MSU	Strong	Negative	Needle- or rod-shaped	2–15
CPPD	Weak or not birefringent	Positive	Rhomboid- or rod-shaped	2–15
Ca oxalate (rare)†	Weak or strong	Positive or indeterminate	Bipyramidal	5–30
BCP	Not birefringent with polarized light	—	Shiny, coinlike, or slightly irregular	3–65 (aggregates)

*Crystals that have negative elongation are yellow parallel to the axis of slow vibration marked on the compensator; positive elongation appears blue in the same direction.

†These crystals occur primarily in patients with renal failure.

BCP = basic Ca phosphate; CPPD = Ca pyrophosphate dihydrate; MSU = monosodium urate.

radiopaque deposits are present in fibrocartilage, hyaline articular cartilage (particularly the knee), or both.

Urate deposition can sometimes be identified by experienced ultrasonographers, even before the patient has any attacks.

Diagnosis of chronic gouty arthritis: Chronic gouty arthritis should be suspected in patients with persistent joint disease or subcutaneous or bony tophi. Plain x-rays of the 1st metatarsophalangeal joint or other affected joint may be useful. These x-rays may show punched-out lesions of subchondral bone with overhanging bony margins, most commonly in the 1st metatarsophalangeal joint; lesions must be ≥ 5 mm in diameter to be visible on x-ray. Joint space is typically preserved until very late in the course of disease.

Bone lesions are not specific or diagnostic but nearly always precede the appearance of subcutaneous tophi.

Diagnostic ultrasonography is increasingly used to detect a typical double-contour sign suggesting urate crystal deposition, but sensitivity is operator-dependent and differentiation from Ca pyrophosphate crystal deposits may be difficult.

Prognosis

With early gout diagnosis, therapy enables most patients to live a normal life. For many patients with advanced disease, aggressive lowering of the serum urate level can resolve tophi and improve joint function. Gout is generally more severe in patients whose initial symptoms appear before age 30. The high prevalence of metabolic syndrome and cardiovascular disease probably increases mortality in patients with gout.

Some patients do not improve sufficiently with treatment. The usual reasons include nonadherence, alcoholism, and undertreatment by physicians.

Treatment

- Termination of an acute attack with NSAIDs, corticosteroids, or colchicine
- Prevention of recurrent acute attacks with daily colchicine or an NSAID
- Prevention of further deposition of MSU crystals, reduction in flare incidence, and resolution of existing tophi by lowering the serum urate level (by decreasing urate production with allopurinol, febuxostat, or uricase, or increasing urate excretion with probenecid or sulfinpyrazone)
- Treatment of coexisting hypertension, hyperlipidemia, and obesity and sometimes avoidance of excess dietary purines

Treatment of acute attacks: NSAIDs are effective in treating acute attacks and are generally well-tolerated. However, they can have adverse effects, including GI upset or bleeding, hyperkalemia, increases in creatinine, and fluid retention. Elderly and dehydrated patients are at particular risk, especially if there is a history of renal disease. Virtually any NSAID used in anti-inflammatory (high) doses is effective and is likely to exert an analgesic effect in a few hours. Treatment should be continued for several days after the pain and signs of inflammation have resolved to prevent relapse.

Oral colchicine, a traditional therapy, often produces a dramatic response if begun soon after the onset of symptoms; it is most effective if started within 12 to 24 h of an acute attack. A dose of 1.2 mg can be followed with 0.6 mg 1 h later; joint pain tends to decrease after 12 to 24 h and sometimes ceases within 3 to 7 days, but usually > 3 doses are needed to achieve resolution. If colchicine is tolerated, 0.6 to 1.2 mg once/day can be continued as the attack subsides. Renal insufficiency and drug interactions, especially with clarithromycin, may warrant reduction of dosage or use of other treatments.

IV colchicine is no longer available in the US because of major toxicity, usually related to inappropriate use or dosing.

Corticosteroids are sometimes used to treat acute attacks. Aspiration of affected joints, followed by instillation of corticosteroid ester crystal suspension, is very effective, particularly for monarticular symptoms; prednisolone tebutate 4 to 40 mg or prednisolone acetate 5 to 25 mg can be used, with dose depending on the size of the affected joint. Oral prednisone (about 0.5 mg/kg once/day), IM or IV corticosteroids, or single-dose ACTH 80 U IM is also very effective, particularly if multiple joints are involved. As with NSAID therapy, corticosteroids should be continued until after the attack fully resolves to prevent relapse.

In addition to NSAIDs or corticosteroids, supplementary analgesics, rest, ice application, and splinting of the inflamed joint may be helpful. Because lowering the serum urate level during an attack may prolong the attack or predispose to recurrence, drugs that lower the serum urate level should not be initiated until acute symptoms have been completely controlled. If patients are taking urate-lowering drugs when an acute attack begins, the drugs should be continued at the same dose; dose adjustments are deferred until the attack has subsided.

If corticosteroids, colchicine, and NSAIDs are contraindicated, an IL-1 antagonist, such as anakinra, can be used. Although it is expensive, it may hasten resolution of an attack and shorten the hospital stay of a patient with multiple comorbidities that limit the use of the other drugs.

Prevention of recurrent attacks: The frequency of acute attacks is reduced by taking one to two 0.6-mg tablets of colchicine daily (depending on tolerance and severity). An extra two 0.6-mg tablets of colchicine taken at the first suggestion of an attack may abort flares. If the patient is taking prophylactic doses of colchicine and has had higher doses of colchicine to treat an acute attack within the past 2 wk, an NSAID should be used instead to try to abort the attack.

A (reversible) neuropathy or myopathy can develop during chronic colchicine ingestion. This condition may occur in patients with renal insufficiency, in patients also receiving a statin or macrolide, or in patients with none of these risk factors.

Attack frequency can also be decreased with daily low-dose NSAIDs.

Lowering the serum urate level: Colchicine, NSAIDs, and corticosteroids do not retard the progressive joint damage caused by tophi. Such damage can be prevented and, if present, reversed with urate-lowering drugs. Tophaceous deposits are resorbed by lowering serum urate. Lowering serum urate may also decrease the frequency of acute arthritic attacks. This decrease is accomplished by

- Blocking urate production with allopurinol or febuxostat
- Increasing urate excretion with a uricosuric drug
- Using both types of drugs together in severe tophaceous gout

Hypouricemic therapy is indicated for patients with

- Tophaceous deposits
- Frequent or disabling attacks of gouty arthritis despite prophylactic colchicine, an NSAID, or both
- Urolithiasis
- Multiple comorbidities (eg, peptic ulcer disease, chronic kidney disease) that are relative contraindications to the drugs used to treat acute attacks (NSAIDs or corticosteroids)

Hyperuricemia is not usually treated in the absence of gout.

The goal of hypouricemic therapy is to lower the serum urate level. If tophi are not present, a reasonable target level is < 6 mg/dL (0.36 mmol/L), which is below the level of saturation (> 7.0 mg/dL [> 0.41 mmol/L] at normal core body temperature and pH). If tophi are present, the goal is to dissolve them, and this requires a lower target level. A reasonable target level is 5 mg/dL (0.30 mmol/L), and the lower the urate level, the faster tophi resolve. These target levels should be maintained indefinitely. Low levels are often difficult to maintain.

Drugs are effective in lowering serum urate; dietary restriction of purines is less effective, but high intake of high-purine food, alcohol (beer in particular), and nonalcoholic beer should be avoided. Carbohydrate restriction and weight loss can lower serum urate in patients with insulin resistance because high insulin levels suppress urate excretion. Intake of low-fat dairy products should be encouraged. Because acute attacks tend to develop during the first months of hypouricemic therapy, such therapy should be started in conjunction with once or twice daily colchicine or NSAIDs and during a symptom-free period.

Resolution of tophi may take many months even with maintenance of serum urate at low levels. Serum urate should be measured periodically, usually monthly while determining required drug dosage and then yearly to confirm the effectiveness of therapy.

Allopurinol, which inhibits urate synthesis, is the most commonly prescribed hypouricemic therapy. Uric acid stones or gravel may dissolve during allopurinol treatment. Treatment begins with 50 to 100 mg po once/day and can be increased up to 800 mg po once/day, or even higher, to achieve target serum urate levels. Some clinicians recommend decreasing the starting dose in patients with renal insufficiency to decrease the incidence of rare but severe systemic hypersensitivity reactions; however, data that confirm the effectiveness of this intervention are limited. The final dose of allopurinol should be determined by the target serum urate level. The most commonly used daily dose is 300 mg, but this dose is adequate for < 50% of patients with gout.

Adverse effects of allopurinol include mild GI distress and rash, which can be a harbinger of Stevens-Johnson syndrome, life-threatening hepatitis, vasculitis, or leukopenia. Adverse effects are more common among patients with renal dysfunction. Some ethnic groups (eg, Koreans with renal disease, Thai, and Han Chinese) are at high risk of allopurinol reactions; HLA B*5801 is a marker for that risk in these ethnic groups. Allopurinol is contraindicated in patients taking azathioprine or mercaptopurine because it can decrease metabolism of and thus potentiate the immunosuppressive and cytolytic effects of these drugs.

Febuxostat is a far more costly (in the US) but potent inhibitor of urate synthesis. It is especially useful in patients who do not tolerate allopurinol, who have contraindications to allopurinol, or in whom allopurinol does not sufficiently decrease urate levels. It is begun at 40 mg po once/day and increased to 80 mg po once/day if urate does not decrease to < 6 mg/dL. Febuxostat (like allopurinol) is contraindicated in patients taking azathioprine or mercaptopurine because it can decrease metabolism of these drugs. Transaminase levels can become elevated and should be measured periodically.

Uricase can also be given but is not yet routinely used. Uricase is an enzyme that converts urate to allantoin, which is more soluble. IV uricase transiently lowers serum urate by a large amount. It decreases urate so much that crystal deposits are partially solubilized, leading to intra-articular release and acute flares in up to 70% of uricase treatment courses. Allergic infusion reactions (anaphylaxis in 6.5% of patients and other infusion reactions in 25 to 40% of patients) may occur with uricase treatment despite pretreatment with corticosteroids and/or antihistamines.

Pegloticase (a pegylated form of recombinant uricase) is the formulation usually used but is very expensive. It is given every 2 wk for many months to several years to totally deplete the excess urate deposits; it often lowers the serum urate level to < 1 mg/dL. Pegloticase is contraindicated in patients with G6PD deficiency because it can cause hemolysis and methemoglobinemia. Failure of urate levels to decrease to < 6 mg/dL after pegloticase treatment predicts pegloticase antibodies and an increased risk of future allergic reactions. To prevent other urate-lowering drugs from masking the ineffectiveness of pegloticase, other urate-lowering drugs should not be used with pegloticase.

Uricosuric therapy is useful in patients who underexcrete uric acid, have normal renal function, and have not had renal stones. It usually involves probenecid or sulfinpyrazone.

- Probenecid treatment begins with 250 mg po bid, with doses increased as needed, to a maximum of 1 g po tid.
- Sulfinpyrazone treatment begins with 50 to 100 mg po bid, with doses increased as needed, to a maximum of 100 mg po qid.

Sulfinpyrazone is more potent than probenecid but is more toxic. Low doses of salicylates may worsen hyperuricemia but only trivially.

Other treatments: Fluid intake ≥ 3 L/day is desirable for all patients, especially those who chronically pass urate gravel or stones.

Alkalinization of urine (with K citrate 20 to 40 mEq po bid or acetazolamide 500 mg po at bedtime) is also occasionally effective for patients with persistent uric acid urolithiasis despite hypouricemic therapy and adequate hydration. However, excessive urine alkalinization may cause deposition of Ca phosphate and oxalate crystals.

Extracorporeal shock wave lithotripsy may be needed to disintegrate renal stones.

Large tophi in areas with healthy skin may be removed surgically; all others should slowly resolve under adequate hypouricemic therapy. Losartan has mild uricosuric effects.

KEY POINTS

- Although increased purine intake and increased production can contribute to hyperuricemia, the most common cause of gout is decreased urate excretion secondary to diuretics, kidney disorders, or hereditary variations.
- Suspect gout in patients with sudden, unexplained acute monoarticular or oligoarticular arthritis, particularly if the great toe is affected or there is a prior history of sudden, unexplained acute arthritis with spontaneous remission.
- Confirm the diagnosis by finding needle-shaped, strongly negatively birefringent urate crystals in joint fluid.
- Treat acute attacks of gout with oral colchicine, another NSAID, or a corticosteroid.
- Decrease the risk of future attacks by prescribing colchicine, another NSAID, or, when indicated, drugs to decrease the serum urate level.
- Give drugs that decrease serum urate if patients have tophi, frequent or severe attacks despite appropriate prophylaxis, urolithiasis, or multiple comorbidities that contraindicate the drugs used to relieve acute attacks.
- Decrease urate levels usually by prescribing allopurinol or febuxostat.

Asymptomatic Hyperuricemia

Asymptomatic hyperuricemia is elevation of serum urate > 7 mg/dL (> 0.42 mmol/L) in the absence of clinical gout.

Generally, treatment is not required. However, patients with overexcretion of urate who are at risk of urolithiasis may receive allopurinol.

Accumulating data suggest that hyperuricemia may contribute to the progression of chronic kidney disease and, in adolescents, primary hypertension.

CALCIUM PYROPHOSPHATE DIHYDRATE CRYSTAL DEPOSITION DISEASE

(Calcium Pyrophosphate Arthritis; Pseudogout)

Calcium pyrophosphate dihydrate (CPPD) crystal deposition disease involves intra-articular and/or extra-articular deposition of CPPD crystals. Manifestations are protean and may be minimal or include intermittent attacks of acute arthritis, termed pseudogout or acute Ca pyrophosphate crystal disease, and a degenerative arthropathy that is often severe. Diagnosis requires identification of CPPD crystals in synovial fluid. Treatment of pseudogout attacks is with intra-articular corticosteroids or oral glucocorticoids, NSAIDs, or colchicine.

CPPD crystal deposition (chondrocalcinosis), whether symptomatic and asymptomatic, becomes more common with age.

Asymptomatic chondrocalcinosis is common in the knee, metacarpophalangeal joints, wrist, symphysis pubis, and spine. Men and women are affected about equally.

Etiology

The cause of CPPD crystal deposition disease is unknown. Frequent association with other conditions, such as trauma (including surgery), hypomagnesemia, hyperparathyroidism, gout, hemochromatosis, and old age, suggests that CPPD crystal deposits are secondary to degenerative or metabolic changes in the affected tissues.

Some cases are familial, usually transmitted in an autosomal dominant pattern, with complete penetration by age 40.

Recent studies indicate that the ANK protein is a central factor in producing excess extracellular pyrophosphate, which promotes CPPD crystal formation. ANK protein is a putative transporter of intracellular pyrophosphate to the extracellular location where CPPD crystals form.

Symptoms and Signs

Acute, subacute, or chronic arthritis can occur, usually in the knee or other large peripheral joints; thus, Ca pyrophosphate crystal disease can mimic many other forms of arthritis. Acute attacks are sometimes similar to gout but are usually less severe. There may be no symptoms of CPPD crystal deposition disease between attacks or continuous low-grade symptoms in multiple joints, similar to RA or osteoarthritis. These patterns tend to persist for life.

Diagnosis

- Synovial fluid analysis
- Identification of crystals microscopically

CPPD crystal deposition disease should be suspected in older patients with arthritis, particularly inflammatory arthritis.

Diagnosis of CPPD crystal deposition disease is established by identifying rhomboid or rod-shaped crystals in synovial fluid that are not birefringent or are weakly positively birefringent on polarized light microscopy. Joint fluid in acute attacks has findings typical of inflammation; thus, coincident infectious arthritis and gout (other common causes of inflammatory joint fluid) must also be excluded. Infectious arthritis is ruled out based on Gram stain and culture findings. Gout is usually best ruled out by the absence of urate crystals in fluid from the inflamed joint. X-rays or ultrasonography are indicated if synovial fluid cannot be obtained for analysis; findings of multiple linear or punctate calcification in articular cartilage, especially fibrocartilages, support the diagnosis but do not exclude gout or infection. Typical ultrasonographic findings of gout (double contour sign) may simulate findings of Ca pyrophosphate crystal deposits.

Prognosis

The prognosis for individual attacks of acute CPPD crystal deposition disease is usually excellent. However, chronic arthritis can occur, and severe destructive arthropathy resembling neurogenic arthropathy (Charcot joints) occasionally occurs.

Treatment

- Intra-articular corticosteroids
- NSAIDs
- Colchicine maintenance

Symptoms of acute synovial effusion abate with synovial fluid drainage and instillation of a microcrystalline corticosteroid ester suspension into the joint space (eg, 40 mg prednisolone acetate or prednisolone tertiary butylacetate into a knee).

Indomethacin, naproxen, or another NSAID given at anti-inflammatory doses often stops acute attacks promptly. Colchicine treatment of acute attacks is identical to that of gout. Colchicine 0.6 mg po once/day or bid may decrease the frequency of recurrent acute attacks.

KEY POINTS

- Asymptomatic chondrocalcinosis becomes common with age, particularly in the knee, hip, wrist, anulus fibrosus, and symphysis pubis.
- Arthritis can affect the knee and large peripheral joints and mimic other forms of arthritis.
- Examine joint fluid for characteristic rhomboid or rod-shaped crystals in synovial fluid that are not birefringent or are weakly positively birefringent, and exclude joint infection.
- For acute symptoms, treat with an intra-articular corticosteroid or an oral NSAID.

BASIC CALCIUM PHOSPHATE CRYSTAL DEPOSITION DISEASE AND CALCIUM OXALATE CRYSTAL DEPOSITION DISEASE

Basic Ca phosphate (BCP; apatite) and Ca oxalate crystal disorders tend to cause clinical manifestations similar to those of other crystal-induced arthritides.

BCP crystal deposition disease: Most pathologic calcifications throughout the body contain mixtures of carbonate-substituted hydroxyapatite and octacalcium phosphate. Because these ultramicroscopic crystals are nonacidic Ca phosphates, the term *basic Ca phosphate* (BCP) is much more precise than *apatite*. These ultramicroscopic crystals occur in snowball-like clumps in rheumatic conditions (eg, calcific tendinitis, calcific periarthritis, some cases of progressive systemic sclerosis and dermatomyositis). They also occur in joint fluids and cartilages of patients with all degenerative arthropathies sufficiently advanced to cause joint space narrowing on x-ray.

BCP crystals can destroy joints and can cause severe intra-articular or periarticular inflammation.

Milwaukee shoulder syndrome, a profoundly destructive arthropathy affecting predominantly elderly women that usually develops in the shoulders and (often) knees, is one example.

Acute podagra due to periarticular BCP deposition can mimic gout; it occurs as a discrete syndrome in young women (less often in young men) and is treated the same as acute gout.

Besides synovial fluid analysis, x-rays should be taken of symptomatic joints. On x-ray, BCP crystals may be visible as periarticular cloudlike opacities; the crystals often spontaneously resolve over months or occasionally within days. Definitive assay for BCP crystals in synovial fluid is not readily available. Clumped crystals can be identified only with transmission electron microscopy. The clumps are not birefringent under polarized light.

Treatment with oral colchicine, an NSAID, or, if a large joint is involved, intra-articular corticosteroid ester crystal suspension is helpful. Treatment is the same as that for acute gout.

Ca oxalate crystal deposition disease: Ca oxalate crystal deposition is rare. It occurs most often in azotemic patients receiving hemodialysis or peritoneal dialysis, particularly those treated with ascorbic acid (vitamin C), which is metabolized to oxalate.

Crystals may deposit in blood vessel walls and skin, as well as joints. The crystals appear as birefringent bipyramidal structures. Synovial fluid may have > 2000 WBC/μL. On x-ray, Ca oxalate crystals are indistinguishable from BCP periarticular calcifications or CPPD crystal deposits in cartilage.

Treatment is the same as that for CPPD crystals.

36 Foot and Ankle Disorders

Most foot problems result from anatomic disorders or abnormal function of articular or extra-articular structures (see Fig. 36–1). Less commonly, foot problems reflect a systemic disorder (see Table 36–1).

In people with diabetes and people with peripheral vascular disease, careful examination of the feet, with evaluation of vascular sufficiency and neurologic integrity, should be done at least twice/yr. People with these diseases should examine their own feet at least once/day.

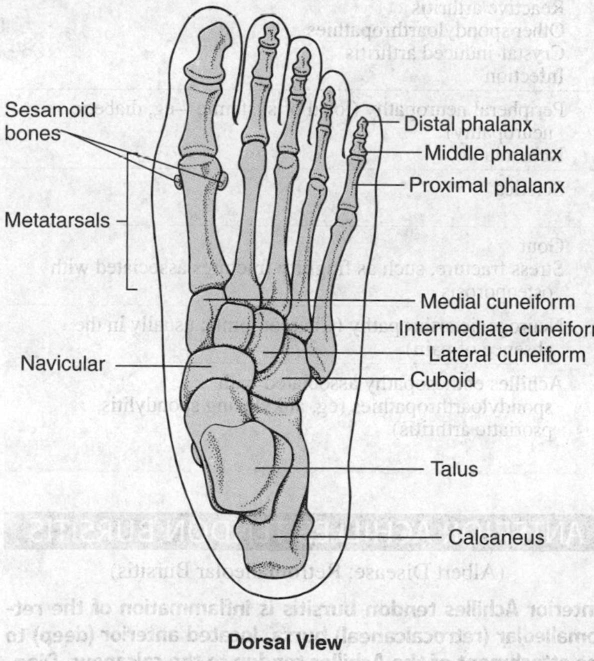

The feet are also common sites for corns and calluses and infections by fungus, bacteria, and viruses.

For foot and ankle disorders according to anatomic site, see Table 36–2. For common causes of heel pain according to location, see Table 36–3.

Fig. 36–1. Bones of the foot.

ACHILLES TENDON ENTHESOPATHY

Achilles tendon enthesopathy is pain at the insertion of the Achilles tendon at the posterosuperior aspect of the calcaneus. Diagnosis is clinical. Treatment is with stretching, splinting, and heel lifts.

The cause of Achilles tendon enthesopathy is chronic traction of the Achilles tendon on the calcaneus. Contracted or shortened calf muscles (resulting from a sedentary lifestyle and obesity) and athletic overuse are factors. Enthesopathy may be caused by a spondyloarthropathy.

Pain at the posterior heel below the top of the shoe counter during ambulation is characteristic. Pain on palpation of the tendon at its insertion in a patient with these symptoms is diagnostic. Manual dorsiflexion of the ankle during palpation usually exacerbates the pain. Recurrent and especially multifocal enthesitis should prompt evaluation (history and examination) for a spondyloarthropathy.

Treatment

- Stretching, splinting, and heel lifts

Physical therapy is essential for home exercise programs aimed at calf muscle–stretching techniques, which should be done for about 10 min 2 to 3 times/day. The patient can exert pressure posteriorly to stretch the calf muscle while facing a wall at arms' length, with knees extended and foot dorsiflexed by the patient's body weight. To minimize stress to the Achilles tendon with weight bearing, the patient should move the foot and ankle actively through their range of motion for about

Table 36–1. FOOT MANIFESTATIONS OF SYSTEMIC DISORDERS

FOOT SYMPTOMS OR SIGNS	POSSIBLE CAUSE
Pain at rest (feet elevated), relieved by dependency	End-stage peripheral arterial disease
Cold, red, or cyanotic feet	Advanced arterial ischemia
Episodically red, hot, very painful, burning feet	Erythromelalgia—idiopathic (most commonly) or secondary to various disorders (eg, myeloproliferative disorders, which are rare)
Foot pain that becomes severe within seconds or possibly minutes, particularly in patients with atrial fibrillation; foot often cool	Embolic arterial occlusion
Cyanosis of a single toe (blue toe syndrome)	Thromboembolic disease due to aortic-iliac stenosis, arrhythmia, or cholesterol embolization (after coronary artery bypass or catheterization) Warfarin therapy
Bilateral episodic digital discomfort, pallor, and cyanosis	Raynaud syndrome
Bilateral painless cyanosis	Acrocyanosis, drug-induced discoloration (eg, minocycline)
Bilateral edema	Renal, hepatic, or cardiac dysfunction Drugs (eg, calcium channel blockers)
Unilateral edema	Deep venous thrombosis Lymphatic obstruction
Firm nonpitting foot and leg edema	Lymphedema Systemic sclerosis
Firm, nonpitting edema with nodular appearance above the malleoli	Pretibial myxedema
Edema with hemosiderin deposition and brownish discoloration	Venous insufficiency Recurrent or prior small-vessel vasculitis
Edema of feet and toes, numbness and pain at the ankle and heel (tarsal tunnel syndrome)	Hypothyroidism Relapsing symmetric seronegative synovitis (rare)
Red, dusky patches on the dorsum with flaccid bullae (necrolytic acral erythema)	Hepatitis C Vasculitis Emboli
Isolated toe swelling and deformity (dactylitis, or sausage digits) with pain	Psoriatic arthritis Reactive arthritis Other spondyloarthropathies Crystal-induced arthritis Infection
Painful feet with paresthesias	Peripheral neuropathy (local or systemic—eg, diabetic neuropathy) Ischemia
Pain or paresthesias in the leg and foot; pain in the foot and back when the leg is extended, relieved when the knee is flexed	Sciatica
Toe, foot, or ankle pain with warmth and redness	Gout Stress fracture, such as fragility fractures associated with osteoporosis
Foot swelling, redness, and warmth with little or no pain	Neurogenic arthropathy (Charcot joints; usually in the absence of pain)
Posterior heel pain below the top of the shoe counter during ambulation Tendon tenderness at its insertion (diagnostic) Exacerbation of tendon pain by passive ankle dorsiflexion	Achilles enthesopathy associated with spondyloarthropathies (eg, ankylosing spondylitis, psoriatic arthritis)

1 min when rising after extended periods of rest. Night splints may also be prescribed to provide passive stretch during sleep and help prevent contractures.

Heel lifts should be used temporarily to decrease tendon stress during weight bearing and relieve pain. Even if the pain is only in one heel, heel lifts should be used bilaterally to prevent gait disturbance and possible secondary (compensatory) hip and or low back pain.

ANTERIOR ACHILLES TENDON BURSITIS

(Albert Disease; Retromalleolar Bursitis)

Anterior Achilles tendon bursitis is inflammation of the retromalleolar (retrocalcaneal) bursa, located anterior (deep) to the attachment of the Achilles tendon to the calcaneus. Diagnosis is mainly clinical. Treatment may include local injection.

Table 36–2. COMMON FOOT AND ANKLE DISORDERS BY ANATOMIC SITE

Ankle (anterolateral)
Meniscoid body
Neuralgia of the intermediate dorsal cutaneous nerve
Peroneal tenosynovitis
Ankle (medial)
Tarsal tunnel syndrome
Tibialis posterior tendinosis
Tibialis posterior tenosynovitis
Ball of the foot
Corns and calluses
Freiberg disease
Interdigital nerve pain (Morton neuroma)
Metatarsophalangeal joint pain
Sesamoiditis
Heel (plantar)
Inferior calcaneal bursitis
Medial or lateral plantar nerve entrapment
Plantar fasciosis
Heel (posterior)
Achilles tendon enthesopathy
Anterior Achilles tendon bursitis
Posterior Achilles tendon bursitis
Heel (sides)
Epiphysitis of the calcaneus (Sever disease)
Tarsal tunnel syndrome
Plantar arch (sole)
Cuboid subluxation syndrome
Plantar fascial sprain
Plantar fibromatosis
Posterior tibial tendon rupture with arch collapse
Toe
Bunion
Dactylitis (painful, isolated toe swelling due to inflammatory arthritis)
Hallux rigidus
Hammer toe
Ingrown toenail
Onychomycosis
Paronychia

Bursitis is due to trauma (eg, caused by rigid or poorly fitting shoes) or inflammatory arthritis (eg, RA, gout). On occasion, small calcaneal erosions may result from severe inflammation (see Fig. 36–2 on p. 280).

Symptoms and Signs

Symptoms and signs caused by trauma or gout develop rapidly; those caused by another systemic disorder develop gradually. Pain, swelling, and warmth around the heel are common, as are difficulty walking and wearing shoes. The bursa is tender. Initially, the swelling is localized anterior to the Achilles tendon but in time extends medially and laterally.

Diagnosis

- Clinical evaluation and x-rays

Fracture of the posterolateral talar tubercle usually causes tenderness anterior to the insertion of the Achilles tendon. Bursitis is often differentiated from the fracture by the localization of warmth and swelling contiguous to the tendon and pain localized primarily in the soft tissue. Also, using the thumb and index finger, compressing side-to-side anterior to the Achilles tendon causes pain. X-rays are taken to rule out fracture and to reveal erosive calcaneal changes characteristic of chronic RA or other rheumatic disorders.

Treatment

- Intrabursal injection of a soluble corticosteroid/anesthetic solution

A corticosteroid/anesthetic injection, NSAIDs, and warm or cold compresses may be effective. Care must be taken to inject only the bursal sac and not the tendon proper because tendon injection may lead to tendon weakening or tearing, predisposing to subsequent rupture.

BUNION

Bunion is a prominence of the medial portion of the head of the 1st metatarsal bone. The cause is often variations in position of the 1st metatarsal bone or great toe, such as lateral angulation of the great toe (hallux valgus). Secondary osteoarthritis and spur formation are common. Symptoms may include pain and redness, bursitis medial to the joint, and mild synovitis. Diagnosis is usually clinical. Treatment is usually a shoe with a wide toe box, protective pads, and orthotics. For bursitis or synovitis, corticosteroid injection may be helpful.

Contributing factors may include excessive foot pronation, wearing tight and pointed-toe shoes, and occasionally trauma.

Table 36–3. DISORDERS ASSOCIATED WITH HEEL PAIN ACCORDING TO LOCATION

LOCATION OF PAIN	ASSOCIATED DISORDER
Plantar surface of the heel	Inferior calcaneal bursitis Plantar fasciosis (plantar fasciitis, calcaneal spur syndrome)
Medial and lateral margins of the heel	In children, epiphysitis of the calcaneus (Sever disease) Medial or lateral plantar nerve entrapment Sometimes tarsal tunnel syndrome
Anterior to the Achilles tendon at the retromalleolar space	Anterior Achilles tendon bursitis Fracture of the posterolateral talar tubercle Tarsal tunnel syndrome Tibialis posterior tendinosis
Posterior to the Achilles tendon	Posterior Achilles tendon bursitis Tendon nodules
Calcaneal insertion or body of the Achilles tendon	Achilles tendon enthesopathy Tendon tear (due to trauma or associated with fluoroquinolone use—see Achilles Tendon Tears on p. 3005)

Joint misalignment causes osteoarthritis with cartilage erosion and exostosis formation, resulting in joint motion being limited (hallux limitus) or eliminated (hallux rigidus). In late stages, synovitis occurs, causing joint swelling. In reaction to pressure from tight shoes, an adventitious bursa can develop medial to the joint prominence, which can become painful, swollen, and inflamed (see Fig. 36–3).

Symptoms and Signs

The initial symptom of bunion may be pain at the joint prominence when wearing certain shoes. The joint capsule may be tender at any stage. Later symptoms may include a painful, warm, red, cystic, movable, fluctuant swelling located medially (adventitial bursitis) and swellings and mild inflammation affecting the entire joint (osteoarthritic synovitis), which is more circumferential. With hallux limitus or rigidus, there is restriction of passive joint motion, tenderness at the dorsolateral aspect of the joint, and increased dorsiflexion of the distal phalanx.

Diagnosis

- Clinical evaluation

Clinical findings are usually specific. Acute circumferential intense pain, warmth, swelling, and redness suggest gouty arthritis or infectious arthritis, sometimes mandating examination of synovial fluid. If multiple joints are affected, gout or another systemic rheumatic disease should be considered.

If clinical diagnosis of osteoarthritic synovitis is equivocal, x-rays are taken. Suggestive findings include joint space narrowing and bony spurs extending from the metatarsal head or sometimes from the base of the proximal phalanx. Periarticular erosions (Martel sign) seen on imaging studies suggest gout.

Treatment

- Wide toe box, bunion pads, orthotics, or a combination
- Treatment of complications

Mild discomfort may lessen by wearing a shoe with a wide toe box or with stretchable material. If not, bunion pads purchased in most pharmacies can shield the painful area. Orthotics can also be prescribed to redistribute and relieve pressure from the affected articulation. If conservative therapy fails, surgery aimed at correcting abnormal bony alignments and restoring

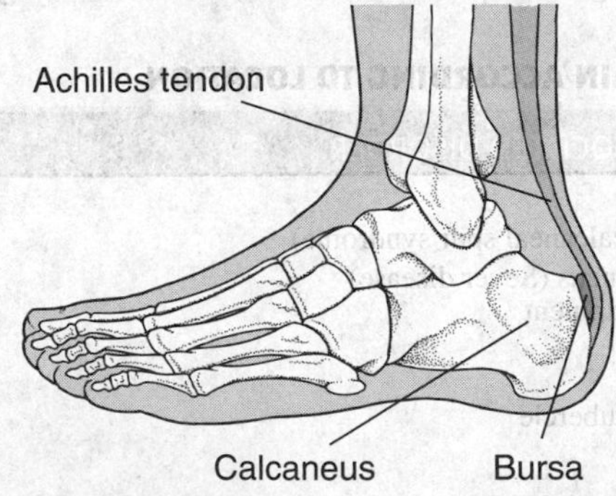

Fig. 36–2. Bursitis in the heel. Normally, only one bursa is in the heel, between the Achilles tendon and the calcaneus. This bursa may become inflamed, swollen, and painful, resulting in anterior Achilles tendon bursitis.

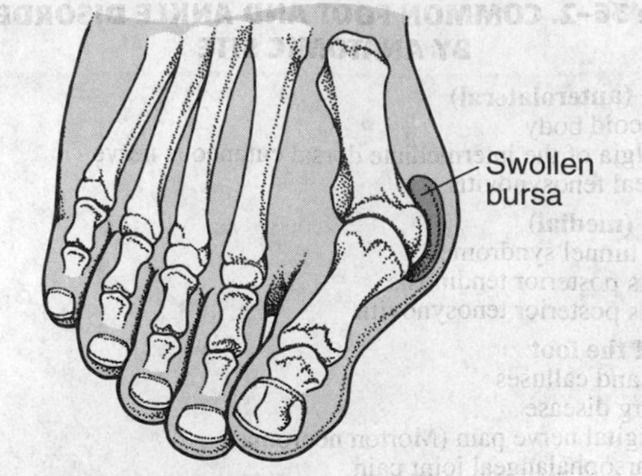

Fig. 36–3. Bunion. A bunion is often caused by hallux valgus. A bursa may result from pressure caused by tight-fitting shoes.

joint mobility should be considered. If the patient is unwilling to wear larger, wider shoes to accommodate the bunion because they are unattractive, surgery can be considered; however, patients should be told that orthotic devices should be worn after surgery to reduce the risk of recurrence.

For bursitis, bursal aspiration and injection of a corticosteroid are indicated.

For osteoarthritic synovitis, oral NSAIDs or an intra-articular injection of a corticosteroid/anesthetic solution reduces symptoms.

For hallux limitus or hallux rigidus, treatment aims to preserve joint mobility by using passive stretching exercises, which occasionally require injection of a local anesthetic to relieve muscle spasm. Sometimes surgical release of contractures is necessary.

KEY POINTS

- Excessive turning in (supination) of the ankles, wearing tight and pointed-toe shoes, and occasionally trauma increase the risk of prominences at the medial 1st metatarsal joints (bunions).
- Symptoms can include pain, synovial or cystic swelling, and limitation of passive joint motion.
- Use clinical findings to confirm the diagnosis.
- Treat initially with a wide or expansile toe box, bunion pads, orthotics, or a combination.

EPIPHYSITIS OF THE CALCANEUS

(Sever Disease)

Epiphysitis of the calcaneus is painful disruption between the calcaneal apophysis and the body of the heel that occurs before calcaneal ossification is complete. Diagnosis is clinical. Treatment is with heel pads and splinting or casting.

The calcaneus develops from two centers of ossification: one begins at birth, the other usually after age 8. Ossification is usually complete by age 15. The cartilaginous disruption in calcaneal epiphysitis may result from an excessive pull on the apophysis by contracted or shortened calf muscles. Bone growth spurts without adaptive calf muscle lengthening may play a role.

Pain develops in patients (usually aged 9 to 14) with a history of athletic activity, especially those who wear footwear without elevation of the heel (such as track flats or soccer cleats); it affects the sides or margins of the heel and is aggravated by standing on tip toes or running. Warmth and swelling are occasionally present.

The diagnosis is clinical. X-rays are not usually helpful.

Treatment

- Heel pads and splinting or casting

Pads that elevate the heel relieve symptoms by reducing the pull of the Achilles tendon on the heel. Night splints may be used to passively stretch the calf muscles, helping maintain flexibility. Rest, ice, activity modifications, and the use of heel pads usually relieve pain. In more severe or recalcitrant cases, cast immobilization may be used to relieve pain and stretch the calf muscles. Reassurance is important because symptoms may last several months but are self-limiting.

FREIBERG DISEASE

(Freiberg Infraction)

Freiberg disease is avascular necrosis of the metatarsal head. Pain is most pronounced with weight bearing. Diagnosis is confirmed with x-rays. Treatment includes corticosteroid injections, immobilization, and orthotics.

Freiberg disease is a common cause of metatarsalgia. Freiberg disease is caused by microtrauma at the metaphysis and growth plate. Avascular necrosis flattens the metatarsal head. The 2nd metatarsal head is most often affected. Freiberg disease is thought to occur more frequently among pubertal females and among people who have a short 1st metatarsal bone or long 2nd metatarsal bone, which increases stress on the 2nd metatarsal head and joint. The metatarsal joint tends to collapse, and activities that repetitively stress this joint, such as dancing, jogging, or running, may accelerate this process.

Symptoms and Signs

The pain is most pronounced in the forefoot at the metatarsal head with weight bearing, particularly when pushing off or when wearing high-heeled footwear. The metatarsophalangeal joint may also be swollen and have limited and painful passive range of motion.

Diagnosis

- X-rays

The diagnosis of Freiberg disease is confirmed with x-rays. Typically, the head of the 2nd metatarsal is widened and flattened, and the metatarsal joint is sclerotic and irregular.

Treatment

- Immobilization and weight unloading if acute, then modification of footwear

Corticosteroid injections and immobilization may help to alleviate acutely painful flare-ups. Long-term management of Freiberg disease may require orthoses with metatarsal bars and low-heeled footwear, possibly with rocker sole modifications, to help reduce stress on the 2nd metatarsal head and joint. Rarely, surgical excision of the metatarsal head may be necessary to relieve recalcitrant pain.

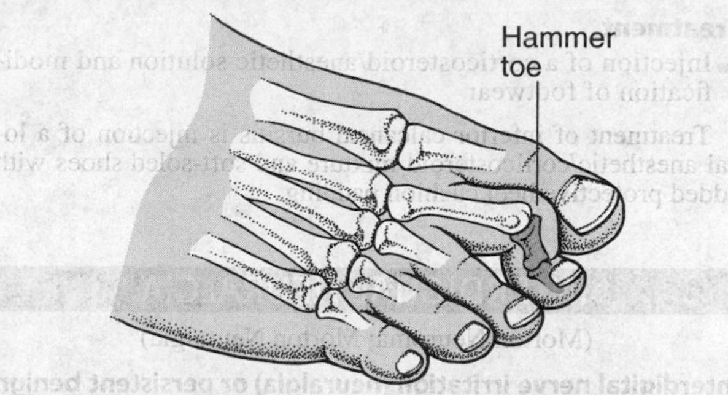

Fig. 36–4. Hammer toe. In hammer toe, usually the 2nd toe, or sometimes another lesser toe, develops a fixed Z-shaped deformity.

HAMMER TOE DEFORMITY

Hammer toe is a Z-shaped deformity caused by dorsal subluxation at the metatarsophalangeal joint. Diagnosis is clinical. Treatment is modification of footwear and/or orthotics.

The usual cause of hammer toe deformity is misalignment of the joint surfaces due to a genetic predisposition toward aberrant foot biomechanics and tendon contractures. RA and neurologic disorders such as Charcot-Marie-Tooth disease (see Hereditary Neuropathies on p. 1984) are other causes. The 2nd toe is the most common digit to develop a hammer toe deformity (see Fig. 36–4). Second toe hammer toes commonly result from an elongated 2nd metatarsal and from pressure due to an excessively abducted great toe (hallux valgus deformity) causing a bunion. Unusually long toes often develop hammer toe deformities. Painful corns often develop in hammer toe deformity, particularly of the 5th toe. Reactive adventitial bursas often develop beneath corns, which may become inflamed.

Symptoms of hammer toe deformity include pain while wearing shoes, especially shoes with low and narrow toe boxes, and sometimes metatarsalgia.

Diagnosis is clinical. Joints are examined for coexistent arthritis (eg, RA—see p. 304).

Treatment

- Wide toe box, toe pads, orthotics, or a combination

Shoes should have a wide toe box. Toe pads sold in pharmacies also help by shielding the affected toes from the overlying shoe. If conservative measures are ineffective, surgical correction of the deformity often relieves symptoms. If there is accompanying metatarsalgia, OTC or prescription orthotic devices with metatarsal pads and cushioning may help alleviate the pain.

INFERIOR CALCANEAL BURSITIS

Bursitis can develop at the inferior calcaneus, near the insertion of the plantar fascia.

Symptoms and signs of inferior calcaneal bursitis include throbbing heel pain, particularly when the shoes are removed; mild warmth; and swelling. The pain is most pronounced when the heel first contacts the ground during walking or running activity.

Treatment

- Injection of a corticosteroid/anesthetic solution and modification of footwear

Treatment of inferior calcaneal bursitis is injection of a local anesthetic/corticosteroid mixture and soft-soled shoes with added protective heel cushion padding.

INTERDIGITAL NEURALGIA

(Morton Neuroma; Morton Neuralgia)

Interdigital nerve irritation (neuralgia) or persistent benign enlargement of the perineurium (neuroma) can cause pain, which may be nonspecific, burning, or lancinating, or a foreign body sensation. Diagnosis is usually clinical. Treatment may involve correction of footwear, local injection, or sometimes surgical excision.

Interdigital neuralgia is a common cause of metatarsalgia. The interdigital nerves of the foot travel beneath and between the metatarsals, extending distally to innervate the toes. Neuralgia of the interdigital nerve along its distal innervation near the ball of the foot develops primarily as a result of improper or constrictive footwear or, less commonly, nerve traction resulting from abnormal foot structure (eg, splayfoot deformity). As a result of chronic repetitive trauma, a benign thickening of the nerve develops (Morton neuroma).

Symptoms and Signs

Interdigital neuralgia is characterized by pain around the metatarsal heads or the toes. Early interdigital neuralgia often causes an occasional mild ache or discomfort in the ball of the foot, usually when wearing a specific shoe, such as those that are too narrow at the front. Neuralgia is usually unilateral. As the condition progresses, the nerve thickens. The pain becomes worse, often with a burning or lancinating quality or paresthesias. In time, patients are unable to wear most closed-toe shoes. While walking, patients often falsely sense a pebble in their shoes, which they take off for relief. Neuroma most frequently affects the 3rd interspace. Only slightly less common is involvement of the 2nd interspace. Sometimes both interspaces or feet are involved simultaneously.

Diagnosis

- Clinical evaluation

The symptoms of interdigital neuralgia are often specific, and the diagnosis is confirmed by tenderness on plantar palpation of the interdigital space and by reproduction of the radiating burning pain, often accompanied by a notable click, by squeezing the space (Mulder sign). Although MRI does not usually confirm neuroma, it may be useful to rule out other interspace lesions or arthritis causing similar symptoms.

Treatment

- Modification of footwear and injection

Neuralgia of recent onset usually resolves quickly with properly fitting shoes and insoles or with local anesthetic injection. Using a metatarsal pad placed proximally to the metatarsal heads of the affected interspace may also help reduce symptoms.

Neuromas may require one or more perineural infiltrations of long-acting corticosteroids with a local anesthetic. Injection is at a 45° angle to the foot, into the interspace at the level of the dorsal aspect of the metatarsophalangeal joints. Orthotics with neuroma pads, rest, cold packs, and properly fitting shoes often relieve symptoms. Nerve ablation techniques, such as injecting 20% alcohol with a local anesthetic directly into the nerve with ultrasonographic guidance, or cryogenic freezing of the nerve may help relieve symptoms. If other treatments are ineffective, excision often brings complete relief. Another neuroma occasionally develops at the site of nerve excision (amputation or stump neuroma), which may require additional surgery.

KEY POINTS

- Metatarsal pain can result from irritation or benign thickening of the interdigital nerves.
- Initially, mild pain caused by wearing narrow shoes can worsen and become lancinating, sometimes with paresthesias and/or a foreign body sensation.
- Diagnose the disorder by clinical findings, including tenderness and reproduction of symptoms with palpation of the interdigital space.
- Treat by modifying footwear, giving local anesthetic injections and sometimes corticosteroid injections, doing nerve ablation techniques, or doing surgery.

MEDIAL AND LATERAL PLANTAR NERVE ENTRAPMENT

Medial and lateral plantar nerve entrapment is symptomatic compression of the medial and/or lateral branches of the posterior tibial nerve at the medial heel and proximal arch. Diagnosis is clinical. Treatment involves orthotics and immobilization.

Symptoms of medial and lateral plantar nerve entrapment include almost constant pain, with and without weight bearing, which helps to differentiate medial and lateral plantar nerve entrapment from plantar fasciosis. The pain is often chronic, intractable, and aggravated by high-impact activities such as running. However, simple standing is often difficult. Burning, numbness, and paresthesias are usually absent.

Diagnosis

- Clinical evaluation

Medial and lateral plantar nerve entrapment may be confused with plantar fasciosis and heel spur pain as well as tarsal tunnel syndrome. In plantar nerve entrapment, the following are often present:

- Other signs of tarsal tunnel syndrome (eg, Tinel sign) are often absent.
- Symptoms can be reproduced by palpation over the proximal aspect of the abductor hallucis, the origin of the plantar fascia, or both at the medial tubercle of the calcaneus.
- With medial nerve entrapment, there is tenderness of the proximal medial arch beneath the navicular bone, sometimes with pain that radiates to the medial toes.
- With lateral plantar nerve entrapment, there is tenderness over the plantar medial heel and abductor hallucis muscle.

Treatment

- Orthoses, immobilization, and physical therapy

Immobilization and foot orthoses to prevent irritating motion and pressure may be helpful, as may physical therapy and cryotherapy. If these treatments are ineffective, injection with a sclerosing agent that contains alcohol or careful surgical decompression of the nerve may help relieve pain.

METATARSALGIA

Metatarsalgia is a general term for pain in the area of the metatarsophalangeal joints. Most common causes include

- Freiberg disease
- Interdigital nerve pain (Morton neuroma)
- Metatarsophalangeal joint pain
- Sesamoiditis
- Submetatarsal head fat pad atrophy typically associated with aging

METATARSOPHALANGEAL JOINT PAIN

Metatarsophalangeal joint pain usually results from tissue changes due to aberrant foot biomechanics. Symptoms and signs include pain with walking and tenderness. Diagnosis is clinical; however, infection or systemic rheumatic diseases (eg, RA) may need to be excluded by testing. Treatment includes orthotics, sometimes local injection, and occasionally surgery.

Metatarsophalangeal joint pain is a common cause of metatarsalgia. Metatarsophalangeal joint pain most commonly results from misalignment of the joint surfaces with altered foot biomechanics, causing joint subluxations, flexor plate tears, capsular impingement, and joint cartilage destruction (osteoarthrosis). Misaligned joints may cause synovial impingement, with minimal if any heat and swelling (osteoarthritic synovitis).

The 2nd metatarsophalangeal joint is most commonly affected. Usually, inadequate 1st ray (1st cuneiform and 1st metatarsal) function results from excessive pronation (the foot rolling inward and the hindfoot turning outward or everted), often leading to capsulitis and hammer toe deformities. Overactivity of the anterior shin muscles in patients with pes cavus (high arch) and ankle equinus (shortened Achilles tendon that restricts ankle dorsiflexion) deformities tends to cause dorsal joint subluxations with retracted (clawed) digits and retrograde, increased submetatarsal head pressure and pain.

Metatarsophalangeal joint subluxations also occur as a result of chronic inflammatory arthropathy, particularly RA. Metatarsophalangeal joint pain with weight bearing and a sense of stiffness in the morning can be significant early signs of early RA. Inflammatory synovitis and interosseous muscle atrophy in RA lead to subluxations of the lesser metatarsophalangeal joints as well, resulting in hammer toe deformities. Consequently, the metatarsal fat pad, which usually cushions the stress between the metatarsals and interdigital nerves during walking, moves distally under the toes; interdigital neuralgia or Morton neuroma may result. To compensate for the loss of cushioning, adventitial calluses and bursae may develop. Coexisting rheumatoid nodules beneath or near the plantarflexed metatarsal heads may increase pain.

Metatarsophalangeal joint pain may also result from functional hallux limitus, which limits passive and active joint motion at the 1st metatarsophalangeal joint. Patients usually have foot pronation disorders that result in elevation of the 1st ray with lowering of the medial longitudinal arch during weight bearing. As a result of the 1st ray elevation, the proximal phalanx of the great toe cannot freely extend on the 1st metatarsal head; the result is jamming at the dorsal joint leading to osteoarthritic changes and loss of joint motion. Over time, pain may develop. Another cause of 1st metatarsophalangeal joint pain due to limited motion is direct trauma with stenosis of the flexor hallucis brevis, usually occurring within the tarsal tunnel. If pain is chronic, the joint may become less mobile with an arthrosis (hallux rigidus), which can be debilitating.

Acute arthritis can occur secondary to systemic arthritides such as gout, RA, and spondyloarthropathy.

Symptoms and Signs

Symptoms of metatarsophalangeal joint pain include pain on walking. Dorsal and plantar joint tenderness is usually present on palpation and during passive range of motion. Mild swelling with minimal heat occurs in osteoarthritic synovitis. Significant warmth, swelling, or redness suggests inflammatory arthropathies or infection.

Diagnosis

- Mainly clinical evaluation
- Exclusion of infection or arthropathy if signs of inflammation

Metatarsophalangeal joint pain can usually be differentiated from neuralgia or neuroma of the interdigital nerves by the absence of burning, numbness, tingling, and interspace pain, but these symptoms may result from joint inflammation; if so, palpation can help with differentiation.

Monarticular heat, redness, and swelling indicate infection until proven otherwise, although gout is more likely. When warmth, redness, and swelling involve multiple joints, evaluation for a systemic cause of joint inflammation (eg, gout, RA, viral-associated arthritis, enteropathic arthritis) with a rheumatic disease assessment (eg, anticyclic citrullinated peptide antibody [anti-CCP], rheumatoid factor [RF], ESR) is indicated.

Treatment

- Orthoses

Foot orthoses with metatarsal pads may help redistribute and relieve pressure from the noninflamed joints. With excess subtalar eversion or when the feet are highly arched, an orthotic that corrects these abnormal alignments should be prescribed. Shoes with rocker sole modifications may also help. For functional hallux limitus, orthosis modifications may further help to plantarflex the 1st ray to improve metatarsophalangeal joint motion and reduce pain. If the 1st ray elevation cannot be reduced by these means, an extended 1st ray elevation pad may be helpful. For more severe limitation of 1st metatarsophalangeal motion or pain, the use of rigid orthoses, carbon fiber plates, or external shoe bars or rocker soles may be necessary to reduce motion at the joint.

Surgery may be needed if conservative therapies are ineffective. If inflammation (synovitis) is present, injection of a local corticosteroid/anesthetic mixture may be useful.

KEY POINTS

- Metatarsophalangeal joint pain most often results from misalignment of joint surfaces, causing synovial impingement with only minimal warmth and swelling, but may be the initial manifestation of RA.
- Patients have dorsal and plantar joint tenderness with usually minimal signs of acute inflammation.

- Diagnose metatarsophalangeal joint pain by the absence of burning, numbness, tingling, and interspace pain (suggesting interdigital nerve pain) and by palpation.
- Correct foot biomechanics with orthoses.

PLANTAR FASCIOSIS

(Plantar Fasciitis)

Plantar fasciosis is pain at the site of the attachment of the plantar fascia and the calcaneus (calcaneal enthesopathy), with or without accompanying pain along the medial band of the plantar fascia. Diagnosis is mainly clinical. Treatment involves calf muscle and plantar soft-tissue foot-stretching exercises, night splints, orthotics, and shoes with appropriate heel elevation.

Syndromes of pain in the plantar fascia have been called plantar fasciitis; however, because there is usually no inflammation, plantar fasciosis is more correct. Other terms used include calcaneal enthesopathy pain or calcaneal spur syndrome; however, there may be no bone spurs on the calcaneus. Plantar fasciosis may involve acute or chronic stretching, tearing, and degeneration of the fascia at its attachment site.

Etiology

Recognized causes of plantar fasciosis include shortening or contracture of the calf muscles and plantar fascia. Risk factors for such shortening include a sedentary lifestyle, occupations requiring sitting, very high or low arches in the feet, and chronic wearing of high-heel shoes. The disorder is also common among runners and dancers and may occur in people whose occupations involve standing or walking on hard surfaces for prolonged periods.

Disorders that may be associated with plantar fasciosis are obesity, RA, reactive arthritis, and psoriatic arthritis. Multiple injections of corticosteroids may contribute by causing degenerative changes of the fascia and possible loss of the cushioning subcalcaneal fat pad.

Symptoms and Signs

Plantar fasciosis is characterized by pain at the bottom of the heel with weight bearing, particularly when first arising in the morning; pain usually abates within 5 to 10 min, only to return later in the day. It is often worse when pushing off of the heel (the propulsive phase of gait) and after periods of rest. Acute, severe heel pain, especially with mild local puffiness, may indicate an acute fascial tear. Some patients describe burning or sticking pain along the plantar medial border of the foot when walking.

Diagnosis

- Pain reproduced by calcaneal pressure during dorsiflexion

Other disorders causing heel pain can mimic plantar fasciosis:

- Throbbing heel pain, particularly when the shoes are removed or when mild heat and puffiness are present, is more suggestive of calcaneal bursitis.
- Acute, severe retrocalcaneal pain, with redness and heat, may indicate gout.
- Pain that radiates from the low back to the heel may be an S1 radiculopathy due to an L5 disk herniation.

Plantar fasciosis is confirmed if firm thumb pressure applied to the calcaneus when the foot is dorsiflexed elicits pain. Fascial pain along the plantar medial border of the fascia may also be present. If findings are equivocal, demonstration of a heel spur on x-ray may support the diagnosis; however, absence does not rule out the diagnosis, and visible spurs are not generally the cause of plantar fasciosis symptoms. Also, infrequently, calcaneal spurs appear ill-defined on x-ray, exhibiting fluffy new bone formation, suggesting spondyloarthropathy (eg, ankylosing spondylitis, reactive arthritis). If an acute fascial tear is suspected, MRI is done.

Treatment

- Splinting, stretching, and cushioning or orthotics

To alleviate the stress and pain on the fascia, the person can take shorter steps and avoid walking barefoot. Activities that involve foot impact, such as jogging, should be avoided. The most effective plantar fasciosis treatments include the use of in-shoe heel and arch cushioning with calf-stretching exercises and night splints that stretch the calf and plantar fascia while the patient sleeps. Prefabricated or custom-made foot orthotics may also alleviate fascial tension and symptoms. Other treatments may include activity modifications, NSAIDs, weight loss in obese patients, cold and ice massage therapy, and occasional corticosteroid injections. However, because corticosteroid injections can predispose to plantar fasciosis, many clinicians limit these injections.

For recalcitrant cases, physical therapy, oral corticosteroids, and cast immobilization should be used before surgical intervention is considered. A newer form of treatment for recalcitrant types of plantar fasciosis is extracorporeal pulse activation therapy (EPAT), in which low-frequency pulse waves are delivered locally using a handheld applicator. The pulsed pressure wave is a safe, noninvasive technique that stimulates metabolism and enhances blood circulation, which helps regenerate damaged tissue and accelerate healing. EPAT is being used at major medical centers.[1]

1. Gerdesmeyer L, Frey C, Vester J, et al: Radial extracorporeal shock wave therapy is safe and effective in the treatment of chronic recalcitrant plantar fasciitis: Results of a confirmatory randomized placebo-controlled multicenter study. *Am J Sports Med* 36:2100–2109, 2008. doi: 10.1177/0363546508324176.

KEY POINTS

- Plantar fasciosis involves various syndromes causing pain in the plantar fascia.
- Various lifestyle factors and disorders increase risk by leading to shortened calf muscles and plantar fascia.
- Pain at the bottom of the heel worsens with weight bearing, particularly when pushing off the heel and over the course of the day.
- Confirm the diagnosis by reproducing pain with calcaneal pressure exerted by the thumb during dorsiflexion.
- Treat at first with in-shoe heel and arch cushioning, calf-stretching exercises, and splinting devices worn at night.

PLANTAR FIBROMATOSIS

Plantar fibromatosis is a benign proliferative neoplasia of the plantar fascia.

In plantar fibromatosis, nodules are displayed most easily when the foot is dorsiflexed against the leg. Most patients also have palmar nodules, usually located at the 4th metacarpophalangeal joint. Reported associations with diabetes, epilepsy, and alcoholism may be anecdotal.

Treatment

- If symptomatic, orthoses

Treatment of plantar fibromatosis is usually not indicated unless the nodules become large enough to cause pressure-related pain with weight bearing. If so, orthoses can help redistribute pressure away from the fibrotic nodular lesions. Surgery usually results in recurrence and sometimes painful scar tissue necessitating further surgery. Excessive fascial removal may also result in unintentional instability of the foot.

POSTERIOR ACHILLES TENDON BURSITIS

Posterior Achilles tendon bursitis is inflammation of a bursa that forms in response to shoe pressure and is located at the top edge of the posterior shoe counter between the skin and Achilles tendon. Diagnosis is clinical. Treatment is footwear modification.

This disorder occurs mainly in young women. Wearing high-heeled shoes is a risk factor. Another risk factor is a bony prominence (Haglund deformity) on the calcaneus. This deformity predisposes to bursa formation if repeatedly irritated by the shoe counter.

Symptoms and Signs

Symptoms and signs of posterior Achilles tendon bursitis develop at the top edge of the posterior shoe counter. Early symptoms may be limited to redness, pain, and warmth. Later, superficial skin erosion may occur. After months or longer, a fluctuant, tender, cystic nodule 1- to 3-cm in diameter develops. It is red or skin-colored. In chronic cases, the bursa becomes fibrotic and calcified.

Diagnosis

- Symptoms and a small, tender, and skin-colored or red nodule

The presence of the small, tender, and skin-colored or red nodule in a patient with compatible symptoms is diagnostic. Rarely, an Achilles tendon xanthoma develops at the top edge of the posterior shoe counter but tends to be pink and asymptomatic. Achilles tendon enthesopathy causes pain mainly at the tendon's insertion but may also cause pain at the top edge of the posterior shoe counter. Enthesopathy is differentiated by the absence of a soft-tissue lesion.

Treatment

- Modification of footwear

Properly fitting shoes with low heels are essential. A foam rubber or felt heel pad may be needed to lift the heel high enough so that the bursa does not contact the shoe counter. Protective gel wraps, padding around the bursa, or the wearing of a backless shoe until inflammation subsides is indicated. Foot orthotics may enhance rear foot stability and help reduce irritating motion on the posterior calcaneus while walking. Warm or cool compresses, NSAIDs, and intrabursal injection of a local anesthetic/corticosteroid solution offer temporary relief; the Achilles tendon itself must not be injected. Surgical removal of a portion of the underlying bone may rarely be necessary to reduce soft-tissue impingement.

SESAMOIDITIS

Sesamoiditis is pain at the sesamoid bones beneath the head of the 1st metatarsal, with or without inflammation or fracture. Diagnosis is usually clinical. Treatment is usually modification of footwear and orthotics.

Sesamoiditis is a common cause of metatarsalgia. The 2 semilunar-shaped sesamoid bones aid the foot in locomotion. The medial bone is the tibial sesamoid, and the lateral bone is the fibular sesamoid. Direct trauma or positional change of the sesamoids due to alterations in foot structure (eg, lateral displacement of a sesamoid due to lateral deviation of the great toe) can make the sesamoids painful. Sesamoiditis is particularly common among dancers, joggers, and people who have high-arched feet or wear high heels. Many people with bunions have tibial sesamoiditis.

Symptoms and Signs

The pain of sesamoiditis is beneath the head of the 1st metatarsal; the pain is usually made worse by ambulation and may be worse when wearing flexible thin-soled or high-heeled shoes. Occasionally, inflammation occurs, causing mild warmth and swelling or occasionally redness that may extend medially and appear to involve the 1st metatarsophalangeal joint. Sesamoid fracture can also cause pain, moderate swelling, and possibly inflammation.

Diagnosis

- Clinical evaluation
- Arthrocentesis if there is circumferential joint swelling
- Imaging if fracture, osteoarthritis, or displacement is suspected

With the foot and 1st (big) toe dorsiflexed, the examiner inspects the metatarsal head and palpates each sesamoid. Tenderness is localized to a sesamoid, usually the tibial sesamoid. Hyperkeratotic tissue may indicate that a wart or corn is causing pain. If inflammation causes circumferential swelling around the 1st metatarsophalangeal joint, arthrocentesis is usually indicated to exclude gout and infectious arthritis. If fracture, osteoarthritis, or displacement is suspected, x-rays are taken. Sesamoids separated by cartilage or fibrous tissue (bipartite sesamoids) may appear fractured on x-rays. If plain x-rays are equivocal, MRI may be done.

Treatment

- New shoes, orthotics, or both

Simply not wearing the shoes that cause pain may be sufficient. If symptoms of sesamoiditis persist, shoes with a thick sole and orthotics are prescribed and help by reducing sesamoid pressure. If fracture without displacement is present, conservative therapy may be sufficient and may also involve immobilization of the joint with the use of a flat, rigid, surgical shoe. NSAIDs and injections of a corticosteroid/local anesthetic solution can be helpful. Although surgical removal of the sesamoid may help in recalcitrant cases, it is controversial because of the potential for disturbing biomechanics and mobility of the foot. If inflammation is present, treatment includes conservative measures plus local infiltration of a corticosteroid/anesthetic solution to help reduce symptoms.

KEY POINTS

- Dancers, joggers, and people who have high-arched feet, wear high heels, or have bunions can develop pain at the sesamoids beneath the head of the 1st metatarsal.
- Pain is worse when weight-bearing, particularly when wearing certain shoes.
- Diagnose based on clinical findings; exclude infection with synovial fluid analysis when swelling is present and exclude suspected fracture with x-rays.
- Prescribe new, thick-soled shoes, orthotics that decrease pressure on the sesamoids, or both.

TARSAL TUNNEL SYNDROME

(Posterior Tibial Nerve Neuralgia)

Tarsal tunnel syndrome is pain along the course of the posterior tibial nerve, usually resulting from nerve compression within the tarsal tunnel.

At the level of the ankle, the posterior tibial nerve passes through a fibro-osseous canal and divides into the medial and lateral plantar nerves. Tarsal tunnel syndrome refers to compression of the nerve within this canal, but the term has been loosely applied to neuralgia of the posterior tibial nerve resulting from any cause. Synovitis of the flexor tendons of the ankle caused by abnormal foot function, inflammatory arthritis (eg, RA), fibrosis, ganglionic cysts, fracture, and ankle venous stasis edema are contributing factors. Patients with hypothyroidism may develop tarsal tunnel–like symptoms as a result of perineural mucin deposition.

Symptoms and Signs

Pain (occasionally burning and tingling) is usually retromalleolar and sometimes in the plantar medial heel and may extend along the plantar surface as far as the toes. Although the pain is worse during standing and walking, pain at rest may occur as the disorder progresses, which helps to distinguish it from plantar fasciosis.

Diagnosis

- Examination and electrodiagnostic testing

Tapping or palpating the posterior tibial nerve below the medial malleolus at a site of compression or injury often causes distal tingling (Tinel sign). Although false-negative results on electrodiagnostic tests are somewhat common, a positive history combined with supportive physical findings and positive electrodiagnostic results makes the diagnosis of tarsal tunnel syndrome highly likely. Plantar heel and arch pain lasting > 6 mo also strongly suggests distal tibial plantar nerve compression with entrapment. The cause of any swelling near the nerve should be determined.

Treatment

- Foot inversion with braces or orthoses, corticosteroid injections, surgery, or a combination

Strapping the foot in a neutral or slightly inverted position and elevating the heel or wearing a brace or orthotic that keeps the foot inverted reduces nerve tension. NSAIDs may be used initially and may relieve some symptoms. Local infiltration of an insoluble corticosteroid/anesthetic mixture may be effective if the cause is inflammation or fibrosis. Surgical decompression may be necessary to relieve suspected fibro-osseus compression with recalcitrant symptoms.

TIBIALIS POSTERIOR TENDINOSIS AND TIBIALIS POSTERIOR TENOSYNOVITIS

(Posterior Tibial Tendon Dysfunction)

Tibialis posterior tendinosis, which is degeneration of the tibialis posterior tendon, and tibialis posterior tenosynovitis are the most common causes of pain behind the medial malleolus.

The posterior tibial tendon lies immediately behind the medial malleolus. Degeneration results from long-standing biomechanical problems, such as excessive pronation (often in obese people) or chronic tenosynovitis.

Tenosynovitis of the tendon sheath begins with acute inflammation. The tendon can be involved by primary inflammatory disorders, such as RA or gout.

Symptoms and Signs

Early on, patients experience occasional pain behind the medial malleolus. Over time, the pain becomes severe, with painful swelling behind the medial malleolus. Normal standing, walking, and standing on the toes become difficult. If the tendon ruptures (eg, with chronic tendinosis), the foot may acutely flatten (arch collapse) and pain may extend into the sole.

In tenosynovitis, pain is typically more acute and the tendon may feel thick and swollen as it courses around the medial malleolus.

Diagnosis

- MRI

Clinical findings suggest the diagnosis. Palpation of the tendon with the foot in an inverted plantar flexed position with applied resistance is usually painful. Standing on the toes is usually painful and may not be possible if the tendon is ruptured or severely dysfunctional. Pain and swelling with tenderness of the tibialis posterior tendon behind the medial malleolus is suggestive of tenosynovitis. Unilateral arch collapse with medial ankle bulging and forefoot abduction (too many toes sign) is particularly suggestive of advanced tendon pathology and warrants testing for tendon rupture. MRI or ultrasonography can confirm a fluid collection around the tendon (indicating tenosynovitis) or the extent of chronic degradation or tearing to the tendon with associated tendinosis.

Treatment

- Orthotics and braces or surgery

Complete rupture requires surgery if normal function is the goal. Surgery is especially important in young active patients with acute tears. Conservative therapy consists of mechanically off-loading the tendon by using custom-molded ankle braces or orthotics modified with a deepened heel cup and appropriate medial wedging or posting. Corticosteroid injections exacerbate the degenerative process (see Sidebar 36–1).

For tenosynovitis, rest and aggressive anti-inflammatory therapy are warranted.

Sidebar 36–1. Considerations for Using Corticosteroid Injections

Corticosteroid injections should be used judiciously to avoid adverse effects. Injectable corticosteroids should be reserved for inflammation (such as gout and disorders such as RA), which is not present in most foot disorders. Because the tarsus, ankle, retrocalcaneal space, and dorsum of the toes have little connective tissue between the skin and underlying bone, injection of insoluble corticosteroids into these structures may cause depigmentation, atrophy, or ulceration, especially in elderly patients with peripheral arterial disease.

Insoluble corticosteroids can be given deeply rather than superficially with greater safety (eg, in the heel pad, tarsal canal, or metatarsal interspaces). The foot should be immobilized for a few days after tendon sheaths are injected. Unusual resistance to injection suggests injection into a tendon. Repeated injection into a tendon should be avoided because the tendon may weaken (partially tear), predisposing to subsequent rupture.

37 Hand Disorders

Common hand disorders include a variety of deformities, ganglia, infections, Kienböck disease, nerve compression syndromes, noninfectious tenosynovitis, and osteoarthritis. Complex regional pain syndrome (reflex sympathetic dystrophy) and hand injuries are discussed elsewhere.

Hand deformities: Deformities of the hand can result from generalized disorders (eg, arthritis) or dislocations, fractures, and other localized disorders. Most nontraumatic localized disorders can be diagnosed by physical examination. Once a hand deformity becomes firmly established, it cannot be significantly altered by splinting, exercise, or other nonsurgical treatment.

Hand infections: Common bacterial hand infections include paronychia, infected bite wounds, felon, palm abscess, and infectious flexor tenosynovitis. Herpetic whitlow is a viral hand infection. Infections often begin with constant, intense, throbbing pain and are usually diagnosed by physical examination. X-rays are taken in some infections (eg, bite wounds, infectious flexor tenosynovitis) to detect occult foreign bodies but may not detect small or radiolucent objects.

Treatment of hand infections involves surgical measures and antibiotics. The increased incidence of community-acquired and nosocomial methicillin-resistant *Staphylococcus aureus* (MRSA) should be taken into consideration.[1] Uncomplicated MRSA infections are best treated with incision and drainage.[2] If there is a high incidence of MRSA and the infection is severe, hospitalization and vancomycin or daptomycin (for IV therapy) are recommended, as is consultation with an infectious disease specialist. For outpatients, trimethoprim/sulfamethoxazole, clindamycin, doxycycline, or linezolid (for oral therapy) can be given. Once culture and sensitivity results rule out MRSA, nafcillin, cloxacillin, dicloxacillin, or a 1st- or 2nd-generation cephalosporin can be given.

1. O'Malley M, Fowler J, Ilyas AM: Community-acquired methicillin-resistant *Staphylococcus aureus* infections of the hand: Prevalence and timeliness of treatment. *J Hand Surg Am* 34(3):504–508, 2009. doi: 10.1016/j.jhsa.2008.11.021.
2. Chen WA, Plate JF, Li Z: Effect of setting of initial surgical drainage on outcome of finger infections. *J Surg Orthop Adv* 24(1):36–41, 2015.

Nerve compression syndromes of the hand: Common nerve compression syndromes include carpal tunnel syndrome, cubital tunnel syndrome, and radial tunnel syndrome. Compression of nerves often causes paresthesias; these paresthesias can often be reproduced by tapping the compressed nerve, usually with the examiner's fingertip (Tinel sign). Suspected nerve compression can be confirmed by testing nerve conduction velocity and distal latencies, which accurately measure motor and sensory nerve conduction. Initial treatment is usually conservative (eg, rest, modified work environment, splinting, corticosteroid injection), but surgical decompression may be necessary if conservative measures fail or if there are significant motor or sensory deficits.

Noninfectious tenosynovitis: Tenosynovitis may involve any of the tendons in or around the hand. Common conditions include digital flexor tendinitis and tenosynovitis (trigger finger) and De Quervain syndrome.

Evaluation

History and physical examination findings are often diagnostic in hand disorders.

History: The history should include information about the trauma or other events that may be associated with symptoms. The presence and duration of deformity and difficulty with motion are noted. The presence, duration, severity, and factors that exacerbate or relieve pain are elicited. Associated symptoms, such as fever, swelling, rashes, Raynaud syndrome, paresthesias, and weakness, are also recorded.

Physical examination: Examination should include inspection for redness, swelling, or deformity and palpation for tenderness. Active range of motion should be tested for any possible tendon injury. Passive range of motion can detect the presence of fixed deformities and assess whether specific motions aggravate pain. Sensation may be tested by 2-point discrimination, using 2 ends of a paper clip. Motor function testing involves muscles innervated by the radial, median, and ulnar nerves. Vascular examination should include evaluation of capillary refill, radial and ulnar pulses, and the Allen test (see p. 396). Stress testing is helpful when specific ligament injuries are suspected (eg, ulnar collateral ligament in gamekeeper's thumb). Provocative testing can aid in the diagnosis of tenosynovitis and nerve compression syndromes.

Laboratory testing: Laboratory testing can aid the diagnosis of inflammatory arthropathies (eg, rheumatoid arthritis) but otherwise has a limited role. Plain x-rays and MRI are helpful for detecting injuries, arthritis, and Kienböck disease or to rule out hidden foreign bodies that could be sources of infections. MRI and ultrasonography can help assess tendon structure and integrity and detect deep abscesses. High-resolution ultrasonography allows imaging in real-time motion and is especially helpful for evaluating tendons and synovitis. Nerve conduction testing can help diagnose nerve compression syndromes. Bone scan is an alternative to MRI for the diagnosis of occult fractures and can aid the diagnosis of complex regional pain syndrome.

BOUTONNIÈRE DEFORMITY

(Buttonhole Deformity)

A boutonnière deformity consists of flexion of the proximal interphalangeal (PIP) joint accompanied by hyperextension of the distal interphalangeal (DIP) joint (see Fig. 37–3 on p. 293).

This deformity can result from tendon laceration, dislocation, fracture, osteoarthritis, or rheumatoid arthritis. Classically, the deformity is caused by disruption of the central slip attachment of the extensor tendon to the base of the middle phalanx, allowing the proximal phalanx to protrude ("buttonhole") between the lateral bands of the extensor tendon.

Initial treatment of boutonnière deformity consists of splinting, but it must occur before scarring and fixed deformities develop. Surgical reconstruction often cannot restore normal motion but may decrease the deformity and improve hand function.

CARPAL TUNNEL SYNDROME

Carpal tunnel syndrome is compression of the median nerve as it passes through the carpal tunnel in the wrist. Symptoms include pain and paresthesias in the median nerve distribution. Diagnosis is suggested by symptoms and signs and is confirmed by nerve conduction velocity testing. Treatments include ergonomic improvements, analgesia, splinting, and sometimes corticosteroid injection or surgery.

Carpal tunnel syndrome is very common and most often occurs in women aged 30 to 50. Risk factors include rheumatoid arthritis or other wrist arthritis (sometimes the presenting manifestation), diabetes mellitus, hypothyroidism, acromegaly, primary or dialysis-associated amyloidosis, and pregnancy-induced edema in the carpal tunnel. Activities or jobs that require repetitive flexion and extension of the wrist may contribute, but rarely. Most cases are idiopathic.

Symptoms and Signs

Symptoms of carpal tunnel syndrome include pain of the hand and wrist associated with tingling and numbness, classically distributed along the median nerve (the palmar side of the thumb, the index and middle fingers, and the radial half of the ring finger) but possibly involving the entire hand. Typically, the patient wakes at night with burning or aching pain and with numbness and tingling and shakes the hand to obtain relief and restore sensation. Thenar atrophy and weakness of thumb opposition and abduction may develop late.

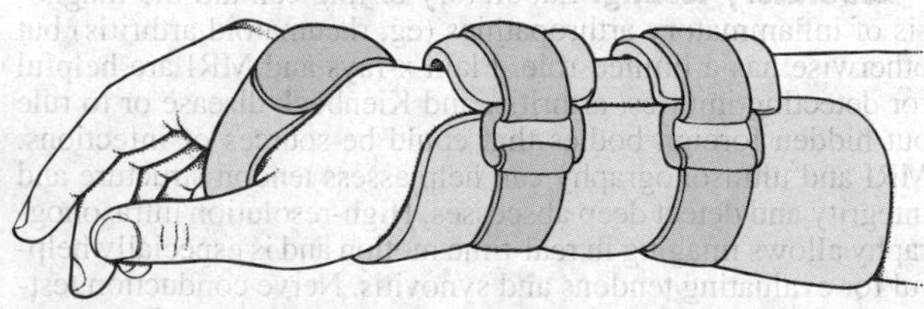

Fig. 37–1. Neutral wrist splint.

Diagnosis

- Clinical evaluation
- Sometimes nerve conduction testing

The diagnosis of carpal tunnel syndrome is strongly suggested by the Tinel sign, in which median nerve paresthesias are reproduced by tapping at the volar surface of the wrist over the site of the median nerve in the carpal tunnel. Reproduction of tingling with wrist flexion (Phalen sign) or with direct pressure on the nerve at the wrist in a neutral position (median nerve compression test) is also suggestive. The median nerve compression test is positive if symptoms develop within 30 sec. However, clinical differentiation from other types of peripheral neuropathy may sometimes be difficult.

If symptoms are severe or the diagnosis is uncertain, nerve conduction testing should be done on the affected arm for diagnosis and to exclude a more proximal neuropathy.

Treatment

- Splinting
- Treatment of underlying disorders
- Sometimes corticosteroid/anesthetic injection
- Sometimes surgical decompression

Changing the position of computer keyboards and making other ergonomic corrections may occasionally provide relief. Otherwise, treatment of carpal tunnel syndrome includes wearing a lightweight neutral wrist splint (see Fig. 37–1), especially at night, and taking mild analgesics (eg, acetaminophen, NSAIDs).

Treating any underlying disorders (eg, diabetes, rheumatoid arthritis, hypothyroidism) can help relieve symptoms.

If these measures do not control symptoms, a mixture of an anesthetic and a corticosteroid (eg, 1.5 mL of a 4-mg/mL dexamethasone solution mixed with 1.5 mL of 1% lidocaine) should be injected into the carpal tunnel at a site just ulnar to the palmaris longus tendon and proximal to the distal crease at the wrist.

If bothersome symptoms persist or recur or if hand weakness and thenar wasting develop, the carpal tunnel can be surgically decompressed by using an open or endoscopic technique.

KEY POINTS

- Although carpal tunnel syndrome has many risk factors, most cases are idiopathic.
- Typical symptoms include wrist and hand pain with tingling and numbness along the palmar side of the thumb, the index and middle fingers, and the radial half of the ring finger.
- Reproducing symptoms with wrist flexion or pressure over the median nerve can provide helpful diagnostic clues.
- Treat first with ergonomic corrections, then try splinting and analgesics, corticosteroid injection, and, for weakness, muscle wasting, and/or severe unresponsive symptoms, surgical decompression.

CUBITAL TUNNEL SYNDROME

(Ulnar Neuropathy)

Cubital tunnel syndrome is compression or traction of the ulnar nerve at the elbow. Symptoms include elbow pain and paresthesias in the ulnar nerve distribution. Diagnosis

is suggested by symptoms and signs and sometimes nerve conduction studies. Treatments include splinting and sometimes surgical decompression.

The ulnar nerve is commonly irritated at the elbow or, rarely, the wrist. Cubital tunnel syndrome is most often caused by leaning on the elbow or by prolonged and excessive elbow flexion. It is less common than carpal tunnel syndrome. Baseball pitching (particularly sliders), which can injure the medial elbow ligaments, confers risk.

Symptoms and Signs

Symptoms of cubital tunnel syndrome include numbness and paresthesia along the ulnar nerve distribution (in the ring and little fingers and the ulnar aspect of the hand) and elbow pain. In advanced stages, weakness of the intrinsic muscles of the hand and the flexors of the ring and little fingers may develop. Weakness interferes with pinch between the thumb and index finger and with hand grip. Patients with chronic cubital tunnel syndrome may present with an ulnar claw hand. An ulnar claw hand is metacarpophalangeal (MCP) joint extension and interphalangeal joint flexion of the small and ring fingers caused by an imbalance between intrinsic and extrinsic hand muscles.

Diagnosis

- Clinical evaluation
- Sometimes nerve conduction studies

Diagnosis of cubital tunnel syndrome is often possible clinically. However, if clinical diagnosis is equivocal and when surgery is being considered, nerve conduction studies are done. Cubital tunnel syndrome is differentiated from ulnar nerve entrapment at the wrist (in Guyon canal) by the presence of sensory deficits over the ulnar dorsal hand, by the presence of ulnar nerve deficits proximal to the wrist on muscle testing or nerve conduction velocity testing, and by the elicitation of ulnar hand paresthesias by tapping the ulnar nerve at the cubital tunnel (positive Tinel sign) elbow.

Treatment

- Splinting
- Sometimes surgical decompression

Treatment of cubital tunnel syndrome involves splinting at night, with the elbow extended at 45°, and use of an elbow pad during the day. Surgical decompression can help if conservative treatment fails.

DE QUERVAIN SYNDROME

(Washerwoman's Sprain)

De Quervain syndrome is stenosing tenosynovitis of the short extensor tendon (extensor pollicis brevis) and long abductor tendon (abductor pollicis longus) of the thumb within the first extensor compartment.

De Quervain syndrome usually occurs after repetitive use (especially wringing) of the wrist, although it occasionally occurs in association with rheumatoid arthritis. It commonly manifests in parents of newborns because of repetitive lifting with wrists in radial deviation.

The major symptom of De Quervain syndrome is aching pain at the wrist and thumb, aggravated by motion. Tenderness can be elicited just proximal to the radial styloid process over the site of the involved tendon sheaths.

Diagnosis of De Quervain syndrome is highly suggested by the Finkelstein test. The patient adducts the involved thumb into the palm and wraps the fingers over the thumb. The test is positive if gentle passive ulnar deviation of the wrist provokes severe pain at the affected tendon sheaths.

Treatment

- Corticosteroid injection
- Thumb spica splint
- Sometimes surgery

Rest, warm soaks, and NSAIDs may help in very mild cases.

Local corticosteroid injections and a thumb spica splint help 70 to 80% of cases. Tendon rupture is a rare complication of injection and can be prevented by confining infiltration to the tendon sheath and avoiding injection of the corticosteroid into the tendon. Intratendinous location of the needle is likely if injection is met with moderate or severe resistance.

Surgical release of the first extensor compartment is very effective when conservative therapy fails.

DIGITAL FLEXOR TENDINITIS AND TENOSYNOVITIS

(Trigger Finger)

Digital flexor tendinitis and tenosynovitis are inflammation, sometimes with subsequent fibrosis, of tendons and tendon sheaths of the digits.

These conditions are idiopathic but are common among patients with rheumatoid arthritis or diabetes mellitus. Repetitive use of the hands (as may occur when using heavy gardening shears) may contribute. In diabetes, they often coexist with carpal tunnel syndrome and occasionally with fibrosis of the palmar fascia. Pathologic changes begin with a thickening or nodule within the tendon; when located at the site of the tight first annular pulley, the thickening or nodule blocks smooth extension or flexion of the finger. The finger may lock in flexion, or "trigger," suddenly extending with a snap.

Treatment

- Conservative measures
- Sometimes corticosteroid injection
- Sometimes surgery

Treatment of acute inflammation and pain includes splinting, moist heat, and anti-inflammatory doses of NSAIDs.

If these measures fail, injection of a corticosteroid suspension into the flexor tendon sheath, along with splinting, may provide safe, rapid relief of pain and triggering. Operative release can be done if corticosteroid therapy fails.

DUPUYTREN CONTRACTURE

(Palmar Fibromatosis)

Dupuytren contracture is progressive contracture of the palmar fascial bands, causing flexion deformities of the fingers. Treatment is with corticosteroid injection, surgery, or injections of clostridial collagenase.

Dupuytren contracture is one of the more common hand deformities; the incidence is higher among men and increases after age 45. This autosomal dominant condition with variable penetrance may occur more commonly among patients with diabetes, alcoholism, or epilepsy. However, the specific factors that cause the palmar fascia to thicken and contract are unknown.

Symptoms and Signs

The earliest manifestation is usually a tender nodule in the palm, most often near the middle or ring finger; it gradually becomes painless. Next, a superficial cord forms and contracts the metacarpophalangeal (MCP) joints and interphalangeal joints of the fingers. The hand eventually becomes arched. The disease is occasionally associated with fibrous thickening of the dorsum of the proximal interphalangeal (PIP) joints (Garrod pads), Peyronie disease (penile fibromatosis) in about 7 to 10% of patients, and rarely nodules on the plantar surface of the feet (plantar fibromatosis). Other types of flexion deformities of the fingers can also occur in diabetes, systemic sclerosis, and chronic reflex sympathetic dystrophy, which need to be differentiated.

Treatment

- Corticosteroid injection (before contractures develop)
- Surgery for disabling contractures
- Injection of clostridial collagenase for certain contractures

Injection of a corticosteroid suspension into the nodule may relieve local tenderness if begun before contractures develop. However, this tenderness is self-limiting and often resolves with no intervention.

If the hand cannot be placed flat on a table or, especially, when significant contracture develops at the PIP joints, surgery is usually indicated. Surgical options include percutaneous needle fasciotomy, temporary application of a dynamic external fixator for PIP joint contractures, and open palmar/digital fasciectomy. For severe disease with multiple finger involvement, open surgery with excision of the diseased fascia is the best treatment; excision must be meticulous because the tissue surrounds neurovascular bundles and tendons. Incomplete excision or new disease results in recurrent contracture, especially in patients who are young at disease onset or who have a family history, Garrod pads, Peyronie disease, or plantar foot involvement.

Injectable collagenase may reverse some contractures,[1,2] particularly those at the MCP joint. Collagenase injections and surgical fasciectomy result in similar improvements at the MCP joint, but injections lead to more rapid recovery with fewer complications.[3]

1. Hurst LC, Badalamente MA, Hentz VR, et al: Injectable collagenase *Clostridium histolyticum* for Dupuytren's contracture. *N Engl J Med* 361(10):968–979, 2009. doi: 10.1056/NEJMoa0810866.
2. Witthaut J, Jones G, Skrepnik N, et al: Efficacy and safety of collagenase *Clostridium histolyticum* injection for Dupuytren contracture: short-term results from 2 open-label studies. *J Hand Surg Am* 38(1):2–11, 2013. doi: 10.1016/j.jhsa.2012.10.008.
3. Zhou C, Hovius SE, Slijper HP, et al: Collagenase *Clostridium histolyticum* versus limited fasciectomy for Dupuytren's contracture: outcomes from a multicenter propensity score matched study. *Plast Reconstr Surg* 136(1):87–97, 2015. doi: 10.1097/PRS.0000000000001320.

FELON

A felon is an infection of the pulp space of the fingertip, usually with staphylococci and streptococci.

The most common site is the distal pulp, which may be involved centrally, laterally, or apically. The septa between pulp spaces ordinarily limit the spread of infection, resulting in an abscess, which creates pressure and necrosis of adjacent tissues. The underlying bone, joint, or flexor tendons may become infected. There is intense throbbing pain and a swollen, warm, extremely tender pulp.

Treatment of felon involves prompt incision and drainage (using a midlateral incision that adequately divides the fibrous septa) and oral antibiotic therapy. Empiric treatment with a cephalosporin is adequate. In areas where methicillin-resistant *Staphylococcus aureus* (MRSA) is prevalent, trimethoprim/sulfamethoxazole, clindamycin, doxycycline, or linezolid should be used instead of a cephalosporin.

GANGLIA

(Ganglion Cysts)

Ganglia are cystic swellings occurring usually on the hands, especially on the dorsal aspect of the wrists. Aspiration or excision is indicated for symptomatic ganglia.

Ganglia constitute about 60% of chronic soft-tissue swellings affecting the hand and wrist. They usually develop spontaneously in adults aged 20 to 50, with a female:male preponderance of 3:1. The size of a ganglion may vary over time and with use of the hand.

Etiology

The cause of most ganglia is unknown. The cystic structures are near or attached (often by a pedicle) to tendon sheaths and joint capsules. The wall of the ganglion is smooth, fibrous, and of variable thickness. The cyst is filled with clear gelatinous, sticky, or mucoid fluid of high viscosity. The fluid in the cyst is sometimes almost pure hyaluronic acid.

Most ganglia are isolated abnormalities. The dorsal wrist ganglion arises from the scapholunate joint and constitutes about 65% of ganglia of the wrist and hand. The volar wrist ganglion arises over the distal aspect of the radius and constitutes about 20 to 25% of ganglia. Flexor tendon sheath ganglia and mucous cysts (arising from the dorsal distal interphalangeal joint) make up the remaining 10 to 15%. Ganglia may spontaneously regress.

Diagnosis

- Examination

Ganglia are evident on examination. Another type of ganglion on the dorsal wrist occurs in patients with RA; it is easily differentiated by its soft irregular appearance and association with proliferative rheumatoid extensor tenosynovitis.

Treatment

- Aspiration or excision if troublesome

Most ganglia do not require treatment. However, if the patient is disturbed by its appearance or if the ganglion is painful or tender, a single aspiration with a large-bore needle is effective in about 50% of patients. Attempting to rupture the ganglion by hitting it with a hard object risks local injury without likely benefit.

Nonsurgical treatment fails in about 40 to 70% of patients, necessitating surgical excision. Excision can be done via arthroscopic or standard open surgery. Recurrence rates after surgical excision are about 5 to 15%.

HERPETIC WHITLOW

Herpetic whitlow is a cutaneous infection of the distal aspect of the finger caused by herpes simplex virus.

Herpetic whitlow may cause intense pain. The digital pulp is not very tense. Vesicles develop on the volar or dorsal distal phalanx but often not until 2 to 3 days after pain begins. The intense pain can simulate a felon, but herpetic whitlow can usually be differentiated by the absence of tenseness in the pulp or the presence of vesicles. Herpetic whitlow can also mimic paronychia or other viral infections in the hand (eg, coxsackievirus). The condition is self-limited but may recur.

Incision and drainage are contraindicated. Topical acyclovir 5% can shorten the duration of a first episode. Oral acyclovir (800 mg po bid) may prevent recurrences if given immediately after onset of symptoms. Open or draining vesicles should be covered to prevent transmission.

PEARLS & PITFALLS

- Before incising a suspected felon or paronychia, consider viral infections such as herpetic whitlow, which should *not* be incised.

INFECTED BITE WOUNDS OF THE HAND

A small puncture wound, particularly from a human or cat bite, may involve significant injury to the tendon, joint capsule, or articular cartilage. The most common cause of human bites is a tooth-induced injury to the metacarpophalangeal joint as a result of a punch to the mouth (clenched fist injury). The oral flora of humans includes *Eikenella corrodens,* staphylococci, streptococci, and anaerobes. Patients with clenched fist injuries tend to wait hours or days after the wound occurs before seeking medical attention, which increases the severity of the infection. Animal bites usually contain multiple potential pathogens, including *Pasteurella multocida* (particularly in cat bites), staphylococci, streptococci, and anaerobes. Serious complications include infectious arthritis and osteomyelitis.

Diagnosis

- Clinical evaluation
- X-rays
- Usually wound cultures

Erythema and pain localized to the bite suggest infection. Tenderness along the course of a tendon suggests spread to the tendon sheath. Pain worsening significantly with motion suggests infection of a joint or tendon sheath.

The diagnosis of infected bite wounds of the hand is clinical, but if the skin is broken, x-rays should be taken to detect fracture or teeth or other foreign bodies that could be a nidus of continuing infection.

Treatment

- Debridement
- Antibiotics

Treatment of infected bite wounds of the hand includes surgical debridement, with the wound left open, and antibiotics.

For outpatient treatment, empiric antibiotics usually include monotherapy with amoxicillin/clavulanate 500 mg po tid or combined therapy with a penicillin 500 mg po qid (for *E. corrodens, P. multocida,* streptococci, and anaerobes) plus either a cephalosporin (eg, cephalexin 500 mg po qid) or semisynthetic penicillin (eg, dicloxacillin 500 mg po qid) for staphylococci. In areas where MRSA is prevalent, trimethoprim/sulfamethoxazole, clindamycin, doxycycline, or linezolid should be used instead of a cephalosporin. If the patient is allergic to penicillin, clindamycin 300 mg po q 6 h can be used.

The hand should be splinted in the functional position and elevated (see Fig. 37–2).

Noninfected bite wounds may require surgical debridement and prophylaxis with 50% of the dose of antibiotic used to treat infected wounds.

INFECTIOUS FLEXOR TENOSYNOVITIS

Infectious flexor tenosynovitis is an acute infection within the flexor tendon sheath. Diagnosis is suggested by Kanavel signs and confirmed with x-rays. Treatment is surgical drainage and antibiotics.

The usual cause of infectious flexor tenosynovitis is a penetration and bacterial inoculation of the sheath.

Diagnosis

- Kanavel signs
- X-rays
- Culture of drainage or surgical sample

Infectious flexor tenosynovitis causes Kanavel signs:

- Flexed resting position of the digit
- Fusiform swelling
- Tenderness along the flexor tendon sheath
- Pain with passive extension of the digit

X-rays should be taken to detect occult foreign bodies. Acute calcific tendinitis and RA can restrict motion and cause pain in the tendon sheath but can usually be differentiated from infectious flexor tenosynovitis by a more gradual onset and the absence of some Kanavel signs. Disseminated gonococcal infection can cause tenosynovitis but often involves multiple joints (particularly those of the wrists, fingers, ankles, and toes), and patients often have recent fever, rash, polyarthralgias, and often risk factors for an STD. Infection of the tendon sheath may involve atypical mycobacteria, but these infections are usually indolent and chronic.

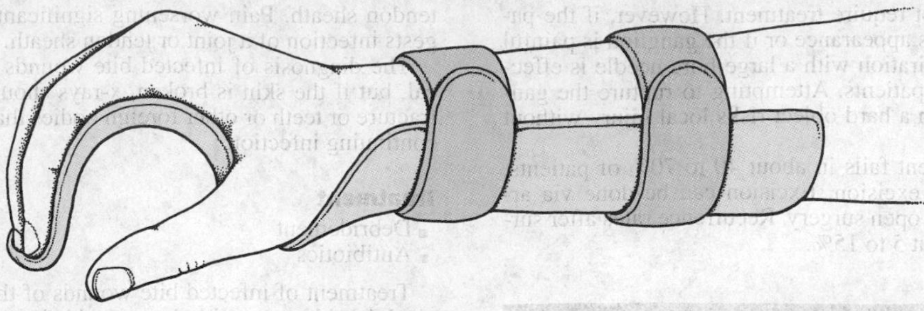

Fig. 37–2. Splint in the functional position (20° wrist extension, 60° MCP joint flexion, slight interphalangeal joint flexion).

Treatment

- Surgical drainage and antibiotics

Treatment of infectious flexor tenosynovitis is surgical drainage (eg, irrigation of the tendon sheath by inserting a cannula into one end and allowing the irrigating fluid to pass along the tendon sheath to the other end). Antibiotic therapy (beginning empirically with a cephalosporin) and cultures are also required. In areas where methicillin-resistant *Staphylococcus aureus* (MRSA) is prevalent, trimethoprim/sulfamethoxazole, clindamycin, doxycycline, or linezolid should be used instead of a cephalosporin.

KIENBÖCK DISEASE

Kienböck disease is avascular necrosis of the lunate bone. Symptoms include wrist pain and tenderness. Diagnosis is with imaging. Treatment is with various surgical procedures.

Kienböck disease occurs most commonly in the dominant hand of men aged 20 to 45, usually in workers doing heavy manual labor. Overall, Kienböck disease is relatively rare. Its cause is unknown. The lunate can eventually collapse and cause fixed rotation of the scaphoid and subsequent degeneration of the carpal joints.

Symptoms and Signs

Symptoms of Kienböck disease generally start with insidious onset of wrist pain, localized to the region of the lunate carpal bone; patients have no recollection of trauma. Kienböck disease is bilateral in 10% of cases. There is localized tenderness in the lunate bone, most commonly over the dorsal wrist along the midline.

Diagnosis

- Imaging

MRI and CT are the most sensitive; plain x-rays show abnormalities later, usually beginning with a sclerotic lunate, then later cystic changes, fragmentation, and collapse.

Differential diagnosis of mid-dorsal wrist pain includes dorsal wrist ganglion, synovitis or arthritis, or extensor tendinitis.

Treatment

- Surgical procedures

Treatment of Kienböck disease is aimed at relieving pressure on the lunate by surgically shortening the radius or lengthening the ulna.[1] Alternative treatments are done in an attempt to revascularize the lunate (eg, implanting a blood vessel or bone graft on a vascular pedicle).[2] For advanced involvement of the lunate, some surgeons have tried to preserve the bone by using free-vascularized bone grafts from the knee.[3]

Salvage procedures (eg, proximal row carpectomy or intercarpal fusions) may help preserve some wrist function if the carpal joints have degenerated.

Total wrist arthrodesis can be done as a last resort to relieve pain. Nonsurgical treatments are not effective.

1. Salmon J, Stanley JK, Trail IA: Kienböck's disease: Conservative management versus radial shortening. *J Bone Joint Surg Br* 82(6):820–823, 2000.
2. Afshar A, Eivaziatashbeik K. Long-term clinical and radiological outcomes of radial shortening osteotomy and vascularized bone graft in Kienböck disease. *J Hand Surg Am* 38(2):289-296, 2013. doi: 10.1016/j.jhsa.2012.11.016.
3. Bürger HK, Windhofer C, Gaggl AJ, et al: Vascularized medial femoral trochlea osteochondral flap reconstruction of advanced Kienböck disease. *J Hand Surg Am* 39(7):1313-22, 2014. doi: 10.1016/j.jhsa.2014.03.040.

OSTEOARTHRITIS OF THE HAND

Hand involvement is extremely common in osteoarthritis.

Osteoarthritis affecting the hand may include asymptomatic enlargement of nodules at the proximal interphalangeal joint (Bouchard nodules) or distal interphalangeal joint (Heberden nodes) or angulation at these joints. Pain and stiffness of these joints and the base of the thumb are also common. The wrist usually is spared (unless there was preexisting trauma), and there is usually minimal or no metacarpophalangeal joint involvement unless the patient also has a metabolic disorder (eg, hemochromatosis). To differentiate hand changes in osteoarthritis from those in rheumatoid arthritis, see Table 32–1 on p. 252.

Treatment

- Conservative measures
- Occasionally corticosteroid injection or surgery

Treatment of osteoarthritis of the hand is symptomatic with analgesics, appropriate rest, splinting, and occasionally corticosteroid injection as needed.

Surgical procedures can help relieve pain and correct deformity for severe changes at the base of the thumb and, less commonly, for advanced degeneration of the interphalangeal joints.

PALM ABSCESS

A palm abscess is a purulent infection of deep spaces in the palm, typically with staphylococci or streptococci.

Palm abscesses can include collar-button abscesses (arising in the web space between two fingers), thenar space abscesses, and midpalmar space abscesses. An abscess can occur in any of the deep palmar compartments and spread between the metacarpals, from the midpalmar space to the dorsum, manifesting as an infection on the dorsum of the hand. Intense throbbing pain occurs with swelling and severe tenderness on palpation. X-rays should be taken to detect occult foreign bodies.

Incision and drainage in the operating room (with cultures), with care to avoid the many important anatomic structures, and antibiotics (eg, a cephalosporin) are required. In areas where MRSA is prevalent, trimethoprim/sulfamethoxazole, clindamycin, doxycycline, or linezolid should be used instead of a cephalosporin.

RADIAL TUNNEL SYNDROME

(Posterior Interosseous Nerve Syndrome)

Radial tunnel syndrome is compression of the radial nerve in the proximal forearm. Symptoms include forearm and elbow pain. Diagnosis is clinical. Treatments include splinting and sometimes surgical decompression.

Compression at the elbow can result from trauma, ganglia, lipomas, bone tumors, or radiocapitellar (elbow) synovitis.

Symptoms and Signs

Symptoms of radial tunnel syndrome include lancinating pain in the dorsum of the forearm and lateral elbow. Pain is precipitated by attempted extension of the wrist and fingers and forearm supination. Sensory loss is rare because the radial nerve is principally a motor nerve at this level. This disorder is sometimes confused with backhand tennis elbow (lateral epicondylitis). When weakness of the extensor muscles is the primary finding, the condition is referred to as posterior interosseus nerve palsy.

Diagnosis

- Clinical evaluation

Lateral epicondylitis can cause similar tenderness around the lateral epicondyle but does not cause the Tinel sign (paresthesia elicited by percussion over a nerve) or tenderness along the course of the radial nerve (which travels under the mobile wad group of muscles in the proximal radial forearm).

Treatment

- Splinting

Splinting allows avoidance of the forceful or repeated motion of supination or wrist dorsiflexion, reducing pressure on the nerve.

If wristdrop or weakened digital extension develops, or conservative treatment fails to provide relief after 3 mo, surgical decompression may be needed.

SWAN-NECK DEFORMITY

A swan-neck deformity consists of hyperextension of the proximal interphalangeal (PIP) joint, flexion of the distal interphalangeal (DIP) joint, and sometimes flexion of the metacarpophalangeal (MCP) joint (see Fig. 37–3).

Although characteristic in rheumatoid arthritis, swan-neck deformity has several causes, including untreated mallet finger, laxity of the ligaments of the volar aspect of the PIP joint (eg, as can occur after rheumatic fever or in SLE as Jaccoud arthropathy), spasticity of intrinsic hand muscles, rupture of the flexor tendon of the PIP joint, and malunion of a fracture of the middle or proximal phalanx. The inability to correct or compensate for hyperextension of the PIP joint makes finger closure impossible and can cause severe disability.

Treatment of swan-neck deformity is aimed at correcting the underlying disorder when possible (eg, correcting the mallet finger or any bony malalignment, releasing spastic intrinsic muscles). Mild deformities in patients with RA may be treated with a functional ring splint.

True swan-neck deformity does not affect the thumb, which has only one interphalangeal joint. However, severe hyperextension of the interphalangeal joint of the thumb with flexion of the MCP joint can occur; this is called a duck bill, Z (zigzag) type, or 90°-angle deformity. With simultaneous thumb instability, pinch is greatly impaired. This deformity can usually be corrected by interphalangeal arthrodesis along with tendon reconstruction at the MCP joint.

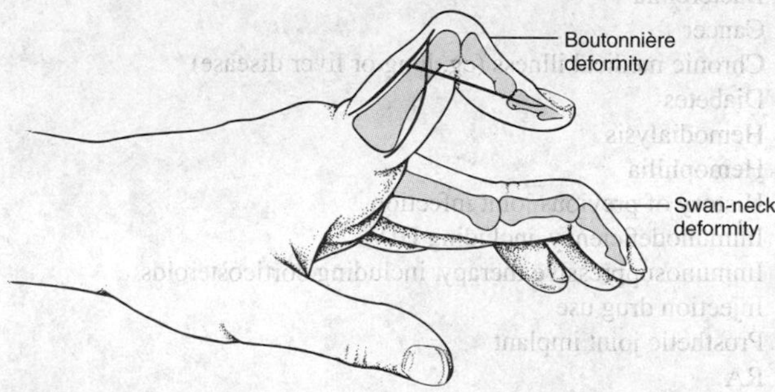

Fig. 37–3. Boutonnière and swan-neck deformities.

38 Infections of Joints and Bones

ACUTE INFECTIOUS ARTHRITIS

Acute infectious arthritis is a joint infection that evolves over hours or days. The infection resides in synovial or periarticular tissues and is usually bacterial—in younger adults, frequently *Neisseria gonorrhoeae*. However, nongonococcal bacterial infections can also occur and can rapidly destroy joint structures. Symptoms include rapid onset of pain, effusion, and restriction of both active and passive range of motion, usually within a single joint. Diagnosis requires synovial fluid analysis and culture. Treatment is IV antibiotics and drainage of pus from joints.

Acute infectious arthritis may occur in children. About 50% of children with joint infection are < 3 yr. However, routine childhood vaccination for *Haemophilus influenzae* and *Streptococcus pneumoniae* is decreasing the incidence of joint infection in this age group.

Risk factors are listed in Table 38–1.

Risk is substantially increased in patients with RA and other disorders causing chronic joint damage, a past history of joint infection, injection drug use, or a prosthetic joint (see p. 298). RA patients are at particular risk of bacterial arthritis (prevalence 0.3 to 3.0%; annual incidence 0.5%). Most children who develop infectious arthritis do not have identified risk factors.

Table 38–1. RISK FACTORS FOR INFECTIOUS ARTHRITIS

Advanced age (50% of adults are > 60 yr)
Alcoholism
Arthrocentesis or joint surgery
Bacteremia
Cancer
Chronic medical illness (eg, lung or liver disease)
Diabetes
Hemodialysis
Hemophilia
History of previous joint infection
Immunodeficiency, including HIV
Immunosuppressive therapy, including corticosteroids
Injection drug use
Prosthetic joint implant
RA
Risk factors for sexually transmitted diseases (eg, multiple sex partners, absence of barrier precautions)
Sickle cell disease
Skin infections
SLE

Etiology

Infectious organisms reach joints by direct penetration (eg, trauma, surgery, arthrocentesis, bites), extension from an adjacent infection (eg, osteomyelitis, a soft-tissue abscess, an infected wound), or hematogenous spread from a remote site of infection. Common organisms are listed in Table 38–2.

In **adults,** most cases result from bacteria and are classified as gonococcal or nongonococcal. This distinction is important because gonococcal infections are far less destructive to the joint. In adults overall, *Staphylococcus aureus* tends to be the most frequent cause of infectious arthritis. Methicillin resistance has become more common among community isolates of *S. aureus.*

In **young adults and adolescents,** *Neisseria gonorrhoeae* is the most common cause and results when *N. gonorrhoeae* spreads from infected mucosal surfaces (cervix, urethra, rectum, pharynx) via the bloodstream. Affected patients often have simultaneous genital infections with *Chlamydia trachomatis* (see p. 1701). *Streptococcus* species are also frequent causes, particularly in patients with polyarticular infections. Patients receiving immunosuppressive therapy (eg, with TNF inhibitors or corticosteroids) may have septic arthritis from less common pathogens (mycobacteria, fungi).

Pathophysiology

Infecting organisms multiply in the synovial fluid and synovial lining. Some bacteria (eg, *S. aureus*) produce virulence factors (adhesins), which allow bacteria to penetrate, remain within, and infect joint tissues. Other bacterial products (eg, endotoxin from gram-negative organisms, cell wall fragments, exotoxins from gram-positive organisms, immune complexes formed by bacterial antigens and host antibodies) augment the inflammatory reaction.

PMNs migrate into the joint and phagocytose the infecting organisms. Phagocytosis of bacteria also results in PMN autolysis with release of lysosomal enzymes into the joint, which damage synovia, ligaments, and cartilage. Therefore, PMNs are both the major host defense system and the cause of joint damage. Articular cartilage can be destroyed within hours or days.

Inflammatory synovitis may occasionally persist even after the infection has been eradicated by antibiotics. Particularly in gonococcal cases, persistent antigen debris from bacteria or infection may alter cartilage, causing it to become antigenic, and—together with the adjuvant effects of bacterial components and immune complexes—immune-mediated, "sterile," chronic inflammatory synovitis may develop.

Symptoms and Signs

Over a few hours to a few days, patients develop moderate to severe joint pain, warmth, tenderness, effusion, restricted active and passive motion, and sometimes redness. Systemic symptoms may be minimal or absent.

Infants and children may present with limited spontaneous movement of a limb (pseudoparalysis), irritability, feeding disturbances, and a high, low-grade, or no fever.

Gonococcal arthritis: Gonococcal arthritis can cause a distinctive dermatitis-polyarthritis-tenosynovitis syndrome.

Classic manifestations are fever (for 5 to 7 days); multiple skin lesions (petechiae, papules, pustules, hemorrhagic vesicles or bullae, necrotic lesions) on mucosal surfaces and on the skin of the trunk, hands, or lower extremities; and migratory arthralgias, arthritis, and tenosynovitis, which evolves into persistent

Table 38–2. ORGANISMS THAT COMMONLY CAUSE ACUTE INFECTIOUS ARTHRITIS

PATIENT GROUP	ORGANISM	TYPICAL SOURCES
Adults and adolescents	Gonococci (in young adults of reproductive age), nongonococcal bacteria (*Staphylococcus aureus,* streptococci), *Neisseria meningitidis* in unusual cases	Cervical, urethral, rectal, or pharyngeal infection with bacteremic dissemination (for gonococci); bacteremia (for staphylococci and streptococci)
Neonates	Group B streptococci, *Escherichia coli* (and other gram-negative enteric bacteria), *S. aureus*	Maternal-fetal transmission; IV punctures or catheters with bacteremic dissemination
Children ≤ 3 yr	*Streptococcus pyogenes, Streptococcus pneumoniae, S. aureus*	Bacteremia (eg, otitis media, URIs, skin infections, meningitis)
Age 3 yr to adolescence	*S. aureus,* streptococci, *Neisseria gonorrhoeae, Pseudomonas aeruginosa, Kingella kingae*	Bacteremia or contiguous spread
Children with meningitis, bacteremia, or palpable purpura	*N. meningitidis* (uncommon)	Bacteremia
All ages	Viruses (eg, parvovirus B19; hepatitis B or hepatitis C virus; rubella virus [active infection and after immunization]; togavirus; chikungunya virus; varicella virus; mumps virus [in adults]; adenovirus; coxsackieviruses A9, B2, B3, B4, and B6; retroviruses, including HIV; Epstein-Barr virus)	Viremia or immune complex deposition
Patients with possible tick exposure	*Borrelia burgdorferi* (causing Lyme disease)	Bacteremia
Patients with bite wounds (human, dog or cat, rat)	Often polymicrobial Human: *Eikenella corrodens,* group B streptococci, *S. aureus,* oral anaerobes (eg, *Fusobacterium* sp, peptostreptococci, *Bacteroides* sp) Dog or cat: *S. aureus, Pasteurella multocida, Pseudomonas* sp, *Moraxella* sp, *Haemophilus* sp Rat: *S. aureus, Streptobacillus moniliformis, Spirillum minus*	Direct joint penetration, usually of the small joints of the hands
The elderly Patients with severe joint trauma or serious disease (eg, immunosuppression, hemodialysis, SLE, RA, diabetes, cancer)	Staphylococci (particularly in RA), gram-negative bacteria (eg, *Enterobacter, P. aeruginosa, Serratia marcescens*), *Salmonella* sp (particularly in SLE*)	Urinary tract, skin
Patients with polyarticular infections Patients with joint penetration (caused by injury, arthrocentesis, or arthrotomy), contiguous infection, diabetes, or cancer	Streptococci Anaerobes (eg, *Propionibacterium acnes, Peptostreptococcus magnus, Fusobacterium* sp, *Clostridium* sp, *Bacteroides* sp); often as mixed infections with facultative or aerobic bacteria such as *S. aureus, Staphylococcus epidermidis, E. coli*	Pharyngitis, cellulitis, GI and GU infections Abdomen, genitals, odontogenic infections, sinuses, ischemic limbs, decubitus ulcers
HIV-infected patients	*S. aureus,* streptococci, *Salmonella* sp, mycobacteria	Skin, mucous membranes, catheters
Injection drug use, indwelling vascular catheters (eg, for hemodialysis, apheresis, or parenteral nutrition)	Gram-negative bacteria, *S. aureus,* streptococci	Bacteremia

*Signs of inflammation can be blunted, so physicians need to have a lower threshold for aspiration and culture; serious conditions (eg, immunosuppression, hemodialysis, SLE, RA, diabetes, cancer) may increase risk of unusual infections (eg, fungal, mycobacterial).

inflammatory arthritis in one or more joints, most often the small joints of the hands, wrists, elbows, knees, and ankles, and rarely the axial skeletal joints.

Symptoms of the original mucosal infection (eg, urethritis, cervicitis) may not be present.

Nongonococcal bacterial arthritis: Nongonococcal bacterial arthritis causes progressive moderate to severe joint pain that is markedly worsened by movement or palpation. Most infected joints are swollen, red, and warm. Fever is absent or low grade in up to 50% of patients; only 20% of patients report a shaking chill. Virulent organisms (eg, *S. aureus, Pseudomonas aeruginosa*) generally cause a more fulminant arthritis, whereas less virulent organisms (eg, coagulase-negative staphylococci, *Propionibacterium acnes*) cause a less fulminant arthritis.

In 80% of **adults,** nongonococcal bacterial arthritis is monarticular and usually occurs in a peripheral joint: knee, hip, shoulder, wrist, ankle, or elbow. In **children,** ≥ 90% is monarticular: knee (39%), hip (26%), and ankle (13%).

Polyarticular involvement is somewhat more common among patients who are immunosuppressed, who have an underlying chronic arthritis (eg, RA, osteoarthritis), or who have a streptococcal infection. In injection drug users and patients with indwelling vascular catheters, axial joints (eg, sternoclavicular, costochondral, hip, shoulder, vertebral, symphysis pubis, sacroiliac) are often involved. *H. influenza* may cause a dermatitis-arthritis syndrome similar to gonococcal infection.

Infectious arthritis secondary to bite wounds: Infection due to human, dog, or cat bites usually develops within 48 h (see p. 2940).

Rat bites cause systemic symptoms such as fever, rash, and joint pain or true arthritis with regional adenopathy within about 2 to 10 days.

Viral infectious arthritis: Viral infectious arthritis sometimes causes symptoms similar to acute nongonococcal bacterial arthritis and is more likely to be polyarticular than bacterial arthritis.

***Borrelia burgdorferi* arthritis:** Patients with *B. burgdorferi* arthritis may have other symptoms of Lyme disease (see p. 1716) or present only with acute monarthritis or oligoarthritis.

A polyarticular RA-like syndrome is distinctly unusual and more likely to be from another diagnosis.

Diagnosis

- Arthrocentesis with synovial fluid examination and culture
- Blood culture
- Sometimes imaging studies
- Usually CBC and ESR (or C-reactive protein)

Infectious arthritis is suspected in patients with acute monarticular arthritis and in patients with other combinations of symptoms characteristic of particular infectious arthritis syndromes (eg, migratory polyarthritis, tenosynovitis, and skin lesions typical of disseminated gonococcal infection; erythema migrans or other symptoms and signs of Lyme disease—see p. 1716).

Even mild monarticular joint symptoms should arouse suspicion in patients taking immunosuppressive therapy (eg, corticosteroids, TNF inhibitors) with risk factors (eg, RA), a prosthetic joint, or an extra-articular infection capable of spreading to a joint (eg, genital gonococcal infection, pneumonia, bacteremia, any anaerobic infection).

PEARLS & PITFALLS

- Do an arthrocentesis and culture synovial fluid to exclude joint infection in patients with joint effusion and findings compatible with bacterial infectious arthritis, even if a known joint disorder (eg, RA) seems like a more likely cause.

General arthritis: Synovial fluid examination is the cornerstone of diagnosis. Fluid is examined grossly and sent for cell count and differential, Gram stain, aerobic and anaerobic culture, and crystals. Foul-smelling synovial fluid suggests anaerobic infection. Fluid from an acutely infected joint usually reveals a WBC count > 20,000/μL (sometimes > 100,000/μL) consisting of > 95% PMNs. WBC counts tend to be higher in nongonococcal bacterial than in gonococcal infectious arthritis. WBC counts may also be lower in early or partially treated infections. Gram stain reveals organisms in only 50 to 75% of joints with acute bacterial arthritis, most often with staphylococci. If positive, Gram stain is suggestive, but cultures are definitive. The presence of crystals does not exclude coexisting infectious arthritis. Sometimes synovial fluid analysis cannot differentiate between infectious and other inflammatory synovial fluid. If differentiation is impossible by clinical means or synovial fluid examination, infectious arthritis is assumed, pending culture results.

Blood tests, such as blood cultures, CBC, and ESR (or C-reactive protein), are usually obtained. However, normal results do not exclude infection. Likewise, WBC count, ESR, or C-reactive protein may be increased in noninfectious joint inflammation (including gout) as well as infectious joint inflammation. The serum urate level should not be used to diagnose or exclude gout as the cause of the arthritis because the level can be normal or even low.

Plain x-rays of the involved joint are not diagnostic of acute infection but can exclude other conditions under consideration (eg, fractures). Abnormalities in early acute bacterial arthritis are limited to soft-tissue swelling and signs of synovial effusions. After 10 to 14 days of untreated bacterial infection, destructive changes of joint space narrowing (reflecting cartilage destruction) and erosions or foci of subchondral osteomyelitis may appear. Gas visible within the joints suggests infection with *Escherichia coli* or anaerobes.

MRI is considered if the joint is not easily accessible for examination and aspiration (eg, an axial joint). MRI or ultrasonography can identify sites of effusion or abscess that can be aspirated or drained for both diagnosis and therapy. MRI can provide early suggestion of associated osteomyelitis. Bone scans using technetium-99m can be falsely negative in infectious arthritis. Also, because they show increased uptake with increased blood flow in inflamed synovial membranes and in metabolically active bone, they can be falsely positive in noninfectious inflammatory arthritis such as gout. Nuclear imaging and MRI do not distinguish infection from crystal-induced arthritis.

Gonococcal arthritis: If gonococcal arthritis is suspected, blood and synovial fluid samples should be *immediately* plated on nonselective chocolate agar, and specimens from the urethra, endocervix, rectum, and pharynx should be plated on selective Thayer-Martin medium. The nucleic acid–based tests often used to diagnose genital gonococcal infection are done on synovial fluid only in specialized laboratories. Genital cultures or DNA testing is also done. Blood cultures may be positive during the first week and may assist in microbiologic diagnosis.

Synovial fluid cultures from joints with frank purulent arthritis are usually positive, and fluid from skin lesions may be positive. If disseminated gonococcal infection is suspected based on clinical criteria, it is assumed to be present even if all gonococcal cultures are negative. Clinical response to antibiotics (anticipated within 5 to 7 days) can help confirm the diagnosis.

Prognosis

Acute nongonococcal bacterial arthritis can destroy articular cartilage, permanently damaging the joint within hours or days.

Gonococcal arthritis does not usually damage joints permanently. Factors that increase susceptibility to infectious arthritis may also increase disease severity. In patients with RA, functional outcome is particularly poor, and the mortality rate is increased.

Treatment

- IV antibiotics
- Drainage of pus from infected joints (for acute nongonococcal bacterial arthritis or any septic arthritis with persistent effusion)

Antibiotic therapy: Initial antibiotic selection is directed at the most likely pathogens. The regimen is adjusted based on the results of culture and susceptibility testing.

Gonococcal arthritis is treated with ceftriaxone 1 g IV once/day until at least 24 h after symptoms and signs resolve, followed by cefixime 400 mg po bid for 7 days. Fluoroquinolones, such as ciprofloxacin 750 mg po bid, may be used in patients who are allergic to beta-lactams if the isolated organism is proven susceptible. Joint drainage and debridement may be unnecessary. Coexisting genital infection with *C. trachomatis* is also treated, often with doxycycline 100 mg po bid for 7 days or azithromycin 1 g orally once; sexual contacts of the patient are treated as necessary (see p. 1702).

If **nongonococcal gram-positive infection** is suspected by Gram stain in an **adult,** the empiric choice is one of the following:

- A semisynthetic penicillin (eg, nafcillin 2 g IV q 4 h)
- A cephalosporin (eg, cefazolin 2 g IV q 8 h)
- Vancomycin 1 g IV q 12 h (if methicillin resistance is common among local community isolates of *S. aureus*)

If gram-negative infection is suspected (eg, in patients with immunosuppression or serious comorbid disorders, injection drug use, a recent infection with antibiotic use, or an indwelling vascular catheter), empiric treatment includes a parenteral 3rd-generation cephalosporin with antipseudomonal activity (eg, ceftazidime 2 g IV q 8 h) and, if infection is severe, an aminoglycoside.

Neonates should be treated initially with an antibiotic that covers gram-positive infection (eg, nafcillin, vancomycin) plus an antibiotic that covers gram-negative infection (eg, gentamicin or a 3rd-generation cephalosporin such as cefotaxime).

Children > 3 mo of age should be treated initially similarly to adults.

Parenteral antibiotics are continued until clinical improvement is clear (usually 2 to 4 wk), and oral antibiotics should be given at high doses for another 2 to 6 wk according to the clinical response.

Infections caused by streptococci and *Haemophilus* are usually eradicated after 2 wk of oral antibiotics after IV treatment.

Staphylococcal infections are treated with antibiotics for at least 3 wk and often 6 wk or longer, especially in patients with prior arthritis or whose diagnosis was delayed.

Other therapies: In addition to antibiotics, **acute nongonococcal bacterial arthritis** requires large-bore needle aspiration of intra-articular pus at least once/day, or tidal irrigation lavage, arthroscopic lavage, or arthrotomy for debridement. Infected RA joints should generally undergo early and aggressive surgical debridement and drainage.

For **gonococcal arthritis** with persistent effusion, pus is aspirated and drainage may need to be repeated as necessary. Acute bacterial arthritis requires joint splinting for the first few days to reduce pain, followed by passive and active range-of-motion exercises to limit contractures, with muscle strengthening as soon as it can be tolerated. NSAIDs can help decrease pain and inflammation. Intra-articular corticosteroids should be avoided during the acute infection.

Viral arthritis and arthritis secondary to bite wounds: Viral arthritis is treated supportively.

Bite wounds are treated with antibiotics and surgical drainage as necessary (see p. 2940).

KEY POINTS

- Gonococcal arthritis manifests with less severe acute inflammation than does acute nongonococcal bacterial arthritis.
- Suspect infectious arthritis if patients have acute monarticular arthritis, particularly patients at risk, or findings suggesting other particular infectious arthritis syndromes.
- Test and culture synovial fluid to confirm or exclude the diagnosis; x-rays and routine laboratory studies are usually of little help.
- Diagnose and treat infectious arthritis, particularly nongonococcal bacterial arthritis, as soon as possible.
- Direct initial antibiotic therapy at pathogens suspected based on clinical and Gram stain findings.

CHRONIC INFECTIOUS ARTHRITIS

Chronic infectious arthritis develops over weeks and is usually caused by mycobacteria, fungi, or bacteria with low pathogenicity.

Chronic infectious arthritis accounts for 5% of infectious arthritis. It can develop in healthy people, but patients at increased risk include those with

- RA
- HIV infection
- Immunosuppression (eg, hematologic or other cancers, immunosuppressive drug use)
- Prosthetic joints

Examples of possible causes are *Mycobacterium tuberculosis, M. marinum, M. kansasii, Candida* sp, *Coccidioides immitis, Histoplasma capsulatum, Cryptococcus neoformans, Blastomyces dermatitidis, Sporothrix schenckii, Aspergillus fumigatus, Actinomyces israelii,* and *Brucella* sp.

The arthritis of Lyme disease is usually acute but may be chronic and recurrent.

Unusual opportunistic organisms are possible in patients with hematologic cancers or HIV infection or who are taking immunosuppressive drugs. A prolonged illness and lack of response to conventional antibiotics suggest a mycobacterial or fungal cause.

In chronic infectious arthritis, the synovial membrane can proliferate and can erode articular cartilage and subchondral bone. Onset is often indolent, with gradual swelling, mild warmth, minimal or no redness of the joint area, and aching pain that may be mild. Usually a single joint is involved.

Patients should have fungal and mycobacterial cultures taken of synovial fluid or synovial tissue, as well as routine studies.

Plain x-ray findings may differ from those of acute infectious arthritis in that joint space is preserved longer, and marginal erosions and bony sclerosis may occur.

Mycobacterial and fungal joint infections require prolonged treatment. Mycobacterial infections are often treated with multiple antibiotics, guided by sensitivity testing results.

PROSTHETIC JOINT INFECTIOUS ARTHRITIS

Prosthetic joints are at risk of acute and chronic infection, which can cause sepsis, morbidity, or mortality.

Etiology

Infections are more common in prosthetic joints than in natural joints. They are frequently caused by perioperative inoculations of bacteria into the joint or by postoperative bacteremia resulting from skin infection, pneumonia, dental procedures, invasive instrumentation, UTI, or possibly falls.

They develop within 1 yr of surgery in two thirds of cases. During the first few months after surgery, the causes are *Staphylococcus aureus* in 50% of cases, mixed flora in 35%, gram-negative organisms in 10%, and anaerobes in 5%. *Propionibacterium acnes* is especially common in infected prosthetic shoulder joints and may require prolonged culture (up to 2 wk) to detect. *Candida* spp infect prosthetic joints in < 5% of cases.

Symptoms and Signs

There is a history of a fall within 2 wk of symptom onset in about 25% of patients and of prior surgical revisions in about 20%.

Some patients have had a postoperative wound infection that appeared to resolve, satisfactory postoperative recovery for many months, and then development of persistent joint pain at rest and during weight bearing.

Symptoms and signs may include pain, swelling, and limited motion; temperature may be normal.

Diagnosis

- Clinical, microbiologic, pathologic, and imaging criteria

The diagnosis often uses a combination of clinical, microbiologic, pathologic, and imaging criteria. Communication between a sinus tract and the prosthesis may also be considered diagnostic of infection.

Synovial fluid should be sampled for cell count and culture. X-rays may show loosening of the prosthesis or periosteal reaction but are not diagnostic. Technetium-99m bone scanning and indium-labeled WBC scanning are more sensitive than plain x-rays but may lack specificity in the immediate postoperative period. Ultimately, periprosthetic tissue collected at the time of surgery may be sent for culture and histologic analysis.

Treatment

- Arthrotomy with debridement
- Long-term systemic antibiotic therapy

Treatment must be prolonged and usually involves arthrotomy for prosthesis removal with meticulous debridement of all cement, abscesses, and devitalized tissues. Debridement is followed by immediate prosthesis revision or placement of an antibiotic-impregnated spacer and then delayed (2 to 4 mo) implantation of a new prosthesis using antibiotic-impregnated cement.

Long-term systemic antibiotic therapy is used in either case; empiric therapy is initiated after intraoperative culture is done and usually combines coverage for methicillin-resistant gram-positive organisms (eg, vancomycin 1 g IV q 12 h) and aerobic gram-negative organisms (eg, piperacillin/tazobactam 3.375 g IV q 6 h or ceftazidime 2 g IV q 8 h) and is revised based on results of culture and sensitivity testing.

Infection develops in 38% of new prostheses, whether replaced immediately or after delay.

If patients cannot tolerate surgery, long-term antibiotic therapy alone can be tried. Excision arthroplasty with or without fusion usually is reserved for patients with uncontrolled infection and insufficient bone stock.

Prevention

In the absence of other indications (eg, valvular heart disease), whether patients with prosthetic joints need prophylactic antibiotics before procedures such as dental work and urologic instrumentation is currently unresolved. Detailed recommendations are available at www.aaos.org and www.idsociety.org.

At many centers, patients are screened for *S. aureus* colonization using nasal cultures. Carriers are decolonized with mupirocin ointment before surgery to implant a prosthetic joint.

OSTEOMYELITIS

Osteomyelitis is inflammation and destruction of bone caused by bacteria, mycobacteria, or fungi. Common symptoms are localized bone pain and tenderness with constitutional symptoms (in acute osteomyelitis) or without constitutional symptoms (in chronic osteomyelitis). Diagnosis is by imaging studies and cultures. Treatment is with antibiotics and sometimes surgery.

Etiology

Osteomyelitis is caused by

- Contiguous spread from infected tissue or an infected prosthetic joint
- Bloodborne organisms (hematogenous osteomyelitis)
- Open wounds (from contaminated open fractures or bone surgery)

Trauma, ischemia, and foreign bodies predispose to osteomyelitis. Osteomyelitis may form under deep pressure ulcers.

About 80% of osteomyelitis results from contiguous spread or from open wounds; it is often polymicrobial. *Staphylococcus aureus* (including both methicillin-sensitive and methicillin-resistant strains) is present in ≥ 50% of patients; other common bacteria include streptococci, gram-negative enteric organisms, and anaerobic bacteria. Osteomyelitis that results from contiguous spread is common in the feet (in patients with diabetes or peripheral vascular disease), at sites where bone was penetrated during trauma or surgery, at sites damaged by radiation therapy, and in bones contiguous to pressure ulcers, such as the hips and sacrum. A sinus, gum, or tooth infection may spread to the skull.

Hematogenously spread osteomyelitis usually results from a single organism. In children, gram-positive bacteria are most common, usually affecting the metaphyses of the tibia, femur, or humerus. In adults, hematogenously spread osteomyelitis usually affects the vertebrae. Risk factors in adults are older age, debilitation, hemodialysis, sickle cell disease, and injection drug use. Common infecting organisms include the following:

- In adults who are older, debilitated, or receiving hemodialysis: *S. aureus* (methicillin-resistant *S. aureus* [MRSA] is common) and enteric gram-negative bacteria
- In injection drug users: *S. aureus, Pseudomonas aeruginosa,* and *Serratia* sp
- In patients with sickle cell disease, liver disease, or immunocompromise: *Salmonella* sp

Fungi and mycobacteria can cause hematogenous osteomyelitis, usually in immunocompromised patients or in areas of endemic infection with histoplasmosis, blastomycosis, or coccidioidomycosis. The vertebrae are often involved.

Pathophysiology

Osteomyelitis tends to occlude local blood vessels, which causes bone necrosis and local spread of infection. Infection may expand through the bone cortex and spread under the periosteum, with formation of subcutaneous abscesses that may drain spontaneously through the skin.

In vertebral osteomyelitis, paravertebral or epidural abscess can develop.

If treatment of acute osteomyelitis is only partially successful, low-grade chronic osteomyelitis develops.

Symptoms and Signs

Patients with **acute osteomyelitis** of peripheral bones usually experience weight loss, fatigue, fever, and localized warmth, swelling, erythema, and tenderness.

Vertebral osteomyelitis causes localized back pain and tenderness with paravertebral muscle spasm that is unresponsive to conservative treatment. More advanced disease may cause compression of the spinal cord or nerve roots, with radicular pain and extremity weakness or numbness. Patients are often afebrile.

Chronic osteomyelitis causes intermittent (months to many years) bone pain, tenderness, and draining sinuses.

Diagnosis

- ESR or C-reactive protein
- X-rays, MRI, or radioisotopic bone scanning
- Culture of bone, abscess, or both

Acute osteomyelitis is suspected in patients with localized peripheral bone pain, fever, and malaise or with localized refractory vertebral pain, particularly in patients with recent risk factors for bacteremia.

Chronic osteomyelitis is suspected in patients with persistent localized bone pain, particularly if they have risk factors.

If osteomyelitis is suspected, CBC and ESR or C-reactive protein, as well as plain x-rays of the affected bone, are obtained. Leukocytosis and elevations of the ESR and C-reactive protein support the diagnosis of osteomyelitis. However, the ESR and C-reactive protein may be elevated in inflammatory conditions, such as RA, or normal in infection caused by indolent pathogens. Thus, the results of these tests must be considered in the context of physical examination and imaging study results.

X-rays become abnormal after 2 to 4 wk, showing periosteal elevation, bone destruction, soft-tissue swelling, and, in the vertebrae, loss of vertebral body height or narrowing of the adjacent infected intervertebral disk space and destruction of the end plates above and below the disk.

If x-rays are equivocal or symptoms are acute, CT and MRI are the current imaging techniques of choice to define abnormalities and reveal abscesses (eg, paravertebral or epidural abscesses).

Alternatively, a radioisotope bone scan with technetium-99m can be done. The bone scan shows abnormalities earlier than plain x-rays but does not distinguish between infection, fractures, and tumors.

A white blood cell scan using indium-111–labeled cells may help to better identify areas of infection seen on bone scan.

Bacteriologic diagnosis is necessary for optimal therapy of osteomyelitis; bone biopsy with a needle or surgical excision and aspiration or debridement of abscesses provides tissue for culture and antibiotic sensitivity testing. Culture of sinus drainage does not necessarily reveal the bone pathogen. Biopsy and culture should precede antibiotic therapy unless the patient is in shock or has neurologic dysfunction.

Treatment

- Antibiotics
- Surgery for abscess, constitutional symptoms, potential spinal instability, or much necrotic bone

Antibiotics: Antibiotics effective against both gram-positive and gram-negative organisms are given until culture results and sensitivities are available.

For **acute hematogenous osteomyelitis,** initial antibiotic treatment should include a penicillinase-resistant semisynthetic penicillin (eg, nafcillin or oxacillin 2 g IV q 4 h) or vancomycin 1 g IV q 12 h (when MRSA is prevalent in a community) and a 3rd- or 4th-generation cephalosporin (such as ceftazidime 2 g IV q 8 h or cefepime 2 g IV q 12 h).

For **chronic osteomyelitis** arising from a contiguous soft-tissue focus, particularly in patients with diabetes, empiric treatment must be effective against anaerobic organisms in addition to gram-positive and gram-negative aerobes. Ampicillin/sulbactam 3 g IV q 6 h or piperacillin/tazobactam 3.375 g IV q 6 h is commonly used; vancomycin 1 g IV q 12 h is added when infection is severe or MRSA is prevalent. Antibiotics must be given parenterally for 4 to 8 wk and tailored to results of appropriate cultures.

Surgery: If any constitutional findings (eg, fever, malaise, weight loss) persist or if large areas of bone are destroyed, necrotic tissue is debrided surgically. Surgery may also be needed to drain coexisting paravertebral or epidural abscesses or to stabilize the spine to prevent injury. Skin or pedicle grafts may be needed to close large surgical defects. Broad-spectrum antibiotics should be continued for > 3 wk after surgery. Long-term antibiotic therapy may be needed.

KEY POINTS

- Most osteomyelitis results from contiguous spread or open wounds and is often polymicrobial and/or involves *S. aureus*.
- Suspect osteomyelitis in patients with localized peripheral bone pain, fever, and malaise or with localized refractory vertebral pain and tenderness, particularly in patients with risk factors for recent bacteremia.
- Do CT or MRI because evidence of osteomyelitis on x-rays typically takes > 2 wk to develop.
- Treat initially with a broad-spectrum antibiotic regimen.
- Base treatment on the results of cultured bone tissue to obtain the best outcome.

39 Joint Disorders

Joint disorders may be inflammatory (RA, spondyloarthropathies, crystal-induced arthritis) or relatively less inflammatory (osteoarthritis, neurogenic arthropathy). Crystal-induced arthritis and infectious arthritis are discussed elsewhere in The Manual.

NEUROGENIC ARTHROPATHY

(Neuropathic Arthropathy; Charcot Joints)

Neurogenic arthropathy is a rapidly destructive arthropathy due to impaired pain perception and position sense, which can result from various underlying disorders, most commonly diabetes and stroke. Common manifestations include joint swelling, effusion, deformity, and instability. Pain may be disproportionately mild due to the underlying neuropathy. Diagnosis requires x-ray confirmation. Treatment consists of joint immobilization, which slows disease progression, and sometimes surgery if the disease is advanced.

Pathophysiology

Many conditions predispose to neurogenic arthropathy (see Table 39–1). Impaired deep pain sensation or proprioception affects the joint's normal protective reflexes, often allowing trauma (especially repeated minor episodes) and small periarticular fractures to go unrecognized. Increased blood flow to bone from reflex vasodilation, resulting in active bone resorption, contributes to bone and joint damage.

Table 39–1. CONDITIONS UNDERLYING NEUROGENIC ARTHROPATHY

Amyloid neuropathy (secondary amyloidosis)
Arnold-Chiari malformation
Congenital insensitivity to pain
Degenerative spinal disease with nerve root compression
Diabetes mellitus
Familial-hereditary neuropathies:
• Familial amyloid polyneuropathy
• Familial dysautonomia (Riley-Day syndrome)
• Hereditary sensory neuropathy
• Hypertrophic interstitial neuropathy (Dejerine-Sottas disease)
• Peroneal muscular atrophy (Charcot-Marie-Tooth disease)
Gigantism with hypertrophic neuropathy
Leprosy
Spina bifida with meningomyelocele (in children)
Stroke
Subacute combined degeneration of the spinal cord
Syringomyelia
Tabes dorsalis
Tumors and injuries of the peripheral nerves (see p. 1991) and spinal cord (see Spinal Trauma on p. 3098 and Spinal Cord Tumors on p. 1916))

Each new injury sustained by the joint causes more distortion as it heals. Hemorrhagic joint effusions and multiple small fractures can occur, accelerating disease progression. Ligamentous laxity, muscular hypotonia, and rapid destruction of joint cartilage are common, predisposing to joint dislocations, which also accelerate disease progression. Advanced neurogenic arthropathy can cause hypertrophic changes, destructive changes, or both.

Symptoms and Signs

Arthropathy does not usually develop until years after onset of the neurologic condition but can then progress rapidly and lead to complete joint disorganization in a few months. Pain is a common early symptom. However, because the ability to sense pain is commonly impaired, the degree of pain is often unexpectedly mild for the degree of joint damage. A prominent, often hemorrhagic, effusion and subluxation and instability of the joint are usually present during early stages. Acute joint dislocation sometimes occurs also.

During later stages, pain may be more severe if the disease has caused rapid joint destruction (eg, periarticular fractures or tense hematomas). During advanced stages, the joint is swollen from bony overgrowth and massive synovial effusion. Deformity results from dislocations and displaced fractures. Fractures and bony healing may produce many loose pieces of cartilage or bone that can slough into the joint, causing a coarse, grating, often audible crepitus usually more unpleasant for the observer than for the patient. The joint may feel like a "bag of bones."

Although many joints can be involved, the knee and the ankle are most often affected. Distribution depends largely on the underlying disease. Thus, tabes dorsalis affects the knee and hip, and diabetes mellitus affects the foot and ankle. Syringomyelia commonly affects the spine and upper limb joints, especially the elbow and shoulder. Frequently, only one joint is affected and usually no more than two or three (except for the small joints of the feet), in an asymmetric distribution.

Infectious arthritis may develop with or without systemic symptoms (eg, fever, malaise), particularly with diabetes. Structures such as blood vessels, nerves, and the spinal cord can become compressed due to the tissue overgrowth.

Diagnosis

- X-rays

The diagnosis of neurogenic arthropathy should be considered in a patient with a predisposing neurologic disorder who develops a destructive but unexpectedly painless arthropathy, usually several years after the onset of the underlying neurologic condition. If neurogenic arthropathy is suspected, x-rays should be taken. Diagnosis is established by characteristic x-ray abnormalities in a patient with a predisposing condition and typical symptoms and signs.

X-ray abnormalities in early neurogenic arthropathy are often similar to those in osteoarthritis (OA—see p. 301). The cardinal signs are

- Bone fragmentation
- Bone destruction
- New bone growth
- Loss of joint space

There may also be synovial effusion and joint subluxation. Later, the bones are deformed, and new bone forms adjacent to the cortex, starting within the joint capsule and often extending up the shaft, particularly in long bones. Rarely, calcification and ossification occur in the soft tissues. Large, bizarrely shaped osteophytes may be present at the joint margins or within joints. Large curved (parrot's beak) osteophytes frequently develop in the spine in the absence of clinical spinal disease.

In its early stages, neurogenic arthropathy can simulate OA. However, neurogenic arthropathy progresses more rapidly than OA and frequently causes proportionately less pain.

Treatment

- Treatment of cause
- Sometimes surgery

Early diagnosis of asymptomatic or minimally symptomatic fractures facilitates early treatment; immobilization (with splints, special boots, or calipers) protects the joint from further injury, possibly stopping disease evolution. Prevention of neurogenic arthropathy may even be possible in a patient at risk.

Treatment of the underlying neurologic condition may slow progression of the arthropathy and, if joint destruction is still in the early stages, partially reverse the process. For a grossly disorganized joint, arthrodesis using internal fixation, compression, and an adequate bone graft may be successful. For grossly disorganized hip and knee joints, if neurogenic arthropathy is not expected to be progressive, good results can be obtained with total hip and knee replacements. However, loosening and dislocation of the prosthesis are major hazards.

KEY POINTS

- Neurogenic arthropathy is a rapidly destructive arthropathy that occurs when perception of pain and position sense are impaired (eg, due to diabetes or stroke).
- Joint destruction out of proportion to pain is typical, often with rapid progression to joint disorganization in advanced stages.
- Confirm the diagnosis with x-ray evidence of joint destruction (similar to changes seen in OA) out of proportion to pain in patients with a predisposing neurologic disorder.
- Treat the cause when possible and protect the joint from further injury by physical means (eg, by immobilization).
- Refer patients for surgery when appropriate.

OSTEOARTHRITIS

(Degenerative Joint Disease; Osteoarthrosis; Hypertrophic Osteoarthritis)

Osteoarthritis (OA) is a chronic arthropathy characterized by disruption and potential loss of joint cartilage along with other joint changes, including bone hypertrophy (osteophyte formation). Symptoms include gradually developing pain aggravated or triggered by activity, stiffness lasting < 30 min on awakening and after inactivity, and occasional joint swelling. Diagnosis is confirmed by x-rays. Treatment includes physical measures, rehabilitation, patient education, and drugs.

OA, the most common joint disorder, often becomes symptomatic in the 40s and 50s and is nearly universal (although not always symptomatic) by age 80. Only half of patients with pathologic changes of OA have symptoms. Below age 40, most OA occurs in men and results from trauma. Women predominate from age 40 to 70, after which men and women are equally affected.

Classification

OA is classified as primary (idiopathic) or secondary to some known cause.

Primary OA may be localized to certain joints (eg, chondromalacia patellae is a mild OA that occurs in young people). Primary OA is usually subdivided by the site of involvement (eg, hands and feet, knee, hip). If primary OA involves multiple joints, it is classified as primary generalized OA.

Secondary OA results from conditions that change the microenvironment of the cartilage. These conditions include significant trauma, congenital joint abnormalities, metabolic defects (eg, hemochromatosis, Wilson disease), infections (causing postinfectious arthritis), endocrine and neuropathic diseases, and disorders that alter the normal structure and function of hyaline cartilage (eg, RA, gout, chondrocalcinosis).

Pathophysiology

Normal joints have little friction with movement and do not wear out with typical use, overuse, or most trauma. Hyaline cartilage is avascular, aneural, and alymphatic. It is 95% water and extracellular cartilage matrix and only 5% chondrocytes. Chondrocytes have the longest cell cycle in the body (similar to CNS and muscle cells). Cartilage health and function depend on compression and release of weight bearing and use (ie, compression pumps fluid from the cartilage into the joint space and into capillaries and venules, whereas release allows the cartilage to reexpand, hyperhydrate, and absorb necessary electrolytes and nutrients).

The trigger of OA is most often unknown, but OA sometimes begins with tissue damage from mechanical injury (eg, torn meniscus), transmission of inflammatory mediators from the synovium into cartilage, or defects in cartilage metabolism. The tissue damage stimulates chondrocytes to attempt repair, which increases production of proteoglycans and collagen. However, efforts at repair also stimulate the enzymes that degrade cartilage, as well as inflammatory cytokines, which are normally present in small amounts. Inflammatory mediators trigger an inflammatory cycle that further stimulates the chondrocytes and synovial lining cells, eventually breaking down the cartilage. Chondrocytes undergo programmed cell death (apoptosis). Once cartilage is destroyed, exposed bone becomes eburnated and sclerotic.

All articular and some periarticular tissues become involved in OA. Subchondral bone stiffens, then undergoes infarction, and develops subchondral cysts. Attempts at bony repair cause subchondral sclerosis and osteophytes at the joint margins. The osteophytes seem to develop in an attempt to stabilize the joint. The synovium becomes inflamed and thickened and produces synovial fluid with less viscosity and greater volume. Periarticular tendons and ligaments become stressed, resulting in tendinitis and contractures. As the joint becomes less mobile, surrounding muscles thin and become less supportive. Menisci fissure and may fragment.

OA of the spine can, at the disk level, cause marked thickening and proliferation of the posterior longitudinal ligaments, which are posterior to the vertebral body but anterior to the spinal cord. The result can be transverse bars that encroach on the anterior spinal cord. Hypertrophy and hyperplasia of the ligamenta flava, which are posterior to the spinal cord, often compress the posterior canal, causing lumbar spinal stenosis. In contrast, the anterior and posterior nerve roots, ganglia, and common spinal nerve are relatively well protected in the intervertebral foramina, where they occupy only 25% of the available and well-cushioned space.

Symptoms and Signs

Onset of OA is most often gradual, usually beginning with one or a few joints. Pain is the earliest symptom of OA, sometimes described as a deep ache. Pain is usually worsened by weight bearing and relieved by rest but can eventually become constant. Stiffness follows awakening or inactivity but lasts < 30 min and lessens with movement. As OA progresses, joint motion becomes restricted, and tenderness and crepitus or grating sensations develop. Proliferation of cartilage, bone, ligament, tendon, capsules, and synovium, along with varying amounts of joint effusion, ultimately cause the joint enlargement characteristic of OA. Flexion contractures may eventually develop. Acute and severe synovitis is uncommon.

Tenderness on palpation and pain on passive motion are relatively late signs. Muscle spasm and contracture add to the pain. Mechanical block by intra-articular loose bodies or abnormally placed menisci can occur and cause locking or catching. Deformity and subluxations can also develop.

The joints most often affected in **generalized OA** include the following:

- Distal interphalangeal (DIP) and proximal interphalangeal (PIP) joints (causing Heberden and Bouchard nodes)
- Thumb carpometacarpal joint
- Intervertebral disks and zygapophyseal joints in the cervical and lumbar vertebrae
- First metatarsophalangeal joint
- Hip
- Knee

Cervical and lumbar spinal OA may lead to myelopathy or radiculopathy. However, the clinical signs of myelopathy are usually mild. Lumbar spinal stenosis may cause lower back or leg pain that is worsened by walking (neurogenic claudication, sometimes called pseudoclaudication) or back extension. Radiculopathy can be prominent but is less common because the nerve roots and ganglia are well protected. Insufficiency of the vertebral arteries, infarction of the spinal cord, and dysphagia due to esophageal impingement by cervical osteophytes occasionally occur. Symptoms and signs caused by OA in general may also derive from subchondral bone, ligamentous structures, synovium, periarticular bursae, capsules, muscles, tendons, disks, and periosteum, all of which are pain sensitive. Venous pressure may increase within the subchondral bone marrow and cause pain (sometimes called bone angina).

Hip OA causes gradual loss of range of motion and is most often symptomatic during weight-bearing activities. Pain may be felt in the inguinal area or greater trochanter or referred to the knee.

Knee OA causes cartilage to be lost (medial loss occurs in 70% of cases). The ligaments become lax and the joint becomes less stable, with local pain arising from the ligaments and tendons.

Erosive OA causes synovitis and cysts in the hand. It primarily affects the DIP or PIP joints. The thumb carpometacarpal joints are involved in 20% of hand OA, but the metacarpophalangeal joints and wrists are usually spared. At this time, it is uncertain whether erosive interphalangeal OA is a variant of hand OA or whether it represents a separate entity.

OA is usually sporadically progressive but occasionally, with no predictability, stops or reverses.

Diagnosis

- X-rays

OA should be suspected in patients with gradual onset of symptoms and signs, particularly in older adults. If OA is suspected, plain x-rays should be taken of the most symptomatic joints. X-rays generally reveal marginal osteophytes, narrowing of the joint space, increased density of the subchondral bone, subchondral cyst formation, bony remodeling, and joint effusions. Standing weight-bearing Merchant view (tangential view with knee flexed 30°) x-rays of the knees are more sensitive in detecting joint space narrowing.

Laboratory studies are normal in OA but may be required to rule out other disorders (eg, RA) or to diagnose an underlying disorder causing secondary OA. If OA causes joint effusions, synovial fluid analysis can help differentiate it from inflammatory arthritides; in OA, synovial fluid is usually clear, viscous, and has ≤ 2000 WBC/μL.

OA involvement outside the usual joints suggests secondary OA; further evaluation may be required to determine the underlying primary disorder (eg, endocrine, metabolic, neoplastic, or biomechanical disorders).

Treatment

- Nondrug therapy (eg, education, rehabilitative and supportive measures)
- Drug therapy

OA treatment goals are relieving pain, maintaining joint flexibility, and optimizing joint and overall function. Primary treatments include physical measures that involve rehabilitation; support devices; exercise for strength, flexibility, and endurance; patient education; and modifications in activities of daily living. Adjunctive therapies include drug treatment and surgery. (See also the European League Against Rheumatism's [EULAR] guidelines for nondrug management of hip and knee OA.)

Physical measures: Moderate weight loss in overweight patients often reduces pain and may even reduce progression of knee OA. Rehabilitation techniques are best begun before disability develops. Exercises (range of motion, isometric, isotonic, isokinetic, postural, strengthening—see p. 3249) maintain range of motion and increase the capacity for tendons and muscles to absorb stress during joint motion. Exercise can sometimes arrest or even reverse hip and knee OA. Aquatic exercises are recommended because they spare the joints from stress. Stretching exercises should be done daily. Immobilization for any prolonged period of time can promote contractures and worsen the clinical course. However, a few minutes of rest (every 4 to 6 h in the daytime) can help if balanced with exercise and use.

Modifying activities of daily living can help. For example, a patient with lumbar spine, hip, or knee OA should avoid soft deep chairs and recliners in which posture is poor and from which rising is difficult. The regular use of pillows under the knees while reclining encourages contractures and should also be avoided. However, pillows placed between the knees can often help relieve radicular back pain. Patients should sit in straight-back chairs without slumping, sleep on a firm bed (perhaps with a bed board), use a car seat shifted forward and designed for comfort, do postural exercises, wear well-supported shoes or athletic shoes, and continue employment and physical activity.

In OA of the spine, knee, or thumb carpometacarpal joint, various supports can relieve pain and increase function, but to preserve flexibility, they should be accompanied by specific exercise programs. In erosive OA, range-of-motion exercises done in warm water can help prevent contractures.

Drugs: Drug therapy is an adjunct to the physical program. Acetaminophen in doses of up to 1 g po qid may relieve pain and is generally safe. More potent analgesics, such as tramadol or rarely opioids, may be required; however, these drugs can cause confusion in older patients. Duloxetine, a serotonin norepinephrine reuptake inhibitor, reduces pain caused by OA. Topical capsaicin has been helpful in relieving pain in superficial joints by disrupting pain transmission.

NSAIDs, including cyclooxygenase-2 (COX-2) inhibitors or coxibs, may be considered if patients have refractory pain or signs of inflammation (eg, redness, warmth). NSAIDs may be used simultaneously with other analgesics (eg, tramadol, opioids) to provide better relief of symptoms. Topical NSAIDs may be of value for superficial joints, such as the hands and knees. Topical NSAIDS may be of particular value in the elderly, because NSAID absorption is reduced, minimizing risk of drug adverse effects.

Muscle relaxants (usually in low doses) occasionally relieve pain that arises from muscles strained by attempting to support OA joints. In the elderly, however, they may cause more adverse effects than relief.

Oral corticosteroids should not be given chronically. Intra-articular depot corticosteroids can help relieve pain and increase joint flexibility in some patients; however, a strong placebo effect has been shown in clinical trials.

Hyaluronic acid formulations can be injected into the knee and provide some pain relief in some patients for prolonged periods of time. They should not be used more often than every 6 mo. The treatment is a series of 1 to 5 weekly injections. Efficacy in patients with x-ray evidence of severe disease is absent or limited and, in some patients, local injection can cause an acute severe inflammatory synovitis. Studies have shown these agents have a strong placebo effect.

Glucosamine sulfate 1500 mg po once/day has been suggested to relieve pain and slow joint deterioration; chondroitin sulfate 1200 mg once/day has also been suggested for pain relief. Studies to date have shown mixed efficacy in terms of pain relief and no strong effect on preservation of cartilage.

Other adjunctive and experimental therapies: Other adjunctive measures can relieve pain, including massage, heating pads, weight loss, acupuncture, and transcutaneous electrical nerve stimulation (TENS). Laminectomy, osteotomy, and total joint replacement should be considered if all nonsurgical approaches fail.

Experimental therapies that may preserve cartilage or allow chondrocyte grafting are being studied. It is not clear whether using a topical lidocaine 5% patch relieves pain. Flavocoxid, a plant-derived compound, can be tried. Little information supports injections of platelet-rich plasma for OA.

KEY POINTS

- OA, the most common joint disorder, becomes particularly common with age.
- Key pathophysiologic features include disruption and loss of joint cartilage and bony hypertrophy.
- OA can affect particular joints (sometimes secondary to injury or another joint problem) or be generalized (often as a primary disorder).
- Symptoms include gradual onset of joint pain that is worsened by weight-bearing or stress and relieved by rest, and stiffness that lessens with activity.
- Confirm the diagnosis with x-ray findings such as marginal osteophytes, narrowing of the joint space, increased density of the subchondral bone, bony remodeling, and sometimes subchondral cyst formation and joint effusion.
- Treat primarily with physical measures that involve rehabilitation; support devices; exercise for strength, flexibility, and endurance; patient education; and modifications in activities of daily living.
- Treat adjunctively with drugs (eg, analgesics, NSAIDs, muscle relaxants) and surgery.

RHEUMATOID ARTHRITIS

Rheumatoid arthritis (RA) is a chronic systemic autoimmune disease that primarily involves the joints. RA causes damage mediated by cytokines, chemokines, and metalloproteases. Characteristically, peripheral joints (eg, wrists, metacarpophalangeal joints) are symmetrically inflamed, leading to progressive destruction of articular structures, usually accompanied by systemic symptoms. Diagnosis is based on specific clinical, laboratory, and imaging features. Treatment involves drugs, physical measures, and sometimes surgery. Disease-modifying antirheumatic drugs help control symptoms and slow disease progression.

RA affects about 1% of the population. Women are affected 2 to 3 times more often than men. Onset may be at any age, most often between 35 yr and 50 yr, but can be during childhood (see Juvenile Idiopathic Arthritis on p. 2694) or old age.

Etiology

Although RA involves autoimmune reactions, the precise cause is unknown; many factors may contribute. A genetic predisposition has been identified and, in white populations, localized to a shared epitope in the HLA-DR β_1 locus of class II histocompatibility antigens. Unknown or unconfirmed environmental factors (eg, viral infections, cigarette smoking) are thought to play a role in triggering and maintaining joint inflammation.

Pathophysiology

Prominent immunologic abnormalities include immune complexes produced by synovial lining cells and in inflamed blood vessels. Plasma cells produce antibodies (eg, rheumatoid factor [RF], anticyclic citrullinated peptide [anti-CCP] antibody) that contribute to these complexes, but destructive arthritis can occur in their absence. Macrophages also migrate to diseased synovium in early disease; increased macrophage-derived lining cells are prominent along with vessel inflammation. Lymphocytes that infiltrate the synovial tissue are primarily CD4+ T cells. Macrophages and lymphocytes produce proinflammatory cytokines and chemokines (eg, TNF-alpha, granulocyte-macrophage colony-stimulating factor [GM-CSF], various ILs, interferon-gamma) in the synovium. Released inflammatory mediators and various enzymes contribute to the systemic and joint manifestations of RA, including cartilage and bone destruction.

In seropositive RA, accumulating evidence suggests that anti-CCP antibodies appear long before any signs of inflammation.[1] Additionally, anti-carbamylated protein (anti-CarP) antibodies predict more radiologic progression in anti-CCP–negative RA patients.[2] Progression to RA in the preclinical phase depends on autoantibody epitope spreading.[3]

In chronically affected joints, the normally thin synovium proliferates, thickens, and develops many villous folds. The synovial lining cells produce various materials, including collagenase and stromelysin, which contribute to cartilage destruction, and IL-1 and TNF-alpha, which stimulate cartilage destruction, osteoclast-mediated bone absorption, synovial inflammation, and prostaglandins (which potentiate inflammation). Fibrin deposition, fibrosis, and necrosis are also present. Hyperplastic synovial tissue (pannus) releases these inflammatory mediators, which erode cartilage, subchondral bone, articular capsule, and ligaments. Polymorphonuclear leukocytes (PMNs) on average make up about 60% of WBCs in the synovial fluid.

Rheumatoid nodules develop in about 30% of patients with RA. They are granulomas consisting of a central necrotic area surrounded by palisaded histiocytic macrophages, all enveloped by lymphocytes, plasma cells, and fibroblasts. Nodules and vasculitis can also develop in visceral organs.

1. Rantapaa-Dahlqvist S, de Jong BA, Berglin E, et al: Antibodies against cyclic citrullinated peptide and IgA rheumatoid factor predict the development of rheumatoid arthritis. *Arthritis Rheum* 48:2741–2749, 2003. doi: 10.1002/art.11223.
2. Brink M, Verheul MK, Rönnelid J, et al: Anti-carbamylated protein antibodies in the pre-symptomatic phase of rheumatoid arthritis, their relationship with multiple anti-citrulline peptide antibodies and association with radiological damage. *Arthritis Res Ther* 17:25, 2015. doi: 10.1186/s13075-015-0536-2.
3. Sokolove J, Bromberg R, Deane KD, et al: Autoantibody epitope spreading in the pre-clinical phase predicts progression to rheumatoid arthritis. *PLoS ONE* 7(5):e35296, 2012. doi: 10.1371/journal.pone.0035296. Clarification and additional information. *PLoS ONE* 7(8), 2012.

Symptoms and Signs

Onset of rheumatoid arthritis is usually insidious, often beginning with systemic and joint symptoms. Systemic symptoms include early morning stiffness of affected joints, generalized afternoon fatigue and malaise, anorexia, generalized weakness, and occasionally low-grade fever. Joint symptoms include pain, swelling, and stiffness. Occasionally, the disease begins abruptly, mimicking an acute viral syndrome.

The disease progresses most rapidly during the first 6 yr, particularly the first year; 80% of patients develop some permanent joint abnormalities within 10 yr. The course is unpredictable in individual patients.

Joint symptoms are characteristically symmetric. Typically, stiffness lasts > 60 min after rising in the morning but may occur after any prolonged inactivity (called gelling). Involved joints become tender, with erythema, warmth, swelling, and limitation of motion. The joints primarily involved include the following:

- Wrists and the index (2nd) and middle (3rd) metacarpophalangeal joints (most commonly involved)
- Proximal interphalangeal joints
- Metatarsophalangeal joints
- Shoulders
- Elbows
- Hips
- Knees
- Ankles

However, virtually any joint, except uncommonly the distal interphalangeal (DIP) joints, may be involved. The axial skeleton is rarely involved except for the upper cervical spine. Synovial thickening is detectable. Joints are often held in flexion to minimize pain, which results from joint capsular distention.

Fixed deformities, particularly flexion contractures, may develop rapidly; ulnar deviation of the fingers with an ulnar slippage of the extensor tendons off the metacarpophalangeal joints is typical, as are swan-neck deformities and boutonnière deformities (see Fig. 37–3 on p. 293). Joint instability due to stretching of the joint capsule can also occur. Carpal tunnel syndrome can result from wrist synovitis compressing the median nerve. Popliteal (Baker) cysts can develop, causing calf swelling and tenderness suggestive of deep venous thrombosis.

Extra-articular manifestations: Subcutaneous rheumatoid nodules are not usually an early sign but eventually develop in up to 30% of patients, usually at sites of pressure and chronic irritation (eg, the extensor surface of the forearm, metacarpophalangeal joints, occiput). Visceral nodules (eg, pulmonary nodules), usually asymptomatic, occur in severe RA. Pulmonary nodules of RA cannot be distinguished from pulmonary nodules of other etiology without biopsy.

Other extra-articular signs include vasculitis causing leg ulcers or mononeuritis multiplex, pleural or pericardial effusions, pulmonary infiltrates or fibrosis, pericarditis, myocarditis, lymphadenopathy, Felty syndrome, Sjögren syndrome, scleromalacia, and episcleritis. Involvement of the cervical spine can cause atlantoaxial subluxationand spinal cord compression; subluxation may worsen with extension of the neck (eg, during endotracheal intubation). Importantly, cervical spine instability is most often asymptomatic.

Diagnosis

- Clinical criteria
- Serum rheumatoid factor (RF), anti-CCP, and ESR or C-reactive protein (CRP)
- X-rays

RA should be suspected in patients with polyarticular, symmetric arthritis, particularly if the wrists and 2nd and 3rd metacarpophalangeal joints are involved. Classification criteria serve as a guide for establishing the diagnosis of RA and are helpful in defining standardized treatment populations for study purposes. Criteria include laboratory test results for RF, anti-CCP, and ESR or CRP (see Table 39–2). Other causes of symmetric polyarthritis, particularly hepatitis C, must be excluded. Patients should have a serum RF test, hand and wrist x-rays, and baseline x-rays of affected joints to document future erosive changes. In patients who have prominent lumbar symptoms, alternative diagnoses should be investigated.

RFs, antibodies to human gamma-globulin, are present in about 70% of patients with RA. However, RF, often in low titers (levels can vary between laboratories), occurs in patients with other diseases, including other connective tissue diseases (eg, SLE), granulomatous diseases, chronic infections (eg, viral hepatitis, bacterial endocarditis, TB), and cancers. Low RF titers can also occur in 3% of the general population and 20% of the elderly. Very high RF titers can occur in patients with hepatitis C infection and sometimes in patients with other chronic infections. An RF titer measured by latex agglutination of > 1:80 or a positive anti-CCP test supports the diagnosis of RA in the appropriate clinical context, but other causes must be excluded.

Anti-CCP antibodies have high specificity (90%) and sensitivity (about 77 to 86%) for RA and, like RF, predict a worse prognosis. RF and anti-CCP values do not fluctuate with disease activity. Anti-CCP antibodies are notably absent in patients with hepatitis C who may have a positive RF titer.

Table 39–2. CLASSIFICATION CRITERIA FOR RHEUMATOID ARTHRITIS*

FINDING	SCORE
Criteria for evaluation: • At least 1 joint with definite clinical synovitis (swelling) • Synovitis not better explained by another disorder	
Classification criteria for RA is a score-based algorithm. Scores for categories A–D are added; a score ≥ 6 (highest possible total 10) is needed to classify a patient as having definite RA.*	
A. Joint involvement†	
1 large joint‡	0
2–10 large joints	1
1–3 small joints§ (with or without involvement of large joints)	2
4–10 small joints (with or without involvement of large joints)	3
>10 joints‖ (at least 1 small joint)	5
B. Serology (at least 1 test result is needed for classification)	
Negative RF and negative anti-CCP	0
Low-positive RF or low-positive anti-CCP	2
High-positive RF or high-positive anti-CCP	3
C. Acute-phase reactants (at least 1 test result is needed for classification)	
Normal CRP and normal ESR	0
Abnormal CRP or abnormal ESR	1
D. Duration of symptoms (based on patient's report)	
< 6 wk	0
≥ 6 wk	1

*Patients with a score of < 6 can be reassessed; they may meet the criteria for RA cumulatively over time.

†Distal interphalangeal joints, first carpometacarpal joints, and first metatarsophalangeal joints are excluded from assessment.

‡Large joints are the shoulders, elbows, hips, knees, and ankles.

§Small joints are the metacarpophalangeal joints, PIP joints, 2nd–5th metatarsophalangeal joints, thumb interphalangeal joints, and wrists.

‖These joints may include other joints not specifically listed elsewhere (eg, temporomandibular, acromioclavicular, sternoclavicular).

Anti-CCP = anticitrullinated protein antibody; CRP = C-reactive protein; RF = rheumatoid factor.

Adapted from Aletaha D, Neogi T, Silman AJ, et al: Rheumatoid arthritis classification criteria: an American College of Rheumatology/European League Against Rheumatism collaborative initiative. *Arthritis Rheum* 62 (9):2569–2581, 2010.

X-rays show only soft-tissue swelling during the first months of disease. Subsequently, periarticular osteoporosis, joint space (articular cartilage) narrowing, and marginal erosions may become visible. Erosions often develop within the first year but may occur any time. MRI seems to be more sensitive and detects earlier articular inflammation and erosions. In addition, abnormal subchondral bone signals (eg, bone marrow lesions, bone marrow edema) around the knee suggest progressive disease.

If RA is diagnosed, additional tests help detect complications and unexpected abnormalities. CBC with differential should be obtained. A normochromic (or slightly hypochromic)-normocytic anemia occurs in 80%; Hb is usually > 10 g/dL. If Hb is ≤ 10 g/dL, superimposed iron deficiency or other causes of anemia should be considered. Neutropenia occurs in 1 to 2% of cases, often with splenomegaly (Felty syndrome). Acute-phase reactants (eg, thrombocytosis, elevated ESR, elevated CRP) reflect disease activity. A mild polyclonal hypergammaglobulinemia often occurs. ESR is elevated in 90% of patients with active disease.

Validated measures of disease activity include the Rheumatoid Arthritis Disease Activity Score DAS-28 and Rheumatoid Arthritis Clinical Disease Activity Index.

Synovial fluid examination is necessary with any new-onset effusion to rule out other disorders and differentiate RA from other inflammatory arthritides (eg, septic and crystal-induced arthritis). In RA, during active joint inflammation, synovial fluid is turbid, yellow, and sterile, and usually has 10,000 to 50,000 WBCs/μL; PMNs typically predominate, but > 50% may be lymphocytes and other mononuclear cells. Crystals are absent.

Differential diagnosis: Many disorders can simulate RA:

- Crystal-induced arthritis
- SLE
- Sarcoidosis
- Reactive arthritis
- Psoriatic arthritis
- Ankylosing spondylitis
- Hepatitis C-related arthritis
- Osteoarthritis

RF can be nonspecific and is often present in several autoimmune diseases; the presence of anti-CCP antibodies is more specific for RA. For example, hepatitis C can be associated with an arthritis similar to RA clinically and that is RF-positive; however, anti-CCP is negative.

Some patients with crystal-induced arthritis may meet criteria for RA; however, synovial fluid examination should clarify the diagnosis. The presence of crystals makes RA unlikely. Joint involvement and subcutaneous nodules can result from gout, cholesterol, and amyloidosis as well as RA; aspiration or biopsy of the nodules may occasionally be needed.

SLE usually can be distinguished if there are skin lesions on light-exposed areas, hair loss, oral and nasal mucosal lesions, absence of joint erosions in even long-standing arthritis, joint fluid that often has < 2000 WBCs/μL (predominantly mononuclear cells), antibodies to double-stranded DNA, renal disease, and low serum complement levels. In contrast to RA, deformities in SLE are usually reducible and lack erosions and bone or cartilage damage on imaging studies.

Arthritis similar to RA can also occur in other rheumatic disorders (eg, polyarteritis, systemic sclerosis, dermatomyositis, or polymyositis), or there can be features of more than one disease, which suggests an overlap syndrome or mixed connective tissue disease.

Sarcoidosis, Whipple disease, multicentric reticulohistiocytosis, and other systemic diseases may involve joints; other clinical features and tissue biopsy sometimes help differentiate these conditions. Acute rheumatic fever has a migratory pattern of joint involvement and evidence of antecedent streptococcal infection (culture or changing antistreptolysin O titer); in contrast, RA tends to involve additional joints over time.

Reactive arthritis can be differentiated by antecedent GI or GU symptoms; asymmetric involvement and pain at the Achilles insertion of the heel, sacroiliac joints, and large joints of the leg; conjunctivitis; iritis; painless buccal ulcers; balanitis circinata; or keratoderma blennorrhagicum on the soles and elsewhere.

Psoriatic arthritis tends to be asymmetric and is not usually associated with RF, but differentiation may be difficult in the absence of nail or skin lesions. DIP joint involvement and severely mutilating arthritis (arthritis mutilans) is strongly suggestive, as is the presence of a diffusely swollen (sausage) digit.

Ankylosing spondylitis may be differentiated by spinal and axial joint involvement, absence of subcutaneous nodules, and a negative RF test. The HLA-B27 allele is present in 90% of patients with ankylosing spondylitis.

OA can be differentiated by the joints involved; the absence of rheumatoid nodules, systemic manifestations, or significant amounts of RF; and by synovial fluid WBC counts < 2000/μL. OA of the hands most typically involves the DIP joints, bases of the thumbs, and PIP joints and may involve the metacarpophalangeal joints but typically spares the wrist. RA does not affect the DIP joints.

Prognosis

RA decreases life expectancy by 3 to 7 yr, with heart disease, infection, and GI bleeding accounting for most excess mortality; drug treatment, cancer, as well as the underlying disease may be responsible. Disease activity should be controlled to lower cardiovascular disease risk in all patients with RA. (See also the European League Against Rheumatism's [EULAR] recommendations for cardiovascular disease risk management in patients with RA and other forms of inflammatory joint disorders.)

At least 10% of patients are eventually severely disabled despite full treatment. Whites and women have a poorer prognosis, as do patients with subcutaneous nodules, advanced age at disease onset, inflammation in ≥ 20 joints, early erosions, cigarette smoking, high ESR, and high levels of RF or anti-CCP.

Treatment

- Supportive measures (eg, smoking cessation, nutrition, rest, physical measures, analgesics)
- Drugs that modify disease progression
- NSAIDs as needed for analgesia

Treatment of RA involves a balance of rest and exercise, adequate nutrition, physical measures, drugs, and sometimes surgery. (See also the American College of Rheumatology's 2015 guidelines for the treatment of rheumatoid arthritis and the European League Against Rheumatism's 2013 update EULAR Recommendations for the Management of Rheumatoid Arthritis with Synthetic and Biological Disease-Modifying Antirheumatic Drugs.)

Lifestyle measures: Complete bed rest is rarely indicated, even for a short time; however, a program including judicious rest should be encouraged.

An ordinary nutritious diet is appropriate. Rarely, patients have food-associated exacerbations; no specific foods have reproducibly been shown to exacerbate RA. Food and diet quackery is common and should be discouraged. Substituting omega-3 fatty acids (in fish oils) for dietary omega-6 fatty acids (in meats) partially relieves symptoms in some patients by transiently decreasing production of inflammatory prostaglandins and possibly by modifying the gut microbiome. Smoking cessation can increase life expectancy.

Physical measures: Joint splinting reduces local inflammation and may relieve severe symptoms of pain or compressive neuropathies. Cold may be applied to reduce joint pain and swelling. Orthopedic or athletic shoes with good heel and arch support are frequently helpful; metatarsal supports placed posteriorly (proximal) to painful metatarsophalangeal joints decrease the pain of weight bearing. Molded shoes may be needed for severe deformities. Occupational therapy and self-help devices enable many patients with debilitating RA to perform activities of daily living.

Exercise should proceed as tolerated. During acute inflammation, passive range-of-motion exercise helps prevent flexion contractures. Heat therapy can be applied to help alleviate stiffness. Range-of-motion exercises done in warm water are helpful because heat improves muscle function by reducing stiffness and muscle spasm. However, contractures can be prevented and muscle strength can be restored more successfully after inflammation begins to subside; active exercise (including walking and specific exercises for involved joints) to restore muscle mass and preserve range of joint motion should not be fatiguing. Flexion contractures may require intensive exercise, casting, or immobilization (eg, splinting) in progressively more stretched-open positions. Paraffin baths can warm digits and facilitate finger exercise.

Massage by trained therapists, traction, and deep heat treatment with diathermy or ultrasonography may be useful adjunctive therapies to anti-inflammatory drugs.

Surgery: Surgery may be considered if drug therapy is unsuccessful. Surgery must always be considered in terms of the total disease and patient expectations. For example, deformed hands and arms limit crutch use during rehabilitation; seriously affected knees and feet limit benefit from hip surgery. Reasonable objectives for each patient must be determined, and function must be considered; straightening ulnar-deviated fingers may not improve hand function. Surgery may be done while the disease is active.

Arthroplasty with prosthetic joint replacement is indicated if damage severely limits function; total hip and knee replacements are most consistently successful. Prosthetic hips and knees cannot tolerate vigorous activity (eg, competitive athletics). Excision of subluxed painful metatarsophalangeal joints may greatly aid walking. Thumb fusions may provide stability for pinch. Neck fusion may be needed for C1-2 subluxation with severe pain or potential for spinal cord compression. Arthroscopic or open synovectomy can relieve joint inflammation but only temporarily unless disease activity can be controlled.

Drugs for RA

The goal is to reduce inflammation as a means of preventing erosions, progressive deformity, and loss of joint function. Disease-modifying antirheumatic drugs (DMARDs) are used early, often in combination. Other drug classes, including biologic agents such as TNF-alpha antagonists, IL-1 receptor antagonists, IL-6 blockers, B-cell depleters, T-cell costimulatory molecules, and Janus kinase (JAK) inhibitors, seem to slow the progression of RA. NSAIDs are of some help for the pain of RA but do not prevent erosions or disease progression and thus should be used only as adjunctive therapy. Low-dose systemic corticosteroids (prednisone < 10 mg once/day) may be added to control severe polyarticular symptoms, usually with the objective of replacement with a DMARD. Intra-articular depot corticosteroids can control severe monarticular or even oligoarticular symptoms but may have adverse metabolic effects, even in low doses.

The optimal combinations of drugs are not yet clear. However, some data suggest that certain combinations of drugs from different classes (eg, methotrexate plus other DMARDs, a rapidly tapered corticosteroid plus a DMARD, methotrexate plus a TNF-alpha antagonist, or a TNF-alpha antagonist plus a DMARD) are more effective than using DMARDs alone sequentially or in combination with other DMARDs. In general, biologic agents are not given in combination with each other due to increased frequency of infections. An example of initial therapy is

- Methotrexate 7.5 mg po once/wk (with folic acid 1 mg po once/day) is given.
- If tolerated and not adequate, the dose of methotrexate is increased after 3- to 5-wk intervals to a maximum of 25 mg po or by injection once/wk.
- If response is not adequate, a biologic agent should be added; alternatively, triple therapy with methotrexate, hydroxychloroquine, and sulfasalazine is an option.

Leflunomide may be used instead of methotrexate or added to methotrexate with close monitoring of liver function test results and CBC.

NSAIDs: Aspirin is no longer used for RA because effective doses are often toxic. Only one NSAID should be given at a time (see Table 39–3), although patients may also take aspirin at ≤ 325 mg/day for its antiplatelet cardioprotective effect. Because the maximal response for NSAIDs can take up to 2 wk, doses should be increased no more frequently than this. Doses of drugs with flexible dosing can be increased until response is maximal or maximum dosage is reached. All NSAIDs treat the symptoms of RA and decrease inflammation but do not alter the course of the disease; thus, they are only used adjunctively.

NSAIDs inhibit cyclooxygenase (COX) enzymes and thus decrease production of prostaglandins. Some prostaglandins under COX-1 control have important effects in many parts of the body (ie, they protect gastric mucosa and inhibit platelet adhesiveness). Other prostaglandins are induced by inflammation and are produced by COX-2. Selective COX-2 inhibitors, also called coxibs (eg, celecoxib), seem to have efficacy comparable to nonselective NSAIDs and are slightly less likely to cause GI toxicity; however, they are not less likely to cause renal toxicity. Celecoxib 200 mg po once/day has a comparable cardiovascular safety profile to nonselective NSAIDs. It remains unclear whether full-dose celecoxib (200 mg po bid) has cardiovascular risks comparable to the nonselective NSAIDs.

NSAIDs other than perhaps coxibs should be avoided in patients with previous peptic ulcer disease or dyspepsia. Other possible adverse effects of all NSAIDs include headache, confusion and other CNS symptoms, increased BP, worsening of hypertension, edema, and decreased platelet function; however, celecoxib has no significant antiplatelet effect. NSAIDs increase cardiovascular risk (see p. 1968). Creatinine levels can rise reversibly because of inhibited renal prostaglandins; less frequently, interstitial nephritis can occur. Patients with urticaria, rhinitis, or asthma caused by aspirin can have the same problems with these other NSAIDs, but celecoxib may not cause these problems.

NSAIDs should be used at the lowest possible dose needed to mitigate their adverse effects.

Table 39–3. NSAID TREATMENT OF RHEUMATOID ARTHRITIS

DRUG	USUAL DOSAGE (ORAL)	MAXIMUM RECOMMENDED DAILY DOSE
Nonselective NSAIDs		
Diclofenac	75 mg bid or 50 mg tid 100 mg once/day sustained-release	150 mg
Etodolac	300–500 mg bid	1200 mg
Fenoprofen	300–600 mg qid	3200 mg
Flurbiprofen	100 mg bid or tid	300 mg
Ibuprofen	400–800 mg qid	3200 mg
Indomethacin	25 mg tid to qid 75 mg bid sustained-release	200 mg
Ketoprofen	50–75 mg qid 200 mg once/day sustained-release	300 mg
Meclofenamate	50 mg tid or qid	400 mg
Nabumetone	1000–2000 mg/day in 1 dose or in divided doses	2000 mg
Naproxen	250–500 mg bid	1500 mg
Oxaprozin	1200 mg once/day	1800 mg
Piroxicam	20 mg once/day	20 mg
Sulindac	150–200 mg bid	400 mg
Tolmetin	400 mg tid	1800 mg
COX-2 selective NSAIDs		
Celecoxib	200 mg once/day or bid	400 mg
Meloxicam*	7.5 mg once/day	15 mg

*COX-2 specificity of this drug is unclear.
COX = cyclooxygenase.

Traditional disease-modifying antirheumatic drugs (DMARDs): (See Table 39–4 for specific dosage information and adverse effects of other drugs used to treat RA.)

DMARDs seem to slow the progression of RA and are indicated for nearly all patients with RA. They differ from each other chemically and pharmacologically. Many take weeks or months to have an effect. About two thirds of patients improve overall, and complete remissions are becoming more common. Many DMARDs result in evidence of decreased damage on imaging studies, presumably reflecting decreased disease activity. Patients should be fully apprised of the risks of DMARDs and monitored closely for evidence of toxicity.

When choosing DMARDs, the following principles should be considered:

- Combinations of DMARDs may be more effective than single drugs. For example, hydroxychloroquine, sulfasalazine, and methotrexate together are more effective than methotrexate alone or the other two together.
- Combining a DMARD with another drug, such as methotrexate plus a TNF-alpha antagonist or a rapidly tapered corticosteroid, may be more effective than using DMARDs alone.

Methotrexate is a folate antagonist with immunosuppressive effects at high dose. It is anti-inflammatory at doses used in RA. It is very effective and has a relatively rapid onset (clinical benefit often within 3 to 4 wk). Methotrexate should be used with caution, if at all, in patients with hepatic dysfunction or renal failure. Alcohol should be avoided. Supplemental folate, 1 mg po once/day, reduces the likelihood of adverse effects. CBC, AST, ALT, and albumin and creatinine level should be determined about every 8 wk. When used early in the course of RA, efficacy may equal the biologic agents. Rarely, a liver biopsy is needed if liver function test findings are persistently twice the upper limit of normal or more and the patient needs to continue to use methotrexate. Severe relapses of arthritis can occur after withdrawal of methotrexate. Paradoxically, rheumatoid nodules may enlarge with methotrexate therapy.

Hydroxychloroquine can also control symptoms of mild RA. Funduscopic examination should be done and visual fields should be assessed before and every 12 mo during treatment. The drug should be stopped if no improvement occurs after 9 mo.

Sulfasalazine can alleviate symptoms and slow development of joint damage. It is usually given as enteric-coated tablets. Benefit should occur within 3 mo. Enteric coating or dose reduction may increase tolerability. Because neutropenia may occur early, CBCs should be obtained after 1 to 2 wk and then about every 12 wk during therapy. AST and ALT should be obtained at about 6-mo intervals and whenever the dose is increased.

Table 39–4. OTHER DRUGS USED TO TREAT RHEUMATOID ARTHRITIS

DRUG	DOSAGE	ADVERSE EFFECTS
Traditional disease-modifying antirheumatic drugs (DMARDs)		
Hydroxychloroquine	5 mg/kg po once/day (eg, with breakfast or dinner) or in 2 divided doses (eg, 2.5 mg q 12 h) If improvement occurs, 200–400 mg once/day as long as effective	Usually mild dermatitis Myopathy Corneal opacity (generally reversible) Occasionally irreversible retinal degeneration
Leflunomide	20 mg po once/day or, if adverse effects occur, reduced to 10 mg once/day	Skin reactions Hepatic dysfunction Alopecia Diarrhea
Methotrexate	Single oral dose once/wk, starting at 7.5 mg and gradually increased as needed to a maximum of 25 mg Doses > 20 mg/wk best given sc to ensure bioavailability	Liver fibrosis (dose-related, often reversible) Nausea Possibly bone marrow suppression Stomatitis Rarely pneumonitis (potentially fatal)
Sulfasalazine*	500 mg po in the evening, increased to 500 mg in the morning and 1000 mg in the evening, then increased to 1000–1500 mg bid	Bone marrow suppression Gastric symptoms Neutropenia Hemolysis Hepatitis
Corticosteroids, intra-articular injections		
Methylprednisolone acetate Triamcinolone acetonide Triamcinolone hexacetonide	Depends on the joint Depends on the joint 10–40 mg, depending on the joint	With long-term use: Rarely infection at the injection site
Corticosteroids, systemic		
Prednisone Prednisolone	Attempts should be made to avoid exceeding 7.5 mg po once/day (except in patients with severe systemic manifestations)	With long-term use: • Weight gain • Diabetes • Hypertension • Osteoporosis

Table 39–4. OTHER DRUGS USED TO TREAT RHEUMATOID ARTHRITIS (*Continued*)

DRUG	DOSAGE	ADVERSE EFFECTS
Immunomodulatory, cytotoxic, or immunosuppressive drugs		
Azathioprine	1 mg/kg (50–100 mg) po once/day or bid, increased† by 0.5 mg/kg/day after 6–8 wk, then q 4 wk to a maximum of 2.5 mg/kg/day	Liver toxicity Bone marrow suppression Possibly increased risk of cancers (eg, lymphoma, nonmelanoma skin cancers)
Cyclosporine (an immunomodulatory drug)	50 mg po bid, not to exceed 1.75 mg/kg po bid	With cyclosporine, impaired renal function, hypertension, and risk of diabetes
Biologic agents		
Abatacept	500 mg IV for patients weighing < 60 kg, 750 mg IV for patients weighing 60–100 kg, and 1 g IV for patients weighing > 100 kg *or* 125 mg sc once/wk	Pulmonary toxicity Susceptibility to infection Headache URI Sore throat Nausea
Rituximab	1 g IV at baseline and at 2 wk (methylprednisolone 60–125 mg IV is given with each dose of rituximab to prevent hypersensitivity reactions)	When the drug is being given: • Mild itching at the injection site • Rashes • Back pain • Hypertension or hypotension • Fever After the drug is given: • Slightly increased risk of infection and possibly cancer • Hypogammaglobulinemia • Neutropenia
IL-1 receptor antagonists‡		
Anakinra	100 mg sc once/day	Injection site reactions Immunosuppression Neutropenia
Tocilizumab	8 mg/kg IV q 4 wk, to a maximum 800 mg/dose *or* 162 mg sc every other week followed by an increase to every week based on clinical response in patients weighing < 100 kg 162 mg sc q wk in patients weighing > 100 kg	Potential risk of infection (particularly opportunistic organisms) Neutropenia Thrombocytopenia GI perforation Anaphylaxis Demyelinating neurologic disorders
TNF-alpha antagonists‡		
Adalimumab	40 mg sc once q 1–2 wk	Potential risk of infection (particularly TB and fungal infections) Nonmelanoma skin cancers Reactivation of hepatitis B Antinuclear antibodies with or without clinical SLE Demyelinating neurologic disorders
Certolizumab pegol	400 mg sc (as 2 sc injections of 200 mg) once and then repeat at wk 2 and wk 4, followed by 200 mg sc q 2 wk (or 400 mg sc q 4 wk)	
Etanercept Etanercept-szzs (biosimilar)	50 mg sc once/wk	
Golimumab	50 mg sc once q 4 wk	
Infliximab Infliximab-dyyb (biosimilar)	3-mg/kg IV infusion in saline at baseline, at 2 wk, and at 6 wk with subsequent injections q 8 wk (dosage may be increased to 10 mg/kg)	
JAK inhibition‡		
Tofacitinib	5 mg po bid	Risk of infection, particularly varicella-zoster virus reactivation Nonmelanoma skin cancers Hypercholesterolemia

*Sulfasalazine is usually given as enteric-coated tablets.
†During dosage increases for azathioprine, CBC, AST, and ALT are monitored.
‡These drugs are biologic agents.
JAK = Janus kinase.

Leflunomide interferes with an enzyme involved with pyrimidine metabolism. It is about as effective as methotrexate but is less likely to suppress bone marrow, cause abnormal liver function, or cause pneumonitis. Alopecia and diarrhea are fairly common at the onset of therapy but may resolve with continuation of therapy.

Parenteral **gold compounds** are not commonly used anymore.

Corticosteroids: Systemic corticosteroids decrease inflammation and other symptoms more rapidly and to a greater degree than other drugs. They also seem to slow bone erosion. However, they may not prevent joint destruction, and their clinical benefit often diminishes with time. Furthermore, rebound often follows the withdrawal of corticosteroids in active disease. Because of their long-term adverse effects, some doctors recommend that corticosteroids are given to maintain function only until another DMARD has taken effect.

Corticosteroids may be used for severe joint or systemic manifestations of RA (eg, vasculitis, pleurisy, pericarditis). Relative contraindications include peptic ulcer disease, hypertension, untreated infections, diabetes mellitus, and glaucoma. The risk of latent TB should be considered before corticosteroid therapy is begun.

Intra-articular injections of depot corticosteroids may temporarily help control pain and swelling in particularly painful joints. Triamcinolone hexacetonide may suppress inflammation for the longest time. Triamcinolone acetonide and methylprednisolone acetate are also effective. No single joint should be injected with a corticosteroid more than 3 to 4 times a year, as too-frequent injections may accelerate joint destruction (although there are no specific data from humans to support this effect). Because injectable corticosteroid esters are crystalline, local inflammation transiently increases within a few hours in < 2% of patients receiving injections. Although infection occurs in only < 1:40,000 patients, it must be considered if pain occurs > 24 h after injection.

Immunomodulatory, cytotoxic, and immunosuppressive drugs: Treatment with azathioprine or cyclosporine (an immunomodulatory drug) provides efficacy similar to DMARDs. However, these drugs are more toxic. Thus, they are used only for patients in whom treatment with DMARDs has failed or to decrease the need for corticosteroids. They are used infrequently unless there are extra-articular complications. For maintenance therapy with azathioprine, the lowest effective dose should be used. Low-dose cyclosporine may be effective alone or when combined with methotrexate but is rarely used anymore. It may be less toxic than azathioprine. Cyclophosphamide is no longer recommended due to its toxicity.

Biologic agents: Biologic response modifiers other than TNF-alpha antagonists can be used to target B cells or T cells. These agents are typically not combined with each other.

Rituximab is an anti-CD 20 antibody that depletes B cells. It can be used in refractory patients. Response is often delayed but may last 6 mo. The course can be repeated after 6 mo. Mild adverse effects are common, and analgesia, corticosteroids, diphenhydramine, or a combination may need to be given concomitantly. Rituximab is usually restricted to patients who have not improved after using a TNF-alpha inhibitor and methotrexate. Rituximab therapy has been associated with progressive multifocal leukoencephalopathy, mucocutaneous reactions, delayed leukopenia, and hepatitis B reactivation.

Abatacept, a soluble fusion cytotoxic T lymphocyte-associated antigen 4 (CTLA-4) Ig, is indicated for patients with RA with an inadequate response to other DMARDs.

Anakinra is a recombinant IL-1 receptor antagonist. IL-1 is heavily involved in the pathogenesis of RA. Infection and leukopenia can be problems. It is used less often because it must be given every day.

TNF-alpha antagonists (eg, adalimumab, etanercept, etanercept-szzs, golimumab, certolizumab pegol, infliximab, and infliximab-dyyb) reduce the progression of erosions and reduce the number of new erosions. Although not all patients respond, many have a prompt, dramatic feeling of well being, sometimes with the first injection. Inflammation is often dramatically reduced. These drugs are often added to methotrexate therapy to increase the effect and possibly prevent the development of drug-neutralizing antibodies.

Tocilizumab blocks the effect of IL-6 and has clinical efficacy in patients who have responded incompletely to other biologic agents.

Tofacitinib is a JAK inhibitor that is given orally with or without concomitant methotrexate to patients who do not respond to methotrexate alone or other biologic agents.

Although there are some differences among agents, the most serious problem is infection, particularly with reactivated TB. Patients should be screened for TB with PPD or an interferon-gamma release assay. Other serious infections can occur, including sepsis, invasive fungal infections, and infections due to other opportunistic organisms. Risk of lymphomas is not increased in RA patients who are treated with TNF inhibitors.[1] Recent information suggests safety during pregnancy with TNF inhibitors and anakinra. TNF-alpha antagonists should probably be stopped before major surgery to decrease the risk of perioperative infection. Etanercept, infliximab, and adalimumab can be used with or without methotrexate. TNF inhibitors may predispose to heart failure and thus are relatively contraindicated in stage 3 and stage 4 heart failure.

1. Leombruno JP, Einarson TR, Keystone EC: The safety of anti-tumour necrosis factor treatments in rheumatoid arthritis: meta and exposure-adjusted pooled analyses of serious adverse events. *Ann Rheum Dis* 68(7):1136–1145, 2009. doi: 10.1136/ard.2008.091025.

KEY POINTS

- RA is a systemic inflammatory disorder.
- The most characteristic manifestation is a symmetric polyarthritis involving peripheral joints such as wrists and metacarpophalangeal and metatarsophalangeal joints, often with constitutional symptoms.
- Extra-articular findings can include rheumatoid nodules, vasculitis causing leg ulcers or mononeuritis multiplex, pleural or pericardial effusions, pulmonary nodules, pulmonary infiltrates or fibrosis, pericarditis, myocarditis, lymphadenopathy, Felty syndrome, Sjögren syndrome, scleromalacia, and episcleritis.
- Take x-rays but diagnose primarily by specific clinical criteria and laboratory test results, including autoantibodies (serum rheumatoid factor and anti-cyclic citrullinated peptide antibody) and acute-cellphase reactants (ESR or CRP).
- RA decreases life expectancy by 3 to 7 yr (eg, due to GI bleeding, infection, or heart disease) and causes severe disability in 10% of patients.
- Treat almost all patients early and primarily with drugs that modify disease activity.
- Drugs that modify disease activity include traditional DMARDs (particularly methotrexate), biologic agents such as TNF-alpha antagonists or other non-TNF biologic agents, and other drugs that are immunomodulatory, cytotoxic, or immunosuppressive.

OVERVIEW OF SERONEGATIVE SPONDYLOARTHROPATHIES

(Seronegative Spondyloarthritides)

Seronegative spondyloarthropathies (seronegative spondyloarthritides) share certain clinical characteristics (eg, back pain, uveitis, GI symptoms, rashes). Some are strongly associated with the HLA-B27 allele. Clinical and genetic similarities suggest that they also share similar causes or pathophysiologies. RF is usually negative in the spondyloarthropathies (hence, why they are called seronegative spondyloarthropathies). They include ankylosing spondylitis, reactive arthritis, psoriatic arthritis, and other disorders.

Spondyloarthropathy can develop in association with GI conditions (sometimes called enteropathic arthritis) such as inflammatory bowel disease, intestinal bypass surgery, or Whipple disease.

Juvenile-onset spondyloarthropathy is an asymmetric, mostly lower extremity spondyloarthropathy that begins most commonly in boys aged 7 to 16.

Spondyloarthropathy can also develop in people without characteristics of other specific spondyloarthropathy (undifferentiated spondyloarthropathy). Treatment of the arthritis of these other spondyloarthropathies is similar to the treatment of reactive arthritis.

ANKYLOSING SPONDYLITIS

Ankylosing spondylitis is the prototypical spondyloarthropathy and a systemic disorder characterized by inflammation of the axial skeleton, large peripheral joints, and digits; nocturnal back pain; back stiffness; accentuated kyphosis; constitutional symptoms; aortitis; cardiac conduction abnormalities; and anterior uveitis. Diagnosis requires showing sacroiliitis on x-ray. Treatment is with NSAIDs and/or tumor necrosis factor antagonists or IL-17 antagonists or physical measures that maintain joint flexibility.

Ankylosing spondylitis (AS) is 3 times more frequent in men than in women and begins most often between ages 20 and 40. It is 10 to 20 times more common among 1st-degree relatives of AS patients than in the general population. The HLA-B27 allele is present in 90% of AS patients, but it is also present in up to 10% of the general population depending on ethnicity. The risk of AS in 1st-degree relatives with the HLA-B27 allele is about 20%. Increased prevalence of HLA-B27 in whites or HLA-B7 in blacks supports a genetic predisposition. However, the concordance rate in identical twins is only about 50%, suggesting that environmental factors contribute. The pathophysiology probably involves immune-mediated inflammation.

Classification

Most patients with AS have predominantly axial involvement (called axial AS). Some have predominately peripheral involvement. Among those with axial involvement, some have no evidence of sacroiliitis on plain x-rays. Thus, some experts have classified AS as follows:

- Axial AS: Has predominantly axial involvement and x-ray findings typical of sacroiliitis
- Nonradiographic AS: Clinically similar to axial AS but without x-ray findings typical of sacroiliitis
- Peripheral AS: AS with predominantly peripheral involvement

Symptoms and Signs

The most frequent manifestation of AS is back pain, but disease can begin in peripheral joints, especially in children and women, and rarely with acute iridocyclitis (iritis or anterior uveitis). Other early symptoms and signs are diminished chest expansion from diffuse costovertebral involvement, low-grade fever, fatigue, anorexia, weight loss, and anemia.

Back pain—often nocturnal and of varying intensity—eventually becomes recurrent. Morning stiffness, typically relieved by activity, and paraspinal muscle spasm develop. A flexed or bent-over posture eases back pain and paraspinal muscle spasm; thus, kyphosis is common in untreated patients. Severe hip arthritis can eventually develop. In late stages, the patient has accentuated kyphosis, loss of lumbar lordosis, and fixed bent-forward posturing, with compromised pulmonary function and inability to lie flat. There may be peripheral potentially deforming joint involvement, sometimes involving the digits (dactylitis). Achilles and patellar tendinitis can occur.

Systemic manifestations of AS occur in one third of patients. Recurrent, acute anterior uveitis is common and usually responds to local therapy; less commonly it becomes protracted and severe enough to impair vision. Neurologic signs occasionally result from compression radiculitis or sciatica, vertebral fracture or subluxation, or cauda equina syndrome. Cardiovascular manifestations can include aortic insufficiency, aortitis, angina, pericarditis, and cardiac conduction abnormalities (which may be asymptomatic). Dyspnea, cough, or hemoptysis can rarely result from nontuberculous fibrosis or cavitation of an upper lobe of the lung; cavitary lesions can become secondarily infected with *Aspergillus*. Rarely, AS results in secondary amyloidosis. Subcutaneous nodules do not develop.

Diagnosis

- Lumbosacral spine and sacroiliac joint radiography
- Blood tests (ESR, C-reactive protein [CRP], HLA-B27, and CBC) or explicit clinical criteria (modified New York criteria or Assessment of SpondyloArthritis International Society criteria)
- Pelvic MRI in select patients

AS should be suspected in patients, particularly young men, with nocturnal back pain and kyphosis, diminished chest expansion, Achilles or patellar tendinitis, or unexplained anterior uveitis. A 1st-degree relative with AS should heighten suspicion.

Patients should generally be tested with ESR, HLA-B27, CRP, and CBC. Rheumatoid factor (RF) and antinuclear antibodies are needed only if peripheral arthritis suggests other diagnoses. The HLA-B27 allele is present in 90% of AS patients, but it is also present in up to 10% of the general population depending on ethnicity. No laboratory test is diagnostic, but results can increase suspicion for the disorder or rule out other disorders that can simulate AS. If, after these tests, AS is still suspected, patients should undergo x-ray of the lumbosacral spine and sacroiliac joint; demonstration of sacroiliitis on x-ray strongly supports the diagnosis.

Some patients should undergo pelvic MRI to look for sacroiliitis that is not seen on x-rays. In these patients, MRI shows osteitis or early erosions.

AS has traditionally been diagnosed by the modified New York criteria. Using these criteria, the patient must have imaging study evidence of sacroiliitis and one of the following:

- Restriction of lumbar spinal motion in both the sagittal (looking from the side) and frontal (looking from the back) planes
- Restriction of chest expansion, adjusted for age
- A history of inflammatory back pain

To diagnose patients earlier in the disease process, particularly those without spondyloarthritis on imaging, the novel Assessment of Spondyloarthritis International Society (ASAS) criteria have been established.[1] The ASAS criteria for axial spondyloarthritis are applied to patients who have had back pain for > 3 mo and who are < 45 yr of age at onset.

Diagnosis can be done using ASAS imaging or clinical criteria. To fulfill the imaging criteria, patients must have radiographic or MRI evidence of sacroiliitis plus at least 1 spondyloarthritis feature. To fulfill the clinical criteria, patients must have HLA-B27 plus at least 2 separate spondyloarthritis features. ASAS spondyloarthritis features include the following:

- Dactylitis
- Enthesitis of the heel
- Family history of spondyloarthritis
- History of inflammatory back pain
- Psoriasis
- IBD
- Presence of HLA-B27
- Uveitis
- Elevated CRP
- Good response to NSAIDs

Historical features that distinguish inflammatory back pain from noninflammatory back pain include onset at ≤ 40 yr, gradual onset, morning stiffness, improvement with activity, and duration ≥ 3 mo before seeking medical attention.

ESR and other acute-phase reactants (eg, CRP) are inconsistently elevated in patients with active AS. Tests for RF and antinuclear antibodies are negative. The HLA-B27 genetic marker is not usually helpful because positive and negative predictive values are low.

The earliest x-ray abnormalities are pseudowidening caused by subchondral erosions, followed by sclerosis or later narrowing and eventually fusion in the sacroiliac joints. Changes are symmetric. Early changes in the spine are upper lumbar vertebral squaring with sclerosis at the corners; spotty ligamentous calcification; and one or two evolving syndesmophytes. Late changes result in a "bamboo spine" appearance, resulting from prominent syndesmophytes, diffuse paraspinal ligamentous calcification, and osteoporosis; these changes develop in some patients on average over 10 yr.

Changes typical of AS may not become visible on plain x-rays for years. MRI shows changes earlier, but there is no consensus regarding its role in routine diagnosis given the lack of prospective, validated data in regard to its diagnostic utility. Pelvic MRI should be done if the index of suspicion of spondyloarthritis is high or if there is a need to rule out other causes of the patient's symptoms.

A herniated intervertebral disk can cause back pain and radiculopathy similar to AS, but the pain is limited to the spine and nerve roots, usually causes more sudden symptoms, and causes no systemic manifestations or laboratory test abnormalities. If necessary, CT or MRI can differentiate it from AS. Involvement of a single sacroiliac joint suggests a different spondyloarthropathy, possibly infection. Tuberculous spondylitis can simulate AS (see TB of bones and joints on p. 1659).

Diffuse idiopathic skeletal hyperostosis (DISH) occurs primarily in men > 50 yr and may resemble AS clinically and on x-ray. Patients uncommonly have spinal pain, stiffness, and insidious loss of motion. X-ray findings in DISH include large ossifications anterior to spinal ligaments (the calcification appears as if someone poured candle wax in front and on the sides of the vertebrae), bridging several vertebrae and usually starting at the lower thoracic spine, eventually affecting the cervical and lumbar spine. There is often subperiosteal bone growth along the pelvic brim and at insertion of tendons (such as the Achilles tendon insertion). However, the anterior spinal ligament is intact and frequently bulging, and sacroiliac and spinal apophyseal joints are not eroded. Additional differentiating features are stiffness that is usually not markedly accentuated in the morning and a normal ESR.

1. Sepriano A, Landewé R, van der Heijde D, et al: Predictive validity of the ASAS classification criteria for axial and peripheral spondyloarthritis after follow-up in the ASAS cohort: a final analysis. *Ann Rheum Dis* 75(6):1034–1042, 2016. doi: 10.1136/annrheumdis-2015-208730.

Prognosis

AS is characterized by mild or moderate flares of active inflammation alternating with periods of little or no inflammation. Proper treatment in most patients results in minimal or no disability and in a full, productive life despite back stiffness. Occasionally, the course is severe and progressive, resulting in pronounced incapacitating deformities.

Treatment

- NSAIDs
- Sulfasalazine, methotrexate, TNF-alpha antagonists, or IL-17 antagonists (eg, secukinumab)
- Exercises and supportive measures

The goals of treatment of AS are relieving pain, maintaining joint range of motion, and preventing end-organ damage. Because the condition may cause lung fibrosis, cigarette smoking is discouraged. (See the American College of Rheumatology/Spondylitis Association of America/Spondyloarthritis Research and Treatment Network's 2015 recommendations for the treatment of ankylosing spondylitis and nonradiographic axial spondyloarthritis.)

NSAIDs reduce pain and suppress joint inflammation and muscle spasm, thereby increasing range of motion, which facilitates exercise and prevents contractures. Most NSAIDs work in AS, and tolerance and toxicity dictate drug choice. The daily dose of NSAIDs should be as low as possible, but maximum doses may be needed with active disease. Drug withdrawal should be attempted only slowly, after systemic and joint signs of active disease have been suppressed for several months.

Sulfasalazine may help reduce peripheral joint symptoms and laboratory markers of inflammation in some patients. Dosage should be started at 500 mg/day and increased by 500 mg/day at 1-wk intervals to 1 to 1.5 g bid maintenance; because acute neutropenia can occur, cell counts must be monitored when initiating therapy or increasing drug dose. Peripheral joint symptoms may also abate with methotrexate, but spinal symptoms are usually not reduced.

TNF-alpha antagonists (eg, etanercept, infliximab, adalimumab, certolizumab, golimumab) are often strikingly effective treatments for inflammatory back pain.

Secukinumab, an IL-17 antagonist, has also been effective in reducing inflammation and joint symptoms. Secukinumab can be given at a dose of 150 mg sc at wk 0, 1, 2, 3, and 4 and every 4 wk thereafter. Without the loading (weekly) doses, secukinumab is 150 mg sc q 4 wk. Adverse effects include urticaria, URIs, fungal infections due to *Candida*, diarrhea, herpes zoster, and inflammatory bowel disease.

Systemic corticosteroids, immunosuppressants, and most disease-modifying antirheumatic drugs (DMARDs) have no proven benefit and should generally not be used.

For proper posture and joint motion, daily exercise and other supportive measures (eg, postural training, therapeutic exercise) are vital to strengthen muscle groups that oppose the direction of potential deformities (ie, the extensor rather than flexor muscles). Reading while lying prone and pushing up on the elbows or pillows and thus extending the back may help keep the back flexible. Because chest wall motion can be restricted, which impairs lung function, cigarette smoking, which also impairs lung function, is strongly discouraged.

Intra-articular depot corticosteroids may be beneficial, particularly when one or two peripheral joints are more severely inflamed than others, thereby compromising exercise and rehabilitation. They may also help if systemic drugs are ineffective. Imaging-guided corticosteroid injections into the sacroiliac joints may occasionally help severe sacroiliitis.

For acute uveitis, topical corticosteroids and mydriatics are usually adequate.

If severe hip arthritis develops, total hip arthroplasty may lessen pain and improve flexibility dramatically.

KEY POINTS

- AS is a systemic disorder that affects the joints and can cause constitutional symptoms, cardiac symptoms, and anterior uveitis.
- Initial manifestation is usually back pain and stiffness sometimes along with peripheral joint symptoms and/or anterior uveitis.
- Diagnose based on the results of lumbosacral spine imaging, sacroiliac joint imaging, pelvic MRI, blood tests (ESR, CRP, HLA-B27, and CBC), and/or explicit clinical criteria.
- Use NSAIDs to help reduce symptom severity and improve function.
- Use sulfasalazine, methotrexate, TNF-alpha antagonists, or IL-17 antagonists to relieve joint symptoms.

PSORIATIC ARTHRITIS

Psoriatic arthritis is a spondyloarthropathy and chronic inflammatory arthritis that occurs in people with psoriasis of the skin or nails. The arthritis is often asymmetric, and some forms involve the distal interphalangeal (DIP) joints. Diagnosis is clinical. Treatment involves disease-modifying antirheumatic drugs (DMARDs) and biologic agents.

Psoriatic arthritis develops in about 30% of patients with psoriasis. Prevalence is increased in patients with AIDS. Risk is increased in patients with HLA-B27 or some other specific alleles and in family members. Etiology and pathophysiology of psoriatic arthritis are unknown.

Symptoms and Signs

Psoriasis of the skin or nails may precede or follow joint involvement. Severity of the joint and skin disease is often discordant. Also, skin lesions may be hidden in the scalp, gluteal folds, or umbilicus and go unrecognized by the patient.

The DIP joints of fingers and toes are especially affected. Asymmetric involvement of large and small joints, including the sacroiliacs and spine, is common. Joint and skin symptoms may lessen or worsen simultaneously. Inflammation of the fingers, toes, or both may lead to sausage-shaped deformities, which are not present in patients with RA. Rheumatoid nodules are absent. Arthritic remissions tend to be more frequent, rapid, and complete than in RA, but progression to chronic arthritis and crippling may occur. There may be arthritis mutilans (destruction of multiple hand joints with telescoping of the digits).

Enthesopathy (inflammation at tendinous insertion into bone—eg, Achilles tendinitis, patellar tendinitis, elbow epicondyles, spinous processes of the vertebrae) can develop and cause pain.

Back pain may be present. It is often accompanied by asymmetric syndesmophytes of the spine.

Diagnosis

- Clinical evaluation
- Rheumatoid factor (RF)

Psoriatic arthritis should be suspected in patients with both psoriasis and arthritis. Because psoriasis may be overlooked or hidden or develop only after arthritis occurs, psoriatic arthritis should be considered in any patient with seronegative inflammatory arthritis; these patients should be examined for psoriasis and nail pitting and should be questioned about a family history of psoriasis. Patients suspected of having psoriatic arthritis should be tested for RF. Occasionally, RF test results can be positive. However, anticyclic citrullinated peptide antibodies (anti-CCP) are highly specific for RA.

Psoriatic arthritis is diagnosed clinically and by excluding other disorders that can cause such similar manifestations. X-ray findings common in psoriatic arthritis include DIP joint involvement; resorption of terminal phalanges; arthritis mutilans; and extensive destruction, proliferative bone reaction, a sausage-like appearance to digits, and dislocation of large and small joints.

Treatment

- Arthritis treated with disease-modifying antirheumatic drugs (DMARDs—particularly methotrexate) and biologic agents (TNF-alpha antagonists, ustekinumab, secukinumab, and apremilast)

Treatment is directed at controlling skin lesions and at reducing joint inflammation. Drug therapy is similar to that for RA, particularly the DMARD methotrexate. Hydroxychloroquine is inconsistently of benefit and may cause exfoliative dermatitis or aggravate underlying psoriasis. Benefit may be gained from NSAIDs, cyclosporine, TNF-alpha antagonists (see Biologic agents on p. 310), ustekinumab, secukinumab, and apremilast. TNF-alpha antagonists have been particularly effective. (See also European League Against Rheumatism's [EULAR] recommendations for the management of psoriatic arthritis with pharmacologic therapies.)

Phototherapy using long-wave psoralen plus ultraviolet A (PUVA) combined with oral methoxsalen 600 mcg/kg po 2 h before PUVA twice/wk has been used for psoriatic lesions and is somewhat effective for peripheral arthritis, but not for spine involvement.

Ustekinumab is an IL-12 and IL-23 antagonist. The dose is 45 mg IM at wk 0 and 4 (loading doses) followed by 45 mg every 12 wk thereafter. The dose is 90 mg IM if the patient weighs > 100 kg. Adverse effects are similar to those of the other biologic agents.

Secukinumab is an IL-17 inhibitor. Secukinumab can be given at doses of 150 mg sc at wk 0, 1, 2, 3, and 4 and every 4 wk thereafter. Without the loading (weekly) doses, secukinumab is given at 150 mg sc q 4 wk. If patients continue to have active psoriatic arthritis, a dose of 300 mg should be considered. Secukinumab may be given with or without methotrexate. Adverse effects include urticaria, URIs, fungal infections due to *Candida*, diarrhea, herpes zoster, and inflammatory bowel disease.

Apremilast is a phosphodiesterase-4 inhibitor. The initial dose is 10 mg po once/day, titrated to the maintenance dose of 30 mg bid as tolerated. Adverse effects include diarrhea, nausea, headache, depression, and weight loss.

KEY POINTS

- Psoriatic arthritis is chronic inflammatory arthritis that occurs in patients with psoriasis; however, psoriasis may be mild or overlooked or may have not yet developed.
- Arthritis is commonly asymmetric, involves large and small joints (including axial joints), and typically affects the finger and toe DIP joints more than others.
- Diagnose based on clinical findings.
- Treat with DMARDs and biologic agents.

REACTIVE ARTHRITIS

Reactive arthritis is an acute spondyloarthropathy that often seems precipitated by an infection, usually GU or GI. Common manifestations include asymmetric arthritis of variable severity that tends to affect the lower extremities with sausage-shaped deformities of fingers or toes or both, constitutional symptoms, enthesitis, tendinitis, and mucocutaneous ulcers, including hyperkeratotic or crusted vesicular lesions (keratoderma blennorrhagicum). Diagnosis is clinical. Treatment involves NSAIDs and sometimes sulfasalazine or immunosuppressants.

Spondyloarthropathy associated with urethritis or cervicitis, conjunctivitis, and mucocutaneous lesions (previously called Reiter syndrome) is one type of reactive arthritis.

Etiology

Two forms of reactive arthritis are common: sexually transmitted and dysenteric. The sexually transmitted form occurs primarily in men aged 20 to 40. Genital infections with *Chlamydia trachomatis* are most often implicated. Men or women can acquire the dysenteric form after enteric infections, primarily *Shigella, Salmonella, Yersinia,* or *Campylobacter*. Reactive arthritis probably results from joint infection or postinfectious inflammation. Although there is evidence of microbial antigens in the synovium, organisms cannot be cultured from joint fluid.

Epidemiology

The prevalence of the HLA-B27 allele in patients is 63 to 96% vs 6 to 15% in healthy white controls, thus supporting a genetic predisposition.

Symptoms and Signs

Reactive arthritis can range from transient monarticular arthritis to a severe, multisystem disorder. Constitutional symptoms may include fever, fatigue, and weight loss. Arthritis may be mild or severe. Joint involvement is generally asymmetric and oligoarticular or polyarticular, occurring predominantly in the large joints of the lower extremities and in the toes. Back pain may occur, usually with severe disease.

Enthesopathy (inflammation at tendinous insertion into bone—eg, plantar fasciitis, digital periostitis, Achilles tendinitis) is common and characteristic.

Mucocutaneous lesions—small, transient, relatively painless, superficial ulcers—commonly occur on the oral mucosa, tongue, and glans penis (balanitis circinata). Particularly characteristic are vesicles (sometimes identical to pustular psoriasis) of the palms and soles and around the nails that become hyperkeratotic and form crusts (**keratoderma blennorrhagicum**). Rarely, cardiovascular complications (eg, aortitis, aortic insufficiency, cardiac conduction defects), pleuritis, and CNS or peripheral nervous system symptoms develop.

Urethritis may develop 7 to 14 days after sexual contact (or occasionally after dysentery); low-grade fever, conjunctivitis, and arthritis develop over the next few weeks. Not all features may occur, so incomplete forms need to be considered. In men, the urethritis is less painful and productive of purulent discharge than acute gonococcal urethritis and may be associated with hemorrhagic cystitis or prostatitis. In women, urethritis and cervicitis may be mild (with dysuria or slight vaginal discharge) or asymptomatic.

Conjunctivitis is the most common eye lesion. It usually causes mild eye redness and grittiness, but keratitis and anterior uveitis can develop also, causing eye pain, photophobia, and tearing.

Diagnosis

- Typical arthritis
- Symptoms of antecedent GI or GU infection
- One other extra-articular feature

Reactive arthritis should be suspected in patients with acute, asymmetric arthritis affecting the large joints of the lower extremities or toes, particularly if there is tendinitis or a history of an antecedent diarrhea or dysuria. Diagnosis is ultimately clinical and requires the typical peripheral arthritis with symptoms of GU or GI infection or one of the other extra-articular features. Because these features may manifest at different times, definitive diagnosis may require several months. Serum and synovial fluid complement levels are high, but these findings are not usually diagnostic and need not be measured.

Disseminated gonococcal infection can closely simulate reactive arthritis. Arthrocentesis may fail to differentiate them, owing to inflammatory characteristics of synovial fluid in both disorders and the difficulty of culturing gonococci from this fluid. Clinical characteristics may help; disseminated gonococcal infection tends to involve upper and lower extremities equally, be more migratory, and not cause back pain, and vesicles tend not to be hyperkeratotic. A positive gonococcal culture from blood or skin lesions helps differentiate the two disorders, but a positive culture from the urethra or cervix does not. If differentiation is still difficult, ceftriaxone may be required for simultaneous diagnosis and treatment.

Psoriatic arthritis can simulate reactive arthritis, causing similar skin lesions, uveitis, and asymmetric arthritis. However, psoriatic arthritis often affects mostly the upper extremities and especially the distal interphalangeal joints, may be abrupt in onset but may also develop gradually, causes less enthesopathy, and tends not to cause mouth ulcers or symptoms of GU or GI infection.

Prognosis

Reactive arthritis often resolves in 3 to 4 mo, but up to 50% of patients experience recurrent or prolonged symptoms over several years. Joint, spinal, or sacroiliac inflammation or deformity may occur with chronic or recurrent disease. Some patients are disabled.

Treatment

- NSAIDs
- Sometimes sulfasalazine, doxycycline, azathioprine or methotrexate, or a combination
- Supportive measures

NSAIDs (eg, indomethacin 25 to 50 mg po tid) usually help relieve symptoms. If induced by infection with *C. trachomatis*, doxycycline 100 mg po bid for up to 3 mo may accelerate recovery, but this is controversial. Sulfasalazine as used to treat RA may also be helpful (see p. 308). If symptoms are severe despite NSAIDs and sulfasalazine, azathioprine or methotrexate may be considered.

Local injection of depot corticosteroids for enthesopathy or resistant oligoarthritis may relieve symptoms. Physical therapy aimed at maintaining joint mobility is helpful during the recovery phase. Anterior uveitis is treated as usual, with corticosteroid and mydriatic eye drops to prevent scarring. Conjunctivitis and mucocutaneous lesions require only symptomatic treatment.

KEY POINTS

- Reactive arthritis is an acute spondyloarthropathy that typically occurs after a sexually transmitted or enteric infection.
- Manifestations can include arthritis (usually asymmetric and involving large lower extremity joints and toes), enthesopathy, mucocutaneous lesions, conjunctivitis, and nonpurulent genital discharge (eg, urethritis, cervicitis).
- Confirm the diagnosis with typical arthritic findings plus either symptoms of GU or GI infection or a characteristic extra-articular finding.
- Treat with NSAIDs and sometimes sulfasalazine or immunosuppressants.

40 Neck and Back Pain

Neck pain and back pain are among the most common reasons for physician visits. This discussion covers neck pain involving the posterior neck (not pain limited to the anterior neck) and does not cover most major traumatic injuries (eg, fractures, dislocations, subluxations).

Pathophysiology

Depending on the cause, neck or back pain may be accompanied by neurologic symptoms.

If a nerve root is affected, pain may radiate distally along the distribution of that root (radicular pain). Strength, sensation, and reflexes of the area innervated by that root may be impaired (see Table 236–5 on p. 1989).

If the spinal cord is affected, strength, sensation, and reflexes may be impaired at the affected spinal cord level and all levels below (called segmental neurologic deficits).

If the cauda equina is affected, segmental deficits develop in the lumbosacral region, typically with disruption of bowel function (constipation or fecal incontinence) and bladder function (urinary retention or incontinence), loss of perianal sensation, erectile dysfunction, and loss of rectal tone and sphincter (eg, bulbocavernosus, anal wink) reflexes.

Any painful disorder of the spine may also cause reflex tightening (spasm) of paraspinal muscles, which can be excruciating.

Etiology

Most neck and back pain is caused by disorders of the spine. Fibromyalgia is also a common cause and may be superimposed on a chronic primary spinal disorder. Occasionally, pain is referred from extraspinal disorders (particularly vascular, gastrointestinal, or genitourinary). Some uncommon causes—spinal and extraspinal—are serious.

Most spinal disorders are mechanical. Only a few involve infection, inflammation, cancer, or fragility fractures due to osteoporosis or cancer and are considered nonmechanical.

Common causes: Most mechanical spine disorders that cause neck or back pain involve a nonspecific mechanical derangement:

- Muscle strain, ligament sprain, spasm, or a combination
- Poor posture, decreased strength of stabilizing muscles, or decreased flexibility

Only about 15% involve specific structural lesions of the spine that clearly cause the symptoms, primarily the following:

- Disk herniation
- Compression fracture
- Lumbar spinal stenosis (LSS)
- Osteoarthritis
- Spondylolisthesis

In the other mechanical disorders, there are no specific lesions, or the findings (eg, disk bulging or degeneration, osteophytes, spondylolysis, congenital facet abnormalities) are common among people without neck or back pain, and thus are questionable as the etiology of pain. However, etiology of back pain, particularly if mechanical, is often multifactorial, with an underlying disorder exacerbated by fatigue, physical deconditioning, and sometimes psychosocial stress or psychiatric abnormality. Thus, identifying a single cause is often difficult or impossible.

Neck and back pain can sometimes be attributed to a generalized myofascial pain syndrome, such as fibromyalgia, rather than a primary spinal disorder.

Serious uncommon causes: Serious causes may require timely treatment to prevent disability or death.

Serious **extraspinal** disorders include the following:

- Abdominal aortic aneurysm
- Aortic dissection
- Carotid or vertebral artery dissection
- Acute meningitis
- Angina or MI
- Certain GI disorders (eg, cholecystitis, diverticulitis, diverticular abscess, pancreatitis, penetrating peptic ulcer, retrocecal appendicitis)
- Certain pelvic disorders (eg, ectopic pregnancy, ovarian cancer, salpingitis)
- Certain pulmonary disorders (eg, pleuritis, pneumonia)
- Certain urinary tract disorders (eg, prostatitis, pyelonephritis, nephrolithiasis)

Serious **spinal** disorders include the following:

- Infections (eg, diskitis, epidural abscess, osteomyelitis)
- Primary tumors (of spinal cord or vertebrae)
- Metastatic vertebral tumors (most often from breasts, lungs, or prostate)

Mechanical spine disorders can be serious if they compress the spinal nerve roots or, particularly, the spinal cord. Spinal cord compression may result from disorders such as tumors and spinal epidural abscess or hematoma.

Other uncommon causes: Neck or back pain can result from many other disorders, such as

- Paget disease of bone
- Torticollis
- Thoracic outlet syndrome
- Temporomandibular joint syndrome
- Herpes zoster (even before the rash)
- Retroperitoneal fibrosis
- Spondyloarthropathies (ankylosing spondylitis most often, but also enteropathic arthritis, psoriatic arthritis, reactive arthritis, and undifferentiated spondyloarthropathy)

Evaluation

General: Because the cause is often multifactorial, a definitive diagnosis cannot be established in many patients. However, clinicians should determine the following if possible:

- Whether pain has a spinal or extraspinal cause
- Whether the cause is a serious disorder

If serious causes have been ruled out, back pain is sometimes classified as follows:

- Nonspecific low back pain
- Low back pain with radicular symptoms or spinal stenosis
- Low back pain associated with another spinal cause

History: History of present illness should include quality, onset, duration, severity, location, radiation, and time course of pain, as well as modifying factors such as rest, activity, changes in position, weight bearing, and time of day (eg, at night, when awakening). Accompanying symptoms to note include stiffness, numbness, paresthesias, weakness, urinary retention, constipation, and fecal incontinence.

Review of systems should note symptoms suggesting a cause, including fever, sweats, and chills (infection); weight loss and poor appetite (infection or cancer); fatigue, depressive symptoms, and headaches (multifactorial mechanical back pain); worsening of neck pain during swallowing (esophageal disorders); anorexia, nausea, vomiting, melena or hematochezia, and change in bowel function or stool (GI disorders); urinary symptoms and flank pain (urinary tract disorders), especially if intermittent, colicky, and recurrent (nephrolithiasis); cough, dyspnea, and worsening during inspiration (pulmonary disorders); vaginal bleeding or discharge and pain related to menstrual cycle phase (pelvic disorders).

Past medical history includes known neck or back disorders (including osteoporosis, osteoarthritis, disk disorders, and recent or remote injury) and surgery, risk factors for back disorders (eg, cancer, osteoporosis), risk factors for aneurysm (eg, smoking, hypertension), risk factors for infection (eg, immunosuppression; IV drug use; recent surgery, hemodialysis, penetrating trauma, or bacterial infection); and extra-articular features of an underlying systemic disorder (eg, diarrhea or abdominal pain, uveitis, psoriasis).

Physical examination: Temperature and general appearance are noted. When possible, patients should be unobtrusively observed as they move into the examination room, undress, and climb onto the table. If symptoms are exacerbated by psychologic issues, true functional level can be assessed more accurately when patients are not aware they are being evaluated.

The examination focuses on the spine and the neurologic examination. If no mechanical spinal source of pain is obvious, patients are checked for sources of localized or referred pain.

In the **spinal examination**, the back and neck are inspected for any visible deformity, area of erythema, or vesicular rash. The spine and paravertebral muscles are palpated for tenderness, muscle spasm, and features of myofascial pain syndrome (taut bands, trigger points, and generalized pressure sensitivity). Gross range of motion is tested. In patients with neck pain, the shoulders are examined. In patients with low back pain, the hips are examined.

The **neurologic examination** should at least assess function of the entire spinal cord. Strength and deep tendon reflexes are tested. In patients with neurologic symptoms, sensation and sacral nerve function (eg, rectal tone, anal wink reflex, bulbocavernosus reflex) are tested. Reflex tests are among the most reliable physical tests for confirming normal spinal cord function. Corticospinal tract dysfunction is indicated by the extensor plantar response and Hoffman sign.

To test for the Hoffman sign, clinicians tap the nail or flick the volar surface of the 3rd finger; if the distal phalanx of the thumb flexes, the test is positive, usually indicating corticospinal tract dysfunction caused by stenosis of the cervical cord or a brain lesion. Sensory findings are subjective and may be unreliable.

The straight leg raise test helps confirm sciatica. The patient is supine with both knees extended and the ankles dorsiflexed. The clinician slowly raises the affected leg, keeping the knee extended. If sciatica is present, 10 to 60° of elevation typically causes symptoms.

For the crossed straight leg raise test, the unaffected leg is raised; the test is positive if sciatica occurs in the affected leg. A positive straight leg test is sensitive but not specific for herniated disk; the crossed straight leg raise test is less sensitive but 90% specific.

The seated straight leg raise test is done while patients are seated with the hip joint flexed at 90°; the lower leg is slowly raised until the knee is fully extended. If sciatica is present, the pain in the spine (and often the radicular symptoms) occurs as the leg is extended.

In the **general examination**, the lungs are auscultated. The abdomen is checked for tenderness, masses, and, particularly in patients > 55, a pulsatile mass (which suggests abdominal aortic aneurysm). With a fist, clinicians percuss the costovertebral angle for tenderness, suggesting pyelonephritis.

Rectal examination, including stool testing for occult blood and, in men, prostate examination, is done. In women with symptoms suggesting a pelvic disorder or with unexplained fever, pelvic examination is done.

Lower-extremity pulses are checked.

Red flags: The following findings are of particular concern:

- Abdominal aorta that is > 5 cm (particularly if tender) or lower-extremity pulse deficits
- Acute, tearing midback pain
- Cancer, diagnosed or suspected
- Duration of pain > 6 wk

- Neurologic deficit
- Fever
- GI findings such as localized abdominal tenderness, peritoneal signs, melena, or hematochezia
- Infection risk factors (eg, immunosuppression; IV drug use; recent surgery, penetrating trauma, or bacterial infection)
- Meningismus
- Severe nocturnal or disabling pain
- Unexplained, new-onset pain after age 55
- Unexplained weight loss

Interpretation of findings: Although serious extraspinal disorders (eg, cancers, aortic aneurysms, epidural abscesses, osteomyelitis) are uncommon causes of back pain, they are not rare, particularly in high-risk groups.

A spinal cause is more likely (but not definitive) than referred pain from an extraspinal cause when

- Pain is worsened by movement or weight bearing and is relieved by rest or recumbency
- Vertebral or paravertebral tenderness is present

Red flag findings should heighten suspicion of a serious cause (see Table 40–1).

Other findings are also helpful. Erythema and tenderness over the spine suggest infection, particularly in patients with risk factors. Worsening of pain with flexion is consistent with intervertebral disk disease; worsening with extension suggests spinal stenosis, arthritis affecting the facet joints, or retroperitoneal inflammation or infiltration (eg, pancreatic or kidney inflammation or tumor). Tenderness over certain specific trigger points suggests fibromyalgia. Deformities of the proximal interphalangeal (PIP) and distal interphalangeal (DIP) finger joints and stiffness that lessens within 30 min after awakening suggest osteoarthritis. Neck pain that is unrelated to swallowing and is exertional may indicate angina.

Testing: Usually, if duration of pain is short (< 4 to 6 wk), no testing is required unless red flag findings are present, patients have had a serious injury (eg, vehicular crash, fall from a height, penetrating trauma), or evaluation suggests a specific nonmechanical cause (eg, pyelonephritis).

Plain x-rays can identify most osteoporotic fractures and osteoarthritis. However, they do not identify abnormalities in soft tissue (the most common cause of back and neck pain) or nerve tissue (as occurs in many serious disorders). Thus, x-rays are usually unnecessary and do not change management. Sometimes x-rays are done to identify obvious bone abnormalities (eg, those due to infection or tumors) and to avoid MRI and CT, which are harder to obtain but which are much more accurate and usually necessary.

Testing is guided by findings and suspected cause. Testing is also indicated in patients who have failed initial treatment or in those whose symptoms have changed. Testing for specific suspected causes includes the following:

- Neurologic deficits, particularly those consistent with spinal cord compression: MRI or CT myelography, done as soon as possible
- Possible infection: WBC count, ESR, imaging (usually MRI or CT), and culture of infected tissue
- Possible cancer: CT or MRI and possibly biopsy
- Possible aneurysm: CT, angiography, or sometimes ultrasonography
- Possible aortic dissection: Angiography, CT, or MRI
- Symptoms that are disabling or that persist > 6 wk: Imaging (usually MRI or CT) and, if infection is suspected, WBC count and ESR (some clinicians begin with anteroposterior and lateral x-rays of the spine to help localize and sometimes diagnose abnormalities)
- Other extraspinal disorders: Testing as appropriate (eg, chest x-ray for pulmonary disorders, urinalysis for urinary tract disorders or for back pain with no clear mechanical cause)

Table 40–1. INTERPRETATION OF RED FLAG FINDINGS IN PATIENTS WITH BACK PAIN

FINDING	CAUSES TO CONSIDER
Abdominal aorta that is > 5 cm (particularly if tender) or lower-extremity pulse deficits	Abdominal aortic aneurysm
Acute, tearing midback pain	Thoracic aortic dissection
Cancer, diagnosed or suspected	Metastases
Duration of pain > 6 wk	Cancer Subacute infection Spondyloarthropathy
Fever	Cancer Infection
GI findings such as localized abdominal tenderness, peritoneal signs (rebound tenderness or abdominal rigidity), melena, or hematochezia	Possible GI emergency (eg, peritonitis, abscess, GI bleeding)
Infection risk factors	Infection
Meningismus	Meningitis
Neurologic deficit	Spinal cord or nerve root compression
Severe nocturnal or disabling pain	Cancer Infection
Unexplained pain after age 55	Abdominal aortic aneurysm Cancer
Unexplained weight loss	Cancer Subacute infection

Treatment

Underlying disorders are treated.

Acute musculoskeletal pain (with or without radiculopathy) is treated with

- Analgesics
- Lumbar stabilization and exercise
- Heat and cold
- Reassurance

In patients with acute nonspecific (nonradicular) back pain, treatment can be started without extensive evaluation to identify a specific etiology.

PEARLS & PITFALLS

- Treat patients with nonspecific, nonradicular back pain who have no red flag findings symptomatically, without first requiring extensive evaluation.

Analgesics: Acetaminophen or NSAIDs are the initial choice of analgesics, but opioids may be necessary, using appropriate precautions, for severe acute pain. Adequate analgesia is important immediately after acute injury to help limit the cycle of pain and spasm. Evidence of benefit for chronic use is weak or absent, so duration of opioid use should be limited.

Lumbar stabilization and exercise: When acute pain decreases enough that motion is possible, a lumbar stabilization program is begun under the supervision of a physical therapist. This program should be started as soon as practical and includes exercises that strengthen abdominal and low back muscles plus instruction in work posture; the aim is to strengthen the supporting structures of the back and reduce the likelihood of the condition becoming chronic or recurrent.

Heat and cold: Acute muscle spasms may also be relieved by cold or heat. Cold is usually preferred to heat during the first 2 days after an injury. Ice and cold packs should not be applied directly to the skin. They should be enclosed (eg, in plastic) and placed over a towel or cloth. The ice is removed after 20 min, then later reapplied for 20 min over a period of 60 to 90 min. This process can be repeated several times during the first 24 h. Heat, using a heating pad, can be applied for the same periods of time. Because the skin on the back may be insensitive to heat, heating pads must be used cautiously to prevent burns. Patients are advised not to use a heating pad at bedtime to avoid prolonged exposure due to falling asleep with the pad still on their back. Diathermy may help reduce muscle spasm and pain after the acute stage.

Corticosteroids: In patients with severe radicular symptoms and lower back pain, some clinicians recommend a course of oral corticosteroids or early referral to a specialist for epidural injection therapy. However, evidence supporting the use of systemic and epidural corticosteroid use is controversial. If injection is planned, clinicians should consider doing MRI before injection so that the pathology can be identified, localized, and optimally treated.

Muscle relaxants: Oral muscle relaxants (eg, cyclobenzaprine, methocarbamol, metaxalone) are controversial. Benefits of these drugs should be weighed against their CNS effects and other adverse effects, particularly in elderly patients, who may have more severe adverse effects. Muscle relaxants should be restricted to patients with visible and palpable muscle spasm and used for no more than 72 h.

Rest and immobilization: Although a brief initial period (eg, 1 to 2 days) of decreased activity is sometimes needed for comfort, prolonged bed rest, spinal traction, and corsets are not beneficial. Patients with torticollis and sometimes cervical strains may benefit from a cervical collar and contour pillow until pain is relieved and they can participate in a stabilization program.

Spinal manipulation: Spinal manipulation may help relieve pain caused by muscle spasm or an acute neck or back injury; however, some forms of manipulation may have risks for patients with disk disorders or osteoporosis.

Reassurance: Clinicians should reassure patients with acute nonspecific musculoskeletal back pain that the prognosis is good and that activity and exercise are safe even when they cause some discomfort. Clinicians should be thorough, kind, firm, and nonjudgmental. If depression persists for several months or secondary gain is suspected, psychologic evaluation should be considered.

Geriatrics Essentials

Low back pain affects 50% of adults > 60.

Abdominal aortic aneurysm (and CT or ultrasonography to detect it) should be considered in older patients with atraumatic low back pain, particularly those who smoke or have hypertension, even if no physical findings suggest this diagnosis.

Imaging of the spine may be appropriate for elderly patients (eg, to rule out cancer) even when the cause appears to be uncomplicated musculoskeletal back pain.

Use of oral muscle relaxants (eg, cyclobenzaprine, methocarbamol, metaxalone) and opioids is controversial; anticholinergic, CNS, and other adverse effects may outweigh potential benefits in elderly patients.

KEY POINTS

- Low back pain affects 50% of adults > 60.
- Most neck and back pain is caused by mechanical spinal disorders, usually nonspecific, self-limited musculoskeletal derangements.
- Most mechanical disorders are treated with analgesics, early mobilization, and exercises; prolonged bed rest and immobilization are avoided.
- Back pain is often multifactorial, making diagnosis difficult.
- Serious spinal or extraspinal disorders are unusual causes.
- Red flag findings often indicate a serious disorder and the need for testing.
- Patients with segmental neurologic deficits suggesting spinal cord compression require MRI or CT myelography as soon as possible.
- Normal spinal cord function during physical examination is best confirmed by tests of sacral nerve function (eg, rectal tone, anal wink reflex, bulbocavernosus reflex), knee and ankle jerk reflexes, and motor strength.
- Pain not worsened by movement is often extraspinal, particularly if no vertebral or paravertebral tenderness is detected.
- Abdominal aortic aneurysm should be considered in any elderly patient with low back pain that is not clearly mechanical, even if no physical findings suggest this diagnosis.
- In patients with acute nonradicular back pain, treatment can be started without extensive evaluation to identify a specific etiology.

ATLANTOAXIAL SUBLUXATION

(C1–C2 Subluxation)

Atlantoaxial subluxation is misalignment of the 1st and 2nd cervical vertebrae, which may occur only with neck flexion.

Atlantoaxial subluxation can result from major trauma or can occur without trauma in patients with rheumatoid arthritis, juvenile idiopathic arthritis, or ankylosing spondylitis.

Atlantoaxial subluxation is usually asymptomatic but may cause vague neck pain, occipital headache, or occasionally intermittent (and potentially fatal) cervical spinal cord compression.

Diagnosis

- Plain x-rays
- MRI if cord compression suspected

Atlantoaxial subluxation is usually diagnosed with plain cervical x-rays; however, flexion views may be required to show intermittent subluxation. Views during flexion, as tolerated by the patient, show dynamic instability of the entire cervical spine. If x-rays are normal and subluxation is still suspected, MRI, which is more sensitive, should be done. MRI also provides the most sensitive evaluation of spinal cord compression and is done immediately if cord compression is suspected.

Treatment

- Treatment of symptoms
- Cervical immobilization
- Surgery

Indications for treatment include pain, neurologic deficits, and potential spinal instability. Treatment includes symptomatic measures and cervical immobilization, usually beginning with a rigid cervical collar. Surgery may be needed to stabilize the spine.

LUMBAR SPINAL STENOSIS

Lumbar spinal stenosis (LSS) is narrowing of the lumbar spinal canal, which puts pressure on the cord or sciatic nerve roots before their exit from the foramina. It causes positional back pain, symptoms of nerve root compression, and lower-extremity pain during walking or weight bearing.

Spinal stenosis can be congenital or acquired. It may involve the cervical or lumbar spine. Acquired LSS is a common cause of sciatica in middle-aged or elderly patients. The most common causes of LSS are osteoarthritis, degenerative disk disorders, spondylosis, and spondylolisthesis with compression of the cauda equina. Other causes include Paget disease of bone, rheumatoid arthritis, and ankylosing spondylitis.

Symptoms and Signs

Pain occurs in the buttocks, thighs, or calves during walking, running, climbing stairs, or even standing. The pain is not relieved by standing still but by flexing the back or by sitting (although paresthesias may continue). Walking up hills is less painful than walking down because the back is slightly flexed. Patients may have pain, paresthesias, weakness, and diminished reflexes in the affected nerve root distribution. Rarely, spinal cord compression may cause cauda equina syndrome.

Diagnosis

- Clinical evaluation
- Sometimes MRI, electrodiagnostic studies, or both

Spinal stenosis is suspected based on characteristic symptoms. Diagnostic tests are the same as for sciatica (see p. 320). Calf symptoms may simulate those of intermittent claudication. Claudication can be differentiated by relief with rest (not position change), skin atrophy, and abnormalities in pulses, capillary refill, and vascular tests.

Treatment

- Activity as tolerated, analgesics, and sometimes drugs that relieve neuropathic pain
- Physical therapy
- Possibly epidural corticosteroid injections
- Surgery for severe cases

Conservative treatments and indications for surgery are similar to those for sciatica. For advanced spinal stenosis, surgery involves decompression of nerve root entrapment by vertebral canal and foraminal encroachments, which sometimes requires laminectomy at 2 or 3 levels plus foraminotomies.

Spinal stability must be preserved. Spinal fusion may be indicated if there is instability or severe, well-localized arthritic changes in 1 or 2 vertebral interspaces.

NONTRAUMATIC SPINAL SUBLUXATION

Spinal dislocation and subluxation (partial dislocation) are usually due to trauma. For example, atlantoaxial subluxation and spondylolisthesis can result from obvious major trauma, such as a high-speed deceleration injury. However, these disorders can occur with minimal, unrecognized, or no trauma. Rarely, cervical disk disorders can cause nontraumatic spinal subluxation.

SCIATICA

Sciatica is pain along the sciatic nerve. It usually results from compression of nerve roots in the lower back. Common causes include intervertebral disk herniation, osteophytes, and narrowing of the spinal canal (spinal stenosis). Symptoms include pain radiating from the buttocks down the leg. Diagnosis sometimes involves MRI or CT. Electromyography and nerve conduction studies can identify the affected level. Treatment includes symptomatic measures and sometimes surgery, particularly if there is a neurologic deficit.

Etiology

Sciatica is typically caused by nerve root compression, usually due to intervertebral disk herniation, bony irregularities (eg, osteoarthritic osteophytes, spondylolisthesis), spinal stenosis, or, much less often, intraspinal tumor or abscess. Compression may occur within the spinal canal or intervertebral foramen. The nerves can also be compressed outside the vertebral column, in the pelvis or buttocks. L5-S1, L4-L5, and L3-L4 nerve roots are most often affected (see Table 240–1 on p. 2027).

Symptoms and Signs

Pain radiates along the course of the sciatic nerve, most often down the buttocks and posterior aspect of the leg to below the knee. The pain is typically burning, lancinating, or stabbing. It may occur with or without low back pain. The Valsalva maneuver or coughing may worsen pain due to disk herniation. Patients may complain of numbness and sometimes weakness in the affected leg.

Nerve root compression can cause sensory, motor, or, the most objective finding, reflex deficits. L5-S1 disk herniation may affect the ankle jerk reflex; L3-L4 herniation may affect the knee jerk.

Straight leg raising may cause pain that radiates down the leg when the leg is slowly raised above 60° and sometimes less. This finding is sensitive for sciatica; pain radiating down the affected leg when the contralateral leg is lifted (crossed straight leg raising) is more specific for sciatica. The straight leg raise test can be done while patients are seated with the hip joint flexed at 90°; the lower leg is slowly raised until the knee is fully extended. If sciatica is present, the pain in the spine (and often the radicular symptoms) occurs as the leg is extended.

Diagnosis

- Clinical evaluation
- Sometimes MRI, electrodiagnostic studies, or both

Sciatica is suspected based on the characteristic pain. If it is suspected, strength, reflexes, and sensation should be tested. If there are neurologic deficits or if symptoms persist for > 6 wk, imaging and electrodiagnostic studies should be done. Structural abnormalities causing sciatica (including spinal stenosis) are most accurately diagnosed by MRI or CT.

Electrodiagnostic studies can confirm the presence and degree of nerve root compression and can exclude conditions that may mimic sciatica, such as polyneuropathy. These studies may help determine whether the lesion involves single or multiple nerve levels and whether the clinical findings correlate with MRI abnormalities (especially valuable before surgery). However, abnormalities may not be evident on electrodiagnostic studies for up to a few weeks after symptoms begin.

Treatment

- Activity as tolerated, analgesics, and sometimes drugs that relieve neuropathic pain
- Physical therapy
- Sometimes oral or epidural corticosteroids
- Surgery for severe cases

Acute pain relief can come from 24 to 48 h of bed rest in a recumbent position with the head of the bed elevated about 30° (semi-Fowler position). Measures used to treat low back pain, including nonopioid analgesics (eg, NSAIDs, acetaminophen), can be tried for up to 6 wk. Drugs that decrease neuropathic pain (see p. 1976), such as gabapentin or other anticonvulsants or low-dose tricyclic antidepressants (no tricyclic is superior to another), may relieve symptoms. Gabapentin 100 to 300 mg po at bedtime is used initially, but doses typically have to be much higher, up to 3600 mg/day. As with all sedating drugs, care should be taken in the elderly, patients at risk of falls, patients with arrhythmias, and those with chronic kidney disease.

Muscle spasm may be relieved with therapeutic heat or cold (see p. 3254), and physical therapy may be useful. Whether corticosteroids should be used to treat acute radicular pain is controversial. Given epidurally, corticosteroids may accelerate pain relief, but they probably should not be used unless pain is severe or persistent. Some clinicians try oral corticosteroids.

Surgery is indicated only for cauda equina syndrome or for unequivocal disk herniation plus one of the following:

- Muscular weakness
- Progressive neurologic deficit
- Intolerable, intractable pain that interferes with job or personal functions in an emotionally stable patient and that has not lessened after 6 wk of conservative treatment; however, in such cases, alternative diagnoses should be considered and evaluated, such as a generalized myofascial pain syndrome

Classic diskectomy with limited laminotomy for intervertebral disk herniation is the standard procedure. If herniation is localized, microdiskectomy may be done; with it, the skin incision and laminotomy can be smaller. Chemonucleolysis, using intradiskal injection of chymopapain, is no longer used.

Predictors of poor surgical outcome include

- Prominent psychiatric factors
- Persistence of symptoms for > 6 mo
- Heavy manual labor
- Prominence of back pain (nonradicular)
- Secondary gain (ie, litigation and compensability)

KEY POINTS

- Sciatica is typically caused by nerve root compression, usually due to intervertebral disk herniation, osteoarthritic osteophytes, spinal stenosis, or spondylolisthesis.
- Classically, burning, lancinating, or stabbing pain radiates along the course of the sciatic nerve, most often down the buttocks and posterior aspect of the leg to below the knee.
- Loss of sensation, weakness, and reflex deficits can occur.
- Do MRI and electrodiagnostic studies if there are neurologic deficits or symptoms persist for > 6 wk.
- Conservative treatment is usually sufficient, but consider surgery for disk herniation with a progressive neurologic deficit, or persistent, intractable pain.

SPONDYLOLISTHESIS

Spondylolisthesis is subluxation of lumbar vertebrae, usually occurring during adolescence. It usually results from a congenital defect in the pars interarticularis (spondylolysis).

Spondylolisthesis is usually fixed. It usually involves the L3-L4, L4-L5, or L5-S1 vertebrae.

Spondylolisthesis often occurs in adolescents or young adults who are athletes and who have had only minimal trauma; the cause is a lumbar vertebra weakened by a congenital defect in the pars interarticularis (spondylolysis). This defect is easily fractured; separation of the fracture fragments causes the subluxation. Spondylolisthesis can also occur with minimal trauma in patients who are > 60 and have osteoarthritis.

If mild to moderate (subluxation of ≤ 50%), spondylolisthesis, particularly in the young, may cause little or no pain. Spondylolisthesis can predispose to later development of spinal stenosis. If due to major trauma, spondylolisthesis can cause spinal cord compression or other neurologic deficits; these deficits rarely occur.

Spondylolisthesis is staged according to the percentage of vertebral body length that one vertebra subluxes over the adjacent vertebra:

- Stage I: 0 to 25%
- Stage II: 25 to 50%
- Stage III: 50 to 75%
- Stage IV: 75 to 100%

Spondylolisthesis is evident on plain lumbar x-rays. The lateral view is usually used for staging. Flexion and extension views may be done to check for instability.

Treatment is usually symptomatic. Physical therapy with lumbar stabilization exercises may be helpful.

41 Osteonecrosis

(Aseptic Necrosis; Avascular Necrosis; Ischemic Necrosis of Bone)

Osteonecrosis (ON) is a focal infarct of bone that may be caused by specific etiologic factors or may be idiopathic. It can cause pain, limitation of motion, joint collapse, and osteoarthritis. Diagnosis is by x-rays and MRI. In early stages, surgical procedures may slow or prevent progression. In later stages, joint replacement may be required for relief of pain and maintenance of function.

In the US, ON affects about 20,000 new patients annually. The hip (femoral head) is most commonly affected, followed by the knee and shoulder (humeral head). The wrist and ankle are less often involved. It is unusual for ON to involve the shoulder or other less commonly affected sites without the hip also being involved. ON of the jaw has certain characteristics that differ from ON at other sites

Etiology

The most common cause of ON is trauma. Nontraumatic ON affects men more often than women, is bilateral in > 60% of cases, and occurs primarily in patients between ages 30 and 50.

Traumatic ON: The most common cause of traumatic ON is a displaced subcapital fracture of the hip; ON is uncommon after intertrochanteric fractures. The incidence of ON after hip dislocation is related primarily to the severity of the initial injury but may be higher if the dislocation is not promptly reduced. Fracture or dislocation may cause ON by grossly disrupting or compressing nearby blood vessels.

Nontraumatic ON: Factors causing or contributing to nontraumatic ON are listed in Table 41–1. The most common factors are the following:

- Chronic corticosteroid use
- Excessive alcohol consumption

The risk of ON is increased when the dose of prednisone or an equivalent corticosteroid is > 20 mg/day for several weeks or months, resulting in a cumulative dose usually > 2000 mg. The risk of ON is also increased when > 3 drinks/day (> 500 mL ethanol/wk) are consumed for several years. Some genetic factors increase susceptibility to ON. Subtle clotting abnormalities due to deficiencies in protein C, protein S, or antithrombin III or to anticardiolipin antibodies (see p. 1206) can be detected in a high percentage of patients with ON.

Table 41–1. NONTRAUMATIC RISK FACTORS FOR OSTEONECROSIS

Alcohol
Chemotherapy
Coagulation disorders (eg, antiphospholipid antibody syndrome, inherited thrombophilia, hypofibrinolytic disorders)
Corticosteroids
Cushing syndrome
Decompression sickness
Dyslipidemia
Gaucher disease
Hemoglobinopathy
Liver disease
Miscellaneous disorders (eg, chronic kidney disease, rare inherited metabolic disorders)
Organ transplantation
Pancreatitis
Radiation
SLE and other autoimmune connective tissue disorders
Smoking
Tumors

Some disorders that are associated with ON are treated with corticosteroids (eg, SLE). Evidence suggests that the risk of ON in many of these disorders is related primarily to the corticosteroid use rather than to the disorder. About 20% of cases are idiopathic. ON of the jaw has been reported in several patients who have received high-dose IV bisphosphonate therapy. Nontraumatic ON of the hip is bilateral in 60% of patients.

Spontaneous ON of the knee (SPONK or SONK) is a process localized to the femoral condyle or tibial plateau in elderly women (occasionally men). SPONK is thought to be caused by an insufficiency fracture (a type of fragility fracture caused by normal wear and tear on osteoporotic bone that occurs without direct trauma).

Pathophysiology

ON involves the death of osteocytes and bone marrow. Mechanisms of nontraumatic ON may include embolization by blood clots or lipid droplets, intravascular thrombosis, and extravascular compression.

After the vascular insult, the repair processes attempt to remove necrotic bone and marrow and replace them with viable tissue. If the infarct is small, particularly if it is not subject to major weight bearing, these processes may succeed. However, in about 80% of patients, these processes are not successful and the infarct gradually collapses.

Because ON usually affects the ends of long bones, the overlying articular surface becomes flattened and irregular, with areas of bone collapse that may eventually lead to osteoarthritis and increased pain.

Symptoms and Signs

General symptoms: Affected areas may remain asymptomatic for weeks to months after the vascular insult. Usually pain then develops gradually, although it may be acute. With progressive collapse of the joint, pain increases and is exacerbated by motion and weight bearing and is relieved by rest.

Joint-specific symptoms: ON of the hip causes groin pain that may radiate down the thigh or into the buttock. Motion becomes limited, and a limp usually develops.

SPONK usually causes sudden knee pain without preceding trauma; the sudden onset and the location of pain may help differentiate it from classical ON. This pain is most often on the medial side of the femoral condyle or tibial plateau and manifests with tenderness, joint effusion, painful motion, and a limp.

ON of the humeral head often causes less pain and disability than hip and knee involvement.

With advanced ON, patients have pain and decreased motion, although passive range of motion is less affected than active range of motion. Symptomatic synovial effusions can occur, especially in the knee, and the fluid is noninflammatory.

Diagnosis

- X-rays
- MRI

ON should be suspected in patients with the following:

- Fractures associated with an increased incidence of ON, particularly if pain persists or worsens
- Persistent spontaneous hip, knee, or shoulder pain, particularly if risk factors for ON are present

Plain x-rays should be done initially. They may show no abnormalities for months. The earliest findings are localized areas of sclerosis and lucency. Later, a subchondral crescent sign may appear. Then, gross collapse and flattening of the articular surface is seen, followed by advanced degenerative changes.

When x-rays are normal or nondiagnostic, an MRI, which is much more sensitive and more specific, should be done. Both hips should be imaged. Bone scans are less sensitive and less specific than MRI and are seldom done today. CT is rarely needed, although it may occasionally be of value to detect joint collapse, which does not appear on plain x-rays and sometimes may not appear on MRI.

Laboratory studies are usually normal and of little value in detecting ON. However, they might help detect an underlying disorder (eg, coagulation defects, hemoglobinopathies, lipid abnormalities).

Treatment

- Symptomatic measures (eg, rest, physical therapy, NSAIDs)
- Surgical decompression or other procedures to stimulate healing
- Hip replacement

Nonsurgical treatments: Small, asymptomatic lesions may heal spontaneously and may not need treatment.

Larger lesions, both symptomatic and asymptomatic, have a poor prognosis if untreated, especially when in the femoral head. Therefore, early treatment to slow or prevent progression and save the joint is desirable. No completely effective treatment is yet available. Nonsurgical treatments include drugs (eg, bisphosphonates) and physical modalities (eg, electromagnetic fields and acoustic waves). Drug therapy and physical modalities have shown promise in limited studies but are not currently in general use. Limited weight bearing or non–weight bearing alone has not been shown to improve outcome.

SPONK is usually treated without surgery, and pain usually resolves.

Surgical treatments: Surgical treatments are most effective when done before joint collapse. They have been used most often in treating ON of the hip where the prognosis without treatment is worse than that for other regions.

Core decompression is the procedure most frequently done; one or more cores of bone are removed from the necrotic region or multiple small tracks or perforations are made in an attempt to decrease intraosseous pressure and stimulate repair. Core decompression is technically simple, and the complication rate is very low if the procedure is done correctly. Protected weight bearing (bearing weight only as tolerated and with a mobility aid, such as crutches or a walker) is needed for about 6 wk. Most reports indicate satisfactory or good results in 65% of patients overall and in 80% of patients whose hips have small, early lesions; however, reported outcomes can vary widely.

Other established procedures include various proximal femoral osteotomies and bone grafting, both vascularized and nonvascularized. These procedures are technically demanding, require protected weight bearing for up to 6 mo, and have not been done often in the US. Reports vary as to their indications and effectiveness. They should be done primarily at selected centers that have the surgical experience and facilities to achieve optimal results. An approach currently being evaluated is injection of autologous marrow into the necrotic lesion; early results are promising.

If extensive collapse of the femoral head and degenerative changes in the acetabulum cause sufficient pain and disability, an arthroplasty usually is the only way to effectively relieve pain and increase range of motion. The conventional approach is total hip replacement. Good to excellent results are achieved in 95% of total hip and total knee replacements, complication rates are low, and patients resume most activities of daily living within 3 mo. Most prosthetic hips and knees last > 15 to 20 yr.

Two alternatives to total hip replacement include surface replacement arthroplasty (SRA) and hemi-SRA. SRA involves the insertion of two metal caps, one into the acetabulum and one onto the femoral head, producing a metal-on-metal articulation. Hemi-SRA involves placement of a metal cap onto only the femoral head. It is done only if disease is limited to the femoral head and is considered a temporizing procedure. These procedures are done less often now than a few years ago because of an increasing incidence of local complications, prosthesis failure, and concerns about possible long-term systemic effects of metal ions.

ON of the knee and shoulder can be managed nonsurgically more often than ON of the hip. Limited experience with core decompression has been promising. In advanced stages, partial or total joint replacement may be indicated.

Prevention

Risk of ON caused by corticosteroids can be minimized by using them only when essential and by giving them in as low a dose as needed and for as short a duration as possible.

To prevent ON caused by decompression sickness, people should follow accepted rules for decompression when diving and when working in pressurized environments.

Excessive alcohol use and smoking should be discouraged. Various drugs (eg, anticoagulants, vasodilators, lipid-lowering drugs) are being evaluated for prevention of ON in patients at high risk.

KEY POINTS

- ON is most often a complication of displaced hip fracture, but factors that compromise bone blood flow (eg, chronic corticosteroid use, excessive alcohol use) increase risk of nontraumatic ON.
- ON should be suspected in patients with unexplained nontraumatic pain in the hip, knee, or shoulder (sometimes the wrist or ankle) and after certain fractures if pain persists or worsens.
- Although x-rays may be diagnostic, MRI is more sensitive and specific.
- Smaller lesions may heal spontaneously, but most larger lesions, especially in the hip, progress without treatment.
- Nonsurgical treatments are not widely used because efficacies are not clearly proved.
- Surgical treatment is often indicated to limit progression and/or relieve symptoms, particularly for ON of the hip.

OSTEONECROSIS OF THE JAW

Osteonecrosis of the jaw (ONJ) is an oral lesion involving bare mandibular or maxillary bone. It may cause pain or may be asymptomatic. Diagnosis is by the presence of exposed bone for at least 8 wk. Treatment is limited debridement, antibiotics, and oral rinses.

ONJ has no unanimously accepted definition or etiology but is generally held to be an oral lesion involving bare mandibular or maxillary bone.

ONJ may occur spontaneously or after dental extraction or trauma, radiation therapy to the head and neck (osteoradionecrosis), or high-dose IV bisphosphonate therapy (eg, for cancer treatment). ONJ may be a refractory osteomyelitis rather than true ON, particularly when associated with bisphosphonate use.

There is no evidence that routine use of oral bisphosphonates for treatment or prevention of osteoporosis increases risk of ONJ. Currently, otherwise appropriate bisphosphonate use should not be discouraged. However, it seems reasonable to do any necessary oral surgery before beginning bisphosphonate therapy and to encourage good oral hygiene while patients are taking bisphosphonates.[1]

Symptoms and Signs

ONJ may be asymptomatic for long periods. Symptoms tend to develop along with signs, although pain may precede signs. ONJ usually manifests with pain and purulent discharge from exposed bone in the mandible or, less often, the maxilla. The teeth and gingiva may be involved. Intraoral or extraoral fistulas may develop.

Diagnosis

- Clinical evaluation

ON of the jaw is diagnosed when exposed, necrotic bone is present in the maxilla or mandible for at least 8 wk.

Treatment

- Limited debridement, antibiotics, and oral rinses

Once established, ONJ is challenging to treat and should be managed by an oral surgeon with experience treating ONJ. Treatment of ONJ typically involves limited debridement, antibiotics, and oral rinses.[1]

Surgical resection of the affected area may worsen the condition and should not be the initial treatment.

1. Edwards BJ, Hellstein JW, Jacobsen PL, et al: Updated recommendations for managing the care of patients receiving oral bisphosphonate therapy: an advisory statement from the American Dental Association Council on Scientific Affairs. *J Am Dent Assoc* 139:1674–1677, 2008.

42 Osteoporosis

Osteoporosis is a progressive metabolic bone disease that decreases bone density (bone mass per unit volume), with deterioration of bone structure. Skeletal weakness leads to fractures with minor or inapparent trauma, particularly in the thoracic and lumbar spine, wrist, and hip (called fragility fractures). Diagnosis is by dual-energy x-ray absorptiometry (DXA) scan or by confirmation of a fragility fracture. Prevention and treatment involve risk factor modification, Ca and vitamin D supplements, exercises to maximize bone and muscle strength, improve balance, and minimize the risk of falls, and drug therapy to preserve bone mass or stimulate new bone formation.

Pathophysiology

Bone is continually being formed and resorbed. Normally, bone formation and resorption are closely balanced. Osteoblasts (cells that make the organic matrix of bone and then mineralize bone) and osteoclasts (cells that resorb bone) are regulated by parathyroid hormone (PTH), calcitonin, estrogen, vitamin D, various cytokines, and other local factors such as prostaglandins.

Peak bone mass in men and women occurs around age 30. Blacks reach higher peak bone mass than whites and Asians, whereas Hispanics have intermediate values. Men have higher bone mass than women. After achieving peak, bone mass plateaus for about 10 yr, during which time bone formation approximately equals bone resorption. After this, bone loss occurs at a rate of about 0.3 to 0.5%/yr. Beginning with menopause, bone loss accelerates in women to about 3 to 5%/yr for about 5 to 7 yr and then the rate of loss decelerates.

Osteoporotic bone loss affects cortical and trabecular (cancellous) bone. Cortical thickness and the number and size of trabeculae decrease, resulting in increased porosity. Trabeculae may be disrupted or entirely absent. Trabecular bone loss occurs more rapidly than cortical bone loss because trabecular bone is more porous and bone turnover is higher. However, loss of both types contributes to skeletal fragility.

Fragility fractures: A fragility fracture occurs after less trauma than might be expected to fracture a normal bone. Falls from a standing height or less, including falls out of bed, are typically considered fragility fractures. The most common sites for fragility fractures are the following:

- Distal radius
- Spine (vertebral compression fractures—the most common osteoporosis-related fracture)
- Femoral neck
- Greater trochanter

Other sites include the proximal humerus and pelvis.

Classification

Osteoporosis can develop as a primary disorder or secondarily due to some other factor. The sites of fracture are similar in primary and secondary osteoporosis.

Primary osteoporosis: More than 95% of osteoporosis in women and about 80% in men is primary. Most cases occur in postmenopausal women and older men. Gonadal insufficiency is an important factor in both men and women. Other contributing factors may include decreased Ca intake, low vitamin D levels, certain drugs, and hyperparathyroidism. Some patients have an inadequate intake of Ca during the bone growth years of adolescence and thus never achieve peak bone mass.

The major mechanism of bone loss is increased bone resorption, resulting in decreased bone mass and microarchitectural deterioration, but sometimes bone formation is impaired. The mechanisms of bone loss may involve the following:

- Local changes in the production of bone-resorbing cytokines, such as increases in cytokines that stimulate bone resorption
- Impaired formation response during bone remodeling (probably caused by age-related decline in the number and activity of osteoblasts)
- Other factors such as a decline in local and systemic growth factors

Fragility fractures rarely occur in children, adolescents, premenopausal women, or men < 50 yr with normal gonadal function and no detectable secondary cause, even in those with low bone mass (low Z-scores on DXA). Such uncommon cases are considered idiopathic osteoporosis.

Secondary osteoporosis: Secondary osteoporosis accounts for < 5% of osteoporosis in women and about 20% in men. The causes (see Table 42–1) may also further accelerate bone loss and increase fracture risk in patients with primary osteoporosis.

Table 42–1. CAUSES OF SECONDARY OSTEOPOROSIS

Cancer (eg, multiple myeloma)
COPD (due to the disorder itself, as well as tobacco use and/or treatment with glucocorticoids)
Chronic kidney disease
Drugs (eg, glucocorticoids, anticonvulsants, medroxyprogesterone, aromatase inhibitors, rosiglitazone, pioglitazone, thyroid replacement therapy, heparin, ethanol, tobacco)
Endocrine disease (eg, glucocorticoid excess, hyperparathyroidism, hyperthyroidism, hypogonadism, hyperprolactinemia, diabetes mellitus)
Hypercalciuria
Hypervitaminosis A
Hypophosphatasia
Immobilization
Liver disease
Malabsorption syndromes
Prolonged weightlessness (as occurs in space flight)
RA

Patients with chronic kidney disease may have several reasons for low bone mass, including secondary hyperparathyroidism, renal osteodystrophy, and adynamic bone.

Risk Factors

Because stress, including weight bearing, is necessary for bone growth, immobilization or extended sedentary periods result in bone loss. A low body mass index predisposes to decreased bone mass. Certain ethnicities, including whites and Asians, have a higher risk of osteoporosis. Insufficient dietary intake of Ca, P, Mg, and vitamin D predisposes to bone loss, as does endogenous acidosis. Tobacco and alcohol use also adversely affect bone mass. A family history of osteoporosis, particularly a parental history of hip fracture, also increases risk. Patients who have had one fragility fracture are at increased risk of having other clinical (symptomatic) fractures and clinically asymptomatic vertebral compression fractures.

Symptoms and Signs

Patients with osteoporosis are asymptomatic unless a fracture has occurred. Nonvertebral fractures are typically symptomatic, but about two-thirds of vertebral compression fractures are asymptomatic (although patients may have underlying chronic back pain due to other causes such as osteoarthritis). A vertebral compression fracture that is symptomatic begins with acute onset of pain that usually does not radiate, is aggravated by weight bearing, may be accompanied by point spinal tenderness, and typically begins to subside in 1 wk. However, residual pain may last for months or be constant.

Multiple thoracic compression fractures eventually cause dorsal kyphosis, with exaggerated cervical lordosis (dowager's hump). Abnormal stress on the spinal muscles and ligaments may cause chronic, dull, aching pain, particularly in the lower back. Patients may have shortness of breath due to the reduced intrathoracic volume and/or abdominal discomfort due to the compression of the abdominal cavity as the rib cage approaches the pelvis.

Diagnosis

- DXA

Bone density should be measured using DXA to screen people at risk and to follow patients with documented low bone density, including those undergoing treatment.

A DXA scan is recommended for the following patients:

- All women ≥ 65 yr
- Women between menopause and age 65 who have risk factors, including a family history of osteoporosis, a low body mass index (eg, previously defined as body weight < 127 lb), and use of tobacco and/or drugs with a high risk of bone loss (eg, glucocorticoids)
- Patients (men and women) of any age who have had fragility fractures
- Patients with evidence on imaging studies of decreased bone density or asymptomatic vertebral compression fractures incidentally noted on imaging studies
- Patients at risk of secondary osteoporosis

Although low bone density (and the associated increased risk of fracture) can be suggested by plain x-rays, it should be confirmed by a bone density measurement. It is not clear how often DXA should be repeated. For example, it can be done frequently (eg, every 2 to 3 yr) in women being treated for osteoporosis or who are at high risk, and can be done less frequently, sometimes much less frequently, in women who are at low risk (eg, T-scores > −2.00 and no risk factors).

Plain x-rays: Bones show decreased radiodensity and loss of trabecular structure, but not until about 30% of bone has been lost. Loss of vertebral body height and increased biconcavity characterize vertebral compression fractures. Thoracic vertebral fractures may cause anterior wedging. In long bones, although the cortices may be thin, the periosteal surface remains smooth. Vertebral fractures at T4 or above raise concern of cancer rather than osteoporosis. Plain x-rays of the spine should be considered in older patients with severe back pain and localized vertebral spinous tenderness.

Glucocorticoid-induced osteoporosis is likely to cause rib fractures as well as fractures at other sites where osteoporotic fractures are common. Osteomalacia may cause abnormalities on imaging tests similar to those of osteoporosis (see Sidebar 42–1). Hyperparathyroidism can be differentiated when it causes subperiosteal resorption or cystic bone lesions (rarely).

Bone density measurement: DXA is used to measure bone mineral density (g/cm^2); it is suggestive of osteopenia or osteoporosis (in the absence of osteomalacia), predicts the risk of fracture, and can be used to follow treatment response. Bone density of the lumbar spine, hip, distal radius, or the entire body can be measured. (Quantitative CT scanning can produce similar measurements of the spine or hip but is currently not widely available.) Bone density is ideally measured at two sites, including the lumbar spine and one hip; however, at some centers, measurements are taken of the spine and both hips.

If the spine or a hip is not available for scanning (eg, because of hardware from prior total hip arthroplasty), the distal radius can be scanned (called "1/3 radius" on the DXA scan report). The distal radius should also be scanned in a patient with hyperparathyroidism because this is the most common site of bone loss in hyperparathyroidism.

DXA results are reported as T-scores and Z-scores. The T-score corresponds to the number of standard deviations that the patient's bone density differs from the peak bone mass of a healthy, young person of the same sex and ethnicity. The WHO establishes cutoff values for T-scores that define osteopenia and osteoporosis. A T-score < −1.0 and > −2.5 defines osteopenia. A T-score ≤ −2.5 defines osteoporosis.

The Z-score corresponds to the number of standard deviations that the patient's bone mineral density differs from that of a person of the same age and sex and should be used for children, premenopausal women, or men < 50 yr. If the Z-score is ≤ −2.0, bone density is low for the patient's age and secondary causes of bone loss should be considered.

Current central DXA systems can also assess vertebral deformities in the lower thoracic and lumbar spine, a procedure termed vertebral fracture analysis (VFA). Vertebral deformities, even those clinically silent, are diagnostic of osteoporosis and are predictive of an increased risk of future fractures. VFA is more likely to be useful in patients with height loss ≥ 3 cm.

The need for drug therapy is based on the probability of fracture, which depends on DXA results as well as other factors. The **fracture risk assessment (FRAX) score** (WHO Fracture Risk Assessment Tool) predicts the 10-yr probability of a major osteoporotic (hip, spine, forearm, or humerus) or hip fracture in untreated patients. The score accounts for significant risk factors for bone loss and fracture. If the FRAX score is above certain thresholds (in the US, a ≥ 20% probability of major osteoporotic fracture or 3% probability of hip fracture), drug therapy should be recommended.

Monitoring for ongoing bone loss or the response to treatment with serial DXA scans should be done using the same DXA machine, and the comparison should use actual bone mineral density (g/cm^2) rather than T-score. In patients being treated for osteoporosis, DXA should be repeated, usually about every 2 to 3 yr, but sometimes more frequently in patients taking glucocorticoids. A stable or improved bone mineral density predicts a lower fracture risk. Patients with a significantly decreased bone mineral density on serial DXA examinations should be evaluated for drug adherence and secondary causes of bone loss.

Other testing: An evaluation for secondary causes of bone loss should be considered in a patient with a Z-score ≤ −2.0 or if a cause of secondary bone loss is clinically suspected. Laboratory testing should usually include the following:

- Serum Ca, Mg, and P
- 25-Hydroxy vitamin D level

Sidebar 42–1. Osteopenia: Differentiating Osteoporosis and Osteomalacia

Osteopenia is decreased bone mass. Two metabolic bone diseases decrease bone mass: osteoporosis and osteomalacia.

In **osteoporosis,** bone mass decreases, but the ratio of bone mineral to bone matrix is normal.

In **osteomalacia,** the ratio of bone mineral to bone matrix is low.

Osteoporosis results from a combination of low peak bone mass, increased bone resorption, and impaired bone formation. Osteomalacia is due to impaired mineralization, usually because of severe vitamin D deficiency or abnormal vitamin D metabolism (see p. 49). Osteoporosis is much more common than osteomalacia in the US. The two disorders may coexist, and their clinical expression is similar; moreover, mild to moderate vitamin D deficiency can occur in osteoporosis.

Osteomalacia should be suspected if the vitamin D level is consistently very low. To definitively differentiate between the two disorders, clinicians can do a tetracycline-labeled bone biopsy.

- Liver function tests, including an alkaline phosphatase (hypophosphatasia)
- Intact PTH level (hyperparathyroidism)
- Serum testosterone in men (hypogonadism)
- 24-h urine for Ca and creatinine (hypercalciuria)

Other tests such as thyroid-stimulating hormone or free thyroxine to check for hyperthyroidism, measurements of urinary free cortisol, and blood counts and other tests to rule out cancer, especially myeloma (eg, serum and urine protein electrophoresis), should be considered depending on the clinical presentation. Patients with chronic kidney disease can have low bone mass due to hyperparathyroidism, renal osteodystrophy, and adynamic bone, so they may need other tests.

Patients with weight loss should be screened for GI disorders (eg, malabsorption, celiac disease, inflammatory bowel disease) as well as cancer. Bone biopsy is reserved for unusual cases (eg, young patients with fragility fractures and no apparent cause, patients with chronic kidney disease who may have other bone disorders, patients with persistently very low vitamin D levels suspected of having osteomalacia).

Levels of fasting serum C-telopeptide cross-links (CTX) or urine N-telopeptide cross-links (NTX) reflect increased bone resorption, and although reliability varies for routine clinical use, CTX and NTX may be helpful in monitoring response to therapy or with the timing of a drug holiday.

Treatment

- Risk factor modification
- Ca and vitamin D supplements
- Antiresorptive drugs (eg, bisphosphonates, hormone replacement therapy, selective estrogen receptor modulators, receptor activator of nuclear factor kappa-B ligand [RANKL] inhibitors)
- Anabolic drugs

The goals of treatment are to preserve bone mass, prevent fractures, decrease pain, and maintain function.

Preserving bone mass: The rate of bone loss can be slowed with drugs. Adequate Ca and vitamin D and physical activity are keys to optimal bone density. Modifiable risk factors should also be addressed.

Risk factor modification can include increasing weight-bearing exercise, minimizing caffeine and alcohol intake, and smoking cessation. The optimal amount of weight-bearing exercise is not established, but an average of 30 min/day is recommended. A physical therapist can develop a safe exercise program and demonstrate how to safely perform daily activities to minimize the risk of falls and spine fractures.

All men and women should consume at least 1000 mg of elemental Ca daily. An intake of 1200 to 1500 mg/day (including dietary consumption) is recommended for postmenopausal women and older men and for periods of increased requirements, such as pubertal growth, pregnancy, and lactation. Ca intake should ideally be from dietary sources, with supplements used if dietary intake is insufficient. Ca supplements are taken most commonly as Ca carbonate or Ca citrate. Ca citrate is better absorbed in patients with achlorhydria, but both are well absorbed when taken with meals. Patients taking proton pump inhibitors or those who have had gastric bypass surgery should take Ca citrate to ensure maximum absorption. Ca should be taken in divided doses of 500 to 600 mg bid or tid.

Vitamin D supplementation is recommended with 800 to 1000 IU/day. Patients with vitamin D deficiency may need even higher doses. Supplemental vitamin D is usually given as cholecalciferol, the natural form of vitamin D, although ergocalciferol, the synthetic plant-derived form, is probably also acceptable. The 25-hydroxy vitamin D level should be ≥ 30 ng/mL.

Bisphosphonates are first-line drug therapy. By inhibiting bone resorption, bisphosphonates preserve bone mass and can decrease vertebral and hip fractures by up to 50%. Bone turnover is reduced after 3 mo of bisphosphonate therapy and fracture risk reduction is evident as early as 1 yr after beginning therapy. DXA scanning, when done serially to monitor response to treatment, need not normally be done at intervals < 2 yr. Bisphosphonates can be given orally or IV. Bisphosphonates include the following:

- Alendronate (10 mg once/day or 70 mg po once/wk)
- Risedronate (5 mg po once/day, 35 mg po once/wk, or 150 mg po once/mo)
- Zoledronic acid (5 mg IV once/yr)
- Ibandronate po (150 mg once/mo) or IV (3 mg once every 3 mo)

Oral bisphosphonates must be taken on an empty stomach with a full (8-oz, 250 mL) glass of water, and the patient must remain upright for at least 30 min (60 min for ibandronate) and not take anything else by mouth during this time period. These drugs are safe to use in patients with a creatinine clearance > 35 mL/min. Bisphosphonates can cause esophageal irritation. Esophageal disorders that delay transit time and symptoms of upper GI disorders are relative contraindications to oral bisphosphonates. IV bisphosphonates are indicated if a patient is unable to tolerate or is nonadherent with oral bisphosphonates.

Osteonecrosis of the jaw has been associated with use of bisphosphonates; however, this condition is rare in patients taking oral bisphosphonates. Risk factors include invasive dental procedures, IV bisphosphonate use, and cancer. The benefits of reduction of osteoporosis-related fractures far outweigh this small risk.

Long-term bisphosphonate use may also increase the risk of atypical femoral fractures. These fractures occur in the midshaft of the femur with minimal or no trauma and may be preceded by weeks or months of thigh pain. The fractures may also be bilateral. To minimize fracture incidence, consideration should be given to stopping bisphosphonates (a bisphosphonate holiday) after about

- 3 to 5 yr of use in patients with osteoporosis (by DXA scan) but few or no other risk factors for bone loss (3 yr for IV zoledronic acid and 5 yr for oral bisphosphonates)
- 5 to 10 yr of use in patients with osteoporosis (by DXA scan) and more risk factors

Patients on a bisphosphonate holiday should be closely monitored for a new fracture or accelerated bone loss evident on a DXA scan. During therapy with an antiresorptive drug, such as a bisphosphonate, bone turnover is suppressed as evidenced by low fasting NTX (< 40 nmol/L) or CTX. These markers may remain low for ≥ 2 yr of a drug holiday.

In untreated patients, an increase in levels of bone turnover markers indicates an increased risk of fracture. However, it is not clear whether levels of bone turnover markers should be used as criteria for when to start or end a drug holiday. The decision to begin or end a drug holiday is complex and should take into account the patient's risk factors.

Intranasal salmon calcitonin should not regularly be used for treating osteoporosis. Salmon calcitonin may provide short-term analgesia after an acute fracture, such as a painful vertebral fracture, due to an endorphin effect. It has not been shown to reduce fractures.

Estrogen can preserve bone density and prevent fractures. Most effective if started within 4 to 6 yr of menopause, estrogen may slow bone loss and possibly reduce fractures even when started much later. Use of estrogen increases the risk of thromboembolism and endometrial cancer and may increase the risk of breast cancer. The risk of endometrial cancer can be reduced in women with an intact uterus by taking a progestin with estrogen (see p. 2276). However, taking a combination of a progestin and estrogen increases the risk of breast cancer, coronary artery disease, stroke, and biliary disease. Because of these risks and the availability of other treatments for osteoporosis, the potential harms of estrogen treatment for osteoporosis treatment outweigh its potential benefits for most women; when treatment is initiated, a short course with close monitoring should be considered.

Raloxifene is a selective estrogen receptor modulator (SERM) that may be appropriate for treatment of osteoporosis in women who cannot take bisphosphonates. It reduces vertebral fractures by about 50% but has not been shown to reduce hip fractures. Raloxifene does not stimulate the uterus and antagonizes estrogen effects in the breast. It has been shown to reduce the risk of invasive breast cancer.

PTH, which stimulates new bone formation, is generally indicated in patients who have the following characteristics:

- Cannot tolerate antiresorptive drugs or have contraindications to their use
- Fail to respond (ie, develop new fractures or lose bone mineral density) to antiresorptive drugs, as well as Ca, vitamin D, and exercise
- Possibly have severe osteoporosis (eg, T-score < –3.5) or multiple vertebral fragility fractures
- Have glucocorticoid-induced osteoporosis

When given daily by injection for an average of 20 mo, synthetic PTH (PTH 1-34; teriparatide) increases bone mass and reduces risk of fractures. Patients taking teriparatide should have a creatinine clearance > 35 mL/min.

Preventing fractures: Many elderly patients are at risk of falls because of poor coordination, poor vision, muscle weakness, confusion, and use of drugs that cause postural hypotension or alter the sensorium. Strengthening exercises may increase stability. Educating patients about the risks of falls and fractures, modifying the home environment for safety, and developing individualized programs to increase physical stability and attenuate risk are important for preventing fractures.

Treating pain and maintaining function: Acute back pain resulting from a vertebral compression fracture should be treated with orthopedic support, analgesics, and (when muscle spasm is prominent) heat and massage (see pp. 3255 and 3256). Chronic backache may be relieved by an orthopedic garment and exercises to strengthen paravertebral muscles. Avoiding heavy lifting can help. Bed rest should be minimized, and consistent, carefully designed weight-bearing exercise should be encouraged.

In some cases, vertebroplasty or kyphoplasty can relieve severe pain due to a new vertebral fragility fracture. In vertebroplasty, methyl methacrylate is injected into the vertebral body. In kyphoplasty, the vertebral body is first expanded with a balloon then injected with methyl methacrylate. These procedures may reduce deformity in the injected vertebrae but do not reduce and may even increase the risk of fractures in adjacent vertebrae. Other risks may include rib fractures, cement leakage, and pulmonary edema or MI. Further study to determine indications for these procedures is warranted.

Prevention

The goals of prevention are 2-fold: preserve bone mass and prevent fractures. Preventive measures are indicated for the following:

- Postmenopausal women
- Older men
- Patients who have osteopenia
- Patients taking long-term systemic glucocorticoids
- Patients with osteoporosis
- Patients with secondary causes for bone loss

Preventive measures for all of these patients include appropriate Ca and vitamin D intake, weight-bearing exercise, fall prevention, and other ways to reduce risk (eg, avoiding tobacco and limiting alcohol). In addition, drug therapy is indicated for patients who have osteoporosis or who have osteopenia if they are at increased risk of fracture, such as those with a high FRAX score and patients taking glucocorticoids. Drug therapy tends to involve the same drugs as are given for treatment of osteoporosis. Educating patients and the community about the importance of bone health remains of utmost importance.

KEY POINTS

- Bone is lost at a rate of about 0.3 to 0.5%/yr after age 40, accelerating after menopause in women to about 3 to 5%/yr for about 5 to 7 yr.
- More than 95% of osteoporosis in women and about 80% in men is primary.
- Suspect osteoporosis in patients who have fractures caused by unexpectedly little force (fragility fractures) of the spine, distal radius, femoral neck, or greater trochanter.
- Use DXA to measure bone density in women ≥ 65 yr; women between menopause and 65 who have risk factors (eg, family history of osteoporosis, a low body mass index, and use of tobacco and/or drugs with a high risk of bone loss [including glucocorticoids]); men and women of any age who have fragility fractures; evidence on imaging studies of decreased bone density or asymptomatic vertebral compression fractures; and patients at risk of secondary osteoporosis.
- Consider testing patients for causes of secondary bone loss if the Z-score is ≤ –2.0 or if a cause of secondary bone loss is clinically suspected.
- For treatment and prevention, ensure adequate intake of Ca and vitamin D, using supplements when necessary, and modify risk factors to help preserve bone mass (eg, with weight-bearing exercise and by minimizing use of caffeine, alcohol, and tobacco).
- Treat most patients with an antiresorptive drug (eg, bisphosphonate, selective estrogen receptor modulator, receptor activator of nuclear factor kappa-B ligand [RANKL] inhibitor, a drug used for hormone replacement therapy) or an anabolic drug (eg, PTH).

43 Paget Disease of Bone

(Osteitis Deformans)

Paget disease of bone is a chronic disorder of the adult skeleton in which bone turnover is accelerated in localized areas. Normal matrix is replaced with softened and enlarged bone. The disease may be asymptomatic or cause gradual onset of bone pain or deformity. Diagnosis is by x-ray. Treatment includes symptomatic measures and often drugs, usually bisphosphonates.

About 1% of adults in the US > 40 have Paget disease, with a 3:2 male predominance. Prevalence increases with age. However, overall prevalence seems to be decreasing. The disease is most common in Europe (except Scandinavia), Australia, and New Zealand.

Etiology

Several genetic abnormalities, many affecting receptor activator of nuclear factor kappa-B (RANK-NFk B) signaling for osteoclast generation and activity, have been identified. Mutations of the *Sequestrum 1* gene related to ubiquitin binding from chromosome 6 are present in about 10% of patients with Paget disease. Appearance of involved bone on electron microscopy suggests a viral infection. Although a viral cause has not been established, it is hypothesized that in genetically predisposed patients an as yet unidentified virus triggers abnormal osteoclast activity.

Pathophysiology

Any bone can be involved. The bones most commonly affected are, in decreasing order, the pelvis, femur, skull, tibia, vertebrae, clavicle, and humerus.

Bone turnover is accelerated at involved sites. Pagetic lesions are metabolically active and highly vascular. Excessively active osteoclasts are often large and contain many nuclei. Osteoblastic repair is also hyperactive, causing coarsely woven, thickened lamellae and trabeculae. This abnormal structure weakens the bone, despite bone enlargement and heavy calcification.

Complications: Overgrown bone may compress nerves and other structures passing through small foramina. Spinal stenosis or spinal cord compression may develop. Osteoarthritis may develop in joints adjacent to involved bone.

In about 10 to 15% of patients, increased bone formation and Ca requirement lead to secondary hyperparathyroidism; if this need is not matched by an increase in Ca intake, hypocalcemia may occur. Hypercalcemia (see p. 1289) occasionally develops in patients who are immobile. It also occurs in patients with Paget disease who develop secondary hyperparathyroidism.

Large or numerous lesions may lead to high-output heart failure. Highly vascular bones may bleed excessively during orthopedic surgery.

Symptoms and Signs

There are usually no symptoms for a prolonged period. If symptoms occur, they develop insidiously, with pain, stiffness, fatigue, and bone deformity. Bone pain is aching, deep, and occasionally severe, sometimes worse at night. Pain also may arise from compression neuropathy or osteoarthritis. If the skull is involved, there may be headaches and hearing impairment.

Signs may include skull enlargement bitemporally and frontally (frontal bossing); dilated scalp veins; nerve deafness in one or both ears or vertigo; headaches; angioid streaks in the fundus of the eye; a short kyphotic trunk with simian appearance; hobbling gait; and anterolateral angulation (bowing) of the thigh, leg, or humerus, often with warmth and tenderness. Deformities may develop from bowing of the long bones or osteoarthritis. Pathologic fractures may be the presenting manifestation. Osteosarcoma develops in < 1% and is often suggested by increasingly severe pain.

Diagnosis

- Plain x-rays
- Serum alkaline phosphatase, Ca, and phosphate (PO_4)
- Bone scan after the diagnosis is established

Paget disease should be suspected in patients with the following:

- Unexplained bone pain or deformity
- Suggestive findings on x-ray
- Unexplained elevation of serum alkaline phosphatase on laboratory tests done for other reasons, particularly if γ-glutamyl-transpeptidase (GGT) is normal
- Hypercalcemia that develops during bed rest, particularly among elderly patients
- Bone sarcoma in elderly patients

If Paget disease is suspected, plain x-rays and serum alkaline phosphatase, Ca, and PO_4 levels should be obtained. Confirmation on x-ray is required to establish the diagnosis. Characteristic x-ray findings include the following:

- Increased bone sclerosis
- Abnormal architecture with coarse cortical trabeculation or cortical thickening
- Bowing
- Bone enlargement

There may be lateral stress microfractures of the tibia or femur.

Characteristic laboratory findings include elevated serum alkaline phosphatase (increased anabolic activity of bone) but usually normal GGT and serum PO_4 levels. Serum Ca is usually normal but can increase because of immobilization or hyperparathyroidism or decrease (often transiently) because of increased bone synthesis. If alkaline phosphatase is not elevated or it is unclear whether the increased serum alkaline phosphatase is of bony origin (ie, if GGT is increased in proportion to alkaline phosphatase), a bone-specific fraction can be measured.

PEARLS & PITFALLS

- Consider Paget disease of bone in older adults with elevated alkaline phosphatase but normal GGT levels.

Occasionally, increased catabolic activity of bone, as demonstrated by elevated urine markers of bone collagen turnover (eg, pyridinoline crosslinks), supplements the findings.

Radionuclide bone scan using technetium-labeled phosphonates should be done at baseline to determine the extent of bone involvement.

Table 43–1. DRUG THERAPY FOR PAGET DISEASE

DRUG	DOSAGE	COMMENTS
Alendronate	40 mg po once/day for 6 mo	Taken as a single dose after rising in the morning, at least 30 min before eating
Etidronate	5–10 mg/kg po once/day for 6 mo; higher doses (20 mg/kg po once/day for 3 mo) possibly needed in markedly active disease	Taken as a single dose on an empty stomach at least 2 h before or after eating; can be repeated after a 3- to 6-mo interim if needed
Pamidronate	30–90 mg IV once/day given as a 4-h infusion for 3 consecutive days or once/mo for 3 mo	For patients intolerant of oral bisphosphonates; possibly more frequent doses in patients with resistant disease
Risedronate	30 mg po once/day for 2 mo	Taken the same way as alendronate
Tiludronate	400 mg po once/day for 3 mo	Taken the same way as alendronate
Zoledronate	5 mg IV given as a single 15-min infusion	For patients intolerant of oral bisphosphonates
Synthetic salmon calcitonin	50–100 IU (0.25–0.5 mL) sc or IM once/day	Dose sometimes tapered to 50 IU every other day and perhaps to twice or once weekly after a favorable initial response (often after 1 mo)

Treatment

- Supportive care for symptoms and complications
- Bisphosphonates

Localized, asymptomatic disease requires no treatment. Symptomatic treatment includes analgesics or NSAIDs for pain. Orthotics help correct abnormal gait caused by bowed lower extremities. Some patients require orthopedic surgery (eg, hip or knee replacement, decompression of the spinal cord). Weight bearing should be encouraged, and bed rest should be avoided. Rarely, rapid correction of severe hypercalcemia is necessary, using IV fluids and furosemide (see p. 1292).

Drug therapy: Drug therapy suppresses osteoclast activity. It is indicated for the following:

- To prevent or retard progression of complications (eg, hearing loss, deformity, osteoarthritis, paraparesis or paraplegia related to vertebral Paget disease, or other neurologic deficits, particularly in a poor surgical candidate)
- To treat pain clearly related to the pagetic process and not to another source (eg, osteoarthritis)
- To prevent or minimize bleeding that can occur during orthopedic surgery
- To suppress excessive osteoclast activity when serum alkaline phosphatase (of bony origin) is > 2 times the normal level, even in the absence of symptoms

Although disease progression can be retarded, existing deficits (eg, deformity, osteoarthritis, hearing loss, neural impingement) are not reversed.

Several bisphosphonates are available and are the drugs of choice (see Table 43–1). Synthetic salmon calcitonin is an alternative to bisphosphonates for patients intolerant of or resistant to them. The newer bisphosphonates (amino-containing bisphosphonates, eg, zolendronate) more effectively suppress markers of disease activity and provide more prolonged response.

Because bone turnover is increased, patients should ensure adequate intake of Ca and vitamin D, and supplements are often needed.

KEY POINTS

- Paget disease of bone is a common and often asymptomatic abnormality, particularly among older adults.
- Complications can include neural compression, osteoarthritis, fractures, secondary hyperparathyroidism, and hypocalcemia or hypercalcemia.
- Confirmation is usually by x-rays showing findings such as bone sclerosis, coarse cortical trabeculation or cortical thickening, and bone bowing or enlargement.
- First-line treatment is zolendronate or another newer bisphosphonate.

44 Pain in and Around Joints

PAIN IN AND AROUND A SINGLE JOINT

Patients may report "joint" pain regardless of whether the cause involves the joint itself or surrounding (periarticular) structures such as tendons and bursae; in both cases, pain in or around a single joint will be referred to as monoarticular pain. Pain originating within a joint (arthralgia) may be caused by joint inflammation (arthritis). Inflammation tends to result in accumulation of intra-articular fluid (effusion) and clinical findings of warmth, swelling, and uncommonly, erythema. With effusion, prompt assessment is essential to exclude infection. Acute monoarticular pain is sometimes caused by a disorder that characteristically causes polyarticular pain (eg, RA) and thus may be the initial manifestation of a polyarthritis (eg, psoriatic arthritis, RA—see Pain in Multiple Joints on p. 332).

Pathophysiology

Pain in and around a joint may involve

- Inflammation (due to, eg, infection, crystal-induced arthritis, or autoimmune systemic inflammatory disorders)
- Noninflammatory problems, usually mechanical (eg, trauma, internal derangements)

The synovium and joint capsule are major sources of intra-articular pain. The synovial membrane is the main site affected by inflammation (synovitis). Pain that originates from the menisci is more likely to be a result of injury.

Etiology

The most common causes of acute monoarticular pain overall are the following:

- Injury
- Infection
- Crystal-induced arthritis

With injury, a history of trauma is usually present and suggestive. Injury can affect intra-articular and/or periarticular structures and involve direct injury (eg, twisting during a fall) or overuse (eg, repetitive motion, prolonged kneeling).

Infection most often involves the joint (septic arthritis—see p. 294), but periarticular structures, including bursae, overlying skin, and adjacent bone, also may become infected.

Among young adults, the most common causes are the following:

- Injury (most common)
- Infection
- Primary inflammatory disorders (eg, gout and RA)

Among older adults, the most common nontraumatic causes are the following:

- Osteoarthritis (most common)
- Crystal-induced arthritis (usually gout or pseudogout)

The most dangerous cause of joint pain at any age is acute infectious (septic) arthritis. Prompt drainage, IV antibiotics, and sometimes operative joint lavage may be required to minimize permanent joint damage and prevent sepsis and death.

Rare causes of monoarticular pain include osteonecrosis, pigmented villonodular synovitis, hemarthrosis (eg, in hemophilia or coagulopathies), tumors (see Table 44–1), and disorders that usually cause polyarticular pain, such as reactive arthritis and enteropathic arthritis.

The most common cause of periarticular pain is injury, including overuse. Common periarticular disorders include bursitis and tendinitis; epicondylitis, fasciitis, and tenosynovitis can also develop. Periarticular infection is less common.

Sometimes, pain is referred to a joint. For example, a splenic injury may cause left shoulder pain, and children with a hip disorder may complain of knee pain.

Evaluation

Acute monoarticular joint pain requires rapid diagnosis because infectious (septic) arthritis requires rapid treatment.

Clinical evaluation should determine whether the joint or periarticular structures are the cause of symptoms and whether there is joint inflammation. If signs of inflammation are present or the diagnosis is unclear, symptoms and signs of polyarticular and systemic disorders should be sought.

History: History of present illness should focus on the location of pain, acuity of onset (eg, abrupt, gradual), whether the problem is new or recurrent, and whether other joints have caused pain in the past. Also, temporal patterns (eg, persistent vs intermittent), associated symptoms (eg, swelling), exacerbating and mitigating factors (eg, activity), and any recent or past trauma to the joint should be noted. Patients should also be asked about unprotected sexual contact (indicating risk of sexually transmitted diseases), previous Lyme disease, and possible tick bites in areas where Lyme disease is endemic.

Review of systems may provide clues to systemic disorders. Review of systems should seek extra-articular symptoms of causative disorders, including fever (infection, sometimes crystal-induced arthritis), urethritis (gonococcal arthritis or reactive arthritis), rash or eye redness (reactive or psoriatic arthritis), history of abdominal pain and diarrhea (inflammatory bowel disease), and recent diarrhea or genital lesions (reactive arthritis).

Past medical history is most likely to be helpful if pain is chronic or recurrent. Past medical history should identify known joint disorders (particularly gout and osteoarthritis), conditions that may cause or predispose to monoarticular joint pain (eg, bleeding disorder, bursitis, tendinitis), and disorders that can predispose to a joint disorder (eg, sickle cell disease or chronic corticosteroid use predisposing to osteonecrosis). Drug history should be reviewed, particularly for use of anticoagulants, quinolone antibiotics (tendinitis), or diuretics (gout). A family history should also be obtained (some spondyloarthropathies—see p. 311).

Physical examination: A complete physical examination is done. All major organ systems (eg, skin and nails, eyes, genitals, mucosal surfaces, heart, lungs, abdomen, nose, neck, lymph nodes, neurologic system) should be examined, as well as the musculoskeletal system. Vital signs are reviewed for fever. Examination of the head, neck, and skin should note any signs of conjunctivitis, psoriatic plaques, tophi, or ecchymoses. Genital examination should note any discharge or other findings suggesting sexually transmitted diseases.

Because involvement of other joints can be clues to a polyarthritis and a systemic disorder, all joints should be inspected for tenderness, deformities, erythema, and swelling.

Palpation helps determine the location of tenderness. Palpation also helps detect joint effusion, warmth, and bony hypertrophy. The joint can also be compressed without flexing or extending it. Range of motion is assessed actively and passively, with attention to the presence of crepitus and whether pain is triggered by joint motion (passive as well as active). For injuries, the joint is stressed with various maneuvers (as tolerated) to identify disruption of cartilage or ligaments (eg, in the knee, valgus and varus tests, anterior and posterior drawer tests, Lachman test, McMurray test). Findings should be compared with those in the contralateral unaffected joint to help detect more subtle changes. Noting whether the tenderness is directly over the joint line or adjacent to it or elsewhere is particularly helpful in determining whether pain (particularly when the knee is involved) is articular or periarticular.

Large effusions in the knee are typical and readily apparent. The examiner can check for minor effusions by pushing the suprapatellar pouch inferiorly and then pressing medially on the lateral side of the patella on an extended knee. This maneuver causes swelling to appear (or be palpable) on the medial side. Large knee effusions in obese patients are best detected with ballottement of the patella. In this technique, the examiner uses both hands to push in toward the center of the knee from all four quadrants and then uses 2 or 3 fingers to push the patella down into the trochlear groove and releases it. Clicking or a feeling that the patella is floating suggests an effusion.

Periarticular structures also should be examined for point tenderness, such as at the insertion of a tendon (enthesitis), over a tendon (tendinitis), or over a bursa (bursitis). With some types of bursitis (eg, olecranon, prepatellar), swelling and sometimes erythema may be localized at the bursa.

Table 44–1. SOME CAUSES OF PAIN IN AND AROUND A SINGLE JOINT

CAUSE	SUGGESTIVE FINDINGS	DIAGNOSTIC APPROACH
Crystal-induced arthritis, usually caused by uric acid crystals (gout) or Ca pyrophosphate crystals (pseudogout) and sometimes by Ca hydroxyapatite crystals	Acute, self-limited, recurrent episodes of monarthritis, most often in the first metatarsophalangeal joint, ankle, or knee (gout) or wrist or knee (pseudogout) Sometimes visible gouty tophi (usually on periarticular structures)	Arthrocentesis with examination for crystals
Hemarthrosis	Acute pain and effusion spontaneously or after trauma Typically, a known bleeding disorder	Arthrocentesis
Infectious (septic) arthritis (eg, bacterial, fungal, viral, mycobacterial, spirochetal)	Acute or subacute onset of pain, swelling, and warmth, commonly with decreased range of motion More frequent in immunosuppressed patients, IV drug users, patients with diabetes or prior antibiotic use, and patients with risk factors for sexually transmitted diseases	Arthrocentesis with cell counts, Gram stain, and cultures
Lyme disease	Monarticular or oligoarticular arthritis in later stage of Lyme disease Prior manifestations of Lyme disease, such as erythema migrans, fever, malaise, and/or myalgias following a tick bite	Serologic testing for antibodies against *Borrelia burgdorferi*
Osteoarthritis	Chronic indolent pain with or without swelling, usually in older adults Bony hypertrophy Sometimes obesity, history of joint overuse (eg, in professional athletes), and/or bony enlargement	X-ray
Osteomyelitis adjacent to a joint (uncommon)	Fever and poorly localized pain without joint swelling or erythema	X-ray plus bone scan, CT, or MRI Bone biopsy with culture
Osteonecrosis (avascular necrosis)	Often past or current corticosteroid use or sickle cell disease	X-ray Usually MRI
Periarticular disorders (eg, bursitis, epicondylitis, fasciitis, tendinitis, tenosynovitis)	Pain with active joint movement; minimal pain with passive movement and joint compression Point tenderness and sometimes swelling and/or erythema over the bursa, tendon insertion site, or other periarticular structure (eg, fascia); minimal localized tenderness over joint, no effusion	Clinical evaluation Sometimes aspiration of bursal fluid for Gram stain, cell count, and culture
Psoriatic arthritis (causes polyarticular pain more often than monoarticular pain)	Usually large joint effusion in the painful joint, often in a patient with psoriasis May occur with dactylitis or enthesitis	Clinical evaluation
Trauma (eg, sprain, meniscal tear, fracture)	Onset following significant and usually recent trauma	X-ray Sometimes MRI (eg, if x-ray normal) and/or arthroscopy
Tumor	Insidious, slowly progressive, and eventually constant pain, usually with joint swelling	X-ray MRI

Red flags: The following findings are of particular concern:

- Erythema, warmth, effusion, and decreased range of motion
- Fever with acute joint pain
- Acute joint pain in a sexually active young adult
- Skin breaks with signs of cellulitis adjacent to the affected joint
- Underlying bleeding disorder or use of anticoagulants
- Systemic or extra-articular symptoms

Interpretation of findings: Recent significant trauma suggests that injury is the cause (eg, fracture, meniscal tear, or hemarthrosis). However, trauma does not rule out other causes, and patients often mistakenly attribute newly developed nontraumatic pain to an injury. Testing is often necessary to rule out serious causes and establish the diagnosis.

Acuteness of onset is an important feature. Severe joint pain that develops over hours suggests crystal-induced arthritis or, less often, infectious arthritis. Previous attacks of rapid-onset monarthritis suggest recurrence of crystal-induced arthritis, particularly if that diagnosis had been confirmed previously. Gradual onset of joint pain is more typical of RA or noninfectious arthritis. Gradual onset, although uncommon in acute bacterial infectious arthritis, can occur in certain infectious arthritides (eg, mycobacterial, fungal).

Whether pain is intra-articular, periarticular, or both (eg, in gout, which can affect intra- and extra-articular structures) and whether there is inflammation are key determinations, based mainly on physical findings. Pain during rest and on initiating activity suggests joint inflammation, whereas pain worsened by movement and relieved by rest suggests mechanical or noninflammatory disorders (eg, osteoarthritis). Pain that is worse with passive as well as active joint motion on examination, and that restricts joint motion, usually indicates inflammation. Increased warmth and erythema also suggest inflammation, but these findings are often insensitive, so their absence does not rule out inflammation. Pain that worsens with active but not passive motion may indicate tendinitis or bursitis, as can tenderness or swelling localized over a bursa or tendon insertion site. Tenderness or swelling at only one side of a joint, or away from the joint line, suggests an extra-articular origin (eg, tendons or bursae); localized joint line tenderness or more diffuse involvement of the joint suggests an intra-articular cause. Compressing the joint without flexing or extending it is not particularly painful in patients with tendinitis or bursitis but is quite painful in those with arthritis.

Involvement of the first metatarsophalangeal joint (podagra) suggests gout but can also result from infectious arthritis, reactive arthritis, or psoriatic arthritis.

Symptoms indicating dermatologic, cardiac, or pulmonary involvement suggest disorders that are systemic and more commonly result in polyarticular joint pain.

Testing: Joint aspiration (arthrocentesis) for synovial fluid examination should be done in patients with joint effusion. Synovial fluid examination includes WBC count with differential, Gram stain and cultures, and microscopic examination for crystals using polarized light. Finding crystals in synovial fluid confirms crystal-induced arthritis but does not rule out coexisting infection. A noninflammatory synovial fluid (eg, < 1000/μL WBCs) is more suggestive of osteoarthritis or trauma. Hemorrhagic fluid is consistent with hemarthrosis. Synovial fluid WBC counts can be very high (eg, > 50,000/μL WBCs) in both infectious and crystal-induced arthritis.

For some patients with prior confirmed gouty arthritis, a recurrent episode may not require any testing. However, if infection is a reasonable possibility, or if symptoms do not rapidly resolve after appropriate therapy for gouty arthritis, arthrocentesis should be done.

X-rays rarely change the diagnosis in acute monarthritis unless fracture is suspected. X-rays may reveal signs of joint damage in patients with a long history of recurrent arthritis. Other imaging tests (eg, CT, bone scan, but most often MRI) are rarely necessary acutely but may be indicated for diagnosis of certain specific disorders (eg, osteonecrosis, tumor [see Table 44–1], occult fracture, pigmented villonodular synovitis).

Blood tests (eg, ESR, rheumatoid factor, anti-cyclic citrullinated peptide [anti-CCP] antibody) may help support a clinically suspected diagnosis of a systemic inflammatory disorder (eg, RA). Serum urate level should not be used to diagnose gout because it is neither sensitive nor specific and does not necessarily reflect intra-articular urate levels.

Treatment

Overall treatment is directed at the underlying disorder. IV antibiotics are usually given immediately or as soon as possible if acute bacterial infectious arthritis is suspected.

Joint inflammation is usually treated symptomatically with NSAIDs. Pain without inflammation is usually more safely treated with acetaminophen. Adjunctive treatment for pain can include joint immobilization with a splint or sling and heat or cold therapy.

Physical therapy after the acute symptoms have lessened is useful to increase or maintain range of motion and strengthen adjacent muscles.

KEY POINTS

- Arthrocentesis is mandatory to rule out infection in acute monoarticular joint pain with swelling.
- Infection is the most common cause of acute nontraumatic monarthritis in young adults, whereas osteoarthritis is the most common cause in older adults.
- Crystals in synovial fluid confirm crystal-induced arthritis but do not rule out coexisting infection.
- Do not use serum urate level to diagnose gout.
- Joint pain that is still unexplained after arthrocentesis and x-ray should be evaluated with MRI to rule out uncommon etiologies (eg, occult fracture, osteonecrosis, pigmented villonodular synovitis).

PAIN IN MULTIPLE JOINTS

Joints may simply be painful (arthralgia) or also inflamed (arthritis). Joint inflammation is usually accompanied by warmth, swelling (due to intra-articular fluid, or effusion), and uncommonly erythema. Pain may occur only with use or also at rest. Sometimes what is described by patients as joint pain can have an extra-articular source (eg, a periarticular structure or bone).

Polyarticular pain (polyarthralgia) involves multiple joints (pain in a single joint is discussed elsewhere—see Pain in and Around a Single Joint on p. 329). Polyarticular joint disorders may affect different joints at different times. When multiple joints are affected, the following distinction can be useful in differentiating among different disorders, particularly arthritides:

- Oligoarticular: Involving ≤ 4 joints
- Polyarticular: Involving > 4 joints

Pathophysiology

Articular sources of pain originate within the joint. Periarticular sources of pain originate in structures surrounding the joint (eg, tendons, ligaments, bursae, muscles).

Polyarticular pain caused by articular sources may result from the following:

- Inflammation (eg, infection, crystal-induced arthritis, systemic inflammatory disorders such as RA and psoriatic arthritis)
- Mechanical or other noninflammatory disorders (eg, osteoarthritis, hypermobility syndromes)

The synovium and joint capsule are major sources of pain within a joint. The synovial membrane is the main site affected by inflammation (synovitis). Pain affecting multiple joints in the absence of inflammation may be due to increased joint laxity and excessive trauma, as in benign hypermobility syndrome.

Polyarthritis may involve peripheral joints, axial joints (eg, sacroiliac, apophyseal, discovertebral, costovertebral), or both.

Etiology

Peripheral oligoarticular arthritis and polyarticular arthritis are more commonly associated with a systemic infection (eg, viral) or systemic inflammatory disorder (eg, RA) than is monoarticular arthritis. A specific cause can usually be determined (see Tables 44–2 and 44–3); however, sometimes the arthritis is transient and resolves before a diagnosis can be clearly established.

Table 44–2. SOME CAUSES OF PAIN IN ≥ 5 JOINTS*

CAUSE	SUGGESTIVE FINDINGS	DIAGNOSTIC APPROACH†
Acute rheumatic fever	Severe, migratory pain affecting mainly the large joints in the legs, elbows, and wrists Tenderness more severe than swelling Extra-articular manifestations, such as fever, symptoms and signs of cardiac dysfunction, chorea, subcutaneous nodules, and rash Prior streptococcal pharyngitis	Specific (Jones) clinical criteria Tests for Group A streptococcal infection (eg, culture, rapid strep test, antistreptolysin O and anti-DNase B titers) ECG and sometimes echocardiogram
Hemoglobinopathies (eg, sickle cell disease or trait, thalassemias)	Pain usually near but sometimes in joints, sometimes symmetric Usually in children or young patients of African or Mediterranean descent, often with known diagnosis	Hb electrophoresis
Hypermobility syndromes (eg, Ehlers-Danlos, Marfan, benign hypermobility)	Polyarthralgia, rarely with arthritis Recurrent joint subluxation Sometimes increased skin laxity Usually family history of joint hypermobility For Marfan and Ehlers-Danlos syndromes, possibly a family history of aortic aneurysm or dissection at a young age or during middle age	Clinical evaluation
Infectious bacterial (septic) arthritis (more commonly monoarticular)	Acute arthritis with severe pain and joint effusions Sometimes immunosuppression or risk factors for STDs	Arthrocentesis
Infectious viral arthritis (parvovirus B19, hepatitis B, hepatitis C, enterovirus, rubella, mumps, and HIV)	Acute arthritis Joint pain and swelling usually less severe than infectious bacterial arthritis Other systemic symptoms depending on virus (eg, jaundice with hepatitis B, often generalized lymphadenopathy with HIV)	Arthrocentesis Viral serology testing as clinically indicated (eg, hepatitis B surface antigen and IgM antibody to hepatitis B core for suspected hepatitis B)
Juvenile idiopathic arthritis	Childhood onset of joint symptoms Manifestation with oligoarthritis plus uveitis, or with systemic symptoms (Still disease—fever, rash, adenopathy, splenomegaly, pleural and/or pericardial effusions)	Clinical evaluation ANA, RF, and HLA-B27 testing
Other rheumatic diseases (eg, Sjögren syndrome, polymyositis/dermatomyositis, polymyalgia rheumatica, systemic sclerosis [scleroderma])	Disease-specific manifestations including specific dermatologic manifestations (dermatomyositis), dysphagia (systemic sclerosis), muscle soreness (polymyalgia rheumatica), or dry eyes and dry mouth (Sjögren syndrome)	Clinical evaluation Sometimes x-rays and/or serologic testing (eg, anti-SSA and anti-SSB in Sjögren syndrome, anti-Scl-70 in systemic sclerosis) Sometimes skin or muscle biopsy
Psoriatic arthritis	One of five patterns of joint involvement, which include polyarthritis similar to RA and oligoarthritis Extra-articular manifestations, such as psoriasis, onychodystrophy, uveitis, tendinitis, and dactylitis (sausage digits)	Clinical evaluation Sometimes x-rays
RA	Symmetric arthritis of small and large joints Sometimes initially monoarticular or oligoarticular More common among young adults but can manifest at any age Sometimes joint deformities at late stages	Clinical evaluation RF and anti-CCP testing X-rays
Serum sickness	Arthralgia more often than arthritis Fever, lymphadenopathy, and rash Exposure to blood products within 21 days of symptom onset	Clinical evaluation
SLE	Arthralgia more often than arthritis Systemic manifestations, such as rash (eg, malar rash), mucosal lesions (eg, oral ulcers), serositis (eg, pleuritis, pericarditis), manifestations of glomerulonephritis More common among women	Clinical evaluation ANA, anti-dsDNA, CBC, urinalysis, chemistry profile with renal and liver enzymes
Systemic vasculitides (eg, immunoglobulin A–associated vasculitis [formerly called Henoch-Schönlein purpura], polyarteritis nodosa, granulomatosis with polyangiitis)	Arthralgias, particularly with immunoglobulin A–associated vasculitis Extra-articular symptoms, often involving multiple organ systems (eg, abdominal pain, renal failure, manifestations of pneumonitis, sinonasal symptoms, skin lesions that may include rash, purpura, nodules, and ulcers)	Serologic testing as clinically indicated (eg, ANCA testing with suspected granulomatosis with polyangiitis) Biopsy as indicated (eg, of kidney, skin, or lung)

*These disorders may also manifest as oligoarticular (involving ≤ 4 joints).

†Patients with joint effusion or inflammation should have arthrocentesis (with cell counts, Gram stain, cultures, and crystal examination), and usually ESR and C-reactive protein. X-rays are often unnecessary.

ANA = antinuclear antibodies; ANCA = antineutrophil cytoplasmic antibodies; anti-CCP = anti-cyclic citrullinated peptide; dsDNA = double-stranded DNA; RF = rheumatoid factor; STD = sexually transmitted disease.

Table 44–3. SOME CAUSES OF PAIN IN ≤ 4 JOINTS

CAUSE	SUGGESTIVE FINDINGS	DIAGNOSTIC APPROACH*
Ankylosing spondylitis†	Usually axial pain and stiffness, worse in the morning and relieved with activity Sometimes effusions in large peripheral joints Sometimes extra-articular manifestations (eg, uveitis, enthesitis, aortic insufficiency) More common among young adult males	Lumbosacral spine x-ray Sometimes MRI or CT, blood tests (ESR, C-reactive protein, and CBC), and/or specific (modified New York) clinical criteria
Behçet syndrome	Arthralgia or arthritis Extra-articular manifestations, such as recurrent oral and/or genital lesions, or uveitis Usually begins during a person's 20s	Specific (international) clinical criteria
Crystal-induced arthritis‡, typically caused by uric acid crystals (gout), Ca pyrophosphate crystals (pseudogout), or Ca hydroxyapatite crystals	Acute onset of arthritis with joint warmth and swelling May be clinically indistinguishable from infectious bacterial (septic) arthritis Sometimes fever	Arthrocentesis
Infective endocarditis	Arthralgia or arthritis Systemic symptoms, such as fever, night sweats, rash, weight loss, heart murmur	Blood cultures Echocardiography
Osteoarthritis†	Chronic pain more commonly affecting the base of the thumbs, PIP and DIP joints, knees, and hips Sometimes Heberden nodes	X-rays
Reactive arthritis and enteropathic arthritis†	Arthritis that is asymmetric and more common in large lower extremity joints Reactive arthritis: GI or GU infection 1–3 wk before onset of acute arthritis Enteropathic arthritis: Coexisting GI condition (eg, inflammatory bowel disease, intestinal bypass surgery) with a chronic arthritis	Clinical evaluation Testing for STDs as clinically indicated

*Patients with joint effusion or inflammation should have arthrocentesis (with cell counts, Gram stain, cultures, and crystal examination), and usually ESR and C-reactive protein. X-rays are often not helpful early in the disease course.
†These disorders can manifest with axial involvement.
‡Crystal-induced arthritis is most often monoarticular but sometimes oligoarticular.
DIP = distal interphalangeal; PIP = proximal interphalangeal; STD = sexually transmitted disease.

Axial involvement suggests a seronegative spondyloarthropathy (also called spondyloarthritis—see p. 311) but can also occur in RA (affecting the cervical spine but not the lumbar spine).

Acute polyarticular arthritis is most often due to the following:

- Infection (usually viral)
- Flare-up of a systemic inflammatory disorder
- Gout or pseudogout

Chronic polyarticular arthritis in adults is most often due to the following:

- RA
- Seronegative spondyloarthropathy (usually ankylosing spondylitis, reactive arthritis, psoriatic arthritis, or enteropathic arthritis)

Noninflammatory polyarticular pain in adults is most often due to the following:

- Osteoarthritis

Chronic polyarthralgia in adults is caused most often by RA and osteoarthritis.

Chronic polyarticular arthralgia in children is most often due to the following:

- Juvenile idiopathic arthritis

Evaluation

Evaluation should determine whether the joints, periarticular structures, or both are the cause of symptoms and whether there is inflammation. Extra-articular symptoms and findings, which may suggest specific systemic inflammatory disorders, should also be sought and evaluated, particularly if there is joint inflammation.

History: History of present illness should identify characteristics of joint pain, associated joint symptoms, and systemic symptoms. Among important joint symptom characteristics are the acuity of onset (eg, abrupt, gradual), temporal patterns (eg, diurnal variation, persistent vs intermittent), duration (eg, acute vs chronic), and exacerbating and mitigating factors (eg, rest, activity). Patients should be specifically asked about unprotected sexual contact (indicating risk of infectious bacterial arthritis with disseminated gonococcal infection) and tick bites or residence in or travel to a Lyme-endemic area.

Review of systems should be complete in order to identify extra-articular symptoms that may suggest specific disorders (see Tables 44–2, 44–3, and 44–4).

Past medical history and family history should identify known systemic inflammatory disorders and other conditions capable of causing joint symptoms (see Tables 44–2 and 44–3). Some systemic inflammatory disorders are more prevalent in families with specific genetic profiles.

Physical examination: The physical examination should be reasonably complete, evaluating all major organ systems (eg, skin and nails, eyes, genitals, mucosal surfaces, heart, lungs, abdomen, nose, neck, lymph nodes, and neurologic system) as well as the musculoskeletal system. Vital signs are reviewed for fever.

Examination of the head should note any signs of eye inflammation (eg, uveitis, conjunctivitis) and nasal or oral lesions. Skin should be inspected for rashes and lesions (eg, ecchymoses, skin ulcers, psoriatic plaques, purpura, malar rash). The patient is also evaluated for lymphadenopathy and splenomegaly.

Cardiopulmonary examination should note any signs that suggest pleuritis, pericarditis, or valve abnormalities (eg, murmur, pericardial rub, muffled heart sounds, bibasilar dullness consistent with pleural effusion).

Genital examination should note any discharge, ulcers, or other findings consistent with sexually transmitted diseases.

Musculoskeletal examination should start by distinguishing articular from periarticular or other connective tissue or muscular tenderness. Joint examination begins with inspection for deformities, erythema, swelling, or effusion and then proceeds to palpation for joint effusions, warmth, and point tenderness. Passive and active range of motion should be evaluated. Crepitus may be felt during joint flexion and/or extension. Comparison with the contralateral unaffected joint often helps detect more subtle changes. Examination should note whether the distribution of affected joints is symmetric or asymmetric. Painful joints can also be compressed without flexing or extending them.

Periarticular structures also should be examined for involvement of tendons, bursae, or ligaments, such as discrete, soft swelling at the site of a bursa (bursitis) or point tenderness at the insertion of a tendon (tendinitis).

Red flags: The following findings are of particular concern:

- Joint warmth, swelling, and erythema
- Any extra-articular symptoms (eg, fever, rash, chills, plaques, mucosal ulcers, conjunctivitis, uveitis, murmur, purpura)

Interpretation of findings: An important initial determination, based mainly on carefully done physical examination, is whether pain originates in the joints, in other adjacent structures (eg, bones, tendons, bursae, muscles), both (eg, as in gout), or other structures. Tenderness or swelling at only one side of a joint, or away from the joint line, suggests an extra-articular origin (eg, tendons or bursae); localized joint line tenderness or more diffuse involvement of the joint suggests an intra-articular cause. Compressing the joint without flexing or extending it is not particularly painful in patients with tendinitis or bursitis but is quite painful in those with arthritis. Pain that worsens with active but not passive joint motion may indicate tendinitis or bursitis (extra-articular); intra-articular inflammation generally restricts active and passive range of joint motion significantly.

Another important determination is whether joints are inflamed. Pain during rest and on initiating activity suggests joint inflammation, whereas pain worsened by movement and relieved by rest suggests mechanical or noninflammatory disorders (eg, osteoarthritis). Increased warmth and erythema also suggest inflammation, but these findings are often insensitive, so their absence does not rule out inflammation.

Clinical findings of prolonged morning stiffness, stiffness after prolonged inactivity (gel phenomenon), nontraumatic joint swelling, and fever or unintentional weight loss suggest a systemic inflammatory disorder involving the joints. Pain that is diffuse, vaguely described, and affects myofascial structures without signs of inflammation suggests fibromyalgia.

Symmetry of joint involvement can be a clue. Involvement tends to be symmetric in RA, whereas asymmetric involvement is more suggestive of psoriatic arthritis, gout, and reactive arthritis or enteropathic arthritis.

Examination of the hand joints may yield other clues (see Table 44–4) that help differentiate osteoarthritis from RA (see Table 44–5) or that may suggest other disorders.

Spinal pain in the presence of peripheral arthritis suggests a seronegative spondyloarthropathy (ankylosing spondylitis, reactive arthritis, psoriatic arthritis, or enteropathic arthritis) but can occur in RA (usually with cervical spinal pain). New-onset oligoarthritis plus spinal pain is particularly likely to be a seronegative spondyloarthropathy if the patient has a family history of the same disorder. Eye redness and pain and low back pain suggest ankylosing spondylitis. Prior plaque psoriasis in a patient with new onset of oligoarthritis strongly suggests psoriatic arthritis.

Testing: The following tests are particularly important:

- Arthrocentesis
- Usually ESR and C-reactive protein
- Serologic testing
- In chronic arthritis, x-rays

Arthrocentesis is mandatory in most patients with a new effusion to rule out infection and identify crystals. It can also help distinguish between an inflammatory and a noninflammatory process. Synovial fluid examination includes WBC count with differential, Gram stain and cultures, and microscopic examination for crystals using polarized light. Finding crystals in synovial fluid confirms crystal-induced arthritis but does not rule out coexisting infection. A noninflammatory synovial fluid (eg, WBC count of < 1000/μL) is more suggestive of osteoarthritis or trauma. Hemorrhagic fluid is consistent with hemarthrosis. Synovial fluid WBC counts can be very high (eg, > 50,000/μL) in both infectious and crystal-induced arthritis. Synovial fluid WBC counts in systemic inflammatory disorders causing polyarthritis are most often between about 1000 and 50,000/μL.

If the specific diagnosis cannot be established based on the history and examination, additional tests may be needed. ESR and C-reactive protein can be done to help determine whether the arthritis is inflammatory. Elevated ESR and C-reactive protein levels suggest inflammation but are nonspecific, particularly in older adults. Findings are more specific if values are high during inflammatory flare-ups and normal between flare-ups.

Once a diagnosis of a systemic inflammatory disorder is clinically suspected, supportive serologic testing for antinuclear antibodies, double-stranded DNA, rheumatoid factor, anti-cyclic citrullinated peptide antibody, and antineutrophil cytoplasmic antibodies (ANCA) may assist in making the diagnosis. Specific tests should *only* be ordered to provide support for a specific diagnosis, such as SLE, ANCA-associated vasculitis, or RA.

If arthritis is chronic, x-rays are typically done to look for signs of joint damage.

Other tests may be needed to identify specific disorders (see Tables 44–2 and 44–3).

Treatment

The underlying disorder is treated whenever possible. Systemic inflammatory diseases may require either immunosuppression or antibiotics as determined by the diagnosis. Joint inflammation is usually treated symptomatically with NSAIDs. Pain without inflammation is usually more safely

Table 44–4. SOME SUGGESTIVE FINDINGS IN POLYARTICULAR JOINT PAIN

FINDING	POSSIBLE CAUSE
General findings	
Coexisting tendinitis	RA, disseminated gonococcal infection, psoriatic arthritis, gout, juvenile idiopathic arthritis (when begins at age ≤ 16)
Conjunctivitis, diarrhea, skin and genital lesions	Reactive arthritis
Fever	Infectious arthritis, gout, systemic inflammatory disorders (eg, SLE, RA)
Malaise, weight loss, and lymphadenopathy	Acute HIV infection, systemic juvenile idiopathic arthritis (Still disease)
Oral and genital lesions	Behçet disease, reactive arthritis
Raised silver plaques	Psoriatic arthritis
Recent pharyngitis and migrating arthritis	Rheumatic fever
Recent vaccination or use of a blood product	Serum sickness
Skin lesions, abdominal pain, respiratory symptoms, and mucosal lesions	Systemic vasculitis
Urethritis	Reactive arthritis or disseminated gonococcal infection
Hand findings (see Table 44–5)	
Asymmetric involvement of PIP and DIP joints with diffuse swelling of fingers (dactylitis) and/or nail pitting	Psoriatic arthritis
Tophi plus asymmetric involvement of any hand joints	Chronic gout
Bony enlargement of the PIP (Bouchard nodes) or DIP (Heberden nodes) joints	Osteoarthritis
First carpometacarpal (CMC) involvement	
Raynaud phenomenon	Systemic sclerosis, SLE, or mixed connective tissue disease
Scaling rash, often with plaque formation, over extensor surfaces of MCP and PIP joints (Gottron papules)	Dermatomyositis
Laxity of multiple finger tendons that can result in reducible finger deformities (Jaccoud arthropathy)	SLE
Symmetric involvement of PIP and MCP joints, particularly with swan-neck or boutonnière deformities	RA
Thickening of the skin over the fingers (sclerodactyly) and flexion contractures	Systemic sclerosis

DIP = distal interphalangeal; MCP = metacarpophalangeal; PIP = proximal interphalangeal.

treated with acetaminophen. Joint immobilization with a splint or sling can sometimes relieve pain. Heat or cold therapy may be analgesic in inflammatory joint diseases. Because chronic polyarthritis can lead to inactivity and secondary muscle atrophy, continued physical activity should be encouraged.

Geriatrics Essentials

Osteoarthritis is by far the most common cause of arthritis in older people. RA most commonly begins between ages 30 and 40, but in up to one third of patients, it develops after the age of 60. Because cancers can cause paraneoplastic polyarthritis, cancer should be considered in older adults in whom new-onset

Table 44–5. DIFFERENTIAL FEATURES OF THE HAND IN RHEUMATOID ARTHRITIS AND OSTEOARTHRITIS

CRITERIA	RHEUMATOID ARTHRITIS	OSTEOARTHRITIS
Joint swelling	Common Synovial, capsular, soft tissue	Uncommon Possibly mild swelling with flare-ups
Bony hypertrophy	Only in late stages	Common, often with irregular spurs
DIP involvement	Rare	Frequent
MCP involvement	Frequent	Unusual Possibly significant MCP involvement in hemochromatosis
PIP involvement	Frequent	Frequent
Wrist involvement	Frequent	Rare, however involvement of first CMC joint (common) sometimes perceived as wrist pain

CMC = carpometacarpal; DIP = distal interphalangeal; MCP = metacarpophalangeal; PIP = proximal interphalangeal.
Adapted from Bilka PJ: Physical examination of the arthritic patient. *Bulletin on the Rheumatic Diseases* 20:596–599, 1970.

RA is suspected, particularly if the onset is acute, if the lower extremities are predominantly affected, or if there is bone tenderness. Polymyalgia rheumatica should also be considered in patients > 50 who have hip and shoulder girdle stiffness and pain, even if patients have arthritis of peripheral joints (most often the hands).

KEY POINTS

- The differential diagnosis of polyarticular joint pain can be narrowed by considering which and how many joints are affected, whether inflammation is present, whether joint distribution is symmetric, and whether any extra-articular symptoms or signs are present.
- Chronic polyarthritis is most often caused by juvenile idiopathic arthritis in children and chronic polyarthralgia is most often caused by osteoarthritis and RA in adults.
- Acute polyarticular arthritis is most often due to infection, gout, or a flare of a systemic inflammatory disease.
- Arthrocentesis is mandatory in most cases of a new effusion to rule out infection, diagnose crystal-induced arthropathy, and help distinguish between an inflammatory and noninflammatory process.

45 Tumors of Bones and Joints

Bone tumors may be benign or malignant. Malignant tumors may be primary or metastatic.

In children, most bone tumors are primary and benign; some are malignant primary tumors (eg, osteosarcoma, Ewing sarcoma). Very few are metastatic tumors (eg, neuroblastoma, Wilms tumor). Bone marrow also can be affected by childhood leukemia and lymphomas.

In adults, especially those over age 40, metastatic tumors are about 100 times more common than primary malignant tumors. Excluding marrow cell tumors (eg, multiple myeloma), there are only about 2500 cases of primary malignant bone tumors in the US each year among children and adults.

Synovial tumors are extremely rare in both children and adults. Pigmented villonodular synovitis is a benign, but at times, destructive tumor of synovial cells. Synovial sarcoma (often with both spindle cell and glandular–like components) is a malignant soft-tissue tumor not of synovial origin, which seldom occurs inside of a joint.

Symptoms and Signs

Bone tumors typically cause unexplained, progressive pain and swelling. Pain can occur without weight bearing (pain at rest), particularly at night, or with mechanical stress.

Diagnosis

- Plain x-rays
- MRI usually and sometimes CT
- Bone scan if multicentric or metastatic tumors are suspected
- Biopsy unless imaging studies clearly show benign characteristics or conversely if there are multiple bony lesions in a patient with a confirmed primary cancer

The most common reason that diagnosis of bone tumors is delayed is that physicians fail to suspect the tumor and order appropriate imaging studies. Bone tumors should be considered in patients who have unexplained bone pain, particularly pain at night or at rest. Persistent or progressive unexplained pain of the trunk or extremities, particularly if associated with a mass, is suggestive of a bone tumor.

Plain x-rays are the first test to identify and characterize a bone tumor. Lesions suggestive of tumors, including those found incidentally on x-rays done for other reasons, usually require further assessment, often with additional imaging studies (eg, MRI) and a biopsy.

PEARLS & PITFALLS

- Consider a bone tumor in patients who have unexplained bone pain, particularly pain at night or at rest.

Characteristic findings: Some tumors (eg, nonossifying fibroma, fibrous dysplasia, enchondromas) and tumorlike conditions (eg, Paget disease of bone) may have characteristic radiographic findings and can be diagnosed without biopsy.

Radiographic findings that suggest cancer include the following:

- A lytic, destructive lesion
- Ill-defined, permeative appearance of bone loss
- Irregular tumor borders
- Loculated areas of bone destruction (moth-eaten appearance)
- Cortical destruction
- Soft-tissue extension
- Pathologic fracture

A lytic appearance is characterized by areas of bone destruction that are sharply demarcated. A permeative appearance is characterized by a faint, gradual loss of bone or an infiltrating pattern without clear borders. Certain tumors have a characteristic appearance. For example, Ewing sarcoma typically shows permeative-type bone destruction, including a large soft-tissue mass with aggressive periosteal onion-skin reactive bone often before there is an extensive, lytic, destructive appearance, and a giant cell tumor has a cystic appearance without a sclerotic interface between the tumor and normal bone. The tumor's location may narrow diagnostic possibilities. For example, Ewing sarcoma commonly appears in the shaft of a long bone, osteosarcoma usually appears in the metaphyseal-diaphyseal region toward the end of a long bone, and a giant cell tumor usually occurs in the epiphysis.

Bone marrow affected by childhood leukemia and lymphomas sometimes causes abnormalities on bone x-rays.

Some benign conditions, however, can mimic a malignant tumor:

- Heterotopic ossification (myositis ossificans) and exuberant callus formation after fracture can cause mineralization around bony cortices and in adjacent soft tissues, mimicking malignant tumors.
- Langerhans cell histiocytosis (histiocytosis X, Letterer-Siwe disease, Hand-Schüller-Christian disease, eosinophilic granuloma) can cause solitary or multiple bone lesions that are usually distinguishable on x-ray. In solitary lesions, there

may be periosteal new bone formation, suggesting a malignant bone tumor.

- Osteopoikilosis (spotted bones) is an asymptomatic condition of no clinical consequence but can simulate osteoblastic bone metastases of breast cancer. It is characterized by multiple small, round, or oval foci of bony sclerosis, usually in the tarsal, carpal, or pelvic bones or the metaphyseal-epiphyseal regions of tubular bones.

Other testing: CT and MRI may help define the location and extent of a bone tumor and sometimes suggest a specific diagnosis. MRI is usually done if cancer is suspected. If tumors are suspected of being metastatic or involving multiple foci (multicentric), then radioisotopic technetium bone scanning should be done to search for additional tumors.

Biopsy is usually essential for diagnosis of malignant tumors, unless the imaging studies have a classically benign appearance. The pathologist should be given pertinent details of the clinical history and should review imaging studies. Histopathologic diagnosis may be difficult and requires sufficient viable tissue from a representative portion of the tumor (usually the soft portion). The best results are obtained in centers with extensive experience in bone biopsies. Immediate, accurate, definitive diagnosis is possible in > 90% of cases.

Biopsy may be needed to confirm the diagnosis of suspected metastatic disease in an isolated, single lesion. However, biopsy may not be needed if there are multiple metastatic lesions in a patient with a confirmed primary cancer.

If a malignant diagnosis is suspected on frozen section histology, often the surgeon will wait for the results of permanent histology before treating definitively. Mistakes occur more frequently in hospitals that infrequently encounter patients with malignant primary bone tumors.

KEY POINTS

- In children, most bone tumors are primary and benign, some are primary and malignant, and very few are metastatic.
- In adults, especially those age > 40, metastatic tumors are about 100 times more common than primary malignant tumors.
- Assessment begins with plain x-rays but typically requires MRI and often other studies.
- General radiographic findings suggesting cancer include a destructive appearance (particularly with multiple foci), irregular borders, cortical destruction, soft-tissue extension, and pathologic fracture.
- Biopsy is required for diagnosis of malignant tumors.

BENIGN BONE TUMORS AND CYSTS

Unicameral bone cyst: Simple unicameral bone cysts occur in the long bones starting distal to the epiphyseal plate in children. The cyst causes the cortex to thin and predisposes the area to a buckle-like pathologic fracture, which is usually how the cyst is recognized. Plain x-rays are usually diagnostic. Simple unicameral bone cysts typically appear as well-marginated lesions without reactive sclerosis or an expansile cortex. Smaller cysts sometimes heal without treatment. A nondisplaced fracture through small cysts may be a stimulus for healing. Larger cysts, particularly in children, may require curettage and bone grafting; however, many respond to injections of corticosteroids, demineralized bone matrix, or synthetic bone substitutes. The response may be variable and may require multiple injections. Regardless of treatment, cysts persist in about 10 to 15% of patients.

Aneurysmal bone cyst: An aneurysmal bone cyst is an idiopathic expansile lesion that usually develops before age 25 yr. This cystic lesion usually occurs in the metaphyseal region of the long bones, but almost any bone may be affected. It tends to grow slowly. A periosteal new bone shell forms around the expansile lesion and is often wider than the original bone. Pain and swelling are common. The lesion may be present for a few weeks to a year before diagnosis.

The appearance on x-ray is often characteristic: the rarefied area is usually well circumscribed and eccentric; the periosteum bulges (balloons), extending into the soft tissues, and may be surrounded by new bone formation. MRI typically shows fluid-fluid levels. On imaging, some aneurysmal bone cyst–like lesions may appear more ominous, having characteristics similar to osteosarcoma, and thus should raise suspicion of telangiectatic osteosarcoma.

Surgical removal of the entire lesion is the most successful treatment; regression after incomplete removal sometimes occurs. Radiation should be avoided when possible because sarcomas occasionally develop. However, radiation may be the treatment of choice in completely surgically inaccessible vertebral lesions that are compressing the spinal cord.

Fibrous dysplasia: Fibrous dysplasia involves abnormal bone development during childhood. It may affect one or several bones. Multiple fibrous dysplasias, cutaneous pigmentation, and endocrine abnormalities may be present (Albright syndrome or McCune-Albright syndrome). The abnormal bone lesions of fibrous dysplasia commonly stop developing at puberty. They rarely undergo malignant degeneration.

On x-ray, the lesions can appear cystic and may be extensive and deforming. On imaging, the lesions have a classic ground-glass appearance.

Bisphosphonates may help relieve pain. Progressive deformities, fractures that do not heal with immobilization, or intractable pain may be effectively treated surgically.

Osteochondroma: Osteochondromas (osteocartilaginous exostoses), the most common benign bone tumors, may arise from any bone but tend to occur near the ends of long bones. These tumors manifest most often in people aged 10 to 20 and may be single or multiple. Multiple osteochondromas tend to run in families. Secondary malignant chondrosarcoma develops in well under 1% of patients with single osteochondromas, but in about 10% of patients with multiple osteochondromas. Patients with multiple hereditary osteochondromas have more tumors and are more likely to develop a chondrosarcoma than patients with a single osteochondroma. Osteochondromas rarely cause the bone to fracture.

On imaging studies, the lesion appears as a bony prominence with a cartilage cap (usually < 2 cm) off the surface of the bone with no underlying cortex under the prominence. The medullary canal is in continuity with the base of the exostosis. The medullary canal and exostosis are confluent, and there is no true underlying cortex at the base of the exostosis. Occasionally, a painful bursa may form over the cartilage cap.

Excision is needed if the tumor is compressing a large nerve; causes pain (especially when impinging on muscle and creating an inflammatory bursa); disturbs growth; or on imaging study has a destructive appearance, soft-tissue mass, or thickened cartilaginous cap (> 2 cm) suggesting transformation into malignant chondrosarcoma. An enlarging tumor in an adult should raise concern of chondrosarcoma and the possible need for excision or biopsy.

Enchondroma: Enchondromas may occur at any age but tend to manifest in people aged 10 to 40. They are usually located within the medullary bone metaphyseal-diaphyseal region. These tumors are usually asymptomatic but may enlarge and become painful. They are often found when x-rays are taken for another reason. Periosteal chondromas are similar cartilage lesions that occur on the surface of bones.

On x-ray, the tumor may appear as a lobulated calcified area within bone; some lesions are less calcified, with areas of stippled calcification on either plain films or CT. If adjacent to the cortex, enchondromas show minor endosteal scalloping. Almost all enchondromas have increased uptake on a bone scan and thus create false concern of cancer. X-ray findings, including MRI and CT, may be diagnostic; if they are not, and especially if the tumor (not the associated joint) is painful, the diagnosis of enchondroma should be confirmed by biopsy. To help differentiate bone pain from joint pain, the joint can be injected, usually with a long-lasting anesthetic (eg, bupivacaine); if pain persists, it may be caused by the bone lesion.

An asymptomatic enchondroma does not need biopsy, excision, or other treatment (usually curettage); however, follow-up imaging studies are indicated to rule out the rare disease progression to chondrosarcoma. These studies are done at 6 mo and again at 1 yr or whenever symptoms develop.

Patients with multiple enchondromas (Ollier disease) and especially multiple enchondromatosis with soft-tissue hemangiomas (Maffucci syndrome) have a much higher risk of chondrosarcoma.

Chondroblastoma: Chondroblastoma is rare and occurs most commonly among people aged 10 to 20. Arising in the epiphysis, this tumor may continue to grow and destroy bone and the joint.

It appears on imaging studies as a sclerotic marginated cyst containing spots of punctate calcification. MRI can help diagnostically by showing significant edema around the lesion.

The tumor must be surgically removed by curettage, and the cavity must be bone grafted. Local recurrence rate is about 10 to 20%, and recurrent lesions often resolve with repeat bone curettage and bone grafting.

Chondromyxofibroma: Chondromyxofibroma is very rare and usually occurs before age 30.

The appearance on imaging studies, which is usually eccentric, sharply circumscribed, lytic, and located near the end of long bones, suggests the diagnosis of chondromyxofibroma.

Treatment of chondromyxofibroma after biopsy is surgical excision or curettage.

Osteoid osteoma: Osteoid osteoma, which tends to affect young people (commonly aged 10 to 35), can occur in any bone but is most common in long bones. It can cause pain (usually worse at night, reflecting increased nocturnal prostaglandin-mediated inflammation). Pain is typically relieved by mild analgesics (particularly aspirin or other NSAIDs) that target prostaglandins. In growing children, the inflammatory response and associated hyperemia, if close to the open growth plate, may cause overgrowth and limb length discrepancy. Physical examination may reveal atrophy of regional muscles because the pain causes muscle disuse.

Characteristic appearance on imaging studies is a small radiolucent zone surrounded by a larger sclerotic zone. If a tumor is suspected, a technetium-99m bone scan should be done; an osteoid osteoma appears as an area of increased uptake. CT with fine image sequences is also done and is most helpful in distinguishing the lesion.

Ablation of the small radiolucent zone with percutaneous radiofrequency energy provides permanent relief in most cases. Most osteoid osteomas are treated by an interventional musculoskeletal radiologist using percutaneous techniques and anesthesia. Less often, osteoid osteomas are surgically curetted or excised. Surgical removal may be preferred when the osteoid osteoma is near a nerve or close to the skin (eg, spine, hands, feet) because the heat produced by radiofrequency ablation may cause damage.

Osteoblastoma: Osteoblastoma is a rare benign tumor that consists of tissue histologically similar to that of an osteoid osteoma. Some experts simply consider them large osteoid osteomas (> 2 cm). Osteoblastoma is much more common among males and appears typically between ages 10 and 35. The tumor develops in the bone of the spine, legs, hands, and feet. It is a slow-growing tumor that destroys normal bone. This tumor is painful.

Imaging is with plain films, CT, and MRI. A biopsy is warranted to make an accurate diagnosis of osteoblastoma.

Treatment of osteoblastoma requires surgery, often curettage and bone grafting. The local recurrence rate for lesions that are treated with intralesional curettage may be as high as 10 to 20%. More aggressive-appearing lesions are treated with surgical en bloc resection and bony reconstruction. A variation called aggressive osteoblastoma is similar to osteosarcoma both radiographically and histologically.

Nonossifying fibroma (fibrous cortical defect, fibroxanthoma): Nonossifying fibroma is a benign fibrous lesion of bone that appears as a well-defined lucent cortical defect on x-ray. A very small nonossifying fibroma is called a fibrous cortical defect. These lesions are developmental defects in which parts of bone that normally ossify are instead filled with fibrous tissue. They commonly affect the metaphyses, and the most commonly affected sites are, in order, the distal femur, distal tibia, and proximal tibia. They can progressively enlarge and become multiloculated. Nonossifying fibromas are common among children. Most lesions eventually ossify and undergo remodeling, often resulting in dense, sclerotic areas. However, some lesions enlarge.

Small nonossifying fibromas are asymptomatic. However, lesions that involve nearly 50% of the bone diameter tend to cause pain and increase the risk of pathologic fracture.

Nonossifying fibromas are generally first noted incidentally on imaging studies (eg, after trauma). They typically are radiolucent, single, < 2 cm in diameter, and have an oblong lucent appearance with a well-defined sclerotic border in the cortex. They can also be multiloculated.

Small nonossifying fibromas require no treatment and limited follow-up. Lesions that cause pain or are close to 50% of the bone diameter may warrant curettage and bone grafting to decrease risk of a pathologic fracture through the lesion.

Benign giant cell tumor of bone: Benign giant cell tumors of bone, which most commonly affect people in their 20s and 30s, occur in the epiphyses. These tumors are considered locally aggressive. They tend to continue to enlarge, destroy bone, and may eventually erode the rest of the bone and extend into the soft tissues. They may cause pain. These tumors are notorious for their tendency to recur. Rarely, a giant cell tumor of bone may metastasize to the lung, even though it remains histologically benign.

Benign giant cell tumors of bone appear as expansile lytic lesions on imaging. On imaging studies, there is a margin without a sclerotic rim where the tumor ends and normal trabecular bone begins. Because a giant cell tumor of bone may metastasize to the lung, a chest CT is done as part of initial staging.

Most benign giant cell tumors of bone are treated by curettage and packing with methyl methacrylate or by bone graft. To reduce recurrence rate, surgeons often prefer using an adjuvant such as thermal heat (provided by the hardening of methyl methacrylate) or treating the tumors chemically with phenol or freezing with liquid nitrogen. If a tumor is very large and destructive to the joint, complete excision with joint reconstruction may be necessary. The monoclonal antibody denosumab, a receptor activator of nuclear factor kappa-B ligand (RANKL) inhibitor, can be used in the treatment of benign giant cell tumor of bone for large, potentially nonoperable tumors.

PRIMARY MALIGNANT BONE TUMORS

Multiple myeloma: Multiple myeloma is the most common primary malignant bone tumor but is often considered a marrow cell tumor within the bone rather than a bone tumor because it is of hematopoietic derivation. It occurs mostly in older adults. Tumor development and progression is usually multicentric and often involves the bone marrow so diffusely that bone marrow aspiration is diagnostic. Unlike in metastatic disease, a radionuclide bone scan may not reliably show lesions and skeletal surveys should be done. Skeletal surveys typically show sharply circumscribed lytic lesions (punched-out lesions) or diffuse demineralization. Rarely, the lesion can appear as sclerotic or as diffuse osteopenia, especially in a vertebral body. An isolated single myeloma lesion without systemic marrow involvement is called a plasmacytoma. Certain bony lesions respond quite well to radiation therapy.

Osteosarcoma (osteogenic sarcoma): Osteosarcoma is the 2nd most common primary bone tumor and is highly malignant. It is most common among people aged 10 to 25, although it can occur at any age. Osteosarcoma produces malignant osteoid (immature bone) from tumor bone cells. Osteosarcoma usually develops around the knee (distal femur more often than proximal tibia) or in other long bones, particularly the metaphyseal-diaphyseal area, and may metastasize, usually to lung or other bone. Pain and swelling are the usual symptoms.

Findings on imaging studies vary and may include sclerotic or lytic features. Diagnosis of osteosarcoma requires biopsy. Patients need a chest x-ray and CT to detect lung metastases and a bone scan to detect bone metastases. MRI is done of the entire involved extremity to detect metachronous lesions if present. PET-CT may show distant metastases or metachronous lesions.

Treatment of osteosarcoma is a combination of chemotherapy and surgery. Use of adjuvant chemotherapy increases survival from < 20% to > 65% at 5 yr. Neoadjuvant chemotherapy usually begins before any surgery. Decreased tumor size on x-ray, decreased pain level, and decreased serum alkaline phosphatase indicate some response, but the desired response is for > 95% tumor necrosis on mapping of the resected specimen. After several courses of chemotherapy (over several months), limb-sparing surgery and limb reconstruction can proceed.

In limb-sparing surgery, the tumor is resected en bloc, including all surrounding reactive tissue and a rim of surrounding normal tissue; to avoid microscopic spillage of tumor cells, the tumor is not violated. More than 85% of patients can be treated with limb-sparing surgery without decreasing the long-term survival rate.

Continuation of chemotherapy after surgery is usually necessary. If there is nearly complete tumor necrosis (about 95%) from preoperative chemotherapy, 5-yr survival rate is > 90%. Limited metastatic disease to the lungs sometimes may be treated with thoracotomy.

Variants of conventional osteosarcoma that occur much less frequently include surface cortical lesions, such as parosteal osteosarcoma and periosteal osteosarcoma. Parosteal osteosarcomas most often involve the posterior cortex of the distal femur and usually are fairly well differentiated. Periosteal osteosarcoma is more of a cartilage surface tumor that is malignant. It is often located on the mid-shaft femur and appears as a sunburst on x-ray. Likelihood of metastases for periosteal osteosarcomas is much greater than for well-differentiated parosteal osteosarcomas, but somewhat less than for typical osteosarcomas. Parosteal osteosarcomas require surgical en bloc resection but no chemotherapy. Most of the time, periosteal osteosarcomas are treated similarly to conventional osteosarcomas with chemotherapy and surgical en bloc resection.

Fibrosarcoma and undifferentiated pleomorphic sarcoma (formerly malignant fibrous histiocytoma of bone): Fibrosarcomas and undifferentiated pleomorphic sarcoma have similar characteristics to osteosarcomas but produce fibrous tumor cells (rather than bone tumor cells), affect the same age group, and pose similar problems. Treatment and outcome for high-grade lesions are similar to osteosarcoma.

Chondrosarcoma: Chondrosarcomas are malignant tumors of cartilage. They differ from osteosarcomas clinically, therapeutically, and prognostically. Of chondrosarcomas, 90% are primary tumors. Chondrosarcomas can also arise in other preexisting conditions, particularly multiple osteochondromas and multiple enchondromatosis (eg, in Ollier disease and Maffucci syndrome). Chondrosarcomas tend to occur in older adults. They often develop in flat bones (eg, pelvis, scapula) but can develop in any portion of any bone and can implant in surrounding soft tissues.

X-rays often reveal punctate calcifications. Chondrosarcomas often also exhibit cortical bone destruction and loss of normal bone trabeculae. MRI may show a soft-tissue mass. Biopsy is required for chondrosarcoma diagnosis and can also determine the tumor's grade (probability of metastasizing). Needle biopsy may provide an inadequate tissue sample.

It is often difficult to differentiate low-grade chondrosarcomas from enchondromas by imaging and sometimes even histology.

Low-grade chondrosarcomas (grade 1/2 or grade 1) are often treated intralesionally (wide curettage) with addition of an adjuvant (often freezing liquid nitrogen, argon beam, heat of methyl methacrylate, radiofrequency, or phenol). Some surgeons prefer surgical en bloc resection for low-grade tumors to reduce risk of recurrence. Higher grade tumors are treated with surgical en bloc resection. When surgical resection with maintenance of function is impossible, amputation may be necessary. Because of the potential to implant the tumor, meticulous care must be taken to avoid spillage of tumor cells into the soft tissues during a biopsy or surgery. Recurrence is inevitable if tumor cells spill. If no spillage occurs, the cure rate depends on the tumor grade. Low-grade tumors are nearly all cured with adequate treatment. Because these tumors have limited vascularity, chemotherapy and radiation therapy have little efficacy.

Ewing sarcoma of bone: Ewing sarcoma of bone is a round-cell bone tumor with a peak incidence between 10 yr and 25 yr. Most tumors develop in the extremities, but any bone may be involved. Ewing sarcoma tends to be extensive, sometimes involving the entire bone shaft, most often the diaphyseal region. About 15 to 20% occur around the metaphyseal region. Pain and swelling are the most common symptoms.

Lytic destruction, particularly a permeative infiltrating pattern without clear borders, is the most common finding on imaging, but multiple layers of subperiosteal reactive new bone formation may give an onion-skin appearance. X-rays do not usually reveal the full extent of bone involvement, and a large soft-tissue mass usually surrounds the affected bone. MRI better defines disease extent, which can help guide treatment. Many other benign and malignant tumors can appear very similarly, so diagnosis of Ewing sarcoma is made by biopsy. At times this type of tumor may be confused with an infection. Accurate histologic diagnosis can be accomplished with molecular markers, including evaluation for a typical clonal chromosomal abnormality.

Treatment of Ewing sarcoma includes various combinations of surgery, chemotherapy, and radiation therapy. Currently, > 60% of patients with primary localized Ewing sarcoma may be cured by this multimodal approach. Cure is sometimes possible even with metastatic disease. Chemotherapy in conjunction with surgical en bloc resection, if applicable, often yields better long-term results.

Lymphoma of bone: Lymphoma of bone (previously known as reticulum cell sarcoma) affects adults, usually in their 40s and 50s. It may arise in any bone. The tumor consists of small round cells, often with a mixture of reticulum cells, lymphoblasts, and lymphocytes. It can develop as an isolated primary bone tumor, in association with similar tumors in other tissues, or as a metastasis from known soft-tissue lymphomatous disease. Pain and swelling are the usual symptoms of lymphoma of bone. Pathologic fracture is common.

Imaging studies reveal bone destruction, which may be in a mottled or patchy or even infiltrating, permeative pattern, often with a clinical and radiographic large soft-tissue mass. In advanced disease, the entire outline of the affected bone may be lost.

In isolated primary bone lymphoma, the 5-yr survival rate is ≥ 50%.

Bone lymphomas are typically treated with systemic chemotherapy. Radiation therapy can be used as an adjuvant in some cases. Stabilization of long bones is often necessary to prevent pathologic fracture. Amputation is indicated only rarely, when function is lost because of pathologic fracture or extensive soft-tissue involvement that cannot be managed otherwise.

Malignant giant cell tumor: Malignant giant cell tumor, which is rare, is usually located at the extreme end of a long bone.

X-ray reveals classic features of malignant destruction (predominantly lytic destruction, cortical destruction, soft-tissue extension, and pathologic fracture). A malignant giant cell tumor that develops in a previously benign giant cell tumor is characteristically radioresistant.

Treatment of malignant giant cell tumor is similar to that of osteosarcoma, but the cure rate is low.

Chordoma: Chordoma, which is rare, develops from the remnants of the primitive notochord. It tends to occur at the ends of the spinal column, usually in the middle of the sacrum or near the base of the skull. A chordoma in the sacrococcygeal region causes nearly constant pain. A chordoma in the base of the skull can cause deficits in a cranial nerve, most commonly in nerves to the eye.

Symptoms of chordoma may exist for months to several years before diagnosis.

A chordoma appears on imaging studies as a destructive bone lesion that may be associated with a soft-tissue mass. Metastasis is unusual, but local recurrence is not.

Chordomas in the sacrococcygeal region may be cured by radical en bloc excision. Chordomas in the base of the skull are usually inaccessible to surgery but may respond to radiation therapy.

METASTATIC BONE TUMORS

Any cancer may metastasize to bone, but metastases from carcinomas are the most common, particularly those arising in the following areas:

- Breast
- Lung
- Prostate
- Kidney
- Thyroid
- Colon

Prostate cancer in men and breast cancer in women are the most common types of cancers. Lung cancer is the most common cause of cancer death in both sexes. Breast cancer is the most common cancer to metastasize to bone. Any bone may be involved with metastases. Metastatic disease does not commonly spread to bone below the mid forearm or mid calf, but when it occurs in those sites, it results most often from lung or sometimes kidney cancer.

Symptoms and Signs

Metastases manifest as bone pain, although they may remain asymptomatic for some time. Bone metastases may cause symptoms before the primary tumor is suspected or may appear in patients with a known diagnosis of cancer.

Diagnosis

- X-ray
- Radionuclide scanning to identify all metastases
- Clinical evaluation and testing to diagnose the primary tumor (if unknown)
- Often biopsy if the primary tumor is unknown after assessment

Metastatic bone tumors are considered in all patients with unexplained bone pain, but particularly in patients who have

- Known cancer
- Pain at more than one site
- Findings on imaging studies that suggest metastases

Prostate cancer is most often blastic, lung cancer is most often lytic, and breast cancer may be blastic or lytic.

CT and MRI are highly sensitive for specific metastases. However, if metastases are suspected, a radionuclide whole-body scan, which is not quite as sensitive, is usually done. Bone scan is more sensitive for early and asymptomatic bone metastases than plain x-rays and can be used to scan the entire body. Lesions on the scan are usually presumed to be metastases if the patient has a known primary cancer. Metastases should be suspected in patients who have multiple lesions on bone scan. Although metastases are suspected in patients with known cancer and a single bone lesion, the lesion may not be a metastasis; thus, a needle biopsy of the lesion is often done to confirm the diagnosis of a metastasis. Whole-body PET-CT is now often used for some tumors; it is more specific for bone metastases than is radionuclide bone scan and can identify many extraskeletal metastases.

If bone metastases are suspected because multiple lytic lesions are found, assessment for the primary tumor can begin with clinical evaluation for primary cancers (particularly focused on the breast, prostate, and thyroid), chest x-ray, mammography, and measurement of prostate-specific antigen level. Initial CT of the chest, abdomen, and pelvis may also reveal the primary tumor.

However, bone biopsy, especially fine-needle or core biopsy, is necessary if metastatic tumor is suspected and the primary tumor has not been otherwise diagnosed. Biopsy with use of immunohistologic stains may give clues to the primary tumor type.

Treatment

- Usually radiation therapy
- Surgery to stabilize bone at risk of pathologic fracture or resect highly diseased bone (with joint reconstruction if needed)
- Kyphoplasty or vertebraplasty for certain painful vertebral fractures

Treatment of metastatic bone tumors depends on the type of tissue involved (which organ tissue type). Radiation therapy, combined with selected chemotherapeutic or hormonal drugs, is the most common treatment modality. Early use of radiation (30 Gy) and bisphosphonates (eg, zoledronate, pamidronate) slows bone destruction. Some tumors are more likely to heal after radiation therapy; eg, blastic lesions of prostate and breast cancer are more likely to heal than lytic destructive lesions of lung cancer and renal cell carcinoma. Drugs used to treat receptor activator of nuclear factor kappa-B ligand (RANKL) are now being used to reduce bone destruction.

If bone destruction is extensive, resulting in imminent or actual pathologic fracture, surgical fixation or resection and reconstruction may be required to provide stabilization and help minimize morbidity. When the primary cancer has been removed and only limited bone metastasis remains (especially if the metastatic lesion appears ≥ 1 yr after the primary tumor), en bloc excision sometimes combined with radiation therapy, chemotherapy, or both rarely may be curative. Insertion of methyl methacrylate into the spine (kyphoplasty or vertebraplasty) relieves pain and expands and stabilizes compression fractures that do not have epidural soft-tissue extension.

KEY POINTS

- Carcinomas of breast, lung, and prostate are the most common sources of metastatic bone tumors.
- Bone metastases should be suspected in patients with known cancer, when pain is at more than one site, and/or when findings on imaging studies suggest metastases.
- Bone biopsy is needed if the primary tumor is unknown after clinical and radiographic evaluation.
- Patients with known solid organ cancer and limited bone lesions may require a needle biopsy to confirm metastatic disease and exclude a second primary tumor.
- Most often, radiation therapy and a bisphosphonate are used to slow bone destruction.
- Pathologic fractures may require treatment with surgery, kyphoplasty, or vertebraplasty.

JOINT TUMORS

Tumors rarely affect joints, unless by direct extension of an adjacent bone or soft-tissue tumor. However, two conditions—synovial chondromatosis and pigmented villonodular synovitis—occur in the lining (synovium) of joints. These conditions are benign but locally aggressive. Both usually affect one joint, most often the knee and second most often the hip, and can cause pain and effusion. Both are treated by synovectomy and removal of any intra-articular bodies.

Synovial chondromatosis: Synovial chondromatosis (previously called synovial osteochondromatosis) is considered metaplastic synovium. It is characterized by numerous calcified cartilaginous bodies in the synovium, which often become loose. Each body may be no larger than a grain of rice, in a swollen, painful joint. Malignant change is very rare. Recurrence is common.

Diagnosis of synovial chondromatosis is by imaging, usually CT or MRI.

Treatment of synovial chondromatosis may be symptomatic, but if mechanical symptoms are prominent, arthroscopic or open removal of the bodies or synovium is warranted.

Pigmented villonodular synovitis: Pigmented villonodular synovitis is considered neoplastic synovium. The synovium becomes thickened and contains hemosiderin, which gives the tissue its blood-stained appearance and characteristic appearance on MRI. This tissue tends to invade adjacent bone, causing cystic destruction and damage to the cartilage. Pigmented villonodular synovitis is usually monarticular but may be polyarticular.

Late management of pigmented villonodular synovitis, especially after recurrence, may require total joint replacement. On rare occasions after several synovectomies, radiation therapy is sometimes used.

46 Vasculitis

Vasculitis is inflammation of blood vessels, often with ischemia, necrosis, and organ inflammation. Vasculitis can affect any blood vessel—arteries, arterioles, veins, venules, or capillaries. Clinical manifestations of specific vasculitic disorders are diverse and depend on the size and location of the involved vessels, the extent of the organ involvement, and the degree and pattern of inflammation.

Etiology

Vasculitis may be

- Primary
- Secondary

Primary vasculitis results from an inflammatory response that targets the vessel walls and has no known cause.

Secondary vasculitis may be triggered by an infection, a drug, or a toxin or may occur as part of another inflammatory disorder or cancer.

Pathophysiology

Histologic description of an affected vessel should include the following:

- A description of vessel wall damage (eg, type and location of inflammatory infiltrate, extent and type of damage, presence or absence of fibrinoid necrosis)
- A description of healing responses (eg, intimal hypertrophy, fibrosis)

Table 46–1. HISTOLOGIC CLUES TO DIAGNOSIS OF VASCULITIC DISORDERS

FINDINGS	POSSIBLE DIAGNOSES
Predominantly nonnecrotizing granulomatous inflammatory infiltrate with lymphocytes, macrophages, and multinucleated giant cells	Giant cell arteritis Primary angiitis of the CNS (certain types) Takayasu arteritis
Fibrinoid vascular necrosis of the vessel wall with a mixed infiltrate consisting of various combinations of leukocytes and lymphocytes	EGPA (formerly Churg-Strauss syndrome) GPA (formerly Wegener granulomatosis) Immune complex–associated vasculitis MPA Polyarteritis nodosa RA
IgA deposits*	IgAV
Scant or complete absence of immunoglobulins and complement deposition in the vessel walls*,†	EGPA GPA MPA

*These findings are detected using immunofluorescence staining.
†Disorders thus characterized are called pauci-immune vasculitic disorders.
EGPA = eosinophilic granulomatosis with polyangiitis; GPA = granulomatosis with polyangiitis; MPA = microscopic polyangiitis.

Certain features (eg, predominant inflammatory cells, location of inflammation) suggest particular vasculitic processes and may aid in the diagnosis (see Table 46–1). For example, in many acute lesions, the predominant inflammatory cells are polymorphonuclear leukocytes; in chronic lesions, lymphocytes predominate.

Inflammation may be segmental or involve the entire vessel. At sites of inflammation, varying degrees of cellular inflammation and necrosis or scarring occur in one or more layers of the vessel wall. Inflammation in the media of a muscular artery tends to destroy the internal elastic lamina. Some forms of vasculitis are characterized by giant cells in the vessel wall.

Leukocytoclastic vasculitis is a histopathologic term used to describe findings in small-vessel vasculitis. It refers to breakdown of inflammatory cells that leaves small nuclear fragments (nuclear debris) in and around the vessels. Inflammation is transmural and nongranulomatous. Polymorphonuclear leukocytes predominate early; later, lymphocytes predominate. Resolution of the inflammation tends to result in fibrosis and intimal hypertrophy. Intimal hypertrophy or secondary clot formation can narrow the vessel lumen and cause tissue ischemia or necrosis.

Classification

Vasculitic disorders can be classified according to the size of the predominant vessel affected. However, there is often substantial overlap (see Table 46–2).

Symptoms and Signs

Size of the affected vessels helps determine clinical presentation (see Table 46–2).

Regardless of the size of the vessels involved, patients can present with symptoms and signs of systemic inflammation (eg, fever, night sweats, fatigue, anorexia, weight loss, arthralgias, arthritis). Some manifestations are life-threatening or organ-threatening and require immediate treatment:

- Alveolar hemorrhage
- Rapidly progressive glomerulonephritis
- Mesenteric ischemia
- Vision loss in patients with giant cell arteritis

Small- and medium-sized vasculitides often manifest with skin lesions such as palpable purpura, urticaria, ulcers, livedo reticularis, and nodules.

Diagnosis

- Clinical evaluation
- Basic laboratory tests to detect inflammation or organ dysfunction (eg, CBC, ESR or C-reactive protein, serum albumin and total protein, AST and ALT, BUN and creatinine, urinalysis)
- Laboratory tests to diagnose the type of vasculitis (eg, antineutrophil cytoplasmic antibodies [ANCA])
- Laboratory and imaging studies that determine the cause of vasculitis and extent of organ involvement
- Biopsy

Systemic vasculitis is suspected in patients with the following:

- Symptoms or signs suggestive of vasculitis (eg, temporal headache and jaw claudication suggesting giant cell arteritis)
- Ischemic manifestations (eg, ischemic stroke, limb claudication, mesenteric ischemia) out of proportion to a patient's risk factors for atherosclerosis
- Unexplained combinations of symptoms in more than one organ system that are compatible with vasculitis (eg, hypertension, myalgias), particularly when symptoms of a systemic illness are present

Primary vasculitic disorders are diagnosed based on the presence of characteristic symptoms, physical findings, compatible laboratory test results, and exclusion of other causes (ie, secondary vasculitis). Histologic examination is done whenever possible and may point to a particular vasculitic disorder (see Table 46–1).

Routine laboratory tests are done first. Most tests yield results that are nonspecific; however, results can often help support the diagnosis, determine the degree of organ involvement, or suggest alternative diagnoses. Tests usually include CBC, ESR or C-reactive protein, serum albumin and total protein, AST, and ALT. Often, patients present with elevated ESR or C-reactive protein, anemia due to chronic inflammation, elevated platelets, and low serum albumin. Freshly voided urine must be tested for RBCs, RBC casts, and protein to identify renal involvement.

Table 46–2. CLASSIFICATION OF VASCULITIC DISORDERS

SIZE OF AFFECTED VESSELS	DISORDERS	SYMPTOMS AND SIGNS
Large	Behçet disease Giant cell arteritis Polymyalgia rheumatica Takayasu arteritis	Limb claudication Unequal BP measurements or unequal pulse strength/absent pulse in the limbs CNS ischemic symptoms (eg, strokes)
Medium	Medium-vessel cutaneous vasculitis Polyarteritis nodosa	Symptoms of tissue infarction in affected organs, such as • Muscles: Myalgias • Nerves: Multiple mononeuropathy (mononeuritis multiplex) • GI tract: Mesenteric ischemia • Kidneys: New-onset hypertension • Skin: Ulcers, nodules, and livedo reticularis
Small	Eosinophilic granulomatosis with polyangiitis (formerly called Churg-Strauss syndrome) Cyroglobulinemic vasculitis Granulomatosis with polyangiitis (formerly called Wegener granulomatosis) Immunoglobulin A–associated vasculitis (formerly called Henoch-Schönlein purpura) Microscopic polyangiitis Small-vessel cutaneous vasculitis	Symptoms of tissue infarction in affected organs similar to those for medium-sized vessels, except skin lesions more likely to be purpuric

Serum creatinine levels should be checked and monitored. Leukopenia and thrombocytopenia are not typical of primary vasculitis and suggest an alternate diagnosis.

Detection of ANCA may support the diagnosis of granulomatosis with polyangiitis (GPA—formerly known as Wegener granulomatosis), eosinophilic granulomatosis with polyangiitis (EGPA—formerly known as Churg-Strauss syndrome), or microscopic polyangiitis (sometimes called collectively ANCA-associated vasculitides). Standardized tests for ANCA include immunofluorescence staining and enzyme-linked immunosorbent assay (ELISA). Immunofluorescence staining of ethanol-fixed neutrophils can detect the cytoplasmic pattern of c-ANCA or the perinuclear pattern of p-ANCA. Then ELISA is used to check for antibodies specific for the major autoantigens: proteinase-3 (PR3), which produces the c-ANCA staining pattern, or myeloperoxidase (MPO), which produces the p-ANCA staining pattern seen on ethanol-fixed neutrophils. Because ANCA-associated vasculitides are rare, and the ANCA test is not completely specific, ANCA testing should be done only when the pretest probability for ANCA-associated vasculitis is moderately high.

Other useful laboratory tests include hepatitis B and C serologic testing, serum and urine protein electrophoresis, antinuclear antibody and anti-extractable nuclear antigens panel, testing for the presence of cryoglobulins, and complement levels to diagnose viral vasculitis, cryoglobulinemic vasculitis, lymphoproliferative disorders, or vasculitis secondary to other autoimmune diseases.

Further testing is determined by clinical findings. If indicated based on clinical findings, a chest x-ray should be done to check for infiltrates, but high-resolution noncontrast CT of the chest may be needed to check for subtle findings, such as small nodules or cavities. Bilateral diffuse infiltrates suggest possible alveolar hemorrhage, which requires immediate diagnosis and treatment. Other imaging tests may be required. For example, magnetic resonance angiography of large blood vessels and the aorta is useful for diagnosis and monitoring when such vessels appear affected. If symptoms and examination suggest a neuropathy, electromyography may be helpful.

Because vasculitic disorders are rare and treatment may have severe adverse effects, tissue biopsy is done to confirm the diagnosis whenever possible. Clinical findings suggest the best site for biopsy. Biopsy results are most likely to be positive if taken from affected lung, skin, and kidney tissue. Blind biopsies of organs without clinical manifestations or laboratory suggestion of involvement have a low likelihood of providing positive results.

Treatment

- Induction of remission for life-threatening or organ-threatening vasculitis with corticosteroids, often with cyclophosphamide or rituximab
- Induction of remission for less severe vasculitis with corticosteroids plus a less potent immunosuppressant (eg, methotrexate, azathioprine, mycophenolate mofetil) or rituximab
- Maintenance of remission with methotrexate, azathioprine, or rituximab, plus tapering of corticosteroids

Treatment depends on the etiology, the type of vasculitis, and extent and severity of disease. For secondary vasculitic disorders, removing the cause (eg, infection, drug, cancer) can help.

For primary vasculitic disorders, treatment aims to induce and maintain remission. Remission is induced by using cytotoxic immunosuppressants and high-dose corticosteroids, usually for 3 to 6 mo, until remission occurs or disease activity is acceptably reduced. The duration of remission is hard to predict and may depend on the type of vasculitis. For many patients, maintaining remission requires continuation of immunosuppressive therapy with or without a low dose of corticosteroids. During this period, the goal is to eliminate corticosteroids or reduce their dose and to use less potent (and less toxic) immunosuppressants as long as needed.

All patients treated with immunosuppressants should be monitored for opportunistic and other infections. Testing for TB and hepatitis B, which can become exacerbated by immunosuppressive therapy, should be considered. Prophylaxis against *Pneumocystis jirovecii* should be considered for patients receiving potent or prolonged immunosuppressive therapy.

Induction of remission: For less severe forms of vasculitis, low doses of corticosteroids and less potent immunosuppressants (eg, methotrexate, azathioprine, mycophenolate mofetil) or rituximab may be used.

Severe, rapidly progressive and life- or organ-threatening vasculitis (eg, causing alveolar hemorrhage, rapidly progressive glomerulonephritis, or mesenteric ischemia) is a medical emergency requiring hospital admission and immediate treatment. Treatment typically consists of the following:

- **Corticosteroids:** High-dose corticosteroids (also called pulse corticosteroids) are often prescribed. Methylprednisolone 15 mg/kg or 1 g IV once/day for 3 days may be used, followed by 1 mg/kg prednisone or methylprednisolone po (or, if hospitalized, sometimes IV) once/day for about 4 wk. The dose is then tapered slowly, as tolerated, usually by 10 mg every week to 40 mg/day, by 5 mg every 2 wk to 20 mg/day, by 2.5 mg every 2 wk to 10 mg/day, and by 1 mg every month from there on until the drug is stopped. Changes in this tapering schedule may be necessary if the patient fails to improve or relapses.
- **Cyclophosphamide:** A dose of 2 mg/kg po once/day is usually recommended for at least 3 mo or until remission occurs. The WBC count must be closely monitored, and the dose must be adjusted to avoid leukopenia. (WBC count should be maintained at > 3500/μL.) Alternatively, an IV cyclophosphamide regimen of 0.5 to 1 g/m^2 at 2- to 4-wk intervals is used. The dose should be reduced in patients with significant renal insufficiency, and WBC counts should be monitored frequently. Patients taking chronic high-dose corticosteroids, particularly with cyclophosphamide, should also be given prophylactic treatment against *Pneumocystis jirovecii*.
- **Mesna:** Mesna is mixed with IV cyclophosphamide to bind acrolein, a product of cyclophosphamide degradation that is toxic to the bladder epithelium and can lead to hemorrhagic cystitis and sometimes transitional cell carcinoma of the bladder. Long-term use of cyclophosphamide increases the risk of bladder cancer. One milligram of mesna is added for each milligram of cyclophosphamide. Recurrence of hematuria, especially without casts and dysmorphic red cells, should prompt a referral for urologic evaluation. Cystoscopy and renal imaging should be done to exclude cancer.
- **Rituximab:** Rituximab, a B cell-depleting anti-CD20 monoclonal antibody, has been shown to be noninferior to cyclophosphamide in inducing remission of severe ANCA-associated vasculitis. Rituximab is given as 375 mg/m^2 IV once/wk for 4 wk. A widely used alternative regimen is two 1000-mg infusions given 2 wk apart.

Remission maintenance: Corticosteroids are tapered to zero or to the lowest dose that can maintain remission. For some forms of vasculitis (most clearly demonstrated in ANCA-associated disease), weekly methotrexate (with folate) or daily azathioprine is prescribed to replace cyclophosphamide because these drugs have a better adverse effects profile. Periodic IV rituximab may also be used to maintain remission. The duration of this treatment varies, from one year to several years, depending on the patient, specific diagnosis, and propensity for relapse. Patients with frequent relapses may need to take immunosuppressants indefinitely.

Long-term use of corticosteroids can have significant adverse effects. Patients who are taking ≥ 7.5 mg of prednisone daily or equivalent doses of other corticosteroids should be given Ca and vitamin D supplements and bisphosphonates to help prevent or minimize osteoporosis; bone density monitoring should be considered.

KEY POINTS

- Vasculitis can be a primary disorder or secondary to other causes.
- Clinical manifestations can be systemic and/or organ-specific, depending on how vessels are affected.
- Vasculitis tends to affect small-, medium-, or large-sized vessels, each with certain patterns of organ involvement.
- Do blood tests, imaging studies, and tissue biopsy as indicated to determine the cause of vasculitis (including disorders such as infections and cancer) and extent of organ involvement.
- Treat with corticosteroids and immunosuppressants.
- Address increased risks of infection and osteoporosis caused by vasculitis treatment with monitoring and/or prophylactic treatments.

BEHÇET DISEASE

Behçet disease is a multisystem, relapsing, chronic vasculitic disorder with mucosal inflammation. Common manifestations include recurrent oral ulcers, ocular inflammation, genital ulcers, and skin lesions. The most serious manifestations are blindness, neurologic or GI manifestations, venous thromboses, and arterial aneurysms. Diagnosis is clinical, using international criteria. Treatment is mainly symptomatic but may involve corticosteroids with or without other immunosuppressants for more severe manifestations.

Behçet disease is an inflammatory disorder that can include a vasculitis of small and large arteries and/or veins. Arterial and venous thrombosis may occur as well.

The disease occurs nearly equally in men and women but tends to be more severe in men, typically beginning during their 20s. Occasionally, the disease develops in children. Incidence varies by location. Behçet disease is most common along the silk route from the Mediterranean to China; it is uncommon in the US.

The cause is unknown. Immunologic (including autoimmune) and viral or bacterial triggers have been suggested, and HLA-B51 is a major risk factor. Prevalence of an HLA-B51 allele is > 15% among people from Europe, the Middle East, and the Far East but is low or absent among people from Africa, Oceania, and South America.

Neutrophil infiltration is detected in biopsy specimens from oral aphthous ulcers and erythema nodosum and pathergy lesions, but no histologic changes are pathognomonic.

Symptoms and Signs

Mucocutaneous: Almost all patients have recurrent, painful oral ulcers resembling those of aphthous stomatitis; in most, these ulcers are the first manifestations. The ulcers are round or oval, 2 to 10 mm in diameter, and shallow or deep with a central yellowish necrotic center; they can occur anywhere in the oral cavity, often in clusters. Ulcers last 1 to 2 wk. Similar ulcers occur on the penis and scrotum, on the vulva where they are painful, or in the vagina where they may cause little or no pain.

Cutaneous lesions are common and may include acneiform lesions, nodules, erythema nodosum, superficial thrombophlebitis, pyoderma gangrenosum–type lesions, and palpable purpura.

Pathergy (an erythematous papular or pustular response to local skin injury) is defined as a papule > 2 mm that appears 24 to 48 h after oblique insertion of a 20- to 25-gauge needle into the skin.

Ocular: The eyes are affected in 25 to 75% of patients. Eye manifestations may be associated with neurologic manifestations. The following may occur:

- Relapsing uveitis or iridocyclitis (most common) often manifests as pain, photophobia, and red eye.
- Hypopyon (a layer of pus visible in the anterior chamber) may occur.
- Uveitis is typically bilateral and episodic, often involves the entire uveal tract (panuveitis), and may not resolve completely between episodes.
- Choroiditis, retinal vasculitis, vascular occlusion, and optic neuritis may irreversibly impair vision and even progress to blindness.

Musculoskeletal: Relatively mild, self-limiting, and nondestructive arthralgias or frank arthritis, especially in the knees and other large joints, occur in 50% of patients. Sacroiliac inflammation can occur.

Vascular: Perivascular and endovascular inflammation may develop in arteries and veins. In arteries, thrombosis, aneurysm, pseudoaneurysm, hemorrhage, and stenosis can develop. Large-vessel arterial involvement is recognized during life in 3 to 5% of patients; however, at autopsy, one-third of patients have evidence of large-vessel involvement that was asymptomatic during life. Aortic and pulmonary artery aneurysms can rupture. In situ thrombosis can cause pulmonary artery occlusion. Hemoptysis may occur if fistulas develop between the pulmonary artery and bronchus.

Venous involvement can cause superficial and deep venous thromboses. More than one vein may be affected, including the inferior and superior vena cava, the hepatic veins (causing Budd-Chiari syndrome), and the dural venous sinuses.

In situ arterial or venous thromboses, aneurysms, and pseudoaneurysms are more common than stenoses and occlusions.

Neurologic and psychiatric: CNS involvement is less common but is serious. Onset may be sudden or gradual. The first manifestations may be parenchymal involvement with pyramidal signs, small-vessel disease with a multiple sclerosis–like pattern, or nonparenchymal with aseptic meningitis or meningoencephalitis, or dural sinus thrombosis.

Psychiatric disorders including personality changes and dementia may develop years later. Peripheral neuropathy, common in other vasculitic disorders, is uncommon in Behçet disease.

GI: Abdominal discomfort, abdominal pain, and diarrhea with intestinal ulcers, occurring primarily in the ileum and colon and closely resembling Crohn disease, may occur.

Constitutional: Fever and malaise may occur.

Diagnosis

- Clinical criteria

Behçet disease should be suspected in young adults with recurrent oral aphthous ulcers, unexplained ocular findings, or genital ulcers. Diagnosis is clinical and often delayed because many of the manifestations are nonspecific and can be insidious.

International criteria for diagnosis include recurrent oral ulcers (3 times in 1 yr) and 2 of the following:

- Recurrent genital ulcers
- Eye lesions
- Skin lesions
- Positive pathergy test with no other clinical explanation

Laboratory tests (eg, CBC, ESR or C-reactive protein, serum albumin and total protein levels) are done. Results are nonspecific but characteristic of inflammatory disease (elevated ESR, C-reactive protein, and α_2- and γ-globulins; mild leukocytosis).

Differential diagnosis: Differential diagnosis includes

- Reactive arthritis
- SLE
- Crohn disease
- Ulcerative colitis
- Ankylosing spondylitis
- Periodic fever syndromes
- Herpes simplex infection

Behçet disease has no single pathognomonic finding but may be distinguished by its combinations of relapsing symptoms with spontaneous remissions and multiple organ involvement, particularly in patients with recurrent, deep mucosal ulcers.

Prognosis

Behçet disease typically has a waxing and waning course characterized by exacerbations and remissions. Prognosis tends to be worse if patients are young men. Risk also appears to be higher if patients have an HLA-B51 allele. Mucocutaneous and ocular lesions and arthralgias are often worse early in the disease. CNS and large-vessel manifestations, if they develop, typically occur later. Occasionally, the disease results in death, usually due to neurologic, vascular (eg, aneurysms), or GI manifestations. Risk of death is highest for young men and patients with arterial disease or a high number of flare-ups. Many patients eventually go into remission.

Treatment

- Colchicine, apremilast, thalidomide, anti-TNF drugs, and/or interferon for mucosal disease
- Azathioprine or cyclosporine for eye disease
- Anti-TNF drugs, cyclophosphamide, and chlorambucil for refractory or life-threatening disease

Treatment depends on the clinical manifestations. Treatment recommendations are limited by incomplete data from clinical studies (eg, cross-sectional studies, usually not prospective, limited statistical power).

Topical corticosteroids may temporarily relieve ocular manifestations and most oral lesions. However, topical or systemic corticosteroids do not alter the frequency of relapses. A few patients with severe uveitis or CNS manifestations respond to high-dose systemic corticosteroids (eg, prednisone 60 to 80 mg po once/day).

Anti-TNF drugs appear to be effective for a wide range of manifestations, including GI manifestations and ocular disease (eg, severe refractory uveitis), and decrease the number of attacks. In severe cases of GI and ocular attacks, an anti-TNF drug can be used in combination with another drug such as azathioprine. Infliximab, in particular, has the advantage of rapid onset of action.

Immunosuppressants, including anti-TNF drugs, improve the prognosis for patients with vascular involvement. Immunosuppressants help prevent recurrence of venous thrombosis, but it is unclear whether anticoagulation does. Anticoagulation is contraindicated in patients with pulmonary arterial aneurysms.

Mucosal disease: Mucosal disease can be managed symptomatically. Topical corticosteroids, local anesthetics, and sucralfate are helpful.

Colchicine 0.6 mg po bid may decrease the frequency and severity of oral or genital ulcers and may be effective for erythema nodosum and arthralgias. Colchicine, which was hypothesized to decrease the need for later immunosuppressive therapy when used early in the disease course, has not been shown to do so.

Apremilast, an oral phosphodiesterase type 4 inhibitor, has been shown to decrease the number of oral ulcers and pain.

Thalidomide 100 to 300 mg po once/day may be used to treat oral, genital, and skin lesions, but lesions may recur when treatment is stopped.

The anti-TNF drug etanercept, 50 mg sc once/wk or 25 mg sc twice/wk, may suppress mucocutaneous lesions. Etanercept can be given if colchicine is ineffective. Sometimes another anti-TNF drug (infliximab or possibly adalimumab) is used instead of etanercept.

Interferon alfa-2a 6 million units 3 times/wk can also be given if colchicine is ineffective.

Ocular disease: Azathioprine 2.5 mg/kg po once/day helps preserve visual acuity and prevent new eye lesions. Azathioprine is also useful for mucocutaneous lesions and arthralgia.

Cyclosporine 5 to 10 mg/kg po once/day may be reserved for patients with severe ocular manifestations and may be used with azathioprine to treat refractory uveitis.

Interferon alfa-2a 6 million units sc 3 times/wk and infliximab (a TNF inhibitor) 3 to 10 mg/kg IV at 0, 2, and 4 wk and then every 8 wk show promise for patients with ocular manifestations.

Refractory or life-threatening disease: Cyclophosphamide and chlorambucil are used in patients with refractory disease, life-threatening conditions (eg, pulmonary aneurysms), or CNS manifestations. A trend toward longer event-free survival has been observed in patients with severe neurologic manifestations after treatment with IV cyclophosphamide than with azathioprine.

KEY POINTS

- Behçet disease is a relapsing inflammatory disorder characterized by prominent mucosal inflammation and usually vasculitis of large and small vessels.
- Among the many organ systems involved, oral and genital ulcers, skin lesions, and ocular findings, particularly in combination, are very characteristic.
- Diagnose based on specific clinical criteria.
- Risk factors for early death are male sex, frequent disease flare-ups, and arterial complications (eg, thrombosis, aneurysms, pseudoaneurysms).
- Treat with cyclophosphamide and chlorambucil (for life-threatening disease), azathioprine or cyclosporine (for eye disease), and colchicine, apremilast, thalidomide, or an anti-TNF drug (for mucosal disease).

CUTANEOUS VASCULITIS

(Cutaneous Leukocytoclastic Angiitis; Cutaneous Leukocytoclastic Vasculitis; Cutaneous Necrotizing Venulitis; Hypersensitivity Vasculitis; Leukoclastic Vasculitis)

Cutaneous vasculitis refers to vasculitis affecting small- or medium-sized vessels in the skin and subcutaneous tissue but not the internal organs. Purpura, petechiae, or ulcers may develop. Diagnosis requires biopsy. Treatment depends on etiology and extent of disease.

Vasculitis can affect the small- or medium-sized vessels of the skin. Vasculitis affecting the small vessels of the skin (eg, arterioles, capillaries, postcapillary venules) tends to cause lesions such as purpura, petechiae, and possibly shallow ulcers. Livedo reticularis, nodules, and deep ulcers are usually caused by vasculitis of deeper, medium or large vessels. Any primary or secondary vasculitis can affect the skin, including that due to serum sickness, infections (eg, hepatitis C), cancers, rheumatologic or other autoimmune disorders, and hypersensitivity to drugs.

Terms used to describe cutaneous vasculitis can overlap and may be used inconsistently:

- Cutaneous vasculitis: This term describes vasculitis that affects the skin but not the internal organs.
- Cutaneous small-vessel vasculitis (CSVV): This term describes vasculitis that affects the small vessels of the skin but not the internal organs. CSVV sometimes refers to small-vessel vasculitis of unknown cause (also called idiopathic CSVV).
- Leukocytoclastic vasculitis: This term describes a common type of CSVV, so-called because inflammation consists initially of neutrophils, which after degranulation result in deposition of nuclear debris (leukocytoclasis) in the vessel wall.
- Hypersensitivity vasculitis: This term previously used to mean CSVV but is now usually not used because the cause of CSVV is usually not hypersensitivity. However, hypersensitivity vasculitis is sometimes used to refer to CSVV caused by a known drug or infection.

Symptoms and Signs

Patients may present with skin symptoms such as lesions, including palpable purpura, petechiae, urticaria, ulcers, livedo reticularis, and nodules. If skin involvement is secondary to a systemic vasculitis, symptoms may also include fever, arthralgias, other organ involvement, or a combination.

Diagnosis

- Exclusion of clinically evident causes of systemic vasculitis
- Routine tests (eg, CBC, ESR, urinalysis, serum creatinine, chest x-ray)
- Biopsy
- Tests to identify the type and etiology of vasculitis (eg, cryoglobulins, antineutrophil cytoplasmic antibodies, hepatitis B and C antibodies, C3 and C4 complement levels, rheumatoid factor, blood cultures, protein electrophoresis)

A diagnosis of vasculitis limited to the skin requires a complete history and physical examination. History is focused at identifying causes, such as new drugs or infections. Evaluation is also focused on excluding manifestations of inflammation or vasculitis in other organs, such as

- Lungs: Shortness of breath, cough, hemoptysis, and signs of consolidation
- Kidneys: New-onset hypertension or edema
- Nerves: New-onset asymmetric weakness or paresthesias
- Intestine: New-onset abdominal pain, diarrhea, and bloody stools

Urinalysis should exclude blood, protein, and RBC casts. A chest x-ray is needed to check for infiltrates (suggesting alveolar hemorrhage). CBC and other blood tests are needed to check for anemia, to determine platelet count and serum creatinine level, and to check for elevated levels of acute-phase reactants (eg, ESR, C-reactive protein).

Skin biopsy should be done, optimally within 24 to 48 h after vasculitic lesions appear. Diagnostic yield depends on the depth and timing of the biopsy. Generally, deep punch biopsy or excision biopsy into the subcutis is preferred; these biopsies can sample small- and medium-sized vessels. Shave biopsy is usually inadequate.

If histologic examination detects the following, cutaneous vasculitis is confirmed:

- Infiltration of the vessel wall by inflammatory cells, resulting in disruption and destruction of the vessel wall
- Intramural and intraluminal fibrin deposition (fibrinoid necrosis)
- Extravasation of RBCs
- Nuclear debris (leukocytoclasis)

Direct immunofluorescence staining is needed to check for IgA, IgM, and IgG and complement deposition in and around the vessel wall, which suggests an immune complex–mediated process, a lymphoproliferative disorder, or other neoplastic disorder, especially in adults. IgA deposition has been associated with renal, joint, and GI manifestations, but IgG and IgM have not. Direct immunofluorescence staining may be positive for IgM or IgG in cryoglobulinemic vasculitis or RA and for IgA in immunoglobulin A–associated vasculitis.

Tests done to identify the cause of vasculitis include cryoglobulins, antineutrophil cytoplasmic antibodies (ANCA), hepatitis B and C antibodies, C3 and C4 levels, rheumatoid factor, blood cultures, and serum and urine protein electrophoresis. Other tests are done as needed to identify clinically suspected causes of vasculitis.

Treatment

- Treatment of the cause
- Drugs, beginning with antihistamines and progressing to colchicine, hydroxychloroquine or dapsone, or a short course of low-dose corticosteroids as needed

Treatment is first directed at any identified cause. If no cause is identified and vasculitis is limited to the skin, treatment is minimal and conservative. Support hose and antihistamines may be sufficient. If this treatment is ineffective, colchicine, hydroxychloroquine or dapsone, or a short course of low-dose corticosteroids can be tried.

Rarely, stronger immunosuppressants (eg, azathioprine, methotrexate) are used, particularly if lesions ulcerate or if corticosteroids must be taken indefinitely to control symptoms.

KEY POINTS

- Cutaneous vasculitis affects small- and medium-sized vessels and can be primary or secondary.
- Manifestations can include palpable purpura, petechiae, urticaria, ulcers, livedo reticularis, and nodules.
- Exclude other causes of vasculitis.
- Do routine laboratory tests and biopsy.
- Treat the cause when possible.

EOSINOPHILIC GRANULOMATOSIS WITH POLYANGIITIS

(Churg-Strauss Syndrome)

Eosinophilic granulomatosis with polyangiitis (EGPA—formerly known as Churg-Strauss syndrome) is a systemic small- and medium-vessel necrotizing vasculitis, characterized by extravascular granulomas, eosinophilia, and tissue infiltration by eosinophils. It occurs in people with adult-onset asthma, allergic rhinitis, nasal polyposis, or a combination. Diagnosis is best confirmed by biopsy. Treatment is primarily with corticosteroids and, for severe disease, addition of other immunosuppressants.

EGPA occurs in about 3 people/million. Mean age at onset is 48.

EGPA is characterized by extravascular necrotizing granulomas (usually rich in eosinophils), eosinophilia, and tissue infiltration by eosinophils. However, these abnormalities do not always coexist. The vasculitis typically affects small- and medium-sized arteries. Any organ can be affected, but the lungs, skin, sinuses, cardiovascular system, kidneys, peripheral nervous system, CNS, joints, and GI tract are most commonly affected. Occasionally, pulmonary capillaritis may cause alveolar hemorrhage.

Etiology

The cause of EGPA is unknown. However, an allergic mechanism, with tissue directly injured by eosinophils and neutrophil degranulation products, may be involved. Activation of T lymphocytes seems to help maintain eosinophilic inflammation. The syndrome occurs in patients who have adult-onset asthma, allergic rhinitis, nasal polyposis, or a combination. Antineutrophil cytoplasmic autoantibodies (ANCA) are present in about 40% of cases.

Symptoms and Signs

The syndrome has 3 phases, which may overlap:

- Prodromal: This phase may persist for years. Patients have allergic rhinitis, nasal polyposis, asthma, or a combination.
- 2nd phase: Peripheral blood and tissue eosinophilia is typical. Clinical presentation, which may resemble Löffler syndrome, includes chronic eosinophilic pneumonia and eosinophilic gastroenteritis.
- 3rd phase: Potentially life-threatening vasculitis develops. Systemic symptoms (eg, fever, malaise, weight loss, fatigue) are common in this phase.

However, the phases do not necessarily follow one another consecutively, and the time interval between them varies greatly.

Various organs and systems may be affected:

- **Respiratory:** Asthma, often with onset during adulthood, occurs in most patients and tends to be severe and corticosteroid-dependent. Sinusitis is common, but not destructive, without severe necrotizing inflammation. Patients may be short of breath. Cough and hemoptysis, due to alveolar hemorrhage, may be present. Transient patchy pulmonary infiltrates are common.
- **Neurologic:** Neurologic manifestations are very common. Multiple mononeuropathy (mononeuritis multiplex) occurs in up to three fourths of patients. CNS involvement is rare but can include hemiparesis, confusion, seizures, and coma, with or without cranial nerve palsies or evidence of cerebral infarction.
- **Cutaneous:** The skin is affected in about one half of patients. Nodules and papules appear on extensor surfaces of extremities. They are caused by extravascular palisading granulomatous lesions with central necrosis. Purpura or erythematous papules, due to leukocytoclastic vasculitis with or without prominent eosinophilic infiltration, may develop.
- **Musculoskeletal:** Occasionally, arthralgias, myalgias, or even arthritis can occur, usually during the vasculitic phase.
- **Cardiac:** Cardiac involvement, a major cause of mortality, includes heart failure due to myocarditis and endomyocardial fibrosis, coronary artery vasculitis (possibly with MI), valvular disorders, and pericarditis. The predominant histopathologic finding is eosinophilic myocarditis.
- **GI:** Up to one-third of patients present with GI symptoms (eg, abdominal pain, diarrhea, bleeding, acalculous cholecystitis) due to eosinophilic gastroenteritis or mesenteric ischemia due to vasculitis.
- **Renal:** The kidneys are affected less often than in other vasculitic disorders associated with ANCA. Typically, pauci-immune (few if any immune complexes), focal segmental necrotizing glomerulonephritis with crescent formation is present; eosinophilic or granulomatous inflammation of the kidneys is rare.

Renal, cardiac, or neurologic involvement indicates a worse prognosis.

Diagnosis

- Clinical criteria
- Routine laboratory tests
- Biopsy

The 2012 Chapel Hill Consensus Conference defined EGPA as an eosinophil-rich and necrotizing granulomatous inflammation involving the respiratory tract with necrotizing vasculitis of small- and medium-sized vessels in association with asthma and eosinophilia. Criteria for classification from the American College of Rheumatology consist of the following:

- Asthma
- Eosinophilia of > 10% in peripheral blood
- Paranasal sinusitis
- Pulmonary infiltrates, sometimes transient
- Histologic evidence of vasculitis with extravascular eosinophils
- Multiple mononeuropathy or polyneuropathy

If ≥ 4 criteria are present, sensitivity is 85%, and specificity is 99.7%.

Testing aims to establish the diagnosis and the extent of organ involvement and to distinguish EGPA from other eosinophilic disorders (eg, parasitic infections, drug reactions, acute and chronic eosinophilic pneumonia, allergic bronchopulmonary aspergillosis, hypereosinophilic syndrome). Diagnosis of EGPA is suggested by clinical findings and results of routine laboratory tests but should usually be confirmed by biopsy of lung or other affected tissue.

Blood tests and chest x-rays are done, but results are not diagnostic. CBC with differential is done to check for eosinophilia, which is also a marker of disease activity. IgE and C-reactive protein levels and ESR are determined periodically to evaluate inflammatory activity. Urinalysis and creatinine are done to screen for renal disease and monitor its severity. Electrolyte levels are measured.

Serologic testing is done and detects ANCA in up to 40% of patients; if ANCA is detected, ELISA is done to check for specific antibodies. Perinuclear ANCA (p-ANCA) with antibodies against myeloperoxidase is the most common result, but ANCA is not a specific or sensitive test for EGPA.

Although used as markers of disease activity, eosinophilia, IgE, ANCA, ESR, and C-reactive protein levels accomplish this and predict flare-ups only with significant limitations.

Chest x-ray often shows transient patchy pulmonary infiltrates.

Biopsy of the most accessible affected tissue should be done if possible.

Treatment

- Corticosteroids

Systemic corticosteroids are the mainstay of treatment. However, corticosteroids alone often do not maintain remission, even if there are no poor prognostic factors. Other immunosuppressants (eg, cyclophosphamide, methotrexate, azathioprine) may be added, depending on the severity and the type of organ involvement, using the same general criteria for treatment of granulomatosis with polyangiitis or microscopic polyangiitis. In a retrospective study of 41 patients with EGPA treated with rituximab, 49% were in remission at 12 mo and rituximab decreased the need for corticosteroids. These results compare favorably to other treatments.

KEY POINTS

- EGPA is a rare small- and medium-sized vessel vasculitis.
- Phases include upper respiratory symptoms and wheezing, eosinophilic pneumonia and gastroenteritis, and life-threatening vasculitis.
- Phases may occur in or out of order and may overlap.
- Renal, cardiac, or neurologic involvement can occur and indicate a poor prognosis.
- Diagnose by clinical criteria, routine laboratory testing, and sometimes biopsy.
- Treat with corticosteroids and sometimes other immunosuppressants, based on severity of disease, and use the same criteria for treatment of granulomatosis with polyangiitis or microscopic polyangiitis.
- Consider treatment with rituximab because possible high rates of response and reduced requirement for corticosteroids.

GIANT CELL ARTERITIS

(Temporal Arteritis; Cranial Arteritis; Horton Disease)

Giant cell arteritis involves predominantly the thoracic aorta, large arteries emerging from the aorta in the neck, and extracranial branches of the carotid arteries. Simultaneous polymyalgia rheumatica is common. Symptoms and signs may include headaches, visual disturbances, temporal artery tenderness, and pain in the jaw muscles during chewing. Fever, weight loss, malaise, and fatigue are also common. ESR and C-reactive protein are typically elevated. Diagnosis is clinical and confirmed by temporal artery biopsy. Treatment with high-dose corticosteroids and aspirin is usually effective and prevents vision loss.

Giant cell arteritis is a relatively common form of vasculitis in the US and Europe. Incidence varies depending on ethnic background. Autopsy studies suggest that the disorder may be more common than is clinically apparent. Women are affected more often. Mean age at onset is about 70, with a range of 50 to > 90. About 40 to 60% of patients with giant cell arteritis have polymyalgia rheumatica. The intracranial vessels are usually not affected.

Pathophysiology

Vasculitis may be localized, multifocal, or widespread. The disorder tends to affect arteries containing elastic tissue, most often the temporal, cranial, or other carotid system arteries. The aortic arch branches, coronary arteries, and peripheral arteries can also be affected. Mononuclear cell infiltrates in the adventitia form granulomas containing activated T cells and macrophages. Multinucleated giant cells, when present, cluster near the disrupted elastic lamina. The intimal layer is markedly thickened, with concentric narrowing and occlusion of the lumen.

Symptoms and Signs

Symptoms may begin gradually over several weeks or abruptly.

Patients may present with systemic symptoms such as fever (usually low-grade), fatigue, malaise, unexplained weight loss, and sweats. Some patients are initially diagnosed as having FUO. Eventually, most patients develop symptoms related to the affected arteries.

Severe, sometimes throbbing headache (temporal, occipital, frontal, or diffuse) is the most common symptom. It may be accompanied by scalp pain elicited by touching the scalp or combing the hair.

Visual disturbances include diplopia, scotomas, ptosis, blurred vision, and loss of vision (which is an ominous sign). Brief periods of partial or complete vision loss (amaurosis fugax) in one eye may be rapidly followed by permanent irreversible loss of vision. If untreated, the other eye may also be affected. However, complete bilateral blindness is uncommon. Vision loss is caused by arteritis of branches of the ophthalmic artery or posterior ciliary arteries, which leads to ischemia of the optic nerve. Funduscopic findings may include ischemic optic neuritis with pallor and edema of the optic disk, scattered cotton-wool patches, and small hemorrhages. Later, the optic nerve atrophies. Rarely, central blindness results from infarction in the occipital cortex caused by arterial lesions in the distal cervical region or base of the brain. The incidence of visual disturbances has declined over the past 5 decades, and rates of recovery have improved, likely because of giant cell arteritis is recognized and treated before visual disturbances develop.

Intermittent claudication (ischemic muscle pain) may occur in jaw muscles and muscles of the tongue or extremities. Jaw claudication is noted especially when firm foods are chewed. Jaw claudication is associated with a higher risk of visual symptoms.

Neurologic manifestations, such as strokes and transient ischemic attacks, can result when the carotid or vertebrobasilar arteries or branches are narrowed or occluded.

Thoracic aortic aneurysms and dissection of the aorta are serious, often late, complications and may progress in the absence of other symptoms.

Diagnosis

- ESR, C-reactive protein, and CBC
- Biopsy, usually of the temporal artery

Giant cell arteritis is suspected in patients > 55 if any of the following develops, especially if they also have symptoms of systemic inflammation:

- A new type of headache
- Any new symptom or sign compatible with ischemia of an artery above the neck
- Jaw pain during chewing
- Temporal artery tenderness
- Unexplained subacute fever or anemia

The diagnosis is more likely if patients also have symptoms of polymyalgia rheumatica.

Physical examination may detect swelling and tenderness, with or without nodularity or erythema, over the temporal arteries. Temporal arteries can become prominent. A temporal artery that rolls under the examiner's fingers, rather than collapses, is abnormal. The large arteries of the neck and limbs and the aorta should be evaluated for bruits.

If the diagnosis is suspected, ESR, C-reactive protein, and CBC are determined. In most patients, ESR and C-reactive protein are elevated; anemia of chronic disease is common. Occasionally, platelets are elevated, and serum albumin and total protein, if measured, are low. Mild leukocytosis is commonly detected but is nonspecific.

If the diagnosis of giant cell arteritis is suspected, biopsy of an artery is recommended. Because inflamed segments often alternate with normal segments, a segment that appears abnormal should be sampled if possible. Usually, the temporal artery is biopsied from the side that is symptomatic, but the occipital artery can also be biopsied if it appears abnormal. The optimal length of temporal artery to remove is unclear, but longer samples, up to 5 cm, increase the yield. The added diagnostic value of contralateral biopsy is small. Treatment should not be delayed to do the biopsy. Because inflammation resolves slowly, the temporal artery biopsy can be done up to 2 wk after treatment is started.

Imaging of the aorta and its branches should be done at the time of diagnosis and then periodically after, even in the absence of suggestive symptoms or signs (see Table 46–3 on p. 359).

Treatment

- Corticosteroids
- Low-dose aspirin

Treatment should be started as soon as giant cell arteritis is suspected, even if biopsy is going to be delayed for several days.

PEARLS & PITFALLS

- If patients > 55 have new-onset headache, jaw claudication, sudden visual disturbances, and/or temporal artery tenderness, consider immediate treatment with corticosteroids for giant cell arteritis.

Corticosteroids are the cornerstone of treatment. Corticosteroids rapidly reduce symptoms and prevent vision loss in most patients. The optimal initial dose, tapering schedule, and total length of treatment are debated. For most patients, an initial dose of prednisone 40 to 60 mg po once/day (or equivalent) for 4 wk, followed by gradual tapering, is effective.

If patients have visual disturbances, an initial dose of IV methylprednisolone 500 to 1000 mg once/day for 3 to 5 days can be tried in an attempt to help prevent further decline in vision, particularly in the contralateral eye. Saving vision probably depends more on how rapidly corticosteroids are started than their dose. Optic nerve infarction, once started, cannot be reversed regardless of corticosteroid dose.

If symptoms lessen, prednisone can be tapered gradually from doses of up to 60 mg/day based on the patient's response, usually as follows: by 5 to 10 mg/day every week to 40 mg/day, by 2 to 5 mg/day every week to 10 to 20 mg/day, then by 1 mg/day every month thereafter until the drug is stopped. ESR alone should not be used to evaluate patient response (and disease activity). For example, in elderly patients, other factors, such as monoclonal gammopathies, can elevate ESR. Clinical symptoms must also be used. C-reactive protein can sometimes be more useful than ESR.

Most patients require at least 2 yr of treatment with corticosteroids. Long-term use of corticosteroids can have significant adverse effects and thus should be limited if possible. More than one half of patients taking these drugs have drug-related complications. Consequently, alternative therapies are being studied. If patients cannot tolerate corticosteroids or if symptoms return when the dose is tapered, methotrexate 0.3 mg/kg/wk may be useful. In some patients, methotrexate can have a corticosteroid-sparing effect and reduce flare-ups. Elderly patients taking prednisone long term should be given a bisphosphonate to prevent osteoporosis.

In a systematic review, evidence for biologic agents has been shown to be weak. In a randomized controlled trial, the anti-TNF drug infliximab had no benefit and potential harms were recognized.

Low-dose aspirin (81 to 100 mg po once/day) may help prevent ischemic events and should be prescribed for all patients unless contraindicated.

KEY POINTS

- Giant cell arteritis is a common large artery vasculitis affecting the aorta and its branches in the head and neck.
- Many patients have polymyalgia rheumatica.
- Manifestations include headache, jaw claudication, temporal artery tenderness, and constitutional symptoms.
- Obtain CBC, ESR, and C-reactive protein and do temporal artery biopsy.
- Treat with corticosteroids (started immediately) and low-dose aspirin.

GRANULOMATOSIS WITH POLYANGIITIS

(Wegener Granulomatosis)

Granulomatosis with polyangiitis (GPA—formerly known as Wegener granulomatosis) is characterized by necrotizing granulomatous inflammation, small- and medium-sized vessel vasculitis, and focal necrotizing glomerulonephritis, often with crescent formation. Typically, the upper and lower respiratory tract and the kidneys are affected, but any organ may be. Symptoms vary depending on the organs and systems affected. Patients may present with upper and lower respiratory tract symptoms (eg, recurrent nasal discharge or epistaxis, cough), followed by hypertension and edema, or with symptoms reflecting multiorgan involvement. Diagnosis usually requires biopsy. Treatment is with corticosteroids plus an immunosuppressant. Remission is usually possible, although relapses are common.

GPA occurs in about 1/25,000 people; it is most common among whites but can occur in all ethnic groups and at any age. Mean age at onset is 40.

The cause is unknown, although immunologic mechanisms play a role. Most patients with active generalized disease have ANCA.

Pathophysiology

Characteristically, granulomas form with histiocytic epithelioid cells and often with giant cells. Plasma cells, lymphocytes, neutrophils, and eosinophils are present. Inflammation affects tissues as well as vessels; vasculitis may be a small or large component of the disease. Micronecrosis, usually with neutrophils (microabscesses), occurs early. Micronecrosis progresses to macronecrosis. A central area of necrosis (called geographic necrosis) is rimmed by lymphocytes, plasma cells, macrophages, and giant cells. A zone of fibroblastic proliferation with palisading histiocytes may surround the area.

Nonspecific chronic inflammation and tissue necrosis occur in the nose. The lungs are most likely to display the full spectrum of histopathologic abnormalities, but diagnostic features are not typically identified on the small tissue samples obtained by transbronchial biopsy. In the kidneys, the most common finding is a proliferative crescentic focal glomerulonephritis with necrosis and thrombosis of individual loops or larger segments of the glomerulus. Vasculitic lesions and disseminated granulomas occur only occasionally.

Symptoms and Signs

Onset may be insidious or acute; the full spectrum of the disease may take years to evolve. Some patients present initially with upper and lower respiratory tract symptoms; at some point later, the kidneys are affected. In other patients, onset of systemic manifestations is relatively acute; several organs and systems, such as the upper respiratory tract, peripheral nervous system (causing multiple mononeuropathy [mononeuritis multiplex]), kidneys (causing glomerulonephritis), and lower respiratory tract (causing hemorrhage, lung nodules, cavities, or a combination), are simultaneously affected.

- **Upper respiratory tract:** Sinus pain, serosanguineous or purulent discharge, and epistaxis may occur. The mucosa appears granular (like cobblestones) and is friable; ulcers, thick dark crusts, and septal perforation are common. Nasal chondritis can occur with swelling, pain, and collapse of the nasal bridge (saddle nose). Patients may report recurrent sinusitis that has responded inadequately to multiple antibiotic regimens and has required one or more sinus operations before diagnosis. Secondary infections (eg, due to *Staphylococcus aureus*) may develop. Subglottic stenosis may develop, causing symptoms such as pain in the larynx, hoarseness, dyspnea, wheezing, and stridor.

- **Ears:** Otitis, sensorineural hearing loss, vertigo, and chondritis may occur. The middle ear, inner ear, and mastoids are often affected.
- **Eyes:** Eyes may appear red and swollen. Nasolacrimal duct inflammation and obstruction, conjunctivitis, scleritis, uveitis, or retinal vasculitis may also occur. Inflammatory infiltrates in the retro-orbital space (orbital pseudotumor) can cause proptosis, compression of the optic nerve, and blindness. Extension into the extraocular muscles leads to diplopia. If serious eye symptoms develop, evaluation and treatment are required immediately to prevent permanent vision loss.
- **Lower respiratory tract:** Respiratory manifestations are common. Inflammation of the major bronchi and branches can cause localized wheezing, postobstructive pneumonia, and atelectasis. Single or multiple pulmonary nodules, with or without cavitation, and parenchymal infiltrates, sometimes cause symptoms, such as chest pain, shortness of breath, and productive cough. Dyspnea with bilateral infiltrates, with or without hemoptysis, may indicate alveolar hemorrhage and must be evaluated immediately.
- **Heart:** Coronary artery disease may occur, but rarely.
- **Musculoskeletal system:** Patients may present with myalgias, arthralgias, or nonerosive inflammatory arthritis.
- **Skin:** Leukocytoclastic vasculitis, tender subcutaneous nodules, papules, livedo reticularis, or pyoderma gangrenosum may develop.
- **Nervous system:** Vasculitis may cause ischemic peripheral neuropathy, brain lesions, or extension of lesions from contiguous sites. Lesions that originate in the sinuses or middle ear may extend directly to the retropharyngeal area and base of the skull, leading to cranial neuropathy, proptosis, diabetes insipidus, or meningitis.
- **Kidneys:** Symptoms and signs of glomerulonephritis develop. Urinary sediment may be abnormal, and serum creatinine may increase rapidly. Edema and hypertension may result. Rapidly progressive glomerulonephritis, which is life threatening, can develop.
- **Venous system:** Deep venous thrombosis can affect the lower extremities mostly when GPA is active.
- **Other organs:** Occasionally, an inflammatory mass occurs in the breasts, kidneys, prostate, or other organs.

Diagnosis

- Routine laboratory tests, including urinalysis
- Tests for ANCA
- Biopsy for definitive diagnosis

GPA should be suspected in patients with chronic, unexplained respiratory symptoms and signs (including otitis media in adults), particularly if manifestations in other organ systems, especially the kidneys, also suggest the disorder. Routine laboratory tests are done, but ANCA testing and biopsy yield the most specific findings.

Routine laboratory tests include ESR, C-reactive protein, CBC with differential, serum albumin and total protein, serum creatinine, urinalysis, 24-h urine protein, and chest x-ray. In most patients with active disease, ESR and C-reactive protein are elevated, and serum albumin and total protein are decreased; anemia, thrombocytosis, and mild-to-moderate eosinophilia are detected. Dysmorphic RBCs and RBC casts, detected during urinalysis, indicate glomerular involvement. Proteinuria may be detected. Serum creatinine may be increased.

Serologic testing to detect ANCA is followed by ELISA to check for specific antibodies. Most patients with active disease have cytoplasmic ANCA (c-ANCA), with antibodies against proteinase-3 (PR3); these findings plus characteristic clinical findings suggest GPA.

Some patients with other disorders (eg, bacterial endocarditis, cocaine abuse, SLE, amebiasis, TB) test positive for ANCA. Because tests for rare diseases are likely to be falsely positive when ordered for the general population and the positive predictive value of a positive ANCA test is around 50%, ANCA testing should be reserved for patients in whom the pretest probability for GPA or another ANCA-associated vasculitis is at least moderately high (eg, patients with alveolar hemorrhage, glomerulonephritis, or multiple mononeuropathy plus other features of microscopic polyangiitis or GPA).

A positive ANCA test does not rule out mycobacterial and fungal infections; thus, patients with positive ANCA results and cavitary lung lesions still require bronchoscopy and adequate cultures and other tests for TB and fungal infections. ANCA testing (titre) should not be used to guide subsequent treatment. During apparent remission, ANCA may increase or ANCA test results may change from negative to positive. In some of these patients, symptoms do not recur; in others, symptoms recur or worsen soon after the test is done or during the next few weeks, months, or sometimes years.

Biopsy should be done if possible to confirm the diagnosis. Clinically abnormal sites may be biopsied first. Biopsy of affected lung tissue is most likely to reveal characteristic findings; open thoracotomy provides the best access. Biopsies of lung or sinus tissue are cultured to exclude infection. Renal biopsy that shows pauci-immune necrotizing focal crescentic or noncrescentic glomerulonephritis strongly supports the diagnosis. Biopsy results of various tissues may also provide histologic information that can help guide treatment (eg, renal fibrosis).

Differential diagnosis includes other vasculitic disorders that affect small- and medium-sized vessels. Infections, especially those due to slow-growing fungi or acid-fast organisms, should be ruled out by staining and culture of the sampled tissues.

Prognosis

Prognosis depends on the extent of disease (how limited or diffuse) and at least as much on how rapidly treatment occurs.

Use of immunosuppressants for severe disease has dramatically improved prognosis. With treatment, complete remission is possible for about 70% of patients, but about half of them eventually relapse; relapse may occur during remission maintenance therapy or after treatment is stopped (sometimes many years later). Resuming or increasing treatment can usually control the disorder. However, 90% of patients develop significant morbidity due to the disease and/or the treatments.

Treatment

- To induce remission in life- or organ-threatening GPA, high-dose corticosteroids plus either cyclophosphamide or rituximab
- To induce remission in less severe GPA, corticosteroids and either methotrexate or rituximab

- To maintain remission, use rituximab alone, another drug (eg, methotrexate, azathioprine, mycophenolate mofetil), or rituximab plus another of these drugs, sometimes with a low dose of a corticosteroid
- Kidney transplantation if necessary

Treatment of GPA depends on the severity of disease. A multidisciplinary approach is required for multiorgan disease, often including a rheumatologist, otorhinolaryngologist, pulmonologist, and nephrologist.

Patients who have severe life-threatening or organ-threatening manifestations (eg, alveolar hemorrhage, rapidly progressive glomerulonephritis, multiple mononeuropathy with motor involvement) require immediate hospital admission for treatment to induce remission. These patients require high-dose corticosteroids and cyclophosphamide or rituximab (see Induction of remission on p. 345). Efficacies of rituximab and cyclophosphamide appear to be similar for inducing and maintaining remission. Although the evidence supporting use of plasma exchange is weaker than that for the other interventions, plasma exchange can be added to the standard treatment regimen in patients with severe acute renal insufficiency (particularly if the anti–glomerular basement membrane antibody test is not known to be negative, so that rapidly progressive glomerulonephritis has not been excluded) or alveolar hemorrhage.

Rituximab seems to be particularly helpful in patients with recurrent disease. In one study, major relapses occurred in only 5% of patients treated with rituximab but occurred in 29% of patients treated with azathioprine. Whether rituximab should be given alone or in combination with another drug and the dose and frequency of rituximab are not entirely clear. However, in one retrospective study, relapse rates were lower when rituximab was combined with methotrexate, azathioprine, or mycophenolate mofetil than when rituximab was used alone. A corticosteroid, given at a low dose, is often used to help maintain remission.

For less severe disease, corticosteroids and methotrexate are used to induce remission. Rituximab may be used instead of methotrexate. For upper respiratory tract manifestations, rituximab appears to maintain remission better than cyclophosphamide, methotrexate, or azathioprine.

Corticosteroids are tapered to as low a dose as possible or discontinued.

Irrigation of sinuses with saline, with or without mupirocin 2% nasal ointment, helps minimize crusting and secondary staphylococcal infections.

Treatment of subglottic stenosis is difficult. Systemic immunosuppressants may not be effective. Intralesional injection of long-acting corticosteroids, with gentle progressive dilation, markedly improves outcome and limits the need for tracheostomy.

Patients should be taught about the disorder so that relapses can be detected early. Patients should learn how to test their urine for blood and protein and be instructed to notify their physician of any sign of hematuria.

Kidney transplantation has been successful; the risk of relapse after transplantation is reduced compared with maintenance dialysis treatment (possibly due in part to use of immunosuppressants to prevent rejection).

KEY POINTS

- In GPA, vasculitis affects small- and medium-sized vessels in any organ, typically the kidneys (with glomerulonephritis), and upper and lower respiratory tracts.
- Manifestations can affect various organ systems and may include upper and lower respiratory tract symptoms (eg, recurrent nasal discharge or epistaxis, cough), followed by hypertension and edema.
- Confirm the diagnosis with ANCA testing and biopsy.
- Relapses are common, and treatments can contribute to morbidity.
- Induce remission with corticosteroids plus an immunosuppressant.
- Maintain remission with methotrexate, azathioprine, or rituximab and by tapering the corticosteroid dose.

IMMUNOGLOBULIN A–ASSOCIATED VASCULITIS

(Henoch-Schönlein Purpura)

Immunoglobulin A–associated vasculitis (IgAV—formerly called Henoch-Schönlein purpura) is vasculitis that affects primarily small vessels. It occurs most often in children. Common manifestations include palpable purpura, arthralgias, GI symptoms and signs, and glomerulonephritis. Diagnosis is clinical in children but usually warrants biopsy in adults. Disease is usually self-limited. Corticosteroids can relieve arthralgias and GI symptoms but do not alter the course of the disease. Progressive glomerulonephritis may require high-dose corticosteroids and cyclophosphamide.

IgA-containing immune complexes are deposited in small vessels of the skin and other sites. Possible inciting antigens include viruses that cause URIs, streptococcal infection, drugs, foods, insect bites, and immunizations. Focal, segmental proliferative glomerulonephritis is typical but mild.

Symptoms and Signs

The disease begins with a sudden palpable purpuric rash typically occurring on the feet, legs, and, occasionally, the trunk and arms. The purpura may start as small areas of urticaria that become palpable and sometimes hemorrhagic and confluent. Crops of new lesions may appear over days to several weeks. Many patients also have fever and polyarthralgia with periarticular tenderness and swelling of the ankles, knees, hips, wrists, and elbows.

GI symptoms are common and include colicky abdominal pain, abdominal tenderness, and melena. Intussusception occasionally develops in children. Stool may test positive for occult blood.

Symptoms of IgAV usually remit after about 4 wk but often recur at least once after a disease-free interval of several weeks. In most patients, the disorder subsides without serious sequelae; however, although rare, some patients develop chronic renal failure.

Diagnosis

- Biopsy of skin lesions

The 2012 Chapel Hill Consensus Conference defined IgAV as vasculitis with IgA1-dominant immune deposits, affecting small vessels in the skin and GI tract and frequently causing arthritis. IgAV is also associated with glomerulonephritis indistinguishable from IgA nephropathy.

The diagnosis of IgAV is suspected in patients, particularly children, with typical skin findings. It is confirmed by biopsy of skin lesions when leukocytoclastic vasculitis with IgA in the vessel walls is identified by immunofluorescence. Biopsy is unnecessary if clinical diagnosis is clear in children.

Urinalysis is done; hematuria, proteinuria, and RBC casts indicate renal involvement.

CBC and renal function tests are done. If renal function is deteriorating, renal biopsy may help define the prognosis. Diffuse glomerular involvement or crescent formation in most glomeruli predicts progressive renal failure.

Treatment

- Primarily corticosteroids and symptomatic measures

If the cause is a drug, it has to be stopped. Otherwise, treatment is primarily symptomatic.

Corticosteroids (eg, prednisone 2 mg/kg up to a total of 50 mg po once/day) may help control abdominal pain and are occasionally needed to treat severe joint pain or renal disease. Pulse IV methylprednisolone followed by oral prednisone and cyclophosphamide can be given to attempt to control inflammation when the kidneys are severely affected. However, the effects of corticosteroids on renal manifestations are not clear.

KEY POINTS

- IgAV is vasculitis that affects primarily small vessels and occurs in children.
- Manifestations can include purpuric rash, arthralgias, fever, abdominal pain, and melena.
- Symptoms usually remit after about 4 wk.
- When necessary to confirm the diagnosis, biopsy skin lesions, looking for IgA deposition.
- Treat symptoms and consider corticosteroids.

MICROSCOPIC POLYANGIITIS

Microscopic polyangiitis (MPA) is a systemic necrotizing vasculitis without immune globulin deposition (pauci-immune) that affects mainly small vessels. It may begin as a pulmonary-renal syndrome with rapidly progressing glomerulonephritis and alveolar hemorrhage, but the pattern of disease depends on the organs affected. Diagnosis is made by clinical findings and sometimes confirmed by biopsy. Treatment, which depends on disease severity, includes corticosteroids and immunosuppressants.

MPA is rare (about 13 to 19 cases/million). Pathogenesis is unknown. MPA affects small vessels and is pauci-immune (ie, immune globulin deposition is not seen on tissue biopsy), similar to granulomatosis with polyangiitis (GPA) and eosinophilic granulomatosis with polyangiitis (EGPA), which differentiates it from immune complex-mediated small-vessel vasculitides (eg, IgAV) and small-vessel cutaneous vasculitis. MPA affects predominantly small vessels (including capillaries and postcapillary venules), unlike polyarteritis nodosa, which affects medium-sized muscular arteries. Older literature (ie, before 1994) did not adequately distinguish between polyarteritis nodosa and MPA—alveolar hemorrhage and glomerulonephritis can occur in MPA but not in polyarteritis nodosa. Rarely, MPA can occur in association with hepatitis B.

Clinical manifestations resemble those of GPA except that granulomatous destructive lesions (eg, pulmonary cavitary lesions) are absent and the upper respiratory tract is usually affected minimally or not at all. In both disorders, ANCA may be present.

Symptoms and Signs

Usually, a prodromal illness with systemic symptoms of fever, weight loss, myalgia, and arthralgia occurs. Other symptoms depend on which organs and systems are affected:

- **Renal:** The kidneys are affected in up to 90% of patients. Hematuria, proteinuria (sometimes > 3 g/24 h), and RBC casts are present. Without prompt diagnosis and treatment, renal failure may follow rapidly.
- **Cutaneous:** About one third of patients have a purpuric rash at the time of the diagnosis. Nail bed infarcts and splinter hemorrhages may occur; digital ischemia occurs rarely.
- **Respiratory:** If the lungs are affected, alveolar hemorrhage may occur and may be followed by pulmonary fibrosis. Rapid-onset dyspnea and anemia, with or without hemoptysis and bilateral patchy infiltrates (seen on chest x-ray) may be due to alveolar hemorrhage, a medical emergency that requires immediate treatment. Mild symptoms of rhinitis, epistaxis, and sinusitis may occur; however, if the upper respiratory tract is severely affected, the cause is more likely to be GPA.
- **GI:** GI symptoms include abdominal pain, nausea, vomiting, diarrhea, and bloody stools.
- **Neurologic:** If the nervous system is affected, multiple mononeuropathy (mononeuritis multiplex) that affects peripheral or cranial nerves usually occurs. Rarely, cerebral hemorrhage, infarction, seizures, or headache results from cerebral vasculitis.
- **Cardiac:** Rarely, the heart is affected.
- **Ocular:** If the eyes are affected, episcleritis usually results.

Diagnosis

- Clinical findings
- Tests for ANCA and C-reactive protein and routine laboratory tests
- Biopsy

MPA should be suspected in patients who have unexplained combinations of fever, weight loss, arthralgias, abdominal pain, alveolar hemorrhage, new-onset nephritic syndrome, new-onset multiple mononeuropathy, or polyneuropathy. Laboratory tests and sometimes x-rays are done, but the diagnosis is usually confirmed by biopsy.

Tests include CBC, ESR, C-reactive protein, urinalysis, serum creatinine, and tests for ANCA. ESR, C-reactive protein levels, and WBC and platelet counts are elevated, reflecting systemic inflammation. Anemia of chronic disease is common. An acute drop in Hct suggests alveolar hemorrhage or hemorrhage in the GI tract. Urinalysis (to check for hematuria, proteinuria, and cellular casts) should be done, and serum creatinine should be measured periodically to check for renal involvement.

Immunofluorescence staining can detect ANCA; this test is followed by an enzyme-linked immunosorbent assay (ELISA) to check for specific antibodies. At least 60% of patients are ANCA-positive, usually perinuclear ANCA (p-ANCA) with antibodies against myeloperoxidase.

Biopsy of the most accessible involved tissue should be done to confirm vasculitis. Renal biopsy may detect focal segmental pauci-immune necrotizing glomerulonephritis with fibrinoid necrosis of the glomerular capillary wall, leading to formation of cellular crescents.

In patients with respiratory symptoms, chest imaging is done to check for infiltrates. Bilateral patchy infiltrates suggest alveolar hemorrhage even in patients without hemoptysis. CT is much more sensitive than x-ray.

If patients have dyspnea and bilateral infiltrates, bronchoscopy should be done immediately to check for alveolar hemorrhages and to exclude infection. Blood coming from both lungs and all bronchi, with more blood coming as the bronchoscope goes deeper in the airways, indicates active alveolar hemorrhage. Hemosiderin-laden macrophages appear within 24 to 72 h after onset of hemorrhage and may persist for up to 2 mo.

Treatment

- When vital organs are affected, high-dose corticosteroids plus cyclophosphamide or rituximab
- For less severe cases, corticosteroids plus azathioprine or methotrexate

Treatment is similar to that of GPA. Cyclophosphamide given daily plus corticosteroids improves survival when vital organs are affected. Rituximab has been shown to be noninferior to cyclophosphamide for inducing remission of severe disease. However, data are limited for patients with very high levels of creatinine. Induction and maintenance regimens vary, and adjunctive therapies such as plasma exchange and pulse IV methylprednisolone may or may not need to be used.

The role of plasma exchange in patients who have impaired renal function due to severe renal involvement or severe alveolar hemorrhage is under investigation.

Less severe cases may be managed with corticosteroids plus azathioprine or methotrexate.

KEY POINTS

- MPA is a rare small-vessel vasculitis.
- Manifestations are variable and may include alveolar hemorrhage, multiple mononeuropathy, and glomerulonephritis.
- Confirm the diagnosis by testing for ANCA and by biopsy.
- Treat with corticosteroids plus an immunosuppressant (eg, cyclophosphamide or rituximab for severe disease).

POLYARTERITIS NODOSA

(Polyarteritis; Periarteritis Nodosa)

Polyarteritis nodosa (PAN) is a systemic necrotizing vasculitis that typically affects medium-sized muscular arteries and occasionally affects small muscular arteries, resulting in secondary tissue ischemia. The kidneys, skin, joints, muscles, peripheral nerves, and GI tract are most commonly affected, but any organ can be. However, the lungs are usually spared. Patients typically present with systemic symptoms (eg, fever, fatigue). Diagnosis requires a biopsy or arteriography. Treatment with corticosteroids and immunosuppressants is often effective.

PAN is rare (about 2 to 33 cases/million). It affects mainly middle-aged adults, and incidence increases with age, peaking in people in their 50s.

Etiology

Most cases are idiopathic. About 20% of patients have hepatitis B or C.

The cause is unknown, but immune mechanisms appear to be involved. The variety of clinical and pathologic features suggests multiple pathogenic mechanisms. Drugs may be a cause. Usually, no predisposing antigen is identified. Patients with certain lymphomas and leukemias, RA, or Sjögren syndrome may develop a systemic vasculitis similar to PAN (sometimes called secondary PAN).

Pathophysiology

PAN is characterized by segmental, transmural necrotizing inflammation of muscular arteries, most commonly at points of bifurcation. Unlike other vasculitic disorders, PAN does not involve postcapillary venules or veins. Lesions in all stages of development and healing are usually present. Early lesions contain polymorphonuclear leukocytes and occasionally eosinophils; later lesions contain lymphocytes and plasma cells.

Granulomatous inflammation does not occur. Intimal proliferation with secondary thrombosis and occlusion leads to organ and tissue infarction. Weakening of the muscular arterial wall may cause small aneurysms and arterial dissection. Healing can result in nodular fibrosis of the adventitia.

Most commonly affected are the kidneys, skin, peripheral nerves, joints, muscles, and GI tract. Often affected are the liver and heart. Renal ischemia and infarction occur, but glomerulonephritis is not a feature of PAN. Purpura (usually resulting from small-vessel inflammation) is not a characteristic of PAN.

Symptoms and Signs

PAN mimics many disorders. The course may be acute and prolonged, subacute and fatal after several months, or insidious, chronic, and debilitating. Symptoms of PAN depend mainly on location and severity of the arteritis and extent of secondary ischemia. Only one organ or organ system may be affected.

Patients typically present with fever, fatigue, night sweats, loss of appetite, weight loss, and generalized weakness. Myalgias with areas of focal ischemic myositis and arthralgias are common. Affected muscles are tender and may be weak. Arthritis may occur.

Symptoms and signs vary, depending on organ or organ system predominantly affected:

- **Peripheral nervous system:** Patients usually present with asymmetric peripheral neuropathy, such as multiple mononeuropathy (mononeuritis multiplex) with signs of motor and sensory involvement of the peroneal, median, or ulnar nerves. As additional nerve branches are affected, patients may appear to have a distal symmetric polyneuropathy.
- **CNS:** Headache and seizures can result. In a few patients, ischemic stroke and cerebral hemorrhage occur, sometimes resulting from hypertension.
- **Renal:** If small- and medium-sized arteries in the kidneys are affected, patients may have hypertension, oliguria, uremia, and a nonspecific urinary sediment with hematuria, proteinuria, and no cellular casts. Hypertension may worsen rapidly. Rupture of renal arterial aneurysms can cause perirenal hematomas. In severe cases, multiple renal infarcts with lumbar pain and gross hematuria may occur. Renal ischemia and infarction can lead to renal failure.
- **GI:** Vasculitis of the liver or gallbladder causes right upper quadrant pain. Perforation of the gallbladder with acute abdomen may occur. Vasculitis of medium-sized mesenteric arteries causes abdominal pain, nausea, vomiting (with or without bloody diarrhea), malabsorption, intestinal perforation, and acute abdomen. Aneurysms may develop in hepatic or celiac arteries.

- **Cardiac:** Some patients have coronary artery disease, which is usually asymptomatic, but may cause angina. Heart failure may result from ischemic or hypertensive cardiomyopathy.
- **Cutaneous:** Livedo reticularis, skin ulcers, tender erythematous nodules, bullous or vesicular eruptions, infarction and gangrene of fingers or toes, or a combination may occur. The nodules in PAN resemble erythema nodosum, but, unlike nodules in erythema nodosum, the nodules in PAN can ulcerate, and have necrotizing vasculitis that is visible on biopsy within the walls of medium-sized arteries, usually located in the deep dermis and subcutaneous fat.
- **Genital:** Orchitis with testicular pain and tenderness can occur.

Diagnosis

- Clinical findings
- Biopsy
- Arteriography if no clinically involved tissue is available for biopsy

PAN can be difficult to diagnose because findings can be nonspecific. The diagnosis should be considered in patients with various combinations of symptoms, such as unexplained fever, arthralgia, subcutaneous nodules, skin ulcers, pain in the abdomen or extremities, new footdrop or wristdrop, or rapidly developing hypertension. The diagnosis is further clarified when clinical findings are combined with certain laboratory results and other causes are excluded.

Diagnosis of PAN is confirmed by biopsy showing necrotizing arteritis or by arteriography showing the typical aneurysms in medium-sized arteries. Magnetic resonance angiography may show microaneurysms, but some abnormalities may be too small for it to detect. Thus, magnetic resonance angiography is not the test used primarily for diagnosis.

Biopsy of clinically uninvolved tissue is often useless because the disease is focal; biopsy should target sites suggested by clinical evaluation. Samples of subcutaneous tissue, sural nerve, and muscle, if thought to be involved, are preferred to samples from the kidneys or liver; kidney and liver biopsies may be falsely negative because of sampling error and may cause bleeding from unsuspected microaneurysms.

If clinical findings are absent or minimal, electromyography and nerve conduction studies may help select the site of muscle or nerve biopsy. If skin lesions are present, surgical skin biopsies that include deeper dermis and subcutaneous fat should be done. (Punch biopsies of the skin that sample the epidermis and superficial dermis miss the lesions of PAN.) Even though microscopic lesions in the testes are common, testicular biopsy should not be done if testicular symptoms are absent and if other possible sites are accessible because the yield is low. Also, men may be reluctant to have testicular biopsy.

Laboratory tests are nonspecific. Leukocytosis up to 20,000 to 40,000/μL, proteinuria, and microscopic hematuria are the most common abnormalities. Patients may have thrombocytosis, markedly elevated ESR, anemia caused by blood loss or renal failure, hypoalbuminemia, and elevated serum immunoglobulins. AST and ALT are often mildly elevated. Testing for hepatitis B and C should be done.

Other testing (eg, ANCA, rheumatoid factor, anticyclic citrullinated peptide antibody [anti-CCP], antinuclear antibodies [ANA], C3 and C4 complement levels, cryoglobulin levels, nuclear antigens and antibodies to extractable nuclear antigens such as anti-Smith, anti-Ro/SSA, anti-La/SSB, and anti-RNP) may suggest other diagnoses, such as RA, SLE, or Sjögren syndrome.

Prognosis

Without treatment, 5-yr survival is < 15%. With treatment, 5-yr survival is > 80% but may be lower for patients with hepatitis B. Prognosis is better if disease remission is achieved within 18 mo after diagnosis. Relapses are less common than in other vasculitic disorders.

The following findings are associated with a poor prognosis:

- Renal insufficiency
- GI involvement
- Neurologic involvement

Treatment

- Corticosteroids alone or with cyclophosphamide, methotrexate, or azathioprine, depending on disease severity
- Addition of lamivudine and plasma exchange for patients with hepatitis B

Treatment of PAN depends on the severity of the disease. For systemic symptoms but no serious neurologic, renal, GI, or cardiac manifestations, corticosteroids may be sufficient, at least initially. For severe disease with neurologic, renal, GI, or cardiac manifestations, cyclophosphamide plus corticosteroids may improve outcome. For moderate disease, corticosteroids plus methotrexate or azathioprine can be used. Hypertension should be treated aggressively.

Hepatitis B–related PAN: Treatment aims at rapidly suppressing inflammation, then eliminating the virus and inducing seroconversion via plasma exchange. A short course of corticosteroids is used for a few weeks. Lamivudine 100 mg po once/day is given for a maximum of 6 mo. A lower dose is used in patients with renal insufficiency.

Plasma exchanges are scheduled as follows: 3 times/wk for 3 wk, 2 times/wk for 2 wk, and once/wk until hepatitis B e antigen (HBeAg) converts to hepatitis B e antibody (anti-HBe) or until clinical recovery is sustained for 2 to 3 mo. Although this approach has not been proved to improve survival when compared with immunosuppressive therapy only, it may reduce the risk of long-term complications of hepatitis B and suppress the side effects of long-term treatment with corticosteroids and immunosuppressants.

Traditional treatment with corticosteroids, sometimes with cytotoxic immunosuppressants (mainly cyclophosphamide), was often effective in the short term but did not prevent relapses and complications (eg, chronic hepatitis, cirrhosis) due to persistence of the hepatitis B virus; immunosuppressive therapy in patients with hepatitis B facilitates viral replication, which can lead to active viral hepatitis and liver failure.

Patients with hepatitis C who develop PAN are treated for hepatitis C.

KEY POINTS

- PAN is a rare systemic vasculitis affecting medium-sized arteries.
- The kidneys, skin, joints, muscles, peripheral nerves, and GI tract are most often affected.
- Suspect PAN if patients have combinations of unexplained fever, arthralgia, subcutaneous nodules, skin ulcers, pain in the abdomen or extremities, new footdrop or wristdrop, or rapidly developing hypertension.
- Confirm the diagnosis by biopsy or arteriography.
- Renal insufficiency, GI involvement, or neurologic involvement portends a less favorable prognosis.
- Treat with corticosteroids alone or with cyclophosphamide, methotrexate, or azathioprine, depending on disease severity.

POLYMYALGIA RHEUMATICA

Polymyalgia rheumatica is a syndrome closely associated with giant cell arteritis (temporal arteritis). It affects adults > 55. It typically causes severe pain and stiffness in proximal muscles, without weakness or atrophy, and nonspecific systemic symptoms. ESR and C-reactive protein are usually elevated. Diagnosis is clinical. Treatment with low-dose corticosteroids is effective. A dramatic and rapid response to low to moderate doses of prednisone or methylprednisolone supports the diagnosis.

Polymyalgia rheumatica affects adults > 55; the female:male ratio is 2:1.

Because polymyalgia rheumatica is closely associated with giant cell arteritis, some authorities consider the two disorders to be different aspects of the same process. Polymyalgia rheumatica appears to be more common. A few patients with polymyalgia rheumatica develop giant cell arteritis, but 40 to 60% of patients with giant cell arteritis have polymyalgia rheumatica. Polymyalgia rheumatica may precede, follow, or occur simultaneously with giant cell arteritis.

Etiology and pathogenesis are unknown. Ultrasound and MRI findings suggest that they probably result from low-grade axial synovitis and bursitis.

Symptoms and Signs

Polymyalgia rheumatica is characterized by bilateral proximal aching of the shoulder and hip girdle muscles and the back (upper and lower) and neck muscles. Stiffness in the morning is typical and lasts > 60 min. Shoulder symptoms reflect proximal bursitis (eg, subdeltoid, subacromial) and less often bicipital tenosynovitis or joint synovitis. Discomfort is worse in the morning and is occasionally severe enough to prevent patients from getting out of bed and from doing simple activities. The pain may make patients feel weak, but objective muscle weakness is not a feature of the disorder.

Diagnosis

- Clinical findings
- Exclusion of other causes

Polymyalgia rheumatica is suspected in elderly patients with typical symptoms, but other possible causes must be excluded.

Tests include ESR, C-reactive protein, CBC, thyroid-stimulating hormone levels, and CK. In > 80% of patients, ESR is markedly elevated, often > 100 mm/h, usually > 50 mm/h (Westergren method). C-reactive protein is also elevated. Electromyography, biopsy, and other tests (eg, rheumatoid factor), which are normal in polymyalgia rheumatica, are sometimes done to rule out other clinically suspected diagnoses.

The following findings in polymyalgia rheumatica distinguish it from

- RA: In polymyalgia rheumatica, chronic small-joint synovitis, erosive or destructive lesions, rheumatoid nodules, and rheumatoid factor are absent in about 80% (although some joint swelling may be present) of patients. Differentiation from RA may be difficult in the remaining 20%.
- Polymyositis: In polymyalgia rheumatica, pain rather than weakness predominates; muscle enzyme levels and electromyography and muscle biopsy results are normal.
- Hypothyroidism: In polymyalgia rheumatica, thyroid function test results and muscle enzyme levels are normal.
- Multiple myeloma: In polymyalgia rheumatica, monoclonal gammopathy is absent.
- Fibromyalgia: In polymyalgia rheumatica, symptoms are more localized, ESR is typically elevated, and pain is present with palpation and range of motion (active and passive) of the shoulders, even when the patient is distracted.

Treatment

- Prednisone

Prednisone started at 15 to 20 mg po once/day results in dramatic improvement, often very rapid (in hours or days), and this response can help support the diagnosis. If giant cell arteritis is thought to be present, the dose of corticosteroids should be higher, and temporal artery biopsy should be done.

Treatment effectiveness is monitored by symptoms, ESR, and C-reactive protein. As symptoms subside, corticosteroids are tapered to the lowest clinically effective dose, regardless of ESR. C-reactive protein is more helpful than ESR in guiding response to treatment because ESR can be persistently elevated in the elderly because of other reasons. Some patients are able to stop corticosteroids in about 2 yr, even sooner without relapse, whereas others require small doses for years. NSAIDs are rarely sufficient.

Some patients who are unable to have their prednisone dose tapered and who have frequent recurrences may benefit from the addition of methotrexate (10 to 15 mg po once/wk, if renal function is normal) or another immunosuppressant such as azathioprine. Adding a second drug in polymyalgia rheumatica or giant cell arteritis is controversial because controlled randomized trials have shown minimal benefit. Trials using anti-TNF drugs (infliximab and adalimumab) and rituximab have not shown benefit.

In elderly patients, physicians should watch for and treat complications of corticosteroid use (eg, diabetes, hypertension). Patients taking prednisone long term should be given a bisphosphonate to prevent osteoporosis.

Giant cell arteritis may develop at the onset of polymyalgia rheumatica or much later, sometimes even after patients appear cured of the disorder. Therefore, all patients should be instructed to immediately report headache, muscle pain during chewing, and, particularly, visual disturbances to their physician.

KEY POINTS

- Polymyalgia rheumatica affects adults > 55, causing proximal myalgias and stiffness.
- It is present in 40 to 60% of patients with giant cell arteritis.
- Diagnose clinically, sometimes with supportive evidence of an elevated ESR and dramatic response to low to moderate doses of corticosteroids.
- Treat with corticosteroids, eventually tapering if possible using methotrexate or azathioprine if necessary.
- Warn patients about symptoms of giant cell arteritis.

TAKAYASU ARTERITIS

(Aortic Arch Syndrome; Occlusive Thromboaortopathy; Pulseless Disease)

Takayasu arteritis is an inflammatory disease affecting the aorta, its branches, and pulmonary arteries. It occurs predominantly in young women. Etiology is unknown. Vascular inflammation may cause arterial stenosis, occlusion, dilation, or aneurysms. Patients may present with

asymmetric pulses or unequal BP measurements between limbs (eg, between limbs on opposite sides or between the arm and leg on the same side), limb claudication, symptoms of decreased cerebral perfusion (eg, transient visual disturbances, transient ischemic attacks, strokes), and hypertension or its complications. Diagnosis is by aortic arteriography or magnetic resonance angiography. Treatment is with corticosteroids and other immunosuppressants and, for organ-threatening ischemia, vascular interventions such as bypass surgery.

Takayasu arteritis is rare. It is more common among Asians but occurs worldwide. Female:male ratio is 8:1, and age at onset is typically 15 to 30. In North America, annual incidence is estimated to be 2.6 cases/million.

Etiology

The cause is unknown. Cell-mediated immune mechanisms may be involved.

Pathophysiology

Takayasu arteritis affects primarily large elastic arteries. The most commonly affected are

- Innominate and subclavian arteries
- Aorta (mainly the ascending aorta and the arch)
- Common carotid arteries
- Renal arteries

Most patients have stenoses or occlusions. Aneurysms occur in about one third of patients. Usually, the wall of the aorta or its branches thickens irregularly, with intimal wrinkling. When the aortic arch is affected, orifices of the major arteries emerging from the aorta may be markedly narrowed or even obliterated by intimal thickening. In one-half of patients, pulmonary arteries are also affected. Sometimes the medium-sized branches of the pulmonary arteries are involved.

Histologically, early changes consist of adventitial mononuclear infiltrate with perivascular cuffing of the vasa vasorum. Later, intense mononuclear inflammation of the media may occur, sometimes accompanied by granulomatous changes, giant cells, and patchy necrosis of the media. Morphologic changes may be indistinguishable from those of giant cell arteritis. Panarteritic inflammatory infiltrates cause marked thickening of the affected artery and subsequent luminal narrowing and occlusion.

Symptoms and Signs

Most patients present with only focal symptoms that reflect hypoperfusion of the affected organ or limb.

About one third of patients report constitutional symptoms such as fever, malaise, night sweats, weight loss, fatigue, and/or arthralgias.

Repetitive arm movements and sustained arm elevation may cause pain and fatigue. Arterial pulses in arms and legs may be diminished and asymmetric. Extremities may have findings of ischemia (eg, coolness, leg claudication). Bruits are often audible over the subclavian arteries, brachial arteries, carotid arteries, abdominal aorta, or femoral arteries. Reduced BP in one or both arms is common.

Involvement of the carotid and vertebral arteries results in reduced cerebral blood flow manifested by dizziness, syncope, orthostatic hypotension, headaches, transient visual disturbances, transient ischemic attacks, or strokes.

Stenotic lesions in a subclavian artery near the origin of a patent vertebral artery can cause posterior circulation ischemic neurologic symptoms or syncope when the arm is used (called subclavian steal syndrome). The mechanisms are retrograde flow through the vertebral artery to supply the subclavian artery distal to the stenosis and vasodilation of the arterial bed in the upper limb during exercise.

Angina pectoris or MI may result from narrowing of the coronary artery orifice due to aortitis or coronary arteritis. Aortic regurgitation may occur if the ascending aorta is markedly dilated. Heart failure can develop.

Obstruction of the descending thoracic aorta sometimes causes signs of aortic coarctation (eg, hypertension, headache, leg claudication). Renovascular hypertension may develop if the abdominal aorta or renal arteries are narrowed. Intermittent arm or leg claudication can develop.

Pulmonary arteries are affected, sometimes causing pulmonary hypertension. Involvement of the medium-sized branches of the pulmonary arteries can cause pulmonary infarcts. Because Takayasu arteritis is chronic, collateral circulation can develop. Thus, ischemic ulcerations or gangrene due to obstruction of the arteries to the extremities is rare.

Diagnosis

- Aortic arteriography, magnetic resonance angiography, or CT angiography
- Monitoring of disease activity

The diagnosis of Takayasu arteritis is suspected when symptoms suggest ischemia of organs supplied by the aorta or its branches or when peripheral pulses are decreased or absent in patients at low risk of atherosclerosis and other aortic disorders, especially in young women. In these patients, arterial bruits and right/left or upper extremity/lower extremity discrepancies in pulses or in BP also suggest the diagnosis.

Confirmation of the diagnosis used to require aortic arteriography; however, now magnetic resonance angiography or CT angiography can be used instead to evaluate all branches of the aorta. Characteristic findings include stenosis, occlusion, irregularities in arterial lumens, poststenotic dilation, collateral arteries around obstructed vessels, and aneurysms (see Table 46-3).

BP is measured in all extremities. However, accurate measurement of BP can be difficult. If both subclavian arteries are severely affected, systemic BP can be accurately measured only in the legs. If the disorder affects both subclavian arteries and patients have coarctation of the descending aorta and/or involvement of both iliac or femoral arteries, BP cannot be accurately measured in any limb. Then, central arterial pressure must be measured via angiography to detect occult hypertension, which can cause complications.

Other clues to occult hypertension can be funduscopic signs of hypertensive retinopathy and/or echocardiographic signs of concentric left ventricular hypertrophy. When severe hypertension is not recognized, complications can be confused with signs of vasculitis causing organ ischemia.

Laboratory tests are nonspecific and not helpful in diagnosis. Common findings include anemia of chronic disease, elevated platelet levels, occasionally elevated WBC counts, and elevated ESR and C-reactive protein.

Table 46–3. IMAGING TESTS USED IN TAKAYASU ARTERITIS

TEST	USES	COMMENTS
Conventional angiography (aortic arteriography)	Preferred when a surgical intervention is being considered and when proximal aortic BP cannot be measured any other way	Provides descriptive anatomic information about the vascular lumen
Magnetic resonance angiography of the aorta and large arteries	Avoids the risk of arterial puncture and of exposure to iodinated contrast or radiation Usually the test of choice in young women, who are less likely to have extensive atherosclerosis and are more susceptible to radiation-induced cancer	Provides some information about arterial wall anatomy Does not provide sufficient information about distal aortic branches because the resolution is too low Provides no information about the content of arterial plaque, making discrimination between vasculitic and atherosclerotic disease difficult
CT angiography	Used to generally survey the aorta and its proximal branches when magnetic resonance angiography is contraindicated or is not available	Can characterize aortic calcification May provide information about arterial wall thickness Unclear whether it is useful in monitoring disease activity
Positron emission tomography with fluorine-18 (^{18}F) deoxyglucose	Used to assess regional differences in glucose metabolism and may help locate regions of inflammation (because inflammatory cells take up more glucose)	Does not provide information about changes in lumen size

The following are indicators of disease activity in Takayasu arteritis:

- Symptoms and signs: New systemic symptoms (eg, fever, fatigue, weight loss, anorexia, night sweats), symptoms suggesting vasculitis involving new arterial territories (eg, claudication), new bruits, and/or new changes in BP measurements
- Laboratory tests: Evidence of inflammation detected by blood tests (although markers of inflammation may miss active arteritis)
- Imaging studies: Development of stenosis or aneurysms in previously unaffected arteries (assessed with periodic imaging [usually magnetic resonance angiography])

However, Takayasu arteritis can progress silently even when clinical and laboratory studies suggest complete remission. Therefore, periodic imaging of the aorta and large arteries is mandatory. BP should be measured regularly in an unaffected limb.

Disorders that mimic Takayasu arteritis must be excluded. They include

- Inherited noninflammatory connective tissue disorders (eg, Ehlers-Danlos syndrome or Marfan syndrome)
- Vascular infections (tuberculous, fungal, or syphilitic)
- Fibromuscular dysplasias
- Disorders causing arterial thrombosis (eg, hypercoagulable states)
- Idiopathic inflammatory conditions (eg, ankylosing spondylitis with aortitis, RA, Cogan syndrome or Behçet syndrome, Kawasaki disease, sarcoidosis)

All of these disorders can affect large vessels.

Prognosis

For 20% of patients, the course is monophasic. For the rest, the course is relapsing and remitting or chronic and progressive. Even when symptoms and laboratory abnormalities suggest quiescence, new vascular lesions occur and are evident on imaging studies. A progressive course and the presence of complications (eg, hypertension, aortic regurgitation, heart failure, aneurysms) predict a less favorable prognosis.

Treatment

- Corticosteroids
- Sometimes other immunosuppressants
- Antihypertensives and/or vascular interventions as needed

Drugs: Corticosteroids are the cornerstone of Takayasu arteritis treatment. The optimal dose, tapering schedule, and length of treatment have not been determined. Treatment with corticosteroids alone induces remission in most patients. Prednisone is usually used. The starting dose is 1 mg/kg po once/day for 1 to 3 mo; the dose is then tapered slowly over several months. Lower starting doses may also induce remission. About half of patients relapse when the drug is tapered or stopped, despite initial response.

Methotrexate, cyclophosphamide, azathioprine, mycophenolate mofetil, and TNF inhibitors (eg, etanercept, infliximab) have been used successfully in some patients. They can be tried if corticosteroids are insufficiently effective or cannot be tapered. Methotrexate is started at a dose of 0.3 mg/kg once/wk, which is increased up to 25 mg/wk. Mycophenolate mofetil can also be tried. Cyclophosphamide should be considered in patients with coronary vasculitis or other serious complications thought to be due to active arteritis.

An antiplatelet drug (eg, aspirin 325 mg po once/day) is frequently used because platelet-mediated occlusion cannot be excluded. Hypertension should be treated aggressively; ACE inhibitors may be effective.

Procedures: Vascular intervention, usually a bypass procedure, may be needed to reestablish blood flow to ischemic tissues if drug therapy is ineffective. Indications include the following:

- Aortic insufficiency
- Coronary artery stenosis causing symptomatic coronary artery disease or ischemic cardiomyopathy
- Dissection of enlarged aortic aneurysm

- Severe hypertension secondary to renal artery stenosis that is refractory to medical management
- Limb ischemia that interferes with daily activities
- Brain ischemia
- Coarctation of the aorta
- Inability to measure blood pressure accurately (in any limb)

Bypass grafting preferably with an autologous graft has the best patency rates. The anastomosis should be made at disease-free sites of the affected arteries to help prevent aneurysm formation and occlusion.

Percutaneous transluminal coronary angioplasty (PTCA) has few risks and may be effective for short lesions. But long-term restenosis rates seem much higher than those with bypass grafting. Vascular stenting is usually not recommended because the restenosis rate is high.

For aortic regurgitation, valvular surgery with aortic root replacement may be necessary.

KEY POINTS

- Takayasu arteritis is a rare arteritis affecting mostly women aged 15 to 30.
- Involvement of the aorta, pulmonary artery, and their branches can cause manifestations such as asymmetric pulses or BP measurements, limb claudication, symptoms of decreased cerebral perfusion (eg, transient visual disturbances, transient ischemic attacks, strokes), and hypertension (systemic and pulmonary) or its complications.
- Diagnose by magnetic resonance angiography or sometimes CT or conventional angiography.
- Treat with corticosteroids, other immunosuppressants, aspirin, and, when indicated, antihypertensive drugs.
- Refer patients for vascular intervention if, despite drug therapy, they have severe vascular complications (eg, end-organ ischemia; aortic dissection coarctation, or insufficiency).

Pulmonary Disorders

47 Approach to the Pulmonary Patient

Key components in the evaluation of patients with pulmonary symptoms are the history, physical examination, and, in most cases, a chest x-ray. These components establish the need for subsequent testing, which may include pulmonary function testing and ABG analysis, CT or other chest imaging tests, and bronchoscopy.

History

The history can often establish whether symptoms of dyspnea, chest pain, wheezing, stridor, hemoptysis, and cough are likely to be pulmonary in origin. When more than one symptom occurs concurrently, the history should focus on which symptom is primary and whether constitutional symptoms, such as fever, weight loss, and night sweats, are also present. Other important information includes

- Occupational and environmental exposures
- Family history, travel history, and contact history
- Previous illnesses
- Use of prescription, OTC, or illicit drugs
- Previous test results (eg, tuberculin skin test, chest x-rays)

Physical Examination

Physical examination starts with assessment of general appearance. Discomfort and anxiety, body habitus, and the effect of talking or movement on symptoms (eg, inability to speak full sentences without pausing to breathe) all can be assessed while greeting the patient and taking a history and may provide useful information relevant to pulmonary status. Next, inspection, auscultation, and chest percussion and palpation are done.

Inspection: Inspection should focus on

- Signs of respiratory difficulty and hypoxemia (eg, restlessness, tachypnea, cyanosis, accessory muscle use)
- Signs of possible chronic pulmonary disease (eg, clubbing, pedal edema)
- Chest wall deformities
- Abnormal breathing patterns (eg, Cheyne-Stokes respiration, Kussmaul respirations)
- Jugular venous distention

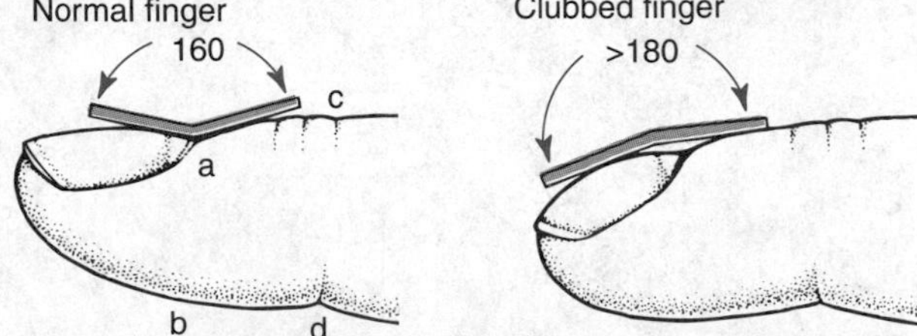

Fig. 47–1. Measuring finger clubbing. The ratio of the anteroposterior diameter of the finger at the nail bed (a–b) to that at the distal interphalangeal joint (c–d) is a simple measurement of finger clubbing. It can be obtained readily and reproducibly with calipers. If the ratio is > 1, clubbing is present. Finger clubbing is also characterized by loss of the normal angle at the nail bed.

Signs of hypoxemia include cyanosis (bluish discoloration of the lips, face, or nail beds), which signifies low arterial oxygen saturation (< 85%); the absence of cyanosis does not exclude the presence of hypoxemia.

Signs of respiratory difficulty include tachypnea, use of accessory respiratory muscles (sternocleidomastoids, intercostals, scalene) to breathe, intercostal retractions, and paradoxical breathing. Patients with COPD sometimes brace their arms against their legs or the examination table while seated (ie, tripod position) in a subconscious effort to provide more leverage to accessory muscles and thereby enhance respiration. Intercostal retractions (inward movement of the rib interspaces) are common among infants and older patients with severe airflow limitation. Paradoxical breathing (inward motion of the abdomen during inspiration) signifies respiratory muscle fatigue or weakness.

Signs of possible chronic pulmonary disease include clubbing, barrel chest (the increased anterior-posterior diameter of the chest present in some patients with emphysema), and pursed lip breathing. Clubbing is enlargement of the fingertips (or toes) due to proliferation of connective tissue between the fingernail and the bone. Diagnosis is based on an increase in the profile angle of the nail as it exits the finger (to > 176°) or on an increase in the phalangeal depth ratio (to > 1—see Fig. 47–1). "Sponginess" of the nail bed beneath the cuticle also suggests clubbing. Clubbing is most commonly observed in patients with lung cancer but is an important sign of chronic pulmonary disease, such as cystic fibrosis and idiopathic pulmonary fibrosis; it also occurs (but less commonly) in cyanotic heart disease, chronic infection (eg, infective endocarditis), stroke, inflammatory bowel disease, and cirrhosis. Clubbing occasionally occurs with osteoarthropathy and periostitis (primary or hereditary hypertrophic osteoarthropathy); in this instance, clubbing may be accompanied by skin changes, such as hypertrophied skin on the dorsa of the hands (pachydermoperiostosis), seborrhea, and coarse facial features. Digital clubbing can also occur as a benign hereditary abnormality that can be distinguished from pathologic clubbing by the absence of pulmonary symptoms or disease and by the presence of clubbing from an early age (by patient report).

Chest wall deformities, such as pectus excavatum (a sternal depression usually beginning over the midportion of the manubrium and progressing inward through the xiphoid process) and kyphoscoliosis, may restrict respirations and exacerbate symptoms of preexisting pulmonary disease. These abnormalities can usually be observed during careful examination after the patient's shirt is removed. Inspection should also include an assessment of the abdomen and the extent of obesity, ascites, or other conditions that could affect abdominal compliance.

Abnormal breathing patterns cause fluctuations in respiratory rate so respiratory rate should be assessed and counted for 1 min.

- **Cheyne-Stokes respiration** (periodic breathing) is a cyclic fluctuation of respiratory rate and depth. From periods of brief apnea, patients breathe progressively faster and deeper (hyperpnea), then slower and shallower until they become apneic and repeat the cycle. Cheyne-Stokes respiration is most often caused by heart failure, a neurologic disorder (eg, stroke, advanced dementia), or drugs. The pattern in heart failure has been attributed to delays in cerebral circulation; respiratory centers lag in recognition of systemic acidosis/

hypoxia (causing hyperpnea) or alkalosis/hypocapnia (causing apnea).

- **Biot respiration** is an uncommon variant of Cheyne-Stokes respiration in which irregular periods of apnea alternate with periods in which 4 or 5 deep, equal breaths are taken. It differs from Cheyne-Stokes respiration in that it is characterized by abrupt starts and stops and lacks periodicity. It results from injury to the CNS and occurs in such disorders as meningitis.
- **Kussmaul respirations** are deep, regular respirations caused by metabolic acidosis.

Pulmonary hypertension, sometimes observed during inspection, indicates an increase in right atrial and usually in right ventricular pressure. The elevated pressure is usually caused by left ventricular dysfunction, but it may also be due to a pulmonary disorder causing pulmonary hypertension. The presence of jugular venous distension should prompt a search for other signs of cardiac disorder (eg, 3rd heart sound [S_3] gallop, dependent edema).

Auscultation: Auscultation is arguably the most important component of the physical examination. All fields of the chest should be listened to, including the flanks and the anterior chest, to detect abnormalities associated with each lobe of the lung. Features to listen for include

- Character and volume of breath sounds
- Presence or absence of vocal sounds
- Pleural friction rubs
- Ratio of inspiration to expiration (I:E ratio)

Cardiac auscultation may reveal signs of pulmonary hypertension, such as a loud pulmonic 2nd heart sound (P_2), and of right heart failure, such as a right ventricular 4th heart sound (S_4) and tricuspid regurgitation.

The character and volume of breath sounds are useful in identifying pulmonary disorders. Vesicular breath sounds are the normal sounds heard over most lung fields. Bronchial breath sounds are slightly louder, harsher, and higher pitched; they normally can be heard over the trachea and over areas of lung consolidation, such as occur with pneumonia.

Adventitious sounds are abnormal sounds, such as crackles, rhonchi, wheezes, and stridor.

- **Crackles** (previously called rales) are discontinuous adventitious breath sounds. Fine crackles are short high-pitched sounds; coarse crackles are longer-lasting low-pitched sounds. Crackles have been compared to the sound of crinkling plastic wrap and can be simulated by rubbing strands of hair together between 2 fingers near one's ear. They occur most commonly with atelectasis, alveolar filling processes (eg, pulmonary edema), and interstitial lung disease (eg, pulmonary fibrosis); they signify opening of collapsed airways or alveoli.
- **Rhonchi** are low-pitched respiratory sounds that can be heard during inspiration or expiration. They occur in various conditions, including chronic bronchitis. The mechanism may relate to variations in obstruction as airways distend with inhalation and narrow with exhalation.
- **Wheezes** are whistling, musical breath sounds that are worse during expiration than inspiration. Wheezing can be a physical finding or a symptom and is usually associated with dyspnea.
- **Stridor** is a high-pitched, predominantly inspiratory sound formed by extrathoracic upper airway obstruction. It usually can be heard without a stethoscope. Stridor is usually louder than wheezing, is predominantly inspiratory, and is heard loudly over the larynx. It should trigger a concern for life-threatening upper airway obstruction.
- **Decreased breath sounds** signify poor air movement in airways, as occurs with asthma and COPD where bronchospasm or other mechanisms limit airflow. Breath sounds may also be decreased in the presence of a pleural effusion, pneumothorax, or obstructing endobronchial lesion.

Vocal sounds involve auscultation while patients vocalize.

- **Bronchophony** and **whispered pectoriloquy** occur when the patient's spoken or whispered voice is clearly transmitted through the chest wall. Voice transmission results from alveolar consolidation, as occurs with pneumonia.
- **Egophony** (E to A change) is said to occur when, during auscultation, a patient says the letter "E" and the examiner hears the letter "A," again as occurs with pneumonia.

Friction rubs are grating or creaking sounds that fluctuate with the respiratory cycle and sound like skin rubbing against wet leather. They are a sign of pleural inflammation and are heard in patients with pleuritis or empyema and after thoracotomy.

I:E ratio is normally 1:2 but is prolonged to ≥ 1:3 when airflow is limited, such as in asthma and COPD, even in the absence of wheezing.

Percussion and palpation: Percussion is the primary physical maneuver used to detect the presence and level of pleural effusion. Finding areas of dullness during percussion signifies underlying fluid or, less commonly, consolidation.

Palpation includes tactile fremitus (vibration of the chest wall felt while a patient is speaking); it is decreased in pleural effusion and pneumothorax and increased in pulmonary consolidation (eg, lobar pneumonias). Point tenderness on palpation may signal underlying rib fracture or pleural inflammation.

In cor pulmonale, a right ventricular impulse at the left lower sternal border may become evident and may be increased in amplitude and duration (right ventricular heave).

48 Symptoms of Pulmonary Disorders

COUGH IN ADULTS

Cough is an explosive expiratory maneuver that is reflexively or deliberately intended to clear the airways. It is one of the most common symptoms prompting physician visits.

Likely causes of cough (see Table 48–1) differ depending on whether the symptom is acute (present < 3 wk) or chronic.

In acute cough, the most common causes are

- URI (including acute bronchitis)
- Postnasal drip
- COPD exacerbation
- Pneumonia

In chronic cough, the most common causes are

- Chronic bronchitis
- Postnasal drip

- Airway hyperresponsiveness after resolution of a viral or bacterial respiratory infection (ie, postinfection cough)
- Gastroesophageal reflux

The causes of cough in children are similar to those in adults, but asthma and foreign body aspiration may be more common.

Very rarely, impacted cerumen or a foreign body in the external auditory canal triggers reflex cough through stimulation of the auricular branch of the vagus nerve. Psychogenic cough is even rarer and is a diagnosis of exclusion.

Patients with chronic cough may develop a secondary reflex or psychogenic component to their cough. Also, protracted coughing may injure the bronchial mucosa, which may trigger more coughing.

Evaluation

History: History of present illness should cover the duration and characteristics of the cough (eg, whether dry or productive of sputum or blood, and whether it is accompanied by dyspnea, chest pain, or both). Asking about precipitating factors (eg, cold air, strong odors) and the timing of the cough (eg, primarily at night) can be revealing.

Review of systems should seek symptoms of possible cause, including runny nose and sore throat (URI, postnasal drip); fever, chills, and pleuritic chest pain (pneumonia); night sweats and weight loss (tumor, TB); heartburn (gastroesophageal reflux); and difficulty swallowing or choking episodes while eating or drinking (aspiration).

Past medical history should note recent respiratory infections (ie, within previous 1 to 2 mo); history of allergies, asthma, COPD, and gastroesophageal reflux disease; risk factors for (or known) TB or HIV infection; and smoking history. Drug history should specifically include use of ACE inhibitors. Patients with chronic cough should be asked about exposure to potential respiratory irritants or allergens and travel to or residence in regions with endemic fungal illness.

Physical examination: Vital signs should be reviewed for the presence of tachypnea and fever.

General examination should look for signs of respiratory distress and chronic illness (eg, wasting, lethargy).

Examination of the nose and throat should focus on appearance of the nasal mucosa (eg, color, congestion) and presence of discharge (external or in posterior pharynx). Ears should be examined for triggers of reflex cough.

The cervical and supraclavicular areas should be inspected and palpated for lymphadenopathy.

A full lung examination is done, particularly including adequacy of air entry and exit; symmetry of breath sounds; and presence of crackles, wheezes, or both. Signs of consolidation (eg, egophony, dullness to percussion) should be sought.

Red flags: The following findings are of particular concern:

- Dyspnea
- Hemoptysis
- Weight loss
- Persistent fever
- Risk factors for TB or HIV infection

Interpretation of findings: Some findings point to particular diagnoses (see Table 48–1).

Other important findings are less specific. For example, the color (eg, yellow, green) and thickness of sputum do not help differentiate bacterial from other causes. Wheezing may occur with several causes. Hemoptysis in small amounts may occur with severe cough of many etiologies, although larger amounts of hemoptysis suggest bronchitis, bronchiectasis, TB, or primary lung cancer. Fever, night sweats, and weight loss may occur with many chronic infections as well as with cancer.

Testing: Patients with red flag findings of dyspnea or hemoptysis and patients in whom suspicion of pneumonia is high should have pulse oximetry and chest x-ray. Patients with weight loss or risk factors should have a chest x-ray and testing for TB and HIV infection.

For many patients without red flag findings, clinicians can base the diagnosis on history and physical examination findings and begin treatment without testing. For patients without a clear cause but no red flag findings, many clinicians empirically begin treatment for postnasal drip (eg, antihistamine and decongestant combinations, nasal corticosteroid sprays) or gastroesophageal reflux disease (eg, proton pump inhibitors, H_2 blockers). An adequate response to these interventions usually precludes the need for further evaluation.

Patients with chronic cough in whom presumptive treatment is ineffective should have a chest x-ray. If the x-ray findings are unremarkable, many clinicians sequentially test for asthma (pulmonary function tests with methacholine challenge), sinus disease (sinus CT), and gastroesophageal reflux disease (esophageal pH monitoring).

Sputum culture is helpful for patients with a possible indolent infection, such as pertussis, TB, or nontuberculous mycobacterial infection. Sputum cytology is noninvasive and should be done if cancer is suspected and the patient is producing sputum or having hemoptysis.

Chest CT and possibly bronchoscopy should be done in patients in whom lung cancer or another bronchial tumor is suspected (eg, patients with a long smoking history, nonspecific constitutional signs) and in patients in whom empiric therapy has failed and who have inconclusive findings on preliminary testing.

Treatment

Treatment is management of the cause.

There is little evidence to support the use of cough suppressants or mucolytic agents. Coughing is an important mechanism for clearing secretions from the airways and can assist in recovery from respiratory infections. Therefore, although patients often expect or request cough suppressants, such treatment should be given with caution and reserved for patients with a URI and for patients receiving therapy for the underlying disorder for whom cough is still troubling. Cough suppressants may help some patients with chronic cough who have a reflex or psychogenic component to their cough or who develop bronchial mucosal injury.

Antitussives depress the medullary cough center (dextromethorphan and codeine) or anesthetize stretch receptors of vagal afferent fibers in bronchi and alveoli (benzonatate). Dextromethorphan, a congener of the opioid levorphanol, is effective as a tablet or syrup at a dose of 15 to 30 mg po 1 to 4 times/day for adults or 0.25 mg/kg po qid for children. Codeine has antitussive, analgesic, and sedative effects, but dependence is a potential problem, and nausea, vomiting, constipation, and tolerance are common adverse effects. Usual doses are 10 to 20 mg po q 4 to 6 h as needed for adults and 0.25 to 0.5 mg/kg po qid for children. Other opioids (hydrocodone,

Table 48–1. SOME CAUSES OF COUGH

CAUSE	SUGGESTIVE FINDINGS	DIAGNOSTIC APPROACH
Acute		
URI (including acute bronchitis)	Rhinorrhea Red, swollen nasal mucosa Sore throat Malaise	Clinical evaluation
Pneumonia (viral, bacterial, aspiration, rarely fungal)	Fever Productive cough Dyspnea Pleuritic chest pain Bronchial breath sounds or egophony	Chest x-ray Cultures (eg, pleural fluid, blood, possibly bronchial washings) in seriously ill patients and patients with hospital-acquired pneumonia
Postnasal drip (allergic, viral, or bacterial origin)	Headache Sore throat Nausea Cobblestoning of posterior oropharynx Pale, boggy, swollen nasal mucosa	Clinical evaluation Sometimes response to empiric antihistamine and decongestant therapy CT of the sinuses if diagnosis is unclear
COPD exacerbation	Known diagnosis of COPD Poor breath sounds Wheezing Dyspnea Pursed lip breathing Use of accessory muscles Tripod positioning of the arms against the legs or examination table	Chest x-ray
Foreign body*	Sudden onset in a toddler who has no URI or constitutional symptoms	Chest x-ray (inspiratory and expiratory views) Bronchoscopy
Pulmonary embolism*	Pleuritic chest pain Dyspnea Tachycardia	CT angiography Less often, ventilation/perfusion scanning and possibly pulmonary arteriography
Heart failure*	Dyspnea Fine crackles Extrasystolic heart sound Dependent peripheral edema	Chest x-ray Brain (B-type) natriuretic peptide level
Chronic		
Chronic bronchitis (in smokers)	Productive cough on most days of the month or for 3 mo of the year for 2 successive years in a patient with known COPD or smoking history Frequent clearing of the throat Dyspnea	Chest x-ray Pulmonary function testing
Postnasal drip (allergic most likely)	Headache Sore throat Cobblestoning of posterior oropharynx Pale, boggy, swollen nasal mucosa	Clinical evaluation Sometimes response to empiric antihistamine and decongestant therapy Allergy testing
Gastroesophageal reflux	Burning chest or abdominal pain that tends to worsen with consumption of certain foods, certain activities, or certain positions Sour taste, particularly on awakening Hoarseness Chronic nocturnal or early morning cough	Clinical evaluation Response to empiric H_2 blocker or proton pump inhibitor therapy Sometimes 24-h esophageal pH probe if diagnosis is unclear
Asthma (cough variant)	Cough in response to various provoking factors (eg, allergens, cold, exercise) Possibly wheezing and dyspnea	Pulmonary function testing Methacholine challenge Response to empiric bronchodilator therapy
Hyperresponsive airways after resolution of respiratory tract infection	Dry, nonproductive cough that may persist for weeks or months after an acute respiratory tract infection	Typically chest x-ray
ACE inhibitors	Dry, persistent cough that may occur within days or months after initiation of ACE inhibitor therapy	Response to stopping ACE inhibitor

Table continues on the following page.

Table 48–1. SOME CAUSES OF COUGH (*Continued*)

CAUSE	SUGGESTIVE FINDINGS	DIAGNOSTIC APPROACH
Pertussis	Repeated bouts of ≥ 5 rapidly consecutive, forceful coughs during a single expiration, followed by a hurried and deep inspiration (whoop) or posttussive emesis	Cultures of nasopharyngeal specimens
Aspiration	Wet-sounding cough after eating or drinking	Chest x-ray Sometimes modified barium pharyngography Bronchoscopy
Tumor*	Atypical symptoms (eg, weight loss, fever, hemoptysis, night sweats) Lymphadenopathy	Chest x-ray If positive, chest CT and bronchoscopic biopsy
TB or fungal infections*	Atypical symptoms (eg, weight loss, fever, hemoptysis, night sweats) Exposure history Immunocompromise	Chest x-ray Skin testing; if positive, sputum cultures and stains for acid-fast bacilli and fungi Sometimes chest CT or bronchoalveolar lavage

*Indicates rare causes.

hydromorphone, methadone, morphine) have antitussive properties but are avoided because of high potential for dependence and abuse. Benzonatate, a congener of tetracaine that is available in liquid-filled capsules, is effective at a dose of 100 to 200 mg po tid.

Expectorants are thought to decrease viscosity and facilitate expectoration (coughing up) of secretions but are of limited, if any, benefit in most circumstances. Guaifenesin (200 to 400 mg po q 4 h in syrup or tablet form) is most commonly used because it has no serious adverse effects, but multiple expectorants exist, including bromhexine, ipecac, and saturated solution of potassium iodide (SSKI). Aerosolized expectorants such as *N*-acetylcysteine and DNase are generally reserved for hospital-based treatment of cough in patients with bronchiectasis or cystic fibrosis. Ensuring adequate hydration may facilitate expectoration, as may inhalation of steam, although neither technique has been rigorously tested.

Topical treatments, such as acacia, licorice, glycerin, honey, and wild cherry cough drops or syrups (demulcents), are locally and perhaps emotionally soothing, but their use is not supported by scientific evidence.

Protussives, which stimulate cough, are indicated for such disorders as cystic fibrosis and bronchiectasis, in which a productive cough is thought to be important for airway clearance and preservation of pulmonary function. DNase or hypertonic saline is given in conjunction with chest physical therapy and postural drainage to promote cough and expectoration. This approach is beneficial in cystic fibrosis but not in most other causes of chronic cough.

Bronchodilators, such as albuterol and ipratropium or inhaled corticosteroids, can be effective for cough after URI and in cough-variant asthma.

KEY POINTS

- Danger signs include respiratory distress, chronic fever, weight loss, and hemoptysis.
- Clinical diagnosis is usually adequate.
- Occult gastroesophageal reflux disease should be remembered as a possible cause.
- Antitussives and expectorants should be used selectively.

DYSPNEA

Dyspnea is unpleasant or uncomfortable breathing. It is experienced and described differently by patients depending on the cause.

Pathophysiology

Although dyspnea is a relatively common problem, the pathophysiology of the uncomfortable sensation of breathing is poorly understood. Unlike those for other types of noxious stimuli, there are no specialized dyspnea receptors (although recent MRI studies have identified a few specific areas in the midbrain that may mediate perception of dyspnea).

The experience of dyspnea likely results from a complex interaction between chemoreceptor stimulation, mechanical abnormalities in breathing, and the perception of those abnormalities by the CNS. Some authors have described the imbalance between neurologic stimulation and mechanical changes in the lungs and chest wall as neuromechanical uncoupling.

Etiology

Dyspnea has many pulmonary, cardiac, and other causes,[1] which vary by acuity of onset (see Tables 48–2, 48–3, and 48–4). The most common causes include

- Asthma
- Pneumonia
- COPD
- Myocardial ischemia
- Physical deconditioning

The most common cause of dyspnea in patients with chronic pulmonary or cardiac disorders is

- Exacerbation of their disease

However, such patients may also acutely develop another condition (eg, a patient with long-standing asthma may have a myocardial infarction, a patient with chronic heart failure may develop pneumonia).

1. Pratter MR, Curley FJ, Dubois J, Irwin RS: Cause and evaluation of chronic dyspnea in a pulmonary disease clinic. *Arch Intern Med* 149(10):2277–2282, 1989.

Table 48–2. SOME CAUSES OF ACUTE* DYSPNEA

CAUSE	SUGGESTIVE FINDINGS	DIAGNOSTIC APPROACH†
Pulmonary causes		
Pneumothorax	Abrupt onset of sharp chest pain, tachypnea, diminished breath sounds, and hyperresonance to percussion May follow injury or occur spontaneously (especially in tall, thin patients and in patients with COPD)	Chest x-ray
Pulmonary embolism	Abrupt onset of sharp chest pain, tachypnea, and tachycardia Often risk factors for pulmonary embolism (eg, cancer, immobilization, DVT, pregnancy, use of oral contraceptives or other estrogen-containing drugs, recent surgery or hospitalization, family history)	CT angiography less often, V/Q scanning and possibly pulmonary arteriography
Asthma, bronchospasm, or reactive airway disease	Wheezing and poor air exchange that arise spontaneously or after exposure to specific stimuli (eg, allergen, URI, cold, exercise) Possibly pulsus paradoxus Often a preexisting history of reactive airway disease	Clinical evaluation Sometimes pulmonary function testing or peak flow measurement
Foreign body inhalation	Sudden onset of cough or stridor in a patient (typically an infant or young child) without URI or constitutional symptoms	Inspiratory and expiratory chest x-rays Sometimes bronchoscopy
Toxin-induced airway damage (eg, due to inhalation of chlorine or hydrogen sulfide)	Sudden onset after occupational exposure or inappropriate use of cleaning agents	Inhalation usually obvious by history Chest x-ray Sometimes ABGs and observation to determine severity
Cardiac causes		
Acute myocardial ischemia or infarction	Substernal chest pressure or pain that may or may not radiate to the arm or jaw, particularly in patients with risk factors for CAD	ECG Cardiac enzyme testing
Papillary muscle dysfunction or rupture	Sudden onset of chest pain, new or loud holosystolic murmur, and signs of heart failure, particularly in patients with recent MI	Auscultation Echocardiography
Heart failure	Crackles, S_3 gallop, and signs of central or peripheral volume overload (eg, elevated neck veins, peripheral edema) Dyspnea while lying flat (orthopnea) or appearing 1–2 h after falling asleep (paroxysmal nocturnal dyspnea)	Auscultation Chest x-ray BNP measurement Echocardiography
Other causes		
Diaphragmatic paralysis	Sudden onset after trauma affecting the phrenic nerve Frequent orthopnea	Chest x-ray Fluoroscopic sniff test
Anxiety disorder causing hyperventilation	Situational dyspnea often accompanied by psychomotor agitation and paresthesias in the fingers or around the mouth Normal examination findings and pulse oximetry measurements	Clinical evaluation Diagnosis of exclusion

*Acute dyspnea occurs within minutes of triggering event.

†Most patients should have pulse oximetry and, unless symptoms are clearly a mild exacerbation of known chronic disease, chest x-ray.

BNP = brain (B-type) natriuretic peptide; CAD = coronary artery disease; DVT = deep venous thrombosis; S_3 = 3rd heart sound; V/Q = ventilation/perfusion.

Evaluation

History: History of present illness should cover the duration, temporal onset (eg, abrupt, insidious), and provoking or exacerbating factors (eg, allergen exposure, cold, exertion, supine position). Severity can be determined by assessing the activity level required to cause dyspnea (eg, dyspnea at rest is more severe than dyspnea only with climbing stairs). Physicians should note how much dyspnea has changed from the patient's usual state.

Review of systems should seek symptoms of possible causes, including chest pain or pressure (pulmonary embolism, myocardial ischemia, pneumonia); dependent edema, orthopnea, and paroxysmal nocturnal dyspnea (heart failure); fever, chills, cough, and sputum production (pneumonia); black, tarry stools or heavy menses (occult bleeding possibly causing anemia); and weight loss or night sweats (cancer or chronic lung infection).

Table 48–3. SOME CAUSES OF SUBACUTE* DYSPNEA

CAUSE	SUGGESTIVE FINDINGS	DIAGNOSTIC APPROACH†
Pulmonary causes		
Pneumonia	Fever, productive cough, dyspnea, sometimes pleuritic chest pain Focal lung findings, including crackles, decreased breath sounds, and egophony	Chest x-ray Sometimes blood and sputum cultures WBC count
COPD exacerbation	Cough, productive or nonproductive Poor air movement Accessory muscle use or pursed lip breathing	Clinical evaluation Sometimes chest x-ray and ABGs
Cardiac causes		
Angina or CAD	Substernal chest pressure with or without radiation to the arm or jaw, often provoked by physical exertion, particularly in patients with risk factors for CAD	ECG Cardiac stress testing Cardiac catheterization
Pericardial effusion or tamponade	Muffled heart sounds or enlarged cardiac silhouette in patients with risk factors for pericardial effusion (eg, cancer, pericarditis, SLE) Possibly pulsus paradoxus	Echocardiography

*Subacute dyspnea occurs within hours or days.
†Most patients should have pulse oximetry and, unless symptoms are clearly a mild exacerbation of a known chronic disease, chest x-ray.
CAD = coronary artery disease.

Past medical history should cover disorders known to cause dyspnea, including asthma, COPD, and heart disease, as well as risk factors for the different etiologies:

- Smoking history—for cancer, COPD, and heart disease
- Family history, hypertension, and high cholesterol levels—for coronary artery disease
- Recent immobilization or surgery, recent long-distance travel, cancer or risk factors for or signs of occult cancer, prior or family history of clotting, pregnancy, oral contraceptive use, calf pain, leg swelling, and known deep venous thrombosis—for pulmonary embolism

Occupational exposures (eg, gases, smoke, asbestos) should be investigated.

Physical examination: Vital signs are reviewed for fever, tachycardia, and tachypnea.

Examination focuses on the cardiovascular and pulmonary systems.

A full lung examination is done, particularly including adequacy of air entry and exit, symmetry of breath sounds, and presence of crackles, rhonchi, stridor, and wheezing. Signs of consolidation (eg, egophony, dullness to percussion) should be sought. The cervical, supraclavicular, and inguinal areas should be inspected and palpated for lymphadenopathy.

Neck veins should be inspected for distention, and the legs and presacral area should be palpated for pitting edema (both suggesting heart failure).

Heart sounds should be auscultated with notation of any extra heart sounds, muffled heart sounds, or murmur. Testing for pulsus paradoxus (a > 12-mm Hg drop of systolic BP during inspiration) can be done by inflating a BP cuff to 20 mm Hg above the systolic pressure and then slowly deflating until the first Korotkoff sound is heard only during expiration. As the cuff is further deflated, the point at which the first Korotkoff sound is audible during both inspiration and expiration is recorded. If the difference between the first and second measurement is > 12 mm Hg, then pulsus paradoxus is present.

Conjunctiva should be examined for pallor. Rectal examination and stool guaiac testing should be done.

Red flags: The following findings are of particular concern:

- Dyspnea at rest during examination
- Decreased level of consciousness or agitation or confusion
- Accessory muscle use and poor air excursion
- Chest pain
- Crackles
- Weight loss
- Night sweats
- Palpitations

Interpretation of findings: The history and physical examination often suggest a cause and guide further testing (see Tables 48–2, 48–3, and 48–4). Several findings are of note. Wheezing suggests asthma or COPD. Stridor suggests extrathoracic airway obstruction (eg, foreign body, epiglottitis, vocal cord dysfunction). Crackles suggest left heart failure, interstitial lung disease, or, if accompanied by signs of consolidation, pneumonia.

However, the symptoms and signs of life-threatening conditions such as myocardial ischemia and pulmonary embolism can be nonspecific. Furthermore, the severity of symptoms is not always proportional to the severity of the cause (eg, pulmonary embolism in a fit, healthy person may cause only mild dyspnea). Thus, a high degree of suspicion for these common conditions is prudent. It is often appropriate to rule out these conditions before attributing dyspnea to a less serious etiology.

A clinical prediction rule (see Table 61–2 on p. 492) can help estimate the risk of pulmonary embolism. Note that normal oxygen saturation does not exclude pulmonary embolism.

Hyperventilation syndrome is a diagnosis of exclusion. Because hypoxia may cause tachypnea and agitation, it is

Table 48–4. SOME CAUSES OF CHRONIC* DYSPNEA

CAUSE	SUGGESTIVE FINDINGS	DIAGNOSTIC APPROACH†
Pulmonary causes		
Obstructive lung disease	Extensive smoking history, barrel chest, and poor air entry and exit	Chest x-ray Pulmonary function testing (at initial evaluation)
Restrictive lung disease	Progressive dyspnea in patients with known occupational exposure or neurologic condition	Chest x-ray Pulmonary function testing (at initial evaluation)
Interstitial lung disease	Fine crackles, frequently accompanied by dry cough	High-resolution chest CT
Pleural effusion	Pleuritic chest pain, lung field that is dull to percussion and has diminished breath sounds Sometimes history of cancer, heart failure, RA, SLE, or acute pneumonia	Chest x-ray Often chest CT and thoracentesis
Cardiac causes		
Heart failure	Crackles, S_3 gallop, and signs of central or peripheral volume overload (eg, elevated neck veins, peripheral edema) Orthopnea or paroxysmal nocturnal dyspnea	Auscultation Chest x-ray Echocardiography
Stable angina or CAD	Substernal chest pressure with or without radiation to the arm or jaw, often provoked by physical exertion, particularly in patients with risk factors for CAD	ECG Cardiac stress testing Sometimes cardiac catheterization
Other causes		
Anemia	Dyspnea on exertion progressing to dyspnea at rest Normal lung examination and pulse oximetry measurement Sometimes systolic heart murmur due to increased flow	CBC
Physical deconditioning	Dyspnea only on exertion in patients with sedentary lifestyle	Clinical evaluation

*Chronic dyspnea occurs within hours to years.
†Most patients should have pulse oximetry and, unless symptoms are clearly a mild exacerbation of a known chronic disease, chest x-ray.
CAD = coronary artery disease; S_3 = 3rd heart sound.

unwise to assume every rapidly breathing, anxious young person merely has hyperventilation syndrome.

Testing: Pulse oximetry should be done in all patients, and a chest x-ray should be done as well unless symptoms are clearly caused by a mild or moderate exacerbation of a known condition. For example, patients with asthma or heart failure do not require an x-ray for each flare-up, unless clinical findings suggest another cause or an unusually severe attack. Most adults should have an ECG to detect myocardial ischemia (and serum cardiac marker testing if suspicion is high) unless myocardial ischemia can be excluded clinically.

In patients with severe or deteriorating respiratory status, ABGs should be measured to more precisely quantify hypoxemia, measure $Paco_2$, diagnose any acid-base disorders stimulating hyperventilation, and calculate the alveolar-arterial gradient.

Patients who have no clear diagnosis after chest x-ray and ECG and are at moderate or high risk of having pulmonary embolism (from the clinical prediction rule—see Table 61–2 on p. 492) should undergo CT angiography or ventilation/perfusion scanning. Patients who are at low risk may have D-dimer testing (a normal D-dimer level effectively rules out pulmonary embolism in a low-risk patient).

Chronic dyspnea may warrant additional tests, such as CT, pulmonary function tests, echocardiography, and bronchoscopy.

Treatment

Treatment is correction of the underlying disorder.

Hypoxemia is treated with supplemental oxygen as needed to maintain oxygen saturation > 88% or PaO_2 > 55 mm Hg because levels above these thresholds provide adequate oxygen delivery to tissues. Levels below these thresholds are on the steep portion of the oxygen–Hb dissociation curve, where even a small decline in arterial oxygen tension can result in a large decline in Hb saturation. Oxygen saturation should be maintained at > 93% if myocardial or cerebral ischemia is a concern.

Morphine 0.5 to 5 mg IV helps reduce anxiety and the discomfort of dyspnea in various conditions, including myocardial infarction, pulmonary embolism, and the dyspnea that commonly accompanies terminal illness. However, opioids can be deleterious in patients with acute airflow limitation (eg, asthma, COPD) because they suppress the ventilatory drive and can worsen respiratory acidemia.

KEY POINTS

- Pulse oximetry is a key component of the examination.
- Low oxygen saturation (< 90%) indicates a serious problem, but normal saturation does not rule one out.

- Accessory muscle use, a sudden decrease in oxygen saturation, or a decreased level of consciousness requires emergency evaluation and hospitalization.
- Myocardial ischemia and pulmonary embolism are relatively common, but symptoms and signs can be nonspecific.
- Exacerbation of known conditions (eg, asthma, COPD, heart failure) is common, but patients may also develop new problems.

HEMOPTYSIS

Hemoptysis is coughing up of blood from the respiratory tract. Massive hemoptysis is production of ≥ 600 mL of blood (about a full kidney basin's worth) within 24 h.

Pathophysiology

Most of the lung's blood (95%) circulates through low-pressure pulmonary arteries and ends up in the pulmonary capillary bed, where gas is exchanged. About 5% of the blood supply circulates through high-pressure bronchial arteries, which originate at the aorta and supply major airways and supporting structures. In hemoptysis, the blood generally arises from this bronchial circulation, except when pulmonary arteries are damaged by trauma, by erosion of a granulomatous or calcified lymph node or tumor, or, rarely, by pulmonary arterial catheterization or when pulmonary capillaries are affected by inflammation.

Etiology

Blood-streaked sputum is common in many minor respiratory illnesses, such as URI and viral bronchitis.

The differential diagnosis is broad (see Table 48–5). In adults, 70 to 90% of cases are caused by

- Bronchitis
- Bronchiectasis
- Necrotizing pneumonia
- TB

Primary lung cancer is an important cause in smokers ≥ 40 yr, but metastatic cancer rarely causes hemoptysis. Cavitary *Aspergillus* infection is increasingly recognized as a cause but is not as common as cancer.

In children, common causes are

- Lower respiratory tract infection
- Foreign body aspiration

Massive hemoptysis: The most common causes have changed over time and vary by geographic region but include the following:

- Bronchogenic carcinoma
- Bronchiectasis
- TB and other pneumonias

Evaluation

History: History of present illness should cover the duration and temporal patterns (eg, abrupt onset, cyclical recurrence), provoking factors (eg, allergen exposure, cold, exertion, supine position), and approximate volume of hemoptysis (eg, streaking, teaspoon, cup). Patients may need specific prompting to differentiate between true hemoptysis, pseudohemoptysis (ie, bleeding originating in the nasopharynx that is subsequently coughed up), and hematemesis. A sensation of postnasal drip

Table 48–5. SOME CAUSES OF HEMOPTYSIS

CAUSE	SUGGESTIVE FINDINGS	DIAGNOSTIC APPROACH*
Tracheobronchial source		
Tumor (bronchogenic, bronchial metastatic, Kaposi sarcoma)	Night sweats Weight loss History of heavy smoking Risk factors for Kaposi sarcoma (eg, HIV)	Chest x-ray CT Bronchoscopy
Bronchitis (acute or chronic)	*Acute:* Productive or nonproductive cough *Chronic:* Cough on most days of the month or for 3 mo per year for 2 successive years in patients with known COPD or smoking history	*Acute:* Clinical evaluation *Chronic:* Chest x-ray
Bronchiectasis	Chronic cough and mucus production in patients with a history of recurrent infections	High-resolution chest CT Bronchoscopy
Broncholithiasis	Calcified lymph nodes in patients with history of prior granulomatous disease	Chest CT Bronchoscopy
Foreign body (typically chronic and undiagnosed)	Chronic cough (typically in an infant or young child) without URI symptoms Sometimes fever	Chest x-ray Sometimes bronchoscopy
Pulmonary parenchymal source		
Lung abscess	Subacute fever Cough Night sweats Anorexia Weight loss	Chest x-ray or CT showing irregularly shaped cavity with air-fluid levels

Table 48–5. SOME CAUSES OF HEMOPTYSIS (*Continued*)

CAUSE	SUGGESTIVE FINDINGS	DIAGNOSTIC APPROACH*
Pneumonia	Fever, productive cough, dyspnea, pleuritic chest pain Decreased breath sounds or egophony Elevated WBC count	Chest x-ray Blood and sputum cultures in hospitalized patients
Active granulomatous disease (tuberculous, fungal, parasitic, syphilitic) or mycetoma (fungus ball)	Fever, cough, night sweats, and weight loss in patients with known exposures Often history of immunosuppression	Chest x-ray Chest CT Microbiologic testing of sputum samples or bronchoscopy washings
Goodpasture syndrome	Fatigue Weight loss Often hematuria Sometimes edema	Urinalysis Creatinine levels Renal biopsy Antiglomerular basement membrane testing cANCA testing
Granulomatosis with polyangiitis	Often chronic, bloody nasal discharge and nasal ulcerations Often joint pain and skin manifestations (nodules, purpura) Gingival thickening and mulberry gingivitis Saddle nose and nasal septum perforation Sometimes renal insufficiency	Biopsy of any affected area (eg, kidney, skin) with cANCA testing and demonstration of vasculitis in small to medium-sized arteries Bronchoscopy
Lupus pneumonitis	Fever, cough, dyspnea, and pleuritic chest pain in patients with a history of SLE	Chest CT (showing alveolitis) Sometimes bronchoscopy washings (showing lymphocytosis or granulocytosis)
Primary vascular source		
Arteriovenous malformation	Presence of mucocutaneous telangiectasia or peripheral cyanosis	Chest CT angiography Pulmonary angiography
Pulmonary embolism	Abrupt onset of sharp chest pain, increased respiratory rate and heart rate, particularly in patients with known risk factors for pulmonary embolism	CT angiography or V/Q scanning Doppler or duplex studies of extremities showing findings of DVT
Elevated pulmonary venous pressure (especially mitral stenosis, left-sided heart failure)	Crackles Signs of central or peripheral volume overload (eg, elevated neck veins, peripheral edema) Dyspnea while lying flat (orthopnea) or appearing 1–2 h after falling asleep (paroxysmal nocturnal dyspnea)	ECG BNP measurement Echocardiography
Aortic aneurysm with leakage into the pulmonary parenchyma	Back pain	Chest x-ray showing widened mediastinum Chest CT angiography
Pulmonary artery rupture	Recent placement or manipulation of a pulmonary artery catheter	Emergency chest CT angiography or emergency pulmonary angiography
Tracheal-innominate artery fistula	Placement of tracheostomy tube within the previous 3 days to 6 wk	Clinical evaluation (eg, identifying hemorrhage from endotracheal tube in compatible clinical setting)
Miscellaneous		
Pulmonary endometriosis (catamenial hemoptysis)	Recurrent hemoptysis during menstruation	Clinical evaluation Sometimes therapeutic trial of oral contraceptives
Systemic coagulopathy or use of anticoagulants or thrombolytics	Patients receiving systemic anticoagulants for treatment of pulmonary embolism, DVT, or atrial fibrillation Patients receiving thrombolytics for treatment of stroke or MI Sometimes a family history	PT/PTT or anti-factor Xa levels Cessation of hemoptysis with correction of coagulation deficit

*All patients with hemoptysis should have chest x-ray and pulse oximetry.

BNP = brain (B-type) natriuretic peptide; cANCA = antineutrophil cytoplasmic antibody; DVT = deep venous thrombosis; V/Q = ventilation/perfusion.

or any bleeding from the nares without coughing is suggestive of pseudohemoptysis. Concomitant nausea and vomiting with black, brown, or coffee-ground–colored blood is characteristic of hematemesis. Frothy sputum, bright red blood, and (if massive) a sensation of choking are characteristic of true hemoptysis.

Review of systems should seek symptoms suggesting possible causes, including fever and sputum production (pneumonia); night sweats, weight loss, and fatigue (cancer, TB); chest pain and dyspnea (pneumonia, pulmonary embolism); leg pain and leg swelling (pulmonary embolism); hematuria (Goodpasture syndrome); and bloody nasal discharge (granulomatosis with polyangiitis).

Patients should be asked about risk factors for causes. These risk factors include HIV infection, use of immunosuppressants (TB, fungal infection); exposure to TB; long smoking history (cancer); and recent immobilization or surgery, known cancer, prior or family history of clotting, pregnancy, use of estrogen-containing drugs, and recent long-distance travel (pulmonary embolism).

Past medical history should cover known conditions that can cause hemoptysis, including chronic lung disease (eg, COPD, bronchiectasis, TB, cystic fibrosis), cancer, bleeding disorders, heart failure, thoracic aortic aneurysm, and pulmonary-renal syndromes (eg, Goodpasture syndrome, granulomatosis with polyangiitis). Exposure to TB is important, particularly in patients with HIV infection or another immunocompromised state.

A history of frequent nosebleeds, easy bruising, or liver disease suggests possible coagulopathy. The drug profile should be reviewed for use of anticoagulants and antiplatelet drugs.

Physical examination: Vital signs are reviewed for fever, tachycardia, tachypnea, and low oxygen saturation. Constitutional signs (eg, cachexia) and level of patient distress (eg, accessory muscle use, pursed lip breathing, agitation, decreased level of consciousness) should also be noted.

A full lung examination is done, particularly including adequacy of air entry and exit, symmetry of breath sounds, and presence of crackles, rhonchi, stridor, and wheezing. Signs of consolidation (eg, egophony, dullness to percussion) should be sought. The cervical and supraclavicular areas should be inspected and palpated for lymphadenopathy (suggesting cancer or TB).

Neck veins should be inspected for distention, and the legs and presacral area should be palpated for pitting edema (suggesting heart failure). Heart sounds should be auscultated with notation of any extra heart sounds or murmur that might support a diagnosis of heart failure and elevated pulmonary pressure.

The abdominal examination should focus on signs of hepatic congestion or masses, which could suggest either cancer or hematemesis from potential esophageal varices.

The skin and mucous membranes should be examined for ecchymoses, petechiae, telangiectasia, gingivitis, or evidence of bleeding from the oral or nasal mucosa.

If the patient can reproduce hemoptysis during examination, the color and amount of blood should be noted.

Red flags: The following findings are of particular concern:

- Massive hemoptysis
- Back pain
- Presence of a pulmonary artery catheter or tracheostomy
- Malaise, weight loss, or fatigue
- Extensive smoking history
- Dyspnea at rest during examination or absent or decreased breath sounds

Interpretation of findings: The history and physical examination often suggest a diagnosis and guide further testing (see Table 48–5).

Despite the many possibilities, some generalities can be made. A previously healthy person with a normal examination and no risk factors (eg, for TB, pulmonary embolism) who presents with acute-onset cough and fever most likely has hemoptysis due to an acute respiratory illness; chronic disorders are much lower on the list of possibilities. However, if risk factors are present, those specific disorders must be strongly suspected. A clinical prediction rule (see Table 61–2 on p. 492) can help estimate the risk of pulmonary embolism. A normal oxygen saturation does not exclude pulmonary embolism.

Patients whose hemoptysis is due to a lung disorder (eg, COPD, cystic fibrosis, bronchiectasis) or heart disease (eg, heart failure) typically have a clear history of those disorders. Hemoptysis is not an initial manifestation.

Patients with known immunocompromise should be suspected of having TB or a fungal infection.

Patients with symptoms or signs of chronic illness but no known disorders should be suspected of having cancer or TB, although hemoptysis can be the initial manifestation of lung cancer in a patient who is otherwise asymptomatic.

Several specific findings are of note. Known renal failure or hematuria suggests a pulmonary-renal syndrome (eg, Goodpasture syndrome, granulomatosis with polyangiitis). Patients with granulomatosis with polyangiitis may have nasal mucosal lesions. Visible telangiectasias suggest arteriovenous malformations. Patients with hemoptysis due to a bleeding disorder usually have cutaneous findings (petechiae, purpura, or both) or a history of anticoagulant or antiplatelet drug use. Recurrent hemoptysis coinciding with menses strongly suggests pulmonary endometriosis.

Testing: Patients with massive hemoptysis require treatment and stabilization, usually in an ICU, before testing. Patients with minor hemoptysis can undergo outpatient testing.

Imaging is always done. A chest x-ray is mandatory. Patients with normal results, a consistent history, and nonmassive hemoptysis can undergo empiric treatment for bronchitis. Patients with abnormal results and patients without a supporting history should undergo CT and bronchoscopy. CT may reveal pulmonary lesions that are not apparent on the chest x-ray and can help locate lesions in anticipation of bronchoscopy and biopsy. CT angiography or, less commonly, ventilation/perfusion scanning with or without pulmonary arteriography can confirm the diagnosis of pulmonary embolism. CT and pulmonary angiography can also detect pulmonary arteriovenous fistulas.

Fiberoptic inspection of the pharynx, larynx, and airways may be indicated along with esophagogastric endoscopy when the etiology is obscure to distinguish hemoptysis from hematemesis and from nasopharyngeal or oropharyngeal bleeding.

Laboratory testing is also done. Patients usually should have a CBC, a platelet count, and measurement of PT and PTT. Anti-factor Xa testing can be used to detect supratherapeutic anticoagulation in patients receiving low molecular weight heparin. Urinalysis should be done to look for signs of glomerulonephritis (hematuria, proteinuria, casts). TB skin testing and sputum culture should be done as the initial tests for active TB, but negative results do not preclude the need to induce sputum or do fiberoptic bronchoscopy to obtain samples for further acid-fast bacillus testing if an alternative diagnosis is not found.

Cryptogenic hemoptysis: The cause of hemoptysis remains unknown in 30 to 40% of patients, but the prognosis for patients with cryptogenic hemoptysis is generally favorable, usually with resolution of bleeding within 6 mo of evaluation.

Treatment

Massive hemoptysis: Initial treatment of massive hemoptysis has two objectives:

- Prevent aspiration of blood into the uninvolved lung (which can cause asphyxiation)
- Prevent exsanguination due to ongoing bleeding

It can be difficult to protect the uninvolved lung because it is often initially unclear which side is bleeding. Once the bleeding side is identified, strategies include positioning the patient with the bleeding lung in a dependent position and selectively intubating the uninvolved lung and/or obstructing the bronchus going to the bleeding lung.

Prevention of exsanguination involves reversal of any bleeding diathesis and direct efforts to stop the bleeding. Clotting deficiencies can be reversed with fresh frozen plasma and factor-specific or platelet transfusions. Laser therapy, cauterization, or direct injection with epinephrine or vasopressin can be done bronchoscopically.

Massive hemoptysis is one of the few indications for rigid (as opposed to flexible) bronchoscopy, which provides control of the airway, allows for a larger field of view than flexible bronchoscopy, allows better suctioning, and is more suited to therapeutic interventions, such as laser therapy.

Embolization via bronchial artery angiography is becoming the preferred method with which to stop massive hemoptysis, with reported success rates of up to 90%.[1] Emergency surgery is indicated for massive hemoptysis not controlled by rigid bronchoscopy or embolization and is generally considered a last resort.

Once a diagnosis is made, further treatment is directed at the cause.[2, 3]

Minor hemoptysis: Treatment of minor hemoptysis is directed at the cause.

Early resection may be indicated for bronchial adenoma or carcinoma. Broncholithiasis (erosion of a calcified lymph node into an adjacent bronchus) may require pulmonary resection if the stone cannot be removed via rigid bronchoscopy. Bleeding secondary to heart failure or mitral stenosis usually responds to specific therapy for heart failure. In rare cases, emergency mitral valvulotomy is necessary for life-threatening hemoptysis due to mitral stenosis.

Bleeding from a pulmonary embolism is rarely massive and almost always stops spontaneously. If emboli recur and bleeding persists, anticoagulation may be contraindicated, and placement of an inferior vena cava filter is the treatment of choice.

Because bleeding from bronchiectatic areas usually results from infection, treatment of the infection with appropriate antibiotics and postural drainage is essential.

1. Mal H, Rullon I, Mellot F, et al: Immediate and long-term results of bronchial artery embolization for life-threatening hemoptysis. *Chest* 150(4):996–1001, 1999.
2. Lordan JL, Gascoigne A, Corris PA. The pulmonary physician in critical care. Illustrative case 7: Assessment and management of massive haemoptysis. *Thorax* 58:814–819, 2003.
3. Jean-Baptiste E. Clinical assessment and management of massive hemoptysis. *Critical Care Medicine* 28(5):1642–1647, 2000.

KEY POINTS

- Hemoptysis needs to be distinguished from hematemesis and nasopharyngeal or oropharyngeal bleeding.
- Bronchitis, bronchiectasis, TB, and necrotizing pneumonia or lung abscess are the most common causes in adults.
- Lower respiratory tract infection and foreign body aspiration are the most common causes in children.
- Patients with massive hemoptysis require treatment and stabilization before testing.
- With massive hemoptysis, if the side of bleeding is known, patients should be positioned with the affected lung in the dependent position.
- Bronchial artery embolization is the preferred treatment for massive hemoptysis.

HYPERVENTILATION SYNDROME

Hyperventilation syndrome is anxiety-related dyspnea and tachypnea often accompanied by systemic symptoms.

Hyperventilation syndrome most commonly occurs among young women but can affect either sex at any age. It is sometimes precipitated by emotionally stressful events. Hyperventilation syndrome is separate from panic disorder, although the two conditions overlap; about half of patients with panic disorder have hyperventilation syndrome and one quarter of patients with hyperventilation syndrome have panic disorder.

Hyperventilation syndrome occurs in 2 forms:

- Acute: Acute form is easier to recognize than the chronic.
- Chronic: Chronic hyperventilation is more common than acute.

Symptoms and Signs

Acute hyperventilation syndrome: Patients with acute hyperventilation syndrome present with dyspnea sometimes so severe that they liken it to suffocation. It is accompanied by agitation and a sense of terror or by symptoms of chest pain, paresthesias (peripheral and perioral), peripheral tetany (eg, stiffness of fingers or arms), and presyncope or syncope or sometimes by a combination of all of these findings. Tetany occurs because respiratory alkalosis causes both hypophosphatemia and hypocalcemia. On examination, patients may appear anxious, tachypneic, or both; lung examination is unremarkable.

Chronic hyperventilation syndrome: Patients with chronic hyperventilation syndrome present far less dramatically and often escape detection; they sigh deeply and frequently and often have nonspecific somatic symptoms in the context of mood and anxiety disorders and emotional stress.

Diagnosis

- Testing to exclude other diagnoses (chest x-ray, ECG, pulse oximetry)

Hyperventilation syndrome is a diagnosis of exclusion; the challenge is to use tests and resources judiciously to distinguish this syndrome from more serious diagnoses.

Basic testing includes

- Pulse oximetry
- Chest x-ray
- ECG

Pulse oximetry in hyperventilation syndrome shows oxygen saturation at or close to 100%. Chest x-ray is normal. ECG is done to detect cardiac ischemia, although hyperventilation syndrome itself can cause ST-segment depressions, T-wave inversions, and prolonged QT intervals.

ABGs are needed when other causes of hyperventilation are suspected, such as metabolic acidosis.

Occasionally, acute hyperventilation syndrome is indistinguishable from acute pulmonary embolism, and tests for pulmonary embolism (eg, D-dimer, ventilation/perfusion scanning, CT angiography) may be necessary.

Treatment

- Supportive counseling
- Sometimes psychiatric or psychologic treatment

Treatment is reassurance. Some physicians advocate teaching the patient maximal exhalation and diaphragmatic breathing. Most patients require treatment for underlying mood or anxiety disorders; such treatment includes cognitive therapy, stress reduction techniques, drugs (eg, anxiolytics, antidepressants, lithium), or a combination of these techniques.

SOLITARY PULMONARY NODULE

A solitary pulmonary nodule is defined as a discrete lesion < 3 cm in diameter that is completely surrounded by lung parenchyma (ie, does not touch the hilum, mediastinum, or pleura) and is without associated atelectasis or pleural effusion. (Evaluation of a mediastinal mass is discussed on p. 468.)

Solitary pulmonary nodules are most often detected incidentally when a chest x-ray is taken for other reasons. Nonpulmonary soft-tissue densities caused by nipple shadows, warts, cutaneous nodules, and bone abnormalities are often confused for a nodule on chest x-ray.

Etiology

Although cancer is usually the primary concern, solitary pulmonary nodules have many causes (see Table 48–6). Of these, the most common vary by age and risk factors, but typically include

- Granulomas
- Pneumonia
- Bronchogenic cysts

Table 48–6. SOME CAUSES OF A SOLITARY PULMONARY NODULE

CAUSE	EXAMPLES
Malignant causes*	
Primary lung cancer	Adenocarcinoma Small cell carcinoma
Metastatic cancer	Breast cancer Melanoma Colon carcinoma Head and neck cancer Renal carcinoma Testicular carcinoma Sarcoma
Nonmalignant causes	
Autoimmune disorders	Granulomatosis with polyangiitis Rheumatoid nodules
Benign tumors	Fibroma Hamartoma Lipoma
Granulomatous infection	Atypical mycobacterial infection Blastomycosis Coccidioidomycosis Cryptococcosis Histoplasmosis TB
Infection	Ascariasis Aspergilloma Bacterial abscess Dirofilariasis (dog heartworm infection) *Echinococcus* cyst *Pneumocystis jirovecii*
Pulmonary vascular abnormalities	Cavernous angioma Hemangioma Pulmonary arteriovenous malformation Pulmonary telangiectasis
Other	Amyloidosis Bronchogenic cyst Hematoma Intrapulmonary lymph node Loculated fluid Mucoid impaction Rounded atelectasis

*The likelihood of a malignant cause increases with age.

Evaluation

The primary goal of evaluation is to detect cancer and active infection.

History: History may reveal information that suggests malignant and nonmalignant causes of a solitary pulmonary nodule and includes

- Current or past cigarette smoking
- History of cancer or an autoimmune disorder
- Occupational risk factors for cancer (eg, exposure to asbestos, vinyl chloride, radon)
- Travel to, or living in, areas with endemic mycosis or a high prevalence of TB
- Risk factors for opportunistic infections (eg, HIV, immune deficiency)

Older age, cigarette smoking, and history of cancer all increase the probability of cancer and are used along with the nodule diameter to estimate likelihood ratios for cancer (see Table 48–7).

Physical examination: A thorough physical examination may uncover findings that suggest an etiology (eg, a breast lump or skin lesion suggestive of cancer) for a pulmonary nodule but cannot definitely establish the cause.

Testing: The goal of initial testing is to estimate the malignant potential of the solitary pulmonary nodule. The first step is a review of plain x-rays and then usually CT.

Table 48–7. ESTIMATING THE PROBABILITY OF CANCER IN A SOLITARY PULMONARY NODULE

I. Establish likelihood ratios (LRs)* for cancer with the following table:

FINDING	LR FOR CANCER
Diameter of nodule (cm)	
< 1.5	0.1
1.5–2.2	0.5[†]
2.3–3.2	1.7
3.3–4.2	4.3
4.3–5.2	6.6
5.3–6.0	29.4
Patient's age (yr)	
≤ 35	0.1
36–44	0.3
45–49	0.7
50–59	1.5
60–69	2.1[†]
70–83	5.7
Smoking history	
Never smoked	0.15
Pipe or cigar only	0.3
Ex-cigarette smoker	1.5
Current smoker or one who quit within past 9 yr (average number of cigarettes/day)	
1–9	0.3
10–20	1.0[†]
21–40	2.0
≥ 41	3.9
Quit smoking (yr)	
≤ 3	1.4
4–6	1.0
7–12	0.5
≥ 13	0.1
Overall prevalence	
Clinical settings	0.7[†]
Community surveys	0.1

II. Multiply the LRs for nodule diameter, patient's age, smoking history, and cancer prevalence to obtain an estimate of the odds of cancer in a solitary pulmonary nodule (OddsCA):

OddsCA = LR Size × LR Age × LR Smoking × LR Prev
In the example: OddsCA = (1.5 × 2.1 × 1.0 × 0.7) = 2.21:1

III. Convert the odds into a probability of cancer:

Probability of cancer (PCA) = OddsCA / (1 + OddsCA) × 100 = %
In the example: PCA (as %) = 2.21/(1 + 2.21) × 100 = 69%

*The LR is a measure of how predictive a finding is of disease and is defined as the probability of the finding being present in a patient with disease divided by the probability of the finding being present in a patient without disease; ie, it is the ratio of true positives to false positives or of sensitivity to 1– specificity.
[†]The example is a 65-yr-old who smokes 20 cigarettes/day and has a 2.0-cm nodule.
Adapted from Cummings SR, Lillington GA, Richard RJ: Estimating the probability of malignancy in solitary pulmonary nodules. A Bayesian approach. *The American Review of Respiratory Disease* 134(3):449–452, 1986.

Radiographic characteristics help define the malignant potential of a solitary pulmonary nodule:

- **Growth rate** is determined by comparison with previous chest x-ray or CT, if available. A lesion that has not enlarged in ≥ 2 yr suggests a benign etiology. Tumors that have volume doubling times from 21 to 400 days are likely to be malignant. Small nodules (< 1 cm) should be monitored at 3 mo, 6 mo, and then yearly for 2 yr.
- **Calcification** suggests benign disease, particularly if it is central (tuberculoma, histoplasmoma), concentric (healed histoplasmosis), or in a popcorn configuration (hamartoma).
- **Margins** that are spiculated or irregular (scalloped) are more indicative of cancer.
- **Diameter** < 1.5 cm strongly suggests a benign etiology; diameter > 5.3 cm strongly suggests cancer. However, nonmalignant exceptions include lung abscess, granulomatosis with polyangiitis, and hydatid cyst.

These characteristics are sometimes evident on the original plain film but usually require CT. CT can also distinguish pulmonary from pleural radiopacities. CT has a sensitivity of 70% and a specificity of 60% for detecting cancer.

PET imaging can help differentiate cancerous and benign nodules. PET is most often used to image nodules whose probability of being cancerous is intermediate or high. It has a sensitivity > 90% and a specificity of about 78% for detecting cancer. PET activity is quantified by the standardized uptake value (SUV) of (18)F-2-deoxy-2-fluoro-D-glucose (FDG). SUV > 2.5 suggests cancer, while nodules with SUV < 2.5 are more likely to be benign. However, both false-positive and false-negative results occur. False-negative results are more likely if nodules are < 8 mm. False-negative PET scans can result from metabolically inactive tumors, and false-positive results can occur in various infectious and inflammatory conditions.

Cultures may be useful when historical information suggests an infectious cause (eg, TB, coccidioidomycosis) as a possible diagnosis.

Invasive testing options include

- CT- or ultrasound-guided transthoracic needle aspiration
- Fiberoptic bronchoscopy
- Surgical biopsy

Although cancers can be diagnosed by biopsy, definitive treatment is resection, and so patients with a high likelihood of cancer with a resectable lesion should proceed to surgical resection. However, bronchoscopic endobronchial ultrasound-guided mediastinal lymph node biopsy is being used increasingly and is recommended by some experts as a less invasive way to diagnose and stage lung cancers before nodules are surgically resected.

Transthoracic needle aspiration is best for peripheral lesions and is particularly useful if infectious etiologies are strongly considered because using the transthoracic approach, as opposed to bronchoscopy, avoids the possibility of contamination of the specimen with upper airway organisms. The main disadvantage of transthoracic needle aspiration is the risk of pneumothorax, which is about 10%.

Fiberoptic bronchoscopy allows for endobronchial washing, brushing, needle aspiration, and transbronchial biopsy. Yield is higher for larger, more centrally located lesions, but very experienced operators using specially designed thin scopes can successfully biopsy peripheral lesions that are < 1 cm in diameter. In cases in which nodules are not accessible from these less invasive approaches, open surgical biopsy is necessary.

Treatment

- Sometimes surgery
- Sometimes observation

If the suspicion of cancer is very low, the lesions are very small (< 1 cm), or the patient refuses or is not a candidate for surgical intervention, observation is reasonable. Monitoring with follow-up at 3 mo, 6 mo, and then yearly for 2 yr is recommended. If the lesion has not grown for > 2 yr, it is likely benign.

When cancer is the most likely cause or when nonmalignant causes are unlikely, patients should undergo resection unless surgery is contraindicated due to poor pulmonary function, comorbidities, or withholding of consent.

STRIDOR

Stridor is a high-pitched, predominantly inspiratory sound. It is most commonly associated with acute disorders, such as foreign body aspiration, but can be due to more chronic disorders, such as tracheomalacia.

Pathophysiology

Stridor is produced by the rapid, turbulent flow of air through a narrowed or partially obstructed segment of the extrathoracic upper airway. Involved areas include the pharynx, epiglottis, larynx, and the extrathoracic trachea.

Etiology

Most causes manifest acutely, but some patients present with chronic or recurrent symptoms (see Table 48–8).

Acute causes are usually infectious except for foreign body and allergy. Chronic causes are usually congenital or acquired structural abnormalities of the upper airway. Transient or intermittent stridor can result from aspiration with acute laryngospasm or from vocal cord dysfunction.

Children: The most common causes of acute stridor in children include

- Croup
- Foreign body aspiration

Epiglottitis has historically been a common cause of stridor in children, but its incidence has decreased since the introduction of the *Haemophilus influenzae* type B (HiB) vaccine. Various congenital airway disorders can manifest as recurrent stridor in neonates and infants.

Adults: Common causes in adults include

- Vocal cord dysfunction (also called paradoxical vocal cord motion)
- Postextubation laryngeal edema
- Vocal cord edema or paralysis
- Laryngeal tumors
- Allergic reactions

Vocal cord dysfunction often mimics asthma, so many patients with vocal cord dysfunction are incorrectly given drugs for asthma but do not respond. Epiglottitis may be becoming more common among adults, but adults with epiglottitis are less likely than children to have stridor.

Evaluation

History: History of present illness should first identify whether symptoms are acute or chronic and whether transient or intermittent. If acute, any symptoms of URI (runny nose, fever, sore throat) or allergy (itching, sneezing, facial swelling, rash, potential allergen exposure) are noted. Recent intubation or neck surgery should be clinically obvious. If chronic, the age at onset (eg, since birth, since infancy, only in adulthood) and duration are determined, as well as whether symptoms are continuous or intermittent. For intermittent symptoms, provoking or exacerbating factors (eg, position, allergen exposure, cold, anxiety, feeding, crying) are sought. Important associated symptoms in all cases include cough, pain, drooling, respiratory distress, cyanosis, and difficulty feeding.

Review of systems should seek symptoms suggesting causative disorders, including heartburn or other reflux symptoms (laryngospasm); night sweats, weight loss, and fatigue (cancer); and voice change, trouble swallowing, and recurrent aspiration (neurologic disorders).

Past medical history in children should cover perinatal history, particularly regarding need for endotracheal intubation, presence of known congenital anomalies, and vaccination

Table 48–8. SOME CAUSES OF STRIDOR

CAUSE	SUGGESTIVE FINDINGS	DIAGNOSTIC APPROACH
Acute stridor		
Allergic reaction (severe)	Sudden onset after exposure to allergen Usually accompanied by wheezing and sometimes orofacial edema; itching No fever or sore throat; cough rare	Clinical evaluation
Croup	Age 6–36 mo Barking cough that is worse at night, URI symptoms, no difficulty swallowing, low-grade fever	Clinical evaluation Sometimes anteroposterior neck x-ray showing subglottic narrowing (steeple sign)
Epiglottitis	Mainly adults, as well as children who missed HiB vaccination Abrupt onset of high fever, sore throat, drooling, and often respiratory distress and marked anxiety Toxic appearance	Lateral neck x-ray if the patient is stable Examination in operating room if any signs of distress
Foreign body	Sudden onset in a toddler or young child who has no URI or constitutional symptoms In adults, foreign body in upper airway typically apparent by history	Direct or indirect laryngoscopy or bronchoscopy
Inhalation injury (eg, due to cleaning agents or smoke inhalation)	Clinically apparent recent toxic inhalation	Clinical evaluation Sometimes bronchoscopy
Postextubation complications (eg, laryngeal edema, laryngospasm, arytenoid dislocation)	Recent intubation and respiratory distress	Clinical evaluation Sometimes direct laryngoscopy
Retropharyngeal abscess	Mainly in children < 4 yr High fevers, severe throat pain, drooling, trouble swallowing, sometimes respiratory distress Swelling that may or may not be visible in the pharynx	Lateral neck x-ray Sometimes neck CT with contrast
Bacterial tracheitis (rare)	Barking cough that is worse at night, high fever, and respiratory distress Toxic appearance	Neck x-rays Sometimes direct or indirect laryngoscopy with visualization and culture of purulent tracheal secretions
Laryngospasm	Recurrent episodes, associated with gastroesophageal reflux or recent drug use or occurring after endotracheal intubation	Direct or indirect laryngoscopy
Vocal cord dysfunction	Recurrent episodes of unexplained stridor often with hoarseness, throat tightness, a choking sensation, and/or cough	Direct laryngoscopy
Chronic stridor		
Congenital anomalies (numerous; laryngomalacia most common)	Usually in neonates or infants Sometimes other congenital anomalies present Sometimes trouble feeding or sleeping Sometimes worse with URI	CT of neck and chest Direct laryngoscopy Spirometry with flow-volume loops
External compression	History of head and neck cancer or obvious mass, night sweats, and weight loss	X-ray of neck and chest CT of neck and chest Direct or indirect laryngoscopy
Laryngeal tumors (eg, squamous cell carcinoma, hemangiomas, small cell carcinoma)	Inspiratory or biphasic stridor that may progressively worsen as tumor enlarges	Direct or indirect laryngoscopy Spirometry with flow-volume loops
Congenital tracheomalacia	Chronic symptoms Stridor or barky cough during coughing, crying, or feeding May worsen in the supine position	CT or MRI Spirometry with flow-volume loops Sometimes bronchoscopy
Bilateral vocal cord paralysis or dysfunction	Recent trauma (eg, during birth, thyroid or other neck surgery, intubation, or deep airway suctioning) Various neurodegenerative or neuromuscular disorders present Good voice quality but limited intensity	Direct or indirect laryngoscopy

HiB = *Haemophilus influenzae* type B.

history (particularly HiB). In adults, history of prior endotracheal intubation, tracheotomy, recurrent respiratory infections, and tobacco and alcohol use should be elicited.

Physical examination: The first step is to determine the presence and degree of respiratory distress by evaluating vital signs (including pulse oximetry) and doing a quick examination. Signs of severe distress include cyanosis, decreased level of consciousness, low oxygen saturation (eg, < 90%), air hunger, use of accessory inspiratory muscles, and difficulty speaking. Children with epiglottitis may sit upright with arms braced on the legs or examination table, lean forward, and hyperextend the neck with the jaw thrust forward and mouth open in an effort to enhance air exchange (tripod position). Moderate distress is indicated by tachypnea, use of accessory muscles of respiration, and intercostal retractions. If distress is severe, further examination is deferred until equipment and personnel are arranged for emergency management of the airway.

Oropharyngeal examination of a patient (particularly a child) with epiglottitis may provoke anxiety, leading to functional obstruction and loss of the airway. Thus, if epiglottitis is suspected, a tongue depressor or other instrument should not be placed in the mouth. When suspicion is low and patients are in no distress, they may undergo imaging; others should be sent to the operating room for direct laryngoscopy, which should be done by an otolaryngologist with the patient under anesthesia.

If the patient's vital signs and airway are stable and acute epiglottitis is not suspected, the oral cavity should be thoroughly examined for pooled secretions, hypertrophic tonsils, induration, erythema, or foreign bodies. The neck is palpated for masses and tracheal deviation. Careful auscultation of the nose, oropharynx, neck, and chest may help discern the location of the stridor. Infants should be examined with special attention to craniofacial morphology (looking for signs of congenital malformations), patency of the nares, and cutaneous abnormalities.

Red flags: The following findings are of particular concern:

- Drooling and agitation
- Tripod position
- Cyanosis or hypoxemia on pulse oximetry
- Decreased level of consciousness

Interpretation of findings: The distinction between acute and chronic stridor is important. Other clinical findings are also often helpful (see Table 48–8).

Acute manifestations are more likely to reflect an immediately life-threatening disorder. With these disorders, fever indicates infection. Fever plus barking cough suggests croup or, very rarely, tracheitis. Patients with croup typically have more prominent URI symptoms and less of a toxic appearance. Fever without cough, particularly if accompanied by toxic appearance, sore throat, difficulty swallowing, or respiratory distress, suggests epiglottitis and, in young children, the less common retropharyngeal abscess. Drooling and the tripod position are suggestive of epiglottitis, whereas retropharyngeal abscess may manifest with neck stiffness and inability to extend the neck.

Patients without fever or URI symptoms may have an acute allergic reaction or aspirated foreign body. Acute allergic reaction severe enough to cause stridor usually has other manifestations of airway edema (eg, oral or facial edema, wheezing) or anaphylaxis (itching, urticaria). Foreign body obstruction of the upper airway that causes stridor is always acute but may be occult in toddlers (older children and adults can communicate the event unless there is near-complete airway obstruction, which will manifest as such, not as stridor). Cough is often present with foreign body but rare with allergic reaction.

Chronic stridor that begins early in childhood and without a clear inciting factor suggests a congenital anomaly or an upper airway tumor. In adults, heavy smoking and alcohol use should raise suspicion of laryngeal cancer. Vocal cord paralysis usually has a clear precipitant, such as surgery or intubation, or is associated with other neurologic findings, such as muscle weakness. Patients with tracheomalacia frequently have cough productive of sputum and have a history of recurrent respiratory infections.

Testing: Testing should include pulse oximetry. In patients with minimal respiratory distress, soft-tissue neck x-rays may help. An enlarged epiglottis or retropharyngeal space can be seen on the lateral view, and the subepiglottic narrowing of croup (steeple sign) may be seen on the anteroposterior view. X-rays may also identify foreign objects in the neck or chest.

In other cases, direct laryngoscopy can detect vocal cord abnormalities, structural abnormalities, and tumors. CT of the neck and chest should be done if there is concern about a structural abnormality, such as an upper airway tumor or tracheomalacia. Flow-volume loops can be useful in chronic and intermittent stridor to show the presence of an upper airway obstruction. Abnormal flow-volume loop findings generally require follow up with CT or laryngoscopy.

Treatment

Definitive treatment of stridor involves treating the underlying disorder. As a temporizing measure in patients with severe distress, a mixture of helium and oxygen (heliox) improves airflow and reduces stridor in disorders of the large airways, such as postextubation laryngeal edema, croup, and laryngeal tumors. The mechanism of action is thought to be reduced flow turbulence as a result of lower density of helium compared with oxygen and nitrogen.

Nebulized racemic epinephrine (0.5 to 0.75 mL of 2.25% racemic epinephrine added to 2.5 to 3 mL of normal saline) and dexamethasone (10 mg IV, then 4 mg IV q 6 h) may be helpful in patients in whom airway edema is the cause.

Endotracheal intubation should be used to secure the airway in patients with advanced respiratory distress, impending loss of airway, or decreased level of consciousness. When significant edema is present, endotracheal intubation can be difficult, and emergency surgical airway measures (eg, cricothyrotomy, tracheostomy) may be required.

KEY POINTS

- Inspiratory stridor is often a medical emergency.
- Assessment of vital signs and degree of respiratory distress is the first step.
- In some cases, securing the airway may be necessary before or in parallel with the physical examination.
- Acute epiglottitis is uncommon in children who have received HiB vaccine.

VOCAL CORD DYSFUNCTION

(Paradoxical Vocal Cord Motion)

Paradoxical or dysfunctional movement of the vocal cords is defined as adduction of the true vocal cords on inspiration and abduction on expiration; it causes inspiratory airway obstruction and stridor that is often mistaken for asthma. Vocal cord paralysis (unilateral and bilateral) is discussed elsewhere. The general evaluation of patients with stridor is discussed elsewhere.

Vocal cord dysfunction occurs more commonly among women aged 20 to 40. Etiology is unclear, but it appears to be associated with anxiety, depression, posttraumatic stress disorder, and personality disorders. It is not considered a factitious disorder (ie, patients are not doing it consciously).

Symptoms are usually inspiratory stridor and less often expiratory wheezing. Other manifestations can include hoarseness, throat tightness, a choking sensation, and cough.[1]

Diagnosis is made by observing inspiratory closure of the vocal cords with direct laryngoscopy. Sometimes a diagnosis of vocal cord dysfunction is entertained only after patients have been misdiagnosed as having asthma and then not responded to bronchodilators or corticosteroids.

Treatment involves educating the patient about the nature of the problem; counseling from a speech therapist on special breathing techniques, such as panting, which can relieve episodes of stridor and obstruction; and avoiding asthma misdiagnosis and treatment.

Vocal cord dysfunction associated with psychiatric diagnoses is often resistant to these measures. Referral for psychiatric counseling is indicated in these cases.

1. Christopher KL. Wood, II RP, Eckert RC, et al: Vocal-cord dysfunction presenting as asthma. *N Engl J Med* 308:1566–1570, 1983.

WHEEZING

Wheezing is a relatively high-pitched whistling noise produced by movement of air through narrowed or compressed small airways. It is a symptom as well as a physical finding.

Pathophysiology

Airflow through a narrowed or compressed segment of a small airway becomes turbulent, causing vibration of airway walls; this vibration produces the sound of wheezing.

Wheezing is more common during expiration because increased intrathoracic pressure during this phase narrows the airways. Wheezing during expiration alone indicates milder obstruction than wheezing during both inspiration and expiration, which suggests more severe airway narrowing.

By contrast, turbulent flow of air through a narrowed segment of the large, extrathoracic airways produces a whistling inspiratory noise (stridor).

Etiology

Small airway narrowing may be caused by bronchoconstriction, mucosal edema, or external compression, or partial obstruction by a tumor, foreign body, or thick secretions.

Overall, the most common causes are

- Asthma
- COPD

But wheezing may occur in other disorders affecting the small airways, including heart failure (cardiac asthma), anaphylaxis, and toxic inhalation. Sometimes, healthy patients manifest wheezing during a bout of acute bronchitis. In children, bronchiolitis and foreign body aspiration are also causes (see Table 48–9).

Evaluation

When patients are in significant respiratory distress, evaluation and treatment proceed at the same time.

History: **History of present illness** should determine whether the wheezing is new or recurrent. If recurrent, patients are asked the previous diagnosis and whether current symptoms are different in nature or severity. Particularly when the diagnosis is unclear, the acuity of onset (eg, abrupt or gradual), temporal patterns (eg, persistent vs intermittent, seasonal variations), and provoking or exacerbating factors (eg, current URI, allergen exposure, cold air, exercise, feeding in infants) are noted. Important associated symptoms include shortness of breath, fever, cough, and sputum production.

Review of systems should seek symptoms and signs of causative disorders, including fever, sore throat, and rhinorrhea (respiratory infection); orthopnea, paroxysmal nocturnal dyspnea, and peripheral edema (heart failure); night sweats, weight loss, and fatigue (cancer); nasal congestion, itching eyes, sneezing, and rash (allergic reaction); and vomiting, heartburn, and swallowing difficulties (gastroesophageal reflux disease with aspiration).

Past medical history should ask about conditions known to cause wheezing, particularly asthma, COPD, and heart failure. Sometimes the patient's drug list may be the only indication of such diagnoses (eg, inhaled bronchodilators and corticosteroids in COPD; diuretics and ACE inhibitors in heart failure). Patients with known disease should be asked about indicators of disease severity, such as previous hospitalization, intubation, or ICU admission. Also, conditions that predispose to heart failure are identified, including atherosclerotic or congenital heart disease and hypertension. Smoking history and exposure to secondhand smoke should be noted.

Physical examination: Vital signs are reviewed for presence of fever, tachycardia, tachypnea, and low oxygen saturation.

Any signs of respiratory distress (eg, accessory muscle use, intercostal retractions, pursed lip breathing, agitation, cyanosis, decreased level of consciousness) should be immediately noted.

Examination focuses on the lungs, particularly adequacy of air entry and exit, symmetry of breath sounds, and localization of wheezing (diffuse vs localized; inspiratory, expiratory, or both). Any signs of consolidation (eg, egophony, dullness to percussion) or crackles should be noted.

The cardiac examination should focus on findings that might indicate heart failure, such as murmurs, a 3rd heart sound (S_3 gallop), and jugular venous distention.

The nose and throat examination should note appearance of the nasal mucosa (eg, color, congestion), swelling of the face or tongue, and signs of rhinitis, sinusitis, or nasal polyps.

The extremities are examined for clubbing and edema, and the skin is examined for signs of allergic reactions (eg, urticaria, rash) or atopy (eg, eczema). The patient's general appearance is noted for constitutional signs, such as the cachexia and barrel chest of severe COPD.

Red flags: The following findings are of particular concern:

- Accessory muscle use, clinical signs of tiring, or decreased level of consciousness
- Fixed inspiratory and expiratory wheezing
- Swelling of the face and tongue (angioedema)

Interpretation of findings: **Recurrent** wheezing in a patient with a known history of disorders such as asthma, COPD, or heart failure is usually presumed to represent an exacerbation. In patients who have both lung and heart disease, manifestations may be similar (eg, neck vein distention and peripheral edema in cor pulmonale due to COPD and in heart failure), and testing is often required. When the cause is known asthma or COPD, a history of cough, postnasal drip, or exposure to

Table 48–9. SOME CAUSES OF WHEEZING

CAUSE	SUGGESTIVE FINDINGS	DIAGNOSTIC APPROACH*
Acute bronchitis	URI symptoms No known history of lung disease	Clinical evaluation
Allergic reaction	Sudden onset, usually within 30 min of exposure to known or potential allergen Often nasal congestion, urticaria, itchy eyes, sneezing	Clinical evaluation
Asthma	Often known history of asthma Wheezing arising spontaneously or after exposure to specific stimuli (eg, allergen, URI, cold, exercise)	Clinical evaluation Sometimes pulmonary function testing, peak flow measurement, methacholine challenge, or observation of response to empiric bronchodilators
Bronchiolitis	In children < 18 mo (usually from November to April in the Northern Hemisphere) Usually URI symptoms and tachypnea	Clinical evaluation
COPD exacerbation	In middle-aged or elderly patients Often known history of COPD Extensive smoking history Poor breath sounds Dyspnea Pursed lip breathing Use of accessory muscles	Clinical evaluation Sometimes chest x-ray and ABG measurement
Drugs (eg, ACE inhibitors, aspirin, beta-blockers, NSAIDs)	Recent initiation of a new drug, most often in a patient with a history of reactive airway disease	Clinical evaluation
Endobronchial tumors	Fixed and constant inspiratory and expiratory wheezes, especially in a patient with risk factors for or signs of cancer (eg, smoking history, night sweats, weight loss, hemoptysis) May be focal rather than diffuse	Chest x-ray or CT Bronchoscopy (usually preceded by spirometry with flow volume loops that indicate obstruction)
Foreign body	Sudden onset in a young child who has no URI or constitutional symptoms	Chest x-ray or CT Bronchoscopy
GERD with chronic aspiration	Chronic or recurrent wheezing, often with heartburn and nocturnal cough No URI or allergic symptoms	Trial of acid-suppressing drugs Sometimes esophageal pH monitoring
Inhaled irritants	Sudden onset after occupational exposure or inappropriate use of cleaning agents	Clinical evaluation
Left-sided heart failure with pulmonary edema (cardiac asthma)	Crackles and signs of central or peripheral volume overload (eg, distended neck veins, peripheral edema) Dyspnea while lying flat (orthopnea) or appearing 1–2 h after falling asleep (paroxysmal nocturnal dyspnea)	Chest x-ray ECG BNP measurement Echocardiography

*Most patients should have pulse oximetry. Unless symptoms are very mild or are clearly an exacerbation of a known chronic disease, chest x-ray should be done.

BNP = brain (B type) natriuretic peptide; GERD = gastroesophageal reflux disease.

allergens or to toxic or irritant gases (eg, cold air, dust, tobacco smoke, perfumes) may suggest a trigger.

Clinical findings help suggest a cause of wheezing in patients without a known history (see Table 48–9).

Acute (sudden-onset) wheezing in the absence of URI symptoms suggests an allergic reaction or impending anaphylaxis, especially if urticaria or angioedema is present. Fever and URI symptoms suggest infection, acute bronchitis in older children and adults, and bronchiolitis in children < 2 yr. Crackles, distended neck veins, and peripheral edema suggest heart failure. Association of wheezing with feeding or vomiting in infants can be a result of gastroesophageal reflux.

Patients with asthma usually have paroxysmal or intermittent bouts of acute wheezing.

Persistent, localized wheezing suggests focal bronchial obstruction by a tumor or foreign body. Persistent wheezing manifesting very early in life suggests a congenital or structural abnormality. Persistent wheezing with sudden onset is consistent with foreign body aspiration, whereas the slowly progressive onset of wheezing may be a sign of extraluminal bronchial compression by a growing tumor or lymph node.

Testing: Testing seeks to assess severity, determine diagnosis, and identify complications.

- Pulse oximetry
- Chest x-ray (if diagnosis unclear)
- Sometimes ABGs
- Sometimes pulmonary function testing

Severity is assessed by pulse oximetry and, in patients with respiratory distress or clinical signs of tiring, ABG testing. Patients known to have asthma usually have bedside peak flow measurements (or, when available, forced expiratory volume in 1 sec [FEV_1]).

Patients with new-onset or undiagnosed persistent wheezing should have a chest x-ray. X-ray can be deferred in patients with asthma who are having a typical exacerbation and in patients having an obvious allergic reaction. Cardiomegaly, pleural effusion, and fluid in the major fissure suggest heart failure. Hyperinflation and hyperlucency suggest COPD. Segmental or subsegmental atelectasis or infiltrate suggests an obstructing endobronchial lesion. Radiopacity in the airways or focal areas of hyperinflation suggest a foreign body.

If the diagnosis is unclear in patients with recurrent wheezing, pulmonary function testing can confirm airflow limitation and quantify its reversibility and severity. Methacholine challenge testing and exercise testing can confirm airway hyperreactivity in patients for whom the diagnosis of asthma is in question.

Treatment

Definitive treatment of wheezing is treatment of underlying disorders.

Wheezing itself can be relieved with inhaled bronchodilators (eg, albuterol 2.5 mg nebulized solution or 180 mg metered dose inhalation). Long-term control of persistent asthmatic wheezing may require inhaled corticosteroids and leukotriene inhibitors.

Intravenous H_2 blockers (diphenhydramine), corticosteroids (methylprednisolone), and subcutaneous and inhaled racemic epinephrine are indicated in cases of anaphylaxis.

KEY POINTS

- Asthma is the most common cause, but not all wheezing is asthma.
- Acute onset of wheezing in a patient without a lung disorder may be due to aspiration, allergic reaction, or heart failure.
- Reactive airway disease can be confirmed via spirometry.
- Inhaled bronchodilators are the mainstay of acute treatment.

49 Diagnostic and Therapeutic Pulmonary Procedures

Diagnostic tests besides pulmonary function testing include various types of

- Chest imaging
- Electrocardiography (ECG)
- Ventilation/perfusion scanning

Diagnostic and therapeutic procedures include

- Bronchoscopy
- Mediastinoscopy and mediastinotomy
- Needle thoracostomy
- Pleural biopsy
- Thoracentesis
- Thoracoscopy and video-assisted thoracoscopic surgery (VATS)
- Thoracotomy
- Transthoracic needle biopsy
- Tube thoracostomy

Pulmonary artery catheterization is discussed elsewhere.

Chest physiotherapy and pulmonary rehabilitation are also discussed elsewhere (see p. 507).

BRONCHOSCOPY

Bronchoscopy is the introduction of an endoscope into the airways. Flexible fiberoptic bronchoscopy has replaced rigid bronchoscopy for virtually all diagnostic, and most therapeutic, indications.

Rigid bronchoscopy is now used only when a wider aperture and channels are required for better visualization and instrumentation, such as when

- Investigating vigorous pulmonary hemorrhage (in which the rigid bronchoscope can better identify the bleeding source and, with its larger suction channel, can better suction the blood and prevent asphyxiation)
- Viewing and removing aspirated foreign bodies in young children
- Viewing obstructive endobronchial lesions for possible laser debulking or stent placement

Flexible bronchoscopes are nearly all color video–compatible, facilitating airway visualization and documentation of findings.

Diagnostically, flexible fiberoptic bronchoscopy (see Table 49–1) allows for

- Direct airway visualization down to, and including, subsegmental bronchi
- Sampling of respiratory secretions and cells via bronchial washings, brushings, and lavage of peripheral airways and alveoli
- Biopsy of endobronchial, parenchymal, and mediastinal structures

Therapeutic uses include suctioning of retained secretions, endobronchial stent placement, removal of foreign objects, and balloon dilation of airway stenoses.

Contraindications: Absolute contraindications include

- Untreatable life-threatening arrhythmias
- Inability to adequately oxygenate the patient during the procedure
- Acute respiratory failure with hypercapnia (unless the patient is intubated and ventilated)
- High-grade tracheal obstruction

Relative contraindications include

- Uncooperative patient
- Recent myocardial infarction
- Uncorrectable coagulopathy

Transbronchial biopsy should be done with caution in patients with uremia, superior vena cava obstruction, or pulmonary

Table 49–1. INDICATIONS FOR FLEXIBLE FIBEROPTIC BRONCHOSCOPY

PROCEDURE	INDICATION
Diagnostic	Abnormal chest radiograph: To diagnose the etiology of pneumonia* in an immunocompromised patient; in an immunocompetent patient with recurrent or nonresolving disease; or in a patient with a paratracheal/mediastinal/hilar mass, parenchymal mass, or nodule, especially in a proximal lung section
	Atelectasis (persistent)*
	Cough (persistent, unexplained)*
	Diffuse lung process (transbronchial lung biopsy)
	Evaluation for rejection in lung transplant recipient
	Evaluation of airway in a burn patient
	Evaluation for bronchial disruption in a patient with chest trauma
	Hemoptysis
	Lung abscess in an edentulous patient (suspect endobronchial lesion)
	Lung cancer staging
	Positive sputum cytology in a patient with a normal chest x-ray*
	Suspected tracheoesophageal fistula
	Unexplained hoarseness or vocal cord paralysis
	Wheeze (localized/fixed)
Therapeutic	Aspiration of retained secretions*, †
	Bronchopulmonary lavage (pulmonary alveolar proteinosis)
	Laser resection of tumor‡
	Management of bronchopleural fistula
	Photodynamic therapy‡
	Placement of airway stent‡
	Placement of endotracheal tube in a difficult situation (cervical injury, abnormal anatomy)
	Removal of foreign body‡

*Flexible fiberoptic bronchoscopy is indicated only after failure of less invasive investigations and treatments.

†Flexible fiberoptic bronchoscopy is not a substitute for chest physiotherapy, bronchodilator nebulization, and nasotracheal suctioning; it should be reserved for hypoxemia (in a ventilated patient) and/or lobar atelectasis secondary to impacted secretions refractory to conventional therapy.

‡Rigid bronchoscopy provides more control for instrumentation than flexible bronchoscopy and may be helpful.

hypertension because of increased risk of bleeding. Inspection of the airways is safe in these patients, however.

Procedure: Bronchoscopy should be done only by a pulmonologist or trained surgeon in a monitored setting, typically a bronchoscopy suite, operating room, or ICU (for ventilated patients).

Patients should receive nothing by mouth for at least 6 h before bronchoscopy and have IV access, intermittent BP monitoring, continuous pulse oximetry, and cardiac monitoring. Supplemental oxygen should be used. Premedication with atropine 0.01 mg/kg IM or IV to decrease secretions and vagal tone is common, although this practice has been called into question by recent studies.

Patients usually receive conscious sedation with short-acting benzodiazepines, opioids, or both before the procedure to decrease anxiety, discomfort, and cough. In some centers, general anesthesia (eg, deep sedation with propofol and airway control via endotracheal intubation or use of a laryngeal mask airway) is commonly used before bronchoscopy.

The pharynx and vocal cords are anesthetized with nebulized or aerosolized lidocaine (1 or 2%, to a maximum of 250 to 300 mg for a 70-kg patient). The bronchoscope is lubricated and passed either through the nostril, the mouth with use of an oral airway or bite block, or an artificial airway such as an endotracheal tube. After inspecting the nasopharynx and larynx, the clinician passes the bronchoscope through the vocal cords during inspiration, into the trachea and then further distally into the bronchi.

Several ancillary procedures can be done as needed, with or without fluoroscopic guidance:

- **Bronchial washing:** Saline is injected through the bronchoscope and subsequently aspirated from the airways.
- **Bronchial brushing:** A brush is advanced through the bronchoscope and used to abrade suspicious lesions to obtain cells.
- **Bronchoalveolar lavage:** 50 to 200 mL of sterile saline is infused into the distal bronchoalveolar tree and subsequently suctioned out, retrieving cells, protein, and microorganisms located at the alveolar level. Local areas of pulmonary edema created by lavage may cause transient hypoxemia.
- **Transbronchial biopsy:** Forceps are advanced through the bronchoscope and airway to obtain samples from one or more sites in the lung parenchyma. Transbronchial biopsy can be done without x-ray guidance, but evidence supports increased diagnostic yields and lower incidence of pneumothorax when fluoroscopic guidance is used.
- **Transbronchial needle aspiration:** A retractable needle is inserted through the bronchoscope and can be used to sample enlarged mediastinal lymph nodes or masses. Endobronchial ultrasonography (EBUS) can be used to help guide the needle biopsy.

Patients are typically given supplemental oxygen and observed for 2 to 4 h after the procedure. Return of a gag reflex and maintenance of oxygen saturation when not receiving supplemental oxygen are the two primary indices of recovery.

Standard practice is to obtain a posteroanterior chest x-ray after transbronchial lung biopsy to exclude pneumothorax.

Complications: Serious complications are uncommon; minor bleeding from a biopsy site and fever occur in 10 to 15% of patients. Premedication can cause oversedation with respiratory depression, hypotension, and cardiac arrhythmias. Rarely, topical anesthesia causes laryngospasm, bronchospasm, seizures, methemoglobinemia with refractory cyanosis, or cardiac arrhythmias or arrest.

Bronchoscopy itself may cause

- Minor laryngeal edema or injury with hoarseness
- Hypoxemia in patients with compromised gas exchange
- Arrhythmias (most commonly premature atrial contractions, ventricular premature beats, or bradycardia)
- Transmission of infection from suboptimally sterilized equipment (very rare)

Mortality is 1 to 4/10,000 patients. The elderly and patients with serious comorbidities (severe COPD, coronary artery disease, pneumonia with hypoxemia, advanced cancers, mental dysfunction) are at greatest risk.

Transbronchial biopsy can cause pneumothorax (2 to 5%), significant hemorrhage (1 to 1.5%), or death (0.1%), but doing the procedure can often avoid the need for thoracotomy.

CHEST IMAGING

Imaging includes use of x-rays, MRI, nuclear scanning, and ultrasonography.

There are no absolute contraindications to undergoing noninvasive imaging procedures except for MRI. The presence of metallic objects in the patient's eye or brain precludes MRI.

Presence of a permanent pacemaker or internal cardioverter-defibrillator is a relative contraindication. Additionally, gadolinium, when used as a contrast agent for MRI, increases risk of nephrogenic systemic fibrosis in patients with stage 4 or 5 chronic kidney disease.

X-Ray Techniques

X-ray techniques that are used to image the chest include plain x-rays, fluoroscopy, high-resolution and helical (spiral) CT, and CT angiography.

Chest x-ray: Plain chest x-rays and fluoroscopy are used to provide images of the lungs and surrounding structures.

Plain chest x-rays provide images of structures in and around the thorax and are most useful for identifying abnormalities in the heart, lung parenchyma, pleura, chest wall, diaphragm, mediastinum, and hilum. They are usually the initial test done to evaluate the lungs.

The standard chest x-ray is taken from back to front (posteroanterior view) to minimize x-ray scatter that could artifactually enlarge the cardiac silhouette and from the side of the thorax (lateral view). Lordotic or oblique views can be obtained to evaluate pulmonary nodules or to clarify abnormalities that may be due to superimposed structures, although chest CT provides more information and has largely superseded these views. Lateral decubitus views may be used to distinguish free-flowing from loculated pleural effusion, but CT or ultrasonography can provide more information. End-expiratory views can be used to detect small pneumothoraxes.

Screening chest x-rays are often done but are almost never indicated; one exception is in asymptomatic patients with positive tuberculin skin test results, in whom a single posteroanterior chest x-ray without a lateral view is used to make decisions regarding additional diagnostic studies and/or treatment for pulmonary TB. Portable (usually anteroposterior) chest x-rays are almost always suboptimal and should be used only when patients are too ill to be transported to the radiology department.

Chest fluoroscopy is the use of a continuous x-ray beam to image movement. It is useful for detecting unilateral diaphragmatic paralysis. During a sniff test, in which the patient is instructed to forcibly inhale through the nose (or sniff), a paralyzed hemidiaphragm moves cranially (paradoxically) while the unaffected hemidiaphragm moves caudally.

Computed tomography: CT defines intrathoracic structures and abnormalities more clearly than does a chest x-ray. Conventional (planar) CT provides multiple 10-mm–thick cross-sectional images through the thorax. Its main advantage is wide availability. Disadvantages are motion artifact and limited detail from volume averaging of tissue within each 10-mm slice.

Chest CT is normally done at full inspiration. Aeration of the lungs during imaging provides the best views of the lung parenchyma, airways, and vasculature, and of abnormal findings such as masses, infiltrates, or fibrosis.

High-resolution CT (HRCT) provides 1-mm–thick cross-sectional images. HRCT is particularly helpful in evaluating

- Interstitial lung diseases (eg, lymphangitic carcinomatosis, sarcoidosis, fibrosing alveolitis)
- Bronchiectasis

Obtaining HRCT images at full expiration as well as full inspiration can help. Expiratory imaging can document air trapping, which is typical of obliterative bronchiolitis and other airway diseases. Images obtained with the patient in the prone position can help differentiate dependent atelectasis (which changes with changes in body position) due to lung disorders that cause ground-glass attenuation in the dependent posterior parts of the lungs, which persists despite changes in patient position (eg, fibrosis due to idiopathic pulmonary fibrosis, asbestosis, or systemic sclerosis).

Helical (spiral) CT provides multiplanar images of the entire chest as patients hold their breath for 8 to 10 sec while being moved continuously through the CT gantry. Helical CT is thought to be at least equivalent to conventional CT for most purposes. Its main advantages are speed, less radiation exposure, and an ability to construct 3-dimensional images. Software can also generate images of bronchial mucosa (virtual bronchoscopy). Its main disadvantages are less availability and the requirement for breath-holding, which can be difficult for patients with symptomatic pulmonary disease. Newer multidetector CT technology allows more rapid scanning of the entire chest with imaging of thin slices at high resolution.

CT angiography uses a bolus of IV radiopaque contrast agent to highlight the pulmonary arteries, which is useful in diagnosis of pulmonary embolism. Contrast agent load is comparable to that with conventional angiography, but the test is quicker and less invasive. Several studies have confirmed CT angiography provides sufficient accuracy for the detection of pulmonary emboli, so it has largely replaced conventional pulmonary angiography and, except in patients unable to tolerate contrast agents, ventilation/perfusion (V/Q) scanning.

Magnetic Resonance Imaging

MRI has a relatively limited role in pulmonary imaging but is preferred over CT in specific circumstances, such as assessment of superior sulcus tumors, possible cysts, and other lesions that abut the chest wall.

In patients with suspected pulmonary embolism in whom IV contrast agents cannot be used, MRI can sometimes identify large proximal emboli but usually is limited in this disorder.

Advantages include absence of radiation exposure, excellent visualization of vascular structures, lack of artifact due to bone, and excellent soft-tissue contrast.

Disadvantages include respiratory and cardiac motion, the time it takes to do the procedure, the expense of MRI, and the occasional presence of contraindications, which include implanted devices, certain metallic foreign bodies, and pregnancy.

Ultrasonography

Ultrasonography is often used to facilitate procedures such as thoracentesis and central venous catheter insertion.

Ultrasonography is also very useful for evaluating presence and size of pleural effusions and is now commonly used at the bedside to guide thoracentesis. Bedside ultrasound is also becoming popular to diagnose pneumothoraxes.

EBUS is increasingly being used in conjunction with fiberoptic bronchoscopy to help localize masses and enlarged lymph nodes. Diagnostic yield of transbronchial lymph node aspiration is higher using EBUS than conventional unguided techniques.

Nuclear Scanning

Nuclear scanning techniques used to image the chest include

- Ventilation/perfusion (V/Q) scanning
- Positron emission tomography (PET)

V/Q scanning: V/Q scanning uses inhaled radionuclides to detect ventilation and IV radionuclides to detect perfusion. Areas of ventilation without perfusion, perfusion without ventilation, or matched increases and decreases in both can be detected with 6 to 8 views of the lungs.

V/Q scanning is most commonly used for diagnosing pulmonary embolism but has largely been replaced by CT angiography. However, V/Q scanning is still indicated in the diagnostic evaluation for chronic thromboembolic pulmonary hypertension.

Split-function ventilation scanning, in which the degree of ventilation is quantified for each lobe, is used to predict the effect of lobar or lung resection on pulmonary function; post-surgical forced expiratory volume in 1 sec (FEV_1) is estimated as the percentage of uptake of ventilation tracer in the healthy fraction of the lungs multiplied by preoperative FEV_1 (in liters). A value of < 0.8 L (or < 40% of that predicted for the patient) indicates limited pulmonary reserve and a high likelihood of unacceptably high perioperative morbidity and mortality.

PET: PET uses radioactively labeled glucose (fluorodeoxyglucose) to measure metabolic activity in tissues. It is used in pulmonary disorders to determine

- Whether lung nodules or mediastinal lymph nodes harbor tumor (metabolic staging)
- Whether cancer is recurrent in previously irradiated, scarred areas of the lung

PET is superior to CT for mediastinal staging because PET can identify tumor in normal-sized lymph nodes and at extrathoracic sites, thereby decreasing the need for invasive procedures such as mediastinoscopy and needle biopsy.

Current spatial resolution of PET is 7 to 8 mm; thus, the test is not useful for lesions < 1 cm. PET reveals metastatic disease in up to 14% of patients in whom it would not otherwise be suspected. The sensitivity of PET (80 to 95%) is comparable to that of histologic tissue examination. False-positive results can occur with inflammatory lesions, such as granulomas. Slowly growing tumors (eg, bronchoalveolar carcinoma, carcinoid tumor, some metastatic cancers) may cause false-negative results.

Newer combined CT-PET scanners may become the most cost-effective technology for lung cancer diagnosis and staging.

ELECTROCARDIOGRAPHY IN PULMONARY DISORDERS

ECG is a useful adjunct to other pulmonary tests because it provides information about the right side of the heart and therefore pulmonary disorders such as chronic pulmonary hypertension and pulmonary embolism.

Chronic pulmonary hypertension leading to chronic right atrial and ventricular hypertrophy and dilation may manifest as prominent P waves (P pulmonale) and ST-segment depression in leads II, III, and aVF; rightward shift in QRS axis; inferior shift of the P wave vector; and decreased progression of R waves in precordial leads.

COPD patients commonly have low voltage due to interposition of hyperexpanded lungs between the heart and ECG electrodes.

Pulmonary embolism (submassive or massive) may cause acute right ventricle overload or failure, which manifests classically (but not commonly) as right axis deviation (R > S in V_1), with S-wave deepening in lead I, Q-wave deepening in lead III, and ST-segment elevation and T-wave inversion in lead III and the precordial leads ($S_1Q_3T_3$ pattern). Right bundle branch block also sometimes occurs.

MEDIASTINOSCOPY AND MEDIASTINOTOMY

Mediastinoscopy is introduction of an endoscope into the mediastinum.

Mediastinotomy is surgical opening of the mediastinum.

The two procedures are complementary. Mediastinotomy gives direct access to aortopulmonary window lymph nodes, which are inaccessible by mediastinoscopy.

Indications: Both procedures are done to evaluate or excise mediastinal lymphadenopathy or masses and to stage cancers (eg, lung cancer, esophageal cancer), although PET scanning and endobronchial ultrasound-guided transbronchial needle aspiration are decreasing the need for these procedures for cancer staging.

Contraindications: Contraindications include the following:

- Superior vena cava syndrome
- Previous mediastinal irradiation
- Median sternotomy
- Tracheostomy
- Aneurysm of the aortic arch

Mediastinoscopy and mediastinotomy are done by surgeons in an operating room using general anesthesia.

For **mediastinoscopy,** an incision is made in the suprasternal notch, and the soft tissue of the neck is bluntly dissected down to the trachea and distally to the carina. A mediastinoscope is inserted into the space allowing access to the paratracheal, tracheobronchial, azygous, and subcarinal nodes and to the superior posterior mediastinum.

Anterior mediastinotomy (the Chamberlain procedure) is surgical entry to the mediastinum through an incision in the parasternal 2nd left intercostal space, allowing access to anterior mediastinal and aortopulmonary window lymph nodes, common sites of metastases for left upper lobe lung cancers.

Complications: Complications occur in < 1% of patients and include bleeding, infection, vocal cord paralysis due to recurrent laryngeal nerve damage, chylothorax due to duct injury, esophageal perforation, and pneumothorax.

HOW TO DO NEEDLE THORACOSTOMY

Needle thoracostomy is insertion of a needle into the pleural space to decompress a tension pneumothorax. This is an emergency, potentially life-saving, procedure that can be done if tube thoracostomy cannot be done quickly enough.

Indications:

- Tension pneumothorax that must be decompressed before tube thoracostomy can be done

Contraindications: There are no **absolute contraindications** because this procedure should be done only in life-threatening conditions. Relative contraindications include hemodynamic stability or a bleeding disorder.

Complications:

- Pulmonary or diaphragmatic laceration
- Intercostal neuralgia due to injury of the neurovascular bundle below a rib
- Bleeding
- Infection
- Rarely perforation of other structures in the chest or abdomen

Equipment:

- A 14- or 16-gauge needle (an over-the-needle catheter is best); 8-cm needles are more successful than 5-cm needles but increase the risk of injury to underlying structures
- Sterile gown, mask, gloves
- Cleansing solution such as 2% chlorhexidine solution

Additional considerations:

- The urgency of the procedure is determined by the patient's condition. Hypotension suggests a more advanced tension pneumothorax requiring more urgent treatment.

Positioning:

- Patient should be supine, lying on the back

Relevant anatomy:

- Neurovascular bundles are located at the lower edge of each rib. Therefore, the needle must be placed over the upper edge of the rib to avoid damage to the neurovascular bundle.

Step-by-step description of procedure and key teaching points:

- The preferred insertion site is the 2nd intercostal space in the mid-clavicular line in the affected hemithorax. However, insertion of the needle virtually anywhere in the correct hemothorax will decompress a tension pneumothorax.
- If time permits, prepare the area at and around the insertion site using an antiseptic solution such as chlorhexidine.
- There is rarely time to provide local anesthesia, but if there is, inject 1% lidocaine into the skin, subcutaneous tissue, rib periosteum (of the rib below the insertion site), and the parietal pleura. Inject a large amount of local anesthetic around the highly pain-sensitive periosteum and parietal pleura. Aspirate with the syringe before injecting lidocaine to avoid injection into a blood vessel. Proper location is confirmed by return of air in the anesthetic syringe when entering the pleural space.
- Insert the thoracostomy needle, piercing the skin over the rib below the target interspace, then directing the needle cephalad over the rib until the pleura is punctured (usually indicated by a pop and/or sudden decrease in resistance).
- After doing a needle thoracostomy, insert a chest tube as soon as possible.

Warnings and common errors:

- Depending on the thickness of the chest wall, a longer needle may be needed.

Tips and tricks:

- After removing the needle, the catheter may become blocked by kinking. Kinking is especially likely with smaller catheters, such as 14 and 16 gauges. Some sources recommend using a larger 10-gauge needle and catheter.[1-3]

1. Aho JM, Thiels CA, El Khatib MM, et al: Needle thoracostomy: clinical effectiveness is improved using a longer angiocatheter. *J Trauma Acute Care Surg* 80(2):272–277, 2016. doi: 10.1097/TA.0000000000000889.
2. Clemency BM, Tanski CT, Rosenberg M, et al: Sufficient catheter length for pneumothorax needle decompression: a meta-analysis. *Prehosp Disaster Med* 30(3):249–253, 2015. doi: 10.1017/S1049023X15004653.
3. Beckett A, Savage E, Pannell D, et al: Needle decompression for tension pneumothorax in Tactical Combat Casualty Care: do catheters placed in the midaxillary line kink more often than those in the midclavicular line? *J Trauma* 71(5 Suppl 1):S408–412, 2011. doi: 10.1097/TA.0b013e318232e558.

PLEURAL BIOPSY

Pleural biopsy is done to determine the cause of an exudative pleural effusion when thoracentesis is not diagnostic.

The yield of closed pleural biopsy is about twice as high for TB than it is for pleural cancers. Improved laboratory techniques, newer diagnostic tests for pleural fluid (eg, adenosine deaminase levels, interferon-gamma, PCR studies for suspected TB), and more widespread availability of thoracoscopy have made the procedure less necessary and therefore uncommonly done.

Percutaneous pleural biopsy should be done only by a pulmonologist or surgeon trained in the procedure and should be done only in patients who are cooperative and have no coagulation abnormalities. Technique is essentially the same as that for thoracentesis and can be done at the bedside; no specific additional patient preparation is necessary. At least 3 specimens obtained from one skin location, with 3, 6, and 9 o'clock positioning of the needle-cutting chamber, are needed for histology and culture.

Chest x ray should be done after biopsy because of increased risk of complications, which are the same as those for thoracentesis but with higher incidence of pneumothorax and hemothorax.

HOW TO DO THORACENTESIS

Thoracentesis is needle aspiration of fluid from a pleural effusion. It may be done for diagnosis or therapy.

Indications:

- Diagnostic thoracentesis: Indicated for almost all patients who have pleural fluid that is new or of uncertain etiology and is ≥ 10 mm in thickness on CT scan, ultrasonography, or lateral decubitus x-ray (see Fig. 59–2 on p. 473)
- Therapeutic thoracentesis: Indicated to relieve symptoms in patients with dyspnea caused by a large pleural effusion

Diagnostic thoracentesis is usually not needed when the etiology of the pleural fluid is apparent (eg, viral pleurisy, typical heart failure).

Selection of laboratory tests typically done on pleural fluid is discussed in pleural effusion.

If pleural fluid continues to reaccumulate after several therapeutic thoracenteses, pleurodesis (injection of an irritating substance into the pleural space) may help prevent recurrence. Pleurodesis is most commonly done to prevent reaccumulation of malignant effusions.

Contraindications: There are no **absolute contraindications** to thoracentesis.

Relative contraindications include

- Bleeding disorder or anticoagulation
- Uncertain fluid location
- Minimal fluid volume
- Altered chest wall anatomy
- Pulmonary disease severe enough to make complications life threatening
- Uncontrolled coughing

Complications: Major complications include

- Pneumothorax
- Bleeding (hemoptysis due to lung puncture)
- Re-expansion pulmonary edema and/or hypotension[1]
- Hemothorax due to damage to intercostal vessels
- Puncture of the spleen or liver
- Vasovagal syncope

Bloody fluid that does not clot in a collecting tube indicates that blood in the pleural space was not iatrogenic, because free blood in the pleural space rapidly defibrinates.

Equipment:

- Local anesthetic (eg, 10 mL of 1% lidocaine), 25-gauge and 20- to 22-gauge needles, and 10-mL syringe
- Antiseptic solution with applicators, drapes, and gloves
- Thoracentesis needle and plastic catheter
- 3-way stopcock
- 30- to 50-mL syringe
- Wound dressing materials
- Bedside table for patient to lean on
- Appropriate containers (eg, red top and purple top tubes, blood culture bottles) for collection of fluid for laboratory tests
- Evacuated containers (vacuum bottle) or collection bags for removal of larger volumes during therapeutic thoracentesis
- Ultrasound machine (if the procedure is ultrasonically guided)

Additional considerations:

- Thoracentesis can be safely done at the patient's bedside or in an outpatient setting.
- Ample local anesthetic is necessary, but procedural sedation is not required in cooperative patients.
- Thoracentesis needle should not be inserted through infected skin (eg, cellulitis or herpes zoster).
- Positive pressure ventilation can increase the risk of complications.
- If the patient is receiving anticoagulant drugs (eg, warfarin), consider giving fresh frozen plasma or another reversal agent prior to the procedure.
- Bloody fluid that does not clot in a collecting tube indicates that blood in the pleural space was not iatrogenic, because free blood in the pleural space rapidly defibrinates.
- Only unstable patients and patients at high risk of decompensation due to complications require monitoring (eg, pulse oximetry, ECG).

Positioning:

- Best done with the patient sitting upright and leaning slightly forward with arms supported.
- Recumbent or supine thoracentesis (eg, in a ventilated patient) is possible but best done with ultrasound or CT guidance.

Relevant anatomy:

- The intercostal neurovascular bundle is located along the lower edge of each rib. Therefore, the needle must be placed over the upper edge of the rib to avoid damage to the neurovascular bundle.
- The liver and spleen rise during exhalation and can go as high as the 5th intercostal space on the right (liver) and 9th intercostal space on the left (spleen).

Step-by-step description of procedure and key teaching points:

- Explain the procedure to the patient and obtain written informed consent.
- Confirm the extent of the pleural effusion by chest percussion and consider an imaging study; bedside ultrasonography is very helpful when available.[2] If the effusion is small or loculated, ultrasound should be used to identify the location of the fluid.
- Select a needle insertion point in the mid-scapular line at the upper border of the rib one intercostal space below the top of the effusion.
- Mark the insertion point and prepare the area with a skin cleansing agent such as chlorhexidine and apply a sterile drape while wearing sterile gloves.
- Using a 25-gauge needle, place a wheal of local anesthetic over the insertion point. Switch to a larger (20- or 22-gauge) needle and inject anesthetic progressively deeper until reaching the parietal pleura, which should be infiltrated the most because it is very sensitive. Continue advancing the needle until pleural fluid is aspirated and note the depth of the needle at which this occurs.
- Attach a large-bore (16- to 19-gauge) thoracentesis needle-catheter device to a 3-way stopcock, place a 30- to 50-mL syringe on one port of the stopcock and attach drainage tubing to the other port.
- Insert the needle along the upper border of the rib while aspirating and advance it into the effusion.
- When fluid or blood is aspirated, insert the catheter over the needle into the pleural space and withdraw the needle, leaving the catheter in the pleural space. While preparing to insert the catheter, cover the needle opening during inspiration to prevent entry of air into the pleural space.
- Withdraw 30 mL of fluid into the syringe and place the fluid in appropriate tubes and bottles for testing.
- If a larger amount of fluid is to be drained, turn the stopcock and allow fluid to drain into a collection bag or bottle. Alternatively, aspirate fluid using the syringe, taking care to periodically release pressure on the plunger.
- If a large amount of fluid (eg, > 500 mL) is withdrawn, monitor patient symptoms and blood pressure and stop drainage if the patient develops chest pain, dyspnea, or hypotension. Some clinicians recommend withdrawing no more than 1.5 L in 24 h, although there is little evidence that the risk of re-expansion pulmonary edema is directly proportional to the volume of fluid removed. Thus it may be reasonable for experienced operators to completely drain effusions in one procedure in properly monitored patients.
- Remove the catheter while patient is holding breath or expiring. Apply a sterile dressing to the insertion site.

Aftercare:

- Sometimes chest x-ray
- Analgesia with oral NSAIDs or acetaminophen if needed

- Advise patients to report any shortness of breath or chest pain; coughing is common after fluid removal and not a cause for concern.

It has been standard practice to obtain a chest x-ray after thoracentesis to rule out pneumothorax, document the extent of fluid removal, and view lung fields previously obscured by fluid, but evidence suggests that routine chest x-ray is not necessary in asymptomatic patients. A chest x-ray is needed for any of the following:

- The patient is ventilated
- Air was aspirated
- The needle was passed more than once
- Symptoms or signs of pneumothorax develop

Warnings and common errors:

- Be sure to adequately anesthetize the parietal pleura.
- Be sure to insert the thoracentesis needle just above the upper edge of the rib and not below the rib, to avoid the intercostal blood vessels and nerves at the lower edge of each rib.

Tips and tricks:

- When marking the insertion point, use a skin marking pen or make an impression with a pen so that the skin cleansing prep will not remove the mark.

1. Feller-Kopman D, Berkowitz D, Boiselle P, et al: Large-volume thoracentesis and the risk of reexpansion pulmonary edema. *Ann Thoracic Surg* 84:1656–1662, 2007.
2. Barnes TW, Morgenthaler TI, Olson EJ, et al: Sonographically guided thoracentesis and rate of pneumothorax. *J Clin Ultrasound* 33(9):1656–1661, 2005.

THORACOSCOPY AND VIDEO-ASSISTED THORACOSCOPIC SURGERY

Thoracoscopy is introduction of an endoscope into the pleural space. Thoracoscopy can be used for visualization (pleuroscopy) or for surgical procedures.

Surgical thoracoscopy is more commonly referred to as video-assisted thoracoscopic surgery (VATS).

Pleuroscopy can be done with the patient under conscious sedation in an endoscopy suite, whereas VATS requires general anesthesia and is done in the operating room. Both procedures induce a pneumothorax to create a clear view.

Indications: Thoracoscopy is used for

- Evaluating exudative effusions and various pleural and lung lesions when noninvasive testing is inconclusive
- Pleurodesis in patients with recurrent malignant effusions
- Breaking up loculations in patients with empyema

The diagnostic accuracy for malignant and tuberculous disease of the pleura is 95%.

Indications for VATS include

- Correction of spontaneous primary pneumothorax
- Bullectomy and lung volume reduction surgery in emphysema
- Wedge resection
- Lung parenchymal biopsy
- In some medical centers, lobectomy and even pneumonectomy

Less common indications for VATS are excision of benign mediastinal masses; biopsy and staging of esophageal cancer; sympathectomy for severe hyperhidrosis or causalgia; and repair of traumatic injuries to the lung, pleura, and diaphragm.

Contraindications: Contraindications are the same as those for thoracentesis.

An **absolute contraindication** is

- Adhesive obliteration of the pleural space

Biopsy is relatively contraindicated in patients with highly vascular cancers, severe pulmonary hypertension, and severe bullous lung disease.

Procedure: Although some pulmonologists do pleuroscopy, VATS is done by thoracic surgeons. Both procedures are similar to chest tube insertion; a trocar is inserted into an intercostal space through a skin incision, through which a thoracoscope is inserted. Additional incisions permit the use of video cameras and accessory instruments.

After thoracoscopy, a chest tube is usually required for 1 to 2 days.

Complications: Complications are similar to those of thoracentesis and include

- Postprocedural fever (16%)
- Pleural tears causing air leak (2%) and/or subcutaneous emphysema (2%)

Serious but rare complications include

- Hemorrhage
- Lung perforation
- Gas embolism

Patients are also at risk of the complications of general anesthesia.

THORACOTOMY

Thoracotomy is surgical opening of the chest. It is done to evaluate and treat pulmonary problems when noninvasive procedures are nondiagnostic or unlikely to be definitive.

Contraindications: Contraindications are those general to surgery and include

- Bleeding disorder or anticoagulation that cannot be corrected
- Acute cardiac ischemia
- Instability or insufficiency of major organ systems

Procedure: Three basic approaches are used:

- Limited anterior or lateral thoracotomy: A 6- to 8-cm intercostal incision is made to approach the anterior structures.
- Posterolateral thoracotomy: The posterolateral approach gives access to pleurae, hilum, mediastinum, and the entire lung.
- Sternal splitting incision (median sternotomy): When access to both lungs is desired, as in lung volume reduction surgery, a sternal splitting incision is used.

Patients undergoing limited thoracotomy require a chest tube for 1 to 2 days and in many cases can leave the hospital in 3 to 4 days.

Indications: The principal indications for thoracotomy are

- Lobectomy
- Pneumonectomy

Both lobectomy and pneumonectomy are done most commonly to treat lung cancer.

VATS has largely replaced thoracotomy for open pleural and lung biopsies.

Complications: Complications are greater than those for any other pulmonary biopsy procedure because of the risks of general anesthesia, surgical trauma, and a longer hospital stay with more postoperative discomfort. The greatest hazards are

- Hemorrhage
- Infection
- Pneumothorax
- Bronchopleural fistula
- Reactions to anesthetics

Mortality for exploratory thoracotomy ranges from 0.5 to 1.8%.

TRANSTHORACIC NEEDLE BIOPSY

Transthoracic needle biopsy of thoracic or mediastinal structures uses a cutting needle to aspirate a core of tissue for histologic analysis.

Indications: Transthoracic needle biopsy is done to evaluate

- Peripheral lung nodules or masses
- Hilar, mediastinal, and pleural abnormalities
- Undiagnosed infiltrates or pneumonias when bronchoscopy is contraindicated or nondiagnostic

When done with the use of CT guidance and with a skilled cytopathologist in attendance, transthoracic needle biopsy confirms the diagnosis of cancer with > 95% accuracy. Needle biopsy yields an accurate diagnosis in benign processes only 50 to 60% of the time.

Contraindications: Contraindications are similar to those of thoracentesis. Additional contraindications include the following:

- Mechanical ventilation
- Contralateral pneumonectomy
- Suspected vascular lesions
- Putrid lung abscess
- Hydatid cyst
- Pulmonary hypertension
- Bullous lung disease
- Intractable coughing
- Bleeding disorder or anticoagulation that cannot be corrected and platelet count < 50,000/μL

Procedure: Transthoracic needle biopsy is usually done by an interventional radiologist, often with a cytopathologist present. Under sterile conditions, local anesthesia, and imaging guidance—usually CT but sometimes ultrasonography for pleural-based lesions—a biopsy needle is passed into the suspected lesion while patients hold their breath.

Lesions are aspirated with or without saline.

Two or 3 samples are collected for cytologic and bacteriologic processing.

After the procedure, fluoroscopy and chest x-rays are used to rule out pneumothorax and hemorrhage.

Core needle biopsies are used to obtain a cylinder of tissue suitable for histologic examination.

Complications: Complications include

- Pneumothorax (10 to 37%)
- Hemoptysis (10 to 25%)
- Parenchymal hemorrhage
- Air embolism
- Subcutaneous emphysema

HOW TO DO TUBE THORACOSTOMY

Tube thoracostomy is insertion of a tube into the pleural space to drain air or fluid from the chest.

Indications:

- Pneumothorax that is recurrent, persistent, traumatic, large, under tension, or bilateral
- Pneumothorax in a patient on positive-pressure ventilation
- Symptomatic or recurrent large pleural effusion
- Empyema
- Hemothorax
- Chylothorax

Contraindications: There are no **absolute contraindications** to tube thoracostomy.

Relative contraindications include

- Coagulopathy or bleeding disorder (may require blood products or coagulation factors)

Complications:

- Malpositioning of the tube in the lung parenchyma, in the lobar fissure, under the diaphragm, or subcutaneously
- Blockage of the tube due to blood clots, debris, or kinking
- Dislodgement of the tube, requiring replacement
- Re-expansion pulmonary edema
- Subcutaneous emphysema
- Infection of residual pleural fluid or recurrent effusion
- Pulmonary or diaphragmatic laceration
- Intercostal neuralgia due to injury of the neurovascular bundle below a rib
- Bleeding
- Rarely perforation of other structures in the chest or abdomen

Equipment:

- Sterile gown, mask, gloves, and drapes
- Petroleum-based and regular gauze dressings and tape
- Cleansing solution such as 2% chlorhexidine solution
- 25- and 21-gauge needles
- 10-mL and 20-mL syringes
- Local anesthetic such as 1% lidocaine
- 2 Hemostat or Kelly clamps
- Nonabsorbable, strong silk or nylon suture (eg, 0 or 1-0)
- Scalpel (size 11 blade)
- Chest tube: Size ranges from 16 to 36 French (Fr) and depends on intended use (20 to 24 Fr for pneumothorax; 20 to 24 Fr for malignant pleural effusion; 28 to 36 Fr for complicated parapneumonic effusions, empyema, and bronchopleural fistula; 32 to 36 Fr for hemothorax)
- Suction
- Water seal drainage apparatus and connecting tubing

Additional considerations:

- Elective chest tube insertion is best done by a physician trained in the procedure. Other physicians can relieve a tension pneumothorax with needle thoracostomy.
- Chest tube placement is an inpatient procedure. If done in the emergency department, the patient is then admitted to the hospital.

Positioning:

- In a spontaneously breathing patient, the head of the bed is elevated 30 to 60° to limit the elevation of the diaphragm that occurs during expiration and thus decrease the risk of inadvertent intra-abdominal tube placement.
- The arm of the affected side can also be placed in a position over the patient's head or otherwise abducted.
- The hand can be placed behind the head.

Relevant anatomy:

- Neurovascular bundles are located at the lower edge of each rib. Therefore, the tube must be placed over the upper edge of the rib to avoid damage to the neurovascular bundle.

Step-by-step description of procedure and key teaching points:

- If there is time, explain the procedure and obtain consent whenever possible from the patient or next of kin.
- Connect a water seal suction apparatus sealed with sterile water to a source of suction. Usually, a commercially available apparatus that connects to wall suction and the thoracostomy tube with plastic connectors is used.
- The insertion site can vary based on whether air or fluid is being drained. For pneumothorax, the tube is usually inserted in the 4th intercostal space, and for other indications in the 5th intercostal space, in the mid-axillary or anterior axillary line.
- Mark the insertion site.
- Prepare the area at and around the insertion site using an antiseptic solution such as chlorhexidine.
- Drape the area.
- Inject a local anesthetic such as 1% lidocaine into the skin, subcutaneous tissue, rib periosteum (of the rib below the insertion site), and the parietal pleura. Inject a large amount of local anesthetic around the highly pain-sensitive periosteum and parietal pleura. Aspirate with the syringe before injecting lidocaine to avoid injection into a blood vessel. Proper location is confirmed by return of air or fluid in the anesthetic syringe when entering the pleural space.
- Estimate how deep the tube needs to be inserted so that all of the tube's holes are inside the pleural space, accounting for all subcutaneous and fat tissue, particularly in obese patients. Note or record the mark on the tube that should be then visible at the skin.
- Make a 1.5- to 2-cm skin incision, and then bluntly dissect the intercostal soft tissue down to the pleura by advancing a clasped hemostat or Kelly clamp and opening it. Identify the rib below the insertion site and move over the rib to find the pleural space above the rib. Then perforate the pleura with the clamped instrument (usually indicated by a pop and/or sudden decrease in resistance) and open in the same way.
- Use a finger to widen the tract and confirm entry into the pleural space and the absence of adhesions.
- Clamp the chest tube on the outside end.
- Insert the chest tube, with another clamp grasping the tip, through the tract and direct it inferoposteriorly for effusions, or apically for pneumothorax, until all of the tube's holes are inside the chest wall.
- Suture the chest tube to the skin of the chest wall using one of many suture methods. One way is to use a purse-string suture. In addition, place an interrupted suture next to the tube across the incision and tie the suture around the tube. Another method is to substitute a second interrupted suture across the incision on the other side of the tube for the purse string suture and tie that suture to the tube as well.
- Place a sterile dressing with petroleum gauze to help seal the wound over the site.
- Cut 2 sterile gauze pads halfway across and place them around the tube.
- Remove the draping.
- Tape the dressing in place using pressure dressings. Consider taping the outside part of the tube to the dressing or the patient separately.
- Connect the tube to the water seal suction apparatus to prevent air from entering the chest through the tube and to allow drainage with or without suction.

Aftercare:

- An anteroposterior chest x-ray should be obtained at the bedside to check the tube's position. If there are concerns about positioning or functioning of the chest tube, posteroanterior and lateral x-rays or a chest CT should be obtained.[1]
- The chest tube is removed when the condition for which it was placed resolves. With a pneumothorax, suction is stopped and the tube is placed on just water seal for several hours to ensure that the air leak has stopped and that the lung remains expanded. Chest x-ray is often repeated 12 to 24 h after the last evidence of an air leak before removing the tube. For pleural effusions or hemothorax, the tube is typically removed when the drainage is < 100 to 200 mL/day of serous fluid.
- Removal of a chest tube in patients on mechanical ventilation, especially those with high oxygen requirements, positive pressure ventilation, chronic lung disease, or increased risk of recurrent pneumothorax, should be done only after consultation with the pulmonary specialist.
- To remove the tube, the patient should be semi-erect. After removal of the sutures, at the moment of removal, the patient is asked to take a deep breath and then to forcibly exhale; the tube is removed during exhalation and the site is covered with petroleum gauze, a sequence that reduces the chance of pneumothorax during removal.
- The purse-string suture, if inserted during tube insertion, is closed, and/or additional sutures may be needed to close the incision.
- A chest x-ray should be repeated several hours after chest tube removal. If no pneumothorax is seen on the x-ray after chest tube removal, there is no need for further chest x-rays except as dictated by clinical changes in the patient's condition.

Warnings and common errors:

- The water seal suction apparatus must be kept 40 in (or 100 cm) below the patient to avoid retrograde flow of fluid or air back into the pleural space.
- Some clinicians recommend draining no more than 1.5 L of pleural fluid in 24 h due to a concern about causing re-expansion pulmonary edema. However, there is little evidence that the risk of re-expansion pulmonary edema is directly proportional to the volume of fluid removed. Thus, it is reasonable to completely drain effusions at the time of chest tube insertion in properly monitored patients.
- If the chest x-ray shows that the chest tube is not far enough into the chest and the aspiration holes in the tube are not in the chest cavity, the chest tube will need to be replaced. Simply advancing the chest tube can introduce non-sterile tubing into the chest.

- Common insertion errors include inadequate quantities of local anesthetic and an initial incision that is too small.[2, 3]
- Lock the stretcher before inserting the tube, which may take significant force.

Tips and tricks:

- Conscious sedation prior to the procedure can be used in selected cases.
- When marking the insertion point, use a skin marking pen or make an impression with a pen so that the skin cleansing prep will not remove the mark.[4]

1. Pacharn P, Heller DN, Kammen BF, et al: Are chest radiographs routinely necessary following thoracostomy tube removal? *Pediatr Radiol* 32(2):138–142, 2002.
2. Kim YW, Byun CS, Cha YS, et al: Differential outcome of fissure-positioned tube in closed thoracostomy for primary spontaneous pneumothorax. *Am Surg* 81(5):463–466, 2015.
3. Menger R, Telford G, Kim P, et al: Complications following thoracic trauma managed with tube thoracostomy. *Injury* 43(1):46–50, 2012.
4. Adrales, G, Huynh T. Broering B, et al: A thoracostomy tube guideline improves management efficiency in trauma patients. *J Trauma* 52(2):210–214, 2002.

50 Tests of Pulmonary Function

Pulmonary function tests provide measures of airflow, lung volumes, gas exchange, response to bronchodilators, and respiratory muscle function. Basic pulmonary function tests available in the ambulatory setting include spirometry and pulse oximetry; these tests provide physiologic measures of pulmonary function and can be used to quickly narrow a differential diagnosis and suggest a subsequent strategy of additional testing or therapy. More complicated testing includes measurement of lung volumes; lung, chest wall, and respiratory system compliance (which requires measurement of esophageal pressure); and complete cardiopulmonary exercise testing. These tests provide a more detailed description of physiologic abnormalities and the likely underlying pathology. The choice and sequence of testing are guided by information taken from the history and physical examination.

AIRFLOW, LUNG VOLUMES, AND FLOW-VOLUME LOOP

Airflow and lung volume measurements can be used to differentiate obstructive from restrictive pulmonary disorders, to characterize severity, and to measure responses to therapy. Measurements are typically reported as absolute flows and volumes and as percentages of predicted values using data derived from large populations of people presumed to have normal lung function. Variables used to predict normal values include age, sex, ethnicity, and height.

Airflow: Quantitative measures of inspiratory and expiratory flow are obtained by forced spirometry. Nose clips are used to occlude the nares.

In assessments of **expiratory flow,** patients inhale as deeply as possible, seal their lips around a mouthpiece, and exhale as forcefully and completely as possible into an apparatus that records the exhaled volume (forced vital capacity [FVC]) and the volume exhaled in the first second (the forced expiratory volume in 1 sec [FEV_1]—see Fig. 50–1). Most currently used devices measure only airflow and integrate time to estimate the expired volume.

In assessments of **inspiratory flow** and volume, patients exhale as completely as possible, then forcibly inhale. These maneuvers provide several measures. The FVC is the maximal amount of air that the patient can forcibly exhale after taking a maximal inhalation. The FEV_1 is the most reproducible flow parameter and is especially useful in diagnosing and monitoring patients with obstructive pulmonary disorders (eg, asthma, COPD). FEV_1 and FVC help differentiate obstructive and restrictive lung disorders. A normal FEV_1 makes irreversible obstructive lung disease unlikely whereas a normal FVC makes restrictive disease unlikely.

The forced expiratory flow averaged over the time during which 25 to 75% of the FVC is exhaled may be a more sensitive marker of mild, small airway airflow limitation than the FEV_1, but the reproducibility of this variable is poor. The peak expiratory flow (PEF) is the peak flow occurring during exhalation. This variable is used primarily for home monitoring of patients with asthma and for determining diurnal variations in airflow.

Interpretation of these measures depends on good patient effort, which is often improved by coaching during the actual

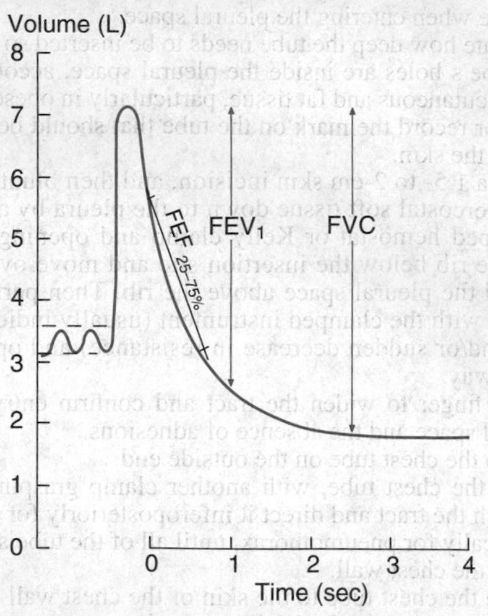

Fig. 50–1. Normal spirogram. $FEF_{25–75\%}$ = forced expiratory flow during expiration of 25 to 75% of the FVC; FEV_1 = forced expiratory volume in the first second of forced vital capacity maneuver; FVC = forced vital capacity (the maximum amount of air forcibly expired after maximum inspiration).

maneuver. Acceptable spirograms demonstrate good test initiation (eg, a quick and forceful onset of exhalation), no coughing, smooth curves, and absence of early termination of expiration (eg, minimum exhalation time of 6 sec with no change in volume for the last 1 sec). Reproducible efforts agree within 5% or 100 mL with other efforts. Results not meeting these minimum acceptable criteria should be interpreted with caution.

Lung volume: Lung volumes (see Fig. 50–2) are measured by determining functional residual capacity (FRC) and with spirometry.

FRC is measured using gas dilution techniques or a plethysmograph (which is more accurate in patients who have airflow limitation and trapped gas).

Gas dilution techniques include

- Nitrogen washout
- Helium equilibration

With nitrogen washout, the patient exhales to FRC and then breathes from a spirometer containing 100% O_2. The test ends when the exhaled nitrogen concentration is zero. The collected volume of exhaled nitrogen is equal to 81% of the initial FRC.

With helium equilibration, the patient exhales to FRC and then is connected to a closed system containing known volumes of helium and O_2. Helium concentration is measured until it is the same on inhalation and exhalation, indicating it has equilibrated with the volume of gas in the lung, which can then be estimated from the change in helium concentration that has occurred.

Both of these techniques may underestimate FRC because they measure only the lung volume that communicates with the airways. In patients with severe airflow limitation, a considerable volume of trapped gas may communicate very poorly or not at all.

Body plethysmography uses Boyle's law to measure the compressible gas volume within the thorax and is more accurate than gas dilution techniques. While sitting in an airtight box, the patient tries to inhale against a closed mouthpiece from FRC. As the chest wall expands, the pressure in the closed box rises. Knowing the pre-inspiratory box volume and the pressure in the box before and after the inspiratory effort allows for calculation of the change in box volume, which must equal the change in lung volume.

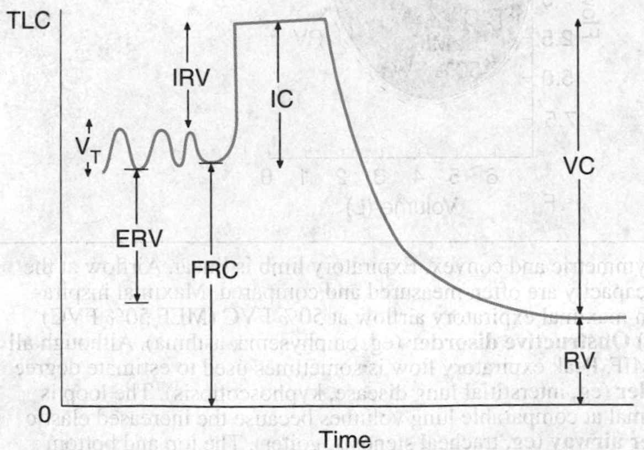

Fig. 50–2. Normal lung volumes. ERV = expiratory reserve volume; FRC = functional residual capacity; IC = inspiratory capacity; IRV = inspiratory reserve volume; RV = residual volume; TLC = total lung capacity; VC = vital capacity; V_T = tidal volume. FRC = RV + ERV; IC = V_T + IRV; VC = V_T + IRV + ERV.

Knowing FRC allows the lungs to be divided into subvolumes that are either measured with spirometry or calculated (see Fig. 50–2). Normally the FRC represents about 40% of total lung capacity (TLC).

Flow-volume loop: In contrast to the spirogram, which displays airflow (in L) over time (in sec), the flow-volume loop (see Fig. 50–3) displays airflow (in L/sec) as it relates to lung volume (in L) during maximal inspiration from complete exhalation (residual volume [RV]) and during maximum expiration from complete inhalation (TLC). The principal advantage of the flow-volume loop is that it can show whether airflow is appropriate for a particular lung volume. For example, airflow is normally slower at low lung volumes because elastic recoil is lower at lower lung volumes. Patients with pulmonary fibrosis have low lung volumes and their airflow appears to be decreased if measured alone. However, when airflow is presented as a function of lung volume, it becomes apparent that airflow is actually higher than normal (as a result of the increased elastic recoil characteristic of fibrotic lungs).

Flow-volume loops require that absolute lung volumes be measured. Unfortunately, many laboratories simply plot airflow against the FVC; the flow-FVC loop does not have an inspiratory limb and therefore does not provide as much information.

Patterns of Abnormalities

Most common respiratory disorders can be categorized as obstructive or restrictive on the basis of airflow and lung volumes (see Table 50–1).

Obstructive disorders: Obstructive disorders are characterized by a reduction in airflow, particularly the FEV_1 and the FEV_1 expressed as a percentage of the FVC (FEV_1/FVC). The degree of reduction in FEV_1 compared with predicted values determines the degree of the obstructive defect (see Table 50–2). Obstructive defects are caused by

- Increased resistance to airflow due to abnormalities within the airway lumen (eg, tumors, secretions, mucosal thickening)
- Changes in the wall of the airway (eg, contraction of smooth muscle, edema)
- Decreased elastic recoil (eg, the parenchymal destruction that occurs in emphysema)

With decreased airflow, expiratory times are longer than usual, and air may become trapped in the lungs due to incomplete emptying, thereby increasing lung volumes (eg, TLC, RV).

Improvement of FEV_1 and FEV_1/FVC by ≥ 12% or 200 mL with the administration of a bronchodilator confirms the diagnosis of asthma or airway hyperresponsiveness. However, some patients with asthma can have normal pulmonary function and normal spirometric parameters between exacerbations. When suspicion of asthma remains high despite normal spirometry results, provocative testing with methacholine, a synthetic analog of acetylcholine that is a nonspecific bronchial irritant, is indicated to detect or exclude bronchoconstriction. In a methacholine challenge test, spirometric parameters are measured at baseline and after inhalation of increasing concentrations of methacholine. Laboratories have different definitions of airway hyperreactivity, but in general patients showing at least a 20% drop in FEV_1 from baseline (PC_{20}) when the concentration of inhaled methacholine is < 1 mg/mL is considered diagnostic of increased bronchial reactivity, whereas a PC_{20} > 16 mg/mL

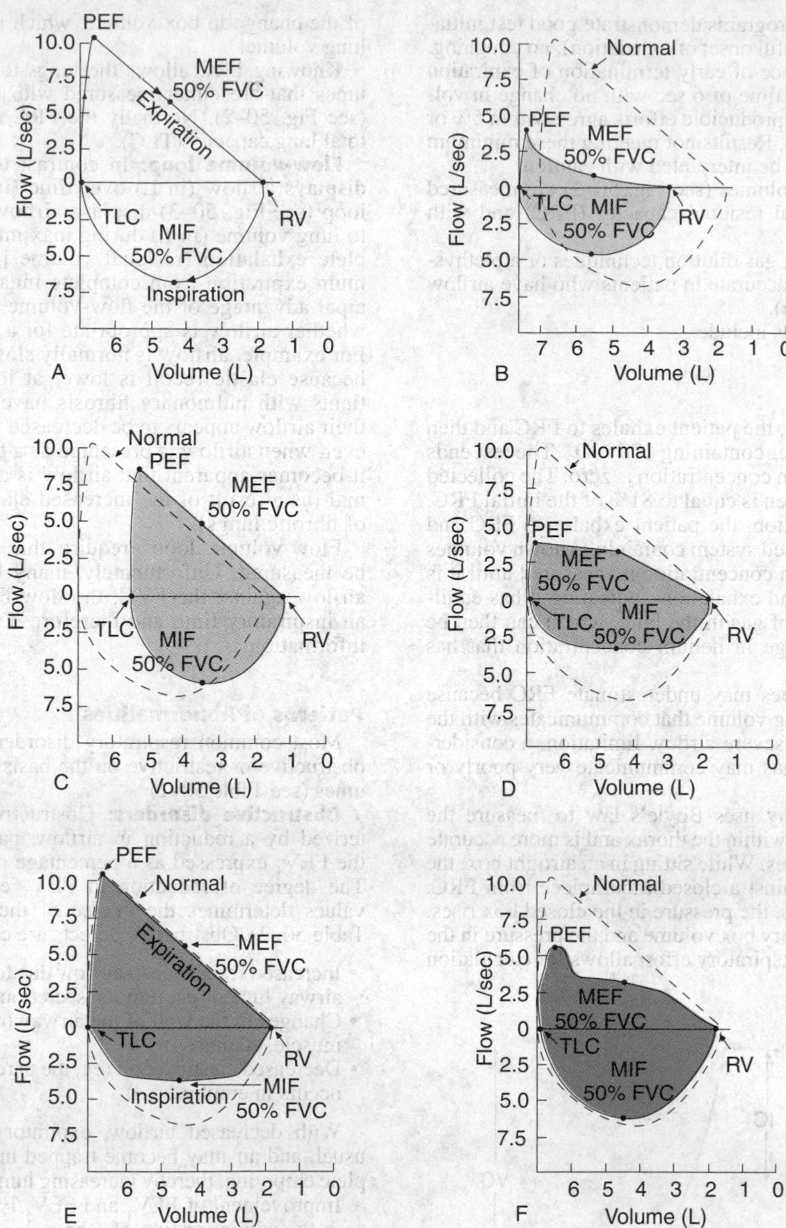

Fig. 50–3. Flow-volume loops. (A) Normal. Inspiratory limb of loop is symmetric and convex. Expiratory limb is linear. Airflow at the midpoint of inspiratory capacity and airflow at the midpoint of expiratory capacity are often measured and compared. Maximal inspiratory airflow at 50% of forced vital capacity (MIF 50% FVC) is greater than maximal expiratory airflow at 50% FVC (MEF 50% FVC) because dynamic compression of the airways occurs during exhalation. **(B) Obstructive disorder** (eg, emphysema, asthma). Although all airflow is diminished, expiratory prolongation predominates, and MEF < MIF. Peak expiratory flow is sometimes used to estimate degree of airway obstruction but depends on patient effort. **(C) Restrictive disorder** (eg, interstitial lung disease, kyphoscoliosis). The loop is narrowed because of diminished lung volumes. Airflow is greater than normal at comparable lung volumes because the increased elastic recoil of lungs holds the airways open. **(D) Fixed obstruction of the upper airway** (eg, tracheal stenosis, goiter). The top and bottom of the loops are flattened so that the configuration approaches that of a rectangle. Fixed obstruction limits flow equally during inspiration and expiration, and MEF = MIF. **(E) Variable extrathoracic obstruction** (eg, unilateral vocal cord paralysis, vocal cord dysfunction). When a single vocal cord is paralyzed, it moves passively with pressure gradients across the glottis. During forced inspiration, it is drawn inward, resulting in a plateau of decreased inspiratory flow. During forced expiration, it is passively blown aside, and expiratory flow is unimpaired. Therefore, MIF 50% FVC < MEF 50% FVC. **(F) Variable intrathoracic obstruction** (eg, tracheomalacia). During a forced inspiration, negative pleural pressure holds the floppy trachea open. With forced expiration, loss of structural support results in tracheal narrowing and a plateau of diminished flow. Airflow is maintained briefly before airway compression occurs.

Table 50–1. CHARACTERISTIC PHYSIOLOGIC CHANGES ASSOCIATED WITH PULMONARY DISORDERS

MEASURE	OBSTRUCTIVE DISORDERS	RESTRICTIVE DISORDERS	MIXED DISORDERS
FEV_1/FVC	Decreased	Normal or increased	Decreased
FEV_1	Decreased	Decreased, normal, or increased	Decreased
FVC	Decreased or normal	Decreased	Decreased or normal
TLC	Normal or increased	Decreased	Decreased, normal, or increased
RV	Normal or increased	Decreased	Decreased, normal, or increased

FEV_1 = forced expiratory volume in 1 sec; FVC = forced vital capacity; RV = residual volume; TLC = total lung capacity.

excludes the diagnosis. PC_{20} values between 1 and 16 mg/mL are inconclusive.

Exercise testing may be used to detect exercise-induced bronchoconstriction but is less sensitive than methacholine challenge testing for detecting general airway hyperresponsiveness. The patient does a constant level of work on a treadmill or cycle ergometer for 6 to 8 min at an intensity selected to produce a heart rate of 80% of predicted maximum heart rate. The FEV_1 and FVC are measured before and 5, 15, and 30 min after exercise. Exercise-induced bronchospasm reduces FEV_1 or FVC ≥ 15% after exercise. Eucapnic voluntary hyperventilation (EVH) may also be used to diagnose exercise-induced bronchoconstriction and is the method accepted by the International Olympic Committee. EVH involves hyperventilation of a gas mixture of 5% CO_2 and 21% O_2 at 85% of maximum voluntary ventilation for 6 min. FEV_1 is then measured at specified intervals after the test. As with other bronchial provocation tests, the drop in FEV_1 that is diagnostic of exercise-induced bronchospasm varies by laboratory.

Restrictive disorders: Restrictive disorders are characterized by a reduction in lung volume, specifically a TLC < 80% of the predicted value. The decrease in TLC determines the severity of restriction (see Table 50–2). The decrease in lung volumes causes a decrease in airflow (reduced FEV_1—see Fig. 50–3B). However, airflow relative to lung volume is increased, so the FEV_1/FVC ratio is normal or increased.

Restrictive defects are caused by the following:

- Loss in lung volume (eg, lobectomy)
- Abnormalities of structures surrounding the lung (eg, pleural disorder, kyphosis, obesity)
- Weakness of the inspiratory muscles of respiration (eg, neuromuscular disorders)
- Abnormalities of the lung parenchyma (eg, pulmonary fibrosis)

The feature common to all is a decrease in the compliance of the lungs, the chest wall, or both.

MEASUREMENT OF GAS EXCHANGE

Gas exchange is measured through several means, including diffusing capacity for carbon monoxide, pulse oximetry, and arterial blood gas sampling.

Diffusing Capacity for Carbon Monoxide

The diffusing capacity for carbon monoxide (DLco) is a measure of the ability of gas to transfer from the alveoli across the alveolar epithelium and the capillary endothelium to the RBCs. The DLco depends not only on the area and thickness of the blood-gas barrier but also on the volume of blood in the pulmonary capillaries. The distribution of alveolar volume and ventilation also affects the measurement.

DLco is measured by sampling end-expiratory gas for carbon monoxide (CO) after patients inspire a small amount of CO, hold their breath, and exhale. Measured DLco should be adjusted for alveolar volume (which is estimated from dilution of helium) and the patient's Hct. DLco is reported as mL/min/mm Hg and as a percentage of a predicted value.

Conditions that decrease DLco: Conditions that primarily affect the pulmonary vasculature, such as primary pulmonary

Table 50–2. SEVERITY OF OBSTRUCTIVE AND RESTRICTIVE LUNG DISORDERS*

	OBSTRUCTIVE		RESTRICTIVE
SEVERITY	FEV_1/FVC (% PREDICTED)	FEV_1 (% PREDICTED)	TLC (% PREDICTED)
Normal	≥ 70	≥ 80	≥ 80
Mild	< 70	≥ 80	70–79
Moderate	< 70	$50 \le FEV_1 < 80$	50–69
Severe	< 70	$30 \le FEV_1 < 50$	< 50
Very severe	< 70	< 30 *or* < 50 with chronic respiratory failure	—[†]

*Severity is based primarily on FEV_1/FVC and FEV_1 for obstructive disorders and on TLC for restrictive disorders.

[†]Criteria vary by guideline.

FEV_1 = forced expiratory volume in 1 sec; FVC = forced vital capacity; TLC = total lung capacity.

hypertension and pulmonary embolism, decrease DLco. Conditions that affect the lung diffusely, such as emphysema and pulmonary fibrosis, decrease both DLco and alveolar ventilation (V_A). Reduced DLco also occurs in patients with previous lung resection because total lung volume is smaller, but DLco corrects to or even exceeds normal when adjusted for V_A because increased additional vascular surface area is recruited in the remaining lung. Anemic patients have lower DLco values that correct when adjusted for Hb.

Conditions that increase DLco: DLco may be higher than predicted in patients with heart failure, presumably because the increased pulmonary venous and arterial pressure recruits additional pulmonary microvessels. DLco is also increased in patients with erythrocythemia, in part because of increased Hct and because of the vascular recruitment that occurs with increased pulmonary pressures due to increased viscosity. DLco is increased in patients with alveolar hemorrhage because RBCs in the alveolar space can also bind CO. DLco is also increased in patients with asthma. Although this increase is attributed to presumed vascular recruitment, some data suggest it may also be due to growth factor–stimulated neovascularization.

Pulse Oximetry

Transcutaneous pulse oximetry estimates O_2 saturation (Spo_2) of capillary blood based on the absorption of light from light-emitting diodes positioned in a finger clip or adhesive strip probe. The estimates are generally very accurate and correlate to within 5% of measured arterial O_2 saturation (Sao_2). Results may be less accurate in patients with highly pigmented skin; patients wearing nail polish; and patients with arrhythmias, hypotension, or profound systemic vasoconstriction, in whom the amplitude of the signal may be dampened. Also, pulse oximetry is able to detect only oxyhemoglobin or reduced Hb but not other types of Hb (eg, carboxyhemoglobin, methemoglobin); those types are assumed to be oxyhemoglobin and falsely elevate the Spo_2 measurement.

Arterial Blood Gas Sampling

ABG sampling is done to obtain accurate measures of Pao_2, $Paco_2$, and arterial pH; these variables adjusted for the patient's temperature allow for calculation of HCO_3 level (which can also be measured directly from venous blood) and Sao_2. ABG sampling can also accurately measure carboxyhemoglobin and methemoglobin.

The radial artery is usually used. Because arterial puncture in rare cases leads to thrombosis and impaired perfusion of distal tissue, Allen test may be done to assess adequacy of collateral circulation. With this maneuver, the radial and ulnar pulses are simultaneously occluded until the hand becomes pale. The ulnar pulse is then released while the pressure on the radial pulse is maintained. A blush across the entire hand within 7 sec of release of the ulnar pulse suggests adequate flow through the ulnar artery.

Under sterile conditions, a 22- to 25-gauge needle attached to a heparinized syringe is inserted just proximal to the maximal impulse of the radial arterial pulse and advanced slightly distally into the artery until pulsatile blood is returned. Systolic BP is usually sufficient to push back the syringe plunger. After 3 to 5 mL of blood is collected, the needle is quickly withdrawn, and firm pressure is applied to the puncture site to facilitate hemostasis. Simultaneously, the ABG specimen is placed on ice to reduce O_2 consumption and CO_2 production by WBCs and is sent to the laboratory.

Oxygenation

Hypoxemia is a decrease in Po_2 in arterial blood; hypoxia is a decrease in the Po_2 in the tissue. ABGs accurately assess the presence of hypoxemia, which is generally defined as a Pao_2 low enough to reduce the Sao_2 below 90% (ie, $Pao_2 < 60$ mm Hg). Abnormalities in Hb (eg, methemoglobin), higher temperatures, lower pH, and higher levels of 2,3-diphosphoglycerate reduce Hb O_2 saturation despite an adequate Pao_2, as indicated by the oxyhemoglobin dissociation curve (see Fig. 50–4).

Causes of hypoxemia can be classified based on whether the alveolar-arterial Po_2 gradient [(A-a)Do_2], defined as the difference between alveolar O_2 tension (PAo_2) and Pao_2, is elevated or normal. PAo_2 is calculated as follows:

$$PAO_2 = \left[FIO_2 \times \left(P_{atm} - P_{H_2O}\right)\right] - PaCO_2/R$$

where FIo_2 is the fraction of inspired O_2 (eg, 0.21 at room air), P_{atm} is the ambient barometric pressure (eg, 760 mm Hg at sea level), P_{H2O} is the partial pressure of water vapor (eg, usually 47 mm Hg), $Paco_2$ is the measured partial pressure of arterial CO_2, and R is the respiratory quotient, which is assumed to be 0.8 in a resting patient eating a normal diet.

For patients at sea level and breathing room air, $FIo_2 = 0.21$, and the (A-a)Do_2 can be simplified as follows:

$$(A - a)DO_2 = 150 - PaCO_2/0.8 - PaCO_2$$

where (A-a)Do_2 is typically < 20 but increases with age (because of age-related decline in pulmonary function) and with increasing FIo_2 (because, although Hb becomes 100% saturated at a Pao_2 of about 150 mm Hg, O_2 is soluble in blood, and the O_2 content of plasma continues to increase at increasing FIo_2). Estimations of normal (A-a)Do_2 values as < (2.5 + [FIo_2 × age in years]) or as less than the absolute value of the FIo_2 (eg, < 21 on room air; < 30 on 30% FIo_2) correct for these effects.

Hypoxemia with increased (A-a)Do_2: This situation is caused by

- Low ventilation/perfusion (V/Q) ratio (a type of V/Q mismatch)
- Right-to-left shunting
- Severely impaired diffusing capacity

Low V/Q ratio is one of the more common reasons for hypoxemia and contributes to the hypoxemia occurring in COPD and asthma. In normal lungs, regional perfusion closely matches regional ventilation because of the arteriolar vasoconstriction that occurs in response to alveolar hypoxia. In disease states, dysregulation leads to perfusion of alveolar units that are receiving less than complete ventilation (V/Q mismatch). As a result, systemic venous blood passes through the pulmonary capillaries without achieving normal levels of Pao_2. Supplemental O_2 can correct hypoxemia due to low V/Q

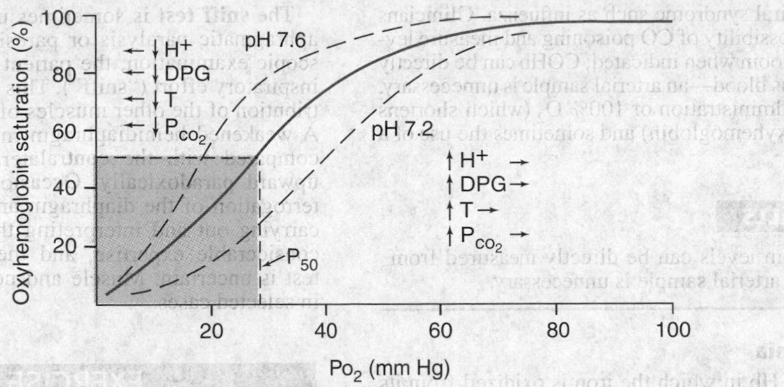

Fig. 50–4. Oxyhemoglobin dissociation curve. Arterial oxyhemoglobin saturation is related to Po_2. Po_2 at 50% saturation (P_{50}) is normally 27 mm Hg. The dissociation curve is shifted to the right by increased hydrogen ion (H^+) concentration, increased RBC 2,3-diphosphoglycerate (DPG), increased temperature (T), and increased Pco_2. Decreased levels of H^+, DPG, temperature, and Pco_2 shift the curve to the left. Hb characterized by a rightward shifting of the curve has a decreased affinity for O_2, and Hb characterized by a leftward shifting of the curve has an increased affinity for O_2.

ratio by increasing the Pao_2, although the increased (A-a)Do_2 persists.

Right-to-left shunting is an extreme example of low V/Q ratio. With shunting, deoxygenated pulmonary arterial blood arrives at the left side of the heart without having passed through ventilated lung segments. Shunting may occur through lung parenchyma, through abnormal connections between the pulmonary arterial and venous circulations, or through intracardiac communications (eg, patent foramen ovale). Hypoxemia due to right-to-left shunting does not respond to supplemental O_2.

Impaired diffusing capacity only rarely occurs in isolation; usually it is accompanied by low V/Q ratio. Because O_2 completely saturates Hb after only a fraction of the time that blood is in contact with alveolar gas, hypoxemia due to impaired diffusing capacity occurs only when cardiac output is increased (eg, with exercise), when barometric pressure is low (eg, at high altitudes), or when > 50% of the pulmonary parenchyma is destroyed. As with low V/Q ratio, the (A-a)Do_2 is increased, but Pao_2 can be increased by increasing the Fio_2. Hypoxemia due to impaired diffusing capacity responds to supplemental O_2.

Hypoxemia with normal (A-a)Do_2: This situation is caused by

- Hypoventilation
- Low partial pressures of inspired O_2 (Pio_2)

Hypoventilation (reduced alveolar ventilation) decreases the P_{AO_2} and increases the $Paco_2$, thereby decreasing Pao_2. In cases of pure hypoventilation, the (A-a)Do_2 is normal. Causes of hypoventilation include decreased respiratory rate or depth (eg, due to neuromuscular disorders, severe obesity, or drug overdose, or in compensation for metabolic alkalosis) or an increase in the fraction of dead space ventilation in patients already at their maximal ventilatory limit (eg, an exacerbation of severe COPD). Hypoventilatory hypoxemia responds to supplemental O_2.

Decreased Pio_2 is a final uncommon cause of hypoxemia that in most cases occurs only at high altitude. Although Fio_2 does not change with altitude, ambient air pressure decreases exponentially; thus, Pio_2 decreases as well. For example, Pio_2 is only 43 mm Hg at the summit of Mt. Everest (altitude, 8848 m [29,028 ft]). The (A-a)Do_2 remains normal. Hypoxic stimulation of respiratory drive increases alveolar ventilation and decreases $Paco_2$ level. This type of hypoxemia responds to supplemental O_2.

Carbon Dioxide

Pco_2 normally is maintained between 35 and 45 mm Hg. A dissociation curve similar to that for O_2 exists for CO_2 but is nearly linear over the physiologic range of $Paco_2$. Abnormal Pco_2 is almost always linked to disorders of ventilation (unless occurring in compensation for a metabolic abnormality) and is always associated with acid-base changes.

Hypercapnia: Hypercapnia is $Pco_2 > 45$ mm Hg. Causes of hypercapnia are the same as those of hypoventilation (see above). Disorders that increase CO_2 production (eg, hyperthyroidism, fever) when combined with an inability to increase ventilation also cause hypercapnia.

Hypocapnia: Hypocapnia is $Pco_2 < 35$ mm Hg. Hypocapnia is always caused by hyperventilation due to pulmonary (eg, pulmonary edema or embolism), cardiac (eg, heart failure), metabolic (eg, acidosis), drug-induced (eg, aspirin, progesterone), CNS (eg, infection, tumor, bleeding, increased intracranial pressure), or physiologic (eg, pain, pregnancy) disorders or conditions. Hypocapnia is thought to directly increase bronchoconstriction and lower the threshold for cerebral and myocardial ischemia, perhaps through its effects on acid-base status.

Carboxyhemoglobinemia

CO binds to Hb with an affinity 210 times that of O_2 and prevents O_2 transport. Clinically toxic carboxyhemoglobin levels are most often the result of exposure to exhaust fumes or from smoke inhalation, although cigarette smokers have detectable levels. Patients with CO poisoning (see p. 3060) may present with nonspecific symptoms such as malaise, headache, and nausea. Because poisoning often occurs during colder months (because of indoor use of combustible fuel heaters), symptoms may be confused with a viral syndrome such as influenza. Clinicians must be alert to the possibility of CO poisoning and measure levels of carboxyhemoglobin when indicated; COHb can be directly measured from venous blood—an arterial sample is unnecessary.

Treatment is the administration of 100% O_2 (which shortens the half-life of carboxyhemoglobin) and sometimes the use of a hyperbaric chamber.

PEARLS & PITFALLS

- Carboxyhemoglobin levels can be directly measured from venous blood—an arterial sample is unnecessary.

Methemoglobinemia

Methemoglobin is Hb in which the iron is oxidized from its ferrous (Fe^{2+}) to its ferric (Fe^{3+}) state. Methemoglobin does not carry O_2 and shifts the normal HbO_2 dissociation curve to the left, thereby limiting the release of O_2 to the tissues. Methemoglobinemia is caused by certain drugs (eg, dapsone, local anesthetics, nitrates, primaquine, sulfonamides) or, less commonly, by certain chemicals (eg, aniline dyes, benzene derivatives). Methemoglobin level can be directly measured by co-oximetry (which emits 4 wavelengths of light and is capable of detecting methemoglobin, COHb, Hb, and HbO_2) or may be estimated by the difference between the O_2 saturation calculated from the measured PaO_2 and the directly measured SaO_2. Patients with methemoglobinemia most often have asymptomatic cyanosis. In severe cases, O_2 delivery is reduced to such a degree that symptoms of tissue hypoxia result, such as confusion, angina, and myalgias. Stopping the causative drug or chemical exposure is often sufficient. Rarely, methylene blue (a reducing agent; a 1% solution is given 1 to 2 mg/kg slowly IV) or exchange transfusion is needed.

TESTS OF RESPIRATORY MUSCLE FUNCTION

Maximal inspiratory pressure (MIP) and maximal expiratory pressure (MEP) measurements may aid in evaluating respiratory muscle weakness.

MIP is the pressure generated during maximal inspiratory effort against a closed system. It is usually measured at residual volume (RV) because inspiratory muscle strength is inversely related to lung volume (in a curvilinear fashion).

MEP is measured during a similar maneuver at TLC because expiratory muscle strength is directly related to lung volume (again in a curvilinear fashion). The information available from these maneuvers is nonspecific, however, and cannot distinguish between insufficient effort, muscle weakness, and a neurologic disorder.

The **maximal voluntary ventilation** (MVV) is another measure of the neuromuscular and respiratory systems. The MVV is the total volume of air exhaled during 12 sec of rapid, deep breathing, which can be compared with a predicted MVV defined as the forced expiratory volume in 1 sec (FEV_1) × 35 or 40. A significant difference between the predicted and measured MVV may indicate insufficient neuromuscular reserve, abnormal respiratory mechanics, or an inadequate effort. Progressive reduction of tidal volumes during the test is consistent with neuromuscular abnormalities but also occurs with gas trapping as a result of disorders that cause airflow limitation.

The **sniff test** is sometimes used in suspected cases of diaphragmatic paralysis or paresis. During continuous fluoroscopic examination, the patient makes a quick, short, strong inspiratory effort ("sniff"). This maneuver minimizes the contribution of the other muscles of respiration (eg, intercostals). A weakened hemidiaphragm may have decreased excursion compared with the contralateral diaphragm or may move upward paradoxically. Occasionally, electromyographic interrogation of the diaphragm and phrenic nerve is done, but carrying out and interpreting the results of this test require considerable expertise, and the diagnostic accuracy of the test is uncertain. Muscle and nerve biopsies may be helpful in selected cases.

EXERCISE TESTING

The two most common forms of exercise testing used to evaluate pulmonary disorders are the 6-min walk test and full cardiopulmonary exercise testing.

Six-minute walk test: This simple test measures the maximal distance that patients can walk at their own pace in 6 min. The test assesses global functional capacity but does not provide specific information on the individual systems involved in exercise capacity (ie, cardiac, pulmonary, hematologic, musculoskeletal). Neither does it assess patient effort. This test is used for preoperative and postoperative evaluation of patients undergoing lung transplantation and lung volume reduction surgery, to monitor response to therapeutic interventions and pulmonary rehabilitation, and to predict mortality and morbidity in patients with cardiac and pulmonary vascular disorders.

Cardiopulmonary exercise testing (CPET): This computerized test provides a breath-by-breath analysis of respiratory gas exchange and cardiac function at rest and during a period of exercise, the intensity of which is increased incrementally until symptoms limit testing. Information on airflow, O_2 consumption, CO_2 production, and heart rate are collected and used for computation of other variables; ABGs may also be sampled. Exercise is done on a treadmill or on a bicycle ergometer; the ergometer may be preferable because work rate can be directly measured and the test is affected less by obesity.

CPET primarily determines whether patients have normal or reduced maximal exercise capacity (VO_2max) and, if so, suggests probable causes. CPET is used to define which organ systems contribute to a patient's symptoms of exertional dyspnea and exercise intolerance and to what extent. The test is also more sensitive for detecting early or subclinical disease than are less comprehensive tests that are done at rest. Examples of applications include

- Assessment of exercise capacity for disability evaluation
- Preoperative assessment
- Determination of whether dyspnea symptoms result from cardiac or pulmonary problems in patients who have disorders of both organ systems
- Selection of candidates for cardiac transplantation
- Assessment of prognosis in selected disorders (eg, heart disease, pulmonary vascular disorders, and cystic fibrosis)

CPET can also help gauge responses to therapeutic interventions and guide prescription of exercise in rehabilitation programs. In following the response to therapy or disease progression, a steady-state CPET involving at least 6 min of constant work at 50 to 70% of the maximal work rate achieved during a maximal CPET may be more useful than an incremental, maximal CPET. Repeated evaluation at this work rate over time provides comparable data and is sensitive to improvement or decline in cardiopulmonary function.

Several variables are assessed during CPET, and no single one is diagnostic of a cause for exercise limitation. Instead, an integrative approach using clinical data, trends during exercise, and recognition of underlying patterns of physiologic responses is used.

51 Acute Bronchitis

Acute bronchitis is inflammation of the tracheobronchial tree, commonly following a URI, that occurs in patients without chronic lung disorders. The cause is almost always a viral infection. The pathogen is rarely identified. The most common symptom is cough, with or without fever, and possibly sputum production. Diagnosis is based on clinical findings. Treatment is supportive; antibiotics are usually unnecessary. Prognosis is excellent.

Acute bronchitis is frequently a component of a URI caused by rhinovirus, parainfluenza, influenza A or B virus, respiratory syncytial virus, coronavirus, or human metapneumovirus. Less common causes may be *Mycoplasma pneumoniae*, *Bordetella pertussis*, and *Chlamydia pneumoniae*. Less than 5% of cases are caused by bacteria, sometimes in outbreaks.

Acute inflammation of the tracheobronchial tree in patients with underlying chronic bronchial disorders (eg, COPD, bronchiectasis, cystic fibrosis) is considered an acute exacerbation of that disorder rather than acute bronchitis. In these patients, the etiology, treatment, and outcome differ from those of acute bronchitis (see also p. 431).

PEARLS & PITFALLS

- Acute cough in patients with COPD, bronchiectasis, or cystic fibrosis should typically be considered an exacerbation of that disorder rather than simple acute bronchitis.

Symptoms and Signs

Symptoms are a nonproductive or mildly productive cough accompanied or preceded by URI symptoms, usually by > 5 days. Subjective dyspnea results from chest pain or tightness with breathing, not from hypoxia. Signs are often absent but may include scattered rhonchi and wheezing. Sputum may be clear, purulent, or occasionally contain blood. Sputum characteristics do not correspond with a particular etiology (ie, viral vs bacterial). Mild fever may be present, but high or prolonged fever is unusual and suggests influenza or pneumonia.

On resolution, cough is the last symptom to subside and often takes 2 to 3 wk or even longer to do so.

Diagnosis

- Clinical evaluation
- Sometimes chest x-ray to exclude other disorders

Diagnosis is based on clinical presentation. Testing is usually unnecessary. However, patients who complain of dyspnea should have pulse oximetry to rule out hypoxemia. Chest x-ray is done if findings suggest serious illness or pneumonia (eg, ill appearance, mental status change, high fever, tachypnea, hypoxemia, crackles, signs of consolidation or pleural effusion). Elderly patients are the occasional exception, as they may have pneumonia without fever and auscultatory findings, presenting instead with altered mental status and tachypnea.

Sputum Gram stain and culture usually have no role. Nasopharyngeal samples can be tested for influenza and pertussis if these disorders are clinically suspected (eg, for pertussis, persistent and paroxysmal cough after 10 to 14 days of illness, only sometimes with the characteristic whoop and/or retching, exposure to a confirmed case—see p. 1589).

Cough resolves within 2 wk in 75% of patients. Patients with persistent cough should undergo a chest x-ray. Evaluation for noninfectious causes, including postnasal drip and gastroesophageal reflux disease, can usually be done clinically. Differentiation of cough-variant asthma may require pulmonary function testing.

PEARLS & PITFALLS

- Treat most cases of acute bronchitis in healthy patients without using antibiotics.

Treatment

- Symptom relief (eg, acetaminophen, hydration, possibly antitussives)
- Inhaled β-agonist or anticholinergic for wheezing

Acute bronchitis in otherwise healthy patients is a major reason that antibiotics are overused. Nearly all patients require only symptomatic treatment, such as acetaminophen and hydration. Evidence supporting efficacy of *routine* use of other symptomatic treatments, such as antitussives, mucolytics, and bronchodilators, is weak. Antitussives should be considered only if the cough is interfering with sleep (see p. 365). Patients with wheezing may benefit from an inhaled β_2-agonist (eg, albuterol) or an anticholinergic (eg, ipratropium) for a few days. Oral antibiotics are typically not used except in patients with pertussis or during known outbreaks of bacterial infection. A macrolide such as azithromycin 500 mg po once, then 250 mg po once/day for 4 days or clarithromycin 500 mg po bid for 14 days is given.

KEY POINTS

- Acute bronchitis is viral in > 95% of cases, often part of a URI.
- Diagnose acute bronchitis mainly by clinical evaluation; do chest x-ray and/or other tests only in patients who have manifestations of more serious illness.
- Treat most patients only to relieve symptoms.

52 Asthma and Related Disorders

ASTHMA

Asthma is a disease of diffuse airway inflammation caused by a variety of triggering stimuli resulting in partially or completely reversible bronchoconstriction. Symptoms and signs include dyspnea, chest tightness, cough, and wheezing. The diagnosis is based on history, physical examination, and pulmonary function tests. Treatment involves controlling triggering factors and drug therapy, most commonly with inhaled beta-2 agonists and inhaled corticosteroids. Prognosis is good with treatment.

Epidemiology

The prevalence of asthma has increased continuously since the 1970s, and the WHO estimates that 235 million people worldwide are affected. More than 25 million people in the US are affected. Asthma is one of the most common chronic diseases of childhood, affecting more than 6 million children in the US; it occurs more frequently in boys before puberty and in girls after puberty. It also occurs more frequently in non-Hispanic blacks and Puerto Ricans.

Despite its increasing prevalence, however, there has been a recent decline in mortality. In the US, about 3400 deaths occur annually as a result of asthma. However, the death rate is 2 to 3 times higher for blacks than for whites. Asthma is the leading cause of hospitalization for children and is the number one chronic condition causing elementary school absenteeism. Asthma is estimated to cost the US $56 billion/yr in medical care and lost productivity.

Etiology

Development of asthma is multifactorial and depends on the interactions among multiple susceptibility genes and environmental factors.

Susceptibility genes are thought to include those for T-helper cells types 1 and 2 (TH1 and TH2), IgE, interleukins (IL-3, -4, -5, -9, -13), granulocyte-monocyte colony-stimulating factor (GM-CSF), tumor necrosis factor-alpha (TNF-α), and the *ADAM33* gene, which may stimulate airway smooth muscle and fibroblast proliferation or regulate cytokine production.

Environmental factors may include the following:

- Allergen exposure
- Diet
- Perinatal factors

Evidence clearly implicates household allergens (eg, dust mite, cockroach, pet) and other environmental allergens in disease development in older children and adults. Diets low in vitamins C and E and in omega–3 fatty acids have been linked to asthma, as has obesity. Asthma has also been linked to perinatal factors, such as young maternal age, poor maternal nutrition, prematurity, low birthweight, and lack of breastfeeding.

On the other hand, endotoxin exposure early in life can induce tolerance and may be protective. Air pollution is not definitively linked to disease development, although it may trigger exacerbations. The role of childhood exposure to cigarette smoke is controversial, with some studies finding a contributory and some a protective effect.

Genetic and environmental components may interact, thereby determining the balance between TH1 and TH2 cell lineages. Infants may be born with a predisposition toward proallergic and proinflammatory TH2 immune responses, characterized by growth and activation of eosinophils and IgE production. Early childhood exposure to bacterial and viral infections and endotoxins may shift the body to TH1 responses, which suppresses TH2 cells and induce tolerance. Trends in developed countries toward smaller families with fewer children, cleaner indoor environments, and early use of vaccinations and antibiotics may deprive children of these TH2-suppressing, tolerance-inducing exposures and may partly explain the continuous increase in asthma prevalence in developed countries (the hygiene hypothesis).

Reactive airways dysfunction syndrome (RADS): Indoor exposures to nitrogen oxide and volatile organic compounds (eg, from paints, solvents, adhesives) are implicated in the development of RADS, a persistent asthma-like syndrome in people with no history of asthma (see p. 444). RADS appears to be distinct from asthma and may be, on occasion, a form of environmental lung disease. However, RADS and asthma have many clinical similarities (eg, wheezing, dyspnea, cough), and both may respond to corticosteroids.

Pathophysiology

Asthma involves

- Bronchoconstriction
- Airway edema and inflammation
- Airway hyperreactivity
- Airway remodeling

In patients with asthma, TH2 cells and other cell types—notably, eosinophils and mast cells, but also other CD4+ subtypes and neutrophils—form an extensive inflammatory infiltrate in the airway epithelium and smooth muscle, leading to airway remodeling (ie, desquamation, subepithelial fibrosis, angiogenesis, smooth muscle hypertrophy). Hypertrophy of smooth muscle narrows the airways and increases reactivity to allergens, infections, irritants, parasympathetic stimulation (which causes release of pro-inflammatory neuropeptides, such as substance P, neurokinin A, and calcitonin gene-related peptide), and other triggers of bronchoconstriction.

Additional contributors to airway hyperreactivity include loss of inhibitors of bronchoconstriction (epithelium-derived relaxing factor, prostaglandin E_2) and loss of other substances called endopeptidases that metabolize endogenous bronchoconstrictors. Mucus plugging and peripheral blood eosinophilia are additional classic findings in asthma and may be epiphenomena of airway inflammation. However, not all patients with asthma have eosinophilia.

Asthma triggers: Common triggers of an asthma exacerbation include

- Environmental and occupational allergens (numerous)
- Infections
- Exercise
- Inhaled irritants

- Emotion
- Aspirin
- Gastroesophageal reflux disease (GERD)

Infectious triggers in young children include respiratory syncytial virus, rhinovirus, and parainfluenza virus infection. In older children and adults, URIs (particularly with rhinovirus) and pneumonia are common infectious triggers. Exercise can be a trigger, especially in cold or dry environments. Inhaled irritants, such as air pollution, cigarette smoke, perfumes, and cleaning products, are often involved. Emotions such as anxiety, anger, and excitement sometimes trigger exacerbations.

Aspirin is a trigger in up to 30% of patients with severe asthma and in < 10% of all patients with asthma. Aspirin-sensitive asthma is typically accompanied by nasal polyps with nasal and sinus congestion.

GERD is a common trigger among some patients with asthma, possibly via esophageal acid-induced reflex bronchoconstriction or by microaspiration of acid. However, treatment of asymptomatic GERD (eg, with proton pump inhibitors) does not seem to improve asthma control.

Allergic rhinitis often coexists with asthma; it is unclear whether the two are different manifestations of the same allergic process or whether rhinitis is a discrete asthma trigger.

Response: In the presence of triggers, there is reversible airway narrowing and uneven lung ventilation. Relative perfusion exceeds relative ventilation in lung regions distal to narrowed airways; thus, alveolar oxygen tensions fall and alveolar carbon dioxide tensions rise. Most patients can compensate by hyperventilating, but in severe exacerbations, diffuse bronchoconstriction causes severe gas trapping, and the respiratory muscles are put at a marked mechanical disadvantage so that the work of breathing increases. Under these conditions, hypoxemia worsens and $Paco_2$ rises. Respiratory acidosis and metabolic acidosis may result and, if left untreated, cause respiratory and cardiac arrest.

Classification

Unlike hypertension (eg, in which one parameter [BP] defines the severity of the disorder and the efficacy of treatment), asthma causes a number of clinical and testing abnormalities. Also, unlike most types of hypertension, asthma manifestations typically wax and wane. Thus, monitoring (and studying) asthma requires a consistent terminology and defined benchmarks.

The term status asthmaticus describes severe, intense, prolonged bronchospasm that is resistant to treatment.

Severity: Severity is the intrinsic intensity of the disease process (ie, how bad it is—see Table 52–1). Severity can usually be assessed directly only before treatment is started, because patients who have responded well to treatment by definition have few symptoms. Asthma severity is categorized as

- Intermittent
- Mild persistent
- Moderate persistent
- Severe persistent

It is important to remember that the severity category does not predict how serious an exacerbation a patient may have. For example, a patient who has mild asthma with long periods of no or mild symptoms and normal pulmonary function may have a severe, life-threatening exacerbation.

Control: Control is the degree to which symptoms, impairments, and risks are minimized by treatment. Control is the parameter assessed in patients receiving treatment. The goal is for all patients to have well controlled asthma regardless of disease severity. Control is classified as

- Well controlled
- Not well controlled
- Very poorly controlled

Severity and control are assessed in terms of patient impairment and risk (see Tables 52–1 and 52–2).

Impairment: Impairment refers to the frequency and intensity of patients' symptoms and functional limitations (see Table 52–1). Impairment differs from severity by its emphasis on symptoms and functional limitations rather than the intrinsic intensity of the disease process. Impairment can be measured by spirometry, mainly forced expiratory volume in 1 sec (FEV_1), and the ratio of FEV_1 to forced vital capacity (FVC), but is manifested as clinical features such as

- How often symptoms are experienced
- How often the patient awakens at night
- How often the patient uses a short-acting beta-2 agonist for symptom relief
- How often asthma interferes with normal activity

Risk: Risk refers to the likelihood of future exacerbations or decline in lung function and the risk of adverse drug effects. Risk is assessed by long-term trends in spirometry and clinical features such as

- Frequency of need for oral corticosteroids
- Need for hospitalization
- Need for ICU admission
- Need for intubation

Symptoms and Signs

Patients with mild asthma are typically asymptomatic between exacerbations. Patients with more severe disease and those with exacerbations experience dyspnea, chest tightness, audible wheezing, and coughing. Coughing may be the only symptom in some patients (cough-variant asthma). Symptoms can follow a circadian rhythm and worsen during sleep, often around 4 AM. Many patients with more severe disease waken during the night (nocturnal asthma).

Signs include wheezing, pulsus paradoxus (ie, a fall of systolic BP > 10 mm Hg during inspiration), tachypnea, tachycardia, and visible efforts to breathe (use of neck and suprasternal [accessory] muscles, upright posture, pursed lips, inability to speak). The expiratory phase of respiration is prolonged, with an inspiratory:expiratory ratio of at least 1:3. Wheezes can be present through both phases or just on expiration, but patients with severe bronchoconstriction may have no audible wheezing because of markedly limited airflow.

Patients with a severe exacerbation and impending respiratory failure typically have some combination of altered consciousness, cyanosis, pulsus paradoxus > 15 mm Hg, oxygen saturation < 90%, $Paco_2$ > 45 mm Hg, or hyperinflation. Rarely, pneumothorax or pneumomediastinum is seen on chest x-ray.

Symptoms and signs disappear between exacerbations, although soft wheezes may be audible during forced expiration at rest, or after exercise in some asymptomatic patients. Hyperinflation of the lungs may alter the chest wall in patients with long-standing uncontrolled asthma, causing a barrel-shaped thorax.

All symptoms and signs are nonspecific, are reversible with timely treatment, and typically are brought on by exposure to one or more triggers.

Table 52–1. CLASSIFICATION OF ASTHMA SEVERITY*

COMPONENTS OF SEVERITY	INTERMITTENT	MILD PERSISTENT	MODERATE PERSISTENT	SEVERE PERSISTENT
Symptoms and risk measures	All ages: ≤ 2 days/week	All ages: > 2 days/week, not daily	All ages: Daily	All ages: Throughout the day
Nighttime awakenings	Adults and children ≥ 5 yr: ≤ 2x/month Children 0–4 yr: 0	Adults and children ≥ 5 yr: 3–4x/month Children 0–4 yr: 1–2x/month	Adults and children ≥ 5 yr: > 1x/week but not nightly Children 0–4 yr: 3–4x/month	Adults and children ≥ 5 yr: Often 7x/week Children 0–4 yr: > 1x/week
SABA rescue inhaler use for symptoms (not to prevent EIB)	≤ 2 days/week	Adults and children ≥ 5 yr: > 2 days/week but not daily Children 0–4 yr: > 2 days/week but not daily	Daily	Several times per day
Interference with normal activity	None	Minor limitation	Some limitation	Extreme limitation
FEV_1	Adults and children ≥ 5 yr: > 80% Children 0–4 yr: Not applicable	Adults and children ≥ 5 yr: > 80% Children 0–4 yr: Not applicable	Adults and children ≥ 5 yr: 60–80% Children 0–4 yr: Not applicable	Adults and children ≥ 5 yr: < 60% Children 0–4 yr: Not applicable
FEV_1/FVC	Adults and children ≥ 12 yr: Normal† Children 5–11 yr: > 85% Children 0–4 yr: Not applicable	Adults and children ≥ 12 yr: Normal† Children 5–11 yr: > 80% Children 0–4 yr: Not applicable	Adults and children ≥ 12 yr: Reduced 5%† Children 5–11 yr: 75–80% Children 0–4 yr: Not applicable	Adults and children ≥ 12 yr: Reduced > 5%† Children 5–11 yr: < 75% Children 0–4 yr: Not applicable
Risk of an asthma exacerbations requiring oral corticosteroid bursts‡	0–1/year	Adults and children ≥ 5 yr: ≥ 2/year Children 0–4 yr: ≥ 2 in 6 months or wheezing ≥ 4x/year lasting > 1 day AND risk factors for persistent asthma	More frequent and intense events indicate greater severity	More frequent and intense events indicate greater severity

*Severity is categorized based on degree of impairment and risk of exacerbations requiring oral corticosteroids. Impairment is assessed over the previous 2–4 weeks, and risk is assessed over the past year. Severity is best classified at the first visit before a controller therapy is initiated (not SABA or systemic corticosteroid bursts for symptoms or exacerbations).

†Evidence for airflow obstruction is based on an FEV_1/FVC ratio less than expected normal values by age group. Normal FEV_1/FVC ratios by age group: 8–19 years = 85%; 20–39 years = 80%; 40–59 years = 75%; 60–80 years = 70%.

‡At present, there are inadequate data to correlate frequencies of exacerbations with different levels of asthma severity. In general, more frequent and intense exacerbations (eg, requiring urgent, unscheduled care, hospitalization, or ICU admission) indicate greater underlying disease severity. For treatment purposes, patients with ≥ 2 exacerbations may be considered to have persistent asthma.

EIB = exercise-induced bronchospasm; FEV_1 = forced expiratory volume in 1 second; FVC = forced vital capacity; ICS = inhaled corticosteroid; SABA = short-acting beta-2 agonist.

Adapted from National Heart, Lung, and Blood Institute: Expert Panel Report 3: Guidelines for the diagnosis and management of asthma—full report 2007. August 28, 2007. Available at http://www.nhlbi.nih.gov/guidelines/asthma/asthgdln.htm.

Diagnosis

- Clinical evaluation
- Pulmonary function testing

Diagnosis is based on history and physical examination and is confirmed with pulmonary function tests. Diagnosis of causes and the exclusion of other disorders that cause wheezing are also important. Asthma and COPD are sometimes easily confused; they cause similar symptoms and produce similar results on pulmonary function tests but differ in important biologic ways that are not always clinically apparent.

Asthma that is difficult to control or refractory to commonly used controller therapies should be further evaluated for alternative causes of episodic wheezing, cough, and dyspnea such as allergic bronchopulmonary aspergillosis, bronchiectasis, or vocal cord dysfunction.

Pulmonary function tests: Patients suspected of having asthma should undergo pulmonary function testing to confirm and quantify the severity and reversibility of airway obstruction. Pulmonary function data quality is effort-dependent and requires patient education before the test. If it is safe to do so, bronchodilators should be stopped before the test: 8 h for short-acting beta-2 agonists, such as albuterol; 24 h for ipratropium; 12 to 48 h for theophylline; 48 h for long-acting beta-2 agonists, such as salmeterol and formoterol; and 1 week for tiotropium.

Spirometry should be done before and after inhalation of a short-acting bronchodilator. Signs of airflow limitation before bronchodilator inhalation include reduced FEV_1 and a reduced

Table 52–2. CLASSIFICATION OF ASTHMA CONTROL*, †

COMPONENT	WELL-CONTROLLED	NOT WELL-CONTROLLED	VERY POORLY CONTROLLED
Symptoms	All ages except children 5–11 yr: ≤ 2 days/wk Children 5–11 yr: ≤ 2 days/wk but not > once/day	All ages except children 5–11 yr: > 2 days/wk Children 5–11 yr: > 2 days/wk or multiple times on ≤ 2 days/wk	For all ages: Throughout the day
Nighttime awakenings	Adults and children ≥ 12 yr: ≤ 2/mo Children 5–11 yr: ≤ 1 /mo Children 0–4 yr: ≤ 1 /mo	Adults and children ≥ 12 yr: 1–3/wk Children 5–11 yr: ≥ 2/mo Children 0–4 yr: > 1/mo	Adults and children ≥ 12 yr: ≥ 4/wk Children 5–11 yr: ≥ 2/wk Children 0–4 yr: > 1/wk
Interference with normal activity	None	Some limitation	Extreme limitation
Use of short-acting beta-2 agonist for symptom control (not prevention of exercise-induced asthma)	≤ 2 days/wk	> 2 days/wk	Several times/day
FEV_1 or peak flow	> 80% predicted/personal best	60–80% predicted/personal best	< 60% predicted/personal best
FEV_1/FVC (children 5–11 yr)	> 80%	75–80%	< 75%
Exacerbations requiring oral systemic corticosteroids‡	0–1/yr	Adults and children ≥ 5 yr: ≥ 2/yr Children 0–4 yr: 2–3/yr	Adults and children ≥ 5 yr: ≥ 2/yr Children 0–4 yr: > 3/yr
Validated questionnaires:			
• ATAQ	0	1–2	3–4
• ACQ	≤ 0.75†	≥ 1.5	N/A
• ACT	≥ 20	16–19	≤ 15
Recommended action	Maintain current step Follow up every 1–6 mo Consider step down if well controlled for ≥ 3 mo	Step up 1 step Reevaluate in 2–6 wk For adverse effects, consider treatment options	Consider short course of systemic corticosteroids Step up 1 or 2 steps Re-evaluate in 2 wk For adverse effects, consider treatment options

*All ages unless specified differently.

†Level of control is based on the most severe impairment or risk category. Additional factors to consider are progressive loss of lung function on pulmonary function tests, significant adverse effects, and severity and interval between exacerbations (ie, one exacerbation requiring intubation or 2 hospitalizations within 1 mo may be considered very poor control).

‡At present, there are inadequate data to correlate frequencies of exacerbations with different levels of asthma control. In general, more frequent and intense exacerbations (eg, requiring urgent, unscheduled care, hospitalization, or ICU admission) indicate poorer asthma control.

ACQ = asthma control questionnaire; ACT = asthma control test; ATAQ = asthma therapy assessment questionnaire; FEV_1 = forced expiratory volume in 1 sec; FVC = forced vital capacity.

Adapted from National Heart, Lung, and Blood Institute: Expert Panel Report 3: Guidelines for the diagnosis and management of asthma—full report 2007. August 28, 2007. Available at http://www.nhlbi.nih.gov/guidelines/asthma/asthgdln.htm.

FEV_1/FVC ratio. The FVC may also be decreased because of gas trapping, such that lung volume measurements may show an increase in the residual volume, the functional residual capacity, or both. An improvement in FEV_1 of > 12% or an increase ≥ 10% of predicted FEV_1 in response to bronchodilator treatment confirms reversible airway obstruction, although absence of this finding should not preclude a therapeutic trial of long-acting bronchodilators.

Flow-volume loops should also be reviewed to diagnose vocal cord dysfunction, a common cause of upper airway obstruction that mimics asthma.

Provocative testing, in which inhaled methacholine (or alternatives, such as inhaled histamine, adenosine, or bradykinin, or exercise testing) is used to provoke bronchoconstriction, is indicated for patients suspected of having asthma who have normal findings on spirometry and flow-volume testing and for patients suspected of having cough-variant asthma, provided there are no contraindications. Contraindications include FEV_1 < 1 L or < 50% predicted, recent myocardial infarction or stroke, and severe hypertension (systolic BP > 200 mm Hg; diastolic BP > 100 mm Hg). A decline in FEV_1 of > 20% on a provocative testing protocol is relatively specific for the diagnosis of asthma. However, FEV_1 may decline in response to drugs used in provocative testing in other disorders, such as COPD. If FEV_1 decreases by < 20% by the end of the testing protocol, asthma is less likely to be present.

Other tests: Other tests may be helpful in some circumstances:

- Diffusing capacity for carbon monoxide (DLco)
- Chest x-ray
- Allergy testing

DLco testing can help distinguish asthma from chronic obstructive pulmonary disease. Values are normal or elevated in asthma and usually reduced in COPD, particularly in patients with emphysema.

A chest x-ray may help exclude some causes of asthma or alternative diagnoses, such as heart failure or pneumonia. The chest x-ray in asthma is usually normal but may show hyperinflation or segmental atelectasis, a sign of mucous plugging. Infiltrates, especially those that come and go and that are associated with findings of central bronchiectasis, suggest allergic bronchopulmonary aspergillosis.

Allergy testing may be indicated for children whose history suggests allergic triggers (particularly for allergic rhinitis) because these children may benefit from immunotherapy. It should be considered for adults whose history indicates relief of symptoms with allergen avoidance and for those in whom a trial of therapeutic anti-IgE antibody therapy (see p. 413) is being considered. Skin testing and measurement of allergen-specific IgE via radioallergosorbent testing (RAST) can identify specific allergic triggers.

Blood tests may be done. Elevated blood eosinophils (> 400 cells/μL) and nonspecific IgE (> 150 IU) are suggestive but not diagnostic of allergic asthma because they can be elevated in other conditions. However, eosinophilia is not sensitive.

Sputum evaluation for eosinophils is not commonly done; finding large numbers of eosinophils is suggestive of asthma but is neither sensitive nor specific.

Peak expiratory flow (PEF) measurements with inexpensive handheld flow meters are recommended for home monitoring of disease severity and for guiding therapy.

Evaluation of exacerbations: Patients with asthma with an acute exacerbation are evaluated based primarily on clinical criteria but should also have certain tests:

- Pulse oximetry
- Peak expiratory flow (or FEV_1) measurement

These measures can help establish the severity of an exacerbation but are usually used to monitor response to treatment. PEF values are interpreted in light of the patient's personal best, which may vary widely among patients who are equally well controlled. A 15 to 20% reduction from this baseline indicates a significant exacerbation. When baseline values are not known, the percent predicted FEV_1 value gives a general idea of airflow limitation but not the individual patient's degree of worsening.

When measuring FEV_1 is impractical (eg, in an emergency department) and baseline PEF is unknown, percent of predicted PEF based on age, height, and sex may be used. Although percent predicted PEF is less accurate than comparison to a personal best, it may be helpful as a baseline to evaluate treatment response. However, the decision to treat an exacerbation should be based primarily on an assessment of signs and symptoms, reserving spirometric and PEF determination for monitoring treatment or when objective measures are required (eg, when an exacerbation appears to be more severe than perceived by the patient or is not recognized).

Chest x-ray is not necessary for most exacerbations but should be done in patients with symptoms or signs suggestive of pneumonia, pneumothorax, or pneumomediastinum.

Arterial blood gas measurements should be done in patients with marked respiratory distress or symptoms and signs of impending respiratory failure.

Prognosis

Asthma resolves in many children, but for as many as 1 in 4, wheezing persists into adulthood or relapse occurs in later years. Female sex, smoking, earlier age of onset, sensitization to household dust mites, and airway hyperresponsiveness are risk factors for persistence and relapse.

Although a significant number of deaths each year are attributable to asthma, most of these deaths are preventable with treatment. Thus, the prognosis is good with adequate access and adherence to treatment. Risk factors for death include increasing requirements for oral corticosteroids before hospitalization, previous hospitalization for acute exacerbations, and lower PEF values at presentation. Several studies show that use of inhaled corticosteroids decreases hospital admission and mortality rates.

Over time, the airways in some patients with asthma undergo permanent structural changes (remodeling) that prevent return to normal lung functioning. Early aggressive use of anti-inflammatory drugs may help prevent this remodeling.

Treatment

- Control of triggers
- Drug therapy
- Monitoring
- Patient education
- Treatment of acute exacerbations

Treatment objectives are to minimize impairment and risk, including preventing exacerbations and minimizing chronic symptoms, including nocturnal awakenings; to minimize the need for emergency department visits or hospitalizations; to maintain baseline (normal) pulmonary function and activity levels; and to avoid adverse treatment effects.

Control of triggering factors: Triggering factors in some patients may be controlled with use of synthetic fiber pillows and impermeable mattress covers and frequent washing of bed sheets, pillowcases, and blankets in hot water. Ideally, upholstered furniture, soft toys, carpets, curtains, and pets should be removed, at least from the bedroom, to reduce dust mites and animal dander. Dehumidifiers should be used in basements and in other poorly aerated, damp rooms to reduce mold. Steam treatment of homes diminishes dust mite allergens. House cleaning and extermination to eliminate cockroach exposure is especially important. Although control of triggering factors is more difficult in urban environments, the importance of these measures is not diminished.

High-efficiency particulate air (HEPA) vacuums and filters may relieve symptoms, but no beneficial effects on pulmonary function and on the need for drugs have been observed.

Sulfite-sensitive patients should avoid sulfite-containing wine.

Nonallergenic triggers, such as cigarette smoke, strong odors, irritant fumes, cold temperatures, high humidity, and exercise, should also be avoided or controlled when possible. Limiting exposure to people with viral URIs is also important.

Patients with aspirin-sensitive asthma can use acetaminophen, choline magnesium salicylate, or celecoxib in place of NSAIDs.

Asthma is a relative contraindication to the use of nonselective beta-blockers, including topical formulations, but cardioselective drugs (eg, metoprolol, atenolol) probably have no adverse effects.

Drug therapy: Major drug classes commonly used in the treatment of asthma and asthma exacerbations include

- Bronchodilators (beta-2 agonists, anticholinergics)
- Corticosteroids
- Leukotriene modifiers
- Mast cell stabilizers
- Methylxanthines
- Immunomodulators

Drugs in these classes (see Table 52–4 on pp. 408–412) are inhaled, taken orally, or injected subcutaneously or intravenously; inhaled drugs come in aerosolized and powdered forms. Use of aerosolized forms with a spacer or holding chamber facilitates deposition of the drug in the airways rather than the pharynx; patients are advised to wash and dry their spacers after each use to prevent bacterial contamination. In addition, use of aerosolized forms requires coordination between actuation of the inhaler (drug delivery) and inhalation; powdered forms reduce the need for coordination, because drug is delivered only when the patient inhales. For details, see Drug Treatment of Asthma on p. 407.

Bronchial thermoplasty: Bronchial thermoplasty (BT) is a bronchoscopic technique in which heat is applied through a device that transfers localized controlled radiofrequency waves to the airways. The heat decreases the amount of airway smooth muscle remodeling (and thus the smooth muscle mass) that occurs with asthma. In clinical trials in patients with severe asthma not controlled with multiple therapies, there have been modest decreases in exacerbation frequency and improvement in asthma symptom control. However, some patients have experienced an immediate worsening of symptoms, sometimes requiring hospitalization immediately after the procedure.

Criteria for consideration of BT include severe asthma not controlled with inhaled corticosteroids and long-acting beta agonists, intermittent or continuous use of oral corticosteroids, $FEV_1 \geq 50\%$ of predicted and no history of life-threatening exacerbations. Patients should understand the risk of post-procedure asthma exacerbation and need for hospitalization before proceeding with BT. The long-term efficacy and safety of BT is not known. There are no data in patients with > 3 exacerbations per year or an $FEV_1 < 50\%$ of predicted because these patients were excluded from the clinical trials.

Monitoring response to treatment: Guidelines recommend office use of spirometry (FEV_1, FEV_1/FVC, FVC) to measure airflow limitation and assess impairment and risk. Spirometry should be repeated at least every 1 to 2 yr in patients with asthma to monitor disease progression, and a step-up in therapy might be required if lung function declines or becomes impaired with evidence of airflow obstruction (see Table 52–2). Outside the office, home PEF monitoring, in conjunction with patient symptom diaries and the use of an asthma action plan, is especially useful for charting disease progression and response to treatment in patients with moderate to severe persistent asthma. When asthma is quiescent, one PEF measurement in the morning suffices. Should PEF measurements fall to < 80% of the patient's personal best, then twice/day monitoring to assess circadian variation is useful. Circadian variation of > 20% indicates airway instability and the need to re-evaluate the therapeutic regimen.

Patient education: The importance of patient education cannot be overemphasized. Patients do better when they know more about asthma—what triggers an exacerbation, what drug to use when, proper inhaler technique, how to use a spacer with a metered-dose inhaler (MDI), and the importance of early use of corticosteroids in exacerbations. Every patient should have a written action plan for day-to-day management, especially for management of acute exacerbations, that is based on the patient's best personal peak flow rather than on a predicted normal value. Such a plan leads to much better asthma control, largely attributable to improved adherence to therapies.

Treatment of acute asthma exacerbation: The goal of asthma exacerbation treatment is to relieve symptoms and return patients to their best lung function. Treatment includes

- Inhaled bronchodilators (beta-2 agonists and anticholinergics)
- Usually systemic corticosteroids

Details of the treatment of acute asthma exacerbations are discussed elsewhere.

Treatment of chronic asthma: Current asthma guidelines recommend treatment based on the severity classification. Continuing therapy is based on assessment of control (see Table 52–2). Therapy is increased in a stepwise fashion (see Table 52–3) until the best control of impairment and risk is achieved (step-up). Before therapy is stepped up, adherence, exposure to environmental factors (eg, trigger exposure), and presence of comorbid conditions (eg, obesity, allergic rhinitis, GERD, COPD, obstructive sleep apnea, vocal cord dysfunction) are reviewed. These factors should be addressed before increasing drug therapy. Once asthma has been well controlled for at least 3 mo, drug therapy is reduced if possible to the minimum that maintains good control (step-down). For specific drugs and doses, see Table 52–4.

Exercise-induced asthma: Exercise-induced asthma can generally be prevented by inhalation of a short-acting beta-2 agonist or mast cell stabilizer before starting the exercise. If beta-2 agonists are not effective or if exercise-induced asthma causes severe symptoms, the patient likely has more severe asthma than was initially recognized and requires controller therapy.

Aspirin-sensitive asthma: The primary treatment for aspirin-sensitive asthma is avoidance of NSAIDs. Celecoxib does not appear to be a trigger. Leukotriene modifiers can blunt the response to NSAIDs. Alternatively, inpatient desensitization has been successful in a few patients.

Future therapies: Multiple therapies are being developed to target specific components of the inflammatory cascade. Therapies directed at IL-4, IL-13, tumor necrosis factor-alpha, other chemokines, and cytokines or their receptors are all under investigation or consideration as therapeutic targets.

Special Populations

Infants, children, and adolescents: Asthma is difficult to diagnose in infants; thus, under-recognition and undertreatment are common (see also p. 2827). Empiric trials of inhaled bronchodilators and anti-inflammatory drugs may be helpful for both. Drugs may be given by nebulizer or MDI with a holding chamber with or without a face mask. Infants and children < 5 yr requiring treatment > 2 times/wk should be given daily anti-inflammatory therapy with inhaled corticosteroids (preferred), leukotriene receptor antagonists, or cromolyn.

Children > 5 yr and adolescents with asthma can be treated similarly to adults. They should be encouraged to maintain physical activities, exercise, and sports participation. Predicted norms for pulmonary function tests in adolescents are closer

Table 52–3. STEPS OF ASTHMA MANAGEMENT*

STEP	PREFERRED TREATMENT	ALTERNATE TREATMENT
1 (starting point for intermittent asthma)	Short-acting beta-2 agonist prn†	—
2 (starting point for mild persistent asthma)	Low-dose inhaled corticosteroid	Mast cell stabilizer, leukotriene receptor antagonist, or theophylline
3 (starting point for moderate persistent asthma)	Medium-dose inhaled corticosteroid *or* Low-dose inhaled corticosteroid plus long-acting beta-2 agonist	Low-dose inhaled corticosteroid plus one of the following: a leukotriene receptor antagonist, theophylline, or zileuton
4	Medium-dose inhaled corticosteroid plus long-acting beta-2 agonist	Medium-dose inhaled corticosteroid plus one of the following: leukotriene receptor antagonist, theophylline, or zileuton
5 (starting point for severe persistent asthma)	High-dose inhaled corticosteroid plus long-acting beta-2 agonist *and* possibly omalizumab for patients with allergic asthma	—
6	High-dose inhaled corticosteroid plus long-acting beta-2 agonist plus oral corticosteroid *and* possibly omalizumab, mepolizumab, or reslizumab for patients with evidence of allergic asthma	

*Before stepping up, adherence, environmental factors (eg, trigger exposure), and comorbid conditions should be reviewed and managed if needed.

†A short-acting beta-2 agonist is indicated to provide quick relief at all steps and to prevent exercise-induced asthma.

to childhood (not adult) standards. Adolescents and mature younger children should participate in developing their own asthma management plans and establishing their own goals for therapy to improve adherence. The action plan should be understood by teachers and school nurses to ensure reliable and prompt access to rescue drugs. Cromolyn and nedocromil are often tried in this group but are not as beneficial as inhaled corticosteroids. Long-acting drugs prevent the problems (eg, inconvenience, embarrassment) of having to take drugs at school.

Pregnant women: About one-third of women with asthma who become pregnant notice relief of symptoms, one-third notice worsening (at times to a severe degree), and one-third notice no change. GERD may be an important contributor to symptomatic disease in pregnancy. Asthma control during pregnancy is crucial because poorly controlled maternal disease can result in increased prenatal mortality, premature delivery, and low birth weight.

Asthma drugs have not been shown to have adverse fetal effects, but safety data are lacking. (See also guidelines from the National Asthma Education and Prevention Program, Managing Asthma During Pregnancy: Recommendations for Pharmacologic Treatment–Update 2004.) In general, uncontrolled asthma is more of a risk to mother and fetus than adverse effects due to asthma drugs. During pregnancy, normal blood PCO_2 level is about 32 mm Hg. Therefore, carbon dioxide retention is probably occurring if PCO_2 approaches 40 mm Hg.

PEARLS & PITFALLS

- Suspect carbon dioxide retention and respiratory failure in pregnant women with uncontrolled asthma and PCO_2 levels near 40 mm Hg.

Elderly patients: The elderly have a high prevalence of other obstructive lung disease (eg, COPD), so it is important to determine the magnitude of the reversible component of airflow obstruction (eg, by a 2- to 3-wk trial of inhaled corticosteroids or pulmonary function testing with bronchodilator challenge). The elderly may be more sensitive to adverse effects of beta-2 agonists and inhaled corticosteroids. Patients requiring inhaled corticosteroids, particularly those with risk factors for osteoporosis, may benefit from measures to preserve bone density (eg, calcium and vitamin D supplements, bisphosphonates).

KEY POINTS

- Asthma triggers range from environmental allergens and respiratory irritants to infections, aspirin, exercise, emotion, and GERD.
- Consider asthma in patients who have unexplained persistent coughing, particularly at night.
- If asthma is suspected, arrange pulmonary function testing, with methacholine provocation if necessary.
- Educate patients on how to avoid triggers.
- Control chronic asthma with drugs that modulate the allergic and immune response—usually inhaled corticosteroids—with other drugs (eg, long-acting bronchodilators, mast cell stabilizers, leukotriene inhibitors) added based on asthma severity.
- Treat acute exacerbations with inhaled beta-2 agonists and anticholinergic drugs, systemic corticosteroids, and sometimes injected epinephrine.
- If mechanical ventilation is necessary, consider using high inspiratory flow rates (to prolong expiration) with low tidal volumes, even at the cost of a slight increase in PCO_2 (permissive hypercapnia).
- Treat asthma aggressively during pregnancy.

DRUG TREATMENT OF ASTHMA

Major drug classes commonly used in the treatment of asthma and asthma exacerbations include

- Bronchodilators (beta-2 agonists, anticholinergics)
- Corticosteroids
- Leukotriene modifiers
- Mast cell stabilizers
- Methylxanthines
- Immunomodulators

Drugs in these classes (see Table 52–4) are inhaled, taken orally, or injected subcutaneously or intravenously; inhaled drugs come in aerosolized and powdered forms. Use of aerosolized forms with a spacer or holding chamber facilitates deposition of the drug in the airways rather than the pharynx; patients are advised to wash and dry their spacers after each use to prevent bacterial contamination. In addition, use of aerosolized forms requires coordination between actuation of the inhaler (drug delivery) and inhalation; powdered forms reduce the need for coordination, because drug is delivered only when the patient fully inhales with a good effort.

Beta-2 agonists: Beta-2 agonists relax bronchial smooth muscle, decrease mast cell degranulation and histamine release, inhibit microvascular leakage into the airways, and increase mucociliary clearance. Beta-2 agonist preparations may be short-acting, long-acting, or ultra–long-acting (see Tables 52–4 and 52–5 on pp. 414–415).

Short-acting beta-2 agonists (eg, albuterol) 2 puffs q 4 h inhaled prn are the drug of choice for relieving acute bronchoconstriction and preventing exercise-induced asthma. They should not be used alone for long-term maintenance of chronic asthma. They take effect within minutes and are active for up to 6 to 8 h, depending on the drug. Tachycardia and tremor are the most common acute adverse effects of inhaled beta-2 agonists and are dose-related. Mild hypokalemia occurs uncommonly. Use of levalbuterol (a solution containing the *R*-isomer of albuterol) theoretically minimizes adverse effects, but its long-term efficacy and safety are unproved. Oral beta-2 agonists have more systemic effects and generally should be avoided.

Long-acting beta-2 agonists (eg, salmeterol) are active for up to 12 h and ultra–long-acting beta-2 agonists are active for up to 24 h. They are used for moderate and severe asthma but should never be used as monotherapy. They interact synergistically with inhaled corticosteroids and permit lower dosing of corticosteroids.

The safety of regular long-term use of beta-2 agonists remains unclear. Long-acting beta-2 agonists may increase the risk of asthma-related death when used as monotherapy. Therefore, when treating patients with asthma, these drugs (salmeterol, formoterol, and vilanterol) should be used only in combination with an inhaled corticosteroid for patients whose condition is not adequately controlled with other asthma controllers (eg, low- to medium-dose inhaled corticosteroids) or whose disease severity clearly warrants additional maintenance therapies. Daily use or diminishing effects of short-acting beta-2 agonists or use of ≥ 1 canister per month suggests inadequate control and the need to begin or intensify other therapies.

Anticholinergics: Anticholinergics relax bronchial smooth muscle through competitive inhibition of muscarinic (M_3) cholinergic receptors. Ipratropium may have an additive effect when combined with short-acting beta-2 agonists. Adverse effects include pupillary dilation, blurred vision, and dry mouth. Tiotropium soft mist inhaler (1.25 mcg/puff) is a 24-h inhaled anticholinergic that can be used for patients with asthma. In patients with asthma, recent clinical trials of tiotropium added to either inhaled corticosteroids or to a combination of an inhaled long-acting beta-2 agonist plus a corticosteroid have shown improved pulmonary function and decreased asthma exacerbations.

Corticosteroids: Corticosteroids inhibit airway inflammation, reverse beta-receptor down-regulation, and inhibit cytokine production and adhesion protein activation. They block the late response (but not the early response) to inhaled allergens. Routes of administration include oral, IV, and inhaled. In acute asthma exacerbations, early use of systemic corticosteroids often aborts the exacerbation, decreases the need for hospitalization, prevents relapse, and speeds recovery. Oral and IV routes are equally effective.

Inhaled corticosteroids have no role in acute exacerbations but are indicated for long-term suppression, control, and reversal of inflammation and symptoms. They substantially reduce the need for maintenance oral corticosteroid therapy. Adverse local effects of inhaled corticosteroids include dysphonia and oral candidiasis, which can be prevented or minimized by having the patient use a spacer, gargle with water after corticosteroid inhalation, or both. Systemic effects are all dose related, can occur with oral or inhaled forms, and occur mainly with inhaled doses > 800 mcg/day. They include suppression of the adrenal-pituitary axis, osteoporosis, cataracts, skin atrophy, hyperphagia, and easy bruisability. Whether inhaled corticosteroids suppress growth in children is unclear. Most children treated with inhaled corticosteroids eventually reach their predicted adult height. Latent TB may be reactivated by systemic corticosteroid use.

Mast cell stabilizers: Mast cell stabilizers inhibit histamine release from mast cells, reduce airway hyperresponsiveness, and block the early and late responses to allergens. They are given by inhalation prophylactically to patients with exercise-induced or allergen-induced asthma. They are ineffective once symptoms have occurred. They are the safest of all antiasthmatic drugs but the least effective.

Leukotriene modifiers: Leukotriene modifiers are taken orally and can be used for long-term control and prevention of symptoms in patients with mild persistent to severe persistent asthma. The main adverse effect is liver enzyme elevation (which occurs with zileuton). Although rare, patients have developed a clinical syndrome resembling eosinophilic granulomatosis with polyangiitis.

Methylxanthines: Methylxanthines relax bronchial smooth muscle (probably by inhibiting phosphodiesterase) and may improve myocardial and diaphragmatic contractility through unknown mechanisms. Methylxanthines appear to inhibit intracellular release of calcium, decrease microvascular leakage into the airway mucosa, and inhibit the late response to allergens. They decrease the infiltration of eosinophils into bronchial mucosa and of T cells into epithelium.

The methylxanthine theophylline is used for long-term control as an adjunct to beta-2 agonists. Extended-release theophylline helps manage nocturnal asthma. Theophylline has fallen into disuse because of its many adverse effects and interactions compared with other drugs. Adverse effects include headache, vomiting, cardiac arrhythmias, and seizures.

Methylxanthines have a narrow therapeutic index; multiple drugs (any metabolized by the cytochrome P-450 pathway, eg, macrolide antibiotics) and conditions (eg, fever, liver disease, heart failure) alter methylxanthine metabolism and elimination. Serum theophylline levels should be monitored periodically and maintained between 5 and 15 μg/mL (28 and 83 μmol/L).

Immunomodulators: Immunomodulators include omalizumab, an anti-IgE antibody, and two antibodies to IL-5

Table 52–4. DRUG TREATMENT OF ASTHMA*

DRUG	FORM	DOSAGE: CHILDREN	DOSAGE: ADULTS	COMMENTS
Short-acting beta-agonists				
Albuterol	HFA: 90 mcg/puff	Same as adults	2 puffs q 4–6 h prn and 2 puffs 15–30 min before exercise	Albuterol is used mainly as a rescue drug. It is not recommended for maintenance treatment. Regular use indicates diminishing asthma control and need for additional drug. MDI-DPI is as effective as nebulized therapy if patients can coordinate the inhalation maneuver using the spacer and holding chamber. Nebulized albuterol can be mixed with other nebulizer solutions.
	DPI: 90 mcg/puff	≥ 4 yr: Same as adults < 4 yr: Not used	2 puffs q 4–6 h prn and 2 puffs 15–30 min before exercise	
	Nebulized solution: 5 mg/mL and 0.63, 1.25, and 2.5 mg/3 mL	< 5 yr: 0.63–2.5 mg in 3 mL of saline q 4–6 h prn ≥ 5 yr: 0.05 mg/kg in 3 mL saline q 4–6 h prn (minimum 1.25 mg, maximum 2.5 mg)	1.25–5 mg in 3 mL saline q 4–6 h prn	
Levalbuterol	HFA: 45 mcg/puff	< 5 yr: Not established ≥ 5 yr: Same as adults	2 puffs q 4–6 hr prn	Levalbuterol is the *R*-isomer of albuterol. 0.63 mg is equivalent to 1.25 mg racemic albuterol. Levalbuterol may have fewer adverse effects.
	Nebulized solution: 0.31, 0.63, and 1.25 mg/3 mL and 1.25 mg/0.5 mL	< 5 yr: 0.31–1.25 mg in 3 mL q 4–6 h prn 5–11 yr: 0.31–0.63 mg q 8 h prn (maximum 0.63 mg q 8 h) ≥ 12 yr: Same as adults	0.63–1.25 mg q 6–8 h prn	
Long-acting beta-2 agonists (not to be used as monotherapy)				
Arformoterol	Nebulized solution: 15 mcg/2 mL	Not established	15–25 mcg q 12 h	Arformoterol is the *R*-isomer of formoterol.
Formoterol	Nebulized solution: 20 mcg/2 mL	Not established	20 mcg q 12 h	DPI form is no longer available.
Salmeterol	HFA: 21 mcg/puff	≥ 12 yr: Same as adults	2 puffs q 12 h; when taken before exercise, should be taken 30–60 min before exercise	Duration of action is 12 h. One dose nightly is helpful for nocturnal asthma. Salmeterol is not to be used for acute symptom relief in an exacerbation.
	DPI: 50 mcg/puff	< 4 yr: Not established ≥ 4 yr: Same as adults	1 puff q 12 h and 30 min before exercise	
Ultra–long-acting beta-2 agonists (not to be used as monotherapy)				
Indacaterol	DPI: 75 mcg/puff	Not established	1 puff once/day	—
Olodaterol	SMI: 2.5 mcg/puff	Not established	2 puffs once/day	—
Vilanterol	DPI: 25 mcg/puff	Not established	1 puff once/day	Vilanterol is available only in combination with fluticasone 100 mcg or 200 mcg.
Anticholinergics				
Ipratropium	HFA: 17 mcg/puff	< 12 yr: Not established ≥ 12 yr: Same as adults	2 puffs q 6 h prn (maximum 12 puffs/day)	Ipratropium may be mixed in the same nebulizer as albuterol. It should not be used as first-line therapy. Regular use provides no clear benefit for long-term maintenance therapy but should be added for treatment of acute symptoms.
	Nebulized solution: 500 mcg (0.02%, 2 mL)	< 12 yr: Not established ≥ 12 yr: Same as adults	500 mcg q 6–8 h prn	
Tiotropium	SMI: 1.25 mcg/puff	< 6 yr: Not established ≥ 6 yr: Same as adults	2 puffs once/day (max 2 puffs/day)	Tiotropium is longer acting than ipratropium. The lower dose SMI tiotropium is the only dose recommended for use in asthma.
	DPI: 18 mcg/capsule	Not established	18 mcg (1 capsule) once/day	

Table 52–4. DRUG TREATMENT OF ASTHMA* (*Continued*)

DRUG	FORM	DOSAGE: CHILDREN	DOSAGE: ADULTS	COMMENTS
Corticosteroids (inhaled)				
Beclomethasone	HFA: 40–80 mcg/puff	< 5 yr: Not established 5–11 yr: 1 puff q 12 h (usual maximum 80 mcg bid) ≥ 12 yr: Same as adults	1–2 puffs q 12 h (usual maximum 320 mcg bid)	Doses depend on severity and range from 1–2 puffs to whatever dose is needed to control asthma.
Budesonide	DPI: 90 or 180 mcg/puff	< 6 yr: Not recommended ≥ 6 yr: Initial dose of 180 mcg bid (maximum 360 mcg bid)	Initial dose of 360 mcg bid (maximum 720 mcg bid)	All may have systemic effects when used long term. Maximum threshold is that above which hypothalamic-pituitary-adrenal suppression is produced.
	Nebulized solution: 0.25, 0.5, or 1.0 mg (each in 2 mL solution)	1–8 yr only: If previously taking bronchodilators alone, initial dose of 0.5 mg once/day or 0.25 mg bid (maximum 0.5 mg/day) If previously taking inhaled corticosteroids, initial dose of 0.5 mg once/day or 0.25 mg bid If previously taking oral corticosteroids, initial dose of 0.5 mg bid or 1 mg once/day (maximum 1 mg/day)	Not indicated for adults	If higher doses are necessary for asthma control, specialist consultation should be considered.
Ciclesonide	HFA: 80 or 160 mcg/puff	≤ 5 yr: 160 mcg daily 6–11 yr: Low dose = 80 mcg once/day, medium dose > 80 to 160 mcg once/day, high dose > 160 mcg once/day ≥ 12 yr: Same as adult	If previously taking bronchodilators alone, initial dose of 80 mcg bid (maximum 320 mcg bid) If previously taking inhaled corticosteroids, initial dose of 80 mcg bid (maximum 640 mcg bid) If previously taking oral corticosteroids, initial dose of 320 mcg bid (maximum 640 mcg bid)	
Flunisolide	HFA: 80 mcg/puff	< 5 yr: Not established 5–11 yr: 1 puff bid (maximum 2 puffs bid [320 mcg/day]) ≥ 12 yr: Same as adults	2 puffs bid (maximum 4 puffs bid [640 mcg/day])	
Fluticasone propionate	HFA: 44, 110, or 220 mcg/puffs	0–4 yr: Initially, 88–176 mcg bid (usual maximum 176 mcg bid) 5–11 yr: Initially, 88–176 mcg bid (usual maximum 176 mcg bid) ≥ 12 yr: Same as adults	If previously taking bronchodilators alone, initial dose of 88 mcg bid (maximum 440 mcg bid) If previously taking inhaled corticosteroids, initial dose of 88–220 mcg bid (maximum 440 mcg bid) If previously taking oral corticosteroids, initial dose of 440–880 mcg bid (maximum 880 mcg bid)	
	DPI: 50, 100, or 250 mcg/puff	0–4 yr: not established 5–11 yr: Initial dose of 50 mcg bid (maximum 100 mcg bid) ≥ 12 yr: Same as adults	If previously taking bronchodilators alone, initial dose of 100 mcg bid (maximum 500 mcg bid) If previously taking inhaled corticosteroids, initial dose of 100–250 mcg bid (maximum 500 mcg bid) If previously taking oral corticosteroids, initial dose of 500–1000 mcg bid (maximum 1000 mcg bid)	

Table continues on the following page.

Table 52–4. DRUG TREATMENT OF ASTHMA* (*Continued*)

DRUG	FORM	DOSAGE: CHILDREN	DOSAGE: ADULTS	COMMENTS
Fluticasone furoate	DPI: 100 or 200 mcg/puff	< 12 yr: Not established. ≥ 12 yr: Same as adults	If previously taking bronchodilators alone, initial dose of 100 mcg once/day (maximum 200 mcg/day) If previously taking inhaled corticosteroids, initial dose of 100–200 mcg once/day (maximum 200 mcg/day)	
Mometasone	DPI: 110 or 220 mcg/puff	< 4 yr: Not established 4–11 yr: 110 mcg once/day in the evening ≥ 12 yr: Same as adults	If previously taking bronchodilators alone or inhaled corticosteroids, initial dose of 220 mcg once/day in the evening (maximum 220 mcg bid or 440 mcg once/day in the evening) If previously taking oral corticosteroids, initial dose of 440 mcg bid (maximum 880 mcg bid)	
	HFA: 100 or 200 mcg/puff	< 12 yr: Not established ≥ 12 yr: Same as adults	If previously taking bronchodilators alone, initial dose of 220 mcg (delivering 200 mcg) once/day or bid (maximum 440 mcg/day) If previously taking inhaled corticosteroids, initial dose of 110–220 mcg (delivering 100 or 200 mcg) bid, (maximum 800 mcg/day) If previously taking oral corticosteroids, initial dose of 440 mcg (delivering 400 mcg) bid (maximum 800 mcg/day)	
Systemic corticosteroids (oral)				
Methylprednisolone	Tablets: 2, 4, 8, 16, or 32 mg	0–11 yr: Short-course burst: 1–2 mg/kg once/day (maximum 60 mg) for 3–10 days ≥ 12 yr: Same as adults	7.5–60 mg once/day in the morning or every other day in the morning Short-course burst: 40–60 mg once/day (or 20–30 mg bid) for 3–10 days	Maintenance doses should be given in a single dose in the morning every day or every other day as needed for control. Some evidence suggests clinical effectiveness increases with no increase in adrenal suppression when dose is given at 3 PM. Short-course burst doses are effective for establishing control when initiating therapy or during a period of gradual deterioration. The burst should be continued until PEF = 80% of personal best or symptoms resolve, possibly requiring > 3–10 days of therapy.
Prednisolone	Tablets: 5 mg Solution: 5 mg/5 mL or 15 mg/5 mL			
Prednisone	Tablets: 1, 2.5, 5, 10, 20, or 50 mg Solution: 5 mg/mL or 5 mg/5 mL			
Combination drugs				
Ipratropium and albuterol	SMI: 20 mcg/puff ipratropium and 100 mcg/puff albuterol	Not established	1 puff qid (maximum 6 puffs/day)	Ipratropium prolongs bronchodilator effect of albuterol.
	Nebulized solution: 0.5 mg ipratropium and 2.5 mg albuterol in a 3-mL vial		3-mL vial via nebulization qid for ambulatory rescue therapy (maximum 6 doses/24 h)	—

Table 52–4. DRUG TREATMENT OF ASTHMA* (*Continued*)

DRUG	FORM	DOSAGE CHILDREN	DOSAGE ADULTS	COMMENTS
Fluticasone and salmeterol	DPI: 100, 250, or 500 mcg fluticasone and 50 mcg salmeterol	< 4 yr: Not established 4–11 yr: 1 puff (100/50) bid ≥ 12 yr: Same as adults	1 puff bid	The 250/50 dose is indicated for asthma not controlled by low-to-medium doses of inhaled corticosteroids. The 500/50 dose is indicated for asthma not controlled by medium-to-high doses of inhaled corticosteroids.
	HFA: 45, 115, or 230 mcg fluticasone and 21 mcg salmeterol	< 12 yr: Not established ≥ 12 yr: Same as adults	2 puffs bid	—
Budesonide and formoterol	HFA: 80 or 160 mcg budesonide and 4.5 mcg formoterol	< 12 yr: Not established ≥ 12 yr: Same as adults	2 puffs bid (maximum 2 puffs of 160/4.5 mcg bid)	The 80/4.5 dose is indicated for asthma not controlled by low-to-medium doses of inhaled corticosteroids. The 160/4.5 dose is indicated for asthma not controlled by medium-to-high doses of inhaled corticosteroids.
Mometasone and formoterol	HFA: 100 mcg or 200 mcg mometasone and 5 mcg formoterol	< 5 yr: Not established ≥ 5 yr: Same as adults	2 puffs bid	The 100/5 dose is recommended for asthma not controlled by low-to-medium-dose inhaled corticosteroids. The 200/5 dose is recommended for asthma not controlled by high-dose inhaled corticosteroids.
Fluticasone and vilanterol	DPI: 100 or 200 mcg fluticasone and 25 mcg vilanterol	Not established	1 puff once/day	Recommended starting dose is based on asthma severity.
Mast cell stabilizers				
Cromolyn	Nebulized solution: 20 mg/ampule	< 2 yr: Not established ≥ 2 yr: Same as adults	1 ampule tid–qid	Cromolyn should be taken before exercise or allergen exposure. One dose provides effective prophylaxis for 1–2 h.
Leukotriene modifiers				
Montelukast	Tablets, chewable tablets, and granules: 4, 5, or 10 mg	12 mo–5 yr: 4 mg po once/day in the evening 6–14 yr: 5 mg po once/day in the evening ≥ 15 yr: Same as adults	10 mg po once/day in the evening Exercise-induced asthma: 10 mg po 2 h before exercise	Montelukast is a leukotriene receptor antagonist that is a competitive inhibitor of leukotrienes D4 and E4.
Zafirlukast	Tablet: 10 or 20 mg	< 5 yr: Not established 5–11 yr: 10 mg po bid ≥ 12 yr: Same as adults	20 mg po in the evening	Zafirlukast is a leukotriene receptor antagonist that is a competitive inhibitor of leukotrienes D4 and E4. It must be taken 1 h before or 2 h after meals.

Table continues on the following page.

Table 52–4. DRUG TREATMENT OF ASTHMA* (*Continued*)

DRUG	FORM	DOSAGE: CHILDREN	DOSAGE: ADULTS	COMMENTS
Zileuton	Tablet, immediate-release: 600 mg	< 12 yr: Not established ≥ 12 yr: Same as adults	600 mg po qid	Zileuton inhibits 5-lipoxygenase. Dosing may limit adherence. Zileuton may cause liver enzyme elevations and inhibit metabolism of drugs processed by CYP3A4, including theophylline.
	Extended-release: 1200 mg	< 12 yr: Not established ≥ 12 yr: Same as adults	1200 mg po bid within 1 h after morning and evening meals	
Methylxanthines				
Theophylline	Capsule, extended-release: 100, 200, 300, and 400 mg Elixir: 80 mg/15 mL Tablet, extended-release: 100, 200, 400, 450, or 600 mg	Initial dose of 10 mg/kg/day up to 600 mg/day, then adjusted to achieve a serum concentration of 5–15 mcg/mL at steady state	Initial dose of 10 mg/kg/day up to 600 mg/day, then adjusted to achieve a serum concentration of 5–15 mcg/mL at steady state	The wide variability in metabolic clearance, drug interactions, and potential for adverse effects mandate routine serum level monitoring. Availability of safer alternatives has led to declining use of this drug. Safety may be better with a target level < 10 mcg/mL.
Immunomodulators				
Mepolizumab	Subcutaneous injection: 100 mg	< 12 yr: Not established ≥ 12 yr: Same as adults	100 mg sc once q 4 wk	—
Omalizumab	Injection sc: 150 mg/1.2 mL	< 12 yr: 75–375 mg sc q 2–4 wk, depending on body weight and serum IgE level ≥ 12 yr: Same as adults	150–375 mg sc q 2–4 wk, depending on body weight and pretreatment serum IgE level	Maximum dose per injection site is 150 mg.
Reslizumab	Intravenous: 100 mg/10 mL	Not established	3 mg/kg IV once q 4 wk	—

*All ages unless specified differently.
DPI = dry-powder inhaler; HFA = hydrofluoroalkane; MDI = metered-dose inhaler; SMI = soft mist inhaler; PEF = peak expiratory flow.
Adapted from the National Heart, Lung, and Blood Institute: Expert Panel Report 3, Guidelines for the diagnosis and management of asthma—full report 2007. August 28, 2007. Available at www.nhlbi.nih.gov/guidelines/asthma/asthgdln.pdf.

(mepolizumab and reslizumab), which are used for the management of severe allergic asthma.

Omalizumab is indicated for patients with severe, allergic asthma who have elevated IgE levels. Omalizumab may decrease asthma exacerbations, corticosteroid requirements, and symptoms. Dosing is determined by a dosing chart based on the patient's weight and IgE levels. The drug is administered sc q 2 to 4 wk.

Mepolizumab and reslizumab were developed for use in patients with eosinophilic asthma and are monoclonal antibodies that block IL-5. IL-5 is a cytokine that promotes eosinophilic inflammation in the airways. Mepolizumab reduces exacerbation frequency, decreases asthma symptoms, and reduces the need for systemic corticosteroid therapy in patients with asthma who are dependent on chronic systemic corticosteroid therapy. Based on data from clinical trials, efficacy occurs with blood absolute eosinophil counts > 150/μL; however, for patients on chronic systemic corticosteroid therapy, the threshold for efficacy is unclear. Mepolizumab is administered subcutaneously 100 mg every 4 weeks.

Reslizumab also appears to reduce frequency of exacerbations and decrease asthma symptoms. In clinical trials, patients had blood absolute eosinophil counts of about 400/μL. In patients treated with chronic systemic corticosteroids, the eosinophil count threshold for efficacy is unclear. Reslizumab is administered 3 mg/kg IV over 20 to 50 minutes.

Clinicians who give any of these immunomodulators should be prepared to identify and treat anaphylaxis or allergic hypersensitivity reactions. Anaphylaxis may occur after any dose of omalizumab or reslizumab even if previous doses have been well tolerated. Allergic hypersensitivity reactions have been reported with mepolizumab. Mepolizumab use has been associated with herpes zoster infection; therefore, zoster vaccination should be considered prior to initiation of therapy.

PEARLS & PITFALLS

- Prepare for possible anaphylactic or hypersensitivity reactions in patients being treated with omalizumab, mepolizumab, or reslizumab regardless of how such treatments have been tolerated previously.

Other drugs: Other drugs are used in asthma treatment uncommonly and in specific circumstances. Magnesium is often used in the emergency department, but it is not recommended in the management of chronic asthma. Immunotherapy may be indicated when symptoms are triggered by allergy, as suggested by history and confirmed by allergy testing. Immunotherapy is generally more effective in children than adults. If symptoms are not significantly relieved after 24 mo, then therapy is stopped. If symptoms are relieved, therapy should continue for ≥ 3 yr, although the optimum duration is unknown.

Other drugs that suppress the immune system are occasionally given to reduce dependence on high-dose oral corticosteroids, but these drugs have a significant risk of toxicity. Low-dose methotrexate (5 to 15 mg po or IM once/wk) can lead to modest improvements in FEV_1 and modest decreases in daily oral corticosteroid use. Gold and cyclosporine are also modestly effective, but toxicity and need for monitoring limit their use.

Other therapies for management of chronic asthma include nebulized lidocaine, nebulized heparin, colchicine, and high-dose IV immune globulin. Limited evidence supports the use of any of these therapies, and their benefits are unproved, so none is currently recommended for routine clinical use.

TREATMENT OF ACUTE ASTHMA EXACERBATIONS

The goal of asthma exacerbation treatment is to relieve symptoms and return patients to their best lung function. Treatment includes

- Inhaled bronchodilators (beta-2 agonists and anticholinergics)
- Usually systemic corticosteroids

Patients having an asthma exacerbation are instructed to self-administer 2 to 4 puffs of inhaled albuterol or a similar short-acting beta-2 agonist up to 3 times spaced 20 min apart for an acute exacerbation and to measure PEF if possible. When these short-acting rescue drugs are effective (symptoms are relieved and PEF returns to > 80% of baseline), the acute exacerbation may be managed in the outpatient setting. Patients who do not respond, have severe symptoms, or have a PEF persistently < 80% should follow a treatment management program outlined by the physician or should go to the emergency department (see Table 52–5 for specific dosing information).

Emergency department care: Inhaled bronchodilators (beta-2 agonists and anticholinergics) are the mainstay of asthma treatment in the emergency department. In adults and older children, albuterol given by an MDI and spacer is as effective as that given by nebulizer. Nebulized treatment is preferred for younger children because of difficulties coordinating MDIs and spacers; evidence suggests that bronchodilator response improves when the nebulizer is powered with a mixture of helium and oxygen (heliox) rather than with oxygen.

Subcutaneous epinephrine 1:1000 solution or terbutaline is an alternative for children. Terbutaline may be preferable to epinephrine because of its lesser cardiovascular effects and longer duration of action, but it is no longer produced in large quantities and is expensive.

Subcutaneous administration of beta-2 agonists in adults raises concerns of adverse cardiostimulatory effects. However, clinically important adverse effects are few, and subcutaneous administration may benefit patients unresponsive to maximal inhaled therapy or patients unable to receive effective nebulized treatment (eg, those who cough excessively, have poor ventilation, or are uncooperative).

Nebulized ipratropium can be co-administered with nebulized albuterol for patients who do not respond optimally to albuterol alone; some evidence favors simultaneous high-dose beta-2 agonist and ipratropium as first-line treatment, but no data favor continuous beta-2 agonist nebulization over intermittent administration. Theophylline has very little role in treatment.

Systemic corticosteroids (prednisone, prednisolone, methylprednisolone) should be given for all but the mildest acute exacerbation; they are unnecessary for patients whose PEF normalizes after 1 or 2 bronchodilator doses. IV and oral routes of administration are probably equally effective. IV methylprednisolone can be given if an IV line is already in place and can be switched to oral dosing whenever necessary or convenient. In general, higher doses (prednisone 50 to 60 mg once/day) are recommended for the management of more severe exacerbations requiring in-patient care while lower doses (40 mg once/day) are reserved for outpatient treatment of milder exacerbations. Although evidence about optimal dose and duration is weak, a treatment duration of 3 to 5 days in children and 5 to 7 days in adults is recommended as adequate by most guidelines and should be tailored to the severity and duration of an exacerbation.[1, 2]

Antibiotics are indicated only when history, examination, or chest x-ray suggests underlying bacterial infection; most infections underlying asthma exacerbations are probably viral in origin.

Supplemental oxygen is indicated for hypoxemia and should be given by nasal cannula or face mask at a flow rate or concentration sufficient to maintain oxygen saturation > 90%.

Reassurance is the best approach when anxiety is the cause of asthma exacerbation. Anxiolytics and morphine are relatively contraindicated because they are associated with increased mortality and the need for mechanical ventilation.

Hospitalization: Hospitalization generally is required if patients have not returned to their baseline within 4 h of aggressive emergency department treatment. Criteria for hospitalization vary, but definite indications are

- Failure to improve
- Worsening fatigue
- Relapse after repeated beta-2 agonist therapy
- Significant decrease in $Pa{O_2}$ (< 50 mm Hg)
- Significant increase in $Pa{CO_2}$ (> 40 mm Hg)

A significant increase in $PaCO_2$ indicates progression to respiratory failure.

Noninvasive positive pressure ventilation (NIPPV) may be needed in patients whose condition continues to deteriorate despite aggressive treatment, to alleviate the work of breathing. Endotracheal intubation and invasive mechanical ventilation may be needed for respiratory failure. NIPPV can be used to prevent intubation if used early in the course of a severe exacerbation and should be considered in patients with acute respiratory distress with a level of $PaCO_2$ that is inappropriately high in relation to the degree of tachypnea. NIPPV should be

Table 52–5. DRUG TREATMENT OF ASTHMA EXACERBATIONS*, †

DRUG	FORM	DOSAGE IN CHILDREN	DOSAGE IN ADULTS	COMMENTS
Systemic beta-2 agonists				
Epinephrine	Injectable solution: 1 mg/mL (1:1000)	0.01 mL/kg /dose sc (maximum 0.4–0.5 mL q 20 min for 3 doses or q 4 h prn)	0.2–0.5 mg sc q 20 min (for maximum of 3 doses) or q 2 h prn	Subcutaneous administration is no more effective than inhalation and may have more adverse effects. Use in adults is controversial and may be contraindicated if significant cardiovascular disease is present.
Terbutaline	Injectable solution: 1 mg/mL	< 12 yr: 0.005–0.01 mg/kg q 20 min up to 3 doses; may repeat q 2–6 h prn ≥ 12 yr: Same as adults	0.25 mg sc once May repeat in 15–30 min (maximum 0.5 mg over 4 h)	—
Short-acting beta-2 agonists				
Albuterol	HFA: 90 mcg/puff	Same as adults	4–8 puffs q 20 min for 3 doses, then q 1–4 h prn	MDI is as effective as nebulized solution if patients can coordinate inhalation maneuver using spacer and holding chamber.
	Nebulized solution: 5 mg/mL and 0.63, 1.25, and 2.5 mg/3 mL	0.15 mg/kg (minimum 2.5 mg) q 20 min for 3 doses, then 0.15–0.3 mg/kg up to 10 mg q 1–4 h prn Alternatively, 0.5 mg/kg/h continuous nebulization	2.5–5 mg q 20 min for 3 doses, then 2.5–10 mg q 1–4 h prn (Alternatively, 10–15 mg/h continuous nebulization is similarly effective but increases frequency of adverse effects.)	—
Levalbuterol	HFA: 90 mcg/puff	Same as adults	4–8 puffs q 20 min for 3 doses, then q 1–4 h prn	Levalbuterol is the *R*-isomer of albuterol. 0.63 mg is equivalent to 1.25 mg racemic albuterol. Levalbuterol may have fewer adverse effects than albuterol.
	Nebulized solution: 0.63 and 1.25 mg/3 mL	0.075 mg/kg (minimum 1.25 mg) q 20 min for 3 doses, then 0.075–0.15 mg/kg up to 5 mg q 1–4 h prn Alternatively, 0.25 mg/kg/h continuous nebulization	1.25–2 mg q 20 min for 3 doses, then 1.25–5 mg q 1–4 h prn Alternatively, 5–7.5 mg/h continuous nebulization	—
Anticholinergics				
Ipratropium	Nebulized solution: 500 mcg/2.5 mL (0.02%)	0.25–0.5 mg q 20 min for 3 doses, then q 2–4 h prn	0.5 mg q 20 min for 3 doses, then q 2–4 h prn	Ipratropium should be added to beta-2 agonists and not used as first-line therapy. It may be mixed in same nebulizer as albuterol. Dose delivered from MDI is low and has not been studied in exacerbations.
Combination drugs				
Ipratropium and albuterol	SMI: 20 mcg ipratropium and 100 mcg albuterol/puff	Same as adults	1 puff q 30 min for 3 doses, then q 2–4 h prn	Ipratropium prolongs bronchodilator effect of albuterol.

Table 52–5. DRUG TREATMENT OF ASTHMA EXACERBATIONS*, † (*Continued*)

DRUG	FORM	DOSAGE IN CHILDREN	DOSAGE IN ADULTS	COMMENTS
	Nebulized solution: 0.5 mg ipratropium and 2.5 mg albuterol in a 3-mL vial	1.5 mL q 20 min for 3 doses, then q 2–4 h prn	3 mL q 30 m for 3 doses, then q 2–4 h prn	
Systemic corticosteroids				
Methylprednisolone	Tablets: 2, 4, 8, 16, and 32 mg	Inpatient:1 mg/kg q 6 h for 48 h, then 0.5–1.0 mg/kg bid (maximum, 60 mg/day) until PEF = 70% of predicted or personal best Outpatient burst: 0.5–1.0 mg/kg bid (maximum 60 mg/day for 3–5 days)	Inpatient: 40–60 mg q 6 h or q 8 h for 48 h, then 60–80 mg/day until PEF = 70% of predicted or personal best Outpatient burst: 40–60 mg in single or 2 divided doses for 5–7 days	IV has no advantage over oral administration if GI function is normal. Higher doses provide no advantage in severe exacerbations. Usual regimen is to continue frequent multiple daily doses until FEV_1 or PEF = 50% of predicted or personal best and then lower the dose to bid, usually within 48 h. Therapy after a hospitalization or ED visit may last 5–10 days. Tapering the dose is not needed if patients are also given inhaled corticosteroids.
Prednisolone	Tablets: 5 mg Orally disintegrating tablets: 10, 15, and 30 mg Solution: 5, 10, 15, 20, and 25 mg/5 mL			
Prednisone	Tablets: 1, 2.5, 5, 10, 20, and 50 mg Solution: 5 mg/mL and 5 mg/5 mL			

*All ages unless specified differently.
†Amount and timing of ongoing doses are dictated by clinical response.
ED = emergency department; FEV_1 = forced expiratory volume in 1 sec; HFA = hydrofluoroalkane; MDI = metered-dose inhaler; PEF = peak expiratory flow.
Adapted from National Heart, Lung, and Blood Institute: Expert Panel Report 3: Guidelines for the diagnosis and management of asthma—full report 2007. August 28, 2007. Available at www.nhlbi.nih.gov/guidelines/asthma/asthgdln.pdf.

reserved for exacerbations that, despite immediate therapy with bronchodilators and systemic corticosteroids, result in respiratory distress, using criteria such as tachypnea (respiratory rate > 25 per minute), use of accessory respiratory muscles, $PaCO_2$ > 40 but < 60 mm Hg, and hypoxemia. Mechanical ventilation should be used rather than NIPPV if patients have any of the following:

- $PaCO_2$ > 60 mm Hg
- Decreased level of consciousness
- Excessive respiratory secretions
- Facial abnormalities (ie, surgical, traumatic) that could impede noninvasive ventilation

Mechanical ventilation should be strongly considered if there is no convincing improvement after 1 h of NIPPV.

Intubation and mechanical ventilation allow the provision of sedation to further alleviate the work of breathing, but the routine use of neuromuscular blocking agents should be avoided because of possible interactions with corticosteroids that can cause prolonged neuromuscular weakness.

Generally, volume-cycled ventilation in assist-control mode is used because it provides constant alveolar ventilation when airway resistance is high and changing. The ventilator should be set to a relatively low frequency with a relatively high inspiratory flow rate (> 80 L/min) to prolong exhalation time, minimizing auto positive end-expiratory pressure (PEEP). Initial tidal volumes can be set to 6 to 8 mL/kg of ideal body weight. High peak airway pressures will generally be present because they result from high airway resistance and inspiratory flow rates. In these patients, peak airway pressure does not reflect the degree of lung distention caused by alveolar pressure. However, if plateau pressures exceed 30 to 35 cm water, then tidal volume should be reduced to limit the risk of pneumothorax. When reduced tidal volumes are necessary, a moderate degree of hypercapnia is acceptable, but if arterial pH falls below 7.10, a slow sodium bicarbonate infusion is indicated to maintain pH between 7.20 and 7.25. Once airflow obstruction is relieved and $Paco_2$ and arterial pH normalize, patients can usually be quickly weaned from the ventilator. (For further details, see Ch. 70.)

Other therapy: Other therapies are reportedly effective for asthma exacerbation, but none have been thoroughly studied. A mixture of helium and oxygen (heliox) is used to decrease the work of breathing and improve ventilation through a decrease in turbulent flow attributable to helium, a gas less dense than oxygen. Despite the theoretical benefits of heliox, studies have reported conflicting results concerning its efficacy; lack of ready availability and inability to concurrently provide high concentrations of oxygen (due to the fact that 70 to 80% of the inhaled gas is helium) may also limit its use. Magnesium sulfate relaxes smooth muscle, but efficacy in management of asthma exacerbation in the emergency department is debated. General anesthesia in patients with status asthmaticus causes bronchodilation by an unclear mechanism, perhaps by a direct relaxant effect on airway smooth muscle or attenuation of cholinergic tone.

1. Global Initiative for Asthma 2017 Report, Global Strategy for Asthma Management and Prevention
2. British Thoracic Society Asthma Guidelines 2016

ALLERGIC BRONCHOPULMONARY ASPERGILLOSIS

Allergic bronchopulmonary aspergillosis (ABPA) is a hypersensitivity reaction to *Aspergillus* species (generally *A. fumigatus*) that occurs almost exclusively in patients with asthma or, less commonly, cystic fibrosis. Immune responses to *Aspergillus* antigens cause airway obstruction and, if untreated, bronchiectasis and pulmonary fibrosis. Symptoms and signs are those of asthma with the addition of productive cough and, occasionally, fever and anorexia. Diagnosis is suspected based on history and imaging tests and confirmed by *Aspergillus* skin testing and measurement of IgE levels, circulating precipitins, and *A. fumigatus*–specific antibodies. Treatment is with corticosteroids and, in patients with refractory disease, itraconazole.

ABPA develops when airways of patients with asthma or cystic fibrosis become colonized with *Aspergillus* sp (ubiquitous fungi in the soil).

Pathophysiology

For unclear reasons, colonization in these patients prompts vigorous antibody (IgE and IgG) and cell-mediated immune responses (type I, III, and IV hypersensitivity reactions) to *Aspergillus* antigens, leading to frequent, recurrent asthma exacerbations. Over time, the immune reactions, combined with direct toxic effects of the fungus, lead to airway damage with dilation and, ultimately, bronchiectasis and fibrosis. The disorder is characterized histologically by mucoid impaction of airways, eosinophilic pneumonia, infiltration of alveolar septa with plasma and mononuclear cells, and an increase in the number of bronchiolar mucous glands and goblet cells.

Rarely, other fungi, such as *Penicillium*, *Candida*, *Curvularia*, *Helminthosporium*, and *Drechslera* spp, cause an identical syndrome called allergic bronchopulmonary mycosis in the absence of underlying asthma or cystic fibrosis.

Aspergillus is present intraluminally but is not invasive. Thus, ABPA must be distinguished from invasive aspergillosis, which occurs in immunocompromised patients; from aspergillomas, which are collections of *Aspergillus* in patients with established cavitary lesions or cystic airspaces; and from the rare *Aspergillus* pneumonia, which occurs in patients who take low doses of prednisone long term (eg, patients with COPD). Although the distinction can be clear, overlap syndromes have been reported.

Symptoms and Signs

Symptoms are those of asthma or pulmonary cystic fibrosis exacerbation, with the addition of cough productive of dirty-green or brown plugs and, occasionally, hemoptysis. Fever, headache, and anorexia are common systemic symptoms in severe disease. Signs are those of airway obstruction, specifically, wheezing and prolonged expiration, which are indistinguishable from asthma exacerbation.

Diagnosis

- History of asthma
- Chest x-ray or high-resolution CT
- Skin prick test with *Aspergillus* antigen
- *Aspergillus* precipitins in blood
- Positive sputum culture for *Aspergillus* species (or, rarely, other fungi)
- IgE levels

The diagnosis is suspected in patients with asthma with recurrent asthma exacerbations, migratory or nonresolving infiltrates on chest x-ray (often due to atelectasis resulting from mucoid plugging and bronchial obstruction), evidence of bronchiectasis on imaging studies, sputum cultures positive for *A. fumigatus*, or notable peripheral eosinophilia.

Several criteria have been proposed for the diagnosis (see Table 52–6), but in practice not all criteria are assessed in every case.

When the diagnosis is suspected, a skin prick test with *Aspergillus* antigen is the best first step. An immediate wheal-and-flare reaction should prompt measurement of serum IgE and *Aspergillus* precipitins because up to 25% of patients with asthma without ABPA may have a positive skin test. An IgE level > 1000 ng/mL (> 417 IU/mL) and positive precipitins suggest the diagnosis, which should be confirmed by measurement of specific anti-*Aspergillus* immunoglobulins (up to 10% of healthy patients have circulating precipitins). When ABPA is suspected, a finding of *A. fumigatus*–specific IgG and IgE antibodies in concentrations at least twice those found in patients without ABPA establishes the diagnosis.

Whenever test results diverge, such as when serum IgE is elevated but no *A. fumigatus*–specific immunoglobulins are found, testing should be repeated and the patient should be monitored over time to definitively establish or exclude the diagnosis.

Table 52–6. DIAGNOSTIC CRITERIA FOR ALLERGIC BRONCHOPULMONARY ASPERGILLOSIS

Essential criteria
• Asthma or cystic fibrosis • Elevated *Aspergillus*-specific IgE or *Aspergillus* skin test positivity • Elevated serum IgE (> 1000 ng/mL or > 417 IU/mL)*
Other criteria
• Precipitating serum antibodies to *A. fumigatus* or elevated serum *Aspergillus* IgG by immunoassay • Radiographic pulmonary opacities consistent with ABPA • Blood eosinophilia (> 500 cells/μL) currently or previously while corticosteroid-naive)

*May be lower if patient meets all other criteria for diagnosis

Adapted from Agarwal R, Chakrabarti A, Shah A, et al: Allergic bronchopulmonary aspergillosis: review of literature and proposal of new diagnostic` and classification criteria. *Clin Exp Allergy* 43:850, 2013.

Table 52–7. STAGES OF ALLERGIC BRONCHOPULMONARY ASPERGILLOSIS*

STAGE	DESCRIPTION	CRITERIA
I	Acute	All diagnostic criteria present
II	Remission	Symptoms resolved for > 6 mo
III	Relapse	Recurrence of ≥ 1 of the diagnostic criteria
IV	Refractory	Corticosteroid-dependent or refractory to treatment
V	Fibrosis	Diffuse fibrosis and bronchiectasis

*Stages do not progress sequentially.

Treatment

- Prednisone
- Sometimes antifungal drugs

Treatment is based on disease stage (see Table 52–7).

Stage I is treated with prednisone 0.5 to 0.75 mg/kg po once/day for 2 to 4 wk, then tapered over 4 to 6 mo. Chest x-ray, blood eosinophil count, and IgE levels should be checked quarterly for improvement, defined as resolution of infiltrates, ≥ 50% decline in eosinophils, and 33% decline in IgE. Patients who achieve stage II disease require annual monitoring only.

Stage II patients who relapse (stage III) are given another trial of prednisone. Stage I or III patients who do not improve with prednisone (Stage IV) are candidates for antifungal treatment. Itraconazole 200 mg po bid for 16 weeks is recommended as a substitute for prednisone and as a corticosteroid-sparing drug. Itraconazole therapy requires checking drug levels and monitoring liver enzymes and triglyceride and potassium levels.

All patients should be optimally treated for their underlying asthma or cystic fibrosis. In addition, patients taking long-term corticosteroids should be monitored for complications, such as cataracts, diabetes mellitus, and osteoporosis, and possibly prescribed treatments to prevent bone demineralization and *Pneumocystis jirovecii* lung infection.

KEY POINTS

- Consider allergic bronchopulmonary aspergillosis (ABPA) if a patient with asthma or cystic fibrosis develops frequent exacerbations for unclear reasons, has migratory or nonresolving infiltrates on chest x-ray, evidence of bronchiectasis on imaging studies, persistent blood eosinophilia, or if a sputum culture reveals *Aspergillus*.
- Begin testing with a skin prick using *Aspergillus* antigen, followed usually by serologic testing.
- Treat initially with prednisone.
- If ABPA persists despite prednisone, treat with an antifungal such as itraconazole.

53 Bronchiectasis and Atelectasis

BRONCHIECTASIS

Bronchiectasis is dilation and destruction of larger bronchi caused by chronic infection and inflammation. Common causes are cystic fibrosis, immune defects, and recurrent infections, though some cases seem to be idiopathic. Symptoms are chronic cough and purulent sputum expectoration; some patients may also have fever and dyspnea. Diagnosis is based on history and imaging, usually involving high-resolution CT, though standard chest x-rays may be diagnostic. Treatment and prevention of acute exacerbations are with antibiotics, drainage of secretions, and management of complications, such as superinfection and hemoptysis. Treatment of underlying disorders is important whenever possible.

Etiology

Bronchiectasis is best considered the common end-point of various disorders that cause chronic airway inflammation. Bronchiectasis may affect many areas of the lung (diffuse bronchiectasis), or it may appear in only one or two areas (focal bronchiectasis).

Diffuse bronchiectasis develops most often in patients with genetic, immunologic, or anatomic defects that affect the airways. In developed countries, many cases appear initially to be idiopathic, probably partly because onset is so slow that the triggering problem cannot be identified by the time bronchiectasis is recognized. With newer, improved genetic and immunologic testing, an increasing number of reports describe finding an etiology in these idiopathic cases after careful, systematic evaluation.

Cystic fibrosis (CF—see p. 2549) is the most common identified cause, and previously undiagnosed CF may account for up to 20% of idiopathic cases. Even heterozygous patients, who typically have no clinical manifestations of CF, may have an increased risk of bronchiectasis.

Immunodeficiencies such as common variable immunodeficiency (CVID) may also lead to diffuse disease, as may rare abnormalities in airway structure. Undernutrition and HIV infection also appear to increase risk.

Congenital defects in mucociliary clearance such as primary ciliary dyskinesia (PCD) syndromes may also be a cause, possibly also explaining some idiopathic cases.

Diffuse bronchiectasis sometimes complicates common autoimmune disorders, such as RA or Sjögren syndrome.

Allergic bronchopulmonary aspergillosis, a hypersensitivity reaction to *Aspergillus* spp (see p. 416) that occurs most commonly in people with asthma, but sometimes in patients with CF, can cause or contribute to bronchiectasis.

In developing countries, most cases are probably caused by TB, particularly in patients with impaired immune function due to undernutrition and HIV infection.

Focal bronchiectasis typically develops as a result of untreated pneumonia or obstruction (eg, due to foreign bodies, tumors, postsurgical changes, lymphadenopathy). Mycobacteria (tuberculous or nontuberculous) can both cause focal bronchiectasis and colonize the lungs of patients with bronchiectasis due to other disorders (see Table 53–1).

Pathophysiology

The pathophysiology of bronchiectasis is not fully understood, likely in part because it is the common end-point of a heterogenous group of disorders predisposing to chronic airway inflammation.

Diffuse bronchiectasis appears to start when a causative disorder triggers inflammation of small and medium-sized airways, releasing inflammatory mediators from intraluminal neutrophils. The inflammatory mediators destroy elastin, cartilage, and muscle in larger airways, resulting in irreversible bronchodilation. Simultaneously, in the inflamed small and medium-sized airways, macrophages and lymphocytes form infiltrates that thicken mucosal walls. This thickening causes the airway obstruction frequently noted during pulmonary function testing. With disease progression, inflammation spreads beyond the airways, causing fibrosis of the surrounding lung parenchyma. What inflames the small airways depends on the etiology of bronchiectasis. Common contributors include impaired airway clearance (due to production of thick, viscous mucus in CF, lack of ciliary motility in PCD, or damage to the cilia and/or airways secondary to infection or injury) and impaired host defenses; these factors predispose patients to chronic infection and inflammation. In the case of immune deficiency (particularly CVID), autoimmune inflammation may also contribute.

Focal bronchiectasis usually occurs when a large airway becomes obstructed. The resulting inability to clear secretions leads to a cycle of infection, inflammation, and airway wall damage. The right middle lobe is involved most often because its bronchus is small and angulated and has lymph nodes in close proximity. Lymphadenopathy due to nontuberculous mycobacterial infection sometimes causes bronchial obstruction and focal bronchiectasis.

As ongoing inflammation changes airway anatomy, pathogenic bacteria (sometimes including mycobacteria) colonize the airways. Common organisms include *Haemophilus influenzae* (35%), *Pseudomonas aeruginosa* (31%), *Moraxella catarrhalis* (20%), *Staphylococcus aureus* (14%), and *Streptococcus pneumoniae* (13%). *S. aureus* colonization is strongly associated with CF; a culture finding of *S. aureus* should raise concern for undiagnosed CF. Also, colonization with *P. aeruginosa* tends to indicate severe disease and portends a rapid decline in lung function. Colonization by multiple organisms is common, and antibiotic resistance is a concern in patients who require frequent courses of antibiotics for treatment of exacerbations.

Complications: As the disease progresses, chronic inflammation and hypoxemia cause neovascularization of the bronchial (not the pulmonary) arteries. Bronchial artery walls rupture easily, leading to massive hemoptysis. Other vascular complications include pulmonary hypertension due to vasoconstriction, arteritis, and sometimes shunt from bronchial to pulmonary vessels. Colonization with multidrug-resistant organisms can lead to chronic, low-grade airway inflammation. This inflammation can progress to recurrent exacerbations and worsen airflow limitation on pulmonary function tests.

Symptoms and Signs

Symptoms characteristically begin insidiously and gradually worsen over years, accompanied by episodes of acute exacerbation.

The most common presenting symptom is chronic cough that produces thick, tenacious, often purulent sputum. Dyspnea and wheezing are common, and pleuritic chest pain can develop. In advanced cases, hypoxemia and right-sided heart failure due to pulmonary hypertension may increase dyspnea. Hemoptysis, which can be massive, occurs due to airway neovascularization.

Acute exacerbations are common and frequently result from new or worsened infection. Exacerbations are marked by a worsening cough and increases in dyspnea and the volume and purulence of sputum. Low-grade fever and constitutional symptoms (eg, fatigue, malaise) may also be present.

Halitosis and abnormal breath sounds, including crackles, rhonchi, and wheezing, are typical physical examination findings. Digital clubbing may be present. In advanced cases, signs of hypoxemia, pulmonary hypertension (eg, dyspnea, dizziness), and right-sided heart failure are common. Chronic rhinosinusitis and nasal polyps may be present, particularly in patients with CF or PCD. Lean body mass commonly decreases, possibly due to inflammation and cytokine excess and, in patients with CF, malabsorption.

Diagnosis

- History and physical examination
- Chest x-ray
- High-resolution chest CT
- Pulmonary function tests for baseline evaluation and monitoring disease progression
- Specific tests for suspected causes

Diagnosis is based on history, physical examination, and radiologic testing, beginning with a chest x-ray. Chronic bronchitis may mimic bronchiectasis clinically, but bronchiectasis is distinguished by increased purulence and volume of daily sputum and by dilated airways shown on imaging studies.

Imaging: Chest x-ray is usually abnormal and may be diagnostic. X-ray findings suggestive of bronchiectasis involve thickening of the airway walls and/or airway dilation; typical findings include ill-defined linear perihilar densities with indistinctness of the central pulmonary arteries, indistinct rings due to thickened airways seen in cross section (parallel to the x-ray beam), and "tram lines" (or tram-track sign) caused by thickened, dilated airways perpendicular to the x-ray beam. Dilated airways filled with mucous plugs can also cause scattered elongated, tubular opacities. Radiographic patterns may differ depending on the underlying disease; bronchiectasis due to CF develops predominantly in the upper lobes, whereas bronchiectasis due to an endobronchial obstruction causes more focal x-ray abnormalities.

High-resolution CT is the test of choice for defining the extent of bronchiectasis and is nearly 100% sensitive and specific. Typical CT findings include airway dilation (in which the inner lumen of two or more airways exceed the diameter of the adjacent artery) and the signet ring sign (in which a thickened, dilated airway appears adjacent to a smaller artery in transaxial view). Lack of normal bronchial tapering can result in visible medium-sized bronchi extending almost to the pleura. "Tram lines" are easily visible on CT. As airway damage increases over time, bronchiectasis changes progress from cylindrical to varicose and then cystic findings on imaging. Atelectasis,

Table 53–1. FACTORS PREDISPOSING TO BRONCHIECTASIS

CATEGORY	EXAMPLES AND COMMENTS
Infections	
Bacterial	*Bordetella pertussis* *Haemophilus influenzae* *Klebsiella* spp. *Moraxella catarrhalis* *Mycoplasma pneumoniae* *Pseudomonas aeruginosa* *Staphylococcus aureus*
Fungal	*Aspergillus* spp. *Histoplasma capsulatum*
Mycobacterial	*Mycobacterium tuberculosis* Nontuberculous mycobacteria
Viral	Adenovirus Herpes simplex virus Influenza Measles Respiratory syncytial virus
Congenital disorders	
α_1-Antitrypsin deficiency	If severe, can cause bronchiectasis
Ciliary defects	Can cause bronchiectasis, sinusitis, otitis media, and male infertility 50% of patients with primary ciliary dyskinesia have situs inversus Kartagener syndrome (clinical triad of dextrocardia, sinus disease, situs inversus)
Cystic fibrosis	Causes viscous secretions due to defects in Na and Cl transport Often complicated by *P. aeruginosa* or *S. aureus* colonization
Immunodeficiencies	
Primary	Chronic granulomatous disease Complement deficiencies Hypogammaglobulinemia, particularly common variable immunodeficiency
Secondary	HIV infection Immunosuppressants
Airway obstruction	
Cancer	Endobronchial lesion
Extrinsic compression	Due to tumor mass or lymphadenopathy
Foreign body	Aspirated or intrinsic (eg, broncholith)
Mucoid impaction	Allergic bronchopulmonary aspergillosis
Postoperative	After lobar resection, due to kinking or twisting of remaining lobes
Connective tissue and systemic disorders	
RA	Commonly causes bronchiectasis (frequently subclinical), more often in men and in patients with long-standing RA
Sjögren syndrome	Bronchiectasis possibly due to increased viscosity of bronchial mucous, which leads to obstruction, poor clearance, and chronic infection
SLE	Bronchiectasis in up to 20% of patients via unclear mechanisms
Inflammatory bowel disease	Bronchopulmonary complications occurring after onset of inflammatory bowel disease in up to 85% and before onset in 10 to 15% Bronchiectasis more common in ulcerative colitis but can occur in Crohn disease
Relapsing polychondritis	—
Congenital structural defects	
Lymphatic	Yellow nail syndrome
Tracheobronchial	Williams-Campbell syndrome (cartilage deficiency) Tracheobronchomegaly (eg, Mounier-Kuhn syndrome)
Vascular	Pulmonary sequestration (a congenital malformation in which a nonfunctioning mass of lung tissue lacks normal communication with the tracheobronchial tree and receives its arterial blood supply from the systemic circulation)

Table continues on the following page.

Table 53–1. FACTORS PREDISPOSING TO BRONCHIECTASIS (*Continued*)

CATEGORY	EXAMPLES AND COMMENTS
Toxic inhalation	
Ammonia Chlorine Nitrogen dioxide	Direct airway damage altering structure and function
Other	
Transplantation	May be secondary to frequent infection due to immunosuppression

Adapted from Barker, AF: Bronchiectasis. *New Engl J Med* 346:1383–1393, 2002.

consolidation, mucus plugs, and decreased vascularity are nonspecific findings. In traction bronchiectasis, pulmonary fibrosis pulls or distorts airways in ways that simulate bronchiectasis on imaging.

Pulmonary function tests: Pulmonary function tests can be helpful for documenting baseline function and for monitoring disease progression. Bronchiectasis causes airflow limitation (reduced forced expiratory volume in 1 sec [FEV_1], forced vital capacity [FVC], and FEV_1/FVC); the FEV_1 may improve in response to β-agonist bronchodilators. Lung volume measurements may be increased or decreased, and diffusing capacity for carbon monoxide (DLco) may be decreased.

Diagnosis of cause: During an exacerbation-free period, all patients should have expectorated or induced sputum cultured to determine the predominant colonizing bacteria and their sensitivities. This information helps with antibiotic selection during exacerbations. A CBC and differential can help determine the severity of disease activity and identify eosinophilia, which may suggest complicating diagnoses. Staining and cultures for bacterial, mycobacterial (*Mycobacterium avium* complex and *M. tuberculosis*), and fungal (*Aspergillus* spp) organisms may also help identify the cause of chronic airway inflammation. Clinically significant nontuberculous mycobacterial infection is diagnosed by finding high colony counts of these mycobacteria in cultures from serial sputum samples or from bronchoalveolar lavage fluid in patients who have granulomas on biopsy or concurrent radiologic evidence of disease.

When the cause of bronchiectasis is unclear, additional testing based on the history and imaging findings may be done. Tests may include the following:

- Serum immunoglobulins (IgG IgA, IgM) and serum electrophoresis to diagnose CVID
- Targeted assessment of baseline and specific antibody responses to peptide and polysaccharide antigens (ie, tetanus, capsular polysaccharide of *S. pneumoniae* and *H. influenzae* type b) done to assess immune responsiveness
- Two sweat chloride tests and *CFTR* gene mutation analysis to diagnose CF (including in adults > 40 yr without an identifiable cause of bronchiectasis, especially if they have upper lobe involvement, malabsorption, or male infertility)
- Rheumatoid factor, ANA, and antineutrophil cytoplasmic antibody testing if an autoimmune condition is being considered
- Serum IgE and *Aspergillus* precipitins if patients have eosinophilia, to rule out allergic bronchopulmonary aspergillosis
- α_1-Antitrypsin level to evaluate for α_1-antitrypsin deficiency if high resolution CT shows lower lobe emphysema

PCD should be considered if adults with bronchiectasis also have chronic sinus disease or otitis media, particularly if problems have persisted since childhood. Bronchiectasis in such patients may have right middle lobe and lingular predominance, and infertility or dextrocardia may be present. Diagnosis requires examination of a nasal or bronchial epithelial sample for abnormal ciliary structure using transmission electron microscopy. The diagnosis of PCD should typically be done in specialized centers because evaluation can be challenging. Nonspecific structural defects can be present in up to 10% of cilia in healthy people and in patients with pulmonary disease, and infection can cause transient dyskinesia. Ciliary ultrastructure may also be normal in some patients with PCD syndromes, requiring further testing to identify abnormal ciliary function.

Bronchoscopy is indicated when an anatomic or obstructive lesion is suspected.

Evaluation of exacerbations: The degree of testing depends on the severity of the clinical presentation. For patients with mild to moderate exacerbations, repeat sputum cultures to confirm the causative organism and sensitivity patterns may be sufficient. These help narrow antibiotic coverage and exclude opportunistic pathogens. For more severely ill patients, a CBC, chest x-ray, and possibly other tests may be warranted to exclude common complications of serious pulmonary infection, such as lung abscess and empyema.

Prognosis

Prognosis varies widely. Mean yearly decrease in FEV_1 is about 50 to 55 mL (normal decrease in healthy people is about 20 to 30 mL). Patients with CF have the poorest prognosis, with a median survival of 36 yr, and most patients continue to have intermittent exacerbations.

Treatment

- Prevention of exacerbations with regular vaccinations and sometimes suppressive antibiotics
- Measures to help clear airway secretions
- Bronchodilators and often inhaled corticosteroids if reversible airway obstruction is present
- Antibiotics and bronchodilators for acute exacerbations
- Sometimes surgical resection for localized disease with intractable symptoms or bleeding

The key treatment goals are to control symptoms and improve quality of life, reduce the frequency of exacerbations, and preserve lung function.

As for all patients with chronic pulmonary disease, smoking cessation and annual influenza vaccination and pneumococcal polysaccharide vaccination are recommended. Revaccination is recommended 5 yr later in patients who are < 65 at the time of their initial pneumococcal vaccination and for patients who are asplenic or immunosuppressed.

Airway clearance techniques are used to reduce chronic cough in patients with significant sputum production and mucus plugging and to reduce symptoms during exacerbations. Such techniques include postural drainage and chest percussion, positive expiratory pressure devices, intrapulmonary percussive ventilators, pneumatic vests, and autogenic drainage (a breathing technique thought to help move secretions from peripheral to central airways). Patients should be taught these techniques by a respiratory therapist and should use whichever one is most effective and sustainable for them; no evidence favors one particular technique.

For patients with reversible airway obstruction, bronchodilator therapy (eg, with some combination of a long-acting β-adrenergic agonist, tiotropium, and a short-acting β-adrenergic drug as indicated by symptoms, as used in patients with COPD) can help improve function and quality of life. Inhaled corticosteroids may also be used in patients with frequent exacerbations or marked variability in lung function measurements. Pulmonary rehabilitation can be helpful.

In patients with CF, a variety of nebulized treatments, including a mucolytic (rhDNase) and hypertonic (7%) saline, can help reduce sputum viscosity and enhance airway clearance. In patients without CF, evidence of benefit with these agents is inconclusive, so only humidification and saline are recommended as inhaled treatments. Inhaled terbutaline, dry powder mannitol, and mucolytics such as carbocysteine and bromhexine have mechanisms that might be expected to accelerate tracheobronchial clearance. However, most of these agents have had mixed results in limited trials in patients with and without CF.

There is no consensus on the best use of antibiotics to prevent or limit the frequency of acute exacerbations. Use of suppressive antibiotics regularly or on a rotating schedule reduces symptoms and exacerbations but may increase the risk that future infections will involve resistant organisms. Current guidelines suggest using antibiotics in patients with ≥ 3 exacerbations per year and possibly also in those with fewer exacerbations who have culture-proven *P. aeruginosa* colonization. Chronic therapy with azithromycin 500 mg po 3 times/wk reduces acute exacerbations in patients with or without CF. Macrolides are thought to be beneficial mainly due to their anti-inflammatory or immunomodulatory effects. Patients with *P. aeruginosa* may benefit from inhaled tobramycin, 300 mg bid given for a month every other month.

Additional treatment depends on the cause. For CF, see p. 2549. Allergic bronchopulmonary aspergillosis is treated with corticosteroids and sometimes azole antifungals (see p. 417). Patients with immunoglobulin or α_1-antitrypsin deficiencies should receive replacement therapy.

Acute exacerbations: Acute exacerbations are treated with antibiotics, inhaled bronchodilators (particularly if patients are wheezing), and increased attempts at mucus clearance, using mechanical techniques, humidification, and nebulized saline (and mucolytics for patients with CF). Inhaled or oral corticosteroids are given to treat airway inflammation. Antibiotic choice depends on previous culture results and whether or not patients have CF.

Initial antibiotics for patients without CF and with no prior culture results should be effective against *H. influenzae*, *M. catarrhalis*, *S. aureus*, and *S. pneumoniae*. Examples include amoxicillin/clavulanate, azithromycin, clarithromycin, and trimethoprim/sulfamethoxazole. Antibiotics should be adjusted based on culture results and given for a typical duration of 14 days. Patients with known *P. aeruginosa* colonization or more severe exacerbations should receive antibiotics effective against this organism (eg, ciprofloxacin 500 mg po bid, levofloxacin 500 mg po once/day for 7 to 14 days) until repeat culture results are available.

Initial antibiotic selection for patients with CF is guided by previous sputum culture results (done routinely in all patients with CF). During childhood, common infecting organisms are *S. aureus* and *H. influenzae*, and quinolone antibiotics such as ciprofloxacin and levofloxacin may be used. In the later stages of CF, infections involve highly resistant strains of certain gram-negative organisms including *P. aeruginosa*, *Burkholderia cepacia*, and *Stenotrophomonas maltophilia*. In patients with infections caused by these organisms, treatment is with multiple antibiotics (eg, tobramycin, aztreonam, ticarcillin/clavulanate, ceftazidime, cefepime). IV administration is frequently required.

Complications: Significant hemoptysis is usually treated with bronchial artery embolization, but surgical resection may be considered if embolization is ineffective and pulmonary function is adequate.

Superinfection with mycobacterial organisms such as *M. avium* complex almost always requires multiple drug regimens that include clarithromycin 500 mg po bid or azithromycin 250 mg po once/day; rifampin 600 mg po once/day or rifabutin 300 mg po once/day; and ethambutol 25 mg/kg po once/day for 2 mo followed by 15 mg/kg po once/day. Drug therapy is modified based on culture and sensitivity results. All drugs should be taken until sputum cultures have been negative for 12 mo.

Surgical resection is rarely needed but may be considered when bronchiectasis is localized, medical therapy has been optimized, and the symptoms are intolerable. In certain patients with diffuse bronchiectasis, lung transplantation is also an option. Five-year survival rates as high as 65 to 75% have been reported when a heart-lung or double lung transplantation is done. Pulmonary function usually improves within 6 mo, and improvement may be sustained for at least 5 yr.

KEY POINTS

- In bronchiectasis, chronic inflammation from various causes destroys elastin, cartilage, and muscle in larger airways, resulting in irreversible bronchodilation; dilated airways are chronically colonized by infectious organisms.
- Patients have chronic productive cough with intermittent acute exacerbations, usually 2 to 3 times/yr.
- Diagnosis is with imaging, usually CT; cultures should be done to identify colonizing organism(s).
- Prevent exacerbations using appropriate immunizations, airway clearance measures, and sometimes macrolide antibiotics.
- Treat exacerbations with antibiotics, bronchodilators, more frequent airway clearance measures, and corticosteroids.

ATELECTASIS

Atelectasis is collapse of lung tissue with loss of volume. Patients may have dyspnea or respiratory failure if atelectasis is extensive. They may also develop pneumonia. Pleuritic chest pain may be present with certain causes of atelectasis. Diagnosis is by chest x-ray. Treatment includes maintaining coughing and deep breathing and treating the cause.

The natural tendency for open air spaces such as the alveoli to collapse is countered by the following:

- Surfactant (which maintains surface tension)
- Continuous breathing (which keeps the alveoli open)
- Intermittent deep breathing (which releases surfactant into the alveoli)
- Periodic coughing (which clears the airways of secretions)
- Major consequences of atelectasis include under ventilation (with hypoxia and ventilation/perfusion [V/Q] mismatch) and pneumonia.

Etiology

The most common factors that can cause atelectasis include the following:

- Intrinsic obstruction of airways (eg, by foreign body, tumor, mucous plug)
- Extrinsic compression of airways (eg, by tumor, lymphadenopathy)
- Suppression of respiration or cough (eg, by general anesthesia, oversedation, severe pleuritic pain)
- Supine positioning, particularly in obese patients
- Compression or collapse of lung parenchyma (eg, by large pleural effusion or pneumothorax)

Thoracic and abdominal surgeries are very common causes because they involve general anesthesia, opioid use (with possible secondary respiratory depression), and often painful respiration. A malpositioned endotracheal tube can cause atelectasis by occluding a mainstem bronchus.

Less common causes of atelectasis include surfactant dysfunction and lung parenchymal scarring or tumor.

Symptoms and Signs

Atelectasis itself is asymptomatic unless hypoxemia or pneumonia develops. Symptoms of hypoxemia tend to be related to acuity and severity of atelectasis. With rapid, extensive atelectasis, dyspnea or even respiratory failure can develop. With slowly developing, less extensive atelectasis, symptoms may be mild or absent.

Pneumonia may cause cough, dyspnea, and pleuritic pain. Pleuritic pain may also be due to the disorder that caused atelectasis (eg, chest trauma or surgery).

Signs are often absent. Decreased breath sounds in the region of atelectasis and possibly dullness to percussion and decreased chest excursion are detectable if the area of atelectasis is large.

Diagnosis

- Chest x-ray

Atelectasis should be suspected in patients who have any unexplained respiratory symptoms and who have risk factors, particularly recent major surgery. Atelectasis that is clinically significant (eg, that causes symptoms, increases risk of complications, or meaningfully affects pulmonary function) is generally visible on chest x-ray; findings can include lung opacification and/or loss of lung volume. If the cause of atelectasis is not clinically apparent (eg, if it is not recent surgery or pneumonia seen on chest x-ray) or another disorder is suspected (eg, pulmonary embolism, tumor), other tests, such as bronchoscopy or chest CT, may be necessary.

Treatment

- Maximizing cough and deep breathing
- If obstruction by tumor or foreign body is suspected, bronchoscopy

Evidence for the efficacy of most treatments for atelectasis is weak or absent. Nonetheless, commonly recommended measures include chest physiotherapy to help maintain ventilation and clearance of secretions, and encouragement of lung expansion techniques such as directed cough, deep breathing exercises, and use of an incentive spirometer. For patients who are not intubated and do not have excessive secretions, continuous positive airway pressure may help. For patients who are intubated, positive end-expiratory pressure and/or higher tidal volume ventilation may help.

Avoiding oversedation helps ensure ventilation and sufficient deep breathing and coughing. However, severe pleuritic pain may impair deep breathing and coughing and may be relieved only with opioids. Thus, many clinicians prescribe opioid analgesics in doses sufficient to relieve pain and advise patients to consciously cough and take deep breaths periodically. In certain postoperative patients, epidural analgesia or an intercostal nerve block may be used to relieve pain without causing respiratory depression. Antitussive therapy should be avoided.

Most importantly, the cause of atelectasis (eg, mucous plug, foreign body, tumor, mass, pulmonary effusion) should be treated. For persistent mucous plugging, nebulized dornase alfa and sometimes bronchodilators are tried. *N*-Acetylcysteine is usually avoided because it can cause bronchoconstriction. If other measures are ineffective or if a cause of obstruction other than mucus plugging is suspected, bronchoscopy should be done.

Prevention

Smokers can decrease their risk of postoperative atelectasis by stopping smoking, ideally 6 to 8 wk before surgery. Drug treatment for patients with chronic lung disorders (eg, COPD) should be optimized before surgery. Preoperative inspiratory muscle training (including incentive spirometry) should be considered for patients scheduled for thoracic or upper abdominal surgery. After surgery, early ambulation and lung expansion techniques (eg, coughing, deep breathing exercises, incentive spirometry) may also decrease risk.

KEY POINTS

- Atelectasis is reversible collapse of lung tissue with loss of volume; common causes include intrinsic or extrinsic airway compression, hypoventilation, and a malpositioned endotracheal tube.
- A large area of atelectasis may cause symptomatic hypoxemia, but any other symptoms are due to the cause or a superimposed pneumonia.
- Diagnosis is by chest x-ray; if the cause is not clinically apparent, bronchoscopy or chest CT may be needed.
- Treatment involves maximizing coughing and deep breathing.

54 Chronic Obstructive Pulmonary Disease and Related Disorders

CHRONIC OBSTRUCTIVE PULMONARY DISEASE

Chronic obstructive pulmonary disease (COPD) is airflow limitation caused by an inflammatory response to inhaled toxins, often cigarette smoke. Alpha-1 antitrypsin deficiency and various occupational exposures are less common causes in nonsmokers. Symptoms are productive cough and dyspnea that develop over years; common signs include decreased breath sounds, prolonged expiratory phase of respiration, and wheezing. Severe cases may be complicated by weight loss, pneumothorax, frequent acute decompensation episodes, right heart failure, and/or acute or chronic respiratory failure. Diagnosis is based on history, physical examination, chest x-ray, and pulmonary function tests. Treatment is with bronchodilators, corticosteroids, and, when necessary, oxygen and antibiotics. About 50% of patients with severe COPD die within 10 yr of diagnosis.

COPD comprises

- Chronic obstructive bronchitis (clinically defined)
- Emphysema (pathologically or radiologically defined)

Many patients have features of both.

Chronic obstructive bronchitis is chronic bronchitis with airflow obstruction. Chronic bronchitis is defined as productive cough on most days of the week for at least 3 mo total duration in 2 successive years. Chronic bronchitis becomes chronic obstructive bronchitis if spirometric evidence of airflow obstruction develops. Chronic asthmatic bronchitis is a similar, overlapping condition characterized by chronic productive cough, wheezing, and partially reversible airflow obstruction; it occurs predominantly in smokers with a history of asthma. In some cases, the distinction between chronic obstructive bronchitis and chronic asthmatic bronchitis is unclear and may be referred to as asthma COPD overlap syndrome (ACOS).

Emphysema is destruction of lung parenchyma leading to loss of elastic recoil and loss of alveolar septa and radial airway traction, which increases the tendency for airway collapse. Lung hyperinflation, airflow limitation, and air trapping follow. Airspaces enlarge and may eventually develop blebs or bullae.

Epidemiology

In the US, about 24 million people have airflow limitation, of whom about 12 million have a diagnosis of COPD. COPD is the 3rd leading cause of death, resulting in 135,000 deaths in 2010—compared with 52,193 deaths in 1980. From 1980 to 2000, the COPD mortality rate increased 64% (from 40.7 to 66.9/100,000) and has remained steady since then. Prevalence, incidence, and mortality rates increase with age. Prevalence is now higher in women, but total mortality is similar in both sexes. COPD seems to aggregate in families independent of alpha-1 antitrypsin deficiency (alpha-1antiprotease inhibitor deficiency).

COPD is increasing worldwide because of the increase in smoking in developing countries, the reduction in mortality due to infectious diseases, and the widespread use of biomass fuels such as wood, grasses, or other organic materials. COPD mortality may also affect developing nations more than developed nations. COPD affects 64 million people and caused > 3 million deaths worldwide in 2005 and is projected to become the 3rd leading cause of death globally by the year 2030.

Etiology

There are several causes of COPD:

- Smoking (and less often other inhalational exposures)
- Genetic factors

Inhalational exposure: Of all inhalational exposures, cigarette smoking is the primary risk factor in most countries, although only about 15% of smokers develop clinically apparent COPD; an exposure history of 40 or more pack-years is especially predictive. Smoke from indoor cooking and heating is an important causative factor in developing countries. Smokers with preexisting airway reactivity (defined by increased sensitivity to inhaled methacholine), even in the absence of clinical asthma, are at greater risk of developing COPD than are those without.

Low body weight, childhood respiratory disorders, and exposure to passive cigarette smoke, air pollution, and occupational dust (eg, mineral dust, cotton dust) or inhaled chemicals (eg, cadmium) contribute to the risk of COPD but are of minor importance compared with cigarette smoking.

Genetic factors: The best-defined causative genetic disorder is alpha-1 antitrypsin deficiency, which is an important cause of emphysema in nonsmokers and influences susceptibility to disease in smokers.

In recent years, > 30 genetic variants have been found to be associated with COPD or decline in lung function in selected populations, but none has been shown to be as consequential as alpha-1 antitrypsin.

Pathophysiology

Various factors cause the airflow limitation and other complications of COPD.

Inflammation: Inhalational exposures can trigger an inflammatory response in airways and alveoli that leads to disease in genetically susceptible people. The process is thought to be mediated by an increase in protease activity and a decrease in antiprotease activity. Lung proteases, such as neutrophil elastase, matrix metalloproteinases, and cathepsins, break down elastin and connective tissue in the normal process of tissue repair. Their activity is normally balanced by antiproteases, such as alpha-1 antitrypsin, airway epithelium–derived secretory leukoproteinase inhibitor, elafin, and matrix metalloproteinase tissue inhibitor. In patients with COPD, activated neutrophils and other inflammatory cells release proteases as part of the inflammatory process; protease activity exceeds antiprotease activity, and tissue destruction and mucus hypersecretion result.

Neutrophil and macrophage activation also leads to accumulation of free radicals, superoxide anions, and hydrogen peroxide, which inhibit antiproteases and cause bronchoconstriction, mucosal edema, and mucous hypersecretion. Neutrophil-induced oxidative damage, release of profibrotic neuropeptides (eg, bombesin), and reduced levels of vascular endothelial growth factor may contribute to apoptotic destruction of lung parenchyma.

The inflammation in COPD increases as disease severity increases, and, in severe (advanced) disease, inflammation does not resolve completely despite smoking cessation. This chronic inflammation does not seem to respond to corticosteroids.

Infection: Respiratory infection (which COPD patients are prone to) may amplify progression of lung destruction.

Bacteria, especially *Haemophilus influenzae*, colonize the lower airways of about 30% of patients with COPD. In more severely affected patients (eg, those with previous hospitalizations), colonization with *Pseudomonas aeruginosa* or other gram-negative bacteria is common. Smoking and airflow obstruction may lead to impaired mucus clearance in lower airways, which predisposes to infection. Repeated bouts of infection increase the inflammatory burden that hastens disease progression. There is no evidence, however, that long-term use of antibiotics slows the progression of COPD.

Airflow limitation: The cardinal pathophysiologic feature of COPD is airflow limitation caused by airway narrowing and/or obstruction, loss of elastic recoil, or both.

Airway narrowing and obstruction are caused by inflammation-mediated mucus hypersecretion, mucus plugging, mucosal edema, bronchospasm, peribronchial fibrosis, and destruction of small airways or a combination of these mechanisms. Alveolar septa are destroyed, reducing parenchymal attachments to the airways and thereby facilitating airway closure during expiration.

Enlarged alveolar spaces sometimes consolidate into bullae, defined as airspaces ≥ 1 cm in diameter. Bullae may be entirely empty or have strands of lung tissue traversing them in areas of locally severe emphysema; they occasionally occupy the entire hemithorax. These changes lead to loss of elastic recoil and lung hyperinflation.

Increased airway resistance increases the work of breathing. Lung hyperinflation, although it decreases airway resistance, also increases the work of breathing. Increased work of breathing may lead to alveolar hypoventilation with hypoxia and hypercapnia, although hypoxia is also caused by ventilation/perfusion (V/Q) mismatch.

Complications: In addition to airflow limitation and sometimes respiratory insufficiency, complications include

- Pulmonary hypertension
- Respiratory infection
- Weight loss and other comorbidities

Chronic hypoxemia increases pulmonary vascular tone, which, if diffuse, causes pulmonary hypertension and cor pulmonale. The increase in pulmonary vascular pressure may be augmented by the destruction of the pulmonary capillary bed due to destruction of alveolar septa.

Viral or bacterial respiratory infections are common among patients with COPD and cause a large percentage of acute exacerbations. It is currently thought that acute bacterial infections are due to acquisition of new strains of bacteria rather than overgrowth of chronic colonizing bacteria.

Weight loss may occur, perhaps in response to decreased caloric intake and increased levels of circulating tumor necrosis factor (TNF)-alpha.

Other coexisting or complicating disorders that adversely affect quality of life and survival include osteoporosis, depression, anxiety, coronary artery disease, lung cancer and other cancers, muscle atrophy, and gastroesophageal reflux. The extent to which these disorders are consequences of COPD, smoking, and the accompanying systemic inflammation is unclear.

Symptoms and Signs

COPD takes years to develop and progress. Most patients have smoked ≥ 20 cigarettes/day for > 20 yr.

- Productive cough usually is the initial symptom, developing among smokers in their 40s and 50s.
- Dyspnea that is progressive, persistent, exertional, or worse during respiratory infection appears when patients are in their late 50s or 60s.

Symptoms usually progress quickly in patients who continue to smoke and in those who have a higher lifetime tobacco exposure. Morning headache develops in more advanced disease and signals nocturnal hypercapnia or hypoxemia.

Signs of COPD include wheezing, a prolonged expiratory phase of breathing, lung hyperinflation manifested as decreased heart and lung sounds, and increased anteroposterior diameter of the thorax (barrel chest). Patients with advanced emphysema lose weight and experience muscle wasting that has been attributed to immobility, hypoxia, or release of systemic inflammatory mediators, such as TNF-alpha.

Signs of advanced disease include pursed-lip breathing, accessory respiratory muscle use, paradoxical inward movement of the lower intercostal interspaces during inspiration (Hoover sign), and cyanosis. Signs of cor pulmonale include neck vein distention, splitting of the 2nd heart sound with an accentuated pulmonic component, tricuspid insufficiency murmur, and peripheral edema. Right ventricular heaves are uncommon in COPD because the lungs are hyperinflated.

Spontaneous pneumothorax may occur (possibly related to rupture of bullae) and should be suspected in any patient with COPD whose pulmonary status abruptly worsens.

Acute exacerbations: Acute exacerbations occur sporadically during the course of COPD and are heralded by increased symptom severity. The specific cause of any exacerbation is almost always impossible to determine, but exacerbations are often attributed to viral URIs, acute bacterial bronchitis, or exposure to respiratory irritants. As COPD progresses, acute exacerbations tend to become more frequent, averaging about 1 to 3 episodes/yr.

Diagnosis

- Chest x-ray
- Pulmonary function testing

Diagnosis is suggested by history, physical examination, and chest imaging and is confirmed by pulmonary function tests. Similar symptoms can be caused by asthma, heart failure, and bronchiectasis (see Table 54–1). COPD and asthma are sometimes easily confused and may overlap (called asthma-COPD overlap syndrome, or ACOS).

Systemic disorders that may have a component of airflow limitation may suggest COPD; they include HIV infection, abuse of IV drugs (particularly cocaine and amphetamines), sarcoidosis, Sjögren syndrome, bronchiolitis obliterans, lymphangioleiomyomatosis, and eosinophilic granuloma. COPD can be differentiated from interstitial lung diseases (ILD) by chest imaging, which shows increased interstitial markings in ILD, and pulmonary function testing, which shows a restrictive ventilatory defect rather than an obstructive ventilatory defect. In some patients, COPD and ILD coexist (combined pulmonary fibrosis and emphysema [CPFE]) in which lung volumes are relatively preserved, but gas exchange is severely impaired.

Pulmonary function tests: Patients suspected of having COPD should undergo pulmonary function testing to confirm airflow limitation, to quantify its severity and reversibility, and

Table 54–1. DIFFERENTIAL DIAGNOSIS OF COPD

DIAGNOSIS	ONSET	IMAGING RESULTS	OTHER FEATURES
COPD	Middle age	Sometimes lung hyperinflation, bullae, increased retrosternal air space, and/or bronchial wall thickening (seen on chest x-ray); however, usually not helpful diagnostically and done mainly to exclude other disorders	Slowly progressive symptoms History of smoking or exposure to tobacco or other types of smoke
Asthma	Early in life (often during childhood)	Usually normal, possibly hyperinflation or segmental atelectasis	Symptoms vary widely from day to day Symptoms often worse at night or early morning History of allergies, rhinitis, or eczema Often family history of asthma
Bronchiectasis	All ages, but most often in older or middle age	Bronchial dilation and bronchial wall thickening (seen on chest x-ray or chest CT)	Often large amounts of purulent sputum Often history of recent bacterial infection
Diffuse panbronchiolitis	Usually between ages 10 and 60 yr (mean age of 40)	Diffuse small centrilobular nodular opacities and hyperinflation seen on chest x-ray and high-resolution CT	Mostly male nonsmokers Almost all have chronic sinusitis Predominately in those of Asian descent
Heart failure	All ages, but most often in older or middle age	Enlarged heart, pleural effusion, fluid in major fissure, sometimes pulmonary edema (seen on chest x-ray)	Volume restriction without airflow limitation (detected by pulmonary function tests)
Obliterative bronchiolitis	Onset at younger age	Hypodense areas (seen on CT during expiration)	Nonsmokers who may have a history of rheumatoid arthritis or acute fume exposure History of lung or bone marrow transplantation
TB	All ages	Lung infiltrates, typically multinodular, sometimes calcified hilar nodes (seen on chest x-ray)	Confirmed by microbiologic testing Usually in areas with high prevalence of TB

Data adapted from The Global Strategy for the Diagnosis, Management and Prevention of COPD Global Initiative for Chronic Obstructive Lung Disease (GOLD), 2016.

to distinguish COPD from other disorders. Pulmonary function testing is also useful for following disease progression and monitoring response to treatment. The primary diagnostic tests are

- FEV_1: The volume of air forcefully expired during the first second after taking a full breath
- Forced vital capacity (FVC): The total volume of air expired with maximal force
- Flow-volume loops: Simultaneous spirometric recordings of airflow and volume during forced maximal expiration and inspiration

Reductions of FEV_1, FVC, and the ratio of FEV_1/FVC are the hallmarks of airflow limitation. Flow-volume loops show a concave pattern in the expiratory tracing (see Fig. 50–3 on p. 394). There are 2 basic pathways by which COPD can develop and manifest with symptoms in later life. In the first, patients may have normal lung function in early adulthood, which is followed by an increased decline in FEV_1 (about ≥ 60 mL/yr). With the second pathway, patients have impaired lung function in early adulthood, often associated with asthma or other childhood respiratory disease. In these patients, COPD may present with a normal age-related decline in FEV_1 (about 30 mL/yr). Although this 2 pathway model is conceptually helpful, a wide range of individual trajectories is possible.[1] When the FEV_1 falls below about 1 L, patients develop dyspnea during activities of daily living (although dyspnea is more closely related to the degree of dynamic hyperinflation [progressive hyperinflation due to incomplete exhalation] than to the degree of airflow limitation). When the FEV_1 falls below about 0.8 L, patients are at risk of hypoxemia, hypercapnia, and cor pulmonale.

FEV_1 and FVC are easily measured with office spirometry and define severity of disease (see Table 54–2) because they correlate with symptoms and mortality. Normal reference values are determined by patient age, sex, and height.

Additional pulmonary function testing is necessary only in specific circumstances, such as before lung volume reduction surgery. Other test abnormalities may include

- Increased total lung capacity
- Increased functional residual capacity
- Increased residual volume
- Decreased vital capacity
- Decreased single-breath diffusing capacity for carbon monoxide (DLco)

Findings of increased total lung capacity, functional residual capacity, and residual volume can help distinguish COPD from restrictive pulmonary disease, in which these measures are diminished.

Table 54–2. CLASSIFICATION AND TREATMENT OF COPD

PATIENT GROUP	FINDINGS	TREATMENT	ALTERNATIVE TREATMENTS
All patients	—	Avoidance of risk factors (eg, smoking) Influenza vaccine annually Pneumococcal polysaccharide vaccine Exercise training as directed by pulmonary rehabilitation Treatment of complications	—
A (low risk, few symptoms)	$FEV_1 \geq 50\%$ predicted 0–1 exacerbation/yr mMRC*: 0–1	SABA or SAC, as needed	LAC *or* LABA *or* SABA plus SAC
B (low risk, more symptoms)	$FEV_1 \geq 50\%$ predicted 0–1 exacerbation/yr mMRC ≥ 2	LAC *or* LABA	LABA plus LAC *or* SABA and/or SAC
C (high risk, few symptoms)	$FEV_1 < 50\%$ predicted ≥ 2 exacerbations/yr mMRC: 0–1	ICS plus LABA *or* LAC	LABA plus LAC *or* LAC plus PDE4I *or* LABA plus PDE4I
D (high risk, more symptoms)	$FEV_1 < 50\%$ predicted ≥ 2 exacerbations/yr mMRC: ≥ 2	ICS plus LABA *and/or* LAC	ICS plus LABA plus LAC *or* ICS plus LABA plus PDE4I *or* LABA plus LAC *or* LAC plus PDE4I

*The COPD Assessment Test (CAT) may be used instead of the mMRC to evaluate symptoms. For MRC definitions, see Table 54–3.

FEV_1 = forced expiratory volume in 1 sec; ICS = inhaled corticosteroid; LABA = long-acting beta-agonist; LAC = long-acting anticholinergic; mMRC = Breathlessness measurement using the Modified British Medical Research Council (mMRC) Questionnaire; PDE4I = phosphodiesterase-4 inhibitor; SABA = short-acting beta-agonist; SAC = short-acting anticholinergic.

Data from the Global Strategy for the Diagnosis, Management, and Prevention of Chronic Obstructive Pulmonary Disease.

Decreased DLco is nonspecific and is reduced in other disorders that affect the pulmonary vascular bed, such as interstitial lung disease, but can help distinguish emphysema from asthma, in which DLco is normal or elevated.

Imaging tests: Chest x-ray may have characteristic findings. In patients with emphysema, changes can include lung hyperinflation manifested as a flat diaphragm (ie, increase in the angle formed by the sternum and anterior diaphragm on a lateral film from the normal value of 45° to > 90°), rapid tapering of hilar vessels, and bullae (ie, radiolucencies > 1 cm surrounded by arcuate, hairline shadows). Other typical findings include widening of the retrosternal airspace and a narrow cardiac shadow. Emphysematous changes occurring predominantly in the lung bases suggest alpha-1 antitrypsin deficiency. The lungs may look normal or have increased lucency secondary to loss of parenchyma. Among patients with chronic obstructive bronchitis, chest x-rays may be normal or may show a bibasilar increase in bronchovascular markings as a result of bronchial wall thickening.

Prominent hila suggest large central pulmonary arteries that may signify pulmonary hypertension. Right ventricular enlargement that occurs in cor pulmonale may be masked by lung hyperinflation or may manifest as encroachment of the heart shadow on the retrosternal space or by widening of the transverse cardiac shadow in comparison with previous chest x-rays.

Chest CT may reveal abnormalities that are not apparent on the chest x-ray and may also suggest coexisting or complicating disorders, such as pneumonia, pneumoconiosis, or lung cancer. CT helps assess the extent and distribution of emphysema, estimated either by visual scoring or with analysis of the distribution of lung density. Indications for obtaining CT in patients with COPD include evaluation for lung volume reduction surgery, suspicion of coexisting or complicating disorders that are not clearly evident or excluded by chest x-ray, suspicion of lung cancer, and screening for lung cancer.

Adjunctive tests: Alpha-1 antitrypsin levels should be measured in patients < 50 yr with symptomatic COPD and in nonsmokers of any age with COPD to detect alpha-1 antitrypsin deficiency. Other indications of possible alpha-1 antitrypsin deficiency include a family history of premature COPD or unexplained liver disease, lower-lobe distribution of emphysema, and COPD associated with antineutrophil cytoplasmic antibody (ANCA)-positive vasculitis. If levels of alpha-1 antitrypsin are low, the diagnosis should be confirmed by genetic testing to establish the alpha-1 antitrypsin phenotype.

ECG, often done to exclude cardiac causes of dyspnea, typically shows diffusely low QRS voltage with a vertical heart axis caused by lung hyperinflation and increased P-wave voltage or rightward shifts of the P-wave vector caused by right atrial enlargement in patients with advanced emphysema. Findings of right ventricular hypertrophy include an R or R′ wave as tall as or taller than the S wave in lead V_1; an R wave smaller than the S wave in lead V_6; right-axis deviation >110° without right bundle branch block; or some combination of these. Multifocal atrial tachycardia, an arrhythmia that can accompany COPD, manifests as a tachyarrhythmia with polymorphic P waves and variable PR intervals.

Echocardiography is occasionally useful for assessing right ventricular function and pulmonary hypertension, although air trapping makes it technically difficult in patients with COPD. Echocardiography is most often indicated when coexistent left ventricular or valvular heart disease is suspected.

CBC is of little diagnostic value in the evaluation of COPD but may show erythrocythemia (Hct > 48%) if the patient has chronic hypoxemia. Patients with anemia (for reasons other than COPD) have disproportionately severe dyspnea.

Serum electrolytes are of little value but may show an elevated bicarbonate level if patients have chronic hypercapnia.

Evaluation of exacerbations: Patients with acute exacerbations usually have combinations of increased cough, sputum, dyspnea, and work of breathing, as well as low oxygen saturation on pulse oximetry, diaphoresis, tachycardia, anxiety, and cyanosis. Patients with exacerbations accompanied by retention of carbon dioxide may be lethargic or somnolent, a very different appearance.

All patients requiring hospitalization for an acute exacerbation should undergo testing (eg, ABG sampling) to quantify hypoxemia and hypercapnia. Hypercapnia may exist without hypoxemia.

Findings of $Pa{O_2} < 50$ mm Hg or $Pa{CO_2} > 50$ mm Hg in patients with respiratory acidemia define acute respiratory failure. However, some patients chronically manifest such levels of PaO_2 and $PaCO_2$ in the absence of acute respiratory failure.

A chest x-ray is often done to check for pneumonia or pneumothorax. Very rarely, among patients receiving chronic systemic corticosteroids, infiltrates may represent *Aspergillus* pneumonia.

Yellow or green sputum is a reliable indicator of neutrophils in the sputum and suggests bacterial colonization or infection. Culture is usually done in hospitalized patients but is not usually necessary in outpatients. In samples from outpatients, Gram stain usually shows neutrophils with a mixture of organisms, often gram-positive diplococci (*Streptococcus pneumoniae*), gram-negative bacilli (*H. influenzae*), or both. Other oropharyngeal commensal organisms, such as *Moraxella* (*Branhamella*) *catarrhalis*, occasionally cause exacerbations. In hospitalized patients, cultures may show resistant gram-negative organisms (eg, *Pseudomonas*) or, rarely, *Staphylococcus*.

1. Lange P, Celli B, Agusti A, et al: Lung-function trajectories leading to chronic obstructive pulmonary disease. *N Engl J Med* 373(2):111–122, 2015.

Prognosis

Severity of airway obstruction predicts survival in patients with COPD. The mortality rate in patients with an $FEV_1 \geq 50\%$ of predicted is slightly greater than that of the general population. If the FEV_1 is 0.75 to 1.25 L, 5-yr survival is about 40 to 60%; if < 0.75 L, about 30 to 40%.

More accurate prediction of death risk is possible by simultaneously measuring body mass index (*B*), the degree of airflow obstruction (*O*, which is the FEV_1), dyspnea (*D*, which is measured using Modified British Medical Research Council (mMRC) Questionnaire—see Table 54–3), and exercise capacity (*E*, which is measured with a 6-min walking test); this is the BODE index. Also, older age, heart disease, anemia, resting tachycardia, hypercapnia, and hypoxemia decrease survival, whereas a significant response to bronchodilators predicts improved survival. Risk factors for death in patients with acute exacerbation requiring hospitalization include older age, higher $PaCO_2$, and use of maintenance oral corticosteroids. (Details for calculating the BODE index are available at Medical Criteria.)

Table 54–3. BREATHLESSNESS MEASUREMENT USING THE MODIFIED BRITISH MEDICAL RESEARCH COUNCIL (MMRC) QUESTIONNAIRE

GRADE	SHORTNESS OF BREATH
0	None except during strenuous exercise
1	Occurring when hurrying on level ground or walking up a slight incline
2	Resulting in walking more slowly than people of the same age on level ground *or* Resulting in stopping for breath when walking at own pace on level ground
3	Resulting in stopping for breath after walking about 100 meters or after a few minutes on level ground
4	Severe enough to prevent the person from leaving the house *or* Occurring when dressing or undressing

Adapted from Mahler DA, Wells CK: Evaluation of clinical methods for rating dyspnea. *Chest* 93:580–586, 1988.

Patients at high risk of imminent death are those with progressive unexplained weight loss or severe functional decline (eg, those who experience dyspnea with self-care, such as dressing, bathing, or eating). Mortality in COPD may result from intercurrent illnesses rather than from progression of the underlying disorder in patients who have stopped smoking. Death is generally caused by acute respiratory failure, pneumonia, lung cancer, heart disease, or pulmonary embolism.

Treatment

- Smoking cessation
- Inhaled bronchodilators, corticosteroids, or both
- Supportive care (eg, oxygen therapy, pulmonary rehabilitation)

COPD management involves treatment of chronic stable disease and treatment of exacerbations. Treatment of cor pulmonale, a common complication of long-standing, severe COPD, is discussed on p. 725.

Smoking cessation is critical in treatment of COPD.

Treatment of chronic stable COPD aims to prevent exacerbations and improve lung and physical function. Relieve symptoms rapidly with primarily short-acting beta-adrenergic drugs and decrease exacerbations with inhaled corticosteroids, long-acting beta-adrenergic drugs, long-acting anticholinergic drugs, or a combination (see Table 54–2).

Treatment of exacerbations ensures adequate oxygenation and near-normal blood pH, reverses airway obstruction, and treats any cause.

KEY POINTS

- Cigarette smoking in susceptible people is the major cause of COPD in the developed world.
- Diagnose COPD and differentiate it from disorders that have similar characteristics (eg, asthma, heart failure) primarily by routine clinical information, such as symptoms (particularly time course), age at onset, risk factors, and results of routine tests (eg, chest x-ray, pulmonary function tests).

- Reductions of FEV_1, FVC, and the ratio of FEV_1/FVC are characteristic findings.
- Categorize patients based on symptoms and exacerbation risk into one of 4 groups and use that category to guide drug treatment.
- Relieve symptoms rapidly with primarily short-acting beta-adrenergic drugs and decrease exacerbations with inhaled corticosteroids, long-acting beta-adrenergic drugs, long-acting anticholinergic drugs, or a combination.
- Encourage smoking cessation using multiple interventions.

TREATMENT OF STABLE COPD

COPD management involves treatment of chronic stable disease and treatment of exacerbations.

Treatment of chronic stable COPD aims to prevent exacerbations and improve lung and physical function through

- Smoking cessation
- Drug therapy
- Oxygen therapy
- Enhancement of nutrition
- Pulmonary rehabilitation, including exercise

Surgical treatment of COPD is indicated for selected patients.

Smoking Cessation

Smoking cessation is both extremely difficult and extremely important; it slows but does not halt the rate of FEV_1 decline (see Fig. 54–1) and increases long-term survival. Simultaneous use of multiple strategies is most effective:

- Establishment of a quit date
- Behavior modification techniques
- Group sessions
- Nicotine replacement therapy (by gum, transdermal patch, inhaler, lozenge, or nasal spray)
- Varenicline or bupropion
- Physician encouragement

Quit rates > 50% at 1 yr have not been demonstrated even with the most effective interventions, such as use of bupropion combined with nicotine replacement or use of varenicline alone.

Drug Therapy

Recommended drug therapy is summarized in Table 54–2.

Inhaled bronchodilators are the mainstay of COPD management; drugs include

- Beta-agonists
- Anticholinergics (antimuscarinics)

These two classes of drugs are equally effective. Patients with mild (group A—see Table 54–2) disease are treated only when symptomatic. Patients with moderate to severe (group B, C, or D—see Table 54–2) COPD should be taking drugs from one or both of these classes regularly to improve pulmonary function and increase exercise capacity.

The frequency of exacerbations can be reduced with the use of anticholinergics, inhaled corticosteroids, or long-acting beta-agonists. However, there is no evidence that regular bronchodilator use slows deterioration of lung function. The initial choice among short-acting beta-agonists, long-acting beta-agonists, anticholinergics, and combination beta-agonist and anticholinergic therapy is often a matter of tailoring cost and convenience to the patient's preferences and symptoms.

For home treatment of chronic stable disease, drug administration by metered-dose inhaler or dry-powder inhaler is preferred over administration by nebulizer; home nebulizers are prone to contamination due to incomplete cleaning and drying. Therefore, nebulizers should be reserved for people who cannot coordinate activation of the metered-dose inhaler with inhalation or cannot develop enough inspiratory flow for dry powder inhalers.

For metered-dose inhalers, patients should be taught to exhale to functional residual capacity, inhale the aerosol slowly to total lung capacity, and hold the inhalation for 3 to 4 sec before exhaling. Spacers help ensure optimal delivery of drug to the distal airways and reduce the importance of coordinating activation of the inhaler with inhalation. Some spacers alert

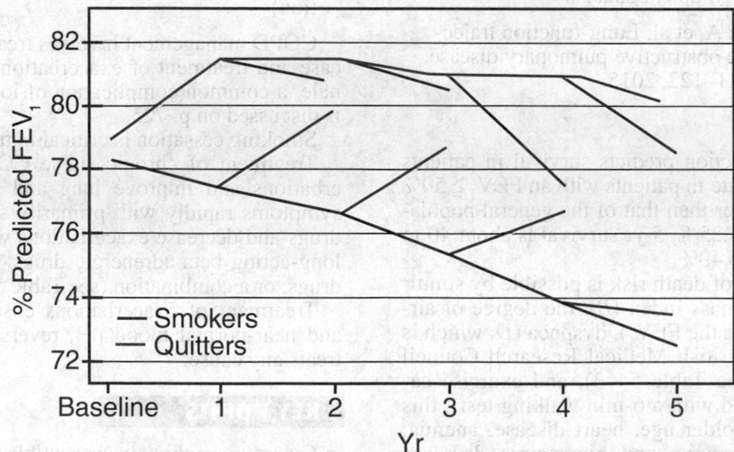

Fig. 54–1. Changes in lung function (percentage of predicted FEV_1) in patients who quit smoking compared with those who continue. During the first year, lung function improved in patients who quit smoking and declined in those who continued. Subsequently, the rate of decline in those who continued was twice that of those who quit. Function declined in those who relapsed and improved in those who quit regardless of when the change occurred. Based on data from Scanlon PD, et al: Smoking cessation and lung function in mild-to-moderate chronic obstructive pulmonary disease; the Lung Health Study. *American Journal of Respiratory and Critical Care Medicine* 161:381–390, 2000.

patients if they are inhaling too rapidly. New or not recently used metered-dose inhalers require 2 to 3 priming doses (different manufacturers have slightly different recommendations for what is considered "not recently used," ranging from 3 to 14 days).

Beta-agonists: Beta-agonists relax bronchial smooth muscle and increase mucociliary clearance. Albuterol aerosol, 2 puffs (90 to 100 mcg/puff) inhaled from a metered-dose inhaler 4 to 6 times/day prn, is usually the drug of choice.

Long-acting beta-agonists are preferable for patients with nocturnal symptoms or for those who find frequent dosing inconvenient. Options include salmeterol powder, 1 puff (50 mcg) inhaled bid, indacaterol 1 puff (75 mcg) inhaled once/day (150 mcg once/day in Europe), and olodaterol 2 puffs once/day at the same time each day. Also available are nebulized forms of arformoterol and formoterol. The dry-powder formulations may be more effective for patients who have trouble coordinating use of a metered-dose inhaler.

Patients should be taught the difference between short-acting and long-acting drugs, because long-acting drugs that are used as needed or more than twice/day increase the risk of cardiac arrhythmias.

Adverse effects commonly result from use of any beta-agonist and include tremor, anxiety, tachycardia, and mild, temporary hypokalemia.

Anticholinergics: Anticholinergics (antimuscarinics) relax bronchial smooth muscle through competitive inhibition of muscarinic receptors (M_1, M_2, and M_3).

Ipratropium is a short-acting anticholinergic; dose is 2 to 4 puffs (18 mcg/puff) from a metered-dose inhaler q 4 to 6 h. Ipratropium has a slower onset of action (within 30 min; peak effect in 1 to 2 h), so a beta-agonist is often prescribed with it in a single combination inhaler or as a separate as-needed rescue drug.

Tiotropium is a long-acting quaternary anticholinergic inhaled as a powder formulation. Dose is 1 puff (18 mcg) once/day. Aclidinium bromide is available as a multidose dry-powder inhaler. Dose is 1 puff (400 mcg/puff) bid. Umeclidinium can be used as a once/day combination with vilanterol (a long-acting beta-agonist) in a dry-powder inhaler. Glycopyrrolate (an anticholinergic) can be used bid in combination with indacaterol or formoterol (long-acting beta-agonists) in a dry powder or metered dose inhaler.

Adverse effects of all anticholinergics are pupillary dilation (and risk of triggering or worsening acute angle closure glaucoma), urinary retention, and dry mouth.

Inhaled corticosteroids: Corticosteroids are often part of treatment. Inhaled corticosteroids seem to reduce airway inflammation, reverse beta-receptor down-regulation, and inhibit leukotriene and cytokine production. They do not alter the course of pulmonary function decline in patients with COPD who continue to smoke, but they do relieve symptoms and improve short-term pulmonary function in some patients, are additive to the effect of bronchodilators, and may diminish the frequency of COPD exacerbations. They are indicated for patients who have repeated exacerbations or symptoms despite optimal bronchodilator therapy. Dose depends on the drug; examples include fluticasone 500 to 1000 mcg/day and beclomethasone 400 to 2000 mcg/day.

The long-term risks of inhaled corticosteroids in elderly people are not proved but probably include osteoporosis, cataract formation, and an increased risk of nonfatal pneumonia. Long-term users therefore should undergo periodic ophthalmologic and bone densitometry screening and should possibly receive supplemental calcium, vitamin D, and a bisphosphonate as indicated.

Combinations of a long-acting beta-agonist (eg, salmeterol) and an inhaled corticosteroid (eg, fluticasone) are more effective than either drug alone in the treatment of chronic stable disease.

Oral or systemic corticosteroids should usually not be used to treat chronic stable COPD.

Theophylline: Theophylline plays only a small role in the treatment of chronic stable COPD now that safer, more effective drugs are available. Theophylline decreases smooth muscle spasm, enhances mucociliary clearance, improves right ventricular function, and decreases pulmonary vascular resistance and arterial pressure. Its mode of action is poorly understood but appears to differ from that of beta-2-agonists and anticholinergics. Its role in improving diaphragmatic function and dyspnea during exercise is controversial.

Theophylline can be used for patients who have not adequately responded to inhaled drugs and who have shown symptomatic benefit from a trial of the drug. Serum levels need not be monitored unless the patient does not respond to the drug, develops symptoms of toxicity, or is questionably adherent; slowly absorbed oral theophylline preparations, which require less frequent dosing, enhance adherence.

Toxicity is common and includes sleeplessness and GI upset, even at low blood levels. More serious adverse effects, such as supraventricular and ventricular arrhythmias and seizures, tend to occur at blood levels > 20 mg/L.

Hepatic metabolism of theophylline varies greatly and is influenced by genetic factors, age, cigarette smoking, hepatic dysfunction, and some drugs, such as macrolide and fluoroquinolone antibiotics and nonsedating histamine$_2$ blockers.

Phosphodiesterase-4 inhibitors: Phosphodiesterase-4 inhibitors are more specific than theophylline for pulmonary phosphodiesterase and have fewer adverse effects. They have anti-inflammatory properties and are mild bronchodilators. Phosphodiesterase-4 inhibitors such as roflumilast can be used in addition to other bronchodilators for reduction of exacerbations in patients with COPD. The dose is 500 mcg po once/day.

Common adverse effects include nausea, headache, and weight loss, but these effects may subside with continued use.

Oxygen Therapy

Long-term oxygen therapy prolongs life in patients with COPD whose Pao_2 is chronically < 55 mm Hg. Continual 24-h use is more effective than a 12-h nocturnal regimen. Oxygen therapy brings Hct toward normal levels; improves neuropsychologic factors, possibly by facilitating sleep; and ameliorates pulmonary hemodynamic abnormalities. Oxygen therapy also increases exercise tolerance in many patients.

Oxygen saturation should be measured during exercise and while at rest. Similarly, a sleep study should be considered for patients with advanced COPD who do not meet the criteria for long-term oxygen therapy while they are awake (see Table 54–4) but whose clinical assessment suggests pulmonary hypertension in the absence of daytime hypoxemia. Nocturnal oxygen may be prescribed if a sleep study shows episodic desaturation to ≤ 88%. Such treatment prevents progression of pulmonary hypertension, but its effects on survival are unknown. Patients with moderate hypoxemia above 88% or exercise desaturation may benefit symptomatically from oxygen, but there is no improvement in survival or reduction in hospitalizations.[1]

Some patients need supplemental oxygen during air travel because flight cabin pressure in commercial airliners is below sea level air pressure (often equivalent to 1830 to 2400 m [6000 to 8000 ft]). Eucapnic COPD patients who have a

Table 54–4. INDICATIONS FOR LONG-TERM OXYGEN THERAPY IN COPD

$Pao_2 \leq 55$ mm Hg or $Sao_2 \leq 88\%$* in patients receiving optimal medical regimen for at least 30 days†
$Pao_2 = 55$ to 59 mm Hg or $Sao_2 \leq 89\%$* for patients with cor pulmonale or erythrocytosis (Hct > 55%)
Can be considered for patients with exercise desaturation if there is symptomatic improvement; however, there is no improvement in survival or hospitalization. May also be considered for patients with nocturnal desaturation.‡

*Arterial oxygen levels are measured at rest during air breathing.

†Patients who are recovering from an acute respiratory illness and who meet the listed criteria should be given oxygen and rechecked while breathing room air after 60 to 90 days.

‡See also Long-Term Oxygen Treatment Trial Research Group: A randomized trial of long-term oxygen for COPD with moderate desaturation. *New Engl J Med* 375:1617–1627, 2016.

$Pao_2 > 68$ mm Hg at sea level generally have an in-flight $Pao_2 > 50$ mm Hg and do not require supplemental oxygen. All patients with COPD with a $Pao_2 \leq 68$ mm Hg at sea level, hypercapnia, significant anemia (Hct < 30), or a coexisting heart or cerebrovascular disorder should use supplemental oxygen during long flights and should notify the airline when making their reservation. Airlines can provide supplemental oxygen, and most require a minimum notice of 24 h, a physician's statement of necessity, and an oxygen prescription before the flight. Patients should bring their own nasal cannulas, because some airlines provide only face masks. Patients are not permitted to transport or use their own liquid oxygen, but many airlines now permit use of portable battery-operated oxygen concentrators, which also provide a suitable oxygen source on arrival.

Oxygen administration: Oxygen is administered by nasal cannula at a flow rate sufficient to achieve a $Pao_2 > 60$ mm Hg (oxygen saturation > 90%), usually ≤ 3 L/min at rest. Oxygen is supplied by electrically driven oxygen concentrators, liquid oxygen systems, or cylinders of compressed gas. Stationary concentrators, which limit mobility but are the least expensive, are preferable for patients who spend most of their time at home. Such patients require small oxygen tanks for backup in case of an electrical failure and for portable use. Portable concentrators that allow mobility can be used for patients who do not require high flow rates.

A liquid system is preferable for patients who spend much time out of their home. Portable canisters of liquid oxygen are easier to carry and have more capacity than portable cylinders of compressed gas. Large compressed-air cylinders are the most expensive way of providing oxygen and should be used only if no other source is available. All patients must be taught the dangers of smoking during oxygen use.

Various oxygen-conserving devices can reduce the amount of oxygen used by the patient, either by using a reservoir system or by permitting oxygen flow only during inspiration. Systems with these devices correct hypoxemia as effectively as do continuous flow systems.

Vaccinations

All patients with COPD should be given annual influenza vaccinations. If a patient is unable to receive a vaccination or if the prevailing influenza strain is not included in the annual vaccine formulation, prophylactic treatment with a neuraminidase inhibitor (oseltamivir or zanamivir) is sometimes used if there is close exposure to influenza-infected people. Treatment with a neuraminidase inhibitor should be started at the first sign of an influenza-like illness.

Pneumococcal polysaccharide vaccine, although of unproven efficacy in COPD, has minimal adverse effects and should also be given.

Nutrition

COPD patients are at risk of weight loss and nutritional deficiencies because of a higher energy cost of daily activities; reduced caloric intake relative to need because of dyspnea; and the catabolic effect of inflammatory cytokines such as TNF-alpha. Generalized muscle strength and efficiency of oxygen use are impaired. Patients with poorer nutritional status have a worse prognosis, so it is prudent to recommend a balanced diet with adequate caloric intake in conjunction with exercise to prevent or reverse undernutrition and muscle atrophy.

Excessive weight gain should be avoided, and obese patients should strive to gradually reduce body fat.

Studies of nutritional supplementation alone have not shown improvement in pulmonary function or exercise capacity. Trials of appetite stimulants, anabolic steroids, growth hormone supplementation, and TNF antagonists in reversing undernutrition and improving functional status and prognosis in COPD have been disappointing.

Pulmonary Rehabilitation

Pulmonary rehabilitation programs serve as adjuncts to drug treatment to improve physical function; many hospitals and health care organizations offer formal multidisciplinary rehabilitation programs. Pulmonary rehabilitation includes exercise, education, and behavioral interventions. Treatment should be individualized; patients and family members are taught about COPD and medical treatments, and patients are encouraged to take as much responsibility for personal care as possible.

The benefits of rehabilitation are greater independence and improved quality of life and exercise capacity. Pulmonary rehabilitation typically does not improve pulmonary function. A carefully integrated rehabilitation program helps patients with severe COPD accommodate to physiologic limitations while providing realistic expectations for improvement. Patients with severe disease require a minimum of 3 mo of rehabilitation to benefit and should continue with maintenance programs.

An exercise program can be helpful in the home, in the hospital, or in institutional settings. Graded exercise can ameliorate skeletal muscle deconditioning resulting from inactivity or prolonged hospitalization for respiratory failure. Specific training of respiratory muscles is less helpful than general aerobic conditioning.

A typical training program begins with slow walking on a treadmill or unloaded cycling on an ergometer for a few minutes. Duration and exercise load are progressively increased over 4 to 6 wk until the patient can exercise for 20 to 30 min nonstop with manageable dyspnea. Patients with very severe COPD can usually achieve an exercise regimen of walking for 30 min at 1 to 2 mph. Maintenance exercise should be done 3 to 4 times/wk to maintain fitness levels. Oxygen saturation is monitored, and supplemental oxygen is provided as needed.

Upper extremity resistance training helps the patient in doing daily tasks (eg, bathing, dressing, house cleaning). The usual benefits of exercise are modest increases in lower extremity strength, endurance, and maximum oxygen consumption.

Patients should be taught ways to conserve energy during activities of daily living and to pace their activities. Difficulties in sexual function should be discussed and advice should be given on using energy-conserving techniques for sexual gratification.

Surgery

Surgical options for treatment of severe COPD include

- Lung volume reduction
- Lung transplantation

Lung volume reduction surgery: Lung volume reduction surgery consists of resecting nonfunctioning emphysematous areas. The procedure improves lung function, exercise tolerance, and quality of life in patients with severe, predominantly upper-lung emphysema who have low baseline exercise capacity after pulmonary rehabilitation. Mortality is increased in the first 90 days after lung volume reduction surgery, but survival is higher at 5 yr.

The effect on ABGs is variable and not predictable, but most patients who require oxygen therapy before surgery continue to need it. Improvement is less than that with lung transplantation. The mechanism of improvement is believed to be enhanced lung recoil and improved diaphragmatic function.

Operative mortality is about 5%. The best candidates for lung volume reduction surgery are patients with an FEV_1 20 to 40% of predicted, a DL CO > 20% of predicted, significantly impaired exercise capacity, heterogeneous pulmonary disease on CT with an upper-lobe predominance, $Paco_2 < 50$ mm Hg, and absence of severe pulmonary hypertension and coronary artery disease.

Rarely, patients have extremely large bullae that compress the functional lung. These patients can be helped by surgical resection of these bullae, with resulting relief of symptoms and improved pulmonary function. Generally, resection is most beneficial for patients with bullae affecting more than one third of a hemithorax and an FEV_1 about half of the predicted normal value. Improved pulmonary function is related to the amount of normal or minimally diseased lung tissue that was compressed by the resected bullae. Serial chest x-rays and CT scans are the most useful procedures for determining whether a patient's functional status is due to compression of viable lung by bullae or to generalized emphysema. A markedly reduced DLco (< 40% predicted) indicates widespread emphysema and suggests a poorer outcome from surgical resection.

Lung transplantation: Lung transplantation can be single or double. Perioperative complications tend to be lower with single-lung transplantation, but some evidence shows that survival time is increased with double-lung transplantation. Candidates for transplantation are patients < 65 yr with an FEV_1 < 25% predicted after bronchodilator therapy or with severe pulmonary hypertension. The goal of lung transplantation is to improve quality of life, because survival time is not necessarily increased. The 5-yr survival after transplantation for emphysema is 45 to 60%. Lifelong immunosuppression is required, with the attendant risk of opportunistic infections.

1. Long-Term Oxygen Treatment Trial Research Group: A randomized trial of long-term oxygen for COPD with moderate desaturation. *New Engl J Med* 375:1617–1627, 2016.

KEY POINTS

- Relieve symptoms rapidly with primarily short-acting beta-adrenergic drugs and decrease exacerbations with inhaled corticosteroids, long-acting beta-adrenergic drugs, long-acting anticholinergic drugs, or a combination.
- Encourage smoking cessation using multiple interventions (eg, behavior modification, support groups, nicotine replacement, drug therapy).
- Optimize use of supportive treatments (eg, nutrition, pulmonary rehabilitation, self-directed exercise).

TREATMENT OF ACUTE COPD EXACERBATION

COPD management involves treatment of chronic stable disease and treatment of exacerbations.

Treatment of acute exacerbations involves

- Oxygen supplementation
- Bronchodilators
- Corticosteroids
- Antibiotics
- Sometimes ventilatory assistance

The immediate objectives are to ensure adequate oxygenation and near-normal blood pH, reverse airway obstruction, and treat any cause.

The cause of an acute exacerbation is usually unknown, although some acute exacerbations result from bacterial or viral infections. Smoking, irritative inhalational exposure, and high levels of air pollution also contribute.

Mild exacerbations often can be treated on an outpatient basis in patients with adequate home support. Elderly, frail patients and patients with comorbidities, a history of respiratory failure, or acute changes in ABG measurements are admitted to the hospital for observation and treatment. Patients with life-threatening exacerbations manifested by uncorrected moderate to severe acute hypoxemia, acute respiratory acidosis, new arrhythmias, or deteriorating respiratory function despite hospital treatment should be admitted to the ICU and their respiratory status monitored frequently.

Oxygen Supplementation

Most patients require oxygen supplementation during a COPD exacerbation, even those who do not need it chronically. Hypercapnia may worsen in patients given oxygen. This worsening has traditionally been thought to result from an attenuation of hypoxic respiratory drive. However, increased ventilation/perfusion (V/Q) mismatch probably is a more important factor.

Before oxygen administration, pulmonary vasoconstriction minimizes V/Q mismatch by decreasing perfusion of the most poorly ventilated areas of the lungs. Increased V/Q mismatch occurs because oxygen administration attenuates this hypoxic pulmonary vasoconstriction.

The Haldane effect may also contribute to worsening hypercapnia, although this theory is controversial. The Haldane effect is a decrease in Hb's affinity for carbon dioxide, which results in increased amounts of carbon dioxide dissolved in plasma. Oxygen administration, even though it may worsen hypercapnia, is recommended; many patients with COPD have chronic as well as acute hypercapnia and thus severe CNS depression is unlikely unless $Paco_2$ is > 85 mm Hg. The target level for Pao_2

is about 60 mm Hg; higher levels offer little advantage and increase the risk of hypercapnia.

Oxygen is given via Venturi mask so it can be closely regulated, and the patient is closely monitored. Patients whose condition deteriorates with oxygen therapy (eg, those with severe acidemia or CNS depression) require ventilatory assistance.

Many patients who require home oxygen for the first time when they are discharged from the hospital after an exacerbation improve within 30 days and no longer require oxygen. Thus, the need for home oxygen should be reassessed 60 to 90 days after discharge.

Ventilatory Assistance

Noninvasive positive-pressure ventilation (eg, pressure support or bilevel positive airway pressure ventilation by face mask) is an alternative to full mechanical ventilation. Noninvasive ventilation appears to decrease the need for intubation, reduce hospital stay, and reduce mortality in patients with severe exacerbations (defined as a pH < 7.30 in hemodynamically stable patients not at immediate risk of respiratory arrest).

Noninvasive ventilation appears to have no effect in patients with less severe exacerbation. However, it may be indicated for patients with less severe exacerbations whose ABGs worsen despite initial drug or oxygen therapy or who appear to be imminent candidates for full mechanical ventilation but who do not require intubation for control of the airway or sedation for agitation. Patients who have severe dyspnea, hyperinflation, and use of accessory muscles of respiration may also gain relief from positive airway pressure. Deterioration while receiving noninvasive ventilation necessitates invasive mechanical ventilation.

Deteriorating ABG values, deteriorating mental status, and progressive respiratory fatigue are indications for endotracheal intubation and mechanical ventilation. Ventilator settings, management strategies, and complications are discussed elsewhere. Risk factors for ventilatory dependence include an $FEV_1 < 0.5$ L, stable ABGs with a $Pao_2 < 50$ mm Hg, or a $Paco_2 > 60$ mm Hg, severe exercise limitation, and poor nutritional status. Therefore, if patients are at high risk, discussion of their wishes regarding intubation and mechanical ventilation should be initiated and documented (see p. 3212) while they are stable outpatients. However, overconcern about possible ventilator dependence should not delay management of acute respiratory failure; many patients who require mechanical ventilation can return to their pre-exacerbation level of health. High-flow nasal oxygen therapy has also been tried for patients with acute respiratory failure due to a COPD exacerbation and would be considered experimental at this time.

In patients who require prolonged intubation (eg, > 2 wk), a tracheostomy is indicated to facilitate comfort, communication, and eating. With a good multidisciplinary pulmonary rehabilitation program, including nutritional and psychologic support, many patients who require prolonged mechanical ventilation can be successfully removed from a ventilator and can return to their former level of function. Specialized programs are available for patients who remain ventilator-dependent after acute respiratory failure. Some patients can remain off the ventilator during the day. For patients with adequate home support, training of family members can permit some patients to be sent home with ventilators.

PEARLS & PITFALLS

• Overconcern about possible ventilator dependence should not delay management of acute respiratory failure; many patients who require mechanical ventilation can return to their pre-exacerbation level of health.

Drug Therapy

Beta-agonists and anticholinergics, with or without corticosteroids, should be started concurrently with oxygen therapy (regardless of how oxygen is administered) with the aim of reversing airway obstruction. Methylxanthines, once considered essential to treatment of acute COPD exacerbations, are no longer used; toxicities exceed benefits.

Beta-agonists: Short-acting beta-agonists are the cornerstone of drug therapy for acute exacerbations. The most widely used drug is albuterol 2.5 mg by nebulizer or 2 to 4 puffs (100 mcg/puff) by metered-dose inhaler q 2 to 6 h. Inhalation using a metered-dose inhaler causes rapid bronchodilation; there are no data indicating that doses taken with nebulizers are more effective than the same doses correctly taken with metered-dose inhalers. In cases of severe unresponsive bronchospasm, continuous nebulizer treatments may sometimes be administered.

Anticholinergic drugs: Ipratropium, an anticholinergic, is effective in acute COPD exacerbations and should be given concurrently or alternating with beta-agonists. Dosage is 0.25 to 0.5 mg by nebulizer or 2 to 4 inhalations (17 to 18 mcg of drug delivered per puff) by metered-dose inhaler q 4 to 6 h. Ipratropium generally provides bronchodilating effect similar to that of usual recommended doses of beta-agonists.

The role of the longer-acting anticholinergic drugs in treating acute exacerbations has not been defined.

Corticosteroids: Corticosteroids should be begun immediately for all but mild exacerbations. Options include prednisone 30 to 60 mg po once/day for 5 days or tapered over 7 to 14 days and methylprednisolone 60 to 500 mg IV once/day for 3 days and then tapered over 7 to 14 days. Alternatively, a 5-day course of 40 mg of prednisone appears to be equally effective. These drugs are equivalent in their acute effects; inhaled corticosteroids have no role in the treatment of acute exacerbations.

Antibiotics: Antibiotics are recommended for exacerbations in patients with purulent sputum. Some physicians give antibiotics empirically for change in sputum color or for nonspecific chest x-ray abnormalities. Routine cultures and Gram stains are not necessary before treatment unless an unusual or resistant organism is suspected (eg, in hospitalized, institutionalized, or immunosuppressed patients). Drugs directed against oral flora are indicated. Examples of antibiotics that are effective and inexpensive are

- Trimethoprim/sulfamethoxazole 160 mg/800 mg po bid
- Amoxicillin 250 to 500 mg po tid
- Tetracycline 250 mg po qid
- Doxycycline 50 to 100 mg po bid

These antibiotics are given for 7 to 14 days. Choice of drug is dictated by local patterns of bacterial sensitivity and patient history.

When patients are seriously ill or clinical evidence suggests that the infectious organisms are resistant, broader spectrum 2nd-line drugs can be used. These drugs include amoxicillin/clavulanate 250 to 500 mg po tid, fluoroquinolones (eg, ciprofloxacin, levofloxacin), 2nd-generation cephalosporins (eg, cefuroxime, cefaclor), and extended-spectrum macrolides (eg, azithromycin, clarithromycin). These drugs are effective against beta-lactamase–producing strains of *H. influenzae* and *M. catarrhalis* but have not been shown to be more effective than first-line drugs for most patients.

Patients can be taught to recognize a change in sputum from normal to purulent as a sign of impending exacerbation and to start a 10- to 14-day course of antibiotic therapy. Long-term antibiotic prophylaxis is recommended only for patients with underlying structural changes in the lung, such as bronchiectasis or infected bullae. In patients with frequent exacerbations, long-term macrolide use reduces exacerbation frequency but may have adverse effects.

Other drugs: Antitussives, such as dextromethorphan and benzonatate, have little role.

Opioids (eg, codeine, hydrocodone, oxycodone) should be used judiciously for relief of symptoms (eg, severe coughing paroxysms, pain) insofar as these drugs may suppress a productive cough, impair mental status, and cause constipation.

End-of-Life Care

With very severe disease exercise is unwarranted and activities of daily living are arranged to minimize energy expenditure. For example, patients may arrange to live on one floor of the house, have several small meals rather than fewer large meals, and avoid wearing shoes that must be tied. End-of-life care should be discussed, including whether to pursue mechanical ventilation, the use of palliative sedation, and appointment of a surrogate medical decision-maker in the event of the patient's incapacitation.

KEY POINTS

- Most patients require oxygen supplementation during an exacerbation.
- Inhaled short-acting beta-agonists are the cornerstone of drug therapy for acute exacerbations.
- Use antibiotics if patients have acute exacerbations and purulent sputum.
- For patients with end stage COPD, address end-of-life care proactively, including preferences regarding mechanical ventilation and palliative sedation.

ALPHA-1 ANTITRYPSIN DEFICIENCY

Alpha-1 antitrypsin deficiency is congenital lack of a primary lung antiprotease, alpha-1 antitrypsin, which leads to increased protease-mediated tissue destruction and emphysema in adults. Hepatic accumulation of abnormal alpha-1 antitrypsin can cause liver disease in both children and adults. Serum alpha-1 antitrypsin level < 11 μmol/L (< 80 mg/dL) confirms the diagnosis. Treatment is smoking cessation, bronchodilators, early treatment of infection, and, in selected cases, alpha-1 antitrypsin replacement. Severe liver disease may require transplantation. Prognosis is related mainly to degree of lung impairment.

Pathophysiology

Alpha-1 antitrypsin is a neutrophil elastase inhibitor (an antiprotease), the major function of which is to protect the lungs from protease-mediated tissue destruction. Most alpha-1 antitrypsin is synthesized by hepatocytes and monocytes and passively diffuses through the circulation into the lungs; some is secondarily produced by alveolar macrophages and epithelial cells. The protein conformation (and hence functionality) and quantity of circulating alpha-1 antitrypsin are determined by codominant expression of parental alleles; > 90 different alleles have been identified and described by protease inhibitor (PI*) phenotype.

Liver: Inheritance of some variant alleles causes a change in conformation of the alpha-1 antitrypsin molecule, leading to polymerization and retention within hepatocytes. The hepatic accumulation of aberrant alpha-1 antitrypsin molecules causes neonatal cholestatic jaundice in 10 to 20% of patients; the remaining patients are probably able to degrade the abnormal protein, although the exact protective mechanism is unclear. About 20% of cases of neonatal hepatic involvement result in development of cirrhosis in childhood. About 10% of patients without childhood liver disease develop cirrhosis as adults. Liver involvement increases the risk of liver cancer.

Lungs: In the lungs, alpha-1 antitrypsin deficiency increases neutrophil elastase activity, which facilitates tissue destruction leading to emphysema (especially in smokers, because cigarette smoke also increases protease activity). Alpha-1 antitrypsin deficiency accounts for 1 to 2% of all cases of COPD. Alpha-1 antitrypsin deficiency most commonly causes early emphysema; symptoms and signs of lung involvement occur earlier in smokers than in nonsmokers but in both cases are rare before age 25. Some patients with bronchiectasis have alpha-1 antitrypsin deficiency.

Other tissues: Other disorders possibly associated with alpha-1 antitrypsin allele variants include panniculitis (an inflammatory disorder of the subcutaneous tissue), life-threatening hemorrhage (through a mutation that converts alpha-1 antitrypsin from a neutrophil elastase to a coagulation factor inhibitor), aneurysms, ulcerative colitis, antineutrophilic cytoplasmic antibody (ANCA)-positive vasculitis, and glomerular disease.

Classification

The normal PI phenotype is PI*MM. More than 95% of people with severe alpha-1 antitrypsin deficiency and emphysema are homozygous for the Z allele (PI*ZZ) and have alpha-1 antitrypsin levels of about 30 to 40 mg/dL (5 to 6 μmol/L). Prevalence in the general population is 1/1500 to 1/5000. Most are whites of Northern European descent; the Z allele is rare in people of Asian descent and blacks. Though emphysema is common among PI*ZZ patients, many nonsmoking patients who are homozygous for PI*ZZ do not develop emphysema; patients who do typically have a family history of COPD. PI*ZZ smokers have a lower life expectancy than PI*ZZ nonsmokers, who have a lower life expectancy than PI*MM nonsmokers and smokers. Nonsmoking people who are PI*MZ heterozygous are more likely to experience more rapid decreases in forced expiratory volume in 1 sec (FEV_1) over time than do people in the general population.

Other rare phenotypes include PI*SZ and two types with nonexpressing alleles, PI*Z-null and PI*null-null (see Table 54–5). The null phenotype leads to undetectable serum levels of alpha-1 antitrypsin. Normal serum levels of malfunctioning alpha-1 antitrypsin may occur with rare mutations.

Table 54–5. EXPRESSION OF PHENOTYPE IN ALPHA-1 ANTITRYPSIN DEFICIENCY

PHENOTYPE	ALPHA-1 ANTITRYPSIN SERUM LEVEL	RISK OF EMPHYSEMA
PI*ZZ	13.6–38 mg/dL (2.5–7 μmol/L)	High
PI*MZ	92–179 mg/dL (17–33 μmol/L)	Minimally increased
PI*SZ	43.5–87 mg/dL (8–16 μmol/L)	Slightly increased
PI*SS	81.5–179 mg/dL (15–33 μmol/L)	Minimally increased
PI*null-null	0	High
PI*Z-null	0–27 mg/dL (0–5 μmol/L)	High
PI*MM	109–261 mg/dL (20–48 μmol/L)	Normal

Symptoms and Signs

Neonates with hepatic involvement present with cholestatic jaundice and hepatomegaly during the first week of life; jaundice usually resolves by 2 to 4 mo of age. Cirrhosis may develop in childhood or adulthood (symptoms and signs of cirrhosis and hepatocellular carcinoma are discussed elsewhere in The Manual). Adults with emphysema have symptoms and signs of COPD, including dyspnea, cough, wheezing, and prolonged expiration.

Severity of pulmonary disease varies greatly depending on phenotype, smoking status, and other factors. Pulmonary function is well preserved in some PI*ZZ smokers and can be severely impaired in some PI*ZZ nonsmokers. PI*ZZ people identified in population surveys (ie, those without symptoms or pulmonary disease) tend to have better pulmonary function, whether they smoke or not, than do index people (those identified because they have pulmonary disease). Airflow obstruction occurs more frequently in men and in people with asthma, recurrent respiratory infections, occupational dust exposure, and a family history of pulmonary disease.

Panniculitis, an inflammatory disorder of subcutaneous soft tissue, manifests as indurated, tender, discolored plaques or nodules, typically on the lower abdomen, buttocks, and thighs.

Diagnosis

- Serum alpha-1 antitrypsin level
- Genotyping

Alpha-1 antitrypsin deficiency is suspected in the following:

- Smokers who develop emphysema before age 45
- Nonsmokers without occupational exposures who develop emphysema at any age
- Patients whose chest x-ray shows predominately lower lung emphysema
- Patients with a family history of emphysema or unexplained cirrhosis
- People with a family history of alpha-1-antitrypsin deficiency
- Patients with panniculitis
- Neonates with jaundice or liver enzyme elevations
- Patients with unexplained bronchiectasis or liver disease

Diagnosis is made by identifying serum alpha-1 antitrypsin levels < 80 mg/dL (< 15 μmol/L) if measured by the radial immunodiffusion method or levels < 50 mg/dL (< 9 μmol/L) if measured by nephelometry. Patients with low levels should have confirmation by genotyping.

Prognosis

As a group, people with severe alpha-1 antitrypsin deficiency who have never smoked have a normal life expectancy and only moderate impairment of pulmonary function. The most common cause of death in alpha-1 antitrypsin deficiency is emphysema, followed by cirrhosis, often with hepatic carcinoma.

Treatment

- Supportive care
- For pulmonary disease, often alpha-1 antitrypsin replacement

Treatment of pulmonary disease is with purified human alpha-1 antitrypsin (60 mg/kg IV over 45 to 60 min given once/wk or 250 mg/kg over 4 to 6 h given once/mo [pooled only]), which can maintain the serum alpha-1 antitrypsin level above a target protective level of 80 mg/dL (35% of normal). Because emphysema causes permanent structural change, therapy cannot repair damaged lung structure or improve lung function but is given to halt progression. Treatment is expensive and is therefore reserved for nonsmoking patients who have two abnormal alleles, mild to moderately abnormal pulmonary function, and confirmation of diagnosis by low serum alpha-1 antitrypsin levels. It is not indicated for patients who have severe disease or for patients in whom one or both alleles are normal.

Smoking cessation, use of bronchodilators, and early treatment of respiratory infections are particularly important for patients with alpha-1 antitrypsin deficiency and emphysema.

For severely impaired people < 60 yr, lung transplantation should be considered. Lung volume reduction in treating the emphysema of alpha-1 antitrypsin deficiency is controversial.

Gene therapy is under study.

Treatment of liver disease is supportive. Enzyme replacement does not help because the disease is caused by abnormal processing rather than by enzyme deficiency. Liver transplantation may be used for patients with liver failure.

Treatment of panniculitis is not well defined. Corticosteroids, antimalarials, and tetracyclines have been used.

KEY POINTS

- Suspect alpha-1 antitrypsin deficiency if patients have unexplained emphysema, liver disease (particularly in neonates), panniculitis, or bronchiectasis.
- Diagnose using serum alpha-1 antitrypsin levels < 80 mg/dL (< 15 μmol/L) and confirm by genotyping.
- Treat selected patients (nonsmoking patients in whom both alleles are abnormal and who have mild to moderately abnormal pulmonary function and low serum alpha-1 antitrypsin levels) with purified human alpha-1 antitrypsin.
- Consider liver transplantation if liver failure develops.

55 Diffuse Alveolar Hemorrhage and Pulmonary-Renal Syndrome

DIFFUSE ALVEOLAR HEMORRHAGE

Diffuse alveolar hemorrhage is persistent or recurrent pulmonary hemorrhage. There are numerous causes, but autoimmune disorders are most common. Most patients present with dyspnea, cough, hemoptysis, and new alveolar infiltrates on chest imaging. Diagnostic tests are directed at the suspected cause. Treatment is with immunosuppressants for patients with autoimmune causes and respiratory support if needed.

Diffuse alveolar hemorrhage is not a specific disorder, but a syndrome that suggests a differential diagnosis and a specific sequence of testing. Some disorders that cause diffuse alveolar hemorrhage are associated with glomerulonephritis; then the disorder is defined as a pulmonary-renal syndrome.

Pathophysiology

Diffuse alveolar hemorrhage results from widespread damage to the pulmonary small vessels, leading to blood collecting within the alveoli. If enough alveoli are affected, gas exchange is disrupted. The specific pathophysiology and manifestations vary depending on cause. For example, isolated pauci-immune pulmonary capillaritis is a small-vessel vasculitis limited to the lungs; its only manifestation is alveolar hemorrhage affecting people aged 18 to 35 yr.

Etiology

Many disorders can cause alveolar hemorrhage; they include

- Autoimmune disorders (eg, systemic vasculitides, Goodpasture syndrome, antiphospholipid antibody syndrome, connective tissue disorders)
- Pulmonary infections (eg, hantavirus infection)
- Toxic exposures (eg, trimellitic anhydride, isocyanates, crack cocaine, certain pesticides)
- Drug reactions (eg, propylthiouracil, diphenylhydantoin, amiodarone, methotrexate, nitrofurantoin, bleomycin, montelukast, infliximab)
- Cardiac disorders (eg, mitral stenosis)
- Coagulation disorders caused by diseases or anticoagulant drugs
- Isolated pauci-immune pulmonary capillaritis
- Idiopathic pulmonary hemosiderosis
- Hematopoietic stem cell transplantation or solid organ transplantation

Symptoms and Signs

Symptoms and signs of milder diffuse alveolar hemorrhage are dyspnea, cough, and fever; however, many patients present with acute respiratory failure, sometimes leading to death. Hemoptysis is common but may be absent in up to one-third of patients. Most patients have anemia and ongoing bleeding with a decreasing Hct.

There are no specific physical examination findings.

Other manifestations depend on the underlying disorder (eg, diastolic murmur in patients with mitral stenosis).

Diagnosis

- Chest x-ray
- Bronchoalveolar lavage
- Serologic and other tests to diagnose the cause

Diagnosis is suggested by dyspnea, cough, and hemoptysis accompanied by chest x-ray findings of diffuse bilateral alveolar infiltrates if one suspects diffuse alveolar hemorrhage. Bronchoscopy with bronchoalveolar lavage (BAL) is strongly recommended to confirm the diagnosis, particularly when manifestations are atypical or an airway source of hemorrhage has not been excluded. Specimens show blood with numerous erythrocytes and siderophages; lavage fluid typically remains hemorrhagic or becomes increasingly hemorrhagic after sequential sampling.

Evaluation of the cause: Further testing for the cause should be done. Urinalysis is indicated to exclude glomerulonephritis and the pulmonary-renal syndromes; serum BUN and creatinine also should be measured.

Other routine tests include

- CBC
- Coagulation studies
- Platelet count
- Serologic tests (antinuclear antibody, anti–double-stranded DNA [anti-dsDNA], antiglomerular basement membrane [anti-GBM] antibodies, antineutrophil cytoplasmic antibodies [ANCA], antiphospholipid antibody)

Serologic tests are done to look for underlying disorders. Perinuclear-ANCA (p-ANCA) titers are elevated in some cases of isolated pauci-immune pulmonary capillaritis.

Other tests depend on clinical context. When patients are stable, pulmonary function tests may be done to document lung function. They may show increased diffusing capacity for carbon monoxide (DLco) due to increased uptake of carbon monoxide by intra-alveolar Hb; however, this finding, which is consistent with hemorrhage, does not assist with establishing a diagnosis.

Echocardiography may be indicated to exclude mitral stenosis. Lung biopsy or, if the urinalysis is abnormal, kidney biopsy is frequently needed when a cause remains unclear or the progression of disease is too rapid to await the results of serologic testing.

Prognosis

Patients can require mechanical ventilation and even die as a result of hemorrhage-associated respiratory failure. Recurrent alveolar hemorrhage causes pulmonary hemosiderosis and fibrosis, both of which develop when ferritin aggregates within alveoli and exerts toxic effects. COPD occurs in some patients with recurrent diffuse alveolar hemorrhage secondary to microscopic polyarteritis.

Treatment

- Corticosteroids
- Sometimes cyclophosphamide or plasma exchange
- Supportive measures

Treatment involves correcting the cause. Corticosteroids and possibly cyclophosphamide are used to treat vasculitides, connective tissue disorders, and Goodpasture syndrome.

Effectiveness of rituximab in diffuse alveolar hemorrhage has not been studied. Plasma exchange may be used to treat Goodpasture syndrome. Several studies have reported successful use of recombinant activated human factor VII in treating severe unresponsive alveolar hemorrhage, but such therapy is controversial because of possible thrombotic complications.

Other possible management measures include supplemental oxygen, bronchodilators, reversal of any coagulopathy, and intubation with protective strategies as for acute respiratory distress syndrome (ARDS) and mechanical ventilation.

KEY POINTS

- Although diffuse alveolar hemorrhage can have various causes (eg, infection, toxins, drugs, hematologic or cardiac disorders), autoimmune disorders are the most common causes.
- Symptoms, signs, and chest-x-ray findings are not specific.
- Confirm diffuse alveolar hemorrhage by doing BAL to show persistent hemorrhage with sequential lavage samples.
- Test for the cause by doing routine laboratory tests, autoantibody testing, and sometimes other tests.
- Treat the cause (eg, with corticosteroids, cyclophosphamide, plasma exchange, and/or immunosuppressants for autoimmune causes).

GOODPASTURE SYNDROME

(Anti-GBM Antibody Disease)

Goodpasture syndrome, a subtype of pulmonary-renal syndrome, is an autoimmune syndrome of alveolar hemorrhage and glomerulonephritis caused by circulating anti-glomerular basement membrane (anti-GBM) antibodies. Goodpasture syndrome most often develops in genetically susceptible people who smoke cigarettes, but hydrocarbon exposure and viral respiratory infections are additional possible triggers. Symptoms are dyspnea, cough, fatigue, hemoptysis, and hematuria. Goodpasture syndrome is suspected in patients with hemoptysis or hematuria and is confirmed by the presence of anti-GBM antibodies in the blood or in a renal biopsy specimen. Prognosis is good when treatment is begun before onset of respiratory or renal failure. Treatment includes plasma exchange, corticosteroids, and immunosuppressants, such as cyclophosphamide.

Pathophysiology

Goodpasture syndrome is the combination of glomerulonephritis with alveolar hemorrhage and anti-GBM antibodies. Goodpasture syndrome most often manifests as diffuse alveolar hemorrhage and glomerulonephritis together but can occasionally cause glomerulonephritis (10 to 20%) or pulmonary disease (10%) alone. Men are affected more often than women.

Anti-GBM antibodies are directed against the noncollagenous (NC-1) domain of the $\alpha3$ chain of type IV collagen, which occurs in highest concentration in the basement membranes of renal and pulmonary capillaries.

Environmental exposures—cigarette smoking, viral URI, and hydrocarbon solvent inhalation most commonly and pneumonia less commonly—expose alveolar capillary antigens to circulating antibody in genetically susceptible people, most notably those with HLA-DRw15, -DR4, and -DRB1 alleles. Circulating anti-GBM antibodies bind to basement membranes, fix complement, and trigger a cell-mediated inflammatory response, causing glomerulonephritis, pulmonary capillaritis, or both.

Symptoms and Signs

Hemoptysis is the most prominent symptom; however, hemoptysis may not occur in patients with alveolar hemorrhage, and patients may present with only chest x-ray infiltrates or with infiltrates and respiratory distress, respiratory failure, or both.

Other common symptoms include

- Dyspnea
- Cough
- Fatigue
- Fever
- Weight loss
- Hematuria

Up to 40% of patients have gross hematuria, although pulmonary hemorrhage may precede renal manifestations by weeks to years.

Signs vary over time and range from clear lungs on auscultation to crackles and rhonchi. Some patients have peripheral edema due to renal failure and pallor due to anemia.

Diagnosis

- Serum anti-GBM antibody tests
- Sometimes renal biopsy

Patients are tested for serum anti-GBM antibodies by indirect immunofluorescence testing or, when available, direct enzyme-linked immunosorbent assay (ELISA) with recombinant or human NC-1 $\alpha3$. Presence of these antibodies confirms the diagnosis. Antineutrophil cytoplasmic antibodies (ANCA) testing is positive (in a peripheral pattern) in only 25% of patients with Goodpasture syndrome.

If anti-GBM antibodies are absent and patients have evidence of glomerulonephritis (hematuria, proteinuria, red cell casts detected with urinalysis, renal insufficiency, or a combination of these findings), renal biopsy is indicated to confirm the diagnosis. A rapidly progressive focal segmental necrotizing glomerulonephritis with crescent formation is found in biopsy specimens in patients with Goodpasture syndrome and all other causes of pulmonary-renal syndrome (PRS). Immunofluorescence staining of renal or lung tissue classically shows linear IgG deposition along the glomerular or alveolar capillaries. IgG deposition also occurs in the kidneys of patients with diabetes or with fibrillary glomerulonephritis (a rare disorder causing PRS), but GBM binding of antibodies in these disorders is nonspecific and does not occur in linear patterns.

Prognosis

Goodpasture syndrome is often rapidly progressive and can be fatal if prompt recognition and treatment are delayed. Prognosis is good when treatment begins before onset of respiratory or renal failure. Long-term morbidity is related to the degree of renal impairment at diagnosis. Patients requiring dialysis right away and those with > 50% crescents in the biopsy specimen (who often will require dialysis) usually survive for < 2 yr unless kidney transplantation is done.

Hemoptysis may be a good prognostic sign because it leads to earlier detection; the minority of patients who are ANCA-positive respond better to treatment. Relapse occurs in a small number and is linked to continued tobacco use and respiratory infection. In patients with end-stage renal disease who receive kidney transplantation, disease can recur in the graft.

Treatment

- Plasma exchange
- Corticosteroids and cyclophosphamide

Immediate survival in patients with pulmonary hemorrhage and respiratory failure is linked to airway control; endotracheal intubation and mechanical ventilation are recommended for patients with borderline ABGs and impending respiratory failure. Patients with significant renal impairment may require dialysis or kidney transplantation.

Treatment is daily or every-other-day plasma exchange for 2 to 3 wk using 4-L exchanges to remove anti-GBM antibodies, combined with a corticosteroid (usually methylprednisolone 1 g IV over 20 min once/day or every other day for 3 doses followed by prednisone (1 mg/kg po once/day for 3 wk, then titrated down to 20 mg po once/day for 6 to 12 mo) and cyclophosphamide (2 mg/kg po or IV once/day for 6 to 12 mo) to prevent formation of new antibodies. Therapy can be tapered when pulmonary and renal function stop improving.

Rituximab could be used in some patients who have severe adverse effects due to cyclophosphamide or refuse cyclophosphamide as treatment, but it has not been studied in patients with Goodpasture syndrome.

KEY POINTS

- Patients with Goodpasture syndrome may have both pulmonary hemorrhage and glomerulonephritis or either one separately.
- Pulmonary findings can be mild or nonspecific.
- Test serum for anti-GBM antibodies.
- Do a renal biopsy if patients have glomerulonephritis.
- Diagnose and treat Goodpasture syndrome before organ failure develops whenever possible.
- Treat using plasma exchange, a corticosteroid, and cyclophosphamide.

IDIOPATHIC PULMONARY HEMOSIDEROSIS

Idiopathic pulmonary hemosiderosis (IPH) is a rare disease that causes recurrent diffuse alveolar hemorrhage with no detectable underlying disorder; it occurs mainly in children < 10 yr. It is thought to be due to a defect in the alveolar capillary endothelium, possibly due to autoimmune injury. Many affected patients have celiac disease.

Symptoms and Signs

Symptoms and signs of idiopathic pulmonary hemosiderosis in children include recurrent episodes of dyspnea and cough, particularly nonproductive cough initially. Hemoptysis occurs later. Children with IPH may present with only failure to thrive and iron deficiency anemia. The most common symptoms in adults are exertional dyspnea and fatigue due to pulmonary hemorrhage and iron deficiency anemia.

Diagnosis

- Bronchoalveolar lavage

Diagnosis of idiopathic pulmonary hemosiderosis involves demonstration of a combination of characteristic clinical findings, iron deficiency anemia, and hemosiderin-laden macrophages in bronchoalveolar lavage (BAL) fluid or lung biopsy specimens plus no evidence of small-vessel vasculitis (pulmonary capillaritis) or another explanatory diagnosis; it is confirmed by lung biopsy if other findings are inconclusive.

Treatment

- Corticosteroids

Corticosteroids may reduce the morbidity and mortality of acute episodes of alveolar bleeding and may control the disease progression of pulmonary fibrosis. Some patients may require additional immunosuppressive drugs.

Patients with celiac disease should be on a gluten-free diet.

PULMONARY-RENAL SYNDROME

Pulmonary-renal syndrome (PRS) is diffuse alveolar hemorrhage plus glomerulonephritis, often occurring simultaneously. Cause is almost always an autoimmune disorder. Diagnosis is by serologic tests and sometimes lung and renal biopsy. Treatment typically includes immunosuppression with corticosteroids and cytotoxic drugs.

PRS is not a specific entity but is a syndrome that suggests a differential diagnosis and a specific sequence of testing.

Pulmonary pathology is small-vessel vasculitis involving arterioles, venules, and, frequently, alveolar capillaries.

Renal pathology is small-vessel vasculitis resulting in a form of focal segmental proliferative glomerulonephritis.

Etiology

Pulmonary-renal syndrome is almost always a manifestation of an underlying autoimmune disorder. Goodpasture syndrome is the prototype cause, but PRS can also be caused by SLE, granulomatosis with polyangiitis, microscopic polyangiitis, and, less commonly, by other vasculitides, connective tissue disorders, and drug-induced vasculitides (eg, propylthiouracil—see Table 55–1).

PRS is less commonly a manifestation of immunoglobulin A (IgA)-mediated disorders, such as IgA nephropathy or IgA–associated vasculitis, and of immune complex–mediated renal disease, such as essential mixed cryoglobulinemia. Rarely, rapidly progressive glomerulonephritis alone can cause PRS through a mechanism involving renal failure, volume overload, and pulmonary edema with hemoptysis.

Table 55–1. CAUSES OF PULMONARY-RENAL SYNDROME

DISORDER	EXAMPLES
Connective tissue disorders	Dermatomyositis Polymyositis Progressive systemic sclerosis RA SLE
Goodpasture syndrome	—
Renal disorders	Idiopathic immune complex glomerulonephritis Immunoglobulin A nephropathy Rapidly progressive glomerulonephritis with heart failure
Systemic vasculitis	Behçet disease Cryoglobulinemia Eosinophilic granulomatosis with polyangiitis Granulomatosis with polyangiitis IgA–associated vasculitis Microscopic polyarteritis
Other	Drugs (eg, propylthiouracil) Heart failure

Symptoms and Signs

Symptoms and signs typically include

- Dyspnea
- Cough
- Fever
- Hemoptysis
- Peripheral edema
- Hematuria

Patients may also have other signs of glomerulonephritis. Pulmonary and renal manifestations can occur weeks to months apart.

PEARLS & PITFALLS

- Consider pulmonary-renal syndrome in patients with findings compatible with alveolar hemorrhage and glomerulonephritis even when pulmonary and renal findings occur at different times.

Diagnosis

- Serologic testing
- Sometimes lung and renal biopsies

Pulmonary-renal syndrome is suspected in patients with hemoptysis not obviously attributable to other causes (eg, pneumonia, carcinoma, bronchiectasis), particularly when hemoptysis is accompanied by diffuse parenchymal infiltrates and findings suggesting renal disease.

Initial testing includes urinalysis for evidence of hematuria and red cell casts (suggesting glomerulonephritis), serum creatinine for renal function assessment, and CBC for evidence of anemia. Chest x-ray is done if not yet obtained.

Serum antibody testing may help distinguish some causes, as in the following:

- Antiglomerular basement membrane antibodies: Goodpasture syndrome
- Antibodies to double-stranded DNA and reduced serum complement levels: SLE
- Antineutrophil cytoplasmic antibodies (ANCA) to proteinase-3 (PR3-ANCA or cytoplasmic ANCA [c-ANCA]): granulomatosis with polyangiitis
- ACNA to myeloperoxidase (MPO-ANCA, or perinuclear ANCA [p-ANCA]): Microscopic polyangiitis

Definitive diagnosis requires lung biopsy with findings of small-vessel vasculitis or renal biopsy with findings of glomerulonephritis with or without antibody deposition.

Pulmonary function tests and bronchoalveolar lavage are not diagnostic of PRS but can be used to help confirm diffuse alveolar hemorrhage in patients with glomerulonephritis and pulmonary infiltrates but without hemoptysis. Lavage fluid that remains hemorrhagic after sequential sampling establishes diffuse alveolar hemorrhage, especially in the context of falling Hct.

Treatment

- Corticosteroids
- Sometimes cyclophosphamide
- Plasma exchange

Immunosuppression is the cornerstone of treatment of pulmonary-renal syndrome. Standard induction-remission regimens include pulse IV methylprednisolone (500 to 1000 mg IV once/day for 3 to 5 days). As life-threatening features subside, the corticosteroid dose can be reduced; 1 mg/kg prednisone (or equivalent) po once/day is given for the first month, then tapered over the next 3 to 4 mo. Cyclophosphamide should be added to corticosteroid therapy in critically ill patients with generalized disease, at a dose of 0.5 to 1 g/m^2 IV given as a pulse once/mo or orally (1 to 2 mg/kg once/day). Rituximab may be used instead of cyclophosphamide; it is non-inferior and causes fewer adverse effects.

Plasma exchange is also often used, particularly in Goodpasture syndrome and certain vasculitides.

Transition to maintenance therapy may occur 6 to 12 mo after the initiation of induction therapy or after clinical remission. Maintenance therapy includes low-dose corticosteroids coupled with cytotoxic agents. However, relapse may occur despite ongoing therapy.

KEY POINTS

- The most suggestive clue to PRS is often that patients have both unexplained pulmonary and renal symptoms, even when such symptoms occur at different times.
- Do routine laboratory tests (including urinalysis and chest x-ray) as well as autoantibody testing.
- Confirm the diagnosis when necessary with lung or renal biopsy.
- Treat underlying autoimmune disorders.

56 Environmental Pulmonary Diseases

Environmental pulmonary diseases result from inhalation of dusts, allergens, chemicals, gases, and environmental pollutants. The lungs are continually exposed to the external environment and are susceptible to a host of environmental diseases. Pathologic processes can involve any part of the lungs, including the airways (eg, in occupational asthma, reactive airways dysfunction syndrome (RADS), or toxic inhalations), interstitium (eg, in pneumoconioses or hypersensitivity pneumonitis), and pleura (eg, in asbestos-related diseases).

Environmental inhalation exposure has long been known to be a risk factor for asthma (see Occupational Asthma on p. 444), but it is also increasingly being recognized as a non-smoking cause of COPD (see p. 423). The American Thoracic Society estimates the population-attributable fraction of COPD related to occupational and environmental exposures to be about 20% (ie, COPD incidence and mortality would decline by about 20% if environmental exposures were reduced to zero).

Clinicians should take an occupational and environmental history in all patients, asking specifically about past and current exposure to vapors, gases, dust, fumes, and/or biomass smoke (ie, from burning wood, animal waste, crops). Any positive response is followed by more detailed questions.

Prevention of occupational and environmental pulmonary diseases centers on reducing exposure (primary prevention). Exposure can be limited by the use of

- Administrative controls (eg, limiting the number of people exposed to hazardous conditions)

- Engineering controls (eg, enclosures, ventilation systems, safe clean-up procedures)
- Product substitution (eg, using safer, less toxic materials)
- Respiratory protection devices (eg, respirator, dust mask, gas mask)

Many clinicians erroneously assume that a patient who has used a respirator or another respiratory protection device has been well protected. Although respirators do afford a degree of protection, especially when fresh air is provided by tank or air hose, the benefit is limited and varies from person to person. When recommending use of a respirator, clinicians should consider several factors. Workers with cardiovascular disease may be unable to carry out jobs that require strenuous work if they must wear a self-contained breathing apparatus (tank). Respirators that are tight-fitting and that require the wearer to draw air through filter cartridges can increase the work of breathing, which can be especially difficult for patients with asthma, COPD, or interstitial lung diseases.

Medical surveillance is a form of secondary prevention. Workers can be offered medical tests that identify disorders early when treatment might help reduce long-term consequences.

AIR POLLUTION–RELATED ILLNESS

The major components of air pollution in developed countries are nitrogen dioxide (from combustion of fossil fuels), ozone (from the effect of sunlight on nitrogen dioxide and hydrocarbons), and suspended solid or liquid particles. Indoors, passive smoking is an additional source, as is burning of biomass fuel (eg, wood, animal waste, crops) in developing countries (eg, for cooking and heating).

High levels of air pollution can adversely affect lung function and trigger asthma and COPD exacerbations. Air pollution also increases risk of acute cardiovascular events (eg, MI) and development of coronary artery disease. People living in areas with a large amount of traffic, especially when stagnant air is created by thermal inversions, are at particular risk. All of the so-called criteria air pollutants (oxides of nitrogen, oxides of sulfur, ozone, carbon monoxide, lead, particulates), except carbon monoxide and lead, cause airway hyperreactivity. Long-term exposure may increase respiratory infections and symptoms in the general population, especially in children, and can decrease lung function in children.

Ozone, which is the major component of smog, is a strong respiratory irritant and oxidant. Ozone levels tend to be highest in the summer and in the late morning and early afternoon. Short-term exposures can cause dyspnea, chest pain, and airway reactivity. Children who regularly participate in outdoor activities during days on which ozone pollution is high are more likely to develop asthma. Long-term exposure to ozone produces a small, permanent decrease in lung function.

Oxides of sulfur, resulting from combustion of fossil fuels that are high in sulfur content, can create acid aerosols with high solubility, which are likely to be deposited in the upper airways. Sulfur oxides can induce airway inflammation, possibly increasing the risk of chronic bronchitis as well as inducing bronchoconstriction.

Particulate air pollution is a complex mixture, derived from fossil fuel combustion (especially diesel). The particles can have both local and systemic inflammatory effects, suggesting an explanation for their impact on both pulmonary and cardiovascular health. So-called PM2.5 (particulate matter $< 2.5\ \mu m$ diameter) produce a greater inflammatory response per mass than do larger particles. Data suggest that particulate air pollution increases death rates from all causes, especially cardiovascular and respiratory illness.

Air pollution data have raised concerns regarding the potential health effects of even smaller particles, so-called nanoparticles, but clinical evidence of disorders related to exposure to nanoparticles has yet to be reported.

OVERVIEW OF ASBESTOS-RELATED DISORDERS

Asbestos is a family of naturally occurring silicates whose heat-resistant and structural properties made it useful for inclusion in construction and shipbuilding materials, automobile brakes, and some textiles. Chrysotile (a serpentine fiber), crocidolite, and amosite (amphibole, or straight fibers) are the 3 main types of asbestos that cause disease. Asbestos can affect the lung, the pleura, or both.

Asbestos-related disorders are caused by inhalation of asbestos fibers. The disorders include

- Asbestosis
- Lung carcinoma
- Nonmalignant pleural plaque formation and thickening
- Benign pleural effusions
- Mesothelioma

Asbestosis and mesothelioma both cause progressive dyspnea, as do extensive effusions and plaques.

ASBESTOSIS

Asbestosis is a form of interstitial pulmonary fibrosis caused by asbestos exposure. Diagnosis is based on history and chest x-ray or CT findings. Treatment is supportive.

Asbestos is a family of naturally occurring silicates whose heat-resistant and structural properties made it useful for inclusion in construction and shipbuilding materials, automobile brakes, and some textiles. Chrysotile (a serpentine fiber), crocidolite, and amosite (amphibole, or straight fibers) are the 3 main types of asbestos that cause disease.

Asbestosis is a much more common consequence of asbestos exposure than cancer. Shipbuilders, textile and construction workers, home remodelers, workers who do asbestos abatement, and miners who are exposed to asbestos fibers are among the many workers at risk. Secondhand exposure may occur among family members of exposed workers and among people who live close to mines.

Pathophysiology

Alveolar macrophages attempting to engulf inhaled fibers release cytokines and growth factors that stimulate inflammation, oxidative injury, collagen deposition, and ultimately fibrosis. Asbestos fibers may also be directly toxic to lung tissue. Risk of disease is generally related to the duration and intensity of exposure and the type, length, and thickness of inhaled fibers.

Symptoms and Signs

Asbestosis is initially asymptomatic but can cause progressive dyspnea, nonproductive cough, and fatigue. The disorder progresses in > 10% of patients even after cessation of exposure. Advanced asbestosis may cause clubbing, dry bibasilar crackles, and, in severe cases, symptoms and signs of right ventricular failure (cor pulmonale).

Diagnosis

- Chest x-ray, preferably chest CT
- Sometimes bronchoalveolar lavage or lung biopsy

Diagnosis is based on history of exposure and chest x-ray or chest CT. Chest x-ray shows linear reticular opacities signifying fibrosis, usually in the peripheral lower lobes. Opacities are often bilateral and are often accompanied by pleural changes (see p. 441). Honeycombing signifies more advanced disease, which may involve the mid and lower lung fields. As with silicosis, severity is graded on the International Labor Organization scale (International Classification of Radiographs of Pneumoconioses) based on size, shape, location, and profusion of opacities. In contrast to silicosis, asbestosis produces reticular opacities with a lower lobe predominance. Hilar and mediastinal adenopathy and nodular opacities are uncharacteristic and suggest a different diagnosis. Chest x-ray is insensitive; high-resolution (thin-section) chest CT is useful when asbestosis is a likely diagnosis. CT is also superior to chest x-ray in identifying pleural abnormalities.

Pulmonary function tests, which may show reduced lung volumes and diffusing capacity for carbon monoxide (DLco), are nonspecific but help characterize changes in lung function over time. Pulse oximetry done at rest and during exertion is nonspecific but sensitive for detecting asbestos-induced impairment.

Bronchoalveolar lavage or lung biopsy is indicated only when noninvasive measures fail to provide conclusive diagnosis; demonstration of asbestos fibers indicates asbestosis in patients with pulmonary fibrosis, although such fibers can occasionally be found in lungs of exposed people without disease and may not be present in specimens from patients with asbestosis. Thus, demonstration of asbestos fibers may be helpful but is not necessary for diagnosis.

Prognosis

Prognosis varies; many patients have no or mild symptoms and do well, whereas some develop progressive dyspnea and a few develop respiratory failure, right ventricular failure, and cancer.

Lung cancer (usually non–small cell lung carcinoma) develops in patients with asbestosis at 8 to 10 times the rate of those without asbestosis and is especially common among workers exposed to amphibole fibers, although all forms of inhaled asbestos have been associated with an elevated cancer risk. Asbestos and smoking have a synergistic effect on lung cancer risk (see p. 518).

Treatment

- Supportive care

No specific treatment exists. Early detection of hypoxemia and right ventricular failure leads to use of supplemental O_2 and treatment of heart failure. Pulmonary rehabilitation can be helpful for patients with impairment.

Prevention

Preventive measures include eliminating exposure, asbestos abatement in occupational and nonoccupational settings, smoking cessation, and pneumococcal and influenza vaccination. Smoking cessation is particularly important in light of the multiplicative risk of lung cancer in patients who have both tobacco smoke and asbestos exposures.

KEY POINTS

- Asbestosis is a much more common consequence of asbestos exposure than cancer, but patients with asbestosis are at increased risk of lung cancer.
- Diagnosis usually requires high-resolution chest CT.
- Treat asbestosis supportively; smoking cessation is important.

MESOTHELIOMA

Pleural mesothelioma is the only known pleural cancer and is caused by asbestos exposure in nearly all cases. Diagnosis is based on history and chest x-ray or CT findings and tissue biopsy. Treatment is supportive, which may require surgery, chemotherapy, or both.

Asbestos is a family of naturally occurring silicates whose heat-resistant and structural properties made it useful for inclusion in construction and shipbuilding materials, automobile brakes, and some textiles. Chrysotile (a serpentine fiber), crocidolite, and amosite (amphibole, or straight fibers) are the 3 main types of asbestos that cause disease.

Asbestos workers have up to a 10% lifetime risk of developing mesothelioma, with an average latency of 30 yr. Risk is independent of smoking. Mesothelioma can spread locally, or it can metastasize to the hilar and mediastinal lymph nodes, pericardium, diaphragm, peritoneum, liver, adrenals, or kidneys and, rarely, the tunica vaginalis of the testis.

Symptoms and Signs

Patients most often present with dyspnea and nonpleuritic chest pain. Constitutional symptoms are uncommon at presentation. Invasion of the chest wall and other adjacent structures may cause severe pain, hoarseness, dysphagia, Horner syndrome, brachial plexopathy, or ascites.

Diagnosis

- Chest x-ray
- Pleural fluid cytology or pleural biopsy
- Sometimes video-assisted thoracoscopic surgery (VATS) or thoracotomy
- Staging with chest CT, mediastinoscopy, and MRI or sometimes with PET and bronchoscopy

The pleural form of mesothelioma, which represents > 90% of all cases (the other 10% include pericardial and peritoneal mesotheliomas), appears on x-ray as diffuse unilateral or bilateral pleural thickening that appears to encase the lungs, usually producing blunting of the costophrenic angles. Pleural effusions are present in 95% of cases and are typically unilateral, large, and hemorrhagic. Diagnosis is based on pleural fluid cytology or pleural biopsy. Increased levels of hyaluronidase in pleural fluid are suggestive but not diagnostic of mesothelioma. If diagnosis is uncertain after these procedures, biopsy by VATS or thoracotomy is done. Soluble mesothelin-related proteins released into the serum by mesothelial cells are being studied as possible tumor markers for disease detection and monitoring, but the false-positive rate may limit their effectiveness.

Staging is done with chest CT, mediastinoscopy, and MRI. Sensitivity and specificity of MRI and CT are comparable, although MRI is helpful in determining tumor extension into the spine or spinal cord. PET may have better sensitivity and specificity for distinguishing benign from malignant pleural thickening. Bronchoscopy should be done to exclude coexisting endobronchial lung cancers.

Prognosis

Mesothelioma remains an incurable cancer, and long-term survival is uncommon. Surgery to remove the pleura, ipsilateral lung, phrenic nerve, hemidiaphragm, and pericardium combined with chemotherapy or radiation therapy may be considered, although it does not substantially change prognosis or survival time. No treatment substantially prolongs survival. Median survival from time of diagnosis is 9 to 12 mo, depending on the location and cell type. A few patients, usually younger patients with shorter duration of symptoms, have a more favorable prognosis, sometimes surviving for several years after diagnosis.

Treatment

- Supportive care
- Pleurodesis or pleurectomy for pleural effusions and relief of dyspnea
- Analgesia with opioids and sometimes radiation therapy
- Chemotherapy for tumor shrinkage and symptom relief
- Experimental therapies

The major focus of treatment is supportive care and relief of pain and dyspnea. Given the diffuse nature of the disorder, radiation therapy is usually unsuitable except to treat localized pain or needle-tract metastases. It is not generally used for treatment of nerve root pain. Pleurodesis or pleurectomy can be used to help reduce dyspnea caused by pleural effusions. Adequate analgesia is important but difficult to achieve. Usually, opioids, both transdermal and delivered via indwelling epidural catheters, are used.

Because morbidity and mortality are high with extrapleural pneumonectomy, pleurectomy and decortication are used increasingly if all grossly visible tumor can be removed. However, complete resection is usually not feasible. Nonsurgical therapies include chemotherapy (eg, with pemetrexed and a platinum compound) and radiation therapy. Chemotherapy can relieve symptoms in most cases and sometimes decreases tumor size. Single-modality therapies do not prolong survival. The effect of multimodal therapies overall and the contribution of each mode have not been established. Therapies under investigation include immunotherapy, gene therapy, photodynamic therapy, and hyperthermic intrapleural chemotherapy.

KEY POINTS

- Mesothelioma is almost always asbestos-related and is pleural in > 90% of cases.
- Median survival from time of diagnosis is 9 to 12 mo, and cure is not possible.
- Treatment focuses on supportive care, but many surgical and nonsurgical treatments are under investigation.

ASBESTOS-RELATED PLEURAL DISEASE

Pleural disease, a hallmark of asbestos exposure, includes formation of pleural plaques, calcification, thickening, rounded atelectasis, adhesions, effusion, and mesothelioma. Diagnosis is based on history and chest x-ray or CT findings. Treatment is supportive.

Asbestos is a family of naturally occurring silicates whose heat-resistant and structural properties made it useful for inclusion in construction and shipbuilding materials, automobile brakes, and some textiles. Chrysotile (a serpentine fiber), crocidolite, and amosite (amphibole, or straight fibers) are the 3 main types of asbestos that cause disease.

Asbestos can cause pleural disease other than mesothelioma (see p. 440). Such pleural disease causes effusion but few symptoms. All pleural changes are diagnosed by chest x-ray or CT, though chest CT is more sensitive than chest x-ray for detecting pleural disorders. Treatment is rarely needed.

Discrete plaques, which occur in up to 60% of workers exposed to asbestos, typically affect the parietal pleura between the 5th and 9th ribs bilaterally and adjacent to the diaphragm. Plaque calcification is common and can lead to misdiagnosis of severe pulmonary disease when radiographically superimposed on lung fields. CT can distinguish pleural from parenchymal disease in this setting. Fat stripes may be mistaken for pleural plaques on chest x-ray. CT can distinguish pleural disease from fat.

Diffuse thickening affects visceral as well as parietal pleurae. It may be an extension of pulmonary fibrosis from parenchyma to the pleurae or a nonspecific reaction to pleural effusion. With or without calcification, pleural thickening can cause a restrictive defect.

Rounded atelectasis is a benign manifestation of pleural thickening in which invagination of pleura into the parenchyma can entrap lung tissue, causing atelectasis. On chest x-ray and CT, it typically appears as a curvilinear, scar-like mass, often in the lower lung zones, and can be confused with a pulmonary cancer.

BERYLLIUM DISEASE

(Berylliosis)

Acute beryllium disease and chronic beryllium disease are caused by inhalation of dust or fumes from beryllium compounds and products. Acute beryllium disease is now rare; chronic beryllium disease is characterized by formation of granulomas throughout the body, especially in the lungs, intrathoracic lymph nodes, and skin. Chronic beryllium disease causes progressive dyspnea, cough, and fatigue. Diagnosis is by history, beryllium lymphocyte proliferation test, and biopsy. Treatment is with corticosteroids.

Etiology

Beryllium exposure is a common but underrecognized cause of illness in many industries, including beryllium mining and extraction, alloy production, metal alloy machining, electronics, telecommunications, nuclear weapon manufacture, defense, aircraft, automotive, aerospace, and metal scrap, computer, and electronics recycling. Because small amounts of beryllium are toxic and are added to many copper, aluminum, nickel, and magnesium alloys, workers are often unaware of their exposure and its risks.

Pathophysiology

Acute beryllium disease is a chemical pneumonitis causing diffuse parenchymal inflammatory infiltrates and nonspecific intra-alveolar edema. Other tissues (eg, skin, conjunctivae) may be affected. Acute beryllium disease is now rare because most industries have reduced exposure levels, but cases were common between 1940 and 1970, and many cases progressed from acute to chronic beryllium disease.

Chronic beryllium disease remains a common illness in industries that use beryllium and beryllium alloy. It differs from most pneumoconioses in that it is a cell-mediated hypersensitivity disease. Beryllium is presented to CD4+ T lymphocytes by antigen-presenting cells, principally in HLA-DP molecules. T lymphocytes in the blood, lungs, or other organs, in turn, recognize the beryllium, proliferate, and form T-lymphocyte clones. These clones then release proinflammatory cytokines, such as tumor necrosis factor-α, IL-2, and interferon-γ. These cytokines amplify the immune response, resulting in formation of mononuclear cell infiltrates and noncaseating granulomas in target organs where beryllium has deposited. On average, about 2% to 6% of beryllium-exposed people develop beryllium sensitization (defined by positive blood lymphocyte proliferation to beryllium salts in vitro), with most progressing to disease. In certain high-risk groups, such as beryllium metal and alloy machinists, chronic beryllium disease prevalence is > 17%. Workers with bystander exposures, such as secretaries and security guards, also develop sensitization and disease but at lower rates. The typical pathologic consequence is a diffuse pulmonary, hilar, and mediastinal lymph node granulomatous reaction that is histologically indistinguishable from sarcoidosis. Early granuloma formation with mononuclear and giant cells can also occur. Many lymphocytes are found when cells are washed from the lungs (bronchoalveolar lavage [BAL]) during bronchoscopy. These T lymphocytes proliferate when exposed to beryllium in vitro, much as the blood cells do (a test called beryllium lymphocyte proliferation test [BeLPT]).

Symptoms and Signs

Patients with chronic beryllium disease often have dyspnea, cough, weight loss, and a variable chest x-ray pattern, typically showing nodular opacities in the mid and upper lung zones, frequently with hilar and mediastinal adenopathy. Patients complain of insidious and progressive exertional dyspnea, cough, chest pain, weight loss, night sweats, and fatigue. Symptoms may develop within months of first exposure or > 40 yr after exposure has ceased. Some people remain asymptomatic.

Diagnosis

- Beryllium lymphocyte proliferation test (using blood or bronchoalveolar lavage cells)
- Chest x-ray or CT

Diagnosis depends on a history of exposure, the appropriate clinical manifestations, and an abnormal blood or BAL BeLPT or both. BAL BeLPT is highly sensitive and specific, helping to distinguish chronic beryllium disease from sarcoidosis and other forms of diffuse pulmonary disease. Chest x-ray may be normal or show diffuse infiltrates that can be nodular, reticular, or have a hazy ground-glass appearance, often with hilar adenopathy resembling the pattern seen in sarcoidosis. A miliary pattern also occurs. High-resolution (thin-section) CT is more sensitive than x-ray, although cases of biopsy-proven disease occur even in people with normal imaging test results.

Prognosis

Acute beryllium disease can be fatal, but prognosis is usually excellent unless progression to chronic beryllium disease occurs. Chronic beryllium disease often results in progressive loss of respiratory function. Early abnormalities include air flow obstruction and decreased oxygenation on ABG at rest and during exercise testing. Decreased diffusing capacity for carbon monoxide (DLco) and restriction appear later. Pulmonary hypertension and right ventricular failure develop in about 10% of cases, with death due to cor pulmonale. Beryllium sensitization progresses to chronic beryllium disease at a rate of about 6%/yr after initial detection through workplace medical surveillance programs. Subcutaneous granulomatous nodules caused by inoculation with beryllium splinters or dust usually persist until excised.

Treatment

- Corticosteroids
- In acute beryllium disease, sometimes mechanical ventilation
- In chronic beryllium disease, sometimes supplemental O_2, pulmonary rehabilitation, and treatment for right ventricular failure
- In end-stage chronic beryllium disease, sometimes lung transplantation

In acute disease, the lungs often become edematous and hemorrhagic. Mechanical ventilation is necessary in severely affected patients.

Some patients with chronic beryllium disease never require treatment because the disease progresses relatively slowly. When needed, treatment is with corticosteroids, which decrease symptoms and improve oxygenation. Treatment is generally started only in patients with significant symptoms and evidence of abnormal gas exchange or evidence of an accelerated decline in lung function or oxygenation. In symptomatic patients with abnormal pulmonary function, prednisone 40 to 60 mg po once/day or every other day is given for 3 to 6 mo. Then, measures of pulmonary physiology and gas exchange are repeated to document a response to therapy, and the dose is gradually tapered to the lowest dose that maintains symptomatic and objective improvement (usually about 10 to 15 mg po once/day or every other day). Lifelong treatment with corticosteroids is usually required. There is anecdotal evidence that the addition of methotrexate (10 to 25 mg po once/wk) reduces the need for corticosteroids as it does in sarcoidosis.

Spontaneous remission of chronic beryllium disease is rare. In patients with end-stage disease, lung transplantation can be lifesaving. Other supportive measures, such as supplemental O_2 therapy, pulmonary rehabilitation, and drugs for treatment of right ventricular failure, are used as needed.

Prevention

Industrial dust suppression is the basis for preventing beryllium exposure. Exposures must be reduced to levels that are as low as reasonably achievable—preferably more than 50-fold below current Occupational Safety and Health Administration (OSHA) standards—to reduce the risk of sensitization and chronic beryllium disease. Medical surveillance, using blood BeLPT and chest x-ray, is recommended for all exposed workers, including those with indirect contact. Both acute and chronic disease must be promptly recognized and affected workers removed from further beryllium exposure.

KEY POINTS

- Beryllium disease is under recognized and affects workers in many industries.
- Consider high resolution CT and beryllium lymphocyte proliferation test (using blood or bronchoalveolar lavage cells) to confirm the diagnosis.
- Treat symptomatic patients with corticosteroids.
- Prevention involves suppression of beryllium dust and surveillance of exposed workers.

BUILDING-RELATED ILLNESSES

Building-related illnesses (BRIs) are a heterogeneous group of disorders whose etiology is linked to the environment of modern airtight buildings. Such buildings are characterized by sealed windows and dependence on heating, ventilation, and air conditioning systems for circulation of air. Most cases occur in nonindustrial office buildings, but cases can occur in apartment buildings, single-family homes, schools, museums, and libraries.

BRIs can be specific or nonspecific. Diagnosis is based on history of exposure and clinical findings. Treatment is generally supportive.

Specific BRIs: Specific BRIs are those for which a link between building-related exposure and illness is proved. Examples include

- *Legionella* infection (see p. 1587)
- Occupational asthma (see p. 444)
- Hypersensitivity pneumonitis (see p. 452)
- Inhalational fever

Inhalational fever is a febrile reaction caused by exposure to organic aerosols or dusts. Names used to describe this type of BRI include humidifier fever, grain fever, swine confinement fever, and mycotoxicosis, depending on the causative agent. Metal fumes and polymer fumes can also cause febrile illness. The term organic dust toxic syndrome (ODTS) has been used to encompass the subacute febrile and respiratory reaction to organic dust that is typically highly contaminated with bacterial endotoxin. Toxic pneumonitis is a commonly used but less specific term.

Humidifier fever occurs in nonindustrial buildings as a consequence of humidifiers or other types of ventilation units serving as a reservoir for the growth of bacteria or fungi and as a method of aerosolizing these contaminants. The disorder usually manifests as low-grade fever, malaise, cough, and dyspnea. Improvement after removal from exposure (eg, weekend away from the office building) is often one of the first indications of etiology. Humidifier fever has an acute onset and is self-limiting (usually 2 to 3 days). Physical signs may be absent or subtle. Clusters of cases are common.

A recent outbreak of interstitial lung disease in Korea has been attributed to use of toxic inhalants in humidifier disinfectants.

Unlike immunologically mediated conditions (eg, hypersensitivity pneumonitis, building-related asthma), inhalational fevers do not require a period of sensitization. The disorder can occur after initial exposure. Acute episodes do not generally require treatment apart from antipyretics and removal from the contaminated environment. If symptoms persist, evaluation may be required to rule out infection, hypersensitivity pneumonitis, or other conditions. Biologic sampling to detect airborne microbials in the work environment can be costly and time consuming but is sometimes necessary to document the source of contaminated air. Inhalational fevers of all types are usually prevented by good maintenance of ventilation systems.

Nonspecific BRIs: Nonspecific BRIs are those for which a link between building-related exposure and illness is more difficult to prove.

The term **sick building syndrome** has been used to refer to illnesses that occur in clusters within a building and that cause often nonspecific symptoms, including

- Itchy, irritated, dry or watery eyes
- Rhinorrhea or nasal congestion
- Throat soreness or tightness
- Dry itchy skin or unexplained rashes
- Headache, lethargy, or difficulty concentrating

Some building-related factors appear to account for symptoms in some instances. These factors include higher building temperature, higher humidity, and poor ventilation, typically with a failure to incorporate sufficient fresh air from outdoors. Patient factors, including female sex, history of atopy, increased attention to body sensations, worry about the meaning of symptoms, anxiety, depression, and occasionally mass hysteria, also seem to underlie experience of symptoms.

BYSSINOSIS

Byssinosis is a form of reactive airways disease characterized by bronchoconstriction in cotton, flax, and hemp workers. The etiologic agent is bacterial endotoxin in cotton dust. Symptoms are chest tightness and dyspnea that worsen on the first day of the work week and subside as the week progresses. Diagnosis is based on history and pulmonary function test findings. Treatment includes avoidance of exposure and use of asthma drugs.

Etiology

Byssinosis occurs almost entirely in workers who contact unprocessed, raw cotton, especially those who are exposed to open bales or who work in cotton spinning or in the carding room. Byssinosis can occur after acute exposure but usually occurs in workers with a history of chronic exposure. Evidence suggests that the cause is bacterial endotoxin in the cotton dust. The endotoxin leads to bronchoconstriction, chronic bronchitis, and gradual decreases in pulmonary function, particularly in genetically susceptible people. Prolonged exposure to cotton dust was once thought to cause emphysema, a theory now disproved.

Symptoms and Signs

Symptoms are chest tightness and dyspnea that lessen with repeated exposure. Symptoms develop on the first day of work after a weekend or vacation and diminish or disappear by the end of the week. With repeated exposure over a period of years, chest tightness tends to return and persist through midweek and occasionally to the end of the week or as long as the person continues to work. This typical temporal pattern distinguishes byssinosis from asthma.

Signs of acute exposure are tachypnea and wheezing. Patients with more chronic exposure may have crackles.

Diagnosis

Diagnosis is based on history and pulmonary function tests that show typical airflow obstruction and a reduction in ventilatory capacity, especially if measured at the start and end of a first work shift. Hyperresponsiveness to methacholine is also often observed. Surveillance measures, including symptom reporting and spirometry in textile workers, can aid in early detection.

Treatment

Treatment includes avoidance or reduction of exposure and use of asthma drugs.

COAL WORKERS' PNEUMOCONIOSIS

(Anthracosis; Black Lung Disease; Coal Miner's Pneumoconiosis)

Coal workers' pneumoconiosis (CWP) is caused by inhalation of coal dust. Deposition of dust produces dust-laden

macrophages around bronchioles (coal macules), occasionally causing focal bronchiolar emphysema. CWP usually causes no symptoms but can progress to progressive massive fibrosis (PMF) with impaired lung function. Diagnosis is based on history and chest x-ray findings. Treatment is generally supportive.

Etiology

CWP is caused by chronic inhalation of dust from high-carbon coal (anthracite and bituminous) and rarely graphite, typically over ≥ 20 yr. Inhalation of silica contained in coal may also contribute to clinical disease.

Pathophysiology

Alveolar macrophages engulf the dust, release cytokines that stimulate inflammation, and collect in lung interstitium around bronchioles and alveoli (coal macules). Coal nodules develop as collagen accumulates, and focal emphysema develops as bronchiole walls weaken and dilate. Fibrosis can occur but is usually limited to areas adjacent to coal macules. Distortion of lung architecture, airflow obstruction, and functional impairment are usually mild but can be highly destructive in some patients.

Two forms of CWP are described:

- Simple, with individual coal macules
- Complicated, with coalescence of macules and PMF

Patients with simple CWP develop PMF at a rate of about 1 to 2% /yr. Recently, rapid progression of CWP to PMF has been recognized in young miners, especially in the eastern US.

In PMF, nodules coalesce to form black, rubbery parenchymal masses usually in the upper posterior fields. The masses may encroach on and destroy vascular supply and airways or may cavitate. PMF can develop and progress even after exposure to coal dust has ceased. Despite the similarity of coal-induced PMF and conglomerate silicosis, the development of PMF in coal workers is unrelated to the silica content of the coal.

Complications: An association between CWP and features of rheumatoid arthritis (RA) is well-described. It is unclear whether CWP predisposes miners to developing RA, whether RA takes on a unique form in patients with CWP, or whether RA alters the response of miners to coal dust. Multiple rounded nodules in the lung appearing over a relatively short time (Caplan syndrome) represent an immunopathologic response related to rheumatoid diathesis. Histologically, they resemble rheumatoid nodules but have a peripheral region of more acute inflammation. Patients with CWP are at a slightly increased risk of developing active TB and non-TB mycobacterial infections. Weak associations have been reported between CWP and progressive systemic sclerosis and stomach cancer.

Symptoms and Signs

CWP does not usually cause symptoms. Most chronic pulmonary symptoms in coal miners are caused by other conditions, such as industrial bronchitis due to coal dust or coincident emphysema due to smoking. Cough can be chronic and problematic in patients even after they leave the workplace, even in those who do not smoke.

PMF causes progressive dyspnea. Occasionally, patients cough up black sputum (melanoptysis), which occurs when PMF lesions rupture into the airways. PMF often progresses to pulmonary hypertension with right ventricular and respiratory failure.

Diagnosis

- History of exposure to coal dust
- Chest CT or chest x-ray

Diagnosis is based on a history of exposure and chest x-ray or chest CT appearance. In patients with CWP, x-ray or CT reveals diffuse, small, rounded opacities or nodules. The finding of at least one opacity > 10 mm suggests PMF. The specificity of the chest x-ray for PMF is low because up to one third of the lesions identified as being PMF turn out to be cancers, scars, or other disorders. Chest CT is more sensitive and specific than chest x-ray for detecting coalescing nodules, early PMF, and cavitation.

Pulmonary function tests are nondiagnostic but are useful for characterizing lung function in patients in whom obstructive, restrictive, or mixed defects may develop. Because abnormalities of gas exchange occur in some patients with extensive simple CWP and in those with complicated CWP, baseline and periodic measures of diffusing capacity for carbon monoxide (DLco) and ABG at rest and during exercise are recommended.

Because patients with CWP often have had exposure to both silica dust and coal dust, surveillance for TB is usually done. Patients with CWP should have annual tuberculin skin testing. In those with positive test results, sputum culture and cytology, CT, and bronchoscopy may be needed to confirm TB.

Treatment

- Sometimes supplemental O_2 and pulmonary rehabilitation
- Restriction from further exposure

Treatment is rarely necessary in simple CWP, although smoking cessation and TB surveillance are recommended. Patients with pulmonary hypertension, hypoxemia, or both are given supplemental O_2 therapy. Pulmonary rehabilitation can help more severely affected workers carry out activities of daily living. Workers with CWP, especially those with PMF, should be restricted from further exposure, especially to high concentrations of dust. TB is treated in accordance with current recommendations (see p. 1654).

Prevention

Preventive measures include eliminating exposure, stopping smoking, and giving pneumococcal and influenza vaccinations. CWP can be prevented by suppressing coal dust at the coal face. Despite long-standing regulations, exposures continue to occur in the mining trade, resulting in increased rates of disease, including severe forms. Respiratory masks provide only limited protection.

KEY POINTS

- CWP is caused by chronic inhalation of dust from high-carbon coal (anthracite and bituminous) and rarely graphite, typically over ≥ 20 yr.
- Most patients have simple CWP, with small, asymptomatic nodules seen on imaging.
- Some patients with CWP develop progressive massive fibrosis, with deterioration of pulmonary function, dyspnea, and marked abnormalities on imaging studies.
- Base the diagnosis on history of exposure as well as chest imaging.
- Treat supportively, encourage smoking cessation, and restrict further exposure.

OCCUPATIONAL ASTHMA

Occupational asthma is reversible airway obstruction that develops after months to years of sensitization to an allergen encountered in the workplace. Symptoms are dyspnea, wheezing, cough, and, occasionally, upper respiratory

allergy symptoms. Diagnosis is based on occupational history, including assessment of job activities, allergens in the work environment, and a temporal association between work and symptoms. Allergen skin testing and provocative inhalational challenge may be used in specialized centers but are usually unnecessary. Treatment involves removing the person from the work environment and using asthma drugs as needed.

Occupational asthma is development of asthma (or worsening of preexisting asthma) by occupational exposure. Symptoms typically develop over months to years because of sensitization to an allergen encountered in the workplace. Once sensitized, the worker invariably responds to much lower concentrations of the allergen than that which initiated the response.

Several other airway diseases caused by inhalational workplace exposures can be distinguished from occupational and occupationally aggravated asthma.

In **RADS,** which is nonallergenic, people with no history of asthma develop persistent, reversible airway obstruction after acute overexposure to irritant dust, fumes, or gas. Airway inflammation persists even after removal of the acute irritant, and the syndrome is indistinguishable from asthma.

In **reactive upper airways syndrome,** upper airway (ie, nasal, pharyngeal) mucosal symptoms develop after acute or repeated exposure to airways irritants.

In **irritant-associated vocal cord dysfunction,** which mimics asthma, abnormal apposition and closure of the vocal cords, especially during inspiration, occur after acute irritant inhalation.

In **industrial bronchitis** (irritant-induced chronic bronchitis), bronchial inflammation causes cough after acute or chronic irritant inhalation.

In **bronchiolitis obliterans,** bronchiolar damage occurs after acute inhalation of gases (eg, anhydrous ammonia). The 2 major forms are proliferative and constrictive. The constrictive form is more common and may or may not be associated with other forms of diffuse lung injury. Recently, cases of bronchiolitis obliterans have been reported in workers exposed to the chemical diacetyl during the manufacture of butter-flavored microwave popcorn. So-called popcorn workers' lung may occur in workers exposed to other flavorings and in some consumers exposed to this chemical.

Etiology

Occupational asthma is caused by both immune- and non–immune-mediated mechanisms. Immune mechanisms involve IgE- and non–IgE-mediated hypersensitivity to workplace allergens. Hundreds of occupational allergens exist, ranging from low molecular weight chemicals to large proteins. Examples include grain dust, proteolytic enzymes used in detergent manufacturing, red cedar wood, isocyanates, formalin (rarely), antibiotics (eg, ampicillin, spiramycin), epoxy resins, and tea.

Non-immune-mediated inflammatory mechanisms cause direct irritation of the respiratory epithelium and upper airway mucosae.

US military personnel deployed to Iraq and Afghanistan have been found to be at increased risk for asthma (and also bronchiolitis obliterans). Possible causes include emissions from open-air burn pits and industrial fires, desert dust, and vehicular exhaust.

Symptoms and Signs

Symptoms include shortness of breath, chest tightness, wheezing, and cough, often with upper respiratory symptoms such as sneezing, rhinorrhea, and tearing. Upper airway and conjunctival symptoms may precede the typical asthmatic symptoms by months or years. Symptoms may develop during work hours after specific dust or vapor exposure but often do not become apparent until several hours after leaving work, thereby making the association with occupational exposure less obvious. Nocturnal wheezing may be the only symptom. Often, symptoms disappear on weekends or during vacations, although with ongoing exposure temporal exacerbations and relief become less apparent.

Diagnosis

- Occupational history of allergen exposure
- Immunologic testing
- Sometimes inhalation challenge test

Diagnosis depends on recognizing the link between workplace allergens and asthma. Diagnosis is suspected on the basis of an occupational history of allergen exposure. A safety data sheet (mandatory at all work sites) can be used to identify potential allergens, and substances listed can be used to direct immunologic testing (eg, skin prick, puddle, or patch testing) of suspected antigens to demonstrate that an agent in the workplace is affecting a worker. An increase in bronchial hyperresponsiveness after exposure to the suspected antigen is also helpful in making the diagnosis.

PEARLS & PITFALLS

- Consider reviewing workplace safety data sheets for potential allergens if workers develop new respiratory symptoms.

In difficult cases, a carefully controlled inhalation challenge test done in the laboratory confirms the cause of the airway obstruction. Such procedures should be done only at centers experienced in inhalation challenge testing and capable of monitoring and treating the sometimes severe reactions that can occur. Pulmonary function tests or peak expiratory flow measurements that show decreasing airflow during work are further evidence that occupational exposure is causative. Methacholine challenge tests can be used to establish the degree of airway hyperreactivity. Sensitivity to methacholine may decrease after exposure to the occupational allergen has ceased.

Differentiation from idiopathic asthma is generally based on the pattern of symptoms, demonstration that allergens are present in the workplace, and the relationship between exposure to allergens and symptoms and physiologic worsening.

Treatment

Treatment is the same as that for idiopathic asthma, including inhaled bronchodilators and corticosteroids (see Table 52–4 on p. 408). Treatment should also include removal of the patient from ongoing exposure to the causative agent.

Prevention

Dust suppression is essential. However, elimination of all instances of sensitization and clinical disease may not be possible. Once sensitized, patients with occupational asthma may react to extremely low levels of airborne allergen. Patients who return to environments in which the allergen persists generally have a poorer prognosis, with more respiratory symptoms, more abnormal lung physiology, a greater need for drugs, and more frequent and severe exacerbations. Whenever possible, a symptomatic person should be removed from a setting known to cause symptoms. If exposure continues, symptoms tend to persist. Occupational asthma can sometimes be cured if it is diagnosed early and exposure ceases.

KEY POINTS

- Occupational asthma can be non-immune-mediated or develop after months or years of sensitization.
- Consider reviewing workplace safety data sheets for potential allergens if workers develop new respiratory symptoms.
- Consider immunologic testing and an inhalation challenge test.
- Treat as for asthma and remove the patient from the environment containing the allergen.

SILICOSIS

Silicosis is caused by inhalation of unbound (free) crystalline silica dust and is characterized by nodular pulmonary fibrosis. Chronic silicosis initially causes no symptoms or only mild dyspnea but over years can advance to involve most of the lung and cause dyspnea, hypoxemia, pulmonary hypertension, and respiratory impairment. Diagnosis is based on history and chest x-ray findings. No effective treatment exists except supportive care and, for severe cases, lung transplantation.

Etiology

Silicosis, the oldest known occupational pulmonary disease, is caused by inhalation of tiny particles of silicon dioxide in the form of unbound (free) crystalline silica (usually quartz) or, less commonly, by inhalation of silicates, minerals containing silicon dioxide bound to other elements, such as talc. Workers at greatest risk are those who move or blast rock and sand (miners, quarry workers, stonecutters) or who use silica-containing rock or sand abrasives (sand blasters; glass makers; foundry, gemstone, and ceramic workers; potters). Coal miners are at risk of mixed silicosis and CWP (see p. 443).

Factors that influence the likelihood of development of silicosis include

- Duration and intensity of exposure
- Form of silicon (exposure to the crystalline form poses greater risk than the bound form)
- Surface characteristics (exposure to the uncoated form poses greater risk than the coated form)
- Rapidity of inhalation after the dust is fractured and becomes airborne (exposure immediately after fracturing poses greater risk than delayed exposure)

Pathophysiology

Alveolar macrophages engulf inhaled free silica particles and enter lymphatics and interstitial tissue. The macrophages cause release of cytokines (tumor necrosis factor-α, IL-1), growth factors (tumor growth factor-β), and oxidants, stimulating parenchymal inflammation, collagen synthesis, and, ultimately, fibrosis.

When the macrophages die, they release the silica into interstitial tissue around the small bronchioles, causing formation of the pathognomonic silicotic nodule. These nodules initially contain macrophages, lymphocytes, mast cells, fibroblasts with disorganized patches of collagen, and scattered birefringent particles that are best seen with polarized light microscopy. As they mature, the centers of the nodules become dense balls of fibrotic scar with a classic onion-skin appearance and are surrounded by an outer layer of inflammatory cells. In low-intensity or short-term exposures, these nodules remain discrete and do not compromise lung function (simple chronic silicosis). But with higher-intensity or more prolonged exposures (complicated chronic silicosis), these nodules coalesce and cause progressive fibrosis and reduction of lung volumes (total lung capacity, ventilatory capacity) on pulmonary function tests, or they coalesce, sometimes forming large conglomerate masses (called progressive massive fibrosis).

Chronic silicosis is the most common form of the disorder and generally develops only after exposure over decades.

Acute silicosis and the rarer **accelerated silicosis** are caused by intense silica dust exposure over short periods (several months or years). Mononuclear cells infiltrate alveolar septa, and alveolar spaces fill with a proteinaceous material that stains periodic acid-Schiff (PAS) positive and is similar to that found in pulmonary alveolar proteinosis (silicoproteinosis—see p. 464). The occupational history of acute exposure is needed to distinguish silicoproteinosis from the idiopathic variety.

Conglomerate (complicated) silicosis is the advanced form of chronic or accelerated silicosis and is characterized by widespread masses of fibrosis, typically in the upper lung zones.

Complications: Patients with silicosis are at risk of other disorders:

- TB
- Nocardiosis
- Lung cancer
- Progressive systemic sclerosis (scleroderma)
- Possibly RA

All patients with silicosis are at about a 30-fold increased risk of pulmonary TB or nontubercular mycobacterial disease and are more likely to develop both pulmonary and extrapulmonary manifestations. Increased risk may result from impaired macrophage function and an increased risk of activation of latent infection. People exposed to silica but without silicosis have 3 times the risk of developing TB compared with the nonexposed general population.

Other complications include spontaneous pneumothorax, broncholithiasis, and tracheobronchial obstruction. Emphysema is a common finding in areas immediately peripheral to conglomerate nodules and in areas of progressive massive fibrosis.

Symptoms and Signs

Chronic silicosis is often asymptomatic, but many patients eventually develop dyspnea during exertion that progresses to dyspnea at rest. Productive cough, when present, may be due to silicosis, coexisting chronic occupational (industrial) bronchitis, or smoking. Breath sounds diminish as the disorder progresses, and pulmonary consolidation, pulmonary hypertension, and respiratory failure with or without right ventricular failure may develop in advanced disease.

Patients with accelerated silicosis experience the same symptoms as those with chronic silicosis, but symptoms develop over a shorter period.

Acute silicosis patients experience rapid progression of dyspnea, weight loss, and fatigue with diffuse bilateral crackles. Respiratory failure often develops within 2 yr.

Conglomerate silicosis causes severe, chronic respiratory symptoms.

Diagnosis

- Occupational history of silica exposure
- Chest CT or chest x-ray
- Sometimes tissue biopsy for confirmation
- Adjunctive tests for distinguishing silicosis from other disorders

Imaging: Silicosis is usually recognized on the basis of chest x-ray or CT appearance in patients with a history of exposure. CT is more sensitive than x-ray, especially when helical CT and high-resolution (thin-section) techniques are used. In most cases, chest CT is preferable because it is more sensitive for detecting silicosis as well as the transition from simple to conglomerate silicosis. Chest CT can also better distinguish asbestosis from silicosis, although this differentiation can usually be made on the basis of chest x-ray and exposure history. In patients who develop RA, 3- to 5-mm pulmonary rheumatoid nodules are visible on chest x-ray or CT.

Chronic silicosis produces multiple 1- to 3-mm rounded opacities or nodules recognized on chest x-ray or CT, usually in upper lung fields. Severity is graded on a standardized scale developed by the International Labor Organization (International Classification of Radiographs of Pneumoconioses), in which specially trained readers examine the chest x-ray for size and shape of opacities, concentration of opacities (profusion), and pleural changes. An equivalent scale does not exist for CT appearance. Calcified hilar and mediastinal lymph nodes are common and occasionally resemble eggshells. Pleural thickening is uncommon unless a severe parenchymal disease abuts the pleura. Rarely, calcified pleural thickening occurs in patients with little parenchymal involvement. Bullae commonly form around the conglomerate masses. Tracheal deviation may occur when the masses become large and cause volume loss. True cavities may indicate TB.

Numerous disorders resemble chronic silicosis on x-ray; they include welders' siderosis, hemosiderosis, sarcoidosis, chronic beryllium disease, hypersensitivity pneumonitis, coal workers' pneumoconiosis, miliary TB, fungal pulmonary diseases, and metastatic cancer. Eggshell calcifications in hilar and mediastinal lymph nodes may help distinguish silicosis from other pulmonary disorders but are not a pathognomonic finding and are not commonly present.

Accelerated silicosis resembles chronic silicosis on x-ray but develops more rapidly.

Acute silicosis is recognized by rapid progression of symptoms. X-ray findings include diffuse alveolar bibasilar opacities representing fluid-filled alveoli. On CT, areas of ground-glass density consisting of reticular infiltration and areas of patchy increased attenuation and inhomogeneity occur. These areas are best observed on high-resolution (thin-section), spiral CT views. The multiple rounded opacities of chronic and accelerated silicosis are not characteristic of acute silicosis.

Conglomerate silicosis is recognizable by confluent opacities > 10 mm in diameter against a background of chronic silicosis findings.

Adjunctive tests: Sputum culture and cytology, PET, and bronchoscopy all may assist in distinguishing silicosis from disseminated TB or cancer.

Pulmonary function tests and measures of gas exchange (diffusing capacity for carbon monoxide [DLco], ABGs) are not diagnostic but help monitor progression. Early chronic silicosis may manifest with reduced lung volumes that are at the lower end of the predicted range and with normal functional residual capacity and residual volume. In conglomerate silicosis, pulmonary function tests reveal decreased lung volumes, decreased DLco, and airway obstruction. ABGs show hypoxemia usually without CO_2 retention. Measurement of gas exchange during exercise, using pulse oximetry or preferably an indwelling arterial catheter, is one of the most sensitive measures of pulmonary impairment.

Antinuclear antibodies and elevated rheumatoid factor are detectable in some patients and are suggestive but not diagnostic of a coexisting connective tissue disorder (eg, systemic sclerosis, RA).

Treatment

- Sometimes whole lung lavage
- Sometimes oral corticosteroids
- Rarely lung transplantation
- Empiric use of bronchodilators and inhaled corticosteroids for obstruction
- Removal from further exposure

Whole lung lavage may be useful in some cases of acute silicosis. Whole lung lavage can reduce the total mineral dust load in the lungs of patients with chronic silicosis. Some studies have shown short-term reduction in symptoms after lavage, but controlled trials have not been done. Anecdotal evidence supports the use of oral corticosteroids in acute and accelerated silicosis. Lung transplantation is a last resort.

Patients with airway obstruction may be treated empirically with bronchodilators and inhaled corticosteroids. Patients should be monitored and treated for hypoxemia to forestall pulmonary hypertension. Pulmonary rehabilitation may help patients carry out activities of daily living. Workers who develop silicosis should be removed from further exposure.

Management of TB is the same as for other patients with TB except that longer courses are usually recommended because relapse is more common in patients with silicotuberculosis.

Prevention

The most effective preventive interventions occur at an industrial rather than clinical level and include dust suppression, process isolation, ventilation, and use of non-silica-containing abrasives. Respiratory masks provide imperfect protection and, although helpful, are not an adequate solution. Surveillance of exposed workers with respiratory questionnaires, spirometry, and chest x-rays is recommended. Frequency of surveillance depends to some degree on the expected intensity of the exposure. (See also guidelines from the American College of Occupational and Environmental Medicine: Medical Surveillance of Workers Exposed to Crystalline Silica.) Other preventive measures include smoking cessation and pneumococcal and influenza vaccination.

Physicians must be alert to the risk of TB and nontuberculous mycobacterial infections in silica-exposed patients, especially miners. People exposed to silica should have annual tuberculin testing. Those with a positive skin test should have sputum culture for TB. In some cases, CT and bronchoscopy may be needed to confirm TB. Patients with a positive tuberculin test and negative TB cultures should be given isoniazid chemoprophylaxis in keeping with standard guidelines for tuberculin reactors.

KEY POINTS

- Silicosis is usually chronic, but acute, accelerated, and conglomerate forms are possible.
- Patients who have silicosis are at risk for pulmonary complications and other disorders (eg, TB, nocardiosis, lung cancer, progressive systemic sclerosis).
- Base the diagnosis on chest imaging (eg, multiple 1- to 3-mm rounded opacities) in patients with a history of exposure.
- Consider whole lung lavage and treat supportively.
- Monitor silica-exposed patients (eg, miners) for TB and nontuberculous mycobacterial infections.

IRRITANT GAS INHALATION INJURY

Irritant gases are those which, when inhaled, dissolve in the water of the respiratory tract mucosa and cause an inflammatory response, usually due to the release of acidic or alkaline radicals. Irritant gas exposures predominantly affect the airways, causing tracheitis, bronchitis, and bronchiolitis. Other inhaled agents may be directly toxic (eg, cyanide, carbon monoxide) or cause harm simply by displacing O_2 and causing asphyxia (eg, methane, carbon dioxide).

The effect of inhaling irritant gases depends on the extent and duration of exposure and on the specific agent. Chlorine, phosgene, sulfur dioxide, hydrogen chloride or sulfide, nitrogen dioxide, ozone, and ammonia are among the most important irritant gases. Hydrogen sulfide is also a potent cellular toxin, blocking the cytochrome system and inhibiting cellular respiration. A common exposure involves mixing household ammonia with cleansers containing bleach; the irritant gas chloramine is released.

Acute Exposure

Acute exposure to high concentrations of toxic gas over a short time is characteristic of industrial accidents resulting from a faulty valve or pump in a gas tank or occurring during gas transport. Many people may be exposed and affected. The release of methyl isocyanate from a chemical plant in Bhopal, India in 1984 killed > 2000 people.

Respiratory damage is related to the concentration of the gas and its solubility.

More water-soluble gases (eg, chlorine, ammonia, sulfur dioxide, hydrogen chloride) dissolve in the upper airway and immediately cause mucous membrane irritation, which may alert people to the need to escape the exposure. Permanent damage to the upper respiratory tract, distal airways, and lung parenchyma occurs only if escape from the gas source is impeded.

Less soluble gases (eg, nitrogen dioxide, phosgene, ozone) may not dissolve until they are well into the respiratory tract, often reaching the lower airways. These agents are less likely to cause early warning signs (phosgene in low concentrations has a pleasant odor), are more likely to cause severe bronchiolitis, and often have a lag of ≥ 12 h before symptoms of pulmonary edema develop.

Complications: The most serious immediate complication is acute respiratory distress syndrome (ARDS), which usually occurs within 24 h. Patients with significant lower airway involvement may develop bacterial infection.

Ten to 14 days after acute exposure to some agents (eg, ammonia, nitrogen oxides, sulfur dioxide, mercury), some patients develop bronchiolitis obliterans progressing to ARDS. Bronchiolitis obliterans with organized pneumonia can ensue when granulation tissue accumulates in the terminal airways and alveolar ducts during the body's reparative process. A minority of these patients develop late pulmonary fibrosis.

Symptoms and Signs

Soluble irritant gases cause severe burning and other manifestations of irritation of the eyes, nose, throat, trachea, and major bronchi. Marked cough, hemoptysis, wheezing, retching, and dyspnea are common. The upper airway may be obstructed by edema, secretions, or laryngospasm. Severity is generally dose-related. Nonsoluble gases cause fewer immediate symptoms but can cause dyspnea or cough.

Patients who develop ARDS have worsening dyspnea and increasing O_2 requirements.

Diagnosis

- History of exposure
- Chest x-ray
- Spirometry and lung volume testing

Diagnosis is usually obvious from the history. Patients should have a chest x-ray and pulse oximetry. Chest x-ray findings of patchy or confluent alveolar consolidation usually indicate pulmonary edema. Spirometry and lung volume testing are done. Obstructive abnormalities are most common, but restrictive abnormalities can predominate after exposure to high doses of chlorine.

CT is used to evaluate patients with late-developing symptoms. Those with bronchiolitis obliterans that progresses to respiratory failure manifest a pattern of bronchiolar thickening and a patchy mosaic of hyperinflation.

Prognosis

Most people recover fully, but some have persistent lung injury with reversible airway obstruction (RADS) or restrictive abnormalities and pulmonary fibrosis; smokers may be at greater risk.

Treatment

- Removal from exposure and 24-h observation
- Bronchodilators and supplemental O_2
- Sometimes inhaled racemic epinephrine, endotracheal intubation, and mechanical ventilation

Management does not differ by specific inhaled agent but rather by symptoms. Patients should be moved into fresh air and given supplemental O_2. Treatment is directed toward ensuring adequate oxygenation and alveolar ventilation. Bronchodilators and O_2 therapy may suffice in less severe cases. Severe airflow obstruction is managed with inhaled racemic epinephrine, endotracheal intubation or tracheostomy, and mechanical ventilation. The efficacy of corticosteroid therapy (eg, prednisone 45 to 60 mg once/day for 1 to 2 wk) is unproved, but it is frequently used.

Because of the risk of ARDS, any patient with respiratory tract symptoms after toxic inhalation should be observed for 24 h.

After the acute phase has been managed, physicians must remain alert to the development of RADS, bronchiolitis obliterans with or without organized pneumonia, pulmonary fibrosis, and delayed-onset ARDS.

Prevention

Care in handling gases and chemicals is the most important preventive measure. The availability of adequate respiratory protection (eg, gas masks with a self-contained air supply) for rescuers is also very important; rescuers without protective gear who rush in to extricate a victim often succumb themselves.

Chronic Exposure

Low-level continuous or intermittent exposure to irritant gases or chemical vapors may lead to chronic bronchitis, although the role of such exposure is especially difficult to substantiate in smokers.

Chronic inhalational exposure to some agents (eg, bis[chloromethyl]ether, certain metals) causes lung and other cancers (eg, liver angiosarcomas after vinyl chloride monomer exposure).

KEY POINTS

- Irritant gas exposures predominantly affect the airways, causing tracheitis, bronchitis, and bronchiolitis.
- Complications of acute exposure may include ARDS, bacterial infections, and bronchiolitis obliterans (sometimes leading to pulmonary fibrosis).
- Diagnosis of acute exposure is usually obvious by history, but do pulse oximetry, chest x-ray, spirometry, and lung volume assessment.
- Treat acute exposure supportively and observe patients for 24 h.

57 Interstitial Lung Diseases

(Diffuse Parenchymal Lung Diseases)

Interstitial lung diseases are a heterogeneous group of disorders characterized by alveolar septal thickening, fibroblast proliferation, collagen deposition, and, if the process remains unchecked, pulmonary fibrosis. Interstitial lung diseases can be classified using various criteria (eg, acute vs chronic, granulomatous vs nongranulomatous, known cause vs unknown cause, primary lung disease vs secondary to systemic disease).

Among the numerous possible causes are most connective tissue disorders and occupational lung exposures and many drugs (see Table 57–1). A number of interstitial lung diseases

Table 57–1. CAUSES OF INTERSTITIAL LUNG DISEASE

CATEGORY	EXAMPLES
Connective tissue disorders	Ankylosing spondylitis (rare) Behçet syndrome (very rare) Dermatomyositis and polymyositis Goodpasture syndrome IgG-4 related disease Mixed connective tissue disease RA Sjögren syndrome SLE Systemic sclerosis Undifferentiated connective tissue disease
Drugs	**Selected list:** Amphotericin B, bleomycin, busulfan, carbamazepine, chlorambucil, cocaine, cyclophosphamide, diphenylhydantoin, flecainide, heroin, melphalan, methadone, methotrexate, methylphenidate, methysergide, mineral oil (via chronic microaspiration), nitrofurantoin, nitrosoureas, procarbazine, silicone (sc injection), tocainide, vinca alkaloids (with mitomycin)
Occupational and environmental exposure	**Inorganic (selected):** Aluminosis (caused by exposure to metallic aluminum powder), asbestosis, baritosis, berylliosis, coal workers' pneumoconiosis, exposure to hard metals (eg, cadmium, cobalt, titanium oxide, tungsten, vanadium carbides), radiation fibrosis, siderosis, silicosis, stannosis, talc pneumoconiosis **Organic (selected):** Bagassosis, bird fancier's lung, coffee worker's lung, farmer's lung, hot tub lung, humidifier lung, malt worker's lung, maple bark stripper's lung, mushroom worker's lung, tea grower's lung
Infections	Aspergillosis Histoplasmosis Parasitic infection Mycobacterial infection Viral infection
Vasculitis	Eosinophilic granulomatosis with polyangiitis Giant cell arteritis (rare) Granulomatosis with polyangiitis Microscopic polyangiitis Polyarteritis nodosa (rare) Takayasu arteritis (rare)
Idiopathic interstitial pneumonias	Acute interstitial pneumonia Cryptogenic organizing pneumonia Desquamative interstitial pneumonia Idiopathic pleuroparenchymal fibroelastosis Idiopathic pulmonary fibrosis Lymphocytic interstitial pneumonia Nonspecific interstitial pneumonia Respiratory bronchiolitis–associated interstitial lung disease
Miscellaneous disorders	Amyloidosis Chronic aspiration Eosinophilic pneumonia Gaucher disease (rare) Lipoid pneumonia Lymphangioleiomyomatosis Microlithiasis Neurofibromatosis Niemann-Pick disease (rare) Pulmonary alveolar proteinosis Pulmonary Langerhans cell histiocytosis (granulomatosis) Pulmonary lymphoma Sarcoidosis Tuberous sclerosis

of unknown etiology have characteristic histology, clinical features, or presentation and thus are considered unique diseases, including

- Eosinophilic pulmonary diseases
- Pulmonary Langerhans cell histiocytosis (granulocytosis)
- Lymphangioleiomyomatosis (LAM)
- Pulmonary alveolar proteinosis
- Sarcoidosis

In up to 30% of patients who have interstitial lung diseases with no clear cause, the disorders are distinguished primarily by characteristic histopathologic features; these disorders are termed the idiopathic interstitial pneumonias (IIPs).

DRUG-INDUCED PULMONARY DISEASE

Drug-induced pulmonary disease is not a single disorder, but rather a common clinical problem in which a patient without previous pulmonary disease develops respiratory symptoms, chest x-ray changes, deterioration of pulmonary function, histologic changes, or several of these findings in association with drug therapy. Over 150 drugs or categories of drugs have been reported to cause pulmonary disease; the mechanism is rarely known, but many drugs are thought to provoke a hypersensitivity response. Some drugs (eg, nitrofurantoin) can cause different injury patterns in different patients.

Depending on the drug, drug-induced syndromes can cause interstitial fibrosis, organizing pneumonia, asthma, noncardiogenic pulmonary edema, pleural effusions, pulmonary eosinophilia, pulmonary hemorrhage, or veno-occlusive disease (see Table 57–2).

Diagnosis is based on observation of responses to withdrawal from and, if practical, reintroduction to the suspected drug.

Treatment

- Stopping the drug

Treatment is stopping the drug that is causing pulmonary disease.

Prevention

A screening pulmonary function test is commonly done in patients about to begin or already taking drugs with pulmonary toxicities, but the benefits of screening for prediction or early detection of toxicity are unproved.

OVERVIEW OF EOSINOPHILIC PULMONARY DISEASES

Eosinophilic pulmonary diseases are a heterogeneous group of disorders characterized by the accumulation of eosinophils in alveolar spaces, the interstitium, or both. Peripheral blood eosinophilia is also common. Known causes of eosinophilic pulmonary disease include

- Infections (especially helminthic infections)
- Drug-induced pneumonitis (eg, therapeutic drugs, such as antibiotics, phenytoin, or L-tryptophan)
- Inhaled toxins (eg, recreational drugs, such as cocaine)
- Systemic disorders (eg, eosinophilic granulomatosis with polyangiitis [formerly Churg-Strauss syndrome])
- Allergic bronchopulmonary aspergillosis

Often the cause is unknown.

The two primary eosinophilic pulmonary diseases of unknown etiology are

- Acute eosinophilic pneumonia
- Chronic eosinophilic pneumonia

Table 57–2. SUBSTANCES WITH TOXIC PULMONARY EFFECTS

CONDITION	DRUG OR AGENT
Asthma	Aspirin, beta-blockers (eg, timolol), cocaine, dipyridamole, IV hydrocortisone (rarely in aspirin-sensitive patients with asthma), IL-2, methylphenidate, nitrofurantoin, protamine, sulfasalazine, vinca alkaloids (with mitomycin-C)
Organizing pneumonia	Amiodarone, bleomycin, cocaine, cyclophosphamide, methotrexate, minocycline, mitomycin-C, penicillamine, sulfasalazine, tetracycline
Hypersensitivity pneumonitis	Azathioprine plus 6-mercaptopurine, busulfan, fluoxetine, radiation
Interstitial pneumonia or fibrosis	Amphotericin B, bleomycin, busulfan, carbamazepine, chlorambucil, cocaine, cyclophosphamide, diphenylhydantoin, flecainide, heroin, melphalan, methadone, methotrexate, methylphenidate, methysergide, mineral oil (via chronic microaspiration), nitrofurantoin, nitrosoureas, procarbazine, silicone (sc injection), tocainide, vinca alkaloids (with mitomycin-C)
Noncardiac pulmonary edema	Beta-adrenergic agonists (eg, ritodrine, terbutaline), chlordiazepoxide, cocaine, cytarabine, ethiodized oil (IV, and via chronic microaspiration), gemcitabine, heroin, hydrochlorothiazide, methadone, mitomycin-C, phenothiazines, protamine, sulfasalazine, tocolytic agents, tricyclic antidepressants, tumor necrosis factor, vinca alkaloids (with mitomycin-C)
Parenchymal hemorrhage	Anticoagulants, azathioprine plus 6-mercaptopurine, cocaine, mineral oil (via chronic microaspiration), nitrofurantoin, radiation
Pleural effusion	Amiodarone, anticoagulants, bleomycin, bromocriptine, busulfan, granulocyte-macrophage colony-stimulating factor, IL-2, methotrexate, methysergide, mitomycin-C, nitrofurantoin, para-aminosalicylic acid, procarbazine, radiation, tocolytic agents
Pulmonary infiltrate with eosinophilia	Amiodarone, amphotericin B, bleomycin, carbamazepine, diphenylhydantoin, ethambutol, etoposide, granulocyte-macrophage colony-stimulating factor, isoniazid, methotrexate, minocycline, mitomycin-C, nitrofurantoin, para-aminosalicylic acid, procarbazine, radiation, sulfasalazine, sulfonamides, tetracycline, trazodone
Pulmonary vascular disease	Appetite suppressants (eg, dexfenfluramine, fenfluramine, phentermine), busulfan, cocaine, heroin, methadone, methylphenidate, nitrosoureas, radiation

Hypereosinophilic syndrome, a systemic disease affecting multiple organs, is discussed elsewhere.

Löffler syndrome, a syndrome of fleeting pulmonary findings and peripheral blood eosinophilia, is another eosinophilic pulmonary disease.

Diagnosis

- Chest-x-ray
- Demonstrating eosinophilia in peripheral blood, bronchoalveolar lavage fluid, or lung tissue

Diagnosis is based on demonstration of opacities on chest x-ray and identification of eosinophilia (> 450/μL) in peripheral blood, bronchoalveolar lavage fluid, or lung biopsy tissue. However, pulmonary eosinophilia may occur in the absence of peripheral eosinophilia. Pulmonary opacities on chest x-ray associated with blood eosinophilia are sometimes called PIE (pulmonary infiltrates with eosinophilia) syndrome.

Eosinophils are primarily tissue-dwelling and are several hundred–fold more abundant in tissues than in blood. Consequently, blood eosinophil numbers do not necessarily indicate the extent of eosinophilic involvement in affected tissues. Eosinophils are most numerous in tissues with a mucosal epithelial interface with the environment, such as the respiratory, GI, and lower GU tracts. Eosinophils are not present in the lungs of healthy people, so their presence in tissue or bronchoalveolar lavage fluid (> 5% of differential count) identifies a pathologic process.

Eosinophils are exquisitely sensitive to corticosteroids and completely disappear from the bloodstream within a few hours after administration of corticosteroids. This rapid disappearance from the blood may obscure the diagnosis in patients who receive corticosteroids before the diagnostic assessment is instituted.

ACUTE EOSINOPHILIC PNEUMONIA

Acute eosinophilic pneumonia (AEP) is a disorder of unknown etiology characterized by rapid eosinophilic infiltration of the lung interstitium.

In contrast to chronic eosinophilic pneumonia, AEP is an acute illness that does not usually recur. Incidence and prevalence are unknown. AEP can occur at any age but most often affects patients between 20 and 40 yr, with a male-to-female ratio of 2:1. The cause is unknown, but AEP may be an acute hypersensitivity reaction to an unidentified inhaled antigen in an otherwise healthy person. Cigarette or other smoke exposure may be involved.

Symptoms and Signs

AEP causes an acute febrile illness of short duration (usually < 7 days). Symptoms are nonproductive cough, dyspnea, malaise, myalgias, night sweats, and pleuritic chest pain. Signs include tachypnea, fever (often > 38.5° C), and bibasilar inspiratory crackles and, occasionally, rhonchi on forced exhalation. Patients with AEP frequently present with acute respiratory failure requiring mechanical ventilation. Rarely, distributive (hyperdynamic) shock can occur.

Diagnosis

- High-resolution CT (HRCT)
- Usually CBC, pleural fluid analysis, and pulmonary function testing
- Bronchoscopy for lavage and, sometimes, biopsy

The diagnosis is suspected in patients with symptoms of acute pneumonia that progresses to respiratory failure and does not respond to antibiotics. Diagnosis is based on findings from routine testing and is confirmed by bronchoscopy. AEP is a diagnosis of exclusion and requires the absence of known causes of eosinophilic pneumonia (eg, drug- and toxin-induced, helminthic and fungal infection–related, eosinophilic granulomatosis with polyangiitis [Churg-Strauss syndrome], idiopathic hypereosinophilic syndrome, tumors). The CBC often fails to demonstrate markedly elevated eosinophil counts, unlike in chronic eosinophilic pneumonia. ESR and IgE levels are high but are nonspecific.

The chest x-ray initially may show only subtle reticular or ground-glass opacities, often with Kerley B lines. Isolated alveolar (about 25% of cases) or reticular (about 25% of cases) opacities may also be observed. Unlike in chronic eosinophilic pneumonia, in AEP opacities are not characteristically localized to the lung periphery. Small pleural effusions occur in two-thirds of patients and are frequently bilateral.

HRCT is always abnormal with bilateral, random, patchy ground-glass or reticular opacities.

Pleural fluid examination shows marked eosinophilia with high pH. Pulmonary function tests often show a restrictive process with reduced diffusing capacity for carbon monoxide (DLco).

Bronchoscopy should be done for lavage and, occasionally, biopsy. Bronchoalveolar lavage fluid often shows a high number and percentage (> 25%) of eosinophils. The most common histopathologic features on biopsy include eosinophilic infiltration with acute and organizing diffuse alveolar damage, but few patients have undergone lung biopsy.

Treatment

- Systemic corticosteroids

Some patients improve spontaneously. Most are treated with prednisone 40 to 60 mg po once/day. In patients with respiratory failure, methylprednisolone 60 to 125 mg IV q 6 h is preferred. The prognosis is usually good; response to corticosteroids and complete recovery is common. Pleural effusions resolve more slowly than parenchymal opacities.

CHRONIC EOSINOPHILIC PNEUMONIA

Chronic eosinophilic pneumonia (CEP) is a disorder of unknown etiology characterized by an abnormal, chronic accumulation of eosinophils in the lung.

CEP is not truly chronic; rather it is an acute or subacute illness that recurs (thus, a better name might be recurrent eosinophilic pneumonia). The prevalence and incidence of CEP are unknown. Etiology is suspected to be an allergic diathesis. Most patients are nonsmokers.

Symptoms and Signs

Patients often present with fulminant illness characterized by cough, fever, progressive breathlessness, wheezing, and night sweats. The clinical presentation may suggest a community-acquired pneumonia. Asthma accompanies or precedes the illness in > 50% of cases. Patients with recurrent symptoms may have weight loss.

Diagnosis

- Chest x-ray
- Exclusion of infectious causes of pneumonia
- Bronchoalveolar lavage

Diagnosis is suspected in patients with characteristic symptoms and typical radiographic appearance. Diagnosis also requires CBC, ESR, sometimes iron studies, and exclusion of infectious causes by appropriate cultures. Peripheral blood eosinophilia, a very high ESR, iron deficiency anemia, and thrombocytosis are all frequently present.

Chest x-ray findings of bilateral peripheral or pleural-based opacities, most commonly in the middle and upper lung zones, are described as the photographic negative of pulmonary edema and are virtually pathognomonic (although present in < 25% of patients). A similar pattern can be present on CT, but the distribution of consolidation can vary and even include unilateral lesions. Bronchoalveolar lavage is usually done to confirm the diagnosis.

Eosinophilia > 40% in bronchoalveolar lavage fluid is highly suggestive of CEP; serial bronchoalveolar lavage examinations may help document the course of disease.

Treatment

- Systemic corticosteroids
- Sometimes maintenance therapy with inhaled corticosteroids, oral corticosteroids, or both

Patients with CEP are uniformly responsive to IV or oral corticosteroids; failure to respond suggests another diagnosis. Initial treatment is prednisone 40 to 60 mg once/day. Clinical improvement is frequently striking and rapid, often occurring within 48 h. Complete resolution of symptoms and x-ray abnormalities occurs within 14 days in most patients and by 1 mo in almost all. Symptoms and plain chest x-rays are both reliable and efficient guides to therapy. Although CT is more sensitive for the detection of imaging abnormalities, there is no benefit gained by repeating CT. Peripheral eosinophil counts, ESR, and IgE levels can also be used to follow the clinical course during treatment. However, not all patients have abnormal laboratory test results.

Symptomatic or radiographic relapse occurs in many cases either after cessation of therapy or, less commonly, with tapering of the corticosteroid dose. Relapse can occur months to years after the initial episode. Thus, corticosteroid therapy may be required for long periods of time (years). Inhaled corticosteroids (eg, fluticasone or beclomethasone 500 to 750 mcg bid) may be effective, especially in reducing the maintenance dose of oral corticosteroid.

Relapse does not appear to indicate treatment failure, a worse prognosis, or greater morbidity. Patients continue to respond to corticosteroids as during the initial episode. Fixed airflow obstruction can occur in some patients who recover, but the abnormalities are usually of borderline clinical significance.

CEP occasionally leads to physiologically important restrictive lung function abnormalities as a result of irreversible fibrosis, but abnormalities are usually mild enough that CEP is an extremely unusual cause of morbidity or death.

LÖFFLER SYNDROME

Löffler syndrome, a form of eosinophilic pulmonary disease, is characterized by absent or mild respiratory symptoms (most often dry cough), fleeting migratory pulmonary opacities, and peripheral blood eosinophilia.

Parasitic infections, especially *Ascaris lumbricoides*, may be the cause, but an identifiable etiologic agent is not found in up to one third of patients.

The disease usually resolves within 1 mo.

Treatment is symptomatic and consists of corticosteroids.

HYPERSENSITIVITY PNEUMONITIS

(Extrinsic Allergic Alveolitis)

Hypersensitivity pneumonitis is a syndrome of cough, dyspnea, and fatigue caused by sensitization and subsequent hypersensitivity to environmental (frequently occupational) antigens. Acute, subacute, and chronic forms exist; all are characterized by acute interstitial inflammation and development of granulomas and fibrosis with long-term exposure. Diagnosis is based on a combination of history, physical examination, imaging tests, bronchoalveolar lavage, and biopsy. Short-term treatment is with corticosteroids; long-term treatment is antigen avoidance.

Etiology

Over 300 antigens have been identified as triggers for hypersensitivity pneumonitis, although farming, birds, and water contamination account for about 75% of cases. Antigens are commonly categorized by type and occupation (see Table 57–3); farmer's lung, caused by inhalation of hay dust containing

Table 57–3. EXAMPLES OF HYPERSENSITIVITY PNEUMONITIS

PNEUMONITIS	ANTIGEN	SOURCE
Farming		
Bagassosis	Thermophilic actinomycetes	Moldy bagasse (sugar cane)
Cheese washer's lung	*Aspergillus clavatus* *Penicillium casei*	Moldy cheese
Coffee worker's lung	Coffee bean dust	Coffee beans
Compost lung	*Aspergillus* sp	Compost
Farmer's lung	Fungi, especially *Aspergillus* sp Thermophilic actinomycetes	Vegetable compost (moldy grain, hay, silage)
Mushroom worker's lung	*Hypsizigus marmoreus* Thermophilic actinomycetes	Mushroom compost
Potato riddler's lung	*Aspergillus* sp Thermophilic actinomycetes	Moldy hay around potatoes
Tobacco grower's lung	*Aspergillus* sp *Scopulariopsis brevicaulis*	Tobacco plants
Wine grower's lung	*Botrytis cinerea*	Moldy grapes

Table 57–3. EXAMPLES OF HYPERSENSITIVITY PNEUMONITIS (*Continued*)

PNEUMONITIS	ANTIGEN	SOURCE
Water		
Hot tub lung	*Cladosporium* sp *Mycobacterium avium* complex	Contaminated mist and mold on ceilings and around tub
Humidifier lung	*Aureobasidium* sp *Candida albicans* Thermophilic actinomycetes	Contaminated water in humidification or air-conditioning systems
Sauna taker's lung	*Aureobasidium* sp	Contaminated sauna water
Sewer worker's lung	*Cephalosporium* sp	Contaminated basement (sewage)
Birds		
Bird fancier's lung	Parakeet, pigeon, chicken, turkey, and duck proteins	Bird droppings or feathers
Animals		
Fish food lung	Unknown	Fish food
Fish meal worker's lung	Fish meal dust	Fish meal dust
Furrier's lung	Animal fur dust	Animal pelts
Laboratory worker's hypersensitivity pneumonitis	Rodent proteins	Male rat urine and fur
Mummy handler's lung	Unknown	Cloth mummy wrappings
Pituitary snuff taker's lung	Animal proteins	Heterologous (bovine, porcine) pituitary snuff
Sausage worker's lung	*Penicillium nalgiovense*	Dry sausage mold
Grains		
Malt worker's lung	*Aspergillus* sp	Moldy barley
Miller's lung	*Sitophilus granarius* (wheat weevil)	Weevil-infested wheat flour
Milling and construction		
Scquoiosis	*Aureobasidium* sp *Graphium* sp	Redwood sawdust
Thatched-roof worker's disease	*Saccharomonospora viridis*	Dried grass and leaves
Wood pulp worker's disease	*Penicillium* sp	Oak and maple tree pulp
Wood trimmer's disease	*Rhizopus* sp *Mucor* sp	Contaminated wood trimmings
Woodworker's lung	*Alternaria* sp *Bacillus subtilis*	Oak, cedar, pine, spruce, and mahogany dusts
Industry		
Chemical worker's lung	Isocyanates	Polyurethane foam, varnishes, lacquer
Detergent worker's lung	*Bacillus subtilis*	*B. subtilis* enzymes in detergent
Vineyard sprayer's lung	Copper sulfate	Copper sulfate use
Other		
Byssinosis (brown lung)	Mill dust (possibly endotoxin related)	Cotton, flax, and hemp dust
Lycoperdonosis	Spores from puffball (*Lycoperdon*) mushrooms	Alternative medicine or recreational use (mistaking puffballs for hallucinogenic mushrooms)

thermophilic actinomycetes, is the prototype. Substantial overlap exists between hypersensitivity pneumonitis and chronic bronchitis in farmers, in whom chronic bronchitis is far more common, occurs independently of smoking status, is linked to thermophilic actinomycete exposure, and leads to findings similar to those of hypersensitivity pneumonitis on diagnostic testing.

Pathophysiology

The disorder seems to represent a type IV hypersensitivity reaction, in which repeated exposure to antigen in genetically susceptible people leads to acute neutrophilic and mononuclear alveolitis, followed by interstitial lymphocytic infiltration and granulomatous reaction. Fibrosis with bronchiolar obliteration occurs with continued exposure.

Circulating precipitins (antibodies sensitized to antigen) seem not to have a primary etiologic role, and clinical history of allergy (such as asthma and seasonal allergies) is not a predisposing factor. Cigarette smoking seems to delay or prevent development, perhaps through down-regulation of the lung's immune response to inhaled antigens. However, smoking may exacerbate the disease once established.

Hypersensitivity pneumonitis has clinical similarities to other disorders that have different pathophysiologies.

- Organic dust toxic syndrome (pulmonary mycotoxicosis, grain fever), for example, is a syndrome consisting of fever, chills, myalgias, and dyspnea that does not require prior sensitization and is thought to be caused by inhalation of toxins produced by fungi or other contaminants of organic dust.
- Silo filler's disease may lead to respiratory failure, acute respiratory distress syndrome (ARDS), and bronchiolitis obliterans or bronchitis but is caused by inhalation of toxic nitrogen oxides produced by freshly fermented corn or alfalfa silage.
- Occupational asthma causes dyspnea in people previously sensitized to an inhaled antigen, but features such as airflow obstruction, airway eosinophilia, and differences in triggering antigens distinguish it from hypersensitivity pneumonitis.

Symptoms and Signs

Symptoms and signs tend to depend on whether onset is

- Acute
- Subacute
- Chronic

Only a small proportion of exposed people develop symptoms and in most cases only after weeks to months of exposure and sensitization.

Acute hypersensitivity pneumonitis: Acute disease occurs in previously sensitized people with acute high-level antigen exposure and manifests as fever, chills, cough, bilateral vice-like chest tightness (as can occur in asthma), and dyspnea 4 to 8 h after exposure. Anorexia, nausea, and vomiting may also be present. Physical examination shows tachypnea, diffuse fine-to-medium inspiratory crackles, and, in almost all cases, absence of wheezing.

Chronic hypersensitivity pneumonitis: Chronic disease occurs in people with long-term low-level antigen exposure (such as owners of birds) and manifests as onset over months to years of exertional dyspnea, productive cough, fatigue, and weight loss. There are few physical findings; clubbing uncommonly occurs and fever is absent. In advanced cases, pulmonary fibrosis causes symptoms and signs of right heart failure, respiratory failure, or both.

Subacute hypersensitivity pneumonitis: Subacute disease falls between the acute and chronic forms and manifests either as cough, dyspnea, fatigue, and anorexia that develops over days to weeks or as acute superimposed on chronic symptoms.

Diagnosis

- Chest x-ray and HRCT
- Pulmonary function tests
- Bronchoalveolar lavage
- Histologic examination and serologic tests

Diagnosis requires a high index of suspicion in patients with compatible symptoms and a compatible occupational, avocational, or domestic exposure history. Chest x-ray, HRCT, and pulmonary function tests are done routinely. Bronchoalveolar lavage and biopsy may be necessary if results are inconclusive. The differential diagnosis is broad and includes environmental pulmonary diseases, sarcoidosis, bronchiolitis obliterans, connective tissue–associated pulmonary disease, and other interstitial lung diseases.

Clues in the history include

- Recurring atypical pneumonias
- Symptom onset after moving to a new job or home
- A hot tub, a sauna, a swimming pool, or other sources of standing water or water damage in the home or regular exposure to them elsewhere
- Having birds as pets
- Exacerbation and relief of symptoms in and away from specific settings

Examination often is not useful in making the diagnosis, although abnormal lung sounds and clubbing may be present.

Imaging tests: Imaging tests are typically done for patients with appropriate history, symptoms, and signs.

Chest x-ray is neither sensitive nor specific for detecting disease and is frequently normal in patients with acute and subacute forms. It may show reticular or nodular opacities, usually when symptoms are present. Chest x-rays of patients with chronic disease are more likely to show reticular or nodular opacities in the upper lobes with reduced lung volumes and honeycombing, similar to that of idiopathic pulmonary fibrosis (IPF).

HRCT is far more likely to show abnormalities and is considered standard for evaluating parenchymal changes in hypersensitivity pneumonitis. The most typical HRCT finding in acute and subacute disease is the presence of profuse, poorly defined centrilobular micronodules. Occasionally, ground-glass opacification (attenuation) is the predominant or only finding. It is usually diffuse but sometimes spares the periphery of the secondary lobule. Focal areas of hyperlucency, similar to those present in obliterative bronchiolitis, may be a prominent feature in some patients (eg, mosaic attenuation with air trapping on expiratory HRCT). In chronic hypersensitivity pneumonitis, there are findings of lung fibrosis (eg, lobar volume loss, linear or reticular opacities, or honeycombing), and centrilobular nodules may be absent. Some nonsmoking patients with chronic hypersensitivity pneumonitis have findings of upper lobe emphysema. Mediastinal lymphadenopathy is uncommon, thereby distinguishing hypersensitivity pneumonitis from sarcoidosis.

Pulmonary function tests: These should be done as part of the standard evaluation of suspected cases of hypersensitivity pneumonitis. The syndrome can cause obstructive, restrictive, or a mixed pattern of airway changes. Advanced disease most commonly causes a restrictive defect (decreased lung volumes), a decreased diffusing capacity for carbon monoxide (DL_{CO}), and hypoxemia. Airway obstruction is unusual in acute disease but may develop in chronic disease.

Bronchoalveolar lavage: Results are rarely specific for the diagnosis but are often a component of the diagnostic assessment for chronic respiratory symptoms and pulmonary function abnormalities. A lymphocytosis in lavage fluid (> 60%) with CD4+/CD8+ ratio < 1.0 (the normal ratio ± standard error of the mean = 2.3 ± 0.2) is characteristic of the disorder; by contrast, lymphocytosis with CD4+ predominance (ratio > 1.0) is more characteristic of sarcoidosis. Other findings may include mast cells > 1% (after acute exposure) and increased neutrophils and eosinophils.

Lymphocyte transformation testing is an in vitro test of sensitization and is particularly useful in detecting sensitization to metals. The test can be done on peripheral blood but is better done on bronchial lavage fluid. In this test, the patient's lymphocytes are exposed to potential antigens. If the lymphocytes transform into blasts and proliferate, they (and hence the patient) were previously sensitized to that antigen.

Lung biopsy: Surgical lung biopsy is indicated when noninvasive testing is inconclusive. Findings vary but typically include peribronchiolocentric lymphocytic alveolitis, poorly formed non-necrotizing granulomas, and organizing pneumonia. Interstitial fibrosis may be present in chronic cases.

Other tests: Additional testing is indicated when additional support for the diagnosis is required or to detect other causes of interstitial lung disease. Circulating precipitins (specific precipitating antibodies to the suspected antigen) are suggestive of an exposure that may be the cause of the illness. However, the presence of circulating precipitins is neither sensitive nor specific. Identification of a specific precipitating antigen may require that industrial hygiene specialists do detailed aerobiologic and/or microbiologic assessment of the workplace, but workplace assessments usually are guided by known sources of inciting antigens (eg, *Bacillus subtilis* in detergent factories). Skin tests are not helpful, and eosinophilia is absent. Tests helpful in detecting other disorders include serologic tests and cultures (for psittacosis and other pneumonias) and autoantibodies (for connective tissue disease). Elevated eosinophil levels may suggest CEPs. Hilar and paratracheal lymph node enlargement is more characteristic of sarcoidosis.

Prognosis

Pathologic changes are completely reversible if detected early and if antigen exposure is eliminated. Acute disease is self-limiting with antigen avoidance; symptoms usually lessen within hours. Chronic disease has a more complicated prognosis: fibrosis is usually irreversible but may not progress if the patient is no longer exposed to the antigen.

Treatment

- Corticosteroids

Treatment of acute or subacute hypersensitivity pneumonitis is with corticosteroids, usually prednisone 60 mg po once/day for 1 to 2 wk, then tapered over the next 2 to 4 wk to 20 mg once/day, followed by weekly decrements of 2.5 mg until the drug is stopped. This regimen relieves initial symptoms but does not appear to alter long-term outcome. Treatment of chronic hypersensitivity pneumonitis is usually with longer courses of prednisone 30 to 40 mg po once/day with tapering dependent on clinical response.

Prevention

The most important aspect of long-term management is avoidance of exposure to antigens. A complete change of environment is rarely realistic, especially for farmers and other workers, in which case dust control measures (such as wetting down compost before disturbing it) or using air filters or protective masks may be effective. Fungicides may be used to prevent the growth of antigenic microorganisms (eg, in hay or on sugar cane), but the long-term safety of this approach is unknown. Extensive cleaning of wet ventilation systems, removal of moist carpets, and maintenance of low humidity are also effective in some settings. Patients must be told, however, that these measures may be inadequate if exposure continues.

KEY POINTS

- Hypersensitivity pneumonitis is a type IV type hypersensitivity reaction that can be triggered with a wide variety of allergens.
- In patients at risk and who have compatible symptoms, elicit a thorough history of occupational, avocational, and domestic exposure.
- Do chest x-ray, HRCT, and pulmonary function tests and, if the diagnosis is unclear, possibly bronchoalveolar lavage and biopsy.
- Treat most patients with oral prednisone.

OVERVIEW OF IDIOPATHIC INTERSTITIAL PNEUMONIAS

Idiopathic interstitial pneumonias (IIPs) are interstitial lung diseases of unknown etiology that share similar clinical and radiologic features and are distinguished primarily by the histopathologic patterns on lung biopsy. Classified into 8 histologic subtypes, all are characterized by varying degrees of inflammation and fibrosis and all cause dyspnea. Diagnosis is based on history, physical examination, HRCT imaging, pulmonary function tests, and lung biopsy. Treatment varies by subtype. Prognosis varies by subtype and ranges from excellent to nearly always fatal.

The 8 histologic subtypes of IIP in decreasing order of frequency are

- IPF (identified histologically as usual interstitial pneumonia)
- Desquamative interstitial pneumonia
- Nonspecific interstitial pneumonia
- Cryptogenic organizing pneumonia
- Respiratory bronchiolitis–associated interstitial lung disease (RBILD)
- Acute interstitial pneumonia (AIP)
- Lymphoid interstitial pneumonia
- Idiopathic pleuroparenchymal fibroelastosis (PPFE)

These subtypes are characterized by varying degrees of interstitial inflammation and fibrosis.[1] All cause dyspnea; diffuse abnormalities on HRCT; and inflammation, fibrosis, or both on biopsy. The subtypes are important to distinguish, however, because they have different clinical features (see Table 57–4) and respond differently to treatment.

1. Travis WD, Costabel U, Hansell DM, et al: An Official American Thoracic Society/European Respiratory Society Statement: Update of the International Multidisciplinary Classification of the Idiopathic Interstitial Pneumonias. *Am J Respir Crit Care Med* 188(6):733–748, 2013.

Symptoms and Signs

Symptoms and signs are usually nonspecific. Cough and dyspnea on exertion are typical, with variable onset and progression. Common signs include tachypnea, reduced chest expansion, bibasilar end-inspiratory dry crackles, and digital clubbing.

Diagnosis

- HRCT
- Pulmonary function tests
- Sometimes surgical lung biopsy

IIP should be suspected in any patient with unexplained interstitial lung disease. Clinicians, radiologists, and pathologists should exchange information to determine the diagnosis in individual patients. Potential causes (see Table 57–1) are assessed systematically. For maximum diagnostic yield, history should address the following criteria:

- Symptom duration
- Family history of lung disease, especially lung fibrosis
- History of tobacco use (because some diseases occur mostly among current or former smokers)
- Current and prior drug use
- Detailed review of home and work environments, including those of family members

Table 57–4. KEY FEATURES OF IDIOPATHIC INTERSTITIAL PNEUMONIAS

DISORDER	PEOPLE MOST OFTEN AFFECTED	PRODROME	CHEST X-RAY FINDINGS	HIGH-RESOLUTION CT FINDINGS	CT DIFFERENTIAL DIAGNOSIS	HISTOLOGIC PATTERN
Idiopathic pulmonary fibrosis	More frequently men > 50 (> 60% smoke)	Chronic (> 12 mo)	Basal-predominant reticular abnormality with volume loss and honeycombing	Peripheral, subpleural, and basal reticular honeycombing Traction bronchiectasis or bronchiolectasis Architectural distortion	Asbestosis Connective tissue disorders Hypersensitivity pneumonitis	Usual interstitial pneumonia
Desquamative interstitial pneumonia	More frequently men, aged 30–50 (> 90% smoke)	Subacute to chronic (weeks to years)	Ground-glass opacification	Lower zone, peripheral predominance in most cases Ground-glass opacification Reticular lines	Hypersensitivity pneumonitis *Pneumocystis jirovecii* pneumonia Respiratory bronchiolitis–associated interstitial lung disease Sarcoidosis	Desquamative interstitial pneumonia
Nonspecific interstitial pneumonia	More frequently women, usually age 40–60 (< 40% smoke)	Subacute to chronic (months to years)	Ground-glass and reticular opacity	Peripheral, basal, symmetric Reticular opacities Variable ground-glass opacification Irregular lines	Cryptogenic organizing pneumonia Desquamative interstitial pneumonia Hypersensitivity pneumonitis Idiopathic pulmonary fibrosis	Nonspecific interstitial pneumonia
Cryptogenic organizing pneumonia	People of any age, usually aged 40–50 (< 50% smoke)	Subacute (< 3 mo)	Patchy bilateral consolidation	Peribronchial Patchy consolidation, nodules, or both	Alveolar cell carcinoma Eosinophilic pneumonia Lymphoma Infection Nonspecific interstitial pneumonia Sarcoidosis Vasculitis	Organizing pneumonia
Respiratory bronchiolitis–associated interstitial lung disease	Slightly more men, aged 30–50 (> 90% smoke)	Subacute (weeks to months)	Bronchial wall thickening Ground-glass opacification	Diffuse pattern Bronchial wall thickening Centrilobular nodules Patchy ground-glass opacification	Desquamative interstitial pneumonia Hypersensitivity pneumonitis Nonspecific interstitial pneumonia Infection	Respiratory bronchiolitis–associated interstitial lung disease

Table 57–4. KEY FEATURES OF IDIOPATHIC INTERSTITIAL PNEUMONIAS (*Continued*)

DISORDER	PEOPLE MOST OFTEN AFFECTED	PRODROME	CHEST X-RAY FINDINGS	HIGH-RESOLUTION CT FINDINGS	CT DIFFERENTIAL DIAGNOSIS	HISTOLOGIC PATTERN
Acute interstitial pneumonia	People of any age[†]	Abrupt (1–2 wk)	Progressive, diffuse ground-glass opacification	Diffuse consolidation, ground-glass opacification, often with lobular sparing Traction bronchiectasis later	Acute eosinophilic pneumonia Acute respiratory distress syndrome Hydrostatic edema Pneumonia	Diffuse alveolar damage
Lymphoid interstitial pneumonia	Mostly women, of any age[†]	Chronic (> 12 mo)	Reticular opacities Nodules	Diffuse pattern Centrilobular nodules Ground-glass opacification Septal and bronchovascular thickening Thin-walled cysts	Langerhans cell histiocytosis Lymphangitic carcinoma Sarcoidosis	Lymphoid interstitial pneumonia
Idiopathic pleuroparenchymal fibroelastosis	No sex predilection, median age of 57 years	Chronic (> 12 months)	Bilateral apical irregular pleural thickening	Dense subpleural consolidation Traction bronchiectasis Architectural distortion Upper lobe volume loss	Hypersensitivity pneumonitis Nonspecific interstitial pneumonia Asbestosis Connective tissue disorders Sarcoidosis Radiation induced lung disease Drug induced lung disease	Pleuroparenchymal fibroelastosis

*Listed in order of decreasing frequency.
[†]History of smoking unknown.

A chronologic listing of the patient's entire employment history, including specific duties and known exposures to organic and inorganic agents (see Table 57-1 on p. 449), is obtained. The degree of exposure, duration of exposure, latency of exposure, and the use of protective devices is elicited.

Chest x-ray is done and is typically abnormal, but findings are not specific enough to differentiate between the various types.

Pulmonary function tests are often done to estimate the severity of physiologic impairment, but they do not help differentiate between the various types. Typical results are restrictive physiology, with reduced lung volumes and diffusion capacity. Hypoxemia is common during exercise and may be present at rest.

HRCT, which distinguishes airspace from interstitial disease, is the most useful test and is always done. It provides assessment of the etiology, extent, and distribution of disease, and is more likely to detect underlying or coexisting disease (eg, occult mediastinal adenopathy, cancer, emphysema). HRCT should be done with the patient supine and prone and should include dynamic expiratory imaging to accentuate evidence of small airway involvement.

Laboratory tests are done for patients who have clinical features suggesting a connective tissue disorder, vasculitis, or environmental exposure. Such tests may include antinuclear antibodies, rheumatoid factor, other more specific serologic tests for connective tissue diseases (eg, RNP, SSA, SSB, scl70, Jo-1), hypersensitivity panel (a collection of tests for antibodies to common antigens from microbial, fungal, and animal sources), antineutrophil cytoplasmic antibodies, and anti-basement membrane antibody.

Bronchoscopic transbronchial biopsy can help differentiate certain interstitial lung diseases, such as sarcoidosis and hypersensitivity pneumonitis, but the biopsy does not yield enough tissue to diagnose the IIPs. Bronchoalveolar lavage helps narrow the differential diagnosis in some patients and can provide information about disease progression and response to therapy. The usefulness of this procedure in the initial clinical assessment and follow-up of most patients with these diseases has not been established, however.

Surgical lung biopsy is needed to confirm the diagnosis when the history and HRCT are nondiagnostic. Biopsy of multiple sites with a video-assisted thoracoscopic surgery (VATS) procedure is preferred.

Treatment

- Varies by disorder
- Often corticosteroids
- Sometimes lung transplantation

Treatment varies by disorder (see Table 57–5). Smoking cessation is always recommended to avoid potentially accelerating disease progression and to limit respiratory comorbidities.

Corticosteroids are typically recommended for cryptogenic organizing pneumonia, lymphoid interstitial pneumonia, and nonspecific interstitial pneumonia (NSIP) but not for IPF.

Lung transplantation may be recommended for selected patients with end-stage disorders.

KEY POINTS

- There are 8 histologic subtypes of IIP.
- Symptoms, signs, and chest x-ray findings are nonspecific.
- Diagnose IIPs initially based primarily on history and HRCT.
- When clinical evaluation and HRCT are not diagnostic, do surgical lung biopsy.
- Treatment varies by subtype.

ACUTE INTERSTITIAL PNEUMONIA

(Accelerated Interstitial Pneumonia; Hamman-Rich Syndrome)

Acute interstitial pneumonia (AIP) is an idiopathic version of the acute respiratory distress syndrome (ARDS).

AIP, a form of idiopathic interstitial pneumonia (IIP), equally affects apparently healthy men and women usually > 40 yr.

AIP is defined histologically by organizing diffuse alveolar damage, a nonspecific pattern that occurs in other causes of lung injury unrelated to IIP. The hallmark of organizing diffuse alveolar damage is diffuse, marked alveolar septal edema with inflammatory cell infiltration, fibroblast proliferation, occasional hyaline membranes, and thickening of the alveolar walls. Septa are lined with atypical, hyperplastic type II pneumocytes, and airspaces are collapsed. Thrombi develop in small arteries but are nonspecific.

Table 57–5. TREATMENT AND PROGNOSIS OF IDIOPATHIC INTERSTITIAL PNEUMONIAS*

DISORDER	TREATMENT	PROGNOSIS
Idiopathic pulmonary fibrosis	Pirfenidone or nintedanib; lung transplantation	Mortality rate: 50–70% in 5 yr
Desquamative interstitial pneumonia	Smoking cessation	Mortality rate: 5% in 5 yr
Nonspecific interstitial pneumonia	Corticosteroids with or without immunosuppressive therapies (eg, azathioprine, mycophenolate mofetil)	Mortality rate: widely variable, but generally better than idiopathic pulmonary fibrosis. In purely cellular disease (rare), extremely low
Cryptogenic organizing pneumonia	Corticosteroids	Complete recovery rate: > 65% Relapses: In many Mortality rate: Rare
Respiratory bronchiolitis–associated interstitial lung disease	Smoking cessation	Mortality rate: Rare
Acute interstitial pneumonia	Supportive care	Mortality rate: 60% in < 6 mo
Lymphoid interstitial pneumonia	Corticosteroids	Not well defined
Idiopathic pleuroparenchymal fibroelastosis	Appropriate treatment unknown; often corticosteroids	Disease progression occurs in 60%

*Listed in order of decreasing frequency.

Symptoms consist of the abrupt onset of fever, cough, and shortness of breath, which in most patients increase in severity over 7 to 14 days, progressing to respiratory failure.

Diagnosis

- High resolution CT
- Usually lung biopsy

Diagnosis is suspected in patients with symptoms, signs, and chest x-ray findings of ARDS (eg, diffuse bilateral airspace opacification).

Diagnosis is supported by HRCT but usually requires biopsy. HRCT shows bilateral patchy symmetric areas of ground-glass attenuation and sometimes bilateral areas of airspace consolidation in a predominantly subpleural distribution. Mild honeycombing, usually affecting < 10% of the lung, may be present. Routine laboratory tests are nonspecific and generally not helpful.

Diagnosis is confirmed by surgical lung biopsy showing diffuse alveolar damage in the absence of known causes of ARDS and diffuse alveolar damage (eg, sepsis, drugs, toxins, radiation, viral infection). Acute exacerbation of underlying lung disease (in particular acute exacerbation of IPF) must be considered and may explain some cases previously characterized as AIP. Biopsy is often required to distinguish AIP from diffuse alveolar hemorrhage syndrome, acute eosinophilic pneumonia, and cryptogenic organizing pneumonia.

Treatment

- Supportive

Treatment is supportive and usually requires mechanical ventilation, often using the same methods as used for ARDS (including low tidal volume ventilation). Corticosteroid therapy is generally used, but efficacy has not been established.

Mortality is > 60%; most patients die within 6 mo of presentation, and death is usually due to respiratory failure. Patients who survive the initial acute episode may recover complete pulmonary function, although the disease may recur.

CRYPTOGENIC ORGANIZING PNEUMONIA

(Bronchiolitis Obliterans Organizing Pneumonia)

Cryptogenic organizing pneumonia (COP) is an idiopathic condition in which granulation tissue obstructs alveolar ducts and alveolar spaces with chronic inflammation occurring in adjacent alveoli.

COP, a form of idiopathic interstitial pneumonia, affects men and women equally, usually in their 40s or 50s. Cigarette smoking does not seem to be a risk factor.

About one half of patients recall having a community-acquired pneumonia-like syndrome (ie, a nonresolving flu-like illness characterized by cough, fever, malaise, fatigue, and weight loss) at the onset of the illness. Progressive cough and exertional dyspnea are what usually prompt the patient to seek medical attention.

Chest examination demonstrates fine, dry, inspiratory crackles (Velcro crackles).

Diagnosis

- HRCT
- Sometimes surgical lung biopsy

Diagnosis requires imaging tests and, if the diagnosis is not otherwise clear, surgical lung biopsy.

Chest x-ray shows bilateral, diffuse, peripherally distributed alveolar opacities with normal lung volumes; a peripheral distribution similar to CEP may occur. Rarely, alveolar opacities are unilateral. Recurrent and migratory pulmonary opacities are common. Rarely, irregular linear or nodular interstitial opacities or honeycombing are visible at presentation.

HRCT of the lung shows patchy airspace consolidation (present in 90% of patients), ground-glass opacities, small nodular opacities, and bronchial wall thickening and dilation. The patchy opacities are more common in the periphery of the lung, often in the lower lung zone. HRCT may show much more extensive disease than is expected from review of the chest x-ray.

Pulmonary function tests usually show a restrictive defect, although an obstructive defect (ratio of forced expiratory volume in 1 sec to forced vital capacity [FEV_1/FVC] < 70%) is found in 21% of patients, and pulmonary function is occasionally normal.

Routine laboratory test results are nonspecific. Leukocytosis without an increase in eosinophils occurs in about one-half of patients. The initial ESR often is elevated.

Lung biopsy shows excessive proliferation of granulation tissue within small airways and alveolar ducts, with chronic inflammation in the surrounding alveoli. Foci of organizing pneumonia are nonspecific and can occur secondary to other pathologic processes, including infections, vasculitis, lymphoma, and other interstitial lung diseases such as IPF, NSIP, connective tissue–related interstitial lung disease, drug induced pulmonary disease, hypersensitivity pneumonitis, and eosinophilic pneumonia.

Treatment

- Corticosteroids

Clinical recovery follows treatment with corticosteroids in most patients, often within 2 wk.

COP recurs occur in up to 50% of patients. Recurrences appear related to the duration of treatment, so treatment should usually be given for 6 to 12 mo. Recurrent disease is generally responsive to additional courses of corticosteroids.

Recovery after treatment is common when COP appears on HRCT as parenchymal consolidation, ground-glass opacity, or nodules. In contrast, recovery is less common when COP appears on HRCT as linear and reticular opacities.

DESQUAMATIVE INTERSTITIAL PNEUMONIA

Desquamative interstitial pneumonia is chronic lung inflammation characterized by mononuclear cell infiltration of the airspaces; it occurs almost exclusively in current or former cigarette smokers.

Desquamative interstitial pneumonia is a type of IIP. The vast majority of adult patients with desquamative interstitial pneumonia are smokers, who tend to develop the disease in their 30s or 40s.

The disease tends to affect the lung parenchyma uniformly. The alveolar walls are lined with plump cuboidal pneumocytes; there is moderate infiltration of the alveolar septum by lymphocytes, plasma cells, and, occasionally, eosinophils. Alveolar septal fibrosis, if present, is mild. The most striking feature is the presence of numerous pigmented macrophages within distal airspaces, mistaken as desquamated pneumocytes when the disease was first described. Honeycombing is rare. Similar but much less extensive findings occur in respiratory bronchiolitis-associated interstitial lung disease (RBILD), leading to the suggestion that desquamative interstitial pneumonia and RBILD are different manifestations of the same disease caused by cigarette smoking.

Diagnosis

- HRCT
- Sometimes surgical lung biopsy

Chest x-ray can show bibasilar hazy opacities without honeycombing, but is normal in up to 20% of cases. HRCT shows multifocal or diffuse, basilar, subpleural ground-glass opacities. Cysts may be present, often in areas of ground-glass opacity. Irregular linear and reticular opacities are common but are not usually the dominant features. Honeycombing may be visible, occurs in the minority of patients, and is usually limited. Surgical lung biopsy is sometimes necessary.

Treatment

- Smoking cessation
- Sometimes corticosteroids or cytotoxic drugs

Smoking cessation results in clinical improvement in an estimated 75% of patients. Patients who do not improve may respond to corticosteroids or cytotoxic drugs.

Prognosis is good, with about 70% survival at 10 yr.

IDIOPATHIC PLEUROPARENCHYMAL FIBROELASTOSIS

Idiopathic pluroparenchymal fibroelastosis (PPFE) is a rare idiopathic interstitial pneumonia that predominantly involves the upper lobes of the lungs and is slowly progressive. Patients often have recurrent infections, shortness of breath, and dry cough. Diagnosis is with HRCT. Corticosteroids may be given.

Idiopathic PPFE is a rare condition that is classified as an IIP.[1] It involves upper lobe fibrosis of the pleura and subpleural lung parenchyma.

1. Travis WD, Costabel U, Hansell DM, et al: An Official American Thoracic Society/European Respiratory Society Statement: Update of the International Multidisciplinary Classification of the Idiopathic Interstitial Pneumonias. *Am J Respir Crit Care Med* 188(6):733–748, 2013.

Etiology

The cause is unknown, but clinical data suggest a link to recurrent pulmonary infection. Genetic and autoimmune mechanisms are also thought to play a role in this disease.

Symptoms and Signs

The median age of presentation is around 57 years, with no sex predilection. Most patients are nonsmokers. Patients often report a history of recurrent infections, shortness of breath, and dry cough. Pneumothorax is common during the course of the disease.

Diagnosis

- HRCT
- For confirmation, surgical lung biopsy

The imaging findings include upper lobe thickening of the pleura and subpleural regions. They can have co-existing findings of other interstitial pneumonias, including usual interstitial pneumonia and nonspecific interstitial pneumonia pattern. Patients can also have areas of consolidation and bronchiectasis.

The pathology is characterized by intra-alveolar fibrosis with the alveolar walls in these areas showing prominent elastosis and dense fibrous thickening of the visceral pleura. In some patients, there is co-existent interstitial pneumonia in the lower lobes. Surgical lung biopsy is required for confirmation of the diagnosis.

Prognosis

The clinical course in patients with PPFE tends to be progressive in the majority of patients. Disease progression occurs in 60% of patients.

Treatment

- Possibly corticosteroids

The appropriate treatment for this condition is unknown. The majority of the literature reports the use of corticosteroids.

IDIOPATHIC PULMONARY FIBROSIS

Idiopathic pulmonary fibrosis (IFP), the most common form of idiopathic interstitial pneumonia (IIP), causes progressive pulmonary fibrosis. Symptoms and signs develop over months to years and include exertional dyspnea, cough, and fine (Velcro) crackles. Diagnosis is based on history, physical examination, HRCT, and/or lung biopsy, if necessary. Treatment may include antifibrotic drugs and oxygen therapy. Most patients deteriorate; median survival is about 3 yr from diagnosis.

IPF, identified histologically as usual interstitial pneumonia, accounts for most cases of IIP. IPF affects men and women > 50 in a ratio of 2:1, with a markedly increased incidence with each decade of age. Current or former cigarette smoking is most strongly associated with the disorder. There is some genetic predisposition; familial clustering occurs in up to 20% of cases.

Etiology

A combination of environmental, genetic, and other unknown factors probably contribute to alveolar epithelial cell dysfunction or reprogramming, which leads to abnormal fibroproliferation in the lung. There is ongoing research into the contributions of genetics, environmental stimuli, inflammatory cells, the alveolar epithelium, mesenchyme, and matrix.

Pathology

The key histologic findings are subpleural fibrosis with sites of fibroblast proliferation (fibroblast foci) and dense scarring, alternating with areas of normal lung tissue (heterogeneity). Scattered interstitial inflammation occurs with lymphocyte, plasma cell, and histiocyte infiltration. Cystic abnormality (honeycombing) occurs in all patients and increases with advanced disease. A similar histologic pattern uncommonly occurs in cases of interstitial lung diseases of known etiology (see Table 57–4).

Symptoms and Signs

Symptoms and signs typically develop over 6 mo to several years and include dyspnea on exertion and nonproductive cough. Constitutional symptoms, such as low-grade fever and myalgias, are uncommon. The classic sign of IPF is fine, dry, inspiratory crackles (Velcro crackles) at both bases. Clubbing is present in about 50% of cases. The remainder of the examination is normal until disease is advanced, at which time signs of pulmonary hypertension and right ventricular systolic dysfunction may develop.

Diagnosis

- HRCT
- Sometimes surgical lung biopsy

Diagnosis is suspected in patients with subacute dyspnea, nonproductive cough, and Velcro crackles on chest examination. However, IPF is commonly overlooked initially because of clinical similarities to other more common diseases, such as bronchitis, asthma, and heart failure. Diagnosis requires HRCT and in some cases surgical lung biopsy.

Chest x-ray typically shows diffuse reticular opacities in the lower and peripheral lung zones. Small cystic lesions (honeycombing) and dilated airways due to traction bronchiectasis are additional findings.

HRCT shows diffuse, patchy, subpleural, reticular opacities with irregularly thickened interlobular septa and intralobular lines; subpleural honeycombing; and traction bronchiectasis. Ground-glass opacities affecting > 30% of the lung suggest an alternative diagnosis.

Laboratory testing plays little role in diagnosis.

Prognosis

Most patients have moderate to advanced clinical disease at the time of diagnosis and deteriorate despite treatment. Median survival is about 3 yr from time of diagnosis. Several prognostic models have been proposed. Among the factors that portend a worse prognosis are older age, male sex, lower forced vital capacity, and lower DLco.

Causes of acute deterioration include infections, pulmonary embolism, pneumothorax, and heart failure. Also, acute exacerbations without an identifiable cause may occur. All acute exacerbations have a high morbidity and mortality. Lung cancer occurs more frequently in patients with IPF, but cause of death is usually respiratory failure. Because of the poor prognosis of IPF, early discussions with the patient and family about advance care planning and end-of-life care are important.

Treatment

- Pirfenidone or nintedanib
- Oxygen and pulmonary rehabilitation
- Sometimes lung transplantation

Pirfenidone and nintedanib are new antifibrotic drugs available in some countries that slow disease progression.[1, 2] Supportive measures include oxygen and pulmonary rehabilitation. Patients may find that joining a support group helps reduce the stress of the illness.

Many novel therapies for IPF are under development or being tested as treatments for IPF, and patients should be encouraged to participate in clinical trials when appropriate.

Lung transplantation is successful for otherwise healthy IPF patients, generally those < 65 yr old. Otherwise healthy IPF patients should be evaluated for lung transplantation at the time of diagnosis.

1. King TE, Bradford WZ, Castro-Bernardini S, et al: A phase 3 trial of pirfenidone in patients with idiopathic pulmonary fibrosis. *N Eng J Med* 370:2083–2092, 2014.
2. Raghu G, Rochwerg B, Zhang Y, et al: An Official ATS/ERS/JRS/ALAT Clinical Practice Guideline: Treatment of Idiopathic Pulmonary Fibrosis. An Update of the 2011 Clinical Practice Guideline. *Am J Respir Crit Care Med* 192(2):e3–e19, June 15, 2015.

KEY POINTS

- IPF accounts for most IIP and tends to affect older people.
- Symptoms and signs (eg, subacute dyspnea, nonproductive cough, and Velcro crackles) are nonspecific and usually caused by other, more common disorders.
- HRCT can help in diagnosis by showing findings such as diffuse, patchy, subpleural, reticular opacities with irregularly thickened interlobular septa and intralobular lines; subpleural honeycombing; and traction bronchiectasis.
- Treat supportively and, if available, use pirfenidone or nintedanib.
- Encourage participation in clinical trials and, if patients are < 65 yr and otherwise healthy, consider lung transplantation at the time of diagnosis.

LYMPHOID INTERSTITIAL PNEUMONIA

(Lymphocytic Interstitial Pneumonitis)

Lymphoid interstitial pneumonia (LIP) is lymphocytic infiltration of the alveolar interstitium and air spaces. The cause is unknown. Symptoms and signs are cough, progressive dyspnea, and crackles. Diagnosis is based on history, physical examination, imaging tests, and lung biopsy. Treatment is with corticosteroids, cytotoxic drugs, or both, although efficacy is unknown. Five-year survival is 50 to 66%.

LIP is a rare idiopathic interstitial pneumonia characterized by infiltration of alveoli and alveolar septa with small lymphocytes and varying numbers of plasma cells. Non-necrotizing, poorly formed granulomas may be present but are usually rare and inconspicuous.

LIP is the most common cause of pulmonary disease after *Pneumocystis* infection in HIV-positive children and is the AIDS-defining illness in up to one half of HIV-positive children. LIP affects < 1% of adults with or without HIV infection. Women and girls are affected more commonly.

The cause is postulated to be an autoimmune disease or a nonspecific response to infection with Epstein-Barr virus, HIV, or other viruses. Evidence of an autoimmune etiology includes its frequent association with Sjögren syndrome (25% of cases of LIP) and other disorders (eg, SLE, RA, Hashimoto thyroiditis—14% of cases). Evidence of an indirect viral etiology includes frequent association with immunodeficient states (HIV/AIDS, combined variable immunodeficiency, agammaglobulinemia—14% of cases) and findings of Epstein-Barr virus DNA and HIV RNA in lung tissue of patients with LIP. According to this theory, LIP is an extreme manifestation of the normal ability of lymphoid tissue in the lung to respond to inhaled and circulating antigens.

Symptoms and Signs

In adults, LIP causes symptoms of progressive dyspnea and cough. These manifestations progress over months or, in some cases, years and appear at a mean age of 54. Weight loss, fever, arthralgias, and night sweats occur but are less common.

Examination may reveal crackles. Findings such as hepatosplenomegaly, arthritis, and lymphadenopathy are uncommon and suggest an accompanying or alternative diagnosis.

Diagnosis

- HRCT
- For confirmation, biopsy

Diagnosis is usually suspected in at-risk patients with compatible symptoms. Imaging tests and sometimes lung biopsy are done.

Chest x-ray shows bibasilar linear reticular or nodular opacities, a nonspecific finding that is present in a number of pulmonary infections. Alveolar opacities, cysts, or both may be present in more advanced disease. HRCT of the chest is done and helps establish the extent of disease, define the hilar anatomy, and identify pleural involvement.

HRCT findings are highly variable. Characteristic findings are centrilobular and subpleural nodules, thickened bronchovascular bundles, nodular ground-glass opacities, and cystic structures.

Marked hypoxemia may occur.

Bronchoalveolar lavage should be done to rule out infection and may reveal an increased number of lymphocytes.

Routine laboratory testing and serum protein electrophoresis (SPEP) are done because about 80% of patients have a serum protein abnormality, most commonly a polyclonal gammopathy and hypogammaglobulinemia, the significance of which is unknown.

Lung biopsy with demonstration of expansion of the alveolar septae due to lymphocytic and other immune cell (plasma cell, immunoblastic, histiocytic) infiltrates is required for diagnosis in adults. Infiltrates appear occasionally along bronchi and vessels but most commonly along alveolar septa. Immunohistochemical staining and flow cytometry must be done on the tissue to distinguish LIP from primary lymphomas. In LIP, the infiltrate is polyclonal (both T and B cells), whereas other lymphomas produce monoclonal infiltrates. Other common findings include germinal centers and multinucleated giant cells with noncaseating granulomas.

Prognosis

The natural history and prognosis of LIP are poorly understood. Spontaneous resolution, resolution after treatment with corticosteroids or other immunosuppressive drugs, progression to lymphoma, or development of pulmonary fibrosis with respiratory insufficiency may ensue. Five-year survival is 50 to 66%. Common causes of death are infection, development of malignant lymphoma (5%), and progressive fibrosis.

Treatment

- Corticosteroids or cytotoxic drugs

Treatment is with corticosteroids, cytotoxic drugs, or both, but, as with many other causes of interstitial lung diseases, the efficacy of this approach is unknown.

KEY POINTS

- LIP is rare overall, but is one of the most common lung disorders in HIV-positive children.
- Symptoms and signs tend to be nonspecific.
- Do HRCT, bronchoalveolar lavage, and sometimes lung biopsy.
- Treat patients with corticosteroids, cytotoxic drugs, or both.

NONSPECIFIC INTERSTITIAL PNEUMONIA

Nonspecific interstitial pneumonia (NSIP) is an idiopathic interstitial pneumonia (IIP) that occurs mainly in women, nonsmokers, and patients < 50 yr.

Compared to idiopathic pulmonary fibrosis (IPF), NSIP is an uncommon IIP. Most patients are women, are between the ages of 40 and 50, and have no known cause or association. However, a similar pathologic process can occur in patients with a connective tissue disorder (in particular, systemic sclerosis or polymyositis/dermatomyositis), in some forms of drug-induced pulmonary disease, and in patients with hypersensitivity pneumonitis.

Clinical presentation is similar to that of IPF. Cough and dyspnea are present for months to years. Constitutional symptoms are unusual, although a low-grade fever and malaise are possible.

Diagnosis

- HRCT
- Surgical lung biopsy

The diagnosis should be considered in patients with unexplained subacute or chronic cough and dyspnea. Diagnosis requires HRCT and always requires confirmation by surgical lung biopsy. NSIP is a diagnosis of exclusion that requires careful clinical review for possible alternative disorders, in particular connective tissue disorders, hypersensitivity pneumonitis, and drug toxicity.

Chest x-ray primarily shows lower-zone reticular opacities. Bilateral patchy opacities are also possible.

HRCT findings include bilateral patchy ground-glass attenuation, irregular lines, and bronchial dilation (traction bronchiectasis), generally with a lower lung zone distribution. Subpleural sparing is possible. Honeycombing is rare.

More than half of patients have an increased percentage of lymphocytes in bronchoalveolar lavage fluid, but this finding is nonspecific.

Surgical lung biopsy is done. Histologically, most patients have some degree of fibrosis. The main feature of NSIP is temporally homogenous inflammation and fibrosis, as opposed to the heterogeneity in usual interstitial pneumonia. Although the changes are temporally uniform, the process may be patchy, with intervening areas of unaffected lung.

Treatment

- Corticosteroids with or without immunosuppressive drugs

Many patients respond to treatment with corticosteroids, with or without immunosuppressive drugs (eg, azathioprine, mycophenolate mofetil, cyclophosphamide). Prognosis seems to depend most on the degree of fibrosis found during surgical lung biopsy. In patients with primarily cellular disease, almost all patients survive at least 10 yr. However, with increasing fibrosis, survival worsens and in some series median survival for fibrotic NSIP is 3 to 5 yr.

KEY POINTS

- NSIP is uncommon; most patients are women, are between the ages of 40 and 50, and have no known risk.
- Exclude connective tissue disorders (particularly systemic sclerosis and polymyositis/dermatomyositis), drug-induced lung injury, and hypersensitivity pneumonitis and do surgical lung biopsy.
- Treat with corticosteroids, with or without immunosuppressive drugs (eg, azathioprine, mycophenolate mofetil, cyclophosphamide).
- Prognosis is worse if biopsy shows more fibrosis.

RESPIRATORY BRONCHIOLITIS–ASSOCIATED INTERSTITIAL LUNG DISEASE

RBILD is a syndrome of small airway inflammation and interstitial lung disease occurring in smokers.

RBILD is a form of idiopathic interstitial pneumonia.

Most smokers develop a subclinical bronchiolitis characterized by mild or moderate inflammation of the small airways. The few patients who develop more severe inflammation with clinically significant interstitial disease are said to have RBILD. Male-to-female ratio is 2:1.

RBILD is characterized histologically by submucosal inflammation of the membranous and respiratory bronchioles manifested by the presence of tan-brown pigmented macrophages (resulting from increased iron content, as occurs in smokers), mucus stasis, and metaplastic cuboidal epithelium in bronchioles and alveoli. Alveolar septal scarring always occurs. Similar findings, however, occur in some hypersensitivity reactions, occupational lung exposures (usually due to mineral dusts), viral infections, and drug reactions.

RBILD also resembles desquamative interstitial pneumonia histologically, but in RBILD, inflammation is patchier and less extensive. The similarity of the 2 conditions has led to the suggestion that they are different manifestations of the same disease caused by cigarette smoking.

Symptoms of cough and breathlessness during exertion resemble those of other interstitial lung diseases, especially IPF, but are milder. Crackles on examination are the only physical finding.

Diagnosis

- Chest x-ray, HRCT
- Sometimes surgical lung biopsy

Diagnosis is considered in patients being evaluated for interstitial lung disease. Diagnostic testing includes imaging tests and biopsy.

Chest x-ray findings include the following:

- Diffuse, fine reticular or nodular opacities
- Bronchial wall thickening
- Prominent peribronchovascular interstitium
- Small regular and irregular opacities
- Small peripheral ring shadows

HRCT often shows centrilobular nodules and patchy areas of hazy ground-glass opacities.

A mixed obstructive-restrictive pattern is a common pulmonary function test finding, although results may be normal or show an isolated increase in residual volume. Routine laboratory tests are not helpful.

Treatment

- Smoking cessation

Treatment is smoking cessation and avoidance of even passive cigarette smoke exposure, which may prevent improvement or lead to recurrence of the illness. There is only anecdotal evidence of the efficacy of corticosteroids. The natural clinical course of the disease is unknown, but prognosis is good with smoking cessation.

LYMPHANGIOLEIOMYOMATOSIS

Lymphangioleiomyomatosis (LAM) is an indolent, progressive growth of smooth muscle cells throughout the lungs, pulmonary blood vessels, lymphatics, and pleurae. It is rare and occurs exclusively in young women. Symptoms are dyspnea, cough, chest pain, and hemoptysis; spontaneous pneumothorax is common. Diagnosis is suspected on the basis of symptoms and chest x-ray and is confirmed by HRCT. Prognosis is uncertain, but the disorder is slowly progressive and over years often leads to respiratory failure and death. Treatment is with sirolimus or lung transplantation.

LAM is not an interstitial lung disease, but patients are occasionally misdiagnosed as having interstitial lung disease (and also asthma or COPD).

LAM is a rare disease exclusive to women, typically affecting those between 20 and 40 yr. Whites are at greatest risk. LAM affects < 1 in 1 million people. It is characterized by proliferation of atypical smooth muscle cells throughout the chest, including lung parenchyma, vasculature, lymphatics, and pleurae, leading to distortion of lung architecture, cystic emphysema, and progressive deterioration of lung function.

Etiology

The cause of LAM is unknown. The tempting hypothesis that female sex hormones play a role in pathogenesis remains unproved. The disease usually arises spontaneously, but LAM bears many similarities to the pulmonary findings of tuberous sclerosis (TS); LAM occurs in some patients with TS and is thought by some to be a forme fruste of TS. Mutations in the TS complex-2 gene (*TSC-2*) have been described in LAM cells and angiomyolipomas (benign renal hamartomas made of smooth muscle, blood vessels, and adipose). Angiomyolipomas occur in up to 50% of patients with LAM. These observations suggest 1 of 2 possibilities:

1. Somatic mosaicism for *TSC-2* mutations within the lungs and kidneys results in foci of disease superimposed against a background of normal cells within these tissues (although multiple discrete sites of disease might be expected).
2. LAM represents a low-grade, destructive, metastasizing neoplasm, perhaps of uterine origin, that spreads through the lymphatic system.

Symptoms and Signs

Initial symptoms are dyspnea and, less commonly, cough, chest pain, and hemoptysis. There are few signs of disease, but some women have crackles and rhonchi. Many patients present with spontaneous pneumothorax. They may also present with manifestations of lymphatic obstruction, including chylothorax, chylous ascites, and chyluria. Symptoms are thought to worsen during pregnancy.

Renal angiomyolipomas, although usually asymptomatic, can cause bleeding if they grow large (eg, > 4 cm), usually manifesting as hematuria or flank pain.

Diagnosis

- Chest x-ray and HRCT
- Lung biopsy if HRCT is nondiagnostic

Diagnosis is suspected in young women with dyspnea plus interstitial changes with normal or increased lung volumes on chest x-ray, spontaneous pneumothorax, or chylous effusion. HRCT is done in all patients suspected of having the disorder; findings of multiple, small, diffusely distributed cysts are generally pathognomonic for LAM.

Biopsy (surgical) is indicated only when HRCT findings are nondiagnostic. Findings of an abnormal proliferation of smooth muscle cells (LAM cells) associated with cystic changes on histologic examination confirm disease.

Pulmonary function tests support the diagnosis and are especially useful for monitoring. Typical findings are of an obstructive or mixed obstructive and restrictive pattern. The lungs are usually hyperinflated with an increase in the total lung capacity (TLC) and thoracic gas volume. Gas trapping (an increase in residual volume [RV] and RV/TLC ratio) is commonly present. The Pao_2 and diffusing capacity for carbon monoxide (DLco) are commonly reduced. Exercise performance is decreased in most patients.

Prognosis

Prognosis is unclear because the disorder is so rare and because the clinical course of patients with LAM is variable. In general, the disease is slowly progressive, leading eventually to respiratory failure and death, but the time to death varies widely among reports. Median survival is likely > 8 yr from diagnosis. Lung function declines 2 to 3 times faster than it does in healthy people. Women should be advised that progression may accelerate during pregnancy.

Treatment

- Sirolimus or lung transplantation

Standard treatment is lung transplantation, but the disorder can recur in transplanted lungs.

Recent data suggest that sirolimus (an mTOR inhibitor) can help stabilize or slow the decline in pulmonary function among patients with moderate lung impairment (forced expiratory volume in 1 sec [FEV_1] < 70% predicted). Alternative treatments, such as hormonal manipulation with progestins, tamoxifen, and oophorectomy, are largely ineffective.

Pneumothoraxes may be difficult to manage because they are often recurrent, bilateral, and less responsive to standard measures. Recurrent pneumothorax requires pleural abrasion, talc or chemical pleurodesis, or pleurectomy. Embolization to prevent bleeding should be considered for angiomyolipomas > 4 cm.

Air travel is well-tolerated by most patients.

In the US, patients can receive education and psychologic support from the LAM Foundation.

KEY POINTS

- LAM can mimic interstitial lung disease but is actually a rare, slowly progressive growth of smooth muscle cells in various organs.
- Consider the diagnosis in young women with unexplained dyspnea plus interstitial changes with normal or increased lung volumes on chest x-ray, spontaneous pneumothorax, or chylous effusion.
- Do HRCT and, if results are inconclusive, biopsy.
- Consider sirolimus treatment for LAM with progressively decreasing pulmonary function.

PULMONARY ALVEOLAR PROTEINOSIS

Pulmonary alveolar proteinosis is accumulation of surfactant in alveoli. Etiology is almost always unknown. Symptoms are dyspnea, fatigue, and malaise. Diagnosis is based on bronchoalveolar lavage, although characteristic x-ray and laboratory test abnormalities occur. Treatment is with whole lung lavage or, in some cases, recombinant granulocyte-macrophage colony stimulating factor. Five-year survival is about 80% with treatment.

Etiology

Pulmonary alveolar proteinosis is most often idiopathic and occurs in otherwise healthy men and women between 30 and 50 yr. Rare secondary forms occur in patients with acute silicosis, *Pneumocystis jirovecii* infection, hematologic cancers, or immunosuppression by drugs and in patients with significant inhalation exposures to aluminum, titanium, cement, and cellulose dusts. Rare congenital forms that cause neonatal respiratory failure also exist. It is unclear whether idiopathic and secondary cases share a common pathophysiology.

Pathophysiology

Impaired alveolar macrophage processing of surfactant due to abnormal granulocyte-macrophage colony-stimulating factor (GM-CSF) signaling is thought to contribute to the disorder, perhaps due to reduced or absent function of the common beta chain of the GM-CSF/IL-13/IL-5 receptor on mononuclear cells (present in some children but not in adults with the disorder). Anti–GM-CSF antibodies have also been found in most patients. Toxic lung injury is suspected but not proved in secondary inhalation causes.

Alveoli are filled with acellular lipoprotein surfactant that stains periodic acid–Schiff (PAS) positive. Alveolar and interstitial cells remain normal. Posterobasal lung segments are mostly affected. The pleura and mediastinum are unaffected.

Symptoms and Signs

Most patients present with progressive exertional dyspnea and weight loss, fatigue, malaise, or low-grade fever. Cough, occasionally producing chunky or gummy sputum, occurs but is less common. Clubbing and cyanosis are uncommon. Inspiratory crackles are rare because alveoli are fluid-filled; when crackles are present, they suggest infection.

Diagnosis

- Bronchoalveolar lavage
- Sometimes biopsy

Pulmonary alveolar proteinosis is usually first suspected when a chest x-ray is taken for nonspecific respiratory symptoms. The x-ray shows bilateral mid- and lower-lung field opacities in a butterfly distribution with normal hila.

Bronchoalveolar lavage is done. Lavage fluid is milky or opaque, stains PAS-positive, and is characterized by scattered surfactant-engorged macrophages, an increase in T cells, and high levels of surfactant apoprotein-A.

Thoracoscopic or open lung biopsy is done when bronchoscopy is contraindicated or when specimens from lavage fluid are nondiagnostic. Tests typically done before treatment begins include

- HRCT
- Pulmonary function tests
- ABGs
- Laboratory tests

HRCT shows ground-glass opacification, thickened intralobular structures, and interlobular septa in typical polygonal shapes (crazy-paving). This finding is not specific, however, as it may also occur in patients with lipoid pneumonia, bronchoalveolar cell carcinoma, and *Pneumocystis jirovecii* pneumonia.

Pulmonary function tests show reduction in diffusing capacity for carbon monoxide (DLco) that is disproportionate to the decreases in vital capacity, residual volume, functional residual capacity, and total lung capacity.

Laboratory test abnormalities include polycythemia, hypergammaglobulinemia, increased serum LDH levels, and increased serum surfactant proteins A and D. Abnormalities are suggestive but nondiagnostic.

ABGs may show hypoxemia with mild to moderate exercise or at rest if disease is more severe.

Prognosis

Without treatment, pulmonary alveolar proteinosis remits spontaneously in up to 10% of patients. A single whole lung lavage is curative in up to 40%; other patients require lavage every 6 to 12 mo for many years. Five-year survival is about 80%; the most common cause of death is respiratory failure, typically occurring within the first year after diagnosis. Secondary pulmonary infections with bacterial (eg, *Mycobacteria*, *Nocardia*) and other organisms (*Aspergillus*, *Cryptococcus*, and other opportunistic fungi) occasionally develop because of impaired macrophage function; these infections require treatment.

Treatment

- Whole lung lavage

Treatment is unnecessary for patients without symptoms or for those with only mild symptoms. In patients with troubling dyspnea, whole lung lavage is done by using general anesthesia and a double-lumen endotracheal tube. Lavage of one lung is done up to 15 times with 1 to 2 L saline while the other lung is ventilated. The process is then reversed. Lung transplantation is not done because the disorder recurs in the transplanted lung.

Systemic corticosteroids play no role in management and may increase the risk of secondary infection. The role of GM-CSF (IV or sc) in management remains to be determined. An open-label study showed clinical improvement in 57% of the patients studied.

KEY POINTS

- Consider pulmonary alveolar proteinosis in otherwise healthy patients between ages 30 and 50 if the chest x-ray shows bilateral mid- and lower-lung field opacities in a butterfly distribution with normal hila.
- Do bronchoalveolar lavage; if contraindicated or when results are not diagnostic, do lung biopsy.
- If dyspnea is moderate or severe, treat with whole lung lavage.

PULMONARY LANGERHANS CELL HISTIOCYTOSIS

(Eosinophilic Granuloma; Histiocytosis X; Pulmonary Granulomatosis X)

Pulmonary Langerhans cell histiocytosis (PLCH) is proliferation of monoclonal Langerhans cells in lung interstitium and airspaces. Etiology is unknown, but cigarette smoking plays a primary role. Symptoms are dyspnea, cough, fatigue, and pleuritic chest pain. Diagnosis is based on history and imaging tests and sometimes on bronchoalveolar lavage and biopsy findings. Treatment is smoking cessation. Corticosteroids are given in many cases, but efficacy is unknown. Lung transplantation is usually curative when combined with smoking cessation. Five-year survival is about 74%. Patients are at increased risk of cancer.

PLCH is a disease in which monoclonal CD1a-positive Langerhans cells (a type of histiocyte) infiltrate the bronchioles and alveolar interstitium, accompanied by lymphocytes, plasma cells, neutrophils, and eosinophils. PLCH is one manifestation of Langerhans cell histiocytosis, which can affect organs in isolation (most notably the lungs, skin, bones, pituitary, and lymph nodes) or simultaneously. PLCH occurs in isolation ≥ 85% of the time.

The etiology of PLCH is unknown, but the disease occurs almost exclusively in whites 20 to 40 yr of age who smoke. Men and women are affected equally. Women develop disease later, but differences in age at onset by sex may represent differences in smoking behavior. Pathophysiology may involve recruitment and proliferation of Langerhans cells in response to cytokines and growth factors secreted by alveolar macrophages in response to cigarette smoke.

Symptoms and Signs

Typical symptoms and signs of PLCH are dyspnea, nonproductive cough, fatigue, fever, weight loss, and pleuritic chest pain. Ten percent to 25% of patients have sudden, spontaneous pneumothorax.

About 15% of patients are asymptomatic, with disease noted incidentally on a chest x-ray taken for another reason.

Bone pain due to bone cysts (18%), rash (13%), and polyuria due to diabetes insipidus (5%) are the most common manifestations of extrapulmonary involvement and occur in up to 15% of patients, rarely being the presenting symptoms of PLCH. There are few signs of PLCH; the physical examination results are usually normal.

Diagnosis

- HRCT
- Pulmonary function tests
- Sometimes bronchoscopy and biopsy

PLCH is suspected based on history and chest x-ray and is confirmed by HRCT and bronchoscopy with biopsy and bronchoalveolar lavage.

Chest x-ray classically shows bilaterally symmetric nodular opacities in the middle and upper lung fields with cystic changes and normal or increased lung volumes. The lung bases are often spared. Appearance may mimic COPD or lymphangioleiomyomatosis.

Confirmation on HRCT of middle and upper lobe cysts (often with bizarre shapes) and/or nodules with interstitial thickening is considered diagnostic of PLCH.

Pulmonary function test findings are normal, restrictive, obstructive, or mixed depending on when the test is done during the course of the disease. Most commonly, the diffusing capacity for carbon monoxide (DLco) is reduced and exercise is impaired.

Bronchoscopy and biopsy are indicated when imaging and pulmonary function tests are inconclusive. Finding > 5% of CD1a cells in bronchoalveolar lavage fluid is highly suggestive of the disease. Biopsy shows proliferation of Langerhans cells with occasional clustering of eosinophils (the origin of the outdated term eosinophilic granuloma) in the midst of cellular and fibrotic nodules that may take on a stellate configuration. Immunohistochemical staining is positive for CD1a, S-100 protein, and HLA-DR antigens.

Prognosis

Spontaneous resolution of symptoms occurs in some patients with minimally symptomatic disease; 5-yr survival is about 75%, and median survival is 12 yr. However, some patients develop slowly progressive disease, for which the clinical markers include continued smoking, age extremes, multiorgan involvement, persistent constitutional symptoms, numerous cysts on chest x-ray, reduced DLco, low forced expiratory volume in 1 sec (FEV_1)/ forced vital capacity (FVC) ratio (< 66%), high residual volume (RV)/total lung capacity (TLC) ratio (> 33%), and need for prolonged corticosteroid use. Cause of death is respiratory insufficiency or cancer. Lung cancer risk is increased because of cigarette smoking.

Treatment

- Smoking cessation
- Possibly corticosteroids and cytotoxic drugs or lung transplantation

The main treatment is smoking cessation, which leads to symptom resolution in up to one-third of patients.

Empiric use of corticosteroids and cytotoxic drugs is common practice even though their effectiveness is unproved.

Lung transplantation is an option for otherwise healthy patients with accelerating respiratory insufficiency, but the disorder may recur in the transplanted lung if the patient continues or resumes smoking.

KEY POINTS

- In PLCH, monoclonal Langerhans cells proliferate in alveolar interstitium and bronchioles.
- Consider PLCH in patients age 20 to 40 who smoke and in whom chest x-ray shows bilaterally symmetric nodular opacities in the middle and upper lung fields with cystic changes.
- Confirm the diagnosis with HRCT or, if results are inconclusive, lung biopsy.
- Recommend smoking cessation.
- Consider corticosteroids and cytotoxic drugs and, if smoking has ceased, lung transplantation.

58 Lung Abscess

Lung abscess is a necrotizing lung infection characterized by a pus-filled cavitary lesion. It is most commonly caused by aspiration of oral secretions by patients who have impaired consciousness. Symptoms are persistent cough, fever, sweats, and weight loss. Diagnosis is based primarily on chest x-ray. Treatment usually is with clindamycin or combination β-lactam/β-lactamase inhibitors.

Etiology

- Aspiration of oral secretions (most common)
- Endobronchial obstruction
- Hematogenous seeding of the lungs (less common)

Most lung abscesses develop after aspiration of oral secretions by patients with gingivitis or poor oral hygiene. Typically, patients have altered consciousness as a result of alcohol intoxication, illicit drugs, anesthesia, sedatives, or opioids. Older patients and those unable to handle their oral secretions, often because of neurologic disease, are also at risk. Lung abscesses can also develop secondary to endobronchial obstruction (eg, due to bronchial carcinoma) or to immunosuppression (eg, due to HIV/AIDS or after transplantation and use of immunosuppressive drugs).

A less common cause of lung abscess is necrotizing pneumonia that may develop from hematogenous seeding of the lungs due to suppurative thromboembolism (eg, septic embolism due to IV drug use) or right-sided endocarditis. In contrast to aspiration and obstruction, these conditions typically cause multiple rather than isolated lung abscesses.

Pathogens: The most common pathogens of lung abscesses due to aspiration are anaerobic bacteria, but about half of all cases involve both anaerobic and aerobic organisms (see Table 58–1). The most common anaerobic pathogens are *Peptostreptococcus, Fusobacterium, Prevotella,* and *Bacteroides*. The most common aerobic pathogens are streptococci and staphylococci—sometimes methicillin-resistant *Staphylococcus aureus* (MRSA). Occasionally, cases are due to gram-negative bacteria, especially *Klebsiella*. Immunocompromised patients with lung abscess are most commonly infected with *Pseudomonas aeruginosa* and other gram-negative bacilli but also may have infection with *Nocardia*, *Mycobacteria* sp, or fungi. Rare cases of pulmonary gangrene or fulminant pneumonia with sepsis have been reported with pathogens such as MRSA, *Pneumococcus*, and *Klebsiella*. Some patients, especially those from developing countries, are at risk of abscess due to *Mycobacterium tuberculosis*, and rare cases are due to amebic infection (eg, with *Entamoeba histolytica*), paragonimiasis, or infection with *Burkholderia pseudomallei*.

Introduction of these pathogens into the lungs first causes inflammation, which, over a week or two, leads to tissue necrosis and then abscess formation. The abscess usually ruptures into a bronchus, and its contents are expectorated, leaving an air- and fluid-filled cavity. In about one-third of cases, direct or indirect extension (via bronchopleural fistula) into the pleural cavity results in empyema.

Symptoms and Signs

Symptoms of abscess due to anaerobic bacteria or mixed anaerobic and aerobic bacteria are usually chronic (eg, occurring over weeks or months) and include productive cough, fever, night sweats, and weight loss. Patients may also present with hemoptysis and pleuritic chest pain. Sputum may be purulent or blood-streaked and classically smells or tastes foul.

Symptoms of abscess due to aerobic bacteria develop more acutely and resemble bacterial pneumonia. Abscesses due to organisms other than anaerobes (eg, *Mycobacteria, Nocardia*) lack putrid respiratory secretions and may be more likely to occur in nondependent lung regions.

Signs of lung abscess, when present, are nonspecific and resemble those of pneumonia: decreased breath sounds indicating consolidation or effusion, temperature ≥ 38° C, crackles over the affected area, egophony, and dullness to percussion in the presence of effusion. Patients typically have signs of periodontal disease and a history of a predisposing cause of aspiration, such as dysphagia or a condition causing impaired consciousness.

Table 58–1. INFECTIOUS CAUSES OF CAVITARY LUNG LESIONS

CAUSES	EXAMPLES (DISORDER)
Aerobic organisms	*Burkholderia pseudomallei**
	*Klebsiella pneumonia**
	Nocardia sp†
	*Pseudomonas aeruginosa**
	Staphylococcus aureus‡
	Streptococcus milleri‡
	Other streptococci‡
Anaerobic organisms	*Actinomyces* sp†
	Bacteroides sp*
	Clostridium sp†
	Fusobacterium sp*
	Peptostreptococcus sp‡
	Prevotella sp*
Fungi	*Aspergillus* sp (aspergillosis)
	Blastomyces dermatitidis (blastomycosis)
	Coccidioides immitis (coccidioidomycosis)
	Cryptococcus neoformans (cryptococcosis)
	Histoplasma capsulatum (histoplasmosis)
	Pneumocystis jirovecii
	Rhizomucor (mucormycosis)
	Rhizopus sp (mucormycosis)
	Sporothrix schenckii (sporotrichosis)
Mycobacteria	*Mycobacterium avium-cellulare*
	Mycobacterium kansasii
	Mycobacterium tuberculosis
Parasites	*Entamoeba histolytica* (amebiasis)
	Echinococcus granulosus (echinococcosis)
	Echinococcus multilocularis (echinococcosis)
	Paragonimus westermani (paragonimiasis)

*Gram-negative bacilli.
†Gram-positive bacilli.
‡Gram-positive cocci.

Diagnosis

- Chest x-ray
- Sometimes CT
- Sputum cultures (unless anaerobic infection is very likely), including for fungi and mycobacteria
- Bronchoscopy as needed to exclude cancer, detect unusual pathogens such as fungi or mycobacteria, and in immunocompromised patients
- Culture of any pleural fluid

Lung abscess is suspected based on history in a patient who is aspiration-prone due to altered consciousness or dysphagia and is confirmed by chest x-ray showing cavitation.

Cavitary pulmonary lesions are not always caused by infection. Noninfectious causes of cavitary pulmonary lesions include the following:

- Empyema or bulla with air-fluid level
- Cystic (saccular) bronchiectasis
- Lung cancer
- Lung infarction
- Nodular silicosis nodule with central necrosis
- Pulmonary embolism
- Pulmonary sequestration
- Sarcoidosis
- Granulomatosis with polyangiitis (Wegener granulomatosis)

In an anaerobic infection due to aspiration, chest x-ray classically shows consolidation with a single cavity containing an air-fluid level in portions of the lung that would be dependent when the patient is recumbent (eg, the posterior segments of the upper lobes or the superior or lateral basal segments of the lower lobes). This pattern helps distinguish anaerobic abscess from other causes of cavitary pulmonary disease, because diffuse or embolic pulmonary disease often causes multiple cavitations, and TB typically involves the apices.

CT is not routinely needed (eg, if cavitation is clear on chest x-ray in a patient who has risk factors for lung abscess). However, CT may be useful when cavitation is suggested but not clearly seen on the chest x-ray, when an underlying pulmonary mass obstructing the drainage of a lung segment is suspected, or when abscess needs to be differentiated from empyema or bulla with an air-fluid level.

Bronchial carcinoma can lead to obstruction that causes pneumonia and abscess formation. Bronchial carcinoma should be suspected in patients who do not respond to antimicrobial treatment or have atypical findings such as a cavitary lesion and no fever. Bronchoscopy is sometimes done to exclude cancer or the presence of a foreign body or to detect unusual pathogens, such as fungi or mycobacteria. Bronchoscopy is done if patients are immunocompromised.

Cultures: Anaerobic bacteria are rarely identifiable on culture because uncontaminated specimens are difficult to obtain and because most laboratories do not culture anaerobes well or often. If sputum is putrid, then anaerobic infection is assumed to be the cause. However, if empyema is present, pleural fluid provides a good source for anaerobic culture.

When clinical findings make anaerobic infection less likely, aerobic, fungal, or mycobacterial infection should be suspected, and attempts should be made to identify a pathogen. Cultures of sputum, bronchoscopic aspirates, or both are helpful.

Treatment

- IV antibiotics or, for less seriously affected patients, oral antibiotics
- Percutaneous or surgical drainage of any abscess that does not respond to antibiotics or of any empyema

Treatment is with antibiotics. Clindamycin 600 mg IV q 6 to 8 h is usually the drug of choice because it has excellent activity against streptococci and anaerobic organisms. The primary alternative is a combination β-lactam/β-lactamase inhibitor (eg, ampicillin/sulbactam 1 to 2 g IV q 6 h). Other alternatives include a carbapenem (eg, imipenem/cilastatin 500 mg IV q 6 h) or combination therapy with metronidazole 500 mg q 8 h plus penicillin 2 million units IV q 6 h. Less seriously ill patients may be given oral antibiotics such as clindamycin 300 mg po q 6 h or amoxicillin/clavulanate 875/125 mg po q 12 h. IV regimens can be converted to oral ones when the patient defervesces. For very serious infections involving MSRA, the best treatment is vancomycin or linezolid.

Optimal duration of treatment is unknown, but common practice is to treat until the chest x-ray shows complete resolution or a small, stable, residual scar, which generally takes 3 to 6 wk or longer. In general, the larger the abscess, the longer it will take for x-rays to show resolution.

Most authorities do not recommend chest physical therapy and postural drainage because of the potential for spillage of infection into other bronchi with extension of the infection or acute obstruction.

An accompanying empyema must be drained. Surgical removal or drainage of lung abscesses is necessary in the roughly

10% of patients in whom lesions do not respond to antibiotics, and those who develop pulmonary gangrene. Resistance to antibiotic treatment is most common with large cavities and with post-obstructive abscesses. If patients fail to defervesce or to improve clinically after 7 to 10 days, they should be evaluated for resistant or unusual pathogens, airway obstruction, and noninfectious causes of cavitation.

When surgery is necessary, lobectomy is the most common procedure; segmental resection may suffice for small lesions (< 6 cm diameter cavity). Pneumonectomy may be necessary for multiple abscesses unresponsive to drug therapy or for pulmonary gangrene. In patients likely to have difficulty tolerating surgery, percutaneous drainage or, rarely, bronchoscopic placement of a pigtail catheter can help facilitate drainage.

KEY POINTS

- Lung abscesses are most often caused by aspiration of oral secretions by patients who have impaired consciousness; thus, anaerobic bacteria are among the common pathogens.
- Suspect lung abscess in patients prone to aspiration, who have subacute constitutional and pulmonary symptoms, and whose chest x-ray shows compatible lesions such as cavities.
- Treat initially with antibiotics; if patients do not respond within 7 to 10 days, evaluate them for unusual or resistant pathogens, bronchial obstructive lesions, and noninfectious causes of lung cavitation.
- Drain empyemas and consider surgical removal or drainage of lung abscesses that do not respond to drug therapy and for pulmonary gangrene.

59 Mediastinal and Pleural Disorders

MEDIASTINAL MASSES

Mediastinal masses are caused by a variety of cysts and tumors; likely causes differ by patient age and by location of the mass (anterior, middle, or posterior mediastinum). The masses may be asymptomatic (in adults) or cause obstructive respiratory symptoms (in children). Testing involves CT with biopsy and adjunctive tests as needed. Treatment differs by cause.

Etiology

Mediastinal masses are divided into those that occur in the anterior, middle, and posterior mediastinum. The anterior mediastinum extends from the sternum to the pericardium and brachiocephalic vessels posteriorly. The middle mediastinum lies between the anterior and posterior mediastinum. The posterior mediastinum is bounded by the pericardium and trachea anteriorly and the vertebral column posteriorly.

Adults: In adults, the **most common** causes vary by location:

- Anterior mediastinum: Thymomas and lymphomas (both Hodgkin and non-Hodgkin)
- Middle mediastinum: Lymph node enlargement and vascular masses
- Posterior mediastinum: Neurogenic tumors and esophageal abnormalities

For other causes, see Fig. 59–1.

Children: In children, the most common mediastinal masses are neurogenic tumors and cysts. For other causes, see Table 59–1.

Symptoms and Signs

Many mediastinal masses are asymptomatic. In general, malignant lesions and masses in children are much more likely to cause symptoms. The most common symptoms are chest pain and weight loss. Lymphomas may manifest with fever and weight loss. In children, mediastinal masses are more likely to cause tracheobronchial compression and stridor or symptoms of recurrent bronchitis or pneumonia.

Symptoms and signs also depend on location. Large anterior mediastinal masses may cause dyspnea when patients are lying supine. Lesions in the middle mediastinum may compress blood vessels or airways, causing the superior vena cava syndrome or airway obstruction. Lesions in the posterior mediastinum may encroach on the esophagus, causing dysphagia or odynophagia.

Diagnosis

- Chest x-ray
- CT
- Sometimes tissue examination

Mediastinal masses are most often incidentally discovered on chest x-ray or other imaging tests during an examination for chest symptoms. Additional diagnostic testing, usually imaging and biopsy, is indicated to determine etiology.

CT with IV contrast is the most valuable imaging technique. With thoracic CT, normal variants and benign tumors, such as fat- and fluid-filled cysts, can be distinguished from other processes.

A definitive diagnosis can be obtained for many mediastinal masses with needle aspiration or needle biopsy. Fine-needle aspiration techniques usually suffice for carcinomatous lesions, but a cutting-needle biopsy should be done whenever lymphoma, thymoma, or a neural mass is suspected. If ectopic thyroid tissue is considered, thyroid-stimulating hormone is measured.

Treatment

- Depends on cause

Treatment depends on etiology. Some benign lesions, such as pericardial cysts, can be observed. Most malignant tumors should be removed surgically, but some, such as lymphomas, are best treated with chemotherapy. Granulomatous disease should be treated with the appropriate antimicrobial drug.

KEY POINTS

- In adults, thymomas and lymphomas (both Hodgkin and non-Hodgkin) are the most common anterior lesions, lymph node enlargement and vascular masses are the most common middle lesions, and neurogenic tumors and esophageal abnormalities are the most common posterior lesions.

- In children, the most common mediastinal masses are neurogenic tumors and cysts.
- The most common symptoms are chest pain and weight loss, but many masses are asymptomatic.
- Obstructive respiratory symptoms can occur in children.
- CT with IV contrast is the most valuable imaging technique.

Table 59–1. SOME CAUSES OF MEDIASTINAL MASSES IN CHILDREN

LOCATION	CAUSE
Anterior	Ectopic thyroid Lymphoma Sarcoma Teratoma
Middle	Bronchogenic cyst Cardiac tumor Cystic hygroma Lymphadenopathy Lymphoma Pericardial cyst Vascular abnormalities
Posterior	Esophageal duplication Meningomyelocele Neuroenteric abnormalities Neurogenic tumors

MEDIASTINITIS

Mediastinitis is inflammation of the mediastinum. Acute mediastinitis usually results from esophageal perforation or median sternotomy. Symptoms include severe chest pain, dyspnea, and fever. The diagnosis is confirmed by chest x-ray or CT. Treatment is with antibiotics (eg, clindamycin plus ceftriaxone) and sometimes surgery.

The 2 most common causes of acute mediastinitis are

- Esophageal perforation
- Median sternotomy

Esophageal perforation: Esophageal perforation may complicate esophagoscopy or insertion of a Sengstaken-Blakemore or Minnesota tube (for esophageal variceal bleeding). Rarely, it results from forceful vomiting (Boerhaave syndrome). Another possible cause is swallowing caustic substances (eg, lye, certain button batteries). Certain pills or esophageal ulcers (eg, in AIDS patients with esophagitis) can contribute.

Patients with esophageal perforation become acutely ill within hours, with severe chest pain and dyspnea due to mediastinal inflammation.

Diagnosis is usually obvious from clinical presentation and a history of instrumentation or of another risk factor. The diagnosis should also be considered in patients who are very ill, have chest pain, and may have a risk factor that they cannot describe (eg, in intoxicated patients who may have vomited forcefully but do not remember and in preverbal children who may have ingested a button battery). The diagnosis is confirmed by chest x-ray or CT showing air in the mediastinum.

Treatment is with parenteral antibiotics selected to be effective against oral and GI flora (eg, clindamycin 450 mg IV q 6 h plus ceftriaxone 2 g once/day, for at least 2 wk). Patients who have severe mediastinitis with pleural effusion or pneumothorax require emergency exploration of the mediastinum with primary repair of the esophageal tear and drainage of the pleural space and mediastinum.

Median sternotomy: This procedure is complicated by mediastinitis in about 1% of cases. Patients most commonly present with wound drainage or sepsis. Diagnosis is based on finding infected fluid obtained by a needle aspiration through the sternum. Treatment consists of immediate surgical drainage, debridement, and parenteral broad-spectrum antibiotics. Mortality approaches 50% in some series.

Chronic fibrosing mediastinitis: This condition usually is due to TB or histoplasmosis but can be due to sarcoidosis,

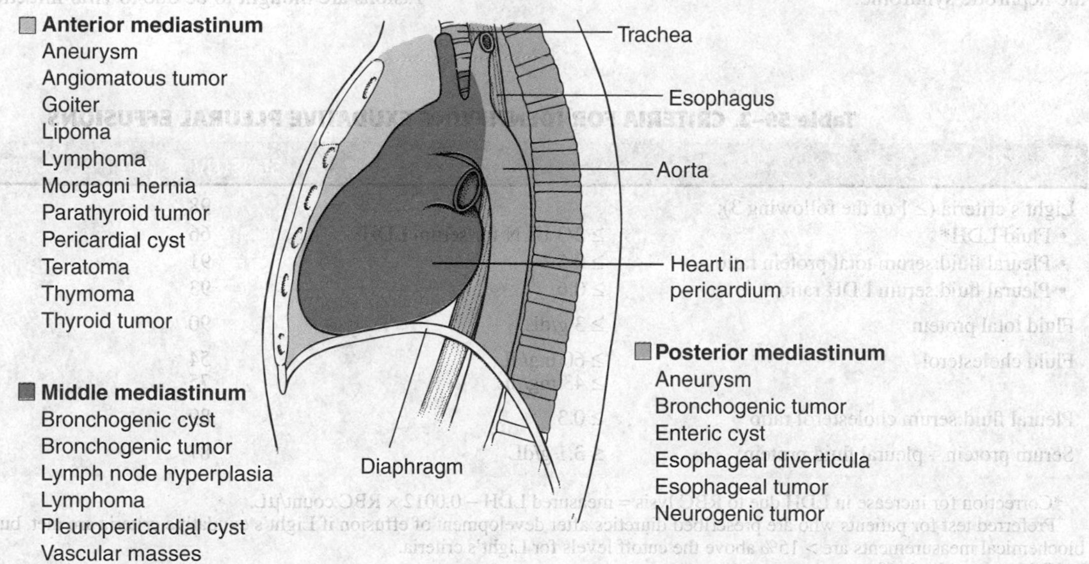

Fig. 59–1. Some causes of mediastinal masses in adults.

silicosis, or other fungal diseases. An intense fibrotic process develops, leading to compression of mediastinal structures that can cause the superior vena cava syndrome, tracheal narrowing, or obstruction of the pulmonary arteries or veins.

Diagnosis is based on CT. If the cause is TB, anti-TB therapy is indicated. Otherwise, no known treatment is beneficial, but insertion of vascular or airway stents can be considered.

PLEURAL EFFUSION

Pleural effusions are accumulations of fluid within the pleural space. They have multiple causes and usually are classified as transudates or exudates. Detection is by physical examination and chest x-ray; thoracentesis and pleural fluid analysis are often required to determine cause. Asymptomatic transudates require no treatment. Symptomatic transudates and almost all exudates require thoracentesis, chest tube drainage, pleurodesis, pleurectomy, or a combination.

Normally, 10 to 20 mL of pleural fluid, similar in composition to plasma but lower in protein (< 1.5 g/dL), is spread thinly over visceral and parietal pleurae, facilitating movement between the lungs and chest wall. The fluid enters the pleural space from systemic capillaries in the parietal pleurae and exits via parietal pleural stomas and lymphatics. Pleural fluid accumulates when too much fluid enters or too little exits the pleural space.

Etiology

Pleural effusions are usually categorized as transudates or exudates based on laboratory characteristics of the fluid (see Table 59–2). Whether unilateral or bilateral, a transudate can usually be treated without extensive evaluation, whereas the cause of an exudate requires investigation. There are numerous causes (see Table 59–3).

Transudative effusions are caused by some combination of increased hydrostatic pressure and decreased plasma oncotic pressure. Heart failure is the most common cause, followed by cirrhosis with ascites and by hypoalbuminemia, usually due to the nephrotic syndrome.

Exudative effusions are caused by local processes leading to increased capillary permeability resulting in exudation of fluid, protein, cells, and other serum constituents. Causes are numerous; the most common are pneumonia, cancer, pulmonary embolism, viral infection, and TB. Yellow nail syndrome is a rare disorder causing chronic exudative pleural effusions, lymphedema, and dystrophic yellow nails—all thought to be the result of impaired lymphatic drainage.

Chylous effusion (chylothorax) is a milky white effusion high in triglycerides caused by traumatic or neoplastic (most often lymphomatous) damage to the thoracic duct. Chylous effusion also occurs with the superior vena cava syndrome.

Chyliform (cholesterol or pseudochylous) effusions resemble chylous effusions but are low in triglycerides and high in cholesterol. Chyliform effusions are thought to be due to release of cholesterol from lysed RBCs and neutrophils in long-standing effusions when absorption is blocked by the thickened pleura.

Hemothorax is bloody fluid (pleural fluid Hct > 50% peripheral Hct) in the pleural space due to trauma or, rarely, as a result of coagulopathy or after rupture of a major blood vessel, such as the aorta or pulmonary artery.

Empyema is pus in the pleural space. It can occur as a complication of pneumonia, thoracotomy, abscesses (lung, hepatic, or subdiaphragmatic), or penetrating trauma with secondary infection. Empyema necessitatis is soft-tissue extension of empyema leading to chest wall infection and external drainage.

Trapped lung is a lung encased by a fibrous peel caused by empyema or tumor. Because the lung cannot expand, the pleural pressure becomes more negative than normal, increasing transudation of fluid from parietal pleural capillaries. The fluid characteristically is borderline between a transudate and an exudate; ie, the biochemical values are within 15% of the cutoff levels for Light's criteria (see Table 59–2).

Iatrogenic effusions can be caused by migration or misplacement of a feeding tube into the trachea or perforation of the superior vena cava by a central venous catheter, leading to infusion of tube feedings or IV solution into the pleural space.

Effusions with no obvious cause are often due to occult pulmonary emboli, TB, or cancer. Etiology is unknown for about 15% of effusions even after extensive study; many of these effusions are thought to be due to viral infection.

Table 59–2. CRITERIA FOR IDENTIFYING EXUDATIVE PLEURAL EFFUSIONS

TEST	EXUDATE	SENSITIVITY (%)	SPECIFICITY (%)
Light's criteria (≥ 1 of the following 3):		98	77
• Fluid LDH*	≥ 2/3 ULN for serum LDH	66	100
• Pleural fluid:serum total protein ratio	≥ 0.5	91	89
• Pleural fluid:serum LDH ratio	≥ 0.6	93	82
Fluid total protein	≥ 3 g/dL	90	90
Fluid cholesterol	≥ 60 mg/dL	54	92
	≥ 43 mg/dL	75	80
Pleural fluid:serum cholesterol ratio	≥ 0.3	89	71
Serum protein – pleural fluid protein†	≤ 3.1 g/dL	87	92

*Correction for increase in LDH due to RBC lysis = measured LDH – 0.0012 × RBC count/μL.

†Preferred test for patients who are prescribed diuretics after development of effusion if Light's exudative criteria are met, but none of the biochemical measurements are > 15% above the cutoff levels for Light's criteria.

ULN = upper limit of normal.

Data modified from Light RW: Pleural effusion. *New England Journal of Medicine* 346:1971–1977, 2002.

Table 59–3. CAUSES OF PLEURAL EFFUSION

CAUSE	COMMENTS
Transudate	
Heart failure	Bilateral effusions in 81%; right-sided in 12%; left-sided in 7% With left ventricular failure, there is increased interstitial fluid, which crosses the visceral pleura and enters the pleural space
Cirrhosis with ascites (hepatic hydrothorax)	Right-sided effusions in 70%; left-sided in 15%; bilateral in 15% Ascitic fluid migration to the pleural space through diaphragmatic defects Effusion present in about 5% of patients with clinically apparent ascites
Hypoalbuminemia	Uncommon Bilateral effusions in > 90% Decreased intravascular oncotic pressure causing transudation into the pleural space Associated with edema or anasarca elsewhere
Nephrotic syndrome	Usually bilateral effusions; commonly subpulmonic Decreased intravascular oncotic pressure plus hypervolemia causing transudation into the pleural space
Hydronephrosis	Retroperitoneal urine dissection into the pleural space, causing urinothorax
Constrictive pericarditis	Increases IV hydrostatic pressure In some patients, accompanied by massive anasarca and ascites due to a mechanism similar to that for hepatic hydrothorax
Atelectasis	Increases negative intrapleural pressure
Peritoneal dialysis	Mechanism similar to that for hepatic hydrothorax Pleural fluid with characteristics similar to dialysate
Trapped lung	Encasement with fibrous peel increasing negative intrapleural pressure May be exudative or borderline effusion
Systemic capillary leak syndrome	Rare Accompanied by anasarca and pericardial effusion
Myxedema	Effusion present in about 5% Usually transudate if pericardial effusion is also present; either transudate or exudate if pleural effusion is isolated
Exudate	
Pneumonia (parapneumonic effusion)	May be uncomplicated or loculated and/or purulent (empyema) Thoracentesis necessary to differentiate
Cancer	Most commonly lung cancer, breast cancer, or lymphoma but possible with any tumor metastatic to pleurae Typically causing dull, aching chest pain
Pulmonary embolism	Effusion present in about 30%: Almost always exudative; bloody in < 50% Pulmonary embolism suspected when dyspnea is disproportionate to size of effusion
Viral infection	Effusion usually small with or without parenchymal infiltrate Predominantly systemic symptoms rather than pulmonary symptoms
Coronary artery bypass surgery	Effusions left-sided or larger on the left in 73%; bilateral and equal in 20%; right-sided or larger on the right in 7% > 25% of the hemithorax filled with fluid 30 days postoperatively in 10% of patients Bloody effusions related to postoperative bleeding likely to resolve Nonbloody effusions likely to recur; etiology unknown but probably with an immunologic basis
TB	Effusion usually unilateral and ipsilateral to parenchymal infiltrates if present Effusion due to hypersensitivity reaction to TB protein Pleural fluid TB cultures positive in < 20%
Sarcoidosis	Effusion in 1–2% Extensive parenchymal sarcoid and often extrathoracic sarcoid Pleural fluid predominantly lymphocytic
Uremia	Effusion in about 3% In > 50%, symptoms secondary to effusion: Most commonly fever (50%), chest pain (30%), cough (35%), and dyspnea (20%) Diagnosis of exclusion

Table continues on the following page.

Table 59–3. CAUSES OF PLEURAL EFFUSION (*Continued*)

CAUSE	COMMENTS
Infradiaphragmatic abscess	Causes sympathetic subpulmonic effusion Neutrophils predominant in pleural fluid pH and glucose normal
HIV infection	Many possible etiologic factors: Pneumonias (parapneumonic), including *Pneumocystis jirovecii* pneumonia, other opportunistic infections, TB, and pulmonary Kaposi sarcoma
RA	Effusion typically in elderly men with rheumatoid nodules and deforming arthritis Must differentiate from parapneumonic effusion
SLE	Effusion possibly first manifestation of SLE Common with drug-induced SLE Diagnosis established by serologic tests of blood, not of pleural fluid
Drugs	Many drugs, most notably bromocriptine, dantrolene, nitrofurantoin, IL-2 (for treatment of renal cell cancer and melanoma), and methysergide
Ovarian hyperstimulation syndrome	Syndrome occurring as a complication of ovulation induction with human chorionic gonadotropin (hCG) and occasionally clomiphene Effusion developing 7–14 days after hCG injection Effusion right-sided in 52%; bilateral in 27%
Pancreatitis	**Acute:** Effusion present in about 50%: Bilateral in 77%; left-sided in 16%; right-sided in 8% Effusion due to transdiaphragmatic transfer of the exudative inflammatory fluid and diaphragmatic inflammation **Chronic:** Effusion due to sinus tract from pancreatic pseudocyst through diaphragm into pleural space Predominantly chest symptoms rather than abdominal symptoms Patients presenting with cachexia that resembles cancer
Superior vena cava syndrome	Effusion usually caused by blockage of intrathoracic venous and lymphatic flow by cancer or thrombosis in a central catheter May be an exudate or a chylothorax
Esophageal rupture	Patients extremely sick Medical emergency Morbidity and mortality due to infection of the mediastinum and pleural space
Benign asbestos pleural effusion	Effusion occurring > 30 yr after initial exposure Frequently asymptomatic Tends to come and go Must rule out mesothelioma
Benign ovarian tumor (Meigs syndrome)	Mechanism similar to that for hepatic hydrothorax Surgery sometimes indicated for patients with ovarian mass, ascites, and pleural effusion For diagnosis, disappearance of ascites and effusion postoperatively required
Yellow nail syndrome	Triad of pleural effusion, lymphedema, and yellow nails, sometimes appearing decades apart Pleural fluid with relatively high protein but low LDH Tendency for effusion to recur No pleuritic chest pain

Symptoms and Signs

Some pleural effusions are asymptomatic and are discovered incidentally during physical examination or on chest x-ray. Many cause dyspnea, pleuritic chest pain, or both. Pleuritic chest pain, a vague discomfort or sharp pain that worsens during inspiration, indicates inflammation of the parietal pleura. Pain is usually felt over the inflamed site, but referred pain is possible. The posterior and peripheral portions of the diaphragmatic pleura are supplied by the lower 6 intercostal nerves, and irritation there may cause pain in the lower chest wall or abdomen that may simulate intra-abdominal disease. Irritation of the central portion of the diaphragmatic pleura, innervated by the phrenic nerves, causes pain referred to the neck and shoulder.

Physical examination reveals absent tactile fremitus, dullness to percussion, and decreased breath sounds on the side of the effusion. These findings can also be caused by pleural thickening. With large-volume effusions, respiration is usually rapid and shallow. A pleural friction rub, although infrequent, is the classic physical sign. The friction rub varies from a few intermittent sounds that may simulate crackles to a fully developed harsh grating, creaking, or leathery sound synchronous with respiration, heard during inspiration and expiration. Friction sounds adjacent to the heart (pleuropericardial rub) may vary with the heartbeat and may be confused with the friction rub of pericarditis. Pericardial rub is best heard over the left border of the sternum in the 3rd and 4th intercostal spaces, is characteristically a to-and-fro sound synchronous with the heartbeat, and is not influenced significantly by respiration. Sensitivity and specificity of the physical examination for detecting effusion are probably low.

Diagnosis

- Chest x-ray
- Pleural fluid analysis
- Sometimes CT angiography or other tests

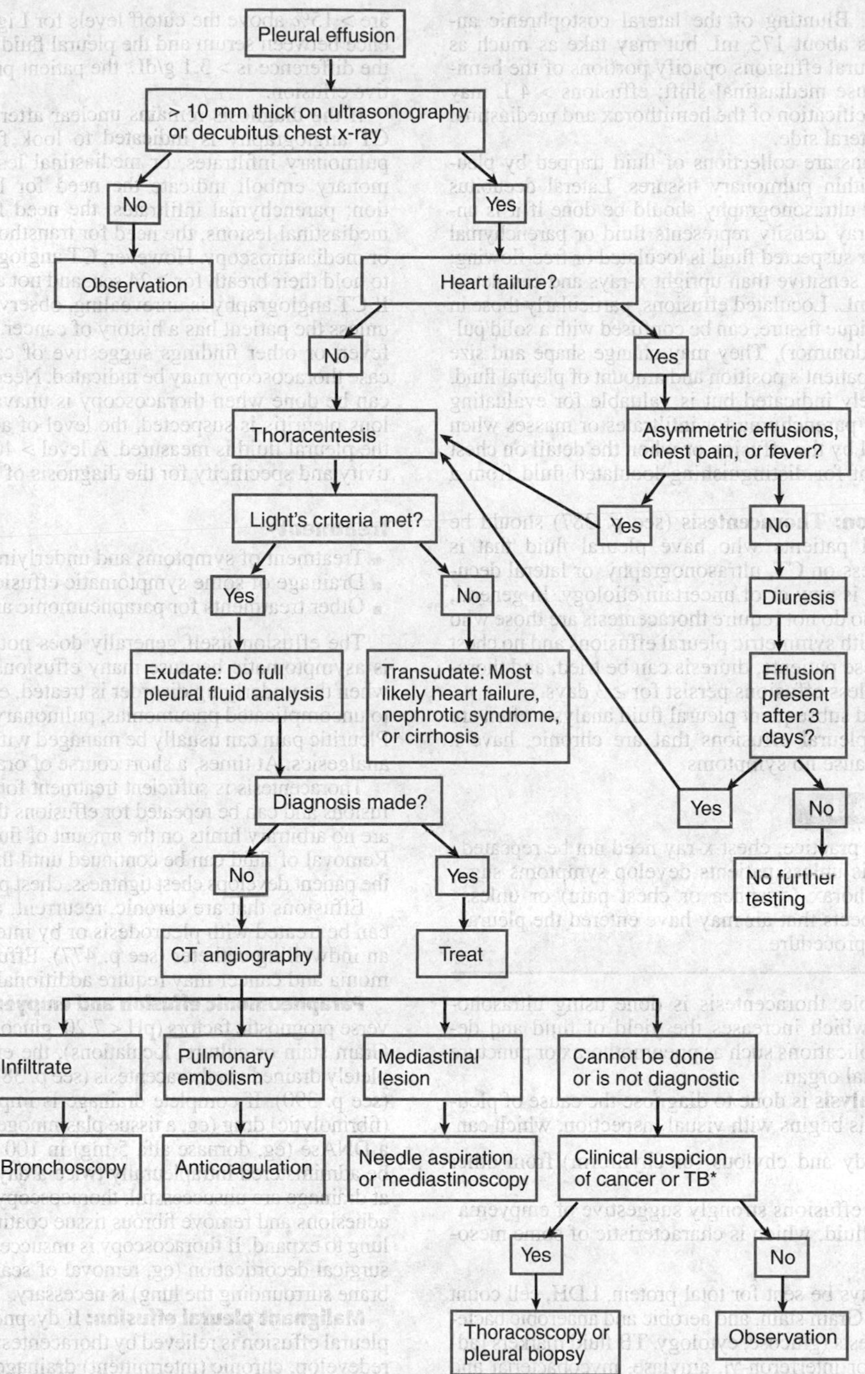

*Based on presence of fever, weight loss, history of cancer, or other suggestive symptoms.

Fig. 59–2. Diagnosis of pleural effusion.

Pleural effusion is suspected in patients with pleuritic pain, unexplained dyspnea, or suggestive signs. Diagnostic tests are indicated to document the presence of pleural fluid and to determine its cause (see Fig. 59–2).

Presence of effusion: Chest x-ray is the first test done to confirm the presence of pleural fluid. The lateral upright chest x-ray should be examined when a pleural effusion is suspected. In an upright x-ray, 75 mL of fluid blunts the posterior costophrenic angle. Blunting of the lateral costophrenic angle usually requires about 175 mL but may take as much as 500 mL. Larger pleural effusions opacify portions of the hemithorax and may cause mediastinal shift; effusions > 4 L may cause complete opacification of the hemithorax and mediastinal shift to the contralateral side.

Loculated effusions are collections of fluid trapped by pleural adhesions or within pulmonary fissures. Lateral decubitus x-rays, chest CT, or ultrasonography should be done if it is unclear whether an x-ray density represents fluid or parenchymal infiltrates or whether suspected fluid is loculated or free-flowing; these tests are more sensitive than upright x-rays and can detect fluid volumes < 10 mL. Loculated effusions, particularly those in the horizontal or oblique fissure, can be confused with a solid pulmonary mass (pseudotumor). They may change shape and size with changes in the patient's position and amount of pleural fluid.

CT is not routinely indicated but is valuable for evaluating the underlying lung parenchyma for infiltrates or masses when the lung is obscured by the effusion or when the detail on chest x-rays is insufficient for distinguishing loculated fluid from a solid mass.

Cause of effusion: **Thoracentesis** (see p. 387) should be done in almost all patients who have pleural fluid that is ≥ 10 mm in thickness on CT, ultrasonography, or lateral decubitus x-ray and that is new or of uncertain etiology. In general, the only patients who do not require thoracentesis are those who have heart failure with symmetric pleural effusions and no chest pain or fever; in these patients, diuresis can be tried, and thoracentesis avoided unless effusions persist for ≥ 3 days.

Thoracentesis and subsequent pleural fluid analysis often are not necessary for pleural effusions that are chronic, have a known cause, and cause no symptoms.

PEARLS & PITFALLS

- Despite common practice, chest x-ray need not be repeated after thoracentesis unless patients develop symptoms suggesting pneumothorax (dyspnea or chest pain) or unless the clinician suspects that air may have entered the pleural space during the procedure.

Whenever possible, thoracentesis is done using ultrasonographic guidance, which increases the yield of fluid and decreases risk of complications such as pneumothorax or puncture of an intra-abdominal organ.

Pleural fluid analysis is done to diagnose the cause of pleural effusion. Analysis begins with visual inspection, which can

- Distinguish bloody and chylous (or chyliform) from other effusions
- Identify purulent effusions strongly suggestive of empyema
- Identify viscous fluid, which is characteristic of some mesotheliomas

Fluid should always be sent for total protein, LDH, cell count and cell differential, Gram stain, and aerobic and anaerobic bacterial cultures. Other tests (glucose, cytology, TB fluid markers [adenosine deaminase or interferon-γ], amylase, mycobacterial and fungal stains and cultures) are used in appropriate clinical settings.

Fluid chemistries help distinguish transudates from exudates; multiple criteria exist, but not one perfectly discriminates between the 2 types. When Light's criteria are used (see Table 59–2 on p. 470), serum LDH and total protein levels should be measured as close as possible to the time of thoracentesis for comparison with those in pleural fluid. Light's criteria correctly identify almost all exudates but misidentify about 20% of transudates as exudates. If transudative effusion is suspected (eg, due to heart failure or cirrhosis) and none of the biochemical measurements are > 15% above the cutoff levels for Light's criteria, the difference between serum and the pleural fluid protein is measured. If the difference is > 3.1 g/dL, the patient probably has a transudative effusion.

If the diagnosis remains unclear after pleural fluid analysis, CT angiography is indicated to look for pulmonary emboli, pulmonary infiltrates, or mediastinal lesions. Findings of pulmonary emboli indicate the need for long-term anticoagulation; parenchymal infiltrates, the need for bronchoscopy; and mediastinal lesions, the need for transthoracic needle aspiration or mediastinoscopy. However, CT angiography requires patients to hold their breath for ≥ 24 sec, and not all patients can comply. If CT angiography is unrevealing, observation is the best course unless the patient has a history of cancer, weight loss, persistent fever, or other findings suggestive of cancer or TB, in which case thoracoscopy may be indicated. Needle biopsy of the pleura can be done when thoracoscopy is unavailable. When tuberculous pleuritis is suspected, the level of adenosine deaminase in the pleural fluid is measured. A level > 40 U/L has a 95% sensitivity and specificity for the diagnosis of tuberculous pleuritis.

Treatment

- Treatment of symptoms and underlying disorder
- Drainage of some symptomatic effusions
- Other treatments for parapneumonic and malignant effusions

The effusion itself generally does not require treatment if it is asymptomatic because many effusions resorb spontaneously when the underlying disorder is treated, especially effusions due to uncomplicated pneumonias, pulmonary embolism, or surgery. Pleuritic pain can usually be managed with NSAIDs or other oral analgesics. At times, a short course of oral opioids is required.

Thoracentesis is sufficient treatment for many symptomatic effusions and can be repeated for effusions that reaccumulate. There are no arbitrary limits on the amount of fluid that can be removed. Removal of fluid can be continued until the effusion is drained or the patient develops chest tightness, chest pain, or severe coughing.

Effusions that are chronic, recurrent, and causing symptoms can be treated with pleurodesis or by intermittent drainage with an indwelling catheter (see p. 477). Effusions caused by pneumonia and cancer may require additional specific measures.

Parapneumonic effusion and empyema: In patients with adverse prognostic factors (pH < 7.20, glucose < 60 mg/dL, positive Gram stain or culture, loculations), the effusion should be completely drained via thoracentesis (see p. 387) or tube thoracostomy (see p. 390). If complete drainage is impossible, a thrombolytic (fibrinolytic) drug (eg, a tissue plasminogen activator 10 mg) plus a DNAse (eg, dornase alfa 5 mg) in 100 mL saline solution can be administered intrapleurally twice a day for 3 days. If attempts at drainage are unsuccessful, thoracoscopy should be done to lyse adhesions and remove fibrous tissue coating the lung to allow the lung to expand. If thoracoscopy is unsuccessful, thoracotomy with surgical decortication (eg, removal of scar, clot, or fibrous membrane surrounding the lung) is necessary.

Malignant pleural effusion: If dyspnea caused by malignant pleural effusion is relieved by thoracentesis but fluid and dyspnea redevelop, chronic (intermittent) drainage or pleurodesis is indicated. Asymptomatic effusions and effusions causing dyspnea unrelieved by thoracentesis do not require additional procedures.

Indwelling catheter drainage is the preferred approach for ambulatory patients because hospitalization is not necessary for catheter insertion and the pleural fluid can be drained intermittently into vacuum bottles. Pleurodesis is done by instilling a sclerosing agent into the pleural space to fuse the visceral and parietal pleura and eliminate the space. The most effective and commonly used sclerosing agents are talc, doxycycline, and bleomycin delivered via chest tube or thoracoscopy.

Pleurodesis is contraindicated if the mediastinum has shifted toward the side of the effusion or if the lung does not expand after a chest tube is inserted.

Shunting of pleural fluid to the peritoneum (pleuroperitoneal shunt) is useful for patients with malignant effusion in whom pleurodesis is unsuccessful and in patients who have trapped lung.

KEY POINTS

- Transudative effusions are caused by some combination of increased hydrostatic pressure and decreased plasma oncotic pressure.
- Exudative effusions result from increased capillary permeability, leading to leakage of protein, cells, and other serum constituents.
- The most common causes of transudative effusions are heart failure, cirrhosis with ascites, and hypoalbuminemia (usually due to the nephrotic syndrome).
- The most common causes of exudative effusions are pneumonia, cancer, pulmonary embolism, and TB.
- Evaluation requires imaging (usually chest x-ray) to confirm presence of fluid and pleural fluid analysis to help determine cause.
- Lateral decubitus x-rays, chest CT, or ultrasonography should be done if it is unclear whether an x-ray density represents fluid or parenchymal infiltrates or whether suspected fluid is loculated or free-flowing.
- Effusions that are chronic or recurrent and causing symptoms can be treated with pleurodesis or by intermittent drainage with an indwelling catheter.

PLEURAL FIBROSIS AND CALCIFICATION

Pleural fibrosis and calcification are usually benign sequelae of pleural inflammation or asbestos exposure.

Pleural fibrosis and calcification can be either postinflammatory or asbestos related (see p. 441). These disorders are suspected and diagnosed based on imaging studies.

Postinflammatory: Pleural inflammation commonly causes acute pleural thickening due to fibrosis. In most cases, the thickening resolves almost completely. Some patients are left with minor degrees of pleural thickening, which usually causes no symptoms or impairment of lung function. Occasionally, the lung becomes encased with a thick, fibrous pleural peel that limits expansion, pulls the mediastinum toward the side of disease, and impairs pulmonary function. Chest x-ray shows asymmetry of the lungs with thickened pleura (trapped lung). Differentiating localized pleural thickening from loculated pleural fluid may be difficult on x-ray, but this differentiation is easily made with CT.

Pleural fibrosis after inflammation can, on occasion, calcify. Calcification produces a dense image on the chest x-ray and almost always involves the visceral pleura. Postinflammatory calcifications are invariably unilateral.

Asbestos-related: Exposure to asbestos can lead to focal, plaquelike pleural fibrosis, at times with calcification, occurring up to ≥ 20 yr after the initial exposure. Diagnosis is usually by chest x-ray. The diameter of the plaques can vary from several millimeters to 10 cm. Any pleural or pericardial surface can be affected, but asbestos-related pleural plaques are usually in the lower two thirds of the thorax and are bilateral. Calcification most often affects the parietal and diaphragmatic pleura and spares the costophrenic sulci and apices. Calcification may be the only evidence of exposure. Dense pleural fibrosis surrounding the entire lung and > 1 cm in thickness can also follow asbestos exposure.

PNEUMOMEDIASTINUM

Pneumomediastinum is air in mediastinal interstices.

The **3 main causes** of pneumomediastinum are

- Alveolar rupture with dissection of air into the mediastinum
- Esophageal perforation
- Esophageal or bowel rupture with dissection of air from the neck or the abdomen into the mediastinum

The primary symptom is substernal chest pain which can, on occasion, be severe. Physical examination may show subcutaneous emphysema, usually in the suprasternal notch, along with a crunching or clicking noise synchronous with the heartbeat; this noise is best heard over the heart when the patient is in the left lateral decubitus position (Hamman sign).

The diagnosis is confirmed by chest x-ray, which shows air in the mediastinum.

PEARLS & PITFALLS

- Although pneumomediastinum may produce dramatic findings on examination and/or x-ray and may indicate a serious disorder, treatment of pneumomediastinum itself is usually unnecessary.

Treatment

Treatment usually is not necessary, although tension pneumomediastinum with compression of mediastinal structures (rare) can be relieved with needle aspiration, leaving the needle open to the atmosphere as is done with tension pneumothorax. Hospital admission is required if pneumomediastinum is secondary to esophageal or bowel rupture but not necessarily if secondary to alveolar rupture.

PNEUMOTHORAX

Pneumothorax is air in the pleural space causing partial or complete lung collapse. Pneumothorax can occur spontaneously or result from trauma or medical procedures. Diagnosis is based on clinical criteria and chest x-ray. Most pneumothoraces require transcatheter aspiration or tube thoracostomy.

Etiology

Primary spontaneous pneumothorax occurs in patients without underlying pulmonary disease, classically in tall, thin young men in their teens and 20s. It is thought to be due to spontaneous rupture of subpleural apical blebs or bullae that result from smoking or that are inherited. It generally occurs at rest, although some cases occur during activities involving reaching or stretching. Primary spontaneous pneumothorax also occurs during diving and high-altitude flying because of unequally transmitted pressure changes in the lung.

Secondary spontaneous pneumothorax occurs in patients with underlying pulmonary disease. It most often results from rupture of a bleb or bulla in patients with severe COPD (forced expiratory volume in 1 sec [FEV_1] < 1 L), HIV-related *Pneumocystis jirovecii* infection, cystic fibrosis, or any underlying pulmonary parenchymal disease (see Table 59–4). Secondary spontaneous pneumothorax is more serious than primary spontaneous pneumothorax because it occurs in patients whose underlying lung disease decreases their pulmonary reserve.

Table 59–4. CAUSES OF SECONDARY SPONTANEOUS PNEUMOTHORAX

TYPE	DISORDER
More common	
Pulmonary	Asthma COPD Cystic fibrosis Necrotizing pneumonia *Pneumocystis jirovecii* infection TB
Less common	
Pulmonary	Idiopathic pulmonary fibrosis Langerhans cell histiocytosis Lung cancer Lymphangioleiomyomatosis Sarcoidosis
Connective tissue disorders	Ankylosing spondylitis Ehlers-Danlos syndrome Marfan syndrome Polymyositis and dermatomyositis RA Systemic sclerosis
Other	Sarcoma Thoracic endometriosis Tuberous sclerosis

Catamenial pneumothorax is a rare form of secondary spontaneous pneumothorax that occurs within 48 h of the onset of menstruation in premenopausal women and sometimes in postmenopausal women taking estrogen. The cause is intrathoracic endometriosis, possibly due to migration of peritoneal endometrial tissue through diaphragmatic defects or embolization through pelvic veins.

Traumatic pneumothorax is a common complication of penetrating or blunt chest injuries (see p. 3115).

Iatrogenic pneumothorax is caused by medical interventions, including transthoracic needle aspiration, thoracentesis, central venous catheter placement, mechanical ventilation, and cardiopulmonary resuscitation.

Pathophysiology

Intrapleural pressure is normally negative (less than atmospheric pressure) because of inward lung and outward chest wall recoil. In pneumothorax, air enters the pleural space from outside the chest or from the lung itself via mediastinal tissue planes or direct pleural perforation. Intrapleural pressure increases, and lung volume decreases.

Tension pneumothorax (see also p. 3115) is a pneumothorax causing a progressive rise in intrapleural pressure to levels that become positive throughout the respiratory cycle and collapses the lung, shifts the mediastinum, and impairs venous return to the heart. Air continues to get into the pleural space but cannot exit. Without appropriate treatment, the impaired venous return can cause systemic hypotension and respiratory and cardiac arrest (pulseless electrical activity) within minutes. Tension pneumothorax most commonly occurs in patients receiving positive-pressure ventilation (with mechanical ventilation or particularly during resuscitation). Rarely, it is a complication of traumatic pneumothorax, when a chest wound acts as a one-way valve that traps increasing volumes of air in the pleural space during inspiration.

Symptoms and Signs

Small pneumothoraces are occasionally asymptomatic. Symptoms of pneumothorax include dyspnea and pleuritic chest pain. Dyspnea may be sudden or gradual in onset depending on the rate of development and size of the pneumothorax. Pain can simulate pericarditis, pneumonia, pleuritis, pulmonary embolism, musculoskeletal injury (when referred to the shoulder), or an intra-abdominal process (when referred to the abdomen). Pain can also simulate cardiac ischemia, although typically the pain of cardiac ischemia is not pleuritic.

Physical findings classically consist of absent tactile fremitus, hyperresonance to percussion, and decreased breath sounds on the affected side. If the pneumothorax is large, the affected side may be enlarged with the trachea visibly shifted to the opposite side. With tension pneumothorax, hypotension can occur.

Diagnosis

- Chest x-ray

The diagnosis is suspected in stable patients with dyspnea or pleuritic chest pain and is confirmed with upright inspiratory chest x-ray. Radiolucent air and the absence of lung markings juxtaposed between a shrunken lobe or lung and the parietal pleura are diagnostic of pneumothorax. Tracheal deviation and mediastinal shift occur with large pneumothoraces.

The size of a pneumothorax is defined as the percentage of the hemithorax that is vacant. This percentage is estimated by taking 1 minus the ratio of the cubes of the width of the lung and hemithorax. For example, if the width of the hemithorax is 10 cm and the width of the lung is 5 cm, the ratio is $5^3/10^3 = 0.125$. Thus, the size of the pneumothorax is about 1 minus 0.125, or 87.5%. If adhesions are present between the lung and the chest wall, the lung does not collapse symmetrically, the pneumothorax may appear atypical or loculated, and the calculation is not accurate.

Small pneumothoraces (eg, < 10%) are sometimes overlooked on chest x-ray. In patients with possible pneumothorax, lung markings should be traced to the edge of the pleura on chest x-ray. Conditions that mimic pneumothorax radiographically include emphysematous bullae, skinfolds, folded bed sheets, and overlap of stomach or bowel markings on lung fields.

PEARLS & PITFALLS

- Sudden hypotension in a mechanically ventilated patient should prompt consideration of tension pneumothorax. If the patient also has decreased breath sounds and hyperresonance to percussion, tension pneumothorax should be presumed and treated immediately without awaiting confirmation by chest x-ray.

Treatment

- Immediate needle decompression for tension pneumothoraces
- Observation and follow-up x-ray for small, asymptomatic, primary spontaneous pneumothoraces
- Catheter aspiration for large or symptomatic primary spontaneous pneumothoraces
- Tube thoracostomy for secondary and traumatic pneumothoraces

Patients should receive supplemental O_2 until chest x-ray results are available because O_2 accelerates pleural reabsorption of air. Treatment then depends on the type, size, and effects of the pneumothorax. Primary spontaneous pneumothorax that is < 20% and that does not cause respiratory or cardiac symptoms can be safely observed without treatment if follow-up chest x-rays done at about 6 and 48 h show no progression. Larger or symptomatic primary spontaneous pneumothoraces should be evacuated by catheter aspiration. Tube thoracostomy is an alternative.

Catheter aspiration is accomplished by insertion of a small-bore (about 7 to 9 French) IV or pigtail catheter into the chest in the 2nd intercostal space at the midclavicular line. The catheter is attached to a 3-way stopcock and syringe. Air is withdrawn from the pleural space through the stopcock into the syringe and expelled into the room. The process is repeated until the lung re-expands or until 4 L of air are removed. If the lung expands, the catheter can be removed or kept in place attached to a one-way Heimlich valve (thus permitting ambulation), and the patient need not be hospitalized. If the lung does not expand, a chest tube should be inserted, and the patient should be hospitalized. Primary spontaneous pneumothoraces can also be managed initially with a chest tube attached to a water seal without or with suction. Patients with primary spontaneous pneumothoraces should also undergo smoking cessation counseling.

Secondary and traumatic pneumothoraces are generally treated with tube thoracostomy (see p. 390). Symptomatic patients with iatrogenic pneumothoraces are best managed initially with aspiration.

Tension pneumothorax is a medical emergency and should be diagnosed clinically; time should not be wasted confirming the diagnosis with a chest x-ray. It should be treated immediately by inserting a 14- or 16-gauge needle with a catheter through the chest wall in the 2nd intercostal space at the midclavicular line. The sound of high-pressure air escaping confirms diagnosis. The catheter can be left open to air or attached to a Heimlich valve. Emergency decompression must be followed immediately by tube thoracostomy, after which the catheter is removed.

Complications

The 3 main problems encountered when treating pneumothorax are

- Air leaks
- Failure of the lung to expand
- Re-expansion pulmonary edema

Air leaks are usually due to the primary defect—ie, continued leakage of air from the lung into the pleural space—but can be due to air leaking around the chest tube insertion site if the site is not properly sutured and sealed. Air leaks are more common in secondary than in primary spontaneous pneumothorax. Most resolve spontaneously in < 1 wk.

Failure of the lung to re-expand is usually due to one of the following:

- Persistent air leak
- Endobronchial obstruction
- Trapped lung
- Malpositioned chest tube

Blood pleurodesis (a blood patch), thoracoscopy, or thoracotomy should be considered if an air leak or an incompletely expanded lung persists beyond 1 wk.

Re-expansion pulmonary edema occurs when the lung is rapidly expanded, as occurs when a chest tube is connected to negative pressure after the lung has been collapsed for > 2 days. Treatment is supportive, with O_2, diuretics, and cardiopulmonary support as needed.

Prevention

Recurrence approaches 50% in the 3 yr after initial spontaneous pneumothorax. The best preventive procedure is video-assisted thoracic surgery (VATS) in which blebs are stapled and pleurodesis is done with pleural abrasion, parietal pleurectomy, or talc insufflation; in some medical centers, thoracotomy is still used. These procedures are recommended when catheter aspiration fails to resolve spontaneous pneumothorax, when pneumothorax recurs, or when patients have secondary spontaneous pneumothorax. Recurrence after these procedures is < 5%. If thoracoscopy cannot be done or is contraindicated, chemical pleurodesis through a chest tube may be done (see p. 474); this procedure, though much less invasive, reduces the recurrence rate to only about 25%.

KEY POINTS

- Primary spontaneous pneumothorax occurs in patients without underlying pulmonary disease, classically in tall, thin young men in their teens and 20s.
- Secondary spontaneous pneumothorax occurs in patients with underlying pulmonary disease; it most often results from rupture of a bleb or bulla in patients with severe COPD.
- Diagnosis is by upright chest x-ray, except for tension pneumothorax, which is diagnosed clinically as soon as suspected.
- Primary spontaneous pneumothorax that is < 20% and that does not cause respiratory or cardiac symptoms can be safely observed without treatment if follow-up chest x-rays done at about 6 and 48 h show no progression.
- Larger or symptomatic primary spontaneous pneumothoraces should be evacuated by catheter aspiration or tube thoracostomy.
- Secondary and traumatic pneumothoraces are generally treated with tube thoracostomy.
- Video-assisted thoracic surgery (VATS) and other procedures can help prevent recurrences of spontaneous pneumothorax, which otherwise occur in 50% of patients within 3 yr.

VIRAL PLEURITIS

Viral pleuritis is a viral infection of the pleurae.

Viral pleuritis is most commonly caused by infection with coxsackie B virus. Occasionally, echovirus causes a rare condition known as epidemic or Bornholm pleurodynia, manifesting as pleuritis, fever, and chest muscle spasms. The condition occurs in the late summer and affects adolescents and young adults.

The primary symptom of viral pleuritis is pleuritic pain; pleural friction rub may be a sign (see p. 472).

Diagnosis is suspected in patients with pleuritic chest pain with or without systemic symptoms of viral infection. Chest x-ray is usually done. Other causes of pleuritic chest pain, such as pulmonary emboli and pneumonia, need to be considered and sometimes ruled out with testing.

Treatment is symptomatic with oral NSAIDs or a short course of oral opioids if needed.

60 Pneumonia

Pneumonia is acute inflammation of the lungs caused by infection. Initial diagnosis is usually based on chest x-ray and clinical findings. Causes, symptoms, treatment, preventive measures, and prognosis differ depending on whether the infection is bacterial, mycobacterial, viral, fungal, or parasitic; whether it is acquired in the community, hospital, or other health care–associated location; and whether it develops in a patient who is immunocompetent or immunocompromised.

An estimated 2 to 3 million people in the US develop pneumonia each year, of whom about 60,000 die. In the US, pneumonia, along with influenza, is the 8th leading cause of death and is the leading infectious cause of death. Pneumonia is the most common fatal hospital-acquired infection and the most common overall cause of death in developing countries.

The **most common cause** of pneumonia in adults > 30 yr is

- Bacterial infection

Streptococcus pneumoniae is the most common pathogen in all age groups, settings, and geographic regions. However, pathogens of every sort, from viruses to parasites, can cause pneumonia.

The airways and lungs are constantly exposed to pathogens in the external environment; the upper airways and oropharynx in particular are colonized with so-called normal flora. Microaspiration of these pathogens from the upper respiratory tract is a regular occurrence, but these pathogens are readily dealt with by lung host defense mechanisms. Pneumonia develops when

- Defense mechanisms are compromised
- Macroaspiration leads to a large inoculum of bacteria that overwhelms normal host defenses
- A particularly virulent pathogen is introduced

Occasionally, infection develops when pathogens reach the lungs via the bloodstream or by contiguous spread from the chest wall or mediastinum.

Upper airway defenses include salivary IgA, proteases, and lysozymes; growth inhibitors produced by normal flora; and fibronectin, which coats the mucosa and inhibits adherence.

Nonspecific **lower airway defenses** include cough, mucociliary clearance, and airway angulation preventing infection in airspaces. Specific lower airway defenses include various pathogen-specific immune mechanisms, including IgA and IgG opsonization, antimicrobial peptides, anti-inflammatory effects of surfactant, phagocytosis by alveolar macrophages, and T-cell–mediated immune responses. These mechanisms protect most people against infection.

Numerous conditions alter the normal flora (eg, systemic illness, undernutrition, hospital or nursing home exposure, antibiotic exposure) or impair these defenses (eg, altered mental status, cigarette smoking, nasogastric or endotracheal intubation). Pathogens that then reach airspaces can multiply and cause pneumonia.

Specific pathogens causing pneumonia cannot be found in < 50% of patients, even with extensive diagnostic investigation, primarily because of the limitations of currently available diagnostic tests. But because pathogens and outcomes tend to be similar in patients in similar settings and with similar risk factors, pneumonias can be categorized as

- Community-acquired
- Hospital-acquired (including ventilator-acquired and postoperative pneumonia)
- Health care–associated (including nursing home-acquired pneumonia)
- Occurring in immunocompromised patients, including patients with HIV infection (see p. 489)
- Aspiration pneumonia, which occurs when large volumes of upper airway or gastric secretions enter into the lungs

These categorizations allow treatment to be selected empirically.

The term interstitial pneumonia refers to various unrelated conditions of varied and sometimes unknown causes characterized by inflammation and fibrosis of the pulmonary interstitium (see p. 455).

ASPIRATION PNEUMONITIS AND PNEUMONIA

Aspiration pneumonitis and pneumonia are caused by inhaling toxic substances, usually gastric contents, into the lungs. Chemical pneumonitis, bacterial pneumonia, or airway obstruction can occur. Symptoms include cough and dyspnea. Diagnosis is based on clinical presentation and chest x-ray findings. Treatment and prognosis differ by aspirated substance.

Aspiration can cause lung inflammation (chemical pneumonitis), infection (bacterial pneumonia or lung abscess), or airway obstruction. However, most episodes of aspiration cause minor symptoms or pneumonitis rather than infection or obstruction, and some patients aspirate with no sequelae. Drowning may also cause inflammation of the lungs and is discussed elsewhere (see p. 2962).

Risk factors for aspiration include

- Impaired cognition or level of consciousness
- Impaired swallowing (such as occurs after some strokes or other neurologic diseases)
- Vomiting
- GI devices and procedures (eg, nasogastric tube placement)
- Dental procedures
- Respiratory devices and procedures (eg, endotracheal tube placement)
- Gastroesophageal reflux disease

Pathophysiology

Chemical pneumonitis: Multiple substances are directly toxic to the lungs or stimulate an inflammatory response when aspirated; gastric acid is the most common such aspirated substance, but others include petroleum products (particularly of low viscosity, such as petroleum jelly) and laxative oils (such as mineral, castor, and paraffin oil), all of which cause lipoid pneumonia. Aspirated gasoline and kerosene also cause a chemical pneumonitis (see p. 3064).

Gastric contents cause damage mainly due to gastric acid, although food and other ingested material (eg, activated charcoal as in treatment of overdose) are injurious in quantity. Gastric acid causes a chemical burn of the airways and lungs, leading to rapid bronchoconstriction, atelectasis, edema, and alveolar hemorrhage. This syndrome may resolve spontaneously, usually within a few days, or may progress to acute respiratory distress syndrome. Sometimes bacterial superinfection occurs.

Oil or petroleum jelly aspiration causes exogenous lipoid pneumonia, which is characterized histologically by chronic granulomatous inflammation with fibrosis.

Aspiration pneumonia: Healthy people commonly aspirate small amounts of oral secretions, but normal defense mechanisms usually clear the inoculum without sequelae. Aspiration of larger amounts, or aspiration in a patient with impaired pulmonary defenses, often causes pneumonia and/or a lung abscess. Elderly patients tend to aspirate because of conditions associated with aging that alter consciousness, such as sedative use and disorders (eg, neurologic disorders, weakness). Empyema (see p. 470) also occasionally complicates aspiration.

Gram-negative enteric pathogens and oral anaerobes are the most frequent cause of aspiration pneumonia.

Symptoms and Signs

Symptoms and signs include

- Cough
- Fever
- Dyspnea
- Chest discomfort

Chemical pneumonitis caused by gastric contents causes acute dyspnea with cough that is sometimes productive of pink frothy sputum, tachypnea, tachycardia, fever, diffuse crackles, and wheezing. When oil or petroleum jelly is aspirated, pneumonitis may be asymptomatic and detected incidentally on chest x-ray or may manifest with low-grade fever, gradual weight loss, and crackles.

Diagnosis

- Chest x-ray

For aspiration pneumonia, chest x-ray shows an infiltrate, frequently but not exclusively, in the dependent lung segments, ie, the superior or posterior basal segments of a lower lobe or the posterior segment of an upper lobe. For aspiration-related lung abscess, chest x-ray may show a cavitary lesion. Contrast-enhanced CT is more sensitive and specific for lung abscess and will show a round lesion filled with fluid or with an air-fluid level. In patients with oil or petroleum jelly aspiration, chest x-ray findings vary; consolidation, cavitation, interstitial or nodular infiltrates, pleural effusion, and other changes may be slowly progressive.

Signs of ongoing aspiration may include frequent throat clearing or a wet-sounding cough after eating. Sometimes no signs are present, and ongoing aspiration is only diagnosed via modified barium esophagography done to rule out an underlying swallowing disorder.

Treatment

- Antibiotics

Treatment is supportive, often involving supplemental oxygen and mechanical ventilation. Antibiotics (a beta-lactam/beta-lactamase inhibitor or clindamycin) often are given to patients with witnessed or known gastric aspiration because of the difficulty in excluding bacterial infection as a contributing or primary factor; however, if no infiltrate develops after 48 to 72 h, antibiotics can be stopped.

Potentially causative toxic substances should be avoided. Anecdotal reports suggest systemic corticosteroids may be beneficial in patients with oil or petroleum jelly aspiration.

For aspiration pneumonia, Infectious Diseases Society of America (IDSA) guidelines recommend a beta-lactam/beta-lactamase inhibitor, clindamycin, or a carbapenem. Some examples include clindamycin 600 mg IV q 8 h (followed by 300 mg po qid) and amoxicillin/clavulanate 875 mg IV q 12 h. Duration of treatment is usually 1 to 2 wk (see also Infectious Diseases Society of America Clinical Guidelines on Community-Acquired Pneumonia).

Treatment of lung abscess is with antibiotics and sometimes percutaneous or surgical drainage (see p. 467).

Prevention

Strategies to prevent aspiration are important to care and overall clinical outcome. For patients with decreased level of consciousness, avoidance of oral feeding and oral drugs and elevation of the head of the bed to > 30 degrees may help. Sedating drugs should be stopped. Patients with dysphagia (due to stroke or other neurologic conditions) may require diets with specialized textures to reduce the risk of aspiration. A speech pathologist may be able to train patients in specific strategies (chin tuck, etc.) to reduce the risk of aspiration. For patients with severe dysphagia, a percutaneous gastrostomy or jejunostomy tube is often used, although it is not clear whether this strategy truly reduces the risk of aspiration.

Optimization of oral hygiene and regular care by a dentist may help prevent development of pneumonia or abscess in patients who repeatedly aspirate.

KEY POINTS

- Patients with aspiration pneumonitis and aspiration pneumonia should be tested for an underlying swallowing disorder.
- Aspiration pneumonia should be treated with antibiotics; treatment of aspiration pneumonitis is primarily supportive.
- Secondary prevention of aspiration using various measures is a key component of care for affected patients.

COMMUNITY-ACQUIRED PNEUMONIA

Community-acquired pneumonia develops in people with limited or no contact with medical institutions or settings. The most commonly identified pathogens are *Streptococcus pneumoniae, Haemophilus influenzae*, atypical bacteria (ie, *Chlamydia pneumoniae, Mycoplasma pneumoniae, Legionella* sp), and viruses. Symptoms and signs are fever, cough, sputum production, pleuritic chest pain, dyspnea, tachypnea, and tachycardia. Diagnosis is based on clinical presentation and chest x-ray. Treatment is with empirically chosen antibiotics. Prognosis is excellent for relatively young or healthy patients, but many pneumonias, especially when caused by *S. pneumoniae*, Legionella, *Staphylococcus aureus*, or influenza virus, are serious or even fatal in older, sicker patients.

Etiology

Many organisms cause community-acquired pneumonia, including bacteria, viruses, and fungi. Pathogens vary by patient age and other factors (see Table 60–1), but the relative importance of each as a cause of community-acquired pneumonia is uncertain, because most patients do not undergo thorough testing, and because even with testing, specific agents are identified in < 50% of cases.

S. pneumoniae, *H. influenzae*, *C. pneumoniae*, and *M. pneumoniae* are the most common bacterial causes. Pneumonias caused by chlamydia and mycoplasma are often clinically indistinguishable from other pneumonias. Common viral agents include respiratory syncytial virus (RSV), adenovirus, influenza viruses, metapneumovirus, and parainfluenza viruses. Bacterial superinfection can make distinguishing viral from bacterial infection difficult.

C. pneumoniae accounts for 2 to 5% of community-acquired pneumonia and is the 2nd most common cause of lung infections in healthy people aged 5 to 35 yr. *C. pneumoniae* is commonly responsible for outbreaks of respiratory infection within families, in college dormitories, and in military training camps. It causes a relatively benign form of pneumonia that infrequently requires

Table 60–1. COMMUNITY-ACQUIRED PNEUMONIA IN ADULTS

GROUP	LIKELY ORGANISMS	EMPIRIC TREATMENT
I. Outpatients—no modifying factors present†	*Streptococcus pneumoniae*, *Mycoplasma pneumoniae*, *Chlamydia pneumoniae*, *Haemophilus influenzae*, respiratory viruses, miscellaneous organisms (eg, *Legionella* sp, *Mycobacterium tuberculosis*, endemic fungi)	Macrolide (azithromycin 500 mg po once, then 250 mg once/day; clarithromycin 250 to 500 mg po bid; or extended-release clarithromycin 1 g once/day) *or* Doxycycline 100 mg po bid (if allergic to macrolide)
II. Outpatients—modifying factors present†	*S. pneumoniae*, including antibiotic-resistant forms; *M. pneumoniae*; *C. pneumoniae*; mixed infection (bacteria + atypical pathogen or virus); *H. influenzae*; enteric gram-negative organisms; respiratory viruses; miscellaneous organisms (eg, *Moraxella catarrhalis, Legionella* sp, anaerobes [aspiration], *M. tuberculosis*, endemic fungi)	Beta-lactam (cefpodoxime 200 mg po q 12 h; cefuroxime 500 mg po q 12 h; amoxicillin 1 g q 8 h; amoxicillin/clavulanate 875/125 mg q 12 h) *plus* Macrolide po *or* Antipneumococcal fluoroquinolone po or IV (alone; eg, moxifloxacin [400 mg po/IV q 24 h], gemifloxacin [320 mg po/IV q 24 h], levofloxacin [750 mg po/IV q 24 h])
III. Inpatient—not in ICU	*S. pneumoniae*; *H. influenzae*; *M. pneumoniae*; *C. pneumoniae*; mixed infection (bacteria + atypical pathogen or virus); respiratory viruses; *Legionella* sp, miscellaneous organisms (eg, *M. tuberculosis*, endemic fungi, *Pneumocystis jirovecii*)	Azithromycin 500 mg IV q 24 h *plus* Beta-lactam IV (cefotaxime 1 to 2 g q 8 to 12 h; ceftriaxone 1 g q 24 h) *or* Antipneumococcal fluoroquinolone po or IV (alone)
IVA. ICU patient—no *Pseudomonas* risk factors	*S. pneumoniae*, including antibiotic-resistant forms; *Legionella* sp; *H. influenzae*; enteric gram-negative organisms; *Staphylococcus aureus*; *M. pneumoniae*; respiratory viruses miscellaneous organisms (eg, *C. pneumoniae*, *M. tuberculosis*, endemic fungi)	Beta-lactam IV (cefotaxime 1 to 2 g IV q 8 to 12 h; ceftriaxone 1 g IV q 24 h) *plus either* Antipneumococcal fluoroquinolone IV *or* Azithromycin 500 mg IV q 24 h
IVB. ICU patient—*Pseudomonas* risk factors present	Same as those for category IVA (above) plus *Pseudomonas* sp	Antipseudomonal beta-lactam‡ or aztreonam (if allergic to or intolerant of beta-lactams) 1 to 2 g q 8 h *plus either* Ciprofloxacin 400 mg IV q 12 h or levofloxacin 750 mg po or IV q 24 h Alternatively: Antipseudomonal beta-lactam‡ *plus* An aminoglycoside *plus either* Ciprofloxacin 400 mg IV q 12 h or levofloxacin 750 mg po or IV q 24 h

*These guidelines do not apply to patients with immunosuppression, influenza, aspiration pneumonia, or health care–associated pneumonia.

†Modifying factors:

- *Increased risk of antibiotic-resistant organisms:* Age > 65, alcoholism, antibiotic within 3 mo, exposure to child in day care center, multiple coexisting illnesses.
- *Increased risk of enteric gram-negative organisms:* Antibiotic use within 3 mo, cardiopulmonary disease (including COPD and heart failure), multiple coexisting illnesses.
- *Increased risk of Pseudomonas aeruginosa:* Broad-spectrum antibiotics > 7 days in past month, corticosteroid use, undernutrition, structural pulmonary disease.

‡Antipseudomonal beta-lactams = cefepime 1 to 2 g IV q 12 h, imipenem 500 mg IV q 6 h, meropenem 500 mg to 1 g IV q 8 h, piperacillin/tazobactam 3.375 g IV q 4 h.

Data from Mandell A, Wunderink R, Azueto A, et al: Infectious Disease Society of America and American Thoracic Society Guidelines for the management of adults with community-acquired pneumonia. *Clinical Infectious Diseases* 44:S27–S72, 2007.

hospitalization. *Chlamydia psittaci* pneumonia (psittacosis) is rare and occurs in patients who own or are often exposed to birds.

Since the year 2000, the incidence of community-acquired methicillin-resistant *Staphylococcus aureus* (CA-MRSA) skin infections has increased markedly. This pathogen can rarely cause severe, cavitating pneumonia and tends to affect young adults.

P. aeruginosa is an especially common cause of pneumonia in patients with cystic fibrosis, neutropenia, advanced AIDS, and/or bronchiectasis.

A host of other organisms causes lung infection in immunocompetent patients. In patients with pneumonia, a thorough history of exposures, travel, pets, hobbies, and other exposures is essential to raise suspicion of less common organisms.

Q fever, tularemia, anthrax, and plague are uncommon bacterial syndromes in which pneumonia may be a prominent feature. Tularemia, anthrax, and plague should raise the suspicion of bioterrorism.

Adenovirus, Epstein-Barr virus, and coxsackievirus are common viruses that rarely cause pneumonia. Seasonal influenza can rarely cause a direct viral pneumonia but often predisposes to the development of a serious secondary bacterial pneumonia. Varicella virus and hantavirus cause lung infection as part of adult chickenpox and hantavirus pulmonary syndrome. A coronavirus causes severe acute respiratory syndrome (SARS) and the Middle East respiratory syndrome (MERS).

Common fungal pathogens include *Histoplasma capsulatum* (histoplasmosis) and *Coccidioides immitis* (coccidioidomycosis). Less common fungal pathogens include *Blastomyces dermatitidis* (blastomycosis) and *Paracoccidioides braziliensis* (paracoccidioidomycosis). *Pneumocystis jirovecii* commonly causes pneumonia in patients who have HIV infection or are immunosuppressed (see p. 487).

Parasites causing lung infection in developed countries include *Toxocara canis* or *T. catis* (visceral larva migrans), *Dirofilaria immitis* (dirofilariasis), and *Paragonimus westermani* (paragonimiasis). (For a discussion of pulmonary TB or of specific microorganisms, see p. 1650.)

In children, the most common causes depend on age:

- < 5 yr: Most often viruses; among bacteria, *S. pneumoniae*, *S. aureus*, and *S. pyogenes*, are common
- ≥ 5 yr: Most often the bacteria *S. pneumoniae*, *M. pneumoniae*, or *Chlamydia pneumoniae*

S. pneumoniae and MRSA can cause necrotizing pneumonia. For pneumonia in neonates, see p. 2635.

Symptoms and Signs

Symptoms include malaise, chills, rigor, fever, cough, dyspnea, and chest pain. Cough typically is productive in older children and adults and dry in infants, young children, and the elderly. Dyspnea usually is mild and exertional and is rarely present at rest. Chest pain is pleuritic and is adjacent to the infected area. Pneumonia may manifest as upper abdominal pain when lower lobe infection irritates the diaphragm. GI symptoms (nausea, vomiting, diarrhea) are also common. Symptoms become variable at the extremes of age. Infection in infants may manifest as nonspecific irritability and restlessness; in the elderly, manifestation may be as confusion and obtundation.

Signs include fever, tachypnea, tachycardia, crackles, bronchial breath sounds, egophony (E to A change—said to occur when, during auscultation, a patient says the letter "E" and the examiner hears the letter "A"), and dullness to percussion. Signs of pleural effusion may also be present. Nasal flaring, use of accessory muscles, and cyanosis are common among infants. Fever is frequently absent in the elderly.

Symptoms and signs were previously thought to differ by type of pathogen. For example, factors thought to suggest viral pneumonia included gradual onset, preceding URI symptoms, diffuse findings on auscultation, and absence of a toxic appearance. Atypical pathogens were considered more likely when onset was less acute and are more likely during known community outbreaks. However, manifestations in patients with typical and atypical pathogens overlap considerably. In addition, no single symptom or sign is sensitive or specific enough to predict the organism. Symptoms and signs are even similar for other noninfective inflammatory lung diseases such as hypersensitivity pneumonitis and organizing pneumonia.

Diagnosis

- Chest x-ray
- Consideration of alternative diagnoses (eg, heart failure, pulmonary embolism)
- Sometimes identification of pathogen

Diagnosis is suspected on the basis of clinical presentation and infiltrate seen on chest x-ray. When there is high clinical suspicion of pneumonia and the chest x-ray does not reveal an infiltrate, doing CT or repeating the chest x-ray in 24 to 48 h is recommended.

Differential diagnosis in patients presenting with pneumonia-like symptoms includes heart failure and COPD exacerbation. Other disorders should be considered, particularly when findings are inconsistent or not typical. The most serious common misdiagnosis is pulmonary embolism, which may be more likely in patients with minimal sputum production, no accompanying URI or systemic symptoms, and risk factors for thromboembolism (see Table 61–1 on p. 490); thus, testing for pulmonary embolism should be considered.

Quantitative cultures of bronchoscopic or suctioned specimens, if they are obtained before antibiotic administration, can help distinguish between bacterial colonization (ie, presence of microorganisms at levels that provoke neither symptoms nor an immune response) and infection. However, bronchoscopy is usually done only in patients receiving mechanical ventilation or for those with other risk factors for unusual microorganisms or complicated pneumonia (eg, immunocompromise, failure of empiric therapy).

Distinguishing between bacterial and viral pneumonias is challenging. Many studies have investigated the utility of clinical, imaging, and routine blood tests, but no test is reliable enough to make this differentiation.

In outpatients with mild or moderate pneumonia, no further diagnostic testing is needed (see Table 60–2). In patients with moderate or severe pneumonia, a WBC count and electrolytes, BUN, and creatinine are useful to classify risk and hydration status. Pulse oximetry or ABG testing should also be done to assess oxygenation. For patients with moderate or severe pneumonia who require hospitalization, 2 sets of blood cultures are obtained to assess for bacteremia and sepsis. The Infectious Diseases Society of America (IDSA) provides a guide to recommended testing based on patient demographic and risk factors (Infectious Diseases Society of America Clinical Guidelines on Community-Acquired Pneumonia).

Pathogen identification: Identification of the pathogen can be useful to direct therapy and verify bacterial susceptibilities to antibiotics. However, because of the limitations of current diagnostic tests and the success of empiric antibiotic treatment, experts recommend limiting attempts at microbiologic identification (eg, cultures, specific antigen testing) unless patients are at high risk or have complications (eg, severe pneumonia,

Table 60–2. RISK STRATIFICATION FOR COMMUNITY-ACQUIRED PNEUMONIA (THE PNEUMONIA SEVERITY INDEX)

FACTOR	POINTS
Patient demographics	
• Men	Age (in yr)
• Women	Age (in yr) – 10
Nursing home resident	10
Coexisting illness	
Cancer	30
Liver disease	20
Heart failure	10
Cerebrovascular disease	10
Renal disease	10
Physical examination	
Altered mental status	20
Respiratory rate ≥ 30 breaths/min	20
Systolic BP < 90 mm Hg	20
Temperature ≥ 40° C or < 35° C	15
Heart rate ≥ 125 beats/min	10
Test results	
Arterial pH < 7.35	30
BUN ≥ 30 mg/dL (11 mmol/L)	20
Sodium < 130 mmol/L	20
Glucose ≥ 250 mg/dL (14 mmol/L)	10
Hct < 30%	10
Pao_2 < 60 mm Hg or Oxygensaturation < 90%*	10
Pleural effusion	10

Points	Mortality	Recommendation
≤ 70	< 1%	Outpatient treatment†
71–90	< 5%	Outpatient treatment†
91–130	5–15%	Admit
> 130	> 15%	Admit

*Many consider hypoxemia an absolute indication for admission.

†Acute care admission, subacute care admission, observation period, home IV antibiotics, or home nursing visits should be considered for patients who are frail, isolated, or living in unstable environments.

Adapted from Pneumonia: New prediction model proves promising (AHCPR Publication No. 97-R031).

immunocompromise, asplenia, failure to respond to empiric therapy). In general, the milder the pneumonia, the less such diagnostic testing is required. Critically ill patients require the most intensive testing, as do patients in whom a antibiotic-resistant or unusual organism is suspected (eg, TB, *P. jirovecii*) and patients whose condition is deteriorating or who are not responding to treatment within 72 h.

Chest x-ray findings generally cannot distinguish one type of infection from another, although the following findings are suggestive:

- Multilobar infiltrates suggest *S. pneumoniae* or *Legionella pneumophila* infection.
- Interstitial pneumonia (on chest x-ray, appearing as increased interstitial markings, subpleural reticular opacities that increase from the apex to the bases of the lungs, and peripheral honeycombing) suggests viral or mycoplasmal etiology.
- Cavitating pneumonia suggests *S. aureus* or a fungal or mycobacterial etiology.

Blood cultures, which are often obtained in patients hospitalized for pneumonia, can identify causative bacterial pathogens if bacteremia is present. About 12% of all patients hospitalized with pneumonia have bacteremia; *S. pneumoniae* accounts for two thirds of these cases.

Sputum testing can include Gram stain and culture for identification of the pathogen, but the value of these tests is uncertain because specimens often are contaminated with oral flora and overall diagnostic yield is low. Regardless, identification of a bacterial pathogen in sputum cultures allows for susceptibility testing. Obtaining sputum samples also allows for testing for viral pathogens via direct fluorescence antibody testing or PCR, but caution needs to be exercised in interpretation because 15% of healthy adults carry a respiratory virus or potential bacterial pathogen. In patients whose condition is deteriorating and in those unresponsive to broad-spectrum antibiotics, sputum should be tested with mycobacterial and fungal stains and cultures.

Sputum samples can be obtained noninvasively by simple expectoration or after hypertonic saline nebulization (induced sputum) for patients unable to produce sputum. Alternatively, patients can undergo bronchoscopy or endotracheal suctioning, either of which can be easily done through an endotracheal tube in mechanically ventilated patients. Otherwise, bronchoscopic sampling is usually done only for patients with other risk factors (eg, immunocompromise, failure of empiric therapy).

Urine testing for *Legionella* antigen and pneumococcal antigen is now widely available. These tests are simple and rapid and have higher sensitivity and specificity than sputum Gram stain and culture for these pathogens. Patients at risk of *Legionella* pneumonia (eg, severe illness, failure of outpatient antibiotic treatment, presence of pleural effusion, active alcohol abuse, recent travel) should undergo testing for urinary *Legionella* antigen, which remains present long after treatment is initiated, but the test detects only *L. pneumophila* serogroup 1 (70% of cases).

The **pneumococcal antigen test** is recommended for patients who are severely ill; have had unsuccessful outpatient antibiotic treatment; or who have pleural effusion, active alcohol abuse, severe liver disease, or asplenia. This test is especially useful if adequate sputum samples or blood cultures were not obtained before initiation of antibiotic therapy. A positive test can be used to tailor antibiotic therapy, though it does not provide antimicrobial susceptibility.

Prognosis

Short-term mortality is related to severity of illness. Mortality is < 1% in patients who are candidates for outpatient treatment. Mortality in hospitalized patients is 8%. Death may be caused by pneumonia itself, progression to sepsis syndrome, or exacerbation of coexisting conditions. In patients hospitalized for pneumonia, risk of death is increased during the year after hospital discharge.

Mortality varies to some extent by pathogen. Mortality rates are highest with gram-negative bacteria and CA-MRSA. However, because these pathogens are relatively infrequent causes of pneumonia, *S. pneumoniae* remains the most common cause of death in patients with community-acquired pneumonia. Atypical pathogens such as *Mycoplasma* have a good prognosis. Mortality is higher in patients who do not respond to initial empiric antibiotics and in those whose treatment regimen does not conform with guidelines.

Treatment

- Risk stratification for determination of site of care
- Antibiotics
- Antivirals for influenza or varicella
- Supportive measures

Risk stratification: Risk stratification via risk prediction rules may be used to estimate mortality risk and can help guide decisions regarding hospitalization. These rules have been used to identify patients who can be safely treated as outpatients and those who require hospitalization because of high risk of complications (see Table 60–2). However, these rules should supplement, not replace, clinical judgment because many unrepresented factors, such as likelihood of adherence, ability to care for self, and wish to avoid hospitalization, should also influence triage decisions. An ICU admission is required for patients who

- Need mechanical ventilation
- Have hypotension (systolic BP ≤ 90 mm Hg) that is unresponsive to volume resuscitation

Other criteria that mandate consideration of ICU admission include

- Respiratory rate > 30/min
- Pa_{O_2}/fraction of inspired oxygen (F_{IO_2}) < 250
- Multilobar pneumonia
- Diastolic BP < 60 mm Hg
- Confusion
- BUN > 19.6 mg/dL

The Pneumonia Severity Index (PSI) is the most studied and validated prediction rule. However, because the PSI is complex and requires several laboratory assessments, simpler rules such as CURB-65 are usually recommended for clinical use. Use of these prediction rules has led to a reduction in unnecessary hospitalizations for patients who have milder illness.

In CURB-65, 1 point is allotted for each of the following risk factors:

- **C**onfusion
- **U**remia (BUN ≥19 mg/dL)
- **R**espiratory rate > 30 breaths/min
- Systolic **BP** < 90 mm Hg or diastolic BP ≤ 60 mm Hg
- Age ≥ **65** yr

Scores can be used as follows:

- 0 or 1 points: Risk of death is < 3%. Outpatient therapy is usually appropriate.
- 2 points: Risk of death is 9%. Hospitalization should be considered.
- ≥ 3 points: Risk of death is 15 to 40%. Hospitalization is indicated, and, particularly with 4 or 5 points, ICU admission should be considered.

Antimicrobials: Antibiotic therapy is the mainstay of treatment for community-acquired pneumonia. Appropriate treatment involves starting empiric antibiotics as soon as possible, preferably ≤ 8 h after presentation. Because organisms are difficult to identify, the empiric antibiotic regimen is selected based on likely pathogens and severity of illness. Consensus guidelines have been developed by many professional organizations; one widely used set is detailed in Table 60–1 (see also Infectious Diseases Society of America Clinical Guidelines on Community-Acquired Pneumonia). Guidelines should be adapted to local susceptibility patterns, drug formularies, and individual patient circumstances. If a pathogen is subsequently identified, the results of antibiotic susceptibility testing can help guide any changes in antibiotic therapy.

For children, treatment depends on age, previous vaccinations, and whether treatment is outpatient or inpatient. For outpatient treatment, treatments are dictated by age:

- < 5 yr: Amoxicillin or amoxicillin/clavulanate is usually the drug of choice. If epidemiology suggests an atypical pathogen as the cause and clinical findings are compatible, a macrolide (eg, azithromycin or clarithromycin) can be used instead. Some experts suggest not using antibiotics if clinical features strongly suggest viral pneumonia.
- ≥ 5 yr: Amoxicillin or (particularly if an atypical pathogen cannot be excluded) amoxicillin plus a macrolide. Amoxicillin/clavulanate is an alternative. If the cause appears to be an atypical pathogen, a macrolide alone can be used.

For children treated as inpatients, antibiotic therapy tends to be more broad-spectrum and depends on the child's previous vaccinations:

- Fully immunized (against *S. pneumoniae* and *H. influenzae*-type b): Ampicillin or penicillin G (alternatives are ceftriaxone or cefotaxime). If MRSA is suspected, vancomycin or clindamycin is added. If an atypical pathogen cannot be excluded, a macrolide is added.
- Not fully immunized: Ceftriaxone or cefotaxime (alternative is levofloxacin). If MRSA is suspected, vancomycin or clindamycin is added. If an atypical pathogen cannot be excluded, a macrolide is added.

Full details are described in the Clinical Practice Guidelines by the Pediatric Infectious Diseases Society and the Infectious Diseases Society of America.

With empiric treatment, 90% of patients with bacterial pneumonia improve. Improvement is manifested by decreased cough and dyspnea, defervescence, relief of chest pain, and decline in WBC count. Failure to improve should trigger suspicion of

- An unusual organism
- Resistance to the antimicrobial used for treatment
- Empyema
- Coinfection or superinfection with a 2nd infectious agent
- An obstructive endobronchial lesion
- Immunosuppression
- Metastatic focus of infection with reseeding (in the case of pneumococcal infection)
- Nonadherence to treatment (in the case of outpatients)

If none of these conditions can be proved, treatment failure is likely due to inadequate host defenses. When therapy has failed, consultation with a pulmonary and/or infectious disease specialist is indicated.

Antiviral therapy may be indicated for select viral pneumonias. Ribavirin is not used routinely for RSV pneumonia in children or adults, but may be used in occasional high-risk children age < 24 mo.

Oseltamivir 75 mg po bid or zanamivir 10 mg inhaled bid started within 48 h of symptom onset and given for 5 days reduces the duration and severity of symptoms in patients who develop influenza infection. In patients hospitalized with confirmed influenza infection, observational studies suggest benefit even 48 h after symptom onset.

Acyclovir 5 to 10 mg/kg IV q 8 h for adults or 250 to 500 mg/m^2 body surface area IV q 8 h for children is recommended for varicella lung infections. Though pure viral pneumonia does occur, superimposed bacterial infections are common and require antibiotics directed against *S. pneumoniae*, *H. influenzae*, and *S. aureus*.

Follow-up x-rays should be obtained 6 wk after treatment in patients > 35; persistence of an infiltrate at ≥ 6 wk raises suspicions of TB or an underlying, possibly malignant endobronchial lesion.

Supportive care: Supportive care includes fluids, antipyretics, analgesics, and, for patients with hypoxemia, oxygen. Prophylaxis against thromboembolic disease and early mobilization improve outcomes for patients hospitalized with pneumonia. Cessation counseling should also be done for smokers.

Prevention

Some forms of community-acquired pneumonia are preventable with vaccination. Pneumococcal conjugate vaccine (PCV13) is recommended for children age 2 mo to 2 yr and for adults ≥ 19 yr with certain comorbid (including immunocompromising) conditions. Pneumococcal polysaccharide vaccine (PPSV23) is given to all adults ≥ 65 yr and to any patient ≥ 2 yr who has risk factors for pneumococcal infections, including but not limited to those with underlying heart, lung, or immune system disorders and those who smoke (see Table 180–2 on p. 1450). The full list of indications for both pneumococcal vaccines can be seen at the CDC website. Recommendations for other vaccines, such as *H. influenzae* type b (Hib) vaccine (for patients < 2 yr), varicella vaccine (for patients < 18 mo and a later booster vaccine), and influenza vaccine (annually for everyone ≥ 6 mo and especially for those at higher risk of developing serious flu-related complications), can also be found at the CDC website. This higher risk group includes people ≥ 65 years and people of any age with certain chronic medical conditions (such as diabetes, asthma, or heart disease), pregnant women, and young children (see Table 291–2 on p. 2462).

In high-risk patients who are not vaccinated against influenza and household contacts of patients with influenza, oseltamivir 75 mg po once/day or zanamivir 10 po mg once/day can be given for 2 wk and started within 48 h of exposure may prevent influenza (although resistance has recently been described for oseltamivir).

Smoking cessation can reduce the risk of developing pneumonia.

KEY POINTS

- Community-acquired pneumonia is a leading cause of death in the US and around the world.
- Common symptoms and signs include cough, fever, chills, fatigue, dyspnea, rigors, sputum production, and pleuritic chest pain.
- Treat patients with mild or moderate risk pneumonia with empiric antibiotics without testing designed to identify the underlying pathogen.
- Hospitalize patients with multiple risk factors, as delineated by the risk assessment tools.
- Consider alternate diagnoses, including pulmonary embolism, particularly if pneumonia-like signs and symptoms are not typical.

HEALTH CARE–ASSOCIATED PNEUMONIA

Health care–associated pneumonia (HCAP) occurs in nonhospitalized patients who reside in a nursing home or other long-term care facility, have undergone IV therapy (including chemotherapy) or wound care within the previous 30 days, have been hospitalized in an acute care hospital for ≥ 2 days within the previous 90 days, or have attended a hospital or hemodialysis center within the previous 30 days. In addition to the usual community-acquired pathogens, HCAP pathogens include gram-negative bacilli (including *Pseudomonas aeruginosa*) and *Staphylococcus aureus* (including methicillin-resistant *S. aureus*) and various antibiotic-resistant pathogens. Symptoms and signs are similar to those of pneumonia that occurs in other settings, except many elderly patients have less prominent changes in vital signs. Diagnosis is based on clinical presentation and chest x-ray. Treatment is with broad-spectrum antibiotics. Mortality is moderately high but may be due in part to coexisting disorders.

The definition of health care–associated pneumonia is designed to identify patients who are at higher risk of developing pneumonia due to antibiotic-resistant organisms and who, therefore, might require broader spectrum empiric antibiotic therapy (see p. 478). Nursing home–acquired pneumonia is the most common subset of HCAP. Risk factors are common among debilitated nursing home residents; they include

- Poor functional status
- Mood disorder
- Altered mental status
- Difficulty swallowing
- Immunosuppression
- Older age
- Use of tube feedings
- Influenza or other viral respiratory infections
- Conditions that predispose to bacteremia (eg, indwelling bladder catheter, pressure ulcers)
- Presence of a tracheostomy tube

Pathogens: In addition to the usual community-acquired pathogens, HCAP pathogens include gram-negative bacilli (including *P. aeruginosa*) and *Staphylococcus aureus* (including methicillin-resistant *S. aureus*) and various antibiotic-resistant pathogens.

The **most common** pathogens are

- *Streptococcus pneumoniae*
- Gram-negative bacilli

These organisms may be responsible for roughly equal numbers of infections; it is not clear whether gram-negative bacilli are sometimes bacteria that are colonizing the patient rather than causative pathogens. *Haemophilus influenzae* and *Moraxella catarrhalis* are next most common. *Chlamydia*, *Mycoplasma*, and *Legionella* spp are rarely identified.

Polymicrobial infection, as well as infection with antibiotic-resistant organisms, particularly methicillin-resistant *S. aureus* and *Pseudomonas* infection, is much more likely with prior antibiotic treatment (within the previous 90 days). Infection with a resistant organism markedly worsens mortality and morbidity. Other risk factors for polymicrobial infection and antibiotic-resistant organisms include

- Current hospitalization of ≥ 5 days
- High incidence of antibiotic resistance in the community, hospital, or specific hospital unit
- Hospitalization for ≥ 2 days within the previous 90 days
- Residence in a nursing home or extended care facility
- Home infusion therapy (including antibiotics)
- Dialysis treatments
- Home wound care
- Family member with infection due to an antibiotic-resistant pathogen
- Immunosuppressive disease or therapy

However, new evidence indicates several of these factors may overestimate the risk of polymicrobial and antibiotic-resistant organisms and thus drive overuse of broad-spectrum antibiotics. Revised guidelines for HCAP are being written and will likely recommend limiting broad-spectrum antibiotics to patients with prior antibiotic treatment in the previous 90 days, while individualizing therapy for the other HCAP-associated factors.

Symptoms and Signs

Symptoms of health care–associated pneumonia often resemble those of community-acquired pneumonia but may be more subtle. Cough and altered mental status are common, as are nonspecific symptoms of anorexia, weakness, restlessness and agitation, falling, and incontinence. Subjective dyspnea occurs but is less common.

Signs include diminished or absent responsiveness, fever, tachycardia, tachypnea, sputum production, wheezes or crackles, and stertorous, wet breathing.

Diagnosis

- Clinical manifestations
- Chest x-ray
- Assessment of renal function and oxygenation

Diagnosis of health care–associated pneumonia is based on clinical manifestations (eg, fever, cough, sputum production) and a chest x-ray demonstrating an infiltrate. Blood tests may show leukocytosis. Because detection of physical changes may be delayed in a nursing home setting and because these patients are at greater risk of complications, evaluation for hypoxemia with pulse oximetry and for decreased intravascular volume with serum BUN and creatinine should be done.

X-rays are often difficult to obtain in nursing home patients, so it may be necessary to transfer them to a hospital at least for initial evaluation. In some cases (eg, if clinical diagnosis is clear, if illness is mild, or if aggressive care is not the goal), treatment may be started without x-ray confirmation. It is thought that nursing home patients may initially lack a radiographic infiltrate, presumably because of the dehydration that commonly accompanies febrile pneumonia in the elderly or a blunted immune response.

Prognosis

Mortality rate for patients with health care–associated pneumonia requiring admission for treatment is 13 to 41%.

Treatment

- Antibiotics

Few data are available to guide decisions about where treatment should take place. In general, patients should be hospitalized if they have ≥ 2 unstable vital signs and if the nursing home cannot administer acute care. Some nursing home patients, such as those undergoing end-of-life care or who have advance directives asking for limited medical measures, are not candidates for aggressive treatment or hospital transfer under any circumstances.

Antibiotics are the mainstay of treatment of health care–associated pneumonia. An antibiotic regimen should be chosen that is effective against *S. pneumoniae*, *H. influenzae*, and common gram-negative bacilli. A common regimen is an oral antipneumococcal quinolone (eg, levofloxacin 750 mg once/day or moxifloxacin 400 mg once/day). Ceftriaxone, ertapenem, and ampicillin/sulbactam (each as monotherapy) are alternatives. For patients who are to be hospitalized, one dose of an appropriate antibiotic should be given before transfer.

KEY POINTS

- Health care–associated pneumonia (HCAP) occurs in non-hospitalized patients who have had recent contact with the health care system, including nursing homes, dialysis centers, and infusion centers.
- The causative pathogen profile of health care–associated pneumonia differs from that of community-acquired pneumonia and requires broader empiric antibiotic therapy that is active against antibiotic-resistant organisms.

HOSPITAL-ACQUIRED PNEUMONIA

Hospital-acquired pneumonia (HAP) develops at least 48 h after hospital admission. The most common pathogens are gram-negative bacilli and *Staphylococcus aureus*; antibiotic-resistant organisms are an important concern. Symptoms and signs include malaise, fever, chills, rigor, cough, dyspnea, and chest pain, but in ventilated patients, pneumonia usually manifests as worsening oxygenation and increased tracheal secretions. Diagnosis is suspected on the basis of clinical presentation and chest x-ray and is confirmed by blood culture or bronchoscopic sampling of the lower respiratory tract. Treatment is with antibiotics. Overall prognosis is poor, due in part to comorbidities.

Hospital-acquired pneumonia includes ventilator-associated pneumonia (VAP), postoperative pneumonia, and pneumonia that develops in unventilated hospitalized inpatients.

Etiology

The most common cause of hospital-acquired pneumonia is microaspiration of bacteria that colonize the oropharynx and upper airways in seriously ill patients. Seeding of the lung due to bacteremia or inhalation of contaminated aerosols (ie, airborne particles containing *Legionella* sp, *Aspergillus* sp, or influenza virus) are less common causes (see p. 478).

Risk factors: Endotracheal intubation with mechanical ventilation poses the greatest overall risk of hospital-acquired pneumonia; ventilator-associated pneumonia constitutes > 85% of all cases, with pneumonia occurring in 9 to 27% of mechanically ventilated patients. The highest risk of VAP occurs during the first 10 days after intubation. Endotracheal intubation breaches airway defenses, impairs cough and mucociliary clearance, and facilitates microaspiration of bacteria-laden secretions that pool above the inflated endotracheal tube cuff. In addition, bacteria form a biofilm on and within the endotracheal tube that protects them from antibiotics and host defenses.

In nonintubated patients, risk factors include previous antibiotic treatment, high gastric pH (due to stress ulcer prophylaxis or therapy with H2 blockers or proton pump inhibitors), and coexisting cardiac, pulmonary, hepatic, or renal insufficiency.

Major risk factors for postoperative pneumonia are age > 70, abdominal or thoracic surgery, and functional debilitation.

Pathogens: Pathogens and antibiotic resistance patterns vary significantly among institutions and can vary within institutions over short periods (eg, month to month). Local antibiograms at the institutional level that are updated on a regular basis are essential in determination of appropriate empiric antibiotic therapy. In general, the most important pathogens are *Pseudomonas aeruginosa*, methicillin-sensitive *Staphylococcus aureus*, and methicillin-resistant *S. aureus* (MRSA).

Other important pathogens include enteric gram-negative bacteria (mainly *Enterobacter* sp, *Klebsiella pneumoniae*, *Escherichia coli*, *Serratia marcescens*, *Proteus* sp, and *Acinetobacter* sp).

Methicillin-sensitive *S. aureus*, *Streptococcus pneumoniae*, and *Haemophilus influenzae* are most commonly implicated when pneumonia develops within 4 to 7 days of hospitalization, whereas *P. aeruginosa*, MRSA, and enteric gram-negative organisms become more common with increasing duration of intubation or hospitalization.

Prior intravenous antibiotic treatment (within the previous 90 days) greatly increases the likelihood of antibiotic-resistant organisms, particularly MRSA and *Pseudomonas* infection in VAP and HAP.[1] Infection with a resistant organism markedly worsens mortality and morbidity. Other risk factors for antibiotic-resistant organisms specific to VAP include

- Septic shock at time of VAP
- ARDS preceding VAP
- Five or more days of hospitalization prior to the occurrence of VAP
- Acute renal replacement therapy prior to VAP onset

High-dose corticosteroids increase the risk of *Legionella* and *Pseudomonas* infections. Chronic suppurative lung diseases such as cystic fibrosis and bronchiectasis increase the risk of Gram-negative pathogens, including antibiotic-resistant strains.

1. Kalil AC, Metersky ML, Klompas M, et al: Management of adults with hospital-acquired and ventilator-associated pneumonia: 2016 clinical practice guidelines by the Infectious Diseases Society of America and the American Thoracic Society. *Clinical Infectious Diseases* 63(5):e61–111, 2016.

Symptoms and Signs

Symptoms and signs of hospital-acquired pneumonia in nonintubated patients are generally the same as those for community-acquired pneumonia and include malaise, fever, chills, rigor, cough, dyspnea, and chest pain. Pneumonia in critically ill, mechanically ventilated patients more typically causes fever and increased respiratory rate or heart rate or changes in respiratory parameters, such as an increase in purulent secretions or worsening hypoxemia.

Diagnosis

- Chest x-ray and clinical criteria (limited accuracy)
- Sometimes bronchoscopy or blood cultures

Diagnosis is imperfect. In practice, hospital-acquired pneumonia is often suspected on the basis of the appearance of a new infiltrate on a chest x-ray that is taken for evaluation of new symptoms or signs (eg, fever, increased secretions, worsening hypoxemia) or of leukocytosis. However, no symptom, sign, or x-ray finding is sensitive or specific for the diagnosis, because all can be caused by atelectasis, pulmonary embolism, or pulmonary edema and may be part of the clinical findings in acute respiratory distress syndrome.

Gram stain and semiquantitive cultures of endotracheal aspirates, though not definitive for identifying infection, are recommended for guiding treatment in VAP. Bronchoscopic sampling of lower airway secretions for quantitative culture yields more reliable specimens that can differentiate colonization from infection. Information gained from bronchoscopic sampling reduces antibiotic use and assists in switching from broader to narrower antibiotic coverage. However, it has not been shown to improve outcomes.

Measurement of inflammatory mediators in bronchoalveolar lavage fluid or serum has not been shown to be reliable in deciding on initiation of antibiotics. The only finding that reliably identifies both pneumonia and the responsible organism is a pleural fluid culture (obtained via thoracentesis in a patient with pleural effusion) that is positive for a respiratory pathogen.

Blood cultures are relatively specific if a respiratory pathogen is identified but are insensitive.

Prognosis

The mortality associated with hospital-acquired pneumonia ranges from 25 to 50% despite the availability of effective antibiotics. However, not all mortality is attributable to the pneumonia itself; many of the deaths are related to the patient's other underlying illness. Adequacy of initial antimicrobial therapy clearly improves prognosis. Infection with antibiotic-resistant gram-negative or gram-positive bacteria worsens prognosis.

Treatment

- Empirically chosen antibiotics active against resistant organisms

If hospital-associated pneumonia is suspected, treatment is with antibiotics that are chosen empirically based on

- Local sensitivity patterns
- Patient risk factors for antibiotic-resistant pathogens

In the 2007 guidelines, the Infectious Diseases Society of America and the American Thoracic Society used very broad criteria for defining the population at risk of infection with antibiotic-resistant pathogens, which resulted in the majority of patients with HAP/VAP requiring broad-spectrum antibiotic therapy for MRSA and resistant *Pseudomonas*. New recommendations in 2016[1] emphasize use of a narrower spectrum of empiric antibiotics when possible. Empiric therapy for HAP/VAP without risk factors for antibiotic-resistant organisms and high mortality (mechanical ventilation for pneumonia or septic shock), in an institution where MRSA incidence is < 20% (of *S. aureus* isolates) and *P. aeruginosa* resistance is < 10% for commonly used empiric antipseudomonal antibiotics, could include any one of the following:

- Piperacillin/tazobactam
- Cefepime
- Levofloxacin
- Imipenem
- Meropenem

Doses depend on renal function (see Table 184–3 on p. 1497).

In treatment settings where MRSA rates are > 20%, vancomycin or linezolid should be added. In patients who are at high risk for mortality or who have risk factors for antibiotic-resistant organisms, or in the absence of reliable local antibiograms, recommendations include triple therapy using 2 drugs with activity against *Pseudomonas* and 1 drug with activity against MRSA:

- An antipseudomonal cephalosporin (cefepime or ceftazidime) *or* an antipseudomonal carbapenem (imipenem, meropenem) *or* a beta-lactam/beta-lactamase inhibitor (piperacillin/tazobactam)
- An antipseudomonal fluoroquinolone (ciprofloxacin or levofloxacin) *or* an aminoglycoside (amikacin, gentamicin, tobramycin)
- Linezolid or vancomycin

While indiscriminate use of antibiotics is a major contributor to development of antimicrobial resistance, adequacy of initial empiric antibiotics is a major determinant of a favorable outcome. Therefore, treatment must begin with initial use of broad-spectrum drugs, which are then changed to the narrowest regimen possible based on clinical response and the results of cultures and antibiotic susceptibility testing.

1. Kalil AC, Metersky ML, Klompas M, et al: Management of adults with hospital-acquired and ventilator-associated pneumonia: 2016 clinical practice guidelines by the Infectious Diseases Society of America and the American Thoracic Society. *Clinical Infectious Diseases* 63(5):e61–111, 2016.

Prevention

Among cases of hospital-acquired infection, the most effective preventative measures are those that focus on ventilator-associated pneumonia. Semiupright or upright positioning reduces risk of aspiration and pneumonia compared with recumbent positioning and is the simplest and most effective preventive method. Noninvasive ventilation using continuous positive airway pressure (CPAP) or bilevel positive airway pressure (BiPAP) prevents the breach in airway defense that occurs with endotracheal intubation and eliminates the need for intubation in some patients.

Continuous aspiration of subglottic secretions using a specially designed endotracheal tube attached to a suction device seems to reduce the risk of aspiration.

Selective decontamination of the oropharynx (using topical gentamicin, colistin, chlorhexidine, vancomycin cream, or a combination) or of the entire GI tract (using polymyxin, an aminoglycoside or quinolone, and either nystatin or amphotericin B) is controversial because of concerns about resistant strains and because decontamination, although it decreases incidence of VAP, has not been shown to decrease mortality.

Surveillance cultures and routinely changing ventilator circuits or endotracheal tubes have not been shown to decrease VAP.

Incentive spirometry is recommended to help prevent postoperative pneumonia.

KEY POINTS

- Hospital-acquired pneumonia (HAP) includes ventilator-associated pneumonia, postoperative pneumonia, and pneumonia that develops in unventilated patients who have been hospitalized for at least 48 h.
- Mechanical ventilation is the most important risk factor for HAP.
- Likely pathogens differ from those causing community-acquired pneumonia and require initial empiric antibiotic therapy that is active against antibiotic-resistant organisms.
- Diagnosis is difficult, with culture of a potential pathogen from pleural fluid or blood being the most specific finding.
- Reassess patients 2 to 3 days after initiation of treatment, and change antibiotics based on available culture and clinical data.

PNEUMONIA IN IMMUNOCOMPROMISED PATIENTS

Pneumonia in immunocompromised patients is often caused by unusual pathogens but may also be caused by the same pathogens as those that cause community-acquired pneumonia. Symptoms and signs depend on the pathogen and on the conditions compromising the immune system. Diagnosis is based on blood cultures and bronchoscopic sampling of respiratory secretions, sometimes with quantitative cultures. Treatment depends on the immune system defect and the pathogen.

The potential pathogens in patients with compromised immune system defenses are legion; they include those that cause community-acquired pneumonia as well as unusual pathogens. Likely pathogens depend on the type of defect in immune system defenses (see Table 60–3). However, respiratory symptoms and changes on chest x-rays in immunocompromised patients may be due to various processes other than infection, such as pulmonary hemorrhage, pulmonary edema, radiation injury, pulmonary toxicity due to cytotoxic drugs, and tumor infiltrates.

Symptoms and Signs

Symptoms and signs may be the same as those that occur with community-acquired pneumonia in immunocompetent patients. Symptoms may include malaise, chills, fever, rigor, cough, dyspnea, and chest pain. However, immunocompromised patients may have no fever or respiratory signs and are less likely to have purulent sputum if they are neutropenic. In some patients, the only sign is fever.

PEARLS & PITFALLS

- Have a high index of suspicion for pneumonia in immunocompromised patients because symptoms can be atypical or muted.

Diagnosis

- Chest x-ray
- Assessment of oxygenation
- Induction or bronchoscopy to obtain sputum
- Blood cultures
- Pathogens predicted based on symptoms, x-ray changes, and type of immunodeficiency

Chest x-ray and assessment of oxygenation (usually by pulse oximetry) are done in immunocompromised patients with respiratory symptoms, signs, or fever. If an infiltrate or hypoxemia is present, diagnostic studies should be done. Chest x-ray may be normal in *Pneumocystis jirovecii* pneumonia, but hypoxia is usually present.

Sputum testing and blood cultures are done. Sputum testing should include Gram stain, mycobacterial and fungal stains and cultures, and sometimes testing for viruses (eg, PCR for cytomegalovirus in a transplant patient or in a patient with AIDS). If signs, symptoms, or risk factors for *Aspergillus* infection are present, serum galactomannan assay should be done.

Optimally, a firm diagnosis is made with induced sputum, bronchoscopy, or both, especially in patients with mild pneumonia, severe defects in immune function, or failure to respond to broad-spectrum antibiotics.

Pathogen identification: Likely pathogens can often be predicted based on symptoms, x-ray changes, and the type of immunodeficiency. In patients with acute symptoms, the differential diagnosis includes bacterial infection, hemorrhage, pulmonary edema, a leukocyte agglutinin reaction to transfusion of blood products, and pulmonary emboli. An indolent time course is more suggestive of a fungal or mycobacterial infection, an opportunistic viral infection, *P. jirovecii* pneumonia, tumor, a cytotoxic drug reaction, or radiation injury.

Table 60–3. PNEUMONIA IN IMMUNOCOMPROMISED PATIENTS

IMMUNE SYSTEM DEFECT	DISORDERS OR THERAPY ASSOCIATED WITH DEFECT*	LIKELY PATHOGENS
Defective PMNs		
Neutropenia	Acute leukemia, aplastic anemia, cancer chemotherapy	Gram-negative bacteria *Staphylococcus aureus* *Aspergillus* sp *Candida* sp
Defective chemotaxis	Diabetes mellitus	*S. aureus* Gram-negative aerobes
Defective intracellular killing	Chronic granulomatous disease	*S. aureus*
Defective alternative pathway	Sickle cell disease	*Streptococcus pneumoniae* *Haemophilus influenzae*
C5 deficiency	Congenital disorder	*S. pneumoniae* *S. aureus* Gram-negative bacteria
Cell-mediated immunity		
T-cell deficiency or dysfunction	Hodgkin lymphoma, cancer chemotherapy, corticosteroid therapy	Mycobacteria Viruses (eg, herpes simplex virus, cytomegalovirus) *Strongyloides* sp Opportunistic fungi (eg, *Aspergillus*, *Mucor*, *Cryptococcus* spp) *Nocardia* sp *Toxoplasma* sp
	AIDS	*Pneumocystis jirovecii* *Toxoplasma* sp Cytomegalovirus Herpes simplex virus Opportunistic fungi (eg, *Aspergillus*, *Mucor*, *Cryptococcus* spp) Mycobacteria
Humoral immunodeficiency		
B-cell deficiency or dysfunction	Multiple myeloma, agammaglobulinemia	*S. pneumoniae* *H. influenzae* *Neisseria meningitidis*
	Selective deficiency: IgA, IgG, IgM	*S. pneumoniae* *H. influenzae*
	Hypogammaglobulinemia	*P. jirovecii* Cytomegalovirus *S. pneumoniae* *H. influenzae*

*Examples. Many disorders cause multiple defects.
PMN = polymorphonuclear leukocytes.

X-rays showing localized consolidation usually indicate an infection involving bacteria, mycobacteria, fungi, or *Nocardia* sp. A diffuse interstitial pattern is more likely to represent a viral infection, *P. jirovecii* pneumonia, drug or radiation injury, or pulmonary edema. Diffuse nodular lesions suggest mycobacteria, *Nocardia* sp, fungi, or tumor. Cavitary disease suggests mycobacteria, *Nocardia* sp, fungi, or bacteria, particularly *S. aureus*.

In organ or bone marrow transplantation recipients with bilateral interstitial pneumonia, the usual cause is cytomegalovirus, or the disease is idiopathic. A pleural-based consolidation is usually *Aspergillus* infection. In patients with AIDS, bilateral pneumonia is usually *P. jirovecii* pneumonia. About 30% of patients with HIV infection have *P. jirovecii* pneumonia as the initial AIDS-defining diagnosis, and > 80% of AIDS patients have this infection at some time if prophylaxis is not given (see p. 1642). Patients with HIV infection become vulnerable to *P. jirovecii* pneumonia when the CD4+ T lymphocyte count is < 200/μL.

Treatment

- Broad-spectrum antimicrobial therapy

The antimicrobial therapy depends on the immune system defect and the risk factors for specific pathogens. Consultation with an infectious diseases specialist is usually indicated. In patients with neutropenia, empiric treatment depends on the immune system defect, x-ray findings, and severity of illness. Generally, broad-spectrum antibiotics that are effective against gram-negative bacilli, *Staphylococcus aureus*, and anaerobes are needed, as for hospital-acquired pneumonia. If patients with conditions other than HIV infection do not improve with

5 days of antibiotic therapy, antifungal therapy is frequently added empirically.

Therapies to enhance immune system function (see below) are an important adjunct for the treatment of pneumonia in immunocompromised patients.

Prevention

Therapies to enhance immune system function are indicated for the prevention of pneumonia in immunocompromised patients. For example, patients with chemotherapy-induced neutropenia should receive granulocyte-colony stimulating factor (G-CSF, or filgrastim), and patients with hypogammaglobulinemia due to an inherited or acquired disease (eg, multiple myeloma, leukemia) should receive IV immune globulin.

Patients with HIV and CD4+ T lymphocyte count < 200/μL should receive daily prophylactic therapy with trimethoprim/sulfamethoxazole or other appropriate therapy.

Vaccination is also important in these patients. For example, patients at risk of pneumonia with encapsulated bacteria (eg, hypogammaglobulinemia, asplenia) should receive vaccinations again pneumococcus and *H. influenzae*.

KEY POINTS

- Consider typical as well as unusual pathogens in immunocompromised patients who have pneumonia.
- If patients have hypoxemia or an abnormal chest x-ray, do further testing, including sputum testing, ideally with induced or bronchoscopically obtained sample.
- Begin with broad-spectrum antimicrobial therapy.

PNEUMOCYSTIS JIROVECII PNEUMONIA

***Pneumocystis jirovecii* is a common cause of pneumonia in immunosuppressed patients, especially in those infected with HIV and in those receiving systemic corticosteroids. Symptoms include fever, dyspnea, and dry cough. Diagnosis requires demonstration of the organism in an induced sputum specimen or bronchoscopic sample. Treatment is with antibiotics, usually trimethoprim/sulfamethoxazole or dapsone/trimethoprim, clindamycin/primaquine, atovaquone, or pentamidine. Patients with Pao_2 < 70 mm Hg receive systemic corticosteroids. Prognosis is generally good with timely treatment.**

P. jirovecii is a ubiquitous organism transmitted by aerosol route and causes no disease in immunocompetent patients. However, some patients are at risk of developing *P. jirovecii* pneumonia:

- Patients with HIV infection and CD4+ T lymphocyte counts < 200/μL
- Organ transplant recipients
- Patients with hematologic cancers
- Patients taking corticosteroids

Most patients have fever, dyspnea, and a dry, nonproductive cough that evolves over several weeks (HIV infection) or over several days (other causes of compromised cell-mediated immunity). Dyspnea is common.

Diagnosis

- Chest x-ray
- Pulse oximetry
- Histopathologic confirmation

Patients should have chest x-ray and assessment of oxygenation by pulse oximetry.

Chest x-ray characteristically shows diffuse, bilateral perihilar infiltrates, but 20 to 30% of patients have normal x-rays.

Hypoxemia may be present even when chest x-ray shows no infiltrate; this finding can be an important clue to diagnosis. When pulse oximetry is abnormal, ABGs are often obtained to show severity of hypoxemia (including an increase in the alveolar-arterial oxygen gradient).

PEARLS & PITFALLS

- In immunosuppressed patients who have a dry, nonproductive cough and abnormal chest x-ray or pulse oximetry, pursue further testing for *P. jirovecii* pneumonia.

If done, pulmonary function tests show altered diffusing capacity (although this is rarely done as a diagnostic test).

Histopathologic demonstration of the organism is needed for confirmation of the diagnosis. Methenamine silver, Giemsa, Wright-Giemsa, modified Grocott, Weigert-Gram, or monoclonal antibody stain is used. Sputum specimens are usually obtained by induced sputum or bronchoscopy. Sensitivity ranges from 30 to 80% for induced sputum and is > 95% for bronchoscopy with bronchoalveolar lavage.

Prognosis

Overall mortality for *P. jirovecii* pneumonia in hospitalized patients is 15 to 20%. Risk factors for death may include previous history of *P. jirovecii* pneumonia, older age, and, in HIV-infected patients, CD4+ T lymphocyte count < 50/μL.

Treatment

- Trimethoprim/sulfamethoxazole
- Corticosteroids if Pao_2 < 70 mm Hg

Treatment is with trimethoprim/sulfamethoxazole (TMP/SMX) 4 to 5 mg/kg IV or po tid for 14 to 21 days. Treatment can be started before diagnosis is confirmed because *P. jirovecii* cysts persist in the lungs for weeks. Adverse effects of treatment are more common among patients with AIDS and include rash, neutropenia, hepatitis, and fever.

Alternative regimens, which are also given for 21 days, are

- Pentamidine 4 mg/kg IV once/day
- Atovaquone 750 mg po bid
- Trimethoprim 5 mg/kg po qid with dapsone 100 mg po once/day
- Clindamycin 300 to 900 mg IV q 6 to 8 h with primaquine base 15 to 30 mg/day po

The major limitation of pentamidine is the high frequency of toxic adverse effects, including acute kidney injury, hypotension, and hypoglycemia.

Adjunctive therapy with corticosteroids is recommended for patients with a Pao_2 < 70 mm Hg. The suggested regimen is prednisone 40 mg po bid (or its equivalent) for the first 5 days, 40 mg po once/day for the next 5 days (or 20 mg bid), and then 20 mg po once/day for the duration of treatment.

Prevention

HIV-infected patients who have had *P. jirovecii* pneumonia or who have a CD4+ T lymphocyte count < 200/μL should receive prophylaxis with TMP/SMX 80/400 mg once/day; if this regimen is not tolerated, dapsone 100 mg po once/day or aerosolized pentamidine 300 mg once/month can be used. These prophylactic regimens are also probably indicated for non–HIV-infected patients at risk of *P. jirovecii* pneumonia.

KEY POINTS

- Consider *P. jirovecii* pneumonia in patients who are immunosuppressed, even if they have mild respiratory symptoms and even if the chest x-ray is normal.
- Do histopathologic examination on induced sputum or bronchoscopically obtained sputum.
- Treat patients with trimethoprim/sulfamethoxazole, adding a corticosteroid if Pao_2 is < 70 mm Hg.

61 Pulmonary Embolism

Pulmonary embolism is the occlusion of ≥ 1 pulmonary arteries by thrombi that originate elsewhere, typically in the large veins of the legs or pelvis. Risk factors for pulmonary embolism are conditions that impair venous return, conditions that cause endothelial injury or dysfunction, and underlying hypercoagulable states. Symptoms of pulmonary embolism are nonspecific and include dyspnea, pleuritic chest pain, and, in more severe cases, light-headedness, presyncope, syncope, or cardiorespiratory arrest. Signs are also nonspecific and may include tachypnea, tachycardia, and in more severe cases, hypotension. Diagnosis of pulmonary embolism is accomplished with CT angiography, ventilation/perfusion scanning, or occasionally, pulmonary arteriography. Pulmonary embolism treatment is with anticoagulants and, sometimes, clot dissolution with thrombolytics or surgical removal. When anticoagulation is contraindicated, an inferior vena caval filter should be placed. Preventive measures include anticoagulants and/or mechanical compression devices that are applied to the legs in hospitalized patients.

Pulmonary embolism affects an estimated 117 people per 100,000 person years, resulting in about 350,000 cases yearly (probably at least 100,000 in the US), and causes up to 85,000 deaths/yr. It affects mainly adults.

Etiology

Nearly all pulmonary emboli arise from thrombi in the veins of the legs or pelvis (deep venous thrombosis). Risk of embolization is higher with thrombi proximal to the calf veins. Thromboemboli can also originate in arm veins or central veins of the chest (caused by central venous catheters or resulting from thoracic outlet syndromes).

Risk factors for deep venous thrombosis and pulmonary embolism (see Table 61–1) are similar in children and adults and include

- Conditions that impair venous return, including bed rest and confinement without walking
- Conditions that cause endothelial injury or dysfunction
- Underlying hypercoagulable (thrombophilic) disorders

Pathophysiology

Once deep venous thrombosis develops, clots may dislodge and travel through the venous system and the right side of the heart to lodge in the pulmonary arteries, where they partially or completely occlude one or more vessels. The consequences depend on the size and number of emboli, the underlying condition of the lungs, how well the right ventricle (RV) is functioning, and the ability of the body's intrinsic thrombolytic system to dissolve the clots. Death occurs due to right ventricular failure.

Table 61–1. RISK FACTORS FOR DEEP VENOUS THROMBOSIS AND PULMONARY EMBOLISM

Age > 60 yr
Cancer
Hormonal modulation
- Estrogen receptor modulators (eg, raloxifene, tamoxifen)
- Exogenous estrogens and progestins, including oral contraceptives and estrogen therapy
- Exogenous testosterone

Heart failure
Immobilization
Indwelling venous catheters
Myeloproliferative disorders (hyperviscosity)
Nephrotic syndrome
Obesity
Pregnancy/postpartum period
Prior thromboembolism
Sickle cell disease
Smoking
Stroke
Thrombotic disorders (thrombophilias)
- Antiphospholipid antibody syndrome
- Antithrombin III deficiency
- Factor V Leiden mutation (activated protein C resistance)
- Heparin-induced thrombocytopenia
- Hereditary fibrinolytic defects
- Hyperhomocystinemia
- Increase in factor VIII levels
- Increase in factor XI levels
- Increase in von Willebrand factor levels
- Paroxysmal nocturnal hemoglobinuria
- Protein C deficiency
- Protein S deficiency
- Prothrombin G20210A gene variant
- Tissue factor pathway inhibitor deficiency or impaired function

Trauma/surgery
Other conditions associated with reduced mobility, venous injury, or hypercoagulability

Small emboli may have no acute physiologic effects and may begin to lyse immediately and resolve within hours or days. Larger emboli can cause a reflex increase in ventilation (tachypnea), hypoxemia due to ventilation/perfusion (V/Q) mismatch, and low mixed venous oxygen content as a result of low cardiac output, atelectasis due to alveolar hypocapnia and abnormalities in surfactant, and an increase in pulmonary vascular resistance caused by mechanical obstruction and vasoconstriction. Endogenous lysis reduces most emboli, even those of moderate size, and physiologic alterations decrease over hours or days. Some emboli resist lysis and may organize and persist.

PE may be designated according to the physiologic effects as

- Massive: Impaired right ventricular function with hypotension, as defined by systolic BP < 90 mm Hg or a drop in systolic BP of ≥ 40 mm Hg from baseline for a period of 15 min and predicts a significant risk of death within hours or days
- Submassive: Impaired right ventricular function without hypotension
- Small: Absence of right ventricular impairment and absence of hypotension

Saddle PE describes a pulmonary embolus that lodges in the bifurcation of the main pulmonary artery and into the right and left pulmonary arteries; saddle PEs are usually submassive or massive.

In 3 to 4% of cases, chronic residual obstruction leads to pulmonary hypertension (chronic thromboembolic pulmonary hypertension) that evolves over months to years and can result in chronic right heart failure.

When large emboli occlude major pulmonary arteries, or when many small emboli occlude > 50% of the more distal vessels, RV pressure increases, which may lead to acute RV failure, shock, or sudden death. The risk of death depends on the degree and rate of rise of right-sided pressures and on the patient's underlying cardiopulmonary status. Patients with preexisting cardiopulmonary disease are at higher risk of death, but young and/or otherwise healthy patients may survive a PE that occludes > 50% of the pulmonary bed.

Pulmonary infarction (interruption of pulmonary artery blood flow leading to necrosis of lung tissue, sometimes represented by a pleural-based [peripherally located], often wedge-shaped, pattern on chest x-ray [Hampton hump] or other imaging modalities) occurs in < 10% of patients diagnosed with PE. This low rate has been attributed to the dual blood supply to the lung (ie, bronchial and pulmonary). Generally, pulmonary infarction is due to smaller emboli that become lodged in more distal pulmonary arteries.

PE can also arise from nonthrombotic sources.

Symptoms and Signs

Many pulmonary emboli are small, physiologically insignificant, and asymptomatic. Even when present, symptoms are nonspecific and vary in frequency and intensity, depending on the extent of pulmonary vascular occlusion and preexisting cardiopulmonary function.

Emboli often cause

- Acute dyspnea
- Pleuritic chest pain

Dyspnea may be minimal at rest and can worsen during activity.

Less common symptoms include

- Cough
- Hemoptysis

In elderly patients, the first symptom may be altered mental status.

Massive PE may manifest with hypotension, tachycardia, light-headedness/presyncope, syncope, or cardiac arrest.

The most common signs of PE are

- Tachycardia
- Tachypnea

Less commonly, patients have hypotension, a loud 2nd heart sound (S_2) due to a loud pulmonic component (P_2), and crackles or wheezing. In the presence of right ventricular failure, distended internal jugular veins and a RV heave may be evident, and a RV gallop (3rd heart sound [S_3]), with or without tricuspid regurgitation, may be audible.

Fever, when present, is usually low-grade unless caused by an underlying condition.

Pulmonary infarction is typically characterized by chest pain (mainly pleuritic) and, occasionally, hemoptysis.

Chronic thromboembolic pulmonary hypertension causes symptoms and signs of right heart failure, including exertional dyspnea, easy fatigue, and peripheral edema that develops over months to years.

Patients with acute PE may also have symptoms of deep venous thrombosis (ie, pain, swelling, and/or erythema of a leg or an arm). Such leg symptoms are often not present, however.

Diagnosis

- High index of suspicion
- Assessment of pretest probability (based on clinical findings, including pulse oximetry and chest x-ray)
- Subsequent testing based on pretest probability

The diagnosis is challenging because symptoms and signs are nonspecific and diagnostic tests are not 100% sensitive and specific. It is important to include PE in the differential diagnosis when nonspecific symptoms, such as dyspnea, pleuritic chest pain, hemoptysis, light-headedness, or syncope are encountered. Thus, PE should be considered in the differential diagnosis of patients suspected of having

- Cardiac ischemia
- Heart failure
- COPD exacerbation
- Pneumothorax
- Pneumonia
- Sepsis
- Acute chest syndrome (in patients with sickle cell disease)
- Acute anxiety with hyperventilation

Significant, unexplained tachycardia may be a clue. PE also should be considered in any elderly patient with tachypnea and altered mental status.

Initial evaluation should include pulse oximetry and chest x-ray. ECG, ABG, or both may help to exclude other diagnoses (eg, acute myocardial infarction). The chest x-ray usually is nonspecific but may show atelectasis, focal infiltrates, an elevated hemidiaphragm, or a pleural effusion. The classic findings of focal loss of vascular markings (Westermark sign), a peripheral wedge-shaped density (Hampton hump), or enlargement of the right descending pulmonary artery (Palla sign) are suggestive but uncommon (ie, insensitive) and have an unknown specificity. Chest x-ray can also help exclude pneumonia. Pulmonary infarction due to PE may be mistaken for pneumonia.

Pulse oximetry provides a quick way to assess oxygenation; hypoxemia is one sign of PE, and it requires further evaluation. ABG measurement may show an increased alveolar to arterial oxygen (A-a) difference (sometimes called A-a gradient) or hypocapnia; one or both of these tests are moderately sensitive for PE, but neither is specific. ABG testing should be considered particularly for patients with dyspnea or tachypnea who do not have hypoxemia detected with pulse oximetry. Oxygen saturation may be normal due to a small clot burden, or to compensatory hyperventilation; a very low pCO_2 detected with ABG measurement can confirm hyperventilation.

ECG most often shows tachycardia and various ST-T wave abnormalities, which are not specific for PE (see Fig. 61–1). An $S_1Q_3T_3$ or a new right bundle branch block may indicate the effect of abrupt rise in RV pressure on RV conduction; these findings are moderately specific but insensitive, occurring in only about 5% of patients. Right axis deviation (R > S in V_1) and P-pulmonale may be present. T-wave inversion in leads V_1 to V_4 also occurs.

Clinical probability: Clinical probability of PE can be assessed by combining ECG and chest x-ray findings with findings from the history and physical examination (see Table 61–2). Clinical prediction scores, such as the Wells score, the revised Geneva score, or the Pulmonary Embolism Rule-Out Criteria (PERC) score, may aid clinicians in assessing the chance that acute PE is present. These systems assign points to a variety of clinical factors, with cumulative scores corresponding to designations of the probability of PE before testing (pretest probability). For example, the Wells score result is classified as likely or unlikely for PE. However, judgment of whether PE is more likely than an alternate diagnosis is somewhat subjective. Also, clinical judgment of experienced clinicians may be as sensitive, or even more sensitive, than results from such prediction scores. PE should probably be considered more likely if one or more of the symptoms and signs, particularly dyspnea, hemoptysis, tachycardia, or hypoxemia, cannot be explained clinically or by chest x-ray results.

Pretest probability guides testing strategy and the interpretation of test results. Patients whose probability for PE is unlikely may need only minimal additional testing (ie, D-dimer testing). In such cases, a negative D-dimer test (< 0.4 μg/mL) is highly indicative of the *absence* of PE. If there is a high clinical suspicion of PE and the risk of bleeding is low, patients are immediately given anticoagulants while the diagnosis is confirmed with additional tests.

Diagnostic testing:

- Screening with D-dimer testing if pre-test probability is unlikely
- If pre-test probability is likely or if D-dimer result is elevated, CT angiography, or V/Q scanning when CT contrast is contraindicated
- Sometimes (eg, to avoid lung imaging) ultrasonography of the legs or arms alone

There is no universally accepted algorithm for the approach to suspected acute pulmonary embolism. Tests most useful for diagnosing or excluding PE are

- D-dimer testing
- CT angiography
- V/Q scanning
- Duplex ultrasonography

D-Dimer is a by-product of intrinsic fibrinolysis; thus, elevated levels occur in the presence of a recent thrombus. When pretest probability is considered unlikely, a negative D-dimer level (< 0.4 μg/mL) is highly sensitive for the *absence* of PE with a negative predictive value of > 95%; in most cases, this makes such a result sufficiently reliable for excluding the diagnosis of PE in routine practice. However, elevated levels are not specific for venous thrombus because many patients without deep venous thrombosis (DVT) or PE also have elevated levels, and therefore, further testing is required when the D-dimer level is elevated or when the pretest probability for PE is likely.

CT angiography is the preferred imaging technique for diagnosing acute PE. It is rapid, accurate, and highly sensitive and specific. It can also give more information about other lung pathology (eg, demonstration of pneumonia rather than PE as a cause of hypoxia or pleuritic chest pain). Although poor quality scans due to motion artifact or poor contrast boluses can limit the sensitivity of the examination, improvements in CT technology have shortened acquisition times to less than 2 sec, providing relatively motion-free images in patients who are

Table 61–2. CLINICAL PREDICTION RULE FOR DIAGNOSING PULMONARY EMBOLISM

Establish clinical probability—add points to determine total score and thus probability.

CLINICAL RISK	POINTS
Clinical signs and symptoms of DVT (objective leg swelling, pain with palpation)	3
PE as likely as or more likely than alternative diagnosis	3
Heart rate > 100 beats/min	1.5
Immobilization ≥ 3 days or surgery in previous 4 wk	1.5
Previous DVT or PE	1.5
Hemoptysis	1
Malignancy (including in patients stopping cancer treatment within 6 mo)	1
TOTAL SCORE	**PROBABILITY**
> 6	High
2–6	Moderate
< 2	Low

Simplified clinical probability assessment:
> 4 = likely
< 4 = unlikely

DVT = deep venous thrombosis; PE = pulmonary embolism; V/Q = ventilation/perfusion.

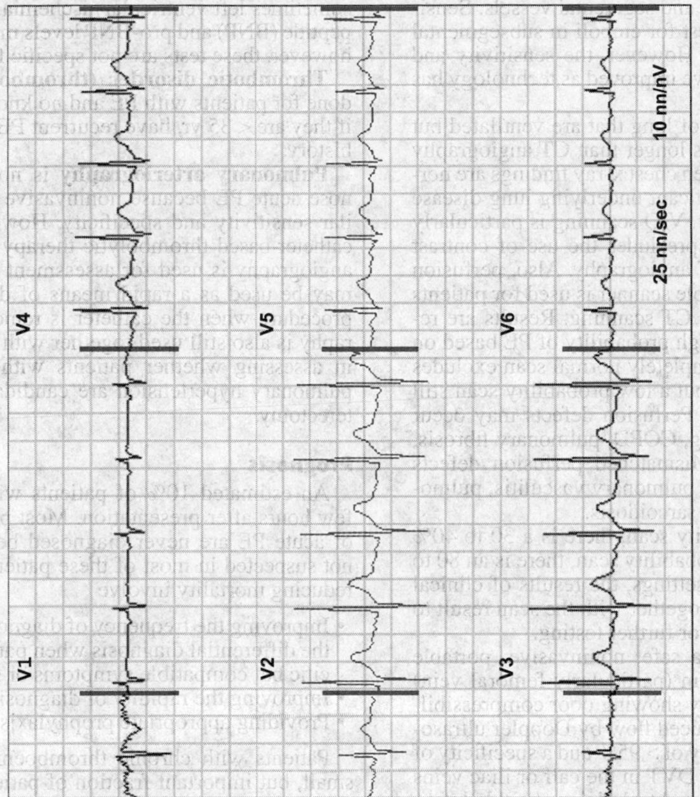

Fig. 61–1. An ECG in pulmonary embolism. The ECG shows sinus tachycardia at a rate of 110 beats/min, an $S_1Q_3T_3$ and R = S in V_1 in a patient with proven acute pulmonary embolism.

dyspneic. Fast scanning times allow the use of smaller volumes of iodinated contrast media, which reduces the risk of acute kidney injury.

The sensitivity of CT angiography is highest for PE in the main pulmonary artery and lobar and segmental vessels. Sensitivity of CT angiography is lowest for emboli in subsegmental vessels (about 30% of all PEs). However, the sensitivity and specificity of CT angiography have improved as technology has evolved.

V/Q scans in PE detect areas of lung that are ventilated but not perfused. V/Q scanning takes longer than CT angiography and is less specific. However, when chest x-ray findings are normal or near normal and no significant underlying lung disease exists, it is a highly sensitive test. V/Q scanning is particularly useful when renal insufficiency precludes the use of contrast that is otherwise required for CT angiography. Also, perfusion scans can be useful when a portable scanner is used for patients who are too unstable to undergo CT scanning. Results are reported as low, intermediate, or high probability of PE based on patterns of V/Q mismatch. A completely normal scan excludes PE with nearly 100% accuracy, but a low probability scan still carries a 15% likelihood of PE. Perfusion defects may occur in many other lung conditions (eg, COPD, pulmonary fibrosis, pneumonia, pleural effusion). Mismatched perfusion defects that may mimic PE may occur in pulmonary vasculitis, pulmonary veno-occlusive disease, and sarcoidosis.

With an intermediate probability scan, there is a 30 to 40% probability of PE; with a high probability scan, there is an 80 to 90% probability of PE. In such settings, the results of clinical probability testing must be used together with the scan result to determine the need for treatment or further testing.

Duplex ultrasonography is a safe, noninvasive, portable technique for detecting leg or arm (particularly femoral vein) thrombi. A clot can be detected by showing poor compressibility of the vein or by showing reduced flow by Doppler ultrasonography. The test has a sensitivity of > 95% and a specificity of > 95% for thrombus. Confirming DVT in the calf or iliac veins can be more difficult. The ultrasound technician should always attempt to image below the popliteal vein into its trifurcation.

Absence of thrombi in the femoral veins does not exclude the possibility of thrombus from other sources, but patients with suspected DVT and negative results on Doppler duplex ultrasonography have > 95% event-free survival, because thrombi from other sources are so much less common.

Although ultrasonography of the legs or arms is not diagnostic for PE, a study that reveals leg or axillary-subclavian thrombus establishes the need for anticoagulation and may obviate the need for further diagnostic testing unless more aggressive therapy (eg, thrombolytic therapy) is being considered. Therefore, stopping the diagnostic evaluation after detection of DVT on ultrasonography of the legs or arms is most appropriate for stable patients with contraindications to CT contrast and in whom V/Q scanning is expected to have low sensitivity (eg, in patients with an abnormal chest x-ray). In suspected acute PE, a negative ultrasound does not negate the need for additional studies.

PEARLS & PITFALLS

- In suspected acute pulmonary embolism, absence of venous thrombosis on ultrasonography does not rule out PE.

Echocardiography may show a clot in the right atrium or ventricle, but it is most commonly used for risk stratification in acute PE. The presence of RV dilation and hypokinesis may suggest the need for more aggressive therapy.

Cardiac marker testing is evolving as a useful means of stratifying mortality risk in patients with acute PE. Cardiac marker testing can be used adjunctively if PE is suspected or proven. Elevated troponin levels signify right ventricular (or sometimes left ventricular) ischemia. Elevated brain natriuretic peptide (BNP) and pro-BNP levels may signify RV dysfunction; however, these tests are not specific for RV strain or for PE.

Thrombotic disorder (thrombophilia) testing should be done for patients with PE and no known risk factors, especially if they are < 35 yr, have recurrent PE, or have a positive family history.

Pulmonary arteriography is now rarely needed to diagnose acute PE because noninvasive CT angiography has similar sensitivity and specificity. However, in patients in whom catheter-based thrombolytic therapy is being used, pulmonary angiography is used for assessment of catheter placement and may be used as a rapid means of determining success of the procedure when the catheter is removed. Pulmonary arteriography is also still used together with right-heart catheterization in assessing whether patients with chronic thromboembolic pulmonary hypertension are candidates for pulmonary endarterectomy.

Prognosis

An estimated 10% of patients with PE die within the first few hours after presentation. Most patients who die as a result of acute PE are never diagnosed before death. In fact, PE is not suspected in most of these patients. The best prospects for reducing mortality involve

- Improving the frequency of diagnosis (eg, by including PE in the differential diagnosis when patients present with nonspecific but compatible symptoms or signs)
- Improving the rapidity of diagnosis and initiation of therapy
- Providing appropriate prophylaxis in at-risk patients

Patients with chronic thromboembolic disease represent a small, but important fraction of patients with PE who survive. Anticoagulant therapy reduces the rate of recurrence of PE to about 5% in all patients.

General Treatment

- Supportive therapy
- Anticoagulation
- Sometimes inferior vena cava filter placement
- Sometimes rapid clot burden reduction

Rapid assessment for the need for supportive therapy should be undertaken. In patients with hypoxemia, oxygen should be given. In patients with hypotension due to massive PE, 0.9% saline can be given IV. Vasopressors may also be given if IV fluids fail to sufficiently increase blood pressure.

Anticoagulation is the mainstay of therapy for PE, and rapid reduction of clot burden via thrombolytic therapy or embolectomy is indicated for patients with hypotension, and for selected patients with impaired RV function. Placement of a removable percutaneous inferior vena cava filter (IVCF) should be considered for patients with contraindications to anticoagulation or for those with recurrent PE despite anticoagulation.

Most patients with strongly suspected or confirmed PE should be hospitalized for at least 24 to 48 h. Patients with abnormal vital signs or massive or submassive PE require longer periods of hospitalization. There should be a very low threshold for ICU admission in patients with extensive clot burdens, RV compromise, and/or significant tachycardia.

Massive PE always requires ICU admission. Patients with incidentally discovered PE or those with very small clot burdens and minimal symptoms can be managed as outpatients if their vital signs are stable and if a reasonable plan for outpatient treatment and follow-up is in place.

Anticoagulation

Initial anticoagulation followed by maintenance anticoagulation is indicated for patients with acute PE to prevent clot extension and further embolization as well as new clot formation. Anticoagulant therapy for acute PE should be started whenever PE is strongly suspected, as long as the risk of bleeding is deemed low. Otherwise, anticoagulation should be started as soon as the diagnosis is made. The likelihood of benefits and harms in treatment of emboli in smaller, subsegmental vessels (particularly asymptomatic and incidentally discovered emboli) is currently unknown, and concern has been expressed over the possibility that harms may outweigh benefits. Still, however, treatment is currently recommended. The primary complication of anticoagulation therapy is bleeding, and patients should be closely observed for bleeding during hospitalization.

Initial anticoagulation: Initial anticoagulation choices for acute PE include

- Intravenous unfractionated heparin
- Subcutaneous low molecular weight heparin
- Subcutaneous fondaparinux
- Factor Xa inhibitors (apixaban and rivaroxaban)
- Intravenous argatroban for patients with heparin-induced thrombocytopenia

Intravenous unfractionated heparin has a short half-life (useful when the potential for bleeding is deemed higher than usual) and is reversible with protamine. An initial bolus of unfractionated heparin is given, followed by an infusion of heparin dosed by protocol to achieve an activated PTT 1.5 to 2.5 times that of normal control (see Fig. 61–2). Therefore, unfractionated heparin requires ongoing hospitalization to administer. Further, the pharmacokinetics of unfractionated heparin are relatively unpredictable, resulting in frequent periods of over-anticoagulation and under-anticoagulation and necessitating frequent dose adjustments. Regardless, many clinicians prefer this IV unfractionated heparin regimen, particularly when thrombolytic therapy is given or contemplated or when patients are at risk of bleeding because if bleeding occurs, the short half-life means that anticoagulation is quickly reversed after the infusion is stopped.

Subcutaneous low molecular weight heparin has several advantages over unfractionated heparin including

- Superior bioavailability
- Weight-based dosing results in a more predictable anticoagulation effect than does weight-based dosing of unfractionated heparin
- Ease of administration (can be given sc once or twice daily)
- Decreased incidence of bleeding
- Potentially better outcomes
- The potential for patients to self-inject (thereby allowing earlier discharge from the hospital)
- Lower risk of heparin-induced thrombocytopenia compared with standard, unfractionated heparin

In patients with renal insufficiency, dose reductions are needed (see Table 61–3), and subsequent verification of appropriate dosing should be done by checking serum factor Xa levels (target: 0.5 to 1.2 IU/mL measured at 3 to 4 h after the 4th dose). Low molecular weight heparins are generally contraindicated in patients with severe renal insufficiency (creatinine clearance < 30 mL/min). Low molecular weight heparins are partially reversible with protamine.

Adverse effects of all heparins include

- Bleeding
- Thrombocytopenia (including heparin-induced thrombocytopenia with the potential for thromboembolism)
- Urticaria
- Anaphylaxis (rare)

Bleeding caused by over-heparinization with unfractionated heparin can be stopped with a maximum of 50 mg of protamine per 5000 units unfractionated heparin infused over 15 to 30 min. Over-heparinization with a low molecular weight heparin can be treated with protamine 1 mg in 20 mL normal saline infused over 10 to 20 min, although the precise dose is undefined because protamine only partially neutralizes low molecular weight heparin inactivation of factor Xa.

Fondaparinux is a newer factor Xa antagonist. It can be used in acute DVT instead of heparin or low molecular weight heparin. It has also been shown to prevent recurrences in patients with superficial venous thrombosis. Outcomes appear to be similar to those of unfractionated heparin. Advantages include once or twice daily fixed-dose administration, no need for monitoring of the degree of anticoagulation, and lower risk of thrombocytopenia. The dose (in mg/kg once/day) is 5 mg for patients < 50 kg, 7.5 mg for patients 50 to 100 kg, and 10 mg for patients >100 kg. Fondaparinux dose is decreased by 50% if creatinine clearance is 30 to 50 mL/min. The drug is contraindicated if creatinine clearance is < 30mL/min.

The other newer **factor Xa inhibitors,** apixaban and rivaroxaban have the advantages of oral fixed dosing, the ability to be used as maintenance anticoagulants, and the lack of need for laboratory monitoring of the anticoagulant effect. They also cause few adverse interactions with other drugs, although azole antifungal therapy and certain HIV therapies will increase certain factor Xa inhibitor drug levels and certain anticonvulsants and rifampin will decrease some factor Xa inhibitor drug levels.

Dose reductions are indicated for patients with renal insufficiency. However (unlike heparin), there is no readily available antidote to reverse their anticoagulation effect if bleeding occurs. Still, the drug half-lives are much shorter than for warfarin. If bleeding develops that requires reversal, use of 4-factor prothrombin complex concentrate should be considered and hematology consultation is recommended. The safety and efficacy of these drugs in patients with PE complicated by cardiopulmonary decompensation have not yet been studied.

The **direct thrombin inhibitor** dabigatran and the factor Xa inhibitor edoxaban have also proven effective for treatment of acute DVT. However, they must be used in transition after 5 to 10 days of parenteral therapy, and not yet been studied for use as monotherapy for initial anticoagulation in patients with PE.

Finally, in patients with suspected or proven heparin-induced thrombocytopenia, intravenous argatroban or subcutaneous fondaparinux can be used for anticoagulation; lepirudin is no longer available. Use of the newer oral anticoagulants has not yet been studied in patients with heparin-induced thrombocytopenia.

Maintenance anticoagulation: Maintenance anticoagulation is indicated to reduce the risk of clot extension or embolization and to reduce the risk of new clot formation. Drug choices for maintenance anticoagulation include

- Oral vitamin K antagonist (warfarin in the US)
- Oral factor Xa inhibitors (apixaban, rivaroxaban, edoxaban)
- Oral direct thrombin inhibitor (dabigatran)
- Subcutaneous low molecular weight heparin, primarily for high-risk cancer patients or patients with recurrent PE despite other anticoagulants

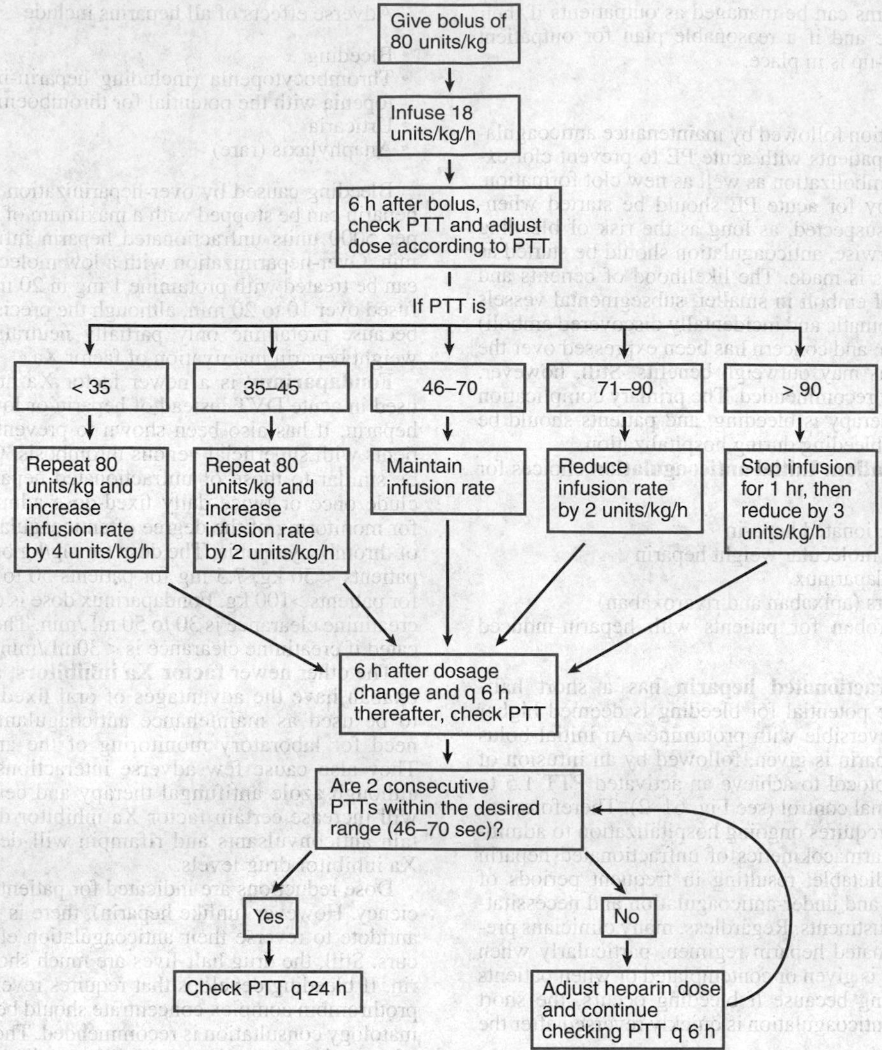

Fig. 61–2. Weight-based heparin dosing.

Warfarin is an effective long-term oral anticoagulant option that has been used for decades. In most patients, warfarin is started on the same day as heparin (or fondaparinux) therapy used for initial anticoagulation. Heparin (or fondaparinux) therapy should be overlapped with warfarin therapy for a minimum of 5 days *and* until the INR has been within the therapeutic range (2.0 to 3.0) for at least 24 h.

The major disadvantages of warfarin are the need for periodic INR monitoring, with frequent dose adjustments, and drug interactions. Physicians prescribing warfarin should be wary of drug interactions; in a patient taking warfarin, virtually any new drug should be checked.

Bleeding is the most common complication of warfarin treatment; patients > 65 yr and those with comorbidities (especially diabetes, recent myocardial infarction, Hct < 30%, or creatinine > 1.5 mg/dL) and a history of stroke or GI bleeding seem to be at greatest risk. Bleeding can be reversed with vitamin K 2.5 to 10 mg IV or po and, in an emergency, with fresh frozen plasma or a new concentrate formulation (prothrombin complex concentrates) containing factor II (prothrombin), factor VII, factor IX, factor X, protein C, and protein S. Vitamin K may cause flushing, local pain, and, rarely, anaphylaxis.

Warfarin-induced necrosis, a devastating complication of warfarin therapy, can occur in patients with heparin-induced thrombocytopenia if warfarin is started before platelet recovery. Based on these considerations and the development of more convenient oral anticoagulants, it is likely that warfarin use will decline substantially over the coming years.

PEARLS & PITFALLS

- In a patient taking warfarin, virtually any new drug should be checked for potential interactions.

The **oral factor Xa inhibitor anticoagulants** apixaban and rivaroxaban can be used for both initial and maintenance

Table 61–3. SOME LOW MOLECULAR WEIGHT HEPARIN* OPTIONS IN THROMBOEMBOLIC DISEASE

LOW MOLECULAR WEIGHT HEPARIN	TREATMENT DOSE	PROPHYLACTIC DOSE
Dalteparin	100 units/kg sc q 12 h or 200 units/kg once/day[†,‡]	2500–5000 units once/day
Enoxaparin	1 mg/kg sc q 12 h or 1.5 mg/kg sc once/day[§]	After abdominal surgery: 40 mg sc once/day After hip replacement surgery: 40 mg sc once/day or 30 mg sc q 12 h; after knee replacement: 30 mg sc q 12h For unstable angina or non-Q wave MI: 1 mg/kg sc q 12 h For other (medical) patients not undergoing surgery: 40 mg sc once/day
Tinzaparin	175 units/kg sc once/day (in patients with or without PE)[¶]	3500 units once/day

*For dosing for unfractionated heparin, see Fig. 61–2.

NOTE: Although low molecular weight heparins can be given by continuous IV infusion, this form of administration is rarely necessary or indicated. They are given by sc injection in the abdominal area while the patient is supine.

†In patients with cancer, dalteparin is dosed as 200 units/kg once/day for the first 30 days of treatment.

‡In patients who develop renal insufficiency, dalteparin dosing should be re-evaluated.

§In patients with renal insufficiency (creatinine clearance < 30 mL/min), the dose of enoxaparin must be reduced or the drug stopped.

¶In patients with renal insufficiency, tinzaparin is given cautiously, although there are no specific recommendations.

PE = pulmonary embolism; sc = subcutaneous

anticoagulation therapy (see Table 61–4). These drugs are more convenient than warfarin due to their fixed dosing and lack of need for laboratory monitoring of their anticoagulant effect; however (unlike heparin and warfarin), there is no readily available antidote to reverse anticoagulation if bleeding occurs. In clinical trials, rates of major bleeding were significantly lower with both rivaroxaban and apixaban compared with warfarin.

Edoxaban, another factor Xa inhibitor, can be used for treatment of acute deep venous thrombosis and PE and for maintenance anticoagulation therapy. After a 5 to 10 days of initial treatment with heparin or low molecular weight heparin, edoxaban is given.

The direct thrombin inhibitor dabigatran can also be used for maintenance anticoagulation therapy. After 5 to 10 days of treatment with unfractionated heparin or low molecular weight heparin, dabigatran is given.

The need for initial heparin treatment with edoxaban and dabigatran may simply be a reflection of the way the clinical trials were conducted. Clinically relevant bleeding was lower with dabigatran or edoxaban than with warfarin. The use of edoxaban or dabigatran as maintenance therapy has the same advantages and disadvantages as the factor Xa inhibitors apixaban and rivaroxaban.

Aspirin has been studied for long-term maintenance therapy. It appears more effective than placebo but less effective than all other available anticoagulants.

Duration of anticoagulation: Duration of maintenance anticoagulation for PE is dependent on a variety of factors

Table 61–4. ORAL ANTICOAGULANTS

DRUG	DOSE	COMMENTS
Factor Xa inhibitors		
Apixaban	10 mg po bid for 7 days Then 5 mg po bid	—
Edoxaban	60 mg po once/day If creatinine clearance is 15–50 mL/min or if body weight ≤ 60 kg, 30 mg po once/day	Initial treatment with heparin is needed for 5–10 days. Edoxaban should not be used if creatinine clearance is < 15 mL/min.
Fondaparinux	Patients < 50 kg: 5 mg Patients 50–100 kg: 7.5 mg Patients > 100 kg: 10 mg	Fondaparinux dose is decreased by 50% if creatinine clearance is 30–50 mL/min. The drug is contraindicated if creatinine clearance is < 30mL/min.
Rivaroxaban	15 mg po bid for 21 days taken with food Then 20 mg po once/day taken with food	Rivaroxiban should not be used for DVT if creatinine clearance is < 30 mL/min.
Factor IIa (thrombin) inhibitor		
Dabigatran	150 mg po bid	Initial treatment with heparin is needed for 5–10 days. Dabigatran should not be used for DVT if creatinine clearance is < 30 mL/min.

(eg, risk factors for PE, bleeding risk) and can range from 3 mo to lifelong therapy. Clearly transient risk factors (eg, immobilization, recent surgery, trauma) require only 3 mo. Patients with unprovoked PE, those with more durable risk factors for PE (eg, cancer, thrombophilic disorder), and those with recurrent PE might benefit from lifelong anticoagulation provided the bleeding risk is low or moderate.

Risk factors for bleeding include

- Age > 65 years
- Previous bleeding
- Thrombocytopenia
- Antiplatelet therapy
- Poor anticoagulant control
- Frequent falls
- Liver failure
- Alcohol abuse
- Recent surgery
- Reduced functional capacity
- Previous stroke
- Diabetes
- Anemia
- Cancer
- Renal failure

Low risk for bleeding is defined as no bleeding risk factors, moderate risk for bleeding is defined as one risk factor, and high risk for bleeding is defined as two or more risk factors.

Rapid Reduction of Clot Burden

Clot elimination by means of embolectomy or dissolution with IV or catheter-based thrombolytic therapy should be considered for acute PE associated with hypotension (massive PE). Patients who are hypotensive and require vasopressor therapy are obvious candidates. Patients with a systolic BP < 90 mm Hg lasting at least 15 min are hemodynamically compromised and are also candidates.

Although only anticoagulation is generally recommended for patients with very mild RV dysfunction (based on clinical, ECG or echocardiographic findings), thrombolytic therapy or embolectomy may be needed when RV compromise is severe, even when hypotension is not present.

Systemic thrombolytic therapy: Systemic thrombolytic therapy with alteplase (tissue plasminogen activator [tPA]), streptokinase, or urokinase offers a noninvasive way to rapidly restore pulmonary blood flow but is controversial because long-term benefits do not clearly outweigh the risk of hemorrhage. Regardless, most experts agree that systemic thrombolytic therapy should be given to patients with hemodynamic compromise, particularly when it is severe. Although no single prospective randomized trial of systemic thrombolytic therapy has shown improved survival in patients with submassive PE, some experts recommend thrombolytics, particularly when patients also have numerous or large clots, very severe RV dysfunction, marked tachycardia, significant hypoxemia, and other concomitant findings such as residual clot in the leg, positive troponin values, and/or elevated BNP values. Others reserve thrombolytic therapy only for patients with massive PE.

Absolute contraindications to thrombolytics include

- Prior hemorrhagic stroke
- Ischemic stroke within 1 yr
- Active external or internal bleeding from any source
- Intracranial injury or surgery within 2 mo
- Intracranial tumor

Relative contraindications include

- Recent surgery (≤ 10 days)
- Hemorrhagic diathesis (as in hepatic insufficiency)
- Pregnancy
- Recent punctures of large noncompressible veins (eg, subclavian or internal jugular veins)
- Recent femoral artery catheterization (eg, ≤ 10 days)
- Peptic ulcer disease or other conditions that increase the risk of bleeding
- Severe hypertension (systolic BP > 180 mm Hg or diastolic BP > 110 mm Hg)

Except for concurrent intracerebral hemorrhage, thrombolytic therapy is sometimes given to patients with massive PE who have "absolute contraindications" to such therapy if death is otherwise expected. In patients with relative contraindications, the decision to give systemic thrombolytics depends on individual patient factors.

Options for systemic thrombolysis include streptokinase, urokinase, and alteplase (see Table 61–5).

Although no drug has proved superior to the others, streptokinase is now rarely used because of the risk of allergic and pyrogenic reactions and because administration requires constant infusion for up to 12 to 24 h. Further, alteplase is more commonly used due to the shorter infusion time when compared with other drugs. Tenecteplase continues to be studied for acute PE. In the US, when systemic thrombolytics are given, heparin is usually stopped after the initial loading dose. However, in Europe, heparin is often continued, and there is no clear determination as to which method is preferred.

Bleeding, if it occurs, can be reversed with cryoprecipitate or fresh frozen plasma. Accessible vascular access sites that are bleeding can be compressed. The potential for bleeding after systemic thrombolysis has led to increased implementation of catheter-based thrombolysis, because much lower doses of thrombolytic agents are used.

Catheter-directed therapy: Catheter-directed PE therapy (thrombolytics, embolectomy) uses catheter placement in the pulmonary arteries for disruption and/or lysis of clot. It is used to treat massive PE. Indications for the treatment of submassive PE are evolving. Studies to date, including prospective randomized clinical trials, have demonstrated that this approach leads to an improved RV/LV ratio at 24 h compared with anticoagulation alone. Other outcomes and safety of catheter-based therapy compared to systemic thrombolysis are under investigation.

In **catheter-based PE thrombolytic therapy,** the pulmonary arteries are accessed via a typical right-heart catheterization/ pulmonary arteriography procedure, and thrombolytics are delivered directly to large proximal emboli via the catheter. The most widely studied technique uses high-frequency, low-power

Table 61–5. REGIMENS FOR SYSTEMIC THROMBOLYSIS

DRUG	STANDARD REGIMEN
Alteplase*	100 mg continuous infusion over 2 h
Streptokinase	250,000 units IV over 30 min Then, 100,000 units/h IV for 24 h
Urokinase	4400 units/kg IV over 10 min Then, 4400 units/kg/h IV for 12 h

*Some data suggest that lower doses of alteplase (50 mg IV) are as effective as the standard dose of 100 mg IV and cause fewer bleeding complications.

ultrasonography to facilitate delivery of the thrombolytics. Ultrasonography accelerates the thrombolytic process by disaggregating fibrin strands and increasing permeability of lytic drug into the clot.

Other techniques involve **catheter-directed vortex suction embolectomy,** sometimes in combination with extracorporeal bypass. Catheter-directed vortex suction embolectomy differs from systemic thrombolysis and catheter-based PE thrombolytic therapy in that a larger bore catheter is required and blood that is suctioned out must be redirected out back into a vein (usually femoral). Patients with venal caval, right atrial, or right ventricular thrombi-in-transit, and very proximal acute PE are the best candidates. Veno-arterial extracorporeal membrane oxygenation (ECMO) may be used as a rescue procedure in severely ill patients with acute PE, regardless of what other therapies are used.

Surgical embolectomy: **Surgical embolectomy** is reserved for patients with PE who are hypotensive despite supportive measures (persistent systolic BP ≤ 90 mm Hg after fluid therapy and oxygen or if vasopressor therapy is required) or on the verge of cardiac or respiratory arrest. Surgical embolectomy should be considered if use of thrombolysis is contraindicated; in such cases, catheter-directed vortex embolectomy may also be considered and, depending on local resources and expertise, tried before surgical embolectomy. Surgical embolectomy appears to increase survival in patients with massive PE but is not widely available. As with catheter-based thrombosis/clot extraction, the decision to proceed with embolectomy and the choice of technique depend on local resources and expertise.

Prevention

Prevention of acute venous thromboembolism: Prevention of PE means prevention of deep venous thrombosis (DVT); the need depends on the patient's risks, including

- Type and duration of surgery
- Comorbid conditions, including cancer and hypercoagulable disorders
- Presence of a central venous catheter
- Prior history of DVT or PE

Bedbound patients and patients undergoing surgical, especially orthopedic, procedures benefit, and most of these patients can be identified before a thrombus forms (see Table 61–6). Preventive measures include low-dose unfractionated heparin, low molecular weight heparin, warfarin, fondaparinux, oral anticoagulants (rivaroxaban, apixaban, dabigatran), compression devices, and elastic compression stockings.

Choice of drug or device depends on various factors, including the patient population, the perceived risk, contraindications (eg, bleeding risk), relative costs, and ease of use. The American College of Chest Physicians has published comprehensive evidence-based recommendations for prophylaxis of acute DVT, including the duration of prophylaxis, in surgical and nonsurgical patients and during pregnancy. The need for prophylaxis has been studied in numerous patient populations.

The type of surgery as well as patient-specific factors determine the risk of DVT. Independent risk factors include

- Age ≥ 60 yr
- Prior DVT or PE
- Cancer
- Anesthesia ≥ 2 h
- Bed rest ≥ 4 days
- Male sex
- Hospital stay ≥ 2 days
- Sepsis
- Pregnancy or the postpartum state
- Central venous access
- BMI > 40

The Caprini score is commonly used for DVT risk stratification and determination of the need for DVT prophylaxis in surgical patients (see Table 61–7).

The need for DVT prophylaxis is based on the risk assessment score (see Table 61–6). Appropriate preventive measures, ranging from early ambulation to use of heparin, depend on the total score.

Drug regimens for pulmonary embolism prevention: Drug therapy to prevent DVT is usually begun after surgery, to help prevent intraoperative bleeding. However, preoperative prophylaxis is also effective.

In general surgery patients, **low dose unfractionated heparin** is given in doses of 5000 units sc q 8 to 12 h for 7 to 10 days or until the patient is fully ambulatory. Immobilized patients not undergoing surgery should receive 5000 units sc q 8 to 12 h until they are ambulatory.

Low molecular weight heparin dosing for DVT prophylaxis depends on the specific drug (enoxaparin, dalteparin, tinzaparin). Low molecular weight heparins are at least as effective as low dose unfractionated heparin for preventing DVT and PE.

Fondaparinux 2.5 mg sc once/day is as effective as low molecular weight heparin for orthopedic surgery and in some other settings. It is a selective factor Xa inhibitor.

Warfarin is usually effective and safe at a dose of 2 to 5 mg po once/day or at a dose adjusted to maintain an INR of 2 to 3 in patients who have undergone total hip or knee replacement. It is still used by some orthopedic surgeons for prophylaxis in these patients but is increasingly being supplanted by the use of the newer oral anticoagulants.

Rivaroxaban, an oral factor Xa inhibitor, is used for prevention of acute DVT/PE in patients undergoing total knee or hip arthroplasty. The dose is 10 mg po once/day. Its use in other patients (surgical and nonsurgical) is currently under investigation.

Apixaban, an oral factor Xa inhibitor, is also used for prevention of acute DVT/PE in patients undergoing total knee or hip arthroplasty. The dose is 2.5 mg po bid. Like rivaroxaban, its use in other types of patients is currently under investigation.

Prophylactic devices for pulmonary embolism: Inferior vena cava filters, intermittent pneumatic compression (also known as sequential compression devices [SCD]), and graded elastic compression stockings may be used alone or in combination with drugs to prevent PE. Whether these devices are used alone or in combination depends on the specific indication.

An **inferior vena cava filter** (IVCF) may help prevent PE in patients with DVT in the leg, but IVCF placement may risk long-term complications. Benefits outweigh risk if a second PE is predicted to be life-threatening; however, few clinical trial data are available. A filter is most clearly indicated in patients who have:

- Proven DVT and contraindications to anticoagulation
- Recurrent DVT (or emboli) despite adequate anticoagulation
- Undergone pulmonary thromboendarterectomy
- Marginal cardiopulmonary function, causing concern for their ability to tolerate additional small emboli (occasionally)

Because venous collaterals can develop, providing a pathway for emboli to circumvent the IVCF, and because filters occasionally thrombose, patients with recurrent DVT or nonmodifiable

Table 61–6. RISK ASSESSMENT FOR THROMBOSIS

RISK FACTOR	SCORE
Age (yr)	
41–60	1
60–74	2
≥ 75	3
Surgery	
Minor surgery during current hospitalization	1
Major surgery within the past 1 mo	1
Arthroscopic surgery during current hospitalization	2
Major surgery lasting > 45 min during current hospitalization	1
Laparoscopic surgery lasting > 45 min during current hospitalization	2
Elective major arthroplasty of the leg during current hospitalization	5
Coexisting conditions	
Varicose veins	1
Inflammatory bowel disease	1
Edema, leg (current)	1
Obesity (BMI > 25)	1
Acute MI	1
Heart failure within the preceding 1 mo	1
Sepsis within the preceding 1 mo	1
Serious lung disease* within the preceding 1 mo	1
Abnormal pulmonary function (eg, COPD)	1
Central venous access	2
Cancer (present or previous)	2
History of DVT/PE	3
Family history of thrombosis†	3
Factor V Leiden mutation	3
Prothrombin 20210A mutation	3
Elevated serum homocysteine	3
Positive lupus anticoagulant	3
Elevated anticardiolipin antibodies	3
Heparin-induced thrombocytopenia	3
Other congenital or acquired thrombophilia	3
Stroke within the preceding 1 mo	5
Multiple trauma within the preceding 1 mo	5
Acute spinal cord injury/paralysis within the preceding 1 mo	5
Immobilization	
Current bed rest (medical patient)	1
Bed rest > 72 h	2
Immobilizing plaster cast within the preceding 1 mo	2
Hip, pelvis, or leg fracture within the preceding 1 mo	5
Additional risk factors for women	
Oral contraceptive use or hormone replacement therapy	1
Pregnancy or postpartum within the preceding 1 mo	1
History of unexplained stillbirth, recurrent spontaneous abortion (≥ 3), premature birth with toxemia or growth-restricted infant	1
Other	
Other risk factors‡	1

*Serious lung disease includes pneumonia.
†Family history of thrombosis is the most frequently missed risk factor.
‡Other risk factors include BMI > 40, smoking, diabetes requiring insulin, chemotherapy, blood transfusions, and length of surgery > 2 h.
Data from Gould MK, Garcia DA, Wren SM, et al: Prevention of VTE in Nonorthopedic Surgical Patients Antithrombotic Therapy and Prevention of Thrombosis, 9th ed: American College of Chest Physicians Evidence-Based Clinical Practice Guidelines. *Chest* 141(2_suppl): e227S, 2012.
BMI = body mass index; COPD = chronic obstructive pulmonary disease; DVT = deep vein thrombosis; PE = pulmonary embolism.

Table 61–7. PROPHYLAXIS BASED ON CAPRINI SCORE

POINTS	RISK	PROPHYLAXIS
0	Very low	Early ambulation
1–2	Low	Sequential compression device (SCD)
3–4	Moderate	Heparin q 8 h or low molecular weight heparin +/− SCD
≥ 5	High	Heparin or low molecular weight heparin + SCD

risk factors for DVT may still require anticoagulation. An IVCF is placed in the inferior vena cava just below the renal veins via catheterization of an internal jugular or femoral vein. Most IVCFs are removable. Occasionally, a filter dislodges and may migrate up the venous bed, even to the heart, and needs to be removed or replaced. A filter can also become thrombosed, causing bilateral venous congestion (including acute phlegmasia cerulea dolens) in the leg, lower body ischemia, and acute kidney injury.

Intermittent pneumatic compression (IPC) with SCDs provides rhythmic external compression to the legs or to the legs and thighs. It is more effective for preventing calf than proximal DVT. It is insufficient as sole prophylaxis after hip or knee replacement but is often used in low-risk patients after other types of surgery or in medical patients who have a low-risk of DVT or who are at high risk of bleeding. IPC can theoretically trigger PE in immobilized patients who have developed occult DVT while not receiving DVT prophylaxis.

Graded elastic compression stockings are likely less effective than external pneumatic leg compression, but one systematic meta-analysis suggested that they reduced the incidence of DVT in postoperative patients from 26% in the control group to 13% in the compression stockings group.

Choice of prevention in pulmonary embolism: After surgical procedures with a high incidence of DVT/PE, low dose unfractionated heparin, low molecular weight heparin, or adjusted-dose warfarin is recommended.

After orthopedic surgery of the hip or knee, additional options include the newer oral anticoagulants, rivaroxaban and apixaban. These drugs are safe and effective and do not require laboratory tests to monitor the level of anticoagulation as is needed for warfarin.

For **total hip arthroplasty,** patients should continue to take anticoagulants for 35 days postoperatively. In selected patients at very high risk of both DVT/PE and bleeding, temporary placement of an IVCF is an option for prophylaxis.

A high risk of DVT/PE also occurs in patients undergoing elective neurosurgery and those with acute spinal cord injury and multiple trauma. Although physical methods (SCDs and elastic stockings) have been used in neurosurgical patients because of concern about intracranial bleeding, low molecular weight heparin appears to be an acceptable alternative. The combination of SCDs and low molecular weight heparin may be more effective than either alone in high-risk patients. Limited data support the combination of SCDs, elastic compression stockings, and low molecular weight heparin in patients with spinal cord injury or in multiple trauma. For very high-risk patients, a temporary IVCF may be considered.

In **acutely ill medical patients,** low dose unfractionated heparin, low molecular weight heparin, or fondaparinux can be given. SCDs, elastic compression stockings, or both may be used when anticoagulants are contraindicated. For ischemic stroke patients, low dose unfractionated heparin or low molecular weight heparin can be used; SCD, elastic compression stockings, or both may be beneficial.

KEY POINTS

- Acute PE is a common and potentially devastating medical condition.
- Clinical suspicion and a confirmatory diagnosis are essential because in most patients who die from acute PE, PE is not even suspected.
- Because anticoagulation improves survival, patients should be anticoagulated when PE is diagnosed or strongly suspected.
- Patients with massive PE and certain patients with submassive PE should be considered for thrombolytic therapy or embolectomy.
- Prevention of deep vein thrombosis (and thus PE) should be considered in all at-risk hospitalized patients.

NONTHROMBOTIC PULMONARY EMBOLISM

Nonthrombotic sources of pulmonary embolism include air, fat, amniotic fluid, infected material, foreign bodies, and tumors.

Pulmonary embolism can arise from nonthrombotic sources. PE caused by nonthrombotic sources results in clinical syndromes that differ from those caused by thrombotic PE. Diagnosis is usually based in part or completely on clinical criteria, including in particular the patient's risk. Treatment includes supportive measures.

Air embolism: Air embolism is caused by introduction of large amounts of air into systemic veins or into the right side of the heart, which then move to the pulmonary arterial system. Pulmonary outflow tract obstruction may occur, which can be rapidly fatal. Causes include surgery, blunt trauma, defective or uncapped venous catheters, and errors occurring during the insertion or removal of central venous catheters.

Treatment includes placement of the patient in the left lateral decubitus position, preferably in the Trendelenburg position (ie, head lower than the feet), to trap air in the apex of the right ventricle and thus prevent brain embolism and main pulmonary artery outflow obstruction. Supportive measures are also needed.

Rapid decompression after underwater diving may cause microbubble formation in the pulmonary circulation, a different problem, which results in endothelial damage, hypoxemia, and diffuse infiltrates (see p. 3024).

Fat embolism: Fat embolism is caused by introduction of fat or bone marrow particles into the systemic venous system and then into pulmonary arteries. Causes include fractures of long bones, orthopedic procedures, microvascular occlusion or necrosis of bone marrow in patients with sickle cell crisis, and, rarely, toxic modification of native or parenteral serum lipids.

Fat embolism causes a pulmonary syndrome similar to acute respiratory distress syndrome (ARDS), with severe hypoxemia of rapid onset often accompanied by neurologic changes and a petechial rash.

Early splinting of fractures of long bones and operative rather than external fixation are thought to help prevent fat embolism.

Amniotic fluid embolism: Amniotic fluid embolism is a rare syndrome caused by introduction of amniotic fluid into the maternal venous and then pulmonary arterial system. The syndrome occurs around the time of labor (amniotic fluid embolism) or, even less often, during prepartum uterine manipulations.

Patients can have cardiac and respiratory distress due to anaphylaxis, vasoconstriction causing acute severe pulmonary hypertension, and direct pulmonary microvascular toxicity with hypoxemia and pulmonary infiltrates.

Septic embolism: Septic embolism occurs when infected material embolizes to the lung. Causes include IV drug use, right-sided infective endocarditis, and septic thrombophlebitis.

Septic embolism causes symptoms and signs of pneumonia (eg, fever, cough, sputum production, pleuritic chest pain, dyspnea, tachypnea, and tachycardia) or sepsis (eg, fever, hypotension, oliguria, tachypnea, tachycardia, and confusion). Initially, nodular opacities appear on the chest x-ray; the appearance may progress to peripheral infiltrates, and emboli may cavitate (particularly emboli caused by *Staphylococcus aureus*).

Treatment includes that of the underlying infection.

Foreign body embolism: Foreign body embolism caused by introduction of particulate matter into the pulmonary arterial system, usually by IV injection of inorganic substances, such as talc by heroin users or elemental mercury by patients with mental disorders.

Focal pulmonary infiltrates may result.

Tumor embolism: Tumor embolism is a rare complication of cancer (usually adenocarcinoma) in which neoplastic cells from an organ enter the systemic venous and pulmonary arterial system, where they lodge, proliferate, and obstruct flow.

Patients typically present with dyspnea and pleuritic chest pain and signs of cor pulmonale that develop over weeks to months.

The diagnosis, which is suggested by micronodules or diffuse pulmonary infiltrates on chest x-ray, can be confirmed by biopsy or occasionally by cytologic aspiration and histologic study of pulmonary capillary blood.

62 Pulmonary Hypertension

Pulmonary hypertension is increased pressure in the pulmonary circulation. It has many secondary causes; some cases are idiopathic. In pulmonary hypertension, pulmonary vessels become constricted and/or obstructed. Severe pulmonary hypertension leads to right ventricular overload and failure. Symptoms are fatigue, exertional dyspnea, and, occasionally, chest discomfort and syncope. Diagnosis is made by finding elevated pulmonary artery pressure (estimated by echocardiography and confirmed by right heart catheterization). Treatment is with pulmonary vasodilators and diuretics. In some advanced cases, lung transplantation is an option. Prognosis is poor overall if a treatable secondary cause is not found.

Pulmonary hypertension is defined as a mean pulmonary arterial pressure ≥ 25 mm Hg at rest and a normal (≤ 15 mm Hg) pulmonary artery occlusion pressure (pulmonary capillary wedge pressure) as measured by right heart catheterization.

Etiology

Many conditions and drugs cause pulmonary hypertension. The most common overall causes of pulmonary hypertension are

- Left heart failure, including diastolic dysfunction
- Parenchymal lung disease with hypoxia
- Miscellaneous: Sleep apnea, connective tissue disorders, and recurrent pulmonary embolism

Pulmonary hypertension is currently classified into 5 groups (see Table 62–1) based on a number of pathologic, physiologic, and clinical factors. In the first group (pulmonary arterial hypertension), the primary disorder affects the small pulmonary arterioles.

A small number of cases of pulmonary arterial hypertension (PAH) occur sporadically, unrelated to any identifiable disorder; these cases are termed idiopathic pulmonary arterial hypertension. Hereditary forms of PAH (autosomal dominant with incomplete penetrance) have been identified; 75% of cases are caused by mutations in bone morphogenetic protein receptor type 2 (*BMPR2*). Other identified mutations include activin-like kinase type 1 receptor (*ALK-1*), caveolin 1 (*CAV1*), endoglin (*ENG*), potassium channel subfamily K member 3 (*KCNK3*), and mothers against decapentaplegic homologue 9 (*SMAD9*) but are much less common, occurring in ~1% of cases. In about 20% of cases of hereditary pulmonary arterial hypertension, the causative mutations are unidentified. A newly identified mutation in the *EIF2AK4* gene has been linked to pulmonary veno-occlusive disease, a form of PAH Group 1'.[1]

Certain drugs and toxins are risk factors for PAH. Those definitely associated with PAH are appetite suppressants (fenfluramine, dexfenfluramine, aminorex), toxic rapeseed oil, and benfluorex. SSRIs taken by pregnant women are a risk for development of persistent pulmonary hypertension of the newborn (PPHN). Drugs that are likely associated with PAH are amphetamines, methamphetamines, L-tryptophan, and dasatinib.[2]

Patients with hereditary causes of hemolytic anemia, such as sickle cell disease, are at high risk of developing pulmonary hypertension (10% of cases based on right heart catheterization criteria). The mechanism is related to intravascular hemolysis and release of cell-free Hb into the plasma, which scavenges nitric oxide, generates reactive oxygen species, and activates the hemostatic system. Other risk factors for pulmonary hypertension in sickle cell disease include iron overload, liver dysfunction, thrombotic disorders, and chronic kidney disease.

1. Eyries M, Montani D, Girerd B, et al: EIF2AK4 mutations cause pulmonary veno-occlusive disease, a recessive form of pulmonary hypertension. *Nat Genet* 46(1):65–69, 2014. doi: 10.1038/ng.2844.
2. Simonneau G, Gatzoulis MA, Adatial I, et al: Updated clinical classification of pulmonary hypertension. *J Am Coll Cardiol* 62(25 Suppl):D34–41, 2013. doi: 10.1038/ng.2844. Erratum in *J Am Coll Cardiol* 63(7):746, 2014.

Pathophysiology

Pathophysiologic mechanisms that cause pulmonary hypertension include

- Increased pulmonary vascular resistance
- Increased pulmonary venous pressure

Increased pulmonary vascular resistance is caused by obliteration of the pulmonary vascular bed and/or by pathologic vasoconstriction. Pulmonary hypertension is characterized by variable and sometimes pathologic vasoconstriction and by endothelial and smooth muscle proliferation, hypertrophy, and chronic inflammation, resulting in vascular wall remodeling. Vasoconstriction is thought to be due in part to enhanced activity of thromboxane and endothelin-1 (both vasoconstrictors) and reduced activity of prostacyclin and nitric oxide (both vasodilators). The increased pulmonary vascular pressure that results from vascular obstruction further injures the endothelium. Injury activates coagulation at the intimal surface, which may worsen the hypertension. Thrombotic coagulopathy due to platelet dysfunction, increased activity of plasminogen activator inhibitor type 1 and fibrinopeptide A, and decreased tissue plasminogen activator activity may also contribute. Platelets, when stimulated, may also play a key role by secreting substances that increase proliferation of fibroblasts and smooth muscle cells such as platelet-derived growth factor (PDGF), vascular endothelial growth factor (VEGF), and transforming growth factor-beta (TGF-β). Focal coagulation at the endothelial surface should not be confused with chronic thromboembolic pulmonary hypertension, in which pulmonary hypertension is caused by organized pulmonary emboli.

Increased pulmonary venous pressure is typically caused by disorders that affect the left side of the heart and raise left chamber pressures, which ultimately lead to elevated pressure in the pulmonary veins. Elevated pulmonary venous pressures can cause acute damage to the alveolar-capillary wall and subsequent edema. Persistently high pressures may eventually lead to irreversible thickening of the walls of the alveolar-capillary membrane, decreasing lung diffusion capacity. The most common setting for pulmonary venous hypertension is in left heart failure with preserved ejection fraction (HF-PEF), typically in older women who have hypertension and metabolic syndrome. When the transpulmonary gradient (mean pulmonary artery pressure to pulmonary artery occlusion pressure gradient) is > 12 mm Hg or the pulmonary artery diastolic pressure to pulmonary artery occlusion pressure gradient is > 6 mm Hg, prognosis is poor.

In most patients, pulmonary hypertension eventually leads to right ventricular hypertrophy followed by dilation and right ventricular failure. Right ventricular failure limits cardiac output during exertion.

Symptoms and Signs

Progressive exertional dyspnea and easy fatigability occur in almost all patients. Atypical chest discomfort and exertional light-headedness or presyncope may accompany dyspnea and indicate more severe disease. These symptoms are due primarily to insufficient cardiac output caused by right heart failure. Raynaud syndrome occurs in about 10% of patients with idiopathic pulmonary arterial hypertension; the majority are women. Hemoptysis is rare but may be fatal. Hoarseness due to recurrent laryngeal nerve compression by an enlarged pulmonary artery (ie, Ortner syndrome) also occurs rarely.

In advanced disease, signs of right heart failure may include right ventricular heave, widely split 2nd heart sound (S_2), an accentuated pulmonic component (P_2) of S_2, a pulmonary ejection click, a right ventricular 3rd heart sound (S_3), tricuspid regurgitation murmur, and jugular vein distention. Liver congestion and peripheral edema are common late manifestations. Pulmonary auscultation is usually normal. Patients also may have manifestations of causative or associated disorders.

Diagnosis

- Exertional dyspnea
- Initial confirmation: Chest x-ray, spirometry, ECG, echocardiography, and CBC
- Identification of underlying disorder: Ventilation/perfusion scan or CT angiography, high-resolution CT (HRCT) of the chest, pulmonary function testing, polysomnography, HIV testing, liver function testing, and autoantibody testing

Table 62–1. CLASSIFICATION OF PULMONARY HYPERTENSION

GROUP	TYPE	SPECIFIC DISORDERS
1	Pulmonary arterial hypertension (PAH)	Idiopathic PAH Heritable PAH: • *BMPR2* • *ALK-1, ENG, SMAD9, CAV1, KCNK3* • Unknown Drug- and toxin-induced PAH Disorders associated with PAH: • Connective tissue disorders • HIV infection • Portal hypertension • Congenital heart disorders • Schistosomiasis
1'	Pulmonary veno-occlusive disease (PVOD) and/or pulmonary capillary hemangiomatosis	Immune mediated: • Connective tissue disorders Heritable PVOD: • *EIF2AK4* Infectious: • Measles • Epstein-Barr virus (EBV) • Cytomegalovirus (CMV) • HIV Drug- and toxin-induced PVOD Coagulopathic

Table continues on the following page.

Table 62–1. CLASSIFICATION OF PULMONARY HYPERTENSION (*Continued*)

GROUP	TYPE	SPECIFIC DISORDERS
1"	Persistent pulmonary hypertension of the newborn (PPHN)	—
2	Pulmonary hypertension with left-heart disease	Left heart systolic dysfunction Left heart diastolic dysfunction, including left heart failure with preserved ejection fraction Valvular heart disorders Congenital or acquired left heart inflow or outflow tract obstruction and congenital cardiomyopathies
3	Pulmonary hypertension associated with lung disorders, hypoxemia, or both	Alveolar hypoventilation disorders COPD Chronic exposure to high altitude Developmental abnormalities Interstitial lung disease Sleep-disordered breathing Other pulmonary disorders with a mixed restrictive and obstructive pattern
4	Pulmonary hypertension due to chronic thrombotic or embolic disorders	Nonthrombotic pulmonary embolism (eg, due to tumors, parasites, or foreign materials) Thromboembolic obstruction of distal or proximal pulmonary arteries
5	Miscellaneous (unclear or multifactorial mechanisms)	Hematologic disorders: • Chronic hemolytic anemia • Myeloproliferative disorders • Splenectomy Systemic disorders: • Sarcoidosis • Pulmonary Langerhans cell histiocytosis • Lymphangioleiomyomatosis Metabolic disorders: • Glycogen storage disease • Gaucher disease • Thyroid disorders Other disorders: • Fibrosing mediastinitis • Tumor, causing obstruction • Chronic kidney disease • Segmental pulmonary hypertension

Adapted from the Fifth World Symposium on PAH, Nice, 2013; Simonneau G, Gatzoulis MA, Adatial, et al: Updated clinical classification of pulmonary hypertension. *Journal of the American College of Cardiology* 62 (supplement D):D34–D41, 2013.

- Confirmation of the diagnosis and gauging severity: Pulmonary artery (right heart) catheterization
- Additional studies to determine severity: 6-min walk distance and plasma levels of N-terminal brain natriuretic peptide (BNP) or pro-BNP

Pulmonary hypertension is suspected in patients with significant exertional dyspnea who are otherwise relatively healthy and have no history or signs of other disorders known to cause pulmonary symptoms.

Patients initially undergo chest x-ray, spirometry, and ECG to identify more common causes of dyspnea, followed by transthoracic Doppler echocardiography to assess right ventricular function and pulmonary artery systolic pressures as well as to detect structural left heart disease that might be causing pulmonary hypertension. CBC is obtained to document the presence or absence of erythrocytosis, anemia, and thrombocytopenia.

The most common x-ray finding in pulmonary hypertension is enlarged hilar vessels that rapidly prune into the periphery and a right ventricle that fills the anterior airspace on lateral view. Spirometry and lung volumes may be normal or detect mild restriction, and diffusing capacity for carbon monoxide (DLco) is usually reduced. Common ECG findings include right axis deviation, R > S in V_1, $S_1Q_3T_3$ (suggesting right ventricular hypertrophy), and peaked P waves (suggesting right atrial dilation).

Additional tests are obtained as indicated to diagnose secondary causes that are not apparent clinically. These tests can include

- Ventilation/perfusion scanning or CT angiography to detect thromboembolic disease
- HRCT for detailed information about lung parenchymal disorders
- Pulmonary function tests to identify obstructive or restrictive lung disease

- Serum autoantibody tests (eg, antinuclear antibodies [ANA], rheumatoid factor [RF], Scl-70 [topoisomerase I], anti-Ro (anti-SSA), antiribonucleoprotein [anti-RNP], and anticentromere antibodies) to gather evidence for or against associated autoimmune disorders

Chronic thromboembolic pulmonary hypertension is suggested by CT or ventilation/perfusion (VQ) scan findings and is confirmed by arteriography. CT angiography is useful to evaluate proximal clot and fibrotic encroachment of the vascular lumen. Other tests, such as HIV testing, liver function tests, and polysomnography, are done in the appropriate clinical context.

When the initial evaluation suggests a diagnosis of pulmonary hypertension, pulmonary artery catheterization is necessary to measure right atrial, right ventricular, pulmonary artery, and pulmonary artery occlusion pressures; cardiac output; and left ventricular diastolic pressure. Right-sided oxygen saturation should be measured to exclude atrial septal defect. Although finding a mean pulmonary arterial pressure of > 25 mm Hg and a pulmonary artery occlusion pressure ≤ 15 mm Hg in the absence of an underlying disorder identifies pulmonary arterial hypertension, most patients with pulmonary arterial hypertension present with substantially higher pressure (eg, mean of 60 mm Hg). Vasodilating drugs, such as inhaled nitric oxide, IV epoprostenol, or adenosine, are often given during catheterization. Decreasing right-sided pressures in response to these drugs may help in the choice of drugs for treatment. Lung biopsy, once widely done, is neither needed nor recommended because of its associated high morbidity and mortality.

Echocardiography findings of right heart systolic dysfunction (eg, tricuspid annular plane systolic excursion) and certain right heart catheterization results (eg, low cardiac output, high mean pulmonary artery pressures, and high right atrial pressures) indicate that pulmonary hypertension is severe. Other indicators of severity in pulmonary hypertension are assessed to evaluate prognosis and to help monitor responses to therapy. They include a low 6-min walk distance and high plasma levels of N-terminal pro-brain natriuretic peptide (NT-pro-BNP) or brain natriuretic peptide (BNP).

Once pulmonary hypertension is diagnosed, the patient's family history should be reviewed to detect possible genetic transmission (eg, premature deaths in otherwise healthy members of the extended family). In familial pulmonary arterial hypertension, genetic counseling is needed to advise mutation carriers of the risk of disease (about 20%) and to advocate serial screening with echocardiography. Testing for mutations in the *BMPR2* gene in idiopathic pulmonary arterial hypertension can help identify family members at risk.

Prognosis

Five-year survival for treated patients is about 50%. However, some patient registries suggest lower mortality (eg, 20 to 30% at 3 to 5 yr in the French registry and 10 to 30% at 1 to 3 yr in the REVEAL registry), presumably because currently available treatments are superior. Indicators of a poorer prognosis include

- Lack of response to vasodilators
- Hypoxemia
- Reduced overall physical functioning
- Low 6-min walk distance
- High plasma levels of NT-pro-BNP or BNP
- Echocardiographic indicators of right heart systolic dysfunction (eg, tricuspid annular plane systolic excursion)
- Right heart catheterization showing low cardiac output, high mean pulmonary artery pressures, and/or high right atrial pressures

Patients with systemic sclerosis, sickle cell disease, or HIV infection with pulmonary arterial hypertension have a worse prognosis than those without pulmonary arterial hypertension. For example, patients with sickle cell disease and pulmonary hypertension have a 40% 4-yr mortality rate.

Treatment

- Avoidance of activities that may exacerbate the condition (eg, cigarette smoking, high altitude, pregnancy, use of sympathomimetics)
- Idiopathic and familial pulmonary arterial hypertension: IV epoprostenol; inhaled, oral, sc, or IV prostacyclin analogs; oral endothelin-receptor antagonists; oral phosphodiesterase 5 inhibitors, and/or soluble guanylate cyclase stimulators
- Secondary pulmonary arterial hypertension: Treatment of the underlying disorder
- Lung transplantation
- Adjunctive therapy: Supplemental oxygen, diuretics, and/or anticoagulants

Pulmonary arterial hypertension, group 1: Treatment is rapidly evolving.

IV epoprostenol, a prostacyclin analog, improves function and lengthens survival even in patients who are unresponsive to a vasodilator during catheterization. Epoprostenol is currently the most effective therapy for pulmonary arterial hypertension. Disadvantages are the need for continuous central catheter infusion and frequent, troubling adverse effects, including flushing, diarrhea, and bacteremia associated with the indwelling central catheter. Prostacyclin analogs that are inhaled, taken orally, or given sc or IV (iloprost and treprostinil), are available. Selexipag became available in 2015 and is an orally bioavailable small molecule that activates the prostaglandin I2 receptor and lowers mortality and morbidity rates.[1]

Three oral endothelin-receptor antagonists, bosentan, ambrisentan, and macitentan, are now available. Sildenafil, tadalafil, and vardenafil, which are oral phosphodiesterase 5 inhibitors, can also be used. Riociguat is the first available soluble guanylate cyclase stimulator. A 2015 study compared the efficacy of monotherapy with oral ambrisentan 10 mg and oral tadalafil 40 mg to combination therapy of these same 2 drugs all taken once daily.[2] Adverse clinical outcomes (death, hospitalization, disease progression, or poor long-term outcome) were fewer with combination therapy than with monotherapy. Combination therapy also significantly reduced NT-proBNP levels and increased 6-min walk distances and the percentage of satisfactory clinical responses. This study supports targeting multiple pathways by beginning treatment of pulmonary arterial hypertension with combination therapy. However, phosphodiesterase 5 inhibitors cannot be combined with riociguat because both drug classes increase cyclic guanosine monophosphate (cGMP) levels, and the combination can lead to dangerous hypotension. Patients with severe right heart failure who are at high risk of sudden death may benefit from early therapy with an intravenous or subcutaneous prostacyclin analog.

Sequential combination therapy is an alternative to initial combination therapy. Studies confirm that morbidity and mortality decreased with macitentan, whether used alone or when combined with other drugs to treat PAH. Morbidity and mortality are lower with selexipag than with placebo, whether selexipag is used alone or combined with a phosphodiesterase 5 inhibitor, an endothelin-receptor antagonist, or both.[3,4] Finally, riociguat increased 6-min walk distance, decreased pulmonary vascular resistance, and improved functional class, whether used as monotherapy or as sequential combination therapy in patients receiving an endothelin-receptor antagonist or prostanoid.[5]

Prostacyclin analogs, endothelin-receptor antagonists, and guanylate cyclase stimulators have been studied primarily in idiopathic PAH; however, these drugs can be used cautiously (attending to drug metabolism and drug-drug interactions) in patients with PAH due to connective tissue disease, HIV, or portopulmonary hypertension. Vasodilators should be avoided in patients with PAH due to pulmonary veno-occlusive disease due to the risk of catastrophic pulmonary edema.[6]

Lung transplantation offers the only hope of cure but has high morbidity because of rejection (bronchiolitis obliterans syndrome) and infection. The 5-yr survival rate is 50%. Lung transplantation is reserved for patients with New York Heart Association class IV disease (defined as dyspnea associated with minimal activity, leading to bed to chair limitations) or complex congenital heart disease in whom all therapies have failed and who meet other health criteria to be a transplant candidate.

Many patients require adjunctive therapies to treat heart failure, including diuretics, and most should receive warfarin unless there is a contraindication.

Pulmonary hypertension, groups 2 to 5: Primary treatment involves management of the underlying disorder. Patients with left-sided heart disease may need surgery for valvular disease. Patients with lung disorders and hypoxia benefit from supplemental oxygen as well as treatment of the primary disorder. Traditional PAH therapies should be used cautiously because they may contribute to V/Q mismatch by reversing underlying hypoxic vasoconstriction. The first-line treatment for patients with severe pulmonary hypertension secondary to chronic thromboembolic disease includes surgical intervention with pulmonary thromboendarterectomy. During cardiopulmonary bypass, an organized endothelialized thrombus is dissected along the pulmonary vasculature in a procedure more complex than acute surgical embolectomy. This procedure cures pulmonary hypertension in a substantial percentage of patients and restores cardiopulmonary function; operative mortality is < 10% in centers that have extensive experience. Riociguat has improved exercise capacity and pulmonary vascular resistance in patients who are not surgical candidates or for whom the risk to benefit ratio is too high.[5]

Patients with **sickle cell disease** who have pulmonary hypertension are aggressively treated using hydroxyurea, iron chelation, and supplemental oxygen as indicated. In patients with pulmonary arterial hypertension and elevated pulmonary vascular resistance confirmed by right heart catheterization, selective pulmonary vasodilator therapy (with epoprostenol or an endothelin-receptor antagonist) can be considered. Sildenafil increases incidence of painful crises in patients with sickle cell disease and so should be used only if patients have limited vaso-occlusive crises and are being treated with hydroxyurea or transfusion therapy.

1. Sitbon O, Channick R, Chin KM, et al: Selexipag for the treatment of pulmonary arterial hypertension. *N Engl J Med* 373:2522–2533, 2015. doi: 10.1056/NEJMoa1503184.
2. Galie N, Barbera JA, Frost AE, et al: Initial use of Ambrisentan plus Tadalafil in Pulmonary Arterial Hypertension. *N Engl J Med* 373:834–844, 2015. doi: 10.1056/NEJMoa1413687.
3. Tamura Y, Channick RN: New paradigm for pulmonary arterial hypertension treatment. *Curr Opin Pulm Med* 22(5):429–433, 2016. doi: 10.1097/MCP.0000000000000308.
4. McLaughlin VV, Channick R, Chin K, et al: Effect of selexipag on morbidity/mortality in pulmonary arterial hypertension: Results of the GRIPHON study. *J Am Coll Cardiol* 65 (suppl):A1538, 2015.
5. Ghofrani HA, Galiè N, Grimminger F, et al: Riociguat for the treatment of pulmonary arterial hypertension. *N Engl J Med* 369(4):330–340, 2013. doi: 10.1056/NEJMoa1209655.
6. Galiè N, Humbert M, Vachiery JL, et al: 2015 ESC/ERS Guidelines for the diagnosis and treatment of pulmonary hypertension: The Joint Task Force for the Diagnosis and Treatment of Pulmonary Hypertension of the European Society of Cardiology (ESC) and the European Respiratory Society (ERS): Endorsed by: Association for European Paediatric and Congenital Cardiology (AEPC), International Society for Heart and Lung Transplantation (ISHLT). *Eur Heart J* 37(1):67–119, 2016. doi: 10.1093/eurheartj/ehv317.

KEY POINTS

- Pulmonary hypertension is classified into 5 groups.
- Suspect pulmonary hypertension if patients have dyspnea unexplained by another clinically evident cardiac or pulmonary disorder.
- Begin diagnostic testing with chest x-ray, spirometry, ECG, and transthoracic Doppler echocardiography.
- Confirm the diagnosis by right heart catheterization.
- Treat group 1 by giving pulmonary vasodilators and, if these are ineffective, considering lung transplantation.
- Treat groups 2 to 5 by managing the underlying disorder, treating symptoms, and sometimes other measures.

PORTOPULMONARY HYPERTENSION

Portopulmonary hypertension is pulmonary arterial hypertension associated with portal hypertension without other secondary causes.

Pulmonary hypertension occurs in patients with various conditions that involve portal hypertension with or without cirrhosis. Portopulmonary hypertension occurs less commonly than hepatopulmonary syndrome in patients with chronic liver disease (3.5 vs 12%).

Presenting symptoms are dyspnea and fatigue. Chest pain and hemoptysis can also occur. Patients have physical findings and ECG abnormalities consistent with pulmonary hypertension and may develop evidence of cor pulmonale (elevated jugular venous pulse, edema). Tricuspid regurgitation is common.

The diagnosis is suspected based on echocardiography findings and confirmed by right heart catheterization.

Treatment is the same as that of pulmonary arterial hypertension except that hepatotoxic drugs and anticoagulants should be avoided. Beta-blockers, frequently used in portal hypertension, should also be avoided in portopulmonary hypertension due to hemodynamic instability.[1] Some patients benefit from vasodilator therapy. The underlying liver disease is a major determinant of outcome. Portopulmonary hypertension is a relative contraindication to liver transplantation because of increased morbidity and mortality from the procedure. However, in some patients who receive a transplant, particularly those with mild pulmonary hypertension, pulmonary hypertension regresses. Some centers consider transplantation in patients who have mean pulmonary arterial pressures < 35 mm Hg after a trial of vasodilator therapy.

1. Galiè N, Humbert M, Vachiery JL, et al: 2015 ESC/ERS Guidelines for the diagnosis and treatment of pulmonary hypertension: The Joint Task Force for the Diagnosis and Treatment of Pulmonary Hypertension of the European Society of Cardiology (ESC) and the European Respiratory Society (ERS): Endorsed by: Association for European Paediatric and Congenital Cardiology (AEPC), International Society for Heart and Lung Transplantation (ISHLT). *Eur Heart J* 37(1):67–119, 2016. doi: 10.1093/eurheartj/ehv317.

HEPATOPULMONARY SYNDROME

Hepatopulmonary syndrome is hypoxemia caused by pulmonary microvascular vasodilation in patients with portal hypertension; dyspnea and hypoxemia are worse when the patient is upright.

Hepatopulmonary syndrome results from the formation of microscopic intrapulmonary arteriovenous dilations in patients with chronic liver disease. The mechanism is unknown but is thought to be due to increased hepatic production or decreased hepatic clearance of vasodilators. The vascular dilations cause overperfusion relative to ventilation, leading to hypoxemia, particularly because patients have an increased cardiac output resulting from systemic vasodilation. Because the lesions frequently are more numerous at the lung bases, hepatopulmonary syndrome can cause platypnea (dyspnea) and orthodeoxia (hypoxemia), which occur when the patient is seated or standing and are relieved by recumbency. Most patients also have characteristic findings of chronic liver disease, such as spider angiomas. About 20% of patients present with pulmonary symptoms alone.

Diagnosis

- Pulse oximetry
- Contrast echocardiography and sometimes other imaging

Hepatopulmonary syndrome should be suspected in patients with known liver disease who report dyspnea (particularly platypnea). Patients with such symptoms should have pulse oximetry. If the symptoms are severe (eg, dyspnea at rest), ABGs should be measured with the patient breathing room air and 100% oxygen to determine shunt fraction.

PEARLS & PITFALLS

- If patients have portal hypertension and dyspnea is relieved by recumbency, consider hepatopulmonary syndrome.

A useful diagnostic test is contrast echocardiography. Intravenous microbubbles from agitated saline that are normally trapped in the pulmonary capillaries rapidly (ie, within 7 heartbeats) traverse the lung and appear in the left atrium. Similarly, IV technetium-99m–labeled albumin may traverse the lungs and appear in the kidneys and brain. Pulmonary angiography may reveal a diffusely fine or blotchy vascular configuration. Angiography is generally not needed unless thromboembolism is suspected.

Treatment

- Supplemental oxygen

The main treatment is supplemental oxygen for symptoms. Other therapies, such as somatostatin to inhibit vasodilation, are of modest benefit in only some patients. Coil embolization is virtually impossible because of the number and size of the lesions. Inhaled nitric oxide synthesis inhibitors may be a future treatment option. Hepatopulmonary syndrome may regress after liver transplantation or if the underlying liver disease subsides. Prognosis is poor without treatment (survival < 2 yr).

KEY POINTS

- Patients with hepatopulmonary syndrome tend to have findings of chronic liver disease and may have platypnea.
- If the diagnosis is suspected, do pulse oximetry and consider ABG and imaging (eg, contrast echocardiography).
- Treat with supplemental oxygen.

63 Pulmonary Rehabilitation

CHEST PHYSIOTHERAPY

Chest physiotherapy consists of external mechanical maneuvers, such as chest percussion, postural drainage, and vibration, to augment mobilization and clearance of airway secretions. It is indicated for patients in whom cough is insufficient to clear thick, tenacious, copious, or loculated secretions. Examples include patients with

- Cystic fibrosis
- Bronchiectasis
- Lung abscess
- Neuromuscular disorders
- Pneumonias in dependent lung regions

Despite relatively few high-quality clinical trials providing strong evidence-based support, chest physiotherapy remains an important component of care in patients with cystic fibrosis.

Contraindications: Contraindications to chest physiotherapy all are relative and include the following:

- Discomfort due to physical positions or manipulations
- Anticoagulation
- Rib fractures
- Vertebral fractures or osteoporosis
- Recent hemoptysis

Procedure: Chest physiotherapy may be administered by a respiratory therapist, although the techniques can often be taught to family members of patients.

The **most common** procedure used is

- Postural drainage and chest percussion

In postural drainage and chest percussion, the patient is rotated to facilitate drainage of secretions from a specific lung lobe or segment while being clapped with cupped hands to loosen and mobilize retained secretions that can then be expectorated or drained. The procedure is somewhat uncomfortable and tiring for the patient. Alternatives to chest percussion by hand include use of mechanical vibrators and inflatable vests.

Other methods that help clear airways include using controlled patterns of breathing, positive expiratory pressure devices to maintain airway patency, and ultra-low-frequency airway oscillation devices to mobilize sputum. The methods of airway clearance are comparable, and methods should be selected based on individual patient needs and preferences.

Complications: Complications are unusual but include position-related hypoxia and aspiration of freed secretions in other lung regions.

PULMONARY REHABILITATION

Pulmonary rehabilitation is the use of exercise, education, and behavioral intervention to improve functional capacity and enhance quality of life in patients with chronic respiratory disorders.

For many patients with chronic respiratory disorders, medical therapy only partially allays the symptoms and complications of the disorder. A comprehensive program of pulmonary rehabilitation may lead to significant clinical improvement by

- Reducing shortness of breath
- Increasing exercise tolerance
- To a lesser extent, decreasing the number of hospitalizations

However, these programs do not improve survival.

Indications: In the past, pulmonary rehabilitation was reserved for patients with severe chronic obstructive pulmonary disease (COPD). However, an increasing body of evidence suggests a benefit to patients with interstitial lung disease (ILD), cystic fibrosis (CF), bronchiectasis, asthma, and lung cancer. Patients undergoing lung transplantation and lung volume reduction surgery also have benefited from pulmonary rehabilitation both before and after surgery.

Studies done in patients with COPD have suggested that pulmonary rehabilitation should start before COPD becomes severe (ie, as identified by degree of airflow obstruction) because there appears to be a poor correlation between disease severity and exercise performance. Furthermore, even patients with less severe disease are likely to benefit from reduced dyspnea, improved exercise tolerance, improved muscle strength, conditioning, improvement of cardiac and pulmonary physiology, reduced dynamic hyperinflation, and the psychosocial benefits that accompany pulmonary rehabilitation.[1]

Contraindications: Contraindications are relative and include comorbidities (eg, untreated angina, left ventricular dysfunction) that could complicate attempts to increase a patient's level of exercise. However, these comorbidities do not preclude application of other components of pulmonary rehabilitation.

Complications: There are no complications of pulmonary rehabilitation beyond those expected from physical exertion and exercise.

Procedure: Pulmonary rehabilitation is best administered as part of an integrated program of

- Exercise training
- Education
- Psychosocial and behavioral interventions

Pulmonary rehabilitation is delivered by a team of physicians, nurses, respiratory therapists, physical and occupational therapists, and psychologists or social workers. The intervention should be individualized and targeted to the patient's needs. Pulmonary rehabilitation can be started at any stage of disease with the goal of minimizing disease burden and symptoms.

Exercise training involves aerobic exercise and respiratory muscle and upper and lower extremity strength training. There is increasing evidence to support doing both strength training and interval training of the extremities.

Inspiratory muscle training (IMT) is an important component of pulmonary rehabilitation. IMT strengthens respiratory muscles using devices that impose a resistive load that is set at a fraction of an individual's maximal inspiratory pressure. When used alone, IMT may decrease dyspnea, but it is not clear whether it can improve exercise tolerance and performance of activities of daily living. However, using IMT in addition to traditional pulmonary rehabilitation exercise does result in clinically meaningful reduction in dyspnea during activities of daily living and improvement in walk distance.

Neuromuscular electrical stimulation (NMES) uses a device that applies transcutaneous electrical impulses to selected muscles to stimulate contraction and thus strengthen them. NMES can be effective in patients with severe lung disease because it minimizes circulatory demand and does not cause the dyspnea that often limits these patients from participating in typical exercise training. Thus, neuromuscular electrical stimulation is uniquely suited for patients with significant deconditioning or for patients with an acute exacerbation of respiratory failure.

Education has many components. Counseling about the need for smoking cessation is important. Teaching breathing strategies (such as pursed-lip breathing, in which exhalations are begun against closed lips to decrease respiratory rate, thereby decreasing gas trapping) and the principles of conserving physical energy are helpful. Explaining treatment, including using drugs correctly and planning for end of life care, are needed.

Psychosocial interventions involve counseling and feedback for the depression, anxieties, and fear that hinder the patient's full participation in activities. Behavioral modification strategies and an emphasis on self-management are critical components of pulmonary rehabilitation. Strategies include techniques for goal-setting and problem solving, decision-making, medication adherence, and the maintenance of routine exercise and physical activity.[1]

Although the most optimal maintenance strategy is unknown, continued participation in an exercise program is essential to maintain the benefits of pulmonary rehabilitation.

1. Rochester CL, Vogiatzis I, Holland AE, et al: An Official American Thoracic Society/European Respiratory Society Policy Statement: Enhancing Implementation, Use, and Delivery of Pulmonary Rehabilitation. *Am J Respir Crit Care Med* 192:1373–1386, 2015. doi: 10.1164/rccm.201510-1966ST.

64 Sarcoidosis

Sarcoidosis is a disorder resulting in noncaseating granulomas in one or more organs and tissues; etiology is unknown. The lungs and lymphatic system are most often affected, but sarcoidosis may affect any organ. Pulmonary symptoms range from none to exertional dyspnea and, rarely, lung or other organ failure. Diagnosis usually is first suspected because of pulmonary involvement and is confirmed by chest x-ray, biopsy, and exclusion of other causes of granulomatous inflammation. First-line treatment is corticosteroids. Prognosis is excellent for limited disease but poor for more advanced disease.

Sarcoidosis most commonly affects people aged 20 to 40 but occasionally affects children and older adults. Worldwide, prevalence is greatest in black Americans and ethnic northern Europeans, especially Scandinavians. Disease presentation varies widely by racial and ethnic background, with black Americans and Puerto Ricans having more frequent extrathoracic manifestations. Sarcoidosis is more prevalent in women. The incidence increases in winter and early spring for unknown reasons.

Löfgren syndrome: Löfgren syndrome manifests as a triad of acute polyarthritis, erythema nodosum, and hilar adenopathy. It often causes fever, malaise, and uveitis, and sometimes parotitis. It is more common among Scandinavian and Irish women.

Löfgren syndrome is often self-limited. Patients usually respond to NSAIDs. Rate of relapse is low.

Heerfordt syndrome: Heerfordt syndrome (uveoparotid fever) manifests as swelling of the parotid gland (due to sarcoid infiltration), uveitis, chronic fever, and less often palsy of the facial nerve. Heerfordt syndrome can be self-limited. Treatment is the same as for sarcoidosis.

Blau syndrome: Blau syndrome is sarcoidosis inherited in a autosomal dominant fashion that manifests in children. In Blau syndrome, children present before the age of 4 yr with arthritis, rash, and uveitis. Blau syndrome is often self-limited. Symptoms usually are relieved with NSAIDs.

Etiology

Sarcoidosis is thought to be due to an inflammatory response to an environmental antigen in a genetically susceptible person. Proposed triggers include

- *Propionibacterium acnes* and mycobacteria (potentially the *Mycobacterium tuberculosis* catalase-peroxidase [mKatG] protein)
- Mold or mildew and certain unidentified substances present in workplaces with musty odors and pesticides

Tobacco use is inversely correlated with sarcoidosis.

Evidence supporting genetic susceptibility includes the following:

- Higher rate of disease concordance in monozygotic than dizygotic twins
- Increased prevalence of sarcoidosis (about 3.6 to 9.6%) among 1st- or 2nd-degree relatives of patients who have sarcoidosis
- Fivefold increase in relative risk of developing sarcoidosis in siblings of patients who have sarcoidosis
- Identification of several possible HLA and non-HLA genes associated with sarcoidosis

Pathophysiology

The unknown antigen triggers a cell-mediated immune response that is characterized by the accumulation of T cells and macrophages, release of cytokines and chemokines, and organization of responding cells into granulomas. Clusters of disease in families and communities suggest a genetic predisposition, shared exposures, or, less likely, person-to-person transmission.

The inflammatory process leads to formation of noncaseating granulomas, the pathologic hallmark of sarcoidosis. Granulomas are collections of mononuclear cells and macrophages that differentiate into epithelioid and multinucleated giant cells and are surrounded by lymphocytes, plasma cells, fibroblasts, and collagen. Granulomas occur most commonly in the lungs and lymph nodes but can involve any organ and cause significant dysfunction. Granulomas in the lungs are distributed along lymphatics, with most occurring in peribronchiolar, subpleural, and perilobular regions.

Hypercalcemia may occur because vitamin D analogs are produced by activated macrophages. Hypercalciuria may be present, even in patients with normal serum Ca levels. Nephrolithiasis and nephrocalcinosis may occur, sometimes leading to chronic kidney disease.

Symptoms and Signs

Symptoms and signs depend on the site and degree of involvement and vary over time, ranging from spontaneous remission to chronic indolent illness. Accordingly, frequent reassessment for new symptoms in different organs is needed. Most cases are probably asymptomatic and thus go undetected. Pulmonary disease occurs in > 90% of adult patients.

Symptoms and signs may include dyspnea, cough, chest discomfort, and crackles. Fatigue, malaise, weakness, anorexia, weight loss, and low-grade fever are also common. Sarcoidosis can manifest as fever of unknown origin. Systemic involvement causes various symptoms (Table 64–1), which vary by race, sex, and age. Blacks are more likely than whites to have involvement of the eyes, liver, bone marrow, peripheral lymph nodes, and skin; erythema nodosum is an exception. Women are more likely to have erythema nodosum and eye or nervous system involvement. Men and older patients are more likely to be hypercalcemic.

Children with sarcoidosis may present with Blau syndrome (arthritis, rash, uveitis), or manifestations similar to those of adults. Sarcoidosis may be confused with juvenile idiopathic arthritis (juvenile RA) in this age group.

Diagnosis

- Chest imaging
- Biopsy
- Exclusion of other granulomatous disorders

Sarcoidosis is most often suspected when hilar adenopathy is incidentally detected on chest x-ray. These changes are the most common abnormality. Therefore, if sarcoidosis is suspected, a chest x-ray should be the first test if it has not already been done. The x-ray appearance tends to roughly predict the likelihood of spontaneous remission (Table 64–2) in patients with only pulmonary involvement. However, staging sarcoidosis by chest x-ray can be misleading; for example, extrapulmonary sarcoidosis, such as cardiac or neurologic sarcoidosis, can portend a serious prognosis in the absence of pulmonary involvement. Also, chest x-rays findings predict pulmonary function poorly, so that chest x-ray appearance may not accurately indicate the severity of pulmonary sarcoidosis.

A normal chest x-ray (stage 0) does not exclude the diagnosis, particularly when cardiac or neurologic involvement is suspected. A high-resolution CT is more sensitive for detecting hilar and mediastinal lymphadenopathy and parenchymal abnormalities. CT findings in more advanced stages (II to IV) include thickening of the bronchovascular bundles and bronchial walls; beading of the interlobular septa; ground-glass opacification; parenchymal nodules, cysts, or cavities; and traction bronchiectasis.

When imaging suggests sarcoidosis, the diagnosis is confirmed by demonstration of noncaseating granulomas on biopsy and exclusion of alternative causes of granulomatous disease (see Table 64–3). Löfgren syndrome does not require confirmation by biopsy.

The diagnostic evaluation, therefore, requires the following:

- Selection of a biopsy site
- Exclusion of other causes of granulomatous disease
- Assessment of the severity and extent of disease to determine whether therapy is indicated

Sites for biopsy: Appropriate biopsy sites may be obvious from physical examination and initial assessment; peripheral lymph nodes, skin lesions, and conjunctivae are all easily accessible. Endobronchial ultrasound-guided transbronchial needle aspiration (EBUS-TBNA) of mediastinal or hilar lymph node has a reported diagnostic yield of about 90%. It is usually the diagnostic procedure of choice in patients with intrathoracic involvement. Bronchoscopic transbronchial biopsy can be tried when EBUS-TBNA is nondiagnostic; if the bronchoscopic transbronchial biopsy is nondiagnostic, it can be tried a second time. If EBUS-TBNA and bronchoscopic transbronchial biopsies are nondiagnostic or if bronchoscopy cannot be tolerated, mediastinoscopy can be done to biopsy mediastinal or hilar lymph nodes, or video-assisted thoracoscopic (VAT) lung biopsy or open-lung biopsy can be done to obtain lung tissue. If sarcoidosis is strongly suspected but a biopsy site is not evident based on examination or imaging findings, PET scanning can help identify sites such as heart and brain.

Exclusion of other diagnoses: Exclusion of other diagnoses is critical, especially when symptoms and x-ray signs are minimal, because many other disorders and processes can cause granulomatous inflammation (see Table 64–3). Biopsy tissue should be cultured for fungi and mycobacteria. Exposure history to occupational (silicates, beryllium), environmental (moldy hay, birds, and other antigenic triggers of hypersensitivity pneumonitis), and infectious (TB, coccidioidomycosis, histoplasmosis) antigens should be explored. PPD skin testing should be done early in the assessment along with anergy controls.

Disease severity assessment: Severity is assessed with

- Pulmonary function tests
- Exercise pulse oximetry

Table 64–1. SYSTEMIC INVOLVEMENT IN SARCOIDOSIS

SYSTEM	ESTIMATED FREQUENCY	COMMENTS
Pulmonary	> 90%	Causes granulomas to form in alveolar septa and bronchiolar and bronchial walls, causing diffuse pulmonary disease; pulmonary arteries and veins also involved Often asymptomatic Spontaneously resolves in many patients but can cause progressive pulmonary dysfunction, leading to limitations in physical function, respiratory failure, and death in a few
Pulmonary lymphatic	90%	Hilar or mediastinal involvement incidentally detected by chest x-ray in most patients; nontender peripheral or cervical lymphadenopathy in others
Muscle	50–80%	Asymptomatic disease with or without enzyme elevations in most patients Sometimes insidious or acute myopathy with muscle weakness
Hepatic	40–75%	Usually asymptomatic Manifests with mild elevations in liver function test results, hypolucent lesions on CT scans with radiopaque dye Rarely, clinically significant cholestasis or cirrhosis Unclear distinction between sarcoidosis and granulomatous hepatitis when sarcoidosis affects the liver only
Joint	25–50%	Ankle, knee, wrist, and elbow arthritis (most common) May cause chronic arthritis with Jaccoud deformities or dactylitis Löfgren syndrome (triad of acute polyarthritis, erythema nodosum, and hilar adenopathy)
Hematologic	< 5–30%	Lymphocytopenia Anemia of chronic disease Anemia due to granulomatous infiltration of bone marrow, sometimes causing pancytopenia Splenic sequestration causing thrombocytopenia Leukopenia
Dermatologic	25%	Erythema nodosum: • Red, indurated, tender nodules on anterior legs • More common among Europeans, Puerto Ricans, and Mexicans • Usually remits in 1–2 mo • Surrounding joints often arthritic (Löfgren syndrome) • May be good prognostic sign

Table 64–1. SYSTEMIC INVOLVEMENT IN SARCOIDOSIS (*Continued*)

SYSTEM	ESTIMATED FREQUENCY	COMMENTS
		Biopsy of erythema nodosum lesions is unnecessary because granulomas characteristic of sarcoidosis are absent Common skin lesions: Plaques, macules and papules, subcutaneous nodules, hypopigmentation and hyperpigmentation Lupus pernio: • Violaceous plaques on the nose, cheeks, lips, and ears • More common among black Americans and Puerto Ricans • Often associated with lung fibrosis Poor prognostic sign
Ocular	25%	Uveitis (most common), causing blurred vision, photophobia, and tearing Can cause blindness Spontaneously resolves in most patients May manifest with conjunctivitis, iridocyclitis, chorioretinitis, dacryocystitis, lacrimal gland infiltration causing dry eyes, optic neuritis, glaucoma, or cataracts Ocular involvement more common among black Americans and people of Japanese descent Annual screening indicated for early disease detection
Psychiatric	10%	Depression (common), but uncertain whether it is a primary manifestation of sarcoidosis or a response to the prolonged course of disease and frequent recurrences
Renal	10%	Asymptomatic hypercalciuria (most common) Interstitial nephritis Chronic renal failure caused by nephrolithiasis and nephrocalcinosis and requiring renal replacement (dialysis or transplantation) in some patients
Splenic	10%	Usually asymptomatic Manifests with left upper quadrant pain and thrombocytopenia or as an incidental finding on x-ray or CT
Neurologic	< 10%	Cranial neuropathy, especially the 7th nerve (causing facial nerve palsy) or 8th nerve (causing hearing loss) Optic and peripheral neuropathy (common) May affect any cranial nerve CNS involvement, with nodular lesions or diffuse meningeal inflammation typically in the cerebellum and brain stem Hypothalamic diabetes insipidus, polyphagia and obesity, and thermoregulatory and libidinal changes
Nasal sinus	< 10%	Acute and chronic granulomatous inflammation of sinus mucosa with symptoms indistinguishable from common allergic and infectious sinusitis Diagnosis confirmed by biopsy More common in patients with lupus pernio
Cardiac	5%	Conduction blocks and arrhythmias (most common), sometimes causing sudden death Heart failure due to restrictive cardiomyopathy (primary) or pulmonary hypertension (secondary) Transient papillary muscle dysfunction and pericarditis (rare) More common among Japanese, in whom cardiomyopathy is the most frequent cause of sarcoidosis-related death
Bone	5%	Osteolytic or cystic lesions Osteopenia
Oral	< 5%	Asymptomatic parotid swelling (most common) Parotitis with xerostomia Heerfordt syndrome (uveoparotid fever), characterized by uveitis, bilateral parotid swelling, facial palsy, and chronic fever Oral lupus pernio, which may disfigure the hard palate and may involve the cheek, tongue, and gums
Gastric or intestinal	Rare	Rarely gastric granulomas Rarely intestinal involvement Mesenteric lymphadenopathy that may cause abdominal pain
Endocrine	Rare	Hypothalamic and pituitary stalk infiltration, possibly causing panhypopituitarism May cause thyroid infiltration without dysfunction Secondary hypoparathyroidism due to hypercalcemia
Pleural	Rare	Causes lymphocytic exudative effusions, usually bilateral
Reproductive	Rare	Case reports of endometrial, ovarian, epididymal, and testicular involvement No effect on fertility May subside during pregnancy and relapse postpartum

Table 64–2. CHEST X-RAY STAGING OF SARCOIDOSIS

STAGE	DEFINITION	INCIDENCE OF SPONTANEOUS REMISSION
0	Normal chest x-ray	—
I	Bilateral hilar, paratracheal, and mediastinal lymphadenopathy without parenchymal infiltrates	60–80%
II	Bilateral hilar and mediastinal adenopathy with interstitial infiltrates (usually in upper lung fields)	50–65%
III	Diffuse interstitial infiltrates without hilar adenopathy	< 30%
IV	Diffuse fibrosis, often associated with fibrotic-appearing conglomerate masses, traction bronchiectasis, and traction cysts	0%

Pulmonary function test results are often normal in early stages but demonstrate restriction and reduced diffusing capacity for carbon monoxide (DLco) in advanced disease. Airflow obstruction also occurs and may suggest involvement of the bronchial mucosae. Pulse oximetry is often normal when measured at rest but may show effort desaturation in patients with more extensive lung involvement. ABG analysis at rest and during exercise is more sensitive than pulse oximetry.

Recommended routine screening tests for extrapulmonary disease include

- ECG
- Slit-lamp ophthalmologic examination
- Routine blood tests to evaluate renal and hepatic function
- Serum Ca levels and 24 h urinary Ca excretion

Echocardiography, cardiac MRI with gadolinium contrast, neuroimaging, bone scans, and electromyography may be appropriate in patients with cardiac, neurologic, or rheumatologic symptoms. PET scanning appears to be the most sensitive test for detecting bone and other extrapulmonary sarcoidosis. Abdominal CT with radiopaque dye is not routinely recommended but can provide evidence of hepatic or splenic involvement (eg, enlargement, hypolucent lesions).

Laboratory testing plays an adjunctive role in establishing the diagnosis and extent of organ involvement. CBC may show anemia, eosinophilia, or leukopenia. Serum Ca should be measured to detect hypercalcemia. BUN, creatinine, and liver function test results may be elevated in renal and hepatic sarcoidosis. Total protein may be elevated because of hypergammaglobulinemia. Elevated ESR is common but nonspecific. Measurement of Ca in a urine specimen collected over 24 h is recommended to exclude hypercalciuria, even in patients with normal serum Ca levels. Elevated serum ACE levels also suggest sarcoidosis but are nonspecific and may be elevated in patients with various other conditions (eg, hyperthyroidism, Gaucher disease, silicosis, mycobacterial disease, fungal infections, hypersensitivity pneumonitis, lymphoma). However, ACE levels may be useful for monitoring adherence with corticosteroid treatment. ACE levels plummet with even low-dose corticosteroids.

Bronchoalveolar lavage (BAL) is used to help exclude other forms of interstitial lung disease if the diagnosis of sarcoidosis is in doubt and to rule out infection. The findings on BAL vary considerably, but lymphocytosis (lymphocytes > 10%), a CD4+/CD8+ ratio of > 3.5 in the lavage fluid cell differential, or both suggest the diagnosis in the proper clinical context. However, absence of these findings does not exclude sarcoidosis.

Whole-body gallium scanning has been largely replaced by PET scanning. If gallium scanning is available, it may provide useful supportive evidence in the absence of tissue confirmation. Symmetric increased uptake in mediastinal and hilar nodes (lambda sign) and in lacrimal, parotid, and salivary glands (panda sign) are patterns highly suggestive of sarcoidosis. A negative result in patients taking prednisone is unreliable.

Table 64–3. DIFFERENTIAL DIAGNOSIS OF SARCOIDOSIS

TYPE	SPECIFIC DISORDER
Mycobacterial infection	Atypical mycobacteria TB
Fungal infection	Aspergillosis Blastomycosis Coccidioidomycosis Cryptococcal infection Histoplasmosis
Other infections	Brucellosis Cat-scratch disease (lymph nodes only) Mycoplasmal infection *Pneumocystis jirovecii* infection Syphilis
Rheumatologic disorders	Juvenile idiopathic arthritis (juvenile RA) Kikuchi-Fujimoto disease (lymph nodes only) RA Sjögren syndrome Granulomatosis with polyangiitis (Wegener granulomatosis)
Hematologic cancer	Castleman disease (a lymphoproliferative disorder associated with infection by HIV or human herpesvirus 8) Hodgkin lymphoma Non-Hodgkin lymphoma Splenic lymphoma
Hypersensitivity	Metals encountered in occupational settings: Aluminum, beryllium, titanium, zirconium Organic antigens causing hypersensitivity pneumonitis: Actinomycetes, atypical mycobacterial antigens, fungi, mushroom spores, other bioaerosols Inorganic antigens causing hypersensitivity pneumonitis: Isocyanate, pyrethrins Drug reaction
Other	Inflammatory bowel disease Foreign body aspiration or inoculation Granulomatous hepatitis Granulomatous lesion of unknown significance Lymphoid interstitial pneumonia

Prognosis

Although spontaneous remission is common, disease manifestations and severity are highly variable, and many patients require corticosteroids at some time during the course of their disease. Thus, serial monitoring for evidence of relapse is imperative. In about 90% of patients who have spontaneous remission, remission occurs within the first 2 yr after diagnosis; < 10% of these patients have relapses after 2 yr. Patients who do not experience remission within 2 yr are likely to have chronic disease.

Sarcoidosis is thought to be chronic in up to 30% of patients, and 10 to 20% experience permanent sequelae. The disease is fatal in 1 to 5% of patients, typically due to respiratory failure caused by pulmonary fibrosis, and less often due to pulmonary hemorrhage caused by aspergilloma. However, in Japan, infiltrative cardiomyopathy causing arrhythmias and heart failure is the most common cause of death.

Prognosis is worse for patients with extrapulmonary sarcoidosis and for blacks. Remission occurs in 89% of whites and 76% of blacks with no extrathoracic disease and in 70% of whites and 46% of blacks with extrathoracic disease.

Good prognostic signs include

- Löfgren syndrome (triad of acute polyarthritis, erythema nodosum, and hilar adenopathy)

Poor prognostic signs include

- Chronic uveitis
- Lupus pernio
- Chronic hypercalcemia
- Neurosarcoidosis
- Cardiac involvement
- Extensive pulmonary involvement

Little difference is demonstrable in long-term outcome between treated and untreated patients, and relapse is common when treatment ends.

Treatment

- NSAIDs
- Corticosteroids
- Occasionally immunosuppressants

Because sarcoidosis often spontaneously resolves, asymptomatic patients and patients with mild symptoms do not require treatment, although they should be monitored for signs of deterioration. These patients can be followed with serial x-rays, pulmonary function tests (including diffusing capacity), and markers of extrathoracic involvement (eg, routine renal and liver function testing, annual slit-lamp ophthalmologic examination). The frequency of follow-up testing is determined by the severity of disease. Patients who require treatment regardless of stage include those with the following:

- Worsening symptoms
- Limitation of activity
- Markedly abnormal or deteriorating lung function
- Worrisome x-ray changes (cavitation, fibrosis, conglomerate masses, signs of pulmonary hypertension)
- Heart, nervous system, or eye involvement
- Renal or hepatic insufficiency or failure
- Moderate to severe hypercalcemia
- Disfiguring skin or joint disease

NSAIDS are used to treat musculoskeletal discomfort.

Disease-modifying treatment begins with corticosteroids. A standard protocol is prednisone 0.3 to 1 mg/kg po once/day depending on symptoms and severity of findings. Alternate-day regimens may be used: eg, prednisone 40 to 60 mg po once every other day. Although patients rarely require > 40 mg/day, higher doses may be needed to reduce complications in patients with heart involvement or ocular or neurologic disease. Response usually occurs within 2 to 4 wk, so symptoms and pulmonary function tests may be reassessed between 4 and 12 wk. Chronic, insidious cases may respond more slowly. Corticosteroids are tapered to a maintenance dose (eg, prednisone 10 to 15 mg/day) after evidence of response and are continued for a minimum of 6 to 12 mo if improvement occurs. The optimal duration of treatment is unknown. Premature taper can result in relapse. The drug is slowly stopped if response is absent or equivocal. Corticosteroids can ultimately be stopped in most patients, but because relapse occurs up to 50% of the time, monitoring should be repeated, usually every 3 to 6 mo. Corticosteroid treatment should be resumed for recurrence of symptoms and signs, including dyspnea, arthralgia, fever, hepatic insufficiency, cardiac arrhythmia, CNS involvement, hypercalcemia, ocular disease uncontrolled by local drugs, and disfiguring skin lesions. Because ACE production is suppressed with low doses of corticosteroids, serial serum ACE levels may be useful in assessing adherence with corticosteroid treatment in patients who have elevated ACE levels.

Inhaled corticosteroids can relieve cough in patients with endobronchial involvement. Topical corticosteroids may be useful in dermatologic, nasal sinus, and ocular disease.

About 10% of patients requiring therapy are unresponsive to tolerable doses of a corticosteroid and should be given a 6-mo trial of methotrexate 10 to 15 mg/wk. Initially, methotrexate and corticosteroids are both given; over 8 wk, the corticosteroid dose can be tapered and, in many cases, stopped. The maximal response to methotrexate, however, may take 6 to 12 mo. In such cases, prednisone must be tapered more slowly. Serial blood counts and liver enzyme tests should be done every 1 to 2 wk initially and then every 4 to 6 wk once a stable dose is achieved. Folate (1 mg po once/day) is recommended for patients treated with methotrexate.

Prophylaxis against *Pneumocystis jirovecii* pneumonia should be considered if patients are taking corticosteroids or immunosuppressants.

Other drugs reported to be effective in small numbers of patients who are corticosteroid-resistant or who experience complicating adverse effects include azathioprine, cyclophosphamide, chlorambucil, chloroquine or hydroxychloroquine, thalidomide, pentoxifylline, and infliximab. Immunosuppressants are often more effective in refractory cases; relapse is common after cessation. Infliximab, a TNF inhibitor, can be effective for treatment of chronic corticosteroid-dependent pulmonary sarcoidosis, refractory lupus pernio, and neurosarcoidosis. It is given intravenously 3 to 5 mg/kg once, again 2 wk later, then once/mo.

Hydroxychloroquine 200 mg po bid can be as effective as corticosteroids for treating hypercalcemia, disfiguring skin sarcoidosis, or enlarged uncomfortable or disfiguring peripheral lymph nodes.

Patients who have heart block or ventricular arrhythmias due to cardiac involvement should have an implantable cardiac defibrillator and pacemaker placed as well as drug therapy.

No available drugs have consistently prevented pulmonary fibrosis.

Organ transplantation is an option for patients with end-stage pulmonary, cardiac, or liver involvement, although disease may recur in the transplanted organ.

KEY POINTS

- Systemic and extrapulmonary involvement are common with sarcoidosis, but > 90% of adult patients have pulmonary involvement.

- Obtain a chest imaging study but confirm the diagnosis by biopsy, usually endobronchial ultrasound-guided transbronchial needle aspiration of a mediastinal or hilar lymph node.
- Assess pulmonary severity with pulmonary function testing and exercise pulse oximetry.
- Test for extrapulmonary involvement with ECG, slit-lamp examination, renal and hepatic function tests, and serum and urinary Ca testing.
- Treat patients with systemic corticosteroids when indicated (eg, severe symptoms, hypercalcemia, progressive decline in organ function, cardiac or neurologic involvement).
- Treat with immunosuppressants if patients cannot tolerate moderate doses of corticosteroids, sarcoidosis is resistant to corticosteroids, or if corticosteroids are required long term.

65 Sleep Apnea

CENTRAL SLEEP APNEA

Central sleep apnea (CSA) is a heterogeneous group of conditions characterized by changes in ventilatory drive without airway obstruction. Most of these conditions cause asymptomatic changes in breathing pattern during sleep. The diagnosis is based on clinical findings and, when necessary, confirmed by polysomnography. Treatment is supportive.

Etiology

Patients with CSA fall into 2 groups based on their carbon dioxide level and ventilatory drive.

- Hypercapnia with decreased ventilatory drive
- Eucapnia or hypocapnia with increased ventilatory drive but with episodes of apnea, periodic breathing, or both

Causes of hypercapnia with decreased ventilatory drive include hypothyroidism and central lesions (eg, brain stem infarctions, encephalitis, Chiari II type malformation).

Cheyne-Stokes breathing, a discrete pattern of the second form of CSA, is thought to be caused by intrinsic properties of the respiratory control center in the response to hypoxia and acidosis with hyperpnea, causing reoxygenation and alkalosis, leading to hypoventilation by hypopnea and apnea.

High altitude is another cause of recurrent CSA manifesting with hypocapnia.

Chronic use of opioids (eg, patients on methadone maintenance, cancer patients with chronic pain) triggers CSA with an erratic rate and depth of breathing and episodes of apnea; CSA can be hypercapneic or hypocapneic.

Congenital central hypoventilation (a form of Ondine curse) is a rare form of idiopathic CSA in neonates and may be associated with Hirschsprung disease. A mutation in the *PHOX2* gene is responsible for 80 to 90% of cases. This mutation produces variable phenotypes, and clinically evident cases are inherited in a dominant pattern.

Symptoms and Signs

CSA is usually asymptomatic and is detected by caretakers or bed partners who notice long respiratory pauses, shallow breaths, or restless sleep. Patients with hypercapnic forms may experience daytime somnolence, lethargy, and morning headache.

Diagnosis

- Clinical evaluation
- Often polysomnography

Diagnosis of CSA is suspected on the basis of history and is confirmed by polysomnography. However, testing may not be necessary if CSA causes no symptoms or is clearly related to an identifiable disorder. To diagnose causes of CSA, brain or brain stem imaging may be indicated.

Treatment

- Supportive care

Primary treatment of CSA is optimal management of underlying conditions and avoidance of opioids and other sedatives. Secondary treatment of symptomatic patients can be a trial of supplemental oxygen or, in patients with hypercapnic CSA who have symptoms despite other treatments, noninvasive continuous or bilevel positive airway pressure.

For patients who have CSA and Cheyne-Stokes breathing, continuous positive airway pressure (CPAP) may decrease apneic and hypopneic episodes, but effects on clinical outcomes are not clear. Acetazolamide is effective in CSA caused by high altitude.

Electrode pacing of the phrenic nerve and/or diaphragm is an option, such as for children > 2 yr with congenital central hypoventilation syndrome.

OBSTRUCTIVE SLEEP APNEA

Obstructive sleep apnea (OSA) consists of episodes of partial or complete closure of the upper airway that occur during sleep and lead to breathing cessation (defined as a period of apnea or hypopnea > 10 sec). Symptoms include excessive daytime sleepiness, restlessness, snoring, recurrent awakening, and morning headache. Diagnosis is based on sleep history and polysomnography. Treatment is with nasal CPAP, oral appliances, and, in refractory cases, surgery. Prognosis is good with treatment. Most cases remain undiagnosed and untreated and are often associated with hypertension, atrial fibrillation and other arrhythmias, heart failure, and injury or death due to motor vehicle crashes and other accidents resulting from hypersomnolence.

In at-risk patients, sleep destabilizes patency of the upper airway, leading to partial or complete obstruction of the nasopharynx, oropharynx, or both.

Obstructive sleep hypopnea occurs when breathing is diminished, even if it is not absent.

The prevalence of OSA is 2 to 9% in adults; the condition is under-recognized and often undiagnosed even in symptomatic patients. OSA is up to 4 times more common among men and 7 times more common among people who are obese (ie, body mass index [BMI] > 30). Severe OSA (apnea-hypopnea index [AHI] > 30/h) increases the risk of death in middle-aged men.

OSA can cause excessive daytime sleepiness, increasing risks of automobile crashes, loss of employment, and sexual dysfunction. Relationships with bed partners and roommates and/or housemates may also be adversely affected because these people may also have difficulty sleeping.

Long-term cardiovascular sequelae of untreated OSA include poorly controlled hypertension, heart failure, and atrial fibrillation (even after catheter ablation) and other arrhythmias. OSA also increases the risk for nonalcoholic steatohepatitis, likely due to intermittent nocturnal hypoxia.[1]

1. Musso G, Cassader M, Olivetti C, et al: Association of obstructive sleep apnoea with the presence and severity of non-alcoholic fatty liver disease. A systematic review and meta-analysis. *Obes Rev* 14:417–431, 2013.

Etiology

Anatomic risk factors for OSA include

- An oropharynx "crowded" by a short or retracted mandible
- A prominent tongue base or tonsils
- A rounded head shape and a short neck
- A neck circumference > 43 cm (> 17 in)
- Thick lateral pharyngeal walls
- Lateral parapharyngeal fat pads

Anatomic risk factors are common among obese people.

Other identified risk factors include postmenopausal status, aging, and alcohol or sedative use. A family history of OSA is present in 25 to 40% of cases, perhaps reflective of heritable factors affecting ventilatory drive or craniofacial structure. The risk of OSA in a family member is proportional to the number of affected family members.

Acromegaly, hypothyroidism, and sometimes stroke can cause or contribute to OSA. Disorders that occur more commonly in patients with OSA include hypertension, stroke, diabetes, hyperlipidemia, gastroesophageal reflux disease, nocturnal angina, heart failure, and atrial fibrillation or other arrhythmias.

Because obesity is a common risk factor for both OSA and obesity-hypoventilation syndrome, the conditions frequently coexist.

Inspiratory efforts against a closed upper airway cause paroxysms of inspiration, reductions in gas exchange, disruption of normal sleep architecture, and partial or complete arousals from sleep. These factors may interact to cause the characteristic symptoms and signs, including hypoxia, hypercapnia, and sleep fragmentation.

OSA is an extreme form of sleep-related upper airway resistance. Less severe forms that do not cause oxygen desaturation include

- Snoring
- Upper airway airflow resistance causing noisy inspiration but without sleep arousals
- Upper airway resistance syndrome, characterized by crescendo snoring terminated by respiratory effort-related arousals (RERAs)

Patients with upper airway resistance syndrome are typically younger and less obese than those with OSA, and they complain of daytime sleepiness more than do patients with primary snoring. Frequent arousals occur, but strict criteria for apneas and hypopneas may not be present. Symptoms, diagnostic evaluation, and treatment of snoring and upper airway resistance syndrome are otherwise the same as for OSA.

Symptoms and Signs

Although loud disruptive snoring is reported by 85% of OSA patients, most people who snore do not have OSA. Other symptoms of OSA may include

- Choking, gasping, or snorting during sleep
- Restless and unrefreshing sleep
- Difficulty staying asleep

Most patients are unaware of these symptoms (because they occur during sleep) but are informed of them by bed partners, roommates, or housemates. Some patients may awake with a sore throat or a dry mouth. A morning headache is a common symptom.

When awake, patients may experience hypersomnolence, fatigue, and impaired concentration. The frequency of sleep complaints and the degree of daytime sleepiness do not correlate well with number of events or arousals from sleep.

Diagnosis

- Symptom criteria
- Sleep studies

The diagnosis of OSA is suspected in patients with identifiable risk factors, symptoms, or both.

Pretest questionnaires, such as STOP-Bang, Berlin, and Epworth Sleepiness Scale, can be used to assess risk. However, these questionnaires have low specificity and so have high false-positive rates.[1, 2] The STOP-BANG appears to have better predictive value than the Epworth Sleepiness Scale and possibly the Berlin questionnaire.[3]

Criteria for diagnosis consist of daytime symptoms, nighttime symptoms, and sleep monitoring that documents > 5 episodes of hypopnea and/or apnea per hour with symptoms, or >15 episodes per hour in the absence of symptoms. Specifically, in regard to symptoms, there should be ≥ 1 of the following:

- Daytime sleepiness, unintentional sleep episodes, unrefreshing sleep, fatigue, or difficulty staying asleep
- Awakening with breath holding, gasping, or choking
- Reports by a bed partner of loud snoring, breathing interruptions, or both in the patient's sleep

The patient and any bed partners, roommates, or housemates should be interviewed. The differential diagnosis of excessive daytime sleepiness is broad and includes

- Reduced quantity or quality of sleep due to poor sleep hygiene
- Sedation or mental status changes due to drugs, chronic diseases (including cardiovascular or respiratory diseases), or metabolic disturbances and accompanying therapies
- Depression
- Alcohol or drug abuse
- Narcolepsy
- Other primary sleep disorders (eg, periodic limb movement disorder, restless legs syndrome)

An extended sleep history should be taken in all patients who

- Are about age 65 or older
- Report daytime fatigue, sleepiness, or difficulty staying asleep
- Are overweight
- Have poorly controlled hypertension (which may be caused or exacerbated by OSA), atrial fibrillation or other arrhythmias, heart failure (which may cause OSA), stroke, or diabetes

Most patients who report only snoring, without other symptoms or cardiovascular risks, do not need an extensive evaluation for OSA.

The physical examination should include evaluation for nasal obstruction, tonsillar hypertrophy, and pharyngeal structure and identification of clinical features of hypothyroidism and acromegaly.

Polysomnography is best for confirming the diagnosis of OSA and quantifying the severity of OSA. Polysomnography includes continuous measurement of breathing effort by plethysmography, airflow at the nose and mouth using flow sensors, oxygen saturation by oximetry, sleep architecture by EEG, chin electromyography (looking for hypotonia), and electro-oculography to assess the occurrence of rapid eye movements. Polysomnography records and helps classify stages of sleep and the occurrence and duration of apneic and hypopneic periods. The patient is also observed by video, and ECG monitoring is used to determine whether arrhythmias occur in conjunction with the apneic episodes. Other variables evaluated include limb muscle activity (to assess nonrespiratory causes of sleep arousal, such as restless legs syndrome and periodic limb movements disorder) and body position (apnea may occur only in the supine position).

The **apnea-hypopnea index** (AHI), which is the total number of episodes of apnea and hypopnea occurring during sleep divided by the hours of sleep time, is the common summary measure used to describe respiratory disturbances during sleep. AHI values can be computed for different sleep stages.

The **respiratory disturbance index** (RDI), a similar measure, describes the number of episodes of certain arousals related to respiratory effort (called respiratory effort-related arousals or RERAs) plus the number of apnea and hypopnea episodes per hour of sleep.

An **arousal index** (AI), which is the number of arousals per hour of sleep, can be computed if EEG monitoring is used. The AI may be correlated with AHI or RDI, but about 20% of apneas and desaturation episodes are not accompanied by arousals, or other causes of arousals are present.

An AHI > 5 is required for the diagnosis of OSA; a value > 15 indicates a moderate level of sleep apnea, and a value > 30 indicates a severe level of sleep apnea. Snoring loudly enough to be heard in the next room confers a 10-fold increase in the likelihood of having AHI > 5. The AI and RDI correlate only moderately with a patient's symptoms.

Portable diagnostic tools are being used more often to diagnose OSA. Portable monitors can measure heart rate, pulse oximetry, effort, position, and nasal airflow to provide fair estimates of respiratory disturbances during self-reported sleep, thereby estimating AHI/RDI. Portable diagnostic tools are often used in combination with questionnaires (eg, STOP-Bang, Berlin Questionnaire) to calculate patients' risk (the sensitivity and specificity of the test depend on pretest probability). When portable tools are used, coexisting sleep disorders (eg, restless legs syndrome) are not excluded. Follow-up polysomnography may still be needed to determine AHI/RDI values in the different stages of sleep and with changes in position, especially when surgery or therapy other than positive airway pressure is being considered.

Measurement of thyroid-stimulating hormone can be done based on clinical suspicion. No other adjunctive testing (eg, upper airway imaging) has sufficient diagnostic accuracy to be recommended routinely.

1. Chung F, Yegneswaran B, Liao P, et al: STOP questionnaire: A tool to screen patients for OSA. *Anesthesiology* 108:812–821, 2008.
2. Netzer NC, Stoohs RA, Netzer CM, et al: Using the Berlin Questionnaire to identify patients at risk for the sleep apnea syndrome. *Ann Intern Med* 131(7):485–491, 1999.
3. Luo J, Huang R, Zhong X, et al: STOP-Bang questionnaire is superior to Epworth sleepiness scales, Berlin questionnaire, and STOP questionnaire in screening OSA hypopnea syndrome patients. *Chin Med J (Engl)* 127(17):3065–3070, 2014.

Prognosis

Prognosis of OSA is excellent if effective treatment is instituted.

Untreated or unrecognized OSA can lead to cognitive impairment as a result of sleeplessness, which, in turn, can lead to serious injury or death caused by accidents, especially motor vehicle crashes. Sleepy patients should be warned of the risks of driving, operating heavy machinery, or engaging in other activities during which unintentional sleep episodes would be hazardous.

Adverse effects of hypersomnolence, such as loss of employment and sexual dysfunction, can affect families considerably.

In addition, perioperative complications, including cardiac arrest, have been attributed to OSA, probably because anesthesia can cause airway obstruction after a mechanical airway is removed. Patients should therefore inform their anesthesiologist of the diagnosis before undergoing any surgery and should expect to receive CPAP when they receive preoperative drugs and during recovery.

Treatment

- Control of risk factors
- CPAP or oral appliances
- For anatomic encroachment or intractable disease, consideration of airway surgery or possibly electrical stimulation of the hypoglossal nerve

The aim of treatment is to reduce episodes of hypoxia and sleep fragmentation; treatment is tailored to the patient and to the degree of impairment. Cure is defined as a resolution of symptoms with AHI reduction below a threshold, usually 10/h.

Treatment is directed at both risk factors and at OSA itself. Specific treatments for OSA include CPAP, oral appliances, and airway surgery.

Control of risk factors: Initial treatment aims at optimal control of modifiable risk factors for OSA, including obesity, alcohol and sedative use, hypothyroidism, acromegaly, and other chronic disorders. Although modest weight loss (15%) may result in clinically meaningful improvement, weight loss is extremely difficult for most people, especially those who are fatigued or sleepy. Bariatric surgery frequently reverses symptoms and improves AHI in morbidly obese (BMI > 40) patients; however, the degree of these improvements may not be as great as the degree of weight loss. Weight loss, with or without bariatric surgery, should not be considered a cure for OSA.

CPAP: Nasal CPAP is the treatment of choice for most patients with OSA and subjective daytime sleepiness; adherence is lower in patients who do not experience sleepiness. CPAP improves upper airway patency by applying positive pressure to the collapsible upper airway segment. Effective pressures typically range from 3 to 15 cm water. Disease severity does not correlate with pressure requirements. Many CPAP devices monitor CPAP efficacy and titrate pressures automatically, according to internal algorithms. If clinical improvement is not apparent, CPAP efficacy should be reviewed and patients should be reassessed for a second sleep disorder (eg, upper airway obstruction) or a comorbid disorder. If necessary, pressure can be titrated manually during monitoring with repeat polysomnography. Regardless of improvement in the AHI, CPAP will reduce cognitive impairment and improve quality of life, and it may reduce BP. If CPAP is withdrawn, symptoms recur over several days, though short interruptions of therapy for acute medical conditions are usually well tolerated. Duration of therapy is indefinite.[1–4]

Failures of nasal CPAP are common because of limited patient adherence. Adverse effects include dryness and nasal irritation, which can be alleviated in some cases with the use of warm humidified air, and discomfort resulting from a poorly fitting mask.

CPAP can be augmented with inspiratory assistance (bilevel positive airway pressure) for patients with obesity-hypoventilation syndrome to increase their tidal volumes.

Oral appliances: Oral appliances are designed to advance the mandible or, at the very least, prevent retrusion with sleep. Some are also designed to pull the tongue forward. Use of these appliances to treat both snoring and mild to moderate OSA is gaining acceptance. Comparisons of appliances to CPAP show equivalence in mild to moderate OSA, but results of cost-effectiveness studies are not available.

Surgery: Surgical procedures to correct anatomic factors such as enlarged tonsils and nasal polyps contributing to upper airway obstruction (called anatomic procedures) should be considered. Surgery for macroglossia or micrognathia is also an option. Surgery is a first-line treatment if anatomic encroachment is identified. However, in the absence of encroachment, evidence to support surgery as a first-line treatment is lacking.

Uvulopalatopharyngoplasty (UPPP) is the most commonly used procedure. It involves resection of submucosal tissue from the tonsillar pillars to the arytenoepiglottic folds, including resection of the adenoids, to enlarge the upper airway. Equivalence with CPAP was shown in one study using CPAP as a bridge to surgery, but the interventions have not been directly compared. UPPP may not be successful in patients who are morbidly obese or who have anatomic narrowing of the airway. Moreover, after UPPP, recognition of sleep apnea is more difficult because of a lack of snoring. Such silent obstructions may cause apneic episodes as severe as those occurring before surgical intervention.

Adjunctive surgical procedures include midline glossectomy, hyoid advancement, and mandibulomaxillary advancement. Mandibulomaxillary advancement is sometimes offered as a 2nd-stage procedure if UPPP is not curative. The optimal multistage approach is not known.

Tracheostomy is the most effective therapeutic maneuver for OSA but is done as a last resort. It bypasses the site of obstruction and is indicated for patients most severely affected (eg, those with cor pulmonale).

Laser-assisted uvuloplasty, uvular splints, and radiofrequency tissue ablation have been promoted as treatments for loud snoring in patients without OSA. Although they may transiently decrease snoring loudness, efficacy declines over months to years.

Hypoglossal nerve stimulation: A new nonanatomic procedure is upper airway stimulation. In upper airway stimulation, an implanted device is used to activate a branch of the hypoglossal nerve. This therapy can be successful in highly selected patients with moderate to severe disease who are unable to tolerate CPAP therapy.[5]

Adjunctive treatments: Adjunctive treatments are commonly used but have no proven role as first-line treatment for OSA.

Modafinil can be used for residual sleepiness in OSA in patients who are effectively using CPAP.

Supplemental oxygen improves blood oxygenation, but a beneficial clinical effect cannot be predicted. Also, oxygen may provoke respiratory acidosis and morning headache in some patients.

A number of drugs have been used to stimulate ventilatory drive (eg, tricyclic antidepressants, theophylline) but cannot be routinely advocated because of limited efficacy, a low therapeutic index, or both.

Nasal dilatory devices and throat sprays sold OTC for snoring have not been studied sufficiently to prove benefits for OSA.

Patient education and support: An informed patient and family are better able to cope with a treatment strategy, including tracheostomy. Patient support groups provide helpful information and effectively support timely treatment and follow-up.

1. McEvoy RD, Antic NA, Heeley E, et al: CPAP for prevention of cardiovascular events in obstructive sleep apnea. *N Engl J Med* 375(10):919–931, 2016. doi: 10.1056/NEJMoa1606599.
2. Gottlieb DJ, Punjabi NM, Mehra R, et al: CPAP versus oxygen in obstructive sleep apnea. *N Engl J Med* 370(24):2276–2285, 2014. doi: 10.1056/NEJMoa1306766.
3. Chirinos JA, Gurubhagavatula I, Teff K, et al: CPAP, weight loss, or both for obstructive sleep apnea. *N Engl J Med* 370(24):2265–2275, 2014. doi: 10.1056/NEJMoa1306187.
4. Pépin JL, Tamisier R, Barone-Rochette G, et al: Comparison of CPAP and valsartan in hypertensive patients with sleep apnea. *Am J Respir Crit Care Med* 182(7):954–60, 2010. doi: 10.1164/rccm.200912-1803OC. Epub 2010 Jun 3.
5. Woodson BT, Soose RJ, Gillespie MB, et al: Three-year outcomes of cranial nerve stimulation for obstructive sleep apnea: The STAR Trial. *Otolaryngol Head Neck Surg* 154(1):181–188, 2016. doi: 10.1177/0194599815616618.

KEY POINTS

- Obesity, anatomic abnormalities in the upper airway passages, family history, certain disorders (eg, hypothyroidism, stroke), and use of alcohol or sedatives increase the risk of OSA.
- Patients typically snore, have restless and unrefreshing sleep, and often feel daytime sleepiness and fatigue.
- Most people who snore do not have OSA.
- Disorders that occur more commonly in patients with OSA include hypertension, stroke, diabetes, gastroesophageal reflux disease, nonalcoholic steatohepatitis, nocturnal angina, heart failure, and atrial fibrillation or other arrhythmias.
- Confirm the diagnosis by polysomnography.
- Control modifiable risk factors and treat most patients with CPAP and/or oral appliances designed to open the airway.
- Consider surgery for abnormalities causing airway encroachment or if the disorder is intractable.

OBSTRUCTIVE SLEEP APNEA IN CHILDREN

OSA is episodes of partial or complete closure of the upper airway that occur during sleep and lead to breathing cessation. Symptoms include snoring and sometimes restless sleep, nocturnal sweating, and morning headache. Complications may include learning or behavioral disturbances, growth disturbance, cor pulmonale, and pulmonary hypertension. Diagnosis is by polysomnography. Treatment is usually adenotonsillectomy.

The prevalence of OSA in children is about 2%. The condition is underdiagnosed and can lead to serious sequelae.

Etiology

Risk factors for OSA in children include the following:

- Enlarged tonsils or adenoids
- Obesity (now the most common cause)
- Craniofacial abnormalities (eg, micrognathia, retrognathia, midfacial hypoplasia, excessively angled skull base)
- Certain drugs (eg, sedatives, opioids)
- Mucopolysaccharidoses
- Disorders causing hypotonia or hypertonia (eg, Down syndrome, cerebral palsy, muscular dystrophies)

- Possibly genetic factors (eg, congenital central hypoventilation disorders that can include obstructive and central apneas and possibly Prader-Willi syndrome and others)

Symptoms and Signs

In most affected children, parents note snoring; however, snoring may not be reported even when OSA is severe. Other sleep symptoms may include restless sleep, sweating at night, and observed apnea. Children may have nocturnal enuresis. Daytime signs and symptoms may include nasal obstruction, mouth breathing, morning headache, and problems concentrating. Excessive daytime sleepiness is less common than among adults with OSA.

Complications of OSA may include problems with learning and behavior, cor pulmonale, pulmonary hypertension, and growth disturbance.

Examination may reveal no abnormalities or may show anatomic facial, nasal, or oral abnormalities contributing to obstruction, increase in the pulmonic component of the 2nd heart sound, or growth disturbance.

Diagnosis

- Polysomnography with oximetry and end-tidal carbon dioxide monitoring

OSA is considered in children with snoring or risk factors. If symptoms of OSA are present, diagnostic testing is done in a sleep laboratory using overnight polysomnography that includes oximetry and end-tidal carbon dioxide monitoring. Home polysomnography is under evaluation.

Polysomnography can help confirm the diagnosis of OSA, but diagnosis also requires that the child not have a cardiac or pulmonary disorder that could explain the polysomnographic abnormalities. Analysis of sleep stage and the effects of position during polysomnography can help indicate the contribution of upper airway obstruction. Thus, results of polysomnography can help determine initial treatment (eg, CPAP with autotitration or oral or surgical appliances).

Patients with OSA are evaluated with other tests based on clinical judgement. Other testing may include ECG, chest x-ray, ABG, and imaging of the upper airway.

Treatment

- Adenotonsillectomy or correction of congenital micrognathia
- Sometimes CPAP and/or weight loss

Adenotonsillectomy is usually effective in children with OSA who are otherwise healthy and have enlarged tonsils and/or adenoids. Adenoidectomy alone is often ineffective. The risk of perioperative airway obstruction is higher among children with OSA than among children without OSA who undergo adenotonsillectomy; thus, close monitoring is important.

For children who are not otherwise healthy, who have complex anatomic abnormalities or genetic conditions altering respiratory control, or who have cardiopulmonary complications, a physician experienced in management of OSA in children should be consulted. Adenotonsillectomy may be effective or may provide some relief. Depending on the anatomic abnormality causing OSA, an alternate surgical procedure may be indicated (eg, uvulopalatopharyngoplasty, tongue or midface surgeries).

CPAP can be used for children who are not candidates for corrective surgery or who continue to have OSA after adenotonsillectomy.

Weight loss can decrease OSA severity in obese children and has other health benefits but is rarely sufficient treatment for OSA as monotherapy.

Nocturnal oxygen supplementation may help prevent hypoxemia until definitive treatment can be accomplished.

Corticosteroids and antibiotics are not usually indicated.

KEY POINTS

- Risk factors for childhood OSA include obesity, enlarged tonsils or adenoids, anatomic (including craniofacial) abnormalities, genetic abnormalities, drugs, and disorders causing hypertonia or hypotonia.
- Problems with learning and behavior are potentially serious complications.
- Diagnose childhood OSA based on caregiver-confirmed symptoms and the results of polysomnography.
- Correct anatomic causes of obstruction (eg, by adenotonsillectomy or correction of micrognathia).
- Consider CPAP and/or weight loss if surgery is not indicated or not completely effective.

66 Tumors of the Lungs

Lung tumors may be

- Primary
- Metastatic from other sites in the body

Primary tumors of the lung may be

- Malignant (see Table 66–1)
- Benign (see Table 66–2)

The most common lung cancer is non–small cell lung cancer (SCLC).

LUNG CARCINOMA

(Lung Cancer)

Lung carcinoma is the leading cause of cancer-related death worldwide. About 85% of cases are related to cigarette smoking. Symptoms can include cough, chest discomfort or pain, weight loss, and, less commonly, hemoptysis; however, many patients present with metastatic disease without any clinical symptoms. The diagnosis is typically made by chest x-ray or CT and confirmed by biopsy. Depending on the stage of the disease, treatment includes surgery, chemotherapy, radiation therapy, or a combination. For the past several decades, the prognosis for a lung cancer patient was poor, with only 15% of patients surviving > 5 yr from the time of diagnosis. For patients with stage IV (metastatic) disease, the 5-yr overall survival rate was < 1%. However, outcomes have improved because of the identification of certain mutations that can be targeted for therapy.

Epidemiology

In 2014, an estimated 224,210 new cases of lung cancer were diagnosed in the US, and 159,260 people died from the disease. The incidence of lung cancer has been declining in men over

Table 66–1. CLASSIFICATION OF PRIMARY MALIGNANT LUNG TUMORS

TYPE	EXAMPLE
Carcinoma	
Small cell lung cancer	Oat cell Intermediate cell Combined
Non–small cell lung cancer	Adenocarcinoma Acinar Bronchioloalveolar Papillary Solid Adenosquamous Large cell Clear cell Giant cell Squamous cell Spindle cell
Other	
Bronchial gland carcinoma	Adenoid cystic Mucoepidermoid
Carcinoid	–
Lymphoma	Primary pulmonary Hodgkin Primary pulmonary non-Hodgkin

the past 2 decades and has leveled off and begun a slight decline in women.

Etiology

Cigarette smoking is the most important cause of lung cancer, accounting for about 85% of cases. The risk of cancer differs by age, smoking intensity, and smoking duration.

The risk of lung cancer increases with combined exposure to toxins and cigarette smoking. Other confirmed or possible risk factors include air pollution, exposure to cigar smoke and second-hand cigarette smoke, and exposure to carcinogens (eg, asbestos, radiation, radon, arsenic, chromates, nickel, chloromethyl ethers, polycyclic aromatic hydrocarbons, mustard gas, coke-oven emissions, primitive cooking, heating huts).

The risk of cancer declines after smoking cessation, but it never returns to baseline. About 15 to 20% of people who develop lung cancer have never smoked or have smoked minimally.

Whether and how much exposure to household radon increases risk of lung cancer is controversial.

It is also suspected that COPD, alpha-1 antitrypsin deficiency, and pulmonary fibrosis may increase susceptibility to lung cancer. People whose lungs are scarred by other lung diseases (eg, TB) are potentially at increased risk of lung cancer. Also, active smokers who take beta-carotene supplements may have an increased risk of developing lung cancer.

Respiratory epithelial cells require prolonged exposure to cancer-promoting agents and accumulation of multiple genetic mutations before becoming neoplastic (an effect called field carcinogenesis). In some patients with lung cancer, secondary or additional mutations in genes that stimulate cell growth (*K-ras*, *MYC*), cause abnormalities in growth factor receptor signaling (EGFR, *HER2/neu*), and inhibit apoptosis contribute to proliferation of abnormal cells. In addition, mutations that inhibit tumor-suppressor genes (*p53*, *APC*) can lead to cancer. Other mutations that may be responsible include the *EML-4-ALK* translocation and mutations

Table 66–2. CLASSIFICATION OF BENIGN LUNG TUMORS

TYPE	EXAMPLE
Laryngotracheobronchial	Adenoma Hamartoma Myoblastoma Papilloma
Parenchymal	Fibroma Hamartoma Leiomyoma Lipoma Neurofibroma Schwannoma Sclerosing hemangioma

in *ROS-1*, *BRAF*, and *PI3KCA*. Genes such as these that are primarily responsible for lung cancer are called oncogenic driver mutations. Although oncogenic driver mutations can cause or contribute to lung cancer among smokers, these mutations are particularly likely to be a cause of lung cancer among nonsmokers. In 2014, the Lung Cancer Mutation Consortium (LCMC) found driver mutations in 64% of 733 lung cancers among smokers and nonsmokers (25% *K-ras* mutations, 17% *EGFR* mutations, 8% *EML-4-ALK*, and 2% *BRAF* mutations[1]). Novel therapies aimed at oncogenic driver mutations are being developed.

1. Kris MG, Johnson BE, Berry LD, et al: Using multiplexed assays of oncogenic drivers in lung cancers to select targeted drugs. *JAMA* 311(19):1998–2006, 2014.

Classification

Lung cancer is classified into 2 major categories:

- SCLC, about 15% of cases
- Non–small cell lung cancer (NSCLC), about 85% of cases

SCLC is highly aggressive and almost always occurs in smokers. It is rapidly growing, and roughly 80% of patients have metastatic disease at the time of diagnosis.

The clinical behavior of **NSCLC** is more variable and depends on histologic type, but about 40% of patients will have metastatic disease outside of the chest at the time of diagnosis. Oncogenic driver mutations have been identified primarily in adenocarcinoma, although attempts are being made to identify similar mutations in squamous cell carcinoma.

Other features of the 2 categories (eg, location, risks, treatment, complications) also vary (see Table 66–3).

Symptoms and Signs

About 25% of lung cancers are asymptomatic and are detected incidentally with chest imaging. Symptoms and signs can result from local tumor progression, regional spread, or distant metastases. Paraneoplastic syndromes and constitutional symptoms may occur at any stage of the disease. Although symptoms are not specific to the classification or histology of the cancer, certain complications may be more likely with different types (see Table 66–3).

Local tumor: The local tumor can cause cough and, less commonly, dyspnea due to airway obstruction, postobstructive atelectasis, and parenchymal loss due to lymphangitic spread. Fever may occur with postobstructive pneumonia. Up to half of patients report vague or localized chest pain. Hemoptysis is less common, and blood loss is minimal, except in rare instances when the tumor erodes into a major artery, causing massive hemorrhage and often death by asphyxiation or exsanguination.

Regional spread: Regional spread of tumor may cause pleuritic chest pain or dyspnea due to development of a pleural effusion, hoarseness due to tumor encroachment on the recurrent laryngeal nerve, and dyspnea and hypoxia from diaphragmatic paralysis due to involvement of the phrenic nerve.

Superior vena cava (SVC) syndrome results from compression or invasion of the SVC and can cause headache or a sensation of head fullness, facial or upper-extremity swelling, breathlessness when supine, dilated veins in the neck, face, and upper trunk, and facial and truncal flushing (plethora).

Pancoast syndrome occurs when apical tumors, usually NSCLC (Pancoast tumor), invade the brachial plexus, pleura, or ribs, causing shoulder and upper-extremity pain and weakness or atrophy of the ipsilateral hand. Pancoast syndrome can also include Horner syndrome.

Horner syndrome (ptosis, miosis, anhidrosis) results when the paravertebral sympathetic chain or cervical stellate ganglion is involved.

Spread of the tumor to the pericardium may be asymptomatic or lead to constrictive pericarditis or cardiac tamponade. In rare cases, esophageal compression by the tumor leads to dysphagia.

Metastases: Metastases eventually cause symptoms that vary by location. Metastases can spread to the

- Liver, causing pain, nausea, early satiety, and ultimately hepatic insufficiency
- Brain, causing behavioral changes, confusion, aphasia, seizures, paresis or paralysis, nausea and vomiting, and ultimately coma and death
- Bones, causing severe pain and pathologic fractures
- Adrenal glands, rarely causing adrenal insufficiency

Paraneoplastic syndromes: Paraneoplastic syndromes are symptoms that occur at sites distant from a tumor or its metastases. Common paraneoplastic syndromes in patients with lung cancer include

- Hypercalcemia (in patients with squamous cell carcinoma, which results because the tumor produces parathyroid hormone–related protein)
- Syndrome of inappropriate antidiuretic hormone (SIADH) secretion
- Finger clubbing with or without hypertrophic pulmonary osteoarthropathy
- Hypercoagulability with migratory superficial thrombophlebitis (Trousseau syndrome)
- Myasthenia-like symptoms (Eaton-Lambert syndrome)
- Cushing syndrome
- Various other neurologic syndromes

Other neurologic syndromes include neuropathies, encephalopathies, encephalitides, myelopathies, and cerebellar disease. Mechanisms for neuromuscular syndromes involve tumor expression of autoantigens with production of autoantibodies, but the cause of most other syndromes is unknown.

Diagnosis

- Chest x-ray
- CT or combined PET–CT

Table 66–3. FEATURES OF LUNG CANCER

FEATURE	SMALL CELL	NON–SMALL CELL: ADENOCARCINOMA	NON–SMALL CELL: SQUAMOUS CELL	NON–SMALL CELL: LARGE CELL
% of lung cancers	13–15%	35–40%	25–30%	10–15%
Location	Submucosa of airways, perihilar mass	Peripheral nodule or mass	Central, endobronchial	Peripheral nodule or mass
Risk factors	Smoking	Smoking (for 80–85% of patients; 15–20% never smoked or smoked only minimally), smokers and particularly nonsmokers often have oncogenic driver mutations Environmental and occupational exposures (mainly to radon, asbestos, radiation, secondhand smoke, polycyclic aromatic hydrocarbons, arsenic, chromates, or nickel)		
Treatment	Etoposide plus cisplatin or carboplatin Sometimes irinotecan or topotecan rather than etoposide in extensive-stage disease Concurrent radiation therapy in limited-stage disease No role for surgery	Stage I and II: Surgery with or without adjuvant chemotherapy Stage IIIA: Surgery with or without adjuvant chemotherapy or concurrent chemotherapy or radiation therapy, chemotherapy plus radiation therapy and surgery, chemotherapy with surgery, or chemotherapy plus radiation therapy Stage IIIB: Radiation therapy with or without chemotherapy Stage IV: Systemic targeted therapy or chemotherapy with or without palliative radiation therapy		
Complications	SVC syndrome Paraneoplastic syndromes	Hemoptysis, airway obstruction, pneumonia, pleuritic involvement with pain, pleural effusion, SVC syndrome, Pancoast tumor (causing shoulder or arm pain), hoarseness due to laryngeal nerve involvement, neurologic symptoms due to brain metastasis, pathologic fractures due to bone metastasis, jaundice due to liver metastasis		
5-yr survival with treatment	Limited: 20% Extensive: < 1%	Stage I: 60–70% Stage II: 39–55% Stage III: 5–25% Stage IV: < 1%		

SVC = superior vena cava.

- Cytopathology examination of pleural fluid or sputum
- Usually bronchoscopy-guided biopsy and core biopsy
- Sometimes open lung biopsy

Imaging: Chest x-ray is often the initial imaging test. It may show clearly defined abnormalities, such as a single mass or multifocal masses or a solitary pulmonary nodule, an enlarged hilum, widened mediastinum, tracheobronchial narrowing, atelectasis, nonresolving parenchymal infiltrates, cavitary lesions, or unexplained pleural thickening or effusion. These findings are suggestive but not diagnostic of lung cancer and require follow-up with CT scans or combined PET–CT scans and cytopathologic confirmation.

CT shows many characteristic anatomic patterns and appearances that may strongly suggest the diagnosis. CT also can guide core needle biopsy of accessible lesions and is useful for staging. If a lesion found on a plain x-ray is highly likely to be lung cancer, PET–CT may be done. This study combines anatomic imaging from CT with functional imaging from PET. The PET images can help differentiate inflammatory and malignant processes.

Cytology: The method used to obtain cells or tissue for confirmation depends on the accessibility of tissue and the location of lesions. Sputum or pleural fluid cytology is the least invasive method. In patients with productive cough, sputum specimens obtained on awakening may contain high concentrations of malignant cells, but yield for this method is < 50% overall. Pleural fluid is another convenient source of cells; a malignant effusion is a poor prognostic sign.

In general, false-negative cytology readings can be minimized by obtaining as large a volume of sputum or pleural fluid as possible early in the day and sending the sample to the pathology laboratory immediately to minimize delays in processing because such delays lead to cell breakdown. Molecular (genetic) studies can be done on paraffin-embedded tumor cell pellets from pleural fluid if the fluid is spun down and the cell pellet preserved in a timely fashion. Biopsy, when done, is core biopsy; fine-needle biopsy retrieves too little tissue for accurate genetic studies.

Procedures: Percutaneous biopsy is the next least invasive procedure. It is more useful for metastatic sites (eg, supraclavicular or other peripheral lymph nodes, pleura, liver, adrenals) than for lung lesions. Risks include a 20 to 25% chance of pneumothorax (primarily in patients with significant emphysema) and the risk of obtaining a false-negative result.

Bronchoscopy is the procedure most often used for diagnosing lung cancer. In theory, the procedure of choice for obtaining tissue is the one that is least invasive; however, in practice, bronchoscopy is often done in addition to or instead of less invasive procedures because diagnostic yields are greater and because bronchoscopy is important for staging. A combination of washings, brushings, and biopsies of visible endobronchial lesions and of paratracheal, subcarinal, mediastinal, and hilar lymph nodes often yields a tissue diagnosis.

Mediastinoscopy is the standard test for evaluating mediastinal lymph nodes but is a higher risk procedure that is usually used before thoracic surgery to confirm or exclude the presence of tumor in enlarged mediastinal lymph nodes. Endobronchial ultrasound-guided biopsy (EBUS) can be done in a fashion similar to bronchoscopy.

Open lung biopsy, done via open thoracotomy or using video assistance, is indicated when less invasive methods do not provide a diagnosis in patients whose clinical characteristics and radiographic features strongly suggest that the tumor is resectable.

Screening: To date, no screening studies are universally accepted. Screening chest x-rays and sputum cytologies in asymptomatic high-risk patients (smokers) are not recommended. Screening CT is being evaluated because it is more sensitive. However, CT may produce more false-positive results, which increase the number of unnecessary invasive diagnostic procedures needed to verify the CT findings. Such procedures are costly and risk additional complications.

Recent studies have suggested a 20% decrease in lung cancer deaths among former or active smokers (mainly ages 55 to 74 and with a heavy smoking history) when annual screening is done using low-dose helical CT (LDCT) as compared to chest x-ray. However, screening LDCT may not be appropriate for patients not at high risk.

Screening is believed to benefit patients with early disease, especially early NSCLC treatable with surgical resection. The U.S. Preventive Services Task Force (USPSTF) recommends, because of "moderate net benefit," annual LDCT screening of asymptomatic smokers age 55 to 80 with a ≥ 30 pack-year history who currently smoke or have quit for less than 15 years. Screening should exclude patients who would not benefit from early detection, such as those who would refuse treatment or be unable to complete treatment due to serious other medical conditions. Additionally, it is recommended that LDCT screening be done at facilities with demonstrated LDCT proficiency and adherence to established protocols for follow-up diagnosis and treatment.

In the future, lung cancer screening may involve some combination of molecular analysis for genetic markers (eg, *K-ras*, *p53*, *EGFR*), sputum cytometry, and detection of cancer-related volatile organic compounds (eg, alkane, benzene) in exhaled breath.

Staging

SCLC has 2 stages:

- Limited
- Extensive

Limited-stage SCLC disease is cancer confined to one hemithorax (including ipsilateral lymph nodes) that can be encompassed within one tolerable radiation therapy port, unless there is a pleural or pericardial effusion.

Extensive-stage disease is cancer outside a single hemithorax or the presence of malignant cells detected in pleural or pericardial effusions. Less than one third of patients with SCLC will present with limited-stage disease; the remainder of patients often have extensive distant metastases.

NSCLC has 4 stages, I through IV (using the TNM system). TNM staging is based on tumor size, tumor and lymph node location, and the presence or absence of distant metastases (see Table 66–4).

Tests for initial evaluation and staging: All lung cancer patients need whole-body imaging. Different combinations of tests can be done. Some tests are done routinely, and others are done depending on whether the results would impact treatment decisions:

- PET or integrated PET–CT
- CT from neck to pelvis and bone scan (done if PET–CT is not available)
- MRI of chest (for tumors near apex or diaphragm to evaluate vascular supply)
- Biopsy of questionable nodes (if PET is indeterminate)
- Head CT or brain MRI

If PET–CT is not available, thin-section high-resolution CT (HRCT) from the neck to the upper abdomen (to detect cervical and supraclavicular and hepatic and adrenal metastases) is one of the first staging tests for both SCLC and NSCLC. However, CT often cannot distinguish postinflammatory changes from malignant intrathoracic lymph node enlargement or benign lesions from malignant hepatic or adrenal lesions (distinctions that determine stage). Thus, other tests are usually done when abnormalities are present in these areas.

PET scanning is a reasonably accurate, noninvasive test used to identify malignant mediastinal lymph nodes and other distant metastases (metabolic staging). Integrated PET–CT scanning, in which PET and CT images are combined into a single image by scanners in a single gantry, is more accurate for NSCLC staging than CT or PET alone or than visual correlation of the 2 tests. The use of PET and integrated PET–CT is limited by cost, availability, and specificity (ie, the test is quite sensitive and has an excellent negative predictive value, but its positive predictive value is not as high). When PET scan results are indeterminate, bronchoscopy, mediastinoscopy, or video-assisted thoracoscopic surgery (VATS) can be used to biopsy questionable mediastinal lymph nodes. Without PET scanning, hepatic or adrenal lesions must be evaluated by needle biopsy.

MRI of the chest is slightly more accurate than high-chest HRCT for staging apical tumors and cancers close to the diaphragm and provides an evaluation of the vasculature surrounding the tumors.

Blood tests are usually done. Calcium and alkaline phosphatase levels, if elevated, suggest possible bone metastases. Other blood tests, such as CBC, serum albumin levels, AST, ALT, total bilirubin, electrolytes, and creatinine levels, have no role in staging but provide important prognostic information about the patient's ability to tolerate treatment and may demonstrate the presence of paraneoplastic syndromes.

After diagnosis, all patients with lung cancer should undergo brain imaging; MRI is preferred to CT. Brain imaging is especially necessary in patients with headache or neurologic abnormalities.

Patients with bone pain or elevated serum calcium or alkaline phosphatase levels should undergo PET–CT or radionuclide bone scanning if PET–CT is not available.

Prognosis

For SCLC, the overall prognosis is poor. The median survival time for limited-stage SCLC is 20 mo, with a 5-yr survival rate of 20%. Patients with extensive-stage SCLC do especially poorly, with a 5-yr survival rate of < 1%.

For NSCLC, the 5-yr survival rate varies by stage, from 60 to 70% for patients with stage I disease to < 1% for patients with stage IV disease. On average, untreated patients with metastatic NSCLC survive 6 mo, whereas the median survival for treated patients is about 9 mo. Recently, patient survival has improved in both early and later stage NSCLC. Evidence shows improved survival in early-stage disease (stages IB to IIIB) when platinum-based chemotherapy regimens are used after surgical resection. In addition, targeted therapies have improved survival in patients with stage IV disease, in particular patients with an *EGFR* mutation, *EML-4-ALK* and *ROS-1* translocations.

Treatment

- Surgery (depending on cell type and stage)
- Chemotherapy
- Radiation therapy

Treatment varies by cell type and by stage of disease. Many patient factors not related to the tumor affect treatment choice. Poor cardiopulmonary reserve, undernutrition, frailty or poor physical performance status (assessed by, eg, Karnofsky performance status [KPS] or Eastern Cooperative Oncology Group performance status [ECOGPS]), comorbidities, including cytopenias, and psychiatric or cognitive illness all may lead to a decision for palliative over curative treatment or for no treatment at all, even though a cure with aggressive therapy might technically be possible.

Radiation therapy carries the risk of radiation pneumonitis when large areas of the lung are exposed to high doses of radiation over time. Radiation pneumonitis can occur up to 3 mo after treatment is completed. Cough, dyspnea, low-grade fever, or pleuritic chest pain may signal the condition, as may crackles or a pleural friction rub detected on chest auscultation. Chest x-ray may have nonspecific findings; CT may show a nonspecific infiltrate without an obvious mass. The diagnosis is often one of exclusion. Radiation pneumonitis can be treated with a corticosteroid taper over several weeks and bronchodilators for symptom relief.

Radiofrequency ablation, in which high-frequency electrical current is used to destroy tumor cells, is a newer technique that can sometimes be used in patients who have small, early-stage tumors or small tumors that have recurred in a previously irradiated chest. This procedure may preserve more lung function than open surgery does and, because it is less invasive, may be appropriate for patients who are not candidates for open surgery.

SCLC: SCLC of any stage is typically initially responsive to treatment, but responses are usually short-lived. Chemotherapy, with or without radiation therapy, is given depending on the stage of disease. In many patients, chemotherapy prolongs survival and improves quality of life enough to warrant its use. Surgery generally plays no role in treatment of SCLC, although it may be curative in the rare patient who has a small focal tumor without spread (such as a **solitary pulmonary nodule**) who underwent surgical resection before the tumor was identified as SCLC.

Chemotherapy regimens of etoposide and a platinum compound (either cisplatin or carboplatin) are commonly used, as are other drugs, such as irinotecan, topotecan, vinca alkaloids (vinblastine, vincristine, vinorelbine), alkylating agents (cyclophosphamide, ifosfamide), doxorubicin, taxanes (docetaxel, paclitaxel), and gemcitabine.

In limited-stage disease, when disease is confined to a hemithorax, radiation therapy further improves clinical outcomes; such response to radiation therapy was the basis for the definition of limited-stage disease. The use of cranial radiation to prevent brain metastases is also advocated in certain cases; micrometastases are common in SCLC, and chemotherapy has less ability to cross the blood-brain barrier.

In extensive-stage disease, treatment is based on chemotherapy rather than radiation therapy, although radiation therapy is often used as palliative treatment for metastases to bone or brain. In patients with an excellent response to chemotherapy, prophylactic brain irradiation is sometimes used as in limited-stage SCLC to prevent growth of SCLC in the brain. In rare, selected patients who have a near-complete response to chemotherapy, thoracic radiation therapy is sometimes thought to improve disease control. It is unclear whether replacing etoposide with topoisomerase inhibitors (irinotecan or topotecan) improves survival. These drugs alone or in combination with other drugs are also commonly used in refractory disease and in cancer of either stage that has recurred.

In general, **recurrent SCLC** carries a poor prognosis, although patients who maintain a good performance status should be offered a clinical trial.

NSCLC: Treatment for NSCLC typically involves assessment of eligibility for surgery followed by choice of surgery, chemotherapy, radiation therapy, or a combination of modalities as appropriate, depending on tumor type and stage.

For **stage I and II disease,** the standard approach is surgical resection with either lobectomy or pneumonectomy combined with mediastinal lymph node sampling or complete lymph node dissection. Lesser resections, including segmentectomy and

Table 66–4. NEW INTERNATIONAL STAGING SYSTEM FOR LUNG CANCER

CATEGORY	DESCRIPTION
Primary tumor (T)	
Tis	Carcinoma in situ
T1	Tumor ≤ 3 cm without invasion more proximal than the lobar bronchus
T1a	Tumor ≤ 2 cm
T1b	Tumor > 2 but ≤ 3 cm
T2	Tumor > 3 cm but ≤ 7 cm *or* with any of the following: • Involves the main bronchus ≥ 2 cm distal to carina • Invades the visceral pleura • Associated with atelectasis or obstructive pneumonia that extends to the hilar region but does not involve the whole lung
T2a	Tumor > 3 but ≤ 5 cm
T2b	Tumor > 5 but ≤ 7 cm
T3	Tumor > 7 cm *or* with any of the following: • Invades the chest wall, diaphragm, phrenic nerve, mediastinal pleura, parietal pericardium, or main bronchus < 2 cm distal to carina but not the carina • Atelectasis or obstructive pneumonitis of the entire lung • Separate tumor nodules in the same lobe
T4	Tumor of any size with either of the following: • Invades the mediastinum, heart, great vessels, trachea, recurrent laryngeal nerve, esophagus, vertebral body, or carina • ≥ 1 Satellite tumors in a different ipsilateral lobe
Regional lymph nodes (N)	
N0	No regional lymph node metastasis
N1	Metastasis to ipsilateral peribronchial or ipsilateral hilar lymph node or both and to intrapulmonary nodes, including that by direct extension of the primary tumor
N2	Metastasis to ipsilateral mediastinal or subcarinal lymph node or both
N3	Metastasis to contralateral mediastinal, contralateral hilar, ipsilateral or contralateral scalene, or supraclavicular lymph node or a combination
Distant metastasis (M)	
M0	No distant metastasis
M1	Distant metastasis
M1a	Tumor with any of the following: • ≥ 1 Tumor nodules in the contralateral lung • Pleural nodules • Malignant pleural or pericardial effusion
M1b	Distant metastasis (extrathoracic)
Stage groupings	
• Stage 0: Tis N0 M0 • Stage IA: T1a–T1b N0 M0 • Stage IB: T2a N0 M0 • Stage IIA: T1a–T2a N1 M0 *or* T2b N0 M0 • Stage IIB: T2b N1 M0 *or* T3 N0 M0 • Stage IIIA: T1a–T2b N2 M0 *or* T3 N1–N2 M0 *or* T4 N0–N1 M0 • Stage IIIB: T1a–T3 N3 M0 *or* T4 N2–N3 M0 • Stage IV: T (any) N (any) M1a–M1b	

Adapted from Edge SB, Byrd DR, Compton CC, et al: *AJCC Cancer Staging Manual,* 7th edition. New York, Springer, 2010.

wedge resection, are considered for patients with poor pulmonary reserve. Surgery is curative in about 55 to 70% of patients with stage I and in 35 to 55% of patients with stage II disease.

Preoperative pulmonary function is assessed. Surgery is done only if NSCLC patients will have adequate pulmonary reserve once a lobe or lung is resected. Patients with preoperative forced expiratory volume in 1 sec (FEV_1) > 2 L generally tolerate pneumonectomy. Patients with FEV_1 < 2 L should have a quantitative xenon radionuclide perfusion scan to determine the proportion of function they can expect to lose as a result of resection. Postoperative FEV_1 can be predicted by multiplying percent perfusion of the nonresected lung by the preoperative FEV_1. A predicted FEV_1 > 800 mL or > 40% of the predicted normal FEV_1 suggests adequate postoperative lung function, although studies of lung volume reduction surgery in COPD patients suggest that patients with FEV_1 < 800 mL can tolerate resection if the cancer is located in poorly functional, bullous (generally apical) lung regions. Patients undergoing resection at hospitals that do more resections have fewer complications and are more likely to survive than those who undergo surgery at hospitals that do fewer lung cancer procedures.

Adjuvant chemotherapy after surgery is now standard practice for patients with stage II or stage III disease and possibly also for patients with stage IB disease and tumors > 4 cm. Clinical trials have shown an increase in 5-yr survival rates with the use of adjuvant chemotherapy. However, the decision to use adjuvant chemotherapy depends on the patient's comorbidities and risk assessment. A commonly used chemotherapy regimen is a cisplatin-based doublet (combination of a cisplatin and another chemotherapy drug, such as vinorelbine, docetaxel, paclitaxel). Neoadjuvant (preoperative) chemotherapy in early-stage NSCLC is also commonly used and consists of 4 cycles of a cisplatin-doublet. In patients who cannot receive cisplatin, carboplatin can be substituted.

Stage III disease is treated with either chemotherapy, radiation therapy, surgery, or a combination of therapies; the sequence and choice of treatment depend on the location of the patient's disease and comorbidities. In general, concurrent chemotherapy and radiation therapy are considered standard treatment for unresectable clinically staged IIIA disease, but the survival remains poor (median survival, 10 to 14 mo). Patients with stage IIIB disease with contralateral mediastinal nodal disease or supraclavicular nodal disease are offered either radiation therapy or chemotherapy or both. Patients with locally advanced tumors invading the heart, great vessels, mediastinum, or spine usually receive radiation therapy. In some patients (ie, those with T4 N0 M0 tumors), surgical resection with either neoadjuvant or adjuvant combined chemotherapy and radiation therapy may be feasible. The 5-yr survival rate for patients with treated stage IIIB disease is 5%.

In **stage IV** disease, palliation of symptoms is the goal. Chemotherapy, targeted drugs, and radiation therapy may be used to reduce tumor burden, relieve symptoms, and improve quality of life. However, if no mutation treatable with a targeted drug is identified, median survival is only 9 mo, and < 25% of patients survive 1 yr. Surgical palliative procedures may be required and may include thoracentesis and pleurodesis of recurrent effusions, placement of indwelling pleural drainage catheters, bronchoscopic fulguration of tumors involving the trachea and mainstem bronchi, placement of stents to prevent airway occlusion, and, in some cases, spinal stabilization for impending spinal cord compression.

In patients with nonsquamous NSCLC without an oncogenic driver mutation, bevacizumab, a vascular endothelial growth factor inhibitor, can be used in combination with standard chemotherapy (eg, a platinum-based doublet, such as carboplatin plus paclitaxel) to improve outcomes. Necitumumab is now available for use in combination with cisplatin plus gemcitabine for first-line treatment of NSCLC squamous cell carcinoma. For NSCLC, second-line therapy now includes immunotherapies (nivolumab, pembrolizumab) and docetaxel plus ramucirumab.

For tumors bearing an oncogenic driver mutation, inhibitors are used first. In stage IV patients with sensitive *EGFR* mutations (ie, deletion exon 19, exon 21 L858 mutation), EGFR tyrosine kinase inhibitors (TKIs) may be given as first-line therapy; response rates and progression-free survival are better than those obtained using standard chemotherapy. EGFR TKIs include gefitinib and erlotinib. Patients who have *EML-4-ALK* translocations should receive crizotinib, an *ALK* and *ROS-1* inhibitor. Patients with *ALK*mutations can be given alectinib or ceritinib. Patients with *ROS-1*mutations can be given crizotinib or erlotinib. Patients with *BRAF* mutations may benefit from the BRAF inhibitors (eg, vemurafenib). Similarly, patients with *PI3K* mutations may be expected to respond to PI3K inhibitors, which are being developed. Many other biologic agents are under investigation, including some that specifically target cancer cell signal transduction pathways or the angiogenesis pathways that supply oxygen and nutrition to growing tumor cells.

Recurrent lung cancer: Treatment options for lung cancer that recurs after treatment vary by location and include repeat chemotherapy or targeted drugs for metastases, radiation therapy for local recurrence or pain caused by metastases, and brachytherapy for endobronchial disease when additional external radiation cannot be tolerated. Rarely, surgical resection of a solitary metastasis or for palliative purposes is considered.

The treatment of a locally recurrent NSCLC follows the same guidelines as for primary tumor stages I to III. If surgery was used initially, radiation therapy is the main modality. If the recurrence manifests as distant metastases, patients are treated as if they have stage IV disease with a focus on palliation.

Treatment for recurrent or metastatic stage IV NSCLC includes chemotherapy or novel targeted drugs. The choice depends on tumor histology, patient functional status, and patient preference. For example, an EGFR TKI, such as gefitinib or erlotinib, can be used as second- or third-line therapy even among patients who do not have sensitive *EGFR* mutations.

Complications of lung cancer: Asymptomatic malignant pleural effusions require no treatment. Initial treatment of a symptomatic effusion is with thoracentesis. Symptomatic effusions that recur despite multiple thoracenteses are drained through a chest tube. Infusion of talc (or occasionally, tetracycline or bleomycin) into the pleural space (a procedure called pleurodesis) scars the pleura, eliminates the pleural space, and is effective in > 90% of cases.

Treatment of SVC syndrome is the same as treatment of lung cancer, with chemotherapy (SCLC), radiation therapy (NSCLC), or both (NSCLC). Corticosteroids are commonly used but are of unproven benefit.

Treatment of Horner syndrome caused by apical tumors is with surgery with or without preoperative radiation therapy or with radiation therapy with or without adjuvant chemotherapy.

Treatment of paraneoplastic syndromes varies by syndrome.

End-of-life care: Because many patients with lung cancer die, the need for end-of-life care should be anticipated. Studies have reported that early palliative care intervention leads to less end-of-life chemotherapy use and may even extend life (ie, by avoiding adverse effects of aggressive treatments).

Symptoms of breathlessness can be treated with supplemental oxygen and bronchodilators. Preterminal breathlessness can be treated with opioids.

Pain, anxiety, nausea, and anorexia are especially common and can be treated with parenteral morphine; oral, transdermal, or parenteral opioids; and antiemetics.

The care provided by hospice programs is extremely well-accepted by patients and families, yet this intervention is markedly underused.

Prevention

No active interventions to prevent lung cancer are proven to be effective except for smoking cessation.

Remediation of high radon levels in private residences removes known cancer-promoting radiation, but a reduction in lung cancer incidence is unproven.

Increasing dietary intake of fruits and vegetables high in retinoids and beta-carotene appears to have no effect on lung cancer incidence. Vitamin supplementation is either unproven (vitamin E) or harmful (beta-carotene) in smokers. Preliminary evidence hinting that NSAIDs and vitamin E supplementation may protect former smokers from lung cancer requires confirmation.

New molecular approaches targeting cell signaling and cell cycle pathways and tumor-associated antigens are under investigation.

KEY POINTS

- The main factor contributing to lung cancer is smoking.
- About 15% of all lung cancer patients have never smoked cigarettes and have suspected driver mutations.
- Lung cancer can be small cell lung carcinoma (SCLC) or non–small cell lung carcinoma (NSCLC).
- Several genetic driver mutations that are amenable to targeted drugs have been identified in NSCLC.
- Manifestations can include cough fever, hoarseness, pleural effusion, pneumonia, Pancoast tumor, paraneoplastic syndromes, SVC syndrome, Horner syndrome, and metastases to the brain, liver, and bone.
- Suspect the diagnosis based on clinical information and imaging studies (eg, CT, PET-CT), and confirm it histologically (eg, by cytology of sputum or pleural fluid or core biopsy).
- Consider yearly screening with low-dose helical CT for smokers ≥ 55 yr at high risk.
- Do testing, beginning with whole-body imaging, to stage cancer.
- Treat early-stage NSCLC with resection when pulmonary reserve is adequate, often followed by chemotherapy.
- Treat advanced stage SCLC and NSCLC with chemotherapy.

AIRWAY TUMORS

The airway can be affected by primary tracheobronchial tumors, primary tumors that are adjacent to and invade or compress the airway, or cancers that metastasize to the airway.

Primary tracheal tumors are rare (0.1/100,000 people). They are often malignant and found at a locally advanced stage. The most common malignant tracheal tumors include adenoid cystic carcinoma, squamous cell carcinoma, carcinoid, and mucoepidermoid carcinomas. The most common benign airway tumor is a squamous papilloma, although pleomorphic adenomas and granular cell and benign cartilaginous tumors also occur.

Symptoms and Signs

Patients often present with

- Dyspnea
- Cough
- Wheezing
- Hemoptysis
- Stridor

Hemoptysis may occur with a squamous cell carcinoma and can potentially lead to earlier diagnosis, whereas wheezing or stridor occurs more often with the adenoid cystic variant. Dysphagia and hoarseness can also be present initially and usually indicate advanced disease.

Diagnosis

- Bronchoscopic biopsy

Symptoms of airway narrowing (eg, stridor, dyspnea, wheezing) can herald life-threatening airway obstruction. An airway tumor should be considered a possible cause if such symptoms are unexplained, are of gradual onset, are associated with other symptoms of airway tumors (eg, unexplained hemoptysis), and respond poorly to standard treatments (eg, if asthma treatments do not relieve wheezing).

If an airway tumor is suspected, patients require immediate evaluation with bronchoscopy. Bronchoscopy can both treat airway obstruction and allow specimens to be obtained for diagnosis. If cancer is found, more extensive testing for staging is done.

Prognosis

Prognosis depends on the histology.

Squamous cell carcinomas tend to metastasize to regional lymph nodes and directly invade mediastinal structures, leading to high local and regional recurrence rates. Even with definitive surgical resection, the 5-yr survival is only 20 to 40%.

Adenoid cystic carcinomas are typically indolent but tend to metastasize to the lungs and to spread perineurally, leading to high recurrence rates after resection. However, these patients have a higher 5-yr survival of 60 to 75% because of the slow rate of growth.

Treatment

- Surgery
- Sometimes radiation therapy
- Obstruction reduction techniques

Primary airway tumors should be treated definitively with surgical resection if possible. Tracheal, laryngotracheal, or carinal resections are the most common procedures. Up to 50% of the length of the trachea can be safely resected with primary reanastomosis. If a lung or thyroid cancer invades the airway, surgery is sometimes still feasible if assessment indicates sufficient tissue is available for airway reconstruction. Adjuvant radiation therapy is recommended if adequate surgical margins cannot be obtained.

Most primary airway tumors are not resectable because of metastasis, locally advanced stage, or patient comorbidities. In cases of endoluminal tumors, therapeutic bronchoscopy can mechanically core-out the tumor. Other techniques to eliminate obstruction include laser vaporization, photodynamic therapy, cryotherapy, and endobronchial brachytherapy. Tumors that compress the trachea are treated with airway stenting, radiation therapy, or both.

KEY POINTS

- Primary tracheal tumors are rare, often malignant, and commonly locally advanced when recognized.
- Suspect airway tumors in patients with gradual, unexplained, or intractable dyspnea, cough, wheezing, hemoptysis, and stridor.
- Treat with local resection or, if resection is not indicated, other locally destructive therapies.

BRONCHIAL CARCINOID

Bronchial carcinoids are rare, slow-growing neuroendocrine tumors arising from bronchial mucosa; they affect patients in their 40s to 60s.

Half of patients are asymptomatic, and half present with symptoms of airway obstruction, including dyspnea, wheezing, and cough, which often leads to a misdiagnosis of asthma. Recurrent pneumonia, hemoptysis, and chest pain are also common.

Paraneoplastic syndromes, including Cushing syndrome due to ectopic ACTH, acromegaly due to ectopic growth hormone–releasing factor, and Zollinger-Ellison syndrome due to ectopic gastrin production, are more common than carcinoid syndrome, which occurs in < 3% of patients with the tumor.

A left-sided heart murmur (mitral stenosis or regurgitation) due to serotonin-induced valvular damage occurs rarely with bronchial carcinoids (as opposed to the right-sided valvular lesions of GI carcinoid).

Diagnosis

- Bronchoscopic biopsy

Diagnosis is based on bronchoscopic biopsy, but evaluation often initially involves chest CT, which reveals tumor calcifications in up to one third of patients.

Indium-111–labeled octreotide scans are useful for determining regional and metastatic spread.

Increased urinary serotonin and 5-hydroxyindoleacetic acid levels support the diagnosis, but these substances are not commonly elevated.

Treatment

- Surgery

Treatment is with surgical removal with or without adjuvant chemotherapy and/or radiation therapy. Prognosis depends on tumor type. Five-year survival for well-differentiated carcinoids is > 90%; for atypical tumors, it is 50 to 70%.

CHEST WALL TUMORS

Chest wall tumors are benign or malignant tumors that can interfere with pulmonary function.

Primary chest wall tumors account for 5% of all thoracic tumors and 1 to 2% of all primary tumors. Almost half are benign. The **most common benign** chest wall tumors are

- Osteochondroma
- Chondroma
- Fibrous dysplasia

A wide range of malignant chest wall tumors exist. Over half are metastases from distant organs or direct invasions from adjacent structures (breast, lung, pleura, mediastinum). The most common malignant primary tumors arising from the chest wall are sarcomas; about 45% originate from soft tissue, and 55% originate from cartilaginous tissue or bone.

Chondrosarcomas are the most common primary chest wall sarcoma and arise from the anterior tract of ribs and less commonly from the sternum, scapula, or clavicle. Bone tumors include osteosarcoma and small-cell malignant tumors (eg, Ewing sarcoma, Askin tumor).

The most common soft-tissue primary malignant tumors are fibrosarcomas (desmoids, neurofibrosarcomas) and malignant fibrous histiocytomas. Other primary tumors include chondroblastomas, osteoblastomas, melanomas, lymphomas, rhabdomyosarcomas, lymphangiosarcomas, multiple myeloma, and plasmacytomas.

Symptoms and Signs

Soft-tissue chest wall tumors often manifest as a localized mass without other symptoms. Some patients have fever. Patients usually do not have pain until the tumor is advanced. In contrast, primary cartilaginous and bone tumors are often painful.

Diagnosis

- Imaging
- Biopsy

Patients with chest wall tumors require chest x-ray, CT, MRI, and sometimes PET–CT to determine the original site and extent of the tumor and whether it is a primary chest wall tumor or a metastasis. Biopsy and histologic evaluation confirm the diagnosis.

Prognosis

Prognosis varies by cancer type, cell differentiation, and stage; firm conclusions are limited by the low incidence of any given tumor. Sarcomas have been the most well studied, and primary chest wall sarcomas have a reported 5-yr survival of 17%. Survival is better with early-stage disease.

Treatment

- Surgery
- Sometimes combination chemotherapy, radiation therapy, and surgery

Most chest wall tumors are treated with surgical resection and reconstruction. Reconstruction often uses a combination of myocutaneous flaps and prosthetic materials. The presence of a malignant pleural effusion is a contraindication to surgical resection.

In cases of multiple myeloma or isolated plasmacytoma, chemotherapy and radiation therapy should be the primary therapy.

Small-cell malignant tumors such as Ewing sarcoma and Askin tumor should be treated with a multimodality approach, combining chemotherapy, radiation therapy, and surgery.

In cases of chest wall metastasis from distant tumors, a palliative chest wall resection is recommended only when nonsurgical options do not alleviate symptoms.

KEY POINTS

- Almost half of chest wall tumors are benign.
- Less than half of malignant chest wall tumors are primary.
- Consider the diagnosis if patients have a chest mass or unexplained chest wall pain, with or without fever.
- Diagnose chest wall tumors with imaging, followed by biopsy.
- Treat most with surgical resection and reconstruction (unless malignant pleural effusion is present), and sometimes chemotherapy and/or radiation therapy.

SECTION 6

Critical Care Medicine

CRC 6

67 Approach to the Critically Ill Patient

Critical care medicine specializes in caring for the most seriously ill patients. These patients are best treated in an ICU staffed by experienced personnel. Some hospitals maintain separate units for special populations (eg, cardiac, surgical, neurologic, pediatric, or neonatal patients). ICUs have a high nurse:patient ratio to provide the necessary high intensity of service, including treatment and monitoring of physiologic parameters.

Supportive care for the ICU patient includes provision of adequate nutrition and prevention of infection, stress ulcers and gastritis, and pulmonary embolism. Because 15 to 25% of patients admitted to ICUs die there, physicians should know how to minimize suffering and help dying patients maintain dignity (see p. 3175).

MONITORING AND TESTING THE CRITICAL CARE PATIENT

Some monitoring is manual (ie, by direct observation and physical examination) and intermittent, with the frequency depending on the patient's illness. This monitoring usually includes measurement of vital signs (temperature, BP, pulse, and respiration rate), quantification of all fluid intake and output, and often daily weight. BP may be recorded by an automated sphygmomanometer; a transcutaneous sensor for pulse oximetry is used as well.

Other monitoring is ongoing and continuous, provided by complex devices that require special training and experience to operate. Most such devices generate an alarm if certain physiologic parameters are exceeded. Every ICU should strictly follow protocols for investigating alarms.

Blood Tests

Although frequent blood draws can destroy veins, cause pain, and lead to anemia, ICU patients typically have routine daily blood tests to help detect problems early. Placement of a central venous catheter or arterial catheter can facilitate easy blood sampling without the need for repeated peripheral needle sticks, but the risk of complications must be considered. Generally, patients need a daily set of electrolytes and a CBC. Patients with arrhythmias should also have magnesium, phosphate, and calcium levels measured. Patients receiving TPN need weekly liver enzymes and coagulation profiles. Other tests (eg, blood culture for fever, CBC after a bleeding episode) are done as needed.

Point-of-care testing uses miniaturized, highly automated devices to do certain blood tests at the patient's bedside or unit (particularly ICU, emergency department, and operating room). Commonly available tests include blood chemistries, glucose, ABGs, CBC, cardiac markers, and coagulation tests. Many are done in < 2 min and require < 0.5 mL blood.

Cardiac Monitoring

Most critical care patients have cardiac activity monitored by a 3-lead system; signals are usually sent to a central monitoring station by a small radio transmitter worn by the patient. Automated systems generate alarms for abnormal rates and rhythms and store abnormal tracings for subsequent review.

Some specialized cardiac monitors track advanced parameters associated with coronary ischemia, although their clinical benefit is unclear. These parameters include continuous ST segment monitoring and heart rate variability. Loss of normal beat-to-beat variability signals a reduction in autonomic activity and possibly coronary ischemia and increased risk of death.

Pulmonary Artery Catheter Monitoring

Use of a pulmonary artery catheter (PAC) is becoming less common in ICU patients. This balloon-tipped, flow-directed catheter is inserted via central veins through the right side of the heart into the pulmonary artery. The catheter typically contains several ports that can monitor pressure or inject fluids. Some PACs also include a sensor to measure central (mixed) venous oxygen saturation. Data from PACs are used mainly to determine cardiac output and preload. Preload is most commonly estimated by the pulmonary artery occlusion pressure. However, preload may be more accurately determined by right ventricular end-diastolic volume, which is measured using fast-response thermistors gated to heart rate.

Despite longstanding use, PACs have not been shown to reduce morbidity and mortality. Rather, PAC use has been associated with excess mortality. This finding may be explained by complications of PAC use and misinterpretation of the data obtained. Nevertheless, some physicians believe PACs, when combined with other objective and clinical data, aid in the management of certain critically ill patients. As with many physiologic measurements, a changing trend is typically more significant than a single abnormal value. Possible indications for PACs are listed in Table 67–1.

Procedure: The PAC is inserted through a special catheter in the subclavian or internal jugular vein with the balloon (at

Table 67–1. POTENTIAL INDICATIONS FOR PULMONARY ARTERY CATHETERIZATION

Cardiac disorders
Acute valvular regurgitation
Cardiac tamponade
Complicated heart failure
Complicated MI
Ventricular septal rupture
Hemodynamic instability*
Assessment of volume status
Shock
Hemodynamic monitoring
Cardiac surgery
Postoperative care in critically ill patients
Surgery and postoperative care in patients with significant heart disease
Pulmonary disorders
Complicated pulmonary embolism
Pulmonary hypertension

*Particularly if inotropic drugs are required.

the tip of the catheter) deflated. Once the catheter tip reaches the superior vena cava, inflation of the balloon permits blood flow to guide the catheter. The position of the catheter tip is usually determined by pressure monitoring (see Table 67–2 for intracardiac and great vessel pressures) or occasionally by fluoroscopy. Entry into the right ventricle is indicated by a sudden increase in systolic pressure to about 30 mm Hg; diastolic pressure remains unchanged from right atrial or vena caval pressure. When the catheter enters the pulmonary artery, systolic pressure does not change, but diastolic pressure rises above right ventricular end-diastolic pressure or central venous pressure (CVP); ie, the pulse pressure (the difference between the systolic and diastolic pressures) narrows. Further movement of the catheter wedges the balloon in a distal pulmonary artery. Once in place in the pulmonary artery, the balloon should be deflated. A chest x-ray confirms proper placement.

The systolic pressure (normal, 15 to 30 mm Hg) and diastolic pressure (normal, 5 to 13 mm Hg) are recorded with the catheter balloon deflated. The diastolic pressure corresponds well to the occlusion pressure, although diastolic pressure can exceed occlusion pressure when pulmonary vascular resistance is elevated secondary to primary pulmonary disease (eg, pulmonary fibrosis, pulmonary hypertension).

Pulmonary artery occlusion pressure (pulmonary artery wedge pressure): With the balloon inflated, pressure at the tip of the catheter reflects the static back pressure of the pulmonary veins. The balloon must not remain inflated for > 30 sec to prevent pulmonary infarction. Normally, pulmonary artery occlusion pressure (PAOP) approximates mean left atrial pressure, which in turn approximates left ventricular end-diastolic pressure (LVEDP). LVEDP reflects left ventricular end-diastolic volume (LVEDV). The LVEDV represents preload, which is the actual target parameter. Many factors cause PAOP to reflect LVEDV inaccurately. These factors include mitral stenosis, high levels of positive end-expiratory pressure (> 10 cm H_2O), and changes in left ventricular compliance (eg, due to MI, pericardial effusion, or increased afterload). Technical difficulties result from excessive balloon inflation, improper catheter position, alveolar pressure exceeding pulmonary venous pressure, or severe pulmonary hypertension (which may make the balloon difficult to wedge).

Elevated PAOP occurs in left-sided heart failure. Decreased PAOP occurs in hypovolemia or decreased preload.

Mixed venous oxygenation: Mixed venous blood comprises blood from the superior and inferior vena cava that has passed through the right heart to the pulmonary artery. The blood may be sampled from the distal port of the PAC, but some catheters have embedded fiberoptic sensors that directly measure oxygen saturation.

Causes of low mixed venous oxygen content ($SmvO_2$) include anemia, pulmonary disease, carboxyhemoglobin, low cardiac output, and increased tissue metabolic needs. The ratio of SaO_2 to (SaO_2 − $SmvO_2$) determines the adequacy of oxygen delivery. The ideal ratio is 4:1, whereas 2:1 is the minimum acceptable ratio to maintain aerobic metabolic needs.

Cardiac output: Cardiac output (CO) is measured by intermittent bolus injection of ice water or, in new catheters, continuous warm thermodilution. The cardiac index divides the CO by body surface area to correct for patient size (see Table 75–3 on p. 608).

Other variables can be calculated from CO. They include systemic and pulmonary vascular resistance and right ventricular stroke work (RVSW) and left ventricular stroke work (LVSW).

Complications and precautions: PACs may be difficult to insert. Cardiac arrhythmias, particularly ventricular arrhythmias, are the most common complication. Pulmonary infarction secondary to overinflated or permanently wedged balloons, pulmonary artery perforation, intracardiac perforation, valvular injury, and endocarditis may occur. Rarely, the catheter may curl into a knot within the right ventricle (especially in patients with heart failure, cardiomyopathy, or increased pulmonary pressure).

Pulmonary artery rupture occurs in < 0.1% of PAC insertions. This catastrophic complication is often fatal and occurs immediately on wedging the catheter either initially or during a subsequent occlusion pressure check. Thus, many physicians prefer to monitor pulmonary artery diastolic pressures rather than occlusion pressures.

Table 67–2. NORMAL PRESSURES IN THE HEART AND GREAT VESSELS

TYPE OF PRESSURE	AVERAGE (mm Hg)	RANGE (mm Hg)
Right atrium	3	0–8
Right ventricle		
Peak-systolic	25	15–30
End-diastolic	4	0–8
Pulmonary artery		
Mean	15	9–16
Peak-systolic	25	15–30
End-diastolic	9	4–14
Pulmonary artery occlusion (pulmonary artery wedge)		
Mean	9	2–12
Left atrium		
Mean	8	2–12
A wave	10	4–16
V wave	13	6–12
Left ventricle		
Peak-systolic	130	90–140
End-diastolic	9	5–12
Brachial artery		
Mean	85	70–150
Peak-systolic	130	90–140
End-diastolic	70	60–90

Adapted from Fowler NO: *Cardiac Diagnosis and Treatment*, ed 3. Philadelphia, JB Lippincott, 1980, p. 11.

Noninvasive Cardiac Output

Other methods of determining CO, such as thoracic bioimpedance and the esophageal Doppler monitor, are being developed to avoid the complications of PACs. Although these methods are potentially useful, neither is yet as reliable as a PAC.

Thoracic bioimpedance: These systems use topical electrodes on the anterior chest and neck to measure electrical impedance of the thorax. This value varies with beat-to-beat changes in thoracic blood volume and hence can estimate CO. The system is harmless and provides values quickly (within 2 to 5 min); however, the technique is very sensitive to alteration of the electrode contact with the patient. Thoracic bioimpedance is more valuable in recognizing changes in a given patient than in precisely measuring CO.

Esophageal Doppler monitor (EDM): This device is a soft 6-mm catheter that is passed nasopharyngeally into the esophagus and positioned behind the heart. A Doppler flow probe at its tip allows continuous monitoring of CO and stroke volume. Unlike the invasive PAC, the EDM does not cause pneumothorax, arrhythmia, or infection. An EDM may actually be more accurate than a PAC in patients with cardiac valvular lesions, septal defects, arrhythmias, or pulmonary hypertension. However, the EDM may lose its waveform with only a slight positional change and produce dampened, inaccurate readings.

Hand-held echocardiography: Assessment of LV function is particularly important because decreased cardiac contractility is a common cause of hemodynamic instability in critically ill patients, including those with sepsis. Bedside transthoracic echocardiography (TTE) provides rapid and noninvasive assessment of cardiac function in critically ill patients, but delays can result if an experienced sonographer or cardiologist is not immediately available.

Intensivists who have completed brief training in the use of hand-held sonographic equipment that is now available can provide point-of-care, bedside TTE when formal TTE is not immediately available. Unlike formal TTE, the limited examination focuses primarily on assessment for hemodynamically significant pericardial effusions and impaired global LV function, which can affect treatment. Results of such limited bedside TTE by intensivists have been shown to be highly concordant with results of formal TTE.

Intracranial Pressure Monitoring

Intracranial pressure (ICP) monitoring is standard for patients with severe closed head injury and is occasionally used for some other brain disorders, such as in selected cases of hydrocephalus and pseudotumor cerebri or in postoperative or postembolic management of arteriovenous malformations. These devices are used to optimize cerebral perfusion pressure (mean arterial pressure minus ICP). Typically, the cerebral perfusion pressure should be kept > 60 mm Hg.

Several types of ICP monitors are available. The most useful method places a catheter through the skull into a cerebral ventricle (ventriculostomy catheter). This device is preferred because the catheter can also drain CSF and hence decrease ICP. However, the ventriculostomy is also the most invasive method, has the highest infection rate, and is the most difficult to place. Occasionally, the ventriculostomy becomes occluded due to severe brain edema.

Other types of intracranial devices include an intraparenchymal monitor and an epidural bolt. Of these, the intraparenchymal monitor is more commonly used. All ICP devices should usually be changed or removed after 5 to 7 days because infection is a risk.

Other Types of Monitoring

Sublingual capnometry uses a similar correlation between elevated sublingual P_{CO_2} and systemic hypoperfusion to monitor shock states using a noninvasive sensor placed under the tongue. This device is easier to use than gastric tonometry and responds quickly to perfusion changes with resuscitation.

Tissue spectroscopy uses a noninvasive near infrared (NIR) sensor usually placed on the skin above the target tissue to monitor mitochondrial cytochrome redox states, which reflect tissue perfusion. NIR may help diagnose acute compartment syndromes (eg, in trauma) or ischemia after free tissue transfer and may be helpful in postoperative monitoring of lower-extremity vascular bypass grafts. NIR monitoring of small-bowel pH may be used to gauge the adequacy of resuscitation.

CRITICAL CARE SCORING SYSTEMS

Several scoring systems have been developed to grade the severity of illness in critically ill patients. These systems are moderately accurate in predicting individual survival. However, these systems are more valuable for monitoring quality of care and for conducting research studies because they allow comparison of outcomes among groups of critically ill patients with similar illness severity.

One of the most common systems is the 2nd version of the Acute Physiologic Assessment and Chronic Health Evaluation II (APACHE II) score introduced in 1985. It generates a point score ranging from 0 to 71 based on 12 physiologic variables, age, and underlying health (see Table 67–3). The APACHE III system was developed in 1991, and the APACHE IV system was developed in 2006. These systems are more complex with a greater number of physiologic variables but are more cumbersome and are somewhat less used. There are many other systems, including the 2nd Simplified Acute Physiology Score (SAPS II), the Mortality Prediction Model (MPM), and the Sequential Organ Failure Assessment (SOFA) score.

VASCULAR ACCESS

A number of procedures are used to gain vascular access.

Peripheral Vein Catheterization

Most patients' needs for IV fluid and drugs can be met with a percutaneous peripheral venous catheter. Venous cutdown can be used when percutaneous catheter insertion is not feasible. Typical cutdown sites are the cephalic vein in the arm and the saphenous vein at the ankle. However, venous cutdown is rarely needed because of the popularity of peripherally inserted central catheter (PICC) lines and intraosseous lines in both adults and children.

Common complications (eg, local infection, venous thrombosis, thrombophlebitis, interstitial fluid extravasation) can be reduced by using a meticulous sterile technique during insertion and by replacing or removing the catheters within 72 h.

Central Venous Catheterization

Patients needing secure or long-term vascular access (eg, to receive antibiotics, chemotherapy, or TPN) and those with poor peripheral venous access require a central venous catheter (CVC). CVCs allow infusion of solutions that are too concentrated or irritating for peripheral veins and allow monitoring of CVP.

CVCs can be inserted through the jugular, subclavian, or femoral veins or via the upper arm peripheral veins (PICC line). Although the type of catheter and site chosen are often determined by individual clinical and patient characteristics, a jugular CVC or PICC line is usually preferred to a subclavian CVC (associated with a higher risk of bleeding and pneumothorax) or femoral CVC (associated with a higher risk of infection). During cardiac arrest, fluid and drugs given through a femoral vein CVC often fail to circulate above the diaphragm because of the increased intrathoracic pressure generated by CPR. In this case, a subclavian or internal jugular approach may be preferred (see Fig. 67–1).

Ultrasound guidance for placement of internal jugular lines and PICC lines is now standard care and reduces the risk of complications. Coagulopathy should be corrected whenever feasible prior to CVC insertion, and the subclavian approach should not be used in patients with uncorrected coagulopathy because the venipuncture site cannot be monitored or compressed.

Table 67–3. ACUTE PHYSIOLOGIC ASSESSMENT AND CHRONIC HEALTH EVALUATION (APACHE) II SCORING SYSTEM*

	PHYSIOLOGIC VARIABLE†	POINT SCORE								
		+4	+3	+2	+1	0	+1	+2	+3	+4
1	Temperature, core (° C)	≥41°	39–40.9°	—	38.5–38.9°	36–38.4°	34–35.9°	32–33.9°	30–31.9°	≤29.9°
2	Mean arterial pressure (mm Hg)	≥ 160	130–159	110–129	—	70–109	—	50–69	—	≤ 49
3	Heart rate	≥ 180	140–179	110–139	—	70–109	—	55–69	40–54	≤ 39
4	Respiratory rate (nonventilated or ventilated)	≥ 50	35–49	—	25–34	12–24	10–11	6–9	—	≤ 5
5	Oxygenation: a) $FIO_2 \geq 0.5$: use A-aDO_2	≥ 500	350–499	200–349	—	< 200	—	—	—	—
	b) $FIO_2 < 0.5$: use PAO_2 (mm Hg)	—	—	—	—	> 70	61–70	—	55–60	< 55
6	Arterial pH	≥ 7.7	7.6–7.69	—	7.5–7.59	7.33–7.49	—	7.25–7.32	7.15–7.24	< 7.15
7	Serum Na (mmol/L)	≥ 180	160–179	155–159	150–154	130–149	—	120–129	111–119	≤110
8	Serum K (mmol/L)	≥ 7	6–6.9	—	5.5–5.9	3.5–5.4	3–3.4	2.5–2.9	—	< 2.5
9	Serum creatinine (mg/dL); double point score for **acute** renal failure	≥ 3.5	2–3.4	1.5–1.9	—	0.6–1.4	—	< 0.6	—	—
10	Hct (%)	≥ 60	—	50–59.9	46–49.9	30–45.9	—	20–29.9	—	< 20
11	WBC (in 1000s)	≥ 40	—	20–39.9	15–19.9	3–14.9	—	1–2.9	—	< 1
12	Glasgow coma score (GCS)	Score = 15 minus actual GCS (see Table 224–1 on p. 1862)								
(13)§	Serum HCO_3 (venous–mmol/L)	≥ 52	41–51.9	—	32–40.9	22–31.9	—	18–21.9	15–17.9	< 15

Acute physiology score is the sum of the 12 individual variable points.

Add 0 points for age < 44; 2 points, 45–54 yr; 3 points, 55–64 yr; 5 points, 65–74 yr; 6 points ≥ 75 yr.

Add chronic health status points: 2 points for elective postoperative patient with immunocompromise or history of severe organ insufficiency; 5 points for nonoperative patient or emergency postoperative patient with immunocompromise or severe organ insufficiency.‡

*APACHE II score = acute physiology score + age points + chronic health points. Minimum score = 0; maximum score = 71. Increasing score is associated with increasing risk of hospital death.

†Choose worst value in the past 24 h.

‡Chronic health status: Organ insufficiency (eg, hepatic, cardiovascular, renal, pulmonary) or immunocompromised state must have preceded current admission.

§This variable is optional; use only if no ABGs are available.

A-a DO_2 = alveolar–arterial oxygen gradient; FIO_2 = fractional inspired O_2.

Adapted from Knaus WA, Draper EA, Wagner DP, Zimmerman JE: APACHE II: A severity of disease classification system. *Critical Care Medicine* 13:818–829, 1985.

Procedure: CVCs are inserted using sterile technique and a local anesthetic (eg, 1% lidocaine) and a series of well-defined steps:

- Needle puncture of the target vessel
- Advancement of a guidewire through the needle
- Removal of the needle
- Advancement and then removal of a tissue dilator over the guidewire
- Placement of the CVC over the guidewire and into the target vessel with subsequent removal of the guidewire

The catheter is flushed with saline and sutured in place, and an occlusive dressing is applied. For jugular and subclavian vein CVCs, a chest x-ray is done to confirm that the tip of the CVC is at the junction between the superior vena cava and the right atrium (the catheter can be advanced or retracted if not in the appropriate position) and to confirm that pneumothorax has not occurred. To prevent cardiac arrhythmias, clinicians should withdraw catheters in the right atrium or ventricle until the tip is within the superior vena cava.

Percutaneous femoral lines must be inserted below the inguinal ligament. Otherwise, laceration of the external iliac vein or

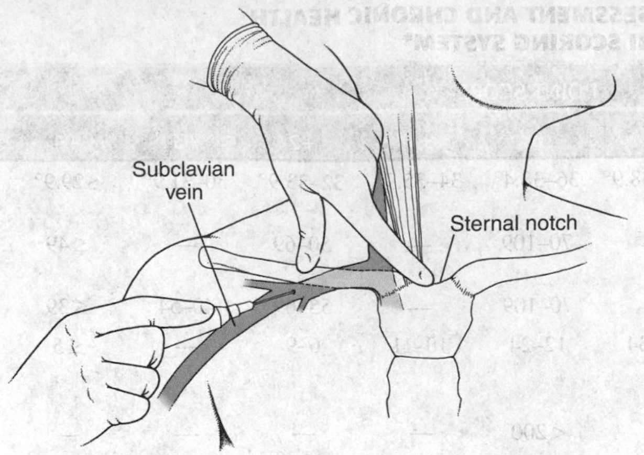

Fig. 67–1. Subclavian venipuncture. This figure shows hand position during subclavian venipuncture (infraclavicular approach).

artery above the inguinal ligament may result in retroperitoneal hemorrhage; external compression of these vessels is nearly impossible.

To reduce the risk of venous thrombosis and catheter sepsis, clinicians should remove CVCs as soon as possible. The skin entry site must be cleansed and inspected daily for local infection; the catheter must be replaced if local or systemic infection occurs. Some clinicians feel it is beneficial to change CVC catheters at regular intervals (eg, every 5 to 7 days) in patients with sepsis who remain febrile; this approach may reduce the risk of bacterial colonization of the catheter. (See also Guidelines for Prevention of Intravascular Catheter-Related Infections at the CDC web site [www.cdc.gov].)

Complications: CVCs can cause many complications (see Table 67–4). Pneumothorax occurs in 1% of patients after CVC insertion. Atrial or ventricular arrhythmias frequently occur during catheter insertion but are generally self-limited and subside when the guide wire or catheter is withdrawn from within the heart. The incidence of catheter bacterial colonization without systemic infection may be as high as 35%, whereas that of true sepsis is 2 to 8%. Catheter-related venous thrombosis is an increasingly recognized complication, particularly in the upper extremities. Rarely, accidental arterial catheterization requires surgical repair of the artery. Hydrothorax and hydromediastinum may occur when catheters are positioned extravascularly. Catheter damage to the tricuspid valve, bacterial endocarditis, and air and catheter embolism occur rarely.

Table 67–4. COMPLICATIONS ASSOCIATED WITH CENTRAL VENOUS CATHETERS

COMPLICATION	POSSIBLE SEQUELAE
Common	
Carotid artery injury	Bleeding, respiratory compromise, neurologic complications (eg, stroke)
Puncture of pleura or lung	Pneumothorax
Puncture of vein resulting in a leak	Bleeding, extravasation of fluid, hemodynamic compromise
Subclavian, carotid, or femoral artery injury	Bleeding, vascular compromise of an extremity, hemothorax, hemodynamic compromise
Thrombosis	Limb edema Pulmonary embolism
Less common	
Air embolism	Cardiac arrest
Arrhythmias	Cardiac arrest
Brachial plexus injury	Compromise of an extremity
Erosion of catheter	Bleeding, extravasation of fluid, hemodynamic compromise
Infection	Sepsis
Injury to clavicle, rib, or vertebra	Osteomyelitis
Lymphatic injury	Chylothorax
Valvular injury	Endocarditis

Arterial Catheterization

The use of automated noninvasive BP devices has diminished the use of arterial catheters simply for pressure monitoring. However, these catheters are beneficial in unstable patients who require minute-to-minute pressure measurement and in those requiring frequent ABG sampling. Indications include refractory shock and respiratory failure. BP is frequently somewhat higher when measured by an arterial catheter than by sphygmomanometry. Initial upstroke, maximum systolic pressure, and pulse pressure increase the more distal the point of measurement, whereas the diastolic and mean arterial pressures decline. Vessel calcification, atherosclerosis, proximal occlusion, and extremity position can all affect the value of arterial catheter measurements.

Procedure: Arterial catheters are inserted using sterile technique and a local anesthetic (eg, 1% lidocaine). They are typically inserted percutaneously into the radial, femoral, axillary, brachial, dorsalis pedis, and (in children) temporal arteries. The radial artery is most frequently used; insertion into the femoral artery has fewer complications but should be avoided after vascular bypass surgery (due to potential injury to the bypass graft) and in patients with distal vascular insufficiency (to avoid precipitating ischemia). Ultrasound guidance may be beneficial in difficult cases.

Before radial artery catheterization, the Allen test (digital compression of both ulnar and radial arteries causes palmar blanching followed by hyperemia when either artery is released) can determine whether there is sufficient ulnar collateral flow to perfuse the hand in the event of radial artery occlusion. If reperfusion does not occur within 8 sec of releasing the compressed ulnar artery, arterial catheterization should not be done or another arterial site is chosen.

Complications: At all sites, bleeding, infection, thrombosis, and distal embolism may occur. Catheters should be removed if signs of local or systemic infection are present.

Radial arterial complications include ischemia of the hand and forearm due to thrombosis or embolism, intimal dissection, or spasm at the site of catheterization. The risk of arterial thrombosis is higher in small arteries (explaining the greater incidence in women) and with increased duration of catheterization. Occluded arteries nearly always recanalize after catheter removal.

Femoral arterial complications include atheroembolism during guide wire insertion. The incidence of thrombosis and distal ischemia is much lower than that for radial arterial catheterization.

Axillary arterial complications include hematomas, which are infrequent but may require urgent care because brachial plexus compression can result in permanent peripheral neuropathy. Flushing the axillary arterial catheter may introduce air or a clot. To avoid neurologic sequelae of these emboli, clinicians should select the left axillary artery for catheterization (the left axillary artery branches further distal to the carotid vessels than does the right).

Intraosseous Infusion

Any fluid or substance routinely given IV (including blood products) may be given via a sturdy needle inserted in the medullary cavity of select long bones. Fluids reach the central circulation as quickly as with venous infusion. This technique is used more commonly in infants and young children, whose bony cortices are thin and easily penetrated and in whom peripheral and central venous access can be quite difficult, particularly in shock or cardiac arrest. However, this technique can be used in older patients at various sites (eg, sternum, proximal tibia, humerus) via special devices (eg, pressure-loaded puncture device, drilling device) that are now more readily available. Thus, intraosseous infusion is becoming more common in adults.

Intraosseous delivery systems should be removed within 24 h of insertion or as soon as practical after peripheral or central IV access has been achieved.

Procedure: A special-purpose intraosseous needle with stylet is used (see Fig. 67–2). The preferred insertion sites in children are the proximal tibia and distal femur; both areas are given a sterile preparation and are included in the operative field. For tibial insertion, the needle is placed on the broad, flat anteromedial surface 1 to 2 cm distal to the tibial tubercle. For the femur, the site is 3 cm above the lateral condyle in the midline. For older children, the medial surface of the distal tibia 2 cm above the medial malleolus may be easier. For adults, the upper humerus also can be used.

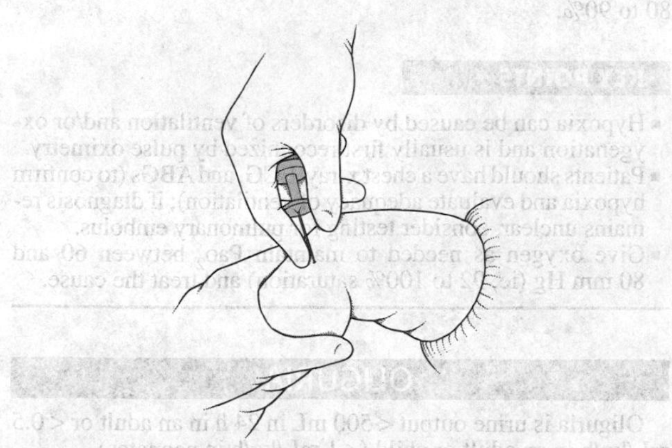

Fig. 67–2. Intraosseous (IO) needle insertion. The physician's fingers and thumb are wrapped around the proximal tibia to stabilize it; the hand should not be placed directly behind the insertion site (to avoid self-puncture). Instead, a towel may be placed behind the knee to support it. The physician holds the needle firmly in the palm of the other hand, directing the point slightly away from the joint space and growth plate. The needle is inserted with moderate pressure and a rotary motion, stopped as soon as a pop indicates penetration of the cortex. Some needles have a plastic sleeve, which can be adjusted to prevent them from being pushed too deeply into or through the bone.

For all sites, the needle is inserted with a rotary, coring motion. Stabilizing the needle shaft at the skin surface with a gloved fingertip aids control, allowing advancement to be stopped once the cortex is penetrated. On entering the medullary cavity, the stylet is removed and infusion is begun. Several semiautomatic insertion devices are available, including spring-powered and battery-powered devices.

Complications: Poor control during insertion may result in the needle exiting the opposite cortex; then, subsequent infusion largely enters the soft tissues, so a site on another bone should be tried. Osteomyelitis may occur but is uncommon (eg, < 2 to 3%). Growth plate damage has not been reported. Other complications include bleeding and compartment syndrome.

OXYGEN DESATURATION

(Hypoxia)

ICU (and other) patients without respiratory disorders may develop hypoxia (oxygen saturation < 90%) during a hospital stay. Hypoxia in patients with known respiratory conditions is discussed under those disorders.

Etiology

Numerous disorders cause hypoxia (eg, dyspnea, respiratory failure—see Table 67–5); however, acute hypoxia developing in a patient hospitalized with a nonrespiratory illness usually has a more limited set of causes. These causes can be divided into

- Disorders of ventilation
- Disorders of oxygenation

Evaluation

Total fluid volume given during the hospital stay and, in particular, the previous 24 h should be ascertained to identify volume overload. Drugs should be reviewed for sedative administration and dosage. In significant hypoxia (oxygen saturation < 85%), treatment begins simultaneously with evaluation.

History: Very sudden onset dyspnea and hypoxia suggest pulmonary embolus (PE) or pneumothorax (mainly in a patient on positive pressure ventilation). Fever, chills, and productive cough (or increased secretions) suggest pneumonia. A history of cardiopulmonary disease (eg, asthma, COPD, heart failure) may indicate an exacerbation of the disease. Symptoms and signs of MI may indicate acute valvular insufficiency, pulmonary edema, or cardiogenic shock. Unilateral extremity pain suggests deep venous thrombosis (DVT) and hence possible PE. Preceding major trauma or sepsis requiring significant resuscitation suggests acute respiratory distress syndrome. Preceding chest trauma suggests pulmonary contusion.

Physical examination: Patency of the airway and strength and adequacy of respirations should be assessed immediately. For patients on mechanical ventilation, it is important to determine that the endotracheal tube is not obstructed or dislodged. Findings are suggestive as follows:

- Unilateral decreased breath sounds with clear lung fields suggest pneumothorax or right mainstem bronchus intubation; with crackles and fever, pneumonia is more likely.
- Distended neck veins with bilateral lung crackles suggest volume overload with pulmonary edema, cardiogenic shock, pericardial tamponade (often without crackles), or acute valvular insufficiency.
- Distended neck veins with clear lungs or unilateral decrease in breath sounds and tracheal deviation suggest tension pneumothorax.

Table 67–5. SOME CAUSES OF OXYGEN DESATURATION

MECHANISM	EXAMPLES
Disorders of ventilation	
Decreased ventilatory drive	Decreased mental status (eg, caused by head injury, oversedation, sepsis, shock, or stroke)
Obstructed ventilation	Bronchospasm Dislodgement of endotracheal tube Mucus plugging of the airways or endotracheal tube
Severe pain in the chest, abdomen, or both	Rib fractures Thoracic or abdominal surgery
Disorders of oxygenation	
Pulmonary causes	Acute respiratory distress syndrome Atelectasis, pneumonia, pneumothorax, pulmonary embolus, pulmonary contusion, aspiration pneumonitis
Nonpulmonary causes	Iatrogenic fluid overload Heart failure (eg, due to exacerbation of underlying disease or to acute MI)

- Bilateral lower-extremity edema suggests heart failure, but unilateral edema suggests DVT and hence possible PE.
- Wheezing represents bronchospasm (typically asthma or allergic reaction, but it occurs rarely with PE or heart failure).
- Decreased mental status suggests hypoventilation.

Testing: Hypoxia is generally recognized initially by pulse oximetry. Patients should have the following:

- A chest x-ray (eg, to assess for pneumonia, pleural effusion, pneumothorax, or atelectasis)
- ECG (to assess for arrhythmia or ischemia)
- ABGs (to confirm hypoxia and evaluate adequacy of ventilation)

Bedside intensivist-performed echocardiography (see p. 530) may be used to assess for hemodynamically significant pericardial effusion or reduced global left ventricular function until formal echocardiography can be done. Elevated serum levels of brain (B-type) natriuretic peptide (BNP) may help differentiate heart failure from other causes of hypoxia. If diagnosis remains unclear after these tests, testing for PE should be considered. Bronchoscopy may be done in intubated patients to rule out (and remove) a tracheobronchial plug.

Treatment

Identified causes are treated as discussed elsewhere in The Manual. If hypoventilation persists, mechanical ventilation via noninvasive positive pressure ventilation or endotracheal intubation is necessary (see p. 559). Persistent hypoxia requires supplemental oxygen.

Oxygen therapy: The amount of oxygen given is guided by ABG or pulse oximetry to maintain PaO_2 between 60 and 80 mm Hg (ie, 92 to 100% saturation) without causing oxygen toxicity. This level provides satisfactory tissue oxygen delivery; because the oxyhemoglobin dissociation curve is sigmoidal, increasing PaO_2 to > 80 mm Hg increases oxygen delivery very little and is not necessary. The lowest fractional inspired O_2 (FIO_2) that provides an acceptable PaO_2 should be provided. Oxygen toxicity is both concentration- and time-dependent. Sustained elevations in FIO_2 > 60% result in inflammatory changes, alveolar infiltration, and, eventually, pulmonary fibrosis. An FIO_2 > 60% should be avoided unless necessary for survival. An FIO_2 < 60% is well tolerated for long periods.

An FIO_2 < 40% can be given via nasal cannula or simple face mask. A nasal cannula uses an oxygen flow of 1 to 6 L/min. Because 6 L/min is sufficient to fill the nasopharynx, higher flow rates are of no benefit. Simple face masks and nasal cannulas do not deliver a precise FIO_2 because of inconsistent admixture of oxygen with room air from leakage and mouth breathing. However, Venturi-type masks can deliver very accurate oxygen concentrations.

An FIO_2 > 40% requires use of an oxygen mask with a reservoir that is inflated by oxygen from the supply. In the typical nonrebreather mask, the patient inhales 100% oxygen from the reservoir, but during exhalation, a rubber flap valve diverts exhaled breath to the environment, preventing admixture of CO_2 and water vapor with the inspired O_2. Nonetheless, because of leakage, such masks deliver an FIO_2 of at most 80 to 90%.

KEY POINTS

- Hypoxia can be caused by disorders of ventilation and/or oxygenation and is usually first recognized by pulse oximetry.
- Patients should have a chest x-ray, ECG, and ABGs (to confirm hypoxia and evaluate adequacy of ventilation); if diagnosis remains unclear, consider testing for pulmonary embolus.
- Give oxygen as needed to maintain PaO_2 between 60 and 80 mm Hg (ie, 92 to 100% saturation) and treat the cause.

OLIGURIA

Oliguria is urine output < 500 mL in 24 h in an adult or < 0.5 mL/kg/h in an adult or child (< 1 mL/kg/h in neonates).

Etiology

Causes of oliguria are typically divided into 3 categories:

- Prerenal (blood-flow related)
- Renal (intrinsic kidney disorders)
- Postrenal (outlet obstruction)

There are numerous such entities (see p. 2075), but a limited number cause most cases of acute oliguria in hospitalized patients (see Table 67–6).

Evaluation

History: In communicative patients, a marked urge to void suggests outlet obstruction, whereas thirst and no urge to void suggest volume depletion. In obtunded (and presumably catheterized) patients, a sudden decrease in urine flow in a normotensive patient suggests catheter occlusion (eg, caused by a clot or kinking) or displacement, whereas a gradual decrease is more likely due to acute tubular necrosis (ATN) or a prerenal cause.

Recent medical events are helpful; they include review of recent BP readings, surgical procedures, and drug and x-ray contrast administration. Recent surgery or trauma may be consistent with hypovolemia. A severe crush injury, deep electrical burn, or heatstroke suggests rhabdomyolysis.

Physical examination: Vital signs are reviewed, particularly for hypotension, tachycardia, or both (suggesting hypovolemia or sepsis) and fever (suggesting sepsis). Signs of focal infection and cardiac failure should be sought. Palpable bladder distention indicates an outlet obstruction. Dark brown urine suggests myoglobinuria.

Testing: In all catheterized patients (and those with an ileal conduit), patency should be ascertained by irrigation before further testing; this approach may solve the problem. In many of the remaining patients, etiology (eg, shock, sepsis) is clinically apparent. In others, particularly those with multiple disorders, testing is needed to differentiate prerenal from renal (ATN) causes. In patients without a urinary catheter, placement of a catheter should be considered; this will diagnose and treat obstruction and provide continuous monitoring of output.

If a central venous or PAC is in place, volume status (and with a PAC, cardiac output) can be determined by measuring CVP (see End Point and Monitoring on p. 577) or PAOP. However, many physicians would not insert such a line for acute oliguria unless other indications were present. An alternative in the patient without signs of volume overload is to rapidly give a test bolus of IV fluid, 500 mL 0.9% saline (20 mL/kg in children); an increase in output suggests a prerenal cause.

Laboratory tests should be done. Serum electrolytes, BUN, and creatinine are standard; often urine sodium and creatinine concentration are also done. Prerenal conditions typically result in a BUN/creatinine ratio > 20, vs ≤ 10 in both normal states and ATN. In prerenal conditions, urine sodium is < 20 mEq/L as the kidney attempts to retain maximum sodium to preserve intravascular volume. In ATN, urine sodium is usually > 40 mEq/L. The fractional sodium excretion (FE_{Na}) is a more accurate representation of the kidney's ability to retain sodium and is defined as

$$\frac{\text{urine NA/plasma NA}}{\text{urine creatinine/plasma creatinine}} \times 100$$

A ratio < 1 indicates the kidney is able to reabsorb sodium, and hence the problem is prerenal. A ratio > 2 indicates a probable renal cause.

Table 67–6. SOME CAUSES OF OLIGURIA

MECHANISM	EXAMPLES
Prerenal*	
Hypovolemia	Bleeding Fluid loss Inadequate fluid replacement
Low cardiac output	MI Heart failure Pulmonary embolism
Decreased systemic vascular resistance	Sepsis
Renal	
Acute tubular necrosis	Hypoperfusion (prolonged, eg, > 4 h) X-ray contrast dye Rhabdomyolysis Nephrotoxic drugs (eg, aminoglycosides and other antibiotics, NSAIDs)
Postrenal	
Mechanical urinary obstruction	Blocked urinary catheter Prostatic hypertrophy Urinary calculi
Bladder or sphincter dysfunction	Anticholinergic drug use Postoperative urinary retention Fecal impaction if severe

*These prerenal conditions often coexist and rapidly (ie, in < 1 h) reduce urine output.

Treatment

Identified causes are treated; outflow obstruction is corrected, volume is replaced, and cardiac output is normalized. Nephrotoxic drugs are stopped, and another drug is substituted. Hypotension should be avoided to prevent further renal insults. Patients with renal failure that cannot be reversed may require renal replacement therapy (eg, continuous venovenous hemofiltration or hemodialysis).

KEY POINTS

- Categories of causes of oliguria include decreased renal blood flow, renal insufficiency, and urinary outflow obstruction.
- History and physical examination often suggest a mechanism (eg, recent hypotension, nephrotoxic drug use).
- Measure serum electrolytes, BUN, and creatinine.
- Measure urine sodium and creatinine concentration, and calculate fractional sodium excretion if it is unclear whether the cause is prerenal or renal; a ratio < 1 indicates the problem is prerenal, whereas a ratio > 2 indicates a probable renal cause.

AGITATION, CONFUSION, AND NEUROMUSCULAR BLOCKADE IN CRITICALLY ILL PATIENTS

ICU patients are often agitated, confused, and uncomfortable. They can become delirious (ICU delirium). These symptoms are unpleasant for patients and often interfere with care and safety. At worst, they may be life threatening (eg, patients dislodge the endotracheal tube or IV lines).

Etiology

In a critically ill patient, agitation, confusion, or both can result from the original medical condition, from medical complications, or from treatment or the ICU environment (see Table 67–7). It is important to remember that neuromuscular blockade merely masks pain and agitation, it does not prevent it; paralyzed patients may be suffering significantly.

Table 67–7. SOME CAUSES OF AGITATION OR CONFUSION IN CRITICAL CARE PATIENTS

MECHANISM	EXAMPLES
Underlying disorder	Head injury Shock Toxin ingestion Pain and discomfort (eg, caused by injuries, surgical procedures, endotracheal intubation, IVs, blood drawing, or NGT)
Complications	Hypoxia (see p. 533) Hypotension Sepsis Organ failure (eg, hepatic encephalopathy) Pulmonary embolism
Drugs	Sedatives and other CNS-active drugs, particularly opioids, benzodiazepines, H_2 blockers, and antihistamines Withdrawal from alcohol, drugs, or both
ICU environment*	Sleep deprivation (eg, due to noise, bright lights, or round-the-clock medical interventions) Fear of death Anxiety about unpleasant medical procedures

*Particularly a problem for the elderly.

Evaluation

The chart should be reviewed and the patient examined before sedatives are ordered for "agitation."

History: The presenting injury or illness is a prime causative suspect. Nursing notes and discussion with personnel may identify downward trends in BP and urine output (suggesting CNS hypoperfusion) and dysfunctional sleep patterns. Drug administration records are reviewed to identify inadequate or excessive analgesia and sedation.

Past medical history is reviewed for potential causes. Underlying liver disease suggests possible hepatic encephalopathy. Known substance dependency or abuse suggests a withdrawal syndrome.

Awake, coherent patients are asked what is troubling them and are questioned specifically about pain, dyspnea, and previously unreported substance dependency.

Physical examination: Oxygen saturation < 90% suggests a hypoxic etiology. Low BP and urine output suggest CNS hypoperfusion. Fever and tachycardia suggest sepsis or delirium tremens. Neck stiffness suggests meningitis, although this finding may be difficult to demonstrate in an agitated patient. Focal findings on neurologic examination suggest stroke, hemorrhage, or increased ICP.

The degree of agitation can be quantified using a scale such as the Riker Sedation-Agitation Scale (see Table 67–8) or the Ramsay Sedation Scale. The Confusion Assessment Method (see Table 67–9) can be used to screen for delirium as a cause of agitation. Use of such scales allows better consistency between observers and the identification of trends. Patients who are under neuromuscular blockade are difficult to evaluate because they may be highly agitated and uncomfortable despite appearing motionless. It is typically necessary to allow paralysis to wear off periodically (eg, daily) so that the patient can be assessed.

Testing: Identified abnormalities (eg, hypoxia, hypotension, fever) should be clarified further with appropriate testing. Head CT need not routinely be done unless focal neurologic findings are present or no other etiology is found. A bispectral index (BIS) monitor may be helpful in determining the level of sedation/agitation of patients under neuromuscular blockade.

Treatment

Underlying conditions (eg, hypoxia, shock, drugs) should be addressed. The environment should be optimized (eg, darkness, quiet, and minimal sleep interruption at night) as much as is compatible with medical care. Clocks, calendars, outside windows, and TV or radio programs also help connect the patient with the world, lessening confusion. Family presence and consistent nursing personnel may be calming.

Drug treatment is dictated by the most vexing symptoms. Pain is treated with analgesics; anxiety and insomnia are treated with sedatives; and psychosis and delirium are treated with small doses of an antipsychotic drug. Intubation may be needed

Table 67–8. RIKER SEDATION-AGITATION SCALE

SCORE	DESCRIPTION	EXPLANATION
7	Dangerous agitation	Tries to remove monitors and devices or climb out of bed; tosses and turns; lashes out at staff
6	Very agitated	Remains restless despite frequent verbal reassurance; bites endotracheal tube; requires restraint
5	Agitated	Anxious or restless; attempts to move; calms down with reassurance
4	Calm and cooperative	Calm; easy to arouse; able to follow instructions
3	Sedated	Difficult to awaken; responds to verbal prompts or gentle shaking but drifts off again
2	Very sedated	Incommunicative; responds to physical stimuli but not verbal instructions; may move spontaneously
1	Unarousable	Incommunicative; little or no response to painful stimuli

Table 67–9. CONFUSION ASSESSMENT METHOD (CAM) FOR DIAGNOSING DELIRIUM*

FEATURE	ASSESSMENT†
Required features	
Acute onset and fluctuating course	Shown by positive responses to the following questions: "Has the patient's mental status changed abruptly from baseline?" "Did the abnormal behavior fluctuate during the day (ie, tend to come and go or increase and decrease in severity)?"
Inattention	Shown by a positive response to the following question: "Did the patient have difficulty focusing attention (eg, was easily distracted or had difficulty following what was being said)?"
One of the following features required	
Disorganized thinking	Shown by a positive response to the following question: "Was the patient's thinking disorganized or incoherent (eg, evidenced by rambling or irrelevant conversation, unclear or illogical flow of ideas, or unpredictable switching from subject to subject)?"
Altered level of consciousness	Shown by any answer other than "alert" to the following question: "Overall, how would you rate this patient's level of consciousness?" • Normal = alert • Hyperalert = vigilant • Drowsy, easily aroused = lethargic • Difficult to arouse = stupor • Unarousable = coma

*The diagnosis of delirium requires the presence of the first 2 features *plus* one of the second 2 features.
†This information is usually obtained from a family member or nurse.

when sedative and analgesic requirements are high enough to jeopardize the airway or respiratory drive. Many drugs are available; generally, short-acting drugs are preferred for patients who need frequent neurologic examination or who are being weaned to extubation.

Analgesia: Pain should be treated with appropriate doses of IV opioids; conscious patients with painful conditions (eg, fractures, surgical incisions) who are unable to communicate should be assumed to have pain and receive analgesics accordingly. Mechanical ventilation is somewhat uncomfortable, and patients generally should receive a combination of opioid and amnestic sedative drugs. Fentanyl is the opioid of choice for short-term treatment because of its potency, short duration of action, and minimal cardiovascular effects. A common regimen can be 30 to 100 mcg/h of fentanyl; individual requirements are highly variable.

Sedation: Despite analgesia, many patients remain sufficiently agitated as to require sedation. A sedative can also provide patient comfort at a lower dose of analgesic. Benzodiazepines (eg, lorazepam, midazolam) are most common, but propofol, a sedative-hypnotic drug, may be used for short-term sedation. A common regimen for sedation is lorazepam 1 to 2 mg IV q 1 to 2 h or a continuous infusion at 1 to 2 mg/h if the patient is intubated. These drugs pose risks of respiratory depression, hypotension, delirium, and prolonged physiologic effects in some patients. Long-acting benzodiazepines such as diazepam, flurazepam, and chlordiazepoxide should be avoided in the elderly. Antipsychotics with less anticholinergic effect, such as haloperidol 1 to 3 mg IV, may work best when combined with benzodiazepines.

Dexmedetomidine is a newer drug that has anxiolytic, sedative, and some analgesic properties and that does not affect respiratory drive. The risk of delirium is lower than with benzodiazepines. Because of these lower rates, dexmedetomidine is an increasingly used alternative to benzodiazepines for patients requiring mechanical ventilation. The character and depth of sedation caused by dexmedetomidine may permit mechanically ventilated patients to interact or be easily awakened, yet remain comfortable. The most common adverse effects are hypotension and bradycardia. Typical dosing is 0.2 to 0.7 mcg/kg/h, but some patients require doses up to 1.5 mcg/kg/h. Because dexmedetomidine is expensive, it is usually used only for brief periods (eg, < 48 h).

Neuromuscular blockade: For intubated patients, neuromuscular blockade is *not* a substitute for sedation; it only removes visible manifestations of the problem (agitation) without correcting it. However, neuromuscular blockade may be required during tests (eg, CT, MRI) or procedures (eg, central line placement) that require patients to be motionless or in patients who cannot be ventilated despite adequate analgesia and sedation. When newer sedative drugs (including dexmedetomidine) are used, neuromuscular blockade is rarely required.

Prolonged neuromuscular blockade should be avoided unless patients have severe lung injury and cannot do the work of breathing safely. Use for > 1 to 2 days may lead to prolonged weakness, particularly when corticosteroids are concomitantly given. Common regimens include vecuronium (continuous infusion as directed by stimulation).

KEY POINTS

- Agitation, confusion, or both can result from the original medical condition, from complications of the acute illness, from treatment, or from the ICU environment.
- History and physical examination often suggest a cause and direct subsequent testing.
- Treat the cause (including giving analgesics for pain and optimizing the environment to minimize confusion) and manage any remaining agitation with a sedative drug such as lorazepam or propofol.
- Neuromuscular blockade merely masks pain and agitation; paralyzed patients may be suffering significantly.

68 Cardiac Arrest and Cardiopulmonary Resuscitation

CARDIAC ARREST

Cardiac arrest is the cessation of cardiac mechanical activity resulting in the absence of circulating blood flow. Cardiac arrest stops blood from flowing to vital organs, depriving them of oxygen, and, if left untreated, results in death. Sudden cardiac arrest is the unexpected cessation of circulation within a short period of symptom onset (sometimes without warning). Sudden cardiac arrest occurs outside the hospital in more than 350,000 people/yr in the US, with a 90% mortality.

Respiratory arrest and cardiac arrest are distinct, but without treatment, one inevitably leads to the other. (See also respiratory failure, dyspnea, and hypoxia.)

(See also the American Heart Association's 2017 update and 2013 update of heart disease and stroke statistics and the statistical update for out-of-hospital and in-hospital cardiac arrest.)

Etiology

In adults, sudden cardiac arrest results primarily from cardiac disease (of all types, but especially coronary artery disease). In a significant percentage of patients, sudden cardiac arrest is the first manifestation of heart disease. Other causes include circulatory shock due to noncardiac disorders (especially pulmonary embolism, GI hemorrhage, or trauma), ventilatory failure, and metabolic disturbance (including drug overdose).

In infants and children, cardiac causes of sudden cardiac arrest are less common than in adults. The predominant cause of sudden cardiac arrest in infants and children is respiratory failure due to various respiratory disorders (eg, airway obstruction, smoke inhalation, drowning, infection, SIDS). Other causes of sudden cardiac arrest include trauma and poisoning.

Pathophysiology

Cardiac arrest causes global ischemia with consequences at the cellular level that adversely affect organ function after resuscitation. The main consequences involve direct cellular damage and edema formation. Edema is particularly harmful in the brain, which has minimal room to expand, and often results in increased intracranial pressure and corresponding decreased cerebral perfusion postresuscitation. A significant proportion of successfully resuscitated patients have short-term or long-term cerebral dysfunction manifested by altered alertness (from mild confusion to coma), seizures, or both.

Decreased ATP production leads to loss of membrane integrity with efflux of potassium and influx of sodium and calcium. Excess sodium causes cellular edema. Excess calcium damages mitochondria (depressing ATP production), increases nitric oxide production (leading to formation of damaging free radicals), and, in certain circumstances, activates proteases that further damage cells.

Abnormal ion flux also results in depolarization of neurons, releasing neurotransmitters, some of which are damaging (eg, glutamate activates a specific calcium channel, worsening intracellular calcium overload).

Inflammatory mediators (eg, IL-1B, TNF-alpha) are elaborated; some of them may cause microvascular thrombosis and loss of vascular integrity with further edema formation. Some mediators trigger apoptosis, resulting in accelerated cell death.

Symptoms and Signs

In critically or terminally ill patients, cardiac arrest is often preceded by a period of clinical deterioration with rapid, shallow breathing, arterial hypotension, and a progressive decrease in mental alertness. In sudden cardiac arrest, collapse occurs without warning, occasionally accompanied by a brief (< 5 sec) seizure.

Diagnosis

- Clinical evaluation
- Cardiac monitor and ECG
- Sometimes testing for cause (eg, echocardiography, chest x-ray, or chest ultrasonography)

Diagnosis of cardiac arrest is by clinical findings of apnea, pulselessness, and unconsciousness. Arterial pressure is not measurable. Pupils dilate and become unreactive to light after several minutes.

A cardiac monitor should be applied; it may indicate ventricular fibrillation (VF), ventricular tachycardia (VT), or asystole. Sometimes a perfusing rhythm (eg, extreme bradycardia) is present; this rhythm may represent true pulseless electrical activity (PEA, or electromechanical dissociation) or extreme hypotension with failure to detect a pulse.

The patient is evaluated for potentially treatable causes; a useful memory aid is "Hs and Ts":

- **H:** *H*ypoxia, *h*ypovolemia, acidosis (*h*ydrogen ion), *h*yperkalemia or *h*ypokalemia, *h*ypothermia, *h*ypoglycemia
- **T:** *T*ablet or *t*oxin ingestion, cardiac *t*amponade, *t*ension pneumothorax, *t*hrombosis (pulmonary embolus or myocardial infarction), *t*rauma

Unfortunately, many causes are not identified during CPR. Clinical examination, chest ultrasonography, and chest x-ray can detect tension pneumothorax. Cardiac ultrasonography can detect cardiac contractions and recognize cardiac tamponade, extreme hypovolemia (empty heart), right ventricular overload suggesting pulmonary embolism, and focal wall motion abnormalities suggesting MI. Rapid bedside blood tests can detect abnormal levels of potassium or glucose. History given by family or rescue personnel may suggest overdose.

Prognosis

Survival to hospital discharge, particularly neurologically intact survival, is a more meaningful outcome than simply return of spontaneous circulation.

Survival rates vary significantly; favorable factors include

- Early and effective bystander-initiated CPR
- Witnessed arrest
- In-hospital location (particularly a monitored unit)
- Initial rhythm of VF or VT
- Early defibrillation (of VT or VF after initial chest compression)
- Postresuscitative care, including circulatory support and access to cardiac catheterization
- In adults, targeted temperature management (body temperature of 32 to 36° C) and avoidance of hyperthermia[1,2]

If many factors are favorable (eg, VF is witnessed in an ICU or emergency department), about 40% of patients survive to hospital discharge. Overall, in-hospital arrest (VT/VF and asystole/PEA) survival is about 25%.

When factors are uniformly unfavorable (eg, patient in asystole after unwitnessed, out-of-hospital arrest), survival is unlikely. Overall, reported survival after out-of-hospital arrest is about 10%.

Only about 10% of all cardiac arrest survivors have good CNS function at hospital discharge.

1. Bernard SA, Gray TW, Buist MD, et al: Treatment of comatose survivors of out-of-hospital cardiac arrest with induced hypothermia. *N Engl J Med* 346:557–563, 2002. doi 10.1056/NEJMoa003289.
2. Nielsen N, Wetterslev J, Cronberg T, et al: Targeted temperature management at 33° C versus 36° C after cardiac arrest. *N Engl J Med* 369:2197–2206, 2013. doi: 10.1056/NEJMoa1310519.

Treatment

- CPR
- When possible, treatment of primary cause
- Postresuscitative care

Rapid intervention is essential.

(See also the American Heart Association's guidelines for CPR and emergency cardiovascular care available online at http://circ.ahajournals.org.)

Cardiopulmonary resuscitation (CPR) is an organized, sequential response to cardiac arrest; rapid initiation of uninterrupted chest compressions ("push hard and push fast") and early defibrillation of patients who are in VF or VT (more commonly adults) are the keys to success.

In children, who most often have asphyxial causes of cardiac arrest, the presenting rhythm is typically a bradyarrhythmia followed by asystole. However, about 15 to 20% of children (particularly when sudden cardiac arrest has not been preceded by respiratory symptoms) present with VT or VF and thus also require prompt defibrillation. The incidence of VF as the initial recorded rhythm increases in children > 12 yr.

Primary causes must be promptly treated. If no treatable conditions are present but cardiac motion is detected or pulses are detected by Doppler, severe circulatory shock is identified, and IV fluid (eg, 1 L 0.9% saline, whole blood, or a combination for blood loss) is given. If response to IV fluid is inadequate, most clinicians give one or more vasopressor drugs (eg, norepinephrine, epinephrine, dopamine, vasopressin); however, there is no firm proof that they improve survival.

In addition to treatment of cause, postresuscitative care typically includes methods to optimize oxygen delivery, rapid coronary angiography in patients with suspected cardiac etiology, and targeted temperature management (32 to 36° C in adults) and therapeutic normothermia (36 to 37.5° C in children and infants).[1,2]

1. Moler FW, Silverstein FS, Holubkov R, et al: Therapeutic hypothermia after in-hospital cardiac arrest in children. *N Engl J Med* 376:318–332, 2017. doi: 10.1056/NEJMoa1610493.
2. Moler FW, Silverstein FS, Holubkov R, et al: Therapeutic hypothermia after out-of-hospital cardiac arrest in children. *N Engl J Med* 372:1898–1908, 2015. doi: 10.1056/NEJMoa1411480.

CARDIOPULMONARY RESUSCITATION IN ADULTS

Cardiopulmonary resuscitation (CPR) is an organized, sequential response to cardiac arrest, including

- Recognition of absent breathing and circulation
- Basic life support with chest compressions and rescue breathing
- Advanced cardiac life support (ACLS) with definitive airway and rhythm control
- Postresuscitative care

Prompt initiation of uninterrupted chest compression and early defibrillation (when indicated) are the keys to success. Speed, efficiency, and proper application of CPR with the least possible interruptions determine successful outcome; the rare exception is profound hypothermia caused by cold water immersion, when successful resuscitation may be accomplished even after prolonged arrest (up to 60 min).

Overview of CPR: Guidelines for health care professionals from the American Heart Association are followed (see Fig. 68–1). If a person has collapsed with possible cardiac arrest, a rescuer first establishes unresponsiveness and confirms absence of breathing or the presence of only gasping respirations. Then, the rescuer calls for help. Anyone answering is directed to activate the emergency response system (or appropriate in-hospital resuscitation personnel) and, if possible, obtain a defibrillator.

If no one responds, the rescuer first activates the emergency response system and then begins basic life support by giving 30 chest compressions at a rate of 100 to 120/min and then opening the airway (lifting the chin and tilting back the forehead) and giving 2 rescue breaths. The cycle of compressions and breaths is continued (see Table 68–1) without interruption; preferably each rescuer is relieved every 2 min.

When a defibrillator (manual or automated) becomes available, a person in VF or pulseless VT is given an unsynchronized shock (see also Defibrillation on p. 541). If the cardiac arrest is witnessed and a defibrillator is on the scene, a person in VF or VT is immediately defibrillated; early defibrillation may promptly convert VF or pulseless VT to a perfusing rhythm. It is recommended that untrained bystanders begin and maintain continuous chest compressions until skilled help arrives.

Airway and Breathing

Opening the airway is given 2nd priority (see Clearing and Opening the Upper Airway on p. 551) after beginning chest compressions. For mechanical measures regarding resuscitation in children, see Table 68–4 on p. 549.

Mouth-to-mouth (adults, adolescents, and children) or combined mouth-to-mouth-and-nose (infants) rescue breathing or bag-valve-mask ventilation is begun for asphyxial cardiac arrest. If available, an oropharyngeal airway may be inserted. Cricoid pressure is no longer recommended.

If abdominal distention develops, the airway is rechecked for patency and the amount of air delivered during rescue breathing is reduced. Nasogastric intubation to relieve gastric distention is delayed until suction equipment is available because regurgitation with aspiration of gastric contents may occur during insertion. If marked gastric distention interferes with ventilation and cannot be corrected by the above methods, patients are positioned on their side, the epigastrium is compressed, and the airway is cleared.

When qualified providers are present, an advanced airway (endotracheal tube or supraglottic device) is placed *without interruption of chest compression* as described under Airway Establishment and Control on p. 550. A breath is given every 6 sec (10 breaths/min) without interrupting chest compression. However, chest compression and defibrillation take precedence over endotracheal intubation. Unless highly experienced providers are available, endotracheal intubation may be delayed in favor of ventilation with bag-valve-mask, laryngeal mask airway, or similar device.

Circulation

Chest compression: In witnessed cardiac arrest, chest compression should be done until defibrillation is available. In an unresponsive patient whose collapse was unwitnessed,

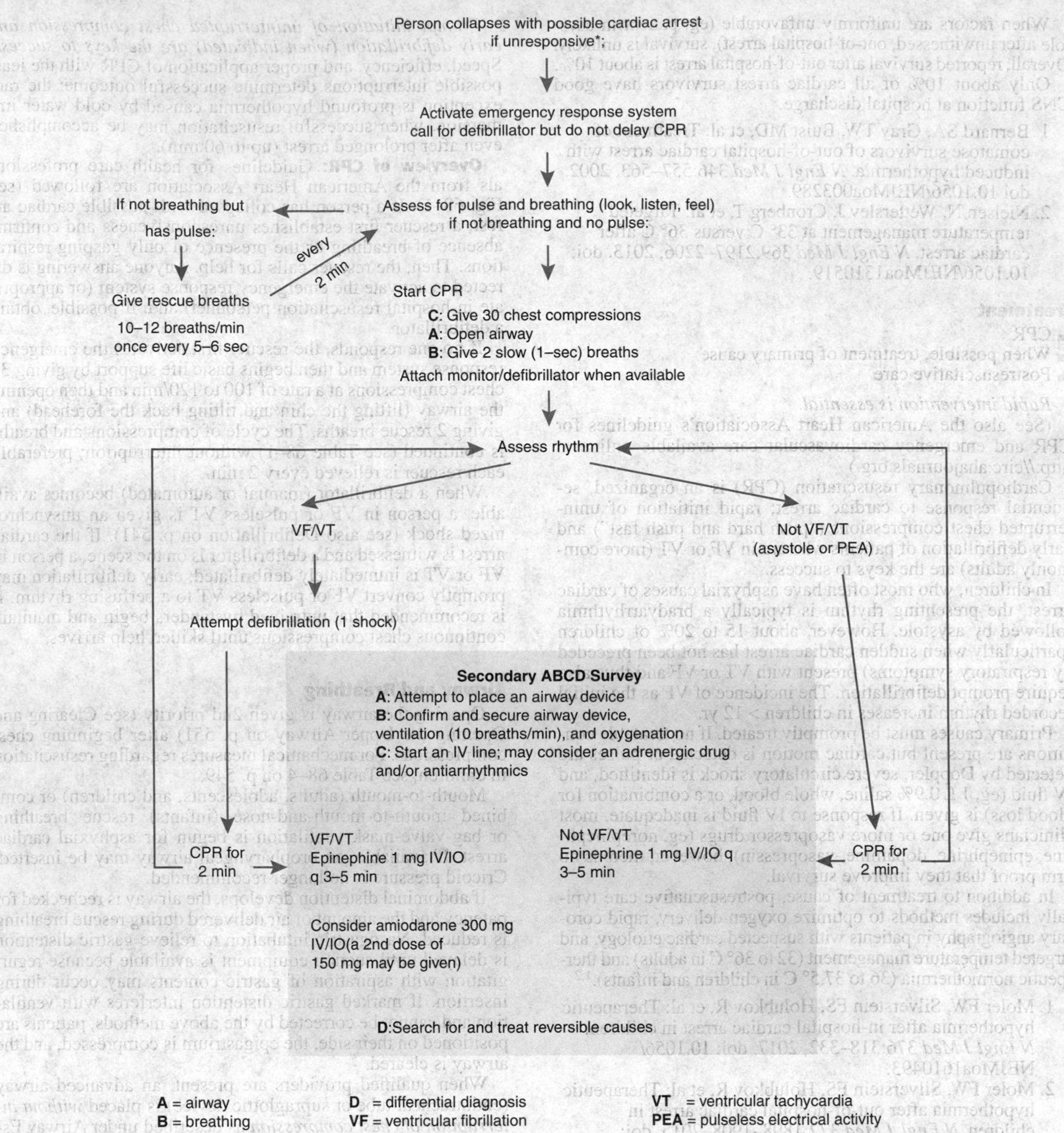

Person collapses with possible cardiac arrest
if unresponsive*;
Activate emergency response system
call for defibrillator but do not delay CPR
If not breathing but
has pulse:
Assess for pulse and breathing (look, listen, feel)
if not breathing and no pulse:
every
2 min
Give rescue breaths
10–12 breaths/min
once every 5–6 sec
Start CPR
C: Give 30 chest compressions
A: Open airway
B: Give 2 slow (1–sec) breaths
Attach monitor/defibrillator when available
Assess rhythm
VF/VT
Not VF/VT
(asystole or PEA)
Attempt defibrillation (1 shock)
Secondary ABCD Survey
A: Attempt to place an airway device
B: Confirm and secure airway device,
ventilation (10 breaths/min), and oxygenation
C: Start an IV line; may consider an adrenergic drug
and/or antiarrhythmics
CPR for
2 min
VF/VT
Epinephine 1 mg IV/IO
q 3–5 min
Not VF/VT
Epinephrine 1 mg IV/IO q
3–5 min
CPR for
2 min
Consider amiodarone 300 mg
IV/IO(a 2nd dose of
150 mg may be given)
D:Search for and treat reversible causes
A = airway
B = breathing
C = circulation
D = differential diagnosis
VF = ventricular fibrillation
IO = intraosseously
VT = ventricular tachycardia
PEA = pulseless electrical activity

Fig. 68–1. Adult comprehensive emergency cardiac care.

*If an adequate number of trained personnel are available, patient assessment, CPR, and activation of the emergency response system should occur simultaneously.

Based on the Comprehensive Emergency Cardiac Care Algorithm from the American Heart Association.

The techniques used in basic 1- and 2-rescuer CPR are listed in Table 68–1. Mastery is best acquired by hands-on training such as that provided in the US under the auspices of the American Heart Association (1-800-AHA-USA1) or corresponding organizations in other countries.

Table 68–1. CPR TECHNIQUES FOR HEALTH CARE PRACTITIONERS

AGE GROUP	ONE-RESCUER CPR*	TWO-RESCUER CPR	BREATH SIZE
Adults and adolescents	2 breaths (1 sec each) after every 30 chest compressions at 100–120/min	2 breaths (1 sec each) after every 30 chest compressions at 100–120/min†	Each breath about 500 mL (caution against hyperventilation)
Children (1 yr—puberty)‡	2 breaths (1 sec each) after every 30 chest compressions at 100–120/min	2 breaths (1 sec each) after every 15 chest compressions at 100–120/min†	Smaller breaths than for adults (enough to make chest rise)
Infants (< 1 yr, excluding newborns)	2 breaths (1 sec each) after every 30 chest compressions at 100–120/min	2 breaths (1 sec each) after every 15 chest compressions at 100–120/min†	Only small puffs from the rescuer's cheeks

*For a single lay rescuer, compression-only CPR is recommended in adults and adolescents.
†Breaths are given without stopping chest compressions.
‡Puberty is defined as the appearance of breasts in females and axillary hair in males.

the trained rescuer should immediately begin external (closed chest) cardiac compression, followed by rescue breathing. Chest compressions must not be interrupted for >10 sec (eg, for intubation, central IV catheter placement, or transport). A compression cycle should consist of 50% compression and 50% release; during the release phase, it is important to allow the chest to recoil fully. Rhythm interpretation and defibrillation (if appropriate) are done as soon as a defibrillator is available.

The recommended chest compression depth for adults is between 2 and 2.4 in (about 5 to 6 cm). Ideally, external cardiac compression produces a palpable pulse with each compression, although cardiac output is only 20 to 30% of normal. However, palpation of pulses during chest compression is difficult, even for experienced clinicians, and often unreliable. End-tidal carbon dioxide monitoring provides a better estimate of cardiac output during chest compression; patients with inadequate perfusion have little venous return to the lungs and hence a low end-tidal carbon dioxide. Restoration of spontaneous breathing or eye opening indicates restoration of spontaneous circulation.

Mechanical chest compression devices are available; these devices are no more effective than properly executed manual compressions but can minimize effects of performance error and fatigue and can be helpful in some circumstances, such as during patient transport or in the cardiac catheterization laboratory.

Open-chest cardiac compression may be effective but is used only in patients with penetrating chest injuries, shortly after cardiac surgery (ie, within 48 h), in cases of cardiac tamponade, and most especially after cardiac arrest in the operating room when the patient's chest is already open. However, thoracotomy requires training and experience and is best done only within these limited indications.

Complications of chest compression: Laceration of the liver is a rare but potentially serious (sometimes fatal) complication and is usually caused by compressing the abdomen below the sternum. Rupture of the stomach (particularly if the stomach is distended with air) is also a rare complication. Delayed rupture of the spleen is very rare. An occasional complication, however, is regurgitation followed by aspiration of gastric contents, causing life-threatening aspiration pneumonia in resuscitated patients.

Costochondral separation and fractured ribs often cannot be avoided because it is important to compress the chest deeply enough to produce sufficient blood flow. Fractures are quite rare in children because of the flexibility of the chest wall. Bone marrow emboli to the lungs have rarely been reported after external cardiac compression, but there is no clear evidence that they contribute to mortality. Lung injury is rare, but pneumothorax after a penetrating rib fracture may occur. Serious myocardial injury caused by compression is very unlikely, with the possible exception of injury to a preexisting ventricular aneurysm. Concern for these injuries should not deter the rescuer from doing CPR.

Defibrillation

The most common rhythm in witnessed adult cardiac arrest is VF; rapid conversion to a perfusing rhythm is essential. Pulseless VT is treated the same as VF.

Prompt direct-current cardioversion is more effective than antiarrhythmic drugs; however, the success of defibrillation is time dependent, with about a 10% decline in success after each minute of VF (or pulseless VT). Automated external defibrillators (AEDs) allow minimally trained rescuers to treat VT or VF. Their use by first responders (police and fire services) and their prominent availability in public locations has increased the likelihood of resuscitation.

Defibrillating paddles or pads are placed between the clavicle and the 2nd intercostal space along the right sternal border and over the 5th or 6th intercostal space at the apex of the heart (in the mid-axillary line). Conventional defibrillator paddles are used with conducting paste; pads have conductive gel incorporated into them. Only 1 initial countershock is now advised (the previous recommendation was 3 stacked shocks), after which chest compression is resumed. Energy level for biphasic defibrillators is between 120 and 200 joules (2 joules/kg in children) for the initial shock; monophasic defibrillators are set at 360 joules for the initial shock. Postshock rhythm is not checked until after 2 min of chest compression. Subsequent shocks are delivered at the same or higher energy level (maximum 360 joules in adults, or 10 joules/kg in children). Patients remaining in VF or VT receive continued chest compression and ventilation and optional drug therapy.

Monitor and IV

ECG monitoring is established to identify the underlying cardiac rhythm. An IV line may be started; 2 lines minimize the risk of losing IV access during CPR. Large-bore peripheral lines in the antecubital veins are preferred. In adults and children, if a peripheral line cannot be established, a subclavian or internal jugular central line (see Procedure on p. 531) can be placed provided it can be done without stopping chest compression (often difficult). Intraosseous and femoral lines (see Intraosseous Infusion on p. 533) are the preferred alternatives, especially in children. Femoral vein catheters (see p. 531), preferably long catheters advanced centrally, are an option because CPR does not need to be stopped and they have less potential for lethal complications; however, they may have a lower rate of successful placement because no discrete femoral arterial pulsations are available to guide insertion.

The type and volume of fluids or drugs given depend on the clinical circumstances. Usually, IV 0.9% saline is given slowly (sufficient only to keep an IV line open); vigorous volume replacement (crystalloid and colloid solutions, blood) is required only when arrest results from hypovolemia (see p. 577).

Special Circumstances

In **accidental electrical shock,** rescuers must be certain that the patient is no longer in contact with the electrical source to avoid shocking themselves. Use of nonmetallic grapples or rods and grounding of the rescuer allows for safe removal of the patient before starting CPR.

In near drowning, rescue breathing may be started in shallow water, although chest compression is not likely to be effectively done until the patient is placed horizontally on a firm surface, such as a surfboard or float.

If **cardiac arrest follows traumatic injury,** airway opening maneuvers and a brief period of external ventilation after clearing the airway have the highest priority because airway obstruction is the most likely treatable cause of arrest. To minimize cervical spine injury, jaw thrust, but not head tilt and chin lift, is advised. Other survivable causes of traumatic cardiac arrest include cardiac tamponade and tension pneumothorax, for which immediate needle decompression is lifesaving. However, most patients with traumatic cardiac arrest have severe hypovolemia due to blood loss (for which chest compression may be ineffective) or nonsurvivable brain injuries.

Drugs for ACLS

Despite widespread and long-standing use, no drug or drug combination has been definitively shown to increase survival to hospital discharge in patients with cardiac arrest. Some drugs do seem to improve the likelihood of restoration of spontaneous circulation (ROSC) and thus may reasonably be given (for dosing, including pediatric, see Table 68–2). Drug therapy for shock and cardiac arrest continues to be researched.

In a patient with a peripheral IV line, drug administration is followed by a fluid bolus ("wide open" IV in adults; 3 to 5 mL in young children) to flush the drug into the central circulation. In a patient without IV or intraosseous access, naloxone, atropine, and epinephrine, when indicated, may be given via the endotracheal tube at 2 to 2.5 times the IV dose. During administration of a drug via endotracheal tube, compression should be briefly stopped.

First-line drugs: The main first-line drug used in cardiac arrest is

- Epinephrine

Epinephrine may be given 1 mg IV q 3 to 5 min. It has combined alpha-adrenergic and beta-adrenergic effects. The alpha-adrenergic effects may augment coronary diastolic pressure, thereby increasing subendocardial perfusion during chest compressions. Epinephrine also increases the likelihood of successful defibrillation. However, beta-adrenergic effects may be detrimental because they increase oxygen requirements (especially of the heart) and cause vasodilation. Intracardiac injection of epinephrine is not recommended because, in addition to interrupting precordial compression, pneumothorax, coronary artery laceration, and cardiac tamponade may occur.

Amiodarone 300 mg can be given once if defibrillation is unsuccessful after epinephrine, followed by 1 dose of 150 mg. It is also of potential value if VT or VF recurs after successful defibrillation; a lower dose is given over 10 min followed by a continuous infusion. There is no persuasive proof that it increases survival to hospital discharge.

A single dose of vasopressin 40 units, which has a duration of activity of 40 min, is an alternative to epinephrine (adults only). However, it is no more effective than epinephrine and is therefore no longer recommended in the American Heart Association's guidelines. However, in the unlikely case of a lack of epinephrine during CPR, vasopressin may be substituted.

Other drugs: A range of additional drugs may be useful in specific settings.

Atropine sulfate is a vagolytic drug that increases heart rate and conduction through the atrioventricular node. It is given for symptomatic bradyarrhythmias and high-degree atrioventricular nodal block. It is no longer recommended for asystole or PEA.

Calcium chloride is recommended for patients with hyperkalemia, hypermagnesemia, hypocalcemia, or calcium channel blocker toxicity. In other patients, because intracellular calcium is already higher than normal, additional calcium is likely to be detrimental. Because cardiac arrest in patients on renal dialysis is often a result of or accompanied by hyperkalemia, these patients may benefit from a trial of calcium if bedside potassium determination is unavailable. Caution is necessary because calcium exacerbates digitalis toxicity and can cause cardiac arrest.

Magnesium sulfate has not been shown to improve outcome in randomized clinical studies. However, it may be helpful in patients with torsades de pointes or known or suspected magnesium deficiency (ie, alcoholics, patients with protracted diarrhea).

Procainamide is a 2nd-line drug for treatment of refractory VF or VT. However, procainamide is not recommended for pulseless arrest in children.

Phenytoin may rarely be used to treat VF or VT, but only when VF or VT is due to digitalis toxicity and is refractory to other drugs. A dose of 50 to 100 mg/min q 5 min is given until rhythm improves or the total dose reaches 20 mg/kg.

Sodium bicarbonate is no longer recommended unless cardiac arrest is caused by hyperkalemia, hypermagnesemia, or tricyclic antidepressant overdose with complex ventricular arrhythmias. In children, sodium bicarbonate may be considered when cardiac arrest is prolonged (> 10 min); it is given only if there is good ventilation. When sodium bicarbonate is used, arterial pH should be monitored before infusion and after each 50-mEq dose (1 to 2 mEq/kg in children).

Lidocaine is not recommended for routine use during cardiac arrest. However, it may be helpful as an alternative to amiodarone for VF or VT that is unresponsive to defibrillation (in children) or after ROSC due to VF or VT (in adults).

Bretylium is no longer recommended for management of cardiac arrest.

Table 68–2. DRUGS FOR RESUSCITATION*

DRUG[†]	ADULT DOSE	PEDIATRIC DOSE	COMMENTS
Adenosine	6 mg initially, then 12 mg × 2	0.1 mg/kg initially, then 0.2 mg/kg × 2	Rapid IV push is followed by flush (maximum single dose 12 mg).
Amiodarone	For VF/pulseless VT: 300 mg	For VF/pulseless VT: 5 mg/kg	For VF/pulseless VT: Give as IV push over 2 min.
	For perfusing VT: Loading dose: 150 mg Infusion (drip): 1 mg/min × 6 h, then 0.5 mg/min × 24 h	For perfusing VT: 5 mg/kg over 20–60 min, repeated to a maximum of 15 mg/kg/day	For perfusing VT: Give initial dose as IV push over 10 min.
Amrinone	Loading dose: 0.75 mg/kg over 2–3 min Infusion (drip): 5–10 mcg/kg/min	Loading dose: 0.75–1 mg/kg over 5 min (may be repeated up to 3 mg/kg) Infusion: 5–10 mcg/kg/min	500 mg in 250 mL 0.9% saline gives 2 mg/mL.
Atropine	0.5–1 mg	0.02 mg/kg	Repeat q 3–5 min to effect or total dose of 0.04 mg/kg (minimum dose 0.1 mg).
Calcium chloride	1 g	20 mg/kg	10% solution contains 100 mg/mL.
Calcium gluceptate	0.66 g	N/A	22% solution contains 220 mg/mL.
Calcium gluconate	0.6 g	60–100 mg/kg	10% solution contains 100 mg/mL.
Dobutamine	2–20 mcg/kg/min (starting at 2–5 mcg/kg/min)	Same as adult dose	500 mg in 250 mL 5% D/W gives 2000 mcg/mL.
Dopamine	2–20 mcg/kg/min (starting at 2–5 mcg/kg/min)	Same as adult dose	400 mg in 250 mL 5% D/W gives 1600 mcg/mL.
Epinephrine	Bolus: 1 mg Infusion: 2–10 mcg/min	Bolus: 0.01 mg/kg Infusion: 0.1–1.0 mcg/kg/min	Repeat q 3 to 5 min as needed. 8 mg in 250 mL 5% D/W gives 32 mcg/mL.
Glucose	25 g 50% D/W	0.5–1 g/kg	Avoid high concentrations in infants and young children. 5% D/W: Give 10–20 mL/kg. 10% D/W: Give 5–10 mL/kg. 25% D/W: Give 2–4 mL/kg. For older children, use a large vein.
Lidocaine	1–1.5 mg/kg; repeat q 5–10 min to a maximum of 3 mg/kg	1 mg/kg loading dose, then 20–50 mcg/kg/min infusion	In adults, lidocaine may be considered after ROSC for VF/VT. In children, lidocaine may be used instead of amiodarone for refractory VF/VT.
Magnesium sulfate	1–2 g	25–50 mg/kg to a maximum of 2 g	Give over 2–5 min.
Milrinone	Loading dose: 50 mcg/kg over 10 min Infusion: 0.5 mcg/kg/min	Loading dose: 50–75 mcg/kg over 10 min Infusion: 0.5–0.75 mcg/kg/min	50 mg in 250 mL 5% D/W gives 200 mcg/mL.
Naloxone	2 mg intranasal or 0.4 mg IM	0.1 mg/kg if patients are < 20 kg or < 5 yr	Repeat as needed.
Norepinephrine	Infusion: 2–16 mcg/min	Infusion: Starting with 0.05–0.1 mcg/kg/min (maximum dose 2 mcg/kg/min)	8 mg in 250 mL 5% D/W gives 32 mcg/mL.
Phenylephrine	Infusion: 0.1–1.5 mcg/kg/min	Infusion: 0.1–0.5 mcg/kg/min	10 mg in 250 mL 5% D/W gives 40 mcg/mL.
Procainamide	30 mg/min to effect or a maximum of 17 mg/kg	Same as adult dose	Procainamide is not recommended for pulseless arrest in children.
Sodium bicarbonate ($NaHCO_3$)	50 mEq	1 mEq/kg	Infuse slowly and only when ventilation is adequate. 4.2% contains 0.5 mEq/mL; 8.4% contains 1 mEq/mL.
Vasopressin	No longer recommended	Not recommended	Vasopressin is no more effective than epinephrine.

*For indications and use, see text.
[†]IV or intraosseous.
ROSC = restoration of spontaneous circulation; VF = ventricular fibrillation; VT = ventricular tachycardia.

Dysrhythmia Treatment

VF or pulseless VT is treated with one direct-current shock, preferably with biphasic waveform, as soon as possible after those rhythms are identified. Despite some laboratory evidence to the contrary, it is not recommended to delay defibrillation to administer a period of chest compressions. Chest compression should be interrupted as little as possible and for no more than 10 sec at a time for defibrillation. Recommended energy levels for defibrillation vary: 120 to 200 joules for biphasic waveform and 360 joules for monophasic. If this treatment is unsuccessful, epinephrine 1 mg IV is administered and repeated q 3 to 5 min. Defibrillation at the same energy level or higher is attempted 1 min after each drug administration. If VF persists, amiodarone 300 mg IV is given. Then, if VF/VT recurs, 150 mg is given followed by infusion of 1 mg/min for 6 h, then 0.5 mg/min. Current versions of AEDs provide a pediatric cable that effectively reduces the energy delivered to children. (For pediatric energy levels, see Defibrillation on p. 548; for drug doses, see Table 68–2.)

Asystole can be mimicked by a loose or disconnected monitor lead; thus, monitor connections should be checked and the rhythm viewed in an alternative lead. If asystole is confirmed, the patient is given epinephrine 1 mg IV repeated q 3 to 5 min. Defibrillation of apparent asystole (because it "might be fine VF") is discouraged because electrical shocks injure the nonperfused heart.

PEA is circulatory collapse that occurs despite satisfactory electrical complexes on the ECG. Patients with PEA receive 500- to 1000-mL (20 mL/kg) infusion of 0.9% saline. Epinephrine may be given in amounts of 0.5 to 1.0 mg IV repeated q 3 to 5 min. Cardiac tamponade can cause PEA, but this disorder usually occurs in patients after thoracotomy and in patients with known pericardial effusion or major chest trauma. In such settings, immediate pericardiocentesis or thoracotomy is done (see Fig. 86–2 on p. 748). Tamponade is rarely an occult cause of cardiac arrest but, if suspected, can be confirmed by ultrasonography or, if ultrasonography is unavailable, pericardiocentesis.

Termination of Resuscitation

CPR should be continued until the cardiopulmonary system is stabilized, the patient is pronounced dead, or a lone rescuer is physically unable to continue. If cardiac arrest is thought to be due to hypothermia, CPR should be continued until the body is rewarmed to 34° C.

The decision to terminate resuscitation is a clinical one, and clinicians take into account duration of arrest, age of the patient, and prognosis of underlying medical conditions. The decision is typically made when spontaneous circulation has not been established after CPR and ACLS measures have been done. In intubated patients, an end-tidal carbon dioxide ($ETCO_2$) level of < 10 mm Hg is a poor prognostic sign.

Postresuscitative Care

ROSC is only an intermediate goal in resuscitation. The ultimate goal is survival to hospital discharge with good neurologic function, which is achieved by only a minority of patients with ROSC. To maximize the likelihood of a good outcome, clinicians must provide good supportive care (eg, manage blood pressure, temperature, and cardiac rhythm) and treat underlying conditions, particularly acute coronary syndromes.

Postresuscitation laboratory studies include ABG, CBC, and blood chemistries, including electrolytes, glucose, BUN, creatinine, and cardiac markers. (Creatine kinase is usually elevated because of skeletal muscle damage caused by CPR; troponins, which are unlikely to be affected by CPR or defibrillation, are preferred.) Arterial Pao_2 should be kept near normal values (80 to 100 mm Hg). Hct should be maintained at ≥ 30 (if cardiac etiology is suspected), and glucose at 140 to 180 mg/dL; electrolytes, especially potassium, should be within the normal range.

Coronary angiography: When indicated, coronary angiography should be done emergently (rather than later during the hospital course) so that if percutaneous coronary intervention (PCI) is needed, it is done as soon as possible. The decision to do cardiac catheterization after resuscitation from cardiac arrest should be individualized based on the ECG, the interventional cardiologist's clinical impression, and the patient's prognosis. However, guidelines suggest doing emergency angiography for adult patients in whom a cardiac cause is suspected and who have

- ST-segment elevation on the ECG
- Coma with no ST-segment elevation

Neurologic support: Only about 10% of all cardiac arrest survivors have good CNS function (cerebral performance index 1 or 2) at hospital discharge. Hypoxic brain injury is a result of ischemic damage and cerebral edema. Both damage and recovery may evolve over 48 to 72 h after resuscitation.

Maintenance of oxygenation and cerebral perfusion pressure (avoiding hypotension) may reduce cerebral complications. Both hypoglycemia and hyperglycemia may damage the post-ischemic brain and should be treated.

In adults, **targeted temperature management** (maintaining body temperature of 32 to 36° C) is recommended for patients who remain unresponsive after spontaneous circulation has returned.[1,2] Cooling is begun as soon as spontaneous circulation has returned. Techniques to induce and maintain hypothermia can be either external or invasive. External cooling methods are easy to apply and range from the use of external ice packs to several commercially available external cooling devices that circulate high volumes of chilled water over the skin. For internal cooling, chilled IV fluids (4° C) can be rapidly infused to lower body temperature, but this method may be problematic in patients who cannot tolerate much additional fluid volume. Also available are external heat-exchange devices that circulate chilled saline to an indwelling IV heat-exchange catheter using a closed-loop design in which chilled saline circulates through the catheter and back to the device, rather than into the patient. Another invasive method for cooling uses an extracorporeal device that circulates and cools blood externally then returns it to the central circulation. Regardless of the method chosen, the goal is to cool the patient rapidly and to maintain the core temperature between 32° C and 36° C. Currently, there is no evidence that any specific temperature within this range is superior, but it is imperative to avoid hyperthermia.

Numerous pharmacologic treatments, including free radical scavengers, antioxidants, glutamate inhibitors, and calcium channel blockers, are of theoretic benefit; many have been successful in animal models, but none have proved effective in human trials.

Blood pressure support: Current recommendations are to maintain a mean arterial pressure (MAP) of > 80 mm Hg in older adults or > 60 mm Hg in younger and previously healthy patients. In patients known to be hypertensive, a reasonable target is systolic BP 30 mm Hg below prearrest level. MAP is best measured with an intra-arterial catheter. Use of a flow-directed pulmonary artery catheter for hemodynamic monitoring has been largely discarded.

BP support includes

- IV 0.9% saline
- Sometimes inotropic or vasopressor drugs
- Rarely intra-aortic balloon counterpulsation

Patients with low MAP and low central venous pressure should have IV fluid challenge with 0.9% saline infused in 250-mL increments.

Although use of inotropic and vasopressor drugs has not proved to enhance long-term survival, older adults with moderately low MAP (70 to 80 mm Hg) and normal or high central venous pressure may receive an infusion of an inotrope (eg, dobutamine started at 2 to 5 mcg/kg/min). Alternatively, amrinone or milrinone is used (see Table 68–2).

If this therapy is ineffective, the inotrope and vasoconstrictor dopamine may be considered. Alternatives are epinephrine and the peripheral vasoconstrictors norepinephrine and phenylephrine (see Table 68–2). However, vasoactive drugs should be used at the minimal dose necessary to achieve low-normal MAP because they may increase vascular resistance and decrease organ perfusion, especially in the mesenteric bed. They also increase the workload of the heart at a time when its capability is decreased because of postresuscitation myocardial dysfunction.

If MAP remains < 70 mm Hg in patients who may have sustained an MI, intra-aortic balloon counterpulsation should be considered. Patients with normal MAP and high central venous pressure may improve with either inotropic therapy or afterload reduction with nitroprusside or nitroglycerin.

Intra-aortic balloon counterpulsation can assist low-output circulatory states due to left ventricular pump failure that is refractory to drugs. A balloon catheter is introduced via the femoral artery, percutaneously or by arteriotomy, retrograde into the thoracic aorta just distal to the left subclavian artery. The balloon inflates during each diastole, augmenting coronary artery perfusion, and deflates during systole, decreasing afterload. Its primary value is as a temporizing measure when the cause of shock is potentially correctable by surgery or percutaneous intervention (eg, acute MI with major coronary obstruction, acute mitral insufficiency, ventricular septal defect).

Dysrhythmia treatment: Although VF or VT may recur after resuscitation, prophylactic antiarrhythmic drugs do not improve survival and are no longer routinely used. However, patients manifesting such rhythms may be treated with procainamide or amiodarone.

Postresuscitation rapid supraventricular tachycardias occur frequently because of high levels of beta-adrenergic catecholamines (both endogenous and exogenous) during cardiac arrest and resuscitation. These rhythms should be treated if extreme, prolonged, or associated with hypotension or signs of coronary ischemia. An esmolol IV infusion is given, beginning at 50 mcg/kg/min.

Patients who had arrest caused by VF or VT not associated with acute MI are candidates for an implantable cardioverter-defibrillator (ICD). Current ICDs are implanted similarly to pacemakers and have intracardiac leads and sometimes subcutaneous electrodes. They can sense arrhythmias and deliver either cardioversion or cardiac pacing as indicated.

1. Bernard SA, Gray TW, Buist MD, et al: Treatment of comatose survivors of out-of-hospital cardiac arrest with induced hypothermia. *N Engl J Med* 346:557–563, 2002. doi 10.1056/NEJMoa003289.
2. Nielsen N, Wetterslev J, Cronberg T, et al: Targeted temperature management at 33° C versus 36° C after cardiac arrest. *N Engl J Med* 369:2197–2206, 2013. doi: 10.1056/NEJMoa1310519.

CARDIOPULMONARY RESUSCITATION IN INFANTS AND CHILDREN

Despite the use of CPR, mortality rates for out-of-hospital cardiac arrest are 80 to 97% for infants and children. Mortality rates for in-hospital cardiac arrest for infants and children range between 40% and 65%. The mortality rate is 20 to 25% for respiratory arrest alone. Neurologic outcome is often severely compromised.

Pediatric resuscitation protocols apply to infants < 1 yr of age and children up to the age of puberty (defined as appearance of breasts in females and axillary hair in males) or children weighing < 55 kg. Adult resuscitation protocols apply to children past the age of puberty or children weighing > 55 kg. Neonatal resuscitation is discussed elsewhere (see p. 2791).

About 50 to 65% of children requiring CPR are < 1 yr; of these, most are < 6 mo. About 6% of neonates require resuscitation at delivery; the incidence increases significantly if birth weight is < 1500 g.

Standardized outcome guidelines should be followed in reporting outcomes of CPR in children; eg, the modified Pittsburgh Outcome Categories Scale reflects cerebral and overall performance (see Table 68–3).

Standards and guidelines for CPR from the American Heart Association are followed (see Table 68–1). For protocol after an infant or child has collapsed with possible cardiac arrest, see Fig. 68–2.

After CPR has been started, defibrillation and identification of the underlying cardiac rhythm (see p. 541) are done.

Major Differences Between Pediatric and Adult CPR

Prearrest: *Bradycardia in a distressed child is a sign of impending cardiac arrest.* Neonates, infants, and young children are more likely to develop bradycardia caused by hypoxemia, whereas older children initially tend to have tachycardia. An infant or child with a heart rate < 60/min and signs of poor perfusion that do not rise with ventilatory support should have cardiac compressions (see Fig. 68–3). Bradycardia secondary to heart block is unusual.

Chest compressions: During chest compressions in infants and children (below the age of puberty or < 55 kg), the chest should be depressed one third of the anteroposterior diameter. This is about 1.5 in (4 cm) to 2 in (5 cm). In adolescents or children > 55 kg, the recommended compression depth is the same as in adults, ie, 2 in (5 cm) to 2.4 in (6 cm).

Method of chest compression is also different in infants and children and is illustrated below. The rate of compression in infants and children is similar to that of adults at 100 to 120 compressions/min.

Drugs: After adequate oxygenation and ventilation, epinephrine is the drug of choice (see First-line drugs on p. 542). Epinephrine dose is 0.01 mg/kg IV, which can be repeated q 3 to 5 min.

Amiodarone 5 mg/kg IV bolus can be given if defibrillation is unsuccessful after epinephrine. It may be repeated up to 2 times for refractory VF or pulseless VT. If amiodarone is not

Table 68–3. PEDIATRIC CEREBRAL PERFORMANCE CATEGORY SCALE*

SCORE	CATEGORY	DESCRIPTION
1	Normal	Age-appropriate level of functioning In preschool-aged children, appropriate development In school-aged children, attendance in regular classes
2	Mild disability	Can interact at an age-appropriate level Minor neurologic disease that is controlled and does not interfere with daily functioning (eg, seizure disorder) In preschool-aged children, possibly minor developmental delays, but with > 75% of all daily living developmental milestones above the 10th percentile In school-aged children, attendance in regular school but in a grade that is not appropriate for age or in the appropriate grade but failing because of cognitive difficulties
3	Moderate disability	Below age-appropriate functioning Neurologic disease that is not controlled and severely limits activities In preschool-aged children, most daily living developmental milestones below the 10th percentile In school-aged children, can do activities of daily living but attend special classes because of cognitive difficulties or a learning deficit
4	Severe disability	In preschool-aged children, activities of daily living milestones below the 10th percentile and excessive dependence on others for activities of daily living In school-aged children, possibly severe impairment that prevents school attendance and dependence on others for activities of daily living In preschool-aged and school-aged children, possibly abnormal motor movements, including nonpurposeful, decorticate, or decerebrate responses to pain
5	Coma or vegetative state	Unawareness
6	Death	—

*Worst level of performance for any single criterion is used for categorizing. Deficits are scored only if they result from a neurologic disorder. Assessments are based on medical records or an interview with the caretaker.

From *Recommended guidelines for uniform reporting of pediatric advanced life support: The pediatric Utstein style; statement for health care professionals* from the Task Force of the American Academy of Pediatrics, the American Heart Association, and the European Resuscitation Council; *Pediatrics* 96(4):765–779, 1995.

available, lidocaine may be given at a loading dose of 1 mg/kg IV followed by a maintenance infusion of 20 to 50 mcg/kg/min. Neither amiodarone nor lidocaine have been shown to improve survival to hospital discharge.

Blood pressure: BP should be measured with an appropriate-sized cuff, but direct invasive arterial BP monitoring is mandatory in severely compromised children.

Because BP varies with age, an easy guideline to remember the lower limits of normal for systolic BP (< 5th percentile) by age is as follows:

- < 1 mo: 60 mm Hg
- 1 mo to 1 yr: 70 mm Hg
- > 1 yr: 70 + (2 × age in yr)

Thus, in a 5-yr-old child, hypotension would be defined by a BP of < 80 mm Hg (70 + [2 × 5]). Of significant importance is that children maintain BP longer because of stronger compensatory mechanisms (increased heart rate, increased systemic vascular resistance). Once hypotension occurs, cardiorespiratory arrest may rapidly follow. All effort should be made to start treatment when compensatory signs of shock (eg, increased heart rate, cool extremities, capillary refill > 2 sec, poor peripheral pulses) are present but before hypotension develops.

Equipment and environment: Equipment size, drug dosage, and CPR parameters vary with patient age and weight (see Tables 68–1, 68–2, and 68–4).). Size-variable equipment includes defibrillator paddles or electrode pads, masks, ventilation bags, airways, laryngoscope blades, endotracheal tubes, and suction catheters. Weight should be measured rather than guessed; alternatively, commercially available measuring tapes that are calibrated to read standard patient weight based on body length can be used. Some tapes are printed with the recommended drug dose and equipment size for each weight. Dosages should be rounded down; eg, a 2 ½-yr-old child should receive the dose for a 2-yr-old child.

Temperature management: Susceptibility to heat loss is greater in infants and children because of a large surface area relative to body mass and less subcutaneous tissue. A neutral external thermal environment is crucial during CPR and post-resuscitation. Hypothermia with core temperature < 35° C makes resuscitation more difficult.

For comatose children resuscitated from in-hospital and out-of-hospital cardiac arrest, there is no evidence that therapeutic hypothermia is beneficial. In comatose children resuscitated from cardiac arrest, therapeutic normothermia (36° C to 37.5° C) should be pursued and fever should be treated aggressively.[1,2]

Airway and ventilation: Upper airway anatomy is different in children. The head is large with a small face, mandible, and external nares, and the neck is relatively short. The tongue is large relative to the mouth, and the larynx lies higher in the neck and is angled more anteriorly. The epiglottis is long, and the narrowest portion of the trachea is inferior to the vocal cords at the cricoid ring, allowing the use of uncuffed endotracheal tubes. In younger children, a straight laryngoscope blade generally allows better visualization of the vocal cords than a curved blade because the larynx is more anterior and the epiglottis is more floppy and redundant.

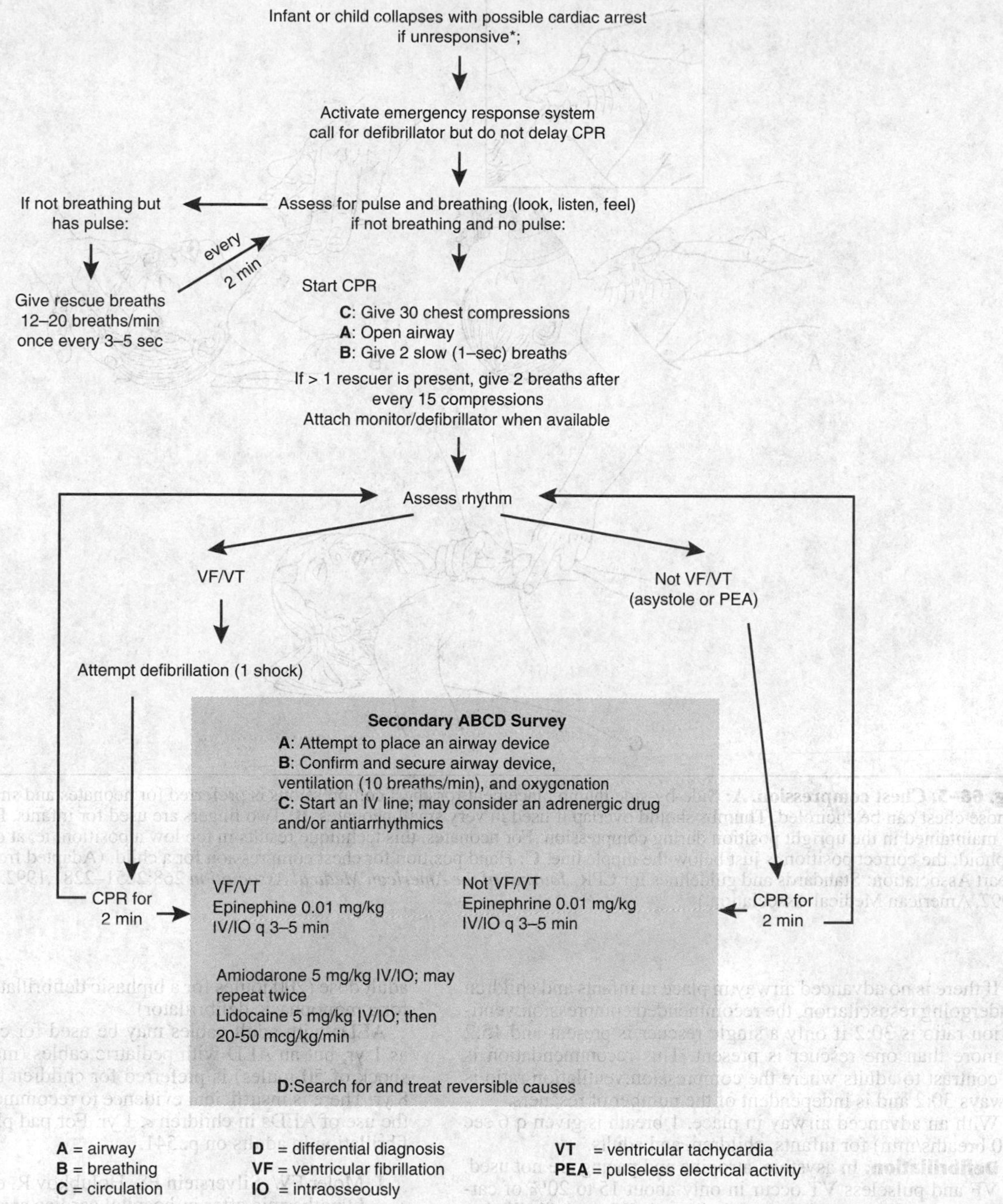
Infant or child collapses with possible cardiac arrest
if unresponsive*;
Activate emergency response system
call for defibrillator but do not delay CPR
Assess for pulse and breathing (look, listen, feel)
if not breathing and no pulse:
If not breathing but
has pulse:
Give rescue breaths
12–20 breaths/min
once every 3–5 sec
every
2 min
Start CPR
C: Give 30 chest compressions
A: Open airway
B: Give 2 slow (1–sec) breaths
If > 1 rescuer is present, give 2 breaths after
every 15 compressions
Attach monitor/defibrillator when available
Assess rhythm
VF/VT
Not VF/VT
(asystole or PEA)
Attempt defibrillation (1 shock)
Secondary ABCD Survey
A: Attempt to place an airway device
B: Confirm and secure airway device,
ventilation (10 breaths/min), and oxygenation
C: Start an IV line; may consider an adrenergic drug
and/or antiarrhythmics
CPR for
2 min
VF/VT
Epinephine 0.01 mg/kg
IV/IO q 3–5 min
Not VF/VT
Epinephrine 0.01 mg/kg
IV/IO q 3–5 min
CPR for
2 min
Amiodarone 5 mg/kg IV/IO; may
repeat twice
Lidocaine 5 mg/kg IV/IO; then
20-50 mcg/kg/min
D:Search for and treat reversible causes
A = airway
B = breathing
C = circulation
D = differential diagnosis
VF = ventricular fibrillation
IO = intraosseously
VT = ventricular tachycardia
PEA = pulseless electrical activity

Fig. 68–2. Pediatric comprehensive emergency cardiac care.

*If an adequate number of trained personnel are available, patient assessment, CPR, and activation of the emergency response system should occur simultaneously.

Based on the Comprehensive Emergency Cardiac Care Algorithm from the American Heart Association.

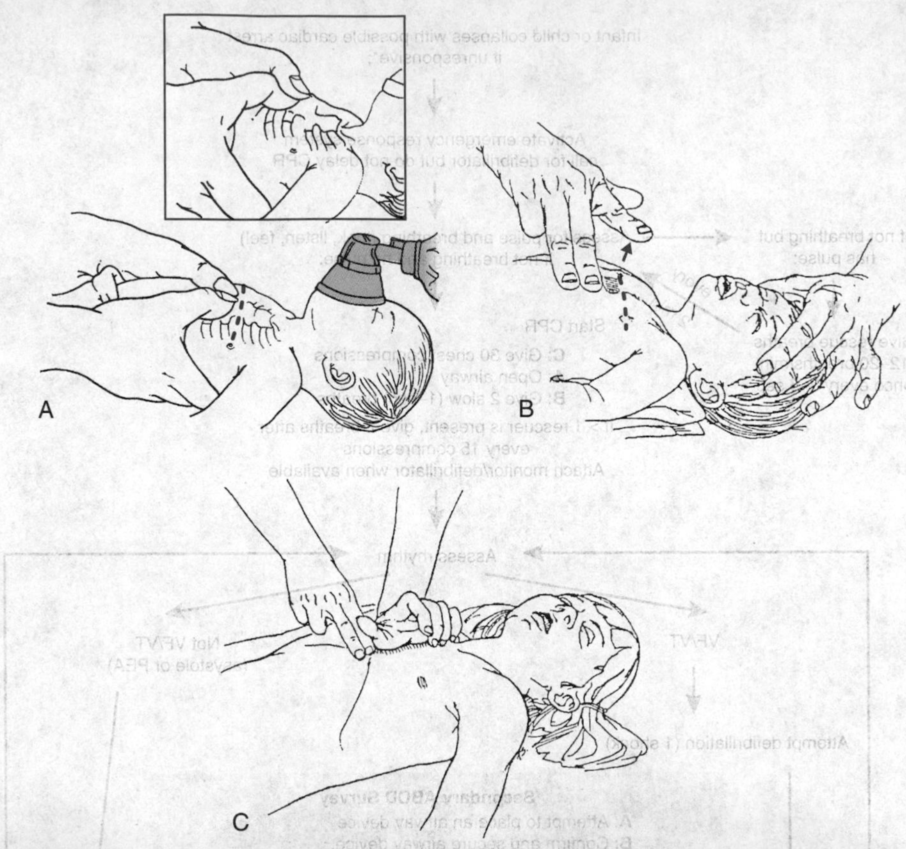

Fig. 68–3. Chest compression. A: Side-by-side thumb placement for chest compressions is preferred for neonates and small infants whose chest can be encircled. Thumbs should overlap if used in very small neonates. **B:** Two fingers are used for infants. Fingers should be maintained in the upright position during compression. For neonates, this technique results in too low a position, ie, at or below the xiphoid; the correct position is just below the nipple line. **C:** Hand position for chest compression for a child. (Adapted from American Heart Association: Standards and guidelines for CPR. *Journal of the American Medical Association* 268:2251–2281,1992. Copyright 1992, American Medical Association.)

If there is no advanced airway in place in infants and children undergoing resuscitation, the recommended compression:ventilation ratio is 30:2 if only a single rescuer is present and 15:2 if more than one rescuer is present. This recommendation is in contrast to adults where the compression:ventilation ratio is always 30:2 and is independent of the number of rescuers.

With an advanced airway in place, 1 breath is given q 6 sec (10 breaths/min) for infants, children, and adults.

Defibrillation: In asystole, atropine and pacing are not used. VF and pulseless VT occur in only about 15 to 20% of cardiac arrests. Vasopressin is not indicated. When defibrillation is used, the absolute energy dose is less than that for adults; waveform can be biphasic (preferred) or monophasic. For either waveform, the recommended energy dose is 2 joules/kg for the first shock, increasing to 4 joules/kg for subsequent attempts (if necessary—see defibrillation in adults on p. 541). The maximum recommended dose is 10 joules/kg or the maximum adult dose (200 joules for a biphasic defibrillator and 360 joules for a monophasic defibrillator).

AEDs with adult cables may be used for children as young as 1 yr, but an AED with pediatric cables (maximum biphasic shock of 50 joules) is preferred for children between 1 yr and 8 yr. There is insufficient evidence to recommend for or against the use of AEDs in children < 1 yr. For pad placement, see defibrillation in adults on p. 541.

1. Moler FW, Silverstein FS, Holubkov R, et al: Therapeutic hypothermia after in-hospital cardiac arrest in children. *N Engl J Med* 376:318–332, 2017. doi: 10.1056/NEJMoa1610493.
2. Moler FW, Silverstein FS, Holubkov R, et al: Therapeutic hypothermia after out-of-hospital cardiac arrest in children. *N Engl J Med* 372:1898–1908, 2015. doi: 10.1056/NEJMoa1411480.

Table 68–4. GUIDE TO PEDIATRIC RESUSCITATION—MECHANICAL MEASURES

AGE (YR)	TERM NEONATE	< 12 MO	1	2	3	4	5	6	7	8	9	10	11	12	13	14	15	16
Weight, typical (kg)	3.5	< 10	10	12	14	16	18	20	22	25	28	30	35	40	45	50	55	60
Compression techniques	Thumb compression, hands around chest (preferred) or 2 fingers		←——— 1 hand ———→							←——— 2 hands ———→								
Airway size (Portex) in cm	000	00	00	0	0	7	7	7	7	7	7	7	7	7	8	8	8	8
	3.5	5	5	6	6													
Masks in Laerdal sizes or equivalent	Circular 0/1	Rendell-Baker type # 1		Rendell-Baker type # 2			←——— Dome cuff mask # 3 ———→					←——— Dome cuff mask # 4 ———→						
Ventilation bag with reservoir for 100% O_2 delivery	Infant 240 mL	←——— Child 400–500 mL ———→									←——— Adult 1600 mL ———→							
Laryngoscope blade size (Miller, Straight)	0	1	1	1	2	2	2	2	2	2	2	3	3	3	3	3	3	3
	←——— Straight blade (preferred) or curved blade ———→									←——— Curved or straight blade ———→								
ETT size (Portex) in mm	3	3.5	4	4.5	4.5	5	5	5.5	5.5	6	6	6	6	6.5	6.5	6.5	6.5	7
	←——— Uncuffed ———→									←——— Cuffed ———→								
Suction catheter Direct oropharyngeal	10 F	←— Pediatric tonsil suction —→				←——— Adult tonsil suction ———→												
Suction catheter Through ETT	←——— 8 Fr ———→					←——— 10 Fr ———→												

*Pause for ventilation.
ETT = endotracheal tube; Fr = French.
Courtesy of Dr. B. Paes and Dr. M. Sullivan, the Departments of Pediatrics and Medicine, St. Joseph's Hospital, The Children's Hospital, Hamilton Health Sciences Corporation, McMaster University, Hamilton, Ontario, Canada.

69 Respiratory Arrest

Respiratory arrest and cardiac arrest are distinct, but inevitably if untreated, one leads to the other.

Interruption of pulmonary gas exchange for > 5 min may irreversibly damage vital organs, especially the brain. Cardiac arrest almost always follows unless respiratory function is rapidly restored. However, aggressive ventilation may also have negative hemodynamic consequences, particularly in the periarrest period and in other circumstances when cardiac output is low. In most cases, the ultimate goal is to restore adequate ventilation and oxygenation without further compromising a tentative cardiovascular situation.

Etiology

Respiratory arrest (and impaired respiration that can progress to respiratory arrest) can be caused by

- Airway obstruction
- Decreased respiratory effort
- Respiratory muscle weakness

Airway obstruction: Obstruction may involve the

- Upper airway
- Lower airway

Infants < 3 mo are usually nose breathers and thus may have upper airway obstruction secondary to nasal blockage. At all ages, loss of muscular tone with decreased consciousness may cause upper airway obstruction as the posterior portion of the tongue displaces into the oropharynx. Other causes of upper airway obstruction include blood, mucus, vomitus, or foreign body; spasm or edema of the vocal cords; and pharyngolaryngeal tracheal inflammation (eg, epiglottitis, croup), tumor, or trauma. Patients with congenital developmental disorders often have abnormal upper airways that are more easily obstructed.

Lower airway obstruction may result from aspiration, bronchospasm, airspace filling disorders (eg, pneumonia, pulmonary edema, pulmonary hemorrhage), or drowning.

Decreased respiratory effort: Decreased respiratory effort reflects CNS impairment due to one of the following:

- Central nervous system disorder
- Adverse drug effect
- Metabolic disorder

CNS disorders that affect the brain stem (eg, stroke, infection, tumor) can cause hypoventilation. Disorders that increase intracranial pressure usually cause hyperventilation initially, but hypoventilation may develop if the brain stem is compressed.

Drugs that decrease respiratory effort include opioids and sedative-hypnotics (eg, barbiturates, alcohol; less commonly, benzodiazepines). Usually, an overdose (iatrogenic, intentional, or unintentional) is involved, although a lower dose may decrease effort in patients who are more sensitive to the effects of these drugs (eg, the elderly, deconditioned patients, patients with chronic respiratory insufficiency).

CNS depression due to severe hypoglycemia or hypotension ultimately compromises respiratory effort.

Respiratory muscle weakness: Weakness may be caused by

- Neuromuscular disorders
- Fatigue

Neuromuscular causes include spinal cord injury, neuromuscular diseases (eg, myasthenia gravis, botulism, poliomyelitis, Guillain-Barré syndrome), and neuromuscular blocking drugs.

Respiratory muscle fatigue can occur if patients breathe for extended periods at a minute ventilation exceeding about 70% of their maximum voluntary ventilation (eg, because of severe metabolic acidosis or hypoxemia).

Symptoms and Signs

With respiratory arrest, patients are unconscious or about to become so.

Patients with hypoxemia may be cyanotic, but cyanosis can be masked by anemia or by carbon monoxide or cyanide intoxication. Patients being treated with high-flow oxygen may not be hypoxemic and therefore may not exhibit cyanosis or desaturation until after respiration ceases for several minutes. Conversely, patients with chronic lung disease and polycythemia may exhibit cyanosis without respiratory arrest. If respiratory arrest remains uncorrected, cardiac arrest follows within minutes of onset of hypoxemia, hypercarbia, or both.

Impending respiratory arrest: Before complete respiratory arrest, patients with intact neurologic function may be agitated, confused, and struggling to breathe. Tachycardia and diaphoresis are present; there may be intercostal or sternoclavicular retractions. Patients with CNS impairment or respiratory muscle weakness have feeble, gasping, or irregular respirations and paradoxical breathing movements. Patients with a foreign body in the airway may choke and point to their necks, exhibit inspiratory stridor, or neither. Monitoring end-tidal CO_2 can alert practitioners to impending respiratory arrest in decompensating patients.

Infants, especially if < 3 mo, may develop acute apnea without warning, secondary to overwhelming infection, metabolic disorders, or respiratory fatigue. Patients with asthma or with other chronic lung diseases may become hypercarbic and fatigued after prolonged periods of respiratory distress and suddenly become obtunded and apneic with little warning, despite adequate oxygen saturation.

Diagnosis

- Clinical evaluation

Respiratory arrest is usually clinically obvious; treatment begins simultaneously with diagnosis. The first consideration is to exclude a foreign body obstructing the airway; if a foreign body is present, resistance to ventilation is marked during mouth-to-mask or bag-valve-mask ventilation. Foreign material may be discovered during laryngoscopy for endotracheal intubation (see p. 551 for removal).

Treatment

- Clearing the airway
- Mechanical ventilation

Treatment is clearing the airway, establishing an alternate airway, and providing mechanical ventilation.

AIRWAY ESTABLISHMENT AND CONTROL

Airway management consists of

- Clearing the upper airway
- Maintaining an open air passage with a mechanical device
- Sometimes assisting respirations

Table 69–1. SITUATIONS REQUIRING AIRWAY CONTROL

CLASSIFICATION	EXAMPLES
Emergencies	Cardiac arrest Respiratory arrest or apnea (eg, due to CNS disease, drugs, or hypoxia) Deep coma, when the tongue relaxes to occlude the glottis Acute laryngeal edema Laryngospasm Foreign body at the larynx (eg, "cafe coronary") Drowning Upper airway trauma Head or high spinal cord injuries
Urgencies	Respiratory failure Need for ventilatory support (eg, in acute respiratory distress syndrome, smoke or toxic inhalation, respiratory burns, gastric aspiration, exacerbations of COPD or asthma, diffuse infectious or other parenchymal lung problems, neuromuscular diseases, respiratory center depression, or extreme respiratory muscle fatigue) Need to relieve the work of breathing in patients in shock or with low cardiac output or myocardial stress that must be decreased Before gastric lavage in patients with an oral drug overdose and altered consciousness Before esophagogastroscopy in patients with upper GI bleeding Before bronchoscopy in patients with marginal respiratory status Before radiologic procedures in patients with altered sensorium, particularly if sedation is required

There are many indications for airway control (see Table 69–1) and many methods of establishing an airway, including

- Basic techniques such as head and neck positioning, abdominal thrusts, and back blows
- Supraglottic methods such as bag-valve-mask and laryngeal mask airways
- Infraglottic techniques (tracheal intubation)
- Surgical airways

Whatever airway management techniques are used, tidal volume should be 6 to 8 mL/kg (significantly less than previously recommended) and ventilatory rate should be 8 to 10 breaths/min (significantly slower than previously recommended to avoid negative hemodynamic consequences). Slower rates are commonly used in patients with severe air trapping (eg, acute asthma, COPD), and passive oxygenation without positive pressure ventilation shows promise in the first minutes after cardiac arrest. Smaller volumes and slower respiratory rates are also desirable in any state of hemodynamic instability; however, it is important to keep in mind that positive pressure ventilation is the opposite of physiologically normal negative pressure ventilation. In cardiac arrest, physiologic demands are significantly less, and in non-arrest, the benefits of hypoventilation in hemodynamic stability and lung protection often outweigh the negative effects of permissive hypercapnia and moderate hypoxia.

Clearing and Opening the Upper Airway

To relieve airway obstruction caused by soft tissues of the upper airway and provide optimal position for bag-valve-mask ventilation and laryngoscopy, the operator flexes the patient's neck to elevate the head until the external auditory meatus is in the same plane as the sternum and positions the face roughly parallel to the ceiling (see Fig. 69–1). This position is slightly different from the previously taught head tilt position. The mandible should be displaced upward by lifting the lower jaw and submandibular soft tissue or by pushing the rami of the mandible upward (see Fig. 69–2).

Anatomic restriction, various abnormalities, or considerations caused by trauma (eg, inadvisability of moving a possibly fractured neck) may obviate the operator's ability to properly position the neck, but careful attention to optimal positioning when possible can maximize airway patency and improve bag-valve-mask ventilation and laryngoscopy.

Obstruction by dentures and oropharyngeal foreign material (eg, blood, secretions) may be removed by finger sweep of the oropharynx and suction, taking care not to push the material

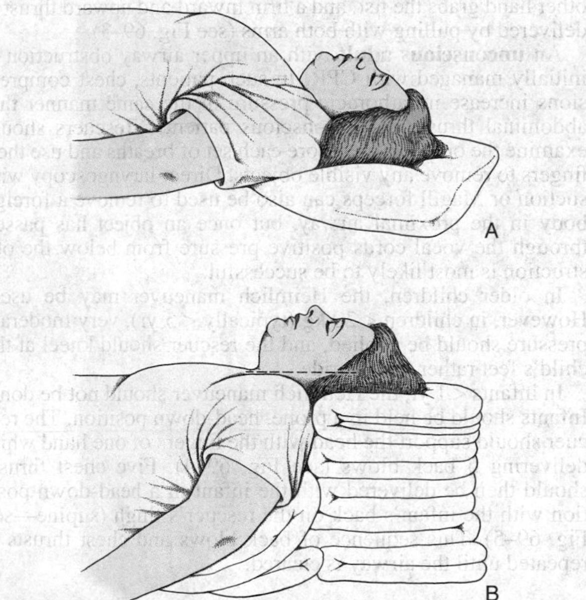

Fig. 69–1. Head and neck positioning to open the airway. **A:** The head is flat on the stretcher; the airway is constricted. **B:** The ear and sternal notch are aligned, with the face parallel to the ceiling, opening the airway. Adapted from Levitan RM, Kinkle WC: *The Airway Cam Pocket Guide to Intubation*, ed. 2. Wayne (PA), Airway Cam Technologies, 2007.

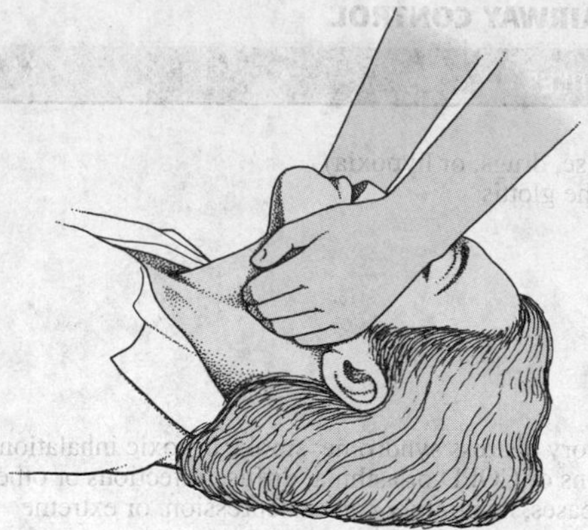

Fig. 69–2. Jaw lift.

deeper (more likely in infants and young children, in whom a blind finger sweep is contraindicated). Deeper material can be removed with Magill forceps or by suction.

Heimlich maneuver (subdiaphragmatic abdominal thrusts): The Heimlich maneuver (for more detailed instructions, see How to do the Heimlich Maneuver on p. 558) consists of manual thrusts to the upper abdomen or, in the case of pregnant or extremely obese patients, chest thrusts until the airway is clear or the patient becomes unconscious; it is the preferred initial method in the awake, choking patient..

In **conscious adults,** the rescuer stands behind the patient with arms encircling the patient's midsection. One fist is clenched and placed midway between the umbilicus and xiphoid. The other hand grabs the fist, and a firm inward and upward thrust is delivered by pulling with both arms (see Fig. 69–3).

An **unconscious adult** with an upper airway obstruction is initially managed with CPR. In such patients, chest compressions increase intrathoracic pressure in the same manner that abdominal thrusts do in conscious patients. Rescuers should examine the oropharynx before each set of breaths and use their fingers to remove any visible objects. Direct laryngoscopy with suction or Magill forceps can also be used to remove a foreign body in the proximal airway, but once an object has passed through the vocal cords positive pressure from below the obstruction is most likely to be successful.

In older children, the Heimlich maneuver may be used. However, in children < 20 kg (typically < 5 yr), very moderate pressure should be applied, and the rescuer should kneel at the child's feet rather than astride.

In infants < 1 yr, the Heimlich maneuver should not be done. Infants should be held in a prone, head-down position. The rescuer should support the head with the fingers of one hand while delivering 5 back blows (see Fig. 69–4). Five chest thrusts should then be delivered with the infant in a head-down position with the infant's back on the rescuer's thigh (supine—see Fig. 69–5). This sequence of back blows and chest thrusts is repeated until the airway is cleared.

AIRWAY AND RESPIRATORY DEVICES

If no spontaneous respiration occurs after airway opening and no respiratory devices are available, rescue breathing (mouth-to-mask or mouth-to-barrier device) is started; mouth-to-mouth ventilation is rarely recommended. Exhaled air contains 16 to

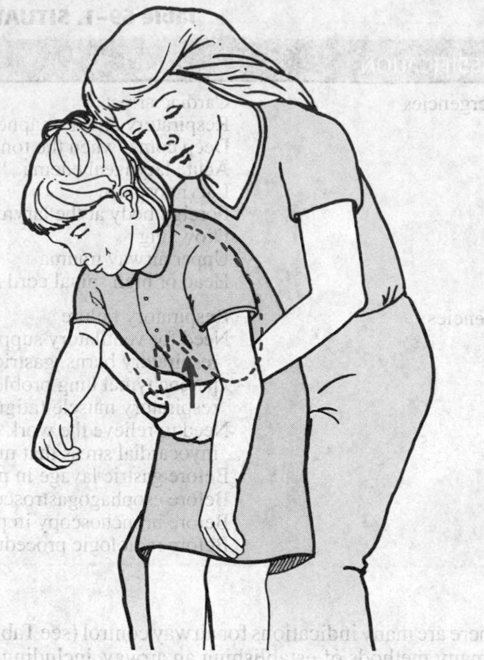

Fig. 69–3. Abdominal thrusts with victim standing or sitting (conscious).

18% oxygen and 4 to 5% carbon dioxide, which is adequate to maintain blood oxygen and carbon dioxide values close to normal. Larger-than-necessary volumes of air may cause gastric distention with associated risk of aspiration.

Bag-Valve-Mask (BVM) Devices

These devices consist of a self-inflating bag (resuscitator bag) with a nonrebreathing valve mechanism and a soft mask that conforms to the tissues of the face; when connected to an oxygen supply, they deliver from 60 to 100% inspired oxygen. In the hands of experienced practitioners, a BVM device provides adequate temporary ventilation in many situations, allow-

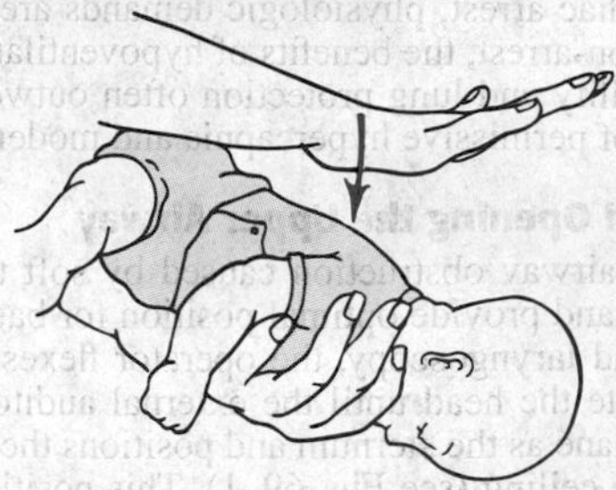

Fig. 69–4. Back blows—infant. Back blows are delivered with the infant in a head-down position to dislodge foreign bodies from the tracheobronchial tube. (Adapted from Standards and Guidelines for Cardiopulmonary Resuscitation [CPR] and Emergency Cardiac Care [ECC], in the *Journal of the American Medical Association* 25:2956 and 2959, June 6, 1986. Copyright 1986, American Medical Association.)

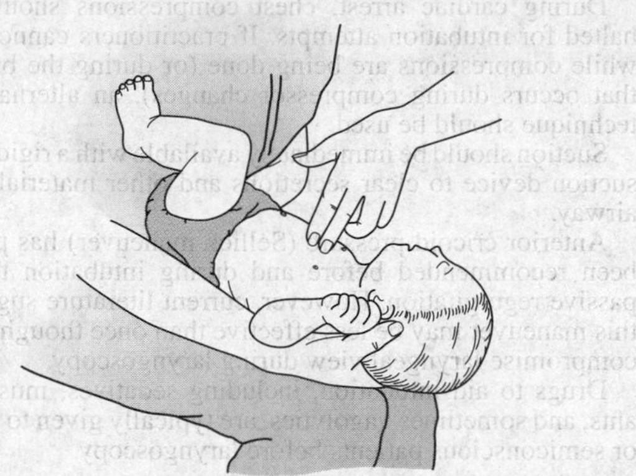

Fig. 69–5. Chest thrusts—infant. Chest thrusts are delivered on the lower half of the sternum, just below the nipple level.

ing time to systematically achieve definitive airway control. However, if BVM ventilation is used for > 5 min, air is typically introduced into the stomach, and an NGT should be inserted to evacuate the accumulated air.

BVM devices do not maintain airway patency, so patients with soft-tissue relaxation require careful positioning and manual maneuvers (see Figs. 69–1 and 69–2), as well as additional devices to keep the airway open.

An oropharyngeal airway or a nasopharyngeal airway may be used during BVM ventilation to keep soft tissues of the oropharynx from blocking the airway. These devices cause gagging and the potential for vomiting and aspiration in conscious patients and so should be used with caution.

Several methods are used to select the proper size oropharyngeal airway, the most common being the distance between the corner of the patient's mouth and the angle of the jaw.

Resuscitator bags are also used with artificial airways, including endotracheal tubes and supraglottic and pharyngeal airways. Pediatric bags have a pressure relief valve that limits peak airway pressures (usually to 35 to 45 cm water); practitioners must monitor the valve setting to avoid inadvertent hypoventilation. The relief valve can be shut off if necessary to provide sufficient pressure.

Laryngeal Mask Airways (LMAs)

A laryngeal mask airway or other supraglottic airway can be inserted into the lower oropharynx to prevent airway obstruction by soft tissues and to create an effective channel for ventilation (see Fig. 69–6). A variety of available LMAs allow passage of an endotracheal tube (ETT) or a gastric decompression tube. As the name implies, these devices seal the laryngeal inlet (rather than the face-mask interface) and thus avoid the difficulty of maintaining an adequate face-mask seal and the risk of displacing the jaw and tongue. LMAs have become the standard rescue ventilation technique for situations in which endotracheal intubation cannot be accomplished, as well as for certain elective anesthesia cases and emergencies. Complications include vomiting and aspiration in patients who have an intact gag reflex, who are receiving excessive ventilation, or both.

There are numerous techniques for LMA insertion. The standard approach is to press the deflated mask against the hard palate (using the long finger of the dominant hand) and rotate it past the base of the tongue until the mask reaches the hypopharynx so that the tip then sits in the upper esophagus. Once in the correct position, the mask is inflated. Inflating the mask with half the recommended volume before insertion stiffens the tip, possibly making insertion easier. Newer mask versions replace the inflatable cuff with a gel that molds to the airway.

Although a laryngeal mask airway does not isolate the airway from the esophagus as well as an ETT, it has some advantages over BVM ventilation:

- It minimizes gastric inflation
- It provides some protection against passive regurgitation

Newer versions of LMAs have an opening through which a small tube can be inserted to decompress the stomach.

The efficacy of the airway seal with an LMA, unlike ETTs, is not directly correlated with the mask inflation pressure. With ETTs, higher balloon pressure causes a tighter seal; with an LMA, overinflation makes the mask more rigid and *less* able to adapt to the patient's anatomy. If the seal is inadequate, mask pressure should be *lowered* somewhat; if this approach does not work, a larger mask size should be tried.

In emergencies, LMAs should be viewed as bridging devices. Prolonged placement, overinflation of the mask, or both may

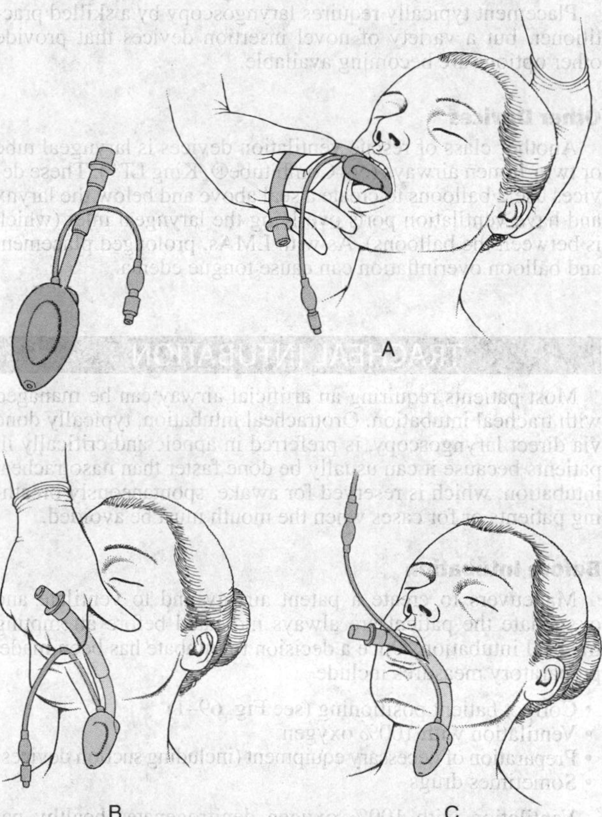

Fig. 69–6. Laryngeal mask airway (LMA). The LMA is a tube with an inflatable cuff that is inserted into the oropharynx. **A:** The deflated cuff is inserted into the mouth. **B:** With the index finger, the cuff is guided into place above the larynx. **C:** Once in place, the cuff is inflated. Some newer cuffs use a gel that molds to the airway rather than an inflatable cuff.

compress the tongue and cause tongue edema. Also, if noncomatose patients are given muscle relaxants before LMA insertion (eg, for laryngoscopy), they may gag and possibly aspirate when such drugs wear off. Either the device should be removed (assuming ventilation and gag reflexes are adequate), or drugs should be given to eliminate the gag response and provide time for an alternative intubation technique.

Endotracheal Tubes

An ETT is inserted directly into the trachea via the mouth or, less commonly, the nose. ETTs have high-volume, low-pressure balloon cuffs to prevent air leakage and minimize the risk of aspiration. Cuffed tubes were traditionally used only in adults and children > 8 yr; however, cuffed tubes are increasingly being used in infants and younger children to limit air leakage or aspiration (particularly during transport). Sometimes cuffs are not inflated or inflated only to the extent needed to prevent obvious leakage.

An ETT is the definitive method to secure a compromised airway, limit aspiration, and initiate mechanical ventilation in comatose patients, in patients who cannot protect their own airways, and in patients who need prolonged mechanical ventilation. An ETT also permits suctioning of the lower respiratory tract. Although drugs can be delivered via an ETT during cardiac arrest, this practice is discouraged.

Placement typically requires laryngoscopy by a skilled practitioner, but a variety of novel insertion devices that provide other options are becoming available.

Other Devices

Another class of rescue ventilation devices is laryngeal tube or twin-lumen airways (eg, Combitube®, King LT®). These devices use 2 balloons to create a seal above and below the larynx and have ventilation ports overlying the laryngeal inlet (which is between the balloons). As with LMAs, prolonged placement and balloon overinflation can cause tongue edema.

TRACHEAL INTUBATION

Most patients requiring an artificial airway can be managed with tracheal intubation. Orotracheal intubation, typically done via direct laryngoscopy, is preferred in apneic and critically ill patients because it can usually be done faster than nasotracheal intubation, which is reserved for awake, spontaneously breathing patients or for cases when the mouth must be avoided.

Before Intubation

Maneuvers to create a patent airway and to ventilate and oxygenate the patient are always indicated before attempting tracheal intubation. Once a decision to intubate has been made, preparatory measures include

- Correct patient positioning (see Fig. 69–1)
- Ventilation with 100% oxygen
- Preparation of necessary equipment (including suction devices)
- Sometimes drugs

Ventilation with 100% oxygen denitrogenates healthy patients and significantly prolongs the safe apneic time (effect is less in patients with severe cardiopulmonary disorders).

Strategies to predict difficult laryngoscopy (eg, Mallampati scoring, thyromental distance testing) are of limited value in emergencies. Practitioners should always be prepared to use an alternate technique (eg, laryngeal mask airway, BVM ventilation, surgical airway) if laryngoscopy does not work.

During cardiac arrest, chest compressions should not be halted for intubation attempts. If practitioners cannot intubate while compressions are being done (or during the brief pause that occurs during compressor changes), an alternate airway technique should be used.

Suction should be immediately available with a rigid tonsil-tip suction device to clear secretions and other material from the airway.

Anterior cricoid pressure (Sellick maneuver) has previously been recommended before and during intubation to prevent passive regurgitation. However, current literature suggests that this maneuver may be less effective than once thought and may compromise laryngeal view during laryngoscopy.

Drugs to aid intubation, including sedatives, muscle relaxants, and sometimes vagolytics, are typically given to conscious or semiconscious patients before laryngoscopy.

Tube Selection and Preparation for Intubation

Most adults can accept a tube with an internal diameter of ≥ 8 mm; these tubes are preferable to smaller ones because they

- Have lower airflow resistance (reducing the work of breathing)
- Facilitate suctioning of secretions
- Allow passage of a bronchoscope
- May aid in liberation from mechanical ventilation

For infants and children ≥ 1 yr, uncuffed tube size is calculated by (patient's age + 16)/4; thus, a 4-yr-old should have a $(4 + 16)/4 = 5$ mm ETT. The tube size suggested by this formula should be reduced by 0.5 (1 tube size) if a cuffed tube is to be used. Reference charts (see Table 68-4 on p. 549) or devices such as the Broselow pediatric emergency tape or Pedi-Wheel can rapidly identify appropriate-sized laryngoscope blades and ETTs for infants and children.

For adults (and sometimes in children), a rigid stylet should be placed in the tube, taking care to stop the stylet 1 to 2 cm before the distal end of the ETT, so that the tube tip remains soft. The stylet should then be used to make the tube straight to the beginning of the distal cuff; from that point, the tube is bent upward about 35° to form a hockey stick shape. This straight-to-cuff shape improves tube delivery and avoids blocking the operator's view of the vocal cords during tube passage. Routinely filling the distal ETT cuff with air to check the balloon is not required; if this technique is used, care must be taken to remove all the air before tube insertion.

Insertion Technique for Intubation

Successful intubation on the first attempt is important. Repeated laryngoscopy (≥ 3 attempts) is associated with much higher rates of significant hypoxemia, aspiration, and cardiac arrest. In addition to correct positioning, several other general principles are critical for success:

- Visualizing the epiglottis
- Visualizing the posterior laryngeal structures (ideally, the vocal cords)
- Not passing the tube unless tracheal insertion is ensured

The laryngoscope is held in the left hand, and the blade is inserted into the mouth and used as a retractor to displace the mandible and tongue up and away from the laryngoscopist, revealing the posterior pharynx. Avoiding contact with the incisors and not placing undue pressure on laryngeal structures are important.

The importance of identifying the epiglottis cannot be overstated. Identifying the epiglottis allows the operator to recognize critical airway landmarks and correctly position the laryngoscope blade. The epiglottis may rest against the posterior pharyngeal wall, where it blends in with the other pink mucus membranes or gets lost in the pool of secretions that invariably exists in the cardiac arrest patient's airway.

Once the epiglottis is found, the operator may pick it up with the tip of the blade (the typical straight blade approach) or advance the tip of the blade into the vallecula, pressing against the hyoepiglottic ligament, to indirectly lift the epiglottis up and out of the line of sight (the typical curved blade approach). Success with the curved blade depends on the proper positioning of the blade tip in the vallecula and the direction of the lifting force (see Fig. 69–7). Lifting the epiglottis by either technique reveals the posterior laryngeal structures (arytenoid cartilages, interarytenoid notch), glottis, and vocal cords. If the tip of the blade is too deep, laryngeal landmarks may be entirely bypassed, and the dark, round hole of the esophagus may be mistaken for the glottis opening.

If identifying structures is difficult, manipulating the larynx with the right hand placed on the anterior neck (allowing the right and left hands to work together) may optimize the laryngeal view (see Fig. 69–7). Another technique involves lifting the head higher (lifting at the occiput, not atlanto-occipital extension), which distracts the jaw and improves the line of sight. Head elevation is inadvisable in patients with potential cervical spine injury and is difficult in the morbidly obese (who must be placed in a ramped or head-elevated position beforehand).

In an optimal view, the vocal cords are clearly seen. If the vocal cords are not seen, at a minimum, the posterior laryngeal landmarks must be viewed and the tip of the tube must be seen passing above the interarytenoid notch and posterior cartilages. Operators must clearly identify laryngeal landmarks to avoid potentially fatal esophageal intubation. If operators are not confident that the tube is going into the trachea, the tube should not be inserted.

Oncc an optimal view has been achieved, the right hand inserts the tube through the larynx into the trachea (if operators have been applying anterior laryngeal pressure with the right hand, an assistant should continue applying this pressure). If the tube does not pass easily, a 90° clockwise twist of the tube may help it pass more smoothly over the anterior tracheal rings. Before withdrawing the laryngoscope, operators should

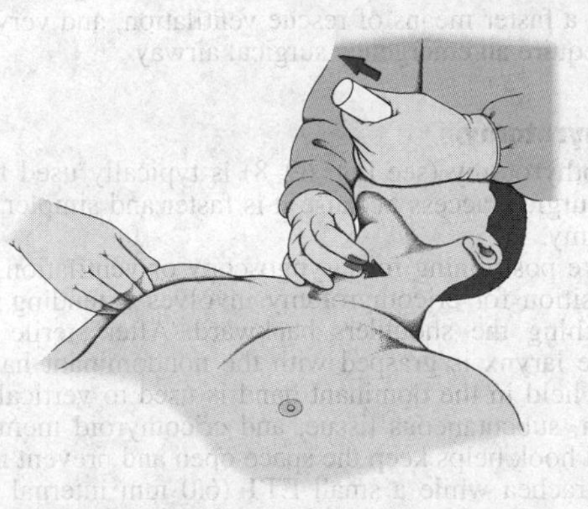

Fig. 69–7. Bimanual laryngoscopy. Pressure is applied on the neck opposite the direction of lift of the laryngoscope. Arrows show the direction for lift of the laryngoscope and for anterior neck pressure.

confirm that the tube is passing between the cords. Appropriate tube depth is usually 21 to 23 cm in adults and 3 times the ETT size in children (for a 4.0-mm ETT, 12 cm; for a 5.5-mm ETT, 16.5 cm). In adults, the tube, if inadvertently advanced, typically migrates into the right mainstem bronchus.

Alternative Intubation Devices

A number of devices and techniques are increasingly used for intubation after failed laryngoscopy or as a primary means of intubation. Devices include

- Video laryngoscopes
- Mirror laryngoscopes
- LMAs with a passage that allows tracheal intubation
- Fiberoptic scopes and optical stylets
- Tube introducers

Each device has its own subtleties; practitioners who are skilled in standard laryngoscopic intubation techniques should not assume they can use one of these devices (especially after use of muscle relaxants) without becoming thoroughly familiarized with it.

Video and mirror laryngoscopes enable practitioners to look around the curvature of the tongue and usually provide excellent laryngeal views. However, the tube requires an exaggerated bend angle to go around the tongue and thus may be more difficult to manipulate and insert.

To pass an ETT through a laryngeal mask airway, practitioners must understand how to optimally position the mask over the laryngeal inlet; there are sometimes mechanical difficulties passing the ETT.

Flexible fiberoptic scopes and optical stylets are very maneuverable and can be used in patients with abnormal anatomy. However, practice is required to recognize laryngeal landmarks from a fiberoptic perspective. Compared with video and mirror laryngoscopes, fiberoptic scopes are more difficult to master and are more susceptible to problems with blood and secretions; also, they do not separate and divide tissue but instead must be moved through open channels.

Tube introducers (commonly called gum elastic bougies) are semirigid stylets that can be used when laryngeal visualization is suboptimal (eg, the epiglottis is visible, but the laryngeal opening is not). In such cases, the introducer is passed along the undersurface of the epiglottis; from this point, it is likely to enter the trachea. Tracheal entry is suggested by the tactile feedback, noted as the tip bounces over the tracheal rings. An ETT is then advanced over the introducer. During passage over a tube introducer or bronchoscope, the tube tip sometimes catches the right aryepiglottic fold. Rotating the tube 90° counterclockwise often frees the ETT tip and allows it to pass smoothly.

Postinsertion

The stylet is removed and the balloon cuff is inflated with air using a 10-mL syringe; a manometer is used to verify that balloon pressure is < 30 cm water. Properly sized ETTs may need considerably < 10 mL of air to create the correct pressure.

After balloon inflation, tube placement should be checked using a variety of methods, including

- Inspection and auscultation
- Carbon dioxide detection
- Esophageal detector devices
- Sometimes chest x-ray

When a tube is correctly placed, manual ventilation should produce symmetric chest rise, good breath sounds over both lungs, and no gurgling over the upper abdomen.

Exhaled air should contain carbon dioxide and gastric air should not; detecting carbon dioxide with a colorimetric end-tidal carbon dioxide device or waveform capnography confirms tracheal placement. However, in prolonged cardiac arrest (ie, with little or no metabolic activity), carbon dioxide may not be detectable even with correct tube placement. In such cases, an esophageal detector device may be used. These devices use an inflatable bulb or a large syringe to apply negative pressure to the ETT. The flexible esophagus collapses, and little or no air flows into the device; in contrast, the rigid trachea does not collapse, and the resultant airflow confirms tracheal placement.

In the absence of cardiac arrest, tube placement is typically also confirmed with a chest x-ray.

After correct placement is confirmed, the tube should be secured using a commercially available device or adhesive tape. Adapters connect the ETT to a resuscitator bag, T-piece supplying humidity and oxygen, or a mechanical ventilator.

ETTs can be displaced, particularly in chaotic resuscitation situations, so tube position should be rechecked frequently. If breath sounds are absent on the left, right mainstem bronchus intubation is probably more likely than a left-sided tension pneumothorax, but both should be considered.

Nasotracheal Intubation

If patients are spontaneously breathing, this technique can be used in certain emergency situations—eg, when patients have severe oral or cervical disorders (eg, injuries, edema, limitation of motion) that make laryngoscopy difficult. Historically, nasal intubation was also used when muscle relaxants were unavailable or forbidden (eg, prehospital settings, certain emergency departments) and when patients with tachypnea, hyperpnea, and upright positioning (eg, those with heart failure) might literally inhale a tube. However, availability of noninvasive means of ventilation (eg, bilevel positive airway pressure [BiPAP]), improved access to and training in pharmacologic adjuncts to intubation, and newer airway devices have markedly decreased the use of nasal intubation. Additional considerations are problems with nasal intubation, including sinusitis (universal after 3 days), and the fact that tubes large enough to permit bronchoscopy (eg, ≥ 8 mm) can rarely be inserted nasotracheally.

When nasotracheal intubation is done, a vasoconstrictor (eg, phenylephrine) and topical anesthetic (eg, benzocaine, lidocaine) must be applied to the nasal mucosa and the larynx to prevent bleeding and to blunt protective reflexes. Some patients may also require IV sedatives, opioids, or dissociative drugs. After the nasal mucosa is prepared, a soft nasopharyngeal airway should be inserted to ensure adequate patency of the selected nasal passage and to serve as a conduit for topical drugs to the pharynx and larynx. The nasopharyngeal airway may be placed using a plain or anesthetic (eg, lidocaine) lubricant. The nasopharyngeal airway is removed after the pharyngeal mucosa has been sprayed.

The nasotracheal tube is then inserted to about 14 cm depth (just above the laryngeal inlet in most adults); at this point, air movement should be audible. As the patient breathes in, opening the vocal cords, the tube is promptly passed into the trachea. A failed initial insertion attempt often prompts the patient to cough. Practitioners should anticipate this event, which allows a second opportunity to pass the tube through a wide open glottis. More flexible ETTs with a controllable tip improve likelihood of success. Some practitioners soften tubes by placing them in warm water to lessen the risk of bleeding and make insertion easier. A small commercially available whistle can also be attached to the proximal tube connector to accentuate the noise of air movement when the tube is in the correct position above the larynx and in the trachea.

Complications of Tracheal Intubation

Complications include

- Direct trauma
- Esophageal intubation
- Tracheal erosion or stenosis

Laryngoscopy can damage lips, teeth, tongue, and supraglottic and subglottic areas.

Tube placement in the esophagus, if unrecognized, causes failure to ventilate and potentially death or hypoxic injury. Insufflating a tube in the esophagus causes regurgitation, which can result in aspiration, compromise subsequent bag mask valve ventilation, and obscure visualization in subsequent intubation attempts.

Any translaryngeal tube injures the vocal cords somewhat; sometimes ulceration, ischemia, and prolonged cord paralysis occur. Subglottic stenosis can occur later (usually 3 to 4 wk).

Erosion of the trachea is uncommon. It results more commonly from excessively high cuff pressure. Rarely, hemorrhage from major vessels (eg, innominate artery), fistulas (especially tracheoesophageal), and tracheal stenosis occur. Using high-volume, low-pressure cuffs with tubes of appropriate size and measuring cuff pressure frequently (every 8 h) to maintain it at < 30 cm water decrease the risk of ischemic pressure necrosis, but patients in shock, with low cardiac output, or with sepsis remain especially vulnerable.

SURGICAL AIRWAY

If the upper airway is obstructed because of a foreign body or massive trauma or if ventilation cannot be accomplished by other means, surgical entry into the trachea is required. Historically, a surgical airway was also the response to failed intubation. However, surgical airways require on average about 100 sec from initial incision to ventilation; LMAs and other devices provide a faster means of rescue ventilation, and very few patients require an emergency surgical airway.

Cricothyrotomy

Cricothyrotomy (see Fig. 69–8) is typically used for emergency surgical access because it is faster and simpler than tracheostomy.

Unlike positioning for laryngoscopy or ventilation, the correct position for cricothyrotomy involves extending the neck and arching the shoulders backward. After sterile preparation, the larynx is grasped with the nondominant hand while a blade held in the dominant hand is used to vertically incise the skin, subcutaneous tissue, and cricothyroid membrane. A tracheal hook helps keep the space open and prevent retraction of the trachea while a small ETT (6.0 mm internal diameter [ID]) or small tracheotomy tube (cuffed 4.0 Shiley preferred) is advanced through the surgical site into the trachea.

Complications include hemorrhage, subcutaneous emphysema, pneumomediastinum, and pneumothorax. Various commercial products allow rapid surgical access to the cricothyroid

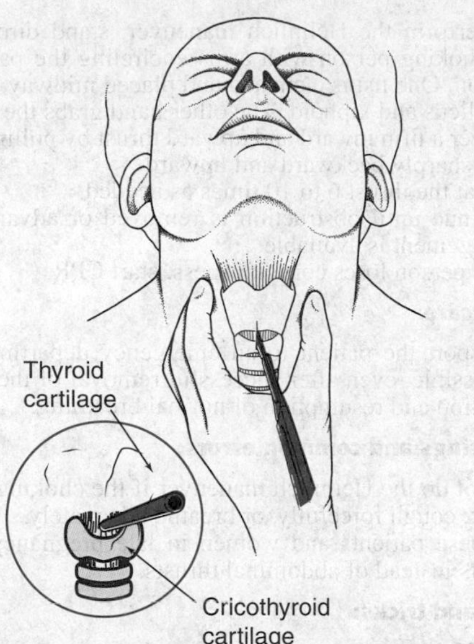

Fig. 69–8. Emergency cricothyrotomy. The patient lies supine with the neck extended. After sterile preparation, the larynx is grasped with one hand while a blade is used to incise the skin, subcutaneous tissue, and cricothyroid membrane precisely in the midline, accessing the trachea. A hollow tube is used to keep the airway open.

space and provide a tube that allows adequate oxygenation and ventilation. Contrary to prior recommendations, needle cricothyrotomy with large bore IV catheters cannot provide adequate ventilation unless a 50-psi driving source (jet insufflator or jet ventilator) is readily available.

Tracheostomy

Tracheostomy is a more complex procedure because the trachea rings are very close together and part of at least one ring usually must be removed to allow tube placement. Tracheostomy is preferably done in an operating room by a surgeon. In emergencies, the procedure has a higher rate of complications than cricothyrotomy and offers no advantage. However, it is the preferred procedure for patients requiring long-term ventilation.

Percutaneous tracheostomy is an attractive alternative for mechanically ventilated, critically ill patients. This bedside technique uses skin puncture and dilators to insert a tracheostomy tube. Fiberoptic assistance (within the trachea) is usually used to prevent puncture of the membranous (posterior) trachea and esophagus.

Rarely, tracheostomy insertion causes hemorrhage, thyroid damage, pneumothorax, recurrent laryngeal nerve paralysis, injury to major vessels, or late tracheal stenosis at the insertion site.

Erosion of the trachea is uncommon. It results more commonly from excessively high cuff pressure. Rarely, hemorrhage from major vessels (eg, innominate artery), fistulas (especially tracheoesophageal), and tracheal stenosis occur. Using high-volume, low-pressure cuffs with tubes of appropriate size and measuring cuff pressure frequently (every 8 h) to maintain it at < 30 cm water decrease the risk of ischemic pressure necrosis, but patients in shock, with low cardiac output, or with sepsis remain especially vulnerable.

DRUGS TO AID INTUBATION

Pulseless and apneic or severely obtunded patients can (and should) be intubated without pharmacologic assistance. Other patients are given sedating and paralytic drugs to minimize discomfort and facilitate intubation (termed rapid sequence intubation).

Pretreatment before intubation: Pretreatment typically includes

- 100% oxygen
- Lidocaine
- Sometimes atropine, a neuromuscular blocker, or both

If time permits, patients should be placed on 100% oxygen for 3 to 5 min; this measure may maintain satisfactory oxygenation in previously healthy patients for up to 8 min. However, oxygen demand and safe apnea times are very dependent on pulse rate, pulmonary function, RBC count, and numerous other metabolic factors.

Laryngoscopy causes a sympathetic-mediated pressor response with an increase in heart rate, BP, and possibly intracranial pressure. To blunt this response, when time permits, some practitioners give lidocaine 1.5 mg/kg IV 1 to 2 min before sedation and paralysis.

Children and adolescents often have a vagal response (marked bradycardia) in response to intubation and are given atropine 0.02 mg/kg IV (minimum: 0.1 mg in infants, 0.5 mg in children and adolescents) at the same time.

Some physicians include a small dose of a neuromuscular blocker (NMB), such as vecuronium 0.01 mg/kg IV, in patients > 4 yr to prevent muscle fasciculations caused by full doses of succinylcholine. Fasciculations may result in muscle pain on awakening and cause transient hyperkalemia; however, the actual benefit of such pretreatment is unclear.

Sedation and analgesia for intubation: Laryngoscopy and intubation are uncomfortable; in conscious patients, a short-acting IV drug with sedative or combined sedative and analgesic properties is mandatory.

Etomidate 0.3 mg/kg, a nonbarbiturate hypnotic, may be the preferred drug. Fentanyl 5 mcg/kg (2 to 5 mcg/kg in children; NOTE: this dose is higher than the analgesic dose) also works well and causes no cardiovascular depression. Fentanyl is an opioid and thus has analgesic as well as sedative properties. However, at higher doses, chest wall rigidity may occur. Ketamine 1 to 2 mg/kg is a dissociative anesthetic with cardiostimulatory properties. It is generally safe but may cause hallucinations or bizarre behavior on awakening. Thiopental 3 to 4 mg/kg and methohexital 1 to 2 mg/kg are effective but tend to cause hypotension and are used less often.

Drugs to cause paralysis for intubation: Skeletal muscle relaxation with an IV NMB markedly facilitates intubation.

Succinylcholine (1.5 mg/kg IV, 2.0 mg/kg for infants), a depolarizing NMB, has the most rapid onset (30 sec to 1 min) and shortest duration (3 to 5 min). It should be avoided in patients with burns, muscle crush injuries > 1 to 2 days old, spinal cord injury, neuromuscular disease, renal failure, or possibly penetrating eye injury. About 1/15,000 children (and fewer adults) have a genetic susceptibility to malignant hyperthermia due to succinylcholine. Succinylcholine should always be given with atropine in children because pronounced bradycardia may occur.

Alternative nondepolarizing NMBs have longer duration of action (> 30 min) but also have slower onset unless used in high doses that prolong paralysis significantly. Drugs include atracurium 0.5 mg/kg, mivacurium 0.15 mg/kg, rocuronium 1.0 mg/kg, and vecuronium 0.1 to 0.2 mg/kg injected over 60 sec.

Topical anesthesia for intubation: Intubation of an awake patient (typically not done in children) requires anesthesia of the nose and pharynx. A commercial aerosol preparation of benzocaine, tetracaine, butyl aminobenzoate (butamben), and benzalkonium is commonly used. Alternatively, 4% lidocaine can be nebulized and inhaled via face mask.

HOW TO DO THE HEIMLICH MANEUVER IN THE CONSCIOUS ADULT

(Abdominal Thrusts; Subdiaphragmatic Abdominal Thrusts)

The Heimlich maneuver is a rapid first aid procedure to treat choking due to upper airway obstruction by foreign objects such as food, a toy, or other object.

Indications:

- Choking due to severe upper airway obstruction due to a foreign object. Choking is signaled by inability to speak, cough, or breathe adequately.

The Heimlich maneuver should only be used when the airway obstruction is severe and life is endangered. Do not interfere if the choking person can speak, cough forcefully, or breathe adequately.

Contraindications: Absolute contraindications:

- Age < 1 yr

Relative contraindications:

- Children < 20 kg (typically < 5 yr) should receive only moderate pressure thrusts.
- Obese patients and women in late pregnancy should receive chest thrusts instead of abdominal thrusts.

Complications:

- Rib injury or fracture
- Internal organ injury

Equipment:

- None

Additional considerations:

- This rapid first aid procedure is done immediately wherever the person is choking.

Positioning:

- In general, the rescuer is standing behind the choking person.
- For children < 20 kg (typically < 5 yr), the rescuer should kneel at the child's feet rather than stand astride them.

Relevant anatomy:

- The vocal cords in the larynx protect the airway. Food and foreign objects that are aspirated and cause severe airway obstruction are usually stopped at this level.

Step-by-step description of procedures and key teaching points:

- Determine if there is severe airway obstruction, which may endanger the person's life. Look for signs of severe airway obstruction such as inability to speak, cough, or breathe adequately.
- Look for hands clutching the throat, which is the Universal Distress Signal of severe airway obstruction.
- Ask: "Are you choking?" If the choking person nods yes and cannot speak, cough, or breathe adequately, that suggests severe airway obstruction and the need for assistance.
- To perform the Heimlich maneuver, stand directly behind the choking person with arms encircling the patient's midsection. One fist is clenched and placed midway between the umbilicus and xiphoid. The other hand grabs the fist.
- Deliver a firm inward and upward thrust by pulling with both arms sharply backward and upward.
- Repeat the thrust 6 to 10 times as needed.
- Continue until obstruction is removed or advanced airway management is available.
- If the person loses consciousness, start CPR.

Aftercare:

- Transport the patient to an emergency department as soon as possible, even after successful removal of the airway obstruction and resumption of normal breathing.

Warnings and common errors:

- Do not do the Heimlich maneuver if the choking person can speak, cough forcefully, or breathe adequately.
- In obese patients and women in late pregnancy, use chest thrusts instead of abdominal thrusts.

Tips and tricks:

- The Heimlich maneuver may induce vomiting. Although vomiting may assist in dislodging a tracheal foreign body, it does not necessarily mean that the airway has been cleared.

Reference: American Heart Association: Basic Life Support (BLS) Provider Manual. Dallas, American Heart Association, 2016.

HOW TO TREAT THE CHOKING CONSCIOUS INFANT

Choking in an infant is usually caused by inhaling a small object the baby has placed in their mouth, such as food, a toy, or other small object (eg, a button, coin, or balloon). If the airway obstruction is severe, then back blows followed by chest thrusts are administered to dislodge the object.

Indications:

- Choking due to severe upper airway obstruction due to a foreign object.

A choking infant with severe airway obstruction, as indicated by the following:

- Cyanosis
- Retractions
- Inability to cry or make much sound
- Weak, ineffective coughing
- Stridor

Do not interfere if the infant can cry and make significant sounds, cough effectively, or breathe adequately, as they do not have severe airway obstruction. Furthermore, strong coughs and cries can help push the object out of the airway.

Contraindications: Absolute contraindications:

- Do not do back blows or chest thrusts if the infant stops breathing for reasons other than an obstructed airway such as asthma, infection, swelling, or a blow to the head.

Relative contraindications:

- None

Complications:

- Rib injury or fracture
- Internal organ injury

Equipment:

- None

Additional considerations:

- This rapid first aid procedure is done immediately whenever the infant is choking.

Positioning:

- For back blows, hold the infant face down along your forearm using the thigh or lap for support. Hold the infant's chest in your hand and the jaw with your fingers. Point the infant's head downward and lower than the body.
- For chest thrusts, hold the infant facing upward and with the head down, along your forearm, using the thigh or lap for support. Hold the infant's head in your hand.

Relevant anatomy:

- The vocal cords in the larynx protect the airway. Food and foreign objects that are aspirated and cause upper airway obstruction are usually stopped at this level.
- In infants and children, the cricoid cartilage is the most narrow part of the upper airway. Objects can become trapped between the vocal cords and the cricoid ring, resulting in an obstruction that is particularly difficult to clear.

Step-by-step description of procedures and key teaching points:

- Determine if there is severe airway obstruction which may endanger the infant's life. Look for signs of severe airway obstruction such as the inability to cry audibly, cough effectively, or breathe adequately (eg, stridor, retractions, cyanosis).
- If the infant has a strong cry or is coughing hard, do not perform these procedures. If you have determined that the infant has severe airway obstruction, proceed with the following procedures.
- Tell someone to call 911 while you begin first aid. If you are alone, shout for help and begin first aid.
- Hold the infant's face down along your forearm using the thigh or lap for support. Hold the infant's chest in your hand and open the jaw by pulling the mandible with your fingers. Point the infant's head downward and lower than the body.
- Give up to 5 quick, forceful back blows between the infant's shoulder blades using the palm of your free hand.
- Check the mouth to see whether the aspirated foreign body is visible; if it can be easily removed, remove it.
- If the object does not come out of the airway after 5 back blows, turn the infant face-up.
- Hold the infant face-up along your forearm using the thigh or lap for support. Hold the head in your hand with the head lower than the torso.
- Place 2 fingers on the middle of the infant's sternum just below the nipples. Avoid the lower ribs or the tip of the sternum.
- Give up to 5 quick thrusts, compressing the chest about 1/3 to ½ the depth of the chest—usually about 1.5 to 4 cm (0.5 to 1.5 inches) for each thrust.
- Continue to deliver 5 back blows followed by 5 chest thrusts until the object is dislodged or the infant becomes unconscious.
- Do not try to grasp and pull out the object if the infant is conscious.
- If the infant becomes unresponsive (unconscious), shout for help and begin infant CPR. If you are alone, after 1 minute of CPR call 911.
- If the infant is unconscious, if you can see the object blocking the airway, try to remove it with a finger. Try to remove the object only if you can see it.

Aftercare:

- The infant should be examined by a physician as soon as possible, even after successful removal of the airway obstruction and resumption of normal breathing.

Warnings and common errors:

- Do not do back blows or chest thrusts if the choking infant can cry audibly, cough forcefully, or breathe adequately.
- Do not do back blows or chest thrusts if the infant stops breathing for reasons other than an obstructed airway (eg, asthma, infection, angioedema, head injury). Do give CPR in these cases.
- Do not perform blind finger sweeps on infants.
- Do not perform abdominal thrusts (Heimlich maneuver) on infants.

Tips and tricks:

- It is important to use gravity as an ally. Keep the infant's head lower than its torso during the procedure.

Reference: American Heart Association: Basic Life Support (BLS) Provider Manual. Dallas, American Heart Association, 2016.

70 Respiratory Failure and Mechanical Ventilation

Respiratory failure is a life-threatening impairment of oxygenation, CO_2 elimination, or both. Respiratory failure may occur because of impaired gas exchange, decreased ventilation, or both. Common manifestations include dyspnea, use of accessory muscles of respiration, tachypnea, tachycardia, diaphoresis, cyanosis, altered consciousness, and, without treatment, eventually obtundation, respiratory arrest, and death. Diagnosis is clinical, supplemented by ABGs and chest x-ray. Treatment is usually in an ICU and involves correction of the underlying cause, supplemental O_2, control of secretions, and ventilatory assistance if needed.

The respiratory system oxygenates and eliminates CO_2 from venous blood. Thus, a useful classification of respiratory failure is whether the principal abnormality is inadequate oxygenation or inadequate CO_2 elimination (which means inadequate ventilation), although many disorders affect both. Although temporizing measures exist, respiratory failure frequently necessitates mechanical ventilation.

OVERVIEW OF MECHANICAL VENTILATION

Mechanical ventilation can be noninvasive, involving various types of face masks, or invasive, involving endotracheal intubation. Selection and use of appropriate techniques require an understanding of respiratory mechanics.

Indications: There are numerous indications for endotracheal intubation and mechanical ventilation (see Table 69–1 on p. 551), but, in general, mechanical ventilation should be considered when there are clinical or laboratory signs that the patient cannot maintain an airway or adequate oxygenation or ventilation. Concerning findings include respiratory rate > 30/min, inability to maintain arterial O_2 saturation > 90% with fractional inspired O_2 (FIO_2) >0.60, and $PaCO_2$ > 50 mm Hg with pH < 7.25. The decision to initiate mechanical ventilation should be based on clinical judgment that considers the entire clinical situation and should not be delayed until the patient is in extremis.

Respiratory Mechanics

Normal inspiration generates negative intrapleural pressure, which creates a pressure gradient between the atmosphere and the alveoli, resulting in air inflow. In mechanical ventilation, the pressure gradient results from increased (positive) pressure of the air source.

Peak airway pressure is measured at the airway opening (Pao) and is routinely displayed by mechanical ventilators. It represents the total pressure needed to push a volume of gas into the lung and is composed of pressures resulting from inspiratory flow resistance (resistive pressure), the elastic recoil of the lung and chest wall (elastic pressure), and the alveolar pressure present at the beginning of the breath (positive end-expiratory pressure [PEEP]—see Fig. 70–1). Thus

Peak airway pressure = resistive pressure + elastic pressure + PEEP

Resistive pressure is the product of circuit resistance and airflow. In the mechanically ventilated patient, resistance to airflow occurs in the ventilator circuit, the endotracheal tube, and, most importantly, the patient's airways. NOTE: Even when these factors are constant, an increase in airflow increases resistive pressure.

Elastic pressure is the product of the elastic recoil of the lungs and chest wall (elastance) and the volume of gas delivered. For a given volume, elastic pressure is increased by increased lung stiffness (as in pulmonary fibrosis) or restricted excursion of the chest wall or diaphragm (eg, in tense ascites or massive obesity). Because elastance is the inverse of compliance, high elastance is the same as low compliance.

End-expiratory pressure in the alveoli is normally the same as atmospheric pressure. However, when the alveoli fail to empty completely because of airway obstruction, airflow limitation, or shortened expiratory time, end-expiratory pressure may be positive relative to the atmosphere. This pressure is called intrinsic PEEP or autoPEEP to differentiate it from externally applied (therapeutic) PEEP, which is created by adjusting the mechanical ventilator or by placing a tight-fitting mask that applies positive pressure throughout the respiratory cycle.

Any elevation in peak airway pressure (eg, > 25 cm H_2O) should prompt measurement of the end-inspiratory pressure (plateau pressure) by an end-inspiratory hold maneuver to determine the relative contributions of resistive and elastic pressures. The maneuver keeps the exhalation valve closed for an additional 0.3 to 0.5 sec after inspiration, delaying exhalation. During this time, airway pressure falls from its peak value as airflow ceases. The resulting end-inspiratory pressure represents

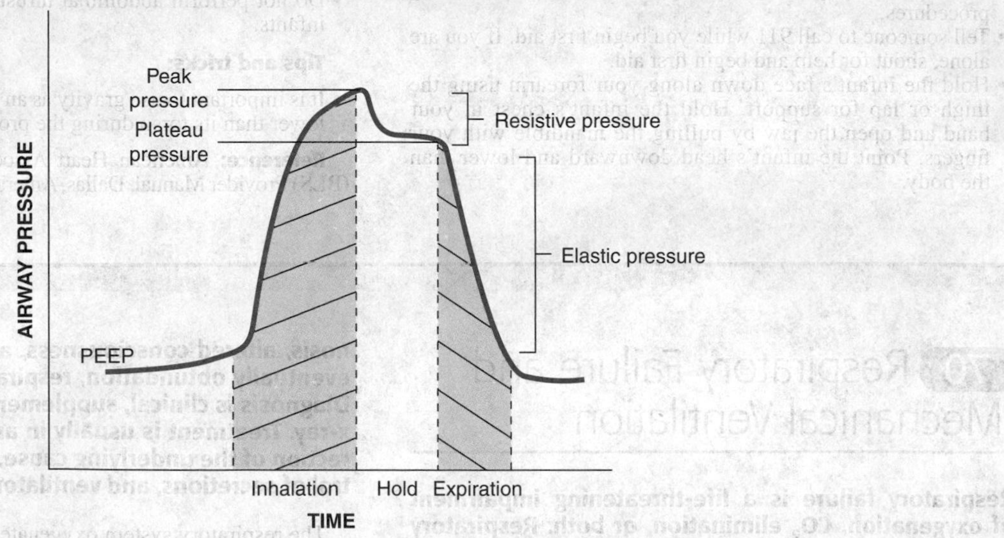

Fig. 70–1. Components of airway pressure during mechanical ventilation, illustrated by an inspiratory-hold maneuver. PEEP = positive end-expiratory pressure.

the elastic pressure once PEEP is subtracted (assuming the patient is not making active inspiratory or expiratory muscle contractions at the time of measurement). The difference between peak and plateau pressure is the resistive pressure.

Elevated resistive pressure (eg, > 10 cm H_2O) suggests that the endotracheal tube has been kinked or plugged with secretions or that an intraluminal mass or bronchospasm is present. An increase in elastic pressure (eg, > 10 cm H_2O) suggests decreased lung compliance due to edema, fibrosis, or lobar atelectasis; large pleural effusions, pneumothorax or fibrothorax; extrapulmonary restriction as may result from circumferential burns or other chest wall deformity, ascites, pregnancy, or massive obesity; or a tidal volume too large for the amount of lung being ventilated (eg, a normal tidal volume being delivered to a single lung because the endotracheal tube is malpositioned).

Intrinsic PEEP can be measured in the passive patient through an end-expiratory hold maneuver. Immediately before a breath, the expiratory port is closed for 2 sec. Flow ceases, eliminating resistive pressure; the resulting pressure reflects alveolar pressure at the end of expiration (intrinsic PEEP). Although accurate measurement depends on the patient being completely passive on the ventilator, it is unwarranted to use neuromuscular blockade solely for the purpose of measuring intrinsic PEEP. A nonquantitative method of identifying intrinsic PEEP is to inspect the expiratory flow tracing. If expiratory flow continues until the next breath or the patient's chest fails to come to rest before the next breath, intrinsic PEEP is present. The consequences of elevated intrinsic PEEP include increased inspiratory work of breathing and decreased venous return, which may result in decreased cardiac output and hypotension.

The demonstration of intrinsic PEEP should prompt a search for causes of airflow obstruction (eg, airway secretions, decreased elastic recoil, bronchospasm); however, a high minute ventilation (> 20 L/min) alone can result in intrinsic PEEP in a patient with no airflow obstruction. If the cause is airflow limitation, intrinsic PEEP can be reduced by shortening inspiratory time (ie, increasing inspiratory flow) or reducing the respiratory rate, thereby allowing a greater fraction of the respiratory cycle to be spent in exhalation.

Means and Modes of Mechanical Ventilation

Mechanical ventilators are set to deliver a constant volume (volume cycled), a constant pressure (pressure cycled), or a combination of both with each breath. Modes of ventilation that maintain a minimum respiratory rate regardless of whether or not the patient initiates a spontaneous breath are referred to as assist-control (A/C). Because pressures and volumes are directly linked by the pressure-volume curve, any given volume will correspond to a specific pressure, and vice versa, regardless of whether the ventilator is pressure or volume cycled.

Adjustable ventilator settings differ with mode but include respiratory rate, tidal volume, trigger sensitivity, flow rate, waveform, and inspiratory/expiratory (I/E) ratio.

Volume-cycled ventilation: In this mode, which includes volume-control (V/C) and synchronized intermittent mandatory ventilation (SIMV), the ventilator delivers a set tidal volume. The resultant airway pressure is not fixed but varies with the resistance and elastance of the respiratory system and with the flow rate selected.

V/C ventilation is the simplest and most effective means of providing full mechanical ventilation. In this mode, each inspiratory effort beyond the set sensitivity threshold triggers delivery of the fixed tidal volume. If the patient does not trigger the ventilator frequently enough, the ventilator initiates a breath, ensuring the desired minimum respiratory rate.

SIMV also delivers breaths at a set rate and volume that is synchronized to the patient's efforts. In contrast to V/C, patient efforts above the set respiratory rate are unassisted, although the intake valve opens to allow the breath. This mode remains popular, despite the fact that it neither provides full ventilator support as does V/C, facilitates liberating the patient from mechanical ventilation, nor improves patient comfort.

Pressure-cycled ventilation: This form of mechanical ventilation includes pressure control ventilation (PCV), pressure support ventilation (PSV), and several noninvasive modalities applied via a tight-fitting face mask. In all of these modalities, the ventilator delivers a set inspiratory pressure. Hence, tidal volume varies depending on the resistance and elastance of the respiratory system. In this mode, changes in respiratory system mechanics can result in unrecognized changes in minute ventilation. Because it limits the distending pressure of the lungs, this mode can theoretically benefit patients with acute respiratory distress syndrome (ARDS—see p. 563); however, no clear clinical advantage over A/C has been shown, and, if the volume delivered by PCV is the same as that delivered by A/C, the distending pressures will be the same.

Pressure control ventilation is a pressure-cycled form of A/C. Each inspiratory effort beyond the set sensitivity threshold delivers full pressure support maintained for a fixed inspiratory time. A minimum respiratory rate is maintained.

In **pressure support ventilation,** a minimum rate is not set; all breaths are triggered by the patient. The ventilator assists the patient by delivering a pressure that continues at a constant level until the patient's inspiratory flow falls below a preset algorithm. Thus, a longer or deeper inspiratory effort by the patient results in a larger tidal volume. This mode is commonly used to liberate patients from mechanical ventilation by letting them assume more of the work of breathing. However, no studies indicate that this approach is more successful.

Noninvasive positive pressure ventilation (NIPPV): NIPPV is the delivery of positive pressure ventilation via a tight-fitting mask that covers the nose or both the nose and mouth. Helmets that deliver NIPPV are being studied as an alternative for patients who cannot tolerate the standard tight-fitting face masks. Because of its use in spontaneously breathing patients, it is primarily applied as a form of PSV or to deliver end-expiratory pressure, although volume control can be used.

NIPPV can be given as continuous positive airway pressure (CPAP) or bilevel positive airway pressure (BiPAP). In CPAP, constant pressure is maintained throughout the respiratory cycle with no additional inspiratory support. With BiPAP, the physician sets both the expiratory positive airway pressure (EPAP) and the inspiratory positive airway pressure (IPAP), with respirations triggered by the patient. Because the airway is unprotected, aspiration is possible, so patients must have adequate mentation and airway protective reflexes and no imminent indication for surgery or transport off the floor for prolonged procedures. NIPPV should be avoided in patients who are hemodynamically unstable and in those with evidence of impaired gastric emptying, as occurs with ileus, bowel obstruction, or pregnancy. In such circumstances, swallowing large quantities of air may result in vomiting and life-threatening aspiration. Indications for conversion to endotracheal intubation and conventional mechanical ventilation include the development of shock or frequent arrhythmias, myocardial ischemia, and transport to a cardiac catheterization laboratory or surgical suite where control of the airway and full ventilatory support are desired. Obtunded patients and patients with copious secretions are not good candidates. Also, IPAP must be set below esophageal opening pressure (20 cm H_2O) to avoid gastric insufflation.

NIPPV can be used in the outpatient setting. For example, CPAP is often used for patients with obstructive sleep apnea (see p. 517), whereas BiPAP can be used for those with concomitant obesity-hypoventilation syndrome or for chronic ventilation in patients with neuromuscular or chest wall diseases.

Ventilator settings: Ventilator settings are tailored to the underlying condition, but the basic principles are as follows.

Tidal volume and respiratory rate set the minute ventilation. Too high a volume risks overinflation; too low a volume allows for atelectasis. Too high a rate risks hyperventilation and respiratory alkalosis along with inadequate expiratory time and autoPEEP; too low a rate risks inadequate minute ventilation and respiratory acidosis. A tidal volume of 8 to 10 mL/kg ideal body weight (IBW—see Sidebar 70–1 on p. 565) is usually appropriate, although some patients with normal lung mechanics (particularly those with neuromuscular disease) benefit from tidal volumes on the high end of this range to prevent atelectasis, whereas patients with ARDS or acute exacerbations of COPD or asthma may require lower volumes (see p. 565). IBW rather than actual body weight is used to determine the appropriate tidal volume for patients who have lung disease and who are receiving mechanical ventilation:

Males: IBW (kg) =
$50 + 2.3$ (height in inches $- 60$)
or $50 + 0.91$ (height in cm $- 152.4$)

Females: IBW (kg) =
$45.5 + 2.3$ (height in inches $- 60$)
or $45.5 + 0.91$ (height in cm $- 152.4$)

Sensitivity adjusts the level of negative pressure required to trigger the ventilator. A typical setting is –2 cm H_2O. Too high a setting (eg, more negative than –2 cm H_2O) causes weak patients to be unable to trigger a breath. Too low a setting (eg, less negative than –2 cm H_2O) may lead to overventilation by causing the machine to auto-cycle. Patients with high levels of autoPEEP may have difficulty inhaling deeply enough to achieve a sufficiently negative intra-airway pressure.

The ratio of time spent in inhalation versus that spent in exhalation (I:E ratio) can be adjusted in some modes of ventilation. A normal setting for patients with normal mechanics is 1:3. Patients with asthma or COPD exacerbations should have ratios of 1:4 or even more to limit the degree of autoPEEP.

The inspiratory flow rate can be adjusted in some modes of ventilation (ie, either the flow rate or the I:E ratio can be adjusted, not both). The inspiratory flow should generally be set at about 60 L/min but can be increased up to 120 L/min for patients with airflow limitation to facilitate having more time in exhalation, thereby limiting autoPEEP.

F_{IO_2} is initially set at 1.0 and is subsequently decreased to the lowest level necessary to maintain adequate oxygenation.

PEEP can be applied in any ventilator mode. PEEP increases end-expired lung volume and reduces airspace closure at the end of expiration. Most patients undergoing mechanical ventilation may benefit from the application of PEEP at 5 cm H_2O to limit the atelectasis that frequently accompanies endotracheal intubation, sedation, paralysis, and/or supine positioning. Higher levels of PEEP improve oxygenation in disorders such as cardiogenic pulmonary edema and ARDS. PEEP permits use of lower levels of F_{IO_2} while preserving adequate arterial oxygenation. This effect may be important in limiting the lung injury that may result from prolonged exposure to a high F_{IO_2} (≥ 0.6). PEEP increases intrathoracic pressure and thus may impede venous return, provoking hypotension in a hypovolemic patient, and may overdistend portions of the lung, thereby causing ventilator-associated lung injury (VALI). By contrast, if PEEP is too low, it may result in cyclic airspace opening and closing, which in turn may also cause VALI from the resultant repetitive shear forces. It is important to keep in mind that the pressure-volume curve varies for different regions of the lung. This variation means that, for a given PEEP, the increase in volume will be lower for dependent regions compared to nondependent regions of the lung.

Patient positioning: Mechanical ventilation is typically done with the patient in the semiupright position. However, in patients with ARDS, prone positioning may result in better oxygenation primarily by creating more uniform ventilation. Uniform ventilation reduces the amount of lung that has no ventilation (ie, the amount of shunt), which is generally greatest in the dorsal and caudal lung regions, while having minimal effects on perfusion distribution.

Although many investigators advocate a trial of prone positioning in patients with ARDS who require high levels of PEEP (eg, > 12 cm H_2O) and F_{IO_2} (eg, > 0.6), until recently trials have not shown any improvement in mortality with this strategy (however, these trials have typically been underpowered). A recent, large, multicenter, prospective trial assessed patients who had severe ARDS (PaO_2:FIO_2 < 150 mm Hg on an FIO_2 ≥ 0.6, PEEP > 5 cm H_2O) and who were on a tidal volume of about 6 mL/kg. These patients were randomized to undergo ≥ 16 h of prone positioning or be left in the supine position during ventilation. The study, which included a total of 466 patients, identified lower 28- and 90-day mortality in the prone-positioning group without a significant incidence of associated complications. Prone positioning is contraindicated in patients with spinal instability or increased intracranial pressure. This position also requires careful attention by the ICU staff to avoid complications, such as dislodgement of the endotracheal tube or intravascular catheters.

Sedation and comfort: Although many patients tolerate mechanical ventilation via endotracheal tube without sedatives, some require IV administration of sedatives (eg, propofol, lorazepam, midazolam) and analgesics (eg, morphine, fentanyl) to minimize stress and anxiety. These drugs can also reduce energy expenditure to some extent, thereby reducing CO_2 production and O_2 consumption. Doses should be titrated to the desired effect, guided by standard sedation/analgesia scoring systems. Patients undergoing mechanical ventilation for ARDS typically require higher levels of sedation and analgesia. The use of propofol for longer than 24 to 48 h requires periodic monitoring of serum triglyceride levels. There is evidence that continuously administered IV sedation prolongs the duration of mechanical ventilation. Thus, the goal is to achieve adequate but not excessive sedation, which can be accomplished by using continuous sedation with daily interruption or by using intermittent infusions.

Neuromuscular blocking agents are not used routinely in patients undergoing mechanical ventilation because of the risk of prolonged neuromuscular weakness and the need for continuous heavy sedation; however, one study did show reduced mortality at 90 days in patients who received 48 h of neuromuscular blockade. Exceptions include patients who fail to tolerate some of the more sophisticated and complicated modes of mechanical ventilation and to prevent shivering when cooling is used after cardiac arrest.

Complications and safeguards: Complications can be divided into those resulting from endotracheal intubation, from mechanical ventilation itself, or from prolonged immobility and inability to eat normally.

The presence of an endotracheal tube causes risk of sinusitis (which is rarely of clinical importance), ventilator-associated pneumonia (see p. 485), tracheal stenosis, vocal cord injury, and, very rarely, tracheal-esophageal or tracheal-vascular fistula. Purulent tracheal aspirate in a febrile patient who has an elevated WBC count > 48 h after ventilation has begun suggests ventilator-associated pneumonia.

Complications of ongoing mechanical ventilation itself include pneumothorax, O_2 toxicity, hypotension, and VALI.

If acute hypotension develops in a mechanically ventilated patient, particularly when it is accompanied by tachycardia and/or a sudden increase in peak inspiratory pressure, tension pneumothorax must always be considered; patients with such findings should immediately have a chest examination and a chest x-ray (or immediate treatment if examination is confirmatory). More commonly, however, hypotension is a result of sympathetic lysis caused by sedatives or opioids used to facilitate intubation and ventilation. Hypotension can also be caused by decreased venous return due to high intrathoracic pressure in patients receiving high levels of PEEP or in those with high levels of intrinsic PEEP due to asthma or COPD. If there are no physical findings suggesting tension pneumothorax, and if ventilation-related causes of hypotension are a possible etiology, pending a portable chest x-ray, the patient may be disconnected from the ventilator and gently bagged manually at 2 to 3 breaths/min with 100% O_2 while fluids are infused (eg, 500 to 1000 mL of 0.9% saline in adults, 20 mL/kg in children). An immediate improvement suggests a ventilation-related cause, and ventilator settings should be adjusted accordingly.

Relative immobility increases the risk of venous thromboembolic disease, skin breakdown, and atelectasis.

Most hospitals have standardized protocols to reduce complications. Elevating the head of the bed to > 30° decreases risk of ventilator-associated pneumonia, and routine turning of the patient every 2 h decreases the risk of skin breakdown. All patients receiving mechanical ventilation should receive deep venous thrombosis prophylaxis, either heparin 5000 units sc bid to tid or low molecular weight heparin or, if heparin is contraindicated, sequential compression devices. To prevent GI bleeding, patients should receive an H_2 blocker (eg, famotidine 20 mg enterally or IV bid) or sucralfate (1 g enterally qid). Proton pump inhibitors should be reserved for patients with a preexisting indication or active bleeding. Routine nutritional evaluations are mandatory, and enteral tube feedings should be initiated if ongoing mechanical ventilation is anticipated.

The most effective way to reduce complications of mechanical ventilation is to limit its duration. Daily "sedation vacations" and spontaneous breathing trials help determine the earliest point at which the patient may be liberated from mechanical support.

ACUTE HYPOXEMIC RESPIRATORY FAILURE

Acute hypoxemic respiratory failure (AHRF), which includes acute respiratory distress syndrome (ARDS), is severe arterial hypoxemia that is refractory to supplemental O_2. It is caused by intrapulmonary shunting of blood resulting from airspace filling or collapse. Findings include dyspnea and tachypnea. Diagnosis is by ABGs and chest x-ray. Treatment usually requires mechanical ventilation.

Etiology

Airspace filling in AHRF may result from

- Elevated alveolar capillary hydrostatic pressure, as occurs in left ventricular failure or hypervolemia
- Increased alveolar capillary permeability, as occurs in any of the conditions predisposing to ARDS
- Blood (as occurs in diffuse alveolar hemorrhage) or inflammatory exudates (as occur in pneumonia or other inflammatory lung conditions)

Pathophysiology

ARDS: In ARDS, pulmonary or systemic inflammation leads to release of cytokines and other proinflammatory molecules. The cytokines activate alveolar macrophages and recruit neutrophils to the lungs, which in turn release leukotrienes, oxidants, platelet-activating factor, and proteases. These substances damage capillary endothelium and alveolar epithelium, disrupting the barriers between capillaries and airspaces. Edema fluid, protein, and cellular debris flood the airspaces and interstitium, causing disruption of surfactant, airspace collapse, ventilation-perfusion mismatch, shunting, and pulmonary hypertension. The airspace collapse more commonly occurs in dependent lung zones.

ARDS is divided into 3 categories of severity: mild, moderate, and severe based on oxygenation defects and clinical criteria (Table 70–1). The mild category corresponds to the previous category termed acute lung injury (ALI).

Causes of ARDS (Table 70–2) may involve direct lung injury (eg, pneumonia, acid aspiration) or indirect lung injury (eg, sepsis, pancreatitis, massive blood transfusion, nonthoracic trauma). Sepsis and pneumonia account for about 60% of cases.

Table 70–1. BERLIN DEFINITION OF ARDS

ARDS CATEGORY	OXYGENATION
Level of severity	
Mild	200 mm Hg < PaO_2/FIO_2 ≤ 300 mm Hg* with PEEP or CPAP ≥ 5 cm H_2O
Moderate	100 mm Hg < PaO_2/FIO_2 ≤ 200 mm Hg with PEEP ≥ 5 cm H_2O
Severe	PaO_2/FIO_2 ≤ 100 mm Hg with PEEP ≥ 5 cm H_2O
Clinical criteria	
Timing	Onset within 1 wk of known insult or of new or worsening respiratory symptoms
Imaging (x-ray or CT of chest)	Bilateral opacities not fully explained by effusions, lobar or lung collapse, or nodules
Origin of edema	Respiratory failure not fully explained by heart failure or fluid overload

*PaO_2 in mm Hg; FIO_2 in decimal fraction (eg, 0.5).

ARDS = acute respiratory distress syndrome; CPAP = continuous positive airway pressure; FIO_2 = fraction of inspired O_2; PaO_2 = partial pressure of arterial O_2; PEEP = positive end-expiratory pressure.

Adapted from ARDS Definition Task Force, Ranieri VM, Rubenfeld GD, et al: Acute respiratory distress syndrome: the Berlin definition. *Journal of the American Medical Association* 307:2526–2533, 2012.

Table 70–2. CAUSES OF ARDS

DIRECT LUNG INJURY	INDIRECT LUNG INJURY
Common causes	
Acid aspiration	Sepsis
Pneumonia	Trauma with prolonged hypovolemic shock
Less common causes	
Diffuse alveolar hemorrhage	Bone marrow transplantation
Fat embolism	Burns
Lung transplantation	Cardiopulmonary bypass
Near drowning	Drug overdose (eg, aspirin, cocaine, opioids, phenothiazines, tricyclics)
Pulmonary contusion	Massive blood transfusion (> 15 units)
Toxic gas inhalation	Neurogenic pulmonary edema due to stroke, seizure, head trauma, anoxia
—	Pancreatitis
—	Radiographic contrast (rare)

ARDS = acute respiratory distress syndrome.

Refractory hypoxemia: In both types of AHRF, flooded or collapsed airspaces allow no inspired gas to enter, so the blood perfusing those alveoli remains at the mixed venous O_2 content no matter how high the fractional inspired O_2 (FIO_2). This effect ensures constant admixture of deoxygenated blood into the pulmonary vein and hence arterial hypoxemia. In contrast, hypoxemia that results from ventilating alveoli that have less ventilation than perfusion (ie, low ventilation-to-perfusion ratios as occurs in asthma or COPD and, to some extent, in ARDS) is readily corrected by supplemental O_2.

Symptoms and Signs

Acute hypoxemia (see also p. 533) may cause dyspnea, restlessness, and anxiety. Signs include confusion or alteration of consciousness, cyanosis, tachypnea, tachycardia, and diaphoresis. Cardiac arrhythmia and coma can result. Airway closure causes crackles, detected during chest auscultation; the crackles are typically diffuse but sometimes worse at the lung bases. Jugular venous distention occurs with high levels of PEEP or right ventricular failure.

Diagnosis

- Chest x-ray and ABGs
- Clinical definition (see Table 70–1)

Hypoxemia is usually first recognized using pulse oximetry. Patients with low O_2 saturation should have a chest x-ray and ABGs and be treated with supplemental O_2 while awaiting test results.

If supplemental O_2 does not improve the O_2 saturation to > 90%, right-to-left shunting of blood should be suspected. An obvious alveolar infiltrate on chest x-ray implicates alveolar flooding as the cause, rather than an intracardiac shunt. However, at the onset of illness, hypoxemia can occur before changes are seen on x-ray.

Once AHRF is diagnosed, the cause must be determined, considering both pulmonary and extrapulmonary causes. Sometimes a known ongoing disorder (eg, acute MI, pancreatitis, sepsis) is an obvious cause. In other cases, history is suggestive; pneumonia should be suspected in an immunocompromised patient, and alveolar hemorrhage is suspected after bone marrow transplantation or in a patient with a connective tissue disease. Frequently, however, critically ill patients have received a large volume of IV fluids for resuscitation, and high-pressure AHRF (eg, caused by ventricular failure or fluid overload) resulting from treatment must be distinguished from an underlying low-pressure AHRF (eg, caused by sepsis or pneumonia).

High-pressure pulmonary edema is suggested by a 3rd heart sound, jugular venous distention, and peripheral edema on examination and by the presence of diffuse central infiltrates, cardiomegaly, and an abnormally wide vascular pedicle on chest x-ray. The diffuse, bilateral infiltrates of ARDS are generally more peripheral. Focal infiltrates are typically caused by lobar pneumonia, atelectasis, or lung contusion. Although echocardiography may show left ventricular dysfunction, implying a cardiac origin, this finding is not specific because sepsis can also reduce myocardial contractility.

When ARDS is diagnosed but the cause is not obvious (eg, trauma, sepsis, severe pulmonary infection, pancreatitis), a review of drugs and recent diagnostic tests, procedures, and treatments may suggest an unrecognized cause, such as use of a radiographic contrast agent, air embolism, or transfusion. When no predisposing cause can be uncovered, some experts recommend doing bronchoscopy with bronchoalveolar lavage to exclude alveolar hemorrhage and eosinophilic pneumonia and, if this procedure is not revealing, a lung biopsy to exclude other disorders (eg, extrinsic allergic alveolitis, acute interstitial pneumonitis).

Prognosis

Prognosis is highly variable and depends on a variety of factors, including etiology of respiratory failure, severity of disease, age, and chronic health status. Overall, mortality in ARDS was very high (40 to 60%) but has declined in recent years to 25 to 40%, probably because of improvements in mechanical ventilation and in treatment of sepsis. However, mortality remains very high (> 40%) for patients with severe ARDS (ie, those with a PaO_2:FIO_2 < 100 mm Hg). Most often, death is not caused by respiratory dysfunction but by sepsis and multiorgan failure. Persistence of neutrophils and high cytokine levels in bronchoalveolar lavage fluid predict a poor prognosis. Mortality otherwise increases with age, presence of sepsis, and severity of preexisting organ insufficiency or coexisting organ dysfunction. Pulmonary function returns to close to normal in 6 to 12 mo in most ARDS patients who survive; however, patients with a protracted clinical course or severe disease may have residual pulmonary symptoms, and many have persistent neuromuscular weakness.

Treatment

- Mechanical ventilation if saturation is < 90% on high-flow O_2

Underlying conditions must be addressed as discussed elsewhere in THE MANUAL. AHRF is initially treated with high flows of 70 to 100% O_2 by a nonrebreather face mask. If O_2 saturation > 90% is not obtained, mechanical ventilation probably should be instituted. Specific management varies by condition.

Mechanical ventilation in cardiogenic pulmonary edema: Mechanical ventilation benefits the failing left ventricle in several ways. Positive inspiratory pressure reduces left and right ventricular preload and left ventricular afterload and reduces the work of breathing. Reducing the work of breathing may allow redistribution of a limited cardiac output away from overworked respiratory muscles. Expiratory pressure (expiratory positive airway pressure [EPAP] or PEEP) redistributes pulmonary edema from alveoli to the interstitium, allowing more alveoli to participate in gas exchange.

Noninvasive positive pressure ventilation (NIPPV), whether continuous positive pressure ventilation or bilevel ventilation, is useful in averting endotracheal intubation in many patients because drug therapy often leads to rapid improvement. Typical settings are inspiratory positive airway pressure (IPAP) of 10 to 15 cm H_2O and EPAP of 5 to 8 cm H_2O.

Conventional mechanical ventilation can use several ventilator modes. Most often, A/C is used in the acute setting, when full ventilatory support is desired. Initial settings are tidal volume of 6 to 8 mL/kg IBW, respiratory rate of 25/min, FIO_2 of 1.0, and PEEP of 5 to 8 cm H_2O. PEEP may then be titrated upward in 2.5-cm H_2O increments while the FIO_2 is decreased to nontoxic levels. PSV can also be used (with similar levels of PEEP). The initial pressure delivered should be sufficient to fully rest the respiratory muscles as judged by subjective patient assessment, respiratory rate, and accessory muscle use. Typically, a pressure support level of 10 to 20 cm H_2O over PEEP is required.

Mechanical ventilation in ARDS: Nearly all patients require mechanical ventilation, which, in addition to improving oxygenation, reduces O_2 demand by resting respiratory muscles. Targets include

- Plateau alveolar pressures < 30 cm H_2O (factors that potentially decrease chest wall and abdominal compliance considered)
- Tidal volume 6 mL/kg predicted body weight to minimize further lung injury
- FIO_2 as low as is allowed to maintain adequate SaO_2 to minimize possible O_2 toxicity

PEEP should be high enough to maintain open alveoli and minimize FIO_2 until a plateau pressure of 28 to 30 cm H_2O is reached. Patients with moderate to severe ARDS are the most likely to have mortality reduced by use of higher PEEP.

NIPPV is occasionally useful with ARDS. However, compared with treatment of cardiogenic pulmonary edema, higher levels of support for a longer duration are often required, and EPAP of 8 to 12 cm H_2O is often necessary to maintain adequate oxygenation. Achieving this expiratory pressure requires inspiratory pressures > 18 to 20 cm H_2O, which are poorly tolerated; maintaining an adequate seal becomes difficult, the mask becomes more uncomfortable, and skin necrosis and gastric insufflation may occur. Also, NIPPV-treated patients who subsequently need intubation have generally progressed to a more advanced condition than if they had been intubated earlier; thus, critical desaturation is possible at the time of intubation. Intensive monitoring and careful selection of patients (see p. 561) are required.

Conventional mechanical ventilation in ARDS previously focused on normalizing ABG values. It is now clear that ventilating with lower tidal volumes reduces mortality. Accordingly, in most patients, tidal volume should be set at 6 mL/kg IBW (see Sidebar 70–1 for equation). This setting necessitates an increase in respiratory rate, even up to 35/min, to produce sufficient alveolar ventilation to allow for adequate CO_2 removal. On occasion, however, respiratory acidosis develops, some degree of which is accepted for the greater good of limiting VALI and is generally well tolerated, particularly when pH is ≥ 7.15. If pH drops below 7.15, bicarbonate infusion or tromethamine may be helpful. Because hypercapnia may cause dyspnea and cause

Sidebar 70–1. Initial Ventilator Management in ARDS

Generally, the following approach is recommended for ventilator management in ARDS:

- Assist-control mode is used initially with a tidal volume 6 mL/kg ideal body weight, respiratory rate 25/min, flow rate 60 L/min, FIO_2 1.0, and PEEP 15 cm H_2O.
- Once O_2 saturation is > 90%, FIO_2 is decreased.
- Then, PEEP is decreased in 2.5-cm H_2O increments as tolerated to find the least PEEP associated with an arterial O_2 saturation of 90% on an FIO_2 of ≤ 0.6.
- The respiratory rate is increased up to 35/min to achieve a pH of > 7.15, or until the expiratory flow tracing shows end-expiratory flow.

Ideal body weight (IBW) rather than actual body weight is used to determine the appropriate tidal volume for patients with lung disease receiving mechanical ventilation:

Males: IBW (kg) =
$$50 + 2.3\,(\text{height in inches} - 60)$$
or $$50 + 0.91\,(\text{height in cm} - 152.4)$$

Females: IBW (kg) =
$$45.5 + 2.3\,(\text{height in inches} - 60)$$
or $$45.5 + 0.91\,(\text{height in cm} - 152.4)$$

the patient to breathe in a fashion that is not coordinated with the ventilator, analgesics (fentanyl or morphine) and sedatives may be needed (eg, propofol initiated at 5 mcg/kg/min and increasing to effect up to 50 mcg/kg/min; because of the risk of hypertriglyceridemia, triglyceride levels should be checked every 48 h). Sedation is preferred to neuromuscular blockade because blockade still requires sedation and may cause residual weakness.

PEEP improves oxygenation in ARDS by increasing the volume of aerated lung through alveolar recruitment, permitting the use of a lower FIO_2. The optimal level of PEEP and the way to identify it have been debated. Many clinicians simply use the least amount of PEEP that results in an adequate arterial O_2 saturation on a nontoxic FIO_2. In most patients, this level is a PEEP of 8 to 15 cm H_2O, although, occasionally, patients with severe ARDS require levels > 20 cm H_2O. In these cases, close attention must be paid to other means of optimizing O_2 delivery and minimizing O_2 consumption (see p. 562).

The best indicator of alveolar overdistention is measurement of a plateau pressure through an end-inspiratory hold maneuver (see p. 560); it should be checked every 4 h and after each change in PEEP or tidal volume. The target plateau pressure is < 30 cm H_2O. If the plateau pressure exceeds this value and there is no problem with the chest wall that could be contributing (eg, ascites, pleural effusion, acute abdomen, chest trauma), the physician should reduce the tidal volume in 0.5- to 1.0-mL/kg increments as tolerated to a minimum of 4 mL/kg, raising the respiratory rate to compensate for the reduction in minute ventilation and inspecting the ventilator waveform display to ensure that full exhalation occurs. The respiratory rate may often be raised as high as 35/min before overt gas trapping due to incomplete exhalation results. If plateau pressure is < 25 cm H_2O and tidal volume is < 6 mL/kg, tidal volume may be increased to 6 mL/kg or until plateau pressure is > 25 cm H_2O. Some investigators believe PCV protects the lungs better, but supportive data are lacking, and it is the peak pressure rather than the plateau pressure that is being controlled. With PCV, because the tidal volume will vary as the patient's lung compliance evolves, it is necessary to continually monitor the tidal volume and adjust the inspiratory pressure to ensure that the patient is not receiving too high or too low a tidal volume.

Prone positioning (see p. 562) improves oxygenation in some patients by allowing recruitment of nonventilating lung regions. A recent study suggests this positioning may improve survival.

Optimal fluid management of patients with ARDS balances the requirement for an adequate circulating volume to preserve end-organ perfusion with the goal of lowering preload and thereby limiting transudation of fluid in the lungs. Recently, a large multicenter trial has shown that a conservative approach to fluid management, in which less fluid is given, shortens the duration of mechanical ventilation and ICU length of stay when compared with a more liberal strategy. However, there was no difference in survival between the 2 approaches, and use of a pulmonary artery catheter also did not improve outcome. Patients not in shock are candidates for such an approach but should be monitored closely for evidence of decreased end-organ perfusion, such as hypotension, oliguria, thready pulses, or cool extremities (see p. 572).

A definitive pharmacologic treatment for ARDS that reduces morbidity and mortality remains elusive. Inhaled nitric oxide, surfactant replacement, activated protein C (drotrecogin alfa) and many other agents directed at modulating the inflammatory response have been studied and found not to reduce morbidity or mortality. Some small studies suggest that systemic corticosteroids may be beneficial in late-stage ARDS, but a larger, prospective, randomized trial found no reduction in mortality. Corticosteroids may be deleterious when given early in the course of the condition.

VENTILATORY FAILURE

Ventilatory failure is a rise in $Paco_2$ (hypercapnia) that occurs when the respiratory load can no longer be supported by the strength or activity of the system. The most common causes are acute exacerbations of asthma and COPD, overdoses of drugs that suppress ventilatory drive, and conditions that cause respiratory muscle weakness (eg, Guillain-Barré syndrome, myasthenia gravis, botulism). Findings include dyspnea, tachypnea, and confusion. Death can result. Diagnosis is by ABGs and patient observation; chest x-ray and clinical evaluation may help delineate cause. Treatment varies by condition but often includes mechanical ventilation.

Pathophysiology

Hypercapnia occurs when alveolar ventilation either falls or fails to rise adequately in response to increased CO_2 production. A fall in alveolar ventilation results from a decrease in minute ventilation or an increase in dead space ventilation without appropriate compensation by increasing minute ventilation.

Ventilatory failure can occur when there is excessive load on the respiratory system (eg, resistive loads or lung and chest wall elastic loads) versus neuromuscular competence for an effective inspiratory effort. When the minute ventilation load increases (eg, as occurs in sepsis) a compromised respiratory system may not be able to meet this increased demand (for causes, see Fig. 70–2).

Physiologic dead space is the part of the respiratory tree that does not participate in gas exchange. It includes the anatomic dead space (oropharynx, trachea, and airways) and alveolar dead space (ie, alveoli that are ventilated but not perfused). Physiologic dead space can also result from shunt or low ventilation/perfusion (V/Q) if patients cannot increase their minute ventilation appropriately. The physiologic dead space normally is about 30 to 40% of tidal volume but increases to 50% in intubated patients and to >70% in massive pulmonary embolism, severe emphysema, and status asthmaticus. Thus, for any given minute ventilation, the greater the dead space, the poorer the CO_2 elimination.

Increased CO_2 production, as occurs with fever, sepsis, trauma, burns, hyperthyroidism, and malignant hyperthermia, is not a primary cause of ventilatory failure because patients should increase their ventilation to compensate. Ventilatory failure caused by these problems results only when the ability to compensate is compromised.

Hypercapnia lowers arterial pH (respiratory acidosis). Severe acidemia (pH < 7.2) contributes to pulmonary arteriolar vasoconstriction, systemic vascular dilation, reduced myocardial contractility, hyperkalemia, hypotension, and cardiac irritability, with the potential for life-threatening arrhythmias. Acute hypercapnia also causes cerebral vasodilation and increased intracranial pressure, a major problem in patients with acute head injury. Over time, tissue buffering and renal compensation can largely correct the acidemia. However, sudden increases in $Paco_2$ can occur faster than compensatory changes ($Paco_2$ rises 3 to 6 mm Hg/min in a totally apneic patient).

Symptoms and Signs

The predominant symptom is dyspnea. Signs include vigorous use of accessory ventilatory muscles, tachypnea, tachycardia, diaphoresis, anxiety, declining tidal volume, irregular or gasping breathing patterns, and paradoxical abdominal motion.

CNS manifestations range from subtle personality changes to marked confusion, obtundation, or coma. Chronic hypercapnia is better tolerated than acute and has fewer symptoms.

Diagnosis

- ABGs
- Chest x-ray
- Tests to determine etiology

Ventilatory failure should be suspected in patients with respiratory distress, visible ventilatory fatigue or cyanosis, or changes in sensorium and in those with disorders causing neuromuscular weakness. Tachypnea is also a concern; respiratory rates > 28 to 30/min cannot be sustained for very long, particularly in elderly or weakened patients.

If ventilatory failure is suspected, ABG analysis, continuous pulse oximetry, and a chest x-ray should be done. Respiratory acidosis on the ABG (eg, pH < 7.35 and PCO_2 > 50) confirms the diagnosis. Patients with chronic ventilatory failure often have quite elevated PCO_2 (eg, 60 to 90 mm Hg) at baseline, typically with a pH that is only slightly acidemic. In such patients, the degree of acidemia rather than the PCO_2 must serve as the primary marker for acute hypoventilation.

Because ABGs can be normal in patients with incipient ventilatory failure, certain bedside pulmonary function tests can

Chest wall elastic loads
Abdominal distention
Ascites
Obesity
Pleural effusion
Pneumothorax
Rib fracture
Tumor

Lung elastic loads
Alveolar edema
Atelectasis
Infection
Intrinsic PEEP

Minute ventilation loads
Excess calories
Hypovolemia
Pulmonary embolus
Sepsis

Resistive loads
Bronchospasm (eg, asthma, bronchiolitis, COPD)
Edema, secretions, or scarring of airway
Obstructive sleep apnea
Upper airway obstruction (eg, croup, epiglottitis)

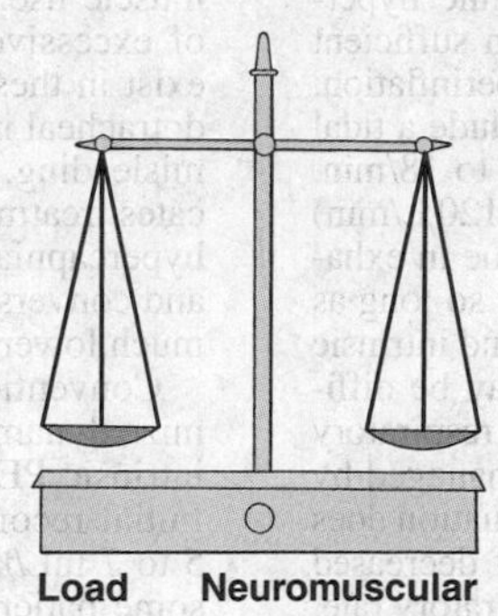

Impaired respiratory drive
Brain stem lesion
Drug overdose
Hypothyroidism
Sleep-disordered breathing

Impaired neurotransmission
Aminoglycosides
Amyotrophic lateral sclerosis
Botulism
Spinal cord lesion
Guillain-Barré syndrome
Myasthenia gravis
Neuromuscular blockers
Phrenic nerve injury

Muscle weakness
Electrolyte abnormalities
Fatigue
Hypoperfusion states
Hypoxemia
Myopathy
Undernutrition

Fig. 70–2. The balance between load (resistive, elastic, and minute ventilation) and neuromuscular competence (drive, transmission, and muscle strength) determines the ability to sustain alveolar ventilation. PEEP = positive end-expiratory pressure.

help predict ventilatory failure, particularly in patients with neuromuscular weakness who may succumb to ventilatory failure without exhibiting respiratory distress. Vital capacity < 10 to 15 mL/kg and an inability to generate a negative inspiratory force of 15 cm H_2O suggest imminent ventilatory failure.

Once ventilatory failure is diagnosed, the cause must be identified. Sometimes a known ongoing disorder (eg, coma, acute asthma, COPD exacerbation, myxedema, myasthenia gravis, botulism) is an obvious cause. In other cases, history is suggestive; sudden onset of tachypnea and hypotension after surgery suggests pulmonary embolism, and focal neurologic findings suggest a CNS or neuromuscular cause. Neuromuscular competence may be assessed through measurement of inspiratory muscle strength (negative inspiratory force and positive expiratory force), neuromuscular transmission (nerve conduction tests and electromyography), and investigations into causes of diminished drive (toxicology screens, brain imaging, and thyroid function tests).

Treatment

- Treatment of cause
- Often positive pressure ventilation

Treatment aims to correct the imbalance between the strength of the respiratory system and its load and varies with etiology. Obvious precipitants (eg, bronchospasm, mucus plugging, foreign bodies) should be corrected if possible.

The 2 most common causes are acute exacerbation of asthma (ie, status asthmaticus) and COPD. Respiratory failure due to COPD is termed acute-on-chronic respiratory failure (ACRF).

Status asthmaticus (SA): Patients should be treated in an ICU by personnel skilled in airway management.

NIPPV can immediately reduce the work of breathing and may forestall endotracheal intubation until drug therapy can take effect. In contrast to patients with COPD, who often welcome NIPPV, the mask often increases the perception of dyspnea in asthmatic patients, so introduction must be done carefully, perhaps starting with titration of expiratory positive airway pressure (EPAP) alone because one of the major functions of IPAP is to increase tidal volume, and, in these patients, end-expiratory lung volume approaches total lung capacity. After an explanation of its benefit, patients hold the mask against their face while modest amounts of pressure are applied (CPAP 3 to 5 cm H_2O). Once tolerated, the mask is strapped in place while pressures are increased to patient comfort and reduced work of breathing as assessed by respiratory rate and accessory muscle use. Final settings are typically IPAP 10 to 15 cm H_2O and EPAP 5 to 8 cm H_2O. Patients should be selected carefully (see p. 561).

Conventional mechanical ventilation via endotracheal intubation is indicated for impending respiratory failure as indicated clinically by obtundation, monosyllabic speech, slumped posture, and shallow breathing. ABGs showing worsening hypercapnia are also an indication, although blood gas confirmation is not required and should not replace the physician's judgment. Oral intubation is preferred over nasal because a larger endotracheal tube, which decreases airway resistance and permits easier suctioning, can be used.

Hypotension and pneumothorax occasionally occur after intubation for SA (see also p. 562). These complications and their corresponding mortality have declined significantly because of a ventilator strategy that emphasizes limiting dynamic hyperinflation over achieving eucapnia. In SA, ventilation sufficient to achieve a normal pH typically causes severe hyperinflation. To avoid hyperinflation, initial ventilator settings include a tidal volume of 5 to 7 mL/kg and a respiratory rate of 10 to 18/min. Inspiratory flows may need to be quite high (eg, 70 to 120 L/min) with a square wave pattern to facilitate maximum time in exhalation. Dangerous dynamic hyperinflation is unlikely so long as the measured plateau pressure is < 30 to 35 cm H_2O and intrinsic PEEP is < 15 cm H_2O (although these pressures may be difficult to measure because of inspiratory and expiratory respiratory muscle activity). Plateau pressure > 35 cm H_2O is managed by reducing the tidal volume (assuming that clinical evaluation does not indicate that the high pressures are the result of decreased compliance of the chest wall or abdomen) or the respiratory rate.

Although it is possible to reduce peak airway pressure by reducing peak flow rate or by changing the waveform to a descending profile, it should *not* be done. Although high flow rates require a high pressure to overcome the high airway resistance of SA, this pressure is dissipated across robust, cartilage-containing airways. Lower flow rates (eg, < 60 L/min) reduce time available for exhalation, thereby increasing the end-expiratory volume (and the resultant intrinsic PEEP) and allowing a greater inspiratory volume during the next breath.

Using low tidal volumes often results in hypercapnia, which is permitted for the greater good of reducing dynamic hyperinflation. An arterial pH > 7.15 is generally well tolerated but often requires large doses of sedatives and opioids. Neuromuscular blockers should be avoided after the peri-intubation period because use of these agents in combination with corticosteroids can cause a severe and occasionally irreversible myopathy, particularly after 24 h of combined use. Patient agitation should be managed with sedation rather than paralysis, but ideally ventilation can be adjusted to patients' needs so as to reduce the need for sedation.

Most patients with SA improve to the point of liberation from mechanical ventilation within 2 to 5 days, although a minority experience protracted severe airflow obstruction. For the discussion on the general approach to liberation see p. 569.

ACRF: In patients with ACRF caused by COPD, the O_2 cost of breathing is several times that of patients without underlying lung disease. This increased respiratory load occurs in the setting of barely adequate neuromuscular competence, so patients easily become too tired to maintain ventilation. These patients are vulnerable to respiratory failure from seemingly trivial insults, and recovery requires systematic identification and correction of these precipitants (see also p. 423). To restore the balance between neuromuscular competence and load, clinicians reduce airflow obstruction and dynamic hyperinflation with bronchodilators and corticosteroids and treat infection with antibiotics. Low serum levels of K, phosphorus, and Mg may exacerbate muscle weakness, frustrating recovery, and must be identified and treated.

NIPPV is the preferred initial treatment for many patients with ACRF, resulting in decreased rates of ventilator-associated pneumonia, length of stay, and mortality compared with endotracheal intubation. Perhaps 75% of patients managed with NIPPV do not require endotracheal intubation. Advantages include the ease of application and removal; once initial stabilization has occurred, NIPPV may be stopped temporarily to allow oral intake in selected patients. Trials of unassisted breathing are easily done, and NIPPV can be reapplied as indicated.

Typical settings are IPAP of 10 to 15 cm H_2O and EPAP of 5 to 8 cm H_2O, titrated to the work of breathing as assessed by patient report, respiratory rate and tidal volume, and accessory muscle use. The same concerns regarding the potential effect of excessive IPAP on total lung capacity as discussed above exist in these patients as well. Deterioration (and need for endotracheal intubation) is best assessed clinically; ABGs may be misleading. Although worsening hypercapnia typically indicates treatment failure, patients differ markedly in tolerance of hypercapnia. Some patients with $Paco_2$ > 100 mm Hg are alert and conversant on NIPPV, whereas others require intubation at much lower levels.

Conventional mechanical ventilation in ACRF aims to minimize dynamic hyperinflation and counter the adverse effects of intrinsic PEEP while resting the fatigued respiratory muscles. Initial recommended settings are A/C with a tidal volume of 5 to 7 mL/kg and a respiratory rate of 20 to 24/min, although some patients need lower initial rates to limit intrinsic PEEP. This intrinsic PEEP represents an inspiratory threshold load that must be overcome by the patient to trigger the ventilator, further increasing the work of breathing and preventing full rest on the ventilator. To counterbalance the effect of intrinsic PEEP, external PEEP should be applied to a level ≤ 85% of intrinsic PEEP (typical setting 5 to 10 cm H_2O). This application decreases the inspiratory work of breathing without increasing dynamic hyperinflation. High inspiratory flow rates should be used to maximize the time for expiration. These settings minimize the risk of alkalemia that follows overly vigorous initial ventilation. Hypotension may also occur immediately after intubation (see p. 562).

Most patients require full ventilatory support for 24 to 48 h before spontaneous breathing trials are considered. It has not been determined whether this duration of treatment is needed to rest the respiratory muscles or to allow hyperinflation to diminish, thereby increasing respiratory muscle strength. The patient often sleeps heavily during this time and, in contrast to patients with asthma, typically requires little sedation. Adequate rest is often not achieved unless sufficient attention is paid to ongoing patient effort. This effort may manifest as accessory muscle use, inappropriately low airway pressures at the onset or throughout inspiration, or frequent failures to trigger the ventilator, indicating high intrinsic PEEP, weakness, or both.

OTHER TYPES OF RESPIRATORY FAILURE

Perioperative respiratory failure is usually caused by atelectasis. Effective means of preventing or treating atelectasis include incentive spirometry, ensuring adequate analgesia for chest and abdominal incisions, upright positioning, and early mobilization. Atelectasis caused by abdominal distention should be alleviated according to the cause (eg, nasogastric suction for excessive intraluminal air, paracentesis to evacuate tense ascites).

Hypoperfusion, regardless of cause, may result in respiratory failure through inadequate delivery of O_2 to respiratory muscles coupled with excess respiratory muscle load (eg, acidosis, sepsis). Mechanical ventilation is useful for diverting blood flow from overworked respiratory muscles to critical organs such as the brain, kidney, and gut.

LIBERATION FROM MECHANICAL VENTILATION

The discontinuation of ventilatory support is best achieved not by gradually reducing the level of ventilatory support (weaning) but by systematically identifying and eliminating the precipitants of respiratory failure. Once this goal has been achieved, the ventilator is no longer necessary. However, if precipitants are still present or recovery is incomplete, reducing needed ventilatory support is more likely to delay recovery. It is now clear that daily spontaneous breathing trials on a T-piece reduce the duration of mechanical ventilation compared with gradual reduction of the respiratory rate using SIMV and, in some studies, compared with pressure support trials.

Once the patient is no longer in shock, has an adequate arterial saturation on a fractional inspired O_2 (FIO_2) ≤ 0.5 with a PEEP ≤ 7.5 cm H_2O, and does not have an obviously unsustainable respiratory load (eg, minute ventilation > 20 L/min), a daily spontaneous breathing trial is done using a T-piece or CPAP of 5 cm H_2O. Patients capable of sustaining spontaneous breathing generally breathe slowly and deeply, instead of rapidly and shallowly. This observation has been formalized as the rapid shallow breathing (RSB) index, determined by dividing the patient's unassisted respiratory rate (in breaths/min) by the tidal volume (in L). A value < 105 suggests that spontaneous breathing is likely to be successful, although a single isolated measurement is not perfectly predictive of success. Recently, the decision of whether to extubate a patient after a spontaneous breathing trial has shifted away from the use of the RSB index and has relied more on clinical assessment during the course of the trial, supplemented by measuring ABGs. Patients who fare well during a brief 1- to 2-h spontaneous breathing trial and who have favorable ABGs are good candidates for extubation. The decision to extubate is a separate one from the decision to stop ventilatory support and requires evaluation of the patient's mentation and airway protective reflexes, as well as the patency of the airway.

Sedatives and opioids may prolong mechanical ventilation. Such drugs may accumulate and cause protracted sedation, frustrating attempts to do spontaneous breathing trials even when the cause of respiratory failure has been corrected. The level of sedation should be continually assessed, and progressive sedative withdrawal should be begun as soon as possible. Formal protocols can be used, or simple daily interruption can be carried out. The infusion is stopped until the patient is either awake and following commands or needs re-sedation for agitation, breathing asynchronously with the ventilator, or other physiologic derangements. If sedation is still needed, it is restarted at half the previous dose and titrated as necessary. Several studies have shown that the mean duration of mechanical ventilation is reduced in institutions that use either daily "sedation vacations" or other sedation protocols, as well as daily spontaneous breathing trials.

71 Sepsis and Septic Shock

Sepsis is a clinical syndrome of life-threatening organ dysfunction caused by a dysregulated response to infection. In septic shock, there is critical reduction in tissue perfusion; acute failure of multiple organs, including the lungs, kidneys, and liver, can occur. Common causes in immunocompetent patients include many different species of gram-positive and gram-negative bacteria. Immunocompromised patients may have uncommon bacterial or fungal species as a cause. Signs include fever, hypotension, oliguria, and confusion. Diagnosis is primarily clinical combined with culture results showing infection; early recognition and treatment is critical. Treatment is aggressive fluid resuscitation, antibiotics, surgical excision of infected or necrotic tissue and drainage of pus, and supportive care.

Sepsis represents a spectrum of disease with mortality risk ranging from moderate (eg, 10%) to substantial (eg, > 40%) depending on various pathogen and host factors along with the timeliness of recognition and provision of appropriate treatment.

Septic shock is a subset of sepsis with significantly increased mortality due to severe abnormalities of circulation and/or cellular metabolism. Septic shock involves persistent hypotension (defined as the need for vasopressors to maintain mean arterial pressure ≥ 65 mm Hg, and a serum lactate level > 18 mg/dL [2 mmol/L] despite adequate volume resuscitation).[1]

The concept of the systemic inflammatory response syndrome (SIRS), defined by certain abnormalities of vital signs and laboratory results, has long been used to identify early sepsis. However, SIRS criteria have been found to lack sensitivity and specificity for increased mortality risk, which is the main consideration for using such a conceptual model. The lack of specificity may be because the SIRS response is often adaptive rather than pathologic.

1. Singer M, Deutschman CS, Seymour CW, et al: The third international consensus definitions for sepsis and septic shock (sepsis-3). *JAMA* 315:801–810, 2016.

Etiology

Most cases of septic shock are caused by hospital-acquired gram-negative bacilli or gram-positive cocci and often occur in immunocompromised patients and patients with chronic and debilitating diseases. Rarely, it is caused by *Candida* or other fungi. A postoperative infection (deep or superficial) should be suspected as the cause of septic shock in patients who have recently had surgery. A unique, uncommon form of shock caused by staphylococcal and streptococcal toxins is called toxic shock syndrome.

Septic shock occurs more often in neonates (see p. 2636), the elderly, and pregnant women. Predisposing factors include

- Diabetes mellitus
- Cirrhosis
- Leukopenia (especially that associated with cancer or treatment with cytotoxic drugs)
- Invasive devices (including endotracheal tubes, vascular or urinary catheters, drainage tubes, and other foreign materials)
- Prior treatment with antibiotics or corticosteroids

Common causative sites of infection include the lungs and the urinary, biliary, and GI tracts.

Pathophysiology

The pathogenesis of septic shock is not completely understood. An inflammatory stimulus (eg, a bacterial toxin) triggers production of proinflammatory mediators, including TNF and IL-1. These cytokines cause neutrophil–endothelial cell adhesion, activate the clotting mechanism, and generate microthrombi. They also release numerous other mediators, including leukotrienes, lipoxygenase, histamine, bradykinin, serotonin, and IL-2. They are opposed by anti-inflammatory mediators, such as IL-4 and IL-10, resulting in a negative feedback mechanism.

Initially, arteries and arterioles dilate, decreasing peripheral arterial resistance; cardiac output typically increases. This stage has been referred to as warm shock. Later, cardiac output may decrease, BP falls (with or without an increase in peripheral resistance), and typical features of shock appear.

Even in the stage of increased cardiac output, vasoactive mediators cause blood flow to bypass capillary exchange vessels (a distributive defect). Poor capillary flow from this shunting along with capillary obstruction by microthrombi decreases delivery of O_2 and impairs removal of CO_2 and waste products. Decreased perfusion causes dysfunction and sometimes failure of one or more organs, including the kidneys, lungs, liver, brain, and heart.

Coagulopathy may develop because of intravascular coagulation with consumption of major clotting factors, excessive fibrinolysis in reaction thereto, and more often a combination of both.

Symptoms and Signs

Symptoms and signs of sepsis can be subtle and often easily mistaken for manifestations of other disorders (eg, delirium, primary cardiac dysfunction, pulmonary embolism), especially in postoperative patients. With sepsis, patients typically have fever, tachycardia, diaphoresis, and tachypnea; BP remains normal. Other signs of the causative infection may be present. As sepsis worsens or septic shock develops, an early sign, particularly in the elderly or very young, may be confusion or decreased alertness. BP decreases, yet the skin is paradoxically warm. Later, extremities become cool and pale, with peripheral cyanosis and mottling. Organ dysfunction causes additional symptoms and signs specific to the organ involved (eg, oliguria, dyspnea).

Diagnosis

- Clinical manifestations
- BP, heart rate, and O_2 monitoring
- CBC with differential, electrolyte panel and creatinine, lactate
- Invasive central venous pressure (CVP), PaO_2, and central venous O_2 saturation ($ScvO_2$) readings
- Cultures of blood, urine, and other potential sites of infection, including wounds in surgical patients

Sepsis is suspected when a patient with a known infection develops systemic signs of inflammation or organ dysfunction. Similarly, a patient with otherwise unexplained signs of systemic inflammation should be evaluated for infection by history, physical examination, and tests, including urinalysis and urine culture (particularly in patients who have indwelling catheters), blood cultures, and cultures of other suspect body fluids. In patients with a suspected surgical or occult cause of sepsis, ultrasonography, CT, or MRI may be required, depending on the suspected source. Blood levels of C-reactive protein and procalcitonin are often elevated in severe sepsis and may facilitate diagnosis but they are not specific. Ultimately, the diagnosis is clinical.

Other causes of shock (eg, hypovolemia, MI) should be ruled out via history, physical examination, ECG, and serum cardiac markers. Even in the absence of MI, hypoperfusion caused by sepsis may result in ECG findings of ischemia including nonspecific ST-T wave abnormalities, T-wave inversions, and supraventricular and ventricular arrhythmias.

It is important to detect organ dysfunction as early as possible. A number of scoring systems have been devised, but the sequential organ failure assessment score (SOFA score) and the quick SOFA score (qSOFA) have been validated with respect to mortality risk and are relatively simple to use.

The **qSOFA criteria** identify patients who should have further clinical and laboratory investigation (all 3 criteria must be present):

- Respiratory rate ≥ 22/min
- Altered mentation
- Systolic BP ≤ 100 mm Hg

The **SOFA score** is somewhat more robust but requires laboratory testing (see Table 71–1).

CBC, ABGs, chest x-ray, serum electrolytes, BUN and creatinine, Pco_2, and liver function are monitored. Serum lactate levels, central venous O_2 saturation ($ScvO_2$), or both can be done to help guide treatment. WBC count may be decreased (< 4,000/μL) or increased (> 15,000/μL), and PMNs may be as low as 20%. During the course of sepsis, the WBC count may increase or decrease, depending on the severity of sepsis or shock, the patient's immunologic status, and the etiology of the infection. Concurrent corticosteroid use may elevate WBC count and thus mask WBC changes due to trends in the illness.

Hyperventilation with respiratory alkalosis (low $Paco_2$ and increased arterial pH) occurs early, in part as compensation for lactic acidemia. Serum HCO_3 is usually low, and serum and blood lactate levels increase. As shock progresses, metabolic acidosis worsens, and blood pH decreases. Early hypoxemic respiratory failure leads to a decreased PaO_2:FIO_2 ratio and sometimes overt hypoxemia with $Pao_2 < 70$ mm Hg. Diffuse infiltrates may appear on the chest x-ray due to acute respiratory distress syndrome (ARDS). BUN and creatinine usually increase progressively as a result of renal insufficiency. Bilirubin and transaminases may rise, although overt hepatic failure is uncommon in patients with normal baseline liver function.

Many patients with severe sepsis develop relative adrenal insufficiency (ie, normal or slightly elevated baseline cortisol levels that do not increase significantly in response to further stress or exogenous ACTH). Adrenal function may be tested by measuring serum cortisol at 8 AM; a level < 5 mg/dL is inadequate. Alternatively, cortisol can be measured before and after injection of 250 mcg of synthetic ACTH; a rise of < 9 mcg/dL is considered insufficient. However, in refractory septic shock, no cortisol testing is required before starting corticosteroid therapy.

Hemodynamic measurements with a central venous or pulmonary artery catheter (see p. 528) can be used when the specific type of shock is unclear or when large fluid volumes (eg, > 4 to 5 L 0.9% saline over 6 to 8 h) are needed. Bedside echocardiography in the ICU is a practical and noninvasive alternative method of hemodynamic monitoring. In septic shock, cardiac output is increased and peripheral vascular resistance is decreased, whereas in other forms of shock, cardiac output is typically decreased and peripheral resistance is increased. Neither CVP nor pulmonary artery occlusive pressure (PAOP) is

Table 71–1. SEQUENTIAL ORGAN FAILURE ASSESSMENT (SOFA) SCORE

PARAMETER	SCORE: 0	SCORE: 1	SCORE: 2	SCORE: 3	SCORE: 4
Pao_2/FIO_2	≥ 400 mm Hg (53.3 kPa)	< 400 mm Hg (53.3 kPa)	< 300 mm Hg (40 kPa)	< 200 mm Hg (26.7 kPa) with respiratory support	< 100 mm Hg (13.3 kPa) with respiratory support
Platelets	≥ 150 × 10³/μL	< 150	< 100	< 50	< 20
Bilirubin	≥ 1.2 mg/dL (20 μmol/L)	1.2–1.9 mg/dL (20–32 μmol/L)	2.0–5.9 mg/dL (33–101 μmol/L)	6.0–11.9 mg/dL (102–204 μmol/L)	> 12.0 mg/dL (204 μmol/L)
Cardiovascular	MAP ≥ 70 mm Hg	MAP < 70 mm Hg	Dopamine < 5 mcg/kg/min for ≥ 1 h *or* Any dose of dobutamine	Dopamine 5.1–15 mcg/kg/min for ≥ 1 h *or* Epinephrine ≤ 0.1 mcg/kg/min for ≥ 1 h *or* Norepinephrine ≤ 0.1 mcg/kg/min for ≥ 1 h	Dopamine > 15 mcg/kg/min for ≥ 1 h *or* Epinephrine > 0.1 mcg/kg/min for ≥ 1 h *or* Norepinephrine > 0.1 mcg/kg/min for ≥ 1 h
Glasgow Coma Scale score*	15 points	13–14 points	10–12 points	6–9 points	< 6 points
Creatinine	< 1.2 mg/dL (110 μmol/L)	1.2-1.9 mg/dL (110–170 μmol/L)	2.0-3.4 mg/dL (171–299 μmol/L)	3.5-4.9 mg/dL (300–400 μmol/L)	> 5.0 mg/dL (440 μmol/L)
Urine output	—	—	—	< 500 mL/day	< 200 mL/day

*A higher score indicates better neurologic function.

FIO_2 = fractional inspired O_2; kPa = kilopascals; MAP = mean arterial pressure; Pao_2 = arterial oxygen partial pressure.

Adapted from Singer M, Deutschman CS, Seymour CW, et al: The third international consensus definitions for sepsis and septic shock (sepsis-3). *JAMA* 315:801–810, 2016.

likely to be abnormal in septic shock, unlike in hypovolemic, obstructive, or cardiogenic shock.

Prognosis

Overall mortality in patients with septic shock is decreasing and now averages 30 to 40% (range 10 to 90%, depending on patient characteristics). Poor outcomes often follow failure to institute early aggressive therapy (eg, within 6 h of suspected diagnosis). Once severe lactic acidosis with decompensated metabolic acidosis becomes established, especially in conjunction with multiorgan failure, septic shock is likely to be irreversible and fatal.

Treatment

- Perfusion restored with IV fluids and sometimes vasopressors
- O_2 support
- Broad-spectrum antibiotics
- Source control
- Sometimes other supportive measures (eg, corticosteroids, insulin)

Patients with septic shock should be treated in an ICU. The following should be monitored hourly:

- CVP, PAOP, or $ScvO_2$
- Pulse oximetry
- ABGs
- Blood glucose, lactate, and electrolyte levels
- Renal function

Urine output, a good indicator of renal perfusion, should be measured, usually with an indwelling catheter. The onset of oliguria (eg, < about 0.5 mL/kg/h) or anuria, or rising creatinine may signal impending renal failure.

Following evidence-based guidelines and formal protocols for timely diagnosis and treatment of sepsis has recently been shown to decrease mortality and length of stay in the hospital.

Perfusion restoration: IV fluids are the first method used to restore perfusion. Isotonic crystalloid (eg, 0.9% saline) is preferred. Some clinicians add albumin to the initial fluid bolus in patients with severe sepsis or septic shock; albumin is more expensive than crystalloid but is generally a safe complement to crystalloid. Starch-based fluids (eg, hydroxyethyl starch) are associated with increased mortality and should not be used. Initially, 1 L of crystalloid is given rapidly. Most patients require a minimum of 30 mL/kg in the first 4 to 6 h. However, the goal of therapy is not to administer a specific volume of fluid but to achieve tissue reperfusion without causing pulmonary edema due to fluid overload.

Estimates of successful reperfusion include $ScvO_2$ and lactate clearance (ie, percent change in serum lactate levels). Target $ScvO_2$ is ≥ 70%. Lactate clearance target is 10 to 20%. Risk of pulmonary edema can be controlled by optimizing preload; fluids should be given until CVP reaches 8 mm Hg (10 cm H_2O) or PAOP reaches 12 to 15 mm Hg; however, patients on mechanical ventilation may require higher CVP levels. The quantity of fluid required often far exceeds the normal blood volume and may reach 10 L over 4 to 12 h. PAOP or echocardiography can identify limitations in left ventricular function and incipient pulmonary edema due to fluid overload.

If a patient with septic shock remains hypotensive after CVP or PAOP has been raised to target levels, norepinephrine or vasopressin (0.03 units/min) may be given to increase mean BP to at least 60 mm Hg. Epinephrine may be added if a second drug is needed. However, vasoconstriction caused by higher doses of these drugs may cause organ hypoperfusion and acidosis.

Oxygen support: O_2 is given by mask or nasal prongs. Tracheal intubation and mechanical ventilation may be needed subsequently for respiratory failure (see Mechanical ventilation in ARDS on p. 565).

Antibiotics: Parenteral antibiotics should be given as soon as possible after specimens of blood, body fluids, and wound sites have been taken for Gram stain and culture. Very prompt empiric therapy, started immediately after suspecting sepsis, is essential and may be lifesaving. Antibiotic selection requires an educated guess based on the suspected source (eg, pneumonia, urinary tract infection), clinical setting, knowledge or suspicion of causative organisms and of sensitivity patterns common to that specific inpatient unit or institution, and previous culture results.

Typically, broad-spectrum gram-positive and gram-negative bacterial coverage is used initially; immunocompromised patients should also receive an empiric antifungal drug. There are many possible starting regimens; when available, institutional trends for infecting organisms and their antibiotic susceptibility patterns (antibiograms) should be used to select empiric treatment. In general, common antibiotics for empiric gram-positive coverage include vancomycin and linezolid. Empiric gram-negative coverage has more options and includes broad-spectrum penicillins (eg, piperacillin/tazobactam), 3rd- or 4th-generation cephalosporins, imipenems, and aminoglycosides. Initial broad coverage is narrowed based on culture and sensitivity data.

Source control: The source of infection should be controlled as early as possible. IV and urinary catheters and endotracheal tubes should be removed if possible or changed. Abscesses must be drained, and necrotic and devitalized tissues (eg, gangrenous gallbladder, necrotizing soft-tissue infection) must be surgically excised. If excision is not possible (eg, because of comorbidities or hemodynamic instability), surgical drainage may help. If the source is not controlled, the patient's condition will continue to deteriorate despite antibiotic therapy.

Other supportive measures: Normalization of blood glucose improves outcome in critically ill patients, even those not known to be diabetic, because hyperglycemia impairs the immune response to infection. A continuous IV insulin infusion (starting dose 1 to 4 units/h) is titrated to maintain glucose between 110 and 180 mg/dL (7.7 to 9.9 mmol/L). This approach necessitates frequent (eg, every 1 to 4 h) glucose measurement.

Corticosteroid therapy may be beneficial in patients who remain hypotensive despite treatment with IV fluids, source control, antibiotics, and vasopressors. There is no need to measure cortisol levels before starting therapy. Treatment is with replacement rather than pharmacologic doses. One regimen consists of hydrocortisone 50 mg IV q 6 h (or 100 mg q 8 h). Continued treatment is based on patient response.

Trials of monoclonal antibodies and activated protein C (drotrecogin alfa—no longer available) have been unsuccessful.

KEY POINTS

- Sepsis and septic shock are increasingly severe clinical syndromes of life-threatening organ dysfunction caused by a dysregulated response to infection.
- An important component is critical reduction in tissue perfusion, which can lead to acute failure of multiple organs, including the lungs, kidneys, and liver.
- Early recognition and treatment is the key to improved survival.
- Resuscitate with IV fluids and sometimes vasopressors titrated to optimize central venous oxygen saturation ($ScvO_2$) and preload, and to lower serum lactate levels.
- Control the source of infection by removing catheters, tubes, and infected and/or necrotic tissue and by draining abscesses.
- Give empiric broad-spectrum antibiotics directed at most likely organisms and switch quickly to more specific drugs based on culture and sensitivity results.

72 Shock and Fluid Resuscitation

(See also Ch. 73.)

The fundamental defect in shock is reduced perfusion of vital tissues. Definitive treatment restores adequate tissue perfusion.

SHOCK

Shock is a state of organ hypoperfusion with resultant cellular dysfunction and death. Mechanisms may involve decreased circulating volume, decreased cardiac output, and vasodilation, sometimes with shunting of blood to bypass capillary exchange beds. Symptoms include altered mental status, tachycardia, hypotension, and oliguria. Diagnosis is clinical, including BP measurement and sometimes markers of tissue hypoperfusion (eg, blood lactate, base deficit). Treatment is with fluid resuscitation, including blood products if necessary, correction of the underlying disorder, and sometimes vasopressors.

Pathophysiology

The fundamental defect in shock is reduced perfusion of vital tissues. Once perfusion declines and O_2 delivery to cells is inadequate for aerobic metabolism, cells shift to anaerobic metabolism with increased production of CO_2 and accumulation of lactic acid. Cellular function declines, and if shock persists, irreversible cell damage and death occur.

During shock, both the inflammatory and clotting cascades may be triggered in areas of hypoperfusion. Hypoxic vascular endothelial cells activate WBCs, which bind to the endothelium and release directly damaging substances (eg, reactive O_2 species, proteolytic enzymes) and inflammatory mediators (eg, cytokines, leukotrienes, tumor necrosis factor [TNF]). Some of these mediators bind to cell surface receptors and activate nuclear factor kappa B (NFκB), which leads to production of additional cytokines and nitric oxide (NO), a potent vasodilator. Septic shock (see p. 569) may be more proinflammatory than other forms of shock because of the actions of bacterial toxins, especially endotoxin.

In septic shock, vasodilation of capacitance vessels leads to pooling of blood and hypotension because of "relative" hypovolemia (ie, too much volume to be filled by the existing amount of blood). Localized vasodilation may shunt blood past the capillary exchange beds, causing focal hypoperfusion despite normal cardiac output and BP. Additionally, excess NO is converted to peroxynitrite, a free radical that damages mitochondria and decreases ATP production.

Blood flow to microvessels including capillaries is reduced even though large-vessel blood flow is preserved in settings of septic shock. Mechanical microvascular obstruction may, at least in part, account for such limiting of substrate delivery. Leukocytes and platelets adhere to the endothelium, and the clotting system is activated with fibrin deposition.

Multiple mediators, along with endothelial cell dysfunction, markedly increase microvascular permeability, allowing fluid and sometimes plasma proteins to escape into the interstitial space. In the GI tract, increased permeability possibly allows translocation of the enteric bacteria from the lumen, potentially leading to sepsis or metastatic infection.

Neutrophil apoptosis may be inhibited, enhancing the release of inflammatory mediators. In other cells, apoptosis may be augmented, increasing cell death and thus worsening organ function.

BP is not always low in the early stages of shock (although hypotension eventually occurs if shock is not reversed). Similarly, not all patients with "low" BP have shock. The degree and consequences of hypotension vary with the adequacy of physiologic compensation and the patient's underlying diseases. Thus, a modest degree of hypotension that is well tolerated by a young, relatively healthy person might result in severe cerebral, cardiac, or renal dysfunction in an older person with significant arteriosclerosis.

Compensation: Initially, when O_2 delivery (DO_2) is decreased, tissues compensate by extracting a greater percentage of delivered O_2. Low arterial pressure triggers an adrenergic response with sympathetic-mediated vasoconstriction and often increased heart rate. Initially, vasoconstriction is selective, shunting blood to the heart and brain and away from the splanchnic circulation. Circulating β-adrenergic amines (epinephrine, norepinephrine) also increase cardiac contractility and trigger release of corticosteroids from the adrenal gland, renin from the kidneys, and glucose from the liver. Increased glucose may overwhelm ailing mitochondria, causing further lactate production.

Reperfusion: Reperfusion of ischemic cells can cause further injury. As substrate is reintroduced, neutrophil activity may increase, increasing production of damaging superoxide and hydroxyl radicals. After blood flow is restored, inflammatory mediators may be circulated to other organs.

Multiple organ dysfunction syndrome (MODS): The combination of direct and reperfusion injury may cause MODS—the progressive dysfunction of ≥ 2 organs consequent to life-threatening illness or injury. MODS can follow any type of shock but is most common when infection is involved; organ failure is one of the defining features of septic shock (see p. 569). MODS also occurs in > 10% of patients with severe traumatic injury and is the primary cause of death in those surviving > 24 h.

Any organ system can be affected, but the most frequent target organ is the lung, in which increased membrane permeability leads to flooding of alveoli and further inflammation. Progressive hypoxia may be increasingly resistant to supplemental O_2 therapy. This condition is termed acute lung injury or, if severe, acute respiratory distress syndrome (ARDS—see p. 563).

The kidneys are injured when renal perfusion is critically reduced, leading to acute tubular necrosis and renal insufficiency manifested by oliguria and progressive rise in serum creatinine.

In the heart, reduced coronary perfusion and increased mediators (including TNF and IL-1) may depress contractility, worsen myocardial compliance, and down-regulate β-receptors. These factors decrease cardiac output, further worsening both myocardial and systemic perfusion and causing a vicious circle often culminating in death. Arrhythmias may occur.

In the GI tract, ileus and submucosal hemorrhage can develop. Liver hypoperfusion can cause focal or extensive hepatocellular necrosis, transaminase and bilirubin elevation, and decreased production of clotting factors.

Etiology and Classification

There are several mechanisms of organ hypoperfusion and shock. Shock may be due to a low circulating volume (hypovolemic shock), vasodilation (distributive shock), a primary decrease in cardiac output (both cardiogenic and obstructive shock), or a combination.

Hypovolemic shock: Hypovolemic shock is caused by a critical decrease in intravascular volume. Diminished venous return (preload) results in decreased ventricular filling and reduced stroke volume. Unless compensated for by increased heart rate, cardiac output decreases.

A common cause is bleeding (hemorrhagic shock), typically due to trauma, surgical interventions, peptic ulcer, esophageal varices, or ruptured aortic aneurysm. Bleeding may be overt (eg, hematemesis, melena) or concealed (eg, ruptured ectopic pregnancy).

Hypovolemic shock may also follow increased losses of body fluids other than blood (Table 72–1).

Hypovolemic shock may be due to inadequate fluid intake (with or without increased fluid loss). Water may be unavailable, neurologic disability may impair the thirst mechanism, or physical disability may impair access.

Table 72–1. HYPOVOLEMIC SHOCK CAUSED BY BODY FLUID LOSS

SITE OF FLUID LOSS	MECHANISM OF LOSS
Skin	Thermal or chemical burn, sweating due to excessive heat exposure
GI tract	Vomiting, diarrhea
Kidneys	Diabetes mellitus or insipidus, adrenal insufficiency, salt-losing nephritis, the polyuric phase after acute tubular damage, use of potent diuretics
Intravascular fluid lost to the extravascular space	Increased capillary permeability secondary to inflammation or traumatic injury (eg, crush), anoxia, cardiac arrest, sepsis, bowel ischemia, acute pancreatitis

In hospitalized patients, hypovolemia can be compounded if early signs of circulatory insufficiency are incorrectly ascribed to heart failure and fluids are withheld or diuretics are given.

Distributive shock: Distributive shock results from a relative inadequacy of intravascular volume caused by arterial or venous vasodilation; circulating blood volume is normal. In some cases, cardiac output (and DO_2) is high, but increased blood flow through arteriovenous shunts bypasses capillary beds; this bypass plus uncoupled cellular O_2 transport cause cellular hypoperfusion (shown by decreased O_2 consumption). In other situations, blood pools in venous capacitance beds and cardiac output falls.

Distributive shock may be caused by anaphylaxis (anaphylactic shock—see p. 1378); bacterial infection with endotoxin release (septic shock—see p. 569); severe injury to the spinal cord, usually above T4 (neurogenic shock); and ingestion of certain drugs or poisons, such as nitrates, opioids, and adrenergic blockers. Anaphylactic shock and septic shock often have a component of hypovolemia as well.

Cardiogenic and obstructive shock: Cardiogenic shock is a relative or absolute reduction in cardiac output due to a primary cardiac disorder. Obstructive shock is caused by mechanical factors that interfere with filling or emptying of the heart or great vessels. Causes are listed in Table 72–2.

Symptoms and Signs

Lethargy, confusion, and somnolence are common. The hands and feet are pale, cool, clammy, and often cyanotic, as are the earlobes, nose, and nail beds. Capillary filling time is prolonged, and, except in distributive shock, the skin appears grayish or dusky and moist. Overt diaphoresis may occur. Peripheral pulses are weak and typically rapid; often, only femoral or carotid pulses are palpable. Tachypnea and hyperventilation may be present. BP tends to be low (< 90 mm Hg systolic) or unobtainable; direct measurement by intra-arterial catheter, if done, often gives higher and more accurate values. Urine output is low.

Distributive shock causes similar symptoms, except the skin may appear warm or flushed, especially during sepsis. The pulse may be bounding rather than weak. In septic shock, fever, usually preceded by chills, is typically present. Some patients with anaphylactic shock have urticaria or wheezing.

Numerous other symptoms (eg, chest pain, dyspnea, abdominal pain) may be due to the underlying disease or secondary organ failure.

Diagnosis

- Clinical evaluation
- Test result trends

Diagnosis is mostly clinical, based on evidence of insufficient tissue perfusion (obtundation, oliguria, peripheral cyanosis) and signs of compensatory mechanisms (tachycardia, tachypnea, diaphoresis). Specific criteria include obtundation, heart rate > 100, respiratory rate > 22, hypotension (systolic BP < 90 mm Hg) or a 30-mm Hg fall in baseline BP, and urine output < 0.5 mL/kg/h. Laboratory findings that support the diagnosis include lactate > 3 mmol/L, base deficit < −4 mEq/L, and $Paco_2$ < 32 mm Hg. However, none of these findings alone is diagnostic, and each is evaluated by its trend (ie, worsening or improving) and in the overall clinical context, including physical signs. Recently, measurement of sublingual PCO_2 and near-infrared spectroscopy have been introduced as noninvasive and rapid techniques that may measure the degree of shock; however, these techniques have yet to be validated on a larger scale.

Diagnosis of cause: Recognizing the cause of shock is more important than categorizing the type. Often, the cause is obvious or can be recognized quickly based on the history and physical examination, aided by simple testing.

Chest pain (with or without dyspnea) suggests MI, aortic dissection, or pulmonary embolism. A systolic murmur may indicate ventricular septal rupture or mitral insufficiency due to acute MI. A diastolic murmur may indicate aortic regurgitation due to aortic dissection involving the aortic root. Cardiac tamponade is suggested by jugular venous distention, muffled heart sounds, and a paradoxical pulse. Pulmonary embolism severe enough to cause shock typically produces decreased O_2 saturation and occurs more often in special settings, including prolonged bed rest and after a surgical procedure. Tests include ECG, troponin I, chest x-ray, ABGs, lung scan, helical CT, and echocardiography.

Abdominal or back pain or a tender abdomen suggests pancreatitis, ruptured abdominal aortic aneurysm, peritonitis, and, in women of childbearing age, ruptured ectopic pregnancy. A pulsatile midline mass suggests ruptured abdominal aortic aneurysm. A tender adnexal mass suggests ectopic pregnancy. Testing typically includes abdominal CT (if the patient is unstable, bedside ultrasound can be helpful), CBC, amylase, lipase, and, for women of childbearing age, urine pregnancy test.

Fever, chills, and focal signs of infection suggest septic shock, particularly in immunocompromised patients. Isolated fever, contingent on history and clinical settings, may point to heatstroke. Tests include chest x-ray; urinalysis; CBC; and cultures of wounds, blood, urine, and other relevant body fluids.

In a few patients, the cause is occult. Patients with no focal symptoms or signs indicative of cause should have ECG, cardiac enzymes, chest x-ray, and ABGs. If results of these tests are normal, the most likely causes include drug overdose, occult infection (including toxic shock), anaphylaxis, and obstructive shock.

Table 72–2. MECHANISMS OF CARDIOGENIC AND OBSTRUCTIVE SHOCK

TYPE	MECHANISM	CAUSE
Obstructive	Mechanical interference with ventricular filling	Tension pneumothorax, cava compression, cardiac tamponade, atrial tumor or clot
	Interference with ventricular emptying	Pulmonary embolism
Cardiogenic	Impaired myocardial contractility	Myocardial ischemia or MI, myocarditis, drugs
	Abnormalities of cardiac rhythm	Tachycardia, bradycardia
	Cardiac structural disorder	Acute mitral or aortic regurgitation, ruptured interventricular septum, prosthetic valve malfunction

Table 72–3. INOTROPIC AND VASOACTIVE CATECHOLAMINES

DRUG	DOSAGE	HEMODYNAMIC ACTIONS
Norepinephrine	4 mg/250 mL or 500 mL 5% D/W continuous IV infusion at 8–12 mcg/min initially, then at 2–4 mcg/min as maintenance, with wide variations	α-Adrenergic: Vasoconstriction β-Adrenergic: Inotropic and chronotropic effects*
Dopamine	400 mg/500 mL 5% D/W continuous IV infusion at 0.3–1.25 mL (250–1000 mcg)/min 2–10 mcg/kg/min for low dose 20 mcg/kg/min for high dose	α-Adrenergic: Vasoconstriction† β-Adrenergic: Inotropic and chronotropic effects and vasodilation† Nonadrenergic: Renal and splanchnic vasodilation
Dobutamine	250 mg/250 mL 5% D/W continuous IV infusion at 2.5–10 mcg/kg/min	β-Adrenergic: Inotropic effects‡

*Effects are not apparent if arterial pressure is elevated too much.
†Effects depend on dosage and underlying pathophysiology.
‡Chronotropic, arrhythmogenic, and direct vascular effects are minimal at lower doses.

Ancillary testing: If not already done, ECG, chest x-ray, CBC, serum electrolytes, BUN, creatinine, PT, PTT, liver function tests, and fibrinogen and fibrin split products are done to monitor patient status and serve as a baseline. If the patient's volume status is difficult to determine, monitoring of central venous pressure (CVP) or pulmonary artery occlusion pressure (PAOP) may be useful. CVP < 5 mm Hg (< 7 cm H_2O) or PAOP < 8 mm Hg may indicate hypovolemia, although CVP may be greater in hypovolemic patients with preexisting pulmonary hypertension. Rapid bedside echocardiography (done by the treating physician) to assess adequacy of cardiac filling and function is being increasingly used to assess shock.

Prognosis and Treatment

Untreated shock is usually fatal. Even with treatment, mortality from cardiogenic shock after MI (60 to 65%) and septic shock (30 to 40%) is high. Prognosis depends on the cause, preexisting or complicating illness, time between onset and diagnosis, and promptness and adequacy of therapy.

General management: First aid involves keeping the patient warm. External hemorrhage is controlled, airway and ventilation are checked, and respiratory assistance is given if necessary. Nothing is given by mouth, and the patient's head is turned to one side to avoid aspiration if emesis occurs.

Treatment begins simultaneously with evaluation. Supplemental O_2 by face mask is provided. If shock is severe or if ventilation is inadequate, airway intubation with mechanical ventilation is necessary. Two large (14- to 16-gauge) IV catheters are inserted into separate peripheral veins. A central venous line or an intraosseous needle, especially in children, provides an alternative when peripheral veins cannot promptly be accessed (see also p. 533).

Typically, 1 L (or 20 mL/kg in children) of 0.9% saline is infused over 15 min. In major hemorrhage, Ringer's lactate is commonly used. Unless clinical parameters return to normal, the infusion is repeated. Smaller volumes (eg, 250 to 500 mL) are used for patients with signs of high right-sided pressure (eg, distention of neck veins) or acute MI. A fluid challenge should probably not be done in a patient with signs of pulmonary edema. Further fluid therapy is based on the underlying condition and may require monitoring of CVP or PAOP. Bedside cardiac ultrasonography to assess contractility and vena caval respiratory variability may help determine the need for additional fluid vs the need for inotropic support.

Patients in shock are critically ill and should be admitted to an ICU. Monitoring includes ECG; systolic, diastolic, and mean BP, preferably by intra-arterial catheter; respiratory rate and depth; pulse oximetry; urine flow by indwelling bladder catheter; body temperature; and clinical status, including sensorium (eg, Glasgow Coma Scale—see Table 224–4 on p. 1862), pulse volume, skin temperature, and color. Measurement of CVP, PAOP, and thermodilution cardiac output using a balloon-tipped pulmonary arterial catheter may be helpful for diagnosis and initial management of patients with shock of uncertain or mixed etiology or with severe shock, especially when accompanied by oliguria or pulmonary edema. Echocardiography (bedside or transesophageal) is a less invasive alternative. Serial measurements of ABGs, Hct, electrolytes, serum creatinine, and blood lactate are obtained. Sublingual CO_2 measurement (see p. 530), if available, is a noninvasive monitor of visceral perfusion. A well-designed flow sheet is helpful.

Because tissue hypoperfusion makes intramuscular absorption unreliable, all parenteral drugs are given IV. Opioids generally are avoided because they may cause vasodilation, but severe pain may be treated with morphine 1 to 4 mg IV given over 2 min and repeated q 10 to 15 min if necessary. Although cerebral hypoperfusion may cause anxiety, sedatives or tranquilizers are not routinely given.

After initial resuscitation, specific treatment is directed at the underlying condition. Additional supportive care is guided by the type of shock.

Hemorrhagic shock: In hemorrhagic shock, surgical control of bleeding is the first priority. Volume replacement (see also p. 576) accompanies rather than precedes surgical control. Blood products and crystalloid solutions are used for resuscitation; however, packed RBCs and plasma are being considered earlier and in a ratio of 1:1 in patients likely to require massive transfusion (see p. 1212). Failure to respond usually indicates insufficient volume administration or unrecognized ongoing hemorrhage. Vasopressor agents are not indicated for treatment of hemorrhagic shock unless cardiogenic, obstructive, or distributive causes are also present.

Distributive shock: Distributive shock with profound hypotension after initial fluid replacement with 0.9% saline may be treated with inotropic or vasopressor agents (eg, dopamine, norepinephrine—Table 72–3). Patients with septic shock also receive broad-spectrum antibiotics (see p. 572). Patients with anaphylactic shock unresponsive to fluid challenge (especially if accompanied by bronchoconstriction) receive epinephrine 0.05 to 0.1 mg IV, followed by epinephrine infusion of 5 mg in 500 mL 5% D/W at 10 mL/h or 0.02 mcg/kg/min (see also p. 1378).

Cardiogenic shock: In cardiogenic shock, structural disorders (eg, valvular dysfunction, septal rupture) are repaired surgically. Coronary thrombosis is treated either by percutaneous interventions (angioplasty, stenting), coronary artery bypass surgery, or thrombolysis (see also p. 665). Tachydysrhythmia (eg, rapid atrial fibrillation, ventricular tachycardia) is slowed by cardioversion or with drugs. Bradycardia is treated with a transcutaneous or transvenous pacemaker; atropine 0.5 mg IV up to 4 doses q 5 min may be given pending pacemaker placement. Isoproterenol (2 mg/500 mL 5% D/W at 1 to 4 mcg/min [0.25 to 1 mL/min]) is occasionally useful if atropine is ineffective, but it is not advised in patients with myocardial ischemia due to coronary artery disease.

Shock after acute MI is treated with volume expansion if PAOP is low or normal; 15 to 18 mm Hg is considered optimal. If a pulmonary artery catheter is not in place, cautious volume infusion (250- to 500-mL bolus of 0.9% saline) may be tried while auscultating the chest frequently for signs of fluid overload. Shock after right ventricular MI usually responds partially to volume expansion; however, vasopressor agents may be needed. Bedside cardiac ultrasonography to assess contractility and vena caval respiratory variability can help determine the need for additional fluid vs vasopressors; inotropic support is a better approach for patients with normal or above-normal filling.

If hypotension is moderate (eg, mean arterial pressure [MAP] 70 to 90 mm Hg), dobutamine infusion may be used to improve cardiac output and reduce left ventricular filling pressure. Tachycardia and arrhythmias occasionally occur during dobutamine administration, particularly at higher doses, necessitating dose reduction. Vasodilators (eg, nitroprusside, nitroglycerin), which increase venous capacitance or lower systemic vascular resistance, reduce the workload on the damaged myocardium and may increase cardiac output in patients without severe hypotension. Combination therapy (eg, dopamine or dobutamine with nitroprusside or nitroglycerin) may be particularly useful but requires close ECG and pulmonary and systemic hemodynamic monitoring.

For more serious hypotension (MAP < 70 mm Hg), norepinephrine or dopamine may be given, with a target systolic pressure of 80 to 90 mm Hg (and not > 110 mm Hg). Intra-aortic balloon counterpulsation is valuable for temporarily reversing shock in patients with acute MI. This procedure should be considered as a bridge to permit cardiac catheterization and coronary angiography before possible surgical intervention in patients with acute MI complicated by ventricular septal rupture or severe acute mitral regurgitation who require vasopressor support for > 30 min.

In obstructive shock, nontraumatic cardiac tamponade requires immediate pericardiocentesis, which can be done at the bedside. Trauma-related cardiac tamponade requires surgical decompression and repair. Tension pneumothorax should be immediately decompressed with a catheter inserted into the 2nd intercostal space, midclavicular line; a chest tube is then inserted. Massive pulmonary embolism resulting in shock is treated with anticoagulation and thrombolysis, surgical embolectomy, or extracorporeal membrane oxygenation in select cases.

INTRAVENOUS FLUID RESUSCITATION

Almost all circulatory shock states require large-volume IV fluid replacement, as does severe intravascular volume depletion (eg, due to diarrhea or heatstroke). Intravascular volume deficiency is acutely compensated for by vasoconstriction, followed over hours by migration of fluid from the extravascular compartment to the intravascular compartment, maintaining circulating volume at the expense of total body water. However, this compensation is overwhelmed after major losses. See Ch. 167 on p. 1298 for maintenance fluid requirement discussion, and see p. 2554 for mild dehydration discussion.

Fluids

Choice of resuscitation fluid depends on the cause of the deficit.

Hemorrhage: Loss of RBCs diminishes O_2-carrying capacity. However, the body increases cardiac output to maintain O_2 delivery (DO_2) and increases O_2 extraction. These factors provide a safety margin of about 9 times the resting O_2 requirement. Thus, non–O_2-carrying fluids (eg, crystalloid or colloid solutions) may be used to restore intravascular volume in mild to moderate blood loss. However, in severe shock, blood products are required. Early administration of plasma and platelets probably helps minimize the dilutional and consumptive coagulopathy that accompanies major hemorrhage. A ratio of 1 unit of plasma for each 1 to 2 units of blood has been recommended, but the optimal ratio has not been confirmed. When the patient is stable, once Hb declines to < 7 g/dL, in the absence of cardiac or cerebral vascular disease, O_2-carrying capacity should be restored by infusion of blood (or in the future by blood substitutes). Patients with active coronary or cerebral vascular disease or ongoing hemorrhage require blood for Hb < 10 g/dL.

Crystalloid solutions for intravascular volume replenishment are typically isotonic (eg, 0.9% saline or Ringer's lactate [RL]). H_2O freely travels outside the vasculature, so as little as 10% of isotonic fluid remains in the intravascular space. With hypotonic fluid (eg, 0.45% saline), even less remains in the vasculature, and, thus, this fluid is not used for resuscitation. Both 0.9% saline and RL are equally effective; RL may be preferred in hemorrhagic shock because it somewhat minimizes acidosis and will not cause hyperchloremia. For patients with acute brain injury, 0.9% saline is preferred. Hypertonic saline is not recommended for resuscitation because the evidence suggests there is no difference in outcome when compared to isotonic fluids.

Colloid solutions (eg, hydroxyethyl starch, albumin, dextrans) are also effective for volume replacement during major hemorrhage. Colloid solutions offer no major advantage over crystalloid solutions, and albumin has been associated with poorer outcomes in patients with traumatic brain injury. Both dextrans and hydroxyethyl starch may adversely affect coagulation when > 1.5 L is given.

Blood typically is given as packed RBCs, which should be cross-matched, but in an urgent situation, 1 to 2 units of type O Rh-negative blood are an acceptable alternative. When > 1 to 2 units are transfused (eg, in major trauma), blood is warmed to 37° C. Patients receiving > 6 units may require replacement of clotting factors with infusion of fresh frozen plasma or cryoprecipitate and platelet transfusion (see also p. 1212).

Blood substitutes are O_2-carrying fluids that can be Hb-based or perfluorocarbons. Hb-based fluids may contain free Hb that is liposome-encapsulated or modified (eg, by surface modification or cross-linking with other molecules) to limit renal excretion and toxicity. Because the antigen-bearing RBC membrane is not present, these substances do not require cross-matching. They can also be stored > 1 yr, providing a more stable source than banked blood. Perfluorocarbons are IV carbon-fluorine emulsions that carry large amounts of O_2. However, no blood substitutes have yet proved to increase survival and some have significant adverse effects (eg, hypotension). Currently, no blood substitutes are commercially available for use.

Nonhemorrhagic hypovolemia: Isotonic crystalloid solutions are typically given for intravascular repletion during shock and hypovolemia. Colloid solutions are generally not used. Patients with dehydration and adequate circulatory volume typically have a free water deficit, and hypotonic solutions (eg, 5% D/W 0.45% saline) are used.

Route and Rate of Fluid Administration

Standard, large (eg, 14- to 16-gauge) peripheral IV catheters are adequate for most fluid resuscitation. With an infusion pump, they typically allow infusion of 1 L of crystalloid in 10 to 15 min and 1 unit of packed RBCs in 20 min. For patients at risk of exsanguination, a large (eg, 8.5 French) central venous catheter provides more rapid infusion rates; a pressure infusion device can infuse 1 unit of packed RBCs in < 5 min.

Patients in shock typically require and tolerate infusion at the maximum rate. Adults are given 1 L of crystalloid (20 mL/kg in children) or, in hemorrhagic shock, 5 to 10 mL/kg of colloid or packed RBCs, and the patient is reassessed. An exception is a patient with cardiogenic shock who typically does not require large volume infusion.

Patients with intravascular volume depletion without shock can receive infusion at a controlled rate, typically 500 mL/h. Children should have their fluid deficit calculated (see p. 2556) and replacement given over 24 h (half in the first 8 h).

End Point and Monitoring

The actual end point of fluid therapy in shock is to optimize tissue perfusion. However, this parameter is not measured directly. Surrogate end points include clinical indicators of end-organ perfusion and measurements of preload.

Adequate end-organ perfusion is best indicated by urine output of > 0.5 to 1 mL/kg/h. Heart rate, mental status, and capillary refill may be affected by the underlying disease process and are less reliable markers. Because of compensatory vasoconstriction, mean arterial pressure (MAP) is only a rough guideline; organ hypoperfusion may be present despite apparently normal values. An elevated arterial blood lactate level reflects hypoperfusion; however, levels do not decline for several hours after successful resuscitation. The trend of the base deficit can help indicate whether resuscitation is adequate. Other investigational methods such as sublingual tissue CO_2 or near-infrared spectroscopy may also be considered.

Central venous pressure: Because urine output does not provide a minute-to-minute indication, measures of preload may be helpful in guiding fluid resuscitation for critically ill patients. Central venous pressure (CVP) is the mean pressure in the superior vena cava, reflecting right ventricular end-diastolic pressure or preload. Normal CVP ranges from 2 to 7 mm Hg (3 to 9 cm H_2O). A sick or injured patient with a CVP < 3 mm Hg is presumed to be volume depleted and may be given fluids with relative safety. When the CVP is within the normal range, volume depletion cannot be excluded, and the response to 100- to 200-mL fluid boluses should be assessed; a modest increase in CVP in response to fluid generally indicates hypovolemia. An increase of > 3 to 5 mm Hg in response to a 100-mL fluid bolus suggests limited cardiac reserve. A CVP > 12 to 15 mm Hg casts doubt on hypovolemia as the sole etiology of hypoperfusion, and fluid administration risks fluid overload.

Because CVP may be unreliable in assessing volume status or left ventricular function, pulmonary artery catheterization (see p. 528) may be considered for diagnosis or for more precise titration of fluid therapy if there is no cardiovascular improvement after initial therapy. Care must be taken when interpreting filling pressures in patients during mechanical ventilation, particularly when positive end-expiratory pressure (PEEP) levels exceeding 10 cm H_2O are being used or during respiratory distress when pleural pressures fluctuate widely. Measurements are made at the end of expiration, and the transducer is referenced to atrial zero levels (mid chest) and carefully calibrated.

Traumatic hemorrhagic shock: Patients with traumatic hemorrhage shock may require a slightly different approach. Experimental and clinical evidence indicates that internal hemorrhage (eg, due to visceral or vascular laceration or crush) may be worsened by resuscitation to normal or supranormal MAP. Some physicians advocate a systolic blood pressure of 80 to 90 mm Hg as the resuscitation end point in such patients pending surgical control of bleeding, unless higher pressure is needed to provide adequate brain perfusion.

After blood loss is controlled, Hb is used to guide the need for further transfusion. A target Hb of 8 to 9 g/dL is suggested to minimize the use of blood products. Patients who may have difficulty tolerating moderate anemia (eg, those with coronary or cerebral artery disease) are kept above 30% Hct. A higher Hct does not improve outcome and, by causing increased blood viscosity, may impair perfusion of capillary beds.

Complications

Overly rapid infusion of any type of fluid may precipitate pulmonary edema, acute respiratory distress syndrome, or even a compartment syndrome (eg, abdominal compartment syndrome, extremity compartment syndrome).

Hemodilution resulting from crystalloid infusion is not of itself injurious, although Hct must be monitored to note whether threshold values for transfusion are met.

RBC transfusion has a low risk of directly transmitting infection, but in critically ill patients, it seems to cause a slightly higher rate of hospital-acquired infection. This risk may be minimized by using blood < 12 days old; such RBCs are more plastic and less likely to cause sludging in the microvasculature. For other complications of massive transfusion, see p. 1213.

SECTION 7

Cardiovascular Disorders

73 Approach to the Cardiac Patient

Symptoms or the physical examination may suggest a cardiovascular disorder. For confirmation, selected noninvasive and invasive cardiac tests are usually done.

History

A thorough history is fundamental; it cannot be replaced by testing. The history must include a thorough systems review because many symptoms apparently occurring in other systems (eg, dyspnea, indigestion) are often caused by cardiac disease. A family history is taken because many cardiac disorders (eg, coronary artery disease, systemic hypertension, bicuspid aortic valve, hypertrophic cardiomyopathy, mitral valve prolapse) have a heritable basis.

Serious cardiac symptoms include chest pain or discomfort, dyspnea, weakness, fatigue, palpitations, light-headedness, sense of an impending faint, syncope, and edema. These symptoms commonly occur in more than one cardiac disorder and in noncardiac disorders.

Physical Examination

The general cardiovascular examination and cardiac auscultation are discussed in other topics. Despite the ever-increasing use of cardiac imaging, bedside examination remains useful as it is always available and can be repeated as often as desired without cost.

CARDIOVASCULAR EXAMINATION

Complete examination of all systems is essential to detect peripheral and systemic effects of cardiac disorders and evidence of noncardiac disorders that might affect the heart. Examination includes the following:

- Vital sign measurement
- Pulse palpation and auscultation
- Vein observation
- Chest inspection, and palpation
- Cardiac percussion, palpation, and auscultation
- Lung examination, including percussion, palpation, and auscultation
- Extremity and abdomen examination

Cardiac auscultation is discussed in a separate topic. Despite the ever-increasing use of cardiac imaging, bedside auscultation remains useful as it is always available and can be repeated as often as desired without cost.

Vital Signs

Vital signs include

- Blood pressure
- Heart rate and rhythm
- Respiratory rate
- Temperature

Blood pressure is measured in both arms and, for suspected congenital cardiac disorders or peripheral vascular disorders, in both legs. The bladder of an appropriately sized cuff encircles 80% of the limb's circumference, and the bladder's width is 40% of the circumference. The first sound heard as the Hg column falls is systolic pressure; disappearance of the sound is diastolic pressure (5th-phase Korotkoff sound). Up to a 15 mm Hg pressure differential between the right and left arms is normal; a greater differential suggests a vascular abnormality (eg, dissecting thoracic aorta) or a peripheral vascular disorder. Leg pressure is usually 20 mm Hg higher than arm pressure.

Heart rate and rhythm are assessed by palpating the carotid or radial pulse or by cardiac auscultation if arrhythmia is suspected; some heartbeats during arrhythmias may be audible but do not generate a palpable pulse.

Respiratory rate, if abnormal, may indicate cardiac decompensation or a primary lung disorder. The rate increases in patients with heart failure or anxiety and decreases or becomes intermittent in the moribund. Shallow, rapid respirations may indicate pleuritic pain.

Temperature may be elevated by acute rheumatic fever or cardiac infection (eg, endocarditis). After a myocardial infarction, low grade fever is very common. Other causes are sought only if fever persists > 72 h.

Ankle-brachial index: The ankle-brachial index is the ratio of systolic BP in the ankle to that in the arm. This ratio is normally > 1. A Doppler probe may be used to measure blood pressure at the ankle if the pedal pulses are not easily palpable.

A low (≤ 0.90) ankle-brachial index suggests peripheral arterial disease, which can be classified as mild (index 0.71 to 0.90), moderate (0.41 to 0.70), or severe (≤ 0.40). A high index (> 1.30) may indicate noncompressible leg vessels (as occurs in Mönckeberg arteriosclerosis with calcification of the arterial wall).

Orthostatic changes: BP and heart rate are measured with the patient supine, seated, and standing; a 1-min interval is needed between each change in position. A difference of ≤ 10 mm Hg is normal; the difference tends to be a little greater in the elderly due to loss of vascular elasticity.

Pulsus paradoxus: Normally during inspiration, systolic arterial blood pressure can decrease as much as 10 mm Hg, and pulse rate increases to compensate. A greater decrease in systolic BP or weakening of the pulse during inspiration is considered pulsus paradoxus. Pulsus paradoxus occurs in

- Cardiac tamponade (commonly)
- Constrictive pericarditis, severe asthma, and COPD (occasionally)
- Restrictive cardiomyopathy, severe pulmonary embolism, and hypovolemic shock (rarely)

BP decreases during inspiration because negative intrathoracic pressure increases venous return and hence right ventricular (RV) filling; as a result, the interventricular septum bulges slightly into the left ventricular (LV) outflow tract, decreasing cardiac output and thus BP. This mechanism (and the drop in systolic BP) is exaggerated in disorders that cause high negative intrathoracic pressure (eg, asthma) or that restrict RV filling (eg, cardiac tamponade, cardiomyopathy) or outflow (eg, pulmonary embolism).

Pulsus paradoxus is quantified by inflating a BP cuff to just above systolic BP and deflating it very slowly (eg, ≤ 2 mm Hg/heartbeat). The pressure is noted when Korotkoff sounds are first heard (at first, only during expiration) and when Korotkoff sounds are heard continuously. The difference between the pressures is the "amount" of pulsus paradoxus.

Pulses

Peripheral pulses: Major peripheral pulses in the arms and legs are palpated for symmetry and volume (intensity); elasticity of the arterial wall is noted. Absence of pulses may suggest an arterial disorder (eg, atherosclerosis) or systemic embolism. Peripheral pulses may be difficult to feel in obese or muscular people. The pulse has a rapid upstroke, then collapses in disorders with a rapid runoff of arterial blood (eg, arteriovenous communication, aortic regurgitation). The pulse is rapid and bounding in hyperthyroidism and hypermetabolic states; it is slow and sluggish in hypothyroidism. If pulses are asymmetric, auscultation over peripheral vessels may detect a bruit due to stenosis.

Carotid pulses: Observation, palpation, and auscultation of both carotid pulses may suggest a specific disorder (see Table 73–1). Aging and arteriosclerosis lead to vessel rigidity, which tends to eliminate the characteristic findings. In very young children, the carotid pulse may be normal, even when severe aortic stenosis is present.

Auscultation over the carotid arteries can distinguish murmurs from bruits. Murmurs originate in the heart or great vessels and are usually louder over the upper precordium and diminish toward the neck. Bruits are higher-pitched, are heard only over the arteries, and seem more superficial. An arterial bruit must be distinguished from a venous hum. Unlike an arterial bruit, a venous hum is usually continuous, heard best with the patient sitting or standing, and is eliminated by compression of the ipsilateral internal jugular vein.

Veins

Peripheral veins: The peripheral veins are observed for varicosities, arteriovenous malformations (AVMs) and shunts, and overlying inflammation and tenderness due to thrombophlebitis. An AVM or a shunt produces a continuous murmur (heard on auscultation) and often a palpable thrill (because resistance is always lower in the vein than in the artery during systole and diastole).

Neck veins: The neck veins are examined to estimate venous wave height and waveform. Height is proportional to right atrial pressure, and waveform reflects events in the cardiac cycle; both are best observed in the internal jugular vein.

Table 73–1. CAROTID PULSE AMPLITUDE AND ASSOCIATED DISORDERS

CAROTID PULSE AMPLITUDE	ASSOCIATED DISORDER
Bounding and prominent	Hypertension Hypermetabolic states Disorders with a rapid rise and fall of pressure (eg, patent ductus arteriosus)
Jerky, with full expansion followed by sudden collapse (Corrigan's or water-hammer pulse)	Aortic valve regurgitation
Low in amplitude and volume with a delayed peak	Aortic stenosis (obstructing left ventricular outflow) Shock
Double-peaked (bifid) with a rapid rise	Hypertrophic cardiomyopathy
Bifid with normal or delayed rise	Combined aortic stenosis and aortic regurgitation
Diminished unilaterally or bilaterally, often with a systolic bruit	Extracranial carotid stenosis due to atherosclerosis

The jugular veins are usually examined with the patient reclining at 45°. The top of the venous column is normally just above the clavicles (upper limit of normal: 4 cm above the sternal notch in a vertical plane). The venous column is elevated in heart failure, volume overload, cardiac tamponade, constrictive pericarditis, tricuspid stenosis, superior vena cava obstruction, or reduced compliance of the RV. If such conditions are severe, the venous column can extend to jaw level, and its top can be detected only when the patient sits upright or stands. The venous column is low in hypovolemia.

Normally, the venous column can be briefly elevated by firm hand pressure on the abdomen (hepatojugular or abdominojugular reflux); the column falls back in a few seconds (maximum 3 respiratory cycles or 15 sec) despite continued abdominal pressure (because a compliant RV increases its stroke volume via the Frank-Starling mechanism). However, the column remains elevated (> 3 cm) during abdominal pressure in disorders that cause a dilated and poorly compliant RV or in obstruction of RV filling by tricuspid stenosis or right atrial tumor.

Normally, the venous column falls slightly during inspiration as lowered intrathoracic pressure draws blood from the periphery into the vena cava. A rise in the venous column during inspiration (Kussmaul sign) occurs typically in chronic constrictive pericarditis, right ventricular MI, and COPD, and usually in heart failure and tricuspid stenosis.

Jugular vein waves (see Fig. 73–1) can usually be discerned clinically but are better seen on the screen during central venous pressure monitoring.

The *a* waves are increased in pulmonary hypertension and tricuspid valve stenosis. Giant *a* waves (Cannon waves) are seen in atrioventricular dissociation when the atrium contracts while the tricuspid valve is closed. The *a* waves disappear in atrial fibrillation and are accentuated when RV compliance is poor (eg, in pulmonary hypertension or pulmonic stenosis). The *v* waves are very prominent in tricuspid regurgitation. The *x* descent is steep in cardiac tamponade. When RV compliance is poor, the *y* descent is very abrupt because the elevated column of venous blood rushes into the RV when the tricuspid valve opens, only to be stopped abruptly by the rigid RV wall (in restrictive myopathy) or the pericardium (in constrictive pericarditis).

Chest Inspection and Palpation

Chest contour and any visible cardiac impulses are inspected. The precordium is palpated for pulsations (determining apical impulse and thus cardiac situs) and thrills.

Inspection: Chest deformities, such as shield chest and pectus carinatum (a prominent birdlike sternum), may be associated with Marfan syndrome (which may be accompanied by aortic root or mitral valve disease) or Noonan syndrome. Rarely, a localized upper chest bulge indicates aortic aneurysm due to syphilis. Pectus excavatum (depressed sternum) with a narrow anteroposterior chest diameter and an abnormally straight thoracic spine may be associated with hereditary disorders involving congenital cardiac defects (eg, Turner syndrome, Noonan syndrome) and sometimes Marfan syndrome.

Palpation: A central precordial heave is a palpable lifting sensation under the sternum and anterior chest wall to the left of the sternum; it suggests severe RV hypertrophy. Occasionally, in congenital disorders that cause severe RV hypertrophy, the precordium visibly bulges asymmetrically to the left of the sternum.

A sustained thrust at the apex (easily differentiated from the less focal, somewhat diffuse precordial heave of RV hypertrophy) suggests LV hypertrophy. Abnormal focal systolic impulses in the precordium can sometimes be felt in patients with a dyskinetic ventricular aneurysm. An abnormal diffuse systolic impulse lifts the precordium in patients with severe mitral regurgitation. The lift occurs because the left atrium expands, causing anterior cardiac displacement. A diffuse and inferolaterally displaced apical impulse is found when the LV is dilated and hypertrophied (eg, in mitral regurgitation).

Location of thrills (palpable buzzing sensation present with particularly loud murmurs) suggests the cause (see Table 73–2).

A sharp impulse at the 2nd intercostal space to the left of the sternum may result from exaggerated pulmonic valve closure in pulmonary hypertension. A similar early systolic impulse at the cardiac apex may represent closure of a stenotic mitral valve; opening of the stenotic valve sometimes can be felt at the beginning of diastole. These findings coincide with an augmented 1st heart sound and an opening snap of mitral stenosis, heard on auscultation.

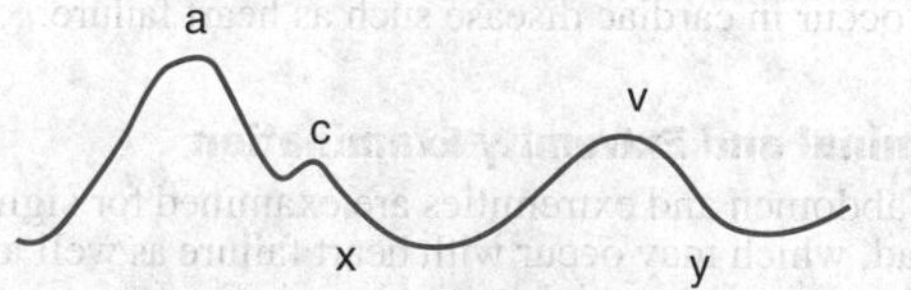

Fig. 73–1. Normal jugular vein waves. The *a* wave is caused by right atrial contraction (systole) and is followed by the *x* descent, which is caused by atrial relaxation. The *c* wave, an interruption of the *x* descent, is caused by the transmitted carotid pulse and bulging of the tricuspid valve into the right atrium as it closes; it is seldom discerned clinically. The *v* wave is caused by right atrial filling during ventricular systole (tricuspid valve is closed). The *y* descent is caused by rapid filling of the right ventricle during ventricular diastole before atrial contraction.

Table 73–2. LOCATION OF THRILLS AND ASSOCIATED DISORDERS

LOCATION OF THRILL	ASSOCIATED DISORDER
Over the base of the heart at the 2nd intercostal space, just to the right of the sternum, during systole	Aortic stenosis
At the apex during systole	Mitral regurgitation
To the left of the sternum at the 2nd intercostal space	Pulmonic stenosis
To the left of the sternum at the 4th intercostal space	Small muscular ventricular septal defect (Roger disease)

Lung Examination

The lungs are examined for signs of pleural effusion and pulmonary edema, which may occur with cardiac disease such as heart failure. The lung examination includes percussion, palpation, and auscultation.

Percussion is the primary physical maneuver used to detect the presence and level of pleural effusion. Finding areas of dullness during percussion signifies underlying fluid or, less commonly, consolidation. Palpation includes tactile fremitus (vibration of the chest wall felt while a patient is speaking); fremitus is decreased in pleural effusion and pneumothorax and increased in pulmonary consolidation (eg, lobar pneumonias).

Auscultation of the lungs is an important component of the examination of patients with suspected cardiac disease.

The character and volume of breath sounds are useful in differentiating cardiac from pulmonary disorders. Adventitious sounds are abnormal sounds, such as crackles, rhonchi, wheezes, and stridor. Crackles (previously called rales) and wheezes are abnormal lung sounds that may occur in heart failure as well as non-cardiac diseases.

- Crackles are discontinuous adventitious breath sounds. Fine crackles are short high-pitched sounds; coarse crackles are longer-lasting low-pitched sounds. Crackles have been compared to the sound of crinkling plastic wrap and can be simulated by rubbing strands of hair together between 2 fingers near one's ear. They occur most commonly with atelectasis, alveolar filling processes (eg, pulmonary edema in heart failure), and interstitial lung disease (eg, pulmonary fibrosis); they signify opening of collapsed airways or alveoli.
- Wheezes are whistling, musical breath sounds that are worse during expiration than inspiration. Wheezing can be a physical finding or a symptom and is usually associated with dyspnea. Wheezes occur most commonly with asthma but can also occur in cardiac disease such as heart failure.

Abdominal and Extremity Examination

The abdomen and extremities are examined for signs of fluid overload, which may occur with heart failure as well as noncardiac disorders (eg, renal, hepatic, lymphatic).

Abdomen: In the abdomen, significant fluid overload manifests as ascites. Marked ascites causes visible abdominal distention, which is tense and nontender to palpation, with shifting dullness on abdominal percussion and a fluid wave. The liver may be distended and slightly tender, with a hepatojugular reflux (see p. 583) present.

Extremities: In the extremities (primarily the legs), fluid overload is manifest as edema, which is swelling of soft tissues due to increased interstitial fluid. Edema may be visible on inspection, but modest amounts of edema in very obese or muscular people may be difficult to recognize visually. Thus, extremities are palpated for presence and degree of pitting (visible and palpable depressions caused by pressure from the examiner's fingers, which displaces the interstitial fluid). The area of edema is examined for extent, symmetry (ie, comparing both extremities), warmth, erythema, and tenderness. With significant fluid overload, edema may also be present over the sacrum, genitals, or both.

Tenderness, erythema, or both, particularly when unilateral, suggests an inflammatory cause (eg, cellulitis or thrombophlebitis). Nonpitting edema is more suggestive of lymphatic or vascular obstruction than fluid overload.

CARDIAC AUSCULTATION

Auscultation of the heart requires excellent hearing and the ability to distinguish subtle differences in pitch and timing. Hearing-impaired health care practitioners can use amplified stethoscopes. High-pitched sounds are best heard with the diaphragm of the stethoscope. Low-pitched sounds are best heard with the bell. Very little pressure should be exerted when using the bell. Excessive pressure converts the underlying skin into a diaphragm and eliminates very low-pitched sounds.

The entire precordium is examined systematically, typically beginning over the apical impulse with the patient in the left lateral decubitus position. The patient rolls supine, and auscultation continues at the lower left sternal border, proceeds cephalad with auscultation of each interspace, then caudad from the right upper sternal border. The clinician also listens over the left axilla and above the clavicles. The patient sits upright for auscultation of the back, then leans forward to aid auscultation of aortic and pulmonic diastolic murmurs or pericardial friction rub.

Major auscultatory findings include

- Heart sounds
- Murmurs
- Rubs

Heart sounds are brief, transient sounds produced by valve opening and closure; they are divided into systolic and diastolic sounds.

Murmurs are produced by blood flow turbulence and are more prolonged than heart sounds; they may be systolic, diastolic, or continuous. They are graded by intensity (see Table 73–3) and are described by their location and when they occur within the cardiac cycle.

Rubs are high-pitched, scratchy sounds often with 2 or 3 separate components; during tachycardia, the sound may be almost continuous.

The clinician focuses attention sequentially on each phase of the cardiac cycle, noting each heart sound and murmur. Intensity, pitch, duration, and timing of the sounds and the intervals between them

Table 73–3. HEART MURMUR INTENSITY

GRADE	DESCRIPTION
1	Barely audible
2	Soft but easily heard
3	Loud without a thrill
4	Loud with a thrill
5	Loud with minimal contact between stethoscope and chest
6	Loud with no contact between stethoscope and chest

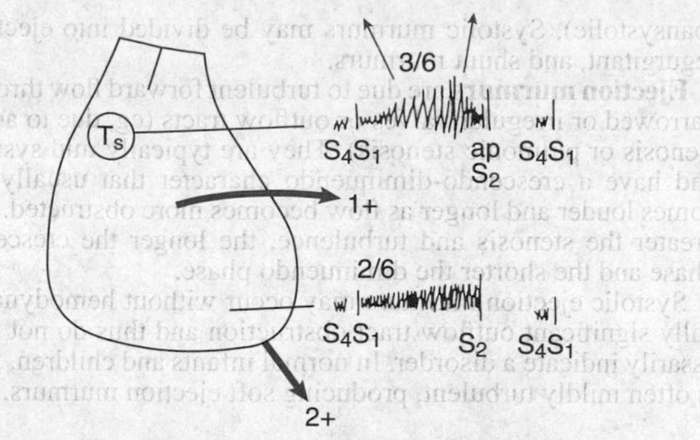

Fig. 73–2. Diagram of physical findings in a patient with aortic stenosis and mitral regurgitation. Murmur, character, intensity, and radiation are depicted. Sound of pulmonic closure exceeds that of aortic closure. Left ventricular (LV) thrust and right ventricular (RV) lift (heavy arrows) are identified. A 4th heart sound (S_4) and systolic thrill (T_S) are present. a = aortic closure sound; p = pulmonic closure sound; S_1 = 1st heart sound; S_2 = 2nd heart sound; 3/6 = grade of crescendo-diminuendo murmur (radiates to both sides of neck); 2/6 = grade of pansystolic apical crescendo murmur; 1 + = mild precordial lift of RV hypertrophy (arrow shows direction of lift); 2 + = moderate LV thrust (arrow shows direction of thrust).

are analyzed, often providing an accurate diagnosis. A diagram of the major auscultatory and palpatory findings of the precordium should be routinely drawn in the patient's chart each time the patient's cardiovascular system is examined (see Fig. 73–2). With such diagrams, findings from each examination can be compared.

Systolic heart sounds: Systolic sounds include the following:

- 1st heart sound (S_1)
- Clicks

S_1 and the 2nd heart sound (S_2, a diastolic heart sound) are normal components of the cardiac cycle, the familiar "lub-dub" sounds.

S_1 occurs just after the beginning of systole and is predominantly due to mitral closure but may also include tricuspid closure components. It is often split and has a high pitch. S_1 is loud in mitral stenosis. It may be soft or absent in mitral regurgitation due to valve leaflet sclerosis and rigidity but is often distinctly heard in mitral regurgitation due to myxomatous degeneration of the mitral apparatus or due to ventricular myocardial abnormality (eg, papillary muscle dysfunction, ventricular dilation).

Clicks occur only during systole; they are distinguished from S_1 and S_2 by their higher pitch and briefer duration. Some clicks occur at different times during systole as hemodynamics change. Clicks may be single or multiple.

Clicks in congenital aortic or pulmonic stenosis are thought to result from abnormal ventricular wall tension. These clicks occur early in systole (very near S_1) and are not affected by hemodynamic changes. Similar clicks occur in severe pulmonary hypertension. Clicks in mitral or tricuspid valve prolapse, typically occurring in mid to late systole, are thought to result from abnormal tension on redundant and elongated chordae tendineae or valve leaflets.

Clicks due to myxomatous degeneration of valves may occur any time during systole but move toward S_1 during maneuvers that transiently decrease ventricular filling volume (eg, standing, Valsalva maneuver). If ventricular filling volume is increased (eg, by lying supine), clicks move toward S_2, particularly in mitral valve prolapse. For unknown reasons, characteristics of the clicks may vary greatly between examinations, and clicks may come and go.

Diastolic heart sounds: Diastolic sounds include the following:

- 2nd, 3rd, and 4th heart sounds (S_2, S_3, and S_4)
- Diastolic knocks
- Mitral valve sounds

Unlike systolic sounds, diastolic sounds are low-pitched; they are softer in intensity and longer in duration. Except for S_2, these sounds are usually abnormal in adults, although an S_3 may be physiologic up to age 40 and during pregnancy.

S_2 occurs at the beginning of diastole, due to aortic and pulmonic valve closure. Aortic valve closure normally precedes pulmonic valve closure unless the former is late or the latter is early. Aortic valve closure is late in left bundle branch block or aortic stenosis; pulmonic valve closure is early in some forms of preexcitation phenomena. Delayed pulmonic valve closure may result from increased blood flow through the right ventricle (eg, in atrial septal defect of the common secundum variety) or complete right bundle branch block. Increased right ventricular flow in atrial septal defect also abolishes the normal respiratory variation in aortic and pulmonic valve closure, producing a fixed split S_2. Left-to-right shunts with normal right ventricular volume flow (eg, in membranous ventricular septal defects) do not cause fixed splitting. A single S_2 may occur when the aortic valve is regurgitant, severely stenotic, or atretic (in truncus arteriosus when there is a common valve).

S_3 occurs in early diastole, when the ventricle is dilated and noncompliant. It occurs during passive diastolic ventricular filling and usually indicates serious ventricular dysfunction in adults; in children, it can be normal, sometimes persisting even to age 40. S_3 also may be normal during pregnancy. Right ventricular S_3 is heard best (sometimes only) during inspiration (because negative intrathoracic pressure augments right ventricular filling volume) with the patient supine. Left ventricular S_3 is best heard during expiration (because the heart is nearer the chest wall) with the patient in the left lateral decubitus position.

S_4 is produced by augmented ventricular filling, caused by atrial contraction, near the end of diastole. It is similar to S_3 and heard best or only with the bell of the stethoscope. During inspiration, right ventricular S_4 increases and left ventricular S_4 decreases. S_4 is heard much more often than S_3 and indicates a lesser degree of ventricular dysfunction, usually diastolic. S_4 is absent in atrial fibrillation (because the atria do not contract) but is almost always present in active myocardial ischemia or soon after myocardial infarction.

S_3, with or without S_4, is usual in significant systolic left ventricular dysfunction; S_4 without S_3 is usual in diastolic left ventricular dysfunction.

A **summation gallop** occurs when S_3 and S_4 are present in a patient with tachycardia, which shortens diastole so that the 2 sounds merge. Loud S_3 and S_4 may be palpable at the apex when the patient is in the left lateral decubitus position.

A **diastolic knock** occurs at the same time as S_3, in early diastole. It is not accompanied by S_4 and is a louder, thudding sound, which indicates abrupt arrest of ventricular filling by a noncompliant, constricting pericardium.

An **opening snap** may occur in early diastole in mitral stenosis or, rarely, in tricuspid stenosis. Mitral opening snap is very high pitched, brief, and heard best with the diaphragm of the stethoscope. The more severe mitral stenosis is (ie, the higher the left atrial pressure), the closer the opening snap is to the pulmonic component of S_2. Intensity is related to the compliance of the valve leaflets: The snap sounds loud when leaflets remain elastic, but it gradually softens and ultimately disappears as sclerosis, fibrosis, and calcification of the valve develop. Mitral opening snap, although sometimes heard at the apex, is often heard best or only at the lower left sternal border.

Approach to murmurs: Timing of the murmur in the cardiac cycle correlates with the cause (see Table 73–4); auscultatory findings correlate with specific heart valve disorders. Various maneuvers (eg, inspiration, Valsalva, handgrip, squatting, amyl nitrate inhalation) can modify cardiac physiology slightly, making differentiation of causes of heart murmur possible (see Table 73–5).

All patients with heart murmurs are evaluated by chest x-ray and ECG. Most require echocardiography to confirm the diagnosis, determine severity, and track severity over time. Usually, a cardiac consultation is obtained if significant disease is suspected.

Systolic murmurs: Systolic murmurs may be normal or abnormal. They may be early, mid, or late systolic, or holosystolic (pansystolic). Systolic murmurs may be divided into ejection, regurgitant, and shunt murmurs.

Ejection murmurs are due to turbulent forward flow through narrowed or irregular valves or outflow tracts (eg, due to aortic stenosis or pulmonic stenosis). They are typically mid systolic and have a crescendo-diminuendo character that usually becomes louder and longer as flow becomes more obstructed. The greater the stenosis and turbulence, the longer the crescendo phase and the shorter the diminuendo phase.

Systolic ejection murmurs may occur without hemodynamically significant outflow tract obstruction and thus do not necessarily indicate a disorder. In normal infants and children, flow is often mildly turbulent, producing soft ejection murmurs. The

Table 73–4. ETIOLOGY OF MURMURS BY TIMING

TIMING	ASSOCIATED DISORDERS
Mid systolic (ejection)	Aortic obstruction (supravalvular stenosis, coarctation of the aorta, aortic stenosis, aortic sclerosis, hypertrophic cardiomyopathy, subvalvular stenosis) Increased blood flow across the aortic valve (hyperkinetic states, aortic regurgitation) Dilation of ascending aorta (atheroma, aortitis, aneurysm of aorta) Pulmonic obstruction (supravalvular pulmonary artery stenosis, pulmonic stenosis, infundibular stenosis) Increased blood flow across the pulmonic valve (hyperkinetic states, left-to-right shunt due to atrial septal defect, ventricular septal defect) Dilation of pulmonary artery
Mid-late systolic	Mitral valve prolapse Papillary muscle dysfunction
Holosystolic	Mitral regurgitation Tricuspid regurgitation Ventricular septal defect
Early diastolic (regurgitant)	Aortic regurgitation: • Acquired or congenital valve abnormality (eg, myxomatous or calcific degeneration, rheumatic fever, endocarditis), dilation of valve ring (eg, aortic dissection, annuloaortic ectasia, cystic medial necrosis, hypertension), widening of commissures (eg, syphilis) • Congenital bicuspid valve with or without ventricular septal defect Pulmonic regurgitation: • Acquired or congenital valve abnormality • Dilation of valve ring (eg, pulmonary hypertension, Marfan syndrome) • Tetralogy of Fallot • Ventricular septal defect
Mid diastolic	Mitral stenosis (eg, rheumatic fever, congenital stenosis, cor triatriatum) Increased blood flow across nonstenotic mitral valve (eg, mitral regurgitation, ventricular septal defect, patent ductus arteriosus, high-output states, complete heart block) Tricuspid stenosis Increased blood flow across nonstenotic tricuspid valve (eg, tricuspid regurgitation, atrial septal defect, anomalous pulmonary venous return) Left or right atrial tumors Atrial ball-valve thrombi
Continuous	Patent ductus arteriosus Coarctation of the pulmonary artery Coronary or intercostal arteriovenous fistula Ruptured aneurysm of sinus of Valsalva Aortic septal defect Cervical venous hum Anomalous left coronary artery Proximal coronary artery stenosis Mammary souffle (venous hum from engorged breast vessels during pregnancy) Pulmonary artery branch stenosis Bronchial collateral circulation Small (restrictive) atrial septal defect with mitral stenosis Coronary-cameral fistula, Aortic–right ventricular or atrial fistula

Table 73–5. MANEUVERS THAT AID IN DIAGNOSIS OF MURMURS

MANEUVER	EFFECT ON BLOOD FLOW	EFFECT ON HEART SOUNDS
Inspiration	Simultaneously increases venous flow into the right ventricle (RV), decreases venous flow into the left heart	Augments right heart sounds (eg, murmurs of tricuspid stenosis and regurgitation, those of pulmonic stenosis* [immediately] and regurgitation [usually]) Reduces left heart sounds
Valsalva maneuver	Reduces size of left ventricle (LV); decreases venous return to the right heart and subsequently to the left heart	Augments murmur of hypertrophic obstructive cardiomyopathy and mitral valve prolapse Reduces murmurs of aortic stenosis, mitral regurgitation, and tricuspid stenosis
Release of Valsalva maneuver	Increases volume of RV and LV	Augments murmurs of aortic stenosis, aortic regurgitation (after 4 or 5 beats), and pulmonic regurgitation or pulmonic stenosis* (immediately) Reduces murmur of tricuspid stenosis
Isometric handgrip	Increases afterload and peripheral arterial resistance	Reduces murmurs of aortic stenosis, hypertrophic obstructive cardiomyopathy, mitral valve prolapse, or papillary muscle dysfunction Augments murmurs of mitral regurgitation and aortic regurgitation and diastolic murmur of mitral stenosis
Squatting	Simultaneously increases venous return to the right heart and increases afterload and peripheral resistance	Augments murmurs of aortic regurgitation, aortic stenosis, mitral regurgitation and diastolic murmur of mitral stenosis Reduces murmur of hypertrophic obstructive cardiomyopathy and mitral valve prolapse
Amyl nitrite	Causes intense venodilation, which reduces venous return to the right heart	Augments murmurs of hypertrophic obstructive cardiomyopathy, aortic stenosis and mitral valve prolapse Reduces murmur of mitral regurgitation.

*Patient may need to be standing for effect on pulmonic stenosis to be heard.

elderly often have ejection murmurs due to valve and vessel sclerosis.

During pregnancy, many women have soft ejection murmurs at the 2nd intercostal space to the left or right of the sternum. The murmurs occur because a physiologic increase in blood volume and cardiac output increases flow velocity through normal structures. The murmurs may be greatly exaggerated if severe anemia complicates the pregnancy.

Regurgitant murmurs represent retrograde or abnormal flow (eg, due to mitral regurgitation, tricuspid regurgitation, or ventricular septal defects) into chambers that are at lower resistance. They are typically holosystolic and tend to be louder with high-velocity, low-volume regurgitation or shunts and softer with high-volume regurgitation or shunts. Late systolic murmurs, which may or may not be preceded by a click, are typical of mitral valve prolapse or papillary muscle dysfunction. Various maneuvers are usually required for more accurate diagnosis of timing and type of murmur (see Table 73–5).

Shunt murmurs may originate at the site of the shunt (eg, patent ductus arteriosus, ventricular septal defects) or result from altered hemodynamics remote from the shunt (eg, pulmonic systolic flow murmur due to an atrial septal defect with left-to-right shunt).

Diastolic murmurs: Diastolic murmurs are always abnormal; most are early or mid diastolic, but they may be late diastolic (presystolic). Early diastolic murmurs are typically due to aortic regurgitation or pulmonic regurgitation. Mid diastolic (or early to mid diastolic) murmurs are typically due to mitral stenosis or tricuspid stenosis. A late diastolic murmur may be due to rheumatic mitral stenosis in a patient in sinus rhythm.

A mitral or tricuspid murmur due to an atrial tumor or thrombus may be evanescent and may vary with position and from one examination to the next because the position of the intracardiac mass changes.

Continuous murmurs: Continuous murmurs occur throughout the cardiac cycle. They are always abnormal, indicating a constant shunt flow throughout systole and diastole. They may be due to various cardiac defects (see Table 73–4). Some defects produce a thrill; many are associated with signs of right ventricular hypertrophy and left ventricular hypertrophy. As pulmonary artery resistance increases in shunt lesions, the diastolic component gradually decreases. When pulmonary and systemic resistance equalize, the murmur may disappear.

Patent ductus arteriosus murmurs are loudest at the 2nd intercostal space just below the medial end of the left clavicle.Aorticopulmonary window murmurs are central and heard at the 3rd intercostal space level. Murmurs of systemic arteriovenous fistulas are best heard directly over the lesions; those of pulmonic arteriovenous fistulas and pulmonary artery branch stenosis are more diffuse and heard throughout the chest.

When circulation is increased, as occurs during pregnancy, anemia, and hyperthyroidism, a continuous venous hum is often heard in the right supraclavicular fossa; this venous hum also occurs normally in children. The sound generated by increased flow in a dilated internal mammary artery (mammary souffle), may be mistaken for a continuous cardiac murmur. Mammary souffle is typically heard best over the breast at the level of the right and/or left 2nd or 3rd intercostal space and, although often classified as continuous, is usually louder during systole.

Pericardial friction rub: A pericardial friction rub is caused by movement of inflammatory adhesions between visceral and parietal pericardial layers. It is a high-pitched or squeaking sound; it may be systolic, diastolic and systolic, or triphasic (when atrial contraction accentuates the diastolic component during late diastole). The rub sounds like pieces of leather squeaking as they are rubbed together. Rubs are best heard with the patient leaning forward or on hands and knees with breath held in expiration.

74 Symptoms of Cardiovascular Disorders

CHEST PAIN

Chest pain is a very common complaint. Many patients are well aware that it is a warning of potential life-threatening disorders and seek evaluation for minimal symptoms. Other patients, including many with serious disease, minimize or ignore its warnings. Pain perception (both character and severity) varies greatly between individuals as well as between men and women. However described, chest pain should never be dismissed without an explanation of its cause.

Pathophysiology

The heart, lungs, esophagus, and great vessels provide afferent visceral input through the same thoracic autonomic ganglia. A painful stimulus in these organs is typically perceived as originating in the chest, but because afferent nerve fibers overlap in the dorsal ganglia, thoracic pain may be felt (as referred pain) anywhere between the umbilicus and the ear, including the upper extremities.

Painful stimuli from thoracic organs can cause discomfort described as pressure, tearing, gas with the urge to eructate, indigestion, burning or aching. Uncommonly, other descriptions of chest pain are given such as stabbing or sharp needle-like pain. When the sensation is visceral in origin, many patients deny they are having pain and insist it is merely "discomfort."

Etiology

Many disorders cause chest pain or discomfort. These disorders may involve the cardiovascular, GI, pulmonary, neurologic, or musculoskeletal systems (see Table 74–1).

Some disorders are immediately life threatening:

- Acute coronary syndromes (acute myocardial infarction/unstable angina)
- Thoracic aortic dissection
- Tension pneumothorax
- Esophageal rupture
- Pulmonary embolism (PE)

Other causes range from serious, potential threats to life to causes that are simply uncomfortable. Often no cause can be confirmed even after full evaluation.

Overall, the most common causes are

- Chest wall disorders (ie, those involving muscle, rib, or cartilage)
- Pleural disorders
- GI disorders (eg, gastroesophageal reflux disease, esophageal spasm, ulcer disease, cholelithiasis)
- Acute coronary syndromes and stable angina

In some cases, no etiology of the chest pain can be determined.

Evaluation

History: History of present illness should note the location, duration, character, and quality of the pain. The patient should be asked about any precipitating events (eg, straining or overuse of chest muscles), as well as any triggering and relieving factors. Specific factors to note include whether pain is present during exertion or at rest, presence of psychologic stress, whether pain occurs during respiration or coughing, difficulty swallowing, relationship to meals, and positions that relieve or exacerbate pain (eg, lying flat, leaning forward). Previous similar episodes and their circumstances should be noted with attention to the similarity or lack thereof. Important associated symptoms to seek include dyspnea, palpitations, syncope, diaphoresis, nausea or vomiting, cough, fever, and chills.

Review of systems should seek symptoms of possible causes, including leg pain, swelling, or both (deep venous thrombosis [DVT] and therefore possible PE) and chronic weakness, malaise, and weight loss (cancer).

Past medical history should document known causes, particularly cardiovascular and GI disorders, and any cardiac investigations or procedures (eg, stress testing, catheterization). Risk factors for coronary artery disease (CAD—eg, hypertension, hyperlipidemia, diabetes, cerebrovascular disease, tobacco use) or PE (eg, lower extremity injury, recent surgery, immobilization, known cancer, pregnancy) should also be noted.

Drug history should note use of drugs that can trigger coronary artery spasm (eg, cocaine, triptans, phosphodiesterase inhibitors) or GI disease (particularly alcohol, NSAIDs).

Family history should note history of myocardial infarction (particularly among 1st-degree relatives at an early age—< 55 in men and < 60 in women) and hyperlipidemia.

Physical examination: Vital signs and weight are measured, and body mass index (BMI) is calculated. Pulses are palpated in both arms and both legs, BP is measured in both arms, and pulsus paradoxus is measured.

General appearance is noted (eg, pallor, diaphoresis, cyanosis, anxiety).

Neck is inspected for venous distention and hepatojugular reflux, and the venous wave forms are noted. The neck is palpated for carotid pulses, lymphadenopathy, or thyroid abnormality. The carotid arteries are auscultated for bruit.

Lungs are percussed and auscultated for presence and symmetry of breath sounds, signs of congestion (dry or wet rales, rhonchi), consolidation (pectoriloquy), pleural friction rubs, and effusion (decreased breath sounds, dullness to percussion).

The cardiac examination notes the intensity and timing of the 1st heart sound (S_1) and 2nd heart sound (S_2), the respiratory movement of the pulmonic component of S_2, pericardial friction rubs, murmurs, and gallops. When murmurs are detected, the timing, duration, pitch, shape, and intensity and the response to changes of position, handgrip, and the Valsalva maneuver should be noted. When gallops are detected, differentiation should be made between the 4th heart sound (S_4), which is often present with diastolic dysfunction or myocardial ischemia, and the 3rd heart sound (S_3), which is present with systolic dysfunction.

The chest is inspected for skin lesions of trauma or herpes zoster infection and palpated for crepitance (suggesting subcutaneous air) and tenderness. The abdomen is palpated for tenderness, organomegaly, and masses or tenderness, particularly in the epigastric and right upper quadrant regions.

The legs are examined for arterial pulses, adequacy of perfusion, edema, varicose veins, and signs of DVT (eg, swelling, erythema, tenderness).

Red flags: Certain findings raise suspicion of a more serious etiology of chest pain:

- Abnormal vital signs (tachycardia, bradycardia, tachypnea, hypotension)
- Signs of hypoperfusion (eg, confusion, ashen color, diaphoresis)
- Shortness of breath
- Hypoxemia on pulse oximetry
- Asymmetric breath sounds or pulses
- New heart murmurs
- Pulsus paradoxus > 10 mm Hg

Table 74–1. SOME CAUSES OF CHEST PAIN

CAUSE*	SUGGESTIVE FINDINGS	DIAGNOSTIC APPROACH†
Cardiovascular		
[1]Myocardial ischemia (acute myocardial infarction/unstable angina/angina)	Acute, crushing pain radiating to the jaw or arm Exertional pain relieved by rest (angina pectoris) S_4 gallop Sometimes systolic murmurs of mitral regurgitation Often red flag findings‡	Serial ECGs and cardiac markers; admit or observe Stress imaging test or CT angiography considered in patients with negative ECG findings and no cardiac marker elevation Often heart catheterization and coronary angiography if findings are positive
[1]Thoracic aortic dissection	Sudden, tearing pain radiating to the back Some patients have syncope, stroke, or leg ischemia Pulse or BP that may be unequal in extremities Age > 55 Hypertension Red flag findings‡	Chest x-ray with findings suggesting diagnosis Enhanced CT scan of aorta for confirmation Transesophageal echocardiography
[2]Pericarditis	Constant or intermittent sharp pain often aggravated by breathing, swallowing food, or supine position and relieved by sitting or leaning forward Pericardial friction rub Jugular venous distention	ECG usually diagnostic Serum cardiac markers (sometimes showing minimal elevation of troponin and CK-MB levels) Transthoracic echocardiography
[2]Myocarditis	Fever, dyspnea, fatigue, chest pain (if myopericarditis), recent viral or other infection Sometimes findings of heart failure, pericarditis, or both	ECG Serum cardiac markers ESR C-reactive protein Usually echocardiography
GI		
[1]Esophageal rupture	Sudden, severe pain following vomiting or instrumentation (eg, esophagogastroscopy or transesophageal echocardiography) Subcutaneous crepitus detected during auscultation Multiple red flag findings‡	Chest x-ray Esophagography with water-soluble contrast for confirmation
[2]Pancreatitis	Pain in the epigastrium or lower chest that is often worse when lying flat and is relieved by leaning forward Vomiting Upper abdominal tenderness Shock Often history of alcohol abuse or biliary tract disease	Serum lipase Sometimes abdominal CT
[3]Peptic ulcer	Recurrent, vague epigastric or right upper quadrant discomfort in a patient who smokes or uses alcohol excessively that is relieved by food, antacids, or both No red flag findings‡	Clinical evaluation Sometimes endoscopy Sometimes testing for *Helicobacter pylori*
[3]Esophageal reflux (GERD)	Recurrent burning pain radiating from epigastrium to throat that is exacerbated by bending down or lying down and relieved by antacids	Clinical evaluation Sometimes endoscopy Sometimes motility studies
[3]Biliary tract disease	Recurrent right upper quadrant or epigastric discomfort following meals (but not exertion)	Ultrasonography of gallbladder
[3]Esophageal motility disorders	Long-standing pain of insidious onset that may or may not accompany swallowing Usually also difficulty swallowing	Barium swallow Esophageal manometry
Pulmonary		
[1]Pulmonary embolism	Often pleuritic pain, dyspnea, tachycardia Sometimes mild fever, hemoptysis, shock More likely when risk factors are present	Varies with clinical suspicion

Table continues on the following page.

Table 74–1. SOME CAUSES OF CHEST PAIN (*Continued*)

CAUSE*	SUGGESTIVE FINDINGS	DIAGNOSTIC APPROACH†
[1]Tension pneumothorax	Significant dyspnea, hypotension, neck vein distention, unilateral diminished breath sounds and hyperresonance to percussion Sometimes subcutaneous air	Usually clinical Obvious on chest x-ray
[2]Pneumonia	Fever, chills, cough, and purulent sputum Often dyspnea, tachycardia, signs of consolidation	Chest x-ray
[2]Pneumothorax	Sometimes, unilateral diminished breath sounds, subcutaneous air	Chest x-ray
[3]Pleuritis	May have preceding pneumonia, pulmonary embolism, or viral respiratory infection Pain with breathing, cough Sometimes a pleural rub, but otherwise examination unremarkable	Usually clinical evaluation
Other		
[3]Musculoskeletal chest wall pain (eg, due to trauma, overuse, or costochondritis)	Often suggested by history Pain typically persistent (typically days or longer), worsened with passive and active motion Diffuse or focal tenderness	Clinical evaluation
[3]Fibromyalgia	Nearly constant pain, affecting multiple areas of the body as well as the chest Typically, fatigue and poor sleep Multiple trigger points	Clinical evaluation
[2]Various thoracic cancers	Variable but sometimes pleuritic pain Sometimes chronic cough, smoking history, signs of chronic illness (weight loss, fever), cervical lymphadenopathy	Chest x-ray Chest CT if x-ray findings are suggestive Bone scan considered for persistent, focal rib pain
[3]Herpes zoster infection	Sharp, band-like pain in the thorax unilaterally Classic linear, vesicular rash Pain may precede rash by several days	Clinical evaluation
[3]Idiopathic	Various features No red flag findings‡	Diagnosis of exclusion

*Seriousness of causes varies as indicated:
[1]Immediate life threats.
[2]Potential life threats.
[3]Uncomfortable but usually not dangerous.
†Most patients with chest pain should have pulse oximetry, ECG, and chest x-ray (basic tests). If there is suspicion of coronary ischemia, serum cardiac markers (troponin, CK-MB) should also be checked.
‡Red flag findings include abnormal vital signs (tachycardia, bradycardia, tachypnea, hypotension), signs of hypoperfusion (eg, confusion, ashen color, diaphoresis), shortness of breath, asymmetric breath sounds or pulses, new heart murmurs, or pulsus paradoxus > 10 mm Hg.
S_4 = 4th heart sound.

Interpretation of findings: Symptoms and signs of thoracic disorders vary greatly, and those of serious and nonserious conditions often overlap. Although red flag findings indicate a high likelihood of serious disease, and many disorders have "classic" manifestations (see Table 74–1), many patients who have serious illness do not present with these classic symptoms and signs. For example, patients with myocardial ischemia may complain only of indigestion or have a very tender chest wall on palpation. A high index of suspicion is important when evaluating patients with chest pain. Nonetheless, some distinctions and generalizations are possible.

Duration of pain can provide clues to the severity of the disorder. Long-standing pain (ie, for weeks or months) is not a manifestation of a disorder that is immediately life threatening. Such pain is often musculoskeletal in origin, although GI origin or a cancer should be considered, particularly in patients who are elderly. Similarly, brief (< 5 sec), sharp, intermittent pains rarely result from serious disorders. Serious disorders typically manifest pain lasting minutes to hours, although episodes may be recurrent (eg, unstable angina may cause several bouts of pain over 1 or more days).

Patient age is helpful in evaluating chest pain. Chest pain in children and young adults (< 30 yr) is less likely to result from myocardial ischemia, although MI can occur in people in their 20s. Musculoskeletal and pulmonary disorders are more common causes in these age groups.

Exacerbation and relief of symptoms also are helpful in evaluating chest pain. Although angina can be felt anywhere between the ear and the umbilicus (and often not in the chest), it is typically consistently related to physical or emotional stress, ie, patients do not experience angina from climbing one flight of stairs one day and tolerate 3 flights the next day. Nocturnal angina is characteristic of acute coronary syndromes, heart failure, or coronary artery spasm.

Pain from many disorders, both serious and minor, can be exacerbated by respiration, movement, or palpation of the chest. These findings are not specific for origin in the chest wall; about 15% of patients with acute MI have chest tenderness on palpation.

Nitroglycerin may relieve pain of both myocardial ischemia and noncardiac smooth muscle spasm (eg, esophageal or biliary disorders); its efficacy or lack thereof should not be used for diagnosis.

Associated findings may also suggest a cause. Fever is nonspecific but, if accompanied by cough, suggests a pulmonary cause. Patients with Raynaud syndrome or migraine headaches sometimes have coronary spasm.

The presence or absence of risk factors for CAD (eg, hypertension, hypercholesterolemia, smoking, obesity, diabetes, positive family history) alters the probability of underlying CAD but does not help diagnose the cause of a given episode of acute chest pain. Patients with those factors may well have another cause of chest pain, and patients without them may have an acute coronary syndrome. However, known CAD in a patient with chest pain raises the likelihood of that diagnosis as the cause (particularly if the patient describes the symptoms as "like my angina" or "like my last heart attack"). A history of peripheral vascular disease also raises the likelihood that angina is the cause of chest pain.

Testing: For adults with acute chest pain, immediate life threats must be ruled out. Most patients should initially have pulse oximetry, ECG, and chest x-ray. If symptoms suggest an acute coronary syndrome or if no other cause is clear (particularly in at-risk patients), troponin levels are measured. If a PE is considered possible, D-dimer testing is done. Expeditious evaluation is essential because if MI or other acute coronary syndrome is present, the patient should be considered for urgent heart catheterization (when available).

Some abnormal findings on these tests confirm a diagnosis (eg, acute myocardial infarction, pneumothorax, pneumonia). Other abnormalities suggest a diagnosis or at least the need to pursue further investigation (eg, abnormal aortic contour on chest x-ray suggests need for testing for thoracic aortic dissection). Thus, if these initial test results are normal, thoracic aortic dissection, tension pneumothorax, and esophageal rupture are highly unlikely. However, in acute coronary syndromes, ECG may not change for several hours or sometimes not at all, and in PE, oxygenation may be normal. Thus, other studies may need to be obtained based on findings from the history and physical examination (see Table 74–1).

Because a single normal set of cardiac markers does not rule out a cardiac cause, patients whose symptoms suggest an acute coronary syndrome should have serial measurement of the cardiac marker troponin and ECGs at least 6 h apart. Some clinicians follow these tests (acutely or within several days) with a stress ECG or a stress imaging test. Drug treatment is begun while awaiting results of the 2nd troponin level unless there is a clear contraindication. A diagnostic trial of sublingual nitroglycerin or an oral liquid antacid does not adequately differentiate myocardial ischemia from gastroesophageal reflux disease or gastritis. Either drug may relieve symptoms of either disorder. Troponin will be elevated in all acute coronary syndromes causing cardiac injury and often in other disorders that damage the myocardium (eg, myocarditis, pericarditis, aortic dissection involving coronary artery flow, PE, heart failure, severe sepsis). CK may be elevated due to damage to any muscle tissue, but CK-MB elevation is specific to damage to the myocardium. However, troponin is now the standard marker of cardiac muscle injury. ST-segment abnormality on the ECG may be nonspecific or due to antecedent disorders, so comparison with previous ECGs is important.

The likelihood of PE is affected by a number of factors, which can be used in an algorithm to derive an approach to testing.

In patients with chronic chest pain, immediate threats to life are unlikely. Most clinicians initially obtain a chest x-ray and do other tests based on symptoms and signs.

Treatment

Specific identified disorders are treated. If etiology is not clearly benign, patients are usually admitted to the hospital or an observation unit for cardiac monitoring and more extensive evaluation. Pain is treated with acetaminophen or opioids as needed, pending a diagnosis. Pain relief following opioid treatment should not diminish the urgency of ruling out serious and life-threatening disease.

Geriatrics Essentials

The probability of serious and life-threatening disease increases with age. Many elderly patients recover more slowly than younger patients but survive for significant time if properly diagnosed and treated. Drug doses are usually lower, and rapidity of dose escalation is slower. Chronic disorders (eg, decreased renal function) are often present and may complicate diagnosis and treatment.

KEY POINTS

- Immediate life threats must be ruled out first.
- Some serious disorders, particularly coronary ischemia and PE, often do not have a classic presentation.
- Most patients should have pulse oximetry, ECG, cardiac markers, and chest x-ray.
- Evaluation must be prompt so that patients with ST-elevation MI can be in the heart catheterization laboratory (or have thrombolysis) within the 90-min standard.
- If PE is highly likely, antithrombin drugs should be given while the diagnosis is pursued; another embolus in a patient who is not receiving anticoagulants may be fatal.

EDEMA

Edema is swelling of soft tissues due to increased interstitial fluid. The fluid is predominantly water, but protein and cell-rich fluid can accumulate if there is infection or lymphatic obstruction.

Edema may be generalized or local (eg, limited to a single extremity or part of an extremity). It sometimes appears abruptly; patients complain that an extremity suddenly swells. More often, edema develops insidiously, beginning with weight gain, puffy eyes at awakening in the morning, and tight shoes at the end of the day. Slowly developing edema may become massive before patients seek medical care.

Edema itself causes few symptoms other than occasionally a feeling of tightness or fullness; other symptoms are usually related to the underlying disorder. Patients with edema due to heart failure (a common cause) often have dyspnea during exertion, orthopnea, and paroxysmal nocturnal dyspnea. Patients with edema due to DVT often have pain.

Edema due to extracellular fluid volume expansion is often dependent. Thus, in ambulatory patients, edema is in the feet and lower legs; patients requiring bed rest develop edema in the buttocks, genitals, and posterior thighs. Women who lie on only one side may develop edema in the dependent breast. Lymphatic obstruction causes edema distal to the site of obstruction.

Pathophysiology

Edema results from increased movement of fluid from the intravascular to the interstitial space or decreased movement of water from the interstitium into the capillaries or lymphatic vessels. The mechanism involves one or more of the following:

- Increased capillary hydrostatic pressure
- Decreased plasma oncotic pressure
- Increased capillary permeability
- Obstruction of the lymphatic system

As fluid shifts into the interstitial space, intravascular volume is depleted. Intravascular volume depletion activates the renin-angiotensin-aldosterone-vasopressin (ADH) system, resulting in renal sodium retention. By increasing osmolality, renal sodium retention triggers water retention by the kidneys and helps maintain plasma volume. Increased renal sodium retention also may be a primary cause of fluid overload and hence edema. Excessive exogenous sodium intake may also contribute.

Less often, edema results from decreased movement of fluid out of the interstitial space into the capillaries due to lack of adequate plasma oncotic pressure as in nephrotic syndrome, protein-losing enteropathy, liver failure, or starvation.

Increased capillary permeability occurs in infections or as the result of toxin or inflammatory damage to the capillary walls.

The lymphatic system is responsible for removing protein and WBCs (along with some water) from the interstitium. Lymphatic obstruction allows these substances to accumulate in the interstitium.

Etiology

Generalized edema is most commonly caused by

- Heart failure
- Liver failure
- Kidney disorders (especially nephrotic syndrome)

Localized edema is most commonly caused by

- DVT or another venous disorder or venous obstruction (eg, by tumor)
- Infection
- Angioedema
- Lymphatic obstruction

Chronic venous insufficiency may involve one or both legs.

Common causes are listed by primary mechanism (see Table 74–2).

Evaluation

History: History of present illness should include location and duration of edema and presence and degree of pain or discomfort. Female patients should be asked whether they are pregnant and whether edema seems related to menstrual periods. Having patients with chronic edema keep a log of weight gain or loss is valuable.

Review of systems should include symptoms of causative disorders, including dyspnea during exertion, orthopnea, and paroxysmal nocturnal dyspnea (heart failure); alcohol or hepatotoxin exposure, jaundice, and easy bruising (a liver disorder); malaise and anorexia (cancer or a liver or kidney disorder); and immobilization, extremity injury, or recent surgery (DVT).

Past medical history should include any disorders known to cause edema, including heart, liver, and kidney disorders and cancer (including any related surgery or radiation therapy). The history should also include predisposing conditions for these causes, including streptococcal infection, recent viral infection (eg, hepatitis), chronic alcohol abuse, and hypercoagulable disorders. Drug history should include specific questions about drugs known to cause edema (see Table 74–2). Patients are asked about the amount of sodium used in cooking and at the table.

Physical examination: The area of edema is identified and examined for extent, warmth, erythema, and tenderness; symmetry or lack of it is noted. Presence and degree of pitting (visible and palpable depressions caused by pressure from the examiner's fingers on the edematous area, which displaces the interstitial fluid) are noted.

In the general examination, the skin is inspected for jaundice, bruising, and spider angiomas (suggesting a liver disorder).

Lungs are examined for dullness to percussion, reduced or exaggerated breath sounds, crackles, rhonchi, and pleural friction rub.

The internal jugular vein height, waveform, and reflux are noted.

The heart is palpated for thrills, thrust, parasternal lift, and asynchronous abnormal systolic bulge. Auscultation for loud pulmonic component of 2nd heart sound (P_2), 3rd (S_3) or 4th (S_4) heart sounds, murmurs, and pericardial rub or knock is done; all suggest cardiac origin.

The abdomen is inspected, palpated, and percussed for ascites, hepatomegaly, and splenomegaly to check for a liver disorder or heart failure. The kidneys are palpated, and the bladder is percussed. An abnormal abdominal mass, if present, should be palpated.

Red flags: Certain findings raise suspicion of a more serious etiology of edema:

- Sudden onset
- Significant pain
- Shortness of breath
- History of a heart disorder or an abnormal cardiac examination
- Hemoptysis, dyspnea, or pleural friction rub
- Hepatomegaly, jaundice, ascites, splenomegaly, or hematemesis
- Unilateral leg swelling with tenderness

Interpretation of findings: Potential acute life threats, which typically manifest with sudden onset of focal edema, must be identified. Such a presentation suggests acute DVT, soft-tissue infection, or angioedema. Acute DVT may lead to PE, which can be fatal. Soft-tissue infections range from minor to life threatening, depending on the infecting organism and the patient's health. Acute angioedema sometimes progresses to involve the airway, with serious consequences.

Dyspnea may occur with edema due to heart failure, DVT if PE has occurred, acute respiratory distress syndrome, or angioedema that involves the airways.

Generalized, slowly developing edema suggests a chronic heart, kidney, or liver disorder. Although these disorders can also be life threatening, complications tend to take much longer to develop.

These factors and other clinical features help suggest the cause (see Table 74–2).

Testing: For most patients with generalized edema, testing should include CBC, serum electrolytes, BUN, creatinine, liver function tests, serum protein, and urinalysis (particularly noting the presence of protein and microscopic hematuria). Other tests should be done based on the suspected cause (see Table 74–2)—eg, brain natriuretic peptide (BNP) for suspected heart failure or D-dimer for suspected PE.

Patients with isolated lower-extremity swelling should usually have venous obstruction excluded by ultrasonography.

Table 74–2. SOME CAUSES OF EDEMA

CAUSE	SUGGESTIVE FINDINGS	DIAGNOSTIC APPROACH*
Increased hydrostatic pressure, fluid overload		
Right heart failure (primary or secondary to left-sided disease or to constrictive pericarditis) directly increasing venous pressure	Symmetric, dependent, painless, pitting edema, often with dyspnea during exertion, orthopnea, and paroxysmal nocturnal dyspnea Commonly, lung crackles, S_3 or S_4 gallop or both, and jugular venous distention, hepatojugular reflux, and Kussmaul sign	Chest x-ray and ECG Usually echocardiography
Pregnancy and premenstrual state	Apparent by history	Clinical evaluation
Drugs (eg, minoxidil, NSAIDs, estrogens, fludrocortisone, dihydropyridine, diltiazem, other calcium channel blockers)	Symmetric, dependent, painless, usually mild pitting edema	Clinical evaluation
Iatrogenic (eg, excessive IV fluids)	Apparent by history and medical record	Clinical evaluation
Increased hydrostatic pressure, venous obstruction		
DVT	Acute, pitting edema in a single, usually lower extremity, usually with pain; sometimes Homans sign (pain in the calf when the foot is dorsiflexed) Redness, warmth, and tenderness; possibly less marked than in soft-tissue infection Sometimes a predisposing factor (eg, recent surgery, trauma, immobilization, hormone replacement, cancer)	Ultrasonography
Chronic venous insufficiency	Chronic edema in one or both lower extremities, with brownish discoloration, discomfort but not marked pain, and sometimes skin ulcers Often associated with varicose veins	Clinical evaluation
Extrinsic venous compression (by tumor, a gravid uterus, or marked abdominal obesity)	Nonpainful, slowly developing edema If tumor compresses the superior vena cava, usually facial plethora, distended neck veins, and absent venous pulse waves above the obstruction	Clinical evaluation Ultrasonography or CT if tumor is suspected
Prolonged absence of skeletal muscle pumping activity on extremity veins	Prolonged immobility (eg, being bedbound or on a long airline flight) Painless, symmetric, dependent edema	Clinical evaluation
Decreased plasma oncotic pressure†		
Nephrotic syndrome	Diffuse edema, often significant ascites, and sometimes periorbital edema	24-h urine collection to check for protein loss Plasma protein assay
Protein-losing enteropathy	Significant diarrhea	Testing for cause
Reduced albumin synthesis (eg, in liver disorders or undernutrition)	Often with significant ascites Causes often apparent by history If cause is a chronic liver disorder, often jaundice, spider angiomas, gynecomastia, palmar erythema, and testicular atrophy	Serum albumin, liver function tests, PT/PTT
Increased capillary permeability		
Angioedema (allergic, idiopathic, hereditary)	Sudden, focal, asymmetric, nondependent, pink or skin-colored edema that is sometimes uncomfortable	Clinical evaluation
Injury (eg, burns, chemicals, toxins, blunt trauma)	Apparent by history	Clinical evaluation
Severe sepsis (causing vascular endothelial leakage)	Obvious sepsis syndrome with fever, tachycardia, focal infection Painless, symmetrical edema	Cultures Imaging studies as needed
Soft-tissue infection (eg, cellulitis, necrotizing myofasciitis)	If due to cellulitis, usually redder and more painful and tender than that due to angioedema and more circumscribed than that due to DVT With necrotizing infections, severe pain, constitutional symptoms	Clinical evaluation Cultures Sometimes ultrasonography to rule out DVT

Table continues on the following page.

Table 74–2. SOME CAUSES OF EDEMA (*Continued*)

CAUSE	SUGGESTIVE FINDINGS	DIAGNOSTIC APPROACH*
Lymphatic obstruction		
Iatrogenic (eg, after lymph node dissection in cancer surgery or after radiation therapy)	Etiology usually apparent by history Initially pitting edema, with fibrosis developing later	Clinical evaluation
Congenital (rare)	Often onset in childhood, but for some types, only later onset May be familial	Sometimes lymphoscintigraphy
Lymphatic filariasis	History of being in an endemic area in a developing country Usually focal edema, sometimes involving the genitals	Microscopic examination of blood smear

*Most patients with generalized edema require CBC, electrolytes, BUN, creatinine, liver function tests, serum protein measurement, and urinalysis (to check for proteinuria).

†Decreased plasma oncotic pressure often triggers secondary Na and water retention, leading to fluid overload.

DVT = deep venous thrombosis; S_3 = 3rd heart sound; S_4 = 4th heart sound.

Treatment

Specific causes are treated.

Patients with sodium retention often benefit from restriction of dietary sodium. Patients with heart failure should eliminate salt in cooking and at the table and avoid prepared foods with added salt.

Patients with advanced cirrhosis or nephrotic syndrome often require more severe sodium restriction (≤ 1 g/day). Potassium salts are often substituted for sodium salts to make sodium restriction tolerable; however, care should be taken, especially in patients receiving potassium-sparing diuretics, ACE inhibitors, or angiotensin II receptor blockers and in those with a kidney disorder because potentially fatal hyperkalemia can result.

People with conditions involving sodium retention may also benefit from loop or thiazide diuretics. However, diuretics should not be given only to improve the appearance caused by edema. When diuretics are used, potassium wasting can be dangerous in some patients; potassium-sparing diuretics (eg, amiloride, triamterene, spironolactone, eplerenone) inhibit sodium reabsorption in the distal nephron and collecting duct. When used alone, they modestly increase sodium excretion. Both triamterene and amiloride have been combined with a thiazide to prevent potassium wasting. An ACE inhibitor–thiazide combination also reduces potassium wasting.

Geriatrics Essentials

In the elderly, use of drugs that treat causes of edema requires special caution, such as the following:

- Starting doses low and evaluating patients thoroughly when the dose is changed
- Monitoring for orthostatic hypotension if diuretics, ACE inhibitors, angiotensin II receptor blockers, or beta-blockers are used
- Evaluating for bradycardia or heart block if digoxin, rate-limiting calcium channel blockers, or beta-blockers are used
- Frequently testing for hypokalemia or hyperkalemia
- Not stopping calcium channel blockers because of pedal edema, which is benign

Logging daily weight helps in monitoring clinical improvement or deterioration immensely.

KEY POINTS

- Edema may result from a generalized or local process.
- Main causes of generalized edema are chronic heart, liver, and kidney disorders.
- Sudden onset should trigger prompt evaluation.
- Edema may occur anywhere in the body, including the brain.
- Not all edema is harmful; consequences depend mainly on the cause.

LIMB PAIN

Limb pain may affect all or part of an extremity (for joint pain, see p. 329). Pain may be constant or intermittent, and unrelated to motion or precipitated by it. Accompanying symptoms and signs often suggest a source.

Etiology

Musculoskeletal injuries and overuse are the most common causes of pain in a limb but are readily apparent by history. This discussion covers extra-articular limb pain unrelated to injury or strain. Pain that is in only one joint or in multiple joints is discussed elsewhere. There are many causes (see Table 74–3) but the most common are the following:

- DVT
- Cellulitis
- Radiculopathy

Uncommon but serious causes that require immediate diagnosis and treatment include

- Acute arterial occlusion
- Deep soft-tissue infection
- Acute coronary ischemia (manifesting with only referred arm pain)

Evaluation

It is important to exclude acute arterial occlusion.

History: History of present illness should address the duration, intensity, location, quality, and temporal pattern of pain.

Table 74–3. SOME CAUSES OF NONTRAUMATIC LIMB PAIN

CAUSE	SUGGESTIVE FINDINGS	DIAGNOSTIC APPROACH
Musculoskeletal and soft tissue		
Cellulitis	Focal redness, warmth, tenderness, swelling Sometimes fever	Clinical evaluation Sometimes blood and tissue cultures (eg, when patients are immunocompromised)
Deep soft-tissue infection (eg, myonecrosis, necrotizing subcutaneous infection)	Deep, constant pain, typically out of proportion to other findings Redness, warmth, tenderness, tense swelling, fever Sometimes crepitation, foul discharge, bullae or necrotic areas, signs of systemic toxicity (eg, delirium, tachycardia, pallor, shock)	Blood and tissue cultures X-ray Sometimes MRI
Osteomyelitis	Deep, constant, often nocturnal pain Bone tenderness, fever Often risk factors (eg, immunocompromise, parenteral drug use, known contiguous or remote source for infection)	X-ray, MRI, and/or CT Sometimes bone culture
Bone tumor (primary or metastatic)	Deep, constant, often nocturnal pain Bone tenderness Often a known cancer	X-ray, MRI, and/or CT
Vascular		
Deep venous thrombosis	Swelling, often warmth and/or redness, sometimes venous distension Often risk factors (eg, hypercoagulable state, recent surgery or immobility, cancer)	Ultrasonography Possibly D-dimer testing
Chronic venous stasis	Mild discomfort with swelling, erythema, and warmth of distal lower extremity Sometimes shallow ulcerations	Clinical evaluation
Acute ischemia (typically due to arterial embolism, dissection, or thrombosis but sometimes due to massive iliofemoral venous thrombosis that completely obstructs flow in the limb)	Sudden, severe pain Signs of distal limb ischemia (eg, coolness, pallor, pulse deficits, delayed capillary refill) Sometimes chronic ischemic skin changes (eg, atrophy, hair loss, pale color, ulceration) After several hours, neurologic deficits and muscle tenderness Sometimes known peripheral vascular disease	Immediate arteriography
Peripheral arterial insufficiency	Intermittent leg pain triggered predictably by exertion and relieved by rest (intermittent claudication), sometimes rest pain which may worsen with leg elevation Low ankle-brachial BP index, chronic ischemic skin changes	Ultrasonography Sometimes arteriography
Neurologic		
Plexopathy (brachial or lumbar)	Pain; usually weakness, decreased reflexes Sometimes numbness in a nerve plexus distribution	Usually electrodiagnostic testing (electromyography and nerve conduction velocity) Sometimes MRI
Thoracic outlet syndrome	Pain and paresthesias beginning in neck or shoulder and extending to medial aspect of arm and hand	Unclear, but possibly electrodiagnostic testing and/or MRI
Radiculopathy (eg, caused by herniated intervertebral disk or bone spurs)	Pain and sometimes sensory deficits following a dermatomal distribution and often worsening with movement Often neck or back pain Usually weakness and diminished deep tendon reflexes in a nerve root distribution	Usually MRI
Painful polyneuropathy (eg, alcoholic neuropathy)	Chronic, burning pain, typically in both hands or both feet Sometimes sensory abnormalities such as hypoesthesia, hyperesthesia, and/or allodynia (pain with non-noxious stimuli)	Clinical evaluation

Table continues on the following page.

Table 74–3. SOME CAUSES OF NONTRAUMATIC LIMB PAIN (*Continued*)

CAUSE	SUGGESTIVE FINDINGS	DIAGNOSTIC APPROACH
Complex regional pain syndrome (CRPS)	Burning pain, hyperesthesia, allodynia, vasomotor abnormalities Typically a prior injury (may be remote)	Clinical evaluation
Other		
Acute coronary ischemia (causing referred arm pain)	Absence of explanatory physical findings at the site of pain; other suggestive findings (eg, history suggesting coronary artery disease, sweating and/or dyspnea occurring simultaneously with arm pain)	ECG and serum troponin Sometimes stress testing or coronary angiography
Myofascial pain syndrome	Chronic pain and tenderness along a taut band of muscle, worsening with movement and with pressure on a trigger point (focal area separate from site of pain)	Clinical evaluation

Recent injury, excessive and/or unusual use, and factors that worsen pain (eg, limb movement, walking) and relieve pain (eg, rest, certain positions) should be noted. Any associated neurologic symptoms (eg, numbness, paresthesias) should be identified.

Review of systems should seek symptoms of possible causes, including back or neck pain (radiculopathy), fever (infections such as osteomyelitis, cellulitis, or deep soft-tissue infection), dyspnea (DVT with PE, MI), and chest pain or sweating (cardiac ischemia).

Past medical history should identify known risk factors, including cancer (metastatic bone tumors); immunocompromising disorders or drugs (infections); hypercoagulable states (DVT); diabetes (peripheral vascular disease with limb ischemia); peripheral vascular disease, hypercholesterolemia, and/or hypertension (acute or chronic ischemia); osteoarthritis or RA (radiculopathy); and prior injury (complex regional pain syndrome [CRPS]). Family and social history should address family history of early vascular disease and cigarette smoking (limb or cardiac ischemia) and illicit use of parenteral drugs (infections).

Physical examination: Vital signs are reviewed for fever (suggesting infection) and tachycardia and/or tachypnea (compatible with DVT with PE, MI, and infection with sepsis).

The painful limb is inspected for color, edema, and any skin or hair changes, and palpated for pulses, temperature, tenderness, and crepitation (a subtle crackling sensation indicating soft-tissue gas). Strength, sensation and deep tendon reflexes are compared between affected and unaffected sides. Systolic BP is measured in the ankle of the affected extremity and compared with systolic BP of an arm; the ratio of the two is the ankle-brachial index.

Red flags:

- Sudden, severe pain
- Signs of acute limb ischemia (eg, coolness, pallor, pulse deficits, delayed capillary refill)
- Dyspnea, chest pain, and/or sweating
- Signs of systemic toxicity (eg, delirium, tachycardia, shock, pallor)
- Crepitation, tenseness, foul discharge, bullae, necrosis
- Risk factors for DVT
- Neurologic deficits

Interpretation of findings: It can be helpful to categorize patients by acuity of symptoms and then further narrow the differential diagnosis based on presence or absence of findings of

- Ischemia
- Inflammation
- Neurologic abnormalities

Sudden, severe pain suggests acute ischemia or acute radiculopathy (eg, from sudden disc herniation). Acute ischemia causes generalized limb pain and manifests with weak or absent pulse, delayed capillary refill, coolness, and pallor; ankle-brachial index is typically < 0.3. Such vascular signs are absent with radiculopathy, in which pain instead follows a dermatomal distribution and is often accompanied by back or neck pain and diminished deep tendon reflexes. However, in both cases, weakness may be present. Acute ischemia due to massive venous thrombosis (phlegmasia cerulea dolens) usually causes edema, which is not present in ischemia due to arterial occlusion.

In **subacute pain** (ie, of 1 to a few days' duration), redness and tenderness, often accompanied by swelling, and/or warmth, suggest an inflammatory cause. If these findings are focal or circumscribed, cellulitis is likely. Generalized, circumferential swelling is more suggestive of DVT or, much less commonly, deep tissue infection. Patients with a deep tissue infection typically appear quite ill and may have blisters, necrosis, or crepitation. Findings in DVT vary widely; swelling and warmth may be minimal or absent. Neurologic findings of weakness, paresthesias, and/or sensory abnormalities suggest radiculopathy or plexopathy. If neurologic findings follow a dermatomal pattern, radiculopathy is more likely.

Chronic pain can be difficult to diagnose. If neurologic findings are present, causes include radiculopathy (dermatomal distribution), plexopathy (plexus distribution), neuropathy (stocking-glove distribution), and CRPS (variable distribution). CRPS should be suspected if vasomotor changes (eg, pallor, mottling, coolness) are present, particularly in those with previous injury to the affected extremity. Myofascial pain syndrome causes no neurovascular abnormalities and classically manifests with a palpably tense band of muscle in the area of pain, and pain may be reproduced by pressure on a trigger point near but not overlying the area of pain. In those with essentially no clinical findings, cancer and osteomyelitis should be considered, particularly in those with risk factors.

Intermittent pain occurring consistently with a given degree of exertion (eg, whenever walking > 3 blocks) and relieved with a few minutes of rest suggests peripheral arterial disease. Such patients typically have an ankle-brachial BP index of ≤ 0.9; an index ≤ 0.4 indicates severe disease. Those with peripheral arterial disease may have chronic skin changes (eg, atrophy, hair loss, pale color, ulceration).

Testing: Cellulitis, myofascial pain, painful polyneuropathy, and CRPS can often be diagnosed clinically. Testing (see Table 74–3) is usually necessary for other suspected causes of pain.

Treatment

Primary treatment is directed at the cause. Analgesics can help relieve pain.

KEY POINTS

- Acute limb ischemia should be considered in patients with sudden, severe pain.
- Presence or absence of findings of ischemia, inflammation, and neurologic abnormalities plus the acuity of onset help narrow the differential diagnosis.

ORTHOSTATIC HYPOTENSION

Orthostatic (postural) hypotension is an excessive fall in BP when an upright position is assumed. The consensus definition is a drop of > 20 mm Hg systolic, 10 mm Hg diastolic, or both. Symptoms of faintness, light-headedness, dizziness, confusion, or blurred vision occur within seconds to a few minutes of standing and resolve rapidly on lying down. Some patients experience falls, syncope, or even generalized seizures. Exercise or a heavy meal may exacerbate symptoms. Most other associated symptoms and signs relate to the cause. Orthostatic hypotension is a manifestation of abnormal BP regulation due to various conditions, not a specific disorder.

Postural orthostatic tachycardia syndrome (POTS): POTS (also called postural autonomic tachycardia or chronic or idiopathic orthostatic intolerance) is a syndrome of orthostatic intolerance in younger patients. Various symptoms (eg, fatigue, light-headedness, exercise intolerance, cognitive impairment) and tachycardia occur upon standing; however, there is little or no fall in BP. The reason for symptoms is unclear.

Pathophysiology

Normally, the gravitational stress of suddenly standing causes blood (½ to 1 L) to pool in the capacitance veins of the legs and trunk. The subsequent transient decrease in venous return reduces cardiac output and thus BP. In response, baroreceptors in the aortic arch and carotid bodies activate autonomic reflexes to rapidly return BP to normal. The sympathetic nervous system increases heart rate and contractility and increases vasomotor tone of the capacitance vessels. Simultaneous parasympathetic (vagal) inhibition also increases heart rate. In most people, changes in BP and heart rate upon standing are minimal and transient, and symptoms do not occur.

With continued standing, activation of the renin-angiotensin-aldosterone system and vasopressin (ADH) secretion cause sodium and water retention and increase circulating blood volume.

Etiology

Homeostatic mechanisms may be inadequate to restore low BP if afferent, central, or efferent portions of the autonomic reflex arc are impaired by disorders or drugs, if myocardial contractility or vascular responsiveness is depressed, if hypovolemia is present, or if hormonal responses are faulty (see Table 74–4).

Causes differ depending on whether symptoms are acute or chronic.

The most common causes of acute orthostatic hypotension include

- Hypovolemia
- Drugs
- Prolonged bed rest
- Adrenal insufficiency

Table 74–4. CAUSES OF ORTHOSTATIC HYPOTENSION

CAUSE	EXAMPLES
Neurologic (involving autonomic dysfunction)	
Central	Multiple system atrophy Parkinson disease Strokes (multiple)
Spinal cord	Tabes dorsalis Transverse myelitis Tumors
Peripheral	Amyloidosis Diabetic, alcoholic, or nutritional neuropathy Familial dysautonomia (Riley-Day syndrome) Guillain-Barré syndrome Paraneoplastic syndromes Pure autonomic failure Surgical sympathectomy
Cardiovascular	
Hypovolemia	Adrenal insufficiency Dehydration Hemorrhage
Impaired vasomotor tone	Bed rest (prolonged) Hypokalemia
Impaired cardiac output	Aortic stenosis Constrictive pericarditis Heart failure Myocardial infarction Tachyarrhythmias or bradyarrhythmias
Other	Hyperaldosteronism* Peripheral venous insufficiency Pheochromocytoma*
Drugs	
Vasodilators	Calcium channel blockers Nitrates
Autonomically active	Alpha-blockers (prazosin, phenoxybenzamine) Antihypertensives (clonidine, methyldopa, reserpine, [rarely] beta-blockers)† Antipsychotics (particularly phenothiazines) Monoamine oxidase inhibitors (MAOIs) Tricyclic or tetracyclic antidepressants
Other	Alcohol Barbiturates Levodopa (in Parkinson disease [rarely]) Loop diuretics (eg, furosemide) Quinidine Vincristine (neurotoxic)

*Disorder causes supine hypertension.
†Symptoms are more common when treatment is begun.

The most common causes of chronic orthostatic hypotension include

- Age-related changes in BP regulation
- Drugs
- Autonomic dysfunction

Postprandial orthostatic hypotension is also common. It may be caused by the insulin response to high-carbohydrate meals and blood pooling in the GI tract; this condition is worsened by alcohol intake.

Evaluation

Orthostatic hypotension is diagnosed when a marked fall in measured BP and symptoms suggesting hypotension are provoked by standing and relieved by lying down. A cause must be sought.

History: History of present illness should identify the duration and severity (eg, whether associated with syncope or falls) of symptoms. The patient is asked about known triggers (eg, drugs, bed rest, fluid loss) and the relationship of symptoms to meals.

Review of symptoms seeks symptoms of causative disorders, particularly symptoms of autonomic insufficiency such as visual impairment (due to mydriasis and loss of accommodation), incontinence or urinary retention, constipation, heat intolerance (due to impaired sweating), and erectile dysfunction. Other important symptoms include tremor, rigidity, and difficulty walking (Parkinson disease, multiple system atrophy); weakness and fatigue (adrenal insufficiency, anemia); and black, tarry stool (GI hemorrhage). Other symptoms of neurologic and cardiovascular disorders and cancer are noted.

Past medical history should identify known potential causes, including diabetes, Parkinson disease, and cancer (ie, causing a paraneoplastic syndrome). The drug profile should be reviewed for offending prescription drugs (see Table 74–4), particularly antihypertensives and nitrates. A family history of orthostatic symptoms suggests possible familial dysautonomia.

Physical examination: BP and heart rate are measured after 5 min supine and at 1 and 3 min after standing; patients unable to stand may be assessed while sitting upright. Hypotension without a compensatory increase in heart rate (< 10 beats/min) suggests autonomic impairment. Marked increase (to > 100 beats/min or by > 30 beats/min) suggests hypovolemia or, if symptoms develop without hypotension, POTS.

The skin and mucosae are inspected for signs of dehydration and for pigment changes suggestive of Addison disease (eg, hyperpigmented areas, vitiligo). A rectal examination is done to detect GI bleeding.

During the neurologic examination, GU and rectal reflexes can be tested to evaluate autonomic function; assessment includes the cremasteric reflex (normally, stroking the thigh results in retraction of the testes) and the anal wink reflex (normally, stroking perianal skin results in contraction of the anal sphincter). Signs of peripheral neuropathy (eg, abnormalities of strength, sensation, and deep tendon reflexes) are assessed.

Red flags: Certain findings suggest a more serious etiology:

- Bloody or heme-positive stool
- Abnormal neurologic examination

Interpretation of findings: In patients with acute symptoms, the most common causes—drugs, bed rest, and volume depletion—are often apparent clinically.

In patients with chronic symptoms, an important goal is to detect any neurologic disorder causing autonomic dysfunction. Patients with movement abnormalities may have Parkinson disease or multiple system atrophy. Patients with findings of peripheral neuropathy may have an apparent cause (eg, diabetes, alcoholism), but a paraneoplastic syndrome due to an occult cancer and amyloidosis must be considered. Patients who have only peripheral autonomic symptoms may have pure autonomic failure.

Testing: ECG and serum electrolytes and glucose are routinely checked. However, these and other tests are usually of little benefit unless suggested by specific symptoms.

The dose of a suspected drug may be reduced or the drug stopped to confirm the drug as the cause.

Tilt table testing may be done when autonomic dysfunction is suspected; it gives more consistent results than supine and upright BP assessment and eliminates augmentation of venous return by leg muscle contraction. The patient may remain upright for 30 to 45 min of BP assessment.

Patients with autonomic symptoms or signs require further evaluation for diabetes, Parkinson disease, and possibly multiple system atrophy and pure autonomic failure. Testing for pure autonomic failure may require plasma norepinephrine or vasopressin (ADH) measurements with the patient supine and upright.

Autonomic function can also be evaluated with bedside cardiac monitoring, although this test is not often done. When the autonomic system is intact, heart rate increases in response to inspiration. The heart is monitored as the patient breathes slowly and deeply (about a 5-sec inspiration and a 7-sec expiration) for 1 min. The longest inter-beat (R-R) interval during expiration is normally at least 1.15 times the minimum R-R interval during inspiration; a shorter interval suggests autonomic dysfunction, but this response to inspiration may decrease with aging. A similar variation in R-R interval should exist between rest and a 10- to 15-sec Valsalva maneuver.

Treatment

Nondrug treatment: Patients requiring prolonged bed rest should sit up each day and exercise in bed when possible. Patients should rise slowly from a recumbent or sitting position, consume adequate fluids, limit or avoid alcohol, and exercise regularly when feasible. Regular modest-intensity exercise promotes overall vascular tone and reduces venous pooling. Elderly patients should avoid prolonged standing. Sleeping with the head of the bed raised may relieve symptoms by promoting sodium retention and reducing nocturnal diuresis.

Postprandial hypotension can often be prevented by reducing the size and carbohydrate content of meals, minimizing alcohol intake, and avoiding sudden standing after meals.

Waist-high fitted elastic hose may increase venous return, cardiac output, and BP after standing. In severe cases, inflatable aviator-type antigravity suits, although often poorly tolerated, may be needed to produce adequate leg and abdominal counterpressure.

Increasing sodium and water intake may expand intravascular volume and lessen symptoms. In the absence of heart failure or hypertension, sodium intake can be increased to 6 to 10 g daily by liberally salting food or taking sodium chloride tablets. This approach risks heart failure, particularly in elderly patients and in patients with impaired myocardial function; development of dependent edema without heart failure does not contraindicate continuing this approach.

Drug treatment: Fludrocortisone, a mineralocorticoid, causes sodium retention, which expands plasma volume, and often lessens symptoms but is effective only when sodium intake is adequate. Dosage is 0.1 mg po at bedtime, increased weekly to 1 mg or until peripheral edema occurs. This drug may also improve the peripheral vasoconstrictor response to sympathetic stimulation. Supine hypertension, heart failure, and hypokalemia may occur; potassium supplements may be needed.

Midodrine, a peripheral alpha-agonist that is both an arterial and a venous constrictor, is often effective. Dosage is 2.5 mg to 10 mg po tid. Adverse effects include paresthesias and itching (probably secondary to piloerection). This drug is not recommended for patients with coronary artery or peripheral arterial disease.

NSAIDs (eg, indomethacin 25 to 50 mg po tid) may inhibit prostaglandin-induced vasodilation, increasing peripheral vascular resistance. However, NSAIDs may cause GI symptoms and unwanted vasopressor reactions (reported with concurrent use of indomethacin and sympathomimetic drugs).

L-Dihydroxyphenylserine, a norepinephrine precursor, may be beneficial for autonomic dysfunction (reported in limited trials).

Propranolol or other beta-blockers may enhance the beneficial effects of sodium and mineralocorticoid therapy. Beta-blockade with propranolol leads to unopposed alpha-adrenergic peripheral vascular vasoconstriction, preventing the vasodilation that occurs when some patients stand.

Geriatrics Essentials

Orthostatic hypotension occurs in about 20% of the elderly; it is more common among people with coexisting disorders, especially hypertension, and among residents of long-term care facilities. Many falls may result from unrecognized orthostatic hypotension.

The increased incidence in the elderly is due to decreased baroreceptor responsiveness plus decreased arterial compliance. Decreased baroreceptor responsiveness delays cardioacceleration and peripheral vasoconstriction in response to standing. Paradoxically, hypertension may contribute to poor baroreceptor sensitivity, increasing vulnerability to orthostatic hypotension. The elderly also have decreased resting parasympathetic tone, so that cardioacceleration due to reflex vagal withdrawal is lessened.

KEY POINTS

- Orthostatic hypotension typically involves volume depletion or autonomic dysfunction.
- Some degree of autonomic dysfunction is common in the elderly, but neurologic disorders must be ruled out.
- Tilt table testing is sometimes done.
- Treatment involves physical measures to reduce venous pooling, increased Na intake, and sometimes fludrocortisone or midodrine.

PALPITATIONS

Palpitations are the perception of cardiac activity. They are often described as a fluttering, racing, or skipping sensation. They are common; some patients find them unpleasant and alarming. Palpitations can occur in the absence of heart disease or can result from life-threatening heart disorders. The key to diagnosis and treatment is to "capture" the rhythm on ECG and make careful observations during the palpitations.

Pathophysiology

The mechanisms responsible for the sensation of palpitations are unknown. Ordinarily, sinus rhythm at a normal rate is not perceived, and palpitations thus usually reflect changes in cardiac rate or rhythm. In all cases, it is the abnormal movement of the heart within the chest that is felt. In cases of isolated extrasystoles, the patient may actually perceive the augmented postextrasystolic beat as the "skipped" beat rather than the premature beat itself, probably because the extrasystole blocks the next sinus beat and allows longer ventricular filling and thus a higher stroke volume.

The clinical perception of cardiac phenomena is highly variable. Some patients are aware of virtually every premature ventricular beat, but others are unaware of even complex atrial or ventricular tachyarrhythmias. Awareness is heightened in sedentary, anxious, or depressed patients and reduced in active, happy patients. In some cases, palpitations are perceived in the absence of any abnormal cardiac activity.

Etiology

Some patients simply have heightened awareness of normal cardiac activity, particularly when exercise, febrile illness, or anxiety increases heart rate. However, in most cases, palpitations result from arrhythmia. Arrhythmias range from benign to life threatening.

The **most common arrhythmias** include

- Premature atrial contractions (PACs)
- Premature ventricular contractions (PVCs)

Both of these arrhythmias usually are harmless.

Other common arrhythmias include

- Paroxysmal supraventricular tachycardia (PSVT)
- Atrioventricular nodal reentrant tachycardia
- Atrial fibrillation or atrial flutter
- Ventricular tachycardia

Bradyarrhythmias rarely cause a complaint of palpitations although some patients are aware of the slow rate.

Causes of arrhythmias: Some arrhythmias (eg, PACs, PVCs, PSVT) often occur spontaneously in patients without serious underlying disorders, but others are often caused by a serious cardiac disorder.

Serious cardiac causes include myocardial ischemia or other myocardial disorders, congenital heart disease (eg, Brugada syndrome, arrhythmogenic right ventricular cardiomyopathy, congenital long QT syndrome), valvular heart disease, and conduction system disturbances (eg, disturbances that cause bradycardia or heart block). Patients with orthostatic hypotension commonly sense palpitations caused by sinus tachycardia upon standing.

Noncardiac disorders that increase myocardial contractility (eg, thyrotoxicosis, pheochromocytoma, anxiety) may cause palpitations.

Some drugs, including digitalis, caffeine, alcohol, nicotine, and sympathomimetics (eg, albuterol, amphetamines, cocaine, dobutamine, epinephrine, ephedrine, isoproterenol, norepinephrine, and theophylline), frequently cause or exacerbate palpitations.

Metabolic disturbances, including anemia, hypoxia, hypovolemia, and electrolyte abnormalities (eg, diuretic-induced hypokalemia), can trigger or exacerbate palpitations.

Consequences: Many arrhythmias that cause palpitations have no adverse physiologic consequences of their own (ie, independent of the underlying disorder). However, bradyarrhythmias, tachyarrhythmias, and heart blocks can be unpredictable and may adversely affect cardiac output and cause hypotension or death. Ventricular tachycardia sometimes degenerates to ventricular fibrillation.

Evaluation

A complete history and physical examination are essential. Observations by other medical personnel or reliable observers should be sought.

History: History of present illness should cover the frequency and duration of palpitations and provoking or exacerbating factors (eg, emotional distress, activity, change in position, intake of caffeine or other drugs). Important associated symptoms include syncope, light-headedness, tunnel vision, dyspnea, and chest pain. Asking the patient to tap out the rate and cadence of palpitations is better than a verbal description and often allows a definitive diagnosis, as in the "missed beat" of atrial or ventricular extrasystoles or the rapid total irregularity of atrial fibrillation.

Review of systems should cover symptoms of causative disorders, including heat intolerance, weight loss, and tremor (hyperthyroidism); chest pain and dyspnea on exertion (myocardial ischemia); and fatigue, weakness, heavy vaginal bleeding, and dark tar-like stools (anemia).

Past medical history should identify known potential causes, including documented arrhythmias and heart or thyroid disorders. Family history should note occurrences of syncope (sometimes mistakenly described as seizures) or sudden death at an early age.

The drug profile should be reviewed for offending prescription drugs (eg, antiarrhythmics, digitalis, beta-agonists, theophylline, and rate-limiting drugs); OTC drugs (eg, cold and sinus drugs, dietary supplements containing stimulants), including alternative medicines; and illicit drugs (eg, cocaine, methamphetamines). Caffeine (eg, coffee, tea, numerous soft drinks and energy drinks), alcohol, and tobacco use should be determined.

Physical examination: The **general examination** should note whether an anxious demeanor or psychomotor agitation is present. Vital signs are reviewed for fever, hypertension, hypotension, tachycardia, bradycardia, tachypnea, and low oxygen saturation. Orthostatic changes in BP and heart rate should be measured.

Examination of the head and neck should note any abnormality or dyssynchrony of the jugular pulse waves compared with the carotid pulse or auscultated heart rhythm and findings of hyperthyroidism, such as thyroid enlargement or tenderness and exophthalmos. The conjunctivae, palmar creases, and buccal mucosa should be inspected for pallor.

Cardiac auscultation should note the rate and regularity of the rhythm as well as any murmurs or extra heart sounds that might indicate underlying valvular or structural heart disease.

Neurologic examination should note whether resting tremors or brisk reflexes are present (suggesting excess sympathetic stimulation). An abnormal neurologic finding suggests that seizures rather than a cardiac disorder may be the cause if syncope is one of the symptoms.

Red flags: Certain findings suggest a more serious etiology:

- Light-headedness or syncope (particularly if injury occurs from syncope)
- Chest pain
- Dyspnea
- New onset of irregularly irregular heart rhythm
- Heart rate > 120 beats/min or < 45 beats/min while at rest
- Significant underlying heart disease
- Family history of recurrent syncope or sudden death
- Exercise-induced palpitations or, particularly, syncope

Interpretation of findings: History (see Table 74–5) and, to a lesser extent, physical examination provide clues to the diagnosis.

Palpation of the arterial pulse and cardiac auscultation may reveal a rhythm disturbance. However, the examination is not always diagnostic of a specific rhythm, except when it identifies the unique irregular irregularity of some cases of rapid atrial fibrillation, the regular irregularity of coupled atrial or ventricular extrasystoles, the regular tachycardia at 150 beats/min of PSVT, and the regular bradycardia of < 35 beats/min of complete atrioventricular block. Careful examination of the jugular venous pulse waves simultaneously with cardiac auscultation and palpation of the carotid artery allows diagnosis of most arrhythmias if an ECG is not available because the jugular waves will show the atrial rhythm while the auscultated sounds or the pulse in the carotids are the product of ventricular contraction.

Thyroid enlargement or tenderness with exophthalmos suggests thyrotoxicosis. Marked hypertension and regular tachycardia suggest pheochromocytoma.

Testing: Testing typically is done.

- ECG, sometimes with ambulatory monitoring
- Laboratory testing
- Sometimes imaging studies, stress testing, or both

ECG is done, but unless the recording is done while symptoms are occurring, it may not provide a diagnosis. Many cardiac arrhythmias are intermittent and show no fixed ECG abnormalities; exceptions include

- Wolff-Parkinson-White syndrome
- Long QT syndrome
- Arrhythmogenic right ventricular dysplasia cardiomyopathy
- Brugada syndrome and its variants

If no diagnosis is apparent and symptoms are frequent, Holter monitoring for 24 to 48 h is useful; for intermittent symptoms, an event recorder worn for longer periods and activated by the patient when symptoms are felt is better. These tests are used mainly when a sustained arrhythmia is suspected, rather than when symptoms suggest only occasional skipped beats. Patients with very infrequent symptoms that clinicians suspect represent a serious arrhythmia may have a device implanted beneath the skin of the upper chest. This device continuously records the rhythm and can be interrogated by an external machine that allows the cardiac rhythm to be printed.

Laboratory testing is needed in all patients. All patients should have measurement of CBC and serum electrolytes, including magnesium and calcium. The cardiac marker troponin should be measured in patients with ongoing arrhythmias, chest discomfort, or other symptoms suggesting active or recent coronary ischemia, myocarditis, or pericarditis.

Thyroid function tests are indicated when atrial fibrillation is newly diagnosed or there are symptoms of hyperthyroidism. Patients with paroxysms of high BP should be evaluated for pheochromocytoma.

Sometimes tilt-table testing is done in patients with postural syncope.

Imaging is often needed. Patients with findings suggesting cardiac dysfunction or structural heart disease require echocardiography and sometimes cardiac MRI. Patients with symptoms on exertion require stress testing sometimes with stress echocardiography, nuclear scanning, or PET.

Treatment

Precipitating drugs and substances are stopped. If dangerous or debilitating arrhythmias are caused by a necessary therapeutic drug, a different drug should be tried.

For isolated PACs and PVCs in patients without structural heart disease, simple reassurance is appropriate. For otherwise healthy patients in whom these phenomena are disabling, a beta-blocker can be given provided efforts are made to avoid reinforcing the perception by anxious patients that they have a serious disorder.

Table 74–5. SUGGESTIVE HISTORICAL FINDINGS IN PATIENTS WITH PALPITATIONS

FINDING	POSSIBLE CAUSE
Occasional skipped beats	PACs, PVCs
Rapid, regular palpitations with sudden onset and termination Often history of recurrence	PSVT, atrial flutter with 2:1 atrioventricular block, ventricular tachycardia
Syncope following palpitations	Sinus node dysfunction, atrioventricular bypass tract (such as in Wolff-Parkinson-White syndrome), congenital long QT syndrome
Palpitations during exercise or an emotional episode	Sinus tachycardia (particularly in healthy people) Ventricular arrhythmia from exercise-induced ischemia (particularly in people with congenital arrhythmic disorders or CAD)
Palpitations following episodic* drug use	Drug-induced cause
Sense of doom, anxiety, or panic	Suggests (but does not confirm) a psychologic cause
Postoperative patient	Sinus tachycardia (eg, due to infection, bleeding, pulmonary embolism, pain)
Recurrent episodes since childhood	Supraventricular arrhythmia (eg, atrioventricular nodal reentrant bypass tract, Wolff-Parkinson-White syndrome) Congenital long QT syndrome (usually manifests during adolescence)
Family history of syncope or sudden death	Brugada syndrome, congenital long QT syndrome, inherited dilated or hypertrophic cardiomyopathy

*The role of regular use of drugs (particularly therapeutic drugs) or substances (eg, daily caffeine) can be hard to determine; sometimes a trial of withdrawal is diagnostic. All drugs with cardiovascular effects, most psychoactive drugs, and drugs capable of causing hypokalemia or hypomagnesemia must be suspected.

CAD = coronary artery disease; PACs = premature atrial contractions; PSVT = paroxysmal supraventricular tachycardia; PVCs = premature ventricular contractions.

Identified rhythm disturbances and underlying disorders are investigated and treated (see Table 74–6).

Geriatrics Essentials

Elderly patients are at particular risk of adverse effects of antiarrhythmics; reasons include lower GFR and concomitant use of other drugs. When drug treatment is needed, lower doses should be used to start. Subclinical conduction abnormalities may be present (recognized on ECG or other studies), which might worsen with use of antiarrhythmics; such patients may require a pacemaker to allow the use of antiarrhythmics.

Table 74–6. SOME TREATMENTS FOR ARRHYTHMIAS

DISORDER	TREATMENT*
Narrow complex tachycardias	
Multifocal atrial extrasystoles	Reassurance or beta-blocker
Atrial fibrillation	Aspirin, warfarin, enoxaparin, unfractionated heparin, DC cardioversion, flecainide, beta-blocker, digoxin, verapamil, diltiazem, ibutilide, amiodarone, radioablation, or Maze procedure depending on clinical circumstances
Atrial flutter	Radioablation (often the best treatment) Sometimes DC cardioversion, digoxin, beta-blocker, verapamil, and/or anticoagulation
Supraventricular tachycardia	Radioablation (often the best treatment) Sometimes vagotonic maneuvers, adenosine, DC cardioversion, beta-blocker, verapamil, flecainide, amiodarone, or digoxin
Atrioventricular nodal reentrant tachycardia	Radioablation (often the best treatment) Sometimes beta-blocker or verapamil
Broad complex tachycardias	
Ventricular tachycardia	DC cardioversion, amiodarone, sotalol, lidocaine, mexiletine, flecainide, radioablation, or an implanted defibrillator
Torsade de pointes	Magnesium, potassium, DC cardioversion, beta-blocker, overdrive pacemaker, or an implanted defibrillator
Ventricular fibrillation	DC cardioversion, amiodarone, lidocaine, or an implanted defibrillator
Brugada syndrome	DC cardioversion or an implanted defibrillator

*Always identify and correct causes and exacerbating factors (eg, electrolyte abnormalities, hypoxemia, drugs).
DC = direct current.

KEY POINTS

- Palpitations are a frequent but relatively nonspecific symptom.
- Palpitations are not a reliable indicator of a significant arrhythmia, but palpitations in a patient with structural heart disease or an abnormal ECG may be a sign of a serious problem and warrant investigation.
- An ECG or other recording done during symptoms is essential; a normal ECG in a symptom-free interval does not rule out significant disease.
- Most antiarrhythmics themselves can cause arrhythmias.
- If in doubt about a rapid tachyarrhythmia in a patient in hemodynamic distress, cardiovert first and ask questions later.

SYNCOPE

Syncope is a sudden, brief loss of consciousness (LOC) with loss of postural tone followed by spontaneous revival. The patient is motionless and limp and usually has cool extremities, a weak pulse, and shallow breathing. Sometimes brief involuntary muscle jerks occur, resembling a seizure.

Near-syncope is light-headedness and a sense of an impending faint without LOC. It is usually classified and discussed with syncope because the causes are the same.

Seizures can cause sudden LOC but are not considered syncope. However, seizures must be considered in patients presenting for apparent syncope because history may be unclear or unavailable, and some seizures do not cause tonic-clonic convulsions. Furthermore, a brief (< 5 sec) seizure sometimes occurs with true syncope.

Diagnosis depends on a careful history, eyewitness accounts, or fortuitous examination during the event.

Pathophysiology

Most syncope results from insufficient cerebral blood flow. Some cases involve adequate flow but with insufficient cerebral substrate (oxygen, glucose, or both).

Insufficient cerebral blood flow: Most deficiencies in cerebral blood flow result from decreased cardiac output (CO).

Decreased CO can be caused by

- Cardiac disorders that obstruct outflow
- Cardiac disorders of systolic dysfunction
- Cardiac disorders of diastolic dysfunction
- Arrhythmias (too fast or too slow)
- Conditions that decrease venous return

Outflow obstruction can be exacerbated by exercise, vasodilation, and hypovolemia (particularly in aortic stenosis and hypertrophic cardiomyopathy), which may precipitate syncope.

Arrhythmias cause syncope when the heart rate is too fast to allow adequate ventricular filling (eg > 150 to 180 beats/min) or too slow to provide adequate output (eg, < 30 to 35 beats/min).

Venous return can be decreased by hemorrhage, increased intrathoracic pressure, increased vagal tone (which can also decrease heart rate), and loss of sympathetic tone (eg, from drugs, carotid sinus pressure, autonomic dysfunction). Syncope involving these mechanisms (except for hemorrhage) is often termed **vasovagal** or neurocardiogenic and is common and benign.

Orthostatic hypotension, a common benign cause of syncope, results from failure of normal mechanisms (eg, sinus tachycardia, vasoconstriction, or both) to compensate for the temporary decrease in venous return that occurs with standing.

Cerebrovascular disorders (eg, strokes, transient ischemic attacks) rarely cause syncope because most of them do not involve the centrencephalic structures that must be affected to produce LOC. However, basilar artery ischemia, due to transient ischemic attack or migraine, may cause syncope. Rarely, patients with severe cervical arthritis or spondylosis develop vertebrobasilar insufficiency with syncope when the head is moved in certain positions.

Insufficient cerebral substrate: The CNS requires oxygen and glucose to function. Even with normal cerebral blood flow, a significant deficit of either will cause LOC. In practice, hypoglycemia is the primary cause because hypoxia rarely develops in a manner causing abrupt LOC (other than in flying or diving incidents). LOC due to hypoglycemia is seldom as abrupt as in syncope or seizures because warning symptoms occur (except in patients taking beta-blockers); however, the onset may be unclear to the examiner unless the event was witnessed.

Etiology

Causes are usually classified by the mechanism (see Table 74–7).

The **most common causes** are

- Vasovagal (neurocardiogenic)
- Idiopathic

Many cases of syncope never have a firm diagnosis but lead to no apparent harm. A smaller number of cases have a serious cause, usually cardiac.

Evaluation

Evaluation should be done as soon as possible after the event. The more remote the syncopal event, the more difficult the diagnosis. Information from witnesses is quite helpful and best obtained as soon as possible.

History: History of present illness should ascertain events leading up to the syncope, including the patient's activity (eg, exercising, arguing, in a potentially emotional situation), position (eg, lying or standing), and, if standing, for how long. Important associated symptoms immediately before or after the event include whether there was a sense of impending LOC, nausea, sweating, blurred or tunnel vision, tingling of lips or fingertips, chest pain, or palpitations. Length of time recovering should also be ascertained. Witnesses, if any, should be sought and asked to describe events, particularly the presence and duration of any seizure activity.

Review of systems should ask about any areas of pain or injury, episodes of dizziness or near-syncope upon arising, and episodes of palpitations or chest pain with exertion. Patients should be asked about symptoms suggesting possible causes, including bloody or tarry stools, heavy menses (anemia); vomiting, diarrhea, or excess urination (dehydration or electrolyte abnormalities); and risk factors for PE (recent surgery or immobilization, known cancer, previous clots or hypercoagulable state).

Past medical history should ask about previous syncopal events, known cardiovascular disease, and known seizure disorders. Drugs used should be identified (particularly antihypertensives, diuretics, vasodilators, and antiarrhythmics—see Table 74–8). Family history should note presence at a young age of heart disease or sudden death in any family member.

Physical examination: Vital signs are essential. Heart rate and BP are measured with the patient supine and after 3 min of standing. Pulse is palpated for irregularity.

General examination notes patient's mental status, including any confusion or hesitancy suggesting a postictal state and any signs of injury (eg, bruising, swelling, tenderness, tongue bite).

The heart is auscultated for murmurs; if present, any change in the murmur with a Valsalva maneuver, standing, or squatting is noted.

Table 74–7. SOME CAUSES OF SYNCOPE

CAUSE	SUGGESTIVE FINDINGS	DIAGNOSTIC APPROACH*
Cardiac outflow or inflow obstruction		
Valvular disease: Aortic stenosis, mitral stenosis, tetralogy of Fallot, prosthetic valve dehiscence or thrombosis	Young or old patient Syncope often exertional; recovery prompt Heart murmur	Echocardiography
Hypertrophic cardiomyopathy, restrictive cardiomyopathy, cardiac tamponade, myocardial rupture	Young or old patient Syncope often exertional; recovery prompt Heart murmur	Echocardiography
Cardiac tumors or thrombi	Syncope may be positional Usually a murmur (possibly variable) Peripheral embolic phenomena	Echocardiography
Pulmonary embolism, amniotic fluid embolism, or, rarely, air embolism	Usually from large embolus, accompanied by dyspnea, tachycardia, or tachypnea Often risk factors for pulmonary embolism	D-Dimer CT angiography or nuclear scan
Cardiac arrhythmia		
Bradyarrhythmias (eg, due to sinus node dysfunction, high-grade atrioventricular block, drugs[†])	Syncope occurring without warning; recovery immediate on awakening May occur in any position Bradyarrhythmias more common in the elderly Patient taking drugs, especially antiarrhythmics or other drugs that prolong the QT interval in susceptible patients Structural heart disease	If ECG unclear, consider Holter monitor, event recorder, or occasionally an implantable loop recorder Electrophysiologic testing if abnormalities detected or high suspicion Serum electrolytes if clinical reason for abnormality (eg, diuretic use, vomiting, diarrhea)
Tachyarrhythmias, either supraventricular or ventricular (eg, due to ischemia, heart failure, myocardial disease, drugs[†], electrolyte abnormalities, arrhythmogenic right ventricular dysplasia, long QT syndrome, Brugada syndrome, preexcitation)	Syncope occurring without warning; recovery immediate on awakening May occur in any position Patient taking drugs, especially antiarrhythmics or other cardiac drugs Structural heart disease	If ECG unclear, consider Holter monitor or event recorder Electrophysiologic testing if abnormalities detected or high suspicion Serum electrolytes if clinical reason for abnormality (eg, diuretic use, vomiting, diarrhea)
Ventricular dysfunction		
Acute myocardial infarction, myocarditis, systolic or diastolic dysfunction, cardiomyopathy	Syncope a rare presenting symptom of myocardial infarction (most such patients are elderly), with arrhythmia or shock	Serum troponin ECG Echocardiography Sometimes cardiac MRI
Pericardial tamponade or constriction	Jugular venous elevation; pulsus paradoxus > 10	Echocardiography Sometimes CT
Vasovagal (neurocardiogenic)		
Increased intrathoracic pressure (eg, tension pneumothoraxh, cough, straining to urinate or defecate, Valsalva maneuver)	Warning symptoms (eg, dizziness, nausea, sweating); recovery usually prompt but not immediate (5 to 15 min or longer, but sometimes up to hours) Precipitant usually apparent	Clinical evaluation
Strong emotion (eg, pain, fear, sight of blood)	Warning symptoms (eg, dizziness, nausea, sweating); recovery prompt but not immediate (5 to 15 min, but sometimes up to hours) Precipitant usually apparent	Clinical evaluation
Carotid sinus pressure	Warning symptoms (eg, dizziness, nausea, sweating); recovery prompt but not immediate (5 to 15 min, but sometimes up to hours) Precipitant usually apparent	Clinical evaluation

Table continues on the following page.

Table 74–7. SOME CAUSES OF SYNCOPE (*Continued*)

CAUSE	SUGGESTIVE FINDINGS	DIAGNOSTIC APPROACH*
Swallowing	Warning symptoms (eg, dizziness, nausea, sweating); recovery prompt but not immediate (5 to 15 min, but sometimes up to hours) Precipitant usually apparent	Clinical evaluation
Anaphylaxis	Drug administration, insect bite, allergy history	Allergy testing
Orthostatic hypotension		
Drugs†	Symptoms developing within several minutes of assuming upright position Drop in BP with standing during examination	Clinical evaluation Sometimes tilt table testing
Autonomic dysfunction	Symptoms developing within several minutes of assuming upright position Drop in BP with standing during examination	Clinical evaluation Sometimes tilt table testing
Deconditioning caused by prolonged bed rest	Symptoms developing within several minutes of assuming upright position Drop in BP with standing during examination	Clinical evaluation Sometimes tilt table testing
Anemia	Chronic fatigue, sometimes dark stools, heavy menses	CBC
Cerebrovascular		
Basilar artery transient ischemic attack or stroke	Sometimes cranial nerve deficits and ataxia	CT or MRI
Migraine	Aura with visual symptoms, photophobia; unilateral	Clinical evaluation
Other		
Prolonged standing	Apparent by history; no other symptoms	Clinical evaluation
Pregnancy	Healthy woman of childbearing age; no other symptoms Usually an early or unrecognized pregnancy	Urine pregnancy test
Hyperventilation	Often tingling around mouth or on fingers prior to syncope Usually in context of an emotional situation	Clinical evaluation
Hypoglycemia	Altered mental status until treated, onset seldom abrupt, sweating, piloerection Usually history of diabetes or insulinoma	Fingerstick glucose Response to glucose infusion
Psychiatric disorders	Not true syncope (patient may be partially or inconsistently responsive during events) Normal examination Often history of psychiatric disorder	Clinical evaluation

*ECG and pulse oximetry are done for all.
†See Table 74–8.

Careful evaluation of the jugular venous waves (see Fig. 73–1 on p. 583) while palpating the carotid or auscultating the heart may allow diagnosis of an arrhythmia if an ECG is not available.

Some clinicians carefully apply unilateral carotid sinus pressure during ECG monitoring with the patient supine to detect bradycardia or heart block, suggesting carotid sinus hypersensitivity. Carotid sinus pressure should not be applied if a carotid bruit is present.

Abdomen is palpated for tenderness, and a rectal examination is done to check for gross or occult blood.

A full neurologic examination is done to identify any focal abnormalities, which suggest a CNS cause (eg, seizure disorder).

Red flags: Certain findings suggest a more serious etiology:

- Syncope during exertion
- Multiple recurrences within a short time
- Heart murmur or other findings suggesting structural heart disease (eg, chest pain)
- Older age
- Significant injury during syncope
- Family history of sudden unexpected death, exertional syncope, or unexplained recurrent syncope or seizures

Interpretation of findings: Although the cause is often benign, it is important to identify the occasional life-threatening cause (eg, tachyarrhythmia, heart block) because sudden death is a risk. Clinical findings (see Table 74–7) help suggest a cause in 40 to 50% of cases. A few generalizations are useful.

Benign causes often lead to syncope.

- Syncope precipitated by unpleasant physical or emotional stimuli (eg, pain, fright), usually occurring in the upright position and often preceded by vagally mediated warning symptoms (eg, nausea, weakness, yawning, apprehension, blurred vision, diaphoresis), suggests vasovagal syncope.
- Syncope that occurs most often when assuming an upright position (particularly in elderly patients after prolonged bed

Table 74–8. SOME DRUG CAUSES OF SYNCOPE

MECHANISM	EXAMPLE
Bradyarrhythmia	Amiodarone, other rate-limiting drugs
	Beta-blockers
	Calcium channel blockers (not dihydropyridines)
	Digoxin
Tachyarrhythmia	Any antiarrhythmic drug that prolongs repolarization (eg, procainamide, disopyramide)
	Quinidine
Orthostatic hypotension	Most antihypertensives (rarely beta-blockers)
	Antipsychotics (mainly phenothiazines)
	Doxorubicin
	Levodopa
	Loop diuretics
	Nitrates (with or without a phosphodiesterase inhibitor for erectile dysfunction)
	Quinidine
	Tricyclic antidepressants
	Vincristine

rest or in patients taking drugs in certain classes) suggests orthostatic syncope.

- Syncope that occurs after standing for long periods without moving is usually due to venous pooling.
- LOC that is abrupt in onset; is associated with muscular jerking or convulsions that last more than a few seconds, incontinence, drooling, or tongue biting; and is followed by postictal confusion or somnolence suggests a seizure.

Dangerous causes are suggested by red flag findings.

- Syncope with exertion suggests cardiac outflow obstruction or exercise-induced arrhythmia. Such patients sometimes also have chest pain, palpitations, or both. Cardiac findings may help identify a cause. A harsh, late-peaking, basal murmur radiating to the carotid arteries suggests aortic stenosis; a systolic murmur that increases with the Valsalva maneuver and disappears with squatting suggests hypertrophic cardiomyopathy.
- Syncope that begins and ends suddenly and spontaneously is typical of cardiac causes, most commonly an arrhythmia.
- Syncope while lying down also suggests an arrhythmia because vasovagal and orthostatic mechanisms do not cause syncope in the recumbent position.
- Syncope accompanied by injury during the episode increases the likelihood of a cardiac cause or seizure somewhat, and therefore the event is of greater concern. The warning signs and slower LOC that accompany benign vasovagal syncope somewhat reduce the likelihood of injury.

Testing: Testing typically is done.

- ECG
- Pulse oximetry
- Sometimes echocardiography
- Sometimes tilt table testing
- Blood tests only if clinically indicated
- CNS imaging rarely indicated

In general, if syncope results in an injury or is recurrent (particularly within a brief period), more intensive evaluation is warranted.

Patients with suspected arrhythmia, myocarditis, or ischemia should be evaluated as inpatients. Others may be evaluated as outpatients.

ECG is done for all patients. The ECG may reveal arrhythmia, a conduction abnormality, ventricular hypertrophy, preexcitation, QT prolongation, pacemaker malfunction, myocardial ischemia, or MI. If there are no clinical clues, measuring cardiac markers and obtaining serial ECGs to rule out MI in older patients plus ECG monitoring for at least 24 h are prudent. Any detected arrhythmia must be associated with altered consciousness in order to be implicated as the cause, but most patients do not experience syncope during monitoring. On the other hand, the presence of symptoms in the absence of rhythm disturbance helps rule out a cardiac cause. An event recorder may be useful if warning symptoms precede syncope. A signal-averaged ECG may identify predisposition to ventricular arrhythmias in patients with ischemic heart disease or in post-myocardial infarction patients. If syncopal episodes are infrequent (eg, < 1/mo), an implantable loop recorder can be used for longer term recording.

Pulse oximetry should be done during or immediately after an episode to identify hypoxemia (which may indicate PE). If hypoxemia is present, CT or a lung scan is indicated to rule out PE.

Laboratory tests are done based on clinical suspicion; reflexively obtained laboratory panels are of little use. However, all females of childbearing age should have a pregnancy test. Hct is measured if anemia is suspected. Electrolytes are measured only if an abnormality is clinically suspected (eg, by symptoms or drug use). Serum troponin is measured if acute MI is suspected.

Echocardiography is indicated for patients with exercise-induced syncope, cardiac murmurs, or suspected intracardiac tumors (eg, those with positional syncope).

Tilt table testing may be done if history and physical examination indicate vasodepressor or other reflex-induced syncope. It is also used to evaluate exercise-induced syncope if echocardiography or exercise stress testing is negative.

Stress testing (exercise or pharmacologic) is done when intermittent myocardial ischemia is suspected. It is often done for patients with exercise-induced symptoms.

Invasive electrophysiologic testing is considered if noninvasive testing does not identify arrhythmia in patients with unexplained recurrent syncope; a negative response defines a low-risk subgroup with a high rate of remission of syncope. The use of electrophysiologic testing is controversial in other patients. Exercise testing is less valuable unless physical activity precipitated syncope.

EEG is warranted if a seizure disorder is suspected.

CT and **MRI** of the head and brain are indicated only if signs and symptoms suggest a focal CNS disorder.

Treatment

In witnessed syncope, pulses are checked immediately. If the patient is pulseless, CPR is begun and cardiac resuscitation is done. If pulses are present, severe bradycardia is treated with atropine or external transthoracic pacing. Isoproterenol can be used to maintain adequate heart rate while a temporary pacemaker is placed.

Tachyarrhythmias are treated; a direct-current synchronized shock is quicker and safer for unstable patients. Inadequate venous return is treated by keeping the patient supine, raising the legs, and giving IV normal saline. Tamponade is relieved by pericardiocentesis. Tension pneumothorax requires insertion of a pleural cannula and drainage. Anaphylaxis is treated with parenteral epinephrine.

Placing the patient in a horizontal position with legs elevated typically ends the syncopal episode if life-threatening disorders are ruled out. If the patient sits upright too rapidly, syncope may recur; propping the patient upright or transporting the patient in an upright position may prolong cerebral hypoperfusion and prevent recovery.

Specific treatment depends on the cause and its pathophysiology.

Geriatrics Essentials

The most common cause of syncope in the elderly is postural hypotension due to a combination of factors. Factors include rigid, noncompliant arteries, reduced skeletal muscle pumping of venous return due to physical inactivity, and degeneration of the sinoatrial node and conduction system due to progressive structural heart disease.

In the elderly, syncope often has more than one cause. For example, the combination of taking several heart and BP drugs and standing in a hot church during a long or emotional service may lead to syncope even though no single factor might cause syncope.

KEY POINTS

- Syncope results from global CNS dysfunction, usually from insufficient cerebral blood flow.
- Most syncope results from benign causes.
- Some less common causes involve cardiac arrhythmia or outflow obstruction and are serious or potentially fatal.
- Vasovagal syncope usually has an apparent trigger, warning symptoms, and a few minutes or longer of postrecovery symptoms.
- Syncope due to cardiac arrhythmias typically occurs abruptly and with quick recovery.
- Seizures have a prolonged (eg, hours) recovery period.
- If a benign etiology is not clear, driving and use of machinery should be prohibited until the etiology is determined and treated—the next manifestation of an unrecognized cardiac cause may be fatal.

75 Cardiovascular Tests and Procedures

Many noninvasive and invasive tests can delineate cardiac structure and function (see Table 75–1). Also, treatments can be administered during certain invasive diagnostic tests (eg, percutaneous coronary intervention during cardiac catheterization, radiofrequency ablation during electrophysiologic testing).

CARDIAC CATHETERIZATION

Cardiac catheterization is the passage of a catheter through peripheral arteries or veins into cardiac chambers, the pulmonary artery, and coronary arteries and veins.

Cardiac catheterization can be used to do various tests, including

- Angiography
- Intravascular ultrasonography
- Measurement of cardiac output (CO)
- Detection and quantification of shunts
- Endomyocardial biopsy
- Measurements of myocardial metabolism

These tests define coronary artery anatomy, cardiac anatomy, cardiac function, and pulmonary arterial hemodynamics to establish diagnoses and help select treatment.

Cardiac catheterization is also the basis for several therapeutic interventions (see Percutaneous Coronary Interventions on p. 615).

Procedure

Patients must be npo for 4 to 6 h before cardiac catheterization. Most patients do not require overnight hospitalization unless a therapeutic intervention is also done.

Left heart catheterization: Left heart catheterization is most commonly used to assess

- Cardiac anatomy

Left heart catheterization is also used to assess

- Aortic blood pressure
- Systemic vascular resistance

Table 75–1. TESTS FOR ASSESSING CARDIAC ANATOMY AND FUNCTION

APPLICATION	TESTS
Left ventricular function	Echocardiography Multiple-gated acquisition (MUGA) radionuclide imaging Gated MRI Contrast ventriculography
Coronary artery disease diagnosis and prognosis	Exercise or pharmacologic stress testing with ECG, myocardial perfusion imaging, or echocardiography Magnetic resonance angiography Coronary angiography Intravascular ultrasonography Multidetector CT coronary angiography
Myocardial viability	Resting single-photon emission CT (SPECT) myocardial perfusion imaging Stress testing (using low-dose dobutamine) with echocardiography Positron emission tomography (PET) Gated MRI

- Aortic valve function
- Mitral valve function
- Left ventricular pressure and function

The procedure is done via femoral, subclavian, radial, or brachial artery puncture, with a catheter passed into the coronary artery ostia or across the aortic valve into the LV.

Catheterization of the left atrium (LA) and LV is occasionally done using transseptal perforation during right heart catheterization.

Right heart catheterization: Right heart catheterization is most commonly used to assess

- Right atrial (RA) pressure
- Right ventricular (RV) pressure
- Pulmonary artery pressure
- Pulmonary artery occlusion pressure (PAOP—see Fig. 75–1)

PAOP approximates left atrial and left ventricular end-diastolic pressure. In seriously ill patients, PAOP helps assess volume status and, with simultaneous measurements of CO, can help guide therapy.

Right heart catheterization is also useful for assessing pulmonary vascular resistance, tricuspid or pulmonic valve function, intracardiac shunts, and right ventricular pressure.

Right heart pressure measurements may help in the diagnosis of cardiomyopathy, constrictive pericarditis, and cardiac tamponade when noninvasive testing is nondiagnostic, and it is an essential part of the assessment for cardiac transplantation or mechanical cardiac support (eg, use of a ventricular assist device).

The procedure is done via femoral, subclavian, internal jugular, or antecubital vein puncture. A catheter is passed into the RA, through the tricuspid valve, into the RV, and across the pulmonary valve into the pulmonary artery.

Selective catheterization of the coronary sinus can also be done.

Specific Tests During Cardiac Catheterization

Angiography: Injection of radiopaque contrast agent into coronary or pulmonary arteries, the aorta, and cardiac chambers is useful in certain circumstances. Digital subtraction angiography is used for nonmoving arteries and for chamber cineangiography.

Coronary angiography via left heart catheterization is used to evaluate coronary artery anatomy in various clinical situations, as in patients with suspected coronary atherosclerotic or congenital disease, valvular disorders before valvular replacement, or unexplained heart failure.

Pulmonary angiography via right heart catheterization can be used to diagnose pulmonary embolism. Intraluminal filling defects or arterial cutoffs are diagnostic. Radiopaque contrast agent is usually selectively injected into one or both pulmonary arteries and their segments. However, computed tomographic pulmonary angiography (CTPA) has largely replaced right heart catheterization for diagnosis of pulmonary embolism.

Aortic angiography via left heart catheterization is used to assess aortic regurgitation, coarctation, patent ductus arteriosus, and dissection.

Ventriculography is used to visualize ventricular wall motion and ventricular outflow tracts, including subvalvular, valvular, and supravalvular regions. It is also used to estimate severity of mitral valve regurgitation and determine its pathophysiology. After LV mass and volume are determined from single planar or biplanar ventricular angiograms, end-systolic and end-diastolic volumes and ejection fraction (EF) can be calculated.

Intravascular ultrasonography: Miniature ultrasound transducers on the end of coronary artery catheters can produce images of coronary vessel lumina and walls and delineate blood

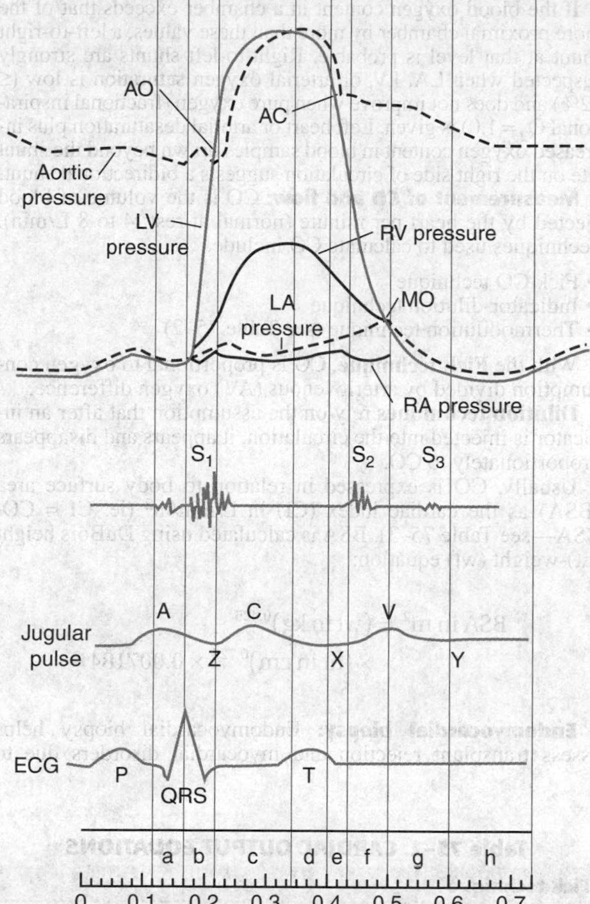

Fig. 75–1. Diagram of the cardiac cycle, showing pressure curves of the cardiac chambers, heart sounds, jugular pulse wave, and the ECG. The phases of the cardiac cycle are atrial systole (a), isometric contraction (b), maximal ejection (c), reduced ejection (d), protodiastolic phase (e), isometric relaxation (f), rapid inflow (g), and diastasis, or slow LV filling (h). For illustrative purposes, time intervals between valvular events have been modified, and the z point has been prolonged.AO = aortic valve opening; AC = aortic valve closing; LV = left ventricle; LA = left atrium; RV = right ventricle; RA = right atrium; MO = mitral valve opening.

flow. This technique is being increasingly used at the same time as coronary angiography.

Optical coherence tomography: Optical coherence tomography (OCT) is an optical analog of intracoronary ultrasound imaging that measures the amplitude of backscattered light to determine the temperature of coronary plaques and can help determine whether lesions are at high risk of future rupture (leading to acute coronary syndromes).

Tests for cardiac shunts: Measuring blood oxygen content at successive levels in the heart and great vessels can help determine the presence, direction, and volume of central shunts. The maximal normal difference in oxygen content between structures is as follows:

- The pulmonary artery and right ventricle: 0.5 mL/dL
- The right ventricle and right atrium: 0.9 mL/dL
- The right atrium and superior vena cava: 1.9 mL/dL

If the blood oxygen content in a chamber exceeds that of the more proximal chamber by more than these values, a left-to-right shunt at that level is probable. Right-to-left shunts are strongly suspected when LA, LV, or arterial oxygen saturation is low (≤ 92%) and does not improve when pure oxygen (fractional inspirational $O_2 = 1.0$) is given. Left heart or arterial desaturation plus increased oxygen content in blood samples drawn beyond the shunt site on the right side of circulation suggests a bidirectional shunt.

Measurement of CO and flow: CO is the volume of blood ejected by the heart per minute (normal at rest: 4 to 8 L/min). Techniques used to calculate CO include.

- Fick CO technique
- Indicator-dilution technique
- Thermodilution technique (see Table 75–2)

With the **Fick technique,** CO is proportional to oxygen consumption divided by arteriovenous (AV) oxygen difference.

Dilution techniques rely on the assumption that after an indicator is injected into the circulation, it appears and disappears proportionately to CO.

Usually, CO is expressed in relation to body surface area (BSA) as the cardiac index (CI) in L/min/m² (ie, CI = CO/BSA—see Table 75–3). BSA is calculated using DuBois height (ht)-weight (wt) equation:

$$\text{BSA in m}^2 = (\text{wt in kg})^{0.425} \times (\text{ht in cm})^{0.725} \times 0.007184$$

Endomyocardial biopsy: Endomyocardial biopsy helps assess transplant rejection and myocardial disorders due to infection or infiltrative diseases. The biopsy catheter (bioptome) can be passed into either ventricle, usually the right. Three to 5 samples of myocardial tissue are removed from the septal endocardium. The main complication of endomyocardial biopsy, cardiac perforation, occurs in 0.3 to 0.5% of patients; it may cause hemopericardium leading to cardiac tamponade. Injury to the tricuspid valve and supporting chordae may also occur and can lead to tricuspid regurgitation.

Coronary artery flow measurements: Coronary angiography shows the presence and degree of stenosis but not the functional significance of the lesion (ie, how much blood flows across the stenosis) or whether a specific lesion is likely to be causing symptoms.

Extremely thin guidewires are available with pressure sensors or Doppler flow sensors. Data from these sensors can be used to estimate coronary artery blood flow, which is expressed as fractional flow reserve (FFR). FFR is the ratio of maximal flow through the stenotic area to normal maximal flow; an FFR of < 0.75 to 0.8 is considered abnormal.

These flow estimates correlate well with the need for intervention and long-term outcome; lesions with FFR > 0.8 do not seem to benefit from stenting. These flow measurements are most useful with intermediate lesions (40 to 70% stenosis) and with multiple lesions (to identify those that are clinically most significant).

Table 75–2. CARDIAC OUTPUT EQUATIONS

Fick technique

$$CO = \frac{\text{Ambient } O_2 - \text{expired } O_2 \text{ (mL/min)}}{(1.36)\ (\text{Hb g/dL}) \times (SaO_2 - SvO_2)}$$

Numerator is O_2 absorbed by lungs (mL/min).

Indicator-dilution technique

$$CO = \frac{\text{Injectate mass (mg)}}{\int_{\infty} C(t)\ dt}$$

Denominator is the sum of dye concentrations (C) at each time interval (t).

Thermodilution technique

$$CO = \frac{(T_B - T_I) \times \text{Injectate volume (mL)} \times 53.5}{\int_{\infty} T_B(t)\ dt}$$

$T_B - T_I$ is the difference between body and injectate temperatures; injectate is usually dextrose or saline. Denominator is the sum of changes in temperature at each time interval (t).

SaO_2 = arterial O_2 saturation (%); SvO_2 = mixed venous O_2 saturation (%), measured in the pulmonary artery.

Contraindications to Cardiac Catheterization

Relative contraindications to cardiac catheterization include

- Renal insufficiency
- Coagulopathy
- Fever
- Systemic infection
- Uncontrolled arrhythmia or hypertension
- Uncompensated heart failure
- Radiopaque contrast agent allergies in patients who have not been appropriately premedicated

Table 75–3. NORMAL VALUES FOR CARDIAC INDEX AND RELATED MEASUREMENTS

MEASUREMENT	NORMAL VALUE	SD
Oxygen uptake	143 mL/min/m²*	14.3
Arteriovenous oxygen difference	4.1 dL	0.6
Cardiac index	3.5 L/min/m²	0.7
Stroke index	46 mL/beat/m²	8.1
Total systemic resistance	1130 dynes-sec-cm^{-5}	178
Total pulmonary resistance	205 dynes-sec-cm^{-5}	51
Pulmonary arteriolar resistance	67 dynes-sec-cm^{-5}	23

*Varies with body mass index.

SD = standard deviation.

Adapted from Barratt-Boyes BG, Wood EH: Cardiac output and related measurements and pressure values in the right heart and associated vessels, together with an analysis of the hemodynamic response to the inhalation of high oxygen mixtures in healthy subjects. *Journal of Laboratory and Clinical Medicine* 51:72–90, 1958.

Complications of Cardiac Catheterization

The incidence of complications after cardiac catheterizations ranges from 0.8 to 8%, depending on patient factors, technical factors, and the experience of the operator. Patient factors that increase risk of complications include

- Increasing age
- Heart failure
- Valvular heart disease
- Peripheral arterial disease
- COPD
- Chronic kidney disease
- Insulin-dependent diabetes

Most complications are minor and can be easily treated. Serious complications (eg, cardiac arrest, anaphylactic reactions, shock, seizures, cyanosis, renal toxicity) are rare. Mortality rate is 0.1 to 0.2%. Myocardial infarction (0.1%) and stroke (0.1%) may result in significant morbidity. Incidence of stroke is higher in patients > 80 yr.

In general, complications involve

- The contrast agent
- Effects of the catheter
- The access site

Contrast agent complications: Injection of radiopaque contrast agent produces a transient sense of warmth throughout the body in many patients. Tachycardia, a slight fall in systemic pressure, an increase in CO, nausea, vomiting, and coughing may occur. Rarely, bradycardia occurs when a large amount of a contrast agent is injected; asking the patient to cough often restores normal rhythm.

More serious reactions (see also Radiographic Contrast Agents and Contrast Reactions on p. 3222) include

- Allergic-type contrast reactions
- Contrast nephropathy

Allergic reactions may include urticaria and conjunctivitis, which usually respond to diphenhydramine 50 mg IV. Anaphylaxis, with bronchospasm, laryngeal edema, and dyspnea are rare reactions; they are treated with inhaled albuterol or epinephrine 0.3 to 0.4 mL sc. Anaphylactic shock is treated with epinephrine and other supportive measures. Patients with a history of allergic reaction to contrast may be premedicated with prednisone (50 mg po 13 h, 7 h, and 1 h before injection of contrast) and diphenhydramine (50 mg po or IM 1 h before the injection). If patients require imaging immediately, they can be given diphenhydramine 50 mg po or IM 1 h before injection of contrast and hydrocortisone 200 mg IV q 4 h until imaging is completed.

Contrast nephropathy is defined as impairment of renal function (either a 25% increase in serum creatinine from baseline or a 0.5 mg/dL increase in absolute value) within 48 to 72 h of IV contrast administration. For patients at risk, use of low-osmolar or iso-osmolar contrast, and infusion of normal saline IV for 4 to 6 h before angiography and 6 to 12 h afterward reduces this risk. In such patients, assess serum creatinine 48 h after injection of contrast.

Catheter-related complications: If the catheter tip contacts the ventricular endocardium, ventricular arrhythmias commonly occur, but ventricular fibrillation is rare. If it occurs, direct current (DC) cardioversion is administered immediately.

Disruption of an atherosclerotic plaque by the catheter can release a shower of atheroemboli. Emboli from the aorta may cause stroke or nephropathy. Emboli from the coronary arteries may cause myocardial infarction.

Coronary artery dissection is possible.

Access site complications: Access site complications include

- Bleeding
- Hematoma
- Pseudoaneurysm
- AV fistula
- Limb ischemia

Bleeding from the access site may occur and usually resolves with compression. Mild bruises and small hematomas are common and do not require specific investigation or treatment.

A large or enlarging lump should be investigated using ultrasonography to distinguish hematoma from pseudoaneurysm. A bruit at the site (with or without pain) suggests an AV fistula, which can be diagnosed using ultrasonography. Hematomas usually resolve with time and do not require specific therapy. Pseudoaneurysms and AV fistulas usually resolve with compression; those that persist may require surgical repair.

Radial artery access is in general more comfortable for the patient and carries a much lower risk of hematoma or pseudoaneurysm or AV fistula formation when compared with femoral artery access.

CORONARY ARTERY BYPASS GRAFTING

Coronary artery bypass grafting (CABG—see also p. 674) involves bypassing native coronary arteries that have high-grade stenosis or occlusion not amenable to angioplasty with stent insertion. Indications are changing as percutaneous interventions are being increasingly used.

Traditional CABG Procedure

Traditional CABG involves thoracotomy via a midline (median) sternotomy. A heart-lung machine is used to establish cardiopulmonary bypass (CPB), allowing the heart to be stopped and emptied of blood to maximize operative exposure and facilitate vessel anastomosis; stopping the heart also markedly decreases myocardial oxygen demand.

Before initiation of CPB, the patient is given a very high dose of heparin to prevent clotting in the bypass circuit. Then the aorta is cross-clamped and the heart is stopped by injection of a cardioplegic solution (crystalloid or more commonly blood-based) that also contains substances that help myocardial cells tolerate ischemia and reperfusion. The cardioplegic solution and the heart are sometimes cooled slightly to enhance tolerance of ischemia; the patient's body is cooled via the CPB machine for similar reasons.

The left internal mammary artery is typically used as a pedicled graft to the left anterior descending coronary artery. Other grafts consist of segments of saphenous vein removed from the leg. Occasionally, the right internal mammary artery or radial artery from the nondominant arm can be used.

On completion of the vascular anastomoses, the aorta is unclamped, allowing the coronary arteries to be perfused by oxygenated blood, which typically restores cardiac activity. Heparin anticoagulation is reversed by giving protamine. Despite cardioprotective measures, stopping the heart is not without consequences. During reperfusion, myocardial dysfunction is common and can lead to bradycardia, arrhythmias (eg, ventricular fibrillation), and low CO; these events are treated by standard measures, such as pacing, defibrillation, and inotropic drugs.

Typically, hospital stays are 4 to 5 days unless prolonged by complications or concomitant illnesses.

Complications of CABG: Complications and disadvantages of traditional CABG involve mainly

- Sternotomy
- Cardiopulmonary bypass

Median sternotomy is surprisingly well tolerated; however, healing takes 4 to 6 wk. Also, wound infections occasionally cause mediastinitis or sternal osteomyelitis, which can be vexing to treat.

CPB causes several complications, including

- Bleeding
- Organ dysfunction
- Neuropsychiatric effects
- Stroke

Post-CPB bleeding is a common problem caused by various factors, including hemodilution, heparin use, platelet dysfunction due to exposure to the bypass pump, disseminated intravascular coagulation, and induced hypothermia.

Organ dysfunction may result from a systemic inflammatory response caused by the CPB machine (probably due to exposure of blood components to the foreign material of the bypass circuit); this response can cause organ dysfunction in any system (eg, pulmonary, renal, brain, GI). Aortic cannulation, cross-clamping, and release can trigger release of emboli, causing stroke in about 1.5%; microemboli may contribute to post-CPB neuropsychiatric effects, which appear in about 5 to 10%.

Other common complications of CABG include

- Focal myocardial ischemia
- Global myocardial ischemia
- Dysrhythmias

Perioperative myocardial infarction occurs in about 1% of patients. Atrial fibrillation occurs in 15 to 40% of patients, typically 2 to 4 days after surgery. Beta-blockers (including sotalol) and amiodarone appear to reduce the likelihood of the development of atrial arrhythmias after cardiac surgery. Nonsustained ventricular tachycardia may occur in up to 50% of patients.

Mortality depends mainly on patients' underlying health; operator and institutional experience (ie, number of annual procedures) also is important. In an experienced program, periprocedural mortality in otherwise healthy patients is typically < 1 to 3%.

A simple calculator can categorize risk of CABG into three groups (low, intermediate, high). A more advanced online cardiac surgery risk calculator is published by the Society of Thoracic Surgeons.

Alternative CABG Procedures

Newer techniques seek to limit the complications of traditional CABG by

- Avoiding cardiopulmonary bypass (off-pump CABG)
- Avoiding median sternotomy (minimally invasive CABG)
- Both

Off-pump CABG: Cardiopulmonary bypass can be avoided in select patients by using techniques that allow the surgeon to revascularize the beating heart. Various devices and methods stabilize a portion of the myocardium, holding the operative site relatively motionless.

Off-pump CABG procedures are more commonly done through small parasternal or intercostal incisions (minimally invasive CABG), sometimes with endoscopy or even robotic assistance, but they may be done through a traditional median sternotomy, which provides better operative exposure.

Allowing the heart to beat means that the myocardium requires more oxygen than when CPB is used. Thus, the heart is sensitive to the interruption of blood flow necessitated while the vascular anastomosis is done; this interruption can cause ischemia or infarction in the myocardium supplied by the affected vessel. Some surgeons place a temporary coronary artery shunt to provide distal perfusion.

Minimally invasive CABG: The minimally invasive CABG technique is somewhat more difficult to do and may not be suitable when multiple bypass grafts, particularly those involving vessels behind the heart, are required. Transfusion requirements, length of stay, and costs are typically less with off-pump CABG, but in some studies, the rate of the more serious complications of death, myocardial infarction, and stroke are similar to that of CABG using CPB. Thus, the theoretic advantages of avoiding CPB do not seem to have been fully realized.

Minimally invasive CABG is usually done off-pump but may be done using CPB. In such cases, CPB is done endovascularly using special catheters inserted into the arterial and venous systems; the aorta is occluded by a balloon at the end of the aortic catheter rather than an external clamp. Although avoiding median sternotomy complications, this technique otherwise has similar rates of mortality and major perioperative complications as conventional techniques.

ECHOCARDIOGRAPHY

Echocardiography uses ultrasound waves to produce an image of the heart, the heart valves, and the great vessels. It helps assess heart wall thickness (eg, in hypertrophy or atrophy) and motion and provides information about ischemia and infarction. It can be used to assess systolic function as well as diastolic filling patterns of the left ventricle, which can help in the assessment of left ventricular hypertrophy, hypertrophic or restrictive cardiomyopathy, severe heart failure, constrictive pericarditis, and severe aortic regurgitation. It also is used to assess the structure and function of the heart valves; detect valvular vegetations and intracardiac thrombus; and provide an estimate of pulmonary arterial pressure and central venous pressure.

Techniques: There are 2 techniques for doing echocardiography:

- Transthoracic
- Transesophageal

Transthoracic echocardiography (TTE) is the most common echocardiography technique. In TTE, a transducer is placed along the left or right sternal border, at the cardiac apex, at the suprasternal notch (to allow visualization of the aortic valve, left ventricular outflow tract, and descending aorta), or over the subxiphoid region. TTE provides 2- or 3-dimensional tomographic images of most major cardiac structures. A limited TTE (focused on detecting significant pericardial effusion and ventricular dysfunction) is sometimes done at the bedside of critically ill patients in the ICU and emergency department (ED); many intensivists and ED physicians have training to do this procedure when experienced radiologists or cardiologists are not available.

In **transesophageal echocardiography** (TEE), a transducer on the tip of an endoscope allows visualization of the heart via the stomach and esophagus. TEE is used to assess cardiac disorders when transthoracic study is technically difficult, as in obese patients and in patients with COPD. It reveals better detail of small abnormal structures (eg, endocarditic vegetations or patent foramen ovale) and posterior cardiac structures (eg, left atrium, left atrial appendage, interatrial septum, pulmonary vein anatomy) because they are closer to the esophagus than to the anterior chest wall. TEE can also produce images of the ascending aorta, which arises behind the 3rd costal cartilage; of structures < 3 mm (eg, thrombi, vegetations); and of prosthetic valves.

Methodology: Two-dimensional (cross-sectional) echocardiography is most commonly used; contrast and spectral Doppler echocardiography provide additional information. Three-dimensional echocardiography is particularly useful in evaluating the mitral valve apparatus for surgical correction.

Contrast echocardiography is 2-dimensional TTE done while agitated saline (or another ultrasonographic contrast agent) is rapidly injected into the cardiac circulation. Agitated saline develops microbubbles, which produce a cloud of echoes in the right cardiac chambers and which, if a septal defect is present, appear on the left side of the heart. Usually, the microbubbles do not traverse the pulmonary capillary bed; however, one agent, sonicated albumin microbubbles, can do so and can enter left heart structures after IV injection and can therefore be used to delineate the heart chambers, especially the left ventricle.

Spectral Doppler echocardiography can record velocity, direction, and type of blood flow. This technique is useful for detecting abnormal blood flow (eg, due to regurgitant lesions) or velocity (eg, due to stenotic lesions). Spectral Doppler echocardiography does not provide spatial information about the size or shape of the heart or its structures.

Color Doppler echocardiography combines 2-dimensional and spectral Doppler echocardiography to provide information about the size and shape of the heart and its structures as well as the velocity of and direction of blood flow around the valves and outflow tracts. Color is used to code blood flow information; by convention, red is toward and blue away from the transducer.

Tissue Doppler imaging uses Doppler techniques to measure the velocity of myocardial tissue contraction (rather than of blood flow). These data can be used to calculate myocardial strain (percentage change in length between contraction and relaxation) and myocardial strain rate (rate of change in length). Strain and strain rate measurements can help assess systolic and diastolic function and identify ischemia during stress testing.

Three-dimensional echocardiography incorporates M-mode echocardiography, Doppler flow measurement, and Doppler tissue imaging to give a real-time, 3-dimensional display of cardiac anatomy and function. This technique continues to evolve; its widespread acceptance and use have been hampered by lack of 3rd-party reimbursement.

Stress echocardiography: TTE is an alternative to radionuclide imaging to identify myocardial ischemia during and after exercise or pharmacologic stress testing. Stress echocardiography shows regional wall motion abnormalities that result from an imbalance in blood flow in epicardial coronary vessels during stress. Computer programs can provide side-by-side assessment of ventricular contraction during systole and diastole at rest and under stress. Exercise and pharmacologic protocols are the same as those used in radionuclide stress testing, except that dobutamine tends to be preferred over dipyridamole or adenosine as the pharmacologic agent.

Stress echocardiography is valuable in evaluating the hemodynamic severity of aortic valve stenosis in patients with significant symptoms but whose resting transvalvular pressure gradient is not markedly high. Stress echocardiography and radionuclide stress testing detect ischemia equally well. The choice between tests is often based on availability, the provider's experience, and cost.

ELECTROCARDIOGRAPHY

The standard ECG provides 12 different vector views of the heart's electrical activity as reflected by electrical potential differences between positive and negative electrodes placed on the limbs and chest wall. Six of these views are vertical (using frontal leads I, II, and III and limb leads aVR, aVL, and aVF), and 6 are horizontal (using precordial leads V_1, V_2, V_3, V_4, V_5, and V_6). The 12-lead ECG is crucial for establishing many cardiac diagnoses (see Table 75–4), including

- Arrhythmias
- Myocardial ischemia
- Atrial enlargement
- Ventricular hypertrophy (see Table 75–5)
- Conditions that predispose to syncope or sudden death (eg, Wolff-Parkinson-White syndrome, long QT syndrome, Brugada syndrome)

For more information on ECG interpretation, see under Diagnosis on p. 621 and under ECG on p. 677.

Standard ECG Components

By convention, the ECG tracing is divided into the P wave, PR interval, QRS complex, QT interval, ST segment, T wave, and U wave (see Fig. 75–2).

P wave: The P wave represents atrial depolarization. It is upright in most leads except aVR. It may be biphasic in leads II and V_1; the initial component represents right atrial activity, and the 2nd component represents left atrial activity.

An increase in amplitude of either or both components occurs with atrial enlargement. Right atrial enlargement produces a P wave > 2 mm in leads II, III, and aVF (P pulmonale); left atrial enlargement produces a P wave that is broad and double-peaked in lead II (P mitrale). Normally, the P axis is between 0° and 75°.

PR interval: The PR interval is the time between onset of atrial depolarization and onset of ventricular depolarization. Normally, it is 0.10 to 0.20 sec; prolongation defines 1st-degree atrioventricular block.

QRS complex: The QRS complex represents ventricular depolarization.

The Q wave is the initial downward deflection; normal Q waves last < 0.05 sec in all leads except V_{1-3}, in which any Q wave is considered abnormal, indicating past or current infarction.

The R wave is the first upward deflection; criteria for normal height or size are not absolute, but taller R waves may be caused by ventricular hypertrophy. A 2nd upward deflection in a QRS complex is designated R′.

The S wave is the 2nd downward deflection if there is a Q wave and the first downward deflection if not.

The QRS complex may be R alone, QS (no R), QR (no S), RS (no Q), or RSR′, depending on the ECG lead, vector, and presence of heart disorders.

Normally, the QRS interval is 0.07 to 0.10 sec. An interval of 0.10 to 0.11 sec is considered incomplete bundle branch block or a nonspecific intraventricular conduction delay, depending on QRS morphology. An interval ≥ 0.12 sec is considered complete bundle branch block or an intraventricular conduction delay.

Normally, the QRS axis is 90° to −30°. An axis of −30° to −90° is considered left axis deviation and occurs in left anterior fascicular block (−60°) and inferior myocardial infarction.

An axis of 90° to 180° is considered right axis deviation; it occurs in any condition that increases pulmonary pressures and causes right ventricular hypertrophy (cor pulmonale, acute

Table 75–4. INTERPRETATION OF ABNORMAL ECGs

ABNORMAL COMPONENT	DESCRIPTION	POSSIBLE CAUSES
P waves	Abnormal	Left or right atrial hypertrophy, atrial escape (ectopic) beats
P waves	Absent	Atrial fibrillation, sinus node arrest or exit block, hyperkalemia (severe)
P-P interval	Varying	Sinus arrhythmia
PR interval	Long	First-degree atrioventricular block
PR interval	Varying	Mobitz type I atrioventricular block, multifocal atrial tachycardia
QRS complex	Wide	Right or left bundle branch block, ventricular flutter or fibrillation, hyperkalemia
QT interval	Long	Myocardial infarction, myocarditis, hypocalcemia, hypokalemia, hypomagnesemia, hypothyroidism, subarachnoid or intracerebral hemorrhage, stroke, congenital long QT syndrome, antiarrhythmics (eg, sotalol, amiodarone, quinidine), tricyclic antidepressants, phenothiazines, other drugs
QT interval	Short	Hypercalcemia, hypermagnesemia, Graves disease, digoxin
ST segment	Depression	Myocardial ischemia; acute posterior myocardial infarction; digoxin; ventricular hypertrophy; pulmonary embolism; left bundle branch block; right bundle branch block in leads V_1–V_3 and possibly in II, III, and aVF; hyperventilation; hypokalemia
ST segment	Elevation	Myocardial ischemia, acute myocardial infarction, left bundle branch block, acute pericarditis, left ventricular hypertrophy, hyperkalemia, pulmonary embolism, digoxin, normal variation (eg, athlete's heart), hypothermia
T wave	Tall	Hyperkalemia, acute myocardial infarction, left bundle branch block, stroke, ventricular hypertrophy
T wave	Small, flattened, or inverted	Myocardial ischemia, myocarditis, age, race, hyperventilation, anxiety, drinking hot or cold beverages, left ventricular hypertrophy, certain drugs (eg, digoxin), pericarditis, pulmonary embolism, conduction disturbances (eg, right bundle branch block), electrolyte disturbances (eg, hypokalemia)
U wave	Prominent	Hypokalemia, hypomagnesemia, ischemia

pulmonary embolism, pulmonary hypertension), and it sometimes occurs in right bundle branch block or left posterior fascicular block.

QT interval: The QT interval is the time between onset of ventricular depolarization and end of ventricular repolarization. The QT interval must be corrected for heart rate using the formula:

$$QTc = \frac{QT}{\sqrt{RR}}$$

where QT_c is the corrected QT interval and R-R interval is the time between 2 QRS complexes. All intervals are recorded in seconds. QT_c prolongation is strongly implicated in development of torsades de pointe ventricular tachycardia. QT_c is often difficult to calculate because the end of the T wave is often unclear or followed by a U wave with which it merges. Numerous drugs are implicated in prolonging the QT interval.

ST segment: The ST segment represents completed ventricular myocardial depolarization. Normally, it is horizontal along the baseline of the PR (or TP) intervals or slightly off baseline.

ST segment elevation can be caused by

- Early repolarization
- Left ventricular hypertrophy
- Myocardial ischemia and infarction
- Left ventricular aneurysm
- Pericarditis
- Hyperkalemia
- Hypothermia
- Pulmonary embolism

ST segment depression can be caused by

- Hypokalemia
- Digoxin
- Subendocardial ischemia
- Reciprocal changes in acute myocardial infarction

T wave: The T wave reflects ventricular repolarization. It usually takes the same direction as the QRS complex (concordance); opposite polarity (discordance) may indicate past or current infarction. The T wave is usually smooth and rounded but may be of low amplitude in hypokalemia and hypomagnesemia and may be tall and peaked in hyperkalemia, hypocalcemia, and left ventricular hypertrophy.

U wave: The U wave appears commonly in patients who have hypokalemia, hypomagnesemia, or ischemia. It is often present in healthy people.

Specialized ECG Tests

A standard 12-lead ECG represents only a single brief period of cardiac activity; enhanced techniques can provide additional information.

Additional precordial leads: Additional precordial leads are used to help diagnose right ventricular and posterior wall myocardial infarction.

Right-sided leads are placed across the right side of the chest to mirror standard left-sided leads. They are labeled V_1R to V_6R; sometimes only V_4R is used, because it is the most sensitive for right ventricular myocardial infarction.

Additional left-sided leads can be placed in the 5th intercostal space, with V_7 at the posterior axillary line, V_8 at the midscapular line, and V_9 at the left border of the spine. These leads are rarely used but may help diagnose a true posterior myocardial infarction.

Table 75–5. CRITERIA FOR ECG DIAGNOSIS OF LEFT VENTRICULAR HYPERTROPHY

CRITERION	FINDING	POINTS
Romhilt-Estes (5 points = definite LVH; 4 points = probable LVH)	R or S wave ≥ 20 mm in any limb lead *or* S wave in V_1 or V_2 ≥ 30 mm *or* R wave in V_5 or V_6 ≥ 30 mm	3
	ST-T changes typical of LVH	—
	• Digitalis	1
	• No digitalis	3
	Left atrial changes: P terminal wave in V_1, amplitude ≥ 1 mm, and duration ≥ 0.04 sec	3
	Left axis deviation ≥ −30°	2
	QRS duration ≥ 90 msec	1
	Interval between QRS and R-wave peak in V_5 or V_6 ≥ 0.05 sec	1
Sokolow-Lyon	V_1 S wave + V_5 or V_6 R wave ≥ 35 mm *or* aVL R wave ≥ 11 mm	N/A
Cornell	Men: V_3 S wave + aVL R wave > 28 mm	N/A
	Women: V_3 S wave + aVL R wave > 20 mm	N/A

LVH = left ventricular hypertrophy.

Esophageal lead: An esophageal lead is much closer to the atria than surface leads; it is an option when the presence of P waves on a standard recording is uncertain and when detecting atrial electrical activity is important, as when atrial or ventricular origin of wide-complex tachycardia must be differentiated or when atrioventricular dissociation is suspected. An esophageal lead may also be used to monitor intraoperative myocardial ischemia or to detect atrial activity during cardioplegia. The lead is placed by having the patient swallow an electrode, which is then connected to a standard ECG machine, often in the lead II port.

Signal averaging: Signal averaging of QRS waveforms creates a digital composite of several hundred cardiac cycles to detect high-frequency, low-amplitude potentials and microcurrents

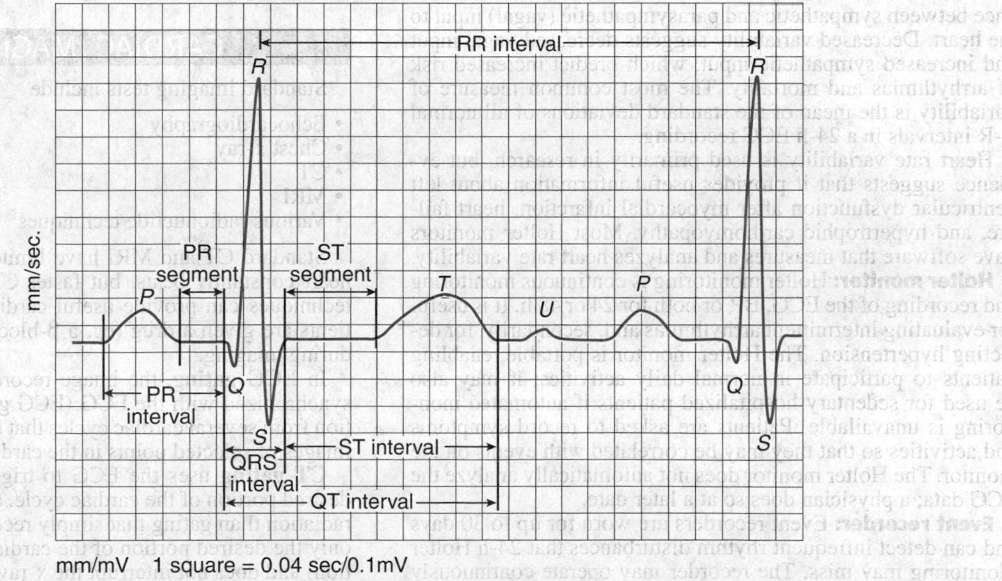

Fig. 75–2. ECG waves. P wave = activation (depolarization) of atria. PR interval = time interval between onset of atrial depolarization and onset of ventricular depolarization. QRS complex = depolarization of ventricles, consisting of the Q, R, and S waves. QT interval = time interval between onset of ventricular depolarization and end of ventricular repolarization. R-R interval = time interval between 2 QRS complexes. T wave = ventricular repolarization. ST segment plus T wave (ST-T) = ventricular repolarization. U wave = probably after-depolarization (relaxation) of ventricles.

at the terminal part of the QRS complex. These findings represent areas of slow conduction through abnormal myocardium, indicating increased risk of reentrant ventricular tachycardia.

Signal-averaged ECG is still largely a research technique but is occasionally used to assess risk of sudden cardiac death (eg, in patients with known significant heart disease). It seems most useful in identifying patients at *low* risk of sudden death. Its value for identifying patients at *high* risk of sudden death has not been established.

Signal averaging is also being investigated in various other cardiac disorders, ranging from the post-myocardial infarction state and cardiomyopathies to Brugada syndrome and ventricular aneurysms, and to assess efficacy of surgery to correct the arrhythmia. This technique may also be useful for assessing the proarrhythmic effects of antiarrhythmic drugs and for detecting rejection of heart transplants.

Signal averaging of P waves is being studied as a way to identify patients at risk of atrial fibrillation.

Continuous ST-segment monitoring: This type of monitoring is used for early detection of ischemia and serious arrhythmias. Monitoring can be automated (dedicated electronic monitoring units are available) or done clinically using serial ECGs. Applications include emergency department monitoring of patients with crescendo angina, evaluation after percutaneous intervention, intraoperative monitoring, and postoperative care.

QT dispersion: QT dispersion (the difference between the longest and shortest QT intervals on a 12-lead ECG) has been proposed as a measure of myocardial repolarization heterogeneity. Increased dispersion (≥ 100 ms) suggests electrically heterogeneous myocardium caused by ischemia or fibrosis, with increased risk of reentrant arrhythmias and sudden death. QT dispersion predicts mortality risk but is not widely measured because measurement error is common, values in patients with and without disease overlap substantially, there is no reference standard, and other validated risk predictors are available.

Heart rate variability: This measurement reflects the balance between sympathetic and parasympathetic (vagal) input to the heart. Decreased variability suggests decreased vagal input and increased sympathetic input, which predict increased risk of arrhythmias and mortality. The most common measure of variability is the mean of the standard deviations of all normal R-R intervals in a 24-h ECG recording.

Heart rate variability is used primarily in research, but evidence suggests that it provides useful information about left ventricular dysfunction after myocardial infarction, heart failure, and hypertrophic cardiomyopathy. Most Holter monitors have software that measures and analyzes heart rate variability.

Holter monitor: Holter monitoring is continuous monitoring and recording of the ECG, BP, or both for 24 or 48 h. It is useful for evaluating intermittent arrhythmias and, secondarily, for detecting hypertension. The Holter monitor is portable, enabling patients to participate in normal daily activities; it may also be used for sedentary hospitalized patients if automated monitoring is unavailable. Patients are asked to record symptoms and activities so that they may be correlated with events on the monitor. The Holter monitor does not automatically analyze the ECG data; a physician does so at a later date.

Event recorder: Event recorders are worn for up to 30 days and can detect infrequent rhythm disturbances that 24-h Holter monitoring may miss. The recorder may operate continuously and also be activated by the patient when symptoms occur. A memory loop enables information to be stored for seconds or minutes before and after activation. The patient can transmit ECG data by telephone or satellite to be read by a physician; some recorders automatically transmit serious events. If patients have serious events (eg, syncope) at intervals of > 30 days, an event recorder may be placed subcutaneously (implantable loop recorder); it can be activated by a small magnet. Battery life for subcutaneous recorders is 36 mo.

Wireless adhesive monitor: A new option for single-channel rhythm monitoring is a small, adhesive, water-resistant, wireless, and disposable device worn on the chest. One type of this device continuously records cardiac rhythms for up to 2 wk. Another similar device functions as an event recorder; a patient pushes a button on the device when experiencing any potential arrhythmia-related symptoms (eg, palpitations, dizziness) to record stored ECG data 45 sec before the event plus 15 sec after the event. However, unlike with event recorders, automated, real-time reporting is not available.

ELECTROPHYSIOLOGIC STUDIES

In electrophysiologic studies, recording and stimulating electrodes are inserted into all 4 cardiac chambers via right- or left-sided cardiac catheterization. Atria are paced from the right or left atrium, ventricles are paced from the right ventricular apex or right ventricular outflow tract, and cardiac conduction is recorded. Various mapping techniques are available. Programmed stimulation techniques may be used to trigger and terminate a reentrant arrhythmia.

Electrophysiologic studies are indicated primarily for evaluation and treatment of arrhythmias that are

- Serious
- Sustained
- Difficult to capture

These studies may be used to make a primary diagnosis, to evaluate the efficacy of antiarrhythmic drugs, or to map arrhythmia foci before radiofrequency catheter ablation.

CARDIAC IMAGING TESTS

Standard imaging tests include

- Echocardiography
- Chest x-ray
- CT
- MRI
- Various radionuclide techniques

Standard CT and MRI have limited application because the heart constantly beats, but faster CT and magnetic resonance techniques can provide useful cardiac images; sometimes patients are given a drug (eg, a β-blocker) to slow the heart rate during imaging.

In **ECG gating,** the image recording (or reconstruction) is synchronized with the ECG (ECG gating), providing information from several cardiac cycles that can be used to create single images of selected points in the cardiac cycle.

CT gating uses the ECG to trigger the x-ray beam at the desired portion of the cardiac cycle, exposing the patient to less radiation than gating that simply reconstructs information from only the desired portion of the cardiac cycle (gated reconstruction) and does not interrupt the x-ray beam.

Chest x-rays: Chest x-rays are often useful as a starting point in a cardiac diagnosis. Posteroanterior and lateral views provide a gross view of atrial and ventricular size and shape and pulmonary vasculature, but additional tests are almost always required for precise characterization of cardiac structure and function.

CT: Spiral (helical) CT may be used to evaluate pericarditis, congenital cardiac disorders (especially abnormal AV connections), disorders of the great vessels (eg, aortic aneurysm, aortic dissection), cardiac tumors, acute pulmonary embolism, chronic pulmonary thromboembolic disease, and arrhythmogenic right ventricular dysplasia. However, CT requires a radiopaque dye, which may limit its use in patients with renal impairment.

Electron beam CT, formerly called ultrafast CT or cine CT, unlike conventional CT, does not use a moving x-ray source and target. Instead, the direction of the x-ray beam is guided by a magnetic field and detected by an array of stationary detectors. Because mechanical motion is not required, images can be acquired in a fraction of a second (and recorded at a specific point in the cardiac cycle).

Electron beam CT is used primarily to detect and quantify coronary artery calcification, an early sign of atherosclerosis. However, spatial resolution is poor and the equipment cannot be used for noncardiac disorders, so newer standard CT techniques are becoming preferred for cardiac use.

Multidetector CT (MDCT), with ≥ 64 detectors, has a very rapid scan time; some advanced machines may generate an image from a single heartbeat, although typical acquisition times are 30 sec. Dual-source CT uses 2 x-ray sources and 2 multidetector arrays on a single gantry, which cuts scan time in half. Both of these modalities appear able to identify coronary calcifications and flow-limiting (ie, > 50% stenosis) coronary artery obstruction. Typically, an IV contrast agent is used, although nonenhanced scans can detect coronary artery calcification.

MDCT is currently used mainly for patients with indeterminate stress imaging test results as a noninvasive alternative to coronary angiography. The primary benefit of MDCT appears to be to rule out clinically significant coronary vascular disease in patients who are at low or intermediate risk of coronary artery disease (CAD). Although the radiation dose can be significant, about 15 mSv (vs 0.1 mSv for a chest x-ray and 7 mSv for coronary angiography), newer imaging protocols can reduce the exposure to 5 to 10 mSv. The presence of high-density calcified plaques creates imaging artifacts that interfere with interpretation.

MRI: Standard MRI is useful for evaluating areas around the heart, particularly the mediastinum and great vessels (eg, for studying aneurysms, dissections, and stenoses). With ECG-gated data acquisition, image resolution can approach that of CT or echocardiography, clearly delineating myocardial wall thickness and motion, chamber volumes, intraluminal masses or clot, and valve planes.

Sequential MRI after injecting a paramagnetic contrast agent (gadolinium-diethylenetriamine pentaacetic acid [Gd-DTPA]) produces higher resolution of myocardial perfusion patterns than does radionuclide imaging. MRI is generally considered the most accurate and reliable measure of ventricular volumes as well as EF. However, patients with impaired renal function can develop nephrogenic systemic fibrosis, a potentially life-threatening disorder, after use of gadolinium contrast.

When MRI is done with contrast, 3-dimensional information on infarct size and location can be obtained, and blood flow velocities in cardiac chambers can be measured. MRI can assess tissue viability by assessing the contractile response to inotropic stimulation with dobutamine or by using a contrast agent (eg, Gd-DTPA, which is excluded from cells with intact membranes). MRI discriminates myocardial scar from inflammation with edema. In patients with Marfan syndrome, MRI measurements of ascending aorta dilation are more accurate than echocardiographic measurements.

Magnetic resonance angiography (MRA) is used to assess blood volumes of interest (eg, blood vessels in the chest or abdomen); all blood flow can be assessed simultaneously. MRA can be used to detect aneurysms, stenosis, or occlusions in the carotid, coronary, renal, or peripheral arteries. Use of this technique to detect deep venous thrombosis is being studied.

Positron emission tomography (PET): PET can demonstrate myocardial perfusion and metabolism and is sometimes used to assess myocardial viability or to assess myocardial perfusion after an equivocal single-photon emission CT (SPECT) study or in very obese patients.

Perfusion agents are radioactive nuclides that are used to trace the amount of blood flow entering a specific region and are therefore useful in unmasking myocardial perfusion deficits not evident at rest. They include carbon-11 (^{11}C) CO_2, oxygen-15 (^{15}O) water, nitrogen-13 (^{13}N) ammonia, and rubidium-82 (^{82}Rb). Only ^{82}Rb does not require an on-site cyclotron.

Metabolic agents are radioactive analogs of normal biologic substances that are taken up and metabolized by cells. They include

- Fluorine-18 (^{18}F)–labeled deoxyglucose (FDG)
- ^{11}C acetate

FDG detects the enhancement of glucose metabolism under ischemic conditions, and can thus distinguish ischemic but still viable myocardium from scar tissue. Sensitivity is greater than with myocardial perfusion imaging, possibly making FDG imaging useful for selecting patients for revascularization and for avoiding such procedures when only scar tissue is present. This use may justify the greater expense of PET. Half-life of ^{18}F is long enough (110 min) that FDG can often be produced off-site. Techniques that enable FDG imaging to be used with conventional SPECT cameras may make this type of imaging widely available. FDG has also been used to detect inflammatory cardiovascular disorders (eg, infected pacemaker wires, aortic vasculitis, cardiac sarcoidosis).

Carbon-11 acetate uptake appears to reflect overall oxygen metabolism by myocytes. Uptake does not depend on such potentially variable factors as blood glucose levels, which can affect FDG distribution. ^{11}C acetate imaging may better predict postintervention recovery of myocardial function than FDG imaging. However, because of a 20-min half-life, ^{11}C must be produced by an on-site cyclotron.

PERCUTANEOUS CORONARY INTERVENTIONS

Percutaneous coronary interventions (PCI—see also p. 667) include percutaneous transluminal coronary angioplasty (PTCA) with or without stent insertion. Primary indications are treatment of

- Angina pectoris (stable or unstable)
- Myocardial ischemia
- Acute myocardial infarction (particularly in patients with developing or established cardiogenic shock)

PTCA and stent placement within 90 min of onset of pain is the optimal treatment of transmural ST-segment–elevation myocardial infarction (STEMI). Elective PCI may be appropriate for post-MI patients who have recurrent or inducible angina before hospital discharge and for patients who have angina and remain symptomatic despite medical treatment.

Percutaneous transluminal angioplasty (PTA) is used to treat peripheral arterial disease.

Procedure: PTCA is done via percutaneous femoral, radial, or brachial artery puncture. The radial approach is technically demanding compared to the femoral approach but may reduce patient discomfort, improve time to ambulation, and reduce the incidence of some complications (eg, bleeding, pseudoaneurysm formation).

A guiding catheter is inserted into a large peripheral artery and threaded to the appropriate coronary ostium. A balloon-tipped catheter, guided by fluoroscopy or intravascular ultrasonography, is aligned within the stenosis, then inflated to disrupt the atherosclerotic plaque and dilate the artery. Angiography is repeated after the procedure to document any changes. The procedure is commonly done in 2 or 3 vessels as needed.

Stents: Stents are most useful for

- Short lesions in large native coronary arteries not previously treated with PTCA
- Focal lesions in saphenous vein grafts
- Treatment of abrupt closure during PTCA

Stents are now used frequently for acute myocardial infarction, ostial or left main disease, chronic total occlusions, and bifurcation lesions.

Types of stents: Bare metal stents (BMS) are made of nickel-titanium alloy. Drug eluting stents (DES) have drugs (eg, 1st-generation: sirolimus, paclitaxel; 2nd-generation: everolimus, zotarolimus) bonded to the metal that limit neointimal proliferation to reduce the risk of restenosis. Radioactive stents or pre-stent intracoronary radiation using radioactive pellets (brachytherapy) have not proven effective at limiting restenosis. Biodegradable stents are currently in clinical trials.

Anticoagulation and ancillary therapy: Various anticoagulation regimens are used during and after angioplasty to reduce the incidence of thrombosis at the site of balloon dilation. Thienopyridines (clopidogrel, prasugrel, ticagrelor) and glycoprotein IIb/IIIa inhibitors (abciximab, eptifibatide, tirofiban) are the standard of care for patients with unstable non-ST-segment elevation myocardial infarction. Thienopyridines (often in combination with aspirin) are continued for at least 9 to 12 mo after PCI to decrease the risk of in-stent thrombosis until endothelialization of the stent has occurred. Calcium channel blockers and nitrates may also reduce risk of coronary spasm.

Contraindications

Relative contraindications to PCI include

- Lack of cardiac surgical support
- Critical left main coronary stenosis without collateral flow from a native vessel or previous bypass graft to the left anterior descending artery
- Coagulopathy
- Hypercoagulable states
- Diffusely diseased vessels without focal stenoses
- A single diseased vessel providing all perfusion to the myocardium
- Total occlusion of a coronary artery
- Stenosis < 50%

Although lack of cardiac surgical support is sometimes considered an absolute contraindication to PCI, many experts advocate that when revascularization is required urgently in STEMI, experienced operators in approved catheterization laboratories should proceed with PCI even if surgical backup is not available.

Although bypass is typically preferred for patients with critical left main coronary stenosis without collateral flow from either a native vessel or previous bypass graft, PCI is increasingly being used in this scenario in selected patients.

Complications

The main complications of balloon angioplasty and stent placement are

- Standard complications of cardiac catheterization and coronary angiography
- Thrombosis and distal embolization
- Restenosis
- Arterial dissection
- Bleeding caused by adjunctive anticoagulation

Of all angiographic procedures, PCI has the highest risk of contrast nephropathy (due to increased contrast load and procedural time); this risk can be reduced by preprocedural hydration and possibly by use of a nonionic contrast agent or hemofiltration in patients with preexisting renal insufficiency.

Compared to coronary angiography without angioplasty or stenting, risk of death, MI, and stroke is greater.

The mortality rate following PCI varies according to patient and technical factors. Mortality scoring systems have been developed to help clinicians determine the risk of death following PCI and can be useful when counseling patients regarding available treatment options (PCI vs medical management alone).

Thrombosis: Stent thrombosis causes complete blockage and may occur at any time:

- Acutely (immediately during or after the procedure)
- Subacutely (within 30 days)
- Late (> 30 days)

Stent thrombosis may be due to inadequate stent expansion or apposition at the time of the procedure, discontinuation of dual antiplatelet therapy (eg, due to nonadherence, need for noncardiac surgery), or both. Rarely, the stent may break up an intracoronary clot (ie, as may be present in acute MI), which may embolize distally and cause myocardial infarction. Use of protection strategies (eg, temporarily blocking blood flow within the artery using a balloon and then aspirating the emboli, deploying a small filter distal to the site of PCI to capture emboli) may improve outcome in PCI done on a previous saphenous vein graft but is not commonly done.

With balloon angioplasty alone, risk of acute thrombosis is about 5 to 10%.

Use of stents has almost eliminated the need for emergency CABG following PCI; the rate of acute and subacute thrombosis is < 1%. However, using a drug-eluting stent increases risk of late stent thrombosis, about 0.6%/yr up to 3 yr.

Restenosis: Restenosis is typically due to collagen deposition and thus does not occur until several weeks after the procedure or later; it may cause partial or, less commonly, complete vessel blockage.

With balloon angioplasty alone, the risk of subacute restenosis is about 5%, and the overall restenosis rate is about 30 to 45%.

With stent use, the rate of subacute restenosis is < 1%. With bare-metal stents, risk of late restenosis is 20 to 30%. Use of a drug-eluting stent lowers late restenosis risk to about 5 to 10%.

Arterial dissection: Arterial dissection is usually detected immediately as various abnormal patterns of contrast filling within the coronary arteries. Insertion of another stent often reopens the dissected segment.

RADIONUCLIDE IMAGING

Radionuclide imaging uses a special detector (gamma camera) to create an image following injection of radioactive material. This test is done to evaluate

- CAD
- Valvular cardiac disorders
- Congenital cardiac disorders
- Cardiomyopathy
- Other cardiac disorders

Radionuclide imaging exposes patients to less radiation than do comparable x-ray studies. However, because the radioactive material is retained in the patient briefly, sophisticated radiation alarms (eg, in airports) may be triggered by the patient for several days after such testing

Single-Photon Emission Computed Tomography (SPECT)

Planar techniques, which produce a 2-dimensional image, are rarely used; SPECT, which uses a rotating camera system and tomographic reconstruction to produce a 3-dimensional image, is more common in the US. With multihead SPECT systems, imaging can often be completed in ≤ 10 min. Visual comparison of stress and delayed images can be supplemented by quantitative displays. With SPECT, the following can be identified:

- Inferior and posterior abnormalities
- Small areas of infarction
- Vessels responsible for infarction

The mass of infarcted and viable myocardium can be quantified, helping determine prognosis.

Myocardial Perfusion Imaging

In myocardial perfusion imaging, IV radionuclides are taken up by cardiac tissues in rough proportion to perfusion; thus, areas of decreased uptake represent areas of relative or absolute ischemia.

Attenuation of myocardial activity by overlying soft tissue may cause false-positive results. Attenuation by breast tissue in women is especially common. Attenuation by the diaphragm and abdominal contents may produce spurious inferior wall defects in both sexes but is more common among men. Attenuation is more likely with technetium-99m (^{99m}Tc) than with radioactive thallium-201 (^{201}Tl).

Indications: Myocardial perfusion imaging is used with stress testing to

- Evaluate patients with chest pain of uncertain origin
- Determine the functional significance of coronary artery stenosis seen on angiography
- Determine the functional significance of collateral vessels seen on angiography
- Evaluate the success of reperfusion interventions (eg, CABG, percutaneous intervention, thrombolysis)
- Estimate prognosis after myocardial infarction

After acute myocardial infarction, myocardial perfusion imaging can help estimate prognosis because it can show extent of the perfusion abnormality due to acute myocardial infarction, extent of scarring due to previous infarcts, and residual peri-infarct or other areas of reversible ischemia.

Protocols and imaging agents: Various protocols are used depending on the imaging agent, which include

- Radioactive thallium-201 (^{201}Tl)
- Technetium-99m (^{99m}Tc) markers (sestamibi, tetrofosmin, and teboroxime)
- Iodine-123 (^{123}I)–labeled fatty acids
- ^{123}I-metaiodobenzylguanidine

Radioactive thallium-201 (^{201}Tl), which acts as a potassium analog, was the original tracer used in stress testing. It is injected at peak stress and imaged with SPECT, followed 4 h later by injection of half the original dose during rest and by repeat SPECT. The goal of this protocol is to evaluate reversible perfusion defects that may warrant intervention. After stress testing, the perfusion imbalance between normal coronary arteries and those distal to a stenosis appears as a relative decrease in ^{201}Tl uptake in the areas perfused by the stenosed arteries. Sensitivity of stress testing with ^{201}Tl for CAD is similar whether imaging is done after exercise stress or pharmacologic stress.

Several **technetium-99m** (^{99m}Tc) myocardial perfusion markers have been developed because the imaging characteristics of ^{201}Tl are not ideal for the gamma camera. Markers include sestamibi (commonly used), tetrofosmin, and teboroxime (see Table 75–6). Protocols include 2-day stress-rest, 1-day rest-stress, and 1-day stress-rest. Some protocols use dual isotopes (^{201}Tl and ^{99m}Tc), although this approach is expensive. With either of these markers, sensitivity is about 90%, and specificity is about 71%.

For 2-day protocols, imaging at rest may be omitted if the initial stress test shows no evidence of abnormal perfusion. When higher doses of ^{99m}Tc (> 30 mCi) are used, first-transit function studies (with ventriculography) may be used with perfusion imaging.

Other radionuclides include iodine-123 (^{123}I)–labeled fatty acids, which produces cold spots where myocardium is ischemic; gallium citrate-67 (^{67}Ga), which accumulates in sites of active inflammation (eg, in acute inflammatory cardiomyopathy); and ^{123}I metaiodobenzylguanidine, a neurotransmitter analog taken up and stored in neurons of the sympathetic nervous system

Table 75–6. TECHNETIUM-99M MYOCARDIAL PERFUSION MARKERS

MARKER	CHARACTERISTICS
^{99m}Tc sestamibi	Myocardial uptake is slower than that with thallium, but there is little myocardial washout, allowing timing flexibility; patients with acute symptoms can be injected with sestamibi immediately and imaged several hours later.
	Uptake depends more on blood flow than on viable myocardium; viable regions with low blood flow may be misclassified as scar.
	Studies may be done on a single or on separate days, with a low initial dose during stress followed by a much higher dose at rest.
	With ECG-gated imaging, ventricular wall motion, wall thickening, and ejection fraction can be estimated.
^{99m}Tc tetrofosmin	Characteristics are similar to those of sestamibi.
^{99m}Tc teboroxime	First-pass extraction from the myocardium is high, with rapid washout; half of peak myocardial activity is gone by 10 min.
	Because of its rapid dynamics, use with treadmill exercise is difficult.
	Preliminary studies suggest that stress-redistribution testing may be completed within 15 min of pharmacologic stress. Coronary artery disease may be detectable by analyzing myocardial washout of the tracer after injection at rest, without the need for stress.

and used in research to evaluate heart failure, diabetes, pheochromocytoma, certain arrhythmias, and arrhythmogenic right ventricular dysplasia.

Infarct Avid Imaging

Infarct avid imaging uses radiolabeled markers that accumulate in areas of damaged myocardium, such as ^{99m}Tc pyrophosphate and antimyosin (indium-111 [^{111}In]–labeled antibodies to cardiac myosin). Images usually become positive 12 to 24 h after acute myocardial infarction and remain positive for about 1 wk; they may remain positive if myocardial necrosis continues post-MI or if aneurysms develop. This technique is rarely used now because other diagnostic tests for myocardial infarction (eg, biomarkers) are more readily available and less expensive and because it provides no prognostic information other than infarct size.

Radionuclide Ventriculography

Radionuclide ventriculography is used to evaluate ventricular function. It is useful for measuring testing and exercise ejection fraction (EF) in CAD, valvular heart disease, and congenital heart disease. Some clinicians prefer it for serial assessment of ventricular function in patients taking cardiotoxic cancer chemotherapy (eg, anthracyclines). However, radionuclide ventriculography has been largely replaced by echocardiography, which is less expensive, does not require radiation exposure, and theoretically can measure EFs as accurately.

^{99m}Tc-labeled RBCs are injected intravenously. Left ventricular (LV) and right ventricular (RV) function can be evaluated by or by

- First-transit studies (a type of beat-to-beat evaluation)
- Gated (ECG-synchronized) blood pool imaging done over several minutes (multiple-gated acquisition [MUGA])

Either study can be done during rest or after exercise. First-transit studies are rapid and relatively easy, but MUGA provides better images and is more widely used.

In **first-transit studies,** 8 to 10 cardiac cycles are imaged as the marker mixes with blood and passes through the central circulation. First-transit studies are ideal for assessing RV function and intracardiac shunts.

In **MUGA,** imaging is synchronized with the R wave of the ECG. Multiple images are taken of short, sequential portions of each cardiac cycle for 5 to 10 min. Computer analysis generates an average blood pool configuration for each portion of the cardiac cycle and synthesizes the configurations into a continuous cinematic loop resembling a beating heart.

MUGA can quantitate numerous indexes of ventricular function, including regional wall motion, EF; ratio of stroke volume to end-diastolic volume, ejection and filling rates, LV volume, and indexes of relative volume overload (eg, LV:RV stroke volume ratios). EF is used most commonly.

MUGA during rest has virtually no risk. It is used for serially evaluating RV and LV function in various disorders (eg, valvular heart disorders); for monitoring patients taking potentially cardiotoxic drugs (eg, doxorubicin); and for assessing the effects of angioplasty, CABG, thrombolysis, and other procedures in patients with CAD or MI. Arrhythmias are a relative contraindication because there may be few normal cardiac cycles.

Left ventriculography: MUGA is useful for detecting left ventricular aneurysms; sensitivity and specificity are > 90% for typical anterior or anteroapical true aneurysms. Conventional gated blood pool imaging shows inferoposterior LV aneurysms less well than it shows anterior and lateral aneurysms; additional views are required. Gated SPECT imaging takes longer (about 20 to 25 min with a multihead camera) than a single planar gated view (5 to 10 min) but shows all portions of the ventricles.

Right ventriculography: MUGA is used to assess right ventricular function in patients who have a lung disorder or an inferior left ventricular infarct that may involve the RV. Normally, right ventricular EF (40 to 55% with most techniques) is lower than left ventricular EF. RVEF is subnormal in many patients with pulmonary hypertension and in patients with RV infarction or cardiomyopathy affecting the RV. Idiopathic cardiomyopathy is usually characterized by biventricular dysfunction, unlike typical CAD, which usually causes more left ventricular than right ventricular dysfunction.

Valve assessment: MUGA can be used with rest-stress protocols to assess valvular disorders that result in left ventricular volume overload. In aortic regurgitation, a reduction in resting EF or no increase in EF with exercise is a sign of deteriorating cardiac function and may indicate a need for valvular repair. MUGA also can be used to calculate the regurgitant fraction in regurgitation of any valve. Normally, the stroke volume of the 2 ventricles is equal. However, in patients with left-sided valvular regurgitation, LV stroke volume exceeds that of the right ventricle by an amount proportional to the regurgitant fraction. Thus, if the RV is normal, the regurgitant fraction of the LV can be calculated from the LV:RV stroke volume ratio.

Shunt assessment: With MUGA and commercially available computer programs, size of a congenital shunt can be quantified by the stroke volume ratio or, during the first transit of the marker, by the ratio of abnormal early pulmonary recirculation of radioactivity to total pulmonary radioactivity.

STRESS TESTING

In stress testing, the heart is monitored by ECG and often imaging studies during an induced episode of increased cardiac demand so that ischemic areas potentially at risk of infarction can be identified. Heart rate is increased to 85% of age-predicted maximum (target heart rate) or until symptoms develop, whichever occurs first.

Stress testing is used for

- Diagnosing CAD
- Stratifying risk in patients with known CAD
- Monitoring patients with known CAD

In patients with CAD, a blood supply that is adequate at rest may be inadequate when cardiac demands are increased by exercise or other forms of stress.

Stress testing is less invasive and less expensive than cardiac catheterization, and it detects pathophysiologic abnormalities of blood flow; however, it is less accurate for diagnosis in patients with a low pretest likelihood of CAD. It can define the functional significance of abnormalities in coronary artery anatomy identified with coronary angiography during catheterization. Because coronary artery plaques that are not significantly stenotic (ie, do not result in ischemia during stress testing) may nonetheless rupture and cause an acute coronary syndrome, a normal stress test result does not guarantee future freedom from myocardial infarction.

Risks of stress testing include infarction and sudden death, which occur in about 1/5000 patients tested. Stress testing has several absolute and relative contraindications

Absolute contraindications to exercise stress testing are

- Acute coronary syndrome (myocardial infarction within 48 h or uncontrolled unstable angina)
- Aortic dissection if acute

- Aortic stenosis if symptomatic or severe
- Arrhythmias if symptomatic or hemodynamically significant
- Heart failure if decompensated
- Myocarditis if acute
- Pericarditis if acute
- Pulmonary embolism if acute
- Pulmonary infarction if acute

Relative contraindications to exercise stress testing include

- Atrioventricular block if high-degree
- Bradyarrhythmias
- Electrolyte imbalance
- Hypertension (systolic BP > 200 mm Hg or diastolic BP > 110 mm Hg)
- Hypertrophic obstructive cardiomyopathy
- Inability to exercise adequately due to mental or physical impairment
- Stenosis of heart valve if moderate or severe
- Stenosis of left main coronary artery
- Systemic illness
- Tachyarrhythmias

Stress Test Methodology

Cardiac demand can be increased by

- Exercise
- Drugs

Patients must be npo for 4 to 6 h before the test. When dipyridamole is used for pharmacologic stress, xanthine compounds (eg, aminophylline, theophylline, caffeine) may produce a false-negative result, so such substances (including tea, coffee, cocoa, chocolate, certain energy supplements and drinks, and caffeinated sodas) should be avoided for 24 h before testing.

Exercise stress testing: Exercise is preferred to drugs for increasing cardiac demand because it more closely replicates ischemia-inducing stressors. Usually, a patient walks on a conventional treadmill, following the Bruce protocol or a similar exercise schedule, until the target heart rate is reached or symptoms occur. The Bruce protocol (most commonly used) increases treadmill speed and slope incrementally at roughly 3-min intervals.

Pharmacologic stress testing: Pharmacologic stress testing is usually used when patients cannot walk on a treadmill long enough to reach their target heart rate because of deconditioning, musculoskeletal disorders, obesity, peripheral arterial disease, or other disorders. Drugs used include IV dipyridamole, adenosine, regadenoson, and dobutamine.

Dipyridamole augments endogenous adenosine, causing coronary artery vasodilation. It increases myocardial blood flow in normal coronary arteries but not in arteries distal to a stenosis, creating a "steal" phenomenon from stenosed arteries and an imbalance in perfusion. Dipyridamole-induced ischemia or other adverse effects (eg, nausea, vomiting, headache, bronchospasm) occur in about 10% of patients, but these effects can be reversed by IV aminophylline. Severe reactions occur in < 1% of patients. Contraindications include asthma, acute phase MI, unstable angina pectoris, critical aortic stenosis, and systemic hypotension (systolic BP < 90 mm Hg).

Adenosine has the same effect as dipyridamole but must be given in a continuous IV infusion because it is rapidly degraded in the plasma. Adverse effects include transient flushing, chest pain, and tachycardia, which can be reversed by terminating the infusion.

Regadenoson is a more selective adenosine agonist than either dipyridamole or adenosine and is non-inferior for the diagnosis of ischemia with fewer adverse effects and greater ease of administration.

Dobutamine is an inotrope, chronotrope, and vasodilator used mainly when dipyridamole and adenosine are contraindicated (eg, in patients with asthma or 2nd-degree atrioventricular block) and when echocardiography is used to image the heart. Dobutamine must be used with caution in patients who have severe hypertension or arrhythmia, left ventricular outflow tract obstruction, multiple previous MIs, or acute MI.

Diagnostic Stress Test Methodology

Several imaging tests can detect ischemia after exercise or pharmacologic stress:

- ECG
- Radionuclide perfusion imaging
- Echocardiography

ECG: ECG is always used with stress testing to diagnose CAD and help determine prognosis. Stress ECG alone (ie, without radionuclide imaging or echocardiography) is most useful in patients with

- Intermediate likelihood of CAD based on age and sex
- Normal ECG at rest

Diagnosis involves assessment of ST-segment response (a measure of global subendocardial ischemia), BP response, and the patient's symptoms.

Average sensitivity is 67%; average specificity is 72%. Sensitivity and specificity are lower in women partly because incidence of CAD is lower in young and middle-aged women. Prognosis worsens with depth of ST depression.

Radionuclide myocardial perfusion imaging: Radionuclide myocardial perfusion imaging is more sensitive (85 to 90%) and specific (70 to 80%) than ECG stress testing. Combining findings from both tests increases sensitivity for CAD.

Myocardial perfusion imaging is particularly useful for patients with

- Baseline ECG abnormalities that may interfere with interpretation of ECG changes during a stress test (eg, bundle branch block, fixed-rate pacemakers, digitalis effects).
- High probability of false-positive results on exercise ECGs (eg, premenopausal women, patients with mitral valve prolapse)

This imaging test can help determine the functional significance of coronary artery stenosis, identified by coronary angiography, when surgeons are choosing lesions to bypass or dilate via percutaneous transluminal coronary angioplasty (PTCA).

Echocardiography: Echocardiography is useful when information about more than just perfusion is needed. Echocardiography detects wall motion abnormalities that are a sign of regional ischemia and, using Doppler techniques, helps evaluate valvular disorders that may contribute to or result from ischemia or valvular disorders unrelated to ischemia but which deserve concomitant evaluation.

The echocardiogram is typically obtained immediately before and after an exercise treadmill test or during dobutamine infusion.

Echocardiography is relatively portable, does not use ionizing radiation, has a rapid acquisition time, and is inexpensive, but it is difficult to carry out in obese patients and in patients with COPD and lung hyperinflation. Done by experts, stress echocardiography has a predictive value similar to that of stress myocardial radionuclide perfusion testing.

Radionuclide ventriculography: Radionuclide ventriculography is occasionally used with exercise stress testing instead of echocardiography to assess exercise ejection fraction (EF), the best prognostic indicator in patients with CAD.

Normally, EF is ≥ 5 percentage points higher during exercise than at rest. Ventricular dysfunction (eg, due to valvular heart disorders, cardiomyopathy, or CAD) can decrease exercise EF below baseline or prevent it from increasing.

In patients with CAD, the 8-yr survival rate is 80% with an exercise EF of 40 to 49%, 75% with an exercise EF of 30 to 39%, and 40% with an exercise EF of < 30%.

TILT TABLE TESTING

Tilt table testing is used to evaluate syncope in

- Younger, apparently healthy patients
- Elderly patients when cardiac and other tests have not provided a diagnosis

Tilt table testing produces maximal venous pooling, which can trigger vasovagal (neurocardiogenic) syncope and reproduce the symptoms and signs that accompany it (nausea, light-headedness, pallor, hypotension, bradycardia).

Procedure

After an overnight fast, a patient is placed on a motorized table with a foot board at one end and is held in place by a single strap over the stomach; an IV line is inserted. After the patient remains supine for 15 min, the table is tilted nearly upright to 60 to 80° for 45 min during which symptoms and vital signs are monitored.

Contraindications: Relative contraindications include

- Severe aortic valve stenosis
- Severe mitral valve stenosis
- Hypertrophic cardiomyopathy
- Severe CAD

Interpretation

If vasovagal symptoms develop, vasovagal syncope is confirmed. If they do not occur, a drug (eg, isoproterenol) may be given to induce them. (NOTE: *Isoproterenol should not be used in patients with hypertrophic cardiomyopathy or severe CAD*). Sensitivity varies from 30 to 80% depending on the protocol used. The false-positive rate is 10 to 15%.

With vasovagal syncope, heart rate and BP usually decrease. Some patients have only a decrease in heart rate (cardioinhibitory); others have only a decrease in BP (vasodepressor). Other responses that suggest alternative diagnoses include a gradual decrease in systolic and diastolic BP with little change in heart rate (dysautonomic pattern), significant increase in heart rate (> 30 beats/min) with little change in BP (postural orthostatic tachycardia syndrome), and report of syncope with no hemodynamic changes (psychogenic syncope).

76 Arrhythmias and Conduction Disorders

The normal heart beats in a regular, coordinated way because electrical impulses generated and spread by myocytes with unique electrical properties trigger a sequence of organized myocardial contractions. Arrhythmias and conduction disorders are caused by abnormalities in the generation or conduction of these electrical impulses or both.

Any heart disorder, including congenital abnormalities of structure (eg, accessory atrioventricular [AV] connection) or function (eg, hereditary ion channelopathies), can disturb rhythm. Systemic factors that can cause or contribute to a rhythm disturbance include electrolyte abnormalities (particularly low potassium or magnesium), hypoxia, hormonal imbalances (eg, hypothyroidism, hyperthyroidism), and drugs and toxins (eg, alcohol, caffeine).

Anatomy of the Cardiac Conduction System

At the junction of the superior vena cava and high lateral right atrium is a cluster of cells that generates the initial electrical impulse of each normal heart beat, called the sinoatrial (SA) or sinus node. Electrical discharge of these pacemaker cells stimulates adjacent cells, leading to stimulation of successive regions of the heart in an orderly sequence. Impulses are transmitted through the atria to the AV node via preferentially conducting internodal tracts and unspecialized atrial myocytes. The AV node is located on the right side of the interatrial septum. It has a slow conduction velocity and thus delays impulse transmission. AV nodal transmission time is heart-rate-dependent and is modulated by autonomic tone and circulating catecholamines to maximize cardiac output at any given atrial rate.

The atria are electrically insulated from the ventricles by the annulus fibrosus except in the anteroseptal region. There, the bundle of His, the continuation of the AV node, enters the top of the interventricular septum, where it bifurcates into the left and right bundle branches, which terminate in Purkinje fibers. The right bundle branch conducts impulses to the anterior and apical endocardial regions of the right ventricle. The left bundle branch fans out over the left side of the interventricular septum. Its anterior portion (left anterior hemifascicle) and its posterior portion (left posterior hemifascicle) stimulate the left side of the interventricular septum, which is the first part of the ventricles to be electrically activated. Thus, the interventricular septum depolarizes left to right, followed by near-simultaneous activation of both ventricles from the endocardial surface through the ventricular walls to the epicardial surface.

Cardiac Physiology

An understanding of normal cardiac physiology is essential before rhythm disturbances can be understood.

Electrophysiology: The passage of ions across the myocyte cell membrane is regulated through specific ion channels that cause cyclical depolarization and repolarization of the cell, called an action potential. The action potential of a working myocyte begins when the cell is depolarized from its diastolic −90 mV transmembrane potential to a potential of about −50 mV. At this threshold potential, voltage-dependent fast sodium channels open, causing rapid depolarization mediated by sodium influx down its steep concentration gradient. The fast sodium channel is rapidly inactivated and sodium influx stops, but other time- and voltage-dependent ion channels open, allowing calcium to enter through slow calcium channels (a depolarizing event) and potassium to leave through potassium channels (a repolarizing event).

At first, these 2 processes are balanced, maintaining a positive transmembrane potential and prolonging the plateau phase of the action potential. During this phase, calcium entering the cell is responsible for electromechanical coupling and myocyte contraction. Eventually, calcium influx ceases, and potassium efflux increases, causing rapid repolarization of the cell back to the −90 mV resting transmembrane potential. While depolarized, the cell is resistant (refractory) to a subsequent depolarizing event. Initially, a subsequent depolarization is not possible (absolute refractory period), and after partial but incomplete repolarization, a subsequent depolarization is possible but occurs slowly (relative refractory period).

There are 2 general types of cardiac tissue:

- Fast-channel tissues
- Slow-channel tissues

Fast-channel tissues (working atrial and ventricular myocytes, His-Purkinje system) have a high density of fast sodium channels and action potentials characterized by little or no spontaneous diastolic depolarization (and thus very slow rates of pacemaker activity), very rapid initial depolarization rates (and thus rapid conduction velocity), and loss of refractoriness coincident with repolarization (and thus short refractory periods and the ability to conduct repetitive impulses at high frequencies).

Slow-channel tissues (SA and AV nodes) have a low density of fast sodium channels and action potentials characterized by more rapid spontaneous diastolic depolarization (and thus more rapid rates of pacemaker activity), slow initial depolarization rates (and thus slow conduction velocity), and loss of refractoriness that is delayed after repolarization (and thus long refractory periods and the inability to conduct repetitive impulses at high frequencies).

Normally, the SA node has the most rapid rate of spontaneous diastolic depolarization, so its cells produce spontaneous action potentials at a higher frequency than other tissues. Thus, the SA node is the dominant automatic tissue (pacemaker) in a normal heart. If the SA node does not produce impulses, tissue with the next highest automaticity rate, typically the AV node, functions as the pacemaker. Sympathetic stimulation increases the discharge frequency of pacemaker tissue, and parasympathetic stimulation decreases it.

Normal cardiac rhythm: The resting sinus heart rate in adults is usually 60 to 100 beats/min. Slower rates (sinus bradycardia) occur in young people, particularly athletes, and during sleep. Faster rates (sinus tachycardia) occur with exercise, illness, or emotion through sympathetic neural and circulating catecholamine drive. Normally, a marked diurnal variation in heart rate occurs, with lowest rates just before early morning awakening. A slight increase in rate during inspiration with a decrease in rate during expiration (respiratory sinus arrhythmia) is also normal; it is mediated by oscillations in vagal tone and is particularly common among healthy young people. The oscillations lessen but do not entirely disappear with age. Absolute regularity of the sinus rhythm rate is pathologic and occurs in patients with autonomic denervation (eg, in advanced diabetes) or with severe heart failure.

Most cardiac electrical activity is represented on the ECG (see Fig. 75–1 on p. 607), although SA node, AV node, and His-Purkinje depolarization does not involve enough tissue to be detected. The P wave represents atrial depolarization. The QRS complex represents ventricular depolarization, and the T wave represents ventricular repolarization.

The PR interval (from the beginning of the P wave to the beginning of the QRS complex) is the time from the beginning of atrial activation to the beginning of ventricular activation. Much of this interval reflects slowing of impulse transmission in the AV node. The R-R interval (time between 2 QRS complexes) represents the ventricular rate. The QT interval (from the beginning of the QRS complex to the end of the T wave) represents the duration of ventricular depolarization. Normal values for the QT interval are slightly longer in women; they are also longer with a slower heart rate. The QT interval is corrected (QTc) for influence of heart rate. The most common formula (all intervals in sec) is

$$QTc = \frac{QT}{\sqrt{RR}}$$

Pathophysiology

Rhythm disturbances result from abnormalities of impulse formation, impulse conduction, or both. Bradyarrhythmias result from decreased intrinsic pacemaker function or blocks in conduction, principally within the AV node or the His-Purkinje system. Most tachyarrhythmias are caused by reentry; some result from enhanced normal automaticity or from abnormal mechanisms of automaticity.

Reentry is the circular propagation of an impulse around 2 interconnected pathways with different conduction characteristics and refractory periods (see Fig. 76–1).

Under certain conditions, typically precipitated by a premature beat, reentry can cause continuous circulation of an activation wavefront, causing a tachyarrhythmia (see Fig. 76–2). Normally, reentry is prevented by tissue refractoriness following stimulation. However, 3 conditions favor reentry: shortening of tissue refractoriness (eg, by sympathetic stimulation), lengthening of the conduction pathway (eg, by hypertrophy or abnormal conduction pathways), and slowing of impulse conduction (eg, by ischemia).

Symptoms and Signs

Arrhythmia and conduction disturbances may be asymptomatic or cause palpitations (sensation of skipped beats or rapid or forceful beats), symptoms of hemodynamic compromise (eg, dyspnea, chest discomfort, presyncope, syncope), or cardiac arrest. Occasionally, polyuria results from release of atrial natriuretic peptide during prolonged supraventricular tachycardias (SVTs).

Palpation of pulse and cardiac auscultation can determine ventricular rate and its regularity or irregularity. Examination of the jugular venous pulse waves may help in the diagnosis of AV blocks and tachyarrhythmias. For example, in complete AV block, the atria intermittently contract when the AV valves are closed, producing large *a* (cannon) waves in the jugular venous pulse. Other physical findings of arrhythmias are few.

Diagnosis

- ECG

History and physical examination may detect an arrhythmia and suggest possible causes, but diagnosis requires a 12-lead ECG or, less reliably, a rhythm strip, preferably obtained during symptoms to establish the relationship between symptoms and rhythm.

The ECG is approached systematically; calipers measure intervals and identify subtle irregularities. The key diagnostic features are rate of atrial activation, rate and regularity of ventricular activation, and the relationship between the two. Irregular activation signals are classified as regularly irregular or irregularly irregular (no detectable pattern). Regular

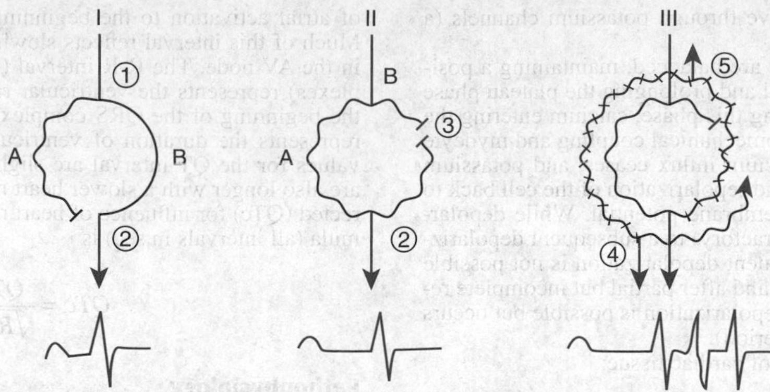

Fig. 76–1. Mechanism of typical reentry. AV nodal reentry is used here as an example. Two pathways connect the same points. Pathway A has slower conduction and a shorter refractory period. Pathway B conducts normally and has a longer refractory period. I. A normal impulse arriving at 1 goes down both A and B pathways. Conduction through pathway A is slower and finds tissue at 2 already depolarized and thus refractory. A normal sinus beat results. II. A premature impulse finds pathway B refractory and is blocked, but it can be conducted on pathway A because its refractory period is shorter. On arriving at 2, the impulse continues forward and retrograde up pathway B, where it is blocked by refractory tissue at 3. A premature supraventricular beat with an increased PR interval results. III. If conduction over pathway A is sufficiently slow, a premature impulse may continue retrograde all the way up pathway B, which is now past its refractory period. If pathway A is also past its refractory period, the impulse may reenter pathway A and continue to circle, sending an impulse each cycle to the ventricle (4) and retrograde to the atrium (5), producing a sustained reentrant tachycardia.

irregularity is intermittent irregularity in an otherwise regular rhythm (eg, premature beats) or a predictable pattern of irregularity (eg, recurrent relationships between groups of beats).

A narrow QRS complex (< 0.12 sec) indicates a supraventricular origin (above the His bundle bifurcation). A wide QRS complex (≥ 0.12 sec) indicates a ventricular origin (below the His bundle bifurcation) or a supraventricular rhythm conducted with an intraventricular conduction defect or with ventricular preexcitation in the Wolff-Parkinson-White (WPW) syndrome.

Bradyarrhythmias: ECG diagnosis of bradyarrhythmias depends on the presence or absence of P waves, morphology of the P waves, and the relationship between P waves and QRS complexes.

A bradyarrhythmia with no relationship between P waves and QRS complexes and more P waves than QRS complexes indicates AV block; the escape rhythm can be junctional (narrow QRS complex) or ventricular (wide QRS complex).

A regular QRS bradyarrhythmia with a 1:1 relationship between P waves and QRS complexes indicates absence of AV block. P waves preceding QRS complexes indicate sinus bradycardia (if P waves are normal) or sinus arrest with an escape atrial bradycardia (if P waves are abnormal). P waves after QRS complexes indicate sinus arrest with a junctional or ventricular escape rhythm and retrograde atrial activation. A ventricular escape rhythm results in a wide QRS complex; a junctional escape rhythm usually has a narrow QRS (or a wide QRS with bundle branch block or preexcitation).

When the QRS rhythm is irregular, P waves usually outnumber QRS complexes; some P waves produce QRS complexes, but some do not (indicating 2nd-degree AV block. An irregular QRS rhythm with a 1:1 relationship between P waves and the following QRS complexes usually indicates sinus arrhythmia with gradual acceleration and deceleration of the sinus rate (if P waves are normal).

Pauses in an otherwise regular QRS rhythm may be caused by blocked P waves (an abnormal P wave can usually be discerned just after the preceding T wave or distorting the morphology of the preceding T wave), sinus arrest, or sinus exit block, as well as by 2nd-degree AV block.

Tachyarrhythmias: Tachyarrhythmias may be divided into 4 groups, defined by being visibly regular vs irregular and by having a narrow vs wide QRS complex.

Irregular, narrow QRS complex tachyarrhythmias include atrial fibrillation (AF), atrial flutter or true atrial tachycardia with variable AV conduction, and multifocal atrial tachycardia. Differentiation is based on atrial ECG signals, which are best seen in the longer pauses between QRS complexes. Atrial ECG signals that are continuous, irregular in timing and morphology, and very rapid (> 300 beats/min) without discrete P waves indicate AF. Discrete P waves that vary from beat to beat with at least 3 different morphologies suggest multifocal atrial tachycardia. Regular, discrete, uniform atrial signals without intervening isoelectric periods (usually at rates > 250 beats/min) suggest atrial flutter. Regular, discrete, uniform, abnormal atrial

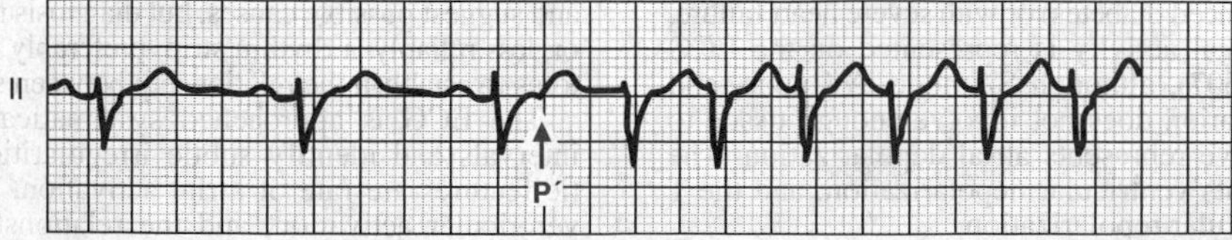

Fig. 76–2. Initiation of an atrioventricular nodal reentry tachycardia. There is an abnormal P wave (P′) and atrioventricular nodal delay (long P′R interval) before onset of the tachycardia.

signals with intervening isoelectric periods (usually at rates < 250 beats/min) suggest true atrial tachycardia.

Irregular, wide QRS complex tachyarrhythmias include the above 4 atrial tachyarrhythmias, conducted with either bundle branch block or ventricular preexcitation, and polymorphic ventricular tachycardia (VT—see Fig. 76-3). Differentiation is based on atrial ECG signals and the presence in polymorphic VT of a very rapid rate (> 250 beats/min).

Regular, narrow QRS complex tachyarrhythmias include sinus tachycardia, atrial flutter or true atrial tachycardia with a consistent AV conduction ratio, and paroxysmal SVTs (AV nodal reentrant SVT, orthodromic reciprocating AV tachycardia in the presence of an accessory AV connection, and SA nodal reentrant SVT). Vagal maneuvers or pharmacologic AV nodal blockade can help distinguish among these tachycardias. With these maneuvers, sinus tachycardia is not terminated, but it slows or

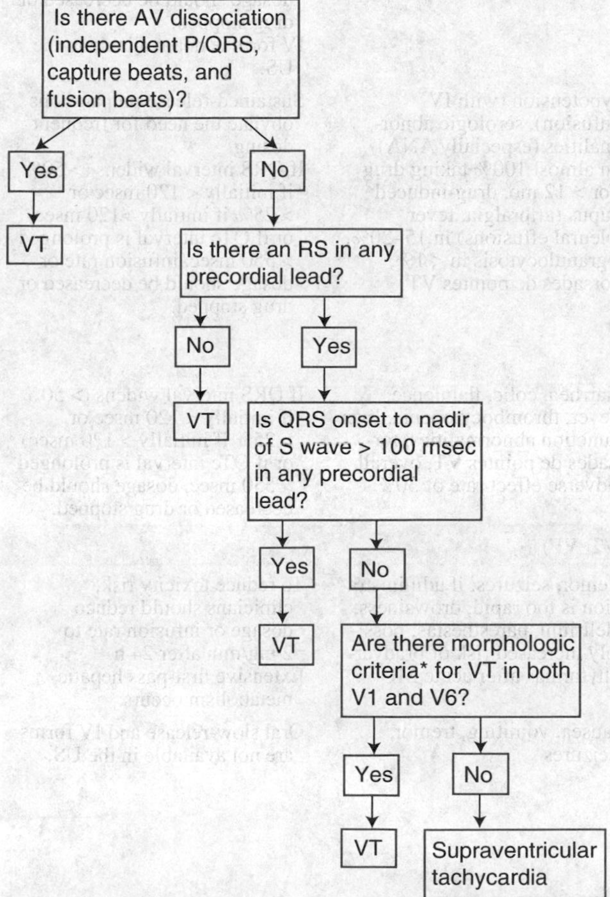

Fig. 76–3. Modified Brugada criteria for ventricular tachycardia.

**With RBBB QRS:*

- In V_1, monophasic R, or QR, or RS
- In V_6, R/S < 1 or monophasic R or QR

With LBBB QRS:

- In V_1, R > 30 msec wide or RS > 60 msec wide
- In V_6, QR or QS

AV = atrioventricular; LBBB = left bundle branch block; RBBB = right bundle branch block; VT = ventricular tachycardia.

AV block develops, disclosing normal P waves. Similarly, atrial flutter and true atrial tachycardia are usually not terminated, but AV block discloses flutter waves or abnormal P waves. The most common forms of paroxysmal SVT (AV nodal reentry and orthodromic reciprocating tachycardia) must terminate if AV block occurs.

Regular, wide QRS complex tachyarrhythmias include those listed for a regular, narrow QRS complex tachyarrhythmia, each with bundle branch block or ventricular preexcitation, and monomorphic VT. Vagal maneuvers can help distinguish among them. ECG criteria to distinguish between VT and SVT with an intraventricular conduction defect are often used (see Table 76–3 on p. 633). When in doubt, the rhythm is assumed to be VT because some drugs for SVTs can worsen the clinical state if the rhythm is VT; however, the reverse is not true.

PEARLS & PITFALLS

- Assume a regular, wide-complex tachyarrhythmia is VT until proven otherwise.

Treatment

- Treatment of cause
- Sometimes antiarrhythmic drugs, pacemakers, cardioversion-defibrillation, catheter ablation, or electrosurgery

The need for treatment varies; it is guided by symptoms and risks of the arrhythmia. Asymptomatic arrhythmias without serious risks do not require treatment even if they worsen. Symptomatic arrhythmias may require treatment to improve quality of life. Potentially life-threatening arrhythmias require treatment.

Treatment is directed at causes. If necessary, direct antiarrhythmic therapy, including antiarrhythmic drugs, cardioversion-defibrillation, implantable cardioverter-defibrillators (ICDs), pacemakers (and a special form of pacing, cardiac resynchronization therapy), or a combination, is used. Patients with arrhythmias that have caused or are likely to cause symptoms of hemodynamic compromise may have to be restricted from driving until response to treatment has been assessed.

Surgery for cardiac arrhythmias: Surgery to remove a focus of a tachyarrhythmia is becoming less necessary as the less invasive radiofrequency ablation techniques evolve. But it is still indicated when an arrhythmia is refractory to radiofrequency ablation or when another indication requires a cardiac surgical procedure, most commonly when patients with AF require valve replacement or repair or when patients with VT require revascularization or resection of a left ventricular aneurysm.

DRUGS FOR ARRHYTHMIAS

The need for treatment of arrhythmias depends on the symptoms and the seriousness of the arrhythmia. Treatment is directed at causes. If necessary, direct antiarrhythmic therapy, including antiarrhythmic drugs, cardioversion-defibrillation, ICDs, pacemakers (and a special form of pacing, cardiac resynchronization therapy), or a combination, is used.

Most antiarrhythmic drugs are grouped into 4 main classes (Vaughan Williams classification) based on their dominant cellular electrophysiologic effect (see Table 76–1).

- Class I: Class I drugs are subdivided into subclasses a, b, and c. Class I drugs are sodium channel blockers (membrane-stabilizing drugs) that block fast sodium channels, slowing

Table 76–1. ANTIARRHYTHMIC DRUGS (VAUGHAN WILLIAMS CLASSIFICATION)

DRUG	DOSAGE	TARGET LEVELS	SELECTED ADVERSE EFFECTS	COMMENTS
Class Ia	Uses: APB and VPB suppression, SVT and VT suppression, AF or atrial flutter, and VF suppression			
Disopyramide	IV: Initially, 1.5 mg/kg over > 5 min followed by an infusion of 0.4 mg/kg/h Oral immediate-release: 100 or 150 mg q 6 h Oral controlled-release: 200 or 300 mg q 12 h	2–7.5 µg/mL	Anticholinergic effects (urinary retention, glaucoma, dry mouth, blurred vision, intestinal upset), hypoglycemia, torsades de pointes VT; negative inotropic effects (which may worsen heart failure or hypotension)	Drug should be used cautiously in patients with impaired LV function. Dosage should be decreased in patients with renal insufficiency. Adverse effects may contribute to nonadherence. If QRS interval widens (> 50% if initially < 120 msec or > 25% if initially > 120 msec) or if QTc interval is prolonged > 550 msec, infusion rate or dosage should be decreased or drug stopped. IV form is not available in the US.
Procainamide*	IV: 10–15 mg/kg bolus at 25–50 mg/min, followed by a constant IV infusion of 1–4 mg/min Oral: 250–625 mg (rarely, up to 1 g) q 3 or 4 h Oral controlled-release: For patients < 55 kg, 500 mg; for patients 55–91 kg, 750 mg; or for patients > 91 kg, 1000 mg q 6 h	4–8 µg/mL	Hypotension (with IV infusion), serologic abnormalities (especially ANA) in almost 100% taking drug for > 12 mo, drug-induced lupus (arthralgia, fever, pleural effusions) in 15–20%, agranulocytosis in < 1%, torsades de pointes VT	Sustained-release preparations obviate the need for frequent dosing. If QRS interval widens (> 50% if initially < 120 msec or > 25% if initially >120 msec) or if QTc interval is prolonged > 550 msec, infusion rate or dosage should be decreased or drug stopped.
Quinidine*	Oral: 200–400 mg q 4–6 h	2–6 µg/mL	Diarrhea, colic, flatulence, fever, thrombocytopenia, liver function abnormalities, torsades de pointes VT; overall adverse effect rate of 30%	If QRS interval widens (> 50% if initially < 120 msec or > 25% if initially > 120 msec) or if QTc interval is prolonged > 550 msec, dosage should be decreased or drug stopped.
Class Ib	Uses: Suppression of ventricular arrhythmias (VPB, VT, VF)			
Lidocaine	IV: 100 mg over 2 min, followed by continuous infusion of 4 mg/min (2 mg/min in patients > 65) and 5 min after first dose, a 2nd 50-mg bolus	2–5 µg/L	Tremor, seizures; if administration is too rapid, drowsiness, delirium, paresthesias; possibly increased risk of bradyarrhythmias after acute MI	To reduce toxicity risk, clinicians should reduce dosage or infusion rate to 2 mg/min after 24 h. Extensive first-pass hepatic metabolism occurs.
Mexiletine	Oral immediate-release: 100–250 mg q 8 h Oral slow-release: 360 mg q 12 h IV: 2 mg/kg at 25 mg/min, followed by 250-mg infusion over 1 h, 250-mg infusion over next 2 h, and maintenance infusion of 0.5 mg/min	0.5–2 µg/mL	Nausea, vomiting, tremor, seizures	Oral slow-release and IV forms are not available in the US.
Class Ic	Uses: APB and VPB suppression, SVT and VT suppression, AF or atrial flutter, and VF suppression			
Flecainide	Oral: 100 mg q 8 or 12 h IV: 1–2 mg/kg over 10 min	0.2–1 µg/mL	Occasionally, blurred vision and paresthesias	If QRS complex widens (> 50% if initially < 120 msec and > 25% if initially > 120 msec), dose must be decreased or drug stopped. IV form is not available in US.

Table 76–1. ANTIARRHYTHMIC DRUGS (VAUGHAN WILLIAMS CLASSIFICATION) (*Continued*)

DRUG	DOSAGE	TARGET LEVELS	SELECTED ADVERSE EFFECTS	COMMENTS
Propafenone	Oral: Initially, 150 mg tid, titrated up to 150–300 mg tid IV: 2-mg/kg bolus, followed by 2 mg/min infusion	0.1–1.0 μg/mL	Beta-blocking activity, possible worsening of reactive airway disorders; occasionally GI upset	Pharmacokinetics are nonlinear; increases in dose should not exceed 50% of previous dose. Bioavailability and protein binding vary; drug has saturable first-pass metabolism. IV form is not available in the US.
Class II (beta-blockers)	Uses: Supraventricular tachyarrhythmias (APB, ST, SVT, AF, atrial flutter) and ventricular arrhythmias (often in a supportive role)			
Acebutolol	Oral: 200 mg bid	Beta-blocker levels not measured; dose adjusted to reduce heart rate by > 25%	Typically for beta-blockers, GI disturbances, insomnia, nightmares, lethargy, erectile dysfunction, possible AV block in patients with AV node dysfunction	Beta-blockers are contraindicated in patients with bronchospastic airway disorders.
Atenolol	Oral: 50–100 mg once/day			
Betaxolol	Oral: 20 mg once/day			
Bisoprolol	Oral: 5–10 mg once/day			
Carvedilol	Oral: Initially, 6.25 mg bid, followed by titration to 25 mg bid			
Esmolol	IV: 50–200 μg/kg/min			
Metoprolol	Oral: 50–100 mg bid IV: 5 mg q 5 min up to 15 mg			
Nadolol	Oral: 60–80 mg once/day			
Propranolol	Oral: 10–30 mg tid or qid IV: 1–3 mg (may repeat once after 5 min if needed)			
Timolol	Oral:10–20 mg bid			
Class III (membrane-stabilizing drugs)	Uses: Any tachyarrhythmia except torsades de pointes VT			
Amiodarone	Oral: 600–1200 mg/day for 7–10 days, then 400 mg/day for 3 wk, followed by a maintenance dose (ideally, ≤ 200 mg/day) IV: 150–450 mg over 1–6 h (depending on urgency), followed by a maintenance dose of 0.5–2.0 mg/min	1–2.5 μg/mL	Pulmonary fibrosis (in up to 5% of patients treated for > 5 yr), which may be fatal; QTc prolongation; torsades de pointes VT (rare); bradycardia; gray or blue discoloration of sun-exposed skin; sun sensitivity; hepatic abnormalities; peripheral neuropathy; corneal microdeposits (in almost all treated patients), usually without serious visual effects and reversed by stopping the drug; changes in thyroid function; serum creatinine increased up to 10% without change in GFR; slow clearance possibly prolonging adverse effects	Drug has noncompetitive beta-blocking, calcium channel blocking, and sodium channel blocking effects, with a long delay in onset of action. By prolonging refractoriness, drug may cause homogeneous conditions of repolarization throughout the heart. IV form can be used for conversion.
Azimilide*	Oral: 100–200 mg once/day	200–1000 ng/mL	Torsades de pointes VT	—
Bretylium*	IV: Initially, 5 mg/kg, followed by 1–2 mg/min as a constant infusion IM: Initially, 5–10 mg/kg, which may be repeated to a total dose of 30 mg/kg IM maintenance dose of 5 mg/kg q 6–8 h	0.8–2.4 μg/mL	Hypotension	Drug has class II properties. Effects may be delayed 10–20 min. Drug is used to treat potentially lethal refractory ventricular tachyarrhythmias (intractable VT, recurrent VF), for which it is usually effective within 30 min of injection.

Table continues on the following page.

Table 76–1. ANTIARRHYTHMIC DRUGS (VAUGHAN WILLIAMS CLASSIFICATION) (*Continued*)

DRUG	DOSAGE	TARGET LEVELS	SELECTED ADVERSE EFFECTS	COMMENTS
Dofetilide	Oral: 500 mcg bid if CrCl is > 60 mL/min; 250 mcg bid if CrCl is 40–60 mL/min; 125 mcg bid if CrCl is 20–40 mL/min	N/A	Torsades de pointes VT	Drug is contraindicated if QTc is > 440 msec or if CrCl is < 20 mL/min.
Dronedarone	Oral: 400 mg bid	N/A	QTc prolongation, torsades de pointes VT (rare), bradycardia, GI upset, possible hepatotoxicity (rare), serum creatinine increased up to 20% without change in GFR	Drug is a modified amiodarone molecule (including deiodination) with shorter half-life, smaller volume of distribution, fewer adverse effects, and less efficacy. Drug should not be used in patients with history of heart failure or with permanent AF.
Ibutilide	IV: For patients ≥ 60 kg, 1 mg infusion or, for patients < 60 kg, 0.01 mg/kg over 10 min, with dose repeated after 10 min if the first infusion is unsuccessful	N/A	Torsades de pointes VT (in 2%)	Drug is used to terminate AF (success rate, about 40%) and atrial flutter (success rate, about 65%).
Sotalol	Oral: 80–160 mg q 12 h IV: 10 mg over 1–2 min	0.5–4 μg/mL	Similar to class II; possible depressed left ventricular function and torsades de pointes VT	Racemic [D-L] form has class II (beta-blocking) properties, [D] form does not. Both forms have class III activity. Only racemic sotalol is available for clinical use. Drug should not be used in patients with renal insufficiency.
Class IV (Calcium channel blockers)	Uses: Termination of SVT and slowing of rapid AF or atrial flutter			
Diltiazem	Oral slow-release (diltiazem CD): 120–360 mg once/day IV: 5–15 mg/h for up to 24 h	0.1–0.4 μg/mL	Possible precipitation of VF in patients with VT, negative inotropy	IV form is most commonly used to slow ventricular response rate to AF or atrial flutter.
Verapamil	Oral: 40–120 mg tid or, for sustained-release form, 180 mg once/day to 240 mg bid IV: 5–15 mg over 10 min Oral prophylaxis: 40–120 mg tid	N/A	Possible precipitation of VF in patients with VT, negative inotropy	IV form is used to terminate narrow-complex tachycardias involving the AV node (success rate, almost 100% with 5–10 mg IV over 10 min).
Other antiarrhythmics				
Adenosine	6 mg rapid IV bolus, repeated twice at 12 mg if needed; flush bolus with additional 20 mL saline	N/A	Transient dyspnea, chest discomfort, and flushing (in 30–60%), transient bronchospasm	Drug slows or blocks AV nodal conduction. Duration of action is extremely short. Contraindications include asthma and high-grade heart block. Dipyridamole potentiates effects.

Table 76–1. ANTIARRHYTHMIC DRUGS (VAUGHAN WILLIAMS CLASSIFICATION) (*Continued*)

DRUG	DOSAGE	TARGET LEVELS	SELECTED ADVERSE EFFECTS	COMMENTS
Digoxin	IV loading dose: 0.5 mg Oral maintenance dose: 0.125–0.25 mg/day	0.8–1.6 μg/mL	Anorexia, nausea, vomiting, and often serious arrhythmias (VPBs, VT, APBs, atrial tachycardia, 2nd-degree or 3rd-degree AV block, combinations of these arrhythmias)	Contraindications include antegrade conduction over an accessory AV connection pathway (manifest Wolff-Parkinson-White syndrome) because if AF occurs, ventricular responses may be excessive (digoxin shortens refractory periods of the accessory connection).

*Availability uncertain.

AF = atrial fibrillation; ANA = antinuclear antibody; APB = atrial premature beat; AV = atrioventricular; CrCl = creatinine clearance; LV = left ventricular; QTc = QT interval corrected for heart rate; SVT = supraventricular tachycardia; VF = ventricular fibrillation; VPB = ventricular premature beat; VT = ventricular tachycardia.

conduction in fast-channel tissues (working atrial and ventricular myocytes, His-Purkinje system).

- Class II: Class II drugs are beta-blockers, which affect predominantly slow-channel tissues (SA and AV nodes), where they decrease rate of automaticity, slow conduction velocity, and prolong refractoriness.
- Class III: Class III drugs are primarily potassium channel blockers, which prolong action potential duration and refractoriness in slow- and fast-channel tissues.
- Class IV: Class IV drugs are the nondihydropyridine calcium channel blockers, which depress calcium-dependent action potentials in slow-channel tissues and thus decrease the rate of automaticity, slow conduction velocity, and prolong refractoriness.

Digoxin and adenosine are not included in the Vaughan Williams classification. Digoxin shortens atrial and ventricular refractory periods and is vagotonic, thereby prolonging AV nodal conduction and AV nodal refractory periods. Adenosine slows or blocks AV nodal conduction and can terminate tachyarrhythmias that rely upon AV nodal conduction for their perpetuation.

Class I Antiarrhythmic Drugs

Sodium channel blockers (membrane-stabilizing drugs) block fast sodium channels, slowing conduction in fast-channel tissues (working atrial and ventricular myocytes, His-Purkinje system). In the ECG, this effect may be reflected as widening of the P wave, widening of the QRS complex, prolongation of the PR interval, or a combination.

Class I drugs are subdivided based on the kinetics of the sodium channel effects:

- Class Ib drugs have fast kinetics.
- Class Ic drugs have slow kinetics.
- Class Ia drugs have intermediate kinetics.

The kinetics of sodium channel blockade determine the heart rates at which their electrophysiologic effects become manifest. Because class Ib drugs have fast kinetics, they express their electrophysiologic effects only at fast heart rates. Thus, an ECG obtained during normal rhythm at normal rates usually shows no evidence of fast-channel tissue conduction slowing. Class Ib drugs are not very potent antiarrhythmics and have minimal effects on atrial tissue. Because class Ic drugs have slow kinetics, they express their electrophysiologic effects at all heart rates. Thus, an ECG obtained during normal rhythm at normal heart rates usually shows fast-channel tissue conduction slowing. Class Ic drugs are more potent antiarrhythmics. Because class Ia drugs have intermediate kinetics, their fast-channel tissue conduction slowing effects may or may not be evident on an ECG obtained during normal rhythm at normal rates. Class Ia drugs also block repolarizing potassium channels, prolonging the refractory periods of fast-channel tissues. On the ECG, this effect is reflected as QT-interval prolongation even at normal rates. Class Ib drugs and class Ic drugs do not block potassium channels directly.

The kinetics of sodium channel blockade determine the heart rates at which their electrophysiologic effects become manifest. The primary indications are supraventricular tachycardia (SVT) for class Ia and Ic drugs and ventricular tachycardias (VTs) for all class I drugs.

Adverse effects of class I drugs include proarrhythmia, a drug-related arrhythmia worse than the arrhythmia being treated, which is the most worrisome adverse effect. All class I drugs may worsen VTs. Class I drugs also tend to depress ventricular contractility. Because these adverse effects are more likely to occur in patients with a structural heart disorder, class I drugs are not generally recommended for such patients. Thus, these drugs are usually used only in patients who do not have a structural heart disorder or in patients who have a structural heart disorder but who have no other therapeutic alternatives. There are other adverse effects of class I drugs that are specific to the subclass or individual drug.

Class Ia antiarrhythmic drugs: Class Ia drugs have kinetics that are intermediate between the fast kinetics of class Ib and the slow kinetics of class Ic. Their fast-channel tissue conduction slowing effects may or may not be evident on an ECG obtained during normal rhythm at normal rates. Class Ia drugs block repolarizing potassium channels, prolonging the refractory periods of fast-channel tissues. On the ECG, this effect is reflected as QT-interval prolongation even at normal rates.

Class Ia drugs are used for suppression of atrial premature beats (APB), ventricular premature beats (VPB), SVTs and VTs, atrial fibrillation (AF), atrial flutter, and ventricular fibrillation (VF). The primary indications are SVTs and VTs.

Class Ia drugs may cause torsades de pointes ventricular tachycardia. Class Ia drugs may organize and slow atrial tachyarrhythmias enough to permit 1:1 AV conduction with marked acceleration of the ventricular response rate.

Class Ib antiarrhythmic drugs: Class Ib drugs have fast kinetics; they express their electrophysiologic effects only at fast heart rates. Thus, an ECG obtained during normal rhythm at normal rates usually shows no evidence of fast-channel tissue conduction slowing. Class Ib drugs are not very potent antiarrhythmics and have minimal effects on atrial tissue. Class Ib drugs do not block potassium channels directly.

Class Ib drugs are used for the suppression of ventricular arrhythmias (ventricular premature beats, VT,VF).

Class Ic antiarrhythmic drugs: Class Ic drugs have slow kinetics; they express their electrophysiologic effects at all heart rates. Thus, an ECG obtained during normal rhythm at normal heart rates usually shows fast-channel tissue conduction slowing. Class Ic drugs are more potent antiarrhythmics than either class Ia or class Ib drugs. Class Ic drugs do not block potassium channels directly.

Class Ic drugs may organize and slow atrial tachyarrhythmias enough to permit 1:1 AV conduction with marked acceleration of the ventricular response rate.

Class Ic drugs are used for suppression of atrial and ventricular premature beats, SVTs and VTs, AF, atrial flutter, and VF.

Class II Antiarrhythmic Drugs

Class II antiarrhythmic drugs are beta-blockers, which affect predominantly slow-channel tissues (SA and AV nodes), where they decrease rate of automaticity, slow conduction velocity, and prolong refractoriness. Thus, heart rate is slowed, the PR interval is lengthened, and the AV node transmits rapid atrial depolarizations at a lower frequency.

Class II drugs are used primarily to treat SVTs, including sinus tachycardia, AV nodal reentry, AF, and atrial flutter. These drugs are also used to treat VTs to raise the threshold for VF and reduce the ventricular proarrhythmic effects of beta-adrenoceptor stimulation.

Beta-blockers are generally well tolerated; adverse effects include lassitude, sleep disturbance, and GI upset. These drugs are contraindicated in patients with asthma.

Class III Antiarrhythmic Drugs

Class III drugs are membrane stabilizing drugs, primarily potassium channel blockers, which prolong action potential duration and refractoriness in slow- and fast-channel tissues. Thus, the capacity of all cardiac tissues to transmit impulses at high frequencies is reduced, but conduction velocity is not significantly affected. Because the action potential is prolonged, rate of automaticity is reduced. The predominant effect on the ECG is QT-interval prolongation.

These drugs are used to treat SVTs and VTs. Class III drugs have a risk of ventricular proarrhythmia, particularly torsades de pointes VT and are not used in patients with torsades de pointes VT.

Class IV Antiarrhythmic Drugs

Class IV drugs are the nondihydropyridine calcium channel blockers, which depress calcium-dependent action potentials in slow-channel tissues and thus decrease the rate of automaticity, slow conduction velocity, and prolong refractoriness. Heart rate is slowed, the PR interval is lengthened, and the AV node transmits rapid atrial depolarizations at a lower frequency. These drugs are used primarily to treat SVTs. They may also be used to slow rapid AF or atrial flutter. One form of VT (left septal or Belhassen VT) can be treated with verapamil.

DIRECT-CURRENT CARDIOVERSION-DEFIBRILLATION

The need for treatment of arrhythmias depends on the symptoms and the seriousness of the arrhythmia. Treatment is directed at causes. If necessary, direct antiarrhythmic therapy, including antiarrhythmic drugs, cardioversion-defibrillation, ICDs, pacemakers (and a special form of pacing, cardiac resynchronization therapy), or a combination, is used.

A transthoracic DC shock of sufficient magnitude depolarizes the entire myocardium, rendering the entire heart momentarily refractory to repeat depolarization. Thereafter, the most rapid intrinsic pacemaker, usually the SA node, reassumes control of heart rhythm. Thus, DC cardioversion-defibrillation very effectively terminates tachyarrhythmias that result from reentry. However, it is less effective for terminating tachyarrhythmias that result from automaticity because the return rhythm is likely to be the automatic tachyarrhythmia. For tachyarrhythmias other than ventricular fibrillation (VF) or pulseless VT, the DC shock must be synchronized to the QRS complex (called DC cardioversion) because a shock that falls during the vulnerable period (near the peak of the T wave) can induce VF. In VF, synchronization of a shock to the QRS complex is neither necessary nor possible. A DC shock applied without synchronization to a QRS complex is DC defibrillation.

Procedure for DC cardioversion: When DC cardioversion is elective, patients should fast for 6 to 8 h to avoid the possibility of aspiration. Because the procedure is frightening and painful, brief general anesthesia or IV analgesia and sedation (eg, fentanyl 1 mcg/kg, then midazolam 1 to 2 mg q 2 min to a maximum of 5 mg) is necessary. Equipment and personnel to maintain the airways must be present.

The electrodes (pads or paddles) used for cardioversion may be placed anteroposteriorly (along the left sternal border over the 3rd and 4th intercostal spaces and in the left infrascapular region) or anterolaterally (between the clavicle and the 2nd intercostal space along the right sternal border and over the 5th and 6th intercostal spaces at the apex of the heart). After synchronization to the QRS complex is confirmed on the monitor, a shock is given. The most appropriate energy level varies with the tachyarrhythmia being treated. Cardioversion efficacy increases with use of biphasic shocks, in which the current polarity is reversed part way through the shock waveform.

DC cardioversion-defibrillation can also be applied directly to the heart during a thoracotomy or through use of an intracardiac electrode catheter; then, much lower energy levels are required.

Complications of DC cardioversion: Complications are usually minor and include atrial and ventricular premature beats and muscle soreness. Less commonly, but more likely if patients have marginal left ventricular function or multiple shocks are used, cardioversion precipitates myocyte damage and electromechanical dissociation.

CARDIAC PACEMAKERS

The need for treatment of arrhythmias depends on the symptoms and the seriousness of the arrhythmia. Treatment is directed at causes. If necessary, direct antiarrhythmic therapy, including antiarrhythmic drugs, cardioversion-defibrillation, ICDs, pacemakers (and a special form of pacing, cardiac resynchronization therapy), or a combination, is used.

Pacemakers sense electrical events and respond when necessary by delivering electrical stimuli to the heart. Permanent pacemaker leads are placed via thoracotomy or transvenously, but some temporary emergency pacemaker leads can be placed on the chest wall.

Indications for pacemaker placement: Indications are numerous (see Table 76–2) but generally involve symptomatic bradycardia or high-grade AV block. Some tachyarrhythmias may be terminated by overdrive pacing with a brief period of pacing at a faster rate; the pacemaker is then slowed to the desired rate. Nevertheless, ventricular tachyarrhythmias are better treated with devices that can cardiovert and defibrillate as well as pace (implantable cardioverter defibrillators).

Types of pacemakers: Types of pacemakers are designated by 3 to 5 letters (see Table 76–3), representing which cardiac chambers are paced, which chambers are sensed, how the pacemaker responds to a sensed event (inhibits or triggers pacing), whether it can increase heart rate during exercise (rate-modulating), and whether pacing is multisite (in both atria, both ventricles, or more than one pacing lead in a single chamber). For example, a VVIR pacemaker paces (V) and senses (V) events in the ventricle, inhibits pacing in response to sensed event (I), and can increase its rate during exercise (R).

VVI and DDD pacemakers are the devices most commonly used. They offer equivalent survival benefits. Compared with VVI pacemakers, physiologic pacemakers (AAI, DDD, VDD) appear to reduce risk of atrial fibrillation (AF) and heart failure and slightly improve quality of life.

Advances in pacemaker design include lower-energy circuitry, new battery designs, and corticosteroid-eluting leads (which reduce pacing threshold), all of which increase pacemaker longevity. Mode switching refers to an automatic change in the mode of pacing in response to sensed events (eg, from DDDR to VVIR during AF).

Complications of pacemaker use: Pacemakers may malfunction by oversensing or undersensing events, failing to pace or capture, or pacing at an abnormal rate. Tachycardias are an especially common complication. Rate-modulating pacemakers may increase stimuli in response to vibration, muscle activity, or voltage induced by magnetic fields during MRI. In pacemaker-mediated tachycardia, a normally functioning dual-chamber pacemaker senses a ventricular premature or paced beat transmitted to the atrium through the AV node or a retrograde-conducting accessory pathway, which triggers ventricular stimulation in a rapid, repeating cycle.

Additional complications associated with normally functioning devices include cross-talk inhibition, in which sensing of the atrial pacing impulse by the ventricular channel of a dual-chamber pacemaker leads to inhibition of ventricular pacing, and pacemaker syndrome, in which AV asynchrony induced by ventricular pacing causes fluctuating, vague cerebral (eg, light-headedness), cervical (eg, neck pulsations), or respiratory (eg, dyspnea) symptoms. Pacemaker syndrome is managed by restoring AV synchrony by atrial pacing (AAI), single-lead atrial sensing ventricular pacing (VDD), or dual-chamber pacing (DDD), most commonly the latter.

Environmental interference comes from electromagnetic sources such as surgical electrocautery and MRI, although MRI may be safe when the pacemaker generator and leads are not inside the magnet. Cellular telephones and electronic security devices are a potential source of interference; telephones should not be placed close to the device but are not a problem when used normally for talking. Walking through metal detectors does not cause pacemaker malfunction as long as patients do not linger.

CARDIAC RESYNCHRONIZATION THERAPY

The need for treatment of arrhythmias depends on the symptoms and the seriousness of the arrhythmia. Treatment is directed at causes. If necessary, direct antiarrhythmic therapy, including antiarrhythmic drugs, cardioversion-defibrillation, ICDs, pacemakers (and a special form of pacing, cardiac resynchronization therapy), or a combination, is used.

In some patients, the normal, orderly, sequential relationship between contraction of the cardiac chambers is disrupted (becomes dyssynchronous). Dyssynchrony may be

- AV: Between atrial and ventricular contraction
- Interventricular: Between left and right ventricular contraction
- Intraventricular: Between different segments of left ventricular contraction

Patients at risk for dyssynchrony include those with the following:

- Ischemic or nonischemic dilated cardiomyopathy
- Prolonged QRS interval (≥ 130 msec)
- Left ventricular end-diastolic dimension ≥ 55 mm
- Left ventricular ejection fraction ≤ 35% in sinus rhythm

Cardiac resynchronization therapy (CRT) involves use of a pacing system to resynchronize cardiac contraction. Such systems usually include a right atrial lead, right ventricular lead, and left ventricular lead. Leads may be placed transvenously or surgically via thoracotomy. In heart failure patients with New York Heart Association (NYHA) class II, III, and IV symptoms, CRT can reduce hospitalization for heart failure and reduce all-cause mortality. However, there is little to no benefit in patients with permanent AF, right bundle branch block (RBBB), nonspecific intraventricular conduction delay, or only mild prolongation of QRS duration (< 150 msec).

IMPLANTABLE CARDIOVERTER-DEFIBRILLATORS

The need for treatment of arrhythmias depends on the symptoms and the seriousness of the arrhythmia. Treatment is directed at causes. If necessary, direct antiarrhythmic therapy, including antiarrhythmic drugs, cardioversion-defibrillation, implantable cardioverter-defibrillators (ICDs), pacemakers (and a special form of pacing, cardiac resynchronization therapy), or a combination, is used.

ICDs cardiovert or defibrillate the heart in response to ventricular tachycardia (VT) or ventricular fibrillation (VF). Contemporary tiered-therapy ICDs also provide antibradycardia pacing and antitachycardia pacing (to terminate responsive atrial or VTs) and store intracardiac electrograms.

ICDs are implanted subcutaneously or subpectorally, with electrodes inserted transvenously into the right ventricle and sometimes also the right atrium. A biventricular ICD also has a left ventricular epicardial lead placed via the coronary sinus venous system or via thoracotomy.

ICDs are the preferred treatment for patients who have had an episode of VF or hemodynamically significant VT not due to

Table 76–2. INDICATIONS FOR PERMANENT PACEMAKERS

ARRHYTHMIA	INDICATED (ESTABLISHED BY EVIDENCE)	POSSIBLY INDICATED AND SUPPORTED BY BULK OF EVIDENCE	POSSIBLY INDICATED BUT LESS WELL SUPPORTED BY EVIDENCE	NOT INDICATED
Sinus node dysfunction	Symptomatic bradycardia, including symptomatic frequent sinus pauses and bradycardia due to essential drugs (alternatives contraindicated) Symptomatic chronotropic incompetence (heart rate cannot meet physiologic demands)	Heart rate of < 40 beats/min when symptoms have not been clearly associated with the bradycardia Syncope of unexplained origin with significant sinus node dysfunction seen on ECG or triggered in an electrophysiologic study	Heart rate of < 40 beats/min in minimally symptomatic patients while awake	Asymptomatic bradycardia Symptoms consistent with bradycardia but clearly shown not to be associated with it Symptomatic bradycardia due to nonessential drugs
AV block	Any 3rd-degree or 2nd-degree AV block associated symptomatic bradycardia or ventricular arrhythmia Third-degree or advanced 2nd-degree AV block at any anatomic level if associated with one of the following: • Arrhythmias and other disorders requiring drugs that cause symptomatic bradycardia • Documented asystole ≥ 3.0 sec (≥ 5.0 sec in atrial fibrillation), any escape rate of < 40 beats/min, or escape rhythm below the AV node in awake, asymptomatic patients • Escape ventricular rates of > 40 beats/min in patients with cardiomegaly or LV dysfunction • Catheter ablation of the AV junction • Postoperative block not expected to resolve after surgery • Neuromuscular disorders with AV block (eg, myotonic muscular dystrophy, Kearns-Sayre syndrome, limb-girdle dystrophy, Charcot-Marie-Tooth disease [peroneal atrophy]) • Exercise (ie, occurring during) in patients without myocardial ischemia	Asymptomatic 3rd-degree AV block at any anatomic level when average ventricular rates during waking are ≥ 40 beats/min in patients without cardiomegaly Asymptomatic type II 2nd-degree AV block with narrow QRS complex (pacemaker is indicated if QRS complex is wide) Asymptomatic 2nd-degree AV block within or below His bundle level, detected during an electrophysiologic study First- or 2nd-degree AV block with symptoms suggesting pacemaker syndrome	AV block in patients who are taking a causative drug or have drug toxicity if block is expected to recur even after drug is withdrawn AV block of any degree (including 1st) associated with neuromuscular disorders in which conduction abnormalities may progress unpredictably (eg, myotonic muscular dystrophy, limb-girdle dystrophy, Charcot-Marie-Tooth disease [peroneal atrophy] with or without symptoms)	Asymptomatic 1st-degree AV block Asymptomatic type I 2nd-degree AV block at the AV node level or not known to be within or below His bundle level AV block expected to resolve or unlikely to recur (eg, due to drug toxicity or Lyme disease or occurring asymptomatically during transient increases in vagal tone or during hypoxia in sleep apnea syndrome)
Tachyarrhythmias	Sustained, pause-dependent VT, with or without prolonged QT interval	High-risk patients with congenital long QT syndrome Symptomatic recurrent SVT reproducibly terminated by pacing when ablation and/or drugs fail (except when there is an accessory AV connection capable of high-frequency antegrade conduction)	Prevention of symptomatic, recurrent atrial fibrillation refractory to drugs when sinus node dysfunction coexists	Frequent or complex ventricular ectopy without sustained VT when long QT syndrome is absent Torsades de pointes VT with reversible causes Prevention of AF in patients without another indication for pacing

Table 76–2. INDICATIONS FOR PERMANENT PACEMAKERS (*Continued*)

ARRHYTHMIA	INDICATED (ESTABLISHED BY EVIDENCE)	POSSIBLY INDICATED AND SUPPORTED BY BULK OF EVIDENCE	POSSIBLY INDICATED BUT LESS WELL SUPPORTED BY EVIDENCE	NOT INDICATED
After acute MI	Persistent 2nd-degree AV block in the His-Purkinje system with bilateral BBB or 3rd-degree AV block within or below the His-Purkinje system Transient advanced 2nd- or 3rd-degree AV block below the AV node level and associated with BBB Persistent symptomatic 2nd- or 3rd-degree AV block	None	Persistent 2nd- or 3rd-degree AV block at the AV node level	Transient AV block without intraventricular conduction defects Transient AV block with isolated left anterior fascicular block Acquired BBB or fascicular block without AV block Persistent 1st-degree AV block with BBB or fascicular block
Multifascicular block	Advanced 2nd-degree or intermittent 3rd-degree AV block Type II 2nd-degree AV block Alternating BBB	Syncope not shown to be due to AV block after other likely causes (especially VT) are excluded Very prolonged HV interval (≥ 100 msec) in asymptomatic patients, detected incidentally during an electrophysiologic study Nonphysiologic, infra-His block induced by pacing, detected incidentally during an electrophysiologic study	Neuromuscular disorders in which conduction abnormalities may progress unpredictably (eg, myotonic muscular dystrophy, limb-girdle dystrophy, Charcot-Marie-Tooth disease [peroneal atrophy] with or without symptoms)	Fascicular block without AV block or symptoms Fascicular block with 1st-degree AV block and without symptoms
Congenital heart disorders	Advanced 2nd- or 3rd-degree AV block causing symptomatic bradycardia, ventricular dysfunction, or low cardiac output Sinus node dysfunction correlated with symptoms during age-inappropriate bradycardia Postoperative high-grade 2nd- or 3rd-degree AV block that is not expected to resolve or that persists ≥ 7 days after surgery Congenital 3rd-degree AV block with a wide QRS escape rhythm, complex ventricular ectopy, or ventricular dysfunction Congenital 3rd-degree AV block in infants with a ventricular rate of < 55 beats/min or with a congenital heart disorder and a ventricular rate of < 70 beats/min Sustained pause-dependent VT, with or without prolonged QT, when pacing has been documented as effective	Congenital heart disorder and sinus bradycardia to prevent recurrent episodes of intra-atrial reentrant tachycardia Congenital 3rd-degree AV block persisting after age 1 yr if average heart rate is < 50 beats/min, ventricular rate pauses abruptly for 2 or 3 times the basic cycle length, or associated symptoms due to chronotropic incompetence occur Asymptomatic sinus bradycardia in children with a complex congenital heart disorder and resting heart rate of < 40 beats/min or pauses in ventricular rate of > 3 sec Patients with a congenital heart disorder and impaired hemodynamics due to sinus bradycardia or loss of AV synchrony Unexplained syncope in patients who have had congenital heart disorder surgery that was complicated by transient 3rd-degree AV block with residual fascicular block	Transient postoperative 3rd-degree AV block that converts to sinus rhythm with residual bifascicular block Congenital 3rd-degree AV block in asymptomatic infants, children, adolescents, or young adults with an acceptable ventricular rate, a narrow QRS complex, and normal ventricular function Asymptomatic sinus bradycardia after biventricular repair of a congenital heart disorder in patients with resting heart rate of < 40 beats/min or pauses in ventricular rate of > 3 sec	Transient postoperative AV block when AV conduction returns to normal Asymptomatic postoperative bifascicular block with or without 1st-degree AV block and without prior transient 3rd-degree AV block Asymptomatic type I 2nd-degree AV block Asymptomatic sinus bradycardia when the longest RR interval is < 3 sec and minimum heart rate is > 40 beats/min

Table continues on the following page.

Table 76–2. INDICATIONS FOR PERMANENT PACEMAKERS (*Continued*)

ARRHYTHMIA	INDICATED (ESTABLISHED BY EVIDENCE)	POSSIBLY INDICATED AND SUPPORTED BY BULK OF EVIDENCE	POSSIBLY INDICATED BUT LESS WELL SUPPORTED BY EVIDENCE	NOT INDICATED
Hypersensitive carotid sinus syndrome and neurocardiogenic syncope	Recurrent syncope due to spontaneously occurring carotid sinus stimulation or to carotid sinus pressure that induces asystole of > 3 sec	Recurrent syncope without obvious triggering events and with a hypersensitive cardioinhibitory response (ie, carotid sinus pressure induces asystole of > 3 sec)	Significantly symptomatic neurocardiogenic syncope associated with bradycardia documented clinically or during tilt-table testing	Hyperactive cardioinhibitory response to carotid sinus stimulation without symptoms or with vague symptoms (eg, dizziness, light-headedness) Situational vasovagal syncope that can be averted by avoidance
Postcardiac transplantation	Persistent inappropriate or symptomatic bradycardia expected to persist Other established indications for permanent pacing	None	Prolonged or recurrent relative bradycardia limiting rehabilitation or discharge after postoperative recovery Syncope after transplantation even when bradyarrhythmia has not been demonstrated	None
Hypertrophic cardiomyopathy	Same as established indications for sinus node dysfunction or AV block	None	Medically refractory, symptomatic hypertrophic cardiomyopathy when resting or induced LV outflow is significantly obstructed	Asymptomatic or medically controlled hypertrophic cardiomyopathy Symptomatic hypertrophic cardiomyopathy with no evidence of LV outflow obstruction
Cardiac resynchronization therapy (CRT) for patients with severe systolic heart failure	CRT (with or without an ICD) for patients with LVEF ≤ 35%, LBBB, QRS duration ≥ 0.15 sec, sinus rhythm, and NYHA class II, class III, or ambulatory class IV heart failure symptoms during optimal medical therapy	CRT (with or without an ICD) for patients with LVEF ≤ 35%, sinus rhythm, LBBB, QRS duration 0.12–0.149 sec, and NYHA class II, class III, or ambulatory class IV heart failure symptoms during optimal medical therapy CRT for patients with LVEF ≤ 35%, sinus rhythm, non-LBBB, QRS duration ≥ 0.15 sec, and NYHA class III or ambulatory class IV heart failure symptoms during optimal medical therapy CRT for patients with LVEF ≤ 35% in AF who otherwise meet criteria for CRT and AV node ablation or pharmacologic therapy will allow near 100% ventricular pacing CRT for patients with LVEF ≤ 35% who are undergoing new or replacement device with anticipated > 40% ventricular pacing	LVEF ≤ 30% caused by ischemic heart disease) in sinus rhythm, QRS duration ≥ 0.15 sec, and NYHA class I heart failure symptoms during optimal medical therapy LVEF ≤ 35%, sinus rhythm, non-LBBB, QRS duration 0.12–0.149 sec, and NYHA class III or ambulatory class IV heart failure symptoms during optimal medical therapy LVEF ≤ 35%, sinus rhythm, non-LBBB, QRS duration ≥ 0.15 sec, and II heart failure symptoms during optimal medical therapy	NYHA class I or II symptoms and non-LBBB QRS pattern with QRS duration < 0.15 sec Comorbidity and/or frailty that will limit survival with good functional status to < 1 yr

AF = atrial fibrillation; AV = atrioventricular; BBB = bundle branch block; EF = ejection fraction; HV interval = interval from the start of the HIS signal to the beginning of the 1st ventricular signal; ICD = implantable cardioverter-defibrillator; LBBB = left bundle branch block; LV = left ventricular; NYHA = New York Heart Association; SVT = supraventricular tachycardia; VT = ventricular tachycardia.

Data from Epstein AE, DiMarco JP, Ellenbogen KA, et al: 2012 ACCF/AHA/HRS focused update incorporated into the ACCF/AHA/HRS 2008 Guidelines for device-based therapy of cardiac rhythm abnormalities. *Circulation* 117(21):e350–e408, 2008 and *Circulation* 127(3):e283–e352, 2013.

Table 76–3. PACEMAKER CODES

I	II	III	IV	V
CHAMBER PACED	CHAMBER SENSED	RESPONSE TO SENSED EVENT	RATE MODULATION	MULTISITE PACING
A = Atrium	A = Atrium	O = None	O = Not programmable	O = None
V = Ventricle	V = Ventricle	I = Inhibits pacemaker	R = Rate-modulated	A = Atrium
D = Dual (both)	D = Dual (both)	T = Triggers pacemaker to stimulate ventricles		V = Ventricle
		D = Dual (both): For events sensed in ventricles, inhibits; for events sensed in atria, triggers		D = Dual (both)

reversible or transient conditions (eg, electrolyte disturbance, antiarrhythmic drug proarrhythmia, acute MI). ICDs may also be indicated for patients with VT or VF inducible during an electrophysiologic study and for patients with idiopathic or ischemic cardiomyopathy, a left ventricular ejection fraction of < 35%, and a high risk of VT or VF. Other indications are less clear (see Table 76–4).

Because ICDs treat rather than prevent VT or VF, patients prone to these arrhythmias may require both an ICD and antiarrhythmic drugs to reduce the number of episodes and need for uncomfortable shocks; this approach also prolongs the life of the ICD.

Impulse generators for ICDs typically last about 5 yr. ICDs may malfunction by delivering inappropriate pacing or shocks in response to sinus rhythm, supraventricular tachycardias (SVTs), or nonphysiologically generated impulses (eg. due to lead fracture). They also may malfunction by not delivering appropriate pacing or shocks when needed because of factors such as lead or impulse generator migration, undersensing, an increase in pacing threshold due to fibrosis at the site of prior shocks, and battery depletion.

In patients who report that the ICD has discharged but that no associated symptoms of syncope, dyspnea, chest pain or persistent palpitations occurred, follow up with the ICD clinic and/or the electrophysiologist within the week is appropriate. The ICD can then be electronically interrogated to determine the reason for discharge. If such associated symptoms were present, or the patient received multiple shocks, emergency department referral is indicated to look for a treatable cause (eg, coronary ischemia, electrolyte abnormality) or device malfunction.

RADIOFREQUENCY ABLATION FOR CARDIAC ARRHYTHMIA

The need for treatment of arrhythmias depends on the symptoms and the seriousness of the arrhythmia. Treatment is directed at causes. If necessary, direct antiarrhythmic therapy, including antiarrhythmic drugs, cardioversion-defibrillation, (ICDs), pacemakers (and a special form of pacing, cardiac resynchronization therapy), or a combination, is used.

If a tachyarrhythmia depends on a specific pathway or ectopic site of automaticity, the site can be ablated by low-voltage, high-frequency (300 to 750 MHz) electrical energy, applied through an electrode catheter. This energy heats and necroses an area < 1 cm in diameter and up to 1 cm deep. Before energy can be applied, the target site or sites must be mapped during an electrophysiologic study.

Success rate is > 90% for reentrant supraventricular tachycardias (via the AV node or an accessory pathway), focal atrial tachycardia and flutter, and focal idiopathic ventricular tachycardia (right ventricular outflow tract, left septal, or bundle branch reentrant VT). Because atrial fibrillation (AF) often originates or is maintained by an arrhythmogenic site in the pulmonary veins, this source can be electrically isolated by ablations at the pulmonary vein–left atrial junction or in the left atrium. Alternatively, in patients with refractory AF and rapid ventricular rates, the AV node may be ablated after permanent pacemaker implantation. Radiofrequency ablation is sometimes successful in patients with VT refractory to drugs particularly when ischemic heart disease is present.

Radiofrequency ablation is safe; mortality is < 1/2000. Complications include valvular damage, pulmonary vein stenosis or occlusion (if used to treat AF), stroke or other embolism, cardiac perforation, tamponade (1%), and unintended AV node ablation.

ATRIAL FIBRILLATION

Atrial fibrillation (AF) is a rapid, irregularly irregular atrial rhythm. Symptoms include palpitations and sometimes weakness, effort intolerance, dyspnea, and presyncope. Atrial thrombi often form, causing a significant risk of embolic stroke. Diagnosis is by ECG. Treatment involves rate control with drugs, prevention of thromboembolism with anticoagulation, and sometimes conversion to sinus rhythm by drugs or cardioversion.

AF has been attributed to multiple wavelets with chaotic reentry within the atria. However, in many cases, firing of an ectopic focus within venous structures *adjacent* to the atria (usually the pulmonary veins) is responsible for initiation and perhaps maintenance of AF. In AF, the atria do not contract, and the AV conduction system is bombarded with many electrical stimuli, causing inconsistent impulse transmission and an irregularly irregular ventricular rate, which is usually in the tachycardia rate range.

AF is one of the most common arrhythmias, affecting about 2.3 million adults in the US. Men and whites are more likely to have AF than women and blacks. Prevalence increases with age; almost 10% of people > 80 yr are affected. AF tends to occur in patients with a heart disorder.

Complications: The absent atrial contractions predispose to thrombus formation; annual risk of cerebrovascular embolic

Table 76–4. INDICATIONS FOR IMPLANTABLE CARDIOVERTER-DEFIBRILLATORS IN VENTRICULAR TACHYCARDIA AND VENTRICULAR FIBRILLATION

LEVEL OF EVIDENCE	SPECIFIC INDICATIONS
Indicated (established by evidence)	Hemodynamically unstable VT or VF when there is no transient or reversible cause Hemodynamically stable sustained VT in patients with a structural heart disorder Syncope of undetermined origin with hemodynamically significant sustained VT or VF induced during an electrophysiologic study Ischemic cardiomyopathy, NYHA class II or III heart failure symptoms during optimal medical therapy, and LV ejection fraction ≤ 0.35 measured at least 40 days post-MI Ischemic cardiomyopathy, NYHA class I heart failure symptoms during optimal medical therapy, and LV ejection fraction ≤ 30% measured at least 40 days post-MI Nonischemic dilated cardiomyopathy, NYHA class II or III heart failure symptoms during optimal medical therapy, and LV ejection fraction ≤ 0. 35 Ischemic cardiomyopathy, nonsustained VT, LV ejection fraction ≤ 40% measured at least 40 days post-MI, and inducible VF or sustained VT detected during an electrophysiologic study
Possibly indicated and supported by bulk of evidence	Patients with idiopathic dilated cardiomyopathy, significant LV dysfunction during optimal medical therapy, with unexplained syncope Patients with sustained VT and normal or near-normal ventricular function Patients with HCM with one or more high risk factors other than sustained VT/VF (family history of premature sudden death, unexplained syncope, LV thickness ≥ 30 mm, abnormal exercise BP response, nonsustained VT) Patients with ARVC with one or more high risk factors other than sustained VT/VF (extensive RV disease, affected family member with sudden death, undiagnosed syncope, nonsustained VT, inducible VT detected during an electrophysiologic study) Long QT syndrome, syncope or VT while receiving a beta-blocker Nonhospitalized patients awaiting cardiac transplantation Brugada syndrome and syncope or documented VT that has not resulted in cardiac arrest Patients with catecholaminergic polymorphic VT with syncope and/or documented sustained VT while receiving a beta-blocker Patients with cardiac sarcoidosis, giant cell myocarditis, or Chagas disease
Possibly indicated but less well supported by evidence	Patients with idiopathic dilated cardiomyopathy, NYHA class I heart failure symptoms during optimal medical therapy, LV ejection fraction ≤ 0.35 Patients with long QT syndrome, without syncope or VT and with one or more high risk factors (QTc > 0.5 sec, LQT1 with 2 abnormal copies of the abnormal gene and deafness [formerly Jervell and Lange-Neilsen syndrome], LQT2, LQT3) Patients with syncope and an advanced structural heart disorder if invasive and noninvasive investigations have not identified a cause Patients with familial cardiomyopathy associated with sudden death Patients with LV noncompaction
Not indicated	Syncope of unknown etiology in absence of inducible VT or VF and without a structural heart disorder Incessant VT or VF VT or VF with mechanisms amenable to catheter or surgical ablation VT or VF due to transient or reversible disorders when correction is feasible and likely to prevent recurrence Psychiatric disorders that may worsen with ICD implantation or that preclude follow-up Patients with no reasonable expectation of survival and with an acceptable functional status for ≥ 1 yr Patients with NYHA class IV drug-refractory heart failure symptoms who are not candidates for cardiac transplantation or a CRT ICD

ARVC = arrhythmogenic right ventricular cardiomyopathy; CRT = cardiac resynchronization therapy; HCM = hypertrophic cardiomyopathy; ICD = implantable cardioverter defibrillator; LQT1 = long QT syndrome type 1; LQT2 = long QT syndrome type 2; LQT3 = long QT syndrome type 3; LV = left ventricular; NYHA = New York Heart Association; QTc = corrected QT interval; RV = right ventricular; VF = ventricular fibrillation; VT = ventricular tachycardia.

Adapted from Epstein AE, DiMarco JP, Ellenbogen KA, et al: 2012 ACCF/AHA/HRS focused update incorporated into the ACCF/AHA/HRS 2008 Guidelines for device-based therapy of cardiac rhythm abnormalities. *Circulation* 127(3):e283–e352, 2013.

events is about 7%. Risk of stroke is higher in patients with a rheumatic valvular disorder, hyperthyroidism, hypertension, diabetes, left ventricular systolic dysfunction, or previous thromboembolic events. Systemic emboli can also cause malfunction or necrosis of other organs (eg, heart, kidneys, GI tract, eyes) or a limb.

AF also may impair cardiac output; loss of atrial contraction can lower cardiac output at normal heart rate by about 10%. Such a decrease is usually well tolerated except when the ventricular rate becomes too fast (eg, > 140 beats/min), or when patients have borderline or low cardiac output to begin with. In such cases, heart failure may develop.

Etiology

The **most common causes** of AF are hypertension, ischemic or nonischemic cardiomyopathy, mitral or tricuspid valvular disorders, hyperthyroidism, and binge alcohol drinking (holiday heart).

Less common causes include pulmonary embolism, atrial septal and other congenital heart defects, COPD, myocarditis, and pericarditis. AF without an identifiable cause in patients < 60 yr is called lone AF.

Classification

Paroxysmal AF is recurrent AF that typically lasts < 1 wk and that converts spontaneously to normal sinus rhythm.

Persistent AF lasts > 1 wk or requires treatment to convert to normal sinus rhythm.

Long-standing persistent AF lasts > 1 yr, but there is still the possibility of restoring sinus rhythm.

Permanent AF cannot be converted to sinus rhythm. The longer AF is present, the less likely is spontaneous conversion and the more difficult is cardioversion because of atrial remodeling (rapid atrial rate-induced changes in atrial electrophysiology that are dominated by a decrease in atrial refractoriness and may also include increase in spatial dispersion of atrial refractoriness slowed atrial conduction velocity, or both).

Symptoms and Signs

AF is often asymptomatic, but many patients have palpitations, vague chest discomfort, or symptoms of heart failure (eg, weakness, light-headedness, dyspnea), particularly when the ventricular rate is very rapid (often 140 to 160 beats/min). Patients may also present with symptoms and signs of acute stroke or of other organ damage due to systemic emboli.

The pulse is irregularly irregular with loss of *a* waves in the jugular venous pulse. A pulse deficit (the apical ventricular rate is faster than the rate palpated at the wrist) may be present because left ventricular stroke volume is not always sufficient to produce a peripheral pressure wave at fast ventricular rates.

Diagnosis

- ECG
- Echocardiography
- Thyroid function tests

Diagnosis of AF is by ECG. Findings include absence of P waves, f (fibrillatory) waves between QRS complexes (irregular in timing, irregular in morphology; baseline undulations at rates > 300/min not always apparent in all leads), and irregularly irregular R-R intervals (see Fig. 76–4).

Other irregular rhythms may resemble AF on ECG but can be distinguished by the presence of discrete P or flutter waves, which can sometimes be made more visible with vagal maneuvers. Muscle tremor or electrical interference may resemble f waves, but the underlying rhythm is regular. AF may also cause a phenomenon that mimics ventricular extrasystoles or VT (Ashman phenomenon). This phenomenon typically occurs when a short R-R interval follows a long R-R interval; the longer interval lengthens the refractory period of the infra-Hisian conduction system, and subsequent QRS complexes are conducted aberrantly, typically with right bundle branch morphology.

Echocardiography and thyroid function tests are important in the initial evaluation. Echocardiography is done to assess structural heart defects (eg, left atrial enlargement, left ventricular wall motion abnormalities suggesting past or present ischemia, valvular disorders, cardiomyopathy) and to identify additional risk factors for stroke (eg, atrial blood stasis or thrombus, complex aortic plaque). Atrial thrombi are more likely in the atrial appendages, where they are best detected by transesophageal rather than transthoracic echocardiography.

PEARLS & PITFALLS

- AF with a wide QRS complex may indicate WPW syndrome; in such cases, use of AV node-blocking drugs may be fatal.

Treatment

- Rate control with drugs or AV node radiofrequency ablation
- Sometimes rhythm control with cardioversion, drugs, or AF substrate ablation
- Prevention of thromboembolism

If a significant underlying disorder is suspected, patients with new-onset AF may benefit from hospitalization, but those with recurrent episodes do not require hospitalization unless other symptoms suggest the need for it. Once causes have been managed, treatment of AF focuses on ventricular rate control, rhythm control, and prevention of thromboembolism.

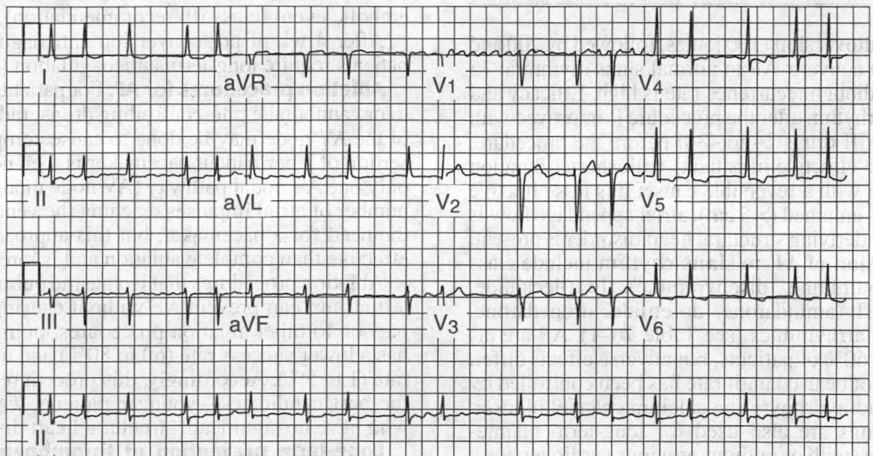

Fig. 76–4. Atrial fibrillation.

Ventricular rate control: Patients with AF of any duration require rate control (typically to < 100 beats/min at rest) to control symptoms and prevent tachycardia-induced cardiomyopathy.

For acute paroxysms of rapid rate (eg, 140 to 160 beats/min), IV AV node blockers are used (for doses, see Table 76–1). CAUTION: *AV node blockers should not be used in patients with WPW syndrome when an accessory AV pathway is involved (indicated by wide QRS duration); these drugs increase frequency of conduction via the bypass tract, possibly causing VF.* Beta-blockers (eg, metoprolol, esmolol) are preferred if excess catecholamines are suspected (eg, in thyroid disorders, exercise-triggered cases). Nondihydropyridine calcium channel blockers (eg, verapamil, diltiazem) are also effective. Digoxin is the least effective but may be preferred if heart failure is present. These drugs may be used orally for long-term rate control. When beta-blockers, nondihydropyridine calcium channel blockers, and digoxin—separately or in combination—are ineffective, amiodarone may be required.

Rhythm control: In patients with heart failure or other hemodynamic compromise directly attributable to new-onset AF, restoration of normal sinus rhythm is indicated to improve cardiac output. In other cases, conversion of AF to normal sinus rhythm is optimal, but the antiarrhythmic drugs that are capable of doing so (class Ia, Ic, III) have a risk of adverse effects and may increase mortality. Conversion to sinus rhythm does not eliminate the need for chronic anticoagulation.

For acute conversion, synchronized cardioversion or drugs can be used. Before conversion is attempted, the ventricular rate should be controlled to < 120 beats/min, and, many patients should be anticoagulated (see Prevention of thromboembolism during rhythm control, below, for criteria and methods). if AF has been present > 48 h, patients should typically be given an oral anticoagulant (conversion, regardless of method used, increases risk of thromboembolism). Anticoagulation should be maintained for > 3 wk before conversion when possible and for at least 4 wk after cardioversion. Many patients need chronic anticoagulation, although the specific criteria are still being debated (see Long-term measures to prevent thromboembolism, below).

PEARLS & PITFALLS

- When possible, give anticoagulation before attempting to convert atrial fibrillation to sinus rhythm. Conversion to sinus rhythm does not eliminate the need for chronic anticoagulation in patients who meet criteria for it.

Synchronized cardioversion (100 joules, followed by 200 and 360 joules as needed) converts AF to normal sinus rhythm in 75 to 90% of patients, although recurrence rate is high. Efficacy and maintenance of sinus rhythm after the procedure is improved with use of class Ia, Ic, or III drugs 24 to 48 h before the procedure. Cardioversion is more effective in patients with shorter duration of AF, lone AF, or AF with a reversible cause; it is less effective when the left atrium is enlarged (> 5 cm), atrial appendage flow is low, or a significant underlying structural heart disorder is present.

Drugs for conversion of AF to sinus rhythm include class Ia (procainamide, quinidine, disopyramide), Ic (flecainide, propafenone), and III (amiodarone, dofetilide, dronedarone, ibutilide, sotalol) antiarrhythmics (see Table 76–1). All are effective in about 50 to 60% of patients, but adverse effects differ. These drugs should not be used until rate has been controlled by a beta-blocker or nondihydropyridine calcium channel blocker. These converting drugs are also used for long-term maintenance of sinus rhythm (with or without previous cardioversion). Choice depends on patient tolerance. However, for paroxysmal AF that occurs only or almost only at rest or during sleep when vagal tone is high, drugs with vagolytic effects (eg, disopyramide) may be particularly effective. Exercise-induced AF may be better prevented with a beta-blocker.

For certain patients with recurrent paroxysmal AF who also can identify its onset by symptoms, some clinicians provide a single oral loading dose of flecainide (300 mg for patients ≥ 70 kg, otherwise 200 mg) or propafenone (600 mg for patients ≥ 70 kg, otherwise 450 mg) that patients carry and self-administer when palpitations develop ("pill-in-the-pocket" approach). This approach must be limited to patients who have no SA or AV node dysfunction, bundle branch block, QT prolongation, Brugada syndrome, or structural heart disease. Its hazard (estimated at 1%) is the possibility of converting AF to a slowish atrial flutter that conducts 1:1 in the 200 to 240 beat/min range. This potential complication can be reduced in frequency by coadministration of an AV nodal suppressing medication (eg, a beta-blocker or a nondihydropyridine calcium antagonist).

ACE inhibitors, angiotensin II receptor blockers, and aldosterone blockers may attenuate the myocardial fibrosis that provides a substrate for AF in patients with heart failure, but the role of these drugs in routine AF treatment has yet to be defined.

Prevention of thromboembolism during rhythm control: Patients, particularly those in whom the current episode of AF has been present > 48 h, have a high risk of thromboembolism for several weeks after pharmacologic or direct current cardioversion. If the onset of the current episode of AF is not clearly within 48 h, the patient should be anticoagulated for 3 wk before and at least 4 wk after cardioversion regardless of the patient's predicted risk of a thromboembolic event (class I recommendation).

Alternatively, therapeutic anticoagulation is started, transesophageal echocardiography (TEE) is done, and, if no left atrial or left atrial appendage clot is seen, cardioversion may be done, followed by at least 4 wk of anticoagulation therapy (class IIa recommendation).

If urgent cardioversion is required because of hemodynamic compromise, cardioversion is done and anticoagulation is started as soon as is practical and continued for at least 4 wk.

If the onset of the current episode of AF is clearly within 48 h, cardioversion may be done without prior anticoagulation if the patient has nonvalvular AF and is not at high risk of a thromboembolic event. After cardioversion, therapeutic anticoagulation is given for 4 wk (class I recommendation); although this may not be necessary in patients at low risk of a thromboembolic event (class IIb recommendation).

After 4 wk of postconversion anticoagulation therapy, some patients require long-term anticoagulation (see p. 637).

Ablation procedures for AF: For patients who do not respond to or cannot take rate-controlling drugs, radiofrequency ablation of the AV node may be done to cause complete heart block; insertion of a permanent pacemaker is then necessary. Ablation of only one AV nodal pathway (AV node modification) reduces the number of atrial impulses reaching the ventricles and eliminates the need for a pacemaker, but this approach is considered less effective than complete ablation and is rarely used.

Ablation procedures that isolate the pulmonary veins from the left atrium can prevent AF without causing AV block. In comparison to other ablation procedures, pulmonary vein isolation has a lower success rate (60 to 80%) and a higher complication rate (1 to 5%). Accordingly, this procedure is often reserved for the best candidates—younger patients with drug-resistant AF who have no significant structural heart disease.

Long-term prevention of thromboembolism: Long-term measures to prevent thromboembolism are taken for certain

Table 76–5. CHADS2 SCORE

VARIABLE	POINTS
Congestive heart failure	1
Hypertension	1
Age ≥ 75 yr	1
Diabetes mellitus	1
Prior stroke/TIA	2

patients with AF during long-term treatment depending on their estimated risk of stroke vs risk of bleeding.

Patients with rheumatic mitral stenosis and patients with mechanical artificial heart valves are considered to be at high risk of a thromboembolic event as are patients with nonvalvular AF who have additional risk factors. The additional risk factors are identified by the CHADS2 score (see Table 76–5) or the CHA2DS2-VASc score (see Table 76–6).

The guidelines for antithrombotic therapy are in a state of flux and differ in different regions. The current guidelines in the United States are as follows:

- Long-term oral anticoagulant therapy is recommended for patients with rheumatic mitral stenosis, artificial heart valve, and for nonvalvular AF patients with a CHA2DS2-VASc score of ≥ 2 (level I recommendation).
- No antithrombotic therapy is recommended for patients with nonvalvular AF and a CHA2DS2-VASc score of 0 (level IIa recommendation).
- No antithrombotic therapy, aspirin therapy, or oral anticoagulant therapy is recommended for patients with nonvalvular AF and a CHA2DS2-VASc score of 1 (level IIb recommendation).
- Patients with AF and a mechanical heart valve(s) are treated with warfarin. Patients with AF and significant mitral stenosis are treated with warfarin. For patients with nonvalvular AF who are to be treated with an oral anticoagulant, a class I indication is given for warfarin with a target INR of 2.0-3.0 (level of evidence A), apixaban (level of evidence B), dabigatran (level of evidence B), and rivaroxaban (level of evidence B).

These general guidelines are altered in patients with more than moderate renal impairment.

The left atrial appendage may be surgically ligated or closed with a transcatheter device when appropriate antithrombotic therapy is absolutely contraindicated.

An individual patient's risk of bleeding may be estimated with any of a number of prognostic tools of which the most commonly used is HAS-BLED (see Table 76–7). The HAS-BLED score serves best in identifying conditions that, if modified, reduce bleeding risk rather than in identifying patients with a higher risk of bleeding who should not receive anticoagulation

Table 76–6. CHA2DS2-VASc SCORE

VARIABLE	POINTS
Congestive heart failure	1
Hypertension	1
Age ≥ 75 yr	2
Diabetes mellitus	1
Prior stroke/TIA	2
Vascular disease	1
Age 65–74 yr	1
Sex (female)	1

Table 76–7. HAS-BLED TOOL FOR PREDICTING RISK OF BLEEDING IN PATIENTS WITH ATRIAL FIBRILLATION

VARIABLE	POINTS
Uncontrolled hypertension	1
Abnormal kidney function	1
Abnormal liver function	1
Prior stroke	1
Prior bleeding	1
Labile INRs if being treated with warfarin (defined as a time in the therapeutic range less than 60%)	1
Elderly (> 65 yr)	1
Drug use (defined as concomitant use of an NSAID or an antiplatelet drug)	1
Alcohol use (defined as > 8 alcohol units per week)	1

KEY POINTS

- AF is an irregularly irregular atrial rhythm that may be episodic or continuous; paroxysms of tachycardia may occur.
- QRS complexes should be narrow; a wide complex occurs with intraventricular conduction defects or WPW syndrome.
- Patients should have echocardiography and thyroid function testing.
- Heart rate is controlled (typically to < 100 beats/min at rest); first-line drugs include beta-blockers and nondihydropyridine calcium channel blockers (eg, verapamil, diltiazem).
- Restoration of sinus rhythm is not as important as rate control and does not eliminate the need for anticoagulation but may help patients with continuing symptoms or hemodynamic compromise (eg, heart failure); synchronized cardioversion or drugs can be used.
- Anticoagulation is usually necessary before cardioversion.
- Long-term oral anticoagulation to prevent stroke is required for patients with risk factors for thromboembolism; aspirin is used for those with no risk factors.

ATRIAL FIBRILLATION AND WOLFF-PARKINSON-WHITE SYNDROME

AF is a medical emergency when rapid antegrade conduction over an accessory pathway occurs in WPW syndrome.

In manifest WPW syndrome, antegrade conduction occurs over the accessory pathway. If AF develops, the normal rate-limiting effects of the AV node are bypassed, and the resultant excessive ventricular rates (sometimes 200 to 240 beats/min) may lead to ventricular fibrillation (VF) (see Fig. 76–5) and sudden death. Patients with concealed WPW syndrome are not at risk because in them, antegrade conduction does not occur over the accessory connection.

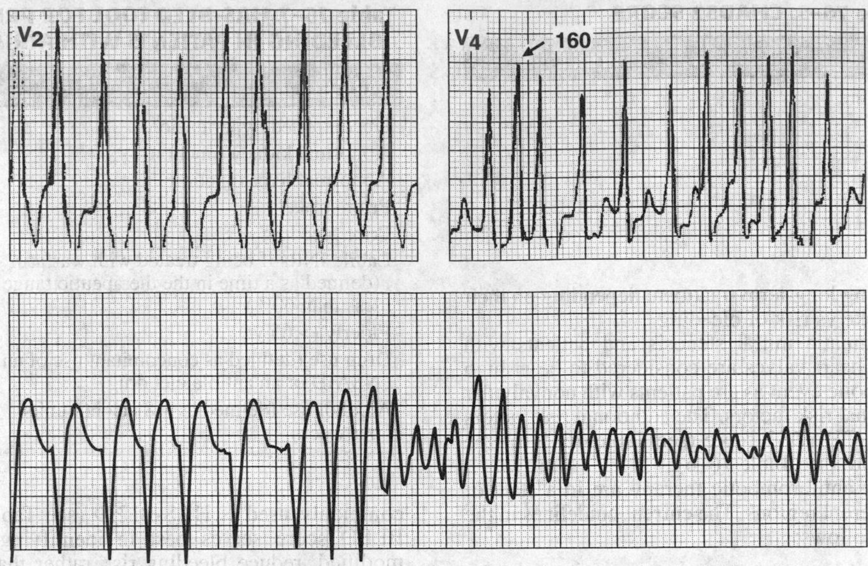

Fig. 76–5. Atrial fibrillation in Wolff-Parkinson-White syndrome. Ventricular response is very fast (RR intervals minimum of 160 msec). Shortly thereafter, ventricular fibrillation develops (lead II continuous rhythm strip at bottom).

PEARLS & PITFALLS

- Do not give digoxin or nondihydropyridine calcium channel blockers (eg, verapamil, diltiazem) to patients with atrial fibrillation and WPW because these drugs may trigger ventricular fibrillation.

Treatment

The treatment of choice is direct-current cardioversion. The usual rate-slowing drugs used in AF are not effective, and digoxin and the nondihydropyridine calcium channel blockers (eg, verapamil, diltiazem) are contraindicated because they may increase the ventricular rate and cause VF. If cardioversion is impossible, drugs that prolong the refractory period of the accessory connection should be used. IV procainamide or amiodarone is preferred, but any class Ia, class Ic, or class III antiarrhythmic can be used.

ATRIAL FLUTTER

Atrial flutter is a rapid regular atrial rhythm due to an atrial macroreentrant circuit. Symptoms include palpitations and sometimes weakness, effort intolerance, dyspnea, and presyncope. Atrial thrombi may form and embolize. Diagnosis is by ECG. Treatment involves rate control with drugs, prevention of thromboembolism with anticoagulants, and often conversion to sinus rhythm with drugs, cardioversion, or atrial flutter substrate ablation.

Atrial flutter is much less common than atrial fibrillation (AF), but its causes and hemodynamic consequences are similar. Many patients with atrial flutter also have periods of AF.

Typical atrial flutter is due to a large reentrant circuit involving most of the right atrium. The atria depolarize at a rate of 250 to 350 beats/min (typically 300 beats/min). Because the AV node cannot usually conduct at this rate, typically half of the impulses get through (2:1 block), resulting in a regular ventricular rate of 150 beats/min. Sometimes the block varies from moment to moment, causing an irregular ventricular rhythm. Less commonly, a fixed 3:1, 4:1, or 5:1 block may be present.

The probability of a thromboembolic event, once considered rare in atrial flutter, is now thought to be about half of that in AF (unless AF is also occurring).

Symptoms and Signs

Symptoms depend primarily on ventricular rate and the nature of any underlying heart disorder. If ventricular rate is < 120 beats/min and regular, there are likely to be few or no symptoms. Faster rates and variable AV conduction usually cause palpitations, and decreased cardiac output may cause symptoms of hemodynamic compromise (eg, chest discomfort, dyspnea, weakness, syncope). Close inspection of the jugular venous pulse reveals flutter *a* waves.

Diagnosis

- ECG

The diagnosis is by ECG. In typical flutter, ECG shows continuous and regular atrial activation with a sawtooth pattern, most obvious in leads II, III, and aVF (see Fig. 76–6).

Carotid sinus massage can increase AV block and better expose the typical flutter waves. A similar response may follow pharmacologic AV nodal blockade (eg, with adenosine), but such therapy does not terminate atrial flutter.

Treatment

- Rate control with drugs
- Rhythm control with cardioversion, drugs, or ablation
- Prevention of thromboembolism

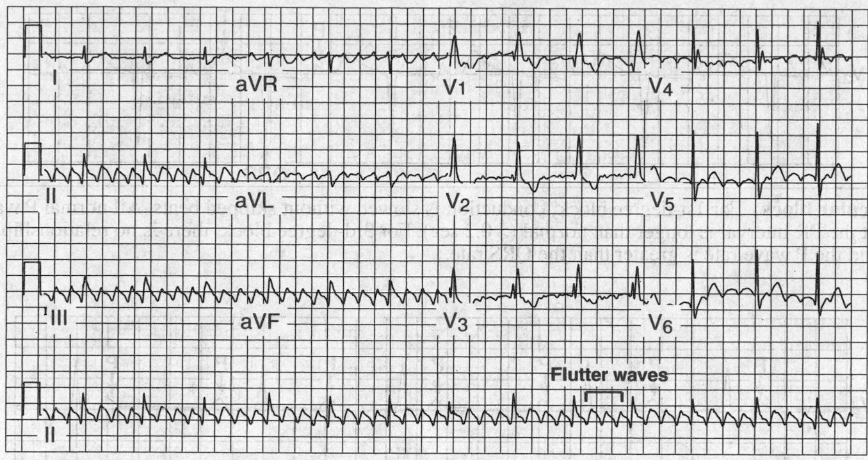

Fig. 76–6. Atrial flutter. (Note: Conducted with right bundle branch block.)

Treatment focuses on ventricular rate control, rhythm control, and prevention of thromboembolism. However, pharmacologic rate control is more difficult to achieve in atrial flutter than in AF. Thus, for most patients, electrical conversion (using synchronized cardioversion or overdrive pacing) is the treatment of choice for an initial episode and is mandatory with 1:1 AV conduction or hemodynamic compromise. Typically, low-energy (50 joules) conversion is effective. Anticoagulation, as in AF, is necessary before cardioversion.

If drugs are used to restore sinus rhythm, rate must first be controlled with beta-blockers or nondihydropyridine calcium channel blockers (eg, verapamil, diltiazem). Many of the antiarrhythmics that can restore sinus rhythm (especially class Ia and Ic) can slow atrial flutter, shorten AV nodal refractoriness (by their vagolytic effects), or do both enough to allow 1:1 conduction with paradoxical increase in ventricular rate and hemodynamic compromise. These drugs may be used for long-term maintenance as required to prevent recurrence.

An antitachycardia pacing system is an alternative to long-term use of antiarrhythmics in selected patients. Also, ablation procedures designed to interrupt the atrial reentrant circuit may effectively prevent atrial flutter, particularly typical atrial flutter.

Patients with chronic or recurrent atrial flutter require an oral anticoagulant (warfarin titrated to an INR of 2 to 3, a direct thrombin inhibitor, or a factor Xa inhibitor) or aspirin therapy long-term. The choice among the therapies is based on the same considerations as for AF.

KEY POINTS

- Atrial flutter is a rapid, regular atrial rhythm that rarely may cause an irregular or nontachycardic QRS response, depending on the degree and type of block present.
- After initial rate control with drugs such as beta-blockers and nondihydropyridine calcium channel blockers (eg, verapamil, diltiazem), most patients should have synchronized cardioversion.
- Anticoagulation is necessary before cardioversion.
- Long-term oral anticoagulation to prevent stroke is required for patients with chronic or recurrent atrial flutter.

ATRIOVENTRICULAR BLOCK

AV block is partial or complete interruption of impulse transmission from the atria to the ventricles. The most common cause is idiopathic fibrosis and sclerosis of the conduction system. Diagnosis is by ECG; symptoms and treatment depend on degree of block, but treatment, when necessary, usually involves pacing.

The **most common causes of AV block** are

- Idiopathic fibrosis and sclerosis of the conduction system (about 50% of patients)
- Ischemic heart disease (40%)

The remaining cases of AV block are caused by

- Drugs (eg, beta-blockers, calcium channel blockers, digoxin, amiodarone)
- Increased vagal tone
- Valvulopathy
- Congenital heart, genetic, or other disorders

AV block may be partial or complete. First-degree and second-degree blocks are partial. Third degree blocks are complete.

First-degree AV block: All normal P waves are followed by QRS complexes, but the PR interval is longer than normal (> 0.20 sec—see Fig. 76–7).

First-degree AV block may be physiologic in younger patients with high vagal tone and in well-trained athletes. First-degree AV block is rarely symptomatic and no treatment is required, but further investigation may be indicated when it accompanies another heart disorder or appears to be caused by drugs.

Second-degree AV block: Some normal P waves are followed by QRS complexes, but some are not. Three types exist.

In **Mobitz type I** 2nd-degree AV block, the PR interval progressively lengthens with each beat until the atrial impulse is not conducted and the QRS complex is dropped (Wenckebach phenomenon); AV nodal conduction resumes with the next beat, and the sequence is repeated (see Fig. 76–8).

Mobitz type I 2nd-degree AV block may be physiologic in younger and more athletic patients. The block occurs at the AV node in about 75% of patients with a narrow QRS complex and

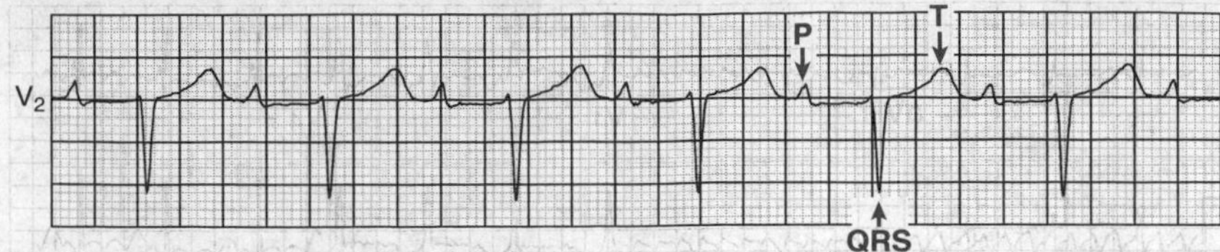

Fig. 76–7. Atrioventricular block. For 1st-degree block, conduction is slowed without skipped beats. All normal P waves are followed by QRS complexes, but the PR interval is longer than normal (> 0.2 sec). For 3rd-degree block, there is no relationship between P waves and QRS complexes, and the P wave rate is greater than the QRS rate.

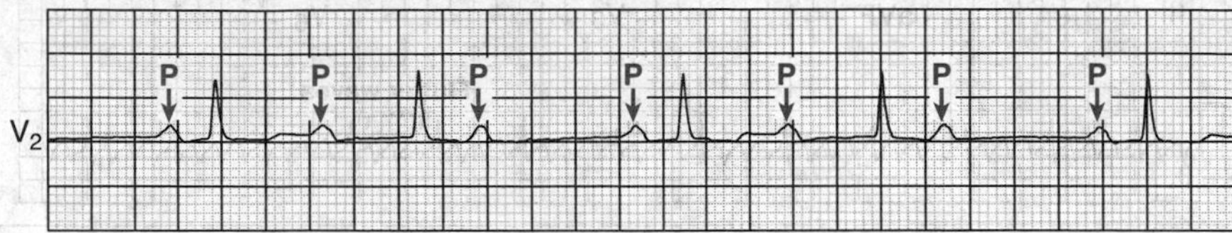

Fig. 76–8. Mobitz type I 2nd-degree atrioventricular block. The PR interval progressively lengthens with each beat until the atrial impulse is not conducted and the QRS complex is dropped (Wenckebach phenomenon); AV nodal conduction resumes with the next beat, and the sequence is repeated.

at infranodal sites (His bundle, bundle branches, or fascicles) in the rest. If the block becomes complete, a reliable junctional escape rhythm typically develops. Treatment is therefore unnecessary unless the block causes symptomatic bradycardia and transient or reversible causes have been excluded. Treatment is pacemaker insertion, which may also benefit asymptomatic patients with Mobitz type I 2nd-degree AV block at infranodal sites detected by electrophysiologic studies done for other reasons.

In **Mobitz type II** 2nd-degree AV block, the PR interval remains constant. Beats are intermittently nonconducted and QRS complexes dropped, usually in a repeating cycle of every 3rd (3:1 block) or 4th (4:1 block) P wave (see Fig. 76–9).

Mobitz type II 2nd-degree AV block is always pathologic; the block occurs at the His bundle in 20% of patients and in the bundle branches in the rest. Patients may be asymptomatic or experience light-headedness, presyncope, and syncope, depending on the ratio of conducted to blocked beats. Patients are at risk of developing symptomatic high-grade or complete AV block, in which the escape rhythm is likely to be ventricular and thus too slow and unreliable to maintain systemic perfusion; therefore, a pacemaker is indicated.

In high-grade 2nd-degree AV block, every 2nd (or more) P wave is blocked (see Fig. 76–10).

The distinction between Mobitz type I and Mobitz type II block is difficult to make because 2 P waves are never conducted in a row. Risk of complete AV block is difficult to predict, and a pacemaker is indicated.

Patients with any form of 2nd-degree AV block and a structural heart disorder should be considered candidates for permanent pacing unless there is a transient or reversible cause.

Third-degree AV block: Heart block is complete (see Fig. 76–11).

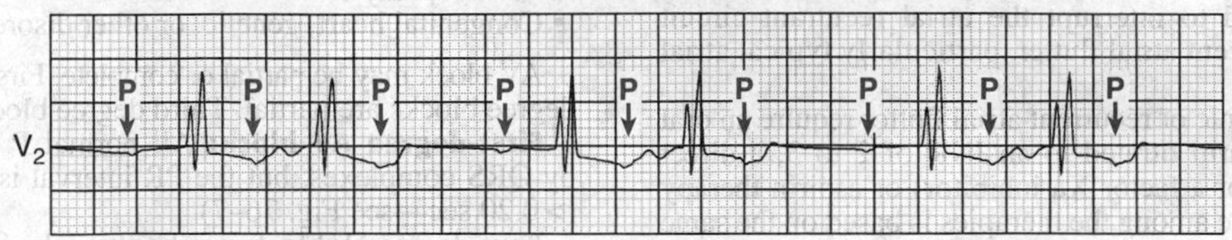

Fig. 76–9. Mobitz type II 2nd-degree atrioventricular block. The PR interval remains constant. Beats are intermittently nonconducted, and QRS complexes dropped, usually in a repeating cycle of every 3rd (3:1 block) or 4th (4:1 block) P wave.

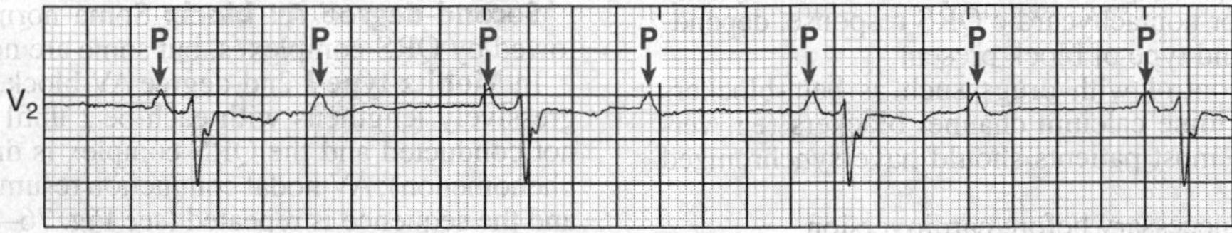

Fig. 76–10. Second-degree atrioventricular block (high grade).

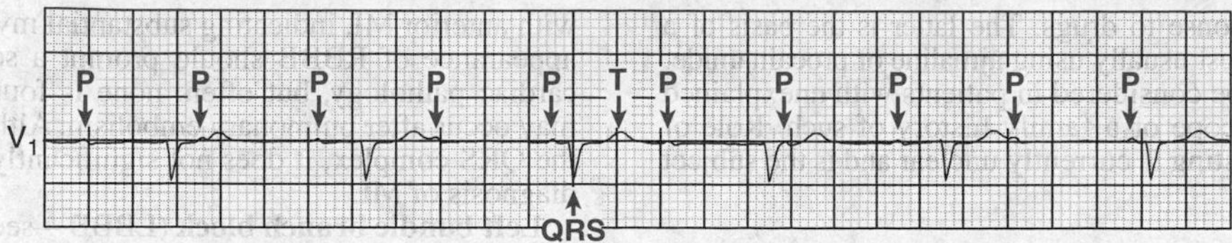

Fig. 76–11. Third-degree atrioventricular block.

There is no electrical communication between the atria and ventricles and no relationship between P waves and QRS complexes (AV dissociation). Cardiac function is maintained by an escape junctional or ventricular pacemaker. Escape rhythms originating above the bifurcation of the His bundle produce narrow QRS complexes, relatively rapid (> 40 beats/min) and reliable heart rates, and mild symptoms (eg, fatigue, postural light-headedness, effort intolerance). Escape rhythms originating below the bifurcation produce wider QRS complexes, slower and unreliable heart rates, and more severe symptoms (eg, presyncope, syncope, heart failure). Signs include those of AV dissociation, such as cannon *a* waves, BP fluctuations, and changes in loudness of the 1st heart sound (S_1). Risk of asystole-related syncope and sudden death is greater if low escape rhythms are present.

Most patients require a pacemaker (see Table 76–3 on p. 633). If the block is caused by antiarrhythmic drugs, stopping the drug may be effective, although temporary pacing may be needed. A block caused by acute inferior MI usually reflects AV nodal dysfunction and may respond to atropine or resolve spontaneously over several days. A block caused by anterior MI usually reflects extensive myocardial necrosis involving the His-Purkinje system and requires immediate transvenous pacemaker insertion with interim external pacing as necessary. Spontaneous resolution may occur but warrants evaluation of AV nodal and infranodal conduction (eg, electrophysiologic study, exercise testing, 24-h ECG).

Most patients with congenital 3rd-degree AV block have a junctional escape rhythm that maintains a reasonable rate, but they require a permanent pacemaker before they reach middle age. Less commonly, patients with congenital AV block have a slow escape rhythm and require a permanent pacemaker at a young age, perhaps even during infancy.

BRUGADA SYNDROME

Brugada syndrome is an inherited disorder of cardiac electrophysiology causing an increased risk of syncope and sudden death.

Several different mutations are involved, most affecting the *SCN5A* gene that encodes the α-subunit of the voltage-dependent cardiac sodium channel. Typically, patients have no structural heart disease. Nevertheless, relationships with other genetic and acquired structural heart diseases are increasingly being recognized, as are overlap syndromes with long QT syndrome type 3 and with arrhythmogenic right ventricular dysplasia (ARVD).

In some patients, Brugada syndrome has no clinical expression. However, in many patients it leads to syncope or sudden cardiac death due to polymorphic VT and VF. Events occur more often at night and are not usually related to exercise. Events may also be brought on by fever and by treatment with certain drugs including sodium channel blockers, beta-blockers, tricyclic antidepressants, lithium, and cocaine.

Diagnosis

- ECG

Initial diagnosis of Brugada syndrome is based on a characteristic ECG pattern (type 1 Brugada ECG pattern—see Fig. 76–12) with prominent ST elevation in V_1 and V_2 (sometimes involving V_3) that causes the QRS complex in these leads to resemble RBBB. The ST segment is coved and descends to an inverted T-wave. Lesser degrees of these patterns (type 2 and type 3 Brugada ECG patterns) are not considered diagnostic. The type 2 and type 3 patterns may change to a type 1 pattern spontaneously,

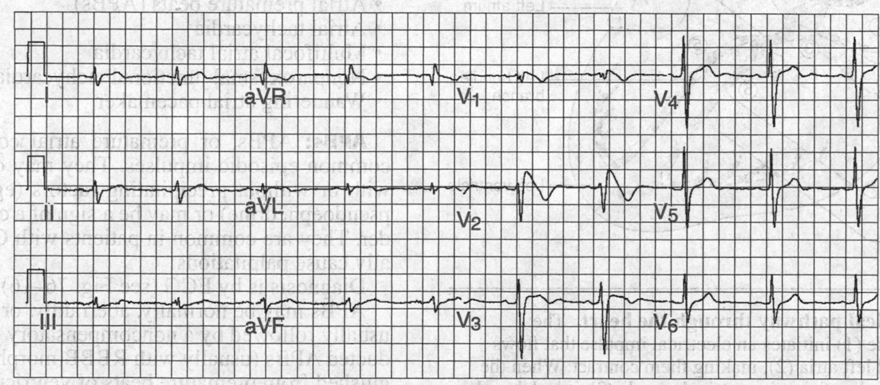

Fig. 76–12. Type 1 Brugada syndrome. Prominent J-point elevation to a coved ST segment, leading to an inverted T-wave in leads V_1 and V_2.

with fever, or in response to drugs. The latter is the basis of a challenge diagnostic test usually using ajmaline or procainamide.

Diagnosis should be considered in patients with unexplained cardiac arrest or syncope or a family history of such. Role of electrophysiologic testing is currently unclear and is the subject of ongoing study.

Treatment

- ICD

Patients presenting with syncope and patients resuscitated from arrest should receive an ICD. Best treatment of Brugada syndrome in patients diagnosed based on ECG changes and family history is unclear, although they do have increased risk of sudden death.

BUNDLE BRANCH AND FASCICULAR BLOCK

Bundle branch block is partial or complete interruption of impulse conduction in a bundle branch; fascicular block is similar interruption in a hemifascicle of the bundle. The 2 disorders often coexist. There are usually no symptoms, but presence of either suggests a heart disorder. Diagnosis is by ECG. No specific treatment is indicated.

Conduction blocks can be caused by many heart disorders, including intrinsic degeneration without another associated heart disorder.

Right bundle branch block (RBBB—see Figs. 76–13 and 76–14) can occur in apparently normal people. It may also occur with anterior MI, indicating substantial myocardial injury. New appearance of RBBB should prompt a search for underlying cardiac pathology, but often, none is found. Transient RBBB may occur after pulmonary embolism. Although RBBB distorts the QRS complex, it does not significantly interfere with ECG diagnosis of MI.

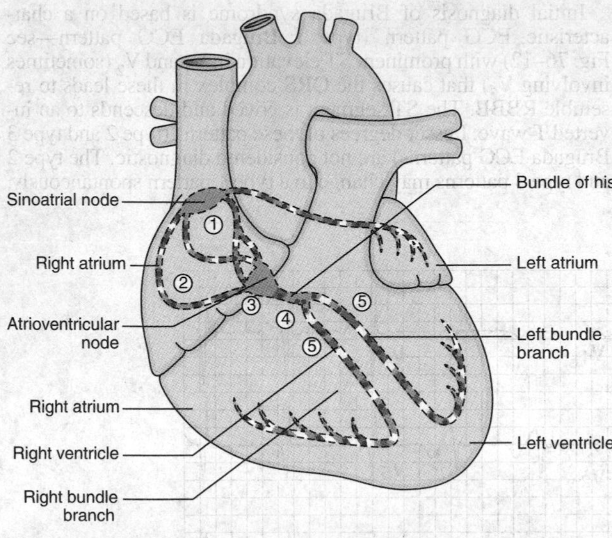

Fig. 76–13. Electrical pathway through the heart. The sinoatrial (sinus) node (1) initiates an electrical impulse that flows through the right and left atria (2), making them contract. When the electrical impulse reaches the atrioventricular node (3), it is delayed slightly. The impulse then travels down the bundle of His (4), which divides into the right bundle branch for the right ventricle (5), and the left bundle branch for the left ventricle (5). The impulse then spreads through the ventricle, making them contract.

Left bundle branch block (LBBB—see Fig. 76–15) is associated with a structural heart disorder more often than is RBBB. LBBB usually precludes use of ECG for diagnosis of MI.

Fascicular block involves the anterior or posterior fascicle of the left bundle branch. Interruption of the left anterior fascicle causes left anterior hemiblock characterized by modest QRS prolongation (< 120 msec) and a frontal plane QRS axis more negative than −30° (left axis deviation). Left posterior hemiblock is associated with a frontal plane QRS axis more positive than +120°. The associations between hemiblocks and a structural heart disorder are the same as for LBBB.

Hemiblocks may coexist with other conduction disturbances: RBBB and left anterior or posterior hemiblock (bifascicular block); and left anterior or posterior hemiblock, RBBB, and 1st-degree AV block (incorrectly called trifascicular block; 1st-degree block is usually AV nodal in origin).

Trifascicular block refers to RBBB with alternating left anterior and left posterior hemiblock or alternating LBBB and RBBB. Presence of bifascicular or trifascicular block after MI implies extensive cardiac damage. Bifascicular blocks require no direct treatment unless intermittent 2nd- or 3rd-degree AV block is present. True trifascicular blocks require immediate, then permanent pacing.

Nonspecific intraventricular conduction defects are diagnosed when the QRS complex is prolonged (> 120 msec), but the QRS pattern is not typical of LBBB or RBBB. The conduction delay may occur beyond the Purkinje fibers and result from slow cell-to-cell myocyte conduction.

No specific treatment is indicated.

ECTOPIC SUPRAVENTRICULAR RHYTHMS

Various rhythms result from supraventricular foci (usually in the atria); many are asymptomatic and require no treatment.

Ectopic supraventricular rhythms include

- Atrial premature beats (APBs)
- Atrial tachycardia
- Multifocal atrial tachycardia
- Nonparoxysmal junctional tachycardia
- Wandering atrial pacemaker

APBs: APBs, or premature atrial contractions (PAC), are common episodic impulses. They may occur in normal hearts with or without precipitating factors (eg, coffee, tea, alcohol, pseudoephedrine) or may be a sign of a cardiopulmonary disorder. They are common in patients with COPD. They occasionally cause palpitations.

Diagnosis is by ECG (see Fig. 76–16).

APBs may be normally, aberrantly, or not conducted and are usually followed by a noncompensatory pause. Aberrantly conducted APBs (usually with RBBB morphology) must be distinguished from premature beats of ventricular origin.

Atrial escape beats are ectopic atrial beats that emerge after long sinus pauses or sinus arrest. They may be single or multiple; escape beats from a single focus may produce a continuous rhythm (called ectopic atrial rhythm). Heart rate is typically

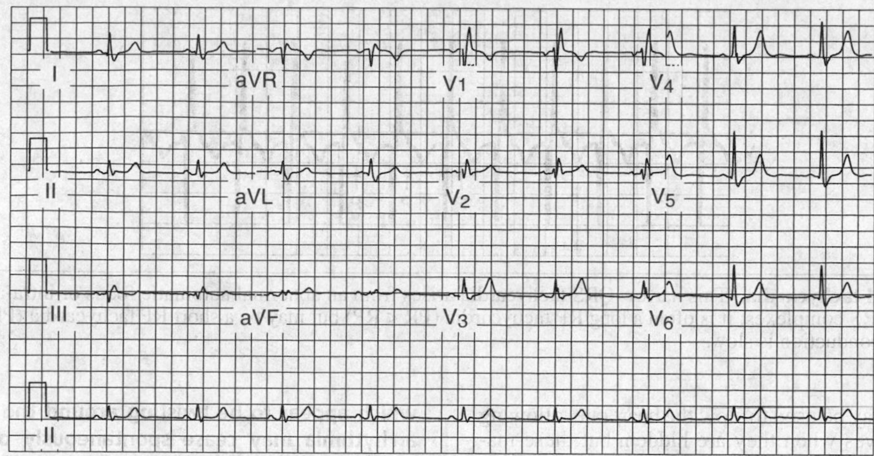

Fig. 76–14. Right bundle branch block.

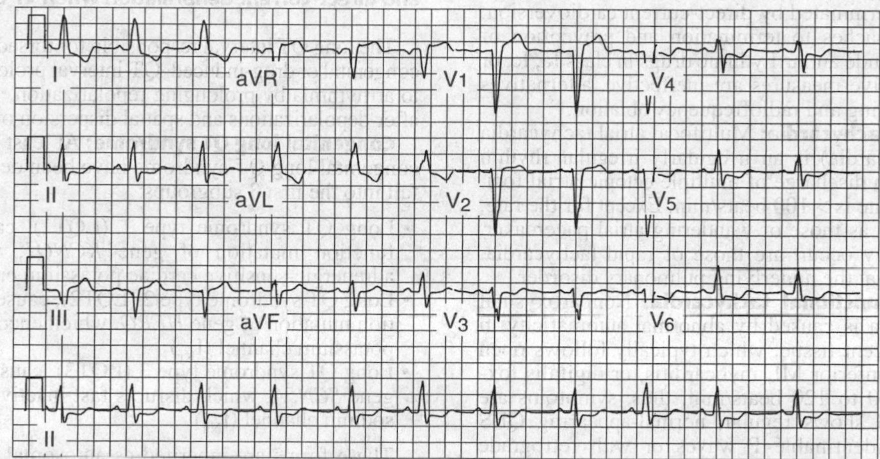

Fig. 76–15. Left bundle branch block.

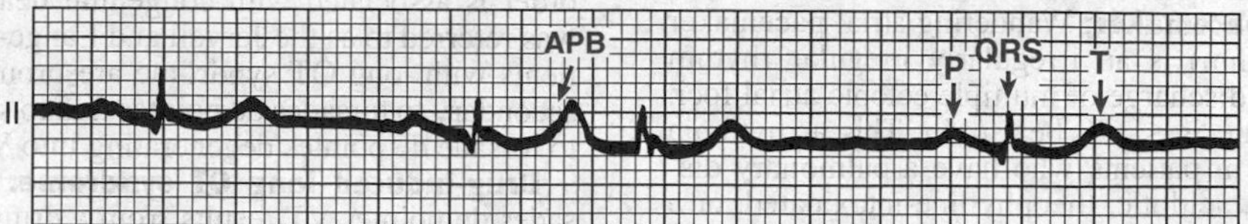

Fig. 76–16. Atrial premature beat (APB). In lead II, after the 2nd beat of sinus origin, the T wave is deformed by an APB. Because the APB occurs relatively early during the sinus cycle, the sinus node pacemaker is reset, and a pause—less than fully compensatory—precedes the next sinus beat.

slower, P wave morphology is typically different, and PR interval is slightly shorter than in sinus rhythm.

Atrial tachycardia: Atrial tachycardia is a regular rhythm caused by the consistent, rapid atrial activation from a single atrial focus. Heart rate is usually 150 to 200 beats/min; however, with a very rapid atrial rate, nodal dysfunction, or digitalis toxicity, AV block may be present, and ventricular rate may be slower. Mechanisms include enhanced atrial automaticity and intra-atrial reentry.

Atrial tachycardia is the least common form (5%) of SVT and usually occurs in patients with a structural heart disorder. Other causes include atrial irritation (eg, pericarditis), drugs (eg, digoxin), alcohol, and toxic gas inhalation.

Symptoms are those of other tachycardias.

Diagnosis is by ECG; P waves, which differ in morphology from normal sinus P waves, precede QRS complexes but may be hidden within the preceding T wave (see Fig. 76–17).

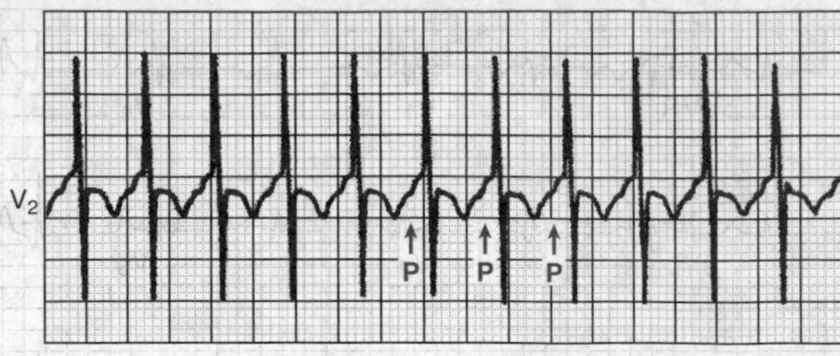

Fig. 76–17. True atrial tachycardia. This narrow QRS tachycardia arises from an abnormal automatic focus or intra-atrial reentry. P waves precede the QRS complexes; it is often a long RP tachycardia (PR < RP) but may be a short RP tachycardia (PR > RP) if atrioventricular nodal conduction is slow.

Vagal maneuvers may be used to slow the heart rate, allowing visualization of P waves when they are hidden, but these maneuvers do not usually terminate the arrhythmia (demonstrating that the AV node is not an obligate part of the arrhythmia circuit). Treatment involves managing causes and slowing ventricular response rate using a beta-blocker or calcium channel blocker. An episode may be terminated by direct-current cardioversion. Pharmacologic approaches to termination and prevention of atrial tachycardia include antiarrhythmic drugs in class Ia, Ic, or III. If these noninvasive measures are ineffective, alternatives include overdrive pacing and radiofrequency ablation.

Multifocal atrial tachycardia: Multifocal atrial tachycardia (chaotic atrial tachycardia) is an irregularly irregular rhythm caused by the random discharge of multiple ectopic atrial foci. By definition, heart rate is > 100 beats/min. Except for the rate, features are the same as those of wandering atrial pacemaker. Symptoms, when they occur, are those of rapid tachycardia. Treatment is directed at the underlying pulmonary disorder.

Nonparoxysmal junctional tachycardia: Nonparoxysmal junctional tachycardia is caused by abnormal automaticity in the AV node or adjacent tissue, which typically follows open heart surgery, acute inferior MI, myocarditis, or digitalis toxicity. Heart rate is 60 to 120 beats/min; thus, symptoms are usually absent. ECG shows regular, normal-appearing QRS complexes without identifiable P waves or with retrograde P waves (inverted in the inferior leads) that occur shortly before (< 0.1 sec) or after the QRS complex. The rhythm is distinguished from paroxysmal SVT by the lower heart rate and gradual onset and offset. Treatment is directed at causes.

Wandering atrial pacemaker: Wandering atrial pacemaker (multifocal atrial rhythm) is an irregularly irregular rhythm caused by the random discharge of multiple ectopic atrial foci. By definition, heart rate is ≤ 100 beats/min. This arrhythmia most typically occurs in patients who have a pulmonary disorder and are hypoxic, acidotic, theophylline-intoxicated, or a combination. On ECG, P-wave morphology differs from beat to beat, and there are ≥ 3 distinct P-wave morphologies. The presence of P waves distinguishes wandering atrial pacemaker from AF.

LONG QT SYNDROME AND TORSADES DE POINTES VENTRICULAR TACHYCARDIA

Torsades de pointes is a specific form of polymorphic ventricular tachycardia (VT) in patients with a long QT interval. It is characterized by rapid, irregular QRS complexes, which appear to be twisting around the ECG baseline. This arrhythmia may cease spontaneously or degenerate into ventricular fibrillation (VF). It causes significant hemodynamic compromise and often death. Diagnosis is by ECG. Treatment is with IV magnesium, measures to shorten the QT interval, and direct-current defibrillation when VF is precipitated.

The long QT interval responsible for torsades de pointes can be congenital or drug-induced. QT-interval prolongation predisposes to arrhythmia by prolonging repolarization, which induces early after-depolarizations and spatial dispersion of refractoriness.

Congenital long QT syndrome: At least 10 distinct forms of congenital long QT syndrome have been described. Most cases fall into the first 3 subgroups:

- Long QT syndrome type 1 (LQT1), caused by a loss of function mutation of gene *KCNQ1*, which encodes an adrenergic-sensitive cardiac potassium current I_{Ks}
- Long QT syndrome type 2 (LQT2), caused by a loss of function mutation of gene *HERG*, which encodes another cardiac potassium channel (I_{Kr})
- Long QT syndrome type 3 (LQT3), caused by a mutation in gene *SCN5A*, which disrupts fast inactivation of the cardiac sodium channel (I_{Na})

These forms are inherited as autosomal dominant disorders with incomplete penetrance and, in the past, were referred to as Romano-Ward syndrome. In rare patients with 2 abnormal copies of the genetic abnormality (particularly LQT1), the disorder is associated with congenital deafness and, in the past, was referred to as the Jervell and Lange-Nielsen syndrome. Patients with long QT syndrome are prone to recurrent syncope secondary to torsades de pointes and to sudden death secondary to torsade de pointes degenerating into VF.

Drug-induced long QT syndrome: More commonly, torsades de pointes VT results from a drug, usually a class Ia, Ic, or III antiarrhythmic. Other drugs that can induce torsades de pointes VT include tricyclic antidepressants, phenothiazines, and certain antivirals and antifungals.

Symptoms and Signs

Patients often present with syncope because the underlying rate (200 to 250 beats/min) is nonperfusing. Palpitations are common among conscious patients. Sometimes the long QT interval is detected after resuscitation.

Diagnosis

- ECG

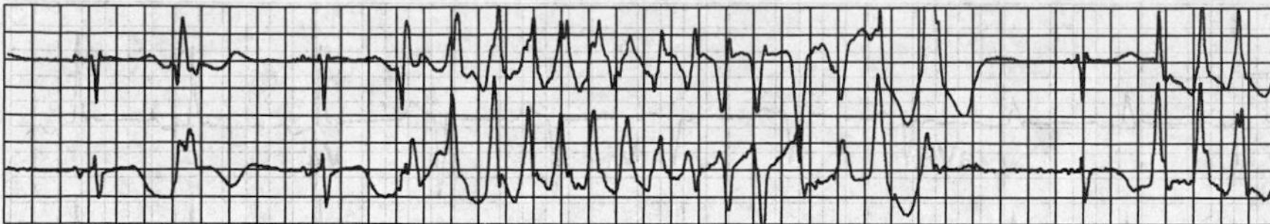

Fig. 76–18. **Torsades de pointes ventricular tachycardia.**

Diagnosis is by ECG showing an undulating QRS axis, with the polarity of complexes shifting around the baseline (see Fig. 76–18). ECG between episodes shows a long QT interval after correction for heart rate (QTc). Normal values average about 0.44 sec, although they vary among individuals and by sex. A family history may suggest a congenital syndrome.

Treatment

- Usually unsynchronized direct-current cardioversion
- Sometimes magnesium sulfate ($MgSO_4$) IV

An acute episode prolonged enough to cause hemodynamic compromise is treated with unsynchronized cardioversion, beginning with 100 joules. Nevertheless, early recurrence is the rule. Patients often respond to magnesium, usually $MgSO_4$ 2 g IV over 1 to 2 min. If this treatment is unsuccessful, a 2nd bolus is given in 5 to 10 min, and a magnesium infusion of 3 to 20 mg/min may be started in patients without renal insufficiency. Lidocaine (a class Ib antiarrhythmic) shortens the QT interval and may be effective especially for drug-induced torsades de pointes. Class Ia, Ic, and III antiarrhythmics are avoided.

If a drug is the cause, it is stopped, but until drug clearance is complete, patients with frequent or long runs of torsades de pointes VT require treatment to shorten the QT interval. Because increasing the heart rate shortens the QT interval, temporary pacing, IV isoproterenol, or both are often effective.

Long-term treatment is required for patients with a congenital long QT-interval syndrome. Treatment choices include beta-blockers, permanent pacing, ICD, or a combination. Family members should be evaluated by ECG.

Patients with congenital long QT syndrome should clearly avoid drugs that prolong the QT interval, and patients with exercise-related symptoms (usually LQT1 or LQT2) should avoid strenuous exercise. Treatment options include beta-blockers, pacing to maintain faster heart rates (which shortens the QT interval), and the ICD, alone or in combinations. Current guidelines recommend the ICD for patients resuscitated from cardiac arrest and those with syncope despite beta-blocker treatment.

KEY POINTS

- The long QT interval responsible for torsades de pointes VT can be congenital or drug-induced.
- Immediate treatment of torsades is unsynchronized cardioversion beginning with 100 joules, although some patients respond to $MgSO_4$ 2 g IV over 1 to 2 min.
- Patients with the congenital syndrome require long-term treatment with beta-blockers, permanent pacing, an ICD, or a combination.
- Family members should be evaluated by ECG.

REENTRANT SUPRAVENTRICULAR TACHYCARDIAS

Reentrant SVTs involve reentrant pathways with a component above the bifurcation of the His bundle. Patients have sudden episodes of palpitations that begin and terminate abruptly; some have dyspnea or chest discomfort. Diagnosis is clinical and by ECG. Treatment is with vagotonic maneuvers and, if they are ineffective, with IV adenosine or nondihydropyridine calcium channel blockers for narrow QRS rhythms or for wide QRS rhythms known to be a reentrant SVT with aberrant conduction that requires AV nodal conduction, procainamide or amiodarone for other wide QRS rhythms, or synchronized cardioversion for all cases.

Pathophysiology

The reentry pathway (see Fig. 76–1 on p. 622) in SVT is within the

- AV node (about 50%)
- Accessory bypass tract (40%)
- Atria or SA node (10%)

AV nodal reentrant tachycardia occurs most often in otherwise healthy patients. It is most commonly triggered by an atrial premature beat.

Accessory pathway reentrant tachycardia involves tracts of conducting tissue that partially or totally bypass normal AV connections (bypass tracts). They run most commonly from the atria directly to the ventricles and less commonly from the atrium to a portion of the conduction system or from a portion of the conduction system to the ventricle. They can be triggered by APBs or ventricular premature beats.

Wolff-Parkinson-White (WPW) syndrome: WPW (preexcitation) syndrome is the most common accessory pathway SVT, occurring in about 1 to 3/1000 people. WPW syndrome is mainly idiopathic, although it is more common among patients with hypertrophic or other forms of cardiomyopathy, transposition of the great vessels, or Epstein anomaly. There are two main forms of WPW syndrome:

- Classic
- Concealed

In **classic (or manifest) WPW syndrome,** antegrade conduction occurs over both the accessory pathway and the normal conducting system during sinus rhythm. The accessory pathway, being faster, depolarizes some of the ventricle early, resulting in a short PR interval and a slurred upstroke to the QRS complex (delta wave—see Fig. 76–19).

The delta wave prolongs QRS duration to > 0.12 sec, although the overall configuration, apart from the delta wave, may appear normal. Depending on the orientation of the delta

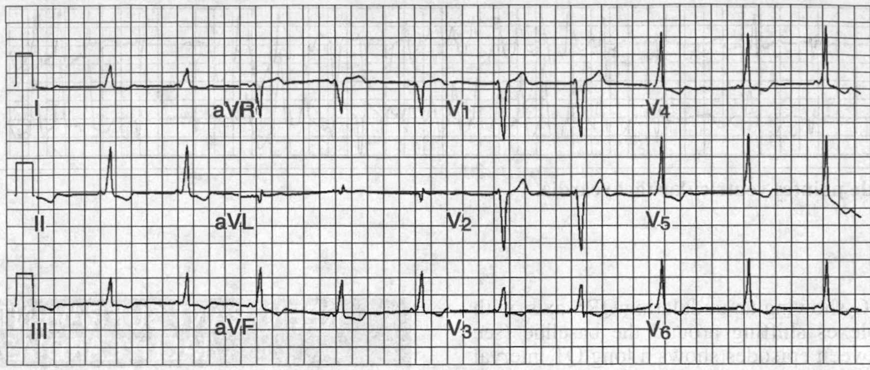

Fig. 76–19. Classic Wolff-Parkinson-White syndrome. Leads I, II, III, V_3 through V_6 show classic features of WPW syndrome, with a short PR interval and a delta wave during sinus rhythm.

wave, a pseudoinfarction pattern Q-wave may be present. Because the early depolarized parts of the ventricle also repolarize early, the T-wave vector may be abnormal.

In **concealed WPW syndrome,** the accessory pathway does not conduct in an antegrade direction; consequently, the above ECG abnormalities do not appear. However, it conducts in a retrograde direction and thus can participate in reentrant tachycardia.

In the most common form of reentrant tachycardia (called orthodromic reciprocating tachycardia), the circuit uses the normal AV conduction pathway to activate the ventricles, returning to the atrium via the accessory AV connection. The resultant QRS complex is thus narrow (unless bundle branch block coexists) and without a delta wave. Orthodromic reciprocating tachycardia is typically a short RP tachycardia with the retrograde P wave in the ST segment.

Rarely, the reentrant circuit revolves in the opposite direction, from the atrium to the ventricle via the accessory AV connection, and returns from the ventricle in the retrograde direction up the normal AV conduction system (called antidromic reciprocating tachycardia). The QRS complex is wide because the ventricles are activated abnormally. In patients with 2 accessory AV connections (not uncommon), a reciprocating tachycardia using one accessory connection in the antegrade direction and the other in the retrograde direction may occur.

Tachycardias in WPW syndrome may begin as or degenerate into atrial fibrillation (AF), which can be very dangerous. Enlarged atria due to hypertrophic cardiomyopathy and other forms of cardiomyopathy makes patients with WPW syndrome more prone to AF.

Symptoms and Signs

Most patients present during young adulthood or middle age. They typically have episodes of sudden-onset, sudden-offset, rapid, regular palpitations often associated with symptoms of hemodynamic compromise (eg, dyspnea, chest discomfort, light-headedness). Attacks may last only a few seconds or persist for several hours (rarely, > 12 h).

Infants present with episodic breathlessness, lethargy, feeding problems, or rapid precordial pulsations. If the episode of tachycardia is protracted, they may present with heart failure.

Examination is usually unremarkable except for a heart rate of 160 to 240 beats/min.

Diagnosis

- ECG

Diagnosis of SVT is by ECG showing rapid, regular tachycardia. Previous tracings, if available, are reviewed for signs of manifest WPW syndrome.

P waves vary. In most cases of AV node reentry, retrograde P waves are in the terminal portion of the QRS complex (often producing a pseudo-R′ deflection in lead V_1); about one-third occur just after the QRS complex, and very few occur before. P waves always follow the QRS complex in orthodromic reciprocating tachycardia of WPW syndrome (see Fig. 76–20).

QRS complex is narrow except with coexisting bundle branch block, antidromic tachycardia, or dual accessory connection reciprocating tachycardia. Wide-complex tachycardia must be distinguished from VT (see Fig 76.3 on p. 623).

PEARLS & PITFALLS

- Although most supraventricular tachycardias have a narrow QRS complex, some have a wide QRS complex and must be distinguished from ventricular tachycardia.

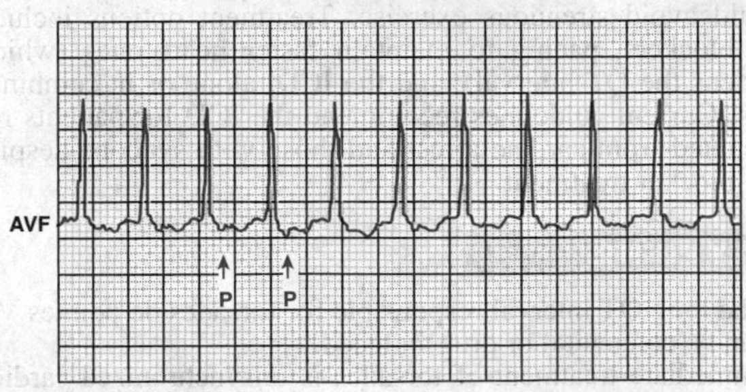

Fig. 76–20. Narrow QRS tachycardia: Orthodromic reciprocating tachycardia using an accessory pathway in Wolff-Parkinson-White syndrome. Activation is as follows: atrioventricular node, His-Purkinje system, ventricle, accessory pathway, atria. The P wave closely follows the QRS complex; it is a short RP tachycardia (PR > RP).

Treatment

- Vagotonic maneuvers
- Adenosine
- Verapamil or diltiazem if narrow QRS complex
- For frequent recurrence, radiofrequency ablation

Many episodes stop spontaneously before treatment.

Vagotonic maneuvers (eg, Valsalva maneuver, unilateral carotid sinus massage, ice water facial immersion, swallowing of ice-cold water), particularly if used early, may terminate the tachyarrhythmia; some patients use these maneuvers at home.

AV node blockers are used if vagotonic maneuvers are ineffective and the QRS complex is narrow (indicating orthodromic conduction); blocking conduction through the AV node for one beat interrupts the reentrant cycle. Adenosine is the first choice. Dose is 6 mg by rapid IV bolus (0.05 to 0.1 mg/kg in children), followed by a 20-mL saline bolus. If this dosage is ineffective, 2 subsequent 12-mg doses are given q 5 min. Adenosine sometimes causes a brief (2- to 3-sec) period of cardiac standstill, which may distress patient and physician. Verapamil 5 mg IV or diltiazem 0.25 to 0.35 mg/kg IV are alternatives.

For a regular, wide QRS complex tachycardia known to be an antidromic reciprocating tachycardia not involving double accessory pathways (which must be identified by the history; they cannot be established acutely), AV nodal blockers may also be effective. However, if the mechanism of the tachycardia is unknown and VT has not been excluded, AV nodal blockers should be avoided because they may worsen VTs. In such cases (or those in which drugs are ineffective), IV procainamide or amiodarone can be used. Alternatively, synchronized cardioversion with 50 joules (0.5 to 2 joules/kg for children) is quick and safe and may be preferred to these more toxic drugs.

When episodes of AV nodal reentrant tachycardia are frequent or bothersome, options include long-term antiarrhythmics or transvenous catheter radiofrequency ablation. Generally, ablation is recommended, but if it is not acceptable, drug prophylaxis usually begins with digoxin and proceeds, as required, to beta-blockers, nondihydropyridine calcium channel blockers, or both, then to one or more class Ia, class Ic, or class III antiarrhythmics. However, postadolescent patients with manifest WPW syndrome (in whom AF becomes more likely) should not receive digoxin or a nondihydropyridine calcium channel blocker alone (see p. 637).

KEY POINTS

- Symptoms begin and end suddenly.
- QRS complexes are typically narrow, rapid, and regular; however, wide complexes may occur and must be differentiated from VT.
- Vagotonic maneuvers (eg, Valsalva maneuver) sometimes help.
- Use AV nodal blockers for narrow complex tachycardia; adenosine is the first choice, and if ineffective, verapamil or diltiazem are alternatives.
- Avoid AV nodal blockers for wide complex tachycardia; use synchronized cardioversion or procainamide or amiodarone.

SINUS NODE DYSFUNCTION

(Sick Sinus Syndrome)

Sinus node dysfunction refers to a number of conditions causing physiologically inappropriate atrial rates. Symptoms may be minimal or include weakness, effort intolerance, palpitations, and syncope. Diagnosis is by ECG. Symptomatic patients require a pacemaker.

Sinus node dysfunction includes

- Inappropriate sinus bradycardia
- Alternating bradycardia and atrial tachyarrhythmias (bradycardia-tachycardia syndrome)
- Sinus pause or arrest
- SA exit block

Sinus node dysfunction affects mainly the elderly, especially those with another cardiac disorder or diabetes.

Sinus pause is temporary cessation of sinus node activity, seen on ECG as disappearance of P waves for seconds to minutes. The pause usually triggers escape activity in lower pacemakers (eg, atrial or junctional), preserving heart rate and function, but long pauses cause dizziness and syncope.

In **SA exit block,** the SA node depolarizes, but conduction of impulses to atrial tissue is impaired.

- In 1st-degree SA block, the SA node impulse is merely slowed, and ECG is normal.
- In type I 2nd-degree SA (SA Wenckebach) block, impulse conduction slows before blocking, seen on the ECG as a P-P interval that decreases progressively until the P wave drops altogether, creating a pause and the appearance of grouped beats; the duration of the pause is less than 2 P-P cycles.
- In type II 2nd-degree SA block, conduction of impulses is blocked without slowing beforehand, producing a pause that is a multiple (usually twice) of the P-P interval and the appearance of grouped beats.
- In 3rd-degree SA block, conduction is blocked; P waves are absent, giving the appearance of sinus arrest.

Etiology

The **most common cause** of sinus node dysfunction is idiopathic SA node fibrosis, which may be accompanied by degeneration of lower elements of the conducting system.

Other causes include drugs, excessive vagal tone, and many ischemic, inflammatory, and infiltrative disorders.

Symptoms and Signs

Many patients are asymptomatic, but depending on the heart rate, all the symptoms of bradycardias and tachycardias can occur.

Diagnosis

- ECG

A slow, irregular pulse suggests the diagnosis of sinus node dysfunction, which is confirmed by ECG, rhythm strip, or continuous 24-h ECG recording. Some patients present with atrial fibrillation (AF), and the underlying sinus node dysfunction manifests only after conversion to sinus rhythm.

Prognosis

Prognosis is mixed; without treatment, mortality is about 2%/yr, primarily resulting from an underlying structural heart disorder. Each year, about 5% of patients develop AF with its risks of heart failure and stroke.

Treatment

- Pacemaker

Treatment is pacemaker implantation. Risk of AF is greatly reduced when a physiologic (atrial or atrial and ventricular) pacemaker rather than a ventricular pacemaker is used. Newer dual chamber pacemakers that minimize ventricular pacing may further reduce risk of AF. Antiarrhythmic drugs may prevent paroxysmal tachyarrhythmias after pacemaker insertion.

Theophylline and hydralazine are options to increase heart rate in healthy, younger patients who have bradycardia without syncope.

VENTRICULAR FIBRILLATION

Ventricular fibrillation (VF) causes uncoordinated quivering of the ventricle with no useful contractions. It causes immediate syncope and death within minutes. Treatment is with cardiopulmonary resuscitation, including immediate defibrillation.

VF is due to multiple wavelet reentrant electrical activity and is manifested on ECG by ultrarapid baseline undulations that are irregular in timing and morphology.

VF is the presenting rhythm for about 70% of patients in cardiac arrest and is thus the terminal event in many disorders. Overall, most patients with VF have an underlying heart disorder (typically ischemic cardiomyopathy, but also hypertrophic or dilated cardiomyopathies, arrhythmogenic right ventricular dysplasia, or Brugada syndrome). Risk of VF in any disorder is increased by electrolyte abnormalities, acidosis, hypoxemia, or ischemia.

VF is much less common among infants and children, in whom asystole is the more common presentation of cardiac arrest.

Treatment

- Defibrillation
- ICD

Treatment is with cardiopulmonary resuscitation, including defibrillation. The success rate for immediate (within 3 min) defibrillation is about 95%, provided that overwhelming pump failure does not preexist. When it does, even immediate defibrillation is only 30% successful, and most resuscitated patients die of pump failure before hospital discharge.

Patients who have VF without a reversible or transient cause are at high risk of future VF events and of sudden death. Most of these patients require an ICD; many require concomitant antiarrhythmic drugs to reduce the frequency of subsequent episodes of VT and VF.

VENTRICULAR PREMATURE BEATS

(Premature Ventricular Contractions)

Ventricular premature beats (VPB) are single ventricular impulses caused by reentry within the ventricle or abnormal automaticity of ventricular cells. They are extremely common in healthy patients and in patients with a heart disorder. VPB may be asymptomatic or cause palpitations. Diagnosis is by ECG. Treatment is usually not required.

VPBs, also called premature ventricular contractions (PVC), may occur erratically or at predictable intervals (eg, every 3rd [trigeminy] or 2nd [bigeminy] beat). VPBs may increase with stimulants (eg, anxiety, stress, alcohol, caffeine, sympathomimetic drugs), hypoxia, or electrolyte abnormalities.

VPBs may be experienced as missed or skipped beats; the VPB itself is not sensed but rather the following augmented sinus beat. When VPBs are very frequent, particularly when they occur at every 2nd heart beat, mild hemodynamic symptoms are possible because the sinus rate has been effectively halved. Existing ejection murmurs may be accentuated because of increased cardiac filling and augmented contractility after the compensatory pause.

Diagnosis

- ECG

Diagnosis is by ECG showing a wide QRS complex without a preceding P wave, typically followed by a fully compensatory pause.

Prognosis

VPBs are not significant in patients without a heart disorder, and no treatment is required beyond avoiding obvious triggers. Beta-blockers are offered only if symptoms are intolerable. Other antiarrhythmics that suppress VPBs increase risk of more serious arrhythmias.

Treatment

- Beta-blockers for patients with symptomatic heart failure and after MI

In patients with a structural heart disorder (eg, aortic stenosis, post MI), treatment is controversial even though frequent VPBs (> 10/h) correlate with increased mortality, because no studies have shown that pharmacologic suppression reduces mortality. In post-MI patients, mortality rate is higher with class I antiarrhythmics than with placebo. This finding probably reflects adverse effects of the antiarrhythmics. Beta-blockers are beneficial in symptomatic heart failure and post MI. If VPBs increase during exercise in a patient with coronary artery disease, evaluation for percutaneous transluminal coronary angioplasty or coronary artery bypass graft surgery should be considered.

VENTRICULAR TACHYCARDIA

Ventricular tachycardia (VT) is ≥ 3 consecutive ventricular beats at a rate ≥ 120 beats/min. Symptoms depend on duration and vary from none to palpitations to hemodynamic collapse and death. Diagnosis is by ECG. Treatment of more than brief episodes is with cardioversion or antiarrhythmics depending on symptoms. If necessary, long-term treatment is with an implantable cardioverter defibrillator.

Some experts use a cutoff rate of ≥ 100 beats/min for VT. Repetitive ventricular rhythms at slower rates are called accelerated idioventricular rhythms or slow VT; they are usually benign and are not treated unless associated with hemodynamic symptoms.

Most patients with VT have a significant heart disorder, particularly prior MI or a cardiomyopathy. Electrolyte abnormalities (particularly hypokalemia or hypomagnesemia), acidemia, hypoxemia, and adverse drug effects contribute. The long QT syndrome (congenital or acquired) is associated with a particular form of VT, torsades de pointes.

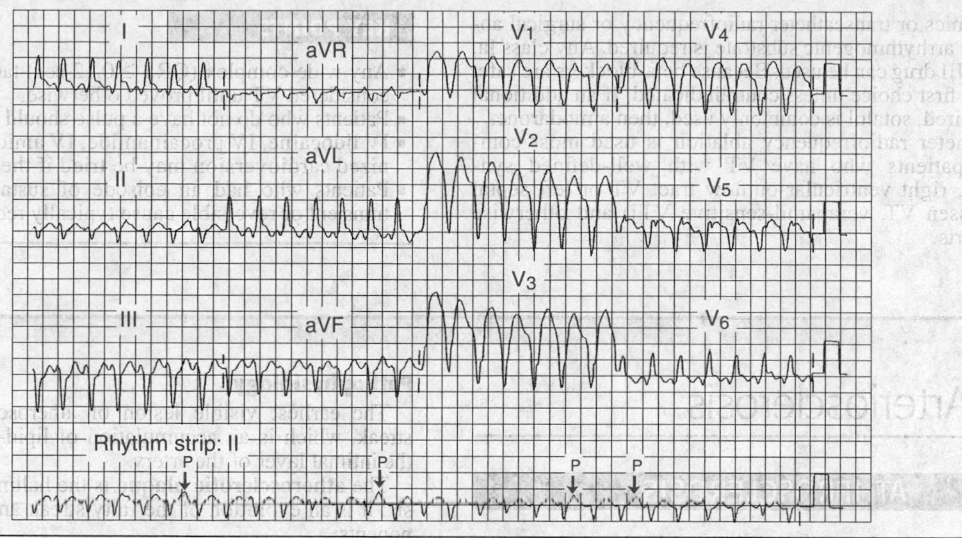

Fig. 76–21. Broad QRS ventricular tachycardia. The QRS duration is 160 msec. An independent P wave can be seen in II (arrows). There is a leftward mean frontal axis shift.

VT may be monomorphic or polymorphic and nonsustained or sustained.

- Monomorphic VT: Single abnormal focus or reentrant pathway and regular, identical-appearing QRS complexes
- Polymorphic VT: Several different foci or pathways and irregular, varying QRS complexes
- Nonsustained VT: Lasts < 30 sec
- Sustained VT: Lasts ≥ 30 sec or is terminated sooner because of hemodynamic collapse

VT frequently deteriorates to VF and thus cardiac arrest.

Symptoms and Signs

VT of short duration or slow rate may be asymptomatic. Sustained VT is almost always symptomatic, causing palpitations, symptoms of hemodynamic compromise, or sudden cardiac death.

Diagnosis

- ECG

Diagnosis of VT is by ECG (see Fig. 76–21). Any wide QRS complex tachycardia (QRS ≥ 0.12 sec) should be considered VT until proved otherwise.

Diagnosis is supported by ECG findings of dissociated P-wave activity, fusion or capture beats, uniformity of QRS vectors in the V leads (concordance) with discordant T-wave vector (opposite QRS vectors), and a frontal-plane QRS axis in the northwest quadrant. Differential diagnosis includes SVT conducted with bundle branch block or via an accessory pathway (see Fig. 76–3 on p. 623). However, because some patients tolerate VT surprisingly well, concluding that a well-tolerated wide QRS complex tachycardia must be of supraventricular origin is a mistake. Using drugs appropriate for SVT (eg, verapamil, diltiazem) in patients with VT may cause hemodynamic collapse and death.

Treatment

- Acute: Sometimes synchronized direct-current cardioversion, sometimes class I or class III antiarrhythmics
- Long-term: Usually an ICD

Acute: Treatment of acute VT depends on symptoms and duration of VT.

Pulseless VT requires defibrillation.

Hypotensive VT requires synchronized direct-current cardioversion with ≥ 100 joules.

Stable sustained VT can be treated with IV class I or class III antiarrhythmic drugs (see Table 76–1 on p. 624). Lidocaine acts quickly but is frequently ineffective. If lidocaine is ineffective, IV procainamide may be given, but it may take up to 1 h to work. IV amiodarone is frequently used but does not usually work quickly. Failure of IV procainamide or IV amiodarone is an indication for cardioversion.

Nonsustained VT does not require immediate treatment unless the runs are frequent or long enough to cause symptoms. In such cases, antiarrhythmics are used as for sustained VT.

Long-term: The primary goal is preventing sudden death, rather than simply suppressing the arrhythmia. It is best accomplished by use of an ICD. However, the decision about whom to treat is complex and depends on the estimated probability of life-threatening VTs and the severity of underlying heart disorders (see Table 76–4 on p. 634).

Long-term treatment is not required when the index episode of VT resulted from a transient cause (eg, during the 48 h after onset of MI) or a reversible cause (acid-base disturbances, electrolyte abnormalities, proarrhythmic drug effect).

In the absence of a transient or reversible cause, patients who have had an episode of sustained VT typically require an ICD. Most patients with sustained VT and a significant structural heart disorder should also receive a beta-blocker. If an ICD cannot be used, amiodarone may be the preferred antiarrhythmic for prevention of sudden death.

Because nonsustained VT is a marker for increased risk of sudden death in patients with a structural heart disorder, such patients (particularly those with an ejection fraction < 0.35) require further evaluation. Such patients should receive an ICD.

When prevention of VTs is important (usually in patients who have an ICD and are having frequent episodes of VT), antiarrhythmics or transcatheter radiofrequency or surgical ablation of the arrhythmogenic substrate is required. Any class Ia, Ib, Ic, II, or III drug can be used. Because beta-blockers are safe, they are the first choice unless contraindicated. If an additional drug is required, sotalol is commonly used, then amiodarone.

Transcatheter radiofrequency ablation is used most commonly in patients who have VT with well-defined syndromes (eg, right ventricular outflow tract VT or left septal VT [Belhassen VT, verapamil-sensitive VT]) and otherwise healthy hearts.

KEY POINTS

- Any wide-complex (QRS ≥ 0.12 sec) tachycardia should be considered VT until proved otherwise.
- Patients who do not have a pulse should be defibrillated.
- IV lidocaine, IV procainamide, IV amiodarone or synchronized cardioversion may be tried if the patient is stable.
- Patients who had an episode of sustained VT without a transient or reversible cause typically require an ICD.

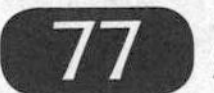

77 Arteriosclerosis

ATHEROSCLEROSIS

Atherosclerosis is characterized by patchy intimal plaques (atheromas) that encroach on the lumen of medium-sized and large arteries; the plaques contain lipids, inflammatory cells, smooth muscle cells, and connective tissue. Risk factors include dyslipidemia, diabetes, cigarette smoking, family history, sedentary lifestyle, obesity, and hypertension. Symptoms develop when growth or rupture of the plaque reduces or obstructs blood flow; symptoms vary by artery affected. Diagnosis is clinical and confirmed by angiography, ultrasonography, or other imaging tests. Treatment includes risk factor, lifestyle, and dietary modification, physical activity, antiplatelet drugs, and antiatherogenic drugs.

Atherosclerosis is the most common form of arteriosclerosis, which is a general term for several disorders that cause thickening and loss of elasticity in the arterial wall. Atherosclerosis is also the most serious and clinically relevant form of arteriosclerosis because it causes coronary artery disease and cerebrovascular disease. Nonatheromatous forms of arteriosclerosis include arteriolosclerosis and Mönckeberg arteriosclerosis.

Atherosclerosis can affect all large and medium-sized arteries, including the coronary, carotid, and cerebral arteries; the aorta; its branches; and major arteries of the extremities. It is the leading cause of morbidity and mortality in the US and in most developed countries. In recent years, age-related mortality attributable to atherosclerosis has been decreasing, but in 2015, cardiovascular disease (CVD), primarily coronary and cerebrovascular atherosclerosis still caused almost 15 million deaths worldwide (> 25% of all deaths).[1] In the US, > 800,000 people died of CVD in 2014, corresponding to almost 1 in 3 of all deaths.[2] Atherosclerosis is rapidly increasing in prevalence in developing countries, and as people in developed countries live longer, incidence will increase. Atherosclerosis is the leading cause of death worldwide.

1. WHO Global Health Estimates 2000-2015. http://www.who.int/healthinfo/global_burden_disease/estimates/en/index1.html
2. Benjamin EJ, Blaha MJ, Chiuve SE, et al: Heart Disease and Stroke Statistics—2017 update: A report From the American Heart Association. *Circulation* 135:1–459, 2017. doi.org/10.1161/CIR.0000000000000048.

Pathophysiology

The earliest visible lesion of atherosclerosis is the fatty streak, which is an accumulation of lipid-laden foam cells in the intimal layer of the artery.

The **atherosclerotic plaque** is the hallmark of atherosclerosis; it is an evolution of the fatty streak and has 3 major components:

- Lipids
- Inflammatory and smooth muscle cells
- A connective tissue matrix that may contain thrombi in various stages of organization and calcium deposits

Atherosclerotic plaque formation: All stages of atherosclerosis—from initiation and growth to complication of the plaque—are considered an inflammatory response to injury mediated by specific cytokines. Endothelial injury is thought to have a primary initiating or inciting role.

Atherosclerosis preferentially affects certain areas of the arterial tree. Nonlaminar or turbulent blood flow (eg, at branch points in the arterial tree) leads to endothelial dysfunction and inhibits endothelial production of nitric oxide, a potent vasodilator and anti-inflammatory molecule. Such blood flow also stimulates endothelial cells to produce adhesion molecules, which recruit and bind inflammatory cells.

Risk factors for atherosclerosis (eg, dyslipidemia, diabetes, cigarette smoking, hypertension), oxidative stressors (eg, superoxide radicals), angiotensin II, and systemic infection and inflammation also inhibit nitric oxide production and stimulate production of adhesion molecules, proinflammatory cytokines, chemotactic proteins, and vasoconstrictors; exact mechanisms are unknown. The net effect is endothelial binding of monocytes and T cells, migration of these cells to the subendothelial space, and initiation and perpetuation of a local vascular inflammatory response. Monocytes in the subendothelium transform into macrophages. Lipids in the blood, particularly low-density lipoprotein (LDL) and very-low-density lipoprotein (VLDL), also bind to endothelial cells and are oxidized in the subendothelium. Uptake of oxidized lipids and macrophage transformation into lipid-laden foam cells result in the typical early atherosclerotic lesions called fatty streaks. Degraded erythrocyte membranes that result from rupture of vasa vasorum and intraplaque hemorrhage may be an important additional source of lipids within plaques.

Macrophages elaborate proinflammatory cytokines that recruit smooth muscle cell migration from the media and that further attract and stimulate growth of macrophages. Various factors promote smooth muscle cell replication and increase production of dense extracellular matrix. The result is a subendothelial fibrous plaque with a fibrous cap, made of intimal smooth muscle cells surrounded by connective tissue and intracellular and extracellular lipids. A process similar to bone formation causes calcification within the plaque.

A link between infection and atherosclerosis has been observed, specifically an association between serologic evidence of certain infections (eg, *Chlamydia pneumoniae*, cytomegalovirus) and coronary artery disease (CAD). Putative mechanisms include indirect effects of chronic inflammation in the bloodstream, cross-reactive antibodies, and inflammatory effects of infectious pathogens on the arterial wall.

Plaque stability and rupture: Atherosclerotic plaques may be stable or unstable.

Stable plaques regress, remain static, or grow slowly over several decades until they may cause stenosis or occlusion.

Unstable plaques are vulnerable to spontaneous erosion, fissure, or rupture, causing acute thrombosis, occlusion, and infarction long before they cause hemodynamically significant stenosis. Most clinical events result from unstable plaques, which do not appear severe on angiography; thus, plaque stabilization may be a way to reduce morbidity and mortality.

The strength of the fibrous cap and its resistance to rupture depend on the relative balance of collagen deposition and degradation. Plaque rupture involves secretion of metalloproteinases, cathepsins, and collagenases by activated macrophages in the plaque. These enzymes digest the fibrous cap, particularly at the edges, causing the cap to thin and ultimately rupture. T cells in the plaque contribute by secreting cytokines. Cytokines inhibit smooth muscle cells from synthesizing and depositing collagen, which normally reinforces the plaque.

Once the plaque ruptures, plaque contents are exposed to circulating blood, triggering thrombosis; macrophages also stimulate thrombosis because they contain tissue factor, which promotes thrombin generation in vivo. One of 5 outcomes may occur:

- The resultant thrombus may organize and be incorporated into the plaque, changing the plaque's shape and causing its rapid growth.
- The thrombus may rapidly occlude the vascular lumen and precipitate an acute ischemic event.
- The thrombus may embolize.
- The plaque may fill with blood, balloon out, and immediately occlude the artery.
- Plaque contents (rather than thrombus) may embolize, occluding vessels downstream.

Plaque stability depends on multiple factors, including plaque composition (relative proportion of lipids, inflammatory cells, smooth muscle cells, connective tissue, and thrombus), wall stress (cap fatigue), size and location of the core, and configuration of the plaque in relation to blood flow. By contributing to rapid growth and lipid deposition, intraplaque hemorrhage may play an important role in transforming stable into unstable plaques. In general, unstable coronary artery plaques have a high macrophage content, a thick lipid core, and a thin fibrous cap; they narrow the vessel lumen by < 50% and tend to rupture unpredictably. Unstable carotid artery plaques have the same composition but typically cause problems through severe stenosis and occlusion or deposition of platelet thrombi, which embolize rather than rupture. Low-risk plaques have a thicker cap and contain fewer lipids; they often narrow the vessel lumen by > 50% and may produce predictable exercise-induced stable angina.

Clinical consequences of plaque rupture in coronary arteries depend not only on plaque anatomy but also on relative balance of procoagulant and anticoagulant activity in the blood and on the vulnerability of the myocardium to arrhythmias.

Risk Factors

There are numerous risk factors for atherosclerosis (see Table 77–1).[1] Certain factors tend to cluster as the metabolic syndrome, which is becoming increasingly prevalent. This syndrome includes abdominal obesity, atherogenic dyslipidemia, hypertension, insulin resistance, a prothrombotic state, and a proinflammatory state in sedentary patients. Insulin resistance is not synonymous with the metabolic syndrome but may be key in its etiology.

Dyslipidemia (high total, high LDL, or low high-density lipoprotein [HDL] cholesterol), hypertension, and diabetes promote atherosclerosis by amplifying or augmenting endothelial dysfunction and inflammatory pathways in vascular endothelium.

In dyslipidemia, subendothelial uptake and oxidation of LDL increases; oxidized lipids stimulate production of adhesion molecules and inflammatory cytokines and may be antigenic, inciting a T cell–mediated immune response and inflammation in the arterial

Table 77–1. RISK FACTORS FOR ATHEROSCLEROSIS

STATUS	RISK FACTOR
Nonmodifiable	Age Family history of premature atherosclerosis* Male sex
Modifiable, established	Certain dyslipidemias (high total or LDL level, low HDL level, increased total-to-HDL cholesterol ratio) Diabetes mellitus Hypertension Tobacco smoking
Modifiable, under study or emerging	Alcohol intake (other than moderate) *Chlamydia pneumoniae* infection Heart transplantation High apolipoprotein B (apoB) level High CRP level High level of small, dense LDL High lipoprotein (a) level Hyperhomocysteinemia Hyperinsulinemia Hypertriglyceridemia 5-Lipoxygenase polymorphisms Low intake of fruits and vegetables Obesityor the metabolic syndrome Prothrombotic states (eg, hyperfibrinogenemia, high plasminogen activator inhibitor level) Psychosocial factors (eg, type A personality, depression, anxiety, work characteristics, socioeconomic status) Radiation therapy to thorax Renal insufficiency Sedentary lifestyle†

*Atherosclerosis is premature when it occurs in a male 1st-degree relative before age 55 and in a female 1st-degree relative before age 65.

†How much this factor contributes independent of other frequently associated risk factors (eg, diabetes, dyslipidemia) is unclear.

CRP = C-reactive protein, HDL = high-density lipoprotein, LDL= low-density lipoprotein.

wall. HDL protects against atherosclerosis via reverse cholesterol transport (see p. 1302); it may also protect by transporting antioxidant enzymes, which can break down and neutralize oxidized lipids. The role of hypertriglyceridemia in atherogenesis is complex, although it may have a small independent effect.[2]

Hypertension may lead to vascular inflammation via angiotensin II–mediated mechanisms. Angiotensin II stimulates endothelial cells, vascular smooth muscle cells, and macrophages to produce proatherogenic mediators, including proinflammatory cytokines, superoxide anions, prothrombotic factors, growth factors, and lectin-like oxidized LDL receptors.

Diabetes leads to the formation of advanced glycation end products, which increase the production of proinflammatory cytokines from endothelial cells. Oxidative stress and reactive oxygen radicals, generated in diabetes, directly injure the endothelium and promote atherogenesis.

Tobacco smoke contains nicotine and other chemicals that are toxic to vascular endothelium. Smoking, including passive smoking, increases platelet reactivity (possibly promoting platelet thrombosis) and plasma fibrinogen levels and hematocrit (increasing blood viscosity). Smoking increases LDL and decreases HDL; it also promotes vasoconstriction, which is particularly dangerous in arteries already narrowed by atherosclerosis. HDL increases by about 6 to 8 mg/dL (0.16 to 0.21 mmol/L) within 1 mo of smoking cessation.

Lipoprotein (a)[Lp(a)] is pro-atherogenic and is an independent risk factor for cardiovascular disease, including myocardial infarction, stroke, and aortic valve stenosis.[3, 4] It has a structure similar to LDL, but it also has a hydrophilic apolipoprotein(a) component that is covalently bound to a hydrophobic apolipoprotein B100.[5] Lp(a) levels are genetically determined and remain fairly stable throughout life. Lp(a) levels above 50 mg/dL are considered pathogenic.

Apolipoprotein (B) (apoB) is a particle with two isoforms: apoB-100, which is synthesized in the liver, and apoB-46, which is synthesized in the intestine. ApoB-100 is able to bind the LDL receptor and is responsible for cholesterol transport. It is also responsible for transport of oxidized phospholipids and has proinflammatory properties. Presence of the apoB particle within the arterial wall is thought to be the initiating event for the development of atherosclerotic lesions.

A **high level of small, dense LDL,** characteristic of diabetes, is highly atherogenic. Mechanisms may include increased susceptibility to oxidation and nonspecific endothelial binding.

A **high C-reactive protein (CRP) level** does not reliably predict extent of atherosclerosis but can predict increased likelihood of ischemic events. In the absence of other inflammatory disorders, elevated levels may indicate increased risk of atherosclerotic plaque rupture, ongoing ulceration or thrombosis, or increased activity of lymphocytes and macrophages. CRP itself does not appear to have a direct role in atherogenesis.

***C. pneumoniae* infection** or other infections (eg, viral, *Helicobacter pylori*) may cause endothelial dysfunction through direct infection, exposure to endotoxin, or stimulation of systemic or subendothelial inflammation.

Chronic kidney disease promotes development of atherosclerosis via several pathways, including worsening hypertension and insulin resistance; decreased apolipoprotein A-I levels; and increased lipoprotein(a), homocysteine, fibrinogen, and C-reactive protein levels.

Heart transplantation is often followed by accelerated coronary atherosclerosis, which is likely related to immune-mediated endothelial injury. Accelerated coronary atherosclerosis is also observed after thoracic radiation therapy and is likely the result of radiation-induced endothelial injury.

Prothrombotic states (see p. 1206) increase likelihood of atherothrombosis.

Several common and rare **genetic variants** have been robustly associated with atherosclerosis and cardiovascular events. Although each variant has a small effect individually, genetic risk scores that sum the total number of risk variants have been shown to strongly associate with more advanced atherosclerosis as well as both primary and recurrent cardiovascular events

Patients with **hyperhomocysteinemia** (eg, due to folate deficiency or a genetic metabolic defect) have an increased risk of atherosclerosis. However, because of results from randomized trials of homocysteine lowering therapies that fail to show a decrease in atherosclerotic disease, as well as evidence from Mendelian randomization trials, it is no longer thought that hyperhomocysteinemia itself causes atherosclerosis. The reason for the association between elevated homocysteine levels and atherosclerosis is unclear.

Documented vascular disease: The presence of atherosclerotic disease in one vascular territory increases the likelihood of disease in other vascular territories. Patients with noncoronary atherosclerotic vascular disease have cardiac event rates comparable to those of patients with known CAD, and they are now considered to have a CAD risk equivalent and should be treated as aggressively.

1. Yusuf S, Hawken S, Ounpuu S, et al: Effect of potentially modifiable risk factors associated with myocardial infarction in 52 countries (the INTERHEART study): case-control study. *The Lancet* 364:937–952, 2004.
2. White J, Swedlow DI, Preiss D, et al: Association of lipid fractions with risks for coronary artery disease and diabetes. *JAMA Cardiol* 1(6):692–699, 2016.
3. Emerging risk factors collaboration, Eroquo S, Kaptoge S, Perry PL, et al: Lipoprotein(a) concentration and the risk of coronary heart disease, stroke, and nonvascular mortality. *JAMA* 302:412–423, 2009.
4. Thanassoulis, G, Campbell CY, Owens DS, et al for the CHARGE Extracoronary Calcium Working Group: Genetic associations with valvular calcification and aortic stenosis. *N Engl J Med* 368:503–512, 2013.
5. Nordestgaard BG, Chapman MJ, Ray K, et al and the European Atherosclerosis Society Consensus Panel: Lipoprotein(a) as a cardiovascular risk factor: current status. *Eur Heart J* 31:2844–2853, 2010.

Symptoms and Signs

Atherosclerosis is initially asymptomatic, often for decades. Symptoms and signs develop when lesions impede blood flow. Transient ischemic symptoms (eg, stable exertional angina, transient ischemic attacks, intermittent claudication) may develop when stable plaques grow and reduce the arterial lumen by > 70%. Vasoconstriction can change a lesion that does not limit blood flow into a severe or complete stenosis. Symptoms of unstable angina or myocardial infarction, ischemic stroke, or rest pain in the limbs may develop when unstable plaques rupture and acutely occlude a major artery, with superimposition of thrombosis or embolism. Atherosclerosis may also cause sudden death without preceding stable or unstable angina pectoris.

Atherosclerotic involvement of the arterial wall can lead to aneurysms and arterial dissection, which can manifest as pain, a pulsatile mass, absent pulses, or sudden death.

Diagnosis

Approach depends on the presence or absence of symptoms.

Symptomatic patients: Patients with symptoms and signs of ischemia are evaluated for the amount and location of vascular occlusion by various invasive and noninvasive tests, depending on the organ involved (see elsewhere in THE MANUAL). Such patients also should be evaluated for atherosclerosis risk factors by using

- History and physical examination
- Fasting lipid profile
- Plasma glucose and glycosylated hemoglobin (HbA_{1c}) levels

Patients with documented disease at one site (eg, peripheral arteries) should be evaluated for disease at other sites (eg, coronary and carotid arteries).

Because not all atherosclerotic plaques have similar risk, various imaging technologies are being studied as a way to identify plaques especially vulnerable to rupture; however, these techniques are not yet used clinically. Three-dimensional vascular ultrasonography, CT angiography, and MR angiography can noninvasively assess plaque morphology and characteristics. Invasive catheter-based tests, including intravascular ultrasonography (which uses an ultrasound transducer on the tip of a catheter to produce images of the arterial lumen and wall), angioscopy, plaque thermography (to detect the increased temperature in plaques with active inflammation), optical coherence tomography (which uses infrared laser light for imaging), and elastography (to identify soft, lipid-rich plaques) are also used. Immunoscintigraphy is a noninvasive alternative using radioactive tracers that localize in vulnerable plaque. PET imaging of the vasculature is another emerging approach to assess vulnerable plaque.

Some clinicians measure serum markers of inflammation. C-reactive protein levels > 3 mg/dL (> 3000 µg/L) are highly predictive of cardiovascular events.

Asymptomatic patients (screening): In patients with risk factors for atherosclerosis but no symptoms or signs of ischemia, the role of additional testing beyond the lipid profile is unclear. Although imaging studies such as carotid ultrasonography to measure intimal medial thickness and other studies that can detect atherosclerotic plaque are being studied, they do not reliably improve prediction of ischemic events over assessment of risk factors or established prediction tools and are not recommended. An exception is CT imaging for coronary artery calcium, for which there is more robust evidence for risk reclassification; it may be useful for refining risk estimates and for deciding on statin therapy in select patients (eg, those with intermediate risk, family history of premature cardiovascular disease).

Most guidelines recommend lipid profile screening in patients with any of the following characteristics:

- Men ≥ 40 yr
- Women ≥ 50 yr and post-menopausal women
- Type 2 diabetes
- Family history of familial hypercholesterolemia or premature cardiovascular disease (ie, age of onset < 55 yr in male 1st degree relative, or < 65 yr in female 1st degree relative)
- Metabolic syndrome
- Hypertension
- Chronic inflammatory conditions

Currently, the American Heart Association (AHA) recommends using the pooled cohort risk assessment equations to estimate lifetime and 10-yr risk of atherosclerotic cardiovascular disease. This calculator has replaced previous risk calculation tools (eg, Framingham score). The new risk calculator is based on sex, age, race, total and HDL cholesterol, systolic BP (and whether BP is being treated), diabetes, and smoking status.[1] The European Cardiovascular Society (ESC) and the European Atherosclerosis Society (EAS) 2016 guideline suggests using the Systemic Coronary Risk Estimation (SCORE), which calculates risk based on age, gender, smoking, systolic blood pressure, and total cholesterol, to estimate the 10-yr risk of the first fatal atherosclerotic event.[2] For patients deemed at intermediate risk, lipoprotein(a) measurement has been suggested to help refine classification.[3]

Urinary albuminuria (> 30 mg albumin/24 h) is a marker for renal disorders and their progression, as well as a strong predictor of cardiovascular and noncardiovascular morbidity and mortality; however, the direct relationship between albuminuria and atherosclerosis has not been established.

1. Goff DC Jr, Lloyd-Jones DM, Bennett G, et al: 2013 ACC/AHA guideline on the assessment of cardiovascular risk: A report of the American College of Cardiology/ American Heart Association Task Force on Practice Guidelines. *Circulation* 129:S49–S73, 2014.
2. Catapano AL, Graham I, De Backe G, et al: 2016 ESC/ EAS guidelines for the management of dyslipidaemias: The task force for the management of dyslipidaemias of the European Society of Cardiology (ESC) and European Atherosclerosis Society (EAS) developed with the special contribution of the European Association for Cardiovascular Prevention and Rehabilitation (EACPR). *Eur Heart J* 37:2999–3058, 2016. doi:10.1093/eurheartj/ehw272. Epub ahead of print.
3. Willeit P, Kiechl S, Kronenberg F, et al: Discrimination and net reclassification of cardiovascular risk with lipoprotein(a): prospective 15-year outcomes in the Bruneck Study. *J Am Coll Cardiol* 64:851–860, 2014. doi: 10.1016/j.jacc.2014.03.061.

Treatment

- Lifestyle changes (diet, smoking, physical activity)
- Drug treatment of diagnosed risk factors
- Antiplatelet drugs
- Statins, possibly ACE inhibitors, beta-blockers

Treatment involves aggressive modification of risk factors to slow progression and induce regression of existing plaques. Lowering LDL to below a certain target is no longer recommended, and "the lower the better" approach is currently favored.

Lifestyle changes include diet modification, smoking cessation, and regular participation in physical activity. Drugs to treat dyslipidemia, hypertension, and diabetes are often required. These lifestyle changes and drugs directly or indirectly improve endothelial function, reduce inflammation, and improve clinical outcome. Statins can decrease atherosclerosis-related morbidity and mortality even when serum cholesterol is normal or slightly high. Antiplatelet drugs help all patients with atherosclerosis. Patients with coronary artery disease may benefit additionally from ACE inhibitors and beta-blockers.

Diet: Several changes are beneficial:

- Less saturated fat
- No trans fats
- More fruits and vegetables
- More fiber
- Moderate (if any) alcohol

Substantial decreases in saturated fat and refined and processed carbohydrates and increases in carbohydrates with fiber (eg, fruits, vegetables) are recommended. These dietary changes are a prerequisite for lipid control and weight reduction and are essential for all patients. Calorie intake should be limited to keep weight within the normal range.

Small decreases in fat intake do not appear to lessen or stabilize atherosclerosis. Effective change requires limiting fat intake to 20 g/day, consisting of 6 to 10 g of polyunsaturated fat with omega-6 (linoleic acid) and omega-3 (eicosapentaenoic acid, docosahexaenoic acid) fatty acids in equal proportion, ≤ 2 g of saturated fat, and the rest as monounsaturated fat. Trans fats, which are highly atherogenic, should be avoided.

Increasing carbohydrates to compensate for decreasing saturated fats in the diet increases plasma triglyceride levels and reduces HDL levels. Thus, any caloric deficiency should be made up with proteins and unsaturated fats rather than simple carbohydrates. Excessive fat and refined sugar intake should be avoided especially in people at risk of diabetes, although sugar intake has not been directly related to cardiovascular risk. Instead, consumption of complex carbohydrates (eg, vegetables, whole grains) is encouraged.

Fruits and vegetables (5 daily servings) seem to decrease risk of coronary atherosclerosis, but whether this effect is due to phytochemicals or to a proportional decrease in saturated fat intake and increase in fiber and vitamin intake is unclear. Phytochemicals called flavonoids (in red and purple grapes, red wine, black teas, and dark beers) appear especially protective; high concentrations in red wine may help explain why incidence of coronary atherosclerosis in the French is relatively low, even though they use more tobacco and consume more fat than Americans do. But no clinical data indicate that eating flavonoid-rich foods or using supplements instead of foods prevents atherosclerosis.

Increased fiber intake decreases total cholesterol and may have a beneficial effect on glucose and insulin levels. Daily intake of at least 5 to 10 g of soluble fiber (eg, oat bran, beans, soy products, psyllium) is recommended; this amount decreases LDL by about 5%. Insoluble fiber (eg, cellulose, lignin) does not appear to affect cholesterol but may confer additional health benefits (eg, reduced risk of colon cancer, possibly by stimulating bowel movement or reducing contact time with dietary carcinogens). However, excessive fiber interferes with the absorption of certain minerals and vitamins. In general, foods rich in phytochemicals and vitamins are also rich in fiber.

Alcohol increases HDL and has poorly defined antithrombotic, antioxidant, and anti-inflammatory properties. These effects appear to be the same for wine, beer, and hard liquor, and occur at moderate levels of consumption; about 30 mL of ethanol (1 oz, contained in about 2 average servings of typical alcoholic beverages) 5 to 6 times/wk protects against coronary atherosclerosis. However, at higher doses, alcohol can cause significant health problems. Thus, the relationship between alcohol and total mortality rate is J-shaped; mortality rate is lowest for men who consume < 14 drinks/wk and women who consume < 9 drinks/wk. People who consume greater amounts of alcohol should cut back. However, clinicians are hesitant to recommend that nondrinkers begin consuming alcohol based on any apparent protective effect.

There is little evidence that dietary supplementation with vitamins, phytochemicals, and trace minerals reduces risk of atherosclerosis. The one exception is fish oil supplements. Although alternative medicines and health foods are becoming more popular, and some may have minor effects on blood pressure or cholesterol, these treatments are not always proven safe or effective and may have negative interactions with proven drugs. Levels of coenzyme Q10, which is necessary for the basic functioning of cells, tend to decrease with age and may be low in patients with certain heart and other chronic diseases; thus, coenzyme Q10 supplementation has been used or recommended, but its therapeutic benefit remains controversial.

Physical activity: Regular physical activity (eg, 30 to 45 min of walking, running, swimming, or cycling 3 to 5 times/wk) reduces incidence of some risk factors (hypertension, dyslipidemia, diabetes), coronary artery disease (eg, myocardial infarction), and death attributable to atherosclerosis in patients with and without previous ischemic events. Whether the association is causal or merely indicates that healthier people are more likely to exercise regularly is unclear.

Optimal intensity, duration, frequency, and type of exercise have not been established, but most evidence suggests an inverse linear relationship between aerobic physical activity and risk. Walking regularly increases the distance patients with peripheral vascular disease can walk without pain.

An exercise program that involves aerobic exercise has a clear role in preventing atherosclerosis and promoting weight loss. Before starting a new exercise program, the elderly and people who have risk factors for atherosclerosis or who have had recent ischemic events should be evaluated by a physician. Evaluation includes history, physical examination, and assessment of risk factor control.

Antiplatelet drugs: Oral antiplatelet drugs are essential because most complications result from plaque fissure or rupture, leading to platelet activation and thrombosis. The following are used:

- Aspirin
- Thienopyridine drugs such as clopidogrel, prasugrel, and ticagrelor

Aspirin is most widely used but, despite its proven benefits, remains underused. It is indicated for secondary prevention and recommended for primary prevention of coronary atherosclerosis in patients at high risk (eg, patients with diabetes with or without atherosclerosis, patients with ≥ 20% risk of cardiac events within 10 yr in whom bleeding risk is not prohibitive, and patients at intermediate risk who have a 10 to 20% risk of cardiac events within 10 yr and have low risk of bleeding). Optimal dose and duration are unknown, but 81 to 325 mg po once/day indefinitely is commonly used for primary and secondary prevention. However, 81 mg is preferred because this dose may minimize the risk of bleeding, particularly when aspirin is used in combination with other antithrombotic drugs. In about 10 to 20% of patients taking aspirin for secondary prevention, ischemic events recur. The reason may be aspirin resistance; assays to detect lack of thromboxane suppression (indicated by elevated urinary 11-dehydrothromboxane B_2) are being studied for clinical use.

Some evidence suggests that ibuprofen can interfere with aspirin's antithrombotic effect, so other NSAIDs are recommended for patients taking aspirin for prevention. However, all NSAIDs, some more than others, including COX-2 selective inhibitors, appear to increase cardiovascular risks.

Clopidogrel (usually 75 mg po once/day) is substituted for aspirin when ischemic events recur in patients taking aspirin and in patients intolerant of aspirin. Clopidogrel in combination with aspirin is effective in treating acute ST-segment and non-ST-segment elevation myocardial infarction; the combination is also given for 9 to 12 mo after percutaneous intervention (PCI) to reduce risk of recurrent ischemic events. Resistance to clopidogrel also occurs. Prasugrel and ticagrelor are newer and more effective drugs than clopidogrel for coronary disease prevention in select patient groups.

Ticlopidine is no longer widely used because it causes severe neutropenia in 1% of users and has severe GI adverse effects.

Statins: Statins primarily lower LDL cholesterol. Other potential beneficial effects include enhanced endothelial nitric oxide production, stabilization of atherosclerotic plaques, reduced lipid accumulation in the arterial wall, and regression of plaques. Statins are recommended as preventive therapy in 4 groups of patients,[1] comprised of those with any of the following:

- Clinical atherosclerotic cardiovascular disease
- LDL cholesterol ≥ 190 mg/dL
- Age 40 to 75, with diabetes and LDL cholesterol 70 to 189 mg/dL
- Age 40 to 75, with LDL cholesterol 70 to 189 mg/dL, and estimated 10-yr risk of arteriosclerotic cardiovascular disease ≥ 7.5%

There is also support for the use of statins in patients with other risk factors, including family history of premature arteriosclerotic cardiovascular disease (ie, age of onset < 55 in male 1st degree relative, or < 65 in female 1st degree relative), high-sensitivity C-reactive protein ≥ 2 mg/L, coronary artery calcium score ≥ 300 Agatston units (or ≥ 75th percentile for the patient's demographic), ankle-brachial BP index < 0.9.

Statin treatment is classified as high, moderate, or low intensity and is given based on treatment group and age (see Table 168–4 on p. 1308). Specific LDL cholesterol targets are no longer recommended to guide lipid-lowering therapy. Instead, response to therapy is determined by whether LDL cholesterol levels decrease as expected based on therapy intensity (ie, patients receiving high-intensity therapy should have a ≥ 50% decrease in LDL cholesterol).

Other drugs: ACE inhibitors, angiotensin II receptor blockers, ezetimibe, PCSK9 inhibitors, and thiazolidinediones (eg, pioglitazone) have anti-inflammatory properties that reduce risk of atherosclerosis independent of their effects on BP, lipids, and glucose.

ACE inhibitors inhibit the contributions of angiotensin to endothelial dysfunction and inflammation.

Ezetimibe also lowers LDL cholesterol by blocking the uptake of cholesterol from the small intestine via inhibition of the Niemann-Pick C1-like 1 protein. Ezetimibe, added to standard statin therapy, has been shown to reduce cardiovascular events in patients with prior cardiovascular event and LDL cholesterol > 1.8 mmol/L.

PCSK9 inhibitors are a new class of lipid-lowering drugs. These drugs are monoclonal antibodies that keep PCSK9 from attaching to LDL receptors, leading to increased recycling of these receptors to the plasma membrane leading to further clearance of plasma LDL cholesterol to the liver. LDL cholesterol is lowered by 40 to 70%. Long-term clinical trials have shown reduction in atherosclerosis and cardiovascular events. These drugs are most useful in patients with familial hypercholesterolemia, patients with prior cardiovascular events whose LDL is not at goal despite maximal medical therapy with statins, and patients who require lipid lowering but have documented objective evidence of statin intolerance.

Thiazolidinediones may control expression of proinflammatory genes, although recent studies suggest that they may increase the risk of coronary events.

Folate (folic acid) 0.8 mg po bid has been previously used to treat hyperhomocysteinemia but does not appear to reduce the risk of acute coronary events. Vitamins B6 and B12 also lower homocysteine levels, but current data do not justify their use alone or in combination with folate.

Macrolide and other antibiotics given to treat chronic occult *C. pneumoniae* infections (and thereby suppress inflammation and theoretically alter the course and manifestations of atherosclerosis) have not been shown useful.

1. Stone NJ, Robinson J, Lichtenstein AH, et al: 2013 ACC/AHA guideline on the treatment of blood cholesterol to reduce atherosclerotic cardiovascular risk in adults: A report of the American College of Cardiology/American Heart Association Task Force on Practice Guidelines. *J Am Coll Cardiol* 63:2899–2934, 2014.

KEY POINTS

- Risk factors include dyslipidemia, diabetes, cigarette smoking, family history, psychosocial factors, sedentary lifestyle, obesity, and hypertension.
- Unstable plaques often cause < 50% stenosis yet are more prone to rupture and cause acute thrombosis or embolic phenomena than are larger, stable plaques.
- In asymptomatic patients, imaging tests to detect atherosclerosis probably do not help predict ischemic events better than standard assessment of risk factors.
- Stopping smoking, exercising, eating a diet low in saturated fat and refined carbohydrates and high in fiber and possibly consuming omega-3 fatty acids and moderate amounts of alcohol help in prevention and treatment.
- Antiplatelet drugs, and depending on patient factors, statins and/or ACE inhibitors also are helpful.

NONATHEROMATOUS ARTERIOSCLEROSIS

Nonatheromatous arteriosclerosis is age-related fibrosis in the aorta and its major branches.

Arteriosclerosis is a general term for several disorders that cause thickening and loss of elasticity in the arterial wall. Atherosclerosis, the most common form, is also the most serious and clinically relevant because it causes coronary artery disease and cerebrovascular disease. Atheromatous disease is characterized by the atherosclerotic plaque, which is a vascular lesion composed of lipids, inflammatory and smooth muscle cells, and a connective tissue matrix that may contain thrombi in various stages of organization and calcium deposits.

Nonatheromatous forms of arteriosclerosis include

- Arteriolosclerosis
- Mönckeberg arteriosclerosis

Nonatheromatous arteriosclerosis causes intimal thickening and weakens and disrupts the elastic lamellae. The smooth muscle (media) layer atrophies, and the lumen of the affected artery widens (becomes ectatic), predisposing to aneurysm or dissection. Hypertension is a major factor in development of aortic arteriosclerosis and aneurysm. Intimal injury, ectasia, and ulceration may lead to thrombosis, embolism, or complete arterial occlusion.

Arteriolosclerosis: Arteriolosclerosis affects distal arteries in patients with diabetes or hypertension.

Hyaline arteriolosclerosis affects small arteries and arterioles in patients with diabetes; typically, hyaline thickening occurs, the arteriolar wall degenerates, and the lumen narrows, causing diffuse ischemia, especially in the kidneys.

Hyperplastic arteriolosclerosis occurs more often in patients with hypertension; typically, laminated, concentric thickening and luminal narrowing occur, sometimes with fibrinoid deposits and vessel wall necrosis (necrotizing arteriolitis). Hypertension promotes these changes, and arteriolosclerosis, by increasing arteriolar rigidity and increasing peripheral resistance, may help sustain the hypertension.

Mönckeberg arteriosclerosis: Mönckeberg arteriosclerosis (medial calcific sclerosis) affects patients > 50; age-related medial degeneration occurs with focal calcification and even bone formation within the arterial wall. Segments of the artery may become a rigid calcified tube without luminal narrowing. The diagnosis is usually obvious by plain x-ray. This disorder is clinically important only because it can greatly reduce arterial compressibility, causing extremely but falsely elevated BP readings.

78 Cardiac Tumors

Cardiac tumors may be primary (benign or malignant) or metastatic (malignant). Myxoma, a benign primary tumor, is the most common type. Cardiac tumors may occur in any cardiac tissue. They can cause valvular or inflow-outflow tract obstruction, thromboembolism, arrhythmias, or pericardial disorders. Diagnosis is by echocardiography and frequently cardiac MRI. Treatment of benign tumors is usually surgical resection; tumors may recur. Treatment of metastatic cancer depends on tumor type and origin; prognosis is generally poor.

Primary cardiac tumors are found in < 1/2000 people at autopsy. Metastatic tumors are 30 to 40 times more common. Usually, primary cardiac tumors originate in the myocardium or endocardium; they may also originate in valve tissue, cardiac connective tissue, or the pericardium.

Classification

Some of the more common primary and secondary cardiac tumors are listed (see Table 78–1). Primary cardiac tumors may be

- Benign (nearly 80% of cases)
- Malignant (the remaining 20%)

Benign primary tumors: Examples are myxomas, papillary fibroelastomas, rhabdomyomas, fibromas, hemangiomas, teratomas, lipomas, paragangliomas, and pericardial cysts.

Table 78–1. TYPES OF CARDIAC TUMORS

TYPE	EXAMPLES
Benign primary tumors	Myxomas
	Papillary fibroelastomas
	Rhabdomyomas
	Fibromas
	Hemangiomas
	Teratomas
	Lipomas
	Paraganglionomas*
	Pericardial cysts
Malignant primary tumors	Sarcomas
	Pericardial mesothelioma
	Primary lymphomas
Metastatic tumors	Lung carcinoma
	Breast carcinoma
	Soft-tissue sarcoma
	Renal carcinoma
	Melanoma

*Paragangliomas can also be malignant.

Myxoma is most common, accounting for 50% of all primary cardiac tumors. Incidence in women is 2 to 4 times that in men. In uncommon familial forms (Carney complex), men are affected more often. About 75% of myxomas occur in the left atrium, and the rest occur in the other chambers as a solitary tumor or, less commonly, at several sites. Myxomas may be up to 15 cm in diameter. About 75% are pedunculated and may prolapse through the mitral valve and obstruct ventricular filling during diastole. The remainder of the tumors are broad-based and sessile. Myxomas may be myxoid and gelatinous; smooth, firm, and lobular; or friable and irregular. Friable, irregular myxomas increase risk of systemic embolism.

Carney complex is a familial, autosomal dominant syndrome of recurrent cardiac myxomas with some combination of cutaneous myxomas, myxoid mammary fibroadenomas, pigmented skin lesions (lentigines, ephelides, blue nevi), multiple endocrine neoplasia (primary pigmented nodular adrenocortical disease causing Cushing syndrome, growth hormone and prolactin-producing pituitary adenoma, testicular tumors, thyroid adenoma or carcinoma, and ovarian cysts), psammomatous melanotic schwannoma, breast ductal adenoma, and osteochondromyxoma. Patients are often young at presentation (median age, 20 yr), have multiple myxomas (particularly in the ventricles), and have a higher risk of myxoma recurrence.

Papillary fibroelastomas are the 2nd most common benign primary tumor. They are avascular papillomas that occur on heart valves in > 80% of cases. The papillomas are more likely to occur on the left side of the heart, predominantly on the aortic and mitral valves. Men and women are affected equally. They have papillary fronds branching from a central core, resembling sea anemones. About 45% are pedunculated. They do not cause valvular dysfunction but increase risk of embolism.

Rhabdomyomas account for 20% of all primary cardiac tumors and 90% of those in children. Rhabdomyomas affect mainly infants and children, 80% of whom also have tuberous sclerosis. Rhabdomyomas are usually multiple and located intramurally in the septum or free wall of the left ventricle, where they affect the cardiac conduction system. They are firm white lobules that typically regress with age. A minority of patients develop tachyarrhythmias and heart failure due to left ventricular outflow tract obstruction.

Fibromas occur mainly in children and are associated with adenoma sebaceum of the skin and kidney tumors. They occur primarily on the left side of the heart, are often located within the ventricular myocardium, and may develop in response to inflammation. They can compress or invade the cardiac conduction system, causing arrhythmias and sudden death. Some fibromas occur as part of a syndrome with generalized body overgrowth, jaw keratocytes, skeletal abnormalities, and various benign and malignant tumors (Gorlin, or basal cell nevus syndrome).

Hemangiomas account for 5 to 10% of benign tumors. They cause symptoms in a minority of patients. Most often, they are incidentally detected during examinations done for other reasons.

Teratomas of the pericardium affect mainly infants and children. They are often attached to the base of the great vessels. About 90% are located in the anterior mediastinum; the rest, mainly in the posterior mediastinum.

Lipomas can develop at a wide range of ages. They originate in the endocardium or epicardium and have a large pedunculated base. Many are asymptomatic, but some obstruct flow or cause arrhythmias.

Paragangliomas, including pheochromocytomas, rarely occur in the heart; when they do, they are usually localized to the base of the heart near vagus nerve endings. They may manifest with symptoms due to catecholamine secretion (eg, increased heart rate and BP, excessive sweating, tremor). Paragangliomas may be benign or malignant.

Pericardial cysts may resemble a cardiac tumor or pericardial effusion on chest x-ray. They are usually asymptomatic, although some cause compressive symptoms (eg, chest pain, dyspnea, cough).

Malignant primary tumors: Malignant primary tumors include sarcomas, pericardial mesothelioma, and primary lymphomas.

Sarcoma is the most common malignant and 2nd most common primary cardiac tumor (after myxoma). Sarcomas affect mainly middle-aged adults (mean, 41 yr). Almost 40% are angiosarcomas, most of which originate in the right atrium and involve the pericardium, causing right ventricular inflow tract obstruction, pericardial tamponade, and lung metastasis. Other types include undifferentiated sarcoma (25%), malignant fibrous histiocytoma (11 to 24%), leiomyosarcoma (8 to 9%), fibrosarcoma, rhabdomyosarcoma, liposarcoma, and osteosarcoma; these types are more likely to originate in the left atrium, causing mitral valve obstruction and heart failure.

Pericardial mesothelioma is rare. It affects all ages, males more than females. It causes tamponade and constriction, and can metastasize to the spine, adjacent soft tissues, and brain.

Primary lymphoma is extremely rare. It usually occurs in AIDS patients or other people with immunodeficiency. These tumors grow rapidly and cause heart failure, arrhythmias, tamponade, and superior vena cava (SVC) syndrome.

Metastatic tumors: Melanoma is a tumor with a high propensity for cardiac involvement . Lung and breast carcinoma, soft-tissue sarcoma, and renal cancer are also common sources of metastases to the heart.[1,2] Leukemia and lymphoma often metastasize to the heart, but the metastases may not be clinically significant. When Kaposi sarcoma spreads systemically in immunodeficient (usually AIDS) patients, it may spread to the heart, but clinical cardiac complications are uncommon.

1. Glancy DL, Roberts WC: The heart in malignant melanoma: A study of 70 autopsy cases. *Am J Cardiol* 21:555–571, 1968.
2. Klatt EC, Heitz DR: Cardiac metastases. *Cancer* 65:1456–1459, 1990.

Symptoms and Signs

Cardiac tumors cause symptoms and signs typical of much more common disorders (eg, heart failure, stroke, coronary artery disease). Symptoms and signs of benign primary cardiac tumors depend on tumor type, location, size, and friability.

Types of symptoms and signs: Symptoms can be classified as

- Extracardiac
- Intramyocardial
- Intracavitary

Extracardiac symptoms and signs may be constitutional or mechanical. Constitutional symptoms of fever, chills, lethargy, arthralgias, and weight loss are caused exclusively by myxomas, perhaps as a result of cytokine (eg, IL-6) release. Petechiae may also occur. These and other findings may erroneously suggest bacterial endocarditis, connective tissue disorders, and occult cancer. With some tumors (especially gelatinous myxomas) thrombi or tumor fragments may embolize into the systemic circulation (eg, brain, coronary arteries, kidneys, spleen, extremities) or the lungs and cause manifestations specific to those organs. Mechanical symptoms (eg, dyspnea, chest discomfort) result from compression of cardiac chambers or coronary arteries or from pericardial irritation or tamponade caused by growth or hemorrhage within the pericardium. Pericardial tumors may cause pericardial friction rubs.

Intramyocardial symptoms and signs are caused by arrhythmias, usually atrioventricular or intraventricular block or paroxysmal supraventricular or ventricular tachycardias due to compression or encroachment on the conduction system (notably rhabdomyomas and fibromas).

Intracavitary symptoms and signs are due to tumors that obstruct valvular function, blood flow, or both (causing valvular stenosis, valvular insufficiency, or heart failure). Intracavitary symptoms and signs may vary with body position, which can alter hemodynamics and physical forces associated with the tumor.

Symptoms and signs by tumor type: Myxomas may manifest with the triad of heart failure, embolic disease, and constitutional symptoms. Myxomas may cause a diastolic murmur that mimics that of mitral stenosis but whose loudness and location vary from beat to beat with body position. About 15% of pedunculated left atrial myxomas produce an audible "tumor plop" as they drop into the mitral orifice during diastole. Myxomas may also cause arrhythmias. Raynaud syndrome and finger clubbing are less typical but may occur.

Fibroelastomas, often discovered incidentally at autopsy, are usually asymptomatic; however, they may be a source of systemic emboli.

Rhabdomyomas are usually asymptomatic.

Fibromas cause arrhythmias and sudden death.

Hemangiomas are usually asymptomatic but may cause any of the extracardiac, intramyocardial, or intracavitary symptoms.

Teratomas cause respiratory distress and cyanosis due to compression of the aortic and pulmonary artery or SVC syndrome.

Symptoms and signs of **malignant cardiac tumors** are more acute in onset and progress more rapidly than those of benign tumors. Cardiac sarcomas most commonly cause symptoms of ventricular inflow tract obstruction and pericardial tamponade. Mesothelioma causes symptoms of pericarditis or tamponade. Primary lymphoma causes refractory progressive heart failure, tamponade, arrhythmias, and SVC syndrome. Metastatic cardiac tumors may manifest as sudden cardiac enlargement, tamponade (due to rapid accumulation of hemorrhagic pericardial effusion), heart block, other arrhythmias, or sudden unexplained heart failure. Fever, malaise, weight loss, night sweats, and loss of appetite may also be present.

Diagnosis

- Echocardiography
- Cardiac MRI

Diagnosis, which is often delayed because symptoms and signs mimic those of much more common disorders, is confirmed by echocardiography. Transesophageal echocardiography is better for visualizing atrial tumors, and transthoracic echocardiography is better for ventricular tumors.

Cardiac MRI is frequently used to identify tumor tissue characteristics and provide clues to tumor type. If results are equivocal, gated radionuclide imaging and CT may be helpful.

Biopsy is not usually done because imaging studies can often distinguish benign from malignant tumors.

Extensive testing often precedes echocardiography in patients with myxomas because their symptoms are nonspecific. Anemia; thrombocytopenia; and elevation of WBC count, ESR, C-reactive protein, and gamma-globulins are common. ECG may show left atrial enlargement. Routine chest x-ray may show calcium deposits in right atrial myxomas or in teratomas seen as anterior mediastinal masses. Myxomas are sometimes diagnosed when tumor cells are found in a surgically removed embolus.

Arrhythmias and heart failure with features of tuberous sclerosis suggest rhabdomyomas or fibromas. New cardiac symptoms and signs in a patient with a known extracardiac cancer suggest cardiac metastases. Chest x-ray may show bizarre changes in the cardiac silhouette.

Treatment

- Benign primary: Excision
- Malignant primary: Palliation
- Metastatic: Depends on tumor origin

Treatment of benign primary tumors is surgical excision followed by serial echocardiography over 5 to 6 yr to monitor for recurrence. Tumors are excised unless another disorder (eg, dementia) contraindicates surgery. Surgery is usually curative (95% survival at 3 yr). Exceptions are rhabdomyomas, most of which regress spontaneously and do not require treatment, and pericardial teratoma, which may require urgent pericardiocentesis. Patients with fibroelastoma may also require valvular repair or replacement. When rhabdomyomas or fibromas are multifocal, surgical excision is usually ineffective, and prognosis is poor after the first year of life; survival at 5 yr may be as low as 15%.

Treatment of malignant primary tumors is usually palliative (eg, radiation therapy, chemotherapy, management of complications) because prognosis is poor.

Treatment of metastatic cardiac tumors depends on tumor origin. It may include systemic chemotherapy or palliation.

KEY POINTS

- Most cardiac tumors are metastatic, most commonly from lung and breast carcinoma, soft-tissue sarcoma, and renal carcinoma.
- Primary cardiac tumors are much less common; most originate in the myocardium or endocardium but they can develop in any cardiac tissue and be benign or malignant.
- Manifestations depend on the location and type of tumor but include constitutional symptoms, valvular or inflow-outflow tract obstruction, thromboembolism, and arrhythmias.
- Diagnosis is by echocardiography, and frequently cardiac MRI.
- For benign tumors, treatment is excision; for malignant primary and most metastatic tumors, treatment is palliative.

79 Cardiomyopathies

A cardiomyopathy is a primary disorder of the heart muscle. It is distinct from structural cardiac disorders such as coronary artery disease, valvular disorders, and congenital heart disorders. Cardiomyopathies are divided into 3 main types based on the pathologic features (see Fig. 79–1):

- Dilated
- Hypertrophic
- Restrictive

The term ischemic cardiomyopathy refers to the dilated, poorly contracting myocardium that can occur in patients with severe coronary artery disease (with or without areas of infarction). It is *not* classically considered to be in the above-listed categories because it does not describe a primary myocardial disorder.

Manifestations of cardiomyopathies are usually those of heart failure and vary depending on whether there is systolic dysfunction, diastolic dysfunction, or both. Some cardiomyopathies may also cause chest pain, syncope, arrhythmias, or sudden death.

Evaluation typically includes family history, blood tests, ECG, chest x-ray, echocardiography, and often cardiac MRI if available. Some patients require endomyocardial biopsy (transvenous right ventricular or retrograde left ventricular). Other tests are done as needed to determine the cause. Treatment depends on the specific type and cause of cardiomyopathy (see Table 79–1).

DILATED CARDIOMYOPATHY

Dilated cardiomyopathy (DCM) is myocardial dysfunction causing heart failure in which ventricular dilation and systolic dysfunction predominate. Symptoms include dyspnea, fatigue, and peripheral edema. Diagnosis is clinical and by elevated natriuretic peptides, chest x-ray, echocardiography, and MRI. Treatment is directed at the cause. If heart failure is progressive and severe, cardiac resynchronization therapy (CRT), implantable cardioverter-defibrillator, repair of moderate to severe valvular regurgitation, or heart transplantation may be needed.

Pathophysiology

As a primary myocardial disorder, the myocardial dysfunction occurs in the absence of severe occlusive coronary artery disease or conditions that involve pressure or volume overload of the ventricle (eg, hypertension, valvular heart disease). In some patients, DCM is believed to start with acute myocarditis (probably viral in most cases), followed by a variable latent phase, a phase with diffuse necrosis of myocardial myocytes (due to an autoimmune reaction to virus-altered myocytes), and chronic fibrosis. Regardless of the cause, the myocardium dilates, thins, and hypertrophies in compensation (see Fig. 79–1), often leading to functional mitral regurgitation or tricuspid regurgitation and atrial dilation.

The disorder affects both ventricles in most patients, only the left ventricle (LV) in a few (unless the cause is ischemia), and only the right ventricle (RV) rarely.

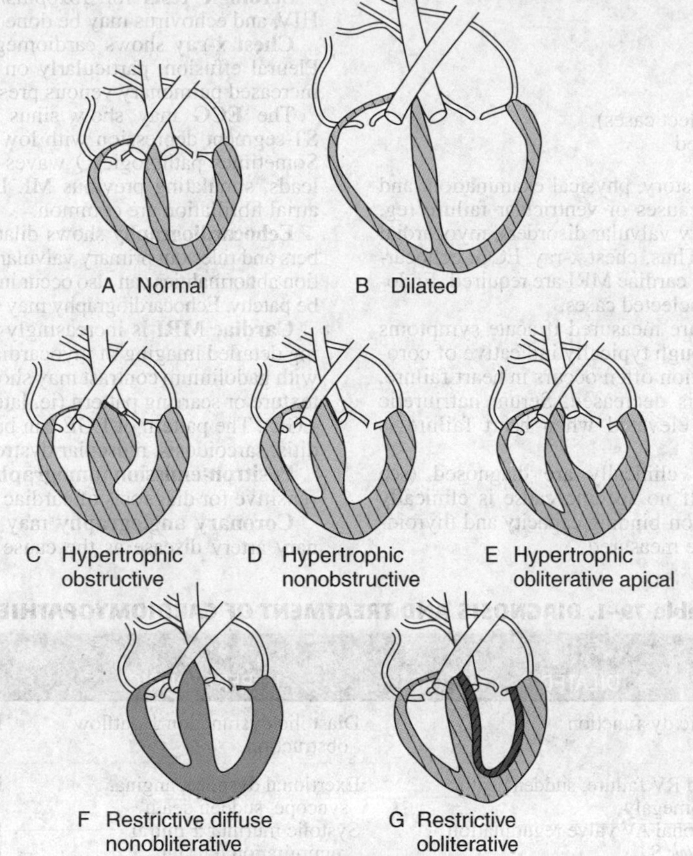

Fig. 79–1. Forms of cardiomyopathy.

Mural thrombi may form once chamber dilation is significant, especially during the acute myocarditis phase. Cardiac tachyarrhythmias often complicate the acute myocarditis and late chronic dilated phases as may atrioventricular block. Atrial fibrillation commonly occurs as the left atrium dilates.

Etiology

DCM has many known and probably many unidentified causes (see Table 79–2). More than 20 viruses can cause DCM; in temperate zones, coxsackievirus B is most common. In Central and South America, Chagas disease due to *Trypanosoma cruzi* is the most common infectious cause, although it is a cause of only 10% of heart failure cases in recent series. DCM is becoming increasingly common among patients with active HIV infection.

Other causes include prolonged tachycardia, toxoplasmosis, thyrotoxicosis, and beriberi. Many toxic substances, particularly alcohol, various organic solvents, iron or heavy metal ions, and certain chemotherapeutic drugs (eg, doxorubicin, trastuzumab), damage the heart. Frequent ventricular ectopy (> 10,000 ventricular premature beats/day) has been associated with left ventricular systolic dysfunction.

Sudden emotional stress and other hyperadrenergic states can trigger acute DCM that is typically reversible (as is that caused by prolonged tachycardia). An example is acute apical ballooning cardiomyopathy (takotsubo cardiomyopathy). In this disorder, usually the apex and occasionally other segments of the LV is affected, causing regional wall dysfunction and sometimes focal dilation (ballooning).

Genetic factors play a role in 20 to 35% of cases; > 60 genes and loci have been implicated.

Symptoms and Signs

Onset of DCM is usually gradual except in acute myocarditis, acute apical ballooning cardiomyopathy, and tachyarrhythmia-induced myopathy. About 25% of all patients with DCM have atypical chest pain. Other symptoms depend on which ventricle is affected.

Left ventricular dysfunction causes exertional dyspnea and fatigue due to elevated LV diastolic pressure and low cardiac output.

Right ventricular failure causes peripheral edema and neck vein distention. Infrequently the RV is predominantly affected in younger patients, and atrial arrhythmias and sudden death due to malignant ventricular tachyarrhythmias are typical.

Diagnosis

- Chest x-ray
- ECG
- Echocardiography
- Cardiac MRI
- Endomyocardial biopsy (select cases)
- Testing for cause as indicated

Diagnosis of DCM is by history, physical examination, and exclusion of other common causes of ventricular failure (eg, systemic hypertension, primary valvular disorders, myocardial infarction—see Table 79–1). Thus, chest x-ray, ECG, echocardiography, and, more recently, cardiac MRI are required. Endomyocardial biopsy is done in selected cases.

Serum cardiac markers are measured if acute symptoms or chest pain is present. Although typically indicative of coronary ischemia,troponin elevation often occurs in heart failure, especially if renal function is decreased. Serum natriuretic peptide levels are typically elevated when heart failure is present.

Specific causes suspected clinically are diagnosed (see elsewhere in The Manual). If no specific cause is clinically apparent, serum ferritin and iron-binding capacity and thyroid-stimulating hormone levels are measured.

Serologic tests for *Toxoplasma*, *T. cruzi*, coxsackievirus, HIV, and echovirus may be done in appropriate cases.

Chest x-ray shows cardiomegaly, usually of all chambers. Pleural effusion, particularly on the right, often accompanies increased pulmonary venous pressure and interstitial edema.

The **ECG** may show sinus tachycardia and nonspecific ST-segment depression with low voltage or inverted T waves. Sometimes pathologic Q waves are present in the precordial leads, simulating previous MI. Left bundle branch block and atrial fibrillation are common.

Echocardiography shows dilated, hypokinetic cardiac chambers and rules out primary valvular disorders. Segmental wall motion abnormalities can also occur in DCM because the process may be patchy. Echocardiography may also show a mural thrombus.

Cardiac MRI is increasingly done and is useful in providing detailed imaging of myocardial structure and function. MRI with gadolinium contrast may show abnormal myocardial tissue texture or scarring pattern (ie, late gadolinium enhancement, or LGE). The pattern of LGE can be diagnostic in active myocarditis, sarcoidosis, muscular dystrophy, or Chagas disease).

Positron-emission tomography (PET) has been shown to be sensitive for diagnosis of cardiac sarcoidosis.

Coronary angiography may be required to exclude coronary artery disease as the cause of LV dysfunction when the

Table 79–1. DIAGNOSIS AND TREATMENT OF CARDIOMYOPATHIES

FEATURE OR METHOD	DILATED	HYPERTROPHIC	RESTRICTIVE
Pathophysiology	Systolic dysfunction	Diastolic dysfunction ± outflow obstruction	Diastolic dysfunction
Clinical findings	LV and RV failure, sudden death, Cardiomegaly Functional AV valve regurgitation S_3 and/or S_4	Exertional dyspnea, angina, syncope, sudden death Systolic murmur ± mitral regurgitation murmur, S_4 Bifid carotid pulse with a brisk upstroke and rapid downstroke	Exertional dyspnea and fatigue LV ± RV failure Functional AV valve regurgitation
ECG	Nonspecific ST- and T-wave abnormalities Q waves ± BBB	LV hypertrophy and ischemia Deep septal Q waves	LV hypertrophy or low QRS voltage
Echocardiography	Dilated hypokinetic ventricles ± mural thrombus Low EF and, frequently, functional AV valve regurgitation	Hypertrophied ventricle, high, normal or low EF, ± mitral systolic anterior motion ± asymmetric hypertrophy ± LV gradient	Increased wall thickness ± cavity obliteration LV diastolic dysfunction
X-ray	Cardiomegaly Pulmonary venous congestion	No cardiomegaly	No or mild cardiomegaly
Hemodynamics	Normal or high EDP, low EF, diffusely dilated hypokinetic ventricles ± AV valve regurgitation Low CO	High EDP ± outflow subvalvular gradient ± mitral regurgitation Normal or low CO	High EDP, dip and plateau diastolic LV pressure curve Normal or low CO
Prognosis	20% mortality in first year, and about 10%/yr thereafter	About 1% annual risk of sudden death	70% 5-yr mortality
Treatment	Diuretics, ACE inhibitors, angiotensin II receptor blockers, beta-blockers, spironolactone or eplerenone, digoxin, ICD, cardiac resynchronization therapy, anticoagulants	Beta-blockers ± verapamil ± disopyramide ± septal myotomy ± catheter alcohol ablation	Phlebotomy for hemochromatosis Endocardial resection Hydroxyurea for hypereosinophilia

AV = atrioventricular; BBB = bundle branch block; CO = cardiac output; EDP = end-diastolic pressure; EF = ejection fraction; ICD = implantable cardioverter-defibrillator; LV = left ventricular; RV = right ventricular; S_3 = 3rd heart sound; S_4 = 4th heart sound; ± = with or without.

Table 79–2. CAUSES OF DILATED CARDIOMYOPATHY

CAUSE	EXAMPLES
Chronic tachycardia	Frequent ventricular ectopy Uncontrolled atrial fibrillation or other persistent tachyarrhythmias
Connective tissue disorders	Rheumatoid arthritis Systemic lupus erythematosus Systemic sclerosis
Drugs and toxins	Anthracyclines Catecholamines Cobalt Cocaine Cyclophosphamide Ethanol Psychotherapeutic drugs (tricyclic and quadricyclic antidepressants, phenothiazine) Radiation Trastuzumab
Eosinophilic myocarditis	—
Genetic abnormality	Familial disease in 20–30% of patients: autosomal dominant, X-linked, autosomal recessive, or mitochondrial inheritance
Granulomatous disorders	Granulomatosis with polyangiitis Granulomatous or giant cell myocarditis Sarcoidosis
Hereditary neuromuscular and neurologic disorders	Duchenne muscular dystrophy Dreyfuss syndrome Emery myotonia congenita Fascioscapulohumeral muscular dystrophy Friedreich ataxia
Infections (acute or chronic)	Bacterial Fungal Helminthic Protozoan Rickettsial Spirochetal Viral (including HIV infection)
Metabolic disorders	Acromegaly Diabetes mellitus Familial storage disorders Hemochromatosis Hyperthyroidism Hypokalemia Hypomagnesemia Hypophosphatemia Hypothyroidism Morbid obesity Nutritional disorders (eg, beriberi, selenium deficiency, carnitine deficiency, kwashiorkor) Pheochromocytoma Uremia
Pregnancy (peripartum period)	—
Tumors	Certain endocrinologically active tumors (eg, pheochromocytoma, adrenal tumors, thyroid tumors)

diagnosis is in doubt after noninvasive tests. Patients with chest pain or several cardiovascular risk factors and elderly patients are more likely to have coronary artery disease. Either ventricle can be biopsied during catheterization in select cases where the results will change management.

Endomyocardial biopsy is indicated if giant cell myocarditis, eosinophilic myocarditis, or sarcoidosis is suspected, as the results will affect management.

Prognosis

Prognosis generally has been poor, although prognosis has improved with current management regimens (eg, use of beta-blockers, ACE inhibitors, mineralocorticoid receptor antagonists, implantable cardioverter-defibrillators, or CRT). About 20% die in the first year and then about 10%/yr thereafter; about 40 to 50% of deaths are sudden, due to a malignant arrhythmia or an embolic event. Prognosis is better if compensatory hypertrophy preserves ventricular wall thickness and is worse if ventricular walls thin markedly and the ventricle dilates. Patients whose DCM is well-compensated with treatment may be stable for many years.

Treatment

- Cause (if any) treated
- Standard therapy for heart failure with reduced ejection fraction (EF)
- Anticoagulants when atrial fibrillation or other indication is present
- Sometimes implantable cardioverter-defibrillator, CRT, or transplantation
- Immunosupression in patients with giant cell myocarditis, eosinophilic myocarditis, or sarcoidosis

Treatable causes (eg, toxoplasmosis, acute Chagas disease, hemochromatosis, thyrotoxicosis, beriberi) are corrected. Patients with HIV infection should have antiretroviral therapy (ART) optimized, Treatment with immunosuppression should be limited to patients with biopsy proven giant cell myocarditis, eosinophilic myocarditis, or sarcoidosis.

Otherwise, treatment is the same as for heart failure with reduced EF: ACE inhibitors, beta-blockers, aldosterone receptor blockers, angiotensin II receptor blockers, valsartan/sacubitril, hydralazine/nitrates, diuretics, and digoxin. Recent studies have shown patients with idiopathic DCM respond particularly well to standard HF treatments and generally do better than patients with ischemic heart disease.

Because mural thrombi may form, prophylactic oral anticoagulation has been used in the past. The use of anticoagulants for patients with reduced LV function and in sinus rhythm remains controversial, and recommendations regarding anticoagulant use in this situation await the results of ongoing clinical trials. Warfarin or a novel oral anticoagulant (NOAC) are recommended when a specific indication is present (eg, previous cerebrovascular embolism, identified cardiac thrombus, atrial fibrillation and/or flutter).

Medical treatment of heart failure reduces risk of arrhythmia, but an implantable cardioverter-defibrillator may be used to prevent death due to sudden arrhythmia in patients who continue to have a reduced EF despite optimal medical therapy. Because atrioventricular (AV) block during acute myocarditis often resolves, a permanent pacemaker is usually not needed acutely. However, a permanent pacemaker may be required if AV block persists or develops during the chronic dilated phase. If patients have a widened QRS interval with a low LV EF and severe symptoms despite optimal medical treatment, CRT should be considered.

Patients with refractory heart failure despite treatment may become candidates for heart transplantation. Selection criteria include absence of associated systemic disorders and psychologic disorders and high, irreversible pulmonary vascular resistance; because donor hearts are scarce, younger patients (usually < 60) are given higher priority. Left ventricular assist devices (LVAD) may also be considered for destination therapy in some patients (eg patients who are not eligible for cardiac transplant). In destination therapy an LVAD is used as a permanent therapy for patients with refractory heart failure (rather than as a temporary measure before cardiac transplant).

KEY POINTS

- In DCM, the myocardium dilates, thins, and hypertrophies.
- Causes include infection (commonly viral), toxins, and metabolic, genetic, or connective tissue disorders.
- Do chest x-ray, ECG, echocardiography, and cardiac MRI to evaluate extent of disease and endomyocardial biopsy in select patients.
- Look for other causes of heart failure if appropriate.
- Treat primary cause if possible and use standard heart failure treatment measures (eg, ACE inhibitors, beta-blockers, aldosterone receptor blockers, angiotensin II receptor blockers, sacubitril/valsartan, hydralazine/nitrates, diuretics, digoxin, implantable cardioverter-defibrillator, and/or CRT).
- Use oral anticoagulants and immunosuppressants in select patients.

HYPERTROPHIC CARDIOMYOPATHY

Hypertrophic cardiomyopathy (HCM) is a congenital or acquired disorder characterized by marked ventricular hypertrophy with diastolic dysfunction but without increased afterload (eg, due to valvular aortic stenosis, coarctation of the aorta, systemic hypertension). Symptoms include dyspnea, chest pain, syncope, and sudden death. A systolic murmur, increased by Valsalva maneuver, is typically present in the hypertrophic obstructive type. Diagnosis is by echocardiography or cardiac MRI. Treatment is with beta-blockers, verapamil, disopyramide, and sometimes chemical reduction or surgical removal of outflow tract obstruction.

HCM is a common cause of sudden death in young athletes. It may cause unexplained syncope and may not be diagnosed before autopsy.

Etiology

Most cases of HCM are inherited. At least 1,500 different mutations that are inherited in an autosomally dominant pattern have been identified; spontaneous mutations can also occur. At least 1 in 500 people are affected; phenotypic expression varies markedly.

Rarely, HCM is acquired. It may develop in patients with acromegaly, pheochromocytoma, and neurofibromatosis.

Pathophysiology

The myocardium is abnormal with cellular and myofibrillar disarray, although this finding is not specific for HCM.

In the most common phenotype, the anterior septum and contiguous anterior free wall below the aortic valve are markedly hypertrophied and thickened, with little or no hypertrophy of the left ventricular posterior wall. Sometimes isolated apical hypertrophy occurs; however, virtually any asymmetric pattern of left ventricular hypertrophy can be observed, and in a small minority of patients even symmetric hypertrophy has been noted.

About two thirds of patients exhibit obstructive physiology at rest or during exercise. Obstruction is the result of mechanical impedance to LV outflow during systole due to systolic anterior motion (SAM) of the mitral valve. During this process (SAM), the mitral valve and valve apparatus are sucked into the LV outflow tract by a Venturi effect of high-velocity blood flow, resulting in obstruction of flow and decrease in cardiac output. Mitral regurgitation can also occur as the result of distortion of leaflet motion by SAM of the mitral valve. This obstruction and valvular regurgitation contribute to the development of symptoms related to heart failure. Less commonly, midventricular hypertrophy leads to an intracavitary gradient at the papillary muscle level.

Contractility is grossly normal, resulting in a normal EF. Later, EF is elevated because the ventricle has a small volume and empties nearly completely to maintain cardiac output.

Hypertrophy results in a stiff, noncompliant chamber (usually the LV) that resists diastolic filling, elevating end-diastolic pressure and thus increasing pulmonary venous pressure. As resistance to filling increases, cardiac output decreases, an effect worsened by any outflow tract gradient present. Because tachycardia allows less time for filling, symptoms tend to appear mainly during exercise or tachyarrhythmias.

Coronary blood flow may be impaired, causing angina pectoris, syncope, or arrhythmias in the absence of epicardial coronary artery disease (CAD). Flow may be impaired because capillary density relative to myocyte size is inadequate (capillary/myocyte imbalance) or lumen diameter of intramyocardial coronary arteries is narrowed by intimal and medial hyperplasia and hypertrophy. A supply-demand mismatch also may be present due to increased oxygen demand caused by the hypertrophy and adverse loading conditions.

In some cases, myocytes gradually die, probably because capillary/myocyte imbalance causes chronic diffuse ischemia. As myocytes die, they are replaced by diffuse fibrosis. Then, the hypertrophied ventricle with diastolic dysfunction gradually dilates and systolic dysfunction develops.

Infective endocarditis can complicate HCM because of the mitral valve abnormality and because of rapid blood flow through the outflow tract during early systole. Atrioventricular block is sometimes a late complication.

Symptoms and Signs

Typically, symptoms appear between ages 20 and 40 and are exertional, but symptoms may be highly variable. They include dyspnea, chest pain (usually resembling typical angina), palpitations, and syncope. Because systolic function is preserved, fatigability is seldom reported. The abnormal diastolic function is responsible for most symptoms. In patients with outflow tract obstruction, differentiation of symptoms due to the obstruction versus those caused by abnormal diastolic function can be difficult.

Syncope may occur during exertion either because outflow obstruction worsens with increased contractility or because of nonsustained ventricular or atrial arrhythmia. *Syncope is a marker of increased risk of sudden death,* which is thought to result from ventricular tachycardia or fibrillation.

Blood pressure and heart rate are usually normal, and signs of increased venous pressure are rare. When the outflow tract is obstructed, the carotid pulse has a brisk upstroke, bifid peak, and rapid downstroke. The apex beat may have a sustained thrust due to LV hypertrophy. A 4th heart sound (S_4) is often present and is associated with a forceful atrial contraction against a poorly compliant LV in late diastole.

In patients with the obstructive form of HCM, a systolic ejection-type murmur can be heard that does not radiate to the neck. This murmur is heard best at the left sternal edge in the 3rd or 4th intercostal space. A mitral regurgitation murmur due to distortion of the mitral apparatus may be heard at the apex. The left ventricular outflow ejection murmur of HCM can be increased by a Valsalva maneuver (which reduces venous return and LV diastolic volume), measures to lower aortic pressure (eg, nitroglycerin), or a postextrasystolic contraction (which increases the outflow tract pressure gradient). Handgrip increases aortic pressure, thereby reducing the murmur's intensity.

Diagnosis

- Clinical suspicion (syncope or murmur)
- Echocardiography and/or MRI

Diagnosis is suspected based on a typical murmur and symptoms. Suspicion is increased if the patient has a history of unexplained syncope or a family history of unexplained sudden death. Unexplained syncope in young athletes should always raise suspicion. HCM must be distinguished from aortic stenosis and coronary artery disease, which cause similar symptoms.

ECG and 2-dimensional echocardiography and/or MRI (the best noninvasive confirmatory tests) are done. Chest x-ray is often done but is usually normal because the ventricles are not dilated (although the left atrium may be enlarged). Patients with syncope or sustained arrhythmias should be evaluated as inpatients. Exercise testing and 24-h ambulatory monitoring may be helpful for patients considered at high risk, although accurately identifying such patients is difficult.

The ECG usually shows voltage criteria for LV hypertrophy (eg, S wave in lead V_1 plus R wave in lead V_5 or $V_6 > 35$ mm). Very deep septal Q waves in leads I, aVL, V_5, and V_6 are often present with asymmetric septal hypertrophy; HCM sometimes produces a QRS complex in V_1 and V_2, simulating previous septal infarction. T waves are usually abnormal; the most common finding is deep symmetric T-wave inversion in leads I, aVL, V_5, and V_6. ST-segment depression in the same leads is common (particularly in the apical obliterative form). The P wave is often broad and notched in leads II, III, and aVF, with a biphasic P wave in leads V_1 and V_2, indicating left atrial hypertrophy. Incidence of preexcitation phenomenon of the Wolff-Parkinson-White syndrome type, which may cause palpitations, is increased. Bundle branch block is common.

Two-dimensional Doppler echocardiography can differentiate the forms of cardiomyopathy (see Fig. 79–1) and quantify the severity of hypertrophy and degree of outflow tract obstruction . These measurements are particularly useful for monitoring the effect of medical or surgical treatment. Midsystolic closure of the aortic valve sometimes occurs when outflow tract obstruction is severe.

Cardiac catheterization is usually done only when invasive therapy is considered. Usually, no significant stenoses are present in the coronary arteries, but elderly patients may have coexisting CAD.

Genetic markers do not influence treatment or identify high-risk individuals. However, genetic testing may be of benefit in screening family members.

Prognosis

Overall, annual mortality is about 1% for adults but is higher for children. Death is usually sudden, and sudden death is the most common sequelae; chronic heart failure occurs less often. A higher risk of sudden cardiac death is predicted by the presence of the following risk factors:

- Family history of sudden cardiac death due to HCM
- Unexplained recent syncope
- Multiple repetitive non-sustained ventricular tachycardia (on ambulatory ECG)
- Hypotensive or attenuated blood pressure response to exercise
- Massive left-ventricular hypertrophy (thickness ≥ 30 mm)
- Extensive and diffuse LGE on MRI

Treatment

- Beta-blockers
- Rate-limiting and negative inotropic calcium channel blockers
- Avoidance of nitrates, diuretics, and ACE inhibitors
- Possibly antiarrhythmics (eg, disopyramide, amiodarone)
- Possibly implantable cardioverter-defibrillator and sometimes surgery or ablative procedures

Treatment is based on the phenotype. Patients without obstruction generally have a stable clinical course without significant symptoms, although some experience heart failure symptoms due to diastolic dysfunction. Beta-blockers and heart rate-limiting calcium channel blockers with a lower arterial dilation capacity (usually verapamil), alone or combined, are the mainstays. By slowing the heart rate, they prolong the diastolic filling period, which may increase left ventricular filling in patients with diastolic dysfunction. Long-term efficacy of such therapy, however, has not been proven.

In patients with the obstructive phenotype, in addition to attempts at improving diastolic function, treatment is directed at reducing the outflow tract gradient. Non-dihydropyridine calcium channel blockers, beta-blockers, and disopyramide reduce the outflow tract gradient through their negative inotropic effects. Disopyramide appears to be most effective for patients with a resting gradient whereas beta-blockers are best at blunting the gradient that occurs during exercise.

Patients who continue to experience symptoms related to significant outflow tract gradients (≥ 50 mm Hg) despite medical therapy are candidates for invasive treatment. When done at an experienced center, surgical myectomy has a low operative mortality with excellent outcomes, making it the preferred therapy in such patients. Percutaneous catheter alcohol septal ablation is an alternative to surgery in elderly patients and others who are at high surgical risk.

Drugs that reduce preload (eg, nitrates, diuretics, ACE inhibitors, angiotensin II receptor blockers) decrease chamber size and worsen symptoms and signs. Vasodilators increase the outflow tract gradient and cause a reflex tachycardia that further worsens ventricular diastolic function. Inotropic drugs (eg, digitalis glycosides, catecholamines) worsen outflow tract obstruction, do not relieve the high end-diastolic pressure, and may induce arrhythmias.

If syncope or sudden cardiac arrest has occurred or if ventricular arrhythmia is confirmed by ECG or 24-h ambulatory monitoring, an implantable cardioverter-defibrillator (ICD) should usually be placed. Controversy exists regarding the need to place a defibrillator in patients without syncope, sudden cardiac arrest, or ventricular arrhythmias. It is generally believed that ICD insertion should be considered in patients with high-risk features, which include a family history of premature sudden cardiac arrest, LV wall thickness > 3 cm, abnormal blood pressure response on exercise treadmill testing (fall in systolic pressure of > 10 mm Hg), left ventricular outflow tract obstructive gradient of > 50 mm Hg, or delayed enhancement on cardiac MR imaging. Competitive sports should be avoided because many sudden deaths occur during increased exertion.

Treatment of the dilated congestive phase of HCM is the same as that of DCM with predominant systolic dysfunction.

Genetic counseling is appropriate for patients with asymmetric septal hypertrophy.

KEY POINTS

- HCM is usually due to one of numerous genetic mutations that cause various types of ventricular hypertrophy that restrict filling (ie, cause diastolic dysfunction) and sometimes obstruct LV outflow.
- Coronary blood flow may be impaired even in the absence of coronary artery atherosclerosis because capillary density is inadequate and the intramyocardial coronary arteries are narrowed by intimal and medial hyperplasia and hypertrophy
- At a young age, patients may have chest pain, dyspnea, palpitations, syncope, and sometimes sudden death, typically triggered by exertion.
- Echocardiography is done, but, if available, MRI best shows the abnormal myocardium.
- Use beta-blockers and/or rate-limiting calcium channel blockers (usually verapamil) to decrease myocardial contractility and slow the heart rate and thus prolong diastolic filling and decrease outflow obstruction.
- Avoid nitrates and other drugs that decrease preload (eg, diuretics, ACE inhibitors, angiotensin II receptor blockers) because these decrease LV size and worsen LV function.
- Place an implantable cardioverter-defibrillator for patients with syncope or sudden cardiac arrest.
- Do surgical myectomy or alcohol septal ablation in patients with symptoms despite medical therapy.

RESTRICTIVE CARDIOMYOPATHY

Restrictive cardiomyopathy (RCM) is characterized by noncompliant ventricular walls that resist diastolic filling; one (most commonly the left) or both ventricles may be affected. Symptoms include fatigue and exertional dyspnea. Diagnosis is by echocardiography and cardiac catheterization. Treatment is often unsatisfactory and is best directed at the cause. Surgery is sometimes useful.

RCM is the least prevalent form of cardiomyopathy. It is classified as

- Nonobliterative (myocardial infiltration by an abnormal substance)
- Obliterative (fibrosis of the endocardium and subendocardium)

Either type may be diffuse or nondiffuse (when the disorder affects only one ventricle or part of one ventricle unevenly).

Etiology

RCM is not always a primary cardiac disorder. Although the cause is usually unknown, it may arise as the consequence of systemic or genetic disorders; identified causes are listed in Table 79–3. Some disorders that cause RCM also affect other tissues (eg, amyloidosis, hemochromatosis). Some myocardial infiltrative disorders also affect other cardiac tissue. Rarely, amyloidosis affects coronary arteries. Sarcoidosis and Fabry disease may also affect nodal conduction tissue. Löffler syndrome (a subcategory of hypereosinophilic syndrome with primary cardiac involvement), which occurs in the tropics, begins as an acute arteritis with eosinophilia, followed by thrombus formation on the endocardium, chordae, and atrioventricular (AV) valves, progressing to fibrosis. Endocardial fibroelastosis (EFE), which occurs in temperate zones, affects only the LV.

Table 79–3. CAUSES OF RESTRICTIVE CARDIOMYOPATHY

CAUSE	EXAMPLES
Genetic abnormalities	Fabry disease Gaucher disease Hemochromatosis
Connective tissue disorders	Amyloidosis Diffuse systemic sclerosis Endocardial fibroelastosis
Other	Carcinoid tumors Endomyocardial fibrosis (EMF) Hypereosinophilic syndrome (including Löffler syndrome) Radiation Sarcoidosis

Pathophysiology

Endocardial thickening or myocardial infiltration (sometimes with death of myocytes, papillary muscle infiltration, compensatory myocardial hypertrophy, and fibrosis) may occur in one, typically the left, or both ventricles. As a result, the mitral or tricuspid valves may malfunction, leading to regurgitation. Functional AV valve regurgitation may result from myocardial infiltration or endocardial thickening. If nodal and conduction tissues are affected, the sinoatrial (SA) and atrioventricular node malfunction, sometimes causing various grades of SA block and AV block.

The main hemodynamic consequence is diastolic dysfunction with a rigid, noncompliant ventricle, impaired diastolic filling, and high filling pressure, leading to pulmonary venous hypertension. Systolic function may deteriorate if compensatory hypertrophy of infiltrated or fibrosed ventricles is inadequate. Mural thrombi can form, resulting in systemic emboli.

Symptoms and Signs

Symptoms are exertional dyspnea, orthopnea, paroxysmal nocturnal dyspnea, and peripheral edema. Fatigue results from a fixed cardiac output due to resistance to ventricular filling. Atrial and ventricular arrhythmias and AV block are common; angina and syncope are uncommon. Symptoms and signs closely mimic those of constrictive pericarditis.

Physical examination detects a quiet precordium, a low-volume and rapid carotid pulse, pulmonary crackles, and pronounced neck vein distention with a rapid *y* descent (see Fig. 73–1 on p. 583). A 3rd and/or 4th heart sound (S_3, S_4) may occur and must be differentiated from the precordial knock of constrictive pericarditis. In some cases, a murmur of functional mitral or tricuspid regurgitation results because myocardial or endocardial infiltration or fibrosis changes chordae or ventricular geometry. Pulsus paradoxus does not occur.

Diagnosis

- Echocardiography
- MRI
- Left and right heart catheterization
- Cardiac biopsy
- Laboratory tests and biopsy of other organ systems as needed

RCM should be considered in patients with heart failure and preserved EF, particularly when a systemic disorder known to lead to RCM has already been diagnosed. However, the underlying disorder may not be obvious on presentation.

ECG, chest x-ray, and echocardiography are required.

The ECG is usually nonspecifically abnormal, showing ST-segment and T-wave abnormalities and sometimes low voltage. Pathologic Q waves, not due to previous myocardial infarction, sometimes occur. Left ventricular hypertrophy due to compensatory myocardial hypertrophy or abnormalities of conduction, including AV block, sometimes occurs.

On chest x-ray, the heart size is often normal or small but can be enlarged in late-stage amyloidosis or hemochromatosis.

Echocardiography shows normal left ventricular EF. Tissue Doppler imaging frequently suggests elevated LV filling pressures, and strain imaging can show impaired longitudinal contraction despite the normal EF. Other common findings include dilated atria and myocardial hypertrophy. In amyloidosis an unusually bright echo pattern from the myocardium may be observed.

If the diagnosis is still in doubt, MRI can show abnormal myocardial texture in disorders with myocardial infiltration (eg, by amyloid or iron). MRI as well as cardiac CT can detect pericardial thickening, which can help diagnose pericardial constriction which can clinically mimic RCM.

If a definitive diagnosis is not evident after noninvasive testing, invasive work-up with cardiac catheterization and endomyocardial biopsy should be considered. Catheterization detects high atrial pressure in RCM with a prominent *y* descent and an early diastolic dip followed by a high diastolic plateau in the ventricular pressure curve. Diastolic pressure is usually a few mm Hg higher in the LV than in the right, in contrast to constrictive pericarditis where pressure in the ventricles is equal. Biopsy can detect endocardial fibrosis and thickening, myocardial infiltration by iron or amyloid, chronic myocardial fibrosis, or in the case of Fabry disease, inclusions in vascular endothelial cytoplasm. Coronary angiography is normal, except when amyloidosis affects epicardial coronary arteries.

Laboratory tests and biopsies of other organ systems for the most common causes of RCM (eg, rectal biopsy for amyloidosis, iron tests or liver biopsy for hemochromatosis) should be done.

Prognosis

Prognosis is poor (see Table 79–1) because the diagnosis is often made at a late stage. No treatment is available for most patients; symptomatic, supportive care can be provided. Standard therapies that are used in DCM (eg, ACE inhibitors, digoxin, beta-blockers) are poorly tolerated in restrictive disease. These patients may also have autonomic dysfunction (especially in amyloid heart disease) or low systemic blood pressure. There is a high rate of conduction system disease, heart block, and sudden death.

Treatment

- Cause treated
- Diuretics considered

Diuretics may be used for patients with edema or pulmonary vascular congestion but must be given cautiously because they can lower preload; the noncompliant ventricles depend on preload to maintain cardiac output. Digoxin does little to alter hemodynamic abnormalities and may cause serious arrhythmias in cardiomyopathy due to amyloidosis, in which extreme digitalis sensitivity is common. If heart rate is elevated, beta-blockers or rate-limiting calcium channel blockers may be used cautiously in low doses. Afterload reducers (eg, nitrates) may cause profound hypotension and usually are not useful.

If the diagnosis is made at an early stage, specific treatment of hemochromatosis, sarcoidosis, and Löffler syndrome may help.

Transplantation is not recommended because the disorder may recur in the transplanted heart.

KEY POINTS

- In RCM, endocardial thickening or myocardial infiltration leads to a rigid, noncompliant ventricle and thus diastolic dysfunction; systolic function is normal until late in the disease.
- Sometimes, valvular tissue or the conduction system is involved, causing valvular regurgitation or heart block and arrhythmias.
- Etiology is usually unknown, but some cases are caused by amyloidosis, hemochromatosis, or sarcoidosis.
- Diagnosis is by echocardiography plus testing for cause.
- Treatment is often unsatisfactory unless the cause can be addressed; diuretics may benefit patients with edema or pulmonary vascular congestion but must be used cautiously to avoid lowering preload.

80 Coronary Artery Disease

Coronary artery disease (CAD) involves impairment of blood flow through the coronary arteries, most commonly by atheromas. Clinical presentations include silent ischemia, angina pectoris, acute coronary syndromes (unstable angina, myocardial infarction), and sudden cardiac death. Diagnosis is by symptoms, ECG, stress testing, and sometimes coronary angiography. Prevention consists of modifying reversible risk factors (eg, hypercholesterolemia, hypertension, physical inactivity, obesity, and smoking). Treatment includes drugs and procedures to reduce ischemia and restore or improve coronary blood flow.

In developed countries, CAD is the leading cause of death in both sexes, accounting for about one-third of all deaths. Mortality rate among white men is about 1/10,000 at ages 25 to 34 and nearly 1/100 at ages 55 to 64. Mortality rate among white men aged 35 to 44 is 6.1 times that among age-matched white women. For unknown reasons, the sex difference is less marked in nonwhites and in patients with diabetes mellitus. Mortality rate among women increases after menopause and, by age 75, equals or even exceeds that of men.

Etiology

Usually, CAD is due to

- Coronary artery atherosclerosis: subintimal deposition of atheromas in large and medium-sized coronary arteries

Less often, CAD is due to

- Coronary artery spasm (see Variant Angina on p. 675)

Vascular endothelial dysfunction can promote atherosclerosis and contribute to coronary artery spasm. Of increasing importance, endothelial dysfunction is now also recognized as a cause of angina in the absence of epicardial coronary artery stenosis or spasm (see Syndrome X on p. 675).

Rare causes include coronary artery embolism, dissection, aneurysm (eg, in Kawasaki disease), and vasculitis (eg, in SLE, syphilis).

Pathophysiology

Coronary atherosclerosis is often irregularly distributed in different vessels but typically occurs at points of turbulence (eg, vessel bifurcations). As the atheromatous plaque grows, the arterial lumen progressively narrows, resulting in ischemia (often causing angina pectoris). The degree of stenosis required to cause ischemia varies with oxygen demand.

Occasionally, an atheromatous plaque ruptures or splits. Reasons are unclear but probably relate to plaque morphology, plaque calcium content, and plaque softening due to an inflammatory process. Rupture exposes collagen and other thrombogenic material, which activates platelets and the coagulation cascade, resulting in an acute thrombus, which interrupts coronary blood flow and causes some degree of myocardial ischemia. The consequences of acute ischemia, collectively referred to as acute coronary syndromes (ACS), depend on the location and degree of obstruction and range from unstable angina to transmural infarction to sudden death.

Coronary artery spasm is a transient, focal increase in vascular tone, markedly narrowing the lumen and reducing blood flow; symptomatic ischemia (variant angina) may result. Marked narrowing can trigger thrombus formation, causing infarction or life-threatening arrhythmia. Spasm can occur in arteries with or without atheroma.

- **In arteries without atheroma,** basal coronary artery tone is probably increased, and response to vasoconstricting stimuli is probably exaggerated. The exact mechanism is unclear but may involve endothelial cell abnormalities of nitric oxide production or an imbalance between endothelium-derived contracting and relaxing factors.
- **In arteries with atheroma,** the atheroma causes endothelial dysfunction, possibly resulting in local hypercontractility. Proposed mechanisms include loss of sensitivity to intrinsic vasodilators (eg, acetylcholine) and increased production of vasoconstrictors (eg, angiotensin II, endothelin, leukotrienes, serotonin, thromboxane) in the area of the atheroma. Recurrent spasm may damage the intima, leading to atheroma formation.

Use of vasoconstricting drugs (eg, cocaine, nicotine) and emotional stress also can trigger coronary spasm.

Risk Factors

Risk factors for CAD are the same as risk factors for atherosclerosis:

- High blood levels of low-density lipoprotein (LDL) cholesterol (see Dyslipidemia on p. 1303)
- High blood levels of lipoprotein a
- Low blood levels of high-density lipoprotein (HDL) cholesterol
- Diabetes mellitus (particularly type 2)
- Smoking
- Obesity
- Physical inactivity
- High level of apoprotein B (apo B)
- High blood levels of C-reactive protein (CRP)

Smoking may be a stronger predictor of MI in women (especially those < 45). Genetic factors play a role, and several systemic disorders (eg, hypertension, hypothyroidism) and metabolic disorders (eg, hyperhomocysteinemia) contribute to risk. A high level of apo B may identify increased risk when total cholesterol or LDL level is normal.

High blood levels of CRP indicate plaque instability and inflammation and may be a stronger predictor of risk of ischemic events than high levels of LDL. High blood levels of triglycerides and insulin (reflecting insulin resistance) may be risk factors, but data are less clear. CAD risk is increased by smoking tobacco; a diet high in fat and calories and low in phytochemicals (found in fruits and vegetables), fiber, and vitamins C, D, and E; a diet relatively low in omega-3 (n-3) polyunsaturated fatty acids (PUFAs—at least in some people); and poor stress management.

Coronary Artery Anatomy

The right and left coronary arteries arise from the right and left coronary sinuses in the root of the aorta just above the aortic valve orifice (see Fig. 80–1). The coronary arteries divide into large and medium-sized arteries that run along the heart's surface (epicardial coronary arteries) and subsequently send smaller arterioles into the myocardium.

The left coronary artery begins as the left main artery and quickly divides into the left anterior descending (LAD), circumflex, and sometimes an intermediate artery (ramus intermedius). The LAD artery usually follows the anterior interventricular groove and, in some people, continues over the apex. This artery supplies the anterior septum (including the proximal conduction system) and the anterior free wall of the left ventricle (LV). The circumflex artery, which is usually smaller than the LAD artery, supplies the lateral LV free wall.

Most people have right dominance: The right coronary artery passes along the atrioventricular (AV) groove over the right side of the heart; it supplies the sinus node (in 55%), right ventricle (RV), and usually the AV node and inferior myocardial wall. About 10 to 15% of people have left dominance: The circumflex artery is larger and continues along the posterior AV groove to supply the posterior wall and AV node.

Treatment

- Medical therapy including antiplatelet drugs, lipid-lowering drugs (eg, statins), and beta-blockers
- Percutaneous coronary intervention (PCI)
- For acute thrombosis, sometimes fibrinolytic drugs
- Coronary artery bypass grafting (CABG)

Treatment generally aims to reduce cardiac workload by decreasing oxygen demand and improving coronary artery blood flow, and, over the long term, to halt and reverse the atherosclerotic process. Coronary artery blood flow can be improved by PCI or CABG. An acute coronary thrombosis may sometimes be dissolved by fibrinolytic drugs.

Medical therapy: Medical management of patients with CAD depends on symptoms, cardiac function, and presence

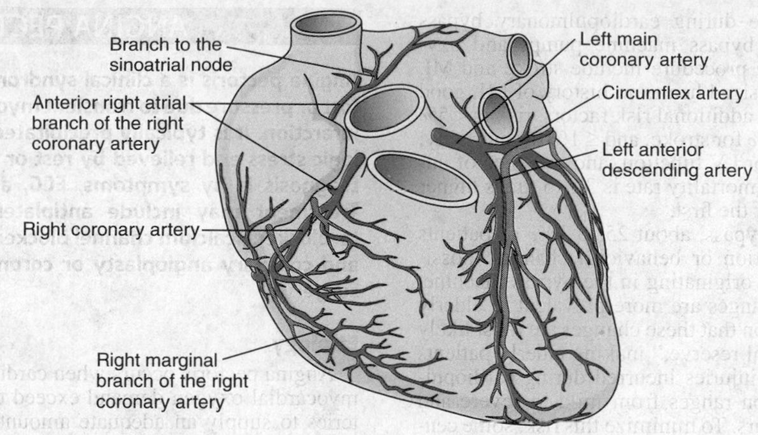

Fig. 80–1. Arteries of the heart.

of other disorders. Recommended therapy includes antiplatelet drugs to prevent clot formation and statins to lower LDL cholesterol levels (improving short-term and long-term outcomes probably by improving atheromatous plaque stability and endothelial function). Beta-blockers are effective in reducing symptoms of angina (by reducing heart rate and contractility, decreasing oxygen demand) and reducing mortality post-infarction, especially in the presence of post-myocardial infarction (MI) LV dysfunction. Calcium channel blockers are also helpful, often combined with beta-blockers in managing angina and hypertension but have not been proven to reduce mortality. Nitrates modestly dilate coronary arteries and decrease venous return, decreasing cardiac work and relieving angina quickly. Longer acting nitrate formulations help decrease angina events but do not decrease mortality. ACE inhibitors and angiotensin II receptor blockers are most effective in CAD patients with LV dysfunction.

Little evidence exists to guide therapy for patients with endothelial dysfunction. Treatment is generally similar to that for typical large-vessel atherosclerosis, but there is concern that use of beta-blockers may enhance endothelial dysfunction.

Percutaneous coronary intervention (see also p. 615): At first, PCI was done with balloon angioplasty alone. However, roughly 30 to 40% of patients developed restenosis within 6 mo, and 1 in 3 ultimately required repeat angioplasty or CABG. Insertion of a bare-metal stent after angioplasty reduced the rate of restenosis, but many patients still required repeat treatment.

Drug-eluting stents, which secrete an antiproliferative drug (eg, sirolimus, paclitaxel, everolimus) over a period of several weeks, have reduced the rate of restenosis to < 10%. When controversy over drug-eluting stents and abrupt stent thrombosis arose in 2006, use of drug-eluting stents decreased in most centers. Subsequent studies have shown that the risk of acute thrombosis is much less than originally believed. With development of new platforms for drug-eluting stents, the incidence of in-stent thrombosis has markedly decreased. Now, most PCI is done with stents, and about three fourths of all stents used in the US are drug-eluting.

Patients without significant infarct or complications may quickly return to work and usual activities after stenting, but strenuous activities should be avoided for 6 wk.

In-stent thrombosis occurs because of the inherent thrombogenicity of metallic stents. Most cases occur within the first 24 to 48 h. However, late stent thrombosis, occurring after 30 days and as late as ≥ 1 yr (rarely), can occur with both bare-metal and drug-eluting stents, especially after cessation of antiplatelet therapy. Progressive endothelialization of the bare-metal stent occurs within the first few months and reduces the risk of thrombosis. However, the antiproliferative drugs secreted by drug-eluting stents inhibit this process and prolong the risk of thrombosis. Thus, patients who undergo stent placement are treated with various antiplatelet drugs. The current standard regimen for patients with a bare-metal or drug-eluting stent consists of aspirin given indefinitely, plus clopidogrel, prasugrel, or ticagrelor for at least 6 to 12 mo, and intraprocedural anticoagulation with heparin or a similar agent (eg, bivalirudin, particularly for those at high risk of bleeding).The best results are obtained when the newer antiplatelet drugs are begun before the procedure.

Glycoprotein (GP) IIb/IIIa inhibitors are no longer routinely used in stable patients (ie, no comorbidities, no acute coronary syndrome) having elective stent placement. Although controversial, they may be beneficial in some patients with an acute coronary syndrome but should not be considered routine. It is unclear whether it is beneficial to give GP IIb/IIIa inhibitors before arrival in the cardiac catheterization laboratory, but most national organizations do not recommend their use in this situation.

After stent insertion, a statin is added if one is not already being used. Patients who receive a statin before the procedure have a lower risk of periprocedural MI.

Overall risk of PCI is comparable with that for CABG. Mortality rate is < 1%; Q wave MI rate is < 2%. In <1%, intimal dissection causes obstruction requiring emergency CABG. Risk of stroke with PCI is clearly less than with CABG (0.34% vs 1.2%).

PCI by itself does not cure or prevent the progression of CAD, so statins should be a part of post-PCI therapy. Such therapy has been shown to improve long-term event-free survival.

Coronary artery bypass grafting (see also p. 609): CABG uses arteries (eg, internal mammary, radial) whenever possible, and if necessary, sections of autologous veins (eg, saphenous) to bypass diseased segments of the coronary arteries. At 1 yr, about 85% of venous bypass grafts are patent, and after 5 yr, one third or more are completely blocked. However, after 10 yr, as many as 97% of internal mammary artery grafts are patent. Arteries also hypertrophy to accommodate increased flow. CABG is superior to PCI in patients with diabetes and in patients with multivessel disease amenable to grafting.

CABG is typically done during cardiopulmonary bypass with the heart stopped; a bypass machine pumps and oxygenates blood. Risks of the procedure include stroke and MI. For patients with a normal-sized heart, no history of MI, good ventricular function, and no additional risk factors, risk is < 5% for perioperative MI, 1 to 2% for stroke, and ≤ 1% for mortality; risk increases with age, poor LV function, and presence of underlying disease. Operative mortality rate is 3 to 5 times higher for a second bypass than for the first.

After cardiopulmonary bypass, about 25 to 30% of patients develop cognitive dysfunction or behavioral changes, possibly caused by microemboli originating in the bypass machine. Cognitive or behavioral changes are more prevalent in elderly patients, prompting suspicion that these changes are most likely due to diminished "neuronal reserve," making elderly patients more susceptible to minor injuries incurred during cardiopulmonary bypass. Dysfunction ranges from mild to severe and may persist for weeks to years. To minimize this risk, some centers use a beating heart technique (off-pump CABG, which uses no cardiopulmonary bypass), in which a device mechanically stabilizes the part of the heart upon which the surgeon is working. However, long-term studies have failed to demonstrate lasting benefits of this approach in comparison to conventional on-pump CABG.

CAD may progress despite bypass surgery. Postoperatively, the rate of proximal obstruction of bypassed vessels increases. Vein grafts become obstructed early if thrombi form and later (several years) if atherosclerosis causes slow degeneration of the intima and media. Aspirin prolongs vein graft patency. Continued smoking has a profound adverse effect on patency. After CABG, a statin should be started or continued at doses required to reach recommended target levels of LDL.

Prevention

Prevention of CAD involves modifying atherosclerosis risk factors:

- Smoking cessation
- Weight loss
- Healthful diet
- Regular exercise
- Modification of serum lipid levels
- Reduction of salt intake
- Control of hypertension and diabetes

Antihypertensives should be used to achieve a goal blood pressure of < 130/80 mm Hg.

Modification of serum lipid levels (particularly with statins) may slow or even partially reverse the progression of CAD. LDL targets are

- ≤ 100 mg/dL(≤ 2.59 mmol/L) for patients with known CAD
- 70 to 80 mg/dL (1.81 to 2.07 mmol/L) for those with a history of an ischemic event

Nicotinic acid or a fibrate may be added for patients with an HDL < 40 mg/dL (< 1.03 mmol/L), although several recent trials have failed to demonstrate a lower risk of ischemia or slowed progression of atherosclerosis when drugs are used to raise HDL.[1]

1. AIM-HIGH Investigators, Boden WE, Probstfield JL, Anderson T, et al. Niacin in patients with low HDL cholesterol levels receiving intensive statin therapy. *N Engl J Med* 365(24):2255–2267, 2011. doi: 10.1056/NEJMoa1107579.

ANGINA PECTORIS

Angina pectoris is a clinical syndrome of precordial discomfort or pressure due to transient myocardial ischemia without infarction. It is typically precipitated by exertion or psychologic stress and relieved by rest or sublingual nitroglycerin. Diagnosis is by symptoms, ECG, and myocardial imaging. Treatment may include antiplatelet drugs, nitrates, beta-blockers, calcium channel blockers, ACE inhibitors, statins, and coronary angioplasty or coronary artery bypass graft surgery.

Etiology

Angina pectoris occurs when cardiac workload and resultant myocardial oxygen demand exceed the ability of coronary arteries to supply an adequate amount of oxygenated blood, as can occur when the arteries are narrowed. Narrowing usually results from coronary artery atherosclerosis but may result from coronary artery spasm or, rarely, coronary artery embolism. Acute coronary thrombosis can cause angina if obstruction is partial or transient, but it usually causes acute MI.

Because myocardial oxygen demand is determined mainly by heart rate, systolic wall tension, and contractility, narrowing of a coronary artery typically results in angina that occurs during exertion and is relieved by rest.

In addition to exertion, cardiac workload can be increased by disorders such as hypertension, aortic stenosis, aortic regurgitation, or hypertrophic cardiomyopathy. In such cases, angina can result whether atherosclerosis is present or not. These disorders can also decrease relative myocardial perfusion because myocardial mass is increased (causing decreased diastolic flow).

A decreased oxygen supply, as in severe anemia or hypoxia, can precipitate or aggravate angina.

Pathophysiology

Angina may be

- Stable
- Unstable

In stable angina, the relationship between workload or demand and ischemia is usually relatively predictable. Unstable angina (see p. 682) is clinically worsening angina (eg, angina at rest or increasing frequency and/or intensity of episodes).

Atherosclerotic arterial narrowing is not entirely fixed; it varies with the normal fluctuations in arterial tone that occur in all people. Thus, more people have angina in the morning, when arterial tone is relatively high. Also, abnormal endothelial function may contribute to variations in arterial tone; eg, in endothelium damaged by atheromas, stress of a catecholamine surge causes vasoconstriction rather than dilation (normal response).

As the myocardium becomes ischemic, coronary sinus blood pH falls, cellular potassium is lost, lactate accumulates, ECG abnormalities appear, and ventricular function (both systolic and diastolic) deteriorates. Left ventricular (LV) diastolic pressure usually increases during angina, sometimes inducing pulmonary congestion and dyspnea. The exact mechanism by which ischemia causes discomfort is unclear but may involve nerve stimulation by hypoxic metabolites.

Symptoms and Signs

Angina may be a vague, barely troublesome ache or may rapidly become a severe, intense precordial crushing sensation. It is rarely described as pain. Discomfort is most commonly felt beneath the sternum, although location varies. Discomfort may radiate to the left shoulder and down the inside of the left arm, even to the fingers; straight through to the back; into the throat, jaws, and teeth; and, occasionally, down the inside of the right arm. It may also be felt in the upper abdomen. The discomfort of angina is never above the ears or below the umbilicus.

Atypical angina (eg, with bloating, gas, abdominal distress) may occur in some patients. These patients often ascribe symptoms to indigestion; belching may even seem to relieve the symptoms. Other patients have dyspnea due to the sharp, reversible increase in LV filling pressure that often accompanies ischemia. Frequently, the patient's description is imprecise, and whether the problem is angina, dyspnea, or both may be difficult to determine. Because ischemic symptoms require a minute or more to resolve, brief, fleeting sensations rarely represent angina.

Between and even during attacks of angina, physical findings may be normal. However, during the attack, heart rate may increase modestly, BP is often elevated, heart sounds become more distant, and the apical impulse is more diffuse. The 2nd heart sound may become paradoxical because LV ejection is more prolonged during an ischemic attack. A 4th heart sound is common, and a 3rd heart sound may develop. A mid or late systolic apical murmur, shrill or blowing—but not especially loud—may occur if ischemia causes localized papillary muscle dysfunction, causing mitral regurgitation.

Angina pectoris is typically triggered by exertion or strong emotion, usually persists no more than a few minutes, and subsides with rest. Response to exertion is usually predictable, but in some patients, exercise that is tolerated one day may precipitate angina the next because of variations in arterial tone. Symptoms are exaggerated when exertion follows a meal or occurs in cold weather; walking into the wind or first contact with cold air after leaving a warm room may precipitate an attack. Symptom severity is often classified by the degree of exertion resulting in angina (see Table 80–1).

Table 80–1. CANADIAN CARDIOVASCULAR SOCIETY CLASSIFICATION SYSTEM OF ANGINA PECTORIS

CLASS	ACTIVITIES TRIGGERING CHEST PAIN
1	Strenuous, rapid, or prolonged exertion
	Not usual physical activities (eg, walking, climbing stairs)
2	Walking rapidly
	Walking uphill
	Climbing stairs rapidly
	Walking or climbing stairs after meals
	Cold
	Wind
	Emotional stress
3	Walking, even 1 or 2 blocks at usual pace and on level ground
	Climbing stairs, even 1 flight
4	Any physical activity
	Sometimes occurring at rest

Adapted from Braunwald E, Antman EM, Beasley JW, et al: ACC/AHA Guidelines for the management of patients with unstable angina and non-ST segment elevation myocardial infarction: A report of the American College of Cardiology/American Heart Association Task Force on Practice Guidelines (Committee on the management of patients with unstable angina). *Journal of American College of Cardiology* 36:970–1062, 2000.

Attacks may vary from several a day to symptom-free intervals of weeks, months, or years. Attacks may increase in frequency (called crescendo angina) leading to a MI or death or gradually decrease or disappear if adequate collateral coronary circulation develops, if the ischemic area infarcts, or if heart failure or intermittent claudication supervenes and limits activity.

Nocturnal angina may occur if a dream causes striking changes in respiration, pulse rate, and BP. Nocturnal angina may also be a sign of recurrent LV failure, an equivalent of nocturnal dyspnea. The recumbent position increases venous return, stretching the myocardium and increasing wall stress, which increases oxygen demand.

Angina decubitus is angina that occurs spontaneously during rest. It is usually accompanied by a modestly increased heart rate and a sometimes markedly higher BP, which increase oxygen demand. These increases may be the cause of rest angina or the result of ischemia induced by plaque rupture and thrombus formation. If angina is not relieved, unmet myocardial oxygen demand increases further, making MI more likely.

Unstable angina: Because angina characteristics are usually predictable for a given patient, any changes (ie, rest angina, new-onset angina, increasing angina) should be considered serious, especially when the angina is severe (ie, Canadian Cardiovascular Society class 3). Such changes are termed unstable angina and require prompt evaluation and treatment.

Silent ischemia: Patients with CAD (particularly patients with diabetes) may have ischemia without symptoms. Silent ischemia sometimes manifests as transient asymptomatic ST-T abnormalities seen during stress testing or 24-h Holter monitoring. Radionuclide studies can sometimes document asymptomatic myocardial ischemia during physical or mental stress. Silent ischemia and angina pectoris may coexist, occurring at different times. Prognosis depends on severity of the CAD.

Diagnosis

- Typical symptoms
- ECG
- Stress testing with ECG or imaging (echocardiographic or nuclear)
- Coronary angiography for significant symptoms or positive stress test

Diagnosis of angina is suspected if chest discomfort is typical and is precipitated by exertion and relieved by rest. Presence of significant risk factors for CAD in the history adds weight to reported symptoms. Patients whose chest discomfort lasts > 20 min or occurs during rest or who have syncope or heart failure are evaluated for an acute coronary syndrome.

Chest discomfort may also be caused by GI disorders (eg, reflux, esophageal spasm, indigestion, cholelithiasis), costochondritis, anxiety, panic attacks, hyperventilation, and other cardiac disorders (eg, aortic dissection, pericarditis, mitral valve prolapse, supraventricular tachycardia, atrial fibrillation), even when coronary blood flow is not compromised.

ECG is always done. More specific tests include stress testing with ECG or with myocardial imaging (eg, echocardiography, radionuclide imaging, MRI) and coronary angiography. Noninvasive tests are considered first.

ECG: If typical exertional symptoms are present, ECG is indicated. Because angina resolves quickly with rest, ECG rarely can be done during an attack except during stress testing. If done during an attack, ECG is likely to show reversible ischemic changes: T wave discordant to the QRS vector, ST-segment depression (typically), ST-segment elevation, decreased R-wave height, intraventricular or bundle branch conduction disturbances, and arrhythmia (usually ventricular extrasystoles). Between attacks, the ECG (and usually LV function) at rest is normal in about 30% of patients with a typical history of angina pectoris, even those with extensive 3-vessel disease. In the remaining 70%, the ECG shows evidence of previous infarction, hypertrophy, or nonspecific ST-segment and T-wave (ST-T) abnormalities. An abnormal resting ECG alone does not establish or refute the diagnosis.

Stress testing: Stress testing is needed to confirm the diagnosis, evaluate disease severity, determine appropriate exercise levels for the patient, and help predict prognosis. If the clinical or working diagnosis is unstable angina, early stress testing is contraindicated.

For CAD, the most accurate tests are stress echocardiography and myocardial perfusion imaging with single-photon emission CT (SPECT) or PET. However, these tests are more expensive than simple stress testing with ECG.

If a patient has a normal resting ECG and can exercise, **exercise stress testing with ECG** is done. In men with chest discomfort suggesting angina, stress ECG testing has a specificity of 70%; sensitivity is 90%. Sensitivity is similar in women, but specificity is lower, particularly in women < 55 (< 70%). However, women are more likely than men to have an abnormal resting ECG when CAD is present (32% vs 23%). Although sensitivity is reasonably high, exercise ECG can miss severe CAD (even left main or 3-vessel disease). In patients with atypical symptoms, a negative stress ECG usually rules out angina pectoris and CAD; a positive result may or may not represent coronary ischemia and indicates need for further testing.

When the resting ECG is abnormal, false-positive ST-segment shifts are common on the stress ECG, so patients should have **stress testing with myocardial imaging**. Exercise or pharmacologic stress (eg, with dobutamine or dipyridamole infusion) may be used. The choice of imaging technique depends on institutional availability and expertise. Imaging tests can help assess LV function and response to stress; identify areas of ischemia, infarction, and viable tissue; and determine the site and extent of myocardium at risk. Stress echocardiography can also detect ischemia-induced mitral regurgitation.

Angiography: Coronary angiography is the standard for diagnosing CAD but is not always necessary to confirm the diagnosis. It is indicated primarily to locate and assess severity of coronary artery lesions when revascularization (PCI or CABG) is being considered. Angiography may also be indicated when knowledge of coronary anatomy is necessary to advise about work or lifestyle needs (eg, discontinuing job or sports activities). Although angiographic findings do not directly show hemodynamic significance of coronary lesions, obstruction is assumed to be physiologically significant when the luminal diameter is reduced > 70%. This reduction correlates well with the presence of angina pectoris unless spasm or thrombosis is superimposed.

Intravascular ultrasonography provides images of coronary artery structure. An ultrasound probe on the tip of a catheter is inserted in the coronary arteries during angiography. This test can provide more information about coronary anatomy than other tests; it is indicated when the nature of lesions is unclear or when apparent disease severity does not match symptom severity. Used with angioplasty, it can help ensure optimal placement of stents.

Guidewires with pressure or flow sensors can be used to estimate blood flow across stenoses. Blood flow is expressed as fractional flow reserve (FFR), which is the ratio of maximal flow through the stenotic area to normal maximal flow. These flow measurements are most useful when evaluating the need for angioplasty or CABG in patients with lesions of questionable severity (40 to 70% stenosis). An FFR of 1.0 is considered normal, while an FFR < 0.75 to 0.8 is associated with myocardial ischemia. Lesions with an FFR > 0.8 are less likely to benefit from stent placement.

Imaging: Electron beam CT can detect the amount of calcium present in coronary artery plaque. The calcium score (from 1 to 100) is roughly proportional to the risk of subsequent coronary events. However, because calcium may be present in the absence of significant stenosis, the score does not correlate well with the need for angioplasty or CABG. Thus, the American Heart Association recommends that screening with electron beam CT should be done only for select groups of patients and is most valuable when combined with historical and clinical data to estimate risk of death or nonfatal MI. These groups may include asymptomatic patients with an intermediate Framingham 10-yr risk estimate of 10 to 20% and symptomatic patients with equivocal stress test results. Electron beam CT is particularly useful in ruling out significant CAD in patients presenting to the emergency department with atypical symptoms, normal troponin levels, and a low probability of hemodynamically significant coronary disease. These patients may have noninvasive testing as outpatients.

Multidetector row CT (MDRCT) coronary angiography can accurately identify coronary stenosis and has a number of advantages. The test is noninvasive, can exclude coronary stenosis with high accuracy, can establish stent or bypass graft patency, can show cardiac and coronary venous anatomy, and can assess calcified and noncalcified plaque burden. However, radiation exposure is significant, and the test is not suitable for patients with a heart rate of > 65 beats/min, those with irregular heart beats, and pregnant women. Patients must also be able to hold their breath for 15 to 20 sec, 3 to 4 times during the study.

Evolving indications for MDRCT coronary angiography include

- Asymptomatic high-risk patients or patients with atypical or typical angina who have inconclusive exercise stress test results, cannot undergo exercise stress testing, or need to undergo major noncardiac surgery
- Patients in whom invasive coronary angiography was unable to locate a major coronary artery or graft

Cardiac MRI has become invaluable in evaluating many cardiac and great vessel abnormalities. It may be used to evaluate CAD by several techniques, which enable direct visualization of coronary stenosis, assessment of flow in the coronary arteries, evaluation of myocardial perfusion and metabolism, evaluation of wall motion abnormalities during stress, and assessment of infarcted myocardium vs viable myocardium.

Current indications for cardiac MRI include evaluation of cardiac structure and function, assessment of myocardial viability, and possibly diagnosis and risk assessment of patients with either known or suspected CAD.

Prognosis

The main adverse outcomes are unstable angina, MI, and sudden death due to arrhythmias. Annual mortality rate is about 1.4% in patients with angina, no history of MI, a normal resting ECG, and normal BP. However, women with CAD tend to have a worse prognosis. Mortality rate is about 7.5% when systolic hypertension is present, 8.4% when the ECG is abnormal, and 12% when both are present. Type 2 diabetes about doubles the mortality rate for each scenario.

Prognosis worsens with increasing age, increasingly severe anginal symptoms, presence of anatomic lesions, and poor ventricular function. Lesions in the left main coronary artery or proximal left anterior descending artery indicate particularly high risk. Although prognosis correlates with number and severity of coronary arteries affected, prognosis is surprisingly good for patients with stable angina, even those with 3-vessel disease, if ventricular function is normal.

Treatment

- Modification of risk factors (smoking, BP, lipids)
- Antiplatelet drugs (aspirin and sometimes clopidogrel, prasugrel, or ticagrelor)
- Beta-blockers
- Nitroglycerin and calcium channel blockers for symptom control
- ACE inhibitors and statins
- Revascularization if symptoms persist despite medical therapy

Reversible risk factors are modified as much as possible (see also p. 653). Smokers should stop smoking; ≥ 2 yr after stopping smoking, risk of MI is reduced to that of people who never smoked. Hypertension is treated diligently because even mild hypertension increases cardiac workload. Weight loss alone often reduces the severity of angina. Sometimes treatment of mild LV failure markedly lessens angina. Paradoxically, digitalis occasionally intensifies angina, presumably because increased myocardial contractility increases oxygen demand, arterial tone is increased, or both. Aggressive reduction of total cholesterol and low-density lipoprotein (LDL) cholesterol (via diet plus drugs as necessary) slows the progression of CAD, may cause some lesions to regress (see p. 1307), and improves endothelial function and thus arterial response to stress. An exercise program emphasizing walking often improves the sense of well-being, reduces risk of acute ischemic events, and improves exercise tolerance.

Drugs: The main goals of angina treatment are to

- Relieve acute symptoms
- Prevent or reduce ischemia
- Prevent future ischemic events

For an acute attack, sublingual nitroglycerin is the most effective drug (see Table 80–2).

To prevent ischemia, all patients diagnosed with CAD or at high risk of developing CAD should take an antiplatelet drug daily. Beta-blockers, unless contraindicated or not tolerated, are given to most patients. For some patients, prevention of symptoms requires calcium channel blockers or long-acting nitrates.

Antiplatelet drugs inhibit platelet aggregation. Aspirin binds irreversibly to platelets and inhibits cyclooxygenase and platelet aggregation. Other antiplatelet drugs (eg, clopidogrel, prasugrel, and ticagrelor) block adenosine diphosphate–induced platelet aggregation. These drugs can reduce risk of ischemic events (MI, sudden death), but the drugs are most effective when given together. Patients unable to tolerate one should receive the other drug alone.

Beta-blockers limit symptoms and prevent infarction and sudden death better than other drugs. Beta-blockers block sympathetic stimulation of the heart and reduce systolic BP, heart rate, contractility, and cardiac output, thus decreasing myocardial oxygen demand and increasing exercise tolerance. Beta-blockers also increase the threshold for ventricular fibrillation (VF). Most patients tolerate these drugs well. Many beta-blockers are available and effective. Dose is titrated upward as needed until limited by bradycardia or adverse effects. Patients who cannot tolerate beta-blockers are given a calcium channel blocker with negative chronotropic effects (eg, diltiazem, verapamil). Those at risk of beta-blocker intolerance (eg, those with asthma) may be tried on a cardioselective beta-blocker (eg, bisoprolol) perhaps with pulmonary function testing before and after drug administration to detect drug-induced bronchospasm.

Nitroglycerin is a potent smooth-muscle relaxant and vasodilator. Its main sites of action are in the peripheral vascular tree, especially in the venous or capacitance system, and in coronary blood vessels. Even severely atherosclerotic vessels may dilate in areas without atheroma. Nitroglycerin lowers systolic BP and dilates systemic veins, thus reducing myocardial wall tension, a major determinant of myocardial oxygen need. Sublingual nitroglycerin is given for an acute attack or for prevention before exertion. Dramatic relief usually occurs within 1.5 to 3 min, is complete by about 5 min, and lasts up to 30 min. The dose may be repeated every 4 to 5 min up to 3 times if relief is incomplete. Patients should always carry nitroglycerin tablets or aerosol spray to use promptly at the onset of an angina attack. Patients should store tablets in a tightly sealed, light-resistant glass container, so that potency is not lost. Because the drug deteriorates quickly, small amounts should be obtained frequently.

Long-acting nitrates (oral or transdermal) are used if symptoms persist after the beta-blocker dose is maximized. If angina occurs at predictable times, a nitrate is given to cover those times. Oral nitrates include isosorbide dinitrate and mononitrate (the active metabolite of the dinitrate). They are effective within 1 to 2 h; their effect lasts 4 to 6 h. Sustained-release formulations of isosorbide mononitrate appear to be effective throughout the day. For transdermal use, cutaneous nitroglycerin patches have largely replaced nitroglycerin ointments primarily because ointments are inconvenient and messy. Patches slowly release the drug for a prolonged effect; exercise capacity improves 4 h after patch application and wanes in 18 to 24 h. Nitrate tolerance may occur, especially when plasma concentrations are kept constant. Because risk of MI is highest in early morning, an afternoon or early evening respite period from nitrates is reasonable unless a patient commonly has angina at that time. For nitroglycerin, an 8- to 10-h respite period seems sufficient. Isosorbide may require a 12-h respite period. If given once/day, sustained-release isosorbide mononitrate does not appear to elicit tolerance.

Calcium channel blockers may be used if symptoms persist despite use of nitrates or if nitrates are not tolerated. Calcium channel blockers are particularly useful if hypertension or coronary spasm is also present. Different types of calcium channel blockers have different effects. Dihydropyridines (eg, nifedipine, amlodipine, felodipine) have no chronotropic effects and vary substantially in their negative inotropic effects. Shorter-acting dihydropyridines may cause reflex tachycardia and are associated with increased mortality in CAD patients; they should not be used alone to treat stable angina. Longer-acting formulations of dihydropyridines have fewer tachycardic effects; they are most commonly used with a beta-blocker. Among longer-acting dihydropyridines, amlodipine has the weakest negative inotropic effects; it may be used in patients with left ventricular systolic dysfunction. Diltiazem and verapamil, other types of calcium channel blockers, have negative chronotropic and inotropic effects. They can be used alone in patients with beta-blocker intolerance or asthma and normal left ventricular systolic function but may increase cardiovascular mortality in patients with left ventricular systolic dysfunction.

Ranolazine is a **sodium channel blocker** that can be used to treat chronic angina. Because ranolazine may also prolong QTc,

Table 80–2. DRUGS FOR CORONARY ARTERY DISEASE*

DRUG	DOSAGE	USE
ACE inhibitors		
Benazepril Captopril Enalapril Fosinopril Lisinopril Moexipril Perindopril Quinapril Ramipril Trandolapril	Variable	All patients with CAD, especially those with large infarctions, renal insufficiency, heart failure, hypertension, or diabetes Contraindications include hypotension, hyperkalemia, bilateral renal artery stenosis, pregnancy, and known allergy
Angiotensin II receptor blockers		
Candesartan Eprosartan Irbesartan Losartan Olmesartan Telmisartan Valsartan	Variable	An effective alternative for patients who cannot tolerate ACE inhibitors (eg, because of cough); currently, not first-line treatment after MI Contraindications include hypotension, hyperkalemia, bilateral renal artery stenosis, pregnancy, and known allergy
Anticoagulants		
Argatroban	350 mcg/kg (IV bolus) followed by 25 mcg/kg/min (IV infusion)	Patients with ACS and a known or suspected history of heparin-induced thrombocytopenia as an alternative to heparin
Bivalirudin	Variable	
Fondaparinux	2.5 mg sc q 24 h	
Low molecular weight heparins: • Dalteparin • Enoxaparin‡ • Tinzaparin	Variable	Patients with unstable angina or NSTEMI Patients < 75 yr receiving tenecteplase Almost all patients with STEMI as an alternative to unfractionated heparin (unless PCI is indicated and can be done in < 90 min); drug continued until PCI or CABG is done or patient is discharged
Unfractionated heparin	60–70 units/kg IV (maximum, 5000 units; bolus), followed by 12–15 units/kg/h (maximum, 1000 units/h) for 3–4 days or until PCI is complete	Patients with unstable angina or NSTEMI as an alternative to enoxaparin
	60 units/kg IV (maximum, 4000 units; bolus) given when alteplase, reteplase, or tenecteplase is started, then followed by 12 units/kg/h (maximum, 1000 units/h) for 48 h or until PCI is complete	Patients who have STEMI and undergo urgent angiography and PCI or patients > 75 yr receiving tenecteplase
Warfarin	Oral dose adjusted to maintain INR of 2.5–3.5	May be useful long-term in patients at high risk of systemic emboli (ie, with large anterior MI, known LV thrombus, or atrial fibrillation)
Antiplatelet drugs		
Aspirin	**For stable angina**†: 75 or 81 mg po once/day (enteric-coated)	All patients with CAD or at high risk of developing CAD, unless aspirin is not tolerated or is contraindicated; used long-term
	For ACS: 160–325 mg po chewed (not enteric-coated) on arrival at emergency department and once/day thereafter during hospitalization and 81 mg† po once/day long-term after discharge	
Clopidogrel (preferred)	75 mg po once/day	Used with aspirin or, in patients who cannot tolerate aspirin, alone
	For patients undergoing PCI: 300–600 mg po once, then 75 mg po once/day for 1–12 mo	For patients undergoing PCI, clopidogrel loading dose to be administered only in cardiac catheterization laboratory after angiography has confirmed that coronary anatomy is amenable to PCI (so as not to delay CABG if indicated) Maintenance therapy required for at least 1 mo for bare-metal stents and for at least 12 mo for drug-eluting stents

Table 80–2. DRUGS FOR CORONARY ARTERY DISEASE* (*Continued*)

DRUG	DOSAGE	USE
Antiplatelet drugs		
Prasugrel	60 mg po once, followed by 10 mg po once/day	Only for patients with ACS undergoing PCI Not used in combination with fibrinolytic therapy
Ticagrelor	**For patients undergoing PCI:** 180 mg po once before the procedure, followed by 90 mg po bid	—
Ticlopidine	250 mg po bid	Rarely used routinely because neutropenia is a risk and WBC count must be monitored regularly
Glycoprotein IIb/IIIa inhibitors		
Abciximab	Variable	Some patients with ACS, particularly those who are having PCI with stent placement and high-risk patients with unstable angina or NSTEMI Therapy started before PCI and continued for 18 to 24 h thereafter
Eptifibatide	Variable	
Tirofiban	Variable	
Beta-blockers		
Atenolol	50 mg po q 12 h acutely; 50–100 mg po bid long-term	All patients with ACS, unless a beta-blocker is not tolerated or is contraindicated, especially high-risk patients; used long-term. Intravenous beta-blockers may be used in patients with ongoing chest pain despite usual measures, or persistent tachycardia, or hypertension in the setting of unstable angina and myocardial infarction. Caution is necessary in the setting of hypotension, or other evidence of hemodynamic instability.
Bisoprolol	2.5–5 mg po once/day, increasing to 10–15 mg once/day depending on heart rate and BP response	
Carvedilol	25 mg po bid (in patients with heart failure or other hemodynamic instability, the starting dose should be as low as 1.625–3.125 mg bid and increased very slowly as tolerated)	
Metoprolol	25–50 mg po q 6 h continued for 48 h; then 100 mg bid or 200 mg once/day given long term	
Calcium channel blockers		
Amlodipine	5–10 mg po once/day	Patients with stable angina if symptoms persist despite nitrates use or if nitrates are not tolerated
Diltiazem (extended-release)	180–360 po once/day	
Felodipine	2.5–20 mg po once/day	
Nifedipine (extended-release)	30–90 mg po once/day	
Verapamil (extended-release)	120–360 mg po once/day	
Statins		
Atorvastatin Fluvastatin Lovastatin Pravastatin Rosuvastatin Simvastatin	Variable	Patients with CAD to achieve a target LDL of 70 mg/dL (1.81 mmol/L)
Nitrates: Short acting		
Sublingual nitroglycerin (tablet or spray)	0.3–0.6 mg q 4–5 min up to 3 doses	All patients for immediate relief of chest pain; used as needed
Nitroglycerin as continuous IV drip	Started at 5 mcg/min and increased 2.5–5.0 mcg every few minutes until required response occurs	Selected patients with ACS: During the first 24 to 48 h, those with heart failure (unless hypotension is present), large anterior MI, persistent angina, or hypertension (BP is reduced by 10–20 mm Hg but not to < 80–90 mm Hg systolic) For longer use, those with recurrent angina or persistent pulmonary congestion

Table continues on the following page.

Table 80–2. DRUGS FOR CORONARY ARTERY DISEASE* (*Continued*)

DRUG	DOSAGE	USE
Nitrates: Long acting		
Isosorbide dinitrate	10–20 mg po tid; can be increased to 40 mg tid	Patients who have unstable angina or persistent severe angina and continue to have anginal symptoms after the beta-blocker dose is maximized A nitrate-free period of 8–10 h (typically at night) recommended to avoid tolerance
Isosorbide dinitrate (sustained-release)	40–80 mg po bid (typically given at 8 AM and 2 PM)	
Isosorbide mononitrate	20 mg po bid, with 7 h between 1st and 2nd doses	
Isosorbide mononitrate (sustained-release)	30 or 60 mg once/day, increased to 120 mg or, rarely, 240 mg	
Nitroglycerin patches	0.2–0.8 mg/h applied between 6:00 and 9:00 AM and removed 12–14 h later to avoid tolerance	
Nitroglycerin ointment 2% preparation (15 mg/2.5 cm)	1.25 cm spread evenly over upper torso or arms q 6 to 8 h and covered with plastic, increased to 7.5 cm as tolerated, and removed for 8–12 h each day to avoid tolerance	
Opioids		
Morphine	2–4 mg IV, repeated as needed	All patients with chest pain due to ACS to relieve pain (but ischemia may persist) Best used after drug therapy has been started or the decision to do revascularization has been made
Other drugs		
Ivabradine	5 mg po bid, increased to 7.5 mg po bid if needed	Inhibits sinus node For symptomatic treatment of chronic stable angina pectoris in patients with normal sinus rhythm who cannot take beta-blockers In combination with beta-blockers in patients inadequately controlled by beta-blocker alone and whose heart rate > 60 beats/min
Ranolazine	500 mg po bid, increased to 1000 mg po bid as needed	Patients in whom symptoms continue despite treatment with other antianginal drugs

*Clinicians may use different combinations of drugs depending on the type of coronary artery disease that is present.
†Higher doses of aspirin do not provide greater protection and increase risk of adverse effects.
‡Of low molecular weight heparins (LMWHs), enoxaparin is preferred.
ACS = acute coronary syndromes; CABG = coronary artery bypass grafting; CAD = coronary artery disease; LV = left ventricular; MI = myocardial infarction; NSTEMI = non–ST-segment elevation MI; PCI = percutaneous intervention; STEMI = ST-segment elevation MI.

it is usually reserved for patients in whom symptoms persist despite optimal treatment with other antianginal drugs. Ranolazine may not be as effective in women as in men. Dizziness, headache, constipation, and nausea are the most common adverse effects.

Revascularization: Revascularization, either with PCI (eg, angioplasty, stenting) or CABG, should be considered if angina persists despite drug therapy and worsens quality of life or if anatomic lesions (noted during angiography) put a patient at high risk of mortality. The choice between PCI and CABG depends on extent and location of anatomic lesions, the experience of the surgeon and medical center, and, to some extent, patient preference.

PCI is usually preferred for 1- or 2-vessel disease with suitable anatomic lesions and is increasingly being used for 3-vessel disease. Lesions that are long or near bifurcation points are often not amenable to PCI. However, as stent technology improves, PCI is being used for more complicated cases.

CABG is very effective in selected patients with angina. CABG is superior to PCI in patients with diabetes and in patients with multivessel disease amenable to grafting. The ideal candidate has severe angina pectoris and localized disease, or diabetes mellitus. About 85% of patients have complete or dramatic symptom relief. Exercise stress testing shows positive correlation between graft patency and improved exercise tolerance, but exercise tolerance sometimes remains improved despite graft closure.

CABG improves survival for patients with left main disease, those with 3-vessel disease and poor left ventricular function, and some patients with 2-vessel disease. However, for patients with mild or moderate angina (CCS class 1 or 2) or 3-vessel disease and good ventricular function, CABG appears to only marginally improve survival. PCI is increasingly being used for unprotected left main stenosis (ie, no left anterior descending or circumflex graft present), with outcomes at one year that are similar to CABG. For patients with 1-vessel disease, outcomes with drug therapy, PCI, and CABG are similar; exceptions are left main disease and proximal left anterior descending disease, for which revascularization appears advantageous.

KEY POINTS

- Angina pectoris occurs when cardiac workload exceeds the ability of coronary arteries to supply an adequate amount of oxygenated blood.
- Symptoms of stable angina pectoris range from a vague, barely troublesome ache to a severe, intense precordial crushing sensation; they are typically precipitated by exertion, last no more than a few minutes, and subside with rest.
- Do stress testing with ECG for patients with normal resting ECG or with myocardial imaging (eg, echocardiography, radionuclide imaging, MRI) for patients with abnormal resting ECG.
- Do coronary angiography when revascularization (percutaneous intervention or CABG) is being considered.
- Give nitroglycerin for immediate relief of angina
- Maintain patients on an antiplatelet drug, a beta-blocker, and a statin, and add a calcium channel blocker for further symptom prevention if needed.
- Consider revascularization if significant angina persists despite drug therapy or if lesions noted during angiography indicate high risk of mortality.

SYNDROME X

(Microvascular Angina)

Syndrome X is cardiac microvascular dysfunction or constriction causing angina in patients with normal epicardial coronary arteries on angiography.

Patients with cardiac syndrome X have

- Typical angina that is relieved by rest or nitroglycerin
- Normal coronary arteriograms (eg, no atherosclerosis, embolism, or inducible arterial spasm)

Some of these patients have ischemia detected during stress testing; others do not. In some patients, the cause of ischemia seems to be reflex intramyocardial coronary constriction and reduced coronary flow reserve. Other patients have microvascular dysfunction within the myocardium: The abnormal vessels do not dilate in response to exercise or other cardiovascular stressors; sensitivity to cardiac pain may also be increased.

This disorder should not be confused with variant angina due to epicardial coronary spasm or with another disorder also called syndrome X, which refers to the metabolic syndrome.

Prognosis is better than for patients with demonstrable CAD, although symptoms of ischemia may recur for years.

In many patients, beta-blockers relieve symptoms.

VARIANT ANGINA

(Prinzmetal Angina)

Variant angina is angina pectoris secondary to epicardial coronary artery spasm. Symptoms include angina at rest and rarely with exertion. Diagnosis is by ECG and provocative testing with ergonovine or acetylcholine. Treatment is with calcium channel blockers and sublingual nitroglycerin.

Most patients with variant angina have significant fixed proximal obstruction of at least one major coronary artery. Spasm usually occurs within 1 cm of the obstruction (often accompanied by ventricular arrhythmia).

Symptoms and Signs

Symptoms are anginal discomfort occurring mainly during rest, often at night, and only rarely and inconsistently during exertion (unless significant coronary artery obstruction is also present). Attacks tend to occur regularly at certain times of day.

Diagnosis

- Provocative testing with ergonovine or acetylcholine during angiography

Diagnosis is suspected if ST-segment elevation occurs during the attack. Between anginal attacks, the ECG may be normal or show a stable abnormal pattern. Confirmation is by provocative testing with ergonovine or acetylcholine, which may precipitate coronary artery spasm. Coronary artery spasm is identified by significant ST-segment elevation or by observation of a reversible spasm during cardiac catheterization. Testing is done most commonly in a cardiac catheterization laboratory and occasionally in a coronary care unit (CCU).

Treatment

- Calcium channel blockers
- Sublingual nitroglycerin

Average survival at 5 yr is 89 to 97%, but mortality risk is greater for patients with both variant angina and atherosclerotic coronary artery obstruction. Usually, sublingual nitroglycerin promptly relieves variant angina. Calcium channel blockers may effectively prevent symptoms. Theoretically, beta-blockers may exacerbate spasm by allowing unopposed alpha-adrenergic vasoconstriction, but this effect has not been proved clinically.

Oral drugs most commonly used are calcium channel blockers:

- Sustained-release diltiazem 120 to 540 mg once/day
- Sustained-release verapamil 120 to 480 mg once/day (dose must be reduced in patients with renal or hepatic dysfunction)
- Amlodipine 15 to 20 mg once/day (dose must be reduced in elderly patients and in patients with hepatic dysfunction)

In refractory cases, amiodarone may be useful. Although these drugs relieve symptoms, they do not appear to alter prognosis.

OVERVIEW OF ACUTE CORONARY SYNDROMES

(Unstable Angina; Acute MI; Myocardial Infarction)

Acute coronary syndromes (ACS) result from acute obstruction of a coronary artery. Consequences depend on degree and location of obstruction and range from unstable angina to non–ST-segment elevation myocardial infarction (NSTEMI), ST-segment elevation myocardial infarction (STEMI), and sudden cardiac death. Symptoms are similar in each of these syndromes (except sudden death) and include chest discomfort with or without dyspnea, nausea, and diaphoresis. Diagnosis is by ECG and the presence or absence of serologic markers. Treatment is antiplatelet drugs, anticoagulants, nitrates, beta-blockers, and, for STEMI, emergency reperfusion via fibrinolytic drugs, percutaneous intervention, or, occasionally, coronary artery bypass graft surgery.

Classification

ACS include

- Unstable angina
- NSTEMI
- STEMI

These syndromes all involve acute coronary ischemia and are distinguished based on symptoms, ECG findings, and cardiac marker levels. It is helpful to distinguish the syndromes because prognosis and treatment vary.

Unstable angina (acute coronary insufficiency, preinfarction angina, intermediate syndrome) is defined as one or more of the following in patients whose cardiac biomarkers do not meet criteria for MI:

- Rest angina that is prolonged (usually > 20 min)
- New-onset angina of at least class 3 severity in the Canadian Cardiovascular Society (CCS) classification (see Table 80–1 on p. 669)
- Increasing angina, ie, previously diagnosed angina that has become distinctly more frequent, more severe, longer in duration, or lower in threshold (eg, increased by ≥ 1 CCS class or to at least CCS class 3)

ECG changes such as ST-segment depression, ST-segment elevation, or T-wave inversion may occur during unstable angina but they are transient. Of cardiac markers, CK is not elevated but cardiac troponin, particularly when measured using high-sensitivity troponin tests (hs-cTn), may be slightly increased. Unstable angina is clinically unstable and often a prelude to MI or arrhythmias or, less commonly, to sudden death.

Non–ST-segment elevation MI (NSTEMI, subendocardial MI) is myocardial necrosis (evidenced by cardiac markers in blood; troponin I or troponin T and CK will be elevated) without acute ST-segment elevation. ECG changes such as ST-segment depression, T-wave inversion, or both may be present.

ST-segment elevation MI (STEMI, transmural MI) is myocardial necrosis with ECG changes showing ST-segment elevation that is not quickly reversed by nitroglycerin or showing new left bundle branch block. Cardiac markers, troponin I or troponin T, and CK are elevated.

Both types of MI may or may not produce Q waves on the ECG (Q wave MI, non-Q wave MI).

Etiology

The **most common cause** of ACS is

- An acute thrombus in an atherosclerotic coronary artery

Atheromatous plaque sometimes becomes unstable or inflamed, causing it to rupture or split, exposing thrombogenic material, which activates platelets and the coagulation cascade and produces an acute thrombus. Platelet activation involves a conformational change in membrane GP IIb/IIIa receptors, allowing cross-linking (and thus aggregation) of platelets. Even atheromas causing minimal obstruction can rupture and result in thrombosis; in > 50% of cases, pre-event stenosis is < 40%. Thus, although the severity of stenosis helps predict symptoms, it does not always predict acute thrombotic events. The resultant thrombus abruptly interferes with blood flow to parts of the myocardium. Spontaneous thrombolysis occurs in about two thirds of patients; 24 h later, thrombotic obstruction is found in only about 30%. However, in virtually all cases, obstruction lasts long enough to cause tissue necrosis.

Rarer causes of ACS are

- Coronary artery embolism
- Coronary spasm

Coronary arterial embolism can occur in mitral or aortic stenosis, infective endocarditis, or marantic endocarditis. Cocaine use and other causes of coronary spasm can sometimes result in MI. Spasm-induced MI may occur in normal or atherosclerotic coronary arteries.

Pathophysiology

Initial consequences vary with size, location, and duration of obstruction and range from transient ischemia to infarction. Measurement of newer, more sensitive markers indicates that some cell necrosis probably occurs even in mild forms; thus, ischemic events occur on a continuum, and classification into subgroups, although useful, is somewhat arbitrary. Sequelae of the acute event depend primarily on the mass and type of cardiac tissue infarcted.

Myocardial dysfunction: Ischemic (but not infarcted) tissue has impaired contractility and relaxation, resulting in hypokinetic or akinetic segments; these segments may expand or bulge during systole (called paradoxical motion). The size of the affected area determines effects, which range from minimal to mild heart failure to cardiogenic shock; usually, large parts of myocardium must be ischemic to cause significant myocardial dysfunction. Some degree of heart failure occurs in about two thirds of hospitalized patients with acute MI. It is termed ischemic cardiomyopathy if low cardiac output and heart failure persist. Ischemia involving the papillary muscle may lead to mitral valve regurgitation. Dysfunctional wall motion can allow mural thrombus formation.

Myocardial infarction: MI is myocardial necrosis resulting from abrupt reduction in coronary blood flow to part of the myocardium. Infarcted tissue is permanently dysfunctional; however, there is a zone of potentially reversible ischemia adjacent to infarcted tissue. MI affects predominantly the LV, but damage may extend into the RV or the atria.

Infarction may be transmural or nontransmural. Transmural infarcts involve the whole thickness of myocardium from epicardium to endocardium and are usually characterized by abnormal Q waves on ECG. Nontransmural or subendocardial infarcts do not extend through the ventricular wall and cause only ST-segment and T-wave (ST-T) abnormalities. Because the transmural depth of necrosis cannot be precisely determined clinically, infarcts are usually classified as STEMI or NSTEMI by the presence or absence of ST-segment elevation or Q waves on the ECG.

Necrosis of a significant portion of the interventricular septum or ventricular wall may rupture, with dire consequences. A ventricular aneurysm or pseudoaneurysm may form,

Electrical dysfunction: Electrical dysfunction can be significant in any form of ACS. Ischemic and necrotic cells are incapable of normal electrical activity, resulting in various ECG changes (predominantly ST-T abnormalities), arrhythmias, and conduction disturbances. ST-T abnormalities of ischemia include ST-segment depression (often downsloping from the J point), T-wave inversion, ST-segment elevation (often referred to as injury current), and peaked T waves in the hyperacute phase of infarction. Conduction disturbances can reflect damage to the sinus node, the atrioventricular (AV) node, or specialized conduction tissues. Most changes are transient; some are permanent.

Symptoms and Signs

Symptoms of ACS depend somewhat on the extent and location of obstruction and are quite variable. Painful stimuli from thoracic organs, including the heart, can cause discomfort described as pressure, tearing, gas with the urge to eructate, indigestion, burning, aching, stabbing, and sometimes sharp needle-like pain. Many patients deny they are having pain and insist it is merely "discomfort." Except when infarction is massive, recognizing the amount of ischemia by symptoms alone is difficult.

Symptoms of ACS are similar to those of angina and are discussed in more detail in sections on unstable angina and acute MI.

After the acute event, many complications can occur. They usually involve

- Electrical dysfunction (eg, conduction defects, arrhythmias)
- Myocardial dysfunction (eg, heart failure, interventricular septum or free wall rupture, ventricular aneurysm, pseudoaneurysm, mural thrombus formation, cardiogenic shock)
- Valvular dysfunction (typically mitral regurgitation)

Electrical dysfunction can be significant in any form of ACS, but usually, large parts of myocardium must be ischemic to cause significant myocardial dysfunction. Other complications of ACS include recurrent ischemia and pericarditis. Pericarditis that occurs 2 to 10 wk after an MI is known as post-MI syndrome or Dressler syndrome.

Diagnosis

- Serial ECGs
- Serial cardiac markers
- Immediate coronary angiography for patients with STEMI or complications (eg, persistent chest pain, hypotension, markedly elevated cardiac markers, unstable arrhythmias)
- Delayed angiography (24 to 48 h) for patients with NSTEMI or unstable angina without complications noted above

ACS should be considered in men > 30 yr and women > 40 yr (younger in patients with diabetes) whose main symptom is chest pain or discomfort. Pain must be differentiated from the pain of pneumonia, pulmonary embolism, pericarditis, rib fracture, costochondral separation, esophageal spasm, acute aortic dissection, renal calculus, splenic infarction, or various abdominal disorders. In patients with previously diagnosed hiatus hernia, peptic ulcer, or a gallbladder disorder, the clinician must be wary of attributing new symptoms to these disorders. (For approach to diagnosis, see also Chest Pain on p. 588.)

The approach is the same when any ACS is suspected: initial and serial ECG and serial cardiac marker measurements, which distinguish among unstable angina, NSTEMI, and STEMI. Every emergency department should have a triage system to immediately identify patients with chest pain for rapid assessment and ECG. Pulse oximetry and chest x-ray (particularly to look for mediastinal widening, which suggests aortic dissection) is also done.

ECG: ECG is the most important test and should be done within 10 min of presentation. It is the center of the decision pathway because fibrinolytics benefit patients with STEMI but may increase risk for those with NSTEMI. Also, urgent cardiac catheterization is indicated for patients with acute STEMI but not for those with NSTEMI.

For STEMI, initial ECG is usually diagnostic, showing ST-segment elevation ≥ 1 mm in 2 or more contiguous leads subtending the damaged area (see Fig. 80–2).

Pathologic Q waves are not necessary for the diagnosis. The ECG must be read carefully because ST-segment elevation may be subtle, particularly in the inferior leads (II, III, aVF); sometimes the reader's attention is mistakenly focused on leads with ST-segment depression. If symptoms are characteristic, ST-segment elevation on ECG has a specificity of 90% and a sensitivity of 45% for diagnosing MI. Serial tracings (obtained every 8 h for 1 day, then daily) showing a gradual evolution toward a stable, more normal pattern or development of abnormal Q waves over a few days (see Fig. 80–3) tends to confirm the diagnosis.

Because nontransmural (non–Q wave) infarcts are usually in the subendocardial or midmyocardial layers, they do not produce diagnostic Q waves or distinct ST-segment elevation on the ECG. Instead, they commonly produce only varying degrees of ST-T abnormalities that are less striking, variable, or nonspecific and sometimes difficult to interpret (NSTEMI). If such abnormalities resolve (or worsen) on repeat ECGs, ischemia is very likely. However, when repeat ECGs are unchanged, acute MI is unlikely and, if still suspected clinically, requires other evidence to make the diagnosis. A normal ECG taken when a patient is pain free does not rule out unstable angina; a normal ECG taken during pain, although it does not rule out angina, suggests that the pain is not ischemic.

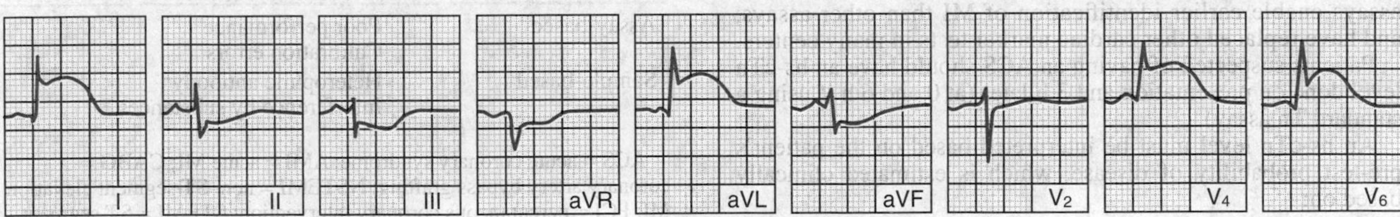

Fig. 80–2. Acute lateral left ventricular infarction (tracing obtained within a few hours of onset of illness). There is striking hyperacute ST-segment elevation in leads I, aVL, V_4, and V_6 and reciprocal depression in other leads.

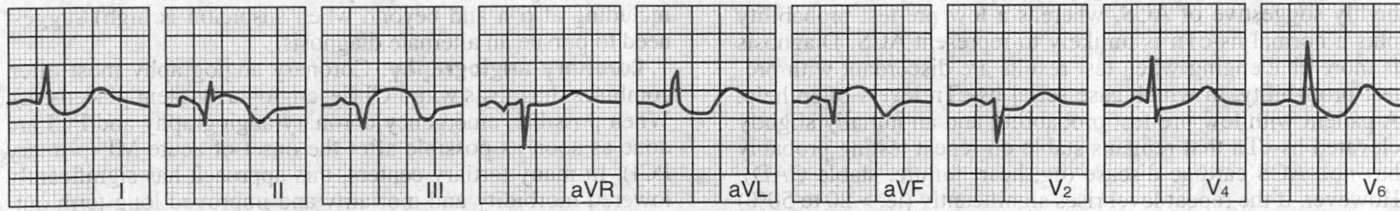

Fig. 80–3. Inferior (diaphragmatic) left ventricular infarction (after the first 24 h). Significant Q waves develop with decreasing ST-segment elevation in leads II, III, and aVF.

If right ventricular (RV) infarction is suspected, a 15-lead ECG is usually recorded; additional leads are placed at V_4R, and, to detect posterior infarction, V_8 and V_9.

ECG diagnosis of MI is more difficult when a left bundle branch block configuration is present because it resembles STEMI changes (see Fig. 76–15 on p. 643). ST-segment elevation concordant with the QRS complex strongly suggests MI as does > 5-mm ST-segment elevation in at least 2 precordial leads. But generally, any patient with suggestive symptoms and new-onset (or not known to be old) left bundle branch block is treated as for STEMI.

Cardiac markers: Cardiac markers (serum markers of myocardial cell injury) are

- Cardiac enzymes (eg, CK-MB)
- Cell contents (eg, troponin I, troponin T, myoglobin)

These markers are released into the bloodstream after myocardial cell necrosis. The markers appear at different times after injury and levels decrease at different rates. Sensitivity and specificity for myocardial cell injury vary significantly among these markers, but the troponins (cTn) are the most sensitive and specific and are now the markers of choice. Recently, several new, highly sensitive assays of cardiac troponin (hs-cTn) that are also very precise have become available. These assays can reliably measure Tn levels (T or I) as low as 0.003 to 0.006 ng/mL (3 to 6 pg/mL); some research assays go as low as 0.001 ng/mL (1 pg/mL).

Previous, less sensitive cTn tests were unlikely to detect Tn except in patients who had an acute cardiac disorder. Thus, a "positive" Tn (ie, above the limit of detection) was very specific. However, the new hs-cTn tests can detect small amounts of Tn in many healthy people. Thus, hs-cTn levels need to be referenced to the normal range, and are defined as "elevated" only when higher than 99% of the reference population. Furthermore, although an elevated troponin level indicates myocardial cell injury, it does not indicate the cause of the damage (although any troponin elevation increases the risk of adverse outcomes in many disorders). In addition to ACS, many other cardiac and non-cardiac disorders can elevate hs-cTn levels (see Table 80–3); not all elevated hs-cTn levels represent MI, and not all myocardial necrosis results from an acute coronary syndrome event even when the etiology is ischemic. However, by detecting lower levels of Tn, hs-cTn assays enable earlier identification of MI than other assays, and have replaced other cardiac marker tests in many centers.

Patients suspected of having an ACS should have an hs-cTn level done on presentation and 3 h later (at 0 and 6 h if using a standard Tn assay).

An hs-cTn level must be interpreted based on the patient's pre-test probability of disease, which is estimated clinically based on:

- Risk factors for ACS
- Symptoms
- ECG

A high pre-test probability plus an elevated hs-cTn level is highly suggestive of ACS, whereas a low pre-test probability plus a normal hs-cTn is unlikely to represent ACS. Diagnosis is more challenging when test results are discordant with pre-test probability, in which case serial hs-cTn levels often help. A patient with low pre-test probability and an initially slightly elevated hs-cTn that remains stable on repeat testing probably has non-ACS cardiac disease (eg, heart failure, stable CAD). However, if the repeat level rises significantly (ie, > 20 to 50%) the likelihood of ACS becomes much higher. If a patient with high pre-test probability has a normal hs-cTn level that rises > 50% on repeat, ACS is likely; continued normal levels (often including at 6 h and beyond when suspicion is high) suggest need to pursue an alternate diagnosis.

Coronary angiography: Coronary angiography most often combines diagnosis with PCI (ie, angioplasty, stent placement). When possible, emergency coronary angiography and PCI are done as soon as possible after the onset of acute MI (primary PCI). In many tertiary centers, this approach has significantly lowered morbidity and mortality and improved long-term outcomes. Frequently, the infarction is actually aborted when the time from pain to PCI is short (< 3 to 4 h).

Table 80–3. CAUSES OF ELEVATED TROPONIN

TYPE	CONDITIONS
MI (ischemic)	
ACS	Classic AMI • STEMI • NSTEMI
Non-ACS (coronary)	Increased demand (stable CAD lesion) Coronary artery spasm, embolism, or dissection Procedure-related (PCI, CABG Cocaine or methamphetamine
Non-ACS (noncoronary)	Hypoxia Global ischemia Hypoperfusion Cardiothoracic surgery
Sudden cardiac death	—
Direct myocardial damage (nonischemic)	
Cardiac disorders	Heart failure Cardiomyopathy (eg, hypertrophic, viral) Hypertension Myocarditis, pericarditis Injury (ablation procedures, cardiac contusion, cardioversion, electrical shock) Cancer Infiltrative disorders (eg, amyloidosis)
Systemic disorders	Pulmonary embolism Toxicity (eg, anthracyclines) Trauma (severe burns) Extreme exertion Renal failure Sepsis Stroke Subarachnoid hemorrhage
Analytical	
Assay-based	Poor performance Calibration errors
Sample-based	Heterophile antibody Interference by substances

ACS = acute coronary syndrome; AMI = acute MI; CABG = coronary artery bypass grafting; NSTEMI = non–ST-segment elevation MI; PCI = percutaneous coronary intervention; STEMI = ST-segment elevation MI.

Angiography is obtained urgently for patients with STEMI, patients with persistent chest pain despite maximal medical therapy, and patients with complications (eg, markedly elevated cardiac markers, presence of cardiogenic shock, acute mitral regurgitation, ventricular septal defect, unstable arrhythmias). Patients with uncomplicated NSTEMI or unstable angina whose symptoms have resolved typically undergo angiography within the first 24 to 48 h of hospitalization to detect lesions that may require treatment.

After initial evaluation and therapy, coronary angiography may be used in patients with evidence of ongoing ischemia (ECG findings or symptoms), hemodynamic instability, recurrent ventricular tachyarrhythmias, and other abnormalities that suggest recurrence of ischemic events. Some experts also recommend that angiography be done before hospital discharge in STEMI patients with inducible ischemia on stress imaging or an ejection fraction < 40%.

Other tests: Routine laboratory tests are nondiagnostic but, if obtained, show nonspecific abnormalities compatible with tissue necrosis (eg, increased ESR, moderately elevated WBC count with a shift to the left). A fasting lipid profile should be obtained within the first 24 h for all patients hospitalized with ACS.

Myocardial imaging (see also p. 614) is not needed to make the diagnosis if cardiac markers or ECG is positive. However, in patients with MI, bedside echocardiography is invaluable for detecting mechanical complications. Before or shortly after discharge, patients with symptoms suggesting an ACS but nondiagnostic ECGs and normal cardiac markers should have a stress imaging test (radionuclide or echocardiographic imaging with pharmacologic or exercise stress). Imaging abnormalities in such patients indicate increased risk of complications in the next 3 to 6 mo and suggest need for angiography, which should be done before discharge or soon thereafter, with PCI or CABG done as necessary.

Right heart catheterization using a balloon-tipped pulmonary artery catheter can be used to measure right heart, pulmonary artery, and pulmonary artery occlusion pressures and cardiac output. This test is not routinely recommended and should be done only if patients have significant complications (eg, severe heart failure, hypoxia, hypotension) and by doctors experienced with catheter placement and management protocols.

Prognosis

Global risk should be estimated via formal clinical risk scores (Thrombosis in Myocardial Infarction [TIMI], Global Registry of Acute Coronary Events [GRACE], Platelet GP IIb/IIIa in Unstable Angina: Receptor Suppression Using Integrilin Therapy [PURSUIT]) or a combination of the following high-risk features:

- Recurrent angina/ischemia at rest or during low-level activity
- Heart failure
- Worsening mitral regurgitation
- High-risk stress test result (test stopped in ≤ 5 min due to symptoms, marked ECG abnormalities, hypotension, or complex ventricular arrhythmias)
- Hemodynamic instability
- Sustained ventricular tachycardia (VT)
- Diabetes mellitus
- PCI within past 6 mo
- Prior CABG
- LV ejection fraction < 0.40

Treatment

- Prehospital care: Oxygen, aspirin, nitrates and/or opioids for pain, and triage to an appropriate medical center
- Drug treatment: Antiplatelet drugs, antianginal drugs, anticoagulants, and in some cases other drugs
- Often, angiography to assess coronary artery anatomy
- Often, reperfusion therapy: Fibrinolytics, PCI or coronary artery bypass surgery
- Supportive care
- Post discharge rehabilitation and chronic management of CAD

Treatment, including drug treatment, is designed to relieve distress, interrupt thrombosis, reverse ischemia, limit infarct size, reduce cardiac workload, and prevent and treat complications. An ACS is a medical emergency; outcome is greatly influenced by rapid diagnosis and treatment.

Treatment occurs simultaneously with diagnosis.

Contributing disorders (eg, anemia, heart failure) are aggressively treated.

Because the chest pain of MI usually subsides within 12 to 24 h, any chest pain that remains or recurs later is investigated. It may indicate such complications as recurrent ischemia, pericarditis, pulmonary embolism, pneumonia, gastritis, or ulcer.

Prehospital care:

- Oxygen
- Aspirin
- Nitrates or morphine
- Triage to appropriate medical center

A reliable IV route must be established, oxygen given (typically 2 L by nasal cannula), and continuous single-lead ECG monitoring started. Prehospital interventions by emergency medical personnel—including ECG, chewed aspirin [325 mg], pain management with nitrates or opioids (see Table 80–2), early thrombolysis when indicated and possible, and triage to the appropriate hospital where primary PCI is available—can reduce risk of mortality and complications. Early diagnostic data and response to treatment can help determine the need for and timing of revascularization (see p. 697) when primary percutaneous coronary intervention is not possible.

Hospital admission:

- Drug therapy with antiplatelet drugs, anticoagulants, and other drugs based on reperfusion strategy
- Risk-stratify patient and choose a reperfusion strategy (fibrinolytics or cardiac angiography with PCI or CABG for patients with STEMI and cardiac angiography with PCI or CABG for patients with unstable angina or NSTEMI

On arrival to the emergency room, the patient's diagnosis is confirmed. Drug therapy and choice of revascularization depend on the type of acute coronary syndrome as well as the clinical picture (see Fig. 80–4). Choice of drug therapy is discussed in Drugs for Acute Coronary Syndrome on p. 694, and choice of reperfusion strategy is further discussed in Revascularization for Acute Coronary Syndromes on p. 697.

When the diagnosis is unclear, bedside cardiac marker tests can help identify low-risk patients with a suspected ACS (eg, those with initially negative cardiac markers and nondiagnostic ECGs), who can be managed in 24-h observation units or chest pain centers. Higher-risk patients should be admitted to a monitored inpatient unit or CCU. Several validated tools can help stratify risk. TIMI risk scores may be the most widely used.

Patients with suspected NSTEMI and intermediate or high risk should be admitted to an inpatient care unit or CCU. Those with STEMI should be admitted to a CCU.

Only heart rate and rhythm recorded by single-lead ECG are consistently useful for routine, continuous monitoring.

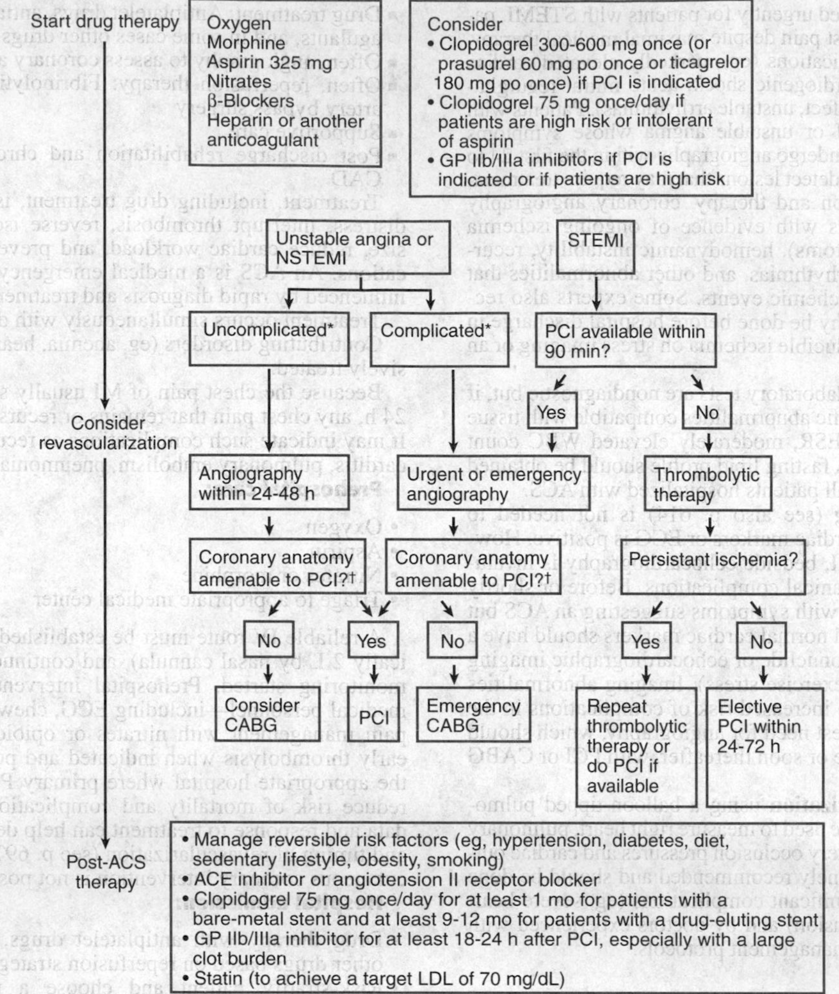

Fig. 80–4. Approach to acute coronary syndromes.

*Complicated means that the hospital course was complicated by recurrent angina or infarction, heart failure, or sustained recurrent ventricular arrhythmias. Absence of any of these events is termed uncomplicated.

†CABG is generally preferred to PCI for patients with the following:

- Left main or left main equivalent disease
- Left ventricular dysfunction
- Treated diabetes

Also, lesions that are long or near bifurcation points are often not amenable to PCI.

CABG = coronary artery bypass grafting; GP = glycoprotein; LDL = low density lipoprotein; NSTEMI = non-ST-segment elevation MI; PCI = percutaneous intervention; STEMI = ST-segment elevation MI.

However, some clinicians recommend routine multilead monitoring with continuous ST-segment recording to identify transient, recurrent ST-segment elevations or depressions. Such findings, even in patients without symptoms, suggest ischemia and identify higher-risk patients who may require more aggressive evaluation and treatment.

Qualified nurses can interpret the ECG for arrhythmia and initiate protocols for its treatment. All staff members should know how to do CPR.

Supportive care: The care unit should be a quiet, calm, restful area. Single rooms are preferred; privacy consistent with monitoring should be ensured. Usually, visitors and telephone calls are restricted to family members during the first few days. A wall clock, a calendar, and an outside window help orient the patient and prevent a sense of isolation, as can access to a radio, television, and newspaper.

Bed rest is mandatory for the first 24 h. On day 1, patients without complications (eg, hemodynamic instability, ongoing ischemia), including those in whom reperfusion with fibrinolytics or PCI is successful, can sit in a chair, begin passive exercises, and use a commode. Walking to the bathroom and doing nonstressful paperwork are allowed shortly thereafter. Recent studies have shown that patients with successful, uncomplicated primary PCI for acute MI may be ambulated quickly and be safely discharged in 3 to 4 days.

If reperfusion is not successful or complications are present, patients require longer bed rest, but they (particularly elderly patients) are mobilized as soon as possible. Prolonged bed rest results in rapid physical deconditioning, with development of orthostatic hypotension, decreased work capacity, increased heart rate during exertion, and increased risk of deep venous thrombosis. Prolonged bed rest also intensifies feelings of depression and helplessness.

Anxiety, mood changes, and denial are common. A mild tranquilizer (usually a benzodiazepine) is often given, but many experts believe such drugs are rarely needed.

Reactive depression is common by the 3rd day of illness and is almost universal at some time during recovery. After the acute phase of illness, the most important tasks are often management of depression, rehabilitation, and institution of long-term preventive programs. Overemphasis on bed rest, inactivity, and the seriousness of the disorder reinforces anxiety and depressive tendencies, so patients are encouraged to sit up, get out of bed, and engage in appropriate activities as soon as possible. The effects of the disorder, prognosis, and individualized rehabilitation program should be explained to the patient.

Maintaining normal bowel function with stool softeners (eg, docusate) to prevent straining is important. Urinary retention is common among elderly patients, especially after several days of bed rest or if atropine was given. A catheter may be required but can usually be removed when the patient can stand or sit to void.

Because smoking is prohibited, a hospital stay should be used to encourage smoking cessation. All caregivers should devote considerable effort to making smoking cessation permanent.

Although acutely ill patients have little appetite, tasty food in modest amounts is good for morale. Patients are usually offered a soft diet of 1500 to 1800 kcal/day with sodium reduction to 2 to 3 g. Sodium reduction is not required after the first 2 or 3 days if there is no evidence of heart failure. Patients are given a diet low in cholesterol and saturated fats, which is used to teach healthy eating.

For patients with diabetes and STEMI, intensive glucose control is no longer recommended; guidelines call for an insulin-based regimen to achieve and maintain glucose levels < 180 mg/dL while avoiding hypoglycemia.

Rehabilitation and Postdischarge Treatment

- Functional evaluation
- Changes in lifestyle: Regular exercise, diet modification, weight loss, smoking cessation
- Drugs: Continuation of antiplatelet drugs, beta-blockers, ACE inhibitors, and statins

Functional evaluation: Patients who did not have coronary angiography during admission, have no high-risk features (eg, heart failure, recurrent angina, VT or VF after 24 h, mechanical complications such as new murmurs, shock), and have an ejection fraction > 40% whether or not they received fibrinolytics usually should have stress testing of some sort before or shortly after discharge (see Table 80–4).

Activity: Physical activity is gradually increased during the first 3 to 6 wk after discharge. Resumption of sexual activity, often of great concern to the patient and partner, and other moderate physical activities may be encouraged. If good cardiac function is maintained 6 wk after acute MI, most patients can return to all their normal activities. A regular exercise program consistent with lifestyle, age, and cardiac status reduces risk of ischemic events and enhances general well-being.

Risk factors: The acute illness and treatment of ACS should be used to strongly motivate the patient to modify risk factors. Evaluating the patient's physical and emotional status and discussing them with the patient, advising about lifestyle (eg, smoking, diet, work and play habits, exercise), and aggressively managing risk factors may improve prognosis.

Drugs: Several drugs clearly reduce mortality risk post-MI and are used unless contraindicated or not tolerated:

- Aspirin and other antiplatelet drugs
- Beta blockers
- ACE inhibitors
- Statins

Aspirin and other antiplatelet drugs reduce mortality and reinfarction rates in post-MI patients. Enteric-coated aspirin 81 mg once/day is recommended long-term. Data suggest that warfarin with or without aspirin reduces mortality and reinfarction rates.

Beta-blockers are considered standard therapy. Most available beta-blockers (eg, acebutolol, atenolol, metoprolol, propranolol, timolol) reduce post-MI mortality rate by about 25% for at least 7 yr.

ACE inhibitors are also considered standard therapy and are given to all post-MI patients if possible. These drugs may provide long-term cardioprotection by improving endothelial function. If an ACE inhibitor is not tolerated because of cough or rash (but not angioedema or renal dysfunction), an angiotensin II receptor blocker may be substituted.

Statins are also standard therapy and are routinely prescribed. Reducing cholesterol levels after MI reduces rates of recurrent ischemic events and mortality in patients with elevated or normal cholesterol levels. Statins appear to benefit post-MI patients regardless of their initial cholesterol level. Post-MI patients whose primary problem is a low HDL level or an elevated triglyceride level may benefit from a fibrate, but evidence of benefit is less clear. A high-dose statin should be continued indefinitely, unless significant adverse effects occur.

Table 80–4. FUNCTIONAL EVALUATION AFTER MI

EXERCISE CAPACITY	IF ECG IS INTERPRETABLE	IF ECG IS NOT INTERPRETABLE
Able to exercise	Submaximal or symptom-limited stress ECG before or after discharge	Exercise echocardiography or nuclear scanning
Unable to exercise	Pharmacologic stress testing (echocardiography or nuclear scanning)	Pharmacologic stress testing (echocardiography or nuclear scanning)

KEY POINTS

- Unstable angina, NSTEMI, and STEMI represent worsening degrees of myocardial ischemia and necrosis; the distinctions help differentiate prognosis and guide treatment.
- Diagnosis is based on serial ECG and cardiac marker levels, particularly using new, highly sensitive troponin T tests.
- Immediate medical treatment depends on the specific syndrome and patient characteristics but typically involves antiplatelet drugs, anticoagulants, beta-blockers, and nitrates as needed (eg, for chest pain, hypertension, pulmonary edema), and a statin to improve prognosis.
- For unstable angina and NSTEMI, do angiography within 24 to 48 h of hospitalization to identify coronary lesions requiring PCI or CABG; fibrinolysis is not helpful.
- For STEMI, do emergency PCI when door to balloon-inflation time is < 90 min; do fibrinolysis if such timely PCI is not available.
- Following recovery, initiate or continue aspirin and other antiplatelet drugs, beta-blockers, ACE inhibitors, and statins in most cases unless contraindicated.

UNSTABLE ANGINA

(Acute Coronary Insufficiency; Preinfarction Angina; Intermediate Syndrome)

Unstable angina results from acute obstruction of a coronary artery without MI. Symptoms include chest discomfort with or without dyspnea, nausea, and diaphoresis. Diagnosis is by ECG and the presence or absence of serologic markers. Treatment is with antiplatelet drugs, anticoagulants, nitrates, statins, and beta-blockers. Coronary angiography with percutaneous intervention or coronary artery bypass surgery is often necessary.

Unstable angina is a type of acute coronary syndrome that is defined as one or more of the following in patients whose cardiac biomarkers do not meet criteria for acute MI:

- Rest angina that is prolonged (usually > 20 min)
- New-onset angina of at least class 3 severity in the Canadian Cardiovascular Society (CCS) classification (see Table 80–1 on p. 669)
- Increasing angina, ie, previously diagnosed angina that has become distinctly more frequent, more severe, longer in duration, or lower in threshold (eg, increased by ≥ 1 CCS class or to at least CCS class 3)

Unstable angina is clinically unstable and often a prelude to MI or arrhythmias or, less commonly, to sudden death.

Symptoms and Signs

Patients have symptoms of angina pectoris (typically chest pain or discomfort) except that the pain or discomfort of unstable angina usually is more intense, lasts longer, is precipitated by less exertion, occurs spontaneously at rest (as angina decubitus), is progressive (crescendo) in nature, or involves any combination of these features.

Unstable angina is classified based on severity and clinical situation (see Table 80–5). Also considered are whether unstable angina occurs during treatment for chronic stable angina and whether transient changes in ST-T waves occur during angina. If angina has occurred within 48 h and no contributory extracardiac condition is present, troponin levels may be measured to help estimate prognosis; troponin-negative results indicate a better prognosis than troponin-positive.

Diagnosis

- Serial ECGs
- Serial cardiac markers
- Immediate coronary angiography for patients with complications (eg, persistent chest pain, hypotension, unstable arrhythmias)
- Delayed angiography (24 to 48 h) for stable patients

Evaluation (see Fig. 80–5) begins with initial and serial ECG and serial measurements of cardiac markers to help distinguish between unstable angina and acute MI—either NSTEMI or STEMI. This distinction is the center of the decision pathway because fibrinolytics benefit patients with STEMI but may increase risk for those with NSTEMI and unstable angina. Also, urgent cardiac catheterization is indicated for patients with acute STEMI but not generally for those with NSTEMI or unstable angina.

ECG: ECG is the most important tesßt and should be done within 10 min of presentation. ECG changes such as ST-segment depression, ST-segment elevation, or T-wave inversion may occur during unstable angina but are transient.

Table 80–5. BRAUNWALD CLASSIFICATION OF UNSTABLE ANGINA*

CLASSIFICATION	DESCRIPTION	DESIGNATION
Severity		
I	New onset of severe angina or increasing† angina No angina during rest	—
II	Angina during rest within past month but not within preceding 48 h	Subacute angina at rest
III‡	Angina during rest within 48 h	Acute angina at rest
Clinical situation		
A	Develops secondary to an extracardiac condition that worsens myocardial ischemia	Secondary unstable angina
B‡	Develops when no contributory extracardiac condition is present	Primary unstable angina
C	Develops within 2 wk of acute MI	Post-MI unstable angina

*Basic classification consists of a Roman numeral and a letter.
†Angina occurs more frequently, is more severe, lasts longer, or is triggered by less exertion.
‡For patients with class IIIB, troponin status (negative or positive) is determined to estimate prognosis.
Adapted from Hamm CW, Braunwald E: APACHE II: A classification of unstable angina revisited. *Circulation* 102:118–122, 2000.

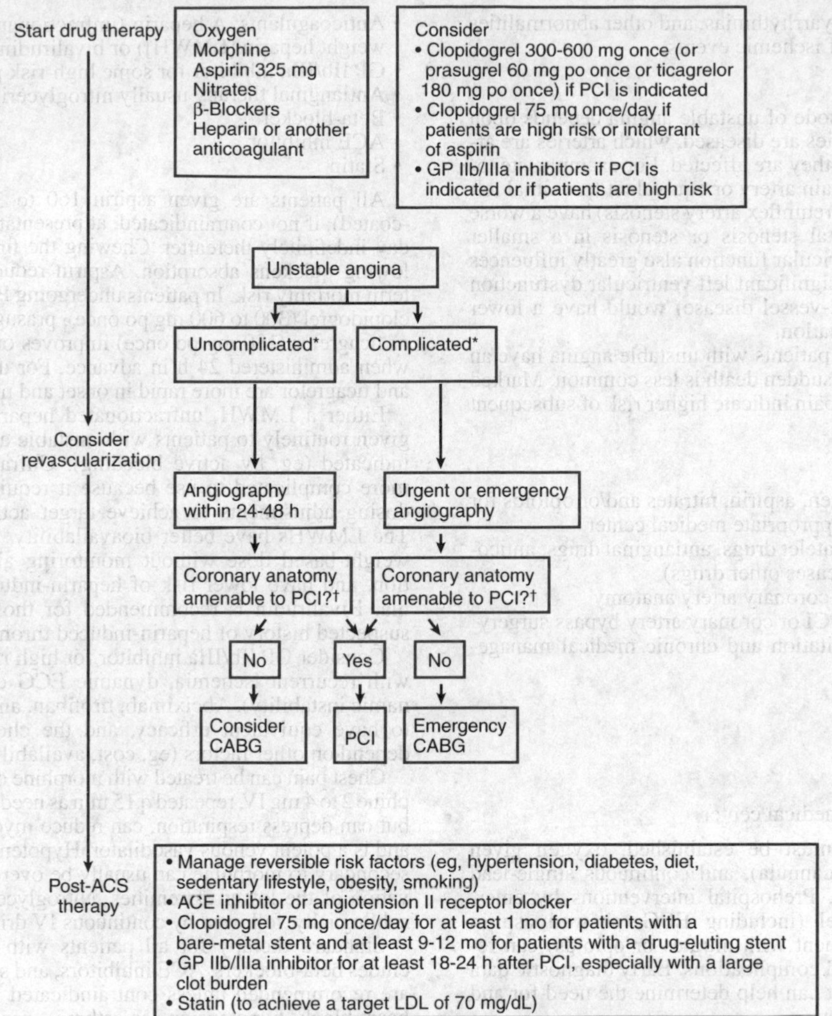

Fig. 80–5. Approach to unstable angina.

*Complicated means that the hospital course was complicated by recurrent angina or infarction, heart failure, or sustained recurrent ventricular arrhythmias. Absence of any of these events is termed uncomplicated.
†CABG is generally preferred to PCI for patients with the following:

- Left main or left main equivalent disease
- Left ventricular dysfunction
- Treated diabetes

Also, lesions that are long or near bifurcation points are often not amenable to PCI.
CABG = coronary artery bypass grafting; GP = glycoprotein; LDL = low density lipoprotein; NSTEMI = non-ST-segment elevation MI; PCI = percutaneous intervention; STEMI = ST-segment elevation MI.

Cardiac markers: Patients suspected of having unstable angina should have a highly sensitive assay of cardiac troponin (hs-cTn) done on presentation and 3 h later (at 0 and 6 h if using a standard Tn assay). Of cardiac markers, CK is not elevated but cardiac troponin, particularly when measured using high-sensitivity troponin tests (hs-cTn), may be slightly increased but do not meet criteria for MI (above the 99th percentile of the upper reference limit or URL).

Coronary angiography: Patients with unstable angina whose symptoms have resolved typically undergo angiography within the first 24 to 48 h of hospitalization to detect lesions that may require treatment. Coronary angiography most often combines diagnosis with PCI (ie, angioplasty, stent placement).

After initial evaluation and therapy, coronary angiography may be used in patients with evidence of ongoing ischemia (ECG findings or symptoms), hemodynamic instability, recurrent ventricular tachyarrhythmias, and other abnormalities that suggest recurrence of ischemic events.

Prognosis

Prognosis after an episode of unstable angina depends upon how many coronary arteries are diseased, which arteries are affected, and how severely they are affected. For example, stenosis of the proximal left main artery or equivalent (proximal left arterial descending and circumflex artery stenosis) have a worse prognosis than does distal stenosis or stenosis in a smaller arterial branch. Left ventricular function also greatly influences prognosis; patients with significant left ventricular dysfunction (even those with 1- or 2-vessel disease) would have a lower threshold for revascularization.

Overall, about 30% of patients with unstable angina have an MI within 3 mo of onset; sudden death is less common. Marked ECG changes with chest pain indicate higher risk of subsequent MI or death.

Treatment

- Prehospital care: Oxygen, aspirin, nitrates and/or opioids for pain, and triage to an appropriate medical center
- Drug treatment: Antiplatelet drugs, antianginal drugs, anticoagulants, and in some cases other drugs)
- Angiography to assess coronary artery anatomy
- Reperfusion therapy: PCI or coronary artery bypass surgery
- Post discharge rehabilitation and chronic medical management of CAD

Prehospital care:

- Oxygen
- Aspirin
- Nitrates and/or opioids
- Triage to appropriate medical center

A reliable IV route must be established, oxygen given (typically 2 L by nasal cannula), and continuous single-lead ECG monitoring started. Prehospital interventions by emergency medical personnel (including ECG, chewed aspirin [325 mg], pain management with nitrates or opioids) can reduce risk of mortality and complications. Early diagnostic data and response to treatment can help determine the need for and timing of revascularization.

Hospital admission:

- Risk-stratify patient and choose timing of reperfusion strategy
- Drug therapy with antiplatelet drugs, anticoagulants and other drugs based on reperfusion strategy

On arrival to the emergency room, the patient's diagnosis is confirmed. Drug therapy and timing of revascularization depend on the clinical picture. In clinically unstable patients (patients with ongoing symptoms, hypotension or sustained arrhythmias), urgent angiography with revascularization is indicated. In clinically stable patients, angiography with revascularization may be deferred for 24 to 48 h (see Fig. 80–5).

Drug treatment of unstable angina: All patients should be given antiplatelet drugs, anticoagulants, and if chest pain is present, antianginals. The specific drugs used depend on the reperfusion strategy and other factors; their selection and use are discussed under Drugs for Acute Coronary Syndrome on p. 694. Other drugs, such as beta-blockers, ACE inhibitors, and statins, should be initiated during admission (see Table 80–2 on p. 672).

Patients with unstable angina should be given the following (unless contraindicated)

- Antiplatelet drugs: Aspirin, clopidogrel, or both (prasugrel or ticagrelor are alternatives to clopidogrel)
- Anticoagulants: A heparin (unfractionated or low molecular weight heparin [LMWH]) or bivalirudin
- GP IIb/IIIa inhibitor for some high-risk patients
- Antianginal therapy usually nitroglycerin
- Beta-blocker
- ACE inhibitor
- Statin

All patients are given aspirin 160 to 325 mg (not enteric -coated), if not contraindicated, at presentation and 81 mg once/day indefinitely thereafter. Chewing the first dose before swallowing quickens absorption. Aspirin reduces short- and long-term mortality risk. In patients undergoing PCI, a loading dose of clopidogrel (300 to 600 mg po once), prasugrel (60 mg po once), or ticagrelor (180 mg po once) improves outcomes, particularly when administered 24 h in advance. For urgent PCI, prasugrel and ticagrelor are more rapid in onset and may be preferred.

Either a LMWH, unfractionated heparin, or bivalirudin is given routinely to patients with unstable angina unless contraindicated (eg, by active bleeding). Unfractionated heparin is more complicated to use because it requires frequent (q 6 h) dosing adjustments to achieve target activated PTT (aPTT). The LMWHs have better bioavailability, are given by simple weight-based dose without monitoring aPTT and dose titration, and have lower risk of heparin-induced thrombocytopenia. Bivalirudin is recommended for those with a known or suspected history of heparin-induced thrombocytopenia.

Consider GP IIb/IIIa inhibitor for high risk patients (patients with recurrent ischemia, dynamic ECG changes or hemodynamic instability). Abciximab, tirofiban, and eptifibatide appear to have equivalent efficacy, and the choice of drug should depend on other factors (eg, cost, availability, familiarity).

Chest pain can be treated with morphine or nitroglycerin. Morphine 2 to 4 mg IV, repeated q 15 min as needed, is highly effective but can depress respiration, can reduce myocardial contractility, and is a potent venous vasodilator. Hypotension and bradycardia secondary to morphine can usually be overcome by prompt elevation of the lower extremities. Nitroglycerin is initially given sublingually, followed by continuous IV drip if needed.

Standard therapy for all patients with unstable angina includes beta-blockers, ACE inhibitors, and statins. Beta-blockers are recommended unless contraindicated (eg, by bradycardia, heart block, hypotension, or asthma), especially for high-risk patients. Beta-blockers reduce heart rate, arterial pressure, and contractility, thereby reducing cardiac workload and oxygen demand. ACE inhibitors may provide long-term cardioprotection by improving endothelial function. If an ACE inhibitor is not tolerated because of cough or rash (but not angioedema or renal dysfunction), an angiotensin II receptor blocker may be substituted. Statins are also standard therapy and should be continued indefinitely.

Reperfusion therapy in unstable angina: Fibrinolytic drugs, which can be helpful in patients with STEMI, do not benefit patients with unstable angina.

Angiography is typically done during admission—within 24 to 48 h of admission if the patient is stable or immediately in unstable patients (eg, with ongoing symptoms, hypotension, sustained arrhythmias). Angiographic findings help determine whether PCI or CABG is indicated. Choice of reperfusion strategy is further discussed under Revascularization for Acute Coronary Syndromes on p. 697.

PEARLS & PITFALLS

- Although fibrinolytic drugs can help patients with STEMI, they are not beneficial in unstable angina

Rehabilitation and postdischarge treatment:

- Functional evaluation
- Changes in lifestyle: Regular exercise, diet modification, weight loss, smoking cessation
- Drugs: Continuation of antiplatelet drugs, beta-blockers, ACE inhibitors, and statins

Patients who did not have coronary angiography during admission, have no high-risk features (eg, heart failure, recurrent angina, VT or VF after 24 h, mechanical complications such as new murmurs, shock), and have an ejection fraction > 40% usually should have stress testing of some sort before or shortly after discharge.

The acute illness and treatment of unstable angina should be used to strongly motivate the patient to modify risk factors. Evaluating the patient's physical and emotional status and discussing them with the patient, advising about lifestyle (eg, smoking, diet, work and play habits, exercise), and aggressively managing risk factors may improve prognosis.

On discharge, all patients should be continued on appropriate antiplatelet drugs, statins, antianginals, and other drugs based on comorbidities.

KEY POINTS

- Unstable angina is new, worsening, or rest angina in patients whose cardiac biomarkers do not meet criteria for MI.
- Symptoms of unstable angina include new or worsening chest pain or chest pain occurring at rest.
- Diagnosis is based on serial ECGs and cardiac markers.
- Immediate treatment includes oxygen, antianginals, antiplatelet drugs, and anticoagulants.
- For patients with ongoing symptoms, hypotension or sustained arrhythmias, do immediate angiography.
- For stable patients, do angiography within 24 to 48 h of hospitalization.
- Following recovery, initiate or continue antiplatelet drugs, beta-blockers, ACE inhibitors, and statins.

ACUTE MYOCARDIAL INFARCTION

Acute MI is myocardial necrosis resulting from acute obstruction of a coronary artery. Symptoms include chest discomfort with or without dyspnea, nausea, and diaphoresis. Diagnosis is by ECG and the presence or absence of serologic markers. Treatment is antiplatelet drugs, anticoagulants, nitrates, beta-blockers, statins, and reperfusion therapy. For ST-segment-elevation MI, emergency reperfusion is via fibrinolytic drugs, percutaneous intervention, or, occasionally, coronary artery bypass graft surgery. For non-ST-segment-elevation MI, reperfusion is via percutaneous intervention or coronary artery bypass graft surgery.

In the US, about 1.5 million MIs occur annually. MI results in death for 400,000 to 500,000 people, with about half dying before they reach the hospital (see Cardiac Arrest on p. 538).

Acute MI, along with unstable angina, is considered an acute coronary syndrome. Acute MI includes both NSTEMI and STEMI. Distinction between NSTEMI and STEMI is vital as treatment strategies are different for these two entities (see Fig. 80–6).

Pathophysiology

MI is defined as myocardial necrosis in a clinical setting consistent with myocardial ischemia.[1] These conditions can be satisfied by a rise of cardiac biomarkers (preferably cardiac troponin [cTn]) above the 99th percentile of the upper reference limit (URL) plus at least one of the following:

- Symptoms of ischemia
- ECG changes indicative of new ischemia (significant ST/T changes or left bundle branch block)
- Development of pathological Q waves
- Imaging evidence of new loss of myocardium or new regional wall motion abnormality
- Angiography or autopsy evidence of intracoronary thrombus

Slightly different criteria are used to diagnose MI during and after PCI or CABG, and as the cause of sudden death.

MI also can be classified into 5 types based on etiology and circumstances:

- Type 1: Spontaneous MI caused by ischemia due to a primary coronary event (eg, plaque rupture, erosion, or fissuring; coronary dissection)
- Type 2: Ischemia due to increased oxygen demand (eg, hypertension), or decreased supply (eg, coronary artery spasm or embolism, arrhythmia, hypotension)
- Type 3: Related to sudden unexpected cardiac death
- Type 4a: Associated with PCI (signs and symptoms of MI with cTn values > 5 × 99th percentile URL)
- Type 4b: Associated with documented stent thrombosis
- Type 5: Associated with CABG (signs and symptoms of MI with cTn values >10 × 99th percentile URL)

Infarct location: MI affects predominantly the LV, but damage may extend into the RV or the atria. RV infarction usually results from obstruction of the right coronary or a dominant left circumflex artery; it is characterized by high RV filling pressure, often with severe tricuspid regurgitation and reduced cardiac output. An inferoposterior infarction causes some degree of RV dysfunction in about half of patients and causes hemodynamic abnormality in 10 to 15%. RV dysfunction should be considered in any patient who has inferoposterior infarction and elevated jugular venous pressure with hypotension or shock. RV infarction complicating LV infarction significantly increases mortality risk.

Anterior infarcts tend to be larger and result in a worse prognosis than inferoposterior infarcts. They are usually due to left coronary artery obstruction, especially in the anterior descending artery; inferoposterior infarcts reflect right coronary or dominant left circumflex artery obstruction.

Infarct extent: Infarction may be

- Transmural
- Nontransmural

Transmural infarcts involve the whole thickness of myocardium from epicardium to endocardium and are usually characterized by abnormal Q waves on ECG. Nontransmural or subendocardial infarcts do not extend through the ventricular wall and cause only ST-segment and T-wave (ST-T) abnormalities. Subendocardial infarcts usually involve the inner one-third of myocardium, where wall tension is highest and myocardial blood flow is most vulnerable to circulatory changes. These infarcts may follow prolonged hypotension. Because the transmural depth of necrosis cannot be precisely determined clinically, infarcts are usually classified as STEMI or NSTEMI by the presence or absence of ST-segment elevation or Q waves on the ECG. Volume of myocardium destroyed can be roughly estimated by the extent and duration of CK elevation or by peak levels of more commonly measured troponins.

NSTEMI (subendocardial MI) is myocardial necrosis (evidenced by cardiac markers in blood; troponin I or troponin

T and CK will be elevated) without acute ST-segment elevation. ECG changes such as ST-segment depression, T-wave inversion, or both may be present.

STEMI (transmural MI) is myocardial necrosis with ECG changes showing ST-segment elevation that is not quickly reversed by nitroglycerin. Cardiac markers, troponin I or troponin T, and CK are elevated.

1. Thygesen K, Alpert JS, Jaffe AS, et al. the Writing Group on behalf of the Joint ESC/ACCF/AHA/WHF Task Force for the Universal Definition of Myocardial Infarction: ESC/ACCF/AHA/WHF Expert Consensus Document Third Universal Definition of Myocardial Infarction. *Circulation* 126:2020–2035, 2012. doi: 10.1161/CIR.0b013e31826e1058

Symptoms and Signs

Symptoms of NSTEMI and STEMI are the same. Days to weeks before the event, about two thirds of patients experience prodromal symptoms, including unstable or crescendo angina, shortness of breath, and fatigue.

Usually, the first symptom of infarction is deep, substernal, visceral pain described as aching or pressure, often radiating to the back, jaw, left arm, right arm, shoulders, or all of these areas. The pain is similar to angina pectoris but is usually more severe and long-lasting; more often accompanied by dyspnea, diaphoresis, nausea, and vomiting; and relieved little or only temporarily by rest or nitroglycerin. However, discomfort may be mild; about 20% of acute MIs are silent (ie, asymptomatic or causing vague symptoms not recognized as illness by the patient), more commonly in patients with diabetes. Patients often interpret their discomfort as indigestion, particularly because spontaneous relief may be falsely attributed to belching or antacid consumption. Some patients present with syncope.

Women are more likely to present with atypical chest discomfort. Elderly patients may report dyspnea more than ischemic-type chest pain. In severe ischemic episodes, the patient often has significant pain and feels restless and apprehensive. Nausea and vomiting may occur, especially with inferior MI. Dyspnea and weakness due to LV failure, pulmonary edema, shock, or significant arrhythmia may dominate.

Skin may be pale, cool, and diaphoretic. Peripheral or central cyanosis may be present. Pulse may be thready, and BP is variable, although many patients initially have some degree of hypertension during pain.

Heart sounds are usually somewhat distant; a 4th heart sound is almost universally present. A soft systolic blowing apical murmur (reflecting papillary muscle dysfunction) may occur. During initial examination, a friction rub or more striking murmurs suggest a preexisting heart disorder or another diagnosis. Detection of a friction rub within a few hours after onset of MI symptoms suggests acute pericarditis rather than MI. However, friction rubs, usually evanescent, are common on days 2 and 3 post-STEMI. The chest wall is tender when palpated in about 15% of patients.

In right ventricular (RV) infarction, signs include elevated RV filling pressure, distended jugular veins (often with Kussmaul sign), clear lung fields, and hypotension.

Diagnosis

- Serial ECGs
- Serial cardiac markers
- Immediate coronary angiography (unless fibrinolytics are given) for patients with STEMI or complications (eg, persistent chest pain, hypotension, markedly elevated cardiac markers, unstable arrhythmias)
- Delayed coronary angiography (within 24 to 48 h) for patients with NSTEMI without complications

Evaluation begins with initial and serial ECG and serial measurements of cardiac markers to help distinguish between unstable angina, ST segment elevation myocardial infarction, and non ST segment elevation myocardial infarction. This distinction is the center of the decision pathway because fibrinolytics benefit patients with STEMI but may increase risk for those with NSTEMI. Also, urgent cardiac catheterization is indicated for patients with acute STEMI but not generally for those with NSTEMI.

ECG: ECG is the most important test and should be done within 10 min of presentation.

For STEMI, initial ECG is usually diagnostic, showing ST-segment elevation ≥ 1 mm in 2 or more contiguous leads subtending the damaged area (see Figs. 80–2, 80–3, 80–7, 80–8, 80–9, and 80–10).

Pathologic Q waves are not necessary for the diagnosis. The ECG must be read carefully because ST-segment elevation may be subtle, particularly in the inferior leads (II, III, aVF); sometimes the reader's attention is mistakenly focused on leads with ST-segment depression. If symptoms are characteristic, ST-segment elevation on ECG has a specificity of 90% and a sensitivity of 45% for diagnosing MI. Serial tracings (obtained every 8 h for 1 day, then daily) showing a gradual evolution toward a stable, more normal pattern or development of abnormal Q waves over a few days tends to confirm the diagnosis.

If right ventricular (RV) infarction is suspected, a 15-lead ECG is usually recorded; additional leads are placed at $V_{4-6}R$, and, to detect posterior infarction, V_8 and V_9.

ECG diagnosis of MI is more difficult when a left bundle branch block configuration is present because it resembles STEMI changes. ST-segment elevation concordant with the QRS complex strongly suggests MI as does > 5-mm ST-segment elevation in at least 2 precordial leads. But generally, any patient with suggestive symptoms and new-onset (or not known to be old) left bundle branch block is treated as for STEMI.

Cardiac markers: Cardiac markers (serum markers of myocardial cell injury) are cardiac enzymes (eg, CK-MB) and cell contents (eg, troponin I, troponin T, myoglobin) that are released into the bloodstream after myocardial cell necrosis. The markers appear at different times after injury, and levels decrease at different rates. Sensitivity and specificity for myocardial cell injury vary significantly among these markers, but the troponins (cTn) are the most sensitive and specific and are now the markers of choice. Recently, several new, highly sensitive assays of cardiac troponin (hs-cTn) that are also very precise have become available. These assays can reliably measure Tn levels (T or I) as low as 0.003 to 0.006 ng/mL (3 to 6 pg/mL); some research assays go as low as 0.001 ng/mL (1 pg/mL).

Previous, less sensitive cTn tests were unlikely to detect Tn except in patients who had an acute cardiac disorder. Thus a "positive" Tn (ie, above the limit of detection) was very specific. However, the new hs-cTn tests can detect small amounts of Tn in many healthy people. Thus, hs-cTn levels need to be referenced to the normal range, and are defined as "elevated" only when higher than 99% of the reference population. Furthermore, although an elevated troponin level indicates myocardial cell injury, it does not indicate the cause of the damage (although any troponin elevation increases the risk of adverse outcomes in many disorders). In addition to acute coronary syndrome (ACS), many other cardiac and non-cardiac disorders can elevate hs-cTn levels (see Table 80–3); not all elevated hs-cTn levels represent MI, and not all myocardial necrosis results from an acute coronary syndrome event even when

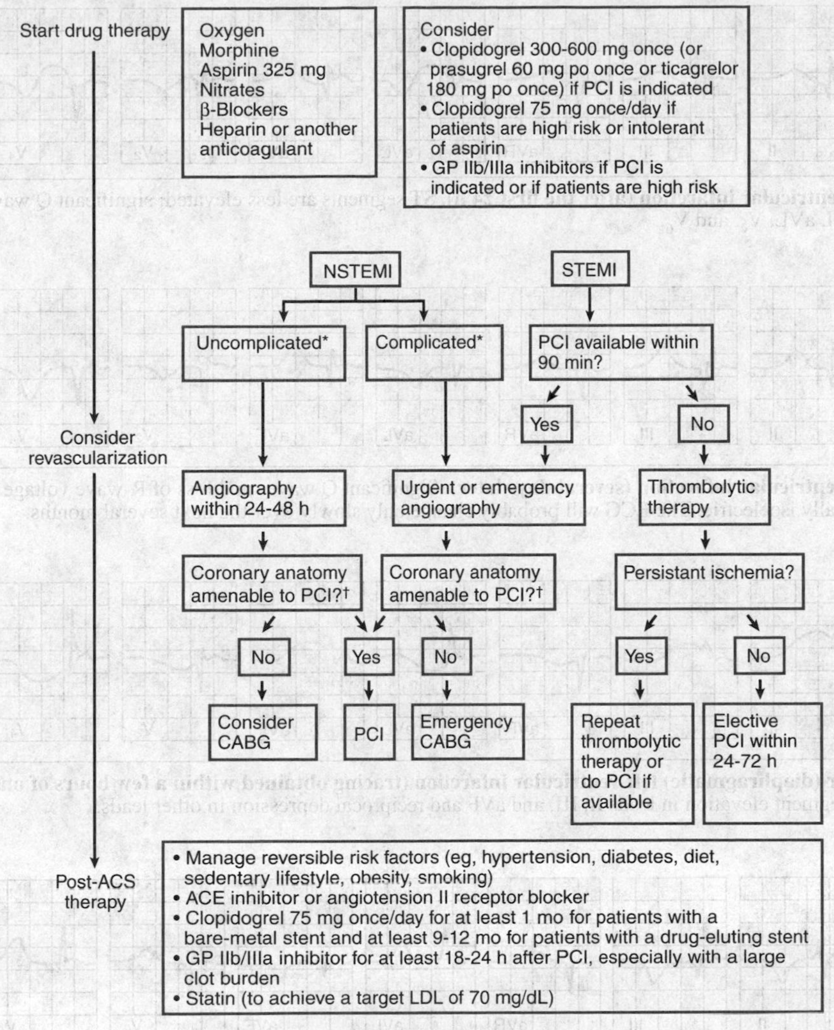

Fig. 80–6. Approach to myocardial infarction.

*Complicated means that the hospital course was complicated by recurrent angina or infarction, heart failure, or sustained recurrent ventricular arrhythmias. Absence of any of these events is termed uncomplicated.

†CABG is generally preferred to PCI for patients with the following:

- Left main or left main equivalent disease
- Left ventricular dysfunction
- Treated diabetes

Also, lesions that are long or near bifurcation points are often not amenable to PCI.

CABG = coronary artery bypass grafting; GP = glycoprotein; LDL = low density lipoprotein; PCI = percutaneous intervention.

the etiology is ischemic. However, by detecting lower levels of Tn, hs-cTn assays enable earlier identification of MI than other assays, and have replaced other cardiac marker tests in many centers.

Patients suspected of having a MI should have an hs-cTn level done on presentation and 3 h later (at 0 and 6 h if using a standard Tn assay).

An hs-cTn level must be interpreted based on the patient's pre-test probability of disease, which is estimated clinically based on:

- Risk factors for ACS
- Symptoms
- ECG

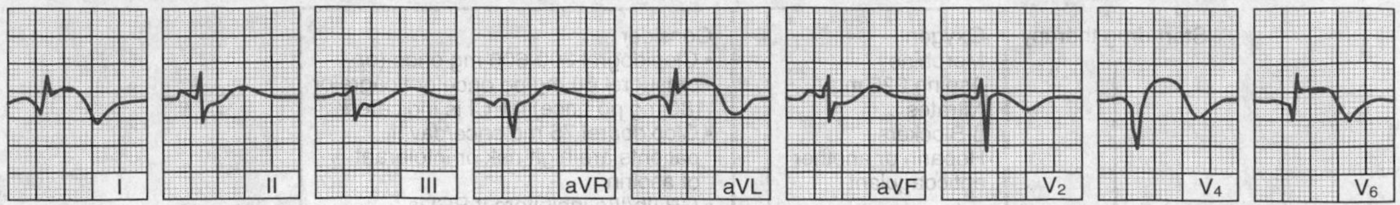

Fig. 80–7. Lateral left ventricular infarction (after the first 24 h). ST segments are less elevated; significant Q waves develop and R waves are lost in leads I, aVL, V_4, and V_6.

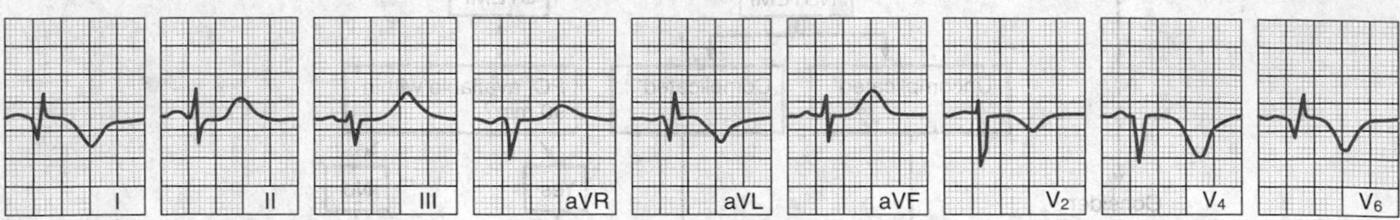

Fig. 80–8. Lateral left ventricular infarction (several days later). Significant Q waves and loss of R-wave voltage persist. ST segments are now essentially isoelectric. The ECG will probably change only slowly over the next several months.

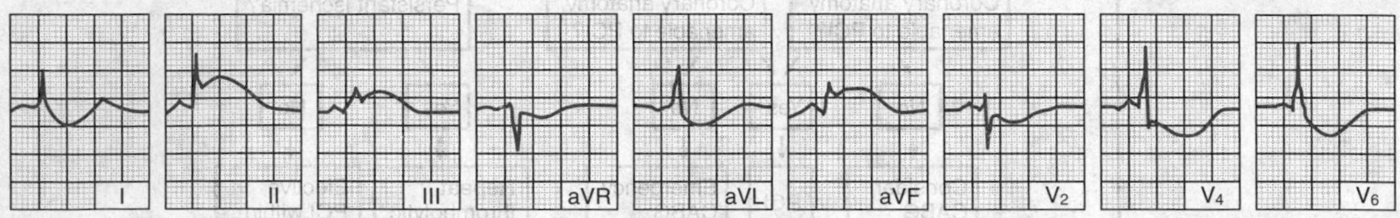

Fig. 80–9. Acute inferior (diaphragmatic) left ventricular infarction (tracing obtained within a few hours of onset of illness). There is hyperacute ST-segment elevation in leads II, III, and aVF and reciprocal depression in other leads.

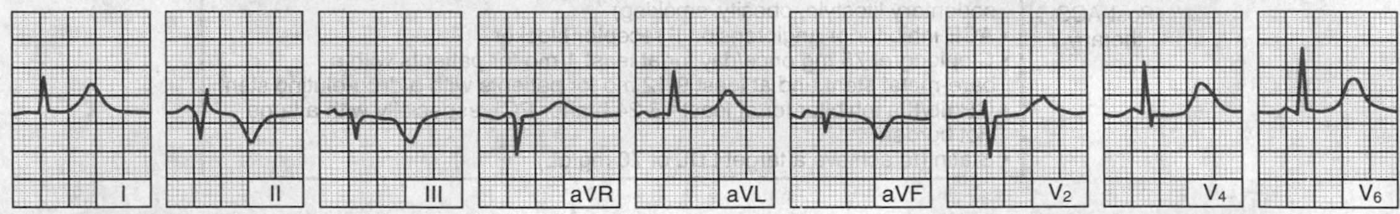

Fig. 80–10. Inferior (diaphragmatic) left ventricular infarction (several days later). ST segments are now isoelectric. Abnormal Q waves in leads II, III, and aVF indicate that myocardial scars persist.

A high pre-test probability plus an elevated hs-cTn level is highly suggestive of MI, whereas a low pre-test probability plus a normal hs-cTn is unlikely to represent MI. Diagnosis is more challenging when test results are discordant with pre-test probability, in which case serial hs-cTn levels often help. A patient with low pre-test probability and an initially slightly elevated hs-cTn that remains stable on repeat testing probably has non-ACS cardiac disease (eg, heart failure, stable CAD). However, if the repeat level rises significantly (ie, > 20 to 50%) the likelihood of MI becomes much higher. If a patient with high pre-test probability has a normal hs-cTn level that rises > 50% when the hs-cTc is re-measured, MI is likely; continued normal levels (often including at 6 h and beyond when suspicion is high) suggest need to pursue an alternate diagnosis.

Coronary angiography: Coronary angiography most often combines diagnosis with PCI (ie, angioplasty, stent placement). When possible, emergency coronary angiography and PCI are done as soon as possible after the onset of acute MI (primary PCI). In many tertiary centers, this approach has significantly lowered morbidity and mortality and improved long-term outcomes. Frequently, the infarction is actually aborted when the time from pain to PCI is short (< 3 to 4 h).

Angiography is obtained urgently for patients with STEMI, patients with persistent chest pain despite maximal medical therapy, and patients with complications (eg, markedly elevated cardiac markers, presence of cardiogenic shock, acute mitral regurgitation, ventricular septal defect, unstable arrhythmias). Patients with uncomplicated NSTEMI whose symptoms have resolved typically undergo angiography within the first 24 to 48 h of hospitalization to detect lesions that may require treatment.

After initial evaluation and therapy, coronary angiography may be used in patients with evidence of ongoing ischemia (ECG findings or symptoms), hemodynamic instability, recurrent ventricular tachyarrhythmias, and other abnormalities that suggest recurrence of ischemic events. Some experts also recommend that angiography be done before hospital discharge in STEMI patients with inducible ischemia on stress imaging or an ejection fraction < 40%.

Prognosis

Global risk should be estimated via formal clinical risk scores or a combination of the following high-risk features:

- Recurrent angina/ischemia at rest or during low-level activity
- Heart failure
- Worsening mitral regurgitation
- High-risk stress test result (test stopped in ≤ 5 min due to symptoms, marked ECG abnormalities, hypotension, or complex ventricular arrhythmias)
- Hemodynamic instability
- Sustained VT
- Diabetes mellitus
- PCI within past 6 mo
- Prior CABG
- LV ejection fraction < 0.40

Overall mortality rate is about 30%, with 25 to 30% of these patients dying before reaching the hospital (typically due to VF). In-hospital mortality rate is about 10% (typically due to cardiogenic shock) but varies significantly with severity of left ventricular failure (see Table 80–6).

For patients receiving reperfusion (fibrinolysis or PCI), in-hospital mortality is 5 to 6%, versus 15% for patients eligible for reperfusion who do not receive reperfusion therapy. In centers with established primary PCI programs, in-hospital mortality is reported to be < 5%.

Most patients who die of cardiogenic shock have an infarct or a combination of scar and new infarct affecting ≥ 50% of LV mass. Five clinical characteristics predict 90% of the mortality in patients who present with STEMI (see Table 80–7): older age (31% of total mortality), lower systolic BP (24%), Killip class > 1 (15%), faster heart rate (12%), and anterior location (6%). Mortality rates of women and patients with diabetes tend to be higher.

Mortality rate of patients who survive initial hospitalization is 8 to 10% in the year after acute MI. Most fatalities occur in the first 3 to 4 mo. Persistent ventricular arrhythmia, heart failure, poor ventricular function, and recurrent ischemia indicate high risk. Many authorities recommend stress ECG before hospital discharge or within 6 wk. Good exercise performance without ECG abnormalities is associated with a favorable prognosis; further evaluation is usually not required. Poor exercise performance is associated with a poor prognosis.

Cardiac performance after recovery depends largely on how much functioning myocardium survives the acute attack. Acute damage adds to scars from previous infarcts. When > 50% of left ventricular mass is damaged, prolonged survival is unusual.

Treatment

- Prehospital care: oxygen, aspirin, nitrates and/or opioids for pain, and triage to an appropriate medical center
- Drug treatment: Antiplatelet drugs, antianginal drugs, anticoagulants, and in some cases other drugs
- Reperfusion therapy: Fibrinolytics or angiography with PCI or coronary artery bypass surgery
- Postdischarge rehabilitation and chronic medical management of CAD

Choice of drug therapy and choice of reperfusion strategy are discussed elsewhere.

Prehospital care:

- Oxygen
- Aspirin
- Nitrates or opioids
- Triage to appropriate medical center

A reliable IV route must be established, oxygen given (typically 2 L by nasal cannula), and continuous single-lead ECG monitoring started. Prehospital interventions by emergency medical personnel (including ECG, chewed aspirin [325 mg], pain management (with nitrates or opioids) can reduce risk of mortality and complications. Early diagnostic data and response to treatment can help determine the need for and timing of revascularization.

Hospital admission:

- Risk-stratify patient and choose reperfusion strategy
- Drug therapy with antiplatelet drugs, anticoagulants and other drugs based on reperfusion strategy

On arrival to the emergency room, the patient's diagnosis is confirmed. Drug therapy and timing of revascularization depend on the clinical picture and diagnosis.

For STEMI, reperfusion strategy can include fibrinolytic therapy or immediate PCI. For patients with NSTEMI, angiography may be done within 24 to 48 h of admission if the patient is clinically stable. If the patient is unstable (eg, ongoing symptoms, hypotension or sustained arrhythmias), then angiography must be done immediately (see Fig. 80–6).

Drug treatment of acute myocardial infarction: All patients should be given antiplatelet drugs, anticoagulants, and if chest pain is present, antianginal drugs. The specific drugs used depend on the reperfusion strategy and other factors; their selection

Table 80–6. KILLIP CLASSIFICATION AND MORTALITY RATE OF ACUTE MYOCARDIAL INFARCTION*

CLASS	PAO_2†	CLINICAL DESCRIPTION	HOSPITAL MORTALITY RATE
1	Normal	No clinical evidence of left ventricular (LV) failure	3–5%
2	Slightly reduced	Mild to moderate LV failure	6–10%
3	Abnormal	Severe LV failure, pulmonary edema	20–30%
4	Severely abnormal	Cardiogenic shock: hypotension, tachycardia, mental obtundation, cool extremities, oliguria, hypoxia	> 80%

*Determined by repeated examination of the patient during the course of illness.
†Determined while the patient is breathing room air.
Modified from Killip T, Kimball JT: Treatment of myocardial infarction in a coronary care unit. A two-year experience with 250 patients. *The American Journal of Cardiology* 20:457–464, 1967.

Table 80–7. MORTALITY RISK AT 30 DAYS IN STEMI

Scoring

RISK FACTOR	POINTS
Age ≥ 75	3
Age 65–74	2
Diabetes mellitus, hypertension, or angina	1
Systolic BP < 100 mm Hg	3
Heart rate > 100 beat/min	2
Killip class II–IV	2
Weight < 67 kg	1
Anterior ST-elevation or left branch bundle block	1
Time to treatment > 4 h	1
Total points possible	0–14

Risk

TOTAL POINTS	MORTALITY RATE AT 30 DAYS (%)
0	0.8
1	1.6
2	2.2
3	4.4
4	7.3
5	12.4
6	16.1
7	23.4
8	26.8
> 8	35.9

STEMI = ST-segment elevation MI; TIMI = thrombolysis in MI.

Based on data from Morrow DA et al: TIMI risk score for ST-elevation myocardial infarction: a convenient, bedside, clinical score for risk assessment at presentation. *Circulation* 102(17):2031–2037, 2000 and ACC/AHA guidelines for the management of patients with acute myocardial infarction.

and use is discussed in Drugs for Acute Coronary Syndrome on p. 694. Other drugs, such as beta-blockers, ACE inhibitors, and statins, should be initiated during admission (see Table 80–2).

Patients with acute MI should be given the following (unless contraindicated):

- Antiplatelet drugs: Aspirin, clopidogrel, or both (prasugrel or ticagrelor are alternatives to clopidogrel)
- Anticoagulants: A heparin (unfractionated or LMWH) or bivalirudin
- GP IIb/IIIa inhibitor for some high risk patients
- Antianginal therapy usually nitroglycerin
- Beta-blocker
- ACE inhibitor
- Statin

All patients are given aspirin 160 to 325 mg (not enteric-coated), if not contraindicated, at presentation and 81 mg once/day indefinitely thereafter. Chewing the first dose before swallowing quickens absorption. Aspirin reduces short-term and long-term mortality risk. In patients undergoing PCI, a loading dose of clopidogrel (300 to 600 mg po once), prasugrel (60 mg po once), or ticagrelor (180 mg po once) improves outcomes, particularly when administered 24 h in advance. For urgent PCI, prasugrel and ticagrelor are more rapid in onset and may be preferred.

Either a LMWH, unfractionated heparin, or bivalirudin is given routinely to patients with unstable angina unless contraindicated (eg, by active bleeding). Unfractionated heparin is more complicated to use because it requires frequent (q 6 h) dosing adjustments to achieve target activated PTT (aPTT). The LMWHs have better bioavailability, are given by simple weight-based dose without monitoring aPTT and dose titration, and have lower risk of heparin-induced thrombocytopenia. Bivalirudin is recommended for those with a known or suspected history of heparin-induced thrombocytopenia.

Consider GP IIb/IIIa inhibitor for high risk patients (patients with recurrent ischemia, dynamic ECG changes or hemodynamic instability). Abciximab, tirofiban, and eptifibatide appear to have equivalent efficacy, and the choice of drug should depend on other factors (eg, cost, availability, familiarity).

Chest pain can be treated with morphine or nitroglycerin. Morphine 2 to 4 mg IV, repeated q 15 min as needed, is highly effective but can depress respiration, can reduce myocardial

Table 80–8. RISK OF ADVERSE EVENTS* AT 14 DAYS IN NSTEMI

Scoring

RISK FACTOR	POINTS
Age > 65	1
CAD risk factors (must have ≥ 3 for 1 point): • Family history • Hypertension • Current smoker • High cholesterol • Diabetes mellitus	1
Known CAD (stenosis ≥ 50%)	1
Previous chronic use of aspirin	1
Two episodes of rest angina in past 24 h	1
Elevated cardiac markers	1
ST elevation ≥ 0.5 mm	1
Risk level is based on total points:	1–2 = low 3–4 = intermediate 5–7 = high

Absolute risk

TOTAL POINTS	RISK OF EVENTS AT 14 DAYS (%)*
0 or 1	4.7
2	8.3
3	13.2
4	19.9
5	26.2
6 or 7	40.9

*Events include all-cause mortality, myocardial infarction, and recurrent ischemia requiring urgent revascularization.

CAD = coronary artery disease; MI = myocardial infarction; NSTEMI = non–ST-segment elevation MI; TIMI = thrombolysis in MI.

Based on data from Antman EM et al: The TIMI risk score for unstable angina/non-ST elevation MI: A method of prognostication and therapeutic decision making. *JAMA* 284:835–842, 2000.

contractility, and is a potent venous vasodilator. Hypotension and bradycardia secondary to morphine can usually be overcome by prompt elevation of the lower extremities. Nitroglycerin is initially given sublingually, followed by continuous IV drip if needed.

Standard therapy for all patients with unstable angina includes beta-blockers, ACE inhibitors, and statins. Beta-blockers are recommended unless contraindicated (eg, by bradycardia, heart block, hypotension, or asthma), especially for high-risk patients. Beta-blockers reduce heart rate, arterial pressure, and contractility, thereby reducing cardiac workload and oxygen demand. ACE inhibitors may provide long-term cardioprotection by improving endothelial function. If an ACE inhibitor is not tolerated because of cough or rash (but not angioedema or renal dysfunction), an angiotensin II receptor blocker may be substituted. Statins are also standard therapy and should be continued indefinitely.

Reperfusion therapy in acute MI:

- For patients with STEMI: Immediate PCI or fibrinolytics
- For patients with NSTEMI: Immediate PCI for unstable patients or within 24 to 48 h for stable patients

For STEMI patients, emergency PCI is the preferred treatment of ST-segment elevation MI when available in a timely fashion (door to balloon-inflation time < 90 min) by an experienced operator. If there is likely to be a significant delay in availability of PCI, thrombolysis should be done for STEMI patients meeting criteria. Reperfusion using fibrinolytics is most effective if given in the first few minutes to hours after onset of MI. The earlier a fibrinolytic is begun, the better. The goal is a door-to-needle time of 30 to 60 min. Greatest benefit occurs within 3 h, but the drugs may be effective up to 12 h. Characteristics and selection of fibrinolytic drugs are discussed elsewhere.

Unstable NSTEMI patients (ie, those with ongoing symptoms, hypotension, or sustained arrhythmias) should proceed directly to the cardiac catheterization laboratory to identify coronary lesions requiring PCI or CABG. Immediate reperfusion is not as urgent in patients with uncomplicated NSTEMI, in whom a completely occluded infarct-related artery at presentation is uncommon. Such patients typically undergo angiography within the first 24 to 48 h of hospitalization to identify coronary lesions requiring PCI or CABG. Fibrinolytics are not indicated for NSTEMI. Risk outweighs potential benefit.

Choice of reperfusion strategy is further discussed under Revascularization for Acute Coronary Syndromes on p. 697.

Rehabilitation and postdischarge treatment:

- Functional evaluation
- Changes in lifestyle: Regular exercise, diet modification, weight loss, smoking cessation
- Drugs: Continuation of antiplatelet drugs, beta-blockers, ACE inhibitors, and statins

Patients who did not have coronary angiography during admission, have no high-risk features (eg, heart failure, recurrent angina, VT or VF after 24 h, mechanical complications such as new murmurs, shock), and have an ejection fraction > 40% whether or not they received fibrinolytics usually should have stress testing of some sort before or shortly after discharge (see Table 80–4).

The acute illness and treatment of MI should be used to strongly motivate the patient to modify risk factors. Evaluating the patient's physical and emotional status and discussing them with the patient, advising about lifestyle (eg, smoking, diet, work and play habits, exercise), and aggressively managing risk factors may improve prognosis.

On discharge, all patients should be on appropriate antiplatelet drugs, statins, antianginals, and other drugs based on comorbidities.

KEY POINTS

- Acute MI is myocardial necrosis resulting from acute obstruction of a coronary artery.
- Symptoms of acute MI include chest pain or discomfort with or without dyspnea, nausea, and diaphoresis.
- Women and patients with diabetes are more likely to present with atypical symptoms, and 20% of acute MI are silent.
- Diagnosis is by ECG and cardiac markers.
- Immediate treatment includes oxygen, antianginals, antiplatelet drugs, and anticoagulants.
- For patients with STEMI, do immediate angiography with PCI; if immediate PCI is not available, give fibrinolytics.
- For patients with NSTEMI who are stable, do angiography within 24 to 48 h; for those who are unstable, do immediate angiography with PCI.
- Following recovery, initiate or continue antiplatelet drugs, beta-blockers, ACE inhibitors, and statins.

COMPLICATIONS OF ACUTE CORONARY SYNDROMES

Numerous complications can occur and increase morbidity and mortality. They can be roughly categorized as

- Electrical dysfunction (conduction disturbance, arrhythmias)
- Mechanical dysfunction (heart failure, myocardial rupture or aneurysm, papillary muscle dysfunction)
- Thrombotic complications (recurrent coronary ischemia, mural thrombosis)
- Inflammatory complications (pericarditis, Dressler syndrome)

Electrical dysfunction occurs in > 90% of MI patients (see also p. 620). Electrical dysfunction that commonly causes mortality in the first 72 h includes tachycardia (from any focus) rapid enough to reduce cardiac output and lower BP, Mobitz type II block (2nd degree) or complete (3rd degree) AV block, VT, and VF. Asystole is uncommon, except as a terminal manifestation of progressive left ventricular failure and shock. Patients with disturbances of cardiac rhythm are checked for hypoxia and electrolyte abnormalities, which can be causative or contributory.

Sinus Node Disturbances

If the artery supplying the sinus node is affected by an acute coronary syndrome, sinus node disturbances can occur; they are more likely if there is a preexisting sinus node disorder (common among the elderly).

Sinus bradycardia: Sinus bradycardia, the most common sinus node disturbance, is usually not treated unless there is hypotension or the heart rate is < 50 beats/min. A lower heart rate, if not extreme, means reduced cardiac workload and possibly reduced infarct size.

For bradycardia with hypotension (which may reduce myocardial perfusion), atropine sulfate 0.5 to 1 mg IV is used; it can be repeated after several minutes if response is inadequate. Several small doses are best because high doses may induce tachycardia. Occasionally, a temporary transvenous pacemaker must be inserted.

Sinus tachycardia: Persistent sinus tachycardia is usually ominous, often reflecting left ventricular failure and low cardiac output. Without heart failure or another evident cause, this arrhythmia may respond to a beta-blocker, given po or IV depending on degree of urgency.

Atrial Arrhythmias

Atrial arrhythmias (atrial ectopic beats, atrial fibrillation, and, less commonly, atrial flutter) occur in about 10% of patients who have had a MI and may reflect left ventricular failure or right atrial infarction.

Paroxysmal atrial tachycardia is uncommon and usually occurs in patients who have had previous episodes of it.

Atrial ectopy is usually benign, but if frequency increases, causes, particularly heart failure, are sought. Frequent atrial ectopic beats may respond to a beta-blocker.

Atrial fibrillation: Atrial fibrillation is usually transient if it occurs within the first 24 h (see Fig. 76–4 on p. 635). Risk factors include age > 70, heart failure, previous history of MI, large anterior infarction, atrial infarction, pericarditis, hypokalemia, hypomagnesemia, a chronic lung disorder, and hypoxia. Fibrinolytics reduce incidence.

Recurrent paroxysmal atrial fibrillation is a poor prognostic sign and increases risk of systemic emboli.

For atrial fibrillation, heparin is usually used because systemic emboli are a risk. IV beta-blockers (eg, atenolol 2.5 to 5.0 mg over 2 min to total dose of 10 mg in 10 to 15 min, metoprolol 2 to 5 mg q 2 to 5 min to a total dose of 15 mg in 10 to 15 min) rapidly slow the ventricular rate. Heart rate and BP are closely monitored. Treatment is withheld when ventricular rate decreases satisfactorily or systolic BP is < 100 mm Hg.

IV digoxin, which is not as effective as beta-blockers, is used cautiously and only in patients with atrial fibrillation and left ventricular systolic dysfunction. Usually, digoxin takes at least 2 h to effectively slow heart rate and may rarely aggravate ischemia in patients with recent acute coronary syndrome. For patients without evident left ventricular systolic dysfunction or conduction delay manifested by a wide QRS complex, IV verapamil or IV diltiazem may be considered. Diltiazem may be given as an IV infusion to control heart rate for long periods.

If atrial fibrillation compromises circulatory status (eg, causing left ventricular failure, hypotension, or chest pain), urgent electrical cardioversion is done. If atrial fibrillation returns after cardioversion, IV amiodarone should be considered.

Atrial flutter: For atrial flutter (see Fig. 76–6 on p. 639), rate is controlled as for atrial fibrillation; heparin is required because the risk of thromboembolism is similar to that with atrial fibrillation. Low-energy direct current (DC) cardioversion will usually terminate atrial flutter.

Conduction Defects

Mobitz type I block (Wenckebach block, progressive prolongation of PR interval with eventual dropped beats) is relatively common with an inferior-diaphragmatic infarction (see Fig. 76–8 on p. 640); it is usually self-limited and rarely progresses to higher grade block.

Mobitz type II block (dropped beats) usually indicates massive anterior MI, as does complete heart block with wide QRS complexes (atrial impulses do not reach the ventricle); both are uncommon.

Frequency of 3rd degree atrioventricular (complete) block depends on site of infarction (see Fig. 76–11 on on p. 641). Complete AV block occurs in 5 to 10% of patients with inferior infarction and is usually transient. It occurs in < 5% with uncomplicated anterior infarction but in up to 26% of those with right bundle branch block and left posterior hemiblock. Even transient complete AV block with an anterior MI is an indication for permanent pacemaker insertion because the risk of sudden death without pacing is significant.

Mobitz type I block usually does not warrant treatment. For true Mobitz type II block with dropped beats or for AV block with slow, wide QRS complexes, temporary transvenous pacing is the treatment of choice. External pacing can be used until a temporary transvenous pacemaker can be placed. Although isoproterenol infusion may restore rhythm and rate temporarily, it is not used because it increases oxygen demand and risk of rhythm abnormalities. Atropine 0.5 mg IV q 3 to 5 min to a total dose of 2.5 mg may be useful for narrow-complex atrioventricular block with a slow ventricular rate but is not recommended for new wide-complex atrioventricular block.

Ventricular Arrhythmias

Ventricular arrhythmias are common and may result from hypoxia, electrolyte imbalance (hypokalemia, possibly hypomagnesemia), or sympathetic overactivity in ischemic cells adjacent to infarcted tissue (which is not electrically active). Treatable causes of ventricular arrhythmias are sought and corrected. Serum potassium should be kept above 4.0 mEq/L. IV potassium chloride is recommended; usually 10 mEq/h can be infused, but for severe hypokalemia (potassium level < 2.5 mEq/L), 20 to 40 mEq/h can be infused through a central venous line.

Ventricular ectopic beats, which are common after MI, do not warrant specific treatment.

An IV beta-blocker early in MI followed by continued oral beta-blockers reduces the incidence of ventricular arrhythmias (including VF) and mortality in patients who do not have heart failure or hypotension. Prophylaxis with other drugs (eg, lidocaine) increases mortality risk and is not recommended.

After the acute phase, the presence of complex ventricular arrhythmias or nonsustained VT, especially with significant left ventricular systolic dysfunction, increases mortality risk. An implantable cardioverter-defibrillator (ICD) should be considered and is indicated when the left ventricular ejection fraction is < 35%. Programmed endocardial stimulation can help select the most effective antiarrhythmics or determine the need for an ICD. Before treatment with an antiarrhythmic or ICD, coronary angiography and other tests are done to look for recurrent myocardial ischemia, which may require PCI or CABG.

Ventricular tachycardia: Nonsustained VT (ie, < 30 sec) and even sustained slow VT (accelerated idioventricular rhythm) without hemodynamic instability do not usually require treatment in the first 24 to 48 h (see Fig. 76–21 on p. 649).

Pulseless VT requires defibrillation. VT without hemodynamic instability may be treated with IV lidocaine, procainamide, amiodarone, or synchronized cardioversion. Some clinicians also treat complex ventricular arrhythmias with magnesium sulfate 2 g IV over 5 min whether or not serum magnesium level is low.

VT may occur months after MI. Late VT is more likely to occur in patients with transmural infarction and to be sustained.

Ventricular fibrillation: VF occurs in 5 to 12% of patients during the first 24 h after MI, usually within 6 h (see p. 648). Late VF usually indicates continued or recurrent myocardial ischemia and, when accompanied by hemodynamic deterioration, is a poor prognostic sign. VF is treated with immediate unsynchronized cardioversion.

Heart Failure

Patients with large infarctions (determined by ECG or cardiac markers) and those with mechanical complications, hypertension, or diastolic dysfunction are more likely to develop heart failure (see p. 712). Clinical findings depend on infarct size, elevation of left ventricular filling pressure, and degree of reduction in cardiac output. Dyspnea, inspiratory crackles at the lung bases, and hypoxemia are common.

Treatment depends on severity. For mild cases, a loop diuretic (eg, furosemide 20 to 40 mg IV once/day or bid) to reduce ventricular filling pressure is often sufficient. For severe cases, vasodilators (eg, IV nitroglycerin, nitroprusside) are often used to reduce preload and afterload; these drugs are effective acutely (eg, in acute pulmonary edema) and may be continued over 24 to 72 h as necessary. During treatment, pulmonary artery occlusion pressure may be measured via right heart (Swan-Ganz) catheterization, especially if the response to therapy is not as desired.

ACE inhibitors are used as long as systolic BP remains > 100 mm Hg. A short-acting ACE inhibitor given in low doses (eg, captopril 3.125 to 6.25 mg po q 4 to 6 h, increasing doses as tolerated) is best for initial treatment. Once the maximum dose is reached (maximum for captopril, 50 mg tid), a longer-acting ACE inhibitor (eg, fosinopril, lisinopril, perindopril, ramipril) is substituted for the long-term. If the patient remains in New York Heart Association class II or worse (see Table 83–2 on p. 716), an aldosterone inhibitor (eg, eplerenone, spironolactone) should be added.

For severe heart failure, an intraarterial counterpulsation balloon pump or an implantable intravascular ventricular assist pump may provide temporary hemodynamic support until the patient stabilizes or the decision is made to provide more advanced support. When revascularization or surgical repair is not feasible, heart transplantation is considered. Long-term left ventricular or biventricular implantable assist devices may be used as a bridge to transplantation. If transplantation is impossible, the left ventricular assist device is increasingly used as permanent treatment (destination therapy). Occasionally, use of such a device results in recovery and can be removed in 3 to 6 mo.

Papillary Muscle Disorders

Functional papillary muscle insufficiency occurs in about 35% of patients during the first few hours of infarction. Papillary muscle ischemic dysfunction causes incomplete coaptation of the mitral valve leaflets, which is transient in most patients. But in some patients, papillary muscle or free wall scarring causes permanent mitral regurgitation. Functional papillary muscle insufficiency is characterized by an apical late systolic murmur and typically resolves without treatment.

Papillary muscle rupture occurs most often after an inferoposterior infarct due to right coronary artery occlusion. It causes acute, severe mitral regurgitation. Papillary muscle rupture is characterized by the sudden appearance of a loud apical holosystolic murmur and thrill, usually with pulmonary edema. Occasionally, severe regurgitation is silent. An abrupt hemodynamic deterioration raises clinical suspicion of papillary muscle rupture; echocardiography should always be done to make the diagnosis. Urgent mitral valve repair or replacement is necessary and effective.

Myocardial Rupture

Interventricular septum or free wall rupture occurs in 1% of patients with acute MI. It causes 15% of hospital mortality.

Interventricular septum rupture, although rare, is 8 to 10 times more common than papillary muscle rupture. Interventricular septum rupture is characterized by the sudden appearance of a loud systolic murmur and thrill medial to the apex along the left sternal border in the 3rd or 4th intercostal space, accompanied by hypotension with or without signs of LV failure. Diagnosis may be confirmed using a balloon-tipped catheter and comparing blood oxygen saturation or Po_2 of right atrial, right ventricular, and pulmonary artery samples. A significant increase in right ventricular Po_2 is diagnostic, as is Doppler echocardiography, which may demonstrate the actual shunt of blood across the ventricular septum.

Treatment is surgery, which should be delayed if possible for up to 6 wk after MI so that infarcted myocardium can heal maximally; if hemodynamic instability persists, earlier surgery is indicated despite a high mortality risk.

Free wall rupture increases in incidence with age and is more common among women. It is characterized by sudden loss of arterial pressure with momentary persistence of sinus rhythm and often by signs of cardiac tamponade. Surgery is rarely successful. Rupture of a free wall is almost always fatal.

Ventricular Aneurysm

A localized bulge in the ventricular wall, usually the left ventricular wall, can occur at the site of a large infarction. Ventricular aneurysms are common, especially with a large transmural infarct (usually anterior). Aneurysms may develop in a few days, weeks, or months. They are unlikely to rupture but may lead to recurrent ventricular arrhythmias, low cardiac output, and mural thrombosis with systemic embolism.

A ventricular aneurysm may be suspected when paradoxical precordial movements are seen or felt, ECG shows persistent ST-segment elevation, and chest x-ray shows a characteristic bulge of the cardiac shadow. Because these findings are not diagnostic of an aneurysm, echocardiography is done to confirm the diagnosis and determine whether a thrombus is present.

Surgical excision may be indicated when left ventricular failure or arrhythmia persists. Early revascularization and probably the use of ACE inhibitors during acute MI modify left ventricular remodeling and have reduced the incidence of aneurysm.

Pseudoaneurysm is incomplete rupture of the free left ventricular wall; it is limited by the pericardium. Pseudoaneurysms may be large, contributing to heart failure, almost always contain a thrombus, and often rupture completely. They are repaired surgically.

Hypotension and Cardiogenic Shock

Hypotension: Hypotension may be due to decreased ventricular filling or loss of contractile force secondary to massive MI. Marked hypotension (eg, systolic BP < 90 mm Hg) with tachycardia and symptoms of end-organ hypoperfusion (reduced urine output, mental confusion, diaphoresis, cold extremities) is termed cardiogenic shock. Pulmonary congestion develops rapidly in cardiogenic shock.

Decreased left ventricular filling is most often caused by reduced venous return secondary to hypovolemia, especially in patients receiving intensive loop diuretic therapy, but it may reflect right ventricular infarction. Marked pulmonary congestion suggests loss of left ventricular contractile force (left ventricular failure) as the cause.

Treatment depends on the cause. In some patients, determining the cause requires use of a pulmonary artery catheter to measure intracardiac pressures. If pulmonary artery occlusion pressure is < 18 mm Hg, decreased filling, usually due to hypovolemia, is likely; if pressure is > 18 mm Hg, left ventricular failure is likely.

For hypotension due to hypovolemia, cautious fluid replacement with 0.9% saline is usually possible without left heart overload (excessive rise in left atrial pressure). However, sometimes left ventricular function is so compromised that adequate fluid replacement sharply increases pulmonary artery occlusion pressure to levels associated with pulmonary edema (> 25 mm Hg). If left atrial pressure is high, hypotension is probably due to left ventricular failure, and if diuretics are ineffective, inotropic therapy or circulatory support may be required.

Cardiogenic shock: Approximately 5 to 10% of patients with acute MI have cardiogenic shock (see also p. 572). In cardiogenic shock, an alpha-agonist or beta-agonist may be temporarily effective. Dopamine, a catecholamine with alpha and beta 1 effects, is given at 0.5 to 1 mcg/kg/min, increased until response is satisfactory or dose is about 10 mcg/kg/min. Higher doses induce vasoconstriction and atrial and ventricular arrhythmias.

Dobutamine, a beta-agonist, may be given IV at 2.5 to 10 mcg/kg/min or in higher doses. It often causes or exacerbates hypotension; it is most effective when hypotension is secondary to low cardiac output with increased peripheral vascular resistance. Dopamine is more effective than dobutamine when a vasopressor effect is also required.

In refractory cases, dobutamine and dopamine may be combined. The combination of dobutamine plus a drug with more alpha-adrenergic effects (phenylephrine, norepinephrine) may be effective without causing excessive arrhythmias.

An intraortic counterpulsation balloon pump may often temporarily support the patient, but recent evidence indicates no short-term or long-term benefit to this approach. Alternatives include a percutaneous or surgically implanted left ventricular assist device and occasionally transplantation.

Definitive treatment for postinfarction cardiogenic shock is revascularization by thrombolysis of the clot, angioplasty, or emergency CABG. Revascularization usually greatly improves ventricular function. PCI of CABG may be considered for persistent ischemia, refractory ventricular arrhythmia, hemodynamic instability, or shock if coronary anatomy is suitable.

Right Ventricular Ischemia or Infarction

Right ventricular infarction rarely occurs in isolation; it usually accompanies inferior left ventricular infarction. The first sign may be hypotension developing in a previously stable patient.

Right-sided ECG leads may show ST-segment changes. Volume loading with 1 to 2 L of 0.9% saline is often effective. Dobutamine or milrinone (which has better dilating effects on the pulmonary circulation) may help. Nitrates and diuretics are not used; they reduce preload (and hence cardiac output), causing severe hypotension. Increased right-sided filling pressure should be maintained by IV fluid infusion, but excessive volume overload may compromise left ventricular filling and cardiac output.

Recurrent Ischemia

Any chest pain that remains or recurs 12 to 24 h after MI may represent recurrent ischemia. Post-MI ischemic pain indicates that more myocardium is at risk of infarction. Usually, recurrent ischemia can be identified by reversible ST-T changes on the ECG; BP may be elevated.

However, because recurrent ischemia may be silent (ECG changes without pain) in up to one-third of patients, serial ECGs are routinely done every 8 h for 1 day and then daily. Recurrent ischemia (which is actually classified as unstable angina class lllC) is treated similarly to unstable angina. Sublingual or IV nitroglycerin is usually effective. Coronary angiography and PCI or CABG should be considered to salvage ischemic myocardium.

Mural Thrombosis

Mural thrombosis occurs in about 20% of patients with acute MI. Systemic embolism occurs in about 10% of patients with left ventricular thrombosis; risk is highest in the first 10 days but persists at least 3 mo. Risk is highest (about 60%) for patients with large anterior infarctions (especially involving the distal septum and apex), a dilated and diffusely hypokinetic LV, or chronic atrial fibrillation.

Anticoagulants are given to reduce risk of emboli. If not contraindicated, full-dose IV heparin followed by warfarin for 3 to 6 mo is given to maintain INR between 2 and 3. Anticoagulants are continued indefinitely when a dilated diffusely hypokinetic LV, left ventricular aneurysm, or chronic atrial fibrillation is present. Aspirin may also be given indefinitely.

Pericarditis

Pericarditis (see also p. 744) results from extension of myocardial necrosis through the wall to the epicardium; it develops in about one third of patients with acute transmural MI, although the rate appears to be much less in patients who have early reperfusion done.

A friction rub usually begins 24 to 96 h after MI onset. Earlier onset of the friction rub is unusual, although hemorrhagic pericarditis occasionally complicates the early phase of MI. Acute tamponade is rare.

Pericarditis is diagnosed by ECG, which shows diffuse ST-segment elevation and sometimes PR-interval depression. Echocardiography is frequently done, but results are usually normal. Occasionally, small pericardial effusions and even unsuspected tamponade are detected.

Aspirin or another NSAID usually relieves symptoms. Colchicine, alone, and especially added to conventional treatment speeds recovery and helps prevent recurrences. High doses or prolonged use of NSAIDs or corticosteroids may impair infarct healing and should be avoided; corticosteroids may also increase the likelihood of recurrence. Anticoagulation is not contraindicated in early peri-infarction pericarditis but is contraindicated in later post-MI (Dressler) syndrome.

Post-MI Syndrome (Dressler Syndrome)

Post-MI syndrome develops in a few patients several days to weeks or even months after acute MI; incidence also appears to have decreased in recent years. It is characterized by fever, pericarditis with a friction rub, pericardial effusion, pleurisy, pleural effusions, pulmonary infiltrates, and joint pain. This syndrome is caused by an autoimmune reaction to material from necrotic myocytes. It may recur.

Differentiating post-MI syndrome from extension or recurrence of infarction may be difficult. However, in post-MI syndrome, cardiac markers do not increase significantly, and ECG changes are nonspecific.

NSAIDs are usually effective, but the syndrome can recur several times. Colchicine is effective for treatment and to prevent recurrences. In severe cases, a short, intensive course of another NSAID or a corticosteroid may be necessary. High doses of an NSAID or a corticosteroid are not used for more than a few days because they may interfere with early ventricular healing after an acute MI.

DRUGS FOR ACUTE CORONARY SYNDROMES

Treatment of ACS is designed to relieve distress, interrupt thrombosis, reverse ischemia, limit infarct size, reduce cardiac workload, and prevent and treat complications. An ACS is a medical emergency; outcome is greatly influenced by rapid diagnosis and treatment. Treatment occurs simultaneously with diagnosis. Treatment includes revascularization (with PCI,

CABG, or fibrinolytic therapy) and drug therapy to treat ACS and underlying CAD.

Drugs used depend on the type of ACS and include

- Aspirin, clopidogrel, or both (prasugrel or ticagrelor is an alternative to clopidogrel if fibrinolytic therapy has not been given)
- Beta-blocker
- GP IIb/IIIa inhibitor considered for certain patients undergoing PCI and for some others at high risk (eg, with markedly elevated cardiac markers, thrombolysis in myocardial infarction (TIMI) risk score ≥ 4, persistent symptoms)
- A heparin (unfractionated or LMWH) or bivalirudin (particularly in STEMI patients at high risk of bleeding)
- IV nitroglycerin (unless low-risk, uncomplicated MI)
- Fibrinolytics for select patients with STEMI when timely PCI unavailable
- ACE inhibitor (as early as possible)
- Statin

Antiplatelet and antithrombotic drugs, which stop clots from forming, are used routinely. Anti-ischemic drugs (eg, beta-blockers, IV nitroglycerin) are frequently added, particularly when chest pain or hypertension is present (see Table 80–2 on p. 672).

Fibrinolytics *should be used if not contraindicated* for STEMI if primary PCI is not immediately available but worsen outcome for unstable angina and NSTEMI.

Chest pain can be treated with morphine or nitroglycerin. Morphine 2 to 4 mg IV, repeated q 15 min as needed, is highly effective but can depress respiration, can reduce myocardial contractility, and is a potent venous vasodilator. Hypotension and bradycardia secondary to morphine can usually be overcome by prompt elevation of the lower extremities. Nitroglycerin is initially given sublingually, followed by continuous IV drip if needed.

BP is normal or slightly elevated in most patients on arrival at the emergency department; BP gradually falls over the next several hours. Continued hypertension requires treatment with antihypertensives, preferably IV nitroglycerin, to lower BP and reduce cardiac workload. Severe hypotension or other signs of shock are ominous and must be treated aggressively with IV fluids and sometimes vasopressors.

Antiplatelet Drugs

Aspirin, clopidogrel, ticagrelor, ticlopidine, and GP IIb/IIIa inhibitors are examples. All patients are given aspirin 160 to 325 mg (not enteric-coated), if not contraindicated, at presentation and 81 mg once/day indefinitely thereafter. Chewing the first dose before swallowing quickens absorption. Aspirin reduces short- and long-term mortality risk.

If aspirin cannot be taken, clopidogrel 75 mg po once/day or ticlopidine 250 mg po bid may be used. Clopidogrel has largely replaced ticlopidine for routine use because neutropenia is a risk with ticlopidine and the WBC count must be monitored regularly.

Patients not undergoing revascularization: Patients with unstable angina or NSTEMI in whom intervention is not possible or recommended are given both aspirin and clopidogrel for at least 1 mo. The optimal duration of double antiplatelet therapy for these patients is the subject of ongoing investigation, but evidence is accumulating that a longer duration (eg, 9 to 12 mo) may be beneficial. In general, the concern with dosage and duration of antiplatelet drugs is to balance the decreased risk of coronary thrombosis with the increased risk of bleeding.

If PCI is not being done, some clinicians give a GP IIb/IIIa inhibitor to all high-risk patients (eg, those with markedly elevated cardiac markers, a TIMI risk score ≥ 4, or persistent symptoms despite adequate drug therapy). The GP IIb/IIIa inhibitor is continued for 24 to 36 h, and angiography is done before the infusion period is over. GP IIb/IIIa inhibitors are not recommended for patients receiving fibrinolytics. Abciximab, tirofiban, and eptifibatide appear to have equivalent efficacy, and the choice of drug should depend on other factors (eg, cost, availability, familiarity).

Patients undergoing revascularization: In patients undergoing PCI, a loading dose of clopidogrel (300 to 600 mg po once), prasugrel (60 mg po once), or ticagrelor (180 mg po once) improves outcomes, particularly when administered 24 h in advance. For urgent PCI, prasugrel and ticagrelor are more rapid in onset and may be preferred. However, delaying PCI for 24 h is not appropriate for many patients. Further, such a loading dose increases risk of perioperative bleeding in patients who require CABG because their coronary anatomy proves unfavorable for PCI. Thus, many clinicians administer a loading dose of one of these drugs only in the catheterization laboratory once coronary anatomy and lesions are determined to be amenable to PCI.

For patients receiving a stent for revascularization, aspirin is continued indefinitely. Clopidogrel 75 mg po once/day, prasugrel 10 mg po once/day, or ticagrelor 90 mg po bid should be used for at least 1 mo in patients with a bare-metal stent. Patients with a drug-eluting stent have a prolonged risk of thrombosis and may benefit from 12 mo of clopidogrel (or prasugrel or ticagrelor) treatment, although the recommended duration is still unclear.

Anticoagulant Drugs

Either a LMWH, unfractionated heparin, or bivalirudin is given routinely to patients with ACS unless contraindicated (eg, by active bleeding or planned use of streptokinase or anistreplase). Choice of agent is somewhat involved.

Patients at high risk of systemic emboli also require long-term therapy with oral warfarin. Conversion to warfarin should begin 48 h after symptom resolution or PCI.

Unfractionated heparin: Unfractionated heparin is more complicated to use because it requires frequent (q 6 h) dosing adjustments to achieve an activated PTT (aPTT) 1.5 to 2 times the control value. In patients undergoing angiography, further dosing adjustment is done to achieve an activated clotting time (ACT) of 200 to 250 sec if the patient is treated with a GP IIb/IIIa inhibitor and 250 to 300 sec if a GP IIb/IIIa inhibitor is not being given. However, if bleeding develops after catheterization, the effects of unfractionated heparin are shorter and can be reversed (by promptly stopping the heparin infusion and giving protamine sulfate).

Low molecular weight heparin: The LMWHs have better bioavailability, are given by simple weight-based dose without monitoring aPTT and dose titration, and have lower risk of heparin-induced thrombocytopenia. They also may produce an incremental benefit in outcomes relative to unfractionated heparin in patients with ACS. Of the LMWHs, enoxaparin appears to be superior to dalteparin or nadroparin. However, enoxaparin may pose a higher bleeding risk in patients with STEMI who are > 75, and its effects are not completely reversible with protamine.

Choice of heparin: Thus, taking all into account, many published guidelines recommend LMWH (eg, enoxaparin) over unfractionated heparin in patients with unstable angina or NSTEMI and in patients < 75 with STEMI who are not undergoing PCI.

By contrast, unfractionated heparin is recommended when emergency PCI is done (eg, patients with acute STEMI who proceed to the catheterization laboratory), when CABG is indicated within the next 24 h, and when patients are at high risk of bleeding complications (eg, history of GI bleeding within the last 6 mo) or have creatinine clearance < 30 mL/min. Ongoing studies should help clarify the choice between LMWH and unfractionated heparin.

For patients undergoing PCI, postprocedure heparin is no longer recommended unless patients are at high risk of thromboembolic events (eg, patients with large anterior MI, known LV thrombus, atrial fibrillation), because postprocedure ischemic events have decreased with the use of stents and antiplatelet drugs. For patients not undergoing PCI, heparin is continued for 48 h (or longer if symptoms persist).

The difficulties with the heparins (including bleeding complications, the possibility of heparin-induced thrombocytopenia, and, with unfractionated heparin, the need for dosing adjustments) have led to the search for better anticoagulants. The direct thrombin inhibitors, bivalirudin and argatroban, may have a lower incidence of serious bleeding and improved outcomes, particularly in patients with renal insufficiency (hirudin, another direct thrombin inhibitor, appears to cause more bleeding than the other drugs). The factor Xa inhibitor, fondaparinux, reduces mortality and reinfarction in patients with NSTEMI who undergo PCI without increasing bleeding but may result in worse outcomes than unfractionated heparin in patients with STEMI. Although routine use of these alternative anticoagulants is thus not currently recommended, they should be used in place of unfractionated heparin or LMWH in patients with a known or suspected history of heparin-induced thrombocytopenia.

Heparin alternatives: Bivalirudin is an acceptable anticoagulant for patients undergoing primary PCI who are at high risk of bleeding and is recommended for those with a known or suspected history of heparin-induced thrombocytopenia. For patients with unstable angina or NSTEMI, dose is an initial bolus of 0.1 mg/kg IV followed by a drip of 0.25 mg/kg/h. For patients with STEMI, initial dose is 0.75 mg/kg IV followed by 1.75 mg/kg/h.

Beta-Blockers

These drugs are recommended unless contraindicated (eg, by bradycardia, heart block, hypotension, or asthma), especially for high-risk patients. Beta-blockers reduce heart rate, arterial pressure, and contractility, thereby reducing cardiac workload and oxygen demand. Infarct size largely determines cardiac performance after recovery. Oral beta-blockers given within the first few hours improve prognosis by reducing infarct size, recurrence rate, incidence of VF, and mortality risk.[1]

Heart rate and BP must be carefully monitored during treatment with beta-blockers. Dosage is reduced if bradycardia or hypotension develops. Excessive adverse effects may be reversed by infusion of the beta-adrenergic agonist isoproterenol 1 to 5 mcg/min.

1. Chen ZM, Pan HC, Chen YP, et al. Early intravenous then oral metoprolol in 45,852 patients with acute MI: randomised placebo controlled trial. *Lancet* 366: 1622–1632, 2005.

Nitrates

A short-acting nitrate, nitroglycerin, is used to reduce cardiac workload in selected patients. Nitroglycerin dilates veins, arteries, and arterioles, reducing left ventricular preload and afterload. As a result, myocardial oxygen demand is reduced, lessening ischemia.

IV nitroglycerin is recommended during the first 24 to 48 h for patients with heart failure, large anterior MI, persistent chest discomfort, or hypertension. BP can be reduced by 10 to 20 mm Hg but not to < 80 to 90 mm Hg systolic.

Longer use may benefit patients with recurrent chest pain or persistent pulmonary congestion. In high-risk patients, nitroglycerin given in the first few hours reduces infarct size and short-term and possibly long-term mortality risk. Nitroglycerin is not routinely given to low-risk patients with uncomplicated MI.

Fibrinolytics

Tenecteplase (TNK), alteplase (rTPA), reteplase (rPA), streptokinase, and anistreplase (anisoylated plasminogen activator complex—APSAC), all given IV, are plasminogen activators. They convert single-chain plasminogen to double-chain plasminogen, which has fibrinolytic activity. They have different characteristics and dosing regimens (see Table 80–9) and are appropriate only for selected patients with STEMI).

TNK and rPA are recommended most often because of their simplicity of administration; TNK is given as a single bolus over 5 sec and rPA as a double bolus 30 min apart. Administration time and drug errors are reduced compared with other fibrinolytics. TNK, like rTPA, has an intermediate risk of intracranial hemorrhage, has a higher rate of recanalization than other fibrinolytics, and is expensive. rPA has the highest risk of intracranial hemorrhage and a recanalization rate similar to that of TNK, and it is expensive.

Streptokinase may induce allergic reactions, especially if it has been used previously, and must be given by infusion over

Table 80–9. IV FIBRINOLYTIC DRUGS AVAILABLE IN THE US

DRUG	DOSAGE (IV)	CIRCULATING HALF-LIFE (min)	CONCURRENT HEPARIN	ALLERGIC REACTIONS
Streptokinase	1.5×10^6 U over 30–60 min	20	No	Yes
Anistreplase	30 mg over 5 min	100	No	Yes
Alteplase	15 mg bolus, then 0.75 mg/kg over next 30 min (maximum 50 mg), followed by 0.50 mg/kg over 60 min (maximum 35 mg) for total dose of 100 mg	6	Yes	Rare
Reteplase	10 unit bolus over 2 min, repeated once after 30 min	13–16	Yes	Rare
Tenecteplase	Weight-adjusted single bolus over 5 sec: < 60 kg: 30 mg 60–69 kg: 35 mg 70–79 kg: 40 mg 80–89 kg: 45 mg ≥ 90 kg: 50 mg	Initial half-life of 20–24 min; terminal phase half-life of 90–130 min	Yes	Rare

30 to 60 min; however, it has a low incidence of intracerebral hemorrhage and is relatively inexpensive. Anistreplase, related to streptokinase, is similarly allergenic and slightly more expensive but can be given as a single bolus. Neither drug requires concomitant heparin use. For both, recanalization rate is lower than that with other plasminogen activators. Because of the possibility of allergic reactions, patients who previously received streptokinase or anistreplase are not given that drug.

rTPA is given in an accelerated or front-loaded dosage over 90 min. rTPA with concomitant IV heparin improves patency, is nonallergenic, has a higher recanalization rate than other fibrinolytics, and is expensive.

Other Drugs

ACE inhibitors reduce mortality risk in MI patients, especially in those with anterior infarction, heart failure, or tachycardia. The greatest benefit occurs in the highest-risk patients early during convalescence. ACE inhibitors are given > 24 h after thrombolysis stabilization and, because of continued beneficial effect, may be prescribed long-term.

Angiotensin II receptor blockers may be an effective alternative for patients who cannot tolerate ACE inhibitors (eg, because of cough). Currently, they are not first-line treatment after MI. Contraindications include hypotension, kidney failure, bilateral renal artery stenosis, and known allergy.

Statins (HMG-CoA reductase inhibitors) have long been used for prevention of CAD and ACS, but there is now increasing evidence that they also have short-term benefits, such as stabilizing plaque, reversing endothelial dysfunction, decreasing thrombogenicity, and reducing inflammation. Thus, all patients without contraindications to therapy should receive a statin as early as possible following ACS.

REVASCULARIZATION FOR ACUTE CORONARY SYNDROMES

Revascularization is the restoration of blood supply to ischemic myocardium in an effort to limit ongoing damage, reduce ventricular irritability, and improve short-term and long-term outcomes. Modes of revascularization include

- Thrombolysis with fibrinolytic drugs
- PCI, with or without stent placement
- CABG

The use, timing, and modality of revascularization depend on which ACS is present, timing of presentation, extent and location of anatomic lesions, and availability of personnel and facilities (see Fig. 80–4).

Unstable Angina and Non-ST-Segment Elevation Myocardial Infarction

Immediate reperfusion is not as urgent in patients with uncomplicated NSTEMI, in whom a completely occluded infarct-related artery at presentation is uncommon, or in patients with unstable angina who respond to medical therapy. Such patients typically undergo angiography within the first 24 to 48 h of hospitalization to identify coronary lesions requiring PCI or CABG.

A **noninterventional approach and a trial of medical management** are used for patients in whom angiography demonstrates

- Only a small area of myocardium at risk
- Lesion morphology not amenable to PCI
- Anatomically insignificant disease (< 50% coronary stenosis)
- Significant left main disease in patients who are candidates for CABG

Further, angiography or PCI should be deferred in favor of medical management for patients with a high risk of procedure-related morbidity or mortality.

By contrast, patients with persistent chest pain despite maximal medical therapy or complications (eg, markedly elevated cardiac markers, presence of cardiogenic shock, acute mitral regurgitation, ventricular septal defect, unstable arrhythmias) should proceed directly to the cardiac catheterization laboratory to identify coronary lesions requiring PCI or CABG.

As in patients with stable angina, CABG is generally preferred over PCI for patients with left main or left main equivalent disease and for those with left ventricular dysfunction or diabetes. CABG must also be considered when PCI is unsuccessful, cannot be used (eg, in lesions that are long or near bifurcation points), or causes acute coronary artery dissection.

Fibrinolytics are not indicated for unstable angina or NSTEMI. Risk outweighs potential benefit.

ST-Segment Elevation Myocardial Infarction

Emergency PCI is the preferred treatment of STEMI when available in a timely fashion (door to balloon-inflation time < 90 min) by an experienced operator. Indications for urgent PCI later in the course of STEMI include hemodynamic instability, malignant arrhythmias requiring transvenous pacing or repeated cardioversion, and age > 75. If the lesions necessitate CABG, there is about 4 to 12% mortality and a 20 to 43% morbidity rate.

If there is likely to be a significant delay in availability of PCI, thrombolysis should be done for STEMI patients meeting criteria (see Table 80–10). Reperfusion using fibrinolytics is

Table 80–10. FIBRINOLYTIC THERAPY FOR STEMI

CRITERIA	SPECIFICS
ECG criteria*	ST-segment elevation in ≥ 2 contiguous leads
	Typical symptoms and left bundle branch block not known to be old
	Strictly posterior MI (large R wave in V_1 and ST depression in V_1–V_4
Absolute contraindications	Aortic dissection
	Previous hemorrhagic stroke (at any time)
	Previous ischemic stroke within 1 yr
	Active internal bleeding (not menses)
	Intracranial tumor
	Pericarditis
Relative contraindications	BP > 180/110 mm Hg after initial antihypertensive therapy
	Trauma or major surgery within 4 wk
	Active peptic ulcer
	Pregnancy
	Bleeding diathesis
	Noncompressible vascular puncture
	Current anticoagulation (INR > 2)

*Patients presenting in the hyperacute phase of MI with giant T waves do not meet current criteria for fibrinolytics; ECG is repeated in 20 to 30 min to see if ST-segment elevation has developed.

most effective if given in the first few minutes to hours after onset of MI. The earlier a fibrinolytic is begun, the better. The goal is a door-to-needle time of 30 to 60 min. Greatest benefit occurs within 3 h, but the drugs may be effective up to 12 h. Used with aspirin, fibrinolytics reduce hospital mortality rate by 30 to 50% and improve ventricular function. Prehospital use of fibrinolytics by trained paramedics can significantly reduce time to treatment and should be considered in situations in which PCI within 90 min is not possible, particularly in patients presenting within 3 h of symptom onset.

Regardless, most patients who undergo thrombolysis will ultimately require transfer to a PCI-capable facility for elective angiography and PCI as necessary before discharge. PCI should be considered after fibrinolytics if chest pain or ST-segment elevation persists ≥ 60 min after initiation of fibrinolytics or if pain and ST-segment elevation recur, but only if PCI can be initiated < 90 min after onset of recurrence. If PCI is unavailable, fibrinolytics can be repeated.

Characteristics and selection of fibrinolytic drugs are discussed in Table 80–9.

81 Diseases of the Aorta and Its Branches

Aneurysms are abnormal dilations of arteries caused by weakening of the arterial wall. Common causes include hypertension, atherosclerosis, infection, trauma, and hereditary or acquired connective tissue disorders (eg, Marfan syndrome, Ehlers-Danlos syndrome). Aneurysms are usually asymptomatic but can cause pain and lead to ischemia, thromboembolism, spontaneous dissection, and rupture, which may be fatal. Diagnosis is by imaging tests (eg, ultrasonography, CT angiography [CTA], magnetic resonance angiography [MRA], aortography). Unruptured aneurysms may be treated with medical management or surgical intervention depending on symptoms and the size and location of the aneurysm. Medical management includes risk factor modification (eg, strict BP control) plus scheduled surveillance imaging. Surgical intervention includes open repair or endovascular stent-graft surgery. Treatment of ruptured aneurysms is immediate repair with either an open surgical synthetic graft or an endovascular stent graft.

The aorta originates at the left ventricle above the aortic valve, travels upward (ascending thoracic aorta) to the first branch of the aorta (brachiocephalic or innominate artery), arches up and behind the heart (aortic arch), then turns downward distal to the left subclavian artery (descending aorta) through the thorax (thoracic aorta) and abdomen (abdominal aorta). The abdominal aorta ends by dividing into the right and left common iliac arteries.

The wall of the aorta is composed of three layers:

- Intima: A thin layer lined with endothelium
- Media: A thick layer of elastic fibers arranged in spiral formation
- Adventitia: A thin fibrous layer containing the nutrients for the media

Aneurysms are abnormal dilations of arteries defined as a ≥ 50% increase in arterial diameter compared with normal segments. They are caused by weakening of the arterial wall, specifically, the media. True aneurysms involve all 3 layers of the artery (intima, media, and adventitia). Aneurysmal disease is not a focal problem and can extend along the aorta with time.

A pseudoaneurysm (false aneurysm) is a communication between the arterial lumen and overlying connective tissue resulting from arterial rupture; a blood-filled cavity forms outside the vessel wall and seals the leak as it thromboses.

Aneurysms are classified as

- Fusiform: Circumferential widening of the artery
- Saccular: Localized, typically asymmetric, outpouchings of the artery wall

Layered (laminated) thrombus may line the walls of either type as the result of alterations in flow within the aneurysmal segment.

Aneurysms may occur in any artery. The most common and significant are

- Abdominal aortic aneurysms
- Thoracic aortic aneurysms (TAAs)

Aneurysms of the major aortic branches (subclavian and splanchnic arteries) are much less common. Aneurysms of peripheral arteries and the cerebrovascular system (causing stroke) are discussed elsewhere.

ABDOMINAL AORTIC ANEURYSMS

Abdominal aortic diameter ≥ 3 cm typically constitutes an abdominal aortic aneurysm (AAA). The cause is multifactorial, but atherosclerosis is often involved. Most aneurysms grow slowly (~10%/year) without causing symptoms, and most are found incidentally. Risk of rupture is proportional to the size of the aneurysm. Diagnosis is made by ultrasonography or CT scan. Treatment is surgery or endovascular stent grafting.

AAAs account for three-fourths of aortic aneurysms and affect 0.5 to 3.2% of the population. Prevalence is 3 times greater in men. AAAs typically begin below the renal arteries (infrarenal) but may include renal arterial ostia; about 50% involve the iliac arteries. Generally, aortic diameter ≥ 3 cm constitutes an AAA. Most AAAs are fusiform. Many are lined with laminated thrombus.

Etiology

Etiology of AAAs is multifactorial but commonly involves a weakening of the arterial wall, usually by atherosclerosis. Other causes include trauma, vasculitis, cystic medial necrosis, and postsurgical anastomotic disruption.

Uncommonly, syphilis and localized bacterial or fungal infection, typically due to sepsis or infective endocarditis, weaken the arterial wall and cause infected (mycotic) aneurysms. Salmonella infection is the number one cause of mycotic aneurysms.

Risk factors: Risk factors include

- Smoking (strongest risk factor)
- Hypertension
- Older age (peak incidence at age 70 to 80)
- Family history (in 15 to 25%)
- Race (more common in whites than in blacks)
- Male sex

Symptoms and Signs

Most AAAs are asymptomatic. Symptoms and signs, when they do occur, may be nonspecific but usually result from compression of adjacent structures. As AAAs expand, they may cause pain, which is steady, deep, boring, visceral, and felt most prominently in the lumbosacral region. Patients may be aware of an abnormally prominent abdominal pulsation. Although most aneurysms grow slowly without symptoms, rapidly enlarging aneurysms that are about to rupture can be tender.

The aneurysm may or may not be palpable as a pulsatile mass, depending on its size and patient habitus. The probability that a patient with a pulsatile palpable mass has an aneurysm > 3 cm is about 40% (positive predictive value). A systolic bruit may be audible over the aneurysm.

Patients with an occult AAA sometimes present with symptoms of complications or of the cause (eg, fever, malaise, or weight loss due to infection or vasculitis).

Complications: The main complications of AAAs include

- Rupture
- Distal embolization
- Disseminated intravascular coagulation (uncommon)

Rupture is most likely to occur on the left posterolateral wall 2 to 4 cm below the renal arteries. If an AAA ruptures, most patients die before reaching a medical facility. Patients who do not die immediately typically present with abdominal or back pain, hypotension, and tachycardia. They may have a history of recent upper abdominal trauma, often minimal, or isometric straining (eg, lifting a heavy object). Even patients who reach the hospital alive have about a 50% mortality.

Distal embolization of thrombus or atheromatous material may dislodge and block arteries of the lower extremities, kidneys, and bowel. Patients typically present with sudden unilateral extremity pain and often pallor and loss of pulses (see also Acute Peripheral Arterial Occlusion on p. 752).

Uncommonly, large AAAs cause disseminated intravascular coagulation, perhaps because large areas of abnormal endothelial surface trigger rapid thrombosis and consumption of coagulation factors.

Diagnosis

- Often incidental
- Confirmation by ultrasonography or abdominal CT
- Sometimes CTA or MRA

Most AAAs are diagnosed incidentally when they are detected during physical examination or when abdominal ultrasonography, CT, or MRI is done for other reasons. An AAA should be considered in elderly patients who present with acute abdominal or back pain whether a palpable pulsatile mass is present or not.

When symptoms or physical examination findings suggest AAA, abdominal ultrasonography or abdominal CT is usually the test of choice. Symptomatic patients should have immediate testing to make the diagnosis before catastrophic rupture. For hemodynamically unstable patients with presumed rupture, ultrasonography provides bedside results more rapidly, but intestinal gas and distention may limit its accuracy. Laboratory tests, including CBC, electrolytes, BUN, creatinine, PT, PTT, and blood type and cross-match, are done in preparation for possible surgery.

If rupture is not suspected, CTA or MRA can more precisely characterize aneurysm size and anatomy. If thrombi line the aneurysm wall, conventional angiography may underestimate true size; CT may provide a more accurate estimate. Aortography is sometimes necessary if renal artery or aortoiliac disease is suspected or if correction with endovascular stent grafts (endografts) is being considered.

Plain abdominal x-rays are neither sensitive nor specific; however, if obtained for other purposes, x-rays may show aortic calcification outlining the aneurysm wall.

If a mycotic aneurysm is suspected, bacterial and fungal blood cultures should be done.

Treatment

- Medical management, particularly BP control and smoking cessation
- Surgery or endovascular stent grafting

Some AAAs enlarge at a rate of 10%/yr. Enlargement often occurs in a stepwise pattern with periods of no growth observed. Other aneurysms enlarge exponentially, and, for unknown reasons, about 20% remain the same size indefinitely.

Control of atherosclerotic risk factors, especially smoking cessation and use of antihypertensives as appropriate, is important. If a small or moderate-sized aneurysm becomes > 5.0 to 5.5 cm and if risk of perioperative complications is lower than estimated risk of rupture, AAA repair is indicated. Risk of rupture vs that of perioperative complications should be discussed frankly with the patient.

The need for surgical treatment is related to size, which is linked to risk of rupture (see Table 81–1). Elective repair should be considered for aneurysms > 5.0 to 5.5 cm.

Ruptured AAAs require immediate open surgery or endovascular stent grafting. Without treatment, mortality rate approaches 100%. With open surgical treatment, mortality rate is about 50%. Mortality with endovascular stent grafting is generally lower (20 to 30%). The mortality remains high because many patients have coexisting coronary, cerebrovascular, and peripheral atherosclerosis.

Table 81–1. ABDOMINAL AORTIC ANEURYSM SIZE AND RUPTURE RISK*

AAA DIAMETER (cm)	RUPTURE RISK (%/yr)
< 4	0
4–4.9	1%
5–5.9*	5–10%
6–6.9	10–20%
7–7.9	20–40%
> 8	30–50%

*Elective surgical repair should be considered for aneurysms > 5.0–5.5 cm.

AAA = abdominal aortic aneurysm.

Patients who present in **hemorrhagic shock** require fluid resuscitation and blood transfusions, but mean arterial pressure should not be elevated to > 70 to 80 mm Hg (permissive hypotension) because bleeding may increase. Preoperative control and avoidance of hypertension is important.

PEARLS & PITFALLS

- In a hypotensive patient with a ruptured AAA, do not raise mean arterial pressure to > 70 to 80 mm Hg because bleeding may increase.

Elective surgical repair is recommended for

- Aneurysms > 5 to 5.5 cm (when risk of rupture increases to > 5 to 10%/yr), unless coexisting medical conditions contraindicate surgery

Additional indications for elective surgery include

- Increase in aneurysm size by > 0.5 cm within 6 mo regardless of size
- Chronic abdominal pain
- Thromboembolic complications
- Iliac or femoral artery aneurysm that causes lower-limb ischemia

Before elective repair, clinical consideration of coronary artery disease (CAD) is often needed and may or may not require further evaluation because some patients with an AAA have significant risk of cardiovascular events. Aggressive medical treatment and risk factor control are essential. Routine preoperative coronary angioplasty or bypass surgery has not been shown to be necessary in most patients who can be prepared with good medical management before aneurysm repair; coronary revascularization should be considered only in patients with unstable CAD.

Surgical repair consists of replacing the aneurysmal portion of the abdominal aorta with a synthetic graft. If the iliac arteries are involved, the graft must be extended to include them. If an aorto-bifemoral repair is done, it is important to ensure flow to at least one internal iliac artery (hypogastric artery) to avoid vasculogenic erectile dysfunction and pelvic ischemia. If the aneurysm extends above the renal arteries, the renal arteries must be reimplanted into the graft, or bypass grafts must be created.

Placement of an **endovascular stent graft** within the aneurysmal lumen via the femoral artery is a less invasive alternative that has been shown to have lower acute morbidity and mortality than open repair. This procedure excludes the aneurysm from systemic blood flow and reduces risk of rupture. The aneurysm eventually thromboses, and 50% of aneurysms decrease in diameter. Short-term results are good and long-term results are favorable. Complications include angulation, kinking, thrombosis, migration of the stent graft, and endoleak (persistent flow of blood into the aneurysm sac after endovascular stent graft placement). Thus, follow-up visits must be more frequent after endovascular stent graft placement than after a traditional repair. If no complications occur, imaging tests are recommended at 1 mo, 6 mo, 12 mo, and every year thereafter. Complex anatomy (eg, short aneurysm neck below renal arteries, severe arterial tortuosity) makes routine endovascular stent grafting difficult in 30 to 40% of patients; however, newer devices have been developed to overcome these issues. In general, for a successful endovascular repair, surgeons should choose a specific device that is appropriate for the patient's anatomic characteristics.

In most cases, repair of aneurysms < 5 cm does not appear to increase survival. Because patients vary in size, it is more precise to offer repair when the aneurysm is larger than twice the diameter of an area of normal aorta in that patient. These aneurysms should be monitored with ultrasonography or abdominal CT every 6 to 12 mo for expansion that warrants treatment.

Treatment of a **mycotic aneurysm** consists of vigorous antimicrobial therapy directed at the pathogen, followed by excision of the aneurysm. Early diagnosis and treatment improve outcome.

Surgical complications: Myocardial infarction is the leading cause of early postoperative death after surgery, and acute kidney injury is the leading cause of late postoperative death after surgery.

Complications following AAA repair include

- Major vein injury due to proximal cross clamping
- Erectile dysfunction (as a result of nerve damage or decreased blood flow)
- Graft infection
- Pseudoaneurysm
- Atherosclerotic occlusion of graft

KEY POINTS

- Abdominal aortic diameter ≥ 3 cm constitutes an AAA.
- AAAs typically enlarge at a rate of 10%/yr, but some enlarge exponentially; about 20% remain the same size indefinitely.
- Risk of rupture is proportional to the size of the aneurysm.
- Diagnose using ultrasonography or abdominal CT; for unruptured aneurysms, CTA or MRA can more precisely characterize aneurysm size and anatomy.
- Ruptured AAAs require immediate open surgery or endovascular stent grafting; even then, mortality is high.
- Elective surgical repair is recommended for aneurysms > 5 to 5.5 cm and for those that are rapidly enlarging or causing ischemic or embolic complications.

THORACIC AORTIC ANEURYSMS

A thoracic aortic diameter ≥ 50% larger than normal is considered an aneurysm (normal diameter varies by location). Most TAAs do not cause symptoms, although some patients have chest or back pain; other symptoms and signs are usually the result of complications (eg, dissection, compression of adjacent structures, thromboembolism, rupture). Risk of rupture is proportional to the size of the aneurysm. Diagnosis is made by CTA or transesophageal echocardiogram (TEE). Treatment is endovascular stent grafting or surgery.

TAAs are abnormal dilatations of the aorta above the diaphragm. TAAs account for one fourth of aortic aneurysms. Men and women are affected equally.

Locations of TAAs include

- Ascending thoracic aorta (between the aortic root and brachiocephalic, or innominate, artery): 40%
- Aortic arch (including the brachiocephalic, carotid, and subclavian arteries): 10%
- Descending thoracic aorta (distal to the left subclavian artery): 35%
- Upper abdomen—thoracoabdominal aneurysms (TAAAs): 15%

Complications: Complications of TAAs include

- Aortic dissection
- Compression or erosion into adjacent structures
- Leak or rupture
- Thromboembolism

Aneurysms of the ascending aorta sometimes affect the aortic root, causing aortic valve regurgitation or occlusion of the coronary arterial ostia, causing angina, myocardial infarction, or syncope.

Etiology

Most TAAs result from

- Atherosclerosis

Risk factors for both TAAs and aortic dissections include prolonged hypertension, dyslipidemia, and smoking. Additional risk factors for TAAs include presence of aneurysms elsewhere in the body, infection, aortitis, and older age (peak incidence at age 65 to 70).

Congenital connective tissue disorders (eg, Marfan syndrome, Ehlers-Danlos syndrome, Loeys-Dietz syndrome) cause cystic medial necrosis, a degenerative change that leads to TAAs complicated by aortic dissection and by widening of the proximal aorta and aortic valve (annuloaortic ectasia), which causes aortic regurgitation. Marfan syndrome causes 50% of cases of annuloaortic ectasia, but cystic medial necrosis and its complications can occur in young people even if no congenital connective tissue disorder is present.

Infected (mycotic) TAAs result from hematogenous spread of systemic or local infections (eg, sepsis, pneumonia), lymphangitic spread (eg, TB), or direct extension (eg, in osteomyelitis or pericarditis). Bacterial endocarditis and tertiary syphilis are uncommon causes. TAAs occur in some inflammatory disorders (eg, giant cell arteritis, Takayasu arteritis, granulomatosis with polyangiitis).

Blunt chest trauma can cause a pseudoaneurysm (false aneurysm) due to injury to the aortic wall resulting in a communication between the arterial lumen and overlying connective tissue and blood leaking outside the confines of the aorta; a blood-filled cavity forms outside the vessel wall and seals the leak as it thromboses).

Symptoms and Signs

Most thoracic abdominal aneurysms are asymptomatic until complications (eg, thromboembolism, rupture, aortic regurgitation, dissection) develop. However, compression of adjacent structures can cause back pain (due to compression of vertebra), cough (due to compression of the trachea), wheezing, dysphagia (due to esophageal compression), hoarseness (due to left recurrent laryngeal or vagus nerve compression), chest pain (due to coronary artery compression), and superior vena cava syndrome.

Erosion of aneurysms into the lungs causes hemoptysis or pneumonitis; erosion into the esophagus (aortoesophageal fistula) causes massive hematemesis.

Dissection manifests with tearing chest pain, often radiating to the back between the shoulder blades.

Thromboembolism may cause stroke, abdominal pain (due to mesenteric ischemia), or extremity pain.

Ruptured TAA that is not immediately fatal manifests with severe chest or back pain and hypotension or shock. Exsanguination due to rupture most commonly occurs into the pleural or pericardial space.

Additional signs include Horner syndrome (miosis, ptosis, anhidrosis) due to compression of sympathetic ganglia, palpable downward pull of the trachea with each cardiac contraction (tracheal tug), and tracheal deviation. Visible or palpable chest wall pulsations, occasionally more prominent than the left ventricular apical impulse, are unusual but may occur.

Syphilitic aneurysms of the aortic root classically lead to aortic regurgitation and inflammatory stenosis of the coronary artery ostia, which may manifest as chest pain due to myocardial ischemia. Syphilitic aneurysms do not dissect.

Diagnosis

- Incidental x-ray finding
- Confirmation by CTA, MRA, or transesophageal echocardiography (TEE)

TAAs are usually first suspected when a chest x-ray incidentally shows a widened mediastinum or enlargement of the aortic knob. However, chest x-ray has poor sensitivity for TAA and is not a reliable diagnostic tool (eg, in patients with chest pain and suspected aortic aneurysm). Chest x-ray abnormalities, or symptoms and signs suggesting an aneurysm, should be followed up with a cross-sectional imaging test; choice among these tests is based on availability and local experience.

If rupture is suspected, TEE (for ascending dissection) or CTA, depending on availability, should be done immediately. Chest CTA can delineate aneurysm size and proximal or distal extent, detect leakage, and identify coincidental pathology. MRA may provide similar detail. Transthoracic echocardiography (TTE) can delineate size and extent and detect leakage of aneurysms of the ascending but not descending aorta. TEE cannot show the entire thoracic aorta, but it can be extremely useful in detecting the entry point in aortic dissection.

Contrast angiography historically has been the standard imaging test. It does provide the best image of the arterial lumen, but it provides no information on extraluminal structures (ie, as an alternative diagnosis). Additionally, angiography is invasive and has a significant risk of renal and extremity atheroembolism and contrast nephropathy.

Aortic root dilation or unexplained ascending aorta aneurysms warrant serologic testing for syphilis. If a mycotic aneurysm is suspected, bacterial and fungal blood cultures are done.

Prognosis

Thoracic abdominal aneurysms enlarge an average of 3 to 5 mm/yr. Risk factors for rapid enlargement include larger size of aneurysm, location in the descending aorta, and presence of mural thrombi.

Annual rupture risk is 2% for aneurysms < 5 cm, 3% for aneurysm of 5 to 5.9 cm, and 8 to 10% for aneurysms > 6 cm. The risk appears to rise abruptly as TAAs reach 6 cm in diameter. Median diameter at aneurysm rupture is 6 cm for ascending aneurysms and 7 cm for descending aneurysms, but rupture of smaller aneurysms may occur, especially in patients with connective tissue disorders or saccular aneurysms.

Survival rate of patients with untreated large TAAs is 65% at 1 yr and 20% at 5 yr. TAAA rupture has a mortality of 97%.

Treatment

- Endovascular stent grafting or open surgical repair
- Control of hypertension and other comorbidities

Medical management with optimal control of hypertension, hypercholesterolemia, diabetes, and respiratory disease is the appropriate treatment until surgery is indicated. Treatment is endovascular stent grafting when anatomically possible and open surgical repair for more complex aneurysms. Immediate control of hypertension is essential.

Ruptured TAAs, if untreated, are universally fatal. They require immediate intervention, as do leaking aneurysms and those that cause acute dissection or acute valvular regurgitation.

Surgery involves a median sternotomy (for ascending and aortic arch aneurysms) or left thoracotomy or thoraco-retroperitoneal exposure (for descending and thoracoabdominal aneurysms) and replacement with a synthetic graft. With emergent open surgery, 1-mo mortality rate is about 40 to 50%. Patients who survive have a high incidence of serious complications (eg, renal failure, respiratory failure, severe neurologic damage).

Transcatheter-placed endovascular stent grafts (endografts) for descending TAAs and TAAAs are being used more frequently as a less invasive alternative to open surgery.

Elective surgery is indicated for aneurysms that are

- Large*
- Rapidly enlarging (> 0.5 cm/year)
- Causing bronchial compression
- Causing aortobronchial or aortoesophageal fistulas
- Symptomatic
- Traumatic
- Mycotic

*Aneurysms of the *ascending aorta* are considered large if the diameter is > 5 to 6 cm or twice the native size of the ascending aorta. In the *descending aorta*, aneurysms are large if they are > 6 to 7 cm and open repair is planned and > 5.5 cm for endovascular repair. In patients with *Marfan syndrome*, large aneurysms are those that are ≥ 4.5 to 5 cm in any location.

Treatment of mycotic aneurysms is aggressive antibiotic therapy directed at the specific pathogen. Generally, these aneurysms must also be surgically repaired.

Although open surgical repair of an intact TAA improves outcome, mortality rate may still exceed 5 to 10% at 30 days and is 40 to 50% at 10 yr. The mortality rate is lower with endovascular stent grafts. Risk of death increases greatly if aneurysms are complicated (eg, located in the aortic arch or thoracoabdominal aorta) or if patients are older or have CAD, symptoms, or preexisting renal insufficiency. Perioperative complications (eg, stroke, spinal injury, renal failure) occur in about 10 to 20%.

Asymptomatic aneurysms that do not meet criteria for elective surgical or endovascular repair are treated with aggressive blood pressure control using a beta-blocker and other antihypertensives if necessary. Smoking cessation is essential. Dyslipidemia, diabetes, and respiratory diseases should all be treated. Patients require frequent follow-ups to check for symptoms and serial CT or ultrasonography every 6 to 12 mo. Imaging frequency depends on aneurysm size.

KEY POINTS

- TAA is a ≥ 50% increase in diameter of the thoracic aorta.
- TAAs may dissect, compress or erode into adjacent structures, cause thromboembolism, leak, or rupture.
- Median diameter at aneurysm rupture is 6 cm for ascending aneurysms and 7 cm for descending aneurysms.
- Diagnosis is often first suspected based on an incidental x-ray or CT finding, and confirmed using CTA, MRA, or TEE.
- Treat small, asymptomatic TAAs with aggressive management of blood pressure and dyslipidemia and smoking cessation.
- Treat larger or symptomatic TAAs with endovascular stent grafting when anatomically possible and open surgical repair for more complex aneurysms.

AORTIC BRANCH ANEURYSMS

Aneurysms may occur in any major aortic branch; such aneurysms are much less common than abdominal or TAAs. Symptoms vary depending on the location and artery affected but may include pain in areas where the aneurysm compresses nearby structures. Diagnosis is made by ultrasonography or CTA. Treatment is endovascular stent grafting or surgery.

Risk factors for aneurysms of aortic branch arteries include atherosclerosis, hypertension, cigarette smoking, and older age. Localized infection can cause mycotic aneurysms.

Subclavian artery aneurysms are sometimes associated with cervical ribs or thoracic outlet compression syndrome.

Aneurysms of the arteries of the splanchnic circulation are uncommon. About 60% occur in the splenic artery, 20% in the hepatic artery, 5.5% in the superior mesenteric artery.

Splenic artery aneurysms are more common in women than men (4:1). Causes include medial fibromuscular dysplasia, portal hypertension, multiple pregnancies, penetrating or blunt abdominal trauma, pancreatitis, and infection.

Hepatic artery aneurysms occur in more men than women (2:1). They may result from previous abdominal trauma, illicit IV drug use, medial degeneration of the arterial wall, or periarterial inflammation.

Renal artery aneurysms may dissect or rupture, causing acute occlusion.

Superior mesenteric artery aneurysms occur equally in men and women. Causes include fibromuscular dysplasia, cystic medial necrosis, and trauma.

Symptoms and Signs

Many aortic branch aneurysm are asymptomatic. Symptoms (when they occur) vary depending on the location and artery affected.

Subclavian aneurysms can cause local pain, a pulsating sensation, venous thrombosis or edema (due to compression of adjacent veins), distal ischemic symptoms, transient ischemic attacks, stroke, hoarseness (due to compression of the recurrent laryngeal nerve), or impaired motor and sensory function (due to compression of the brachial plexus).

Splenic artery aneurysm may cause left upper quadrant abdominal pain. Hepatic artery aneurysm may cause right upper quadrant pain and jaundice. Superior mesenteric aneurysms may cause generalized abdominal pain and ischemic colitis.

Regardless of location, mycotic or inflammatory aneurysms may cause local pain and sequelae of systemic infection (eg, fever, malaise, weight loss).

Diagnosis

- Ultrasonography, CT scan, or other axial imaging study

With the routine availability of axial diagnostic imaging, many aneurysms are now diagnosed before rupture. Calcified asymptomatic or occult aneurysms may be seen on x-rays or other imaging tests done for other reasons. Ultrasonography or CT is typically used to detect or confirm aortic branch aneurysms. Angiography is typically reserved for treatment or to evaluate distal organ perfusion.

Treatment

- Open repair or sometimes endovascular stent grafting

Treatment is surgical removal and replacement with a graft. Endovascular repair is an option for some patients. The decision to repair asymptomatic aneurysms is based on risk of rupture, extent and location of the aneurysm, and perioperative risk.

Surgery for subclavian artery aneurysms may involve removal of a cervical rib (if present) before repair and replacement.

For splanchnic aneurysms, risk of rupture and death is as high as 10% and is particularly high for women of childbearing age and for patients with hepatic aneurysms (> 35%). Elective repair of splanchnic aneurysms is therefore indicated for

- Aneurysms > 2 cm in diameter
- Aneurysms in pregnant women or women of childbearing age
- Symptomatic aneurysms in any age group
- Hepatic aneurysms

For splenic aneurysms, repair may consist of ligation without arterial reconstruction or aneurysm exclusion and vascular reconstruction. Depending on location of the aneurysm, splenectomy may be necessary.

Treatment of mycotic aneurysms is aggressive antibiotic therapy directed at the specific pathogen. Generally, these aneurysms must also be surgically repaired.

AORTIC DISSECTION

Aortic dissection is the surging of blood through a tear in the aortic intima with separation of the intima and media and creation of a false lumen (channel). The intimal tear may be a primary event or secondary to hemorrhage within the media. The dissection may occur anywhere along the aorta and extend proximally or distally into other arteries. Hypertension is an important contributor. Symptoms and signs include abrupt onset of tearing chest or back pain, and dissection may result in aortic regurgitation and compromised circulation in branch arteries. Diagnosis is by imaging tests (eg, transesophageal echocardiography, CTA, MRI, contrast aortography). Treatment always involves aggressive blood pressure control and serial imaging to monitor progression of dissection. Surgical repair of the aorta and placement of a synthetic graft are needed for ascending aortic dissection and for certain descending aortic dissections. Endovascular stent grafts are used for certain patients, especially when dissection involves the descending thoracic aorta. One fifth of patients die before reaching the hospital, and up to one third die of operative or perioperative complications.

Evidence of dissection is found in 1 to 3% of all autopsies. Blacks, men, the elderly, and people with hypertension are especially at risk. Peak incidence occurs at age 50 to 65 in the general population and at age 20 to 40 for patients with congenital connective tissue disorders (eg, Marfan syndrome, Ehlers-Danlos syndrome).

Classification of aortic dissection: Aortic dissections are classified anatomically.

The **DeBakey classification system** is most widely used.

- Type I (50% of dissections): These dissections start in the ascending aorta and extend at least to the aortic arch and sometimes beyond.
- Type II (35%): These dissections start in and are confined to the ascending aorta (proximal to the brachiocephalic or innominate artery).
- Type III (15%): These dissections start in the descending thoracic aorta just beyond the origin of the left subclavian artery and extend distally or, less commonly, proximally. Type IIIa dissections originate distal to the left subclavian artery and are confined to the thoracic aorta. Type IIIb dissections originate distal to the left subclavian artery and extend below the diaphragm.

The **Stanford system** is simpler.

- Type A: These dissections involve the ascending aorta.
- Type B: These dissections are confined to the descending thoracic aorta (distal to the left subclavian artery).

Although dissection may originate anywhere along the aorta, it occurs most commonly at areas of greatest hydraulic stress, which are the

- Right lateral wall of the ascending aorta (within 5 cm of the aortic valve)
- Proximal segment of the descending aorta (just beyond the origin of the left subclavian artery)

Rarely, dissection is confined to individual arteries (eg, coronary or carotid arteries), typically in pregnant or postpartum women.

Etiology

Aortic dissections often occur in patients with preexisting degeneration of the aortic media. Causes and risk factors include connective tissue disorders, atherosclerotic disease, and injury (see Table 81–2).

Atherosclerotic risk factors, notably hypertension, contribute in more than two thirds of patients. After rupture of the intima, which is a primary event in some patients and secondary to hemorrhage within the media in others, blood flows into the media, creating a false channel that extends distally or, less commonly, proximally along the artery.

Pathophysiology

The pathophysiologic sequence of aortic dissections involves aortic wall inflammation, apoptosis of vascular smooth muscle cells, degeneration of aortic media, elastin disruption, and then vessel dissection. Dissections may communicate back with the

Table 81–2. CONDITIONS CONTRIBUTING TO AORTIC DISSECTION

CATEGORY	EXAMPLES
Atherosclerotic risk factors	Cocaine Dyslipidemia Hypertension Smoking
Connective tissue disorders, acquired	Behçet disease Giant cell arteritis Takayasu arteritis
Connective tissue disorders, congenital or hereditary	Bicuspid aortic valve Coarctation of the aorta Cystic medial necrosis Ehlers-Danlos syndrome Marfan syndrome Turner syndrome Familial thoracic aortic aneurysm
Iatrogenic	Aortic catheterization Aortic valve surgery
Trauma	Deceleration injuries

true aortic lumen through intimal rupture at a distal site, maintaining systemic blood flow.

Serious consequences are common and include

- Compromise of the blood supply of arteries that branch off the aorta (including coronary arteries)
- Aortic valvular dilation and regurgitation
- Heart failure
- Fatal rupture of the aorta through the adventitia into the pericardium, right atrium, or left pleural space

Acute dissections and those present < 2 wk are most likely to cause these complications. Risk decreases at ≥ 2 wk if evidence indicates thrombosis of the false lumen and loss of communication between the true and false lumina.

Variants of aortic dissection include separation of the intima and media by intramural hematoma without a clear intimal tear or flap, intimal tear and bulge without hematoma or false lumen, and dissection or hematoma caused by ulceration of atherosclerotic plaque. These variants are thought to be precursors of classic aortic dissection.

Symptoms and Signs

Typically, excruciating precordial or interscapular pain, often described as tearing or ripping, occurs abruptly. The pain frequently migrates from the original location as the dissection extends along the aorta. Up to 20% of patients present with syncope due to severe pain, aortic baroreceptor activation, extracranial cerebral artery obstruction, or cardiac tamponade. Hypotension and tachycardia could indicate active bleeding.

Occasionally, patients present with symptoms of malperfusion (stroke, myocardial infarction, intestinal infarction, renal insufficiency, paraparesis, or paraplegia) due to interruption of the blood supply to a particular vascular bed, including the spinal cord, brain, heart, kidneys, intestine, or extremities. The interruption in blood supply is most often due to acute distal arterial obstruction by the false lumen.

About 20% of patients have partial or complete deficits of major arterial pulses, which may wax and wane. Limb blood pressures may differ, sometimes by > 30 mm Hg; this finding suggests a poor prognosis. A murmur of aortic regurgitation is heard in about 50% of patients with proximal dissection. Peripheral signs of aortic regurgitation may be present. Rarely, heart failure results from severe acute aortic regurgitation. Leakage of blood or inflammatory serous fluid into the left pleural space may lead to signs of pleural effusion. Occlusion of a limb artery may cause signs of peripheral ischemia or neuropathy. Renal artery occlusion may cause oliguria or anuria. Cardiac tamponade may cause pulsus paradoxus and jugular venous distention.

PEARLS & PITFALLS

- Only about 20% of patients with aortic dissection have pulse deficits.

Diagnosis

- Transesophageal echocardiography (TEE), CT angiography (CTA), or magnetic resonance angiography (MRA)

Aortic dissection must be considered in any patient with chest pain, thoracic back pain, unexplained syncope, unexplained abdominal pain, stroke, or acute-onset heart failure, especially when pulses or blood pressures in the limbs are unequal. Such patients require a chest x-ray; in 60 to 90%, the mediastinal shadow is widened, usually with a localized bulge signifying the site of origin. Left pleural effusion is common.

Patients presenting with acute chest pain, ECG changes of acute inferior myocardial infarction, and a previously undocumented murmur of aortic insufficiency (AI) are of particular concern for a type I aortic dissection into the right coronary artery (causing inferior myocardial infarction), and the aortic valve (causing AI).

If chest x-ray suggests dissection, TEE, CTA, or MRA is done immediately after the patient is stabilized. Findings of an intimal flap and double lumina confirm dissection.

Multiplanar TEE is 97 to 99% sensitive and, with M-mode echocardiography, is nearly 100% specific. It can be done at the bedside in < 20 min and does not require contrast agents. However, CTA is typically the first-line imaging modality because it is often available more rapidly and widely than TEE. The sensitivity of CTA exceeds 95% and it has a positive predictive value of 100% and a negative predictive value of 86%.

MRA has nearly 100% sensitivity and specificity for aortic dissection. But it is time-consuming and ill-suited for emergencies. It is probably best used for stable patients with subacute or chronic chest pain when dissection is suspected.

Contrast aortography is an option if surgery is being considered. In addition to identifying the origin and extent of dissection, severity of aortic regurgitation, and extent of involvement of the aorta's major branches, aortography helps determine whether simultaneous coronary artery bypass surgery is needed. Echocardiography should also be done to check for aortic regurgitation and thus determine whether the aortic valve should be repaired or replaced concomitantly.

ECG is nearly universally done. However, findings range from normal to markedly abnormal (in acute coronary artery occlusion or aortic regurgitation), so the test is not diagnostically helpful for dissection itself. Assays for soluble elastin compounds and smooth-muscle myosin heavy-chain protein are being studied; the data appears promising, but the assays are not routinely available. Serum CK-MB and troponin may help distinguish aortic dissection from myocardial infarction, except when dissection causes myocardial infarction.

Routine laboratory tests may detect slight leukocytosis and anemia if blood has leaked from the aorta. Increased LDH may be a nonspecific sign of celiac or mesenteric arterial trunk involvement.

A cardiothoracic surgeon should be consulted early during the diagnostic evaluation.

Prognosis

About 20% of patients with aortic dissection die before reaching the hospital. Without treatment, mortality rate is 1 to 3%/h during the first 24 h, 30% at 1 wk, 80% at 2 wk, and 90% at 1 yr.

Hospital mortality rate for treated patients is about 30% for proximal dissection and 10% for distal. For treated patients who survive the acute episode, survival rate is about 60% at 5 yr and 40% at 10 yr. About one-third of late deaths are due to complications of the dissection; the rest are due to other disorders.

Treatment

- Beta-blockers and other drugs to control BP
- Usually surgery (endovascular or open repair)

Patients who do not immediately die of aortic dissection should be admitted to an ICU with intra-arterial blood pressure monitoring and an indwelling urethral catheter to monitor urine output. Blood should be typed and cross-matched for 4 to 6 units of packed RBCs when surgery is likely. Hemodynamically unstable patients should be intubated.

Medical management: Drugs to decrease arterial pressure, arterial shear stress, ventricular contractility, and pain are started immediately to maintain systolic BP at ≤ 110 mm Hg or the lowest level compatible with adequate cerebral, coronary, and renal perfusion.

A beta-blocker is usually the first-line drug for BP control. Options include metoprolol 5 mg IV up to 4 doses 15 min apart, esmolol 50 to 200 mcg/kg/min in a constant IV infusion, and labetalol (an alpha- and beta-adrenergic blocker) 1 to 2 mg/min in a constant IV infusion or 5 to 20 mg IV initial bolus with additional doses of 20 to 40 mg given q 10 to 20 min until BP is controlled or a total of 300 mg has been given, followed by additional 20- to 40-mg doses q 4 to 8 h prn.

Alternatives to beta-blockers include calcium channel blockers (eg, verapamil 0.05 to 0.1 mg/kg IV bolus or diltiazem 0.25 mg/kg [up to 25 mg] IV bolus or 5 to 10 mg/h by continuous infusion).

If systolic BP remains > 110 mm Hg despite use of beta-blockers, nitroprusside in a constant IV infusion can be started at 0.2 to 0.3 mcg/kg/min and titrated upward (often to 200 to 300 mcg/min) as necessary to control BP. Nitroprusside should not be given without a beta-blocker or calcium channel blocker, because reflex sympathetic activation in response to vasodilation can increase ventricular inotropy and aortic shear stress, worsening the dissection.

PEARLS & PITFALLS

- To manage BP in aortic dissection, do not use a vasodilator (eg, nitroprusside) without a beta-blocker or calcium channel blocker because the vasodilator causes reflex sympathetic activation, which increases aortic shear stress.

Surgical repair: For the **descending aorta,** a trial of drug therapy alone is appropriate for an uncomplicated, stable dissection confined to the descending aorta (type B). Endovascular repair is warranted in patients with complications (malperfusion, persistent hypertension and pain, rapidly enlarging aortic diameter, extension of the dissection, and rupture). Surgery is also best for acute distal dissections in patients with Marfan syndrome.

For the **ascending aorta,** surgery is virtually always indicated due to the risk of life-threatening complications and usually involves open repair and replacement, although endovascular therapy is gaining support in certain circumstances.

The extent of repair depends upon the reason for repair and the anatomic nature of the dissection.

The goal of surgery is to obliterate entry into the false channel and reconstitute the aorta with a synthetic graft. If present, severe aortic regurgitation must be treated by resuspending the aortic leaflets or replacing the valve. Surgical outcomes are best with early, aggressive intervention. Mortality rate ranges from 7 to 36%. Predictors of poor outcome include hypotension, renal failure, age > 70, abrupt onset of chest pain, pulse deficit, and ST-segment elevation on ECG.

Stent grafts that seal entry to the false lumen and improve patency of the true lumen, balloon fenestration (in which an opening is made in the dissection flap that separates the true and false lumina), or both may be less invasive alternatives for patients with type B dissection if peripheral ischemic complications develop. Currently, there are no endovascular stent grafts approved for routine use in type A dissections. However, some endovascular devices are available for compassionate use in patients with type A dissections who have contraindications to open surgical repair.

Complications of surgery include death, stroke (due to emboli), paraplegia (due to spinal cord ischemia), renal failure (especially if dissection includes renal arteries) and endoleak (leakage of blood back into the aneurysmal sac). The most important late complications include redissection, formation of localized aneurysms in the weakened aorta, and progressive aortic regurgitation. These complications may require surgical or endovascular repair.

Long-term management: All patients, including those treated by surgery or endovascular methods, are given long-term antihypertensive drug therapy, usually including beta-blockers, calcium channel blockers, and ACE inhibitors. Almost any combination of antihypertensives is acceptable; exceptions are those that act mainly by vasodilation (eg, hydralazine, minoxidil) and beta-blockers that have intrinsic sympathomimetic action (eg, acebutolol, pindolol). Avoidance of strenuous physical activity is often recommended. CT may be done before discharge and repeated at 6 mo and 1 yr, then every 1 to 2 yr.

After repair of a dissection, the aorta should be monitored for the rest of the patient's life. The weakened aorta may develop aneurysmal degeneration above or below the surgical repair or re-dissect. For these reasons, continued surveillance is indicated.

KEY POINTS

- Aortic dissection may originate anywhere along the aorta but is most common at the proximal ascending aorta (within 5 cm of the aortic valve) or the descending thoracic aorta just beyond the origin of the left subclavian artery.
- Dissection requires preexisting degeneration of the aortic media (eg, caused by connective tissue disorders, injury) but hypertension is commonly also involved.
- Patients typically have excruciating, tearing precordial or interscapular pain.
- Other manifestations depend on whether the aortic root and/or branches of the aorta are affected, and the presence and location of any rupture; heart failure, organ ischemia, and hemorrhagic shock may occur.
- Diagnose using TEE, CTA, or MRA.
- Immediately give beta-blockers and other drugs as needed to control blood pressure.
- Drug therapy alone is appropriate for uncomplicated, stable dissection confined to the descending aorta; other cases require surgery.

AORTITIS

Aortitis is inflammation of the aorta, sometimes causing aneurysm or occlusion.

Aortitis is rare, but potentially life threatening. Its reported incidence is 1 to 3 per one million/year.

Aortitis is caused by

- Connective tissue disorders (eg, Takayasu arteritis, giant cell arteritis, ankylosing spondylitis, relapsing polychondritis)
- Infections (eg, bacterial endocarditis, syphilis, Rocky Mountain spotted fever, fungal infections)

It is also a feature of Cogan syndrome (inflammatory keratitis, vestibular and auditory dysfunction, and aortitis).

Inflammation usually involves all layers of the aorta (intima, media, adventitia) and may lead to occlusion of the aorta or its branches or weakening of the arterial wall, resulting in an aortic aneurysm. Pathogenesis, symptoms and signs, diagnosis, and treatment differ by etiology. However, the general principle for treatment is to treat the underlying disorder.

ABDOMINAL AORTIC BRANCH OCCLUSION

Various branches of the aorta can be occluded by atherosclerosis, fibromuscular dysplasia, or other conditions, causing symptoms and signs of ischemia or infarction. Diagnosis is by imaging tests. Treatment is with embolectomy, angioplasty, or sometimes surgical bypass grafting.

Occlusion of branches of the abdominal aorta may be

- Acute: Resulting from embolism, atherothrombosis, or dissection
- Chronic: Resulting from atherosclerosis, fibromuscular dysplasia, or external compression by mass lesions

Common sites of occlusion include

- Superior mesenteric arteries
- Celiac axis
- Renal arteries
- Aortic bifurcation

Chronic occlusion of the celiac axis is more common among women for unclear reasons.

Symptoms and Signs

Clinical manifestations (eg, pain, organ failure, necrosis) result from ischemia or infarction and vary depending on the artery involved and acuity.

Acute mesenteric occlusioncauses intestinal ischemia and infarction, resulting in severe, diffuse abdominal pain typically out of proportion to the minimal physical findings. Acute occlusion of the celiac axis may cause liver or spleen infarction.

Chronic mesenteric vascular insufficiency rarely causes symptoms unless both the superior mesenteric artery and celiac axis are substantially narrowed or occluded because collateral circulation between the major splanchnic trunks is extensive. Symptoms of chronic mesenteric vascular insufficiency typically occur postprandially (as intestinal angina) because digestion requires increased mesenteric blood flow; pain begins about 30 min to 1 h after eating and is steady, severe, and usually periumbilical and may be relieved by sublingual nitroglycerin. Patients become fearful of eating; weight loss, often extreme, is common. Rarely, malabsorption develops and contributes to weight loss. Patients may have an abdominal bruit, nausea, vomiting, diarrhea or constipation, and dark stools.

Acute renal artery embolismcauses sudden flank pain, followed by hematuria. Chronic occlusion may be asymptomatic or result in new or hard-to-control hypertension and other sequelae of renal insufficiency or failure.

Acute occlusion of the aortic bifurcation or distal branches can cause sudden onset of pain at rest, pallor, paralysis, absence of peripheral pulses, and coldness in the legs (see p. 752). Chronic occlusion can cause intermittent claudication in the legs and buttocks and erectile dysfunction (Leriche syndrome). Femoral pulses are absent. A limb may be jeopardized.

Diagnosis

- Imaging tests

Diagnosis is based primarily on history and physical examination and is confirmed by duplex ultrasonography, CTA, MRA, or traditional angiography.

Treatment

- Embolectomy or percutaneous angioplasty for acute occlusion
- Surgery or angioplasty for chronic, severe occlusion

Acute occlusion is a surgical emergency requiring embolectomy or percutaneous transluminal angioplasty (PTA) with or without stent placement. A laparotomy with bypass graft and bowel resection may be necessary if embolectomy or PTA is unsuccessful.

Chronic occlusion, if symptomatic, may require surgery or angioplasty. Risk factor modification and antiplatelet drugs may help.

Acute mesenteric occlusion (eg, in the superior mesenteric artery), which causes significant morbidity and mortality, requires prompt revascularization. Prognosis is poor if the intestine is not revascularized within 4 to 6 h.

For chronic occlusion of the superior mesenteric artery and celiac axis, dietary modifications may temporarily relieve symptoms. If symptoms are severe, surgical bypass from the aorta to the splanchnic arteries distal to the occlusion usually results in revascularization. Long-term patency of the grafts exceeds 90%. In appropriately selected patients (particularly among older patients who may be poor candidates for surgery), revascularization by PTA with or without stent placement may be successful. Symptoms may resolve rapidly, and weight may be regained.

Acute renal artery occlusion requires embolectomy; sometimes PTA can be done. Initial treatment of chronic occlusion involves antihypertensives. If blood pressure is not controlled adequately or if renal function deteriorates, PTA with stent placement or, when PTA is impossible, open surgical bypass or endarterectomy can improve blood flow.

Occlusion of the aortic bifurcation requires urgent embolectomy, usually done transfemorally. If chronic occlusion of the aortic bifurcation causes claudication, an aortoiliac or aortofemoral graft can be used to surgically bypass the occlusion. PTA is an alternative for selected patients.

KEY POINTS

- Abdominal aortic branch occlusion can be acute or chronic.
- Symptoms vary depending on the acuity of the occlusion and the artery involved.
- Diagnose abdominal aortic branch occlusion based on history and physical examination and confirm with imaging tests.
- Treat acute occlusion as a surgical emergency with embolectomy, PTA, or surgical bypass. Treat chronic occlusion with drugs and lifestyle changes and, if severe, surgery or angioplasty.

82 Endocarditis

Endocarditis usually refers to infection of the endocardium (ie, infective endocarditis). The term can also include noninfective endocarditis, in which sterile platelet and fibrin thrombi form on cardiac valves and adjacent endocardium. Noninfective endocarditis sometimes leads to infective endocarditis. Both can result in embolization and impaired cardiac function.

The diagnosis of infective endocarditis is usually based on a constellation of clinical findings rather than a single definitive test result.

INFECTIVE ENDOCARDITIS

Infective endocarditis is infection of the endocardium, usually with bacteria (commonly, streptococci or staphylococci) or fungi. It causes fever, heart murmurs, petechiae, anemia, embolic phenomena, and endocardial vegetations. Vegetations may result in valvular incompetence or obstruction, myocardial abscess, or mycotic aneurysm. Diagnosis requires demonstration of microorganisms in blood and usually echocardiography. Treatment consists of prolonged antimicrobial treatment and sometimes surgery.

Endocarditis can occur at any age. Men are affected about twice as often as women. IV drug abusers and immunocompromised patients are at highest risk.

Etiology

The normal heart is relatively resistant to infection. Bacteria and fungi do not easily adhere to the endocardial surface, and constant blood flow helps prevent them from settling on endocardial structures. Thus, 2 factors are typically required for endocarditis:

- A predisposing abnormality of the endocardium
- Microorganisms in the bloodstream (bacteremia)

Rarely, massive bacteremia or particularly virulent microorganisms cause endocarditis on normal valves.

Endocardial factors: Endocarditis usually involves the heart valves. Major predisposing factors are congenital heart defects, rheumatic valvular disease, bicuspid or calcific aortic valves, mitral valve prolapse, hypertrophic cardiomyopathy, and prior endocarditis. Prosthetic valves are a particular risk. Occasionally, mural thrombi, ventricular septal defects, and patent ductus arteriosus sites become infected. The actual nidus for infection is usually a sterile fibrin-platelet vegetation formed when damaged endothelial cells release tissue factor.

Infective endocarditis occurs most often on the left side (eg, mitral or aortic valve). About 10 to 20% of cases are right-sided (tricuspid or pulmonic valve). IV drug abusers have a much higher incidence of right-sided endocarditis (about 30 to 70%).

Microorganisms: Microorganisms that infect the endocardium may originate from distant infected sites (eg, cutaneous abscess, inflamed or infected gums, UTI) or have obvious portals of entry such as a central venous catheter or a drug injection site. Almost any implanted foreign material (eg, ventricular or peritoneal shunt, prosthetic device) is at risk of bacterial colonization, thus becoming a source of bacteremia and hence endocarditis. Endocarditis also may result from asymptomatic bacteremia, such as typically occurs during invasive dental, medical, or surgical procedures. Even toothbrushing and chewing can cause bacteremia (usually due to viridans streptococci) in patients with gingivitis.

Causative microorganisms vary by site of infection, source of bacteremia, and host risk factors (eg, IV drug abuse), but overall, streptococci and *Staphylococcus aureus* cause 80 to 90% of cases. Enterococci, gram-negative bacilli, HACEK organisms (*Haemophilus* sp, *Actinobacillus actinomycetemcomitans*, *Cardiobacterium hominis*, *Eikenella corrodens*, and *Kingella kingae*), and fungi cause most of the rest. Why streptococci and staphylococci frequently adhere to vegetations and why gram-negative aerobic bacilli seldom adhere are unclear. However, the ability of *S. aureus* to adhere to fibronectin may play a role, as may dextran production by viridans streptococci.

After colonizing vegetations, microorganisms are covered by a layer of fibrin and platelets, which prevents access by neutrophils, immunoglobulins, and complement and thus blocks host defenses.

Pathophysiology

Endocarditis has local and systemic consequences.

Local consequences: Local consequences include formation of myocardial abscesses with tissue destruction and sometimes conduction system abnormalities (usually with low septal abscesses). Severe valvular regurgitation may develop suddenly, causing heart failure and death (usually due to mitral or aortic valve lesions). Aortitis may result from contiguous spread of infection. Prosthetic valve infections are particularly likely to involve valve ring abscesses, obstructing vegetations, myocardial abscesses, and mycotic aneurysms manifested by valve obstruction, dehiscence, and conduction disturbances.

Systemic consequences: Systemic consequences are primarily due to embolization of infected material from the heart valve and, primarily in chronic infection, immune-mediated phenomena. Right-sided lesions typically produce septic pulmonary emboli, which may result in pulmonary infarction, pneumonia, or empyema. Left-sided lesions may embolize to any tissue, particularly the kidneys, spleen, and CNS. Mycotic aneurysms can form in any major artery. Cutaneous and retinal emboli are common. Diffuse glomerulonephritis may result from immune complex deposition.

Classification

Infective endocarditis may have an indolent, subacute course or a more acute, fulminant course with greater potential for rapid decompensation.

Subacute bacterial endocarditis (SBE), although aggressive, usually develops insidiously and progresses slowly (ie, over weeks to months). Often, no source of infection or portal of entry is evident. SBE is caused most commonly by streptococci (especially viridans, microaerophilic, anaerobic, and nonenterococcal group D streptococci and enterococci) and less commonly by *S. aureus*, *Staphylococcus epidermidis*, *Gemella morbillorum*, *Abiotrophia defectiva* (formerly, *Streptococcus defectivus*), *Granulicatella* sp, and fastidious *Haemophilus* sp. SBE often develops on abnormal valves after asymptomatic bacteremia due to periodontal, GI, or GU infections.

Acute bacterial endocarditis (ABE) usually develops abruptly and progresses rapidly (ie, over days). A source of infection or portal of entry is often evident. When bacteria are virulent or bacterial exposure is massive, ABE can affect normal valves. It is usually caused by *S. aureus*, group A hemolytic streptococci, pneumococci, or gonococci.

Prosthetic valvular endocarditis (PVE) develops in 2 to 3% of patients within 1 yr after valve replacement and in 0.5%/yr thereafter. It is more common after aortic than after mitral valve replacement and affects mechanical and bioprosthetic valves equally. Early-onset infections (< 2 mo after surgery) are caused mainly by contamination during surgery with antimicrobial-resistant bacteria (eg, *S. epidermidis*, diphtheroids, coliform bacilli, *Candida* sp, *Aspergillus* sp). Late-onset infections are caused mainly by contamination with low-virulence organisms during surgery or by transient asymptomatic bacteremias, most often with streptococci; *S. epidermidis*; diphtheroids; and the fastidious gram-negative bacilli, *Haemophilus* sp, *Actinobacillus actinomycetemcomitans*, and *Cardiobacterium hominis*.

Symptoms and Signs

Symptoms and signs vary based on the classification but are nonspecific.

SBE: Initially, symptoms are vague: low-grade fever (< 39° C), night sweats, fatigability, malaise, and weight loss. Chills and arthralgias may occur. Symptoms and signs of valvular insufficiency may be a first clue. Initially, ≤ 15% of patients have fever or a murmur, but eventually almost all develop both. Physical examination may be normal or include pallor, fever, change in a preexisting murmur or development of a new regurgitant murmur, and tachycardia.

Retinal emboli can cause round or oval hemorrhagic retinal lesions with small white centers (Roth spots). Cutaneous manifestations include petechiae (on the upper trunk, conjunctivae, mucous membranes, and distal extremities), painful erythematous subcutaneous nodules on the tips of digits (Osler nodes), nontender hemorrhagic macules on the palms or soles (Janeway lesions—see Plate 4), and splinter hemorrhages under the nails. About 35% of patients have CNS effects, including transient ischemic attacks, stroke, toxic encephalopathy, and, if a mycotic CNS aneurysm ruptures, brain abscess and subarachnoid hemorrhage. Renal emboli may cause flank pain and, rarely, gross hematuria. Splenic emboli may cause left upper quadrant pain. Prolonged infection may cause splenomegaly or clubbing of fingers and toes.

ABE and PVE: Symptoms and signs are similar to those of SBE, but the course is more rapid. Fever is almost always present initially, and patients appear toxic; sometimes septic shock develops. Heart murmur is present initially in about 50 to 80% and eventually in > 90%. Rarely, purulent meningitis occurs.

Right-sided endocarditis: Septic pulmonary emboli may cause cough, pleuritic chest pain, and sometimes hemoptysis. A murmur of tricuspid regurgitation is typical.

Diagnosis

- Blood cultures
- Echocardiography
- Clinical criteria

Because symptoms and signs are nonspecific, vary greatly, and may develop insidiously, diagnosis requires a high index of suspicion. Endocarditis should be suspected in patients with fever and no obvious source of infection, particularly if a heart murmur is present. Suspicion of endocarditis should be very high if blood cultures are positive in patients who have a history of a heart valve disorder, who have had certain recent invasive procedures, or who abuse IV drugs. Patients with documented bacteremia should be examined thoroughly and repeatedly for new valvular murmurs and signs of emboli.

If endocarditis is suspected, 3 blood cultures (20 mL each) should be obtained within 24 h (if presentation suggests ABE, 2 cultures within the first 1 to 2 h). Each set of cultures should be obtained from a separate, fresh venipuncture site (ie, not from preexisting vascular catheters). Blood cultures do not need to be done during chills or fever because most patients have continuous bacteremia. When endocarditis is present and no prior antibiotic therapy was given, all 3 blood cultures usually are positive because the bacteremia is continuous; at least one culture is positive in 99%. Premature use of empiric antibiotic therapy should be avoided in patients with acquired or congenital valvular or shunt lesions to avoid culture-negative endocarditis. If prior antimicrobial therapy was given, blood cultures should still be obtained, but results may be negative.

Echocardiography, typically transthoracic (TTE) rather than transesophageal (TEE), should be done. Although TEE is somewhat more accurate (ie, capable of revealing vegetations too small to be seen on TTE), it is invasive and more costly. TEE should be done when endocarditis is suspected in patients with prosthetic valves, when TTE is nondiagnostic, and when diagnosis of infective endocarditis has been established clinically.

Other than positive blood cultures, there are no specific laboratory findings. Established infections often cause a normocytic-normochromic anemia, elevated WBC count, increased ESR, increased immunoglobulin levels, and the presence of circulating immune complexes and rheumatoid factor, but these findings are not diagnostically helpful. Urinalysis often shows microscopic hematuria and, occasionally, RBC casts, pyuria, or bacteriuria.

Identification of the organism and its antimicrobial susceptibility is vital to guide treatment. Blood cultures may require 3 to 4 wk incubation for certain organisms; however, some proprietary, automated culture monitoring systems can identify positive cultures within a week. Other organisms (eg, *Aspergillus* sp) may not produce positive cultures. Some organisms (eg, *Coxiella burnetii*, *Bartonella* sp, *Chlamydia psittaci*, *Brucella* sp) require serodiagnosis; others (eg, *Legionella pneumophila*) require special culture media or PCR (eg, *Tropheryma whippelii*). Negative blood culture results may indicate suppression due to prior antimicrobial therapy, infection with organisms that do not grow in standard culture media, or another diagnosis (eg, noninfective endocarditis, atrial myxoma with embolic phenomena, vasculitis).

Infective endocarditis is definitively diagnosed when microorganisms are seen histologically in (or cultured from) endocardial vegetations obtained during cardiac surgery, embolectomy, or autopsy. Because vegetations are not usually available for examination, clinical criteria for establishing a diagnosis (with a sensitivity and specificity > 90%) have been developed (see Table 82–1).

Prognosis

Untreated, infective endocarditis is always fatal. Even with treatment, death is more likely and the prognosis is generally poorer for older people and people who have infection with resistant organisms, an underlying disorder, or a long delay in treatment. The prognosis is also poorer for people with aortic or multiple valve involvement, large vegetations, polymicrobial bacteremia, prosthetic valve infections, mycotic aneurysms, valve ring abscess, and major embolic events. Septic shock is more likely in patients with diabetes, acute renal insufficiency, *S. aureus* infection, supraventricular tachycardia, vegetation size > 15 mm, and signs of persistent infection. The mortality rate for viridans streptococcal endocarditis without major

Table 82–1. REVISED DUKE CLINICAL DIAGNOSTIC CRITERIA FOR INFECTIVE ENDOCARDITIS

MAJOR CRITERIA
Two positive blood cultures for organisms typical of endocarditis
Three positive blood cultures for organisms consistent with endocarditis
Serologic evidence of *Coxiella burnetii* (or one positive blood culture)
Echocardiographic evidence of endocardial involvement:
• Oscillating intracardiac mass on a heart valve, on supporting structures, in the path of regurgitant jets, or on implanted material without another anatomic explanation
• Cardiac abscess
• New dehiscence of prosthetic valve
• New valvular regurgitation
MINOR CRITERIA
Predisposing heart disorder
IV drug abuse
Fever ≥ 38° C
Vascular phenomena:
• Arterial embolism
• Septic pulmonary embolism
• Mycotic aneurysm
• Intracranial hemorrhage
• Conjunctival petechiae
• Janeway lesions
Immunologic phenomena:
• Glomerulonephritis
• Osler nodes
• Roth spots
• Rheumatoid factor
Microbiologic evidence of infection consistent with but not meeting major criteria
Serologic evidence of infection with organisms consistent with endocarditis

For definite clinical diagnosis: 2 major criteria *or* 1 major and 3 minor criteria, *or* 5 minor criteria.

For possible clinical diagnosis: 1 major criterion and 1 minor criterion *or* 3 minor criteria.

For rejection of diagnosis: Firm alternative diagnosis explaining the findings of infective endocarditis, resolution of symptoms and signs after antimicrobial therapy for ≤ 4 days, no pathologic evidence of infective endocarditis found during surgery or autopsy, or failure to meet the clinical criteria for possible endocarditis.

Adapted from Li JS, Sexton DJ, Mick N, et al: Proposed modifications to the Duke criteria for the diagnosis of infective endocarditis. *Clinical Infectious Diseases* 30:633–638, 2000.

complications is < 10% but is virtually 100% for *Aspergillus* endocarditis after prosthetic valve surgery.

The prognosis is better with right-sided than left-sided endocarditis because tricuspid valve dysfunction is tolerated better, systemic emboli are absent, and right-sided *S. aureus* endocarditis responds better to antimicrobial therapy.

Treatment

- IV antibiotics (based on the organism and its susceptibility)
- Sometimes valve debridement, repair, or replacement

Treatment consists of a prolonged course of antimicrobial therapy. Surgery may be needed for mechanical complications or resistant organisms. Typically, antimicrobials are given IV. Because they must be given for 2 to 8 wk, home IV therapy is often used.

Any apparent source of bacteremia must be managed: necrotic tissue debrided, abscesses drained, and foreign material and infected devices removed. Existing IV catheters (particularly central venous ones) should be changed. If endocarditis persists in a patient with a newly inserted central venous catheter, that catheter should also be removed. Organisms within biofilms adherent to catheters and other devices may not respond to antimicrobial therapy, leading to treatment failure or relapse. If continuous infusions are used instead of intermittent boluses, infusions should not be interrupted for long periods.

Antibiotic regimens: Drugs and dosages depend on the microorganism and its antimicrobial susceptibility (for typical regimens, see Table 82–2). Initial therapy before organism identification (but after adequate blood cultures have been obtained) should be broad spectrum to cover all likely organisms:

- Native valves and no IV drug abuse: Ampicillin 500 mg/h continuous IV infusion plus nafcillin 2 g IV q 4 h plus gentamicin 1 mg/kg IV q 8 h
- Prosthetic valve: Vancomycin 15 mg/kg IV q 12 h plus gentamicin 1 mg/kg q 8 h plus rifampin 300 po q 8 h.
- IV drug abusers: Nafcillin 2 g IV q 4 h

In all regimens, penicillin-allergic patients require substitution of vancomycin 15 mg/kg IV q 12 h for the penicillin.

IV drug abusers frequently do not adhere to treatment, abuse IV access lines, and tend to leave the hospital too soon. For such patients, short-course IV or (less preferably) oral therapy may be used. For right-sided endocarditis caused by methicillin-sensitive *S. aureus*, nafcillin 2 g IV q 4 h plus gentamicin 1 mg/kg IV q 8 h for 2 wk is effective, as is a 4-wk oral regimen of ciprofloxacin 750 mg po bid plus rifampin 300 mg po bid. Left-sided endocarditis does not respond to 2-wk courses.

Cardiac valve surgery: Surgery (debridement, valve repair or replacement) is frequently required for abscess, persistent infection despite antimicrobial therapy (ie, persistent positive blood cultures or recurrent emboli), or severe valvular regurgitation.

Timing of surgery requires experienced clinical judgment. If heart failure caused by a correctable lesion is worsening (particularly when the organism is *S. aureus*, a gram-negative bacillus, or a fungus), surgery may be required after only 24 to 72 h of antimicrobial therapy. In patients with prosthetic valves, surgery may be required when TEE shows valve dehiscence on a paravalvular abscess, when valve dysfunction precipitates heart failure, when recurrent emboli are detected, or when the infection is caused by an antimicrobial-resistant organism.

Response to treatment: After starting therapy, patients with penicillin-susceptible streptococcal endocarditis usually feel better, and fever is reduced within 3 to 7 days. Fever may continue for reasons other than persistent infection (eg, drug allergy, phlebitis, infarction due to emboli). Patients with staphylococcal endocarditis tend to respond more slowly. Diminution of vegetation size can be followed by serial echocardiography.

Relapse usually occurs within 4 wk. Antibiotic retreatment may be effective, but surgery may also be required. In patients without prosthetic valves, recrudescence of endocarditis after 6 wk usually results from a new infection rather than a relapse. Even after successful antimicrobial therapy, sterile emboli and valve rupture may occur up to 1 yr later.

Table 82–2. SOME ANTIBIOTIC REGIMENS FOR ENDOCARDITIS

TYPE	DRUG AND DOSAGE FOR ADULTS	DRUG AND DOSAGE FOR ADULTS ALLERGIC TO PENICILLIN
Penicillin-susceptible streptococci (penicillin G MIC ≤ 0.1 μg/mL), including most viridans streptococci	Penicillin G 12–18 million units/day IV continuously or 2–3 million units q 4 h for 4 wk or, if gentamicin 1 mg/kg* IV (up to 80 mg) q 8 h is given concurrently, for 2 wk	Ceftriaxone 2 g once/day IV for 4 wk or, if gentamicin 1 mg/kg* IV (up to 80 mg) q 8 h is given concurrently, for 2 wk through a central venous catheter (can be given on outpatient basis) if there is no history of penicillin anaphylaxis *or* Vancomycin† 15 mg/kg IV q 12 h for 4 wk
Streptococci relatively resistant to penicillin (penicillin G MIC > 0.1 μg/mL), including enterococci, some other streptococcal strains, and *Abiotrophia defectiva* (formerly, *Streptococcus defectivus*)	Gentamicin 1 mg/kg* IV q 8 h plus penicillin G 18–30 million units/day IV or ampicillin 12 g/day IV continuously or 2 g q 4 h for 4–6 wk‡	Desensitization to penicillin *or* Vancomycin† 15 mg/kg IV (up to 1 g) q 12 h plus gentamicin 1mg/kg* IV q 8 h for 4–6 wk
Pneumococci or group A streptococci	Penicillin G 12–18 million units/day IV continuously for 4 wk if susceptible to penicillin *or* Vancomycin† 15 mg/kg IV q 12 h for 4 wk for pneumococci with penicillin G MIC ≥ 2 μg/mL	Ceftriaxone 2 g once/day IV for 4 wk through a central venous catheter (can be given on outpatient basis) if there is no history of penicillin anaphylaxis *or* Vancomycin† 15 mg/kg IV q 12 h for 4 wk
Penicillin-resistant *Staphylococcus aureus* strains	For patients with a left-sided native valve: Oxacillin or nafcillin 2 g IV q 4 h for 4–6 wk§ For patients with a right-sided native valve: Oxacillin or nafcillin 2 g IV q 4 h for 2–4 wk plus gentamicin 1 mg/kg* IV q 8 h for 2 wk For patients with a prosthetic valve: Oxacillin or nafcillin 2 g IV q 4 h for 6–8 wk plus gentamicin 1 mg/kg* IV q 8 h for 2 wk plus rifampin 300 mg po q 8 h for 6–8 wk	Cefazolin 2 g IV q 8 h for 4–6 wk if staphylococci are susceptible to oxacillin or nafcillin and if there is no history of penicillin anaphylaxis *or* Cefazolin 2 g IV q 8 h for 2–4 wk plus gentamicin 1 mg/kg* IV q 8 h for 2 wk *or* Cefazolin 2 g IV q 8 h for 4–6 wk plus gentamicin 1 mg/kg* IV q 8 h for 2 wk plus rifampin 300 mg po q 8 h for 6–8 wk *or* Vancomycin† 15 mg/kg IV q 12 h alone if native valve, plus gentamicin 1 mg/kg* IV q 8 h for 2 wk plus rifampin 300 mg po q 8 h for 4–6 wk if prosthetic valve
Oxacillin and nafcillin-resistant *S. aureus* strains	Vancomycin† 15 mg/kg IV q 12 h alone if native valve, plus gentamicin 1 mg/kg IV* q 8 h for 2 wk plus rifampin 300 mg po q 8 h for 6–8 wk if prosthetic valve	—
HACEK microorganisms	Ceftriaxone 2 g once/day IV for 4 wk *or* Ampicillin 12 g/day IV continuously or 2 g q 4 h plus gentamicin 1 mg/kg* IV q 8 h for 4 wk	Ceftriaxone 2 g once/day IV for 4 wk or, if gentamicin 1 mg/kg* IV (up to 80 mg) q 8 h is given concurrently, for 2 wk if there is no history of penicillin anaphylaxis
Coliform bacilli	Sensitivity-proven β-lactam antimicrobial (eg, ceftriaxone 2 g IV q 12–24 h or ceftazidime 2 g IV q 8 h) plus an aminoglycoside (eg, gentamicin 2 mg/kg* IV q 8 h) for 4–6 wk	—
Pseudomonas aeruginosa	Ceftazidime 2 g IV q 8 h or cefepime 2 g IV q 8 h or imipenem 500 mg IV q 6 h plus tobramycin 2.5 mg/kg q 8 h for 6–8 wk; amikacin 5 mg/kg q 12 h substituted for tobramycin if bacteria are susceptible	Ceftazidime 2 g IV q 8 h or cefepime 2 g IV q 8 h plus tobramycin 2.5 mg/kg q 8 h for 6–8 wk; amikacin 5 mg/kg q 12 h substituted for tobramycin if bacteria are susceptible only to amikacin

*Based on ideal rather than actual weight in obese patients.

†With vancomycin, serum levels must be monitored if doses > 2 g/24 h are administered.

‡If enterococcal endocarditis lasts > 3 mo and involves large vegetations or vegetations on prosthetic valves, treatment should last for 6 wk.

§Some clinicians add gentamicin 1 mg/kg IV q 8 h for 3–5 days if patients have a native valve.

HACEK microorganisms: *Haemophilus parainfluenzae*, *H. aphrophilus*, *Actinobacillus actinomycetemcomitans*, *Cardiobacterium hominis*, *Eikenella corrodens*, and *Kingella kingae*.

Table 82–3. PROCEDURES REQUIRING ANTIMICROBIAL ENDOCARDITIS PROPHYLAXIS IN HIGH-RISK PATIENTS

TYPE	EXAMPLES
Oral-dental*	Dental extraction Dental implant placement or reimplantation of avulsed teeth Periodontal procedures, including surgery, scaling, root planing, and probing Prophylactic cleaning of teeth or implants when bleeding is anticipated Root canal instrumentation or surgery beyond the apex
Respiratory tract	Bronchoscopy if mucosa is to be incised Procedures done during an established infection Tonsillectomy, adenoidectomy, or both
GI tract	None, unless procedure is done during an established infection
GU tract	None, unless procedure is done during an established infection (eg, cystoscopy during known enterococcal UTI)
Musculoskeletal	None, unless procedure involves infected tissue
Skin	None, unless procedure involves infected tissue

*Examples of oral-dental procedures that do not require prophylaxis are anesthetic injection through uninfected mucosa and placement of orthodontic brackets.

Data from Wilson W, Taubert KS, Gewitz M, et al: Prevention of infective endocarditis. *Circulation* 116(15):1736–1754, 2007.

Prevention

Preventive dental examination and therapy before surgery to repair heart valves or congenital heart lesions is recommended.

Patients: The American Heart Association (AHA) recommends antimicrobial prophylaxis for patients at high risk of an adverse outcome from infective endocarditis (see AHA Guidelines). Such patients include those with

- Prosthetic heart valves or prosthetic material used for valve repair
- Previous infective endocarditis
- Certain congenital heart diseases (CHD): Unrepaired cyanotic CHD (including palliative shunts and conduits), completely repaired CHD during the first 6 mo after surgery if prosthetic material or device was used, repaired CHD that has residual defects at or adjacent to the site of repair
- Heart transplant recipients with valvulopathy

Procedures: Most procedures for which prophylaxis is required for high-risk patients are oral-dental procedures that manipulate the gingiva or the periapical region of teeth or perforate the oral mucosa. Other procedures include those respiratory tract procedures in which mucosa is incised, and GI, GU, or musculoskeletal procedures that involve an area with an established infection (see Table 82–3).

Antibiotic regimens: For most patients and procedures, a single dose shortly before the procedure is effective. For oral-dental and respiratory procedures, a drug effective against viridans group streptococci is used (see Table 82–4).

For GI, GU, and musculoskeletal procedures on areas involving infected tissue, antibiotics should be selected based on the known organism and its sensitivities. If infection is present but the infecting organism has not been identified, antibiotics for GI and GU prophylaxis should be effective against enterococci (eg, amoxicillin or ampicillin, or vancomycin for patients who are allergic to penicillin). Antibiotics for skin and musculoskeletal prophylaxis should be effective against staphylococci and beta-hemolytic streptococci (eg, a cephalosporin or vancomycin or clindamycin if infection with methicillin-resistant staphylococci is possible).

KEY POINTS

- Because the normal heart is relatively resistant to infection, endocarditis occurs mainly when there is a predisposing abnormality of the endocardium.
- Predisposing cardiac abnormalities include congenital heart defects, rheumatic valvular disease, bicuspid or calcific aortic valves, mitral valve prolapse, hypertrophic cardiomyopathy, prior endocarditis, and presence of a prosthetic valve.
- Local cardiac consequences include myocardial abscess, conduction system abnormalities, and sudden, severe valvular regurgitation.

Table 82–4. RECOMMENDED ENDOCARDITIS PROPHYLAXIS DURING ORAL-DENTAL OR RESPIRATORY TRACT PROCEDURES*

ROUTE	DRUG AND DOSAGE IN ADULTS (AND CHILDREN)	DRUG AND DOSAGE IN ADULTS (AND CHILDREN) ALLERGIC TO PENICILLIN
Oral (given 1 h before procedure)	Amoxicillin 2 g (50 mg/kg) po	Clindamycin 600 mg (20 mg/kg) po *or* Cephalexin or cefadroxil 2 g (50 mg/kg) po *or* Azithromycin or clarithromycin 500 mg (15 mg/kg) po
Parenteral (given 30 min before procedure)	Ampicillin 2 g (50 mg/kg) IM or IV	Clindamycin 600 mg (20 mg/kg) IV *or* Cefazolin 1 g (25 mg/kg) IM or IV

*For patients without active infection.

Adapted from Wilson W, Taubert KS, Gewitz M, et al: Prevention of infective endocarditis. *Circulation* 116(15):1736–1754, 2007.

- Systemic consequences include immune phenomena (eg, glomerulonephritis) and septic emboli, which may affect any organ put particularly the lungs (with right sided endocarditis), kidneys, spleen, CNS, skin, and retina (with left-sided endocarditis).
- Diagnose using blood cultures and Duke criteria.
- Treat with a prolonged course of antimicrobial therapy; surgery may be needed for mechanical complications or resistant organisms.
- Give antimicrobial prophylaxis for patients at high risk of an adverse outcome from infective endocarditis, including those with prosthetic heart valves, previous infective endocarditis, certain congenital heart diseases, or who are heart transplant recipients with valvulopathy.

NONINFECTIVE ENDOCARDITIS

Noninfective endocarditis (nonbacterial thrombotic endocarditis) refers to formation of sterile platelet and fibrin thrombi on cardiac valves and adjacent endocardium in response to trauma, circulating immune complexes, vasculitis, or a hypercoagulable state. Symptoms are those of systemic arterial embolism. Diagnosis is by echocardiography and negative blood cultures. Treatment consists of anticoagulants.

Etiology

Vegetations are caused by physical trauma, not infection. They may be clinically undetectable or become a nidus for infection (leading to infective endocarditis), produce emboli, or impair valvular function.

Catheters passed through the right side of the heart may injure the tricuspid and pulmonic valves, resulting in platelet and fibrin attachment at the site of injury. In disorders such as SLE, circulating immune complexes may result in friable platelet and fibrin vegetations along a valve leaflet closure (Libman-Sacks lesions). These lesions do not usually cause significant valvular obstruction or regurgitation. Antiphospholipid antibody syndrome (lupus anticoagulants, recurrent venous thrombosis, stroke, spontaneous abortions, livdo reticularis) also can lead to sterile endocardial vegetations and systemic emboli. Rarely, granulomatosis with polyangiitis leads to noninfective endocarditis.

Marantic endocarditis: In patients with chronic wasting diseases, disseminated intravascular coagulation, mucin-producing metastatic carcinomas (of lung, stomach, or pancreas), or chronic infections (eg, TB, pneumonia, osteomyelitis), large thrombotic vegetations may form on valves and produce significant emboli to the brain, kidneys, spleen, mesentery, extremities, and coronary arteries. These vegetations tend to form on congenitally abnormal cardiac valves or those damaged by rheumatic fever.

Symptoms and Signs

Vegetations themselves do not cause symptoms. Symptoms result from embolization and depend on the organ affected (eg, brain, kidneys, spleen). Fever and a heart murmur are sometimes present.

Diagnosis

- Blood cultures
- Echocardiography

Noninfective endocarditis should be suspected when chronically ill patients develop symptoms suggesting arterial embolism. Serial blood cultures (see p. 707) and echocardiography should be done. Negative blood cultures and valvular vegetations (but not atrial myxoma) suggest the diagnosis. Examination of embolic fragments after embolectomy can help make the diagnosis. Differentiation from culture-negative infective endocarditis may be difficult but is important. An anticoagulant is often needed in noninfective endocarditis but is contraindicated in infective endocarditis.

Prognosis

Prognosis is generally poor, more because of the seriousness of predisposing disorders than the cardiac lesion.

Treatment

- Anticoagulation

Treatment consists of anticoagulation with heparin or warfarin, although results of such treatment have not been evaluated. Predisposing disorders should be treated whenever possible.

83 Heart Failure

(Congestive Heart Failure)

Heart failure (HF) is a syndrome of ventricular dysfunction. Left ventricular failure causes shortness of breath and fatigue, and right ventricular failure causes peripheral and abdominal fluid accumulation; the ventricles can be involved together or separately. Diagnosis is initially clinical, supported by chest x-ray, echocardiography, and levels of plasma natriuretic peptides. Treatment includes patient education, diuretics, ACE inhibitors, angiotensin II receptor blockers, beta-blockers, aldosterone antagonists, neprilysin inhibitors, specialized implantable pacemakers/defibrillators and other devices, and correction of the cause(s) of the HF syndrome.

HF affects about 6.5 million people in the US; > 960,000 new cases occur each year. About 26 million people are affected worldwide.

Physiology

Cardiac contractility (force and velocity of contraction), ventricular performance, and myocardial oxygen requirements are determined by

- Preload
- Afterload
- Substrate availability (eg, oxygen, fatty acids, glucose)
- Heart rate and rhythm
- Amount of viable myocardium

Cardiac output (CO) is the product of stroke volume and heart rate; it is also affected by venous return, peripheral vascular tone, and neurohumoral factors.

Preload is the loading condition of the heart at the end of its relaxation and filling phase (diastole) just before contraction (systole). Preload represents the degree of end-diastolic fiber stretch and end-diastolic volume, which is influenced by ventricular diastolic pressure and the composition of the myocardial wall. Typically, left ventricular (LV) end-diastolic pressure, especially if higher than normal, is a reasonable measure of preload. LV dilation, hypertrophy, and changes in myocardial distensibility (compliance) modify preload.

Afterload is the force resisting myocardial fiber contraction at the start of systole. It is determined by LV chamber pressure, radius, and wall thickness at the time the aortic valve opens. Clinically, systemic systolic blood pressure at or shortly after the aortic valve opens correlates with peak systolic wall stress and approximates afterload.

The **Frank-Starling principle** describes the relationship between preload and cardiac performance. It states that, normally, systolic contractile performance (represented by stroke volume or CO) is proportional to preload within the normal physiologic range (see Fig. 83–1). Contractility is difficult to measure clinically (because it requires cardiac catheterization with pressure-volume analysis) but is reasonably reflected by the ejection fraction (EF), which is the percentage of end-diastolic volume ejected with each contraction (stroke volume/end-diastolic volume). EF can generally be adequately assessed noninvasively with echocardiography, nuclear imaging, or MRI.

Cardiac reserve is the ability of the heart to increase its performance above resting levels in response to emotional or physical stress; body oxygen consumption may increase from 250 to ≥ 1500 mL/min during maximal exertion. Mechanisms include increasing heart rate, systolic and diastolic volumes, stroke volume, and tissue extraction of oxygen (the difference between oxygen content in arterial blood and in mixed venous or pulmonary artery blood). In well-trained young adults during maximal exercise, heart rate may increase from 55 to 70 beats/min at rest to 180 beats/min, and CO may increase from 6 to ≥ 25 L/min. At rest, arterial blood contains about 18 mL oxygen/dL of blood, and mixed venous or pulmonary artery blood contains about 14 mL/dL. Oxygen extraction is thus about 4 mL/dL. When demand is increased, it may increase to 12 to 14 mL/dL. This mechanism also helps compensate for reduced tissue blood flow in HF.

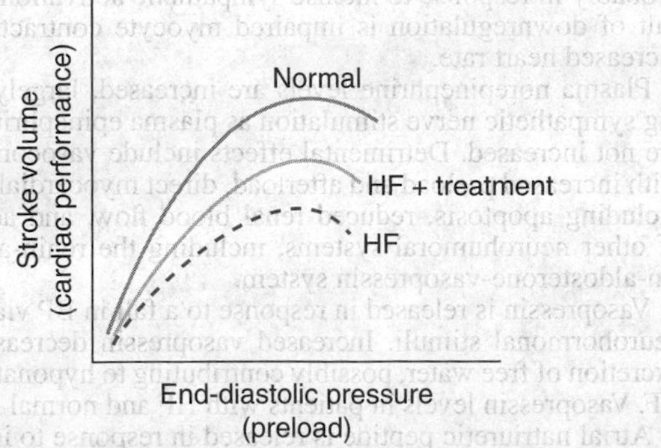

Fig. 83–1. Frank-Starling principle. Normally (top curve), as preload increases, cardiac performance also increases. However at a certain point, performance plateaus, then declines. In heart failure (HF) due to systolic dysfunction (bottom curve), the overall curve shifts downward, reflecting reduced cardiac performance at a given preload, and, as preload increases, there is less of an increase in cardiac performance. With treatment (middle curve), performance is improved, although not normalized.

Pathophysiology

In HF, the heart may not provide tissues with adequate blood for metabolic needs, and cardiac-related elevation of pulmonary or systemic venous pressures may result in organ congestion. This condition can result from abnormalities of systolic or diastolic function or, commonly, both. Although a primary abnormality can be a change in cardiomyocyte function, there are also changes in collagen turnover of the extracellular matrix. Cardiac structural defects (eg, congenital defects, valvular disorders), rhythm abnormalities (including persistently high heart rate), and high metabolic demands (eg, due to thyrotoxicosis) also can cause HF.

Heart failure with reduced ejection fraction (HFrEF): In HFrEF (also called systolic HF), global LV systolic dysfunction predominates. The LV contracts poorly and empties inadequately, leading to increased diastolic volume and pressure and decreased ejection fraction. Many defects in energy utilization, energy supply, electrophysiologic functions, and contractile element interaction occur, with abnormalities in intracellular calcium modulation and cAMP production.

Predominant systolic dysfunction is common in heat failure due to myocardial infarction, myocarditis, and dilated cardiomyopathy. Systolic dysfunction may affect primarily the LV or the right ventricle (RV); LV failure often leads to RV failure.

Heart failure with preserved ejection fraction (HFpEF): In HFpEF (previously known as diastolic HF), LV filling is impaired, resulting in increased LV end-diastolic pressure at rest or during exertion. Global contractility and hence ejection fraction remain normal. In most patients with HFpEF, LV end-diastolic volume is normal. However, in some patients, marked restriction to LV filling can cause inappropriately low LV end-diastolic volume and thus cause low CO and systemic symptoms. Elevated left atrial pressures can cause pulmonary hypertension and pulmonary congestion.

Diastolic dysfunction usually results from impaired ventricular relaxation (an active process), increased ventricular stiffness, valvular disease, or constrictive pericarditis. Acute myocardial ischemia is also a cause of diastolic dysfunction. Resistance to filling increases with age, reflecting both cardiomyocyte dysfunction and cardiomyocyte loss, and increased interstitial collagen deposition; thus, diastolic dysfunction is particularly common among the elderly. Diastolic dysfunction predominates in hypertrophic cardiomyopathy, disorders with ventricular hypertrophy (eg, hypertension, significant aortic stenosis), and amyloid infiltration of the myocardium. LV filling and function may also be impaired if marked increases in RV pressure shift the interventricular septum to the left.

Diastolic dysfunction has increasingly been recognized as a cause of HF. Estimates vary, but about 50% of patients with HF have HFpEF; the prevalence increases with age and in patients with diabetes. It is now known that HFpEF is a complex, heterogenous, multiorgan, systemic syndrome, often with multiple concomitant pathophysiologies. Current data suggest that multiple comorbidities (eg, obesity, hypertension, diabetes, chronic kidney disease) lead to systemic inflammation, widespread endothelial dysfunction, cardiac microvascular dysfunction, and, ultimately, molecular changes in the heart that cause increased myocardial fibrosis and ventricular stiffening. Thus, although HFrEF is typically associated with primary myocardial injury, HFpEF may be associated with secondary myocardial injury due to abnormalities in the periphery.

LV failure: In HF due to left ventricular dysfunction, CO decreases and pulmonary venous pressure increases. When pulmonary capillary pressure exceeds the oncotic pressure of plasma proteins (about 24 mm Hg), fluid extravasates from the capillaries into the interstitial space and alveoli, reducing pulmonary compliance and increasing the work of breathing. Lymphatic drainage increases but cannot compensate for the increase in pulmonary fluid. Marked fluid accumulation in alveoli (pulmonary edema) significantly alters ventilation-perfusion (V/Q) relationships: Deoxygenated pulmonary arterial blood passes through poorly ventilated alveoli, decreasing systemic arterial oxygenation (Pao_2) and causing dyspnea. However, dyspnea may occur before V/Q abnormalities, probably because of elevated pulmonary venous pressure and increased work of breathing; the precise mechanism is unclear.

In severe or chronic LV failure, pleural effusions characteristically develop, further aggravating dyspnea. Minute ventilation increases; thus, $Paco_2$ decreases and blood pH increases (respiratory alkalosis). Marked interstitial edema of the small airways may interfere with ventilation, elevating $Paco_2$—a sign of impending respiratory failure.

RV failure: In HF due to right ventricular dysfunction, systemic venous pressure increases, causing fluid extravasation and consequent edema, primarily in dependent tissues (feet and ankles of ambulatory patients) and abdominal viscera. The liver is most severely affected, but the stomach and intestine also become congested; fluid accumulation in the peritoneal cavity (ascites) can occur. RV failure commonly causes moderate hepatic dysfunction, with usually modest increases in conjugated and unconjugated bilirubin, PT, and hepatic enzymes (particularly alkaline phosphatase and gamma-glutamyl transpeptidase [GGT]). The impaired liver breaks down less aldosterone, further contributing to fluid accumulation. Chronic venous congestion in the viscera can cause anorexia, malabsorption of nutrients and drugs, protein-losing enteropathy (characterized by diarrhea and marked hypoalbuminemia), chronic GI blood loss, and rarely ischemic bowel infarction.

Cardiac response: In HFrEF, left ventricular systolic function is grossly impaired; therefore, a higher preload is required to maintain CO. As a result, the ventricles are remodeled over time: The LV becomes less ovoid and more spherical, dilates, and hypertrophies; the RV dilates and may hypertrophy. Initially compensatory, these changes eventually increase diastolic stiffness and wall tension (ie, diastolic dysfunction develops), compromising cardiac performance, especially during physical stress. Increased wall stress raises oxygen demand and accelerates apoptosis (programmed cell death) of myocardial cells. Dilation of the ventricles can also cause mitral or tricuspid valve regurgitation (due to annular dilation) with further increases in end-diastolic volumes.

Hemodynamic responses: With reduced CO, oxygen delivery to the tissues is maintained by increasing oxygen extraction from the blood and sometimes shifting the oxyhemoglobin dissociation curve (see Fig. 50–4 on p. 397) to the right to favor oxygen release.

Reduced CO with lower systemic blood pressure activates arterial baroreflexes, increasing sympathetic tone and decreasing parasympathetic tone. As a result, heart rate and myocardial contractility increase, arterioles in selected vascular beds constrict, venoconstriction occurs, and sodium and water are retained. These changes compensate for reduced ventricular performance and help maintain hemodynamic homeostasis in the early stages of HF. However, these compensatory changes increase cardiac work, preload, and afterload; reduce coronary and renal perfusion; cause fluid accumulation resulting in congestion; increase potassium excretion; and may cause cardiomyocyte necrosis and arrhythmias.

Renal responses: As cardiac function deteriorates, renal blood flow decreases (due to low CO). In addition, renal venous pressures increase, leading to renal venous congestion. These changes both result in a decrease in GFR, and blood flow within the kidneys is redistributed. The filtration fraction and filtered sodium decrease, but tubular resorption increases, leading to sodium and water retention. Blood flow is further redistributed away from the kidneys during exercise, but renal blood flow improves during rest.

Decreased perfusion of the kidneys (and possibly decreased arterial systolic stretch secondary to declining ventricular function) activates the renin-angiotensin-aldosterone system (RAAS), increasing sodium and water retention and renal and peripheral vascular tone. These effects are amplified by the intense sympathetic activation accompanying HF.

The renin-angiotensin-aldosterone-vasopressin (antidiuretic hormone [ADH]) system causes a cascade of potentially deleterious long-term effects. Angiotensin II worsens HF by causing vasoconstriction, including efferent renal vasoconstriction, and by increasing aldosterone production, which enhances sodium reabsorption in the distal nephron and also causes myocardial and vascular collagen deposition and fibrosis. Angiotensin II increases norepinephrine release, stimulates release of vasopressin, and triggers apoptosis. Angiotensin II may be involved in vascular and myocardial hypertrophy, thus contributing to the remodeling of the heart and peripheral vasculature, potentially worsening HF. Aldosterone can be synthesized in the heart and vasculature independently of angiotensin II (perhaps mediated by corticotropin, nitric oxide, free radicals, and other stimuli) and may have deleterious effects in these organs.

HF that causes progressive renal dysfunction (including that renal dysfunction caused by drugs used to treat HF) contributes to worsening HF and has been termed the cardiorenal syndrome.

Neurohumoral responses: In conditions of stress, neurohumoral responses help increase heart function and maintain BP and organ perfusion, but chronic activation of these responses is detrimental to the normal balance between myocardial-stimulating and vasoconstricting hormones and between myocardial-relaxing and vasodilating hormones.

The heart contains many neurohumoral receptors (alpha-1, beta-1, beta-2, beta-3, angiotensin II type 1 [AT_1] and type 2 [AT_2], muscarinic, endothelin, serotonin, adenosine, cytokine, natriuretic peptides); the roles of all of these receptors are not yet fully defined. In patients with HF, beta-1 receptors (which constitute 70% of cardiac beta receptors) are downregulated, probably in response to intense sympathetic activation. The result of downregulation is impaired myocyte contractility and increased heart rate.

Plasma norepinephrine levels are increased, largely reflecting sympathetic nerve stimulation as plasma epinephrine levels are not increased. Detrimental effects include vasoconstriction with increased preload and afterload, direct myocardial damage including apoptosis, reduced renal blood flow, and activation of other neurohumoral systems, including the renin-angiotensin-aldosterone-vasopressin system.

Vasopressin is released in response to a fall in BP via various neurohormonal stimuli. Increased vasopressin decreases renal excretion of free water, possibly contributing to hyponatremia in HF. Vasopressin levels in patients with HF and normal BP vary.

Atrial natriuretic peptide is released in response to increased atrial volume and pressure; brain (B-type) natriuretic peptide (BNP) is released from the ventricle in response to ventricular stretching. These peptides enhance renal excretion of sodium, but in patients with HF, the effect is blunted by decreased renal perfusion pressure, receptor downregulation, and perhaps enhanced enzymatic degradation. In addition, elevated levels of natriuretic peptides exert a counter-regulatory effect on the RAAS and catecholamine stimulation.

Because endothelial dysfunction occurs in HF, fewer endogenous vasodilators (eg, nitric oxide, prostaglandins) are produced, and more endogenous vasoconstrictors (eg, endothelin) are produced, thus increasing afterload.

The failing heart and other organs produce tumor necrosis factor (TNF) alpha. This cytokine increases catabolism and is possibly responsible for cardiac cachexia (loss of lean tissue ≥ 10%), which may accompany severely symptomatic HF, and for other detrimental changes. The failing heart also undergoes metabolic changes with increased free fatty acid utilization and decreased glucose utilization; these changes may become therapeutic targets.

Changes with aging: Age-related changes in the heart and cardiovascular system lower the threshold for expression of HF. Interstitial collagen within the myocardium increases, the myocardium stiffens, and myocardial relaxation is prolonged. These changes lead to a significant reduction in diastolic left ventricular function, even in healthy elderly people. Modest decline in systolic function also occurs with aging. An age-related decrease in myocardial and vascular responsiveness to beta-adrenergic stimulation further impairs the ability of the cardiovascular system to respond to increased work demands.

As a result of these changes, peak exercise capacity decreases significantly (about 8%/decade after age 30), and CO at peak exercise decreases more modestly. This decline can be slowed by regular physical exercise. Thus, elderly patients are more prone than are younger ones to develop HF symptoms in response to the stress of systemic disorders or relatively modest cardiovascular insults. Stressors include infections (particularly pneumonia), hyperthyroidism, anemia, hypertension, myocardial ischemia, hypoxia, hyperthermia, renal failure, perioperative IV fluid loads, nonadherence to drug regimens or to low-salt diets, and use of certain drugs (particularly NSAIDs).

Table 83–1. CAUSES OF HEART FAILURE

TYPE	EXAMPLES
Cardiac	
Myocardial damage	Myocardial infarction Myocarditis Cardiomyopathy Some chemotherapy drugs
Valvular disorders	Aortic stenosis Mitral regurgitation
Arrhythmias	Bradyarrhythmias Tachyarrhythmias
Conduction defects	AV node block Left bundle branch block
Reduced substrate availability (eg, of free fatty acids or glucose)	Ischemia
Infiltrative or matrix disorders	Amyloidosis Chronic fibrosis (eg, systemic sclerosis) Hemochromatosis
Systemic	
Disorders that increase demand for CO	Anemia Hyperthyroidism Paget disease
Disorders that increase resistance to output (afterload)	Aortic stenosis Hypertension

AV = atrioventricular; CO = cardiac output.

Etiology

Both cardiac and systemic factors can impair cardiac performance and cause or aggravate HF (see Table 83–1).

Classification

The most common classification of HF currently in use stratifies patients into

- HF with reduced ejection fraction ("systolic HF")
- HF with preserved ejection fraction ("diastolic HF")

HFrEF is defined as HF with LVEF ≤ 40%. HFpEF is defined as HF with LVEF ≥ 50%. Patients with LVEF between 40% and 50% are in an intermediate zone, and have recently been categorized as HF with mid-range EF (HFmrEF).[1]

The traditional distinction between left and right ventricular failure is somewhat misleading because the heart is an integrated pump, and changes in one chamber ultimately affect the whole heart. However, these terms indicate the major site of pathology leading to HF and can be useful for initial evaluation and treatment. Other common descriptive terms include acute or chronic; high output or low output; dilated or nondilated; and ischemic, hypertensive, or idiopathic dilated cardiomyopathy. Treatment differs based on whether the presentation is acute or chronic HF.

LV failure characteristically develops in ischemic heart disease, hypertension, mitral regurgitation, aortic regurgitation, aortic stenosis, most forms of cardiomyopathy, and congenital heart disorders (eg, ventricular septal defect, patent ductus arteriosus with large shunts).

RV failure is most commonly caused by previous LV failure (which increases pulmonary venous pressure and leads to pulmonary hypertension, thus overloading the RV) or by a severe lung disorder (in which case it is called cor pulmonale). Other causes are multiple pulmonary emboli, RV infarction, pulmonary arterial hypertension, tricuspid regurgitation, tricuspid stenosis, mitral stenosis, pulmonary artery stenosis, pulmonic valve stenosis, pulmonary venous occlusive disease, arrhythmogenic RV cardiomyopathy, or congenital disorders such as Ebstein anomaly or Eisenmenger syndrome. Some conditions mimic RV failure, except cardiac function may be normal; they include volume overload and increased systemic venous pressure in polycythemia or overtransfusion, acute kidney injury with retention of sodium and water, obstruction of either vena cava, and hypoproteinemia due to any cause resulting in low plasma oncotic pressure and peripheral edema.

Biventricular failure results from disorders that affect the whole myocardium (eg, viral myocarditis, amyloidosis, Chagas disease) or long-standing LV failure causing RV failure.

High-output HF results from a persistently high CO, which may eventually result in an inability of a normal heart to maintain adequate output. Conditions that may increase CO include severe anemia, end-stage liver disease, beriberi, thyrotoxicosis, advanced Paget disease, arteriovenous fistula, and persistent tachycardia.

Cardiomyopathy is a general term reflecting disease of the myocardium. Most commonly, the term refers to a primary disorder of the ventricular myocardium that is not caused by congenital anatomic defects; valvular, systemic, or pulmonary vascular disorders; isolated pericardial, nodal, or conduction system disorders; or epicardial coronary artery disease (CAD). The term is sometimes used to reflect etiology (eg, ischemic vs hypertensive cardiomyopathy). Cardiomyopathy does not always lead to symptomatic HF. It is often idiopathic and is classified as dilated, congestive, hypertrophic, infiltrative-restrictive, or apical-ballooning cardiomyopathy (also known as takotsubo or stress cardiomyopathy).

1. Yancy CW, Jessup M, Bozkurt B, et al: 2013 ACCF/AHA guideline for the management of heart failure: a report of the American College of Cardiology Foundation/ American Heart Association Task Force on Practice Guidelines. *Circulation* 128:e240–327, 2013.

Symptoms and Signs

Manifestations differ depending on the extent to which the LV and RV are initially affected. Clinical severity varies significantly and is usually classified according to the New York Heart Association (NYHA) system (see Table 83–2); the examples of ordinary activity may be modified for elderly, debilitated patients. Because HF has such a broad range of severity, some experts suggest subdividing NYHA class III into IIIA or IIIB. Class IIIB is typically reserved for those patients who recently had a HF exacerbation. The American College of Cardiology/ American Heart Association has advocated a staging system for HF (A, B, C, or D) to highlight the need for HF prevention.

- A: High risk of HF but no structural or functional cardiac abnormalities or symptoms
- B: Structural or functional cardiac abnormalities but no symptoms of HF
- C: Structural heart disease with symptoms of HF
- D: Refractory HF requiring advanced therapies (eg, mechanical circulatory support, cardiac transplantation) or palliative care

Severe LV failure may cause pulmonary edema or cardiogenic shock.

History: In LV failure, the most common symptoms are dyspnea and fatigue due to increased pulmonary venous pressures, and low CO (at rest or inability to augment CO during exertion). Dyspnea usually occurs during exertion and is relieved by rest. As HF worsens, dyspnea can occur during rest and at night, sometimes causing nocturnal cough. Dyspnea occurring immediately or soon after lying flat and relieved promptly by sitting up (orthopnea) is common as HF advances. In paroxysmal nocturnal dyspnea (PND), dyspnea awakens patients several hours after they lie down and is relieved only after they sit up for 15 to 20 min. In severe HF, periodic cycling of breathing (Cheyne-Stokes respiration—a brief period of increased breathing [hyperpnea] followed by a brief period of no breathing [apnea])—can occur during the day or night; the sudden hyperpneic phase may awaken the patient from sleep. Cheyne-Stokes breathing differs from PND in that the hyperpneic phase is short, lasting only 10 to 15 sec, but the cycle recurs regularly, lasting 30 sec to 2 min. PND is associated with pulmonary congestion, and Cheyne-Stokes respiration with low CO. Sleep-related breathing disorders, such as sleep apnea, are common in HF and may aggravate HF. Severely reduced cerebral blood flow and hypoxemia can cause chronic irritability and impair mental performance.

In RV failure, the most common symptoms are ankle swelling and fatigue. Sometimes patients feel a sensation of fullness in the abdomen or neck. Hepatic congestion can cause right upper quadrant abdominal discomfort, and stomach and intestinal congestion can cause early satiety, anorexia, and abdominal bloating.

Less specific HF symptoms include cool peripheries, postural light-headedness, nocturia, and decreased daytime micturition.

Table 83–2. NEW YORK HEART ASSOCIATION (NYHA) CLASSIFICATION OF HEART FAILURE

NYHA CLASS	DEFINITION	LIMITATION	EXAMPLE
I	Ordinary physical activity does not cause undue fatigue, dyspnea, or palpitations.	None	Can complete any activity requiring ≤ 7 MET: • Carry 11 kg up 8 steps • Carry objects weighing 36 kg • Shovel snow • Spade soil • Ski • Play squash, handball, or basketball • Jog or walk 8 km/h
II	Ordinary physical activity causes fatigue, dyspnea, palpitations, or angina.	Mild	Can complete any activity requiring ≤ 5 MET: • Sexual intercourse without stopping • Garden • Roller skate • Walk 7 km/h on level ground • Climb one flight of stairs at a normal pace without symptoms
III	Comfortable at rest; less than ordinary physical activity causes fatigue, dyspnea, palpitations, or angina.	Moderate	Can complete any activity requiring ≤ 2 MET: • Shower or dress without stopping • Strip and make a bed • Clean windows • Play golf • Walk 4 km/h
IV	Symptoms occur at rest; any physical activity increases discomfort.	Severe	Cannot do or cannot complete any activity requiring ≥ 2 MET; cannot do any of the above activities

MET = metabolic equivalent task.

Skeletal muscle wasting can occur in severe biventricular failure and may reflect some disuse but also increased catabolism associated with increased cytokine production. Significant weight loss (cardiac cachexia) is an ominous sign associated with high mortality.

In the elderly, presenting complaints may be atypical, such as confusion, delirium, falls, sudden functional decline, nocturnal urinary incontinence, or sleep disturbance. Coexisting cognitive impairment and depression may also influence assessment and therapeutic interventions and may be worsened by the HF.

Examination: General examination may detect signs of systemic or cardiac disorders that cause or aggravate HF (eg, anemia, hyperthyroidism, alcoholism, hemochromatosis, atrial fibrillation with rapid rate, mitral regurgitation).

In LV failure, tachycardia and tachypnea may occur. Patients with severe LV failure may appear visibly dyspneic or cyanotic, hypotensive, and confused or agitated because of hypoxia and poor cerebral perfusion. Some of these less specific symptoms (eg, confusion) are more common in the elderly.

Central cyanosis (affecting all of the body, including warm areas such as the tongue and mucous membranes) reflects severe hypoxemia. Peripheral cyanosis of the lips, fingers, and toes reflects low blood flow with increased oxygen extraction. If vigorous massage improves nail bed color, cyanosis may be peripheral; increasing local blood flow does not improve color if cyanosis is central.

Cardiac findings in HFrEF include a diffuse, sustained, and laterally displaced apical impulse; audible and occasionally palpable 3rd (S_3) and 4th (S_4) heart sounds, and an accentuated pulmonic component (P_2) of the 2nd heart sound (S_2). These abnormal heart sounds can also occur in HFpEF. A pansystolic murmur of mitral regurgitation at the apex may occur in either HFrEF or HFpEF. Pulmonary findings include early inspiratory basilar crackles that do not clear with coughing and, if pleural effusion is present, dullness to percussion and diminished breath sounds at the lung base(s).

Signs of RV failure include nontender peripheral pitting edema (digital pressure leaves visible and palpable imprints, sometimes quite deep) in the feet and ankles; an enlarged and sometimes pulsatile liver palpable below the right costal margin; abdominal swelling and ascites; and visible elevation of the jugular venous pressure, sometimes with large *a* or *v* waves that are visible even when the patient is seated or standing (see Fig. 73–1 on p. 583). Large V waves in the jugular veins are usually indicative of significant tricuspid regurgitation which is often present in RV failure. A paradoxical increase in the jugular venous pressure during inspiration (Kussmaul sign) is indicative of right-sided HF and can be seen in RV failure, restrictive cardiomyopathy, constrictive pericarditis, and severe tricuspid regurgitation. In severe cases of HF, peripheral edema can extend to the thighs or even the sacrum, scrotum, lower abdominal wall, and occasionally even higher. Severe edema in multiple areas is termed anasarca. Edema may be asymmetric if patients lie predominantly on one side.

With hepatic congestion, the liver may be palpably enlarged or tender, and hepatojugular or abdominal-jugular reflux may be detected (see p. 582). Precordial palpation may detect the left parasternal lift of RV enlargement, and auscultation may detect the murmur of tricuspid regurgitation or the RV S_3 along the left sternal border; both findings are augmented upon inspiration.

Diagnosis

- Sometimes only clinical evaluation
- Chest x-ray
- Echocardiography, cardiac radionuclide scan, and/or MRI
- Sometimes BNP or N-terminal-pro-BNP (NT-pro-BNP) levels
- ECG and other tests for etiology as needed

Clinical findings (eg, exertional dyspnea or fatigue, orthopnea, edema, tachycardia, pulmonary crackles, S_3, jugular venous distention) suggest HF but are usually not apparent early. Similar symptoms may result from COPD or recurrent pneumonia or may be erroneously attributed to obesity or old age. Suspicion for HF should be high in patients with a history of myocardial infarction, hypertension, or valvular disorders or murmurs and should be moderate in any patient who is elderly or has diabetes.

Chest x-ray, ECG, and an objective test of cardiac function, typically echocardiography, should be done. Blood tests, except for BNP levels, are not used for diagnosis but are useful for identifying cause and systemic effects.

Chest x-ray: Chest x-ray findings suggesting HF include an enlarged cardiac silhouette, pleural effusion, fluid in the major fissure, and horizontal lines in the periphery of lower posterior lung fields (Kerley B lines). These findings reflect chronic elevation of left atrial pressure and chronic thickening of the intralobular septa due to edema. Upper lobe pulmonary venous congestion and interstitial or alveolar edema may also be present. Careful examination of the cardiac silhouette on a lateral projection can identify specific ventricular and atrial chamber enlargement. The x-ray may also suggest alternative diagnoses (eg, COPD, pneumonia, idiopathic pulmonary fibrosis, lung cancer).

ECG: ECG findings are not diagnostic, but an abnormal ECG, especially showing previous myocardial infarction, left ventricular hypertrophy, left bundle branch block, or tachyarrhythmia (eg, rapid atrial fibrillation), increases suspicion for HF and may help identify the cause. An entirely normal ECG is uncommon in chronic HF.

Imaging: Echocardiography can help evaluate chamber dimensions, valve function, LVEF, wall motion abnormalities, LV hypertrophy, diastolic function, pulmonary artery pressure, LV and RV filling pressures, RV function, and pericardial effusion. Intracardiac thrombi, tumors, and calcifications within the heart valves, mitral annulus, and aortic wall abnormalities can be detected. Localized or segmental wall motion abnormalities strongly suggest underlying CAD but can also be present with patchy myocarditis. Doppler or color Doppler echocardiography accurately detects valvular disorders and shunts. The combination of Doppler evaluation of mitral inflow with tissue Doppler imaging of the mitral annulus can help identify and quantify LV diastolic dysfunction and LV filling pressures. Measuring LVEF can distinguish between predominant HFpEF (EF $\geq$ 0.50) and HFrEF (EF $\leq$ 0.40). It is important to re-emphasize that HF can occur with a normal LVEF. Speckle-tracking echocardiography (which is useful in detecting subclinical systolic function and specific patterns of myocardial dysfunction) may become important but currently is available only in specialized centers.

Radionuclide imaging also can help assess systolic and diastolic function, previous MI, and inducible ischemia or myocardial hibernation.

Cardiac MRI provides accurate images of cardiac structures and is becoming more widely available. Cardiac MRI is useful to evaluate the cause of myocardial disease and to detect focal and diffuse myocardial fibrosis. Cardiac amyloidosis, sarcoidosis, hemachromatosis, and myocarditis are causes of HF that can be detected with or suspected by cardiac MRI findings.

Blood tests: Serum BNP levels are often high in HF; this finding may help when clinical findings are unclear or other diagnoses (eg, COPD) need to be excluded. It may be particularly useful for patients with a history of both pulmonary and cardiac disorders. NT-pro-BNP, an inactive moiety created when pro BNP is cleaved, can be used similarly to BNP. However, a normal BNP level does not exclude the diagnosis of HF. In HFpEF, 30% of patients have a BNP level below the commonly used threshold of 100 pg/mL. Obesity, which is becoming an increasingly common comorbidity in HF, is associated with reduced BNP production and increased BNP clearance.

Besides BNP, recommended blood tests include CBC, creatinine, BUN, electrolytes (including magnesium and calcium), glucose, albumin, and liver function tests. Thyroid function tests are recommended for patients with atrial fibrillation and for selected, especially elderly, patients.

Other tests: **Thoracic ultrasonography** is a noninvasive method of detecting pulmonary congestion in patients with HF. Sonographic "comet tail artifact" on thoracic ultrasonography corresponds to the x-ray finding of Kerley B lines.

Coronary angiography or **CT coronary angiography** is indicated when CAD is suspected or the etiology of HF is uncertain. Cardiac catheterization with intracardiac pressure measurements (invasive hemodynamics) may be helpful in the diagnosis of restrictive cardiomyopathies and constrictive pericarditis. Invasive hemodynamic measurements are also very helpful when the diagnosis of HF is equivocal, particularly in patients with HFpEF. In addition, perturbing the cardiovascular system (eg, exercise testing, volume challenge, drug challenges [eg, nitroglycerin, nitroprusside]) can be very helpful during invasive hemodynamic testing to help diagnose HF.

Endocardial biopsy is sometimes done when an infiltrative cardiomyopathy is strongly suspected but cannot be confirmed with noninvasive imaging (eg, cardiac MRI).

Prognosis

Generally, patients with HF have a poor prognosis unless the cause is correctable. Five-year survival after hospitalization for HF is about 35% regardless of the patient's EF. In overt chronic HF, mortality depends on severity of symptoms and ventricular dysfunction and can range from 10 to 40%/yr.

Specific factors that suggest a poor prognosis include hypotension, low ejection fraction, presence of CAD, troponin release, elevation of BUN, reduced GFR, hyponatremia, and poor functional capacity (eg, as tested by a 6-min walk test).

BNP, NTproBNP, and risk scores such as the MAGGIC Risk Score and the Seattle Heart Failure model, are helpful to predict prognosis in HF patients as an overall group, although there is significant variation in survival among individual patients.

HF usually involves gradual deterioration, interrupted by bouts of severe decompensation, and ultimately death, although the time course is being lengthened with modern therapies. However, death can also be sudden and unexpected, without prior worsening of symptoms.

End-of-life care: All patients and family members should be taught about disease progression and the risk of sudden cardiac death. For some patients, improving quality of life is as important as increasing quantity of life. Thus, it is important to determine patients' wishes about resuscitation (eg, endotracheal intubation, CPR) if their condition deteriorates, especially when HF is already severe.

All patients should be reassured that symptoms will be relieved, and they should be encouraged to seek medical attention early if their symptoms change significantly. Involvement of pharmacists, nurses, social workers, and clergy (when desired), who may be part of an interdisciplinary team or disease management program already in place, is particularly important in end-of-life care.

Treatment

- Diet and lifestyle changes
- Treatment of cause
- Drugs (numerous classes)
- Sometimes device therapy (eg, implantable cardioverter-defibrillator [ICD], cardiac resynchronization therapy [CRT], mechanical circulatory support)
- Sometimes cardiac transplantation
- Multidisciplinary care

Immediate inpatient treatment is required for patients with acute or worsening HF due to certain disorders (eg, acute myocardial infarction, atrial fibrillation with a very rapid ventricular rate, severe hypertension, acute valvular regurgitation), as well as for patients with pulmonary edema, severe symptoms, new-onset HF, or HF unresponsive to outpatient treatment. Patients with mild exacerbations of previously diagnosed HF can be treated at home.

The primary goal is to diagnose and to correct or treat the disorder that led to HF.

Short-term goals include relieving symptoms and improving hemodynamics; avoiding hypokalemia, renal dysfunction, and symptomatic hypotension; and correcting neurohumoral activation.

Long-term goals include correcting hypertension, preventing myocardial infarction and atherosclerosis, improving cardiac function, reducing hospitalizations, and improving survival and quality of life.

Treatment involves dietary and lifestyle changes, drugs, devices, and sometimes percutaneous coronary interventions or surgery.

Treatment is tailored to the patient, considering causes, symptoms, and response to drugs, including adverse effects. There are currently several evidence-based therapies for chronic HFrEF.[1] There are fewer evidence-based treatments for chronic HFpEF, acute HF syndromes, and RV failure.[2]

Disease management: General measures, especially patient and caregiver education and diet and lifestyle modifications, are important for all patients with HF.

- Education
- Sodium restriction
- Appropriate weight and fitness levels
- Correction of underlying conditions

Patient and caregiver education are critical to long-term success. The patient and family should be involved in treatment choices. They should be taught the importance of drug adherence, warning signs of an exacerbation, and how to link cause with effect (eg, increased salt in the diet with weight gain or symptoms).

Many centers (eg, specialized outpatient clinics) have integrated health care practitioners from different disciplines (eg, HF nurses, pharmacists, social workers, rehabilitation specialists) into multidisciplinary teams or outpatient HF management programs. These approaches can improve outcomes and reduce hospitalizations and are most effective in the sickest patients.

Dietary sodium restriction helps limit fluid retention. All patients should eliminate salt in cooking and at the table and avoid salted foods; the most severely ill should limit sodium to < 2 g/day by consuming only low-sodium foods.

Monitoring daily morning weight helps detect sodium and water accumulation early. If weight increases > 2 kg over a few days, patients may be able to adjust their diuretic dose themselves, but if weight gain continues or symptoms occur, patients should seek medical attention.

Intensive case management, particularly by monitoring drug adherence and frequency of unscheduled visits to the physician or emergency department and hospitalizations, can identify when intervention is needed. Specialized HF nurses are valuable in education, follow-up, and dosage adjustment according to predefined protocols.

Patients with atherosclerosis or diabetes should strictly follow a diet appropriate for their disorder. Obesity may cause and always aggravates the symptoms of HF; patients should attain a body mass index (BMI) ≤ 30 kg/m^2 (ideally 21 to 25 kg/m^2).

Regular light activity (eg, walking), tailored to symptoms, is generally encouraged. Activity prevents skeletal muscle deconditioning, which worsens functional status; however, activity does not appear to improve survival or decrease hospitalizations. Rest is appropriate during acute exacerbations. Formal exercise cardiac rehabilitation is useful for chronic HFrEF and is likely helpful for patients with HFpEF.

Patients should have annual influenza vaccination because influenza can precipitate HF exacerbations, particularly in the elderly.

If hypertension, persistent tachyarrhythmia, severe anemia, hemochromatosis, uncontrolled diabetes, thyrotoxicosis, beriberi, alcoholism, Chagas disease, or toxoplasmosis is successfully treated, patients may dramatically improve. Significant myocardial ischemia should be treated aggressively; treatment may include revascularization by percutaneous coronary intervention or bypass surgery. Management of extensive ventricular infiltration (eg, in amyloidosis) has improved considerably. Treatment of primary (amyloidogenic light chain [AL]) amyloidosis with chemotherapy, and in some cases, autologous stem cell transplantation, has markedly improved prognosis for these patients.

Drug treatment: Drug treatment of HF involves

- Symptom relief: Diuretics, nitrates, or digoxin
- Long-term management and improved survival: ACE inhibitors, beta-blockers, aldosterone antagonists, angiotensin II receptor blockers (ARBs), or angiotensin receptor/neprilysin inhibitors (ARNIs)

(For details on the specific drugs and classes, see Drugs for Heart Failure on p. 720).

In **HFrEF**, all these drug classes have been studied and have shown benefit for long-term management .

In **HFpEF**, fewer drugs have been adequately studied. However, ACE inhibitors, ARBs, and beta-blockers are generally used to treat HFpEF. ARNIs are currently being studied. Randomized, controlled trials suggest aldosterone antagonists are beneficial, but nitrates probably are not. In patients with severe HFpEF, lowering the heart rate (eg, with a beta-blocker) can exacerbate symptoms because they have a relatively fixed stroke volume due to severe diastolic dysfunction. In these patients, CO is heart rate dependent and lowering heart rate can thus lower CO at rest and/or with exertion.

In patients with hypertrophic cardiomyopathy, digoxin is not effective and may be harmful.

All patients should be given clear and explicit information about their drugs, including the importance of timely prescription renewal and adherence to therapy, how to recognize adverse effects, and when to contact their physician.

Arrhythmias: It is important to identify and treat the cause of an arrhythmia.

- Electrolytes are normalized.
- Atrial and ventricular rates are controlled.
- Sometimes antiarrhythmic drugs are given.

Sinus tachycardia, a common compensatory change in HF, usually subsides when HF treatment is effective. If it does not, associated causes (eg, hyperthyroidism, pulmonary emboli, fever, anemia, pain) should be sought. If sinus tachycardia persists despite correction of causes, a beta-blocker, given in gradually increasing doses, may help selected patients. However, lowering heart rate with a beta-blocker can be detrimental to patients with advanced HFpEF (eg, restrictive cardiomyopathy), in whom stroke volume is fixed because of severe diastolic dysfunction. In these patients, CO is heart rate dependent and lowering heart rate can thus lower CO at rest and/or with exertion .

Atrial fibrillation with an uncontrolled ventricular rate must be treated; the target resting ventricular rate is typically < 80 beats/min. Beta-blockers are the treatment of choice, although rate-limiting calcium channel blockers may be used cautiously if systolic function is preserved. Adding digoxin, low-dose amiodarone, or other rhythm and/or rate controlling drugs may help some patients. Routine conversion to and maintenance of sinus rhythm has not been shown to be superior to rate control alone in large clinical trials. However, it is best to make this determination on a case-by-case basis because some patients improve significantly with restoration of normal sinus rhythm. If rapid atrial fibrillation does not respond to drugs, permanent pacemaker insertion with complete or partial ablation of the atrioventricular node, or other atrial fibrillation ablation procedures, may be considered in selected patients to restore a sinus or regular rhythm.

Isolated ventricular premature beats, which are common in HF, do not require specific treatment, although rarely very frequent ventricular premature beats (> 15,000/day) have been shown to precipitate HF. However, optimization of HF treatments and correction of electrolyte abnormalities (especially potassium and magnesium) reduce the risk of ventricular arrhythmias.

Sustained ventricular tachycardia that persists despite correction of cause (eg, low potassium or magnesium, ischemia) and optimal medical treatment of HF may require an antiarrhythmic drug. Amiodarone, beta-blockers, and dofetilide are the drugs of choice because other antiarrhythmics have adverse proarrhythmic effects when LV systolic dysfunction is present. Because amiodarone increases digoxin and warfarin levels, digoxin and/or warfarin doses should be decreased by half or stopped. Serum digoxin level and INR level should be routinely monitored. However, drug toxicity can occur even at therapeutic levels. Because long-term use of amiodarone can cause adverse effects, a low dose (200 mg po once/day) is used when possible; blood tests for liver function and thyroid-stimulating hormone are done every 6 mo. If chest x-ray is abnormal or dyspnea worsens significantly, chest x-ray and pulmonary function tests are done yearly to check for pulmonary fibrosis. For sustained ventricular arrhythmias, amiodarone may be required; to reduce risk of sudden death, a loading dose of 400 to 800 mg po bid is given for 1 to 3 wk until rhythm control is adequate, then dose is decreased over 1 mo to a maintenance dose of 200 mg po once/day.

Device therapy: Use of an ICD or CRT is appropriate for some patients.

An **ICD** is recommended for patients with an otherwise good life expectancy if they have symptomatic sustained ventricular tachycardia or ventricular fibrillation or if they remain symptomatic and have an LVEF persistently < 0.30 while receiving guideline-directed medical therapy. The data for ICD use in HFrEF are stronger for ischemic cardiomyopathy than in nonischemic cardiomyopathy.

CRT may relieve symptoms and reduce HF hospitalizations for patients who have HF, LVEF < 0.35, and a widened QRS complex with a left bundle branch block pattern (> 0.15 sec—the wider the QRS, the greater potential benefit). CRT devices are effective but expensive, and patients should be appropriately selected. Many CRT devices also incorporate an ICD in their mechanism.

An implantable device that remotely monitors invasive hemodynamics (eg, pulmonary artery pressure) may help guide HF management in highly selected patients. For example, drug (eg, diuretic) titration based on readings from one of these devices was associated with a marked reduction in HF hospitalization in one clinical trial that included patients with both HFrEF and HFpEF. The device uses the pulmonary artery diastolic pressure as a surrogate for pulmonary capillary wedge pressure (and hence left atrial pressure) in HF patients. However, it has been evaluated only in NYHA class III patients who had recurrent HF exacerbations. Further evidence will help guide how this technology should be implemented.

Ultrafiltration (venovenous filtration) can be useful in selected hospitalized patients with severe cardiorenal syndrome and volume overload refractory to diuretics. However, ultrafiltration should not be used routinely because clinical trials do not show long-term clinical benefit.

An **intra-aortic counterpulsation balloon pump** is helpful in selected patients with acute HF who have a good chance of recovery (eg, acute HF following myocardial infarction) or in those who need a bridge to a more permanent solution such as cardiac surgery (eg, to fix severe valvular disease or to revascularize multivessel CAD), an LV assist device, or heart transplantation.

LV assist devices are implantable pumps that augment LV output. They are commonly used to maintain patients with severe HF who are awaiting transplantation and are also used as "destination therapy" (ie, as a long-term solution) in some patients who are not transplant candidates.

Surgery: Surgery may be appropriate when certain underlying disorders are present. Surgery in patients with advanced HF should be done in a specialized center.

Surgical closure of congenital or acquired intracardiac shunts can be curative.

Coronary artery bypass grafting (CABG) to reduce ischemia did not improve overall 5 yr survival in a large clinical trial of HF patients with ischemic LV systolic dysfunction; however, CABG was associated with reduced overall 10-yr mortality and with reduced 10-yr mortality and hospitalizations due to cardiovascular causes. Thus, the decision to revascularize a HF patient with multivessel CAD should be made on a case-by-case basis.

If HF is primarily due to a valvular disorder, valve repair or replacement should be considered. Patients with primary mitral regurgitation are more likely to benefit than patients with mitral regurgitation secondary to LV dilation, in whom myocardial function is likely to continue to be poor postoperatively. Surgery is preferably done before myocardial dilation and damage become irreversible.

Heart transplantation is the treatment of choice for patients < 60 who have severe, refractory HF and no other life-threatening conditions and who are highly adherent to management recommendations. Some older patients (about 60 to 70 yrs) with otherwise good health are also typically considered if they meet other criteria for transplantation. Survival is 85 to 90% at 1 yr, and annual mortality thereafter is about 4%/yr; however, mortality rate while waiting for a donor is 12 to 15%. Human organ donation remains low.

Persistent heart failure: After treatment, symptoms often persist. Reasons include persistence of the underlying disorder (eg, hypertension, ischemia/infarction, valvular disease) despite treatment; suboptimal treatment of HF; drug nonadherence; excess intake of dietary sodium or alcohol; and presence of an undiagnosed thyroid disorder, anemia, or supervening arrhythmia (eg, atrial fibrillation with rapid ventricular response, intermittent ventricular tachycardia). Also, drugs used to treat other disorders may interfere with HF treatment. NSAIDs, thiazolidinediones (eg, pioglitazone) for diabetes, and short-acting dihydropyridine or nondihydropyridine calcium channel blockers can worsen HF and should be avoided unless no alternative exists; patients who must take such drugs should be followed closely.

1. Yancy CW, Jessup M, Bozkurt B, et al: 2016 ACC/AHA/HFSA Focused update on new pharmacological therapy for heart failure: An update of the 2013 ACCF/AHA Guideline for the Management of Heart Failure: A report of the American College of Cardiology/American Heart Association Task Force on Clinical Practice Guidelines and the Heart Failure Society of America. *Circulation* 134(13):e282–293, 2016.
2. Shah SJ, Kitzman D, Borlaug B, et al: Phenotype-specific treatment of heart failure With preserved ejection fraction: A multiorgan roadmap. *Circulation* 134(1):73–90, 2016.

KEY POINTS

- HF involves ventricular dysfunction that ultimately leads to the heart not providing tissues with adequate blood for metabolic needs.
- In HF with reduced ejection fraction, the ventricle contracts poorly and empties inadequately; EF is low.
- In HF with preserved ejection fraction, ventricular filling is impaired, resulting in increased end-diastolic pressure at rest and/or during exercise; EF is normal.
- Consider HF in patients with exertional dyspnea or fatigue, orthopnea, and/or edema, particularly in those with a history of myocardial infarction, hypertension, or valvular disorders or murmurs.
- Do chest x-ray, ECG, BNP levels, and an objective test of cardiac function, typically echocardiography.
- Unless adequately treated, HF tends to progress and has a poor prognosis.
- Treatment includes education and lifestyle changes, control of underlying disorders, a variety of drugs, and sometimes implantable devices (CRT, ICDs).

DRUGS FOR HEART FAILURE

Drug treatment of HF involves

- Symptom relief: Diuretics, nitrates, or digoxin
- Long-term management and improved survival: ACE inhibitors, beta-blockers, aldosterone antagonists, ARBs, or ARNIs

Choice of drug depends on the type of HF along with individual patient characteristics. The most common classification of HF currently in use stratifies patients into

- HF with reduced ejection fraction ("systolic HF")
- HF with preserved ejection fraction ("diastolic HF")

In HF with reduced ejection fraction, all these drug classes have been studied and have shown benefit for long-term management.

In HF with preserved ejection fraction, fewer drugs have been adequately studied. However, ACE inhibitors, ARBs, and beta-blockers are generally used to treat HFpEF. ARNIs are currently being studied. Randomized, controlled trials suggest aldosterone antagonists are beneficial, but nitrates probably are not. In patients with severe HFpEF, lowering the heart rate (eg, with a beta-blocker) can exacerbate symptoms because they have a relatively fixed stroke volume due to severe diastolic dysfunction; in these patients, CO is heart rate dependent and lowering heart rate can thus lower CO at rest and/or with exertion.

In patients with hypertrophic cardiomyopathy, digoxin is not effective and may be harmful.

All patients should be given clear and explicit information about their drugs, including the importance of timely prescription renewal and adherence to therapy, how to recognize adverse effects, and when to contact their physician.

Diuretics: Diuretics are given to all patients with HF (regardless of underlying ejection fraction) who have current or previous volume overload; dose is adjusted to the lowest dose that stabilizes weight and relieves symptoms.

Loop diuretics should be used initially for control of volume overload, but their dose should be reduced when possible in favor of aldosterone antagonists.

Commonly used loop diuretics include furosemide, bumetanide, and torsemide. The starting dose of these drugs depends on whether the patient has previously received loop diuretics. Common starting doses are: furosemide 20 to 40 mg po once/day or bid, bumetanide 0.5 to 1.0 mg po once/day, and torsemide 10 to 20 mg po once/day. If needed, loop diuretics can be titrated up to doses of furosemide 120 mg po bid, bumetanide 2 mg po bid, and torsemide 40 mg po bid based on response and renal function. Bumetanide and torsemide have better bioavailability than furosemide. If patients are switched between different loop diuretics, they should be placed on equivalent doses. Furosemide 40 mg is equivalent to bumetanide 1 mg and both are equivalent to torsemide 20 mg.

In refractory cases, IV loop diuretics or metolazone 2.5 to 10 mg po can be used for additive effect. IV infusion of furosemide (5 to 10 mg/hour) or other loop diuretics may be helpful in selected patients with severe edema. A bolus dose of loop diuretic should be given before starting an IV infusion and before each increase in infusion rate.

Loop diuretics (particularly when used with metolazone) may cause hypovolemia with hypotension, hyponatremia, hypomagnesemia, and severe hypokalemia. The dose of diuretic required acutely can usually be gradually reduced; the target is the lowest dose that maintains stable weight and controls symptoms. When HF improves, the diuretic may be stopped if other drugs improve heart function and relieve HF symptoms. Using larger than required doses of diuretics lowers CO, impairs renal function, causes hypokalemia, and increases mortality. Serum electrolytes and renal function are monitored, initially daily (when diuretics are given IV) and subsequently as needed, particularly after a dose increase.

An **aldosterone antagonist,** either spironolactone or eplerenone, should be added early to offset the potassium-losing effects of higher-dose loop diuretics. Hyperkalemia may result, especially when ACE inhibitors or ARBs are also taken, so electrolytes must still be monitored, especially during a dehydrating illness that could cause renal dysfunction. These drugs may have particular benefit in chronic right ventricular failure, in which hepatic congestion results in elevated aldosterone levels as aldosterone metabolism is reduced. To reduce the risk of hyperkalemia, aldosterone antagonists should generally be given only to patients whose potassium level is < 5.0 mEq/L, serum creatinine is < 2.5 mg/dL, and GFR is > 30 ml/min/1.73 m^2. Furthermore, it should be noted that the equivalent dose of eplerenone is twice that of spironolactone (ie, spironolactone 25 mg = eplerenone 50 mg).

Thiazide diuretics are not normally used alone unless being given as treatment of hypertension; however, a thiazide diuretic may be added to a loop diuretic for additional diuresis and to reduce the loop diuretic dose. Hydrochlorothiazide, metolazone, and chlorthalidone can be used in this manner.

Reliable patients are taught to take additional diuretic doses as needed when weight or peripheral edema increases. They should seek medical attention promptly if weight gain persists.

Vasopressin (antidiuretic hormone) receptor antagonists are not frequently used though they may be helpful in cases of severe refractory hyponatremia in patients with HF.

ACE inhibitors: All **patients with HFrEF** should be given oral ACE inhibitors unless contraindicated (eg, by plasma creatinine > 2.8 mg/dL [> 250 μmol/L], bilateral renal artery stenosis, renal artery stenosis in a solitary kidney, or previous angioedema due to ACE inhibitors).

ACE inhibitors reduce production of angiotensin II and breakdown of bradykinin, mediators that affect the sympathetic nervous system, endothelial function, vascular tone, and myocardial performance. Hemodynamic effects include arterial and venous vasodilation, sustained decreases in LV filling pressure during rest and exercise, decreased systemic vascular resistance, and favorable effects on ventricular remodeling. ACE inhibitors prolong survival and reduce HF hospitalizations. For patients with atherosclerosis and a vascular disorder, these drugs reduce the risk of myocardial infarction and stroke. For patients with diabetes, they delay onset of nephropathy. Thus, ACE inhibitors may be used in patients with diastolic dysfunction and any of these disorders.

The starting dose typically should be low (usually one fourth to one half of the target dose depending on BP and renal function); the dose is gradually adjusted upward over 8 wk as tolerated, then continued indefinitely. Usual target doses of representative drugs include enalapril 10 to 20 mg bid, lisinopril 20 to 30 mg once/day, and ramipril 5 mg bid; there are many others.

If the hypotensive effect (more marked in patients with hyponatremia or volume depletion) is troublesome, it can often be minimized by separating administration of other BP-lowering drugs, reducing the dose of concomitant diuretics, using a longer acting ACE inhibitor (eg, perindopril), or giving the dose at bedtime. ACE inhibitors often cause mild to moderate reversible serum creatinine elevation due to vasodilation of the efferent glomerular arteriole. An initial 20 to 30% increase in creatinine is no reason to stop the drug but does require closer monitoring, slower increases in dose, reduction in diuretic dose, or avoidance of NSAIDs. Because aldosterone's effect is reduced, potassium retention may result, especially in patients receiving potassium supplements. Cough occurs in 5 to 15% of patients, probably because bradykinin accumulates, but other causes of cough should also be considered. Occasionally, rash or dysgeusia occurs. Angioedema is rare but can be life threatening and is a contraindication to ACE inhibitors. Alternatively, ARBs can be used, although rarely cross-reactivity is reported. Both are contraindicated in pregnancy.

Serum electrolytes and renal function should be measured before an ACE inhibitor is started, at 1 mo, and after each significant increase in dose or change in clinical condition. If dehydration or poor renal function due to acute illness develops, the ACE inhibitor dose may need to be reduced or the drug may be temporarily stopped.

In **HFpEF,** a randomized controlled trial of the ACE inhibitor perindopril demonstrated improved exercise capacity. It did not improve survival, although there was a high rate of crossover from placebo to ACE inhibitor in this trial.[1] Given the very high prevalence of hypertension in HFpEF, it is reasonable to use an ACE inhibitor to control hypertension in these patients as these drugs may have secondary beneficial effects on exercise capacity in these patients.

Angiotensin II receptor blockers (ARBs): These drugs are not demonstrably superior to ACE inhibitors but are less likely to cause cough and angioedema; they may be used when these adverse effects prohibit ACE inhibitor use.

In **chronic HFrEF,** ACE inhibitors and ARBs are likely equally effective. Usual oral target doses are valsartan 160 mg bid, candesartan 32 mg once/day, and losartan 50 to 100 mg once/day. Introduction, upward titration, and monitoring of ARBs and ACE inhibitors are similar. Like ACE inhibitors, ARBs can cause reversible renal dysfunction, and the dose may need to be reduced or stopped temporarily during an acute dehydrating illness.

Adding an ARB to a regimen of an ACE inhibitor, beta-blocker, and aldosterone antagonist is unlikely to be helpful and should be avoided given the risk of hyperkalemia. If a patient who is taking an ACE inhibitor or ARB is still symptomatic, an aldosterone antagonist should be started and/or an ARNI should be used.

In **HFpEF,** a large randomized controlled trial of candesartan[2] demonstrated reduced number of hospitalizations for recurrent HF; however, hospitalization was a secondary endpoint. In another trial,[3] irbesartan was not associated with any improvement in outcomes in HFpEF. Therefore, ARBs should be used in HFpEF only if they are already being used to treat hypertension, diabetic kidney disease, or microalbuminuria.

ARBs are contraindicated in pregnancy.

Angiotensin receptor/neprilysin inhibitor (ARNI): ARNIs are a new combination drug for the treatment of HF. They include an ARB and a new class of drug, neprilysin inhibitors (sacubitril is the only member currently available). Neprilysin is an enzyme involved in the breakdown of vasoactive substances such as BNP and other peptides. By inhibiting the breakdown of BNP and other beneficial vasoactive peptides, these drugs lower blood pressure, decrease afterload, and enhance natriuresis. Because neprilysin inhibitors increase BNP levels, NTproBNP levels (which are not increased by the drug) should be used instead to help diagnose and manage HF.

A large randomized, controlled trial[4] recently compared sacubitril/valsartan to enalapril in patients with NYHA class II through IV HFrEF. Sacubitril/valsartan reduced the primary endpoints of combined cardiovascular mortality or hospitalizations for HF; the number needed to treat was 21. Sacubitril/valsartan also reduced all-cause mortality. Thus, the ARNI sacubitril/valsartan should be considered in all patients with stable HFrEF, particularly those with NYHA class II or III symptoms on optimal guideline-directed medical therapy.

There are 3 strengths of sacubitril/valsartan: 24/26 mg, 49/51 mg, and 97/103 mg, all are taken po twice/day. The starting dose is 49/51 mg po bid for patients previously taking an ACE inhibitor or ARB, and 24/26 mg for patients previously taking a low dose of an ACE inhibitor or ARB (eg, ≤ 10 mg enalapril daily) or in those patients who are ACE inhibitor/ARB naive or who have low/borderline blood pressure. ACE inhibitors must be discontinued 36 h before initiation of sacubitril/valsartan. Patients previously taking an ARB can simply switch to sacubitril/valsartan without a washout period.

Complications associated with use of ARNI include hypotension, hyperkalemia, renal insufficiency, and angioedema. Sacubitril must be coupled with valsartan (an ARB) because of the increased risk of angioedema with the use of sacubitril alone or in combination with an ACE inhibitor. For this reason, combined ACE/ARNI therapy is absolutely contraindicated.

In **HFpEF**, a phase 2 trial showed that the ARNI valsartan/sacubitril reduced NTproBNP levels at 12 wk and left atrial volume at 36 wk; a large randomized controlled phase 3 trial of this drug is ongoing and should determine whether it improves outcomes in HFpEF.

Aldosterone antagonists: Because aldosterone can be produced independently of the renin-angiotensin system, its adverse effects are not inhibited completely even by maximal use of ACE inhibitors and ARBs. Thus, the aldosterone antagonists (also termed mineralocorticoid receptor antagonists) are often used, particularly for patients with moderate to severe symptoms or signs of HF. Typical drugs include spironolactone 25 to 50 mg po once/day and eplerenone 25 to 100 mg po once/day (does not cause gynecomastia in males). Aldosterone antagonists can reduce mortality, including from sudden death, in patients with LVEF < 30% and chronic HF, or acute HF complicating acute myocardial infarction.

Potassium supplements should be stopped. Serum potassium and creatinine should be checked every 1 to 2 wk for the first 4 to 6 wk and after dose changes. Dose is lowered if potassium is between 5.0 and 5.5 mEq/L and stopped if potassium is > 5.5 mEq/L, if creatinine increases above 2.5 mg/dL (220 μmol/L), or if ECG changes of hyperkalemia are present. Aldosterone antagonists should not be used in patients receiving both an ACE inhibitor and an ARB because of the high risk of hyperkalemia and renal dysfunction.

In **patients with HFrEF,** an aldosterone antagonist plus either an ACE inhibitor or ARB is preferred over the combination of an ACE inhibitor and ARB.

In **patients with HFpEF**, spironolactone reduces hospitalization for HF and likely reduces cardiovascular mortality.[5] Thus, aldosterone antagonists should be used in patients with HFpEF, particularly if they are volume overloaded and/or have a history of HF hospitalization. Loop diuretics can be minimized if necessary to accommodate the use of aldosterone antagonists.

Beta-blockers: In **patients with HFrEF,** beta-blockers, unless otherwise contraindicated (by asthma, 2nd- or 3rd-degree atrioventricular block, or previous significant intolerance), are critical for the treatment, and an important addition to ACE inhibitors in these patients. In HFrEF, beta-blockers are best started when the patient has no evidence of pulmonary congestion. Specific beta-blockers such as carvedilol and metoprolol succinate (ie, long-acting metoprolol) improve LVEF, survival, and other major cardiovascular outcomes in patients with chronic HFrEF, including those with severe symptoms.

In **patients with HFpEF,** beta-blockers have not been adequately tested in clinical trials , but large registries have shown that beta-blocker use is associated with improved outcomes in HFpEF despite the relatively high prevalence of chronotropic incompetence in HFpEF.

The starting dose should be low (one fourth of the target daily dose), then the dose is gradually increased over 8 wk as tolerated. The acute negative inotropic effects of beta-blockade may initially cause cardiac depression and fluid retention. In such cases, a temporary increase in diuretic dose and slower upward titration of the beta-blocker dose is warranted. Tolerance may improve over time, and efforts should be made to reach target doses. Usual oral target doses are carvedilol 25 mg bid (50 mg bid for patients ≥ 85 kg), bisoprolol 10 mg once/day, and metoprolol 50 to 75 mg bid (tartrate) or 200 mg once/day (succinate extended-release). Carvedilol, a 3rd-generation nonselective beta-blocker, is also a vasodilator with alpha-blocking and antioxidant effects; it is the preferred and most widely studied beta-blocker but is more expensive in many countries. Some beta-blockers (eg, bucindolol, xamoterol) do not appear beneficial and may be harmful.

During a severe, acute decompensation, beta-blockers should not be started until patients are stabilized and have little evidence of fluid retention. For HFrEF patients with acute HF exacerbation already taking a beta-blocker, the dose should not be decreased or stopped unless absolutely necessary. Often the beta-blocker dose can be continued in patients with an acute HF exacerbation if the diuretic dose is temporarily increased.

In **HFrEF,** after initial treatment, heart rate and myocardial oxygen consumption decrease, and stroke volume and filling pressure are unchanged. With the slower heart rate, diastolic function improves. Ventricular filling returns to a more normal pattern (increasing in early diastole), which appears less restrictive. Improved myocardial function is measurable in some patients after 6 to 12 mo but may take longer; EF and CO increase, and LV filling pressure decreases. Exercise capacity improves.

Vasodilators: Hydralazine plus isosorbide dinitrate may help patients truly intolerant of ACE inhibitors or ARBs (usually because of significant renal dysfunction), although long-term benefit of this combination is limited. In black patients, when added to standard therapy, this combination has been shown to reduce mortality and hospitalization, and improve quality of life. As vasodilators, these drugs improve hemodynamics, reduce valvular regurgitation, and increase exercise capacity without causing significant renal impairment.

Hydralazine is started at 25 mg po qid and increased every 3 to 5 days to a target total dose of 300 mg/day, although many patients cannot tolerate > 200 mg/day because of hypotension. Isosorbide dinitrate is started at 20 mg po tid (with a 12-h nitrate-free interval) and increased to a target of 40 to 50 mg tid. Whether lower doses (frequently used in clinical practice) provide long-term benefit is unknown. In general, vasodilators have been replaced by ACE inhibitors, which are easier to use, are usually better tolerated, and have greater proven benefit.

Nitrates alone can relieve HF symptoms in patients with HFrEF; patients can be taught to use sublingual nitroglycerin spray as needed for acute dyspnea and a transdermal patch for nocturnal or exertional dyspnea. In HFrEF, nitrates are safe, effective, and well tolerated and are particularly helpful in patients with HF and angina. Adverse effects include hypotension and headache. Isosorbide mononitrate has been tested in HFpEF,[6] where it was shown to be associated with increased adverse effects (eg, headache) and reduced physical activity. Thus, routine use of long-acting nitrates should be avoided in HFpEF.

Other vasodilators such as calcium channel blockers are not used to treat LV systolic dysfunction. Short-acting dihydropyridines (eg, nifedipine) and nondihydropyridines (eg, diltiazem, verapamil) may be deleterious. However, amlodipine and felodipine are better tolerated and may be useful for patients with HF and associated angina or hypertension. Both drugs may cause peripheral edema; rarely, amlodipine causes pulmonary edema. Felodipine should not be taken with grapefruit juice, which significantly increases plasma levels and adverse effects by inhibiting cytochrome P-450 metabolism. In patients with HFpEF, dihydropyridine calcium channel blockers such as amlodipine may be used as needed to treat hypertension or ischemia; nondihydropyridines such as diltiazem or verapamil may be used to control ventricular rate in atrial fibrillation. Verapamil is often used in hypertrophic cardiomyopathy.

Digoxin: Digoxin inhibits the sodium-potassium pump (Na^+, K^+-ATPase). As a result, it causes weak positive inotropy, reduces sympathetic activity, blocks the atrioventricular node (slowing the ventricular rate in atrial fibrillation or prolonging the PR interval in sinus rhythm), reduces vasoconstriction, and improves renal blood flow. Digoxin is excreted by the kidneys; elimination half-life is 36 to 40 h in patients with normal renal function.

Digoxin has no proven survival benefit but, when used with diuretics and an ACE inhibitor, may help control symptoms and reduce the likelihood of hospitalization in patients with HFrEF. However, because of the availability of a large number of evidence-based treatments for HFrEF, digoxin use has dropped significantly and is reserved for patients with significant symptoms despite optimal treatment with other mortality lowering medications. Digoxin should not be used in HFpEF unless it is being used to control heart rate in concomitant atrial fibrillation or to augment RV function in patients with RV failure. Digoxin is most effective in patients with large LV end-diastolic volumes and an S_3. Acute withdrawal of digoxin may increase the hospitalization rate and worsen symptoms.

In patients with normal renal function, digoxin, 0.125 to 0.25 mg po once/day depending on age, sex, and body size, achieves full digitalization in about 1 wk (5 half-lives). More rapid digitalization can be achieved with digoxin 0.5 mg IV over 15 min followed by 0.25 mg IV at 8 and 16 h or with 0.5 mg po followed by 0.25 mg po at 8, 16, and 24 h. Prescription patterns vary widely by physician and by country, but in general, doses are lower than those used in the past, and a trough (8- to 12-h post-dose) digoxin level of 0.8 to 1.2 ng/mL is preferable. In addition, unlike in the treatment of atrial fibrillation, there is typically little reason to rapidly digitalize (ie, digoxin load) patients with HF. Thus, simply starting digoxin at 0.125 mg po once/day (in patients with normal renal function) or digoxin 0.125 mg po every Monday, Wednesday, and Friday (in patients with abnormal renal function) is sufficient in patients with HF.

Digoxin toxicity is a concern, especially in patients with renal dysfunction and perhaps in women. These patients may need a lower oral dose, as may elderly patients, patients with a low lean body mass, and patients also taking amiodarone. Digoxin has a narrow therapeutic window. The most important toxic effects are life-threatening arrhythmias (eg, ventricular fibrillation, ventricular tachycardia, complete atrioventricular block). Bidirectional ventricular tachycardia, nonparoxysmal junctional tachycardia in the presence of atrial fibrillation, and hyperkalemia are serious signs of digitalis toxicity. Nausea, vomiting, anorexia, diarrhea, confusion, amblyopia, and, rarely, xerophthalmia may occur. If hypokalemia or hypomagnesemia (often due to diuretic use) is present, lower doses and serum levels can still cause toxicity. Electrolyte levels should be monitored in patients taking diuretics and digoxin, so that abnormalities can be prevented if possible; potassium-sparing diuretics may be helpful.

When digoxin toxicity occurs, the drug should be stopped; electrolyte abnormalities should be corrected (IV if abnormalities are severe and toxicity is acute). Patients with severe toxicity are admitted to a monitored unit, and digoxin immune Fab (ovine antidigoxin antibody fragments) is given if arrhythmias are present or if significant overingestion is accompanied by a serum potassium of > 5 mEq/L. Digoxin immune Fab is also useful for glycoside toxicity due to plant ingestion. Dose is based on the steady-state serum digoxin level or total amount ingested. Ventricular arrhythmias are treated with lidocaine or phenytoin. Atrioventricular block with a slow ventricular rate may require a temporary transvenous pacemaker. Isoproterenol is contraindicated because it increases risk of ventricular arrhythmia.

Other drugs: Ivabradine is an inward "funny" (I_f) channel blocker that acts at the AV node to slow the heart rate. It is currently approved for use in HFrEF patients who have symptomatic HF, normal sinus rhythm, and heart rate > 70 beats/minute despite guideline-directed medical therapy (which should include beta-blockers). Typically, patients who may benefit from ivabradine are those with HFrEF who have NYHA class II or class III symptoms and heart rate > 70 beats/min who are at target beta-blocker dose or cannot tolerate a further increase in beta-blocker dose.

Various positive inotropic drugs have been evaluated in HF but, except for digoxin, they increase mortality risk. These drugs can be grouped as adrenergic mode of action (norepinephrine, epinephrine, dobutamine, dopamine) or nonadrenergic (enoximone, milrinone, levosimendan [calcium sensitizers]). Regular outpatient IV infusions of inotropes (eg, dobutamine) increase mortality and are not recommended. However, outpatient continuous infusions of inotropes such as dobutamine or milrinone can be used for palliative purposes in patients with severe HFrEF.

Anticoagulant drugs may be considered in patients with very large ventricles at risk of mural thrombus.

1. Cleland JG, Tendera M, Adamus J, et al: The perindopril in elderly people with chronic heart failure (PEP-CHF) study. *Eur Heart J* 27:2338–2345, 2006.
2. Yusuf S, Pfeffer MA, Swedberg K, et al: Effects of candesartan in patients with chronic heart failure and preserved left-ventricular ejection fraction: the CHARM-Preserved Trial. *Lancet* 362:777, 2003.
3. Massie BM, Carson PE, McMurray JJ, et al: Irbesartan in patients with heart failure and preserved ejection fraction. *N Engl J Med* 359:2456–2467, 2008.
4. McMurray JJ, Packer M, Desai AS, et al: Angiotensin-neprilysin inhibition versus enalapril in heart failure. *N Engl J Med* 371:993–1004, 2014.
5. Pitt B, Pfeffer MA, Assmann SF, et al: Spironolactone for heart failure with preserved ejection fraction. *N Engl J Med* 370:1383–1392, 2014.
6. Redfield M, Anstrom KJ, Levine JA, et al: Isosorbide mononitrate in heart failure with preserved ejection fraction. *N Engl J Med* 373:2314–2324, 2015.

PULMONARY EDEMA

Pulmonary edema is acute, severe left ventricular failure with pulmonary venous hypertension and alveolar flooding. Findings are severe dyspnea, diaphoresis, wheezing, and sometimes blood-tinged frothy sputum. Diagnosis is clinical and by chest x-ray. Treatment is with oxygen, IV nitrates, diuretics, and sometimes morphine and, in patients with HF and reduced ejection fraction short-term IV positive inotropes , and assisted ventilation (ie, endotracheal intubation with mechanical ventilation or bilevel positive airway pressure ventilation).

If left ventricular filling pressure increases suddenly, plasma fluid moves rapidly from pulmonary capillaries into interstitial spaces and alveoli, causing pulmonary edema. Although precipitating causes vary by age and country, about one half of cases result from acute coronary ischemia; some from decompensation of significant underlying HF, including HF with preserved ejection fraction due to hypertension; and the rest from arrhythmia, an acute valvular disorder, or acute volume overload often due to IV fluids. Drug or dietary nonadherence is often involved.

Symptoms and Signs

Patients present with extreme dyspnea, restlessness, and anxiety with a sense of suffocation. Cough producing blood-tinged sputum, pallor, cyanosis, and marked diaphoresis are common; some patients froth at the mouth. Frank hemoptysis is uncommon. The pulse is rapid and low volume, and BP is variable. Marked hypertension indicates significant cardiac reserve; hypotension with systolic BP < 100 mg Hg is ominous. Inspiratory fine crackles are widely dispersed anteriorly and posteriorly over both lung fields. Marked wheezing (cardiac asthma) may occur. Noisy respiratory efforts often make cardiac auscultation difficult; a summation gallop—merger of 3rd (S_3) and 4th (S_4) heart sounds—may be present. Signs of right ventricular (RV) failure (eg, neck vein distention, peripheral edema) may be present.

Diagnosis

- Clinical evaluation showing severe dyspnea and pulmonary crackles
- Chest x-ray
- Sometimes serum brain natriuretic peptide (BNP) or N-terminal-pro BNP (NT-pro-BNP)
- ECG, cardiac markers, and other tests for etiology as needed

A COPD exacerbation can mimic pulmonary edema due to LV failure or even that due to biventricular failure if cor pulmonale is present. Pulmonary edema may be the presenting symptom in patients without a history of cardiac disorders, but COPD patients with such severe symptoms usually have a history of COPD, although they may be too dyspneic to relate it.

A chest x-ray, done immediately, is usually diagnostic, showing marked interstitial edema. Bedside measurement of serum BNP/NT-proBNP levels (elevated in pulmonary edema; normal in COPD exacerbation) is helpful if the diagnosis is in doubt. ECG, pulse oximetry, and blood tests (cardiac markers, electrolytes, BUN, creatinine and, for severely ill patients, ABGs) are done. Echocardiography may be helpful to determine the cause of the pulmonary edema (eg, myocardial infarction, valvular dysfunction, hypertensive heart disease, dilated cardiomyopathy) and may influence the choice of therapies. Hypoxemia can be severe. Carbon dioxide retention is a late, ominous sign of secondary hypoventilation.

Treatment

- Treatment of cause
- Oxygen
- IV diuretic
- Nitrates
- IV inotropes
- Morphine
- Ventilatory assistance

Initial treatment includes identifying the cause; 100% oxygen by nonrebreather mask; upright position; furosemide 0.5 to 1.0 mg/kg IV or by continuous infusion 5 to 10 mg/h; nitroglycerin 0.4 mg sublingually q 5 min, followed by an IV drip at 10 to 20 mcg/min, titrated upward at 10 mcg/min q 5 min as needed to a maximum 300 mcg/min if systolic BP is > 100 mm Hg. Morphine, 1 to 5 mg IV once or twice, has long been used to reduce severe anxiety and the work of breathing but is decreasingly used due to observational studies suggesting a poorer outcome with its use. Noninvasive ventilatory assistance with bilevel positive airway pressure (BiPAP) is helpful if hypoxia is significant. If CO_2 retention is present or the patient is obtunded, tracheal intubation and mechanical ventilation are required.

Specific additional treatment depends on etiology:

- For acute myocardial infarction or another acute coronary syndrome, thrombolysis or direct percutaneous coronary angioplasty with or without stent placement
- For severe hypertension, an IV vasodilator
- For supraventricular or ventricular tachycardia, direct-current cardioversion
- For rapid atrial fibrillation, cardioversion is preferred. To slow the ventricular rate, an IV beta-blocker, IV digoxin, or cautious use of an IV calcium channel blocker

In patients with acute MI, fluid status before onset of pulmonary edema is usually normal, so diuretics are less useful than in patients with acute decompensation of chronic HF and may precipitate hypotension. If systolic BP falls < 100 mm Hg or shock develops, IV dobutamine and an intra-aortic balloon pump (counterpulsation) may be required.

Some newer drugs, such as IV BNP (nesiritide), and calcium-sensitizing inotropic drugs (levosimendan, pimobendan), vesnarinone, and ibopamine, may have initial beneficial effects but do not appear to improve outcomes compared to standard therapy, and mortality may be increased. Serelaxin, a recombinant form of the human pregnancy hormone relaxin-2, is currently being investigated in a large phase 3 trial in acute HF.

Once patients are stabilized, long-term HF treatment is begun.

KEY POINTS

- Acute pulmonary edema can result from acute coronary ischemia, decompensation of underlying HF, arrhythmia, an acute valvular disorder, or acute volume overload.
- Patients have severe dyspnea, diaphoresis, wheezing, and sometimes blood-tinged frothy sputum.
- Clinical examination and chest x-ray are usually sufficient for diagnosis; ECG, cardiac markers, and sometimes echocardiography are done to identify cause.
- Treat the cause and give oxygen and IV furosemide and/or nitrates as needed; try noninvasive ventilatory assistance initially but use tracheal intubation and assisted ventilation if necessary.

COR PULMONALE

Cor pulmonale is right ventricular enlargement secondary to a lung disorder that causes pulmonary artery hypertension. Right ventricular failure follows. Findings include peripheral edema, neck vein distention, hepatomegaly, and a parasternal lift. Diagnosis is clinical and by echocardiography. Treatment is directed at the cause.

Cor pulmonale results from a disorder of the lung or its vasculature; it does not refer to right ventricular enlargement secondary to left ventricular failure, a congenital heart disorder (eg, ventricular septal defect), or an acquired valvular disorder. Cor pulmonale is usually chronic but may be acute and reversible. Primary pulmonary hypertension (ie, not caused by a pulmonary or cardiac disorder) is discussed elsewhere.

Pathophysiology

Lung disorders cause pulmonary hypertension by several mechanisms:

- Loss of capillary beds (eg, due to bullous changes in COPD or thrombosis in pulmonary embolism)
- Vasoconstriction caused by hypoxia, hypercapnia, or both
- Increased alveolar pressure (eg, in COPD, during mechanical ventilation)
- Medial hypertrophy in arterioles (often a response to pulmonary hypertension due to other mechanisms)

Pulmonary hypertension increases afterload on the RV, resulting in a cascade of events that is similar to what occurs in LV failure, including elevated end-diastolic and central venous pressure and ventricular hypertrophy and dilation. Demands on the RV may be intensified by increased blood viscosity due to hypoxia-induced polycythemia. Rarely, RV failure affects the LV if a dysfunctional septum bulges into the LV, interfering with filling and thus causing diastolic dysfunction.

Etiology

Acute cor pulmonale has few causes. Chronic cor pulmonale is usually caused by COPD, but there are several less common causes (see Table 83–3). In patients with COPD, an acute exacerbation or pulmonary infection may trigger RV overload. In chronic cor pulmonale, risk of venous thromboembolism is increased.

Symptoms and Signs

Initially, cor pulmonale is asymptomatic, although patients usually have significant symptoms (eg, dyspnea, exertional fatigue) due to the underlying lung disorder. Later, as RV pressures increase, physical signs commonly include a left parasternal systolic lift, a loud pulmonic component of the 2nd heart sound (S_2), and murmurs of functional tricuspid and pulmonic insufficiency. Later, an RV gallop rhythm (3rd [S_3] and 4th [S_4] heart sounds) augmented during inspiration, distended jugular veins (with a dominant *a* wave unless tricuspid regurgitation is present), hepatomegaly, and lower-extremity edema may occur.

Diagnosis

- Clinical suspicion
- Echocardiography

Cor pulmonale should be suspected in all patients with one of its causes. Chest x-ray shows RV and proximal pulmonary

Table 83–3. CAUSES OF COR PULMONALE

ACUITY	CONDITION
Acute	Massive pulmonary embolization Injury due to mechanical ventilation (most commonly in patients with ARDS)
Chronic	COPD* Extensive loss of lung tissue due to surgery or trauma Chronic, unresolved pulmonary emboli Pulmonary veno-occlusive disorders Systemic sclerosis Pulmonary interstitial fibrosis Kyphoscoliosis Obesity with alveolar hypoventilation Neuromuscular disorders involving respiratory muscles Idiopathic alveolar hypotension

*COPD is the most common cause of chronic cor pulmonale.
ARDS = acute respiratory distress syndrome.

artery enlargement with distal arterial attenuation. ECG evidence of RV hypertrophy (eg, right axis deviation, QR wave in lead V_1, and dominant R wave in leads V_1 to V_3) correlates well with degree of pulmonary hypertension. However, because pulmonary hyperinflation and bullae in COPD cause realignment of the heart, physical examination, x-rays, and ECG may be relatively insensitive.

Echocardiography or radionuclide imaging is done to evaluate LV and RV function; echocardiography can assess RV systolic pressure but is often technically limited by the lung disorder; cardiac MRI may be helpful in some patients to assess cardiac chambers and function. Right heart catheterization may be required for confirmation.

Treatment

- Treatment of cause

Treatment is difficult; it focuses on the cause (see elsewhere in THE MANUAL), particularly alleviation or moderation of hypoxia. Early identification and treatment are important before structural changes become irreversible.

If peripheral edema is present, diuretics may seem appropriate, but they are helpful only if LV failure and pulmonary fluid overload are also present. Diuretics may be harmful because small decreases in preload often worsen cor pulmonale. Pulmonary vasodilators (eg, hydralazine, calcium channel blockers, nitrous oxide, prostacyclin, phosphodiesterase inhibitors), although beneficial in primary pulmonary hypertension, are not effective. Bosentan, an endothelin receptor blocker, also may benefit patients with primary pulmonary hypertension, but its use is not well studied in cor pulmonale. Digoxin is effective only if patients have concomitant LV dysfunction; caution is required because patients with COPD are sensitive to digoxin's effects.

Phlebotomy during hypoxic cor pulmonale has been suggested, but the benefits of decreasing blood viscosity are not likely to offset the harm of reducing oxygen-carrying capacity unless significant polycythemia is present. For patients with chronic cor pulmonale, long-term anticoagulants reduce risk of venous thromboembolism.

KEY POINTS

- Cor pulmonale is RV enlargement and eventually failure secondary to a lung disorder that causes pulmonary artery hypertension.
- Cor pulmonale itself is usually asymptomatic but common physical findings include a left parasternal systolic lift, a loud pulmonic component of S_2, functional tricuspid and pulmonic insufficiency murmurs, and later, distended jugular veins, hepatomegaly, and lower-extremity edema.
- Diagnosis usually requires echocardiography or radionuclide imaging, and sometimes right heart catheterization.
- Early identification and treatment of the cause are important before cardiac structural changes become irreversible.
- Although patients may have significant peripheral edema, diuretics are not helpful and may be harmful; small decreases in preload often worsen cor pulmonale.

84 Hypertension

Hypertension is sustained elevation of resting systolic BP (≥ 140 mm Hg), diastolic BP (≥ 90 mm Hg), or both. Hypertension with no known cause (primary; formerly, essential hypertension) is most common. Hypertension with an identified cause (secondary hypertension) is usually due to chronic kidney disease or primary aldosteronism. Usually, no symptoms develop unless hypertension is severe or long-standing. Diagnosis is by sphygmomanometry. Tests may be done to determine cause, assess damage, and identify other cardiovascular risk factors. Treatment involves lifestyle changes and drugs, including diuretics, beta-blockers, ACE inhibitors, angiotensin II receptor blockers, and calcium channel blockers.

In the US, about 75 million people have hypertension. About 81% of these people are aware that they have hypertension, only 73% are being treated, and only 51% have adequately controlled BP. In adults, hypertension occurs more often in blacks (41%) than in whites (28%) or Mexican Americans (28%), and morbidity and mortality are greater in blacks.

Blood pressure increases with age. About two-thirds of people > 65 have hypertension, and people with a normal BP at age 55 have a 90% lifetime risk of developing hypertension. Because hypertension becomes so common with age, the age-related increase in BP may seem innocuous, but higher BP increases morbidity and mortality risk. Hypertension may develop during pregnancy (see pp. 2353 and 2396).

Etiology

Hypertension may be

- Primary (85 to 95% of cases)
- Secondary

Primary hypertension: Hemodynamics and physiologic components (eg, plasma volume, activity of the renin-angiotensin system) vary, indicating that primary hypertension is unlikely to have a single cause. Even if one factor is initially responsible, multiple factors are probably involved in sustaining elevated blood pressure (the mosaic theory). In afferent systemic arterioles, malfunction of ion pumps on sarcolemmal membranes of smooth muscle cells may lead to chronically increased vascular tone. Heredity is a predisposing factor, but the exact mechanism is unclear. Environmental factors (eg, dietary sodium, obesity, stress) seem to affect only genetically susceptible people at younger ages; however, in patients > 65, high sodium intake is more likely to precipitate hypertension.

Secondary hypertension: Causes include primary aldosteronism (thought to be most common), renal parenchymal disease (eg, chronic glomerulonephritis or pyelonephritis, polycystic renal disease, connective tissue disorders, obstructive uropathy), renovascular disease, pheochromocytoma, Cushing syndrome, congenital adrenal hyperplasia, hyperthyroidism, myxedema, and coarctation of the aorta. Excessive alcohol intake and use of oral contraceptives are common causes of curable hypertension. Use of sympathomimetics, NSAIDs, corticosteroids, cocaine, or licorice commonly contributes to worsening of blood pressure control.

Pathophysiology

Because blood pressure equals cardiac output (CO) × total peripheral vascular resistance (TPR), pathogenic mechanisms must involve

- Increased CO
- Increased TPR
- Both

In most patients, CO is normal or slightly increased, and TPR is increased. This pattern is typical of primary hypertension and hypertension due to primary aldosteronism, pheochromocytoma, renovascular disease, and renal parenchymal disease.

In other patients, CO is increased (possibly because of venoconstriction in large veins), and TPR is inappropriately normal for the level of CO. Later in the disorder, TPR increases and CO returns to normal, probably because of autoregulation. Some disorders that increase CO (thyrotoxicosis, arteriovenous fistula, aortic regurgitation), particularly when stroke volume is increased, cause isolated systolic hypertension. Some elderly patients have isolated systolic hypertension with normal or low CO, probably due to inelasticity of the aorta and its major branches. Patients with high, fixed diastolic pressures often have decreased CO.

Plasma volume tends to decrease as BP increases; rarely, plasma volume remains normal or increases. Plasma volume tends to be high in hypertension due to primary aldosteronism or renal parenchymal disease and may be quite low in hypertension due to pheochromocytoma. Renal blood flow gradually decreases as diastolic BP increases and arteriolar sclerosis begins. GFR remains normal until late in the disorder; as a result, the filtration fraction is increased. Coronary, cerebral, and muscle blood flow is maintained unless severe atherosclerosis coexists in these vascular beds.

Abnormal sodium transport: In many cases of hypertension, sodium transport across the cell wall is abnormal, because the sodium-potassium pump (Na^+, K^+-ATPase) is defective or inhibited or because permeability to sodium ions is increased. The result is increased intracellular sodium, which makes the cell more sensitive to sympathetic stimulation. Calcium follows sodium, so accumulation of intracellular calcium may be responsible for the increased sensitivity. Because Na^+, K^+-ATPase may pump norepinephrine back into sympathetic neurons (thus inactivating this neurotransmitter), inhibition of this mechanism could also enhance the effect of norepinephrine, increasing BP. Defects in sodium transport may occur in normotensive children of hypertensive parents.

Sympathetic nervous system: Sympathetic stimulation increases blood pressure, usually more in patients with prehypertension (systolic BP 120 to 139 mm Hg, diastolic BP 80 to 89 mm Hg) or hypertension (systolic BP ≥ 140 mm Hg, diastolic BP ≥ 90 mm Hg, or both) than in normotensive patients. Whether this hyperresponsiveness resides in the sympathetic nervous system or in the myocardium and vascular smooth muscle is unknown. A high resting pulse rate, which may result from increased sympathetic nervous activity, is a well-known predictor of hypertension. In some hypertensive patients, circulating plasma catecholamine levels during rest are higher than normal.

Renin-angiotensin-aldosterone system: This system helps regulate blood volume and therefore blood pressure. Renin, an enzyme formed in the juxtaglomerular apparatus, catalyzes conversion of angiotensinogen to angiotensin I. This inactive product is cleaved by ACE, mainly in the lungs but also in the kidneys and brain, to angiotensin II, a potent vasoconstrictor that also stimulates autonomic centers in the brain to increase sympathetic discharge and stimulates release of aldosterone and vasopressin. Aldosterone and vasopressin cause sodium and water retention, elevating BP. Aldosterone also enhances potassium excretion; low plasma potassium (< 3.5 mEq/L) increases vasoconstriction through closure of potassium channels. Angiotensin III, present in the circulation, stimulates aldosterone release as actively as angiotensin II but has much less pressor activity. Because chymase enzymes also convert angiotensin I to angiotensin II, drugs that inhibit ACE do not fully suppress angiotensin II production.

Renin secretion is controlled by at least 4 mechanisms, which are not mutually exclusive:

- A renal vascular receptor responds to changes in tension in the afferent arteriolar wall
- A macula densa receptor detects changes in the delivery rate or concentration of sodium chloride in the distal tubule
- Circulating angiotensin has a negative feedback effect on renin secretion
- Sympathetic nervous system stimulates renin secretion mediated by beta-receptors (via the renal nerve)

Angiotensin is generally acknowledged to be responsible for renovascular hypertension, at least in the early phase, but the role of the renin-angiotensin-aldosterone system in primary hypertension is not established. However, in black and elderly patients with hypertension, renin levels tend to be low. The elderly also tend to have low angiotensin II levels.

Hypertension due to chronic renal parenchymal disease (renoprival hypertension) results from the combination of a renin-dependent mechanism and a volume-dependent mechanism. In most cases, increased renin activity is not evident in peripheral blood. Hypertension is typically moderate and sensitive to sodium and water balance.

Vasodilator deficiency: Deficiency of a vasodilator (eg, bradykinin, nitric oxide) rather than excess of a vasoconstrictor (eg, angiotensin, norepinephrine) may cause hypertension. If the kidneys do not produce adequate amounts of vasodilators (because of renal parenchymal disease or bilateral nephrectomy), blood pressure can increase. Vasodilators and vasoconstrictors (mainly endothelin) are also produced in endothelial cells. Therefore, endothelial dysfunction greatly affects BP.

Pathology and complications: No pathologic changes occur early in hypertension. Severe or prolonged hypertension damages target organs (primarily the cardiovascular system, brain, and kidneys), increasing risk of

- Coronary artery disease (CAD) and myocardial infarction
- Heart failure (HF)
- Stroke (particularly hemorrhagic)
- Renal failure
- Death

The mechanism involves development of generalized arteriolosclerosis and acceleration of atherogenesis. Arteriolosclerosis is characterized by medial hypertrophy, hyperplasia, and hyalinization; it is particularly apparent in small arterioles, notably in the eyes and the kidneys. In the kidneys, the changes narrow the arteriolar lumen, increasing TPR; thus, hypertension leads to more hypertension. Furthermore, once arteries are narrowed, any slight additional shortening of already hypertrophied smooth muscle reduces the lumen to a greater extent than in normal-diameter arteries. These effects may explain why the longer hypertension has existed, the less likely specific treatment (eg, renovascular surgery) for secondary causes is to restore blood pressure to normal.

Because of increased afterload, the left ventricle gradually hypertrophies, causing diastolic dysfunction. The ventricle eventually dilates, causing dilated cardiomyopathy and HF due to systolic dysfunction often worsened by arteriosclerotic CAD. Thoracic aortic dissection is typically a consequence of hypertension; almost all patients with abdominal aortic aneurysms have hypertension.

Symptoms and Signs

Hypertension is usually asymptomatic until complications develop in target organs. Dizziness, flushed facies, headache, fatigue, epistaxis, and nervousness are not caused by uncomplicated hypertension. Severe hypertension (hypertensive emergencies) can cause severe cardiovascular, neurologic, renal, and retinal symptoms (eg, symptomatic coronary atherosclerosis, HF, hypertensive encephalopathy, renal failure).

A 4th heart sound is one of the earliest signs of hypertensive heart disease.

Retinal changes may include arteriolar narrowing, hemorrhages, exudates, and, in patients with encephalopathy, papilledema (hypertensive retinopathy). Changes are classified (according to the Keith, Wagener, and Barker classification) into 4 groups with increasingly worse prognosis:.

- Grade 1: Constriction of arterioles only
- Grade 2: Constriction and sclerosis of arterioles
- Grade 3: Hemorrhages and exudates in addition to vascular changes
- Grade 4: Papilledema

Diagnosis

- Multiple measurements of BP to confirm
- Urinalysis and urinary albumin:creatinine ratio; if abnormal, consider renal ultrasonography
- Blood tests: Fasting lipids, creatinine, potassium
- Renal ultrasonography if creatinine increased
- Evaluate for aldosteronism if potassium decreased
- ECG: If left ventricular hypertrophy, consider echocardiography
- Sometimes thyroid-stimulating hormone measurement
- Evaluate for pheochromocytoma or a sleep disorder if BP elevation sudden and labile or severe

Hypertension is diagnosed and classified by sphygmomanometry. History, physical examination, and other tests help identify etiology and determine whether target organs are damaged.

Blood pressure must be measured twice—first with the patient supine or seated, then after the patient has been standing for ≥ 2 min—on 3 separate days. The average of these measurements is used for diagnosis. BP is classified as normal, prehypertension, or stage 1 (mild) or stage 2 hypertension (see Table 84–1). Normal blood pressure is much lower for infants and children.

Ideally, BP is measured after the patient rests > 5 min and at different times of day. A BP cuff is applied to the upper arm. An appropriately sized cuff covers two thirds of the biceps; the bladder is long enough to encircle > 80% of the arm, and bladder width equals at least 40% of the arm's circumference. Thus, obese patients require large cuffs. The health care practitioner inflates the cuff above the expected systolic pressure and gradually releases the air while listening over the brachial artery. The pressure at which the first heartbeat is heard as the pressure falls is systolic BP. Total disappearance of the sound marks diastolic BP. The same principles are followed to measure BP in a forearm (radial artery) and thigh (popliteal artery). Sphygmomanometers that contain mercury are most accurate. Mechanical devices should be calibrated periodically; automated readers are often inaccurate.

Table 84–1. JNC 7 CLASSIFICATION OF BLOOD PRESSURE IN ADULTS

CLASSIFICATION	BLOOD PRESSURE
Normal	< 120/80 mm Hg
Prehypertension	120–139/80–89 mm Hg
Stage 1	140–159 mm Hg (systolic) or 90–99 mm Hg (diastolic)
Stage 2	≥ 160 mm Hg (systolic) or ≥ 100 mm Hg (diastolic)

JNC = Joint National Committee on Prevention, Detection, Evaluation, and Treatment of High Blood Pressure.

BP is measured in both arms. BP > 15 mm Hg higher in one arm than the other is associated with higher mortality, and requires evaluation of the upper vasculature when this pattern of measurement is found. BP is also measured in a thigh (with a much larger cuff) to rule out coarctation of the aorta, particularly in patients with diminished or delayed femoral pulses; with coarctation, BP is significantly lower in the legs. If BP is in the low-hypertensive range or is markedly labile, more BP measurements are desirable. BP measurements may be sporadically high before hypertension becomes sustained; this phenomenon probably accounts for "white coat hypertension," in which BP is elevated when measured in the physician's office but normal when measured at home or by ambulatory BP monitoring. However, extreme BP elevation alternating with normal readings is unusual and possibly suggests pheochromocytoma, a sleep disorder such as sleep apnea, or unacknowledged drug use.

History: The history includes the known duration of hypertension and previously recorded levels; any history or symptoms of CAD, HF, or other relevant coexisting disorders (eg, stroke, renal dysfunction, peripheral arterial disease, dyslipidemia, diabetes, gout); and a family history of any of these disorders. Social history includes exercise levels and use of tobacco, alcohol, and stimulant drugs (prescribed and illicit). A dietary history focuses on intake of salt and stimulants (eg, tea, coffee, caffeine-containing sodas, energy drinks).

Physical examination: The physical examination includes measurement of height, weight, and waist circumference; funduscopic examination for retinopathy; auscultation for bruits in the neck and abdomen; and a full cardiac, respiratory, and neurologic examination. The abdomen is palpated for kidney enlargement and abdominal masses. Peripheral arterial pulses are evaluated; diminished or delayed femoral pulses suggest aortic coarctation, particularly in patients < 30. A unilateral renal artery bruit may be heard in slim patients with renovascular hypertension.

Testing: The more severe the hypertension and the younger the patient, the more extensive is the evaluation. Generally, when hypertension is newly diagnosed, routine testing is done to

- Detect target-organ damage
- Identify cardiovascular risk factors

Tests include

- Urinalysis and spot urine albumin:creatinine ratio
- Blood tests (creatinine, potassium, sodium, fasting plasma glucose, lipid profile, and often thyroid-stimulating hormone)
- ECG

Ambulatory blood pressure monitoring, renal radionuclide imaging, chest x-ray, screening tests for pheochromocytoma, and renin-sodium profiling are not routinely necessary. Peripheral plasma renin activity is not helpful in diagnosis or drug selection.

Depending on results of initial tests and examination, other tests may be needed. If urinalysis detects albuminuria (proteinuria), cylindruria, or microhematuria or if serum creatinine is elevated (≥ 1.4 mg/dL [124 μmol/L] in men; ≥ 1.2 mg/dL [106 μmol/L] in women), renal ultrasonography to evaluate kidney size may provide useful information. Patients with hypokalemia unrelated to diuretic use are evaluated for primary aldosteronism and high salt intake.

On ECG, a broad, notched P-wave indicates atrial hypertrophy and, although nonspecific, may be one of the earliest signs of hypertensive heart disease. Left ventricular hypertrophy, indicated by a sustained apical thrust and elevated QRS voltage with or without evidence of ischemia, may occur later. If either of these findings is present, echocardiography is often done. In patients with an abnormal lipid profile or symptoms of CAD, tests for other cardiovascular risk factors (eg, C-reactive protein) may be useful.

If coarctation of the aorta is suspected, chest x-ray, echocardiography, CT, or MRI helps confirm the diagnosis.

Patients with labile, significantly elevated BP and symptoms such as headache, palpitations, tachycardia, excessive perspiration, tremor, and pallor are screened for pheochromocytoma (eg, by measuring plasma free metanephrines). A sleep study should also be strongly considered.

Patients with symptoms suggesting Cushing syndrome, a connective tissue disorder, eclampsia, acute porphyria, hyperthyroidism, myxedema, acromegaly, or CNS disorders are evaluated.

Prognosis

The higher the blood pressure and the more severe the retinal changes and other evidence of target-organ involvement, the worse is the prognosis. Systolic BP predicts fatal and nonfatal cardiovascular events better than diastolic BP. Without treatment, 1-yr survival is < 10% in patients with retinal sclerosis, cotton-wool exudates, arteriolar narrowing, and hemorrhage (grade 3 retinopathy), and < 5% in patients with the same changes plus papilledema (grade 4 retinopathy). CAD is the most common cause of death among treated hypertensive patients. Ischemic or hemorrhagic stroke is a common consequence of inadequately treated hypertension. However, effective control of hypertension prevents most complications and prolongs life.

Treatment

- Weight loss and exercise
- Smoking cessation
- Diet: Increased fruits and vegetables, decreased salt, limited alcohol
- Drugs if BP is initially high (> 160/100 mm Hg) or unresponsive to lifestyle modifications

Primary hypertension has no cure, but some causes of secondary hypertension can be corrected. In all cases, control of blood pressure can significantly limit adverse consequences. Despite the theoretical efficacy of treatment, BP is lowered to the desired level in only one third of hypertensive patients in the US.

JNC 8 (see Fig. 84–1) recommends treatment targets for the general population:

- **For all patients,** including all those with a kidney disorder or diabetes, treatment aims to reduce BP to < 140/90 mm Hg
- **For patients ≥ 60,** treatment aims to reduce BP to < 150/90 mm Hg

However, some clinicians believe that certain patients should have a lower treatment goal of systolic BP 125 to 130 mm Hg (if BP is measured by standard manual office readings) or 120 to 125 mm Hg (if BP is measured with an automatic digital monitor). This includes patients > 50 yr of age who are considered high-risk for cardiovascular events (age > 75 yr, history of CAD or chronic kidney disease, Framingham risk score > 15%). Some clinicians also believe the systolic BP goal of 125 to 130 mm Hg should apply to certain patients with diabetes, eg, those with diabetic nephropathy and proteinuria (500 mg/day).

The benefits of lowering BP to levels approaching 120 mm Hg systolic should be weighed with the higher risk of dizziness and light-headedness and possible worsening of kidney function.

Even the elderly and frail elderly can tolerate a diastolic BP as low as 60 to 65 mm Hg well and without an increase in cardiovascular events. Ideally, patients or family members measure BP at home, provided they have been trained to do so, they are closely monitored, and the sphygmomanometer is regularly calibrated. Treatment of hypertension during pregnancy requires special considerations because some antihypertensive drugs can harm the fetus.

Lifestyle modifications: Recommendations include regular aerobic physical activity at least 30 min/day most days of the week; weight loss to a body mass index of 18.5 to 24.9; smoking cessation; a diet rich in fruits, vegetables, and low-fat dairy products with reduced saturated and total fat content; dietary sodium [Na^+] of < 2.4 g/day (< 6 g sodium chloride); and alcohol consumption of ≤ 1 oz/day [29.5 mL/day] in men and ≤ 0.5 oz/day [15 mL/day] in women.

In stage 1 (mild) hypertension with no signs of target-organ damage, lifestyle changes may make drugs unnecessary. Patients with uncomplicated hypertension do not need to restrict their activities as long as blood pressure is controlled. Dietary modifications can also help control diabetes, obesity, and dyslipidemias. Patients with prehypertension are encouraged to follow these lifestyle recommendations.

Drugs: See also Drugs for Hypertension on p. 732.

If systolic BP remains > 140 mm Hg (> 150 mm Hg for patients ≥ 60) or diastolic BP remains > 90 mm Hg after 6 mo of lifestyle modifications, antihypertensive drugs are required. Unless hypertension is severe, drugs are usually started at low doses. Drugs are initiated simultaneously with lifestyle changes for all patients with hypertension plus diabetes, a kidney disorder, target-organ damage, or cardiovascular risk factors and for those with an initial BP of > 160/100 mm Hg. Signs of hypertensive emergencies require immediate blood pressure reduction with parenteral antihypertensives.

For most patients with hypertension, one drug is given initially. For non-black patients, including those with diabetes, initial treatment should be with either an ACE inhibitor, angiotensin receptor blocker, calcium channel blocker, or a thiazide-like diuretic (chlorthalidone or indapamide). For black patients, including those with diabetes, a calcium channel blocker or a thiazide-like diuretic is recommended initially. Some antihypertensives are contraindicated in certain disorders (eg, beta-blockers in asthma) or are indicated particularly for hypertensive patients with certain disorders (eg, calcium channel blockers for angina pectoris, ACE inhibitors or angiotensin II receptor blockers for diabetes with proteinuria—see Tables 84–1, 84–2, and 84–3).

If the target BP is not achieved in 1 mo, the dose of the initial drug can be increased or a second drug added (selected from the drugs recommended for initial treatment). Note that an ACE inhibitor and an angiotensin receptor blocker should not be used together. Therapy is titrated frequently. If target BP cannot be achieved with 2 drugs, a third drug from the initial

Table 84–2. INITIAL CHOICE OF ANTIHYPERTENSIVE DRUG CLASS

DRUGS	INDICATIONS
ACE inhibitors[†]	Youth Left ventricular failure due to systolic dysfunction* Type 1 diabetes with nephropathy* Severe proteinuria in chronic renal disorders or diabetic glomerulosclerosis Erectile dysfunction due to other drugs
Angiotensin II receptor blockers[†]	Youth Conditions for which ACE inhibitors are indicated but not tolerated because of cough Type 2 diabetes with nephropathy Left ventricular failure with systolic dysfunction Secondary stroke
Long-acting calcium channel blockers	Old age Black race Angina pectoris Arrhythmias (eg, atrial fibrillation, paroxysmal supraventricular tachycardia) Isolated systolic hypertension in elderly patients (dihydropyridines)* High CAD risk (nondihydropyridines)*
Thiazide-like diuretics* (chlorthalidone or indapamide)	Old age Black race Heart failure

*Reduced morbidity and mortality rates in randomized studies.
[†]Contraindicated in pregnancy.
CAD = coronary artery disease.

group is added. If such a third drug is not available (eg, for black patients) or tolerated, a drug from another class (eg, beta-blocker, aldosterone antagonist) can be used. Patients with such difficult to control BP may benefit from consultation with a hypertension specialist.

If initial systolic BP is > 160 mm Hg, 2 drugs are often used from the start. An appropriate combination and dose are determined; many are available as single tablets, which improve compliance. For severe or refractory hypertension, 3 or 4 drugs may be necessary.

Achieving adequate control often requires several evaluations and changes in drug therapy. Reluctance to titrate or add drugs until BP is at an acceptable level must be overcome. Lack of patient adherence, particularly because lifelong treatment is required, can interfere with adequate BP control. Education, with empathy and support, is essential for success.

Devices and physical interventions: Percutaneous catheter-based radiofrequency ablation of the sympathetic nerves in the renal artery is approved in Europe and Australia for resistant hypertension. Hypertension is defined as resistant when BP remains > 160/100 mm Hg despite use of 3 different antihypertensive drugs with complementary mechanisms of action (one of which being a diuretic). Although initial studies appeared promising, a recent large, double-blind study was done.[1] This study for the first time incorporated a sham ablation procedure in the control arm and failed to show a benefit from radiofrequency ablation. Thus, sympathetic ablation should still be considered experimental and done only in European or Australian centers with extensive experience.

A second physical intervention involves stimulating the carotid baroreceptor with a device surgically implanted around the carotid body. A battery attached to the device, much like a pacemaker, is used to stimulate the baroreceptor and, in a dose-dependent manner, lower BP. This procedure has so far proven safe and effective, although experience is limited and trials are ongoing. This device is not yet approved in the US for treatment of hypertension.

1. Bhatt DL, Kandzari DE, O'Neill WW, et al, for the SYMPLICITY HTN-3 Investigators: A controlled trial of renal denervation for resistant hypertension. *N Engl J Med* 370:1393–1401, 2014. DOI: 10.1056/NEJMoa1402670.

KEY POINTS

- Only about three quarters of hypertensive patients in the US are being treated and only half are adequately controlled.
- Most hypertension is primary; only 5 to 15% is secondary to another disorder (eg, renal parenchymal or vascular disease, pheochromocytoma, Cushing syndrome, congenital adrenal hyperplasia, hyperthyroidism).
- Severe or prolonged hypertension damages the cardiovascular system, brain, and kidneys, increasing risk of MI, stroke, and renal failure.
- Hypertension is usually asymptomatic until complications develop in target organs.
- When hypertension is newly diagnosed, do urinalysis, spot urine albumin:creatinine ratio, blood tests (creatinine,

Table 84–3. ANTIHYPERTENSIVES FOR HIGH-RISK PATIENTS

COEXISTING CONDITION	DRUG CLASSES
Cardiovascular risk factors	Beta-blockers ACE inhibitors Diuretics Calcium channel blockers
Chronic kidney disorders	ACE inhibitors Angiotensin II receptor blockers
Diabetes	Diuretics ACE inhibitors Angiotensin II receptor blockers Calcium channel blockers
Heart failure	ACE inhibitors Angiotensin II receptor blockers Beta-blockers Potassium-sparing diuretics Other diuretics*
Post-myocardial infarction	ACE inhibitors Beta-blockers Spironolactone or eplerenone
Risk of recurrent stroke	ACE inhibitors Angiotensin II receptor blockers Calcium channel blockers Diuretics

*Long-term diuretic use may increase mortality in patients with heart failure who do not have pulmonary congestion.

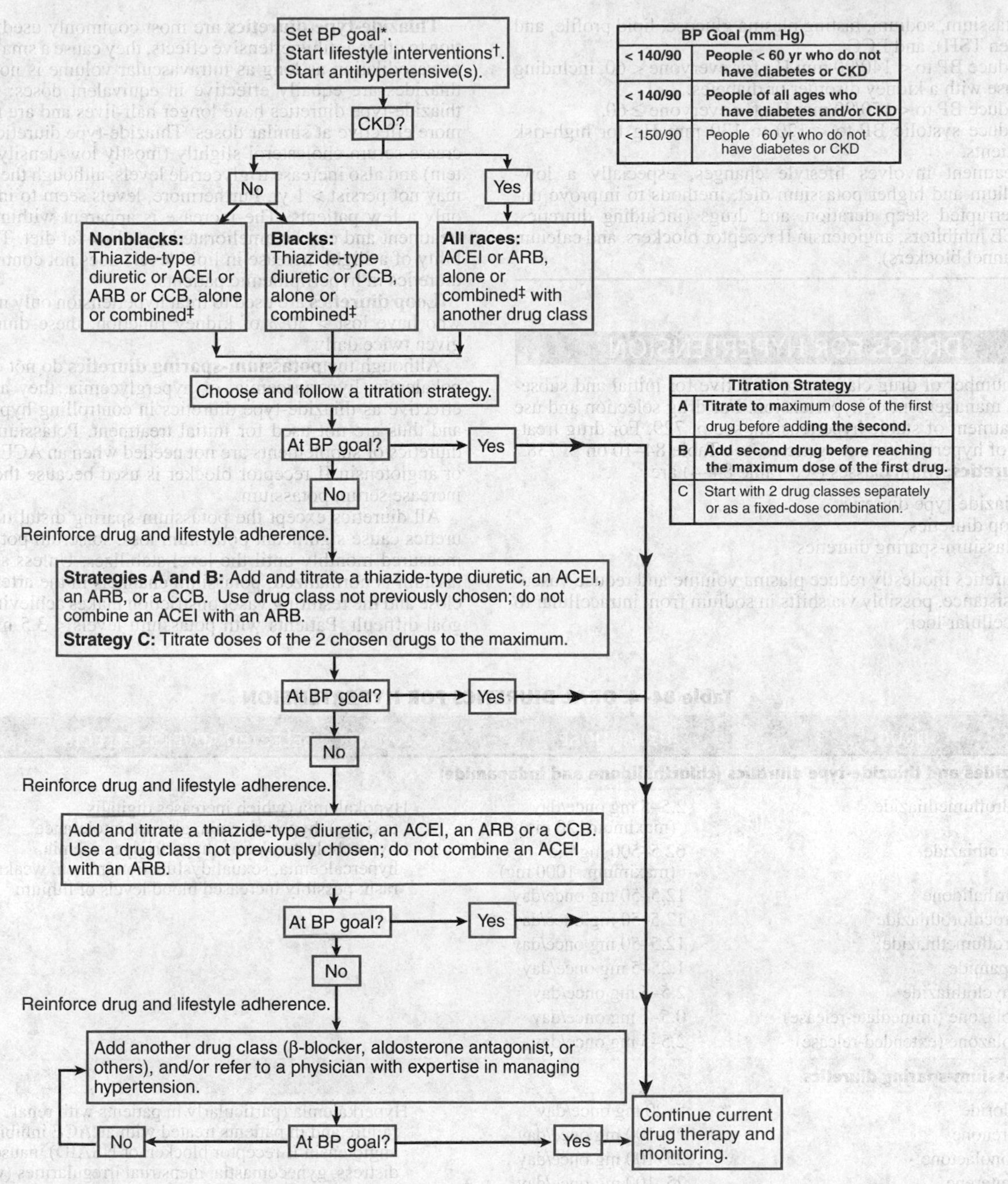
Set BP goal*.
Start lifestyle interventions†.
Start antihypertensive(s).
CKD?
No
Yes
Nonblacks: Thiazide-type diuretic or ACEI or ARB or CCB, alone or combined‡
Blacks: Thiazide-type diuretic or CCB, alone or combined‡
All races: ACEI or ARB, alone or combined‡ with another drug class
Choose and follow a titration strategy.
At BP goal?
Yes
No
Reinforce drug and lifestyle adherence.
Strategies A and B: Add and titrate a thiazide-type diuretic, an ACEI, an ARB, or a CCB. Use drug class not previously chosen; do not combine an ACEI with an ARB.
Strategy C: Titrate doses of the 2 chosen drugs to the maximum.
At BP goal?
Yes
No
Reinforce drug and lifestyle adherence.
Add and titrate a thiazide-type diuretic, an ACEI, an ARB or a CCB. Use a drug class not previously chosen; do not combine an ACEI with an ARB.
At BP goal?
Yes
No
Reinforce drug and lifestyle adherence.
Add another drug class (β-blocker, aldosterone antagonist, or others), and/or refer to a physician with expertise in managing hypertension.
No
At BP goal?
Yes
Continue current drug therapy and monitoring.
BP Goal (mm Hg)
< 140/90 People < 60 yr who do not have diabetes or CKD
< 140/90 People of all ages who have diabetes and/or CKD
< 150/90 People 60 yr who do not have diabetes or CKD
Titration Strategy
A Titrate to maximum dose of the first drug before adding the second.
B Add second drug before reaching the maximum dose of the first drug.
C Start with 2 drug classes separately or as a fixed-dose combination.

Fig. 84–1. Algorithm for treatment of hypertension in patients ≥ 18 yr.

*BP goal and drug therapy are based on age and the presence of diabetes and CKD.
†Lifestyle interventions should be maintained throughout treatment.
‡ACEIs and ARBs should not be used together in the same patient.
ACEI = angiotensin-converting enzyme inhibitor; ARB = angiotensin II receptor blocker; CCB = calcium channel blocker; CKD = chronic kidney disease.
Data from James PA, Oparil S, Carter BL, et al: Evidence-based guideline for the management of high blood pressure in adults: Report from the panel members appointed to the Eighth Joint National Committee (JNC 8). *JAMA* 311(5):507–520, 2014.

potassium, sodium, fasting plasma glucose, lipid profile, and often TSH), and ECG.

- Reduce BP to < 140/90 mm Hg for everyone < 60, including those with a kidney disorder or diabetes.
- Reduce BP to < 150/90 mm Hg for everyone ≥ 60.
- Reduce systolic BP to < 120 to 130 mm Hg for high-risk patients.
- Treatment involves lifestyle changes, especially a low-sodium and higher potassium diet, methods to improve uninterrupted sleep duration, and drugs (including diuretics, ACE inhibitors, angiotensin II receptor blockers, and calcium channel blockers).

DRUGS FOR HYPERTENSION

A number of drug classes are effective for initial and subsequent management of hypertension. For drug selection and use in treatment of stable hypertension, see p. 729. For drug treatment of hypertensive emergencies, see Table 84–10 on p. 738.

Diuretics: Main classes (see Table 84–4) are

- Thiazide-type diuretics
- Loop diuretics
- Potassium-sparing diuretics

Diuretics modestly reduce plasma volume and reduce vascular resistance, possibly via shifts in sodium from intracellular to extracellular loci.

Thiazide-type diuretics are most commonly used. In addition to other antihypertensive effects, they cause a small amount of vasodilation as long as intravascular volume is normal. All thiazides are equally effective in equivalent doses; however, thiazide-type diuretics have longer half-lives and are relatively more effective at similar doses. Thiazide-type diuretics can increase serum cholesterol slightly (mostly low-density lipoprotein) and also increase triglyceride levels, although these effects may not persist > 1 yr. Furthermore, levels seem to increase in only a few patients. The increase is apparent within 4 wk of treatment and can be ameliorated by a low-fat diet. The possibility of a slight increase in lipid levels does not contraindicate diuretics in hyperlipidemic patients.

Loop diuretics are used to treat hypertension only in patients who have lost > 50% of kidney function; these diuretics are given twice daily.

Although the **potassium-sparing diuretics** do not cause hypokalemia, hyperuricemia, or hyperglycemia, they are not as effective as thiazide-type diuretics in controlling hypertension and thus are not used for initial treatment. Potassium-sparing diuretics or supplements are not needed when an ACE inhibitor or angiotensin II receptor blocker is used because these drugs increase serum potassium.

All diuretics except the potassium-sparing distal tubular diuretics cause significant potassium loss, so serum potassium is measured monthly until the level stabilizes. Unless serum potassium is normalized, potassium channels in the arterial walls close and the resulting vasoconstriction makes achieving the BP goal difficult. Patients with potassium levels < 3.5 mEq/L are

Table 84–4. ORAL DIURETICS FOR HYPERTENSION

DRUG	USUAL DOSE*	SELECTED ADVERSE EFFECTS
Thiazides and thiazide-type diuretics (chlorthalidone and indapamide)		
Bendroflumethiazide	2.5–5 mg once/day (maximum: 20 mg)	Hypokalemia (which increases digitalis toxicity), hyperuricemia, glucose intolerance, hypercholesterolemia, hypertriglyceridemia, hypercalcemia, sexual dysfunction in men, weakness, rash; possibly increased blood levels of lithium
Chlorothiazide	62.5–500 mg bid (maximum: 1000 mg)	
Chlorthalidone	12.5–50 mg once/day	
Hydrochlorothiazide	12.5–50 mg once/day	
Hydroflumethiazide	12.5–50 mg once/day	
Indapamide	1.25–5 mg once/day	
Methyclothiazide	2.5–5 mg once/day	
Metolazone (immediate-release)	0.5–1 mg once/day	
Metolazone (extended-release)	2.5–5 mg once/day	
Potassium-sparing diuretics		
Amiloride	5–20 mg once/day	Hyperkalemia (particularly in patients with renal failure and in patients treated with an ACE inhibitor, angiotensin II receptor blocker, or NSAID), nausea, GI distress, gynecomastia, menstrual irregularities (with spironolactone); possibly increased blood levels of lithium
Eplerenone†	25–100 mg once/day	
Spironolactone†	25–100 mg once/day	
Triamterene	25–100 mg once/day	
Loop diuretics		
Bumetanide	0.5–2 mg bid	Hyperkalemia, hyponatremia, hypomagnesemia, dehydration, postural hypotension, tinnitus, hearing loss
Ethacrynic acid	25–100 mg once/day	
Furosemide	20–320 mg bid	
Torsemide	5–100 mg once/day	

*Larger doses may be required in patients with renal failure.
†Aldosterone receptor blockers.

given potassium supplements. Supplements may be continued long-term at a lower dose, or a potassium-sparing diuretic (eg, daily spironolactone 25 to 100 mg, triamterene 50 to 150 mg, amiloride 5 to 10 mg) may be added. Supplements or addition of a potassium-sparing diuretic is also recommended for any patients who are also taking digitalis, have a known heart disorder, have an abnormal ECG, have ectopy or arrhythmias, or develop ectopy or arrhythmias while taking a diuretic.

In most patients with diabetes, thiazide-type diuretics do not affect control of diabetes. Uncommonly, diuretics precipitate or worsen type 2 diabetes in patients with metabolic syndrome.

A hereditary predisposition probably explains the few cases of gout due to diuretic-induced hyperuricemia. Diuretic-induced hyperuricemia without gout does not require treatment or discontinuation of the diuretic.

Diuretics may slightly increase mortality in patients with a history of HF who do not have pulmonary congestion, particularly in those who are also taking an ACE inhibitor or angiotensin II receptor blocker and who do not drink at least 1400 mL (48 oz) of fluid daily. The increased mortality is probably related to diuretic-induced hyponatremia and hypotension.

Beta-blockers: Beta-blockers (see Table 84–5) slow heart rate and reduce myocardial contractility, thus reducing blood pressure. All beta-blockers are similar in antihypertensive efficacy. In patients with diabetes, chronic peripheral arterial disease, or COPD, a cardioselective beta-blocker (acebutolol, atenolol, betaxolol, bisoprolol, metoprolol) may be preferable, although cardioselectivity is only relative and decreases as dose increases. Even cardioselective beta-blockers are contraindicated in patients with asthma or in patients with COPD with a prominent bronchospastic component.

Beta-blockers are particularly useful in patients who have angina, who have had a myocardial infarction, or who have HF, although atenolol may worsen prognosis in patients with CAD. These drugs are no longer considered problematic for the elderly.

Beta-blockers with intrinsic sympathomimetic activity (eg, acebutolol, carteolol, penbutolol, pindolol) do not adversely affect serum lipids; they are less likely to cause severe bradycardia.

Beta-blockers have CNS adverse effects (sleep disturbances, fatigue, lethargy) and exacerbate depression. Nadolol affects the CNS the least and may be best when CNS effects must be avoided. Beta-blockers are contraindicated in patients with 2nd- or 3rd-degree atrioventricular block, asthma, or sick sinus syndrome.

Calcium channel blockers: Dihydropyridines (see Table 84–6) are potent peripheral vasodilators and reduce blood pressure by decreasing TPR; they sometimes cause reflexive tachycardia.

The **nondihydropyridines** verapamil and diltiazem slow the heart rate, decrease atrioventricular conduction, and decrease myocardial contractility. These drugs should not be prescribed for patients with 2nd- or 3rd-degree atrioventricular block or with left ventricular failure.

Long-acting nifedipine, verapamil, or diltiazem is used to treat hypertension, but short-acting nifedipine and diltiazem are associated with a high rate of MI and are not recommended.

A calcium channel blocker is preferred to a beta-blocker in patients with angina pectoris and a bronchospastic disorder, with coronary spasms, or with Raynaud syndrome.

ACE inhibitors: ACE inhibitors (see Table 84–7) reduce blood pressure by interfering with the conversion of angiotensin I to angiotensin II and by inhibiting the degradation of bradykinin, thereby decreasing peripheral vascular resistance without causing reflex tachycardia. These drugs reduce BP in many hypertensive patients, regardless of plasma renin activity. Because these drugs provide renal protection, they are the drugs

Table 84–5. ORAL BETA-BLOCKERS FOR HYPERTENSION

DRUG	USUAL DOSE	SELECTED ADVERSE EFFECTS	COMMENTS
Acebutolol*,†	200–800 mg once/day	Bronchospasm, fatigue, insomnia, sexual dysfunction, exacerbation of heart failure, masking of symptoms of hypoglycemia, triglyceridemia, increased total cholesterol and decreased high- density lipoprotein cholesterol (except for pindolol, acebutolol, penbutolol, carteolol, and labetalol)	Contraindicated in patients with asthma, greater than 1st-degree atrioventricular block, or sick sinus syndrome Should be used cautiously in patients with heart failure or insulin-treated diabetes Should not be stopped abruptly in patients with coronary artery disease Carvedilol and metoprolol approved for treating heart failure
Atenolol*	25–100 mg once/day		
Betaxolol*	5–20 mg once/day		
Bisoprolol*	2.5–20 mg once/day		
Carteolol†	2.5–10 mg once/day		
Carvedilol‡	6.25–25 mg bid		
Carvedilol (controlled-release)‡	20–80 mg once/day		
Labetalol‡,§	100–900 mg bid		
Metoprolol*	25–150 mg bid		
Metoprolol (extended-release)	50–400 mg once/day		
Nadolol	40–320 mg once/day		
Nebivolol	5–40 mg once/day		
Penbutolol†	10–20 mg once/day		
Pindolol†	5–30 mg bid		
Propranolol	20–160 mg bid		
Propranolol, long-acting	60–320 mg once/day		
Timolol	10–30 mg bid		

*Cardioselective.

†With intrinsic sympathomimetic activity.

‡Alpha-beta-blockers. Labetalol can also be given IV for hypertensive emergencies. For IV administration, it is started as 20 mg up to a maximum 300 mg.

§Can also be given for hypertensive emergencies; for IV administration, started as 20 mg up to a maximum 300 mg.

Table 84–6. ORAL CALCIUM CHANNEL BLOCKERS FOR HYPERTENSION

DRUG	USUAL DOSE	SELECTED ADVERSE EFFECTS	COMMENTS
Benzothiazepine derivatives			
Diltiazem, sustained-release Diltiazem, extended-release	60–180 mg bid 120–360 mg once/day	Headache, dizziness, asthenia, flushing, edema, negative inotropic effect; possibly liver dysfunction	Contraindicated in heart failure due to systolic dysfunction, in sick sinus syndrome, or in greater than 1st-degree atrioventricular block
Diphenylalkylamine derivatives			
Verapamil Verapamil, sustained-release	40–120 mg tid 120–480 mg once/day	Same as for benzothiazepine derivatives, plus constipation	Same as for benzothiazepine derivatives
Dihydropyridines			
Amlodipine Felodipine Isradipine Nicardipine Nicardipine, sustained-release Nifedipine, extended-release Nisoldipine	2.5–10 mg once/day 2.5–20 mg once/day 2.5–10 mg bid 20–40 mg tid 30–60 mg bid 30–90 mg once/day 10–60 mg once/day	Dizziness, flushing, headache, weakness, nausea, heartburn, pedal edema, tachycardia	Contraindicated in heart failure, possibly except for amlodipine Use of short-acting nifedipine possibly associated with higher MI rate

of choice for patients with diabetes. They are not recommended for initial treatment in blacks, in whom they appear to increase the risk of stroke when used for initial treatment.

A dry, irritating cough is the most common adverse effect, but angioedema is the most serious and, if it affects the oropharynx, can be fatal. Angioedema is most common among blacks and smokers. ACE inhibitors may increase serum potassium and creatinine levels, especially in patients with chronic kidney disease and those taking potassium-sparing diuretics, potassium supplements, or NSAIDs. ACE inhibitors are the least likely of the antihypertensives to cause erectile dysfunction. ACE inhibitors are contraindicated during pregnancy. In patients with a renal disorder, serum creatinine and potassium levels are monitored at least every 3 mo. Patients who have stage 3 nephropathy

Table 84–7. ORAL ACE INHIBITORS AND ANGIOTENSIN II RECEPTOR BLOCKERS FOR HYPERTENSION

DRUG	USUAL DOSE	SELECTED ADVERSE EFFECTS
ACE inhibitors*		
Benazepril Captopril Enalapril Fosinopril Lisinopril Perindopril Quinapril Ramipril Trandolapril	5–40 mg once/day 12.5–150 mg bid 2.5–40 mg once/day 10–80 mg once/day 5–40 mg once/day 4–8 mg once/day 5–80 mg once/day 1.25–20 mg once/day 1–4 mg once/day	Rash, cough, angioedema, hyperkalemia (particularly in patients with renal insufficiency or taking NSAIDs, potassium-sparing diuretics, or potassium supplements), dysgeusia, reversible acute kidney injury if stenosis affecting one or both kidneys threatens renal function, proteinuria (rare at recommended doses), neutropenia (rare), hypotension with initiation of treatment (particularly in patients with high plasma renin activity or with hypovolemia due to diuretics or other conditions)
Angiotensin II receptor blockers		
Azilsartan	80 mg once/day In patients > 65, initial dose 40 mg once/day	Dizziness, angioedema (very rare); theoretically, same adverse effects as ACE inhibitors on renal function (except proteinuria and neutropenia), serum potassium, and BP
Candesartan Eprosartan Irbesartan Losartan Olmesartan Telmisartan Valsartan	8–32 mg once/day 400–1200 mg once/day 75–300 mg once/day 25–100 mg once/day 20–40 mg once/day 20–80 mg once/day 80–320 mg once/day	

*All ACE inhibitors and angiotensin II receptor blockers are contraindicated in pregnancy (category C during 1st trimester; category D during 2nd and 3rd trimesters).

Table 84–8. ADRENERGIC MODIFIERS FOR HYPERTENSION

DRUG*	USUAL DOSE	SELECTED ADVERSE EFFECTS	COMMENTS
Alpha-2-agonists (central acting)			
Clonidine	0.05–0.3 mg bid	Drowsiness, sedation, dry mouth, fatigue, sexual dysfunction, rebound hypertension with abrupt discontinuance (particularly if doses are high or concomitant beta-blockers are continued), localized skin reaction to clonidine patch; possibly liver damage, Coombs-positive hemolytic anemia with methyldopa	Should be used cautiously in elderly patients because of orthostatic hypotension Interferes with measurements of urinary catecholamine levels by fluorometric methods
Clonidine TTS (patch)	0.1–0.3 mg once/wk		
Guanabenz	2–16 mg bid		
Guanfacine	0.5–3 mg once/day		
Methyldopa	250–1000 mg bid		
Alpha-1-blockers			
Doxazosin	1–16 mg once/day	First-dose syncope, orthostatic hypotension, weakness, palpitations, headache	Should be used cautiously in elderly patients because of orthostatic hypotension Relieves symptoms of benign prostatic hyperplasia
Prazosin	1–10 mg bid		
Terazosin	1–20 mg once/day		

*Peripheral-acting adrenergic blockers (eg, guanadrel, guanethidine, reserpine) are no longer available.
TTS = transdermal therapeutic system.

(estimated GFR of < 60 mL/min to > 30 mL/min) and are given ACE inhibitors can usually tolerate up to a 30 to 35% increase in serum creatinine above baseline. ACE inhibitors can cause acute kidney injury in patients who have hypovolemia, severe HF, severe bilateral renal artery stenosis, or severe stenosis in the artery to a solitary kidney.

Thiazide-type diuretics enhance the antihypertensive activity of ACE inhibitors more than that of other classes of antihypertensives. Spironolactone and eplerenone also appear to enhance the effect of ACE inhibitors.

Angiotensin II receptor blockers: Angiotensin II receptor blockers (see Table 84–7) block angiotensin II receptors and therefore interfere with the renin-angiotensin system. Angiotensin II receptor blockers and ACE inhibitors are equally effective as antihypertensives. Angiotensin II receptor blockers may provide added benefits via tissue ACE blockade. The 2 classes have the same beneficial effects in patients with left ventricular failure or with nephropathy due to type 1 diabetes. An angiotensin II receptor blocker should not be used together with an ACE inhibitor, but when used with a beta-blocker may reduce the hospitalization rate for patients with HF. Angiotensin II receptor blockers may be safely started in people < 60 with initial serum creatinine of ≤ 3 mg/dL.

Incidence of adverse events is low; angioedema occurs but much less frequently than with ACE inhibitors. Precautions for use of angiotensin II receptor blockers in patients with renovascular hypertension, hypovolemia, and severe HF are the same as those for ACE inhibitors (see Table 84–7). Angiotensin II receptor blockers are contraindicated during pregnancy.

Direct renin inhibitor: Aliskiren, a direct renin inhibitor, is used in the management of hypertension. Dosage is 150 to 300 mg po once/day, with a starting dose of 150 mg. Clinical trials are ongoing to assess its efficacy for reducing mortality in HF.

As with ACE inhibitors and angiotensin II receptor blockers, aliskiren causes elevation of serum potassium and creatinine. Aliskiren should not be combined with ACE inhibitors or angiotensin II receptor blockers in patients with diabetes or renal disease (estimated GFR < 60 mL/min).

Adrenergic modifiers: Adrenergic modifiers include central alpha-2-agonists, postsynaptic alpha-1-blockers, and peripheral-acting non-selective adrenergic blockers (see Table 84–8).

Alpha-2-agonists (eg, methyldopa, clonidine, guanabenz, guanfacine) stimulate alpha-2-adrenergic receptors in the brain stem and reduce sympathetic nervous activity, lowering BP. Because they have a central action, they are more likely than other antihypertensives to cause drowsiness, lethargy, and depression; they are no longer widely used. Clonidine can be applied transdermally once/wk as a patch; thus, it may be useful for nonadherent patients (eg, those with dementia).

Postsynaptic alpha-1-blockers (eg, prazosin, terazosin, doxazosin) are no longer used for primary treatment of hypertension because evidence suggests no reduction in mortality. Also, doxazosin used alone or with antihypertensives other than diuretics increases risk of HF. However, they may be used in patients who have prostatic hypertrophy and need a 4th antihypertensive or in people with high sympathetic tone (ie, with high heart rate and spiking blood pressures) already on the maximum dose of a beta-blocker.

Table 84–9. DIRECT VASODILATORS FOR HYPERTENSION

DRUG	USUAL DOSE	SELECTED ADVERSE EFFECTS*	COMMENTS
Hydralazine	10–50 mg qid	Positive antinuclear antibody test, drug-induced lupus (rare at recommended doses)	Augments vasodilating effects of other vasodilating drugs
Minoxidil	1.25–40 mg bid	Sodium and water retention, hypertrichosis; possibly new or worsening pleural and pericardial effusions	Reserved for severe, refractory hypertension

*Both drugs may cause headache, tachycardia, and fluid retention and may precipitate angina in patients with coronary artery disease.

Direct vasodilators: Direct vasodilators, including minoxidil and hydralazine (see Table 84–9), work directly on blood vessels, independently of the autonomic nervous system. Minoxidil is more potent than hydralazine but has more adverse effects, including sodium and water retention and hypertrichosis, which is poorly tolerated by women. Minoxidil should be reserved for severe, refractory hypertension.

Hydralazine is used during pregnancy (eg, for preeclampsia) and as an adjunct antihypertensive. Long-term, high-dose (> 300 mg/day) hydralazine has been associated with a drug-induced lupus syndrome, which resolves when the drug is stopped.

RENOVASCULAR HYPERTENSION

Renovascular hypertension is blood pressure elevation due to partial or complete occlusion of one or more renal arteries or their branches. It is usually asymptomatic unless long-standing. A bruit can be heard over one or both renal arteries in < 50% of patients. Diagnosis is by physical examination and renal imaging with duplex ultrasonography, radionuclide imaging, or magnetic resonance angiography. Angiography is done before definitive treatment with surgery or angioplasty.

Renovascular disease is one of the most common causes of curable hypertension but accounts for < 2% of all cases of hypertension. Stenosis or occlusion of one or both main renal arteries, an accessory renal artery, or any of their branches can cause hypertension by stimulating release of renin from juxtaglomerular cells of the affected kidney (see p. 2157). The area of the arterial lumen must be decreased by ≥ 70% and a significant poststenotic gradient must also be present before stenosis is likely to contribute to BP elevation. For unknown reasons, renovascular hypertension is much less common among blacks than among whites.

Overall, about 80% of cases are caused by atherosclerosis and 20% by fibromuscular dysplasia. Atherosclerosis is more common among men > 50 and affects mainly the proximal one third of the renal artery. Fibromuscular dysplasia is more common among younger patients (usually women) and usually affects the distal two thirds of the main renal artery and the branches of the renal arteries. Rarer causes include emboli, trauma, inadvertent ligation during surgery, and extrinsic compression of the renal pedicle by tumors.

Renovascular hypertension is characterized by high CO and high peripheral resistance.

Symptoms and Signs

Renovascular hypertension is usually asymptomatic. A systolic-diastolic bruit in the epigastrium, usually transmitted to one or both upper quadrants and sometimes to the back, is almost pathognomonic, but it is present in only about 50% of patients with fibromuscular dysplasia and is rare in patients with renal atherosclerosis.

Renovascular hypertension should be suspected if

- Diastolic hypertension develops abruptly in a patient < 30 or > 50
- New or previously stable hypertension rapidly worsens within 6 mo
- Hypertension is initially very severe, associated with worsening renal function, or highly refractory to drug treatment

A history of trauma to the back or flank or acute pain in this region with or without hematuria suggests renovascular hypertension (possibly due to arterial injury), but these findings are rare. Asymmetric renal size (> 1 cm difference) discovered incidentally during imaging tests, and recurrent episodes of unexplained acute pulmonary edema or HF also suggest renovascular hypertension.

Diagnosis

- Initial identification with ultrasonography, magnetic resonance angiography, or radionuclide imaging
- Confirmation with renal angiography (also may be therapeutic)

If renovascular hypertension is suspected, ultrasonography, magnetic resonance angiography (MRA), or radionuclide imaging may be done to identify patients who should have renal angiography, the definitive test.

Duplex Doppler ultrasonography can assess renal blood flow and is a reliable noninvasive method for identifying significant stenosis (eg, > 60%) in the main renal arteries. Sensitivity and specificity approach 90% when experienced technicians do the test. It is less accurate in patients with branch stenosis.

MRA is a more accurate and specific noninvasive test to assess the renal arteries.

Radionuclide imaging is often done before and after an oral dose of captopril 50 mg. The ACE inhibitor causes the affected artery to narrow, decreasing perfusion on the scintiscan. Narrowing also causes an increase in serum renin, which is measured before and after captopril administration. This test may be less reliable in blacks and in patients with decreased renal function.

Renal angiography is done if MRA indicates a lesion amenable to angioplasty or stenting or if other screening tests are positive. Digital subtraction angiography with selective injection of the renal arteries can also confirm the diagnosis, but angioplasty or stent placement cannot be done in the same procedure.

Measurements of renal vein renin activity are sometimes misleading and, unless surgery is being considered, are not necessary. However, in unilateral disease, a renal vein renin activity ratio of > 1.5 (affected to unaffected side) usually predicts a good outcome with revascularization. The test is done when patients are depleted of sodium, stimulating the release of renin.

Treatment

- Aggressive medical management of hypertension, atherosclerosis, and related disorders
- For fibromuscular dysplasia, sometimes angioplasty with or without stent placement
- Rarely bypass graft

Without treatment, the prognosis is similar to that for patients with untreated primary hypertension.

All patients should have aggressive medical management of their hypertension.

Atherosclerotic renal artery stenosis: For patients with atherosclerotic renal artery stenosis, angioplasty with stent placement was previously considered beneficial for many patients. However, data from a recent large, randomized, controlled trial (the cardiovascular outcomes in renal atherosclerotic lesions [CORAL]) showed that stent placement did not improve outcomes compared to medical management alone.[1] Although stent placement did provide a small (–2 mm Hg), statistically significant decrease in systolic BP, there was no significant clinical benefit for prevention of stroke, MI, HF, death due to cardiovascular or renal disease, or progression of kidney disease (including the need for renal replacement therapy). Importantly, all patients in the CORAL study received aggressive medical management of their hypertension and any diabetes, along with antiplatelet drugs and a statin to manage atherosclerosis. Thus, the decision to eschew angioplasty must be accompanied by strict adherence to current medical management guidelines.

Fibromuscular dysplasia: For most patients with fibromuscular dysplasia of the renal artery, percutaneous transluminal angioplasty (PTA) is recommended. Placement of a stent reduces the risk of restenosis; antiplatelet drugs (aspirin, clopidogrel) are given afterward. Saphenous vein bypass grafting is recommended only when extensive disease in the renal artery branches makes PTA technically unfeasible. Sometimes complete surgical revascularization requires microvascular techniques that can only be done ex vivo with autotransplantation of the kidney. Cure rate is 90% in appropriately selected patients; surgical mortality rate is < 1%. Medical treatment is always preferable to nephrectomy in young patients whose kidneys cannot be revascularized for technical reasons.

1. Cooper CJ, Murphy TP, Cutlip DE, et al. Stenting and medical therapy for atherosclerotic renal-artery stenosis. *N Engl J Med* 370:13–22, 2014. DOI: 10.1056/NEJMoa1310753.

KEY POINTS

- Stenosis (> 70%) or occlusion of a renal artery can cause hypertension by stimulating release of renin from juxtaglomerular cells of the affected kidney.
- About 80% of cases are caused by atherosclerosis, and 20% by fibromuscular dysplasia.
- Suspect a renovascular cause if diastolic hypertension develops abruptly in a patient < 30 or > 50; if new or previously stable hypertension rapidly worsens within 6 mo; or if hypertension is initially very severe, associated with worsening renal function, or highly refractory to drug treatment.
- Do ultrasonography, MRA, or radionuclide imaging to identify patients who should have renal angiography, the definitive test.
- Give aggressive medical treatment of hypertension, atherosclerosis, and related disorders.
- For patients with fibromuscular dysplasia, consider percutaneous angioplasty and/or stent placement or rarely a vascular bypass graft.

HYPERTENSIVE EMERGENCIES

A hypertensive emergency is severe hypertension with signs of damage to target organs (primarily the brain, cardiovascular system, and kidneys). Diagnosis is by BP measurement, ECG, urinalysis, and serum BUN and creatinine measurements. Treatment is immediate BP reduction with IV drugs (eg, clevidipine, fenoldopam, nitroglycerin, nitroprusside, nicardipine, labetalol, esmolol, hydralazine).

Target-organ damage includes hypertensive encephalopathy, preeclampsia and eclampsia, acute left ventricular failure with pulmonary edema, myocardial ischemia, acute aortic dissection, and renal failure. Damage is rapidly progressive and often fatal.

Hypertensive encephalopathy may involve a failure of cerebral autoregulation of blood flow. Normally, as blood pressure increases, cerebral vessels constrict to maintain constant cerebral perfusion. Above a mean arterial pressure (MAP) of about 160 mm Hg (lower for normotensive people whose BP suddenly increases), the cerebral vessels begin to dilate rather than remain constricted. As a result, the very high BP is transmitted directly to the capillary bed with transudation and exudation of plasma into the brain, causing cerebral edema, including papilledema.

Although many patients with stroke and intracranial hemorrhage present with elevated BP, elevated BP is often a consequence rather than a cause of the condition. Whether rapidly lowering BP is beneficial in these conditions is unclear; it may even be harmful.

Hypertensive urgencies: Very high blood pressure (eg, diastolic pressure > 120 to 130 mm Hg) without target-organ damage (except perhaps grades 1 to 3 retinopathy) may be considered a hypertensive urgency. BP at these levels often worries the physician; however, acute complications are unlikely, so immediate BP reduction is not required. However, patients should be started on a 2-drug oral combination (see p. 729), and close evaluation (with evaluation of treatment efficacy) should be continued on an outpatient basis.

Symptoms and Signs

Blood pressure is elevated, often markedly (diastolic pressure > 120 mm Hg). CNS symptoms include rapidly changing neurologic abnormalities (eg, confusion, transient cortical blindness, hemiparesis, hemisensory defects, seizures). Cardiovascular symptoms include chest pain and dyspnea. Renal involvement may be asymptomatic, although severe azotemia due to advanced renal failure may cause lethargy or nausea.

Physical examination focuses on target organs, with neurologic examination, funduscopy, and cardiovascular examination. Global cerebral deficits (eg, confusion, obtundation, coma), with or without focal deficits, suggest encephalopathy; normal mental status with focal deficits suggests stroke. Severe retinopathy (sclerosis, cotton-wool spots, arteriolar narrowing, hemorrhage, papilledema) is usually present with hypertensive encephalopathy, and some degree of retinopathy is present in many other hypertensive emergencies. Jugular venous distention, basilar lung crackles, and a 3rd heart sound suggest pulmonary edema. Asymmetry of pulses between arms suggests aortic dissection.

Diagnosis

- Very high BP
- Identify target-organ involvement: ECG, urinalysis, BUN, creatinine; if neurologic findings, head CT

Testing typically includes ECG, urinalysis, and serum BUN and creatinine.

Patients with neurologic findings require head CT to diagnose intracranial bleeding, edema, or infarction.

Patients with chest pain or dyspnea require chest x-ray.

ECG abnormalities suggesting target-organ damage include signs of left ventricular hypertrophy or acute ischemia.

Urinalysis abnormalities typical of renal involvement include RBCs, RBC casts, and proteinuria.

Diagnosis is based on the presence of a very high BP and findings of target-organ involvement.

Treatment

- Admit to ICU
- Short-acting IV drug: nitrates, fenoldopam, nicardipine, or labetalol
- Goal: 20 to 25% reduction MAP in 1 to 2 h

Hypertensive emergencies are treated in an ICU; blood pressure is progressively (although not abruptly) reduced using a short-acting, titratable IV drug. Choice of drug and speed and degree of reduction vary somewhat with the target organ involved, but generally a 20 to 25% reduction in MAP over an hour or so is appropriate, with further titration based on symptoms. Achieving "normal" BP urgently is not necessary. Typical first-line drugs include nitroprusside, fenoldopam, nicardipine, and labetalol (see Table 84–10). Nitroglycerin alone is less potent.

Oral drugs are not indicated because onset is variable and the drugs are difficult to titrate. Although short-acting oral nifedipine reduces BP rapidly, it may lead to acute cardiovascular and cerebrovascular events (sometimes fatal) and is therefore not recommended.

Clevidipine is a new, ultra-short-acting (within 1 to 2 minutes), 3rd-generation calcium channel blocker that reduces peripheral resistance without affecting venous vascular tone and cardiac filling pressures. Clevidipine is rapidly hydrolyzed by blood esterases and, thus, its metabolism is not affected by renal or hepatic function. In recent trials, it has been shown to be effective and safe in the control of perioperative hypertension and hypertensive emergencies and was associated with lower mortality than nitroprusside.

Starting dose of clevidipine is 1 to 2 mg/h, doubling the dose every 90 sec until approaching target BP, at which time dose is increased by less than double every 5 to 10 min. Clevidipine may thus be preferred over nitroprusside for most hypertensive emergencies, although it should be used with caution in acute HF with low ejection fraction as it may have negative inotropic effects. If clevidipine is not available, then fenoldopam, nitroglycerin, or nicardipine are reasonable alternatives.

Nitroprusside is a venous and arterial dilator, reducing preload and afterload; thus, it is the most useful for hypertensive patients with HF. It is also used for hypertensive encephalopathy and, with beta-blockers, for aortic dissection. Starting dose is 0.25 to 1.0 mcg/kg/min titrated in increments of 0.5 mcg/kg to a maximum of 8 to 10 mcg/kg/min; maximum dose is given for ≤ 10 min to minimize risk of cyanide toxicity. The drug is rapidly broken down into cyanide and nitric oxide (the active moiety). Cyanide is detoxified to thiocyanate. However, administration of > 2 mcg/kg/min can lead to cyanide accumulation with toxicity to the CNS and heart; manifestations

Table 84–10. PARENTERAL DRUGS FOR HYPERTENSIVE EMERGENCIES

DRUG	DOSE	SELECTED ADVERSE EFFECTS*	SPECIAL INDICATIONS
Clevidipine	1–21 mg/h IV	Atrial fibrillation, fever, insomnia, nausea, headache	Most hypertensive emergencies Should be used cautiously in patients with acute heart failure
Enalaprilat	0.625–5 mg q 6 h IV	Precipitous fall in BP in high-renin states, variable response	Acute left ventricular failure Should be avoided in acute MI
Esmolol	250–500 mcg/kg/min for 1 min, then 50–100 mcg/kg/min for 4 min; may repeat sequence	Hypotension, nausea	Aortic dissection perioperatively
Fenoldopam	0.1–0.3 mcg/kg/min IV infusion; maximum dose 1.6 mcg/kg/min	Tachycardia, headache, nausea, flushing, hypokalemia, elevation of intraocular pressure in patients with glaucoma	Most hypertensive emergencies Should be used cautiously in patients with myocardial ischemia
Hydralazine	10–40 mg IV 10–20 mg IM	Tachycardia, flushing, headache, vomiting, aggravation of angina	Eclampsia
Labetalol	20 mg IV bolus over 2 min, followed q 10 min by 40 mg, then up to 3 doses of 80 mg; or 0.5–2 mg/min IV infusion	Vomiting, scalp tingling, burning in throat, dizziness, nausea, heart block, orthostatic hypotension	Most hypertensive emergencies, except acute left ventricular failure Should be avoided in patients with asthma
Nicardipine	5–15 mg/h IV	Tachycardia, headache, flushing, local phlebitis	Most hypertensive emergencies, except acute heart failure Should be used cautiously in patients with myocardial ischemia
Nitroglycerin	5–100 mcg/min IV infusion†	Headache, tachycardia, nausea, vomiting, apprehension, restlessness, muscular twitching, palpitations, methemoglobinemia, tolerance with prolonged use	Myocardial ischemia, heart failure
Nitroprusside	0.25–10 mcg/kg/min IV infusion† (maximum dose for 10 min only)	Nausea, vomiting, agitation, muscle twitching, sweating, cutis anserina (if BP is reduced too rapidly), thiocyanate and cyanide toxicity	Most hypertensive emergencies Should be used cautiously in patients with high intracranial pressure or azotemia
Phentolamine	5–15 mg IV	Tachycardia, flushing, headache	Catecholamine excess

*Hypotension may occur with all drugs.
†A special delivery system (eg, infusion pump for nitroprusside, nonpolyvinyl chloride tubing for nitroglycerin) is required.

include agitation, seizures, cardiac instability, and an anion gap metabolic acidosis.

Prolonged administration of nitroprusside (> 1 wk or, in patients with renal insufficiency, 3 to 6 days) leads to accumulation of thiocyanate, with lethargy, tremor, abdominal pain, and vomiting. Other adverse effects include transitory elevation of hair follicles (cutis anserina) if BP is reduced too rapidly. Thiocyanate levels should be monitored daily after 3 consecutive days of therapy, and the drug should be stopped if the serum thiocyanate level is > 12 mg/dL (> 2 mmol/L). Because nitroprusside is broken down by ultraviolet light, the IV bag and tubing are wrapped in an opaque covering. Given some recent data showing increased mortality with nitroprusside compared to clevidipine, nitroglycerin, and nicardipine, nitroprusside should probably not be used when other alternatives are available.

Fenoldopam is a peripheral dopamine-1 agonist that causes systemic and renal vasodilation and natriuresis. Onset is rapid and half-life is brief, making it an effective alternative to nitroprusside, with the added benefit that it does not cross the blood-brain barrier. Initial dosage is 0.1 mcg/kg/min IV infusion, titrated upward by 0.1 mcg/kg q 15 min to a maximum of 1.6 mcg/kg/min.

Nitroglycerin is a vasodilator that affects veins more than arterioles. It can be used to manage hypertension during and after coronary artery bypass graft surgery, acute myocardial infarction, unstable angina pectoris, and acute pulmonary edema. IV nitroglycerin is preferable to nitroprusside for patients with severe CAD because nitroglycerin increases coronary flow, whereas nitroprusside tends to decrease coronary flow to ischemic areas, possibly because of a "steal" mechanism. Starting dose is 10 to 20 mcg/min titrated upward by 10 mcg/min q 5 min to maximum antihypertensive effect.

For long-term BP control, nitroglycerin must be used with other drugs. The most common adverse effect is headache (in about 2%); others include tachycardia, nausea, vomiting, apprehension, restlessness, muscular twitching, and palpitations.

Nicardipine, a dihydropyridine calcium channel blocker with less negative inotropic effects than nifedipine, acts primarily as a vasodilator. It is most often used for postoperative hypertension and during pregnancy. Dosage is 5 mg/h IV, increased q 15 min to a maximum of 15 mg/h. It may cause flushing, headache, and tachycardia; it can decrease GFR in patients with renal insufficiency.

Labetalol is a beta-blocker with some alpha-1-blocking effects, thus causing vasodilation without the typical accompanying reflex tachycardia. It can be given as a constant infusion or as frequent boluses; use of boluses has not been shown to cause significant hypotension. Labetalol is used during pregnancy, for intracranial disorders requiring BP control, and after myocardial infarction. Infusion is 0.5 to 2 mg/min, titrated upward to a maximum of 4 to 5 mg/min. Boluses begin with 20 mg IV followed every 10 min by 40 mg, then 80 mg (up to 3 doses) to a maximum total of 300 mg. Adverse effects are minimal, but because of its beta-blocking activity, labetalol should not be used for hypertensive emergencies in patients with asthma. Low doses may be used for left ventricular failure if nitroglycerin is given simultaneously.

KEY POINTS

- A hypertensive emergency is hypertension that causes target-organ damage; it requires intravenous therapy and hospitalization.
- Target-organ damage includes hypertensive encephalopathy, preeclampsia and eclampsia, acute left ventricular failure with pulmonary edema, myocardial ischemia, acute aortic dissection, and renal failure.
- Do ECG, urinalysis, serum BUN and creatinine, and head CT for patients with neurologic symptoms or signs.
- Reduce MAP by about 20 to 25% over the first hour using a short-acting, titratable IV drug such as clevidipine, nitroglycerin, fenoldopam, nicardipine, or labetalol.
- It is not necessary to achieve "normal" BP urgently (especially true in acute stroke).

85 Lymphatic Disorders

Plasma, along with some WBCs, routinely moves out of capillaries into the interstitial space. Most of the fluid and its constituents is taken up by tissue cells or reabsorbed into the vascular tree, depending on the balance of hydrostatic and oncotic pressures. However, some of the fluid, along with certain cells and cellular debris (eg, from the immune response to local infection, cancer, inflammation) enters the lymphatic system.

Like the venous system, the lymphatic system consists of a multitude of thin-walled vessels that transport fluid throughout the body. Small lymphatic vessels empty into larger ones that ultimately drain into the central venous system via the thoracic duct or the right lymphatic duct. Most lymphatic vessels have valves, similar to those in veins, that keep lymph flowing in one direction (toward the heart). Unlike the venous system, in which fluid (blood) is pumped by the heart, lymph is propelled by pressure generated during muscle contraction.

Before entering the central venous system, lymph passes through lymph nodes, which filter out cellular material, including cancer cells, and foreign particles. Lymph nodes also are key participants in the immune system because they are packed with lymphocytes, macrophages, and dendritic cells that are poised to respond to any antigens transported from tissues in the lymph.

Lymph nodes are categorized as superficial or deep. Superficial nodes are just below the skin; they are present throughout the body, but particular collections are present in the neck, axillae, and groin. Deep lymph nodes are those located in the abdominal or thoracic cavity.

Disorders of the lymphatic system: Disorders of the lymphatic system involve one or more of the following:

- Obstruction
- Infection or inflammation
- Cancer

Obstruction leads to accumulation of lymphatic fluid in tissues (lymphedema) and is usually secondary to surgery, radiation therapy, injury, or, in tropical countries, lymphatic filariasis. Rarely, the cause is a congenital disorder (see p. 742).

Infection may cause reactive lymph node enlargement (lymphadenopathy) or the nodes themselves may become infected (lymphadenitis) by organisms spread through the lymphatic system from the primary site of infection.

Various **cancers** may metastasize to local or regional lymph nodes. Rarely, a primary cancer (eg, lymphangiosarcoma) develops in the lymphatic system.

LYMPHADENOPATHY

Lymphadenopathy is palpable enlargement of ≥ 1 lymph nodes. Diagnosis is clinical. Treatment is of the causative disorder.

Lymph nodes are present throughout the body, but particular collections are present in the neck, axillae, and inguinal region; a few small (< 1 cm) nodes often are palpable in those areas in healthy people (see p. 739).

Lymphadenopathy is palpable enlargement (> 1 cm) of ≥ 1 lymph nodes; it is categorized as

- Localized: When present in only 1 body area
- Generalized: When present in ≥ 2 body areas

Lymphadenitis is lymphadenopathy with pain and/or signs of inflammation (eg, redness, tenderness).

Other symptoms may be present depending on the underlying disorder.

Pathophysiology

Some plasma and cells (eg, cancer cells, infectious microorganisms) in the interstitial space, along with certain cellular material, antigens, and foreign particles enter lymphatic vessels, becoming lymphatic fluid. Lymph nodes filter the lymphatic fluid on its way to the central venous circulation, removing cells and other material. The filtering process also presents antigens to the lymphocytes contained within the nodes. The immune response from these lymphocytes involves cellular proliferation, which can cause the nodes to enlarge (**reactive lymphadenopathy**). Pathogenic microorganisms carried in the lymphatic fluid can directly infect the nodes, causing lymphadenitis, and cancer cells may lodge in and proliferate in the nodes.

Etiology

Because lymph nodes participate in the body's immune response, a large number of infectious and inflammatory disorders and cancers are potential causes (see Table 85–1). Only the more common causes are discussed here. Causes most likely vary depending on patient age, associated findings, and risk factors, but overall the **most common causes** are

- Idiopathic, self-limited
- Upper respiratory infections (URI)
- Local soft-tissue infections

The **most dangerous causes** are

- Cancer
- HIV infection
- TB

However, most cases represent benign disorders or clinically obvious local infections. Probably < 1% of undifferentiated cases presenting for primary care involve cancer.

Evaluation

Adenopathy may be the patient's reason for presenting or be discovered during evaluation for another complaint.

History: History of present illness should determine the location and duration of adenopathy and whether it is accompanied by pain. Recent cutaneous injuries (particularly cat scratches and rat bites) and infections in the area drained by affected nodes are noted.

Review of systems should seek symptoms of possible causes, including runny, congested nose (URI); sore throat (pharyngitis, mononucleosis); mouth, gum, or tooth pain (oral-dental infection); cough and/or dyspnea (sarcoidosis, lung cancer, TB, some fungal infections); fever, fatigue, and malaise (mononucleosis and many other infections, cancers, and connective tissue disorders); genital lesions or discharge (herpes simplex, chlamydia, syphilis); joint pain and/or swelling (SLE or other connective tissue disorders); easy bleeding and/or bruising (leukemia); and dry, irritated eyes (Sjögren syndrome).

Past medical history should identify risk factors for (or known) TB or HIV infection, and cancer (particularly use of alcohol and/or tobacco). Patients are queried about contacts who are ill (to assess risk of TB or viral illnesses, such as Epstein-Barr virus), sexual history (to assess risk of STDs),

Table 85–1. SOME CAUSES OF LYMPHADENOPATHY

CAUSE	SUGGESTIVE FINDINGS	DIAGNOSTIC APPROACH
Infections		
URI	Cervical adenopathy with only little or no tenderness Sore throat, runny nose, cough	Clinical evaluation
Oropharyngeal infection (eg, pharyngitis, stomatitis, dental abscess)	Cervical adenopathy only (often tender) Clinically apparent oropharyngeal infection	Clinical evaluation
Mononucleosis	Symmetric adenopathy, typically cervical but sometimes in axillae and/or inguinal areas Fever, sore throat, severe fatigue Often splenomegaly Typically in adolescents or young adults	Heterophile antibody test Sometimes Epstein-Barr virus serologic test
TB (extrapulmonary—tuberculous lymphadenitis)	Usually cervical or supraclavicular adenopathy, sometimes inflamed or draining Often in patients with HIV infection	Tuberculin skin testing or interferon-gamma release assay Usually node aspiration or biopsy
HIV (primary infection)	Generalized adenopathy Usually fever, malaise, rash, arthralgia Often history of HIV exposure or high-risk activity	HIV antibody testing Sometimes HIV-RNA assay (if early primary infection is suspected)

Table 85–1. SOME CAUSES OF LYMPHADENOPATHY (*Continued*)

CAUSE	SUGGESTIVE FINDINGS	DIAGNOSTIC APPROACH
Sexually transmitted diseases (STDs—particularly herpes simplex, chlamydial infections, and syphilis)	Except for secondary syphilis, only inguinal adenopathy (fluctuant or draining nodes suggest lymphogranuloma venereum) Often urinary symptoms, urethral or cervical discharge Sometimes genital lesions For secondary syphilis, often widespread mucocutaneous lesions, generalized lymphadenopathy	For herpes simplex, culture For chlamydial infections, nucleic acid-based testing For syphilis, serologic testing
Skin and soft-tissue infections (eg, cellulitis, abscess, cat-scratch disease), including direct lymph node infection	Usually a visible local lesion (or recent history of a lesion) distal to site of adenopathy Sometimes only erythema, tenderness of an isolated node (often cervical) without apparent primary site of entry	Usually clinical evaluation For cat scratch disease, serum antibody titers
Toxoplasmosis	Bilateral, nontender cervical or axillary adenopathy Sometimes a flu-like syndrome, hepatosplenomegaly Often history of exposure to cat feces	Serologic testing
Other infections (eg, brucellosis, cytomegalovirus infection, histoplasmosis, paracoccidioidomycosis, plague, rat bite fever, tularemia)	Vary Often risk factors (eg, geographic location, exposure)	Varies
Cancers		
Leukemias (typically chronic and sometimes acute lymphocytic leukemia)	Fatigue, fever, weight loss, splenomegaly With acute leukemia, often easy bruising and/or bleeding	CBC, peripheral smear, flow cytometry, bone marrow examination
Lymphomas	Painless adenopathy (local or generalized), often rubbery, sometimes matted Often fever, night sweats, weight loss, splenomegaly	Lymph node biopsy or flow cytometry
Metastatic cancers (often head and neck, thyroid, breast, or lung)	One or several painless local nodes Nodes often hard, sometimes fixed to adjacent tissue	Usually evaluation to identify the primary tumor
Connective tissue disorders		
Systemic lupus erythematosus (SLE)	Generalized adenopathy Typically arthritis or arthralgias Sometimes malar rash, other skin lesions	Clinical criteria, antibody testing
Sarcoidosis	Painless adenopathy (local or generalized) Often cough and/or dyspnea, fever, malaise, muscle weakness, weight loss, joint pains	Chest imaging (plain x-ray or CT) If imaging results are positive, node biopsy
Kawasaki disease	Tender cervical adenopathy in children Fever (usually > 39° C), truncal rash, strawberry tongue, periungual, palmar and plantar desquamation	Clinical criteria
Other connective tissue disorders (eg, juvenile idiopathic arthritis, Kikuchi lymphadenopathy, RA, Sjögren syndrome)	Vary	Varies
Other conditions		
Drugs such as allopurinol, antibiotics (eg, cephalosporins, penicillin, sulfonamides), atenolol, captopril, carbamazepine, phenytoin, pyrimethamine, and quinidine	History of using a causative drug Except for phenytoin, a serum sickness-type reaction (eg, rash, arthritis and/or arthralgias, myalgia, fever)	Clinical evaluation
Silicone breast implants	Localized adenopathy in patients with breast implants	Exclusion of other causes of adenopathy

travel history to areas of endemic infections (eg, Middle East for brucellosis, American Southwest for plague) and possible exposures (eg, cat feces for toxoplasmosis, farm animals for brucellosis, wild animals for tularemia). Drug history is reviewed for specific known causative agents.

Physical examination: Vital signs are reviewed for fever. Areas of particular lymph node concentration in the neck (including occipital and supraclavicular areas), axillae, and inguinal region are palpated. Node size, tenderness, and consistency are noted as well as whether the nodes are freely mobile or fixed to adjacent tissue.

Skin is inspected for rash and lesions, with particular attention to areas drained by the affected nodes. The oropharynx is inspected and palpated for signs of infection and any lesions that may be cancerous. The thyroid gland is palpated for enlargement and nodularity. Breasts (including in males) are palpated for lumps. Lungs are auscultated for crackles (suggesting sarcoidosis or infection). Abdomen is palpated for hepatomegaly and splenomegaly. Genitals are examined for chancres, vesicles, and other lesions, and for urethral discharge. Joints are examined for signs of inflammation.

Red flags:

- Node > 2 cm
- Node that is draining, hard, or fixed to underlying tissue
- Supraclavicular node
- Risk factors for HIV or TB
- Fever and/or weight loss
- Splenomegaly

Interpretation of findings: Patients with generalized adenopathy usually have a systemic disorder. However, patients with localized adenopathy may have a local or systemic disorder (including one that often causes generalized adenopathy).

Sometimes, history and physical examination suggest a cause (see Table 85–1) and may be diagnostic in patients with a clear viral URI or with local soft-tissue or dental infection. In other cases, findings (such as the red flag findings) are of concern but do not point to a single cause.

Nodes that are hard, markedly enlarged (> 2 to 2.5 cm), and/or fixed to adjacent tissue, particularly nodes in the supraclavicular area or in patients who have had prolonged use of tobacco and/or alcohol, are concerning for cancer. Marked tenderness, erythema, and warmth in a single enlarged node may be due to a suppurative node infection (eg, due to staphylococcus or streptococcus).

Fever may occur with many of the infectious, malignant, and connective tissue disorders. Splenomegaly can occur with mononucleosis, toxoplasmosis, leukemia, and lymphoma. Weight loss occurs with TB and cancer. Risk factors and travel and exposure history are at best suggestive.

Finally, adenopathy sometimes has a serious cause in patients who have no other manifestations of illness.

Testing: If a specific disorder is suspected (eg, mononucleosis in a young patient with fever, sore throat, and splenomegaly), initial testing is directed at that condition (see Table 85–1).

If history and physical examination do not show a likely cause, further evaluation depends on the nodes involved and the other findings present.

Patients with red flag findings and those with generalized adenopathy should have a CBC and chest x-ray. If abnormal WBCs are seen on CBC, a peripheral smear and flow cytometry are done to evaluate for leukemia or lymphoma. For generalized adenopathy, most clinicians usually also do a tuberculin skin test (or interferon-gamma release assay) and serologic tests for HIV, mononucleosis, and perhaps toxoplasmosis and syphilis. Patients with joint symptoms or rash should have antinuclear antibody testing for SLE.

Most clinicians believe patients with localized adenopathy and no other findings can safely be observed for 3 to 4 wk, unless cancer is suspected. If cancer is suspected, patients typically should have node biopsy (patients with a neck mass require a more extensive evaluation prior to biopsy). Biopsy is also done if isolated or generalized adenopathy does not resolve in 3 to 4 wk.

Treatment

Primary treatment is directed at the cause; adenopathy itself is not treated. A trial of corticosteroids is not done for adenopathy of unknown etiology because corticosteroids can reduce adenopathy caused by leukemia and lymphoma and thus delay diagnosis, and corticosteroids can exacerbate TB. A trial of antibiotics is also not indicated, except when a suppurative lymph node infection is suspected.

KEY POINTS

- Most cases are idiopathic and self-limited, or result from clinically apparent local causes
- Initial testing should be done if there are red flag findings, if other manifestations or risk factors suggest a specific disorder, or when generalized adenopathy has no apparent cause.
- Patients with acute localized lymphadenopathy and no other findings can be observed for 3 to 4 wk, after which time biopsy should be considered.

LYMPHEDEMA

Lymphedema is edema of a limb due to lymphatic hypoplasia (primary) or to obstruction or disruption (secondary) of lymphatic vessels (see p. 739). Symptoms and signs are brawny, fibrous, nonpitting edema in one or more limbs. Diagnosis is by physical examination. Treatment consists of exercise, pressure gradient dressings, massage, and sometimes surgery. Cure is unusual, but treatment may lessen symptoms, slow progression, and prevent complications. Patients are at risk of cellulitis, lymphangitis, and, rarely, lymphangiosarcoma.

Etiology

Lymphedema may be

- Primary: Due to lymphatic hypoplasia
- Secondary: Due to obstruction or disruption of lymphatic vessels

Primary lymphedemas: Primary lymphedemas are inherited and uncommon. They vary in phenotype and patient age at presentation.

Congenital lymphedema appears before age 2 yr and is due to lymphatic aplasia or hypoplasia. **Milroy disease** is an autosomal dominant familial form of congenital lymphedema attributed to vascular endothelial growth factor receptor-3 (*VEGFR-3*) gene mutations and sometimes associated with cholestatic jaundice and edema or diarrhea due to a protein-losing enteropathy caused by intestinal lymphangiectasia.

Lymphedema praecox appears between ages 2 and 35, typically in women at the onset of menses or pregnancy. **Meige disease** is an autosomal dominant familial form of lymphedema praecox attributed to mutations in a transcription factor gene (*FOXC2*) and associated with extra eyelashes (distichiasis), cleft palate, and edema of legs, arms, and sometimes the face.

Lymphedema tarda occurs after age 35. Familial and sporadic forms exist; the genetic basis of both is unknown. Clinical findings are similar to those of lymphedema praecox but may be less severe.

Lymphedema is prominent in some other genetic syndromes, including

- **Turner syndrome**
- **Yellow nail syndrome,** characterized by pleural effusions and yellow nails
- **Hennekam syndrome,** a rare congenital syndrome of intestinal and other lymphangiectases, facial anomalies, and intellectual disability

Secondary lymphedema: Secondary lymphedema is far more common than primary.

Most common causes are

- Surgery (especially lymph node dissection, typically for treatment of breast cancer)
- Radiation therapy (especially axillary or inguinal)
- Trauma
- Lymphatic obstruction by a tumor
- Lymphatic filariasis (in developing countries)

Mild lymphedema may also result from leakage of lymph into interstitial tissues in patients with chronic venous insufficiency.

Symptoms and Signs

Symptoms of secondary lymphedema include aching discomfort and a sensation of heaviness or fullness.

The cardinal sign is soft-tissue edema, graded in 3 stages:

- In stage 1, the edema is pitting, and the affected area often returns to normal by morning.
- In stage 2, the edema is nonpitting, and chronic soft-tissue inflammation causes early fibrosis.
- In stage 3, the edema is brawny and irreversible, largely because of soft-tissue fibrosis.

The swelling is most often unilateral and may worsen when the weather is warm, before menstruation occurs, and after the limb remains for a long time in a dependent position. It can affect any part of the limb (isolated proximal or distal) or the entire extremity; it can restrict range of motion when swelling is periarticular. Disability and emotional distress can be significant, especially when lymphedema results from medical or surgical treatment.

Skin changes are common and include hyperkeratosis, hyperpigmentation, verrucae, papillomas, and fungal infections.

Rarely, an affected limb becomes extremely large, and the hyperkeratosis is severe, giving the appearance of elephant skin (**elephantiasis**). This manifestation is more common with filariasis than with other causes of lymphedema.

Complications: Lymphangitis may develop, most often when bacteria enter through skin cracks between the toes as a result of fungal infections or through cuts to the hand. Lymphangitis is almost always streptococcal, causing erysipelas; sometimes it is staphylococcal. The affected limb becomes red and feels hot; red streaks may extend proximally from the point of entry, and lymphadenopathy may develop. Rarely, the skin breaks down.

Rarely, long-standing lymphedema leads to **lymphangiosarcoma** (Stewart-Treves syndrome), usually in postmastectomy patients and in patients with filariasis.

Diagnosis

- Clinical diagnosis
- CT or MRI if cause is not apparent

Primary lymphedema is usually obvious, based on characteristic soft-tissue edema throughout the body and other information from the history and physical examination.

Diagnosis of secondary lymphedema is usually obvious from physical examination. Additional tests are indicated when secondary lymphedema is suspected unless the diagnosis and cause are obvious. CT and MRI can identify sites of lymphatic obstruction; radionuclide lymphoscintigraphy can identify lymphatic hypoplasia or sluggish flow.

Progression can be monitored by measuring limb circumference, measuring water volume displaced by the submerged limb, or using skin or soft-tissue tonometry; these tests have not been validated.

In developing countries, tests for lymphatic filariasis should be done.

If lymphedema seems much greater than expected (eg, on the basis of lymph node dissection) or appears after a delay in a woman treated for breast cancer, cancer recurrence should be considered.

Prognosis

Cure is unusual once lymphedema occurs. Meticulous treatment and possibly preventive measures can lessen symptoms, slow or halt disease progression, and prevent complications.

Treatment

- Sometimes surgical reconstruction for primary lymphedema
- Mobilizing fluid (eg, by elevation and compression, massage, pressure bandages, intermittent pneumatic compression)

Treatment of primary lymphedema may include surgical soft-tissue reduction (removal of subcutaneous fat and fibrous tissue) and reconstruction if quality of life is significantly reduced.

Treatment of secondary lymphedema involves managing its cause. For lymphedema itself, several interventions to mobilize fluid (complex decongestive therapy) can be used. They include

- Manual lymphatic drainage, in which the limb is elevated and compressed ("milked") toward the heart
- Gradient pressure bandages or sleeves
- Limb exercises
- Limb massage, including intermittent pneumatic compression

Surgical soft-tissue reduction, lymphatic reanastomoses, and formation of drainage channels are sometimes tried but have not been rigorously studied.

Preventive measures include avoiding heat, vigorous exercise, and constrictive garments (including blood pressure cuffs) around the affected limb. Skin and nail care require meticulous attention; vaccination, phlebotomy, and IV catheterization in the affected limb should be avoided.

Cellulitis and lymphangitis are treated with beta-lactamase–resistant antibiotics that are effective against gram-positive organisms (eg, dicloxacillin, cephalexin).

PEARLS & PITFALLS

- Avoid vaccination, phlebotomy, and IV catheterization in limbs affected by lymphedema.

86 Pericarditis

Pericarditis is inflammation of the pericardium, often with fluid accumulation. Pericarditis may be caused by many disorders (eg, infection, myocardial infarction (MI), trauma, tumors, metabolic disorders) but is often idiopathic. Symptoms include chest pain or tightness, often worsened by deep breathing. Cardiac output may be greatly reduced if cardiac tamponade or constrictive pericarditis develops. Diagnosis is based on symptoms, a friction rub, ECG changes, and evidence of pericardial fluid accumulation on x-ray or echocardiogram. Finding the cause requires further evaluation. Treatment depends on the cause, but general measures include analgesics, anti-inflammatory drugs, colchicine, and rarely surgery.

Pericarditis is the most common pericardial disorder. Congenital pericardial disorders are rare.

Anatomy

The pericardium has 2 layers. The visceral pericardium is a single layer of mesothelial cells that is attached to the myocardium, folds back (reflects) on itself over the origin of the great vessels, and joins with a tough, fibrous layer to envelop the heart as the parietal pericardium. The sac created by these layers contains a small amount of fluid (< 25 to 50 mL), composed mostly of an ultrafiltrate of plasma. The pericardium limits distention of the cardiac chambers and increases the heart's efficiency.

The pericardium is richly innervated with sympathetic and somatic afferents. Stretch-sensitive mechanoreceptors sense changes in cardiac volume and tension and may be responsible for transmitting pericardial pain. The phrenic nerves are embedded in the parietal pericardium and are vulnerable to injury during surgery on the pericardium.

Pathophysiology

Pericarditis may be

- Acute
- Subacute
- Chronic

Acute pericarditis develops quickly, causing inflammation of the pericardial sac and often a pericardial effusion. Inflammation can extend to the epicardial myocardium (myopericarditis). Adverse hemodynamic effects and rhythm disturbance are rare, although cardiac tamponade is possible.

Acute disease may become subacute or chronic. These forms develop more slowly; their prominent feature is effusion.

Subacute pericarditis occurs within weeks to months of an inciting event.

Chronic pericarditis is defined as pericarditis persisting > 6 mo.

Pericardial effusion is accumulation of fluid in the pericardium. The fluid may be serous fluid (sometimes with fibrin strands), serosanguineous fluid, blood, pus, or chyle.

Cardiac tamponade occurs when a large pericardial effusion impairs cardiac filling, leading to low cardiac output and sometimes shock and death. If fluid (usually blood) accumulates rapidly, even small amounts (eg, 150 mL) may cause tamponade because the pericardium cannot stretch quickly enough to accommodate it. Slow accumulation of up to 1500 mL may not cause tamponade. Loculated effusion may cause localized tamponade on the right or left side of the heart.

Occasionally, pericarditis causes a marked thickening and stiffening of the pericardium (constrictive pericarditis).

Constrictive pericarditis, which is uncommon, results from marked inflammatory, fibrotic thickening of the pericardium. Sometimes the visceral and parietal layers adhere to each other or to the myocardium. The fibrotic tissue often contains calcium deposits. The stiff, thickened pericardium markedly impairs ventricular filling, decreasing stroke volume and cardiac output. Significant pericardial fluid accumulation is rare. Rhythm disturbance is common. The diastolic pressures in the ventricles, atria, and venous beds become virtually the same. Systemic venous congestion occurs, causing considerable transudation of fluid from systemic capillaries, with dependent edema and, later, ascites. Chronic elevation of systemic venous pressure and hepatic venous pressure may lead to liver scarring, called cardiac cirrhosis, in which case, patients may initially present for evaluation of cirrhosis. Constriction of the left atrium, the left ventricle, or both may elevate pulmonary venous pressure. Occasionally, pleural effusion develops.

- Chronic constrictive pericarditis is less common than in the past.
- Subacute constriction (weeks to months after an inciting injury) is increasingly recognized.
- The transient variant of constrictive pericarditis resolves spontaneously or after medical therapy.

Etiology

Acute pericarditis may result from infection, autoimmune or inflammatory disorders, uremia, trauma, MI, cancer, radiation therapy, or certain drugs (see Table 86–1).

Infectious pericarditis is most often viral or idiopathic. Purulent bacterial pericarditis is uncommon but may follow infective endocarditis, pneumonia, septicemia, penetrating trauma, or cardiac surgery. Often, the cause cannot be identified (called nonspecific or idiopathic pericarditis), but many of these cases are probably viral.

Acute MI causes 10 to 15% of cases of acute pericarditis. Post-MI syndrome (Dressler syndrome) is a less common cause now, occurring mainly when reperfusion with percutaneous transluminal coronary angioplasty (PTCA) or thrombolytic drugs is ineffective in patients with transmural infarction. Pericarditis occurs after pericardiotomy (called postpericardiotomy syndrome) in 5 to 30% of cardiac operations. Postpericardiotomy syndrome, post-MI syndrome, and traumatic pericarditis comprise the post-cardiac injury syndrome.

Subacute pericarditis is a prolongation of acute pericarditis and thus has the same causes. For example, some patients have transient constriction occurring days to weeks after recovery from acute pericarditis.

Chronic pericardial effusion or **chronic constrictive pericarditis** may follow acute pericarditis of almost any etiology. In addition, some cases occur without antecedent acute pericarditis.

Hypothyroidism may cause pericardial effusion and cholesterol pericarditis. Cholesterol pericarditis is a rare disorder that may be associated with myxedema, in which a chronic pericardial effusion has a high level of cholesterol that triggers inflammation and pericarditis.

Sometimes no cause of chronic pericarditis is identified.

Table 86–1. CAUSES OF ACUTE PERICARDITIS

Idiopathic
Viral infections (echovirus, influenza virus, coxsackie B virus, HIV*)
Bacterial infections (streptococci; staphylococci; gram-negative bacilli; TB[†]; in children, *Haemophilus influenzae*)
Fungal infections (histoplasmosis, coccidioidomycosis, candidiasis, blastomycosis)
Parasitic infections (toxoplasmosis, amebiasis, echinococcosis)
Autoimmune disorders (RA, SLE, systemic sclerosis)
Cancer (eg, leukemia, breast or lung cancer, and, in people with AIDS, Kaposi sarcoma)
Radiation therapy
Inflammatory disorders (amyloidosis, inflammatory bowel disease, sarcoidosis)
Uremia
Trauma
MI
Post-MI (Dressler) syndrome
Postpericardiotomy syndrome
Drugs (eg, anticoagulants, hydralazine, isoniazid, methysergide, penicillin, phenytoin, procainamide)

*If patients with AIDS develop lymphoma, Kaposi sarcoma, or certain infections (eg, *Mycobacterium avium*, *M. tuberculosis*, or *Nocardia* infections; other fungal or viral infections), pericarditis may follow.

[†]Tuberculous pericarditis accounts for < 5% of cases of acute or subacute pericarditis in the US but the majority of cases in some areas of India and Africa.

Transient constrictive pericarditis is most commonly caused by infection or postpericardiotomy inflammation, or is idiopathic.

Fibrosis of the pericardium may follow purulent pericarditis or accompany a connective tissue disorder. In older patients, common causes are malignant tumors, MI, and TB. Hemopericardium (accumulation of blood within the pericardium) may lead to pericarditis or pericardial fibrosis; common causes include chest trauma, iatrogenic injury (eg, from cardiac catheterization, pacemaker insertion, or central venous line placement), and rupture of a thoracic aortic aneurysm.

Symptoms and Signs

Some patients present with symptoms and signs of inflammation (acute pericarditis); others present with those of fluid accumulation (pericardial effusion). Symptoms and signs vary depending on the severity of inflammation and the amount and rate of fluid accumulation. Even a large amount of pericardial fluid may be asymptomatic if it develops slowly (eg, over months).

Acute pericarditis: Acute pericarditis tends to cause chest pain and a pericardial rub, sometimes with dyspnea. The first evidence can be tamponade, with hypotension, shock, or pulmonary edema.

Because the innervation of the pericardium and myocardium is the same, the chest pain of pericarditis is sometimes similar to that of myocardial inflammation or ischemia: Dull or sharp precordial or substernal pain may radiate to the neck, trapezius ridge (especially the left), or shoulders. Pain ranges from mild to severe. Unlike ischemic chest pain, pain due to pericarditis is usually aggravated by thoracic motion, cough, breathing, or swallowing food; it may be relieved by sitting up and leaning forward. Tachypnea and nonproductive cough may be present; fever, chills, and weakness are common. In 15 to 25% of patients with idiopathic pericarditis, symptoms recur intermittently for months or years (recurrent pericarditis).

The most important physical finding is a triphasic or a systolic and diastolic precordial friction rub. However, the rub is often intermittent and evanescent; it may be present only during systole or, less frequently, only during diastole. If no rub is heard with the patient seated and leaning forward, auscultation may be attempted by listening with the diaphragm of the stethoscope while with the patient is on all fours. Sometimes, a pleural component to the rub is noted during breathing, which is due to inflammation of the pleura adjacent to the pericardium.

Pericardial effusion: Pericardial effusion is often painless, but when it occurs with acute pericarditis, pain may be present. Considerable amounts of pericardial fluid may muffle heart sounds, increase the area of cardiac dullness, and change the size and shape of the cardiac silhouette. A pericardial rub may be heard. With large effusions, compression of the base of the left lung can decrease breath sounds (heard near the left scapula) and cause crackles. Arterial pulse, jugular venous pulse, and BP are normal unless intrapericardial pressure increases substantially, causing tamponade.

In the post-MI syndrome, pericardial effusion can occur with fever, friction rub, pleurisy, pleural effusions, and joint pain. This syndrome usually occurs within 10 days to 2 mo after MI. It is usually mild but may be severe. Occasionally, the heart ruptures post-MI, causing hemopericardium and tamponade, usually 1 to 10 days post-MI and more commonly in women.

Cardiac tamponade: The clinical findings are similar to those of cardiogenic shock: decreased cardiac output, low systemic arterial pressure, tachycardia, and dyspnea. Neck veins are markedly dilated. Severe cardiac tamponade is nearly always accompanied by a fall of > 10 mm Hg in systolic BP during inspiration (pulsus paradoxus). In advanced cases, pulse may disappear during inspiration. (However, pulsus paradoxus can also occur in COPD, bronchial asthma, pulmonary embolism, right ventricular infarction, and noncardiogenic shock.) Heart sounds are muffled unless the effusion is small. Loculated effusions and eccentric or localized hematoma may cause localized tamponade, in which only selected cardiac chambers are compressed. In these cases, physical, hemodynamic, and some echocardiographic signs may be absent.

Constrictive pericarditis: Fibrosis or calcification rarely causes symptoms unless constrictive pericarditis develops. The only early abnormalities may be elevated ventricular diastolic, atrial, pulmonary, and systemic venous pressures. Symptoms and signs of peripheral venous congestion (eg, peripheral edema, neck vein distention, hepatomegaly) may appear with an early diastolic sound (pericardial knock), often best heard during inspiration. This sound is due to abrupt slowing of diastolic ventricular filling by the rigid pericardium. Ventricular systolic function (based on ejection fraction) is usually preserved. Prolonged elevation of pulmonary venous pressure results in dyspnea (particularly during exertion) and orthopnea. Fatigue may be severe. Distention of neck veins with a rise in venous pressure during inspiration (Kussmaul sign) is present; it is absent in tamponade. Pulsus paradoxus is rare and is usually less severe than in tamponade. Lungs are not congested unless severe left ventricular constriction develops.

Diagnosis

- ECG and chest x-ray
- Echocardiography
- Tests to identify cause (eg, pericardial fluid aspiration, pericardial biopsy)

ECG and chest x-ray are done. Echocardiography is done to check for effusion (particularly loculated effusion with localized tamponade, which because of its atypical manifestations may not be suspected, and which may be suggested by indirect findings such as compression of chambers and characteristic respiratory variations), cardiac filling abnormalities, and wall motion abnormalities characteristic of myocardial involvement. Blood tests may detect leukocytosis and an elevated ESR, but these findings are nonspecific.

Acute pericarditis: The diagnosis is based on the presence of the following clinical findings and ECG abnormalities, which are not always present in all cases.

- Characteristic chest pain
- Pericardial rub
- ECG abnormalities
- Pericardial effusion

Serial ECGs may be needed to show abnormalities. The ECG in acute pericarditis may show abnormalities confined to ST and PR segments and T waves, usually in most leads. (ECG changes in lead aVR are generally in the opposite direction of other leads.) Unlike MI, acute pericarditis does not cause reciprocal depression in ST segments (except in leads aVR and V_1), and there are no pathologic Q waves. ECG changes in pericarditis can occur in 4 stages although not all stages are present in all cases.

- Stage I: ST segments show upward concave elevation; the PR segments may be depressed (see Fig. 86–1)
- Stage II: ST segments return to baseline; T waves flatten.
- Stage III: T waves are inverted throughout the ECG; T wave–inversion occurs after the ST segment has returned to baseline and thus differs from the pattern of acute ischemia or MI.
- Stage IV: T wave changes resolve

Echocardiography in acute pericarditis typically shows an effusion, which helps confirm the diagnosis, except in patients with purely fibrinous acute pericarditis in whom echocardiography is often normal. Findings indicating myocardial involvement include new focal or diffuse left ventricular dysfunction.

Because the pain of pericarditis may resemble that of acute MI or pulmonary infarction, additional tests (eg, serum cardiac marker measurement, lung scan) may be required if the history and ECG findings are atypical for pericarditis. Troponin is often elevated in acute pericarditis due to epicardial inflammation, so it cannot discriminate between pericarditis, acute infarction, and pulmonary embolism. Very high levels of troponin may indicate myopericarditis. The CK level, which is less sensitive than the troponin level, is usually normal in acute pericarditis unless myocarditis is also present.

Postpericardiotomy and post-MI syndromes may be difficult to identify and must be distinguished from recent MI, pulmonary embolism, and pericardial infection after surgery. Pain, friction rub, and fever appearing 2 wk to several months after surgery and a rapid response to aspirin, NSAIDs, colchicine, or corticosteroids aid diagnosis.

Pericardial effusion: Diagnosis is suggested by clinical findings but often is suspected only after finding an enlarged cardiac silhouette on chest x-ray. On ECG, QRS voltage is often decreased, and sinus rhythm remains in about 90% of patients. With large, chronic effusions, the ECG may show electrical alternans (ie, P, QRS, or T wave amplitude increases and decreases on alternate beats). Electrical alternans is associated with variation in cardiac position (swinging heart).

Echocardiography estimates the volume of pericardial fluid; identifies cardiac tamponade, acute myocarditis, and/or heart failure; and may suggest the cause of pericarditis.

Patients with a normal ECG, small (< 50 mL) effusion, and no suspicious findings from the history and examination may be observed with serial examination and echocardiography. Other patients must be evaluated further to determine etiology.

Constrictive pericarditis: Diagnosis may be suspected based on clinical, ECG, chest x-ray, and Doppler echocardiography findings, but cardiac catheterization and CT (or MRI) are usually required. Rarely, right heart biopsy is needed to exclude restrictive cardiomyopathy.

ECG changes are nonspecific. QRS voltage is usually low. T waves are usually nonspecifically abnormal. Atrial fibrillation occurs in about one third of patients; atrial flutter is less common.

Lateral chest x-ray often shows pericardial calcification best, but the finding is nonspecific.

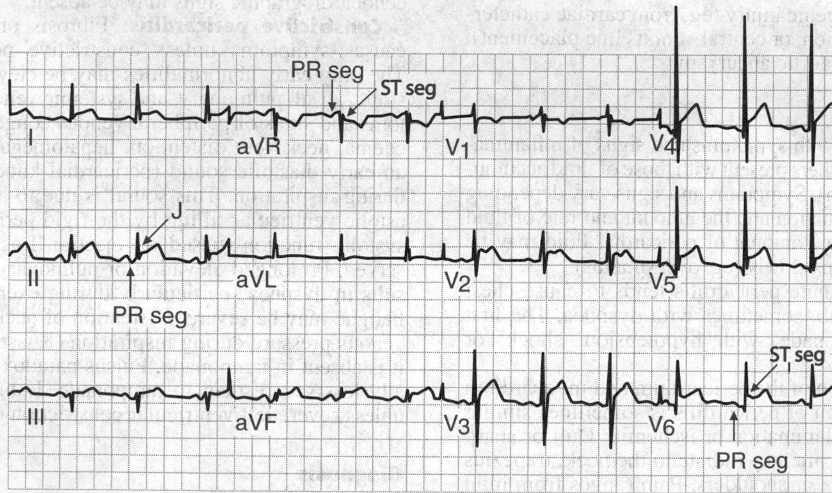

Fig. 86–1. Acute pericarditis: Stage 1 ECG. ST segments, except in aVR and V_1, demonstrate upward concave elevation. T waves are essentially normal PR segments, except aVR and V_1, are depressed.

Echocardiography also is nonspecific. When the right and left ventricular filling pressures are equally elevated, Doppler echocardiography helps distinguish constrictive pericarditis from restrictive cardiomyopathy.

- During inspiration, mitral diastolic flow velocity usually falls > 25% in constrictive pericarditis but < 15% in restrictive cardiomyopathy.
- In constrictive pericarditis, inspiratory tricuspid flow velocity increases more than it normally does, but it does not do so in restrictive cardiomyopathy.

Determining tissue velocities at the mitral annulus may be helpful when excessively high left atrial pressure blunts respiratory variation in transvalvular velocities.

Cardiac catheterization, right and left sided, is done if clinical and echocardiographic findings suggest constrictive pericarditis. Cardiac catheterization helps confirm and quantify the abnormal hemodynamics that define constrictive pericarditis:

- Mean pulmonary artery occlusion pressure (pulmonary capillary wedge pressure), pulmonary artery diastolic pressure, right ventricular end-diastolic pressure, and mean right atrial pressure are all at about 10 to 30 mm Hg.
- The pulmonary artery and right ventricular systolic pressures are normal or modestly elevated, so that pulse pressures are small.
- In the atrial pressure curve, x and y descents are typically accentuated.
- In the ventricular pressure curve, a diastolic dip occurs at the time of rapid ventricular filling.
- During peak inspiration, right ventricular pressure increases when left ventricular pressure is lowest (sometimes called mirror-image discordance, suggesting increased ventricular interdependence).
- Because ventricular filling is restricted, ventricular pressure tracings show a sudden dip followed by a plateau (resembling a square root sign) in early diastole.

Measuring these changes requires simultaneous right and left heart cardiac catheterization, using separate transducers. These hemodynamic changes almost always occur with significant constrictive pericarditis but may be masked during hypovolemia.

Right ventricular systolic pressure of > 50 mm Hg often occurs in restrictive cardiomyopathy but less often in constrictive pericarditis. When the pulmonary artery occlusion pressure equals the right atrial mean pressure and an early diastolic dip in the ventricular pressure curve occurs with large x and y waves in the right atrial curve, either disorder may be present.

CT or MRI can identify pericardial thickening > 5 mm.

- > 5-mm thickening, with typical hemodynamic changes (assessed by echocardiography and catheterization), can confirm constrictive pericarditis.
- When no pericardial thickening or fluid is seen, the diagnosis of restrictive cardiomyopathy is favored but not proved.
- A normal pericardial thickness does not exclude constrictive pericarditis.

Cardiac MRI, specifically the degree of late gadolinium enhancement of the pericardium, may help identify patients in whom constriction will reverse or resolve.

Cardiac tamponade: Low voltage and electrical alternans on the ECG suggest cardiac tamponade, but these findings lack sensitivity and specificity. When tamponade is suspected, echocardiography is done unless even a brief delay might be life threatening. Then pericardiocentesis is done immediately for diagnosis and treatment. On an echocardiogram, respiratory variation of transvalvular and venous flows and compression or collapse of right cardiac chambers in the presence of a pericardial effusion support the diagnosis.

PEARLS & PITFALLS

- Significant cardiac tamponade is a clinical diagnosis; echocardiographic findings alone are not an indication for pericardiocentesis.

If tamponade is suspected, right heart (Swan-Ganz) catheterization may be done. In cardiac tamponade:

- There is no early diastolic dip in the ventricular pressure record.
- Diastolic pressures are elevated (about 10 to 30 mm Hg) and equal in all cardiac chambers and in the pulmonary artery.
- In the atrial pressure curve, x descent is preserved and y descent is lost.

In contrast, in severe congestive states due to dilated cardiomyopathy, pulmonary artery occlusion or left ventricular diastolic pressure usually exceeds right atrial mean pressure and right ventricular diastolic pressure by ≥ 4 mm Hg.

Diagnosis of cause: After pericarditis is diagnosed, tests to determine etiology and the effect on cardiac function are done. In a young, previously healthy adult who presents with a viral infection and acute pericarditis, an extensive evaluation is usually unnecessary. Differentiating viral from idiopathic pericarditis is difficult, expensive, and generally of little practical importance.

In other cases, a biopsy of pericardial tissue or aspiration of pericardial fluid may be needed to establish a diagnosis. Acid-fast stains and cultures of pericardial fluid are essential if TB is considered possible (TB pericarditis can be aggressive and can worsen rapidly with corticosteroid therapy). Samples are examined for malignant cells. However, complete drainage of a newly identified pericardial effusion is usually unnecessary for diagnosis. Persistent (usually > 3 mo) or progressive effusion, particularly when the etiology is uncertain, also warrants pericardiocentesis.

The choice between needle pericardiocentesis and surgical drainage depends on institutional resources and physician experience, the etiology of the effusion, the need for diagnostic tissue samples, and the prognosis of the patient. Needle pericardiocentesis is often best when the etiology is known or the presence of tamponade is in question. Surgical drainage is best when the presence of tamponade is certain but the etiology is unclear.

Laboratory tests of pericardial fluid other than culture and cytology are usually nonspecific. But specific diagnoses are sometimes possible using newer visual, cytologic, and immunologic analysis of fluid obtained via pericardioscopic-guided biopsy.

Cardiac catheterization may be useful for evaluating pericarditis and identifying the cause of reduced cardiac function.

CT or MRI can help identify metastases, although echocardiography is usually sufficient.

Other tests include CBC, acute-phase reactants, routine chemistries, cultures, autoimmune tests, and, when appropriate, tests for HIV, histoplasmosis complement fixation (in endemic areas), and antibody tests for coxsackievirus, influenza virus, echovirus, and streptococcus. Anti-DNA and anti-RNA antibody tests may be useful. A PPD skin test is done, but it can give false negative results; TB pericarditis can be ruled out only by culture of pericardial fluid for acid-fast bacilli.

Treatment

- Varies by cause
- NSAIDs, colchicine, and, infrequently, corticosteroids for pain and inflammation.

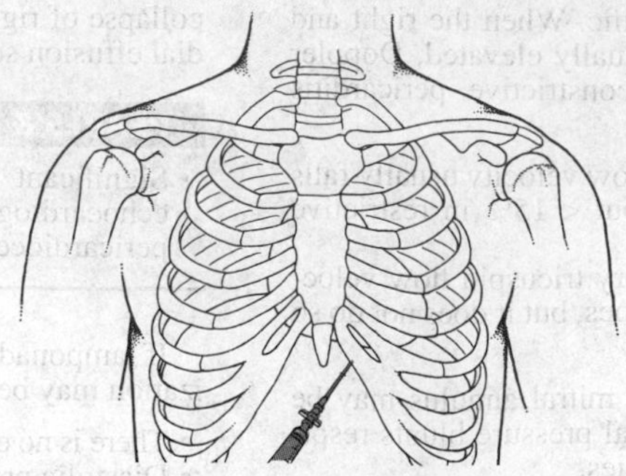

Fig. 86–2. Pericardiocentesis. Except in emergencies (eg, cardiac tamponade), pericardiocentesis, a potentially lethal procedure, should be done using echocardiographic guidance in a cardiac catheterization laboratory and should be supervised by a cardiologist or thoracic surgeon if possible. Resuscitation equipment must be at hand. IV sedation (eg, morphine 0.1 mg/kg or fentanyl 25 to 50 mcg plus midazolam 3 to 5 mg) is desirable. The patient should be recumbent, with the head elevated 30° from the horizontal. Under aseptic conditions, the skin and subcutaneous tissues are infiltrated with lidocaine. A 75-mm short-beveled, 16-gauge needle is attached via a 3-way stopcock to a 30- or 50-mL syringe. The pericardium may be entered via the right or left xiphocostal angle or from the tip of the xiphoid process with the needle directed inward, upward, and close to the chest wall. The needle is advanced with constant suction applied to the syringe. Echocardiography may be used to guide the needle as agitated saline is injected through it. Agitated saline contains microbubbles, facilitating its identification by contrast during echocardiography. Echocardiography is also increasingly used to identify the optimal puncture site and the needle trajectory. Once in place, the needle should be clamped next to the skin to prevent it from entering further than necessary and possibly puncturing the heart or injuring a coronary vessel. ECG monitoring is essential for detecting arrhythmias produced when the myocardium is touched or punctured. As a rule, right atrial pressure and pulmonary artery occlusion pressure (pulmonary capillary wedge pressure) are monitored. Fluid is withdrawn until intrapericardial pressure falls below right atrial pressure, usually to subatmospheric levels. If continued drainage is needed, a plastic catheter may be passed through the needle into the pericardium and the needle withdrawn. The catheter may be left in place for 2 to 4 days.

- Pericardiocentesis for tamponade and some large effusions
- Sometimes intrapericardial drugs (eg, triamcinolone)
- Sometimes pericardial resection for constrictive pericarditis
- Treatment of underlying cause (eg, cancer)

Hospitalization is warranted for some patients with an initial episode of acute pericarditis, particularly those with moderate or large effusions or with high-risk features, such as elevated temperature, subacute onset, immunosuppression, recent trauma, oral anticoagulant therapy, failure to respond to an initial course of aspirin or NSAIDs, and myopericarditis. Hospitalization is needed to determine etiology and to observe for the development of cardiac tamponade. Close, early follow-up is important in patients who are not hospitalized. Possible causative drugs (eg, anticoagulants, procainamide, phenytoin) are stopped. For cardiac tamponade, immediate pericardiocentesis (see Fig. 86–2) is done; removal of even a small volume of fluid may be lifesaving.

Pain can usually be controlled with colchicine or aspirin 325 to 650 mg po q 4 to 6 h or other NSAIDs (eg, ibuprofen 600 to 800 mg po q 6 to 8 h). The intensity of therapy is dictated by the patient's distress. Severe pain may require opioids. Colchicine 0.5 to 1 mg po once/day for 3 mo as an adjunct significantly decreases the recurrence rate and symptom persistence at 72 h in patients with a first episode of acute pericarditis and is increasingly being used as 1st-line therapy.

Although most mild cases of idiopathic and viral pericarditis respond well within a week, the optimal duration of treatment is unclear. Typically, patients should be treated at least until any effusion and evidence of inflammation (eg, ESR or C-reactive protein levels) have resolved.

Corticosteroids (eg, prednisone 60 to 80 mg po once/day for 1 wk, followed by rapid tapering of the dose) may be used in patients with specific indications (eg, connective tissue disorder, autoimmune or uremic pericarditis, failure to respond to colchicine or NSAIDs) but are not given routinely because they enhance viral multiplication and recurrence is common when the dosage is tapered; colchicine may be particularly useful during the taper. Tuberculous and pyogenic pericarditis should be excluded before corticosteroid therapy is initiated. Intrapericardial instillation of triamcinolone 300 mg/m² avoids systemic adverse effects and is highly effective but is typically reserved for patients with recurrent or refractory disease.

Anticoagulants are usually contraindicated in acute pericarditis because they may cause intrapericardial bleeding and even fatal tamponade; however, they can be given in early pericarditis complicating acute MI. Uncommonly, pericardial resection is required.

Painful recurrences of pericarditis may respond to NSAIDs and/or colchicine 0.5 mg po bid for 6 to 12 mo with a gradual taper. If these drugs do not suffice, corticosteroids may be tried, presuming the cause is not infectious.

Infections are treated with specific antimicrobials. Complete drainage is often necessary.

In postpericardiotomy syndrome, post-MI syndrome, or idiopathic pericarditis, antibiotics are not indicated. An NSAID at full doses may control pain and effusion. When required to control pain, fever, and effusion, prednisone 20 to 60 mg po once/day may be given for 3 to 4 days. If the response is satisfactory, the dose is gradually reduced, and the drug may be stopped in 7 to 14 days. But sometimes many months of treatment are needed. Colchicine 1 mg po once/day after a 2 mg load for 30 days, beginning on postoperative day 3 may reduce the incidence of postpericardiotomy syndrome after cardiac surgery

For pericarditis due to rheumatic fever, another connective tissue disorder, or tumor, therapy is directed at the underlying process.

For pericardial effusion due to trauma, surgery is sometimes required to repair the injury and remove blood from the pericardium.

Pericarditis due to uremia may respond to increased frequency of hemodialysis, aspiration, or systemic or intrapericardial corticosteroids. Intrapericardial triamcinolone may be useful.

Chronic effusions are best treated by treating the cause, if known. Recurrent or persistent symptomatic effusions may be treated with balloon pericardiotomy or a surgical pericardial window. Asymptomatic effusions of unknown cause may require only observation.

Congestion in chronic constrictive pericarditis may be alleviated with salt restriction and diuretics. Digoxin is indicated only if atrial arrhythmias or ventricular systolic dysfunction is present. Patients with symptomatic constrictive pericarditis (eg, with dyspnea, unexplained weight gain, a new or increased pleural effusion, or ascites) and those with markers of chronic constriction (eg, cachexia, atrial fibrillation, hepatic dysfunction, pericardial calcification) usually require pericardial resection. However, patients with mild symptoms, heavy calcification, or extensive myocardial damage may be poor surgical candidates.

The mortality rate for pericardial resection may approach 40% in New York Heart Association (NYHA) functional class IV patients (see Table 83–2 on p. 716). Patients who have constrictive pericarditis due to irradiation or a connective tissue disorder are especially likely to have severe myocardial damage and may not benefit from pericardial resection. Patients with newly diagnosed constrictive pericarditis who are hemodynamically stable and without evidence of chronic constriction may be given a 2- to 3-mo trial of anti-inflammatory drugs, rather than pericardiectomy.

KEY POINTS

- Patients may have signs of inflammation and/or fluid accumulation (effusion).
- ECG and echocardiography are usually adequate for diagnosis, but right and left heart catheterization, CT, or MRI may be needed to diagnose constrictive pericarditis.
- Pain is treated with NSAIDs and/or colchicine; corticosteroids may be added for noninfectious causes.
- Effusions usually respond to treatment of the cause, but recurrent or persistently symptomatic effusions may require drainage (percutaneous or surgical).
- Symptomatic chronic constrictive pericarditis usually requires pericardial resection.

87 Peripheral Arterial Disorders

ACROCYANOSIS

Acrocyanosis is persistent, painless, symmetric cyanosis of the hands, feet, or face caused by vasospasm of the small vessels of the skin in response to cold.

Acrocyanosis usually occurs in women and is not associated with occlusive arterial disease. The digits and hands or feet are persistently cold and bluish, sweat profusely, and may swell. In acrocyanosis, unlike Raynaud syndrome, cyanosis persists and is not easily reversed, trophic changes and ulcers do not occur, and pain is absent. Pulses are normal.

Treatment, other than reassurance and avoidance of cold, is usually unnecessary. Vasodilators may be tried but are usually ineffective.

ERYTHROMELALGIA

Erythromelalgia is distressing paroxysmal vasodilation of small arteries in the feet and hands and, less commonly, in the face, ears, or knees; it causes burning pain, increased skin temperature, and redness.

This **rare** disorder may be primary (cause unknown) or secondary to myeloproliferative disorders (eg, polycythemia vera, thrombocythemia), hypertension, venous insufficiency, diabetes mellitus, SLE, RA, lichen sclerosus, gout, spinal cord disorders, or multiple sclerosis. Less commonly, the disorder is related to the use of some drugs (eg, nifedipine, bromocriptine). A rare hereditary form of erythromelalgia starts at birth or during childhood.

Burning pain, heat, and redness in the feet or hands last a few minutes to several hours. In most patients, symptoms are triggered by warmth (temperatures of 29 to 32° C) and are typically relieved by immersion in ice water. Trophic changes do not occur. Symptoms may remain mild for years or become severe enough to cause total disability. Generalized vasomotor dysfunction is common, and Raynaud syndrome may occur.

Diagnosis is clinical. Testing is done to detect causes. Because erythromelalgia may precede a myeloproliferative disorder by several years, repeated blood counts may be indicated. Differential diagnosis includes posttraumatic reflex dystrophies, shoulder-hand syndrome, peripheral neuropathy, causalgia, Fabry disease, and bacterial cellulitis.

Treatment is warmth avoidance, rest, elevation of the extremity, and application of cold. For primary erythromelalgia, gabapentin may be of benefit. For secondary erythromelalgia, the underlying disorder is treated; aspirin may be helpful when a myeloproliferative disorder is involved.

FIBROMUSCULAR DYSPLASIA

Fibromuscular dysplasia includes a heterogenous group of nonatherosclerotic, noninflammatory arterial changes, causing some degree of vascular stenosis, occlusion, or aneurysm.

Fibromuscular dysplasia usually occurs in women aged 40 to 60. The cause is unknown. However, there may be a genetic component, and smoking may be a risk factor. Fibromuscular dysplasia is more common among people with certain connective tissue disorders (eg, Ehlers-Danlos syndrome type 4, cystic medial necrosis, hereditary nephritis, neurofibromatosis).

Medial dysplasia, the most common type, is characterized by alternating regions of thick and thin fibromuscular ridges containing collagen along the media. In perimedial dysplasia, extensive collagen deposition occurs in the outer half of the media. Fibromuscular dysplasia may affect the renal arteries (60 to 75%), carotid and intracranial arteries (25 to 30%), intra-abdominal arteries (9%), or external iliac arteries (5%).

Fibromuscular dysplasia is usually asymptomatic regardless of location. Symptoms, when they occur, vary by location:

- Claudication in the thighs and calves, femoral bruits, and decreased femoral pulses when leg arteries are affected
- Secondary hypertension when renal arteries are affected
- Transient ischemic attack or stroke symptoms when carotid arteries are affected
- Aneurysmal symptoms when intracranial arteries are affected
- Rarely, mesenteric ischemic symptoms when intra-abdominal arteries are affected

Ultrasonography may suggest the diagnosis, but definitive diagnosis is made by angiography showing a beaded appearance (in medial or perimedial dysplasia) or a concentric band or long, smooth narrowing (in other forms).

Treatment varies by location. It may involve percutaneous transluminal angioplasty alone, percutaneous stent angioplasty, bypass surgery, or aneurysm repair. Smoking cessation is important. Control of other risk factors for atherosclerosis (hypertension, dyslipidemia, diabetes) helps prevent accelerated development of flow-limiting arterial stenoses.

PERIPHERAL ARTERIAL ANEURYSMS

Peripheral arterial aneurysms are abnormal dilations of the peripheral arteries caused by weakening of the arterial wall (see also p. 698).

About 70% of peripheral arterial aneurysms are popliteal aneurysms; 20% are iliofemoral aneurysms. Aneurysms at these locations frequently accompany abdominal aortic aneurysms, and > 50% are bilateral. Rupture is relatively infrequent, but these aneurysms may lead to thromboembolism. They occur in men much more often than women (> 20:1); mean age at presentation is 65. Aneurysms in arm arteries are relatively rare; they may cause limb ischemia, distal embolism, and stroke.

Infectious (mycotic) aneurysms may occur in any artery but are most common in the femoral. They are usually due to salmonellae, staphylococci, or *Treponema pallidum* (which causes syphilitic aneurysm).

Common causes include atherosclerosis, popliteal artery entrapment, and septic emboli (which cause mycotic aneurysms).

Peripheral arterial aneurysms are usually asymptomatic at the time of detection. Thrombosis or embolism (or rarely, aneurysm rupture) causes extremities to be painful, cold, pale, paresthetic, or pulseless. Infectious aneurysms may cause local pain, fever, malaise, and weight loss.

Diagnosis is by ultrasonography, magnetic resonance angiography, or CT. Popliteal aneurysms may be suspected when physical examination detects an enlarged, pulsatile artery; the diagnosis is confirmed by imaging tests.

Risk of rupture of extremity aneurysms is low (< 5% for popliteal and 1 to 14% for iliofemoral aneurysms). For leg artery aneurysms, surgical repair is therefore often elective. It is indicated when the arteries are twice normal size or when the patient is symptomatic. However, surgical repair is indicated for all arm artery aneurysms because serious complications (eg, thromboembolism) are a greater risk. The affected segment of artery is excised and replaced with a graft. Limb salvage rate after surgical repair is 90 to 98% for asymptomatic patients and 70 to 80% for symptomatic patients.

In certain patients, an endovascular-covered stent graft is another option for repair.

PERIPHERAL ARTERIAL DISEASE

(Peripheral Vascular Disease)

Peripheral arterial disease (PAD) is atherosclerosis of the extremities (virtually always lower) causing ischemia. Mild PAD may be asymptomatic or cause intermittent claudication; severe PAD may cause rest pain with skin atrophy, hair loss, cyanosis, ischemic ulcers, and gangrene. Diagnosis is by history, physical examination, and measurement of the ankle-brachial index. Treatment of mild PAD includes risk factor modification, exercise, antiplatelet drugs, and cilostazol or possibly pentoxifylline as needed for symptoms. Severe PAD usually requires angioplasty or surgical bypass and may require amputation. Prognosis is generally good with treatment, although mortality rate is relatively high because coronary artery or cerebrovascular disease often coexists.

Etiology

Prevalence of PAD is about 12% in the US; men are affected more commonly. Risk factors are the same as those for atherosclerosis: increasing age, hypertension, diabetes, dyslipidemia (high low-density lipoprotein [LDL] cholesterol, low high-density lipoprotein [HDL] cholesterol), cigarette smoking (including passive smoking) or other forms of tobacco use, and a family history of atherosclerosis. Obesity, male sex, and a high homocysteine level are also risk factors.

Atherosclerosis is a systemic disorder; 50 to 75% of patients with PAD also have clinically significant coronary artery disease (CAD) or cerebrovascular disease. However, CAD may be silent in part because PAD may prevent patients from exerting themselves enough to trigger angina.

Symptoms and Signs

Typically, PAD causes intermittent claudication, which is a painful, aching, cramping, uncomfortable, or tired feeling in the legs that occurs during walking and is relieved by rest. Claudication usually occurs in the calves but can occur in the feet, thighs, hips, buttocks, or, rarely, arms. Claudication is a manifestation of exercise-induced reversible ischemia, similar to angina pectoris. As PAD progresses, the distance that can be walked without symptoms may decrease, and patients with severe PAD may experience pain during rest, reflecting irreversible ischemia. Rest pain is usually worse distally, is aggravated by leg elevation (often causing pain at night), and lessens when the leg is below heart level. The pain may be burning, tightening, or aching, although this finding is nonspecific. About 20% of patients with PAD are asymptomatic, sometimes because they are not active enough to trigger leg ischemia. Some patients have atypical symptoms (eg, nonspecific exercise intolerance, hip or other joint pain).

Mild PAD often causes no signs. Moderate to severe PAD commonly causes diminished or absent peripheral (popliteal, tibialis posterior, dorsalis pedis) pulses; Doppler ultrasonography can often detect blood flow when pulses cannot be palpated.

When below heart level, the foot may appear dusky red (called dependent rubor). In some patients, elevating the foot causes loss of color and worsens ischemic pain; when the foot is lowered, venous filling is prolonged (> 15 sec). Edema is usually not present unless the patient has kept the leg immobile and in a dependent position to relieve pain. Patients with chronic PAD may have thin, pale (atrophic) skin with hair thinning or loss. Distal legs and feet may feel cool. The affected leg may sweat excessively and become cyanotic, probably because of sympathetic nerve overactivity.

As ischemia worsens, ulcers may appear (typically on the toes or heel, occasionally on the leg or foot), especially after local trauma. The ulcers tend to be surrounded by black, necrotic tissue (dry gangrene). They are usually painful, but people with peripheral neuropathy due to diabetes or alcoholism may not feel them. Infection of ischemic ulcers (wet gangrene) occurs readily, causing rapidly progressive cellulitis.

The level of arterial occlusion influences location of symptoms. Aortoiliac PAD may cause buttock, thigh, or calf claudication; hip pain; and, in men, erectile dysfunction (Leriche syndrome). In femoropopliteal PAD, claudication typically occurs in the calf; pulses below the femoral artery are weak or absent. In PAD of more distal arteries, femoropopliteal pulses may be present, but foot pulses are absent.

Arterial occlusive disease occasionally affects the arms, epecially the left proximal subclavian artery, causing arm fatigue with exercise and occasionally embolization to the hands.

Diagnosis

- Ankle-brachial BP index
- Ultrasonography
- Angiography before surgery

PAD is suspected clinically but is underrecognized because many patients have atypical symptoms or are not active enough to have symptoms. Spinal stenosis may also cause leg pain during walking but can be distinguished because the pain (called pseudoclaudication) requires sitting, not just rest, for relief, and distal pulses remain intact.

Diagnosis is confirmed by noninvasive testing. First, bilateral arm and ankle systolic BP is measured; because ankle pulses may be difficult to palpate, a Doppler probe may be placed over the dorsalis pedis or posterior tibial arteries. Doppler ultrasonography is often used, because pressure gradients and pulse volume waveforms can help distinguish isolated aortoiliac PAD from femoropopliteal PAD and below-the-knee PAD.

A low (≤ 0.90) ankle-brachial index (ratio of ankle to arm systolic BP) indicates PAD, which can be classified as mild (0.71 to 0.90), moderate (0.41 to 0.70), or severe (≤ 0.40). If the index is normal (0.91 to 1.30) but suspicion of PAD remains high, the index is determined after exercise stress testing. A high index (> 1.30) may indicate noncompressible leg vessels (as occurs in Mönckeberg arteriosclerosis with calcification of the arterial wall). If the index is > 1.30 but suspicion of PAD remains high, additional tests (eg, Doppler ultrasonography, measurement of BP in the first toe using toe cuffs) are done to check for arterial stenoses or occlusions. Ischemic lesions are unlikely to heal when systolic BP is < 55 mm Hg in patients without diabetes or < 70 mm Hg in patients with diabetes; below-the-knee amputations usually heal if BP is ≥ 70 mm Hg. Peripheral arterial insufficiency can also be assessed by transcutaneous oximetry (TcO_2). A TcO_2 level < 40 mm Hg is predictive of poor healing, and a value < 20 mm Hg is consistent with critical limb ischemia.

Angiography provides details of the location and extent of arterial stenoses or occlusion; it is a prerequisite for surgical correction or percutaneous transluminal angioplasty (PTA). It is not a substitute for noninvasive testing because it provides no information about the functional significance of abnormal findings. Magnetic resonance angiography and CT angiography are noninvasive tests that may eventually supplant contrast angiography.

Treatment

- Risk factor modification
- Exercise
- Antiplatelet drugs
- Sometimes pentoxifylline or cilostazol for claudication
- ACE inhibitors
- PTA or surgery for severe disease

All patients require aggressive risk factor modification, including smoking cessation; control of diabetes, dyslipidemia, hypertension, and hyperhomocysteinemia; and dietary changes (see p. 653). β-Blockers are safe unless PAD is very severe.

Exercise—35 to 50 min of treadmill or track walking in an exercise-rest-exercise pattern 3 to 4 times/wk—is an important but underused treatment. Supervised exercise programs are probably superior to unsupervised programs. Exercise can increase symptom-free walking distance and improve quality of life. Mechanisms probably include increased collateral circulation, improved endothelial function with microvascular vasodilation, decreased blood viscosity, improved RBC filterability, decreased ischemia-induced inflammation, and improved O_2 extraction.

Patients are advised to keep the legs below heart level. For pain relief at night, the head of the bed can be elevated about 10 to 15 cm (4 to 6 inches) to improve blood flow to the feet.

Patients are also advised to avoid cold and drugs that cause vasoconstriction (eg, pseudoephedrine, contained in many sinus and cold remedies).

Preventive foot care is crucial, especially for patients with diabetes. It includes daily foot inspection for injuries and lesions; treatment of calluses and corns by a podiatrist; daily washing of the feet in lukewarm water with mild soap, followed by gentle, thorough drying; and avoidance of thermal, chemical, and mechanical injury, especially that due to poorly fitting footwear. For foot ulcer management, see p. 1067.

Antiplatelet drugs may modestly lessen symptoms and improve walking distance; more importantly, these drugs modify atherogenesis and help prevent acute coronary syndromes and transient ischemic attacks (see also p. 695). Options include aspirin 81 to 162 mg po once/day, aspirin 25 mg plus dipyridamole 200 mg po once/day, and clopidogrel 75 mg po once/day or ticlopidine 250 mg po bid with or without aspirin. Aspirin is typically used alone first, followed by addition or substitution of other drugs if PAD progresses.

For relief of claudication, pentoxifylline 400 mg po tid with meals or cilostazol 100 mg po bid may be used to relieve intermittent claudication by improving blood flow and enhancing tissue oxygenation in affected areas; however, these drugs are no substitute for risk factor modification and exercise. Use of pentoxifylline is controversial because evidence of its effectiveness is mixed. A trial of ≥ 2 mo may be warranted, because adverse effects are uncommon and mild. The most common adverse effects of cilostazol are headache and diarrhea. Cilostazol is contraindicated in patients with severe heart failure.

ACE inhibitors have several beneficial effects. They are antiatherogenic and, by inhibiting the degradation of bradykinin and promoting the release of nitric oxide, are potent vasodilators. Among patients with intermittent claudication, a recent randomized trial of ramipril 10 mg po once/day showed a significant increase in pain-free and maximum treadmill walking times compared to placebo.

Other drugs that may relieve claudication are being studied; they include L-arginine (the precursor of endothelium-dependent vasodilator), nitric oxide, vasodilator prostaglandins, and angiogenic growth factors (eg, vascular endothelial growth factor [VEGF], basic fibroblast growth factor [bFGF]). Gene therapy for PAD is also being studied. In patients with severe limb ischemia, long-term parenteral use of vasodilator prostaglandins may decrease pain and facilitate ulcer healing, and intramuscular gene transfer of DNA encoding VEGF may promote collateral blood vessel growth.

Percutaneous transluminal intervention: PTA with or without stent insertion is the primary nonsurgical method for dilating vascular occlusions. PTA with stent insertion may keep the artery open better than balloon compression alone, with a lower rate of reocclusion. Stents work best in large arteries with high flow (iliac and renal); they are less useful for smaller arteries and for long occlusions.

Indications for PTA are similar to those for surgery: intermittent claudication that inhibits daily activities, rest pain, and gangrene. Suitable lesions are flow-limiting, short iliac stenoses (< 3 cm) and short, single or multiple stenoses of the superficial femoropopliteal segment. Complete occlusions (up to 10 or 12 cm long) of the superficial femoral artery can be successfully dilated, but results are better for occlusions ≤ 5 cm. PTA is also useful for localized iliac stenosis proximal to a bypass of the femoropopliteal artery.

PTA is less useful for diffuse disease, long occlusions, and eccentric calcified plaques. Such lesions are particularly common in patients with diabetes, often affecting small arteries.

Complications of PTA include thrombosis at the site of dilation, distal embolization, intimal dissection with occlusion by a flap, and complications related to heparin use.

With appropriate patient selection (based on complete and adequate angiography), the initial success rate approaches 85 to 95% for iliac arteries and 50 to 70% for thigh and calf arteries. Recurrence rates are relatively high (25 to 35% at ≤ 3 yr); repeat PTA may be successful.

Surgery: Surgery is indicated for patients who can safely tolerate a major vascular procedure and whose severe symptoms do not respond to noninvasive treatments. The goal is to relieve symptoms, heal ulcers, and avoid amputation. Because many patients have underlying CAD, which places them at risk of acute coronary syndromes during surgical procedures for PAD, patients usually undergo cardiac evaluation prior to surgery.

Thromboendarterectomy (surgical removal of an occlusive lesion) is used for short, localized lesions in the aortoiliac, common femoral, or deep femoral arteries.

Revascularization (eg, femoropopliteal bypass grafting) uses synthetic or natural materials (often the saphenous or another vein) to bypass occlusive lesions. Revascularization helps prevent limb amputation and relieve claudication.

In patients who cannot undergo major vascular surgery, sympathectomy may be effective when a distal occlusion causes severe ischemic pain. Chemical sympathetic blocks are as effective as surgical sympathectomy, so the latter is rarely done.

Amputation is a procedure of last resort, indicated for uncontrolled infection, unrelenting rest pain, and progressive gangrene. Amputation should be as distal as possible, preserving the knee for optimal use with a prosthesis.

External compression therapy: External pneumatic compression of the lower limb to increase distal blood flow is an option for limb salvage in patients who have severe PAD and are not candidates for surgery. Theoretically, it controls edema and improves arterial flow, venous return, and tissue oxygenation, but data supporting its use are lacking. Pneumatic cuffs or stockings are placed on the lower leg and inflated rhythmically during diastole, systole, or part of both periods for 1 to 2 h several times/wk.

Bone marrow stem cell transplantation: Bone marrow stem cells can differentiate into small blood vessels. Clinical trials are investigating autologous iliac crest bone marrow stem cell transplantation into legs of patients with critical limb ischemia. Although this therapy may not be appropriate for every patient, it may prove to be an alternative for some who would otherwise need major amputation; current results show that 2 yr post-transplant, 60 to 70% have avoided amputation.

KEY POINTS

- PAD occurs almost always in the lower extremities.
- 50 to 75% of patients also have significant cerebral and/or coronary atherosclerosis.
- When symptomatic, PAD causes intermittent claudication, which is discomfort in the legs that occurs during walking and is relieved by rest; it is a manifestation of exercise-induced reversible ischemia, similar to angina pectoris.
- Severe PAD may cause pain during rest, reflecting irreversible ischemia, or ischemic ulcers on the feet.
- A low (≤ 0.90) ankle-brachial index (ratio of ankle to arm systolic BP) indicates PAD.
- Modify atherosclerosis risk factors; give statins, antiplatelet drugs, and sometimes ACE inhibitors, pentoxifylline, or cilostazol.
- PTA with or without stent insertion may dilate vascular occlusions; sometimes surgery (endarterectomy or bypass grafting) is necessary.

ACUTE PERIPHERAL ARTERIAL OCCLUSION

Peripheral arteries may be acutely occluded by a thrombus, an embolus, aortic dissection, or acute compartment syndrome.

Acute peripheral arterial occlusion may result from:

- Rupture and thrombosis of an atherosclerotic plaque
- Embolus from the heart or thoracic or abdominal aorta
- Aortic dissection
- Acute compartment syndrome (see p. 2997)

Symptoms and signs are sudden onset in an extremity of the 5 P's: severe **p**ain, **p**olar sensation (coldness), **p**aresthesias (or anesthesias), **p**allor, and **p**ulselessness. The occlusion can be roughly localized to the arterial bifurcation just distal to the last palpable pulse (eg, at the common femoral bifurcation when the femoral pulse is palpable; at the popliteal bifurcation when the popliteal pulse is palpable). Severe cases may cause loss of motor function. After 6 to 8 h, muscles may be tender when palpated.

Diagnosis is clinical. Immediate angiography is required to confirm location of the occlusion, identify collateral flow, and guide therapy.

Treatment consists of embolectomy (catheter or surgical), thrombolysis, or bypass surgery. The decision to do surgical thromboembolectomy vs thrombolysis is based on the severity of ischemia, the extent or location of the thrombus, and the general medical condition of the patient.

A thrombolytic (fibrinolytic) drug, especially when given by regional catheter infusion, is most effective for patients with acute arterial occlusions of < 2 wk and intact motor and sensory limb function. Tissue plasminogen activator and urokinase are most commonly used. A catheter is threaded to the occluded area, and the thrombolytic drug is given at a rate appropriate for the patient's size and the extent of thrombosis. Treatment is usually continued for 4 to 24 h, depending on severity of ischemia and signs of thrombolysis (relief of symptoms and return of pulses or improved blood flow shown by Doppler ultrasonography). About 20 to 30% of patients with acute arterial occlusion require amputation within the first 30 days.

RAYNAUD SYNDROME

Raynaud syndrome is vasospasm of parts of the hand in response to cold or emotional stress, causing reversible discomfort and color changes (pallor [see Plate 5], cyanosis, erythema, or a combination) in one or more digits. Occasionally, other acral parts (eg, nose, tongue) are affected. The disorder may be primary or secondary. Diagnosis is clinical; testing focuses on distinguishing primary from secondary disease. Treatment of uncomplicated cases includes avoidance of cold, biofeedback, smoking cessation, and, as needed, vasodilating Ca channel blockers (eg, nifedipine) or prazosin.

Overall prevalence is about 3 to 5%; women are affected more than men, and younger people are affected more than older people. Raynaud syndrome is probably due to an exaggerated α_2-adrenergic response that triggers vasospasm; the mechanism is not defined.

Primary Raynaud syndrome is much more common (> 80% of cases) than secondary; it occurs without symptoms or signs of other disorders. In the remaining 20% of patients with Raynaud symptoms, a causative underlying disease (eg, systemic sclerosis) will be evident at initial presentation or diagnosed subsequently.

Secondary Raynaud syndrome accompanies various disorders and conditions, mostly connective tissue disorders (see Table 87–1).

Nicotine commonly contributes to it but is often overlooked. Raynaud syndrome may accompany migraine headaches, variant angina, and pulmonary hypertension, suggesting that these disorders share a common vasospastic mechanism.

Symptoms and Signs

Sensations of coldness, burning pain, paresthesias, or intermittent color changes of one or more digits are precipitated by exposure to cold, emotional stress, or vibration. All can be reversed by removing the stimulus. Rewarming the hands accelerates restoration of normal color and sensation.

Color changes are clearly demarcated across the digit. They may be triphasic (pallor, followed by cyanosis and after warming by erythema due to reactive hyperemia), biphasic (cyanosis, erythema), or uniphasic (pallor or cyanosis only). Changes are often symmetric. Raynaud syndrome does not occur proximal to the metacarpophalangeal joints; it most commonly affects the middle 3 fingers and rarely affects the thumb. Vasospasm may last minutes to hours but is rarely severe enough to cause tissue loss in primary Raynaud syndrome.

Raynaud syndrome secondary to a connective tissue disorder may progress to painful digital gangrene; Raynaud syndrome secondary to systemic sclerosis tends to cause extremely painful, infected ulcers on the fingertips.

Table 87–1. CAUSES OF SECONDARY RAYNAUD SYNDROME

CAUSE	EXAMPLES
Connective tissue disorders	Mixed or undifferentiated connective tissue disease Polymyositis/dermatomyositis RA Sjögren syndrome SLE Systemic sclerosis
Endocrine disorders	Hypothyroidism
Hematologic disorders	Cold agglutinin disease Polycythemia vera
Neoplastic disorders	Carcinoid Paraneoplastic syndrome
Neurologic disorders	Carpal tunnel syndrome
Trauma	Frost bite Vibration
Vascular disorders	Thoracic outlet syndrome
Drugs	β-Blockers Cocaine Ergot preparations Nicotine Sympathomimetic drugs

Diagnosis

- Clinical criteria
- Examination and testing for underlying disorder

Raynaud syndrome itself is diagnosed clinically. Acrocyanosis (see p. 749) also causes color change of the digits in response to cold but differs from Raynaud syndrome in that it is persistent, not easily reversed, and does not cause trophic changes, ulcers, or pain.

Primary and secondary forms are distinguished clinically, supported by vascular laboratory studies and blood testing. Vascular laboratory testing includes digital pulse wave forms and pressures. The primary blood testing is the panel for collagen vascular diseases (eg, testing for ESR or C-reactive protein, rheumatoid factor, anti-DNA, antinuclear, and anti-CCP antibodies).

Clinical findings: A thorough history and physical examination directed at identifying a causative disorder are helpful but rarely diagnostic.

Findings suggesting primary Raynaud syndrome are the following:

- Age at onset < 40 (in two-thirds of cases)
- Mild symmetric attacks affecting both hands
- No tissue necrosis or gangrene
- No history or physical findings suggesting another cause

Findings suggesting secondary Raynaud syndrome are the following:

- Age at onset > 30
- Severe painful attacks that may be asymmetric and unilateral
- Ischemic lesions
- History and findings suggesting an accompanying disorder

Laboratory testing: Blood tests (eg, measurement of ESR, antinuclear antibodies, rheumatoid factor, anticentromere antibody, anti-SCL-70 antibody) are done to detect accompanying disorders.

Treatment

- Trigger avoidance
- Smoking cessation
- Ca channel blockers or prazosin

Treatment of the primary form involves avoidance of cold, smoking cessation, and, if stress is a triggering factor, relaxation techniques (eg, biofeedback) or counseling. Drugs are used more often than behavioral treatments because of convenience. Vasodilating Ca channel blockers (extended-release nifedipine 60 to 90 mg po once/day, amlodipine 5 to 20 mg po once/day, felodipine 2.5 to 10 mg po bid, or isradipine 2.5 to 5 mg po bid) are most effective, followed by prazosin 1 to 5 mg po once/day or bid. Topical nitroglycerine paste, pentoxifylline 400 mg po bid or tid with meals, or both may be effective, but no evidence supports routine use. β-Blockers, clonidine, and ergot preparations are contraindicated because they cause vasoconstriction and may trigger or worsen symptoms.

Treatment of the secondary form focuses on the underlying disorder. Ca channel blockers or prazosin is also indicated. Antibiotics, analgesics, and, occasionally, surgical debridement may be necessary for ischemic ulcers. Low-dose aspirin may prevent thrombosis but theoretically may worsen vasospasm via prostaglandin inhibition. IV prostaglandins (alprostadil, epoprostenol, iloprost) appear to be effective and may be an option for patients with ischemic digits. However, these drugs are not yet widely available, and their role is yet to be defined. Cervical or local sympathectomy is controversial; it is reserved for patients with progressive disability unresponsive to all other measures, including treatment of underlying disorders. Sympathectomy often abolishes the symptoms, but relief may last only 1 to 2 yr.

KEY POINTS

- Raynaud syndrome is reversible vasospasm of parts of the hand in response to cold or emotional stress.
- Raynaud syndrome may be primary, or secondary to another disorder, typically one affecting connective tissue.
- Primary Raynaud syndrome, unlike the secondary form, rarely causes gangrene or tissue loss.
- Diagnose clinically but consider testing to diagnose a suspected cause.
- Avoid cold, smoking, and any other triggers.
- Give a vasodilating Ca channel blocker or prazosin.

THROMBOANGIITIS OBLITERANS

(Buerger Disease)

Thromboangiitis obliterans is inflammatory thrombosis of small and medium-sized arteries and some superficial veins, causing arterial ischemia in distal extremities and superficial thrombophlebitis. Tobacco use is the primary risk factor. Symptoms and signs include claudication, nonhealing foot ulcers, rest pain, and gangrene. Diagnosis is by clinical findings, noninvasive vascular testing, angiography, and exclusion of other causes. Treatment is cessation of tobacco use. Prognosis is excellent when tobacco use is stopped, but when it is not, the disorder inevitably progresses, often requiring amputation.

Thromboangiitis obliterans occurs almost exclusively in tobacco users (nearly all of them smokers) and predominantly affects men aged 20 to 40; it rarely occurs in women. It occurs more commonly in people with HLA-A9 and HLA-B5 genotypes. Prevalence is highest in Asia and the Far and Middle East.

Thromboangiitis obliterans produces segmental inflammation in small and medium-sized arteries and, frequently, in superficial veins of the extremities. In acute thromboangiitis obliterans, occlusive thrombi accompany neutrophilic and lymphocytic infiltration of the intima; endothelial cells proliferate, but the internal elastic lamina remains intact. In an intermediate phase, thrombi organize and recanalize incompletely; the media is preserved but may be infiltrated with fibroblasts. In older lesions, periarterial fibrosis may occur, sometimes affecting the adjacent vein and nerve.

The cause is unknown, although cigarette smoking is a primary risk factor. The mechanism may involve delayed hypersensitivity or toxic angiitis. According to another theory, thromboangiitis obliterans may be an autoimmune disorder caused by cell-mediated sensitivity to types I and III human collagen, which are constituents of blood vessels.

Symptoms and Signs

Symptoms and signs are those of arterial ischemia and superficial thrombophlebitis. Some patients have a history of migratory phlebitis, usually in the superficial veins of a foot or leg.

Onset is gradual, starting in the most distal vessels of the upper and lower extremities with coldness, numbness, tingling, or burning. These symptoms may develop before objective evidence of disease. Raynaud syndrome (see p. 753) is common. Intermittent claudication occurs in the affected extremity (usually in the arch of the foot or in the leg; rarely in the hand, arm, or thigh) and may progress to rest pain. Frequently, if pain is severe and persistent, the affected leg feels cold, sweats excessively, and becomes cyanotic, probably because of sympathetic nerve overactivity. Later, ischemic ulcers develop in most patients and may progress to gangrene.

Pulses are impaired or absent in one or more pedal arteries and often at the wrist. In young men who smoke and have extremity ulcers, a positive Allen test (the hand remains pale after the examiner simultaneously compresses the radial and ulnar arteries, then alternately releases them) suggests the disorder. Pallor with elevation and rubor with dependency frequently occur in affected hands, feet, or digits. Ischemic ulceration and gangrene, usually of one or more digits, may occur early in the disorder but not acutely. Noninvasive tests show greatly decreased blood flow and pressure in the affected toes, feet, and fingers.

Diagnosis

- Other causes of ischemia excluded by testing
- Angiography

History and physical examination suggest the diagnosis. It is confirmed when the ankle-brachial index (ratio of ankle to arm systolic BP) for legs or segmental pressures for arms indicates distal ischemia, when echocardiography excludes cardiac emboli, when blood tests (eg, measurement of antinuclear antibody, rheumatoid factor, complement, anticentromere antibody, anti-SCL-70 antibody) exclude vasculitis, when tests for antiphospholipid antibodies exclude antiphospholipid antibody syndrome (although these levels may be slightly elevated in thromboangiitis obliterans), and when angiography shows characteristic findings (segmental occlusions of the distal arteries in the hands and feet, tortuous, corkscrew collateral vessels around occlusions, and no atherosclerosis).

Treatment

- Smoking cessation
- Local measures
- Sometimes drug therapy

Treatment is cessation of tobacco use (see p. 3260). Continuing to use tobacco inevitably leads to disease progression and severe ischemia, often requiring amputation.

Other measures include avoiding cold; avoiding drugs that can cause vasoconstriction; and avoiding thermal, chemical, and mechanical injury, especially that due to poorly fitting footwear. For patients in the first phase of smoking cessation, iloprost 0.5 to 3 ng/kg/min IV infusion over 6 h may help prevent amputation. Pentoxifylline, Ca channel blockers, and thromboxane inhibitors may be tried empirically, but no data support their use. Use of antiendothelial cell antibody measurements to follow the course of disease is being studied. When these options fail, lumbar sympathetic chemical ablation or surgical sympathectomy can alleviate ischemic pain and enhance ulcer healing in about 70% of patients with an ankle-brachial pressure index ≥ 0.35 and no diabetes mellitus.

KEY POINTS

- Thromboangiitis obliterans is inflammatory thrombosis of small and medium-sized arteries and sometimes superficial veins in distal upper and lower extremities.
- It occurs almost exclusively in male smokers aged 20 to 40.
- Claudication may occur, and patients may develop ischemic ulceration and gangrene of one or more digits.
- Diagnose clinically but exclude other causes of ischemia by testing.
- Smoking cessation is essential; iloprost infusion may help prevent amputation, but there is little evidence supporting use of other drugs.

88 Peripheral Venous Disorders

ARTERIOVENOUS FISTULA

An arteriovenous fistula is an abnormal communication between an artery and a vein.

An arteriovenous fistula may be congenital (usually affecting smaller vessels) or acquired as a result of trauma (eg, a bullet or stab wound) or erosion of an arterial aneurysm into an adjacent vein.

The fistula may cause symptoms and signs of

- Arterial insufficiency (eg, ulceration due to reduced arterial flow or ischemia)
- Chronic venous insufficiency due to high-pressure arterial flow in the affected veins (eg, peripheral edema, varicose veins, stasis pigmentation)

Emboli (eg, causing ulceration) may pass from the venous to the arterial circulation, although pressure differences make this unlikely. If the fistula is near the surface, a mass can be felt, and the affected area is usually swollen and warm with distended, often pulsating superficial veins.

A thrill can be palpated over the fistula, and a continuous loud, to-and-fro (machinery) murmur with accentuation during systole can be heard during auscultation.

Rarely, if a significant portion of cardiac output is diverted through the fistula to the right heart, high-output heart failure develops.

Diagnosis

- Clinical evaluation
- Sometimes ultrasonography

Fistulas are diagnosed clinically based on presence of thrill, murmur and other signs. Doppler ultrasonography is the best confirmatory test.

Treatment

- Sometimes percutaneous occlusion techniques
- Sometimes surgery

Congenital fistulas need no treatment unless significant complications develop (eg, leg lengthening in a growing child). When necessary, percutaneous vascular techniques can be used to place coils or plugs into the vessels to occlude the fistula. Treatment is seldom completely successful, but complications are often controlled. Acquired fistulas usually have a single large connection and can be effectively treated by surgery.

CHRONIC VENOUS INSUFFICIENCY AND POSTPHLEBITIC SYNDROME

Chronic venous insufficiency is impaired venous return, sometimes causing lower extremity discomfort, edema, and skin changes. Postphlebitic (postthrombotic) syndrome is symptomatic chronic venous insufficiency after deep venous thrombosis (DVT). Causes of chronic venous insufficiency are disorders that result in venous hypertension, usually through venous damage or incompetence of venous valves, as occurs (for example) after DVT. Diagnosis is by history, physical examination, and duplex ultrasonography. Treatment is compression, wound care, and, rarely, surgery. Prevention requires adequate treatment of DVT and compression stockings.

Chronic venous insufficiency affects up to 5% of people in the US. Postphlebitic syndrome may affect one fifth to two thirds of patients with DVT, usually within 1 to 2 yr after acute DVT.

Etiology

Venous return from the lower extremities relies on contraction of calf muscles to push blood from intramuscular (soleal) sinusoids and gastrocnemius veins into and through deep veins. Venous valves direct blood proximally to the heart. Chronic venous insufficiency occurs when venous obstruction (eg, in DVT), venous valvular insufficiency, or decreased contraction of muscles surrounding the veins (eg, due to immobility) decrease forward venous flow and increase venous pressure (venous hypertension). Fluid accumulation in the lower extremities (eg, in right heart failure) can also contribute by causing venous hypertension. Prolonged venous hypertension causes tissue edema, inflammation, and hypoxia, leading to symptoms. Pressure may be transmitted to superficial veins if valves in perforator veins, which connect deep and superficial veins, are ineffective.

The **most common risk factor** for chronic venous insufficiency is

- Deep venous thrombosis

Other risk factors include

- Trauma
- Age
- Obesity

Idiopathic cases are often attributed to a history of occult DVT.

Postphlebitic (or postthrombotic) syndrome is symptomatic chronic venous insufficiency that follows DVT. Risk factors for postphlebitic syndrome in patients with DVT include proximal thrombosis, recurrent ipsilateral DVT, and body mass index (BMI) ≥ 22 kg/m^2. Age, female sex, and estrogen therapy are also associated with the syndrome but are probably nonspecific. Use of compression stockings after DVT decreases risk.

Symptoms and Signs

Clinically evident chronic venous insufficiency may not cause any symptoms but always causes signs; postphlebitic syndrome always causes symptoms. Both disorders are a concern because their symptoms can mimic those of acute DVT and both can lead to substantial reductions in physical activity and quality of life.

Symptoms include a sense of fullness, heaviness, aching, cramps, pain, tiredness, and paresthesias in the legs; these symptoms worsen with standing or walking and are relieved by rest and elevation. Pruritus may accompany skin changes. Signs occur along a continuum: no changes to varicose veins (rare) to stasis dermatitis on the lower legs and at the ankles, with or without ulceration (see Table 88–1 and Plate 53). The calf may be painful when compressed.

Venous stasis dermatitis consists of reddish brown hyperpigmentation, induration, venous ectasia, lipodermatosclerosis (fibrosing subcutaneous panniculitis), and venous stasis ulcers.

Venous stasis ulcers may develop spontaneously or after affected skin is scratched or injured. They typically occur around the medial malleolus, tend to be shallow and moist, and may be malodorous (especially when poorly cared for) or painful. They do not penetrate the deep fascia. In contrast, ulcers due to peripheral arterial disease eventually expose tendons or bone.

Leg edema tends to be unilateral or asymmetric; bilateral symmetric edema is more likely to result from a systemic disorder (eg, heart failure, hypoalbuminemia) or certain drugs (eg, calcium channel blockers).

In general, unless the lower extremities are adequately cared for, patients with any manifestation of chronic venous insufficiency or postphlebitic syndrome are at risk of progression to more advanced forms.

Table 88–1. CLINICAL CLASSIFICATION OF CHRONIC VENOUS INSUFFICIENCY

CLASS	SIGNS
0	No signs of venous disease
1	Ectatic or reticular veins*
2	Varicose veins*
3	Edema
4	Skin changes due to venous stasis (eg, pigmentation, induration, lipodermatosclerosis)
5	Skin changes due to venous stasis and healed ulceration
6	Skin changes due to venous stasis and active ulceration

*May occur idiopathically without chronic venous insufficiency.

Diagnosis

- Clinical evaluation
- Ultrasonography to exclude DVT

Diagnosis is usually based on history and physical examination. A clinical scoring system that ranks 5 symptoms (pain, cramps, heaviness, pruritus, paresthesia) and 6 signs (edema, hyperpigmentation, induration, venous ectasia, blanching hyperemia, pain with calf compression) on a scale of 0 (absent or minimal) to 3 (severe) is increasingly recognized as a standard diagnostic tool of disease severity. Scores of 5 to 14 on 2 visits separated by ≥ 6 mo indicate mild-to-moderate disease, and scores of ≥ 15 indicate severe disease.

Lower-extremity duplex ultrasonography reliably excludes or confirms DVT. Absence of edema and a reduced ankle-brachial index suggest peripheral arterial disease rather than chronic venous insufficiency and postphlebitic syndrome.

Treatment

- Elevation
- Compression
- Topical treatments
- Treatment of secondary infection, when present

Treatment depends on the disorder's severity and involves leg elevation; compression using bandages, stockings, and pneumatic devices; topical wound care; and surgery. Some experts also believe that weight loss, regular exercise, and reduction of dietary sodium may benefit patients with bilateral chronic venous insufficiency. However, all interventions may be difficult to implement.

Elevating the leg above the level of the right atrium decreases venous hypertension and edema, is appropriate for all patients, and should be done a minimum of 3 times/day for ≥ 30 min. However, most patients cannot adhere to this schedule during the day.

Compression is effective for treatment and prevention of the effects of chronic venous insufficiency and postphlebitic syndrome and is indicated for all patients. Elastic bandages are used initially until edema and ulcers resolve and leg size stabilizes; commercial compression stockings are then used. Stockings that provide 20 to 30 mm Hg of distal circumferential pressure are indicated for smaller varicose veins and mild chronic venous insufficiency; 30 to 40 mm Hg is indicated for larger varicose veins and moderate disease; and 40 to > 60 mm Hg is indicated for severe disease. Stockings should be put on when patients awaken, before leg edema worsens with activity, and should exert maximal pressure at the ankles and gradually less pressure proximally. Adherence to this treatment varies; many younger or more active patients consider stockings irritating, restricting, or cosmetically undesirable; elderly patients may have difficulty putting them on.

Intermittent pneumatic compression (IPC) uses a pump to cyclically inflate and deflate hollow plastic leggings. IPC provides external compression, squeezing blood and fluid out of the lower legs. It effectively treats severe postphlebitic syndrome and venous stasis ulcers but may be no more effective than compression stockings alone and is much less practical for patients to adhere to on an ongoing basis.

Topical wound care is important in venous stasis ulcer management (see p. 1067 for full discussion). When an Unna boot (zinc oxide–impregnated bandages) is properly applied, covered by compression bandages, and changed weekly, almost all ulcers heal. Occlusive interactive dressings (eg, hydrocolloids such as aluminum chloride) provide a moist environment for wound healing and promote growth of new tissue; they may be used for ulcers with light to moderate exudate, but they probably add little to simple Unna bandaging and are expensive. Passive dressings are absorptive, making them most appropriate for heavier exudate.

Drugs have no role in routine treatment of chronic venous insufficiency, although many patients are given aspirin, topical corticosteroids, diuretics for edema, or antibiotics.

Surgery (eg, venous ligation, stripping, valve reconstruction) is also typically ineffective. Grafting autologous skin or skin created from epidermal keratinocytes or dermal fibroblasts may be an option for patients with stasis ulcers when all other measures are ineffective, but the graft will reulcerate unless underlying venous hypertension is managed.

Prevention

Primary prevention involves adequate anticoagulation after DVT and use of compression stockings for up to 2 yr after DVT or lower extremity venous trauma. However, a recent study using sham-compression stockings failed to show any decrease in postphlebitic syndrome. Lifestyle changes (eg, weight loss, regular exercise, reduction of dietary sodium) can decrease risk by decreasing lower extremity venous pressure.

KEY POINTS

- Skin changes range on a continuum from normal skin or mildly ectatic veins to severe stasis dermatitis and ulceration.
- Symptoms are more common with postphlebitic syndrome and include heaviness, aching, and paresthesias.
- Diagnosis is based on inspection, but patients should have ultrasonography to rule out DVT.
- Treatment is with elevation and compression; drugs and surgery are typically ineffective.

DEEP VENOUS THROMBOSIS

Deep venous thrombosis (DVT) is clotting of blood in a deep vein of an extremity (usually calf or thigh) or the pelvis. DVT is the primary cause of pulmonary embolism (PE). DVT results from conditions that impair venous return, lead to endothelial injury or dysfunction, or cause hypercoagulability. DVT may be asymptomatic or cause pain and swelling in an extremity; PE is an immediate complication. Diagnosis is by history and physical examination and is confirmed by objective testing, typically with duplex ultrasonography. D-Dimer testing is used when DVT is suspected; a negative result helps to exclude DVT, whereas a positive result is nonspecific and requires additional testing to confirm DVT. Treatment is with anticoagulants. Prognosis is generally good with prompt, adequate treatment. Common long-term complications include venous insufficiency with or without the postphlebitic syndrome.

DVT occurs most commonly in the lower extremities or pelvis (see Fig. 88–1). It can also develop in deep veins of the upper extremities (4 to 13% of DVT cases).

Lower extremity DVT is much more likely to cause PE, possibly because of the higher clot burden. The superficial femoral and popliteal veins in the thighs and the posterior tibial and peroneal veins in the calves are most commonly affected. Calf vein DVT is less likely to be a source of large emboli but can propagate to the proximal thigh veins and from there cause PE. About 50% of patients with DVT have occult PE, and at least 30% of patients with PE have demonstrable DVT.

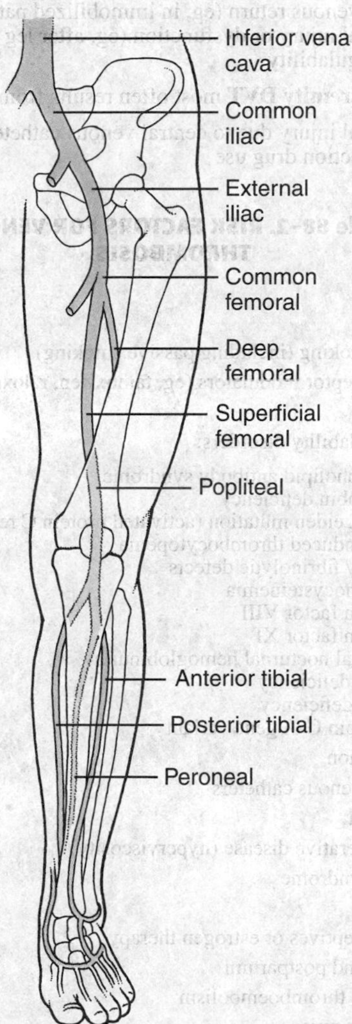

Fig. 88–1. Deep veins of the legs.

PEARLS & PITFALLS

- About 50% of patients with DVT have occult pulmonary emboli.

Etiology

Many factors can contribute to DVT (see Table 88–2). Cancer is a risk factor for DVT, particularly in elderly patients and in patients with recurrent thrombosis. The association is strongest for mucin-secreting endothelial cell tumors such as bowel or pancreatic cancers. Occult cancers may be present in patients with apparently idiopathic DVT, but extensive workup of patients for tumors is not recommended unless patients have major risk factors for cancer or symptoms suggestive of an occult cancer.

Pathophysiology

Lower extremity DVT most often results from

- Impaired venous return (eg, in immobilized patients)
- Endothelial injury or dysfunction (eg, after leg fractures)
- Hypercoagulability

Upper extremity DVT most often results from

- Endothelial injury due to central venous catheters, pacemakers, or injection drug use

Table 88–2. RISK FACTORS FOR VENOUS THROMBOSIS

Age > 60 yr
Cancer
Cigarette smoking (including passive smoking)
Estrogen receptor modulators (eg, tamoxifen, raloxifene)
Heart failure
Hypercoagulability disorders:
• Antiphospholipid antibody syndrome
• Antithrombin deficiency
• Factor V Leiden mutation (activated protein C resistance)
• Heparin-induced thrombocytopenia
• Hereditary fibrinolytic defects
• Hyperhomocysteinemia
• Increase in factor VIII
• Increase in factor XI
• Paroxysmal nocturnal hemoglobinuria
• Protein C deficiency
• Protein S deficiency
• Prothrombin G-A gene variant
Immobilization
Indwelling venous catheters
Limb trauma
Myeloproliferative disease (hyperviscosity)
Nephrotic syndrome
Obesity
Oral contraceptives or estrogen therapy
Pregnancy and postpartum
Prior venous thromboembolism
Sickle cell anemia
Surgery within the past 3 mo
Trauma

Upper extremity DVT occasionally occurs as part of superior vena cava (SVC) syndrome or results from a hypercoagulable state or subclavian vein compression at the thoracic outlet. The compression may be due to a normal or an accessory first rib or fibrous band (thoracic outlet syndrome) or occur during strenuous arm activity (effort thrombosis, or Paget-Schroetter syndrome, which accounts for 1 to 4% of upper extremity DVT cases).

Deep venous thrombosis usually begins in venous valve cusps. Thrombi consist of thrombin, fibrin, and RBCs with relatively few platelets (red thrombi); without treatment, thrombi may propagate proximally or travel to the lungs.

Complications: Common complications of deep venous thrombosis include

- Chronic venous insufficiency
- Postphlebitic syndrome
- PE

Much less commonly, acute DVT leads to phlegmasia alba dolens or phlegmasia cerulea dolens, both of which, unless promptly diagnosed and treated, can result in venous gangrene.

In **phlegmasia alba dolens,** a rare complication of DVT during pregnancy, the leg turns milky white. Pathophysiology is unclear, but edema may increase soft-tissue pressure beyond capillary perfusion pressures, resulting in tissue ischemia and wet gangrene.

In **phlegmasia cerulea dolens,** massive iliofemoral venous thrombosis causes near-total venous occlusion; the leg becomes ischemic, extremely painful, and cyanotic. Pathophysiology may involve complete stasis of venous and arterial blood flow in the lower extremity because venous return is occluded or massive edema cuts off arterial blood flow. Venous gangrene may result.

Rarely, venous clots can become infected. Jugular vein suppurative thrombophlebitis (Lemierre syndrome), a bacterial (usually anaerobic) infection of the internal jugular vein and surrounding soft tissues, may follow tonsillopharyngitis and is often complicated by bacteremia and sepsis. In septic pelvic thrombophlebitis, pelvic thromboses develop postpartum and become infected, causing intermittent fever. Suppurative (septic) thrombophlebitis, a bacterial infection of a superficial peripheral vein, comprises infection and clotting that usually is caused by venous catheterization.

Symptoms and Signs

DVT may occur in ambulatory patients or as a complication of surgery or major medical illness. Among high-risk hospitalized patients, most deep vein thrombi occur in the small calf veins, are asymptomatic, and may not be detected.

When present, symptoms and signs (eg, vague aching pain, tenderness along the distribution of the veins, edema, erythema) are nonspecific, vary in frequency and severity, and are similar in arms and legs. Dilated collateral superficial veins may become visible or palpable. Calf discomfort elicited by ankle dorsiflexion with the knee extended (Homans sign) occasionally occurs with distal leg DVT but is neither sensitive nor specific. Tenderness, swelling of the whole leg, > 3 cm difference in circumference between calves, pitting edema, and collateral superficial veins may be most specific; DVT is likely with a combination of ≥ 3 in the absence of another likely diagnosis (see Table 88–3).

Low-grade fever may be present; DVT may be the cause of fever without an obvious source, especially in postoperative patients. Symptoms of PE, if it occurs, may include shortness of breath and pleuritic chest pain.

Table 88–3. PROBABILITY OF DEEP VENOUS THROMBOSIS BASED ON CLINICAL FACTORS

Factors
Tenderness along distribution of the veins in calf or thigh
Swelling of entire leg
Calf swelling (> 3 cm difference in circumference between calves, measured 10 cm below tibial tuberosity)
Pitting edema greater in affected leg
Dilated collateral superficial veins
Cancer (including cases in which treatment was stopped within 6 mo)
Immobilization of lower extremity (eg, due to paralysis, paresis, casting, or recent long-distance travel)
Surgery leading to immobility for > 3 days within the past 4 wk
Probability
Probability equals the number of factors, subtracting 2 if another diagnosis is as likely as or more likely than DVT.
• High probability: ≥ 3 points
• Moderate probability: 1–2 points
• Low probability: ≤ 0 points

Based on data from Anand SS, Wells PS, Hunt D, et al: Does this patient have deep vein thrombosis? *Journal of the American Medical Association* 279 (14):1094–1099, 1998.

Common causes of asymmetric leg swelling that mimic DVT are soft-tissue trauma, cellulitis, pelvic venous or lymphatic obstruction, and popliteal bursitis (Baker cyst) that obstructs venous return. Abdominal or pelvic tumors that obstruct venous or lymphatic return are less common causes. Use of drugs that cause dependent edema (eg, dihydropyridine Ca channel blockers, estrogen, high-dose opioids), venous hypertension (usually due to right heart failure), and hypoalbuminemia typically cause symmetric bilateral leg swelling; however, swelling may be asymmetric if venous insufficiency coexists and is worse in one leg.

Common causes of calf pain that mimic acute DVT include venous insufficiency and postphlebitic syndrome; cellulitis that causes painful erythema of the calf; ruptured popliteal (Baker) cyst (pseudo-DVT), which causes calf swelling, pain, and sometimes bruising in the region of the medial malleolus; and partial or complete tears of the calf muscles or tendons.

Diagnosis

- Ultrasonography
- Sometimes D-dimer testing

History and physical examination help determine probability of DVT before testing (see Table 88–3). Diagnosis is typically by ultrasonography with Doppler flow studies (duplex ultrasonography). The need for additional tests (eg, D-dimer testing) and their choice and sequence depend on pretest probability and sometimes ultrasonography results. No single testing protocol is best; one approach is described in Fig. 88–2.

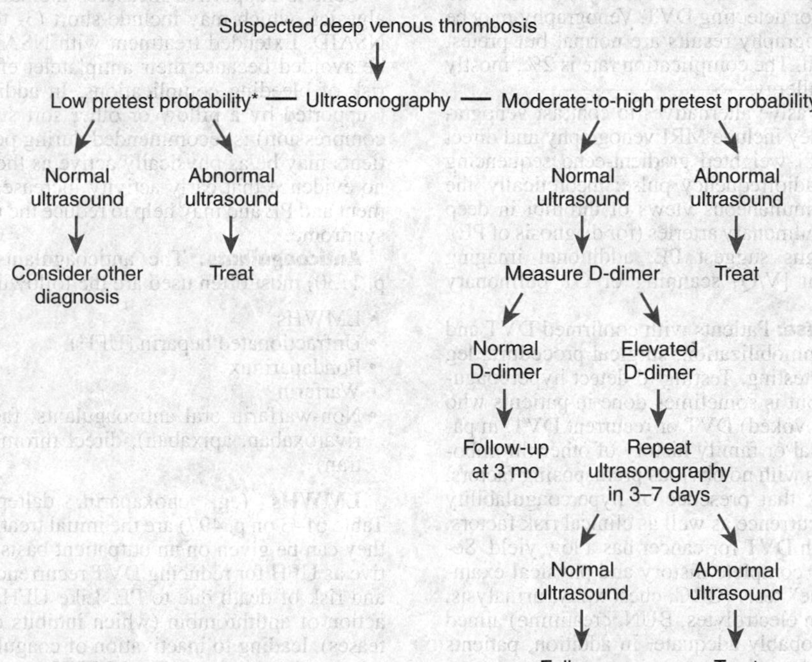

Fig. 88–2. One approach to testing for suspected deep venous thrombosis.

Ultrasonography: Ultrasonography identifies thrombi by directly visualizing the venous lining and by demonstrating abnormal vein compressibility or, with Doppler flow studies, impaired venous flow. The test is > 90% sensitive and > 95% specific for femoral and popliteal vein thrombosis but is less accurate for iliac or calf vein thrombosis.

D-Dimer: D-Dimer is a byproduct of fibrinolysis; elevated levels suggest recent presence and lysis of thrombi. D-Dimer assays vary in sensitivity and specificity; however, most are sensitive and not specific. Only the most accurate tests should be used. For example, a highly sensitive test is enzyme-linked immunosorbent assay (ELISA), which has a sensitivity of about 95%.

If pretest probability of DVT is low, DVT can be safely excluded in patients with a normal D-dimer level on a sensitive test. Thus, a negative D-dimer test can identify patients who have a low probability of DVT and do not require ultrasonography. However, a positive test result is nonspecific; because levels can be elevated by other conditions (eg, liver disease, trauma, pregnancy, positive rheumatoid factor, inflammation, recent surgery, cancer), further testing is necessary.

If pretest probability of DVT is moderate or high, D-dimer testing can be done at the same time as duplex ultrasonography. A positive ultrasound result confirms the diagnosis regardless of the D-dimer level. If ultrasonography does not reveal evidence of DVT, a normal D-dimer level helps exclude DVT. Patients with an elevated D-dimer level should have repeat ultrasonography in a few days or additional imaging, such as venography, depending on clinical suspicion..

Venography: Contrast venography was the definitive test for the diagnosis of DVT but has been largely replaced by ultrasonography, which is noninvasive, more readily available, and almost equally accurate for detecting DVT. Venography may be indicated when ultrasonography results are normal but pretest suspicion for DVT is high. The complication rate is 2%, mostly because of contrast dye allergy.

Other testing: Noninvasive alternatives to contrast venography are being studied. They include MRI venography and direct MRI of thrombi using T1-weighted gradient-echo sequencing and a water-excitation radiofrequency pulse; theoretically, the latter test can provide simultaneous views of thrombi in deep veins and subsegmental pulmonary arteries (for diagnosis of PE).

If symptoms and signs suggest PE, additional imaging (eg, ventilation/perfusion [V/Q] scanning or CT pulmonary angiography) is required.

Determination of cause: Patients with confirmed DVT and an obvious cause (eg, immobilization, surgical procedure, leg trauma) need no further testing. Testing to detect hypercoagulability is controversial but is sometimes done in patients who have idiopathic (or unprovoked) DVT or recurrent DVT, in patients who have a personal or family history of other thromboses, and in young patients with no obvious predisposing factors. Some evidence suggests that presence of hypercoagulability does not predict DVT recurrence as well as clinical risk factors.

Screening patients with DVT for cancer has a low yield. Selective testing guided by complete history and physical examination and basic "routine" tests (CBC, chest x-ray, urinalysis, liver enzymes, and serum electrolytes, BUN, creatinine) aimed at detecting cancer is probably adequate. In addition, patients should have any age- and gender-appropriate cancer screening (eg, mammography, colonoscopy) that is due.

Prognosis

Without adequate treatment, lower extremity DVT has a 3% risk of fatal PE; death due to upper extremity DVT is very rare. Risk of recurrent DVT is lowest for patients with transient risk factors (eg, surgery, trauma, temporary immobility) and greatest for patients with persistent risk factors (eg, cancer), idiopathic DVT, or incomplete resolution of past DVT (residual thrombus). A normal D-dimer level obtained after warfarin is stopped may help predict a relatively low risk of DVT or PE recurrence. Risk of venous insufficiency is difficult to predict. Risk factors for postphlebitic syndrome include proximal thrombosis, recurrent ipsilateral DVT, and body mass index (BMI) ≥ 22 kg/m^2.

Treatment

- Anticoagulation with an injectable heparin followed by an oral anticoagulant (warfarin, or a factor Xa or direct thrombin inhibitor)

Treatment is aimed primarily at PE prevention and secondarily at symptom relief and prevention of DVT recurrence, chronic venous insufficiency, and postphlebitic syndrome. Treatment of lower and upper extremity DVT is generally the same.

All patients with DVT are given anticoagulants, initially an injectable heparin (unfractionated or low molecular weight) for a brief period, followed by longer term treatment with an oral drug (eg, warfarin) started within 24 to 48 h. Select patients may continue treatment with a low molecular weight heparin (LMWH) rather than switching to an oral drug. Inadequate anticoagulation in the first 24 to 48 h may increase risk of recurrence or PE. Acute DVT can be treated on an outpatient basis unless severe symptoms require parenteral analgesics, other disorders preclude safe outpatient discharge, or other factors (eg, functional, socioeconomic) might prevent the patient from adhering to prescribed treatments.

General supportive measures include pain control with analgesics, which may include short (3- to 5-day) courses of an NSAID. Extended treatment with NSAIDs and aspirin should be avoided because their antiplatelet effects may increase the risk of bleeding complications. In addition, elevation of legs (supported by a pillow or other soft surface to avoid venous compression) is recommended during periods of inactivity. Patients may be as physically active as they can tolerate; there is no evidence that early activity increases risk of clot dislodgement and PE and may help to reduce the risk of the postphlebitic syndrome.

Anticoagulants: The anticoagulants (see Fig. 145–2 on p. 1130) most often used are the following:

- LMWHs
- Unfractionated heparin (UFH)
- Fondaparinux
- Warfarin
- Non-warfarin oral anticoagulants: factor Xa inhibitors (eg, rivaroxaban, apixaban), direct thrombin inhibitors (dabigatran)

LMWHs (eg, enoxaparin, dalteparin, tinzaparin—see Table 61–3 on p. 497) are the initial treatment of choice because they can be given on an outpatient basis. LMWHs are as effective as UFH for reducing DVT recurrence, thrombus extension, and risk of death due to PE. Like UFH, LMWHs catalyze the action of antithrombin (which inhibits coagulation factor proteases), leading to inactivation of coagulation factor Xa and, to a lesser degree, factor IIa. LMWHs also have some antithrombin–mediated anti-inflammatory properties, which facilitate clot organization and resolution of symptoms and inflammation.

LMWHs are typically given sc in a standard weight-based dose (eg, enoxaparin 1.5 mg/kg sc once/day or 1 mg/kg sc q 12 h or dalteparin 200 units/kg sc once/day). Patients with renal insufficiency may be treated with UFH or with reduced doses of LMWH.

Monitoring is not reliable because LMWHs do not significantly prolong the results of global tests of coagulation. Furthermore, they have a predictable dose response, and there is no clear relationship between the anticoagulant effect of LMWH and bleeding. Treatment is continued until full anticoagulation is achieved with warfarin (typically about 5 days). However, evidence suggests that LMWH is effective for long-term DVT treatment in high-risk patients, such as those with cancer. Thus, LMWH may become an acceptable alternative to warfarin for some patients, although warfarin is likely to be the treatment of choice for most patients because of its low cost and oral route of administration.

UFH may be used instead of LMWH for hospitalized patients and for patients who have renal insufficiency or failure (creatinine clearance 10 to 30 mL/min) because UFH is not cleared by the kidneys. UFH is given as a bolus and infusion (see Fig. 61–2 on p. 496) to achieve full anticoagulation, (eg, activated PTT [aPTT] 1.5 to 2.5 times that of the reference range). For outpatients, UFH 333 units/kg initial bolus, then 250 units/kg sc q 12 h can be substituted for IV UFH to facilitate mobility; the dose does not appear to need adjustment based on aPTT. Treatment is continued until full anticoagulation has been achieved with warfarin.

Complications of heparins include bleeding, thrombocytopenia (less common with LMWHs), urticaria, and, rarely, thrombosis and anaphylaxis. Long-term use of UFH causes hypokalemia, liver enzyme elevations, and osteopenia. Rarely, UFH given sc causes skin necrosis. Inpatients and possibly outpatients should be screened for bleeding with serial CBCs and, where appropriate, testing for occult blood in stool.

Bleeding due to overheparinization can be stopped with protamine sulfate. The dose is 1 mg protamine for each milligram of LMWH given as 1 mg in 20 mL of normal saline infused slowly over 10 to 20 min. If a 2nd dose is required, it should be one half the first dose. However, the precise dose is undefined because protamine only partially neutralizes LMWH inactivation of factor Xa. During all infusions, patients should be observed for hypotension and a reaction similar to an anaphylactic reaction. Because UFH given IV has a half-life of 30 to 60 min, protamine is not given to patients receiving UFH (eg, if UFH was given > 60 min beforehand) or is given at a dose based on the amount of heparin estimated to be remaining in plasma, based on the half-life of UFH.

Fondaparinux, a parenteral selective factor Xa inhibitor, may be used as an alternative to UFH or LMWH for the initial treatment of DVT or PE. It is given in a fixed dose of 7.5 mg sc once/day (10 mg for patients > 100 kg, 5 mg for patients < 50 kg). It has the advantage of fixed dosing and is less likely to cause thrombocytopenia.

Parenteral direct thrombin inhibitors (argatroban, bivalirudin, desirudin) are available but do not have a role in treatment or prevention of DVT or PE. Argatroban may be useful to treat DVT in patients with heparin-induced thrombocytopenia.

Vitamin K antagonists, including warfarin, are the drugs of choice for long-term anticoagulation for all patients except pregnant women (who should continue to take heparin) and patients who have had new or worsening venous thromboembolism during warfarin treatment (who may be candidates for an inferior vena cava filter [IVCF]). Warfarin 5 to 10 mg can be started immediately with heparin because it takes about 5 days to achieve desired therapeutic effect. The elderly and patients with a liver disorder typically require lower warfarin doses. Therapeutic goal is an INR of 2.0 to 3.0. INR is monitored weekly for the first 1 to 2 mo of warfarin treatment and monthly thereafter; the dose is increased or decreased by 0.5 to 3 mg to maintain the INR within this range. Patients taking warfarin should be informed of possible drug interactions, including interactions with foods and nonprescription medicinal herbs.

Non-warfarin oral anticoagulants, also called direct oral anticoagulants (DOACs), are available as alternatives to warfarin as a 1st-line treatment for the treatment of DVT and PE; not all DOACs are currently FDA-approved for this indication (see Table 61–3 on p. 497). Drugs include factor Xa inhibitors (rivaroxaban, apixaban, edoxaban) and a direct thrombin inhibitor (dabigatran). Compared to warfarin, these drugs have been shown to give similar protection against recurrent DVT and have similar (or with apixaban, perhaps lower) risk of serious bleeding.

Their advantages are that they are effective within several hours (thus, except for dabigatran, do not require parenteral bridging treatment with a heparin), and they are given as a fixed dose (thus do not require ongoing laboratory testing).

Their disadvantages are that they are expensive, and currently (except for dabigatran) there are no available antidotes to reverse their anticoagulant effect in patients with life-threatening bleeding or who need urgent surgery. Idarucizumab is a humanized monoclonal antibody to dabigatran that is an effective antidote to dabigatran. Antidotes for the other DOACs are currently being developed. If life-threatening bleeding occurs, prothrombin complex concentrate (PCC) may be tried to decrease the anticoagulant effect of rivaroxaban and apixaban, and activated PCC may be used for dabigatran (if the antidote is not available). Rarely, hemodialysis or hemoperfusion may help decrease the anticoagulant effect of dabigatran, which is not highly protein bound; such measures are not effective on rivaroxaban and apixaban. Supportive care with intravenous fluids and packed RBC transfusions are sufficient for many bleeding episodes in patients who are receiving a DOAC.

If used, rivaroxaban 15 mg po bid is started immediately upon diagnosis and given for 3 wk followed by 20 mg po once/day for 9 wk. Apixaban 10 mg po bid is started immediately upon diagnosis and given for 7 days followed by 5 mg po bid for 6 mo. Dabigatran 150 mg po bid is given only after an initial 5 to 7 days of treatment with LMWH.

Duration of treatment varies. Patients with transient risk factors for DVT (eg, immobilization, surgery) can usually stop taking warfarin after 3 to 6 mo. Patients with nonmodifiable risk factors (eg, hypercoagulability), idiopathic (or unprovoked) DVT with no known risk factors, or recurrent DVT should take warfarin for at least 6 mo and, in selected patients, probably for life unless complications occur.

Bleeding is the most common complication. Risk factors for severe bleeding (defined as life-threatening hemorrhage or loss of ≥ 2 units of blood in ≤ 7 days) include

- Age ≥ 65
- History of prior GI bleeding or stroke
- Recent MI
- Coexisting anemia (Hct < 30%), renal insufficiency (serum creatinine > 1.5 mg/dL), or diabetes

In patients who are actively bleeding or may be at increased risk of bleeding, anticoagulation can be reversed with vitamin K; the dose is 1 to 2.5 mg po if INR is 5 to 9, 2.5 to 5 mg po if INR is > 9, and 5 to 10 mg IV (given slowly to avoid anaphylaxis) if hemorrhage occurs. If hemorrhage is severe, a transfusion of coagulation factors, fresh frozen plasma, or PCC should also be given. Selected patients with overanticoagulation (INR 5 to 9) who are neither actively bleeding nor at increased risk of bleeding can be managed by omitting 1 or 2 warfarin doses and monitoring INR more frequently, then giving warfarin at a lower dose. Rarely, warfarin causes skin necrosis in patients with protein C or S deficiency or factor V Leiden mutations.

Inferior vena cava filter: An IVCF may help prevent PE in patients with lower extremity DVT who have contraindications to anticoagulant therapy or in patients with recurrent DVT (or emboli) despite adequate anticoagulation. An IVCF is placed in the inferior vena cava just below the renal veins via catheterization of an internal jugular or femoral vein. Some IVCFs are removable and can be used temporarily (eg, until contraindications to anticoagulation subside or resolve).

IVCFs reduce risk of acute embolic complications but can have longer-term complications (eg, venous collaterals can develop, providing a pathway for emboli to circumvent the IVCF, and increased risk of recurrent DVT). Also, IVCFs can dislodge or become obstructed by a clot. Thus, patients with recurrent DVT or nonmodifiable risk factors for DVT may still require anticoagulation despite the presence of an IVCF. A clotted filter may cause bilateral lower extremity venous congestion (including acute phlegmasia cerulea dolens), lower body ischemia, and acute kidney injury. Treatment for a dislodged filter is removal, using angiographic or, if necessary, surgical methods. Despite widespread use of IVCFs, efficacy in preventing PE is unstudied and unproved. IVCFs should be removed whenever possible.

Thrombolytic (fibrinolytic) drugs: Streptokinase, urokinase, and alteplase lyse clots and may be more effective to prevent postphlebitic syndrome than heparin alone, but the risk of bleeding is higher than with heparin. Their use is under ongoing study, especially in patients with PE and right ventricular dysfunction and in combination with percutaneous mechanical thrombectomy for extensive proximal DVT.

Thrombolytic therapy alone may be indicated for large proximal thrombi, especially those in the iliofemoral veins, and for phlegmasia alba or cerulea dolens. Local administration of thrombolytic therapy with an indwelling catheter (during percutaneous thrombectomy) may be preferable to IV administration.

Surgery: Surgery is rarely needed. However, thrombectomy, fasciotomy, or both are mandatory for phlegmasia alba dolens or phlegmasia cerulea dolens unresponsive to thrombolytics to try to prevent limb-threatening gangrene.

Prevention

It is preferable and safer to prevent DVT than to treat it, particularly in high-risk patients (see Table 88–4). The following modalities are used (for a more complete discussion, see DVT Prevention, below).

- Prevention of immobility
- Anticoagulation (eg, LMWH, fondaparinux, adjusted-dose warfarin)
- Intermittent pneumatic compression
- IVCF

KEY POINTS

- Symptoms and signs are nonspecific, so clinicians must be alert, particularly in high-risk patients.
- Low-risk patients may have D-dimer testing, as a normal result essentially excludes DVT; others should have ultrasonography.
- Treatment initially is with an injectable heparin (unfractionated or LMWH) followed by oral warfarin or perhaps a LMWH; the role of oral factor Xa and direct thrombin inhibitors is evolving.
- Duration of treatment is typically 3 or 6 mo depending on the presence and nature of risk factors; certain patients require lifelong treatment.
- Preventive treatment is required for bedbound patients with major illness and/or those undergoing certain surgical procedures.
- Early mobilization, leg elevation, and an anticoagulant are the recommended preventive measures; patients who should not receive anticoagulants may benefit from intermittent pneumatic compression devices, elastic stockings, or both.

DEEP VENOUS THROMBOSIS PREVENTION

DVT prophylaxis begins with

- Risk assessment

Risk, along with other factors, allow the proper modality to be selected. Preventive measures include

- Prevention of immobility
- Anticoagulation (eg, LMWH, fondaparinux, adjusted-dose warfarin)
- Intermittent pneumatic compression
- IVCF

Risk Assessment

Patients at low risk of DVT (eg, those who are undergoing minor surgery but have no clinical risk factors for DVT; those who must be temporarily inactive for long periods, as during an airplane flight) should be encouraged to walk or otherwise move their legs periodically; no medical treatment is needed. Dorsiflexion 10 times/h is probably sufficient.

Patients at higher risk of DVT include those undergoing minor surgery if they have clinical risk factors for DVT; those undergoing major surgery, especially orthopedic surgery, even without risk factors; and bedbound patients with major medical illnesses (eg, most critical care unit patients, other patients with heart failure, COPD, chronic liver disease, stroke). These patients require additional preventive treatment (see Table 88–4). Most of these patients can be identified and should receive DVT prophylaxis; in-hospital thrombosis may be responsible for > 50,000 deaths/yr in the US. Hospitalization itself is not considered a risk factor, and hospitalized patients not in one of these categories do not require routine DVT prophylaxis.

Treatment

DVT prophylaxis can involve one or more of the following:

- Mechanical therapy (eg, compression devices or stockings, venous filters)
- Drug therapy (including low-dose unfractionated heparin, LMWHs, warfarin, fondaparinux, new oral anticoagulants)

Choice depends on patient's risk level, type of surgery (if applicable), projected duration of preventive treatment, contraindications, adverse effects, relative cost, ease of use, and local practice.

Mechanical therapy for DVT prophylaxis: After surgery, elevating the legs and avoiding prolonged immobility, which places the legs in a dependent position thereby impeding venous return, can help.

The benefit of graded compression stockings is questionable except for low-risk surgical patients and selected hospitalized medical patients. However, combining stockings with other preventive measures may be more protective than any single approach.

Intermittent pneumatic compression (IPC) uses a pump to cyclically inflate and deflate hollow plastic leggings, providing

Table 88–4. RISK OF DEEP VENOUS THROMBOSIS AND PULMONARY EMBOLISM IN SURGICAL PATIENTS

RISK CATEGORY	EXAMPLES	PREVENTIVE MEASURES	RISK OF DVT/PE (%)			
			Calf	Proximal	PE	Fatal PE
Low	Nonmajor surgery* in patients < 40 yr with no clinical risk factors	Early and aggressive ambulation	2	0.4	0.2	0.002
Moderate	Nonmajor surgery in patients with risk factors Minor surgery in patients 40–60 yr with no clinical risk factors Major surgery in patients < 40 yr with no other clinical risk factors Immobilized patients with major medical illnesses	LDUH q 12 h, LMWH, fondaparinux, or IPC, with or without elastic stockings	10–20	2–4	1–2	0.1–0.4
High	Nonmajor surgery in patients > 60 yr or 40–60 with risk factors Major surgery in patients > 40 yr or with other clinical risk factors	LDUH q 8 h, LMWH, fondaparinux, or IPC	20–40	4–8	2–4	0.4–1.0
Very high	Major surgery in patients > 40 yr who have had a previous venous thromboembolic, malignant, or hypercoagulability disorder In patients of any age: • Hip or knee arthroplasty • Hip fracture surgery • Elective neurosurgery • Multiple trauma • Spinal cord injury	LMWH, oral anticoagulation, IPC, or elastic stockings plus either LDUH q 8 h or LMWH Fondaparinux if patients have had orthopedic, abdominal, or thoracic surgery or have an acute, severe illness	40–80	10–20	4–10	0.2–5

*Nonmajor surgery is defined here as an operation that does not involve general anesthesia or respiratory assistance.

DVT = deep venous thrombosis; PE = pulmonary embolism; LDUH = low-dose unfractionated heparin; LMWH = low molecular weight heparin; IPC = intermittent pneumatic compression.

Adapted with permission from Geerts WH, Heit JA, Clagett GP, et al: Prevention of venous thromboembolism. *Chest* 119:132S–175S, 2001.

external compression to the lower legs and sometimes thighs. IPC may be used instead of or in combination with anticoagulants after surgery. IPC is recommended for patients undergoing surgery associated with a high risk of bleeding in whom anticoagulant use may be contraindicated. IPC is probably more effective for preventing calf than proximal DVT. IPC is contraindicated in some obese patients who may be unable to apply the devices properly.

For patients who are at very high risk of venous thromboembolism and bleeding (eg, after major trauma) IPC is recommended until the bleeding risk subsides and anticoagulants can be given. The use of IVCFs should be avoided unless DVT has been confirmed, except in highly selected patients.

Drug therapy for DVT prophylaxis: Aspirin is better than placebo but likely worse than LMWH and warfarin for preventing DVT and PE and is not recommended as the first-line method of prevention in most patients (see Table 88–4).

Low-dose UFH 5000 units sc is given 2 h before surgery and q 8 to 12 h thereafter for 7 to 10 days or until patients are fully ambulatory. Bedbound patients who are not undergoing surgery are given 5000 units sc q 12 h until risk factors are reversed.

LMWHs are more effective than low-dose UFH for preventing DVT and PE, but widespread use is limited by cost. Enoxaparin 30 mg sc q 12 h, dalteparin 5000 units sc once/day, and tinzaparin 4500 units sc once/day appear to be are equally effective. Fondaparinux 2.5 mg sc once/day is at least as effective as LMWH in patients who are undergoing nonorthopedic surgery and is possibly more effective than LMWHs after orthopedic surgery.

Warfarin, using a target INR of 2.0 to 3.0, is proven to be effective in orthopedic surgery but is being used less frequently because alternative anticoagulants such as LMWHs and new oral anticoagulants are easier to administer.

New oral anticoagulants (eg, dabigatran, rivaroxaban, apixaban) are at least as effective and safe as LMWH for preventing DVT and PE after hip or knee replacement surgery but are more expensive than warfarin, and their cost-effectiveness requires further study.

DVT prophylaxis in selected populations: For elective neurosurgery, spinal cord injury, or multiple trauma, low-dose UFH (eg, 5000 units sc q 8 h), LMWH, or adjusted-dose warfarin is recommended. For hip and other lower extremity orthopedic surgery, LMWH, fondaparinux, or adjusted-dose warfarin is recommended. For patients undergoing total knee replacement and some other high-risk patients, IPC is also beneficial. For orthopedic surgery, preventive treatment may be started before or after surgery and continued for at least 14 days. Fondaparinux 2.5 mg sc once/day appears to be more effective to prevent DVT than LMWH for orthopedic surgery but may be associated with an increased risk of bleeding.

For neurosurgery patients, physical measures (IPC, elastic stockings) have been used because intracranial bleeding is a concern; however, LMWH appears to be an acceptable alternative. Limited data support the combination of IPC, elastic stockings, and LMWH in patients with spinal cord injury or multiple trauma.

Preventive treatment is also indicated for patients who have a major medical illnesses requiring bed rest (eg, MI, ischemic stroke, heart failure). Low-dose UFH or LMWH is effective in patients who are not already receiving IV heparin or thrombolytics; IPC, elastic stockings, or both may be used when anticoagulants are contraindicated. After a stroke, low-dose UFH or LMWH can be used; IPC, elastic stockings, or both may be beneficial.

Prevention of postphlebitic syndrome: In patients with symptomatic DVT who develop symptoms of postphlebitic syndrome (eg, leg swelling, pain, aching), the use of knee-high compression stockings providing 30 to 40 mm Hg pressure is recommended, although stockings with lower tension (20 to 30 mm Hg) can be considered if patients are unable to tolerate the higher tension stockings. However, the routine use of stockings in all patients who have had a DVT has been questioned by a recent study which randomly allocated patients with a DVT to receive knee-high compression stockings or sham-compression stockings. This study failed to show any decrease in postphlebitic syndrome with use of compression stockings.

KEY POINTS

- Preventive treatment is required for bedbound patients with major illness and/or those undergoing certain surgical procedures.
- Early mobilization, leg elevation, and an anticoagulant are the recommended preventive measures; patients who should not receive anticoagulants may benefit from intermittent pneumatic compression devices, elastic stockings, or both.

IDIOPATHIC TELANGIECTASIAS

Idiopathic telangiectasias are fine, dilated intracutaneous veins that are not clinically significant but may be extensive and unsightly.

Telangiectasias are usually asymptomatic. However, some patients report a burning sensation or pain, and many people consider even the smallest telangiectasias cosmetically unacceptable.

Treatment

- Sclerotherapy
- Laser treatment

Telangiectasias can usually be eliminated by sclerotherapy, intracapillary injections of 0.3% solution of sodium tetradecyl sulfate through a fine-bore needle. Hypertonic saline 23.4% is sometimes used but causes fairly severe, temporary, localized pain; therefore, large areas of spider veins (multiple telangiectasias) may require several treatments. Pigmentation may develop but usually subsides, often completely. Skin ulceration may result if the injection is extravascular or too large.

Laser treatment is effective, but large areas require several treatments. Small telangiectasias may persist or recur after initial treatment.

SUPERFICIAL VENOUS THROMBOSIS

Superficial venous thrombosis is a blood clot in a superficial vein of the upper or lower extremities or, less commonly, in one or more veins of the chest or breast (Mondor disease).

Superficial venous thrombosis in the upper extremity most commonly results from IV infusions or catheterization; varicose veins seem to be the main risk factor for the lower extremity, especially among women. Superficial venous thrombi rarely cause serious complications and rarely become emboli.

Typically, patients present with pain, tenderness, or an indurated cord along a palpable superficial vein. The overlying skin is usually warm and erythematous.

Migratory superficial venous thrombosis, which develops, resolves, and recurs in normal veins of the arms, legs, and torso at various times, is a possible harbinger of pancreatic cancer and other adenocarcinomas (Trousseau syndrome).

Diagnosis is based on history and physical examination. Patients with superficial venous thrombosis above the knee have an increased risk of deep venous thrombosis and should probably have ultrasonography.

Treatment traditionally involves warm compresses and NSAIDs. In patients with extensive superficial phlebitis, anticoagulation (eg, with LMWH, fondaparinux) is often beneficial. The optimal regimen and duration are unknown, but most experts recommend using either LMWH (eg, enoxaparin 40 mg once/day or fondaparinux 2.5 mg once/day) and treating for about one month.

VARICOSE VEINS

Varicose veins are dilated superficial veins in the lower extremities. Usually, no cause is obvious. Varicose veins are typically asymptomatic but may cause a sense of fullness, pressure, and pain or hyperesthesia in the legs. Diagnosis is by physical examination. Treatment may include compression, wound care, sclerotherapy, and surgery.

Varicose veins may occur alone or with chronic venous insufficiency.

Etiology

Etiology is usually unknown, but varicose veins may result from primary venous valvular insufficiency with reflux or from primary dilation of the vein wall due to structural weakness. In some people, varicose veins result from chronic venous insufficiency and venous hypertension. Most people have no obvious risk factors. Varicose veins are common within families, suggesting a genetic component. Varicose veins are more common among women because estrogen affects venous structure, pregnancy increases pelvic and leg venous pressures, or both. Rarely, varicose veins are part of Klippel-Trénaunay-Weber syndrome, which includes congenital arteriovenous fistulas and diffuse cutaneous capillary angiomas.

Symptoms and Signs

Varicose veins may initially be tense and palpable but are not necessarily visible. Later, they may progressively enlarge, protrude, and become obvious; they can cause a sense of fullness, fatigue, pressure, and superficial pain or hyperesthesia in the legs. Varicose veins are most visible when the patient stands.

For unclear reasons, stasis dermatitis and venous stasis ulcers are uncommon. When skin changes (eg, induration, pigmentation, eczema) occur, they typically affect the medial malleolar region. Ulcers may develop after minimal trauma to an affected area; they are usually small, superficial, and painful.

Varicose veins occasionally thrombose, causing pain. Superficial varicose veins may cause thin venous bullae in the skin, which may rupture and bleed after minimal trauma. Very rarely, such bleeding, if undetected during sleep, is fatal.

PEARLS & PITFALLS

- Varicose veins rarely lead to stasis dermatitis or stasis ulcers, but ulceration may develop following minor injury to an affected area.

Diagnosis

- Clinical evaluation
- Sometimes Doppler ultrasonography

Diagnosis is usually obvious from the physical examination. Trendelenburg test (comparing venous filling before and after release of a thigh tourniquet) is no longer commonly used to identify retrograde blood flow past incompetent saphenous valves.

Duplex ultrasonography is an accurate test, but it is not clear whether it is routinely necessary.

Treatment

- Compression stockings
- Sometimes minimally invasive therapy (eg, sclerotherapy) or surgery

Treatment aims to relieve symptoms, improve the leg's appearance, and, in some cases, prevent complications. Treatment includes compression stockings and local wound care as needed.

Minimally invasive therapy (eg, sclerotherapy) and surgery are indicated for prevention of recurrent variceal thrombosis and for skin changes; these procedures are also commonly used for cosmetic reasons.

Sclerotherapy uses an irritant (eg, sodium tetradecyl sulfate) to induce a thrombophlebitic reaction that fibroses and occludes the vein; however, many varicose veins recannulate. Surgery involves ligation or stripping of the long and sometimes the short saphenous veins. These procedures provide good short-term symptom relief, but long-term efficacy is poor (ie, patients often develop recurrent varicose veins).

Thermal ablation with the use of laser or radiofrequency ablation is another minimally invasive tool for the treatment of varicose veins.

Regardless of treatment, new varicose veins develop, and treatment often must be repeated indefinitely.

89 Sports and the Heart

ATHLETE'S HEART

Athlete's heart is a constellation of structural and functional changes that occur in the heart of people who train for > 1 h most days. The changes are asymptomatic; signs include bradycardia, a systolic murmur, and extra heart sounds. ECG abnormalities are common. Diagnosis is clinical or by echocardiography. No treatment is necessary. Athlete's heart is significant because it must be distinguished from serious cardiac disorders.

Intensive, prolonged endurance and strength training causes many physiologic adaptations. Volume and pressure loads in the left ventricle (LV) increase, which, over time, increase LV muscle mass, wall thickness, and chamber size. Maximal stroke volume and cardiac output increase, contributing to a lower resting heart rate and longer diastolic filling time. Lower heart rate results primarily from increased vagal tone, but decreased sympathetic activation and other nonautonomic factors that decrease intrinsic sinus node activity may play a role. Bradycardia decreases myocardial oxygen demand; at the same time, increases in total Hb and blood volume enhance oxygen transport. Despite these changes, systolic function and diastolic function remain normal. Structural changes in women are typically less than those in men of the same age, body size, and level of training.

Symptoms and Signs

There are no symptoms. Signs vary but may include bradycardia; an LV impulse that is laterally displaced, enlarged, and increased in amplitude; a systolic ejection (flow) murmur at the left lower sternal border; a 3rd heart sound (S_3) due to early, rapid diastolic ventricular filling; a 4th heart sound (S_4), heard best during resting bradycardia because diastolic filling time is increased; and hyperdynamic carotid pulses. These signs reflect structural cardiac changes that are adaptive for intense exercise.

Diagnosis

- Clinical evaluation
- Usually ECG
- Sometimes echocardiography
- Rarely, stress testing

Findings are typically detected during routine screening or during evaluation of unrelated symptoms. Most athletes do not require extensive testing, although ECG is often warranted. If symptoms suggest a cardiac disorder (eg, palpitations, chest pain), ECG, echocardiography, and exercise stress testing are done.

Athlete's heart is a diagnosis of exclusion; it must be distinguished from disorders that cause similar findings but are life threatening (eg, hypertrophic or dilated cardiomyopathies, ischemic heart disease, arrhythmogenic right ventricular dysplasia).

ECG: Numerous changes in rhythm and ECG morphology can occur; they correlate poorly with level of training and cardiovascular performance. The most common ECG finding is

- Sinus bradycardia

Rarely, heart rate is < 40 beats/min. Sinus arrhythmia often accompanies the slow heart rate. Resting bradycardia may also predispose to

- Atrial or ventricular ectopy (including couplets and bursts of nonsustained ventricular tachycardia); pauses after ectopic beats do not exceed 4 sec
- Wandering supraventricular pacemaker

Other ECG findings that may occur include

- First-degree atrioventricular (AV) block (in up to one third of athletes)
- Second-degree AV block (mainly type I); this finding occurs during rest and disappears with exercise
- High-voltage QRS with inferolateral T-wave changes (reflecting LV hypertrophy)
- Deep anterolateral T-wave inversion
- Incomplete right bundle branch block

However, 3rd-degree AV block is abnormal and should be investigated thoroughly.

These ECG and rhythm changes have not been associated with adverse clinical events, suggesting that various arrhythmias are not abnormal in athletes. The arrhythmias are usually abolished or substantially reduced after a relatively brief period of deconditioning.

Echocardiography: Echocardiography can usually distinguish athlete's heart from cardiomyopathies (see Table 89–1), but the distinction is not always clear because there is a continuum from physiologic to pathologic cardiac enlargement. The zone of overlap between athlete's heart and cardiomyopathy is left ventricular septal thickness:

- In men, 13 to 15 mm
- In women, 11 to 13 mm

In this overlap area, the presence of mitral valve systolic anterior motion strongly suggests hypertrophic cardiomyopathy. Also, diastolic indexes may be abnormal in cardiomyopathy but are usually normal in athlete's heart. In general, echocardiographic changes correlate poorly with level of training and cardiovascular performance. Trace mitral regurgitation and tricuspid regurgitation are commonly detected. Of note, reduction of physical training will result in regression of cardiac enlargement in patients with athlete's heart but not in those with cardiomyopathy.

Stress testing: During exercise stress testing, heart rate remains lower than normal at submaximal stress and increases appropriately and comparably to heart rate in nonathletes at maximal stress; it rapidly recovers after exercise. BP response is normal:

- Systolic BP increases
- Diastolic BP falls
- Mean BP stays relatively constant

Many resting ECG changes decrease or disappear during exercise; this finding is unique to athlete's heart, distinguishing it from pathologic conditions. However, pseudonormalization of T-wave inversions could reflect myocardial ischemia and thus warrants further investigation in older athletes. However, a normal exercise stress test result does not rule out a cardiomyopathy.

Prognosis

Although gross structural changes resemble those in some cardiac disorders, no adverse effects are apparent. In most cases, structural changes and bradycardia regress with detraining, although up to 20% of elite athletes have residual chamber enlargement, raising questions, in the absence of long-term data, about whether athlete's heart is truly benign.

Treatment

- Possibly a period of deconditioning to monitor LV regression

No treatment is required, although 3 mo of deconditioning may be needed to monitor LV regression as a way of distinguishing this syndrome from cardiomyopathy. Such deconditioning can greatly interfere with an athlete's life and may meet with resistance.

KEY POINTS

- Intensive physical exercise increases LV muscle mass, wall thickness, and chamber size but systolic function and diastolic function remain normal.
- Resting heart rate is slow and there may be a systolic ejection murmur at the left lower sternal border, a 3rd heart sound (S_3), and/or a 4th heart sound (S_4).
- ECG shows bradycardia and signs of hypertrophy and sometimes other findings such as sinus arrhythmia, atrial or ventricular ectopy, and 1st or 2nd degree AV block.

Table 89–1. FEATURES DISTINGUISHING ATHLETE'S HEART FROM CARDIOMYOPATHY

FEATURE	ATHLETE'S HEART	CARDIOMYOPATHY
Left ventricular septal thickness*	In men, < 13 mm In women, < 11 mm	In men, > 15 mm In women, > 13 mm
Left ventricular end-diastolic diameter†	< 60 mm	> 70 mm
Diastolic function	Normal (E:A ratio > 1)	Abnormal (E:A ratio < 1)
Septal hypertrophy	Symmetric	Asymmetric (in hypertrophic cardiomyopathy)
Family history	None	May be present
BP response to exercise	Normal	Normal or reduced systolic BP response
Deconditioning	Left ventricular hypertrophy regression	No left ventricular hypertrophy regression

*A value of 13 to 15 mm in men and 11 to 13 mm in women is indeterminate.
†A value of 60 to 70 mm is indeterminate.
E:A ratio = ratio of early to late atrial transmitral flow velocity.

- Structural and ECG changes due to athlete's heart are asymptomatic; the presence of cardiovascular symptoms (eg, chest pain, dyspnea, palpitations) or 3rd degree AV block should prompt a search for an underlying cardiac disorder.

SUDDEN CARDIAC DEATH IN ATHLETES

An estimated 1 to 3/100,000 apparently healthy young athletes develop abrupt-onset ventricular tachycardia or ventricular fibrillation and die suddenly during exercise. Males are affected 10 times more often than females. Basketball and football players in the US and soccer players in Europe may be at highest risk.[1]

In **young athletes,** sudden cardiac death has many causes (see Table 89–2), but the most common is

- Undetected hypertrophic cardiomyopathy

Commotio cordis (sudden ventricular tachycardia or fibrillation after a blow to the precordium) is a risk in athletes with thin, compliant chest walls even when no cardiovascular disorder is present. The blow may involve a moderate-force projectile (eg, baseball, hockey puck, lacrosse ball) or impact with another player during a vulnerable phase of myocardial repolarization.

Other causes include inherited arrhythmia syndromes (eg, long QT syndrome, Brugada syndrome). Some young athletes die of aortic aneurysm rupture (in Marfan syndrome).

In **older athletes,** sudden cardiac death is typically caused by

- Coronary artery disease

Occasionally, hypertrophic cardiomyopathy, mitral valve prolapse, or acquired valvular disease is involved.

In other conditions underlying sudden death in athletes (eg, asthma, heatstroke, illicit or performance-enhancing drug-related complications), ventricular tachycardia or fibrillation is a terminal, not a primary event.

Table 89–2. CAUSES OF SUDDEN CARDIOVASCULAR DEATH IN YOUNG ATHLETES

Hypertrophic cardiomyopathy
Commotio cordis
Coronary artery anomalies (eg, anomalous left main coronary artery origin, anomalous right coronary artery origin, coronary arterial hypoplasia)
Myocarditis
Ruptured aortic aneurysm
Arrhythmogenic right ventricular dysplasia
Tunneled left anterior descending coronary artery
Aortic stenosis
Premature atherosclerotic coronary artery disease
Dilated cardiomyopathy
Myxomatous degeneration of mitral valve
Long QT syndrome
Brugada syndrome
Wolff-Parkinson-White syndrome (anterograde conduction only)
Catecholaminergic polymorphic tachycardia
Right ventricular outflow tract tachycardia
Coronary vasospasm
Cardiac sarcoidosis
Cardiac trauma
Ruptured cerebral artery aneurysm

Symptoms and signs are those of cardiovascular collapse; diagnosis is obvious.

Immediate treatment with advanced cardiac life support is successful in < 20%; the percentage may increase as distribution of community-based, automated external defibrillators expands. For survivors, treatment is management of the underlying condition. In some cases, an implanted cardioverter-defibrillator may ultimately be required.

1. Maron BJ, Shirani J, Poliac LC, et al: Sudden death in young competitive athletes: Clinical, demographic, and pathological profiles. *JAMA* 276(3):199–204, 1996.

Cardiovascular Screening for Sports Participation

Athletes are commonly screened to identify risk before participation in sports, and they are reevaluated every 2 yr (if high school age) or every 4 yr (if college age or older).

Screening recommendations in the US for college-age young adults—as well as for children and adolescents—include the following:

- Medical, family, and drug history (including use of performance-enhancing drugs and drugs that predispose to long QT syndrome)
- Physical examination (including BP and supine and standing cardiac auscultation)
- Selected testing based on findings on history and physical examination

European guidelines differ from American guidelines in that a screening electrocardiogram (ECG) is recommended for all children, adolescents, and college-age athletes.

Screening for older adults (35 yr or older) may include incremental symptom-limited exercise testing.

History and examination are neither sensitive nor specific; false-negative and false-positive findings are common because prevalence of cardiac disorders in an apparently healthy population is very low. Use of screening ECG or echocardiography would improve disease detection but would produce even more false-positive diagnoses and is impractical at a population level.

Genetic testing for hypertrophic cardiomyopathy or long QT syndrome is not recommended or even feasible for the screening of athletes.

Selected testing: Athletes with a family history or symptoms or signs of hypertrophic cardiomyopathy, long QT syndrome, or Marfan syndrome require further evaluation, typically with ECG, echocardiography, or both. Confirmation of any of these disorders may preclude sports participation.

Athletes with presyncope or syncope can also be evaluated for anomalous coronary arteries (eg, by cardiac catheterization).

If ECG reveals Mobitz type II heart block, complete heart block, true right bundle branch block, or left bundle branch block, or there is clinical or electrocardiographic evidence of supraventricular or ventricular rhythm disorders, a search for cardiac disease is required.

If an enlarged aorta is detected on echocardiography (or incidentally), further assessment is needed.

Recommendations: Athletes should be counseled against use of illicit and performance-enhancing drugs. Patients with mild or moderate valvular heart disease may participate in vigorous activity; however, patients with severe valvular heart disease, particularly of the stenotic variety, should not participate in competitive sports or high-intensity recreational sports. Patients with most structural or arrhythmogenic heart disorders (eg, hypertrophic cardiomyopathy, coronary artery anomalies, arrhythmogenic right ventricular dysplasia) should not participate in competitive sports or high-intensity recreational sports.

KEY POINTS

- Sudden cardiac death during exercise is rare and is most commonly due to hypertrophic cardiomyopathy (younger athletes) and coronary artery disease (older athletes).
- Screen younger participants (children through young adults) with history and physical examination; those with abnormal findings or positive family history typically have ECG and/or echocardiography.
- Screen older participants with history, physical examination, and usually an exercise stress test.

90 Valvular Disorders

Any heart valve can become stenotic or insufficient (also termed incompetent), causing hemodynamic changes long before symptoms. Most often, valvular stenosis or insufficiency occurs in isolation in individual valves, but multiple valvular disorders may coexist, and a single valve may be both stenosed and insufficient.

Heart valve disorders include

- Aortic regurgitation (AR): Insufficiency of the aortic valve causing backflow of blood from the aorta into the left ventricle (LV) during diastole
- Aortic stenosis (AS): Narrowing of the aortic valve, obstructing blood flow from the LV to the ascending aorta during systole
- Mitral regurgitation (MR): Insufficiency of the mitral valve causing flow of blood from the LV into the left atrium (LA) during ventricular systole
- Mitral stenosis: Narrowing of the mitral orifice that impedes blood flow from the LA to the LV
- Mitral valve prolapse (MVP): Billowing of mitral valve leaflets into the LA during systole
- Pulmonic regurgitation: Insufficiency of the pulmonic valve causing blood flow from the pulmonary artery into the right ventricle (RV) during diastole
- Pulmonic stenosis (PS): Narrowing of the pulmonary outflow tract causing obstruction of blood flow from the RV to the pulmonary artery during systole
- Tricuspid regurgitation (TR): Insufficiency of the tricuspid valve causing blood flow from the RV to the right atrium (RA) during systole
- Tricuspid stenosis (TS): Narrowing of the tricuspid orifice that obstructs blood flow from the RA to the RV

Historically, diagnosis of valvular disorders by observation, palpation, and auscultation was a tough test for aspiring clinicians.[1] Today, with the physical examination supplemented by cardiac ultrasonography, diagnosis is comparatively straightforward. Standard 2-dimensional studies show the anatomy. Doppler echocardiography evaluates pressure gradients and blood flow. Evaluation also includes ECG (to detect heart rhythm and chamber alterations) and chest x-ray (to detect chamber alterations, pulmonary congestion, and other lung pathology).

1. Ma I, Tierney LM: Name that murmur—Eponyms for the astute auscultician. *N Engl J Med* 363:2164–2168, 2010.

Treatment

- Valvuloplasty or valve replacement

Management of a valvular lesion commonly requires only periodic observation, with no active treatment for many years. In general, neither lifestyle measures nor drugs alter the natural history of valvular lesions. Intervention is usually indicated only when a moderate or severe valvular lesion causes symptoms or cardiac dysfunction. Because patients may not recognize symptoms due to their slow onset, many clinicians now use exercise testing to help monitor patients.

The intervention may involve valvuloplasty, valve repair, or valve replacement, all of which may be done percutaneously or surgically. Valvular disorders are currently subject to intensive research to develop percutaneous valve replacement. In addition, randomized, controlled trials of different valvular interventions are being done. The result for patients is an increasing number of therapeutic options and better evidence on how to choose one. For clinicians, the increase in complexity now requires a multidisciplinary heart valve team composed of surgeons, cardiologists, and other specialists to help decide which intervention is best for a given patient.

If coronary artery bypass surgery is being done, it is usual to surgically treat (during the same operation) any moderate or severe valve lesions, even if asymptomatic.

Endocarditis prophylaxis is indicated when there is a history of endocarditis and for patients with prosthetic heart valves.

Choice of cardiac valve prosthesis: For replacement, two kinds of valve prosthesis are used:

- Bioprosthetic (porcine or bovine)
- Mechanical (manufactured)

Traditionally, a mechanical valve has been used in patients < 65 and in older patients with a long life expectancy because bioprosthetic valves deteriorate over 10 to 12 yr (more rapidly in younger patients).

Lifelong **anticoagulation with warfarin** is required in patients with a mechanical valve to prevent thromboembolism. Newer novel oral anticoagulants (NOAC) are ineffective and should not be used.

PEARLS & PITFALLS

- Warfarin is the only appropriate oral anticoagulant for thromboembolism prevention in patients with prosthetic valves. Newer oral anticoagulants are ineffective.

An aortic bioprosthetic valve, which does not require anticoagulation beyond the immediate postoperative period, has been used in patients > 65, younger patients with a life expectancy < 10 yr, and those with some right-sided lesions. However, newer bioprosthetic valves may be more durable than 1st-generation valves; thus, patient preference regarding valve type can now be considered.

Women of childbearing age who require valve replacement and plan to become pregnant must balance the teratogenic risk due to warfarin when mechanical valves are used against the risk of accelerated valve deterioration when bioprosthetic valves are used. Teratogenic risks can be reduced by use of heparin instead of warfarin in the first 12 wk and last 2 wk of the pregnancy, but management is difficult and careful discussion is required before surgery.

AORTIC REGURGITATION

Aortic regurgitation (AR) is incompetency of the aortic valve causing backflow from the aorta into the LV during diastole. Causes include valvular degeneration and aortic root dilation (with or without a bicuspid valve), rheumatic fever, endocarditis, myxomatous degeneration, aortic root dissection, and connective tissue (eg, Marfan syndrome) or rheumatologic disorders. Symptoms include exertional dyspnea, orthopnea, paroxysmal nocturnal dyspnea, palpitations, and chest pain. Signs include widened pulse pressure and an early diastolic murmur. Diagnosis is by physical examination and echocardiography. Treatment is surgical aortic valve replacement or repair. Percutaneous valve replacement is being evaluated.

Etiology

AR may be acute (very uncommonly) or chronic.

The primary causes of **acute AR** are

- Infective endocarditis
- Dissection of the ascending aorta

The primary causes of **chronic AR in adults** are

- Degeneration of the aortic valve and root (with or without a bicuspid valve)
- Rheumatic fever
- Infective endocarditis
- Myxomatous degeneration
- Trauma
- Thoracic aortic aneurysm

In children, the most common cause of chronic AR is a ventricular septal defect with aortic valve prolapse.

Rarely, AR is caused by seronegative spondyloarthropathies (ankylosing spondylitis, reactive arthritis, psoriatic arthritis), RA, SLE, arthritis associated with ulcerative colitis, luetic (syphilitic) aortitis, osteogenesis imperfecta, supravalvular or discrete membranous subaortic stenosis, Takayasu arteritis, rupture of a sinus of Valsalva, acromegaly, and giant cell (temporal) arteritis. AR due to myxomatous degeneration may develop in patients with Marfan syndrome or Ehlers-Danlos syndrome.

Pathophysiology

In AR, volume overload of the LV occurs because the LV receives blood regurgitated from the aorta during diastole in addition to blood from the LA.

In acute AR, the LV does not have time to dilate to accommodate the increased volume, which then causes a rapid increase in left ventricular pressure and subsequently pulmonary edema and decreased cardiac output.

In chronic AR, LV hypertrophy and dilation can gradually occur, so normal left ventricular pressures and cardiac output are maintained. But decompensation eventually develops, ultimately causing arrhythmias, LV impairment, and heart failure (HF).

Symptoms and Signs

Acute AR causes symptoms of HF (dyspnea, fatigue, weakness, edema) and cardiogenic shock (hypotension with resultant multisystem organ damage).

Chronic AR is typically asymptomatic for years; progressive exertional dyspnea, orthopnea, paroxysmal nocturnal dyspnea, and palpitations develop insidiously.

Symptoms of HF correlate poorly with objective measures of left ventricular function. Chest pain (angina pectoris) affects only about 5% of patients who do not have coexisting coronary artery disease (CAD) and, when it occurs, is especially common at night. Patients may present with endocarditis (eg, fever, anemia, weight loss, embolic phenomena) because the abnormal aortic valve is predisposed to bacterial seeding.

Signs vary by severity and acuity. Signs in acute AR reflect HF and cardiogenic shock and typically include tachycardia, cool extremities, lung crackles, and low blood pressure. The 1st heart sound (S_1) is usually absent (because aortic and LV diastolic pressures equalize), and a third heart sound (S_3) is common. An AR murmur may be absent even if AR is severe, although an Austin Flint murmur is common.

As chronic disease progresses, systolic blood pressure increases while diastolic BP decreases, creating a widened pulse pressure. With time, the LV impulse may become enlarged, increased in amplitude, and displaced downward and laterally, with systolic depression of the entire left parasternal area, giving a rocking motion to the left chest.

A systolic apical or carotid thrill may become palpable in later stages of AR; it is caused by large forward stroke volumes and low aortic diastolic pressure.

Auscultatory findings include a normal S_1 and a nonsplit, loud, sharp or slapping 2nd heart sound (S_2) caused by increased elastic aortic recoil. The murmur of AR is often unimpressive. The murmur is blowing, high-pitched, diastolic, and decrescendo, beginning soon after the aortic component of S_2 (A_2); it is loudest at the 3rd or 4th left parasternal intercostal space. The murmur is heard best with the diaphragm of the stethoscope when the patient is leaning forward, with breath held at end-expiration. It increases in volume in response to maneuvers that increase afterload (eg, squatting, isometric handgrip). If AR is slight, the murmur may occur only in early diastole. If LV diastolic pressure is very high, the murmur is short because aortic and LV diastolic pressures equalize earlier in diastole.

Other abnormal sounds include a forward ejection and backward regurgitant flow (to-and-fro) murmur, an ejection click soon after the S_1, and an aortic ejection flow murmur. A diastolic murmur heard near the axilla or mid left thorax (Cole-Cecil murmur) is caused by fusion of the aortic murmur with the S_3, which is due to simultaneous filling of LV from the LA and AR. A mid-to-late diastolic rumble heard at the apex (Austin Flint murmur) may result from rapid regurgitant flow into the LV, causing mitral valve leaflet vibration at the peak of atrial flow; this murmur mimics the diastolic murmur of mitral stenosis.

Other signs are unusual; sensitivity and specificity are low or unknown. Visible signs include head bobbing (Musset sign) and pulsation of the fingernail capillaries (Quincke sign, best seen while applying slight pressure) or uvula (Müller sign).

Palpable signs include a large-volume pulse with rapid rise and fall (slapping, water-hammer, or collapsing pulse) and pulsation of the carotid arteries (Corrigan sign), retinal arteries (Becker sign), liver (Rosenbach sign), or spleen (Gerhard sign). BP findings may include popliteal systolic pressure ≥ 60 mm Hg higher than brachial pressure (Hill sign) and a fall in diastolic BP of > 15 mm Hg with arm elevation (Mayne sign). Auscultatory signs include a sharp sound heard over the femoral pulse (pistol-shot sound, or Traube sign) and a femoral systolic bruit distal and a diastolic bruit proximal to arterial compression (Duroziez sign).

Diagnosis

- Echocardiography

Diagnosis of AR is suspected based on history and physical examination findings and confirmed by echocardiography. Doppler echocardiography is the test of choice to detect and quantify the magnitude of regurgitant blood flow and grade overall severity of the AR. Two-dimensional echocardiography can quantify aortic root size and anatomy and LV function.

Severe AR is suggested by any of the following:

- Color Doppler jet width > 65% of the LV outflow tract diameter
- Vena contracta > 6 mm (the narrowest diameter of the fluid stream downstream of the abnormal valve orifice)
- Holodiastolic flow reversal in the abdominal aorta
- Regurgitant volume > 60 mL/beat
- Regurgitation fraction > 50%

In the presence of severe AR, decompensation of the LV (and thus need for surgery) is suggested by any of the following:

- End-systolic LV volume > 60 mL/m^2
- End-systolic LV diameter > 50 mm
- LV ejection fraction (LVEF) < 50%

Echocardiography can also assess severity of pulmonary hypertension secondary to LV failure, detect vegetations or pericardial effusions (eg, in aortic dissection), and provide information about prognosis. Coarctation is associated with bicuspid valve and is detected by placing the ultrasound transducer at the suprasternal notch. Transesophageal echocardiography provides additional delineation of aortic dilatation and valve anatomy, which is especially useful when surgical repair is being considered. If the aorta is enlarged, CT or MRI is recommended to evaluate the entire thoracic aorta. MRI also can help assess LV function and degree of AR when echocardiographic images are suboptimal.

Radionuclide imaging may be used to determine left ventricular ejection fraction if echocardiographic results are borderline abnormal or if echocardiography is technically difficult.

ECG and chest x-ray should be done. ECG may show repolarization abnormalities with or without QRS voltage criteria of LV hypertrophy, left atrial enlargement, and T-wave inversion with ST-segment depression in precordial leads. Chest x-ray may show cardiomegaly and a prominent aortic root in patients with chronic progressive AR. If AR is severe, signs of pulmonary edema and HF may also be present. Exercise testing may help assess functional capacity and symptoms in patients with documented AR and equivocal symptoms.

Coronary angiography should be done before surgery, even if no angina is present because about 20% of patients with severe AR have significant CAD, which may need concomitant coronary artery bypass graft surgery.

First-degree relatives of patients with a bicuspid valve should be screened using echocardiography because 20 to 30% will be similarly affected.

Prognosis

With treatment, the 10-yr survival for patients with mild to moderate AR is 80 to 95%. With appropriately timed valve replacement (ie, before HF and using accepted criteria for intervention), long-term prognosis for patients with moderate to severe AR is good. However, the prognosis for those with severe AR and HF is considerably poorer.

Treatment

- Aortic valve replacement or repair
- Sometimes vasodilators, diuretics, and nitrates

When aortic root dilatation is part of the mechanism of AR, angiotensin-receptor blockers may slow progression, making them favored drugs for patients with concomitant hypertension.

Intervention is either surgical aortic valve replacement or (less commonly) valve repair. Percutaneous options are being developed. An aortic bioprosthetic valve does not require anticoagulation beyond the immediate postoperative period, but a mechanical valve requires lifetime anticoagulation using warfarin. Newer NOAC are ineffective and should not be used.

Patients who are not candidates for surgery benefit from treatment of HF. Intra-aortic balloon pump insertion is contraindicated because the diastolic balloon inflation worsens AR. Beta-blockers should be used with caution because they block compensatory tachycardia and worsen AR by prolonging diastole.

Patients with severe AR who do not meet the criteria for intervention should be reevaluated by physical examination and echocardiography every 6 to 12 mo.

Antibiotic prophylaxis against endocarditis is no longer recommended for AR except for patients who have had valve replacement or repair (see Table 82–4 on p. 711).

Criteria for intervention: Intervention is indicated when

- AR is severe and is causing symptoms
- AR is severe and is causing LV dysfunction (EF < 50%, LV end-systolic dimension > 50 mm, or LV end-diastolic dimension > 65 to 75 mm)

Sometimes, intervention is done before AR becomes severe if the ascending aorta is dilated > 55 mm (> 50 mm in patients with Marfan syndrome and maybe for bicuspid aortic valve).

When cardiac surgery is done for other indications, concomitant aortic valve intervention is indicated if AR is moderate or severe.

KEY POINTS

- The primary causes of acute AR are infective endocarditis and dissection of the ascending aorta; chronic AR in adults is most often caused by degeneration of the aortic valve or root.
- Acute AR causes symptoms of HF and cardiogenic shock, but signs of AR may be absent.
- Chronic AR is typically asymptomatic for years followed by progressive exertional dyspnea, orthopnea, and paroxysmal nocturnal dyspnea.
- Typical heart sounds include a normal S_1 followed by a sharp or slapping S_2 and a blowing, high-pitched, decrescendo diastolic murmur.
- Acute AR requires prompt aortic valve replacement or repair.
- Chronic AR requires aortic valve replacement or repair when symptoms or LV dysfunction develops; patients who meet criteria but are not candidates for surgery benefit from HF treatment.

AORTIC STENOSIS

Aortic stenosis (AS) is narrowing of the aortic valve, obstructing blood flow from the LV to the ascending aorta during systole. Causes include a congenital bicuspid valve, idiopathic degenerative sclerosis with calcification, and rheumatic fever. Untreated AS progresses to become symptomatic with one or more of the classic triad of syncope, angina, and exertional dyspnea; HF and arrhythmias may develop. A crescendo-decrescendo ejection murmur is characteristic. Diagnosis is by physical examination and echocardiography. Asymptomatic AS in adults usually requires no treatment. Once symptoms develop, surgical or percutaneous valve replacement is required. For severe or symptomatic AS in children, balloon valvotomy is effective.

Etiology

In elderly patients, the most common precursor to AS is

- Aortic sclerosis

Aortic sclerosis is a degenerative aortic valve disease with thickening of aortic valve structures by fibrosis and calcification initially without causing significant obstruction. Over years, aortic sclerosis progresses to stenosis in as many as 15% of patients. Aortic sclerosis resembles atherosclerosis, with deposition of lipoproteins and inflammation and calcification of the valves; risk factors are similar. Patients with psoriasis are at increased risk for atherosclerosis, and more recently psoriasis has been tied to an increased risk of AS.

In patients < 70 yr, the most common cause of AS is

- A congenital bicuspid aortic valve

Congenital AS occurs in 3 to 5/1000 live births and affects more males; it is associated with coarctation and progressive dilatation of the ascending aorta, causing dissection.

In developing countries, the most common cause of AS in all age groups is

- Rheumatic fever

Supravalvular AS caused by a discrete congenital membrane or hypoplastic constriction just above the sinuses of Valsalva is uncommon. A sporadic form of supravalvular AS is associated with a characteristic facial appearance (high and broad forehead, hypertelorism, strabismus, upturned nose, long philtrum, wide mouth, dental abnormalities, puffy cheeks, micrognathia, low-set ears). When associated with idiopathic hypercalcemia of infancy, this form is known as Williams syndrome.

Subvalvular AS caused by a congenital membrane or fibrous ring just beneath the aortic valve is uncommon.

Pathophysiology

AR may accompany AS, and about 60% of patients > 60 yr with significant AS also have mitral annular calcification, which may lead to MR.

The increased pressure load imposed by AS results in compensatory hypertrophy of the LV without cavity enlargement (concentric hypertrophy). With time, the ventricle can no longer compensate, causing secondary LV cavity enlargement, reduced ejection fraction (EF), decreased cardiac output, and a misleadingly low gradient across the aortic valve (low-gradient severe AS). Patients with other disorders that also cause LV enlargement and reduced EF (eg, myocardial infarction, intrinsic cardiomyopathy) may generate insufficient flow to fully open a sclerotic valve and have an apparently small valve area even when their AS is not particularly severe (pseudosevere AS). Pseudosevere AS must be differentiated from low-gradient severe AS because only patients with low-gradient severe AS benefit from valve replacement.

Elevated shear stress across the stenosed aortic valve degrades von Willebrand factor multimers. The resulting coagulopathy may cause GI bleeding in patients with angiodysplasia (Heyde syndrome).

Symptoms and Signs

Congenital AS is usually asymptomatic until age 10 or 20 yr, when symptoms develop insidiously. In all forms, progressive untreated AS ultimately results in exertional syncope, angina, and dyspnea (SAD triad). Other symptoms and signs may include those of HF and arrhythmias, including ventricular fibrillation leading to sudden death.

Exertional syncope occurs because cardiac output cannot increase enough to meet the demands of physical activity. Nonexertional syncope may result from altered baroreceptor responses or ventricular tachycardia. Exertional angina pectoris affects about two thirds of patients; about half have significant coronary artery atherosclerosis, and half have normal coronary arteries but have ischemia induced by LV hypertrophy and altered coronary flow dynamics.

There are no visible signs of AS. Palpable signs include carotid and peripheral pulses that are reduced in amplitude and slow rising (pulsus parvus, mollus et tardus) and an apical impulse that is sustained (thrusts with the 1st heart sound [S_1] and relaxes with the 2nd heart sound [S_2]) because of left ventricular hypertrophy. The LV impulse may become displaced when systolic dysfunction develops. A palpable 4th heart sound (S_4), felt best at the apex, and a systolic thrill, corresponding with the murmur of AS and felt best at the left upper sternal border, are occasionally present in severe cases. Systolic BP may be high even when AS is severe but ultimately falls when the LV fails.

On auscultation, S_1 is normal and S_2 is single because aortic valve closing is delayed and merges with the pulmonic (P_2) component of S_2. The aortic component may also be soft. Paradoxical splitting of S_2 may be heard. A normally split S_2 is the only physical finding that reliably excludes severe AS. An S_4 may be audible. An ejection click may also be audible early after S_1 in patients with congenital bicuspid AS when valve leaflets are stiff but not completely immobile. The click does not change with dynamic maneuvers.

The hallmark finding is a crescendo-decrescendo ejection murmur, heard best with the diaphragm of the stethoscope at the right and left upper sternal border when a patient who is sitting upright leans forward. The murmur typically radiates to the right clavicle and both carotid arteries (left often louder than right) and has a harsh or grating quality. But in elderly patients, vibration of the unfused cusps of calcified aortic valve leaflets may transmit a louder, more high-pitched, "cooing" or musical sound to the cardiac apex, with softening or absence of the murmur parasternally (Gallavardin phenomenon), thereby mimicking MR. The murmur is soft when stenosis is less severe, grows louder as stenosis progresses, and becomes longer and peaks in volume later in systole (ie, crescendo phase becomes longer and decrescendo phase becomes shorter) as stenosis becomes more severe. As LV contractility decreases in critical AS, the murmur becomes softer and shorter. The intensity of the murmur may therefore be misleading in these circumstances.

The murmur of AS typically increases with maneuvers that increase LV volume and contractility (eg, leg-raising, squatting, Valsalva release, after a ventricular premature beat) and decreases with maneuvers that decrease LV volume (Valsalva maneuver) or increase afterload (isometric handgrip). These dynamic maneuvers have the opposite effect on the murmur of hypertrophic cardiomyopathy, which can otherwise resemble that of AS. The murmur of MR due to prolapse of the posterior leaflet may also mimic AS.

Diagnosis

- Echocardiography

Diagnosis or AS is suspected clinically and confirmed by echocardiography. Two-dimensional transthoracic echocardiography is used to identify a stenotic aortic valve and possible causes, to quantify LV hypertrophy and degree of systolic dysfunction, and to detect coexisting valvular heart disorders (AR, mitral valve disorders) and complications (eg, endocarditis). Doppler echocardiography is used to quantify degree of stenosis by measuring jet velocity, transvalvular systolic pressure gradient, and aortic valve area

Severity of AS is characterized echocardiographically as

- Moderate: Peak aortic jet velocity 3 to 4 m/sec, mean gradient 20 to 40 mm Hg, valve area 1.0 to 1.5 cm^2
- Severe: Peak aortic jet velocity > 4 m/sec, mean gradient > 40 mm Hg, valve area < 1.0 cm^2
- Very severe: Peak aortic jet velocity > 5 m/sec or mean gradient > 60 mm Hg

Clinical judgment is used to resolve any discordance among these parameters (eg, moderate valve area but severe mean gradient). When LV function is normal, the valve area is the least accurate.

The gradient may be overestimated when AR is present. The gradient may under-represent severity when the stroke volume is low, eg, in patients with LV systolic dysfunction (low-gradient AS with reduced EF) or a small, hypertrophied LV (low-gradient AS with normal EF). Sometimes LV systolic dysfunction results in low ventricular pressure that is inadequate to open nonstenotic valve leaflets, causing echocardiographic appearance of low valve area in the absence of stenosis (pseudostenosis).

Prior to intervention, cardiac catheterization is necessary to determine whether coronary artery disease (CAD) is the cause of angina and, occasionally, to resolve inconsistency between clinical and echocardiographic findings.

An ECG and chest x-ray are obtained. ECG typically shows changes of LV hypertrophy with or without an ischemic ST- and T-wave pattern. Chest x-ray findings may include calcification of the aortic cusps (seen on the lateral projection or on fluoroscopy) and evidence of HF. Heart size may be normal or only mildly enlarged.

In asymptomatic patients with severe AS, closely supervised exercise ECG testing is recommended in an attempt to elicit symptoms of angina, dyspnea, or hypotension—any of these symptoms, when due to the AS, is an indication for intervention. Failure to normally increase BP and development of ST segment depression are less predictive of adverse prognosis. Exercise testing is contraindicated in symptomatic patients. When there is LV dysfunction and the aortic valve gradient is low but the valve area is small, then low-dose dobutamine stress echocardiography distinguishes low-gradient AS from pseudostenosis.

Prognosis

AS progresses faster as severity increases, but the wide variability in progression rates requires regular surveillance, particularly in sedentary elderly patients. In such patients, flow may become significantly compromised without triggering symptoms.

Asymptomatic patients with severe AS and normal systolic function should be reevaluated every 6 mo because 3 to 6% will develop symptoms or LVEF impairment every year. The risk of surgery outweighs the survival benefit in asymptomatic patients, but with the onset of symptoms the mean survival plummets to 2 to 3 yr, and prompt valve replacement is indicated to relieve symptoms and improve survival. Risk of surgery increases for patients who require simultaneous coronary artery bypass graft (CABG) and for those with depressed systolic LV function.

In patients with severe AS, about 50% of deaths occur suddenly, and these patients should be advised to limit physical exertion.

Treatment

- Sometimes aortic valve replacement

Nothing has yet been proved to slow the progression of AS. In randomized trials, statin therapy has been ineffective.

Drugs that can cause hypotension (eg, nitrates) should be used cautiously, although nitroprusside has been used as a temporizing measure to reduce afterload in patients with decompensated HF in the hours before valve replacement. Patients who develop HF but are too high risk for valve intervention benefit from cautious treatment with digoxin, diuretics, and ACE inhibitors.

Timing of intervention: The benefits of intervention do not outweigh the risks until patients develop symptoms and/or meet certain echocardiographic criteria. Thus, patients should have periodic clinical evaluations, including echocardiography and sometimes exercise testing, to determine the optimal time for valve replacement. Valve replacement is recommended for

Symptomatic patients (including those with symptoms or reduced effort tolerance on exercise testing) with

- Severe AS

Asymptomatic patients with any one of the following:

- LV EF < 50%
- Moderate or severe AS when undergoing cardiac surgery for other reasons
- Very severe AS (and low surgical risk)

Choice of intervention: Balloon valvotomy is used primarily in children and very young adults with congenital AS. In older patients who are not candidates for surgery, balloon valvuloplasty may be used as a bridge to valve replacement but it has a high complication rate and provides only temporary relief.

Surgical aortic valve replacement is the best choice for most patients but **transcatheter (percutaneous) valve replacement (TAVR)** may be chosen instead when surgical risk is high (as long as coexisting conditions do not preclude benefit from relieving the AS). TAVR affords better survival and quality of life than medical therapy and is safer than surgery in many high-risk patients.[1,2] Surgery usually involves replacement with a mechanical or bioprosthetic valve, but in younger patients, the patient's own pulmonic valve can be used, and a bioprosthesis is then used to replace the pulmonic valve (Ross procedure). Preoperative evaluation for CAD is indicated so that CABG and valve replacement, if indicated, can be done during the same procedure. An aortic bioprosthetic valve does not require anticoagulation beyond the immediate postoperative period but a mechanical valve requires lifetime anticoagulation using warfarin. Newer NOAC are ineffective and should not be used.

1. Kapadia SR, Leon MB, Makkar RR, et al. Five-year outcomes of transcatheter aortic valve replacement compared with standard treatment for patients with inoperable AS (PARTNER 1): a randomised controlled trial. *Lancet* 385:2485–2491, 2015.
2. Mack MJ, Leon MB, Smith CR, et al. Five-year outcomes of transcatheter aortic valve replacement or surgical aortic valve replacement for high surgical risk patients with AS (PARTNER 1): a randomised controlled trial. *Lancet* 385:2477–2484, 2015.

KEY POINTS

- The most common cause of AS in patients < 70 yr is bicuspid aortic valve; aortic sclerosis is the most common precursor in the elderly.
- Untreated AS ultimately results in exertional syncope, angina, and dyspnea; sudden death may occur.

- Typical heart sounds are a crescendo-decrescendo ejection murmur that increases with maneuvers that increase LV volume and contractility (eg, leg-raising, squatting, Valsalva release) and decreases with maneuvers that decrease LV volume (Valsalva maneuver) or increase afterload (isometric handgrip).
- Nitrates may cause dangerous hypotension and should be used with caution for angina in patients with AS.
- Replacement is indicated once symptoms begin or LV dysfunction occurs.
- Surgical valve replacement is the best option for most patients, but transcatheter replacement is now available for patients at high surgical risk.

MITRAL REGURGITATION

Mitral regurgitation (MR) is incompetency of the mitral valve causing flow from the LV into the LA during ventricular systole. MR can be primary (common causes are MVP and rheumatic fever) or secondary to LV dilation or infarction. Complications include progressive HF, arrhythmias, and endocarditis. Symptoms and signs include palpitations, dyspnea, and a holosystolic apical murmur. Diagnosis is by physical examination and echocardiography. Prognosis depends on LV function and etiology, severity, and duration of MR. Patients with mild, asymptomatic MR may be monitored, but progressive or symptomatic MR requires mitral valve repair or replacement.

Etiology

MR may be acute or chronic.

Causes of acute MR include

- Ischemic papillary muscle dysfunction or rupture
- Infective endocarditis with rupture of the chordae tendineae
- Acute rheumatic fever
- Myxomatous rupture of the chordae tendinae
- Acute dilation of the LV due to myocarditis or ischemia
- Mechanical failure of a prosthetic mitral valve

Common causes of chronic MR are intrinsic valve pathology (primary MR) or distortion of a normal valve by dilatation and impairment of the LV (secondary MR).

Primary MR pathology is most often MVP or rheumatic heart disease. Less common causes are connective tissue disorders, congenital cleft mitral valve, and radiation heart disease.

In secondary MR, ventricular impairment and dilation displace the papillary muscles, which tether the otherwise normal leaflets and prevent them from closing fully. The causes are myocardial infarction (ischemic chronic secondary MR) or intrinsic myocardial disease (nonischemic chronic secondary MR).

In infants, the most likely causes of MR are papillary muscle dysfunction, endocardial fibroelastosis, acute myocarditis, cleft mitral valve with or without an endocardial cushion defect, and myxomatous degeneration of the mitral valve. MR may coexist with mitral stenosis when thickened valvular leaflets do not close.

Pathophysiology

Acute MR may cause acute pulmonary edema and cardiogenic shock or sudden cardiac death.

Complications of chronic MR include gradual enlargement of the LA; LV enlargement and eccentric hypertrophy, which initially compensates for regurgitant flow (preserving forward stroke volume) but eventually decompensates (reducing forward stroke volume); atrial fibrillation (AF), which may be further complicated by thromboembolism; and infective endocarditis.

Symptoms and Signs

Acute MR causes the same symptoms and signs as acute HF (dyspnea, fatigue, weakness, edema) and cardiogenic shock (hypotension with resultant multisystem organ damage). Specific signs of MR may be absent.

Chronic MR in most patients is initially asymptomatic and symptoms develop insidiously as the LA enlarges, pulmonary artery pressure and venous pressure increase, and LV compensation fails. Symptoms include dyspnea, fatigue (due to HF), orthopnea, and palpitations (often due to AF). Rarely, patients present with endocarditis (eg, fever, weight loss, embolic phenomena).

Signs develop only when MR becomes moderate to severe. Inspection and palpation may detect a brisk apical impulse and sustained left parasternal movement due to systolic expansion of an enlarged LA. An LV impulse that is sustained, enlarged, and displaced downward and to the left suggests LV hypertrophy and dilation. A diffuse precordial lift occurs with severe MR because the LA enlarges, causing anterior cardiac displacement, and pulmonary hypertension causes right ventricular hypertrophy. A regurgitant murmur (or thrill) may also be palpable in severe cases.

On auscultation, the 1st heart sound (S_1) may be soft (or occasionally loud). A 3rd heart sound (S_3) at the apex reflects a dilated LV and severe MR.

The cardinal sign of MR is a holosystolic (pansystolic) murmur, heard best at the apex with the diaphragm of the stethoscope when the patient is in the left lateral decubitus position. In mild MR, the systolic murmur may be abbreviated or occur late in systole. The murmur begins with S_1 in conditions causing leaflet incompetency throughout systole, but it often begins after S_1 (eg, when chamber dilation during systole distorts the valve apparatus or when myocardial ischemia or fibrosis alters dynamics). When the murmur begins after S_1, it always continues to the 2nd heart sound (S_2). The murmur radiates toward the left axilla; intensity may remain the same or vary. If intensity varies, the murmur tends to crescendo in volume up to S_2. MR murmurs increase in intensity with handgrip or squatting because peripheral vascular resistance to ventricular ejection increases, augmenting regurgitation into the LA; murmurs decrease in intensity with standing or the Valsalva maneuver. A short rumbling mid-diastolic inflow murmur due to torrential mitral diastolic flow may be heard following an S_3. In patients with posterior leaflet prolapse, the murmur may be coarse and radiate to the upper sternum, mimicking AS.

MR murmurs may be confused with TR, which can be distinguished because TR murmur is augmented during inspiration.

Diagnosis

- Echocardiography

Diagnosis is suspected clinically and confirmed by echocardiography. Doppler echocardiography is used to detect regurgitant flow and pulmonary hypertension. Two-dimensional or 3-dimensional echocardiography is used to determine the cause and severity of MR (see Table 90–1), the presence and extent of annular calcification, and the size and function of the LV and LA and to detect pulmonary hypertension.

When it is acute, severe MR may not be apparent on color Doppler echocardiography, but suspicion is raised when acute HF is accompanied by hyperdynamic LV systolic function.

Table 90–1. GRADING OF MITRAL REGURGITATION

PARAMETER	MODERATE MR*	SEVERE PRIMARY MR	SEVERE SECONDARY MR
Vena contracta†	3–7 mm	> 7 mm	No recognized criteria
Effective regurgitant orifice area	0.20–0.40 cm^2	> 0.40 cm^2	> 0.20 cm^2
Regurgitant volume	30–60 mL	> 60 mL	> 30 mL
Regurgitant fraction	40–50%	> 50%	> 50%

*No recognized criteria exist for moderate secondary MR.
†The narrowest diameter of the fluid stream downstream of an abnormal valve orifice; it is slightly smaller than the anatomic valve orifice.
MR = mitral regurgitation.

If endocarditis or valvular thrombi are suspected, transesophageal echocardiography (TEE) can provide a more detailed view of the mitral valve and LA. TEE is also indicated when mitral valve repair instead of replacement is being considered to evaluate the mechanism of MR in more detail.

An ECG and chest x-ray are usually obtained initially. ECG may show LA enlargement and LV hypertrophy with or without ischemia. Sinus rhythm is usually present when MR is acute because the atria have not had time to stretch and remodel.

Chest x-ray in acute MR may show pulmonary edema; abnormalities in cardiac silhouette are not evident unless an underlying chronic disorder is also present. Chest x-ray in chronic MR may show LA and LV enlargement. It may also show pulmonary vascular congestion and pulmonary edema with HF.

Cardiac catheterization is done before surgery, mainly to determine whether coronary artery disease (CAD) is present. A prominent systolic *c-v* wave is seen on pulmonary artery occlusion pressure (pulmonary capillary wedge pressure) tracings during ventricular systole. Ventriculography can be used to quantify MR. Cardiac MRI can accurately measure regurgitant fraction and determine the cause of dilated myopathy with MR.

Periodic exercise testing (stress ECG) is often done to detect any decrease in effort tolerance, which would prompt consideration of surgical intervention. Periodic echocardiography is done to detect progression of MR.

Prognosis

Prognosis varies by duration, severity, and cause of MR. Some MR worsens and eventually becomes severe. Once MR becomes severe, about 10% of asymptomatic patients become symptomatic each year thereafter. About 10% of patients with chronic MR caused by MVP require surgical intervention.

Treatment

- Mitral valve repair or replacement
- Anticoagulants for patients with AF

ACE inhibitors and other vasodilators do not delay LV dilation or MR progression and so have no role in asymptomatic MR with preserved LV function. However, if LV dilation or dysfunction is present, vasodilators, spironolactone, and vasodilating beta-blockers (eg, carvedilol) are indicated. If the ECG shows left bundle branch block, then biventricular pacing may be beneficial for secondary MR. Loop diuretics such as furosemide are helpful in patients with exertional or nocturnal dyspnea. Digoxin may reduce symptoms in patients with AF or those in whom valve surgery is not appropriate.

Antibiotic prophylaxis is no longer recommended except for patients who have had valve replacement or repair (see Table 82–4 on p. 711).

Anticoagulants are used to prevent thromboemboli in patients with AF.

Timing of intervention: Acute MR requires emergency mitral valve repair or replacement with concomitant coronary revascularization as necessary. Pending surgery, nitroprusside or nitroglycerin infusion and an intra-aortic ballon pump may be used to reduce afterload, thus improving forward stroke volume and reducing ventricular and regurgitant volume.

Chronic primary MR that is severe needs intervention at the onset of symptoms or LV decompensation (LV EF < 60% or LV end-systolic diameter > 40 mm). Even in the absence of these triggers, intervention may be beneficial when valve morphology suggests a high likelihood of successful repair, particularly if there is new onset AF or resting pulmonary systolic pressure is > 50 mm Hg. When the EF falls < 30%, surgical risk is high, necessitating a careful weighing of risk and benefit.

Chronic secondary MR has many fewer indications for intervention. Because the primary pathology involves the LV muscle, correction of MR is not as likely to be beneficial. Additionally, there is no durable way to repair secondary MR, and valve replacement has both early (perioperative complications and mortality) and late risks (thromboembolism and infection). One study of 2-yr outcome in patients with severe secondary MR randomized to repair or chordal-sparing replacement found no difference in LV remodeling or survival. MR recurred more frequently in the repair group (59% vs 4%), resulting in more HF–related adverse events and readmissions.[1]

For patients undergoing cardiac surgery for other indications, concomitant mitral valve surgery should be considered for a repairable valve with MR that is moderate. However, for secondary MR, this practice has been questioned by the 1-yr outcome of a recent randomized comparison with CABG alone. There was no difference in LV remodelling, but an excess of adverse events occurred.[2] Longer term followup is needed. If the valve is not repairable, then replacement is usually done only when MR is severe.

Choice of intervention: In primary MR, the closer the mitral valve intervention mimics the native valve, the better for LV preservation and mortality. Hence, the order of preference is

1. Repair
2. Replacement with chordal preservation
3. Replacement with removal of chordae

Mechanical prostheses are preferred because tissue valves have reduced longevity in the mitral position. Repair of secondary MR with an annuloplasty ring often provides only temporary relief of MR but is usually done at the time of coronary artery bypass grafting if the MR is moderate or severe. Percutaneous mitral valve repair with a device that approximates the mitral leaflets is being developed. One randomized comparison of surgery and the percutaneous device found that after 5 yr, patients with the percutaneously placed device had similar mortality rates but more recurrent MR.[3]

Lifelong **anticoagulation with warfarin** is required in patients with a mechanical valve to prevent thromboembolism. Newer NOAC are ineffective and should not be used.

In about 50% of decompensated patients, prosthetic valve implantation markedly depresses ejection fraction because in such patients, ventricular function has become dependent on the afterload reduction of MR.

Selected patients with AF may benefit from concomitant ablation therapy, although this therapy increases operative morbidity.

1. Goldstein D, Moskowitz AJ, Gelijns AC, et al: Two-year outcomes of surgical treatment of severe ischemic mitral regurgitation. *N Engl J Med* 374:344–353, 2016. doi: 10.1056/NEJMoa1512913.
2. Michler RE, Smith PK, Parides MK, et al: Two-year outcomes of surgical treatment of moderate ischemic mitral regurgitation. *N Engl J Med* 374:1932–1941, 2016. doi: 10.1056/NEJMoa1602003.
3. Feldman T, Kar S, Elmariah S, et al: Randomized comparison of percutaneous repair and surgery for mitral regurgitation: 5-year results of EVEREST II. *J Am Coll Cardiol*. 66:2844–2854, 2015. doi: 10.1016/j.jacc.2015.10.018.

KEY POINTS

- Common causes include MVP, rheumatic fever, and LV dilation or infarction.
- Acute MR may cause acute pulmonary edema and cardiogenic shock or sudden cardiac death.
- Chronic MR causes slowly progressive symptoms of HF and, if AF develops, palpitations.
- Typical heart sounds are a holosystolic murmur that is heard best at the apex, radiates toward the left axilla, increases in intensity with handgrip or squatting, and decreases in intensity with standing or the Valsalva maneuver.
- Symptomatic patients and those meeting certain echocardiographic criteria benefit from valve replacement or repair.

MITRAL STENOSIS

Mitral stenosis (MS) is narrowing of the mitral orifice that impedes blood flow from the LA to the LV. The (almost) invariable cause is rheumatic fever. Common complications are pulmonary hypertension, AF, and thromboembolism. Symptoms are those of HF; signs include an opening snap and a diastolic murmur. Diagnosis is by physical examination and echocardiography. Prognosis is good. Medical treatment includes diuretics, beta-blockers or rate-limiting calcium channel blockers, and anticoagulants. Effective treatment for more severe disease consists of balloon commissurotomy, surgical commissurotomy, or valve replacement.

In mitral stenosis, mitral valve leaflets become thickened and immobile and the mitral orifice becomes narrowed due to fusion of the commissures and the presence of shortened, thickened and matted chordae. The most common cause is rheumatic fever, even though many patients do not recall the disorder. Very rare causes include mitral annular calcification with extension of calcification into the leaflets, causing them to stiffen and not open fully. Occasionally, MS is congenital. If the valve cannot close completely, MR may coexist with MS. Patients with MS due to rheumatic fever may also have lesions of the aortic or tricuspid valve or both.

Left atrial (LA) size and pressure increase progressively to compensate for MS; pulmonary venous and capillary pressures also increase and may cause secondary pulmonary hypertension, leading to right ventricular (RV) HF, TR, and pulmonic regurgitation. Rate of progression varies.

LA enlargement predisposes to AF, a risk factor for thromboembolism. The faster heart rate and loss of atrial contraction with onset of AF often lead to sudden worsening of symptoms.

Symptoms and Signs

Symptoms of mitral stenosis correlate poorly with disease severity because the disease often progresses slowly, and patients unconsciously reduce their activity. Many patients are asymptomatic until they become pregnant or AF develops. Initial symptoms are usually those of HF (eg, exertional dyspnea, orthopnea, paroxysmal nocturnal dyspnea, fatigue).

Symptoms typically do not appear until 15 to 40 yr after an episode of rheumatic fever. In developing countries, young children may become symptomatic because streptococcal infections may not be treated with antibiotics and recurrent infections are common.

Paroxysmal or chronic AF further reduces blood flow into the LV, precipitating pulmonary edema and acute dyspnea when ventricular rate is poorly controlled. AF may also cause palpitations. In up to 15% of patients not taking anticoagulants, it causes systemic embolism with symptoms of stroke or other organ ischemia.

Less common symptoms include hemoptysis due to rupture of small pulmonary vessels and pulmonary edema, particularly during pregnancy when blood volume increases. Hoarseness due to compression of the left recurrent laryngeal nerve by a dilated LA or pulmonary artery (Ortner syndrome) and symptoms of pulmonary hypertension and RV failure may also occur.

Mitral stenosis may cause signs of cor pulmonale. The classic facial appearance in MS, a plum-colored malar flush, occurs only when cardiac output is low and pulmonary hypertension is severe; cause is cutaneous vasodilation and chronic hypoxemia.

Occasionally, the initial symptoms and signs of MS are those of an embolic event such as stroke. Endocarditis is rare in MS unless MR is also present.

Palpation: Palpation may detect palpable 1st and 2nd heart sounds (S_1 and S_2). S_1 is best palpated at the apex, and S_2 at the upper left sternal border. The pulmonic component of S_2 (P_2) is responsible for the impulse and results from pulmonary hypertension. An RV impulse (heave) palpable at the left sternal border may accompany jugular venous distention when pulmonary hypertension is present and RV diastolic dysfunction develops.

Auscultation: Auscultatory findings include a loud S_1 caused by the leaflets of a stenotic mitral valve closing abruptly (M_1); it is heard best at the apex. S_1 may be absent when the valve is heavily calcified and immobile. A normally split S_2 with an exaggerated P_2 due to pulmonary hypertension is also heard.

Most prominent is an early diastolic opening snap as the leaflets billow into the LV, which is loudest close to left lower sternal border; it is followed by a low-pitched decrescendo-crescendo rumbling diastolic murmur, heard best with the bell of the stethoscope at the apex (or over the palpable apex beat) at end-expiration when the patient is in the left lateral decubitus position. The opening snap may be soft or absent if the mitral valve is calcified; the snap moves closer to S_2 (increasing duration of the murmur) as mitral stenosis becomes more severe and LA pressure increases.

The diastolic murmur increases after a Valsalva maneuver (when blood pours into the LA), after exercise, and in response to maneuvers that increase afterload (eg, squatting, isometric handgrip). The murmur may be softer or absent when an enlarged RV displaces the LV posteriorly and when other disorders (pulmonary hypertension, right-sided valve abnormalities, AF with fast ventricular rate) decrease blood flow across the mitral valve. The presystolic crescendo is caused by increased flow with atrial contraction. However, the closing mitral valve leaflets during LV contraction may also contribute to this finding but only at the end of short diastoles when LA pressure is still high.

Diastolic murmurs that may coexist with the MS murmur are:

- Early diastolic murmur of coexisting AR, which may be conducted to the apex
- Graham Steell murmur (a soft decrescendo diastolic murmur heard best along the left sternal border and caused by pulmonic regurgitation secondary to severe pulmonary hypertension)
- Diastolic flow murmur in the presence of severe MR
- Obstructing left atrial myxoma or ball thrombus (rare)

Diagnosis

- Echocardiography

Diagnosis is suspected clinically and confirmed by echocardiography. Typically, 2-dimensional echocardiography shows abnormal valve and subvalve structures. It also provides information about the degree of valvular calcification and stenosis and LA size. Doppler echocardiography provides information about the transvalvular gradient and pulmonary artery pressure. The normal area of the mitral valve orifice is 4 to 5 cm^2.

Severity is characterized echocardiographically as

- Moderate: Valve area 1.5 to 2.5 cm^2
- Severe: Valve area < 1.5 cm^2; symptoms are often present
- Very severe: Valve area < 1.0 cm^2

However, the relationship between the area of the valve orifice and symptoms is not always consistent. Color Doppler echocardiography detects associated MR. TEE can be used to detect or exclude small LA thrombi, especially those in the LA appendage, which usually cannot be seen transthoracically.

An ECG and chest x-ray are usually obtained.

The ECG may show LA enlargement, manifest as a P wave lasting > 0.12 msec with prominent negative deflection of its terminal component (duration: > 0.04 msec; amplitude: > 0.10 mV) in V_1; broad, notched P waves in lead II; or both. Right axis QRS deviation and tall R waves in V_1 suggest RV hypertrophy.

Chest x-ray usually shows straightening of the left cardiac border due to a dilated LA appendage, and widening of the carina. With barium in the esophagus, the lateral chest x-ray will show the dilated LA displacing the esophagus posteriorly. The main pulmonary artery (trunk) may be prominent; the descending right pulmonary artery diameter is ≥ 16 mm if pulmonary hypertension is significant. The upper lobe pulmonary veins may be dilated. A double shadow of an enlarged LA may be seen along the right cardiac border. Horizontal lines in the lower posterior lung fields (Kerley B lines) indicate interstitial edema associated with high LA pressure.

Cardiac catheterization, indicated only for perioperative assessment of coronary artery disease (CAD) before surgical repair, can confirm elevated LA and pulmonary artery pressures, mitral gradient and valve area.

Prognosis

The natural history of mitral stenosis varies, but the interval between onset of symptoms and severe disability is about 7 to 9 yr. Outcome is affected by the patient's preprocedural age and functional status, pulmonary hypertension, and degree of MR. Symptomatic results of balloon or surgical commissurotomy are equivalent in patients with valves that are not calcified. However, after a variable period of time, function deteriorates in most patients due to restenosis, and valve replacement may become necessary. Risk factors for death are AF and pulmonary hypertension. Cause of death is most commonly HF or pulmonary or cerebrovascular embolism.

Treatment

- Diuretics and sometimes beta-blockers or calcium channel blockers
- Anticoagulation for AF
- Commissurotomy or valve replacement

Asymptomatic patients require no treatment other than appropriate prophylaxis against rheumatic fever recurrence.

Mildly symptomatic patients usually respond to diuretics and, if sinus tachycardia or AF is present, to beta-blockers or calcium channel blockers, which can control ventricular rate.

Anticoagulants are indicated to prevent thromboembolism if patients have or have had AF, embolism, or a left atrial clot. Anticoagulation may also be considered in the presence of dense spontaneous contrast or an enlarged LA (M-mode diameter > 50 mm). All patients should be encouraged to continue at least low levels of physical exercise despite exertional dyspnea.

Antibiotic prophylaxis against endocarditis is no longer recommended except for patients who have had valve replacement (see Table 82–4 on p. 711).

Timing of intervention: For **moderate mitral stenosis,** intervention may be indicated when there is ≥ 1 of the following:

- Cardiac surgery is required for other indications
- Patients are symptomatic and have exercise-induced mean transmitral gradient > 15 mm Hg or pulmonary capillary occlusion pressure > 25 mm Hg

For **severe mitral stenosis,** intervention is indicated when there is ≥ 1 of the following:

- Any symptoms if the valve is suitable for percutaneous balloon commissurotomy (may be considered in asymptomatic patients)
- Cardiac surgery is required for other indications

For **very severe mitral stenosis,** intervention is indicated for all patients (with or without symptoms) who are suitable candidates for percutaneous balloon commissurotomy.

Choice of intervention: Percutaneous balloon commissurotomy is the procedure of choice for younger patients and for patients without heavily calcified valve commissures, subvalvular distortion, LA thrombi, or severe MR. In this fluoroscopic- and echocardiographic-guided procedure, a transvenous catheter with an inflatable distal balloon is passed transseptally from the RA to the LA and inflated to separate fused mitral valve commissures. Outcomes are equivalent to those of more invasive procedures. Complications are uncommon but include MR, embolism, and tamponade.

Surgical commissurotomy may be used in patients with severe subvalvular disease, valvular calcification, or LA thrombi. In this procedure, fused mitral valve leaflets are separated using a dilator passed through the LV (closed commissurotomy) via a thoracotomy, or by direct vision (open commissurotomy) via a sternotomy. Choice of procedure is based on surgeon's experience and the morphology of the valve, although closed valvotomy is now done less frequently in Western countries. Because of its greater risks, surgery is usually deferred until symptoms reach New York Heart Association class III (see Table 83–2 on p. 716). During surgery, some clinicians ligate the left atrial appendage to reduce thromboembolism.

Valve replacement is confined to patients with severe morphologic changes that make the valve unsuitable for balloon or surgical commissurotomy. Lifelong anticoagulation with warfarin is required in patients with a mechanical valve to prevent thromboembolism. Newer NOAC are ineffective and should not be used.

When the etiology is annular calcification, there is no benefit from percutaneous balloon commissurotomy because there is no commissural fusion. Furthermore, surgical valve replacement is technically demanding because of the annular calcification and often high risk because many patients are elderly and have comorbidities. Therefore, intervention is delayed until symptoms become severe despite use of diuretic and rate control drugs.

KEY POINTS

- Mitral stenosis is almost always caused by rheumatic fever.
- Pulmonary hypertension and AF (with consequent thromboembolism) may develop.
- Heart sounds include a loud S_1 and an early diastolic opening snap followed by a low-pitched decrescendo-crescendo rumbling diastolic murmur, heard best at the apex at end-expiration when the patient is in the left lateral decubitus position; the murmur increases after a Valsalva maneuver, exercise, squatting, and isometric handgrip.
- Mildly symptomatic patients usually respond to diuretics and, if sinus tachycardia or AF is present, to beta-blockers or calcium channel blockers for rate control.
- Severely symptomatic patients and those with evidence of pulmonary hypertension require commissurotomy or valve replacement.

MITRAL VALVE PROLAPSE

Mitral valve prolapse (MVP) is a billowing of mitral valve leaflets into the LA during systole. The most common cause is idiopathic myxomatous degeneration. MVP is usually benign, but complications include MR, endocarditis, and chordal rupture. MVP is usually asymptomatic in the absence of significant regurgitation, although there are reports that some patients experience chest pain, dyspnea, dizziness, and palpitations. Signs include a crisp midsystolic click, followed by a late systolic murmur if regurgitation is present. Diagnosis is by physical examination and echocardiography. Prognosis is excellent in the absence of significant regurgitation, but chordal rupture and endocarditis may occur. No specific treatment is necessary unless significant MR is present.

MVP is common; prevalence is 1 to 3% in otherwise normal populations, depending on the echocardiographic criteria used. Women and men are affected equally; onset usually follows the adolescent growth spurt.

Etiology

MVP is most often caused by

- Myxomatous degeneration of the mitral valve leaflets and chordae tendineae

In myxomatous degeneration, the fibrous collagen layer of the valve thins and mucoid (myxomatous) material accumulates. The chordae become longer and thinner and the valve leaflets enlarge and become rubbery. These changes result in floppy valve leaflets that can balloon back (prolapse) into the LA when the LV contracts. Rupture of a degenerate chorda can allow part of the valve leaflet to flail into the atrium, which typically causes severe regurgitation.

Degeneration is usually idiopathic, although it may be inherited in an autosomal dominant or, rarely, in an X-linked recessive fashion. Myxomatous degeneration may also be caused by connective tissue disorders (eg, Marfan syndrome, Ehlers-Danlos syndrome, adult polycystic kidney disease, osteogenesis imperfecta, pseudoxanthoma elasticum, SLE, polyarteritis nodosa) and muscular dystrophies. MVP is more common among patients with Graves disease, hypomastia, von Willebrand syndrome, sickle cell disease, and rheumatic heart disease. Myxomatous degeneration may also affect the aortic or tricuspid valve, resulting in aortic or tricuspid prolapse. Primary TR is much less common than secondary TR due to left ventricular pathology.

MR due to MVP may occur in patients with apparently normal mitral valve leaflets (ie, nonmyxomatous) due to ischemic papillary muscle dysfunction or rheumatic chordal rupture. Transient MVP may occur when intravascular volume decreases significantly, as occurs in severe dehydration or sometimes during pregnancy (when the woman is recumbent and the gravid uterus compresses the inferior vena cava, reducing venous return).

Complications: MR is the most common complication of MVP. MR may be acute (due to ruptured chordae tendineae causing flail mitral valve leaflets) or chronic. Sequelae of MVP with MR include HF, infective endocarditis, and AF with thromboembolism. Whether MVP causes stroke or endocarditis independent of MR and AF is unclear.

Symptoms and Signs

Most patients with MVP are asymptomatic. Some experience nonspecific symptoms (eg, chest pain, dyspnea, palpitations, dizziness, near syncope, migraines, anxiety) thought to be due to poorly defined associated abnormalities in adrenergic signaling and sensitivity rather than to mitral valve pathology. In about one third of patients, emotional stress precipitates palpitations, which may be a symptom of benign arrhythmias (atrial premature beats, paroxysmal atrial tachycardia, ventricular premature beats, complex ventricular ectopy).

Occasionally, patients present with MR. Rarely, patients present with endocarditis (eg, fever, weight loss, thromboembolic phenomena) or stroke. Sudden death occurs in < 1%, most often resulting from ruptured chordae tendineae and flail mitral valve leaflets. Death due to a ventricular arrhythmia is rare.

Other physical findings associated with but not diagnostic of MVP include hypomastia, pectus excavatum, straight back syndrome, and a narrow anteroposterior chest diameter.

Auscultation: Typically, MVP causes no visible or palpable cardiac signs.

MVP alone often causes a crisp mid-systolic click as the subvalve apparatus abruptly tightens. The click is heard best with the diaphragm of the stethoscope over the left apex when the patient is in the left lateral decubitus position. MVP with MR causes a click with a late-systolic MR murmur. The click moves closer to the 1st heart sound (S_1) with maneuvers that decrease LV size (eg, sitting, standing, Valsalva maneuver); the same maneuvers cause an MR murmur to appear or become louder and last longer. These effects occur because decreasing LV size causes papillary muscles and chordae tendineae to pull together more centrally beneath the valve, resulting in quicker, more forceful prolapse with earlier, more severe regurgitation. Conversely, squatting or isometric handgrip delays the S_1 click and shortens the MR murmur.

The systolic click may be confused with the click of congenital AS; the latter may be distinguished because it occurs very early in systole and does not move with postural or LV volume changes. Other findings include a systolic honk or whoop, thought to be caused by valvular leaflet vibration; these findings are usually transient and may vary with respiratory phase. An early diastolic opening snap caused by return of the prolapsed valve to its normal position is rarely heard. In some patients, especially children, the findings of MVP may be more noticeable after exertion.

Diagnosis

- Echocardiography

Diagnosis of MVP is suggested clinically and confirmed by echocardiography. Thickened (≥ 5 mm), redundant mitral valve leaflets are thought to indicate more extensive myxomatous degeneration and greater risk of endocarditis and MR.

Prognosis

MVP is usually benign, but severe myxomatous degeneration of the valve can lead to MR. In patients with severe MR, incidence of LV or LA enlargement, arrhythmias (eg, AF), infective endocarditis, stroke, need for valve replacement, and death is about 2 to 4%/yr. Men are less likely to have MVP, but those who do are more likely to progress to severe MR.

Treatment

- Usually none
- Sometimes beta-blockers

MVP does not usually require treatment.

Beta-blockers may be used to relieve symptoms of excess sympathetic tone (eg, palpitations, migraines, dizziness) and to reduce risk of tachyarrhythmias, although no data support this practice. A typical regimen is atenolol 25 to 50 mg po once/day or propranolol 20 to 40 mg po bid.

Treatment of AF may be required.

Treatment of MR depends on severity and associated left atrial and LV changes.

Antibiotic prophylaxis against endocarditis is no longer recommended. Anticoagulants to prevent thromboembolism are recommended only for patients with AF or prior transient ischemic attack or stroke.

KEY POINTS

- MVP is most often caused by idiopathic myxomatous degeneration of the mitral valve and chordae tendineae.
- MR is the most common complication.
- Heart sounds often include a sharp, mid-systolic click that occurs earlier with the Valsalva maneuver.
- Prognosis is usually benign unless MR develops, in which case there is increased risk of HF, AF, stroke, and infective endocarditis,
- Treatment is not needed unless significant MR develops.

PULMONIC REGURGITATION

Pulmonic (pulmonary) regurgitation (PR) is incompetency of the pulmonic valve causing blood flow from the pulmonary artery into the RV during diastole. The most common cause is pulmonary hypertension. PR is usually asymptomatic. Signs include a decrescendo diastolic murmur. Diagnosis is by echocardiography. Usually, no specific treatment is necessary except for management of pulmonary hypertension.

The **most common cause** by far of pulmonic regurgitation is

- Secondary pulmonary hypertension

Less common causes are

- Infective endocarditis
- Surgical repair of tetralogy of Fallot
- Idiopathic pulmonary artery dilation
- Congenital valvular heart disease

Rare causes are

- Carcinoid syndrome
- Rheumatic fever
- Catheter-induced trauma

Severe pulmonic regurgitation is rare and most often results from an isolated congenital defect involving dilation of the pulmonary artery and pulmonary valve annulus.

PR may contribute to development of right ventricular (RV) dilatation and eventually RV dysfunction–induced HF, but in most cases, pulmonary hypertension contributes to this complication much more significantly. Rarely, acute RV dysfunction–induced HF develops when endocarditis causes acute PR.

Symptoms and Signs

PR is usually asymptomatic. A few patients develop symptoms and signs of RV dysfunction–induced HF.

Palpable signs are attributable to pulmonary hypertension and RV hypertrophy. They include a palpable pulmonic component (P_2) of the 2nd heart sound (S_2) at the left upper sternal border and a sustained RV impulse that is increased in amplitude at the left middle and lower sternal border.

On auscultation, the 1st heart sound (S_1) is normal. The S_2 may be split or single. When split, P_2 may be loud and audible shortly after the aortic component of S_2 (A_2) because of pulmonary hypertension, or P_2 may be delayed because of increased RV stroke volume. S_2 may be single because of prompt pulmonic valve closing with a merged A_2-P_2 or, rarely, because of congenital absence of the pulmonic valve. An RV 3rd heart sound (S_3), 4th heart sound (S_4), or both may be audible with RV dysfunction–induced HF or RV hypertrophy; these sounds can be distinguished from left ventricular heart sounds because they are located at the left parasternal 4th intercostal space and because they grow louder with inspiration.

The murmur of PR due to pulmonary hypertension is a high-pitched, early diastolic decrescendo murmur that begins with P_2 and ends before S_1 and that radiates toward the mid-right sternal edge (Graham Steell murmur); it is heard best at the left upper sternal border with the diaphragm of the stethoscope while the patient holds the breath at end-expiration and sits upright.

The murmur of PR without pulmonary hypertension is shorter, lower-pitched (rougher in quality), and begins after P_2. Both murmurs may resemble the murmur of AR but can be distinguished by inspiration (which makes the PR murmur louder) and by Valsalva release. After Valsalva release, the PR murmur immediately becomes loud (because of immediate venous return to the right side of the heart), but the AR murmur requires 4 or 5 beats to do so. Also, a soft PR murmur may sometimes become even softer during inspiration because this murmur is usually best heard at the 2nd left intercostal space, where inspiration pushes the stethoscope away from the heart. In some forms of congenital heart disease, the murmur of severe PR is quite short because the pressure gradient between the pulmonary artery and the RV equalizes rapidly in diastole.

Diagnosis

- Echocardiography

PR is usually incidentally detected during a physical examination or Doppler echocardiography done for other reasons. Mild PR is a normal echocardiographic finding that requires no action.

An ECG and chest x-ray are usually obtained. ECG may show signs of RV hypertrophy; chest x-ray may show RV enlargement and evidence of conditions underlying pulmonary hypertension.

Treatment

- Treatment of cause
- Rarely valve replacement

Treatment is management of the condition causing pulmonic regurgitation. Pulmonic valve replacement is an option if symptoms and signs of RV dysfunction–induced HF develop, but outcomes and risks are unclear because the need for replacement is so infrequent.

KEY POINTS

- Pulmonic regurgitation (PR) is usually caused by pulmonary hypertension.
- Hemodynamic consequences are usually due to the cause rather than PR itself.
- Heart sounds when PR is due to pulmonary hypertension include a high-pitched, early diastolic decrescendo murmur that begins with P_2 and ends before S_1 and that radiates toward the mid-right sternal edge; it is heard best at the left upper sternal border while the patient holds the breath at end-expiration and sits upright. The murmur of PR without pulmonary hypertension is shorter, lower-pitched, and begins after P_2.
- Treatment is directed at the cause; valve replacement is usually not needed.

PULMONIC STENOSIS

Pulmonic stenosis (PS) is narrowing of the pulmonary outflow tract causing obstruction of blood flow from the RV to the pulmonary artery during systole. Most cases are congenital; many remain asymptomatic until adulthood. Signs include a crescendo-decrescendo ejection murmur. Diagnosis is by echocardiography. Symptomatic patients and those with large gradients require balloon valvuloplasty.

Etiology

PS is most often congenital and affects predominantly children; stenosis may be valvular or just below the valve in the outflow tract (infundibular). It commonly is a component of tetralogy of Fallot. Less common causes are Noonan syndrome (a familial syndrome similar to Turner syndrome but with no chromosomal defect) and carcinoid syndrome in adults.

Symptoms and Signs

Many children with PS remain asymptomatic for years and do not present to a physician until adulthood. Even then many patients remain asymptomatic. When symptoms of PS develop, they resemble those of AS (syncope, angina, dyspnea).

Visible and palpable signs reflect the effects of right ventricular (RV) hypertrophy and include a prominent jugular venous *a* wave (due to forceful atrial contraction against a hypertrophied RV), an RV precordial lift or heave, and a left parasternal systolic thrill at the 2nd intercostal space.

Auscultation: On auscultation, the 1st heart sound (S_1) is normal and the normal splitting of the 2nd heart sound (S_2) is widened because of prolonged pulmonic ejection (P_2, the pulmonic component of S_2, is delayed). In RV failure and hypertrophy, the 3rd and 4th heart sounds (S_3 and S_4) are rarely audible at the left parasternal 4th intercostal space. A click in congenital PS is thought to result from abnormal ventricular wall tension. The click occurs early in systole (very near S_1) and is not affected by hemodynamic changes. A harsh crescendo-decrescendo ejection murmur is audible and is heard best at the left parasternal 2nd (valvular stenosis) or 4th (infundibular stenosis) intercostal space with the diaphragm of the stethoscope when the patient leans forward.

Unlike the AS murmur, a PS murmur does not radiate, and the crescendo component lengthens as stenosis progresses. The murmur grows louder immediately with Valsalva release and with inspiration; the patient may need to be standing for this effect to be heard.

Diagnosis

- Echocardiography

Diagnosis of PS is confirmed by Doppler echocardiography, which can characterize the severity as

- Mild: Peak gradient < 36 mm Hg
- Moderate: Peak gradient 36 to 64 mm Hg
- Severe: Peak gradient > 64 mm Hg

ECG may be normal or show RV hypertrophy or right bundle branch block.

Right heart catheterization is indicated only when 2 levels of obstruction are suspected (valvular and infundibular), when clinical and echocardiographic findings differ, or before intervention is done.

Treatment

- Sometimes balloon valvuloplasty

Prognosis of PS without treatment is generally good and improves with appropriate intervention.

Treatment of PS is balloon valvuloplasty, indicated for symptomatic patients and asymptomatic patients with normal systolic function and a peak gradient > 40 to 50 mm Hg.

Percutaneous valve replacement may be offered at highly selected congenital heart centers, especially for younger patients or those with multiple previous procedures, in order to reduce the number of open heart procedures. When surgical replacement is necessary, bioprosthetic valves are preferred due to the high rates of thrombosis of right-sided mechanical heart valves.

KEY POINTS

- PS is usually congenital, but symptoms (eg, syncope, angina, dyspnea) usually do not appear until adulthood.
- Heart sounds include increased splitting of S_2 and a harsh crescendo-decrescendo ejection murmur heard best at the left parasternal 2nd or 4th intercostal space when the patient leans forward; the murmur grows louder immediately with Valsalva release and with inspiration.
- Balloon valvuloplasty is done for symptomatic patients and asymptomatic patients with normal systolic function and a peak gradient > 40 to 50 mm Hg.

TRICUSPID REGURGITATION

Tricuspid regurgitation (TR) is insufficiency of the tricuspid valve causing blood flow from the RV to the RA during systole. The most common cause is dilation of the RV. Symptoms and signs are usually absent, but severe TR can cause neck pulsations, a holosystolic murmur, and right ventricular–induced HF or AF. Diagnosis is by physical examination and echocardiography. TR is usually benign and does not require treatment, but some patients require annuloplasty or valve repair or replacement.

Etiology

TR may be

- Primary
- Secondary (most common)

Primary TR is less common. It can be due to valvular abnormalities caused by infective endocarditis in users of illicit IV drugs, carcinoid syndrome, blunt chest trauma, rheumatic fever, idiopathic myxomatous degeneration, congenital defects (eg, cleft tricuspid valve, endocardial cushion defects), Ebstein anomaly (downward displacement of a congenitally malformed tricuspid cusp into the RV), Marfan syndrome, and use of certain drugs (eg, ergotamine, fenfluramine, phentermine). Iatrogenic causes include pacemaker leads that cross the tricuspid valve and valve damage sustained during RV endomyocardial biopsy.

Secondary TR is most commonly caused by dilation of the RV with malfunction of a normal valve, as occurs in pulmonary hypertension, RV dysfunction–induced HF, and pulmonary outflow tract obstruction.

Long-standing severe TR may lead to RV dysfunction–induced HF and AF.

Symptoms and Signs

TR usually causes no symptoms, but some patients experience neck pulsations due to elevated jugular pressures. Symptoms of severe TR include fatigue, abdominal bloating, and anorexia. Patients may also develop symptoms of AF or atrial flutter.

Signs of moderate to severe TR include jugular venous distention, with a prominent merged *c-v* wave and a steep *y* descent, and sometimes enlarged liver and peripheral edema. In severe TR, a right jugular venous thrill may be palpable, as may systolic hepatic pulsation and an RV impulse at the left lower sternal border.

Auscultation: On auscultation, the 1st heart sound (S_1) may be normal or barely audible if a TR murmur is present; the 2nd heart sound (S_2) may be split (with a loud pulmonic component [P_2] in pulmonary hypertension) or single because of prompt pulmonic valve closing with merger of P_2 and the aortic component (A_2). An RV 3rd heart sound (S_3) may be audible near the sternum with RV dysfunction–induced HF.

The murmur of TR is frequently not heard. When evident, it is a holosystolic murmur heard best at the left middle or lower sternal border or at the epigastrium with the bell of the stethoscope when the patient is sitting upright or standing. The murmur may be high-pitched if TR is trivial and due to pulmonary hypertension, or it may be medium-pitched if TR is severe and has other causes. When the murmur is not present at all, the diagnosis is best made by the appearance of the jugular venous wave pattern and the presence of hepatic systolic pulsations. The murmur varies with respiration, becoming louder with inspiration (Carvallo sign).

Diagnosis

- Echocardiography

Mild TR is most often detected on echocardiography done for other reasons.

More moderate or severe TR may be suggested by history and physical examination. Confirmation is by echocardiography.

Severe TR is characterized echocardiographically by ≥ 1 of the following:

- 2-Dimensional failure of coaptation or flail
- Large regurgitant jet on color Doppler
- Large flow convergence zone proximal to the valve
- Vena contracta width > 7 mm
- Systolic flow reversal in the hepatic veins
- Transtricuspid E wave dominant > 1 cm/sec
- Dense, triangular, early peaking, continuous wave Doppler of TR jet

When TR is moderate or severe, the peak regurgitant velocity will underestimate pulmonary pressure. Two-dimensional echocardiography detects the structural abnormalities present in primary TR.

Cardiac MRI is now the preferred method for evaluating RV size and function, which typically should be done when echocardiographic image quality is inadequate.

An ECG and chest x-ray are often done.

ECG is usually normal but, in advanced cases, may show tall peaked P waves caused by right atrial enlargement, a tall R or QR wave in V_1 characteristic of RV hypertrophy, or AF.

Chest x-ray is usually normal but, in advanced cases with RV hypertrophy or RV dysfunction–induced HF, may show an enlarged superior vena cava, an enlarged right atrial or RV silhouette (behind the upper sternum in the lateral projection), or pleural effusion.

Laboratory testing is not needed but if done may show hepatic dysfunction in patients with severe TR.

Cardiac catheterization is indicated for accurate measurement of pulmonary pressure when TR is severe and to evaluate coronary anatomy when surgery is planned. Catheterization findings include a prominent right atrial *c-v* pressure wave during ventricular systole.

Prognosis

Severe TR ultimately has a poor prognosis, even if it is initially well-tolerated for years. As with left-sided valvular regurgitation, the volume-overloaded ventricle eventually decompensates irreversibly.

Treatment

- Treatment of cause
- Sometimes annuloplasty or valve repair or replacement

Very mild TR is a normal finding and requires no action. Medical treatment of causes (eg, HF, endocarditis) is indicated.

Patients with severe TR should undergo operation as soon as symptoms are present despite medical treatment or when there is moderate, progressive RV enlargement or dysfunction. During surgery for left-sided heart lesions, moderate or mild TR with dilated annulus > 40 mm should also undergo repair.

Surgical options include

- Annuloplasty
- Valve repair
- Valve replacement

Annuloplasty, in which the tricuspid valve annulus is sutured to a prosthetic ring or a tailored reduction in annulus circumferential size is done, is indicated when TR is due to annular dilation.

Valve repair or replacement is indicated when TR is due to primary valve abnormalities or when annuloplasty is not technically feasible. Tricuspid valve replacement is indicated when TR is due to carcinoid syndrome or Ebstein anomaly. A bioprosthetic valve is used to reduce the risk of thromboembolism associated with the low pressures of the right heart; in the right heart, unlike the left heart, bioprosthetic valves last > 10 yr. A bioprosthetic valve does not necessitate anticoagulation beyond the immediate postoperative period.

KEY POINTS

- TR usually occurs in a normal valve affected by RV dilation; less often there is an intrinsic valve disorder (eg, due to infective endocarditis, carcinoid syndrome, certain drugs).
- Jugular venous distention may occur; severe TR may cause abdominal distension, hepatic enlargement, and peripheral edema.
- Heart sounds include a holosystolic murmur heard best at the left middle or lower sternal border or at the epigastrium when the patient is sitting upright or standing; the murmur becomes louder with inspiration.
- TR is usually well tolerated, but severe cases may require annuloplasty, valve repair, or valve replacement.

TRICUSPID STENOSIS

Tricuspid stenosis (TS) is narrowing of the tricuspid orifice that obstructs blood flow from the RA to the RV. Almost all cases result from rheumatic fever. Symptoms include a fluttering discomfort in the neck, fatigue, cold skin, and right upper quadrant abdominal discomfort. Jugular pulsations are prominent, and a presystolic murmur is often heard at the left sternal edge in the 4th intercostal space and is increased during inspiration. Diagnosis is by echocardiography. TS is usually benign, requiring no specific treatment, but symptomatic patients may benefit from surgery.

TS is almost always due to rheumatic fever; TR is almost always also present, as is rheumatic mitral valvulopathy (usually mitral stenosis).

Rare causes of TS include SLE, right atrial (RA) myxoma, congenital malformations, and metastatic tumors.

The RA becomes hypertrophied and distended, and sequelae of right heart disease–induced HF develop but without right ventricular (RV) dysfunction; the RV remains underfilled and small. Uncommonly, AF occurs.

Table 90–2. DISTINGUISHING MURMURS OF TRICUSPID STENOSIS AND MITRAL STENOSIS

FEATURE	TRICUSPID STENOSIS	MITRAL STENOSIS
Character	Scratchy	Rumbling, low-pitched
Duration	Short	Long
Timing	Starts in early diastole and does not increase up to S_1	Increases through diastole
Augmenting factor	Inspiration	Exercise
Site	Lower right and left parasternal borders	Cardiac apex with patient in left lateral decubitus position

S_1 = 1st heart sound.

Symptoms and Signs

The only symptoms of severe TS are fluttering discomfort in the neck (due to giant *a* waves in the jugular pulse), fatigue and cold skin (due to low cardiac output), and right upper quadrant abdominal discomfort (due to an enlarged liver).

The primary visible sign is a giant flickering *a* wave with gradual *y* descent in the jugular veins. Jugular venous distention may occur, increasing with inspiration (Kussmaul sign). The face may become dusky and scalp veins may dilate when the patient is recumbent (suffusion sign). Hepatic congestion and peripheral edema may occur.

Auscultation: On auscultation, TS is often inaudible but may produce a soft opening snap and a mid-diastolic rumble with presystolic accentuation. The murmur becomes louder and longer with maneuvers that increase venous return (exercise, inspiration, leg-raising, Müller maneuver) and softer and shorter with maneuvers that decrease venous return (standing, Valsalva maneuver).

Findings of TS often coexist with those of mitral stenosis and are less prominent. The murmurs can be distinguished clinically (see Table 90–2).

Diagnosis

- Echocardiography

Diagnosis is suspected based on history and physical examination and confirmed by Doppler echocardiography showing a pressure gradient across the tricuspid valve. Severe TS is signified by a mean forward gradient across the valve > 5 mm Hg. Two-dimensional echocardiography shows thickened leaflets with reduced movement and RA enlargement.

ECG may show RA enlargement out of proportion to RV hypertrophy and tall, peaked P waves in inferior leads and V_1.

Chest x-ray may show a dilated superior vena cava and RA enlargement, indicated by an enlarged right heart border.

Liver enzymes are elevated because of passive hepatic congestion.

Cardiac catheterization is rarely indicated for evaluation of TS. When catheterization is indicated (eg, to evaluate coronary anatomy), findings include elevated RA pressure with a slow fall in early diastole and a diastolic pressure gradient across the tricuspid valve.

Treatment

- Diuretics and aldosterone antagonists
- Rarely valve repair or replacement

Evidence to guide treatment of TS is scarce. Symptomatic patients not undergoing intervention should receive a low-salt diet, diuretics, and aldosterone antagonists.

Patients with severe TS should undergo intervention if they are symptomatic or if cardiac surgery is being done for other reasons. Percutaneous balloon tricuspid commissurotomy might be considered for severe TS without accompanying TR.

KEY POINTS

- TS is almost always due to rheumatic fever; TR and mitral stenosis are often also present.
- Heart sounds include a soft opening snap and a mid-diastolic rumble with presystolic accentuation; the murmur becomes louder and longer with maneuvers that increase venous return (eg, exercise, inspiration, leg-raising) and softer and shorter with maneuvers that decrease venous return (standing, Valsalva maneuver).
- Treatment includes diuretics and aldosterone antagonists; surgical repair or replacement is rarely needed.

SECTION 8

Ear, Nose, and Throat Disorders

91 Approach to the Patient with Ear Problems

Earache, hearing loss, otorrhea, tinnitus, and vertigo are the principal symptoms of ear problems. Hearing loss is discussed on p. 809.

In addition to the ears, nose, nasopharynx, and paranasal sinuses, the teeth, tongue, tonsils, hypopharynx, larynx, salivary glands, and temporomandibular joint are examined; pain and discomfort may be referred from them to the ears. It is important to examine cranial nerve function (see p. 1835) and to perform tests of hearing (see p. 810) and of the vestibular apparatus. The patient is also examined for nystagmus (a rhythmic movement of the eyes)—see Sidebar 91–1.

Sidebar 91–1. Nystagmus

Nystagmus is a rhythmic movement of the eyes that can have various causes. Vestibular disorders can result in nystagmus because the vestibular system and the oculomotor nuclei are interconnected. The presence of vestibular nystagmus helps identify vestibular disorders and sometimes distinguishes central from peripheral vertigo. Vestibular nystagmus has a slow component caused by the vestibular input and a quick, corrective component that causes movement in the opposite direction. The direction of the nystagmus is defined by the direction of the quick component because it is easier to see. Nystagmus may be rotary, vertical, or horizontal and may occur spontaneously, with gaze, or with head motion.

Initial inspection for nystagmus is done with the patient lying supine with unfocused gaze (+30 diopter or Frenzel lenses can be used to prevent gaze fixation). The patient is then slowly rotated to a left and then to a right lateral position. The direction and duration of nystagmus are noted. If nystagmus is not detected, the Dix-Hallpike (or Barany) maneuver is done. In this maneuver, the patient sits erect on a stretcher so that when lying back, the head extends beyond the end. With support, the patient is rapidly lowered to horizontal, and the head is extended back 45° below horizontal and rotated 45° to the left. Direction and duration of nystagmus and development of vertigo are noted. The patient is returned to an upright position, and the maneuver is repeated with rotation to the right. Any position or maneuver that causes nystagmus should be repeated to see whether it fatigues.

Nystagmus secondary to peripheral nervous system disorders has a latency period of 3 to 10 sec and fatigues rapidly, whereas nystagmus secondary to CNS has no latency period and does not fatigue. During induced nystagmus, the patient is instructed to focus on an object. Nystagmus caused by peripheral disorders is inhibited by visual fixation. Because Frenzel lenses prevent visual fixation, they must be removed to assess visual fixation.

Caloric stimulation of the ear canal induces nystagmus in a person with an intact vestibular system. Failure to induce nystagmus or a > 20 to 25% difference in duration between sides suggests a lesion on the side of the decreased response. Quantification of caloric response is best done with formal (computerized) electronystagmography.

Ability of the vestibular system to respond to peripheral stimulation can be assessed at the bedside. Care should be taken not to irrigate an ear with a known tympanic membrane perforation or chronic infection. With the patient supine and the head elevated 30°, each ear is irrigated sequentially with 3 mL of ice water. Alternatively, 240 mL of warm water (40 to 44° C) may be used, taking care not to burn the patient with overly hot water. Cold water causes nystagmus to the opposite side; warm water causes nystagmus to the same side. A mnemonic device is COWS (*C*old to the *O*pposite and *W*arm to the *S*ame).

Testing

Patients with abnormal hearing on history or physical examination or with tinnitus or vertigo undergo an audiogram (see p. 813). Patients with nystagmus or altered vestibular function may benefit from computerized electronystagmography (ENG), which quantifies spontaneous, gaze, or positional nystagmus that might not be visually detectable. Computerized ENG caloric testing quantifies the strength of response of the vestibular system to cool and warm irrigations in each ear, enabling the physician to discriminate unilateral weakness. Different components of the vestibular system can be tested by varying head and body position or by presenting visual stimuli.

Posturography uses computerized test equipment to quantitatively assess the patient's control of posture and balance. The patient stands on a platform containing force and motion transducers that detect the presence and amount of body sway while the patient attempts to stand upright. The testing can be done under various conditions, including with the platform stationary or moving, flat or tilted, and with the patient's eyes open or closed, which can help isolate the contribution of the vestibular system to balance.

Primary imaging tests include CT of the temporal bone with or without radiopaque dye and gadolinium-enhanced MRI of the brain, the latter with attention paid to the internal auditory canals to rule out an acoustic neuroma. These tests may be indicated in cases of trauma to the ear, head, or both; chronic infection; hearing loss; vertigo; facial paralysis; and otalgia of obscure origin.

EARACHE

(Otalgia)

Earache may occur in isolation or along with discharge or, rarely, hearing loss.

Pathophysiology

Pain may come from a process within the ear itself or may be referred to the ear from a nearby nonotologic disorder.

Pain from the ear itself may result from a pressure gradient between the middle ear and outside air, from local inflammation, or both. A middle ear pressure gradient usually involves eustachian tube obstruction, which inhibits equilibration between middle ear pressure and atmospheric pressure and also allows fluid to accumulate in the middle ear. Otitis media causes painful inflammation of the tympanic membrane (TM) as well as pain from increased middle ear pressure (causing bulging of the TM).

Referred pain can result from disorders in areas innervated by cranial nerves responsible for sensation in the external and middle ear (5th, 9th, and 10th). Specific areas include the nose, paranasal sinuses, nasopharynx, teeth, gingiva, temporomandibular joint (TMJ), mandible, parotid glands, tongue, palatine tonsils, pharynx, larynx, trachea, and esophagus. Disorders in these areas sometimes also obstruct the eustachian tube, causing pain from a middle ear pressure gradient.

Etiology

Earache results from otologic causes (involving the middle ear or external ear) or from nonotologic causes referred to the ear from nearby disease processes (see Table 91–1).

With **acute pain,** the most common causes are

- Middle ear infection
- External ear infection

With **chronic pain** (> 2 to 3 wk), the most common causes are

- TMJ dysfunction
- Chronic eustachian tube dysfunction
- Chronic otitis externa

Table 91–1. SOME CAUSES OF EARACHE

CAUSE	SUGGESTIVE FINDINGS*	DIAGNOSTIC APPROACH
Middle ear		
Acute eustachian tube obstruction	Less severe discomfort Gurgling, crackling, or popping noises, with or without nasal congestion TM not red but mobility decreased Unilateral conductive hearing loss	Clinical evaluation
Barotrauma	Significant pain History of rapid change in air pressure (eg, air travel, scuba diving) Often hemorrhage on or behind TM	Clinical evaluation
Mastoiditis	Recent history of otitis media May have otorrhea, redness, and tenderness over mastoid process	Clinical evaluation Usually CT to monitor extent and sometimes MRI if intracranial complications suspected
Otitis media (acute or chronic)	Significant pain, often URI symptoms Bulging, red TM More common among children Possible discharge if eardrum perforated	Clinical evaluation
External ear		
Impacted cerumen or foreign body	Visible on otoscopy	Clinical evaluation
Local trauma	Usually history of attempts at ear cleaning Canal lesion visible on otoscopy	Clinical evaluation
Otitis externa (acute or chronic)	Itching and pain (more itching and only mild discomfort in chronic otitis externa) Often history of swimming or recurrent water exposure Sometimes foul-smelling discharge Canal red, swollen; purulent debris TM normal	Clinical evaluation CT of temporal bone if malignant external otitis suspected
Nonotologic causes[†]		
Cancer (nasopharynx, tonsils, base of tongue, larynx)	Chronic discomfort Often long history of tobacco or alcohol use Sometimes middle ear effusion, cervical lymphadenopathy Usually in older patients	Gadolinium-enhanced MRI Biopsy of visible lesions
Infection (tonsils, peritonsillar abscess)	Pain with swallowing Visible pharyngeal erythema Bulging if abscess	Clinical evaluation Sometimes strep culture
Neuralgia (trigeminal, sphenopalatine, glossopharyngeal, geniculate)	Random, brief, severe, lancinating pain	Clinical evaluation
TMJ disorders	Pain worsens with jaw movement, lack of smooth TMJ movement	Clinical evaluation

*Some degree of conductive hearing loss is common in many middle and external ear disorders.
[†]Common feature is normal ear examination.
TM = tympanic membrane; TMJ = temporomandibular joint.

Also with chronic pain, a tumor must be considered, particularly in elderly patients and if the pain is associated with ear drainage. People with diabetes or in other immunocompromised states may develop a particularly severe form of external otitis termed malignant or necrotizing external otitis. In this situation, if abnormal soft tissue is found on examination of the ear canal, the tissue must be biopsied to rule out cancer.

TMJ dysfunction is a common cause of earache in patients with a normal ear examination.

Evaluation

History: History of present illness should assess the location, duration, and severity of pain and whether it is constant or intermittent. If intermittent, it is important to determine whether it is random or occurs mainly with swallowing or jaw movement. Important associated symptoms include ear drainage, hearing loss, and sore throat. The patient should be asked about any attempts at cleaning the ear canal (eg, with cotton swab) or other recent instrumentation, foreign bodies, recent air travel or scuba diving, and swimming or other recurrent water exposure to ears.

Review of systems should ask about symptoms of chronic illness, such as weight loss and fevers.

Past medical history should ask about known diabetes or other immunocompromised state, previous ear disorders (particularly infections), and amount and duration of tobacco and alcohol use.

Physical examination: Vital signs should be checked for fever.

Examination focuses on the ears, nose, and throat.

The pinna and area over the mastoid process should be inspected for redness and swelling. The pinna is gently tugged; significant pain exacerbation with tugging suggests otitis externa. The ear canal should be examined for redness, discharge, swelling, cerumen or foreign body, and any other lesions. The TM should be examined for redness, perforation, and signs of middle ear fluid collection (eg, bulging, distortion, change in normal light reflex). A brief bedside test of hearing (see p. 813) should be conducted.

The throat should be examined for erythema, tonsillar exudate, peritonsillar swelling, and any mucosal lesions suggesting cancer.

TMJ function should be assessed by palpation of the joints on opening and closing of the mouth, and notation should be made of trismus or evidence of bruxism.

The neck should be palpated for lymphadenopathy. In-office fiber-optic examination of the pharynx and larynx should be considered, particularly if no cause for the pain is identified on routine examination and if nonotologic symptoms such as hoarseness, difficulty swallowing, or nasal obstruction are reported.

Red flags: The following findings are of particular concern:

- Diabetes or immunocompromised state
- Redness and fluctuance over mastoid and protrusion of auricle
- Severe swelling at external auditory canal meatus
- Chronic pain, especially if associated with other head/neck symptoms

Interpretation of findings: An important differentiator is whether the ear examination is normal; middle and external ear disorders cause abnormal physical findings, which, when combined with history, usually suggest an etiology (see Table 91–1) For example, patients with chronic eustachian tube dysfunction have abnormalities of the TM, typically a retraction pocket.

Patients with a normal ear examination may have a visible oropharyngeal cause, such as tonsillitis or peritonsillar abscess. Ear pain due to neuralgia has a classic manifestation as brief (usually seconds, always < 2 min) episodes of extremely severe, sharp pain. Chronic ear pain without abnormality on ear examination might be due to a TMJ disorder, but patients should have a thorough head and neck examination (including fiber-optic examination) to rule out cancer.

Testing: Most cases are clear after history and physical examination. Depending on clinical findings, nonotologic causes may require testing (see Table 91–1). Patients with a normal ear examination, particularly with chronic or recurrent pain, may warrant evaluation with an MRI to rule out cancer.

Treatment

Underlying disorders are treated.

Pain is treated with oral analgesics; usually an NSAID or acetaminophen is adequate, but sometimes a brief course of an oral opioid is necessary, particularly for cases of severe otitis externa. In cases of severe otitis externa, effective treatment requires suction of debris from the ear canal and insertion of a wick to allow for delivery of antibiotic ear drops to the infected tissue; oral antibiotics are not used unless part or all of the pinna is erythematous, suggesting spread of infection. Topical analgesics (eg, antipyrine-benzocaine combinations) are generally not very effective but can be used on a limited basis.

Patients should be instructed to avoid digging in their ears with any objects (no matter how soft the objects are or how careful patients claim to be). Also, patients should not irrigate their ears unless instructed by a physician to do so, and then only gently. An oral irrigator should never be used to irrigate the ear.

KEY POINTS

- Most cases are due to infection of the middle or external ear.
- History and physical examination are usually adequate for diagnosis.
- Nonotologic causes should be considered when ear examination is normal.

OTORRHEA

Ear discharge (otorrhea) is drainage exiting the ear. It may be serous, serosanguineous, or purulent. Associated symptoms may include ear pain, fever, pruritus, vertigo, tinnitus, and hearing loss.

Etiology

Causes may originate from the ear canal, the middle ear, or the cranial vault. Certain causes tend to manifest acutely because of the severity of their symptoms or associated conditions. Others usually have a more indolent, chronic course but sometimes manifest acutely (see Table 91–2).

Overall, the most common causes are

- Acute otitis media with perforation
- Chronic otitis media (with a perforation of the eardrum, cholesteatoma, or both)
- Otitis externa

The most serious causes are necrotizing external otitis and cancer of the ear.

Evaluation

History: History of present illness should cover duration of symptoms and whether symptoms have been recurrent. Important associated symptoms include pain, itching, decreased hearing, vertigo, and tinnitus. Patients are questioned about activities that can affect the canal or tympanic membrane (TM—eg, swimming; insertion of objects, including cotton swabs; use of ear drops). Head trauma sufficient to cause a CSF leak is readily apparent.

Review of systems should seek symptoms of cranial nerve deficit and systemic symptoms suggesting granulomatosis with polyangiitis (eg, nasal discharge, cough, joint pains).

Past medical history should note any previous known ear disorders, ear surgery (particularly tympanostomy tube placement), and diabetes or immunodeficiency.

Physical examination: Examination begins with a review of vital signs for fever.

Ear and surrounding tissues (particularly the area over the mastoid) are inspected for erythema and edema. The pinna is pulled and the tragus is pushed gently to see whether pain is

Table 91–2. SOME CAUSES OF EAR DISCHARGE

CAUSE	SUGGESTIVE FINDINGS	DIAGNOSTIC APPROACH
Acute discharge*		
Acute otitis media with perforated TM	Severe pain, with relief on appearance of purulent discharge	Clinical evaluation
Chronic otitis media	Otorrhea in patients with chronic perforation, sometimes with cholesteatoma Can also manifest as chronic discharge	Clinical evaluation Sometimes high-resolution temporal bone CT
CSF leak caused by head trauma	Significant, clinically obvious head injury or recent surgery Fluid ranges from crystal clear to pure blood	Head CT, including skull base
Otitis externa (infectious or allergic)	*Infectious*: Often after swimming, local trauma; marked pain, worse with ear traction Often a history of chronic ear dermatitis with itching and skin changes *Allergic*: Often after use of ear drops; more itching, erythema, less pain than with infectious Typically involvement of earlobe, where drops trickled out of ear canal *Both*: Canal very edematous, inflamed, with debris; normal TM	Clinical evaluation
Post-tympanostomy tube	After tympanostomy tube placement May occur with water exposure	Clinical evaluation
Chronic discharge		
Cancer of ear canal	Discharge often bloody, mild pain Sometimes visible lesion in canal Easy to confuse with otitis externa early on	Biopsy CT MRI in some cases
Cholesteatoma	History of TM perforation Flaky debris in ear canal, pocket in TM filled with caseous debris Sometimes polypoid mass or granulation tissue over the cholesteatoma	CT Culture (No use for MRI unless intracranial extension is suspected)
Chronic purulent otitis media	Long history of ear infections or other ear disorders Less pain than with external otitis Canal macerated, granulation tissue TM immobile, distorted, usually visible perforation	Clinical evaluation Usually culture
Foreign body	Usually in children Drainage foul-smelling, purulent Foreign body often visible on examination unless marked edema or drainage	Clinical evaluation
Mastoiditis	Often fever, history of untreated or unresolved otitis media Redness, tenderness over mastoid	Clinical evaluation Culture Usually CT
Necrotizing otitis externa	Usually history of immune deficiency or diabetes Chronic severe pain Periauricular swelling and tenderness, granulation tissue in ear canal Sometimes facial nerve paralysis	CT or MRI Culture
Granulomatosis with polyangiitis (formerly Wegener granulomatosis)	Often with respiratory tract symptoms, chronic rhinorrhea, arthralgias, and oral ulcers	Urinalysis Chest x-ray Antineutrophilic cytoplasmic antibody testing Biopsy

*< 6 wk.

TM = tympanic membrane.

worsened. The ear canal is inspected with an otoscope; the character of discharge and presence of canal lesions, granulation tissue, or foreign body are noted. Edema and discharge may block visualization of all but the distal canal (irrigation should not be used in case there is a TM perforation), but when possible, the TM is inspected for inflammation, perforation, distortion, and signs of cholesteatoma (eg, canal debris, polypoid mass from TM).

When the ear canal is severely swollen at the meatus (eg, as with severe otitis externa) or there is copious drainage, careful suctioning can permit an adequate examination and also allow treatment (eg, application of drops, with or without a wick).

The cranial nerves are tested. The nasal mucosa is examined for raised, granular lesions, and the skin is inspected for vasculitic lesions, both of which may suggest granulomatosis with polyangiitis.

Red flags: The following findings are of particular concern:

- Recent major head trauma
- Any cranial nerve dysfunction (including sensorineural hearing loss)
- Fever
- Erythema of ear or periauricular tissue
- Diabetes or immunodeficiency

Interpretation of findings: Otoscopic examination can usually diagnose perforated TM, external otitis media, foreign body, or other uncomplicated sources of otorrhea. Some findings are highly suggestive (see Table 91–2). Other findings are less specific but indicate a more serious problem that involves more than a localized external ear or middle ear disorder:

- Vertigo and tinnitus (disorder of the inner ear)
- Cranial nerve deficits (disorder involving the skull base)
- Erythema and tenderness of ear, surrounding tissues, or both (significant infection)

Testing: Many cases are clear after clinical evaluation.

If CSF leakage is in question, discharge can be tested for glucose or β_2-transferrin; these substances are present in CSF but not in other types of discharge.

Patients without an obvious etiology on examination require audiogram and CT of the temporal bone or gadolinium-enhanced MRI. Biopsy should be considered when auditory canal granulation tissue is present.

Treatment

Treatment is directed at the cause. Most physicians do not treat a suspected CSF leak with antibiotics without a definitive diagnosis because drugs might mask the onset of meningitis.

KEY POINTS

- Acute discharge in a patient without chronic ear problems or immunodeficiency is likely the result of otitis externa or perforated otitis media.
- Severe otitis externa may require specialty referral for more extensive cleaning and possible wick placement.
- Patients with recurrent ear symptoms (diagnosed or undiagnosed), cranial nerve findings, or systemic symptoms should have specialty referral.

TINNITUS

Tinnitus is a noise in the ears. It is experienced by 10 to 15% of the population.

Subjective tinnitus is perception of sound in the absence of an acoustic stimulus and is heard only by the patient. Most tinnitus is subjective.

Objective tinnitus is uncommon and results from noise generated by structures near the ear. Sometimes the tinnitus is loud enough to be heard by the examiner.

Characteristics: Tinnitus may be described as buzzing, ringing, roaring, whistling, or hissing and is sometimes variable and complex. Objective tinnitus typically is pulsatile (synchronous with the heartbeat) or intermittent. Tinnitus is most noticeable in quiet environments and in the absence of distracting stimuli and, thus, frequently seems worse at bedtime.

Tinnitus may be intermittent or continuous. Continuous tinnitus is at best annoying and is often quite distressing. Some patients adapt to its presence better than others; depression occasionally results. Stress generally exacerbates tinnitus.

Pathophysiology

Subjective tinnitus is thought to be caused by abnormal neuronal activity in the auditory cortex. This activity results when input from the auditory pathway (cochlea, auditory nerve, brain stem nuclei, auditory cortex) is disrupted or altered in some manner. This disruption may cause loss of suppression of intrinsic cortical activity and perhaps creation of new neural connections. Some believe the phenomenon is similar to the development of phantom limb pain after amputation. Conductive hearing loss (eg, caused by cerumen impaction, otitis media, or eustachian tube dysfunction) may also be associated with subjective tinnitus, by altering sound input to the central auditory system.

Objective tinnitus represents actual noise generated by physiologic phenomena occurring near the middle ear. Usually the noise comes from blood vessels, either normal vessels in conditions of increased or turbulent flow (eg, caused by atherosclerosis) or abnormal vessels (eg, in tumors or vascular malformations). Sometimes muscle spasms or myoclonus of palatal muscles or muscles in the middle ear (stapedius, tensor tympani) cause clicking sounds.

Etiology

Causes may be considered by whether they cause subjective or objective tinnitus (see Table 91–3).

Subjective tinnitus: Subjective tinnitus may occur with almost any disorder affecting the auditory pathways.

The most common disorders are those that involve sensorineural hearing loss, particularly

- Acoustic trauma (noise-induced sensorineural hearing loss)
- Presbycusis (with aging)
- Ototoxic drugs
- Meniere disease

Infections and CNS lesions (eg, caused by tumor, stroke, multiple sclerosis) that affect auditory pathways also may be responsible.

Disorders causing conductive hearing loss also may cause tinnitus. These include obstruction of the ear canal by cerumen, a foreign body, or external otitis. Otitis media, barotrauma, eustachian tube dysfunction, and otosclerosis may also be associated with tinnitus.

Temporomandibular joint dysfunction may be associated with tinnitus in some patients.

Objective tinnitus: Objective tinnitus usually involves noise from vascular flow, which causes an audible pulsating sound synchronous with the pulse. Causes include

- Turbulent flow through the carotid artery or jugular vein
- Highly vascular middle ear tumors
- Dural arteriovenous malformations (AVMs)

Muscle spasms or myoclonus of palatal muscles or those of the middle ear (stapedius, tensor tympani) may cause perceptible noise, typically a rhythmic clicking. Such spasms may be idiopathic or caused by tumors, head trauma, and infectious or demyelinating diseases (eg, multiple sclerosis). Palatal myoclonus causes visible movement of the palate, tympanic membrane, or both that coincides with tinnitus.

Evaluation

History: History of present illness should note duration of tinnitus, whether it is in one or both ears, and whether it is a constant tone or intermittent. If intermittent, the clinician should determine whether it is regular and whether it is about

Table 91–3. SOME CAUSES OF TINNITUS

CAUSE	SUGGESTIVE FINDINGS	DIAGNOSTIC APPROACH
Subjective tinnitus*		
Acoustic trauma (eg, noise-induced hearing loss)	History of occupational or recreational exposure, hearing loss	Clinical evaluation†
Barotrauma	Clear history of exposure	Clinical evaluation*†
CNS tumors (eg, acoustic neuroma, meningioma) and lesions (eg, caused by multiple sclerosis or stroke)	Unilateral tinnitus and often hearing loss Sometimes other neurologic abnormalities	Gadolinium-enhanced MRI Audiometry
Drugs (eg, salicylates; aminoglycosides; loop diuretics; some chemotherapeutic drugs, including cisplatin)	Onset of bilateral tinnitus coincident with use of drug Except with salicylates, hearing loss also possible Aminoglycosides also possibly associated with bilateral vestibular loss (eg, dizziness, dysequilibrium)	Clinical evaluation†
Eustachian tube dysfunction	Often prolonged decreased hearing, preceding URIs, problems clearing ears with air travel or other pressure change Severe allergies can worsen symptoms Unilateral or bilateral (often one ear more of a problem than the other)	Audiometry Tympanometry
Infections (eg, otitis media, labyrinthitis, meningitis, neurosyphilis)	History of infection	Clinical evaluation†
Meniere disease	Episodic unilateral hearing loss, tinnitus, fullness in the ear, and severe vertigo Typically, fluctuating and eventually permanent low-frequency hearing loss	Audiometry Vestibular testing Gadolinium-enhanced MRI to evaluate unilateral sensorineural hearing loss and rule out acoustic neuroma
Obstruction of ear canal (eg, caused by cerumen, foreign body, or external otitis)	Unilateral, with visible, diagnostic abnormalities on ear examination, including discharge with external otitis	Clinical evaluation†
Presbycusis (with aging)	Progressive hearing loss, often with family history	Clinical evaluation†
Objective tinnitus‡		
Dural arteriovenous malformations	Unilateral, constant, pulsatile tinnitus Usually no other symptoms May have bruit over skull Physical examination should always include periauricular auscultation	Angiogram
Myoclonus (palatal muscles, tensor tympani, stapedius)	Irregular clicking or mechanical-sounding noise Possibly other neurologic symptoms (eg, of multiple sclerosis) Movement of the palate, TM, or both seen on examination when symptomatic	Neurology consultation MRI Tympanometry
Turbulent flow in carotid artery or jugular vein	Bruit or venous hum in neck Venous hum possibly ceasing with jugular vein compression or head rotation	Clinical evaluation
Vascular middle ear tumors (eg, glomus tympanicum, glomus jugulare)	Unilateral, constant, pulsatile tinnitus Sometimes bruit on auscultation of ear Tumor usually visible behind TM as a very erythematous, sometimes pulsatile mass, which may blanch (on pneumatoscopy)	CT MRI Angiogram (usually done before surgery)

*Typically a constant tone and accompanied by some degree of hearing loss.
†Most patients should have audiometry.
‡Typically intermittent or pulsatile.
TM = tympanic membrane.

the rate of the pulse or sporadic. Any exacerbating or relieving factors (eg, swallowing, head position) should be noted. Important associated symptoms include hearing loss, vertigo, ear pain, and ear discharge.

Review of systems should seek symptoms of possible causes, including diplopia and difficulty swallowing or speaking (lesions of the brain stem) and focal weakness and sensory changes (peripheral nervous system disorders). The impact of the tinnitus on the patient also should be assessed. Whether the tinnitus is sufficiently distressing to cause significant anxiety, depression, or sleeplessness should be noted.

Past medical history should ask about risk factors for tinnitus, including exposure to loud noise, sudden pressure change (from diving or air travel), history of ear or CNS infections or trauma, radiation therapy to the head, and recent major weight loss (risk of eustachian dysfunction). Drug use should be ascertained, particularly any salicylates, aminoglycosides, or loop diuretics.

Physical examination: Physical examination focuses on the ear and the nervous system.

The ear canal should be inspected for discharge, foreign body, and cerumen. The tympanic membrane should be inspected for signs of acute infection (eg, redness, bulging), chronic infection (eg, perforation, cholesteatoma), and tumor (red or bluish mass). A bedside hearing test should be done.

Cranial nerves, particularly vestibular function (see p. 792), are tested along with peripheral strength, sensation, and reflexes. A stethoscope is used to listen for vascular noise over the course of the carotid arteries and jugular veins and over and adjacent to the ear.

Red flags: The following findings are of particular concern:

- Bruit, particularly over the ear or skull
- Accompanying neurologic symptoms or signs (other than hearing loss)
- Unilateral tinnitus

Interpretation of findings: In some cases, tinnitus may indicate retrocochlear pathology, such as an acoustic neuroma (benign but invasive tumor originating from the vestibular portion of the 8th cranial nerve in the internal auditory canal).

It is important to note whether the tinnitus is unilateral because acoustic neuromas may manifest only with unilateral tinnitus. This diagnosis is more likely if there is also unilateral sensorineural hearing loss or asymmetric hearing loss with worse hearing in the ear with tinnitus.

It also is important to distinguish the uncommon cases of objective tinnitus from the more common cases of subjective tinnitus. Tinnitus that is pulsatile or intermittent is almost always objective (although not always detectable by the examiner), as is that associated with a bruit. Pulsatile tinnitus is nearly always benign. Continuous tinnitus is usually subjective (except perhaps for that caused by a venous hum, which may be identified by presence of a bruit and often by a change in tinnitus with head rotation or jugular vein compression).

Specific causes can often be suspected by findings on examination (see Table 91–3). In particular, exposure to loud noise, barotrauma, or certain drugs before onset suggests those factors as the cause.

Testing: All patients with significant tinnitus should be referred for comprehensive audiologic evaluation to determine the presence, degree, and type of hearing loss.

In patients with unilateral tinnitus and hearing loss, acoustic neuroma should be ruled out by gadolinium-enhanced MRI. In patients with unilateral tinnitus and normal hearing and physical examination, MRI is not necessary unless tinnitus persists > 6 mo.

Other testing depends on patient presentation (see Table 91–3).

Patients with visible evidence of a vascular tumor in the middle ear require CT, gadolinium-enhanced MRI, and referral to a subspecialist if the diagnosis is confirmed.

Patients with pulsatile, objective tinnitus and no ear abnormalities on examination or audiology require further investigation of the vascular system (carotid, vertebral, and intracranial vessels). The usual test sequence is to begin with magnetic resonance angiography (MRA). However, because MRA is not very sensitive for dural AVMs, many clinicians then consider doing an arteriogram. However, because dural AVMs are rare, the significant risks of arteriography must be weighed against the potential benefit of diagnosis and treatment (with embolization) of this vascular anomaly.

Patients who report hearing clicking sounds in one or both ears should be evaluated for the presence of objective tinnitus. This evaluation may be done by auscultation using a stethoscope or with tympanometry to identify clonus of the tensor tympani, stapedius, and/or palatal muscles. Palatal myoclonus should be visible on physical exam of the oral cavity.

Treatment

Treatment of the underlying disorder may lessen tinnitus. Correcting hearing loss (eg, with a hearing aid) relieves tinnitus in about 50% of patients.

Because stress and other mental factors (eg, depression) can exacerbate symptoms, efforts to recognize and treat these factors may help. Many patients are reassured by learning that their tinnitus does not represent a serious medical problem. Tinnitus also can be worsened by caffeine and other stimulants, so patients should try eliminating use of these substances.

Although no specific medical or surgical therapy is available, many patients find that background sound masks the tinnitus and may help them fall asleep. Some patients benefit from a tinnitus masker, a device worn like a hearing aid that provides a low-level sound that can cover up the tinnitus. Tinnitus retraining therapy, offered by programs that specialize in tinnitus treatment, are helpful for some patients. Electrical stimulation of the inner ear, as with a cochlear implant, occasionally reduces the tinnitus but is appropriate only for patients who are profoundly deaf.

Geriatrics Essentials

One out of 4 people > 65 yr have significant hearing impairment. Because tinnitus is common among people with sensorineural hearing loss, tinnitus is a common complaint among the elderly.

KEY POINTS

- Subjective tinnitus is caused by an abnormality somewhere in the auditory pathway.
- Objective tinnitus is caused by an actual noise produced in a vascular structure near the ear.
- Loud noise, aging, Meniere disease, and drugs are the most common causes of subjective tinnitus.
- Unilateral tinnitus with hearing loss or dizziness/dysequilibrium warrants gadolinium-enhanced MRI to rule out acoustic neuroma.
- Any tinnitus accompanied by a neurologic deficit is of concern.

DIZZINESS AND VERTIGO

Dizziness is an imprecise term patients often use to describe various related sensations, including

- Faintness (a feeling of impending syncope)
- Light-headedness
- Feeling of imbalance or unsteadiness
- A vague spaced-out or swimmy-headed feeling
- A spinning sensation

Vertigo is a false sensation of movement of the self or the environment. Usually the perceived movement is rotary—a spinning or wheeling sensation—but some patients simply feel pulled to one side. Vertigo is not a diagnosis—it is a description of a sensation.

Both sensations may be accompanied by nausea and vomiting or difficulty with balance, gait, or both.

Perhaps because these sensations are hard to describe in words, patients often use "dizziness," "vertigo," and other terms interchangeably and inconsistently. Different patients with the same underlying disorder may describe their symptoms very differently. A patient may even give different descriptions of the same "dizzy" event during a given visit depending on how the question is asked. Because of this discrepancy, even though vertigo seems to be a clearly delineated subset of dizziness, many clinicians prefer to consider the two symptoms together.

However they are described, dizziness and vertigo may be disturbing and even incapacitating, particularly when accompanied by nausea and vomiting. Symptoms cause particular problems for people doing an exacting or dangerous task, such as driving, flying, or operating heavy machinery.

Dizziness accounts for about 5 to 6% of physician visits. It may occur at any age but becomes more common with increasing age; it affects about 40% of people over 40 yr at some time. Dizziness may be temporary or chronic. Chronic dizziness, defined as lasting > 1 mo, is more common among elderly people.

Pathophysiology

The **vestibular system** is the main neurologic system involved in balance. This system includes

- The vestibular apparatus of the inner ear
- The 8th (vestibulocochlear) cranial nerve, which conducts signals from the vestibular apparatus to the central components of the system
- The vestibular nuclei in the brain stem and cerebellum

Disorders of the inner ear and 8th cranial nerve are considered peripheral disorders. Those of the vestibular nuclei and their pathways in the brain stem and cerebellum are considered central disorders.

The sense of balance also incorporates visual input from the eyes and proprioceptive input from the peripheral nerves (via the spinal cord). The cerebral cortex receives output from the lower centers and integrates the information to produce the perception of motion.

Vestibular apparatus: Perception of stability, motion, and orientation to gravity originates in the vestibular apparatus, which consists of

- The 3 semicircular canals
- The 2 otolith organs—the saccule and utricle

Rotary motion causes flow of endolymph in the semicircular canal oriented in the plane of motion. Depending on the direction of flow, endolymph movement either stimulates or inhibits neuronal output from hair cells lining the canal. Similar hair cells in the saccule and utricle are embedded in a matrix of Ca carbonate crystals (otoliths). Deflection of the otoliths by gravity stimulates or inhibits neuronal output from the attached hair cells.

Etiology

There are numerous structural (trauma, tumors, degenerative), vascular, infectious, toxic (including drug-related), and idiopathic causes (see Table 91–4), but only a small percentage of cases are caused by a serious disorder.

The **most common causes of dizziness with vertigo** involve some component of the peripheral vestibular system:

- Benign paroxysmal positional vertigo
- Meniere disease
- Vestibular neuronitis
- Labyrinthitis

Less often, the cause is a central vestibular disorder (most commonly migraine), a disorder with a more global effect on cerebral function, a psychiatric disorder, or a disorder affecting visual or proprioceptive input. Sometimes, no cause can be found.

The **most common causes of dizziness without vertigo** are less clear cut, but they are usually not otologic and probably are

- Drug effects
- Multifactorial or idiopathic

Nonneurologic disorders with a more global effect on cerebral function sometimes manifest as dizziness and rarely as vertigo. These disorders typically involve inadequate substrate (eg, O_2, glucose) delivery caused by hypotension, hypoxemia, anemia, or hypoglycemia; when severe, some of these disorders may manifest as syncope. Additionally, certain hormonal changes (eg, as with thyroid disease, menstruation, pregnancy) can cause dizziness. Numerous CNS-active drugs can cause dizziness independent of any toxic effect on the vestibular system.

Occasionally, dizziness and vertigo may be psychogenic. Patients with panic disorder, hyperventilation syndrome, anxiety, or depression may present with complaints of dizziness.

In elderly patients, dizziness is often multifactorial secondary to drug adverse effects and age-diminished visual, vestibular, and proprioceptive abilities. Two of the most common specific causes are disorders of the inner ear: benign paroxysmal positional vertigo and Meniere disease.

Evaluation

History: History of present illness should cover the sensations felt; an open-ended question is best (eg, "Different people use the word 'dizziness' differently. Can you please describe as thoroughly as you can what you feel?"). Brief, specific questioning as to whether the feeling is faintness, light-headedness, loss of balance, or vertiginous may bring some clarity, but persistent efforts to categorize a patient's sensations are unnecessary. Other elements are more valuable and clear-cut:

- Severity of initial episode
- Severity and characteristics of subsequent episodes
- Symptoms continuous or episodic
- If episodic, frequency and duration
- Triggers and relievers (ie, triggered by head/body position change)
- Associated aural symptoms (eg, hearing loss, ear fullness, tinnitus)
- Severity and related disability

Table 91–4. SOME CAUSES OF DIZZINESS AND VERTIGO

CAUSE	SUGGESTIVE FINDINGS	DIAGNOSTIC APPROACH
Peripheral vestibular system disorders[a,b]		
Benign paroxysmal positional vertigo	Severe, brief (< 1 min) spinning triggered by moving head in a specific direction Nystagmus has a latency of 1–10 sec, is fatigable, and is torsional, beating toward the undermost ear Frenzel lenses needed to prevent visual fixation Hearing and neurologic examination intact	Dix-Hallpike maneuver to assess characteristic positional nystagmus
Meniere disease	Recurrent episodes of unilateral tinnitus, hearing loss, ear fullness	Audiogram Gadolinium-enhanced MRI to rule out other causes
Vestibular neuronitis (viral cause suspected)	Sudden, incapacitating, severe vertigo with no hearing loss or other findings Lasts up to 1 wk, with gradual lessening of symptoms Positional vertigo may result	Clinical evaluation Gadolinium-enhanced MRI
Labyrinthitis (viral or bacterial)	Hearing loss, tinnitus	Temporal bone CT if purulent infection suspected Gadolinium-enhanced MRI if unilateral hearing loss and tinnitus
Otitis media (acute or chronic, sometimes with cholesteatoma)	Ear pain, abnormal ear examination, including discharge if chronic otitis History of infection	Clinical evaluation CT if cholesteatoma to rule out semicircular canal fistula formation
Trauma (eg, tympanic membrane rupture, labyrinthine contusion, perilymphatic fistula, temporal bone fracture, postconcussion)	Trauma obvious on history Other findings depending on location and extent of damage	CT depending on cause and findings
Acoustic neuroma	Slowly progressive unilateral hearing loss, tinnitus, dizziness, dysequilibrium Rarely, facial numbness, weakness, or both	Audiogram Gadolinium-enhanced MRI if significant hearing asymmetry or unilateral tinnitus
Ototoxic drugs[c]	Treatment with aminoglycoside drugs recently instituted, usually with bilateral hearing loss and vestibular loss	Clinical evaluation Vestibular evaluation with electronystagmography and rotary chair tests
Herpes zoster oticus (Ramsay Hunt syndrome)	Also affects geniculate ganglion, so facial weakness and taste loss often manifest along with hearing loss Vertigo possible but not typical Vesicles present on pinna and in ear canal	Clinical evaluation
Chronic motion sickness (mal de debarquement)	Persistent symptoms after acute motion sickness	Clinical evaluation
Central vestibular system disorders[d]		
Brain stem hemorrhage or infarction	Sudden onset Involvement of cochlear artery possibly causing ear symptoms	Immediate imaging Gadolinium-enhanced MRI if available, otherwise CT
Cerebellar hemorrhage or infarction	Sudden onset, with ataxia and other cerebellar findings, often headache Deteriorates rapidly	Immediate imaging Gadolinium-enhanced MRI if available, otherwise CT
Migraine	Episodic, recurrent vertigo, usually without unilateral auditory symptoms (may have tinnitus that is usually bilateral) Possibly headache, but often personal or family history of migraine Photophobia, phonophobia, visual or other auras possible, helping make diagnosis	Usually clinical examination but with imaging to rule out other causes Trial of migraine prophylaxis
Multiple sclerosis	Varied CNS motor and sensory deficits, with remissions and recurring exacerbations	Gadolinium-enhanced MRI of brain and spine

Table continues on the following page.

Table 91–4. SOME CAUSES OF DIZZINESS AND VERTIGO (*Continued*)

CAUSE	SUGGESTIVE FINDINGS	DIAGNOSTIC APPROACH
Vertebral artery dissection	Often head and neck pain	Magnetic resonance angiography
Vertebrobasilar insufficiency	Intermittent brief episodes, sometimes with drop attacks, visual disturbance, confusion	Magnetic resonance angiography
Global disturbance of CNS function[e]		
Anemia (numerous causes)	Pallor, weakness, sometimes heme-positive stool	CBC
CNS-active drugs[f] (not ototoxic)	Drug recently instituted or dose increased; multiple drugs, particularly in an elderly patient Symptoms unrelated to movement or position	Sometimes, drug levels (certain anticonvulsants) Trial of withdrawal
Hypoglycemia (usually caused by drugs for diabetes)	Recent dose increase Sometimes sweating	Fingerstick glucose test (during symptoms if possible)
Hypotension (caused by cardiac disorders, antihypertensives, blood loss, dehydration, or orthostatic hypotension syndromes including postural orthostatic tachycardia syndrome and other dysautonomias)	Symptoms on arising, sometimes with vagal stimulation (eg, urination) but not with head motion or while recumbent Manifestation possibly dominated by cause (eg, blood loss, diarrhea)	Orthostatic vital signs, sometimes with tilt table test, ECG Other testing directed at suspected cause
Hypoxemia (numerous causes)	Tachypnea Often history of lung disease	Pulse oximetry
Other causes[e]		
Pregnancy	May be unrecognized	Pregnancy test
Psychiatric (eg, panic attack, hyperventilation syndrome, anxiety, depression)	Symptoms chronic, brief, recurrent Unrelated to movement or position but may occur with stress or upset Neurologic and ENT examinations normal Initially, patient may be diagnosed with peripheral vestibular dysfunction and fail to respond to appropriate management	Clinical evaluation
Syphilis	Chronic symptoms with bilateral hearing loss, fluctuating, with episodic vertigo	Syphilis serology
Thyroid disorders	Weight change Heat or cold intolerance	Thyroid function testing

[a]Symptoms are typically paroxysmal, severe, and episodic rather than continuous. Ear symptoms (eg, tinnitus, fullness, hearing loss) usually indicate a peripheral disorder. Loss of consciousness is not associated with dizziness due to peripheral vestibular pathology.

[b]Peripheral vestibular system disorders are listed in rough order of frequency of occurrence.

[c]Numerous drugs, including aminoglycosides, chloroquine, furosemide, and quinine. Many other drugs are ototoxic but have more effect on the cochlea than the vestibular apparatus.

[d]Ear symptoms are rarely present, but gait/balance disturbance is common. Nystagmus is not inhibited by visual fixation.

[e]These causes should not cause otic symptoms (eg, hearing loss, tinnitus) or focal neurologic deficits (sometimes occurs with hypoglycemia). Vertiginous symptoms are rare but have been reported.

[f]There are numerous drugs, including most antianxiety, anticonvulsant, antidepressant, antipsychotic, and sedative drugs. Drugs used to treat vertigo are also included.

Is the patient having a single, sudden, acute event, or has dizziness been chronic and recurrent? Was the first episode the most severe (vestibular crisis)? How long do episodes last, and what seems to trigger and worsen them? The patient should be asked specifically about movement of the head, arising, being in anxious or stressful situations, and menses. Important associated symptoms include headache, hearing loss, tinnitus, nausea and vomiting, impaired vision, focal weakness, and difficulty walking. The severity of impact on the patient's life should be estimated: Has the patient fallen? Is the patient reluctant to drive or leave the house? Has the patient missed work days?

Review of systems should seek symptoms of causative disorders, including URI symptoms (inner ear disorders); chest pain, palpitations, or both (heart disease); dyspnea (lung disease); dark stools (anemia caused by GI blood loss); and weight change or heat or cold intolerance (thyroid disease).

Past medical history should note presence of recent head trauma (usually obvious by history), migraine, diabetes, heart or lung disease, and drug and alcohol abuse. In addition to identifying all current drugs, drug history should assess recent changes in drugs, doses, or both.

Physical examination: Examination begins with a review of vital signs, including presence of fever, rapid or irregular pulse, and supine and standing BP, noting any drop in BP on standing up (orthostatic hypotension) and whether standing provokes symptoms. If standing does provoke symptoms, postural symptoms should be distinguished from those triggered by head movement by returning the patient supine until symptoms dissipate and then rotating the head.

The ENT and neurologic examinations are fundamental. Specifically, with the patient supine, the eyes are checked for presence, direction, and duration of spontaneous nystagmus (for full description of examination for nystagmus, see Sidebar 91–1). Direction and duration of nystagmus and development of vertigo are noted.

A gross bedside hearing test is done, the ear canal is inspected for discharge and foreign body, and the tympanic membrane is checked for signs of infection or perforation.

Cerebellar function is tested by assessing gait and doing a finger-nose test and the Romberg test. The Unterberger (or Fukuda) stepping test may be done by specialists to help detect a unilateral vestibular lesion. The remainder of the neurologic examination is done, including testing the rest of the cranial nerves.

Red flags: The following findings are of particular concern:

- Head or neck pain
- Ataxia
- Loss of consciousness
- Focal neurologic deficit
- Severe, continuous symptoms for > 1 h

Interpretation of findings: Traditionally, differential diagnosis has been based on the exact nature of the chief complaint (ie, distinguishing dizziness from light-headedness from vertigo). However, the inconsistency of patients' descriptions and the poor specificity of symptoms make this unreliable. A better approach places more weight on the onset and timing of symptoms, the triggers, and associated symptoms and findings, particularly otologic and neurologic ones.

Some constellations of findings are highly suggestive (see Table 91–4), particularly those that help differentiate peripheral from central vestibular disorders.

- Peripheral: Ear symptoms (eg, tinnitus, fullness, hearing loss) usually indicate a peripheral disorder. They are typically associated with vertigo and not generalized dizziness (unless caused by uncompensated peripheral vestibular weakness). Symptoms are usually paroxysmal, severe, and episodic; continuous dizziness is rarely due to peripheral vertigo. Loss of consciousness is not associated with dizziness due to peripheral vestibular pathology.
- Central: Ear symptoms are rarely present, but gait/balance disturbance is common. Nystagmus is not inhibited by visual fixation.

Testing: Patients with a sudden, ongoing attack should have pulse oximetry and fingerstick glucose test. Women should have a pregnancy test. Most clinicians also do an ECG. Other tests are done based on findings (see Table 91–4), but generally gadolinium-enhanced MRI is indicated for patients with acute symptoms who have headache, neurologic abnormalities, or any other findings suggestive of a CNS etiology.

Patients with chronic symptoms should have gadolinium-enhanced MRI to look for evidence of stroke, multiple sclerosis, or other CNS lesions.

Patients for whom results of bedside tests of hearing and vestibular function are abnormal or equivocal should undergo formal testing with audiometry and electronystagmography.

ECG, Holter monitoring for heart rhythm abnormalities, echocardiography, and exercise stress testing may be done to evaluate heart function.

Laboratory tests are rarely helpful, except for patients with chronic vertigo and bilateral hearing loss, for whom syphilis serology is indicated.

Treatment

Treatment is directed at the cause, including stopping, reducing, or switching any causative drugs.

If a vestibular disorder is present and thought to be secondary to active Meniere disease or vestibular neuronitis or labyrinthitis, the most effective vestibular nerve suppressants are diazepam (2 to 5 mg po q 6 to 8 h, with higher doses given under supervision for severe vertigo) or oral antihistamine/anticholinergic drugs (eg, meclizine 25 to 50 mg tid). All of these drugs can cause drowsiness, thereby limiting their use for certain patients. Nausea can be treated with prochlorperazine 10 mg IM qid or 25 mg rectally bid. Vertigo associated with benign paroxysmal positional vertigo is treated with the Epley maneuver (otolith repositioning) done by an experienced practitioner (see Fig. 95–2 on p. 821). Meniere disease is best managed by an otolaryngologist with training in management of this chronic disorder, but initial management consists of a low-salt diet and a K-sparing diuretic.

Patients with persistent or recurrent vertigo secondary to unilateral vestibular weakness (such as secondary to vestibular neuronitis) usually benefit from vestibular rehabilitation therapy done by an experienced physical therapist. Most patients compensate well, although some, especially the elderly, have more difficulty. Physical therapy can also provide important safety information for elderly or particularly disabled patients.

Geriatrics Essentials

As people age, organs involved in balance function less well. For example, seeing in dim light becomes more difficult, inner ear structures deteriorate, proprioception becomes less sensitive, and mechanisms that control BP become less responsive (eg, to postural changes, postprandial demands). Older people also are more likely to have cardiac or cerebrovascular disorders that can contribute to dizziness. They also are more likely to be taking drugs that can cause dizziness, including those for hypertension, angina, heart failure, seizures, and anxiety, as well as certain antibiotics, antihistamines, and sleep aids. Thus, dizziness in elderly patients usually has more than one cause.

Although unpleasant at any age, the consequences of dizziness and vertigo are a particular problem for elderly patients. Patients with frailty are at significant risk of falling with consequent fractures; their fear of moving and falling often significantly decreases their ability to do daily activities.

In addition to treatment of specific causes, elderly patients with dizziness or vertigo may benefit from physical therapy and exercises to strengthen muscles and help maintain independent ambulation as long as possible.

KEY POINTS

- Vague or inconsistently described symptoms may still be associated with a serious condition.
- Cerebrovascular disease and drug effects should be sought, particularly in elderly patients.
- Peripheral vestibular system disorders should be differentiated from central vestibular system disorders.
- Immediate neuroimaging should be done when symptoms are accompanied by headache, focal neurologic abnormalities, or both.

92 Approach to the Patient with Nasal and Pharyngeal Symptoms

The nose and pharynx (consisting of the nasopharynx, oropharynx, and hypopharynx) may be affected by inflammation, infection, trauma, tumors, and several miscellaneous conditions.

Anatomy

Throat: The uvula hangs in the midline at the far end of the soft palate. It varies greatly in length. A long uvula and loose or excess velopharyngeal tissue may cause snoring and occasionally contribute to obstructive sleep apnea.

Tonsils and adenoids are patches of lymphoid tissue surrounding the posterior pharynx in an area termed Waldeyer's ring. Their role is to combat infection.

The larynx is discussed in Ch. 96 on p. 824.

Nose: The nasal cavity is covered with a highly vascular mucosa that warms and humidifies incoming air. Each lateral wall of the cavity has 3 turbinates, which are bony shelves that increase the surface area, thereby allowing more effective heat and moisture exchange. Nasal mucus traps incoming particulate matter. The space between the middle and inferior turbinate is the middle meatus, into which the maxillary and most of the ethmoid sinuses drain. Polyps may develop between the turbinates, often in association with asthma, allergy, aspirin use, and cystic fibrosis.

Sinuses: The paranasal sinuses are mucus-lined bony cavities that connect to the nasopharynx. The 4 types are maxillary, frontal, ethmoid, and sphenoid sinuses. They are located in the facial and cranial bones (see Fig. 92–1). The physiologic role of the sinuses is unclear.

Evaluation

Examination of the nose and pharynx is part of every general physical examination.

History: General information includes use of alcohol or tobacco (both major risk factors for head and neck cancer) and systemic symptoms, such as fever and weight loss. Oropharyngeal symptoms include pain, ulcers, and difficulty swallowing or speaking. Nasal and sinus symptoms include presence and duration of congestion, discharge, loss of smell and/or taste, and bleeding.

Physical examination: Most physicians use a head-mounted light. However, because the light cannot be precisely aligned on the axis of vision, it is difficult to avoid shadowing in narrow areas (eg, nasal cavity). Better illumination results with a head-mounted convex mirror; the physician looks through a hole in the center of the mirror, so the illumination is always on-axis. The head mirror reflects light from a source placed behind the patient and slightly to one side and requires practice to use effectively.

The nose is examined using a nasal speculum, which is held so that the 2 blades open in an anteroposterior (or slightly oblique) direction and do not press against the septum. The physician notes any crusting, discharge, septal deviation, or perforation; whether mucosa is erythematous, boggy, or swollen; and presence of polyps. The skin over the frontal and maxillary sinuses is examined for erythema and tenderness, suggesting sinus inflammation.

If necessary, the nasopharynx and hypopharynx can be examined with a flexible nasopharyngoscope. A topical anesthetic (eg, lidocaine 4%) is sprayed in the nose and throat, and the nose is also sprayed with a decongestant (eg, phenylephrine 0.5%). After several minutes, the scope is gently passed through the nares, and the nasal cavity, hypopharynx, and larynx are inspected. Alternatively, a mirror examination can be done. The mirror should be warmed before use to avoid fogging. A small mirror is used for the nasopharynx. It is held just below the uvula, angling upward; the tongue is pushed down with a tongue blade. A larger mirror is used for the hypopharynx and larynx. The tongue is retracted by grasping it with a gauze pad, and the mirror is placed against the soft palate, angling downward. A nasal endoscopic examination can also be done using a rigid scope, which provides excellent views inside of the nose, but this requires skill to do without causing the patient discomfort.

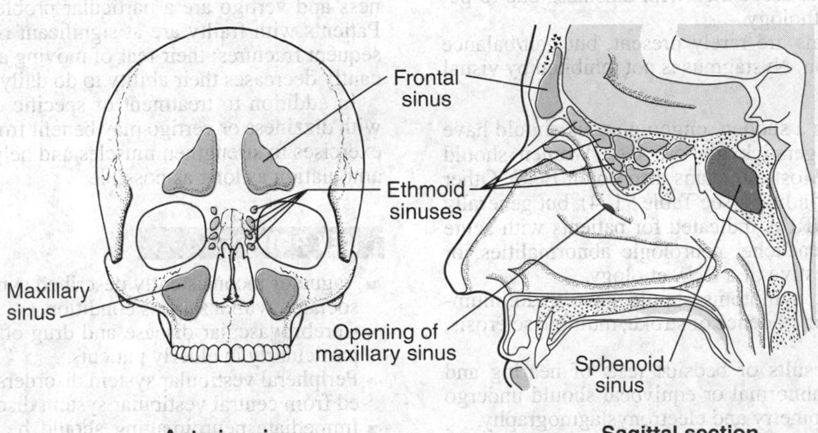

Fig. 92–1. Paranasal sinuses.

Neck examination consists of inspection and palpation for masses. If masses are found, the physician notes whether they are tender; fluctuant, firm, or stony hard; and movable or fixed. Masses caused by infection are tender and mobile; cancers tend to be nontender, hard, and fixed. Particular attention is paid to the cervical lymph nodes and thyroid and parotid glands.

EPISTAXIS

Epistaxis is nose bleeding. Bleeding can range from a trickle to a strong flow, and the consequences can range from a minor annoyance to life-threatening hemorrhage.

Pathophysiology

Most nasal bleeding is anterior, originating from a plexus of vessels in the anteroinferior septum (Kiesselbach's area).

Less common but more serious are posterior nosebleeds, which originate in the posterior septum overlying the vomer bone, or laterally on the inferior or middle turbinate. Posterior nosebleeds tend to occur in patients who have preexisting atherosclerotic vessels or bleeding disorders and have undergone nasal or sinus surgery.

Etiology

The most common causes of epistaxis are

- Local trauma (eg, nose blowing and picking)
- Drying of the nasal mucosa

There are a number of less common causes (see Table 92–1). Hypertension may contribute to the persistence of a nosebleed that has already begun but is unlikely to be the sole etiology.

Evaluation

History: History of present illness should try to determine which side began bleeding first; although major epistaxis quickly involves both nares, most patients can localize the initial flow to one side, which focuses the physical examination. Also, the duration of bleeding should be established, as well as any triggers (eg, sneezing, nose blowing, picking) and attempts by the patient to stop the bleeding. Melena may occur, and swallowed blood is a gastric irritant, so patients also may describe vomiting blood. Important associated symptoms prior to onset include symptoms of a URI, sensation of nasal obstruction, and nasal or facial pain. The time and number of previous nose-bleeding episodes and their resolution should be identified.

Review of systems should ask about symptoms of excessive bleeding, including easy bruising; bloody or tarry stools; hemoptysis; blood in urine; and excess bleeding with toothbrushing, phlebotomy, or minor trauma.

Past medical history should note presence of known bleeding disorders (including a family history) and conditions associated with defects in platelets or coagulation, particularly cancer, cirrhosis, HIV, and pregnancy. Drug history should specifically query about use of drugs that may promote bleeding, including aspirin and other NSAIDs, other antiplatelet drugs (eg, clopidogrel), heparin, and warfarin.

Physical examination: Vital signs should be reviewed for indications of intravascular volume depletion (tachycardia, hypotension) and marked hypertension. With active bleeding, treatment takes place simultaneously with evaluation.

During active bleeding, inspection is difficult, so attempts are first made to stop the bleeding as described below. The nose is then examined using a nasal speculum and a bright head lamp or head mirror, which leaves one hand free to manipulate suction or an instrument.

Anterior bleeding sites are usually apparent on direct examination. If no site is apparent and there have been only 1 or 2 minor nosebleeds, further examination is not needed. If bleeding is severe or recurrent and no site is seen, fiber-optic endoscopy may be necessary.

The general examination should look for signs of bleeding disorders, including petechiae, purpura, and perioral and oral mucosal telangiectasias as well as any intranasal masses.

Red flags: The following findings are of particular concern:

- Signs of hypovolemia or hemorrhagic shock
- Anticoagulant drug use
- Cutaneous signs of a bleeding disorder
- Bleeding not stopped by direct pressure or vasoconstrictor-soaked pledgets
- Multiple recurrences, particularly with no clear cause

Interpretation of findings: Many cases have a clear-cut trigger (particularly nose blowing or picking) as suggested by findings (see Table 92–1).

Testing: Routine laboratory testing is not required. Patients with symptoms or signs of a bleeding disorder and those with severe or recurrent epistaxis should have CBC, PT, and PTT.

CT may be done if a foreign body, a tumor, or sinusitis is suspected.

Treatment

Presumptive treatment for actively bleeding patients is that for anterior bleeding. The need for blood replacement is determined by the Hb level, symptoms of anemia, and vital signs. Any identified bleeding disorders are treated.

Anterior epistaxis: Bleeding can usually be controlled by pinching the nasal alae together for 10 min while the patient sits upright (if possible). If this maneuver fails, a cotton pledget impregnated with a vasoconstrictor (eg, phenylephrine 0.25%) and a topical anesthetic (eg, lidocaine 2%) is inserted and the nose pinched for another 10 min. The bleeding point may then be cauterized with electrocautery or silver nitrate on an applicator stick. Cauterizing 4 quadrants immediately adjacent to the bleeding vessel is most effective. Care must be taken to avoid burning the mucous membrane too deeply; therefore, silver nitrate is the preferred method.

Alternatively, a nasal tampon of expandable foam may be inserted. Coating the tampon with a topical ointment, such as bacitracin or mupirocin, may help. If these methods are ineffective, various commercial nasal balloons can be used to compress bleeding sites.

As another alternative, an anterior nasal pack consisting of ½-in petrolatum gauze may be inserted; up to 72 in of gauze may be required. This procedure is painful, and analgesics usually are needed; it should be used only when other methods fail or are not available.

Posterior epistaxis: Posterior bleeding may be difficult to control. Commercial nasal balloons are quick and convenient; a gauze posterior pack is effective but more difficult to position. Both are very uncomfortable; IV sedation and analgesia may be needed, and hospitalization is required.

Commercial balloons are inserted according to the instructions accompanying the product.

The posterior gauze pack consists of 4-in gauze squares folded, rolled, tied into a tight bundle with 2 strands of heavy silk suture, and coated with antibiotic ointment. The ends of one suture are tied to a catheter that has been introduced through the

Table 92–1. SOME CAUSES OF EPISTAXIS

CAUSE*	SUGGESTIVE FINDINGS	DIAGNOSTIC APPROACH
Common		
Local trauma (eg, nose blowing, picking, blunt impact)	Apparent by history	Clinical evaluation
Drying of the mucosa (eg, in cold weather)	Usually visibly dry on examination	Clinical evaluation
Less common		
Local infections (eg, vestibulitis, rhinitis)	Crusting in the nasal vestibule, often with local pain and dry mucosa	Clinical evaluation
Systemic disorders (eg, AIDS, liver disease)	Presence of known disease Mucosal erosions and hypertrophy	Clinical evaluation
Foreign bodies (mainly in children)	Often recurrent epistaxis with a malodorous discharge	Clinical evaluation
Arteriosclerosis	Usually in older patients	Clinical evaluation
Rendu-Osler-Weber syndrome	Telangiectasias on the face, lips, oral and nasal mucosa, and tips of the fingers and toes Positive family history	Clinical evaluation
Tumor (benign or malignant) of the nasopharynx or paranasal sinuses	Mass seen within the nose or nasopharynx Bulging of the lateral nasal wall	CT
Septal perforation	Visible on examination	Clinical examination
Coagulopathy	History of prior epistaxis or other bleeding sites, such as gingiva	CBC with platelet count, PT/PTT

*Epistaxis of any cause is more common among patients with bleeding disorders (eg, thrombocytopenia, liver disease, coagulopathies) and with anticoagulant use. In such patients, bleeding is also often more severe and difficult to treat.

nasal cavity on the side of the bleeding and brought out through the mouth. As the catheter is withdrawn from the nose, the postnasal pack is pulled into place above the soft palate in the nasopharynx. The 2nd suture hangs down the back of the throat and is trimmed below the level of the soft palate so that it can be used to remove the pack. The nasal cavity anterior to this pack is firmly packed with ½-in petrolatum gauze, and the 1st suture is tied over a roll of gauze at the anterior nares to secure the postnasal pack. The packing remains in place for 4 to 5 days. An antibiotic (eg, amoxicillin/clavulanate 875 mg po bid for 7 to 10 days) is given to prevent sinusitis and otitis media. Posterior nasal packing lowers the arterial Po_2, and supplementary O_2 is given while the packing is in place. This procedure is uncomfortable and should be avoided if possible.

On occasion, the internal maxillary artery and its branches must be ligated to control the bleeding. The arteries may be ligated with clips using endoscopic or microscopic guidance and a surgical approach through the maxillary sinus. Alternatively, angiographic embolization may be done by a skilled radiologist. These procedures, if done in a timely manner, may shorten hospital stay.

Bleeding disorders: In Rendu-Osler-Weber syndrome, a split-thickness skin graft (septal dermatoplasty) reduces the number of nosebleeds and allows the anemia to be corrected. Laser (Nd:YAG) photocoagulation can be done in the operating room. Selective embolization also is very effective, particularly in patients who cannot tolerate general anesthesia or for whom surgical intervention has not been successful. New endoscopic sinus devices have made transnasal surgery more effective.

Blood may be swallowed in large amounts and, in patients with liver disease, should be eliminated promptly with enemas and cathartics to prevent hepatic encephalopathy. The GI tract should be sterilized with nonabsorbable antibiotics (eg, neomycin 1 g po qid) to prevent the breakdown of blood and the absorption of ammonia.

KEY POINTS

- Most nosebleeds are anterior and stop with direct pressure.
- Screening (by history and physical examination) for bleeding disorders is important.
- Patients should always be asked about aspirin or ibuprofen use.

NASAL CONGESTION AND RHINORRHEA

Nasal congestion and rhinorrhea (runny nose) are extremely common problems that commonly occur together but occasionally occur alone.

Etiology

The most common causes (see Table 92–2) are the following:

- Viral infections
- Allergic reactions

Dry air may provoke congestion. Acute sinusitis is slightly less common, and a nasal foreign body is unusual (and occurs predominantly in children).

Patients who use topical decongestants for > 3 to 5 days often experience significant rebound congestion when the effects of the drug wear off, causing them to continue using the decongestant in a vicious circle of persistent, worsening congestion. This situation (rhinitis medicamentosa) may persist for some

Table 92–2. SOME CAUSES OF NASAL CONGESTION AND RHINORRHEA

CAUSE	SUGGESTIVE FINDINGS	DIAGNOSTIC APPROACH
Acute sinusitis	Mucopurulent discharge, often unilateral Red mucosa Sometimes a foul or metallic taste, focal facial pain or headache, and erythema or tenderness over the maxillary or frontal sinus	Clinical evaluation CT considered in patients with diabetes, immunocompromise, or signs of serious illness
Allergies	Watery discharge; sneezing; watery, itchy eyes; pale, boggy nasal mucosa Symptoms often seasonal or with exposure to possible triggers	Clinical evaluation
Decongestant overuse	Rebound congestion as decongestant wears off Pale, markedly swollen mucosa	Clinical evaluation
Nasal foreign body	Unilateral, foul-smelling (sometimes blood-tinged) discharge in a child	Clinical evaluation
Vasomotor rhinitis	Recurrent watery discharge; sneezing; red, swollen mucosa No identifiable triggers	Clinical evaluation
Viral URI	Watery to mucoid discharge; accompanied by sore throat, malaise, erythematous nasal mucosa	Clinical evaluation

time and may be misinterpreted as a continuation of the original problem rather than a consequence of treatment.

Evaluation

History: **History of present illness** should determine the nature of the discharge (eg, watery, mucoid, purulent, bloody) and whether discharge is chronic or recurrent. If recurrent, any relation to patient location, season, or exposure to potential triggering allergens (numerous) should be determined. A unilateral, clear, watery discharge, particularly when following head trauma, can signify cerebrospinal fluid (CSF) leak. CSF discharge also can occur spontaneously in obese women in their 40s, secondary to idiopathic intracranial hypertension.

Review of systems should seek symptoms of possible causes, including fever and facial pain (sinusitis); watery, itchy eyes (allergies); and sore throat, malaise, fever, and cough (viral URI).

Past medical history should seek known allergies and existence of diabetes or immunocompromise. Drug history should ask specifically about topical decongestant use.

Physical examination: Vital signs are reviewed for fever.

Examination focuses on the nose and area over the sinuses. The face is inspected for focal erythema over the frontal and maxillary sinuses; these areas are also palpated for tenderness. Nasal mucosa is inspected for color (eg, red or pale), swelling, color and nature of discharge, and (particularly in children) presence of any foreign body.

Red flags: The following findings are of particular concern:

- Unilateral discharge, particularly if purulent or bloody
- Facial pain, tenderness, or both

Interpretation of findings: Symptoms and examination are often enough to suggest a diagnosis (see Table 92–2).

In children, unilateral foul-smelling discharge suggests a nasal foreign body. If no foreign body is seen, sinusitis is suspected when purulent rhinorrhea persists for > 10 days along with fatigue and cough.

Testing: Testing is generally not indicated for acute nasal symptoms unless invasive sinusitis is suspected in a diabetic or immunocompromised patient; these patients usually should undergo CT. If a CSF leak is suspected, a sample of the discharge should be tested for the presence of beta-2 transferrin, which is highly specific for CSF.

Treatment

Specific conditions are treated. Symptomatic relief of congestion can be achieved with topical or oral decongestants. Topical decongestants include oxymetazoline, 2 sprays each nostril once/day or bid for 3 days. Oral decongestants include pseudoephedrine 60 mg bid. Prolonged use should be avoided.

Viral rhinorrhea can be treated with oral antihistamines (eg, diphenhydramine 25 to 50 mg po bid), which are recommended because of their anticholinergic properties unrelated to their H_2-blocking properties.

Allergic congestion and rhinorrhea can be treated with antihistamines; in such cases, nonanticholinergic antihistamines (eg, fexofenadine 60 mg po bid) as needed provoke fewer adverse effects. Nasal corticosteroids (eg, mometasone 2 sprays each nostril daily) also help allergic conditions.

Antihistamines and decongestants are not recommended for children < 6 yr.

Geriatrics Essentials

Antihistamines can have sedating and anticholinergic effects and should be given in decreased dosage in the elderly. Similarly, sympathomimetics should be used with the lowest dosage that is clinically effective.

KEY POINTS

- Most nasal congestion and rhinorrhea are caused by URI or allergies.
- A foreign body should be considered in children.
- Rebound from topical decongestant overuse should also be considered.

NECK MASS

Patients or their family members may notice a mass on the neck, or one may be discovered during routine examination. A neck mass may be painless or painful depending on the cause.

When a neck mass is painless, much time may pass before patients seek medical care.

Etiology

There are many causes of neck mass, including infectious, cancerous, and congenital causes (see Table 92–3).

The most common causes in younger patients include the following:

- Reactive adenitis
- Primary bacterial lymph node infection
- Systemic infections

Reactive adenitis occurs in response to viral or bacterial infection somewhere in the oropharynx. Some systemic infections (eg, mononucleosis, HIV, TB) cause cervical lymph node enlargement—usually generalized rather than isolated.

Congenital disorders may cause a neck mass, typically longstanding. The most common are thyroglossal duct cysts, branchial cleft cysts, and dermoid or sebaceous cysts.

Cancerous masses are more common among older patients but may occur in younger ones. These masses may represent a local primary tumor or lymph node involvement from a local, regional, or distant primary cancer. About 60% of supraclavicular triangle masses are metastases from distant primary sites. Elsewhere in the neck, 80% of cancerous cervical adenopathy originates in the upper respiratory or alimentary tract. Likely sites of origin are the posterior-lateral border of the tongue and the floor of the mouth followed by the nasopharynx, palatine tonsil, laryngeal surface of the epiglottis, and hypopharynx, including the pyriform sinuses.

The thyroid gland may enlarge in various disorders, including simple nontoxic goiter, subacute thyroiditis, and, less often, thyroid cancer.

Table 92–3. SOME CAUSES OF NECK MASS

CAUSE	SUGGESTIVE FINDINGS	DIAGNOSTIC APPROACH
Infectious disorders		
HIV	High-risk groups Generalized, painless adenopathy	Serologic testing for HIV
Mononucleosis	Multiple, nontender or moderately tender cervical nodes in an adolescent Usually pharyngitis and marked malaise	Serologic testing for Epstein-Barr virus
Oropharyngeal infection, viral or bacterial (most commonly pharyngitis or URI, sometimes a dental infection)	Frequently URI symptoms, sore throat, or toothache Acute, rubbery adenopathy with little or no tenderness Multiple enlarged nodes sometimes present with viral URI	Clinical evaluation Sometimes throat culture
Primary bacterial lymphadenitis	Acute, isolated, tender adenopathy	Clinical evaluation
TB	High-risk groups Matted, painless adenopathy, sometimes fluctuant	PPD Culture
Cancer*		
Local primary (eg, oropharyngeal, thyroid, salivary) Nodes from distant primary (eg, lymphomas, prostate, breast, colon, kidney) Nodes from local or regional primary (eg, lung, upper GI)	For most common local primary cancers, usually in older patients, typically with significant tobacco use, alcohol consumption, or both; may or may not have visible or palpable primary (eg, in oropharynx) Cancerous masses likely to be firm or hard and fixed to underlying tissues rather than mobile Regional or distant metastases with or without local symptoms	Typically laryngoscopy, bronchoscopy, and esophagoscopy with biopsy of all suspect areas CT of the head, neck, and chest and possibly a thyroid scan
Congenital disorders		
Branchial cleft cyst	Lateral mass, usually overlying the sternocleidomastoid muscle, often with a sinus or fistula	In children, ultrasonography In adults, CT
Dermoid or sebaceous cyst	Rubbery and nontender (unless infected)	
Thyroglossal duct cyst	Midline, nontender mass Usually manifests in childhood or adolescence but sometimes not until later	
Other disorders		
Simple, nontoxic goiter	Nontender diffuse thyroid enlargement	Thyroid function testing Thyroid scan Ultrasonography
Subacute thyroiditis	Fever, usually thyroid tenderness and enlargement	
Submandibular salivary gland enlargement (eg, due to sialadenitis or stones)	Typically a painless mass just below the mandible laterally	CT and MRI Biopsy

*Patients suspected of having cancer should undergo a head and neck examination by an otolaryngologist.

A submandibular salivary gland can enlarge if it is blocked by a stone, becomes infected, or develops a cancer.

Evaluation

History: History of present illness should note how long the mass has been present and whether it is painful. Important associated acute symptoms include sore throat, URI symptoms, and toothache.

Review of systems should ask about difficulty swallowing or speaking and symptoms of chronic disease (eg, fever, weight loss, malaise). Regional and distant cancers causing metastases to the neck occasionally cause symptoms in their system of origin (eg, cough in lung cancer, swallowing difficulty in esophageal cancer). Because numerous cancers can metastasize to the neck, a complete review of systems is important to help identify a source.

Past medical history should inquire about known HIV or TB and risk factors for them. Risk factors for cancer are assessed, including consumption of alcohol or use of tobacco (particularly snuff or chewing tobacco), ill-fitting dental appliances, and chronic oral candidiasis. Poor oral hygiene also may be a risk.

Physical examination: The neck mass is palpated to determine consistency (ie, whether soft and fluctuant, rubbery, or hard) and presence and degree of tenderness. Whether the mass is freely mobile or appears fixed to the skin or underlying tissue also needs to be determined.

The scalp, ears, nasal cavities, oral cavity, nasopharynx, oropharynx, hypopharynx, and larynx are closely inspected for signs of infection and any other visible lesions. Teeth are percussed to detect the exquisite tenderness of root infection. The base of the tongue, floor of the mouth, and the thyroid and salivary glands are palpated for masses.

The breasts and prostate gland are palpated for masses, and the spleen is palpated for enlargement. Stool is checked for occult blood, suggestive of a GI cancer.

Other lymph nodes are palpated (eg, axillary, inguinal).

Red flags: The following findings are of particular concern:

- Hard, fixed mass
- Older patient
- Presence of oropharyngeal lesions (other than simple pharyngitis or dental infection)
- A history of persistent hoarseness or dysphagia

Interpretation of findings: Important differentiating factors for a neck mass (see Table 92–3) include acuity, pain and tenderness, and consistency and mobility.

A new mass (ie, developing over only a few days), particularly after symptoms of a URI or pharyngitis, suggests benign reactive lymphadenopathy. An acute tender mass suggests lymphadenitis or an infected dermoid cyst.

A chronic mass in younger patients suggests a cyst. A non-midline mass in older patients, particularly those with risk factors, should be considered cancer until proven otherwise; a midline mass is likely of thyroid origin (benign or malignant).

Pain, tenderness, or both in the mass suggest inflammation (particularly infectious), whereas a painless mass suggests a cyst or tumor. A hard, fixed, nontender mass suggests cancer, whereas rubbery consistency and mobility suggest otherwise.

Generalized adenopathy and splenomegaly suggest infectious mononucleosis or a lymphoreticular cancer. Generalized adenopathy alone may suggest HIV infection, particularly in those with risk factors.

Red and white mucosal patches (erythroplakia and leukoplakia) in the oropharynx may be malignant lesions responsible for the neck mass.

Difficulty swallowing may be noted with thyroid enlargement or cancer originating in various sites in the neck. Difficulty speaking suggests a cancer involving the larynx or recurrent laryngeal nerve.

Testing: If the nature of the mass is readily apparent (eg, lymphadenopathy caused by recent pharyngitis) or is in a healthy young patient with a recent, tender swelling and no other findings, then no immediate testing is required. However, the patient is reexamined regularly; if the mass fails to resolve, further evaluation is needed.

Most other patients should have a CBC and chest x-ray. Those with findings suggesting specific causes should also have testing for those disorders (see Table 92–3).

If examination reveals an oral or nasopharyngeal lesion that fails to begin resolving within 2 wk, testing may include CT or MRI and fine-needle biopsy of that lesion.

In young patients with no risk factors for head and neck cancer and no other apparent lesions, the neck mass may be biopsied.

Older patients, particularly those with risk factors for cancer, should first undergo further testing to identify the primary site; biopsy of the neck mass may simply reveal undifferentiated squamous cell carcinoma without illuminating the source. Such patients should have direct laryngoscopy, bronchoscopy, and esophagoscopy with biopsy of all suspicious areas. Specimens identified as squqmous cell carcinoma should be tested for HPV. CT of the head, neck, and chest and possibly a thyroid scan are done. Ultrasound is preferred for children to avoid radiation exposure and may be used in adults if a thyroid mass is suspected. If a primary tumor is not found, fine-needle aspiration biopsy of the neck mass should be done, which is preferable to an incisional biopsy because it does not leave a transected mass in the neck. If the neck mass is cancerous and a primary tumor has not been identified, random biopsy of the nasopharynx, palatine tonsils, and base of the tongue should be considered.

Treatment

Treatment is directed at the cause.

KEY POINTS

- An acute neck mass in younger patients is usually benign.
- Neck mass in an elderly patient raises concern of cancer.
- Thorough oropharyngeal examination is important.

SORE THROAT

Sore throat is pain in the posterior pharynx that occurs with or without swallowing. Pain can be severe; many patients refuse oral intake.

Etiology

Sore throat results from infection; the most common cause is

- Tonsillopharyngitis

Rarely, an abscess or epiglottitis is involved; although uncommon, these are of particular concern because they may compromise the airway.

Tonsillopharyngitis: Tonsillopharyngitis is predominantly a viral infection; a lesser number of cases are caused by bacteria.

The respiratory viruses (rhinovirus, adenovirus, influenza, coronavirus, respiratory syncytial virus) are the most common viral causes, but occasionally Epstein-Barr virus (the cause of mononucleosis), herpes simplex, cytomegalovirus, or primary HIV infection is involved.

The main bacterial cause is group A β-hemolytic streptococci (GABHS), which, although estimates vary, causes perhaps 10% of cases in adults and slightly more in children. GABHS is a concern because of the possibility of the poststreptococcal sequelae of rheumatic fever, glomerulonephritis, and abscess. Uncommon bacterial causes include gonorrhea, diphtheria, mycoplasma, and chlamydia.

Abscess: An abscess in the pharyngeal area (peritonsillar, parapharyngeal, and, in children, retropharyngeal) is uncommon but causes significant throat pain. The usual causative organism is GABHS.

Epiglottitis: Epiglottitis, perhaps better termed supraglottitis, used to occur primarily in children and usually was caused by *Haemophilus influenzae* type B (HiB). Now, because of widespread childhood vaccination against HiB, supraglottitis/epiglottitis has been almost eradicated in children (more cases occur in adults). Causal organisms in children and adults include *Streptococcus pneumoniae*, *Staphylococcus aureus*, nontypeable *H. influenzae*, *Haemophilus parainfluenzae*, β-hemolytic streptococci, *Branhamella catarrhalis*, and *Klebsiella pneumoniae*. HiB is still a cause in adults and unvaccinated children.

Evaluation

History: History of present illness should note the duration and severity of sore throat.

Review of systems should seek important associated symptoms, such as runny nose, cough, and difficulty swallowing, speaking, or breathing. The presence and duration of any preceding weakness and malaise (suggesting mononucleosis) are noted.

Past medical history should seek history of previous documented mononucleosis (recurrence is highly unlikely). Social history should inquire about close contact with people with documented GABHS infection, risk factors for gonorrhea transmission (eg, recent oral-genital sexual contact), and risk factors for HIV acquisition (eg, unprotected intercourse, multiple sex partners, IV drug abuse).

Physical examination: General examination should note fever and signs of respiratory distress, such as tachypnea, dyspnea, stridor, and, in children, the tripod position (sitting upright, leaning forward with neck hyperextended and jaw thrust forward).

Pharyngeal examination should not be done in children if supraglottitis/epiglottitis is suspected, because it may trigger complete airway obstruction. Adults with no respiratory distress may be examined but with care. Erythema, exudates, and any signs of swelling around the tonsils or retropharyngeal area should be noted. Whether the uvula is in the midline or appears pushed to one side should also be noted.

The neck is examined for presence of enlarged, tender lymph nodes. The abdomen is palpated for presence of splenomegaly.

Red flags: The following findings are of particular concern:

- Stridor or other sign of respiratory distress
- Drooling
- Muffled, "hot potato" voice
- Visible bulge in pharynx

Interpretation of findings: Supraglottitis/epiglottitis and pharyngeal abscess pose a threat to the airway and must be differentiated from simple tonsillopharyngitis, which is uncomfortable but not acutely dangerous. Clinical findings help make this distinction.

With supraglottitis/epiglottitis, there is abrupt onset of severe throat pain and dysphagia, usually with no preceding URI symptoms. Children often have drooling and signs of toxicity. Sometimes (more often in children), there are respiratory manifestations, with tachypnea, dyspnea, stridor, and sitting in the tripod position. If examined, the pharynx almost always appears unremarkable.

Pharyngeal abscess and tonsillopharyngitis both may cause pharyngeal erythema, exudate, or both. However, some findings are more likely in one condition or another:

- Pharyngeal abscess: Muffled, "hot potato" voice (speaking as if a hot object is being held in the mouth); visible focal swelling in the posterior pharyngeal area (often with deviation of the uvula)
- Tonsillopharyngitis: Accompanied by URI symptoms (eg, runny nose, cough)

Although tonsillopharyngitis is easily recognized clinically, its cause is not. Manifestations of viral and GABHS infection overlap significantly, although URI symptoms are more common with a viral cause. In adults, clinical criteria that increase suspicion of GABHS as a cause include

- Tonsillar exudate
- Tender lymphadenopathy
- Fever (including history)
- Absence of cough

Adults with ≤ 1 criterion reasonably may be presumed to have viral illness. If ≥ 2 criteria are present, the likelihood of GABHS is high enough to warrant testing but probably not high enough to warrant antibiotics, but this decision needs to be patient-specific (ie, threshold for testing and treatment may be lower in those at risk because of diabetes or immunocompromise). In children, testing usually is done. Although this approach is reasonable, not all experts agree on when to test for GABHS and when antibiotic treatment is indicated.

Regarding rarer causes of tonsillopharyngitis, infectious mononucleosis should be considered when there is posterior cervical or generalized adenopathy, hepatosplenomegaly, and fatigue and malaise for > 1 wk. Patients with no URI symptoms but recent oral-genital contact may have pharyngeal gonorrhea. A dirty-gray, thick, tough membrane on the posterior pharynx that bleeds if peeled away indicates diphtheria (rare in the US). HIV infection should be considered in patients with risk factors.

Testing: If supraglottitis/epiglottitis is considered possible after evaluation, testing is required. Patients who do not appear seriously ill and have no respiratory symptoms may have plain lateral neck x-rays to look for an edematous epiglottis. However, a child who appears seriously ill or has stridor or any other respiratory symptoms should not be transported to the x-ray suite. Such patients (and those with positive or equivocal x-ray findings) usually should have flexible fiber-optic laryngoscopy. (CAUTION: *Examination of the pharynx and larynx may precipitate complete respiratory obstruction in children, and the pharynx and larynx should not be directly examined except in the operating room, where the most advanced airway intervention is available.*)

PEARLS & PITFALLS

- If epiglottitis is considered, directly examine a child's pharynx only in the operating room to minimize the risk of complete airway obstruction.

Many abscesses are managed clinically, but if location and extent are unclear, immediate CT of the neck should be done.

In tonsillopharyngitis, throat culture is the only reliable way to differentiate viral infection from GABHS. To balance timeliness of diagnosis, cost, and accuracy, one strategy in children is to do a rapid strep screen in the office, treat if positive, and send a formal culture if negative. In adults, because other bacterial pathogens may be involved, throat culture for all bacterial pathogens is appropriate for those meeting clinical criteria described previously.

Testing for mononucleosis, gonorrhea, or HIV is done only when clinically suspected.

Treatment

Specific conditions are treated. Patients with severe symptoms of tonsillopharyngitis may be started on a broad-spectrum antibiotic (eg, amoxicillin/clavulanate) pending culture results.

Symptomatic treatments such as warm saltwater gargles and topical anesthetics (eg, benzocaine, lidocaine, dyclonine) may help temporarily relieve pain in tonsillopharyngitis. Patients in severe pain (even from tonsillopharyngitis) may require short-term use of opioids.

Corticosteroids (eg, dexamethasone, 10 mg IM) are occasionally used, for example, for tonsillopharyngitis that appears to pose a risk of airway obstruction (eg, due to mononucleosis) or very severe tonsillopharyngitis symptoms.

KEY POINTS

- Most sore throats are caused by viral tonsillopharyngitis.
- It is difficult to clinically distinguish viral from bacterial causes of tonsillopharyngitis.
- Abscess and epiglottitis are rare but serious causes.
- Severe sore throat in a patient with a normal-appearing pharynx should raise suspicion of epiglottitis.

OVERVIEW OF SMELL AND TASTE ABNORMALITIES

Because distinct flavors depend on aromas to stimulate the olfactory chemoreceptors, smell and taste are physiologically interdependent (see Fig. 92–2). Dysfunction of one often disturbs the other. Disorders of smell and taste are rarely incapacitating or life threatening, so they often do not receive close medical attention, although their effect on quality of life can be severe.

Taste: Although abnormal taste sensations may be due to mental disorders, local causes should always be sought. Glossopharyngeal and facial nerve integrity can be determined by testing taste on both sides of the dorsum of the tongue with sugar, salt, vinegar (acid), and quinine (bitter).

Drying of the oral mucosa caused by heavy smoking, Sjögren syndrome, radiation therapy of the head and neck, or desquamation of the tongue can impair taste, and various drugs (eg, those with anticholinergic properties and vincristine) alter taste. In all instances, the gustatory receptors are diffusely involved. When limited to one side of the tongue (eg, in Bell palsy), ageusia (loss of the sense of taste) is rarely noticed.

Smell: The inability to detect certain odors, such as gas or smoke, may be dangerous, and several systemic and intracranial disorders should be excluded before dismissing symptoms as harmless. Whether brain stem disease (involvement of the nucleus solitarius) can cause disorders of smell and taste is uncertain, because other neurologic manifestations usually take precedence.

Anosmia (complete loss of the sense of smell) is probably the most common abnormality. Hyperosmia (increased sensitivity to odors) usually reflects a neurotic or histrionic personality but can occur intermittently with seizure disorders. Dysosmia (disagreeable or distorted sense of smell) may occur with infection of the nasal sinuses, partial damage to the olfactory bulbs, or mental depression. Some cases, accompanied by a disagreeable taste, result from poor dental hygiene. Uncinate epilepsy can produce brief, vivid, unpleasant olfactory hallucinations. Hyposmia (partial loss of smell) and hypogeusia (diminished sense of taste) can follow acute influenza, usually temporarily.

ANOSMIA

Anosmia is complete loss of smell. Hyposmia is partial loss of smell. Most patients with anosmia have normal perception of salty, sweet, sour, and bitter substances but lack flavor discrimination, which largely depends on olfaction. Therefore, they often complain of losing the sense of taste (ageusia) and of not enjoying food. If unilateral, anosmia is often unrecognized.

Etiology

Anosmia occurs when intranasal swelling or other obstruction prevents odors from gaining access to the olfactory area; when the olfactory neuroepithelium is destroyed; or when the olfactory nerve fila, bulbs, tracts, or central connections are destroyed (see Table 92–4).

Major causes include

- Head trauma (young adults)
- Viral infections and Alzheimer disease (older adults)

Prior URI, especially influenza infection, is implicated in 14 to 26% of all presenting cases of hyposmia or anosmia.

Drugs can contribute to anosmia in susceptible patients. Other causes include prior head and neck radiation, recent nasal or sinus surgery, nasal and brain tumors, and toxins. The role of tobacco is uncertain.

Evaluation

History: History of present illness should assess the time course of symptoms and their relation to any URI or head injury. Important associated symptoms are nasal congestion, rhinorrhea, or both. The nature of rhinorrhea should be assessed (eg, watery, mucoid, purulent, bloody).

Review of systems should assess neurologic symptoms, particularly those involving mental status (eg, difficulty with recent memory) and cranial nerves (eg, diplopia, difficulty speaking or swallowing, tinnitus, vertigo).

Past medical history should include history of sinus disorders, cranial trauma or surgery, allergies, drugs used, and exposure to chemicals or fumes.

Physical examination: The nasal passages should be inspected for swelling, inflammation, discharge, and polyps. Having the patient breathe through each nostril sequentially (while the other is manually occluded) may help identify obstruction.

A complete neurologic examination, particularly of mental status and cranial nerves, is done.

Red flags: The following findings are of particular concern:

- Previous head injury
- Neurologic symptoms or signs
- Sudden onset

Interpretation of findings: Sudden onset after significant head trauma or toxin exposure strongly implicates that event as the cause.

A history of chronic rhinosinusitis is suggestive, particularly when significant congestion, polyps, or both are visible

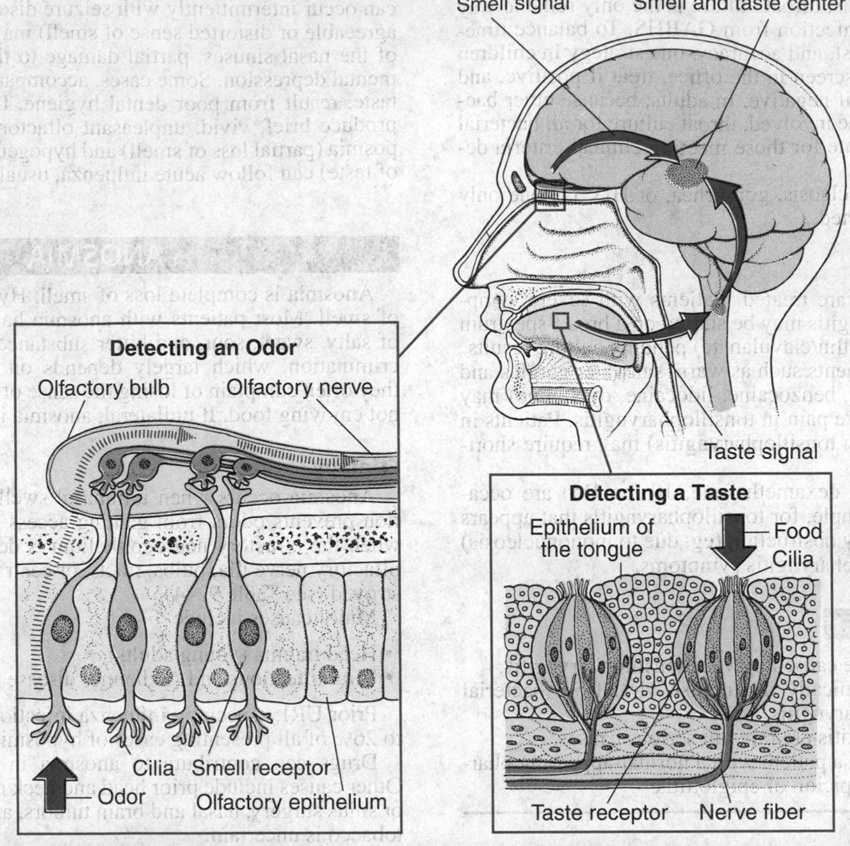

Fig. 92–2. How people sense flavors.

To distinguish most flavors, the brain needs information about both smell and taste. These sensations are communicated to various areas of the brain from receptors in the nose and mouth.

The olfactory epithelium is an area of the nasal mucosa in the upper part of the nasal cavity. The smell receptors in this epithelium are specialized nerve cells with cilia that detect odors. Airborne molecules entering the nasal passage stimulate the cilia, triggering a nerve impulse that is transmitted upward through the cribriform plate and across a synapse within the olfactory bulbs (the distal ends of the 1st cranial nerves—olfactory nerves). The olfactory nerves transmit the impulse to the brain, which interprets the impulse as a distinct odor. Information is also sent to the middle part of the temporal lobe—the smell and taste center, in which memories of odors are stored.

Thousands of tiny taste buds cover most of the tongue's surface. A taste bud contains several types of ciliated taste receptors. Each type detects one of the five basic tastes: sweet, salty, sour, bitter, or savory (also called umami, the taste of monosodium glutamate). These tastes can be detected all over the tongue, but certain areas are more sensitive for each taste. Sweetness is most easily identified by the tip of the tongue, whereas saltiness is best appreciated at the front sides of the tongue. Sourness is best perceived along the sides of the tongue, and bitter sensations are readily detected in the back one third of the tongue. Nerve impulses from the taste buds are transmitted to the brain through the facial and glossopharyngeal nerves (cranial nerves VII and IX).

The brain interprets the combination of impulses from the olfactory and taste receptors along with other sensory information (eg, the food's texture and temperature) to produce a distinct flavor when food enters the mouth and is chewed.

on examination. However, because these findings are common in the population, the physician should be wary of missing another disorder. Progressive confusion and recent memory loss in an elderly patient suggest Alzheimer disease as a cause. Waxing and waning neurologic symptoms affecting multiple areas suggest a neurodegenerative disease such as multiple sclerosis. Slowly progressive anosmia in an elderly patient with no other symptoms or findings suggests normal aging as the cause.

Testing: An in-office test of olfaction can help confirm olfactory dysfunction. Commonly, one nostril is pressed shut, and a pungent odor such as from a vial containing coffee, cinnamon, or tobacco is placed under the open nostril; if the patient can identify the substance, olfaction is presumed intact. The test is repeated on the other nostril to determine whether the response is bilateral. Unfortunately, the test is crude and unreliable.

If anosmia is present and no cause is readily apparent on clinical evaluation (see Table 92–4), patients should have CT of the head (including sinuses) with contrast to rule out a tumor or unsuspected fracture of the floor of the anterior cranial fossa.

Table 92–4. SOME CAUSES OF ANOSMIA

CAUSE	SUGGESTIVE FINDINGS	DIAGNOSTIC APPROACH
Intranasal obstruction		
Allergic rhinitis	History of chronic allergic symptoms (eg, congestion, clear rhinorrhea), no pain	Clinical evaluation
Nasal polyps	Polyps usually visible on examination	Clinical evaluation
Destruction of olfactory neuroepithelium		
Atrophic rhinitis	Chronic rhinitis with atrophic and sclerotic mucous membranes, patency of nasal passages, crust formation, foul odor	Clinical evaluation Sometimes biopsy, which shows the normal ciliated columnar epithelium converted to stratified squamous (squamous metaplasia) and the lamina propria reduced in amount and vascularity
Chronic sinusitis	Chronic mucopurulent drainage, documented infections	Clinical evaluation CT Panograph that shows apices of maxillary teeth to rule out tooth abscess
Some viral URIs	Onset after clinical infection	Clinical evaluation
Tumors (rare cause)	Possibly visual difficulty or only anosmia	CT MRI
Drugs (eg, amphetamines, enalapril, estrogen, naphazoline, phenothiazines, reserpine; prolonged use of decongestants)	Usually, an apparent history of exposure	Clinical evaluation
Toxins (eg, cadmium, manganese)	Usually, an apparent history of exposure	Clinical evaluation
Destruction of central pathways		
Alzheimer disease	Progressive confusion and loss of recent memory	MRI Sequential memory tests
Degenerative neurologic disorders (eg, multiple sclerosis)	Intermittent episodes of other neurologic symptoms (eg, weakness;, numbness; difficulty speaking, seeing, or swallowing)	MRI Sometimes lumbar puncture
Head trauma	Apparent by history	CT
Intracranial surgery, infection, or tumor	Surgery and CNS infection apparent by history Tumors with or without other neurologic symptoms	CT or MRI

MRI is also used to evaluate intracranial disease and may be needed as well, particularly in those patients with no nasal or sinus pathology on CT.

A psychophysical assessment of odor and taste identification and threshold detection is done as well. This assessment commonly involves use of one or several commercially available testing kits. One kit uses a scratch-and-sniff battery of odors, whereas another kit involves sequential dilutions of an odorous chemical.

Treatment

Specific causes are treated; however, smell does not always recover even after successful treatment of sinusitis.

There are no treatments for anosmia. Patients who retain some sense of smell may find adding concentrated flavoring agents to food improves their enjoyment of eating. Smoke alarms, important in all homes, are even more essential for patients with anosmia. Patients should be cautioned about consumption of stored food and use of natural gas for cooking or heating, because they have difficulty detecting food spoilage or gas leaks.

Geriatrics Essentials

There is a significant loss of olfactory receptor neurons with normal aging, leading to a marked diminution of the sense of smell. Changes are usually noticeable by age 60 and can be marked after age 70.

KEY POINTS

- Anosmia may be part of normal aging.
- Common causes include URI, sinusitis, and head trauma.
- Cranial imaging is typically required unless the cause is obvious.

93 External Ear Disorders

DERMATITIS OF THE EAR CANAL

(Chronic Otitis Externa)

Dermatitis of the ear canal is characterized by pruritis, scaling, flaking, and erythema of the skin of the external auditory meatus and ear canal. Dermatitis can be caused by exposure to allergens (contact dermatitis) or can be spontaneous (chronic otitis externa, aural eczematoid dermatitis).

Common contact allergens include nickel-containing earrings and numerous beauty products (eg, hairsprays, lotions, hair dye). Aural eczematoid dermatitis is more common among people with a predisposition toward atopy and with other similar dermatitides (eg, seborrhea, psoriasis).

Both contact dermatitis and aural eczematoid dermatitis cause itching, redness, clear (serous) discharge, desquamation, hyperpigmentation, and, sometimes, fissuring. A secondary bacterial infection can occur (acute otitis externa).

Treatment

- Avoidance of triggers and/or irritants
- Usually topical corticosteroids

Contact dermatitis requires avoidance or withdrawal of allergic triggers, especially earrings. Trial and error may be needed to identify the offending agent. Topical corticosteroids (eg, 1% hydrocortisone cream or a more potent 0.1% betamethasone cream) can decrease inflammation and itching. Patients should avoid using cotton swabs, water, and other potential irritants in the ear, because these will aggravate the inflammatory process. Recalcitrant cases can be treated with a short course of an oral corticosteroid (eg, prednisone).

Aural eczematoid dermatitis can be treated with dilute aluminum acetate solution (Burow solution), which can be applied as often as required for comfort. Itching and inflammation can be reduced with topical corticosteroids (eg, 0.1% betamethasone cream). If acute external otitis ensues, careful debridement of the ear canal and topical antibiotic therapy may be required (see p. 807). Potential irritants, including water and cotton swabs, should be avoided.

EXTERNAL EAR OBSTRUCTIONS

(Ear Foreign Body)

The ear canal may be obstructed by cerumen (earwax), a foreign object, or an insect. Itching, pain, and temporary conductive hearing loss may result. Most causes of obstruction are readily apparent during otoscopic examination. Treatment is careful manual removal.

Before and after attempting to remove cerumen or a foreign body, clinicians should consider doing a hearing assessment if they have the necessary equipment readily available. Hearing loss (compared to the unaffected ear) that does not improve after removal of the obstruction could indicate that the foreign body (or prior attempts to remove it) has damaged the middle or inner ear. Hearing that worsens after removal of the obstruction could indicate damage caused by the removal process. However, practitioners who cannot formally assess hearing need not defer removal of common, easily removable obstructions. An in-office tuning fork test may also document hearing status.

Cerumen: Cerumen may be pushed farther into the ear canal and accumulate during patients' attempts to clean the ear canal with cotton swabs, resulting in obstruction or impaction. Cerumen solvents (hydrogen peroxide, carbamide peroxide, glycerin, triethanolamine, liquid docusate sodium, or mineral oil) may be used to soften very hard wax before direct removal. However, the prolonged use of these agents may lead to canal skin irritation or allergic reactions.

Cerumen is removed by rolling it out of the ear canal with a blunt curet or loop or a small right angle hook, or by removing it with a suction tip (eg, Baron, size 5 French). Proper lighting is essential. These methods are quicker, safer, and more comfortable for the patient than irrigation. Irrigation is sometimes done and should be done carefully to avoid complications. Irrigation may also be combined with cerumenolytic agents such as docusate sodium. Irrigation is contraindicated in patients with one or more of the following factors: anticoagulant therapy, immunocompromised state, diabetes mellitus, prior radiation therapy to the head and neck, ear canal stenosis, exostoses, and non-intact tympanic membrane. Water entering the middle ear through a tympanic membrane perforation may exacerbate chronic otitis media and cause an acute otitis media.

Foreign bodies in the ear: Foreign bodies are common, particularly among children, who often insert objects, particularly beads, erasers, and beans, into the ear canal. Foreign bodies may remain unnoticed until they provoke an inflammatory response, causing pain, itching, infection, and foul-smelling, purulent drainage.

In general, foreign bodies that appear easy to grasp and remove (eg, paper, an insect wing) can be removed with alligator forceps by most practitioners. However, forceps tend to push round, smooth objects (eg, beads, beans) deeper into the canal. Patients with such objects should be referred to an otolaryngologist. A smooth, rounded foreign body is best removed by reaching behind it and rolling it out with a small, blunt hook, which should be done under operating microscope guidance by a specialist. Without a microscope, a foreign body lying at or medial to the isthmus (the bony cartilaginous junction of the external auditory canal) is difficult to remove without injuring the delicate canal skin, tympanic membrane, or ossicular chain. Referral to an otolaryngologist also is indicated for an uncooperative child, who may require sedation, or for failed attempts at removal.

PEARLS & PITFALLS

- Irrigation is not recommended for foreign body removal; hygroscopic foreign bodies (eg, beans or other vegetable matter) swell when water is added, complicating removal.

A general anesthetic or deep sedation may be needed when a child cannot remain still or when removal is difficult, threatening injury to the tympanic membrane or ossicles. Further, if manipulating a presumed foreign object results in bleeding, further attempts at removal should stop and immediate otolaryngologic consultation should be sought. Bleeding may indicate a laceration of the canal skin or that the foreign body is actually a middle ear polyp.

Insects in the canal are most annoying while alive. Filling the canal with viscous lidocaine kills the insect, which provides immediate relief and allows the immobilized insect to be removed with forceps by grasping a wing or leg.

EXTERNAL OTITIS (ACUTE)

External otitis is an acute infection of the ear canal typically caused by bacteria (*Pseudomonas* is most common). Symptoms include pain, discharge, and hearing loss if the ear canal has swollen shut; manipulation of the auricle causes pain. Diagnosis is based on inspection. Treatment is with debridement and topical drugs, including antibiotics, corticosteroids, and acetic acid or a combination.

External otitis may manifest as a localized furuncle or as a diffuse infection of the entire canal (acute diffuse external otitis). The latter is often called swimmer's ear; the combination of water in the canal and use of cotton swabs is the major risk factor. Malignant external otitis (see p. 808) is a severe *Pseudomonas* osteomyelitis of the temporal bone, usually affecting the elderly, diabetics, and immunocompromised patients.

Etiology

Acute diffuse external otitis is usually caused by bacteria, such as *Pseudomonas aeruginosa, Proteus vulgaris, Staphylococcus aureus,* or *Escherichia coli.* Fungal external otitis (otomycosis), typically caused by *Aspergillus niger* or *Candida albicans,* is less common. Furuncles usually are caused by *S. aureus* (and by methicillin-resistant *S. aureus* in recent years).

Predisposing conditions include

- Inadvertent injury to the canal caused by cleaning with cotton swabs or other objects
- Allergies
- Psoriasis
- Eczema
- Seborrheic dermatitis
- Decreased canal acidity (possibly due to the repeated presence of water)
- Irritants (eg, hair spray, hair dye)

Attempts to clean the ear canal with cotton swabs can cause microabrasions of the delicate skin of the ear canal (which act as portals of entry for bacteria) and may push debris and cerumen deeper into the canal. These accumulated substances tend to trap water, resulting in skin maceration that sets the stage for bacterial infection.

Symptoms and Signs

Patients have pain and drainage. Sometimes, a foul-smelling discharge and hearing loss occur if the canal becomes swollen or filled with purulent debris. Exquisite tenderness accompanies traction of the pinna or pressure over the tragus. Otoscopic examination is painful and difficult to conduct. It shows the ear canal to be red, swollen, and littered with moist, purulent debris.

Otomycosis is more pruritic than painful, and patients also complain of aural fullness. Otomycosis caused by *A. niger* usually manifests with grayish black or yellow dots (fungal conidiophores) surrounded by a cottonlike material (fungal hyphae). Infection caused by *C. albicans* does not show any visible fungi but usually contains a thickened, creamy white exudate.

Furuncles cause severe pain and may drain sanguineous, purulent material. They appear as a focal, erythematous swelling (pimple).

Diagnosis

- Clinical evaluation

Diagnosis is based on inspection. When discharge is copious, external otitis can be difficult to differentiate from an acute, purulent otitis media with tympanic membrane perforation; pain elicited by pulling on the pinna may indicate an external otitis. Fungal infection is diagnosed by appearance or culture.

Treatment

- Debridement
- Topical acetic acid and corticosteroids
- Sometimes topical antibiotics

In **mild and moderate acute external otitis,** topical antibiotics and corticosteroids are effective. First, the infected debris should be gently and thoroughly removed from the canal with suction or dry cotton swabs under adequate lighting. Water irrigation of the canal is discouraged.

Mild external otitis can be treated by altering the ear canal's pH with 2% acetic acid and by relieving inflammation with topical hydrocortisone; these are given as 5 drops tid for 7 days.

Moderate external otitis requires the addition of an antibacterial solution or suspension, such as neomycin/polymyxin, ciprofloxacin, or ofloxacin. When inflammation of the ear canal is relatively severe, an ear wick should be placed into the ear canal and wetted with Burow solution (5% aluminum acetate) or a topical antibiotic 4 times/day. The wick helps direct the drops deeper into the external canal when the canal is greatly swollen. The wick is left in place for 24 to 72 h (or may fall out on its own), after which time the swelling may have receded enough to allow the instillation of drops directly into the canal.

Severe external otitis or the presence of cellulitis extending beyond the ear canal may require systemic antibiotics, such as cephalexin 500 mg po qid for 10 days or ciprofloxacin 500 mg po bid for 10 days. An analgesic, such as an NSAID or even an oral opioid, may be necessary for the first 24 to 48 h.

Fungal external otitis requires thorough cleaning of the ear canal and application of an antimycotic solution (eg, gentian violet, cresylate acetate, nystatin, clotrimazole, or even a combination of acetic acid and isopropyl alcohol). However, these solutions should not be used if the tympanic membrane is perforated because they can cause severe pain or damage to the inner ear. Repeated cleanings and treatments may be needed.

Dry ear precautions (eg, wearing shower cap, avoiding swimming) are strongly advised for both external otitis and fungal external otitis.

A furuncle, if obviously pointing, should be incised and drained. Incision is of little value, however, if the patient is seen at an early stage. Topical antibiotics are ineffective; oral antistaphylococcal antibiotics should be given. Analgesics, such as oxycodone with acetaminophen, may be necessary for pain relief. Dry heat can also lessen pain and hasten resolution.

PEARLS & PITFALLS

- Applying a few drops of a 1:1 mixture of rubbing alcohol and vinegar (as long as the eardrum is intact) immediately after swimming can help prevent swimmer's ear (and is also an excellent treatment for otomycosis).

Prevention

External otitis often can be prevented by applying a few drops of a 1:1 mixture of rubbing alcohol and vinegar (as long as the eardrum is intact) immediately after swimming. The alcohol helps remove water, and the vinegar alters the pH of the canal. Use of cotton swabs or other implements in the canal should be strongly discouraged.

KEY POINTS

- Acute external otitis is usually bacterial (pseudomonal); fungal causes are less likely and cause more itching and less pain.
- Severe pain with pulling on the pinna suggests acute external otitis.
- Under close and direct visualization, gently remove infected debris from the canal with suction or dry cotton swabs.
- Do not irrigate the ear.
- For mild cases, apply acetic acid and hydrocortisone drops.
- For more severe cases, debridement is critical along with topical antibiotics (use a wick if the canal is swollen); sometimes give systemic antibiotics.

MALIGNANT EXTERNAL OTITIS

(Necrotizing Otitis Externa; Skull Base Osteomyelitis)

Malignant external otitis, also referred to as skull base osteomyelitis or necrotizing otitis externa, is typically a *Pseudomonas* osteomyelitis of the temporal bone. Methicillin-resistant *Staphylococcus aureus* (MRSA) has also been reported as a cause.

Soft tissue, cartilage, and bone are all affected. The osteomyelitis spreads along the base of the skull and may cause cranial neuropathies (VII usually affected first followed by IX, X, and XI) and may cross the midline.

Malignant external otitis occurs mainly in elderly patients with diabetes or in immunocompromised patients. It is often initiated by *Pseudomonas* external otitis; methicillin-resistant *Staphylococcus aureus* (MRSA) has also been identified as a cause. It is characterized by persistent and severe, deep-seated ear pain (often worse at night), foul-smelling purulent otorrhea, and granulation tissue or exposed bone in the ear canal (usually at the junction of the bony and cartilaginous portions of the canal). Varying degrees of conductive hearing loss may occur. In severe cases, facial nerve paralysis, and even lower cranial nerve (IX, X, or XI) paralysis, may ensue as this erosive, potentially life-threatening infection spreads along the skull base (skull base osteomyelitis) from the stylomastoid foramen to the jugular foramen and beyond.

Diagnosis

- CT scan of the temporal bone

Diagnosis is based on a high-resolution CT scan of the temporal bone, which may show increased radiodensity in the mastoid air-cell system and middle ear radiolucency (demineralization) in some areas. Identifying bony erosion confirms the diagnosis. Cultures are done, and, importantly, the ear canal must be biopsied to differentiate this disorder from a malignant tumor.

Treatment

- Systemic antibiotics, typically a fluoroquinolone and/or an aminoglycoside/semisynthetic penicillin combination
- Topical antibiotic/steroid preparations (eg, ciprofloxacin/dexamethasone)
- Rarely, surgical debridement

Treatment is typically with a 6-wk IV course of a culture-directed fluoroquinolone (eg, ciprofloxacin, 400 mg IV q 8 h) and/or a semisynthetic penicillin (piperacillin–tazobactam or piperacillin)/aminoglycoside combination (for ciprofloxacin resistant *Pseudomonas*). However, mild cases may be treated with a high-dose oral fluoroquinolone (eg, ciprofloxacin, 750 mg po q 12 h) on an outpatient basis with close follow-up. Treatment also includes topical ciprofloxacin/dexamethasone preparations (eg, ear drops, impregnated canal dressings). Hyperbaric oxygen may be a useful adjunctive treatment, but its definitive role remains to be elucidated. Consultation with an infectious disease specialist for optimal antibiotic therapy and duration and with an endocrinologist for strict diabetic control is recommended. Extensive bone disease may require more prolonged antibiotic therapy. Meticulous control of diabetes is essential. Frequent office debridement is necessary to remove granulation tissue and purulent discharge. Surgery usually is not necessary, but surgical debridement may be used for more extensive infections.

PERICHONDRITIS OF THE EAR

Perichondritis of the ear can be a diffuse inflammatory, but not necessarily infectious, process resulting in diffuse swelling, redness, and pain of the pinna, or an abscess between the cartilage and the perichondrium.

Causes of perichondritis include

- Trauma
- Insect bites
- Ear piercings through the cartilage
- Systemic inflammatory conditions (eg, vasculitides such as granulomatosis with polyangiitis, relapsing polychondritis)
- Incision of superficial infections of the pinna

Because the cartilage's blood supply is provided by the perichondrium, separation of the perichondrium from both sides of the cartilage may lead to avascular necrosis and a deformed pinna (called cauliflower ear) in a matter of weeks. Septic necrosis may also ensue, often with infection by gram-negative bacilli.

Symptoms include redness, pain, and swelling. The course of perichondritis can be indolent, recurrent, long-term, and destructive.

Treatment

- Prompt oral antibiotic therapy, typically a fluoroquinolone, sometimes with an aminoglycoside plus a semisynthetic penicillin
- For an abscess, prompt incision and drainage

Patients with diffuse inflammation of the entire pinna are given empiric antibiotics (eg, fluoroquinolones, which have good cartilage penetration) and often a systemic corticosteroid for its anti-inflammatory effects. Any foreign material (eg, ring, splinter) should be removed. If the etiology is not clearly infectious (eg, an infected piercing), patients should be evaluated for an inflammatory disorder.

Perichondrial abscesses are incised, and a drain is left in place for 24 to 72 h. Systemic antibiotics are initiated with a fluoroquinolone or an aminoglycoside plus a semisynthetic penicillin. Subsequent antibiotic choice is guided by culture and sensitivity. Warm compresses may help. It is important to ensure that the perichondrium is reapproximated to the cartilage to maintain the blood supply to the cartilage and prevent necrosis. Reapproximation is ensured by inserting 1 or 2 mattress sutures through the entire thickness of the pinna, preferably through dental rolls on both sides of the pinna.[1]

1. Kesser BW: Assessment and management of chronic otitis externa. *Curr Opin Otolaryngol Head Neck Surg* 19(5):341–347. 2011.

94 Hearing Loss

More than 10% of people in the US have some degree of hearing loss that compromises their daily communication, making it the most common sensory disorder. About 1/800 to 1/1000 neonates are born with severe to profound hearing loss. Two to 3 times as many are born with lesser hearing loss. During childhood, another 2 to 3/1000 children acquire moderate to severe hearing loss. Adolescents are at risk from excessive exposure to noise, head trauma, or both. Older adults typically experience a progressive decrease in hearing (presbycusis—see p. 816), which is directly related to a combination of aging, noise exposure, and genetic factors. It is estimated that about 30 million people in the US are exposed to injurious levels of noise on a daily basis.

Hearing deficits in early childhood can result in lifelong impairments in receptive and expressive language skills. The severity of the handicap is determined by

- The age at which the hearing loss occurred
- The nature of the loss (its duration, the frequencies affected, and the degree)
- The susceptibilities of the individual child (eg, coexisting visual impairment, intellectual disability, primary language deficits, inadequate linguistic environment)

Children who have other sensory, linguistic, or cognitive deficiencies are affected most severely.

Pathophysiology

Hearing loss can be classified as conductive, sensorineural, or both (mixed loss).

Conductive hearing loss occurs secondary to lesions in the external auditory canal, tympanic membrane (TM), or middle ear. These lesions prevent sound from being effectively conducted to the inner ear.

Sensorineural hearing loss is caused by lesions of either the inner ear (sensory) or the auditory (8th) nerve (neural—see Table 94–1). This distinction is important because sensory hearing loss is sometimes reversible and is seldom life threatening. A neural hearing loss is rarely recoverable and may be due to a potentially life-threatening brain tumor—commonly a cerebellopontine angle tumor.

Mixed loss may be caused by severe head injury with or without fracture of the skull or temporal bone, by chronic infection, or by one of many genetic disorders. It may also occur when a transient conductive hearing loss, commonly due to otitis media, is superimposed on a sensorineural hearing loss.

Etiology

Hearing loss can be congenital (see Table 94–2) or acquired (see Table 94–3), progressive or sudden (see p. 817), temporary or permanent, unilateral or bilateral, and mild or profound. Drug-induced ototoxicity is discussed elsewhere (see p. 821).

The **most common causes** overall are the following:

- Cerumen accumulation
- Noise
- Aging
- Infections (particularly among children and young adults)

Cerumen (earwax) accumulation is the most common cause of treatable conductive hearing loss, especially in the elderly. Foreign bodies obstructing the canal are sometimes a problem in children, both because of their presence and because of any damage inadvertently caused during their removal.

Noise can cause sudden or gradual sensorineural hearing loss. In acoustic trauma, hearing loss results from exposure to a single, extreme noise (eg, a nearby gunshot or explosion);

Table 94–1. DIFFERENCES BETWEEN SENSORY AND NEURAL HEARING LOSSES

TEST	SENSORY HEARING LOSS	NEURAL HEARING LOSS
Speech discrimination	Moderate decrement	Severe decrement
Discrimination with increasing sound intensity	Usually improves up to a point, depending on the severity and distribution of loss of sensory elements	Deteriorates
Recruitment in which the perception of sound is exaggerated, especially at high sound levels	Present	Absent
Acoustic reflex decay in which the acoustic reflex response is reduced over time during a measurement	Absent or mild	Present
Waveforms in auditory brain stem responses	Well formed with normal latencies for mild to moderate hearing losses; reduced for more severe losses	Absent or with abnormally long latencies
Otoacoustic emissions	Present	

Table 94–2. CONGENITAL CAUSES OF HEARING LOSS*

ANATOMIC AREA AFFECTED	ETIOLOGY†
Conductive	
External and middle ear	Genetic Developmental (eg, ossicular fixation) Idiopathic malformation Drug-induced malformation (eg, with thalidomide)
Sensory	
Inner ear	Genetic Idiopathic malformation Congenital infection (eg, rubella, cytomegalovirus infection, toxoplasmosis, syphilis) Rh incompatibility Anoxia Maternal ingestion of ototoxic drugs (eg, for TB or severe infection) Drug-induced malformation (eg, with thalidomide)
Neural	
CNS	Anoxia Idiopathic (unknown) malformation Genetic Congenital infection (eg, rubella, cytomegalovirus infection, toxoplasmosis, syphilis) Neurofibromatosis (type 2) Hyperbilirubinemia

*A number of congenital hearing losses may be mixed losses—a combination of conductive and sensory with or without a neural component.

†Causes are listed in approximate order of greatest frequency first.

some patients develop tinnitus as well. The loss is usually temporary (unless there is also blast damage, which may destroy the TM, ossicles, or both). In noise-induced hearing loss, the loss develops over time because of chronic exposure to noise > 85 decibels (dB—see Sidebar 94–1). Although people vary somewhat in susceptibility to noise-induced hearing loss, nearly everyone loses some hearing if they are exposed to sufficiently intense noise for an adequate time. Repeated exposure to loud noise ultimately results in loss of hair cells in the organ of Corti. Hearing loss typically occurs first at 4 kHz and gradually spreads to the lower and higher frequencies as exposure continues. In contrast to most other causes of sensorineural hearing losses, noise-induced hearing loss may be less severe at 8 kHz than at 4 kHz.

Aging, together with noise exposure and genetic factors, is a common risk factor for progressive decrease in hearing. Age-related hearing loss is termed presbycusis. Presbycusis is due to a combination of sensory cell (hair cell) and neuronal loss. Research also strongly suggests that early noise exposure accelerates age-related hearing loss. Higher frequencies are more affected than lower frequencies in age-related hearing loss.

Acute otitis media (AOM—see p. 830) is a common cause of transient mild to moderate hearing loss (mainly in children). However, without treatment, AOM sequelae and chronic otitis media (and the rarer purulent labyrinthitis) can cause permanent loss, particularly if a cholesteatoma forms.

Secretory otitis media (SOM—see p. 832) occurs in several ways. Almost all episodes of AOM are followed by a period of 2 to 4 wk of SOM. SOM can also be caused by eustachian tube dysfunction (eg, resulting from cleft palate, benign or malignant tumors of the nasopharynx, or rapid changes in external air pressure as occur during descent from high altitudes or rapid ascent while scuba diving).

Autoimmune disorders can cause sensorineural hearing loss at all ages and can cause other symptoms and signs as well.

Evaluation

Evaluation consists of detecting and quantifying hearing loss and determining etiology (particularly reversible causes).

Screening: Most adults and older children notice a sudden hearing loss, and caregivers may suspect that a neonate has a severe hearing loss within the first weeks of life when the neonate does not respond to voices or other sounds. However, progressive losses and nearly all losses in infants and young children must be detected by screening. Screening should begin at birth (see p. 2431) so that linguistic input can allow optimal language development.

Suspected hearing loss at any time should prompt referral to a specialist. If screening is not done, severe bilateral losses may not be recognized until age 2 yr, and mild to moderate or severe unilateral losses are often not recognized until children reach school age.

History: History of present illness should note how long hearing loss has been perceived, how it began (eg, gradual, acute), whether it is unilateral or bilateral, and whether sound is distorted (eg, music is off—dull or lifeless) or there is difficulty with speech discrimination. The patient should be asked whether the loss followed any acute event (eg, head injury, loud noise exposure, barotrauma [particularly a diving injury], or starting of a drug). Important accompanying symptoms include other otologic symptoms (eg, ear pain, tinnitus, ear discharge), vestibular symptoms (eg, disorientation in the dark, vertigo), and other neurologic symptoms (eg, headache, weakness or asymmetry of the face, an abnormal sense of taste, fullness of the ear). In children, important associated symptoms include presence of delays in speech or language development, visual changes, or delayed motor development.

Review of systems should seek to determine the impact of hearing difficulty on the patient's life.

Past medical history should note previous possibly causative disorders, including CNS infection, repeated ear infections, chronic exposure to loud noise, head trauma, rheumatic disorders (eg, RA, lupus), and a family history of hearing loss. Drug history should specifically query current or previous use of ototoxic drugs (see p. 821). For young children, a birth history should be sought to determine if there were any intrauterine infections or birth complications.

Physical examination: The focus is examination of the ears and hearing and the neurologic examination. The external ear is inspected for obstruction, infection, congenital malformations, and other lesions. The TM is examined for perforation, drainage, otitis media (pus seen in the middle ear through the TM), and cholesteatoma. During the neurologic examination, particular attention needs to be paid to the 2nd through 7th cranial nerves as well as to vestibular and cerebellar function because abnormalities in these areas often occur with tumors of the brain stem and cerebellopontine angle. The Weber and Rinne tests require a tuning fork to differentiate conductive from sensorineural hearing loss.

Table 94–3. SOME CAUSES OF ACQUIRED HEARING LOSS

CAUSE*	SUGGESTIVE FINDINGS	DIAGNOSTIC APPROACH†
External ear (conductive loss)		
Obstruction (eg, caused by cerumen, a foreign body, otitis externa, or, rarely, tumor)	Visible during examination	Otoscopy Clinical evaluation
Middle ear (conductive loss)		
Otitis media (secretory)	Hearing loss that may fluctuate Sometimes also dizziness, pain, or fullness in the ear Usually abnormal-looking TM Often a history of acute otitis media or other causative event	Otoscopy Audiologic testing with tympanogram
Otitis media (chronic)‡	Chronic ear discharge Usually visible perforation Granulation tissue or polyp in the canal Sometimes cholesteatoma	Otoscopy For cholesteatoma, CT or MRI
Ear trauma‡	Apparent by history Often visible perforation of the TM, blood in the canal or behind the TM (if intact)	Otoscopy Clinical evaluation
Otosclerosis‡	Family history Age at onset in 20's to 30's Slowly progressive	Audiogram, tympanogram, and otoscopy
Tumors (benign and malignant)	Unilateral loss Often lesion visible during otoscopy	CT or MRI
Inner ear (sensory loss)		
Genetic disorders (eg, connexin 26 mutation, Waardenburg syndrome, Usher syndrome, Pendred syndrome)	Sometimes a positive family history (but usually negative) Connexin 26 mutations account for the vast majority of non-syndromic hearing loss cases and should be screened for initially Sometimes a white forelock of hair or different colored eyes suggests Waardenburg syndrome Loss of both vision and hearing can suggest Usher syndrome	Clinical evaluation Genetic testing CT and/or MRI
Noise exposure	Usually apparent by history	Clinical evaluation
Presbycusis	> 55 yr in men, > 65 yr in women Progressive, bilateral loss Normal neurologic examination	Clinical evaluation
Ototoxic drugs (eg, aspirin, aminoglycosides, vancomycin, cisplatinum, furosemide, ethacrynic acid, quinine)	History of use Bilateral loss Variable vestibular symptoms Renal failure	Clinical evaluation
Infections (eg,meningitis, purulent labyrinthitis)	Obvious history of infection Symptoms that begin during or shortly after an infection	Clinical evaluation
Autoimmune disorders (eg, RA, SLE)	Joint inflammation, rash Sometimes a sudden change in vision or eye irritation Pain or swelling in cartilage Often known history of the disorder	Serologic testing
Meniere syndrome	Episodes of unilateral, fluctuating hearing loss accompanied by aural fullness, tinnitus, and vertigo	Gadolinium-enhanced MRI to rule out tumor
Barotrauma (with perilymphatic fistula)‡	History of abrupt pressure change (eg, scuba diving, rapid descent in airplane) or a blow to the ear canal Sometimes severe ear pain or vertigo	Tympanometry and balance function tests Surgical exploration if vertigo persists

Table continues on the following page.

Table 94–3. SOME CAUSES OF ACQUIRED HEARING LOSS (*Continued*)

CAUSE*	SUGGESTIVE FINDINGS	DIAGNOSTIC APPROACH†
Head trauma (with basilar skull fracture or cochlear concussion)‡	History of significant injury Possibly vestibular symptoms, facial weakness Sometimes blood behind the TM, CSF leak, ecchymosis over the mastoid	CT or MRI
CNS (neural loss)		
Tumors of the cerebellopontine angle (eg, acoustic neuroma, meningioma)	Unilateral hearing loss, often with tinnitus Vestibular abnormalities Sometimes facial or trigeminal nerve deficits	Gadolinium-enhanced MRI
Demyelinating disease (eg, multiple sclerosis)	Unilateral loss Multifocal Waxing and waning symptoms	MRI of the brain Sometimes lumbar puncture

*Each group is listed in approximate order of frequency.
†All patients should have otoscopy and audiologic testing.
‡Mixed conductive and sensorineural loss may also be present.
TM = tympanic membrane.

In the **Weber test,** the stem of a vibrating 512-Hz or 1024-Hz tuning fork is placed on the midline of the head, and the patient indicates in which ear the tone is louder. In unilateral conductive hearing loss, the tone is louder in the ear with hearing loss. In unilateral sensorineural hearing loss, the tone is louder in the normal ear because the tuning fork stimulates both inner ears equally and the patient perceives the stimulus with the unaffected ear.

In the **Rinne test,** hearing by bone and by air conduction is compared. Bone conduction bypasses the external and middle ear and tests the integrity of the inner ear, 8th cranial nerve, and central auditory pathways. The stem of a vibrating tuning fork is held against the mastoid (for bone conduction); as soon as the sound is no longer perceived, the fork is removed from the mastoid, and the still-vibrating tines are held close to the pinna

Sidebar 94–1. Sound Levels

Sound intensity and pressure (the physical correlates of loudness) are measured in decibels (dB). A dB is a unitless figure that compares 2 values and is defined as the logarithm of the ratio of a measured value to a reference value, multiplied by a constant:

$$dB = k \log (V_{measured}/V_{ref})$$

By convention, the reference value for sound pressure level (SPL) is taken as the quietest 1000-Hz sound detectable by young, healthy human ears.* The sound may be measured in terms of pressure (N/m^2) or intensity ($watts/m^2$).

Because sound intensity equals the square of sound pressure, the constant (k) for SPL is 20; for sound intensity, 10. Thus, each 20-dB increase represents a 10-fold increase in SPL but a 100-fold increase in sound intensity.

The dB values in the table below give only a rough idea of the risk of hearing loss. Some of them are dB SPL values (referenced to N/m^2), whereas others represent peak dB or dB on the A-scale (a scale that emphasizes the frequencies that are most hazardous to human hearing).

dB	Example
0	Faintest sound heard by human ear
30	Whisper, quiet library
60	Normal conversation, sewing machine, typewriter
90	Lawnmower, shop tools, truck traffic (90 dB for 8 h/day is the maximum exposure without protection†)
100	Chain saw, pneumatic drill, snowmobile (2 h/day is the maximum exposure without protection)
115	Sandblasting, loud rock concert, automobile horn (15 min/day is the maximum exposure without protection)
140	Gun muzzle blast, jet engine (noise causes pain and even brief exposure injures unprotected ears; injury may occur even with hearing protectors)
180	Rocket launching pad

*In audiometric testing, because human ears respond differently at different frequencies, the reference value changes for each frequency tested. Threshold values reported on audiograms take this into account; the normal threshold is always 0 dB, regardless of the actual sound pressure level (SPL).

†This is the mandatory federal standard, but protection is recommended for more than brief exposure to sound levels > 85 dB.

(for air conduction). Normally, the fork can once more be heard, indicating that air conduction is better than bone conduction. With conductive hearing loss, the relationship is reversed; bone conduction is louder than air conduction. With sensorineural hearing loss, both air and bone conduction are reduced, but air conduction remains louder.

Red flags: Findings of particular concern are

- Unilateral sensorineural hearing loss
- Abnormalities of cranial nerves (other than hearing loss)
- Rapidly worsening hearing loss

Interpretation of findings: Many causes of hearing loss (eg, cerumen, injury, significant noise exposure, infectious sequelae, drugs) are readily apparent based on results of the history and examination (see Table 94–3).

Associated findings are helpful in diagnosing the remaining small number of patients in whom no clear cause can be found. Patients who have focal neurologic abnormalities are of particular concern. The 5th or 7th cranial nerve or both are often affected by tumors that involve the 8th nerve, so loss of facial sensation and weak jaw clench (5th) and hemifacial weakness and taste abnormalities (7th) point to a lesion in that area. Signs of autoimmune disorders (eg, joint swelling or pain, eye inflammation) or renal dysfunction may suggest these disorders as a cause. Maxillofacial malformations may suggest a genetic or developmental abnormality.

Any child with delays in speech or language development or difficulty in school should be evaluated for hearing loss. Intellectual disability, aphasia, and autism must also be considered. Delayed motor development may signal vestibular deficit, which is often associated with a sensorineural hearing loss.

Testing: Testing includes

- Audiologic tests
- Sometimes MRI or CT

Audiologic tests are required for all people who have hearing loss; these tests usually include

- Measurement of pure-tone thresholds with air and bone conduction
- Speech reception threshold
- Speech discrimination
- Tympanometry
- Acoustic reflex testing

Information gained from these tests helps determine whether more definitive differentiation of sensory from neural hearing loss is needed.

Pure-tone audiometry quantifies hearing loss. An audiometer delivers sounds of specific frequencies (pure tones) at different intensities to determine the patient's hearing threshold (how loud a sound must be to be perceived) for each frequency. Hearing in each ear is tested from 125 or 250 to 8000 Hz by air conduction (using earphones) and up to 4 kHz by bone conduction (using an oscillator in contact with the mastoid process or forehead). Test results are plotted on graphs called audiograms (see Fig. 94–1), which show the difference between the patient's hearing threshold and normal hearing at each frequency. The difference is measured in dB (see Sidebar 94–1). The normal threshold is considered 0 dB hearing level (Hl); hearing loss is considered present if the patient's threshold is > 25 dB Hl. When hearing loss is such as to require loud test tones, intense tones presented to one ear may be heard in the other ear. In such cases, a masking sound, usually narrow band noise, is presented to the ear not being tested to isolate it.

Speech audiometry includes the speech reception threshold (SRT) and the word recognition score. The SRT is a measure of the intensity at which speech is recognized. To determine the SRT, the examiner presents the patient with a list of words at specific sound intensities. These words usually have 2 equally accented syllables (spondees), such as "railroad," "staircase," and "baseball." The examiner notes the intensity at which the patient repeats 50% of the words correctly. The SRT approximates the average hearing level at speech frequencies (eg, 500 Hz, 1000 Hz, 2000 Hz).

The **word recognition score** tests the ability to discriminate among the various speech sounds or phonemes. It is determined by presenting 50 phonetically balanced one-syllable words at an intensity of 35 to 40 dB above the patient's SRT. The word list contains phonemes in the same relative frequency found in conversational English. The score is the percentage of words correctly repeated by the patient and reflects the ability to understand speech under optimal listening conditions. A normal score ranges from 90 to 100%. The word recognition score is normal with conductive hearing loss, albeit at a higher intensity level, but can be reduced at all intensity levels with sensorineural hearing loss. Discrimination is even poorer in neural than in sensory hearing loss. Testing of words understood within full sentences is another type of recognition test that is often used to assess candidacy for implantable devices (when the benefit from hearing aids is insufficient).

Tympanometry measures the impedance of the middle ear to acoustic energy and does not require patient participation. It is commonly used to screen children for middle ear effusions. A probe containing a sound source, microphone, and air pressure regulator is placed snugly with an airtight seal into the ear canal. The probe microphone records the reflected sound from the TM while pressure in the canal is varied. Normally, maximal compliance of the middle ear occurs when the pressure in the ear canal equals atmospheric pressure. Abnormal compliance patterns suggest specific anatomic disruptions. In eustachian tube obstruction and middle ear effusion, maximal compliance occurs with a negative pressure in the ear canal. When the ossicular chain is disrupted, as in necrosis or dislocation of the long process of the incus, the middle ear is excessively compliant. When the ossicular chain is fixed, as in stapedial ankylosis in otosclerosis, compliance may be normal or reduced.

The **acoustic reflex** is contraction of the stapedius muscle in response to loud sounds, which changes the compliance of the TM, protecting the middle ear from acoustic trauma. The reflex is tested by presenting a tone and measuring what intensity provokes a change in middle ear impedance as noted by movement of the TM. An absent reflex could indicate middle ear disease or a tumor of the auditory nerve. Any conductive hearing loss abolishes the acoustic reflex. Additionally, facial paralysis abolishes the reflex because the facial nerve innervates the stapedius muscle.

Advanced testing is sometimes needed. Gadolinium-enhanced MRI of the head to detect lesions of the cerebellopontine angle may be needed in patients with an abnormal neurologic examination or those whose audiologic testing shows poor word recognition, asymmetric sensorineural hearing loss, or a combination when the etiology is not clear.

CT is done if bony tumors or bony erosion is suspected. Magnetic resonance angiography is done if vascular abnormalities such as glomus tumors are suspected.

The **auditory brain stem response** uses surface electrodes to monitor brain wave response to acoustic stimulation in people who cannot otherwise respond.

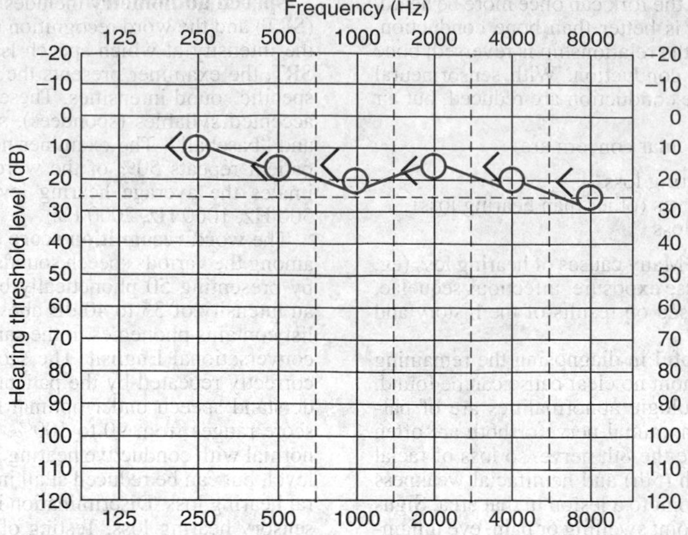

Fig. 94–1. Audiogram of right ear in a patient with normal hearing. Normal audiogram of the right ear. The vertical lines represent the frequencies that are tested from 125 to 8000 Hz. The horizontal lines record the threshold at which the patient states that the sound is heard. Normal thresholds are 0 dB +/– 10 dB. Patients with a hearing threshold below 20 dB are considered to have average or better-than-average hearing. The greater the dB, the louder is the sound and the worse the hearing. "O" is the standard symbol for air conduction of the right ear; "X" is the standard symbol for air conduction for the left ear. The "<" is the standard symbol for unmasked bone conduction for the right ear; ">" is the standard symbol for unmasked bone conduction of the left ear. The reason why both masked and unmasked measures are needed is to make sure one ear is not hearing the sound presented to the other ear (one ear is 'masked' so it does not hear the sound presented to the other ear, giving a false value).

Electrocochleography measures the activity of the cochlea and the auditory nerve with an electrode placed on or through the eardrum. It can be used to assess and monitor patients with dizziness, can be used in patients who are awake, and is useful in intraoperative monitoring.

Otoacoustic emissions testing measures sounds produced by outer hair cells of the cochlea in response to a sound stimulus usually placed in the ear canal. These emissions are essentially low-intensity echoes that occur with cochlear outer hair cell activation. Emissions are used to screen neonates and infants for hearing loss and to monitor the hearing of patients who are using ototoxic drugs (eg, gentamicin, cisplatin).

Central auditory evaluation measures discrimination of degraded or distorted speech, discrimination in the presence of a competing message in the opposite ear, the ability to fuse incomplete or partial messages delivered to each ear into a meaningful message, and the capacity to localize sound in space when acoustic stimuli are delivered simultaneously to both ears. This testing should be done on certain patients, such as children with a reading or other learning problem and elderly people who seem to hear but do not comprehend.

In children with hearing loss, additional testing should include an ophthalmologic examination because many genetic causes of deafness also cause ocular abnormalities. Children with unexplained hearing loss should also have an ECG to look for long QT syndrome and possibly also genetic testing.

Treatment

The causes of a hearing loss should be determined and treated. Ototoxic drugs should be stopped or the dose should be lowered unless the severity of the disease being treated (usually cancer or a severe infection) requires that the risk of additional ototoxic hearing loss be accepted. Attention to peak and trough drug levels may help minimize risk. There are some genetic abnormalities involving the mitochondria that increase the sensitivity to aminoglycoside antibiotics, and these can be identified with genetic screening.

Fluid from middle ear effusion can be drained by myringotomy and prevented from reaccumulating with the insertion of a tympanostomy tube. Benign growths (eg, enlarged adenoids, nasal polyps) and malignant tumors (eg, nasopharyngeal cancers, sinus cancers) blocking the eustachian tube or ear canal can be removed. Hearing loss caused by autoimmune disorders may respond to corticosteroids.

Damage to the TM or ossicles or otosclerosis may require reconstructive surgery. Brain tumors causing hearing loss may in some cases be removed or radiated and hearing preserved.

Many causes of hearing loss have no cure, and treatment involves compensating for the hearing loss with hearing aids and, for severe to profound loss, a cochlear implant. In addition, various coping mechanisms may help.

Hearing aids: Amplification of sound with a hearing aid helps many people. Although hearing aids do not restore hearing to normal, they can significantly improve communication. Advances in amplification circuits provide a more natural, tonal quality to amplified sound and offer features of "smart," responsive amplification that takes into account the listening environment (eg, in noise-challenging and multi-talker environments). Physicians should encourage hearing aid use and help patients overcome a sense of social stigma that continues to obstruct use of these devices, perhaps by making the analogy that a hearing aid is to hearing as eye glasses are to seeing. Other factors that limit more widespread hearing aid use include cost, comfort issues, and for some, the social stigma of wearing a hearing aid.

All hearing aids have a microphone, amplifier, speaker, earpiece, and volume control, although they differ in the location of these components. An audiologist should be involved in selection and fitting of a hearing aid.

The best models are adjusted to a person's particular pattern of hearing loss. People with mainly high-frequency hearing loss do not benefit from simple amplification, which merely makes the garbled speech they hear sound louder. They usually need a hearing aid that selectively amplifies the high frequencies. Some hearing aids contain vents in the ear mold, which facilitate the passage of high-frequency sound waves. Some use digital sound processing with multiple frequency channels so that amplification more precisely matches hearing loss as measured on the audiogram.

Telephone use can be difficult for people with hearing aids. Typical hearing aids cause squealing when the ear is placed next to the phone handle. Some hearing aids have a phone coil with a switch that turns the microphone off and links the phone coil electromagnetically to the speaker magnet in the phone.

For moderate to severe hearing loss, a postauricular (ear-level) aid, which fits behind the pinna and is coupled to the ear mold with flexible tubing, is appropriate. An in-the-ear aid is contained entirely within the ear mold and fits less conspicuously into the concha and ear canal; it is appropriate for mild to moderate hearing loss. Some people with mild hearing loss limited to high frequencies are most comfortably fitted with postauricular aids and completely open ear canals. Canal aids are contained entirely within the ear canal and are cosmetically acceptable to many people who would otherwise refuse to use a hearing aid, but they are difficult for some people (especially the elderly) to manipulate.

The CROS aid (contralateral routing of signals) is occasionally used for severe unilateral hearing loss; a hearing-aid microphone is placed in the nonfunctioning ear, and sound is routed to the functioning ear through a wire or radio transmitter. This device enables the wearer to hear sounds from the nonfunctioning side, allowing for some limited capacity to localize sound. If the better ear also has some hearing loss, the sound from both sides can be amplified with the binaural CROS (BiCROS) aid. The body aid type is appropriate for profound hearing loss. It is worn in a shirt pocket or a body harness and connected by a wire to the earpiece (the receiver), which is coupled to the ear canal by a plastic insert (ear mold).

A bone conduction aid may be used when an ear mold or tube cannot be used, as in atresia of the ear canal or persistent otorrhea. An oscillator is held against the head, usually over the mastoid, with a spring band, and sound is conducted through the skull to the cochlea. Bone conduction hearing aids require more power, introduce more distortion, and are less comfortable to wear than air conduction hearing aids. Some bone conduction aids (bone-anchored hearing aids or BAHAs) are surgically implanted in the mastoid process, avoiding the discomfort and prominence of the spring band.

Cochlear implants: Patients with advanced levels of hearing loss, including those with some hearing but who even with a hearing aid cannot understand more than half of the words contained in connected speech, may benefit from a cochlear implant.

This device provides electrical signals directly into the auditory nerve via multiple electrodes implanted in the cochlea. An external microphone and processor convert sound waves to electrical impulses, which are transmitted through the skin electromagnetically from an external induction coil to an internal coil implanted in the skull above and behind the ear. The internal coil connects to electrodes inserted in the scala tympani.

Cochlear implants help with speech-reading by providing information about the intonation of words and the rhythm of speech. Many if not most adults with cochlear implants can discriminate words without visual clues, allowing them to talk on the telephone. Cochlear implants enable deaf people to hear and distinguish environmental sounds and warning signals. They also help deaf people modulate their voice and make their speech more intelligible.

Outcomes with cochlear implants vary, depending on a number of factors, including the

- Length of time between onset of hearing loss and placement of the implant (shorter duration leads to better outcomes)
- Cause of the underlying hearing loss
- Position of the implant within the cochlea

Brain stem implants: Patients who have had both acoustic nerves destroyed (eg, by bilateral temporal bone fractures or neurofibromatosis) or are born without cochlear nerves can have some hearing restored by means of brain stem implants that have electrodes connected to sound-detecting and sound-processing devices similar to those used for cochlear implants.

Assistive strategies and technologies: Alerting systems that use light let people know when the doorbell is ringing, a smoke detector is sounding, or a baby is crying. Special sound systems transmitting infrared or FM radio signals help people hear in theaters, churches, or other places where competing noise exists. Many television programs carry closed captioning. Telephone communication devices are also available.

Lip-reading or speech-reading is particularly important for people who can hear but have trouble discriminating sounds. Most people get useful speech information from lip-reading even without formal training. Even people with normal hearing can better understand speech in a noisy place if they can see the speaker. To use this information the listener must be able to see the speaker's mouth. Health care personnel should be sensitive to this issue and always position themselves appropriately when speaking to the hearing-impaired. Observing the position of a speaker's lips allows recognition of the consonant being spoken, thereby improving speech comprehension in patients with high-frequency hearing loss. Lip-reading may be learned in aural rehabilitation sessions in which a group of age-matched peers meets regularly for instruction and supervised practice in optimizing communication.

People can gain control over their listening environment by modifying or avoiding difficult situations. For example, people can visit a restaurant during off-peak hours, when it is quieter. They can ask for a booth, which blocks out some extraneous sounds. In direct conversations, people may ask the speaker to face them. At the beginning of a telephone conversation, they can identify themselves as being hearing-impaired. At a conference, the speaker can be asked to use an assistive listening system, which makes use of either inductive loop, infrared, or FM technology that sends sound through the microphone to a patient's hearing aid.

People with profound hearing loss often communicate by using sign language. American Sign Language (ASL) is the most common version in the US. Other forms of linguistic communication that utilize visual inputs include Signed English, Signing Exact English, and Cued Speech.

Single-Sided Deafness

Patients with single-sided deafness (SSD) represent a special challenge. In one-on-one situations, hearing and speech understanding is relatively unaffected. However, with noisy backgrounds or complex acoustic environments (eg, classrooms, parties, meetings), patients with SSD are unable to hear and communicate effectively. Further, patients who hear out of only one ear are unable to localize the origin of sounds. The "head shadow" effect is the skull's ability to block sound coming from the deaf side from reaching the hearing ear. This can result in up to a 30 dB loss of sound energy reaching the hearing ear (as a comparison, a store-bought ear plug results in a 22 to 32 dB drop in hearing, roughly equivalent). For many patients, SSD can be life-altering and lead to significant disability at work and socially.

Treatment for SSD includes contralateral routing of signal (CROS) hearing aids or bone-anchored hearing implants that pick up sound from the deaf side and transfer it to the hearing ear without the loss of sound energy. Although these technologies improve hearing in noisy settings, they do not allow sound localization. Cochlear implants are increasingly being used with success in patients with SSD, particularly if the deaf ear also has severe tinnitus; implants have also been shown to provide sound localization.

Treatment of Hearing Loss in Children

In addition to treatment of any cause and the provision of hearing aids, children with hearing loss require support of language development with appropriate therapy. Because children must hear language to learn it spontaneously, most deaf children develop language only with special training, ideally beginning as soon as the hearing loss is identified (an exception would be a deaf child growing up with deaf parents who are fluent sign language users). Deaf infants must be provided with a form of language input. For example, a visually based sign language can provide a foundation for later development of oral language if a cochlear implant is not available. However, for children, there is no substitute for access to the sounds of speech (phonemes) to enable them to integrate acoustic inputs and develop a refined and nuanced understanding of speech and language.

If infants as young as 1 mo have profound bilateral hearing loss and cannot benefit from hearing aids, they can be candidates for a cochlear implant. Although cochlear implants allow auditory communication in many children with either congenital or acquired deafness, they are generally more effective in children who already have developed language. Children who have postmeningitic deafness eventually develop an ossified inner ear that prevents the placement of an implant; they should receive cochlear implants as soon as possible to allow the implant to be correctly placed and maximize effectiveness. Children whose acoustic nerves have been destroyed by tumors may be helped by implantation of brain stem auditory-stimulating electrodes. Children with cochlear implants may have a slightly greater risk of meningitis than children without cochlear implants or adults with cochlear implants.

Children with unilateral deafness should be allowed to use a special system in the classroom, such as an FM auditory trainer. With these systems, the teacher speaks into a microphone that sends signals to a hearing aid in the child's nonaffected ear, improving the child's greatly impaired ability to hear speech against a noisy background.

Prevention

Prevention of hearing loss consists mainly of limiting duration and intensity of noise exposure. People required to expose themselves to loud noise must wear ear protectors (eg, plastic plugs in the ear canals or glycerin-filled muffs over the ears). The Occupational Safety and Health Administration (OSHA) of the US Department of Labor and similar agencies in many other countries have standards regarding the length of time that a person can be exposed to a noise. The louder the noise, the shorter the permissible time of exposure.

Geriatrics Essentials

Elderly people typically experience a progressive decrease in hearing (presbycusis). In the United States, 40% of those who are hearing impaired are elderly. Hearing impairment is prevalent in over one third of people over age 65 yr and over half of people over age 75 yr, making it the most common sensory disorder in this population. Nonetheless, hearing loss in the elderly should be evaluated and not ascribed simply to aging; elderly patients may have a tumor, a neurologic or autoimmune disorder, or an easily correctable conductive hearing loss. Also, recent research strongly suggests that hearing loss in the elderly can facilitate dementia (which can be mitigated by properly correcting hearing loss).

Presbycusis: Presbycusis is sensorineural hearing loss that probably results from a combination of age-related deterioration and cell death in various components of the hearing system and the effects of chronic noise exposure.

Hearing loss usually affects the highest frequencies (18 to 20 kHz) early on and gradually affects the lower frequencies; it usually becomes clinically significant when it affects the critical 2- to 4-kHz range at about age 55 to 65 (sometimes sooner). The loss of high-frequency hearing significantly affects speech comprehension. Although the loudness of speech seems normal, certain consonant sounds (eg, C, D, K, P, S, T) become harder to hear. Consonant sounds are the most important sounds for speech recognition. For example, when "shoe," "blue," "true," "too," or "new" is spoken, many people with presbycusis can hear the "oo" sound, but most have difficulty recognizing which word has been spoken because they cannot distinguish the consonants. This inability to distinguish consonants causes affected people to often think the speaker is mumbling. A speaker attempting to speak louder usually accentuates vowel sounds (which are low frequency), doing little to improve speech recognition. Speech comprehension is particularly difficult when background noise is present.

Screening: A screening tool is often helpful for elderly people because many do not complain of hearing loss. One tool is the Hearing Handicap Inventory for the Elderly–Screening Version, which asks

- Does a hearing problem cause you to feel embarrassed when you meet people?
- Does a hearing problem cause you to feel frustrated when talking to a family member?
- Do you have difficulty hearing when someone whispers?
- Do you feel handicapped by a hearing problem?
- Does a hearing problem cause you difficulty when visiting friends, relatives, or neighbors?
- Does a hearing problem cause you to attend religious services less often than you would like?
- Does a hearing problem cause you to have arguments with family members?
- Does a hearing problem cause you difficulty when listening to the television or radio?

• Do you feel that any difficulty with your hearing hampers your personal or social life?
• Does a hearing problem cause you difficulty when in a restaurant with relatives or friends?

Scoring is "no" = 0 points, "sometimes" = 2 points, and "yes" = 4 points. Scores > 10 suggest signßificant hearing impairment and necessitate follow-up.

KEY POINTS

- Cerumen, genetic disorders, infections, aging, and noise exposure are the most common causes.
- All patients with hearing loss should have audiologic testing.
- Cranial nerve deficits and other neurologic deficits should raise concern and warrant imaging tests.

SUDDEN HEARING LOSS

Sudden hearing loss is moderate to severe sensorineural hearing loss that develops suddenly, within a few hours or is noticed on awakening. It affects about 1/5000 to 1/10,000 people each year. Initial hearing loss is typically unilateral (unless drug-induced) and may range in severity from mild to profound. Many also have tinnitus, and some have dizziness, vertigo, or both.

Sudden hearing loss has some causes that differ from chronic hearing loss and must be addressed urgently.[1]

1. Stachler RJ, Chandrasekhar SS, Archer SM, et al: Clinical practice guideline: Sudden hearing loss. *Otolaryngol Head Neck Surg* 146(3 Suppl):S1–35, 2012. doi: 10.1177/0194599812436449.

Etiology

The following are common characteristics of sudden hearing loss:

- Most cases (see Table 94–4) are idiopathic.
- Some occur in the course of an obvious explanatory event.
- A few represent the initial manifestation of an occult but identifiable disorder.

Idiopathic: There are numerous theories for which some evidence (although conflicting and incomplete) exists. The most promising possibilities include viral infections (particularly involving herpes simplex), autoimmune attacks, and acute microvascular occlusion.

Obvious event: Some causes of sudden hearing loss are readily apparent.

Blunt head trauma with temporal bone fracture or severe concussion involving the cochlea can cause sudden hearing loss.

Large ambient pressure changes (eg, caused by diving) or strenuous activities (eg, weightlifting) can induce a perilymphatic fistula between the middle and inner ear, causing sudden, severe symptoms. Perilymphatic fistula can also be congenital; it can spontaneously cause a sudden loss or loss may occur after trauma or severe pressure changes.

Ototoxic drugs can result in hearing loss occurring sometimes within a day, especially with an overdose (systemically or when applied to a large wound area, such as a burn). There is a rare genetic mitochondrial-transmitted disorder that increases the susceptibility to aminoglycoside ototoxicity.

A number of **infections** cause sudden hearing loss during or immediately after acute illness. Common causes include bacterial meningitis, Lyme disease, and many viral infections that affect the cochlea (and sometimes the vestibular apparatus). The most common viral causes in the developed world are mumps

Table 94–4. SOME CAUSES OF SUDDEN HEARING LOSS

TYPE	EXAMPLES
Idiopathic	N/A Accounts for a majority of cases
Obvious events	Acute infections (eg, bacterial meningitis, mumps, herpes) Major head or ear trauma (including barotrauma during scuba diving causing perilymphatic fistula) Ototoxic drugs (eg, aminoglycosides, vancomycin, cisplatin, furosemide, ethacrynic acid); these mostly cause hearing loss over a longer time period but can rarely present as a sudden loss)*
Occult disorders	Acoustic neuroma Autoimmune disorders (eg, Cogan syndrome, vasculitides) Cerebellar stroke Meniere disease Multiple sclerosis Reactivation of syphilis in HIV-infected patient Red blood cell abnormalities (eg, sickle cell disease) Vascular disorders (eg, vertebrobasilar insufficiency)

*Loss occurs over 1–2 days.
N/A = not applicable.

and herpes. Measles is a very rare cause because most of the population is immunized.

Occult disorders: Sudden hearing loss rarely can be an isolated first manifestation of some disorders that usually have other initial symptoms. For example, sudden hearing loss rarely may be the first manifestation of an acoustic neuroma, multiple sclerosis, Meniere disease, or a small cerebellar stroke. Syphilis reactivation in HIV-infected patients rarely can cause sudden hearing loss.

Cogan syndrome is a rare autoimmune reaction directed against an unknown common autoantigen in the cornea and inner ear; > 50% of patients present with vestibuloauditory symptoms. About 10 to 30% of patients also have a severe systemic vasculitis, which may include life-threatening aortitis.

Some vasculitic disorders can cause hearing loss, some of which is acute. Hematologic disorders, such as Waldenström macroglobulinemia, sickle cell disease, and some forms of leukemia, rarely can cause sudden hearing loss.

Evaluation

Evaluation consists of detecting and quantifying hearing loss and determining etiology (particularly reversible causes).

History: History of present illness should verify that loss is sudden and not chronic. The history should also note whether loss is unilateral or bilateral and whether there is a current acute event (eg, head injury, barotrauma [particularly a diving injury], infectious illness). Important accompanying symptoms include other otologic symptoms (eg, tinnitus, ear discharge), vestibular symptoms (eg, disorientation in the dark, vertigo), and other neurologic symptoms (eg, headache, weakness or asymmetry of the face, abnormal sense of taste).

Review of systems should seek symptoms of possible causes, including transient, migratory neurologic deficits (multiple sclerosis) and eye irritation and redness (Cogan syndrome).

Past medical history should ask about known HIV or syphilis infection and risk factors for them (eg, multiple sex partners, unprotected intercourse). Family history should note close relatives with hearing loss (suggesting a congenital fistula). Drug history should specifically query current or previous use of ototoxic drugs (see p. 821) and whether the patient has known renal insufficiency or renal failure.

Physical examination: The examination focuses on the ears and hearing and on the neurologic examination.

The tympanic membrane is inspected for perforation, drainage, or other lesions. During the neurologic examination, attention should be paid to the cranial nerves (particularly the 5th, 7th, and 8th) and to vestibular and cerebellar function because abnormalities in these areas often occur with tumors of the brain stem and cerebellopontine angle.

The Weber and Rinne tests require a tuning fork to differentiate conductive from sensorineural hearing loss.

Additionally, the eyes are examined for redness and photophobia (possible Cogan syndrome), and the skin is examined for rash (eg, viral infection, syphilis).

Red flags: Findings of particular concern are

- Abnormalities of cranial nerves (other than hearing loss)
- Significant asymmetry in speech understanding between the 2 ears
- Other neurologic symptoms and signs (eg, motor weakness, aphasia, Horner syndrome, sensory or temperature sensation abnormalities)

Interpretation of findings: Traumatic, ototoxic, and some infectious causes are usually apparent clinically. A patient with perilymphatic fistula may hear an explosive sound in the affected ear when the fistula occurs and may also have sudden vertigo, nystagmus, and tinnitus.

Focal neurologic abnormalities are of particular concern. The 5th cranial nerve, 7th cranial nerve, or both are often affected by tumors that involve the 8th cranial nerve, so loss of facial sensation and weak jaw clench (5th) and hemifacial weakness and taste abnormalities (7th) point to a lesion in that area.

Fluctuating unilateral hearing loss accompanied by aural fullness, tinnitus, and vertigo also suggests Meniere disease. Systemic symptoms suggesting inflammation (eg, fevers, rash, joint pains, mucosal lesions) should raise suspicion of an occult infection or autoimmune disorder.

Testing:

- Audiometry
- MRI and CT

Patients should have an audiogram, and unless the diagnosis is clearly an acute infection or drug toxicity, most clinicians do gadolinium-enhanced MRI to diagnose inapparent causes, particularly for unilateral losses. Patients with an acute traumatic cause also should have MRI. A perilymphatic fistula is typically suspected from an inciting event (eg, excessive strain, barotrauma), and testing may be done by using positive pneumatic pressure to evoke eye movements (nystagmus). CT of the temporal bones is usually done to show the bony characteristics of the inner ear and can help elucidate congenital abnormalities (eg, enlarged vestibular aqueduct), fractures of the temporal bone from trauma, or erosive processes (eg, cholesteatoma).

Patients who have risk factors for or symptoms that suggest causes should have appropriate tests based on clinical evaluation (eg, serologic tests for possible HIV infection or syphilis, CBC and coagulation profile for hematologic disorders, ESR and antinuclear antibodies for vasculitis).

Treatment

Treatment of sudden hearing loss focuses on the causative disorder when known. Fistulas are explored and repaired surgically when bed rest fails to control symptoms.

In viral and idiopathic cases, hearing returns to normal in about 50% of patients and is partially recovered in others.

In patients who recover their hearing, improvement usually occurs within 10 to 14 days.

Recovery from an ototoxic drug varies greatly depending on the drug and its dosage. With some drugs (eg, aspirin, diuretics), hearing loss resolves within 24 h, whereas other drugs (eg, antibiotics, chemotherapy drugs) often cause permanent hearing loss if safe dosages have been exceeded.

For patients with idiopathic loss, many clinicians empirically give a course of glucocorticoids (typically prednisone 80 mg/kg po once/day for 7 to 14 days followed by a 5 day taper). Glucocorticoids can be given orally and/or by transtympanic injection. Direct transtympanic injection avoids the systemic side effects of oral glucocorticoids and appears equally effective except in profound (> 90 decibels) hearing loss. There are data showing that using both oral and intratympanic steroids leads to better outcomes than either alone. Although clinicians often give antiviral drugs effective against herpes simplex (eg, valacyclovir, famciclovir), data show that such drugs do not affect hearing outcomes. There are some limited data suggesting that hyperbaric oxygen therapy may be beneficial in idiopathic sudden hearing loss.

KEY POINTS

- Most cases are idiopathic.
- A few cases have an obvious cause (eg, major trauma, acute infection, drugs).
- A very few cases represent unusual manifestations of treatable disorders.

95 Inner Ear Disorders

The inner ear is in the petrous area of the temporal bone. Within the bone is the osseous labyrinth, which encases the membranous labyrinth. The osseous labyrinth includes the vestibular system (made up of the semicircular canals and the vestibule) and the cochlea (see Fig. 95–1).

The vestibular system, responsible for balance and posture, consists of the saccule, utricle, and semicircular canals. The saccule and utricle contain cells that sense movement of the head in a straight line (sensing acceleration) or up and down (sensing gravity). The 3 semicircular canals sense angular rotation of the head. Depending on the direction the head moves, the fluid movement will be greater in one on the 3 canals than in the others. Hair cells in the canals respond to the fluid movement, initiating nerve impulses so that the brain can take appropriate action to maintain balance.

The cochlea, responsible for hearing, is filled with fluid. Within the cochlea is the organ of Corti, containing about 30,000 hair cells. Cilia from the hair cells extend into the fluid and are embedded in a gelatinous membrane. Sound vibrations are transmitted from the ossicles, through the middle ear and the oval window, into the inner ear where these vibrations cause the fluid and cilia to vibrate. These vibrations are then transformed into an electric signal that is sent to the brain. There are many environmental factors that can damage the cells within the inner ear and cause hearing loss. One of the most important is loud noise exposure. Despite the protective effect of the acoustic reflex which tenses the middle ear bones to blunt loud sounds, loud noise can damage and permanently destroy hair cells. Continued exposure to loud noise causes progressive damage, eventually resulting in hearing loss and sometimes in tinnitus.

Inner ear disorders include

- Acoustic neuroma
- Benign paroxysmal positional vertigo
- Drug-induced ototoxicity
- Herpes zoster oticus
- Meniere disease
- Purulent labyrinthitis
- Vestibular neuronitis

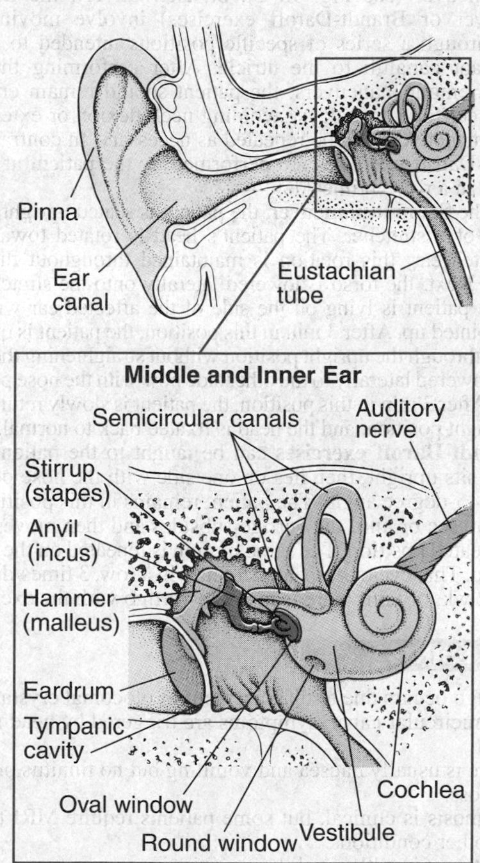

Fig. 95–1. Inside the ear.

ACOUSTIC NEUROMA

(Acoustic Neurinoma; 8th Nerve Tumor; Vestibular Schwannoma)

An acoustic neuroma, also called a vestibular schwannoma, is a Schwann cell–derived tumor of the 8th cranial nerve. Symptoms include unilateral hearing loss. Diagnosis is based on audiology and confirmed by MRI. When required, treatment is surgical removal, stereotactic radiation therapy, or both.

Acoustic neuromas almost always arise from the vestibular division of the 8th cranial nerve and account for about 7% of all intracranial tumors. As the tumor expands, it projects from the internal auditory canal into the cerebellopontine angle, compressing the 7th and 8th cranial nerves. As the tumor continues to enlarge, the cerebellum, brain stem, and nearby cranial nerves (5th and 9th to 12th) can also become compressed.

Bilateral acoustic neuromas are a common feature of neurofibromatosis type 2.

Symptoms and Signs

Slowly progressive unilateral sensorineural hearing loss is the hallmark symptom of acoustic neuroma. However, the onset of hearing loss may be abrupt, and the degree of impairment may fluctuate. Other early symptoms include unilateral tinnitus, dizziness and dysequilibrium, headache, sensation of pressure or fullness in the ear, otalgia, trigeminal neuralgia, and numbness or weakness in the face due to involvement of the facial nerve.

Diagnosis

- Audiogram
- If asymmetric hearing loss, gadolinium-enhanced MRI

Most commonly, an audiogram is the first test done as part of the evaluation to diagnose acoustic neuroma. It usually reveals an asymmetric sensorineural hearing loss and a greater impairment of speech discrimination than would be expected for the degree of hearing loss. Such findings indicate the need for imaging tests, preferably gadolinium-enhanced MRI. However, some tumors are found incidentally when brain imaging is done for another reason.

Other findings include presence of acoustic reflex decay on tympanometry. Auditory brain stem response testing may show the absence of waveforms and/or increased latency of the 5th waveform. Although not usually required in the routine evaluation of a patient with asymmetric sensorineural hearing loss, caloric testing shows marked vestibular hypoactivity (canal paresis) on the affected side.

Treatment

- Observation
- Sometimes surgical removal or stereotactic radiation therapy in selected cases

Small, asymptomatic (ie, discovered incidentally), and nongrowing acoustic neuromas do not require treatment; such tumors may be observed with serial MRI scans and treated if they begin growing or cause symptoms. Whether to use stereotactic radiation therapy (eg, gamma knife or cyberknife radiation therapy) or conventional microsurgery depends on many factors including the amount of residual hearing, tumor size, and patient age and health. Stereotactic radiation therapy tends to be used for patients who are elderly, those with smaller tumors, or those who cannot undergo surgery for medical reasons. Microsurgery can involve a hearing-preservation approach (middle cranial fossa or retrosigmoid approach) or a translabyrinthine approach if there is no useful residual hearing.

KEY POINTS

- Acoustic neuroma is usually unilateral but can be bilateral in neurofibromatosis.
- Unilateral hearing loss, sometimes with tinnitus and dizziness, is typical.
- Larger and/or symptomatic tumors are treated with stereotactic radiosurgery or conventional microsurgery.
- Small or nongrowing tumors can be observed with serial MRI scans.

BENIGN PAROXYSMAL POSITIONAL VERTIGO

(Benign Positional Vertigo; Benign Postural Vertigo; BPPV)

In benign paroxysmal positional vertigo, short (< 60 sec) episodes of vertigo occur with certain head positions. Nausea and nystagmus develop. Diagnosis is clinical. Treatment involves canalith repositioning maneuvers. Drugs and surgery are rarely, if ever, indicated.

Benign paroxysmal positional vertigo (BPPV) is the most common cause of relapsing otogenic vertigo. It affects people increasingly as they age and can severely affect balance in the elderly, leading to potentially injurious falls.

Etiology

The condition is thought to be caused by displacement of otoconial crystals (Ca carbonate crystals normally embedded in the saccule and utricle). This displaced material stimulates hair cells most commonly in the posterior semicircular canal (and rarely in the superior semicircular canal), creating the illusion of motion. Etiologic factors include

- Spontaneous degeneration of the utricular otolithic membranes
- Labyrinthine concussion
- Otitis media
- Ear surgery
- Recent viral infection (eg, viral neuronitis)
- Head trauma
- Prolonged anesthesia or bed rest
- Previous vestibular disorders (eg, Meniere disease)
- Occlusion of the anterior vestibular artery

Symptoms and Signs

Vertigo is triggered when the patient's head moves (eg, when rolling over in bed or bending over to pick up something). Acute paroxysms of vertigo last only a few seconds to minutes; episodes tend to peak in the morning and abate throughout the day. Nausea and vomiting may occur, but hearing loss and tinnitus do not.

Diagnosis

- Clinical evaluation
- Gadolinium-enhanced MRI if findings suggest CNS lesion

The diagnosis of benign positional vertigo is based on characteristic symptoms, on nystagmus as determined by the Dix-Hallpike maneuver (a provocative test for positional nystagmus), and on absence of other abnormalities on neurologic examination. Such patients require no further testing.

Unlike the positional nystagmus caused by BPPV, the positional nystagmus caused by a CNS lesion

- Lacks latency, fatigability, and severe subjective sensation
- May continue for as long as the position is maintained
- May be vertical or change direction
- If rotary, is likely to be in the unexpected direction

Patients with nystagmus suggesting a CNS lesion undergo gadolinium-enhanced MRI.

Treatment

- Provocative maneuvers to fatigue symptoms
- Canalith repositioning maneuvers
- Drug treatment typically not recommended

BPPV usually subsides spontaneously in several weeks or months but may continue for months or years. Because the condition can be long-lasting, drug treatment (like that used in Meniere disease—see p. 822) is not recommended. Often, the adverse effects of drugs worsen dysequilibrium.

Because BPPV is fatigable, one therapy is to have the patient perform provocative maneuvers early in the day in a safe environment. Symptoms are then minimal for the rest of the day.

Canalith repositioning maneuvers (most commonly the Epley maneuver (see Fig. 95–2), or, alternatively, the Semont maneuver or Brandt-Daroff exercises) involve moving the head through a series of specific positions intended to return the errant canalith to the utricle. After performing the Epley or Semont maneuvers, the patient should remain erect or semi-erect for 1 to 2 days, avoiding neck flexion or extension. These maneuvers can be repeated as necessary. In contrast, the Brandt-Daroff exercises are performed by the patient at home 5 times in a row, 3 times/day.

For the **Semont maneuver,** the patient is seated upright in the middle of a stretcher. The patient's head is rotated toward the unaffected ear; this rotation is maintained throughout the maneuver. Next, the torso is lowered laterally onto the stretcher so that the patient is lying on the side of the affected ear with the nose pointed up. After 3 min in this position, the patient is quickly moved through the upright position without straightening the head and is lowered laterally to the other side now with the nose pointed down. After 3 min in this position, the patient is slowly returned to the upright position, and the head is rotated back to normal.

Brandt-Daroff exercises can be taught to the patient. The patient sits upright, then lies on one side with the nose pointed up at a 45-degree angle. The patient remains in this position for about 30 sec or until the vertigo subsides and then moves back to the seated position. The same motion is repeated on the opposite side. This cycle is repeated 5 times in a row, 3 times/day, for about 2 wk, or until there is no more vertigo with the exercise.

KEY POINTS

- Vertigo occurs due to displacement of otoconial crystals into a semicircular canal; symptoms are triggered by head movement.
- There is usually nausea and vomiting but no tinnitus or hearing loss.
- Diagnosis is clinical, but some patients require MRI to rule out other conditions.
- Treatment is with canalith-repositioning maneuvers.
- Drugs rarely help and may worsen symptoms.

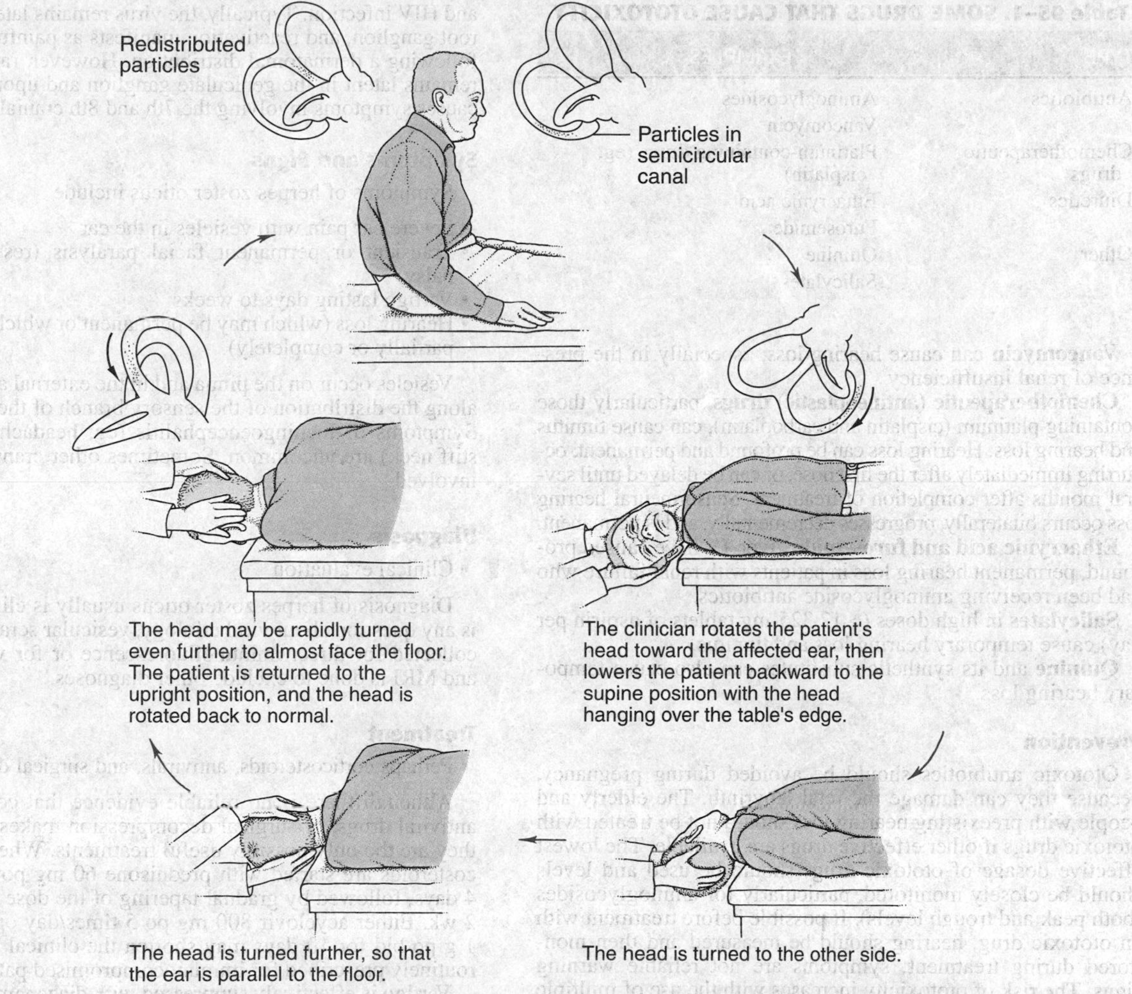

Redistributed particles
Particles in semicircular canal
The head may be rapidly turned even further to almost face the floor. The patient is returned to the upright position, and the head is rotated back to normal.
The clinician rotates the patient's head toward the affected ear, then lowers the patient backward to the supine position with the head hanging over the table's edge.
The head is turned further, so that the ear is parallel to the floor.
The head is turned to the other side.

Fig. 95–2. The Epley maneuver. This maneuver is used to treat benign paroxysmal positional vertigo by returning displaced otoliths from the posterior semicircular canal back to the utricle. If vertigo occurs during any of the positions, that position is held until the vertigo subsides.

DRUG-INDUCED OTOTOXICITY

A wide variety of drugs can be ototoxic (see Table 95–1). Factors affecting ototoxicity include

- Dose
- Duration of therapy
- Concurrent renal failure
- Infusion rate
- Lifetime dose
- Coadministration with other drugs having ototoxic potential
- Genetic susceptibility

Ototoxic drugs should not be used for otic topical application when the tympanic membrane is perforated because the drugs might diffuse into the inner ear.

Streptomycin tends to cause more damage to the vestibular portion than to the auditory portion of the inner ear. Although vertigo and difficulty maintaining balance tend to be temporary, severe loss of vestibular sensitivity may persist, sometimes permanently. Loss of vestibular sensitivity causes difficulty walking, especially in the dark, and oscillopsia (a sensation of bouncing of the environment with each step). About 4 to 15% of patients who receive 1 g/day for > 1 wk develop measurable hearing loss, which usually occurs after a short latent period (7 to 10 days) and slowly worsens if treatment is continued. Complete, permanent deafness may follow.

Neomycin has the greatest cochleotoxic effect of all antibiotics. When large doses are given orally or by colonic irrigation for intestinal sterilization, enough may be absorbed to affect hearing, particularly if diffuse mucosal lesions of the colon are present. Neomycin should not be used for wound irrigation or for intrapleural or intraperitoneal irrigation, because massive amounts of the drug may be retained and absorbed, causing deafness.

Kanamycin and amikacin are close to neomycin in cochleotoxic potential and are both capable of causing profound, permanent hearing loss while sparing balance.

Viomycin has both cochlear and vestibular toxicity.

Gentamicin and tobramycin have vestibular and cochlear toxicity, causing impairment in balance and hearing.

Table 95–1. SOME DRUGS THAT CAUSE OTOTOXICITY

TYPE	EXAMPLES
Antibiotics	Aminoglycosides Vancomycin
Chemotherapeutic drugs	Platinum-containing drugs (eg, cisplatin)
Diuretics	Ethacrynic acid Furosemide
Other	Quinine Salicylates

Vancomycin can cause hearing loss, especially in the presence of renal insufficiency.

Chemotherapeutic (antineoplastic) drugs, particularly those containing platinum (cisplatin and carboplatin), can cause tinnitus and hearing loss. Hearing loss can be profound and permanent, occurring immediately after the first dose, or can be delayed until several months after completion of treatment. Sensorineural hearing loss occurs bilaterally, progresses decrementally, and is permanent.

Ethacrynic acid and furosemide given IV have caused profound, permanent hearing loss in patients with renal failure who had been receiving aminoglycoside antibiotics.

Salicylates in high doses (> 12 325-mg tablets of aspirin per day) cause temporary hearing loss and tinnitus.

Quinine and its synthetic substitutes can also cause temporary hearing loss.

Prevention

Ototoxic antibiotics should be avoided during pregnancy, because they can damage the fetal labyrinth. The elderly and people with preexisting hearing loss should not be treated with ototoxic drugs if other effective drugs are available. The lowest effective dosage of ototoxic drugs should be used and levels should be closely monitored, particularly for aminoglycosides (both peak and trough levels). If possible before treatment with an ototoxic drug, hearing should be measured and then monitored during treatment; symptoms are not reliable warning signs. The risk of ototoxicity increases with the use of multiple drugs with ototoxic potential and the use of ototoxic drugs excreted through the kidneys in patients with renal compromise; in such cases, closer monitoring of drug levels is advised.

KEY POINTS

- Drugs may cause hearing loss, dysequilibrium, and/or tinnitus.
- Common drugs include aminoglycosides, platinum-containing chemotherapy drugs, and high-dose salicylates.
- Symptoms may be transient or permanent.
- Drugs are stopped if possible, but there is no specific treatment.

HERPES ZOSTER OTICUS

(Geniculate Herpes; Ramsay Hunt Syndrome; Viral Neuronitis)

Herpes zoster oticus is an uncommon manifestation of herpes zoster that affects the 8th cranial nerve ganglia and the geniculate ganglion of the 7th (facial) cranial nerve.

Herpes zoster (shingles) is reactivation of varicella-zoster virus infection. Risk factors for reactivation include immunodeficiency secondary to cancer, chemotherapy, radiation therapy, and HIV infection. Typically, the virus remains latent in a dorsal root ganglion, and reactivation manifests as painful skin lesions following a dermatomal distribution. However, rarely the virus remains latent in the geniculate ganglion and upon reactivation causes symptoms involving the 7th and 8th cranial nerves.

Symptoms and Signs

Symptoms of herpes zoster oticus include

- Severe ear pain with vesicles in the ear
- Transient or permanent facial paralysis (resembling Bell palsy)
- Vertigo lasting days to weeks
- Hearing loss (which may be permanent or which may resolve partially or completely)

Vesicles occur on the pinna and in the external auditory canal along the distribution of the sensory branch of the facial nerve. Symptoms of meningoencephalitis (eg, headache, confusion, stiff neck) are uncommon. Sometimes other cranial nerves are involved.

Diagnosis

- Clinical evaluation

Diagnosis of herpes zoster oticus usually is clinical. If there is any question about viral etiology, vesicular scrapings may be collected for direct immunofluorescence or for viral cultures, and MRI is done to exclude other diagnoses.

Treatment

- Perhaps corticosteroids, antivirals, and surgical decompression

Although there is no reliable evidence that corticosteroids, antiviral drugs, or surgical decompression makes a difference, they are the only possibly useful treatments. When used, corticosteroids are started with prednisone 60 mg po once/day for 4 days, followed by gradual tapering of the dose over the next 2 wk. Either acyclovir 800 mg po 5 times/day or valacyclovir 1 g po bid for 10 days may shorten the clinical course and is routinely prescribed for immunocompromised patients.

Vertigo is effectively suppressed with diazepam 2 to 5 mg po q 4 to 6 h. Pain may require oral opioids. Postherpetic neuralgia may be treated with amitriptyline.

Surgical decompression of the fallopian canal may be indicated if the facial palsy is complete (no visible facial movement), but must be performed within 2 wk of onset of the facial paralysis to be effective. Before surgery, however, electroneurography is done and should show a > 90% decrement.

MENIERE DISEASE

(Endolymphatic Hydrops)

Meniere disease is an inner ear disorder that causes vertigo, fluctuating sensorineural hearing loss, and tinnitus. There is no reliable diagnostic test. Vertigo and nausea are treated symptomatically with anticholinergics or benzodiazepines during acute attacks. Diuretics and a low-salt diet, the first line of treatment, often decrease the frequency and severity of episodes. For severe or refractory cases, the vestibular system can be ablated with topical gentamicin or surgery.

In Meniere disease, pressure and volume changes of the labyrinthine endolymph affect inner ear function. The etiology of endolymphatic fluid buildup is unknown. Risk factors include a family history of Meniere disease, preexisting autoimmune disorders, allergies, trauma to the head or ear, and, very rarely, syphilis. Peak incidence is between ages 20 and 50.

Symptoms and Signs

Patients have sudden attacks of vertigo that usually last for 1 to 6 h but that can (rarely) last up to 24 h, usually with nausea and vomiting. Accompanying symptoms include diaphoresis, diarrhea, and gait unsteadiness.

Tinnitus in the affected ear may be constant or intermittent, buzzing or roaring; it is not related to position or motion. Hearing impairment, typically affecting low frequencies, may follow. Before and during an episode, most patients sense fullness or pressure in the affected ear. In a majority of patients, only one ear is affected.

During the early stages, symptoms remit between episodes; symptom-free interludes may last > 1 yr. As the disease progresses, however, hearing impairment persists and gradually worsens, and tinnitus may be constant.

Diagnosis

- Clinical evaluation
- Audiogram and gadolinium-enhanced MRI to rule out other causes

The diagnosis of Meniere disease is made clinically. The simultaneous combination of fluctuating low-frequency sensorineural hearing loss, episodic vertigo, ipsilateral fluctuating aural fullness, and tinnitus is characteristic. Similar symptoms can result from vestibular migraine, viral labyrinthitis or neuronitis, a cerebellopontine angle tumor (eg, acoustic neuroma), or a brain stem stroke. Although bilateral Meniere disease can occur, bilateral symptoms increase the likelihood of an alternate diagnosis (eg, vestibular migraine).

Patients with suggestive symptoms should have an audiogram and an MRI (with gadolinium enhancement) of the CNS with attention to the internal auditory canals to exclude other causes. Audiogram typically shows a low-frequency sensorineural hearing loss in the affected ear that fluctuates between tests. The Rinne test and the Weber test also may indicate sensorineural hearing loss (see p. 809).

On examination during an acute attack, the patient has nystagmus and falls to the affected side. Between attacks, the examination may be entirely normal. However, in long-standing or refractory cases with associated labyrinthine hypofunction, the Fukuda stepping test (marching in place with eyes closed, previously known as the Unterberger test) causes the patient to turn toward the affected ear, consistent with a unilateral labyrinthine lesion.

The **Halmagyi head thrust maneuver**, or head impulse test, is another technique that is used to show unilateral labyrinthine dysfunction. In the Halmagyi maneuver, the examiner has the patient visually fixate on a target straight ahead (eg, the examiner's nose). The examiner then rapidly rotates the patient's head 15 to 30° to one side while observing the patient's eyes. When vestibular function on the side to which the head has been rotated is normal, the patient's eyes remain fixated on the target. When vestibular function is impaired on the side to which the head has been rotated, the vestibulo-ocular reflex fails and the patient's eyes do not remain fixated on the target but instead transiently follow the head rotation and then quickly and voluntarily return back to the target (called delayed catch-up saccades).

Treatment

- Symptom relief with antiemetics, antihistamines, or benzodiazepines
- Diuretics and low-salt diet
- Rarely vestibular ablation by drugs or surgery

Meniere disease tends to be self-limited. Treatment of an acute attack is aimed at symptom relief and done in a staged fashion; the least invasive measures are done first, and then ablative procedures are sometimes done if the measures fail.

Anticholinergic antiemetics (eg, prochlorperazine 25 mg rectally or 10 mg po q 6 to 8 h; promethazine 25 mg rectally or 25 mg po q 6 to 8 h) can minimize vagal-mediated GI symptoms; ondansetron is a 2nd-line antiemetic. Antihistamines (eg, diphenhydramine, meclizine, or cyclizine 50 mg po q 6 h) or benzodiazepines (eg, diazepam 5 mg po q 6 to 8 h) are used to sedate the vestibular system. Neither antihistamines nor benzodiazepines are effective as prophylactic treatment. Some physicians also use an oral corticosteroid burst (eg, prednisone 60 mg po once/day for 1 wk, tapered over another wk) or intratympanic dexamethasone injections for an acute episode.

A low-salt (< 1.5 g/day) diet, avoidance of alcohol and caffeine, and a diuretic (eg, hydrochlorothiazide 25 mg po once/day or acetazolamide 250 mg po bid) may help prevent or reduce the incidence of vertigo attacks and are commonly used first steps. However, there are no well-designed studies that clearly prove the efficacy of these measures for Meniere disease.

Although more invasive, endolymphatic sac decompression relieves vertigo in a majority of patients, spares vestibular function, and poses minimal risk of hearing loss. Thus this procedure is still classified as a vestibular-sparing treatment.

When vestibular-sparing treatments fail, an ablative procedure is considered. Intratympanic gentamicin (chemical labyrinthectomy—typically 0.5 mL of a 40 mg/mL concentration) is injected through the tympanic membrane. Follow up with serial audiometry is recommended to monitor for hearing loss. The injection can be repeated in 4 wk if vertigo persists without hearing loss.

Ablative surgery is reserved for patients with frequent, severely debilitating episodes who are unresponsive to less invasive modalities. Vestibular neurectomy (an intracranial procedure) relieves vertigo in about 95% of patients and usually preserves hearing. A surgical labyrinthectomy is done only if preexisting hearing loss is profound.

Unfortunately, there is no known way to prevent the natural progression of hearing loss. Most patients sustain moderate to severe sensorineural hearing loss in the affected ear within 10 to 15 yr.

KEY POINTS

- Meniere disease typically causes vertigo with nausea and vomiting, unilateral tinnitus, and chronic, progressive hearing loss.
- Testing is with audiogram, and MRI is done to rule out other disorders.
- Antiemetics and antihistamines can help relieve symptoms; some clinicians also use oral or transtympanic corticosteroids.
- More invasive treatments for refractory cases include endolymphatic sac decompression, intratympanic gentamicin, and vestibular neurectomy.
- Diuretics, a low-salt diet, and avoidance of alcohol and caffeine help prevent attacks.

PURULENT LABYRINTHITIS

Purulent (suppurative) labyrinthitis is bacterial infection of the inner ear, often causing deafness and loss of vestibular function.

Purulent labyrinthitis usually occurs when bacteria spread to the inner ear during the course of severe acute otitis media, purulent meningitis, trauma causing a labyrinthine fracture with a subsequent infection, or an enlarging cholesteatoma.

Symptoms and Signs

Symptoms of purulent labyrinthitis include

- Severe vertigo and nystagmus
- Nausea and vomiting
- Tinnitus
- Varying degrees of hearing loss

Pain and fever are common.

Diagnosis

- Temporal bone CT
- Possibly MRI

Purulent labyrinthitis is suspected if vertigo, nystagmus, sensorineural hearing loss, or a combination occurs during an episode of acute otitis media. CT of the temporal bone is done to identify erosion of the otic capsule bone or other complications of acute otitis media, such as coalescent mastoiditis. MRI may be indicated if symptoms of meningitis or brain abscess, such as altered mental status, meningismus, or high fever, are present; in such cases, a lumbar puncture and blood cultures also are done.

Treatment

- IV antibiotics
- Myringotomy
- Sometimes tympanostomy

Treatment is with IV antibiotics appropriate for meningitis (eg, ceftriaxone 50 to 100 mg/kg IV once/day to maximum 2 g). Ceftazidime is often substituted for ceftriaxone in nosocomial infections to cover *P. aeruginosa*. The antibiotics are later adjusted according to results of culture and sensitivity testing. A myringotomy (and sometimes tympanostomy tube placement) is done to drain the middle ear. Mastoidectomy may be required.

VESTIBULAR NEURONITIS

(Viral Labyrinthitis)

Vestibular neuronitis causes a self-limited episode of vertigo, presumably due to inflammation of the vestibular division of the 8th cranial nerve; some vestibular dysfunction may persist.

Sometimes vestibular neuronitis is used synonymously with viral labyrinthitis. However vestibular neuronitis only presents with vertigo, while viral labyrinthitis is also accompanied by tinnitus, hearing loss, or both.

Although etiology is unclear, a viral cause is suspected.

Symptoms and Signs

Symptoms of vestibular neuronitis include a single attack of severe vertigo, with nausea and vomiting and persistent nystagmus toward the affected side, which lasts 7 to 10 days. The nystagmus is unidirectional, horizontal, and spontaneous, with fast-beat oscillations in the direction of the unaffected ear. The absence of concomitant tinnitus or hearing loss is a hallmark of vestibular neuronitis and helps distinguish it from Meniere disease as well as labyrinthitis. The condition slowly subsides over days to weeks after the initial episode. Some patients have residual dysequilibrium, especially with rapid head movements, probably due to permanent vestibular injury.

Diagnosis

- Audiology, electronystagmography, and MRI

Patients suspected of having vestibular neuronitis undergo an audiologic assessment, electronystagmography with caloric testing, and gadolinium-enhanced MRI of the head, with attention to the internal auditory canals to exclude other diagnoses, such as cerebellopontine angle tumor, brain stem hemorrhage, or infarction. MRI may show enhancement of the vestibular nerves, consistent with inflammatory neuritis.

Treatment

- Symptom relief with antiemetics, antihistamines, or benzodiazepines

Symptoms of vestibular neuronitis are symptomatically addressed over the short term as in Meniere disease (see p. 823), ie, with anticholinergics, antiemetics (eg, prochlorperazine or promethazine 25 mg rectally or 10 mg po q 6 to 8 h), antihistamines or benzodiazepines, and a corticosteroid burst with rapid taper. If vomiting is prolonged, IV fluids and electrolytes may be required. Long-term use (ie, for more than several weeks) of vestibular suppressants is highly discouraged because these drugs delay vestibular compensation, particularly in the elderly. Vestibular rehabilitation (usually given by a physical therapist) helps compensate for any residual vestibular deficit.

KEY POINTS

- Patients have severe, constant vertigo with nausea and vomiting and nystagmus towards the affected side lasting days to weeks.
- There is no hearing loss or tinnitus.
- Testing is done to exclude other disorders.
- Treatment is directed at symptoms and includes antiemetics and antihistamines or benzodiazepines; corticosteroids may also be helpful.

96 Laryngeal Disorders

The larynx contains the vocal cords and serves as the opening to the tracheobronchial tree. Laryngeal disorders include

- Benign laryngeal tumors
- Contact ulcers
- Laryngitis
- Laryngoceles
- Malignant laryngeal tumors
- Spasmodic dysphonia
- Vocal cord paralysis
- Vocal cord polyps, nodules, and granulomas

Other disorders that affect the larynx include acute laryngotracheobronchitis (croup—see p. 2826), epiglottitis (see p. 840), and laryngomalacia (see Table 48–8 on p. 379). For removal of a foreign body via the Heimlich maneuver, see p. 551.

Most laryngeal disorders cause dysphonia, which is impairment of the voice (see Sidebar 96–1). A persistent change in the voice (eg, > 3 wk) requires visualization of the vocal cords, including their mobility. Although the voice changes with advancing age, becoming breathy and aperiodic, acute or prominent changes in the elderly should not be presumed to result from aging, and evaluation is required.

The voice should be assessed and recorded, particularly if surgical procedures are planned. Examination of the larynx includes external inspection and palpation of the neck and internal visualization of the epiglottis, false cords, true cords, arytenoids, pyriform sinuses, and subglottic region below the cords. Internal visualization is accomplished by either indirect mirror examination (see Fig. 96–1) or direct flexible fiber-optic laryngoscopy in an outpatient setting with a topical anesthetic. Rigid laryngoscopy with the patient under general anesthesia provides the most thorough examination of the vocal cords, including

- Visualization of the undersurfaces
- Assessment of passive mobility when immobilized by either paralysis or fixation
- Biopsy

BENIGN LARYNGEAL TUMORS

(For malignant laryngeal tumors, see Laryngeal Cancer on p. 849.)

Benign laryngeal tumors include juvenile papillomas, hemangiomas, fibromas, chondromas, myxomas, and neurofibromas. They may appear in any part of the larynx. Papillomas and neurofibromas can become malignant.

Symptoms of benign laryngeal tumors include hoarseness, breathy voice, dyspnea, aspiration, dysphagia, otalgia (ear pain), and hemoptysis. Otalgia represents referred pain to the ear from irritation or distension of the vagus nerve and is more often than not caused by a rapidly growing malignant tumor.

Diagnosis of benign laryngeal tumors is based on direct or indirect visualization of the larynx, supplemented by CT.

Sidebar 96–1. The Professional Voice

People who use their voice professionally for public speaking and singing often experience voice disorders manifesting as hoarseness or breathiness, lowered vocal pitch, vocal fatigue, nonproductive cough, persistent throat clearing, and/or throat ache. These symptoms often have benign causes, such as vocal nodules, vocal fold edema, polyps, or granulomas. Such disorders are usually caused by vocal fold hyperfunction (excessive laryngeal muscular tension when speaking) and possibly gastroesophageal reflux.

Treatment in most cases includes the following:

- Voice evaluation by a speech pathologist or experienced physician, including, when available, use of a computer-assisted program to assess pitch and intensity and to determine parameters of vocal acoustics
- Behavioral treatment (decreasing musculoskeletal laryngeal tension when speaking) using a computer program for visual and auditory biofeedback
- A vocal hygiene program to eliminate vocally abusive behaviors, such as excessive loudness, long duration (continuous speech for > 1 h), vocal tension (excessive muscular strain during phonation), and habitual throat clearing
- An antireflux regimen, when appropriate
- Adequate hydration to promote an adequate glottal mucosal wave
- Diet and behavioral modification before vocal performances, which may include avoidance of alcohol, caffeine, and ambient tobacco smoke and other inhaled irritants

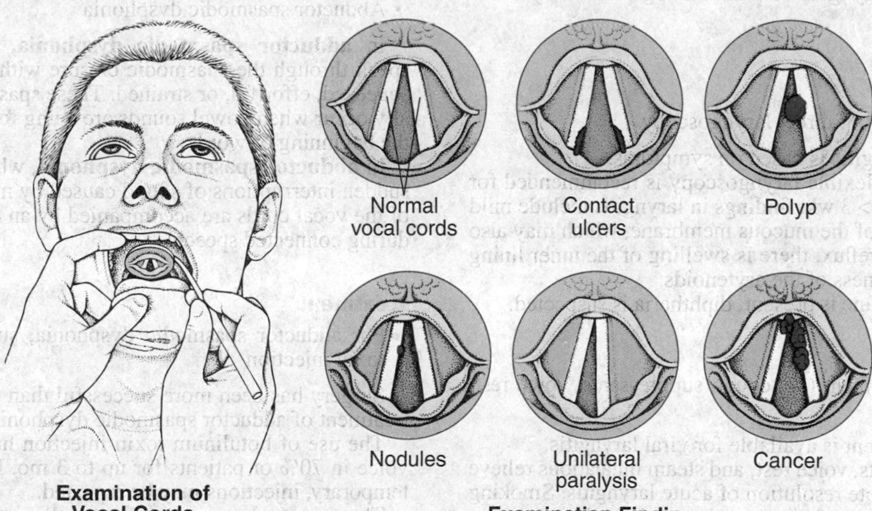

Fig. 96–1. Laryngeal disorders. When relaxed, the vocal cords normally form a V-shaped opening that allows air to pass freely through to the trachea. The cords open during inspiration and close during swallowing or speech. When a mirror is held in the back of a patient's mouth, the vocal cords can often be seen and checked for disorders, such as contact ulcers, polyps, nodules, paralysis, and cancer. Paralysis may affect one (unilateral) or both vocal cords (bilateral—not shown).

Removal restores the voice, the functional integrity of the laryngeal sphincter, and the airway. Smaller lesions may be excised endoscopically by using a CO_2 laser and general anesthesia. Larger lesions extending beyond the laryngeal framework often require pharyngotomy or laryngofissure.

LARYNGITIS

Laryngitis is inflammation of the larynx, usually the result of a virus or overuse. The result is acute change in the voice, with decreased volume and hoarseness. Diagnosis is based on clinical findings. Laryngoscopy is required for symptoms persisting > 3 wk. Viral laryngitis is self-limited. Other infectious or irritating causes may require specific treatment.

The most common cause of acute laryngitis is a viral URI. Coughing-induced laryngitis may also occur in bronchitis, pneumonia, influenza, pertussis, measles, and diphtheria. Excessive use of the voice (especially with loud speaking or singing), allergic reactions, gastroesophageal reflux, bulimia, or inhalation of irritating substances (eg, cigarette smoke or certain aerosolized drugs) can cause acute or chronic laryngitis. Drugs can induce potentially life-threatening laryngeal edema, for example, as a side effect of ACE inhibitors. Bacterial laryngitis is extremely rare. Smoking can cause Reinke edema, which is a watery swelling of both vocal cords.

Symptoms and Signs

The most prominent symptom of laryngitis is usually

- An unnatural change of voice

Volume is typically greatly decreased; some patients have aphonia. Hoarseness, a sensation of tickling, rawness, and a constant urge to clear the throat may occur. Symptoms vary with the severity of the inflammation.

Fever, malaise, dysphagia, and throat pain may occur in more severe infections. Laryngeal edema, although rare, may cause stridor and dyspnea.

Diagnosis

- Clinical evaluation
- Sometimes indirect or direct laryngoscopy

Diagnosis of laryngitis is based on symptoms.

Indirect or direct flexible laryngoscopy is recommended for symptoms persisting > 3 wk; findings in laryngitis include mild to marked erythema of the mucous membrane, which may also be edematous. With reflux, there is swelling of the inner lining of the larynx and redness of the arytenoids.

If a pseudomembrane is present, diphtheria is suspected.

Treatment

- Symptomatic treatment (eg, cough suppressants, voice rest, steam inhalations)

No specific treatment is available for viral laryngitis.

Cough suppressants, voice rest, and steam inhalations relieve symptoms and promote resolution of acute laryngitis. Smoking cessation and treatment of acute or chronic bronchitis may relieve laryngitis.

Depending on the presumed cause, specific treatments to control gastroesophageal reflux, bulimia, or drug-induced laryngitis may be beneficial.

LARYNGOCELES

Laryngoceles are evaginations of the mucous membrane of the laryngeal ventricle.

Internal laryngoceles displace and enlarge the false vocal cords, resulting in hoarseness and airway obstruction. External laryngoceles extend through the thyrohyoid membrane, causing a mass in the neck. Laryngoceles tend to occur in musicians who play wind instruments. Laryngoceles are filled with air and can be expanded by the Valsalva maneuver.

Laryngoceles appear on CT as smooth, ovoid, low-density masses. They may become infected (laryngopyocele) when filled with mucoid fluid.

Treatment of laryngoceles is excision.

SPASMODIC DYSPHONIA

Spasmodic dysphonia (vocal cord spasms) is intermittent spasm of laryngeal muscles that causes an abnormal voice.

Cause is unknown. Patients often describe the onset of symptoms following a URI, a period of excessive voice use, or occupational or emotional stress. As a localized form of movement disorder, spasmodic dysphonia has an onset between ages 30 and 50 yr, and about 60% of patients are women.

There are two forms:

- Adductor spasmodic dysphonia
- Abductor spasmodic dysphonia

In **adductor spasmodic dysphonia,** patients attempt to speak through the spasmodic closure with a voice that sounds squeezed, effortful, or strained. These spasmodic episodes usually occur when vowel sounds are being formed, particularly at the beginning of words.

In **abductor spasmodic dysphonia,** which is less common, sudden interruptions of sound caused by momentary abduction of the vocal cords are accompanied by an audible escape of air during connected speech.

Treatment

- For adductor spasmodic dysphonia, surgery, or botulinum toxin injection

Surgery has been more successful than other approaches for treatment of adductor spasmodic dysphonia.

The use of botulinum toxin injection has restored a normal voice in 70% of patients for up to 3 mo. Because the effect is temporary, injections may be repeated.

There is no known permanent alleviation of the abductor form of this disorder.

VOCAL CORD PARALYSIS

Vocal cord paralysis has numerous causes and can affect speaking, breathing, and swallowing. The left vocal cord is affected twice as often as the right, and females are affected more often than males (3:2). Diagnosis is based on direct visualization. An extensive assessment may be necessary to determine the cause. Several direct surgical approaches are available if treating the cause is not curative.

Vocal cord paralysis may result from lesions at the nucleus ambiguus, its supranuclear tracts, the main trunk of the vagus, or the recurrent laryngeal nerves. The left vocal cord is paralyzed more often than the right because the left recurrent nerve takes a longer course from the brain stem to the larynx, providing more opportunity for compression, traction, or surgical injuries.

Unilateral vocal cord paralysis is most common. About one third of unilateral paralyses are neoplastic in origin, one third are traumatic, and one third are idiopathic. Intracranial tumors, vascular accidents, and demyelinating diseases cause nucleus ambiguus paralysis. Tumors at the base of the skull and trauma to the neck cause vagus paralysis. Recurrent laryngeal nerve paralysis is caused by neck or thoracic lesions (eg, aortic aneurysm; mitral stenosis; mediastinal tuberculous adenitis; tumors of the thyroid gland, esophagus, lung, or mediastinal structures), trauma, thyroidectomy, neurotoxins (eg, lead, arsenic, mercury), neurotoxic infections (eg, diphtheria), cervical spine injury or surgery, Lyme disease, and viral illness. Viral neuronitis probably accounts for most idiopathic cases.

Bilateral vocal cord paralysis is a life-threatening disorder caused by thyroid and cervical surgery, tracheal intubation, trauma, and neurodegenerative and neuromuscular diseases.

Symptoms and Signs

Vocal cord paralysis results in loss of vocal cord abduction and adduction. Paralysis may affect phonation, respiration, and deglutition, and food and fluids may be aspirated into the trachea. The paralyzed cord generally lies 2 to 3 mm lateral to the midline.

In recurrent laryngeal nerve paralysis, the cord may move with phonation but not with inspiration.

In **unilateral paralysis,** the voice may be hoarse and breathy, but the airway is usually not obstructed because the normal cord abducts sufficiently.

In **bilateral paralysis,** both cords generally lie within 2 to 3 mm of the midline, and the voice is of good quality but of limited intensity and pitch modulation. The airway, however, is inadequate, resulting in stridor and dyspnea with moderate exertion as each cord is drawn to the midline glottis by an inspiratory Bernoulli effect. Aspiration is also a danger.

Diagnosis

- Laryngoscopy
- Various tests for possible causes

Diagnosis of vocal cord paralysis is based on laryngoscopy. The cause must always be sought. Evaluation is guided by abnormalities identified on history and physical examination. During the history, the physician asks about all possible causes of peripheral neuropathy, including chronic heavy metal exposure (arsenic, lead, mercury), drug effects from phenytoin and vincristine, and history of connective tissue disorders, Lyme disease, sarcoidosis, diabetes, and alcoholism. Further evaluation may include enhanced CT or MRI of the head, neck, and chest; thyroid scan; barium swallow or bronchoscopy; and esophagoscopy.

Cricoarytenoid arthritis, which may cause fixation of the cricoarytenoid joint, must be differentiated from a neuromuscular etiology. Fixation is best documented by absence of passive mobility during rigid laryngoscopy under general anesthesia. Cricoarytenoid arthritis may complicate such conditions as RA, external blunt trauma, and prolonged endotracheal intubation.

Treatment

- For unilateral paralysis, surgical procedures to move cords closer together
- For bilateral paralysis, surgical procedures and measures to maintain airway

In **unilateral paralysis,** treatment is directed at improving voice quality through augmentation, medialization, or reinnervation.

Augmentation involves injecting a paste of plasticized particles, collagen, micronized dermis, or autologous fat into the paralyzed cord, bringing the cords closer together to improve the voice and prevent aspiration.

Medialization is shifting the vocal cord toward the midline by inserting an adjustable spacer laterally to the affected cord. This can be done with a local anesthetic, allowing the position of the spacer to be "tuned" to the patient's voice.

Reinnervation has only rarely been successful.

In **bilateral paralysis,** an adequate airway must be reestablished. Tracheotomy may be needed permanently or temporarily during a URI. An arytenoidectomy with lateralization of the true vocal cord opens the glottis and improves the airway but may adversely affect voice quality. Posterior laser cordectomy opens the posterior glottis and may be preferred to endoscopic or open arytenoidectomy. Successful laser establishment of a posterior glottic airway usually obviates the need for long-term tracheotomy while preserving a serviceable voice quality.

KEY POINTS

- Vocal cord paralysis can be caused by a lesion anywhere on the neural pathway to the larynx (the nucleus ambiguus, its supranuclear tracts, the main trunk of the vagus, the recurrent laryngeal nerves).
- Most paralyses are unilateral and affect mainly the voice, but bilateral paralysis can occur and obstruct the airway.
- Paralysis is diagnosed by direct laryngoscopy, but identification of the cause typically requires imaging (eg, MRI) and other tests.
- Patients with bilateral paralysis often require tracheal intubation initially.
- Various surgical procedures are available to improve voice quality in unilateral paralysis or to improve airway patency in long-term bilateral paralysis.

VOCAL CORD POLYPS, NODULES, AND GRANULOMAS

Acute trauma or chronic irritation causes changes in the vocal cords that can lead to polyps, nodules, or granulomas. All cause hoarseness and a breathy voice. Persistence

of these symptoms for > 3 wk dictates visualization of the vocal cords. Diagnosis is based on laryngoscopy and on biopsy in selected cases to rule out cancer. Judicious surgical removal restores the voice, and removal of the irritating source prevents recurrence.

Etiology

Polyps and nodules result from injury to the lamina propria of the true vocal cords. Granulomas result from injury to the perichondrium overlying the vocal processes of the arytenoid cartilages (see Table 96–1).

Polyps may occur at the mid third of the membranous cords and are more often unilateral. Polyps tend to be larger and more protuberant than nodules and often have a dominant surface blood vessel. They frequently result from an initiating acute phonatory injury. Other polypoid changes, often bilateral, may have several other causes, including gastroesophageal reflux, untreated hypothyroid states, chronic laryngeal allergic reactions, or chronic inhalation of irritants, such as industrial fumes or cigarette smoke. Acute injury usually causes pedunculated polyps, whereas polypoid edema results from chronic irritation.

Nodules usually occur bilaterally at the junction of the anterior and middle third of the cords. Their main cause is chronic voice abuse—yelling, shouting, singing loudly, or using an unnaturally low frequency.

Granulomas occur in the posterior glottis against the vocal processes. They can be bilateral or unilateral. They usually result from intubation trauma but may be aggravated by reflux disease.

Symptoms and Signs

All result in slowly developing hoarseness and a breathy voice.

Diagnosis

- Laryngoscopy
- Sometimes biopsy

Diagnosis is based on direct or indirect visualization of the larynx with a mirror or laryngoscope. Biopsy of discrete lesions to exclude carcinoma is done by microlaryngoscopy.

Treatment

- Avoidance of cause
- For polyps, usually surgical removal

Correction of the underlying voice abuse cures most nodules and granulomas and prevents recurrence. Removal of the offending irritants (including treatment of any gastroesophageal reflux) allows healing, and voice therapy with a speech therapist reduces the trauma to the vocal cords caused by improper singing or protracted loud speaking. Nodules usually regress with voice therapy alone. Granulomas that do not regress can be removed surgically but tend to recur.

Most polyps must be surgically removed to restore a normal voice. Cold-knife microsurgical excision during direct microlaryngoscopy is preferable to laser excision, which is more likely to cause collateral thermal injury if improperly applied.

In **microlaryngoscopy,** an operating microscope is used to examine, biopsy, and operate on the larynx. Images can be recorded on video as well. The patient is anesthetized, and the airway is secured by high-pressure jet ventilation through the laryngoscope, endotracheal intubation, or, for an inadequate upper airway, tracheotomy. Because the microscope allows observation with magnification, tissue can be removed precisely and accurately, minimizing damage (possibly permanent) to the vocal mechanism. Laser surgery can be done through the optical system of the microscope to allow for precise cuts. Microlaryngoscopy is preferred for almost all laryngeal biopsies, for procedures involving benign tumors, and for many forms of phonosurgery.

KEY POINTS

- Vocal cord polyps result from acute trauma or chronic irritation.
- Symptoms persisting > 3 wk dictate visualization of the vocal cords.
- Biopsy may be necessary to rule out cancer.
- After excision, removal of the irritating source is necessary to prevent recurrence.

LARYNGEAL CONTACT ULCERS

Laryngeal contact ulcers are unilateral or bilateral erosions of the mucous membrane over the vocal process of the arytenoid cartilage.

Laryngeal contact ulcers are usually caused by voice abuse in the form of repeated sharp glottal attacks (abrupt loudness at the onset of phonation), often experienced by singers. They may also occur after endotracheal intubation if an oversized tube

Table 96–1. DIFFERENTIATING VOCAL POLYPS, NODULES, AND GRANULOMAS

TYPE	CAUSES	FEATURES	TREATMENT
Polyps	Acute trauma, gastroesophageal reflux, untreated hypothyroid states, chronic laryngeal allergic reactions, chronic inhalation of irritants (eg, industrial fumes, cigarette smoke)	Unilateral Occur at the membranous cord Larger than nodules Surface blood vessel	Surgical removal of traumatic polyps Medical treatment, initially, of other polypoid lesions
Nodules	Chronic trauma (eg, voice abuse, yelling, shouting, singing loudly, using an unnaturally low frequency)	Bilateral Occur at the membranous cord	Behavior modification (eg, decreasing musculoskeletal laryngeal tension when speaking), voice therapy, antireflux therapy
Granulomas	Repeated vocal abuse, reflux disease, endotracheal intubation	Often bilateral but can be unilateral Occur at both vocal processes (posterior cords) Larger than nodules	Voice therapy, antireflux therapy For granulomas that do not regress, surgical removal

erodes the mucosa overlying the cartilaginous vocal processes. Gastroesophageal reflux may also cause or aggravate contact ulcers. Prolonged ulceration leads to nonspecific granulomas.

Symptoms of laryngeal contact ulcers include varying degrees of hoarseness and mild pain with phonation and swallowing.

Diagnosis of laryngeal contact ulcers is by laryngoscopy. Biopsy to exclude carcinoma or TB is important.

Treatment of laryngeal contact ulcers consists of ≥ 6 wk of voice rest. Patients must recognize the limitations of their voice and learn to adjust their post-recovery vocal activities to avoid recurrence. Suppression of bacterial flora with antibiotics is also recommended.

Risk of recurrence is reduced through vigorous treatment of gastroesophageal reflux (see p. 113).

97 Middle Ear and Tympanic Membrane Disorders

Middle ear disorders may be secondary to infection, eustachian tube obstruction, or trauma. Information about objects placed in the ear and symptoms such as rhinorrhea, nasal obstruction, sore throat, URI, allergies, headache, systemic symptoms, and fever aid diagnosis. The appearance of the external auditory canal and tympanic membrane (see Fig. 97–1) often yields a diagnosis. The nose, nasopharynx, and oropharynx are examined for signs of infection and allergy and for evidence of tumors.

Middle ear function is evaluated with use of pneumatic otoscopy, the Weber and Rinne tuning fork tests, tympanometry, and audiologic tests (see p. 813).

MASTOIDITIS

Mastoiditis is a bacterial infection of the mastoid air cells, which typically occurs after acute otitis media. Symptoms include redness, tenderness, swelling, and fluctuation over the mastoid process, with displacement of the pinna. Diagnosis is clinical. Treatment is with antibiotics, such as ceftriaxone, and mastoidectomy if drug therapy is not effective.

In acute purulent otitis media, inflammation often extends into the mastoid antrum and air cells, resulting in fluid accumulation. In a few patients, bacterial infection develops in the collected fluid, typically with the same organism causing the otitis media; pneumococcus is most common. Mastoid infection can cause osteitis of the septae, leading to coalescence of the air cells.

The infection may decompress through a perforation in the tympanic membrane or extend through the lateral mastoid cortex, forming a postauricular subperiosteal abscess. Rarely, it extends centrally, causing a temporal lobe abscess or a septic thrombosis of the lateral sinus. Occasionally, the infection may erode through the tip of the mastoid and drain into the neck (called a Bezold abscess).

Symptoms and Signs

Symptoms begin days to weeks after onset of acute otitis media and include fever and persistent, throbbing otalgia. Nearly all patients have signs of otitis media (see p. 830) and purulent otorrhea. Redness, swelling, tenderness, and fluctuation may develop over the mastoid process; the pinna is typically displaced laterally and inferiorly.

Diagnosis

- Clinical evaluation
- Rarely CT

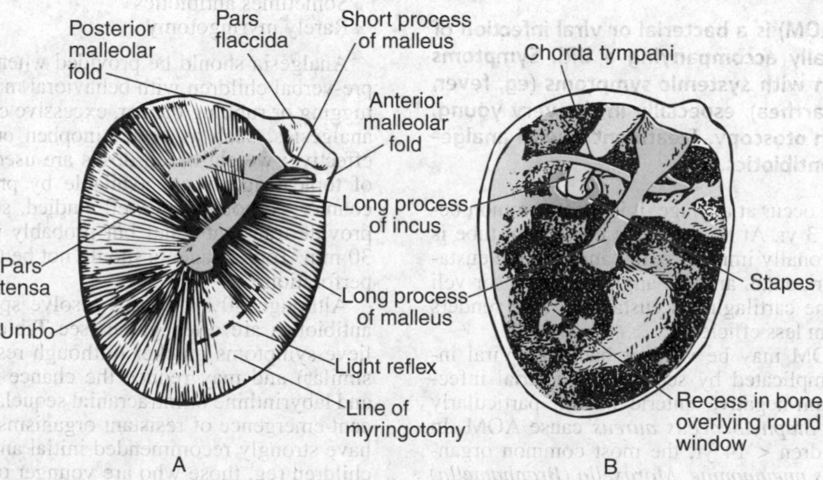

Fig. 97–1. Tympanic membrane of right ear (A); tympanic cavity with tympanic membrane removed (B).

Diagnosis is clinical. CT is rarely necessary but can confirm the diagnosis and show the extent of the infection. Any middle ear drainage is sent for culture and sensitivity. Tympanocentesis for culture purposes can be done if no spontaneous drainage occurs. CBC and ESR may be abnormal but are neither sensitive nor specific and add little to the diagnosis.

Treatment

- IV ceftriaxone

IV antibiotic treatment is initiated immediately with a drug that provides CNS penetration, such as ceftriaxone 1 to 2 g (children, 50 to 75 mg/kg) once/day continued for ≥ 2 wk. Oral treatment with a quinolone may be acceptable. Subsequent antibiotic choice is guided by culture and sensitivity test results.

A subperiosteal abscess usually requires a simple mastoidectomy, in which the abscess is drained, the infected mastoid cells are removed, and drainage is established from the antrum of the mastoid to the middle ear cavity.

MYRINGITIS

(Bullous Myringitis)

Myringitis is a form of acute otitis media in which vesicles develop on the tympanic membrane.

Myringitis can develop with viral, bacterial (particularly *Streptococcus pneumoniae*), or mycoplasmal otitis media. Pain occurs suddenly and persists for 24 to 48 h. Hearing loss and fever suggest a bacterial origin. Diagnosis is based on otoscopic visualization of vesicles on the tympanic membrane.

Because differentiation among a viral, bacterial, and mycoplasmal cause is difficult, antibiotics effective against organisms causing otitis media are prescribed (see Table 97–1). Severe, continued pain may be relieved by rupturing the vesicles with a myringotomy knife or by oral analgesics (eg, oxycodone with acetaminophen). Topical analgesics (eg, benzocaine, antipyrine) may also be beneficial.

OTITIS MEDIA (ACUTE)

Acute otitis media (AOM) is a bacterial or viral infection of the middle ear, usually accompanying a URI. Symptoms include otalgia, often with systemic symptoms (eg, fever, nausea, vomiting, diarrhea), especially in the very young. Diagnosis is based on otoscopy. Treatment is with analgesics and sometimes antibiotics.

Although AOM can occur at any age, it is most common between ages 3 mo and 3 yr. At this age, the eustachian tube is structurally and functionally immature, the angle of the eustachian tube is more horizontal, and the angle of the tensor veli palatini muscle and the cartilaginous eustachian tube renders the opening mechanism less efficient.

The etiology of AOM may be viral or bacterial. Viral infections are often complicated by secondary bacterial infection. In neonates, gram-negative enteric bacilli, particularly *Escherichia coli,* and *Staphylococcus aureus* cause AOM. In older infants and children < 14 yr, the most common organisms are *Streptococcus pneumoniae, Moraxella (Branhamella) catarrhalis,* and nontypeable *Haemophilus influenzae;* less common causes are group A β-hemolytic streptococci and *S. aureus*. In patients > 14 yr, *S. pneumoniae,* group A β-hemolytic streptococci, and *S. aureus* are most common, followed by *H. influenzae*.

Risk factors: The presence of smoking in the household is a significant risk factor for acute otitis media. Other risk factors include a strong family history of otitis media, bottle feeding (ie, instead of breastfeeding), and attending a day care center.

Complications: Complications of acute otitis media are uncommon. In rare cases, bacterial middle ear infection spreads locally, resulting in acute mastoiditis, petrositis, or labyrinthitis. Intracranial spread is extremely rare and usually causes meningitis, but brain abscess, subdural empyema, epidural abscess, lateral sinus thrombosis, or otitic hydrocephalus may occur. Even with antibiotic treatment, intracranial complications are slow to resolve, especially in immunocompromised patients.

Symptoms and Signs

The usual initial symptom is earache, often with hearing loss. Infants may simply be cranky or have difficulty sleeping. Fever, nausea, vomiting, and diarrhea often occur in young children. Otoscopic examination can show a bulging, erythematous tympanic membrane (TM) with indistinct landmarks and displacement of the light reflex. Air insufflation (pneumatic otoscopy) shows poor mobility of the TM. Spontaneous perforation of the TM causes serosanguineous or purulent otorrhea.

Severe headache, confusion, or focal neurologic signs may occur with intracranial spread of infection. Facial paralysis or vertigo suggests local extension to the fallopian canal or labyrinth.

Diagnosis

- Clinical evaluation

Diagnosis of acute otitis media usually is clinical, based on the presence of acute (within 48 h) onset of pain, bulging of the TM and, particularly in children, the presence of signs of middle ear effusion on pneumatic otoscopy. Except for fluid obtained during myringotomy, cultures are not generally done.

Treatment

- Analgesics
- Sometimes antibiotics
- Rarely myringotomy

Analgesia should be provided when necessary, including to pre-verbal children with behavioral manifestations of pain (eg, tugging or rubbing the ear, excessive crying or fussiness). Oral analgesics, such as acetaminophen or ibuprofen, are usually effective; weight-based doses are used for children. A variety of topical agents are available by prescription and over the counter. Although not well studied, some topical agents may provide transient relief but probably not for more than 20 to 30 min. Topical agents should not be used when there is a TM perforation.

Although 80% of cases resolve spontaneously, in the US, antibiotics are often given (see Table 97–1).[1] Antibiotics relieve symptoms quicker (although results after 1 to 2 wk are similar) and may reduce the chance of residual hearing loss and labyrinthine or intracranial sequelae. However, with the recent emergence of resistant organisms, pediatric organizations have strongly recommended initial antibiotics only for certain children (eg, those who are younger or more severely ill—see Table 97–1) or for those with recurrent AOM (eg, ≥ 4 episodes in 6 mo).

Table 97–1. ANTIBIOTICS FOR OTITIS MEDIA

DRUG	DOSE* (BY AGE)	COMMENTS
Initial treatment		
Amoxicillin	< 14 yr: 40–45 mg/kg q 12 h > 14 yr: 500 mg q 8 h	Preferred unless the child has one of the following: • Received amoxicillin in the past 30 days • Purulent conjunctivitis • Recurrent acute otitis media unresponsive to amoxicillin High-dose regimen for possible resistant organisms
Penicillin-allergic†		
Cefdinir	14 mg/kg once/day or 7 mg/kg q 12 h	—
Cefuroxime	< 14 yr: 15 mg/kg q 12 h > 14 yr: 500 mg q 12 h	Maximum 1000 mg/day
Cefpodoxime	5 mg/kg q 12 h	—
Ceftriaxone	50 mg/kg IM or IV once May repeat at 72 h	Consider particularly for children with severe vomiting or who will not swallow antibiotic liquids
Resistant cases‡		
Amoxicillin/clavulanate	< 14 yr: 40–45 mg/kg q 12 h ≥ 14 yr: 500 mg q 12 h	Preferred; dose based on amoxicillin component Use new formulation to limit clavulanate to maximum of 10 mg/kg/day
Ceftriaxone	50 mg/kg IM or IV once/day for 3 days	Can use even if failed on oral cephalosporin Considered if adherence is likely to be poor
Clindamycin	10 to 13 mg/kg q 8 h	2nd-line alternative, consider using along with a cephalosporin

*Treatment duration is typically 10 days for children < 2 yr and 7 days for older children unless otherwise specified. Drugs are given orally unless otherwise specified.

†Cross reactivity of 2nd- and 3rd-generation cephalosporins with penicillin is very low.

‡No improvement after 48 to 72 h of treatment, or previous resistant infection; amoxicillin used in the previous 30 days; or concurrent purulent conjunctivitis

Data from Lieberthal AS, Carroll AE, Chonmaitree T, et al: The diagnosis and management of acute otitis media. *Pediatrics* e964–999, 2013.

Others, provided there is good follow-up, can safely be observed for 48 to 72 h and given antibiotics only if no improvement is seen; if follow-up by phone is planned, a prescription can be given at the initial visit to save time and expense. Decision to observe should be discussed with the caregiver.

All patients receive analgesics (eg, acetaminophen, ibuprofen). In adults, topical intranasal vasoconstrictors, such as phenylephrine 0.25% 3 drops q 3 h, improve eustachian tube function. To avoid rebound congestion, these preparations should not be used > 4 days. Systemic decongestants (eg, pseudoephedrine 30 to 60 mg po q 6 h prn) may be helpful. Antihistamines (eg, chlorpheniramine 4 mg po q 4 to 6 h for 7 to 10 days) may improve eustachian tube function in people with allergies but should be reserved for the truly allergic.

Table 97–2. GUIDELINES FOR USING ANTIBIOTICS IN CHILDREN WITH AOM*

AGE	OTORRHEA	SEVERE SYMPTOMS† (UNILATERAL OR BILATERAL)	BILATERAL DISEASE	UNILATERAL DISEASE, NO SEVERE SYMPTOMS
< 6 mo‡	Antibiotics	Antibiotics	Antibiotics	Antibiotics
6 mo to 2 yr	Antibiotics	Antibiotics	Antibiotics	Antibiotics or observe 48 to 72 h§
≥ 2 yr	Antibiotics	Antibiotics	Antibiotics or observe 48 to 72 h§	Antibiotics or observe 48 to 72 h§

*These guidelines apply only to children who meet the diagnostic criteria for AOM(eg, acute [within 48 h] onset of pain, bulging of the tympanic membrane, and signs of middle ear effusion on pneumatic otoscopy).

†Symptoms include temperature ≥ 39° C rectally any time within previous 24 h or moderate to severe otalgia for > 48 h, or physician's judgment that child is seriously ill.

‡The guidelines in the *Pediatrics* article from which this table was derived do not include this age group in which observation has not been thoroughly studied. Thus it is reasonable to continue to treat with antibiotics.

§Decision making should be shared with parents. Observation is appropriate only if phone or office follow-up can be assured within 48 to 72 h; antibiotics are started if no improvement.

Modified from Lieberthal AS, Carroll AE, Chonmaitree T, et al: The diagnosis and management of acute otitis media. *Pediatrics* e964–999, 2013.

For children, neither vasoconstrictors nor antihistamines are of benefit.

Myringotomy may be done for a bulging TM, particularly if severe or persistent pain, fever, vomiting, or diarrhea is present. The patient's hearing, tympanometry, and TM appearance and movement are monitored until normal.

1. Lieberthal AS, Carroll AE, Chonmaitree T, et al: The diagnosis and management of acute otitis media. *Pediatrics* e964–999, 2013.

Prevention

Routine childhood vaccination against pneumococci (with pneumococcal conjugate vaccine), *H. influenzae* type B, and influenza decreases the incidence of AOM. Infants should not sleep with a bottle, and elimination of household smoking may decrease incidence. Prophylactic antibiotics are not recommended for children who have recurrent episodes of AOM.

KEY POINTS

- Give analgesics to all patients.
- Antihistamines and decongestants are not recommended for children; oral or nasal decongestants may help adults, but antihistamines are reserved for adults with an allergic etiology.
- Antibiotics should be used selectively based on the age of the patient, severity of illness, and availability of follow-up.

OTITIS MEDIA (SECRETORY)

(Serous Otitis Media)

Secretory otitis media is an effusion in the middle ear resulting from incomplete resolution of acute otitis media or obstruction of the eustachian tube without infection. Symptoms include hearing loss and a sense of fullness or pressure in the ear. Diagnosis is based on appearance of the tympanic membrane and sometimes on tympanometry. Most cases resolve in 2 to 3 wk. If there is no improvement in 1 to 3 mo, some form of myringotomy is indicated, usually with insertion of a tympanostomy tube. Antibiotics and decongestants are not effective.

Normally, the middle ear is ventilated 3 to 4 times/min as the eustachian tube opens during swallowing, and O_2 is absorbed by blood in the vessels of the middle ear mucous membrane. If patency of the eustachian tube is impaired, a relative negative pressure develops within the middle ear, which can lead to fluid accumulation. This fluid may cause hearing loss.

Secretory otitis media is a common sequela to acute otitis media in children (often identified on routine ear recheck) and may persist for weeks to months. In other cases, eustachian tube obstruction may be secondary to inflammatory processes in the nasopharynx, allergies, hypertrophic adenoids or other obstructive lymphoid aggregations on the torus of the eustachian tube and in the Rosenmüller fossa, or benign or malignant tumors. The effusion may be sterile or (more commonly) contain pathogenic bacteria sometimes as a biofilm, although inflammation is not observed.

Symptoms and Signs

Patients may report no symptoms, but some (or their family members) note hearing loss. Patients may experience a feeling of fullness, pressure, or popping in the ear with swallowing. Otalgia is rare.

Various possible changes to the tympanic membrane (TM) include an amber or gray color, displacement of the light reflex, mild to severe retraction, and accentuated landmarks. On air insufflation, the TM may be immobile. An air-fluid level or bubbles of air may be visible through the TM.

Diagnosis

- Tympanometry
- Nasopharyngeal examination

Diagnosis of secretory otitis media is clinical. Tympanometry may be done to confirm middle ear effusion (ie, by showing lack of mobility of the tympanic membrane). Adults and adolescents must undergo nasopharyngeal examination to exclude malignant or benign tumors.

Treatment

- Observation
- If unresolved, myringotomy with tympanostomy tube insertion
- If recurrent in childhood, sometimes adenoidectomy

For most patients, watchful waiting is all that is required. Antibiotics and decongestants are not helpful. For patients in whom allergies are clearly involved, antihistamines and topical corticosteroids may be helpful.

If no improvement occurs in 1 to 3 mo, myringotomy may be done for aspiration of fluid and insertion of a tympanostomy tube, which allows ventilation of the middle ear and temporarily ameliorates eustachian tube obstruction, regardless of cause. Tympanostomy tubes may be inserted for persistent conductive hearing loss or to help prevent recurrence of acute otitis media.

Occasionally, the middle ear is temporarily ventilated with the Valsalva maneuver or politzerization. To do the Valsalva maneuver, patients keep their mouth closed and try to forcibly blow air out through their pinched nostrils (ie, popping the ear). To do politzerization, the physician blows air with a special syringe (middle ear inflator) into one of the patient's nostrils and blocks the other while the patient swallows. This forces the air into the eustachian tube and middle ear. Neither procedure should be done if the patient has a cold and rhinorrhea.

Persistent, recurrent secretory otitis media may require correction of underlying nasopharyngeal conditions. In children, particularly adolescent boys, a nasopharyngeal angiofibroma should be ruled out and, in adults, nasopharyngeal carcinoma must be ruled out. Children may benefit from adenoidectomy, including the removal of the central adenoid mass as well as lymphoid aggregations on the torus of the eustachian tube and in the Rosenmüller fossa. Antibiotics should be given for bacterial rhinitis, sinusitis, and nasopharyngitis. Demonstrated allergens should be eliminated from the patient's environment and immunotherapy should be considered.

KEY POINTS

- Secretory otitis media is noninflammatory middle ear effusion usually following acute otitis media.
- Diagnosis is clinical; adults and adolescents must undergo nasopharyngeal examination to exclude malignant or benign tumors.

- Antibiotics and decongestants are not helpful.
- If unresolved in 1 to 3 mo, myringotomy with tympanostomy tube insertion may be needed.

OTITIS MEDIA (CHRONIC)

Chronic otitis media is a persistent, chronically draining (> 6 wk), suppurative perforation of the tympanic membrane. Symptoms include painless otorrhea with conductive hearing loss. Complications include development of aural polyps, cholesteatoma, and other infections. Treatment requires complete cleaning of the ear canal several times daily, careful removal of granulation tissue, and application of topical corticosteroids and antibiotics. Systemic antibiotics and surgery are reserved for severe cases.

Chronic otitis media can result from AOM, eustachian tube obstruction, mechanical trauma, thermal or chemical burns, blast injuries, or iatrogenic causes (eg, after tympanostomy tube placement). Further, patients with craniofacial abnormalities (eg, Down syndrome, cri du chat syndrome, cleft lip and/or cleft palate, velocardiofacial syndrome [Shprintzen syndrome]) have an increased risk.

Chronic otitis media may become exacerbated after a URI or when water enters the middle ear through a tympanic membrane (TM) perforation during bathing or swimming. Infections often are caused by gram-negative bacilli or *Staphylococcus aureus,* resulting in painless, purulent, sometimes foul-smelling otorrhea. Persistent chronic otitis media may result in destructive changes in the middle ear (such as necrosis of the long process of the incus) or aural polyps (granulation tissue prolapsing into the ear canal through the TM perforation). Aural polyps are a serious sign, almost invariably suggesting cholesteatoma.

A cholesteatoma is an epithelial cell growth that forms in the middle ear, mastoid, or epitympanum after chronic otitis media (see Plate 6). Lytic enzymes, such as collagenases, produced by the cholesteatoma can destroy adjacent bone and soft tissue. The cholesteatoma is also a nidus for infection; purulent labyrinthitis, facial paralysis, or intracranial abscess may develop.

Symptoms and Signs

Chronic otitis media usually manifests with conductive hearing loss and otorrhea. Pain is uncommon unless an associated osteitis of the temporal bone occurs. The TM is perforated and draining, and the auditory canal is macerated and littered with granulation tissue.

A patient with cholesteatoma has white debris in the middle ear, a draining polypoid mass protruding through the TM perforation, and an ear canal that appears clogged with mucopurulent granulation tissue.

Diagnosis

- Clinical evaluation

Diagnosis of chronic otitis media is usually clinical. Drainage is cultured. When cholesteatoma or other complications are suspected (as in a febrile patient or one with vertigo or otalgia), CT or MRI is done. These tests may reveal intratemporal or intracranial processes (eg, labyrinthitis, ossicular or temporal erosion, abscesses).

Treatment

- Topical antibiotic drops
- Removal of granulation tissue
- Surgery for cholesteatomas

Ten drops of topical ciprofloxacin solution are instilled in the affected ear 2 times/day for 14 days.

When granulation tissue is present, it is removed with microinstruments or cauterization with silver nitrate sticks. Ciprofloxacin 0.3% and dexamethasone 0.1% is then instilled into the ear canal for 7 to 10 days.

Severe exacerbations require systemic antibiotic therapy with amoxicillin 250 to 500 mg po q 8 h for 10 days or a 3rd-generation cephalosporin, subsequently modified by culture results and response to therapy.

Tympanoplasty is indicated for patients with marginal or attic perforations and chronic central TM perforations. A disrupted ossicular chain may be repaired during tympanoplasty as well.

Cholesteatomas must be removed surgically. Because recurrence is common, reconstruction of the middle ear is usually deferred until a 2nd-look operation (using an open surgical approach or a small-diameter otoscope) is done 6 to 8 mo later.

KEY POINTS

- Chronic otitis media is a persistent perforation of the TM with chronic suppurative drainage.
- Damage to middle ear structures often develops; less commonly, intratemporal or intracranial structures are affected.
- Initial treatment is with topical antibiotics.
- Severe exacerbations require systemic antibiotics.
- Surgery is needed for certain types of perforation and damaged ossicles and to remove any cholesteatomas.

OTIC BAROTRAUMA

(Barotitis Media; Aerotitis Media)

Otic barotrauma is ear pain or damage to the tympanic membrane caused by rapid changes in pressure.

To maintain equal pressure on both sides of the tympanic membrane (TM), gas must move freely between the nasopharynx and middle ear. When a URI, allergy, or other mechanism interferes with eustachian tube functioning during changes in environmental pressure, the pressure in the middle ear either falls below ambient pressure, causing retraction of the TM, or rises above it, causing bulging. With negative middle ear pressure, a transudate of fluid may form in the middle ear. As the pressure differential increases, ecchymosis and subepithelial hematoma may develop in the mucous membrane of the middle ear and the TM. A very large pressure differential may cause bleeding into the middle ear, TM rupture, and the development of a perilymph fistula through the oval or round window.

Symptoms of otic barotrauma are severe pain, conductive hearing loss, and, if there is a perilymph fistula, sensorineural hearing loss and/or vertigo. Symptoms usually worsen during rapid increase in external air pressures, such as a rapid ascent (eg, during scuba diving) or descent (eg, during air travel). Sensorineural hearing loss or vertigo during descent suggests the development of a perilymph fistula; the same symptoms during ascent from a deep-sea dive can additionally suggest an air bubble formation in the inner ear.

Treatment

- Methods to equalize pressure (eg, yawning, swallowing, chewing gum)

Routine self-treatment of pain associated with changing pressure in an aircraft includes chewing gum, attempting to yawn and swallow, blowing against closed nostrils, and using decongestant nasal sprays.

If hearing loss is sensorineural and vertigo is present, a perilymph fistula is suspected and middle ear exploration to close a fistula is considered. If pain is severe and hearing loss is conductive, myringotomy is helpful.

Prevention

A person with nasal congestion due to URI or allergies should avoid flying and diving. When these activities are unavoidable, a topical nasal vasoconstrictor (eg, phenylephrine 0.25 to 1.0%) is applied 30 to 60 min before descent or ascent.

OTOSCLEROSIS

Otosclerosis is a disease of the bone of the otic capsule that causes an abnormal accumulation of new bone within the oval window.

In otosclerosis, the new bone traps and restricts the movement of the stapes, causing conductive hearing loss (see p. 809). Otosclerosis also may cause a sensorineural hearing loss, particularly when the foci of otosclerotic bone are adjacent to the scala media. Half of all cases are inherited. The measles virus plays an inciting role in patients with a genetic predisposition for otosclerosis.

Although about 10% of white adults have some otosclerosis (compared with 1% of African Americans and even less in blacks of primarily African origin), only about 10% of affected people develop conductive hearing loss. Hearing loss caused by otosclerosis rarely may manifest as early as age 7 or 8, but most cases do not become evident until the late adolescent or early adult years, when slowly progressive, asymmetric hearing loss is diagnosed. It is thought that fixation of the stapes may progress during pregnancy.

A hearing aid may improve hearing. Alternatively, stapedectomy to remove some or all of the stapes and to replace it with a prosthesis may be beneficial, but the risks of hearing loss and impaired vestibular function need to be considered.

TRAUMATIC PERFORATION OF THE TYMPANIC MEMBRANE

Traumatic perforation of the tympanic membrane (TM) can cause pain, bleeding, hearing loss, tinnitus, and vertigo. Diagnosis is based on otoscopy. Treatment often is unnecessary. Antibiotics may be needed for infection. Surgery may be needed for perforations persisting > 2 mo, disruption of the ossicular chain, or injuries affecting the inner ear.

Traumatic causes of TM perforation include

- Insertion of objects into the ear canal purposely (eg, cotton swabs) or accidentally
- Concussion caused by an explosion or open-handed slap across the ear
- Head trauma (with or without basilar fracture)
- Sudden negative pressure (eg, strong suction applied to the ear canal)
- Barotrauma (eg, during air travel or scuba diving)
- Iatrogenic perforation during irrigation or foreign body removal

Penetrating injuries of the TM may result in dislocations of the ossicular chain, fracture of the stapedial footplate, displacement of fragments of the ossicles, bleeding, a perilymph fistula from the oval or round window resulting in leakage of perilymph into the middle ear space, or facial nerve injury.

Symptoms and Signs

Traumatic perforation of the TM causes sudden severe pain sometimes followed by bleeding from the ear, hearing loss, and tinnitus. Hearing loss is more severe if the ossicular chain is disrupted or the inner ear is injured. Vertigo suggests injury to the inner ear. Purulent otorrhea may begin in 24 to 48 h, particularly if water enters the middle ear.

Diagnosis

- Otoscopy
- Audiometry

Perforation is generally evident on otoscopy. Any blood obscuring the ear canal is carefully suctioned. Irrigation and pneumatic otoscopy are avoided. Extremely small perforations may require otomicroscopy or middle ear impedance studies for definitive diagnosis. If possible, audiometric studies are done before and after treatment to avoid confusion between trauma-induced and treatment-induced hearing loss.

Patients with marked hearing loss or severe vertigo are evaluated by an otolaryngologist as soon as possible. Exploratory tympanotomy may be needed to assess and repair damage. Patients with a large TM defect should also be evaluated, because the displaced flaps may need to be repositioned.

Treatment

- Ear kept dry
- Oral or topical antibiotics if dirty injury

Often, no specific treatment is needed. The ear should be kept dry; routine antibiotic ear drops are unnecessary. However, prophylaxis with oral broad-spectrum antibiotics or antibiotic ear drops is necessary if contaminants may have entered through the perforation as occurs in dirty injuries.

If the ear becomes infected, amoxicillin 500 mg po q 8 h is given for 7 days.

Although most perforations close spontaneously, surgery is indicated for a perforation persisting > 2 mo. Persistent conductive hearing loss suggests disruption of the ossicular chain, necessitating surgical exploration and repair.

KEY POINTS

- Many perforations are small and heal spontaneously.
- The ear should be kept dry during healing; topical or systemic antibiotics are unnecessary unless there is significant contamination or if infection develops.
- Surgery is done to repair damage to the ossicles and for perforations persisting > 2 mo.

98 Nose and Paranasal Sinus Disorders

BACTERIAL NASAL INFECTIONS

Nasal vestibulitis is bacterial infection of the nasal vestibule, typically with *Staphylococcus aureus*. It may result from nose picking or excessive nose blowing and causes annoying crusts and bleeding when the crusts slough off. Bacitracin or mupirocin ointment applied topically bid for 14 days is effective.

Furuncles of the nasal vestibule are usually staphylococcal; they may develop into spreading cellulitis of the tip of the nose. Systemic antistaphylococcal antibiotics (eg, cephalexin 500 mg po qid) are given and warm compresses and topical mupirocin are applied. Furuncles are incised and drained to prevent local thrombophlebitis and subsequent cavernous sinus thrombosis.

Treatment of community-associated methicillin-resistant *S. aureus* infections should be directed by culture and sensitivity test results. Typically, clindamycin, trimethoprim/sulfamethoxazole, and doxycycline are effective against most strains.

NASAL FOREIGN BODIES

Nasal foreign bodies are found occasionally in young children, the intellectually impaired, and psychiatric patients. Common objects pushed into the nose include cotton, paper, pebbles, beads, beans, seeds, nuts, insects, and button batteries (which may cause chemical burns). When mineral salts are deposited on a long-retained foreign body, the object is called a rhinolith.

A nasal foreign body is suspected in any patient with a unilateral, foul-smelling, bloody, purulent rhinorrhea. Diagnosis is often made through another party's observation of the item being pushed into the nose or through visualization with a nasal speculum.

Nasal foreign bodies can sometimes be removed in the office with a nasal speculum and Hartmann nasal forceps. Pretreatment with topical phenylephrine may aid visualization and removal. To avoid pushing a slippery, round object deeper, it is better to reach behind the object with the bent tip of a blunt probe and pull it forward. Sometimes, general anesthesia is necessary if a rhinolith has formed or if the foreign body may be displaced dorsally and then aspirated, resulting in airway obstruction.

NASAL POLYPS

Nasal polyps are fleshy outgrowths of the nasal mucosa that form at the site of dependent edema in the lamina propria of the mucous membrane, usually around the ostia of the maxillary sinuses (see Plate 7).

Allergic rhinitis, acute and chronic infections, and cystic fibrosis all predispose to the formation of nasal polyps. Bleeding polyps occur in rhinosporidiosis. Unilateral polyps occasionally occur in association with or represent benign or malignant tumors of the nose or paranasal sinuses. They can also occur in response to a foreign body. Nasal polyps are strongly associated with

- Aspirin allergy
- Sinus infections
- Asthma

Symptoms include obstruction and postnasal drainage, congestion, sneezing, rhinorrhea, anosmia, hyposmia, facial pain, and ocular itching.

Diagnosis generally is based on physical examination. A developing polyp is teardrop-shaped; when mature, it resembles a peeled seedless grape.

Treatment

- Topical corticosteroid spray
- Sometimes surgical removal

Corticosteroids (eg, mometasone [30 mcg/spray], beclomethasone [42 mcg/spray], flunisolide [25 mcg/spray] aerosols), given as 1 or 2 sprays bid in each nasal cavity, may shrink or eliminate polyps, as may a 1-wk tapered course of oral corticosteroids.

Surgical removal is required in many cases. Polyps that obstruct the airway or promote sinusitis are removed, as are unilateral polyps that may be obscuring benign or malignant tumors.

Polyps tend to recur unless the underlying allergy or infection is controlled. After removal of nasal polyps, topical beclomethasone or flunisolide therapy tends to retard recurrence. In severe recurrent cases, maxillary sinusotomy or ethmoidectomy may be indicated. These procedures are usually done endoscopically.

NONALLERGIC RHINITIS

Rhinitis is inflammation of the nasal mucous membrane, with resultant nasal congestion, rhinorrhea, and variable associated symptoms depending on etiology (eg, itching, sneezing, watery or purulent rhinorrhea, anosmia). Rhinitis is classified as allergic or nonallergic. The cause of nonallergic rhinitis is usually viral, although irritants can cause it. Diagnosis is usually clinical. Treatment includes humidification of room air, sympathomimetic amines, and antihistamines. Bacterial superinfection requires appropriate antibiotic treatment.

There are several forms of nonallergic rhinitis. For allergic rhinitis, see p. 1376.

Acute rhinitis: Acute rhinitis, manifesting with edema and vasodilation of the nasal mucous membrane, rhinorrhea, and obstruction, is usually the result of a common cold (see p. 1685); other causes include streptococcal, pneumococcal, and staphylococcal infections.

Chronic rhinitis: Chronic rhinitis is generally a prolongation of subacute (resolved in 30 to 90 days) inflammatory or infectious viral rhinitis. It may also rarely occur in syphilis, TB, rhinoscleroma, rhinosporidiosis, leishmaniasis, blastomycosis, histoplasmosis, and leprosy—all of which are characterized by granuloma formation and destruction of soft tissue, cartilage, and bone. Nasal obstruction, purulent rhinorrhea, and frequent bleeding result. Rhinoscleroma causes progressive nasal obstruction from indurated inflammatory tissue in the lamina propria. Rhinosporidiosis is characterized by bleeding polyps. Both low humidity and airborne irritants can result in chronic rhinitis.

Atrophic rhinitis: Atrophic rhinitis, a form of chronic rhinitis, results in atrophy and sclerosis of mucous membrane; the mucous membrane changes from ciliated pseudostratified columnar epithelium to stratified squamous epithelium, and the lamina propria is reduced in amount and vascularity. Atrophic rhinitis is associated with advanced age, granulomatosis with polyangiitis (GPA, formerly known as Wegener granulomatosis), and iatrogenically induced excessive nasal tissue extirpation. Although the exact etiology is unknown, bacterial infection frequently plays a role. Nasal mucosal atrophy often occurs in the elderly.

Vasomotor rhinitis: Vasomotor rhinitis, also called nonallergic rhinitis, is a chronic condition in which intermittent vascular engorgement of the nasal mucous membrane leads to watery rhinorrhea and sneezing. Etiology is uncertain, and no allergy can be identified. A dry atmosphere seems to aggravate the condition.

Symptoms and Signs

Acute rhinitis results in cough, low-grade fever, nasal congestion, rhinorrhea, and sneezing.

Chronic rhinitis manifestations are similar to those of acute rhinitis, but in prolonged or severe cases, patients may also have thick, foul-smelling, mucopurulent drainage; mucosal crusting; and/or bleeding.

Atrophic rhinitis results in enlargement of the nasal cavities, crust formation and malodorous bacterial colonization, nasal congestion, anosmia, and epistaxis that may be recurrent and severe.

Vasomotor rhinitis results in sneezing and watery rhinorrhea. The turgescent mucous membrane varies from bright red to purple. The condition is marked by periods of remission and exacerbation.

Diagnosis

The different forms of rhinitis are diagnosed clinically. Testing is unnecessary.

Vasomotor rhinitis is differentiated from specific viral and bacterial infections of the nose by the lack of purulent exudate and crusting. It is differentiated from allergic rhinitis by the absence of an identifiable allergen.

Treatment

- For viral rhinitis, decongestants, antihistamines, or both
- For atrophic rhinitis, topical treatment
- For vasomotor rhinitis, humidification and sometimes topical corticosteroids and oral pseudoephedrine

Viral rhinitis may be treated symptomatically with decongestants (either topical vasoconstriction with a sympathomimetic amine, such as oxymetazoline q 8 to 12 h or phenylephrine 0.25% q 3 to 4 h for not more than 7 days, or systemic sympathomimetic amines, such as pseudoephedrine 30 mg po q 4 to 6 h). Antihistamines (see Table 175–3 on p. 1376) may be helpful, but those with anticholinergic properties dry mucous membranes and therefore may increase irritation. Decongestants also may relieve symptoms of acute bacterial rhinitis and chronic rhinitis, whereas an underlying bacterial infection requires culture or biopsy, pathogen identification, antibiotic sensitivities, and appropriate antimicrobial treatment.

Treatment of atrophic rhinitis is directed at reducing the crusting and eliminating the odor with nasal irrigation, topical antibiotics (eg, bacitracin, mupirocin), topical or systemic estrogens, and vitamins A and D. Occluding or reducing the patency of the nasal cavities surgically decreases the crusting caused by the drying effect of air flowing over the atrophic mucous membrane.

Treatment of vasomotor rhinitis is by trial and error and is not always satisfactory. Patients benefit from humidified air, which may be provided by a humidified central heating system or a vaporizer in the workroom or bedroom. Topical corticosteroids (eg, mometasone 2 sprays bid) and nasal antihistamines can be of some benefit. Systemic sympathomimetic amines (eg, for adults, pseudoephedrine 30 mg po q 4 to 6 h prn) relieve symptoms but are not recommended for long-term use because they thicken the mucus and may cause tachycardia and nervousness. Topical vasoconstrictors are avoided because they cause the vasculature of the nasal mucous membrane to lose its sensitivity to other vasoconstrictive stimuli—eg, the humidity and temperature of inspired air.

SEPTAL DEVIATION AND PERFORATION

Deviations of the nasal septum due to developmental abnormalities or trauma are common but often are asymptomatic and require no treatment. Symptomatic septal deviation causes nasal obstruction and predisposes the patient to sinusitis (particularly if the deviation obstructs the ostium of a paranasal sinus) and to epistaxis due to drying air currents. Other symptoms may include facial pain, headaches, and noisy night breathing.

Septal deviation is usually evident on examination, although a flashlight and examination of the anterior nasal passage may not be sufficient. Treatment consists of septoplasty (septal reconstruction).

Septal ulcers and perforations may result from nasal surgery; repeated trauma, such as chronic nose picking; cosmetic piercing; toxic exposures (eg, to acids, chromium, phosphorus, or copper vapor); chronic cocaine use; chronic nasal spray use (including corticosteroids and OTC phenylephrine or oxymetazoline sprays); transnasal O_2 use; or diseases such as TB, syphilis, leprosy, SLE, and granulomatosis with polyangiitis (GPA, formerly known as Wegener granulomatosis).

Crusting around the margins and repeated epistaxis, which can be severe, may result. Small perforations may whistle. Anterior rhinoscopy or fiber-optic endoscopy can be used to view septal perforations. Topical bacitracin or mupirocin ointment reduces crusting, as may saline nasal spray. Symptomatic septal perforations are occasionally repaired with buccal or septal mucous membrane flaps; closing the perforation with a silicone septal button is a reliable option.

SINUSITIS

Sinusitis is inflammation of the paranasal sinuses due to viral, bacterial, or fungal infections or allergic reactions. Symptoms include nasal obstruction and congestion, purulent rhinorrhea, and facial pain or pressure; sometimes malaise, headache, and/or fever are present. Treatment

of suspected bacterial infection is with antibiotics, such as amoxicillin/clavulanate or doxycycline, given for 5 to 7 days for acute sinusitis and for up to 6 wk for chronic sinusitis. Decongestants, corticosteroid nasal sprays, and application of heat and humidity may help relieve symptoms and improve sinus drainage. Recurrent sinusitis may require surgery to improve sinus drainage.

Sinusitis may be classified as acute (completely resolved in < 30 days); subacute (completely resolved in 30 to 90 days); recurrent (≥ 4 discrete acute episodes per year, each completely resolved in < 30 days but recurring in cycles, with at least 10 days between complete resolution of symptoms and initiation of a new episode); and chronic (lasting > 90 days).

Etiology

Acute sinusitis in immunocompetent patients in the community is almost always viral (eg, rhinovirus, influenza, parainfluenza). A small percentage develop secondary bacterial infection with streptococci, pneumococci, *Haemophilus influenzae, Moraxella catarrhalis,* or staphylococci. Occasionally, a periapical dental abscess of a maxillary tooth spreads to the overlying sinus. Hospital-acquired acute infections are more often bacterial, typically involving *Staphylococcus aureus, Klebsiella pneumoniae, Pseudomonas aeruginosa, Proteus mirabilis,* and *Enterobacter*. Immunocompromised patients may have acute invasive fungal sinusitis.

Chronic sinusitis involves many factors that combine to create chronic inflammation. Chronic allergies, structural abnormalities (eg, nasal polyps), environmental irritants (eg, airborne pollution, tobacco smoke), mucociliary dysfunction, and other factors interact with infectious organisms to cause chronic sinusitis. The organisms are commonly bacterial (possibly as part of a biofilm on the mucosal surface) but may be fungal. Many bacteria have been implicated, including gram-negative bacilli and oropharyngeal anaerobic microorganisms; polymicrobial infection is common. In a few cases, chronic maxillary sinusitis is secondary to dental infection. Fungal infections (*Aspergillus, Sporothrix, Pseudallescheria*) may be chronic and tend to strike the elderly and immunocompromised patients.

Allergic fungal sinusitis is a form of chronic sinusitis characterized by diffuse nasal congestion, markedly viscid nasal secretions, and, often, nasal polyps. It is an allergic response to the presence of topical fungi, often *Aspergillus,* and is not caused by an invasive infection.

Invasive fungal sinusitis is an aggressive, sometimes fatal, infection in immunocompromised patients, usually caused by *Aspergillus* or *Mucor* species.

Risk factors: Common risk factors for sinusitis include factors that obstruct normal sinus drainage (eg, allergic rhinitis, nasal polyps, nasogastric or nasotracheal tubes), and immunocompromised states (eg, diabetes, HIV infection). Other factors include prolonged ICU stays, severe burns, cystic fibrosis, and ciliary dyskinesia.

Pathophysiology

In a URI, the swollen nasal mucous membrane obstructs the ostium of a paranasal sinus, and the oxygen in the sinus is absorbed into the blood vessels of the mucous membrane. The resulting relative negative pressure in the sinus (vacuum sinusitis) is painful. If the vacuum is maintained, a transudate from the mucous membrane develops and fills the sinus; the transudate serves as a medium for bacteria that enter the sinus through the ostium or through a spreading cellulitis or thrombophlebitis in the lamina propria of the mucous membrane. An outpouring of serum and leukocytes to combat the infection results, and painful positive pressure develops in the obstructed sinus. The mucous membrane becomes hyperemic and edematous.

Complications: The main complication of sinusitis is local spread of bacterial infection, causing periorbital or orbital cellulitis, cavernous sinus thrombosis, or epidural or brain abscess.

Symptoms and Signs

Acute and chronic sinusitis cause similar symptoms and signs, including purulent rhinorrhea, pressure and pain in the face, nasal congestion and obstruction, hyposmia, halitosis, and productive cough (especially at night). Often the pain is more severe in acute sinusitis. The area over the affected sinus may be tender, swollen, and erythematous.

- Maxillary sinusitis causes pain in the maxillary area, toothache, and frontal headache.
- Frontal sinusitis causes pain in the frontal area and frontal headache.
- Ethmoid sinusitis causes pain behind and between the eyes, a frontal headache often described as splitting, periorbital cellulitis, and tearing.
- Sphenoid sinusitis causes less well localized pain referred to the frontal or occipital area.

Malaise may be present. Fever and chills suggest an extension of the infection beyond the sinuses.

The nasal mucous membrane is red and turgescent; yellow or green purulent rhinorrhea may be present. Seropurulent or mucopurulent exudate may be seen in the middle meatus with maxillary, anterior ethmoid, or frontal sinusitis and in the area medial to the middle turbinate with posterior ethmoid or sphenoid sinusitis.

Manifestations of complications include periorbital swelling and redness, proptosis, ophthalmoplegia, confusion or decreased level of consciousness, and severe headache.

Diagnosis

- Clinical evaluation
- Sometimes CT

Sinus infections are usually diagnosed clinically. Imaging is not indicated in acute sinusitis unless there are findings that suggest complications, in which case CT is done. In chronic sinusitis, CT is done more often, and x-rays of the apices of the teeth may be required in chronic maxillary sinusitis to exclude a periapical abscess.

Microbial cultures are rarely done because a valid culture requires a sample obtained by sinus endoscopy or sinus puncture; culturing a swab of nasal secretions is inadequate. Cultures are typically done only when empiric treatment fails and in immunocompromised patients and some hospital-acquired causes of sinusitis.

Pediatrics: Sinusitis in children can initially be difficult to distinguish from a URI. Bacterial sinusitis is suspected when purulent rhinorrhea persists for > 10 days along with fatigue and cough. Fever is uncommon. Local facial pain or discomfort may be present. Nasal examination discloses purulent drainage and should rule out foreign body.

Diagnosis of acute sinusitis in children is clinical. CT is avoided because of concerns about radiation exposure unless there are signs of orbital or intracranial complications (eg, periorbital swelling, vision loss, diplopia, or ophthalmoplegia), there is chronic sinusitis that has not responded to treatment, or there is concern about rare nasopharyngeal cancer (eg, based on unilateral nasal obstruction, pain, epistaxis, facial swelling, or, particularly concerning, diminished vision). Periorbital edema in a child requires prompt assessment for orbital cellulitis and possible surgical intervention to prevent visual impairment and intracranial infection.

Treatment

- Local measures to enhance drainage (eg, steam, topical vasoconstrictors)
- Sometimes antibiotics (eg, amoxicillin/clavulanate, doxycycline)

In acute sinusitis, improved drainage and control of infection are the aims of therapy. Steam inhalation; hot, wet towels over the affected sinuses; and hot beverages help alleviate nasal vasoconstriction and promote drainage.

Topical vasoconstrictors, such as phenylephrine 0.25% spray q 3 h or oxymetazoline q 8 to 12 h, are effective but should be used for a maximum of 5 days or for a repeating cycle of 3 days on and 3 days off until the sinusitis is resolved. Systemic vasoconstrictors, such as pseudoephedrine 30 mg po (for adults) q 4 to 6 h, are less effective.

Saline nasal irrigation may help symptoms slightly but is cumbersome and uncomfortable, and patients require teaching to execute it properly; it may thus be better for patients with recurrent sinusitis, who are more likely to master (and tolerate) the technique.

Corticosteroid nasal sprays can help relieve symptoms but typically take at least 10 days to be effective.

Antibiotic treatment: Although most cases of community-acquired acute sinusitis are viral and resolve spontaneously, previously many patients were given antibiotics because of the difficulty in clinically distinguishing viral from bacterial infection. However, current concerns about creation of antibiotic-resistant organisms have led to a more selective use of antibiotics (see Fig. 98–1). The Infectious Diseases Society of America suggests the following characteristics help identify patients who should be started on antibiotics:

- Mild to moderate sinus symptoms persisting for ≥ 10 days
- Severe symptoms (eg, fever ≥ 39°, severe pain) for ≥ 3 to 4 days
- Worsening sinus symptoms after initially improving from a typical viral URI ("double sickening" or biphasic illness)

Because many causative organisms are resistant to previously used drugs, amoxicillin/clavulanate 875 mg po q 12 h (25 mg/kg po q 12 h in children) is the current first-line drug. Patients at risk of antibiotic resistance are given a higher dose of 2 g po q 12 h (45 mg/kg po q 12 h in children). Patients at risk of resistance include those who are under 2 yr of age or over 65 yr, who have received antibiotics in the previous month, who have been hospitalized within the past 5 days, and those who are immunocompromised.

Adults with penicillin allergy may receive doxycycline or a respiratory fluoroquinolone (eg, levofloxacin, moxifloxacin). Children with penicillin allergy may receive levofloxacin, or clindamycin plus a 3rd-generation oral cephalosporin (cefixime or cefpodoxime).

If there is improvement within 3 to 5 days, the drug is continued. Adults without risk factors for resistance are treated for 5 to 7 days total; other adults are treated for 7 to 10 days. Children are treated for 10 to 14 days. If there is no improvement in 3 to 5 days, a different drug is used. Macrolides, trimethoprim/sulfamethoxazole, and monotherapy with a cephalosporin are no longer recommended because of bacterial resistance. Emergency surgery is needed if there is vision loss or an imminent possibility of vision loss.

In exacerbations of chronic sinusitis in children or adults, the same antibiotics are used, but treatment is given for 4 to 6 wk. The sensitivities of pathogens isolated from the sinus exudate and the patient's response to treatment guide subsequent therapy.

Sinusitis unresponsive to antibiotic therapy may require surgery (maxillary sinusotomy, ethmoidectomy, or sphenoid sinusotomy) to improve ventilation and drainage and to remove inspissated mucopurulent material, epithelial debris, and hypertrophic mucous membrane. These procedures usually are done intranasally with the aid of an endoscope. Chronic frontal sinusitis may be managed either with osteoplastic obliteration of the frontal sinuses or endoscopically in selected patients. The use of intraoperative computer-aided surgery to localize disease and prevent injury to surrounding contiguous structures (such as the eye and brain) has become common.

KEY POINTS

- Most acute sinusitis in immunocompetent patients is viral.
- Immunocompromised patients are at greater risk of aggressive fungal or bacterial infection.
- Diagnosis is clinical; CT and cultures (obtained endoscopically or through sinus puncture) are done mainly for chronic, refractory, or atypical cases.
- Antibiotics may be withheld pending a trial of symptomatic treatment, the duration of which depends on the severity and timing of symptoms.
- The first-line antibiotic is amoxicillin/clavulanate, with doxycycline or respiratory fluoroquinolones as alternatives.

Invasive Sinusitis in Immunocompromised Patients

Aggressive and even fatal fungal or bacterial sinusitis can occur in patients who are immunocompromised because of poorly controlled diabetes, neutropenia, or HIV infection.

Mucormycosis: Mucormycosis (zygomycosis, also sometimes called phycomycosis) is a mycosis due to fungi of the order Mucorales, including species of *Mucor, Absidia,* and *Rhizopus*. This mycosis may develop in patients with poorly controlled diabetes. It is characterized by black, devitalized tissue in the nasal cavity and neurologic signs secondary to retrograde thromboarteritis in the carotid arterial system.

Diagnosis is based on histopathologic demonstration of mycelia in the avascularized tissue. Prompt biopsy of intranasal tissue for histology and culture is warranted.

Treatment requires control of the underlying condition (such as reversal of ketoacidosis in diabetes), surgical debridement of necrotic tissue, and IV amphotericin B therapy.

Aspergillosis and candidiasis: *Aspergillus* and *Candida* spp may infect the paranasal sinuses of patients who are

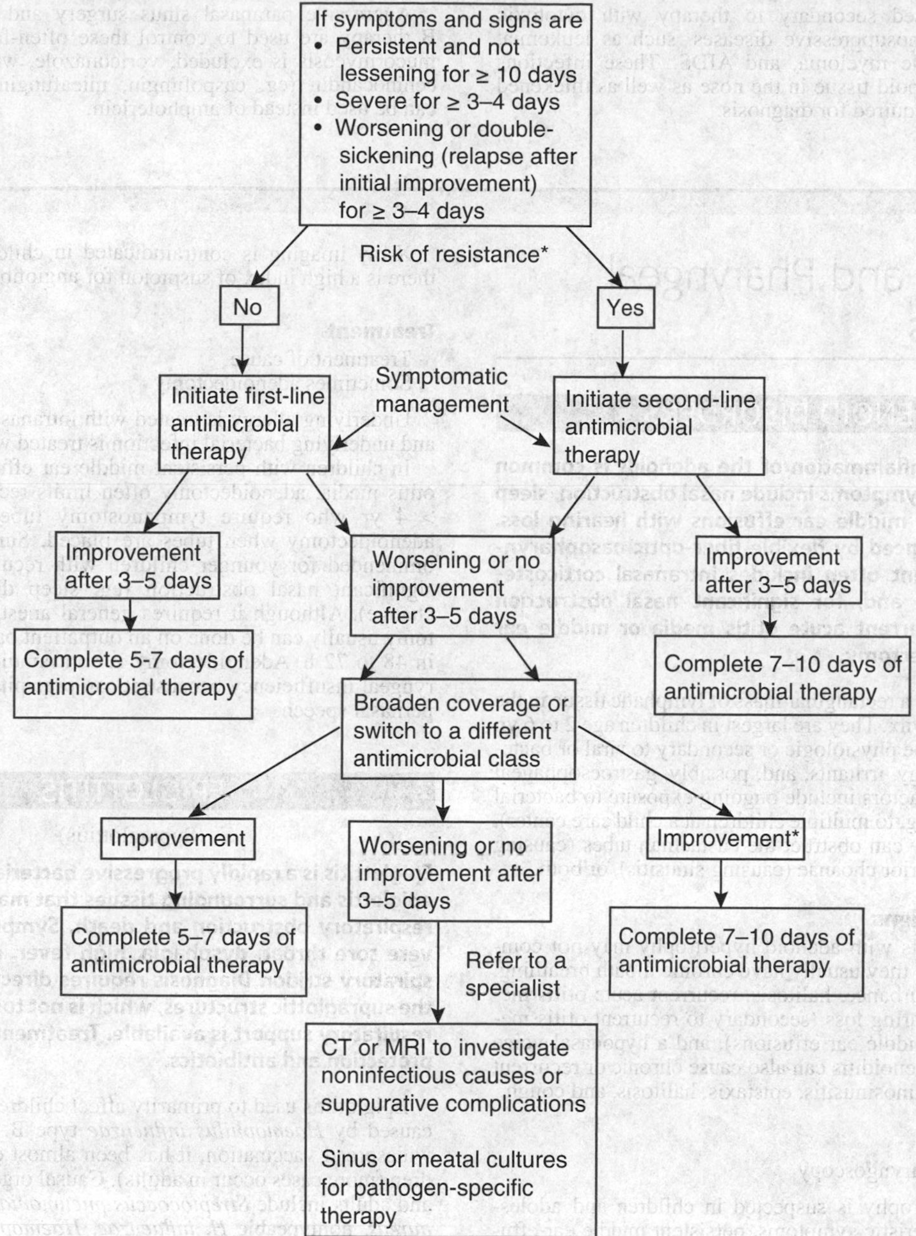

Fig. 98–1. Algorithm for use of antibiotics in acute sinusitis.
Adapted from Chow AW, Benninger MS, Brook I, et al: IDSA clinical practice guideline for acute bacterial rhinosinusitis in children and adults. *Clinical Infectious Diseases* 54 (8):1041–1045 (2012).

immunocompromised secondary to therapy with cytotoxic drugs or to immunosuppressive diseases, such as leukemia, lymphoma, multiple myeloma, and AIDS. These infections can appear as polypoid tissue in the nose as well as thickened mucosa; tissue is required for diagnosis.

Aggressive paranasal sinus surgery and IV amphotericin B therapy are used to control these often-fatal infections. If mucormycosis is excluded, voriconazole, with or without an echinocandin (eg, caspofungin, micafungin, anidulafungin), can be used instead of amphotericin.

99 Oral and Pharyngeal Disorders

ADENOID DISORDERS

Hypertrophy or inflammation of the adenoids is common among children. Symptoms include nasal obstruction, sleep disturbances, and middle ear effusions with hearing loss. Diagnosis is enhanced by flexible fiber-optic nasopharyngoscopy. Treatment often includes intranasal corticosteroids, antibiotics, and, for significant nasal obstruction or persistent recurrent acute otitis media or middle ear effusion, adenoidectomy.

The adenoids are a rectangular mass of lymphatic tissue in the posterior nasopharynx. They are largest in children age 2 to 6 yr. Enlargement may be physiologic or secondary to viral or bacterial infection, allergy, irritants, and, possibly, gastroesophageal reflux. Other risk factors include ongoing exposure to bacterial or viral infection (eg, to multiple children at a child care center). Severe hypertrophy can obstruct the eustachian tubes (causing otitis media), posterior choanae (causing sinusitis), or both.

Symptoms and Signs

Although patients with adenoid hypertrophy may not complain of symptoms, they usually have chronic mouth breathing, snoring, sleep disturbance, halitosis, recurrent acute otitis media, conductive hearing loss (secondary to recurrent otitis media or persistent middle ear effusions), and a hyponasal voice quality. Chronic adenoiditis can also cause chronic or recurrent nasopharyngitis, rhinosinusitis, epistaxis, halitosis, and cough.

Diagnosis

- Flexible nasopharyngoscopy

Adenoid hypertrophy is suspected in children and adolescents with characteristic symptoms, persistent middle ear effusions, or recurrent acute otitis media or rhinosinusitis. Similar symptoms and signs in a male adolescent may result from an angiofibroma.

Children with velopharyngeal insufficiency, eg, due to velocardiofacial syndrome, may produce a hypernasal speech that must be differentiated from the hyponasal speech of adenoid hypertrophy.

The standard for office assessment of the nasopharynx is flexible nasopharyngoscopy. Sleep tape recording, often used to document snoring, is not as accurate or specific. A sleep study may help define the severity of any sleep disturbance due to chronic obstruction.

X-ray imaging is contraindicated in children except when there is a high index of suspicion for angiofibroma or cancer.

Treatment

- Treatment of cause
- Sometimes adenoidectomy

Underlying allergy is treated with intranasal corticosteroids, and underlying bacterial infection is treated with antibiotics.

In children with persistent middle ear effusions or frequent otitis media, adenoidectomy often limits recurrence. Children > 4 yr who require tympanostomy tubes often undergo adenoidectomy when tubes are placed. Surgery is also recommended for younger children with recurrent epistaxis or significant nasal obstruction (eg, sleep disturbance, voice change). Although it requires general anesthesia, adenoidectomy usually can be done on an outpatient basis with recovery in 48 to 72 h. Adenoidectomy is contraindicated in velopharyngeal insufficiency because it can precipitate or worsen hypernasal speech.

EPIGLOTTITIS

(Supraglottitis)

Epiglottitis is a rapidly progressive bacterial infection of the epiglottis and surrounding tissues that may lead to sudden respiratory obstruction and death. Symptoms include severe sore throat, dysphagia, high fever, drooling, and inspiratory stridor. Diagnosis requires direct visualization of the supraglottic structures, which is not to be done until full respiratory support is available. Treatment includes airway protection and antibiotics.

Epiglottitis used to primarily affect children and usually was caused by *Haemophilus influenzae* type B. Now, because of widespread vaccination, it has been almost eradicated in children (more cases occur in adults). Causal organisms in children and adults include *Streptococcus pneumoniae, Staphylococcus aureus,* nontypeable *H. influenzae, Haemophilus parainfluenzae,* β-hemolytic streptococci, *Branhamella catarrhalis,* and *Klebsiella pneumoniae. H. influenzae* type B is still a cause in adults and unvaccinated children.

Bacteria that have colonized the nasopharynx spread locally to cause supraglottic cellulitis with marked inflammation of the epiglottis, vallecula, aryepiglottic folds, arytenoids, and laryngeal ventricles. With *H. influenzae* type B, infection may spread hematogenously.

The inflamed supraglottic structures mechanically obstruct the airway, increasing the work of breathing, ultimately causing respiratory failure. Clearance of inflammatory secretions is also impaired.

Symptoms and Signs

In **children,** sore throat, odynophagia, and dysphagia develop abruptly. Fatal asphyxia may occur within a few hours of onset. Drooling is very common. Additionally, the child has signs of toxicity (poor or absent eye contact, failure to recognize parents, cyanosis, irritability, inability to be consoled or distracted) and is febrile and anxious. Dyspnea, tachypnea, and inspiratory stridor may be present, often causing the child to sit upright, lean forward, and hyperextend the neck with the jaw thrust forward and mouth open in an effort to enhance air exchange (tripod position). Relinquishing this position may herald respiratory failure. Suprasternal, supraclavicular, and subcostal inspiratory retractions may be present.

In **adults,** symptoms are similar to those of children, including sore throat, fever, dysphagia, and drooling, but peak symptoms usually take > 24 h to develop. Because of the larger diameter of the adult airway, obstruction is less common and less fulminant. Often, there is no visible oropharyngeal inflammation. However, severe throat pain with a normal-appearing pharynx raises suspicion of epiglottitis. A delay in diagnosis and treatment increases the risk of airway obstruction and death.

Diagnosis

- Direct inspection (typically in operating room)
- X-ray in milder cases with low suspicion

Epiglottitis is suspected in patients with severe sore throat and no pharyngitis and also in patients with sore throat and inspiratory stridor. Stridor in children may also result from croup (viral laryngotracheal bronchitis—see Table 99–1 and p. 2826), bacterial tracheitis, and airway foreign body. The tripod position may also occur with peritonsillar or retropharyngeal abscess.

The patient is hospitalized if epiglottitis is suspected. Diagnosis requires direct examination, usually with flexible fiber-optic laryngoscopy. (CAUTION: *Examination of the pharynx and larynx may precipitate complete respiratory obstruction in children, and the pharynx and larynx should not be directly examined except in the operating room, where the most advanced airway intervention is available.*) Although plain x-rays may be helpful, a child with stridor should not be transported to the x-ray suite. Direct laryngoscopy that reveals a beefy-red, stiff, edematous epiglottis is diagnostic. Cultures from the supraglottic tissues and blood can then be taken to search for the causative organism.

Adults may, in some cases, safely undergo flexible fiber-optic laryngoscopy.

Table 99–1. DIFFERENTIATING EPIGLOTTITIS FROM CROUP

FEATURE	EPIGLOTTITIS	CROUP*
Onset	Acute and fulminant	More gradual
Age	Commonly, 2–8 yr (if not vaccinated against *Haemophilus influenzae* type B) and adults	Commonly, 6–36 mo
Barking cough	Uncommon	Characteristic
Epiglottis	Edematous and cherry red	May be erythematous
Neck x-ray findings	Enlarged epiglottis (thumb sign) and distention of the hypopharynx	Subglottic narrowing (steeple sign) and a normal-sized epiglottis

*Also called viral laryngotracheal bronchitis.

PEARLS & PITFALLS

- Examination of the pharynx or larynx in children with epiglottitis and stridor may precipitate complete airway obstruction.

Treatment

- Adequate airway ensured
- Antibiotics (eg, ceftriaxone)

In children with stridor, any intervention that could be upsetting (and thus could trigger airway obstruction) should be avoided until an airway is established. In children with epiglottitis, the airway must be secured immediately, preferably by nasotracheal intubation. Securing the airway can be quite difficult and should, if possible, be done by experienced personnel in the operating room. An endotracheal tube is usually required until the patient has been stabilized for 24 to 48 h (usual total intubation time is < 60 h). Alternatively, a tracheotomy is done. If respiratory arrest occurs before an airway is established, bag-mask ventilation may be a life-saving temporary measure. For emergency care of children with epiglottitis, each institution should have a protocol that involves critical care, otolaryngology, anesthesia, and pediatrics.

Adults whose airway is severely obstructed can be endotracheally intubated during flexible fiber-optic laryngoscopy. Other adults may not require immediate intubation but should be observed for airway compromise in an ICU with an intubation set and cricothyrotomy tray at the bedside.

A β-lactamase–resistant antibiotic, such as ceftriaxone 50 to 75 mg/kg IV once/day (maximum 2 g), should be used empirically, pending culture and sensitivity test results.

Epiglottitis caused by *H. influenzae* type B can be effectively prevented with the *H. influenzae* type B (HiB) conjugate vaccine.

KEY POINTS

- The incidence of epiglottitis has decreased significantly, particularly in children, because of widespread vaccination against the most common cause, *Haemophilus influenzae* type B.
- Stridor, as well as sore throat with a normal-appearing pharynx, are important clues.
- Examination of the pharynx or larynx in children with epiglottitis and stridor may precipitate complete airway obstruction.
- If the diagnosis is suspected, do flexible fiber-optic laryngoscopy in the operating room; reserve imaging studies for cases with very low suspicion.
- Children typically should have their airway secured by tracheal intubation; adults often can be observed for signs of airway compromise.
- Give a β-lactamase–resistant antibiotic, such as ceftriaxone.

PARAPHARYNGEAL ABSCESS

A parapharyngeal abscess is a deep neck abscess. Symptoms include fever, sore throat, odynophagia, and swelling in the neck down to the hyoid bone. Diagnosis is by CT. Treatment is antibiotics and surgical drainage.

The parapharyngeal (pharyngomaxillary) space is lateral to the superior pharyngeal constrictor and medial to the masseter muscle. This space connects to every other major fascial neck space and is divided into anterior and posterior compartments by the styloid process. The posterior compartment contains the carotid artery, internal jugular vein, and numerous nerves. Infections in the parapharyngeal space usually originate in the tonsils or pharynx, although local spread from odontogenic sources and lymph nodes may occur.

Abscess swelling can compromise the airway. Posterior space abscess can erode into the carotid artery or cause septic thrombophlebitis of the internal jugular vein (Lemierre syndrome).

Symptoms and Signs

Most patients have fever, sore throat, odynophagia, and swelling in the neck down to the hyoid bone.

Anterior space abscesses cause trismus and induration along the angle of the mandible, with medial bulging of the tonsil and lateral pharyngeal wall.

Posterior space abscesses cause swelling that is more prominent in the posterior pharyngeal wall. Trismus is minimal. Posterior abscesses may involve structures within the carotid sheath, possibly causing rigors, high fever, bacteremia, neurologic deficits, and massive hemorrhage caused by carotid artery rupture.

Diagnosis

- CT

Diagnosis is suspected in patients with poorly defined deep neck infection or other typical symptoms and is confirmed by using contrast-enhanced CT.

Treatment

- Broad-spectrum antibiotics (eg, ceftriaxone, clindamycin)
- Surgical drainage

Treatment may require airway control. Parenteral broad-spectrum antibiotics (eg, ceftriaxone, clindamycin) and surgical drainage are generally needed. Posterior abscesses are drained externally through the submaxillary fossa. Anterior abscesses can often be drained through an intra-oral incision. Several days of parenteral culture-determined antibiotics are required after drainage, followed by 10 to 14 days of oral antibiotics. Occasionally, small abscesses can be treated with IV antibiotics alone.

PERITONSILLAR ABSCESS AND CELLULITIS

Peritonsillar abscess and cellulitis are acute pharyngeal infections most common among adolescents and young adults. Symptoms are severe sore throat, trismus, "hot potato" voice, and uvular deviation. Diagnosis requires needle aspiration. Treatment includes broad-spectrum antibiotics, drainage of any pus, hydration, analgesics, and, occasionally, acute tonsillectomy.

Etiology

Abscess (quinsy) and cellulitis probably represent a spectrum of the same process in which bacterial infection of the tonsils and pharynx spreads to the soft tissues. Infection is virtually always unilateral and is located between the tonsil and the superior pharyngeal constrictor muscle. It usually involves multiple bacteria. *Streptococcus* and *Staphylococcus* are the most frequent aerobic pathogens, whereas *Bacteroides* sp is the predominant anaerobic pathogen.

Symptoms and Signs

Symptoms include gradual onset of severe unilateral sore throat, dysphagia, fever, otalgia, and asymmetric cervical adenopathy. Trismus, "hot potato" voice (speaking as if a hot object was in the mouth), a toxic appearance (eg, poor or absent eye contact, failure to recognize parents, irritability, inability to be consoled or distracted, fever, anxiety) drooling, severe halitosis, tonsillar erythema, and exudates are common. Abscess and cellulitis both have swelling above the affected tonsil, but with abscess there is more of a discrete bulge, with deviation of the soft palate and uvula and pronounced trismus.

Diagnosis

- Needle aspiration
- Sometimes CT

Peritonsillar cellulitis is recognized in patients with severe sore throat who have trismus, "hot potato" voice, and uvular deviation. All such patients require needle aspiration of the tonsillar mass and cultures. Aspiration of pus differentiates abscess from cellulitis.

CT or ultrasonography of the neck can help confirm the diagnosis when the physical examination is difficult or the diagnosis is in doubt, particularly when the condition must be differentiated from a parapharyngeal infection or other deep neck infection.

Treatment

- Antibiotics
- Drainage of abscess

Cellulitis subsides, usually within 48 h, with hydration and high-dose penicillin (eg, 2 million units IV q 4 h or 1 g po qid); alternative drugs include a 1st-generation cephalosporin or clindamycin. Culture-directed antibiotics are then prescribed for 10 days.

Abscesses are incised and drained in the emergency department using thorough local anesthesia and sometimes procedural sedation; many clinicians believe needle aspiration alone provides adequate drainage. Although most patients can be treated as outpatients, some need brief hospitalization for parenteral antibiotics, IV hydration, and airway monitoring. Rarely, an immediate tonsillectomy is done, particularly in a young or uncooperative patient who has other indications for elective tonsillectomy (eg, history of frequently recurrent tonsillitis or obstructive sleep apnea). Otherwise, elective tonsillectomy is done 4 to 6 wk later to prevent abscess recurrence.

RETROPHARYNGEAL ABSCESS

Retropharyngeal abscesses, most common among young children, can cause sore throat, fever, neck stiffness, and

stridor. Diagnosis requires lateral neck x-ray or CT. Treatment is with endotracheal intubation, drainage, and antibiotics.

Retropharyngeal abscesses develop in the retropharyngeal lymph nodes at the back of the pharynx, adjacent to the vertebrae. They can be seeded by infection of the pharynx, sinuses, adenoids, or nose. They occur mainly in children 1 to 8 yr because the retropharyngeal lymph nodes begin to recede by 4 to 5 yr. However, adults may develop infection after foreign body ingestion or after instrumentation. Common organisms include aerobic (*Streptococcus* and *Staphylococcus* sp) and anaerobic (*Bacteroides* and *Fusobacterium*) bacteria and, increasingly in adults and children, HIV and TB.

The most serious consequences include airway obstruction, septic shock, rupture of the abscess into the airway resulting in aspiration pneumonia or asphyxia, mediastinitis, carotid rupture, and suppurative thrombophlebitis of the internal jugular veins (Lemierre syndrome).

Symptoms and Signs

Symptoms and signs are usually preceded in children by an acute URI and in adults by foreign body ingestion or instrumentation. Children may have odynophagia, dysphagia, fever, cervical lymphadenopathy, nuchal rigidity, stridor, dyspnea, snoring or noisy breathing, and torticollis. Adults may have severe neck pain but less often have stridor. The posterior pharyngeal wall may bulge to one side.

Diagnosis

- CT

Diagnosis is suspected in patients with severe, unexplained sore throat and neck stiffness, stridor, or noisy breathing.

Lateral soft-tissue x-rays of the neck, taken in the maximum possible hyperextension and during inspiration, may show focal widening of the prevertebral soft tissues, reversal of normal cervical lordosis, air in the prevertebral soft tissues, or erosion of the adjacent vertebral body.

CT can help diagnose questionable cases, help differentiate cellulitis from an abscess, and assess extent of the abscess.

Treatment

- Antibiotics (eg, ceftriaxone, clindamycin)
- Usually surgical drainage

Antibiotics, such as a broad-spectrum cephalosporin (eg, ceftriaxone 50 to 75 mg/kg IV once/day) or clindamycin, may occasionally be sufficient for children with small abscesses. However, most patients also require drainage through an incision in the posterior pharyngeal wall. Endotracheal intubation is done preoperatively and maintained for 24 to 48 h.

SALIVARY STONES

(Sialolithiasis)

Stones composed of calcium salts often obstruct salivary glands, causing pain, swelling, and sometimes infection. Diagnosis is made clinically or with CT, ultrasonography, or sialography. Treatment involves stone expression with saliva stimulants, manual manipulation, a probe, or surgery.

The major salivary glands are the paired parotid, submandibular, and sublingual glands. Stones in the salivary glands are most common among adults. Eighty percent of stones originate in the submandibular glands and obstruct the Wharton duct. Most of the rest originate in the parotid glands and block the Stensen duct. Only about 1% originate in the sublingual glands. Multiple stones occur in about 25% of patients.

Etiology

Most salivary stones are composed of calcium phosphate with small amounts of magnesium and carbonate. Patients with gout may have uric acid stones. Stone formation requires a nidus on which salts can precipitate during salivary stasis. Stasis occurs in patients who are debilitated, dehydrated, have reduced food intake, or take anticholinergics. Persisting or recurrent stones predispose to infection of the involved gland (sialadenitis—see p. 844).

Symptoms and Signs

Obstructing stones cause glandular swelling and pain, particularly after eating, which stimulates saliva flow. Symptoms may subside after a few hours. Relief may coincide with a gush of saliva. Some stones cause intermittent or no symptoms.

If a stone is lodged distally, it may be visible or palpable at the duct's outlet.

Diagnosis

- Clinical evaluation
- Sometimes imaging (eg, CT, ultrasonography, sialography)

If a stone is not apparent on examination, the patient can be given a sialagogue (eg, lemon juice, hard candy, or some other substance that triggers saliva flow). Reproduction of symptoms is almost always diagnostic of a stone.

CT, ultrasonography, and sialography are highly sensitive and are used if clinical diagnosis is equivocal. Contrast sialography may be done through a catheter inserted into the duct and can differentiate between stone, stenosis, and tumor. This technique is occasionally therapeutic. Because 90% of submandibular calculi are radiopaque and 90% of parotid calculi are radiolucent, plain x-rays are not always accurate. Ultrasonography is being used increasingly and has reported sensitivities for all (radiopaque and radiolucent) stones of about 60 to 95% and specificities between 85 and 100%. The role of MRI is evolving; reported sensitivities and specificities are > 90% and it appears to image small stones and distal ducts more sensitively than ultrasonography or contrast sialography.

Treatment

- Local measures (eg, sialagogues, massage)
- Sometimes manual expression or surgical removal

Analgesics, hydration, and massage can relieve symptoms.

Antistaphylococcal antibiotics can be used to prevent acute sialadenitis if started early.

Stones may pass spontaneously or when salivary flow is stimulated by sialagogues; patients are encouraged to suck a lemon wedge or sour candy every 2 to 3 h. Stones right at the duct orifice can sometimes be expressed manually by squeezing with the fingertips. Dilation of the duct with a small probe may facilitate expulsion.

Surgical removal of stones succeeds if other methods fail. Stones at or near the orifice of the duct may be removed transorally, whereas those in the hilum of the gland often require complete excision of the salivary gland. Stones up to 5 mm in size may be removed endoscopically.

KEY POINTS

- About 80% of salivary stones occur in the submandibular glands.
- Clinical diagnosis is usually adequate but sometimes CT, ultrasonography, or sialography is needed.
- Many stones pass spontaneously or with use of sialagogues and manual expression, but some require endoscopic or surgical removal.

SIALADENITIS

Sialadenitis is bacterial infection of a salivary gland, usually due to an obstructing stone or gland hyposecretion. Symptoms are swelling, pain, redness, and tenderness. Diagnosis is clinical. CT, ultrasonography, and MRI may help identify the cause. Treatment is with antibiotics.

Etiology

Sialadenitis usually occurs after hyposecretion or duct obstruction but may develop without an obvious cause. The major salivary glands are the parotid, submandibular, and sublingual glands.

Sialadenitis is most common in the parotid gland and typically occurs in

- Patients in their 50s and 60s
- Chronically ill patients with xerostomia
- Patients with Sjögren syndrome
- Adolescents and young adults with anorexia

The most common causative organism is *Staphylococcus aureus;* others include streptococci, coliforms, and various anaerobic bacteria.

Inflammation of the parotid gland can also develop in patients who have had radiation therapy to the oral cavity or radioactive iodine therapy for thyroid cancer. Although sometimes described as sialoadenitis, this inflammation is rarely a bacterial infection, particularly in the absence of fever.

Symptoms and Signs

Fever, chills, and unilateral pain and swelling develop. The gland is firm and diffusely tender, with erythema and edema of the overlying skin. Pus can often be expressed from the duct by compressing the affected gland and should be cultured. Focal enlargement may indicate an abscess.

Diagnosis

- CT, ultrasonography, or MRI

CT, ultrasonography, and MRI can confirm sialadenitis or abscess that is not obvious clinically, although MRI may miss an obstructing stone. If pus can be expressed from the duct of the affected gland, it is sent for Gram stain and culture.

Treatment

- Antistaphylococcal antibiotics
- Local measures (eg, sialagogues, warm compresses)

Initial treatment is with antibiotics active against *S. aureus* (eg, dicloxacillin, 250 mg po qid, a 1st-generation cephalosporin, or clindamycin), modified according to culture results. With the increasing prevalence of methicillin-resistant *S. aureus,*especially among the elderly living in extended-care nursing facilities, vancomycin is often required. Chlorhexidine 0.12% mouth rinses three times a day will reduce bacterial burden in the oral cavity and will promote oral hygiene.

Hydration, sialagogues (eg, lemon juice, hard candy, or some other substance that triggers saliva flow), warm compresses, gland massage, and good oral hygiene are also important. Abscesses require drainage.

Occasionally, a superficial parotidectomy or submandibular gland excision is indicated for patients with chronic or relapsing sialadenitis.

Other Salivary Gland Infections

Mumps often causes parotid swelling (see Table 323–1 on p. 2762).

Patients with HIV infection often have parotid enlargement secondary to one or more lymphoepithelial cysts.

Cat-scratch disease caused by *Bartonella* infection often invades periparotid lymph nodes and may infect the parotid glands by contiguous spread. Although cat-scratch disease is self-limited, antibiotic therapy is often provided, and incision and drainage are necessary if an abscess develops.

Atypical mycobacterial infections in the tonsils or teeth may spread contiguously to the major salivary glands. The PPD may be negative, and the diagnosis may require biopsy and tissue culture for acid-fast bacteria. Treatment recommendations are controversial. Options include surgical debridement with curettage, complete excision of the infected tissue, and use of anti-TB drug therapy (rarely necessary).

SUBMANDIBULAR SPACE INFECTION

(Ludwig Angina)

Submandibular space infection is acute cellulitis of the soft tissues below the mouth. Symptoms include pain, dysphagia, and potentially fatal airway obstruction. Diagnosis usually is clinical. Treatment includes airway management, surgical drainage, and IV antibiotics.

Submandibular space infection is a rapidly spreading, bilateral, indurated cellulitis occurring in the suprahyoid soft tissues, the floor of the mouth, and both sublingual and submaxillary spaces without abscess formation. Although not a true abscess, it resembles one clinically and is treated similarly.

The condition usually develops from an odontogenic infection, especially of the 2nd and 3rd mandibular molars, or as an extension of peritonsillar cellulitis. Contributing factors may include poor dental hygiene, tooth extractions, and trauma (eg, fractures of the mandible, lacerations of the floor of the mouth).

Symptoms and Signs

Early manifestations are pain in any involved teeth, with severe, tender, localized submental and sublingual induration. Boardlike firmness of the floor of the mouth and brawny induration of the suprahyoid soft tissues may develop rapidly. Drooling, trismus, dysphagia, stridor caused by laryngeal edema, and elevation of the posterior tongue against the palate may be present. Fever, chills, and tachycardia are usually present as well. The condition can cause airway obstruction within hours and does so more often than do other neck infections.

Diagnosis

- Clinical evaluation and sometimes CT

The diagnosis usually is obvious. If not, CT is done.

Treatment

- Maintenance of airway patency
- Surgical incision and drainage
- Antibiotics active against oral flora

Maintaining airway patency is of the highest priority. Because swelling makes oral endotracheal intubation difficult, fiber-optic nasotracheal intubation done with topical anesthesia in the operating room or ICU with the patient awake is preferable. Some patients require a tracheotomy. Patients without immediate need for intubation require intense observation and may benefit temporarily from a nasal trumpet.

Incision and drainage with placement of drains deep into the mylohyoid muscles relieve the pressure. Antibiotics should be chosen to cover both oral anaerobes and aerobes (eg, clindamycin, ampicillin/sulbactam, high-dose penicillin).

TONSILLOPHARYNGITIS

Tonsillopharyngitis is acute infection of the pharynx, palatine tonsils, or both. Symptoms may include sore throat, dysphagia, cervical lymphadenopathy, and fever. Diagnosis is clinical, supplemented by culture or rapid antigen test. Treatment depends on symptoms and, in the case of group A β-hemolytic streptococcus, involves antibiotics.

The tonsils participate in systemic immune surveillance. In addition, local tonsillar defenses include a lining of antigen-processing squamous epithelium that involves B- and T-cell responses.

Tonsillopharyngitis of all varieties constitutes about 15% of all office visits to primary care physicians.

Etiology

Tonsillopharyngitis is usually viral, most often caused by the common cold viruses (adenovirus, rhinovirus, influenza, coronavirus, and respiratory syncytial virus), but occasionally by Epstein-Barr virus, herpes simplex virus, cytomegalovirus, or HIV.

In about 30% of patients, the cause is bacterial. Group A β-hemolytic streptococcus (GABHS) is most common (see p. 1605), but *Staphylococcus aureus, Streptococcus pneumoniae, Mycoplasma pneumoniae,* and *Chlamydia pneumoniae* are sometimes involved. Rare causes include pertussis, *Fusobacterium,* diphtheria, syphilis, and gonorrhea.

GABHS occurs most commonly between ages 5 and 15 and is uncommon before age 3.

Symptoms and Signs

Pain with swallowing is the hallmark and is often referred to the ears. Very young children who are not able to complain of sore throat often refuse to eat. High fever, malaise, headache, and GI upset are common, as are halitosis and a muffled voice. A scarlatiniform or nonspecific rash may also be present. The tonsils are swollen and red and often have purulent exudates. Tender cervical lymphadenopathy may be present. Fever, adenopathy, palatal petechiae, and exudates are somewhat more common with GABHS than with viral tonsillopharyngitis, but there is much overlap.

GABHS usually resolves within 7 days. Untreated GABHS may lead to local suppurative complications (eg, peritonsillar abscess or cellulitis) and sometimes to rheumatic fever or glomerulonephritis.

Diagnosis

- Clinical evaluation
- GABHS ruled out by rapid antigen test, culture, or both

Pharyngitis itself is easily recognized clinically. However, its cause is not. Rhinorrhea and cough usually indicate a viral cause. Infectious mononucleosis is suggested by posterior cervical or generalized adenopathy, hepatosplenomegaly, fatigue, and malaise for > 1 wk; a full neck with petechiae of the soft palate; and thick tonsillar exudates. A dirty gray, thick, tough membrane that bleeds if peeled away indicates diphtheria (rare in the US).

Because GABHS requires antibiotics, it must be diagnosed early. Criteria for testing are controversial. Many authorities recommend testing with a rapid antigen test or culture for all children. Rapid antigen tests are specific but not sensitive and may need to be followed by a culture, which is about 90% specific and 90% sensitive. In adults, many authorities recommend using the following 4 criteria:

- History of fever
- Tonsillar exudates
- Absence of cough
- Tender anterior cervical lymphadenopathy

Patients who meet 1 or no criteria are unlikely to have GABHS and should not be tested. Patients who meet 2 criteria can be tested. Patients who meet 3 or 4 criteria can be tested or treated empirically for GABHS.

Treatment

- Symptomatic treatment
- Antibiotics for GABHS
- Tonsillectomy considered for recurrent GABHS

Supportive treatments include analgesia, hydration, and rest. Analgesics may be systemic or topical. NSAIDs are usually effective systemic analgesics. Some clinicians also give a single dose of a corticosteroid (eg, dexamethasone 10 mg IM), which may help shorten symptom duration without affecting rates of relapse or adverse effects.[1] Topical analgesics are available as lozenges and sprays; ingredients include benzocaine, phenol, lidocaine, and other substances. These topical analgesics can reduce pain but have to be used repeatedly and often affect taste. Benzocaine used for pharyngitis has rarely caused methemoglobinemia.

Penicillin V is usually considered the drug of choice for GABHS tonsillopharyngitis; dose is 250 mg po bid for 10 days for patients < 27 kg and 500 mg for those > 27 kg. Amoxicillin is effective and more palatable if a liquid preparation is required. If adherence is a concern, a single dose of benzathine penicillin 1.2 million units IM (600,000 units for children ≤ 27 kg) is effective. Other oral drugs include macrolides for patients allergic to penicillin, a 1st-generation cephalosporin, and clindamycin. Diluting over-the-counter hydrogen peroxide with water in a 1:1 mixture and gargling with it will promote debridement and improve oropharyngeal hygiene.

Treatment may be started immediately or delayed until culture results are known. If treatment is started presumptively, it should be stopped if cultures are negative. Follow-up throat cultures are not done routinely. They are useful in patients with multiple GABHS recurrences or if pharyngitis spreads to close contacts at home or school.

Tonsillectomy: Tonsillectomy has often been considered if GABHS tonsillitis recurs repeatedly (> 6 episodes/yr, > 4 episodes/yr for 2 yr, or > 3 episodes/yr for 3 yr) or if acute infection is severe and persistent despite antibiotics. Other criteria for tonsillectomy include obstructive sleep disorder, recurrent peritonsillar abscess, and suspicion of cancer. However, these criteria, and the use of any specific guideline, are being questioned.[2,3] Decisions should be individual, based on patient age, multiple risk factors, and response to infection recurrences.

Numerous effective surgical techniques are used to perform tonsillectomy, including electrocautery dissection, microdebrider, radiofrequency coblation, and sharp dissection. Significant intraoperative or postoperative bleeding occurs in < 2% of patients, usually within 24 h of surgery or after 7 days, when the eschar detaches. Patients with bleeding should go to the hospital. If bleeding continues on arrival, patients generally are examined in the operating room, and hemostasis is obtained. Any clot present in the tonsillar fossa is removed, and patients are observed for 24 h. Postoperative IV rehydration is necessary in ≤ 3% of patients, possibly in fewer patients with use of optimal preoperative hydration, perioperative antibiotics, analgesics, and corticosteroids.

Postoperative airway obstruction occurs most frequently in children < 2 yr who have preexisting severe obstructive sleep disorders and in patients who are morbidly obese or have neurologic disorders, craniofacial anomalies, or significant preoperative obstructive sleep apnea. Complications are generally more common and serious among adults.

1. Hayward G, Thompson MJ, Perera R, et al: Corticosteroids as standalone or add-on treatment for sore throat. *Cochrane Database Syst Rev.*, 2012. doi: 10.1002/14651858.CD008268.pub2.
2. Rosenfeld RM: Talking Points for AAO-HNS Tonsillectomy Guideline. *Otolaryngology—Head and Neck Surgery*, 2011.
3. Ruben RJ: Randomized controlled studies and the treatment of middle-ear effusions and tonsillar pharyngitis: how random are the studies and what are their limitations? *Otolaryngol Head Neck Surg.* 139(3):333–339, 2008. doi: 10.1016.

KEY POINTS

- Pharyngitis itself is easily recognized clinically, but only in 25 to 30% of cases is testing likely to be required to determine if it is due to streptococcal infection.
- Clinical criteria (modified Centor score) can help to select patients for further testing or empiric antibiotic treatment, although some authorities recommend testing all children using a rapid antigen test and sometimes culture.
- Penicillin remains the drug of choice for streptococcal pharyngitis; cephalosporins or macrolides are alternatives for patients allergic to penicillin.

TORNWALDT CYST

(Pharyngeal Bursa)

Tornwaldt cyst is a rare cyst in the midline of the nasopharynx that may become infected.

Tornwaldt cyst is a remnant of the embryonal notochord superficial to the superior constrictor muscle of the pharynx and is covered by the mucous membrane of the nasopharynx. It may become infected, causing persistent purulent drainage with a foul taste and odor, eustachian tube obstruction, and sore throat.

Purulent exudate may be seen at the opening of the cyst.

Diagnosis is based on nasopharyngoscopy supplemented by CT or MRI when the diagnosis is in doubt.

Treatment consists of marsupialization or excision.

VELOPHARYNGEAL INSUFFICIENCY

Velopharyngeal insufficiency is incomplete closure of a sphincter between the oropharynx and nasopharynx, often resulting from anatomic abnormalities of the palate and causing hypernasal speech. Diagnosis is direct inspection with a fiber-optic nasoendoscope. Treatment is with speech therapy and surgery.

Velopharyngeal insufficiency is incomplete closure of the velopharyngeal sphincter between the oropharynx and the nasopharynx. Closure, normally achieved by the sphincteric action of the soft palate and the superior constrictor muscle, is impaired in patients with cleft palate, repaired cleft palate, congenitally short palate, submucous cleft palate, palatal paralysis, and, sometimes, enlarged tonsils. The condition may also result when adenoidectomy or uvulopalatopharyngoplasty is done in a patient with a congenital underdevelopment (submucous cleft) or paralysis of the palate.

Symptoms and Signs

Speech in a patient with velopharyngeal insufficiency is characterized by hypernasal resonant voice, nasal emission of air, nasal turbulence, and inability to produce sounds requiring oral pressure (plosives). Severe velopharyngeal insufficiency results in regurgitation of solid foods and fluids through the nose. Inspection of the palate during phonation may reveal palatal paralysis.

Diagnosis

- Direct inspection with a fiber-optic nasoendoscope

The diagnosis is suspected in patients with the typical speech abnormalities.

Palpation of the midline of the soft palate may reveal an occult submucous cleft. Direct inspection with a fiber-optic nasoendoscope is the primary diagnostic technique.

Multiview videofluoroscopy during connected speech and swallowing (modified barium swallow), done in conjunction with a speech pathologist, should be used only when other diagnostic measures fail to provide necessary information.

Treatment

- Surgical repair and speech therapy

Treatment consists of speech therapy and surgical correction by a palatal elongation pushback procedure, posterior pharyngeal wall implant, pharyngeal flap, or pharyngoplasty, depending on the mobility of the lateral pharyngeal walls, the degree of velar elevation, and the size of the defect. A palatal lift prosthesis (from a prosthodontist) may also be helpful.

100 Tumors of the Head and Neck

Head and neck cancer develops in almost 60,000 people in the United States each year. Excluding skin and thyroid cancers, > 90% of head and neck cancers are squamous cell (epidermoid) carcinomas; most of the rest are adenocarcinomas, sarcomas, and lymphomas.

The **most common sites** of head and neck cancer are the

- Larynx (including the supraglottis, glottis, and subglottis)
- Oral cavity (tongue, floor of mouth, hard palate, buccal mucosa, and alveolar ridges)
- Oropharynx (base of tongue, tonsils, and soft palate)

Less common sites include the nasopharynx, nasal cavity and paranasal sinuses, hypopharynx, and salivary glands.

Additional discussions regarding other sites of head and neck tumors are found elsewhere in THE MANUAL:

- Intracranial tumors in adults
- Intracranial tumors in children
- Thyroid cancers
- Tumors of the orbit and cancers affecting the retina
- Acoustic neuromas
- Skin cancers

The incidence of head and neck cancer increases with age. Although most patients are between 50 yr and 70 yr, the incidence in younger patients is increasing. Head and neck cancer is more common among men than women; however, the incidence by sex varies with anatomic location and has been changing because the number of female smokers has increased.

Etiology

The vast majority of patients, 85% or more, with cancer of the head and neck have a history of alcohol use, smoking, or both. Heavy long-term users of tobacco and alcohol have an almost 40-fold greater risk of developing squamous cell carcinoma. Other suspected causes include use of snuff or chewing tobacco, sunlight exposure, previous x-rays of the head and neck, certain viral infections, ill-fitting dental appliances, chronic candidiasis, and poor oral hygiene. In India, oral cancer is extremely common, probably because of chewing betel quid (a mixture of substances, also called paan). Long-term exposure to sunlight and the use of tobacco products are the primary causes of squamous cell carcinoma of the lower lip.

Patients who in the past were treated with radiation for acne, excess facial hair, enlarged thymus, or hypertrophic tonsils and adenoids are predisposed to thyroid and salivary gland cancers and benign salivary tumors.

Epstein-Barr virus plays a role in the pathogenesis of nasopharyngeal cancer, and serum measures of certain Epstein-Barr virus proteins may be biomarkers of recurrence.

The link between human papillomavirus (HPV) infection and head and neck squamous cell carcinoma, particularly oropharyngeal cancer, has been well established. The increase in HPV-related cancer has caused an overall increase in the incidence of oropharyngeal cancer, which otherwise would have been expected to decrease because of the decrease in smoking over the last 2 decades or so. The mechanism for viral-mediated tumor genesis appears to be distinct from tobacco-related pathways.

Symptoms and Signs

The manifestations of head and neck cancer depend greatly on the location and extent of the tumor. Common initial manifestations of head and neck cancers include an asymptomatic neck mass, painful mucosal ulceration, visible mucosal lesion (eg, leukoplakia, erythroplakia), hoarseness, and dysphagia.

Subsequent symptoms depend on location and extent of the tumor and include pain, paresthesia, nerve palsies, trismus, and halitosis. Otalgia is an often overlooked symptom usually representing referred pain from the primary tumor. Weight loss caused by perturbed eating and odynophagia is also common.

Diagnosis

- Clinical evaluation
- Biopsy
- Imaging tests and endoscopy to evaluate extent of disease

Routine physical examination (including a thorough oral examination) is the best way to detect cancers early before they become symptomatic. Commercially available brush biopsy kits help screen for oral cancers. Any head and neck symptom (eg, sore throat, hoarseness, otalgia) lasting > 2 to 3 wk should prompt referral to a head and neck specialist who will typically do flexible fiber-optic laryngoscopy to evaluate the larynx and pharynx.

Definitive diagnosis usually requires a biopsy. Fine-needle aspiration is used for a neck mass; it is well tolerated, accurate, and, unlike an open biopsy, does not impact future treatment options. Oral lesions are evaluated with an incisional biopsy or a brush biopsy. Nasopharyngeal, oropharyngeal, or laryngeal lesions are biopsied endoscopically.

Imaging (CT, MRI, or PET/CT) is done to help determine the extent of the primary tumor, involvement of adjacent structures, and spread to cervical lymph nodes.

Staging

Head and neck cancers are staged (see Table 100–1) according to size and site of the primary tumor (T), number and size of metastases to the cervical lymph nodes (N), and evidence of distant metastases (M). Staging usually requires imaging with CT, MRI, or both, and often PET.

Prognosis

Prognosis in head and neck cancer varies greatly depending on the tumor size, primary site, etiology, and presence of regional or distant metastases. In general, the prognosis is favorable if diagnosis is early and treatment is timely and appropriate.

Head and neck cancers first invade locally and then metastasize to regional cervical lymph nodes. The spread to regional lymphatics is partially related to tumor size, extent, and aggressiveness and reduces overall survival by nearly half. Distant metastases (most often to the lungs) tend to occur later, usually in patients with advanced-stage disease. Distant metastases greatly reduce survival and are almost always incurable.

Advanced local disease (a criterion for advanced T stage) with invasion of muscle, bone, or cartilage also significantly decreases cure rate. Perineural spread, as evidenced by pain, paralysis, or numbness, indicates a highly aggressive tumor, is associated with nodal metastasis, and has a less favorable prognosis than a similar lesion without perineural invasion.

Table 100–1. STAGING OF HEAD AND NECK CANCER

STAGE	TUMOR (MAXIMUM PENETRATION)	REGIONAL LYMPH NODE METASTASIS	DISTANT METASTASIS
I	T1	N0	M0
II	T2	N0	M0
III	T3 or	N0	M0
	T1–3	N1	M0
IVA	T1–3	N2	M0
	T4a	N0–2	M0
IVB	T4b	Any N	M0
	Any T	N3	M0
IVC	Any T	Any N	M1

TNM classification: T1 ≤ 2 cm in greatest dimension; T2 = 2–4 cm or affects 2 areas within a specific site; T3 > 4 cm or affects 3 areas within a specific site; T4 = invades specific structures (4a is moderately advanced local disease and 4b is very advanced local disease).

N0 = none; N1 = one node ≤ 3 cm; N2 = node between 3 and 6 cm or multiple nodes; N3 = node > 6 cm.

M0 = none; M1 = present.

With appropriate treatment, 5-yr survival can be as high as 90% for stage I, 75 to 80% for stage II, 45 to 75% for stage III, and up to 50% for some stage IV cancers. The survival rates vary greatly depending on the primary site and etiology. Stage I laryngeal cancers have an excellent survival rate when compared to other sites. Oropharyngeal cancers caused by HPV have a significantly better prognosis compared with oropharyngeal tumors caused by tobacco or alcohol. Because the prognosis between HPV-positive and HPV-negative oropharyngeal cancers differs, all tumors of the oropharynx should be routinely tested for HPV.

Treatment

- Surgery, radiation therapy, or both
- Sometimes chemotherapy

The main treatments for head and neck cancer are surgery and radiation. These modalities can be used alone or in combination and with or without chemotherapy. However, chemotherapy is almost never used as primary treatment for cure. Many tumors, regardless of location, respond similarly to surgery and to radiation therapy, allowing other factors such as patient preference or location-specific morbidity to determine choice of therapy.

However, at certain locations, there is clear superiority of one modality. For example, surgery is better for early-stage disease involving the oral cavity because radiation therapy has the potential to cause mandibular osteoradionecrosis. Endoscopic surgery has become more frequently used; in select head and neck cancers, it has cure rates similar to those of open surgery or radiation, and its morbidity is significantly less. Endoscopic approaches are most often used for laryngeal surgery and usually use a laser to make the cuts.

If radiation therapy is chosen for primary therapy, it is delivered to the primary site and sometimes bilaterally to the cervical lymph nodes. The treatment of lymphatics, whether by radiation or surgery, is determined by the primary site, histologic criteria, and risk of nodal disease. Early-stage lesions often do not require treatment of the lymph nodes, whereas more advanced lesions do. Head and neck sites rich in lymphatics (eg, oropharynx, supraglottis) usually require lymph node radiation regardless of tumor stage, whereas sites with fewer lymphatics (eg, larynx) usually do not require lymphatic radiation for early-stage disease. Intensity-modulated radiation therapy (IMRT) delivers radiation to a very specific area, potentially reducing adverse effects without compromising tumor control.

Advanced-stage disease (stages III and IV) often requires multimodality treatment, incorporating some combination of chemotherapy, radiation therapy, and surgery. Bone or cartilage invasion requires surgical resection of the primary site and usually regional lymph nodes because of the high risk of nodal spread. If the primary site is treated surgically, then postoperative radiation to the cervical lymph nodes is delivered if there are high-risk features, such as multiple lymph nodes with cancer or extracapsular extension. Postoperative radiation usually is preferred over preoperative radiation because radiated tissues heal poorly.

Recent studies have shown that adding chemotherapy to adjuvant radiation therapy to the neck improves regional control of the cancer and improves survival. However, this approach causes significant adverse effects, such as increased dysphagia and bone marrow suppression, so the decision to add chemotherapy should be carefully considered.

Advanced squamous cell carcinoma without bony invasion often is treated with concomitant chemotherapy and radiation therapy. Although advocated as organ-sparing, combining chemotherapy with radiation therapy doubles the rate of acute toxicities, particularly severe dysphagia. Radiation may be used alone for debilitated patients with advanced disease who cannot tolerate the sequelae of chemotherapy and are too high a risk for general anesthesia.

Primary chemotherapy is reserved for chemosensitive tumors, such as Burkitt lymphoma, or for patients who have widespread metastases (eg, hepatic or pulmonary involvement). Several drugs—cisplatin, fluorouracil, bleomycin, and methotrexate—provide palliation for pain and shrink the tumor in patients who cannot be treated with other methods. Response may be good initially but is not durable, and the cancer almost always returns.

Because the treatment of head and neck cancer is so complex, multidisciplinary treatment planning is essential. Ideally, each patient should be discussed by a tumor board consisting of members of all treating disciplines, along with radiologists and pathologists, so that a consensus can be reached on the best treatment. Once treatment has been determined, it is best coordinated by a team that includes ENT and reconstructive surgeons, radiation and medical oncologists, speech and language pathologists, dentists, and nutritionists.

Plastic and reconstructive surgeons play an increasingly important role because the use of free-tissue transfer flaps has allowed functional and cosmetic reconstruction of defects to significantly improve a patient's quality of life after procedures that previously caused excessive morbidity have been done. Common donor sites used for reconstruction include the fibula (often used to reconstruct the mandible), the radial forearm (commonly used for the tongue and floor of mouth), and the anterior lateral thigh (often used for laryngeal or pharyngeal reconstruction).

Treatment of tumor recurrence: Managing recurrent tumors after therapy is complex and has potential complications. A palpable mass or ulcerated lesion with edema or pain at the primary site after therapy strongly suggests a persistent tumor. Such patients require CT (with thin cuts) or MRI.

For local recurrence after surgical treatment, all scar planes and reconstructive flaps are excised along with residual cancer. Radiation therapy, chemotherapy, or both may be done but have limited effectiveness. Patients with recurrence after radiation therapy are best treated with surgery. However, some patients may benefit from additional radiation treatments, but this approach has a high risk of adverse effects and should be done with care.

Symptom control: Pain is a common symptom in patients with head and neck cancer and must be adequately addressed. Palliative surgery or radiation may temporarily alleviate pain, and in 30 to 50% of patients, chemotherapy can produce improvement that lasts a mean of 3 mo. A stepwise approach to pain management, as recommended by the WHO, is critical to controlling pain. Severe pain is best managed in association with a pain and palliative care specialist.

Pain, difficulty eating, choking on secretions, and other problems make adequate symptomatic treatment essential. Patient directives regarding such care should be clarified early (see p. 3212).

Adverse effects of treatment: All cancer treatments have potential complications and expected sequelae. Because many treatments have similar cure rates, the choice of modality is based largely on real, or perceived, differences in sequelae.

Although it is commonly thought that surgery causes the most morbidity, many procedures can be done without significantly impairing appearance or function. Increasingly complex reconstructive procedures and techniques, including prostheses, grafts, regional pedicle flaps, and complex free flaps, can restore function and appearance often to near normal.

Toxic effects of chemotherapy include malaise, severe nausea and vomiting, mucositis, transient hair loss, gastroenteritis, hematopoietic and immune suppression, and infection.

Therapeutic radiation for head and neck cancers has several adverse effects. The function of any salivary gland within the beam is permanently destroyed by a dose of about 40 Gy, resulting in xerostomia, which markedly increases the risk of dental caries. Newer radiation techniques, such as intensity-modulated radiation therapy (IMRT), can minimize or eliminate toxic doses to the parotid glands in certain patients.

In addition, the blood supply of bone, particularly in the mandible, is compromised by doses of > 60 Gy, and osteoradionecrosis may occur. In this condition, tooth extraction sites break down, sloughing bone and soft tissue. Therefore, any needed dental treatment, including scaling, fillings, and extractions, should be done before radiation therapy. Any teeth in poor condition that cannot be rehabilitated should be extracted.

Radiation therapy may also cause oral mucositis and dermatitis in the overlying skin, which may result in dermal fibrosis. Loss of taste (ageusia) and impaired smell (dysosmia) often occur but are usually transient.

Prevention

Removing risk factors is critical, and all patients should cease tobacco use and limit alcohol consumption. Removing risk factors also helps prevent disease recurrence in patients treated for cancer. A new primary cancer develops in about 5% of patients/yr (to a maximum risk of about 20%); risk is lower in those who stop using tobacco.

Current vaccines against HPV target some of the HPV strains that cause oropharyngeal cancer, so childhood vaccination as currently recommended could be expected to lower the incidence of these cancers.

Cancer of the lower lip may be prevented by sunscreen use and tobacco cessation. Because 60% of head and neck cancers are well advanced (stage III or IV) at the time of diagnosis, the most promising strategy for reducing morbidity and mortality is diligent routine examination of the oral cavity.

LARYNGEAL CANCER

Ninety percent of laryngeal cancer is squamous cell carcinoma. Smoking, alcohol abuse, lower socioeconomic status, and being male and > 60 yr increase risk. Early diagnosis is common with vocal cord tumors because hoarseness develops early. However, supraglottic tumors (above the vocal cords) and subglottic tumors (below the vocal cords) often manifest at an advanced stage because they can remain asymptomatic for a longer time frame. Diagnosis is based on laryngoscopy and biopsy. Treatment of early-stage tumors is with surgery or radiation. Advanced-stage tumors are often treated with chemotherapy and radiation therapy. Surgery is reserved for salvage treatment or lesions with extralaryngeal extension or cartilage destruction. Reestablishment of speaking ability is needed if a total laryngectomy is done.

Squamous cell carcinoma is the most common cancer of the larynx. In the US, it is 4 times more common among men and is more common among people of lower socioeconomic status. Over 95% of patients are smokers; 15 pack-years of smoking increase the risk 30-fold. The incidence of laryngeal cancer is about 14,000 new cases per year and is decreasing, particularly among men, most likely due to changes in smoking habits. Annual deaths are about 3600.

Sixty percent of patients present with localized disease alone; 25% present with local disease and regional nodal metastatic disease; and 15% present with advanced disease, distant metastases, or both. Lymph node metastasis are more common in supraglottic and subglottic tumors than with glottic cancers due to the minimal lymphatic drainage of the glottis. Distant metastases occur most frequently in the lungs and liver.

Common sites of origin are the true vocal cords (glottis) and the supraglottic larynx. The least common site is the subglottic larynx, where only 1% of primary laryngeal cancers originate. Verrucous carcinoma, a rare variant of squamous cell carcinoma, usually arises in the glottic area and has a better survival rate than standard squamous cell carcinoma.

Symptoms and Signs

Symptoms and signs differ based on the involved portion of the larynx. Hoarseness is common early in glottic cancers but is a late symptom for supraglottic and subglottic cancers. Patients with subglottic cancer often present with airway obstruction, and hoarseness is a common late symptom. Patients with supraglottic cancer often present with dysphagia; other common symptoms include airway obstruction, otalgia, development of a neck mass, or a "hot potato" voice. Patients with these symptoms should be referred for direct laryngoscopy without delay.

Diagnosis

- Laryngoscopy
- Operative endoscopy and biopsy
- Imaging tests for staging

All patients who have hoarseness for > 2 to 3 wk should have their larynx examined by a head and neck specialist. Some practitioners use a mirror to evaluate the larynx, but most prefer a flexible fiber-optic examination. Any lesions discovered require further evaluation, usually with operative endoscopy and biopsy, with concomitant evaluation of the upper airway and GI tract for coexisting cancers. The incidence of a synchronous second primary tumor may be as high as 10%.

Patients with confirmed carcinoma typically have neck CT with contrast and a chest x-ray or chest CT. Most clinicians also do PET of the neck and chest at the time of diagnosis.

Prognosis

Early-stage glottic carcinoma has a 5-yr survival rate of 85 to 95%. The overall 5-yr survival rate for patients with laryngeal cancer is 60%. Patients who present with regional nodal disease have a 43% 5-yr survival rate, and those who present with distant metastases have a 30% 5-yr survival rate.

Treatment

- Early-stage (T1 and T2): Surgery or radiation therapy
- Moderately advanced (T3): Radiation therapy and sometimes chemotherapy
- Advanced (T4): Surgery (often followed by radiation therapy and sometimes chemotherapy) or sometimes chemotherapy and radiation therapy

Early-stage glottic carcinoma (see Table 100–1) is treated with laser excision, radiation therapy, or occasionally open laryngeal surgery. Endoscopic laser resection and radiation therapy usually preserve a normal voice and post-treatment function and have similar cure rates. Whether surgery or radiation is used to treat early-stage glottic cancer usually depends on the preferences of the treating institution and the patient.

For advanced glottic carcinoma, defined by a lack of vocal cord mobility or extension into the tongue, most patients are treated with both chemotherapy and radiation therapy. If the patient presents with extension outside of the larynx or with cartilage invasion, a laryngectomy provides the best oncologic results; the laryngectomy is commonly total, but endoscopic laser resection or open partial laryngectomy can be used in select appropriate cases. A total laryngectomy is also commonly used for salvage situations; however, endoscopic resection or open partial laryngectomy may sometimes be used in these situations.

Early supraglottic carcinoma can be effectively treated with radiation therapy or partial laryngectomy. Laser resection has shown considerable success on early-stage supraglottic squamous cell carcinomas and minimizes functional changes after surgery. If the carcinoma is more advanced but does not affect the true vocal cords, a supraglottic partial laryngectomy can be done to preserve the voice and glottic sphincter. If the true vocal cords also are affected, a supracricoid laryngectomy or a total laryngectomy is required if surgery is chosen.

As with glottic carcinoma, most advanced-stage supraglottic cancers initially are treated with chemotherapy and radiation therapy. The supraglottis has a rich lymphatic network, so the neck must be addressed in all patients with supraglottic cancer.

Treatment of hypopharyngeal carcinomas is similar to that of laryngeal cancer. Early-stage lesions usually are treated with radiation alone, although endoscopic resection is an option. However, the majority of patients with hypopharyngeal cancer have advanced-stage disease because of the silent nature of the disease and frequent regional lymphatic spread; such patients are treated with chemotherapy and radiation therapy primarily, with surgical salvage.

Rehabilitation: Rehabilitation may be required after either surgical or nonsurgical treatment. Significant swallowing problems are common after chemotherapy and radiation therapy and may require esophageal dilation, swallowing therapy, or, in severe cases, surgical replacement of the pharynx or gastrostomy tube feedings. Swallowing also is affected by surgery and may require swallowing therapy or dilation as well.

Speech, on the other hand, is more significantly affected by surgery. After total laryngectomy, the patient requires creation of a new voice by way of

- Esophageal speech
- A tracheoesophageal puncture
- An electrolarynx

In all 3 techniques, sound is articulated into speech by the pharynx, palate, tongue, teeth, and lips.

Esophageal speech involves taking air into the esophagus during inspiration and gradually eructating the air through the pharyngoesophageal junction to produce a sound.

A tracheoesophageal puncture involves placement of a one-way valve between the trachea and esophagus to facilitate phonation. This valve forces air into the esophagus during expiration to produce a sound. Patients receive physical rehabilitation, speech therapy, and appropriate training in the maintenance and use of this valve and must be cautioned against the possible aspiration of food, fluids, and secretions.

An electrolarynx is a battery-powered sound source that is held against the neck to produce sound. Although it carries a great deal of social stigma for many patients, it has the advantage of being functional immediately with little or no training.

KEY POINTS

- Hoarseness is common early in glottic cancers but is a late symptom for supraglottic and subglottic cancers.
- All patients who have hoarseness for > 2 to 3 wk should have their larynx examined by a head and neck specialist.
- Patients with confirmed carcinoma typically have neck CT with contrast and often PET/CT for advanced stages.
- Treat early-stage (T1 and T2) cancer with surgery or radiation therapy.
- Treat moderately advanced (T3) cancer with radiation therapy and sometimes chemotherapy.
- Treat advanced cancer (T4) that extends outside of the larynx with surgery and then postoperative chemotherapy and radiation therapy.

NASOPHARYNGEAL CANCER

Nasopharyngeal cancers are rare in the US but common in the South China Sea region. Symptoms develop late, including unilateral bloody nasal discharge, nasal obstruction, hearing loss, ear pain, facial swelling, and facial numbness. Diagnosis is based on inspection and biopsy, with CT, MRI, or PET to evaluate extent. Treatment is with radiation, chemotherapy, and, rarely, surgery.

Squamous cell carcinoma is the most common malignant tumor of the nasopharynx. It can occur in any age group, including adolescents, and is rare in North America. It is one of the most common cancers among people of Chinese, especially southern Chinese, and Southeast Asian ancestry, including Chinese immigrants to North America. Over several generations, the prevalence among Chinese-Americans gradually decreases to that among non-Chinese Americans, suggesting an environmental component to etiology. Dietary exposure to nitrites and salted fish also is thought to increase risk. Epstein-Barr virus is a significant risk factor, and there is hereditary predisposition.

Other nasopharyngeal cancers include adenoid cystic and mucoepidermoid carcinomas, malignant mixed tumors, adenocarcinomas, lymphomas, fibrosarcomas, osteosarcomas, chondrosarcomas, and melanomas.

Symptoms and Signs

Nasopharyngeal cancer often presents with palpable lymph node metastases in the neck. Another common presenting symptom is hearing loss, usually caused by nasal or eustachian tube obstruction leading to a middle ear effusion. Other symptoms include ear pain, purulent bloody rhinorrhea, frank epistaxis, cranial nerve palsies, and cervical lymphadenopathy. Cranial nerve palsies most often involve the 6th, 4th, and 3rd cranial nerves due to their location in the cavernous sinus, in close proximity to the foramen lacerum, which is the most common route of intracranial spread for these tumors. Because lymphatics of the nasopharynx communicate across the midline, bilateral metastases are common.

Diagnosis

- Nasopharyngeal endoscopy and biopsy
- Imaging tests for staging

Patients suspected of having nasopharyngeal cancer must undergo examination with a nasopharyngeal mirror or endoscope, and lesions are biopsied. Open cervical node biopsy should not be done as the initial procedure (see Neck Mass on p. 799), although a needle biopsy is acceptable and often recommended.

Gadolinium-enhanced MRI (with fat suppression) of the head with attention to the nasopharynx and skull base is done; the skull base is involved in about 25% of patients. CT also is required to accurately assess skull base bony changes, which are less visible on MRI. A PET scan also commonly is done to assess the extent of disease as well as the cervical lymphatics.

Prognosis

Patients with early-stage disease (see Table 100–1) typically have a good outcome (5-yr survival is 60 to 75%), whereas patients with stage IV disease have a poor outcome (5-yr survival is < 40%).

Treatment

- Chemotherapy plus radiation therapy
- Surgery

Because of the location and extent of involvement, nasopharyngeal cancers often are not amenable to surgical resection. They are typically treated with chemotherapy and radiation therapy, which are often followed by adjuvant chemotherapy.

Recurrent tumors can be treated with another course of radiation, commonly with brachytherapy; radionecrosis of the skull base is a risk. An alternative to radiation is skull base resection. Resection is usually done by removing part of the maxilla for access but, in select cases, resection can be done endoscopically, although little data yet exists on endoscopic resection.

ORAL SQUAMOUS CELL CARCINOMA

Oral squamous cell carcinoma affects about 30,000 people in the US each year. Over 95% smoke tobacco, drink alcohol, or both. Early, curable lesions are rarely symptomatic; thus, preventing fatal disease requires early detection by screening. Treatment is with surgery, radiation, or both, although surgery plays a larger role in the treatment of most oral cavity cancer. The overall 5-yr survival rate (all sites and stages combined) is > 50%.

Oral cancer refers to cancer occurring between the vermilion border of the lips and the junction of the hard and soft palates or the posterior one third of the tongue.

In the US, 3% of cancers in men and 2% in women are oral squamous cell carcinomas, most of which occur after age 50. As with most head and neck sites, squamous cell carcinoma is the most common oral cancer.

The chief risk factors for oral squamous cell carcinoma are

- Smoking (especially > 2 packs/day)
- Alcohol use

Risk increases dramatically when alcohol use exceeds 6 oz of distilled liquor, 15 oz of wine, or 36 oz of beer/day. The combination of heavy smoking and alcohol abuse is estimated to raise the risk 100-fold in women and 38-fold in men.

Squamous cell carcinoma of the tongue may also result from any chronic irritation, such as dental caries, overuse of mouthwash, chewing tobacco, or the use of betel quid. Oral human papillomavirus (HPV), typically acquired via oral-genital contact, may have a role in the etiology of some oral cancers; however, the role of HPV is not as clearly defined in oral cancer as it is in oropharyngeal cancer.

About 40% of intraoral squamous cell carcinomas begin on the floor of the mouth or on the lateral and ventral surfaces of the tongue. About 38% of all oral squamous cell carcinomas occur on the lower lip; these are usually solar-related cancers on the external surface.

Symptoms and Signs

Oral lesions are asymptomatic initially, highlighting the need for oral screening. Most dental professionals carefully examine the oral cavity and oropharynx during routine care and may do a brush biopsy of abnormal areas. The lesions may appear as areas of erythroplakia or leukoplakia and may be exophytic or ulcerated. Cancers are often indurated and firm with a rolled border. As the lesions increase in size, pain, dysarthria, and dysphagia may result.

Diagnosis

- Biopsy
- Endoscopy to detect second primary cancer
- Chest x-ray and CT of head and neck

Any suspicious areas should be biopsied. Incisional or brush biopsy can be done depending on the surgeon's preference. Direct laryngoscopy and esophagoscopy are done in all patients with oral cavity cancer to exclude a simultaneous second primary cancer. Head and neck CT usually is done and a chest x-ray is done; however, as in most sites in the head and neck, PET/CT has begun to play a larger role in the evaluation of patients with oral cavity cancer.

Prognosis

If carcinoma of the tongue is localized (no lymph node involvement), 5-yr survival is > 75%. For localized carcinoma of the floor of the mouth, 5-yr survival is 75%. Lymph node metastasis decreases survival rate by about half. Metastases reach the regional lymph nodes first and later the lungs.

For lower lip lesions, 5-yr survival is 90%, and metastases are rare. Carcinoma of the upper lip tends to be more aggressive and metastatic.

Treatment

- Surgery, with postoperative radiation or chemoradiation as needed

For most oral cavity cancers, surgery is the initial treatment of choice. Radiation or chemoradiation is added postoperatively if disease is more advanced or has high-risk features. (See also the National Cancer Institute's summary Lip and Oral Cavity Cancer Treatment.)

Selective neck dissection is indicated if the risk of nodal disease exceeds 15 to 20%. Although there is no firm consensus, neck dissections are typically done for T2 (see Table 100–1) lesions (greatest dimension 2 to 4 cm) and most T1 lesions with a depth of invasion about ≥ 4 mm.

Routine surgical reconstruction is the key to reducing postoperative oral disabilities; procedures range from local tissue flaps to free tissue transfers. Speech and swallowing therapy may be required after significant resections.

Radiation therapy is an alternative treatment. Chemotherapy is not used routinely as primary therapy but is recommended as adjuvant therapy along with radiation in patients with advanced nodal disease.

Treatment of squamous cell carcinoma of the lip is surgical excision with reconstruction to maximize postoperative function. When large areas of the lip exhibit premalignant change, the lip can be surgically shaved, or a laser can remove all affected mucosa. Mohs surgery can be used. Thereafter, appropriate sunscreen application is recommended.

KEY POINTS

- The chief risk factors for oral squamous cell carcinoma are heavy smoking and alcohol use.
- Oral cancer is sometimes asymptomatic initially, so oral screening (typically by dental professionals) is useful for early diagnosis.
- Do direct laryngoscopy and esophagoscopy to exclude a simultaneous second primary cancer.
- Once cancer is confirmed, do head and neck CT and a chest x-ray or PET/CT.
- Initial treatment is usually surgical.

OROPHARYNGEAL SQUAMOUS CELL CARCINOMA

Oropharyngeal squamous cell carcinoma affects over 13,000 people in the US each year. Tobacco and alcohol are major risk factors, and the role of human papillomavirus (HPV) infection as a risk factor is increasing. Symptoms include sore throat and painful and/or difficult swallowing. Treatment is with radiation, chemotherapy, or both, but primary surgery has begun to be used more often. Survival rate is much higher in HPV-positive patients.

Oropharyngeal squamous cell carcinoma refers to cancer of the tonsil, base and posterior one third of the tongue, soft palate, and posterior and lateral pharyngeal walls. Squamous cell carcinoma comprises over 95% of oropharyngeal cancers.

In the US in 2015, there were an expected > 13,000 new cases of oropharyngeal cancer. Although the incidence of oropharyngeal cancer is increasing, its cure rates are also improving.

Like most head and neck cancers, oropharyngeal cancer is more common among older men with a mean age of 63. The male:female ratio is 2.7:1. However, recently, oropharyngeal cancer patients have become younger and more commonly female as HPV infection has emerged as an etiology. The risk of developing oropharyngeal cancer is 16 times higher in HPV-positive patients. In Europe and North America, HPV infection accounts for about 70 to 80% of oropharyngeal cancers. Nonetheless, tobacco and alcohol remain important risk factors for oropharyngeal cancer. Patients who smoke more than 1.5 packs/day have about a 3-fold increased risk of cancer, and patients who drink 4 or more drinks/day have about a 7-fold increased risk. People who both drink and smoke heavily have 30 times the risk of developing oropharyngeal cancer.

Symptoms and Signs

Oropharyngeal cancer symptoms vary slightly depending on the subsite but typically patients present with sore throat, dysphagia, odynophagia, dysarthria, and otalgia. A neck mass, often cystic, is a common presenting symptom of patients with oropharyngeal cancer. Because the symptoms of oropharyngeal cancer mimic those of common URIs, it often takes many months before patients are referred to a specialist.

Diagnosis

- Laryngoscopy
- Operative endoscopy and biopsy
- Imaging tests for staging

All patients should undergo a direct laryngoscopy and biopsy before starting treatment to evaluate the primary lesion and to look for second primary lesions. Patients with confirmed carcinoma typically have neck CT with contrast, and most clinicians also do PET of the neck and chest.

Prognosis

The overall 5-yr survival rate is about 60%. However, prognosis varies with the cause. Patients who are HPV-positive have a 5-yr survival of > 75% (and a 3-yr survival of almost 90%), whereas HPV-negative patients have a 5-yr survival of < 50%.

Treatment

- Surgery, increasingly, transoral laser microsurgery
- Radiation therapy, with or without chemotherapy

Surgery is increasingly being used as primary treatment of oropharyngeal cancer. Transoral laser microsurgery (TLM) is increasingly being used to resect tumors of the tonsil and base of tongue endoscopically, avoiding the morbidity of open surgery. Transoral robotic surgery (TORS) is an increasingly popular means of treating select oropharyngeal lesions. In TORS, a surgical robot with multiple adaptable arms is controlled by a surgeon at a console. The articulating arms of the robot and an endoscopic camera are inserted through the patient's mouth (which is held open by a retractor). The robotic procedure provides better visualization of structures and causes less surgical morbidity compared to open surgery. However, the indications for using TORS are not yet well defined. When TORS is used on patients with more advanced tumors, postoperative radiation or chemoradiation is often done.

Radiation therapy, sometimes combined with chemotherapy (chemoradiation), can be used as primary therapy or postoperatively. Traditionally, radiation has been used for early-stage cancers and chemoradiation has been used for advanced cancers (see Table 100–1). Intensity-modulated radiation therapy (IMRT) has increasingly been used as a way to spare surrounding tissue and decrease long-term adverse effects.

Because the oropharynx is rich in lymphatics, cervical lymph node metastasis is common and must be considered in all patients with oropharyngeal cancer. If a cervical lymph node metastasis does not resolve after radiation or chemoradiation, post-treatment neck dissection is warranted.

JAW TUMORS

Numerous tumor types, both benign and malignant, originate in the jaw. Symptoms are swelling, pain, tenderness, and unexplained tooth mobility; some tumors are discovered on routine dental x-rays, whereas others are found on routine examinations of the oral cavity and teeth. Treatment depends on location and tumor type. Benign tumors may be observed and may not need surgical excision, although most tumors require resection with possible reconstruction.

If not initially detected on x-ray, jaw tumors are diagnosed clinically because their growth causes swelling of the face, palate, or alveolar ridge (the part of the jaw supporting the teeth). They can also cause bone tenderness and severe pain.

Bony outgrowths (torus palatinus, torus mandibularis) may develop on the palate or mandible. These are common growths and may prompt concerns about cancer, although they are benign and of concern only if they interfere with dental care or function of the submandibular gland. When on the palate, they are in the midline and have intact, smooth mucosa.

The most common tumor of the mandible and maxilla is squamous cell carcinoma invading the bone through dental sockets. These can involve any portion of the intraoral mandible or maxilla.

Ameloblastoma, the most common epithelial odontogenic tumor, usually arises in the posterior mandible. It is slowly invasive and rarely metastatic. On x-ray, it typically appears as multiloculated or soap-bubble radiolucency. Treatment is wide surgical excision and reconstruction if appropriate.

Odontoma, the most common odontogenic tumor, affects the dental follicle or the dental tissues and usually appears in the mandibles of young people. Odontomas include fibrous odontomas and cementomas. A clinically absent molar tooth suggests a composite odontoma. Typically, these tumors are excised, particularly when the diagnosis is in doubt.

Osteosarcoma, giant cell tumor, Ewing tumor, multiple myeloma, and metastatic tumors may affect the jaw. Treatment is the same as for those tumors in other bony sites.

OTIC TUMORS

A number of malignant and benign otic tumors occur, usually manifesting with hearing loss. They may also manifest with dizziness, vertigo, or imbalance. These tumors are rare and can be difficult to diagnose.

Malignant otic tumors: Basal cell and squamous cell carcinomas may arise in the ear canal. Persistent inflammation caused by chronic otitis media may predispose to the development of squamous cell carcinoma. Extensive resection is indicated, followed by radiation therapy. En bloc resection of the ear canal with sparing of the facial nerve is done when lesions are limited to the canal and have not invaded the middle ear. Deeper invasion requires a more significant temporal bone resection.

Rarely, squamous cell carcinoma originates in the middle ear. The persistent otorrhea of chronic otitis media may be a predisposing factor. Resection of the temporal bone and postoperative radiation therapy are necessary.

Nonchromaffin paragangliomas (chemodectomas) arise in the temporal bone from glomus bodies in the jugular bulb (glomus jugulare tumors) or the medial wall of the middle ear (glomus tympanicum tumors). They appear as a pulsatile red mass in the middle ear.

The first symptom often is tinnitus that is synchronous with the pulse. Hearing loss develops, followed by vertigo. Cranial nerve palsies of the 9th, 10th, or 11th nerve may accompany glomus jugulare tumors that extend through the jugular foramen.

Excision is the treatment of choice, and radiation is used for nonsurgical candidates.

Benign otic tumors: Sebaceous cysts, osteomas, and keloids may arise in and occlude the ear canal, causing retention of cerumen and conductive hearing loss. Excision is the treatment of choice for all benign otic tumors.

Ceruminomas occur in the outer third of the ear canal. These tumors appear benign histologically and do not metastasize regionally or distantly but they are locally invasive and potentially destructive and should be excised widely.

SALIVARY GLAND TUMORS

Most salivary gland tumors are benign and occur in the parotid glands. A painless salivary mass is the most common sign and is evaluated by fine-needle aspiration biopsy. Imaging with CT and MRI can be helpful. For malignant tumors, treatment is with excision and radiation. Long-term results are related to the grade of the cancer.

About 85% of salivary gland tumors occur in the parotid glands, followed by the submandibular and minor salivary glands, and about 1% occur in the sublingual glands. About 75 to 80% are benign, slow-growing, movable, painless, usually solitary nodules beneath normal skin or mucosa. Occasionally, when cystic, they are soft but most often they are firm.

Benign tumors: The most common type is a pleomorphic adenoma (mixed tumor). Malignant transformation is possible, resulting in carcinoma ex pleomorphic adenoma, but this usually occurs only after the benign tumor has been present for 15 to 20 yr. If malignant transformation occurs, the cure rates are very low, despite adequate surgery and adjuvant therapy.

Other benign tumors include monomorphic adenoma, oncocytoma, and papillary cystadenoma lymphomatosum (previously known as cylindroma). These tumors rarely recur and rarely become malignant.

Malignant salivary gland tumors: Malignant tumors are less common and can be characterized by rapid growth or a sudden growth spurt. They are firm, nodular, and can be fixed to adjacent tissue, often with a poorly defined periphery. Eventually, the overlying skin or mucosa may become ulcerated or the adjacent tissues may become invaded.

Mucoepidermoid carcinoma is the most common salivary gland cancer, typically occurring in people in their 20s to 50s. It can manifest in any salivary gland, most commonly in the parotid gland but also in the submandibular gland or a minor salivary gland of the palate. Intermediate and high-grade mucoepidermoid carcinomas may metastasize to the regional lymphatics.

Adenoid cystic carcinoma is the most common malignant tumor of minor salivary glands (and of the trachea). It is a slowly growing malignant transformation of a much more common benign cylindroma. Its peak incidence is between ages 40 and

60, and symptoms include severe pain and, often, facial nerve paralysis. It has a propensity for perineural invasion and spread, with disease potentially extending many centimeters from the main tumor mass. Lymphatic spread is not a common feature of this tumor. Pulmonary metastases are common, although patients can live quite long with them.

Acinic cell carcinoma, a common parotid tumor, occurs in people in their 40s and 50s. This carcinoma has a more indolent course, as well as an incidence of multifocality.

Carcinoma ex mixed tumor is adenocarcinoma arising in a preexisting benign mixed tumor. Only the carcinomatous element metastasizes.

Symptoms and Signs

Most benign and malignant tumors manifest as a painless mass. However, malignant tumors may invade nerves, causing localized or regional pain, numbness, paresthesia, causalgia, or a loss of motor function.

Diagnosis

- Fine-needle aspiration biopsy
- CT and MRI for extent of disease

CT and MRI locate the tumor and describe its extent. Fine-needle aspiration biopsy of the mass confirms the cell type. A search for spread to regional nodes or distant metastases in the lung, liver, bone, or brain may be indicated before treatment is selected.

Treatment

- Surgery, sometimes plus radiation therapy

Treatment of benign tumors is surgery. The recurrence rate is high when excision is incomplete.

For malignant salivary gland tumors, surgery, sometimes followed by radiation therapy, is the treatment of choice for resectable disease. Currently, there is no effective chemotherapy for salivary cancer.

Treatment of mucoepidermoid carcinoma consists of wide excision and postoperative radiation for high-grade lesions. The 5-yr survival rate is 95% with the low-grade type, primarily affecting mucus cells, and 50% with the high-grade type, primarily affecting epidermoid cells. Metastases to the regional lymphatics must be addressed with surgical resection and postoperative radiation therapy.

Treatment of adenoid cystic carcinoma is wide surgical excision, but local recurrence is common due to the propensity for perineural spread. Elective nodal treatment is less likely to be required because lymphatic spread is less common. Although the 5- and 10-yr survival rates are quite good, the 15- and 20-yr rates are worse with many patients developing distant metastases. Lung metastases and death are common, although many years (usually a decade or more), after the initial diagnosis and treatment.

The prognosis for acinic cell carcinoma is favorable after wide excision.

All surgeries are designed to spare the facial nerve, which is sacrificed only in cases of direct tumor involvement with the nerve.

KEY POINTS

- Only about 20 to 25% of salivary gland tumors are malignant; the parotid gland is most commonly affected.
- Cancers are firm, nodular, and can be fixed to adjacent tissue; pain and nerve involvement (causing numbness and/or weakness) are common.
- Do biopsy and CT and MRI if cancer is confirmed.
- Treat using surgery, sometimes plus radiation therapy for certain cancers.

PARANASAL SINUS CANCER

(Sinus Cancer)

Paranasal sinus (PNS) cancer is rare. It usually is squamous cell carcinoma but can also be adenocarcinoma, and it occurs most often in the maxillary and ethmoid sinuses. In most cases its cause is not known, symptoms develop late, and survival is generally poor.

Although rare in the US, PNS cancer is more common in Japan and among the Bantu people of South Africa. Men over 40 yr are affected most often.

The cause is uncertain, but chronic sinusitis is not believed to be a cause. Human papillomavirus (HPV) and Epstein-Barr virus (EBV) may play a role in some cases. Risk factors include

- Regular inhalation of certain types of wood, leather, and metal dust
- Smoking tobacco

Symptoms and Signs

Because the sinuses provide room for the cancer to grow, symptoms usually do not develop until the cancer is well advanced. Pain, nasal obstruction and discharge, epistaxis, diplopia, ear pain or fullness, facial paresthesias, and loose maxillary teeth below the affected sinus result from local pressure of the cancer on adjacent structures. Tumor is sometimes visible in the oral or nasal cavities.

Diagnosis

- Endoscopy, with biopsy
- CT and MRI

Endoscopy, CT, and MRI are most often used to locate and help stage the tumor. Biopsy confirms the cell type. Staging, which includes assessing tumor spread to the brain, face, neck, lungs, and lymph nodes, helps determine treatment.

Prognosis

The earlier the cancer is treated, the better the prognosis. Prognosis also depends on histology. Survival is improving but remains generally poor. Overall, about 40% of people will have recurrent disease, and 5-yr survival is about 60%.

Treatment

- Surgery
- Often radiation
- Sometimes chemotherapy

Treatment for most early-stage cancers is complete surgical excision. Recent advances in surgical techniques, particularly endoscopic techniques, can sometimes achieve complete tumor excisions, spare surrounding tissues, and achieve reconstruction. If risk of recurrence is high, radiation therapy is given post operatively. If surgical excision is not realistic or would cause excessive morbidity, radiotherapy plus chemotherapy may be used.In some cases, chemotherapy is given to shrink the tumor; if the tumor responds well to the chemotherapy, it is resected surgically. If not, the tumor can be treated with radiation.

SECTION 9

Dental Disorders

101 Approach to the Dental Patient

A physician should always examine the mouth and be able to recognize major oral disorders, particularly possible cancers. However, consultation with a dentist is needed to evaluate patients with nonmalignant changes as well as tooth problems. Likewise, patients with xerostomia or unexplained swelling or pain in the mouth, face, or neck require a dental consultation.

Children with abnormal facies (who also may have dental malformations requiring correction) should be evaluated by a dentist.

In FUO or a systemic infection of unknown cause, a dental disorder should be considered.

A dental consultation is necessary before head and neck radiation therapy and is advisable before chemotherapy.

Common dental disorders (see p. 876), dental emergencies (see p. 879), and other dental and oral symptoms (see p. 864), including toothache, are discussed elsewhere in The Manual. This chapter focuses on

- Systemic disease that manifests in the mouth
- Dental anatomy
- Evaluation of the dental patient
- Geriatric changes that affect oral health

Geriatrics Essentials

Resting salivary secretion rarely diminishes significantly solely due to aging. Xerostomia or hyposalivation in the elderly is almost always a side effect of drugs, although meal-stimulated salivary flow is usually adequate.

The flattened cusps of worn teeth and weakness of the masticatory muscles may make chewing tiresome, impairing food intake.

Loss of bone mass in the jaws (particularly the alveolar portion), dryness of the mouth, thinning of the oral mucosa, and impaired coordination of lip, cheek, and tongue movements may make denture retention difficult.

The taste buds become less sensitive, so the elderly may add abundant seasonings, particularly salt (which is harmful for some), or they may desire very hot foods for more taste, sometimes burning the often atrophic oral mucosa.

Gingival recession and xerostomia contribute to development of root caries.

Despite these changes, improved dental hygiene has greatly decreased the prevalence of tooth loss, and most older people can expect to retain their teeth.

Poor oral health contributes to poor nutritional intake, which impairs general health. Dental disease (particularly periodontitis) is associated with a 2-fold increased risk of coronary artery disease. Edentulous patients cannot have periodontitis because they do not have a periodontium, although periodontitis may have resulted in their tooth loss. Aspiration pneumonia in patients with periodontitis can involve anaerobic organisms and has a high mortality rate. Severe bacteremias secondary to acute or chronic dental infection may contribute to brain abscesses, cavernous sinus thrombosis, endocarditis, prosthetic joint infections, and unexplained fevers.

SYSTEMIC DISORDERS AND THE MOUTH

Clues suggesting systemic disease may be found in the mouth and adjacent structures (see Table 101–1). A dentist should

Table 101–1. ORAL FINDINGS IN SYSTEMIC DISORDERS

ORAL MANIFESTATION	ASSOCIATED DISORDERS
Thrush (oral candidiasis)	Diabetes (see p. 1253), AIDS (see p. 1628), other causes of immunosuppression (eg, agranulocytosis, neutropenia, leukemia, immunoglobulin defects, disorders of leukocyte function), antibiotic use
Atrophic glossitis (a smooth tongue caused by atrophy of filiform papillae)	Iron deficiency
Painful atrophy of the oral mucosa and surface of the tongue, sometimes with aphthous ulcers	Megaloblastic anemias
Magenta tongue	Vitamin B_{12} deficiency
Darkly pigmented areas (if not a racial characteristic)	Hemochromatosis, Addison disease, Peutz-Jeghers syndrome, melanoma (rare, but may be seen on the palate), smoker's melanosis
Linear, grayish discoloration (lead line) in the gingiva adjacent to teeth	Lead, silver, or bismuth poisoning
Violaceous patches	Kaposi sarcoma, AIDS
Keratotic lichenoid patches, sometimes with painful mucosal atrophy	Graft-vs-host disease if in the mouth of an organ transplant recipient
Reddish discoloration of the teeth	Congenital erythropoietic porphyria
High, arched soft palate	Marfan syndrome
Notched incisors, domed or mulberry molars	Congenital syphilis
Hairy leukoplakia (white, vertical folds on lateral border of tongue)	HIV transforming to AIDS
Red or reddish purple collections of oral telangiectases	Hereditary hemorrhagic telangiectasia (Osler-Weber-Rendu syndrome)
Multiple impacted supernumerary teeth and osteomas	Gardner syndrome
Granulomatous gingivitis with cobblestone appearance	Crohn disease

consult a physician when a systemic disorder is suspected, when the patient is taking certain drugs (eg, warfarin, bisphosphonates), and when a patient's ability to withstand general anesthesia or extensive oral surgery must be evaluated.

Patients with certain heart valve abnormalities may require antibiotic prophylaxis to help prevent bacterial endocarditis before undergoing certain dental procedures (see Tables 82–3 and 82–4 on p. 711).

Dental Care of Patients with Systemic Disorders

Certain medical conditions (and their treatment) predispose patients to dental problems or affect dental care.

Hematologic disorders: People who have disorders that interfere with coagulation (eg, hemophilia, acute leukemia, thrombocytopenia) require medical consultation before undergoing dental procedures that might cause bleeding (eg, extraction, mandibular block, tooth cleaning). Patients with hemophilia should have clotting factors given before, during, and after an extraction and restorative dentistry requiring local anesthesia (eg, fillings). Most hematologists prefer that patients with hemophilia, especially those who have developed factor inhibitors, receive infiltrative local anesthetics instead of blocks for restorative dentistry.

Restorative dentistry can be completed in a dental office after consultation with a hematologist; however, if the patient has inhibitor to factor VIII, the dentistry should be done in a hospital under general anesthesia. Oral surgery should be done in the hospital in consultation with a hematologist. All patients with bleeding disorders should maintain a lifelong routine of regular dental visits, which includes cleanings, fillings, topical fluoride, and preventative sealants, to avoid the need for extractions.

Cardiovascular disorders: After an MI, dental procedures should be avoided for 6 mo, if possible, to allow damaged myocardium to become less electrically labile. Patients with pulmonary or cardiac disease who require inhalation anesthesia for dental procedures should be hospitalized.

Endocarditis prophylaxis is required before dental procedures only in patients with

- Prosthetic cardiac valves or prosthetic material used for cardiac valve repair
- Previous history of bacterial endocarditis
- Unrepaired cyanotic congenital heart disease, including palliative shunts and conduits; completely repaired congenital heart defect with prosthetic material or device for 6 mo after the procedure; repaired congenital heart disease with residual defects at the site or adjacent to the site of a prosthetic patch or prosthetic device
- Completely repaired congenital heart defect with prosthetic material or device (for 6 mo after the procedure)
- Repaired congenital heart disease with residual defects at the site or adjacent to the site of a prosthetic patch or prosthetic device
- Cardiac transplantation recipients with a valvulopathy

The heart is better protected against low-grade bacteremias, which occur in chronic dental conditions, when dental treatment is received (with prophylaxis) than when it is not received. Patients who are to undergo cardiac valve surgery or repair of congenital heart defects should have any necessary dental treatment completed before surgery.

Although probably of marginal benefit, antibiotic prophylaxis is sometimes recommended for patients with hemodialysis shunts and within 2 yr of receipt of a major prosthetic joint (hip, knee, shoulder, elbow). The organisms causing infections at these sites are almost invariably of dermal rather than oral origin.

Adrenergic drugs such as epinephrine and levonordefrin are added to local anesthetics to increase the duration of anesthesia. In some cardiovascular patients, excess amounts of these drugs cause arrhythmias, myocardial ischemia, or hypertension. Plain anesthetic can be used for procedures requiring < 45 min, but in longer procedures or where hemostasis is needed, up to 0.04 mg epinephrine (2 dental cartridges with 1:100,000 epinephrine) is considered safe. Generally, no healthy patient should receive > 0.2 mg epinephrine at any one appointment. Absolute contraindications to epinephrine (any dose) are uncontrolled hyperthyroidism; pheochromocytoma; BP > 200 mm Hg systolic or > 115 mm Hg diastolic; uncontrolled arrhythmias despite drug therapy; and unstable angina, MI, or stroke within 6 mo.

Some electrical dental equipment, such as an electrosurgical cautery, a pulp tester, or an ultrasonic scaler, can interfere with early-generation pacemakers.

Cancer: Extracting a tooth adjacent to a carcinoma of the gingiva, palate, or antrum facilitates invasion of the alveolus (tooth socket) by the tumor. Therefore, a tooth should be extracted only during the course of definitive treatment. In patients with leukemia or agranulocytosis, infection may follow an extraction despite the use of antibiotics.

Immunosuppression: People with impaired immunity are prone to severe mucosal and periodontal infections by fungi, herpes and other viruses, and, less commonly, bacteria. The infections may cause hemorrhage, delayed healing, or sepsis. Dysplastic or neoplastic oral lesions may develop after a few years of immunosuppression. People with AIDS may develop Kaposi sarcoma, non-Hodgkin lymphoma, hairy leukoplakia, candidiasis, aphthous ulcers, or a rapidly progressive form of periodontal disease, HIV-associated periodontitis.

Endocrine disorders: Dental treatment may be complicated by some endocrine disorders. For example, people with hyperthyroidism may develop tachycardia and excessive anxiety as well as thyroid storm if given epinephrine. Insulin requirements may be reduced on elimination of oral infection in diabetics; insulin dose may require reduction when food intake is limited because of pain after oral surgery. In people with diabetes, hyperglycemia with resultant polyuria may lead to dehydration, resulting in decreased salivary flow (xerostomia), which, along with elevated salivary glucose levels, contributes to caries.

Patients receiving corticosteroids and those with adrenocortical insufficiency may require supplemental corticosteroids during major dental procedures. Patients with Cushing syndrome or who are taking corticosteroids may have alveolar bone loss, delayed wound healing, and increased capillary fragility.

Neurologic disorders: Patients with seizures who require dental appliances should have nonremovable appliances that cannot be swallowed or aspirated. Patients unable to brush or floss effectively may use 0.12% chlorhexidine rinses in the morning and at bedtime. In many countries outside the US chlorhexidine is available at 0.2%. However, this higher strength has not been shown to be for effective for gingival health and may cause increased tooth staining.

Obstructive sleep apnea: Patients with obstructive sleep apnea who are unable to tolerate treatment with a continuous positive airway pressure (CPAP) or bilevel PAP (BiPAP) mask are sometimes treated with an intraoral device that expands the oropharynx. This treatment is not as effective as CPAP, but more patients tolerate using it.

Drugs: Certain drugs, such as corticosteroids, immunosuppressants, and antineoplastics, compromise healing and host defenses. When possible, dental procedures should not be done while these drugs are being given.

Many drugs cause dry mouth (xerostomia), which is a significant health issue, especially in geriatric patients. Causative drugs often have anticholinergic effects and include certain antidepressants, antipsychotics, diuretics, antihypertensives, anxiolytic and sedative drugs, NSAIDs, antihistamines, and opioid analgesics.

Some antineoplastics (eg, doxorubicin, 5-fluorouracil, bleomycin, dactinomycin, cytosine, arabinoside, methotrexate) cause stomatitis, which is worse in patients with preexisting periodontal disease. Before such drugs are prescribed, oral prophylaxis should be completed, and patients should be instructed in proper toothbrushing and flossing.

Drugs that interfere with clotting may need to be reduced or stopped before oral surgery. Patients taking aspirin, NSAIDs, or clopidogrel should stop taking them 4 days before undergoing dental surgery and can resume taking these drugs after bleeding stops. Most patients taking an oral anticoagulant who have a stable INR < 4 do not need to stop the drug before outpatient dental surgery (including extraction) because the risk of significant bleeding is very small and the risk of thrombosis may be increased when oral anticoagulants are temporarily stopped. For people receiving hemodialysis, dental procedures should be done the day after dialysis, when heparinization has subsided.

Phenytoin, cyclosporine, and calcium channel blockers, particularly nifedipine, contribute to gingival hyperplasia. Gingival hyperplasia develops in about 50% of patients taking phenytoin and 25% of patients taking cyclosporine or a calcium channel blocker. However, hyperplasia is minimized with excellent oral hygiene and frequent cleanings by a dentist.

Bisphosphonates can result in antiresorptive agent-induced osteonecrosis of the jaw (ONJ—see p. 323) after an extraction. ONJ occurs primarily when bisphosphonates are given parenterally to treat bone cancer and to a much lesser extent when they are taken orally to prevent osteoporosis (risk of ONJ about 0.1%). Diligent oral hygiene practices and regular dental care may help lower the risk of ONJ, but there are no validated techniques to determine who is at risk of developing antiresorptive agent–induced ONJ. Stopping bisphosphonate therapy may not lower the risk and may increase the rate of bone loss in people being treated for osteoporosis.

Radiation therapy: (CAUTION: *Extraction of teeth from irradiated tissues [particularly if the total dose was > 65 Gy, especially in the mandible] is commonly followed by osteoradionecrosis of the jaw. This is a catastrophic complication in which extraction sites break down, frequently sloughing bone and soft tissue.*) Thus, if possible, patients should have any necessary dental treatment completed before undergoing radiation therapy of the head and neck region, with time allowed for healing. Teeth that may not survive should be extracted. Necessary sealants and topical fluoride should be applied. After radiation, extraction should be avoided, if possible, by using dental restorations and root canal treatment instead.

Head and neck radiation often damages salivary glands, causing permanent xerostomia, which promotes caries. Patients must therefore practice lifelong good oral hygiene. A fluoride gel and fluoride mouth rinse should be used daily. Rinsing with 0.12% chlorhexidine for 30 to 60 sec, if tolerated, can be done in the morning and at bedtime. Viscous lidocaine may enable a patient with sensitive oral tissues to brush and floss the teeth and eat.

A dentist must be seen at 3-, 4-, or 6-mo intervals, depending on findings at the last examination. Irradiated tissue under dentures is likely to break down, so dentures should be checked and adjusted whenever discomfort is noted. Early caries may also be reversed by calcium phosphopeptides and amorphous calcium phosphate, which can be applied by a dentist or prescribed to a patient for at-home use.

Patients who undergo radiation therapy may develop oral mucosal inflammation and diminished taste as well as trismus due to fibrosis of the masticatory muscles. Trismus may be minimized by such exercises as opening and closing the mouth widely 20 times 3 or 4 times/day. Extractions of teeth in irradiated bone should be avoided (because of possible osteoradionecrosis). Sometimes root canal therapy is done, and the tooth is ground down to the gum line in order to prevent bone atrophy. If extraction is required after radiation, 10 to 20 treatments in a hyperbaric O_2 chamber may forestall or prevent osteoradionecrosis.

DENTAL ANATOMY AND DEVELOPMENT

Teeth

The teeth are categorized as incisors, canines, premolars, and molars and conventionally are numbered beginning with the maxillary right 3rd molar (see Fig. 101–1).

Each tooth has a crown and a root. The canines have the largest and strongest roots. An inner pulp contains blood vessels, lymphatics, and nerves, surrounded by the hard but porous dentin, a very hard enamel coating that covers the crown; it is sensitive to touch and to temperature changes. The bonelike cementum is over the root, which, when healthy, is covered by gingiva (see Fig. 101–2).

Twenty deciduous teeth normally begin appearing at close to age 6 mo and should all be in place by age 30 mo (see Fig. 101–1). These teeth are followed by 32 permanent teeth that begin to appear by about age 6. The period from age 6 to 11 is called the mixed dentition stage, in which both deciduous and permanent teeth are present. Timing of tooth eruption is one indicator of skeletal age and may identify growth retardation or establish age for forensic purposes.

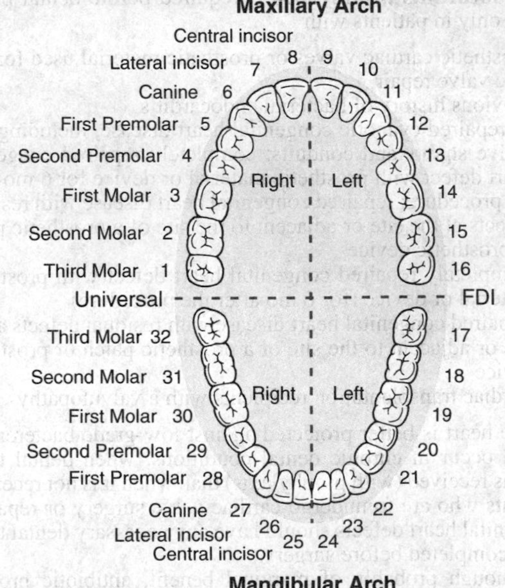

Fig. 101–1. Identifying the teeth. The numbering system shown is the one most commonly used in the US.

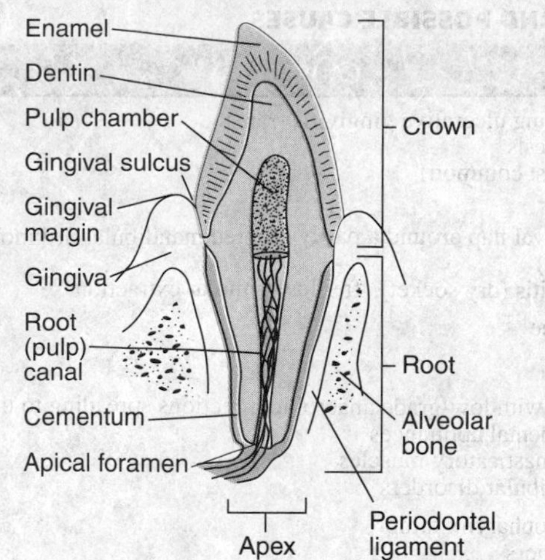

Fig. 101–2. Section of a canine tooth.

Supporting Tissues

The gingiva surrounds the teeth at the base of their crown. The alveolar ridges are trabecular bone containing sockets for the teeth. The periodontium consists of the tissues that support the teeth—the gingiva, epithelial attachment, connective tissue attachment, periodontal ligament, and alveolar bone. The mandible and maxilla support the alveolar ridges and house the teeth. Saliva from the salivary glands bathes and protects the teeth. The tongue directs food between the grinding surfaces and helps clean the teeth. The maxilla receives innervation from the maxillary nerve, the 2nd division of the trigeminal nerve (the 5th cranial nerve). The mandibular nerve, which is the 3rd and most inferior division of the trigeminal nerve, innervates the mandible.

In the elderly, or in some periodontal diseases, gingival recession exposes the dental root adjacent to the crown, making root caries common. If tooth destruction results and the tooth must be removed, the mechanical stimulation necessary for maintaining bone integrity ceases. Consequently, atrophy of the alveolar ridge (senile atrophy) begins when teeth are absent.

Mouth

Normally, keratinized epithelium occurs on the facial aspect of the lips, dorsum of the tongue, hard palate, and gingiva around the teeth. When healthy, the keratinized gingiva extends 5 to 7 mm from the crown of the tooth. Nonkeratinized mucosa occurs over alveolar bone further from the teeth, inside the lips and cheeks, on the sides and undersurface of the tongue, on the soft palate, and covering the floor of the mouth. The skin and mucosa of the lips are demarcated by the vermilion border.

The **buccal mucosa,** including the vestibule and nonkeratinized alveolar mucosa, is usually smooth, moist, and more red than pink (as compared to healthy gingiva). Innocuous entities in this region include linea alba (a thin white line, typically bilateral, on the level of the occlusal plane, where the cheek is bitten), Fordyce granules (aberrant sebaceous glands appearing as < 1 mm light yellow spots that also may occur on the lips), and white sponge nevus (bilateral thick white folds over most of the buccal mucosa). Occasionally, pigmentation of the mucosa may arise from foreign material that is incorporated into the tissue. Most commonly, this occurs as a blue or black area adjacent to a dental amalgam filling. This is known as an amalgam tattoo. The orifices of the parotid (Stensen) ducts are opposite the maxillary 1st molar on the inside of each cheek and should not be mistaken for an abnormality. Recognizing these avoids needless biopsy and apprehension.

The **dorsal surface of the tongue** is covered with numerous whitish elevations called the filiform papillae. Interspersed among them are isolated reddish prominences called the fungiform papillae, occurring mostly on the anterior part of the tongue. The circumvallate papillae, numbering 8 to 12, are considerably larger and lie posteriorly in a V pattern. The circumvallate papillae do not project from the tongue but instead are surrounded by a trench. The foliate papillae appear as a series of parallel, slitlike folds on the lateral borders of the tongue, near the anterior pillars of the fauces. They vary in length and can easily be confused with malignant lesions, as may the foramen cecum, median rhomboid glossitis, and, rarely, a lingual thyroid nodule. Lingual tonsils are components of the Waldeyer ring, are at the back of the tongue, and should not be mistaken for lesions. If an apparent abnormality is bilateral, it is almost always a normal variant.

Innervation is supplied by the lingual nerves (branches of the 5th cranial nerves), for general sensory innervation, and the chorda tympani fibers (of the 7th cranial nerves), which innervate the taste buds of the anterior two thirds of the tongue. Behind the circumvallate papillae, the glossopharyngeal nerves (9th cranial nerves) provide the sensations of touch and taste. The tongue has taste receptors for sweet, salty, sour, bitter, and umami (a savory taste triggered by natural glutamic acid and glutamates such as the flavoring agent monosodium glutamate). Although previously thought to be isolated to particular portions of the tongue, taste receptors are now known to be distributed over the surface of the tongue. The hypoglossal nerves (12th cranial nerves) control movement of the tongue.

The **major salivary glands** are the paired parotid, submandibular, and sublingual glands. Most oral mucosal surfaces contain many minor mucus-secreting salivary glands. Anteriorly and near the midline on each side of the floor of the mouth are the openings of the Wharton ducts, which drain the ipsilateral submandibular and sublingual glands. The parotid glands drain into the cheeks via the Stensen ducts.

EVALUATION OF THE DENTAL PATIENT

The first routine dental examination should take place by age 1 yr or when the first tooth erupts. Subsequent evaluations should take place at 6-mo intervals or whenever symptoms develop. Examination of the mouth is part of every general physical examination. Oral findings in many systemic diseases are unique, sometimes pathognomonic, and may be the first sign of disease. Oral cancer may be detected at an early stage.

History

Important dental symptoms include bleeding, pain, malocclusion, new growths, numbness or paresthesias, and chewing problems (see Table 101–2); prolonged dental symptoms may decrease oral intake, leading to weight loss. General information includes use of alcohol or tobacco (both major risk factors for head and neck cancer) and systemic symptoms, such as fever and weight loss.

Physical Examination

A thorough inspection requires good illumination, a tongue blade, gloves, and a gauze pad. Complete or partial dentures are removed so that underlying soft tissues can be seen.

Table 101–2. SOME ORAL SYMPTOMS AND POSSIBLE CAUSES

SYMPTOM	CAUSES
Bleeding or pain with brushing (common)	Acute necrotizing ulcerative gingivitis (rare) Bleeding diathesis* Gingivitis (most common) Leukemia*
Ear pain, referred (fairly common)	Inflamed gingival flap around a partly erupted mandibular 3rd molar (pericoronitis) Localized osteitis (dry socket) after lower molar extraction
Face, head, or neck pain (uncommon, except with poorly fitting dental appliances or temporomandibular disorders)	Eagle syndrome† Infection Malocclusion Occult lesions with low-grade anaerobic infections spreading to the bone Poorly fitting dental appliances Spasm of the masticatory muscles Temporomandibular disorders
Facial numbness or paresthesias (uncommon, except with stroke)	Antrum or nasopharynx tumor Brain stem tumors Extraction of a mandibular molar causing damage to the inferior alveolar nerve‡ Multiple sclerosis Oral tumor (rare) Stroke Viral infection (facial nerve palsy)
Masticatory fatigue (rare, except with poorly fitting dentures)	Congenital muscular or neuromuscular disorder (in younger people) Myasthenia gravis (a cardinal symptom) Poorly occluding artificial dentures (in older people)
Masticatory pain or jaw claudication (rare)	Giant cell arteritis Polymyalgia rheumatica
Weight loss (fairly common)	Poorly fitting dental appliances Stomatitis Temporomandibular disorder Too loose, too few, or painful teeth

*May first manifest as easily induced gingival hemorrhaging.
†Elongation of the styloid process or ossification of the stylohyoid ligament, causing pain when the head is turned.
‡May cause paresthesia of the lower lip.

Most physicians use a head-mounted light. However, because the light cannot be precisely aligned on the axis of vision, it is difficult to avoid shadowing in narrow areas. Better illumination results with a head-mounted convex mirror; the physician looks through a hole in the center of the mirror, so the illumination is always on-axis. The head mirror reflects light from a source (any incandescent light) placed behind the patient and slightly to one side and requires practice to use effectively.

The face: The examiner initially looks at the face for asymmetry, masses, and skin lesions. Slight facial asymmetry is universal, but more marked asymmetry may indicate an underlying disorder, either congenital or acquired (see Table 101–3).

The teeth: Teeth are inspected for shape, alignment, defects, mobility, color, and presence of adherent plaque, materia alba (dead bacteria, food debris, desquamated epithelial cells), and calculus (tartar).

Teeth are gently tapped with a tongue depressor or mirror handle to assess tenderness (percussion sensitivity). Tenderness to percussion suggests deep caries that has caused a necrotic pulp with periapical abscess or severe periodontal disease. Percussion sensitivity or pain on biting also can indicate an incomplete (green stick) fracture of a tooth. Percussion tenderness in multiple adjacent maxillary teeth may result from maxillary sinusitis. Tenderness to palpation around the apices of the teeth also may indicate an abscess.

Loose teeth usually indicate severe periodontal disease but can be caused by bruxism (clenching or grinding of teeth) or trauma that damages periodontal tissues. Rarely, teeth become loose when alveolar bone is eroded by an underlying mass (eg, ameloblastoma, eosinophilic granuloma). A tumor or systemic cause of alveolar bone loss (eg, diabetes mellitus, hyperparathyroidism, osteoporosis, Cushing syndrome) is suspected when teeth are loose and heavy plaque and calculus are absent.

Calculus is mineralized bacterial plaque—a concretion of bacteria, food residue, saliva, and mucus with calcium and phosphate salts. After a tooth is cleaned, a mucopolysaccharide coating (pellicle) is deposited almost immediately. After about 24 h, bacterial colonization turns the pellicle into plaque. After about 72 h, the plaque starts calcifying, becoming calculus. When present, calculus is deposited most heavily on the lingual (inner, or tongue) surfaces of the mandibular anterior teeth near the submandibular and sublingual duct orifices (Wharton ducts) and on the buccal (cheek) surfaces of the maxillary molars near the parotid duct orifices (Stensen ducts).

Caries (tooth decay) first appears as defects in the tooth enamel. Caries then appears as white spots, later becoming brown.

Attrition (wearing of biting surfaces) can result from chewing abrasive foods or tobacco, from gastric acid exposure due to severe gastroesophageal reflux, or from the wear that accompanies aging, but it usually indicates bruxism. Another common

Table 101–3. SOME DISORDERS OF THE ORAL REGION BY PREDOMINANT SITE OF INVOLVEMENT

SITE	DISORDER OR LESION	DESCRIPTION
Lips	Actinic atrophy	Thin atrophic mucosa with erosive areas; predisposes to neoplasia
	Angioedema	Acute swelling
	Angular cheilitis (cheilosis)	Fissuring at corners of mouth, often with maceration
	Cheilitis glandularis	Enlarged, nodular labial glands with inflamed, dilated secretory ducts; sometimes everted, hypertrophic lips
	Cheilitis granulomatosa	Diffusely swollen lips, primarily the lower
	Erythema multiforme	Multiple bullae that rupture quickly, leaving hemorrhagic ulcers; includes Stevens-Johnson syndrome
	Exfoliative cheilitis	Chronic desquamation of superficial mucosal cells
	Keratoacanthoma	A locally destructive epithelial tumor thought to be a form of squamous cell carcinoma that usually regresses spontaneously
	Peutz-Jeghers syndrome	Brownish black melanin spots, with GI polyposis
	Secondary herpes simplex (cold sore)	Short-lived vesicle (≤1 day) followed by small painful ulcer (≤ 10 days) at the vermillion border (common)
	Verruca vulgaris (wart)	Pebbly surface
Buccal mucosa	Aspirin burn	Painful white area; when wiped off, exposes an inflamed area
	Fordyce granules	Cream-colored macules about 1 mm in diameter; benign; aberrant sebaceous glands
	Hand-foot-and-mouth disease	Small ulcerated vesicles; coxsackievirus strain infection in young children; mild
	Herpangina	Vesicles in posterior of mouth
	Irritation fibroma	Smooth-surfaced, dome-shaped, sessile
	Koplik spots	Tiny, grayish white macules with red margins near orifice of parotid duct; measles precursor
	Linea alba	Thin white line, typically bilateral, on the level of the occlusal plane; benign
	Smokeless tobacco lesion	White or gray corrugated; usually behind lower lip; tends toward cancer
	Verrucous carcinoma	Slow-growing, exophytic, usually well differentiated; at site of snuff application; metastasis unusual, occurs late
	White sponge nevus	Thick white folds over most of buccal mucosa except gingivae; benign
Palate	Granulomatosis with polyangiitis (formerly Wegener granulomatosis)	Lethal midline granuloma, with bone destruction, sequestration, and perforation
	Infectious mononucleosis	Petechiae at junction of hard and soft palate
	Kaposi sarcoma	Red to purple painless macules progressing to painful papules
	Necrotizing sialometaplasia	Large, rapidly developing ulcer, often painless; appears grossly malignant; heals spontaneously in 1–3 mo
	Papillary inflammatory hyperplasia	Red, spongy tissue, succeeded by fibrous tissue folds; velvety texture; benign; occurs under poorly fitting dentures
	Pipe smoker's palate (nicotine stomatitis)	Red punctate areas are ducts of minor salivary glands, appearance is red spots surrounded by leukoplakia (often severe, usually benign)
	Secondary herpes simplex	Small papules quickly coalescing into series of ulcers (uncommon)
	Torus palatinus	Overgrowth of bone in midline; benign
Tongue and floor of mouth	Ankyloglossia	Tongue unable to protrude; speech difficulty Pulling away of the gingiva by the lingual frenulum
	Benign lymphoepithelial cyst	Yellowish nodule on ventral part of tongue or anterior floor of mouth
	Benign migratory glossitis (geographic tongue, erythema migrans)	Changing patterns of hyperkeratosis and erythema on dorsum and edges; desquamated filiform papillae in irregular circinate pattern, often with an inflamed center and a white or yellow border
	Dermoid cyst	Swelling in floor of mouth

Table continues on the following page.

Table 101–3. SOME DISORDERS OF THE ORAL REGION BY PREDOMINANT SITE OF INVOLVEMENT (*Continued*)

SITE	DISORDER OR LESION	DESCRIPTION
	Enlargement of tongue (macroglossia)	Localized or generalized depending on how many teeth are missing; adjacent teeth may indent tongue; posterior enlargement associated with obstructive sleep apnea and snoring
	Fissured (scrotal) tongue	Deep furrows in lateral and dorsal areas
	Glossitis	Red, painful tongue; often secondary to another condition, allergic, or idiopathic
	Hairy tongue	Dark, elongated filiform papillae
	Linea alba	Thin white line on edges of tongue, usually bilateral
	Lingual thyroid nodule	Smooth-surfaced nodular mass of thyroid tissue follicles, on the far posterior dorsum of tongue, usually at the midline
	Ludwig angina	Painful, tender swelling under the tongue resulting from odontogenic infection; can compromise the airway by forcing the tongue superiorly and posteriorly
	Median rhomboid glossitis	Red (usually) patch in midline of tongue, without papillae; asymptomatic
	Neurilemoma	Persistent swelling, sometimes at site of prior trauma; can be painful
	Pernicious anemia	Smooth, pale tongue, often with glossodynia or glossopyrosis
	Ranula	Large mucocele penetrating the mylohyoid muscle; may plunge deep into the neck; swollen floor of mouth
	Thyroglossal duct cyst	Midline swelling that moves upward when tongue protrudes
	TB	Ulcers on dorsum (firm), cervical adenopathy
Salivary glands	Benign lymphoepithelial lesion (Mikulicz disease)	Unilateral or bilateral enlargement of salivary glands; often with dry mouth and eyes
	Sialadenitis	Swelling, often painful; benign
	Sialolithiasis	Swelling (eg, of floor of mouth) that increases at mealtime or when offered a pickle
	Sjögren syndrome	Systemic disease causing dry mucous membranes
	Xerostomia	Dry mouth; usually secondary to drugs
Various	Acute herpetic gingivostomatitis	Widespread ulcerating vesicular lesions; always present on gingiva; other locations may be involved; usually in young children
	Behçet disease	Multiple oral ulcers similar to those of aphthous stomatitis; also includes dry eyes
	Canker sores, recurrent aphthous stomatitis	Small painful ulcers (canker sores) or large, painful scarring ulcers (recurrent aphthous stomatitis)
	Cicatricial pemphigoid	Bullae that rupture quickly, leaving ulcers; ocular lesions develop after oral lesions; found on alveolar mucosa and vestibules
	Condyloma acuminatum	Venereally transmitted wart forming cauliflower-like clumps
	Dyskeratosis	Occurs with erythroplakia (red), leukoplakia (white patch on mucous membrane that does not rub off), and mixed red and white lesions; precancerous
	Hemangioma	Purple to dark-red lesions, similar to port wine stain; benign
	Hereditary hemorrhagic telangiectasia	Localized dilated blood vessels
	Lichen planus	Lacy pattern (Wickham striae), sometimes erosive; may become malignant; most common on buccal mucosa, lateral tongue
	Lymphangioma	Localized swelling or discoloration; benign; most common on tongue
	Mucocele (mucous retention cyst)	Soft nodule resulting from traumatized salivary gland; if superficial, covered by thin epithelium; appears bluish; most common on lips and floor of mouth
	Noma	Small vesicle or ulcer that rapidly enlarges and becomes necrotic
	Pemphigoid	Small yellow or hemorrhagic tense bullae; may last several days before rupture; most common on vestibules and alveolar mucosa
	Pemphigus	Bullae that rupture quickly, leaving ulcers; can be fatal without treatment
	Syphilis	Chancre (red papule rapidly developing into a painless ulcer with a serosanguineous crust), mucous patch, gumma

cause is abrasion of a porcelain crown occluding against opposing enamel because porcelain is considerably harder than enamel. Attrition makes chewing less effective and causes noncarious teeth to become painful when the eroding enamel exposes the underlying dentin. Dentin is sensitive to touch and to temperature changes.

A dentist can desensitize such teeth or restore the dental anatomy by placing crowns or onlays over badly worn teeth. In minor cases of root sensitivity, the exposed root may be desensitized by fluoride application or dentin-bonding agents.

Deformed teeth may indicate a developmental or endocrine disorder. In Down syndrome, teeth are small, sometimes with agenesis of lateral incisors or premolars and conically shaped mandibular incisors. In congenital syphilis, the incisors may be small at the incisal third, causing a pegged or screwdriver shape with a notch in the center of the incisal edge (Hutchinson incisors), and the 1st molar is small, with a small occlusal surface and roughened, lobulated, often hypoplastic enamel (mulberry molar). In ectodermal dysplasia, teeth are absent or conical, so that dentures are needed from childhood.

Dentinogenesis imperfecta, an autosomal dominant disorder, causes abnormal dentin that is dull bluish brown and opalescent and does not cushion the overlying enamel adequately. Such teeth cannot withstand occlusal stresses and rapidly become worn.

People with pituitary dwarfism or with congenital hypoparathyroidism have small dental roots; people with gigantism have large ones. Acromegaly causes excess cementum in the roots as well as enlargement of the jaws, so teeth may become widely spaced. Acromegaly also can cause an open bite, a condition that occurs when the maxillary and mandibular incisors do not come into contact when the jaws are closed.

Congenitally narrow lateral incisors occur in the absence of systemic disease. The most commonly congenitally absent teeth are the 3rd molars, followed in frequency by the maxillary lateral incisors and 2nd mandibular premolars.

Defects in tooth color must be differentiated from the darkening or yellowing that is caused by food pigments, aging, and, most prominently, smoking. A tooth may appear gray because of pulpal necrosis, usually due to extensive caries penetrating the pulp or because of hemosiderin deposited in the dentin after trauma, with or without pulpal necrosis.

Children's teeth darken appreciably and permanently after even short-term use of tetracyclines by the mother during the 2nd half of pregnancy or by the child during odontogenesis (tooth development), specifically calcification of the crowns, which lasts until age 9. Tetracyclines rarely cause permanent discoloration of fully formed teeth in adults. However, minocycline darkens bone, which can be seen in the mouth when the overlying gingiva and mucosa are thin. Affected teeth fluoresce with distinctive colors under ultraviolet light corresponding to the specific tetracycline taken.

In congenital porphyria, both the deciduous and permanent teeth may have red or brownish discoloration but always fluoresce red from the pigment deposited in the dentin. Congenital hyperbilirubinemia causes a yellowish tooth discoloration.

Teeth can be whitened (see Table 101–4).

Defects in tooth enamel may be caused by rickets, which results in a rough, irregular band in the enamel. Any prolonged febrile illness during odontogenesis can cause a permanent narrow zone of chalky, pitted enamel or simply white discoloration visible after the tooth erupts. Thus, the age at which the disease occurred and its duration can be estimated from the location and height of the band.

Enamel pitting also occurs in tuberous sclerosis and Angelman syndrome. Amelogenesis imperfecta, an autosomal dominant disease, causes severe enamel hypoplasia. Chronic vomiting and esophageal reflux can decalcify the dental crowns, primarily the lingual surfaces of the maxillary anterior teeth.

Chronic snorting of cocaine can result in widespread decalcification of teeth because the drug dissociates in saliva into a base and HCl. Chronic use of methamphetamines markedly increases dental caries ("meth mouth").

Swimmers who spend a lot of time in overchlorinated pools may lose enamel from the outer facial/buccal side of the teeth, especially the maxillary incisors, canines, and 1st premolars. If sodium carbonate has been added to the pool water to correct pH, brown calculus develops but can be removed by a dental cleaning.

Fluorosis is mottled enamel that may develop in children who drink water containing > 1 ppm of fluoride during tooth development. Fluorosis depends on the amount of fluoride ingested and the age of the child during exposure. Enamel changes range from irregular whitish opaque areas to severe brown discoloration of the entire crown with a roughened surface. Such teeth are highly resistant to dental caries.

The mouth and oral cavity: The lips are palpated. With the patient's mouth open, the buccal mucosa and vestibules are

Table 101–4. TOOTH WHITENING PROCEDURES

DONE BY	INGREDIENTS	COMMENTS
Dentist		
In office	Concentrated hydrogen peroxide is applied to teeth, which is exposed to a light or laser	Very effective Gingiva, skin, and eyes must be protected
Patient		
At home	6% carbamide peroxide (becomes 3% hydrogen peroxide when applied) and a thickening agent containing copolymers of acrylic acid cross-linked with a polyalkenyl polyether are added to a custom-made tray	Very effective
Patient (OTC products)		
Commercial whitening strips	Composed of carbamide peroxide	Very effective
Whitening toothpaste	Usually contain carbamide or hydrogen peroxide	Moderately effective
Paint-on whitening	Usually composed of titanium dioxide	Not very effective

examined with a tongue blade; then the hard and soft palates, uvula, and oropharynx are viewed. The patient is asked to extend the tongue as far as possible, exposing the dorsum, and to move the extended tongue as far as possible to each side, so that its posterolateral surfaces can be seen. If a patient does not extend the tongue far enough to expose the circumvallate papillae, the examiner grasps the tip of the tongue with a gauze pad and extends it. Then the tongue is raised to view the ventral surface and the floor of the mouth. The teeth and gingiva are viewed.

An abnormal distribution of keratinized or nonkeratinized oral mucosa demands attention. Keratinized tissue that occurs in normally nonkeratinized areas appears white. This abnormal condition, called leukoplakia, requires a biopsy because it may be cancerous or precancerous. More ominous, however, are thinned areas of mucosa. These red areas, called erythroplakia, if present for at least 2 wk, especially on the ventral tongue and floor of the mouth, suggest dysplasia, carcinoma in situ, or cancer.

With gloved hands, the examiner palpates the vestibules and the floor of the mouth, including the sublingual and submandibular glands. To make palpation more comfortable, the examiner asks the patient to relax the mouth, keeping it open just wide enough to allow access.

The temporomandibular joint: The temporomandibular joint (TMJ) is assessed by looking for jaw deviation on opening and by palpating the head of the condyle anterior to the external auditory meatus. Examiners then place their little fingers into the external ear canals with the pads of the fingertips lightly pushing anteriorly while patients open widely and close 3 times. Patients also should be able to comfortably open wide enough to fit 3 of their fingers vertically between the incisors (typically 4 to 5 cm).

Trismus, the inability to open the mouth, may indicate temporomandibular disease (the most common cause), pericoronitis, systemic sclerosis, arthritis, ankylosis of the TMJ, dislocation of the temporomandibular disk, tetanus, or peritonsillar abscess. Unusually wide opening suggests subluxation or type III Ehlers-Danlos syndrome.

Testing

For a new patient or for someone who requires extensive care, the dentist takes a full mouth x-ray series. This series consists of 14 to 16 periapical films to show the roots and bone plus 4 bite-wing films to detect early caries between posterior teeth. Modern techniques reduce radiation exposure to a near-negligible level.

Patients at high risk of caries (ie, those who have had caries detected during the clinical examination, have many restorations, or have recurrent caries on teeth previously restored) should undergo bite-wing x-rays every 12 mo. Otherwise, bite-wings are indicated every 2 to 3 yr.

A panoramic x-ray can yield useful information about tooth development, cysts or tumors of the jaws, supernumerary or congenitally absent teeth, 3rd molar impaction, Eagle syndrome (less frequently), and carotid plaques.

102 Symptoms of Dental and Oral Disorders

BRUXISM

Bruxism is clenching or grinding of teeth. Bruxism can abrade and eventually wear down enamel and dentin in the crowns of teeth, damage metal or ceramic dental crowns, and cause teeth to become mobile. Tooth abrasion and erosion is often worse in patients who also have gastroesophageal reflux disease (GERD—see p. 113) and/or obstructive sleep apnea (see p. 514).

A **bruxism triad** has been described, consisting of

- Arousal-induced tooth grinding
- Airway-associated sleep disorders
- Sleep-related GERD

In some people, bruxism causes headaches, neck pain, and/or jaw pain. The most severe and extensive grinding and clenching occurs during sleep, so the person may be oblivious to it, but family members might notice.

Treatment requires that the patient consciously try to reduce bruxism while awake. Plastic oral appliances (night guards) that prevent occlusal contact by fitting between the teeth can be used while sleeping. When symptoms are severe, a guard can also be used during the day. Usually, such devices are custom-made and fitted by dentists. However, if the only problem is tooth wear, OTC heat-moldable devices fitted at home are available, but a dental evaluation should first be done to assess the severity of wear and determine whether an OTC device is adequate. Mild anxiolytics, particularly benzodiazepines, may help until a night guard is available but should not be used for extended periods.

BURNING MOUTH SYNDROME

(Glossodynia; Oral Dysesthesia)

Burning mouth syndrome (BMS) is intraoral pain, usually involving the tongue, in the absence of intraoral physical signs. There are no specific diagnostic tests, and treatment is symptomatic. BMS can be either idiopathic or caused by a disorder.

BMS usually affects postmenopausal women. It is believed to be neurogenic, affecting nerves of pain and taste. Causes of secondary BMS include

- Nutritional deficiency (Vitamin B_{12}, iron)
- Diabetes mellitus
- *Candida* infection (candidiasis)
- Allergy (foods, dental products)
- Xerostomia (or significant dry mouth)
- ACE inhibitors

BMS may cause burning, tingling, or numbness of the tongue or other areas of the mouth, including the lips. Dry mouth or altered taste may occur. The pain may be constant or increase throughout the day and may be relieved by eating or drinking. Duration of symptoms of BMS is variable and may recur if the cause is not addressed.

Diagnosis

Diagnosis requires oral symptoms as noted above and the absence of oral signs. Pain must occur for > 2 h/day for > 3 mo. There are no diagnostic tests for BMS. Idiopathic BMS is a diagnosis of exclusion; therefore, secondary causes should be sought.

Treatment

- Symptomatic treatment
- Curative treatment for secondary BMS

Pain may be relieved with cold beverages, ice chips, chewing gum (sugarless), and by avoidance of irritants such as tobacco, spicy or acidic foods, and alcohol (in beverages and mouthwash). Tricyclic antidepressants, alpha-lipoic acid, clonazepam, and cognitive-behavioral therapy may sometimes help.

Secondary BMS may be cured by appropriate treatment of the underlying cause.

HALITOSIS

(Fetor Oris; Oral Malodor)

Halitosis is a frequent or persistent unpleasant breath odor.

Pathophysiology

Halitosis most often results from fermentation of food particles by anaerobic gram-negative bacteria in the mouth, producing volatile sulfur compounds such as hydrogen sulfide and methyl mercaptan. Causative bacteria may be present in areas of periodontal disease, particularly when ulceration or necrosis is present. The causative organisms reside deep in periodontal pockets around teeth. In patients with healthy periodontal tissue, these bacteria may proliferate on the dorsal posterior tongue.

Factors contributing to the overgrowth of causative bacteria include decreased salivary flow (eg, due to parotid disease, Sjögren syndrome [SS], or use of anticholinergics), salivary stagnation, and increased salivary pH.

Certain foods or spices, after digestion, release the odor of that substance to the lungs; the exhaled odor may be unpleasant to others. For example, the odor of garlic is noted on the breath by others 2 or 3 h after consumption, long after it is gone from the mouth.

Etiology

About 85% of cases result from oral conditions. A variety of systemic and extraoral conditions account for the remainder (see Table 102–1).

The **most common causes** overall are the following:

- Gingival or periodontal disease
- Smoking
- Ingested foods that have a volatile component

GI disorders rarely cause halitosis because the esophagus is normally collapsed. It is a fallacy that breath odor reflects the state of digestion and bowel function.

Table 102–1. SOME CAUSES OF HALITOSIS

CAUSE	SUGGESTIVE FINDINGS	DIAGNOSTIC APPROACH
Oral conditions		
Bacteria on dorsum of tongue	Malodorous tongue scrapings, healthy oral tissue	Clinical evaluation
Gingival or periodontal disease	Oral disease, often including bleeding and/or purulent exudate Apparent during the examination Often history of poor oral hygiene	Clinical evaluation Dental consultation
Necrotic oral cancer (rare—usually identified before becoming necrotic)	Lesion usually identifiable during the examination In older patients, who often have extensive history of using alcohol, tobacco, or both	Biopsy, CT, or MRI
Extraoral disorders		
Nasal foreign body*	Usually in children Purulent or bloody nasal discharge Visible on examination	Clinical evaluation Sometimes imaging
Necrotic nasopharyngeal cancer*	Discomfort with swallowing	Clinical evaluation
Necrotic pulmonary infection (eg, lung abscess, bronchiectasis, foreign body)	Productive cough Fevers	Chest x-ray Sputum cultures Sometimes CT or bronchoscopy
Psychogenic halitosis	Malodor not detected by others Often history of other hypochondriacal complaints	Clinical evaluation
Sinus infection*	Purulent nasal discharge Facial pain, headache, or both	Clinical evaluation Sometimes CT
Zenker diverticulum GERD	Undigested food regurgitated when lying down or bending over	Video barium swallow or upper GI endoscopy
Ingested substances†		
Alcoholic beverages, garlic, onions, tobacco	Use apparent on history	Clinical evaluation Trial of avoidance

*Malodor typically more prominent from the nose than the mouth.
†Typically, a diagnosis of exclusion after examination rules out other causes.

Other breath odors: Several systemic diseases produce volatile substances detectable on the breath, although not the particularly foul, pungent odors typically considered halitosis. Diabetic ketoacidosis (DKA) produces a sweet or fruity odor of acetone, liver failure produces a mousy or sometimes faintly sulfurous odor, and renal failure produces an odor of urine or ammonia.

Evaluation

History: History of present illness should ascertain duration and severity of halitosis (including whether other people have noticed or complained), adequacy of the patient's oral hygiene, and the relationship of halitosis to ingestion of causative foods (see Table 102–1).

Review of systems should seek symptoms of causative disorders, including nasal discharge and face or head pain (sinusitis, nasal foreign body), productive cough and fevers (pulmonary infection), and regurgitation of undigested food when lying down or bending over (Zenker diverticulum). Predisposing factors such as dry mouth, dry eyes, or both (SS) should be noted.

Past medical history should ask about duration and amount of use of alcohol and tobacco. Drug history should specifically ask about use of drugs that can cause dry mouth (eg, those with anticholinergic effects—see Table 102–5 on p. 874).

Physical examination: Vital signs are reviewed, particularly for presence of fever.

The nose is examined for discharge and foreign body.

The mouth is examined for signs of periodontal disease, dental infection, and cancer. Signs of apparent dryness are noted (eg, whether the mucosa is dry, sticky, or moist; whether saliva is foamy, stringy, or normal in appearance).

The pharynx is examined for signs of infection and cancer.

Sniff test: A sniff test of exhaled air is conducted. In general, oral causes result in a putrefying, pungent smell, whereas systemic conditions result in a more subtle, abnormal odor. Ideally, for 48 h before the examination, the patient avoids eating garlic or onions, and for 2 h before, the patient abstains from eating, chewing, drinking, gargling, rinsing, or smoking. During the test, the patient exhales 10 cm away from the examiner's nose, first through the mouth and then with the mouth closed. Malodor that is perceived as worse through the mouth suggests an oral etiology; malodor that is perceived as worse through the nose suggests a nasal or sinus etiology. Similar malodor through both nose and mouth may suggest a systemic or pulmonary cause.

If site of origin is unclear, the posterior tongue is scraped with a plastic spoon. After 5 sec, the spoon is sniffed 5 cm from the examiner's nose; a bad odor suggests the malodor is caused by bacteria on the tongue.

Red flags: The following findings are of particular concern:

- Fever
- Purulent nasal discharge or sputum
- Visible or palpable oral lesions

Interpretation of findings: Because oral causes are by far the most common, any visible oral disease may be presumed to be the cause in patients with no extraoral symptoms or signs, and a dentist should be consulted. When other disorders are involved, clinical findings often suggest a diagnosis (see Table 102–1).

In patients whose symptoms seem to be related to intake of certain food or drink and who have no other findings, a trial of avoidance (followed by a sniff test) may clarify the diagnosis.

Testing: Extensive diagnostic evaluation should not be undertaken unless the history and physical examination suggest an underlying disease (see Table 102–1). Portable sulfur monitors, gas chromatography, and chemical tests of tongue scrapings are available but best left to research protocols or to specific dental offices that focus on halitosis evaluation and treatment.

Treatment

- Regular oral hygiene and dental care
- Cause treated

Underlying diseases are treated.

If the cause is oral, the patient should see a dentist for professional cleaning and treatment of gingival disease and caries. Home treatment involves enhanced oral hygiene, including thorough flossing, toothbrushing, and brushing of the tongue with the toothbrush or a scraper. Mouthwashes are of limited benefit but some with oxidant formulations (typically containing chlorine dioxide) have shown greater short-term success. If the patient has a history of alcohol abuse, nonalcoholic mouthwashes should be used. Psychogenic halitosis may require psychiatric consultation.

Geriatrics Essentials

Elderly patients are more likely to take drugs that cause dry mouth, which leads to difficulties with oral hygiene and hence to halitosis, but they are otherwise not more likely to have halitosis. Also, oral cancers are more common with aging and are more of a concern among elderly than younger patients.

KEY POINTS

- Most halitosis results from fermentation of food particles by anaerobic gram-negative bacteria that reside around the teeth and on the dorsum of the tongue.
- Extraoral disorders may cause halitosis but are often accompanied by suggestive findings.
- It is a fallacy that breath odor reflects the state of digestion and bowel function.
- Mouthwashes provide only brief benefit.

MALOCCLUSION

Malocclusion is abnormal contact between the maxillary and mandibular teeth.

Normally, each dental arch consists of teeth in side-by-side contact, forming a smooth curve, with the maxillary anterior teeth overlying the upper third of the mandibular anterior teeth (see Fig. 101–1). The buccal (outer) cusps of the maxillary posterior teeth are external to the corresponding cusps of the mandibular posterior teeth. In most cases, the anterior buccal cusp of the maxillary 1st permanent molar fits into the anterior buccal groove of the mandibular 1st molar. Because the outer parts of all maxillary teeth are normally external to the mandibular teeth, the lips and cheeks are displaced from between the teeth so that they are not bitten. The lingual (inner) surfaces of the lower teeth form a smaller arc than those of the upper teeth, confining the tongue and minimizing the likelihood of its being bitten. All the maxillary teeth should contact the corresponding mandibular teeth, so that the masticatory forces (which may be > 150 lb in the molar region and 250 lb when clenching during sleep) are widely distributed. If these forces are applied to only a few teeth, those teeth may eventually become mobile or show abnormal wear.

Etiology

Causes of malocclusion include

- Size mismatch between jaw and teeth
- Certain oral habits (eg, thumb-sucking, tongue thrusting)
- Missing teeth
- Certain congenital defects

Malocclusion most often results from jaw and tooth size discrepancies (ie, the jaw is too small or the teeth are too large for the jaw to accommodate them in proper alignment). People who habitually suck their thumb or push their tongue up against their front teeth may cause gradual protrusion of the upper incisors. When permanent teeth are lost, adjacent teeth may shift and opposing teeth may extrude, causing malocclusion unless a bridge, implant, or partial denture (see p. 878) is worn to prevent these movements. When children lose deciduous teeth prematurely, the teeth more posterior in the arch or the permanent 1st molars often drift forward, leaving insufficient space for other permanent teeth to erupt. Malocclusion after facial trauma may indicate tooth displacement and/or alveolar bone or jaw fractures. In ectodermal dysplasia, cleft palate, or Down syndrome, malocclusions may result from having too few teeth.

Evaluation

- Physical examination

Occlusion is checked on both sides of the mouth by retracting each cheek with a tongue depressor while telling the patient to close on the back teeth; telling patients to bite may mistakenly cause them to close on their incisors (as in biting a piece of fruit), which gives the false appearance of malocclusion of the back teeth. Malocclusion sometimes is identified as early as the first dental visit (age 1 yr). Early identification may make later treatment easier and more effective.

Treatment

- Dental modification
- Orthodontic appliances (braces)
- Sometimes surgery

Malocclusions are corrected primarily for aesthetic and psychologic reasons. However, in some cases, treatment may increase resistance to caries (in specific teeth), to anterior tooth fracture, and, possibly, to periodontal disease or stripping of the gingiva on the palate. Treatment may improve speech and mastication as well. Occlusion can be improved by aligning teeth properly, by selectively grinding teeth and restorations that contact prematurely, and by inserting crowns or onlays to build up tooth surfaces that are below the plane of occlusion.

Orthodontic appliances (braces) apply a continuous mild force to teeth to gradually remodel the surrounding alveolar bone. Extraction of one or more permanent teeth (usually a 1st premolar) may be needed to allow other teeth to be repositioned or to erupt into a stable alignment. After the teeth are properly aligned, the patient wears a plastic-and-wire retainer 24 h/day initially, then only at night for 2 to 3 yr.

When orthodontic treatment alone is insufficient, surgical correction of jaw abnormalities contributing to malocclusion (orthognathic surgery) may be indicated.

ORAL GROWTHS

Growths can originate in any type of tissue in and around the mouth, including connective tissues, bone, muscle, and nerve. Most commonly, growths form on the lips, the sides of the tongue, the floor of the mouth, and the soft palate. Some growths cause pain or irritation. Growths may be noticed by the patient or discovered only during routine examination.

Etiology

Oral growths can be

- Benign
- Premalignant (dysplastic)
- Malignant

Benign oral growths: Most oral growths are benign; there are numerous types.

Chronic irritation can cause a persistent lump or raised area on the gingiva. Benign growths due to irritation are relatively common and, if necessary, can be removed by surgery. In 10 to 40% of people, benign growths on the gingiva reappear because the irritant remains. Occasionally such irritation, particularly if it persists over a long period of time, can lead to premalignant or malignant changes.

Warts may occur in the mouth. Ordinary warts (verrucae vulgaris) can infect the mouth if a person sucks or chews one that is growing on a finger. Genital warts, caused by human papillomavirus infection (HPV), may also occur in the oral cavity when transmitted through oral sex.

Oral candidiasis (thrush) often appears as white, cheesy plaques that stick tightly to the mucous membranes and leave red erosions when wiped off. Thrush is most common among patients with diabetes or immunocompromise and among those who are taking antibiotics.

A **torus** is a slow-growing, rounded projection of bone that forms in the midline of the hard palate (torus palatinus) or on the inner aspect of the mandible (torus mandibularis). This hard growth is both common and harmless. Even a large growth can be left alone unless it gets traumatized during eating or the person needs a denture that covers the area.

Gardner syndrome is a type of familial adenomatous polyposis, a hereditary disorder of the GI tract that involves multiple colorectal polyps. Patients who have Gardner syndrome often present with multiple oral osteomas that may clinically resemble multiple torus lesions, particularly in the body and angle of the lower jaw.

Keratoacanthomas are growths that form on the lips and other sun-exposed areas, such as the face, forearms, and hands. A keratoacanthoma usually reaches its full size of about 1 to 3 cm or more in diameter within 1 or 2 mo, then begins to shrink after another few months and may eventually disappear without treatment. Once, all keratoacanthomas were considered to be noncancerous, but many experts now consider those that do not diminish in size to be low-grade cancerous lesions, and biopsy or excision is currently recommended for such lesions.

Many kinds of **cysts** cause jaw pain and swelling. Often they are associated with an impacted wisdom tooth and can destroy considerable areas of the mandible as they expand. Certain types of cysts are more likely to recur after surgical removal. Various types of cysts may also develop in the floor of the mouth. Often, these cysts are surgically removed because they make swallowing uncomfortable or because they are unattractive. By far the most common cyst occurs in the lip and is called a mucocele or mucus retention cyst. It is usually the result of accidentally biting the (lower) lip and occurs when saliva draining into the mouth from a minor salivary gland is obstructed. Most mucoceles disappear in a week or two but can be surgically removed if annoying.

Odontomas are overgrowths of tooth-forming cells that look like small, misshapen extra teeth. In children, they may get in the way of normal tooth eruption. In adults, they may push teeth out of alignment. They are usually removed surgically.

Salivary gland tumors are mostly (75 to 80%) benign, slow-growing, and painless. They usually occur as a single, soft, movable lump beneath normal-appearing skin or under the buccal mucosa. Occasionally, when hollow and fluid-filled, they are firm. The most common type is a pleomorphic adenoma (mixed tumor) and it occurs mainly in women > age 40. Pleomorphic adenomas can become malignant and are removed surgically. Unless completely removed, this type of tumor is likely to recur. Other types of benign tumors are also removed surgically but are much less likely to become malignant or recur.

Premalignant (dysplastic) changes: White, red, or mixed white-red areas that are not easily wiped away, persist for > 2 wk, and are not definable as some other condition may be dysplastic. The same risk factors are involved in dysplastic changes as in malignant growths, and dysplastic changes may become malignant if not removed.

Leukoplakia is a flat white spot that may develop when the oral mucosa is irritated for a long period. The irritated spot appears white because it has a thickened layer of keratin, which normally is less abundant in the oral mucosa. Factors often associated with the development of idiopathic oral leukoplakia include tobacco use, alcohol consumption, vitamin deficiency, and endocrine disturbances.

Erythroplakia is a red and flat or worn away area that results when the oral mucosa thins. The area appears red because the underlying capillaries are more visible. Erythroplakia is a much more ominous predictor of oral cancer than leukoplakia.

Mixed lesions show intermixed areas of leukoplakia and erythroplakia and also may be precursors of cancer.

Oral cancer: People who use tobacco, alcohol, or both are at much greater risk (up to 15 times) of oral cancer. For people who use chewing tobacco and snuff, the insides of the cheeks and lips are common sites. In other people, the most common sites for cancer include the lateral borders of the tongue, the floor of the mouth, and the oropharynx. Human papillomavirus infection is a risk factor for oral cancer, primarily in the tonsils and at the base of the tongue. Rarely, cancers found in the oral region have metastasized from the lungs, breast, or prostate.

Oral cancer can have many different appearances but typically resembles dysplastic lesions (eg, white, red, or mixed white-red areas that are not easily wiped away).

Evaluation

History: History of present illness includes questions about how long the growth has been present, whether it is painful, and whether there has been any injury to the area (eg, biting a cheek, scraping by a sharp tooth edge or dental restoration). Patients are asked about symptoms of systemic illness, particularly weight loss and malaise.

Past medical history should seek risk factors for candidiasis, including recent antibiotic use, diabetes, and HIV infection (or risk factors for HIV). The amount and duration of use of alcohol and tobacco is noted.

Physical examination: The physical examination focuses on the mouth and neck, inspecting and palpating all areas of the mouth and throat, including under the tongue. The neck is palpated for lymphadenopathy, which suggests possible cancer or chronic infection.

Red flags: The following findings are of particular concern:

- Weight loss
- Neck mass

Interpretation of findings: The main concern is to not mistake an oral cancer or dysplastic lesion for a benign disorder. Clinicians should maintain a high degree of suspicion and refer the patient for biopsy if the lesion does not resolve in a few weeks.

Testing: Suspected candidiasis can be confirmed by finding yeast and pseudohyphae in 10% KOH wet mounts of scrapings from a lesion. Other acute lesions, particularly those that appear related to local trauma or irritation, may be observed. However, most lesions present for more than a few weeks, and those of unknown duration, should be biopsied because cancer is difficult to exclude clinically.

Treatment

- Dependent on cause

Treatment depends on the cause of the growth.

KEY POINTS

- Most oral growths are benign.
- Warts, candidal infections, and repeated trauma are common causes of benign growths.
- Use of alcohol and tobacco is a risk factor for cancer.
- Because cancer is difficult to diagnose by inspection, biopsy is often necessary.

RECURRENT APHTHOUS STOMATITIS

Recurrent aphthous stomatitis (RAS) is a common condition in which round or ovoid painful ulcers recur on the oral mucosa. Etiology is unclear. Diagnosis is clinical. Treatment is symptomatic and usually includes topical corticosteroids.

RAS affects 20 to 30% of adults and a greater percentage of children at some time in their life.

Etiology

Etiology is unclear, but RAS tends to run in families. The damage is predominately cell-mediated. Cytokines, such as IL-2, IL-10, and, particularly, TNF-alpha, play a role.

Predisposing factors include

- Oral trauma
- Stress
- Foods, particularly chocolate, coffee, peanuts, eggs, cereals, almonds, strawberries, cheese, and tomatoes

Allergy does not seem to be involved.

Factors that may, for unknown reasons, be *protective* include oral contraceptives, pregnancy, and tobacco, including smokeless tobacco and nicotine-containing tablets.

Symptoms and Signs

Symptoms and signs usually begin in childhood (80% of patients are < 30 yr) and decrease in frequency and severity with aging. Symptoms may involve as few as one ulcer 2 to 4 times/yr or almost continuous disease, with new ulcers forming as old ones heal. A prodrome of pain or burning for 1 to 2 days precedes ulcers, but there are no antecedent vesicles or bullae. Severe pain, disproportionate to the size of the lesion, can last from 4 to 7 days.

Aphthous ulcers are well-demarcated, shallow, ovoid, or round and have a necrotic center with a yellow-gray pseudomembrane, a red halo, and slightly raised red margins.

Minor aphthous ulcers (Mikulicz disease) account for 85% of cases. They occur on the floor of the mouth, lateral and ventral tongue, buccal mucosa, and pharynx; are < 8 mm (typically 2 to 3 mm); and heal in 10 days without scarring.

Major aphthous ulcers (Sutton disease, periadenitis mucosa necrotica recurrens) constitute 10% of cases. Appearing after puberty, the prodrome is more intense and the ulcers are deeper, larger (> 1 cm), and longer lasting (weeks to months) than minor aphthae. They appear on the lips, soft palate, and throat. Fever, dysphagia, malaise, and scarring may occur.

Herpetiform aphthous ulcers (morphologically resembling but unrelated to herpes virus) account for 5% of cases. They begin as multiple (up to 100) 1- to 3-mm crops of small, painful clusters of ulcers on an erythematous base. They coalesce to form larger ulcers that last 2 wk. They tend to occur in women and at a later age of onset than do other forms of RAS.

Diagnosis

- Clinical evaluation

Evaluation proceeds as described previously under stomatitis. Diagnosis is based on appearance and on exclusion because there are no definitive histologic features or laboratory tests.

Primary oral herpes simplex may mimic RAS but usually occurs in younger children, always involves the gingiva and may affect any keratinized mucosa (hard palate, attached gingiva, dorsum of tongue), and is associated with systemic symptoms. Viral culture can be done to identify herpes simplex. Recurrent herpetic lesions are usually unilateral.

Similar recurrent episodes can occur with Behçet disease, inflammatory bowel disease, celiac disease, HIV infection, periodic fevers with aphthous stomatitis, pharyngitis, and adenitis (PFAPA) syndrome, and nutritional deficiencies; these conditions generally have systemic symptoms and signs. Isolated recurrent oral ulcers can occur with herpes infection, HIV, and, rarely, nutritional deficiency. Viral testing and serum hematologic tests can identify these conditions.

Drug reactions may mimic RAS but are usually temporally related to ingestion. However, reactions to foods or dental products may be difficult to identify; sequential elimination may be necessary.

Treatment

- Topical chlorhexidine and corticosteroids

General treatments for stomatitis (see below) may help patients with RAS.

Chlorhexidine gluconate mouthwashes and topical corticosteroids, the mainstays of therapy, should be used during the prodrome, if possible. The corticosteroid can be dexamethasone 0.5 mg/5 mL tid used as a rinse and then expectorated or clobetasol ointment 0.05% or fluocinonide ointment 0.05% in carboxymethylcellulose mucosal protective paste (1:1) applied tid. Patients using these corticosteroids should be monitored for candidiasis. If topical corticosteroids are ineffective, prednisone (eg, 40 mg po once/day) may be needed for ≤ 5 days.

Continuous or particularly severe RAS is best treated by a specialist in oral medicine. Treatment may require prolonged use of systemic corticosteroids, azathioprine or other immunosuppressants, pentoxifylline, or thalidomide. Intralesional injections can be done with betamethasone, dexamethasone, or triamcinolone. Supplemental B_1, B_2, B_6, B_{12}, folate, or iron lessens RAS in some patients.

STOMATITIS

(Oral Mucositis)

Oral inflammation and ulcers, known as stomatitis, may be mild and localized or severe and widespread. They are invariably painful. Stomatitis may involve swelling and redness of the oral mucosa or discrete, painful ulcers (single or multiple). Less commonly, whitish lesions form, and, rarely, the mouth appears normal (BMS—see p. 864) despite significant symptoms. Symptoms hinder eating, sometimes leading to dehydration and malnutrition. Secondary infection occasionally occurs, especially in immunocompromised patients. Some conditions are recurrent.

Etiology

Stomatitis may be caused by local infection, systemic disease, a physical or chemical irritant, or an allergic reaction (see Table 102–2); many cases are idiopathic. Because the normal flow of saliva protects the mucosa against many insults, xerostomia predisposes the mouth to stomatitis of any cause.

The **most common specific causes** overall include

- RAS—also called recurrent aphthous ulcers (RAU)
- Viral infections, particularly herpes simplex and herpes zoster
- Other infectious agents (*Candida albicans* and bacteria)
- Trauma
- Tobacco or irritating foods or chemicals
- Chemotherapy and radiation therapy

Evaluation

History: History of present illness should ascertain the duration of symptoms and whether the patient ever had them previously. Presence and severity of pain should be noted. The relation of symptoms to food, drugs, oral hygiene materials (eg, toothpaste, mouth rinses), and other substances (particularly occupational exposure to chemicals, metals, fumes, or dust) is sought.

Review of systems seeks symptoms of possible causes, including chronic diarrhea and weakness (inflammatory bowel disease, celiac disease; genital lesions (Behçet disease, syphilis); eye irritation (Behçet disease); and weight loss, malaise, and fever (nonspecific chronic illness).

Past medical history should ascertain known conditions that cause oral lesions, including herpes simplex, Behçet disease, inflammatory bowel disease, and risk factors for oral lesions, including immunocompromised state (eg, cancer, diabetes, organ transplant, use of immunosuppressants, HIV infection). Whether chemotherapy or radiation therapy has ever been used to manage cancer needs to be determined. Drug history should note all recent drugs used. History of tobacco use should be noted. Social history should include sexual contact, particularly oral sex, unprotected sex, and sex with multiple partners.

Physical examination: Vital signs are reviewed for fever. The patient's general appearance is noted for lethargy, discomfort, or other signs of significant systemic illness.

The mouth is inspected for the location and nature of any lesions.

The skin and other mucosal surfaces (including the genitals) are inspected for any lesions, rash, petechiae, or desquamation. Any bullous lesions are rubbed for the Nikolsky sign (upper layers of epidermis move laterally with slight pressure or rubbing of skin adjacent to a blister).

Red flags: The following findings are of particular concern:

- Fever
- Cutaneous bullae
- Ocular inflammation
- Immunocompromise

Interpretation of findings: Occasionally, causes are obvious in the history (eg, cytotoxic chemotherapy; significant occupational exposure to chemicals, fumes, or dust). Recurrent episodes of oral lesions occur with RAS, herpes simplex, and Behçet disease. History of diabetes, HIV infection or other immunocompromise, or recent antibiotic use should increase suspicion of *Candida* infection. Recent drug use (particularly sulfa drugs, other antibiotics, and antiepileptics) should increase suspicion of SJS.

Table 102–2. SOME CAUSES OF STOMATITIS

CATEGORY	EXAMPLES
Bacterial infections	Actinomycosis* Acute necrotizing ulcerative gingivitis Gonorrhea Syphilis, primary or secondary TB*
Fungal infections	Blastomycosis* Candidal infections (most common) Coccidioidomycosis* Cryptococcosis* Mucormycosis* (more common in diabetics)
Viral infections	Herpes simplex infection, primary (mostly in young children) Herpes simplex infection, secondary (cold sores on the lips or palate) Varicella zoster, primary (chickenpox) Varicella zoster reactivation (shingles) Others (eg, infection by coxsackievirus, cytomegalovirus, Epstein-Barr virus, or HIV; condyloma acuminata; influenza; rubeola)
Systemic disorders	Behçet syndrome Celiac disease Cyclic neutropenia Erythema multiforme Inflammatory bowel disease Iron deficiency Kawasaki disease Leukemia Pemphigoid, pemphigus vulgaris Platelet disorders Stevens-Johnson syndrome (SJS) Thrombotic thrombocytopenic purpura Vitamin B deficiency (pellagra) Vitamin C deficiency (scurvy)
Drugs	Antibiotics* Anticonvulsants* Barbiturates* Chemotherapy drugs Gold Iodides* NSAIDs*
Physical irritation	Dentures that fit poorly Broken or jagged teeth Habitual cheek or lip biting
Irritants and allergies	Acidic foods Dental appliances containing nickel or palladium Occupational exposure to dyes, acid fumes, heavy metals, or metal or mineral dusts Tobacco (nicotinic stomatitis, particularly pipe smoker's palate [hyperkeratotic palate with red dots at the openings of minor salivary glands]) Type IV hypersensitivity reaction (eg, to ingredients in toothpaste such as sodium lauryl sulfate, mouthwash, candy, gum, dyes, or lipstick) Aspirin, when applied topically
Other	Lichen planus RAS (most commonly, minor aphthae) Head and neck radiation

*Rare.

Some causes typically have **extraoral, noncutaneous findings,** some of which suggest a cause. Recurrent GI symptoms suggest inflammatory bowel disease or celiac disease. Ocular symptoms can occur with Behçet disease and SJS. Genital lesions may occur with Behçet disease and primary syphilis.

Some causes usually also have **extraoral, cutaneous findings. Cutaneous bullae** suggest SJS, pemphigus vulgaris, or bullous pemphigoid. Prodrome of malaise, fever, conjunctivitis, and generalized macular target lesions suggests SJS. Pemphigus vulgaris starts with oral lesions, then progresses to flaccid cutaneous bullae. Bullous pemphigoid has tense bullae on normal-appearing skin. The Nikolsky sign is usually positive in SJS and pemphigus vulgaris.

Cutaneous vesicles are typical with chickenpox or herpes zoster (see p. 1616). Unilateral lesions in a band along a dermatome suggest herpes zoster. Diffuse, scattered vesicular and pustular lesions in different stages suggest chickenpox.

Kawasaki disease usually has a macular rash, desquamation of hands and feet, and conjunctivitis; it occurs in children, usually those < 5 yr. Oral findings include erythema of the lips and oral mucosa.

Other cutaneous lesions may implicate erythema multiforme, hand-foot-and-mouth disease (resulting from coxsackievirus), or secondary syphilis.

Some causes have **isolated oral findings,** including RAS, most viral infections, acute necrotizing ulcerative gingivitis, primary syphilis, gonorrhea, and *Candida*.

Location of oral lesions may help identify the cause. Interdental ulcers occur with primary herpes simplex or acute necrotizing ulcerative gingivitis. Lesions on keratinized surfaces suggest herpes simplex, RAS, or physical injury. Physical injury typically has an irregular appearance and occurs near projections of teeth, dental appliances, or where biting or an errant toothbrush can injure the mucosa. An aspirin burn next to a tooth and pizza burn on the palate are common.

Primary herpes simplex infection causes multiple vesicular lesions on the intraoral mucosa on both keratinized and nonkeratinized surfaces and always includes the gingiva. These lesions rapidly ulcerate. Clinical manifestation occurs most often in children. Subsequent reactivations (secondary herpes simplex, cold sore) usually appear starting in puberty on the lip at the vermilion border and, rarely, on the hard palate.

Acute necrotizing ulcerative gingivitis causes severe inflammation and punched-out ulcers on the dental papillae and marginal gingivae. A severe variant called **noma** (gangrenous stomatitis) can cause full-thickness tissue destruction (sometimes involving the lips or cheek), typically in a debilitated patient. It begins as a gingival, buccal, or palatal (midline lethal granuloma) ulcer that becomes necrotic and spreads rapidly. Tissue sloughing may occur.

Isolated oral gonorrhea very rarely causes burning ulcers and erythema of the gingiva and tongue, as well as the more common pharyngitis. Primary **syphilis** chancres may appear in the mouth. Tertiary syphilis may cause oral gummas or a generalized glossitis and mucosal atrophy. The site of a gumma is the only time that squamous cell carcinoma develops on the dorsum of the tongue. A common sign of HIV becoming AIDS is **hairy leukoplakia** (vertical white lines on the lateral border of the tongue).

C. albicans and related species, which are normal oral flora, can overgrow in people who have taken antibiotics or corticosteroids or who are immunocompromised, such as patients with AIDS. *C. albicans* can cause whitish, cheesy plaques that leave erosions when wiped off. Sometimes only flat, erythematous areas appear (erosive form of *Candida*).

Testing:

- Bacterial and viral culture
- Laboratory tests
- Biopsy

Patients with acute stomatitis and no symptoms, signs, or risk factors for systemic illness probably require no testing.

If stomatitis is recurrent, viral and bacterial cultures, CBC, serum iron, ferritin, vitamin B_{12}, folate, zinc, and endomysial antibody (for sprue) are done. Biopsy at the periphery of normal and abnormal tissue can be done for persistent lesions that do not have an obvious etiology.

Systematically eliminating foods from the diet can be useful, as can changing brands of toothpaste, chewing gum, or mouthwash.

Treatment

- Cause treated
- Oral hygiene
- Topical agents and rinses
- Chemical or physical cautery

Specific disorders are treated, and any causative substances or drugs are avoided. Mouth rinses that contain ethanol can cause stomatitis and should not be used.

Meticulous oral hygiene (using a soft toothbrush and salt-water rinses) may help prevent secondary infection. A soft diet that does not include acidic or salty foods is followed.

Topical measures: Numerous topical treatments, alone or in combination, are used to ease symptoms. These treatments include

- Anesthetics
- Protective coatings
- Corticosteroids
- Physical measures (eg, cautery)

For topical anesthesia of discomfort that may interfere with eating and drinking, the following may be effective:

- Lidocaine rinse
- Sucralfate plus aluminum-magnesium antacid rinse

A 2-min rinse is done with 15 mL (1 tbsp) 2% viscous lidocaine q 3 h prn; patient expectorates when done (no rinsing with water and no swallowing unless the pharynx is involved). A soothing coating may be prepared with sucralfate (1-g pill dissolved in 15 mL water) plus 30 mL of aluminum-magnesium liquid antacid; the patient should rinse with or without swallowing. Many institutions and pharmacies have their own variation of this formulation (magic mouthwash), which sometimes also contains an antihistamine.

If the physician is certain the inflammation is not caused by an infectious organism, the patient can

- Rinse and expectorate after meals with dexamethasone elixir 0.5 mg/5 mL (1 tsp)
- Apply a paste of 0.1% triamcinolone in an oral emollient
- Wipe amlexanox over the ulcerated area with the tip of a finger

Chemical or physical cautery can ease the pain of localized lesions. Silver nitrate sticks are not as effective as low-power (2- to 3-watt), defocused, pulsed-mode CO_2 laser treatments, after which pain relief is immediate and lesions tend not to recur locally.

KEY POINTS

- Isolated stomatitis in patients with no other symptoms and signs or risk factors for systemic illness is usually caused by a viral infection or RAS.
- Extraoral symptoms, rash, or both suggest more immediate need for diagnosis.

TOOTHACHE AND INFECTION

Pain in and around the teeth is a common problem, particularly among patients with poor oral hygiene. Pain may be constant, felt after stimulation (eg, heat, cold, sweet food or drink, chewing, brushing), or both.

Etiology

The most common causes of toothache (see Table 102–3) are

- Dental caries
- Pulpitis
- Periapical abscess
- Trauma
- Erupting wisdom tooth (causing pericoronitis)

Toothache is usually caused by dental caries and its consequences.

Caries causes pain when the lesion extends through the enamel into dentin. Pain usually occurs after stimulation from cold, heat, sweet food or drink, or brushing; these stimuli cause fluid to move within dentinal tubules to induce a response in the pulp. As long as the discomfort does not persist after the stimulus is removed, the pulp is likely healthy enough to be maintained. This is referred to as normal dentinal sensitivity, reversible pulpalgia, or reversible pulpitis.

Pulpitis is inflammation of the pulp, typically due to advancing caries, cumulative minor pulp damage resulting from previous large restorations, a defective restoration, or trauma. It may be reversible or irreversible. Pressure necrosis frequently results from pulpitis. Pain may be spontaneous or in response to stimulation, particularly heat or cold. In both cases, pain lingers for a minute or longer. Once the pulp becomes necrotic, pain ends briefly (hours to weeks). Subsequently, periapical inflammation (apical periodontitis) or an abscess develops.

Periapical abscess may follow untreated caries or pulpitis. The tooth is exquisitely sensitive to percussion (tapping with a metal dental probe or tongue blade) and chewing. The abscess may point intraorally and eventually drain or may become a cellulitis.

Tooth trauma can damage the pulp. The damage may manifest soon after the injury or up to decades later.

Pericoronitis is inflammation and infection of the tissue between the tooth and its overlying flap of gingiva (operculum). It usually occurs in an erupting wisdom tooth (almost always a lower one).

Complications: Rarely, sinusitis results from untreated maxillary dental infection. More commonly, pain resulting from a sinus infection is perceived as originating in the unaffected teeth adjacent to the sinus, mistakenly creating the impression of a dental origin.

Rarely, cavernous sinus thrombosis (see p. 950) or Ludwig angina (submandibular space infection—see p. 844) develops;

Table 102–3. SOME CAUSES OF TOOTHACHE

CAUSE	SUGGESTIVE FINDINGS	DIAGNOSTIC APPROACH*
Apical abscess	Constant pain that worsens when chewing or biting Normally precise identification of the involved tooth by the patient Tooth tender to percussion (tapping with a metal probe or tongue blade) Sometimes visible fluctuant swelling of mucosa over the affected root, painful swelling of the adjacent cheek and/or lip	Dental evaluation
Apical periodontitis	Symptoms and findings similar to apical abscess but less severe and without swelling over the root	Dental evaluation
Caries (dentinal sensitivity)	Pain after stimulation (eg, heat, cold, sweet food or drink, brushing) Pain is isolated to a single tooth and usually stops when stimulus is removed Usually a visible carious lesion or a root surface exposed by gum recession or abrasion	Dental evaluation
Incomplete fracture of the crown of a vital tooth	Sharp pain on release from a chewing stroke Marked sensitivity to cold	Dental evaluation
Irreversible pulpitis	Pain without stimulation, lingering pain after stimulation, or both Usually difficulty identifying the involved tooth	Dental evaluation
Pericoronitis caused by eruption or partial impaction of a 3rd molar (wisdom tooth)	Constant dull pain, especially with chewing Inflammation around the mandibular wisdom tooth, sometimes with purulent drainage Trismus may occur and limit opening	Dental evaluation
Pulp damage caused by trauma	Tooth discoloration (may be delayed up to many years after injury) Can result in an apical abscess	Dental evaluation
Reversible pulpitis	Similar to caries but with difficulty identifying the involved tooth	Dental evaluation
Sinusitis	Many maxillary posterior teeth (eg, molars, premolars) sensitive when chewing and to percussion Pain during posture changes, especially lowering the head (eg, tying shoe laces) Often nasal discharge and tenderness to percussion over the affected sinus	Sinus CT Dental evaluation if no sinusitis detected
Teething	Discomfort and fussiness during tooth eruption in young children Drooling common, chewing on things (eg, crib rail)	Clinical evaluation
Vertical root fracture	Tooth that is mobile and exquisitely sensitive to touch Isolated deep periodontal probing depth Characteristic "J" appearance on x-ray	Dental evaluation

*Dental evaluation entails referral to a dentist for examination and usually dental x-rays.

these conditions are life threatening and require immediate intervention.

Evaluation

History: **History of present illness** should identify the location and duration of the pain and whether it is constant or present only after stimulation. Specific triggering factors to review include heat, cold, sweet food or drink, chewing, and brushing. Any preceding trauma or dental work should be noted.

Review of systems should seek symptoms of complications, including face pain, swelling, or both (dental abscess, sinusitis); pain below the tongue and difficulty swallowing (submandibular space infection); pain with bending forward (sinusitis); and retro-orbital headache, fever, and vision symptoms (cavernous sinus thrombosis).

Past medical history should note previous dental problems and treatment.

Physical examination: Vital signs are reviewed for fever.

The examination focuses on the face and mouth. The face is inspected for swelling and is palpated for induration and tenderness.

The oral examination includes inspection for gum inflammation and caries and any localized swelling at the base of a tooth that may represent a pointing apical abscess. If no tooth is clearly involved, teeth in the area of pain are percussed for tenderness with a tongue depressor. Also, an ice cube can be applied briefly to each tooth, removing it immediately once pain is felt. In healthy teeth, the pain stops almost immediately. Pain lingering more than a few seconds indicates pulp damage (eg, irreversible pulpitis, necrosis). The floor of the mouth is palpated for induration and tenderness, suggesting a deep space infection.

Neurologic examination, concentrating on the cranial nerves, should be done in patients with fever, headache, or facial swelling.

Red flags: Findings of particular concern are

- Headache
- Fever
- Swelling or tenderness of floor of the mouth
- Cranial nerve abnormalities

Interpretation of findings: Red flag finding of headache suggests sinusitis, particularly if multiple upper molar and premolar (back) teeth are painful. However, presence of vision symptoms or abnormalities of the pupils or of ocular motility suggests cavernous sinus thrombosis.

Fever is unusual with routine dental infection unless there is significant local extension. Bilateral tenderness of the floor of the mouth suggests Ludwig angina.

Difficulty opening the mouth (trismus) can occur with any lower molar infection but is common only with pericoronitis.

Isolated dental condition: Patients without red flag findings or facial swelling likely have an isolated dental condition, which, although uncomfortable, is not serious. Clinical findings, particularly the nature of the pain, help suggest a cause (Tables 102–3 and 102–4). Because of its innervation, the pulp can perceive stimuli (eg, heat, cold, sweets) only as pain. An important distinction is whether there is continuous pain or pain only on stimulation and, if pain is only on stimulation, whether the pain lingers after the stimulus is removed.

Swelling at the base of a tooth, on the cheek, or both indicates infection, either cellulitis or abscess. A tender, fluctuant area at the base of a tooth suggests a pointing abscess.

Testing: Dental x-rays are the mainstay of testing but can be deferred to a dentist.

The rare cases in which cavernous sinus thrombosis or Ludwig angina are suspected require imaging studies, typically CT or MRI.

Table 102–4. CHARACTERISTICS OF PAIN IN TOOTHACHE

FINDING	COMMON CAUSES
Pain only after stimulation, no lingering pain	Reversible pulpitis (dentinal pain)
Pain lingers after stimulation (may have unstimulated pain)	Irreversible pulpitis
No pain with stimulation	Pulp necrosis without apical periodontitis or abscess
Continuous pain (worse when chewing or percussed; easily localized)	Apical periodontitis or abscess

Treatment

- Topical or oral analgesics
- Sometimes rinses or systemic antibiotics

Analgesics (see p. 1968) may be given pending dental evaluation and definitive treatment. For severe dental pain, local nerve block injections with bupivacaine hydrochloride and epinephrine 1:200,000 may relieve pain for many hours until the patient receives definitive dental care. A patient who is seen frequently for emergencies but who never receives definitive dental treatment despite availability may be seeking opioids.

Antibiotics directed at oral flora are given for most disorders beyond irreversible pulpitis (eg, necrotic pulp, abscess, cellulitis). Patients with pericoronitis should also receive an antibiotic. However, antibiotics can be deferred if patients can be seen the same day by a dentist, who may be able to treat the infection by removing the source (eg, by extraction, pulpectomy, or curettage). When antibiotics are used, penicillin or amoxicillin is preferred, with clindamycin the alternative.

An **abscess** associated with well-developed (soft) fluctuance is typically drained through an incision with a #15 scalpel blade at the most dependent point of the swelling. A rubber drain, held by a suture, may be placed.

Pericoronitis or erupting 3rd molars are treated with chlorhexidine 0.12% rinses or hypertonic salt-water soaks (1 tbsp salt mixed in a glass of hot water—no hotter than the coffee or tea a patient normally drinks). The salt water is held in the mouth on the affected side until it cools and then is expectorated and immediately replaced with another mouthful. Three or 4 glasses of salt water a day may control inflammation and pain pending dental evaluation.

Teething pain in young children may be treated with weight-based doses of acetaminophen or ibuprofen. Topical treatments can include chewing hard crackers (eg, biscotti), applying 7.5% or 10% benzocaine gel qid (provided there is no family history of methemoglobinemia), and chewing on anything cold (eg, gel-containing teething rings).

The rare patient with cavernous sinus thrombosis or Ludwig angina requires immediate hospitalization, removal of the infected tooth, and culture-guided parenteral antibiotics.

Geriatrics Essentials

The elderly are more prone to caries of the root surfaces, usually because of gingival recession. Periodontitis often begins in young adulthood; if untreated, tooth pain and loss are common in old age.

KEY POINTS

- Most toothache involves dental caries or its complications (eg, pulpitis, abscess).
- Symptomatic treatment and dental referral are usually adequate.
- Antibiotics are given if signs of an abscess, necrotic pulp, or more severe conditions are present.
- Very rare but serious complications include extension of dental infection to the floor of the mouth or to the cavernous sinus.
- Dental infections rarely cause sinusitis, but sinus infection may cause pain perceived as originating in the teeth.

XEROSTOMIA

Xerostomia is dry mouth caused by reduced or absent flow of saliva. This condition can result in discomfort, interfere with speech and swallowing, make wearing dentures difficult, cause halitosis, and impair oral hygiene by causing a decrease in oral pH and an increase in bacterial growth. Long-standing xerostomia can result in severe tooth decay and oral candidiasis. Xerostomia is a common complaint among older adults, affecting about 20% of the elderly.

Pathophysiology

Stimulation of the oral mucosa signals the salivatory nuclei in the medulla, triggering an efferent response. The efferent nerve impulses release acetylcholine at salivary gland nerve terminals, activating muscarinic receptors (M_3), which increase saliva production and flow. Medullary signals responsible for salivation may also be modulated by cortical inputs from other stimuli (eg, taste, smell, anxiety).

Etiology

Xerostomia is usually caused by the following:

- Drugs
- Radiation to the head and neck (for cancer treatment)

Systemic disorders are less commonly the cause, but xerostomia is common in (SS) and may occur in HIV/AIDS, uncontrolled diabetes, and certain other disorders.

Drugs: Drugs are the most common cause (see Table 102–5); about 400 prescription drugs and many OTC drugs cause decreased salivation. The most common include the following:

- Anticholinergics
- Antiparkinsonian drugs
- Antineoplastics (chemotherapy)

Chemotherapy drugs cause severe dryness and stomatitis while they are being taken; these problems usually end after therapy is stopped.

Other common drug classes that cause xerostomia include antihypertensives, anxiolytics, and antidepressants (less severe with SSRIs than with tricyclics).

The rise of illicit methamphetamine use has resulted in an increasing incidence of meth mouth, which is severe tooth decay caused by methamphetamine-induced xerostomia. The damage is exacerbated by the bruxing and clenching caused by the drug and by the heat of the inhaled vapor. This combination causes very rapid destruction of teeth.

Tobacco use usually causes a decrease of saliva.

Radiation: Incidental radiation to the salivary glands during radiation therapy for head and neck cancer often causes severe xerostomia (5200 cGy causes severe, permanent dryness, but even low doses can cause temporary drying).

Table 102–5. SOME CAUSES OF XEROSTOMIA

CAUSE	EXAMPLES
Drugs	
Anticholinergic	Antidepressants Antiemetics Antihistamines Antipsychotics Antispasmodics Anxiolytics
Recreational/illicit	Cannabis Methamphetamines Tobacco
Other	Antihypertensives Antineoplastics (chemotherapy drugs) Antiparkinsonian drugs Bronchodilators Decongestants Diuretics Meperidine, methadone, and other opioids
Systemic disorders	
—	Amyloidosis HIV infection Leprosy Sarcoidosis SS TB
Other	
—	Excessive mouth breathing Head and neck trauma Radiation treatment Viral infections

Evaluation

History: History of present illness should include acuity of onset, temporal patterns (eg, constant vs intermittent, presence only on awakening), provoking factors, including situational or psychogenic factors (eg, whether xerostomia occurs only during periods of psychologic stress or certain activities), assessment of fluid status (eg, fluid intake habits, recurrent vomiting or diarrhea), and sleeping habits. Use of recreational drugs should be specifically elicited.

Review of systems should seek symptoms of causative disorders, including dry eyes, dry skin, rashes, and joint pain (SS).

Past medical history should inquire about conditions associated with xerostomia, including SS, history of radiation treatment, head and neck trauma, and a diagnosis of or risk factors for HIV infection. Drug profiles should be reviewed for potential offending drugs (see Table 102–5).

Physical examination: Physical examination is focused on the oral cavity, specifically any apparent dryness (eg, whether the mucosa is dry, sticky, or moist; whether saliva is foamy, thick, stringy, or normal in appearance), the presence of any lesions caused by *Candida albicans,* and the condition of the teeth.

The presence and severity of xerostomia can be assessed in several ways. For example, a tongue blade can be held against the buccal mucosa for 10 sec. If the tongue blade falls off immediately when released, salivary flow is considered normal.

The more difficulty encountered removing the tongue blade, the more severe the xerostomia. In women, the lipstick sign, where lipstick adheres to the front teeth, may be a useful indicator of xerostomia.

If there appears to be dryness, the submandibular, sublingual, and parotid glands should be palpated while observing the ductal openings for saliva flow. The openings are at the base of the tongue anteriorly for the submandibular and sublingual glands and on the middle of the inside of the cheek for the parotid glands. Drying the duct openings with a gauze square before palpation aids observation. If a graduated container is available, the patient can expectorate once to empty the mouth and then expectorate all saliva into the container. Normal production is 0.3 to 0.4 mL/min. Significant xerostomia is 0.1 mL/min.

Dental caries may be sought at the margins of restorations or in unusual places (eg, at the gum line, incisal edges, or cusp tips of the teeth).

A common manifestation of *C. albicans* infection is areas of erythema and atrophy (eg, loss of papillae on the dorsum of the tongue). Less common is the better-known white, cheesy curd that bleeds when wiped off.

Red flags: The following findings are of particular concern:

- Extensive tooth decay
- Concomitant dry eyes, dry skin, rash, or joint pain
- Risk factors for HIV

Interpretation of findings: Xerostomia is diagnosed by symptoms, appearance, and absence of salivary flow when massaging the salivary glands.

No further assessment is required when xerostomia occurs after initiation of a new drug and stops after cessation of that drug or when symptoms appear within several weeks of irradiation of the head and neck. Xerostomia that occurs with abrupt onset after head and neck trauma may be caused by nerve damage.

Concomitant presence of dry eyes, dry skin, rash, or joint pain, particularly in a female patient, suggests a diagnosis of SS. Severe tooth discoloration and decay, out of proportion to expected findings, may be indicative of illicit drug use, particularly methamphetamines. Xerostomia that occurs only during nighttime or that is noted only on awakening may be indicative of excessive mouth breathing in a dry environment.

Testing:

- Sialometry
- Salivary gland biopsy

For patients in whom the presence of xerostomia is unclear, sialometry can be conducted by placing collection devices over the major duct orifices and then stimulating salivary production with citric acid or by chewing paraffin. Normal parotid flow is 0.4 to 1.5 mL/min/gland. Flow monitoring can also help determine response to therapy.

The cause of xerostomia is often apparent, but if the etiology is unclear and systemic disease is considered possible, further assessment should be pursued with biopsy of a minor salivary gland (for detection of SS, sarcoidosis, amyloidosis, TB, or cancer) and HIV testing. The lower lip is a convenient site for biopsy.

Treatment

- Cause treated and causative drugs stopped when possible
- Cholinergic drugs
- Saliva substitutes
- Regular oral hygiene and dental care to prevent tooth decay

When possible, the cause of xerostomia should be addressed and treated.

For patients with drug-related xerostomia whose therapy cannot be changed to another drug, drug schedules should be modified to achieve maximum drug effect during the day because nighttime xerostomia is more likely to cause caries. Custom-fitted acrylic night guards carrying fluoride gel may also help limit caries in these patients. For all drugs, easy-to-take formulations, such as liquids, should be considered, and sublingual dosage forms should be avoided. The mouth and throat should be lubricated with water before swallowing capsules and tablets or before using sublingual nitroglycerin. Patients should avoid decongestants and antihistamines.

Patients using continuous positive airway pressure for obstructive sleep apnea may benefit from using the humidifier function of the device. Patients using oral appliance therapy may benefit from a room humidifier.

Symptom control: Symptomatic treatment consists of measures that do the following:

- Increase existing saliva
- Replace lost secretions
- Control caries

Drugs that augment saliva production include cevimeline and pilocarpine, both cholinergic agonists. Cevimeline (30 mg po tid) has less M_2 (cardiac) receptor activity than pilocarpine and a longer half-life. The main adverse effect is nausea. Pilocarpine (5 mg po tid) may be given after ophthalmologic and cardiorespiratory contraindications are excluded; adverse effects include sweating, flushing, and polyuria.

Sipping sugarless fluids frequently, chewing xylitol-containing gum, and using an OTC saliva substitute containing carboxymethylcellulose, hydroxyethylcellulose, or glycerin may help. Petroleum jelly can be applied to the lips and under dentures to relieve drying, cracking, soreness, and mucosal trauma. A cold-air humidifier may aid mouth breathers who typically have their worst symptoms at night.

Meticulous oral hygiene is essential. Patients should brush and floss regularly (including just before bedtime) and use fluoride rinses or gels daily; using newer toothpastes with added calcium and phosphates also may help avoid rampant caries. An increased frequency of preventive dental visits with plaque removal is advised. The most effective way to prevent caries is to sleep with individually fitted carriers containing 1.1% sodium fluoride or 0.4% stannous fluoride. In addition, a dentist can apply a 5% sodium fluoride varnish 2 to 4 times/yr.

Patients should avoid sugary or acidic foods and beverages and any irritating foods that are dry, spicy, astringent, or excessively hot or cold. It is particularly important to avoid ingesting sugar near bedtime.

Geriatrics Essentials

Although xerostomia becomes more common among the elderly, this is probably due to the many drugs typically used by the elderly rather than aging itself.

KEY POINTS

- Drugs are the most common cause, but systemic diseases (most commonly SS) and radiation therapy also can cause xerostomia.
- Symptomatic treatment includes increasing existing saliva flow with stimulants or drugs, and artificial saliva replacement; xylitol-containing gum and sugarless candy may be useful.
- Patients with xerostomia are at high risk of tooth decay; meticulous oral hygiene, additional preventive measures in home care, and professionally applied fluorides are essential.

103 Common Dental Disorders

CARIES

Caries is tooth decay, commonly called cavities. The symptoms—tender, painful teeth—appear late. Diagnosis is based on inspection, probing of the enamel surface with a fine metal instrument, and dental x-rays. Treatment involves removing affected tooth structure and restoring it with various materials. Fluoride, diligent dental hygiene, sealants, and proper diet can prevent virtually all caries.

Etiology

Caries is caused by acids produced by bacteria in dental plaque. Plaque is, at first, a soft, thin film of bacteria, mucin, dead epithelial cells, and food debris that develops on the tooth surface within about 24 h after the tooth is cleaned. *Streptococcus mutans* species are a group of related bacteria that grow in plaque and can cause caries. Some strains are more cariogenic than others. Eventually (commonly, after 72 h), soft plaque mineralizes, mainly with calcium, phosphate, and other minerals, becoming calculus (hard plaque or tartar), which cannot easily be removed with a toothbrush.

Risk factors: There are several risk factors for caries:

- Inadequate plaque control
- Dental defects
- Frequent dietary carbohydrates and sugars
- High-acid and/or low-fluoride environment
- Reduced salivary flow

Many teeth have open enamel pits, fissures, and grooves, which may extend from the surface to the dentin. These defects may be wide enough to harbor bacteria but too narrow to clean effectively. They predispose teeth to caries.

Frequent dietary exposure to carbohydrates and sugars promotes the growth of plaque-forming bacteria. Rampant caries in deciduous teeth suggests prolonged contact with infant formula, milk, or juice, typically when an infant goes to bed with a bottle (baby or nursing bottle caries). Thus, bedtime bottles should contain only water.

A tooth surface is more susceptible to caries when it is poorly calcified, has low fluoride exposure, and/or is in an acidic environment. Typically, decalcification begins when the pH at the tooth falls below 5.5 (eg, when lactic acid–producing bacteria colonize the area or when people drink cola beverages, which contain phosphoric acid).

The elderly often take drugs that reduce salivary flow, predisposing to caries. The elderly also have a higher incidence of root caries because of gingival recession, exposure of root surfaces, and declining manual dexterity (causing ineffective oral hygiene).

Complications: Untreated caries leads to tooth destruction, infections, and the need for extractions and replacement prostheses. Premature loss of deciduous teeth may shift the adjacent teeth, hindering eruption of their permanent successors.

Symptoms and Signs

Caries initially involves only the enamel and causes no symptoms. Caries that invades the dentin causes pain, first when hot, cold, or sweet foods or beverages contact the involved tooth, and later with chewing or percussion. Pain can be intense and persistent when the pulp is severely involved (see Pulpitis on p. 877).

Diagnosis

- Direct inspection
- Sometimes use of x-rays or special testing instruments

Routine, frequent (every 6 to 12 mo) clinical evaluation identifies early caries at a time when minimal intervention prevents its progression. A thin probe, sometimes special dyes, and transillumination by fiberoptic lights are used, frequently supplemented by new devices that detect caries by changes in electrical conductivity or laser reflectivity. However, x-rays are still important for detecting caries, determining the depth of involvement, and identifying caries under existing restorations.

Treatment

- Restorative therapy
- Sometimes a root canal and crown

Remineralization of teeth: Incipient caries (which is confined to the enamel) should be remineralized through improved home care (brushing and flossing), cleanings, prescriptions for high-fluoride toothpastes, and multiple fluoride applications at the dental office.

Restoration of teeth: The primary treatment of caries that has entered dentin is removal by drilling, followed by filling of the resultant defect. For very deep cavities, a temporary filling may be left in place 6 to 10 wk in the hope that a tooth will deposit reparative dentin, preventing exposure of the pulp, which necessitates root canal treatment.

Fillings for occlusal surfaces of posterior teeth, which bear the brunt of mastication, must be composed of strong materials, including

- Silver amalgam (most common)
- Composite resins
- Glass ionomer

Silver amalgam combines silver, mercury, copper, tin, and occasionally zinc, palladium or indium. Amalgam is inexpensive and lasts an average of 14 yr. However, if oral hygiene is good and if amalgam was placed using a rubber dam for isolation from saliva, many amalgam fillings last > 40 yr. Although concern has been raised about mercury poisoning, the number of amalgam fillings a person has bears no relationship to blood mercury levels. Replacing amalgam is not recommended because it is expensive, damages tooth structure, and actually increases patient exposure to mercury.

Composite resins, which have a more acceptable appearance, have long been used in anterior teeth, where aesthetics are primary and the forces of chewing are minimal. Some patients request them in posterior teeth as well, and they are becoming common there. However, composite resins under high occlusal stress generally last less than half as long as amalgam and tend to develop recurrent decay because the composite resin shrinks when it hardens and expands and contracts with heat and cold more than the tooth or other filling materials. The current generation of composites also closely resembles enamel but does not appear to have the same incidence of recurrent caries as earlier materials and may also last longer. However, although long-term results with these newer amalgam substitutes appear good, data equivalent in numbers and duration to those with amalgam are not yet available.

Glass ionomer, a tooth-colored filling, releases fluoride when in place, a benefit for patients especially prone to tooth decay. It is also used to restore areas damaged by overzealous brushing. Glass ionomer is not as aesthetic as composite and it should not be used on chewing surfaces because it has a high wear rate.

If decay leaves too little dentin to hold a restoration, a dentist replaces the missing dentin with cement, amalgam, composite, or other materials. Sometimes a post must be inserted into one or more roots to support a gold, silver, or composite core, which replaces the coronal dentin. This procedure necessitates a root canal filling, in which an opening is made in the tooth and the pulp is removed. The root canal system is thoroughly debrided, shaped, and then filled with gutta-percha. The outer tooth surfaces (what would have been the enamel) are then reduced so that an artificial crown, usually made of gold, porcelain, or both, can be placed. Crowns for anterior teeth are made of, or covered with, porcelain.

Prevention

- Regular brushing and flossing
- Fluoride in water, toothpaste, or both
- Regular professional cleanings
- Rarely chlorhexidine rinses and topical fluoride applications

For most people, caries is preventable. Cavities first form on permanent teeth in the early teens to late 20s. Caries-prone people typically have low exposure to fluoride and a relatively cariogenic microflora acquired from their mothers and through social contact. Maintaining good oral hygiene and minimizing sugar intake are especially important.

Removal of plaque at least every 24 h, usually by brushing and flossing, helps prevent dental caries. The gingival third of the tooth is the most important area to clean but is the area most often neglected. Brushing with an electric toothbrush for 2 min is excellent; brushing with a manual soft toothbrush for 3 to 4 min suffices. Using excess toothpaste, particularly an abrasive type, may erode the teeth. Dental floss is placed between each of the teeth, curved against the side of each tooth, and moved up and down 3 times, going just beneath the gingival margin. Flosses that are very thin or coated with wax or polytetraethylene can be used for exceptionally tight contacts between teeth or rough filling margins.

Teeth with **fluoride** incorporated into their enamel are more resistant to acidic decalcification and more readily recalcify when pH increases. If drinking water is not adequately fluoridated, oral fluoride supplements are recommended for children from shortly after birth through age 8 yr and for pregnant women beginning at 3 mo gestation (when teeth are forming in the fetus). The dose must be selected according to the amount of fluoride present in the drinking water, the age of the child, and whether topical fluoride is being used in toothpaste and/or applied during dental care. The total dose should not be so high as to cause dental fluorosis (see p. 863). Fluoridated toothpaste should also be used by people of all ages. Because young children may swallow toothpaste when brushing, which can lead to fluorosis, they should use children's toothpastes, which contain lower amounts of fluoride.

Fluoridation offers less protection against caries in pits and fissures than against those on smooth surfaces. Pits and fissures require use of sealants (plastic materials that adhere tightly to the surface of the enamel) to prevent nutrients from reaching bacteria, reducing their growth and acid production.

If these measures do not decrease cavity formation, more intensive therapy is aimed at changing the flora. After cavities are treated, pits and fissures, which can harbor *S. mutans,* are sealed. This treatment is followed by a 0.12% chlorhexidine mouth rinse used for 60 sec bid for 2 wk, which may reduce the cariogenic bacteria in plaque and allow repopulation with less cariogenic strains of *S. mutans*. To encourage this repopulation, xylitol in the form of hard candy or chewing gum is used for 5 min tid. Additionally, topical fluoride may be applied by a dentist or used at night in a custom-made fluoride carrier.

For pregnant women with a history of severe caries, the above regimen may be used before the fetus's teeth develop (about 12 weeks' gestation). If this is not feasible, the mother can use xylitol, as mentioned above, from the time of the child's birth to the age at which the mother no longer samples the child's food (the hypothesized mode of transfer).

For prevention of caries in deciduous teeth (once they have erupted) in infants, bedtime bottles should contain only water.

KEY POINTS

- Caries is caused by acids produced by bacteria in dental plaque.
- Risk factors include preexisting tooth defects, low saliva flow, an acidic oral environment, frequent exposure to carbohydrates and sugar in the diet, and inadequate exposure to fluoride.
- Treatment involves drilling out the decayed area and restoring the defect with amalgam or a composite resin.
- Prevention involves meticulous regular brushing, flossing, and professional cleaning; adequate fluoride must be available in toothpaste and, when not present in drinking water, as oral supplements for children and pregnant women.

PULPITIS

Pulpitis is inflammation of the dental pulp resulting from untreated caries, trauma, or multiple restorations. Its principal symptom is pain. Diagnosis is based on clinical findings and is confirmed by x-ray. Treatment involves removing decay, restoring the damaged tooth, and sometimes doing root canal therapy or extracting the tooth.

Pulpitis can occur when

- Caries progresses deeply into the dentin
- A tooth requires multiple invasive procedures
- Trauma disrupts the lymphatic and blood supply to the pulp

Pulpitis is designated as

- Reversible: Pulpitis begins as limited inflammation, and the tooth can be saved by a simple filling.
- Irreversible: Swelling inside the rigid encasement of the dentin compromises circulation, making the pulp necrotic, which predisposes to infection.

Complications: Infectious sequelae of pulpitis include apical periodontitis, periapical abscess, cellulitis, and osteomyelitis of the jaw. Spread from maxillary teeth may cause purulent sinusitis, meningitis, brain abscess, orbital cellulitis, and cavernous sinus thrombosis. Spread from mandibular teeth may cause Ludwig angina, parapharyngeal abscess, mediastinitis, pericarditis, empyema, and jugular thrombophlebitis.

Symptoms and Signs

In **reversible pulpitis,** pain occurs when a stimulus (usually cold or sweet) is applied to the tooth. When the stimulus is removed, the pain ceases within 1 to 2 sec.

In **irreversible pulpitis,** pain occurs spontaneously or lingers minutes after the stimulus is removed. A patient may have difficulty locating the tooth from which the pain originates, even confusing the maxillary and mandibular arches (but not the left and right sides of the mouth). The pain may then cease for several days because of pulpal necrosis. When pulpal necrosis is complete, the pulp no longer responds to hot or cold but often responds to percussion. As infection develops and extends through the apical foramen, the tooth becomes exquisitely sensitive to pressure and percussion. A periapical (dentoalveolar) abscess elevates the tooth from its socket, and the tooth feels "high" when the patient bites down.

Diagnosis

- Clinical evaluation
- Sometimes dental x-rays

Diagnosis is based on the history and physical examination, which makes use of provoking stimuli (application of heat, cold, and/or percussion). Dentists may also use an electric pulp tester, which indicates whether the pulp is alive but not whether it is healthy. If the patient feels the small electrical charge delivered to the tooth, the pulp is alive.

X-rays help determine whether inflammation has extended beyond the tooth apex and help exclude other conditions.

Treatment

- Drilling and filling for reversible pulpitis
- Root canal and crown or extraction for irreversible pulpitis
- Antibiotics (eg, amoxicillin) for infection

In **reversible pulpitis,** pulp vitality can be maintained if the tooth is treated, usually by caries removal, and then restored.

In **irreversible pulpitis,** the pulpitis and its sequelae require endodontic (root canal) therapy or tooth extraction. In endodontic therapy, an opening is made in the tooth and the pulp is removed. The root canal system is thoroughly debrided, shaped, and then filled with gutta-percha. After root canal therapy, adequate healing is manifested clinically by resolution of symptoms and radiographically by bone filling in the radiolucent area at the root apex over a period of months. If patients have systemic signs of infection (eg, fever), an oral antibiotic is prescribed (amoxicillin 500 mg q 8 h; for patients allergic to penicillin, clindamycin 150 mg or 300 mg q 6 h). If symptoms persist or worsen, root canal therapy is usually repeated in case a root canal was missed, but alternative diagnoses (eg, temporomandibular disorder, occult tooth fracture, neurologic disorder) should be considered.

Very rarely, subcutaneous or mediastinal emphysema develops after compressed air or a high-speed air turbine dental drill has been used during root canal therapy or extraction. These devices can force air into the tissues around the tooth socket that dissects along fascial planes. Acute onset of jaw and cervical swelling with characteristic crepitus of the swollen skin on palpation is diagnostic. Treatment usually is not required, although prophylactic antibiotics are sometimes given.

KEY POINTS

- Pulpitis is inflammation of the dental pulp due to deep cavities, trauma, or extensive dental repair.
- Sometimes infection develops (eg, periapical abscess, cellulitis, osteomyelitis).
- Pulpitis may be reversible or irreversible.
- In reversible pulpitis, the pulp is not necrotic, a cold or sweet stimulus causes pain that typically lasts 1 or 2 sec, and repair requires only drilling and filling.
- In irreversible pulpitis, the pulp is becoming necrotic, a cold or sweet stimulus causes pain that typically lasts minutes, and root canal or extraction is needed.
- Pulpal necrosis is a later stage of irreversible pulpitis; the pulp does not respond to hot or cold but often responds to percussion, and root canal or extraction is needed.

DENTAL APPLIANCES

Teeth may be lost to dental caries, periodontal disease, or trauma or may be removed when treatment fails. Missing teeth may cause cosmetic, phonation, and occlusal problems and may allow movement of remaining teeth.

Types of dental appliance: Dental appliances include

- Fixed bridges
- Removable partial dentures
- Removable complete dentures
- Osseo-integrated implants

A **bridge** (fixed partial denture) is composed of false teeth cast or soldered to each other and, at each end, to a crown that is cemented to natural (abutment) teeth, which bear all stress of biting. A bridge is not removed. A bridge is smaller than a removable partial denture, but one or multiple bridges can be made to replace many of the teeth in a dental arch.

A **removable partial denture,** typically an appliance with clasps that snap over abutment teeth, may be removed for cleaning and during sleep. Part of the occlusal stress may be borne by the soft tissues under the denture, often on both sides of the jaw. This appliance commonly is used when many teeth have to be replaced and bridges or implants are not feasible or affordable.

Complete dentures are removable appliances used when no teeth remain. They help a patient chew and improve speech and appearance but do not provide the efficiency or sensation of natural dentition. When teeth are absent, the mandible slowly resorbs, resulting in ill-fitting dentures that require revision (called reline or rebase) or replacement. Alternatives are oral surgical procedures to enlarge the alveolar ridge or dental implants to replace missing teeth.

An **implant** is typically a titanium cylinder or screw that replaces a tooth root. One or more implants are placed into the alveolar bone, where they ankylose. After 2 to 6 mo, artificial teeth are attached to the implants. Implants are not readily removable, although the prostheses they support can be. The potential for infection at these sites warrants scrupulous attention to oral hygiene.

Dental appliances and surgery: Generally, all removable dental appliances are removed before general anesthesia, throat surgery, or convulsive therapy to prevent their breakage or aspiration. They are stored in water to prevent changes in shape. However, some anesthesiologists believe that leaving appliances in place aids the passage of an airway tube, keeps the face in a more normal shape so that the anesthetic mask fits better, prevents natural teeth from injuring the opposing gingiva of a completely edentulous jaw, and does not interfere with laryngoscopy.

Denture problems: Occasionally, the mucosa beneath a denture becomes inflamed (denture sore mouth, inflammatory papillary hyperplasia). Contributing factors to this usually painless condition include candidal infections, poor denture fit, poor hygiene, excessive movement of the denture, and, most frequently, wearing a denture 24 h/day. The mucosa appears red and velvety. Candidal overgrowth may be indicated by adherent cottonlike patches or, more commonly, erosive lesions on the mucosa. The presence of *Candida* can be confirmed by the microscopic appearance of typical branching hyphae. Without *Candida,* inflammatory papillary hyperplasia is unlikely.

A new well-made denture almost always improves the situation. Other treatments consist of improving oral and denture hygiene, refitting the existing denture, removing the denture for extended periods, and using antifungal therapy (nystatin rinses for the mouth and overnight nystatin soaks for the denture). Soaking the denture in a commercial cleanser is sometimes helpful. Other options are applying nystatin suspension to the tissue surface of the denture and clotrimazole troches 10 mg 5 times/day. Ketoconazole 200 mg po once/day may be required. If inflammation persists, biopsy is indicated, and systemic conditions should be ruled out.

104 Dental Emergencies

Emergency dental treatment by a physician is sometimes required when a dentist is unavailable to treat the following conditions:

- Fractured and avulsed teeth
- Mandibular dislocation
- Postextraction problems (eg, bleeding, swelling and pain, alveolitis and osteomyelitis, and osteonecrosis of the jaw [ONJ])

Oral analgesics effective for most dental problems include acetaminophen 650 to 1000 mg q 6 h and NSAIDs such as ibuprofen 400 to 800 mg q 6 h. Ibuprofen and acetaminophen also can be used together for a brief period, alternating the drugs every 3 h. For severe pain, these drugs may be combined with opioids such as codeine 60 mg; hydrocodone 5 mg, 7.5 mg, or 10 mg; or oxycodone 5 mg.

Antibiotics for dental infections include penicillin VK 500 mg po q 6 h and clindamycin 300 mg po q 6 h.

Prophylactic antibiotics: Current American Heart Association guidelines (2007) recommend prophylactic antibiotics for prevention of infective endocarditis (see p. 711) in patients undergoing dental procedures only for patients with prosthetic cardiac valves, previous infective endocarditis, specific congenital heart diseases, and for cardiac transplant recipients with heart valve problems (valvulopathy). Dental procedures requiring prophylaxis are those that require manipulation or perforation of gingival or oral mucosa or that involve the root end area of the teeth (ie, those most likely to cause bacteremia). The preferred drug is amoxicillin 2 g po 30 to 60 min before the procedure. For those who cannot tolerate penicillins, alternatives include clindamycin 600 mg or cephalexin 2 g.

FRACTURED AND AVULSED TEETH

Tooth fracture: Fractures are divided by depth into those that

- Affect only the enamel
- Expose the dentin
- Expose the pulp

If the fracture involves only the enamel, patients notice rough or sharp edges but are otherwise asymptomatic. Dental treatment to smooth the edges and improve appearance is elective.

If dentin is exposed but not the dental pulp, patients usually exhibit sensitivity to cold air and water. Treatment is a mild analgesic and referral to a dentist. Dental treatment consists of restoration of the tooth by a composite (white filling) or, if the fracture is extensive, a dental crown, to cover the exposed dentin.

If the pulp is exposed (indicated by bleeding from the tooth) or if the tooth is mobile, dental referral is urgent. Dental treatment usually involves a root canal.

Root fractures and alveolar fractures are not visible, but the tooth (or several teeth) may be mobile. Dental referral is also urgent for stabilization by bonding an orthodontic arch wire or polyethylene line onto several adjacent teeth.

Tooth avulsion: Avulsed primary teeth are not replaced because they typically will become necrotic, then infected. They may also become ankylosed and do not exfoliate, thereby interfering with the eruption of the permanent tooth.

If a **permanent tooth is avulsed,** the patient should replace it in its socket immediately and seek dental care to stabilize it. If this cannot be done, the tooth should be kept immersed in milk or wrapped in a moistened paper towel and brought to a dentist for replacement and stabilization. The tooth can be rinsed gently under cold water for 10 sec if dirty but should not be scrubbed because scrubbing may remove viable periodontal ligament fibers, which aid in reattachment. A patient with an avulsed tooth should take an antibiotic (eg, penicillin VK 500 mg po q 6 h) for several days. If the avulsed tooth cannot be found, it may have been aspirated, embedded in soft tissue, or swallowed. A chest x-ray may be needed to rule out aspiration, but a swallowed tooth is harmless.

A partially avulsed tooth that is repositioned and stabilized quickly usually is permanently retained. A completely avulsed tooth may be permanently retained if replaced in the socket with minimal handling within 30 min to 1 h. Both partial and complete avulsions usually ultimately require root canal therapy because the pulp tissue becomes necrotic. When replacement of the tooth is delayed, the long-term retention rate drops, and root resorption eventually occurs. Nevertheless, a patient may be able to use the tooth for several years.

KEY POINTS

- Tooth fracture that exposes dentin but not pulp can be treated with a filling or sometimes a dental crown.
- Tooth fracture that exposes the pulp will likely require a root canal.
- An avulsed primary tooth is not replaced.
- An avulsed secondary tooth is gently rinsed (but not scrubbed) and immersed in milk or a wet paper towel for transport to a dentist for replacement in the socket.
- Avulsed teeth that are quickly replaced are often retained but ultimately most likely will require a root canal.

MANDIBULAR DISLOCATION

Spontaneous mandibular dislocation usually occurs in people with a history of such dislocations. Although a dislocated mandible is occasionally caused by trauma, the initiating episode is typically a wide opening followed by biting pressure (eg, biting into a large sandwich with hard bread), a wide yawn, or a dental procedure. People prone to dislocation may have naturally loose temporomandibular joint (TMJ) ligaments.

Patients present with a wide-open mouth that they are unable to close. Pain is secondary to patients' attempts to close the mouth. If the mandibular midline deviates to one side, the dislocation is unilateral. Although rarely used, a local anesthetic (eg, 2% lidocaine 2 to 5 mL) injected into the ipsilateral joint and into the adjacent area of insertion of the lateral pterygoid muscle may allow the mandible to reduce spontaneously.

Manual reduction may be necessary (see Fig. 104–1). Premedication may be used (eg, diazepam 5 to 10 mg IV at 5 mg/min or midazolam 3 to 5 mg IV at 2 mg/min and an opioid such as fentanyl 0.5 to 1 mcg/kg IV) but is usually unnecessary, especially if time will be lost preparing the IV. The longer the mandible is dislocated, the more difficult it is to reduce and the greater the likelihood that dislocation will recur.

A Barton bandage (see Fig. 104–2) may be needed for 2 or 3 days. Most importantly, the patient must avoid opening the mouth wide for at least 6 wk. When anticipating a yawn, the patient should place a fist under the chin to prevent wide opening. Food must be cut into small pieces. If the patient suffers from chronic dislocations and more conservative treatment modalities have been exhausted, an oral and maxillofacial surgeon may be consulted. As last-resort treatments, the ligaments around the TMJ can be surgically tightened (shortened) in an attempt to stabilize the joint or the articular eminence can be reduced (eminectomy).

POSTEXTRACTION PROBLEMS

Swelling and pain: Swelling is normal after oral surgery and is proportional to the degree of manipulation and trauma. An ice pack (or a plastic bag of frozen peas or corn, which adapts to facial contours) should be used for the first day. Cold is applied for 25-min periods every hour or 2. If swelling does not begin to subside by the 3rd postoperative day, infection is likely and

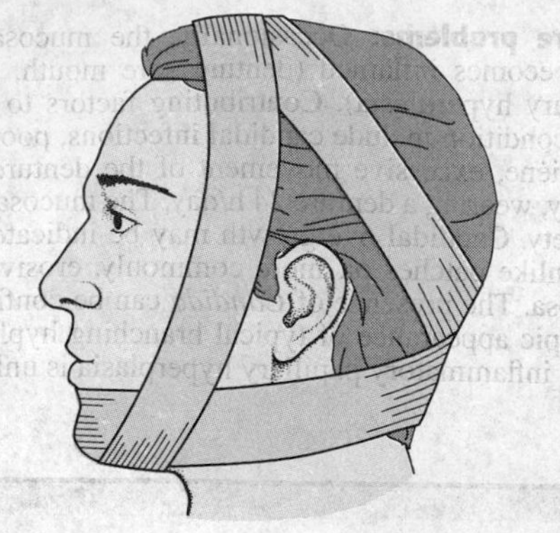

Fig. 104–2. Barton bandage. This figure 8 bandage is wrapped around the head and jaw to provide support below and anterior to the lower jaw.

an antibiotic may be given (eg, penicillin VK 500 mg po q 6 h or clindamycin 300 mg po q 6 h) until 72 h after symptoms subside.

Postoperative pain varies from moderate to severe and is treated with analgesics (see p. 1968).

Alveolitis and osteomyelitis: Postextraction alveolitis (dry socket) is pain emanating from bare bone if the socket's clot lyses. Although assumed to be due to bacterial action, it is much more common among smokers and oral contraceptive users. It is peculiar to the removal of mandibular molars, usually wisdom teeth. Typically, the pain begins on the 2nd or 3rd postoperative day, is referred to the ear, and lasts from a few days to many weeks. Alveolitis is best treated with topical analgesics: a 1- to 2-in iodoform gauze strip saturated in eugenol or coated with an anesthetic ointment, such as lidocaine 2.5% or tetracaine 0.5%, is placed in the socket. The gauze is changed every 1 to 3 days until symptoms do not return after the gauze is left out for a few hours. This procedure eliminates the need for systemic analgesics.

Osteomyelitis, which in rare cases is confused with alveolitis, is differentiated by fever, local tenderness, and swelling. If symptoms last a month, a sequestrum, which is diagnostic of osteomyelitis, should be sought by x-ray. Osteomyelitis

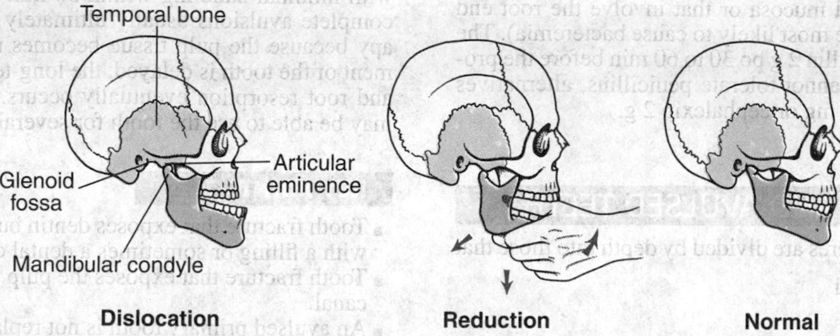

Fig. 104–1. Mandibular reduction. The patient's head is stabilized. The operator's thumbs are placed on the external oblique line of the mandible (lateral to the 3rd molar area) or, after wrapping the thumbs in gauze, on the occlusal surface of the lower molars. The other fingers are curled under the mandible. The patient is asked to open wide, as if yawning, and the operator then applies downward force on the molars while applying upward force over the chin until the mandible reduces.

requires long-term treatment with antibiotics effective against both gram-positive and gram-negative organisms and referral for definitive care.

ONJ: ONJ (see p. 323) is an oral lesion involving persistent exposure of mandibular or maxillary bone, which usually manifests with pain, loosening of teeth, and purulent discharge.[1] ONJ may occur after dental extraction but also may develop after trauma or radiation therapy to the head and neck.

Medication-related ONJ refers to the association discovered between use of antiresorptive agents and ONJ. These agents include bisphosphonates (BP), osteoclast-inhibiting drugs, and cathepsin K inhibitors. Cancer patients receiving IV BP have a 4-fold increased risk of ONJ, perhaps due to greater bioavailability of IV BP. However, oral BP therapy for noncancer patients seems to pose very low risk of ONJ; the prevalence in this population is about 0.1% according to a recent estimate. Stopping oral BP therapy is unlikely to reduce this already low rate of ONJ, and maintaining good oral hygiene is a more effective preventative measure than stopping oral BP before dental procedures. Higher doses and longer duration (therapy > 2 yr) of antiresorptive therapies are associated with ONJ. Other drugs that cause ONJ include the osteoclast inhibitor, denosumab, and some targeted anticancer agents, such as bevacizumab and sunitinib.

Management of ONJ is challenging and typically involves limited debridement, antibiotics, and oral rinses.

Bleeding: Postextraction bleeding usually occurs in the small vessels. Any clots extending out of the socket are removed with gauze, and a 4-in gauze pad (folded) or a tea bag is placed over the socket. Then the patient is instructed to apply continuous pressure by biting for 1 h. The procedure may have to be repeated 2 or 3 times. Patients are told to wait at least 1 h before checking the site so as not to disrupt clot formation. They also are informed that a few drops of blood diluted in a mouth full of saliva appear to be more blood than is actually present.

If bleeding continues, the site may be anesthetized by nerve block or local infiltration with 2% lidocaine containing 1:100,000 epinephrine. The socket is then curetted to remove the existing clot and to freshen the bone and is irrigated with normal saline. Then the area is sutured under gentle tension. Local hemostatic agents, such as oxidized cellulose, topical thrombin on a gelatin sponge, or microfibrillar collagen, may be placed in the socket before suturing.

If possible, patients taking anticoagulants (eg, aspirin, clopidogrel, warfarin) should stop therapy 3 to 4 days before surgery. Therapy can be reinstated that evening. If these measures fail, a systemic cause (eg, bleeding diathesis) is sought.

1. Khan A, Morrison A, Cheung A, et al: Osteonecrosis of the jaw (ONJ): diagnosis and management in 2015. *Osteoporos Int* 27(3):853-859, 2016. doi: 10.1007/s00198-015-3335-3.

105 Periodontal Disorders

PERIODONTITIS

(Pyorrhea)

Periodontitis is a chronic inflammatory disease of the gums resulting from an opportunistic infection of endogenous plaque biofilm. It usually manifests as a worsening of gingivitis and then, if untreated, with loosening and loss of teeth. Other symptoms are rare except in patients with HIV infection or in whom abscesses develop, in which case pain and swelling are common. Diagnosis is based on inspection, periodontal probing, and x-rays. Treatment involves dental cleaning that extends under the gums and a vigorous home hygiene program. Advanced cases may require antibiotics and surgery.

Pathophysiology

Periodontitis usually develops when gingivitis, usually with abundant plaque and calculus beneath the gingival margin, has not been adequately treated. In periodontitis, the deep pockets can harbor anaerobic organisms that do more damage than those usually present in simple gingivitis. The organisms trigger chronic release of inflammatory mediators, including cytokines, prostaglandins, and enzymes from neutrophils and monocytes. The resulting inflammation affects the periodontal ligament, gingiva, cementum, and alveolar bone. The gingiva progressively loses its attachment to the teeth, bone loss begins, and periodontal pockets deepen. With progressive bone loss, teeth may loosen, and gingiva recedes. Tooth migration is common in later stages, and tooth loss can occur.

Risk Factors

Modifiable risk factors that contribute to periodontitis include

- Plaque
- Smoking
- Obesity
- Diabetes (especially type 1)
- Emotional stress
- Vitamin C deficiency (scurvy)

Addressing these conditions can improve the treatment outcomes of periodontitis.

Classification

The classifications described here are based on the American Academy of Periodontology's (AAP) classification system for periodontal diseases and conditions (1999):

- Chronic periodontitis (formerly called adult periodontitis)
- Aggressive periodontitis (formerly the early-onset and juvenile periodontitides)
- Periodontitis as a manifestation of systemic diseases
- Necrotizing ulcerative periodontitis (formerly called HIV periodontitis)

Other AAP designations are abscesses of the peridontium, periodontitis associated with endodontic lesions, and developmental or acquired deformities and conditions. In developmental or acquired deformities and conditions, faulty occlusion, causing an excessive functional load on teeth, plus the requisite plaque and gingivitis may contribute to progression of a particular type of periodontitis characterized by angular bony defects.

Chronic periodontitis: Chronic periodontitis is the most common type of periodontitis. It occurs most often in adults > 35 yr, but adolescents and even children with primary dentition can be affected. It is characterized by its slow rate of progression, with periods of exacerbation and remission, and also by a correlation between the extent of destruction and the presence of local factors such as plaque.

About 85% of the population is affected to a mild degree, but the most advanced cases are seen in < 5% of the population. Because of its slow progression, the patient's age at presentation is not always indicative of when the disease started. Patients with significant disease tend to be > 35 yr, and tooth loss typically starts in a patient's 40s.

Based on the extent of disease, chronic periodontitis is classified further as

- Localized: ≤ 30% of teeth affected
- Generalized: > 30% of teeth affected

Aggressive periodontitis: Aggressive periodontitis is much less common than chronic periodontitis. It usually occurs in children (sometimes before age 3 yr) or young adults but also occurs in older adults. It is characterized by its familial aggregation and rapid progression of bone loss and even tooth loss. The extent of destruction usually is disproportionate to the extent of plaque or calculus. By definition, patients have no systemic illness, whereas in periodontitis as a manifestation of systemic disease, patients do have a systemic illness. Neutrophil and macrophage/monocyte function may be abnormal.

Localized aggressive periodontitis (formerly called localized juvenile periodontitis), occurs mostly in healthy adolescents. Patients often have significant colonization of *Aggregatibacter actinomycetemcomitans* (formerly *Actinobacillus actinomycetemcomitans*), and a strong antibody response to infecting bacteria often occurs. Typically, the signs of inflammation are minor. The disease is detected by periodontal probing or x-rays, which show localized, deep (vertical) bone loss. Disease involves at least two of the 1st molars and incisors and no more than two other teeth. Bone loss progresses faster than in chronic periodontitis, often at a rate of 3 to 4 μm/day; it is unclear whether localized aggressive periodontitis can be self-arresting.

Generalized aggressive periodontitis(formerly called rapidly progressive periodontitis) occurs mostly in patients aged 20 to 35. It is often associated with *A. actinomycetemcomitans, Porphyromonas gingivalis, Eikenella corrodens,* and many gram-negative bacilli, but cause and effect are not clear. A weak antibody response to infecting bacteria often occurs. All teeth may be affected, which must include ≥ 3 that are not 1st molars or incisors.

Prepubertal periodontitis, an uncommon type of aggressive periodontitis (and not recognized in the 1999 AAP classification), can result from one of the genetic disorders listed below (see Periodontitis as a manifestation of systemic disease below) but also may have its own mutation. It affects deciduous teeth, usually shortly after eruption. Generalized acute proliferative gingivitis and rapid alveolar bone destruction are its hallmarks. Patients also have frequent bouts of otitis media and are usually diagnosed by age 4 yr. In some patients, the disease resolves before the permanent teeth erupt.

Periodontitis as a manifestation of systemic disease: Periodontitis as a manifestation of systemic disease is considered in patients who have inflammation disproportionate to plaque or other local factors and who also have a systemic disease. However, distinguishing whether a disease is causing periodontitis or contributing to plaque-induced periodontitis is often difficult.

Systemic diseases associated with hematologic disease that can manifest as periodontitis include

- Acquired neutropenia
- Agranulocytosis
- Leukemias
- Lazy leukocyte syndrome
- Hypogammaglobulinemia

Systemic diseases associated with genetic disorders that can manifest as periodontitis include

- Familial, and cyclic neutropenia
- Down syndrome
- Leukocyte adhesion deficiency syndromes
- Papillon-Lefèvre syndrome
- Chédiak-Higashi syndrome
- Histiocytosis syndromes
- Glycogen storage disease
- Infantile genetic agranulocytosis
- Ehlers-Danlos syndrome (types IV and VIII)
- Hypophosphatasia
- Cohen syndrome
- Crohn disease

Necrotizing ulcerative periodontitis: Necrotizing ulcerative periodontitis is a particularly virulent, rapidly progressing disease. It is often called **HIV-associated periodontitis** because HIV is a common cause. Clinically, it resembles acute necrotizing ulcerative gingivitis combined with generalized aggressive periodontitis. Patients may lose 9 to 12 mm of attachment in as little as 6 mo.

Symptoms and Signs

Pain is usually absent unless an acute infection forms in one or more periodontal pockets or if HIV-associated periodontitis is present. Impaction of food in the pockets can cause pain at meals. Abundant plaque along with redness, swelling, and exudate are characteristic. Gums may be tender and bleed easily, and breath may be foul. As teeth loosen, particularly when only one third of the root is in the bone, chewing becomes painful.

Diagnosis

- Clinical evaluation
- Sometimes dental x-rays

Inspection of the teeth and gingiva combined with probing of the pockets and measurement of their depth are usually sufficient for diagnosis. Pockets deeper than 4 mm indicate periodontitis.

Dental x-rays reveal alveolar bone loss adjacent to the periodontal pockets.

Treatment

- Treatment of risk factors
- Scaling and root planing
- Sometimes oral antibiotics, antibiotic packs, or both
- Surgery or extraction

Treatment of modifiable risk factors such as poor oral hygiene, diabetes, and smoking improves outcomes.

For all forms of periodontitis, the first phase of treatment consists of thorough scaling (professional cleaning with hand or ultrasonic instruments) and root planing (removal of diseased or toxin-affected cementum and dentin followed by smoothing of the root) to remove plaque and calculus deposits. Thorough home oral hygiene is necessary and includes careful brushing, flossing, and use of a rubber tip to help clean. It may include chlorhexidine swabs or rinses. A therapist should help teach the patient how to do these procedures. The patient is reevaluated after 3 wk. If pockets are no deeper than 4 mm at this point, the only treatment needed is regular cleanings. Sometimes a flap of gum tissue is made to allow access for scaling and planing of deeper parts of the root.

If deeper pockets persist, systemic antibiotics can be used. A common regimen is amoxicillin 500 mg po tid for 10 days. In addition, a gel containing doxycycline or microspheres of minocycline can be placed into isolated recalcitrant pockets. These drugs are resorbed in 2 wk.

Another approach is to surgically eliminate the pocket and recontour the bone (pocket reduction/elimination surgery) so that the patient can clean the depth of the normal crevice (sulcus) between the tooth and gingiva. In certain patients, regenerative surgery and bone grafting are done to encourage alveolar bone growth. Splinting of loose teeth and selective reshaping of tooth surfaces to eliminate traumatic occlusion may be necessary. Extractions are often necessary in advanced disease. Contributing systemic factors should be controlled before initiating periodontal therapy.

Ninety percent of patients with necrotizing ulcerative periodontitis due to HIV (HIV-associated periodontitis) respond to combined treatment with scaling and planing, irrigation of the sulcus with povidone-iodine (which the dentist applies with a syringe), regular use of chlorhexidine mouth rinses, and systemic antibiotics, usually metronidazole 250 mg po tid for 14 days.

Localized aggressive periodontitis requires periodontal surgery plus oral antibiotics (eg, amoxicillin 500 mg qid or metronidazole 250 mg tid for 14 days).

KEY POINTS

- Periodontitis is an inflammatory reaction triggered by bacteria in dental plaque.
- There is loss of alveolar bone, formation of deep gum pockets, and eventually loosening of teeth.
- Treatment involves scaling and root planing and sometimes antibiotics and/or surgery.

GINGIVITIS

Gingivitis is inflammation of the gingivae, causing bleeding with swelling, redness, exudate, a change of normal contours, and, occasionally, discomfort. Diagnosis is based on inspection. Treatment involves professional teeth cleaning and intensified home dental hygiene. Advanced cases may require antibiotics or surgery.

Normally, the gingivae are firm, tightly adapted to the teeth, and contoured to a point. Keratinized gingiva near the crowns is pink stippled tissue. This tissue should fill the entire space between the crowns. The gingiva farther from the crowns, called alveolar mucosa, is nonkeratinized, highly vascular, red, movable, and continuous with the buccal mucosa. A tongue depressor should express no blood or pus from normal gingiva.

Inflammation, or gingivitis, the most common gingival problem, may evolve into periodontitis (see p. 881).

Etiology

Gingivitis can be

- Plaque induced (due to poor oral hygiene)
- Non–plaque-induced

Almost all gingivitis is **plaque induced**. Poor oral hygiene allows plaque to accumulate between the gingiva and the teeth; gingivitis does not occur in places where teeth are missing. Irritation due to plaque deepens the normal crevice (sulcus) between the tooth and gingiva, creating gingival pockets. These pockets contain bacteria that may cause gingivitis and root caries. Other local factors, such as malocclusion, dental calculus, food impaction, faulty dental restorations, and xerostomia, play a secondary role.

Plaque-induced gingivitis may be precipitated or exacerbated by hormonal changes, systemic disorders, drugs, or nutritional deficiencies.

Hormonal changes that occur at puberty, during menstrual cycles and pregnancy, and at menopause or that are due to oral (or injectable) contraceptives may exacerbate inflammation.

Systemic disorders (eg, diabetes, AIDS, vitamin deficiency, leukemia, leukopenia) can affect the response to infection. Some patients with Crohn disease have a cobblestone area of granulomatous gingival hypertrophy when intestinal flare-ups occur.

Drugs such as cyclosporin and nifedipine and severe deficiencies (rare in the US) of niacin (causing pellagra) or vitamin C (causing scurvy) can cause gingivitis.

Exposure to heavy metals (eg, lead, bismuth) may cause gingivitis and a dark line at the gingival margin.

Non–plaque-induced gingivitis occurs in a small percentage of people. Causes include bacterial, viral, and fungal infections, allergic reactions, trauma, mucocutaneous disorders (eg, lichen planus, pemphigoid), and hereditary disorders (eg, hereditary gingival fibromatosis).

Symptoms and Signs

Simple gingivitis first causes a deepening of the sulcus between the tooth and gingiva, followed by a band of red, inflamed gingiva along one or more teeth, with swelling of the interdental papillae and easily induced bleeding. Pain is usually absent. The inflammation may resolve, remain superficial for years, or occasionally progress to periodontitis.

Pericoronitis is acute, painful inflammation of the gingival flap (operculum) over a partly erupted tooth, usually around mandibular 3rd molars (wisdom teeth). Infection is common, and an abscess or cellulitis may develop. Pericoronitis often recurs as food gets trapped beneath the flap. The gingival flap disappears when the tooth is fully erupted. Many wisdom teeth do not erupt and are termed impacted.

During menopause, a desquamative gingivitis may occur. It is characterized by deep red, painful gingival tissue that bleeds easily. Vesicles may precede desquamation. The gingivae are soft because the keratinized cells that resist abrasion by food particles are absent. A similar gingival lesion may be associated with pemphigus vulgaris, bullous pemphigoid, benign mucous membrane pemphigoid, or atrophic lichen planus.

During pregnancy, swelling, especially of the interdental papillae, is likely to occur. Soft, reddish pedunculated gingival growths often arise in the interdental papillae during the 1st trimester, may persist throughout pregnancy, and may or may not subside after delivery. Such growths are pyogenic granulomas that are sometimes referred to as pregnancy tumors. They develop rapidly and then remain static. An underlying irritant is common, such as calculus or a restoration with a rough margin. These growths also may occur in nonpregnant women and men.

Uncontrolled diabetes can exaggerate the effects of gingival irritants, making secondary infections and acute gingival abscesses common.

In leukemia, the gingivae may become engorged with a leukemic infiltrate, exhibiting clinical symptoms of edema, pain, and easily induced bleeding.

In scurvy, the gingivae are inflamed, hyperplastic, and engorged, bleeding easily. Petechiae and ecchymoses may appear throughout the mouth.

In pellagra, the gingivae are inflamed, bleed easily, and are susceptible to secondary infection. Additionally, the lips are reddened and cracked, the mouth feels scalded, the tongue is smooth and bright red, and the tongue and mucosa may have ulcerations.

Diagnosis

- Clinical evaluation

Finding erythematous, friable tissue at the gum lines confirms the diagnosis of gingivitis. To detect early gingival disease, some dentists frequently measure the depth of the pocket around each tooth. Depths < 3 mm are normal; deeper pockets are at high risk of gingivitis and periodontitis.

Treatment

- Regular oral hygiene and professional cleaning

Simple gingivitis is controlled by proper oral hygiene with or without an antibacterial mouth rinse. Thorough scaling (professional cleaning with hand or ultrasonic instruments) should be done. If appropriate, poorly contoured restorations are reshaped or replaced and local irritants are removed. Excess gingiva, if present, can be excised. Drugs causing gingival hyperplasia should be stopped if possible; if not, improved home care and more frequent professional cleanings (at least every 3 mo) usually reduce the hyperplasia. Pregnancy tumors are excised.

Pericoronitis treatment consists of

- Removal of debris from under the gingival flap
- Rinses with saline, 1.5% hydrogen peroxide, or 0.12% chlorhexidine
- Extraction (particularly when episodes recur)

If severe infection develops, antibiotics may be given for a day before extraction and continued during healing. A common regimen is amoxicillin 500 mg po q 6 h for 10 days (or until 3 days after all inflammation has subsided). Abscesses associated with pericoronitis require localized incision and drainage, a periodontal flap and root debridement, or extraction.

In gingivitis caused by systemic disorders, treatment is directed at the cause. In desquamative gingivitis during menopause, sequential administration of estrogens and progestins may be beneficial, but adverse effects of this therapy (see p. 2276) limit recommendations for its use. Otherwise, dentists may prescribe a corticosteroid rinse or a corticosteroid paste that is applied directly to the gums. Gingivitis caused by pemphigus vulgaris (see p. 1010) and similar mucocutaneous conditions may require systemic corticosteroid therapy.

Prevention

Daily removal of plaque with dental floss and a toothbrush and routine cleaning by a dentist or hygienist at 6-mo to 1-yr intervals can help minimize gingivitis. Patients with systemic disorders predisposing to gingivitis require more frequent professional cleanings (from every 2 wk to every 3 mo).

KEY POINTS

- Gingivitis is caused mainly by poor oral hygiene but is sometimes due to hormonal changes (eg, pregnancy, menopause) or certain systemic disorders (eg, diabetes, AIDS).
- Professional cleaning with or without an antibacterial rinse is usually adequate treatment.
- Systemic causes must also be treated.

ACUTE NECROTIZING ULCERATIVE GINGIVITIS

(Fusospirochetosis; Trench Mouth; Vincent Infection or Vincent Angina)

Acute necrotizing ulcerative gingivitis (ANUG) is a painful infection of the gums. Symptoms are acute pain, bleeding, and foul breath. Diagnosis is based on clinical findings. Treatment is gentle debridement, improved oral hygiene, mouth rinses, supportive care, and, if debridement must be delayed, antibiotics.

ANUG occurs most frequently in smokers and debilitated patients who are under stress. Other risk factors are poor oral hygiene, nutritional deficiencies, immunodeficiency (eg, HIV/AIDS, use of immunosuppressive drugs), and sleep deprivation. Some patients also have oral candidiasis.

Symptoms and Signs

The usually abrupt onset may be accompanied by malaise or fever. The chief manifestations are

- Acutely painful, bleeding gingivae
- Excessive salivation
- Sometimes overwhelmingly foul breath (fetor oris)

Ulcerations, which are pathognomonic, are present on the dental papillae and marginal gingiva. These ulcerations have a characteristically punched-out appearance and are covered by a gray pseudomembrane. Similar lesions on the buccal mucosa and tonsils are rare. Swallowing and talking may be painful. Regional lymphadenopathy often is present.

Often, ANUG can manifest without a significant odor, and it also may manifest as a localized condition.

Diagnosis

- Clinical evaluation

Rarely, tonsillar or pharyngeal tissues are affected, and diphtheria or infection due to agranulocytosis must be ruled out by throat culture and CBC when the gum manifestations do not respond quickly to conventional therapy.

Treatment

- Debridement
- Rinses (eg, hydrogen peroxide, chlorhexidine)
- Improved oral hygiene
- Sometimes oral antibiotics

Treatment of ANUG consists of gentle debridement with a hand scaler or ultrasonic device. Debridement is done over several days. The patient uses a soft toothbrush or washcloth to wipe the teeth.

Rinses at hourly intervals with warm normal saline or twice/day with 1.5% hydrogen peroxide or 0.12% chlorhexidine may help during the first few days after initial debridement.

Essential supportive measures include improving oral hygiene (done gently at first), adequate nutrition, high fluid intake, rest, analgesics as needed, and avoiding irritation (eg, caused by smoking or hot or spicy foods). Marked improvement usually occurs within 24 to 48 h, after which debridement can be completed.

If debridement is delayed (eg, if a dentist or the instruments necessary for debridement are unavailable), oral antibiotics (eg, amoxicillin 500 mg q 8 h, erythromycin 250 mg q 6 h, or tetracycline 250 mg q 6 h) provide rapid relief and can be continued until 72 h after symptoms resolve.

Treatment of oral candidiasis (see p. 1032) is described elsewhere.

If the gingival contour inverts (ie, if the tips of papillae are lost) during the acute phase, surgery is eventually required to prevent subsequent periodontitis.

106 Temporomandibular Disorders

The term temporomandibular disorders is an umbrella term for conditions causing dysfunction of the jaw joint or pain in the jaw and face, often in or around the temporomandibular joint (TMJ), including masticatory and other muscles of the head and neck, their fascia, or both. A person is considered to have a temporomandibular disorder only if pain or limitation of motion is severe enough to require professional care.

Temporomandibular disorders typically are multifactorial in origin, but most are related to problems with muscles or joints. Internal derangements of the TMJ cause disturbed movement of the mandibular condyle in the glenoid fossa or against the cartilaginous articular disk (see Fig. 106–1). This disk, shaped like a mature red blood cell, serves as a cushion between bone surfaces. Causes for this disturbed movement include clenching and grinding of the teeth, trauma, systemic disorders (eg, arthritis), local or systemic infections, and malocclusion and missing teeth. Even persistent gum chewing can lead to symptoms.

Diagnosis

Disorders of the TMJ must be distinguished from the many conditions that mimic them (see Table 106–1). Pain exacerbated by finger pressure on the joint when the mouth is opened implicates the TMJ.

Patients are asked to describe the pain and designate painful areas. The muscles of mastication (temporalis, masseters, and medial and lateral pterygoids) and cervical and occipital muscles are palpated for general tenderness and trigger points (spots that radiate pain to another area).

Patients are observed opening the mouth as wide as is comfortable. When patients open and close their mouth with the junction of the maxillary and mandibular central incisors (normally in the midline) lined up against a vertical straight edge, the mandibular midline typically deviates toward the painful side. Palpation and auscultation of the joint during opening and closing may reveal tenderness, catching, clicking, crepitus, or popping.

Condylar motion can best be palpated by placing the 5th fingers into the external ear canals and exerting very gentle forward pressure as patients move the jaw. The average-sized patient can open the mouth at least 40 mm (measured between upper and lower central incisors). To account for differences in patient size, a patient should be able to fit 3 fingers (index, middle, ring) in the mouth on top of each other up to the first joint.

ANKYLOSIS OF THE TEMPOROMANDIBULAR JOINT

Ankylosis of the temperomandibular joint (TMJ) is immobility or fusion of the joint.

Ankylosis of the TMJ most often results from trauma or infection, but it may be congenital or a result of RA. Chronic, painless limitation of motion occurs. When ankylosis leads to arrest of condylar growth, facial asymmetry is common. Intra-articular (true) ankylosis must be distinguished from extra-articular (false) ankylosis, which may be caused by enlargement

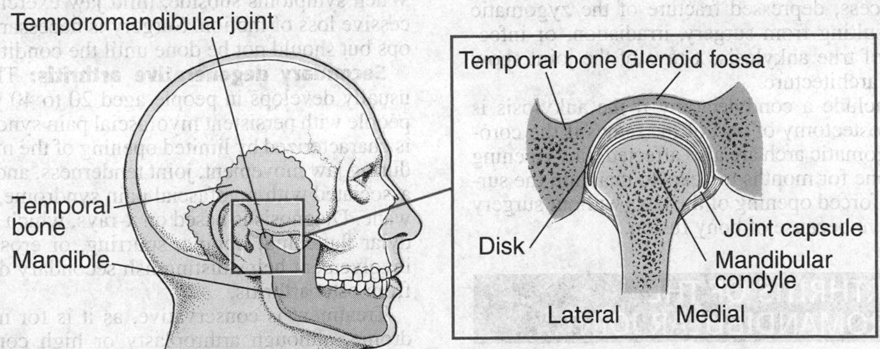

Fig. 106–1. The temporomandibular joint. The joint is formed by the mandibular condyle and the glenoid fossa of the temporal bone; a cartilaginous articular disk functions as a cushion between the joint surfaces.

Table 106–1. SOME CONDITIONS THAT MIMIC TEMPOROMANDIBULAR DISORDERS

SYMPTOM	CONDITION
Headaches	Sinusitis Temporal arteritis Tension, migraine, and cluster headaches Bruxism (causing muscle tension headaches) Referred pain originating from neck disorders
Pain	Postherpetic neuralgia Reflex sympathetic dystrophy or traumatic neuroma after head or neck surgery Head and neck trauma Toothache Trigeminal neuralgia
Pain accompanied by hearing problems	Obstruction of the ear canals or eustachian tubes Otitis media Joint inflammation
Pain in the head, neck, and other areas of the body	Fibromyalgia Generalized myofascial pain
Pain, numbness	Intracranial aneurysm Metastatic tumors
Pain that radiates to theTMJ region	Whiplash injuries affecting muscle or cervical spine
Pain that worsens when the patient swallows or turns the head	Cervical spine or muscle disorders Eagle syndrome (calcified styloid process) Glossopharyngeal neuralgia Subacute thyroiditis
Trismus	Depressed fracture of the zygomatic arch Infection Osteochondroma of the coronoid process Pericoronitis

of the coronoid process, depressed fracture of the zygomatic arch, or scarring resulting from surgery, irradiation, or infection. In most cases of true ankylosis, x-rays of the joint show loss of normal bony architecture.

Treatment may include a condylectomy if the ankylosis is intra-articular or an ostectomy of part of the ramus if the coronoid process and zygomatic arch are also affected. Jaw-opening exercises must be done for months to years to maintain the surgical correction, but forced opening of the jaws without surgery is generally ineffective because of bony fusion.

ARTHRITIS OF THE TEMPOROMANDIBULAR JOINT

Infectious arthritis, traumatic arthritis, osteoarthritis, rheumatoid arthritis (RA), and secondary degenerative arthritis can affect the temperomandibular joint (TMJ).

Infectious arthritis: Infection of the TMJ may result from direct extension of adjacent infection or hematogenous spread of bloodborne organisms (see p. 294). The area is inflamed, and jaw movement is limited and painful. Local signs of infection associated with evidence of a systemic disease or with an adjacent infection suggest the diagnosis. X-ray results are negative in the early stages but may show bone destruction later. If suppurative arthritis is suspected, the joint is aspirated to confirm the diagnosis and to identify the causative organism. Diagnosis must be made rapidly to prevent permanent joint damage.

Treatment includes antibiotics, proper hydration, pain control, and motion restriction. Parenteral penicillin G is the drug of choice until a specific bacteriologic diagnosis can be made on the basis of culture and sensitivity testing. Suppurative infections are aspirated or incised. Once the infection is controlled, jaw-opening exercises help prevent scarring and limitation of motion.

Traumatic arthritis: Rarely, acute injury (eg, due to difficult tooth extraction or endotracheal intubation) may lead to arthritis of the TMJ. Pain, tenderness, and limitation of motion occur. Diagnosis is based primarily on history. X-ray results are negative except when intra-articular edema or hemorrhage widens the joint space. Treatment includes NSAIDs, application of heat, a soft diet, and restriction of jaw movement.

Osteoarthritis: The TMJ may be affected, usually in people > 50 yr. Occasionally, patients complain of stiffness, grating, or mild pain. Crepitus results from a hole worn through the disk, causing bone to grate on bone. Joint involvement is generally bilateral. X-rays or CT may show flattening and lipping of the condyle, suggestive of dysfunctional change. Treatment is symptomatic. A mouth guard worn during the night or day may help alleviate pain and reduce grating sounds in patients with missing teeth (which can cause their jaws to come closer together when biting).

Rheumatoid arthritis: The TMJ is affected in > 17% of adults and children with RA, but it is usually among the last joints involved. Pain, swelling, and limited movement are the most common findings. In children, destruction of the condyle results in mandibular growth disturbance and facial deformity. Ankylosis may follow. X-rays of the TMJ are usually negative in early stages but later show bone destruction, which may result in an anterior open-bite deformity. The diagnosis is suggested by TMJ inflammation associated with polyarthritis and is confirmed by other findings typical of the disease.

Treatment is similar to that of RA in other joints. In the acute stage, NSAIDs may be given, and jaw function should be restricted. A mouth guard or splint worn at night is often helpful. When symptoms subside, mild jaw exercises help prevent excessive loss of motion. Surgery is necessary if ankylosis develops but should not be done until the condition is quiescent.

Secondary degenerative arthritis: This type of arthritis usually develops in people aged 20 to 40 yr after trauma or in people with persistent myofascial pain syndrome (see p. 888). It is characterized by limited opening of the mouth, unilateral pain during jaw movement, joint tenderness, and crepitus. When it is associated with myofascial pain syndrome, symptoms wax and wane. Diagnosis is based on x-rays, which generally show condylar flattening, lipping, spurring, or erosion. Unilateral joint involvement helps distinguish secondary degenerative arthritis from osteoarthritis.

Treatment is conservative, as it is for myofascial pain syndrome, although arthroplasty or high condylectomy may be necessary. An occlusal splint (mouth guard) usually relieves symptoms. The splint is worn constantly, except during meals, oral hygiene, and appliance cleaning. When symptoms resolve, the length of time that the splint is worn each day is gradually reduced. Intra-articular injection of corticosteroids may relieve symptoms but may harm the joint if repeated often.

MANDIBULAR CONDYLAR HYPERPLASIA

Mandibular condylar hyperplasia is a disorder of unknown etiology characterized by persistent or accelerated growth of the condyle when growth should be slowing or ended. Growth eventually stops without treatment.

Slowly progressive unilateral enlargement of the head and neck of the condyle causes crossbite malocclusion, facial asymmetry, and shifting of the midpoint of the chin toward the unaffected side. The patient may appear prognathic. The lower border of the mandible is often convex on the affected side. Chondroma and osteochondroma may cause similar symptoms and signs, but they grow more rapidly and may cause even greater asymmetric condylar enlargement.

Diagnosis

- Plain x-rays
- Usually CT

On plain x-rays, the TMJ may appear normal, or the condyle may be proportionally enlarged and the mandibular neck elongated. CT is usually done to determine whether bone growth is generalized, which confirms the diagnosis, or localized to part of the condylar head. If growth is localized, a biopsy may be necessary to distinguish between tumor and hyperplasia.

Treatment

- During active growth, usually condylectomy
- After growth cessation, orthodontics followed by surgical mandibular repositioning

Treatment usually includes condylectomy during the period of active growth. If growth has stopped, orthodontics and surgical mandibular repositioning are indicated. If the height of the mandibular body is greatly increased, facial symmetry can be further improved by reducing the inferior border.

MANDIBULAR CONDYLAR HYPOPLASIA

Mandibular condylar hypoplasia is facial deformity caused by a short mandibular ramus.

This condition usually results from trauma, infection, or irradiation occurring during the growth period but may be idiopathic. The deformity involves fullness of the face, deviation of the chin toward the affected side, an elongated mandible, and flatness of the face on the unaffected side. (The side to which the ramus is short causes muscles to appear fuller; the muscles on the unaffected side are stretched so that side appears flatter.) Mandibular deviation causes malocclusion.

Diagnosis is based on a history of progressive facial asymmetry during the growth period and x-ray evidence of condylar deformity and antegonial notching (a depression in the inferior border of the mandible just anterior to the angle of the mandible). There is frequently a causative history.

Treatment consists of surgical shortening of the unaffected side of the mandible or lengthening of the affected side. Presurgical orthodontic therapy helps optimize results.

INTERNAL TEMPOROMANDIBULAR JOINT DERANGEMENT

The most common form of internal temperomandibular joint (TMJ) derangement is anterior misalignment or displacement of the articular disk above the condyle. Symptoms are localized joint pain and popping on jaw movement. Diagnosis is based on history and physical examination. Treatment is with analgesics, jaw rest, muscle relaxation, physical therapy, and bite splinting. If these methods fail, surgery may be necessary. Early treatment greatly improves results.

The superior head of the lateral pterygoid muscle may pull the articular disk out of place anteriorly when abnormal jaw mechanics cause it to spasm. Abnormal jaw mechanics can be due to congenital or acquired asymmetries or to the sequelae of trauma or arthritis. If the disk remains anterior, the derangement is said to be without reduction. Restricted jaw opening (locked jaw) and pain in the ear and around the TMJ may result. If at some point in the joint's excursion the disk returns to the head of the condyle, the derangement is said to be with reduction. Derangement with reduction occurs in about one third of the population at some point.

All types of derangement can cause capsulitis (or synovitis), which is inflammation of the tissues surrounding the joint (eg, tendons, ligaments, connective tissue, synovium). Capsulitis can also occur spontaneously or result from arthritis, trauma, or infection.

Symptoms and Signs

Disk derangement with reduction often causes a clicking or popping sound when the mouth is opened. Pain may be present, particularly when chewing hard foods. Patients are often embarrassed because they think others can hear noise when they chew. Indeed, although the sound seems louder to the patient, others can sometimes hear it.

Disk derangement without reduction usually causes no sound, but maximum opening between the tips of the upper and lower incisors is reduced from the normal 45 to 50 mm to ≤ 30 mm. Pain and a change in the patient's perception of their bite generally result. It usually manifests acutely in a patient with a chronically clicking joint; about 8 to 9% of the time, the patient wakes up unable to open the jaw fully.

Capsulitis results in localized joint pain, tenderness, and, sometimes, restricted opening.

Diagnosis

- Clinical evaluation

Diagnosis of disk derangement with reduction requires observation of the jaw when the mouth is opened. When the jaw is opened > 10 mm (measured between upper and lower incisors), a click or pop is heard, or a catch is felt, as the disk pops back over the head of the condyle. The condyle remains on the disk during further opening. Usually, another, more subtle (reciprocal) click is heard during closing when the condyle slips over the posterior rim of the disk and the disk slips forward.

Diagnosis of disk derangement without reduction requires that the patient open as wide as possible. The opening is measured, and gentle pressure is then exerted to open the mouth a little wider. Normally, the jaw opens about 45 to 50 mm; if the disk is deranged, it will open about ≤ 30 mm. Closing or protruding the jaw against resistance worsens the pain.

MRI is usually done to confirm presence of a disk derangement or to determine why a patient is not responding to treatment.

Capsulitis is often diagnosed based on a history of injury or infection along with exquisite tenderness over the joint and by exclusion when pain remains after treatment for myofascial pain syndrome, disk derangement, arthritis, and structural asymmetries. However, capsulitis may be present with any of these conditions.

Treatment

- Analgesics as needed
- Sometimes nonsurgical treatments such as exercising devices (eg, passive jaw motion devices) or repositioning occlusal splints
- Surgery if conservative treatment fails
- Sometimes corticosteroid injection for capsulitis

Disk derangement with reduction does not require treatment if the patient can open reasonably wide (about 40 mm or the width of the index, middle, and ring fingers) without discomfort. If pain occurs, mild analgesics, such as NSAIDs (ibuprofen 400 mg po q 6 h), can be used. Some patients benefit from doing passive jaw-motion exercises using commercially available mechanical devices.

If onset is < 6 mo, an anterior repositioning splint may be used to position the mandible forward and on the disk. This splint is a horseshoe-shaped appliance of hard, transparent acrylic (plastic) made to fit snugly over the teeth of one arch. Its chewing surface is designed to hold the mandible forward when the patient closes on the splint. In this position, the disk is always on the head of the condyle. The splint is gradually adjusted to allow the mandible to move posteriorly. If the disk stays with the condyle as the superior head of the external pterygoid stretches, the disk is said to be captured. The longer the disk is displaced, the more deformed it becomes and the less likely repositioning will succeed. Surgical plication of the disk may be done, with variable success.

Disk derangement without reduction may not require treatment other than analgesics. Splints may help if the articular disk has not been significantly deformed, but long-term use may result in irreversible changes in oral architecture. In some cases, the patient is instructed to slowly stretch the disk out of position, which allows the jaw to open normally. Various arthroscopic and open surgical procedures are available when conservative treatment fails.

Capsulitis is initially treated with NSAIDs, jaw rest, and muscle relaxation. Sometimes a splint worn at night or during the day may be used briefly until the inflammation decreases. If these treatments are unsuccessful, corticosteroids may be injected into the joint, or arthroscopic joint lavage and debridement are used.

KEY POINTS

- The articular disk is pulled out of place anteriorly due to abnormal jaw mechanics; it may remain displaced (without reduction) or return (with reduction).
- Disk displacement with reduction typically causes clicking and pain with chewing.
- Disk displacement without reduction does not cause clicking but reduces maximum jaw opening to ≤ 30 mm.
- Surrounding tissues may become painfully inflamed (capsulitis).
- Analgesics, repositioning splints, and passive jaw-motion exercisers often help, but surgery is occasionally required.

MYOFASCIAL PAIN SYNDROME

Myofascial pain syndrome (previously known as myofascial pain and dysfunction syndrome [MFPDS]) can occur in patients with a normal temperomandibular joint (TMJ). It is caused by tension, fatigue, or spasm in the masticatory muscles (medial or internal and lateral or external pterygoids, temporalis, and masseter). Symptoms include bruxism, pain and tenderness in and around the masticatory apparatus or referred to other locations in the head and neck, and, often, abnormalities of jaw mobility. Diagnosis is based on history and physical examination. Conservative treatment, including analgesics, muscle relaxation, habit modification, and bite splinting, usually is effective.

This syndrome is the most common disorder affecting the temporomandibular region. It is more common among women and has a bimodal age distribution in the early 20s and around menopause.

The muscle spasm causing the disorder usually is the result of nocturnal bruxism (clenching or grinding of the teeth—see p. 864). Whether bruxism is caused by irregular tooth contacts, emotional stress, or sleep disorders is controversial. Bruxism usually has a multifactorial etiology. Myofascial pain syndrome is not limited to the muscles of mastication. It can occur anywhere in the body, most commonly involving muscles in the neck and back.

Symptoms and Signs

Symptoms include pain and tenderness of the masticatory muscles and often pain and limitation of jaw excursion. Both nocturnal bruxism and sleep-disordered breathing (such as obstructive sleep apnea and upper airway resistance syndrome) can lead to headache that is more severe on awakening and gradually subsides during the day. Such pain must be distinguished from giant cell arteritis. Daytime symptoms, including jaw muscle fatigue, jaw pain, and headaches, may worsen if bruxing continues throughout the day.

The jaw deviates when the mouth opens but usually not as suddenly or always at the same point of opening as it does with internal TMJ derangement (see p. 887). Exerting gentle pressure, the examiner can open the patient's mouth another 1 to 3 mm beyond unaided maximum opening.

Diagnosis

- Clinical evaluation
- Sometimes polysomnography

A simple test may aid the diagnosis: two or three tongue blades are placed between the rear molars on each side, and the patient is asked to close the mouth gently. The distraction produced in the joint space may ease the symptoms. X-rays usually do not help except to rule out arthritis. If giant cell arteritis is suspected, ESR is measured.

Polysomnography should be done if sleep-disordered breathing is suspected.

Treatment

- Mild analgesics
- Splint or mouth guard
- An anxiolytic at bedtime can be considered
- Physical therapy modalities considered

A plastic splint or mouth guard from a dentist can keep teeth from contacting each other and prevent the damages caused by bruxism. Comfortable, heat-moldable splints are available from many sporting goods stores or drugstores; however, these types of splints should be used briefly and only as short-term diagnostic tools. Because teeth may move, mouth guards that are properly made and fitted by a dentist are recommended.

Low doses of a benzodiazepine at bedtime are often effective for acute exacerbations and temporary relief of symptoms; however, in patients with associated sleep disorders, such as sleep apnea, anxiolytics and muscle relaxants should be used with caution because they can aggravate these conditions. Mild analgesics, such as NSAIDs or acetaminophen, are indicated. Cyclobenzaprine may help muscle relaxation in some people. Because the condition is chronic, opioids should not be used, except perhaps briefly for acute exacerbations.

The patient must learn to stop clenching the jaw and grinding the teeth when awake. Hard-to-chew foods and chewing gum should be avoided. Physical therapy, biofeedback to encourage relaxation, and counseling help some patients. Physical modalities include transcutaneous electric nerve stimulation (TENS) and "spray and stretch," in which the jaw is stretched open after the skin over the painful area has been chilled with ice or sprayed with a skin refrigerant, such as ethyl chloride. Botulinum toxin has recently been used successfully to relieve muscle spasm in myofascial pain syndrome. Most patients, even if untreated, stop having significant symptoms within 2 to 3 yr.

KEY POINTS

- Myofascial pain syndrome is a more common cause of temporomandibular pain than TMJ derangement.
- Tension, fatigue, and spasm of the masticatory muscles results from nocturnal bruxism.
- Patients have pain and tenderness of the masticatory muscles, painful limitation of jaw excursion, and sometimes headache.
- Bedtime use of splints or mouth guards and a benzodiazepine may help, along with nonopioid analgesics.

SECTION 10

Eye Disorders

107 Approach to the Ophthalmologic Patient

It is important to understand the anatomy of the eye prior to doing an examination (see Fig. 107–1).

The eye can be examined with routine equipment, including a standard ophthalmoscope; thorough examination requires special equipment and evaluation by an ophthalmologist.

History

History includes location, speed of onset, and duration of current symptoms and history of previous ocular symptoms; the presence and nature of pain, discharge, or redness; and changes in visual acuity. Worrisome symptoms besides vision loss and eye pain include flashing lights, showers of floaters (both of which may be symptoms of retinal detachment), diplopia, and loss of peripheral vision.

Physical Examination

Visual acuity: The first step is to record visual acuity. Many patients do not give a full effort. Providing adequate time and coaxing patients tend to yield more accurate results. Visual acuity is measured with and without the patient's own glasses. If patients do not have their glasses, a pinhole refractor is used. If a commercial pinhole refractor is unavailable, one can be made at the bedside by poking holes through a piece of cardboard using an 18-gauge needle and varying the diameter of each hole slightly. Patients choose the hole that corrects vision the most. If acuity corrects with pinhole refraction, the problem is a refractive error. Pinhole refraction is a rapid, efficient way to diagnose refractive errors, which are the most common cause of blurred vision. However, with pinhole refraction, best correction is usually to only about 20/30, not 20/20.

Visual acuity in each eye is tested as the opposite eye is covered with a solid object (not the patient's fingers, which may separate during testing). Patients look at an eye chart 20 ft (6 m) away. If this test cannot be done, acuity can be measured by using a chart held about 36 cm (14 in) from the eye. Normal and abnormal vision is quantified by Snellen notation. A Snellen notation of 20/40 (6/12) indicates that the smallest letter that can be read by someone with normal vision at 40 ft (12 m) has to be brought to 20 ft (6 m) before it is recognized by the patient. Vision is recorded as the smallest line in which the patient can read half of the letters, even if the patient feels that the letters are blurry or they have to guess. If the patient cannot read the top line of the Snellen chart at 20 ft (6 m), acuity is tested at 10 ft (3 m). If nothing can be read from a chart even at the closest distance, the examiner holds up different numbers

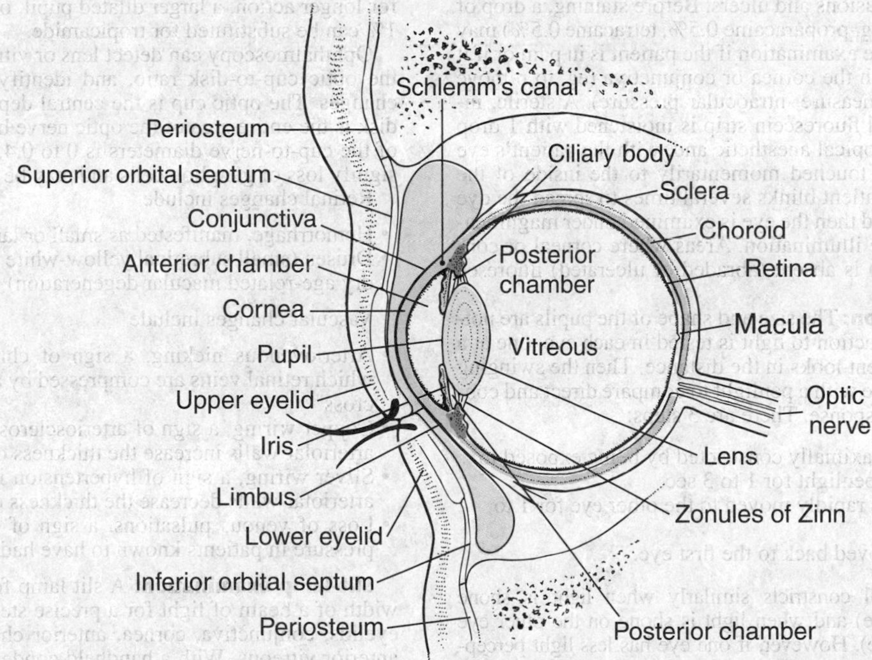

Fig. 107–1. Cross-section of the eye. The zonules of Zinn keep the lens suspended, and the muscles of the ciliary body focus the lens. The ciliary body also secretes aqueous humor, which fills the anterior and posterior chambers, passes through the pupil into the anterior chamber, and drains primarily via the Schlemm canal (see Fig. 112–1 on p. 934). The iris regulates the amount of light entering the eye by adjusting the size of its central opening, the pupil. Visual images are focused on the retina. The conjunctiva covers the eyeball and lines the upper and lower eyelids; it ends at the limbus. The cornea is covered with epithelium that is more sensitive than and differs from the conjunctival epithelium.

of fingers to see whether the patient can accurately count them. If not, the examiner tests whether the patient can perceive hand motion. If not, a light is shined into the eye to see whether light is perceived.

Near vision is checked by asking patients to read a standard near card or newsprint at 14 in (36 cm); patients > 40 yr who require corrective lenses (reading glasses) should wear them during near vision testing.

Refractive error can be estimated roughly with a handheld ophthalmoscope by noting the lens necessary for the examiner to focus on the retina; this procedure requires examiners to use their own corrective lenses and is never a substitute for a comprehensive assessment of refraction. More commonly, refractive error is measured with a standard phoropter or an automated refractor (a device that measures changes in light projected and reflected by the patient's eye). These devices also measure astigmatism (see p. 954).

Eyelid and conjunctival examination: Eyelid margins and periocular cutaneous tissues are examined under a focal light and magnification (eg, provided by loupe, slit lamp, or ophthalmoscope). In cases of suspected dacryocystitis or canaliculitis, the lacrimal sacs are palpated and an attempt is made to express any contents through the canaliculi and puncta. After eyelid eversion, the palpebral and bulbar conjunctivae and the fornices can be inspected for foreign bodies, signs of inflammation (eg, follicular hypertrophy, exudate, hyperemia, edema), or other abnormalities.

Corneal examination: Indistinct or blurred edges of the corneal light reflex (reflection of light from the cornea when illuminated) suggest the corneal surface is not intact or is roughened, as occurs with a corneal abrasion or keratitis. Fluorescein staining reveals abrasions and ulcers. Before staining, a drop of topical anesthetic (eg, proparacaine 0.5%, tetracaine 0.5%) may be added to facilitate examination if the patient is in pain or if it is necessary to touch the cornea or conjunctiva (eg, to remove a foreign body or measure intraocular pressure). A sterile, individually packaged fluorescein strip is moistened with 1 drop of sterile saline or topical anesthetic and, with the patient's eye looking upward, is touched momentarily to the inside of the lower eyelid. The patient blinks several times to spread the dye into the tear film, and then the eye is examined under magnification and cobalt blue illumination. Areas where corneal or conjunctival epithelium is absent (abraded or ulcerated) fluoresce green.

Pupil examination: The size and shape of the pupils are noted, and pupillary reaction to light is tested in each eye, one at a time, while the patient looks in the distance. Then the swinging flashlight test is done with a penlight to compare direct and consensual pupillary response. There are 3 steps:

1. One pupil is maximally constricted by being exposed to light from the penlight for 1 to 3 sec.
2. The penlight is rapidly moved to the other eye for 1 to 3 sec.
3. The light is moved back to the first eye.

Normally, a pupil constricts similarly when light is shone on it (direct response) and when light is shone on the other eye (consensual response). However, if one eye has less light perception than the other, as caused by dysfunction of the afferent limb (from the optic nerve to the optic chiasm) or extensive retinal disease, then the *consensual* response in the affected eye is stronger than the *direct* response. Thus, on step 3 of the swinging light test, when the light is shined back on the affected eye, it paradoxically appears to dilate. This finding indicates a relative afferent pupillary defect (RAPD, or Marcus Gunn pupil).

Extraocular muscles: The examiner guides the patient to look in 8 directions (up, up and right, right, down and right, down, down and left, left, left and up) with a moving finger, penlight, or transillumination light, observing for gaze deviation, limitation of movement, disconjugate gaze, or a combination consistent with cranial nerve palsy, orbital disease, or other abnormalities that restrict movement.

Ophthalmoscopy: Ophthalmoscopy (examination of the posterior segment of the eye) can be done directly by using a handheld ophthalmoscope or with a handheld lens in conjunction with the slit lamp biomicroscope. Indirect ophthalmoscopy can be done by using a head-mounted ophthalmoscope with a handheld lens. With handheld ophthalmoscopy, the examiner dials the ophthalmoscope to zero diopters, then increases or decreases the setting until the fundus comes into focus. The view of the retina is limited with a handheld ophthalmoscope, whereas indirect ophthalmoscopy gives a 3-dimensional view and is better for visualizing the peripheral retina, where retinal detachment most commonly occurs.

The view of the fundus can be improved by dilating the pupils. Before dilation, the anterior chamber depth is estimated because mydriasis can precipitate an attack of acute angle-closure glaucoma if the anterior chamber is shallow. Depth can be estimated with a slit lamp or less accurately with a penlight held at the temporal limbus parallel to the plane of the iris and pointed toward the nose. If the medial iris is in shadow, the chamber is shallow and dilation should be avoided. Other contraindications to dilation include head trauma, suspicion of a ruptured globe, a narrow angle, and angle-closure glaucoma.

Pupils can be dilated using 1 drop of tropicamide 1%, phenylephrine 2.5%, or both (repeated in 5 to 10 min if necessary); for longer action, a larger dilated pupil, or both, cyclopentolate 1% can be substituted for tropicamide.

Ophthalmoscopy can detect lens or vitreous opacities, assess the optic cup-to-disk ratio, and identify retinal and vascular changes. The optic cup is the central depression, and the optic disk is the entire area of the optic nerve head. The normal ratio of the cup-to-nerve diameters is 0 to 0.4. A ratio of ≥ 0.5 may signify loss of ganglion cells and may be a sign of glaucoma.

Retinal changes include

- Hemorrhage, manifested as small or large areas of blood
- Drusen (small subretinal yellow-white spots that may signify dry age-related macular degeneration)

Vascular changes include

- Arteriovenous nicking, a sign of chronic hypertension in which retinal veins are compressed by arteries where the two cross
- Copper wiring, a sign of arteriosclerosis in which thickened arteriolar walls increase the thickness of the light reflex
- Silver wiring, a sign of hypertension in which thin, fibrotic arteriolar walls decrease the thickness of the light reflex
- Loss of venous pulsations, a sign of increased intracranial pressure in patients known to have had pulsations

Slit-lamp examination: A slit lamp focuses the height and width of a beam of light for a precise stereoscopic view of the eyelids, conjunctiva, cornea, anterior chamber, iris, lens, and anterior vitreous. With a handheld condensing lens, it can also be used for detailed examination of the retina and macula. It is especially useful for the following:

- Identifying corneal foreign bodies and abrasions
- Measuring depth of the anterior chamber
- Detecting cells (RBCs or WBCs) and flare (evidence of protein) in the anterior chamber

- Identifying scleral edema, which is seen as a bowing forward of the slit beam when it is focused beneath the conjunctiva and which is usually a sign of scleritis
- Identifying diseases such as macular degeneration, diabetic eye disease, preretinal membranes, macular edema, and retinal tears (when using a condensing lens)

Tonometry and gonioscopy, which quantifies the iridocorneal angle and requires the use of a special lens, may be done.

Visual field testing: Visual fields may be impaired by lesions anywhere in the neural visual pathways from the optic nerves to the occipital lobes (see Table 107–1 and Fig. 114–1 on p. 946). Glaucoma causes loss of peripheral vision. Fields can be assessed grossly by direct confrontation testing or by more precise, more detailed testing.

In **direct confrontation,** patients maintain a fixed gaze at the examiner's eye or nose. The examiner brings a small target (eg, a match or a finger) from the patients' visual periphery into each of the 4 visual quadrants and asks patients to indicate when they first see the object. Slowly wiggling the small target helps patients separate and define it. Another method of direct confrontation visual field testing is to hold a number of fingers in each quadrant and ask patients how many they see. For both methods, each eye is tested separately. Abnormalities in target detection should prompt detailed testing with more precise instruments.

More detailed methods include use of a tangent screen, Goldmann perimeter, or computerized automated perimetry (in which the visual field is mapped out in detail based on patient response to a series of flashing lights in different locations controlled by a standardized computer program). The Amsler grid is used to test central vision. Distortion of the grid (metamorphopsia) or a missing area (central scotoma) may indicate disease of the macula (eg, choroidal neovascularization), as occurs in age-related macular degeneration.

Color vision testing: Twelve to 24 Ishihara color plates, which have colored numbers or symbols hidden in a field of colored dots, are commonly used to test color vision. Color-blind patients or patients with acquired color deficiency (eg, in optic nerve diseases) cannot see some or all of the hidden numbers. Most congenital color blindness is red-green; most acquired (eg, caused by glaucoma or optic nerve disease) is blue-yellow.

Testing

Tonometry: Tonometry measures intraocular pressure by determining the amount of force needed to indent the cornea. Handheld pen-type tonometers are used for screening. This test requires topical anesthesia (eg, proparacaine 0.5%). Another handheld tonometer, the icare tonometer, can be used without topical anesthesia. The icare tonometer is useful in children and is widely used in emergency departments by

Table 107–1. TYPES OF FIELD DEFECTS

TYPE*	DESCRIPTION	CAUSES
Altitudinal field defect	Loss of all or part of the superior or inferior half of the visual field; does not cross the horizontal median	*More common*: Ischemic optic neuropathy, hemibranch retinal artery occlusion, retinal detachment *Less common*: Glaucoma, optic nerve or chiasmal lesion, optic nerve coloboma
Arcuate scotoma	A small, bow-shaped (arcuate) visual field defect that follows the arcuate pattern of the retinal nerve fibers; does not cross the horizontal median	Damage to ganglion cells that feed into a particular part of the optic nerve head *More common*: Glaucoma *Less common*: Ischemic optic neuropathy (usually nonarteritic), optic disk drusen, high myopia
Binasal field defect (uncommon)	Loss of all or part of the medial half of both visual fields; does not cross the vertical median	*More common*: Glaucoma, bitemporal retinal disease (eg, retinitis pigmentosa) *Rare*: Bilateral occipital disease, tumor or aneurysm compressing both optic nerves
Bitemporal hemianopia	Loss of all or part of the lateral half of both visual fields; does not cross the vertical median	*More common*: Chiasmal lesion (eg, pituitary adenoma, meningioma, craniopharyngioma, aneurysm, glioma) *Less common*: Tilted optic disks *Rare*: Nasal retinitis pigmentosa
Blind-spot enlargement	Enlargement of the normal blind spot at the optic nerve head	Papilledema, optic nerve drusen, optic nerve coloboma, myelinated nerve fibers at the optic disk, drugs, myopic disk with a crescent
Central scotoma	A loss of visual function in the middle of the visual field	Macular disease, optic neuropathy (eg, ischemic or Leber hereditary neuropathy, optic neuritis-multiple sclerosis), optic atrophy (eg, due to tumor compressing the nerve or toxic-metabolic disorders) *Rare*: Occipital cortex lesion
Constriction of the peripheral fields, leaving only a small residual central field	Loss of the outer part of the entire visual field in one or both eyes	Glaucoma, retinitis pigmentosa or another peripheral retinal disorder, chronic papilledema after panretinal photocoagulation, central retinal artery occlusion with cilioretinal artery sparing, bilateral occipital lobe infarction with macular sparing, nonphysiologic vision loss, carcinoma-associated retinopathy *Rare*: Drugs
Homonymous hemianopia	Loss of part or all of the left half or right half of both visual fields; does not cross the vertical median	Optic tract or lateral geniculate body lesion; lesion in temporal, parietal, or occipital lobe (more commonly, stroke or tumor; less commonly, aneurysm or trauma); migraine (which may cause transient homonymous hemianopia)

*Migraine can cause various visual field defects, although it most commonly causes homonymous hemianopia.
Adapted from Rhee DJ, Pyfer MF: *The Wills Eye Manual*, ed. 3. Philadelphia, Lippincott Williams & Wilkins, 1999.

nonophthalmologists. Office-based screening with noncontact air-puff tonometry also can be used; it requires less training because it makes no direct corneal contact. Goldmann applanation tonometry is the most accurate method but requires more training and typically is used only by ophthalmologists. Measurement of intraocular pressure alone is not adequate screening for glaucoma; the optic nerve also should be examined.

Angiography: Fluorescein angiography is used to investigate underperfusion and neovascularization in conditions such as diabetes, age-related macular degeneration, retinal vascular occlusion, and ocular inflammation. It is also useful in preoperative assessment for retinal laser procedures. After IV injection of fluorescein solution, the retinal, choroidal, optic disk, or iris vasculature is photographed in rapid sequence.

Indocyanine green angiography is used to image vasculature of the retina and choroid and can sometimes provide more detail on choroidal vasculature than can fluorescein angiography. It is used to image age-related macular degeneration and can be particularly helpful in detection of neovascularization.

Optical coherence tomography: Optical coherence tomography (OCT) provides high-resolution images of posterior eye structures, such as the retina (including retinal pigment epithelium), choroid, and posterior vitreous. Retinal edema can be identified. OCT works in a manner similar to that of ultrasonography but uses light instead of sound; it does not involve contrast use or ionizing radiation and is noninvasive. OCT is useful in imaging retinal disorders that cause macular edema or fibrous proliferation over or underneath the macula, including age-related macular degeneration, diabetic edema, macular holes, and epiretinal membranes. It is also useful for monitoring progression of glaucoma.

Electroretinography: Electrodes are placed on each cornea and on the surrounding skin, and electrical activity in the retina is recorded. This technique evaluates retinal function in patients with retinal degeneration. It does not evaluate vision.

Ultrasonography: B-mode ultrasonography provides 2-dimensional structural information even in the presence of opacities of the cornea and lens. Examples of ophthalmologic applications include assessment of retinal tumors, detachments, and vitreous hemorrhages; location of foreign bodies; detection of posterior scleral edema characteristic of posterior scleritis; and distinction of choroidal melanoma from metastatic carcinoma and subretinal hemorrhage.

A-mode ultrasonography is 1-dimensional ultrasonography used to determine the axial length of the eye, a measurement needed to calculate the power of an intraocular lens for implantation as a part of cataract surgery.

Ultrasonic pachymetry is use of ultrasonography to measure the thickness of the cornea before refractive surgery (eg, laser in situ keratomileusis [LASIK]) and in patients with corneal dystrophies.

CT and MRI: These imaging techniques most often are used for evaluation of ocular trauma, particularly if an intraocular foreign body is suspected, and in the evaluation of orbital tumors, optic neuritis, and optic nerve tumors. MRI should not be done when there is suspicion of a metallic intraocular foreign body.

Electronystagmography: See p. 785.

108 Symptoms of Ophthalmologic Disorders

ACUTE VISION LOSS

Loss of vision is usually considered acute if it develops within a few minutes to a couple of days. It may affect one or both eyes and all or part of a visual field. Patients with small visual field defects (eg, caused by a small retinal detachment) may describe their symptoms as blurred vision.

Pathophysiology

Acute loss of vision has 3 general causes:

- Opacification of normally transparent structures through which light rays pass to reach the retina (eg, cornea, vitreous)
- Retinal abnormalities
- Abnormalities affecting the optic nerve or visual pathways

Etiology

The most common causes of acute loss of vision are

- Vascular occlusions of the retina (central retinal artery occlusion [see Plate 10], central retinal vein occlusion [see Plate 11])
- Ischemic optic neuropathy (often in patients with temporal arteritis)
- Vitreous hemorrhage (caused by diabetic retinopathy or trauma)
- Trauma

In addition, sudden recognition of loss of vision (pseudosudden loss of vision) may manifest initially as sudden onset. For example, a patient with long-standing reduced vision in one eye (possibly caused by a dense cataract) suddenly is aware of the reduced vision in the affected eye when covering the unaffected eye.

Presence or absence of pain helps categorize loss of vision (see Table 108–1).

Most disorders that cause total loss of vision when they affect the entire eye may affect only part of the eye and cause only a visual field defect (eg, branch occlusion of the retinal artery or retinal vein, local retinal detachment).

Less common causes of acute loss of vision include

- Anterior uveitis (a common disorder, but one that usually causes eye pain severe enough to trigger evaluation before vision is lost)
- Aggressive retinitis
- Certain drugs (eg, methanol, salicylates, ergot alkaloids, quinine)

Evaluation

History: History of present illness should describe loss of vision in terms of onset, duration, progression, and location (whether it is monocular or binocular and whether it involves the entire visual field or a specific part and which part). Important associated visual symptoms include floaters, flashing lights, halos around lights, distorted color vision, and jagged or mosaic patterns (scintillating scotomata). The patient should be asked about eye pain and whether it is constant or occurs only with eye movement.

Table 108–1. SOME CAUSES OF ACUTE VISION LOSS

CAUSE	SUGGESTIVE FINDINGS	DIAGNOSTIC APPROACH
Acute loss of vision without eye pain		
Amaurosis fugax	Monocular blindness lasting minutes to hours (typically < 5 min when due to cerebrovascular disease)	Consideration of Carotid ultrasonography Echocardiography MRI or CT ECG Continuous monitoring of cardiac rhythm
Arteritic ischemic optic neuropathy (usually in patients with giant cell [temporal] arteritis)	Sometimes headache, jaw or tongue claudication, temporal artery tenderness or swelling, pale and swollen disk with surrounding hemorrhages, occlusion of retinal artery or its branches Sometimes proximal myalgias with stiffness (due to polymyalgia rheumatica)	ESR, C-reactive protein (CRP), platelet count Temporal artery biopsy
Functional loss of vision (uncommon)	Normal pupillary light reflexes, positive optokinetic nystagmus, no objective abnormalities on eye examination Often inability to write name or bring outstretched hands together Sometimes indifferent affect despite severity of claimed loss of vision	Clinical evaluation If diagnosis is in doubt, ophthalmologic evaluation and visual evoked responses
Macular hemorrhage due to neovascularization in age-related macular degeneration	Blood within or deep to retina in and around the macula	Clinical evaluation
Nonarteritic ischemic optic neuropathy	Optic disk edema and hemorrhages Sometimes loss of inferior and central visual fields Risk factors (eg, diabetes, hypertension, hypotensive episode)	ESR, CRP, and platelet count Consideration of temporal artery biopsy to exclude giant cell arteritis
Ocular migraine	Scintillating scotomata, mosaic patterns, or complete loss of vision lasting usually 10–60 min and often followed by headache Often in young patients	Clinical evaluation
Retinal artery occlusion	Nearly instantaneous onset, pale retina, cherry-red fovea, sometimes Hollenhorst plaque (refractile object at the site of arterial occlusion) Risk factors for vascular disease	ESR, CRP, and platelet count to exclude giant cell arteritis Carotid ultrasonography Echocardiography Consideration of MRI or CT ECG Continuous monitoring of cardiac rhythm
Retinal detachment	Recent increase in floaters, photopsias (flashing lights), or both Visual field defect, retinal folds Risk factors (eg, trauma, eye surgery, severe myopia; in men, advanced age)	Clinical evaluation
Retinal vein occlusion	Frequent, multiple, widely distributed retinal hemorrhages Risk factors (eg, diabetes, hypertension, hyperviscosity syndrome, sickle cell anemia)	Clinical evaluation
Transient ischemic attack or stroke	Bilaterally symmetric (homonymous) field defects, no effect on visual acuity in the intact parts of the visual field (bilateral occipital lesions are the exception and are uncommon but can occur due to basilar artery occlusion) Risk factors for atherosclerosis	Carotid ultrasonography Echocardiography Consideration of MRI or CT ECG Continuous monitoring of cardiac rhythm
Vitreous hemorrhage	Previous floaters or spider web in vision Risk factors (eg, diabetes, retinal tear, sickle cell anemia, trauma)	Possible ocular ultrasonography to assess retina

Table continues on the following page.

Table 108–1. SOME CAUSES OF ACUTE VISION LOSS (*Continued*)

CAUSE	SUGGESTIVE FINDINGS	DIAGNOSTIC APPROACH
Acute loss of vision with eye pain		
Acute angle-closure glaucoma	Halos around lights, nausea, headache, photophobia, conjunctival injection, corneal edema, shallow anterior chamber, intraocular pressure usually > 40	Immediate ophthalmologic evaluation Gonioscopy
Corneal ulcer	Ulcer visible with fluorescein staining, slit-lamp examination, or both Risk factors (eg, injury, contact lens use)	Ophthalmologic evaluation
Endophthalmitis	Floaters, conjunctival injection, decreased red reflex, hypopyon, or a combination Risk factors (infection after eye surgery, traumatic ruptured globe, intraocular foreign body [eg, after hammering metal on metal], fungemia, or bacteremia)	Immediate ophthalmologic evaluation with cultures of anterior chamber and vitreous fluids
Optic neuritis (usually painful but not always)	Mild pain with eye movement, afferent pupillary defect (occurs early) Visual field defects, typically central Abnormal color vision testing results Sometimes optic disk edema	Gadolinium-enhanced MRI to diagnose multiple sclerosis and related disorders

Review of systems should seek extraocular symptoms of possible causes, including jaw or tongue claudication, temporal headache, proximal muscle pain, and stiffness (giant cell arteritis); and headaches (ocular migraine).

Past medical history should seek known risk factors for eye disorders (eg, contact lens use, severe myopia, recent eye surgery or injury), risk factors for vascular disease (eg, diabetes, hypertension), and hematologic disorders (eg, sickle cell anemia or disorders such as Waldenström macroglobulinemia or multiple myeloma that could cause a hyperviscosity syndrome).

Family history should note any family history of migraine headaches.

Physical examination: Vital signs, including temperature, are measured.

If the diagnosis of a transient ischemic attack is under consideration, a complete neurologic examination is done. The temples are palpated for pulses, tenderness, or nodularity over the course of the temporal artery. However, most of the examination focuses on the eye.

Eye examination includes the following:

- Visual acuity is measured.
- Peripheral visual fields are assessed by confrontation.
- Central visual fields are assessed by Amsler grid.
- Direct and consensual pupillary light reflexes are examined using the swinging flashlight test.
- Ocular motility is assessed.
- Color vision is tested with color plates.
- The eyelids, sclera, and conjunctiva are examined using a slit lamp if possible.
- The cornea is examined with fluorescein staining.
- The anterior chamber is examined for cells and flare in patients who have eye pain or conjunctival injection.
- The lens is checked for cataracts using a direct ophthalmoscope, slit lamp, or both.
- Intraocular pressure is measured.
- Ophthalmoscopy is done, preferably after dilating the pupil with a drop of a sympathomimetic (eg, 2.5% phenylephrine), cycloplegic (eg, 1% cyclopentolate or 1% tropicamide), or both; dilation is nearly full after about 20 min. The entire fundus, including the retina, macula, fovea, vessels, and optic disk and its margins, is examined.
- If pupillary light responses are normal and functional loss of vision is suspected (rarely), optokinetic nystagmus is checked. If an optokinetic drum is unavailable, a mirror can be held near the patient's eye and slowly moved. If the patient can see, the eyes usually track movement of the mirror (considered to be the presence of optokinetic nystagmus).

Red flags: Acute loss of vision is itself a red flag; most causes are serious.

Interpretation of findings: Diagnosis of acute vision loss can be begun systematically. Specific patterns of visual field deficit help suggest a cause. Other clinical findings also help suggest a cause for acute vision loss:

- Difficulty seeing the red reflex during ophthalmoscopy suggests opacification of transparent structures (eg, caused by corneal ulcer, vitreous hemorrhage, or severe endophthalmitis).
- Retinal abnormalities that are severe enough to cause acute loss of vision are detectable during ophthalmoscopy, particularly if the pupils are dilated. Retinal detachment may show retinal folds; retinal vein occlusion may show marked retinal hemorrhages; and retinal artery occlusion may show pale retina with a cherry-red fovea.
- An afferent pupillary defect (absence of a direct pupillary light response but a normal consensual response) with an otherwise normal examination (except sometimes an abnormal optic disk) suggests an abnormality of the optic nerve or retina (ie, anterior to the chiasm).

In addition, the following facts may help:

- Monocular symptoms suggest a lesion anterior to the optic chiasm.
- Bilateral, symmetric (homonymous) visual field defects suggest a lesion posterior to the chiasm.
- Constant eye pain suggests a corneal lesion (ulcer or abrasion), anterior chamber inflammation, or increased intraocular pressure, whereas eye pain with movement suggests optic neuritis.
- Temporal headaches suggest giant cell arteritis or migraine.

Testing: ESR, C-reactive protein, and platelet count are done for all patients with symptoms (eg, temporal headaches, jaw claudication, proximal myalgias, stiffness) or signs (eg, temporal artery tenderness or induration, pale retina, papilledema) suggesting optic nerve or retinal ischemia to exclude giant cell arteritis.

Other testing is listed in Table 108–1. The following are of particular importance:

- Ultrasonography is done to view the retina if the retina is not clearly visible with pupillary dilation and indirect ophthalmoscopy done by an ophthalmologist.
- Gadolinium-enhanced MRI is done for patients who have eye pain with movement or afferent pupillary defect, particularly with optic nerve swelling on ophthalmoscopy, to diagnose multiple sclerosis.

Treatment

Causative disorders are treated. Treatment should usually commence immediately if the cause is treatable. In many cases (eg, vascular disorders), treatment is unlikely to salvage the affected eye but can decrease the risk of the same process occurring in the contralateral eye or of a complication caused by the same process (eg, ischemic stroke).

KEY POINTS

- Diagnosis and treatment should occur as rapidly as possible.
- Acute monocular loss of vision with an afferent pupillary defect indicates a lesion of the eye or of the optic nerve anterior to the optic chiasm.
- Optic nerve lesion, particularly ischemia, is considered in patients with acute monocular loss of vision or afferent pupillary defect and in those with or without optic nerve abnormalities on ophthalmoscopy but no other abnormalities on eye examination.
- Corneal ulcer, acute angle-closure glaucoma, endophthalmitis, or severe anterior uveitis is considered in patients with acute monocular loss of vision, eye pain, and conjunctival injection.

ANISOCORIA

(Unequal Pupils)

Anisocoria is unequal pupil sizes. Anisocoria itself does not cause symptoms.

Etiology

The most common cause of anisocoria is

- Physiologic (present in about 20% of people)

See Table 108–2 for other causes of anisocoria.

Many disorders are accompanied by anisocoria due to iris or neurologic dysfunction but usually manifest with other, more bothersome symptoms (eg, uveitis, stroke, subarachnoid hemorrhage, acute angle-closure glaucoma).

Evaluation

The goal of evaluation is to elucidate the physiologic mechanism of anisocoria. By identifying certain mechanisms (eg, Horner syndrome, 3rd cranial nerve palsy), clinicians can diagnose the occasional serious occult disorder (eg, tumor, aneurysm) manifesting with anisocoria.

History: History of present illness includes the presence, nature, and duration of symptoms. Any history of head or ocular trauma is noted.

Review of systems seeks symptoms that may suggest a cause, such as birth defects or chromosomal abnormalities (congenital defects); droopy eyelid, cough, chest pain, or dyspnea (Horner syndrome); genital lesions, adenopathy, rashes, or fever (syphilis); and headaches or other neurologic symptoms (Horner syndrome or 3rd cranial nerve palsy).

Past medical history includes known ocular disorders and surgeries and exposure to drugs.

Physical examination: Pupillary size and light responses should be examined in lighted and dark rooms. Accommodation and extraocular movements should be tested. Ocular structures are inspected by using a slit lamp or other magnification to identify structural abnormalities and ptosis. Other ocular symptoms are evaluated by eye examination as clinically indicated. An old

Table 108–2. SOME COMMON CAUSES OF ANISOCORIA

CAUSE	SUGGESTIVE FINDINGS
Adie tonic pupil (idiopathic impaired constriction)	Pupils that respond more to accommodation than to light; delayed dilation after constriction
Argyll Robertson pupil (due to syphilis)	Pupils that respond more to accommodation than to light; possibly findings suggesting syphilis
Congenital iris defects	Associated ocular abnormalities, chromosomal disorder, nonocular congenital defects, chronicity
Drugs (eg, scopolamine patch; cocaine, pilocarpine, animal flea collars or sprays, organophosphates, or aerosolized ipratropium if they contact the eye; cycloplegic, mydriatic, clonidine, or apraclonidine eye drops)	History of use or exposure
Horner syndrome (eg, congenital, traumatic, postsurgical, due to migraine or lung tumors)	Ptosis, anhidrosis, delayed dilation after constriction, features of causative disorder
Iris or other ocular dysfunction after surgery	History
Physiologic anisocoria	Chronicity, absence of symptoms or associated findings, difference of < 1 mm (usually < 0.4 mm) between pupil sizes, normal pupillary light responses
Third cranial nerve palsy (eg, due to aneurysm or tumor)	Impaired extraocular movements, ptosis
Traumatic mydriasis	History or evidence of trauma

photograph of the patient or the patient's driver's license should be examined (under magnification if possible) to see whether anisocoria was present previously.

Red flags: The following findings are of particular concern:

- Ptosis
- Anhidrosis
- Pupils that respond more to accommodation than light
- Impaired extraocular movements

Interpretation of findings: If the difference in size is greater in the dark, the smaller pupil is abnormal. Common causes include Horner syndrome and physiologic anisocoria. An ophthalmologist can differentiate them because the small pupil in Horner syndrome does not dilate after instillation of an ocular dilating drop (eg, 10% cocaine). In physiologic anisocoria, the difference in pupil size may also be equal in light and dark.

If the difference in pupillary sizes is greater in light, the larger pupil is abnormal. If extraocular movements are impaired, particularly with ptosis, 3rd cranial nerve palsy is likely. If extraocular movements are intact, an ophthalmologist can further differentiate among causes by instilling a drop of a pupillary constrictor (eg, 0.1% pilocarpine). If the large pupil constricts, the cause is probably Adie tonic pupil; if the large pupil does not constrict, the cause is probably drugs or structural (eg, traumatic, surgical) damage to the iris.

Testing: Testing is usually unnecessary but is indicated for clinically suspected disorders. Patients with Horner syndrome or 3rd cranial nerve palsy usually require brain MRI or CT and, with Horner syndrome, chest CT.

Treatment

Treatment of anisocoria is unnecessary.

KEY POINTS

- Physiologic anisocoria is very common and causes < 1 mm of difference between the pupils in size.
- Examining the pupils in light and dark and inspecting an old photograph or the driver's license of the patient provide a great deal of diagnostic information.
- Serious disorders should be considered in patients with Horner syndrome or 3rd cranial nerve palsy.

BLURRED VISION

Blurred vision is the most common visual symptom. It usually refers to decreased visual acuity of gradual onset. For sudden, complete loss of vision in one or both eyes (blindness), see p. 896. Patients with small visual field defects (eg, caused by a small retinal detachment) may describe their symptoms as blurring.

Etiology

The **most common** causes of blurred vision (see Table 108–3) include

- Refractive errors (the most common cause overall)
- Age-related macular degeneration
- Cataracts
- Diabetic retinopathy

Blurred vision has 4 general mechanisms:

- Opacification of normally transparent ocular structures (cornea, lens, vitreous) through which light rays must pass to reach the retina
- Disorders affecting the retina
- Disorders affecting the optic nerve or its connections
- Refractive errors

Certain disorders can have more than one mechanism. For example, refraction can be impaired by early cataracts or the reversible lens swelling caused by poorly controlled diabetes.

Patients with certain disorders that cause blurred vision (eg, acute corneal lesions [such as abrasions], ulcers, herpes simplex keratitis, herpes zoster ophthalmicus, acute angle-closure glaucoma) are more likely to present with other symptoms such as eye pain and red eye.

Rare disorders that can cause blurred vision include hereditary optic neuropathies (eg, dominant optic atrophy, Leber hereditary optic neuropathy) and corneal scarring due to vitamin A deficiency.

Evaluation

History: History of present illness should ascertain the onset, duration, and progression of symptoms, as well as whether they are bilateral or unilateral. The symptom should be defined as precisely as possible by asking an open-ended question or request (eg, "Please describe what you mean by blurred vision"). For example, loss of detail is not the same as loss of contrast. Also, visual field defects may not be recognized as such by patients, who may instead describe symptoms such as missing steps or the inability to see words when reading. Important associated symptoms include eye redness, photophobia, floaters, sensation of lightning-like flashes of light (photopsias), and pain at rest or with eye movement. The effects of darkness (night vision), bright lights (ie, causing blur, star bursts, halos, photophobia), distance from an object, and corrective lenses and whether central or peripheral vision seems to be more affected should be ascertained.

Review of systems includes questions about symptoms of possible causes, such as increased thirst and polyuria (diabetes).

Past medical history should note previous eye injury or other diagnosed eye disorders and ask about disorders known to be risk factors for eye disorders (eg, hypertension, diabetes, HIV/AIDS, SLE, sickle cell anemia, disorders that could cause hyperviscosity syndrome such as multiple myeloma or Waldenström macroglobulinemia). Drug history should include questions about use of drugs that could affect vision (eg, corticosteroids) and treatments for disorders affecting vision (eg, diabetic retinopathy).

Physical examination: Nonvisual symptoms are evaluated as needed; however, examination of the eyes may be all that is necessary.

Testing **visual acuity** is key. Many patients do not give a full effort. Providing adequate time and coaxing patients tend to yield more accurate results.

Acuity ideally is measured while the patient stands 6 m (about 20 ft) from a Snellen chart posted on a wall. If this test cannot be done, acuity can be measured using a chart held about 36 cm (14 in) from the eye. Measurement of near vision should be done with reading correction in place for patients > 40 yr. Each eye is measured separately while the other eye is covered with a solid object (not the patient's fingers, which may separate during testing). If the patient cannot read the top line of the Snellen chart at 6 m, acuity is tested at 3 m. If nothing can be read from a chart even at the closest distance, the examiner holds up different numbers of fingers to see whether the patient can accurately count them. If not, the examiner tests whether the patient can perceive hand motion. If not, a light is shined into the eye to see whether light is perceived.

Table 108–3. SOME CAUSES OF BLURRED VISION

CAUSE	SUGGESTIVE FINDINGS	DIAGNOSTIC APPROACH
Opacification of eye structures		
Cataracts	Gradual onset, often risk factors (eg, aging, corticosteroid use), loss of contrast, glare Lens opacification on ophthalmoscopy or slit-lamp examination	Clinical evaluation
Corneal opacification (eg, posttraumatic or postinfectious scarring)	Corneal abnormalities on slit-lamp examination	Clinical evaluation
Disorders affecting the retina		
Age-related macular degeneration	Gradual onset, central vision affected (central scotoma) without loss of peripheral vision, macular drusen or scarring, neovascular membrane	Fluorescein angiography or other retinal imaging as clinically indicated
Infectious retinitis (eg, cytomegalovirus, *Toxoplasma*)	Usually HIV infection or other immunosuppressive disorder, often eye redness or pain, abnormal retinal findings	Studies as clinically indicated (eg, anti-*Toxoplasma* antibodies)
Retinitis pigmentosa	Primarily night blindness, gradual onset, pigmented retinal lesions	Specialized testing by ophthalmologist (eg, dark adaptation, electroretinography)
Retinopathy associated with systemic disorders (eg, hypertension, SLE, diabetes, Waldenström macroglobulinemia, multiple myeloma, or other disorders that could cause hyperviscosity syndrome)	Risk factors, retinal abnormalities detected during ophthalmoscopy (see Table 108–5)	Testing as indicated for clinically suspected disorders
Epiretinal membrane	Risk factors (eg diabetic retinopathy, uveitis, retinal detachment or ocular injury) Blurry or distorted vision (eg, straight lines appear wavy)	Funduscopy, optical coherence tomography
Macular hole	Blurry vision, initially central	Fundoscopy, optical coherence tomography
Retinal vein occlusion	Risk factors (eg hypertension, age, glaucoma) Painless vision loss (usually sudden) Sometimes, blurry vision	Funduscopy Sometimes, fluorescein angiography Sometimes, optical coherence tomography
Disorders affecting the optic nerve or neural pathways		
Optic neuritis	Gradual onset unless due to multiple sclerosis (in which onset of optic neuritis is rapid) Often unilateral or asymmetric Pain with eye movement, direct pupillary light reflex decreased more than consensual (afferent pupillary defect), sometimes loss of optic disk margins and/or globe tenderness	Often MRI to rule out multiple sclerosis
Disorders affecting focus		
Refractive errors	Visual acuity varying with distance from objects, acuity corrected with refraction	Clinical refraction by an optometrist or ophthalmologist

Visual acuity is measured with and without the patients' own glasses. If acuity is corrected with glasses, the problem is a refractive error. If patients do not have their glasses, a pinhole refractor is used. If a commercial pinhole refractor is unavailable, one can be made at the bedside by poking holes through a piece of cardboard using an 18-gauge needle and varying the diameter of each hole slightly. Patients choose the hole that corrects vision the most. If acuity corrects with pinhole refraction, the problem is a refractive error. Pinhole refraction is a rapid, efficient way to diagnose refractive errors, which are the most common cause of blurred vision. However, with pinhole refraction, best correction is usually to only about 20/30, not 20/20.

Eye examination is also important. Direct and consensual pupillary light responses are examined using the swinging flashlight test. Visual fields are checked using confrontation and an Amsler grid.

The cornea is examined for opacification, ideally using a slit lamp. The anterior chamber is examined for cells and flare using a slit lamp if possible, although results of this examination are unlikely to explain visual blurring in patients without eye pain or redness.

Table 108–4. INTERPRETATION OF SOME RED FLAG FINDINGS

FINDINGS	POSSIBLE CAUSE
A systemic disorder that could cause retinopathy (eg, sickle cell anemia, possible hyperviscosity syndrome, diabetes, hypertension)	Retinopathy
Bilateral symmetric visual field defects	Lesion affecting cortical visual pathways
Eye pain*	Optic neuritis
HIV/AIDS or other immunosuppressive disorder*	Infectious retinitis
Monocular visual field defect*	Retinal detachment, other retinal abnormality, other optic neuropathy
Retinal or optic disk abnormality	Infectious retinitis,* retinitis pigmentosa, worsening retinopathy* (see Table 108–5)
Sudden change in vision*	Optic neuritis, sudden worsening of retinopathy, or other physical eye disorder (see p. 896)

*Urgent or immediate ophthalmologic referral is usually indicated.

The lens is examined for opacities using an ophthalmoscope, slit lamp, or both.

Ophthalmoscopy is done using a direct ophthalmoscope. More detail is visible if the eyes are dilated for ophthalmoscopy with a drop of a sympathomimetic (eg, 2.5% phenylephrine), cycloplegic (eg, 1% tropicamide or 1% cyclopentolate), or both; dilation is nearly full after about 20 min. As much of the fundus as is visible, including the retina, macula, fovea, vessels, and optic disk and its margins, is examined. To see the entire fundus (ie, to see a peripheral retinal detachment), the examiner, usually an ophthalmologist, must use an indirect ophthalmoscope.

Intraocular pressure is measured.

Red flags: The following findings are of particular concern:

- Sudden change in vision
- Eye pain (with or without eye movement)
- Visual field defect (by history or examination)
- Visible abnormality of the retina or optic disk
- HIV/AIDS or other immunosuppressive disorder
- A systemic disorder that could cause retinopathy (eg, sickle cell anemia, possible hyperviscosity syndrome, diabetes, hypertension)

Interpretation of findings: Symptoms and signs help suggest a cause (see Table 108–3).

If visual acuity is corrected with glasses or a pinhole refractor, simple refractive error is likely the cause of blurring. Loss of contrast or glare may still be caused by cataract, which should be considered.

However, red flag findings suggest a more serious ophthalmologic disorder (see Table 108–4) and need for a complete examination, including slit-lamp examination, tonometry, ophthalmoscopic examination with pupillary dilation, and, depending on findings, possibly immediate or urgent ophthalmologic referral.

Specific retinal findings help suggest a cause (see Table 108–5).

Testing: If acuity corrects appropriately with refraction, patients are referred to an optometrist or ophthalmologist for routine formal refraction. If visual acuity is not corrected with refraction but there are no red flag findings, patients are referred to an ophthalmologist for routine evaluation. With certain red flag findings, patients are referred for immediate or urgent ophthalmologic evaluation.

Patients with symptoms or signs of systemic disorders should have appropriate testing:

- Diabetes: Fingerstick or random glucose measurement
- Poorly controlled hypertension and acute hypertensive retinopathy (hemorrhages, exudates, or papilledema): Urinalysis, renal function testing, BP monitoring, and ECG

Table 108–5. INTERPRETATION OF RETINAL FINDINGS

FINDINGS	POSSIBLE CAUSE
Arteriolar narrowing, copper wiring, flame hemorrhages, arteriovenous nicking	Hypertensive retinopathy
Dark-pigmented lesions in bone spicule formation in the midperipheral retina (rarely visible with direct ophthalmoscopy)	Retinitis pigmentosa
Diffuse hemorrhages, venous dilation	Hyperviscosity syndrome
Indistinct optic disk margins, suggesting optic nerve swelling	Optic neuritis
Macular hyperpigmentation, loss of pigment in retinal epithelium, drusen, hemorrhage	Age-related macular degeneration
Microaneurysms and neovascularization at posterior retina	Diabetic retinopathy
White retinal infiltrates, sometimes loss of red reflex or visible vitreous inflammation	Infectious retinitis Toxoplasmosis suggested by retinal infiltrate immediately adjacent to a scar

- HIV/AIDS and retinal abnormalities: HIV serology and CD4+ count
- SLE and retinal abnormality: Antinuclear antibodies, ESR, and CBC
- Waldenström macroglobulinemia, multiple myeloma, or sickle cell anemia: CBC with differential count and other testing (eg, serum protein electrophoresis) as clinically indicated

Treatment

Underlying disorders are treated. Corrective lenses may be used to improve visual acuity, even when the disorder causing blurring is not purely a refractive error (eg, early cataract).

Geriatrics Essentials

Although some decrease in visual acuity in low light or loss of contrast sensitivity can normally occur with aging, acuity normally is correctable to 20/20 with refraction, even in very elderly patients.

KEY POINTS

- If visual acuity is corrected with pinhole refraction, refractive error is likely the problem.
- If pinhole refraction does not correct acuity and there is no obvious cataract or corneal abnormality, ophthalmoscopy should be done after pupillary dilation.
- Many abnormalities on ophthalmoscopy, particularly if symptoms are recently worsening, require urgent or immediate ophthalmologic referral.

DIPLOPIA

(Double Vision)

Diplopia is the perception of 2 images of a single object. Diplopia may be monocular or binocular. Monocular diplopia is present when only one eye is open. Binocular diplopia disappears when either eye is closed.

Etiology

Monocular diplopia can occur when something distorts light transmission through the eye to the retina. There may be > 2 images. One of the images is of normal quality (eg, brightness, contrast, clarity); the rest are of inferior quality. The most common causes of monocular diplopia are

- Cataract
- Corneal shape problems, such as keratoconus or surface irregularity
- Uncorrected refractive error, usually astigmatism

Other causes include corneal scarring and dislocated lens. Complaints also may represent malingering.

Binocular diplopia suggests disconjugate alignment of the eyes. There are only 2 images, and they are of equal quality. There are many possible causes of binocular diplopia (see Table 108–6). The most common are

- Cranial nerve (3rd, 4th, or 6th) palsy
- Myasthenia gravis
- Orbital infiltration (eg, thyroid infiltrative ophthalmopathy, orbital pseudotumor)

Most commonly, the eyes are misaligned because of a disorder affecting the cranial nerves innervating the extraocular muscles (3rd, 4th, or 6th cranial nerves). These palsies may be isolated and idiopathic or the result of various disorders involving the cranial nerve nuclei or the infranuclear nerve or nerves. Whether pain is present depends on the disorder. Other causes involve mechanical interference with ocular motion (which often cause pain) or a generalized disorder of neuromuscular transmission (which typically do not cause pain).

Evaluation

History: History of present illness should determine whether diplopia involves one or both eyes, whether diplopia is intermittent or constant, and whether the images are separated vertically, horizontally, or both. Any associated pain is noted, as well as whether it occurs with or without eye movement.

Review of systems should seek symptoms of other cranial nerve dysfunction, such as vision abnormalities (2nd cranial nerve); numbness of forehead and cheek (5th cranial nerve); facial weakness (7th cranial nerve); dizziness, hearing loss, or gait difficulties (8th cranial nerve); and swallowing or speech difficulties (9th and 12th cranial nerves). Other neurologic symptoms, such as weakness and sensory abnormalities, should be sought, noting whether these are intermittent or constant. Nonneurologic symptoms of potential causes are ascertained. They include nausea, vomiting, and diarrhea (botulism); palpitations, heat sensitivity, and weight loss (Graves disease); and difficulty with bladder control (multiple sclerosis).

Past medical history should seek presence of known hypertension, diabetes, or both; atherosclerosis, particularly including cerebrovascular disease; and alcohol abuse.

Physical examination: Examination begins with a review of vital signs for fever and general appearance for signs of toxicity (eg, prostration, confusion).

Eye examination begins with noting the initial position of the eyes, followed by measuring visual acuity (with correction) in each eye and both together, which also helps determine whether diplopia is monocular or binocular. Eye examination should note presence of bulging of one or both eyes, eyelid droop, pupillary abnormalities, and disconjugate eye movement and nystagmus during ocular motility testing. Ophthalmoscopy should be done, particularly noting any abnormalities of the lens (eg, cataract, displacement) and retina (eg, detachment).

Ocular motility is tested by having the patient hold the head steady and track the examiner's finger, which is moved to extreme gaze to the right, left, upward, downward, diagonally to either side, and finally inward toward the patient's nose (convergence). However, mild paresis of ocular motility sufficient to cause diplopia may escape detection by such examination.

If diplopia occurs in one direction of gaze, the eye that produces each image can be determined by repeating the examination with a red glass placed over one of the patient's eyes. The image that is more peripheral originates in the paretic eye; ie, if the more peripheral image is red, the red glass is covering the paretic eye. If a red glass is not available, the paretic eye can sometimes be identified by having the patient close each eye. The paretic eye is the eye that when closed eliminates the more peripheral image.

The other cranial nerves are tested, and the remainder of the neurologic examination, including strength, sensation, reflexes, cerebellar function, and observation of gait, is completed.

Relevant nonneurophthalmologic components of the examination include palpation of the neck for goiter and inspection of the shins for pretibial myxedema (Graves disease).

Red flags: The following findings are of particular concern:

- More than one cranial nerve deficit
- Pupillary involvement of any degree
- Any neurologic symptoms or signs besides diplopia
- Pain
- Proptosis

Table 108–6. SOME CAUSES OF BINOCULAR DIPLOPIA

CAUSE	SUGGESTIVE FINDINGS	DIAGNOSTIC APPROACH
Disorders affecting cranial nerves to extraocular muscles (presence of pain varies by cause)		
Cerebrovascular disease affecting pons or midbrain	Older patients, risk factors (eg, hypertension, atherosclerosis, diabetes) Sometimes internuclear ophthalmoplegia or other deficits No pain	MRI
Compressive lesion (eg, aneurysm, tumor)	Often pain (sudden if caused by aneurysm) and other neurologic deficits	Immediate imaging (CT, MRI)
Idiopathic (usually microvascular)	Occurs in isolation (no other manifestations)	Ophthalmologic referral to check for other deficits For isolated diplopia, observation for spontaneous resolution Imaging (MRI, CT) if not resolved in several weeks
Inflammatory or infectious lesions (eg, sinusitis, abscess, cavernous sinus thrombosis)	Constant pain Sometimes fever or systemic complaints, facial sensory changes, proptosis	CT or MRI
Wernicke encephalopathy	History of significant alcohol abuse, ataxia, confusion	Clinical diagnosis
Mechanical interference with ocular motion (pain is often present)		
Graves disease (infiltrative ophthalmopathy usually associated with hyperthyroidism)	Local symptoms: Eye pain, exophthalmos, lacrimation, dry eyes, irritation, photophobia, ocular muscle weakness causing diplopia, vision loss caused by optic nerve compression Systemic symptoms: Palpitations, anxiety, increased appetite, weight loss, insomnia, goiter, pretibial myxedema Sometimes eye abnormalities precede thyroid dysfunction	Thyroid function testing
Orbital myositis	Constant eye pain that worsens with eye motion, proptosis, sometimes injection	MRI
Trauma (eg, fracture, hematoma)	Signs of external trauma; apparent by history	CT or MRI
Tumors (near base of skull, in or near sinuses or orbit)	Often pain (unrelated to eye motion), unilateral proptosis, sometimes other neurologic manifestations	CT or MRI
Neuromuscular transmission disorders (typically, pain is absent)		
Botulism	Sometimes preceded by GI symptoms Descending weakness, other cranial nerve dysfunction, dilated pupils, normal sensation	Serum and stool testing for toxin
Guillain-Barré syndrome, Miller Fisher variant	Ataxia, decreased reflexes	Lumbar puncture
Multiple sclerosis	Intermittent, migratory neurologic symptoms, including extremity paresthesias or weakness, visual disturbance, urinary dysfunction Sometimes internuclear ophthalmoplegia	MRI of brain and spinal cord
Myasthenia gravis	Diplopia intermittent, often with ptosis, bulbar symptoms, weakness that worsens with repeated use of muscle	Edrophonium test

Interpretation of findings: Findings sometimes suggest which cranial nerve is involved.

- 3rd: Eyelid droop, eye deviated laterally and down, sometimes pupillary dilation
- 4th: Vertical diplopia worse on downward gaze (patient tilts head to improve vision)
- 6th: Eye deviated medially, diplopia worse on lateral gaze (patient turns head to improve vision)

Other findings help suggest a cause (see Table 108–6).

Intermittent diplopia suggests a waxing and waning neurologic disorder, such as myasthenia gravis or multiple sclerosis, or unmasking of a latent phoria (eye deviation). Patients with latent phoria do not have any other neurologic manifestations.

Internuclear ophthalmoplegia (INO) results from a brain stem lesion in the medial longitudinal fasciculus (MLF). INO manifests on horizontal gaze testing with diplopia, weak adduction on the affected side (usually cannot adduct eye past midline), and nystagmus of the contralateral eye. However, the affected eye adducts normally on convergence testing (which does not require an intact MLF).

Pain suggests a compressive lesion or inflammatory disorder.

Testing: Patients with monocular diplopia are referred to an ophthalmologist for evaluation of ocular pathology; no other tests are required beforehand.

For binocular diplopia, patients with a unilateral, single cranial nerve palsy, a normal pupillary light response, and no other symptoms or signs can usually be observed without testing for a few weeks. Many cases resolve spontaneously. Ophthalmologic evaluation may be done to monitor the patient and help further delineate the deficit.

Most other patients require neuroimaging with MRI to detect orbital, cranial, or CNS abnormalities. CT may be substituted if there is concern about a metallic intraocular foreign body or if MRI is otherwise contraindicated or unavailable. Imaging should be done immediately if findings suggest infection, aneurysm, or acute (< 3 h) stroke.

Patients with manifestations of Graves disease should have thyroid tests (serum thyroxine [T_4] and thyroid-stimulating hormone [TSH] levels). Testing for myasthenia gravis and multiple sclerosis should be strongly considered for patients with intermittent diplopia.

Treatment

Treatment is management of the underlying disorder.

KEY POINTS

- Isolated, pupil-sparing nerve palsy in patients with no other symptoms may resolve spontaneously.
- Imaging is required for patients with red flag findings.
- Focal weakness (in any muscle) may indicate a disorder of neuromuscular transmission.

EYELID SWELLING

Eyelid swelling can be unilateral or bilateral. It may be asymptomatic or accompanied by itching or pain.

Etiology

Eyelid swelling has many causes (see Table 108–7). It usually results from an eyelid disorder but may result from disorders in and around the orbit or from systemic disorders that cause generalized edema.

Table 108–7. SOME CAUSES OF EYELID SWELLING

CAUSE	SUGGESTIVE FINDINGS	DIAGNOSTIC APPROACH
Eyelid disorders		
Allergic reaction, local	Itching, no pain Pale, puffy eyelid or eyelids, conjunctiva, or both Sometimes history of recurrence, exposure to allergen, or both Unilateral or bilateral	Clinical evaluation
Blepharitis	Lash involvement and crusting usually visible grossly or under magnification (eg, with slit lamp) Itching, burning, redness, ulceration, or a combination Sometimes concomitant seborrheic dermatitis Unilateral or bilateral	Clinical evaluation
Chalazion	Focal redness and pain involving only one eyelid Eventual development of localized, nonpainful swelling away from eyelid margin	Clinical evaluation
Conjunctivitis, infectious	Conjunctival injection, discharge Sometimes preauricular node, chemosis, or both Unilateral or bilateral	Clinical evaluation, usually fluorescein staining to rule out herpes simplex keratoconjunctivitis
Herpes simplex blepharitis (primary)	Clusters of vesicles on an erythematous base, ulceration, severe pain Unilateral	Clinical evaluation
Herpes zoster (shingles)	Clusters of vesicles on an erythematous base, ulceration, severe pain Unilateral, V_1 nerve root distribution	Clinical evaluation
Hordeolum	Focal redness and pain involving only one eyelid Eventual development of swelling localized to eyelid margin, sometimes with pustule	Clinical evaluation
Insect bite	Itching, redness, sometimes a papule	Clinical evaluation

Table continues on the following page.

Table 108–7. SOME CAUSES OF EYELID SWELLING (*Continued*)

CAUSE	SUGGESTIVE FINDINGS	DIAGNOSTIC APPROACH
Disorders in and around the orbit		
Cavernous sinus thrombosis (rare)	Headache, proptosis, ophthalmoplegia, ptosis, decreased visual acuity, fever Usually unilateral at first, then bilateral Manifestations of sinusitis or other facial infection	Immediate CT or MRI
Orbital cellulitis	Proptosis, redness, fever, pain Impaired or painful extraocular movements Sometimes decreased visual acuity Usually unilateral Sometimes preceded by manifestations of the source infection (typically sinusitis)	CT or MRI
Preseptal cellulitis (periorbital cellulitis)	Swelling (but not proptosis), redness, sometimes pain, fever Usually unilateral Vision and ocular motility normal Sometimes preceded by manifestations of the source infection (typically local skin infection)	CT or MRI if necessary to exclude orbital cellulitis
Systemic disorders*		
Allergic reaction, systemic (eg, angioedema, rhinitis)	Itching Sometimes extraocular allergic manifestations (eg, urticaria, wheezing, rhinorrhea) Sometimes history of recurrence, exposure to allergen, atopy, or a combination Usually bilateral	Clinical evaluation
Generalized edema	Bilateral asymptomatic eyelid and sometimes facial edema; usually also edema of dependent body parts (eg, feet, presacral region) Usually manifestations of underlying disorder (eg, chronic renal disease, heart failure, liver failure, preeclampsia) Sometimes use of an ACE inhibitor	Testing for cardiac, hepatic, or renal disorders as clinically directed
Hyperthyroidism (with Graves ophthalmopathy)	Stare, eyelid lag, proptosis, impaired extraocular movements Not painful unless cornea is irritated from drying Tachycardia, anxiety, weight loss	Thyroid function tests (TSH, T_4)
Hypothyroidism	Painless, bilateral diffuse facial puffiness Dry, scaly skin; coarse hair Cold intolerance	Thyroid function tests (TSH, T_4)

*Swelling due to systemic disorders is bilateral and not erythematous.
T_4 = thyroxine; TSH = thyroid-stimulating hormone; V_1 = ophthalmic division of the trigeminal nerve.

The **most common** causes are allergic, including

- Local allergy (contact sensitivity)
- Systemic allergy (eg, angioedema, systemic allergy accompanying allergic rhinitis)

Focal swelling of one eyelid is most often caused by a chalazion.

The most immediately dangerous causes are orbital cellulitis and cavernous sinus thrombosis (rare).

In addition to the disorders listed in Table 108–7, eyelid swelling may result from the following:

- Disorders that may involve the eyelid but do not cause swelling unless very advanced (eg, eyelid tumors, including squamous cell carcinomas and melanoma)
- Disorders that cause swelling that begins and is usually most severe in structures near, but not part of, the eyelids (eg, dacryocystitis, canaliculitis)
- Disorders in which swelling occurs but is not the presenting symptom (eg, basilar skull fracture, burns, trauma, postsurgery)

Evaluation

History: History of present illness should ascertain how long swelling has been present, whether it is unilateral or bilateral, and whether it has been preceded by any trauma (including insect bites). Important accompanying symptoms to identify include itching, pain, headache, change in vision, fever, and eye discharge.

Review of systems should seek symptoms of possible causes, including runny nose, itching, rash, and wheezing (systemic allergic reaction); headache, nasal congestion, and purulent nasal discharge (sinusitis); toothache (dental infection); dyspnea, orthopnea, and paroxysmal nocturnal dyspnea (heart failure); cold intolerance and changes in skin texture (hypothyroidism); and heat intolerance, anxiety, and weight loss (hyperthyroidism).

Past medical history should include recent eye injury or surgery; known heart, liver, renal, or thyroid disease; and allergies and exposure to possible allergens. Drug history should specifically include use of ACE inhibitors.

Physical examination: Vital signs should be assessed for fever and tachycardia.

Eye inspection should assess the location and color of swelling (erythematous or pale), including whether it is present on one eyelid, both eyelids, or both eyes and whether it is tender, warm, or both. The examiner should observe whether the finding represents edema of the eyelids, protrusion of the globe (proptosis), or both. Eye examination should particularly note visual acuity and range of extraocular motion (full or limited). This examination can be difficult when swelling is marked but is important because deficits suggest an orbital or retro-orbital disorder rather than an eyelid disorder; an assistant may be required to hold the eyelids open. Conjunctivae are examined for injection and discharge. Any eyelid or eye lesions are evaluated using a slit lamp.

General examination should assess signs of toxicity, suggesting a serious infection, and signs of a causative disorder. Facial skin is inspected for dryness and scales (which may suggest hypothyroidism) and greasy scales or other signs of seborrheic dermatitis. Extremities and the presacral area are examined for edema, which suggests a systemic cause. If a systemic cause is suspected, see p. 591 for further discussion of the evaluation.

Red flags: The following findings are of particular concern:

- Fever
- Loss of visual acuity
- Impaired extraocular movements
- Proptosis

Interpretation of findings: Some findings help distinguish among categories of disorders. The first important distinction is between inflammation or infection and allergy or fluid overload. Pain, redness, warmth, and tenderness suggest inflammation or infection. Painless, pale swelling suggests angioedema. Itching suggests allergic reaction, and absence of itching suggests cardiac or renal dysfunction.

Swelling localized to one eyelid in the absence of other signs is rarely caused by a dangerous disorder. Massive swelling of the eyelids of one or both eyes should raise suspicion of a serious problem. Signs of inflammation, proptosis, loss of vision, and impaired extraocular movements suggest an orbital disorder (eg, orbital cellulitis, cavernous sinus thrombosis) that may be pushing the globe forward or affecting the nerves or muscles. Other suggestive and specific findings are listed in Table 108–7.

Testing: In most cases, diagnosis can be established clinically and no testing is necessary. If orbital cellulitis or cavernous sinus thrombosis is suspected, diagnosis and treatment should proceed as rapidly as possible. Immediate imaging with CT or MRI should be done. If cardiac, liver, renal, or thyroid dysfunction is suspected, organ function is evaluated with laboratory tests and imaging as appropriate for that system.

Treatment

Treatment is directed at the underlying disorder. There is no specific treatment for the swelling.

KEY POINTS

- Proptosis with impaired vision or extraocular movements suggests orbital cellulitis or cavernous sinus thrombosis, and diagnosis and treatment should proceed as rapidly as possible.
- Eyelid disorders should be differentiated from orbital and systemic causes of swelling.

EYE PAIN

Eye pain may be described as sharp, aching, or throbbing and should be distinguished from superficial irritation or a foreign body sensation. In some disorders, pain is worsened by bright light. Eye pain may be caused by a serious disorder and requires prompt evaluation. Many causes of eye pain also cause a red eye.

Pathophysiology

The cornea is richly innervated and highly sensitive to pain. Many disorders that affect the cornea or anterior chamber (eg, uveitis) also cause pain via ciliary muscle spasm; when such spasm is present, bright light causes muscle contraction, worsening pain.

Etiology

Disorders that cause eye pain can be divided into those that affect primarily the cornea, other ocular disorders, and disorders that cause pain referred to the eye (see Table 108–8).

The **most common** causes overall are

- Corneal abrasion
- Foreign bodies

However, most corneal disorders can cause eye pain.

A feeling of scratchiness or of a foreign body may be caused by either a conjunctival or a corneal disorder.

Evaluation

History: **History of present illness** should address the onset, quality, and severity of pain and any history of prior episodes (eg, daily episodes in clusters). Important associated symptoms include true photophobia (shining a light into the unaffected eye causes pain in the affected eye when the affected eye is shut), decreased visual acuity, foreign body sensation and pain when blinking, and pain when moving the eye.

Review of systems should seek symptoms suggesting a cause, including presence of an aura (migraine); fever and chills (infection); and pain when moving the head, purulent rhinorrhea, productive or nocturnal cough, and halitosis (sinusitis).

Past medical history should include known disorders that are risk factors for eye pain, including autoimmune disorders, multiple sclerosis, migraine, and sinus infections. Additional risk factors to assess include use (and overuse) of contact lenses (contact lens keratitis), exposure to excessive sunlight or to welding (ultraviolet keratitis), hammering or drilling metal (foreign body), and recent eye injury or surgery (endophthalmitis).

Physical examination: Vital signs are checked for the presence of fever. The nose is inspected for purulent rhinorrhea, and the face is palpated for tenderness. If the eye is red, the preauricular region is checked for adenopathy. Hygiene during examination must be scrupulous when examining patients who have chemosis, preauricular adenopathy, punctate corneal staining, or a combination; these findings suggest epidemic keratoconjunctivitis, which is highly contagious.

Eye examination should be as complete as possible for patients with eye pain. Best corrected visual acuity is checked. Visual fields are typically tested by confrontation in patients with eye pain, but this test can be insensitive (particularly for small defects) and unreliable because of poor patient cooperation. A light is moved from one eye to the other to check for pupillary size and direct and consensual pupillary light responses. In patients who have unilateral eye pain, a light is shined in the unaffected eye while the affected eye is shut; pain in the affected eye represents true photophobia. Extraocular movements are checked. The orbital and periorbital structures are inspected. Conjunctival injection that seems most intense and confluent around the cornea and limbus is called ciliary flush.

Slit-lamp examination is done if possible. The cornea is stained with fluorescein and examined under magnification with cobalt blue light. If a slit lamp is unavailable, the cornea can be examined after fluorescein staining with a Wood light using magnification. Ophthalmoscopy is done, and ocular pressures are measured (tonometry). In patients with a foreign body sensation or unexplained corneal abrasions, the eyelids are everted and examined for foreign bodies.

Red flags: The following findings are of particular concern:

- Vomiting, halos around lights, or corneal edema
- Signs of systemic infection (eg, fever, chills)
- Decreased visual acuity
- Proptosis
- Impaired extraocular motility

Interpretation of findings: Suggestive findings are listed in Table 108–8. Some findings suggest categories of disorders.

Scratchiness or a foreign body sensation is most often caused by disorders of the eyelids, conjunctivae, or superficial cornea. Photosensitivity is possible.

Surface pain with photophobia is often accompanied by a foreign body sensation and pain when blinking; it suggests a corneal lesion, most often a foreign body or abrasion.

Deeper pain—often described as aching or throbbing—usually indicates a serious disorder such as glaucoma, uveitis, scleritis, endophthalmitis, orbital cellulitis, or orbital pseudotumor. Within this group, eyelid swelling, proptosis, or both and impaired extraocular movements or visual acuity suggest orbital pseudotumor, orbital cellulitis, or possibly severe endophthalmitis. Fever, chills, and tenderness suggest infection (eg, orbital cellulitis, sinusitis).

A red eye suggests that the disorder causing pain is ocular rather than referred.

If pain develops in the affected eye in response to shining light in the unaffected eye when the affected eye is shut (true photophobia), the cause is most often a corneal lesion or uveitis.

If topical anesthetic drops (eg, proparacaine) abolish pain in a red eye, the cause is probably a corneal disorder.

Some findings are more suggestive of particular disorders. Pain and photophobia days after blunt eye trauma suggest post-traumatic uveitis. Hammering or drilling metal is a risk factor for occult metal intraocular foreign body. Pain with movement of extraocular muscles and loss of pupillary light response that is disproportionate to loss of visual acuity suggest optic neuritis.

Testing: Testing is not usually necessary, with some exceptions (see Table 108–8). Gonioscopy is done if glaucoma is suspected based on increased intraocular pressure. Imaging, usually with CT or MRI, is done if orbital pseudotumor or orbital cellulitis is suspected, or if sinusitis is suspected but the diagnosis is not clinically clear. MRI is often done when optic

Table 108–8. SOME CAUSES OF EYE PAIN

CAUSE	SUGGESTIVE FINDINGS*	DIAGNOSTIC APPROACH
Disorders affecting primarily the cornea[†]		
Contact lens keratitis	Ocular ache, grittiness, prolonged wearing of contact lenses, bilateral red eyes, lacrimation, corneal edema	Clinical evaluation
Corneal abrasion or foreign body	Usually clear history of injury, unilateral pain when blinking, foreign body sensation Sometimes a predisposing disorder such as trichiasis Lesion or foreign body visible on slit-lamp examination	Clinical evaluation, including eyelid eversion
Corneal ulcer	Aching, foreign body sensation, photophobia, red eye, grayish opacity on cornea, followed by a visible crater Possibly history of sleeping with contact lenses	Scrapings for culture (done by ophthalmologist)
Epidemic keratoconjunctivitis (adenoviral keratitis) when severe	Ocular ache, grittiness, bilateral red eyes, copious watery discharge, preauricular lymphadenopathy, chemosis (bulging of the conjunctiva), often eyelid edema Punctate corneal staining on fluorescein examination	Clinical evaluation
Herpes zoster ophthalmicus	Early: Unilateral vesicles and crusts on an erythematous base in a V_1 distribution, sometimes affecting the tip of the nose Eyelid edema, red eye Late: Redness, quite severe pain Often associated with uveitis	Clinical evaluation Viral culture if diagnosis is unclear
Herpes simplex keratitis	Acute: Onset after conjunctivitis, blisters on eyelid Late acute or recurrent: Classic dendritic corneal lesion on slit-lamp examination Usually unilateral (may be bilateral in children or patients with atopy)	Clinical evaluation Viral culture if diagnosis is unclear
Welder's or UV keratitis	Onset hours after exposure to excessive UV light (eg, from welding or bright sun on snow) Bilateral; ocular ache, grittiness Marked injection and typical punctate corneal staining on fluorescein examination of the cornea	Clinical evaluation
Other ocular disorders		
Acute angle-closure glaucoma	Severe ocular ache, headache, nausea, vomiting, halos around lights, hazy cornea (caused by edema), marked erythema Intraocular pressure usually > 40 mm Hg	Gonioscopy by ophthalmologist

Table 108–8. SOME CAUSES OF EYE PAIN (*Continued*)

CAUSE	SUGGESTIVE FINDINGS*	DIAGNOSTIC APPROACH
Other ocular disorders		
Anterior uveitis	Ocular ache, ciliary flush, photophobia, often a risk factor (eg, autoimmune disorder, posttrauma) Cells and flare on slit-lamp examination Rarely hypopyon	Clinical evaluation
Endophthalmitis	Ocular ache, intense conjunctival hyperemia, photophobia, severely decreased visual acuity, risk factors (usually recent intraocular surgery or trauma) Unilateral Cells and flare and commonly hypopyon on slit-lamp examination	Clinical evaluation and cultures of aqueous or vitreous humor by ophthalmologist
Optic neuritis	Mild pain, which may worsen with eye movement Vision loss, ranging from a small scotoma to blindness Afferent pupillary defect (a particularly characteristic finding if some visual acuity is preserved) Eyelids and cornea normal, sometimes a swollen optic disk	Consideration of gadolinium-enhanced MRI to look for optic nerve edema and demyelinating lesions within the brain (most commonly due to multiple sclerosis)
Orbital cellulitis	Ocular ache, periocular ache, red and swollen eyelids, proptosis, impaired extraocular movements, decreased visual acuity, fever Unilateral Sometimes preceded by symptoms of sinusitis	CT or MRI
Orbital pseudotumor	Ocular ache, periocular ache (may be very severe), unilateral proptosis Impaired extraocular movements, periorbital edema, gradual onset	CT or MRI Biopsy
Scleritis	Pain very severe (often described as boring), photophobia, lacrimation, red or violaceous patches under bulbar conjunctiva, scleral edema Often history of autoimmune disorder	Clinical evaluation
Disorders causing referred pain		
Cluster headaches or migraine headaches	Prior episodes, characteristic temporal pattern (eg, clusters of episodes at the same time each day) Aura, knifelike quality, throbbing, rhinorrhea, lacrimation, facial flushing, sometimes photosensitivity or photophobia	Clinical evaluation
Sinusitis	Sometimes periorbital edema but eye examination otherwise unremarkable Purulent rhinorrhea, headache, or eye or facial pain that varies with head position Facial tenderness, fever, sometimes productive nocturnal cough, halitosis	Sometimes CT

*Routine evaluation should include slit-lamp examination with fluorescein staining and ocular tonometry.
†Most patients have lacrimation and true photophobia (shining a light into the unaffected eye causes pain in the affected eye when the affected eye is shut).
UV = ultraviolet; V_1 = ophthalmic division of the trigeminal nerve.

neuritis is suspected, looking for demyelinating lesions in the brain suggesting multiple sclerosis.

Intraocular fluids (vitreous and aqueous humor) may be cultured for suspected endophthalmitis. Viral cultures can be used to confirm herpes zoster ophthalmicus or herpes simplex keratitis if the diagnosis is not clear clinically.

Treatment

The cause of pain is treated. Pain itself is also treated. Systemic analgesics are used as needed. Pain caused by uveitis and many corneal lesions is also relieved with cycloplegic eye drops (eg, cyclopentolate 1% qid).

KEY POINTS

- Most diagnoses can be made by clinical evaluation.
- Infection precautions should be maintained when examining patients with bilateral red eyes.
- Important danger signs are vomiting, halos around lights, fever, decreased visual acuity, proptosis, and impaired extraocular motility.
- Pain in the affected eye in response to shining light in the unaffected eye when the affected eye is shut (true photophobia) suggests a corneal lesion or uveitis.
- If a topical anesthetic (eg, proparacaine) relieves pain, the cause of pain is a corneal lesion.
- Hammering or drilling on metal is a risk factor for occult intraocular foreign body.

PROPTOSIS

(Exophthalmos)

Proptosis is protrusion of the eyeball. Exophthalmos means the same thing, and this term is usually used when describing proptosis due to Graves disease. Disorders that may cause

Table 108–9. SOME CAUSES OF PROPTOSIS

CAUSE	SUGGESTIVE FINDINGS	DIAGNOSTIC APPROACH
Graves disease	Eye symptoms: Eye pain, lacrimation, dry eyes, irritation, photophobia, ocular muscle weakness causing diplopia, vision loss caused by optic nerve compression Systemic symptoms: Palpitations, anxiety, increased appetite, weight loss, insomnia, goiter, pretibial myxedema (see p. 1347)	Thyroid function tests
Carotid-cavernous sinus or dural-cavernous sinus fistula	Pulsating proptosis with an orbital bruit	Magnetic resonance angiography
Cavernous sinus thrombosis	Ophthalmoplegia, headache, ptosis, decreased visual acuity, fever	CT or MRI
Congenital glaucoma and unilateral high myopia	Tearing, blepharospasm, redness	Intraocular pressure measurement and funduscopy by ophthalmologist
Orbital cellulitis	Redness, fever, pain, impaired visual acuity, impaired or painful extraocular movements Usually unilateral	CT or MRI
Orbital tumors (eg, lymphoma, hemangioma, vascular malformations)	Decreased visual acuity, diplopia, pain	MRI or CT
Retrobulbar hemorrhage	Decreased visual acuity, diplopia, pain, ophthalmoplegia, risk factors	Immediate CT or treatment based on clinical findings
Spheno-orbital meningioma	Pain, headache, visual field defects, ophthalmoplegia	MRI or CT

changes in the appearance of the face and eyes that resemble proptosis but are not include hyperthyroidism without infiltrative eye disease, Cushing disease, and severe obesity.

Etiology

The **most common cause** is Graves disease (see Table 108–9), which causes edema and lymphoid infiltration of the orbital tissues.

Evaluation

Rate of onset may provide a clue to diagnosis. Sudden unilateral onset suggests intraorbital hemorrhage (which can occur after surgery, retrobulbar injection, or trauma) or inflammation of the orbit or paranasal sinuses. A 2- to 3-wk onset suggests chronic inflammation or orbital inflammatory pseudotumor (non-neoplastic cellular infiltration and proliferation); slower onset suggests an orbital tumor.

Ocular examination findings typical of hyperthyroidism but unrelated to infiltrative eye disease include eyelid retraction, eyelid lag, temporal flare of the upper eyelid, and staring. Other signs include eyelid erythema and conjunctival hyperemia. Prolonged exposure of larger-than-usual areas of the eyeball to air causes corneal drying and can lead to infection and ulceration.

Red flags: The following findings are of particular concern:

- Eye pain or redness
- Headache
- Loss of vision
- Diplopia
- Fever
- Pulsating proptosis
- Neonatal proptosis

Testing: Proptosis can be confirmed with exophthalmometry, which measures the distance between the lateral angle of the bony orbit and the cornea; normal values are < 20 mm in whites and < 22 mm in blacks. CT or MRI is often useful to confirm the diagnosis and to identify structural causes of unilateral proptosis. Thyroid function testing is indicated when Graves disease is suspected.

Treatment

Lubrication to protect the cornea is required in severe cases. When lubrication is not sufficient, surgery to provide better coverage of the eye surface or to reduce proptosis may be required. Systemic corticosteroids (eg, prednisone 1 mg/kg po once/day for 1 wk, tapered over ≥ 1 mo) are often helpful in controlling edema and orbital congestion due to thyroid eye disease or inflammatory orbital pseudotumor. Other interventions vary by etiology. Graves exophthalmos is not affected by treatment of the thyroid condition but may lessen over time. Tumors must be surgically removed. Selective embolization or, rarely, trapping procedures may be effective in cases of arteriovenous fistulas involving the cavernous sinus.

KEY POINTS

- The most common cause of bilateral proptosis is Graves disease.
- Acute unilateral proptosis suggests infection or vascular disorder (eg, hemorrhage, fistula, cavernous sinus thrombosis).
- Chronic unilateral proptosis suggests tumor.
- Do CT or MRI and thyroid function testing when Graves disease is suspected.
- Apply lubrication to exposed cornea.

FLOATERS

Floaters are opacities that move across the visual field and do not correspond to external visual objects.

Pathophysiology

With aging, the vitreous humor can contract and separate from the retina. The age at which this change occurs varies but most often is between 50 and 75 yr. During this separation, the vitreous can intermittently tug on the retina. The mechanical traction stimulates the retina, which sends a signal that is perceived by the brain and interpreted as light. Complete separation of the vitreous leads to an increase in floaters, which may last for years.

However, traction on the retina may create a hole (retinal tear), and if fluid leaks behind the tear, the retina may detach. Retinal detachment may also be caused by other factors (eg, trauma, primary retinal disorders). Lightning-like flashes, common in retinal detachment, are called photopsias. Photopsias can also occur when rubbing the eyes or when looking around after awakening.

Etiology

The **most common** cause of vitreous floaters is

- Idiopathic contraction of the vitreous humor

Less common causes are listed in Table 108–10.

Rare causes of floaters include intraocular tumors (eg, lymphoma) and vitritis (inflammation of the vitreous). Intraocular foreign bodies can cause floaters but usually manifest with other symptoms, such as loss of vision, eye pain, or redness.

Table 108–10. SOME CAUSES OF FLOATERS

CAUSE	SUGGESTIVE FINDINGS*	DIAGNOSTIC APPROACH
Benign disorders		
Idiopathic vitreous floaters	Mild, stable floaters that come into the field of view intermittently and move as the eye moves Often shaped like cells or strands Translucent May be more noticeable under certain lighting conditions (eg, in bright sunlight) Normal vision May occur in both eyes, although not synchronously Normal eye examination	Clinical evaluation
Serious vitreous and retinal disorders		
Retinal detachment	Sudden, spontaneous, continuous shower of lightning-like flashes (photopsias) Curtain of vision loss moving across the visual field, visual field defect (usually peripheral) Abnormal retinal examination (eg, detached retina appears as a pale billowing parachute) Possible risk factors (eg, recent trauma, eye surgery, severe myopia)	Indirect ophthalmoscopy by an ophthalmologist after pupillary dilation
Retinal tear	Sudden, spontaneous photopsias May occur in the periphery of the retina and may be visible only by indirect ophthalmoscopy	Indirect ophthalmoscopy by an ophthalmologist after pupillary dilation
Vitreous detachment	Increase in unilateral floaters over 1 wk–3 mo in patients with average age of 50–75 yr Floaters that are cobweb-like One large floater that moves in and out of central vision Spontaneous photopsias	Indirect ophthalmoscopy by an ophthalmologist after pupillary dilation
Vitreous hemorrhage	History of proliferative diabetic retinopathy or trauma Loss of vision that may affect entire visual field Loss of red reflex	Indirect ophthalmoscopy by an ophthalmologist after pupillary dilation
Vitreous inflammation (eg, cytomegalovirus, *Toxoplasma,* or fungal chorioretinitis)	Pain Loss of visual acuity Loss of vision affecting the entire visual field Retinal lesions (sometimes cotton-like) that do not conform to an arterial or a venous territory Risk factors (eg, AIDS) Decreased red reflex May be bilateral	Evaluation and testing as directed by an ophthalmologist, based on suspected cause
Nonocular disorders		
Ocular migraine	Bilateral, synchronous, flashing lights often zigzagging on the peripheral field for 10–20 min Possible blurring of central vision Possible headache after visual symptoms Possible migraine history	Clinical evaluation

*Unilateral unless otherwise specified.

Evaluation

The most important goal is to identify serious vitreous and retinal disorders. If these disorders cannot be ruled out, patients should be examined by an ophthalmologist using an indirect ophthalmoscope after pupillary dilation. Recognizing ocular migraine is also helpful.

History: History of present illness should ascertain onset and duration of symptoms and the shape and volume of floaters, as well as whether they are unilateral or bilateral and whether they have been preceded by trauma. The patient should try to distinguish floaters from lightning-like flashes of light (as in photopsias) or jagged lines across the visual field (as in migraine). Important associated symptoms include loss of vision (and its distribution in the visual field) and eye pain.

Review of systems should seek symptoms of possible causes, such as headaches (ocular migraine) and eye redness (vitreous inflammation).

Past medical history should note diabetes (including diabetic retinopathy), migraine headaches, eye surgery, severe myopia, and any disorders that could affect the immune system (eg, AIDS).

Physical examination: Eye examination should be reasonably complete. Best corrected visual acuity is measured. The eyes are inspected for redness. Visual fields are assessed in all patients. However, recognition of visual field defects by bedside examination is very insensitive, so inability to show such a defect is not evidence that the patient has full visual fields. Extraocular movements and pupillary light responses are assessed. If patients have a red eye or eye pain, the corneas are examined under magnification after fluorescein staining, and slit-lamp examination is done if possible. Ocular pressure is measured (tonometry).

Ophthalmoscopy is the most important part of the examination; it is done after dilating the pupils. To dilate the pupils, the physician first makes sure to record pupillary size and light responses, then instills drops, usually 1 drop each of a short-acting α-adrenergic agonist (eg, 2.5% phenylephrine) and a cycloplegic (eg, 1% tropicamide or 1% cyclopentolate). The pupils are fully dilated about 20 min after these drops are instilled. Ophthalmoscopy is done by a nonophthalmologist using a direct ophthalmoscope. An ophthalmologist does indirect ophthalmoscopy, which provides a more complete view of the retina, particularly the periphery.

Red flags: The following findings are of particular concern:

- Sudden increase in floaters
- Photopsias
- Loss of vision, diffuse or focal (visual field defect)
- Recent eye surgery or eye trauma
- Eye pain
- Loss of red reflex
- Abnormal retinal findings

Interpretation of findings: Retinal detachment is suggested by sudden increases in floaters, photopsias, or any of its other, more specific characteristics (eg, visual field defects, retinal abnormalities). Bilateral synchronous symptoms suggest ocular migraine, although patients often have difficulty deciphering the laterality of their symptoms (eg, they often interpret scintillating scotoma of the left field of both eyes as left-eyed). Loss of red reflex suggests opacification of the vitreous (eg, vitreous hemorrhage or inflammation), but it also can be caused by advanced cataracts. Loss of vision suggests a serious disorder causing dysfunction of the vitreous or retina.

Testing: Patients who require evaluation by an ophthalmologist may need testing. However, tests can be selected by or in conjunction with the ophthalmologist. For example, patients suspected of having chorioretinitis may require microbiologic testing.

Treatment

Idiopathic vitreous floaters require no treatment. Other disorders causing symptoms are treated.

KEY POINTS

- Floaters by themselves rarely indicate a serious disorder.
- Patients with any abnormal findings on examination require ophthalmologic referral.
- If floaters are accompanied by any other symptoms (eg, persistent flashing lights, visual deficit, sensation of a moving curtain of vision loss) or develop suddenly, patients require ophthalmologic referral, regardless of examination findings.

RED EYE

(Pink Eye)

Red eye refers to a red appearance of the opened eye, reflecting dilation of the superficial ocular vessels.

Pathophysiology

Dilation of superficial ocular vessels can result from

- Infection
- Allergy
- Inflammation (noninfectious)
- Elevated intraocular pressure (less common)

Several ocular components may be involved, most commonly the conjunctiva, but also the uveal tract, episclera, and sclera.

Etiology

The most common causes of red eye include

- Infectious conjunctivitis
- Allergic conjunctivitis

Corneal abrasions and foreign bodies are common causes (see Table 108–11). Although the eye is red, patients usually present with a complaint of injury, eye pain, or both. However, in young children and infants, this information may be unavailable.

Evaluation

Most disorders can be diagnosed by a general health care practitioner.

History: History of present illness should note the onset and duration of redness and presence of any change in vision, itching, scratchy sensation, pain, or discharge. Nature and severity of pain, including whether pain is worsened by light (photophobia), are noted. The clinician should determine whether discharge is watery or purulent. Other questions assess history of injury, including exposure to irritants and use of contact lenses (eg, possible overuse, such as wearing them while sleeping). Prior episodes of eye pain or redness and their time patterns are elicited.

Review of systems should seek symptoms suggesting possible causes, including headache, nausea, vomiting, and halos around lights (acute angle-closure glaucoma); runny nose and sneezing (allergies, URI); and cough, sore throat, and malaise (URI).

Past medical history includes questions about known allergies and autoimmune disorders. Drug history should specifically ask about recent use of topical ophthalmic drugs (including OTC drugs), which might be sensitizing.

Table 108–11. SOME CAUSES OF RED EYE

CAUSE	SUGGESTIVE FINDINGS	DIAGNOSTIC APPROACH
Conjunctival disorders and episcleritis*		
Allergic or seasonal conjunctivitis	Bilateral, prominent itching, possibly conjunctival bulging (chemosis) Known allergies or other features of allergies (eg, seasonal recurrences, rhinorrhea) Sometimes use of topical ophthalmic drugs (particularly neomycin)	Clinical evaluation
Chemical (irritant) conjunctivitis	Exposure to potential irritants (eg, dust, smoke, ammonia, chlorine, phosgene)	Clinical evaluation
Episcleritis	Unilateral focal redness, mild irritation, minimal lacrimation	Clinical evaluation
Infectious conjunctivitis	Scratchy sensation, photosensitivity Sometimes mucopurulent discharge, eyelid edema, or follicles on tarsal conjunctiva	Clinical evaluation
Subconjunctival hemorrhage	Unilateral, asymptomatic focal red patch or confluent redness Possibly prior trauma or Valsalva maneuver Often history of use of anticoagulants or antiplatelet drugs (eg, aspirin, NSAIDs, warfarin)	Clinical evaluation
Vernal conjunctivitis	Intense itching, stringy discharge Usually preadolescent or adolescent males Other atopic disorders Waxing in spring and waning in winter	Clinical evaluation
Corneal disorders†		
Contact lens keratitis	Prolonged wearing of contact lenses, lacrimation, corneal edema	Clinical evaluation
Corneal abrasion or foreign body	Onset after injury (but this history may be inapparent in infants and young children) Foreign body sensation Lesion on fluorescein staining	Clinical evaluation
Corneal ulcer	Often grayish opacity on the cornea, followed by a visible crater Possibly a history of sleeping with contact lenses	Culture of ulcer (scrapings done by an ophthalmologist)
Epidemic keratoconjunctivitis (adenoviral keratitis), if moderate or severe	Copious watery discharge Often eyelid edema, preauricular lymphadenopathy, chemosis (bulging of the conjunctiva) Occasionally severe temporary loss of vision Punctate pattern on fluorescein staining	Clinical evaluation
Herpes simplex keratitis	Onset after conjunctivitis, blisters on eyelid Classic dendritic corneal lesion on fluorescein staining Unilateral	Clinical evaluation Viral culture if diagnosis is unclear
Herpes zoster ophthalmicus	Unilateral vesicles and crusts on an erythematous base in a V_1 distribution, sometimes affecting the tip of the nose Eyelid edema Red eye May be associated with uveitis Possibly severe pain	Clinical evaluation Viral culture if diagnosis is unclear
Other disorders		
Acute angle-closure glaucoma	Severe ocular ache Headache, nausea, vomiting, halos around lights Hazy cornea (caused by edema), marked conjunctival erythema Decreased visual acuity Intraocular pressure usually > 40 mm Hg	Tonometry and gonioscopy

Table continues on the following page.

Table 108–11. SOME CAUSES OF RED EYE (*Continued*)

CAUSE	SUGGESTIVE FINDINGS	DIAGNOSTIC APPROACH
Anterior uveitis	Ocular ache, photophobia Ciliary flush (redness most concentrated and often confluent around the cornea) Often a risk factor (eg, autoimmune disorder, blunt trauma within previous few days) Possibly decreased visual acuity or pus in anterior chamber (hypopyon) Cells and flare on slit-lamp examination	Clinical evaluation
Scleritis	Severe pain, often described as boring Photophobia, lacrimation Red or violaceous patches under bulbar conjunctiva Scleral edema Tenderness of globe when palpated Often history of autoimmune disorder	Clinical evaluation Further testing by or in conjunction with an ophthalmologist

*Unless otherwise described, usually characterized by itching or scratchy sensation, lacrimation, diffuse redness, and often photosensitivity, but no change in vision and absence of pain and true photophobia.

†Unless otherwise described, usually characterized by lacrimation, pain, and true photophobia. Vision affected if the lesion involves the visual axis.

V_1 = ophthalmic division of the trigeminal nerve.

Physical examination: General examination should include head and neck examination for signs of associated disorders (eg, URI, allergic rhinitis, zoster rash).

Eye examination involves a formal measure of visual acuity and usually requires a penlight, fluorescein stain, and slit lamp.

Best corrected visual acuity is measured. Pupillary size and reactivity to light are assessed. True photophobia (sometimes called consensual photophobia) is present if shining light into an unaffected eye causes pain in the affected eye when the affected eye is shut. Extraocular movements are assessed, and the eye and periorbital tissues are inspected for lesions and swelling. The tarsal surface is inspected for follicles. The corneas are stained with fluorescein and examined with magnification. If a corneal abrasion is found, the eyelid is everted and examined for hidden foreign bodies. Inspection of the ocular structures and cornea is best done using a slit lamp. A slit lamp is also used to examine the anterior chamber for cells, flare, and pus (hypopyon). Ocular pressure is measured using tonometry, although it may be permissible to omit this test if there are no symptoms or signs suggesting a disorder other than conjunctivitis.

Red flags: The following findings are of particular concern:

- Sudden, severe pain and vomiting
- Zoster rash
- Decreased visual acuity
- Corneal crater
- Branching, dendritic corneal lesion
- Ocular pressure > 40 mm Hg
- Failure to blanch with phenylephrine eye drop

Interpretation of findings: Conjunctival disorders and **episcleritis** are differentiated from other causes of red eye by the absence of pain, photophobia, and corneal staining. Among these disorders, episcleritis is differentiated by its focality, and subconjunctival hemorrhage is usually differentiated by the absence of lacrimation, itching, and photosensitivity. Clinical criteria do not accurately differentiate viral from bacterial conjunctivitis.

Corneal disorders are differentiated from other causes of red eye (and usually from each other) by fluorescein staining. These disorders also tend to be characterized by pain and photophobia. If instillation of an ocular anesthetic drop (eg, proparacaine 0.5%), which is done before tonometry and ideally before fluorescein instillation, completely relieves pain, the cause is probably limited to the cornea. If pain is present and is not relieved by an ocular anesthetic, the cause may be anterior uveitis, glaucoma, or scleritis. Because patients may have anterior uveitis secondary to corneal lesions, persistence of pain after instillation of the anesthetic does not exclude a corneal lesion.

Anterior uveitis, glaucoma, acute angle-closure glaucoma, and scleritis can usually be differentiated from other causes of red eye by the presence of pain and the absence of corneal staining. Anterior uveitis is likely in patients with pain, true photophobia, absence of corneal fluorescein staining, and normal intraocular pressure; it is definitively diagnosed based on the presence of cells and flare in the anterior chamber. However, these findings may be difficult for general health care practitioners to discern. Acute angle-closure glaucoma can usually be recognized by the sudden onset of its severe and characteristic symptoms, but tonometry is definitive.

Instillation of phenylephrine 2.5% causes blanching in a red eye unless the cause is scleritis. Phenylephrine is instilled to dilate the pupil in patients needing a thorough retinal examination. However, it should not be used in patients who have the following:

- Suspected acute angle-closure glaucoma
- A history of angle-closure glaucoma
- A narrow anterior chamber

Testing: Testing is usually unnecessary. Viral cultures may help if herpes simplex or herpes zoster is suspected and the diagnosis is not clear clinically. Corneal ulcers are cultured by an ophthalmologist. Gonioscopy is done in patients with glaucoma. Testing for autoimmune disorders may be worthwhile in patients with uveitis and no obvious cause (eg, trauma). Patients with scleritis undergo further testing as directed by an ophthalmologist.

Treatment

The cause is treated. Red eye itself does not require treatment. Topical vasoconstrictors are not recommended.

KEY POINTS

- Most cases are caused by conjunctivitis.
- Pain and true photophobia suggest other, more serious diagnoses.
- In patients with pain, slit-lamp examination with fluorescein staining and tonometry are key.
- Persistence of pain despite an ocular anesthetic in a patient with a normal fluorescein examination suggests anterior uveitis, scleritis, or acute angle-closure glaucoma. These diagnoses should not be missed.

TEARING

(Epiphora)

Excess tearing may cause a sensation of watery eyes or result in tears falling down the cheek (epiphora).

Pathophysiology

Tears are produced in the lacrimal gland and drain through the upper and lower puncta into the canaliculi and then into the lacrimal sac and nasolacrimal duct (see Fig. 110–1 on p. 921). Obstruction of tear drainage can lead to stasis and infection. Recurrent infection of the lacrimal sac (dacryocystitis) can sometimes spread, potentially leading to orbital cellulitis.

Etiology

Overall, the **most common** causes of tearing are

- URI
- Allergic rhinitis

Tearing can be caused by increased tear production or decreased nasolacrimal drainage.

Increased tear production: The most common causes are

- URI
- Allergic rhinitis
- Allergic conjunctivitis
- Dry eyes (reflex tearing produced in response to dryness of the ocular surface)
- Trichiasis

Any disorder causing conjunctival or corneal irritation can increase tear production (see Table 108–12). However, most patients with corneal disorders that cause excess tearing (eg, corneal abrasion, corneal ulcer, corneal foreign body, keratitis) or with primary angle-closure glaucoma or anterior uveitis present with eye symptoms other than tearing (eg, eye pain, redness). Most people who have been crying do not present for evaluation of tearing.

Decreased nasolacrimal drainage: The most common causes are

- Idiopathic age-related nasolacrimal duct stenosis
- Dacryocystitis
- Ectropion

Table 108–12. SOME CAUSES OF TEARING

CAUSE	SUGGESTIVE FINDINGS
Disorders causing excess tear production	
Dry eyes with reflex tearing	Worse on cold or windy days or with exposure to cigarette smoke or dry heat Intermittent foreign body sensation In patients with a disorder known to cause dry eyes (eg, blepharitis)
Ocular surface irritation (eg, allergic conjunctivitis, corneal abrasion or erosion or ulcer, foreign body, hordeolum, infectious conjunctivitis, irritant chemicals, keratitis, trichiasis, irritation with punctate lesions due to paresis of blink muscles as in facial nerve palsy)	Grittiness Redness In patients with corneal lesions, pain, constant foreign body sensation, and photophobia
Allergic conjunctivitis	Itching Possibly follicles on tarsal conjunctiva
Nasal irritation and inflammation (eg, allergic rhinitis, URI)	Rhinorrhea, sneezing, nasal congestion
Disorders causing nasolacrimal drainage obstruction	
Congenital nasolacrimal duct obstruction	Symptoms that begin shortly after age 2 wk
Idiopathic age-related nasolacrimal duct stenosis	Usually normal examination except for evidence of obstruction
Dacryocystitis	Nasal pain Often swelling, redness, and warmth over the lacrimal sac and, with palpation, tenderness and expression of pus
Tumors	Hard mass in the nasolacrimal duct system, particularly in the elderly
Other causes of nasolacrimal drainage stricture or obstruction (see text)	Often risk factors Often no characteristic examination findings other than obstruction
Disorders causing decreased drainage without obstruction	
Misalignment between tear film and puncta (eg, ectropion, entropion)	Usually visible on examination

Nasolacrimal drainage system obstruction may be caused by strictures, tumors, or foreign bodies (eg, stones, often associated with subclinical infection by *Actinomyces*). Obstruction can also be a congenital malformation. Many disorders and drugs can cause stricture or obstruction of nasolacrimal drainage.

Other causes of nasolacrimal drainage stricture or obstruction include

- Burns
- Chemotherapy drugs
- Eye drops (particularly echothiophate iodide, epinephrine, and pilocarpine)
- Infection, including canaliculitis (eg, caused by *Staphylococcus aureus, Actinomyces, Streptococcus, Pseudomonas,* herpes zoster virus, herpes simplex conjunctivitis, infectious mononucleosis, human papillomavirus, *Ascaris,* leprosy, TB)
- Inflammatory disorders (sarcoidosis, granulomatosis with polyangiitis [formerly called Wegener granulomatosis])
- Injuries (eg, nasoethmoid fractures; nasal, orbital, or endoscopic sinus surgery)
- Obstruction of nasal outlet despite an intact nasolacrimal system (eg, URI, allergic rhinitis, sinusitis)
- Radiation therapy
- Stevens-Johnson syndrome
- Tumors (eg, primary lacrimal sac tumors, benign papillomas, squamous and basal cell carcinoma, transitional cell carcinoma, fibrous histiocytomas, midline granuloma, lymphoma)

Evaluation

History: History of present illness addresses the duration, onset, and severity of symptoms, including whether tears drip down the cheek (true epiphora). The effects of weather, environmental humidity, and cigarette smoke are ascertained.

Review of symptoms should seek symptoms of possible causes, including itching, rhinorrhea, or sneezing, particularly when occurring perennially or after exposure to specific potential allergens (allergic reaction); eye irritation or pain (blepharitis, corneal abrasion, irritant chemicals); and pain near the medial canthus (dacryocystitis). Other symptoms are of lower yield but should be sought; they include positional headache, purulent rhinorrhea, nocturnal cough, and fever (sinusitis, granulomatosis with polyangiitis); rash (Stevens-Johnson syndrome); cough, dyspnea, and chest pain (sarcoidosis); and epistaxis, hemoptysis, polyarthralgias, and myalgias (granulomatosis with polyangiitis).

Past medical history asks about known disorders that can cause tearing, including granulomatosis with polyangiitis, sarcoidosis, and cancer treated with chemotherapy drugs; disorders that cause dry eyes (eg, RA, sarcoidosis, Sjögren syndrome); and drugs, such as echothiophate, epinephrine, and pilocarpine. Previous ocular and nasal history, including infections, injuries, surgical procedures, and radiation exposure, is ascertained.

Physical examination: Examination focuses on the eye and surrounding structures.

The face is inspected; asymmetry suggests congenital or acquired obstruction of nasolacrimal duct drainage. When available, a slit lamp should be used to examine the eyes. The conjunctivae and corneas are inspected for lesions, including punctate spots, and redness. The cornea is stained with fluorescein and examined. The lids are everted to detect hidden foreign bodies. The eyelids, including the lacrimal puncta, are closely inspected for foreign bodies, blepharitis, hordeola, ectropion, entropion, and trichiasis. The lacrimal sac (near the medial canthus) is palpated for warmth, tenderness, and swelling. Any swellings are palpated for consistency and to see whether pus is expressed.

The nose is examined for congestion, purulence, and bleeding.

Red flags: The following findings are of particular concern:

- Repeated, unexplained episodes of tearing
- Hard mass in or near the nasolacrimal drainage structures

Interpretation of findings: Findings that suggest obstruction of nasolacrimal drainage include

- Tears running down the cheek (true epiphora)
- Absence of signs of a specific cause

A cause is often evident from the clinical evaluation (see Table 108–12).

Testing: Testing is often unnecessary because the cause is usually evident from the examination.

Schirmer test with a large amount of wetting (eg, > 25 mm) suggests an evaporative dry eye as the etiology of tearing. Schirmer test with very little wetting (< 5.5 mm) suggests an aqueous tear-deficient dry eye. Usually, Schirmer test is done by an ophthalmologist to ensure it is done and interpreted correctly.

Probing and saline irrigation of the lacrimal drainage system can help detect anatomic obstruction of drainage, as well as stenosis due to complete obstruction of the nasolacrimal drainage system. Irrigation is done with and without fluorescein dye. Reflux through the opposite punctum or canaliculus signals fixed obstruction; reflux and nasal drainage signify stenosis. This test is considered adjunctive and is done by ophthalmologists.

Imaging tests and procedures (dacryocystography, CT, nasal endoscopy) are sometimes useful to delineate abnormal anatomy when surgery is being considered or occasionally to detect an abscess.

Treatment

Underlying disorders (eg, allergies, foreign bodies, conjunctivitis) are treated.

The use of artificial tears lessens tearing when dry eyes or corneal epithelial defects are the cause.

Congenital nasolacrimal duct obstruction often resolves spontaneously. In patients < 1 yr, manual compression of the lacrimal sac 4 or 5 times/day may relieve the distal obstruction. After 1 yr, the nasolacrimal duct may need probing with the patient under general anesthesia. If obstruction is recurrent, a temporary drainage tube may be inserted.

In acquired nasolacrimal duct obstruction, irrigation of the nasolacrimal duct may be therapeutic when underlying disorders do not respond to treatment. As a last resort, a passage between the lacrimal sac and the nasal cavity can be created surgically (dacryocystorhinostomy).

In cases of punctal or canalicular stenosis, dilation is usually curative. If canalicular stenosis is severe and bothersome, a surgical procedure that places a glass tube leading from the caruncle into the nasal cavity can be considered.

Geriatrics Essentials

Idiopathic age-related nasolacrimal duct stenosis is the most common cause of unexplained epiphora in elderly patients; however, tumors should also be considered.

KEY POINTS

- If tears do not run down the cheek, dry eyes is often the cause.
- If tears run down the cheek, obstruction of nasolacrimal drainage is likely.
- Testing is often unnecessary but is needed in cases of recurrent infectious dacryocystitis, which can progress to more serious conditions such as orbital cellulitis.

OTHER EYE SYMPTOMS

See p. 927 for a discussion of dry eyes. The disorder is most often idiopathic or associated with older age but can also be caused by connective tissue diseases (eg, Sjögren syndrome, RA, SLE).

Eye discharge: Discharge is often accompanied by a red eye (see p. 912) and commonly is caused by allergic or infectious conjunctivitis, blepharitis, and, in infants, ophthalmia neonatorum (neonatal conjunctivitis). Infectious discharge may be purulent in bacterial infection, such as staphylococcal conjunctivitis or gonorrhea. Less common causes include dacryocystitis and canaliculitis.

Diagnosis is usually made clinically. Allergic conjunctivitis can often be distinguished from infectious by predominance of itching, clear discharge, and presence of other allergic symptoms (eg, runny nose, sneezing). Clinical differentiation between viral and bacterial conjunctivitis is difficult. Cultures are not usually done, but are indicated for patients with the following:

- Clinically suspected gonococcal or chlamydial conjunctivitis
- Severe symptoms
- Immunocompromise
- A vulnerable eye (eg, after a corneal transplant, in exophthalmos due to Graves disease)
- Ineffective initial therapy

Halos: Halos around light may result from cataracts; conditions that result in corneal edema, such as acute angle-closure glaucoma or disorders that cause bullous keratopathy; corneal haziness; mucus on the cornea; or drugs, such as digoxin or chloroquine.

Blue hues: Certain conditions may cause a blue tint to the visual field (cyanopsia), such as cataract removal or use of sildenafil. Cyanopsia may occur for a few days after cataract removal or as an adverse effect of sildenafil and possibly other phosphodiesterase-5 (PDE5) inhibitors.

Scotomata: Scotomata are visual field deficits and are divided into

- Negative scotomata (blind spots)
- Positive scotomata (light spots or scintillating flashes)

Negative scotomata may not be noticed by patients unless they involve central vision and interfere significantly with visual acuity; the complaint is most often decreased visual acuity (see p. 896). Negative scotomata have multiple causes that can sometimes be distinguished by the specific type of field deficit as identified by use of a tangent screen, Goldmann perimeter, or computerized automated perimetry (in which the visual field is mapped out in detail based on patient response to a series of flashing lights in different locations controlled by a standardized computer program).

Positive scotomata represent a response to abnormal stimulation of some portion of the visual system, as occurs in migraines.

109 Cataract

A cataract is a congenital or degenerative opacity of the lens. The main symptom is gradual, painless vision blurring. Diagnosis is by ophthalmoscopy and slit-lamp examination. Treatment is surgical removal and placement of an intraocular lens.

Cataracts (see Plate 9) are the leading cause of blindness worldwide. In the US, almost 20% of people aged 65 to 74 have cataracts that interfere with vision. Almost one in two people older than 75 has cataracts.

Lens opacity can develop in several locations:

- Central lens nucleus (nuclear cataract)
- Beneath the posterior lens capsule (posterior subcapsular cataract)
- On the side of the lens (cortical cataract)—these usually do not interfere with central vision

Etiology

Cataracts occur with aging. Other risk factors may include the following:

- Trauma (sometimes causing cataracts years later)
- Smoking
- Alcohol use
- Exposure to x-rays
- Heat from infrared exposure
- Systemic disease (eg, diabetes)
- Uveitis
- Systemic drugs (eg, corticosteroids)
- Undernutrition
- Chronic ultraviolet light exposure

Many people have no risk factors other than age. Some cataracts are congenital, associated with numerous syndromes and diseases.

Estrogen use by women after menopause may be protective, but estrogen should not be used solely for this purpose.

Symptoms and Signs

Cataracts usually develop slowly over years. Early symptoms may be loss of contrast, glare (ie, halos and starbursts around lights, not photophobia), needing more light to see well, and problems distinguishing dark blue from black. Painless blurring eventually occurs. The degree of blurring depends on the location and extent of the opacity. Double vision or ghost images occur rarely.

With a nuclear cataract, distance vision worsens. Near vision may improve in the early stages because of changes in the refractive index of the lens; presbyopic patients may be temporarily able to read without glasses (second sight).

A posterior subcapsular cataract disproportionately affects vision because the opacity is located at the crossing point of incoming light rays. Such cataracts reduce visual acuity more when the pupil constricts (eg, in bright light, during reading). They are also the type most likely to cause loss of contrast as well as glare (halos and starbursts around lights), especially from bright lights or from car headlights while driving at night.

Rarely, the cataract swells, pushing the iris over the trabecular drainage meshwork and causing its occlusion and thus secondary closed-angle glaucoma and pain.

Diagnosis

- Ophthalmoscopy followed by slit-lamp examination

Diagnosis is best made with the pupil dilated. Well-developed cataracts appear as gray, white, or yellow-brown opacities in the lens. Examination of the red reflex through the dilated pupil with the ophthalmoscope held about 30 cm away usually discloses subtle opacities. Small cataracts stand out as dark defects in the red reflex. A large cataract may obliterate the red reflex. Slit-lamp examination provides more details about the character, location, and extent of the opacity.

PEARLS & PITFALLS

- Examination of the red reflex through the dilated pupil with the ophthalmoscope held about 30 cm away can help identify early cataracts if a slit lamp is unavailable.

Treatment

- Surgical removal of the cataract
- Placement of an intraocular lens

Frequent refractions and corrective lens prescription changes may help maintain useful vision during cataract development. Rarely, long-term pupillary dilation (with phenylephrine 2.5% q 4 to 8 h) is helpful for small centrally located cataracts. Indirect lighting while reading minimizes pupillary constriction and may optimize vision for close tasks.

Usual indications for surgery include the following:

- Best vision obtained with glasses is worse than 20/40 (< 6/12), or vision is significantly decreased under glare conditions (eg, oblique lighting while trying to read a chart) in a patient with bothersome halos or starbursts.
- Patients sense that vision is limiting (eg, by preventing activities of daily living such as driving, reading, hobbies, and occupational activities).
- Vision could potentially be meaningfully improved if the cataract is removed (ie, a significant portion of the vision loss must be caused by the cataract).

Far less common indications include cataracts that cause glaucoma or that obscure the fundus in patients who need periodic fundus examinations for management of diseases such as diabetic retinopathy and macular degeneration. There is no advantage to removing a cataract early.

Cataract extraction and lens implant procedures: Cataract extraction is usually done using a topical or local anesthetic and IV sedation. There are 3 extraction techniques:

- In **intracapsular cataract extraction,** the cataract and lens capsule are removed in one piece; this technique is rarely used.
- In **extracapsular cataract extraction,** the hard central nucleus is removed in one piece and then the soft cortex is removed in multiple small pieces.
- In **phacoemulsification,** the hard central nucleus is dissolved by ultrasound and then the soft cortex is removed in multiple small pieces.

Phacoemulsification uses the smallest incision, thus enabling the fastest healing, and is usually the preferred procedure. Femtosecond lasers can be used in refractive laser-assisted cataract surgery to perform certain parts of the cataract surgery prior to phacoemulsification. In extracapsular extraction (including phacoemulsification), the lens capsule is not removed.

A plastic or silicone lens is almost always implanted intraocularly to replace the optical focusing power of the removed crystalline lens. The lens implant is usually placed on or within the lens capsule (posterior chamber lens). The lens can also be placed in front of the iris (anterior chamber lens) or attached to the iris and within the pupil (iris plane lens). Iris plane lenses are rarely used in the US because many designs led to a high frequency of postoperative complications. Multifocal intraocular lenses are newer and have different focusing zones that may reduce dependence on glasses after surgery. Patients occasionally experience glare with these lenses, especially under low-light conditions, and also have problems with reduced contrast sensitivity.

Postsurgical care and complications: In most cases, a tapering schedule of topical antibiotics and topical corticosteroids (eg, prednisolone acetate 1% 1 drop qid) is used for up to 4 wk postsurgery. Antibiotics can also be injected into the eye (intracameral) at the conclusion of cataract surgery, with a reduced need for topical eyedrops postoperatively. Several large, controlled studies show that intracameral antibiotics decrease postoperative endophthalmitis.[1,2] Patients often wear an eye shield while sleeping and should avoid the Valsalva maneuver, heavy lifting, excessive forward bending, and eye rubbing for several weeks.

Major complications of cataract surgery are rare. Complications include the following:

- Intraoperative: Bleeding beneath the retina, causing the intraocular contents to extrude through the incision (choroidal hemorrhage—very rare and could result in irreversible blindness), vitreous prolapsing out of the incision (vitreous loss), fragments of the cataract dislocating into the vitreous, incisional burn, and detachment of corneal endothelium and its basement membrane (Descemet membrane)
- Within the first week: Endophthalmitis (infection within the eye—very rare and could result in irreversible blindness) and glaucoma
- Within the first month: Cystoid macular edema
- Months later: Bullous keratopathy (ie, swelling of the cornea due to damage to the corneal pump cells during cataract surgery), retinal detachment, and posterior capsular opacification (common but treatable with laser)

After surgery, vision returns to 20/40 (6/12) or better in 95% of eyes if there are no preexisting disorders such as amblyopia, retinopathy, macular degeneration, and glaucoma. If an intraocular lens is not implanted, contact lenses or thick glasses are needed to correct the resulting hyperopia.

1. Endophthalmitis Study Group, European Society of Cataract & Refractive Surgeons, Dublin, Ireland. Prophylaxis of postoperative endophthalmitis following cataract surgery: results of the ESCRS multicenter study and identification of risk factors. *J Cataract Refract Surg* 33:978–988; 2007.
2. Shorstein NH, Winthrop KL, Herrinton LJ: Decreased postoperative endophthalmitis rate after institution of intracameral antibiotics in a Northern California eye department. *J Cataract Refract Surg* 39:8–14; 2013.

Prevention

Many ophthalmologists recommend ultraviolet-coated eyeglasses or sunglasses as a preventive measure. Reducing risk factors such as alcohol, tobacco, and corticosteroids and controlling blood glucose in diabetes delay onset. A diet high in vitamin C, vitamin A, and carotenoids (contained in vegetables such as spinach and kale) may protect against cataracts.

KEY POINTS

- Modifiable risk factors for cataract include exposure to ultraviolet light; use of alcohol, tobacco, and systemic corticosteroids; and poor control of blood glucose.
- Symptoms include loss of contrast, glare (halos and starbursts around lights), and eventually visual blurring.
- Diagnosis is by examination with the eye dilated.
- Surgical removal and placement of an intraocular lens are usually indicated if the cataract contributes to visual loss that interferes with activities of daily living, causes bothersome glare, or reaches certain degrees of severity (eg, best-corrected visual acuity worse than 20/40).

110 Eyelid and Lacrimal Disorders

BLEPHARITIS

Blepharitis is inflammation of the eyelid margins that may be acute or chronic. Symptoms and signs include itching and burning of the eyelid margins with redness and edema. Diagnosis is by history and examination. Acute ulcerative blepharitis is usually treated with topical antibiotics or systemic antivirals. Acute nonulcerative blepharitis is occasionally treated with topical corticosteroids. Chronic disease is treated with tear supplements, warm compresses, and occasionally oral antibiotics (eg, a tetracycline) for meibomian gland dysfunction or with eyelid hygiene and tear supplements for seborrheic blepharitis.

Etiology

Blepharitis may be acute (ulcerative or nonulcerative) or chronic (meibomian gland dysfunction, seborrheic blepharitis).

Acute blepharitis: Acute ulcerative blepharitis is usually caused by bacterial infection (usually staphylococcal) of the eyelid margin at the origins of the eyelashes; the lash follicles and the meibomian glands are also involved. It may also be due to a virus (eg, herpes simplex, varicella zoster). Bacterial infections typically have more crusting than the viral type which usually has more of a clear serous discharge.

Acute nonulcerative blepharitis is usually caused by an allergic reaction involving the same area (eg, atopic blepharodermatitis and seasonal allergic blepharoconjunctivitis, which cause intense itching, rubbing, and a rash; or contact sensitivity [dermatoblepharoconjunctivitis]).

Chronic blepharitis: Chronic blepharitis is noninfectious inflammation of unknown cause. Meibomian glands in the eyelid produce lipids (meibum) that reduce tear evaporation by forming a lipid layer on top of the aqueous tear layer. In meibomian gland dysfunction, the lipid composition is abnormal, and gland ducts and orifices become inspissated with hard, waxy plugs. Many patients have rosacea and recurrent hordeola or chalazia.

Many patients with seborrheic blepharitis have seborrheic dermatitis of the face and scalp or acne rosacea. Secondary bacterial colonization often occurs on the scales that develop on the eyelid margin. Meibomian glands can become obstructed.

Most patients with meibomian gland dysfunction or seborrheic blepharitis have increased tear evaporation and secondary keratoconjunctivitis sicca, also known as dry eye.

Symptoms and Signs

Symptoms common to all forms of blepharitis include itching and burning of the eyelid margins and conjunctival irritation with lacrimation, photosensitivity, and foreign body sensation.

Acute blepharitis: In acute ulcerative blepharitis, small pustules may develop in eyelash follicles and eventually break down to form shallow marginal ulcers. Tenacious adherent crusts leave a bleeding surface when removed. During sleep, eyelids can become glued together by dried secretions. Recurrent ulcerative blepharitis can cause eyelid scars and loss of eyelashes.

In acute nonulcerative blepharitis, eyelid margins become edematous and erythematous; eyelashes may become crusted with dried serous fluid.

Chronic blepharitis: In meibomian gland dysfunction, examination reveals dilated, inspissated gland orifices that, when pressed, exude a waxy, thick, yellowish secretion. In seborrheic blepharitis, greasy, easily removable scales develop on eyelid margins. Most patients with seborrheic blepharitis and meibomian gland dysfunction have symptoms of keratoconjunctivitis sicca, such as foreign body sensation, grittiness, eye strain and fatigue, and blurring with prolonged visual effort.

Diagnosis

- Slit-lamp examination

Diagnosis is usually by slit-lamp examination. Chronic blepharitis that does not respond to treatment may require biopsy to exclude eyelid tumors that can simulate the condition.

Prognosis

Acute blepharitis most often responds to treatment but may recur, develop into chronic blepharitis, or both. Chronic blepharitis is indolent, recurrent, and resistant to treatment. Exacerbations are inconvenient, uncomfortable, and cosmetically unappealing but do not usually result in corneal scarring or vision loss.

Treatment

- Supportive measures (eg, treatment of keratoconjunctivitis sicca, warm compresses, cleansing of eyelids) as clinically indicated
- Antimicrobials for acute ulcerative blepharitis

Acute blepharitis: Acute ulcerative blepharitis is treated with an antibiotic ointment (eg, bacitracin/polymyxin B, erythromycin, or gentamicin 0.3% qid for 7 to 10 days). Acute viral ulcerative blepharitis is treated with systemic antivirals (eg, for herpes simplex, acyclovir 400 mg po tid for 7 days; for varicella zoster, famciclovir 500 mg po tid or valacyclovir 1 g po tid for 7 days).

Treatment of acute nonulcerative blepharitis begins with avoiding the offending action (eg, rubbing) or substance (eg, new eye drops). Warm compresses over the closed eyelid may relieve symptoms and speed resolution. If swelling persists > 24 h, topical corticosteroids (eg, fluorometholone ophthalmic ointment 0.1% tid for 7 days) can be used.

Chronic blepharitis: The initial treatment for both meibomian gland dysfunction and seborrheic blepharitis is directed toward the secondary keratoconjunctivitis sicca. Tear supplements during the day, bland ointments at night, and, if necessary, punctal plugs (inserts that obstruct the puncta and thus decrease tear drainage) are effective in most patients.

If needed, additional treatment for meibomian gland dysfunction includes warm compresses to melt the waxy plugs and occasionally eyelid massage to extrude trapped secretions and coat the ocular surface.

If needed, additional treatment for seborrheic blepharitis includes gentle cleansing of the eyelid margin (lid scrubs) 2 times a day with a cotton swab dipped in a dilute solution of baby shampoo (2 to 3 drops in ½ cup of warm water). A topical antibiotic ointment (erythromycin, bacitracin/polymyxin B or sulfacetamide 10% bid for up to 3 mo) may be added to reduce bacterial counts on the eyelid margin when cases are unresponsive to weeks of eyelid hygiene.

In some cases, a tetracycline (eg, doxycycline 100 mg po bid tapered over 3 to 4 mo) may also be effective because it changes the composition of meibomian gland secretions or alters the composition of skin bacteria.

KEY POINTS

- Common forms of blepharitis include acute ulcerative (often secondary to staphylococcal or herpes virus infection), acute nonulcerative (usually allergic), and chronic (often with meibomian gland dysfunction or seborrheic dermatitis).
- Secondary conjunctivitis sicca usually accompanies chronic blepharitis.
- Common symptoms include itching and burning of the eyelid margins and conjunctival irritation with lacrimation, photosensitivity, and foreign body sensation.
- Diagnosis is usually by slit-lamp examination.
- Supportive treatments are indicated (eg, warm compresses, eyelid cleansing, and treatment of keratoconjunctivitis sicca as needed).
- Specific treatments can include antimicrobials for acute ulcerative blepharitis and sometimes chronic blepharitis and topical corticosteroids for persistent acute nonulcerative blepharitis.

BLEPHAROSPASM

Blepharospasm is spasm of muscles around the eye causing involuntary blinking and eye closing.

The cause of blepharospasm is most often unknown. It affects women more than men and tends to occur in families. Rarely, blepharospasm may be secondary to eye disorders, including those that cause ocular irritation (eg, trichiasis, an inward growing eye lash), corneal foreign body, keratoconjunctivitis sicca (dry eye) and systemic neurologic diseases that cause spasm (eg, Parkinson disease).

Symptoms are involuntary blinking and closing of the eyes; in severe cases, people cannot open their eyes. Spasms may be made worse by fatigue, bright light, and anxiety.

Treatment of blepharospasm involves injecting botulinum toxin type A into the eyelid muscles; treatment must be repeated in most instances. Anxiolytics may help. Surgery to cut the periorbital muscles is also effective but, because of potential complications, is considered only if botulinum toxin is ineffective. Sunglasses help decrease the light sensitivity that may cause or accompany blepharospasm.

CANALICULITIS

Canaliculitis is inflammation of the canaliculus.

Etiology

The most common cause of canaliculitis is infection with *Actinomyces israelii,* a gram-positive bacillus with fine branching filaments, but other bacteria, fungi (eg, *Candida albicans*), and viruses (eg, herpes simplex) may be causative. An increasingly common cause of canaliculitis is a retained punctal plug (inserted as treatment for dry eyes) that has migrated into the canaliculus from the punctum.

Symptoms and Signs

Symptoms and signs are tearing, discharge, red eye (especially nasally), and mild tenderness over the involved side.

Diagnosis

- Clinical evaluation

Diagnosis is suspected based on symptoms and signs, expression of turbid secretions with pressure over the lacrimal sac and canaliculus, and a gritty sensation caused by necrotic material that can be felt during probing of the lacrimal system (see Fig. 110–1).

Canaliculitis can be differentiated from dacryocystitis. In canaliculitis, the punctum and canaliculus are red and swollen; in dacryocystitis, the punctum and canaliculus are normal, but a red, swollen, tender mass is located in or near the lacrimal sac.

Treatment

- Supportive measures (eg, warm compresses)
- Antibiotics
- Sometimes, surgery to remove concretions or foreign bodies

Treatment of canaliculitis is warm compresses, irrigation of the canaliculus with antibiotic solution (by an ophthalmologist), and removal of any concretions or foreign bodies, which usually requires surgery. Antibiotic selection is usually empiric with a 1st-generation cephalosporin or penicillinase-resistant synthetic penicillin but may be guided by irrigation samples.

KEY POINTS

- Common causes of canaliculitis are infection or retained punctal plug.
- Patients often have tearing, discharge, red eye (especially nasally), and mild tenderness over the involved side.
- On examination, secretions may be expressed when pressure is applied to the lacrimal sac and canaliculus and a gritty sensation is felt by the patient when the lacrimal system is probed.
- Treatment includes supportive measures, such as compresses, antibiotics, and sometimes surgery.

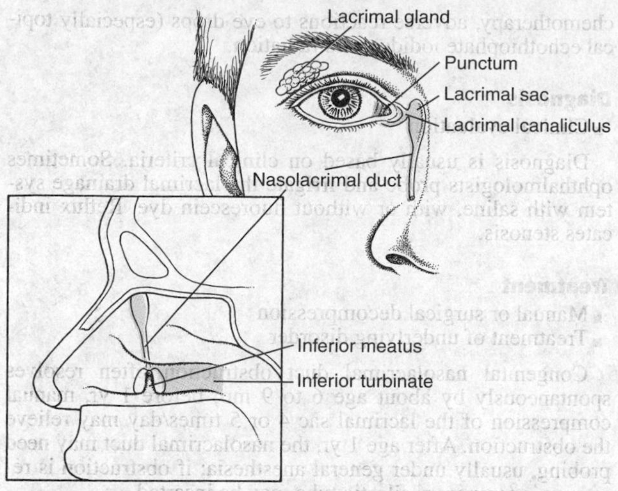

Fig. 110–1. Anatomy of the lacrimal system.

CHALAZION AND HORDEOLUM

(Stye)

Chalazia and hordeola are sudden-onset localized swellings of the eyelid. A chalazion is caused by noninfectious meibomian gland occlusion, whereas a hordeolum usually is caused by infection. Both conditions initially cause eyelid hyperemia and edema, swelling, and pain. With time, a chalazion becomes a small nontender nodule in the eyelid center, whereas a hordeolum remains painful and localizes to an eyelid margin. Diagnosis is clinical. Treatment is primarily with hot compresses. Both conditions improve spontaneously, but incision or, for chalazia, intralesional corticosteroids may be used to hasten resolution.

Chalazion: A chalazion (see Plate 12) is noninfectious obstruction of a meibomian gland causing extravasation of irritating lipid material in the eyelid soft tissues with focal secondary granulomatous inflammation. Disorders that cause abnormally thick meibomian gland secretions (eg, meibomian gland dysfunction, acne rosacea) increase the risk of meibomian gland obstruction.

Hordeolum: A hordeolum (stye—see Plate 20) is an acute, localized swelling of the eyelid that may be external or internal and usually is a pyogenic (typically staphylococcal) infection or abscess. Most hordeola are external and result from obstruction and infection of an eyelash follicle and adjacent glands of Zeis or Moll glands. Follicle obstruction may be associated with blepharitis. An internal hordeolum, which is very rare, results from infection of a meibomian gland. Sometimes cellulitis accompanies hordeola.

Symptoms and Signs

Chalazia and hordeola each cause eyelid redness, swelling, and pain.

Chalazion: Initially the eyelid is diffusely swollen. Occasionally the eyelid can be massively swollen, shutting the eye completely. After 1 or 2 days, a chalazion localizes to the body of the eyelid. Typically, a small nontender nodule or lump develops. A chalazion usually drains through the inner surface of the eyelid or is absorbed spontaneously over 2 to 8 wk; rarely, it persists longer. Depending on its size and location, a chalazion may indent the cornea, resulting in slightly blurred vision.

Hordeolum: After 1 to 2 days, an external hordeolum localizes to the eyelid margin. There may be tearing, photophobia, and a foreign body sensation. Typically, a small yellowish pustule develops at the base of an eyelash, surrounded by hyperemia, induration, and diffuse edema. Within 2 to 4 days, the lesion ruptures and discharges material (often pus), thereby relieving pain and resolving the lesion.

Symptoms of an internal hordeolum are the same as those of a chalazion, with pain, redness, and edema localized to the posterior tarsal conjunctival surface. Inflammation may be severe, sometimes with fever or chills. Inspection of the tarsal conjunctivae shows a small elevation or yellow area at the site of the affected gland. Later, an abscess forms. Spontaneous rupture is rare; however, when it does occur, it usually occurs on the conjunctival side of the eyelid and sometimes erupts through the skin side. Recurrence is common.

Diagnosis

- Clinical assessment

Diagnosis of chalazion and both kinds of hordeola is clinical; however, during the first 2 days, they may be clinically indistinguishable. Because internal hordeola are so rare, they are not usually suspected unless inflammation is severe or fever or chills are present. If the chalazion or hordeolum lies near the inner canthus of the lower eyelid, it must be differentiated from dacryocystitis and canaliculitis, which can usually be excluded by noting the location of maximum induration and tenderness (eg, eyelid for a chalazion, under the medial canthus near the side of the nose for dacryocystitis, and over the punctum for canaliculitis). Chronic chalazia that do not respond to treatment require biopsy to exclude tumor of the eyelid.

Treatment

- Hot compresses
- Sometimes drainage or drug therapy

Hot compresses for 5 to 10 min 2 or 3 times a day can be used to hasten resolution of chalazia and external hordeola.

Chalazion: Incision and curettage or intrachalazion corticosteroid therapy (0.05 to 0.2 mL triamcinolone 25 mg/mL) may be indicated if chalazia are large, unsightly, and persist for more than several weeks despite conservative therapy.

Hordeolum: An external hordeolum that does not respond to hot compresses can be incised with a sharp, fine-tipped blade. Systemic antibiotics (eg, dicloxacillin or erythromycin 250 mg po qid) are indicated when preseptal cellulitis accompanies a hordeolum.

Treatment of an internal hordeolum is oral antibiotics and incision and drainage if needed. Topical antibiotics are usually ineffective.

KEY POINTS

- Chalazia and hordeola initially cause eyelid hyperemia and edema, swelling, and pain and may be clinically indistinguishable for a few days.
- A hordeolum remains painful and localizes to an eyelid margin.
- Hot compresses can hasten resolution of either lesion.
- Other treatments that may be needed include intralesional corticosteroids (for chalazia) and incision and/or antibiotics (for hordeola).

DACRYOCYSTITIS

Dacryocystitis is infection of the lacrimal sac that sometimes leads to abscess formation. The usual cause is a staphyloccocal or streptococcal species, typically as a consequence of nasolacrimal duct obstruction.

In acute dacryocystitis, the patient presents with pain, redness, and edema around the lacrimal sac. Diagnosis is suspected based on symptoms and signs and when pressure over the lacrimal sac causes reflux of mucoid material through the puncta. Initial treatment is with warm compresses and oral antibiotics for mild cases or IV antibiotics for severe cases. The antibiotic is usually a 1st-generation cephalosporin or penicillinase-resistant synthetic penicillin. If the infection does not respond as expected, consideration should be given to methicillin-resistant *Staphylococcus aureus* (MRSA), and antibiotics changed accordingly. The abscess can be drained and the antibiotics can be changed based on culture results if the initial antibiotic proves ineffective.

Patients with chronic dacryocystitis usually present with a mass under the medial canthal tendon and chronic conjunctivitis. Definitive treatment for resolved acute dacryocystitis or chronic conjunctivitis is usually surgery that creates a passage between the lacrimal sac and the nasal cavity (dacryocystorhinostomy).

DACRYOSTENOSIS

Dacryostenosis is obstruction or stenosis of the nasolacrimal duct, causing excess tearing.

Nasolacrimal obstruction may be congenital or acquired. One cause of congenital obstruction is inadequate development of any part of the nasolacrimal ducts. Typically, a membrane at the distal end of the nasolacrimal duct persists. There is tearing and purulent discharge; the condition may manifest as chronic conjunctivitis, usually beginning after the age of 2 wk (most often at age 3 to 12 wk).

There are many causes of acquired nasolacrimal duct obstruction (see Table 110–1). The cause is most often age-related stenosis of the nasolacrimal duct. Other causes include past nasal or facial bone fractures and sinus surgery, which disrupt the nasolacrimal duct; inflammatory diseases (eg, sarcoidosis, granulomatosis with polyangiitis [formerly Wegener granulomatosis]); tumor (eg, maxillary and ethmoid sinus tumors); and dacryocystitis.

Causes of punctal or canalicular stenosis include chronic conjunctivitis (especially herpes simplex), certain types of chemotherapy, adverse reactions to eye drops (especially topical echothiophate iodide), and radiation.

Table 110–1. CAUSES OF ACQUIRED NASOLACRIMAL DUCT OBSTRUCTION

Dacryolith (a concretion)
Granulomatosis with polyangiitis (formerly Wegener granulomatosis)
Idiopathic (usually age-related)
Sarcoidosis
Trauma (including surgical, especially previous sinus surgery)
Tumor

Diagnosis

- Clinical evaluation

Diagnosis is usually based on clinical criteria. Sometimes ophthalmologists probe and irrigate the lacrimal drainage system with saline, with or without fluorescein dye. Reflux indicates stenosis.

Treatment

- Manual or surgical decompression
- Treatment of underlying disorder

Congenital nasolacrimal duct obstruction often resolves spontaneously by about age 6 to 9 mo; before 1 yr, manual compression of the lacrimal sac 4 or 5 times/day may relieve the obstruction. After age 1 yr, the nasolacrimal duct may need probing, usually under general anesthesia; if obstruction is recurrent, a temporary silastic tube may be inserted.

In acquired nasolacrimal duct obstruction, the underlying disorder is treated when possible. If treatment is not possible or is ineffective, a passage between the lacrimal sac and the nasal cavity can be created surgically (dacryocystorhinostomy).

In cases of punctal or canalicular stenosis, dilation is usually curative. If canalicular stenosis is severe and bothersome, a surgical procedure (conjunctivo-dacryocystorhinostomy or C-DCR) that places a tube made of low thermal-expansion borosilicate glass (Jones tube) leading from the caruncle into the nasal cavity can be considered.

KEY POINTS

- Dacryostenosis is either congenital or acquired.
- Symptoms include excessive tearing.
- Reflux of saline or fluorescein dye when flushing the lacrimal drainage system confirms the diagnosis.
- In congenital dacryostenosis, symptoms usually resolve by 9 mo; manual decompression of the lacrimal sac may help.
- In acquired dacryostenosis, treat the underlying disorder.
- For both congenital and acquired dacryostenosis, surgery may be needed if symptoms persist.

ENTROPION AND ECTROPION

Entropion is inversion of an eyelid. Ectropion is eversion of the lower eyelid.

Entropion: Entropion (inversion of an eyelid) is caused by age-related tissue relaxation, postinfectious changes (particularly trachoma), posttraumatic changes, or blepharospasm. Eyelashes rub against the eyeball and may lead to corneal ulceration and scarring. Symptoms can include foreign body sensation, tearing, and red eye. Diagnosis is clinical. Definitive treatment is surgery.

Ectropion: Ectropion (eversion of the lower eyelid—see Plate 16). is caused by age-related tissue relaxation, cranial nerve VII palsy, and posttraumatic or postsurgical changes. Symptoms are tearing (due to poor drainage of tears through the nasolacrimal system, which may no longer contact the eyeball) and symptoms of dry eyes. Diagnosis is clinical. Symptomatic treatment can include tear supplements and, at night, ocular lubricants; definitive treatment is surgery.

EYELID GROWTHS

The skin of the eyelids is a common site for benign and malignant growths.

Xanthelasma: Xanthelasma is a common, benign deposit of yellow-white flat plaques of lipid material that occur subcutaneously on the upper and lower eyelids. Although some people with xanthelasmas have dyslipidemias, most do not. Diagnosis is by appearance. No treatment is necessary, although xanthelasmas can be removed for cosmetic reasons, and underlying dyslipidemias should be treated.

Basal cell carcinoma: Basal cell carcinoma frequently occurs at the eyelid margins, at the inner canthus, and on the upper cheek. Metastasis is rare. Biopsy establishes the diagnosis. Treatment is surgical excision using conventional techniques or by Mohs surgery.

Other malignant growths: Other types of malignant growths are less common; they include squamous cell carcinoma, sebaceous gland carcinoma, and melanomas. Eyelid growths may simulate chronic blepharitis or chronic chalazion. Therefore, chronic blepharitis, chronic chalazion, or similar lesions should be biopsied if unresponsive to initial treatment.

TRICHIASIS

Trichiasis is an anatomic misalignment of eyelashes, which rub against the eyeball, in a patient with no entropion.

Trichiasis is most often idiopathic, but known causes include blepharitis, posttraumatic and postsurgical changes, conjunctival scarring (eg, secondary to cicatricial pemphigoid, atopic keratoconjunctivitis, Stevens-Johnson syndrome, or chemical injury), epiblepharon (an extra lower eyelid skinfold that directs lashes into a vertical position), and distichiasis (a congenital extra row of eyelashes).

Corneal ulceration and scarring can occur in chronic cases. Symptoms are foreign body sensation, tearing, and red eye.

Diagnosis is usually clinical. Trichiasis differs from entropion in that the eyelid position is normal. Evaluation includes fluorescein staining to exclude corneal abrasion or ulceration.

Treatment is eyelash removal with forceps. If eyelashes grow back, electrolysis or cryosurgery is more effective at permanently preventing recurrence.

111 Corneal Disorders

The cornea is subject to infection, noninfectious inflammation, ulceration, mechanical damage, and environmental injury. Infection (keratitis), frequently with secondary conjunctivitis, can be due to viruses, bacteria, *Acanthamoeba,* or fungi. Ulceration usually represents progression of keratitis. Symptoms that suggest corneal involvement rather than simple conjunctivitis include pain, particularly with exposure to light, and decreased visual acuity. Evaluation of the cornea requires slit-lamp examination and sometimes microbial studies.

PEARLS & PITFALLS

- Do a slit-lamp examination and fluorescein staining if patients have a red eye with pain, foreign body sensation, and/or decreased visual acuity.

BULLOUS KERATOPATHY

Bullous keratopathy is the presence of corneal epithelial bullae, resulting from corneal endothelial disease.

Bullous keratopathy is caused by edema of the cornea, resulting from failure of the corneal endothelium to maintain the normally dehydrated state of the cornea. Most frequently, it is due to Fuchs corneal endothelial dystrophy or corneal endothelial trauma. Fuchs dystrophy is a genetic disorder that causes bilateral, progressive corneal endothelial cell loss, sometimes leading to symptomatic bullous keratopathy by age 50 to 60. Fuchs dystrophy may be autosomal dominant with incomplete penetrance. Another frequent cause of bullous keratopathy is corneal endothelial trauma, which can occur during intraocular surgery (eg, cataract removal) or after placement of a poorly designed or malpositioned intraocular lens implant. Bullous keratopathy after cataract removal is called pseudophakic (if an intraocular lens implant is present) or aphakic (if no intraocular lens implant is present) bullous keratopathy.

Subepithelial fluid-filled bullae form on the corneal surface as the corneal stroma (the deeper layers of the cornea) swells, leading to eye discomfort, decreased visual acuity, loss of contrast, glare, and photophobia. Sometimes bullae rupture, causing pain and foreign body sensation. Bacteria can invade a ruptured bulla, leading to a corneal ulcer.

The bullae and swelling of the corneal stroma can be seen on slit-lamp examination.

Treatment requires an ophthalmologist and includes topical dehydrating agents (eg, hypertonic saline and hypertonic sodium chloride 5% ointment), intraocular pressure–lowering agents, occasional short-term use of therapeutic soft contact lenses for some mild to moderate cases, and treatment of any secondary microbial infection. Corneal transplantation is usually curative.

CORNEAL ULCER

A corneal ulcer is a corneal epithelial defect with underlying inflammation (which soon results in necrosis of corneal tissue) due to invasion by bacteria, fungi, viruses, or *Acanthamoeba*. It can be initiated by mechanical trauma or nutritional deficiencies. Symptoms are progressive redness, foreign body sensation, ache, photophobia, and lacrimation. Diagnosis is by slit-lamp examination, fluorescein staining, and microbial studies. Treatment with topical antimicrobials and often dilating drops is urgent and requires an ophthalmologist.

Etiology

Corneal ulcers have many causes (see Table 111–1). Bacterial ulcers (most commonly due to contact lens wear) may occasionally complicate herpes simplex keratitis and, depending

Table 111–1. CAUSES OF CORNEAL ULCERS

CATEGORY	EXAMPLES
Nontraumatic corneal abnormalities	Bullous keratopathy (ie, ruptured bullae) Cicatricial pemphigoid Herpes simplex keratitis with secondary bacterial superinfection Dry eyes, primary Dry eyes, secondary (eg, neurotrophic keratitis) Trachoma
Corneal injury	Corneal abrasion Penetrating corneal trauma Corneal foreign body (rare) Contact lenses (most commonly when worn during sleep and/or inadequately disinfected)
Eyelid abnormalities	Chronic blepharitis Entropion Incomplete eye closure (eg, due to inadequate eye closure [lagophthalmos], peripheral facial nerve palsy, eyelid defects after trauma, or exophthalmos) Trichiasis
Nutritional deficiencies	Protein undernutrition Vitamin A deficiency

on the bacterial species, may be particularly refractory to treatment. The time course for ulcers varies. Ulcers caused by *Acanthamoeba* (also most commonly due to exposure to contaminated water while wearing contact lenses) and fungi (most commonly due to trauma with vegetable material) are indolent but progressive, whereas those caused by *Pseudomonas aeruginosa* (seen almost exclusively in contact lens wearers) develop rapidly, causing deep and extensive corneal necrosis. Wearing contact lenses while sleeping or wearing inadequately disinfected contact lenses can cause corneal ulcers (see p. 955).

Pathophysiology

Ulcers are characterized by corneal epithelial defects with underlying inflammation, and soon necrosis of the corneal stroma develops. Corneal ulcers tend to heal with scar tissue, resulting in opacification of the cornea and decreased visual acuity. Uveitis, corneal perforation with iris prolapse, pus in the anterior chamber (hypopyon), panophthalmitis, and destruction of the eye may occur without treatment and, on occasion, even with the best available treatment, particularly if treatment is delayed. More severe symptoms and complications tend to occur with deeper ulcers.

Symptoms and Signs

Conjunctival redness, eye ache, foreign body sensation, photophobia, and lacrimation may be minimal initially.

A corneal ulcer begins as a corneal epithelial defect that stains with fluorescein and an underlying dull, grayish, circumscribed superficial opacity. Subsequently, the ulcer suppurates and necroses to form an excavated ulcer. Considerable circumcorneal conjunctival hyperemia is usual. In long-standing cases, blood vessels may grow in from the limbus (corneal neovascularization). The ulcer may spread to involve the width of the cornea, may penetrate deeply, or both. Hypopyon (layered WBCs in the anterior chamber) may occur (see Plate 13).

Corneal ulcers due to *Acanthamoeba* are often intensely painful and may show transient corneal epithelial defects, multiple corneal stromal infiltrates, and, later, a large ring-shaped infiltrate. Fungal ulcers, which are more chronic than bacterial ulcers, are densely infiltrated and show occasional discrete islands of infiltrate (satellite lesions) at the periphery.

Diagnosis

- Slit-lamp examination

Diagnosis is made by slit-lamp examination; a corneal infiltrate with an epithelial defect that stains with fluorescein is diagnostic. All but small ulcers should be cultured by scraping with a disposable #15 blade, sterile platinum spatula, or jeweler's forceps (typically by an ophthalmologist). Microscopic examination of scrapings can identify *Acanthamoeba*.

Treatment

- Initially empiric topical broad-spectrum antibiotic therapy
- More specific antimicrobial therapy directed at the cause

Treatment for corneal ulcers, regardless of cause, begins with moxifloxacin 0.5% or gatifloxacin 0.3 to 0.5% for small ulcers and fortified (higher than stock concentration) antibiotic drops, such as tobramycin 15 mg/mL and cefazolin 50 mg/mL, for more significant ulcers, particularly those that are near the center of the cornea. Frequent dosing (eg, q 15 min for 4 doses, followed by q 1 h around the clock) is necessary initially. Patching is contraindicated because it creates a stagnant, warm environment that favors bacterial growth and prevents the administration of topical drugs.

Herpes simplex is treated with trifluridine 1% drops q 2 h while the patient is awake to a total of 9 times/day, ganciclovir 0.15% gel 5 times/day, valacyclovir 1000 mg po bid, or acyclovir 400 mg po 5 times/day (or tid for recurrent herpes simplex keratitis) for about 14 days.

Fungal infections are treated with one of many topical antifungal drops (eg, voriconazole 1%, natamycin 5%, amphotericin B 0.15%), initially q 1 h during the day and q 2 h overnight. Deep infections may require addition of oral voriconazole 200 mg bid, ketoconazole 400 mg once/day, fluconazole 400 mg once then 200 mg once/day, or itraconazole 400 mg once then 200 mg once/day.

If *Acanthamoeba* is identified, therapy can include topical propamidine 0.1%, neomycin 0.175%, and polyhexamethylene biguanide 0.02% or chlorhexidine 0.02% supplemented with miconazole 1%, clotrimazole 1%, or oral ketoconazole 400 mg once/day or itraconazole 400 mg once then 200 mg once/day. The drops are used q 1 to 2 h until clinical improvement is evident, then gradually reduced to 4 times/day and continued for a number of months until all inflammation has resolved. Polyhexamethylene biguanide and chlorhexidine are not commercially available as ocular agents but can be prepared by a compounding pharmacy.

For all ulcers, treatment may also include a cycloplegic, such as atropine 1% or scopolamine 0.25% 1 drop tid, to decrease the ache of a corneal ulcer and to reduce the formation of posterior synechiae. In severe cases, debridement of the infected epithelium or even penetrating keratoplasty may be required. Patients who are poorly compliant or who have large, central, or refractory ulcers may need to be hospitalized. Very selective patients can be treated adjunctively with a corticosteroid drop (eg, prednisolone acetate 1% qid for 1 wk then tapered over 2 to 3 wk). The final appearance of the scar and final visual acuity are not improved with topical corticosteroids. Topical corticosteroids do decrease the pain and photophobia, and speed the increase in visual acuity, significantly. Because there is a very small risk of the ulcer worsening, adding topical corticosteroids is only indicated when a patient needs to get back to normal functioning (e.g., work, driving etc.) as soon as possible. Such treatment should only be prescribed by ophthalmologists and should be restricted to patients in whom clinical and microbiologic evidence indicates a favorable response to antimicrobial treatment and who can be closely followed.

KEY POINTS

- Causes of corneal ulcers include infection of the cornea (including overwearing of contact lenses), eye trauma, abnormalities of the eyelid, and nutritional deficiencies.
- Ulcers may be accompanied by circumcorneal hyperemia and WBC layering in the anterior chamber (hypopyon).
- All but the smallest ulcers are cultured, usually by an ophthalmologist.
- Treatment usually involves frequent (eg, every 1 to 2 h around the clock) application of topical antimicrobials.

HERPES SIMPLEX KERATITIS

(Herpes Simplex Keratoconjunctivitis)

Herpes simplex keratitis is corneal infection with herpes simplex virus. It may involve the iris. Symptoms and signs include foreign body sensation, lacrimation, photophobia, and conjunctival hyperemia. Recurrences are common and may lead to corneal hypoesthesia, ulceration, permanent scarring, and decreased vision. Diagnosis is based on the characteristic dendritic corneal ulcer and sometimes viral culture. Treatment is with topical and occasionally systemic antiviral drugs.

Herpes simplex usually affects the corneal surface but sometimes involves the corneal stroma (the deeper layers of the cornea). Stromal involvement is probably an immunologic response to the virus.

As with all herpes simplex virus infections, there is a primary infection, followed by a latent phase, in which the virus goes into the nerve roots. Latent virus may reactivate, causing recurrent symptoms.

Symptoms and Signs

Primary infection: The initial (primary) infection is usually nonspecific self-limiting conjunctivitis, often in early childhood and usually without corneal involvement. If the cornea is involved, early symptoms include foreign body sensation, lacrimation, photophobia, and conjunctival hyperemia. Sometimes vesicular blepharitis (blisters on the eyelid) follows, symptoms worsen, vision blurs, and blisters break down and ulcerate, then resolve without scarring in about a week.

Recurrent infection: Recurrences usually take the form of epithelial keratitis (also called dendritic keratitis) with tearing, foreign body sensation, and a characteristic branching (dendritic or serpentine) lesion of the corneal epithelium with knoblike terminals that stain with fluorescein (see Plate 18). Multiple recurrences may result in corneal hypoesthesia or anesthesia, ulceration, permanent scarring, and decreased vision.

Stromal involvement: Most patients with disciform keratitis, which involves the corneal endothelium primarily, have a history of epithelial keratitis. Disciform keratitis is a deeper, disc-shaped, localized area of secondary corneal edema and haze accompanied by anterior uveitis. This form may cause pain and vision loss.

Stromal keratitis can cause necrosis of the stroma and severe ache, photophobia, foreign body sensation, and decreased vision.

Diagnosis

- Slit-lamp examination

Slit-lamp examination is mandatory. Finding a dendrite is enough to confirm the diagnosis in most cases. When the appearance is not conclusive, viral culture of the lesion can confirm the diagnosis.

Treatment

- Topical ganciclovir or trifluridine
- Oral or IV acyclovir or valacyclovir
- For stromal involvement or uveitis, topical corticosteroids in addition to antiviral drugs

Most patients are managed by an ophthalmologist. If stromal or uveal involvement occurs, treatment is more involved and referral to an ophthalmologist is mandatory.

Topical therapy (eg, ganciclovir 0.15% gel applied q 3 h while awake [5 times/day] or trifluridine 1% drops q 2 h while awake [9 times/day]) is usually effective. Occasionally, acyclovir 400 mg po 5 times/day (or 3 times/day for recurrent herpes simplex keratitis) or valacyclovir 1000 mg po bid is indicated. Immunocompromised patients may require IV antivirals (eg, acyclovir 5 mg/kg IV q 8 h for 7 days). If the epithelium surrounding the dendrite is loose and edematous, debridement by gentle swabbing with a cotton-tipped applicator before beginning drug therapy may speed healing.

Topical corticosteroids are contraindicated in epithelial keratitis but may be effective when used **with an antiviral** to manage later-stage stromal involvement (disciform or stromal keratitis) or uveitis. In such cases, patients may be given prednisolone acetate 1% instilled q 2 h initially, lengthening the interval to q 4 to 8 h as symptoms improve. Topical drugs to relieve photophobia include atropine 1% or scopolamine 0.25% tid.

KEY POINTS

- Herpes simplex keratitis typically is a recurrence of primary herpes simplex eye infection that was typically a nonspecific, self-limiting conjunctivitis.
- Characteristic findings include a branching dendritic or serpentine corneal lesion (indicating dendritic keratitis) or disc-shaped, localized corneal edema and haze plus anterior uveitis (indicating disciform keratitis).
- Diagnosis is confirmed by finding a dendritic ulcer or by viral culture.
- Treatment requires antivirals, usually topical ganciclovir or trifluridine or oral acyclovir or valacyclovir.

HERPES ZOSTER OPHTHALMICUS

(Herpes Zoster Virus Ophthalmicus; Ophthalmic Herpes Zoster; Varicella-Zoster Virus Ophthalmicus)

Herpes zoster ophthalmicus is reactivation of a varicella-zoster virus infection (shingles) involving the eye. Symptoms and signs, which may be intense, include dermatomal forehead rash and painful inflammation of all the tissues of the anterior and, rarely, posterior structures

of the eye. Diagnosis is based on the characteristic appearance of the anterior structures of the eye plus zoster dermatitis of the first branch of the trigeminal nerve (V1). Treatment is with oral antivirals, mydriatics, and topical corticosteroids.

Herpes zoster of the forehead involves the globe in three fourths of cases when the nasociliary nerve is affected (as indicated by a lesion on the tip of the nose—see Plate 19). and in one third of cases not involving the tip of the nose. Overall, the globe is involved in half of patients.

Symptoms and Signs

A prodrome of tingling of the forehead may occur. During acute disease, in addition to the painful forehead rash, symptoms and signs may include severe ocular pain; marked eyelid edema; conjunctival, episcleral, and circumcorneal conjunctival hyperemia; corneal edema; and photophobia.

Complications: Keratitis and/or uveitis may be severe and followed by scarring. Late sequelae—glaucoma, cataract, chronic or recurrent uveitis, corneal scarring, corneal neovascularization, and hypesthesia—are common and may threaten vision. Postherpetic neuralgia may develop late. Patients may develop episcleritis (without increased risk of visual loss) and/or retinitis (with risk of severe visual loss).

Diagnosis

- Zoster rash on the forehead or eyelid plus eye findings

Diagnosis is based on a typical acute herpes zoster rash on the forehead, eyelid, or both or on a characteristic history plus signs of previous zoster rash (eg, atrophic hypopigmented scars). Vesicular or bullous lesions in this distribution that do not yet involve the eye suggest significant risk and should prompt an ophthalmologic consultation to determine whether the eye is involved. Culture and immunologic or PCR studies of skin at initial evaluation or serial serologic tests are done only when lesions are atypical and the diagnosis uncertain.

Treatment

- Oral antivirals (eg, acyclovir, famciclovir, valacyclovir)
- Sometimes topical corticosteroids

Early treatment with acyclovir 800 mg po 5 times/day or famciclovir 500 mg or valacyclovir 1 g po tid for 7 days reduces ocular complications. Patients with uveitis or keratitis require topical corticosteroids (eg, prednisolone acetate 1% instilled q 1 h for uveitis or qid for keratitis initially, lengthening the interval as symptoms lessen). The pupil should be dilated with atropine 1% or scopolamine 0.25% 1 drop tid. Intraocular pressure must be monitored and treated if it rises significantly above normal values.

Use of a brief course of high-dose oral corticosteroids to prevent postherpetic neuralgia in patients > 60 yr who are in good general health remains controversial.

Prevention

A herpes zoster vaccine is recommended for healthy adults ≥ 60 yr, regardless of whether they have had chickenpox or herpes zoster. This vaccine decreases the chance of getting herpes zoster by half. If herpes zoster develops in people who have been vaccinated, it is less severe than in people who have not been vaccinated.

KEY POINTS

- The eye is affected in about half of cases of V1 varicella-zoster virus reactivation.
- Keratitis and/or uveitis can be severe and cause morbidity.
- Appearance of the typical herpes zoster rash is usually diagnostic.
- Treatment is with oral antivirals and usually topical corticosteroids and pupillary dilation.

INTERSTITIAL KERATITIS

(Parenchymatous Keratitis)

Interstitial keratitis is chronic, nonulcerative inflammation of the mid-stroma (the middle layers of the cornea) that is sometimes associated with uveitis. The cause is usually infectious. Symptoms are photophobia, pain, lacrimation, and vision blurring. Diagnosis is by slit-lamp examination and serologic tests to determine the cause. Treatment is directed at the cause and may require topical corticosteroids.

Interstitial keratitis, a manifestation of certain corneal infections, is rare in the US. Most cases occur in children or adolescents as a late complication of congenital syphilis. Ultimately, both eyes may be involved. A similar but less dramatic bilateral keratitis occurs in Cogan syndrome, Lyme disease, and Epstein-Barr virus infection. Rarely, acquired syphilis, herpes simplex, herpes zoster, or TB may cause a unilateral form in adults.

Symptoms and Signs

Photophobia, pain, lacrimation, and vision blurring are common. The lesion begins as patches of inflammation in the mid-stroma that cause opacification. Typically with syphilis and occasionally with other causes, the entire cornea develops a ground-glass appearance, obscuring the iris. New blood vessels grow in from the limbus (neovascularization) and cause orange-red areas (salmon patches). Anterior uveitis and choroiditis are common in syphilitic interstitial keratitis. Inflammation and neovascularization usually begin to subside after 1 to 2 mo. Some corneal opacity usually remains, causing mild to moderate vision impairment.

Diagnosis

- Corneal opacification and other typical findings on slit-lamp examination
- Serologic testing to determine etiology

The specific etiology must be determined. The stigmas of congenital syphilis, vestibuloauditory symptoms, history of an expanding rash, and tick exposure support specific etiologies. However, all patients should have serologic testing, including all of the following:

- Fluorescent treponemal antibody absorption test or the microhemagglutination assay for *Treponema pallidum*
- Lyme titer
- Epstein-Barr virus panel

Patients with negative serologic test results may have Cogan syndrome, an idiopathic syndrome consisting of interstitial keratitis and vestibular and auditory deficits. To prevent permanent vestibuloauditory damage, symptoms of hearing loss, tinnitus, or vertigo require urgent referral to an otolaryngologist.

Treatment

- Sometimes topical corticosteroids

Keratitis may resolve with treatment of the underlying condition. Additional topical treatment with a corticosteroid, such as prednisolone 1% qid, is often advisable. An ophthalmologist should treat these patients.

KEY POINTS

- Interstitial keratitis, which is rare in the US, involves chronic inflammation of the middle corneal layers.
- Findings include pain, tearing, decreased visual acuity, and often orange-red discoloration of the cornea and anterior uveitis.
- Test patients for syphilis, Lyme disease, and Epstein-Barr virus infection.
- Treatment is by an ophthalmologist; sometimes topical corticosteroids are prescribed.

COGAN SYNDROME

Cogan syndrome is a rare autoimmune disease involving the eye and the inner ear.

Cogan syndrome affects young adults, with 80% of patients between 14 yr and 47 yr. The disease appears to result from an autoimmune reaction directed against an unknown common autoantigen in the cornea and inner ear. About 10 to 30% of patients also have severe systemic vasculitis, which may include life-threatening aortitis.

Symptoms and Signs

The presenting symptoms involve the ocular system in 38% of patients, the vestibuloauditory system in 46%, and both in 15%. By 5 mo, 75% of patients have both ocular and vestibuloauditory symptoms. Nonspecific systemic complaints include fever, headache, joint pain, and myalgia.

Ocular: Ocular involvement includes any combination of the following:

- Bilateral interstitial keratitis or other corneal stromal keratitis
- Episcleritis or scleritis
- Uveitis
- Papillitis
- Other orbital inflammation (eg, vitritis, choroiditis)

Ocular symptoms include irritation, pain, photophobia, and decreased vision. Ocular examination shows a patchy corneal stromal infiltrate typical of interstitial keratitis, ocular redness, optic nerve edema, proptosis, or a combination of these symptoms.

Vestibuloauditory: Vestibuloauditory symptoms include sensorineural hearing loss, tinnitus, and vertigo.

Vascular: A diastolic heart murmur may be present when aortitis is significant. Claudication may be present if limb vessels are affected.

Diagnosis

Diagnosis is based on clinical findings and exclusion of other causes (eg, syphilis, Lyme disease, Epstein-Barr virus infection) by appropriate serologic tests. Urgent evaluation by an ophthalmologist and otolaryngologist is indicated.

Treatment

- Initially topical and sometimes systemic corticosteroids for ocular involvement

Untreated disease may lead to corneal scarring and vision loss and, in 60 to 80% of patients, permanent hearing loss. Keratitis, episcleritis, and anterior uveitis can usually be treated with topical prednisolone acetate 1% q 1 h to qid. To treat deeper ocular inflammation and especially to treat vestibuloauditory symptoms before they become permanent, prednisone 1 mg/kg po once/day is begun as soon as possible and continued for 2 to 6 mo. Some clinicians add cyclophosphamide, methotrexate, or cyclosporine for recalcitrant cases.

KERATOCONJUNCTIVITIS SICCA

(Dry Eyes; Keratitis Sicca)

Keratoconjunctivitis sicca is chronic, bilateral desiccation of the conjunctiva and cornea due to an inadequate tear film. Symptoms include itching, burning, irritation, and photophobia. Diagnosis is clinical; the Schirmer test may be helpful. Treatment is with topical tear supplements and sometimes blockage of the nasolacrimal openings.

Etiology

There are 2 main types:

- Aqueous tear-deficient keratoconjunctivitis sicca is caused by inadequate tear volume.
- Evaporative keratoconjunctivitis sicca (more common) is caused by accelerated tear evaporation due to poor tear quality.

Aqueous tear-deficient keratoconjunctivitis sicca is most commonly an isolated idiopathic condition in postmenopausal women. It is also commonly part of Sjögren syndrome, RA, or SLE. Less commonly, it is secondary to other conditions that scar the lacrimal ducts (eg, cicatricial pemphigoid, Stevens-Johnson syndrome, trachoma). It may result from a damaged or malfunctioning lacrimal gland due to graft-vs-host disease, HIV (diffuse infiltrative lymphocytosis syndrome), local radiation therapy, or familial dysautonomia.

Evaporative keratoconjunctivitis sicca is caused by loss of the tear film due to abnormally rapid evaporation caused by an inadequate oil layer on the surface of the aqueous layer of tears. Symptoms may result from abnormal oil quality (ie, meibomian gland dysfunction) or a degraded normal oil layer (ie, seborrheic blepharitis). Patients frequently have acne rosacea.

Drying can also result from exposure due to inadequate eye closure at night (nocturnal lagophthalmos or Bell or facial nerve palsy) or from inadequate frequency of reapplication of tears to the cornea due to an insufficient blink rate (eg, in Parkinson disease).

Symptoms and Signs

Patients report itching; burning; a gritty, pulling, or foreign body sensation; or photosensitivity. A sharp stabbing pain, eye strain or fatigue, and blurred vision may also occur. Some patients note a flood of tears after severe irritation. Typically, symptoms fluctuate in intensity and are intermittent. Certain factors can worsen symptoms:

- Prolonged visual efforts (eg, reading, working on the computer, driving, watching television)
- Local environments that are dry, windy, dusty, or smoky

- Certain systemic drugs, including isotretinoin, sedatives, diuretics, antihypertensives, oral contraceptives, and all anticholinergics (including antihistamines and many GI drugs)
- Dehydration

Symptoms lessen on cool, rainy, or foggy days or in other high-humidity environments, such as in the shower. Recurrent and prolonged blurring and frequent intense irritation can impair daily function. However, permanent impairment of vision is rare.

With both forms, the conjunctiva is hyperemic, and there is often scattered, fine, punctate loss of corneal epithelium (superficial punctate keratitis), conjunctival epithelium, or both. When the condition is severe, the involved areas, mainly between the eyelids (the intrapalpebral or exposure zone), stain with fluorescein. Patients often blink at an accelerated rate because of irritation.

With the aqueous tear-deficient form, the conjunctiva can appear dry and lusterless with redundant folds. With the evaporative form, abundant tears may be present as well as foam at the eyelid margin. Very rarely, severe, advanced, chronic drying leads to significant vision loss due to keratinization of the ocular surface or loss of corneal epithelium, leading to sequelae such as scarring, neovascularization, infections, ulceration, and perforation.

Diagnosis

- Schirmer test and tear breakup test (TBUT)

Diagnosis is based on characteristic symptoms and clinical appearance. The Schirmer test and TBUT may differentiate type.

The Schirmer test determines whether tear production is normal. After blotting the closed eye to remove excess tears, a strip of filter paper is placed, without topical anesthesia, at the junction of the middle and lateral third of the lower eyelid. If < 5.5 mm of wetting occurs after 5 min on 2 successive occasions, the patient has aqueous tear-deficient keratoconjunctivitis sicca.

With evaporative keratoconjunctivitis sicca, the Schirmer test is usually normal. The tear film can be made visible under cobalt blue light at the slit lamp by instillation of a small volume of highly concentrated fluorescein (made by wetting a fluorescein strip with saline and shaking the strip to remove any excess moisture). Blinking several times reapplies a complete tear film. The patient then stares, and the length of time until the first dry spot develops is determined (TBUT). An accelerated rate of intact tear film breakup (< 10 sec) is characteristic of evaporative keratoconjunctivitis sicca.

If aqueous tear-deficient keratoconjunctivitis sicca is diagnosed, Sjögren syndrome should be suspected, especially if xerostomia is also present. Serologic tests and labial salivary gland biopsy are used for diagnosis. Patients with primary or secondary Sjögren syndrome are at increased risk of several serious diseases (eg, primary biliary cirrhosis, non-Hodgkin lymphoma). Therefore, proper evaluation and monitoring are essential.

Treatment

- Artificial tears
- Sometimes occlusion of nasolacrimal punctum or tarsorrhaphy

Frequent use of artificial tears can be effective for both types. More viscous artificial tears coat the ocular surface longer, and artificial tears that contain polar lipids such as glycerin reduce evaporation; both types are particularly useful in evaporative keratoconjunctivitis sicca. Artificial tear ointments applied before sleep are particularly useful when patients have nocturnal lagophthalmos or irritation on waking. Most cases are treated adequately throughout the patient's life with such supplementation. Staying hydrated, using humidifiers, and avoiding dry, drafty environments can often help. Not smoking and avoiding secondary smoke are important. In recalcitrant cases, occlusion of the nasolacrimal punctum may be indicated. In severe cases, a partial tarsorrhaphy can reduce tear loss through evaporation. Topical cyclosporine and ω-3 fatty acid dietary supplements may be a useful adjunct in some patients.

Patients with evaporative keratoconjunctivitis sicca often benefit from treatment of concomitant blepharitis and associated rosacea with measures such as the following:

- For meibomian gland dysfunction: Warm compresses and/or systemic doxycycline 50 to 100 mg po once or twice daily (contraindicated in pregnant or nursing patients)
- For seborrheic blepharitis: Eyelid margin scrubs and/or intermittent topical eyelid antibiotic ointments (eg, bacitracin at bedtime)

Cyclosporine drops that decrease the inflammation associated with dryness of the eye are available. They lead to meaningful improvement but only in a fraction of patients. These drops sting and take months before an effect is noticed.

KEY POINTS

- Keratoconjunctivitis sicca is chronic, bilateral desiccation of the conjunctiva and cornea caused by too little tear production or accelerated tear evaporation.
- Typical symptoms include intermittent itching; burning; a gritty, pulling, or foreign body sensation; and photosensitivity.
- Findings include conjunctival hyperemia and often scattered, fine, punctate loss of corneal epithelium (superficial punctate keratitis) and conjunctival epithelium.
- The Schirmer test and tear breakup test may help determine whether the cause is deficient tear production or accelerated tear evaporation.
- Using artificial tears and avoiding corneal drying is usually sufficient treatment, but sometimes occlusion of the nasolacrimal punctum or partial tarsorrhaphy is indicated.

KERATOCONUS

Keratoconus is a bulging distortion of the cornea, leading to loss of visual acuity.

Keratoconus is a slowly progressive thinning and bulging of the cornea, usually bilateral, beginning between ages 10 and 25. Its cause is unknown.

Risk factors include the following:

- Family history of keratoconus
- An atopic disorder
- Vigorous eye rubbing
- Lax eyelids
- Certain connective tissue disorders (eg, Ehlers-Danlos syndrome, Marfan syndrome, osteogenesis imperfecta)
- Down syndrome
- Congenital disorders with poor vision (eg, Leber congenital optic neuropathy, retinopathy of prematurity, aniridia)
- Obstructive sleep apnea

The distorted cone shape of the cornea causes major changes in the refractive characteristics of the cornea (irregular astigmatism) that cannot be fully corrected with glasses. Progressing keratoconus necessitates frequent change of eyeglasses. Contact lenses may provide better vision correction and should be tried when eyeglasses are not satisfactory. Corneal transplant surgery may be necessary if visual acuity with contact lenses is inadequate, contact lenses are not tolerated, or a visually significant corneal scar (caused by tearing of stromal fibers) is present.

Newer treatments seem promising. Implantation of corneal ring segments appears to have the potential to improve visual results by increasing tolerance of contact lenses and thus saving selected patients from transplantation. Corneal collagen cross-linking, an ultraviolet light treatment that stiffens the cornea thereby preventing progressive bulging and thinning, is used throughout Europe and has recently been approved for use in the US.

KERATOMALACIA

(Xerophthalmia; Xerotic Keratitis)

Keratomalacia is degeneration of the cornea caused by nutritional deficiency.

Keratomalacia is caused by vitamin A deficiency typically in patients with protein-calorie undernutrition. It is characterized by a hazy, dry cornea. Corneal ulceration with secondary infection is common. The lacrimal glands and conjunctiva are also affected. Lack of tears causes extreme dryness of the eyes, and foamy spots appear on the temporal and often nasal bulbar conjunctiva (Bitot spots). Night blindness may occur. For further details, including specific therapy, see p. 44.

PERIPHERAL ULCERATIVE KERATITIS

(Marginal Keratolysis; Peripheral Rheumatoid Ulceration)

Peripheral ulcerative keratitis is inflammation and ulceration of the cornea that often occurs with chronic connective tissue diseases. Irritation and decreased vision result.

Peripheral ulcerative keratitis is a serious corneal ulceration; it often occurs with autoimmune connective tissue diseases that are active, long-standing, or both, such as RA, granulomatosis with polyangiitis (formerly called Wegener granulomatosis), and relapsing polychondritis.

Patients often have decreased visual acuity, photophobia, and foreign body sensation. A crescentic area of opacification in the periphery of the cornea, due to infiltration by WBCs and ulceration, stains with fluorescein. Infectious causes, such as bacteria, fungi, and herpes simplex virus, must be ruled out by culturing the ulcer and eyelid margins.

Among patients with autoimmune connective tissue disease and peripheral ulcerative keratitis, the 10-yr mortality rate is about 40% (usually due to MI) without treatment and about 8% with systemic cytotoxic therapy.

Any patient with peripheral ulcerative keratitis should be promptly referred to an ophthalmologist. Systemic cyclophosphamide or other immunosuppressants treat the keratitis, life-threatening vasculitis, and underlying autoimmune disease. Treatment also includes local approaches to control inflammation (eg, tissue adhesive and bandage contact lenses) and repair damage (eg, patch grafts). Other possibly helpful drugs include collagenase inhibitors, such as systemic tetracycline or topical 20% *N*-acetylcysteine.

PHLYCTENULAR KERATOCONJUNCTIVITIS

(Phlyctenular Conjunctivitis; Phlyctenulosis)

Phlyctenular keratoconjunctivitis, a hypersensitivity reaction of the cornea and conjunctiva to bacterial antigens, is characterized by discrete nodular areas of corneal or conjunctival inflammation.

Phlyctenular keratoconjunctivitis results from a hypersensitivity reaction to bacterial antigens, primarily staphylococcal, but TB, *Chlamydia,* and other agents have been implicated. It is more common among children. Many patients also have blepharitis.

Patients have multiple lesions, consisting of small yellow-gray nodules (phlyctenules) that appear at the limbus, on the cornea, or on the bulbar conjunctiva and persist from several days to 2 wk. On the conjunctiva, these nodules ulcerate but heal without a scar. When the cornea is affected, severe lacrimation, photophobia, blurred vision, aching, and foreign body sensation may be prominent. Frequent recurrence, especially with secondary infection, may lead to corneal opacity and neovascularization with loss of visual acuity.

Diagnosis is by characteristic clinical appearance. Testing for TB may be indicated (eg, for patients at risk).

Treatment for nontuberculous cases is with a topical corticosteroid–antibiotic combination. If patients have seborrheic blepharitis, eyelid scrubs may help prevent recurrence.

SUPERFICIAL PUNCTATE KERATITIS

Superficial punctate keratitis is corneal inflammation of diverse causes characterized by scattered, fine, punctate corneal epithelial loss or damage. Symptoms are redness, lacrimation, photophobia, and slightly decreased vision. Diagnosis is by slit-lamp examination. Treatment depends on the cause.

Superficial punctate keratitis is a nonspecific finding. Causes may include any of the following:

- Viral conjunctivitis (most commonly adenovirus)
- Blepharitis
- Keratoconjunctivitis sicca
- Trachoma
- Chemical burns
- Ultraviolet (UV) light exposure (eg, welding arcs, sunlamps, snow glare)
- Contact lens overwear
- Systemic drugs (eg, adenine arabinoside)
- Topical drug or preservative toxicity
- Peripheral facial nerve palsy (including Bell palsy)

Symptoms include photophobia, foreign body sensation, lacrimation, redness, and slightly decreased vision. Slit-lamp or ophthalmoscope examination of the cornea reveals a characteristic hazy appearance with multiple punctate speckles that stain with fluorescein. With viral conjunctivitis, preauricular adenopathy is common and chemosis may occur.

Keratitis that accompanies adenovirus conjunctivitis resolves spontaneously in about 3 wk. Blepharitis, keratoconjunctivitis sicca, and trachoma require specific therapy. When caused by overwearing contact lenses, keratitis is treated with discontinuation of the contact lens and an antibiotic ointment (eg, ciprofloxacin 0.3% qid), but the eye is not patched because serious infection may result. Contact lens wearers with superficial punctate keratitis should be examined the next day. Suspected causative topical drugs (active ingredient or preservative) should be stopped.

Ultraviolet keratitis: UVB light (wavelength < 300 nm) can burn the cornea, causing keratitis or keratoconjunctivitis. Arc welding is a common cause; even a brief, unprotected glance at a welding arc may result in a burn. Other causes include high-voltage electric sparks, artificial sun lamps, and sunlight reflected off snow at high altitudes. UV radiation increases 4 to 6% for every 1000-ft (305-m) increase in altitude above sea level, and snow reflects 85% of UVB.

Symptoms are usually not apparent for 8 to 12 h after exposure and last 24 to 48 h. Patients have lacrimation, pain, redness, swollen eyelids, photophobia, headache, foreign body sensation, and decreased vision. Permanent vision loss is very rare.

Diagnosis is by history, presence of superficial punctate keratitis, and absence of a foreign body or infection.

Treatment consists of an antibiotic ointment (eg, bacitracin or gentamicin 0.3% ointment q 8 h) and occasionally a short-acting cycloplegic drug (eg, cyclopentolate 1% drop q 4 h). Severe pain may require systemic analgesics (eg, acetaminophen 500 mg q 4 h for 24 h). The corneal surface regenerates spontaneously in 24 to 48 h. The eye should be rechecked in 24 h. Dark glasses or welder's helmets that block UV light are preventive.

CORNEAL TRANSPLANTATION

(Corneal Graft; Endothelial Keratoplasty; Penetrating Keratoplasty)

Indications: Corneal transplantations are done for several reasons:

- To reconstruct the cornea (eg, replacing a perforated cornea)
- To relieve intractable pain (eg, severe foreign body sensation due to recurrent ruptured bullae in bullous keratopathy)
- To treat a disorder unresponsive to medical management (eg, severe, uncontrolled fungal corneal ulcer)
- To improve the optical qualities of the cornea and thus improve vision (eg, replacing a cornea that is scarred after a corneal ulcer, is clouded because of edema as occurs in Fuchs dystrophy or after cataract surgery, is opaque because of deposits of nontransparent abnormal corneal stromal proteins as occurs in hereditary corneal stromal dystrophy, or has irregular astigmatism as occurs with keratoconus)

The most common indications are the following:

- Bullous keratopathy (pseudophakic or aphakic, Fuchs endothelial dystrophy)
- Keratoconus
- Repeat graft
- Keratitis or postkeratitis (caused by viral, bacterial, fungal, or *Acanthamoeba* infection or perforation)
- Corneal stromal dystrophies

Procedure: Tissue matching is not routinely done. Cadaveric donor tissue can be used unless the donor is suspected of having a communicable disease.

Corneal transplantation can be done using general anesthesia or local anesthesia plus IV sedation.

Topical antibiotics are used for several weeks postoperatively and topical corticosteroids for several months. To protect the eye from inadvertent trauma after transplantation, the patient wears shields, glasses, or sunglasses. If transplantation involves the full thickness of the cornea (as in penetrating keratoplasty, or PKP), achievement of full visual potential may take up to 18 mo because of changing refraction with wound healing and after suture removal. Only the corneal endothelium needs to be transplanted in diseases where the corneal stroma is clear, has a smooth stromal surface with a regular curvature, and only the corneal endothelium is not functioning well (eg, Fuchs dystrophy, bullous keratopathy resulting from cataract surgery). In corneal endothelium transplantation (eg, Descemet stripping endothelial keratoplasty [DSEK]) or the newest technique, Descemet membrane endothelial keratoplasty (DMEK), achievement of full visual potential usually occurs by 6 mo or 3 mo respectively. In many patients, earlier and better vision is attained by wearing a rigid contact lens over the corneal transplant.

Complications: Complications include the following:

- Graft rejection
- Infection (intraocular and corneal)
- Wound leak
- Glaucoma
- Graft failure
- High refractive error (especially astigmatism, myopia, or both)
- Recurrence of disease (with herpes simplex or hereditary corneal stromal dystrophy)

Graft rejection rates are usually < 10% (eg, in patients with early bullous keratopathy), but may be up to 68% in higher-risk patients (eg, those with chemical injury). Rejection symptoms include decreased vision, photosensitivity, ocular ache, and ocular redness. Graft rejection is treated with topical corticosteroids (eg, prednisolone 1% hourly), sometimes with a supplemental periocular injection (eg, triamcinolone acetonide 40 mg). If graft rejection is severe or if graft function is marginal, additional corticosteroids are given orally (eg, prednisone 1 mg/kg once/day) and occasionally IV (eg, methylprednisolone 3 to 5 mg/kg once). Typically, the rejection episode reverses, and graft function returns fully. The graft may fail if the rejection episode is unusually severe or long-standing or if multiple episodes of graft rejection occur. Regraft is possible, but the long-term prognosis is worse than for the original graft. Keratoprosthesis (artificial cornea) can be placed if grafts fail repeatedly.

Prognosis

The chance of long-term transplant success is

- > 90% for keratoconus, traumatic corneal scars, early bullous keratopathy, or hereditary corneal stromal dystrophies
- 80 to 90% for more advanced bullous keratopathy or inactive viral keratitis
- 50% for active corneal infection
- 0 to 50% for chemical or radiation injury

The generally high rate of success of corneal transplantation is attributable to many factors, including the avascularity of the cornea and the fact that the anterior chamber has venous drainage but no lymphatic drainage. These conditions promote low-zone tolerance (an immunologic tolerance that results from constant exposure to low doses of an antigen) and a process termed anterior chamber–associated immune deviation, in which there is active suppression of intraocular lymphocytes and delayed-type hypersensitivity to transplanted intraocular antigens. Another important factor is the effectiveness of the corticosteroids used topically, locally, and systemically to treat graft rejection.

Corneal Limbal Stem Cell Transplantation

Corneal limbal stem cell transplantation surgically replaces critical stem cells at the limbus (the area where the conjunctiva meets the cornea). Host stem cells normally reside in this area.

Transplantation is done when the host stem cells have been too severely damaged to recover from disease or injury.

Conditions such as severe chemical burns, Stevens-Johnson syndrome, and severe damage caused by chronic contact lens overwear may cause persistent nonhealing corneal epithelial defects. These defects result from failure of corneal epithelial stem cells to produce sufficient epithelial cells to repopulate the cornea. If untreated, persistent nonhealing corneal epithelial defects are vulnerable to infection, which can lead to scarring, perforation, or both. Under these circumstances, a corneal transplant, which replaces only the central cornea and not the limbus, is insufficient. Stem cells are needed to produce new cells that repopulate the cornea, restoring the regenerative capacity of the ocular surface.

Corneal limbal stem cells can be transplanted from the patient's own healthy eye or from a cadaveric donor eye. The patient's damaged corneal epithelial stem cells are removed by a partial-thickness dissection of the limbus (ie, all the epithelium and the superficial stroma of the limbus). Donor limbal tissue, which is prepared by a similar dissection, is sutured into the prepared bed. Systemic immunosuppression is required after cadaveric limbal grafts.

112 Glaucoma

Glaucomas are a group of eye disorders characterized by progressive optic nerve damage in which an important part is a relative increase in intraocular pressure (IOP). Glaucoma is the 2nd most common cause of blindness worldwide and the 2nd most common cause of blindness in the US, where it is the leading cause of blindness for people of African ethnicity and Hispanics. About 3 million Americans and 14 million people worldwide have glaucoma, but only half are aware of it. Glaucoma can occur at any age but is 6 times more common among people > 60 yr.

Glaucomas are categorized as

- Open-angle glaucoma
- Closed-angle glaucoma

See Tables 112–1, 112–2, and 112–3.

The "angle" refers to the angle formed by the junction of the iris and cornea at the periphery of the anterior chamber (see Fig. 112–1). The angle is where > 98% of the aqueous humor exits the eye via either the trabecular meshwork and the Schlemm canal (the major pathway, particularly in the elderly) or the ciliary body face and choroidal vasculature. These outflow pathways are not simply a mechanical filter and drain but instead involve active physiologic processes.

Glaucomas are further subdivided into primary (cause of outflow resistance or angle closure is unknown) and secondary (outflow resistance results from a known disorder), accounting for > 20 adult types.

Pathophysiology

Axons of retinal ganglion cells travel through the optic nerve carrying visual information from the eye to the brain. Damage to these axons causes ganglion cell death with resultant optic nerve atrophy and patchy vision loss. Elevated IOP (in unaffected eyes, the average range is 11 to 21 mm Hg) plays a role in axonal damage, either by direct nerve compression or diminution of blood flow. However, the relationship between externally measured pressure and nerve damage is complicated. Of people with IOP > 21 mm Hg (ie, ocular hypertension), only about 1 to 2%/yr (about 10% over 5 yr) develop glaucoma. Additionally, about one third of patients with glaucoma do not have IOP > 21 mm Hg (known as low-tension glaucoma or normal-tension glaucoma).

One factor may be that externally measured IOP does not always reflect true IOP; the cornea may be thinner than average, which leads to a higher IOP measurement, or thicker than average, which leads to a lower IOP measurement, inside the eye than externally measured IOP. Another factor may be that a vascular disorder compromises blood flow to the optic nerve. Also, it is likely that there are factors within the optic nerve that affect susceptibility to damage.

IOP is determined by the balance of aqueous secretion and drainage. Elevated IOP is caused by inhibited or obstructed outflow, not oversecretion; a combination of factors in the trabecular meshwork appear to be involved. In open-angle glaucoma, IOP is elevated because outflow is inadequate despite an angle that appears unobstructed. In angle-closure glaucoma, IOP is elevated when a physical distortion of the peripheral iris mechanically blocks outflow.

Symptoms and Signs

Symptoms and signs vary with the type of glaucoma, but the defining characteristic is optic nerve damage as evidenced by an abnormal optic disk (see p. 934) and certain types of visual field deficits (see p. 935).

IOP may be elevated or within the average range. (For techniques of measurement, see Testing on p. 895.)

Diagnosis

- Characteristic optic nerve changes
- Characteristic visual field defects
- Exclusion of other causes
- IOP usually > 21 mm Hg (but not required for the diagnosis)

Glaucoma should be suspected in a patient with any of the following:

- Abnormal optic nerve on ophthalmoscopy
- Elevated IOP
- Typical visual field defects
- Family history of glaucoma

Such patients (and those with any risk factors) should be referred to an ophthalmologist for a comprehensive examination that includes a thorough history, family history, examination of the optic disks (preferably using a binocular examination technique), formal visual field examination, IOP measurement, measurement of central corneal thickness, and gonioscopy (visualization of the anterior chamber angle with a special mirrored contact lens prism).

Glaucoma is diagnosed when characteristic findings of optic nerve damage are present and other causes (eg, multiple sclerosis) have been excluded. Elevated IOP makes the diagnosis more likely, but elevated IOP can occur in the absence of glaucoma and is not essential for making the diagnosis.

Screening: Screening for glaucoma can be done by primary physicians by checking visual fields with frequency-doubling

Table 112–1. OPEN-ANGLE GLAUCOMA: CLASSIFICATION BASED ON MECHANISMS OF OUTFLOW OBSTRUCTION*

TYPE	MEANS	EXAMPLES
Trabecular		
Idiopathic	—	Chronic open-angle glaucoma Juvenile glaucoma
Obstruction	By RBCs	Ghost cell glaucoma Hemorrhagic glaucoma
	By macrophages	Hemolytic glaucoma Melanomalytic glaucoma Phacolytic glaucoma
	By neoplastic cells	Juvenile xanthogranuloma Malignant tumors Neurofibromatosis Nevus of Ota
	By pigment particles	Exfoliation syndrome (glaucoma capsulare) Pigmentary glaucoma Uveitis
	By protein	Lens-induced glaucoma Uveitis
	By drugs	Corticosteroid-induced glaucoma
	Due to other means	Viscoelastic agents Vitreous hemorrhage
Alterations	Due to edema	Alkali burns Iritis or uveitis causing trabeculitis Scleritis or episcleritis
	Due to trauma	Angle recession
	Due to intraocular foreign bodies	Chalcosis Hemosiderosis
Posttrabecular		
Obstruction	Of the Schlemm canal	Clogging of canal (eg, by sickled RBCs) Collapse of canal
Other	Elevated episcleral venous pressure	Carotid-cavernous fistula Cavernous sinus thrombosis Idiopathic episcleral venous pressure elevation Mediastinal tumors Infiltrative ophthalmopathy (thyrotropic exophthalmos) Retrobulbar tumors Sturge-Weber syndrome Superior vena cava obstruction

*Clinical examples cited; not an inclusive list of glaucomas.
Adapted from Ritch R, Shields MB, Krupin T: *The Glaucomas*, 2nd ed. St. Louis, Mosby; 1996, p. 720; with permission.

technology (FDT) perimetry and ophthalmoscopic evaluation of the optic nerve. FDT perimetry involves use of a desktop device that can screen for visual field abnormalities suggestive of glaucoma in 2 to 3 min per eye. Although IOP should be measured, screening based only on IOP has low sensitivity, low specificity, and low positive predictive value. Patients > 40 yr and those who have risk factors for open-angle or angle-closure glaucoma should receive a comprehensive eye examination every 1 to 2 yr.

Treatment

- Decreasing IOP by using drugs or laser or incisional surgery

Patients with characteristic optic nerve and corresponding visual field changes are treated regardless of IOP measurement. Lowering the IOP is the only clinically proven treatment. For chronic adult and juvenile glaucomas, the initial target IOP measurement is at least 20 to 40% below pretreatment readings.

Three methods are available: drugs, laser surgery, and incisional surgery. The type of glaucoma determines the appropriate method or methods.

Drugs and most laser surgeries (trabeculoplasty) modify the existing aqueous secretion and drainage system.

Traditional incisional surgeries (eg, guarded filtration procedures [trabeculectomy], glaucoma drainage implant devices [tube shunts]) create a new drainage pathway between the anterior chamber and subconjunctival space. Newer incisional surgeries attempt to enhance trabecular or uveoscleral outflow without creating a full-thickness fistula.

Table 112–2. ANGLE-CLOSURE GLAUCOMA: CLASSIFICATION BASED ON MECHANISMS OF OUTFLOW OBSTRUCTION*

TYPE	DISORDERS	EXAMPLES
Anterior (pulling mechanism)		
Contracture of membranes	Iridocorneal endothelial syndrome Neovascular glaucoma Posterior polymorphous dystrophy Surgery (eg, corneal transplant) Trauma (penetrating and nonpenetrating)	—
Contracture of inflammatory precipitates	—	—
Inflammatory membrane	Fuchs heterochromic iridocyclitis Luetic interstitial keratitis	—
Posterior (pushing mechanism)		
With pupillary block	Lens-induced mechanisms	Intumescent lens Subluxation of lens Mobile lens syndrome
	Posterior synechiae	Iris-vitreous block in aphakia Pseudophakia Uveitis
	Pupillary block glaucoma	—
Without pupillary block	Ciliary block (malignant) glaucoma	—
	Cysts of the iris and ciliary body	—
	Forward vitreous shift after lens extraction	—
	Intraocular tumors	Malignant melanoma Retinoblastoma
	Lens-induced mechanisms	Intumescent lens Subluxation of lens Mobile lens syndrome
	Plateau iris syndrome	—
	Uveal edema	After scleral buckling, panretinal photocoagulation, or central retinal vein occlusion
	Retrolenticular tissue contracture	Persistent hyperplastic primary vitreous Retinopathy of prematurity (retrolental fibroplasia)

*Clinical examples cited; not an inclusive list of glaucomas.
Adapted from Ritch R, Shields MB, Krupin T: *The Glaucomas*, 2nd ed. St. Louis, Mosby; 1996, p. 720; with permission.

Prophylactic IOP lowering in patients with ocular hypertension delays the onset of glaucoma. However, because the rate of conversion from ocular hypertension to glaucoma in untreated people is low, the decision to treat prophylactically should be individualized based on the presence of risk factors, magnitude of IOP elevation, and patient factors (ie, preference for drugs vs surgery, drug adverse effects). Generally, treatment is recommended for patients with IOP > 30 mm Hg even if the visual field is full and the optic nerve disk appears healthy because the likelihood of damage is significant at that IOP level.

Table 112–3. DEVELOPMENTAL ABNORMALITIES OF THE ANTERIOR CHAMBER ANGLE CAUSING GLAUCOMA: CLASSIFICATION BASED ON MECHANISMS OF OUTFLOW OBSTRUCTION*

MECHANISM	DISORDERS
High insertion of peripheral iris	Axenfeld-Rieger syndrome Peters anomaly
Incomplete development of trabecular meshwork or the Schlemm canal	Congenital (infantile) glaucoma Glaucomas associated with other developmental abnormalities
Fine strands that contract to close angle	Aniridia

*Clinical examples cited; not an inclusive list of the glaucomas.
Adapted from Ritch R, Shields MB, Krupin T: *The Glaucomas*, 2nd ed. St. Louis, Mosby; 1996, p. 720; with permission.

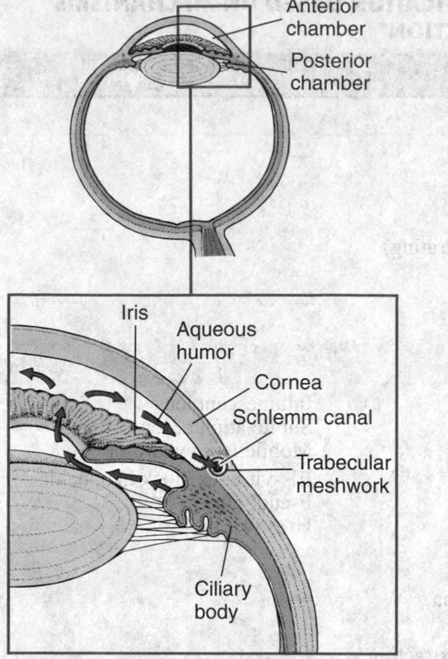

Fig. 112–1. Aqueous humor production and flow. Most of the aqueous humor, produced by the ciliary body, exits the eye at the angle formed by the junction of the iris and cornea. It exits primarily via the trabecular meshwork and the Schlemm canal.

KEY POINTS

- Glaucoma is common, often asymptomatic, and contributes heavily to blindness worldwide.
- Suspect glaucoma if patients have elevated IOP, optic nerve abnormalities on ophthalmoscopy, or a family history of glaucoma.
- Do not rule out glaucoma because IOP is not high.
- Screen patients > 40 yr or with risk factors every 1 to 2 yr, based mainly on results of ophthalmoscopy and FDT (to assess visual fields).
- Treat by decreasing IOP.
- Prophylactically decrease IOP if > 30 mm Hg, even if glaucoma is absent.

PRIMARY OPEN-ANGLE GLAUCOMA

Primary open-angle glaucoma is a syndrome of optic nerve damage associated with an open anterior chamber angle and an elevated or sometimes average intraocular pressure (IOP). Symptoms are a result of visual field loss. Diagnosis is by ophthalmoscopy, gonioscopy, visual field examination, and measurement of central corneal thickness and IOP. Treatment includes topical drugs (eg, prostaglandin analogs, β-blockers) and often requires laser or incisional surgery to increase aqueous drainage.

Etiology

Although open-angle glaucomas can have numerous causes (see Table 112–1), 60 to 70% of cases in the US have no identifiable cause and are termed primary open-angle glaucoma. Both eyes usually are affected, but typically not equally.

Risk factors for primary open-angle glaucoma include

- Older age
- Positive family history
- African ethnicity
- Thinner central corneal thickness
- Systemic hypertension
- Diabetes
- Myopia

In people of African ethnicity, glaucoma is more severe and develops at an earlier age, and blindness is 6 to 8 times more likely.

Pathophysiology

IOP can be elevated or within the average range.

Elevated-pressure glaucoma: Two thirds of patients with glaucoma have elevated (> 21 mm Hg) IOP. Aqueous humor drainage is inadequate, whereas production by the ciliary body is normal. Identifiable mechanisms (ie, secondary open-angle glaucomas) are not present. Secondary mechanisms include developmental anomalies, scarring caused by trauma or infection, and plugging of channels by detached iris pigment (ie, pigment dispersion syndrome) or abnormal protein deposits (eg, pseudoexfoliation syndrome).

Normal-pressure glaucoma or low-pressure glaucoma: In at least one third of patients with glaucoma, IOP is within the average range, but optic nerve damage and visual field loss typical of glaucoma are present. These patients have a higher incidence of vasospastic diseases (eg, migraines, Raynaud syndrome) than the general population, suggesting that a vascular disorder compromising blood flow to the optic nerve may play a role. Glaucoma occurring with average-range IOP is more common among Asians.

Symptoms and Signs

Early primary open-angle glaucoma symptoms are uncommon. Usually, the patient becomes aware of visual field loss only when optic nerve atrophy is marked; the typically asymmetric deficits contribute to delay in recognition. However, some patients have complaints, such as missing stairs if their inferior visual field has been lost, noticing portions of words missing when reading, or having difficulty with driving earlier in the course of the disease.

Examination findings include an unobstructed open angle on gonioscopy and characteristic optic nerve appearance and visual field defects. IOP may be normal or high but is almost always higher in the eye with more optic nerve damage.

Optic nerve appearance: The optic nerve head (ie, disk) is normally a slightly vertically elongated circle with a centrally located depression called the cup. The neurosensory rim is the tissue between the margin of the cup and the edge of the disk and is composed of the ganglion cell axons from the retina.

Characteristic optic nerve changes include

- Increased cup:disk ratio (including an increasing ratio over time)
- Thinning of the neurosensory rim
- Pitting or notching of the rim

- Nerve fiber layer hemorrhage that crosses the disk margin (ie, Drance hemorrhage or splinter hemorrhages)
- Vertical elongation of the cup
- Quick angulations in the course of the exiting blood vessels (called bayoneting)

Thinning of the neurosensory rim (optic nerve or retinal nerve fiber layer) over time alone can be diagnostic of glaucoma regardless of the IOP or visual field and is the initial sign of damage in 40 to 60% of cases (see Plate 17). In other cases, the initial sign of damage is some visual field change.

Visual field defects: Visual field changes caused by lesions of the optic nerve include

- Nasal step defects (which do not cross the horizontal meridian—an imaginary horizontal line between the upper and lower parts of the visual field)
- Arcuate (arc-shaped) scotomata extending nasally from the blind spot
- Temporal wedge defects
- Paracentral scotomata

In contrast, deficits of the more proximal visual pathways (ie, from the lateral geniculate nucleus to the occipital lobe) involve quadrants or hemispheres of the visual field; thus, deficits do not cross the vertical meridian.

Diagnosis

- Visual field testing
- Ophthalmoscopy
- Measurement of central corneal thickness and IOP
- Exclusion of other optic neuropathies

Diagnosis of primary open-angle glaucoma is suggested by the examination, but similar findings can result from other optic neuropathies (eg, caused by ischemia, cytomegalovirus infection, or vitamin B_{12} deficiency).

Before a diagnosis of normal-pressure glaucoma can be established, the following factors may need to be ruled out:

- Inaccurate IOP readings
- Large diurnal fluctuations (causing intermittent normal readings)
- Optic nerve damage caused by previously resolved glaucoma (eg, a previously elevated IOP due to corticosteroid use or uveitis)
- Intermittent angle-closure glaucoma
- Other ocular or neurologic disorders that cause similar visual field defects

Central corneal thickness is measured to help interpret the result of IOP measurement.

Optic disk photography or a detailed optic disk drawing is helpful for future comparison. The frequency of follow-up examinations varies from weeks to years, depending on the patient's reliability, severity of the glaucoma, and response to treatment.

Treatment

- Decreasing IOP 20 to 40%
- Initially, drugs (eg, prostaglandin analogs such latanoprost or tafluprost, beta-blockers such as timolol)
- Sometimes surgery, such as laser trabeculoplasty or guarded filtration procedure

Vision lost by glaucoma cannot be recovered. The goal is to prevent further optic nerve and visual field damage by lowering IOP. The target level is 20 to 40% below pretreatment readings or the IOP at which damage is known to have occurred. In general, the greater the damage caused by glaucoma, the lower the IOP must be to prevent further damage. If damage progresses, the IOP goal is lowered further and additional therapy is initiated.

Initial treatment is usually drug therapy, proceeding to laser therapy and then incisional surgery if the target IOP is not met. Surgery may be the initial treatment if IOP is extremely high, the patient does not wish to use or has trouble adhering to drug therapy, or if there is significant visual field damage at presentation.

Drug therapy: Multiple drugs are available (see Table 112–4). Topical agents are preferred. The most popular are prostaglandin analogs, followed by β-blockers (particularly timolol). Other drugs include α_2-selective adrenergic agonists, carbonic anhydrase inhibitors, and cholinergic agonists. Oral carbonic anhydrase inhibitors are effective, but adverse effects limit their use.

Patients taking topical glaucoma drugs should be taught passive eyelid closure with punctal occlusion to help reduce systemic absorption and associated adverse effects, although the effectiveness of these maneuvers is controversial. Patients who have difficulty instilling drops directly onto the conjunctiva may place the drop on the nose just medial to the medial canthus, then roll the head slightly toward the eye so that the liquid flows into the eye.

Typically, to gauge effectiveness, clinicians start drugs in one (one-eye trial) or both eyes.

Surgery: Surgery for primary open-angle glaucoma and normal-pressure glaucoma includes laser trabeculoplasty, a guarded filtration procedure, and procedures that enhance only a portion of the drainage pathway.

Argon laser trabeculoplasty (ALT) may be the initial treatment for patients who do not respond to or who cannot tolerate drug therapy. Laser energy is applied to either 180° or 360° of the trabecular meshwork to improve the drainage of aqueous humor. Within 2 to 5 yr, about 50% of patients require additional drug therapy or surgery because of insufficient IOP control.

Selective laser trabeculoplasty (SLT) uses a pulsed double-frequency neodymium:yttrium-aluminum-garnet laser. SLT and ALT are equally effective initially, but SLT may have greater effectiveness in subsequent treatments. SLT may also be considered for initial treatment.

A **guarded filtration procedure** is the most commonly used filtration procedure. A hole is made in the limbal sclera (trabeculectomy), which is covered by a partial-thickness scleral flap that controls egress of aqueous from the eye to the subconjunctival space, forming a filtration bleb. Adverse effects of glaucoma filtration surgery include acceleration of cataract growth, pressures that are too low, and transient accumulation of fluid in the choroidal space (ie, choroidal effusion) during the perioperative period. Patients with trabeculectomies are at increased risk of bacterial endophthalmitis and should be instructed to report any symptoms or signs of bleb infection (blebitis) or endophthalmitis (eg, worsening vision, conjunctival hyperemia, pain) immediately.

Partial-thickness procedures bypass portions of the outflow pathways, unlike full-thickness procedures, even if guarded, that create a direct conduit between the anterior chamber and subconjunctival space.

In the ab interno approach (an approach from inside the eye), a device is used to remove (eg, with ab interno trabeculectomy) or bypass (eg, with some stent procedures) the trabecular meshwork, creating direct communication between the anterior chamber and collecting channels. No bleb is formed.

Table 112–4. DRUGS USED TO TREAT GLAUCOMA

DRUG	DOSE/FREQUENCY	MECHANISM OF ACTION ON EYE	COMMENTS
Prostaglandin analogs (topical)			
Bimatoprost	1 drop at bedtime	Increase uveoscleral outflow rather than altering conventional (trabeculocanalicular) aqueous outflow	Increased pigmentation of the iris and skin; possible worsening of uveitis Elongated and thickened eyelashes; muscle, joint, and back pain; rash
Latanoprost	1 drop at bedtime		
Tafluprost	1 drop at bedtime		
Travoprost	1 drop at bedtime		
β-Blockers (topical)			
Timolol	1 drop once/day–bid	Decrease aqueous production; do not affect pupil size	Systemic adverse effects (eg, bronchospasm, depression, fatigue, confusion, erectile dysfunction, hair loss, bradycardia) May develop insidiously and be attributed by patients to aging or other processes
Betaxolol	1 drop once/day–bid*		
Carteolol	1 drop once/day–bid		
Levobetaxolol	1 drop bid*		
Levobunolol	1 drop once/day–bid		
Metipranolol	1 drop once/day–bid		
Carbonic anhydrase inhibitors (oral or IV)			
Acetazolamide	125–250 mg po qid (or 500 mg po bid using extended-release capsules) or 500 mg IV single dose	Decrease aqueous production	Used as adjunctive therapy Cause fatigue, altered taste, anorexia, depression, paresthesias, electrolyte abnormalities, kidney calculi, and blood dyscrasias Possibly nausea, diarrhea, weight loss
Methazolamide	25–50 mg po bid–tid		
Carbonic anhydrase inhibitors (topical)			
Brinzolamide	1 drop bid–qid	—	Low risk of systemic effects, but may cause bad taste in mouth
Dorzolamide	1 drop bid–tid		
Miotics, direct-acting (cholinergic agonists; topical)†			
Carbachol	1 drop bid–tid	Cause miosis, increase aqueous outflow	Less effective as monotherapy than β-blockers Possible need for higher strengths in patients with darker-pigmented pupils Hinder dark adaptation
Pilocarpine	1 drop bid–qid		
Miotic, indirect-acting (cholinesterase inhibitors; topical)†			
Echothiophate iodide	1 drop once/day–bid‡	Causes miosis, increases aqueous outflow	Very long acting: Irreversible inhibition; can cause cataracts and retinal detachment; should be avoided in angle-closure glaucoma because of the extreme miosis; hinders dark adaptation Systemic effects (eg, sweating, headache, tremor, excess saliva production, diarrhea, abdominal cramps, nausea) more likely than with direct-acting miotics May still be an option in pseudophakic patients

Table 112–4. DRUGS USED TO TREAT GLAUCOMA (*Continued*)

DRUG	DOSE/FREQUENCY	MECHANISM OF ACTION ON EYE	COMMENTS
Osmotic diuretics (oral, IV)			
Glycerin	1–1.5 g/kg body weight po (may repeat 8–12 h later)	Cause increased serum osmolarity, which draws fluid from eye	Used for acute angle closure Have adverse systemic effects Can rarely cause cerebral hemorrhage and acute, decompensated heart failure Ineffective in patients with moderate to severe renal failure
Mannitol	0.5–2.0 g/kg body weight IV over 30–45 min (may repeat 8–12 h later)		
α_2-Selective adrenergic agonists (topical)			
Apraclonidine	1 drop bid–tid	Decrease aqueous production; may increase uveoscleral aqueous outflow; may cause mydriasis	With apraclonidine, high rate of allergic reactions and tachyphylaxis; less common with brimonidine, which may cause dry mouth and is contraindicated in children < 2 yr Systemic effects (eg, hypertension, tachycardia) less common than with nonselective agonists
Brimonidine	1 drop bid–tid§		

*β_1-Selective.
†Miotics are rarely used.
‡Irreversible; may be cataractogenic; increased risk of retinal detachment.
§More α_2-selective than apraclonidine.

The ab externo approach (an approach from outside the eye), including viscocanalostomy, deep sclerectomy, and canaloplasty, involves a deep dissection of greater than > 98% thickness of the scleral passage, leaving a window of Descemet membrane and/or the inner wall of the Schlemm canal and trabecular meshwork. The canal is dilated by using a viscoelastic solution (in viscocanalostomy) or a microcatheter (in canaloplasty). Deep sclerectomy generally relies on the formation of a conjunctival bleb.

In general, these procedures appear to be safer but less effective than trabeculectomy.

KEY POINTS

- Primary open-angle glaucoma is usually related to elevated IOP but may occur with normal IOP.
- Vision loss due to glaucoma cannot be recovered.
- Begin diagnostic evaluation with ophthalmoscopy, measurement of IOP, and visual field testing.
- Aim to decrease IOP by 20 to 40%.
- Begin treatment with topical drugs (eg, prostaglandin analogs such latanoprost or tafluprost, β-blockers such as timolol).
- Consider surgical treatment if drugs are not effective or if visual loss is severe.

ANGLE-CLOSURE GLAUCOMA

(Closed-Angle Glaucoma)

Angle-closure glaucoma is glaucoma associated with a physically obstructed anterior chamber angle, which may be chronic or, rarely, acute. Symptoms of acute angle closure are severe ocular pain and redness, decreased vision, colored halos around lights, headache, nausea, and vomiting. Intraocular pressure (IOP) is elevated. Immediate treatment of the acute condition with multiple topical and systemic drugs is required to prevent permanent vision loss, followed by the definitive treatment, iridotomy.

Angle-closure glaucoma accounts for about 10% of all glaucomas in the US.

Etiology

Angle-closure glaucoma is caused by factors that either pull or push the iris up into the angle (ie, junction of the iris and cornea at the periphery of the anterior chamber), physically blocking drainage of aqueous and raising IOP (see Table 112–2). Elevated IOP damages the optic nerve.

Pathophysiology

Angle closure may be primary (cause is unknown) or secondary to another condition (see Table 112–1) and can be acute, subacute (intermittent), or chronic.

Primary angle-closure glaucoma: Narrow angles are not present in young people. As people age, the lens of the eye continues to grow. In some but not all people, this growth pushes the iris forward, narrowing the angle. Risk factors for developing narrow angles include family history, advanced age, and ethnicity; risk is higher among people of Asian and Inuit ethnicity and lower among people of European and African ethnicity.

In people with narrow angles, the distance between the iris at the pupil and the lens is also very narrow. When the iris dilates, forces pull the iris centripetally and posteriorly causing increasing iris–lens contact, which prevents aqueous from passing between the lens and iris, through the pupil, and into the anterior chamber (this mechanism is termed pupillary block). Pressure from the continued secretion of aqueous into the posterior chamber by the ciliary body pushes the peripheral iris anteriorly (causing a forward-bowing iris called iris bombe), closing the angle. This closure blocks aqueous outflow, resulting in rapid (within hours) and severe (> 40 mm Hg) elevation of IOP.

Because of the rapid onset, this condition is called primary acute angle-closure glaucoma and is an ophthalmic emergency requiring immediate treatment. Non-pupillary block mechanisms include plateau iris syndrome in which the central anterior chamber is deep, but the peripheral anterior chamber is made shallow by a ciliary body that is displaced forward.

Intermittent angle-closure glaucoma occurs if the episode of pupillary block resolves spontaneously after several hours, usually after sleeping supine.

Chronic angle-closure glaucoma occurs if the angle narrows slowly, allowing scarring between the peripheral iris and trabecular meshwork; IOP elevation is slow.

Pupillary dilation (mydriasis) can push the iris into the angle and precipitate acute angle-closure glaucoma in any person with narrow angles. This development is of particular concern when applying topical agents to dilate the eye for examination (eg, cyclopentolate, phenylephrine) or for treatment (eg, homatropine) or when giving systemic drugs that have the potential to dilate the pupils (eg, scopolamine, α-adrenergic agonists commonly used to treat urinary incontinence, drugs with anticholinergic effects).

Secondary angle-closure glaucomas: The mechanical obstruction of the angle is due to a coexisting condition, such as proliferative diabetic retinopathy (PDR), ischemic central vein occlusion, uveitis, or epithelial down-growth. Contraction of a neovascular membrane (eg, in PDR) or inflammatory scarring can pull the iris into the angle.

Symptoms and Signs

Acute angle-closure glaucoma: Patients have severe ocular pain and redness, decreased vision, colored halos around lights, headache, nausea, and vomiting. The systemic complaints may be so severe that patients are misdiagnosed as having a neurologic or GI problem. Examination typically reveals conjunctival hyperemia, a hazy cornea, a fixed mid-dilated pupil, and anterior chamber inflammation. Vision is decreased. IOP measurement is usually 40 to 80 mm Hg. The optic nerve is difficult to visualize because of corneal edema, and visual field testing is not done because of discomfort. For primary mechanisms of angle-closure (eg, pupillary block and plateau iris), examination of the uninvolved contralateral eye can indicate the diagnosis.

PEARLS & PITFALLS

- In patients who have sudden headache, nausea, and vomiting, examine the eyes.

Chronic angle-closure glaucoma: This type of glaucoma manifests similarly to open-angle glaucoma. Some patients have ocular redness, discomfort, blurred vision, or headache that lessens with sleep (perhaps because of sleep-induced miosis and posterior displacement of the lens by gravity). On gonioscopy, the angle is narrow, and peripheral anterior synechiae (adhesions between the peripheral iris and angle structure causing blockage of trabecular meshwork and/or ciliary body face), also called PAS, may be seen. IOP may be normal but is usually higher in the affected eye.

Diagnosis

- **Acute:** Measurement of IOP and clinical findings
- **Chronic:** Gonioscopy showing peripheral anterior synechiae and characteristic optic nerve and visual field abnormalities

Diagnosis of acute angle-closure glaucoma is clinical and by measurement of IOP. Gonioscopy may be difficult to do in the involved eye because of a clouded cornea with friable corneal epithelium. However, examination of the other eye reveals a narrow or occludable angle. If the other eye has a wide angle, a diagnosis other than primary angle-closure glaucoma should be considered.

Diagnosis of chronic angle-closure glaucoma is based on the presence of PAS on gonioscopy and characteristic optic nerve and visual field changes (see Symptoms and Signs on p. 934).

Treatment

- **Acute:** Timolol, pilocarpine, and brimonidine drops, oral acetazolamide, and a systemic osmotic drug, followed by laser peripheral iridotomy
- **Chronic:** Similar to primary open-angle glaucoma except that laser peripheral iridotomy may be done if the ophthalmologist feels that the procedure may slow mechanical closing of the angle

Acute angle-closure glaucoma: Treatment must be initiated immediately because vision can be lost quickly and permanently. The patient should receive several drugs at once. A suggested regimen is timolol 0.5% one drop q 30 min for 2 doses, pilocarpine 2 to 4% one drop q 15 min for 2 doses, brimonidine (0.15 or 0.2%) one drop q 15 min for 2 doses, acetazolamide 500 mg po initially (IV if patients are nauseated) followed by 250 mg q 6 h, and an osmotic agent, such as oral glycerol 1 mL/kg diluted with an equal amount of cold water, mannitol 1.0 to 1.5 mg/kg IV, or isosorbide 100 g po (220 mL of a 45% solution). (NOTE: This form of isosorbide is not isosorbide dinitrate.) Response is evaluated by measuring IOP. Miotics (eg, pilocarpine) are generally not effective when IOP is > 40 or 50 mm Hg because of an anoxic pupillary sphincter.

Definitive treatment is with laser peripheral iridotomy (LPI), which opens another pathway for fluid to pass from the posterior to the anterior chamber, breaking the pupillary block. It is done as soon as the cornea is clear and inflammation has subsided. In some cases the cornea clears within hours of lowering the IOP; in other cases, it can take 1 to 2 days. Because the chance of having an acute attack in the other eye is 80%, LPI is done on both eyes.

The risk of complications with LPI is extremely low compared with its benefits. Glare, which can be bothersome, may occur.

Chronic angle-closure glaucoma: Patients with chronic, subacute, or intermittent angle-closure glaucoma should also have LPI. Additionally, patients with a narrow angle, even in the absence of symptoms, should undergo prompt LPI to prevent angle-closure glaucoma.

The drug and surgical treatments are the same as with open-angle glaucoma. Laser trabeculoplasty is relatively contraindicated if the angle is so narrow that additional PAS may form after the laser procedure. Typically, partial-thickness procedures are not indicated.

KEY POINTS

- Angle-closure glaucoma can develop acutely, intermittently, or chronically.
- Suspect acute angle-closure glaucoma based on clinical findings and confirm it by measuring IOP.
- Confirm chronic angle-closure glaucoma by peripheral anterior synechiae and optic nerve and visual field changes.
- Treat acute angle-closure glaucoma as an emergency.
- Consult an ophthalmologist to arrange laser peripheral iridotomy for all patients with angle-closure glaucoma.

113 Conjunctival and Scleral Disorders

The **conjunctiva** lines the back of the eyelids (palpebral or tarsal conjunctiva), crosses the space between the lid and the globe (forniceal conjunctiva), then folds back on itself as it spreads over the sclera to the cornea (bulbar conjunctiva). The conjunctiva helps maintain the tear film and protect the eye from foreign objects and infection.

The **sclera** is the thick white sphere of dense connective tissue that encloses the eye and maintains its shape. Anteriorly, the sclera fuses with the cornea at the limbus, and posteriorly it blends with the meninges where the optic nerve penetrates the globe.

The **episclera** is a thin vascular membrane between the conjunctiva and the sclera.

The most common disorders are inflammatory (eg, conjunctivitis, episcleritis, scleritis). Conjunctivitis can be acute or chronic and is infectious, allergic, or irritant in origin. Episcleritis and scleritis usually result from immune-mediated disease. Episcleritis usually does not threaten vision, but scleritis can destroy vision and the eye. Major symptoms of conjunctivitides (eg, conjunctival hyperemia) are similar. Early, accurate diagnosis is important.

Select eye findings in conjunctival disorders: Edema of the bulbar conjunctiva results in a diffusely translucent, bluish, thickened conjunctiva. Gross edema with ballooning of the conjunctiva, often leading to prolapse of conjunctiva, is known as chemosis.

Edema of the tarsal conjunctiva (typical of allergic conjunctivitis) results in fine, minute projections (papillae), giving the conjunctiva a velvety appearance.

Hyperplasia of lymphoid follicles in the conjunctiva can occur in viral conjunctivitis or chlamydial conjunctivitis. It appears as small bumps with pale centers, resembling cobblestones. It occurs most commonly in the inferior tarsal conjunctiva.

OCULAR MUCOUS MEMBRANE PEMPHIGOID

(Benign Mucous Membrane Pemphigoid; Cicatricial Pemphigoid; Mucous Membrane Pemphigoid; Ocular Cicatricial Pemphigoid; Ocular Mucous Membrane Pemphigoid)

Ocular mucous membrane pemphigoid is a chronic, bilateral, progressive scarring and shrinkage of the conjunctiva with opacification of the cornea. Early symptoms are hyperemia, discomfort, itching, and discharge; progression leads to eyelid and corneal damage and sometimes blindness. Diagnosis is sometimes confirmed by biopsy. Treatment often requires systemic immunosuppression.

Ocular mucous membrane pemphigoid is an autoimmune disease in which binding of anticonjunctival basement membrane antibodies results in conjunctival inflammation. It is unrelated to bullous pemphigoid.

Symptoms and Signs

Usually beginning as a chronic conjunctivitis with nonspecific hyperemia without discharge in certain quadrants, the condition progresses to symblephara (adhesions between the tarsal and bulbar conjunctiva); trichiasis (in-turning eyelashes); keratoconjunctivitis sicca; corneal neovascularization, opacification, and keratinization; and conjunctival shrinkage and keratinization. Chronic corneal epithelial defects can lead to secondary bacterial ulceration, scarring, and blindness. Oral mucous membrane involvement with ulceration and scarring is common, but skin involvement, characterized by scarring bullae and erythematous plaques, is uncommon.

Diagnosis

- Unexplained symblephara or biopsy findings

Diagnosis of ocular mucous membrane pemphigoid is suspected clinically in patients with conjunctival scarring plus corneal changes, symblephara, or both. The differential diagnosis of progressive conjunctival scarring includes previous radiation exposure and atopic disease. Therefore, the clinical diagnosis of cicatricial pemphigoid is made when there is progression of a symblepharon without a history of local radiation or severe perennial allergic conjunctivitis. Diagnosis can be confirmed by conjunctival biopsy showing antibody deposition on the basement membrane. A negative biopsy does not rule out the diagnosis.

Treatment

- Epilation of in-turning lashes
- Often systemic immunosuppression

Tear substitutes and epilation, cryoepilation, or electroepilation of the in-turning eyelashes may increase patient comfort and reduce the risk of ocular infection, secondary corneal scarring, and decreased vision. For progressive trichiasis, conjunctival scarring, or corneal opacification or for nonhealing corneal epithelial defects, systemic immunosuppression (eg, with dapsone, cyclophosphamide, intravenous immunoglobulin (IVIG), or rituximab) is indicated.

KEY POINTS

- Ocular mucous membrane pemphigoid is a chronic, autoimmune scarring of the conjunctiva with opacification of the cornea.
- Findings include symblephara (adhesions between the tarsal and bulbar conjunctiva); trichiasis (in-turning eyelashes); keratoconjunctivitis sicca; corneal neovascularization, opacification, and keratinization; and conjunctival shrinkage and keratinization.
- Diagnosis is usually by finding a symblepharon in a patient without a history of local radiation or severe perennial allergic conjunctivitis.
- Treatment can include tear substitutes, epilation of in-turning lashes, and sometimes systemic immunosuppression.

OVERVIEW OF CONJUNCTIVITIS

Conjunctival inflammation typically results from infection, allergy, or irritation. Symptoms are conjunctival hyperemia and ocular discharge and, depending on the etiology, discomfort and itching. Diagnosis is clinical; sometimes cultures are indicated. Treatment depends on etiology and

may include topical antibiotics, antihistamines, mast cell stabilizers, and corticosteroids.

Infectious conjunctivitis is most commonly viral conjunctivitis or bacterial conjunctivitis and is contagious. Rarely, mixed or unidentifiable pathogens are present. Numerous allergens can cause allergic conjunctivitis. Nonallergic conjunctival irritation can result from foreign bodies; wind, dust, smoke, fumes, chemical vapors, and other types of air pollution; and intense ultraviolet light of electric arcs, sunlamps, and reflection from snow.

Conjunctivitis is typically acute, but both infectious and allergic conditions can be chronic. Additional conditions that cause chronic conjunctivitis include ectropion, entropion, blepharitis, and chronic dacryocystitis.

Symptoms and Signs

Any source of inflammation can cause lacrimation or discharge and diffuse conjunctival vascular dilation. Discharge may cause the eyes to crust overnight. Thick discharge may blur vision, but once discharge is cleared, visual acuity should be unaffected.

Itching and watery discharge predominate in allergic conjunctivitis. Chemosis and papillary hyperplasia also suggest allergic conjunctivitis. Irritation or foreign body sensation, photophobia, and discharge suggest infectious viral conjunctivitis; purulent discharge suggests bacterial conjunctivitis. Severe eye pain suggests scleritis.

Diagnosis

- Clinical evaluation
- Sometimes culture

Usually, diagnosis of conjunctivitis is made by history and examination (see Table 113–1), usually including slit-lamp examination with fluorescein staining of the cornea and, if glaucoma is suspected, measurement of intraocular pressure. In order to prevent transmitting infection to other patients and to staff, meticulous disinfection of equipment that touches the eye is particularly important after examination of patients who could have conjunctivitis.

Other disorders can cause a red eye. Deep pain in the affected eye when a light is shone in the unaffected eye (true photophobia) does not occur in uncomplicated conjunctivitis and suggests a disorder of the cornea or anterior uvea. Circumcorneal conjunctival hyperemia (sometimes described as ciliary flush) is caused by dilated, fine, straight, deep vessels that radiate out 1 to 3 mm from the limbus, without significant hyperemia of the bulbar and tarsal conjunctivae. Ciliary flush occurs with uveitis, acute glaucoma, and some types of keratitis (see p. 926) but not with uncomplicated conjunctivitis.

PEARLS & PITFALLS

- Suspect another cause of red eye (eg, uveitis, glaucoma, keratitis) if patients have true photophobia, loss of vision, or ciliary flush and do not have significant discharge or tearing.

The cause of conjunctivitis is suggested by clinical findings. However, cultures are indicated for patients with severe symptoms, immunocompromise, a vulnerable eye (eg, after a corneal transplant, in exophthalmos due to Graves disease), or poor response to initial therapy.

Clinical differentiation between viral and bacterial infectious conjunctivitis is not highly accurate. However, if the history and examination strongly suggest viral conjunctivitis, withholding antibiotics initially is appropriate. Antibiotics can be prescribed later if the clinical picture changes or if symptoms persist.

Treatment

- Prevention of spread
- Treatment of symptoms

Most infectious conjunctivitis is highly contagious and spreads by droplets, fomites, and hand-to-eye inoculation. To avoid transmitting infection, physicians must use hand sanitizer or wash their hands properly (fully lather hands, scrub hands for at least 20 seconds, rinse well, and turn off the water using a paper towel) and disinfect equipment after examining patients. Patients should use hand sanitizer and/or wash their hands thoroughly after touching their eyes or nasal secretions, avoid touching the noninfected eye after touching the infected eye, avoid sharing towels or pillows, and avoid swimming in pools. Eyes should be kept free of discharge and should not be patched. Small children with conjunctivitis should be kept home from school to avoid spread. Cool washcloths applied to the eyes may help relieve local burning and itching. Antimicrobials are used for certain infections.

KEY POINTS

- Conjunctivitis typically results from infection, allergy, or irritation.
- Infectious conjunctivitis is usually highly contagious.
- Typical findings are redness (without ciliary flush) and discharge, without significant pain or loss of vision.
- Diagnosis is usually clinical.
- Treatment includes measures to prevent spread and treatment of the cause (sometimes antimicrobials).

Table 113–1. DIFFERENTIATING FEATURES IN ACUTE CONJUNCTIVITIS

ETIOLOGY	DISCHARGE/CELL TYPE	EYELID EDEMA	NODE INVOLVEMENT	ITCHING
Bacterial	Purulent/polymorphonuclear leukocytes	Moderate	Usually none	None
Viral	Clear/mononuclear cells	Minimal	Often present	None
Allergic	Clear, mucoid, ropy/eosinophils	Moderate to severe	None	Mild to intense

VIRAL CONJUNCTIVITIS

Viral conjunctivitis is a highly contagious acute conjunctival infection usually caused by adenovirus. Symptoms include irritation, photophobia, and watery discharge. Diagnosis is clinical; sometimes viral cultures or immunodiagnostic testing is indicated. Infection is self-limited, but severe cases sometimes require topical corticosteroids.

Etiology

Conjunctivitis may accompany the common cold and other systemic viral infections (especially measles, but also chickenpox, rubella, and mumps). Localized viral conjunctivitis without systemic manifestations usually results from adenoviruses and sometimes enteroviruses.

Epidemic keratoconjunctivitis usually results from adenovirus serotypes Ad 5, 8, 11, 13, 19, and 37 and tends to cause severe conjunctivitis. Pharyngoconjunctival fever usually results from serotypes Ad 3, 4, and 7. Outbreaks of acute hemorrhagic conjunctivitis, a rare conjunctivitis associated with infection by enterovirus type 70, have occurred in Africa and Asia.

Symptoms and Signs

After an incubation period of about 5 to 12 days, conjunctival hyperemia, watery discharge, and ocular irritation usually begin in one eye and spread rapidly to the other. Follicles may be present on the palpebral conjunctiva. A preauricular lymph node is often enlarged and painful. Many patients have had contact with someone with conjunctivitis, a recent URI, or both.

In severe adenoviral conjunctivitis, patients may have photophobia and foreign body sensation due to corneal involvement. Chemosis may be present. Pseudomembranes of fibrin and inflammatory cells on the tarsal conjunctiva, focal corneal inflammation, or both may blur vision. Even after conjunctivitis has resolved, residual corneal subepithelial opacities (multiple, coin-shaped, 0.5 to 1.0 mm in diameter) may be visible with a slit lamp for up to 2 yr. Corneal opacities occasionally result in decreased vision and significant halos and starbursts.

Diagnosis

- Clinical evaluation

Diagnosis of conjunctivitis and differentiation between bacterial, viral, and noninfectious conjunctivitis (see Table 113–1) are usually clinical; special tissue cultures are necessary for growth of the virus but are rarely indicated. PCR and other rapid, office-based immunodiagnostic tests can be useful especially when the inflammation is severe and other diagnoses (eg, orbital cellulitis) must be ruled out. Features that may help differentiate between viral and bacterial conjunctivitis can include purulence of ocular discharge, presence of preauricular lymphadenopathy, and, in epidemic keratoconjunctivitis, chemosis. Patients with photophobia are stained with fluorescein and examined with a slit lamp. Epidemic keratoconjunctivitis may cause punctate corneal staining. Secondary bacterial infection of viral conjunctivitis is very rare. However, if any signs suggest bacterial conjunctivitis (eg, purulent discharge), cultures or other studies may be useful.

Treatment

- Supportive measures

Viral conjunctivitis is highly contagious, and transmission precautions must be followed as described previously (see p. 939). Children should generally be kept out of school until resolution.

Viral conjunctivitis is self-limiting, lasting 1 wk in mild cases to up to 3 wk in severe cases. It requires only cool compresses for symptomatic relief. However, patients who have severe photophobia or whose vision is affected may benefit from topical corticosteroids (eg, 1% prednisolone acetate qid). Corticosteroids, if prescribed, are usually prescribed by an ophthalmologist. Herpes simplex keratitis must be ruled out first (by fluorescein staining and slit-lamp examination) because corticosteroids can exacerbate it.

KEY POINTS

- Most viral conjunctivitis is caused by adenoviruses or enteroviruses.
- Features that may help differentiate between viral and bacterial conjunctivitis can include purulence of ocular discharge, presence of preauricular lymphadenopathy, and, in epidemic keratoconjunctivitis, chemosis.
- Diagnosis is usually clinical.
- Treatment is usually cool compresses and measures to prevent spread.

ACUTE BACTERIAL CONJUNCTIVITIS

Acute conjunctivitis can be caused by numerous bacteria. Symptoms are hyperemia, lacrimation, irritation, and discharge. Diagnosis is clinical. Treatment is with topical antibiotics, augmented by systemic antibiotics in more serious cases.

Most bacterial conjunctivitis is acute; chronic bacterial conjunctivitis may be caused by *Chlamydia* and rarely *Moraxella*. Chlamydial conjunctivitis includes trachoma and adult or neonatal inclusion conjunctivitis.

Etiology

Bacterial conjunctivitis is usually caused by *Staphylococcus aureus, Streptococcus pneumoniae, Haemophilus* sp, or, less commonly, *Chlamydia trachomatis* (see p. 943). *Neisseria gonorrhoeae* causes gonococcal conjunctivitis, which usually results from sexual contact with a person who has a genital infection.

Ophthalmia neonatorum (neonatal conjunctivitis) results from a maternal gonococcal and/or chlamydial infection. Neonatal conjunctivitis occurs in 20 to 40% of neonates delivered through an infected birth canal.

Symptoms and Signs

Symptoms are typically unilateral but frequently spread to the opposite eye within a few days. Discharge is typically purulent.

The bulbar and tarsal conjunctivae are intensely hyperemic and edematous. Petechial subconjunctival hemorrhages, chemosis, photophobia, and an enlarged preauricular lymph node are typically absent. Eyelid edema is often moderate.

With adult gonococcal conjunctivitis, symptoms develop 12 to 48 h after exposure. Severe eyelid edema, chemosis, and a profuse purulent exudate are typical. Rare complications include corneal ulceration, abscess, perforation, panophthalmitis, and blindness.

Ophthalmia neonatorum caused by gonococcal infection appears 2 to 5 days after delivery. With ophthalmia neonatorum caused by a chlamydial infection, symptoms appear within 5 to 14 days. Symptoms of both are bilateral, intense papillary conjunctivitis with eyelid edema, chemosis, and mucopurulent discharge.

Diagnosis

- Clinical evaluation
- Sometimes culture of conjunctival smear or scrapings

Diagnosis of conjunctivitis and differentiation between bacterial, viral, and noninfectious conjunctivitis (see Table 113–1) are usually clinical. Smears and bacterial cultures should be done in patients with severe symptoms, immunocompromise, ineffective initial therapy, or a vulnerable eye (eg, after a corneal transplant, in exophthalmos due to Graves disease). Smears and conjunctival scrapings should be examined microscopically and stained with Gram stain to identify bacteria and stained with Giemsa stain to identify the characteristic epithelial cell basophilic cytoplasmic inclusion bodies of chlamydial conjunctivitis.

Treatment

- Antibiotics (topical for all causes except gonococcal and chlamydial)

Bacterial conjunctivitis is very contagious, and standard infection control measures (see p. 940) should be followed.

If neither gonococcal nor chlamydial infection is suspected, most clinicians treat presumptively with moxifloxacin 0.5% drops tid for 7 to 10 days or another fluoroquinolone or trimethoprim/polymyxin B qid. A poor clinical response after 2 or 3 days indicates that the cause is resistant bacteria, a virus, or an allergy. Culture and sensitivity studies should then be done (if not done previously); results direct subsequent treatment.

Adult gonococcal conjunctivitis requires a single dose of ceftriaxone 1 g IM. Fluoroquinolones are no longer recommended because resistance is now widespread. Bacitracin 500 U/g or gentamicin 0.3% ophthalmic ointment instilled into the affected eye every 2 h may be used in addition to systemic treatment. Sex partners should also be treated. Because chlamydial genital infection is often present in patients with gonorrhea, patients should also receive a single dose of azithromycin 1 g po or doxycycline 100 mg po bid for 7 days. Patients need to be evaluated for other sexually transmitted diseases and the local public health authorities (at least in the US) need to be notified.

Ophthalmia neonatorum is prevented by the routine use of silver nitrate eye drops or erythromycin ointment at birth. Infections that develop despite this treatment require systemic treatment. For gonococcal infection, ceftriaxone 25 to 50 mg/kg IV or IM (not exceeding 125 mg) is given as a single dose. Chlamydial infection is treated with erythromycin 12.5 mg/kg po or IV qid for 14 days. The parents should also be treated.

KEY POINTS

- Acute bacterial conjunctivitis tends to differ from viral conjunctivitis by the presence of purulent discharge and the absence of chemosis and preauricular adenopathy.
- Forms of bacterial conjunctivitis that need to be treated differently include neonatal conjunctivitis, gonococcal conjunctivitis, trachoma, and inclusion conjunctivitis.
- Diagnosis is usually clinical.
- Treatment includes measures to prevent spread and antibiotics (topical, such as a fluoroquinolone, for causes except gonococcal and chlamydial).

ADULT INCLUSION CONJUNCTIVITIS

(Adult Chlamydial Conjunctivitis; Swimming Pool Conjunctivitis)

Adult inclusion conjunctivitis is caused by sexually transmitted *Chlamydia trachomatis*. Symptoms include chronic unilateral hyperemia and mucopurulent discharge. Diagnosis is clinical. Treatment is with systemic antibiotics.

Adult inclusion conjunctivitis is caused by *Chlamydia trachomatis* serotypes D through K. In most instances, adult inclusion conjunctivitis results from sexual contact with a person who has a genital infection. Usually, patients have acquired a new sex partner in the preceding 2 mo. Rarely, adult inclusion conjunctivitis is acquired from contaminated, incompletely chlorinated swimming pool water.

Symptoms and Signs

Adult inclusion conjunctivitis has an incubation period of 2 to 19 days. Most patients have a unilateral mucopurulent discharge. The tarsal conjunctiva is often more hyperemic than the bulbar conjunctiva. Characteristically, there is a marked tarsal follicular response. Occasionally, superior corneal opacities and vascularization occur. Preauricular lymph nodes may be swollen on the side of the involved eye. Often, symptoms have been present for many weeks or months and have not responded to topical antibiotics.

Diagnosis

- Clinical evaluation
- Laboratory testing

Chronicity (symptoms for > 3 wk), mucopurulent discharge, marked tarsal follicular response, and failure of topical antibiotics differentiate adult inclusion conjunctivitis from other bacterial conjunctivitides. Smears, bacterial cultures, and chlamydial studies should be done. Immunofluorescent staining techniques, PCR, and special cultures are used to detect *C. trachomatis*. Smears and conjunctival scrapings should be examined microscopically and stained with Gram stain to identify bacteria and stained with Giemsa stain to identify the characteristic epithelial cell basophilic cytoplasmic inclusion bodies of chlamydial conjunctivitis.

PEARLS & PITFALLS

- If patients have symptoms of bacterial conjunctivitis plus a marked tarsal follicular response (often with mucopurulent discharge), symptoms for > 3 wk, or failure to respond to topical antibiotics, do smears, bacterial cultures, and chlamydial studies.

Treatment

- Oral azithromycin or doxycycline

Azithromycin 1 g po once only or either doxycycline 100 mg po bid or erythromycin 500 mg po qid for 1 wk cures the conjunctivitis and concomitant genital infection. Sex partners also require treatment.

ALLERGIC CONJUNCTIVITIS

(Atopic Conjunctivitis; Atopic Keratoconjunctivitis; Hay Fever Conjunctivitis; Perennial Allergic Conjunctivitis; Seasonal Allergic Conjunctivitis; Vernal Keratoconjunctivitis)

Allergic conjunctivitis is an acute, intermittent, or chronic conjunctival inflammation usually caused by airborne allergens. Symptoms include itching, lacrimation, discharge, and conjunctival hyperemia. Diagnosis is clinical. Treatment is with topical antihistamines and mast cell stabilizers.

Etiology

Allergic conjunctivitis is due to a type I hypersensitivity reaction to a specific antigen.

Seasonal allergic conjunctivitis (hay fever conjunctivitis) is caused by airborne mold spores, or pollen of trees, grasses, or weeds. It tends to peak during the spring, late summer, or early fall and disappear during the winter months—corresponding to the life cycle of the causative plant.

Perennial allergic conjunctivitis (atopic conjunctivitis, atopic keratoconjunctivitis) is caused by dust mites, animal dander, and other nonseasonal allergens. These allergens, particularly those in the home, tend to cause symptoms year-round.

Vernal keratoconjunctivitis is a more severe type of conjunctivitis most likely allergic in origin. It is most common among males aged 5 to 20 who also have eczema, asthma, or seasonal allergies. Vernal conjunctivitis typically reappears each spring and subsides in the fall and winter. Many children outgrow the condition by early adulthood.

Symptoms and Signs

General: Patients report bilateral mild to intense ocular itching, conjunctival hyperemia, photosensitivity (photophobia in severe cases), eyelid edema, and watery or stringy discharge. Concomitant rhinitis is common. Many patients have other atopic diseases, such as eczema, allergic rhinitis, or asthma.

Findings characteristically include conjunctival edema and hyperemia and a discharge. The bulbar conjunctiva may appear translucent, bluish, and thickened. Chemosis and a characteristic boggy blepharedema of the lower eyelid are common. Chronic itching can lead to chronic eyelid rubbing, periocular hyperpigmentation, and dermatitis.

Seasonal and perennial conjunctivitis: Fine papillae on the upper tarsal conjunctiva give it a velvety appearance. In more severe forms, larger tarsal conjunctival papillae, conjunctival scarring, corneal neovascularization, and corneal scarring with variable loss of visual acuity can occur (see Plate 26).

Vernal keratoconjunctivitis: Usually, the palpebral conjunctiva of the upper eyelid is involved, but the bulbar conjunctiva is sometimes affected. In the palpebral form, square, hard, flattened, closely packed, pale pink to grayish cobblestone papillae are present, chiefly in the upper tarsal conjunctiva. The uninvolved tarsal conjunctiva is milky white. In the bulbar (limbal) form, the circumcorneal conjunctiva becomes hypertrophied and grayish. Discharge may be tenacious and mucoid, containing numerous eosinophils.

Occasionally, a small, circumscribed loss of corneal epithelium occurs, causing pain and increased photophobia. Other corneal changes (eg, central plaques) and white limbal deposits of eosinophils (Horner-Trantas dots) may be seen.

Diagnosis

The diagnosis is usually clinical. Eosinophils are present in conjunctival scrapings, which may be taken from the lower or upper tarsal conjunctiva; however, such testing is rarely indicated.

Treatment

- Symptomatic measures
- Topical antihistamines, NSAIDs, mast cell stabilizers, or a combination
- Topical corticosteroids or cyclosporine for recalcitrant cases

Avoidance of known allergens and use of tear supplements can reduce symptoms; antigen desensitization is occasionally helpful. Topical OTC antihistamines (eg, ketotifen) are useful for mild cases. If these drugs are insufficient, topical prescription antihistamines (eg, olopatadine, bepotastine, alcaftadine), NSAIDs (eg, ketorolac), or mast cell stabilizers (eg, pemirolast, nedocromil, azelastine) can be used separately or in combination. Topical corticosteroids (eg, loteprednol, fluorometholone 0.1%, prednisolone acetate 0.12% to 1% drops tid) can be useful in recalcitrant cases. Because topical corticosteroids can exacerbate ocular herpes simplex virus infections (see p. 925), possibly leading to corneal ulceration and perforation and, with long-term use, to glaucoma and possibly cataracts, their use should be initiated and monitored by an ophthalmologist. Topical cyclosporine may be helpful.

Seasonal allergic conjunctivitis is less likely to require multiple drugs or intermittent topical corticosteroids.

KEY POINTS

- Allergic conjunctivitis is usually caused by airborne allergens and can be seasonal or perennial.
- Symptoms tend to include itching, eyelid edema, stringy or watery discharge, and sometimes a history of seasonal recurrence.
- Diagnosis is usually clinical.
- Treatment includes tear supplements and topical drugs (usually antihistamines, vasoconstrictors, NSAIDs, mast cell stabilizers, or a combination).

TRACHOMA

(Egyptian Ophthalmia; Granular Conjunctivitis)

Trachoma is a chronic conjunctivitis caused by *Chlamydia trachomatis* and is characterized by progressive exacerbations and remissions. It is the leading cause of preventable blindness worldwide. Initial symptoms are conjunctival hyperemia, eyelid edema, photophobia, and lacrimation. Later, corneal neovascularization and scarring of the conjunctiva, cornea, and eyelids occur. Diagnosis is usually clinical. Treatment is with topical or systemic antibiotics.

Trachoma is endemic in poverty-stricken parts of North Africa, the Middle East, the Indian subcontinent, Australia, and Southeast Asia. The causative organism is *Chlamydia trachomatis* (serotypes A, B, Ba, and C). In the US, trachoma is rare, occurring occasionally among Native Americans and immigrants. The disease occurs mainly in children, particularly those between the ages of 3 yr and 6 yr. Older children and adults are much less susceptible because of increased immunity and better personal hygiene. Trachoma is highly contagious in its early stages and is transmitted by eye-to-eye contact, hand-to-eye contact, eye-seeking flies, or the sharing of contaminated articles (eg, towels, handkerchiefs, eye makeup).

Symptoms and Signs

Trachoma usually affects both eyes. Four stages are described.

In **stage 1,** after an incubation period of about 7 days, conjunctival hyperemia, eyelid edema, photophobia, and lacrimation gradually appear, usually bilaterally.

In **stage 2,** after 7 to 10 days, small follicles develop in the upper tarsal conjunctiva and gradually increase in size and number for 3 or 4 wk (see Plate 25). Inflammatory papillae appear on the upper tarsal conjunctiva. Corneal neovascularization begins, with invasion of the upper half of the cornea by loops of vessels from the limbus (called pannus formation). The phase of acute follicular/papillary hypertrophy and corneal neovascularization may last from several months to > 1 yr, depending on response to therapy.

In **stage 3,** the follicles and papillae gradually shrink and are replaced by bands of scar tissue. Without treatment, corneal scarring eventually occurs. The entire cornea may ultimately be involved, reducing vision. Secondary bacterial infection is common, contributing to scarring and disease progression.

In **stage 4,** the conjunctival scar tissue often causes entropion (often with trichiasis) and lacrimal duct obstruction. Entropion and trichiasis lead to further corneal scarring and neovascularization. The corneal epithelium becomes dull and thickened, and lacrimation is decreased. Small corneal ulcers may appear at the site of peripheral corneal infiltrates, stimulating further neovascularization.

Rarely, corneal neovascularization regresses completely without treatment, and corneal transparency is restored. With treatment and healing, the conjunctiva becomes smooth and grayish white. Impaired vision or blindness occurs in about 5% of people with trachoma.

Diagnosis

- Clinical findings (eg, tarsal lymphoid follicles, linear conjunctival scars, corneal pannus)

Diagnosis of trachoma is usually clinical because testing is rarely available in endemic areas. Lymphoid follicles on the tarsal plate or along the corneal limbus, linear conjunctival scarring, and corneal pannus are considered diagnostic in the appropriate clinical setting.

If the diagnosis is uncertain, *C. trachomatis* can be isolated in culture or identified by PCR and immunofluorescence techniques. In the early stage, minute basophilic cytoplasmic inclusion bodies within conjunctival epithelial cells in Giemsa-stained conjunctival scrapings differentiate trachoma from nonchlamydial conjunctivitis. Inclusion bodies are also found in adult inclusion conjunctivitis, but the setting and developing clinical picture distinguish it from trachoma. Palpebral vernal conjunctivitis appears similar to trachoma in its follicular hypertrophic stage, but symptoms are different, milky flat-topped papillae are present, and eosinophils (not basophilic inclusion bodies) are found in the scrapings.

Treatment

- Oral azithromycin
- SAFE (Surgery, Antibiotics, Facial cleanliness, Environmental improvement) program in endemic areas

For individual or sporadic cases of trachoma, azithromycin 20 mg/kg (maximum 1 g) po as a single dose is 78% effective. Alternatives are doxycycline 100 mg bid or tetracycline 250 mg qid for 4 wk. In hyperendemic areas, tetracycline or erythromycin ophthalmic ointment applied bid for 5 consecutive days each month for 6 mo has been effective as treatment and prophylaxis. Endemic trachoma has been dramatically reduced by using community-wide oral azithromycin in a single dose or in repeated doses. Reinfection due to re-exposure is common among endemic areas.

The World Health Organization has endorsed a 4-step program for control of trachoma in endemic areas. This program is known as SAFE:

- Surgery to correct eyelid deformities (eg, entropion and trichiaisis) that place patients at risk of blindness
- Antibiotics to treat individual patients and mass drug administration to reduce the disease burden in the community
- Facial cleanliness to reduce transmission from infected individuals
- Environmental improvement (eg, access to potable water and improved sanitation) to reduce transmission of disease and reinfection of patients

KEY POINTS

- Trachoma is a chronic, exacerbating, and remitting chlamydial conjunctivitis that is common among children ages 3 yr through 6 yr in certain poverty-stricken areas worldwide.
- Manifestations develop in stages and include conjunctivitis, formation of tarsal follicles, corneal neovascularization, and scarring.
- About 5% of patients develop decreased vision or blindness; trachoma is the leading cause of blindness worldwide.
- Diagnosis is usually clinical, but standard methods to detect chlamydia can be done when available.
- Treatment is usually with oral azithromycin.
- For endemic areas, the World Health Organization also advocates corrective surgery, emphasizing facial cleanliness, and environmental interventions to reduce transmission.

PINGUECULA AND PTERYGIUM

Pinguecula and pterygium are benign growths of the conjunctiva that can result from chronic actinic irritation (see Fig. 113–1). Both typically appear adjacent to the cornea at the 3-o'clock position, the 9-o'clock position, or both.

A **pinguecula** is a raised yellowish white mass within the bulbar conjunctiva, adjacent to the cornea. It does not tend to grow onto the cornea. However, it may cause irritation or cosmetic blemish and, although rarely necessary, can easily be removed.

A **pterygium** (see Plate 24) is a fleshy triangular growth of bulbar conjunctiva that may spread across and distort the cornea, induce astigmatism, and change the refractive power of the eye. Symptoms may include decreased vision and foreign body sensation. It is more common in hot, dry climates. To relieve symptoms caused by a pterygium, artificial tears or a short period of treatment with corticosteroid drops or ointments may be prescribed. Removal is often indicated for cosmesis, to reduce irritation, and to improve or preserve vision.

SUBCONJUNCTIVAL HEMORRHAGES

Subconjunctival hemorrhages are extravasations of blood beneath the conjunctiva.

Subconjunctival hemorrhages usually result from minor local trauma, straining, sneezing, or coughing; rarely, they occur

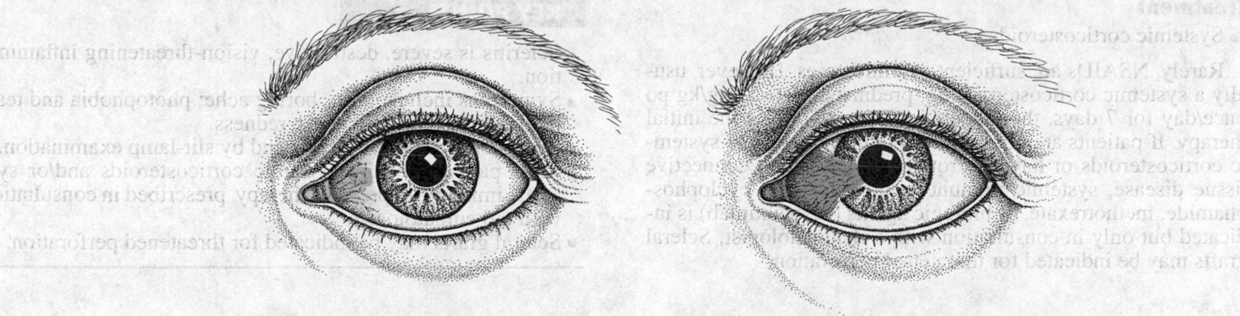

Fig. 113–1. Pinguecula and pterygium Pinguecula and pterygium are conjunctival growths that may result from chronic actinic irritation. Pinguecula (left) is accumulation of conjunctival tissue at the nasal or temporal junction of the sclera and cornea. Pterygium (right) is conjunctival tissue that becomes vascularized, invades the cornea, and may decrease vision.

spontaneously. The extent and location of hyperemia can help determine etiology. Diffuse hyperemia of the bulbar and tarsal conjunctivae is typical of conjunctivitis. Subconjunctival hemorrhages alarm the patient but are of no pathologic significance except when associated with blood dyscrasia, which is rare, or facial or ocular injuries. They are absorbed spontaneously, usually within 2 wk. Topical corticosteroids, antibiotics, vasoconstrictors, and compresses do not speed reabsorption; reassurance is adequate therapy.

EPISCLERITIS

Episcleritis is self-limiting, recurring, idiopathic inflammation of the episcleral tissue that does not threaten vision. Symptoms are a localized area of hyperemia of the globe, irritation, and lacrimation. Diagnosis is clinical. Treatment is symptomatic.

Episcleritis occurs in young adults, more commonly among women. It is usually idiopathic; it can be associated with connective tissue diseases and rarely with serious systemic diseases.

Mild irritation occurs. Additionally, a bright red patch is present just under the bulbar conjunctiva (simple episcleritis). A hyperemic, edematous, raised nodule (nodular episcleritis) may also be present. The palpebral conjunctiva is normal.

Episcleritis is distinguished from conjunctivitis by hyperemia localized to a limited area of the globe, much less lacrimation and no discharge. It is distinguished from scleritis by lack of photophobia and lack of severe pain.

The condition is self-limited, and a diagnostic assessment for systemic disorders is not routinely warranted. A topical corticosteroid (eg, prednisolone acetate, 1% drops qid for 7 days, gradually reduced over 3 wk) or an oral NSAID usually shortens the attack; corticosteroids are usually prescribed by an ophthalmologist. Topical vasoconstrictors (eg, tetrahydrozoline) to improve appearance are optional.

SCLERITIS

Scleritis is a severe, destructive, vision-threatening inflammation involving the deep episclera and sclera. Symptoms are moderate to marked pain, hyperemia of the globe, lacrimation, and photophobia. Diagnosis is clinical. Treatment is with systemic corticosteroids and possibly immunosuppressants.

Scleritis is most common among women aged 30 to 50 yr, and many have connective tissue diseases, such as RA, SLE, polyarteritis nodosa, granulomatosis with polyangiitis (formerly called Wegener granulomatosis), or relapsing polychondritis. A few cases are infectious in origin. About half of the cases of scleritis have no known cause. Scleritis most commonly involves the anterior segment and occurs in 3 types—diffuse, nodular, and necrotizing.

Symptoms and Signs

Pain (often characterized as a deep, boring ache) is severe enough to interfere with sleep and appetite. Photophobia and lacrimation may occur. Hyperemic patches develop deep beneath the bulbar conjunctiva and are more violaceous than those of episcleritis or conjunctivitis. The palpebral conjunctiva is normal. The involved area may be focal (usually one quadrant of the globe) or involve the entire globe and may contain a hyperemic, edematous, raised nodule (nodular scleritis) or an avascular area (necrotizing scleritis). Posterior scleritis is less common and is less likely to cause red eye but more likely to cause blurred or decreased vision.

In severe cases of necrotizing scleritis, perforation of the globe and loss of the eye may result. Connective tissue disease occurs in 20% of patients with diffuse or nodular scleritis and in 50% of patients with necrotizing scleritis. Necrotizing scleritis in patients with connective tissue disease signals underlying systemic vasculitis.

Diagnosis

- Clinical evaluation

Diagnosis of scleritis is made clinically and by slit-lamp examination. Smears or rarely biopsies are necessary to confirm infectious scleritis. CT or ultrasonography may be needed for posterior scleritis.

Prognosis

Of patients with scleritis, 14% lose significant visual acuity within 1 yr, and 30% lose significant visual acuity within 3 yr. Patients with necrotizing scleritis and underlying systemic vasculitis have a mortality rate of up to 50% in 10 yr (mostly due to MI).

Treatment

- Systemic corticosteroids

Rarely, NSAIDs are sufficient for mild cases. However, usually a systemic corticosteroid (eg, prednisone 1 to 2 mg/kg po once/day for 7 days, then tapered off by day 10) is the initial therapy. If patients are unresponsive to or intolerant of systemic corticosteroids or have necrotizing scleritis and connective tissue disease, systemic immunosuppression with cyclophosphamide, methotrexate, or biologic agents (eg, rituximab) is indicated but only in consultation with a rheumatologist. Scleral grafts may be indicated for threatened perforation.

KEY POINTS

- Scleritis is severe, destructive, vision-threatening inflammation.
- Symptoms include deep, boring ache; photophobia and tearing; and focal or diffuse eye redness.
- Diagnosis is made clinically and by slit-lamp examination.
- Most patients require systemic corticosteroids and/or systemic immunosuppressive therapy, prescribed in consultation with a rheumatologist.
- Scleral grafts may be indicated for threatened perforation.

114 Optic Nerve Disorders

The optic pathway includes the retina, optic nerve, optic chiasm, optic radiations, and occipital cortex (see Fig. 114–1). Damage along the optic pathway causes a variety of visual field defects. The type of field defect can help localize the lesion (see Table 107–1 on p. 895).

HEREDITARY OPTIC NEUROPATHIES

Hereditary optic neuropathies result from genetic defects that cause vision loss and occasionally cardiac or neurologic abnormalities. There is no effective treatment.

Hereditary optic neuropathies include dominant optic atrophy and Leber hereditary optic neuropathy, which are both mitochondrial cytopathies. These disorders typically manifest in childhood or adolescence with bilateral, symmetric central vision loss. Optic nerve damage is usually permanent and in some cases progressive. By the time optic atrophy is detected, substantial optic nerve injury has already occurred.

Dominant optic atrophy: Dominant optic atrophy is inherited in an autosomal dominant fashion. It is believed to be the most common of the hereditary optic neuropathies, with prevalence in the range of 1:10,000 to 1:50,000. It is thought to be optic abiotrophy, premature degeneration of the optic nerve leading to progressive vision loss. Onset is in the 1st decade of life.

Leber hereditary optic neuropathy: Leber hereditary optic neuropathy involves a mitochondrial DNA abnormality that affects cellular respiration. Although mitochondrial DNA throughout the body is affected, vision loss is the primary manifestation. Most cases (80 to 90%) occur in males. The disease

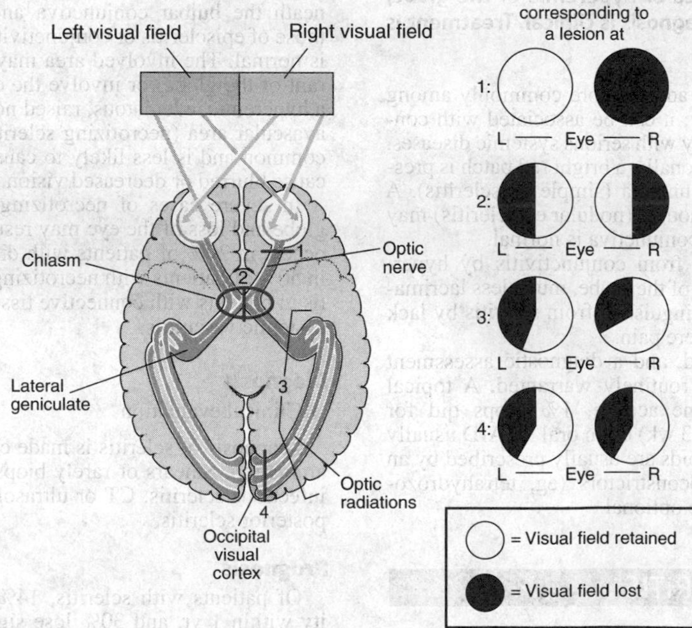

Fig. 114–1. Higher visual pathways—lesion sites and corresponding visual field defects. With retrochiasmal lesions, visual field defects become more symmetric (congruous), as shown with the occipital lesion in #4.

is inherited with a maternal inheritance pattern, meaning that all offspring of a woman with the abnormality inherit the abnormality, but only females can pass on the abnormality because the zygote receives mitochondria only from the mother.

Symptoms and Signs

Dominant optic atrophy: Most patients with dominant optic atrophy have no associated neurologic abnormalities, although nystagmus and hearing loss have been reported. The only symptom is slowly progressive bilateral vision loss, usually mild until late in life. The entire optic disk or, at times, only the temporal portion is pale without visible vessels. A blue-yellow color vision deficit is characteristic.

Leber hereditary optic neuropathy: Vision loss in patients with Leber hereditary optic neuropathy typically begins between 15 and 35 yr (range, 1 to 80 yr). Painless central vision loss in one eye is usually followed weeks to months later by loss in the other eye. Simultaneous vision loss has been reported. Most patients lose vision and develop worse than 20/200 acuity. Ophthalmoscopic examination may show telangiectatic microangiopathy, swelling of the nerve fiber layer around the optic disk, and an absence of leakage on fluorescein angiography. Eventually, optic atrophy supervenes.

Some patients with Leber hereditary optic neuropathy have cardiac conduction defects. Other patients have minor neurologic abnormalities, such as a postural tremor, loss of ankle reflexes, dystonia, spasticity, or a multiple sclerosis–like illness.

Diagnosis

- Clinical evaluation
- Molecular genetic testing

Diagnosis of dominant optic atrophy and Leber hereditary optic atrophy is mainly clinical. Molecular genetic testing is available to confirm many mutations responsible for both disorders. However, results can be falsely negative because mutations may exist for which molecular testing does not yet test.

If Leber hereditary optic neuropathy is suspected, ECG should be done to diagnose occult cardiac conduction defects.

Treatment

- Symptomatic treatment

There is no effective treatment for the hereditary optic neuropathies. Low-vision aids (eg, magnifiers, large-print devices, talking watches) may be helpful. Genetic counseling is suggested.

Leber hereditary optic neuropathy: In patients with Leber hereditary optic neuropathy, corticosteroids, vitamin supplements, and antioxidants have been tried without success. A small study found benefits from quinone analogs (ubiquinone and idebenone) during the early phase. Suggestions to avoid agents that might stress mitochondrial energy production (eg, tobacco, alcohol, particularly if excessive) have no proven benefit but are theoretically reasonable. Patients with cardiac and neurologic abnormalities should be referred to a specialist.

ISCHEMIC OPTIC NEUROPATHY

Ischemic optic neuropathy is infarction of the optic disk. The only constant symptom is painless vision loss. Diagnosis is clinical. Treatment is ineffective.

Two varieties of optic nerve infarction exist: nonarteritic and arteritic. The nonarteritic variant occurs more frequently, typically affecting people about 50 yr and older. Vision loss tends not to be as severe as in the arteritic variant, which usually affects an older group, typically about 70 yr and older.

Most ischemic optic neuropathy is unilateral. Bilateral, sequential cases occur in about 20%, but bilateral simultaneous involvement is uncommon. Bilateral involvement is much more common among arteritic than nonarteritic cases. Atherosclerotic narrowing of the posterior ciliary arteries may predispose to nonarteritic optic nerve infarction, particularly after a hypotensive episode. Any of the inflammatory arteritides, especially giant cell arteritis, can precipitate the arteritic form.

Acute ischemia causes nerve edema, which further worsens ischemia. A small optic cup to optic disk ratio is a risk factor for nonarteritic ischemic optic neuropathy but not for the arteritic variety. Usually, no medical condition is found as the apparent cause of the nonarteritic variety, although factors contributing to atherosclerosis (eg, diabetes, smoking, hypertension), obstructive sleep apnea, certain drugs (eg, amiodarone, possibly phosphodiesterase-5 inhibitors), and hypercoagulable disorders are present in some patients and are thought to be risk factors. Vision loss on awakening leads investigators to suspect nocturnal hypotension as a potential cause of the nonarteritic variety.

Symptoms and Signs

Vision loss with both varieties is typically rapid (over minutes, hours, or days) and painless. Some patients notice the loss on awakening. Symptoms such as general malaise, muscle aches and pains, headaches over the temple, pain when combing hair, jaw claudication, and tenderness over the temporal artery may be present with giant cell arteritis; however, such symptoms may not occur until after vision is lost. Visual acuity is reduced, and an afferent pupillary defect is present.

The optic disk is swollen and elevated, and the swollen nerve fibers obscure the fine surface vessels of the optic nerve. Often hemorrhages surround the optic disk. The optic disk may be pale in the arteritic variety and hyperemic in the nonarteritic variety. In both varieties, visual field examination often shows a defect in the inferior and central visual fields.

Diagnosis

- ESR, C-reactive protein, and CBC
- CT or MRI if vision loss is progressive

Diagnosis is based mainly on clinical evaluation, but ancillary testing may be needed. Most important is to exclude the arteritic variety because the other eye is at risk if treatment is not started quickly. Immediate tests include ESR, CBC, and C-reactive protein. ESR is usually dramatically elevated in the arteritic variety, often exceeding 100 mm/h, and normal in the nonarteritic variety. CBC is done to identify thrombocytosis ($> 400 \times 10^3/\mu L$), which adds to the positive and negative predictive value of using ESR alone.

If giant cell arteritis is suspected, temporal artery biopsy should be done as soon as feasible (at least within 1 to 2 wk because effects of the prednisone therapy may reduce the diagnostic yield of histopathology). Changes in C-reactive protein level are useful for monitoring disease activity and the response to treatment. For isolated cases of progressive vision loss, CT or MRI should be done to rule out compressive lesions.

For nonarteritic ischemic optic neuropathy, additional testing may be indicated based on the suspected cause or risk factor. For example, if patients have excessive daytime sleepiness or snoring or are obese, polysomnography should be considered to diagnose obstructive sleep apnea. If patients have vision loss on awakening, 24-h BP monitoring can be done.

Prognosis

There is no effective treatment for the arteritic variety, and most lost vision is not recovered; however, in the nonarteritic variety, up to 40% of patients spontaneously recover some useful vision.

Treatment

- Corticosteroids for the arteritic variety

The arteritic variety is treated with oral corticosteroids (prednisone 80 mg po once/day and tapered based on ESR) to protect the other eye. If vision loss is imminent, IV corticosteroids should be considered. Treatment should not be delayed while awaiting the biopsy procedure or its results. Treatment of the nonarteritic variety with aspirin or corticosteroids has not been helpful. Risk factors are controlled. Low-vision aids (eg, magnifiers, large-print devices, talking watches) may be helpful in both types.

PEARLS & PITFALLS

- Give systemic corticosteroids as soon as possible to patients 55 yr and older who have sudden, painless loss of vision until giant cell arteritis is excluded.

KEY POINTS

- Ischemic optic neuropathy is usually caused by giant cell arteritis or atherosclerosis.
- Suspect ischemic optic neuropathy in patients 55 yr and older who have sudden, painless loss of vision.
- Unless excluded, treat for giant cell arteritis to decrease the risk of contralateral involvement.
- Prognosis tends to be poor.
- Give corticosteroids if giant cell arteritis is possible.

OPTIC NEURITIS

Optic neuritis is inflammation of the optic nerve. Symptoms are usually unilateral, with eye pain and partial or complete vision loss. Diagnosis is primarily clinical. Treatment is directed at the underlying condition; most cases resolve spontaneously.

Etiology

Optic neuritis is most common among adults 20 to 40 yr. Most cases result from demyelinating disease, particularly multiple sclerosis, in which case there may be recurrences. Optic neuritis is often the presenting manifestation of multiple sclerosis. Other causes include:

- Infectious diseases (eg, viral encephalitis [particularly in children], sinusitis, meningitis, TB, syphilis, HIV)
- Tumor metastasis to the optic nerve
- Chemicals and drugs (eg, lead, methanol, quinine, arsenic, antibiotics)
- Neuromyelitis optica (NMO)

Rare causes include diabetes, pernicious anemia, systemic autoimmune diseases, Graves ophthalmopathy, bee stings, and trauma. Often, the cause remains obscure despite thorough evaluation.

Symptoms and Signs

The main symptom of optic neuritis is vision loss, frequently maximal within 1 or 2 days and varying from a small central or paracentral scotoma to complete blindness. Most patients have mild eye pain, which often feels worse with eye movement.

If the optic disk is swollen, the condition is called papillitis. If the optic disk appears normal, the condition is called retrobulbar neuritis. The most characteristic findings include reduced visual acuity, a visual field deficit, and disturbed color vision (often out of proportion to loss of visual acuity). An afferent pupillary defect is usually detectable if the contralateral eye is unaffected or involved to a lesser degree. Testing of color vision is a useful adjunct. In about two thirds of patients, inflammation is entirely retrobulbar, causing no visible changes to the optic nerve head. In the rest, disk hyperemia, edema in or around the disk, vessel engorgement, or a combination is present. A few exudates and hemorrhages may be present near or on the optic disk.

Diagnosis

- Clinical evaluation
- MRI

Optic neuritis is suspected in patients with characteristic pain and vision loss, particularly if they are young. Neuroimaging, preferably with gadolinium-enhanced MRI, is usually done and may show an enlarged, enhancing optic nerve. MRI may also help diagnose multiple sclerosis and NMO. Fluid attenuating inversion recovery (FLAIR) MRI sequences may show typical demyelinating lesions in a periventricular location if optic neuritis is related to demyelination.

PEARLS & PITFALLS

- Do gadolinium-enhanced MRI for young patients who have eye pain with movement and loss of vision (eg, decreased visual acuity or color vision, field defects) or an afferent pupillary defect.

Prognosis

Prognosis depends on the underlying condition. Most episodes resolve spontaneously, with return of vision in 2 to 3 mo. Most patients with a typical history of optic neuritis and no underlying systemic disease, such as a connective tissue disease, recover vision, but > 25% have a recurrence in the same eye or in the other eye. MRI is used to determine future risk of demyelinating disease.

Treatment

- Corticosteroids

Corticosteroids are an option, especially if multiple sclerosis or neuromyelitis optica are suspected. Treatment with methylprednisolone (500 mg to 1000 mg IV once/day) for 3 days followed by prednisone (1 mg/kg po once/day) for 11 days may speed recovery, but ultimate vision results are no different from those with observation alone. IV corticosteroids have been reported to delay onset of multiple sclerosis for at least 2 yr. Treatment with oral prednisone alone does not improve vision outcome and may increase the rate of recurrent episodes. Low-vision aids (eg, magnifiers, large-print devices, talking watches) may be helpful. Other treatments, such as those used to treat multiple sclerosis, can be given if multiple sclerosis is suspected.

KEY POINTS

- Optic neuritis is most common among adults 20 to 40 yr.
- The most common causes are demyelinating diseases, particularly multiple sclerosis and neuromyelitis optica, but infections, tumors, drugs, and toxins are other possible causes.[1]
- Findings include mild pain with eye movement, visual disturbances (particularly disproportionate loss of color vision), and afferent pupillary defect.
- Do gadolinium-enhanced MRI.
- Corticosteroids and other treatments can be given, particularly if multiple sclerosis is suspected.

1. Pittock SJ, Luccienetti CF: Neuromyelitis optica and the evolving spectrum of autoimmune aquaporin-4 channelopathies: a decade later. *Ann NY Acad Sci* 2015. doi: 10.1111/nyas.12794.

PAPILLEDEMA

Papilledema is swelling of the optic disk due to increased intracranial pressure. Optic disk swelling resulting from causes that do not involve increased intracranial pressure (eg, malignant hypertension, thrombosis of the central retinal vein) is not considered papilledema. There are no early symptoms, although vision may be disturbed for a few seconds. Papilledema requires an immediate search for the cause. Diagnosis is by ophthalmoscopy with further tests, usually brain imaging and sometimes subsequent lumbar puncture, to determine cause. Treatment is directed at the underlying condition.

Papilledema is a sign of elevated intracranial pressure and is almost always bilateral. Causes include the following:

- Brain tumor or abscess
- Cerebral trauma or hemorrhage
- Meningitis
- Arachnoidal adhesions
- Cavernous or dural sinus thrombosis
- Encephalitis
- Idiopathic intracranial hypertension (pseudotumor cerebri), a condition with elevated CSF pressure and no mass lesion

Symptoms and Signs

In patients with papilledema, vision is usually not affected initially, but seconds-long graying out of vision, flickering, or blurred or double vision may occur. Patients may have symptoms of increased intracranial pressure, such as headache or nausea and vomiting. Pain is absent.

Ophthalmoscopic examination reveals engorged and tortuous retinal veins, a hyperemic and swollen optic disk (optic nerve head), and retinal hemorrhages around the disk but not into the retinal periphery (see Plate 23). Isolated disk edema (eg, caused by optic neuritis or ischemic optic neuropathy) without the retinal findings indicative of elevated CSF pressure is not considered papilledema.

In the early stages of papilledema, visual acuity and pupillary response to light are usually normal and become abnormal only after the condition is well advanced. Visual field testing may detect an enlarged blind spot. Later, visual field testing may show defects typical of nerve fiber bundle defects and loss of peripheral vision.

Diagnosis

- Clinical evaluation
- Immediate neuroimaging

The degree of disk swelling can be quantified by comparing the plus lens numbers needed to focus an ophthalmoscope on the most elevated portion of the disk and on the unaffected portion of the retina. Swelling can also be quantified by measuring nerve fiber layer thickness using optical coherence tomography (OCT); OCT is done to quantify the degree of papilledema so that changes can be monitored.

Differentiating papilledema from other causes of a swollen optic disk, such as optic neuritis, ischemic optic neuropathy, hypotony, central retinal vein occlusion, uveitis, or pseudo swollen disks (eg, optic nerve drusen), requires a thorough ophthalmologic evaluation. If papilledema is suspected clinically, MRI with gadolinium contrast or CT with contrast is done immediately to exclude causes such as an intracranial mass. Lumbar puncture with measurement of CSF pressure and analysis of CSF should be done if a mass lesion has been ruled out. Lumbar puncture in patients with intracranial mass lesions can result in brain stem herniation. B-scan ultrasonography and fundus autofluorescence are the best diagnostic tools for the pseudo disk edema of optic nerve drusen.

Treatment

- Treatment of underlying disorder

Urgent treatment of the underlying disorder is indicated to decrease intracranial pressure. If intracranial pressure is not reduced, secondary optic nerve atrophy and vision loss eventually occur, along with other serious neurologic sequelae.

KEY POINTS

- Papilledema indicates increased intracranial pressure.
- In addition to bilateral hyperemic and swollen optic disks (optic nerve heads), patients typically have engorged and tortuous retinal veins, and retinal hemorrhages around the disk but not into the retinal periphery.
- Funduscopic abnormalities usually precede visual disturbances.
- Do immediate neuroimaging and, if no mass lesion is seen, obtain CSF for analysis and measure CSF pressure with a lumbar puncture.
- Treat the underlying disorder.

TOXIC AMBLYOPIA

(Nutritional Amblyopia)

Toxic amblyopia is reduction in visual acuity believed to be the result of a toxic reaction in the orbital portion (papillomacular bundle) of the optic nerve. It can be caused by various toxic and nutritional factors and probably unknown factors. The main symptom is painless vision loss. Diagnosis is by history and visual field examination. Treatment is avoiding suspected toxic agents and improving nutrition.

Etiology

Toxic amblyopia is usually bilateral and symmetric. Undernutrition and vitamin deficiencies (eg, vitamins B_1 or B_{12} or folate) may be the cause, particularly in alcoholics. True tobacco-induced amblyopia is rare. Lead, methanol, chloramphenicol, digoxin, ethambutol, and many other chemicals can damage the optic nerve. Deficiencies of protein and antioxidants are likely risk factors. Toxic amblyopia may occur with other nutritional disorders, such as Strachan syndrome (polyneuropathy and orogenital dermatitis).

Symptoms and Signs

In patients with toxic amblyopia, vision blurring and dimness typically develop over days to weeks. An initially small central or pericentral scotoma slowly enlarges, typically involving both the fixation and the blind spot (centrocecal scotoma), and progressively interferes with vision. Total blindness may occur in methanol ingestion, but other nutritional causes typically do not cause profound vision loss. Retinal abnormalities do not usually occur, but temporal disk pallor may develop late.

Diagnosis

- Mainly clinical evaluation

A history of undernutrition or toxic or chemical exposure combined with typical bilateral scotomata on visual field testing justifies treatment. Laboratory testing for lead, methanol, suspected nutritional deficiencies, and other suspected toxins is done.

Prognosis

Patients with decreased vision may improve if the cause is treated or removed quickly. Once the optic nerve has atrophied, vision usually does not recover.

Treatment

- Treat the cause of the toxic amblyopia
- Low-vision aids

The cause of the patient's toxic amblyopia is treated. Exposure to toxic substances should stop immediately. Alcohol and other potentially causative chemicals or drugs should be avoided. Chelation therapy is indicated in lead poisoning. Dialysis, fomepizole, ethanol, or a combination is used for methanol poisoning. Treatment with oral or parenteral B vitamins and/or folate before vision loss becomes severe may reverse the condition when undernutrition is the presumed cause.

Low-vision aids (eg, magnifiers, large-print devices, talking watches) may be helpful.

The role of antioxidants has not been fully characterized. Their use could be justified on a theoretic basis; however, there is no proof of efficacy, and the at-risk population that should receive such supplements has not been defined.

KEY POINTS

- Toxic amblyopia is reduced visual acuity caused most often by drugs or toxins or nutritional deficiencies, particularly in alcoholics.
- Vision loss is usually gradual and partial.
- Diagnosis is mainly clinical (eg, bilateral scotomata, suggestive history).
- Treat the cause (eg, stopping exposure to a drug or toxin, improving nutrition).

115 Orbital Diseases

CAVERNOUS SINUS THROMBOSIS

Cavernous sinus thrombosis (CST) is a very rare, typically septic thrombosis of the cavernous sinus, usually caused by nasal furuncles or bacterial sinusitis. Symptoms and signs include pain, proptosis, ophthalmoplegia, vision loss, papilledema, and fever. Diagnosis is confirmed by CT or MRI. Treatment is with IV antibiotics. Complications are common, and prognosis is poor.

Etiology

The cavernous sinuses are trabeculated sinuses located at the base of the skull that drain venous blood from facial veins. CST is an extremely rare complication of common facial infections, most notably nasal furuncles (50%), sphenoidal or ethmoidal sinusitis (30%), and dental infections (10%). Most common pathogens are *Staphylococcus aureus* (70%), followed by *Streptococcus* sp; anaerobes are more common when the underlying condition is dental or sinus infection.

Thrombosis of the lateral sinus (related to mastoiditis) and thrombosis of the superior sagittal sinus (related to bacterial meningitis) occur but are rarer than CST.

Pathophysiology

The 3rd, 4th, and 6th cranial nerves and the ophthalmic and maxillary branches of the 5th cranial nerve are adjacent to the cavernous sinus and are commonly affected. Complications include meningoencephalitis, brain abscess, stroke, blindness, and pituitary insufficiency.

Symptoms and Signs

Initial symptoms are progressively severe headache or facial pain, usually unilateral and localized to retro-orbital and frontal regions. High fever is common. Later, ophthalmoplegia (typically the 6th cranial nerve in the initial stage), proptosis, and eyelid edema develop and often become bilateral. Facial sensation may be diminished or absent. Decreased level of consciousness, confusion, seizures, and focal neurologic deficits are signs of CNS spread. Patients may also have anisocoria or mydriasis (3rd cranial nerve dysfunction), papilledema, and vision loss.

Diagnosis

- MRI or CT

CST is often misdiagnosed because it is rare. It should be considered in patients who have signs consistent with orbital cellulitis. Features that distinguish CST from orbital cellulitis include cranial nerve dysfunction, bilateral eye involvement, and mental status changes.

Diagnosis is based on neuroimaging. MRI is the better study, but CT is also helpful. Useful adjunct testing may include blood cultures and lumbar puncture.

Prognosis

Mortality is 30% in all patients and 50% in those with underlying sphenoid sinusitis. An additional 30% develop serious sequelae (eg, ophthalmoplegia, blindness, disability due to stroke, pituitary insufficiency), which may be permanent.

Treatment

- IV high-dose antibiotics
- Sometimes corticosteroids

Initial antibiotics include nafcillin or oxacillin 1 to 2 g q 4 to 6 h combined with a 3rd-generation cephalosporin (eg, ceftriaxone 1 g q 12 h). In areas where methicillin-resistant *S. aureus* is prevalent, vancomycin 1 g IV q 12 h should be substituted for nafcillin or oxacillin. A drug for anaerobes (eg, metronidazole 500 mg q 8 h) should be added if an underlying sinusitis or dental infection is present.

In cases with underlying sphenoid sinusitis, surgical sinus drainage is indicated, especially if there is no clinical response to antibiotics within 24 h.

Secondary treatment may include corticosteroids (eg, dexamethasone 10 mg po q 6 h) for cranial nerve dysfunction; anticoagulation is controversial because most patients respond to antibiotics, and adverse effects may exceed benefits.

INFLAMMATORY ORBITAL DISEASE

(Inflammatory Orbital Pseudotumor)

Inflammatory orbital disease is a benign space-occupying inflammation involving orbital tissues.

Orbital inflammation (inflammatory orbital pseudotumor) can affect any or all structures within the orbit. The inflammatory response can be nonspecific, granulomatous, or vasculitic or due to reactive lymphoid hyperplasia. The inflammation can be part of an underlying medical disorder or can exist in isolation. Patients of all ages can be affected. The process can be acute or chronic and can recur.

Symptoms and Signs

Symptoms and signs typically include a sudden onset of pain along with swelling and erythema of the eyelids. Proptosis, diplopia, and vision loss are also possible. In cases of reactive lymphoid hyperplasia, there are typically few symptoms other than proptosis or swelling.

Diagnosis

- CT or MRI

Similar findings occur with orbital infection, but there is no history of trauma or adjacent focus of infection (eg, sinusitis). Neuroimaging with CT or MRI is required. For chronic or recurrent disease, biopsy may be used to find evidence of an underlying medical condition.

Treatment

Treatment depends on the type of inflammatory response and may include oral corticosteroids, radiation therapy, and one of several immunomodulating drugs. In difficult cases, some initial success has occurred with monoclonal antibodies against TNF-alphaor with another monoclonal antibody that causes lymphocyte depletion.

PRESEPTAL AND ORBITAL CELLULITIS

Preseptal cellulitis (periorbital cellulitis) is infection of the eyelid and surrounding skin anterior to the orbital septum. Orbital cellulitis is infection of the orbital tissues posterior to the orbital septum. Either can be caused by an external focus of infection (eg, a wound), infection that extends from the nasal sinuses or teeth, or metastatic spread from infection elsewhere. Symptoms include eyelid pain, discoloration, and swelling; orbital cellulitis also causes fever, malaise, proptosis, impaired ocular movement, and impaired vision. Diagnosis is based on history, examination, and CT or MRI. Treatment is with antibiotics and sometimes surgical drainage.

Preseptal cellulitis and orbital cellulitis are 2 distinct diseases that share a few clinical symptoms and signs. Preseptal cellulitis usually begins superficial to the orbital septum (see Fig. 115–1). Orbital cellulitis usually begins deep to the orbital septum. Both are more common among children; preseptal cellulitis is far more common than orbital cellulitis.

Etiology

Preseptal cellulitis is usually caused by contiguous spread of infection from local facial or eyelid injuries, insect or animal bites, conjunctivitis, chalazion, or sinusitis.

Orbital cellulitis is most often caused by extension of infection from adjacent sinuses, especially the ethmoid sinus; it is less commonly caused by direct infection accompanying local trauma (eg, insect or animal bite, penetrating eyelid injuries) or contiguous spread of infection from the face or teeth or by hematogenous spread.

Pathogens vary by etiology and patient age. *Streptococcus pneumoniae* is the most frequent pathogen associated with sinus infection, whereas *Staphylococcus aureus* and *S. pyogenes* predominate when infection arises from local trauma. *Haemophilus influenzae* type b, once a common cause, is now less common because of widespread vaccination. Fungi are uncommon pathogens, causing orbital cellulitis in diabetic or immunosuppressed patients. Infection in children < 9 yr is typically with a single aerobic organism; with increasing age, particularly age > 15 yr, infection is more typically polymicrobial with mixed aerobic and anaerobic (*Bacteroides, Peptostreptococcus*) infections.

Pathophysiology

Because orbital cellulitis originates from large adjacent foci of fulminant infection (eg, sinusitis) separated by only a thin bone barrier, orbital infection can be extensive and severe. Subperiosteal fluid collections, some quite large, can accumulate; they are called subperiosteal abscesses, but many are sterile initially.

Complications include vision loss (3 to 11%) due to ischemic retinopathy and optic neuropathy caused by increased intraorbital pressure; restricted ocular movements (ophthalmoplegia) caused by soft-tissue inflammation; and intracranial sequelae from central spread of infection, including CST, meningitis, and cerebral abscess.

Symptoms and Signs

Symptoms and signs of preseptal cellulitis include tenderness, swelling, warmth, redness or discoloration (violaceous in the case of *H. influenzae*) of the eyelid, and sometimes fever. Patients may be unable to open their eyes because of eyelid swelling. The swelling and discomfort can make it difficult to examine the eye, but when accomplished, examination shows that visual acuity is not affected, ocular movement is intact, and the globe is not pushed forward (proptosis).

Symptoms and signs of orbital cellulitis include swelling and redness of the eyelid and surrounding soft tissues, conjunctival

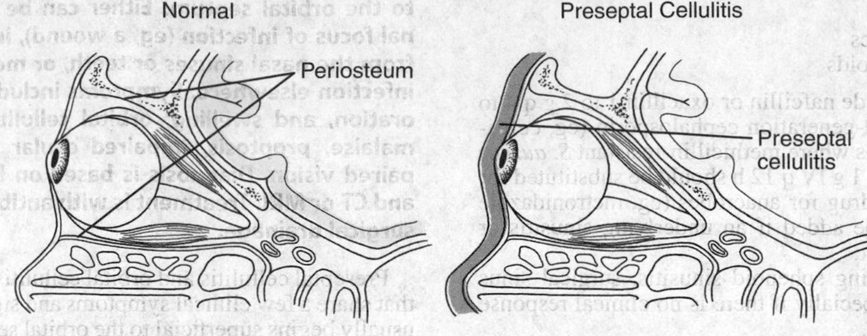

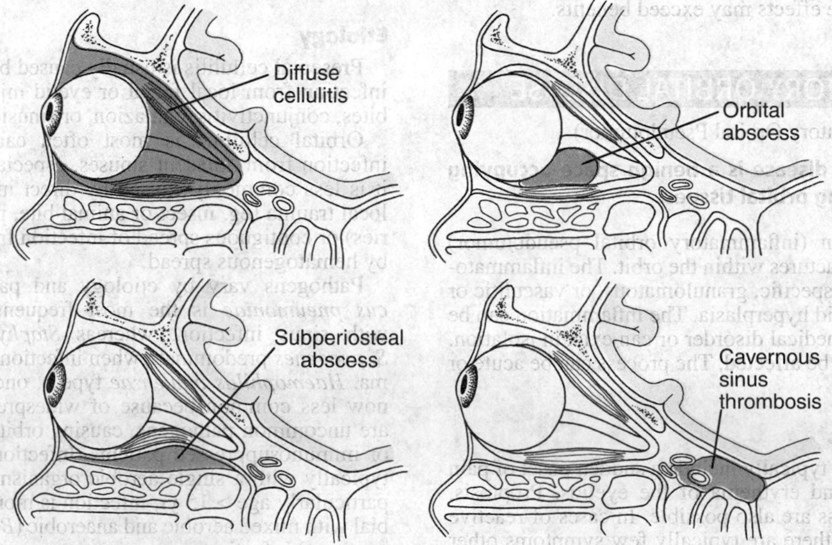

Fig. 115–1. Preseptal and orbital cellulitis.

hyperemia and chemosis, decreased ocular motility, pain with eye movements, decreased visual acuity, and proptosis caused by orbital swelling. Signs of the primary infection are also often present (eg, nasal discharge and bleeding with sinusitis, periodontal pain and swelling with abscess). Fever is usually present. Headache and lethargy should raise suspicion of associated meningitis. Some or all of these findings may be absent early in the course of the infection.

Subperiosteal abscesses, if large enough, can contribute to symptoms of orbital cellulitis such as swelling and redness of the eyelid, decreased ocular motility, proptosis, and decreased visual acuity.

Diagnosis

- Mainly clinical evaluation
- CT or MRI if orbital cellulitis is possible

Diagnosis is primarily clinical. Other disorders to consider include trauma, insect or animal bites without cellulitis, retained foreign bodies, allergic reactions, tumors, and inflammatory orbital pseudotumor.

Eyelid swelling may require the use of lid retractors for evaluation of the globe, and initial signs of complicated infection may be subtle. An ophthalmologist should be consulted when orbital cellulitis is suspected.

Preseptal cellulitis and orbital cellulitis are often distinguishable clinically. Preseptal cellulitis is likely if eye findings are normal except for eyelid swelling. The presence of a local nidus of infection on the skin makes preseptal cellulitis even more likely.

PEARLS & PITFALLS

- Suspect orbital cellulitis and consult an ophthalmologist if there is decreased ocular motility, pain with eye movements, proptosis, or decreased visual acuity.

If findings are equivocal, if the examination is difficult (as in young children), or if nasal discharge is present (suggesting sinusitis), CT or MRI should be done to exclude orbital cellulitis, tumor, and pseudotumor. MRI is better than CT if CST is being considered.

The direction of proptosis may be a clue to the site of infection; eg, extension from the frontal sinus pushes the globe down and out, and extension from the ethmoid sinus pushes the globe laterally and out.

Blood cultures are often done (ideally before beginning antibiotics) in patients with orbital cellulitis, but less than one-third are positive. Lumbar puncture is done if meningitis is suspected. Cultures of the paranasal sinus fluid are done if sinusitis is the suspected source. Other laboratory tests are not particularly helpful.

Treatment

- Antibiotics

Preseptal cellulitis: Initial therapy should be directed against sinusitis pathogens (*S. pneumoniae,* nontypeable *H. influenzae, S. aureus, Moraxella catarrhalis*); however, in areas where methicillin-resistant *S. aureus* is prevalent, clinicians should add appropriate antibiotics (eg, clindamycin, trimethoprim/sulfamethoxazole, or doxycycline for oral treatment and vancomycin for inpatient treatment). In patients with dirty wounds, gram-negative infection must be considered.

Outpatient treatment is an option if orbital cellulitis has been definitively excluded; children should have no signs of systemic infection and should be in the care of responsible parents or guardians. Patients should be closely followed by an ophthalmologist. Outpatient treatment options include amoxicillin/clavulanate 30 mg/kg po q 8 h (for children < 12 yr) or 500 mg po tid or 875 mg po bid (for adults) for 10 days.

For inpatients, ampicillin/sulbactam 50 mg/kg IV q 6 h (for children) or 1.5 to 3 g (for adults) IV q 6 h (maximum 8 g ampicillin/day) for 7 days is an option.

Orbital cellulitis: Patients with orbital cellulitis should be hospitalized and treated with meningitis-dose antibiotics (see Table 231–6 on p. 1923.) A 2nd- or 3rd-generation cephalosporin, such as cefotaxime 50 mg/kg IV q 6 h (for children < 12 yr) or 1 to 2 g IV q 6 h (for adults) for 14 days, is an option when sinusitis is present; imipenem, ceftriaxone, and piperacillin/tazobactam are other options. If cellulitis is related to trauma or foreign body, treatment should cover gram-positive (vancomycin 1 g IV q 12 h) and gram-negative (eg, ertapenem 100 mg IV once/day) pathogens and be taken for 7 to 10 days or until clinical improvement.

Surgery to decompress the orbit, drain an abscess, open infected sinuses, or a combination is indicated in any of the following circumstances:

- Vision is compromised.
- Suppuration or foreign body is suspected.
- Imaging shows orbital or large subperiosteal abscess.
- The infection does not resolve with antibiotics.

KEY POINTS

- Preseptal and orbital cellulitis are differentiated by whether infection is anterior or posterior to the orbital septum.
- Orbital cellulitis is usually caused by contiguous spread of ethmoid or frontal sinusitis, whereas preseptal cellulitis is commonly caused by contiguous spread from local facial or eyelid injuries, insect or animal bites, conjunctivitis, and chalazion.
- Both disorders can cause tenderness, swelling, warmth, redness or discoloration of the eyelid, and fever.
- Orbital cellulitis is likely if there is decreased ocular motility, pain with eye movements, proptosis, or decreased visual acuity.
- Antibiotic therapy is indicated, with surgery reserved for complicated orbital cellulitis (eg, abscess, foreign body, impaired vision, antibiotic failure).

TUMORS OF THE ORBIT

Orbital tumors can be benign or malignant and arise primarily within the orbit or secondarily from an adjacent source, such as the eyelid, paranasal sinus, or intracranial compartment. Orbital tumors can also be metastatic from distant sites.

Some types of orbital tumors usually cause proptosis and displacement of the globe in a direction opposite the tumor. Pain, diplopia, and vision loss may also be present. The diagnosis is suspected based on the history, examination, and neuroimaging (CT, MRI, or both), but confirmation often ultimately requires a biopsy. Causes and treatment vary by age group.

Children: Benign pediatric tumors are most commonly dermoid tumors and vascular lesions such as capillary hemangioma and lymphangioma. Treatment of dermoid tumors is excision. Capillary hemangiomas tend to spontaneously involute and therefore usually do not need any treatment; however, especially when located on the upper eyelid, they may affect vision and require treatment with intralesional injection of corticosteroids or, in exceptional cases, surgical debulking. In recent cases, involution has followed therapy with systemic beta-blockers. Small lymphangiomas that do not cause symptoms may be followed clinically. For larger lymphangiomas or those that are causing symptoms, options include surgical debulking, intralesional sclerotherapy, and, in some cases, sildenafil.

Malignant pediatric tumors are most commonly rhabdomyosarcoma and metastatic lesions related to leukemia or neuroblastoma. If rhabdomyosarcoma is resectable, surgery is done, followed by chemotherapy and orbital radiation therapy. Leukemic disease is usually managed by orbital radiation therapy, chemotherapy, or both.

Adults: Benign adult tumors are most commonly meningiomas, mucoceles, and cavernous venous malformations (also known as cavernous hemangiomas). Pleomorphic adenomas of the lacrimal gland are less common. When symptomatic, sphenoid wing meningiomas are treated with debulking via craniotomy, sometimes followed by a course of radiation therapy. Because meningioma cells infiltrate bone of the skull base, complete resection usually is not possible. Mucoceles are treated by draining them into the nose because they most commonly arise from the ethmoid or frontal sinus. Cavernous venous malformations and lacrimal gland pleomorphic adenomas are excised.

Malignant adult tumors are most commonly lymphoma, squamous cell carcinoma, and metastatic disease. Less commonly, the tumor is an adenoid cystic carcinoma of the lacrimal gland, which is an aggressive tumor.

Lymphomas involving the orbit are typically B-cell and characteristically low grade. Lymphomas can be bilateral and simultaneous and can be part of a systemic process or exist in the orbit in isolation. Radiation therapy effectively treats orbital lymphomas with few adverse effects, but treatment with monoclonal antibodies against a surface receptor (CD20) on the lymphocyte is also effective and should be considered in addition to or instead of radiation therapy, particularly if lymphoma is systemic.

Most squamous cell carcinomas arise from the adjacent paranasal sinuses. Surgery, radiation therapy, or both form the backbone of therapy.

Metastatic disease is usually treated with radiation therapy. Metastatic disease involving the orbit is usually an unfavorable prognostic sign; carcinoid tumors are a notable exception.

Lacrimal gland adenoid cystic carcinoma is treated with surgery and then usually with radiation therapy (sometimes proton beam therapy) or by a protocol using intra-arterial chemotherapy with radiation therapy and surgery.

116 Refractive Error

In the emmetropic (normally refracted) eye, entering light rays are focused on the retina by the cornea and the lens, creating a sharp image that is transmitted to the brain. The lens is elastic, more so in younger people. During accommodation, the ciliary muscles adjust lens shape to properly focus images. Refractive errors are failure of the eye to focus images sharply on the retina, causing blurred vision (see Fig. 116–1).

In **myopia** (nearsightedness), the point of focus is in front of the retina because the cornea is too steeply curved, the axial length of the eye is too long, or both. Distant objects are blurred, but near objects can be seen clearly. To correct myopia, a concave (minus) lens is used. Myopic refractive errors in children frequently increase until the child stops growing.

In **hyperopia** (farsightedness), the point of focus is behind the retina because the cornea is too flatly curved, the axial length is too short, or both. In adults, both near and distant objects are blurred. Children and young adults with mild hyperopia may be able to see clearly because of their ability to accommodate. To correct hyperopia, a convex (plus) lens is used.

In **astigmatism,** nonspherical (variable) curvature of the cornea or lens causes light rays of different orientations (eg, vertical, oblique, horizontal) to focus at different points. To correct astigmatism, a cylindrical lens (a segment cut from a cylinder) is used. Cylindric lenses have no refractive power along one axis and are concave or convex along the other axis.

Presbyopia is loss of the lens' ability to change shape to focus on near objects due to aging. Typically, presbyopia becomes noticeable by the time a person reaches the early or mid-40s. A convex (plus) lens is used for correction when viewing near objects. These lenses may be supplied as separate glasses or built into a lens as bifocals or variable focus lenses.

Anisometropia is a significant difference between the refractive errors of the 2 eyes (usually > 3 diopters). When corrected with eyeglasses, a difference in image size (aniseikonia) is produced; it can lead to difficulties with fusion of the 2 differently sized images and even to suppression of one of the images.

Symptoms and Signs

The primary symptom of refractive errors is blurred vision for distant objects, near objects, or both. Sometimes the excessive ciliary muscle tone can cause headaches. Prolonged squinting and frowning with ocular use can also lead to headaches. Occasionally, excessive staring can lead to ocular surface desiccation, causing eye irritation, itching, visual fatigue, foreign body sensation, and redness. Frowning when reading and excessive blinking or rubbing of the eyes are symptoms of refractive error in children.

Diagnosis

- Visual acuity testing
- Refraction
- Comprehensive eye examination

Visual acuity testing and refraction (determination of refractive error) as needed should be done every 1 or 2 yr. Screening children's visual acuity helps detect refractive errors before they interfere with learning. A comprehensive eye examination, done by an ophthalmologist or an optometrist, should accompany refraction.

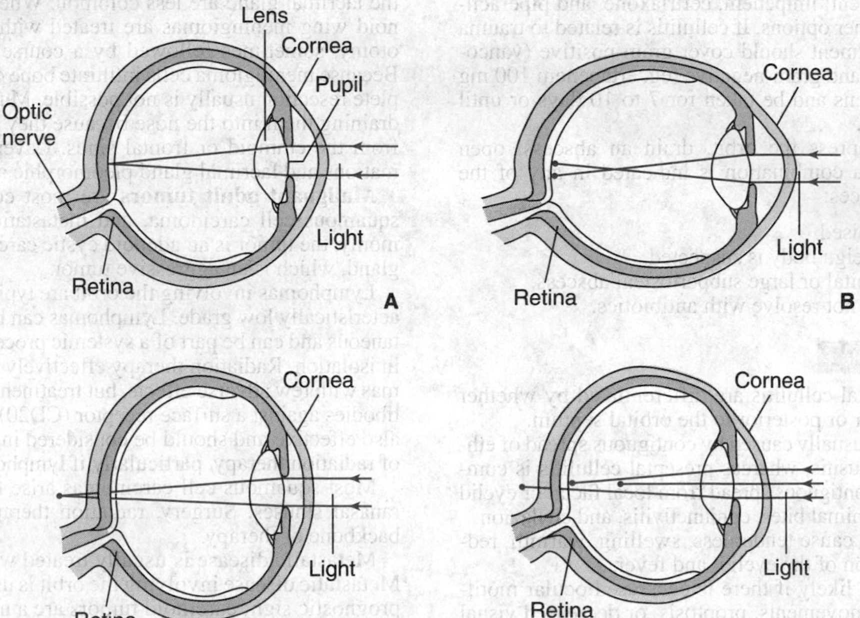

Fig. 116–1. Errors of refraction. (A) Emmetropia; (B) myopia; (C) hyperopia; (D) astigmatism.

Treatment

- Corrective lenses
- Contact lenses
- Refractive surgery

Treatments for refractive errors include corrective lenses, contact lenses, and refractive surgery.

Myopia and hyperopia are corrected with spherical lenses. Concave lenses are used to treat myopia; they are minus or divergent. Convex lenses are used to treat hyperopia; they are plus or convergent. Astigmatism is treated with cylindrical lenses. Corrective lens prescriptions have 3 numbers. The first number is the power (magnitude) of spherical correction required (minus for myopia; plus for hyperopia). The second number is the power of cylindrical correction required (plus or minus). The third number is the axis of the cylinder. As an example, a prescription for a person with myopic astigmatism may read $-4.50 + 2.50 \times 90$, and a prescription for a person with hyperopic astigmatism may read $+3.00 + 1.50 \times 180$.

CONTACT LENSES

Contact lenses often provide better visual acuity and peripheral vision than do eyeglasses and can be prescribed to correct the following:

- Myopia
- Hyperopia
- Astigmatism
- Anisometropia
- Aniseikonia (a difference in image size)
- Aphakia (absence of the lens) after cataract removal
- Keratoconus (a cone-shaped cornea)

Either soft or rigid lenses are used to correct myopia and hyperopia. Toric soft contact lenses (which have different curvatures molded onto the front lens surface) or rigid lenses are used to correct significant astigmatism; they are satisfactory in many cases but require expert fitting.

Contact lenses are also used to correct presbyopia. In one approach, termed monovision, the nondominant eye is corrected for near vision (reading) and the dominant eye is corrected for distant vision. Rigid and soft bifocal and multifocal contact lenses can also be successful, but the fitting procedure is time-consuming because precise alignment is essential.

Neither rigid nor soft contact lenses offer the eyes the protection against blunt or sharp injury that eyeglasses do.

Care and Complications

Instructions for hygiene and handling lenses must be strictly observed. Poor contact lens hygiene may lead to infection of the cornea or persistent inflammation. Contact lenses occasionally cause painless superficial corneal changes. Contact lenses can be painful when

- The corneal epithelium is abraded (see p. 2969), the eye becomes red, and the cornea stains with fluorescein.
- The lenses fit poorly (eg, too tight, too loose, poorly centered).
- There is too little moisture to keep the lens floating above the cornea.
- The lenses are worn in a nonideal environment (eg, O_2-poor, smoky, windy).
- A lens is improperly inserted or removed.
- A small foreign particle (eg, soot, dust) becomes trapped between the lens and the cornea.
- The lenses are worn for a long time (overwear syndrome).

In **overwear syndrome,** spontaneous healing may occur in a day or so if lenses are not worn. In some cases, active treatment is required (eg, topical antibiotic eye drops or ointments). Dilating the eye with mydriatic drops can ease photophobia. Mydriatics work by temporarily paralyzing the muscles of the iris and ciliary body (movement of the inflamed muscles causes pain). In overwear syndrome or any other condition in which pain does not quickly resolve when lenses are removed, an ophthalmologist should be consulted before lenses are worn again.

Risk factors for contact lens–related corneal infection (keratitis) include the following:

- Poor lens hygiene
- Overnight or extended wear
- Use of tap water in the cleaning regimen
- Eyes with a compromised ocular surface (eg, dryness, poor corneal sensation)

Infections require rapid treatment by an ophthalmologist.

Corneal ulcer: A corneal ulcer, which is a potentially vision-threatening infection of the cornea, is suspected when a contact lens wearer has intense eye pain (both foreign body sensation and ache), redness, photophobia, and tearing. Use of contact lenses increases risk of corneal ulcer. The risk increases about 15 times if contact lenses are worn overnight. Corneal ulcers can be caused by bacteria, viruses, fungi, or amebas.

Diagnosis is by slit-lamp examination and fluorescein staining. A corneal epithelial defect (which stains with fluorescein) and a corneal infiltrate (collection of WBCs in the corneal stroma) are present. At times, the corneal defect is large and dense enough to be seen with handheld magnification or even with the naked eye as a white spot on the cornea. Microbiologic analysis of cultures and smears of the corneal infiltrate, contact lens, and contact lens case is indicated.

Contact lens use is stopped. Antibiotic eye drops are given empirically for possible bacterial infection. Initial therapy is broad-spectrum, using a fluoroquinolone antibiotic eye drop every 15 to 60 minutes around the clock for the first 24 to 72 h, then at gradually longer intervals. Additional antibiotic eye drops, such as cefazolin, vancomycin, or concentrated tobramycin, are used if the ulcer is large, deep, or close to the visual axis. The antibiotic may be changed or stopped later based on culture results. Neglected cases may respond poorly or not at all to treatment, and severe vision loss may result.

Rigid Corneal Contact Lenses

A rigid lens is able to revise the natural shape of the cornea into a new, better refracting surface than a soft lens and thus tends to provide more consistent improvement in refraction for people who have astigmatism or an irregular corneal surface. Older polymethyl methacrylate rigid contact lenses have been replaced by gas-permeable contact lenses (GPCLs) made of fluorocarbon and polymethyl methacrylate admixtures. GPCLs are 6.5 to 10 mm in diameter and cover part of the cornea, floating on the tear layer overlying it.

Rigid contact lenses can improve vision in people with myopia, hyperopia, and astigmatism. Rigid contact lenses can also correct corneal irregularities, such as keratoconus. In most cases, patients with keratoconus see better with rigid contact lenses than glasses.

GPCLs can be designed to fit the eye exactly. For complete wearing comfort, they require an adaptation period, typically about 4 to 7 days. During this time, the wearer gradually increases the number of hours the lenses are worn each day. Importantly, no pain should occur at any time. Pain is a sign of an ill-fitting contact lens or corneal irritation. Wearers usually have temporary (< 2 h) blurred vision (spectacle blur) when wearing eyeglasses after removing rigid contact lenses.

Soft Hydrophilic Contact Lenses

Soft contact lenses are made of poly-2-hydroxyethyl methacrylate and other flexible plastics (such as silicone hydrogels) and are 30 to 79% water. They are 13 to 15 mm in diameter and cover the entire cornea. Soft contact lenses are often replaced daily (disposable single-use), every 2 wk, or monthly.

Soft contact lenses can improve vision in people with myopia and hyperopia. Because soft contact lenses mold to the existing corneal curvature, anything greater than minimal astigmatism cannot be treated unless a special toric lens, which has different curvatures molded onto the front lens surface, is used. Weighting the lower aspect of the toric lens maintains its orientation by reducing lens spinning.

Soft contact lenses are also prescribed for treatment of corneal abrasion, recurrent erosions, or other corneal disorders (called bandage or therapeutic contact lenses). Prophylactic antibiotic eye drops (eg, fluoroquinolone qid) may be advisable with a bandage lens. Extended wearing of soft contact lenses, especially in aphakia after cataract surgery, is practical, but an ophthalmologist should examine the patient regularly. The patient should clean the lenses once/wk.

Because of their larger size, soft contact lenses are not as likely as rigid contact lenses to eject spontaneously and are less likely to allow foreign bodies to lodge beneath them. Immediate wearing comfort allows for a brief adaptation period.

Soft contact lenses have a higher incidence of corneal infections than GPCLs, particularly when soft lenses are worn overnight. When dry, soft contact lenses are brittle and break easily. They absorb a certain amount of moisture (based on the water content) from the tear film to retain adequate shape and pliability. Therefore, patients with dry eye are usually more comfortable wearing lenses that have a low water content.

REFRACTIVE SURGERY

Corneal refractive surgery alters the curvature of the cornea to focus light more precisely on the retina. The goal of refractive surgery is to decrease dependence on eyeglasses or contact lenses. Most people who undergo refractive surgery achieve this goal; about 95% do not need corrective lenses for distance vision.

Ideal candidates for refractive surgery are healthy people aged 18 and older with healthy eyes who are not satisfied wearing eyeglasses or contact lenses.

Contraindications to refractive surgery include

- Active ocular diseases, including severe dry eye
- Autoimmune or connective tissue diseases, which can impair wound healing
- Use of isotretinoin or amiodarone

Refraction should be stable for at least 1 yr prior to surgery. Latent herpes simplex virus may be reactivated after surgery; patients should be advised accordingly.

Adverse effects of refractive surgery include temporary symptoms of

- Foreign body sensation
- Glare
- Halos
- Dryness

Occasionally, these symptoms persist.

Potential complications include

- Overcorrection
- Undercorrection
- Infection
- Irregular astigmatism

In excimer laser procedures done on the superficial corneal stroma, haze formation is possible. If infection, irregular astigmatism, or haze formation causes permanent changes in the central cornea, best-corrected acuity could be lost. The overall complication rate is low; chance of vision loss is < 1% if the patient is considered a good candidate for refractive surgery preoperatively.

Types of Refractive Surgery

The two **most common refractive surgery procedures** are

- Laser in situ keratomileusis (LASIK)
- Photorefractive keratectomy (PRK)

Other refractive surgeries include

- Small incision lenticule extraction (SMILE)
- IOL
- Corneal inlays
- Clear lensectomy
- Intracorneal ring segments (INTACS)
- Radial keratotomy
- Astigmatic keratotomy

LASIK

In LASIK, a flap of corneal tissue is created with a femtosecond laser or mechanical microkeratome. The flap is turned back and the underlying stromal bed is sculpted (photoablated) with the excimer laser. The flap is then replaced without suturing. Because surface epithelium is not disrupted centrally, vision returns rapidly. Most people notice a significant improvement the next day. LASIK can be used to treat myopia, hyperopia, and astigmatism.

Advantages of LASIK over PRK include the desirable lack of central stromal healing response (the central corneal epithelium is not removed, thereby decreasing the risk of central haze formation that occurs during healing), the shorter visual rehabilitation period, and minimal postoperative pain.

Disadvantages include possible intraoperative and postoperative flap-related complications, such as irregular flap formation, flap dislocation, and long-term corneal ectasia. Ectasia occurs when the cornea has become so thin that intraocular pressure causes instability and bulging of the thinned and weakened corneal stroma. Blurring, increasing myopia, and irregular astigmatism can result.

PRK

In PRK, the corneal epithelium is removed and then the excimer laser is used to sculpt the anterior curvature of the corneal stromal bed. PRK is used to treat myopia, hyperopia, and astigmatism. The epithelium typically takes 3 to 4 days to regenerate; during this time a bandage contact lens is worn. Unlike LASIK, no corneal flap is created.

PRK may be more suitable for patients with thin corneas or anterior basement membrane dystrophy.

Advantages of PRK include an overall thicker residual stromal bed, which reduces but does not eliminate the risk of ectasia, and lack of flap-related complications.

Disadvantages include the potential for corneal haze formation (if a large amount of corneal tissue is ablated) and the need for postoperative corticosteroid drops for several months. The intraocular pressure of postoperative patients who are using topical corticosteroids should be monitored carefully because corticosteroid-induced glaucoma has been reported after PRK.

SMILE

In SMILE, a femtosecond laser is used to create a thin, intrastromal lenticule of tissue, which is then removed through a small (2–4 mm) peripheral corneal laser incision. SMILE is FDA-approved to treat myopia.

The efficacy, predictability, and safety of SMILE are similar to those of LASIK, with the additional benefit that it eliminates flap creation and the attendant risks. Another benefit of SMILE is the reduced degree of postoperative corneal denervation and higher-order ophthalmologic aberrations and an accelerated rate of corneal nerve regeneration relative to LASIK.

Disadvantages include increased incidence of suction loss (an operative complication during refractive surgery) and difficulty with enhancements (additional ophthalmic surgery).

Phakic Intraocular Lenses (IOLs)

IOLs are lens implants that are used to treat severe myopia in patients who are not suitable candidates for laser vision correction. Unlike in cataract surgery, the patient's natural lens is not removed. The phakic IOL is inserted directly anterior or posterior to the iris through an incision in the eye. This procedure is intraocular surgery and must be done in an operating room.

Risks include cataract formation, glaucoma, infection, inflammation, and loss of corneal endothelial cells with subsequent chronic corneal edema that eventually becomes symptomatic.

Because phakic IOLs do not correct astigmatism, patients can undergo subsequent laser vision correction to refine refractive results in a technique known as bioptics. Because the bulk of the myopia is corrected with the phakic IOL, less corneal tissue is removed with the excimer laser, and the risk of ectasia is thus low.

Corneal Inlays

Corneal inlays are implants placed into the corneal stroma via a lamellar pocket or flap to treat presbyopia. One type of corneal inlay is made of hydrogel material and creates a hyperprolate anterior corneal surface. A prolate shape is one in which the steepest radius of curvature is central. A hyperprolate surface exaggerates this difference and results in sharper central near vision. Another type of corneal inlay is made of polyvinylidene fluoride and carbon and is a small aperture inlay which improves near vision by increasing depth of focus. These inlays are placed only in the non-dominant eye of presbyopic patients.

Advantages of corneal inlays are improved near vision with a 1–2 line decrease in distance vision in the corrected eye. Also, corneal inlays are removable.

Disadvantages include risk of corneal haze or inflammation, which requires long-term topical steroid use and can result in glare, halo, and difficulty reading in dim light. Complications can include inlay decentration, dry eye, and epithelial ingrowth.

Clear Lensectomy

Clear lensectomy can be considered in patients with high hyperopia who are already presbyopic. This procedure is identical to cataract surgery except the patient's lens is clear and not cataractous. An extended depth-of-focus, multifocal or accommodating IOL, which allows the patient to focus over a wide range of distances without external lens correction, can be inserted.

The main risks of clear lensectomy are infection and rupture of the posterior capsule of the lens, which would necessitate further surgery. Clear lensectomy should be done with great caution in young patients with myopia because they have an increased risk of postoperative retinal detachment.

INTACS

INTACS are thin arc-shaped segments of biocompatible plastic that are inserted in pairs through a small radial corneal incision into the peripheral corneal stroma at two-thirds depth. After INTACS are inserted, the central corneal curvature is flattened, reducing myopia. INTACS are used to treat mild myopia (< 3 diopters) and minimal astigmatism (< 1 diopter). INTACS maintain a central, clear, optical zone because the 2 segments are placed in the corneal periphery. INTACS can be replaced or removed if desired.

Risks include induced astigmatism, undercorrection and overcorrection, infection, glare, halo, and incorrect depth placement. Currently, INTACS are mostly used for treatment of corneal ectatic disorders such as keratoconus and post-LASIK ectasia when glasses or contact lenses no longer provide adequate vision or are uncomfortable. Best-corrected vision and contact lens tolerance improve in 70 to 80% of patients.

Radial Keratotomy and Astigmatic Keratotomy

Radial and astigmatic keratotomy procedures change the shape of the cornea by making deep corneal incisions using a diamond blade.

Radial keratotomy has been replaced by laser vision correction and is rarely used because it offers no clear advantages over laser vision correction, has a greater need for subsequent retreatment, can lead to visual and refractive results that change through the day, and can cause a hyperopic shift in the long term.

Astigmatic keratotomy is still commonly done at the time of cataract surgery. The incisions are referred to as limbal relaxing incisions because the optical zone is much larger and closer to the limbus.

117 Retinal Disorders

AGE-RELATED MACULAR DEGENERATION

(Senile Macular Degeneration)

Age-related macular degeneration (AMD) is the most common cause of irreversible central vision loss in elderly patients. Dilated funduscopic findings are diagnostic; color photographs, fluorescein angiography, and optical coherence tomography assist in confirming the diagnosis and in directing treatment. Treatment is with dietary supplements, intravitreal injection of antivascular endothelial growth factor drugs, laser photocoagulation, photodynamic therapy, and low-vision devices.

AMD is the leading cause of permanent, irreversible vision loss in the elderly. It is more common among whites.

Etiology

Risk factors include the following:

- Age
- Genetic variants (eg, abnormal complement factor H)
- Family history
- Smoking
- Cardiovascular disease
- Hypertension
- Obesity
- Sun exposure
- A diet low in omega-3 fatty acids and dark green leafy vegetables

Pathophysiology

Two different forms occur:

- Dry (nonexudative or atrophic): All AMD starts as the dry form. About 85% of people with AMD have only dry AMD.
- Wet (exudative or neovascular):Wet AMD occurs in about 15% of people.

Although only 15% of patients with AMD have the wet form, 80 to 90% of the severe vision loss caused by AMD results from wet AMD.

Dry AMD causes changes of the retinal pigment epithelium, typically visible as dark pinpoint areas. The retinal pigment epithelium plays a critical role in keeping the cones and rods healthy and functioning well. Accumulation of waste products from the rods and cones can result in drusen, which appear as yellow spots. Areas of chorioretinal atrophy (referred to as geographic atrophy) occur in more advanced cases of dry AMD. There is no elevated macular scar (disciform scar), edema, hemorrhage, or exudation.

Wet AMD occurs when new abnormal blood vessels develop under the retina in a process called choroidal neovascularization (abnormal new vessel formation). Localized macular edema or hemorrhage may elevate an area of the macula or cause a localized retinal pigment epithelial detachment (see Plate 8). Eventually, untreated neovascularization causes a disciform scar under the macula.

Symptoms and Signs

Dry AMD: The loss of central vision occurs over years and is painless, and most patients retain enough vision to read and drive. Central blind spots (scotomas) usually occur late in the disease and can sometimes become severe. Symptoms are usually bilateral.

Funduscopic changes include the following:

- Changes in the retinal pigment epithelium
- Drusen
- Areas of chorioretinal atrophy

Wet AMD: Rapid vision loss, usually over days to weeks, is more typical of wet AMD. The first symptom is usually visual distortion, such as a central blind spot (scotoma) or curving of straight lines (metamorphopsia). Peripheral vision and color vision are generally unaffected; however, the patient may become legally blind (< 20/200 vision) in the affected eye, particularly if AMD is not treated. Wet AMD usually affects one eye at a time; thus, symptoms of wet AMD are often unilateral.

Funduscopic changes include the following:

- Subretinal fluid, appearing as localized retinal elevation
- Retinal edema
- Gray-green discoloration under the macula
- Exudates in or around the macula
- Detachment of retinal pigment epithelium (visible as an area of retinal elevation)
- Subretinal hemorrhage in or around the macula

Diagnosis

- Funduscopic examination
- Color fundus photography
- Fluorescein angiography
- Optical coherence tomography

Both forms of AMD are diagnosed by funduscopic examination. Visual changes can often be detected with an Amsler grid (see p. 895). Color photography and fluorescein angiography are done when findings suggest wet AMD. Angiography shows and characterizes subretinal choroidal neovascular membranes and can delineate areas of geographic atrophy. Optical coherence tomography (OCT) aids in identifying intraretinal and subretinal fluid and can help assess response to treatment.

Treatment

- Dietary supplements for high-risk dry or unilateral wet AMD
- Intravitreal antivascular endothelial growth factor drugs or laser treatments for wet AMD
- Supportive measures

Dry AMD: There is no way to reverse damage caused by dry AMD. Patients with extensive drusen, pigment changes, and/or geographic atrophy can reduce the risk of developing advanced AMD by 25% by taking daily supplements of the following:

- Zinc oxide 80 mg
- Copper 2 mg
- Vitamin C 500 mg
- Vitamin E 400 IU
- Lutein 10 mg/zeaxanthin 2 mg (or beta-carotene 15 mg or vitamin A 28,000 IU for patients who have not smoked)

In current and former smokers, beta-carotene can increase the risk of lung cancer. Recently, substitution of beta-carotene with lutein plus zeaxanthin has been shown to have comparable efficacy.[1] Therefore, such a substitution should be considered in current or former smokers. The zinc component of these supplements increases risk of hospitalization for GU tract disorders. Some patients taking beta-carotene also have yellowing of the skin. Reducing cardiovascular risk factors as well as regularly eating foods high in omega-3 fatty acids and dark green leafy vegetables may help slow disease progression; however, recent large trials have not shown that taking supplements of omega-3 fatty acids reduces disease progression.

Wet AMD: Patients with unilateral wet AMD should take the daily nutritional supplements that are recommended for dry AMD to reduce the risk of AMD-induced vision loss in the other eye. The choice of other treatments depends on the size, location, and type of neovascularization. Intravitreal injection of antivascular endothelial growth factor (anti-VEGF) drugs (usually ranibizumab, bevacizumab, or aflibercept) can substantially reduce the risk of vision loss and can help restore reading vision in up to one third of patients. In a small subset of patients, thermal laser photocoagulation of neovascularization outside the fovea may prevent severe vision loss. Photodynamic therapy, a type of laser treatment, also helps under specific circumstances. Corticosteroids (eg, triamcinolone) are sometimes injected intraocularly along with an anti-VEGF drug. Other treatments, including transpupillary thermotherapy, subretinal surgery, and macular translocation surgery, are seldom used.

1. Age-Related Eye Disease Study 2 Research Group: Lutein + zeaxanthin and omega-3 fatty acids for age-related macular degeneration: the age-related eye disease study 2 (AREDS2) randomized clinical trial. *JAMA* 309(19):2005–2015, 2013. doi: 10.1001/jama.2013.4997. Clarification and additional information. *JAMA* 310(2):208, 2013. doi:10.1001/jama.2013.6403.

Supportive measures: For patients who have lost central vision, low-vision devices such as magnifiers, high-power reading glasses, large computer monitors, and telescopic lenses are available. Also, certain types of software can display computer data in large print or read information aloud in a synthetic voice. Low-vision counseling is advised.

KEY POINTS

- AMD is more common among whites and is the leading cause of permanent vision loss in the elderly.
- AMD can be dry (nonexudative or atrophic) or wet (exudative or neovascular).
- Although 85% of AMD is dry, 80 to 90% of severe vision loss caused by AMD results from the wet type.
- Funduscopic changes in dry AMD include drusen, areas of chorioretinal atrophy, and changes to the retinal pigment epithelium.
- Funduscopic changes in wet AMD include retinal edema and localized elevation, detachment of the retinal pigment epithelium, a gray-green discoloration under the macula, and exudates in and around the macula.
- If patients have AMD on funduscopy, do color fundus photography, fluorescein angiography, and optical coherence tomography.
- Prescribe dietary supplements for unilateral wet or high-risk dry AMD.
- Treat wet AMD with intravitreal antivascular endothelial growth factor drugs or laser therapy.

CENTRAL AND BRANCH RETINAL ARTERY OCCLUSION

(Retinal Artery Occlusion)

Central retinal artery occlusion occurs when the central retinal artery becomes blocked, usually due to an embolus. It causes sudden, painless, unilateral, and usually severe vision loss. Diagnosis is by history and characteristic retinal findings on funduscopy. Decreasing intraocular pressure can be done within the first 24 h of occlusion to attempt to dislodge the embolus. If patients present within the first few hours of occlusion, some centers catheterize the carotid/ophthalmic artery and selectively inject thrombolytic drugs.

Etiology

Retinal artery occlusion may be due to embolism or thrombosis.

Emboli may come from any of the following:

- Atherosclerotic plaques
- Endocarditis
- Fat
- Atrial myxoma

Thrombosis is a less common cause of retinal artery occlusion but can be seen with systemic vasculitis such as SLE and giant cell arteritis, which is an important cause of arterial occlusion that requires prompt diagnosis and treatment.

Occlusion can affect a branch of the retinal artery as well as the central retinal artery.

Neovascularization (abnormal new vessel formation) of the retina or iris (rubeosis iridis) with secondary (neovascular) glaucoma occurs in about 20% of patients within weeks to months after occlusion. Vitreous hemorrhage may result from retinal neovascularization.

Symptoms and Signs

Retinal artery occlusion causes sudden, painless, severe vision loss or visual field defect, usually unilaterally.

The pupil may respond poorly to direct light but constricts briskly when the other eye is illuminated (relative afferent pupillary defect). In acute cases, funduscopy shows a pale, opaque fundus with a red fovea (cherry-red spot). Typically, the arteries are attenuated and may even appear bloodless. An embolus (eg, a cholesterol embolus, called a Hollenhorst plaque) is sometimes visible. If a major branch is occluded rather than the entire artery, fundus abnormalities and vision loss are limited to that sector of the retina.

Patients who have giant cell arteritis are 55 or older and may have a headache, a tender and palpable temporal artery, jaw claudication, fatigue, or a combination.

Diagnosis

- Clinical evaluation
- Color fundus photography and fluorescein angiography

The diagnosis is suspected when a patient has acute, painless, severe vision loss. Funduscopy is usually confirmatory. Fluorescein angiography is often done and shows absence of perfusion in the affected artery.

Once the diagnosis is made, carotid Doppler ultrasonography and echocardiography should be done to identify an embolic source so that further embolization can be prevented.

If giant cell arteritis is suspected, ESR, C-reactive protein, and platelet count should be done immediately. These tests may not be necessary if an embolic plaque is visible in the central retinal artery.

Prognosis

Patients with a branch artery occlusion may maintain good to fair vision, but with central artery occlusion, vision loss is often profound, even with treatment. Once retinal infarction occurs (as quickly as 90 min after the occlusion), vision loss is permanent.

If underlying giant cell arteritis is diagnosed and treated promptly, the vision in the uninvolved eye can often be protected and some vision may be recovered in the affected eye.

Treatment

- Sometimes reduction of intraocular pressure

Immediate treatment is indicated if occlusion occurred within 24 h of presentation. Reduction of intraocular pressure with ocular hypotensive drugs (eg, topical timolol 0.5%, acetazolamide 500 mg IV or po), intermittent digital massage over the closed eyelid, or anterior chamber paracentesis may dislodge an embolus and allow it to enter a smaller branch of the artery, thus reducing the area of retinal ischemia. Some centers have tried infusing thrombolytics into the carotid artery to dissolve the obstructing clot. Nonetheless, treatments for retinal artery occlusions rarely improve visual acuity. Surgical or laser-mediated embolectomy is available but not commonly done. These treatments are sometimes shown to be effective in small case series, but none have strong evidence to support efficacy.

PEARLS & PITFALLS

- Consider immediate measures to reduce intraocular pressure in patients who have sudden, painless, severe loss of vision.

Patients with occlusion secondary to giant cell arteritis should receive high-dose systemic corticosteroids.

KEY POINTS

- Central or branch retinal artery occlusion can be caused by an embolus (eg, due to atherosclerosis or endocarditis), thrombosis, or giant cell arteritis.
- Painless, severe loss of vision affects part or all of the visual field.
- Confirm the diagnosis by doing funduscopy (typically showing a pale, opaque fundus with a red fovea and arterial attenuation).
- Do color fundus photography and fluorescein angiography and search for an embolic source by doing Doppler ultrasonography and echocardiography.
- Treat immediately if possible with ocular hypotensive drugs (eg, topical timolol or IV or oral acetazolamide), intermittent digital massage over the closed eyelid, or anterior chamber paracentesis.

CENTRAL AND BRANCH RETINAL VEIN OCCLUSION

(Retinal Vein Occlusion)

Central retinal vein occlusion is a blockage of the central retinal vein by a thrombus. It causes painless vision loss, ranging from mild to severe, and usually occurs suddenly. Diagnosis is by funduscopy. Treatments can include antivascular endothelial growth factor drugs (eg, ranibizumab, pegaptanib, bevacizumab), intraocular injection of a dexamethasone implant or triamcinolone, and laser photocoagulation.

Etiology

Major risk factors include

- Hypertension
- Age

Other risk factors include

- Glaucoma
- Diabetes
- Increased blood viscosity

Occlusion may also be idiopathic. The condition is uncommon among young people. Occlusion may affect a branch of the retinal vein or the central retinal vein.

Neovascularization (abnormal new vessel formation) of the retina or iris (rubeosis iridis) occurs in about 16% of patients with central retinal vein occlusion and can result in secondary (neovascular) glaucoma, which can occur weeks to months after occlusion. Vitreous hemorrhage may result from retinal neovascularization.

Symptoms and Signs

Painless vision loss is usually sudden but it can also occur gradually over a period of days to weeks. Funduscopy reveals hemorrhages throughout the retina, engorged (dilated) and tortuous retinal veins, and, usually, significant retinal edema. These changes are typically diffuse if obstruction involves the central retinal vein and are limited to one quadrant if obstruction involves only a branch of the central retinal vein.

Diagnosis

- Funduscopy
- Color fundus photography
- Fluorescein angiography
- Optical coherence tomography

The diagnosis is suspected in patients with painless vision loss, particularly those with risk factors. Funduscopy, color photography, and fluorescein angiography confirm the diagnosis. Optical coherence tomography is used to determine the degree of macular edema and its response to treatment. Patients with a central retinal vein occlusion are evaluated for hypertension and glaucoma and tested for diabetes. Young patients are tested for increased blood viscosity (with a CBC and other coagulable factors as deemed necessary).

Prognosis

Most patients have some visual deficit. In mild cases, there can be spontaneous improvement to near-normal vision over a variable period of time. Visual acuity at presentation is a good indicator of final vision. If visual acuity is at least 20/40, visual acuity will likely remain good, occasionally near normal. If visual acuity is worse than 20/200, it will remain at that level or worsen in 80% of patients. Central retinal vein occlusions rarely recur.

Treatment

- For macular edema, intraocular injection of antivascular endothelial growth factor (anti-VEGF) drugs, dexamethasone implant, and/or triamcinolone acetonide
- For some cases of macular edema with branch retinal vein occlusion, focal laser photocoagulation
- Panretinal laser photocoagulation if neovascularization develops

Treatment for branch retinal vein occlusion in patients with macular edema that involves the fovea is usually intraocular injection of an anti-VEGF drug (eg, ranibizumab, aflibercept, or bevacizumab) or intraocular injection of triamcinolone or a slow-release dexamethasone implant. These treatments can also be used to treat central retinal vein occlusion in patients with macular edema. With these treatments, vision improves significantly in 30 to 40% of patients.

Focal laser photocoagulation can be used for branch retinal vein occlusion with macular edema but is less effective than intraocular injection of an anti-VEGF drug or a dexamethasone implant. Focal laser photocoagulation is typically not effective for the treatment of macular edema due to a central retinal vein occlusion.

If retinal or anterior segment neovascularization develops secondary to central or branch retinal vein occlusion, panretinal laser photocoagulation should be done promptly to decrease vitreous hemorrhage and prevent neovascular glaucoma.

KEY POINTS

- Retinal vein occlusion involves blockage by a thrombus.
- Patients have painless loss of vision that is typically sudden and may have risk factors (eg, older age, hypertension).
- Fundoscopy characteristically demonstrates macular edema with dilated veins and hemorrhages; additional tests include color fundus photography, fluorescein angiography, and optical coherence tomography.
- Treat patients who have macular edema with an intraocular injection of an anti-VEGF drug (ranibizumab, aflibercept, or bevacizumab) or intraocular injection of a dexamethasone implant or triamcinolone.
- Focal laser photocoagulation is useful in some cases of macular edema secondary to a branch retinal vein occlusion, and panretinal laser photocoagulation should be done for retinal or anterior segment neovascularization.

DIABETIC RETINOPATHY

Manifestations of diabetic retinopathy include microaneurysms, intraretinal hemorrhage, exudates, macular edema, macular ischemia, neovascularization, vitreous hemorrhage, and traction retinal detachment. Symptoms may not develop until late in the disease. Diagnosis is by funduscopy; further details are elucidated by color fundus photography, fluorescein angiography, and optical coherence tomography. Treatment includes control of blood glucose and BP. Ocular treatments included retinal laser photocoagulation, intravitreal injection of antivascular endothelial growth factor drugs (eg, aflibercept, ranibizumab, bevacizumab), intraocular corticosteroids, vitrectomy, or a combination.

Pathophysiology

Diabetic retinopathy is a major cause of blindness, particularly among working-age adults. The degree of retinopathy is highly correlated with

- Duration of diabetes
- Blood glucose levels
- BP levels

Pregnancy can impair blood glucose control and thus worsen retinopathy.

Nonproliferative retinopathy: Nonproliferative retinopathy (also called background retinopathy) develops first and causes increased capillary permeability, microaneurysms, hemorrhages, exudates, macular ischemia, and macular edema (thickening of the retina caused by fluid leakage from capillaries).

Proliferative retinopathy: Proliferative retinopathy develops after nonproliferative retinopathy and is more severe; it may lead to vitreous hemorrhage and traction retinal detachment. Proliferative retinopathy is characterized by abnormal new vessel formation (neovascularization), which occurs on the inner (vitreous) surface of the retina and may extend into the vitreous cavity and cause vitreous hemorrhage. Neovascularization is often accompanied by preretinal fibrous tissue, which, along with the vitreous, can contract, resulting in traction retinal detachment. Neovascularization may also occur in the anterior segment of the eye on the iris; neovascular membrane growth in the anterior chamber angle of the eye at the peripheral margin of the iris can occur, and this growth leads to neovascular glaucoma. Vision loss with proliferative retinopathy may be severe.

Clinically significant macular edema can occur with nonproliferative or proliferative retinopathy and is the most common cause of vision loss due to diabetic retinopathy.

Symptoms and Signs

Nonproliferative retinopathy: Vision symptoms are caused by macular edema or macular ischemia. However, patients may not have vision loss even with advanced retinopathy. The first signs of nonproliferative retinopathy are

- Capillary microaneurysms
- Dot and blot retinal hemorrhages
- Hard exudates
- Cotton-wool spots (soft exudates)

Hard exudates are discrete, yellow particles within the retina (see Plate 14). When present, they suggest chronic edema. Cotton-wool spots are areas of microinfarction of the retinal nerve fiber layer that lead to retinal opacification; they are fuzzy-edged and white and obscure underlying vessels.

Signs in later stages are

- Macular edema (seen on slit-lamp biomicroscopy as elevation and blurring of retinal layers)
- Venous dilation and intraretinal microvascular abnormalities

Proliferative retinopathy: Symptoms may include blurred vision, floaters (black spots) or flashing lights in the field of vision, and sudden, severe, painless vision loss. These symptoms are typically caused by vitreous hemorrhage or traction retinal detachment.

Proliferative retinopathy, unlike nonproliferative retinopathy, causes formation of fine preretinal vessel neovascularization visible on the optic nerve or retinal surface (see Plate 15). Macular edema or retinal hemorrhage may be visible on funduscopy.

Diagnosis

- Funduscopy
- Color fundus photography
- Fluorescein angiography
- Optical coherence tomography

Diagnosis is by funduscopy. Color fundus photography helps grade the level of retinopathy. Fluorescein angiography is used to determine the extent of retinopathy, to develop a treatment plan, and to monitor the results of treatment. Optical coherence tomography is also useful to assess severity of macular edema and treatment response.

Screening: Because early detection is important, all patients with diabetes should have an annual dilated ophthalmologic examination. Pregnant patients with diabetes should be examined every trimester. Vision symptoms (eg, blurred vision) are indications for ophthalmologic referral.

Treatment

- Control of blood glucose and BP
- For macular edema, intraocular injection of antivascular endothelial growth factor (anti-VEGF) drugs, intraocular corticosteroid implants, focal laser, and/or vitrectomy

- For high-risk or complicated proliferative retinopathy, panretinal laser photocoagulation and sometimes vitrectomy

Control of blood glucose and BP are critical; intensive control of blood glucose slows progression of retinopathy. Clinically significant diabetic macular edema is treated with intraocular injection of anti-VEGF drugs (eg, ranibizumab, bevacizumab, aflibercept) and/or with focal laser photocoagulation.[1] The intraocular dexamethasone implant and intravitreal triamcinolone can treat eyes with persistent macular edema. In certain countries, an intraocular fluocinolone implant is available for patients with chronic diabetic macular edema. Vitrectomy can help in recalcitrant diabetic macular edema. In select cases of severe nonproliferative retinopathy, panretinal laser photocoagulation may be used; however, usually panretinal laser photocoagulation can be delayed until proliferative retinopathy develops.

Proliferative diabetic retinopathy with high-risk characteristics of vitreous hemorrhage, extensive preretinal neovascularization, or anterior segment neovascularization/neovascular glaucoma should be treated with panretinal laser photocoagulation. Recent studies have also supported the use of intravitreal anti-VEGF drugs in the treatment of proliferative diabetic retinopathy.[2] This treatment significantly reduces the risk of severe vision loss.

Vitrectomy can help preserve and often restore lost vision in patients with any of the following:

- Persistent vitreous hemorrhage
- Extensive preretinal membrane formation
- Traction retinal detachment
- Recalcitrant diabetic macular edema

1. The Diabetic Retinopathy Clinical Research Network: Aflibercept, bevacizumab, or ranibizumab for diabetic macular edema. *N Engl J M* 372(13):1193–1203, 2015. doi:10.1056/NEJMoa1414264.
2. Beaulieu WT, Bressler NM, Melia M, et al: Panretinal photocoagulation versus ranibizumab for proliferative diabetic retinopathy: patient-centered outcomes from a randomized clinical trial. *Am J Ophthalmol* 170:206–213, 2016. doi: 10.1016/j.ajo.2016.08.008.

Prevention

Control of blood glucose and BP is critical; intensive control of blood glucose delays onset of retinopathy.

KEY POINTS

- Features of diabetic retinopathy can include microaneurysms, intraretinal hemorrhage, exudates, cotton-wool spots, macular edema, macular ischemia, neovascularization, vitreous hemorrhage, and traction retinal detachment.
- Symptoms may not develop until damage is advanced.
- Test patients who have diabetic retinopathy with color fundus photography, fluorescein angiography, and optical coherence tomography.
- Screen all diabetic patients with an annual dilated ophthalmologic examination.
- Treat patients with macular edema with intraocular anti-VEGF drugs (eg, ranibizumab, aflibercept, bevacizumab), intraocular corticosteroid implants, focal laser photocoagulation, and/or vitrectomy.
- Treat patients with high-risk or complicated proliferative retinopathy with panretinal laser photocoagulation and sometimes vitrectomy.

HYPERTENSIVE RETINOPATHY

Hypertensive retinopathy is retinal vascular damage caused by hypertension. Signs usually develop late in the disease. Funduscopic examination shows arteriolar constriction, arteriovenous nicking, vascular wall changes, flame-shaped hemorrhages, cotton-wool spots, yellow hard exudates, and optic disk edema. Treatment is directed at controlling BP and, when vision loss occurs, treating the retina.

Pathophysiology

Acute BP elevation typically causes reversible vasoconstriction in retinal blood vessels, and hypertensive crisis may cause optic disk edema. More prolonged or severe hypertension leads to exudative vascular changes, a consequence of endothelial damage and necrosis. Other changes (eg, arteriole wall thickening, arteriovenous nicking) typically require years of elevated BP to develop. Smoking compounds the adverse effects of hypertensive retinopathy.

Hypertension is a major risk factor for other retinal disorders (eg, retinal artery or vein occlusion, diabetic retinopathy). Also, hypertension combined with diabetes greatly increases risk of vision loss. Patients with hypertensive retinopathy are at high risk of hypertensive damage to other end organs.

Symptoms and Signs

Symptoms usually do not develop until late in the disease and include blurred vision or visual field defects.

In the early stages, funduscopy identifies arteriolar constriction, with a decrease in the ratio of the width of the retinal arterioles to the retinal venules.

Chronic, poorly controlled hypertension causes the following:

- Permanent arterial narrowing
- Arteriovenous crossing abnormalities (arteriovenous nicking)
- Arteriosclerosis with moderate vascular wall changes (copper wiring) to more severe vascular wall hyperplasia and thickening (silver wiring)

Sometimes total vascular occlusion occurs. Arteriovenous nicking is a major predisposing factor to the development of a branch retinal vein occlusion.

If acute disease is severe, the following can develop:

- Superficial flame-shaped hemorrhages
- Small, white, superficial foci of retinal ischemia (cotton-wool spots)
- Yellow hard exudates
- Optic disk edema

Yellow hard exudates represent intraretinal lipid deposition from leaking retinal vessels (see Plate 21). These exudates can develop a star shape within the macula, particularly when hypertension is severe (see Plate 22). In severe hypertension, the optic disk becomes congested and edematous (papilledema indicating hypertensive crisis).

Diagnosis

Diagnosis is by history (duration and severity of hypertension) and funduscopy.

Treatment

Hypertensive retinopathy is managed primarily by controlling hypertension. Other vision-threatening conditions should also be aggressively controlled. If vision loss occurs, treatment of the retinal edema with laser or with intravitreal injection of corticosteroids or antivascular endothelial growth factor drugs (eg, ranibizumab, pegaptanib, bevacizumab) may be useful.

KEY POINTS

- Chronic hypertension progressively damages the retina, causing few or no symptoms until changes are advanced.
- Chronic hypertensive retinopathy is recognized by permanent arterial narrowing, arteriovenous crossing abnormalities (arteriovenous nicking), arteriosclerosis with moderate vascular wall changes (copper wiring), or more severe vascular wall hyperplasia and thickening (silver wiring).
- Hypertensive crisis can cause retinopathy with superficial flame-shaped hemorrhages; small, white, superficial foci of retinal ischemia (cotton-wool spots); yellow hard exudates; and optic disk edema.
- Diagnose patients by history and funduscopy.
- Treat primarily by controlling BP, and, for retinal edema, sometimes laser or intravitreal injection of corticosteroids or antivascular endothelial growth factor drugs.

RETINAL DETACHMENT

Retinal detachment is separation of the neurosensory retina from the underlying retinal pigment epithelium. The most common cause is a retinal break (a tear or, less commonly, a hole) (rhegmatogenous detachment). Symptoms are decreased peripheral or central vision, often described as a curtain or dark cloud coming across the field of vision. Associated symptoms can include painless vision disturbances, including flashing lights and increased floaters. Traction and serous retinal detachments (not involving retinal breaks) cause central or peripheral vision loss. Diagnosis is by funduscopy; ultrasonography may help determine the presence and type of retinal detachment if it cannot be seen with funduscopy. Immediate treatment is imperative if rhegmatogenous retinal detachment is acute and threatens central vision. Treatment of rhegmatogenous detachment may include sealing retinal breaks (by laser or cryotherapy), supporting the breaks with scleral buckling, pneumatic retinopexy, and/or vitrectomy.

Etiology

There are 3 types of detachment: rhegmatogenous (which involves a retinal break), traction, and serous (exudative) detachment. Traction and serous retinal detachments do not involve a break and are called nonrhegmatogenous.

Rhegmatogenous detachment is the most common. Risk factors include the following:

- Myopia
- Previous cataract surgery
- Ocular trauma
- Lattice retinal degeneration

Traction retinal detachment can be caused by vitreoretinal traction due to preretinal fibrous membranes as may occur in proliferative diabetic or sickle cell retinopathy.

Serous detachment results from transudation of fluid into the subretinal space. Causes include severe uveitis, especially in Vogt-Koyanagi-Harada disease, choroidal hemangiomas, and primary or metastatic choroidal cancers (see p. 965).

Symptoms and Signs

Retinal detachment is painless. Early symptoms of rhegmatogenous detachment may include dark or irregular vitreous floaters (particularly a sudden increase, flashes of light (photopsias), and blurred vision. As detachment progresses, the patient often notices a curtain, veil, or grayness in the field of vision. If the macula is involved, central vision becomes poor. Patients may have simultaneous vitreous hemorrhage. Traction and serous (exudative) retinal detachments can cause blurriness of vision, but they may not cause any symptoms in the early stages.

Diagnosis

- Indirect ophthalmoscopy with pupillary dilation

Retinal detachment should be suspected in patients, particularly those at risk, who have any of the following:

- Sudden increase or change in floaters
- Photopsias
- Curtain or veil across the visual field
- Any sudden, unexplained loss of vision
- Vitreous hemorrhage that obscures the retina

Indirect ophthalmoscopy shows the retinal detachment and can differentiate the subtypes of retinal detachment in nearly all cases. Direct funduscopy using a handheld ophthalmoscope can miss some retinal detachments, which may be peripheral. Peripheral fundus examination, using either indirect ophthalmoscopy with scleral depression, the slit lamp with the eye in extreme positions of gaze, or using a 3-mirror lens, should be done.

If vitreous hemorrhage (which may be due to a retinal tear), cataract, corneal opacification, or traumatic injury obscures the retina, retinal detachment should be suspected and B-scan ultrasonography should be done.

Treatment

- Sealing retinal breaks
- Scleral buckling
- Pneumatic retinopexy
- Vitrectomy

Although often localized, retinal detachments due to retinal breaks can expand to involve the entire retina if they are not treated promptly. *Any patient with a suspected or established retinal detachment should be examined urgently by an ophthalmologist.*

PEARLS & PITFALLS

- If patients have a sudden increase or change in floaters; photopsias; a curtain or veil across the visual field; any sudden, unexplained loss of vision; or if vitreous hemorrhage obscures the retina, arrange for an ophthalmologist to do urgent indirect ophthalmoscopy to diagnose retinal detachment.

Rhegmatogenous detachment is treated with one or more methods, depending on the cause and location of the lesion. These methods involve sealing the retinal breaks by laser or cryotherapy. In scleral buckling, a piece of silicone is placed on the sclera, which indents the sclera and pushes the retina inward, thereby relieving vitreous traction on the retina. During this procedure, fluid may be drained from the subretinal space. Pneumatic retinopexy (intravitreal injection of gas) and vitrectomy are other treatments. Retinal breaks without detachment can be sealed by laser photocoagulation or transconjunctival cryopexy. Nearly all rhegmatogenous detachments can be reattached surgically.

Nonrhegmatogenous detachments due to vitreoretinal traction may be treated by vitrectomy; transudative detachments due to uveitis may respond to systemic corticosteroids or systemic immunosuppression (eg, methotrexate, azathioprine, anti-TNF drugs). Alternatively, transudative detachments due to uveitis can be treated locally with a periocular corticosteroid injection, intravitreal corticosteroid injection, or an intravitreal dexamethasone implant. Primary and metastatic choroidal cancers also require treatment. Choroidal hemangiomas may respond to localized photocoagulation or photodynamic therapy.

KEY POINTS

- Risk factors for rhegmatogenous retinal detachments include myopia, previous cataract surgery, ocular trauma, and lattice retinal degeneration.
- All forms of retinal detachment eventually blur vision; early symptoms of rhegmatogenous detachment can include irregular vitreous floaters (particularly with a sudden increase) and flashes of light (photopsias).
- Arrange for urgent indirect ophthalmoscopy by an ophthalmologist to diagnose retinal detachment if patients have a sudden increase or change in floaters; photopsias; a curtain or veil across the visual field; any sudden, unexplained loss of vision; or if vitreous hemorrhage obscures the retina.
- Treat rhegmatogenous detachment by sealing retinal breaks (with laser or cryotherapy), by supporting the breaks with scleral buckling, with pneumatic retinopexy, and/or with vitrectomy.

RETINITIS PIGMENTOSA

Retinitis pigmentosa is a slowly progressive, bilateral degeneration of the retina and retinal pigment epithelium caused by various genetic mutations. Symptoms include night blindness and loss of peripheral vision. Diagnosis is by funduscopy, which shows pigmentation in a bone-spicule configuration in the equatorial retina, narrowing of the retinal arterioles, a waxy pallor of the optic disk, posterior subcapsular cataracts, and cells in the vitreous. Electroretinography helps confirm the diagnosis. Vitamin A palmitate, omega-3 fatty acids, and lutein plus zeaxanthin may help slow progression of vision loss.

Abnormal gene coding for retinal proteins appears to be the cause of retinitis pigmentosa; several genes have been identified. Transmission may be autosomal recessive, autosomal dominant, or, infrequently, X-linked. It may occur as part of a syndrome (eg, Bassen-Kornzweig, Laurence-Moon). One of these syndromes includes congenital hearing loss as well (Usher syndrome).

Symptoms and Signs

Retinal rods are affected, causing defective night vision that becomes symptomatic at varying ages, sometimes in early childhood. Night vision may eventually be lost. A peripheral ring scotoma (detectable by visual field testing) widens gradually, and central vision may also be affected in advanced cases.

Hyperpigmentation in a bone-spicule configuration in the midperipheral retina is the most conspicuous funduscopic finding. Other findings include the following:

- Narrowing of the retinal arterioles
- Cystoid macular edema
- Waxy yellow appearance of the disk
- Posterior subcapsular cataracts
- Cells in the vitreous (less common)
- Myopia

Diagnosis

- Funduscopy
- Electroretinography

The diagnosis is suspected in patients with poor night vision or a family history. Diagnosis is by funduscopy, usually supplemented with electroretinography. Other retinopathies that can simulate retinitis pigmentosa should be excluded; they include retinopathies associated with syphilis, rubella, phenothiazine or chloroquine toxicity, and nonocular cancer.

Family members should be examined and tested as necessary or desired to establish the hereditary pattern. Patients with a hereditary syndrome may wish to seek genetic counseling before having children.

Treatment

- Vitamin A palmitate
- Omega-3 fatty acids
- Lutein plus zeaxanthin
- Carbonic anhydrase inhibitors for cystoid macular edema
- Intraocular computer chip implants

There is no way to reverse damage caused by retinitis pigmentosa, but vitamin A palmitate 15,000 IU po once/day may help slow disease progression in some patients. Patients taking vitamin A palmitate should have regular liver function tests. Dietary supplementation with an omega-3 fatty acid (eg, docosahexaenoic acid) and an oral preparation of lutein plus zeaxanthin may also slow the rate of vision loss. Vision decreases as the macula becomes increasingly involved and can evolve to legal blindness. For patients with cystoid macular edema, carbonic anhydrase inhibitors given orally (eg, acetazolamide) or topically (eg, dorzolamide) may yield mild vision improvement. For patients with total or near total vision loss, epiretinal and subretinal computer chip implants can restore some visual sensations.

EPIRETINAL MEMBRANE

(Cellophane Maculopathy; Macular Pucker; Premacular Fibrosis)

Epiretinal membrane is formation of a thin, fibrotic membrane over the retina that contracts, wrinkling the underlying retina and interfering with vision.

Epiretinal membrane typically occurs after age 50 and is most common among people > 75.

Risk factors for epiretinal membrane are the following:

- Diabetic retinopathy
- Uveitis
- Retinal tear or detachment
- Ocular injury

Most cases are idiopathic.

Symptoms may include blurred vision or distorted vision (eg, straight lines may appear wavy). Many patients say that it seems like they are looking through plastic wrap or cellophane. Diagnosis is by funduscopy. Fluorescein angiography and optical coherence tomography may also be helpful.

Most people need no treatment. If problems with vision are significant, the membrane can be removed surgically with vitrectomy and membrane peel.

CANCERS AFFECTING THE RETINA

Cancers affecting the retina usually begin in the choroid. Because the retina depends on the choroid for its support and half of its blood supply, damage to the choroid by a cancer is likely to affect vision.

Choroidal melanoma: Choroidal melanoma originates from choroidal melanocytes. Choroidal melanoma is the most common cancer originating in the eye, with an incidence of about 1 in 2500 whites. It is less common among darker-skinned people. It occurs most frequently at age 55 to 60. It may spread locally or metastasize and be fatal.

Symptoms tend to develop late and include loss of vision and symptoms of retinal detachment (see p. 963).

Diagnosis is by funduscopy, supplemented, when indicated, by other tests, such as ultrasonography, CT, fluorescein angiography, and serial photographs.

Small cancers are treated with laser, radiation, or radioactive implants, which may preserve vision and save the eye. Rarely, local resection is used. Large cancers may require enucleation.

Choroidal metastases: Choroidal metastases are common because the choroid is highly vascular. The most common primary cancers are those of the breast in women and of the lung and prostate in men.

Symptoms tend to develop late and include loss of vision and symptoms of retinal detachment.

Diagnosis is often incidental during routine ophthalmoscopy. Ultrasonography is usually done, and the diagnosis is confirmed using fine-needle biopsy.

Treatment depends on the primary cancer and usually involves systemic chemotherapy, radiation therapy, or both.

118 Uveitis and Related Disorders

Uveitis is defined as inflammation of the uveal tract—the iris, ciliary body, and choroid. However, the retina and fluid within the anterior chamber and vitreous are often involved as well. About half of cases are idiopathic; identifiable causes include trauma, infection, and systemic diseases, many of which are autoimmune. Symptoms include decreased vision, ocular ache, redness, photophobia, and floaters. Although uveitis is identified clinically, identifying the cause typically requires testing. Treatment depends on cause, but typically includes topical, locally injected, or systemic corticosteroids with a topical cycloplegic-mydriatic drug. Noncorticosteroid immunosuppressive drugs may be used in severe and refractory cases.

Uveitis is classified anatomically as

- **Anterior uveitis:** Localized primarily to the anterior segment of the eye, includes iritis (inflammation in the anterior chamber alone) and iridocyclitis (inflammation in the anterior chamber and anterior vitreous)
- **Intermediate uveitis**: Localized to the vitreous cavity and/or pars plana
- **Posterior uveitis:** Any form of retinitis, choroiditis, or inflammation of the optic disk
- **Panuveitis**: Inflammation involving anterior, intermediate, and posterior strufctures

Uveitis is also classified by onset (sudden or insidious), duration (limited or persistent), and course (acute, recurrent, or chronic).[1]

1. Jabs DA, Nussenblatt RB, Rosenbaum JT, et al: Standardization of uveitis nomenclature for reporting clinical data. Results of the First International Workshop. *Am J Ophthalmol* 140(3):509–516, 2005.

Etiology

Causes of **anterior uveitis** include

- Idiopathic or post-surgical (most common cause)
- Trauma
- Spondyloarthropathies
- Juvenile idiopathic arthritis
- Herpesvirus infection (herpes simplex virus [HSV], varicella-zoster virus [VZV], and cytomegalovirus [CMV])

Causes of **intermediate uveitis** include

- Idiopathic (most common)
- Multiple sclerosis
- Sarcoidosis
- Tuberculosis (TB)
- Syphilis
- Lyme disease (in endemic regions)

Causes of **posterior uveitis** (retinitis) include

- Idiopathic (most common)
- Toxoplasmosis
- CMV (in patients with HIV/AIDS)
- HSV/VZV
- Sarcoidosis

Causes of **panuveitis** include

- Idiopathic (most common)
- Sarcoidosis
- TB

Infrequently, systemic drugs cause uveitis (usually anterior). Examples are sulfonamides, bisphosphonates (inhibitors of bone resorption), rifabutin, and cidofovir.

Systemic diseases causing uveitis and their treatment are discussed elsewhere in THE MANUAL.

Symptoms and Signs

Symptoms and signs may be subtle and vary depending on the site and severity of inflammation.

Anterior uveitis tends to be the most symptomatic (especially when acute), usually manifesting with

- Pain (ocular ache)
- Redness
- Photophobia
- Decreased vision (to a variable degree)

Chronic anterior uveitis may have less dramatic symptoms and present with irritation or decreased vision.

Signs include hyperemia of the conjunctiva adjacent to the cornea (ciliary flush or limbal injection). Slit-lamp findings include keratic precipitates (WBC clumps on the inner corneal surface), cells and flare (a haze) in the anterior chamber (aqueous humor), and posterior synechiae. With severe anterior uveitis, WBCs may layer in the anterior chamber (hypopyon).

Intermediate uveitis is typically painless and manifests with

- Floaters
- Decreased vision

The primary sign is cells in the vitreous humor. Aggregates and condensations of inflammatory cells often occur over the pars plana (near the junction of the iris and sclera), forming "snowballs." Vision may be decreased because of floaters or cystoid macular edema, which results from fluid leakage from blood vessels in the macula. Confluent and condensed vitreous cells and snowballs over the pars plana may cause a classic "snowbank" appearance, which can be associated with neovascularization of the retinal periphery.

Posterior uveitis may give rise to diverse symptoms but most commonly causes floaters and decreased vision as occurs in intermediate uveitis. Signs include

- Cells in the vitreous humor
- White or yellow-white lesions in the retina (retinitis), underlying choroid (choroiditis), or both
- Exudative retinal detachments
- Retinal vasculitis
- Optic disk edema

Panuveitis may cause any combination of the previously mentioned symptoms and signs.

Complications: Serious complications of uveitis include profound and irreversible vision loss, especially when uveitis is unrecognized, inadequately treated, or both.

The **most frequent complications** include

- Cataract
- Glaucoma
- Retinal detachment
- Neovascularization of the retina, optic nerve, or iris
- Cystoid macular edema (the most common cause of decreased vision in patients with uveitis)
- Hypotony (an intraocular pressure that is too low to support the health of the eye)

Diagnosis

- Slit-lamp examination
- Ophthalmoscopy after pupil dilation

Uveitis should be suspected in any patient who has ocular ache, redness, photophobia, floaters, or decreased vision. Patients with unilateral anterior uveitis have ocular ache in the affected eye if light is shined in the unaffected eye (true photophobia), which is uncommon in conjunctivitis.

Diagnosis of anterior uveitis is by recognizing cells and flare in the anterior chamber. Cells and flare are seen with a slit lamp and are most evident when using a narrow, intensely bright light focused on the anterior chamber in a dark room. Findings of intermediate and posterior uveitis are most easily seen after dilating the pupil (see p. 894). Indirect ophthalmoscopy (usually done by an ophthalmologist) is more sensitive than direct ophthalmoscopy. (NOTE: If uveitis is suspected, patients should be referred immediately for complete ophthalmologic evaluation.)

Many conditions that cause intraocular inflammation can mimic uveitis and should be considered in the appropriate clinical settings. Such conditions include severe conjunctivitis (eg, epidemic keratoconjunctivitis), severe keratitis (eg, herpetic keratoconjunctivitis, peripheral ulcerative keratitis), and severe scleritis.

Acute angle closure glaucoma can cause redness and severe pain similar to that of uveitis, which is why it is important to check intraocular pressure at every visit. Uveitis is often (but not always) associated with a low intraocular pressure whereas pressure is typically high in acute angle closure glaucoma. Uveitis also can be distinguished from angle closure glaucoma by the absence of corneal haze and the presence of a deeper anterior chamber.

Other masqueraders include intraocular cancers in the very young (typically retinoblastoma and leukemia) and in the elderly (intraocular lymphoma). Much less commonly, retinitis pigmentosa can manifest with mild inflammation, which may be confused with uveitis.

Treatment

- Corticosteroids (usually topical) and sometimes other immunosuppressive drugs
- Cycloplegic-mydriatic drugs
- Sometimes antimicrobial drugs
- Sometimes surgical therapy

Treatment of active inflammation usually involves corticosteroids given topically (eg, prednisolone acetate 1% 1 drop q 1 h while awake) or by periocular or intraocular injection along with a cycloplegic-mydriatic drug (eg, homatropine 2% or 5% drops [if available] or cyclopentolate 0.5% or 1.0% drops, either drug given bid to qid depending on severity). Antimicrobial drugs are used to treat infectious uveitis. Particularly severe or chronic cases may require systemic corticosteroids (eg, prednisone 1 mg/kg po once/day), systemic noncorticosteroid immunosuppressive drugs (eg, methotrexate 15 to 25 mg po once/wk or adalimumab 40 mg every other week), laser phototherapy, cryotherapy applied transsclerally to the retinal periphery, or surgical removal of the vitreous (vitrectomy).[1]

1. Jaffe GJ, Dick AD, Brézin AP, et al: Adalimumab in Patients with Active Noninfectious Uveitis. *N Engl J Med* 8;375(10):932–943, 2016. doi: 10.1056/NEJMoa1509852.

KEY POINTS

- Inflammation of the uveal tract (uveitis) can affect the anterior segment (including the iris), intermediate uveal tract (including the vitreous), or posterior uvea (including the choroid, retina, and optic nerve).
- Most cases are idiopathic, but known causes include infections, trauma, and autoimmune disorders.
- Findings in acute anterior uveitis include aching eye pain, photophobia, redness closely surrounding the cornea (ciliary flush), and, on slit-lamp examination, cells and flare.
- Chronic anterior uveitis may have less dramatic symptoms and present with eye irritation or decreased vision.

- Intermediate and posterior uveitis tend to cause less pain and eye redness but more floaters and decreased vision.
- Diagnosis is confirmed by slit-lamp examination and ophthalmoscopic examination (often indirect) after pupillary dilation.
- Treatment should be managed by an ophthalmologist and often includes corticosteroids and a cycloplegic-mydriatic drug along with treatment of any specific cause.

UVEITIS CAUSED BY CONNECTIVE TISSUE DISEASE

A number of connective tissue diseases cause inflammation of the uveal tract.

Spondyloarthropathies: The seronegative spondyloarthropathies (see p. 311) are a common cause of anterior uveitis.

Among the seronegative spondyloarthropathies, ocular inflammation is most common with ankylosing spondylitis but also occurs with reactive arthritis, inflammatory bowel disease (ulcerative colitis and Crohn disease), and psoriatic arthritis. Uveitis is classically unilateral, but recurrences are common and active inflammation may alternate between eyes. Men are affected more commonly than women. Most patients, regardless of sex, are HLA-B27 positive.

Treatment requires a topical corticosteroid and a cycloplegic-mydriatic drug. Occasionally, periocular corticosteroids are required. Severe chronic cases may require noncorticosteroid immunosuppressive drugs (eg, methotrexate, mycophenolate mofetil).

Juvenile idiopathic arthritis (JIA, previously known as juvenile RA): JIA characteristically causes chronic bilateral iridocyclitis in children, particularly those with the pauciarticular variety (see p. 2694). Unlike most forms of anterior uveitis, however, JIA tends not to cause pain, photophobia, and conjunctival injection but only blurring and miosis and is, therefore, often referred to as white iritis. JIA-associated uveitis is more common among girls.

Rheumatoid arthritis, in contrast, is not associated with isolated uveitis but can cause scleritis, which may cause secondary uveal tract inflammation.

Recurrent bouts of inflammation are best treated with a topical corticosteroid and a cycloplegic-mydriatic drug. Given the chronic nature of disease and risk of treatment-related cataract and glaucoma development, long-term control often requires use of a noncorticosteroid immunosuppressive drug (eg, methotrexate, mycophenolate mofetil).

Sarcoidosis: Sarcoidosis (see p. 509) accounts for 10 to 20% of cases of uveitis, and about 25% of patients with sarcoidosis develop uveitis. Sarcoid uveitis is more common among blacks and the elderly.

Virtually any symptoms and signs of anterior, intermediate, posterior, or panuveitis can occur. Suggestive findings include conjunctival granulomas, large keratic precipitates on the corneal endothelium (so-called granulomatous or mutton fat precipitates), iris granulomas, and retinal vasculitis. Biopsy of suggestive lesions, which provides the most secure diagnosis, is usually done on the conjunctiva; it is rarely done on intraocular tissues because of the risk associated with the procedure.

Treatment usually involves topical, periocular, intraocular, or systemic corticosteroids, or a combination, along with a topical cycloplegic-mydriatic drug. Patients with moderate to severe inflammation may require a noncorticosteroid immunosuppressive drug (eg, methotrexate, mycophenolate mofetil).

Behçet disease: Behçet disease is rare in North America but is a fairly common cause of uveitis in the Middle East and Far East.

Typical findings include severe anterior uveitis with hypopyon, retinal vasculitis, and optic disk inflammation. The clinical course is usually severe with multiple recurrences.

Diagnosis requires the presence of associated systemic manifestations, such as oral aphthous or genital ulcers; dermatitis, including erythema nodosum; thrombophlebitis; or epididymitis. Oral aphthae may be biopsied to show an occlusive vasculitis. There are no laboratory tests for Behçet disease, but it is associated with HLA-B51 (see also p. 345).

Treatment with local and systemic corticosteroids and a cycloplegic-mydriatic drug may alleviate acute exacerbations, but most patients eventually require systemic corticosteroids and a noncorticosteroid immunosuppressive drug (eg, cyclosporine, chlorambucil) to control the inflammation and avoid the serious complications of long-term corticosteroid treatment. Biologic agents such as interferons and tumor necrosis factor inhibitors have been effective in selected patients unresponsive to other therapies.

Vogt-Koyanagi-Harada (VKH) disease: VKH disease is an uncommon systemic disorder characterized by uveitis accompanied by cutaneous and neurologic abnormalities. VKH disease is particularly common among people of Asian, Asian Indian, and American Indian descent. Women in their 20s and 30s are affected more often than men. The etiology is unknown, although an autoimmune reaction directed against melanin-containing cells in the uveal tract, skin, inner ear, and meninges is strongly suspected.

Neurologic symptoms tend to occur early and include tinnitus, dysacusis (auditory agnosia), vertigo, headache, and meningismus. Cutaneous findings frequently occur later and include patchy vitiligo (especially common on the eyelids, low back, and buttocks), poliosis (a localized patch of white hair, which may involve the eyelashes), and alopecia, often involving the head and neck. Common findings include serous retinal detachment, optic disk edema, and choroiditis. Long-term complications include cataracts, glaucoma, subretinal fibrosis, and choroidal neovascularization.

Early treatment includes local and systemic corticosteroids and a cycloplegic-mydriatic drug. Many patients also require noncorticosteroid immunosuppressive drugs (eg, methotrexate, mycophenolate mofetil).

ENDOPHTHALMITIS

Endophthalmitis is an acute panuveitis resulting most often from bacterial infection.

Most cases of endophthalmitis are caused by gram-positive bacteria, such as *Staphylococcus epidermidis* or *S. aureus*. Endophthalmitis caused by gram-negative organisms tends to be more virulent and has a worse prognosis. Fungal and protozoan causes of endophthalmitis are rare. Most cases occur after intraocular surgery (exogenous) or penetrating ocular trauma. Less commonly, infection reaches the eye via the bloodstream after systemic surgery or dental procedures or when IV lines or IV drugs are used (endogenous).

Endophthalmitis is a medical emergency because vision prognosis is directly related to the time from onset to treatment. Rarely, untreated intraocular infections extend beyond the confines of the eye to involve the orbit and CNS.

Exogenous endophthalmitis typically causes severe ocular ache and decreased vision. Signs include

- Intense conjunctival hyperemia and intraocular inflammation within the anterior chamber and vitreous
- Loss of the red reflex
- Eyelid edema (occasionally)

Diagnosis

- Clinical evaluation
- Microbiologic testing (eg, gram stain and culture of aspirates for endogenous endophthalmitis, blood and urine cultures)

Diagnosis requires a high index of suspicion in at-risk patients, especially those with recent eye surgery or trauma. Gram stain and culture of aspirates from the anterior chamber and vitreous are standard. Patients with suspected endogenous endophthalmitis should also have blood and urine cultures.

Treatment

- Intravitreal antibiotics
- For endogenous endophthalmitis, intravitreal and IV antibiotics
- In severe cases, possible vitrectomy and intraocular corticosteroids

Initial treatment includes broad-spectrum intravitreal antibiotics, most commonly vancomycin and ceftazidime. Patients with endogenous endophthalmitis should receive both intravitreal and IV antibiotics. Therapy is modified based on culture and sensitivity results.

Vision prognosis is often poor, even with early and appropriate treatment. Patients whose vision at presentation is count-fingers or worse should be considered for vitrectomy and use of intraocular corticosteroids. Corticosteroids are, however, contraindicated in fungal endophthalmitis.

INFECTIOUS UVEITIS

A number of infectious diseases cause uveitis (see Table 118–1). The most common are toxoplasmosis, herpes simplex virus, and varicella-zoster virus. Different organisms affect different parts of the uveal tract.

Toxoplasmosis: Toxoplasmosis is the most common cause of retinitis in immunocompetent patients. Most cases are acquired postnatally; however, congenital cases occur as well, particularly in countries where infection is endemic. Symptoms of floaters and decreased vision may be due to cells in the vitreous humor or to retinal lesions or scars. Concurrent anterior segment involvement can occur and may cause ocular ache, redness, and photophobia. Laboratory testing should include serum anti–*Toxoplasma gondii* antibody titers.

Treatment is recommended for patients with posterior lesions that threaten vital visual structures, such as the optic disk or macula, and for immunocompromised patients. Multidrug therapy is commonly prescribed; it includes pyrimethamine, sulfonamides, clindamycin, and, in select cases, systemic corticosteroids. Corticosteroids should not, however, be used without concurrent antimicrobial coverage. Toxoplasmosis can recur, and patients with vision-threatening lesions may require long-term prophylaxis with trimethoprim-sulfamethoxazole. Long-acting periocular and intraocular corticosteroids (eg, triamcinolone acetonide) should be avoided.

Patients with small peripheral lesions that do not directly threaten vital visual structures may be observed without treatment and should begin to show slow improvement in 1 to 2 mo.

Herpesviruses (HSV and VZV): Herpes simplex virus (HSV) causes anterior uveitis. Varicella-zoster virus (VZV) does so less commonly, although the prevalence of zoster-associated anterior uveitis increases with age. Both HSV and VZV can also result in posterior uveitis, although this is less common.

Table 118–1. INFECTIOUS CAUSES OF UVEITIS

FREQUENCY	VIRUSES OR INFECTIONS
More common	Herpes simplex virus
	Toxoplasmosis
	Varicella-zoster virus
Less common	Bartonellosis
	Histoplasmosis
	Lyme disease
	Syphilis
	Toxocariasis
	Tuberculosis
	Cytomegalovirus*
	*Pneumocystis jirovecii**
Rare	*Aspergillus*
	Candida
	Coccidioidomycosis
	Cryptococcus
	Cysticercosis
	Leprosy
	Leptospirosis
	Onchocerciasis
	Tropheryma whippelii

*Particularly in patients with AIDS.

Symptoms of anterior uveitis include

- Ocular aching
- Photophobia
- Decreased vision

Signs include

- Redness
- Conjunctival injection and anterior chamber inflammation (cells and flare), often accompanied by corneal inflammation (keratitis)
- Decreased corneal sensation
- Patchy or sectorial iris atrophy

Intraocular pressure may be elevated as well; elevation can be detected by using applanation tonometry with, for example, a Goldmann tonometer, a pneumotonometer, an electronic indentation tonometer, or, if these are not available, a Schiotz tonometer.

Treatment should generally be initiated by an ophthalmologist and should include a topical corticosteroid and a cycloplegic-mydriatic drug. Acyclovir (400 mg po 5 times/day for herpes simplex virus and 800 mg po 5 times/day for herpes zoster virus) may also be given. Drops to lower intraocular pressure may be required in patients with ocular hypertension.

Acute retinal necrosis (ARN) is a rapidly progressing form of retinitis that is a much less common manifestation of varicella-zoster and herpes simplex virus infection. ARN typically manifests as confluent retinitis, occlusive retinal vasculitis, and moderate to severe vitreous inflammation. One-third of ARN cases become bilateral, and in three fourths of eyes, retinal detachmentoccurs. ARN may also occur in patients with HIV/AIDS, but severely immunocompromised patients can have less prominent vitreous inflammation. Vitreous biopsy for culture and PCR analysis may be useful in diagnosing ARN. Treatment options include IV acyclovir, IV ganciclovir or foscarnet, intravitreal ganciclovir or foscarnet, and oral valacyclovir or valganciclovir.

Herpesviruses (cytomegalovirus): Cytomegalovirus (CMV) is the most common cause of retinitis in immunocompromised patients, but prevalence has decreased among patients with HIV/AIDS receiving antiretroviral therapy (ART). Currently, ≤ 5% of these patients are affected. Most affected patients have a CD4+ count < 100 cells/μL. CMV retinitis may also occur in neonates and in pharmacologically immunosuppressed patients but is uncommon. CMV can rarely cause anterior uveitis in the immunocompetent person.

Symptoms of CMV retinitis include blurry vision, blind spots, floaters, flashing lights, and vision loss.

The diagnosis is largely clinical based on direct or indirect ophthalmoscopic examination; serologic tests are of limited use although analysis of aqueous fluid can be confirmatory if the diagnosis is in question.

Treatment in patients with HIV/AIDS is with systemic or intravitreal ganciclovir, systemic or intravitreal foscarnet, or systemic valganciclovir. Therapy is typically continued indefinitely, unless immune reconstitution is achieved with combination antiretroviral therapy (typically a CD4+ count > 100 cells/μL for at least 3 mo).

SYMPATHETIC OPHTHALMIA

Sympathetic ophthalmia is inflammation of the uveal tract after trauma or surgery to the other eye.

Sympathetic ophthalmia is a rare granulomatous uveitis that occurs after penetrating trauma or surgery to the other eye. Sympathetic ophthalmia has been estimated to occur in up to 0.5% of nonsurgical penetrating eye wounds and in about 0.03% of surgical penetrating eye wounds. The underlying mechanism is thought to be an autoimmune reaction directed against melanin-containing cells in the uvea. Uveitis appears within 2 to 12 wk after trauma or surgery in about 80% of cases. Isolated cases of sympathetic ophthalmia have occurred as early as 1 wk or as late as 30 yr after the initial trauma or surgery.

Symptoms typically include floaters and decreased vision. Choroiditis, often with overlying exudative retinal detachment, is common.

Diagnosis is clinical.

Treatment

- Oral corticosteroids and immunosuppressants
- With severe injuries, possibly early prophylactic enucleation

Treatment typically requires oral corticosteroids (eg, prednisone, 1 mg/kg po once/day) followed by long-term use of a noncorticosteroid immunosuppressive drug. Prophylactic enucleation of a severely injured eye should be considered within 2 wk of vision loss to minimize the risk of sympathetic ophthalmia developing in the other eye, but only when the injured eye has no vision potential.

Dermatologic Disorders

119 Approach to the Dermatologic Patient

History and physical examination are adequate for diagnosing many skin lesions. Some require biopsy or other testing.

Dermatologic history: Important information to obtain from history includes

- Personal or family history of atopy (suggesting atopic dermatitis)
- Occupational exposures (contact dermatitis)
- Long-term exposure to sunlight or other forms of radiation (benign and malignant skin tumors)
- Systemic disease (diabetes and *Candida* or tinea, hepatitis C, and cryoglobulinemia)
- Sexual history (syphilis and gonorrhea)
- Use of drugs (Stevens-Johnson syndrome, toxic epidermal necrolysis)
- Travel history (Lyme disease, skin infections)

A negative history is as important as a positive history. The history of the particular skin lesions is also important, including time and site of initial appearance, spread, change in appearance, and triggering factors.

Dermatologic examination: Visual inspection is the central evaluation tool; many skin disorders are diagnosed by the characteristic appearance or morphology of the lesions (see also below). A full skin examination, including examination of the scalp, nails, and mucous membranes, is done to screen for skin cancers and to detect clues to the diagnosis of a widespread eruption. Magnification with a hand lens can help reveal morphologic detail. A hand-held dermatoscope with built-in lighting is particularly useful in evaluating pigmented lesions. Further information can be gathered by using diascopy or a Wood light.

An extensive language has been developed to standardize the description of skin lesions, including

- Lesion type (sometimes called primary morphology)
- Lesion configuration (sometimes called secondary morphology)
- Texture
- Distribution
- Color

Rash is a general term for a temporary skin eruption.

Lesion Type (Primary Morphology)

Macules are flat, nonpalpable lesions usually < 10 mm in diameter. Macules represent a change in color and are not raised or depressed compared to the skin surface. A patch is a large macule. Examples include freckles, flat moles, tattoos, and port-wine stains, and the rashes of rickettsial infections, rubella, measles (can also have papules and plaques), and some allergic drug eruptions.

Papules are elevated lesions usually < 10 mm in diameter that can be felt or palpated. Examples include nevi, warts, lichen planus, insect bites, seborrheic keratoses, actinic keratoses, some lesions of acne, and skin cancers. The term maculopapular is often loosely and improperly used to describe many red skin rashes; because this term is nonspecific and easily misused, it should be avoided.

Plaques are palpable lesions > 10 mm in diameter that are elevated or depressed compared to the skin surface. Plaques may be flat topped or rounded. Lesions of psoriasis and granuloma annulare commonly form plaques.

Nodules are firm papules or lesions that extend into the dermis or subcutaneous tissue. Examples include cysts, lipomas, and fibromas.

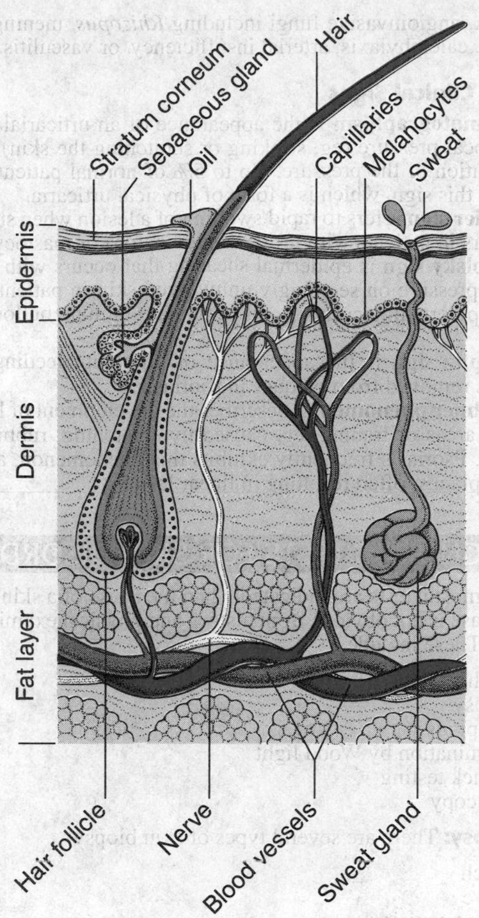

Fig. 119–1. Cross-section of the skin and skin structures.

Vesicles are small, clear, fluid-filled blisters < 10 mm in diameter. Vesicles are characteristic of herpes infections, acute allergic contact dermatitis, and some autoimmune blistering disorders (eg, dermatitis herpetiformis).

Bullae are clear fluid-filled blisters > 10 mm in diameter. These may be caused by burns, bites, irritant or allergic contact dermatitis, and drug reactions. Classic autoimmune bullous diseases include pemphigus vulgaris and bullous pemphigoid. Bullae also may occur in inherited disorders of skin fragility.

Pustules are vesicles that contain pus. Pustules are common in bacterial infections and folliculitis and may arise in some inflammatory disorders including pustular psoriasis.

Urticaria (wheals or hives) is characterized by elevated lesions caused by localized edema. Wheals are pruritic and red (see Plate 61). Wheals are a common manifestation of hypersensitivity to drugs, stings or bites, autoimmunity, and, less commonly, physical stimuli including temperature, pressure, and sunlight. The typical wheal lasts < 24 h.

Scale is heaped-up accumulations of horny epithelium that occur in disorders such as psoriasis, seborrheic dermatitis, and fungal infections. Pityriasis rosea and chronic dermatitis of any type may be scaly.

Crusts (scabs) consist of dried serum, blood, or pus. Crusting can occur in inflammatory or infectious skin diseases (eg, impetigo).

Erosions are open areas of skin that result from loss of part or all of the epidermis. Erosions can be traumatic or can occur with various inflammatory or infectious skin diseases. An excoriation is a linear erosion caused by scratching, rubbing, or picking.

Ulcers result from loss of the epidermis and at least part of the dermis. Causes include venous stasis dermatitis, physical trauma with or without vascular compromise (eg, caused by decubitus ulcers or peripheral arterial disease), infections, and vasculitis.

Petechiae are nonblanchable punctate foci of hemorrhage. Causes include platelet abnormalities (eg, thrombocytopenia, platelet dysfunction), vasculitis, and infections (eg, meningococcemia, Rocky Mountain spotted fever, other rickettsioses).

Purpura is a larger area of hemorrhage that may be palpable. Palpable purpura is considered the hallmark of leukocytoclastic vasculitis. Purpura may indicate a coagulopathy. Large areas of purpura may be called ecchymoses or, colloquially, bruises.

Atrophy is thinning of the skin, which may appear dry and wrinkled, resembling cigarette paper. Atrophy may be caused by chronic sun exposure, aging, and some inflammatory and neoplastic skin diseases, including cutaneous T-cell lymphoma and lupus erythematosus. Atrophy also may result from long-term use of potent topical corticosteroids.

Scars are areas of fibrosis that replace normal skin after injury. Some scars become hypertrophic or thickened and raised. Keloids are hypertrophic scars that extend beyond the original wound margin.

Telangiectases are foci of small, permanently dilated blood vessels that may occur in areas of sun damage, rosacea, systemic diseases (especially systemic sclerosis), or inherited diseases (eg, ataxia-telangiectasia, hereditary hemorrhagic telangiectasia) or after long-term therapy with topical fluorinated corticosteroids.

Lesion Configuration (Secondary Morphology)

Configuration is the shape of single lesions and the arrangement of clusters of lesions.

Linear lesions take on the shape of a straight line and are suggestive of some forms of contact dermatitis, linear epidermal nevi, and lichen striatus. Traumatically induced lesions, including excoriations caused by the patient's fingernails, are typically linear.

Annular lesions are rings with central clearing. Examples include granuloma annulare, some drug eruptions, some dermatophyte infections (eg, ringworm), and secondary syphilis.

Nummular lesions are circular or coin-shaped; an example is nummular eczema.

Target (bull's-eye or iris) lesions appear as rings with central duskiness and are classic for erythema multiforme.

Serpiginous lesions have linear, branched, and curving elements. Examples include some fungal and parasitic infections (eg, cutaneous larva migrans).

Reticulated lesions have a lacy or networked pattern. Examples include cutis marmorata and livedo reticularis.

Herpetiform describes grouped papules or vesicles arranged like those of a herpes simplex infection.

Zosteriform describes lesions clustered in a dermatomal distribution similar to those of herpes zoster.

Texture

Some skin lesions have visible or palpable texture that suggests a diagnosis.

Verrucous lesions have an irregular, pebbly, or rough surface. Examples include warts and seborrheic keratoses.

Lichenification is thickening of the skin with accentuation of normal skin markings; it results from repeated scratching or rubbing.

Induration, or deep thickening of the skin, can result from edema, inflammation, or infiltration, including by cancer. Indurated skin has a hard, resistant feeling. Induration is characteristic of panniculitis, some skin infections, and cutaneous metastatic cancers.

Umbilicated lesions have a central indentation and are usually viral. Examples include molluscum contagiosum and herpes simplex.

Xanthomas, which are yellowish, waxy lesions, may be idiopathic or may occur in patients who have lipid disorders.

Location and Distribution

It is important to note whether

- Lesions are single or multiple
- Particular body parts are affected (eg, palms or soles, scalp, mucosal membranes)
- Distribution is random or patterned, symmetric or asymmetric
- Lesions are on sun-exposed or protected skin

Although few patterns are pathognomonic, some are consistent with certain diseases.

Psoriasis frequently affects the scalp, extensor surfaces of the elbows and knees, umbilicus, and the gluteal cleft.

Lichen planus frequently arises on the wrists, forearms, genitals, and lower legs.

Vitiligo may be patchy and isolated or may group around the distal extremities and face, particularly around the eyes and mouth.

Discoid lupus erythematosus has characteristic lesions on sun-exposed skin of the face, especially the forehead, nose, and the conchal bowl of the ear.

Hidradenitis suppurativa involves skin containing a high density of apocrine glands, including the axillae, groin, and under the breasts.

Color

Red skin (erythema) can result from many different inflammatory or infectious diseases. Cutaneous tumors are often pink or red. Superficial vascular lesions such as port-wine stains may appear red.

Orange skin is most often seen in hypercarotenemia, a usually benign condition of carotene deposition after excess dietary ingestion of beta-carotene.

Yellow skin is typical of jaundice, xanthelasmas and xanthomas, and pseudoxanthoma elasticum.

Green fingernails suggest *Pseudomonas aeruginosa* infection.

Violet skin may result from cutaneous hemorrhage or vasculitis. Vascular lesions or tumors, such as Kaposi sarcoma and hemangiomas, can appear purple. A lilac color of the eyelids or heliotrope eruption is characteristic of dermatomyositis.

Shades of blue, silver, and gray can result from deposition of drugs or metals in the skin, including minocycline, amiodarone, and silver (argyria). Ischemic skin appears purple to gray in color. Deep dermal nevi appear blue.

Black skin lesions may be melanocytic, including nevi and melanoma. Black eschars are collections of dead skin that can arise from infarction, which may be caused by infection (eg, anthrax, angioinvasive fungi including *Rhizopus,* meningococcemia), calciphylaxis, arterial insufficiency, or vasculitis.

Other Clinical Signs

Dermatographism is the appearance of an urticarial wheal after focal pressure (eg, stroking or scratching the skin) in the distribution of the pressure. Up to 5% of normal patients may exhibit this sign, which is a form of physical urticaria.

Darier sign refers to rapid swelling of a lesion when stroked. It occurs in patients with urticaria pigmentosa or mastocytosis.

Nikolsky sign is epidermal shearing that occurs with gentle lateral pressure on seemingly uninvolved skin in patients with toxic epidermal necrolysis and some autoimmune bullous diseases.

Auspitz sign is the appearance of pinpoint bleeding after scale is removed from plaques in psoriasis.

Koebner phenomenon describes the development of lesions within areas of trauma (eg, caused by scratching, rubbing, or injury). Psoriasis frequently exhibits this phenomenon, as may lichen planus, often resulting in linear lesions.

DIAGNOSTIC TESTS FOR SKIN DISORDERS

Diagnostic tests are indicated when the cause of a skin lesion or disease is not obvious from history and physical examination alone. These include

- Patch testing
- Biopsy
- Scrapings
- Examination by Wood light
- Tzanck testing
- Diascopy

Biopsy: There are several types of skin biopsy:

- Punch
- Shave
- Wedge excision

One procedure is a punch biopsy, in which a tubular punch (diameter usually 4 mm) is inserted into deep dermal or subcutaneous tissue to obtain a specimen, which is snipped off at its base. More superficial lesions may be biopsied by shaving with a scalpel or razor blade. Bleeding is controlled by aluminum chloride solution or electrodesiccation; large incisions are closed by sutures. Larger or deeper biopsies can be done by excising a wedge of skin with a scalpel. Pigmented lesions are often excised for histologic evaluation of depth; if too superficial, definitive diagnosis may be impossible. Diagnosis and cure can often be achieved simultaneously for most small tumors by complete excision that includes a small border of normal skin.

Scrapings: Skin scrapings help diagnose fungal infections and scabies. For fungal infection, scale is taken from the border of the lesion and placed onto a microscope slide. Then a drop of 10 to 20% potassium hydroxide is added. Hyphae, budding yeast, or both confirm the diagnosis of tinea or candidiasis. For scabies, scrapings are taken from suspected burrows and placed directly under a coverslip with mineral oil; findings of mites, feces, or eggs confirm the diagnosis.

Wood light: A Wood light (black light) can help clinicians diagnose and define the extent of lesions (eg, borders of pigmented lesions before excision). It can help distinguish hypopigmentation from depigmentation (depigmentation of vitiligo fluoresces ivory-white and hypopigmented lesions do not). Erythrasma fluoresces a characteristic bright orange-red. Tinea capitis caused by *Microsporum canis* and *M. audouinii* fluoresces a light, bright green. (NOTE: Most tinea capitis in the US is caused by *Trichophyton* species, which do not fluoresce.) The earliest clue to cutaneous *Pseudomonas* infection (eg, in burns) may be green fluorescence.

Tzanck testing: Tzanck testing can be used to diagnose viral disease, such as herpes simplex and herpes zoster, and is done when active intact vesicles are present. Tzanck testing cannot distinguish between herpes simplex and herpes zoster infections. An intact blister is the preferred lesion for examination. The blister roof is removed with a sharp blade, and the base of the unroofed vesicle is scraped with a #15 scalpel blade. The scrapings are transferred to a slide and stained with Wright stain or Giemsa stain. Multinucleated giant cells are a sign of herpes infection.

Diascopy: Diascopy is used to determine whether erythema in a lesion is due to blood within superficial vessels (inflammatory or vascular lesions), or is due to hemorrhage (petechiae or purpura). A microscope slide is pressed against a lesion (diascopy) to see whether it blanches. Hemorrhagic lesions do not blanch; inflammatory and vascular lesions do. Diascopy can also help identify sarcoid skin lesions, which, when tested, turn an apple jelly color.

ITCHING

(Pruritus)

Itching is a symptom that can cause significant discomfort and is one of the most common reasons for consultation with a dermatologist. Itching leads to scratching, which can cause inflammation, skin degradation, and possible secondary infection. The skin can become lichenified, scaly, and excoriated.

Pathophysiology

Itch can be prompted by diverse stimuli, including light touch, vibration, and wool fibers. There are a number of chemical mediators as well as different mechanisms by which the sensation of itch occurs. The existence of specific peripheral sensory neurons responsible for mediating the itch sensation was recently demonstrated. These neurons are distinct from those that respond to light touch or pain; they contain a receptor, MrgA3, the stimulation of which causes the sensation of itching.

Mediators: Histamine is one of the most significant mediators. It is synthesized and stored in mast cells in the skin and is released in response to various stimuli. Other mediators (eg, neuropeptides) can either cause the release of histamine or act as pruritogens themselves, thus explaining why antihistamines ameliorate some cases of itching and not others. Opioids have a central pruritic action as well as stimulating the peripherally mediated histamine itch.

Mechanisms: There are 4 mechanisms of itch:

- Dermatologic—typically caused by inflammatory or pathologic processes (eg, urticaria, eczema)
- Systemic—related to diseases of organs other than skin (eg, cholestasis)
- Neuropathic—related to disorders of the CNS or peripheral nervous system (eg, multiple sclerosis)
- Psychogenic—related to psychiatric conditions

Intense itching stimulates vigorous scratching, which in turn can cause secondary skin conditions (eg, inflammation, excoriation, infection), which can lead to more itching through disruption of the skin barrier. Although scratching can temporarily reduce the sensation of itch by activating inhibitory neuronal circuits, it also leads to amplification of itching at the level of the brain, exacerbating the itch scratch cycle.

Etiology

Itching can be a symptom of a primary skin disease or, less commonly, a systemic disease. Also, drugs can cause itching (see Table 119–1).

Skin disorders: Many skin disorders cause itching. The most common include

- Dry skin
- Atopic dermatitis (eczema)
- Contact dermatitis
- Fungal skin infections

Table 119–1. SOME CAUSES OF ITCHING

CAUSE	SUGGESTIVE FINDINGS	DIAGNOSTIC APPROACH
Primary skin disorders		
Atopic dermatitis	Presence of erythema, possible lichenification, keratosis pilaris, xerosis, Dennie-Morgan lines, hyperlinear palms Usually a family history of atopy or chronic recurring dermatitis	Clinical evaluation
Contact dermatitis	Dermatitis secondary to contact with allergen; erythema, vesicles	Clinical evaluation
Dermatophytosis (eg, tinea capitis, tinea corporis, tinea cruris, tinea pedis)	Localized itching, circular lesions with raised scaly borders, areas of alopecia Common sites are genital area and feet in adults; scalp and body in children Sometimes, predisposing factors (eg, moisture, obesity)	KOH examination of lesion scrapings
Lichen simplex chronicus	Areas of skin thickening secondary to repetitive scratching Lesions are discrete, erythematous, scaly plaques, well-circumscribed, rough, lichenified skin	Clinical evaluation
Pediculosis	Common sites are scalp, axillae, waist, and pubic area Areas of excoriation, possible punctate lesions from fresh bites, possible bilateral blepharitis	Visualization of eggs (nits), and sometimes lice
Psoriasis	Plaques with silvery scale typically on extensor surfaces of elbow, knees, scalp, and trunk Itching not necessarily limited to plaques Possibly small-joint arthritis manifesting as stiffness and pain	Clinical evaluation

Table continues on the following page.

Table 119–1. SOME CAUSES OF ITCHING (*Continued*)

CAUSE	SUGGESTIVE FINDINGS	DIAGNOSTIC APPROACH
Scabies	Small erythematous or dark papules at one end of a fine, wavy, slightly scaly line up to 1 cm long (burrow); possibly on web spaces, belt line, flexor surfaces, and areolas of women and genitals of men Family or close community members with similar symptoms Intense nocturnal itching	Clinical evaluation Microscopic examination of skin scrapings from burrows
Urticaria	Evanescent, circumscribed, raised, erythematous lesions with central pallor Can be acute or chronic (≥ 6 wk)	Clinical evaluation
Xerosis (dry skin)	Most common in the winter Itchy, dry, scaly skin, mostly on lower extremities Exacerbated by dry heat	Clinical evaluation
Systemic disorders		
Allergic reaction, internal (numerous ingested substances)	Generalized itching, rash with macules and papules or urticarial rash May or may not have known allergy	Trial of avoidance Sometimes skin-prick testing
Cancer (eg, Hodgkin lymphoma, polycythemia vera, mycosis fungoides)	Itching may precede any other symptoms Burning quality to itching, primarily in lower extremities (Hodgkin lymphoma) Itching after bathing (polycythemia vera) Heterogeneous cutaneous lesions—plaques, patches, tumors, erythroderma (mycosis fungoides)	CBC Peripheral smear Chest x-ray Biopsy (bone marrow for polycythemia vera, lymph node for Hodgkin lymphoma, skin lesion for mycosis fungoides)
Cholestasis	Findings suggestive of liver or gallbladder damage or dysfunction (eg, jaundice, steatorrhea, fatigue, right upper quadrant pain) Usually widespread itching without rash, developing sometimes in late pregnancy	Liver function tests and evaluation for cause of jaundice
Diabetes*	Urinary frequency, thirst, weight loss, vision changes	Urine and blood glucose HbA_{1C}
Iron deficiency anemia	Fatigue, headache, irritability, exercise intolerance, pica, hair thinning	Hb, Hct, red cell indices, serum ferritin, iron, and iron-binding capacity
Multiple sclerosis	Intermittent intense itching, numbness, tingling in limbs, optic neuritis, vision loss, spasticity or weakness, vertigo	MRI CSF analysis Evoked potentials
Psychiatric illness	Linear excoriations, presence of psychiatric condition (eg, clinical depression, delusions of parasitosis)	Clinical evaluation Diagnosis of exclusion
Renal disease	End-stage renal disease Generalized itching, may be worse during dialysis, may be prominent on the back	Diagnosis of exclusion
Thyroid disorders*	Weight loss, heart palpitations, sweating, irritability (hyperthyroidism) Weight gain, depression, dry skin and hair (hypothyroidism)	TSH, T_4
Drugs		
Drugs (eg, opioids, penicillin, ACE inhibitors, statins, antimalarials, epidermal growth factor inhibitors, interleukin 2, vemurafenib, ipilimumab, other anti-neoplastic agents)	History of ingestion	Clinical evaluation

*Itching as the patient's presenting complaint is unusual.
HbA_{1C} = glycosylated Hb; KOH = potassium hydroxide; T_4 = thyroxine; TSH = thyroid-stimulating hormone.

Systemic disorders: In systemic disorders, itching may occur with or without skin lesions. However, when itching is prominent without any identifiable skin lesions, systemic disorders and drugs should be considered more strongly. Systemic disorders are less often a cause of itching than skin disorders, but some of the more common causes include

- Allergic reaction (eg, to foods, drugs, and bites and stings)
- Cholestasis
- Chronic kidney disease

Less common systemic causes of itching include hyperthyroidism, hypothyroidism, diabetes, iron deficiency, dermatitis herpetiformis, and polycythemia vera.

Drugs: Drugs can cause itching as an allergic reaction or by directly triggering histamine release (most commonly morphine, some IV contrast agents).

Evaluation

History: **History of present illness** should determine onset of itching, initial location, course, duration, patterns of itching (eg, nocturnal or diurnal, intermittent or persistent, seasonal variation), and whether any rash is present. A careful drug history should be obtained including both prescription and OTC medications with particular attention paid to recently started drugs. The patient's use of moisturizers and other topicals (eg, hydrocortisone, diphenhydramine) should be reviewed. History should include any factors that make the itching better or worse.

Review of systems should seek symptoms of causative disorders, including

- Irritability, sweating, weight loss, and palpitations (hyperthyroidism)
- Depression, dry skin, and weight gain (hypothyroidism)
- Headache, pica, hair thinning, and exercise intolerance (iron deficiency anemia)
- Constitutional symptoms of weight loss, fatigue, and night sweats (cancer)
- Intermittent weakness, numbness, tingling, and visual disturbances or loss (multiple sclerosis)
- Steatorrhea, jaundice, and right upper quadrant pain (cholestasis)
- Urinary frequency, excessive thirst, and weight loss (diabetes)

Past medical history should identify known causative disorders (eg, renal disease, cholestatic disorder, cancer being treated with chemotherapy) and the patient's emotional state. Social history should focus on family members with similar itching and skin symptoms (eg, scabies, pediculosis); relationship of itching to occupation or exposures to plants, animals, or chemicals; and history of recent travel.

Physical examination: Physical examination begins with a review of clinical appearance for signs of jaundice, weight loss or gain, and fatigue. Close examination of the skin should be done, taking note of presence, morphology, extent, and distribution of lesions. Cutaneous examination also should make note of signs of secondary infection (eg, erythema, swelling, warmth, yellow or honey-colored crusting).

The examination should make note of significant adenopathy suggestive of cancer. Abdominal examination should focus on organomegaly, masses, and tenderness (cholestatic disorder or cancer). Neurologic examination should focus on weakness, spasticity, or numbness (multiple sclerosis).

Red flags: The following findings are of particular concern:

- Constitutional symptoms of weight loss, fatigue, and night sweats
- Extremity weakness, numbness, or tingling
- Abdominal pain and jaundice
- Urinary frequency, excessive thirst, and weight loss

Interpretation of findings: Generalized itching that begins shortly after use of a drug is likely caused by that drug. Localized itching (often with rash) that occurs in the area of contact with a substance is likely caused by that substance. However, many systemic allergies can be difficult to identify because patients typically have consumed multiple different foods and have been in contact with many substances before developing itching. Similarly, identifying a drug cause in a patient taking several drugs may be difficult. Sometimes the patient has been taking the offending drug for months or even years before developing a reaction.

If an etiology is not immediately obvious, the appearance and location of skin lesions can suggest a diagnosis (see Table 119–1).

In the minority of patients in whom no skin lesions are evident, a systemic disorder should be considered. Some disorders that cause itching are readily apparent on evaluation (eg, chronic renal failure, cholestatic jaundice). Other systemic disorders that cause itching are suggested by findings (see Table 119–1). Rarely, itching is the first manifestation of significant systemic disorders (eg, polycythemia vera, certain cancers, hyperthyroidism).

Testing: Many dermatologic disorders are diagnosed clinically. However, when itching is accompanied by discrete skin lesions of uncertain etiology, biopsy can be appropriate. When an allergic reaction is suspected but the substance is unknown, skin testing (either prick or patch testing depending on suspected etiology) is often done. When a systemic disorder is suspected, testing is directed by the suspected cause and usually involves CBC; liver, renal, and thyroid function measurements; and appropriate evaluation for underlying cancer.

Treatment

Any underlying disorder is treated. Supportive treatment involves the following (see also Table 119–2):

- Local skin care
- Topical treatment
- Systemic treatment

Skin care: Itching due to any cause benefits from use of cool or lukewarm (but not hot) water when bathing, mild or moisturizing soap, limited bathing duration and frequency, frequent lubrication, humidification of dry air, and avoidance of irritating or tight clothing. Avoidance of contact irritants (eg, wool clothing) also may be helpful.

Topical drugs: Topical drugs may help localized itching. Options include lotions or creams that contain camphor and/or menthol, pramoxine, capsaicin, or corticosteroids. Corticosteroids are effective in relieving itch caused by inflammation but should be avoided for conditions that have no evidence of inflammation. Topical benzocaine, diphenhydramine, and doxepin should be avoided because they may sensitize the skin.

Systemic drugs: Systemic drugs are indicated for generalized itching or local itching resistant to topical agents. Antihistamines, most notably hydroxyzine, are effective, especially for nocturnal itch, and are most commonly used. Sedating antihistamines must be used cautiously in elderly patients during the day because they can lead to falls; newer nonsedating antihistamines such as loratadine, fexofenadine, and cetirizine can be useful for daytime itching. Other drugs include doxepin (typically taken at night due to high level of sedation), cholestyramine (for renal failure, cholestasis, and polycythemia vera), opioid antagonists

Table 119–2. SOME THERAPEUTIC APPROACHES TO ITCHING

DRUG/AGENT	USUAL REGIMEN	COMMENTS
Topical therapy		
Capsaicin cream	Apply regularly for required period of time to a localized area of neuropathic itch	May require ≥ 2 wk for effect Vegetable oil can help with removal Initial burning sensation dissipates with time
Corticosteroid creams or ointments	Apply to affected area twice daily for 5–7 days	Avoid face, moist skinfolds Should not be used for prolonged periods of time (> 2 wk)
Menthol-containing and/or camphor-containing creams	Apply to affected areas as needed for relief	These preparations have strong odors
Pramoxine cream	Apply as needed, 4–6 times/day	Can cause dryness or irritation at application site
Tacrolimus ointment or pimecrolimus cream	Apply to affected area twice daily for 10 days	Should not be used for long periods of time or on children < 2 yr
Ultraviolet B therapy	1–3 times/wk until itching lessens Treatment often continued for months	Sunburn-like adverse effects can occur Long-term risk of skin cancer, including melanoma
Systemic therapy		
Cetirizine*	5–10 mg po once/day	Rarely can have a sedating effect in elderly patients
Cholestyramine (cholestatic pruritus)	4–16 g po once/day	Adherence can be poor Constipating, unpalatable Can interfere with absorption of other drugs
Cyproheptadine†	4 mg po tid	Sedating, also helpful when given before bedtime
Diphenhydramine†	25–50 mg po q 4–6 h (no more than 6 doses in 24 h)	Sedating, also helpful when given before bedtime
Doxepin	25 mg po once/day	Helpful in severe and chronic itching Very sedating so taken at bedtime
Fexofenadine*	60 mg po bid	Headache can be an adverse effect
Gabapentin (uremic pruritus)	100 mg po after hemodialysis	Sedation can be a problem Low doses to start and titrated up to clinical effect
Hydroxyzine†	25–50 mg po q 4–6 h (no more than 6 doses in 24 h)	Sedating, also helpful when given before bedtime
Loratadine*	10 mg po once/day	Rarely can have a sedating effect in elderly patients
Naltrexone (cholestatic pruritus)	12.5–50 mg po once/day	Can lead to withdrawal symptoms in patients with tolerance to opioids

*Nonsedating antihistamine.
†Sedating antihistamine.

such as naltrexone (for biliary pruritus), and possibly gabapentin (for uremic pruritus).

Physical agents that may be effective for itching include ultraviolet phototherapy.

Geriatrics Essentials

Age-related changes in the immune system and in nerve fibers may contribute to the high prevalence of itch in older adults.

Xerotic eczema is very common among elderly patients. It is especially likely if itching is primarily on the lower extremities.

Severe, diffuse itching in the elderly should raise concern for cancer, especially if another etiology is not immediately apparent.

When treating the elderly, sedation can be a significant problem with antihistamines. Use of nonsedating antihistamines during the day and sedating antihistamines at night, liberal use of topical ointments and corticosteroids (when appropriate), and consideration of ultraviolet phototherapy can help avoid the complications of sedation.

KEY POINTS

- Itching is usually a symptom of a skin disorder or systemic allergic reaction but can result from a systemic disorder.
- If skin lesions are not evident, systemic causes should be investigated.
- Skin care (eg, limiting bathing, avoiding irritants, moisturizing regularly, humidifying environment) should be observed.
- Symptoms can be relieved by topical or systemic drugs.

URTICARIA

(Hives; Wheals)

Urticaria consists of migratory, well-circumscribed, erythematous, pruritic plaques on the skin (see Plate 61).

Urticaria also may be accompanied by angioedema, which results from mast cell and basophil activation in the deeper dermis and subcutaneous tissues and manifests as edema of the face and lips, extremities, or genitals. Angioedema can occur in the bowel and present as colicky abdominal pain. Angioedema can be life-threatening if airway obstruction occurs because of laryngeal edema or tongue swelling.

Pathophysiology

Urticaria results from the release of histamine, bradykinin, kallikrein, and other vasoactive substances from mast cells and basophils in the superficial dermis, resulting in intradermal edema caused by capillary and venous vasodilation and occasionally caused by leukocyte infiltration.

The process can be immune mediated or nonimmune mediated.

Immune-mediated mast cell activation includes

- Type I hypersensitivity reactions, in which allergen-bound IgE antibodies bind to high-affinity cell surface receptors on mast cells and basophils
- Autoimmune disorders, in which antibodies to an IgE receptor functionally cross-link IgE receptors and cause mast cell degranulation

Nonimmune-mediated mast cell activation includes

- Direct nonallergic activation of mast cells by certain drugs
- Drug-induced cyclooxygenase inhibition that activates mast cells by poorly understood mechanisms
- Activation by physical or emotional stimuli; mechanism is poorly understood but possibly involves the release of neuropeptides that interact with mast cells

Etiology

Urticaria is classified as acute (< 6 wk) or chronic (> 6 wk); acute cases (70%) are more common than chronic (30%).

Acute urticaria (see Table 119–3) most often results from

- Type I hypersensitivity reactions

A presumptive trigger (eg, drug, food ingestion, insect bite or sting, infcction) occasionally can bc idcntificd.

Chronic urticaria most often results from

- Idiopathic causes
- Autoimmune disorders

Chronic urticaria often lasts months to years, eventually resolving without a cause being found.

Evaluation

Because there are no definitive diagnostic tests for urticaria, evaluation largely relies on history and physical examination.

History: History of present illness should include a detailed account of the individual episodes of urticaria, including distribution, sizc, and appcarancc of lcsions; frcqucncy of occurrence; duration of individual lesions; and any prior episodes. Activities and exposures during, immediately before, and within the past 24 h of the appearance of urticaria should be noted. Clinicians specifically should ask about recent exercise; exposure to potential allergens (see Table 119–3), insects, or animals; new laundry detergent or soaps; new foods; recent infections; or recent stressful life events. The patient should be asked about the duration between any suspected

Table 119–3. SOME CAUSES OF URTICARIA

CAUSE	SUGGESTIVE FINDINGS	DIAGNOSTIC APPROACH
Acute urticaria		
Contact or inhaled allergens (eg, latex, animal saliva, dust, pollen, molds, dander)	Onset within minutes or hours after contact with offending agent	Clinical evaluation Sometimes allergy testing
Drug effects • Cyclooxygenase inhibition (eg, aspirin, NSAIDs) • Direct mast cell release (eg, opioids, vancomycin, succinylcholine, curare, radiocontrast agents) • IgE mediated (any prescription, OTC, or herbal drug) • Increased bradykinin levels (ACE inhibitors)	Urticaria within 48 h of drug exposure Angioedema common with ACE inhibitors	Clinical evaluation Sometimes allergy testing
Emotional or physical stimuli • Adrenergic (stress, anxiety) • Cholinergic (sweating, eg, while taking a warm bath, while exercising, or during episodes of fever) • Cold • Delayed pressure • Exercise • Focal pressure (dermatographism) • Heat • Sunlight (solar urticaria) • Vibration	Onset typically within seconds or minutes of offending stimulus	Clinical evaluation, including reproducible response to suspected stimulus

Table continues on the following page.

Table 119–3. SOME CAUSES OF URTICARIA (*Continued*)

CAUSE	SUGGESTIVE FINDINGS	DIAGNOSTIC APPROACH
Infections • Bacterial (eg, group A streptococci, *Helicobacter pylori*) • Parasitic (eg, *Toxocara canis, Giardia lamblia, Strongyloides stercoralis, Trichuris trichiura, Blastocystis hominis, Schistosoma mansoni*) • Viral (eg, hepatitis A, B, or C; HIV; CMV; EBV; enterovirus)	Symptoms of systemic infection*	Testing for specific suspected underlying infection Resolution of urticaria after eradication of the infection
Ingested allergens (eg, peanuts, tree nuts, fish, shellfish, wheat, eggs, milk, soybeans)	Urticaria within minutes or hours after ingestion of offending agent	Clinical evaluation Sometimes allergy testing
Insect bites or stings (*Hymenoptera* venom)	Urticaria within seconds or minutes after insect bite or sting	Clinical evaluation
Serum sickness	Urticaria with or without fever, polyarthralgias, polyarthritis, lymphadenopathy, proteinuria, edema, and abdominal pain within 7–10 days after parenteral administration of a biologic-based drug or substance	Clinical evaluation
Transfusion reactions	Urticaria usually within a few minutes after initiating blood product transfusion (or switching to a new unit of blood product)	Clinical evaluation
Chronic urticaria		
Autoimmune disorders (eg, SLE, Sjögren syndrome, autoimmune thyroid disease, cryoglobulinemia, urticarial vasculitis)	Evidence of systemic autoimmune disease, including hypothyroidism or hyperthyroidism (autoimmune thyroiditis); hepatitis, renal failure, and polyarthritis (cryoglobulinemia); malar rash, serositis, and polyarthritis (SLE); dry eyes and dry mouth (Sjögren syndrome); cutaneous ulcers or hypopigmented lesions after resolution of urticaria (urticarial vasculitis)	TSH measurement Thyroid autoantibodies (eg, thyroid peroxidase antibodies, antimicrosomal antibodies) Cryoglobulin titers Rheumatologic serologies (eg, ANA, RF, anti-SS-A, anti-SS-B, anti-Sm, anti-RNP, anti-Jo-1) Skin biopsy (cryoglobulinemia, urticarial vasculitis)
Cancer (typically GI, lung, lymphoma)	Signs of underlying cancer (eg, weight loss, night sweats, abdominal pain, cough, hemoptysis, jaundice, lymphadenopathy, melena)	Specific to the type of suspected underlying cancer
Chronic idiopathic urticaria	Occurrence of daily (or almost daily) wheals, and itching for at least 6 wk, with no obvious cause	Diagnosis of exclusion
Drugs (same as those causing acute urticaria)	Unexplained urticaria in a patient chronically taking prescription, OTC, or herbal drugs	Clinical evaluation Sometimes allergy testing Resolution with stoppage of offending drug
Emotional or physical stimuli (same as those causing acute urticaria)	Urticaria typically within seconds or minutes of offending stimulus	Clinical evaluation, including reproducible response to suspected stimulus
Endocrine abnormalities (eg, thyroid dysfunction, elevated progesterone level)	Heat or cold intolerance, bradycardia or tachycardia, hyporeflexia or hyperreflexia Patients taking progesterone-containing oral contraceptives or hormone replacement therapy or those with cyclic urticaria that appears during the 2nd half of the menstrual cycle and resolves with menstruation	Clinical evaluation TSH measurement
Systemic mastocytosis (urticaria pigmentosa)	Presence of small pigmented papules that turn into wheals with mild trauma (eg, gentle stroking) Possible concomitant anemia, abdominal pain, easy flushing, and recurrent headaches	Skin biopsy Serum tryptase level

*Patients should be asked about recent travel to a developing country.
ANA = antinuclear antibodies; CMV = cytomegalovirus; EBV = Epstein-Barr virus; RF = rheumatoid factor; TSH = thyroid-stimulating hormone.

trigger and the appearance of urticaria and which particular triggers are suspected. Important associated symptoms include pruritus, rhinorrhea, swelling of the face and tongue, and dyspnea.

Review of systems should seek symptoms of causative disorders, including fever, fatigue, abdominal pain, and diarrhea (infection); heat or cold intolerance, tremor, or weight change (autoimmune thyroiditis); joint pain (cryoglobulinemia, SLE); malar rash (SLE); dry eyes and dry mouth (Sjögren syndrome); cutaneous ulcers and hyperpigmented lesions after resolution of urticaria (urticarial vasculitis); small pigmented papules (mastocytosis); lymphadenopathy (viral illness, cancer, serum sickness); acute or chronic diarrhea (viral or parasitic enterocolitis); and fevers, night sweats, or weight loss (cancer).

Past medical history should include a detailed allergy history, including known atopic conditions (eg, allergies, asthma, eczema) and known possible causes (eg, autoimmune disorders, cancer). All drug use should be reviewed, including OTC drugs and herbal products, specifically any agents particularly associated with urticaria (see Table 119–3). Family history should elicit any history of rheumatoid disease, autoimmune disorders, or cancer. Social history should cover any recent travel and any risk factors for transmission of infectious disease (eg, hepatitis, HIV).

Physical examination: Vital signs should note the presence of bradycardia or tachycardia and tachypnea. General examination should immediately seek any signs of respiratory distress and also note cachexia, jaundice, or agitation.

Examination of the head should note any swelling of the face, lips, or tongue; scleral icterus; malar rash; tender and enlarged thyroid; lymphadenopathy; or dry eyes and dry mouth. The oropharynx should be inspected and the sinuses should be palpated and transilluminated for signs of occult infection (eg, sinus infection, tooth abscess).

Abdominal examination should note any masses, hepatomegaly, splenomegaly, or tenderness. Neurologic examination should note any tremor or hyperreflexia or hyporeflexia. Musculoskeletal examination should note the presence of any inflamed or deformed joints.

Skin examination should note the presence and distribution of urticarial lesions as well as any cutaneous ulceration, hyperpigmentation, small papules, or jaundice. Urticarial lesions usually appear as well-demarcated transient swellings involving the dermis. These swellings are typically red and vary in size from pinprick to covering wide areas. Some lesions can be very large. In other cases, smaller urticarial lesions may become confluent. However, skin lesions also may be absent at the time of the visit. Maneuvers to evoke physical urticaria can be done during the examination, including exposure to vibration (tuning fork), warmth (tuning fork held under warm water), cold (stethoscope or chilled tuning fork), water, or pressure (lightly scratching an unaffected area with a fingernail).

Red flags: The following findings are of particular concern:

- Angioedema (swelling of the face, lips, or tongue)
- Stridor, wheezing, or other respiratory distress
- Hyperpigmented lesions, ulcers, or urticaria that persist > 48 h
- Signs of systemic illness (eg, fever, lymphadenopathy, jaundice, cachexia)

Interpretation of findings: Acute urticaria is nearly always due to some defined exposure to a drug or physical stimulus or an acute infectious illness. However, the trigger is not always clear from the history, particularly because allergy may develop without warning to a previously tolerated substance.

Most **chronic urticaria** is idiopathic. The next most common cause is an autoimmune disorder. The causative autoimmune disease is sometimes clinically apparent. Urticarial vasculitis sometimes is associated with connective tissue disorders (particularly SLE or Sjögren syndrome). In urticarial vasculitis, urticaria is accompanied by findings of cutaneous vasculitis; it should be considered when the urticaria is painful rather than pruritic, lasts > 48 h, does not blanch, or is accompanied by vesicles or purpura.

Testing: Usually, no testing is needed for an isolated episode of urticaria unless symptoms and signs suggest a specific disorder (eg, infection).

Unusual, recurrent, or persistent cases warrant further evaluation. Referral for allergy skin testing should be done, and routine laboratory tests should consist of CBC, blood chemistries, liver function tests, and thyroid-stimulating hormone (TSH). Further testing should be guided by symptoms and signs (eg, of autoimmune disorders) and any abnormalities on the screening tests (eg, hepatitis serologies and ultrasonography for abnormal liver function tests; ova and parasites for eosinophilia; cryoglobulin titer for elevated liver function tests or elevated creatinine; thyroid autoantibodies for abnormal TSH).

Skin biopsy should be done if there is any uncertainty as to the diagnosis or if wheals persist > 48 h (to rule out urticarial vasculitis).

Clinicians should not recommend the patient do an empiric challenge (eg, "Try such and such again and see whether you get a reaction") because subsequent reactions may be more severe.

Treatment

Any identified causes are treated or remedied. Implicated drugs or foods should be stopped.

Nonspecific symptomatic treatment (eg, taking cool baths, avoiding hot water and scratching, wearing loose clothing) may be helpful.

Drugs: Antihistamines remain the mainstay of treatment. They must be taken on a regular basis, rather than as needed. Newer oral antihistamines often are preferred because of once-daily dosing and because some are less sedating. Appropriate choices include

- Cetirizine 10 mg once/day
- Fexofenadine 180 mg once/day
- Desloratadine 5 mg once/day
- Levocetirizine 5 mg once/day

Older oral antihistamines (eg, hydroxyzine 10 to 25 mg q 4 to 6 h; diphenhydramine 25 to 50 mg q 6 h) are sedating but inexpensive and sometimes quite effective.

Systemic corticosteroids (eg, prednisone 30 to 40 mg po once/day) are given for severe symptoms but should not be used long term. Topical corticosteroids or topical antihistamines are not beneficial.

Patients with chronic idiopathic urticaria often do not respond to antihistamines or other drugs commonly used. Omalizumab, a monoclonal antibody that can suppress certain allergic reactions, may help relieve symptoms, but experience with this use is limited.

Angioedema: Patients who have angioedema involving the oropharynx or any involvement of the airway should receive epinephrine 0.3 mL of 1:1000 solution sc and be admitted to the hospital. On discharge, patients should be supplied with and trained in the use of an auto-injectable epinephrine pen.

Geriatrics Essentials

The older oral antihistamines (eg, hydroxyzine, diphenhydramine) are sedating and can cause confusion, urinary retention, and delirium. They should be used cautiously to treat urticaria in elderly patients.

KEY POINTS

- Urticaria can be caused by allergic or nonallergic mechanisms.
- Most acute cases are caused by an allergic reaction to a specific substance.
- Most chronic cases are idiopathic or result from autoimmune disease.
- Treatment is based on severity; nonsedating antihistamines and avoidance of triggers are first-line options.
- Topical corticosteroids and topical antihistamines are not beneficial.
- Concomitant systemic symptoms require a thorough evaluation for the etiology.

SKIN MANIFESTATIONS OF INTERNAL DISEASE

The skin frequently serves as a marker for underlying internal disease. The type of lesion typically relates to a specific disease or type of disease.

Internal cancer: Patients with dermatomyositis who are over age 40 have an increased risk of breast, lung, ovarian, and GI cancers.

Acute onset of multiple seborrheic keratoses (Leser-Trélat sign) may indicate underlying internal cancer, particularly adenocarcinoma. However, because of the high prevalence of seborrheic keratoses in healthy adults, this sign may be overdiagnosed.

Acute febrile neutrophilic dermatosis (Sweet syndrome) is sometimes associated with hematologic cancer.

Acanthosis nigricans (see Plate 27) that is associated with cancer can be of rapid onset and particularly widespread. Acquired ichthyosis or pruritus without a clearly associated dermatitis may indicate occult cancer, often lymphoma.

Paraneoplastic pemphigus is a relatively rare autoimmune blistering disease that has been associated with various cancers, including leukemias.

Carcinoid syndrome (flushing and erythema of the neck) is associated with carcinoid tumor.

Erythema gyratum repens is a rare eruption consisting of concentric erythematous lesions, resembling wood grain, which has been associated with various cancers.

Endocrinopathies: Many skin findings are associated with endocrinopathies but are not specific.

Patients with diabetes mellitus may have acanthosis nigricans, necrobiosis lipoidica, perforating disorders, and scleredema.

Thyroid disease, both hypothyroidism and hyperthyroidism, can affect hair, nails, and skin.

Cushing syndrome causes striae distensae, moon facies, and skin fragility.

Addison disease is characterized by hyperpigmentation that is accentuated in skin creases and areas of trauma.

GI disorders: Skin conditions commonly associated with GI disorders include

- Pyoderma gangrenosum: Inflammatory bowel disease
- Lichen planus and porphyria cutanea tarda: Hepatitis C infection
- Diffuse hyperpigmentation in patients with diabetes (known as bronze diabetes): Hemochromatosis
- Erythema nodosum: Inflammatory bowel disease, sarcoidosis, and various infections
- Eruptive xanthomas: Elevated serum triglycerides

120 Principles of Topical Dermatologic Therapy

Topical dermatologic treatments are grouped according to their therapeutic functions and include

- Cleansing agents
- Absorbent dressings (eg, hydrocolloid patches or powder) and super-absorbent powders
- Anti-infective agents
- Anti-inflammatory agents
- Astringents (drying agents that precipitate protein and shrink and contract the skin)
- Drying agents
- Moisturizing agents (emollients, skin hydrators, and softeners)
- Keratolytics (agents that soften, loosen, and facilitate exfoliation of the squamous cells of the epidermis)
- Antipruritics

For certain topical treatments, successful therapy may also depend on

- The vehicle with which an agent is formulated
- The type of dressing used

Vehicles

Topical therapies can be delivered in various vehicles, which include

- Powders
- Liquids
- Combinations of liquid and oil

The vehicle influences a therapy's effectiveness and may itself cause adverse effects (eg, contact or irritant dermatitis). Generally, aqueous and alcohol-based preparations are drying because the liquid evaporates and are used in acute inflammatory conditions. Powders are also drying. Oil-based preparations are moisturizing and are preferred for chronic inflammation. Vehicle selection is guided by location of application, cosmetic effects, and convenience.

Powders: Inert powders may be mixed with active agents (eg, antifungals) to deliver therapy. They are prescribed for lesions in moist or intertriginous areas.

Liquids: Liquid vehicles include

- Baths and soaks
- Foams
- Solutions
- Lotions
- Gels

Baths and soaks are used when therapy must be applied to large areas, such as with extensive contact dermatitis or atopic dermatitis.

Foams are alcohol- or emollient-based aerosolized preparations. They tend to be rapidly absorbed and may be favored in hair-bearing areas of the body.

Solutions are ingredients dissolved in a solvent, usually ethyl alcohol, propylene glycol, polyethylene glycol, or water. Solutions are convenient to apply (especially to the scalp for disorders such as psoriasis or seborrhea) but tend to be drying. Two common solutions are Burow solution and Domeboro® solution.

Lotions are water-based emulsions. They are easily applied to hairy skin. Lotions cool and dry acute inflammatory and exudative lesions, such as contact dermatitis, tinea pedis, and tinea cruris.

Gels are ingredients suspended in a solvent thickened with polymers. Gels are often more effective for controlled release of topical agents. They are often used in acne, rosacea, and psoriasis of the scalp.

Combination vehicles: Combinations include

- Creams
- Ointments

Combination vehicles usually contain oil and water but may also contain propylene or polyethylene glycol.

Creams are semi-solid emulsions of oil and water. They are used for moisturizing and cooling and when exudation is present. They vanish when rubbed into skin.

Ointments are oil based (eg, petrolatum) with little if any water. Ointments are optimal lubricants and increase drug penetration because of their occlusive nature; a given concentration of drug is typically more potent in an ointment. They are preferred for lichenified lesions and lesions with thick crusts or heaped-up scales, including psoriasis and lichen simplex chronicus. Ointments are less irritating than creams for erosions or ulcers. They are usually best applied after bathing or dampening the skin with water.

Dressings

Dressings protect open lesions, facilitate healing, increase drug absorption, and protect the patient's clothing.

Nonocclusive dressings: The most common nonocclusive dressings are gauze dressings. They maximally allow air to reach the wound, which is at times preferred in healing, and allow the lesion to dry.

Wet-to-dry dressings are nonocclusive dressings wetted with solution, usually saline, that are used to help cleanse and debride thickened or crusted lesions. The dressings are applied wet and removed after the solution has evaporated (ie, wet-to-dry), with materials from the skin adhering to the dried dressing.

Occlusive dressings: Occlusive dressings increase the absorption and effectiveness of topical therapy. Most common are transparent films such as polyethylene (plastic household wrap) or flexible, transparent, semi-permeable dressings. Hydrocolloid dressings can be applied with a gauze cover in patients with cutaneous ulceration. Zinc oxide gelatin (Unna paste boot) is an effective occlusive dressing for patients with stasis dermatitis and ulcers. Plastic tape impregnated with flurandrenolide, a corticosteroid, can be used for isolated or recalcitrant lesions.

Occlusive dressings applied over topical corticosteroids to increase absorption are sometimes used to treat psoriasis, atopic dermatitis, skin lesions resulting from systemic lupus erythematosus, and chronic hand dermatitis, among other conditions. Systemic absorption of topical corticosteroids may occur and cause adrenal suppression. Local adverse effects of topical corticosteroids include

- Development of miliaria
- Skin atrophy
- Striae
- Bacterial or fungal infections
- Acneiform eruptions

Other occlusive dressings are used to protect and help heal open wounds, such as burns; special silicone dressings are sometimes used for keloids.

Topical Agents

Major categories of topical agents include

- Cleansing
- Moisturizing
- Drying
- Anti-inflammatory
- Antimicrobial
- Keratolytic
- Astringent
- Antipruritic

Cleansing agents: The principal cleansing agents are soaps, detergents, and solvents. Soap is the most popular cleanser, but synthetic detergents are also used. Baby shampoos are usually well tolerated around the eyes and for cleansing wounds and abrasions; they are useful for removing crusts and scales in psoriasis, eczema, and other forms of dermatitis. However, acutely irritated, weeping, or oozing lesions are most comfortably cleansed with water or isotonic saline.

Water is the principal solvent for cleansing. Organic solvents (eg, acetone, petroleum products, propylene glycol) are very drying, can be irritating, and cause irritant or, less commonly, allergic contact dermatitis. Removal of hardened tar and dried paint from the skin may require a petrolatum-based ointment or commercial waterless cleanser.

Moisturizing agents: Moisturizers (emollients) restore water and oils to the skin and help maintain skin hydration. They typically contain glycerin, mineral oil, or petrolatum and are available as lotions, creams, ointments, and bath oils. Stronger moisturizers contain urea 2%, lactic acid 5 to 12%, and glycolic acid 10% (higher concentrations of glycolic acid are used as keratinolytics, eg, for ichthyosis). They are most effective when applied to already moistened skin (ie, after a bath or shower). Cold creams are moisturizing OTC emulsions of fats (eg, beeswax) and water.

Drying agents: Excessive moisture in intertriginous areas (eg, between the toes; in the intergluteal cleft, axillae, groin, and inframammary areas) can cause irritation and maceration. Powders dry macerated skin and reduce friction by absorbing moisture. However, some powders tend to clump and can be irritating if they become moist. Cornstarch and talc are most often used. Although talc is more effective, talc may cause granulomas if inhaled and is no longer used in baby powders. Cornstarch may promote fungal growth. Aluminum chloride solutions are another type of drying agent (often useful in hyperhidrosis). Super-absorbent powders (extremely absorbent powders) are occassionally required to dry very moist areas (eg, to treat intertrigo).

Anti-inflammatory agents: Topical anti-inflammatory agents are either corticosteroids or noncorticosteroids.

Corticosteroids are the mainstay of treatment for most noninfectious inflammatory dermatoses. Lotions are useful on intertriginous areas and the face. Gels are useful on the scalp and in management of contact dermatitis. Creams are useful on the face and in intertriginous areas and for management of inflammatory dermatoses. Ointments are useful for dry scaly areas and when increased potency is required. Corticosteroid-impregnated tape is useful to protect an area from excoriation. It also increases corticosteroid absorption and therefore potency.

Topical corticosteroids range in potency from mild (class VII) to superpotent (class I—see Table 120–1). Intrinsic differences

Table 120–1. RELATIVE POTENCY OF SELECTED TOPICAL CORTICOSTEROIDS

CLASS*	DRUG
I	Betamethasone dipropionate 0.05% ointment
	Clobetasol propionate 0.05% cream or ointment
	Diflorasone diacetate 0.05% ointment
	Halobetasol propionate 0.05% cream or ointment
II	Amcinonide 0.1% ointment
	Betamethasone dipropionate 0.05% cream
	Betamethasone dipropionate 0.05% ointment
	Desoximetasone 0.25% cream, 0.05% gel, 0.25% ointment
	Diflorasone diacetate 0.05% ointment
	Fluocinonide 0.05% cream, gel, ointment, or solution
	Halcinonide 0.1% cream
	Mometasone furoate 0.1% ointment
III	Amcinonide 0.1% cream or lotion
	Betamethasone dipropionate 0.05% cream
	Betamethasone dipropionate 0.05% lotion
	Betamethasone valerate 0.1% ointment
	Desoximetasone 0.05% cream
	Diflorasone diacetate 0.05% cream
	Fluocinonide cream 0.05%
	Fluticasone propionate 0.005% ointment
	Halcinonide 0.1% ointment or solution
	Triamcinolone acetonide 0.1% ointment
IV	Fluocinolone acetonide 0.025% ointment
	Flurandrenolide 0.05% ointment
	Mometasone furoate 0.1% cream or lotion
	Triamcinolone acetonide 0.1% cream or ointment
V	Betamethasone valerate 0.1% cream
	Desonide 0.05% ointment
	Fluocinolone acetonide 0.025% cream
	Flurandrenolide 0.05% cream
	Fluticasone propionate 0.05% cream
	Hydrocortisone butyrate 0.1% cream, ointment, or solution
	Hydrocortisone valerate 0.2% cream or ointment
	Triamcinolone acetonide 0.1% lotion or 0.025% ointment
VI	Alclometasone dipropionate 0.05% cream or ointment
	Betamethasone valerate 0.1% lotion
	Desonide 0.05% cream
	Flumethasone pivalate 0.03% cream
	Fluocinolone acetonide 0.01% cream or solution
	Triamcinolone acetonide 0.1% cream
	Triamcinolone acetonide 0.025% cream or lotion
VII	Hydrocortisone 1% or 2.5% cream, 1% or 2.5% lotion, 1% or 2.5% ointment
	Hydrocortisone acetate (1% or 2.5% cream, 1% or 2.5% lotion, 1% or 2.5% ointment) and pramoxine hydrochloride 1%

*Class I is the most potent, and class VII is the least potent. Potency depends on many factors, including the drug's characteristics and concentration and the base in which it is used.

in potency are attributable to fluorination or chlorination (halogenation) of the compound.

Topical corticosteroids are generally applied 2 to 3 times daily, but high-potency formulations may require application only once/day or even less frequently. Most dermatoses are treated with mid-potency to high-potency formulations; mild formulations are better for mild inflammation and for use on the face or intertriginous areas, where systemic absorption and local adverse effects are more likely. All agents can cause local skin atrophy, striae, and acneiform eruptions when used for > 1 mo. This effect is particularly problematic on the thinner skin of the face or genitals. Corticosteroids also promote fungal growth. Contact dermatitis in reaction to preservatives and additives is also common with prolonged use. Contact dermatitis to the corticosteroid itself may also occur. Perioral dermatitis occurs with mid-potency or high-potency formulations used on the face but is uncommon with mild formulations. High-potency formulations may cause adrenal suppression when used in children, over extensive skin surfaces, or for long periods. Relative contraindications include conditions in which infection plays an underlying role and acneiform disorders.

Noncorticosteroid anti-inflammatory agents include tar preparations. Tar comes in the form of crude coal tar and is indicated for psoriasis. Adverse effects include irritation, folliculitis, staining of clothes and furniture, and photosensitization. Contraindications include infected skin. Several herbal products are commonly used in commercial products, although their effectiveness has not been well established. Among the most popular are chamomile and calendula.

Antimicrobials: Topical antimicrobials include

- Antibiotics
- Antifungals
- Insecticides
- Nonspecific antiseptic agents

Antibiotics have few indications. Topical clindamycin and erythromycin are used as primary or adjunctive treatment for acne vulgaris in patients who do not warrant or tolerate oral antibiotics. Topical metronidazole and occasionally topical sulfacetamide, clindamycin, or erythromycin are used for rosacea. Mupirocin has excellent gram-positive (mainly *Staphylococcus aureus* and streptococci) coverage and can be used to treat impetigo when deep tissues are not affected.

OTC topical antibiotics such as bacitracin and polymyxin have been replaced by topical petrolatum for postoperative care of a skin biopsy site and to prevent infection in scrapes, minor burns, and excoriations. Topical petrolatum is as effective as these topical antibiotics and does not cause contact dermatitis, which these antibiotics, especially topical neomycin, can cause. Also, the use of topical antibiotics and washing with antiseptic soaps in healing wounds may actually slow healing.

Antifungals are used to treat candidiasis, a wide variety of dermatophytoses, and other fungal infections (see Table 128–1 on p. 1033).

Insecticides (eg, permethrin, malathion) are used to treat lice (see Table 132–1 on p. 1059) and scabies (see Table 132–2 on p. 1060).

Nonspecific antiseptic agents include iodine solutions (eg, povidone iodine, clioquinol), gentian violet, silver preparations (eg, silver nitrate, silver sulfadiazine), and zinc pyrithione. Iodine is indicated for presurgical skin preparation. Gentian violet is used when a chemically and physically stable antiseptic/antimicrobial is needed and must be very inexpensive. Silver preparations are effective in treating burns and ulcers and have strong antimicrobial properties; several wound dressings are impregnated with silver. Zinc pyrithione is an antifungal and a common ingredient in shampoos used to treat dandruff due to psoriasis or seborrheic dermatitis. Healing wounds should generally not be treated with topical antiseptics other than silver because they are irritating and tend to kill fragile granulation tissue.

Keratolytics: Keratolytics soften and facilitate exfoliation of epidermal cells. Examples include 3 to 6% salicylic acid and urea. Salicylic acid is used to treat psoriasis, seborrheic dermatitis, acne, and warts. Adverse effects are burning and, if large areas are covered, systemic toxicity. It should rarely be used in children and infants. Urea is used to treat plantar keratodermas and ichthyosis. Adverse effects are irritation and intractable burning. It should not be applied to large surface areas.

Astringents: Astringents are drying agents that precipitate protein and shrink and contract the skin. The most commonly used astringents are aluminum acetate (Burow solution) and aluminum sulfate plus calcium acetate (Domeboro® solution). Usually applied with dressings or as soaks, astringents are used to treat infectious eczema, exudative skin lesions, and weeping pressure ulcers. Witch hazel is a popular OTC astringent.

Antipruritics: Doxepin is a topical antihistamine that is effective in treating itching of atopic dermatitis, lichen simplex chronicus dermatitis, and nummular dermatitis. Topical benzocaine and diphenhydramine (present in certain OTC lotions) are sensitizing and not recommended. Other antipruritics include camphor 0.5 to 3%, menthol 0.1 to 0.2%, pramoxine hydrochloride, and eutectic mixture of local anesthetics (EMLA), which contain equal parts lidocaine and prilocaine in an oil-in-water vehicle. Topical antipruritics are preferred over systemic drugs (eg, oral antihistamines) when smaller surface areas of skin are affected and pruritus is not intractable. Calamine lotion is soothing but not specifically antipruritic.

121 Acne and Related Disorders

ACNE VULGARIS

(Acne)

Acne vulgaris is the formation of comedones, papules, pustules, nodules, and/or cysts as a result of obstruction and inflammation of pilosebaceous units (hair follicles and their accompanying sebaceous gland). Acne develops on the face and upper trunk. It most often affects adolescents. Diagnosis is by examination. Treatment, based on severity, can involve a variety of topical and systemic agents directed at reducing sebum production, comedone formation, inflammation, and bacterial counts and at normalizing keratinization.

Acne is the most common skin disease in the US and affects 80% of the population at some point in life.

Pathophysiology

Acne occurs through the interplay of 4 major factors:

- Excess sebum production
- Follicular plugging with sebum and keratinocytes
- Colonization of follicles by *Propionibacterium acnes* (a normal human anaerobe)
- Release of multiple inflammatory mediators

Acne can be classified as

- Noninflammatory: Characterized by comedones
- Inflammatory: Characterized by papules, pustules, nodules, and cysts

Noninflammatory acne: Comedones are sebaceous plugs impacted within follicles. They are termed open or closed depending on whether the follicle is dilated or closed at the skin surface. Plugs are easily extruded from open comedones but are more difficult to remove from closed comedones. Closed comedones are the precursor lesions to inflammatory acne.

Inflammatory acne: Papules and pustules occur when *P. acnes* colonizes the closed comedones, breaking down sebum into free fatty acids that irritate the follicular epithelium and eliciting an inflammatory response by neutrophils and then lymphocytes, which further disrupts the epithelium. The inflamed follicle ruptures into the dermis (sometimes precipitated by physical manipulation or harsh scrubbing), where the comedone contents elicit a further local inflammatory reaction, producing papules. If the inflammation is intense, grossly purulent pustules occur.

Nodules and cysts are other manifestations of inflammatory acne. Nodules are deeper lesions that may involve > 1 follicle, and cysts are large fluctuant nodules.

Etiology

The **most common** trigger is

- Puberty

During puberty, surges in androgen stimulate sebum production and hyperproliferation of keratinocytes.

Other triggers include

- Hormonal changes that occur with pregnancy or the menstrual cycle
- Occlusive cosmetics, cleansers, lotions, and clothing
- High humidity and sweating

Associations between acne exacerbation and diet, inadequate face washing, masturbation, and sex are unfounded. Some studies suggest a possible association with milk products and high-glycemic diets. Acne may abate in summer months because of sunlight's anti-inflammatory effects. Proposed associations between acne and hyperinsulinism require further investigation. Some drugs and chemicals (eg, corticosteroids, lithium, phenytoin, isoniazid) worsen acne or cause acneiform eruptions.

Symptoms and Signs

Skin lesions and scarring can be a source of significant emotional distress. Nodules and cysts can be painful. Lesion types frequently coexist at different stages.

Comedones appear as whiteheads or blackheads. Whiteheads (closed comedones) are flesh-colored or whitish palpable lesions 1 to 3 mm in diameter; blackheads (open comedones) are similar in appearance but with a dark center.

Papules and pustules are red lesions 2 to 5 mm in diameter. Papules are relatively deep. Pustules are more superficial.

Nodules are larger, deeper, and more solid than papules. Such lesions resemble inflamed epidermoid cysts, although they lack true cystic structure.

Cysts are suppurative nodules. Rarely, cysts form deep abscesses. Long-term cystic acne can cause scarring that manifests as tiny and deep pits (icepick scars), larger pits, shallow depressions, or hypertrophic scarring or keloids.

Acne conglobata is the most severe form of acne vulgaris, affecting men more than women. Patients have abscesses, draining sinuses, fistulated comedones, and keloidal and atrophic scars. The back and chest are severely involved. The arms, abdomen, buttocks, and even the scalp may be affected.

Acne fulminans is acute, febrile, ulcerative acne, characterized by the sudden appearance of confluent abscesses leading to hemorrhagic necrosis. Leukocytosis and joint pain and swelling may also be present.

Pyoderma faciale (also called rosacea fulminans) occurs suddenly on the midface of young women. It may be analogous to acne fulminans. The eruption consists of erythematous plaques and pustules, involving the chin, cheeks, and forehead. Papules and nodules may develop and become confluent.

Diagnosis

- Assessment for contributing factors (eg, hormonal, mechanical, or drug-related)
- Determination of severity (mild, moderate, severe)
- Assessment of psychosocial impact

Diagnosis of acne vulgaris is by examination.

Differential diagnosis includes rosacea (in which no comedones are seen), corticosteroid-induced acne (which lacks comedones and in which pustules are usually in the same stage of development), perioral dermatitis (usually with a more perioral and periorbital distribution), and acneiform drug eruptions (see Table 130–2 on p. 1046). Acne severity is graded mild, moderate, or severe based on the number and type of lesions; a standardized system is outlined in Table 121–1.

Prognosis

Acne of any severity usually remits spontaneously by the early to mid 20s, but a substantial minority of patients, usually women, may have acne into their 40s; options for treatment may be limited because of childbearing. Many adults occasionally develop mild, isolated acne lesions. Noninflammatory and mild inflammatory acne usually heals without scars. Moderate to severe inflammatory acne heals but often leaves scarring. Scarring is not only physical; acne may be a huge emotional stressor for adolescents who may withdraw, using

Table 121–1. CLASSIFICATION OF ACNE SEVERITY

SEVERITY	DEFINITION
Mild	< 20 comedones, or < 15 inflammatory lesions, or < 30 total lesions
Moderate	20 to 100 comedones, or 15 to 50 inflammatory lesions, or 30 to 125 total lesions
Severe	> 5 cysts, or total comedone count > 100, or total inflammatory lesion count > 50, or > 125 total lesions

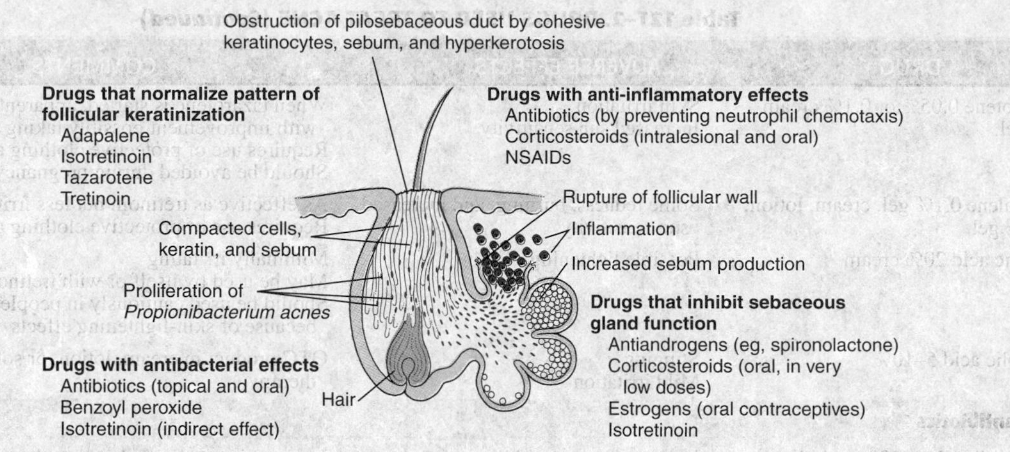

Fig. 121–1. How various drugs work in treating acne.

the acne as an excuse to avoid difficult personal adjustments. Supportive counseling for patients and parents may be indicated in severe cases.

Treatment

- Comedones: Topical tretinoin
- Mild inflammatory acne: Topical retinoid alone or with a topical antibiotic, benzoyl peroxide, or both
- Moderate acne: Oral antibiotic plus topical therapy as for mild acne
- Severe acne: Oral isotretinoin
- Cystic acne: Intralesional triamcinolone

It is important to treat acne to reduce the extent of disease, scarring, and psychologic distress.

Treatment of acne involves a variety of topical and systemic agents directed at reducing sebum production, comedone formation, inflammation, and bacterial counts and at normalizing keratinization (see Fig. 121–1). Selection of treatment is generally based on severity; options are summarized in Table 121–2. See guidelines of care for the management of acne vulgaris from the American Academy of Dermatology.

Affected areas should be cleansed daily, but extra washing, use of antibacterial soaps, and scrubbing confer no added benefit.

A lower glycemic diet and moderation of milk intake might be considered for treatment-resistant adolescent acne.

Peeling agents such as sulfur, salicylic acid, glycolic acid, and resorcinol can be useful therapeutic adjuncts but are no longer commonly used.

Table 121–2. DRUGS USED TO TREAT ACNE

DRUG	ADVERSE EFFECTS	COMMENTS
Topical antibacterials		
Benzoyl peroxide 2.5%, 5%, and 10% gel, lotion, or wash	Dry skin Possible bleaching of clothing and hair Allergic reactions (rarely)	Comedolytic and antibacterial with very low to no development of resistance Should be used in all patients if tolerated Gel product usually preferred
Benzoyl peroxide/erythromycin gel	—	Must be kept refrigerated
Benzoyl peroxide/clindamycin gel	—	—
Clindamycin 1% gel or lotion	Diarrhea (rarely)	Should be avoided in patients with inflammatory bowel disease
Erythromycin 1.5 to 2% (multiple vehicles)	—	Well-tolerated, but frequent development of bacterial resistance
Topical comedolytics and exfoliants		
Tretinoin 0.025%, 0.05%, and 0.1% cream; 0.05% liquid; 0.025% and 0.1% gel	Skin irritation Increased sun sensitivity	Initial strength should be 0.025% and, if ineffective, should be increased; if irritation occurs, strength, frequency, or both should be reduced When tretinoin is started, apparent worsening of acne, with improvement possibly taking 3 to 4 wk to occur Requires use of protective clothing and sunscreen Should be avoided during pregnancy

Table continues on the following page.

Table 121–2. DRUGS USED TO TREAT ACNE (*Continued*)

DRUG	ADVERSE EFFECTS	COMMENTS
Tazarotene 0.05% or 0.1% cream or gel	Skin irritation Increased sun sensitivity	When tazarotene is started, apparent worsening of acne, with improvement possibly taking 3 to 4 wk to occur Requires use of protective clothing and sunscreen Should be avoided during pregnancy
Adapalene 0.1% gel, cream, lotion; 0.3% gel	Some redness, burning, and increased sun sensitivity	As effective as tretinoin but less irritating Requires use of protective clothing and sunscreen
Azelaic acid 20% cream	Possible lightening of skin	Minimally irritating May be used by itself or with tretinoin Should be used cautiously in people with darker skin because of skin-lightening effects
Glycolic acid 5–10%	Stinging Mild irritation	OTC product in cream, lotion, or solution; adjunct therapy
Oral antibiotics		
Tetracycline 250–500 mg bid	Increased sun sensitivity	Inexpensive and safe, but must be taken on an empty stomach Requires use of protective clothing and sunscreen
Doxycycline 50–100 mg bid	Increased sun sensitivity	Good first-line drug in terms of efficacy and cost Requires use of protective clothing and sunscreen
Minocycline 50–100 mg bid	Headache Dizziness Skin discoloration	Most effective antibiotic but is expensive
Erythromycin 250–500 mg bid	Stomach upset	Frequent development of bacterial resistance
Oral retinoid		
Isotretinoin 1–2 mg/kg once/day for 16–20 wk	Possible harm to a developing fetus Possible effect on blood cells, the liver, and fat (triglyceride and cholesterol) levels Dry eyes, chapped lips, drying of mucous membranes Pain or stiffness of large joints and lower back with high dosages Associated with depression, suicidal thoughts, attempted suicide, and (rarely) completed suicide Unclear whether associated with new or worsened inflammatory bowel disease (Crohn disease and ulcerative colitis)	For sexually active women, requires a pregnancy test before the start of therapy with isotretinoin and at monthly intervals during use of the drug plus use of 2 forms of contraception or sexual abstinence, beginning 1 mo before the drug is started, continued during drug use, and for 1 mo after stopping the drug Requires periodic CBC, liver function tests, fasting glucose, and lipid profile

Oral contraceptives are effective in treating inflammatory and noninflammatory acne, and spironolactone (beginning at 50 mg po once/day, increased to 100 mg po once/day after a few mo if needed) is another anti-androgen that is occasionally useful in women. Various light therapies, with and without topical photosensitizers, have been used effectively, mostly for inflammatory acne.

Treatment should involve educating the patient and tailoring the plan to one that is realistic for the patient. Treatment failure can frequently be attributed to lack of adherence to the plan and also to lack of follow-up. Consultation with a specialist may be necessary.

Mild acne: Treatment of mild acne should be continued for 6 wk or until lesions respond. Maintenance treatment may be necessary to maintain control.

Single-agent therapy is generally sufficient for comedonal acne. A mainstay of treatment for comedones is daily topical tretinoin as tolerated. Daily adapalene gel, tazarotene cream or gel, azelaic acid cream, and glycolic or salicylic acid are alternatives for patients who cannot tolerate topical tretinoin. Adverse effects include erythema, burning, stinging, and peeling. Adapalene and tazarotene are retinoids; like tretinoin, they tend to be somewhat irritating and photosensitizing. Azelaic acid has comedolytic and antibacterial properties by an unrelated mechanism and may be synergistic with retinoids.

Dual therapy (eg, a combination of tretinoin with benzoyl peroxide, a topical antibiotic, or both) should be used to treat mild papulopustular (inflammatory) acne. The topical antibiotic is usually erythromycin or clindamycin. Combining benzoyl peroxide with these antibiotics may help limit development of resistance. Glycolic acid may be used instead of or in addition to tretinoin. Treatments have no significant adverse effects other than drying and irritation (and rare allergic reactions to benzoyl peroxide).

Physical extraction of comedones using a comedone extractor is an option for patients unresponsive to topical treatment. Comedone extraction may be done by a physician, nurse, or physician assistant. One end of the comedone extractor is like a blade or bayonet that punctures the closed comedone. The other end exerts pressure to extract the comedone.

Oral antibiotics (eg, tetracycline, minocycline, doxycycline, erythromycin) can be used when wide distribution of lesions makes topical therapy impractical.

Moderate acne: Oral systemic therapy with antibiotics is the best way to treat moderate acne. Antibiotics effective for acne include tetracycline, minocycline, erythromycin, and doxycycline. Full benefit takes ≥ 12 wk.

Topical therapy as for mild acne is usually used concomitantly with oral antibiotics.

Doxycycline and minocycline are first-line drugs; both can be taken with food. Tetracycline is also a good first choice, but it cannot be taken with food and may have lower efficacy than doxycycline and minocycline. Doxycycline and minocycline dosage is 50 to 100 mg po bid. Doxycycline may cause photosensitivity, and minocycline may have more adverse effects with chronic use, including drug-induced lupus and hyperpigmentation. Tetracycline dosage is 250 or 500 mg po bid between meals. To reduce the development of antibiotic resistance after control is achieved (usually 2 to 3 mo), the dose is tapered as much as possible to maintain control. Antibiotics may be discontinued if topical therapy maintains control.

Erythromycin is another option, but it can cause GI adverse effects and antibiotic resistance develops more often.

Long-term use of antibiotics may cause a gram-negative pustular folliculitis around the nose and in the center of the face. This uncommon superinfection may be difficult to clear and is best treated with oral isotretinoin after discontinuing the oral antibiotic. Ampicillin is an alternative treatment for gram-negative folliculitis. In women, prolonged antibiotic use can cause candidal vaginitis; if local and systemic therapy does not eradicate this problem, antibiotic therapy for acne must be stopped.

If the patient is female and unresponsive to oral antibiotics, a trial of oral antiandrogens (oral contraceptives and/or spironolactone) may be considered.

Severe acne: Oral isotretinoin is the best treatment for patients with moderate acne in whom antibiotics are unsuccessful and for those with severe inflammatory acne. Dosage of isotretinoin is usually 1 mg/kg once/day for 16 to 20 wk, but the dosage may be increased to 2 mg/kg once/day. If adverse effects make this dosage intolerable, it may be reduced to 0.5 mg/kg once/day. After therapy, acne may continue to improve. Most patients do not require a 2nd course of treatment; when needed, it should be resumed only after the drug has been stopped for 4 mo. Retreatment is required more often if the initial dosage is low (0.5 mg/kg). With this dosage (which is very popular in Europe), fewer adverse effects occur, but prolonged therapy is usually required. Cumulative dosing has gained support; a total dosage of 120 to 150 mg/kg resulted in lower recurrence rates.

Isotretinoin is nearly always effective, but use is limited by adverse effects, including dryness of conjunctivae and mucosae of the genitals, chapped lips, arthralgias, depression, elevated lipid levels, and the risk of birth defects if treatment occurs during pregnancy. Hydration with water followed by petrolatum application usually alleviates mucosal and cutaneous dryness. Arthralgias (mostly of large joints or the lower back) occur in about 15% of patients. Increased risk of depression and suicide is much publicized but probably rare. It is not clear whether risk of new or worsened inflammatory bowel disease (Crohn disease and ulcerative colitis) is increased.

CBC, liver function, and fasting glucose, triglyceride, and cholesterol levels should be determined before treatment. Each should be reassessed at 4 wk and, unless abnormalities are noted, need not be repeated until the end of treatment. Triglycerides rarely increase to a level at which the drug should be stopped. Liver function is seldom affected. Because isotretinoin is teratogenic, women of childbearing age are told that they are required to use 2 methods of contraception for 1 mo before treatment, during treatment, and for at least 1 mo after stopping treatment. Pregnancy tests should be done before beginning therapy and monthly until 1 mo after therapy stops.

Cystic acne: Intralesional injection of 0.1 mL triamcinolone acetonide suspension 2.5 mg/mL (the 10 mg/mL suspension must be diluted) is indicated for patients with firm (cystic) acne who seek quick clinical improvement with reduced scarring. Local atrophy may occur but is usually transient. For isolated, very boggy lesions, incision and drainage are often beneficial but may result in residual scarring.

Other forms of acne: Pyoderma faciale is treated with oral corticosteroids and isotretinoin.

Acne fulminans is treated with oral corticosteroids and systemic antibiotics.

Acne conglobata is treated with oral isotretinoin if systemic antibiotics fail.

For acne caused by endocrine abnormalities (eg, polycystic ovary syndrome, virilizing adrenal tumors in females), antiandrogens are indicated. Spironolactone, which has some antiandrogen effects, is sometimes prescribed to treat acne at a dose of 50 to 100 mg po once/day. Cyproterone acetate is used in Europe. When other measures fail, an estrogen/progesterone–containing contraceptive may be tried; therapy ≥ 6 mo is needed to evaluate effect.

Scarring: Small scars can be treated with chemical peels, laser resurfacing, or dermabrasion. Deeper, discrete scars can be excised. Wide, shallow depressions can be treated with subcision or collagen injection. Collagen implants are temporary and must be repeated every few years.

KEY POINTS

- If noninflammatory, acne is characterized by comedones and, if inflammatory, by papules, pustules, nodules, and cysts.
- Mild and moderate acne usually heals without scarring by the mid-20s.
- Recommend that patients avoid triggers (eg, occlusive cosmetics and clothing, cleansers, lotions, high humidity, some drugs and chemicals, possibly a high intake of milk or a high-glycemic diet).
- Consider the psychologic as well as the physical effects of acne.
- Prescribe a topical comedolytic (eg, tretinoin) plus, for inflammatory acne, benzoyl peroxide, a topical antibiotic, or both.
- Prescribe an oral antibiotic for moderate acne and oral isotretinoin for severe acne.
- Treat cystic acne with intralesional triamcinolone.

HIDRADENITIS SUPPURATIVA

Hidradenitis suppurativa is a chronic, scarring, acnelike inflammatory process that occurs in the axillae, groin, and around the nipples and anus. Diagnosis is by examination. Treatment depends on stage.

Hidradenitis suppurativa is currently thought to be a chronic inflammatory condition of the hair follicle and associated structures. Follicular inflammation and subsequent occlusion leads to rupture of the follicle and development of abscesses, sinus tracts, and scarring.

Swollen, tender masses resembling cutaneous abscesses develop. These lesions are often sterile. Pain, fluctuance, discharge, and sinus tract formation are characteristic in chronic cases. In chronic cases, bacterial infection may occur in deep abscesses and sinus tracts. In chronic axillary cases, coalescence of inflamed nodules causes palpable cordlike fibrotic bands. The condition may become disabling because of pain and foul odor.

Diagnosis

- Clinical evaluation

Diagnosis of hidradenitis suppurativa is by examination. Cultures should be taken from deep abscesses and sinus tracts in patients who have chronic disease, but often no pathogens will be found. The Hurley staging system describes the severity of disease.

- Stage I: Abscess formation, single or multiple, without sinus tracts or scarring
- Stage II: Single or multiple, widely separated, recurrent abscesses with sinus tract formation or scarring
- Stage III: Diffuse or near diffuse involvement or multiple interconnected sinus tracts and abscesses across the entire area

Treatment

- Stage I: Topical clindamycin, intralesional corticosteroids, and oral antibiotics
- Stage II: Longer courses of oral antibiotics and sometimes drainage or punch debridement
- Stage III: Infliximab or adalimumab and often wide surgical excision and repair or grafting

Hidradenitis suppurative treatment goals are to prevent new lesions, reduce inflammation, and remove sinus tracts.

For **Hurley stage I disease,** typical treatment includes topical 1% clindamycin solution bid, topical resorcinol 15% cream once/day, oral zinc gluconate (90 mg once/day), intralesional corticosteroids (eg, 0.1 to 0.5 mL of a 5 to 10 mg/mL solution of triamcinolone acetonide once/mo), and short (eg, 7 to 10 days) courses of oral antibiotics. Tetracycline (500 mg bid), doxycycline (100 to 200 mg once/day), minocycline (100 mg once/day), or erythromycin (250 to 500 mg qid) are used until the lesions resolve. A typical regimen could include one topical treatment (eg, based on the patient's skin sensitivity) and an antibiotic; however, all treatments can be used in combination or alone.

For **Hurley stage II disease,** treatment is with a longer (eg, 2 to 3 mo) course of the same oral antibiotics used to treat stage I disease; if response is incomplete, clindamycin 300 mg po bid and/or rifampin 600 mg po once/day may be added to the regimen. Adding antiandrogen therapy (eg, with oral estrogen or combination oral contraceptives, spironolactone, cyproterone acetate [not available in the US], finasteride, or combinations) may be helpful in women. Incision and drainage may reduce the pain of an abscess but are insufficient for disease control (unlike in common cutaneous abscesses). For acute inflammatory lesions that are not excessively deep, punch debridement (ie, excision with a 5-mm to 7-mm punch instrument followed by digital debridement and curettage or scrubbing) is preferable. Sinus tracts should be unroofed. Patients whose lesions are deeper should be evaluated by a plastic surgeon for consideration of excision and grafting.

For **Hurley Stage III disease** (see Plate 38), medical and surgical therapy should be more aggressive. Evidence of efficacy in reducing inflammation is strongest for infliximab (5 mg/kg IV at wk 0, 2, and 6). Alternatively, adalimumab may be given (initial dose of 160 mg sc given in 1 day or split over 2 consecutive days, followed by 1 dose of 80 mg sc on day 15 and maintenance doses of 40 mg sc once/wk beginning on day 29). Oral retinoids (isotretinoin 0.25 to 0.4 mg/kg bid for 4 to 6 mo or acitretin 0.6 mg/kg once/day for 9 to 12 mo) have been effective in some patients. Wide surgical excision and repair or grafting of the affected areas is often necessary if the disease persists. Ablative laser therapy (CO_2 or erbium:YAG) is an alternate surgical treatment. Laser hair removal has also been used with some success.

Recommended adjunctive measures for all patients with hidradenitis suppurativa include maintaining good skin hygiene, minimizing trauma, providing psychologic support, and possibly avoiding high glycemic load diets.

KEY POINTS

- Lesions are usually sterile except for deep abscesses and sinus tracts in chronic disease.
- Hidradenitis suppurativa can be disabling.
- Treat hidradenitis suppurativa based on the Hurley staging system.

PERIORAL DERMATITIS

Perioral dermatitis is an erythematous, papulopustular facial eruption that resembles acne and/or rosacea but typically starts around the mouth. Diagnosis is by appearance. Treatment includes avoidance of causes, and topical and sometimes oral antibiotics.

A variety of causes of perioral dermatitis have been proposed, including exposure to topical corticosteroids and/or fluoride in water and toothpaste, but the etiology of perioral dermatitis is unknown. Despite its name, perioral dermatitis is not a true dermatitis. It primarily affects women of childbearing age and children. The eruption classically starts at the nasolabial folds and spreads perioraly, sparing a zone around the vermilion border of the lips. But the eruption can also spread periorbitally and to the forehead.

Diagnosis

- Clinical evaluation

Diagnosis of perioral dermatitis is by appearance; perioral dermatitis is distinguished from acne by the absence of comedones and from rosacea by the latter's lack of lesions around the mouth and eyes. Seborrheic dermatitis and contact dermatitis must be excluded.

Biopsy, which is generally not clinically necessary, shows spongiosis and a lymphohistiocytic infiltrate affecting vellus hair follicles. In the lupoid variant, granulomas may be present.

Treatment

- Avoidance of fluorinated dental products and topical corticosteroids
- Topical or sometimes oral antibiotics

Perioral dermatitis treatment is to stop fluorinated dental products and topical corticosteroids (if being used) and then use topical antibiotics (eg, erythromycin 2% or metronidazole 0.75% gel or cream bid). If there is no response, doxycycline or minocycline 50 to 100 mg po bid or oral tetracycline 250 to

500 mg po bid (between meals) may be given for 4 wk and then tapered to the lowest effective dose.

In contrast to acne, antibiotics can usually be stopped. Topical pimecrolimus (for people > age 2 yr) also reduces disease severity. Isotretinoin has been successfully used to treat granulomatous perioral dermatitis.

ROSACEA

(Acne Rosacea)

Rosacea is a chronic inflammatory disorder characterized by facial flushing, telangiectasias, erythema, papules, pustules, and, in severe cases, rhinophyma (see Plate 49). Diagnosis is based on the characteristic appearance and history. Treatment depends on severity and includes topical metronidazole, topical and oral antibiotics, topical ivermectin, rarely isotretinoin, and, for severe rhinophyma, surgery.

Rosacea most commonly affects patients aged 30 to 50 with fair complexions, most notably those of Irish and Northern European descent, but it affects and is probably under-recognized in darker-skinned patients.

Etiology

The etiology of rosacea is unknown, but some proposed associations include

- Abnormal vasomotor control
- Impaired facial venous drainage
- Increased follicle mites (*Demodex folliculorum*)
- Increased angiogenesis, ferritin expression, and reactive oxygen species
- Dysfunction of antimicrobial peptides (eg, cathelicidin)

Diet plays no consistent role, but some agents (eg, amiodarone, topical and nasal corticosteroids, high doses of B_6 and B_{12}) may worsen rosacea.

Symptoms and Signs

Rosacea is limited to the face and scalp and manifests in 4 phases:

- Pre-rosacea
- Vascular
- Inflammatory
- Late

In the **pre-rosacea phase,** patients describe embarrassing flushing and blushing, often accompanied by uncomfortable stinging. Common reported triggers for these flares include sun exposure, emotional stress, cold or hot weather, alcohol, spicy foods, exercise, wind, cosmetics, and hot baths or hot drinks. These symptoms persist throughout other phases of the disorder.

In the **vascular phase,** patients develop facial erythema and edema with multiple telangiectases, possibly as a result of persistent vasomotor instability.

An **inflammatory phase** often follows, in which sterile papules and pustules (leading to the designation of rosacea as adult acne) develop.

The **late phase** (developing in some patients), is characterized by coarse tissue hyperplasia of the cheeks and nose (rhinophyma) caused by tissue inflammation, collagen deposition, and sebaceous gland hyperplasia.

The phases of rosacea are usually sequential. Some patients go directly into the inflammatory stage, bypassing the earlier stages. Treatment may cause rosacea to return to an earlier stage. Progression to the late stage is not inevitable.

Ocular rosacea often precedes or accompanies facial rosacea and manifests as some combination of blepharoconjunctivitis, iritis, scleritis, and keratitis, causing itching, foreign body sensation, erythema, and edema of the eye.

Diagnosis

- Clinical evaluation

Diagnosis of rosacea is based on the characteristic appearance; there are no specific diagnostic tests. The age of onset and absence of comedones help distinguish rosacea from acne.

Differential diagnosis of rosacea includes acne vulgaris, SLE, sarcoidosis, photodermatitis, drug eruptions (particularly caused by iodides and bromides), granulomas of the skin, and perioral dermatitis.

Treatment

- Avoidance of triggers
- Consideration of topical or oral antibiotics or topical azelaic acid or ivermectin
- For flushing or persistent erythema, consideration of topical brimonidine
- For recalcitrant cases, consideration of oral isotretinoin
- For rhinophyma, consideration of dermabrasion and tissue excision
- For telangiectasia, consideration of laser or electrocautery treatment

Primary initial treatment of rosacea involves avoidance of triggers (including use of sunscreen). Antibiotics and/or azelaic acid may be used for inflammatory disease. The objective of treatment is control of symptoms, not cure. See the Canadian clinical practice guidelines for rosacea at http://journals.sagepub.com.

Metronidazole cream (1%), lotion (0.75%), or gel (0.75%) and azelaic acid 20% cream, applied bid, are equally effective; 2.5% benzoyl peroxide in any form (eg, gel, lotion, cream), applied once/day or bid, can be added for improved control. Less effective alternatives include sodium sulfacetamide 10%/sulfur 5% lotion; clindamycin 1% solution, gel, or lotion; and erythromycin 2% solution, all applied bid. Many patients require indefinite treatment for long-term control. Topical ivermectin 1% cream appears to have efficacy in the treatment of inflammatory lesions of rosacea.

Oral antibiotics are indicated for patients with multiple papules or pustules and for those with ocular rosacea; options include doxycycline 50 to 100 mg bid, tetracycline 250 to 500 mg bid, minocycline 50 to 100 mg bid, and erythromycin 250 to 500 mg bid. Dose should be reduced to the lowest one that controls symptoms once a beneficial response is achieved. Subantimicrobial doses of doxycycline (40 mg once/day in a preparation containing 30 mg of immediate-release and 10 mg of sustained-release doxycycline) are effective for acne and rosacea.

Persistent erythema or flushing may be treated with topical α_2-selective adrenergic agonist brimonidine 0.33% gel applied once/day.

Recalcitrant cases may respond to oral isotretinoin.

Techniques for treatment of rhinophyma include dermabrasion and tissue excision; cosmetic results are good.

Techniques for treatment of telangiectasia include laser and electrocautery.

KEY POINTS

- Consider rosacea if patients have flushing and blushing, with or without stinging, often triggered by sun exposure, emotional stress, cold or hot weather, alcohol, spicy foods, exercise, wind, cosmetics, or hot baths or hot drinks.
- Diagnose rosacea by its typical appearance (eg, central facial erythema and edema with or without pustules, papules, or multiple telangiectases).
- Treat rosacea with avoidance of triggers; treat inflammation, depending on severity, with topical antibiotics and/or azelaic acid, oral antibiotics, isotretinoin, or topical ivermectin.
- Consider brimonidine for persistent erythema or flushing.
- Dermabrasion and tissue excision for rhinophyma give good cosmetic results.
- Consider laser or electrocautery for telangiectasia.

122 Bacterial Skin Infections

Bacterial skin infections may be uncomplicated or complicated. Uncomplicated infections usually respond promptly to systemic antibiotics and local wound care. A skin infection is considered complicated when it meets 2 of the following 5 criteria:

- Involves a preexisting wound or ulceration of the skin
- Involves the deeper soft tissues
- Requires surgical intervention
- Is caused or exacerbated by underlying comorbid disease states (eg, diabetes, systemic immunosuppression)
- Is unresponsive to conventional antibiotic therapy or is recurrent

All uncomplicated skin infections have the potential to become complicated. Complicated skin and soft-tissue infections may require multidrug therapy and the assistance of other consultants (eg, surgeons, infectious disease specialists), particularly in light of resistance in many strains of bacteria and the rapid loss of efficacy among more potent antibiotics. Recurrent skin infections should raise suspicion of colonization (eg, staphylococcal nasal carriage), resistant strains of bacteria (eg, methicillin-resistant *Staphylococcus aureus* [MRSA]), cancer, poorly controlled diabetes, or other reasons for immunocompromise (eg, HIV, hepatitis, advanced age, congenital susceptibility). Bacteria are involved in the pathophysiology of acne, but acne is not primarily considered a bacterial skin infection.

CELLULITIS

Cellulitis is acute bacterial infection of the skin and subcutaneous tissue most often caused by streptococci or staphylococci. Symptoms and signs are pain, rapidly spreading erythema, and edema; fever may occur, and regional lymph nodes may enlarge. Diagnosis is by appearance; cultures are sometimes helpful, but awaiting these results should not delay empiric therapy. Treatment is with antibiotics. Prognosis is excellent with timely treatment.

Etiology

- *Streptococcus pyogenes*
- *Staphylococcus aureus*

Cellulitis is most often caused by group A β-hemolytic streptococci (eg, *Streptococcus pyogenes*) or *Staphylococcus aureus*. Streptococci cause diffuse, rapidly spreading infection because enzymes produced by the organism (streptokinase, DNase, hyaluronidase) break down cellular components that would otherwise contain and localize the inflammation. Staphylococcal cellulitis is typically more localized and usually occurs in open wounds or cutaneous abscesses.

Recently, methicillin-resistant *S. aureus* (MRSA) has become more common in the community (community-associated MRSA [CA-MRSA]). Historically, MRSA was typically confined to patients who were exposed to the organism in a hospital or nursing facility. MRSA infection should now be considered in patients with community-acquired cellulitis, particularly in those with cellulitis that is recurrent or unresponsive to monotherapy.

Less common causes are group B streptococci (eg, *S. agalactiae*) in older patients with diabetes; gram-negative bacilli (eg, *Haemophilus influenzae*) in children; and *Pseudomonas aeruginosa* in patients with diabetes or neutropenia, hot tub or spa users, and hospitalized patients. Animal bites may result in cellulitis; *Pasteurella multocida* is the cause in cat bites, and *Capnocytophaga* sp is responsible in dog bites. Immersion injuries in fresh water may result in cellulitis caused by *Aeromonas hydrophila*; in warm salt water, by *Vibrio vulnificus*.

Immunocompromised patients may become infected by opportunistic organisms, including gram-negative bacteria (such as *Proteus, Serratia, Enterobacter,* or *Citrobacter*), anaerobic bacteria, and *Helicobacter* and *Fusarium* spp. Mycobacteria may rarely cause cellulitis.

Risk factors include skin abnormalities (eg, trauma, ulceration, fungal infection, other skin barrier compromise due to preexisting skin disease), which are common in patients with chronic venous insufficiency or lymphedema. Scars from saphenous vein removal for cardiac or vascular surgery are common sites for recurrent cellulitis, especially if tinea pedis is present. Frequently, no predisposing condition or site of entry is evident.

Symptoms and Signs

Infection is most common in the lower extremities. Cellulitis is typically unilateral; stasis dermatitis closely mimics cellulitis but is usually bilateral. The major findings are local erythema and tenderness, frequently with lymphangitis and regional lymphadenopathy. The skin is hot, red, and edematous (see Plate 34), often with surface appearance resembling the skin of an orange (peau d'orange). The borders are usually indistinct, except in erysipelas (a type of cellulitis with sharply demarcated margins—see p. 995). Petechiae are common; large areas of ecchymosis are rare. Vesicles and bullae may develop and rupture, occasionally with necrosis of the involved skin. Cellulitis may mimic deep venous thrombosis but can often be differentiated by one or more features (see Table 122–1). Fever, chills, tachycardia, headache, hypotension, and delirium may precede cutaneous findings by several hours, but many patients

Table 122–1. DIFFERENTIATING CELLULITIS AND DEEP VENOUS THROMBOSIS

FEATURE	CELLULITIS	DEEP VENOUS THROMBOSIS
Skin temperature	Hot	Normal or cool
Skin color	Red	Normal or cyanotic
Skin surface	Peau d'orange	Smooth
Lymphangitis and regional lymphadenopathy	Frequent	Nonexistent

do not appear ill. Leukocytosis is common. Cellulitis with rapid spread of infection, rapidly increasing pain, hypotension, delirium, or skin sloughing, particularly with bullae and fevers, suggests life-threatening infection.

Diagnosis

- Examination
- Blood and sometimes tissue cultures for immunocompromised patients

Diagnosis is by examination. Skin and (when present) wound cultures are generally not indicated because they rarely identify the infecting organism. Blood cultures are useful in immunocompromised patients to detect or rule out bacteremia. Culture of involved tissue may be required in immunocompromised patients if they are not responding to empiric therapy or if blood cultures do not isolate an organism. Abscess should be ruled out based on clinical findings.

Prognosis

Most cellulitis resolves quickly with antibiotic therapy. Local abscesses occasionally form, requiring incision and drainage. Serious but rare complications include severe necrotizing subcutaneous infection (see p. 999) and bacteremia with metastatic foci of infection.

Recurrences in the same area are common, sometimes causing serious damage to the lymphatics, chronic lymphatic obstruction, and lymphedema.

Treatment

- Antibiotics

Treatment is with antibiotics. When prevalence of local skin pathogens is known, empiric treatment should be directed against the most prevalent ones. For most patients, empiric treatment effective against both group A streptococci and *S. aureus* is used. Oral therapy is usually adequate with dicloxacillin 250 mg or cephalexin 500 mg qid for mild infections. Levofloxacin 500 mg po once/day or moxifloxacin 400 mg po once/day works well for patients who are unlikely to adhere to multiple daily dosing schedules; however, bacteria resistant to fluoroquinolones are becoming more prevalent. In patients allergic to penicillin, clindamycin 300 to 450 mg po tid or a macrolide (clarithromycin 250 to 500 mg po bid or azithromycin 500 mg po on 1st day, then 250 mg po once/day) are alternatives.

Initial use of empiric therapy against MRSA is not typically recommended unless risk is particularly high (eg, contact with a person who has a documented case, exposure to a documented outbreak, culture-documented local prevalence of > 10% or 15%). In high-risk cases, double-strength trimethoprim/sulfamethoxazole (160 mg trimethoprim/800 mg sulfamethoxazole) po bid, clindamycin 300 to 450 mg po tid, and doxycycline 100 mg po bid are reasonable outpatient empiric treatments.

For more serious infections, patients are hospitalized and given oxacillin or nafcillin 1 g IV q 6 h, or a cephalosporin (eg, cefazolin 1 g IV q 8 h). For penicillin-allergic patients or those with suspected or confirmed MRSA infection, vancomycin 15 mg/kg IV q 12 h is the drug of choice (see also p. 1604). Linezolid is another option, usually for the treatment of highly resistant MRSA, at a dose of 600 mg IV q 12 h for 10 to 14 days. Daptomycin 4 to 6 mg/kg IV once/day can be used. Teicoplanin has a mechanism of action similar to vancomycin. It is commonly used outside the US to treat MRSA; the usual dose is 6 mg/kg IV q 12 h for 2 doses, followed by 6 mg/kg (or 3 mg/kg) IV or IM once/day. Immobilization and elevation of the affected area help reduce edema; cool, wet dressings relieve local discomfort.

Cellulitis in a patient with neutropenia requires empiric antipseudomonal antibiotics (eg, tobramycin 1.5 mg/kg IV q 8 h and piperacillin 3 g IV q 4 h) until blood culture results are available.

A patient with mild cellulitis caused by mammalian bites can be treated as an outpatient with amoxicillin/clavulanate (if penicillin allergic, with a fluoroquinolone plus clindamycin or trimethoprim/sulfamethoxazole).

Cellulitis that develops after exposure to brackish or salt water should be treated with doxycycline 100 mg po bid and ceftazidime or a fluoroquinolone. Cellulitis caused by exposure to fresh water should be treated with ceftazidime, cefepime, or a fluoroquinolone. Likely infecting organisms tend to be similar in brackish and fresh water (eg, *Vibrio* sp, *Aeromonas* sp, *Shewanella* sp, *Erysipelothrix rhusiopathiae, Mycobacterium marinum, Streptococcus iniae*).

Recurrent leg cellulitis is prevented by treating concomitant tinea pedis, which often eliminates the source of bacteria residing in the inflamed, macerated tissue. If such therapy is unsuccessful or not indicated, recurrent cellulitis can sometimes be prevented by benzathine penicillin 1.2 million units IM monthly or penicillin V or erythromycin 250 mg po qid for 1 wk/mo. If these regimens prove unsuccessful, tissue culture may be required.

KEY POINTS

- The most common pathogens causing cellulitis overall are *S. pyogenes* and *S. aureus*.
- MRSA should be considered, particularly if there is a known outbreak or local prevalence is high.
- Differentiate leg cellulitis from deep vein thrombosis by the presence of skin warmth, redness, peau d'orange quality, and by the presence of lymphadenopathy.
- Do not culture skin or wounds; however, with severe or complicated infection, culture blood and possibly tissue.
- Direct antibiotic therapy against the most likely pathogens.

ERYSIPELAS

Erysipelas is a type of superficial cellulitis (see p. 994) with dermal lymphatic involvement.

Erysipelas should not be confused with erysipeloid, a skin infection caused by *Erysipelothrix* (see p. 1614). Erysipelas is characterized clinically by shiny, raised, indurated, and tender plaque-like lesions with distinct margins (see Plate 36). There is also a bullous form of erysipelas. Erysipelas is most often caused by group A (or rarely group C or G) β-hemolytic streptococci and occurs most frequently on the legs and face. However, other causes have been reported, including *Staphylococcus aureus* (including methicillin-resistant *S. aureus* [MRSA]), *Klebsiella pneumoniae, Haemophilus influenzae, Escherichia coli, S. warneri, Streptococcus pneumoniae, S. pyogenes,* and *Moraxella* sp. Erysipelas of the face must be differentiated from herpes zoster, angioedema, and contact dermatitis. It is commonly accompanied by high fever, chills, and malaise; MRSA is more common in facial erysipelas than in lower-extremity erysipelas. Erysipelas may be recurrent and may result in chronic lymphedema.

Diagnosis

Diagnosis is by characteristic appearance; blood culture is done in toxic-appearing patients. Diffuse inflammatory carcinoma of the breast may also be mistaken for erysipelas.

Treatment

- Usually penicillin for lower-extremity erysipelas
- Initially vancomycin for facial erysipelas or if MRSA is suspected

Treatment of choice for lower-extremity erysipelas is penicillin V 500 mg po qid for ≥ 2 wk. In severe cases, penicillin G 1.2 million units IV q 6 h is indicated, which can be replaced by oral therapy after 36 to 48 h. An alternative parenteral therapy is ceftriaxone 1 g IV q 24 h or cefazolin 1 to 2 g IV q 8 h. Dicloxacillin 500 mg po qid for 10 days can be used for infections with staphylococci. Erythromycin 500 mg po qid for 10 days may be used in penicillin-allergic patients; however, there is growing macrolide resistance in streptococci. In infections resistant to these antibiotics, cloxacillin or nafcillin can be used. In Europe, pristinamycin and roxithromycin have been shown to be good choices for erysipelas. If facial erysipelas is present or if MRSA is suspected, empiric therapy should be initiated with vancomycin 1 g IV q 12 h (which is active against MRSA). Cold packs and analgesics may relieve local discomfort. Fungal foot infections may be an entry site for infection and may require antifungal treatment to prevent recurrence.

CUTANEOUS ABSCESS

A cutaneous abscess is a localized collection of pus in the skin and may occur on any skin surface. Symptoms and signs are pain and a tender and firm or fluctuant swelling. Diagnosis is usually obvious by examination. Treatment is incision and drainage.

Bacteria causing cutaneous abscesses are typically indigenous to the skin of the involved area. For abscesses on the trunk, extremities, axillae, or head and neck, the most common organisms are *Staphylococcus aureus* and streptococci. In recent years, methicillin-resistant *S. aureus* (MRSA) has become a more common cause.

Abscesses in the perineal (ie, inguinal, vaginal, buttock, perirectal) region contain organisms found in the stool, commonly anaerobes or a combination of aerobes and anaerobes. Carbuncles and furuncles are follicle-based cutaneous abscesses with characteristic features (see p. 997).

Cutaneous abscesses tend to form in patients with bacterial overgrowth, antecedent trauma (particularly when a foreign body is present), or immunologic or circulatory compromise.

Symptoms and Signs

Cutaneous abscesses are painful, tender, indurated, and usually erythematous. They vary in size, typically 1 to 3 cm in length, but are sometimes much larger. Initially the swelling is firm; later, as the abscess points, the overlying skin becomes thin and feels fluctuant. The abscess may then spontaneously drain. Local cellulitis, lymphangitis, regional lymphadenopathy, fever, and leukocytosis are variable accompanying features.

Diagnosis

- Examination
- Culture to identify MRSA

Diagnosis is usually obvious by examination. Culture is recommended, primarily to identify MRSA.

Conditions resembling simple cutaneous abscesses include hidradenitis suppurativa (see p. 991) and ruptured epidermal cysts. Epidermal cysts (often incorrectly referred to as sebaceous cysts) rarely become infected; however, rupture releases keratin into the dermis, causing an exuberant inflammatory reaction sometimes clinically resembling infection. Culture of these ruptured cysts seldom reveals any bacteria. Perineal abscesses may represent cutaneous emergence of a deeper perirectal abscess or drainage resulting from Crohn disease via a fistulous tract. These other conditions are usually recognizable by history and rectal examination.

Treatment

- Incision and drainage
- Sometimes antibiotics

Some small abscesses resolve without treatment, coming to a point and draining. Warm compresses help accelerate the process. Incision and drainage are indicated when significant pain, tenderness, and swelling are present; it is unnecessary to await fluctuance. Under sterile conditions, local anesthesia is given as either a lidocaine injection or a freezing spray.

Patients with large, extremely painful abscesses may benefit from IV sedation and analgesia during drainage. A single puncture with the tip of a scalpel is often sufficient to open the abscess. After the pus drains, the cavity should be bluntly probed with a gloved finger or curette to clear loculations and then irrigated with 0.9% saline solution. Some clinicians pack the cavity loosely with a gauze wick that is removed 24 to 48 h later. Local heat and elevation may hasten resolution of inflammation.

Antibiotics are unnecessary unless the patient has signs of systemic infection, cellulitis, multiple abscesses, immunocompromise, or a facial abscess in the area drained by the cavernous sinus. In these cases, empiric therapy should be started with a drug active against MRSA (eg, trimethoprim/sulfamethoxazole, clindamycin; for severe infection, vancomycin) pending results of bacterial culture.

KEY POINTS

- Pathogens reflect flora of the involved area (eg, *S. aureus* and streptococci in the trunk, axilla, head, and neck), but MRSA has become more common.
- Culture abscesses to identify MRSA.
- Drain abscesses accompanied by significant pain, tenderness, and swelling and provide adequate analgesia and, when indicated, sedation.
- Avoid antibiotics in simple abscesses.

FOLLICULITIS

Folliculitis is a bacterial infection of hair follicles.

Folliculitis is usually caused by *Staphylococcus aureus* but occasionally *Pseudomonas aeruginosa* (hot tub folliculitis) or other organisms. Hot tub folliculitis occurs because of inadequate treatment of water with chlorine or bromine.

Symptoms of folliculitis are mild pain, pruritus, or irritation. Signs of folliculitis are a superficial pustule or inflammatory nodule surrounding a hair follicle. Infected hairs easily fall out or are removed, but new papules tend to develop. Growth of stiff hairs into the skin may cause chronic low-grade irritation or inflammation that may mimic infectious folliculitis (pseudofolliculitis barbae—see p. 1044).

Treatment

- Clindamycin 1% lotion or gel

Because most folliculitis is caused by *S. aureus,* clindamycin 1% lotion or gel may be applied topically bid for 7 to 10 days. Alternatively, benzoyl peroxide 5% wash may be used when showering for 5 to 7 days. Extensive cutaneous involvement may warrant systemic therapy (eg, cephalexin 250 to 500 mg po tid to qid for 10 days). If these measures do not result in a cure, or folliculitis recurs, pustules are Gram stained and cultured to rule out gram-negative or methicillin-resistant *S. aureus* (MRSA) etiology, and nares are cultured to rule out nasal staphylococcal carriage. Potassium hydroxide wet mount should be done on a plucked hair to rule out fungal folliculitis.

Treatment for MRSA usually requires 2 oral antibiotics, and the choice of therapeutic drugs should be based on culture and sensitivity reports.

Hot tub folliculitis usually resolves without treatment. However, adequate chlorination of the hot tub is necessary to prevent recurrences and to protect others from infection.

FURUNCLES AND CARBUNCLES

Furuncles (boils) are skin abscesses caused by staphylococcal infection, which involve a hair follicle and surrounding tissue. Carbuncles are clusters of furuncles connected subcutaneously, causing deeper suppuration and scarring. They are smaller and more superficial than subcutaneous abscesses (see p. 996). Diagnosis is by appearance. Treatment is warm compresses and often oral antistaphylococcal antibiotics.

Both furuncles and carbuncles may affect healthy young people but are more common among the obese, the immunocompromised (including those with neutrophil defects), the elderly, and possibly those with diabetes. Clustered cases may occur among those living in crowded quarters with relatively poor hygiene or among contacts of patients infected with virulent strains. Predisposing factors include bacterial colonization of skin or nares, hot and humid climates, and occlusion or abnormal follicular anatomy (eg, comedones in acne). Methicillin-resistant *Staphylococcus aureus* (MRSA) is a common cause.

Furuncles are common on the neck, breasts, face, and buttocks. They are uncomfortable and may be painful when closely attached to underlying structures (eg, on the nose, ear, or fingers). Appearance is a nodule or pustule that discharges necrotic tissue and sanguineous pus. Carbuncles may be accompanied by fever and prostration.

Diagnosis

Diagnosis is by examination. Material for culture should be obtained.

Treatment

- Drainage
- Often antibiotics effective against MRSA

Abscesses are incised and drained. Intermittent hot compresses are used to facilitate drainage. Antibiotics, when used, should be effective against MRSA, pending culture and sensitivity test results. In afebrile patients, treatment of a single lesion < 5 mm requires no antibiotics. If a single lesion is ≥ 5 mm, an oral antibiotic is given for 5 to 10 days; choices include trimethoprim/sulfamethoxazole (TMP/SMX) 160/800 mg to 320/1600 mg bid, clindamycin 300 to 600 mg q 6 to 8 h, and doxycycline or minocycline 100 mg q 12 h. Patients with fever, multiple abscesses, or carbuncles are given 10 days of TMP/SMX 160/800 mg to 320/1600 mg bid plus rifampin 300 mg bid. Systemic antibiotics are also needed for

- Lesions < 5 mm that do not resolve with drainage
- Evidence of expanding cellulitis
- Immunocompromised patients
- Patients at risk of endocarditis

Furuncles frequently recur and can be prevented by applying liquid soap containing either chlorhexidine gluconate with isopropyl alcohol or 2 to 3% chloroxylenol and by giving maintenance antibiotics over 1 to 2 mo. Patients with recurrent furunculosis should be treated for predisposing factors such as obesity, diabetes, occupational or industrial exposure to inciting factors, and nasal carriage of *S. aureus* or MRSA colonization.

KEY POINTS

- Suspect a furuncle if a nodule or pustule involves a hair follicle and discharges necrotic tissue and sanguineous pus, particularly if on the neck, breasts, face, or buttocks.
- Culture furuncles and carbuncles.
- Drain lesions.
- Prescribe antibiotics effective against MRSA for patients who are immunocompromised or at risk for endocarditis or if lesions are > 5 mm or expanding.

ERYTHRASMA

Erythrasma is an intertriginous infection with *Corynebacterium minutissimum* that is most common among patients with diabetes and among people living in the tropics.

Erythrasma resembles tinea or intertrigo. It is most common in the foot, where it manifests as superficial scaling, fissuring, and maceration most commonly confined to the 3rd and 4th web spaces. Erythrasma is also common in the groin, where it manifests as irregular but sharply marginated pink or brown patches with fine scaling. Erythrasma may also involve the axillae, submammary or abdominal folds, and perineum, particularly in obese middle-aged women and in patients with diabetes.

Erythrasma fluoresces a characteristic coral-red color under a Wood light. Absence of hyphae in skin scrapings also distinguishes erythrasma from tinea.

Treatment is erythromycin or tetracycline 250 mg po qid for 14 days. Topical erythromycin or clindamycin is also effective. Recurrence is common.

IMPETIGO AND ECTHYMA

Impetigo is a superficial skin infection with crusting or bullae caused by streptococci, staphylococci, or both. Ecthyma is an ulcerative form of impetigo.

No predisposing lesion is identified in most patients, but impetigo may follow any type of break in the skin. General risk factors seem to be a moist environment, poor hygiene, or chronic nasopharyngeal carriage of staphylococci or streptococci. Impetigo may be bullous or nonbullous. *Staphylococcus aureus* is the predominant cause of nonbullous impetigo and the cause of all bullous impetigo. Bullae are caused by exfoliative toxin produced by staphylococci. Methicillin-resistant *S. aureus* (MRSA) has been isolated in about 20% of recent cases of impetigo.

Symptoms and Signs

Nonbullous impetigo typically manifests as clusters of vesicles or pustules that rupture and develop a honey-colored crust (exudate from the lesion base) over the lesions (see Plate 39).

Bullous impetigo is similar except that vesicles typically enlarge rapidly to form bullae. The bullae burst and expose larger bases, which become covered with honey-colored varnish or crust.

Ecthyma is characterized by small, purulent, shallow, punched-out ulcers with thick, brown-black crusts and surrounding erythema.

Impetigo and ecthyma cause mild pain or discomfort. Pruritus is common; scratching may spread infection, inoculating adjacent and nonadjacent skin.

Diagnosis

- Clinical evaluation

Diagnosis of impetigo and ecthyma is by characteristic appearance. Cultures of lesions are indicated only when the patient does not respond to empiric therapy. Patients with recurrent impetigo should have nasal culture. Persistent infections should be cultured to identify MRSA.

Treatment

- Topical mupirocin, retapamulin, or fusidic acid
- Sometimes oral antibiotics

The affected area should be washed gently with soap and water several times a day to remove any crusts. Treatment for localized impetigo is topical mupirocin antibiotic ointment tid for 7 days or retapamulin ointment bid for 5 days. Fusidic acid 2% cream tid to qid until lesions resolve is as effective but is not available in the US. Oral antibiotics (eg, dicloxacillin or cephalexin 250 to 500 mg qid [12.5 mg/kg qid for children] for 10 days) may be needed in patients with extensive or resistant lesions; clindamycin 300 mg po q 6 h or erythromycin 250 mg po q 6 h may be used in penicillin-allergic patients, but resistance to both drugs is an increasing problem. Use of initial empiric therapy against MRSA is not typically advised unless there is compelling clinical evidence (eg, contact with a person who has a documented case, exposure to a documented outbreak, culture-documented local prevalence of > 10% or 15%). Treatment of MRSA should be directed by culture and sensitivity test results; typically, clindamycin, TMP/SMX, and doxycycline are effective against most strains of community-associated MRSA.

Other therapy includes restoring a normal cutaneous barrier in patients with underlying atopic dermatitis or extensive xerosis using topical emollients and corticosteroids if warranted. Chronic staphylococcal nasal carriers are given topical antibiotics (mupirocin) for 1 wk each of 3 consecutive months.

Prompt recovery usually follows timely treatment. Delay can cause cellulitis, lymphangitis, furunculosis, and hyperpigmentation or hypopigmentation with or without scarring. Children aged 2 to 4 yr are at risk of acute glomerulonephritis if nephritogenic strains of group A streptococci are involved; nephritis seems to be more common in the southern US than in other regions. It is unlikely that treatment with antibiotics prevents poststreptococcal glomerulonephritis.

KEY POINTS

- *S. aureus* causes most nonbullous impetigo and all bullous impetigo.
- Honey-colored crust is characteristic of bullous and nonbullous impetigo.
- For persistent impetigo, culture the wound (to identify MRSA) and the nose (to identify a causative nasal reservoir).
- Treat most cases with topical antibiotics.

LYMPHADENITIS

Lymphadenitis is an acute infection of one or more lymph nodes.

Lymphadenitis is a feature of many bacterial, viral, fungal, and protozoal infections. Focal lymphadenitis is prominent in streptococcal infection, TB or nontuberculous mycobacterial infection, tularemia, plague, cat-scratch disease, primary syphilis, lymphogranuloma venereum, chancroid, and genital herpes simplex. Multifocal lymphadenitis is common in infectious mononucleosis, cytomegalovirus infection, toxoplasmosis, brucellosis, secondary syphilis, and disseminated histoplasmosis.

Symptoms and Signs

Lymphadenitis typically causes pain, tenderness, and lymph node enlargement. Pain and tenderness typically distinguish lymphadenitis from lymphadenopathy. With some infections, the overlying skin is inflamed, occasionally with cellulitis. Abscesses may form, and penetration to the skin produces draining sinuses. Fever is common.

Diagnosis

The underlying disorder is usually suggested by history and examination. If not, aspiration and culture or excisional biopsy is indicated.

Treatment

- Treatment of cause

Treatment is directed at the cause and is usually empiric. Options include IV antibiotics, antifungals, and antiparasitics depending upon etiology or clinical suspicion. Many patients with lymphadenitis may respond to outpatient therapy with oral antibiotics. However, many also go on to form abscesses, which require surgical drainage; an extensive procedure is done with accompanying IV antibiotics. In children, IV antibiotics are commonly needed. Hot, wet compresses may relieve some pain. Lymphadenitis usually resolves with timely treatment, although residual, persistent, nontender lymphadenopathy is common.

LYMPHANGITIS

Lymphangitis is acute bacterial infection (usually streptococcal) of peripheral lymphatic channels.

Rare causes include staphylococcal infections, *Pasteurella* infections, *Erysipelothrix,* anthrax, herpes simplex infections, lymphogranuloma venereum, rickettsial infections, sporotrichosis, *Nocardia* infections, leishmaniasis, tularemia, *Burkholderia* infections, and atypical mycobacterial infections. Pathogens enter the lymphatic channels from an abrasion, wound, or coexisting infection (usually cellulitis). Patients with underlying lymphedema are at particular risk. Red, irregular, warm, tender streaks develop on an extremity and extend proximally from a peripheral lesion toward regional lymph nodes, which are typically enlarged and tender. Systemic manifestations (eg, fever, shaking chills, tachycardia, headache) may occur and may be more severe than cutaneous findings suggest. Leukocytosis is common. Bacteremia may occur. Rarely, cellulitis with suppuration, necrosis, and ulceration develops along the involved lymph channels as a consequence of primary lymphangitis.

Diagnosis is clinical. Isolation of the responsible organism is usually unnecessary. Most cases respond rapidly to antistreptococcal antibiotics (see Cellulitis on p. 994). If response to treatment is poor or presentation is unusual, rare pathogens should be considered.

NECROTIZING SUBCUTANEOUS INFECTION

(Necrotizing Cellulitis or Fasciitis)

Necrotizing subcutaneous infection (NSI) is typically caused by a mixture of aerobic and anaerobic organisms that cause necrosis of subcutaneous tissue, usually including the fascia. This infection most commonly affects the extremities and perineum. Affected tissues become red, hot, and swollen, resembling severe cellulitis (see p. 994), and pain develops out of proportion to clinical findings. Without timely treatment, the area becomes gangrenous. Patients are acutely ill. Diagnosis is by history and examination and is supported by evidence of overwhelming infection. Treatment involves antibiotics and surgical debridement. Prognosis is poor without early, aggressive treatment.

Etiology

NSI typically results from infection with group A streptococci (eg, *Streptococcus pyogenes*) or a mixture of aerobic and anaerobic bacteria (eg, *Bacteroides* sp). These organisms typically extend to subcutaneous tissue from a contiguous ulcer or an infection or after trauma. Streptococci can arrive from a remote site of infection via the bloodstream. Perineal involvement (also called Fournier gangrene) is usually a complication of recent surgery, perirectal abscess, periurethral gland infection, or retroperitoneal infection resulting from perforated abdominal viscera. Patients with diabetes are at particular risk of NSI.

Pathophysiology

NSI causes tissue ischemia by widespread occlusion of small subcutaneous vessels. Vessel occlusion results in skin infarction and necrosis, which facilitates the growth of obligate anaerobes (eg, *Bacteroides*) while promoting anaerobic metabolism by facultative organisms (eg, *Escherichia coli*), resulting in gangrene. Anaerobic metabolism produces hydrogen and nitrogen, relatively insoluble gases that may accumulate in subcutaneous tissues.

Symptoms and Signs

The primary symptom is intense pain. In patients with normal sensation, pain out of proportion to clinical findings may be an early clue. However, in areas denervated by peripheral neuropathy, pain may be minimal or absent. Affected tissue is red, hot, and swollen and rapidly becomes discolored. Bullae, crepitus (resulting from soft-tissue gas), and gangrene may develop. Subcutaneous tissues (including adjacent fascia) necrose, with widespread undermining of surrounding tissue. Muscles are spared initially. Patients are acutely ill, with high fever, tachycardia, altered mental status ranging from confusion to obtundation, and hypotension. Patients may be bacteremic or septic and may require aggressive hemodynamic support. Streptococcal toxic shock syndrome may develop.

Diagnosis

- Clinical examination
- Blood and wound cultures

Diagnosis, made by history and examination, is supported by leukocytosis, soft-tissue gas on x-ray, positive blood cultures, and deteriorating metabolic and hemodynamic status.

NSI must be differentiated from clostridial soft-tissue infections, in which cellulitis, myositis, and myonecrosis often occur (see p. 1469). Such infections are anaerobic. Anaerobic cellulitis produces lots of gas but little pain, edema, or change in skin; it very seldom travels into the muscle. Necrotizing myositis manifests with fever, pain, and muscle swelling without early skin changes; later, skin may develop redness, warmth, purpura, and bullae.

Prognosis

Mortality rate is about 30%. Old age, underlying medical problems, delayed diagnosis and therapy, and insufficient surgical debridement worsen prognosis.

Treatment

- Surgical debridement
- Antibiotics
- Amputation if necessary

Treatment of early NSI is primarily surgical, which should not be delayed by diagnostic studies. IV antibiotics are adjuncts, usually including 2 or more drugs, but regimens vary depending on results of Gram stain and culture (eg, penicillin G 4 million units q 4 h combined with clindamycin 600 to 900 mg q 8 h or ceftriaxone 2 g q 12 h). Evidence of bullae, ecchymosis, fluctuance, crepitus, and systemic spread of infection requires immediate surgical exploration and debridement. The initial incision should be extended until an instrument or finger can no longer separate the skin and subcutaneous tissue from the deep fascia. The most common error is insufficient surgical intervention; repeat operation every 1 to 2 days, with further incision and debridement as needed, should be carried out routinely. Amputation of an extremity may be necessary.

PEARLS & PITFALLS

- If findings suggest NSI, arrange for surgical treatment without delay for testing and institute IV fluid and antibiotic therapy.

IV fluids may be needed in large volumes before and after surgery. Antibiotic choices should be reviewed based on Gram stain and culture of tissues obtained during surgery. Hyperbaric O_2 therapy as adjuvant therapy may also be of benefit; however, the evidence is inconclusive. IV immune globulin has been suggested for streptococcal toxic shock syndrome with NSI.

KEY POINTS

- NSI can develop from a contiguous ulcer, an infection, or hematogenous spread or after trauma.
- Consider NSI in patients with characteristic findings or pain out of proportion to clinical findings, particularly patients with diabetes or other risk factors.
- Arrange surgical therapy while instituting IV fluid and antibiotic therapy and without delaying for testing.

STAPHYLOCOCCAL SCALDED SKIN SYNDROME

Staphylococcal scalded skin syndrome (SSSS) is an acute epidermolysis caused by a staphylococcal toxin. Infants and children are most susceptible. Symptoms are widespread bullae with epidermal sloughing. Diagnosis is by examination and sometimes biopsy. Treatment is antistaphylococcal antibiotics and local care. Prognosis is excellent with timely treatment.

SSSS almost always affects children < 6 yr (especially infants); it rarely occurs in older patients unless they have renal failure or are immunocompromised. Epidemics may occur in nurseries, presumably transmitted by the hands of personnel who are in contact with an infected infant or who are nasal carriers of *Staphylococcus aureus*. Sporadic cases also occur.

SSSS is caused by group II coagulase-positive staphylococci, usually phage type 71, which elaborate exfoliatin (also called epidermolysin), a toxin that splits the upper part of the epidermis just beneath the granular cell layer (see also p. 1602). The primary infection often begins during the first few days of life in the umbilical stump or diaper area; in older children, the face is the typical site. Toxin produced in these areas enters the circulation and affects the entire skin.

Symptoms and Signs

The initial lesion is usually superficial and crusted. Within 24 h, the surrounding skin becomes painful and scarlet, changes that quickly spread to other areas. The skin may be exquisitely tender and have a wrinkled tissue paper–like consistency. Large, flaccid blisters arise on the erythematous skin and quickly break to produce erosions. Blisters are frequently present in areas of friction, such as intertriginous areas, buttocks, hands, and feet. Intact blisters extend laterally with gentle pressure (Nikolsky sign). The epidermis may peel easily, often in large sheets (see Plate 52). Widespread desquamation occurs within 36 to 72 h, and patients become very ill with systemic manifestations (eg, malaise, chills, fever). Desquamated areas appear scalded. Loss of the protective skin barrier can lead to sepsis and to fluid and electrolyte imbalance.

Diagnosis

- Biopsy
- Cultures from areas of suspected primary infection

Diagnosis is suspected clinically, but confirmation usually requires biopsy (frozen section may give earlier results). Specimens show noninflammatory superficial splitting of the epidermis. In children, skin cultures are seldom positive; in adults, they are frequently positive. Cultures should be taken from the conjunctiva, nasopharynx, blood, urine, and areas of possible primary infection, such as the umbilicus in a neonate or suspect skin lesions. Cultures should not be taken from bullae because they are sterile.

Differential diagnosis: Differential diagnosis includes drug hypersensitivity, viral exanthemas, scarlet fever, thermal burns, genetic bullous diseases (eg, some types of epidermolysis bullosa), acquired bullous diseases (eg, pemphigus vulgaris, bullous pemphigoid), and toxic epidermal necrolysis (see Table 122–2 and p. 1050). Stevens-Johnson syndrome is characterized by mucosal involvement, which is absent in SSSS.

Treatment

- Antibiotics
- Gel dressings for weeping lesions

With prompt diagnosis and therapy, death rarely occurs; the stratum corneum is quickly replaced, and healing usually occurs within 5 to 7 days after start of treatment.

Table 122–2. DIFFERENTIATING STAPHYLOCOCCAL SCALDED SKIN SYNDROME (SSSS) AND TOXIC EPIDERMAL NECROLYSIS (TEN)

FEATURE	SSSS	TEN
Patients affected	Infants, young children, immunocompromised adults	Older patients
Patient history	Recent staphylococcal infection	Drug use, renal failure
Level of epidermal cleavage (blister formation)*	Within the granular cell (outermost) layer of the epidermis	Between the epidermis and dermis or at the level of the basal cell

*Determined by Tzanck test or by a frozen section of a fresh specimen.

Penicillinase-resistant antistaphylococcal antibiotics given IV must be started immediately. Nafcillin 12.5 to 25 mg/kg IV q 6 h for neonates > 2 kg and 25 to 50 mg/kg for older children is given until improvement is noted, followed by oral cloxacillin 12.5 mg/kg q 6 h (for infants and children weighing ≤ 20 kg) and 250 to 500 mg q 6 h (for older children). Vancomycin should be considered in areas with a high prevalence of methicillin-resistant *S. aureus* or in patients failing to respond to initial therapy. Corticosteroids are contraindicated. Emollients (eg, white petrolatum) are sometimes used to prevent further insensible water loss from ulcerated skin. However, topical therapy and patient handling must be minimized.

PEARLS & PITFALLS

- Avoid corticosteroids if SSSS is possible.

If disease is widespread and lesions are weeping, the skin should be treated as for burns (see p. 2956). Hydrolyzed polymer gel dressings may be very useful, and the number of dressing changes should be minimized.

Steps to detect carriers and prevent or treat nursery epidemics are discussed elsewhere (see p. 2631).

KEY POINTS

- Generalized desquamation and systemic illness most often is TEN in older patients and SSSS in infants and young children (and occasionally in immunocompromised adults).
- Complications similar to those that occur with burns can develop (eg, fluid and electrolyte imbalance, sepsis).
- Do a biopsy and culture the conjunctiva, nasopharynx, blood, urine, and areas of possible primary infection, such as the umbilicus and suspect skin lesions.
- Treat patients with antistaphylococcal antibiotics and, if disease is widespread, in a burn unit if possible.

123 Benign Skin Tumors, Growths, and Vascular Lesions

ATYPICAL MOLES

(Atypical Nevus; Dysplastic Nevus)

Atypical moles are benign melanocytic nevi with irregular and ill-defined borders, variegated colors usually of brown and tan tones, and macular or papular components. Patients with atypical moles have an increased risk of melanoma. Management is by close clinical monitoring and biopsy of highly atypical or changed lesions. Patients should reduce sun exposure and conduct regular self-examinations for new moles or changes in existing ones.

Atypical moles (AM) are nevi with a slightly different clinical and histologic appearance (disordered architecture and atypia of melanocytes). Most melanomas arise de novo. Risk factors for melanoma include increased number of AM and increased exposure to ultraviolet radiation and sun. Some patients have only one or a few AM; others have many.

The propensity to develop AM may be inherited (autosomal dominant) or sporadic without apparent familial association. Familial atypical mole–melanoma syndrome refers to the presence of multiple AM and melanoma in ≥ two 1st-degree relatives. These patients are at markedly increased risk (25 times) of melanoma.

Symptoms and Signs

AM are often larger than other nevi (> 6 mm diameter) and primarily round (unlike many melanomas) but with indistinct borders and mild asymmetry. In contrast, melanomas have greater irregularity of color and may have areas that are red, blue, whitish, or depigmented with a scarred appearance.

Diagnosis

- Clinical evaluation
- Sometimes biopsy
- Regular physical examinations

AM must be differentiated from melanoma. Features that suggest melanoma, known as the ABCDEs of melanoma, are

- A: Asymmetry—asymmetric appearance
- B: Borders—irregular borders (ie, not round or oval)
- C: Color—color variation within the mole, unusual colors, or a color significantly different or darker than the patient's other moles
- D: Diameter—> 6 mm
- E: Evolution—a new mole in a patient > 30 yr of age or a changing mole

Although clinical findings can sometimes establish a diagnosis of AM (see Table 123–1), visual differentiation between atypical nevi and melanoma can be difficult; biopsy of the worst-appearing lesions should be done to establish the diagnosis and to determine the degree of atypia. Biopsy should aim to include the complete depth and breadth of the lesion; excisional biopsy is often ideal.

Patients with multiple AM and a personal or family history of melanoma should be examined regularly (eg, yearly for family history of melanoma, more often for personal history of melanoma). Some dermatologists do imaging of the skin using a hand-held instrument (dermoscopy) to see structures not visible to the naked eye. Dermoscopy can reveal certain high-risk characteristics.

Treatment

- Removal by excision or shaving when desired
- Excision of high-risk lesions

If desired, AM can be removed by excision or shaving.

Prophylactic removal of all AM is not effective in preventing melanoma and is not recommended. However, AMs may warrant removal for any of the following conditions:

- A patient has a high-risk history (eg, personal or family history of melanoma).
- A patient cannot guarantee close follow-up.

Table 123–1. CHARACTERISTICS OF ATYPICAL VS TYPICAL MOLES

CRITERIA	TYPICAL MOLES	ATYPICAL MOLES
Age of onset	Childhood or adolescence	Continue to appear after adolescence
Color	Flesh-colored, yellow-brown, or black	Tan to dark brown with a pink background; often resembling a fried egg, with a dark or light target commonly with a flatter rim than center Pigment often blurred at the edges or notched
Diameter	1–10 mm (usually < 6 mm)	5–12 mm
Shape	Symmetric with regular borders	Can be asymmetric or with irregular borders
Location	Anywhere on the body	Most common on sun-exposed skin but may occur on covered areas (eg, buttocks, breasts, scalp)
Number of lesions	≥ 10	One to several dozen

- The mole has high-risk dermatoscopic findings.
- The mole is in a location that makes monitoring the lesion for changes difficult or impossible for the patient.

Prevention

- Sun protection
- Regular self-examination
- Full-body photography
- Sometimes surveillance of family members

Patients with AM should avoid excessive sun exposure and use sunscreens. Patients who are vigilant about sun protection should be counseled to take sufficient supplemental vitamin D. Also, they should be taught self-examination to detect changes in existing moles and to recognize features of melanomas. Full-body photography may help detect new nevi and monitor existing nevi for changes. Regular follow-up examinations are recommended.

If patients have a history of melanoma (whether developing from AM or de novo) or other skin cancers, 1st-degree relatives should be examined. Patients who are from melanoma-prone families (ie, ≥ 2 1st-degree relatives with cutaneous melanomas) have a high lifetime risk of developing melanomas. The entire skin (including the scalp) of members of an at-risk family should be examined at least once to determine risk and needed follow-up.

KEY POINTS

- Risk of melanoma is higher if patients have increased numbers of AM, increased sun exposure, or familial atypical mole–melanoma syndrome.
- Because clinical differentiation from melanoma can be difficult, biopsy the worst-appearing AMs.
- Closely follow patients with AM, particularly those at higher risk of melanoma, and do full-body photography.
- Recommend sun protection (with supplemental vitamin D) and self-examination for high-risk changes.
- Do full-body examinations of all 1st-degree relatives of patients who have melanoma.

CAPILLARY MALFORMATIONS

(Nevi Flammei; Nevus Flammeus; Port-Wine Stain)

Capillary malformations are present at birth and appear as flat, pink, red, or purplish lesions.

Port-wine stains are flat, reddish to purple lesions appearing anywhere on the body. Lesions become darker and more palpable with time (often becoming quite hyperplastic by late middle age), but the lateral extent increases only in proportion to the growth of the patient. Port-wine stains of the trigeminal area may be a component of the Sturge-Weber syndrome (in which a similar vascular lesion appears on the underlying meninges and cerebral cortex and is associated with seizures).

Diagnosis of capillary malformations is made clinically. Imaging studies may be indicated, depending on findings, to diagnose associated syndromes (eg, Sturge-Weber syndrome).

Treatment

- Vascular laser treatment or cosmetic creams

Treatment with vascular lasers produces excellent results in many cases, especially if the lesion is treated as early in life as possible. The lesion can also be hidden with an opaque cosmetic cream prepared to match the patient's skin color.

CUTANEOUS CYSTS

(Epidermal Inclusion Cyst [Epidermoid Cyst]; Milia; Pilar Cyst; Trichilemmal Cyst [Wen])

Epidermal inclusion cysts are the most common cutaneous cysts. Milia are small epidermal inclusion cysts. Pilar cysts are usually on the scalp and may be familial.

Benign cutaneous cysts are classified according to histologic features of the cyst wall or lining and anatomic location. On palpation, a cyst is firm, globular, movable, and nontender; cysts usually range from about 1 to 5 cm in diameter.

Epidermal inclusion cysts (epidermoid cysts) seldom cause discomfort unless they have ruptured internally, causing a rapidly enlarging, painful foreign body reaction and abscess. Epidermal inclusion cysts are often surmounted by a visible punctum or pore; their contents are white, cheesy, and malodorous.

Milia are minute superficial epidermal inclusion cysts that are most often on the face and scalp.

Pilar cysts (trichilemmal cysts) may appear identical to epidermal inclusion cysts, but 90% are on the scalp. There is often a family history of pilar cysts; inheritance is autosomal dominant.

Treatment

- Cyst excision if needed
- Milia evacuation

Troublesome cysts can be removed. To prevent recurrence, the entire cyst and its wall should be removed. Ruptured cysts can be incised and drained but may recur if the wall is not eventually removed. Antibiotics are not needed unless cellulitis is present.

Milia may be evacuated with a #11 blade and comedone extractor.

DERMATOFIBROMAS

(Benign Fibrous Histiocytomas)

Dermatofibromas are firm, red-to-brown, small papules or nodules composed of fibroblastic tissue. They usually occur on the thighs or legs but can occur anywhere.

Dermatofibromas are common among adults, more so in women. Their cause is probably genetic. Lesions are usually 0.5 to 1 cm in diameter, firm, and may dimple inward with gentle pinching. Most lesions are asymptomatic, but some itch or ulcerate after minor trauma.

Diagnosis of dermatofibromas can often be made clinically. Lesions are sometimes biopsied to exclude melanocytic proliferation (eg, nevus, solar lentigo, melanoma) or other tumors.

Treatment

- Excision if troublesome

Dermatofibromas that cause troublesome symptoms can be excised.

INFANTILE HEMANGIOMAS

Infantile hemangiomas are raised, red or purplish, hyperplastic vascular lesions appearing in the first year of life. Most spontaneously involute; those obstructing vision, the airway, or other structures require treatment. Ideal treatment varies based on many patient-specific factors.

Infantile hemangioma (IH) is the most common tumor of infancy, affecting 10 to 12% of infants by age 1 yr. IH is present at birth in 10 to 20% of affected infants and almost always within the first several weeks of life; occasionally, deeper lesions may not be apparent until a few months after birth. Size and vascularity increase rapidly, usually peaking at about age 1 yr.

IH can be classified by general appearance (superficial, deep, or cavernous) or by other descriptive terms (eg, strawberry hemangioma). However, because all of these lesions share a common pathophysiology and natural history, the inclusive term IH is preferred.

Symptoms and Signs

Superficial lesions have a bright red appearance; deeper lesions have a bluish color. Lesions can bleed or ulcerate from minor trauma; ulcers may be painful.

IH in certain locations can interfere with function. Lesions on the face or oropharynx may interfere with vision or obstruct the airway; those near the urethral meatus or anus may interfere with elimination. A periocular hemangioma in an infant is considered an emergency and should be attended to promptly to avoid permanent visual defects. Lumbosacral hemangiomas may be a sign of underlying neurologic or GU anomalies.

Lesions slowly involute starting at 12 to 18 mo, decreasing in size and vascularity. Generally, IH involute by 10%/yr of age (eg, 50% by age 5, 60% by age 6), with maximal involution by age 10. Involuted lesions commonly have a yellowish or telangiectatic color and a wrinkled or lax fibrofatty texture. Residual changes are almost always proportional to the lesion's maximal size and vascularity.

Diagnosis

- Clinical evaluation

Diagnosis of IHs is clinical; the extent can be evaluated by MRI if lesions appear to encroach on vital structures.

Treatment

- Individualized based on location, size, and severity of lesions
- For lesions that require treatment, possibly topical, intralesional, or systemic corticosteroids; laser; or oral propranolol
- General wound care for ulcerated lesions
- Usually avoidance of surgery

There is no universal IH treatment recommendation. Because most lesions resolve spontaneously, observation is usually indicated before initiating treatment. Treatment should be considered for lesions that

- Threaten life
- Threaten function (eg, vision)
- Involve large areas of the face
- Are distributed over the beard area
- Are ulcerated
- Are multiple
- Are lumbosacral

Topical treatments and wound care are useful for ulcerated lesions and help prevent scarring, bleeding, and pain. Compresses, topical mupirocin or metronidazole, barrier dressings (generally polyurethane film dressing or petrolatum-impregnated gauze), or barrier creams may be used.

Unless complications are life threatening or vital organs are compromised, surgical excision or other destructive procedures should be avoided because they frequently cause more scarring than occurs with spontaneous involution. To help parents accept nonintervention, the physician can review the natural history (photographic examples are helpful), provide serial photography of the lesion to document involution, and listen sympathetically to parents' concerns.

KEY POINTS

- IHs affect 10 to 12% of infants by age 1 yr.
- Lesions slowly involute starting at 12 to 18 mo, with maximal involution by age 10 yr.
- Unless complications are life-threatening or vital organs are compromised, avoid surgery.

KELOIDS

Keloids are smooth overgrowths of fibroblastic tissue that arise in an area of injury (eg, lacerations, surgical scars, truncal acne) or, occasionally, spontaneously.

Keloids are more frequent in darker-skinned patients. They tend to appear on the upper trunk, especially the upper back and mid chest, and on deltoid areas. Unlike hypertrophic scars, keloidal scar tissue extends beyond the margins of the wound or injury. They may appear spontaneously.

Keloids are shiny, firm, smooth, usually ovoid but sometimes contracted or webbed, and slightly pink or hyperpigmented (see Plate 41).

Diagnosis of keloids is clinical.

Treatment

- Possibly corticosteroid injection, excision, gel sheeting, and/or immunomodulators

Treatment of keloids is often ineffective.

Monthly corticosteroid injections (eg, triamcinolone acetonide 5 to 40 mg/mL) into the lesion sometimes flatten the keloid.

Surgical or laser excision may debulk lesions, but they usually recur larger than before. Excision is more successful if preceded and followed by a series of intralesional corticosteroid injections. Gel sheeting (applying a soft, semiocclusive dressing made of cross-linked polymethylsiloxane polymer, or silicone) or pressure garments are other adjuncts to prevent recurrence.

More recently, immunomodulators (eg, imiquimod) have been used to prevent keloid development or recurrence.

LIPOMAS

Lipomas are soft, movable, subcutaneous nodules of adipocytes (fat cells); overlying skin appears normal.

Lipomas are very common, benign, and usually solitary, but some patients have multiple lipomas. Common sites are the proximal extremities, trunk, and neck. Multiple lipomas can be familial and/or associated with various syndromes.

Lipomas are usually asymptomatic but can be tender or painful. A lipoma is usually easily movable within the subcutis. Lipomas are generally soft, but some become firmer.

Diagnosis of lipomas is usually clinical, but a rapidly growing lesion should be biopsied.

Treatment

- Excision or liposuction if bothersome

Treatment is not usually required, but bothersome lipomas may be removed by excision or liposuction.

LYMPHATIC MALFORMATIONS

(Cavernous Lymphangioma; Cystic Hygroma; Lymphangioma; Lymphangioma Circumscriptum)

Lymphatic vascular malformations are elevated lesions composed of dilated lymphatic vessels.

Most lymphatic malformations are present at birth or develop within the first 2 yr.

Lesions are usually yellowish tan but occasionally reddish or purple if small blood vessels are intermingled. Puncture of the lesion yields a colorless or blood-tinged fluid.

Diagnosis of lymphatic malformations is made clinically and by MRI.

Treatment

- Usually unnecessary

Treatment of lymphatic malformations is usually not needed. If the lesion is excised, recurrence is common, even when removal of dermal and subcutaneous tissues is extensive.

MOLES

(Melanocytic Nevi)

Moles are flesh- to brown-colored macules, papules, or nodules composed of nests of melanocytes or nevus cells. Their main significance (other than cosmetic) is their resemblance to melanoma. Pigmented lesions are assessed for characteristics of concern (new or changing appearance, irregular borders, multiple colors within one lesion, bleeding, ulceration, or itching) that could suggest atypical nevi or melanoma.

Almost everyone has a few moles, which usually appear in childhood or adolescence. There are different types of moles (see Table 123–2). During adolescence, more moles often appear, and existing ones may enlarge or darken. Nevus cells may be eventually replaced with fat or fibrous tissue. Moles typically change consistency, becoming softer and boggy, or firmer, and less pigmented over the decades.

An individual mole is unlikely to become malignant (lifetime risk is about 1 in 3000 to 10,000); however, patients with large

Table 123–2. CLASSIFICATION OF MOLES

TYPE	CLINICAL CHARACTERISTICS	HISTOLOGY
Blue nevus	Bluish gray Usually flat but may be slightly elevated; 2–4 mm	Deeply pigmented dendritic melanocytes and scattered melanophages in the dermis
Compound nevus	Light brown to dark brown May be slightly or considerably elevated; 3–6 mm	Nests of melanocytes at the epidermodermal junction and within the dermis
Halo nevus	Any type of mole surrounded by a 2- to 6-mm ring of depigmented skin	Same as for other moles but with inflammation and loss of melanocytes in halo skin
Intradermal nevus	Flesh-colored to brown; may be smooth, hairy, or warty Elevated; 3–6 mm	Melanocytes and nevus cells confined almost entirely to the dermis
Junctional nevus	Light brown to nearly black Usually flat but may be slightly elevated; 1–10 mm	Nests of melanocytes at the epidermodermal junction

numbers of benign moles (> about 50) have an increased risk of developing melanoma. These patients should be taught to self-monitor for warning signs and have skin surveillance as part of their primary care (see diagnosis of moles).

Blue nevi are benign moles that appear as bluish gray macules or thin papules. The depth and density of pigment in the skin account for the apparent blue color.

Diagnosis

- Biopsy

Because moles are extremely common and melanomas are uncommon, prophylactic removal is not justifiable. However, biopsy and histologic evaluation should be considered if moles have certain characteristics of concern (known as the ABCDEs of melanoma):

- A: Asymmetry—asymmetric appearance
- B: Borders—irregular borders (ie, not round or oval)
- C: Color—color variation within the mole, unusual colors, or a color significantly different or darker than the patient's other moles
- D: Diameter—> 6 mm
- E: Evolution—a new mole in a patient > 30 yr of age or a changing mole

If a mole becomes painful or itchy or bleeds or ulcerates, biopsy can also be considered.

The biopsy specimen must be deep enough for accurate microscopic diagnosis and should contain the entire lesion if possible, especially if the concern for cancer is strong. However, wide primary excision should not be the initial procedure, even for highly abnormal-appearing lesions. Many such lesions are not melanomas and, even with melanoma, the proper treatment margin and recommendation for lymph node sampling is determined based on histopathologic features. Incisional biopsy does not increase the likelihood of metastasis if the lesion is malignant, and it avoids extensive surgery for a benign lesion.

Treatment

- Sometimes excision

Moles can be removed by shaving or excision for cosmetic purposes, and all moles removed should be examined histologically. If hair growth is a concern for the patient, a hairy mole should be adequately excised rather than removed by shaving. Otherwise, hair will regrow.

KEY POINTS

- Almost everyone has moles, but people with > about 50 are at increased risk of melanoma.
- Consider biopsy if moles have ABCDE characteristics: *A*symmetry; irregular *B*orders; high-risk *C*olors (variations within or between moles or unusual colors); *D*iameter > 6 mm; *E*volution (new moles after age 30 or changes in existing moles).
- Consider excision if a mole is a significant cosmetic problem.

NEVUS ARANEUS

(Spider Angioma; Spider Nevus; Vascular Spider)

Nevus araneus is a bright red, faintly pulsatile vascular lesion consisting of a central arteriole with slender projections resembling spider legs (see Plate 29).

These lesions are acquired. One lesion or small numbers of lesions unrelated to internal disease may occur in children or adults. Patients with cirrhosis develop many spider angiomas that may become quite prominent. Many women develop lesions during pregnancy or while taking oral contraceptives.

The lesions are asymptomatic and usually resolve spontaneously about 6 to 9 mo postpartum or after oral contraceptives are stopped. Lesions are not uncommon on the faces of children. Compression of the central vessel temporarily obliterates the lesion.

Diagnosis of nevus araneus is clinical.

Treatment

- Usually unnecessary

Treatment of nevus araneus is not usually required.

If resolution is not spontaneous or treatment is desired for cosmetic purposes, the central arteriole can be destroyed with fine-needle electrodesiccation; vascular laser treatment may also be done.

PYOGENIC GRANULOMAS

Pyogenic granulomas are fleshy, moist or crusty, usually scarlet vascular nodules composed of proliferating capillaries in an edematous stroma.

The lesion, composed of vascular tissue, is neither of bacterial origin nor a true granuloma. It develops rapidly, often at the site of recent injury (although injury may not be recalled), typically grows no larger than 2 cm in diameter, and probably represents a vascular and fibrous response to injury. There is no sex or age predilection.

The overlying epidermis is thin, and the lesion tends to be friable, bleeds easily, and does not blanch on pressure. The base may be pedunculated and surrounded by a collarette of epidermis.

During pregnancy, pyogenic granulomas may become large and exuberant (called gingival pregnancy tumors or telangiectatic epulis).

Diagnosis of pyogenic granuloma involves biopsy and histologic examination. Histologic analysis is required for all removed tissue because these lesions occasionally resemble and must be differentiated from melanomas or other malignant tumors.

Treatment

- Excision or curettage and electrodesiccation

Treatment of pyogenic granulomas consists of removal by excision or curettage and electrodesiccation, but the lesions may recur.

SEBORRHEIC KERATOSES

Seborrheic keratoses are superficial, often pigmented, epithelial lesions that are usually warty but may occur as smooth papules.

The cause is unknown, but genetic mutations have been identified in certain types. The lesions commonly occur in middle age and later and most often appear on the trunk or temples. In darker-skinned people, multiple 1- to 3-mm lesions can occur on the cheekbones; this condition is termed dermatosis papulosa nigra.

Seborrheic keratoses vary in size and grow slowly. They may be round or oval and flesh-colored, brown, or black. They usually appear stuck on and may have a verrucous, velvety, waxy, scaling, or crusted surface (see Plate 51).

Seborrheic keratoses that are large, multiple, and/or rapidly developing can be a cutaneous paraneoplastic syndrome (Leser-Trélat sign) in patients who have certain cancers (eg, lymphoma, GI cancers).

Diagnosis of seborrheic keratosis is clinical.

Treatment

- Removal only if bothersome

Lesions are not premalignant and need no treatment unless they are irritated, itchy, or cosmetically bothersome.

Lesions may be removed with little or no scarring by cryotherapy (which can cause hypopigmentation) or by electrodesiccation and curettage after local injection of lidocaine.

SKIN TAGS

(Acrochordons; Soft Fibromas)

Skin tags are common, soft, small, flesh-colored or hyperpigmented, pedunculated lesions; there are usually multiple lesions, typically on the neck, axilla, and groin.

Skin tags are usually asymptomatic but may be irritating.

Treatment

- Removal if irritating or unsightly

Irritating or unsightly skin tags can be removed by freezing with liquid nitrogen, light electrodesiccation, or excision with a scalpel or scissors.

VASCULAR LESIONS OF THE SKIN

Vascular lesions include acquired lesions (eg, pyogenic granuloma) and those that are present at birth or arise shortly after birth (vascular birthmarks).

Vascular birthmarks include vascular tumors (eg, IH) and vascular malformations.

Vascular malformations are congenital, life-long, localized defects in vascular morphogenesis and include capillary (eg, nevus flammeus), venous, arteriovenous (eg, cirsoid aneurysm), and lymphatic malformations.

124 Bullous Diseases

Bullae are elevated, fluid-filled blisters ≥ 10 mm in diameter. The autoimmune bullous diseases include

- Bullous pemphigoid
- Dermatitis herpetiformis
- Epidermolysis bullosa acquisita
- Linear Immunoglobulin A disease
- Mucous membrane pemphigoid
- Pemphigoid gestationis
- Pemphigus foliaceus
- Pemphigus vulgaris

Other bullous conditions include staphylococcal scalded skin syndrome, toxic epidermal necrolysis, severe cellulitis, and certain drug eruptions.

BULLOUS PEMPHIGOID

Bullous pemphigoid is a chronic autoimmune skin disorder resulting in generalized, pruritic, bullous lesions in elderly patients. Mucous membrane involvement is rare. Diagnosis is by skin biopsy and immunofluorescence testing of skin and serum. Topical and systemic corticosteroids are used initially. Most patients require long-term maintenance therapy, for which a variety of immunosuppressants can be used.

Bullous pemphigoid occurs more often in patients > 60 yr but can occur in children. IgG autoantibodies bind to certain hemidesmosomal antigens (BPAg1, BPAg2), resulting in the activation of complement to form a subepidermal blister.

Etiology

No cause has been proved; however, the following triggers have been suggested:

- Drugs (including furosemide, spironolactone, sulfasalazine, penicillin, penicillamine, etanercept, and antipsychotics)
- Physical triggers (including trauma, radiation therapy for breast cancer, UV radiation, and anthralin)
- Skin disorders (including psoriasis, lichen planus, and some infections)
- Disorders (diabetes mellitus, rheumatoid arthritis, ulcerative colitis, and multiple sclerosis)

Genetic and environmental factors may play a role.

Triggers may induce an autoimmune reaction by mimicking molecular sequences in the epidermal basement membrane (molecular mimicry, as with drugs and possibly infections), by exposing or altering normally tolerated host antigens (as with physical triggers and certain disorders), or by other mechanisms. Epitope spreading refers to the recruitment of autoreactive lymphocytes against normally tolerated host antigens, which contributes to disease chronicity and course.

Symptoms and Signs

Pruritus is the first symptom. Skin lesions may not develop for several years, but often characteristic tense bullae develop on normal-appearing or erythematous skin of the trunk and in the flexural and intertriginous areas. Localized disease may occur at trauma sites, stomas, and anogenital and lower leg areas. Bullae usually do not rupture, but those that do often rapidly heal.

Polymorphic, annular, dusky-red, edematous lesions, with or without peripheral vesicles, can occur. Rarely, small blisters develop on the mucosa. Leukocytosis and eosinophilia are common, but fever is rare. The Nikolsky sign, where upper layers of epidermis move laterally with slight pressure or rubbing of skin adjacent to a blister, is negative.

Diagnosis

- Skin biopsy and IgG titers

If blisters develop, bullous pemphigoid needs to be differentiated from pemphigus vulgaris, a blistering disorder with a worse prognosis; differentiation is usually possible using clinical criteria (see Table 124–1).

Test results help differentiate bullous pemphigoid from pemphigus vulgaris, linear IgA disease, erythema multiforme,

Table 124–1. DISTINGUISHING PEMPHIGOID FROM PEMPHIGUS VULGARIS

DISORDER	APPEARANCE OF LESION	ORAL INVOLVEMENT	ITCHING	NIKOLSKY SIGN	PROGNOSIS
Pemphigoid	Tense bullae on normal-appearing or erythematous skin	Rare, with small blisters	Common	Generally negative	Usually good; occasionally fatal in the elderly
Pemphigus vulgaris	Flaccid bullae of various sizes Often shearing off of skin or mucosa, leaving painful erosions	Typically starts in the mouth	Absent	Positive	Mortality ≤ 10% with treatment; higher without treatment

drug-induced eruptions, mucous membrane pemphigoid, paraneoplastic pemphigoid, dermatitis herpetiformis, and epidermolysis bullosa acquisita.

If bullous pemphigoid is suspected, skin biopsy is done for histology and direct immunofluorescence testing. Samples from in and around the lesion itself are often used for histology, but samples of uninvolved skin (often about 3 mm from the edge of a lesion) are used for direct immunofluorescence results. The blister in bullous pemphigoid is subepidermal, often containing many neutrophils and eosinophils.

Serum is tested for IgG antibodies to BPAg1 and BPAg2 using an enzyme-linked immunosorbent assay (ELISA). Circulating IgG autoantibodies are present in about three fourths of patients.

Prognosis

Without treatment, bullous pemphigoid usually remits after 3 to 6 yr but can be fatal in about one third of elderly, debilitated patients. High-dose systemic corticosteroid therapy appears to increase the risk.

Treatment

- Corticosteroids, topical or oral

High-potency topical corticosteroids (eg, clobetasol 0.05% cream) should be used for localized disease and may reduce the required dose of systemic drugs. Patients with generalized disease often require prednisone 60 to 80 mg po once/day, which can be tapered to a maintenance level of ≤ 10 to 20 mg/day after several weeks. Most patients achieve remission after 2 to 10 mo. If long-term therapy is necessary, a new blister every few weeks does not require increasing the prednisone dose.

Bullous pemphigoid occasionally responds to a combination of tetracycline or minocycline and nicotinamide. Other treatment options include monotherapy with dapsone, sulfapyridine, or erythromycin. IV immune globulin has been used occasionally. For patients with generalized and recalcitrant disease, and sometimes to decrease corticosteroid dose in chronic disease, immunosuppressants such as methotrexate, azathioprine, cyclophosphamide, mycophenolate mofetil, rituximab, and cyclosporine may be used.

KEY POINTS

- Bullous pemphigoid usually affects patients > 60 yr and is autoimmune and idiopathic.
- Pruritus may precede development of a rash by years, and mucous membrane involvement is rare.
- Biopsy the skin for histology and immunofluorescence testing and measure circulating autoantibodies.
- Treat patients with high-potency topical corticosteroids when possible to avoid or minimize use of systemic corticosteroids.

DERMATITIS HERPETIFORMIS

Dermatitis herpetiformis is an intensely pruritic, chronic, autoimmune, papulovesicular cutaneous eruption in patients who have celiac disease. Typical findings are clusters of intensely pruritic, erythematous, urticarial lesions, as well as vesicles, papules, and bullae, usually distributed symmetrically on extensor surfaces (see Plate 35). Diagnosis is by skin biopsy with direct immunofluorescence testing. Treatment is usually with dapsone or sulfapyridine and a gluten-free diet.

Dermatitis herpetiformis often occurs in young adults but can occur in children and the elderly. It is rare in blacks and Asians.

All patients with dermatitis herpetiformis have celiac disease, but most are asymptomatic. Dermatitis herpetiformis develops in 15 to 25% of patients with celiac disease. Patients may have a higher incidence of other autoimmune disorders (including thyroid disorders, pernicious anemia, and diabetes) and small-bowel lymphoma. IgA deposits collect in the dermal papillary tips and attract neutrophils; they can be eliminated by a gluten-free diet.

The term herpetiformis refers to the clustered appearance of the lesions (similar to that seen in herpesvirus infection) but does not indicate a causal relationship to herpesvirus.

Symptoms and Signs

Onset can be acute or gradual. Vesicles, papules, and urticarial lesions are usually distributed symmetrically on extensor aspects of the elbows and knees and on the sacrum, buttocks, and occiput. Lesions itch and burn. Because itching is intense and skin is fragile, vesicles tend to rupture quickly, often making intact vesicles difficult to detect. Oral lesions may develop but are usually asymptomatic. Iodides and iodine-containing preparations may exacerbate the cutaneous symptoms.

Diagnosis

- Skin biopsy and direct immunofluorescence

Diagnosis of dermatitis herpetiformis is based on skin biopsy and direct immunofluorescence testing of a lesion and adjacent (perilesional) normal-appearing skin. Granular IgA deposition in the dermal papillary tips is invariably present and important for diagnosis. All patients with dermatitis herpetiformis should be evaluated for celiac disease.

Treatment

- Dapsone
- Gluten-free diet

Dapsone generally results in remarkable improvement. Initial dosages of dapsone are 25 to 50 mg po once/day in adults and 0.5 mg/kg in children. Usually, this dose dramatically relieves dermatitis herpetiformis symptoms, including itching and burning, within 1 to 3 days. If improvement occurs, the dose is continued. If no improvement occurs, the dose can be increased every week, up to 300 mg/day. Most patients respond well to 50 to 150 mg/day.

Dapsone can cause hemolytic anemia; risk is highest after 1 mo of treatment and is increased in patients who have G6PD deficiency. Patients suspected of having G6PD deficiency should be tested for this deficiency before being treated with dapsone. Methemoglobinemia is common; hepatitis, agranulocytosis, dapsone syndrome (hepatitis and lymphadenopathy), and a motor neuropathy are more serious complications.

Sulfapyridine 500 mg po tid (or, alternatively, sulfasalazine) is an alternative for patients who cannot tolerate dapsone. Doses of sulfapyridine up to 2000 mg po tid can be used. Sulfapyridine may cause agranulocytosis.

Patients receiving dapsone or sulfapyridine should have a baseline CBC. CBC is then done weekly for 4 wk, then every 2 to 3 wk for 8 wk, and every 12 to 16 wk thereafter.

If patients cannot tolerate dapsone or sulfonamides, heparin may be used alone or in combination with tetracycline and nicotinamide.

Patients are also placed on a strict gluten-free diet. After initial therapy and disease stabilization, most patients can stop drug therapy and be maintained on the gluten-free diet, but this may take months or years. A gluten-free diet also maximizes improvement in the enteropathy and, if strictly followed for 5 to 10 yr, decreases risk of lymphoma.

KEY POINTS

- Patients who have dermatitis herpetiformis, even if they have no GI symptoms, have celiac disease and are at risk of small-bowel lymphoma.
- Because itching is intense and skin is fragile, vesicles may all be broken and thus not evident on examination.
- Confirm the diagnosis with skin biopsy and direct immunofluorescence testing of a lesion and adjacent normal-appearing skin.
- Use dapsone or an alternative drug (eg, sulfapyridine) to control skin manifestations initially.
- Have patients try to maintain long-term control with only a strict gluten-free diet so that drug therapy can be stopped.

EPIDERMOLYSIS BULLOSA ACQUISITA

Epidermolysis bullosa acquisita is a rare, acquired, chronic condition characterized by subepidermal blistering.

Epidermolysis bullosa acquisita can occur in all ages. Collagen type VII, the major component of the anchoring fibrils, is the target antigen of this autoimmune disorder. Multiple myeloma, amyloidosis, lymphoma, inflammatory bowel disease, and systemic lupus erythematosus increase the risk of having epidermolysis bullosa acquisita.

Symptoms and Signs

Initial manifestations are highly variable, sometimes resembling those of bullous pemphigoid. Bullous lesions are most often in areas subject to minor trauma, such as the extensor aspects of the elbows and the dorsal aspects of the hands and feet. Healing usually causes scars, milia (superficial epidermal inclusion cysts), and hyperpigmentation. Some patients have dystrophic nails, mucosal involvement, or ocular lesions leading to blindness.

Diagnosis

- Skin biopsy and direct immunofluorescence

Diagnosis of epidermolysis bullosa acquisita is confirmed by skin biopsy and direct immunofluorescence.

Salt-split skin (skin incubated with sodium chloride to separate the sample into zones) for indirect immunofluorescence may be needed for differentiation from bullous pemphigoid.

Treatment

- Corticosteroids and dapsone

The prognosis is variable, but disease course tends to be prolonged. High-quality evidence about treatments is lacking, and treatment recommendations are often anecdotal. However, in children, corticosteroids in combination with dapsone have shown benefit. In adults and in people with more severe disease, corticosteroids, dapsone, colchicine, cyclosporine, mycophenolate mofetil, IV immune globulin, and azathioprine have been reported to be successful.

LINEAR IMMUNOGLOBULIN A DISEASE

Linear immunoglobulin A (IgA) disease is an uncommon bullous disease distinguished from bullous pemphigoid and dermatitis herpetiformis by linear deposits of IgA in the basement membrane zone.

Linear IgA disease has two main clinical variants—bullous disease of childhood and adult linear IgA disease. Although they vary clinically in minor ways, their immunofluorescence patterns are identical. The IgA autoantibodies target several antigens within the dermal-epidermal junction.

Infections and penicillins trigger more than one-fourth of childhood and adult cases. Vancomycin, diclofenac, and NSAIDs also have been suggested as causes. Risk of linear IgA disease is increased in patients who have inflammatory bowel disease (possibly with a related pathophysiology that involves a generation of autoantibodies) or lymphoproliferative cancers (in adults) but not other autoimmune disorders.

Symptoms and Signs

In linear IgA disease, vesicular or bullous skin lesions occur frequently in a clustered (herpetiform) arrangement. In younger children, the face and perineum are often involved, and spread to the limbs, trunk, hands, feet, and scalp is common. In adults, the trunk is almost always involved, and the scalp, face, and limbs are often involved. Lesions are often pruritic and may burn. Mucosal involvement is common in both age groups; milia are not characteristic.

Diagnosis

- Skin biopsy and direct immunofluorescence

Diagnosis of linear immunoglobulin A disease is by skin biopsy and direct immunofluorescence. The histologic features are not specific, but direct immunofluorescence shows IgA deposited along the basement membrane zone in a linear fashion.

Treatment

- Withdrawal of causative drugs
- For mild disease, topical corticosteroids
- For children, erythromycin

Drug-induced disease may be treated solely with withdrawal of the causative drug.

Mild disease can be treated with topical corticosteroids. Erythromycin can be used in children. Dapsone and sulfonamides (using doses and precautions similar to those for dermatitis herpetiformis) and colchicine are alternatives. Often the cutaneous lesions respond before the mucosal lesions. Spontaneous remission occurs in most patients after 3 to 6 yr.

MUCOUS MEMBRANE PEMPHIGOID

Mucous membrane pemphigoid (MMP) is the designation given to a heterogeneous group of rare chronic autoimmune disorders that tend to cause waxing and waning bullous lesions of the mucous membranes, often with subsequent scarring and morbidity.

(Synonyms of MMP that are no longer used include cicatricial pemphigoid, ocular cicatricial pemphigoid, and benign MMP.)

Oral MMP and ocular MMP are typical, but other mucosal sites and the skin (usually of the head and upper trunk) may be involved. The elderly are most often affected, women more than men.

MMP is characterized by subepithelial lesions caused by autoantibodies against molecules of epithelial basement membranes. The target molecules in MMP lie deep to those of bullous pemphigoid. Several autoantibodies have been identified, including those against BPAG2, laminin-332, and type VII collagen. Antibodies to beta-4 integrin have been identified in generalized MMP and ocular MMP, and antibodies to alpha-6 integrin have been identified in oral MMP.

Diagnosis

- Skin biopsy and direct immunofluorescence

Prevalent mucosal involvement and scarring lesions help distinguish MMP from bullous pemphigoid. Diagnosis of MMP is supported by lesion biopsy and direct immunofluorescence. Linear basement membrane deposits may include IgG, IgA, and C3. Serum autoantibodies tend to be absent or at low titre.

Prognosis

MMP progresses slowly, rarely remits spontaneously, and often responds incompletely to treatment. Depending on the site affected, serious sequelae may include ocular damage and blindness, airway erosions and destruction, and strictures of the esophagus or anogenital regions. Anti-laminin-332 MMP is associated with an increased risk of internal cancer.

Treatment

- For mild disease, corticosteroids and doxycycline plus nicotinamide
- For severe disease, systemic immunosuppression

Treatment of MMP is similar to that for bullous pemphigoid. Topical or intralesional corticosteroids and a combination of oral doxycycline 100 mg po bid and nicotinamide 500 mg po tid may be useful for milder cases. Severe disease may require systemic immunosuppression with dapsone or prednisone or sometimes high-dose prednisone with immunosuppressants (eg, azathioprine, mycophenolate, cyclophosphamide, rituximab) and IV immune globulin.

PEMPHIGUS FOLIACEUS

Pemphigus foliaceus is an autoimmune blistering disorder in which splits in the superficial epidermis result in cutaneous erosions.

Pemphigus foliaceus usually occurs in middle-aged patients, affecting men and women in equal numbers. An endemic form of pemphigus foliaceus, fogo selvagem, occurs in younger adults and children, particularly in South America. Pemphigus erythematosus, a localized form of pemphigus foliaceus, has immunologic features of pemphigus and lupus erythematosus (IgG and C3 deposition on keratinocyte surfaces and basement membrane zone with circulating antinuclear antibodies); however, patients rarely are diagnosed with both diseases concurrently. Pemphigus foliaceus may occur after use of penicillamine, nifedipine, or captopril.

Symptoms and Signs

The primary lesion is a flaccid vesicle or bulla, but due to the superficial location of the epidermal split, lesions tend to rupture, so intact bullae or vesicles are rarely evident on examination. Instead, well-demarcated, scattered, crusted, erythematous lesions are common on the face, scalp, and upper trunk. Mucosal involvement is rare. Skin lesions can burn and cause pain, but patients are typically not severely ill. Pemphigus erythematosus tends to affect the malar cheeks.

Diagnosis

- Skin biopsy and immunofluorescence

Diagnosis of pemphigus foliaceus is by biopsy of a lesion and adjacent (perilesional) unaffected skin that shows IgG autoantibodies against the keratinocyte cell surface via direct immunofluorescence. Autoantibodies to desmoglein 1, a transmembrane glycoprotein that affects cell-cell adhesion and signaling between epidermal cells, can be detected in serum via direct immunofluorescence, indirect immunofluorescence, and ELISA.

Treatment

- Corticosteroids, topical or systemic

If the disease is localized and not severe, high-potency topical corticosteroids are typically effective. More widespread or severe cases require systemic corticosteroids plus, at times, other immunosuppressive therapies, such as rituximab, plasma exchange, methotrexate, mycophenolate mofetil, or azathioprine. Limited studies suggest that addition of a combination of tetracycline 500 mg po qid and nicotinamide 500 mg po tid may be effective in some people.

PEMPHIGUS VULGARIS

Pemphigus vulgaris is an uncommon, potentially fatal, autoimmune disorder characterized by intraepidermal blisters and extensive erosions on apparently healthy skin and mucous membranes. Diagnosis is by skin biopsy with direct immunofluorescence testing. Treatment is with corticosteroids sometimes along with other immunosuppressive therapies.

Pemphigus vulgaris usually occurs in middle-aged patients, affecting men and women in equal numbers. Rarely, cases have been reported in children. One variant, paraneoplastic pemphigus, can occur in patients who have malignant or benign tumors, most commonly non-Hodgkin lymphoma.

Pemphigus vulgaris is characterized by IgG autoantibodies directed against the calcium-dependent cadherins desmoglein 1 and desmoglein 3. These transmembrane glycoproteins affect cell-cell adhesion and signaling between epidermal cells. Acantholysis (loss of intercellular adhesion) results from either direct inhibition of desmoglein function by autoantibody binding or from autoantibody-induced cell signaling that results in down-regulation of cell-cell adhesion and formation of blisters. These autoantibodies are present in both serum and skin during active disease. Any area of stratified squamous epithelium may be affected, including mucosal surfaces.

Symptoms and Signs

Flaccid bullae (see Plate 46), which are the primary lesions of pemphigus vulgaris, cause widespread and painful skin, oral, and other mucosal erosions. About half of patients have only oral erosions, which rupture and remain as chronic, painful lesions for variable periods. Often, oral lesions precede skin involvement. Dysphagia and poor oral intake are common because lesions also may occur in the upper esophagus. Cutaneous bullae typically arise in normal-appearing skin, rupture, and leave a raw area with crusting. Itching is usually absent. Erosions often become infected. If large portions of the body are affected, fluid and electrolyte loss may be significant.

Diagnosis

- Biopsy with immunofluorescence testing

Pemphigus vulgaris should be suspected in patients with unexplained chronic mucosal ulceration, particularly if they have bullous skin lesions. This disorder must be differentiated from other disorders that cause chronic oral ulcers and from other bullous dermatoses (eg, pemphigus foliaceus, bullous pemphigoid, MMP, drug eruptions, toxic epidermal necrolysis, erythema multiforme, dermatitis herpetiformis, bullous contact dermatitis). Two clinical findings, both reflecting lack of epidermal cohesion, that are somewhat specific for pemphigus vulgaris are the following:

- Nikolsky sign: Upper layers of epidermis move laterally with slight pressure or rubbing of skin adjacent to a bulla.
- Asboe-Hansen sign: Gentle pressure on intact bullae causes fluid to spread away from the site of pressure and beneath the adjacent skin.

The diagnosis of pemphigus vulgaris is confirmed by biopsy of lesional and surrounding (perilesional) normal skin. Immunofluorescence testing shows IgG autoantibodies against the keratinocyte's cell surface. Serum autoantibodies to desmoglein 1 and desmoglein 3 transmembrane glycoproteins can be identified via direct immunofluorescence, indirect immunofluorescence, and ELISA.

Prognosis

Without systemic corticosteroid treatment, pemphigus vulgaris is often fatal, usually within 5 yr of disease onset. Systemic corticosteroid and immunosuppressive therapy has improved prognosis, but death may still result from complications of therapy.

Treatment

- Corticosteroids, oral or IV
- Sometimes immunosuppressants
- Sometimes plasma exchange or IV immune globulin (IVIG)

Referral to a dermatologist with expertise in treating this disorder is recommended. Hospitalization is required initially for all but the most minor cases. Cleansing and dressing of open skin lesions is similar to that done to treat partial-thickness burns (eg, reverse isolation, hydrocolloid or silver sulfadiazine dressings).

Treatment of pemphigus vulgaris is aimed at decreasing production of pathogenic autoantibodies. The mainstay of treatment is systemic corticosteroids. Some patients with few lesions may respond to oral prednisone 20 to 30 mg once/day, but most require 1 mg/kg once/day as an initial dose. Some clinicians begin with even higher doses, which may slightly hasten initial response but does not appear to improve outcome. If new lesions continue to appear after 5 to 7 days, IV pulse therapy with methylprednisolone 1 g once/day can be tried.

Immunosuppressants such as methotrexate, cyclophosphamide, azathioprine, gold, mycophenolate mofetil, cyclosporine, or rituximab can reduce the need for corticosteroids and thus minimize the undesirable effects of long-term corticosteroid use. Plasma exchange and high-dose IV immune globulin to reduce antibody titers have also been effective.

Once no new lesions have appeared for 7 to 10 days, corticosteroid dose should be tapered monthly by about 10 mg/day (tapering continues more slowly once 20 mg/day is reached). A relapse requires a return to the starting dose. If the patient has been stable after a year, a trial without treatment can be attempted but must be closely monitored.

KEY POINTS

- About half of patients with pemphigus vulgaris have only oral lesions.
- Use Nikolsky and Asboe-Hansen signs to help clinically differentiate pemphigus vulgaris from other bullous disorders.
- Confirm the diagnosis by immunofluorescence testing of skin samples.
- Treat with systemic corticosteroids, with or without other immunosuppressive therapies (drugs, IV immune globulin, or plasma exchange).

125 Cancers of the Skin

Skin cancer is the most common type of cancer and commonly develops in sun-exposed areas of skin. The incidence is highest among outdoor workers, sportsmen, and sunbathers and is inversely related to the amount of melanin skin pigmentation; fair-skinned people are most susceptible. Skin cancers may also develop years after therapeutic x-rays or exposure to carcinogens (eg, arsenic ingestion).

Over 5.4 million new cases of skin cancer are diagnosed in over 3.3 million people in the US yearly. (See The Skin Cancer Foundation at www.skincancer.org and also the US Preventive Services Task Force summary of recommendations for screening and counseling for skin cancer [www.uspreventiveservicestaskforce.org].)

The most common forms of skin cancer are

- Basal cell carcinoma (about 80%)
- Squamous cell carcinoma (about 16%)
- Melanoma (about 4%)

The less common forms of skin cancer are

- Paget disease of the nipple or extramammary Paget (usually near the anus)
- Kaposi sarcoma
- Merkel cell carcinoma
- Atypical fibroxanthomas
- Tumors of the adnexa
- Cutaneous T-cell lymphoma (mycosis fungoides)

Bowen disease is a superficial squamous cell carcinoma. Keratoacanthoma may be a well-differentiated form of squamous cell carcinoma.

Initially, skin cancers are often asymptomatic. The most frequent presentation is an irregular red or pigmented lesion that does not go away. Any lesion that appears to be enlarging should be biopsied—whether tenderness, mild inflammation, crusting, or occasional bleeding is present or not. If treated early, most skin cancers are curable.

PEARLS & PITFALLS

- Biopsy any skin lesion, whether appearance is typical for cancer or atypical, that enlarges or persists longer than expected.

Screening: Routine screening for skin cancer is by patient self-examination, physician examination, or both.

Prevention: Because many skin cancers seem to be related to ultraviolet (UV) exposure, a number of measures are recommended to limit exposure.

- Sun avoidance: Seeking shade, minimizing outdoor activities between 10 AM and 4 PM (when sun's rays are strongest), and avoiding sunbathing and the use of tanning beds
- Use of protective clothing: Long-sleeved shirts, pants, and broad-brimmed hats
- Use of sunscreen: At least sun protection factor (SPF) 30 with broad-spectrum UVA/UVB protection, used as directed (ie, reapplied every 2 h and after swimming or sweating); should not be used to prolong sun exposure

Current evidence is inadequate to determine whether these measures reduce incidence or mortality of melanoma; in nonmelanoma skin cancers (basal cell carcinoma and squamous cell carcinoma), sun protection does decrease the incidence of new cancers.

ATYPICAL FIBROXANTHOMA

Atypical fibroxanthoma is a low-grade sarcoma of the skin.

Atypical fibroxanthomas most commonly occur on the head and neck of elderly patients. They appear similar to other nonmelanoma skin cancers, as nonhealing or tender pink-red skin papules or nodules.

Diagnosis is with biopsy.

Tumors are excised, or Mohs micrographic surgery—in which tissue borders are progressively excised until specimens are tumor-free (as determined by microscopic examination during surgery)—is done if clinically appropriate. Metastasis is unusual.

Prevention: Because atypical fibroxanthomas seem to be related to UV exposure, a number of measures are recommended to limit exposure.

- Sun avoidance: Seeking shade, minimizing outdoor activities between 10 AM and 4 PM (when sun's rays are strongest), and avoiding sunbathing and the use of tanning beds
- Use of protective clothing: Long-sleeved shirts, pants, and broad-brimmed hats
- Use of sunscreen: At least SPF 30 with broad-spectrum UVA/UVB protection, used as directed (ie, reapplied every 2 h and after swimming or sweating); should not be used to prolong sun exposure

BASAL CELL CARCINOMA

(Rodent Ulcer)

Basal cell carcinoma is a superficial, slowly growing papule or nodule (see Plate 32) that derives from certain epidermal cells. Basal cell carcinomas arise from keratinocytes near the basal layer and can be referred to as basaloid keratinocytes. Metastasis is rare, but local growth can be highly destructive. Diagnosis is by biopsy. Treatment depends on the tumor's characteristics and may involve curettage and electrodesiccation, surgical excision, cryosurgery, topical chemotherapy, or, occasionally, radiation therapy or drug therapy.

Basal cell carcinoma is the most common type of skin cancer, with > 4 million new cases yearly in the US. It is most common among fair-skinned people with a history of sun exposure and is very rare in darkly pigmented people.

Symptoms and Signs

The clinical manifestations and biologic behavior of basal cell carcinomas are highly variable. The most common types are

- Nodular (about 60% of basal cell carcinomas): Small, shiny, firm, almost translucent to pink nodules with telangiectases, usually on the face. Ulceration and crusting are common.

- Superficial (about 30%): Red or pink, marginated, thin papules or plaques, commonly on the trunk, that are difficult to differentiate from psoriasis or localized dermatitis
- Morpheaform (5 to 10%): Flat, scarlike, indurated plaques that can be flesh-colored or light red and have vague borders
- Others: Other types are possible. Nodular and superficial basal cell carcinomas can produce pigment (sometimes called pigmented basal cell carcinomas)

Most commonly, the carcinoma begins as a shiny papule, enlarges slowly, and, after a few months or years, shows a shiny, pearly border with prominent engorged vessels (telangiectases) on the surface and a central dell or ulcer. Recurrent crusting or bleeding is not unusual. Commonly, the carcinomas may alternately crust and heal, which may unjustifiably decrease patients' and physicians' concern about the importance of the lesion.

Diagnosis

- Biopsy

Diagnosis is by biopsy and histologic examination.

Prognosis

Basal cell carcinomas rarely metastasize but may invade healthy tissues. Rarely, patients die because the carcinoma invades or impinges on underlying vital structures or orifices (eg, eyes, ears, mouth, bone, dura mater).

Almost 25% of patients with a history of basal cell carcinoma develop a new basal cell cancer within 5 yr of the original carcinoma. Consequently, patients with a history of basal cell carcinoma should be seen annually for a skin examination.

Treatment

- Usually with local methods

Treatment should be done by a specialist.

The clinical appearance, size, site, and histologic subtype determine choice of treatment—curettage and electrodesiccation, surgical excision, cryosurgery, topical chemotherapy (imiquimod or 5-fluorouracil) and photodynamic therapy, or, occasionally, radiation therapy.

Recurrent or incompletely treated cancers, large cancers, cancers at recurrence-prone sites (eg, head and neck), and morphea-like cancers with vague borders are often treated with Mohs microscopically controlled surgery, in which tissue borders are progressively excised until specimens are tumor-free (as determined by microscopic examination during surgery).

If patients have metastatic or locally advanced disease and are not candidates for surgery or radiation therapy (eg, because lesions are large, recurrent, or metastatic), vismodegib and sonidegib are now available. Both medications inhibits the hedgehog pathway (a pathway that is mutated in most patients with basal cell carcinoma).

Prevention

Because basal cell carcinoma seems to be related to UV exposure, a number of measures are recommended to limit exposure.

- Sun avoidance: Seeking shade, minimizing outdoor activities between 10 AM and 4 PM (when sun's rays are strongest), and avoiding sunbathing and the use of tanning beds
- Use of protective clothing: Long-sleeved shirts, pants, and broad-brimmed hats
- Use of sunscreen: At least SPF 30 with broad-spectrum UVA/UVB protection, used as directed (ie, reapplied every 2 h and after swimming or sweating); should not be used to prolong sun exposure

KEY POINTS

- Basal cell carcinomas, the most common skin cancers, are particularly common among fair-skinned people on sun-exposed skin.
- Consider the diagnosis with typical lesions (eg, shiny, slowly enlarging papule, often with a shiny, pearly border) and lesions that alternately crust and heal.
- Refer patients to specialists for treatment, usually by locally destructive methods.

BOWEN DISEASE

(Intraepidermal Squamous Cell Carcinoma)

Bowen disease is a superficial squamous cell carcinoma in situ.

Bowen disease is most common in sun-exposed areas but may arise at any location.

Symptoms and Signs

Lesions can be solitary or multiple. They are red-brown and scaly or crusted, with little induration; they frequently resemble a localized thin plaque of psoriasis, dermatitis, or a dermatophyte infection.

Diagnosis

- Biopsy

Diagnosis is by biopsy, which shows full-thickness epidermal dysplasia but no dermal involvement.

Treatment

- Removal or ablation via local methods

Treatment depends on the lesion's characteristics and may involve topical chemotherapy, curettage and electrodesiccation, surgical excision, or cryosurgery.

Prevention

Because many skin cancers seem to be related to UV exposure, a number of measures are recommended to limit exposure.

- Sun avoidance: Seeking shade, minimizing outdoor activities between 10 AM and 4 PM (when sun's rays are strongest), and avoiding sunbathing and the use of tanning beds
- Use of protective clothing: Long-sleeved shirts, pants, and broad-brimmed hats
- Use of sunscreen: At least SPF 30 with broad-spectrum UVA/UVB protection, used as directed (ie, reapplied every 2 h and after swimming or sweating); should not be used to prolong sun exposure

KAPOSI SARCOMA

(Multiple Idiopathic Hemorrhagic Sarcoma)

Kaposi sarcoma (KS) is a multicentric vascular tumor caused by herpesvirus type 8. It can occur in classic, AIDS-associated, endemic (in Africa), and iatrogenic (eg, after organ transplantation) forms. Diagnosis is by biopsy. Treatment for indolent superficial lesions involves cryotherapy, electrocoagulation, excision, or electron beam radiation

therapy. Radiation therapy is used for more extensive disease. In the AIDS-associated form, antiretrovirals provide the most improvement.

KS originates from endothelial cells in response to infection by human herpesvirus 8 (HHV-8). Immunosuppression (particularly by AIDS and drugs for organ transplant recipients) markedly increases the likelihood of KS in HHV-8–infected patients. The tumor cells have a spindle shape, resembling smooth muscle cells, fibroblasts, and myofibroblasts.

Classification

Classic KS: This form occurs most often in older (> 60 yr) men of Italian, Jewish, or Eastern European ancestry. The course is indolent, and the disease is usually confined to a small number of lesions on the skin of the lower extremities (see Plate 40); visceral involvement occurs in < 10%. This form is usually not fatal.

AIDS-associated (epidemic) KS: This form is the most common AIDS-associated cancer and is more aggressive than classic KS. Multiple cutaneous lesions are typically present, often involving the face and trunk. Mucosal, lymph node, and GI involvement is common. Sometimes KS is the first manifestation of AIDS.

Endemic KS: This form occurs in Africa independent of HIV infection. There are 2 main types:

- Prepubertal lymphadenopathic form: It predominantly affects children; primary tumors involve lymph nodes, with or without skin lesions. The course is usually fulminant and fatal.
- Adult form: This form resembles classic KS.

Iatrogenic (immunosuppressive) KS: This form typically develops several years after organ transplantation. The course is more or less fulminant, depending on the degree of immunosuppression.

Symptoms and Signs

Cutaneous lesions are asymptomatic purple, pink, or red macules that may coalesce into blue-violet to black plaques and nodules. Some edema may be present. Occasionally, nodules fungate or penetrate soft tissue and invade bone. Mucosal lesions appear as bluish to violaceous macules, plaques, and tumors. GI lesions can bleed, sometimes extensively, but usually are asymptomatic.

Diagnosis

- Biopsy

Diagnosis of KS is confirmed by punch biopsy.

Patients with AIDS or immunosuppression require evaluation for visceral spread by CT of the chest and abdomen. If CT is negative but pulmonary or GI symptoms are present, bronchoscopy or GI endoscopy should be considered.

Treatment

- Surgical excision, cryotherapy, electrocoagulation, or possibly imiquimod for superficial lesions
- Local radiation therapy for multiple lesions or lymph node disease
- Antiretroviral therapy or sometimes IV interferon alfa for AIDS-associated KS
- Reduction of immunosuppressants for iatrogenic KS

Indolent lesions often require no treatment. One or a few superficial lesions can be removed by excision, cryotherapy, or electrocoagulation. Imiquimod has also been reported to be effective. Intralesional vinblastine or interferon alfa is also useful. Multiple lesions and lymph node disease are treated locally with 10 to 20 Gy of radiation therapy.

AIDS-associated KS responds markedly to highly active antiretroviral therapy (HAART), probably because CD4+ count improves and HIV viral load decreases; however, there is some evidence that protease inhibitors in this regimen may block angiogenesis. AIDS patients with indolent disease and CD4+ counts > 150/μL and HIV RNA < 500 copies/mL can be treated with IV interferon alfa. Patients with more extensive or visceral disease can be given liposomal doxorubicin 20 mg/m^2 IV q 2 to 3 wk. If this regimen fails, patients may receive paclitaxel. Other agents being investigated as adjuncts include IL-12, desferrioxamine, and oral retinoids. Treatment of KS does not prolong life in most AIDS patients because infections dominate the clinical course.

Iatrogenic KS responds best to stopping immunosuppressants. In organ transplant patients, reduction of immunosuppressant dosage often results in reduction of KS lesions. If dosage reduction is not possible, conventional local and systemic therapies used in other forms of KS should be instituted. Sirolimus may also improve iatrogenic KS.

Treatment of endemic KS is challenging and typically palliative.

KEY POINTS

- Consider KS in older men, Africans, and patients with organ transplants or AIDS.
- Test patients with immunosuppression (including AIDS) for metastases.
- Treat superficial lesions with locally ablative methods.

KERATOACANTHOMA

Keratoacanthomas are round, firm, usually flesh-colored nodules with sharply sloping borders and a characteristic central crater containing keratinous material; they usually resolve spontaneously, but some may be a well-differentiated form of squamous cell carcinoma.

Etiology is unknown. Most experts consider these lesions to be well-differentiated squamous cell carcinomas with a tendency to involute.

Development is rapid. Usually the lesion reaches its full size, typically 1 to 3 cm but sometimes > 5 cm, within 1 or 2 mo. Common sites are sun-exposed areas, the face, the forearms, and the dorsum of the hands. Spontaneous involution may start within a few months, but involution is not guaranteed.

Diagnosis

- Biopsy or excision

Because this lesion cannot be relied on to involute, biopsy or excision is recommended.

Treatment

- Surgery or injections of methotrexate or 5-fluorouracil

Spontaneous involution may leave substantial scarring; surgery or intralesional injections with methotrexate or 5-fluorouracil usually yield better cosmetic results, and excision allows histologic confirmation of the diagnosis.

Prevention

It is unclear whether keratoacanthoma risk increases with increasing UV exposure. Because it may, a number of measures are often recommended to limit exposure.

- Sun avoidance: Seeking shade, minimizing outdoor activities between 10 AM and 4 PM (when sun's rays are strongest), and avoiding sunbathing and the use of tanning beds
- Use of protective clothing: Long-sleeved shirts, pants, and broad-brimmed hats
- Use of sunscreen: At least SPF 30 with broad-spectrum UVA/UVB protection, used as directed (ie, reapplied every 2 h and after swimming or sweating); should not be used to prolong sun exposure

MELANOMA

(Malignant Melanoma)

Malignant melanoma arises from melanocytes in a pigmented area (eg, skin, mucous membranes, eyes, or CNS). Metastasis is correlated with depth of dermal invasion. With spread, prognosis is poor. Diagnosis is by biopsy. Wide surgical excision is the rule for operable tumors. Metastatic disease requires systemic therapy but is difficult to cure.

In 2016, about 76,380 new cases of melanoma occurred in the US, causing about 10,130 deaths. Lifetime risk is about 1 to 2%. Incidence has remained steady over the last 8 yr (it had previously been increasing at a faster rate than any other malignant tumor). Melanoma accounts for < 5% of total skin cancers diagnosed in the US but causes most skin cancer deaths. On average, one person in the US dies of melanoma every hour.

Melanomas occur mainly on the skin but also on the mucosa of the oral, genital, and rectal regions and conjunctiva. Melanomas may also develop in the choroid layer of the eye, in the leptomeninges (pia or arachnoid mater), and in the nail beds. Melanomas vary in size, shape, and color (usually pigmented) and in their propensity to invade and metastasize. Metastasis occurs via lymphatics and blood vessels. Local metastasis results in the formation of nearby satellite papules or nodules that may or may not be pigmented. Metastasis to skin or internal organs may occur, and, occasionally, metastatic nodules or enlarged lymph nodes are discovered before the primary lesion is identified.

Etiology

Risk factors for melanoma include

- Sun exposure, particularly repeated blistering sunburns
- Repeated tanning with ultraviolet A (UVA) or psoralen plus UVA (PUVA) treatments
- Nonmelanoma skin cancer
- Family and personal history
- Fair skin, freckling
- Atypical moles, particularly > 5
- Increased numbers of melanocytic nevi (particularly > 20, depending on family history)
- Immunosuppression
- Occurrence of lentigo maligna
- Congenital melanocytic nevus > 20 cm (giant congenital nevi)
- Atypical mole syndrome (dysplastic nevus syndrome)
- Familial atypical mole–melanoma syndrome

Patients with a personal history of melanoma have an increased risk of additional melanomas. People who have one or more 1st-degree relatives with a history of melanoma have an increased risk (up to 6 or 8 times) over those without a family history.

Atypical mole syndrome is the presence of > 50 moles, at least one of which is atypical and at least one of which is > 8 mm in diameter.

Familial atypical mole–melanoma syndrome is the presence of multiple atypical moles and melanoma in ≥ 2 1st-degree relatives; such people are at markedly increased risk (25 times) of melanoma.

Melanoma is less common among people with darker pigmentation; when it occurs, the nail beds, palms, and soles are more often affected.

About 30% of melanomas develop from pigmented moles (about half each from typical and atypical moles); almost all the rest arise from melanocytes in normal skin. Atypical moles (dysplastic nevi) may be precursors to melanoma. The very rare melanomas of childhood almost always arise in the leptomeninges or from giant congenital nevi present at birth. Although melanomas occur during pregnancy, pregnancy does not increase the likelihood that a mole will become a melanoma; moles frequently change in size and darken uniformly during pregnancy. However, the following signs of malignant transformation should be carefully sought:

- Change in size
- Change in shape, including irregular or indistinct borders
- Irregular change in color, especially spread of red, white, and blue pigmentation to surrounding normal skin
- Change in surface characteristics or consistency
- Signs of inflammation in surrounding skin, with possible bleeding, ulceration, itching, or tenderness

Recent enlargement, darkening, ulceration, or bleeding usually indicates that the melanoma has invaded the skin deeply. Patients at risk can be taught self-examination to detect changes in existing moles and to recognize features suggesting melanoma (see Diagnosis on p. 1005).

Classification

There are 4 main types of melanoma and a few minor subtypes.

Superficial spreading melanoma: This type accounts for 70% of melanomas. Typically asymptomatic, it occurs most commonly on women's legs and men's torsos. The lesion is usually a plaque with irregular, raised, indurated, and tan or brown areas, which often have red, white, black, and blue spots or small, sometimes protuberant blue-black nodules (see Plate 44). Small notchlike indentations of the margins may be noted, along with enlargement or color change. Histologically, atypical melanocytes characteristically invade the dermis and epidermis. This type of melanoma most commonly has activating mutations in the *BRAF* gene at V600.

Nodular melanoma: This type accounts for 15 to 30% of melanomas. It may occur anywhere on the body as a dark, protuberant papule or a plaque that varies from pearl to gray to black. Occasionally, a lesion contains little if any pigment or may look like a vascular tumor. Unless it ulcerates, nodular melanoma is asymptomatic, but patients usually seek advice because the lesion enlarges rapidly.

Lentigo maligna melanoma: This type accounts for 5% of melanomas. It tends to arise in older patients. It arises from lentigo maligna (Hutchinson freckle or malignant melanoma in situ—a frecklelike tan or brown macule). It usually occurs on the face or other areas of chronic sun exposure as an asymptomatic, flat, tan or brown, irregularly shaped macule or patch with darker brown or black spots scattered irregularly on its surface. In lentigo maligna, both normal and malignant melanocytes are confined to the epidermis. When malignant melanocytes invade the dermis, the lesion is called lentigo maligna melanoma, and the cancer may metastasize. This type of melanoma most commonly has mutations in the *C-kit* gene.

Acral-lentiginous melanoma: This type accounts for only 2 to 10% of melanomas. Incidence is probably the same regardless of skin pigmentation, but because people with darkly pigmented skin infrequently develop other forms of melanoma, acral-lentiginous melanoma is the most common type among them. It arises on palmar, plantar, and subungual skin and has a characteristic histologic picture similar to that of lentigo maligna melanoma. This type of melanoma often has mutations in the *C-kit* gene.

Amelanotic melanoma: Amelanotic melanoma is a type of melanoma that does not produce pigment. It can be any of the 4 main types and is most often grouped with the minor categories of melanoma such as spitzoid melanoma, desmoplastic melanoma, neurotropic melanoma, and others.

Occurring in < 10% of melanomas, amelanotic melanomas may be pink, red, or slightly light-brown and may have well-defined borders. Their appearance may suggest benign lesions, or a form of nonmelanoma skin cancer, and thereby lead to a late diagnosis and possibly a worse prognosis.

Diagnosis

- Biopsy

Differential diagnosis includes basal cell carcinomas and squamous cell carcinomas, seborrheic keratoses, atypical moles, blue nevi, dermatofibromas, moles, hematomas (especially on the hands or feet), venous lakes, pyogenic granulomas, and warts with focal thromboses.

If doubt exists, biopsy should include the full depth of the dermis and extend slightly beyond the edges of the lesion. Biopsy should be excisional for most lesions except those on anatomically sensitive or cosmetically important areas; in these cases, a broad shave biopsy can be done. For broader lesions such as lentigo maligna, representative shave biopsies from several areas can increase the diagnostic yield. By doing step sections, the pathologist can determine the maximal thickness of the melanoma. Definitive radical surgery should not precede histologic diagnosis.

Pigmented lesions with the following features should be excised or biopsied:

- Recent enlargement
- Darkening
- Bleeding
- Ulceration

However, these features usually indicate that the melanoma has already invaded the skin deeply. Earlier diagnosis of melanoma is possible if biopsy specimens can be obtained from lesions having variegated colors (eg, brown or black with shades of red, gray, or blue), irregular elevations that are visible or palpable, and borders with angular indentations or notches. Polarized light and immersion contact dermoscopy, which is used to examine pigmented lesions, may be useful for distinguishing melanomas from benign lesions. Because earlier diagnosis can be lifesaving and features of melanoma can be variable, even slightly suspect lesions should be biopsied.

Tumors, particularly if metastatic, are sometimes tested genetically for mutations, eg, to suggest treatment with vemurafenib, a *BRAF* inhibitor, for metastatic melanomas bearing a V600 mutation in the *BRAF* gene.

Staging: The staging of melanoma is based on clinical and pathologic criteria and closely corresponds to the traditional tumor-node-metastasis (TNM) classification system. The staging system classifies melanomas based on local, regional, or distant disease.

- Stages I and II: Localized primary melanoma
- Stage III: Metastasis to regional lymph nodes
- Stage IV: Distant metastatic disease

Stage strongly correlates with survival. A minimally invasive microstaging technique, the so-called sentinel lymph node biopsy (SLNB), is a major advance in the ability to stage cancers more accurately. Recommended staging studies depend on the Breslow depth (how deeply tumor cells have invaded) and histologic characteristics of the melanoma; dermal mitoses and ulceration indicate higher risk in melanomas that are < 1 mm Breslow depth (see Table 125–1). Staging studies may include SLNB, laboratory tests (eg, CBC, LDH, liver function tests), chest x-ray, CT, and PET and are done by a coordinated team that includes dermatologists, oncologists, general surgeons, plastic surgeons, and dermatopathologists.

Prognosis

Melanoma may spread rapidly, causing death within months of its recognition, yet the 5-yr cure rate of early, very superficial lesions is very high. Thus, cure depends on early diagnosis and early treatment.

For tumors of cutaneous origin (not CNS and subungual melanomas) that have not metastasized, the survival rate varies depending on the thickness of the tumor at the time of diagnosis. The 5-yr survival rates range from 97% for patients with stage IA melanomas to 53% for patients with stage IIC melanomas; 10-yr survival rates range from 93% for patients with stage IA melanomas to 39% for patients with stage IIC melanomas.

Mucosal melanomas (especially anorectal melanomas), which are more common among nonwhites, have a poor prognosis, although they often seem quite limited when discovered.

Once melanoma has metastasized to the lymph nodes, 5-yr survival ranges from 25 to 70% depending on the degree of

Table 125–1. STAGING OF MELANOMA BASED ON THICKNESS AND ULCERATION

STAGE	DESCRIPTION
0	Intraepithelial or in situ melanoma
IA	≤ 1 mm with no ulceration and dermal mitoses < 1/mm^2
IB	≤ 1 mm with ulceration and/or at least 1 dermal mitoses/mm^2 1.01–2 mm with no ulceration
IIA	1.01–2 mm with ulceration 2.01–4 mm with no ulceration
IIB	2.01–4 mm with ulceration ≥ 4 mm with no ulceration
IIC	> 4 mm with ulceration

Adapted from Edge SB, Byrd DR, Compton CC, et al: *AJCC Cancer Staging Manual,* 7th ed. New York, Springer (2010).

ulceration and number of nodes involved. Once melanoma has metastasized to distant sites, 5-yr survival is about 10%.

Degree of lymphocytic infiltration, which represents reaction by the patient's immunologic defense system, may correlate with the level of invasion and prognosis. Chances of cure are maximal when lymphocytic infiltration is limited to the most superficial lesions and decrease with deeper levels of tumor cell invasion, ulceration, and vascular or lymphatic invasion.

A new commercially available test of gene expression (DecisionDx™-Melanoma) helps determine whether patients who have stage I or II melanomas are at high or low risk of metastases. This test has not yet been added to consensus guidelines; using it to determine whether patients should receive immunotherapy is not recommended at this time.

Treatment

- Surgical excision
- Possibly adjuvant radiation therapy, imiquimod, or cryotherapy
- For metastatic or unresectable melanoma, immunotherapy (eg, pembrolizumab, nivolumab), targeted therapy (eg, ipilimumab, vemurafenib, dabrafenib), and radiation therapy

Treatment of melanoma is primarily by surgical excision (wide local excision). Although the width of margins is debated, most experts agree that a 1-cm lateral tumor-free margin is adequate for lesions < 1 mm thick. In tumors < 1 mm thick, but with ulceration or at least 1 dermal mitoses/mm², SLNB can be considered. Thicker lesions may deserve larger margins, more radical surgery, and SLNB.

Lentigo maligna melanoma and lentigo maligna are usually treated with wide local excision and, if necessary, skin grafting. Intensive radiation therapy is much less effective. The ideal treatment of melanoma in situ is surgical excision. Sometimes this can be accomplished with staged excisions or Mohs micrographic surgery, in which tissue borders are progressively excised until specimens are tumor-free (as determined by microscopic examination during surgery). If patients decline or are not candidates for surgical therapy (eg, because of comorbidities or involvement of cosmetically important areas), imiquimod and cryotherapy can be considered. Most other treatment methods usually do not penetrate deeply enough into involved follicles, which must be removed.

Spreading or nodular melanomas are usually treated with wide local excision extending down to the fascia. Lymph node dissection may be recommended when nodes are involved. (See also the American Academy of Dermatology Association's guidelines of care for the management of primary cutaneous melanoma [www.ncbi.nlm.nih.gov].)

Metastatic disease: Treatment of metastatic melanoma typically includes

- Immunotherapy
- Molecular targeted therapy
- Radiation therapy
- Rarely surgical resection

All of these treatments should be considered for all patients who have metastatic melanoma. Final decisions are generally individualized by an oncologist and may depend on availability.

Metastatic disease is generally inoperable, but in certain cases, localized and regional metastases can be excised to help eliminate residual disease.

Immunotherapy with anti-programmed death (PD-1) antibodies (pembrolizumab and nivolumab) lengthens survival. They inhibit the PD-1 receptor that attenuates T-cell effector responses against cancers.

Ipilimumab (a monoclonal antibody to cytotoxic T lymphocyte-associated antigen 4 [CTLA-4]) is another form of immunotherapy that can also lengthen survival. It works by preventing anergy of T cells, thus freeing the immune system to attack tumor cells.

Molecular targeted therapy includes use of vemurafenib and dabrafenib, which function by inhibiting *BRAF* activity, resulting in slowing or stopping of tumor cell proliferation. These drugs have lengthened survival in patients with metastases; adding mitogen-activated protein kinase (MEK) inhibitor enzymes MEK1 and MEK2 (via trametinib) lengthens survival even more.

Cytotoxic chemotherapy has not been shown to improve survival in patients with metastatic disease and is normally reserved for patients who do not have other options.

Adjuvant therapy with recombinant biologic response modifiers (particularly interferon alfa) to suppress clinically inapparent micrometastases may also be used for inoperable metastatic melanoma.

Radiation therapy may be used to palliate brain metastases, but the response is poor.

The following are under study:

- Infusion of lymphokine-activated killer cells or antibodies (for advanced-stage disease)
- Vaccine therapy

Prevention

Because melanoma seems to be related to UV exposure, a number of measures are recommended to limit exposure.

- Sun avoidance: Seeking shade, minimizing outdoor activities between 10 AM and 4 PM (when sun's rays are strongest), and avoiding sunbathing and the use of tanning beds
- Use of protective clothing: Long-sleeved shirts, pants, and broad-brimmed hats
- Use of sunscreen: At least SPF 30 with broad-spectrum UVA/UVB protection, used as directed (ie, reapplied every 2 h and after swimming or sweating); should not be used to prolong sun exposure

Current evidence is inadequate to determine whether these measures reduce incidence or mortality of melanoma; in nonmelanoma skin cancers (basal cell carcinoma and squamous cell carcinoma), sun protection does decrease the incidence of new cancers.

KEY POINTS

- Melanoma accounts for < 5% of total skin cancers diagnosed in the US but causes most skin cancer deaths.
- Melanoma can develop in the skin, mucosa, conjunctiva, choroid layer of the eye, leptomeninges, and nail beds.
- Although melanoma can develop from a typical or atypical mole, most do not.
- Physicians (and patients) should monitor moles for changes in size, shape, borders, color, or surface characteristics and for bleeding, ulceration, itching, and tenderness.
- Biopsy even slightly suspect lesions.
- Excise melanomas whenever feasible, particularly when melanomas have not metastasized.
- Consider immunotherapy (eg, pembrolizumab, nivolumab), targeted therapies (eg, ipilimumab, vemurafenib), radiation therapy, and excision if melanoma is unresectable or metastatic.

MERKEL CELL CARCINOMA

(Anaplastic Skin Cancer; APUDoma of the Skin; Neuroendocrine Skin Carcinoma; Primary Small Cell Skin Carcinoma; Trabecular Cell Carcinoma)

Merkel cell carcinoma is a rare, aggressive skin cancer that tends to affect older white people.

Mean age at diagnosis is about 75. Merkel cell carcinoma also affects younger patients who are immunosuppressed. Other risk factors include cumulative exposure to UV light, exposure to the Merkel cell polyomavirus, and having another cancer (eg, multiple myeloma, chronic lymphocytic leukemia, melanoma). Lymphatic spread is common.

Symptoms and Signs

Skin lesions are typically firm, shiny, flesh-colored or bluish-red, and nodular. Their most characteristic clinical findings are rapid growth and absence of pain and tenderness. Although Merkel cell carcinoma can affect any part of the skin, it is most common on sun-exposed areas (eg, face, upper extremities).

Diagnosis

- Biopsy

Diagnosis is by biopsy.

Most patients have metastatic disease at presentation, and the prognosis is poor.

Treatment

- Determined by staging

Treatment is determined by cancer staging and typically includes wide local excision, often followed by radiation therapy, lymph node dissection, or both.

Chemotherapy may be indicated for metastatic or recurrent cancer.

Prevention

Because Merkel cell carcinoma seems to be related to UV exposure, a number of measures are recommended to limit exposure.

- Sun avoidance: Seeking shade, minimizing outdoor activities between 10 AM and 4 PM (when sun's rays are strongest), and avoiding sunbathing and the use of tanning beds
- Use of protective clothing: Long-sleeved shirts, pants, and broad-brimmed hats
- Use of sunscreen: At least SPF 30 with broad-spectrum UVA/UVB protection, used as directed (ie, reapplied every 2 h and after swimming or sweating); should not be used to prolong sun exposure

PAGET DISEASE OF THE NIPPLE

Paget disease is a rare type of carcinoma that appears as a unilateral eczematous to psoriasiform plaque of the nipple and areola. It results from extension to the epidermis of an underlying ductal adenocarcinoma of the breast.

Paget disease of the nipple should not be confused with the metabolic bone disease that is also called Paget disease. In Paget disease of the nipple, metastatic disease is often present at the time of the diagnosis.

Paget disease of the nipple also occurs at other sites, most often in the groin or perianal area (extramammary Paget disease). Extramammary Paget disease is a rare adenocarcinoma that can either arise from apocrine glands of the skin or extend from a cancer in the bladder, anus, or rectum.

Diagnosis

- Biopsy

The redness, oozing, and crusting closely resemble dermatitis, but physicians should suspect carcinoma because the lesion is sharply marginated, unilateral, and unresponsive to topical therapy. Biopsy shows typical histologic changes.

Because this tumor is associated with underlying cancer, systemic evaluation (eg, history and physical examination, age-appropriate cancer screening, imaging) is required.

Treatment

- Treatment of underlying tumor
- Excision of the nipple-areolar complex

Treatment of Paget disease of the nipple involves appropriate breast cancer treatment for discovered underlying tumors and includes wide excision of the nipple-areolar complex. If no underlying breast cancer is found, either mastectomy or nipple-areolar complex resection followed by radiation treatment may be used.

Treatment of extramammary Paget disease may also involve ablation of overlying cutaneous involvement, either with topical therapies (eg, topical 5-fluorouracil, imiquimod, photodynamic therapy), radiation therapy, surgically, or by CO_2 laser ablation. A thorough work-up to rule out an internal malignancy should be performed.

SQUAMOUS CELL CARCINOMA

Squamous cell carcinoma is a malignant tumor of epidermal keratinocytes that invades the dermis; this cancer usually occurs in sun-exposed areas. Local destruction may be extensive, and metastases occur in advanced stages. Diagnosis is by biopsy. Treatment depends on the tumor's characteristics and may involve curettage and electrodesiccation, surgical excision, cryosurgery, or, occasionally, radiation therapy.

Squamous cell carcinoma is the 2nd most common type of skin cancer after basal cell carcinoma, with > 1 million cases annually in the US, and 2500 deaths. It may develop in normal tissue, in a preexisting actinic keratosis, in a patch of oral leukoplakia, or in a burn scar.

Symptoms and Signs

The clinical appearance is highly variable, but any nonhealing lesion on sun-exposed surfaces should be suspect. The tumor may begin as a red papule or plaque with a scaly or crusted surface and may become nodular or hyperkeratotic, sometimes with a warty surface. In some cases, the bulk of the lesion may lie below the level of the surrounding skin. Eventually the tumor ulcerates and invades the underlying tissue.

Diagnosis

- Biopsy

Biopsy is essential.

Differential diagnosis: Differential diagnosis varies based on the lesion's appearance.

Nonhealing ulcers should be differentiated from pyoderma gangrenosum and venous stasis ulcers.

Nodular and hyperkeratotic lesions should be differentiated from keratoacanthomas (probably squamous cell carcinomas themselves) and verruca vulgaris.

Scaling plaques should be differentiated from basal cell carcinoma, actinic keratosis, verruca vulgaris, seborrheic keratosis, psoriasis, and nummular dermatitis (nummular eczema).

Prognosis

In general, the prognosis for small lesions removed early and adequately is excellent. Regional and distant metastases of squamous cell carcinomas on sun-exposed skin are uncommon but do occur, particularly with poorly differentiated tumors. Characteristics of more aggressive tumors include

- Size > 2 cm in diameter
- Invasion depth of > 2 mm
- Perineural invasion
- Location on the ear or non-hair bearing lip

However, about one-third of lingual or mucosal cancers have metastasized before diagnosis (see p. 851).

Late-stage disease, which may require extensive surgery, is far more likely to metastasize. It spreads initially regionally to surrounding skin and lymph nodes and eventually to nearby organs. Cancers that occur near the ears or the vermilion border, in scars, or that have perineural invasion are more likely to metastasize. The overall 5-yr survival rate for metastatic disease is 34% despite therapy.

Treatment

- Usually locally destructive techniques

Treatment of squamous cell carcinoma is similar to that for basal cell carcinoma treatment and includes curettage and electrodesiccation, surgical excision, cryosurgery, topical chemotherapy (imiquimod or 5-fluorouracil) and photodynamic therapy, or, occasionally, radiation therapy. Treatment and follow-up must be monitored closely because of the greater risk of metastasis compared with a basal cell carcinoma.

Squamous cell carcinoma on the lip or other mucocutaneous junction should be excised; at times, cure is difficult.

Recurrences and large tumors should be treated aggressively with Mohs microscopically controlled surgery, in which tissue borders are progressively excised until specimens are tumor-free (as determined by microscopic examination during surgery), or by a team approach with surgery and radiation therapy. Because tumors with perineural invasion are aggressive, radiation therapy should be considered after surgery.

Metastatic disease is responsive to radiation therapy if metastases can be identified and are isolated. Widespread metastases do not respond well to chemotherapeutic regimens.

Prevention

Because squamous cell carcinoma seems to be related to UV exposure, a number of measures are recommended to limit exposure.

- Sun avoidance: Seeking shade, minimizing outdoor activities between 10 AM and 4 PM (when sun's rays are strongest), and avoiding sunbathing and the use of tanning beds
- Use of protective clothing: Long-sleeved shirts, pants, and broad-brimmed hats
- Use of sunscreen: At least SPF 30 with broad-spectrum UVA/UVB protection, used as directed (ie, reapplied every 2 h and after swimming or sweating); should not be used to prolong sun exposure

KEY POINTS

- Squamous cell carcinoma, because of its high frequency of occurrence and highly variable appearance, should be considered in any nonhealing lesion in a sun-exposed area.
- Metastases are uncommon but are more likely in cancers involving the lingual or mucosal surfaces; that occur near the ears, the vermilion border, or in scars; or that have perineural invasion.
- Treatment is usually with locally destructive methods, sometimes also with radiation therapy (eg, for tumors that are large, recurrent, or have perineural invasion).

126 Cornification Disorders

CALLUSES AND CORNS

(Clavi; Helomas; Tylomas)

Calluses and corns are circumscribed areas of hyperkeratosis at a site of intermittent pressure or friction. Calluses are more superficial, cover broader areas of skin, and usually asymptomatic. Corns are deeper, more focal, and frequently painful. Diagnosis is by appearance. Treatment is with manual abrasion with or without keratolytics. Prevention involves altering biomechanics, such as changing footwear. Rarely, surgery is required.

Calluses and corns are caused by intermittent pressure or friction, usually over a bony prominence (eg, calcaneus, metatarsal heads).

Corns consist of a sharply circumscribed keratinous plug, pea-sized or slightly larger, which extends through most of the underlying dermis. An underlying adventitial bursitis may develop. Hard corns occur over prominent bony protuberances, especially on the toes and plantar surface. Soft corns occur between the toes. Most corns result from poorly fitting footwear, but small seed-sized corns on non-weight-bearing aspects of the soles and palms may represent inherited keratosis punctata.

Calluses lack a central plug and have a more even appearance. They usually occur on the hands or feet but may occur elsewhere, especially in a person whose occupation entails repeated trauma to a particular area (eg, the mandible and clavicle of a violinist).

Symptoms and Signs

Calluses are usually asymptomatic but, if friction is extreme, may become thick and irritated, causing mild burning discomfort. At times, the discomfort may mimic that of interdigital neuralgia.

Corns may be painful or tender when pressure is applied. A bursa or fluid-filled pocket sometimes forms beneath a corn.

Diagnosis

- Clinical evaluation

A corn may be differentiated from a plantar wart or callus by paring away the thickened skin. After paring, a callus shows smooth translucent skin, whereas a wart appears sharply circumscribed, sometimes with soft macerated tissue or with central black dots (bleeding points) representing thrombosed capillaries. A corn, when pared, shows a sharply outlined yellowish to tan translucent core that interrupts the normal architecture of the papillary dermis.

Treatment

- Manual removal
- Keratolytics
- Cushioning
- Altering foot biomechanics
- Sometimes expert foot care

Manual removal: A nail file, emery board, or pumice stone used immediately after bathing is often a practical way to manually remove hyperkeratotic tissue.

Keratolytics: Keratolytics (eg, 17% salicylic acid in collodion, 40% salicylic acid plasters, 40% urea) can also be used, taking care to avoid applying the agents to normal skin. Normal skin may be protected by covering it with petrolatum before application of the keratolytic.

Cushioning and foot biomechanics: Cushioning and altering foot biomechanics can help prevent corns and help treat existing corns. Although difficult to eliminate, pressure on the affected surface should be reduced and redistributed. For foot lesions, soft, well-fitting shoes are important; they should have a roomy toe box so that toes can move freely in the shoe. Stylish shoes often prevent this freedom of motion. Shoes that increase discomfort of a lesion should be eliminated from the wardrobe. Pads or rings of suitable shapes and sizes, moleskin or foam-rubber protective bandages, arch inserts (orthotics), or metatarsal plates or bars may help redistribute the pressure. For corns and calluses on the ball of the foot, an orthotic should not be full length but should extend only to the ball or part of the shoe immediately behind the corn or callus. Surgical off-loading or removal of the offending bone is rarely necessary.

Expert foot care: Patients who have a tendency to develop recalcitrant painful calluses and corns may need regular care from a podiatrist. Patients who also have impaired peripheral circulation, particularly if they also have diabetes, require intensive foot care.

KEY POINTS

- The cause of corns and calluses is usually intermittent pressure or friction, usually over a bony prominence.
- After paring away the thickened overlying skin, a wart will bleed, whereas a corn will not.
- Recommend mechanical abrasion and keratolytics to help remove corns and calluses.
- Recommend cushioning and redistributing pressure in the foot to help prevent corns and calluses.

ICHTHYOSIS

Ichthyosis is scaling and flaking of skin ranging from mild but annoying dryness to severe disfiguring disease. Ichthyosis can also be a sign of systemic disease. Diagnosis is clinical. Treatment involves emollients and sometimes oral retinoids.

Ichthyosis differs from simple dry skin (xeroderma) by its association with a systemic disorder or drug, inheritability, severity, or a combination. Ichthyosis can also be much more severe than xeroderma.

Inherited ichthyoses: Inherited ichthyoses, which are characterized by excessive accumulation of scale on the skin surface, are classified according to clinical and genetic criteria (see Table 126–1). Some occur in isolation and are not part of a syndrome (eg, ichthyosis vulgaris, X-linked ichthyosis, lamellar ichthyosis, congenital ichthyosiform erythroderma [epidermolytic hyperkeratosis]). Other ichthyoses are part of a syndrome that involves multiple organs. For instance, Refsum disease and Sjögren-Larsson syndrome (hereditary intellectual disability and spastic paralysis caused by a defect in fatty aldehyde dehydrogenase) are autosomal recessive conditions with skin and extracutaneous organ involvement. A dermatologist should assist in diagnosis and management, and a medical geneticist should be consulted for genetic counseling.

Acquired ichthyosis: Ichthyosis may be an early manifestation of some systemic disorders (eg, leprosy [Hansen disease], hypothyroidism, lymphoma, AIDS). Some drugs cause ichthyosis (eg, nicotinic acid, triparanol, butyrophenones). The dry scale may be fine and localized to the trunk and legs, or it may be thick and widespread.

Biopsy of ichthyotic skin is usually not diagnostic of the systemic disorder; however, there are exceptions, most notably sarcoidosis, in which a thick scale may appear on the legs, and biopsy usually shows the typical granulomas.

Treatment

- Minimization of exacerbating factors
- Moisturization and keratolytics
- Sometimes infection prophylaxis

When ichthyosis is caused by a systemic disorder, the underlying disorder must be treated for the ichthyosis to abate. Other treatments of ichthyosis include emollients and keratolytics and avoiding drying.

Moisturization and keratolytics: In any ichthyosis, there is impaired epidermal barrier function, and moisturizers should be applied immediately after bathing. Substances that are applied to the skin may have increased absorption. For example, hexachlorophene products should not be used because of increased absorption and toxicity.

An emollient, preferably plain petrolatum, mineral oil, or lotions containing urea or α-hydroxy acids (eg, lactic, glycolic, and pyruvic acids), should be applied twice daily, especially after bathing while the skin is still wet. Blotting with a towel removes excess applied material.

Table 126–1. CLINICAL AND GENETIC FEATURES OF SOME INHERITED ICHTHYOSES

DISORDER	INHERITANCE PATTERN/ PREVALENCE	ONSET	TYPE OF SCALE	DISTRIBUTION	ASSOCIATED CLINICAL FINDINGS
Ichthyosis vulgaris	Autosomal dominant 1:300	Childhood	Fine	Usually back and extensor surfaces but not intertriginous surfaces Usually many markings on palms and soles	Atopy Keratosis pilaris Asthma
X-linked ichthyosis	X-linked 1:6000 (males)	Birth or infancy	Large, dark (may be fine)	Prominent on neck and trunk Normal palms and soles	Corneal opacities Cryptorchidism Testicular cancer
Lamellar ichthyosis (an autosomal recessive congenital ichthyosis)	Autosomal recessive 1:300,000	Birth	Large, coarse, sometimes fine	Variable palm and sole changes Most of body	Ectropion Hypohidrosis with heat intolerance Alopecia
*Congenital ichthyosiform erythroderma (an autosomal recessive congenital ichthyosis)	Autosomal dominant (mutations spontaneous in about 50% of cases) 1:300,000	Birth	Thick, warty At birth: Redness and blisters In adulthood: Scaling	Most of body Especially warty in flexural creases	Bullae, frequent skin infections

*This disorder is also called bullous congenital ichthyosiform erythroderma, or epidermolytic hyperkeratosis.

Ichthyosis typically responds well to the topical keratolytic propylene glycol. To remove scale (eg, if ichthyosis is severe), patients can apply a preparation containing 40 to 60% propylene glycol in water under occlusion (eg, a thin plastic film or bag worn overnight) every night after hydrating the skin (eg, by bathing or showering); in children, the preparation should be applied twice daily without occlusion. After scale has decreased, less frequent application is required. Other useful topical agents include ceramide-based creams, 6% salicylic acid gel, hydrophilic petrolatum and water (in equal parts), and the α-hydroxy acids in various bases. Topical calcipotriol cream has been used with success; however, this vitamin D derivative can result in hypercalcemia when used over broad areas, especially in small children.

Retinoids are effective in treating inherited ichthyosis. Oral synthetic retinoids are effective for most ichthyoses. Acitretin (see p. 1072) is effective in treating most forms of inherited ichthyosis. In lamellar ichthyosis, 0.1% tretinoin cream or oral isotretinoin may be effective. The lowest effective dose should be used. Long-term (1 yr) treatment with oral isotretinoin has resulted in bony exostoses in some patients, and other long-term adverse effects may arise.

PEARLS & PITFALLS

- Oral retinoids are contraindicated in pregnancy because of their teratogenicity, and acitretin should be avoided in women of childbearing potential because of its teratogenicity and long duration of action.

Infection prophylaxis: Patients with epidermolytic hyperkeratosis may need long-term treatment with cloxacillin 250 mg po tid or qid or erythromycin 250 mg po tid or qid, as long as thick intertriginous scale is present, to prevent bacterial superinfection from causing painful, foul-smelling pustules. Regularly using soaps containing chlorhexidine may also reduce the bacteria, but these soaps tend to dry the skin.

KEY POINTS

- Ichthyosis may be acquired or inherited as an isolated disorder or as part of a syndrome.
- Evaluate patients with gradual-onset ichthyosis for an underlying systemic disorder.
- Emollients that speed the shedding of skin (keratolytics) are effective in treating ichthyosis.

KERATOSIS PILARIS

Keratosis pilaris is a disorder of keratinization in which horny plugs fill the openings of hair follicles.

Keratosis pilaris is common. The cause is unknown, but there is often an autosomal dominant inheritance.

Multiple small, pointed, keratotic follicular papules appear mainly on the lateral aspects of the upper arms, thighs, and buttocks. Facial lesions may also occur, particularly in children. Lesions are most prominent in cold weather and sometimes abate in the summer. Skin may appear red. The problem is mainly cosmetic, but the disorder may cause itching or, rarely, follicular pustules.

Treatment

- Symptomatic measures

Treatment of keratosis pilaris is usually unnecessary and often unsatisfactory.

Hydrophilic petrolatum and water (in equal parts) or petrolatum with 3% salicylic acid may help flatten the lesions.

Buffered lactic acid (ammonium lactate) lotions or creams, urea creams, 6% salicylic acid gel, or 0.1% tretinoin cream may also be effective. Acid creams should be avoided in young children because of burning and stinging.

Pulse-dye laser has been used successfully to treat facial redness.

PALMOPLANTAR KERATODERMAS

Palmoplantar keratodermas are rare inherited disorders characterized by palmar and plantar hyperkeratosis.

Most palmoplantar keratodermas are not severe and are autosomal dominant. Secondary infections are common. Examples include the following:

- Howel-Evans syndrome: This autosomal dominant form has extracutaneous manifestations, with onset between ages 5 yr and 15 yr. Esophageal cancer may develop at a young age.
- Unna-Thost disease and Vorner disease: These are autosomal dominant forms.
- Papillon-Lefèvre syndrome: This autosomal recessive form causes manifestations before age 6 mo. Severe periodontitis can result in loss of teeth.
- Vohwinkel syndrome: In this autosomal dominant form, patients may also develop digital autoamputation and high-frequency hearing loss.

Treatment

- Symptomatic treatment

Symptomatic measures can include emollients, keratolytics, and physical scale removal. Secondary infections require treatment with antimicrobials. Oral retinoids are sometimes used.

XERODERMA

(Xerosis)

Xeroderma is dry skin that is neither inherited nor associated with systemic abnormalities.

Xeroderma results from delayed shedding of the superficial cells of the skin, yielding fine white scale. Risk factors for xerosis include the following:

- Residence in a dry, cold climate
- Older age
- Atopic dermatitis
- Frequent bathing, particularly if using harsh soaps

Diagnosis of xeroderma is based on clinical evaluation.

Treatment

- Maximization of skin moisture

Treatment of xeroderma is focused on keeping the skin moist:

- Frequency of bathing should decrease and tepid, rather than hot, water should be used.
- Skin moisturizers should be used frequently, particularly immediately after bathing, to decrease transepidermal water loss. Thicker moisturizers such as petrolatum- or oil-based moisturizers are more effective than water-based lotions, although water-based lotions may be better tolerated in warmer climates. Moisturizers with additives such as ceramides, alpha-glycolic acids (eg, lactic, glycolic, and pyruvic acids), and beta-glycolic acids (eg, salicylic acid) are very commonly used.
- Increasing fluid intake and use of humidifiers also help.

127 Dermatitis

(Eczema)

Dermatitis is superficial inflammation of the skin characterized by

- Redness
- Edema
- Oozing
- Crusting
- Scaling
- Vesicles (sometimes)

Pruritus is common. Eczema is a nonspecific term synonymous with dermatitis, but it is often used to refer to atopic dermatitis, the most common type of dermatitis.

ATOPIC DERMATITIS

(Atopic Eczema; Eczema; Infantile Eczema)

Atopic dermatitis (AD, often referred to as eczema) is a chronic inflammatory skin disorder with a complex pathogenesis involving genetic susceptibility, immunologic and epidermal barrier dysfunction, and environmental factors. Pruritus is the primary symptom; skin lesions range from mild erythema to severe lichenification. Diagnosis is by history and examination. Treatment is moisturizers, avoidance of allergic and irritant triggers, and often topical corticosteroids or immune modulators. Childhood AD frequently resolves or lessens significantly by adulthood.

Etiology

AD primarily affects children in urban areas or developed countries, and prevalence has increased over the last 30 yr; up to 20% of children and 1 to 3% of adults in developed countries are affected. Most people with the disorder develop it before age 5, many of them before age 1. The unproven hygiene hypothesis is that decreased early childhood exposure to infectious agents (ie, because of more rigorous hygiene regimens at home) may increase the development of atopic disorders and autoimmunity to self-proteins; many patients or family members who have AD also have asthma or allergic rhinitis.

Pathophysiology

All of the following contribute to the development of AD:

- Genetic factors
- Epidermal barrier dysfunction

- Immunologic mechanisms
- Environmental triggers

Genes implicated in AD are those encoding epidermal and immunologic proteins. A major predisposing factor for AD is the existence in many patients of a mutation in the gene encoding for the filaggrin protein, which is a component of the cornified cell envelope produced by differentiating keratinocytes.

Known epidermal barrier defects in skin affected by AD also include decreased ceramides and antimicrobial peptides and increased transepidermal water loss, which increase penetration of environmental irritants and allergens, and microbes, triggering inflammation and sensitization.

In acute AD lesions, Th2 T cell cytokines (IL-4, IL-5, IL-13) predominate, whereas in chronic lesions Th1 T cell cytokines (IFN-gamma, IL-12) are present. Numerous other cytokines, including thymic stromal lipoprotein, CCL17, and CCL22, play a role in the inflammatory reaction in AD. New treatments targeting specific cytokines are helping to identify the specific immune pathways in AD.

Common environmental triggers include

- Foods (eg, milk, eggs, soy, wheat, peanuts, fish)
- Airborne allergens (eg, dust mites, molds, dander)
- *Staphylococcus aureus* colonization on skin due to deficiencies in endogenous antimicrobial peptides
- Topical products (eg, cosmetics, fragrances, harsh soaps)
- Sweating
- Rough fabrics

Symptoms and Signs

AD usually appears in infancy, typically by 3 mo.

In the **acute phase** (see Plate 30), lesions are red, edematous, scaly patches or plaques that may be weepy. Occasionally vesicles are present.

In the **chronic phrase** (see Plate 31), scratching and rubbing create skin lesions that appear dry and lichenified.

Distribution of lesions is age specific. In infants, lesions characteristically occur on the face, scalp, neck, and extensor surfaces of the extremities. In older children and adults, lesions occur on flexural surfaces such as the neck, and the antecubital and popliteal fossae.

Intense pruritus is a key feature. Itch often precedes lesions, and itch worsens with allergen exposures, dry air, sweating, local irritation, wool garments, and emotional stress.

Complications: Secondary bacterial infections (superinfections), especially staphylococcal and streptococcal infections (eg, cellulitis and regional lymphadenitis) are common. Exfoliative dermatitis can develop.

Eczema herpeticum (also called Kaposi varicelliform eruption) is a diffuse herpes simplex infection occurring in patients with AD. It manifests as grouped vesicles in areas of active or recent dermatitis, although normal skin can be involved. High fever and adenopathy may develop after several days. Occasionally, this infection can become systemic, which may be fatal. Sometimes the eye is involved, causing a painful corneal lesion.

Fungal and nonherpetic viral skin infections (eg, common warts, molluscum contagiosum) can also occur.

Patients with long-standing AD may develop cataracts in their 20s or 30s.

Frequent use of topical products exposes patients to many potential allergens, and contact dermatitis caused by these products may aggravate and complicate AD, as may the generally dry skin that is common among these patients.

Diagnosis

- Clinical evaluation
- Sometimes testing for allergic triggers with skin prick testing, radioallergosorbent testing levels, or patch testing

Diagnosis is clinical. See Table 127–1 for the modified clinically relevant diagnostic criteria proposed by the American Academy of Dermatology in 2003.

AD is often hard to differentiate from other dermatoses (eg, seborrheic dermatitis, contact dermatitis, nummular dermatitis, psoriasis), although a family history of atopy and the distribution of lesions are helpful. The following distribution patterns can help with differentiation:

- Psoriasis is usually extensoral rather than flexural, may involve the fingernails, and has a thicker and whiter (micaceous) scale.
- Seborrheic dermatitis affects the face (eg, nasolabial folds, eyebrows, glabellar region, scalp) most commonly.
- Nummular dermatitis is not flexural, and lichenification is rare.

Because patients can still develop other skin disorders, not all subsequent skin problems should be attributed to AD.

PEARLS & PITFALLS

- Clues to AD include a flexural distribution and personal or family history of allergic rhinitis, asthma, or allergies.
- Bacterial superinfection is a common complication in AD and may be easily confused with eczema herpeticum.

There is no definitive laboratory test for AD. However, precipitating environmental allergens of AD can be identified with skin testing, measurement of allergen-specific IgE levels, or both. Routine cultures for *S. aureus* are not done because that organism is present in skin lesions of > 75% of AD patients (vs in < 25% of unaffected people). However, nasal and skinfold cultures are done in patients with recurrent, unresponsive, and possibly antimicrobial-resistant infections.

Prognosis

AD in children often abates by age 5 yr, although exacerbations are common throughout adolescence and into adulthood. Girls and patients with severe disease, early age of onset, family history, and associated allergic rhinitis or asthma are more likely to have prolonged disease. Even in these patients, AD frequently resolves or lessens significantly by adulthood. AD may have long-term psychologic sequelae as children confront the many challenges of living with a visible, sometimes disabling, skin disease during their formative years.

Treatment

- Supportive care (eg, moisturizers and dressings, antihistamines for pruritus)
- Avoidance of precipitating factors
- Topical corticosteroids
- Topical immune modulators
- In severe disease, systemic immunosuppressants
- Sometimes ultraviolet (UV) therapy
- Treatment of superinfections

Treatment can usually be given at home, but patients who have exfoliative dermatitis, cellulitis, or eczema herpeticum may need to be hospitalized.

(See also the American Academy of Dermatology Association's Guidelines of Care for Atopic Dermatitis at www.aad.org.)

Table 127–1. DIAGNOSTIC CLINICAL FEATURES IN ATOPIC DERMATITIS*

Essential features
Pruritus Dermatitis (eczema)—acute, subacute, or chronic, with • Typical age-specific patterns† • Chronic or relapsing history
Important features
Early age of onset Personal or family history of atopic disease IgE reactivity Xerosis
Associated features (help to suggest the diagnosis)
White dermatographism Keratosis pilaris Pityriasis alba Hyperlinear palms Ichthyosis Facial pallor Infraorbital folds Nipple dermatitis Perifollicular accentuation Lichenification Prurigo lesions Delayed blanch response Certain regional changes (eg, perioral changes, periauricular changes)

*Derived from: Guidelines of care for the management of atopic dermatitis: section 1. Diagnosis and assessment of atopic dermatitis. *J Am Acad Dermatol* 70(2):338–351, 2014 and Consensus conference on pediatric atopic dermatitis. *J Am Acad Dermatol* 49:1088–1095, 2003.

†On the face, neck, and extensor surfaces in infants and children; flexural surfaces in any age group; spares groin and axillae.

Supportive care: Skin care involves the following measures:

- Hydrating with water
- Use of nonsoap cleansers that are neutral- to low-pH, hypoallergenic, and fragrance free
- Taking baths with diluted bleach or colloidal oatmeal
- Applying moisturizers (eg, white petrolatum ointments or creams)
- Wearing wet wraps

Bathing should not be done more than once daily. Bathing with diluted bleach 2 times/wk plus nasal application of mupirocin can reduce *S. aureus* colonization and decrease the severity of AD.[1] Colloidal oatmeal is sometimes soothing. When toweling dry, the skin should be blotted or patted dry rather than rubbed.

Moisturizers (ointments such as white petrolatum or hydrophilic petrolatum [unless the patient is allergic to lanolin] or thick creams) are applied immediately after bathing to help retain skin moisture and reduce itching.

Wet wraps (a topical corticosteroid or immunomodulator applied to wet skin, wrapped with a moist layer, and then overlaid with a dry layer) are helpful for severe, thick, and recalcitrant lesions.

Antihistamines can help relieve pruritus via their sedating properties. Options include hydroxyzine 25 mg po tid or qid (for children, 0.5 mg/kg q 6 h or 2 mg/kg in a single bedtime dose) and diphenhydramine 25 to 50 mg po at bedtime. Low-sedating H1 receptor blockers (such as loratadine 10 mg po once/day, fexofenadine 60 mg po bid or 180 mg po once/day, and cetirizine 5 to 10 mg po once/day) may be useful, although their efficacy has not been defined. Doxepin (a tricyclic antidepressant also with H1 and H2 receptor blocking activity) 25 to 50 mg po at bedtime may also help, but its use is not recommended for children < 12 yr. Fingernails should be cut short to minimize excoriations and secondary infections.

1. Huang JT, Abrams M, Tlougan B, et al: Treatment of *Staphylococcus aureus* colonization in atopic dermatitis decreases disease severity. *Pediatrics* 123(5):e808–814, 2009. doi: 10.1542/peds.2008-2217.

Avoidance of precipitating factors: Household antigens can be controlled by the following measures:

- Using synthetic fiber pillows and impermeable mattress covers
- Washing bedding in hot water
- Removing upholstered furniture, soft toys, carpets, and pets (to reduce dust mites and animal dander)
- Using air circulators equipped with high-efficiency particulate air (HEPA) filters in bedrooms and other frequently occupied living areas
- Using dehumidifiers in basements and other poorly aerated, damp rooms (to reduce molds)

Reduction of emotional stress is useful but often difficult. Extensive dietary changes intended to eliminate exposure to allergenic foods are unnecessary and probably ineffective; food hypersensitivities rarely persist beyond childhood.

Corticosteroids: Topical corticosteroids are the mainstay of therapy. Creams or ointments applied twice daily are effective for most patients with mild or moderate disease. Moisturizers are liberally applied after corticosteroid applications to all skin. Systemic corticosteroids should be avoided whenever possible, because disease rebound is often severe and topical therapy is safer. Prolonged topical use can lead to thinning of the skin and striae. Prolonged, widespread use of high-potency corticosteroid creams or ointments should be avoided in infants because adrenal suppression may ensue.

Other therapies: Topical tacrolimus and pimecrolimus are T-cell inhibitors effective for AD. They can be used for mild to moderate AD or when corticosteroid adverse effects such as skin atrophy, striae formation, or adrenal suppression is a concern. Tacrolimus ointment or pimecrolimus cream is applied twice daily. Burning or stinging after application is usually transient and abates after a few days. Flushing is less common.

Repair of the stratum corneum and barrier function may help alleviate AD. Research has shown that skin affected by AD is particularly deficient in ceramides and that a deficiency in ceramides increases transepidermal water loss. Several ceramide-containing emollient products are considered helpful for AD control.

Phototherapy is helpful for extensive AD. Natural sun exposure ameliorates disease in many patients, including children. Alternatively, therapy with ultraviolet A (UVA) or B (UVB) may be used. Narrowband UVB therapy is proving more effective than traditional broadband UVB therapy and is also effective in children. Psoralen plus UVA (PUVA—see p. 1072) therapy is reserved for extensive, refractory AD. Adverse effects include sun damage (eg, PUVA lentigines, nonmelanoma skin cancer). Because of these adverse effects, phototherapy, particularly PUVA, is avoided when possible in children or young adults.

Systemic immune modulators effective in at least some patients include cyclosporine, interferon gamma, mycophenolate, methotrexate, and azathioprine. All downregulate or inhibit T-cell function and have anti-inflammatory properties. These agents are indicated for widespread, recalcitrant, or disabling AD that fails to abate with topical therapy and phototherapy.

Antistaphylococcal antibiotics, both topical (eg, mupirocin, fusidic acid [applied for ≤ 2 wk]) and oral (eg, dicloxacillin, cephalexin, erythromycin [all 250 mg qid for 1 to 2 wk]), are used to treat bacterial *skin* superinfections such as impetigo, folliculitis, or furunculosis. Nasal mupirocin can also be used to decrease carriage of *S. aureus* and the severity of AD.

Eczema herpeticum is treated with acyclovir. Infants receive 10 to 20 mg/kg IV q 8 h; older children and adults with mild illness may receive 200 mg po 5 times/day. Involvement of the eye is considered an ophthalmic emergency, and if eye involvement is suspected, an ophthalmology consult should be obtained.

KEY POINTS

- AD is common, particularly in developed nations, affecting 15 to 30% of children and 2 to 10% of adults.
- Common triggers include airborne allergens (eg, pollen, dust), sweat, harsh soaps, rough fabrics, and fragrances.
- Common findings include pruritus and erythematous patches and plaques and lichenification in the antecubital and popliteal fossae and on the eyelids, neck, and wrists.
- Superinfections (particularly *S. aureus* infections and eczema herpeticum) are common.
- AD often improves by adulthood.
- First-line treatments include moisturizers, topical corticosteroids, and antihistamines as needed for pruritus.

CONTACT DERMATITIS

Contact dermatitis (CD) is acute inflammation of the skin caused by irritants or allergens. The primary symptom is pruritus. Skin changes range from erythema to blistering and ulceration, often on or near the hands but occurring on any exposed skin surface. Diagnosis is by exposure history, examination, and sometimes skin patch testing. Treatment entails antipruritics, topical corticosteroids, and avoidance of causes.

Pathophysiology

CD is caused by irritants or allergens.

Irritant contact dermatitis (ICD): ICD accounts for 80% of all cases of CD. It is a nonspecific inflammatory reaction to substances contacting the skin; the immune system is not activated. Numerous substances are involved, including

- Chemicals (eg, acids, alkalis, solvents, metal salts)
- Soaps (eg, abrasives, detergents)
- Plants (eg, poinsettias, peppers)
- Body fluids (eg, urine, saliva)

Properties of the irritant (eg, extreme pH, solubility in the lipid film on skin), environment (eg, low humidity, high temperature, high friction), and patient (eg, very young or old) influence the likelihood of developing ICD. ICD is more common among patients with atopic disorders, in whom ICD also may initiate immunologic sensitization and hence allergic CD.

Phototoxic dermatitis (see p. 1078) is a variant in which topical (eg, perfumes, coal tar) or ingested (eg, psoralens) agents generate damaging free radicals and inflammatory mediators only after absorption of ultraviolet light.

Allergic contact dermatitis (ACD): ACD is a type IV cell-mediated hypersensitivity reaction that has 2 phases:

- Sensitization to an antigen
- Allergic response after reexposure

In the sensitization phase, allergens are captured by Langerhans cells (dendritic epidermal cells), which migrate to regional lymph nodes where they process and present the antigen to T cells. The process may be brief (6 to 10 days for strong sensitizers such as poison ivy) or prolonged (years for weak sensitizers such as sunscreens, fragrances, and glucocorticoids). Sensitized T cells then migrate back to the epidermis and activate on any reexposure to the allergen, releasing cytokines, recruiting inflammatory cells, and leading to the characteristic symptoms and signs of ACD.

In **autoeczematization** (id reaction), epidermal T cells activated by an allergen migrate locally or through the circulation to cause dermatitis at sites remote from the initial trigger. However, contact with fluid from vesicles or blisters cannot trigger a reaction elsewhere on the patient or on another person.

Multiple allergens cause ACD (see Table 127–2), and cross-sensitization among agents is common (eg, between benzocaine and paraphenylenediamine). Cross-sensitization means that exposure to one substance can result in an allergic response after exposure to a different but related substance. *Toxicodendron* sp plants (eg, poison ivy, poison oak, poison sumac) account for a large percentage of ACD, including moderate and severe cases. The offending allergen is urushiol.

ACD variants include photoallergic CD and systemically induced ACD. In photoallergic CD, a substance becomes sensitizing only after it undergoes structural change triggered by ultraviolet light. Typical causes include aftershave lotions, sunscreens, and topical sulfonamides. Reactions may extend to non-sun-exposed skin. In systemically induced ACD, ingestion of an allergen after topical sensitization causes diffuse dermatitis (eg, oral diphenhydramine after sensitization with topical diphenhydramine).

Symptoms and Signs

Irritant CD: ICD is more painful than pruritic. Signs range from mild erythema to hemorrhage, crusting, erosion, pustules, bullae, and edema.

Allergic CD: In ACD, the primary symptom is intense pruritus; pain is usually the result of excoriation or infection. Skin changes range from transient erythema through vesiculation to severe swelling with bullae, ulceration, or both. Changes often occur in a pattern, distribution, or combination that suggests a specific exposure, such as linear streaking on an arm or leg (eg, due to brushing against poison ivy) or circumferential erythema (under a wristwatch or waistband). Linear streaks are almost always indicative of an external allergen or irritant.

Any surface may be involved, but hands are the most common surface due to handling and touching potential allergens. With airborne exposure (eg, perfume aerosols), areas not covered by clothing are predominantly affected. The dermatitis is typically limited to the site of contact but may later spread due to scratching and autoeczematization (id reaction). In systemically induced ACD, skin changes may be distributed over the entire body. The eruption usually begins within 24 to 48 h after exposure to the allergen.

PEARLS & PITFALLS

- Lesion shape or pattern (linear streaks are almost always indicative of an external allergen or irritant) can help differentiate CD from other forms of dermatitis.

Table 127–2. CAUSES OF ALLERGIC CONTACT DERMATITIS

CAUSE	EXAMPLES
Airborne substances	Ragweed pollen, insecticide spray
Chemicals used in shoe or clothing manufacturing	Particularly agents used in leather and rubber processing, tanning agents in shoes, rubber accelerators and antioxidants in apparel (eg, gloves, shoes, underpants), formaldehyde in durable-press finishes
Cosmetics	Depilatories, nail polish, deodorant
Dyes	Paraphenylenediamines (hair and textile dyes)
Fragrances	Various compounds Ubiquitous in toiletries, soaps, and scented household products
Industrial agents	Many compounds, including acrylic monomers, epoxy compounds, vat dyes, rubber accelerators, and formaldehyde (in plastics and adhesives)
Ingredients in topical drugs	Antibiotics (eg, bacitracin, neomycin) Antihistamines (eg, diphenhydramine) Anesthetics (eg, benzocaine) Antiseptics (eg, thimerosal, hexachlorophene) Stabilizers (eg, ethylenediamine and derivatives)
Latex	Latex gloves, condoms, catheters, balloons
Metal compounds Chromates Cobalt Mercury Nickel	Numerous occupational exposures Personal items (eg, belt buckles, watch buckles, jewelry)
Plants	Poison ivy, oak, and sumac; ragweed; primrose; cashew shells; mango peel

Diagnosis

- Clinical evaluation
- Sometimes patch testing

CD can often be diagnosed by skin changes and exposure history. The patient's occupation, hobbies, household duties, vacations, clothing, topical drug use, cosmetics, and spouse's activities must be considered. The "use" test, in which a suspected agent is applied far from the original area of dermatitis, usually on the flexor forearm, is useful when perfumes, shampoos, or other home agents are suspected.

Patch testing is indicated when ACD is suspected and does not respond to treatment, suggesting that the trigger has not been identified (see Table 127–3). In patch testing, standard contact allergens are applied to the upper back using adhesive-mounted patches containing minute amounts of allergen or plastic (Finn®) chambers containing allergen held in place with porous tape. Thin-layer rapid use epicutaneous (TRUE TEST®) patch testing is a simple, easy-to-use kit with the most common contact allergens that can be applied and interpreted by any health care practitioner. Skin under the patches is evaluated 48 and 96 h after application. False-positive results occur when concentrations provoke an irritant rather than an allergic reaction, when reaction to one antigen triggers a nonspecific reaction to others, or with cross-reacting antigens. False-negative results occur when patch allergens do not include the offending antigen. Definitive diagnosis requires a history of exposure to the test agent in the original area of dermatitis.

Prognosis

Resolution may take up to 3 wk. Reactivity is usually lifelong. Patients with photoallergic CD can have flares for years when exposed to sun (persistent light reaction).

Treatment

- Avoidance of offending agents
- Supportive care (eg, cool compresses, dressings, antihistamines)
- Corticosteroids (most often topical but sometimes oral)

CD is prevented by avoiding the trigger; patients with photosensitive CD should avoid exposure to sun.

Topical treatment includes cool compresses (saline or Burow solution) and corticosteroids; patients with mild to moderate ACD are given mid- to high-potency topical corticosteroids (eg, triamcinolone 0.1% ointment or betamethasone valerate cream 0.1%). Oral corticosteroids (eg, prednisone 60 mg once/day for 7 to 14 days) can be used for severe blistering or extensive disease. Systemic antihistamines (eg, hydroxyzine, diphenhydramine) help relieve pruritus; antihistamines with low anticholinergic potency, such as low-sedating H1 blockers, are not as effective. Wet-to-dry dressings can soothe oozing blisters, dry the skin, and promote healing.

KEY POINTS

- CD can be caused by irritants (eg, plants, soaps, chemicals, body fluids), comprising 80% of cases, or by allergens, comprising 20% of cases.
- Symptoms can include predominantly pain (for irritant CD) or pruritus (for allergic CD).
- Diagnosis is usually clinical.
- Patch testing is helpful when ACD is suspected and the trigger has not been identified.
- Treatments commonly include cool compresses, topical corticosteroids, and systemic antihistamines as needed for pruritus.

Table 127–3. COMMON ALLERGENS* USED IN PATCH TESTING

AGENT	SOURCES
Bacitracin	In topical antibiotic preparations
Balsam of Peru (myroxylon)	A flavoring agent for drinks and tobacco, as well as a fixative and fragrance in perfumes; also occurs in many topical drugs, dental agents, and other products Chief allergens: Esters of cinnamic and benzoic acid, vanillin Cross-reactions with colophony (rosin) and balsam of Tolu, cinnamates, benzoates, styrax, and tincture of benzoin Probably also some phototoxicity
Black rubber mix	In rubber May cross-react with hair dyes
Bronopol	A preservative found in cosmetics, shampoos, and skin care products; also in some detergents and cleaning agents
Budesonide	Screens for class B corticosteroid allergy. A corticosteroid drug, used to treat various diseases; can be found in creams and ointments used to treat eczema; in eye drops or inhaled medications
Caine mix	Contains 3 topical anesthetics: Benzocaine, dibucaine hydrochloride, and tetracaine hydrochloride Often used in dentistry but also widely found and used in topical preparations to reduce itching, pain, and stinging and widely used in hemorrhoidal preparations and cough syrups
Carba mix	Used as an accelerator in rubber, rubber glues, vinyl, and some pesticides
Cl+ Me– isothiazolinone and methylisothiazolinone	Occur in cosmetics and skin care products, some drugs, household cleaning products, and certain industrial fluids and greases
Cobalt dichloride	Occurs in some paints, cement, metal, and metal-plated objects Coactivity with nickel (which is not cross-sensitivity)
Colophony (rosin)	Used by string players (violinists are especially prone to rosin allergy), baseball players, and bowlers Derived from several conifer species Occurs in cosmetics, adhesives, lacquers, varnishes, soldering fluxes, paper, and many other industrial products
Diazolidinyl urea	A preservative with broad-spectrum application found in cosmetics, shampoos, skin care products, and cleaning agents
Disperse blue 106	A dark blue textile dye found in fabrics colored dark blue, brown, black, purple, and some greens
Epoxy resin	A low molecular weight (340) epoxy based on bisphenol A and epichlorohydrin Is a sensitizer only when uncured or incompletely cured
Ethylenediamine	Used as an emulsifier and stabilizer in certain topical drugs, eye drops, some industrial solvents, curing agents for certain plastics, and anticorrosion agents
Formaldehyde and formaldehyde releasers	Released by quaternium-15, a germicidal agent, and occasionally by imidazolidinyl urea Used widely in formulation of plastics, resins for clothing, glues, and adhesives
Fragrance mixes	Can contain alpha amyl cinnamic alcohol, cinnamic aldehyde, cinnamic alcohol, oak moss absolute, hydroxycitronellal, eugenol, isoeugenol, geraniol, citral, citronellol, coumarin, farnesol, hexyl cinnamal, hydroxyisohexyl-3-cyclohexene, and carboxaldehyde Occurs in many toiletries, soaps, aftershave lotions, shampoos, and scented household products and in many industrial products (eg, cutting fluids)
Gold sodium thiosulfate	Found in gold or gold-plated jewelry or dental restorations
Hydrocortisone 17-butyrate	A corticosteroid found in creams or lotions used to treat inflammatory skin diseases; also present in some ear and eye drops
Imidazolidinyl urea	A preservative with broad-spectrum application found in cosmetics, shampoos, skin care products, and cleaning agents
Mercaptobenzothiazole	Occurs in rubber, adhesives, and coolants
Mercapto mix	Occurs in rubber, glues, coolants, and other industrial products
Methyldibromo-glutaronitrile	Found in paints, adhesives, and oils
Neomycin sulfate	Found in topical antibiotics, first-aid creams, ear drops, and nose drops; possible delay (about 4–5 days) in patch test reaction (so reading should be done at 7 days when possible)
Nickel sulfate	Occurs in jewelry, dentures, scissors, razors, eyeglass frames, silverware, and foods (eg, canned foods, foods cooked in nickel utensils, herring, oyster, asparagus, beans, mushrooms, onions)

Table 127–3. COMMON ALLERGENS* USED IN PATCH TESTING (*Continued*)

AGENT	SOURCES
Paraben mix	Five parabens: Methyl, ethyl, propyl, butyl, and benzyl parahydroxybenzoates, which are the most common preservatives used worldwide and occur in numerous creams and cosmetics and in some industrial oils, fats, and glues
Parthenolide	A sesquiterpene lactone naturally present in the traditional medicine herb, feverfew (*Tanacetum parthenium*); found in natural medicine and cosmetics Cross-reacts with other genera in Compositae and Magnoliaceae
Potassium dichromate	Occurs in cement (in minute amounts), in tanning solutions for leather, and in safety matches Used in photography, electroplating solutions, many anticorrosives, paints, glues, pigments, and some detergents
p-Phenylenediamine (PPD)	Occurs in hair dyes, some inks, photo developers, and textile dyes
p-Tert-butylphenol formaldehyde resin	A resin formed by condensation between *p*-tert-butylphenol and formaldehyde Occurs in leather finishes (especially shoes), paper, fabrics, rockwood, furniture, and certain glues
Quaternium	Common preservative occurring in cosmetics and in some household cleaners and polishes
Quinolone mix	Contains clioquinol and chlorquinaldol Antimicrobials occurring in certain medicated creams and ointments, medicated bandages, and veterinary products
Thimerosal	Preservative in contact lens solutions, certain cosmetics, nose and ear drops, and injectables Source often not identified
Thiuram mix	Common rubber allergen Also occurs in adhesives, certain pesticides, and drugs (eg, disulfiram)
Tixocortol-21-pivalate	Screens for class A corticosteroid allergy; found in buccal, nasal, throat, and rectal but not topical corticosteroid preparations
Wool alcohols	Part of lanolin; found in many cosmetics, ointments, sunscreens, and prescription and over-the-counter topical medications

Patient information leaflets for TRUE TEST allergens can be found at https://www.diagenics.co.uk/allergy-testing-and-treatment/true-test-patient-information-leaflets.

EXFOLIATIVE DERMATITIS

(Erythroderma)

Exfoliative dermatitis is widespread erythema and scaling of the skin caused by preexisting skin disorders, drugs, cancer, or unknown causes. Symptoms and signs are pruritus, diffuse erythema, and epidermal sloughing. Diagnosis is clinical. Treatment involves corticosteroids and correction of the cause.

Exfoliative dermatitis is a manifestation of rapid epidermal cell turnover. Its cause is unknown, but it most often occurs in the context of

- Preexisting skin disorders (eg, atopic dermatitis [AD], contact dermatitis [CD], seborrheic dermatitis, psoriasis, pityriasis rubra pilaris)
- Use of drugs (eg, penicillin, sulfonamides, isoniazid, phenytoin, barbiturates)
- Cancer (eg, lymphoma, mycosis fungoides, leukemia, and, rarely, adenocarcinomas)

Up to 25% of patients have no identifiable underlying cause. Bacterial superinfection can complicate exfoliative dermatitis.

Symptoms and Signs

Symptoms include pruritus, malaise, and chills. Diffuse erythema initially occurs in patches but spreads and involves all or nearly all of the body. Extensive epidermal sloughing leads to abnormal thermoregulation, nutritional deficiencies because of extensive protein losses, increased metabolic rate with a hypercatabolic state, and hypovolemia due to transdermal fluid losses.

Diagnosis

- Clinical evaluation

Diagnosis is by history and examination. Preexisting skin disease may underlie the extensive erythema and suggest a cause. Biopsy is often nonspecific but is indicated when mycosis fungoides is suspected. Blood tests may reveal hypoproteinemia, hypocalcemia, and iron deficiency; however, these findings are not diagnostic.

Prognosis

The disease may be life threatening; hospitalization is often necessary. Prognosis depends on the cause. Cases related to drug reactions have the shortest duration, lasting 2 to 6 wk after the drug is withdrawn.

Treatment

- Supportive care (eg, rehydration)
- Topical care (eg, emollients, colloidal oatmeal baths)
- Systemic corticosteroids for severe disease

Any known cause is treated. Supportive care consists of correction of dehydration, correction of electrolyte abnormalities and nutritional deficiencies, and comprehensive wound care and dressings to prevent bacterial superinfection. Because drug eruptions and CD cannot be ruled out by history alone, all drugs should be stopped if possible or changed. Skin care is with emollients and colloidal oatmeal baths. Weak topical corticosteroids (eg, 1 to 2.5% hydrocortisone ointment) may be used. Corticosteroids (prednisone 40 to 60 mg po once/day for 10 days, then tapered) are used for severe disease.

KEY POINTS

- Exfoliative dermatitis often occurs with preexisting skin disorders, drugs, and cancer, but the cause may be unknown.
- Symptoms include pruritus, widespread erythema, and epidermal sloughing.
- Diagnosis is clinical.
- Hospitalization is often necessary, because the disease may be life threatening.
- Treatment consists of supportive care, comprehensive wound and skin care, and systemic corticosteroids for severe disease.

HAND AND FOOT DERMATITIS

Hand and foot dermatitis is not a single disorder. Rather, it is a categorization of dermatitis that affects the hands and feet selectively because of one of several causes.

Patients often present with isolated dermatitis of the hands or feet. Causes include

- Contact dermatitis (CD—allergic or irritant)
- Atopic dermatitis (AD)
- Fungal infection
- Dyshidrotic eczema (dyshidrotic dermatitis)
- Psoriasis (may affect only the palms and soles and be mistaken for a dermatitis)
- Scabies (usually web spaces)

Other causes include systemic viral infection in children (hand-foot-and-mouth disease) or certain chemotherapies (hand-foot syndrome). Some cases are idiopathic.

Diagnosis can sometimes be inferred from location and appearance of the skin lesions (see Table 127–4).

Treatment of all forms of hand and foot dermatitis should be directed at the cause when possible. Topical corticosteroids may be tried empirically. Patients should also avoid prolonged contact with water that would otherwise remove protective oils and lead to paradoxical drying of the skin.

Dyshidrotic eczema (dyshidrotic dermatitis): Pruritic vesicles or bullae on the palms, sides of the fingers, or soles are characteristic of this disorder. Scaling, redness, and oozing often follow vesiculation. Symptoms are intermittent and attacks typically last several weeks but are shorter if treated.

Pompholyx is a severe form with bullae. The cause is unknown, but fungal infection, CD, and dermatophytid (id) reactions to tinea pedis can cause a similar clinical appearance and should be ruled out. Treatment includes potent topical corticosteroids, tacrolimus or pimecrolimus, oral antibiotics (if secondarily infected), and ultraviolet light. Wet compresses with potassium permanganate or aluminum acetate can help relieve symptoms.

Keratolysis exfoliativa: Painless patchy peeling of the palms, soles, or both is characteristic of this disorder. The cause is unknown; treatment is unnecessary because the condition is self-resolving.

Hyperkeratotic eczema: Thick yellow-brown plaques on the palms and sometimes soles are characteristic of this disorder. Scaling can occur. The cause is unknown. Treatment is with topical corticosteroids and keratolytics, oral psoralen plus UVA (PUVA), and retinoids.

Dermatophytid reaction (id reaction): The appearance of vesicles usually on the sides of the fingers or on the palms or soles in response to active dermatitis elsewhere is characteristic of this disorder. The cause may be an allergic reaction (see p. 1036). The reaction takes multiple forms and may manifest as vesicles, papules, erysipelas-like plaques, erythema nodosum, erythema annulare centrifugum, or urticaria.

Irritant contact dermatitis (housewives' eczema): This ICD affects people whose hands are frequently immersed in water. It is worsened by washing dishes, clothes, and babies because repeated exposure to even mild detergents and water or prolonged sweating under rubber gloves may irritate dermatitic skin or cause an ICD (see p. 1024).

Hand-foot syndrome: This disorder (also called acral erythema or palmar-plantar erythrodysesthesia) represents cutaneous toxicity caused by certain systemic chemotherapies (eg, capecitabine, cytarabine, fluorouracil, idarubicin, doxorubicin, taxanes, methotrexate, cisplatin, tegafur). Manifestations include pain, swelling, numbness, tingling, redness, and sometimes flaking or blistering of the palms or soles. Treatment is with oral or topical corticosteroids, topical dimethylsulfoxide, oral vitamin B_6 (pyridoxine), OTC analgesics (eg, acetaminophen, ibuprofen), and supportive measures (eg, cool compresses, minimizing manual tasks).

Table 127–4. DIFFERENTIAL DIAGNOSIS OF HAND DERMATITIS

APPEARANCE OF LESION	LOCATION	
	Palm	**Dorsum**
Erythema and scaling	ACD Dyshidrotic eczema ICD Hyperkeratotic eczema Keratolysis exfoliativa Psoriasis Fungal infection (tinea manum)	Atopic dermatitis ACD ICD Nummular dermatitis Psoriasis Fungal infection (tinea manum)
Pustules	Dyshidrotic eczema Infection (bacterial) Psoriasis	Infection (bacterial) Psoriasis Scabies (web spaces) Tinea
Vesicles	ACD Dyshidrotic eczema (dyshidrotic dermatitis) Id reaction	ACD Scabies (web spaces)

ACD = allergic contact dermatitis; ICD = irritant contact dermatitis.

LICHEN SIMPLEX CHRONICUS

(Neurodermatitis)

Lichen simplex chronicus is eczema caused by repeated scratching; by several mechanisms, chronic scratching causes further itching, creating a vicious circle. Diagnosis is by examination. Treatment is through education and behavioral techniques to prevent scratching and corticosteroids and antihistamines.

Etiology

Lichen simplex chronicus is thickened and leathery (lichenified) skin with variable scaling that arises secondary to repetitive scratching or rubbing. Lichen simplex chronicus is not a primary process. Perceived pruritus in a specific area of skin (with or without underlying pathology) provokes rubbing and mechanical trauma, resulting in secondary lichenification and further pruritus. Lichen simplex chronicus frequently occurs in people with anxiety disorders and nonspecific emotional stress as well as in patients with any type of underlying chronic dermatitis.

Pathophysiology

The underlying pathophysiology is unknown but may involve alterations in the way the nervous system perceives and processes itchy sensations. Skin that tends toward eczematous conditions (eg, atopic dermatitis) is more prone to lichenification.

Symptoms and Signs

Lichen simplex chronicus is characterized by pruritic, dry, scaling, hyperpigmented, lichenified plaques in irregular, oval, or angular shapes. It involves easily reached sites, most commonly the legs, arms, neck, upper trunk, and anal region.

Diagnosis

- Clinical evaluation

Diagnosis is by examination. A fully developed plaque is hyperpigmented with varying amounts of erythema that is well-demarcated and has exaggerated skin lines and a thickened and leathery appearance characteristic of lichenification. Look-alike conditions include tinea corporis, lichen planus, and psoriasis; lichen simplex chronicus can be distinguished from these by potassium hydroxide wet mount and biopsy.

Treatment

- Education and behavioral techniques
- Corticosteroids (most often topical but sometimes intralesional)
- Antihistamines

Primary treatment is patient education about the effects of scratching and rubbing. Secondary treatment is topical corticosteroids (eg, triamcinolone acetonide, fluocinonide); surgical tape impregnated with flurandrenolide (applied in the morning and replaced in the evening) may be preferred because occlusion prevents scratching. Small areas may be locally infiltrated (intralesional injections) with a long-acting corticosteroid such as triamcinolone acetonide 2.5 mg/mL (diluted with saline), 0.3 mL/cm^2 of lesion; treatment can be repeated every 3 to 4 wk. Oral H1-blocking antihistamines may be useful. Emollients may also be helpful. Topical capsaicin cream may also be helpful, but the initial burning sensations may make this therapy unacceptable to patients.

KEY POINTS

- Chronic scratching causes further itching, creating a vicious circle.
- Itchy, dry, scaling, hyperpigmented, lichenified plaques occur in irregular, oval, or angular shapes on the legs, arms, neck, and upper trunk and sometimes the anogenital area.
- Diagnosis is clinical, but potassium hydroxide wet mount and biopsy can help in the differential diagnosis.
- Patients need to be educated about the vicious circle of scratching and further itching; topical corticosteroids and antihistamines help control the itching.

NUMMULAR DERMATITIS

(Discoid Dermatitis)

Nummular dermatitis is inflammation of the skin characterized by coin-shaped or discoid eczematous lesions. Diagnosis is clinical. Treatment may include topical corticosteroids and ultraviolet light therapy.

Nummular dermatitis is most common among middle-aged and older patients and is often associated with dry skin, especially during the winter. Dermatophytid (identity, or id) reactions may manifest as nummular dermatitis. The cause is unknown.

Symptoms and Signs

Discoid lesions often start as patches of confluent vesicles and papules that ooze serum and form crusts. Later they become dry, scaly, lichenified, and sometimes annular (central clearing). Lesions are often intensely pruritic. They can number from 1 to about 50 and tend to be from 2 to 10 cm in diameter. They are often more prominent on the extensor aspects of the extremities and on the buttocks but also appear on the trunk. Exacerbations and remissions may occur, and when they do, new lesions tend to reappear at the sites of healed lesions.

Diagnosis

- Clinical evaluation

Diagnosis is clinical based on the characteristic appearance and distribution of the skin lesions. Tests for bacteria and fungi may be done to rule out infection.

Treatment

- Supportive care
- Antibiotics
- Corticosteroids (most often topical, but sometimes intralesional or oral)
- Ultraviolet light therapy

No treatment is uniformly effective. Oral antibiotics (eg, dicloxacillin or cephalexin 250 mg qid) may be given, along with use of tap water compresses, if weeping and pus are present. Mid- to high-potency corticosteroid cream or ointment should be rubbed in 2 times daily. An occlusive dressing with a corticosteroid cream under polyethylene film or with flurandrenolide-impregnated tape can be applied at bedtime. Intralesional corticosteroid injections may be beneficial for the few lesions that do not respond to therapy.

In more widespread, resistant, and recurrent cases, UVB radiation alone or oral psoralen plus ultraviolet A (PUVA) radiation may be helpful. Occasionally, oral corticosteroids are required, but long-term use should be avoided; a reasonable starting dose is prednisone 40 mg every other day. Corticosteroid alternatives for recalcitrant disease include cyclosporine and methotrexate.

KEY POINTS

- The etiology of nummular dermatitis is unknown, but the disorder is most common in middle-aged and older patients.
- Pruritic discoid lesions form in patches of confluent vesicles and papules that later become dry and lichenified.
- Diagnosis is clinical.
- Treatment includes supportive care (eg, corticosteroid cream) for the itching, antibiotics for infection, and ultraviolet light therapy for widespread, resistant, and recurrent lesions.

SEBORRHEIC DERMATITIS

Seborrheic dermatitis (SD) is inflammation of skin regions with a high density of sebaceous glands (eg, face, scalp, upper trunk). The cause is unknown, but species of *Malassezia*, a normal skin yeast, play some role. SD occurs with increased frequency in patients with HIV and in those with certain neurologic disorders. SD causes occasional pruritus, dandruff, and yellow, greasy scaling along the hairline and on the face. Diagnosis is made by examination. Treatment is tar or other medicated shampoo and topical corticosteroids and antifungals.

Despite the name, the composition and flow of sebum are usually normal. The pathogenesis of SD is unclear, but its activity has been linked to the number of *Malassezia* yeasts present on the skin. SD occurs most often in infants, usually within the first 3 mo of life, and in those aged 30 to 70 yr. The incidence and severity of disease seem to be affected by genetic factors, emotional or physical stress, and climate (usually worse in cold weather). SD may precede or be associated with psoriasis (called seborrhiasis). SD may be more common and more severe among patients with neurologic disorders (especially Parkinson disease) or HIV/AIDS. Very rarely, the dermatitis becomes generalized.

Symptoms and Signs

Symptoms develop gradually, and the dermatitis is usually apparent only as dry flakes (dandruff) or greasy diffuse scaling of the scalp (dandruff) with variable pruritus. In severe disease, yellow-red scaling papules appear along the hairline, behind the ears, in the external auditory canals, on the eyebrows, in the axillae, on the bridge of the nose, in the nasolabial folds, and over the sternum. Marginal blepharitis with dry yellow crusts and conjunctival irritation may develop. SD does not cause hair loss.

Newborns may develop SD with a thick, yellow, crusted scalp lesion (cradle cap); fissuring and yellow scaling behind the ears; red facial papules; and stubborn diaper rash. Older children and adults may develop thick, tenacious, scaly plaques on the scalp that may measure 1 to 2 cm in diameter.

Diagnosis

- Clinical evaluation

Diagnosis is made by physical examination. SD may occasionally be difficult to distinguish from other disorders, including psoriasis, AD or CD, tinea, and rosacea.

Treatment

- Topical therapy with antifungals, corticosteroids, and calcineurin inhibitors

Adults and older children: In adults with involvement of the scalp, zinc pyrithione, selenium sulfide, sulfur and salicylic acid, ketoconazole (2% and 1%), and tar shampoo (available OTC) should be used daily or every other day until dandruff is controlled and twice/wk thereafter. A corticosteroid lotion (eg, 0.01% fluocinolone acetonide solution, 0.025% triamcinolone acetonide lotion) can be rubbed into the scalp or other hairy areas twice daily until scaling and redness are controlled.

For SD of the postauricular areas, nasolabial folds, eyelid margins, and bridge of the nose, 1 to 2.5% hydrocortisone cream is rubbed in 2 or 3 times daily, decreasing to once/day when SD is controlled; hydrocortisone cream is the safest corticosteroid for the face because fluorinated corticosteroids may cause adverse effects (eg, telangiectasia, atrophy, perioral dermatitis). In some patients, 2% ketoconazole cream or other topical imidazoles applied twice daily for 1 to 2 wk induce a remission that lasts for months. An imidazole or hydrocortisone can be used as first-line therapy; if necessary, they can be used simultaneously. Calcineurin inhibitors (pimecrolimus and tacrolimus) are also effective particularly when long-term use is necessary. For eyelid margin seborrhea, a dilution of 1 part baby shampoo to 9 parts water is applied with a cotton swab.

Infants and children: In infants, a baby shampoo is used daily, and 1 to 2.5% hydrocortisone cream or fluocinolone 0.01% oil can be used once to twice daily for redness and scaling on the scalp or face. Topical antifungals such as ketoconazole 2% cream or econazole 1% cream can also be helpful in severe cases. For thick lesions on the scalp of a young child, mineral oil, olive oil, or a corticosteroid gel or oil is applied at bedtime to affected areas and rubbed in with a toothbrush. The scalp is shampooed daily until the thick scale is gone.

KEY POINTS

- In adults, SD causes dandruff and sometimes scaling around the eyebrows, nose, and external ear, behind the ears, in the axilla, and on the sternum.
- SD can cause a thick, yellow, crusted scalp lesion in newborns or thick, scaly scalp plaques in older children and adults.
- Treatments can include medicated shampoos and topical corticosteroids.

STASIS DERMATITIS

Stasis dermatitis is inflammation of the skin of the lower legs caused by chronic venous insufficiency. Symptoms are itching, scaling, hyperpigmentation, and sometimes ulceration. Diagnosis is clinical. Treatment is directed at the chronic venous insufficiency and preventing occurrence or progression of associated ulcers.

Stasis dermatitis occurs in patients with chronic venous insufficiency because pooled venous blood in the legs compromises the endothelial integrity in the microvasculature, resulting in fibrin leakage, local inflammation, and local cell necrosis.

Symptoms and Signs

In the early stage, eczematous changes (erythema, scaling, weeping, crusting—see Plate 53) develop, all of which can be made worse by bacterial superinfection or by CD caused by the many topical treatments often applied. Hyperpigmentation and red-brown discoloration can occur secondary to venous stasis and be present before stasis dermatitis develops. Hyperpigmentation can also appear after stasis dermatitis develops, as a secondary change. When chronic venous insufficiency and stasis dermatitis are both inadequately treated, stasis dermatitis progresses to frank skin ulceration (see Plate 54), chronic edema, thickened fibrotic skin, or lipodermatosclerosis (a painful induration resulting from panniculitis, which, if severe, gives the lower leg an inverted bowling pin shape with enlargement of the calf and narrowing at the ankle).

Diagnosis

- Clinical evaluation

Diagnosis is clinical based on the characteristic appearance of the skin lesions and other signs of chronic venous insufficiency. Consultation with a vascular specialist and testing (such as ultrasonography) may be needed.

Treatment

- Elevation, compression, and dressings
- Sometimes topical or oral antibiotics

Chronic venous insufficiency must be adequately treated with leg elevation and compression stockings (see p. 756).

For **acute stasis dermatitis** (characterized by crusts, exudation, and superficial ulceration), continuous and then intermittent tap water compresses should be applied. For **a weeping lesion,** a hydrocolloid dressing may be best. For **less acute dermatitis**, a corticosteroid cream or ointment should be applied 3 times/day or incorporated into zinc oxide paste.

Ulcers are best treated with compresses and bland dressings (eg, zinc oxide paste); other dressings (eg, hydrocolloids) are also effective (see also p. 1067). Ulcers in ambulatory patients may be healed with an Unna paste boot (zinc gelatin), the less messy zinc gelatin bandage, or a colloid dressing (all are available commercially). Colloid-type dressings used under elastic support are more effective than an Unna paste boot. It may be necessary to change the dressing every 2 or 3 days, but as edema recedes and the ulcer heals, once or twice/wk is sufficient. After the ulcer heals, an elastic support should be applied before the patient rises in the morning. Regardless of the dressing used, reduction of edema (usually with compression) is paramount for healing.

Oral antibiotics (eg, cephalosporins, dicloxacillin) are used to treat superimposed cellulitis. Topical antibiotics (eg, mupirocin, silver sulfadiazine) are useful for treating erosions and ulcers. When edema and inflammation subside, split-thickness skin grafts may be needed for large ulcers.

Complex or multiple topical drugs or OTC remedies should not be used. The skin in stasis dermatitis is more vulnerable to direct irritants and to potentially sensitizing topical agents (eg, antibiotics; anesthetics; vehicles of topical drugs, especially lanolin or wool alcohols).

KEY POINTS

- Stasis dermatitis results from chronic venous insufficiency.
- Early signs include erythema, scaling, weeping, and crusting.
- Eventual results can include hyperpigmentation, ulceration, fibrotic skin, chronic edema, and lipodermatosclerosis (a painful induration resulting from panniculitis).
- Treat chronic venous insufficiency with elevation and compression.
- Treat skin lesions with dressings and sometimes antibiotics.

128 Fungal Skin Infections

CANDIDIASIS (MUCOCUTANEOUS)

(Moniliasis)

Candidiasis (moniliasis) is skin infection with *Candida* sp, most commonly *Candida albicans*. Infections can occur anywhere and are most common in skinfolds, digital web spaces, genitals, cuticles, and oral mucosa. Symptoms and signs vary by site. Diagnosis is by clinical appearance and potassium hydroxide wet mount of skin scrapings. Treatment is with drying agents and antifungals.

Most candidal infections are of the skin and mucous membranes, but invasive candidiasis is common among immunosuppressed patients and can be life threatening. Systemic candidiasis is discussed in Ch. 189. Vulvovaginal candidiasis is discussed in Candidal Vaginitis on p. 2314.

Etiology

Candida is a group of about 150 yeast species. *C. albicans* is responsible for about 70 to 80% of all candidal infections. Other significant species include *C. glabrata, C. tropicalis, C. krusei,* and *C. dubliniensis.*

Candida is a ubiquitous yeast that resides harmlessly on skin and mucous membranes until dampness, heat, and impaired local and systemic defenses provide a fertile environment for it to grow.

Risk factors for candidiasis include

- Hot weather
- Restrictive clothing
- Poor hygiene
- Infrequent diaper or undergarment changes in children and elderly patients
- Altered flora resulting from antibiotic therapy
- Inflammatory diseases (eg, psoriasis) that occur in skinfolds
- Immunosuppression resulting from corticosteroids and immunosuppressive drugs, pregnancy, diabetes, other endocrinopathies (eg, Cushing disease, hypoadrenalism, hypothyroidism), blood dyscrasias, or T-cell defects

Candidiasis occurs most commonly in intertriginous areas such as the axillae, groin, and gluteal folds (eg, diaper rash), in digital web spaces, on the glans penis, and beneath the breasts. Vulvovaginal candidiasis is common among women. Candidal nail infections and paronychia may develop after improperly done manicures and in kitchen workers and others whose hands are continually exposed to water (see p. 1053). In obese people, candidal infections may occur beneath the pannus (abdominal fold). Oropharyngeal candidiasis is a common sign of local or systemic immunosuppression.

Chronic mucocutaneous candidiasis typically affects the nails, skin, and oropharynx. Patients have cutaneous anergy to *Candida,* absent proliferative responses to *Candida* antigen (but normal proliferative responses to mitogens), and an intact antibody response to *Candida* and other antigens. Chronic mucocutaneous candidiasis may occur as an autosomal recessive illness associated with hypoparathyroidism and Addison disease (*Candida*-endocrinopathy syndrome).

Symptoms and Signs

Intertriginous infections manifest as pruritic, well-demarcated, erythematous patches of varying size and shape; erythema may be difficult to detect in darker-skinned patients. Primary patches may have adjacent satellite papules and pustules. Perianal candidiasis produces white maceration and pruritus ani. Vulvovaginal candidiasis causes pruritus and discharge (see p. 2314).

Candidal infection is a frequent cause of chronic paronychia, which manifests as painful red periungual swelling. Subungual infections are characterized by distal separation of one or several fingernails (onycholysis), with white or yellow discoloration of the subungual area.

Oropharyngeal candidiasis causes white plaques on oral mucous membranes that may bleed when scraped (see Interpretation of findings on p. 869).

Perlèche is candidiasis at the corners of the mouth, which causes cracks and tiny fissures. It may stem from chronic lip licking, thumb sucking, ill-fitting dentures, or other conditions that make the corners of the mouth moist enough that yeast can grow.

Chronic mucocutaneous candidiasis is characterized by red, pustular, crusted, and thickened plaques resembling psoriasis, especially on the nose and forehead, and is invariably associated with chronic oral candidiasis.

Diagnosis

- Clinical appearance
- Potassium hydroxide wet mounts

Diagnosis of mucocutaneous candidiasis is based on clinical appearance and identification of yeast and pseudohyphae in potassium hydroxide wet mounts of scrapings from a lesion. Positive culture alone is usually meaningless because *Candida* is omnipresent.

Treatment

- Sometimes drying agents
- Topical or oral antifungals

Intertriginous infection is treated with drying agents as needed (eg, Burow solution compresses applied for 15 to 20 min for oozing lesions) and topical antifungals (see Table 128–1). Powdered formulations are also helpful (eg, miconazole powder bid for 2 to 3 wk). Fluconazole 150 mg po once/wk for 2 to 4 wk can be used for extensive intertriginous candidiasis; topical antifungal agents may be used at the same time.

Candidal diaper rash is treated with more frequent changes of diapers, use of super- or ultra-absorbent disposable diapers, and an imidazole cream bid. Oral nystatin is an option for infants with coexisting oropharyngeal candidiasis; 1 mL of suspension (100,000 units/mL) is placed in each buccal pouch qid (see Plate 33).

Candidal paronychia is treated by protecting the area from wetness and giving topical or oral antifungals. These infections are often resistant to treatment. Thymol 4% in alcohol applied to the affected area twice daily is often helpful.

Oral candidiasis can be treated by dissolving 1 clotrimazole 10-mg troche in the mouth 4 to 5 times/day for 14 days. Another option is nystatin oral suspension (4 to 6 mL of a 100,000 unit/mL solution) held in the mouth for as long as possible and then swallowed or expectorated 3 to 4 times/day, continuing for 7 to 14 days after symptoms and signs have resolved. A systemic antifungal may also be used (eg, fluconazole 200 mg po on the first day, then 100 mg po once/day for 2 to 3 wk thereafter; see also Plate 72).

Chronic mucocutaneous candidiasis requires long-term oral antifungal treatment with oral fluconazole.

KEY POINTS

- *Candida* are normal skin flora that can become infective under certain conditions (eg, excessive moisture, alteration of normal flora, host immunosuppression).
- Consider candidiasis with erythematous, scaling, pruritic patches in intertriginous areas and with lesions in the mucous membranes, around the nails, or at the corners of the mouth.
- If clinical appearance is not diagnostic, try to identify yeast and pseudohyphae in potassium hydroxide wet mounts of scrapings from a lesion.
- Treat most intertriginous candidiasis with a drying agent and a topical antifungal.
- Treat most diaper rash with frequent changes of absorbent disposable diapers and an imidazole cream.
- Treat oral candidiasis with clotrimazole troches, nystatin oral suspension, or an oral antifungal.

OVERVIEW OF DERMATOPHYTOSES

Dermatophytoses are fungal infections of keratin in the skin and nails (nail infection is called tinea unguium or onychomycosis). Symptoms and signs vary by site of infection. Diagnosis is by clinical appearance and by examination of skin scrapings on potassium hydroxide wet mount. Treatment varies by site but always involves topical or oral antifungals.

Dermatophytes are molds that require keratin for nutrition and must live on stratum corneum, hair, or nails to survive. Human infections are caused by *Epidermophyton, Microsporum,* and *Trichophyton* spp. These infections differ from candidiasis in that they are rarely if ever invasive. Transmission is person-to-person, animal-to-person, and, rarely, soil-to-person. The organism may persist indefinitely. Most people do not develop clinical infection; those who do may have impaired T-cell responses from an alteration in local defenses (eg, from trauma with vascular compromise) or from primary (hereditary) or secondary (eg, diabetes, HIV) immunosuppression.

Common dermatophytoses include

- Tinea barbae
- Tinea capitis
- Tinea corporis
- Tinea cruris
- Tinea pedis
- Dermatophytid reaction

Symptoms and Signs

Symptoms and signs of dermatophytoses vary by site (skin, hair, nails). Organism virulence and host susceptibility and hypersensitivity determine severity. Most often, there is little or

Table 128–1. OPTIONS FOR TREATMENT OF SUPERFICIAL FUNGAL INFECTIONS*

DRUGS	FORMULATIONS	USES
Allylamines		
Amorolfine	5% solution	Tinea unguium
Naftifine	1% cream or gel	Dermatophytoses, skin candidiasis
Terbinafine	Topical: 1% cream or solution	Dermatophytoses
	Oral: 250-mg tablet	
Benzylamine		
Butenafine	1% cream	Dermatophytoses
Imidazoles		
Butoconazole	2% cream	Vulvovaginal candidiasis
Clotrimazole	Topical: 1% cream, lotion, or solution; 100-, 200-, and 500-mg vaginal suppository tablets	Dermatophytoses, candidiasis (oropharyngeal, skin, vulvovaginal)
	Oral: 10-mg lozenges	
Econazole	1% cream	Dermatophytoses, skin candidiasis, tinea versicolor
Fluconazole	50 and 200 mg/5 mL solution; 50-, 100-, 150-, and 200-mg tablets	Candidiasis (vulvovaginal, skin, oropharyngeal)
Itraconazole	100-mg capsules, 10 mg/mL solution	Tinea unguium, other onychomycoses
Ketoconazole	2% cream, 1 to 2% shampoo	Dermatophytoses, skin candidiasis
Miconazole	1 to 2% liquid (aerosol), 2% powder (aerosol), 1 to 2% cream and lotion, 1% solution, 2% powder or tincture, 100- or 200-mg vaginal suppositories	Dermatophytoses, candidiasis (skin, vulvovaginal)
Oxiconazole	1% cream or lotion	Dermatophytoses, tinea versicolor
Sulconazole	1% cream or solution	Dermatophytoses, tinea versicolor
Terconazole	0.4% and 0.8% cream, 80-mg suppositories	Vulvovaginal candidiasis
Tioconazole	6.5% ointment	Vulvovaginal candidiasis
Polyene		
Nystatin	Topical: 100,000 U/g cream, ointment, powder, or vaginal tablet	Candidiasis (oropharyngeal, skin)
	Oral: 100,000 U/mL suspension, 500,000-U tablets	Candidiasis (oropharyngeal, GI)
Miscellaneous		
Carbolfuchsin	Solution	Chronic dermatophytoses, intertrigo
Ciclopirox	0.77% gel, 8% lacquer solution	Dermatophytoses, candidiasis, tinea versicolor, onychomycosis
Clioquinol	3% cream	Dermatophytoses
Gentian violet	1 or 2% solution	Dermatophytoses, especially tinea pedis; sometimes candidiasis
Griseofulvin	125-, 165-, 250-, 330-, and 500-mg tablets	Dermatophytoses
Tolnaftate	1% liquid, powder, liquid or aerosol spray, cream, or solution	Dermatophytoses, tinea versicolor
Zinc		
Undecylenate/ undecylenic acid	25% solution, 10% tincture	Superficial dermatophyte infections (eg, tinea pedis)

*Advantages of one topical drug over another for most infections are not clear. For skin infections, allylamines have good activity against dermatophytes but weaker activity against *Candida;* imidazoles have better activity against both dermatophytes and *Candida*. Adverse effects are rare, but all topical antifungals can cause skin irritation, burning, and contact dermatitis. Drug doses may vary by indication.

Oral antifungals can cause hepatitis and neutropenia. Periodic laboratory monitoring of hepatic function and of CBC is recommended when oral antifungals (eg, itraconazole, terbinafine) are given for > 1 mo.

Oral itraconazole, terbinafine, and fluconazole are metabolized through the cytochrome P-450 enzyme system and thus have many potential drug interactions. Some interactions may be severe; cardiac arrhythmias are a risk for some people. Care should be taken to minimize the effects of interactions with these drugs.

no inflammation; asymptomatic or mildly itching lesions with a scaling, slightly raised border remit and recur intermittently. Occasionally, inflammation is more severe and manifests as sudden vesicular or bullous disease (usually of the foot) or as an inflamed boggy lesion of the scalp (kerion).

Diagnosis

- Clinical appearance
- Potassium hydroxide wet mount

Diagnosis of dermatophytoses is based on clinical appearance and site of infection and can be confirmed by skin scrapings and demonstration of hyphae on potassium hydroxide (KOH) wet mount or by culture of plucked hairs. For onychomycosis, the most sensitive test is a periodic acid-Schiff stain of nail clippings. For KOH wet mount, the affected area of the nail plate, not subungual debris, should be pared and tested.

Identification of specific organisms by culture is unnecessary except for scalp infection (where an animal source may be identified and treated) and nail infection (which may be caused by a nondermatophyte). Culture may also be useful when overlying inflammation and bacterial infection are severe and/or accompanied by alopecia.

Differential diagnosis of dermatophytoses includes

- Folliculitis decalvans
- Bacterial pyodermas
- Entities that cause scarring alopecia, such as discoid lupus erythematosus, lichen planopilaris, and pseudopelade

Treatment

- Topical or oral antifungals
- Sometimes corticosteroids

Topical antifungals are generally adequate (see Table 128–1). OTC terbinafine is fungicidal and allows for shorter treatment duration. Econazole or ciclopirox may be better if candidal infection cannot be excluded. Other adequate OTC topical treatments include clotrimazole and miconazole.

Oral antifungals are used for most nail and scalp infections, resistant skin infections, and patients unwilling or unable to adhere to prolonged topical regimens; doses and duration differ by site of infection.

Corticosteroids are sometimes used in addition to antifungal creams to help relieve itching and inflammation. However, combining topical corticosteroids and antifungal creams should be avoided when possible because topical corticosteroids promote fungus growth. Commercially available topical corticosteroid and antifungal products should not be used as substitutes for obtaining an accurate diagnosis with a KOH wet mount or culture.

TINEA BARBAE

(Barber's Itch)

Tinea barbae is a dermatophyte infection of the beard area most often caused by *Trichophyton mentagrophytes* or *T. verrucosum*.

Tinea barbae is a dermatophytosis that manifests in the beard area as superficial annular lesions, but deeper infection similar to folliculitis may occur. Tinea barbae may also occur as an inflammatory kerion that can result in scarring hair loss.

Diagnosis

- KOH wet mount

Diagnosis of tinea barbae is by KOH wet mount of involved skin or plucked hairs, culture, or biopsy.

Treatment

- Oral antifungals
- Sometimes prednisone

Treatment of tinea barbae is micronized griseofulvin 500 mg to 1 g po once/day until 2 to 3 wk after clinical clearance. Terbinafine 250 mg po once/day and itraconazole 200 mg po once/day have also been used.

If the lesions are severely inflamed, a short course of prednisone should be added (to lessen symptoms and perhaps reduce the chance of scarring), starting with 40 mg po once/day (for adults) and tapering the dose over 2 wk.

TINEA CAPITIS

(Scalp Ringworm)

Tinea capitis is a dermatophyte infection of the scalp.

Tinea capitis is a dermatophytosis that mainly affects children, is contagious, and can be epidemic. *Trichophyton tonsurans* is the most common cause in the US, followed by *Microsporum canis* and *M. audouinii*; other *Trichophyton* sp (eg, *T. schoenleinii, T. violaceum*) are common elsewhere.

Tinea capitis causes the gradual appearance of round patches of dry scale, alopecia, or both. *T. tonsurans* infection causes black dot ringworm, in which hair shafts break at the scalp surface; *M. audouinii* infection causes gray patch ringworm, in which hair shafts break above the surface, leaving short stubs. Tinea capitis less commonly manifests as diffuse scaling, like dandruff, or in a diffuse pustular pattern.

Kerion: Dermatophyte infection occasionally leads to formation of a kerion, which is a large, boggy, inflammatory scalp mass (see Plate 56) caused by a severe inflammatory reaction to the dermatophyte. A kerion may have pustules and crusting and can be mistaken for an abscess. A kerion may result in scarring hair loss.

Diagnosis

- Clinical appearance
- KOH wet mount
- Sometimes a Wood light examination and sometimes culture

Tinea capitis is diagnosed by clinical appearance and by KOH wet mount of plucked hairs or of hairs and scale obtained by scraping or brushing. Spore size and appearance inside (endothrix) or outside (ectothrix) the hair shaft distinguish organisms and can help guide treatment.

Blue-green fluorescence during a Wood light examination is diagnostic for infection with *M. canis* and *M. audouinii* and can distinguish tinea from erythrasma.

Fungal culture of plucked hairs can be done when necessary. A scalp lesion in a child that appears similar to an abscess may be a kerion; if necessary, cultures can help make the distinction.

PEARLS & PITFALLS

- Before draining a scalp abscess in a child, consider the diagnosis of kerion.

Differential diagnosis of tinea capitis includes

- Seborrheic dermatitis
- Psoriasis

Treatment

- Oral antifungals
- Selenium sulfide shampoo
- Sometimes prednisone

Children are treated with micronized griseofulvin suspension 10 to 20 mg/kg po once/day (doses vary by several parameters, but maximum dose is generally 1 g/day) or, if > 2 yr, with ultramicronized griseofulvin 5 to 10 mg/kg (maximum 750 mg/day) po once/day or in 2 divided doses with meals or milk for 4 to 6 wk or until all signs of infection are gone. Terbinafine also may be used. Children < 20 kg are given terbinafine 62.5 mg po once/day, those 20 to 40 kg are given 125 mg po once/day, and those > 40 kg are given 250 mg po once/day.

An imidazole or ciclopirox cream should be applied to the scalp to prevent spread, especially to other children, until tinea capitis is cured; selenium sulfide 2.5% shampoo should also be used at least twice/wk. Children may attend school during treatment.

Adults are treated with terbinafine 250 mg po once/day for 2 to 4 wk, which is more effective for endothrix infections, or itraconazole 200 mg once/day for 2 to 4 wk or 200 mg bid for 1 wk, followed by 3 wk without the drug (pulsed) for 2 to 3 mo.

For severely inflamed lesions and for kerion, a short course of prednisone should be added (to lessen symptoms and perhaps reduce the chance of scarring), starting with 40 mg po once/day (1 mg/kg for children) and tapering the dose over 2 wk.

KEY POINTS

- Tinea capitis affects mostly children and can be contagious and epidemic.
- Confirm tinea capitis by KOH wet mount, fungal culture, or sometimes Wood light examination.
- Treat with oral griseofulvin or terbinafine in addition to a topical antifungal.
- Add a short course of oral prednisone for a kerion or severe inflammation.

TINEA CORPORIS

(Body Ringworm)

Tinea corporis is a dermatophyte infection of the face, trunk, and extremities.

Tinea corporis is a dermatophytosis that causes pink-to-red annular (O-shaped) patches and plaques with raised scaly borders that expand peripherally and tend to clear centrally (see Plate 57). A rare variant form appears as nummular (circle- or round-shaped) scaling patches studded with small papules or pustules that have no central clearing. Common causes are *Trichophyton mentagrophytes, T. rubrum,* and *Microsporum canis*.

Diagnosis

- Clinical evaluation
- KOH wet mount

Differential diagnosis of tinea corporis includes

- Pityriasis rosea
- Drug eruptions
- Nummular dermatitis
- Erythema multiforme
- Tinea versicolor
- Erythrasma
- Psoriasis
- Secondary syphilis

Treatment

- Topical or oral antifungals

Treatment of mild-to-moderate lesions is an imidazole, ciclopirox, naftifine, or terbinafine in cream, lotion, or gel. The drug should be rubbed in bid continuing at least 7 to 10 days after lesions disappear, typically at about 2 to 3 wk.

Extensive and resistant lesions occur in patients infected with *T. rubrum* and in people with debilitating systemic diseases. For such cases, the most effective therapy is oral itraconazole 200 mg once/day or terbinafine 250 mg once/day for 2 to 3 wk.

TINEA CRURIS

(Jock Itch)

Tinea cruris is a dermatophyte infection of the groin.

Tinea cruris is a dermatophytosis that is commonly caused by *Trichophyton rubrum* or *T. mentagrophytes*. The primary risk factors are associated with a moist environment (ie, warm weather, wet and restrictive clothing, obesity causing constant apposition of skinfolds). Men are affected more than women because of apposition of the scrotum and thigh.

Typically, a pruritic, ringed lesion extends from the crural fold over the adjacent upper inner thigh (see Plate 58). Infection may be bilateral. Lesions may be complicated by maceration, miliaria, secondary bacterial or candidal infection, and reactions to treatment. In addition, scratch dermatitis and lichenification can occur. Recurrence is common because fungi may repeatedly infect susceptible people or people with onychomycosis or tinea pedis, which can serve as a dermatophyte reservoir. Flare-ups occur more often during summer.

Diagnosis

- Clinical evaluation
- Sometimes KOH wet mount

Differential diagnosis of tinea cruris includes

- Contact dermatitis
- Psoriasis
- Erythrasma
- Candidiasis

Scrotal involvement is usually absent or slight; by contrast, the scrotum is often inflamed in candidal intertrigo or lichen simplex chronicus. If the appearance is not diagnostic, a KOH wet mount is helpful.

Treatment

- Topical antifungal cream, lotion, or gel

Antifungal choices include terbinafine, miconazole, clotrimazole, ketoconazole, econazole, naftifine, and (uncommonly) ciclopirox applied bid for 10 to 14 days.

Itraconazole 200 mg po once/day or terbinafine 250 mg po once/day for 3 to 6 wk may be needed in patients who have refractory, inflammatory, or widespread infections.

TINEA PEDIS

(Athlete's Foot)

Tinea pedis is a dermatophyte infection of the feet.

Tinea pedis is the most common dermatophytosis because moisture resulting from foot sweating facilitates fungal growth. Tinea pedis may occur as any of 4 clinical forms or in combination:

- Chronic hyperkeratotic
- Chronic intertriginous
- Acute ulcerative
- Vesiculobullous

Chronic hyperkeratotic tinea pedis due to *Trichophyton rubrum* causes a distinctive pattern of lesion, manifesting as scaling and thickening of the soles, which often extends beyond the plantar surface in a moccasin distribution. Patients who are not responding as expected to antifungal therapy may have another less common cause of plantar rash. Differential diagnosis is sterile maceration (due to hyperhidrosis and occlusive footgear), contact dermatitis (due to type IV delayed hypersensitivity to various materials in shoes, particularly adhesive cement, thiuram compounds in footwear that contains rubber, and chromate tanning agents used in leather footwear), irritant contact dermatitis, and psoriasis.

Chronic intertriginous tinea pedis is characterized by scaling, erythema, and erosion of the interdigital and subdigital skin of the feet, most commonly affecting the lateral 3 toes.

Acute ulcerative tinea pedis (most often caused by *T. mentagrophytes* var. *interdigitale*) typically begins in the 3rd and 4th interdigital spaces and extends to the lateral dorsum and/or the plantar surface of the arch. These toe web lesions are usually macerated and have scaling borders (see Plate 59). Secondary bacterial infection, cellulitis, and lymphangitis are common complications.

Vesiculobullous tinea pedis, in which vesicles develop on the soles and coalesce into bullae, is the less common result of a flare-up of interdigital tinea pedis; risk factors are occlusive shoes and environmental heat and humidity.

Diagnosis

- Clinical evaluation
- KOH wet mount

Diagnosis of tinea pedis is usually obvious based on clinical examination and review of risk factors. If the appearance is not diagnostic, a KOH wet mount is helpful.

Differential diagnosis of tinea pedis includes

- Dyshidrotic eczema
- Palmoplantar psoriasis (see Table 135–1 on p. 1071)
- Allergic contact dermatitis

Treatment

- Topical and oral antifungals
- Moisture reduction and drying agents

The safest tinea pedis treatment is topical antifungals, but recurrence is common and treatment must often be prolonged. Alternatives that provide a more durable response include itraconazole 200 mg po once/day for 1 mo (or pulse therapy with 200 mg bid 1 wk/mo for 1 to 2 mo) and terbinafine 250 mg po once/day for 2 to 6 wk. Concomitant topical antifungal use may reduce recurrences.

Moisture reduction on the feet and in footwear is necessary for preventing recurrence. Permeable or open-toe footwear and sock changes are important especially during warm weather. Interdigital spaces should be manually dried after bathing. Drying agents are also recommended; options include antifungal powders (eg, miconazole), gentian violet, Burow solution (5% aluminum subacetate) soaks, and 20 to 25% aluminum chloride solution nightly for 1 wk then 1 to 2 times/wk as needed.

DERMATOPHYTID REACTION

Dermatophytid reaction is an inflammatory reaction to dermatophytosis at a cutaneous site distant from the primary infection.

Dermatophytid (identity or id) reactions are protean; they are not related to localized growth of the fungus but rather are an inflammatory reaction to a dermatophytosis elsewhere on the body. Lesions are typically pruritic but may manifest as

- Vesicular eruptions on the hands and feet
- Follicular papules
- Erysipelas-like plaques
- Erythema nodosum
- Erythema annulare centrifugum
- Urticaria

Distribution may be extensive.

Diagnosis of dermatophytid reaction is by KOH wet mounts that are negative at the site of the id reaction and positive at the distant site of dermatophyte infection.

Treatment of the primary infection cures dermatophytid; pending cure, topical corticosteroids and/or antipruritics (eg, hydroxyzine 25 mg po qid) can be used to relieve symptoms.

INTERTRIGO

Intertrigo is skin maceration in intertriginous areas caused by moisture and/or infection.

Intertrigo develops when friction and trapped moisture in intertriginous areas cause skin maceration and inflammation with formation of patches or plaques. Infection by bacteria and yeast is also common. Typical locations are the inframammary, infrapannicular, interdigital, axillary, infragluteal, and genitocrural folds.

Diagnosis

- Clinical evaluation

Diagnosis of intertrigo is based on clinical appearance; KOH wet mounts and cultures can guide treatment.

Differential diagnosis of intertrigo includes

- Tinea cruris (for inguinal intertrigo)
- Candidiasis
- Inverse psoriasis (psoriasis of intertriginous areas)

Treatment

- Drying agents and sometimes topical antibacterial lotions or antifungal creams

If no bacteria or yeast are detected, drying agents should be therapeutic. Effective options include talc (rather than cornstarch, which can support fungal growth), Burow solution compresses, and super-absorbent powders.

If bacteria or yeast are present, topical antibacterial lotions or antifungal creams are given in addition to drying agents.

TINEA VERSICOLOR

(Pityriasis Versicolor)

Tinea versicolor is skin infection with *Malassezia furfur* that manifests as multiple asymptomatic scaly patches varying in color from white to tan to brown to pink. Diagnosis is based on clinical appearance and KOH wet mount of skin scrapings. Treatment is with topical or sometimes oral antifungals. Recurrence is common.

Malassezia furfur is a dimorphic fungus that is normally a harmless component of normal skin flora but that in some people causes tinea versicolor. Most affected people are healthy. Factors that may predispose to tinea versicolor include heat and humidity and immunosuppression due to corticosteroids, pregnancy, undernutrition, diabetes, or other disorders. Hypopigmentation in tinea versicolor is due to the inhibition of tyrosinase caused by *M. furfur* production of azelaic acid.

Symptoms and Signs

Tinea versicolor usually is asymptomatic. Classically, it causes the appearance of multiple tan, brown, salmon, pink, or white scaling patches (see Plate 60) on the trunk, neck, abdomen, and occasionally face. The lesions may coalesce. In light-skinned patients, the condition is often diagnosed in summer months because the lesions, which do not tan, become more obvious against tanned skin. Tinea versicolor is benign and is not considered contagious.

Diagnosis

- Clinical appearance
- KOH wet mount
- Sometimes Wood light examination

Diagnosis of tinea versicolor is based on clinical appearance and by identification of hyphae and budding cells ("spaghetti and meatballs") on KOH wet mount of fine scale scrapings.

A Wood light examination reveals golden-white fluorescence.

Treatment

- Topical antifungals
- Sometimes oral antifungals

Treatment of tinea versicolor is any topical antifungal drug. Examples include selenium sulfide shampoo 2.5% (in 10-min applications daily for 1 wk or 24-h applications weekly for 1 mo); topical azoles (eg, ketoconazole 2% daily for 2 wk); and daily bathing with zinc pyrithione soap 2% or sulfur-salicylic shampoo 2% for 1 to 2 wk.

Fluconazole 150 mg/wk po for 2 to 4 wk is indicated for patients with extensive disease and those with frequent recurrences.

Hypopigmentation from tinea versicolor is reversible in months to years after the yeast has cleared.

Recurrence is almost universal after treatment because the causative organism is a normal skin inhabitant. Fastidious hygiene, regular use of zinc pyrithione soap, or once-monthly use of topical antifungal therapy lowers the likelihood of recurrence.

KEY POINTS

- Although tinea versicolor can occur in immunosuppressed patients, most affected patients are healthy.
- The disorder is frequently diagnosed in the summer, but mainly because hypopigmented lesions become more obvious against tanned skin.
- Try to confirm the diagnosis by finding hyphae and budding cells on KOH wet mount of fine scale scrapings.
- Treat with topical or oral antifungals.

129 Hair Disorders

ALOPECIA

(Baldness; Hair Loss)

Alopecia is defined as loss of hair from the body. Hair loss is often a cause of great concern to the patient for cosmetic and psychologic reasons, but it can also be an important sign of systemic disease.

Pathophysiology

Growth cycle: Hair grows in cycles. Each cycle consists of phases:

- A long growing phase (anagen)
- A brief transitional apoptotic phase (catagen)
- A short resting phase (telogen)

At the end of the resting phase, the hair falls out (exogen) and a new hair starts growing in the follicle, beginning the cycle again.

Normally, about 50 to 100 scalp hairs reach the end of resting phase each day and fall out. When significantly more than 100 hairs/day go into resting phase, clinical hair loss (telogen effluvium) may occur. A disruption of the growing phase causing abnormal loss of anagen hairs is an anagen effluvium.

Classification: Alopecia can be classified as focal or diffuse and by the presence or absence of scarring.

Scarring alopecia is the result of active destruction of the hair follicle. The follicle is irreparably damaged and replaced by fibrotic tissue. Several hair disorders show a biphasic pattern in which nonscarring alopecia occurs early in the course of the disease, and then scarring alopecia and permanent hair loss occurs as the disease progresses. Scarring alopecias can be subdivided further into primary forms, where the target of inflammation is the follicle itself, and secondary forms, where the follicle is destroyed as a result of nonspecific inflammation (see Table 129–1).

Nonscarring alopecia results from processes that reduce or slow hair growth without irreparably damaging the hair follicle. Disorders that primarily affect the hair shaft (trichodystrophies) also are considered nonscarring alopecia.

Etiology

The alopecias comprise a large group of disorders with multiple and varying etiologies (see Table 129–1).

The **most common cause** of alopecia is

- Androgenetic alopecia (male-pattern or female-pattern hair loss)

Table 129–1. SOME CAUSES OF ALOPECIA

ALOPECIA DISORDER	CAUSES OR DESCRIPTIONS
Nonscarring diffuse hair loss	
Anagen effluvium (caused by agents that impair or disrupt the anagen cycle)	Chemotherapeutic agents Poisoning (eg, thallium, arsenic, other metals) Radiation (also causes scarring focal hair loss)
Androgenetic alopecia (male-pattern or female-pattern hair loss)	Androgens (eg, dihydrotestosterone) Familial Pathologic hyperandrogenism (virilization in females—see p. 1041)
Congenital disorders	Congenital atrichia with papules Ectodermal dysplasia
Primary hair shaft abnormalities	Easy hair breakage (trichorrhexis nodosa) Genetic disorders Loose anagen hair syndrome Overuse of hair dryers (bubble hair)
Telogen effluvium (increased number of hairs entering resting phase)	Drugs (eg, antimitotic chemotherapeutic agents, anticoagulants, retinoids, oral contraceptives, ACE inhibitors, beta-blockers, lithium, antithyroid drugs, anticonvulsants, vitamin A excess) Endocrine problems (eg, hyperthyroidism, hypothyroidism) Nutritional deficiencies (eg, zinc, biotin, or possibly iron deficiency) Physiologic or psychologic stress (eg, surgery, systemic or febrile illness, pregnancy)
Alopecia areata	Diffuse loss of scalp hair (less common form of alopecia areata) Alopecia totalis (complete scalp hair loss) Alopecia universalis (complete scalp and body hair loss)
Nonscarring focal hair loss	
Alopecia areata	Patchy loss of scalp hair (most common form of alopecia areata) Ophiasis (band pattern hair loss along periphery of temporal and occipital scalp)
Other	Hair loss due to compulsive hair pulling, twisting, or teasing (trichotillomania) Lipedematous alopecia Postoperative (pressure-induced) alopecia Primary hair shaft abnormalities Secondary syphilis SLE (typically causes scarring discoid lesions or non-scarring diffuse alopecia) Temporal triangular alopecia
Tinea capitis*	*Microsporum audouinii* *Microsporum canis* *Trichophyton schoenleinii* *Trichophyton tonsurans*
Traction alopecia	Traction due to braids, rollers, or ponytails (occurs primarily at frontal and temporal hairlines)
Scarring hair loss (focal or diffuse)	
Acne keloidalis nuchae	Folliculitis on the occipital scalp that results in scarring alopecia
Central centrifugal cicatricial alopecia (CCCA)	Progressive scarring alopecia on the crown or vertex of the scalp Most common cause of alopecia in black patients, typically occurring in women of African descent
Chronic cutaneous lupus	Discoid lupus lesions of the scalp
Dissecting cellulitis of the scalp	Boggy inflammatory nodules that coalesce with sinus tract formation Part of the follicular occlusion tetrad†
Lichen planopilaris (lichen planus of the scalp)	Typically perifollicular erythema and follicular hyperkeratosis
Secondary scarring alopecias	Burns Morphea Progressive systemic sclerosis (scleroderma) Radiation therapy (also causes nonscarring diffuse hair loss) Sarcoidosis Skin cancer Superinfected kerion (due to severe primary syphilis or severe tinea capitis) Trauma

*Tinea capitis can cause scarring if the follicle is sufficiently damaged.
†The follicular occlusion tetrad (also called acne inversa) is acne conglobata, hidradenitis suppurativa, dissecting cellulitis of the scalp, and pilonidal sinus—disorders that have follicular hyperkeratinization in common.

Androgenetic alopecia is an androgen-dependent hereditary disorder in which dihydrotestosterone plays a major role. This form of alopecia may eventually affect up to 80% of white men by the age of 70 (male-pattern hair loss) and about half of all women (female-pattern hair loss).

Other common causes of hair loss are

- Drugs (including chemotherapeutic agents)
- Infection (eg, tinea capitis, kerion)
- Systemic disorders (disorders that cause high fever, systemic lupus erythematosus, endocrine disorders, and nutritional deficiencies)
- Alopecia areata
- Trauma

Traumatic causes include trichotillomania, traction alopecia, central centrifugal cicatricial alopecia (CCCA), burns, radiation, and pressure-induced (eg, postoperative) hair loss.

Less common causes are

- Primary hair shaft abnormalities
- Autoimmune diseases
- Heavy metal poisoning
- Rare dermatologic conditions (eg, dissecting cellulitis of the scalp, which most often affects young black men)

Evaluation

History: History of present illness should cover the onset and duration of hair loss, whether hair shedding is increased, and whether hair loss is generalized or localized. Associated symptoms such as pruritus and scaling should be noted. Patients should be asked about typical hair care practices, including use of braids, rollers, and hair dryers, and whether they routinely pull or twist their hair.

Review of systems should include recent exposures to noxious stimuli (eg, drugs, toxins, radiation) and stressors (eg, surgery, chronic illness, fever, psychologic stressors). Symptoms of possible causes should be sought, including fatigue and cold intolerance (hypothyroidism) and, in women, hirsutism deepening of the voice, and increased libido (virilization). Other features, including dramatic weight loss, dietary practices (including various restrictive diets), and obsessive-compulsive behavior, should be noted. In women, a hormonal/gynecologic/obstetric history should be obtained.

Past medical history should note known possible causes of hair loss, including endocrine and skin disorders. Current and recent drug use should be reviewed for offending agents (see Table 129–1). A family history of hair loss should be recorded.

Physical examination: Examination of the scalp should note the distribution of hair loss, the presence and characteristics of any skin lesions, and whether there is scarring. Part widths should be measured. Abnormalities of the hair shafts should be noted.

A full skin examination should be done to evaluate hair loss elsewhere on the body (eg, eyebrows, eyelashes, arms, legs), rashes that may be associated with certain types of alopecia (eg, discoid lupus lesions, signs of secondary syphilis or of other bacterial or fungal infections), and signs of virilization in women (eg, hirsutism, acne, deepening voice, clitoromegaly). Signs of potential underlying systemic disorders should be sought, and a thyroid examination should be done.

Red flags: The following findings are of particular concern:

- Virilization in women
- Signs of systemic illness or constellations of nonspecific findings possibly indicating poisoning

Interpretation of findings: Hair loss that begins at the temples and/or crown (vertex) and spreads to diffuse thinning or nearly complete hair loss is typical of male-pattern hair loss. Hair thinning in the frontal, parietal, and crown regions is typical of female-pattern hair loss (see Fig. 129–1). In androgenetic alopecia, the central part width is wider on the crown of the scalp than it is on the occipital scalp.

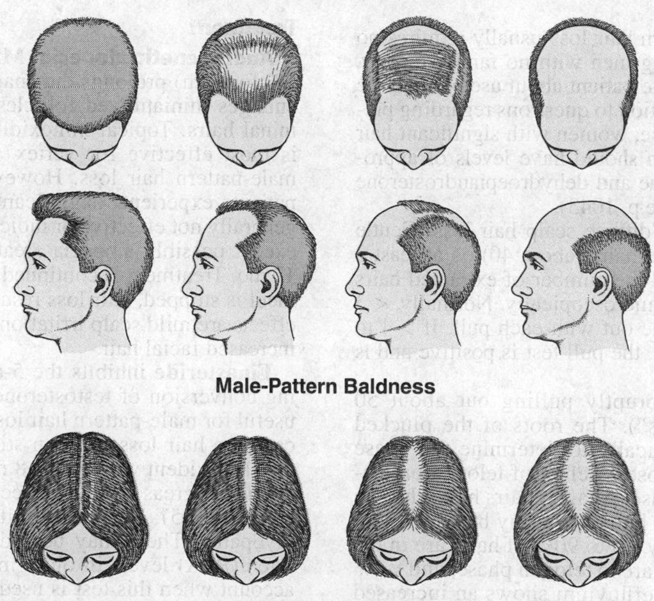

Fig. 129–1. Male- and female-pattern hair loss (androgenetic alopecia).

Table 129–2. INTERPRETING PHYSICAL FINDINGS IN ALOPECIA

FINDING	POSSIBLE CAUSES
Asymmetric, bizarre, irregular hair loss pattern	Trichotillomania
Circular, discrete patches of loss; short, broken hairs; exclamation point hairs at periphery of patches	Alopecia areata
Patchy hair loss that appears moth-eaten	Secondary syphilis
Pruritus, erythema, and scaling	Chronic cutaneous lupus, lichen planopilaris Tinea capitis (particularly if adenopathy present)
Pustules	Scarring dermatologic or infectious process (eg, dissecting cellulitis of the scalp, acne keloidalis nuchae)
Scalp and body hair loss	Alopecia universalis
Unruly or unusually wooly hair	Primary hair shaft abnormality
Virilization (see p. 1041)	Adrenal disorder or tumor Pituitary adenoma Polycystic ovary syndrome (PCOS) or ovarian tumor Anabolic steroid use (sometimes surreptitious)

Hair loss that occurs 2 to 4 wk after chemotherapy or radiation therapy (anagen effluvium) can typically be ascribed to those causes. Hair loss that occurs 3 to 4 mo after a major stressor (pregnancy, major febrile illness, surgery, medication change, or severe psychologic stressor) suggests a diagnosis of telogen effluvium.

Other findings help suggest alternative diagnoses (see Table 129–2).

Other than hair loss, scalp symptoms (eg, itching, burning, tingling) are often absent and, when present, are not specific to any cause.

Signs of hair loss in patterns other than those described above are nondiagnostic and may require microscopic hair examination or scalp biopsy for definitive diagnosis.

Testing: Evaluation for causative disorders (eg, endocrinologic, autoimmune, toxic) should be done based on clinical suspicion.

Male-pattern or female-pattern hair loss usually requires no testing. When it occurs in young men with no family history, the physician should question the patient about use of anabolic steroids and other drugs. In addition to questions regarding prescription drug and illicit drug use, women with significant hair loss and evidence of virilization should have levels of appropriate hormones (eg, testosterone and dehydroepiandrosterone sulfate [DHEAS]) measured (see p. 1043).

The **pull test** helps evaluate diffuse scalp hair loss. Gentle traction is exerted on a bunch of hairs (about 40) on at least 3 different areas of the scalp, and the number of extracted hairs is then counted and examined microscopically. Normally, < 3 telogen-phase hairs should come out with each pull. If > 4 to 6 hairs come out with each pull, the pull test is positive and is suggestive of telogen effluvium.

The **pluck test** involves abruptly pulling out about 50 individual hairs ("by the roots"). The roots of the plucked hairs are examined microscopically to determine the phase of growth and thus help diagnose a defect of telogen or anagen or an occult systemic disease. Anagen hairs have sheaths attached to their roots; telogen hairs have tiny bulbs without sheaths at their roots. Normally, 85 to 90% of hairs are in the anagen phase, about 10 to 15% are in telogen phase, and < 1% are in catagen phase. Telogen effluvium shows an increased percentage of telogen-phase hairs on microscopic examination (typically > 20%), whereas anagen effluvium shows a decrease in telogen-phase hairs and an increased number of broken hairs. Primary hair shaft abnormalities are usually obvious on microscopic examination of the hair shaft.

Scalp biopsy is indicated when alopecia persists and diagnosis is in doubt. Biopsy may differentiate scarring from nonscarring forms. Specimens should be taken from areas of active inflammation, ideally at the border of a bald patch. Fungal and bacterial cultures may be useful.

Daily hair counts can be done by the patient to quantify hair loss when the pull test is negative. Hairs lost during the first morning combing or during washing are collected in clear plastic bags daily for 14 days. The number of hairs in each bag is then recorded. Scalp hair counts of > 100/day are abnormal except after shampooing, when hair counts of up to 250 may be normal. Hairs may be brought in by the patient for microscopic examination.

Treatment

Androgenetic alopecia: Minoxidil (2% for women, 2% or 5% for men) prolongs the anagen growth phase and gradually enlarges miniaturized follicles (vellus hairs) into mature terminal hairs. Topical minoxidil 1 mL bid applied to the scalp is most effective for vertex alopecia in male-pattern or female-pattern hair loss. However, usually only 30 to 40% of patients experience significant hair growth, and minoxidil is generally not effective or indicated for other causes of hair loss except possibly alopecia areata. Hair regrowth can take 8 to 12 mo. Treatment is continued indefinitely because, once treatment is stopped, hair loss resumes. The most frequent adverse effects are mild scalp irritation, allergic contact dermatitis, and increased facial hair.

Finasteride inhibits the 5-alpha-reductase enzyme, blocking conversion of testosterone to dihydrotestosterone, and is useful for male-pattern hair loss. Finasteride 1 mg po once/day can stop hair loss and can stimulate hair growth. Efficacy is usually evident within 6 to 8 mo of treatment. Adverse effects include decreased libido, erectile and ejaculatory dysfunction (see p. 2135), hypersensitivity reactions, gynecomastia, and myopathy. There may be a decrease in prostate-specific antigen (PSA) levels in older men, which should be taken into account when this test is used for cancer screening. Common practice is to continue treatment for as long as positive results persist. Once treatment is stopped, hair loss returns to previous levels. Finasteride is not indicated for women and is contraindicated in pregnant women because it has teratogenic effects in animals.

Hormonal modulators such as oral contraceptives or spironolactone may be useful for female-pattern hair loss.

Surgical options include follicle transplant, scalp flaps, and alopecia reduction. Few procedures have been subjected to scientific scrutiny, but patients who are self-conscious about their hair loss may consider them.

Hair loss due to other causes: Underlying disorders are treated.

Treatment for alopecia areata includes topical, intralesional, or, in severe cases, systemic corticosteroids, topical minoxidil, topical anthralin, topical immunotherapy (diphenylcyclopropenone or squaric acid dibutylester), or psoralen plus ultraviolet A (PUVA).

Treatment for traction alopecia is elimination of physical traction or stress to the scalp.

Treatment for tinea capitis is oral antifungals.

Trichotillomania is difficult to treat, but behavior modification, clomipramine, or a selective serotonin reuptake inhibitor (SSRI—eg, fluoxetine, fluvoxamine, paroxetine, sertraline, citalopram) may be of benefit.

Scarring alopecia as in CCCA or dissecting cellulitis of the scalp is best treated with an oral tetracycline plus a potent topical corticosteroid. Severe or chronic acne keloidalis nuchae can be treated similarly; if mild, topical retinoids, topical antibiotics, and/or topical benzoyl peroxide may suffice.

Lichen planopilaris and chronic cutaneous lupus lesions may be treated with drugs such as oral antimalarials, topical or oral corticosteroids, topical or oral retinoids, topical tacrolimus, or oral immunosuppressants.

Hair loss due to chemotherapy is temporary and is best treated with a wig; when hair regrows, it may be different in color and texture from the original hair. Hair loss due to telogen effluvium or anagen effluvium is usually temporary as well and abates after the precipitating agent is eliminated.

KEY POINTS

- Androgenetic alopecia (male-pattern and female-pattern hair loss) is the most common type of hair loss.
- Concomitant virilization in women or scarring hair loss should prompt a thorough evaluation for an underlying disorder.
- Microscopic hair examination or scalp biopsy may be required for definitive diagnosis.

ALOPECIA AREATA

Alopecia areata is typically sudden patchy nonscarring hair loss in people with no obvious skin or systemic disorder.

The scalp and beard are most frequently affected, but any hairy area may be involved. Hair loss may affect most or all of the body (alopecia universalis). Alopecia areata is thought to be an autoimmune disorder affecting genetically susceptible people exposed to unclear environmental triggers, such as infection or emotional stress. It occasionally coexists with autoimmune vitiligo or thyroiditis.

Diagnosis

- Examination

Diagnosis is by inspection. Alopecia areata typically manifests as discrete circular patches of hair loss characterized by short broken hairs at the margins, which resemble exclamation points. Nails are sometimes pitted or display trachyonychia, a roughness of the nail also seen in lichen planus.

Differential diagnosis includes tinea capitis, trichotillomania, traction alopecia, lupus, and secondary syphilis. If findings are equivocal, further testing can be pursued with KOH preparation, fungal culture, screening for syphilis, or biopsy. Patients with clinical findings suggesting associated autoimmune diseases (particularly thyroid disease) are tested for those diseases.

Treatment

- Corticosteroids
- Sometimes topical anthralin, minoxidil, or both

If therapy is considered, intralesional corticosteroid injection is the treatment of choice in adults. Triamcinolone acetonide suspension (typically in doses of 0.1 to 3 mL of 2.5 to 5 mg/mL concentration q 4 to 8 wk) can be injected intradermally if the lesions are small. Potent topical corticosteroids (eg, clobetasol propionate 0.05% foam, gel, or ointment bid for about 4 wk) can be used; however, they often do not penetrate to the depth of the hair bulb where the inflammatory process is located. Oral corticosteroids are effective, but hair loss often recurs after cessation of therapy and adverse effects limit use.

Topical anthralin cream (0.5 to 1% applied for 10 to 20 min daily then washed off; contact time titrated as tolerated up to 1 h/day) may be used to stimulate a mild irritant reaction. Minoxidil 5% solution may be helpful as an adjuvant to corticosteroid or anthralin treatment.

Induction of allergic contact dermatitis using diphenylcyclopropenone or squaric acid dibutylester (topical immunotherapy) leads to hair growth due to unknown mechanisms, but this treatment is best reserved for patients with diffuse involvement who have not responded to other therapies.

Alopecia areata may spontaneously regress, become chronic, or spread diffusely. Risk factors for chronicity include extensive involvement, onset before adolescence, atopy, and involvement of the peripheral temporal and occipital scalp (ophiasis).

HIRSUTISM

Hirsutism is the excessive growth of thick or dark hair in women in locations that are more typical of male hair growth patterns (eg, mustache, beard, central chest, shoulders, lower abdomen, back, inner thigh). The amount of hair growth that is considered excessive may differ depending on ethnic background and cultural interpretation.

Hypertrichosis is a separate condition. It is simply an increase in the amount of hair growth anywhere on the body. Hypertrichosis may be generalized or localized.

Men vary significantly in amount of body hair, some being quite hairy, but rarely present for medical evaluation.

Pathophysiology

Hair growth depends on the balance between androgens (eg, testosterone, dehydroepiandrosterone sulfate [DHEAS], dihydrotestosterone [DHT]) and estrogens. Androgens promote thick, dark hair growth, whereas estrogens slow hair growth or modulate it toward finer, lighter hairs.

Hirsutism can be due to an increase in circulating androgen levels, or to an enhanced end organ response to androgens. Testosterone stimulates hair growth in the pubic area and underarms. Dihydrotestosterone stimulates beard hair growth and scalp hair loss.

Table 129–3. SOME CAUSES OF HIRSUTISM

CAUSES	EXAMPLES
Adrenal disorders	Adrenal tumor Congenital or delayed-onset adrenal hyperplasia Cushing syndrome
Androgenic drugs	Anabolic steroids (including danazol) Oral contraceptives (high-progesterone type)
Ectopic hormone production	Lung cancer and carcinoid tumors (ectopic ACTH secretion) Choriocarcinomas (beta-human chorionic gonadotropin)
Familial hirsutism	May be secondary to a familial increased end-organ response to normal plasma androgen levels
Ovarian disorders	Ovarian hyperthecosis Ovarian tumors PCOS
Pituitary disorders	Acromegaly Cushing disease Drugs Prolactin-secreting pituitary adenoma

When caused by increased androgen levels, hirsutism is often accompanied by virilization, which may manifest as loss of menses, increased muscle mass, voice deepening, acne, androgenetic alopecia, and clitoromegaly.

Etiology

There are a number of causes of hirsutism (see Table 129–3). Overall, the most common cause is

- Polycystic ovary syndrome (PCOS)

Androgen excess: Hirsutism typically results from abnormally high androgen levels as a result of increased production of androgens (eg, due to ovarian or adrenal disorders) or increased peripheral conversion of testosterone to DHT by 5-alpha-reductase. Free androgen levels also can increase as a result of decreased production of sex hormone–binding globulin, which can occur in a variety of conditions, including hyperinsulinemia, hyperprolactinemia, and in androgen excess itself. However, the severity of hirsutism does not correlate with the level of circulating androgens because of individual differences in androgen sensitivity of the hair follicle.

No androgen excess: Hirsutism not associated with androgen excess may be the result of increased end organ response to normal plasma levels of androgens and manifest as a familial phenomenon in people of Mediterranean, South Asian, or Middle Eastern ancestry. Hirsutism in pregnancy and menopause is due to temporary, physiologic fluctuations in androgen levels.

Hypertrichosis involves nonandrogenic hair growth and is usually caused by a drug, systemic illness (see Table 129–4), or paraneoplastic syndrome. It also occurs in rare familial disorders called congenital hypertrichosis.

Evaluation

History: History of present illness should cover the extent, location, and acuity of hair growth as well as the age of onset.

Review of systems should seek symptoms of virilization and review menstrual and fertility history. Symptoms of causative disorders should be sought, including polyuria (diabetes), bingeing and purging (eating disorders), and weight loss and fevers (cancer).

Past medical history should specifically seek known causative disorders such as endocrine disorders, adrenal or ovarian pathology, and cancer.

Family history should inquire about excess hair growth in family members. Drug history should review all prescribed drugs and specifically query for the surreptitious use of anabolic steroids.

Physical examination: The presence of excess coarse and dark hair growth should be assessed at multiple sites, including

Table 129–4. CAUSES OF HYPERTRICHOSIS

CAUSES	EXAMPLES
Disorders	Acrodynia Anorexia, bulimia, undernutrition CNS disorders Dermatomyositis Familial HIV infection if advanced Paraneoplastic syndromes Porphyria Pretibial myxedema Repeated skin trauma, friction, and/or inflammation (eg, after removal of a cast) Systemic illness Traumatic brain injury Undernutrition
Nonandrogenic drugs	Acetazolamide Benoxaprofen Bimatoprost and latanoprost (prostaglandin eye drops) Cetuximab Corticosteroids (systemic or topical) Cyclosporine Diazoxide Fenoterol Hexachlorobenzene Interferon alfa Minoxidil Penicillamine Phenytoin Prostaglandin E_1 Psoralen Streptomycin

the face, chest, lower abdomen, back, buttocks, and inner thigh. Signs of virilization should be sought, including

- Female-pattern baldness (ie, androgenetic alopecia in women)
- Acne
- Increased muscle mass
- Breast atrophy
- Clitoromegaly

General physical examination should note signs of potentially causative disorders:

- The general habitus should be examined for fat distribution (particularly a round face and accumulation of fat at the base of the neck posteriorly).
- The skin should be examined for velvety, black pigmentation on the axillae and neck and under the breasts (acanthosis nigricans), (listed above), and striae.
- The eyes should be examined for extraocular movements and the visual fields should be assessed.
- The breasts should be examined for galactorrhea.
- The abdomen (including pelvic examination) should be examined for masses.

Red flags: The following findings are of particular concern:

- Virilization
- Abrupt appearance and rapid growth of excess hair
- Pelvic or abdominal mass

Interpretation of findings: Excess hair growth beginning after use of an anabolic steroid or other causative drug (see Tables 129–3 and 129–4) in an otherwise healthy female is likely due to that drug. Symptoms and signs sometimes point to a diagnosis (see Table 129–5).

Abrupt-onset of hirsutism or hypertrichosis may portend cancer. The abrupt onset of hirsutism may be due to adrenal, ovarian, or pituitary tumors or from ectopic hormone production from other types of tumors. Hypertrichosis lanuginosa (malignant down) is fine hair growth that appears over the entire body over a short period of time, although it can be localized to the face in mild forms.

Testing: Diagnostic testing in men with no other signs of illness is unnecessary.

Women should have laboratory measurement of serum hormone levels, including the following:

- Free and total testosterone
- DHEAS
- Follicle-stimulating hormone (FSH) and luteinizing hormone (LH)

Depending on clinical findings, androstenedione and/or prolactin levels may also be measured.

High levels of testosterone accompanied by a normal level of DHEAS indicate that the ovaries, and not the adrenal glands, are producing the excess androgen. High levels of testosterone accompanied by moderate elevations in DHEAS suggest an adrenal origin for the hirsutism.

Often, in women with polycystic ovary syndrome, LH levels are elevated and FSH levels are depressed, which results in elevated LH/FSH ratios (> 3 is common for polycystic ovary syndrome).

Imaging: Pelvic ultrasonography, CT, or both should be done to rule out pelvic or adrenal cancer, particularly when a pelvic mass is suspected, when the total testosterone level is > 150 ng/dL (> 100 ng/dL in postmenopausal women), or when the DHEAS level is > 7000 ng/dL (> 4000 ng/dL in postmenopausal women). However, the majority of patients with elevated DHEAS have adrenal hyperplasia rather than adrenal carcinoma.

Patients with signs of Cushing syndrome or an adrenal mass on imaging studies should have urine cortisol levels measured for 24 h.

Treatment

- Treatment of underlying disorder
- Hair removal
- Hormonal treatment

The underlying disorder should be treated, including stopping or changing causative drugs. Treatment for hirsutism itself is necessary only if the patient finds the excess hair cosmetically objectionable.

Nonandrogen-dependent excess hair growth, such as hypertrichosis, is treated primarily with physical hair removal methods. Patients with androgen-dependent hirsutism require a combination of hair removal and antiandrogen therapy.

Hair removal: There are several techniques.

Depilatory techniques remove hair from the surface of the skin and include shaving and OTC depilatory creams, such as those containing barium sulfate and Ca thioglycolate.

Epilation involves removing intact hairs with their roots and can be achieved via mechanical means (eg, tweezing, plucking, waxing) or home epilating devices. Permanent epilation techniques, including electrolysis, thermolysis, and laser epilation, can result in more long-term hair removal but often require multiple treatments.

As an alternative to hair removal, hair bleaching is inexpensive and works well when hirsutism is not excessive. Bleaches lighten the color of the hair, rendering it less noticeable. There are several types of commercial hair-bleaching products, most of which use hydrogen peroxide as the active ingredient.

Topical eflornithine, applied twice daily, slows the rate of hair growth and, with long-term use, may increase the amount of time between hair removal treatments.

Table 129–5. INTERPRETING FINDINGS IN HIRSUTISM

FINDING	POSSIBLE CAUSES
Abrupt-onset hirsutism, flank or pelvic mass	Adrenal or ovarian cancer
Acanthosis nigricans	Polycystic ovary syndrome (PCOS) or other hyperinsulinemic states Cancer
Central obesity, moon facies, striae, hypertension, proximal muscle wasting and weakness	Cushing syndrome
Galactorrhea, amenorrhea (with or without visual field deficits)	Pituitary disorder causing hyperprolactinemia
Irregular menses or amenorrhea, acne, obesity, hirsutism beginning after puberty	PCOS
Signs of undernutrition, poor dentition (particularly in adolescent females)	Eating disorder
Weight loss, fevers	Paraneoplastic syndromes caused by occult cancer

Hormonal treatment: Hirsutism resulting from androgen excess usually requires long-term therapy because the source of excess androgen rarely can be eliminated permanently. Hormonal treatments include

- Oral contraceptives
- Antiandrogenic drugs
- Sometimes other drugs

Oral contraceptives in standard doses often are the initial treatment for hirsutism caused by ovarian hyperandrogenism. Oral contraceptives reduce ovarian androgen secretion and increase sex hormone–binding globulin, thereby decreasing free testosterone levels.

Antiandrogenic therapy is also used and can include finasteride (5 mg po once/day), spironolactone (25 to 100 mg po bid), or flutamide (125 mg po once/day or bid). These drugs are contraindicated in women of childbearing age unless contraception is used because they may feminize a male fetus.

Insulin sensitizers such as metformin decrease insulin resistance, causing a decline in testosterone levels. However, they are less effective than other antiandrogenic drugs. Corticosteroids are used when necessary to suppress adrenal androgen production. Gonadotropin-releasing hormone agonists (eg, leuprolide acetate, nafarelin, triptorelin) can be used for severe forms of ovarian hyperandrogenism under the direction of a gynecologist or endocrinologist.

KEY POINTS

- Hirsutism may be familial, and the degree of hair growth may vary with ethnicity.
- Polycystic ovary syndrome is the most frequent cause of hirsutism.
- Virilization suggests an androgenic disorder that requires further evaluation.
- Abrupt onset of hirsutism or hypertrichosis may indicate cancer.

PSEUDOFOLLICULITIS BARBAE

Pseudofolliculitis barbae is irritation of the skin due to beard hairs that penetrate the skin before leaving the hair follicle or that leave the follicle and curve back into the skin, causing a foreign-body reaction.

Pseudofolliculitis barbae predominantly affects black men. It is most noticeable around the beard and neck. It causes small papules and pustules that can be confused with bacterial folliculitis. Scarring can eventually result.

Diagnosis is by physical examination.

Treatment

- Warm compresses and ingrown hair removal for acute inflammation
- Cessation of shaving
- Topical or oral drugs as needed for infection and inflammation
- Sometimes hair follicle removal

Acute manifestations of pseudofolliculitis barbae (eg, papules and pustules) can be treated with warm compresses and manual removal of ingrown hairs with a needle or tweezers.

Topical hydrocortisone 1% or topical antibiotics can be used for mild inflammation. Oral doxycycline (50 to 100 mg bid) or oral erythromycin (250 to 500 mg qid, 333 mg tid, 500 mg bid) can be used for moderate to severe inflammation.

Tretinoin (retinoic acid) liquid or cream or benzoyl peroxide cream may also be effective in mild or moderate cases but may irritate the skin.

Topical eflornithine hydrochloride cream may help by slowing hair growth. Hairs should be allowed to grow out; grown hairs can then be cut to about 0.5 cm in length. Depilatories are an alternative but may irritate the skin.

Hair follicles can be permanently removed by electrolysis or laser treatment.

130 Hypersensitivity and Inflammatory Disorders

The immune system plays a significant role in a large number of skin disorders, including dermatitis, sunlight reactions, and bullous diseases. Although all of these disorders involve some level of inflammation, certain skin disorders are primarily characterized by their inflammatory component or as a hypersensitivity reaction, be it to a drug, infection, or cancer.

ACUTE FEBRILE NEUTROPHILIC DERMATOSIS

(Sweet Syndrome)

Acute febrile neutrophilic dermatosis is characterized by tender, indurated, dark-red papules and plaques with prominent edema in the upper dermis and dense infiltrate of neutrophils. The cause is not known. It frequently occurs with underlying cancer, especially hematologic cancers.

Etiology

Acute febrile neutrophilic dermatosis may occur with various disorders. It is often classified into 3 categories: classical, malignancy-associated, and drug-induced (see Table 130–1).

About 25% of patients have an underlying cancer, 75% of which are hematologic cancers, especially myelodysplastic syndromes and acute myeloid leukemia. Classical acute febrile neutrophilic dermatosis affects mostly women ages 30 to 50, with a female:male ratio of 3:1. In contrast, men who develop the condition tend to be older (60 to 90).

The cause is unknown; however, type 1 helper T-cell cytokines, including IL-2 and interferon-γ, are predominant and may play a role in lesion formation.

Symptoms and Signs

Patients are febrile, with an elevated neutrophil count, and have tender, dark-red plaques or papules, most often on the face, neck, and upper extremities, especially the dorsum of

Table 130–1. DISORDERS AND DRUGS ASSOCIATED WITH ACUTE FEBRILE NEUTROPHILIC DERMATOSIS

CLASSIFICATION	DISORDER/DRUG
Classical	Acute respiratory illness GI infection Inflammatory and autoimmune disorders Pregnancy
Malignancy-associated	Acute myeloid leukemia Myelodysplastic syndromes
Drug-induced	Granulocyte colony-stimulating factor (G-CSF, the most common drug cause) Antibiotics Antiepileptics Others (eg, abacavir, furosemide, hydralazine, NSAIDs, oral contraceptives, retinoids)

hands. Oral lesions can also occur. Rarely, bullous and pustular lesions are present. The lesions often develop in crops and may appear annular. Each crop is preceded by fever and persists for days to weeks. Acute febrile neutrophilic dermatosis resulting from a hematologic cancer can cause a subcutaneous form, typically with 2- to 3-cm erythematous nodules, commonly involving the extremities. When on the lower extremities, this form can resemble erythema nodosum.

Extracutaneous manifestations can involve the eyes (eg, conjunctivitis, episcleritis, iridocyclitis), joints (eg, arthralgia, myalgia, arthritis), and internal organs (eg, neutrophilic alveolitis; sterile osteomyelitis; psychiatric or neurologic changes; transient kidney, liver, and pancreatic insufficiency).

Diagnosis

- Clinical evaluation
- Skin biopsy

Diagnosis is suggested by the appearance of the lesions and is supported by the presence of associated conditions or drugs. Differential diagnosis can include erythema multiforme, erythema elevation diutinum, acute cutaneous lupus erythematosus, pyoderma gangrenosum, and erythema nodosum. If diagnosis is unclear, skin biopsy should be done. The histopathologic pattern is that of edema in the upper dermis with a dense infiltrate of neutrophils in the dermis. Vasculitis may be present but is secondary.

Treatment

- Corticosteroids

Treatment involves systemic corticosteroids, chiefly prednisone 0.5 to 1.5 mg/kg po once/day tapered over 3 wk. Colchicine 0.5 mg po tid or K iodide 300 mg po tid are alternative treatments. Antipyretics are also recommended. In difficult cases, dapsone 100 to 200 mg po once/day, indomethacin 150 mg po once/day for 1 wk and 100 mg po once/day for 2 additional wk, clofazimine (eg, 200 mg po once/day for 4 wk then 100 mg/day for 4 wk), or cyclosporine (eg, 2 to 4 mg/kg po bid) can be given. For localized involvement, intralesional corticosteroids (eg, triamcinolone acetonide) may help.

KEY POINTS

- Acute febrile neutrophilic dermatosis can occur in patients who have certain disorders (classical form) or take certain drugs (drug-induced form), but about 25% of patients have an underlying cancer (malignancy-associated form), usually a hematologic cancer.
- Diagnose acute febrile neutrophilic dermatosis based on the appearance of the lesions and presence of an associated disorder or drug, and confirm with biopsy when necessary.
- Treat most patients with systemic corticosteroids or, alternatively, colchicine or K iodide.

DRUG ERUPTIONS AND REACTIONS

Drugs can cause multiple skin eruptions and reactions. The most serious of these are discussed elsewhere in THE MANUAL and include Stevens-Johnson syndrome and toxic epidermal necrolysis, hypersensitivity syndrome, serum sickness, exfoliative dermatitis, angioedema and anaphylaxis, and drug-induced vasculitis. Drugs can also be implicated in hair loss, lichen planus, erythema nodosum, pigmentation changes, SLE, photosensitivity reactions, pemphigus, and pemphigoid. Other drug reactions are classified by lesion type (see Table 130–2).

Symptoms and Signs

Symptoms and signs vary based on the cause and the specific reaction (see Table 130–2).

Diagnosis

- Clinical evaluation and drug exposure history
- Sometimes skin biopsy

A detailed history is often required for diagnosis, including recent use of OTC drugs. Because the reaction may not occur until several days or even weeks after first exposure to the drug, it is important to consider all new drugs and not only the one that has been most recently started. No laboratory tests reliably aid diagnosis, although biopsy of affected skin is often suggestive. Sensitivity can be definitively established only by rechallenge with the drug, which may be hazardous and unethical in patients who have had severe reactions.

Treatment

- Discontinuation of offending drug
- Sometimes antihistamines and corticosteroids

Most drug reactions resolve when drugs are stopped and require no further therapy. Whenever possible, chemically unrelated compounds should be substituted for suspect drugs. If no substitute drug is available and if the reaction is a mild one, it might be necessary to continue the treatment under careful watch despite the reaction. Pruritus and urticaria can be controlled with oral antihistamines and topical corticosteroids.

Table 130–2. TYPES OF DRUG REACTIONS AND TYPICAL CAUSATIVE AGENTS

TYPE OF REACTION	DESCRIPTION AND COMMENTS	TYPICAL CAUSATIVE AGENTS
Acneiform eruptions	Resemble acne but lack comedones and usually begin suddenly	Corticosteroids, iodides, bromides, hydantoins, androgenic steroids, lithium, isoniazid, phenytoin, phenobarbital, vitamins B_2, B_6, and B_{12}
Acral cyanosis	Appears as gray-blue discoloration of tips of the fingers, toes, nose, and ears	Bleomycin
Acute generalized exanthematous pustulosis	Rapidly appearing and spreading pustular eruption	Aminopenicillins (ampicillin, amoxicillin, and bacampicillin), Ca channel blockers, cephalosporins, tetracyclines
Blistering eruptions	Appear with widespread vesicles and bullae resembling autoimmune bullous disorders (see p. 1006)	Penicillamine and other thiol-containing drugs (eg, ACE inhibitors, gold Na thiomalate)
Cutaneous necrosis	Appears as demarcated, painful, erythematous or hemorrhagic lesions progressing to hemorrhagic bullae and full-thickness skin necrosis with eschar formation	Warfarin, heparin, barbiturates, epinephrine, norepinephrine, vasopressin, levamisole (contaminant in street preparations of cocaine)
Drug-induced lupus	Appears as lupuslike syndrome, although often without the rash	Hydrochlorothiazide, minocycline, hydralazine, procainamide, anti-TNF agents
Drug reaction with eosinophilia and systemic symptoms or drug hypersensitivity syndrome	Manifests as fever, facial edema, and rash 2–6 wk after 1st dose of a drug Patients may have elevated eosinophils, atypical lymphocytes, hepatitis, pneumonitis, lymphadenopathy, and myocarditis	Anticonvulsants, allopurinol, sulfonamides
Erythema nodosum	Characterized by tender red nodules, predominantly in the pretibial region, but occasionally involving the arms or other areas	Sulfonamides, oral contraceptives
Exfoliative dermatitis	Characterized by redness and scaling of the entire skin surface (see p. 1027) May be fatal	Penicillin, sulfonamides, hydantoins
Fixed drug eruptions	Appear as frequently isolated, well-circumscribed, circinate or ovoid dusky red or purple lesions on the skin or mucous membranes (especially of the genitals) and reappear at the same sites each time the drug is taken	Tetracyclines, sulfonamides, NSAIDs
Lichenoid or lichen planus–like eruptions	Appear as angular papules that coalesce into scaly plaques (see p. 1073)	Antimalarials, chlorpromazine, thiazides
Morbilliform or maculopapular eruptions (exanthems)	Range in appearance from a morbilliform disease to an eruption resembling pityriasis rosea Mildly pruritic, typically appearing 3 to 7 days after start of the drug	Almost any drug (especially barbiturates, analgesics, sulfonamides, ampicillin, and other antibiotics)
Mucocutaneous eruptions	Vary from a few small oral vesicles or urticaria–like skin lesions to painful oral ulcers with widespread bullous skin lesions (see Erythema Multiforme on p. 1047 and Stevens-Johnson Syndrome and Toxic Epidermal Necrolysis on p. 1050)	Penicillin, barbiturates, sulfonamides (including derivatives used to treat hypertension and diabetes)
Photosensitivity eruptions	Appear as areas of dermatitis or gray-blue hyperpigmentation (phenothiazines and minocycline) on skin exposed to the sun or other ultraviolet light source	Phenothiazines, tetracyclines, sulfonamides, chlorothiazide, artificial sweeteners
Purpuric eruptions	Appear as nonblanching hemorrhagic macules that vary in size Most common on the lower extremities but may occur anywhere and may indicate a more serious purpuric vasculitis May occur as type II cytotoxic reactions, type IV cell-mediated delayed-type allergic reactions, or type III humoral allergic immune complex vasculitis	Chlorothiazide, meprobamate, anticoagulants
Serum sickness–type drug reaction	A type III immune complex reaction Acute urticaria and angioedema more common than morbilliform or scarlatiniform eruptions Possibly polyarthritis, myalgias, polysynovitis, fever, and neuritis	Penicillin, insulin, foreign proteins

Table 130–2. TYPES OF DRUG REACTIONS AND TYPICAL CAUSATIVE AGENTS (*Continued*)

TYPE OF REACTION	DESCRIPTION AND COMMENTS	TYPICAL CAUSATIVE AGENTS
Stevens-Johnson syndrome	Characterized by focal areas of skin necrosis and involvement of mucosa (see p. 1050) Lips develop hemorrhagic crusts and ulcerations Overlaps with toxic epidermal necrolysis	Anticonvulsants, NSAIDs, penicillin, sulfonamides
Toxic epidermal necrolysis	Characterized by large areas of loosened, easily detached epidermis that give the skin a scalded appearance (see p. 1050) May be fatal in 30 to 40% of patients Resembles staphylococcal scalded skin syndrome (see p. 1000), a similar disorder that occurs in infants, young children, and immunosuppressed patients Overlaps with Stevens-Johnson syndrome	Anticonvulsants, barbiturates, hydantoins, penicillin, sulfonamides
Urticaria	Common Classically but not always IgE-mediated Easily recognized by typical well-defined edematous wheals Occasionally the first sign of impending serum sickness, with fever, joint pain, and other systemic symptoms developing within days	Penicillin, aspirin, sulfonamides, ACE inhibitors

For IgE-mediated reactions (eg, urticaria), desensitization (see p. 1384) can be considered when there is critical need for a drug.

If anaphylaxis occurs, treatment is with aqueous epinephrine (1:1000) 0.2 mL sc or IM, parenteral antihistamines, and with the slower-acting but more persistent soluble hydrocortisone 100 mg IV, which may be followed by an oral corticosteroid for a short period.

KEY POINTS

- Because drugs can cause a wide variety of reactions, drugs should be considered as causes of almost any unexplained skin reaction.
- Base the diagnosis primarily on clinical criteria, including a detailed history of prescription and OTC drugs.
- Stop the suspected offending drug and treat symptoms as needed.

ERYTHEMA MULTIFORME

Erythema multiforme (EM) is an inflammatory reaction, characterized by target or iris skin lesions. Oral mucosa may be involved. Diagnosis is clinical. Lesions spontaneously resolve but frequently recur. EM usually occurs as a reaction to an infectious agent such as herpes simplex virus or mycoplasma but may be a reaction to a drug. Suppressive antiviral therapy may be indicated for patients with frequent or symptomatic recurrence due to herpes simplex virus.

For years, EM was thought to represent the milder end of a spectrum of drug hypersensitivity disorders that included Stevens-Johnson syndrome and toxic epidermal necrolysis (see p. 1050). Recent evidence suggests that EM is different from these other disorders.

Etiology

The majority of cases are caused by herpes simplex virus (HSV) infection (HSV-1 more so than HSV-2), although it is unclear whether EM lesions represent a specific or nonspecific reaction to the virus. Current thinking holds that EM is caused by a T-cell-mediated cytolytic reaction to HSV DNA fragments present in keratinocytes. A genetic disposition is presumed given that EM is such a rare clinical manifestation of HSV infection, and several HLA subtypes have been linked with the predisposition to develop lesions. Less commonly, cases are caused by drugs, vaccines, other viral diseases (especially hepatitis C), or possibly SLE. EM that occurs in patients with SLE is sometimes referred to as Rowell syndrome.

Symptoms and Signs

EM manifests as the sudden onset of asymptomatic, erythematous macules, papules, wheals, vesicles, bullae, or a combination on the distal extremities (often including palms and soles) and face. The classic lesion is annular with a violaceous center and pink halo separated by a pale ring (target or iris lesion). Distribution is symmetric and centripetal; spread to the trunk is common. Some patients have itching. Oral lesions include target lesions on the lips and vesicles and erosions on the palate and gingivae (see Plate 55).

Diagnosis

- Clinical evaluation

Diagnosis is by clinical appearance; biopsy is rarely necessary. Differential diagnosis includes essential urticaria, vasculitis, bullous pemphigoid, pemphigus, linear IgA dermatosis, acute febrile neutrophilic dermatosis, and dermatitis herpetiformis; oral lesions must be distinguished from aphthous stomatitis, pemphigus, herpetic stomatitis, and hand-foot-and-mouth disease. Patients with widely disseminated purpuric macules and blisters and prominent involvement of the trunk and face are likely to have Stevens-Johnson syndrome rather than EM.

Treatment

- Supportive care
- Sometimes prophylactic antivirals

EM spontaneously resolves, so treatment is usually unnecessary. Topical corticosteroids and anesthetics may ameliorate symptoms and reassure patients. Recurrences are common, and empiric oral maintenance therapy with acyclovir 400 mg po q 12 h, famciclovir 250 mg po q 12 h, or valacyclovir 1000 mg po q 24 h can be attempted if symptoms recur more than 5 times/yr and HSV association is suspected or if recurrent EM is consistently preceded by herpes flares.

KEY POINTS

- EM is usually caused by HSV but can be caused by a drug.
- Target lesions and lesions on the palms and soles can be relatively specific findings.
- Biopsy is rarely necessary.
- Treat EM supportively and consider prophylactic antiviral drugs if HSV is the suspected cause and recurrences are frequent.

PANNICULITIS

Panniculitis describes inflammation of the subcutaneous fat that can result from multiple causes. Diagnosis is by clinical evaluation and biopsy. Treatment depends on the cause.

Panniculitis can be classified as lobular or septal depending on the principal site of the inflammation within the fat.

Etiology

There are multiple causes of panniculitis, including

- Infections (the most common)
- Physical factors (eg, cold, trauma)
- Proliferative disorders
- Connective tissue disorders (eg, SLE, systemic sclerosis)
- Pancreatic disorders
- Alpha$_1$-antitrypsin deficiency

Idiopathic panniculitis is sometimes referred to as Weber-Christian disease.

Symptoms and Signs

Panniculitis is characterized by tender and erythematous subcutaneous nodules located over the extremities and sometimes over the posterior thorax, abdominal area, breasts, face, or buttocks. Rarely, nodules can involve the mesentery, lungs, scrotum, and cranium. Signs of systemic inflammation can accompany panniculitis. In Weber-Christian disease, systemic involvement can result in fever as well as signs of organ dysfunction, including hepatic, pancreatic, and bone marrow insufficiency, which is potentially fatal.

Diagnosis

- Clinical evaluation
- Excisional biopsy

Diagnosis is by usually by clinical appearance and can be confirmed by excisional biopsy.

Treatment

- Supportive care
- Anti-inflammatory drugs
- Immunosuppressants

There is no specific definitive treatment for panniculitis. Several strategies have been used with modest results, including NSAIDs, antimalarials, dapsone, and thalidomide. Corticosteroids (1 to 2 mg/kg po or IV once/day) and other immunosuppressive or chemotherapeutic drugs have been used to treat patients with progressive symptoms or signs of systemic involvement.

KEY POINTS

- Causes of panniculitis can vary widely.
- Diagnose panniculitis by clinical evaluation (including presence of tender, red, subcutaneous nodules) and confirm with excisional biopsy.
- Treat panniculitis supportively and consider anti-inflammatory orimmunosuppressive drug therapy, particularly if manifestations are severe.

ERYTHEMA NODOSUM

Erythema nodosum (EN) is a specific form of panniculitis characterized by tender, red or violet, palpable, subcutaneous nodules on the shins and occasionally other locations. It often occurs with an underlying systemic disease, notably streptococcal infections, sarcoidosis, and inflammatory bowel disease. Diagnosis is by clinical evaluation and sometimes biopsy. Treatment depends on the cause.

Etiology

EN primarily affects people in their 20s and 30s but can occur at any age; women are more often affected. Etiology is unknown, but an immunologic reaction is suspected because EN is frequently accompanied by other disorders. The most common disorders are

- Streptococcal infection (especially in children)
- Sarcoidosis
- Inflammatory bowel disease

Other possible triggering disorders include

- Other bacterial infections (eg, *Yersinia, Salmonella,* mycoplasma, chlamydia, leprosy, lymphogranuloma venereum)
- Fungal infections (eg, kerion, coccidioidomycosis, blastomycosis, histoplasmosis)
- Rickettsial infections
- Viral infections (eg, Epstein-Barr, hepatitis B)
- Use of drugs (eg, sulfonamides, iodides, bromides, oral contraceptives)
- Hematologic and solid cancers
- Pregnancy
- Behçet disease
- TB

Up to one-third of cases of EN are idiopathic.

Erythema induratum, a similar disorder, manifests with lesions on the calves and classically affects patients with TB.

Symptoms and Signs

EN is a subset of panniculitis that manifests as erythematous, tender nodules or plaques, primarily in the pretibial region (see Plate 37), often preceded or accompanied by fever, malaise, and arthralgia. Lesions may be detected more easily by palpation than inspection and can evolve into bruiselike areas over weeks.

Diagnosis

- Clinical evaluation
- Excisional biopsy

Diagnosis is usually by clinical appearance and can be confirmed by excisional biopsy of a nodule when necessary. A diagnosis of EN should prompt evaluation for causes. Evaluation might include biopsy, skin testing (PPD or anergy panel), antinuclear antibodies, CBC, chest x-ray, and serial antistreptolysin O titers or a pharyngeal culture. ESR is often high.

Treatment

- Supportive care
- Anti-inflammatory drugs (rarely corticosteroids)

EN almost always resolves spontaneously. Treatment includes bed rest, elevation, cool compresses, and NSAIDs. K iodide 300 to 500 mg po tid can be given to decrease inflammation. Systemic corticosteroids are effective but should be used only as a last resort because they can worsen an occult infection. If an underlying disorder is identified, it should be treated.

KEY POINTS

- The most common causes of EN are streptococcal infections (particularly in children), sarcoidosis, and inflammatory bowel disease.
- Diagnose EN primarily by clinical appearance but, when necessary, excise a nodule for biopsy confirmation.
- Treat EN supportively and use NSAIDs or K iodide as needed until the disorder resolves spontaneously.

GRANULOMA ANNULARE

Granuloma annulare is a benign, chronic, idiopathic condition characterized by papules or nodules that spread peripherally to form a ring around normal or slightly depressed skin.

Etiology

Etiology is unclear but proposed mechanisms include cell-mediated immunity (type IV), immune complex vasculitis, and an abnormality of tissue monocytes. Granuloma annulare is not associated with systemic disorders, except that the incidence of abnormal glucose metabolism is increased among adults with many lesions. In some cases, exposure to sunlight, insect bites, TB skin testing, BCG vaccination, trauma, *Borrelia* infection, and viral infections have induced disease flares. The condition is twice as prevalent among women.

Symptoms and Signs

Lesions are erythematous, yellowish tan, bluish, or the color of the surrounding skin; one or more lesions may occur, most often on dorsal feet, legs, hands, or fingers. They are usually asymptomatic but may occasionally be tender. The lesions often expand or join to form rings. The center of each ring may be clear or be slightly depressed and sometimes pale or light brown. In some cases, lesions may become generalized and widespread.

Diagnosis

Diagnosis is usually clinical but can be confirmed by skin biopsy. Unlike tinea corporis (which can cause raised annular lesions with central clearing), granuloma annulare typically has no scale and does not itch.

Treatment

- Sometimes corticosteroids, topical tacrolimus, or psoralen plus ultraviolet A (PUVA) therapy

Usually no treatment is necessary; spontaneous resolution is common. For patients with more widespread or bothersome lesions, quicker resolution may be promoted by the use of high-strength topical corticosteroids under occlusive dressings every night, flurandrenolide-impregnated tape, topical tacrolimus (eg, 0.1% ointment bid, with dosing frequency decreasing as symptoms resolve), and intralesional corticosteroids. PUVA therapy, isotretinoin, dapsone, and cyclosporine have been reported to be successful in treating widespread disease. Recent reports have suggested that TNF-α inhibitors (eg, infliximab, adalimumab), 595-nm pulsed-dye laser, excimer laser, and fractional photothermolysis are useful in managing disseminated and recalcitrant lesions.

KEY POINTS

- Granuloma annulare, which is twice as common among women, is not associated with systemic disorders.
- Diagnose granuloma annulare clinically (eg, by the characteristic rings with central clearing and absence of scaling).
- If symptoms are bothersome, treat with corticosteroids or topical tacrolimus.

PYODERMA GANGRENOSUM

Pyoderma gangrenosum is a chronic, neutrophilic, progressive skin necrosis of unknown etiology often associated with systemic illness.

Etiology

Etiology is unknown, but pyoderma gangrenosum can be associated with various systemic illnesses, including vasculitis, gammopathies, RA, leukemia, lymphoma, hepatitis C virus infection, SLE, sarcoidosis, polyarthritis, Behçet disease, hidradenitis suppurativa, and especially inflammatory bowel disease. It is thought to be mediated by an abnormal immune response. Most patients are age 25 to 55. It can manifest in various subtypes.

Pathophysiology

Pathophysiology is poorly understood but may involve problems with neutrophil chemotaxis. IL-8 is overexpressed in lesions. Ulcerations of pyoderma gangrenosum occur after trauma or injury to the skin in about 30% of patients; this process is termed pathergy.

Symptoms and Signs

Most often, pyoderma gangrenosum begins as an inflamed erythematous papule, pustule, or nodule. The lesion, which may resemble a furuncle or an arthropod bite at this stage, then ulcerates and expands rapidly, developing a swollen necrotic base and a raised dusky to violaceous border. An undermined border (ie, loss of underlying support tissue at the border) is common, if not pathognomonic. Systemic symptoms such as fever and malaise are common. The ulcers can coalesce to form larger ulcers, often with cribriform or sieve-like scarring. Symptoms and signs can vary with the subtype:

- Ulcerative (classic) subtype: In this most common subtype, ulcers form as described above, most commonly on the lower extremities or trunk, particularly the buttocks and perineum.

- Bullous (atypical) subtype: This less common subtype often develops in patients with hematologic disorders. Lesions usually begin as bullae that erode, becoming superficial ulcers. The arms and face are most often involved.
- Pustular subtype: This subtype tends to develop during exacerbations of inflammatory bowel disease. Painful pustules develop, surrounded by erythema. Arthralgias are common.
- Vegetative (superficial granulomatous pyoderma) subtype: In this subtype, a single, indolent, mildly painful plaque or superficial ulcer develops, most often on the head or neck. The border is not undermined and the base is not necrotic.

Pyoderma gangrenosum can also develop at other sites, such as around a stoma in patients who have inflammatory bowel disease (peristomal pyoderma gangrenosum), on the genitals (genital pyoderma gangrenosum), or in sites other than the skin, such as the bones, cornea, CNS, heart, intestine, liver, lungs, or muscle (extracutaneous pyoderma gangrenosum).

Diagnosis

Diagnosis is clinical and is a diagnosis of exclusion after other causes of ulceration have been ruled out. Expansion of ulceration after surgical debridement strongly suggests pyoderma gangrenosum. Biopsies of lesions are not often diagnostic but may be supportive; 40% of biopsies from a leading edge show vasculitis with neutrophils and fibrin in superficial vessels. Patients who have bullous (atypical) pyoderma gangrenosum should be monitored with periodic clinical assessment and CBC for development of a hematologic disorder.

Treatment

- Wound care
- Corticosteroids
- TNF-α inhibitors
- Sometimes other anti-inflammatory drugs or immunosuppressants
- Avoidance of surgical debridement

Wound healing can be promoted with wound care that includes moisture-retaining occlusive dressings for less exudative plaques and absorptive dressings for highly exudative plaques. Wet-to-dry dressings should be avoided. Topical therapy with high-potency corticosteroids or tacrolimus can help with superficial and early lesions. For more severe manifestations, prednisone 60 to 80 mg po once/day is a common first-line therapy. TNF-α inhibitors (eg, infliximab, adalimumab, etanercept) are effective, particularly in patients who have inflammatory bowel disease. Cyclosporine 3 mg/kg po once/day is also quite effective, particularly in rapidly progressive disease. Dapsone, azathioprine, cyclophosphamide, methotrexate, clofazimine, thalidomide, and mycophenolate mofetil have also been used successfully. Antimicrobials such as minocycline have also been used for vegetative (superficial) pyoderma gangrenosum. Surgical treatments are avoided because of the risk of wound extension.

KEY POINTS

- Pyoderma gangrenosum is often associated with a systemic disorder and is probably immune-mediated.
- There are several subtypes; the ulcerative subtype (ie, necrotic base and raised violaceous border with undermined edge on a lower extremity, buttock, or perineum) is most common.
- Diagnose pyoderma gangrenosum clinically.
- Optimize wound care and avoid surgical debridement.
- Use topical potent corticosteroids or tacrolimus to treat early lesions and use systemic corticosteroids, TNF-α inhibitors, or other anti-inflammatories or immunosuppressants to treat more severe manifestations.

STEVENS-JOHNSON SYNDROME AND TOXIC EPIDERMAL NECROLYSIS

Stevens-Johnson syndrome (SJS) and toxic epidermal necrolysis (TEN) are severe cutaneous hypersensitivity reactions. Drugs, especially sulfa drugs, antiepileptics, and antibiotics, are the most common causes. Macules rapidly spread and coalesce, leading to epidermal blistering, necrosis, and sloughing. Diagnosis is usually obvious by appearance of initial lesions and clinical syndrome. Treatment is supportive care; cyclosporine, plasma exchange or IVIG, and early pulse corticosteroid therapy have been used. Mortality can be as high as 7.5% in children and 20 to 25% in adults but tends to be lower with early treatment.

SJS and TEN are clinically similar except for their distribution. By one commonly accepted definition, changes affect < 10% of body surface area in SJS and > 30% of body surface area in TEN; involvement of 15 to 30% of body surface area is considered SJS/TEN overlap.

The disorders affect between 1 and 5 people/million. Incidence, severity, or both of these disorders may be higher in bone marrow transplant recipients, in *Pneumocystis jirovecii*–infected HIV patients, in patients with SLE, and in patients with other chronic rheumatologic diseases.

Etiology

Drugs precipitate over 50% of SJS cases and up to 95% of TEN cases. The most common drug causes include

- Sulfa drugs (eg, cotrimoxazole, sulfasalazine)
- Other antibiotics (eg, aminopenicillins [usually ampicillin or amoxicillin], fluoroquinolones, cephalosporins)
- Antiepileptics (eg, phenytoin, carbamazepine, phenobarbital, valproate, lamotrigine)
- Miscellaneous individual drugs (eg, piroxicam, allopurinol, chlormezanone)

Cases that are not caused by drugs are attributed to

- Infection (mostly with *Mycoplasma pneumoniae*)
- Vaccination
- Graft-vs-host disease

Rarely, a cause cannot be identified.

Pathophysiology

The exact mechanism is unknown; however, one theory holds that altered drug metabolism (eg, failure to clear reactive metabolites) in some patients triggers a T-cell-mediated cytotoxic reaction to drug antigens in keratinocytes. CD8+ T cells have been identified as important mediators of blister formation.

Recent findings suggest that granulysin released from cytotoxic T cells and natural killer cells might play a role in keratinocyte death; granulysin concentration in blister fluid correlates with severity of disease. Another theory is that interactions between Fas (a cell-surface receptor that induces apoptosis) and its ligand, particularly a soluble form of Fas ligand released from mononuclear cells, lead to cell death and blister formation. A genetic predisposition for SJS/TEN has been suggested.

Symptoms and Signs

Within 1 to 3 wk after the start of the offending drug, patients develop a prodrome of malaise, fever, headache, cough, and keratoconjunctivitis. Macules, often in a target configuration, then appear suddenly, usually on the face, neck, and upper trunk. These macules simultaneously appear elsewhere on the body, coalesce into large flaccid bullae, and slough over a period of 1 to 3 days. Nails and eyebrows may be lost along with epithelium. The palms and soles may be involved. In some cases, diffuse erythema is the first skin abnormality of TEN.

In severe cases of TEN, large sheets of epithelium slide off the entire body at pressure points (Nikolsky sign), exposing weepy, painful, and erythematous skin. Painful oral crusts and erosions, keratoconjunctivitis, and genital problems (eg, urethritis, phimosis, vaginal synechiae) accompany skin sloughing in up to 90% of cases. Bronchial epithelium may also slough, causing cough, dyspnea, pneumonia, pulmonary edema, and hypoxemia. Glomerulonephritis and hepatitis may develop.

Diagnosis

- Clinical evaluation
- Often skin biopsy

Diagnosis is often obvious from appearance of lesions and rapid progression of symptoms. Histologic examination of sloughed skin shows necrotic epithelium, a distinguishing feature.

Differential diagnosis in SJS and early TEN includes EM, viral exanthems, and other drug rashes; SJS/TEN can usually be differentiated clinically as the disorder evolves and is characterized by significant pain and skin sloughing. In later stages of TEN, differential diagnosis includes the following:

- Toxic shock syndrome (usually has more prominent multiple organ involvement and different cutaneous manifestations, such as macular rash on palms and soles that evolves to desquamation over about 2 wk)
- Exfoliative erythroderma (usually spares mucous membranes and is not as painful)
- Paraneoplastic pemphigus (sometimes with different mucocutaneous findings or in patients with evidence of cancer)

In children, TEN is less common and must be distinguished from staphylococcal scalded skin syndrome (see p. 1000), usually by noting sparing of mucous membranes and risk factors, such as drug history and clinical suspicion of staphylococcal infection.

Prognosis

Severe TEN is similar to extensive burns; patients are acutely ill, may be unable to eat or open their eyes, and suffer massive fluid and electrolyte losses. They are at high risk of infection, multiorgan failure, and death. With early therapy, survival rates approach 90%. The severity-of-illness score for TEN (see Table 130–3) systematically scores 7 independent risk factors within the first 24 h of presentation to the hospital to determine the mortality rate for a particular patient.

Treatment

- Supportive care
- Cyclosporine
- Possibly plasma exchange or IV immune globulin (IVIG)

Treatment is most successful when SJS or TEN is recognized early and treated in an inpatient dermatologic or ICU setting; treatment in a burn unit may be needed for severe disease. Ophthalmology consultation and specialized eye care are mandatory for patients with ocular involvement. Potentially causative drugs should be stopped immediately. Patients are isolated to minimize exposure to infection and are given fluids, electrolytes, blood products, and nutritional supplements as needed. Skin care includes prompt treatment of secondary bacterial infections and daily wound care as for severe burns. Prophylactic systemic antibiotics are controversial and often avoided.

Drug treatment of STS and TEN is controversial. Cyclosporine (3 to 5 mg/kg po once/day) inhibits CD8 cells and has been

Table 130–3. SEVERITY-OF-ILLNESS SCORE FOR TOXIC EPIDERMAL NECROLYSIS (SCORTEN)

RISK FACTOR*	SCORE	
	0	**1**
Age	< 40 yr	≥ 40 yr
Associated cancer	No	Yes
Heart rate (beats/min)	< 120	≥ 120
Serum BUN (mg/dL)	≤ 28	> 28
Detached or compromised body surface	< 10%	≥ 10%
Serum bicarbonate (mEq/L)	≥ 20	< 20
Serum glucose (mg/dL)	≤ 250	> 250

*More risk factors indicate a higher score and a higher mortality rate (%) as follows:

- 0–1 = 3.2% (CI: 0.1 to 16.7)
- 2 = 12.1% (CI: 5.4 to 22.5)
- 3 = 35.3% (CI: 19.8 to 53.5)
- 4 = 58.3% (CI: 36.6 to 77.9)
- ≥ 5 = > 90% (CI: 55.5 to 99.8)

CI = confidence interval.

Data from Bastuji-Garin S, Fouchard N, Bertocchi M, et al: SCORTEN: A severity-of-illness score for toxic epidermal necrolysis. *Journal of Investigative Dermatology* 115:149–153, 2000.

shown to decrease the duration of active disease by 2 to 3 days in some instances and possibly decrease mortality. The use of systemic corticosteroids has been controversial and is thought by many experts to increase mortality because of increased rates of infection and the risk of masking sepsis. However, recent reports have shown improved ocular outcomes with early pulse corticosteroid therapy. Plasma exchange can remove reactive drug metabolites or antibodies and can be considered. Early high-dose IVIG 2.7 g/kg over 3 days blocks antibodies and Fas ligand. However, despite some remarkable initial results using high-dose IVIG for TEN, further clinical trials involving small cohorts have reported conflicting results, and a retrospective analysis has suggested no improvement or even higher than expected mortality.

KEY POINTS

- Drugs cause > 50% of SJS and up to 95% of TEN cases, but infection, vaccination, and graft-vs-host disease are also potential causes.
- Confirm the diagnosis by biopsy (showing necrotic epithelium) if clinical characteristics (eg, target lesions progressing to bullae, ocular and mucous membrane involvement, Nikolsky sign, desquamation in sheets) are inconclusive.
- Early treatment decreases the often high mortality rate.
- Except for mild cases, treat SJS/TEN in a burn unit and with intensive supportive care.
- Consult ophthalmology if the eyes are affected.
- Consider cyclosporine and possibly plasma exchange for severe cases.

131 Nail Disorders

A variety of disorders can affect nails, including deformities, infections of the nail, paronychia, and ingrown toenails. Nail changes may occur in many systemic conditions and genetic syndromes or result from trauma.

Most nail infections are fungal (onychomycosis), but bacterial and viral infections can occur (eg, green-nail syndrome [*Pseudomonas*], herpetic whitlow [herpes simplex virus-1]). Even parasitic infestation such as crusted scabies can lead to changes in the nail plate. Paronychia is not actually an infection of the nail but rather of periungual tissues.

Common warts (verrucae vulgaris) result from papillomavirus infection and frequently infect the proximal nail fold and sometimes the subungual area. Onychophagia (nail-biting) can help spread this infection. Warts involving these areas are especially difficult to treat.

Toenails require special attention in the elderly and in people with diabetes or peripheral vascular disease; a podiatrist can help avoid local breakdown and secondary infections.

NAIL DEFORMITIES AND DYSTROPHIES

Deformities are often considered together with dystrophies, but the two are slightly different; deformities are generally considered to be gross changes in nail shape, whereas dystrophies are changes in nail texture or composition (eg, onychomycosis).

About 50% of nail dystrophies result from fungal infection. The remainder result from various causes, including trauma, congenital abnormalities, psoriasis, lichen planus, and occasionally cancer. Diagnosis may be obvious on examination, but often fungal scrapings and culture are done. Dystrophies may resolve with treatment of the cause, but if not, manicurists may be able to hide nail changes with appropriate trimming and polishes.

Congenital deformities: In some congenital ectodermal dysplasias, patients have no nails (anonychia). In pachyonychia congenita, the nail beds are thickened, discolored, and transversely hypercurved (pincer nail deformity). Nail-patella syndrome causes triangular lunulae and partially absent thumb nails. Patients with Darier disease can have nails with red and white streaks and a distal V-shaped nick.

Deformities and dystrophies associated with systemic problems: In Plummer-Vinson syndrome (esophageal webs caused by severe, untreated iron deficiency), 50% of patients have koilonychia (concave, spoon-shaped nails).

Yellow nail syndrome (characterized by hard, hypercurved, transversely thickened, yellow nails) occurs in patients with lymphedema of limbs and/or chronic respiratory disorders.

Half-and-half nails (Lindsay nails) occur usually with renal failure; the proximal half of the nail is white, and the distal half is pink or pigmented.

White nails occur with cirrhosis, although the distal third may remain pinker.

Beau lines are horizontal grooves in the nail plate that occur when nail growth temporarily slows, which can occur after infection, trauma, or systemic illness. Onychomadesis similarly results from temporary growth arrest of the nail plate and differs from Beau lines in that the full thickness of the nail is involved, causing a proximal separation of the nail plate from the nail bed. It most frequently occurs several months after hand-foot-and-mouth disease but can occur after other viral infections. Nails affected by Beau lines or onychomadesis regrow normally with time.

Deformities associated with dermatologic conditions: In **psoriasis,** nails may have a number of changes, including irregular pits, oil spots (localized areas of tan-brown discoloration), separation of part of the nail from the nail bed (onycholysis), and thickening and crumbling of the nail plate.

Lichen planus of the nail matrix causes scarring with early longitudinal ridging and splitting of the nail and later leads to pterygium formation or total nail loss, and sometimes scarring nail loss.

Pterygium of the nail is characterized by scarring from the proximal nail outward in a V formation, which leads ultimately to nail loss.

Alopecia areata can be accompanied by regular pits that form a geometric pattern. Pits are small and fine. Alopecia areata may also be associated with severe onychorrhexis (brittleness with nail breakage).

Topical tacrolimus 0.1% and intralesional corticosteroid injections may help treat nail deformities associated with psoriasis and lichen planus.

Discoloration: Cancer chemotherapy drugs (especially the taxanes) can cause melanonychia (nail plate pigmentation), which can be diffuse or may occur in transverse bands. Some drugs can cause characteristic changes in nail coloration:

- Quinacrine: Nails appear greenish yellow or white under ultraviolet light.
- Cyclophosphamide: The onychodermal bands (seal formed at the junction of the nail plate and distal nail bed at the free edge of the nail plate) become slate-gray or bluish.
- Arsenic: Nails may turn diffusely brown.
- Tetracyclines, ketoconazole, phenothiazines, sulfonamides, and phenindione: Nails may have brownish or blue discoloration.
- Gold therapy: Nails may be light or dark brown.
- Silver salts (argyria): Nails may be diffusely blue-gray.

Tobacco smoking or nail polish can result in yellow or brownish discoloration of nails and fingertips.

White transverse lines of the nails (Mees lines) may occur with chemotherapy, acute arsenic intoxication, malignant tumors, MI, thallium and antimony intoxication, fluorosis, and even during etretinate therapy. These lines are not due to changes in the nail bed, but are a true leukonychia and thus can grow out if the insulting exposure has been removed. They also develop with trauma to the finger, although traumatic white lines usually do not span the entire nail. The fungus *Trichophyton mentagrophytes* causes a chalky white discoloration of the surface of the nail plate.

Green-nail syndrome is caused by infection with *Pseudomonas*. It is generally a harmless infection, usually of 1 or 2 nails, and is noteworthy for its striking blue-green color. It often occurs in patients with onycholysis or chronic paronychia whose nails have been immersed in fresh water for a long period. Treatment is most effective with soaks of 1% acetic acid solution or alcohol diluted 1:4 with water or treatment of the underlying cause of onycholysis. If the onycholysis is treated effectively, the *Pseudomonas* infection will resolve. Patients should soak their affected nails twice a day for 10 min and should avoid trauma and excess moisture. Frequent clipping of the nail increases the response to treatment.

Median nail dystrophy: Median nail dystrophy (median canaliform dystrophy) is characterized by small cracks in the nail that extend laterally and look like the branches of an evergreen tree (eg, fir tree, such as a Christmas tree). The cracks and ridges are similar to those seen in habit-tic nail deformity (which is dystrophy of the central nail caused by repetitive trauma to the nail matrix resulting from rubbing or picking with another finger). The cause is unknown in some cases, but trauma is thought to play a role. Frequent use of personal digital devices that subject the nails to repetitive striking has been implicated in several cases. Tacrolimus 0.1% at bedtime without occlusion has been successful when patients stop all activities that might lead to repetitive low-level trauma.

Melanonychia striata: Melanonychia striata are hyperpigmented bands that are longitudinal and extend from the proximal nail fold and cuticle to the free distal end of the nail plate. In dark-skinned people, these bands may be a normal physiologic variant requiring no treatment. Other causes include trauma, pregnancy, Addison disease, post-inflammatory hyperpigmentation, and the use of certain drugs, including doxorubicin, 5-fluorouracil, zidovudine, and psoralens. Hyperpigmented bands can also occur in benign melanocytic nevi and malignant melanoma. Hutchinson sign (extension of hyperpigmentation through the lunula and cuticle and into the proximal nail fold) may signal a melanoma in the nail matrix. Rapid biopsy and treatment are essential.

Onychogryphosis: Onychogryphosis is a nail dystrophy in which the nail, most often on the big toe, becomes thickened and curved. It may be caused by ill-fitting shoes. It is common among the elderly. Treatment consists of trimming the deformed nails.

Onycholysis: Onycholysis is separation of the nail plate from the nail bed or complete nail plate loss. It can occur as a drug reaction in patients treated with tetracyclines (photo-onycholysis), doxorubicin, 5-fluorouracil, cardiovascular drugs (particularly practolol and captopril), cloxacillin and cephaloridine (rarely), trimethoprim/sulfamethoxazole, diflunisal, etretinate, indomethacin, isoniazid, griseofulvin, and isotretinoin. Partial onycholysis may also result from exposure to irritants, such as frequent exposure to water or citrus fruits. Irritant contact dermatitis of the hands and fingers may lead to onycholysis. Colonization of the nail bed with *Candida albicans* may occur, but treating the underlying irritant exposure will lead to resolution of the onycholysis, with or without treating the *Candida*.

Partial onycholysis may also occur in patients with psoriasis or thyrotoxicosis.

Onychotillomania: In this disorder, patients pick at and self-mutilate their nails, which can lead to parallel transverse grooves and ridges (washboard deformity or habit-tic nail deformity). It most commonly manifests in patients who habitually push back the cuticle on one finger, causing dystrophy of the nail plate as it grows. Subungual hemorrhages can also develop in onychotillomania.

Pincer nail deformity: Pincer nail deformity is a transverse over-curvature of the nail plate. It can occur in patients with psoriasis, SLE, Kawasaki disease, cancer, end-stage renal disease, and some genetic syndromes (eg, as paronychia congenita). Patients often have pain at the borders of the nail where the nail plate curves into the tips of the fingers.

Subungual hematoma and nail bed trauma: Subungual hematoma occurs when blood becomes trapped between the nail plate and nail bed, usually as a result of trauma. Subungual hematoma causes significant and throbbing pain, bluish black discoloration, and, unless small, eventual separation of and temporary loss of the nail plate. When the cause is a crush injury, underlying fracture and nail bed damage are common. Nail bed damage may result in permanent nail deformity.

If the injury is acute, nail trephination (eg, creating a hole in the nail plate using a cautery device, 18-gauge needle, or red-hot paperclip) can help relieve pain by draining accumulated blood; after 24 h, blood is coagulated, thus trephination offers no benefit. It is not clear whether removing the nail and repairing any nail bed damage reduces risk of permanent nail deformity.

Trachyonychia: Trachyonychia (rough, opaque nails) may occur with alopecia areata, lichen planus, atopic dermatitis, and psoriasis. It is most common among children. When present in all nails, trachyonychia is often called 20-nail dystrophy.

Tumors: Benign and malignant tumors can affect the nail unit, causing deformity. These tumors include benign myxoid cysts, pyogenic granulomas, and glomus tumors. Malignant tumors include Bowen disease, squamous cell carcinoma, and malignant melanoma. When cancer is suspected, expeditious biopsy followed by referral to a surgeon is strongly advised.

ONYCHOMYCOSIS

(Tinea Unguium)

Onychomycosis is fungal infection of the nail plate, nail bed, or both. The nails typically are deformed and discolored white or yellow. Diagnosis is by appearance, wet mount,

culture, PCR, or a combination. Treatment, when indicated, is with oral terbinafine or itraconazole.

About 10% (range 2 to 14%) of the population has onychomycosis. Risk factors include

- Tinea pedis
- Preexisting nail dystrophy (eg, in patients with psoriasis)
- Older age
- Male sex
- Exposure to someone with tinea pedis or onychomycosis (eg, a family member or through public bathing)
- Peripheral vascular disease or diabetes
- Immunocompromise

Toenails are 10 times more commonly infected than fingernails. About 60 to 80% of cases are caused by dermatophytes (eg, *Trichophyton rubrum*); dermatophyte infection of the nails is called tinea unguium. Many of the remaining cases are caused by nondermatophyte molds (eg, *Aspergillus, Scopulariopsis, Fusarium*). Immunocompromised patients and those with chronic mucocutaneous candidiasis may have candidal onychomycosis (which is more common on the fingers). Subclinical onychomycosis can also occur in patients with recurrent tinea pedis. Onychomycosis may predispose patients to lower extremity cellulitis.

Symptoms and Signs

Nails have asymptomatic patches of white or yellow discoloration and deformity. There are 3 common characteristic patterns:

- Distal subungual, in which the nails thicken and yellow, keratin and debris accumulate distally and underneath, and the nail separates from the nail bed (onycholysis)
- Proximal subungual, a form that starts proximally and is a marker of immunosuppression
- White superficial, in which a chalky white scale slowly spreads beneath the nail surface

Diagnosis

- Clinical evaluation
- Potassium hydroxide wet mount examination
- Histopathologic examination of periodic acid-Schiff–stained nail clippings and subungual debris
- Culture

Onychomycosis is suspected by appearance; predictive clinical features include involvement of the 3rd or 5th toenail, involvement of the 1st and 5th toenails on the same foot, unilateral nail deformity, but only if the patient has tinea pedis. Subclinical onychomycosis should be considered in patients with recurrent tinea pedis.

Differentiation from psoriasis or lichen planus is important because the therapies differ, so diagnosis is typically confirmed by microscopic examination and, unless microscopic findings are conclusive, culture of scrapings or rarely PCR of clippings. Scrapings are taken from the most proximal position that can be accessed on the affected nail and are examined for hyphae on potassium hydroxide wet mount and cultured. Histopathologic examination of periodic acid-Schiff (PAS)–stained nail clippings and subungual debris may also be helpful.

Obtaining an adequate sample of nail for culture can be difficult because the distal subungual debris, which is easy to sample, often does not contain living fungus. Therefore, removing the distal portion of the nail with clippers before sampling or using a small curette to reach more proximally beneath the nail increases the yield. PCR can be done if cultures are negative and the cost of finding a definitive diagnosis is warranted.

Treatment

- Selective use of oral terbinafine or itraconazole
- Occasional use of topical treatments (eg, efinaconazole, tavaborole, ciclopirox 8%, amorolfine)

Onychomycosis is not always treated because many cases are asymptomatic or mild and unlikely to cause complications, and the oral drugs that are the most effective treatments can potentially cause hepatotoxicity and serious drug interactions. Some proposed indications for treatment include the following:

- Previous ipsilateral cellulitis
- Diabetes or other risk factors for cellulitis
- Presence of bothersome symptoms
- Psychosocial impact
- Desire for cosmetic improvement (controversial)

Treatment is typically oral terbinafine or itraconazole. Terbinafine 250 mg once/day for 12 wk (6 wk for fingernail) achieves a cure rate of 75 to 80% and itraconazole 200 mg bid 1 wk/mo for 3 mo achieves a cure rate of 40 to 50%, but the recurrence rate is estimated to be as high as 10 to 50%. It is not necessary to treat until all abnormal nail is gone because these drugs remain bound to the nail plate and continue to be effective after oral administration has ceased. The affected nail will not revert to normal; however, newly growing nail will appear normal.

The newer topical agents efinaconazole and tavaborole can penetrate the nail plate and are more effective than older topical agents.[1–4]

Investigative treatments that have less frequent and/or less severe adverse effects include laser therapy, new formulations of topical agents (including efinaconazole), and new delivery systems for terbinafine.[5,6] Topical antifungal nail lacquer containing ciclopirox 8% or amorolfine 5% (not available in the US) is occasionally effective as primary treatment (cure rate of about 30%) and can improve cure rate when used as an adjunct with oral drugs, particularly in resistant infections.

To limit relapse, the patient should trim nails short, dry feet after bathing, wear absorbent socks, and use antifungal foot powder. Old shoes may harbor a high density of spores and, if possible, should not be worn.

1. Elewski BE, Tosti A: Tavaborole for the treatment of onychomycosis. *Expert Opin Pharmacother* 15(10): 1439–1448, 2014. doi: 10.1517/14656566.2014.921158.
2. Gupta AK, Daigle D: Tavaborole (AN-2690) for the treatment of onychomycosis of the toenail in adults. *Expert Rev Anti Infect Ther* 12(7):735–742, 2014. doi: 10.1586/14787210.2014.915738.
3. Elewski BE, Rich P, Pollak R, et al: Efinaconazole 10% solution in the treatment of toenail onychomycosis: Two phase III multicenter, randomized, double-blind studies. *J Am Acad Dermatol* 68(4):600–608, 2013. doi: 10.1016/j.jaad.2012.10.013.
4. Jo Siu WJ, Tatsumi Y, Senda H, et al: Comparison of in vitro antifungal activities of efinaconazole and currently available antifungal agents against a variety of pathogenic fungi associated with onychomycosis. *Antimicrob Agents Chemother* 57(4):1610-1616, 2013. doi: 10.1128/AAC.02056-12.
5. Adigun CG, Vlahovic TC, McClellan MB, et al: Efinaconazole 10% and tavaborole 5% penetrate across poly-ureaurethane 16%: Results of in vitro release testing

and clinical implications of onychodystrophy in onychomycosis. *J Drugs Dermatol* 1;15(9):1116–1120, 2016.
6. Baker SJ, Zhang YK, Akama T, et al: Discovery of a new boron-containing antifungal agent, 5-fluoro-1, 3-dihydro-1-hydroxy-2,1- benzoxaborole (AN2690), for the potential treatment of onychomycosis. *J Med Chem* 27;49(15):4447–4450, 2006.

KEY POINTS

- Onychomycosis is highly prevalent, particularly among older men and patients with compromised distal circulation, nail dystrophies, and/or tinea pedis.
- Suspect the diagnosis based on appearance and the pattern of nail involvement and confirm it by microscopy and sometimes culture or PCR.
- Treatment is warranted only if onychomycosis causes complications or troublesome symptoms.
- If treatment is warranted, consider terbinafine (the most effective treatment) and measures to prevent recurrence (eg, limiting moisture, discarding old shoes, trimming nails short).

ACUTE PARONYCHIA

Paronychia is infection of the periungual tissues. Acute paronychia causes redness, warmth, and pain along the nail margin. Diagnosis is by inspection. Treatment is with antistaphylococcal antibiotics and drainage of any pus.

Paronychia is usually acute, but chronic cases occur. In acute paronychia, the causative organisms are usually *Staphylococcus aureus* or streptococci and, less commonly, *Pseudomonas* or *Proteus* spp. Organisms enter through a break in the epidermis resulting from a hangnail, trauma to a nail fold, loss of the cuticle, or chronic irritation (eg, resulting from water and detergents). Biting or sucking the fingers can also predispose people to developing the infection. In toes, infection often begins at an ingrown toenail.

Novel drug therapies, such as with inhibitors of epidermal growth factor receptor (EGFR), mammalian target of rapamycin (mTOR), and less commonly *BRAF* gene inhibitors, can cause paronychia along with other skin changes. The mechanism is not completely understood. However, most cases seem to be caused by the drug itself, such as through alterations in retinoic acid metabolism, and not by secondary infection.

In patients with diabetes and those with peripheral vascular disease, toe paronychia can threaten the limb.

Symptoms and Signs

Paronychia develops along the nail margin (lateral and/or proximal nail fold), manifesting over hours to days with pain, warmth, redness, and swelling. Pus usually develops along the nail margin and sometimes beneath the nail. Infection can spread to the fingertip pulp, causing a felon. Rarely, infection penetrates deep into the finger, sometimes causing infectious flexor tenosynovitis.

Diagnosis

Diagnosis is by inspection. Several skin conditions can cause changes that mimic paronychia and should be considered, particularly when treatment is not effective initially. These conditions include squamous cell carcinoma, proximal onychomycosis, pyogenic granuloma, pyoderma gangrenosum, and herpetic whitlow.

Treatment

- Antistaphylococcal antibiotics
- Drainage of pus

Early treatment is warm compresses or soaks and an antistaphylococcal antibiotic (eg, dicloxacillin or cephalexin 250 mg po qid, clindamycin 300 mg po qid). In areas where methicillin-resistant *S. aureus* is common, antibiotics that are effective against this organism (eg, trimethoprim/sulfamethoxazole) should be chosen based on results of local sensitivity testing. In patients with diabetes and others with peripheral vascular disease, toe paronychia should be monitored for signs of cellulitis or more severe infection (eg, extension of edema or erythema, lymphadenopathy, fever).

Fluctuant swelling or visible pus should be drained with a Freer elevator, small hemostat, or #11 scalpel blade inserted between the nail and nail fold. Skin incision is unnecessary. A thin gauze wick can be inserted for 24 to 48 h to allow drainage.

A case caused by EGFR inhibitor therapy and refractory to the usual treatments was treated successfully with autologous platelet-rich plasma.

KEY POINTS

- Acute paronychia can be related to a hangnail, nail fold trauma, loss of the cuticle, chronic irritation, or biting or sucking of the fingers.
- The diagnosis is likely when severe redness, pain, and warmth develop acutely along the nail margin, but consider alternative diagnoses, particularly if treatment is unsuccessful.
- Treat by draining any visible pus or, if none is visible, with an antibiotic and moist heat.

CHRONIC PARONYCHIA

Chronic paronychia is recurrent or persistent nail fold inflammation, typically of the fingers.

Chronic paronychia occurs almost always in people whose hands are chronically wet (eg, dishwashers, bartenders, housekeepers), particularly if they have hand eczema, are diabetic, or are immunocompromised. *Candida* is often present but its role in etiology is unclear; fungal eradication does not always resolve the condition. The condition may be an irritant dermatitis with secondary fungal colonization.

The nail fold is painful and red as in acute paronychia, but there is almost never pus accumulation. There is often loss of the cuticle and separation of the nail fold from the nail plate. This separation leaves a space that allows entry of irritants and microorganisms. The nail becomes distorted.

Diagnosis is clinical.

Treatment

- Keeping hands dry
- Topical corticosteroid or tacrolimus

Primary treatment is to keep the hands dry and to assist the cuticle in reforming to close the space between the nail fold and nail plate. Gloves or barrier creams are used if water contact is necessary. Topical drugs that may help include corticosteroids and tacrolimus 0.1% (a calcineurin inhibitor). Antifungal treatments are added to therapy only when fungal colonization is a concern. Thymol 3% in ethanol applied several times a day to the space left by loss of cuticle aids in keeping this space dry and free of microorganisms. If there is no response to therapy and a single digit is affected, squamous cell carcinoma should be considered and a biopsy should be done.

INGROWN TOENAIL

(Onychocryptosis)

An ingrown toenail is incurvation or impingement of a nail border into its adjacent nail fold, causing pain.

Causes include tight shoes, abnormal gait (eg, toe-walking), bulbous toe shape, excessive trimming of the nail plate, or congenital variations in nail contour (eg, congenital pincer nail deformity). Sometimes an underlying osteochondroma is responsible, especially in the young. In the elderly, peripheral edema is a risk factor. Eventually, infection can occur along the nail margin (paronychia).

Symptoms and Signs

Pain occurs at the corner of the nail fold or, less commonly, along its entire lateral margin. Initially only mild discomfort may be present, especially when wearing certain shoes. In chronic cases, granulation tissue becomes visible, more often in the young.

Diagnosis

- Clinical evaluation

Redness, swelling, and pain may also suggest concurrent paronychia. In young patients (eg, < 20 yr) with recurrent ingrown toenails, x-rays should be considered to exclude underlying osteochondroma. In the absence of an ingrown toenail, apparent granulation tissue around the toe suggests the possibility of amelanotic melanoma, which is often overlooked; biopsy is necessary.

Treatment

- Usually nail excision and destruction of adjacent nail matrix

In mild cases, inserting cotton between the ingrown nail plate and painful fold (using a thin toothpick) may provide immediate relief and, if continued, correct the problem. If the shoes are too tight, a larger toe box is indicated. In most cases, however, particularly with paronychia, excision of the ingrown toenail after injecting a local anesthetic is the only effective treatment. After excision, a flexible tube can be used to separate the nail plate and painful fold and allow healing. If ingrown toenails recur, phenol is applied to permanently destroy the nearby lateral nail matrix. Phenol should not be used if there is arterial insufficiency.

132 Parasitic Skin Infections

BEDBUGS

Bedbug bites are usually painless but cause reactions, often pruritic, in susceptible patients.

Etiology

Bedbug infestations have become more common in the developed world in recent years. The most common bedbugs affecting humans are *Cimex lectularis* (in temperate climates) and *C. hemipterus* (mainly in tropical climates). Bedbugs hide in cracks and crevices of mattresses, other structures (eg, bedframes, cushions, and walls; in developing nations, mud houses and thatched roofs). They move slowly and are attracted to people by warmth and carbon dioxide. Bedbugs bite exposed skin, usually at night. A feeding is completed in 5 to 10 min.

Symptoms and Signs

Lesions are generally on exposed skin. They develop sometime between the morning after and 10 days after being bitten. Lesions can be any of the following:

- Puncta only
- Purpuric macules
- Erythematous macules, papules, or wheals, often pruritic, each with a central hemorrhagic punctum
- Bullae

Lesions may form linear patterns or may be seen in groups. Older adults develop symptoms less often than do younger people. Lesions resolve after about 1 wk. Secondary infection can develop.

Patients may be anxious about the difficulty and expense of eradicating a bedbug infestation and about the social stigma that can result from infestation. They may isolate themselves to avoid spreading infestation.

Diagnosis

- Clinical evaluation

Diagnosis based on lesion appearance may be difficult because the appearance is usually nonspecific. However, most bedbug bites are larger and more edematous than other bites (eg, flea bites).

Identification of bedbugs can help confirm the diagnosis. Bedbugs have flat, oval, reddish-brown bodies. After a blood meal, the body is less flat and more reddish. Adult *C. lectularis* are about 5 to 7 mm in length, and *C. hemipterus* are slightly longer. Bedbug feces or blood may be evident on bed linens or behind wallpaper.

Treatment

- Symptomatic treatment

Bedbug bites are treated symptomatically (eg, with topical corticosteroids and/or systemic antihistamines) as needed.

Bedbugs should be eradicated using physical and usually chemical means. Physical means include vacuuming affected areas and laundering suspect articles, then drying them on the dryer's hottest setting. In addition, entire rooms should be treated professionally, when possible, by heating to temperatures ≥3 times/wk. After 50 ° C (122 ° F) or with multiple insecticides.

KEY POINTS

- Consider bedbug bites particularly if initially asymptomatic lesions cluster linearly on exposed skin.

- Search for evidence of infestation to help confirm the diagnosis.
- Recommend professional assistance to help eradicate bedbugs.

CUTANEOUS LARVA MIGRANS

(Creeping Eruption)

Cutaneous larva migrans (CLM, also creeping eruption) is the skin manifestation of hookworm infestation.

CLM is caused by *Ancylostoma* sp, most commonly dog or cat hookworm *Ancylostoma braziliense*. Hookworm ova in dog or cat feces develop into infective larvae when left in warm moist ground or sand; transmission occurs when skin directly contacts contaminated soil or sand and larvae penetrate unprotected skin, usually of the feet, legs, buttocks, or back. CLM occurs worldwide but most commonly in tropical environments.

CLM causes intense pruritus; signs are erythema and papules at the site of entry, followed by a winding, threadlike subcutaneous trail of reddish-brown inflammation. Patients may also develop papules and vesicles resembling folliculitis, called hookworm folliculitis. Diagnosis is by history and clinical appearance.

Although the infection resolves spontaneously after a few weeks, discomfort and the risk of secondary bacterial infection warrant treatment. Topical thiabendazole 15% liquid or cream (compounded) bid to tid for 5 days is extremely effective. Oral thiabendazole is not well tolerated and not usually used. Albendazole (400 mg po once/day for 3 to 7 days) and ivermectin (200 mcg/kg once/day for 1 to 2 days) can cure the infestation and are well tolerated.

CLM may be complicated by a self-limiting pulmonary reaction called Löffler syndrome (patchy pulmonary infiltrates and peripheral blood eosinophilia).

CUTANEOUS MYIASIS

Cutaneous myiasis is skin infestation by the larvae of certain fly species.

Myiasis involves the larvae (maggots) of two-winged (dipterous) flies. Three types of cutaneous infestation exist, depending on the species involved:

- Furuncular
- Wound
- Migratory

Other organs sometimes are involved (eg, nasopharynx, GI tract, GU tract). Infestation usually occurs in tropical countries, so most cases in the US occur in people who have recently arrived from endemic areas.

Furuncular myiasis: Many of the common sources are known as bot flies. *Dermatobia hominis,* native to South and Central America, is the most common cause in travelers returning to the US. Other species include *Cordylobia anthropophaga* (in sub-Saharan Africa), various *Cuterebra* sp (in North America), and *Wohlfahrtia* sp (in North America, Europe, and Pakistan). Many of the flies do not lay their eggs on humans but on other insects (eg, mosquitoes) or objects (eg, drying laundry) that may contact skin. Eggs on the skin hatch into larvae, which burrow into the skin and develop through successive stages (instars) into mature larvae; mature larvae may be 1 to 2 cm long, depending on the species. If the infestation is untreated, larvae eventually emerge from the skin and drop to the ground to continue their life cycle.

Typical symptoms include itching, a sensation of movement, and sometimes lancinating pain. The initial lesion may resemble an arthropod bite or bacterial furuncle but may be distinguished by the presence of a central punctum with serosanguineous drainage; sometimes a small portion of the end of the larva is visible. *D. hominis* lesions are more common on the face, scalp, and extremities, whereas *C. anthropophaga* lesions tend to occur in areas that are covered by clothing and appear on the head, neck, and back.

Because larvae require atmospheric O_2, occlusion of the skin opening may cause them to depart or at least come closer to the surface, facilitating manual removal. The numerous occlusive methods include use of petrolatum, nail polish, bacon, or a paste of tobacco. However, larvae that die during occlusion are difficult to remove and often trigger an intense inflammatory reaction. Larvae may be extracted through a small incision. Ivermectin, oral (200 mcg/kg, 1 dose) or topical, may kill the larvae or induce migration.

Wound myiasis: Open wounds and mucous membranes, typically in the homeless, alcoholics, and other people in poor social circumstances, may be infested by fly larvae, most often from green or black blowflies. Unlike larvae of common houseflies, most agents of wound myiasis invade healthy as well as necrotic tissue. Treatment is usually with irrigation and manual debridement.

Migratory myiasis: The most common flies are *Gasterophilus intestinalis* and *Hypoderma* sp. These flies typically infest horses and cattle; people acquire them via contact with infested animals or, less often, via direct egg-laying on their skin. Larvae of these flies burrow under the skin, causing pruritic, advancing lesions, which may be mistaken for CLM; however, fly larvae are much larger than nematodes, and the lesions created by fly larvae last longer. Treatment is similar to that of furuncular myiasis.

DELUSIONAL PARASITOSIS

In delusional parasitosis, patients mistakenly believe that they are infested with parasites.

Patients have an unshakable belief that they are infested with insects, worms, mites, lice, or other organisms. They often provide vivid descriptions of how the organisms enter their skin and move around their bodies, and bring samples of hair, skin, and debris such as dried scabs, dust, and lint on slides or in containers (the matchbox sign) to prove that the infestation is real. The condition is considered a somatoform type of delusional disorder. Patients may have other psychiatric or physical disorders (eg, structural brain disorders, toxic psychosis).

Diagnosis

- Clinical evaluation

Diagnosis is suspected by history and clinical examination. Evaluation requires ruling out true infestations and other physiologic disease by physical examination and judicious testing, such as skin scrapings and other tests as clinically indicated.

Treatment

- Psychologic support and possibly antipsychotic drugs

It is important to establish an empathetic and supportive relationship with the patient. Although often rejected, the most effective treatment is with antipsychotic drugs (see Table 213–1 on p. 1792). Typically, the patient seeks confirmation that the drug treats the infestation itself, and any suggestion that the treatment is for something else is met with resistance, rejection, or both. Thus, effective treatment often requires diplomacy and a delicate balance between offering proper treatment and respecting the patient's right to know.

LICE

(Pediculosis)

Lice (pediculosis) can infect the scalp, body, pubis, and eyelashes. Head lice are transmitted by close contact; body lice are transmitted in cramped, crowded conditions; and pubic lice are transmitted by sexual contact. Symptoms, signs, diagnosis, and treatment differ by location of infestation.

Lice are wingless, blood-sucking insects that infest the head (*Pediculus humanus* var. *capitis*), body (*P. humanus* var. *corporis*), or pubis (*Phthirus pubis*). The 3 kinds of lice differ substantially in morphology and clinical features. Head lice and pubic lice live directly on the host; body lice live in garments. All types occur worldwide.

Head lice: Head lice are most common among girls aged 5 to 11 but can affect almost anyone; infestations are rare in blacks. Head lice are easily transmitted from person to person with close contact (as occurs within households and classrooms) and may be ejected from hair by static electricity or wind; transmission by these routes (or by sharing of combs, brushes, and hats) is likely but unproved. There is no association between head lice and poor hygiene or low socioeconomic status.

Infestation typically involves the hair and scalp but may involve other hair-bearing areas. Active infection usually involves ≤ 20 lice and causes severe pruritus. Examination is most often normal but may reveal scalp excoriations and posterior cervical adenopathy.

Diagnosis depends on demonstration of living lice. Lice are detected by a thorough combing-through of wet hair from the scalp with a fine-tooth comb (teeth of comb about 0.2 mm apart); lice are usually found at the back of the head or behind the ears. Nits are more commonly seen and are ovoid, grayish white eggs fixed to the base of hair shafts (see Plate 42). Each adult female louse lays 3 to 5 eggs/day, so nits typically vastly outnumber lice and are not a measure of severity of infestation.

Treatment is outlined in see Table 132–1. Drug resistance is common and should be managed with use of oral ivermectin and by attempting to rotate pediculicides. After applying a topical pediculicide, nits are removed by using a fine-tooth comb on wet hair (wet combing). Termination or removal of live (viable) nits is important in preventing reinfestation; live nits fluoresce on illumination with a Wood lamp. Most pediculicides also kill nits. Dead nits remain after successful treatment and do not signify active infection; they do not have to be removed. Nits grow away from the scalp with time; the absence of nits less than one fourth of an inch from the scalp rules out current active infection. Hot air has been shown to kill > 88% of nits but has been variably effective in killing hatched lice. Thirty minutes of hot air, slightly cooler than a blow drier, may be an effective adjunctive measure to treat head lice.

Controversy surrounds the need to clean the personal items of people with lice or nits and the need to exclude children with head lice or nits from school; there are no conclusive data supporting either approach. However, some experts recommend replacement of personal items or thorough cleaning, followed by drying at 130 ° F for 30 min. Items that cannot be washed may be placed in airtight plastic bags for 2 wk to kill the lice, which live only about 10 days.

Body lice: Body lice primarily live on bedding and clothing, not people, and are most frequently found in cramped, crowded conditions (eg, military barracks) and in people of low socioeconomic status. Transmission is by sharing of contaminated clothing and bedding. Body lice are main vectors of epidemic typhus, trench fever, and relapsing fever.

Body lice cause pruritus; signs are small red puncta caused by bites, usually associated with linear scratch marks, urticaria, or superficial bacterial infection. These findings are especially common on the shoulders, buttocks, and abdomen. Nits may be present on body hairs.

Diagnosis is by demonstration of lice and nits in clothing, especially at the seams.

Primary treatment is thorough cleaning (eg, cleaning, followed by drying at 149 ° F) or replacement of clothing and bedding, which is often difficult because affected people often have few resources and little control over their environment.

Pubic lice: Pubic lice ("crabs") are sexually transmitted in adolescents and adults and may be transmitted to children by close parental contact. They may also be transmitted by fomites (eg, towels, bedding, clothing). They most commonly infest pubic and perianal hairs but may spread to thighs, trunk, and facial hair (beard, mustache, and eyelashes).

Pubic lice cause pruritus. Physical signs are few, but some patients have excoriations and regional lymphadenopathy and/or lymphadenitis. Pale, bluish gray skin macules (maculae ceruleae) on the trunk, buttocks, and thighs are caused by anticoagulant activity of louse saliva while feeding; they are unusual but characteristic of infestation. Eyelash infestation manifests as eye itching, burning, and irritation.

Diagnosis is by demonstration of nits, lice, or both by close inspection (Wood light) or microscopic analysis (see Plate 45). A supporting sign of infestation is scattering of dark brown specks (louse excreta) on skin or undergarments.

Treatment is outlined in Table 132–1. Treatment of eyelid and eyelash infestation is often difficult and involves use of petrolatum, physostigmine ointment, oral ivermectin, or physical removal of lice with forceps. Sex partners should also be treated.

KEY POINTS

- Head and pubic lice live on people, whereas body lice live in garments.
- Confirm the diagnosis of lice by finding live lice or live nits.
- Treat head or pubic lice with a topical drug (eg, a pyrethroid) or oral ivermectin.
- Treat body lice symptomatically and by eliminating the source of lice.

SCABIES

Scabies is an infestation of the skin with the mite *Sarcoptes scabiei*. Scabies causes intensely pruritic lesions with erythematous papules and burrows in web spaces, wrists, waistline, and genitals. Diagnosis is based on examination and scrapings. Treatment is with topical scabicides or, sometimes, oral ivermectin.

Table 132–1. TREATMENT OPTIONS FOR LICE

THERAPY	INSTRUCTIONS	COMMENTS
Lice, head		
Malathion 0.5%	Apply to dry hair and scalp, wash and rinse in 8–12 h, shampoo scalp, and remove nits May repeat in 7–9 days if live nits (nits closer than a 1/4 inch away from the scalp) are seen	Highly effective but not 1st-line treatment because of flammability and unpleasant odor
Permethrin, other pyrethroids, pyrethrins*	Wash hair and apply to wet hair, behind ears a nd on nape; wash off in 10 min May repeat in 7 days if live nits (closer than a 1/4 inch away from the scalp) are seen	Contraindicated in patients sensitive to the chrysanthemum family of plants
Wet combing with a metal nit comb	Should be combined with all of the therapies	—
Lindane 1% shampoo	Apply shampoo, lather for 4–5 min, rinse, and comb with fine-tooth comb Repeat in 1 wk	Increasing resistance to drug Toxicity (eg, seizures) not typical with treatment of head lice but not recommended for children < 2 yr, people with an uncontrolled seizure disorder, or for pregnant or lactating women Cannot be used on eyelashes
Ivermectin	200 mcg/kg po for 1 dose Repeat in 7–10 days	Useful for resistant lice
Cetaphil® cleanser	Apply, wait 2 min, comb out excess, blow dry hair, wait 8 h, then shampoo and remove nits with wet combing Repeat weekly as necessary	—
Lice, body		
—	Treatment of pruritus and secondary infection	Topical measures not used because body lice are found in clothing Wash clothes and linens and dry them at at least 149° F Dry cleaning or ironing clothes
Lice, pubic		
Lindane 1% (60 mL) shampoo	Same as for head lice	Same as for head lice
Pyrethrins* with piperonyl butoxide (60 mL) shampoo	Apply to dry hair and skin, leave on for 10 min, rinse, and repeat in 7–10 days	Cannot be applied more than twice in 24 h
Permethrin 1% (60 mL) cream	Same as for head lice Must repeat in 10 days	—
Lice, eyelashes		
Petrolatum ointment	Apply 3–4 times/day for 8–10 days	—
Fluorescein drops 10–20%	Applied to the eyelids	Provides immediate pediculicidal effect

*Pyrethrins are natural components of chrysanthemum flowers, with strong insecticidal activity, pyrethroids are synthetic and natural relatives of pyrethrin, and permethrin is a commonly used synthetic pyrethroid. Pyrethrins are combined with a piperic acid derivative (piperonyl butoxide) to enhance efficacy.

Etiology

Scabies is caused by the mite *Sarcoptes scabiei* var. *hominis,* an obligate human parasite that lives in burrowed tunnels in the stratum corneum. Scabies is easily transmitted from person to person through physical contact; animal and fomite transmission probably also occurs. The primary risk factor is crowded conditions (as in schools, shelters, barracks, and some households); there is no clear association with poor hygiene.

For unknown reasons, crusted scabies (see Plate 50) is more common among immunosuppressed patients (eg, those with HIV infection, hematologic cancer, chronic corticosteroid or other immunosuppressant use), patients with severe physical disabilities or intellectual disability, and Australian Aborigines. Infestations occur worldwide. Patients in warm climates develop small erythematous papules with few burrows. Severity is related to the patient's immune status, not geography.

Symptoms and Signs

The primary symptom is intense pruritus, classically worse at night, although that timing is not specific to scabies.

Classic scabies: Erythematous papules initially appear in finger web spaces, flexor surfaces of the wrist and elbow, axillary folds, along the belt line, or on the lower buttocks. Papules can affect any area of the body, including the breasts and penis. The face remains uninvolved in adults. Burrows, usually on the wrists, hands, or feet, are pathognomonic for disease, manifesting as fine, wavy, and slightly scaly lines several mm to 1 cm long. A tiny dark papule—the mite—is often visible at one end. In classic scabies, people usually have only 10 to 12 mites. Secondary bacterial infection commonly occurs.

Signs of classic scabies may be atypical. In blacks and other people with dark skin, scabies can manifest as granulomatous nodules. In infants, the palms, soles, face, and scalp may be involved, especially in the posterior auricular folds. In elderly patients, scabies can cause intense pruritus with subtle skin findings, making it a challenge to diagnose. In immunocompromised patients, there may be widespread nonpruritic scaling (particularly on the palms and soles in adults and on the scalp in children).

Other forms: Crusted (Norwegian) scabies is due to an impaired host immune response, allowing mites to proliferate and number in the millions; scaling erythematous patches often involve the hands, feet, and scalp and can become widespread.

Nodular scabies is more common among infants and young children and may be due to hypersensitivity to retained organisms; nodules are usually erythematous, 5 to 6 mm, and involve the groin, genitals, axillary folds, and buttocks. Nodules are hypersensitivity reactions and may persist for months after eradication of mites.

Bullous scabies occurs more commonly among children. When it occurs in the elderly, it can mimic bullous pemphigoid, resulting in a delay in diagnosis.

Scalp scabies occurs in infants and immunocompromised people and can mimic dermatitis, particularly atopic dermatitis or seborrheic dermatitis.

Scabies incognito is a widespread atypical form resulting from application of topical corticosteroids.

Diagnosis

- Clinical evaluation
- Burrow scrapings

Diagnosis is suspected by physical findings, especially burrows, and itching that is out of proportion to physical findings and similar symptoms among household contacts. Confirmation is by finding mites, ova, or fecal pellets on microscopic examination of burrow scrapings; failure to find mites is common and does not exclude scabies. Scrapings should be obtained by placing glycerol, mineral oil, or immersion oil over a burrow or papule (to prevent dispersion of mites and material during scraping), which is then unroofed with the edge of a scalpel. The material is then placed on a slide and covered with a coverslip; potassium hydroxide should be avoided because it dissolves fecal pellets.

Treatment

- Topical permethrin or lindane
- Sometimes oral ivermectin

Primary treatment is topical or oral scabicides (see Table 132–2). Permethrin is the 1st-line topical drug.

Older children and adults should apply permethrin or lindane to the entire body from the neck down and wash it off after 8 to 14 h. Permethrin is often preferred because lindane can be neurotoxic. Treatments should be repeated in 7 days.

For infants and young children, permethrin should be applied to the head and neck, avoiding periorbital and perioral regions. Special attention should be given to intertriginous areas, fingernails, toenails, and the umbilicus. Mittens on infants can keep permethrin out of the mouth. Lindane is not recommended in children < 2 yr and in patients with a seizure disorder because of potential neurotoxicity.

Table 132–2. TREATMENT OPTIONS FOR SCABIES

THERAPY	INSTRUCTIONS	COMMENTS
Permethrin* 5% (60 g) cream	Apply to whole body; wash off after 8–14 h Repeat in 1 wk	1st-line treatment Can cause stinging and itching
Lindane 1% (60 mL) lotion	Apply to whole body; wash off after 8–12 h in adults and 6 h in children Repeat in 1 wk	Not recommended for children < 2 yr, pregnant or lactating women, people with extensive dermatitis, people with an uncontrolled seizure disorder, and those with severe skin conditions involving skin barrier compromise Potentially neurotoxic
Ivermectin	200 mcg/kg po for 1 dose Repeat in 7–10 days	Indicated as a 2nd-line treatment to permethrin For use in institutional epidemics and immunocompromised patients Caution required when given to elderly patients with hepatic, renal, or cardiac disorders Not recommended for pregnant or lactating women; unproven safety in children < 15 kg or < 5 yr May cause tachycardia
Crotamiton 10% cream/lotion	Apply after bath to whole body, apply 2nd dose after 24 h, and bathe 48 h after 2nd dose Repeat both doses in 7–10 days	—
Sulfur ointment 6–10%	Apply to whole body at bedtime for 3 nights and leave each application on for 24 h	Very effective and safe May be limited by its malodor

*Pyrethrins are natural components of chrysanthemum flowers, with strong insecticidal activity; pyrethroids are synthetic and natural relatives of pyrethrin; and permethrin is a commonly used synthetic pyrethroid. Pyrethrins are combined with a piperic acid derivative (piperonyl butoxide) to enhance efficacy.

Precipitated sulfur 6 to 10% in petrolatum, applied for 24 h for 3 consecutive days, is safe and effective and usually used in infants < 2 mo of age.

Ivermectin is indicated for patients who do not respond to topical treatment, are unable to adhere to topical regimens, or are immunocompromised with Norwegian scabies. Ivermectin has been used with success in epidemics involving close contacts, such as nursing homes.

Close contacts should also be treated simultaneously, and personal items (eg, towels, clothing, bedding) should be washed in hot water and dried in a hot drier or isolated (eg, in a closed plastic bag) for at least 3 days.

Pruritus can be treated with corticosteroid ointments and/or oral antihistamines (eg, hydroxyzine 25 mg po qid). Secondary infection should be considered in patients with weeping, yellow-crusted lesions and treated with the appropriate systemic or topical antistaphylococcal or antistreptococcal antibiotic.

Symptoms and lesions take up to 3 wk to resolve despite killing of the mites, making failed treatment due to resistance, poor penetration, incompletely applied therapy, reinfection, or nodular scabies difficult to recognize. Skin scrapings can be done periodically to check for persistent scabies.

KEY POINTS

- Risk factors for scabies include crowded living conditions and immunosuppression; poor hygiene is not a risk factor.
- Suggestive findings include burrows in characteristic locations, intense itching (particularly at night), and clustering of cases among household contacts.
- Confirm scabies when possible by finding mites, ova, or fecal pellets.
- Treat scabies usually with topical permethrin or, when necessary, oral ivermectin.

133 Pigmentation Disorders

Pigmentation disorders involve hypopigmentation, depigmentation, or hyperpigmentation. Areas may be focal or diffuse. In hypopigmentation, pigment is decreased, whereas in depigmentation, pigment is completely lost, leaving white skin.

Focal hypopigmentation is most commonly a consequence of

- Injury
- Inflammatory dermatoses (eg, atopic dermatitis, psoriasis)
- Burns
- Chemical exposure (especially to hydroquinones and phenols)

Focal hypopigmentation or depigmentation is also a feature of vitiligo (which may involve large areas of skin), leprosy, nutritional deficiencies (kwashiorkor), and genetic conditions (eg, tuberous sclerosis, piebaldism, Waardenburg syndrome).

Diffuse hypopigmentation or depigmentation is most often caused by

- Albinism
- Vitiligo

Hyperpigmentation typically occurs after inflammation due to various causes. This postinflammatory hyperpigmentation is usually focal in distribution. Hyperpigmentation may also be caused by a systemic disorder, drug, or cancer; distribution is usually more diffuse.

ALBINISM

Oculocutaneous albinism is an inherited defect in melanin formation that causes diffuse hypopigmentation of the skin, hair, and eyes. Ocular albinism affects the eyes and usually not the skin. Ocular involvement causes strabismus, nystagmus, and decreased vision (see Plate 28). Diagnosis of oculocutaneous albinism is usually obvious from the skin examination, but ocular evaluation is necessary. No treatment for the skin involvement is available other than protection from sunlight.

Pathophysiology

Oculocutaneous albinism (OCA) is a group of rare inherited disorders in which a normal number of melanocytes are present but melanin production is absent or greatly decreased. OCA occurs in people of all races throughout the world. Cutaneous and ocular pathologies (ocular involvement) are both present. Findings in ocular involvement include abnormal optic tract development manifested by foveal hypoplasia with decreased photoreceptors and misrouting of optic chiasmal fibers. Ocular albinism (OA) does not usually affect the skin.

Most cases of OCA are autosomal recessive; autosomal dominant inheritance is rare. There are 4 main genetic forms:

- Type I is caused by absent (OCA1A; 40% of all OCA) or reduced (OCA1B) tyrosinase activity; tyrosinase catalyzes several steps in melanin synthesis.
- Type II (50% of all OCA) is caused by mutations in the *P* (pink-eyed) gene. The function of the P protein is not yet known but may involve regulation of organelle pH and accumulation of vacuolar glutathione. Tyrosinase activity is present.
- Type III occurs only in people with otherwise dark skin (skin types III to V). It is caused by mutations in a *tyrosinase-related protein 1* gene whose product is important in eumelanin synthesis.
- Type IV is an extremely rare form in which the defect is in a gene (SLC45A2) that codes a membrane transporter protein involved in tyrosinase processing and trafficking of proteins to melanosomes. Type IV is the most common form of OCA in Japan.

OA types Nettleship-Falls (OA1) and Forsius-Eriksson (OA2) are extremely rare compared to OCA. They are inherited in an X-linked dominant fashion. Usually findings are confined to the eyes, but skin may be hypopigmented. Patients with OA1 may have late-onset sensorineural deafness.

In another group of inherited diseases, a clinical phenotype of OCA occurs in conjunction with bleeding disorders. In Hermansky-Pudlak syndrome, OCA-like findings occur with platelet abnormalities and a ceroid-lipofuscin lysosomal storage disease. This syndrome is rare except in people with family origin in Puerto Rico, where its incidence is 1 in 1800. In Chédiak-Higashi syndrome, OCA-like cutaneous and ocular findings occur, hair is silvery gray, and a decrease in platelet-dense granules results in a bleeding diathesis. Patients have severe immunodeficiency due to abnormal lymphocyte lytic granules. Progressive neurologic degeneration occurs.

Symptoms and Signs

The different genetic forms have a variety of phenotypes.

Type I (OCA1A) is classic tyrosinase-negative albinism; skin and hair are milky white, and eyes are blue-gray. Pigmentary dilution in OCA1B ranges from obvious to subtle.

Type II has phenotypes with pigmentary dilution that ranges from minimal to moderate. Pigmented nevi and lentigines may develop if skin is exposed to the sun; some lentigines become large and dark. Eye color varies greatly.

In type III, skin is brown, hair is rufous (reddish), and eye color can be blue or brown.

In type IV, the phenotype is similar to that for type II.

Patients with ocular involvement may have decreased retinal pigmentation, leading to sensitivity to light and light avoidance. In addition, nystagmus, strabismus, reduced visual acuity, and loss of binocular stereopsis likely result from defective routing of the optic fibers.

Diagnosis

- Clinical evaluation

Diagnosis of all types of OCA and OA is based on examination of the skin and eyes. Early ocular examination may detect iris translucency, reduced retinal pigmentation, foveal hypoplasia, reduced visual acuity, strabismus, and nystagmus.

Treatment

- Strict sun protection
- Sometimes surgical intervention for strabismus

There is no treatment for albinism. Patients are at high risk of sunburn and skin cancers (especially squamous cell carcinoma) and should avoid direct sunlight, use sunglasses with ultraviolet (UV) filtration, wear protective clothing, and use sunscreen with a sun protection factor (SPF) as high as possible (eg, 50 or higher) that protects against UVA and UVB wavelengths (see p. 1077). Some surgical interventions may lessen strabismus.

KEY POINTS

- OCA is a group of rare, usually autosomal recessive disorders, resulting in hypopigmentation of the skin, hair, and eyes.
- Ocular involvement causes photosensitivity and often nystagmus, strabismus, reduced visual acuity, and loss of binocular stereopsis.
- Examine the eyes and skin to make the diagnosis.
- Instruct patients on how to strictly protect the skin and eyes from sun exposure.

VITILIGO

Vitiligo is a loss of skin melanocytes that causes areas of skin depigmentation of varying sizes. Cause is unknown, but genetic and autoimmune factors are likely. Diagnosis is usually clear based on skin examination. Common treatments include topical corticosteroids (often combined with calcipotriene), calcineurin inhibitors (tacrolimus and pimecrolimus), and narrowband ultraviolet (UV) B or psoralen plus UVA. Widespread disease may be responsive to narrowband UVB treatments. For severe widespread pigment loss, residual patches of normal skin may be permanently depigmented (bleached) with monobenzyl ether of hydroquinone. Surgical skin-grafting may also be considered.

Vitiligo affects up to 2% of the population.

Etiology

Etiology is unclear, but melanocytes are lacking in affected areas. Proposed mechanisms include autoimmune destruction of melanocytes, reduced survival of melanocytes, and primary melanocyte defects.

Vitiligo can be familial (autosomal dominant with incomplete penetrance and variable expression) or acquired. Some patients have antibodies to melanin. Up to 30% have other autoimmune antibodies (to thyroglobulin, adrenal cells, and parietal cells) or clinical autoimmune endocrinopathies (Addison disease, diabetes mellitus, pernicious anemia, and thyroid dysfunction). However, the relationship is unclear and may be coincidental. The strongest association is with hyperthyroidism (Graves disease) and hypothyroidism (Hashimoto thyroiditis).

Occasionally, vitiligo occurs after a direct physical injury to the skin (eg, as a response to sunburn). Patients may associate the onset of vitiligo with emotional stress.

Symptoms and Signs

Vitiligo is characterized by hypopigmented or depigmented areas (see Plate 62), usually sharply demarcated and often symmetric. Depigmentation may be localized, involving 1 or 2 spots or entire body segments (segmental vitiligo); rarely, it may be generalized, involving most of the skin surface (universal vitiligo). However, vitiligo most commonly involves the face (especially around the orifices), digits, dorsal hands, flexor wrists, elbows, knees, shins, dorsal ankles, armpits, inguinal area, anogenital area, umbilicus, and nipples. Cosmetic disfigurement can be especially severe and emotionally devastating in dark-skinned patients. Hair in vitiliginous areas is usually white.

Diagnosis

- Clinical evaluation

Depigmented skin is typically obvious on examination. Subtle hypopigmented or depigmented lesions are accentuated under a Wood light. Differential diagnosis includes postinflammatory hypopigmentation, piebaldism (a rare autosomal dominant disorder in which depigmented patches surrounded by hyperpigmented areas occur most often on the forehead, neck, anterior trunk, and mid-extremities), morphea (localized scleroderma, in which skin is usually sclerotic), leprosy (in which lesions are usually hypoesthetic), lichen sclerosus, pityriasis alba, chemical leukoderma, and leukoderma due to melanoma. Although there are no evidence-based guidelines, it is reasonable for physicians to do CBC, fasting blood glucose, and thyroid function tests.

Treatment

- Protection of affected areas from sunlight
- Topical corticosteroids and calcipotriene
- Topical calcineurin inhibitors with face or groin involvement
- Narrowband UVB or psoralen plus ultraviolet A (PUVA) therapy

Treatment is supportive and cosmetic. Physicians must be aware of individual and ethnic sensibilities regarding uniform skin coloring; the disease can be psychologically devastating. All depigmented areas are prone to severe sunburn and must be protected with clothing or sunscreen.

Small, scattered lesions may be camouflaged with makeup. With more extensive involvement, treatment is usually aimed at repigmentation. However, little is known about comparative efficacies of such treatments. Traditional first-line therapy is potent topical corticosteroids, which may cause hypopigmentation or atrophy in normal surrounding skin. Calcineurin inhibitors (tacrolimus and pimecrolimus) may be particularly useful for treating areas of the skin (such as the face and groin) where adverse effects of topical corticosteroid therapy most commonly occur. Calcipotriene blended with betamethasone dipropionate may also be helpful and more successful than monotherapy with either drug. Oral and topical PUVA is often successful, but hundreds of treatment sessions may be necessary. Narrowband UVB is as effective as topical PUVA and has few adverse effects, making narrowband UVB preferable to PUVA. Narrowband UVB is often the preferred initial treatment for widespread vitiligo. Excimer laser may be useful, particularly for localized disease that does not respond to initial topical therapy.

Surgery is reasonable only for patients with stable, limited disease when medical therapy has failed. Therapies include autologous micrografting,[1] suction blister grafting, and tattooing; tattooing is especially useful for difficult-to-repigment areas such as the nipples, lips, and fingertips.

Depigmentation of unaffected skin to achieve homogeneous skin tone is possible with 20% monobenzyl ether of hydroquinone applied twice daily. This treatment is indicated only when most of the skin is involved and the patient is prepared for permanent pigment loss and the subsequent increased risks of photo-induced skin damage (eg, skin cancers, photoaging). This treatment can be extremely irritating, so a smaller test area should be treated before widespread use. Treatment for ≥ 1 yr may be required.

1. Gan EY, Kong YL, Tan WD, et al: Twelve-month and sixty-month outcomes of noncultured cellular grafting for vitiligo. *J Am Acad Dermatol* 75(3):564–571, 2016. doi: 10.1016/j.jaad.2016.04.007.

KEY POINTS

- Some cases of vitiligo may involve genetic mutations or autoimmune disorders.
- Vitiligo can be focal, segmental, or, rarely, generalized.
- Diagnose by skin examination and consider testing with CBC, fasting blood glucose, and thyroid function tests.
- Consider treatments such as topical calcipotriene plus betamethasone dipropionate, corticosteroid topical monotherapy, narrowband UVB, or a calcineurin inhibitor (tacrolimus and pimecrolimus).

HYPERPIGMENTATION

Hyperpigmentation has multiple causes and may be focal or diffuse. Most cases are due to an increase in melanin production and deposition.

Focal hyperpigmentation is most often postinflammatory in nature, occurring after injury (eg, cuts and burns) or other causes of inflammation (eg, acne, lupus). Focal linear hyperpigmentation is commonly due to phytophotodermatitis, which is a phototoxic reaction that results from ultraviolet light combined with psoralens (specifically furocoumarins) in plants (eg, limes, parsley, celery—see p. 1078). Focal hyperpigmentation can also result from neoplastic processes (eg, lentigines, melanoma), melasma, freckles, or café-au-lait macules. Acanthosis nigricans causes focal hyperpigmentation and a velvety plaque most often on the axillae and posterior neck.

Diffuse hyperpigmentation can result from drugs and also has systemic and neoplastic causes (especially lung carcinomas and melanoma with systemic involvement). After eliminating drugs as a cause of diffuse hyperpigmentation, patients should be tested for the most common systemic causes. These causes are Addison disease, hemochromatosis, and primary biliary cholangitis. Skin findings are nondiagnostic; therefore, a skin biopsy is not necessary or helpful.

Melasma (chloasma): Melasma consists of dark brown, sharply marginated, roughly symmetric patches of hyperpigmentation on the face (usually on the forehead, temples, cheeks, upper lip, or nose). It occurs primarily in pregnant women (melasma gravidarum, or the mask of pregnancy) and in women taking oral contraceptives. Ten percent of cases occur in nonpregnant women and dark-skinned men. Melasma is more prevalent among and lasts longer in people with dark skin.

Because melasma risk increases with increasing sun exposure, the mechanism probably involves overproduction of melanin by hyperfunctional melanocytes. Other than sun exposure, aggravating factors include

- Autoimmune thyroid disorders
- Photosensitizing drugs

In women, melasma fades slowly and incompletely after childbirth or cessation of hormone use. In men, melasma rarely fades.

Treatment depends on whether the pigmentation is epidermal or dermal; epidermal pigmentation becomes accentuated with a Wood light or can be diagnosed with biopsy. Only epidermal pigmentation responds to treatment. First-line therapy, often effective, includes a combination of hydroquinone 2 to 4%, tretinoin 0.05 to 1%, and a class V to VII topical corticosteroid (see Table 120–1 on p. 986). Hydroquinone 3 to 4% applied twice daily is usually required for long courses; 2% hydroquinone is useful as maintenance. Hydroquinone should be tested behind one ear or on a small patch on the forearm for 1 wk before use on the face because it may cause irritation or an allergic reaction. Azelaic acid 15 to 20% cream, can be used in place of or with hydroquinone and/or tretinoin. Hydroquinone, tretinoin, and azaleic acid are bleaching agents.

Chemical peeling with glycolic acid or 30 to 50% trichloroacetic acid is an option for patients with severe melasma unresponsive to topical bleaching agents. Laser treatments have been used, but none has been established yet as standard therapy. Two promising technologies are the Q-switched Nd:YAG (1064 nm) laser and nonablative fractional resurfacing in conjunction with triple topical therapy. During and after therapy, strict sun protection must be maintained.

Lentigines: Lentigines (singular: lentigo) are flat, tan to brown, oval macules. They are commonly due to chronic sun exposure (solar lentigines; sometimes called liver spots) and occur most frequently on the face and back of the hands. They typically first appear during middle age and increase in number with age. Although progression from lentigines to melanoma has not been established, lentigines are an independent risk factor for melanoma. If lentigines are a cosmetic concern, they are treated with cryotherapy or laser; hydroquinone is not effective.

Table 133–1. HYPERPIGMENTATION EFFECTS OF SOME DRUGS AND CHEMICALS

SUBSTANCE	EFFECT
Drugs	
Amiodarone	Slate-gray to violaceous discoloration of sun-exposed areas; yellowish brown deposits in the dermis
Antimalarials	Yellow-brown to gray to bluish black discoloration of pretibial areas, face, oral cavity, and nails; drug–melanin complexes in the dermis; hemosiderin around capillaries
Bleomycin	Flagellate hyperpigmented streaks on the back, often in areas of scratching or minor trauma
Cancer chemotherapy drugs, including busulfan, cyclophosphamide, dactinomycin, daunorubicin, and 5-fluorouracil (5-FU)	Diffuse hyperpigmentation
Desipramine Imipramine	Grayish blue discoloration on sun-exposed areas; golden-brown granules in upper dermis
Hydroquinone	Bluish black discoloration of ear cartilage and face after years of use
Phenothiazines, including chlorpromazine	Grayish blue discoloration on sun-exposed areas; golden-brown granules in upper dermis
Tetracyclines, particularly minocycline	Grayish discoloration of teeth, nails, sclerae, oral mucosa, acne scars, face, forearms, and lower legs
Heavy metals	
Bismuth	Blue-gray discoloration of face, neck, and hands
Gold	Blue-gray deposits around the eyes (chrysiasis)
Mercury	Slate-gray discoloration of skinfolds
Silver	Diffuse slate-gray discoloration (argyria), especially in sun-exposed areas

Nonsolar lentigines are sometimes associated with systemic disorders, such as Peutz-Jeghers syndrome (in which profuse lentigines of the lips occur), multiple lentigines syndrome (Leopard syndrome), or xeroderma pigmentosum.

Drug-induced hyperpigmentation: Changes are usually diffuse but sometimes have drug-specific distribution patterns or hues (see Table 133–1). Mechanisms include

- Increased melanin in the epidermis (tends to be more brown)
- Melanin in the epidermis and high dermis (mostly brown with hints of gray or blue)
- Increased melanin in the dermis (tends to be more grayish or blue)
- Dermal deposition of the drug, metabolite, or drug–melanin complexes (usually slate or bluish gray)

Drugs may cause secondary hyperpigmentation. For example, focal hyperpigmentation frequently occurs after drug-induced lichen planus (also known as lichenoid drug eruption).

In fixed drug eruptions, red plaques or blisters form at the same site each time a drug is taken; residual postinflammatory hyperpigmentation usually persists. Typical lesions occur on the face (especially the lips), hands, feet, and genitals. Typical inciting drugs include sulfonamides, tetracycline, NSAIDs, barbiturates, and carbamazepine.

KEY POINTS

- Common causes of focal hyperpigmentation include injury, inflammation, phytophotodermatitis, lentigines, melasma, freckles, café-au-lait macules, and acanthosis nigricans.
- Common causes of widespread hyperpigmentation include melasma, drugs, cancers, and other systemic disorders.
- Test patients who have widespread hyperpigmentation not caused by drugs for primary biliary cholangitis, hemochromatosis, and Addison disease.
- Treat melasma initially with a combination of hydroquinone 2 to 4%, tretinoin 0.05 to 1%, and a class V to VII topical corticosteroid.
- If lentigines are a cosmetic concern, treat with cryotherapy or laser.

134 Pressure Ulcers

(Bedsores; Decubiti; Decubitus Ulcers; Pressure Sores)

Pressure ulcers (PUs) are areas of necrosis and ulceration where tissues are compressed between bony prominences and hard surfaces. They are caused by pressure in combination with friction, shearing forces, and moisture. Risk factors include age > 65, impaired circulation, immobilization, undernutrition, and incontinence. Severity ranges from nonblanchable skin erythema to full-thickness skin loss with extensive soft-tissue necrosis. Diagnosis is clinical. Prognosis is excellent for early-stage ulcers; neglected and late-stage ulcers pose risk of serious infection and are difficult to heal. Treatment includes pressure reduction, avoidance of friction and shearing

Patient's Name		Evaluator's Name		Date of Assessment				
SENSORY PERCEPTION Ability to respond meaningfully to pressure-related discomfort	1. *Completely limited:* Unresponsive (does not moan, flinch, or grasp) to painful stimuli, owing to diminished level of consciousness or sedation or limited ability to feel pain over most of body surface	2. *Very limited:* Responds only to painful stimuli; cannot communicate discomfort except by moaning or restlessness or has a sensory impairment that limits the ability to feel pain or discomfort over half of body	3. *Slightly limited:* Responds to verbal commands but cannot always communicate discomfort or need to be turned or has some sensory impairment that limits ability to feel pain or discomfort in 1 or 2 extremities	4. *No impairment:* Responds to verbal commands; has no sensory deficit that would limit ability to feel or voice pain or discomfort				
MOISTURE Degree to which skin is exposed to moisture	1. *Constantly moist:* Skin is kept moist almost constantly by perspiration, urine, etc: dampness is detected every time patient is moved or turned	2. *Moist:* Skin is often but not always moist; linen must be changed at least once a shift	3. *Occasionally moist:* Skin is occasionally moist, requiring extra linen change about once a day	4. *Rarely moist:* Skin is usually dry; linen changes required only at routine intervals				
ACTIVITY Degree of physical activity	1. *Bedfast:* Confined to bed	2. *Chairfast:* Ability to walk severely limited or nonexistent; cannot bear own weight or must be assisted into chair or wheelchair	3. *Walks occasionally:* Walks occasionally during day but for very short distances, with or without assistance; spends most of each shift in bed or chair	4. *Walks frequently:* Walks outside the room at least twice a day and inside room at least once every 2 h during waking hours				
MOBILITY Ability to change and control body position	1. *Completely immobile:* Does not make even slight changes in body or extremity position without assistance	2. *Very limited:* Makes occasional slight changes in body or extremity position but unable to make frequent or significant changes independently	3. *Slightly limited:* Makes frequent though slight changes in body or extremity position independently	4. *No limitations:* Makes major and frequent changes in position without assistance				
NUTRITION Usual food intake pattern	1. *Very poor:* Never eats a complete meal; rarely eats > 1/3 of any food offered; eats ≤ 2 servings of protein (meat or dairy products) per day; takes fluids poorly; does not take a liquid dietary supplement or is NPO or maintained on clear liquids or IV for > 5 days	2. *Probably inadequate:* Rarely eats a complete meal and generally eats only about half of any food offered; protein intake includes only 3 servings of meat or dairy products per day; occasionally takes a dietary supplement or receives less than optimum amount of liquid diet or tube feeding	3. *Adequate:* Eats > 1/2 of most meals; eats a total of 4 servings of protein (meat, dairy products) each day; occasionally refuses a meal, but usually takes a supplement if offered or is on a tube feeding or TPN regimen, which probably meets most of nutritional needs	4. *Excellent:* Eats most of every meal; never refuses a meal; usually eats a total of ≥ 4 servings of meat and dairy products; occasionally eats between meals; does not require supplementation				
FRICTION AND SHEAR	1. *Problem:* Requires moderate to maximum assistance in moving; complete lifting without sliding against sheets is impossible; frequently slides down in bed or chair, requiring frequent repositioning with maximum assistance; spasticity, contrac-tures, or agitation leads to almost constant friction	2. *Potential problem:* Moves feebly or requires minimum assistance; during a move skin probably slides to some extent against sheets, chair, restraints, or other devices; maintains relatively good position in chair or bed most of the time but occasionally slides down	3. *No apparent problem:* Moves in bed and in chair independently and has sufficient muscle strength to lift up completely during move; maintains good position in bed or chair at all times					
				Total Score				

Fig. 134–1. Braden scale for predicting risk for pressure ulcers. The patient is evaluated in 6 categories: sensory perception, moisture, activity, mobility, nutrition, and friction and shear. Pressure sore risk increases as the score decreases: 15–16 = mild risk; 12–14 = moderate risk; < 12 = serious risk. Adapted from Braden B, Bergstrom N: Pressure ulcers in adults: Prediction and prevention. *Clinical Practice Guideline*, no. 3, pp 14–17, May 1992. US Department of Health and Human Services.

forces, and diligent wound care. Sometimes, skin grafts or myocutaneous flaps are needed to facilitate healing.

Between 1993 and 2006, the number of hospitalized patients with PUs increased by > 75%, a rate over 5 times the increase of hospital admissions overall. The rate increased most in patients who developed PUs during hospitalization. Today, an estimated 1.3 to 3 million patients in the US have PUs, resulting in a significant financial burden to patients and health care institutions.

Etiology

Risk factors for PUs include the following:

- Age > 65 (possibly due to reduced subcutaneous fat and capillary blood flow)
- Decreased mobility (eg, due to prolonged hospital stay, bed rest, spinal cord injury, sedation, weakness that decreases spontaneous movement, and/or cognitive impairment)
- Exposure to skin irritants (eg, due to incontinence)

- Impaired capacity for wound healing (eg, due to undernutrition, diabetes, peripheral arterial disease, and/or venous insufficiency)

Several scales (see Fig. 134–1) have been developed to predict risk. Although use of these scales is considered standard care, they have not been shown to result in fewer PUs than skilled clinical assessment alone. Therefore, use of a risk assessment scale along with skilled clinical assessment is recommended.

Pathophysiology

The main factors contributing to PUs are

- Pressure: When soft tissues are compressed between bony prominences and contact surfaces, microvascular occlusion with tissue ischemia and hypoxia occurs; if compression is not relieved, a PU can develop in 3 to 4 h. This most commonly occurs over the sacrum, ischial tuberosities, trochanters, malleoli, and heels, but PUs can develop anywhere.
- Friction: Friction (rubbing against clothing or bedding) can help trigger skin ulceration by causing local erosion and breaks in the epidermis and superficial dermis.
- Shearing forces: Shearing forces (eg, when a patient is placed on an incline) stress and damage supporting tissues by causing forces of muscles and subcutaneous tissues that are drawn down by gravity to oppose the more superficial tissues that remain in contact with external surfaces. Shearing forces contribute to PUs but are not direct causes.
- Moisture: Moisture (eg, perspiration, incontinence) leads to tissue breakdown and maceration, which can initiate or worsen PUs.

Because muscle is more susceptible to ischemia with compression than skin, muscle ischemia and necrosis may underlie PUs resulting from prolonged compression.

Symptoms and Signs

PUs at any stage may be painful or pruritic but may not be noticed by patients with blunted awareness or sensation.

Staging systems: Several staging systems exist. The most widely used system, developed by the National Pressure Ulcer Advisory Panel (NPUAP), classifies ulcers according to the depth of soft-tissue damage.

Stage I PUs manifest as nonblanchable erythema, usually over a bony prominence. Color changes may not be as visible in darkly pigmented skin. The lesion may also be warmer, cooler, firmer, softer, or more tender than adjacent or contralateral tissue. This stage is a misnomer in the sense that an actual ulcer (a defect of skin into the dermis) is not yet present. However, ulceration will occur if the course is not arrested and reversed.

Stage II PUs manifest as a loss of epidermis (erosion) with or without true ulceration (defect beyond the level of the epidermis); subcutaneous tissue is not exposed. The ulcer is shallow with a pink to red base. Stage II also includes intact or partially ruptured blisters secondary to pressure. (NOTE: Non-pressure-related causes of erosion, ulceration, or blistering, such as skin tears, tape burns, maceration, and excoriation, are excluded from stage II.)

Stage III PUs manifest as full-thickness loss without underlying muscle or bone exposure.

Stage IV PUs manifest as full-thickness loss with exposure of underlying bone, tendon, or muscle.

Unstageable PUs are those covered with debris or eschar, which does not allow assessment of depth. Stable, nonfluctuant heel lesions with dry eschar should never be debrided for the sake of staging.

Suspected deep tissue injury is a newer category of findings that suggest damage to underlying tissue. Findings include purple to maroon areas of intact skin, and blood-filled vesicles or bullae. The area may feel firmer, boggier, warmer, or cooler compared with surrounding tissue.

PUs do not always present as stage I and then progress to higher stages. Sometimes, the first sign of a PU is a deep, necrotic stage III or IV ulcer. In a rapidly developing PU, subcutaneous tissue can become necrotic before the epidermis erodes. Thus, a small ulcer may in fact represent extensive subcutaneous necrosis and damage.

PEARLS & PITFALLS

- Suspect deeper tissue damage than is clinically evident in patients who have PUs.

Complications

PUs are a reservoir for hospital-acquired antibiotic-resistant organisms. High bacteria counts within the wound can hinder tissue healing. If wound healing is delayed despite proper treatment, underlying osteomyelitis (present in up to 32% of patients) or rarely squamous cell carcinoma within the ulcer (Marjolin ulcer) should be considered. Other local complications of nonhealing PUs include sinus tracts, which can be superficial or connect the ulcer to deep adjacent structures (eg, sinus tracts from a sacral ulcer to the bowel), cellulitis, and tissue calcification. Systemic or metastatic infectious complications can include bacteremia, meningitis, and endocarditis.

Diagnosis

- Clinical evaluation
- Nutritional assessment

Diagnosis is based on clinical evaluation. Ulcers caused by arterial and venous insufficiency or diabetic neuropathy may mimic PUs, particularly on the lower extremities, and can also be worsened by the same forces that cause or worsen PUs.

Depth and extent of PUs can be difficult to determine. Serial staging and photography of wounds is essential for monitoring ulcer progression or healing. Many healing scales are available. The PUSH scale, designed as a companion to the NPUAP staging scale, has been adopted by many institutions.

Routine wound culture is not recommended because all PUs are heavily colonized by bacteria.

A nutritional assessment is recommended in patients with PUs, particularly those with stage III or IV PUs. Recommended tests include Hct, transferrin, prealbumin, albumin, and total and CD4+ lymphocyte counts. Undernutrition requires further evaluation and treatment (see pp. 34 and 35).

Nonhealing ulcers may be due to inadequate treatment but should raise suspicion of a complication. Tenderness, erythema of surrounding skin, exudate, or foul odor suggests an underlying infection. Fever and leukocytosis should raise suspicion of cellulitis, bacteremia, or underlying osteomyelitis. If osteomyelitis is suspected, CBC, blood cultures, and ESR or C-reactive protein is recommended. Osteomyelitis is confirmed ideally by bone biopsy and culture, but this is not always feasible. Imaging tests lack the combination of high sensitivity and specificity. MRI is sensitive but not specific and can help define the extent of PU spread. MRI with gadolinium can help identify draining or communicating sinus tracts.

Prognosis

Prognosis for early-stage PUs is excellent with timely, appropriate treatment, but healing typically requires weeks. After 6 mo of treatment, > 70% of stage II PUs, 50% of stage III PUs, and 30% of stage IV PUs resolve. PUs often develop in patients who are receiving suboptimal care. If care cannot be improved, long-term outcome is poor, even if short-term wound healing is accomplished.

Treatment

- Pressure reduction
- Direct ulcer care
- Management of pain
- Control of infection
- Assessment of nutritional needs
- Adjunctive therapy or surgery

Pressure reduction: Reducing tissue pressure is accomplished through careful positioning of the patient, protective devices, and use of support surfaces.

Frequent repositioning (and selection of the proper position) is most important. A written schedule should be used to direct and document repositioning. Bedbound patients should be turned a minimum of every 2 h and should be placed at a 30° angle to the mattress when on their side (lateral decubitus) to avoid direct trochanteric pressure. Elevation of the head of the bed should be minimal to avoid the effects of shearing forces. When repositioning patients, lifting devices (eg, a Stryker frame) or bed linen should be used instead of dragging patients to avoid unnecessary friction. Patients placed in chairs should be repositioned every hour and encouraged to change position on their own every 15 min.

Protective padding such as pillows, foam wedges, and heel protectors can be placed between the knees, ankles, and heels when patients are supine or on their side. Windows should be cut out of plaster casts at pressure sites in patients immobilized by fractures. Soft seat cushions should be provided for patients able to sit in a chair.

Support surfaces under bedbound patients can be changed to reduce pressure. They are often combined with other measures when treating PUs.

Support surfaces are classified based on whether they require electricity to operate. Static surfaces do not require electricity, whereas dynamic surfaces do. Although dynamic surfaces are usually recommended for more severe PUs, no conclusive evidence favors dynamic over static surfaces.

Static surfaces include air, foam, gel, and water overlays and mattresses. Egg-crate mattresses offer no advantage. In general, static surfaces increase surface support area and decrease pressure and shearing forces. Static surfaces have traditionally been used for PU prevention or stage I PUs.

Dynamic surfaces include alternating-air mattresses, low-air-loss mattresses, and air-fluidized mattresses. Alternating-air mattresses have air cells that are alternately inflated and deflated by a pump, thus shifting supportive pressure from site to site. Low-air-loss mattresses are giant air-permeable pillows that are continuously inflated with air; the air flow has a drying effect on tissues. These specialized mattresses are indicated for patients with stage I PUs who develop hyperemia on static surfaces and for patients with stage III or IV PUs. Air-fluidized (high-air-loss) mattresses contain silicone-coated beads that liquefy when air is pumped through the bed. Advantages include reduction of moisture and cooling. These mattresses are indicated for patients with nonhealing stages III and IV PUs or numerous truncal ulcers (see Table 134–1).

Direct ulcer care: Appropriate ulcer care involves cleaning, debridement, and dressings.

Cleaning should be done initially and with each dressing change. Normal saline is usually the best choice. Cleaning often involves irrigation at pressures sufficient to remove bacteria without traumatizing tissue; commercial syringes, squeeze bottles, or electrically pressurized systems can be used. Irrigation may also help remove necrotic tissue (debridement). Alternatively, a 35-mL syringe and an 18-gauge IV catheter can be used. Irrigation should continue until no further debris can be loosened. Antiseptics (iodine, hydrogen peroxide) and antiseptic washes can destroy healthy granulation tissue and thus should be avoided.

Debridement is necessary to remove necrotic tissue. Necrotic tissue serves as a medium for bacterial growth and blocks normal wound healing. Methods include

- **Mechanical debridement:** This method includes hydrotherapy (whirlpool baths) and most commonly wet-to-dry dressings. Cleaning wounds by irrigation at sufficient pressures can also accomplish mechanical debridement. Mechanical debridement removes necrotic debris on the

Table 134–1. OPTIONS FOR SUPPORT SURFACES

	STATIC			DYNAMIC		
	Standard Hospital Mattress	**Foam**	**Static Flotation (Air or Water)**	**Alternating Air**	**Low Air Loss**	**Air Fluidized (High Air Loss)**
Support area increase	No	Yes	Yes	Yes	Yes	Yes
Pressure reduction	No	Yes	Yes	Yes	Yes	Yes
Shear reduction	No	No	Yes	Yes	Unknown	Yes
Heat reduction	No	No	No	No	Yes	Yes
Low moisture retention	No	No	No	No	Yes	Yes
Cost	Low	Low	Low	Moderate	High	High

Adapted from Bergstrom N et al: US Agency for Health Care Policy and Research. Pressure Ulcer Treatment (Quick Reference Guideline Number 15). AHCPR Publication No. 95-0653, December 1994.

wound's surface and should only be done on wounds with very loose exudate. Wet-to-dry dressings must be used cautiously because changing them is often painful and may remove underlying healthy granulation tissue.

- **Sharp (surgical) debridement:** This method involves using a sterile scalpel or scissors to remove eschar and thick necrosis. Modest amounts of eschar or tissue can be debrided at the patient's bedside, but extensive or deep areas (eg, if underlying bone, tendon, or joints are exposed) should be debrided in the operating room. Sharp debridement should be done urgently for advancing cellulitis or lesions suspected of causing sepsis.
- **Autolytic debridement:** Synthetic occlusive (hydrocolloids/hydrogels) or semi-occlusive (transparent film) dressings are used to facilitate the digestion of dead tissues by the enzymes already normally present in the wound. Autolytic debridement may be used for smaller wounds with little exudate. This method should not be used if a wound infection is suspected.
- **Enzymatic debridement:** This technique (using collagenase, papain, fibrinolysin, deoxyribonuclease, or streptokinase/streptodornase) can be used for patients with mild fibrotic or necrotic tissue within the ulcer. It can also be used for patients whose caretakers are not trained to do mechanical debridement or for patients unable to tolerate surgery. It is most effective after careful and judicious cross-hatching of the wound with a scalpel to improve penetration.
- **Biosurgery:** Medical maggot therapy is useful for selectively removing dead necrotic tissue. This method is most helpful in patients who have exposed bone, tendons, and joints in the wound where sharp debridement is contraindicated.

Dressings are helpful for protecting the wound and facilitating the healing process (see Table 134–2).

Dressings should be used for stage I PUs that are subject to friction or incontinence and for all other PUs (see Table 134–2). In stage I PUs subject to increased friction, transparent films are sufficient. For PUs with minimal exudate, transparent films or hydrogels, which are cross-linked polymer dressings that come in sheets or gels, are used to protect the wound from infection and create a moist environment. Transparent films or hydrogels should be changed every 3 to 7 days. Hydrocolloids, which combine gelatin, pectin, and carboxymethylcellulose in the form of wafers and powders, are indicated for PUs with light-to-moderate exudate and must be changed every 3 days. Alginates (polysaccharide seaweed derivatives containing alginic acid), which come as pads, ropes, and ribbons, are indicated for absorbing extensive exudate and for controlling bleeding after surgical debridement. Alginates can be placed for up to 7 days but must be changed earlier if they become saturated. Foam dressings can be used in wounds with various levels of exudate and provide a moist environment for wound healing. Foam dressings must be changed every 3 to 4 days. Waterproof versions protect the skin from incontinence.

Management of pain: PUs can cause significant pain. Pain should be monitored regularly using a pain scale. Primary treatment of pain is treatment of the PU itself, but an NSAID or acetaminophen is useful for mild-to-moderate pain. Opioids should be avoided, if possible, because sedation promotes immobility. However, opioids or topical nonopioid preparations such as mixtures of local anesthetics may be necessary during dressing changes and debridement. In cognitively impaired patients, changes in vital signs can be used as indicators of pain.

Control of infection: PUs should be continually assessed for signs of bacterial infection such as increased erythema, foul odor, warmth, drainage, fever, and elevated WBC count. Impaired wound healing should also raise concern of infection. These abnormal findings indicate a wound culture should be

Table 134–2. OPTIONS FOR PRESSURE ULCER DRESSINGS

ULCER TYPE*	DESCRIPTION	OBJECTIVE	USE	OPTIONS
Shallow (stage II)	Dry with minimal exudate	Create or retain moisture Protect from infection	Transparent films or hydrogels	*Cover with:* Transparent film, thin hydrocolloid, or thin polyurethane foam *Wrap with:* Nonadherent gauze dressing
	Wet with moderate-to-extensive exudate	Absorb exudate Facilitate autolysis Maintain moisture Protect from infection	Hydrocolloid (if light-to-moderate exudate) or foam dressings	*Cover with:* Alginates (if extensive exudate), hydrocolloids (with or without paste or powder), or polyurethane foam *Wrap with:* Nonstick gauze dressing or absorptive contact layer
Deep (stages III–IV)	Dry with minimal exudate	Fill cavities Create or maintain moisture Protect from infection	Hydrocolloids, hydrogels, or foam dressings	*Fill with:* Copolymer starch, hydrogel, or damp gauze *Cover with:* Transparent thin film, polyurethane foam, or gauze pad
	Wet with moderate-to-extensive exudate	Fill cavities Absorb exudate Maintain moisture Protect from infection	Alginates or foam dressings	*Fill with:* Copolymer starch, dextranomer beads, calcium alginates, hydrofibers, or hydrocellular gauze or foam *Cover with:* Transparent thin film or polyurethane foam

*Dressings are not usually needed for stage I pressure ulcers.

done. However, because all PUs are colonized, results should be interpreted with caution; bacterial count rather than bacterial presence should guide treatment.

Local wound infection can be treated topically with agents such as silver sulfadiazine, mupirocin, polymyxin B, and metronidazole. Silver sulfadiazine and similar opaque topical agents should be used cautiously because they can impair visualization of the underlying wound and can be difficult to remove. A 2-wk trial of topical antibiotics for all clean PUs that do not heal despite 2 to 4 wk of proper PU treatment is recommended. Systemic antibiotics should be given for cellulitis, bacteremia, or osteomyelitis; usage should be guided by tissue culture, blood culture, or both or clinical suspicion and not by surface culture.

Assessment of nutritional needs: Undernutrition is common among patients with PUs and is a risk factor for delayed healing. Markers of undernutrition include albumin < 3.5 mg/dL or weight < 80% of ideal. Protein intake of 1.25 to 1.5 g/kg/day, sometimes requiring oral, nasogastric, or parenteral supplementation, is desirable for optimal healing. Current evidence does not support supplementing vitamins or calories in patients who have no signs of nutritional deficiency.

Adjunctive therapy: Multiple adjunctive therapies are being tried to promote PU healing:

- **Negative-pressure therapy:** Negative-pressure therapy (vacuum-assisted closure, or VAC) applies suction to the wound. It can be applied to clean wounds. High-quality evidence of efficacy does not yet exist, but negative-pressure therapy has shown some promise in small studies.
- **Topical recombinant growth factors:** Some evidence suggests that topical recombinant growth factors (eg, nerve growth factor, platelet-derived growth factor) and skin equivalents facilitate wound healing.
- **Electrical stimulation therapy:** Electrical stimulation therapy combined with standard wound therapy can increase wound healing.
- **Therapeutic ultrasonography:** Ultrasonography is sometimes used, but there is no good evidence of benefit or harm.
- **Electrical magnetic, heat, massage, and hyperbaric O_2** therapies: No evidence supports efficacy of these treatments.

Surgery: Large defects, especially with exposure of musculoskeletal structures, require surgical closure. Skin grafts are useful for large, shallow defects. However, because grafts do not add to blood supply, measures must be taken to prevent pressure from developing to the point of ischemia and further breakdown. Myocutaneous flaps, because of their pressure-sharing bulk and rich vasculature, are the closures of choice over large bony prominences (usually the sacrum, ischia, and trochanters). Surgery may rapidly improve the quality of life in patients with PUs. Surgical outcomes are best if preceded by optimal treatment of undernutrition and comorbid disorders.

Prevention

Prevention requires

- Identification of high-risk patients
- Repositioning
- Conscientious skin care and hygiene
- Avoidance of immobilization

Patient risk should be estimated based on the assessment of skilled clinicians and use of risk assessment scales (see Fig. 134-1).

Treatment and prevention overlap considerably. The mainstay of prevention is frequent repositioning. Pressure should not continue over any bony surface for > 2 h. Patients who cannot move themselves must be repositioned and cushioned with pillows. Patients must be turned even when they are lying on low-pressure mattresses. Pressure points should be checked for erythema or trauma at least once per day under adequate lighting. Patients and family members must be taught a routine of daily visual inspection and palpation of sites for potential ulcer formation.

Daily attention to hygiene and dryness is necessary to prevent maceration and secondary infection. Protective padding, pillows, or sheepskin can be used to separate body surfaces. Bedding and clothing should be changed frequently. In incontinent patients, ulcers should be protected from contamination; synthetic dressings can help. Skin breakdown can be prevented with careful cleansing and drying (patting and not rubbing the skin) and using anticandidal creams and moisture barrier creams or skin-protective wipes. Use of adhesive tape should be minimized, because it can irritate and even tear fragile skin. Areas subject to friction may be powdered with plain talc. Use of cornstarch is discouraged because it may allow microbial growth.

Most importantly, immobilization should be avoided. Sedatives should be minimized, and patients should be mobilized as quickly and safely as possible.

KEY POINTS

- PUs can develop secondary to immobilization and hospitalization, particularly in patients who are elderly, incontinent, or undernourished.
- Base risk of PUs on standardized scales as well as the assessment of skilled clinicians.
- PUs are staged according to ulcer depth, but tissue damage may be deeper and more severe than is evident from the physical examination.
- Assess patients with PUs for local wound infection (sometimes manifesting as failure to heal), sinus tracts, cellulitis, bacteremic spread (eg, with endocarditis or meningitis), osteomyelitis, and undernutrition.
- Treat and help prevent PUs by reducing skin pressure, repositioning frequently, and using protective padding and support surfaces that can be dynamic (powered electrically) or static (not powered electrically).
- Clean and dress PUs frequently to reduce bacterial counts and facilitate wound healing.
- Apply transparent films or hydrogels (if exudate is minimal), hydrocolloids (if exudate is light to moderate), alginates (if exudate is extensive), or foam dressings (for various amounts of exudate).
- Treat pain with analgesics, local wound infection with topical antibiotics, and cellulitis or systemic infections with systemic antibiotics.
- Surgically close large defects, especially those with exposed musculoskeletal structures.
- Optimize nutritional status and treatment of comorbid disorders before surgery.
- Help prevent PUs in patients at risk with meticulous wound care, pressure reduction, and avoiding any unnecessary immobilization.

135 Psoriasis and Scaling Diseases

PSORIASIS

Psoriasis is an inflammatory disease that manifests most commonly as well-circumscribed, erythematous papules and plaques covered with silvery scales. Multiple factors contribute, including genetics. Common triggers include trauma, infection, and certain drugs. Symptoms are usually minimal, but mild to severe itching may occur. Cosmetic implications may be major. Some people develop severe disease with painful arthritis. Diagnosis is based on appearance and distribution of lesions. Treatment can include topical treatments (eg, emollients, vitamin D analogs, retinoids, coal tar, anthralin, corticosteroids), phototherapy, and, when severe, systemic drugs (eg, methotrexate, oral retinoids, cyclosporine, immunomodulatory agents [biologics]).

Psoriasis is hyperproliferation of epidermal keratinocytes combined with inflammation of the epidermis and dermis. It affects about 1 to 5% of the population worldwide; light-skinned people are at higher risk, and blacks are at lower risk. Peak onset is roughly bimodal, most often at ages 16 to 22 and at ages 57 to 60, but the disorder can occur at any age.

Etiology

The cause of psoriasis is unclear but involves immune stimulation of epidermal keratinocytes; T cells seem to play a central role. Family history is common, and certain genes and HLA antigens (Cw6, B13, B17) are associated with psoriasis. Genomewide linkage analysis has identified numerous psoriasis susceptibility loci; the *PSORS1* locus on chromosome 6p21 plays the greatest role in determining a patient's susceptibility of developing psoriasis. An environmental trigger is thought to evoke an inflammatory response and subsequent hyperproliferation of keratinocytes.

Well-identified triggers include

- Injury (Koebner phenomenon)
- Sunburn
- HIV infection
- Beta-hemolytic streptococcal infection
- Drugs (especially beta-blockers, chloroquine, lithium, ACE inhibitors, indomethacin, terbinafine, and interferon-alfa)
- Emotional stress
- Alcohol consumption
- Tobacco smoking
- Obesity

Symptoms and Signs

Lesions are either asymptomatic or pruritic and are most often localized on the scalp, extensor surfaces of the elbows and knees, sacrum, buttocks (commonly the gluteal cleft), and genitals. The nails, eyebrows, axillae, umbilicus, and perianal region may also be affected. The disease can be widespread, involving confluent areas of skin extending between these regions. Lesions differ in appearance depending on type.

Among the various psoriasis subtypes, plaque psoriasis (psoriasis vulgaris or chronic plaque psoriasis) accounts for about 90%; lesions are discrete, erythematous papules or plaques covered with thick, silvery, shiny scales. Lesions appear gradually and remit and recur spontaneously or with the appearance and resolution of triggers (see Table 135–1).

Arthritis develops in 5 to 30% of patients and can be disabling (psoriatic arthritis); joint destruction may ultimately occur.

Psoriasis is rarely life-threatening but can affect a patient's self-image. Besides the patient's appearance, the sheer amount of time required to treat extensive skin or scalp lesions and to maintain clothing and bedding may adversely affect quality of life.

Diagnosis

- Clinical evaluation
- Rarely biopsy

Diagnosis of psoriasis is most often by clinical appearance and distribution of lesions.

Differential diagnosis includes

- Seborrheic dermatitis
- Dermatophytoses (potassium hydroxide wet mount should be done for any scaly plaques, especially if they do not have a classic appearance of eczema or psoriasis)
- Cutaneous lupus erythematosus
- Eczema
- Lichen planus
- Allergic contact dermatitis
- Pityriasis rosea
- Squamous cell carcinoma in situ (Bowen disease, especially when on the trunk; this diagnosis should be considered for isolated plaques that do not respond to usual therapy)
- Lichen simplex chronicus
- Secondary syphilis

Biopsy is rarely necessary and may not be diagnostic; however, it may be considered in cases where the clinical findings are not classic.

Disease is graded as mild, moderate, or severe based on the body surface area affected and how the lesions affect the patient's quality of life. To be considered mild, usually < 10% of the skin surface should be involved. There are many more complex scoring systems for disease severity (eg, the Psoriasis Area and Severity Index), but these systems are useful mainly in research protocols.

Treatment

- Topical treatments
- Ultraviolet (UV) light therapy
- Systemic treatments

Treatment options are extensive and range from topical treatments (eg, emollients, salicylic acid, coal tar, anthralin, corticosteroids, vitamin D_3 analogs, calcineurin inhibitors, tazarotene) to UV light therapy to systemic treatments (eg, methotrexate, oral retinoids, cyclosporine, immunomodulatory agents [biologics]. (See the American Academy of Dermatology's clinical guideline for psoriasis at www.aad.org.)

Topical treatments: Corticosteroids are usually used topically but may be injected into small or recalcitrant lesions. (CAUTION: *Systemic corticosteroids may precipitate exacerbations or development of pustular psoriasis and should not be used to treat psoriasis.*) Topical corticosteroids are used twice

Table 135–1. SUBTYPES OF PSORIASIS

SUBTYPE	DESCRIPTION	TREATMENT AND PROGNOSIS
Plaque psoriasis	Gradual appearance of discrete, erythematous papules or plaques covered with thick, silvery, shiny scales Lesions that remit and recur spontaneously or with appearance and resolution of triggers	*Treatment:* Topical corticosteroids of minimal effective potency, with or without vitamin D_3 analogs (eg, calcipotriol) Systemic immunosuppressant or immunomodulatory drugs (eg, methotrexate, cyclosporine, TNF-α inhibitor) *Prognosis:* Waxes and wanes, without cure
Inverse psoriasis	Psoriasis of intertriginous areas (usually the inguinal, gluteal, axillary, inframammary, and retroauricular folds and the glans of the uncircumcised penis) Possibly formation of cracks or fissures in the center or edge of involved areas Possibly absence of scales	*Treatment:* Topical corticosteroids of minimal effective potency, with or without vitamin D_3 analogs (eg, calcipotriol) Possibly tacrolimus 0.1% ointment in recalcitrant cases Tar and anthralin possibly irritating *Prognosis:* Waxes and wanes
Guttate psoriasis	Abrupt appearance of multiple plaques 0.5 to 1.5 cm in diameter, usually on the trunk in children and young adults after streptococcal pharyngitis	*Treatment:* Antibiotics for underlying streptococcal infection *Prognosis:* Excellent, often with permanent cure May progress to plaque psoriasis
Palmoplantar psoriasis	Hyperkeratotic, discrete plaques on palms and/or soles that tend to become confluent	*Treatment:* Systemic retinoids, topical corticosteroids, vitamin D_3 analogs (eg, calcipotriol), systemic immunosuppressant or immunomodulatory drugs (eg methotrexate, cyclosporine, TNF-α inhibitor) *Prognosis:* Waxes and wanes Rarely resolves completely, even with treatment
Nail psoriasis	Pitting, stippling, fraying, discoloration (oil spot sign), and thickening of the nails, with or without separation of the nail plate (onycholysis) May resemble a fungal nail infection Affects 30–50% of patients with other forms of psoriasis	*Treatment:* Responds best to systemic therapy For brave or stoic patients, possibly intralesional injection with corticosteroids *Prognosis:* Often unresponsive to treatment
Pustular psoriasis of the palms and soles	Gradual appearance of deep pustules on palms and soles Flare-ups that may be painful and disabling Typical psoriatic lesions possibly absent	*Treatment:* Systemic retinoids or psoralen plus ultraviolet A (PUVA) therapy *Prognosis:* Waxes and wanes
Acrodermatitis continua of Hallopeau	Pustular psoriasis confined to distal fingers or toes, sometimes just one digit Replaced by scale and crust when it resolves	*Treatment:* Systemic retinoids, vitamin D_3 analogs (eg, calcipotriol), topical corticosteroids *Prognosis:* Waxes and wanes
Generalized pustular psoriasis	Explosive onset of widespread erythema and sterile pustules	*Treatment:* Systemic retinoids or methotrexate *Prognosis:* If untreated, can be fatal due to high-output heart failure
Erythrodermic psoriasis	Gradual or sudden onset of diffuse erythema, usually in patients with plaque psoriasis (possibly the first manifestation of erythrodermic psoriasis); typical psoriatic plaques less prominent or absent Most commonly triggered by inappropriate use of topical or systemic corticosteroids or light therapy	*Treatment:* Potent systemic drugs (eg, methotrexate, cyclosporine, TNF-α inhibitor) or intense topical therapy, sometimes as inpatient therapy Tars, anthralin, and phototherapy likely to exacerbate the condition *Prognosis:* Good with elimination of triggering factors

daily. Corticosteroids are most effective when used overnight under occlusive polyethylene coverings or incorporated into tape; a corticosteroid cream is applied without occlusion during the day. Corticosteroid potency is selected according to the extent of involvement.

As lesions abate, the corticosteroid should be applied less frequently or at a lower potency to minimize local atrophy, striae formation, and telangiectases. Ideally, after about 3 wk, an emollient should be substituted for the corticosteroid for 1 to 2 wk (as a rest period); this substitution limits corticosteroid dosage and prevents tachyphylaxis. Topical corticosteroid use can be expensive because large quantities (about 1 oz or 30 g) are needed for each application when a large body surface area is affected. Topical corticosteroids applied for long duration to large areas of the body may cause systemic effects and exacerbate psoriasis. For small, thick, localized, or recalcitrant lesions, high-potency corticosteroids are used with an occlusive dressing or flurandrenolide tape; these dressings are left on overnight and changed in the morning. Relapse after topical corticosteroids are stopped is often faster than with other agents.

Vitamin D_3 analogs (eg, calcipotriol [calcipotriene], calcitriol) are topical vitamin D analogs that induce normal keratinocyte proliferation and differentiation; they can be used alone or in combination with topical corticosteroids. Some clinicians have patients apply calcipotriol on weekdays and corticosteroids on weekends.

Calcineurin inhibitors (eg, tacrolimus, pimecrolimus) are available in topical form and are generally well-tolerated. They are not as effective as corticosteroids but may avoid the complications of corticosteroids when treating facial and intertriginous psoriasis. It is not clear whether they increase the risk of lymphoma and skin cancer.

Tazarotene is a topical retinoid. It is less effective than corticosteroids as monotherapy but is a useful adjunct.

Other adjunctive topical treatments include emollients, salicylic acid, coal tar, and anthralin.

Emollients include emollient creams, ointments, petrolatum, paraffin, and even hydrogenated vegetable (cooking) oils. They reduce scaling and are most effective when applied twice daily and immediately after bathing. Lesions may appear redder as scaling decreases or becomes more transparent. Emollients are safe and should probably always be used for mild to moderate plaque psoriasis.

Salicylic acid is a keratolytic that softens scales, facilitates their removal, and increases absorption of other topical agents. It is especially useful as a component of scalp treatments; scalp scale can be quite thick.

Coal tar preparations are anti-inflammatory and decrease keratinocyte hyperproliferation via an unknown mechanism. Ointments or solutions are typically applied at night and washed off in the morning. Coal tar products can be used in combination with topical corticosteroids or with exposure to natural or artificial broad-band UVB light (280 to 320 nm) in slowly increasing increments (Goeckerman regimen). Shampoos should be left in for 5 to 10 min and then rinsed out.

Anthralin is a topical antiproliferative, anti-inflammatory agent. Its mechanism of action is unknown. Effective dose is 0.1% cream or ointment increased to 1% as tolerated. Anthralin may be irritating and should be used with caution in intertriginous areas; it also stains. Irritation and staining can be avoided by washing off the anthralin 20 to 30 min after application. Using a liposome-encapsulated preparation may also avoid some disadvantages of anthralin.

Phototherapy: UV light therapy is typically used in patients with extensive psoriasis. The mechanism of action is unknown, although UVB light reduces DNA synthesis and can induce mild systemic immunosuppression. In PUVA, oral methoxypsoralen, a photosensitizer, is followed by exposure to long-wave UVA light (330 to 360 nm). PUVA has an antiproliferative effect and also helps to normalize keratinocyte differentiation. Doses of light are started low and increased as tolerated. Severe burns can result if the dose of drug or UVA is too high.

Although the treatment is less messy than topical treatment and may produce remissions lasting several months, repeated treatments may increase the incidence of UV-induced skin cancer and melanoma. Less UV light is required when used with oral retinoids (the so-called re-PUVA regimen). NBUVB light (311 to 312 nm), which is used without psoralens, is similar in effectiveness to PUVA. Excimer laser therapy is a type of phototherapy using a 308-nm laser directed at focal psoriatic plaques.

Systemic treatments: Methotrexate taken orally is an effective treatment for severe disabling psoriasis, especially severe psoriatic arthritis or widespread erythrodermic or pustular psoriasis unresponsive to topical agents or UV light therapy (narrowband UVB [NBUVB]) or psoralen plus ultraviolet A (PUVA). Methotrexate seems to interfere with the rapid proliferation of epidermal cells. Hematologic, renal, and hepatic function should be monitored. Dosage regimens vary, so only physicians experienced in its use for psoriasis should undertake methotrexate therapy.

Systemic retinoids (eg, acitretin, isotretinoin) may be effective for severe and recalcitrant cases of psoriasis vulgaris, pustular psoriasis (in which isotretinoin may be preferred), and hyperkeratotic palmoplantar psoriasis. Because of the teratogenic potential and long-term retention of acitretin in the body, women who use it must not be pregnant and should be warned against becoming pregnant for at least 2 yr after treatment ends. Pregnancy restrictions also apply to isotretinoin, but the agent is not retained in the body beyond 1 mo. Long-term treatment may cause diffuse idiopathic skeletal hyperostosis (DISH).

Immunosuppressants can be used for severe psoriasis. Cyclosporine is a commonly used immunosuppressant. It should be limited to courses of several months (rarely, up to 1 yr) and alternated with other therapies. Its effect on the kidneys and potential long-term effects on the immune system preclude more liberal use. Other immunosuppressants (eg, hydroxyurea, 6-thioguanine, mycophenolate mofetil) have narrow safety margins and are reserved for severe, recalcitrant psoriasis.

Immunomodulatory agents (biologics—see Immunotherapeutics on p. 1366) include TNF-α inhibitors (etanercept, adalimumab, infliximab). TNF-α inhibitors lead to clearing of psoriasis, but their safety profile is still under study. Efalizumab is no longer available in the US due to increased risk of progressive multifocal leukoencephalopathy. Ustekinumab, a human monoclonal antibody that targets IL-12 and IL-23, can be used for moderate to severe psoriasis. IL-17 inhibitors (secukinumab and ixekizumab) are the most recently available biologics for moderate to severe psoriasis. Apremilast (inhibitor of phosphodiesterase 4) is the only available oral drug for psoriasis; however, early post-marketing data suggest it is not as effective as the TNF-α inhibitors.

Choice of therapy: Choice of specific agents and combinations requires close cooperation with the patient, always keeping in mind the untoward effects of the treatments. There is no single ideal combination or sequence of agents, but treatment should be kept as simple as possible. Monotherapy is preferred, but combination therapy is the norm. First-line treatment for psoriasis includes topical corticosteroids and topical vitamin D_3 analogs (either as monotherapy or in combination).

Rotational therapy refers to the substitution of one therapy for another after 1 to 2 yr to reduce the adverse effects caused by chronic use and to circumvent disease resistance. Sequential therapy refers to initial use of potent agents (eg, cyclosporine) to quickly gain control followed by use of agents with a better safety profile. Immunomodulatory agents achieve clearance or near clearance of lesions more often than methotrexate or NBUVB.

Mild plaque psoriasis can be treated with emollients, keratolytics, tar, topical corticosteroids, vitamin D_3 analogs, or anthralin alone or in combination. Moderate exposure to sunlight is beneficial, but sunburn can induce exacerbations.

Moderate to severe plaque psoriasis (see Plate 48) should be treated with topical agents and either phototherapy or systemic agents. Immunosuppressants are used for quick, short-term control (eg, in allowing a break from other modalities) and for the most severe disease. Immunomodulatory agents are used for moderate to severe disease unresponsive to other agents.

Scalp plaques are notoriously difficult to treat because they resist systemic therapy, and because hair blocks application of topical agents and scale removal and shields skin from UV light. A suspension of 10% salicylic acid in mineral oil may be rubbed into the scalp at bedtime manually or with a toothbrush, covered with a shower cap (to enhance penetration and avoid messiness), and washed out the next morning with a tar (or other) shampoo. More cosmetically acceptable corticosteroid solutions can be applied to the scalp during the day. These treatments are continued until the desired clinical response is achieved. Resistant skin or scalp patches may respond to local superficial intralesional injection of triamcinolone acetonide suspension diluted with saline to 2.5 or 5 mg/mL, depending on the size and severity of the lesion. Injections may cause local atrophy, which is usually reversible.

Special treatment needs for subtypes of psoriasis are described above.

For psoriatic arthritis, treatment with systemic therapy is important to prevent joint destruction; methotrexate or a TNF-α inhibitor may be effective.

KEY POINTS

- Psoriasis is a common inflammatory disorder affecting the skin that has a genetic component and several triggers (eg, trauma, infection, certain drugs).
- Skin findings are usually well-circumscribed, erythematous papules and plaques covered with silvery scales.
- Psoriatic arthritis develops in 5 to 30% of patients and can cause joint destruction and disability.
- Diagnose based on the appearance and distribution of lesions.
- Use topical treatments (eg, emollients, salicylic acid, coal tar preparations, anthralin, corticosteroids, vitamin D_3 analogs, calcineurin inhibitors, tazarotene), particularly for mild disease.
- Use ultraviolet (UV) light therapy, usually for moderate or severe psoriasis.
- For extensive psoriasis, use systemic treatments, such as immunomodulatory (biologic) agents, methotrexate, cyclosporine, retinoids, and/or other immunosuppressants.

LICHEN PLANUS

Lichen planus is a recurrent, pruritic, inflammatory eruption characterized by small, discrete, polygonal, flat-topped, violaceous papules that may coalesce into rough scaly plaques, often accompanied by oral and/or genital lesions. Diagnosis is usually clinical and supported by skin biopsy. Treatment generally requires topical or intralesional corticosteroids. Severe cases may require phototherapy or systemic corticosteroids, retinoids, or immunosuppressants.

Etiology

Lichen planus (LP) is thought to be caused by a T-cell-mediated autoimmune reaction against basal epithelial keratinocytes in people with genetic predisposition. Drugs (especially beta-blockers, NSAIDs, ACE inhibitors, sulfonylureas, gold, antimalarial drugs, penicillamine, and thiazides) can cause LP; drug-induced LP (sometimes called lichenoid drug eruption) may be indistinguishable from non-drug-induced LP or may have a pattern that is more eczematous.

Associations with hepatitis (hepatitis B infection, hepatitis B vaccine, and, particularly, hepatitis C–induced liver insufficiency), primary biliary cirrhosis, and other forms of hepatitis have been reported.

Symptoms and Signs

Typical lesions are pruritic, violaceous (purple), polygonal, flat-topped papules and plaques (see Plate 43). Lesions initially are 2 to 4 mm in diameter, with angular borders and a distinct sheen in cross-lighting. They are usually symmetrically distributed, most commonly on the flexor surfaces of the wrists, legs, trunk, glans penis, and oral and vaginal mucosae but can be widespread. The face is rarely involved. Onset may be abrupt or gradual. Children are affected infrequently.

During the acute phase, new papules may appear at sites of minor skin injury (Koebner phenomenon), such as a superficial scratch. Lesions may coalesce or change over time, becoming hyperpigmented, atrophic, hyperkeratotic (hypertrophic LP), or vesiculobullous. Although pruritic, lesions are rarely excoriated or crusted. If the scalp is affected, patchy scarring alopecia (lichen planopilaris) may occur.

The oral mucosa is involved in about 50% of cases; oral lesions may occur without cutaneous lesions. Reticulated, lacy, bluish white, linear lesions (Wickham striae) are a hallmark of oral LP, especially on the buccal mucosae. Tongue margins and gingival mucosae in edentulous areas may also be affected. An erosive form of LP may occur in which the patient develops shallow, often painful, recurrent oral ulcers, which, if long-standing, rarely become cancerous. Chronic exacerbations and remissions are common.

Vulvar and vaginal mucosae are often involved. Up to 50% of women with oral mucosal findings have undiagnosed vulvar LP. In men, genital involvement is common, especially of the glans penis.

Nails are involved in up to 10% of cases. Findings vary in intensity with nail bed discoloration, longitudinal ridging and lateral thinning, and complete loss of the nail matrix and nail, with scarring of the proximal nail fold onto the nail bed (pterygium formation).

Diagnosis

- Clinical evaluation
- Biopsy

Although the diagnosis of lichen planus is suggested by appearance of the lesions, similar lesions may result from any of the papulosquamous disorders, lupus erythematosus, and secondary syphilis, among others. Oral or vaginal LP may resemble leukoplakia, and the oral lesions must also be distinguished from candidiasis, carcinoma, aphthous ulcers, pemphigus, mucous membrane (cicatricial) pemphigoid, and chronic erythema multiforme. Typically, biopsy is done.

If LP is diagnosed, laboratory testing for liver dysfunction, including hepatitis B and C infections, should be considered.

Prognosis

Many cases resolve without intervention, presumably because the inciting agent is no longer present. Recurrence after years may be due to reexposure to the trigger or some change in the triggering mechanism. Sometimes treatment of a previously occult infection, such as a dental abscess, results in resolution.

Vulvovaginal LP may be chronic and refractory to therapy, causing decreased quality of life and vaginal or vulvar scarring. Oral mucosal lesions usually persist for life.

Treatment

- Local treatments
- Systemic treatments
- Sometimes light therapy

Asymptomatic LP does not require treatment. Drugs suspected of triggering LP should be stopped; it can takes weeks to months after the offending drug has been stopped for the lesions to resolve.

Local treatments: Few controlled studies have evaluated treatments. Options differ by location and extent of disease. Most cases of LP on the trunk or extremities can be treated with topical treatments. Topical corticosteroids are first-line treatment for most cases of localized disease. High-potency ointments or creams (eg, clobetasol, fluocinonide) may be used on the thicker lesions on the extremities; lower-potency drugs (eg, hydrocortisone, desonide) may be used on the face, groin, and axillae. As always, courses should be limited to reduce risk of corticosteroid atrophy. Potency may be enhanced with use of polyethylene wrapping or flurandrenolide tape. Intralesional corticosteroids (triamcinolone acetonide solution diluted with saline to 5 to 10 mg/mL) can be used every 4 wk for hyperkeratotic plaques, scalp lesions, and lesions resistant to other therapies.

Systemic treatments and phototherapy: Local therapy is impractical for generalized LP; oral drugs or phototherapy is used. Oral corticosteroids (eg, prednisone 20 mg once/day for 2 to 6 wk followed by a taper) may be used for severe cases. The disease may rebound when therapy ceases; however, long-term systemic corticosteroids should not be used.

Oral retinoids (eg, acitretin 30 mg once/day for 8 wk) are indicated for otherwise recalcitrant cases. Griseofulvin 250 mg po bid given for 3 to 6 mo may be effective. Cyclosporine (1.25 to 2.5 mg/kg bid) can be used when corticosteroids or retinoids fail. Light therapy using psoralen plus ultraviolet A (PUVA) or narrowband ultraviolet B (NBUVB) is an alternative to oral therapies, especially if they have failed or are contraindicated.

Dapsone, hydroxychloroquine, azathioprine, systemic cyclosporine, and topical tretinoin may also be useful. As with any disease with so many therapies, individual drugs have not been uniformly successful.

Oral lichen planus: Treatment of oral LP differs slightly. Viscous lidocaine may help relieve symptoms of erosive ulcers; because inflamed mucous membranes can absorb high amounts, dose should not exceed 200 mg (eg, 10 mL of a 2% solution) or 4 mg/kg (in children) qid. Tacrolimus 0.1% ointment applied twice daily may induce lasting remission, although it has not been fully evaluated.

Other treatment options include topical (in an adhesive base), intralesional, and systemic corticosteroids.

Erosive oral LP may respond to oral dapsone, hydroxychloroquine, or cyclosporine. Cyclosporine rinses also may be helpful.

KEY POINTS

- Lichen planus is thought to be an autoimmune disorder in patients with a genetic predisposition but may be caused by drugs or be associated with disorders such as hepatitis C.
- LP is characterized by recurrent, pruritic papules that are polygonal, flat-topped, and violaceous and can coalesce into plaques.
- Oral and genital lesions can develop, become chronic, and cause morbidity.
- Diagnose LP by clinical appearance and, if necessary, biopsy.
- Treat localized LP with topical or injected corticosteroids.
- Treat generalized LP with oral drugs or phototherapy.

LICHEN SCLEROSUS

Lichen sclerosus is an inflammatory dermatosis of unknown cause, possibly autoimmune, that usually affects the anogenital area.

The earliest signs are skin fragility, bruising, and sometimes blistering. Lesions typically cause mild to severe itching. When lichen sclerosus manifests in children, the appearance may be confused with sexual abuse. With time, the involved tissue becomes atrophic, thinned, hypopigmented (there may be flecks of postinflammatory hyperpigmentation), fissured, and scaly. Hyperkeratotic and fibrotic forms exist.

Severe and longstanding cases cause scarring and distortion or absorption of normal anogenital architecture. In women, this distortion can even lead to total destruction of the labia minora and clitoris. In men, phimosis or fusion of the foreskin to the coronal sulcus can occur.

Diagnosis

- Clinical evaluation
- Sometimes biopsy

Diagnosis of lichen sclerosus can usually be based on appearance, especially in advanced cases; however, biopsy should be done on any anogenital dermatosis that does not resolve with mild conventional therapy (eg, topical hydrocortisone, antifungal drug). It is especially important to biopsy any area that becomes thickened or ulcerated, because lichen sclerosus is associated with an increased frequency of squamous cell carcinoma.

Treatment

- Topical corticosteroids

Treatment of lichen sclerosus consists of potent topical corticosteroids (drugs that otherwise should be used with extreme caution in this area). The disease is generally intractable, so long-term treatment and follow-up are necessary.

Monitoring for squamous cell carcinoma and sexual dysfunction and providing psychologic support are indicated.

PARAPSORIASIS

Parapsoriasis refers to a group of skin diseases characterized by maculopapular or scaly lesions.

Parapsoriasis describes a poorly understood and poorly distinguished group of diseases that share clinical features. Parapsoriasis is not related to psoriasis; it is so-called because the scaly plaques sometimes appear similar.

There are 2 general forms:

- Small-plaque type: Usually benign
- Large-plaque type: A precursor of cutaneous T-cell lymphoma (CTCL)

Small-plaque parapsoriasis transforms into CTCL extremely rarely. Large-plaque parapsoriasis transforms into CTCL in about 10% of patients per decade.

Symptoms and Signs

The plaques are usually asymptomatic; their typical appearance is thin, scaling, dull, pink patches and plaques with a slightly atrophic or wrinkled appearance. In contrast, the plaques in psoriasis are well-demarcated and pink with thicker silvery scale.

Small-plaque parapsoriasis is defined by lesions < 5 cm in diameter, whereas large-plaque parapsoriasis has lesions > 5 cm in diameter.

Sometimes digitate plaques develop along the dermatomes, especially on the flanks and abdomen, in small-plaque parapsoriasis.

Although digitate plaques of parapsoriasis may be > 5 cm, transformation into CTCL is extremely rare in small-plaque parapsoriasis.

Prognosis

Course for both types is unpredictable; periodic clinical follow-up and biopsies give the best indication of risk of developing CTCL.

Treatment

Treatment of **small-plaque parapsoriasis** is unnecessary but can include emollients, topical tar preparations or corticosteroids, phototherapy, or a combination.

Treatment of **large-plaque parapsoriasis** is phototherapy (narrowband ultraviolet B [NBUVB]) or topical corticosteroids.

PITYRIASIS LICHENOIDES

Pityriasis lichenoides is a clonal T-cell disorder that may develop in response to foreign antigens (eg, infections or drugs) and may be associated with cutaneous T-cell lymphoma. Treatment may include various topical and oral drugs.

Pityriasis lichenoides has distinct acute and chronic forms, which are usually distinct entities; however, lesions may evolve from the acute to chronic type. The acute form typically appears in children and young adults, with crops of asymptomatic chickenpox-like lesions that typically resolve, often with scarring, within weeks to months. Antibiotics (eg, tetracycline, erythromycin) or phototherapy may help.

The chronic form of pityriasis lichenoides initially manifests as flatter, reddish brown, scaling papules that may take months or longer to resolve.

Treatment

- Various topical and oral treatments

Treatment of pityriasis lichenoides is often ineffective, but sunlight, topical corticosteroids, topical tacrolimus, oral antibiotics, phototherapy, and immunosuppressants have been used with varying success.[1]

1. Bowers S, Warshaw EM: Pityriasis lichenoides and its subtypes. *J Am Acad Dermatol* 55:557–572, 2006. doi: 10.1016/j.jaad.2005.07.058.

PITYRIASIS ROSEA

Pityriasis rosea (PR) is a self-limited, inflammatory disease characterized by diffuse, scaling papules or plaques. Treatment is usually unnecessary.

PR most commonly occurs between ages 10 and 35. It affects women more often. The cause may be viral infection (some research has implicated human herpesviruses 6, 7, and 8). Drugs may cause a PR-like reaction.

Symptoms and Signs

The condition classically begins with a single, primary, 2- to 10-cm herald patch that appears on the trunk or proximal limbs (see Plate 47). A general centripetal eruption of 0.5- to 2-cm rose- or fawn-colored oval papules and plaques follows within 7 to 14 days. The lesions have a scaly, slightly raised border (collarette) and resemble ringworm (tinea corporis). Most patients itch, occasionally severely. Papules may dominate with little or no scaling in children and pregnant women. The rose or fawn color is not as evident in patients with darker skin; children more commonly have inverse PR (lesions in the axillae or groin that spread centrifugally).

Classically, lesions orient along skin lines, giving PR a Christmas tree–like distribution when multiple lesions appear on the back. A prodrome of malaise, headache, and sometimes arthralgia precedes the lesions in a minority of patients.

Diagnosis

- Clinical evaluation

Diagnosis of pityriasis rosea is based on clinical appearance and distribution.

Differential diagnosis includes

- Tinea corporis
- Tinea versicolor
- Drug eruptions
- Psoriasis
- Parapsoriasis
- Pityriasis lichenoides chronica
- Lichen planus
- Secondary syphilis

Serologic testing for syphilis is indicated when the palms or soles are affected, when a herald patch is not seen, or when lesions occur in an unusual sequence or distribution.

Treatment

- Antipruritic therapy

No specific treatment is necessary because the eruption usually remits within 5 wk and recurrence is rare.

Artificial or natural sunlight may hasten resolution.

Antipruritic therapy such as topical corticosteroids, oral antihistamines, or topical measures may be used as needed.

Some data suggest that acyclovir 800 mg po 5 times a day for 7 days may be helpful in patients who present early and have widespread disease, or present with flu-like symptoms. Of note, PR during pregnancy (especially during the first 15 wk of gestation) is associated with premature birth or fetal demise. Pregnant women should be offered acyclovir; however, antiviral therapy has not proved to reduce obstetric complications.

KEY POINTS

- Pityriasis rosea is a self-limited, inflammatory disorder of the skin possibly caused by human herpesvirus types 6, 7, or 8 or drugs.
- An initial 2- to 10-cm herald patch is followed by centripetal eruption of oval papules and plaques with a slightly raised and scaly border, typically appearing along skin lines.
- Diagnose based on clinical appearance and distribution.
- Treat with antipruritic drugs as needed and possibly topical corticosteroids and/or sunlight.
- Pityriasis rosea during the first 15 wk of pregnancy is associated with premature birth or fetal demise.
- Pregnant women should be offered antiviral therapy, even though this has not proved to reduce obstetric complications.

PITYRIASIS RUBRA PILARIS

Pityriasis rubra pilaris is a rare chronic disorder that causes hyperkeratotic yellowing of the skin, including the trunk, extremities, and, particularly, the palms and soles. Red follicular papules typically merge to form red-orange scaling plaques and confluent areas of erythema with islands of normal skin between lesions.

The cause of pityriasis rubra pilaris is unknown.

The 2 most common forms of the disorder are

- Juvenile classic (characterized by autosomal dominant inheritance and childhood onset)
- Adult classic (characterized by no apparent inheritance and adult onset)

Atypical (nonclassic) forms exist in both age groups. Sunlight, HIV or another infection, minor trauma, or an autoimmune disorder may trigger a flare-up.

Diagnosis

- Clinical evaluation

Diagnosis of pityriasis rubra pilaris is by clinical appearance and may be supported by biopsy.

Differential diagnosis includes seborrheic dermatitis (in children) and psoriasis when disease occurs on the scalp, elbows, and knees.

Treatment

- Symptom relief (eg, with emollients, topical lactic acid and topical corticosteroids, or oral retinoids)

Treatment of pityriasis rubra pilaris is exceedingly difficult and empiric. The disorder may be ameliorated but almost never cured; classic forms of the disorder resolve slowly over 3 yr, whereas nonclassic forms persist. Scaling may be reduced with emollients or 12% lactic acid under occlusive dressing, followed by topical corticosteroids. Oral vitamin A may be effective. Oral acitretin (a retinoid) or methotrexate is an option when a patient is resistant to topical treatment.

Phototherapy, immunomodulatory agents (biologics), cyclosporine, mycophenolate mofetil, azathioprine, and corticosteroids have also been used.[1]

1. Eastham AB, Femia A, Qureshi A, et al: Treatment options for pityriasis rubra pilaris including biologic agents: a retrospective analysis from an academic medical center. *JAMA Dermatol* 150(1):92–94, 2014. doi:10.1001/jamadermatol.2013.4773.

136 Reactions to Sunlight

The skin may respond to sunlight with chronic (eg, dermatoheliosis [photoaging], actinic keratosis) or acute (eg, photosensitivity, sunburn) changes.

Ultraviolet (UV) radiation: The sun emits a wide range of electromagnetic radiation. Most of the dermatologic effects of sunlight are caused by UV radiation, which is divided into 3 bands (UVA, 320 to 400 nm; UVB, 280 to 320 nm; and UVC, 100 to 280 nm). Because the atmosphere filters the radiation, only UVA and UVB reach the earth's surface. The character and amount of sunburn-producing rays (primarily wavelengths < 320 nm) reaching the earth's surface vary greatly with the following factors:

- Atmospheric and surface conditions
- Latitude
- Season
- Time of day
- Altitude
- Ozone layer

Exposure of skin to sunlight also depends on multiple lifestyle factors (eg, clothing, occupation, recreational activities).

Sunburn-producing rays are filtered out by glass and to a great extent by heavy clouds, smoke, and smog; however, they may still pass through light clouds, fog, or 30 cm of clear water, potentially causing severe burns. Snow, sand, and water enhance exposure by reflecting the rays. Exposure is increased at low latitudes (nearer the equator), in the summer, and during midday (10 AM to 3 PM) because sunlight passes through the atmosphere more directly (ie, at less of an angle) in these settings. Exposure is also increased at high altitudes primarily because of a thinner atmosphere. Stratospheric ozone, which filters out UV radiation, especially shorter wavelengths, is depleted by man-made chlorofluorocarbons (eg, in refrigerants and aerosols). A decreased ozone layer increases the amount of UVA and UVB reaching the earth's surface.

Sun-tanning lamps use artificial light that is more UVA than UVB. This UVA use is often advertised as a "safer" way to tan; however, many of the same long-term deleterious effects occur as with UVB exposure, including photoaging and skin cancer. UV light emitted from tanning beds has been classified as a human carcinogen, and indoor tanning has been shown to increase the risk of melanoma. Quite simply, there is no "safe" tan.

Pathophysiology

Adverse effects of UV exposure include acute sunburn and several chronic changes. Chronic changes include skin thickening, wrinkling, and certain lesions such as actinic keratosis and cancer. Exposure also leads to inactivation and loss of epidermal Langerhans cells, which are an important part of the skin's immune system.

As a protective response after exposure to sunlight, the epidermis thickens, and melanocytes produce the pigment melanin at an increased rate, causing what is commonly referred to as a "tan." Tanning provides some natural protection against UV radiation but otherwise has no health benefits.

People differ greatly in their sensitivity and response to sunlight, based mainly on the amount of melanin in the skin. The skin has been classified into 6 types (I to VI) in order of decreasing susceptibility to sun injury. Classification is based on the interrelated variables of skin color, UV sensitivity, and response to sun exposure. Skin type I is white to very lightly pigmented, very sensitive to UV light, has no immediate pigment darkening, always burns easily, and never tans. Skin type VI is dark brown or black, is most protected from UV light, and is a deep dark (black-brown) color with or without sun exposure. However, dark-skinned people are not immune to the effects of the sun, and darkly pigmented skin can develop sun damage with strong or prolonged exposure. Long-term effects of UV exposure in dark-skinned people are the same as those in light-skinned people but are often delayed and less severe because the melanin in their skin provides built-in UV protection.

People with blonde or red hair are especially susceptible to the acute and chronic effects of UV radiation. Uneven melanocyte activation occurs in many of these fair-haired people and results in freckling.

There is no skin pigmentation in people with albinism because of a defect in melanin metabolism. Patchy areas of depigmentation are present in patients with vitiligo because of immunologic destruction of melanocytes. These and any other group of people who are unable to produce melanin at a rapid and complete rate are especially susceptible to sun damage.

Prevention

Avoiding the sun, wearing protective clothing, and applying sunscreen help minimize UV exposure.

Avoiding the sun: Simple precautions help prevent sunburn and the chronic effects of sunlight. These precautions are recommended for people of all skin types, particularly those who are fair skinned and burn easily. Exposure to bright midday sun and other high-UV environments (see p. 1076) should be minimized (30 min or less), even for people with dark skin. In temperate zones, UV ray intensity is less before 10 AM and after 3 PM because more sunburn-producing wavelengths are filtered out. Fog and clouds do not reduce risk significantly, and risk is increased at high altitudes and low latitudes (eg, at the equator).

Although sun exposure helps generate vitamin D, most experts recommend maintaining adequate vitamin D levels by consuming supplements if needed rather than by intentional sunlight exposure.

Protective clothing: Skin exposure to UV radiation can be minimized through the use of protective coverings such as hats, shirts, pants, and sunglasses. Fabrics with a tight weave block the sun better than fabrics with a loose weave. Special clothing that provides high sun protection is commercially available. This type of clothing is labeled with UV protection factor (UPF) followed by a number that indicates the level of protection (similar to sunscreen labeling). Broad-brimmed hats help protect the face, ears, and neck, but these areas still need supplemental protection with a topical sunscreen. Regular use of UV-protective, wrap-around sunglasses helps shield the eyes and eyelids.

Sunscreens: Sunscreens help protect the skin from sunburn and chronic sun damage by absorbing or reflecting the sun's UV rays. Older sunscreens tended to filter only UVB light, but most newer sunscreens now effectively filter UVA light as well and are labeled "broad spectrum." In the US, the FDA rates sunscreens by sun protection factor (SPF): the higher the number, the greater the protection. The SPF only quantifies the protection against UVB exposure; there is no scale for UVA protection. People should typically use a broad-spectrum sunscreen with an SPF rating of 30 or higher.

Sunscreens are available in a wide variety of formulations, including creams, gels, foams, sprays, and sticks. Self-tanning products do not provide significant protection from UV exposure.

Most sunscreens contain several agents that function as chemical screens, absorbing light or providing a physical screen that reflects or scatters light. Sunscreen ingredients that absorb UVB radiation include cinnamates, salicylates, and PABA derivatives. Benzophenones are commonly used to provide UVB and short-wave UVA protection. Avobenzone and ecamsule filter in the UVA range and may be added to provide further UVA protection.

Other sunscreens, called sunblocks, contain zinc oxide and titanium dioxide, which physically reflect both UVB and UVA rays (thus blocking them from reaching the skin). Although previously very white and pasty when applied, micronized formulations of these products have significantly improved their cosmetic acceptability.

Sunscreen failure is common and usually results from insufficient application of the product, too-late application (sunscreens should optimally be applied 30 min before exposure), failure to reapply after swimming or exercise, or failure to apply every 2 to 3 h during sun exposure.

Allergic or photoallergic reactions can occur to sunscreens and must be distinguished from other photosensitive skin eruptions. Patch or photopatch testing with sunscreen components may be necessary to make the diagnosis. This testing is usually done by dermatologists with expertise in allergic contact dermatitis.

CHRONIC EFFECTS OF SUNLIGHT

Photoaging: Chronic exposure to sunlight ages the skin (photoaging, dermatoheliosis, extrinsic aging), primarily by causing destruction of skin collagen due to various biochemical and DNA disruptions. Skin changes include both fine and coarse wrinkles, rough leathery texture, mottled pigmentation, lentigines (large frecklelike spots), sallowness, and telangiectasia.

Actinic keratoses: Actinic keratoses are precancerous changes in skin cells (keratinocytes) that are a frequent, disturbing consequence of many years of sun exposure. People with blonde or red hair, blue eyes, and skin type I or II are particularly susceptible.

Actinic keratoses are usually pink or red, poorly marginated, and feel rough and scaly on palpation, although some are light gray or pigmented, giving them a brown appearance. They should be differentiated from seborrheic keratoses, which increase in number and size with age. Seborrheic keratoses tend to appear waxy and stuck-on but can take on an appearance similar to actinic keratoses. Close inspection usually reveals distinguishing characteristics of the lesion. Unlike actinic keratoses, seborrheic keratoses also occur on non–sun-exposed areas of the body and are not premalignant.

Skin cancers: The incidence of squamous cell carcinoma and basal cell carcinoma in fair, light-skinned people is directly proportional to the total annual sunlight in the area. Such lesions are especially common among people who were extensively exposed to sunlight as children and adolescents and among those who are chronically exposed to the sun as part of their profession or recreational activities (eg, athletes, farmers, ranchers, sailors, frequent sunbathers). Sun exposure also substantially increases the risk of malignant melanoma.

Treatment

- Minimization of UV light exposure
- Topical treatments for photoaged skin

Treatment begins with preventive efforts to minimize UV light exposure—avoiding the sun and tanning beds and wearing protective clothing and sunscreen.

Photoaging: Various combination therapies, including chemical peels, 5-fluorouracil (5-FU), topical alpha-hydroxy acids, imiquimod, photodynamic therapy, and tretinoin, have been used to reduce carcinogenic changes and improve the cosmetic appearance of chronically sun-damaged skin. These therapies are often effective in ameliorating superficial skin changes (eg, fine wrinkles, irregular pigmentation, sallowness, roughness, minor laxity) but have a much less pronounced effect on deeper changes (eg, telangiectasias). Many ingredients are used in OTC cosmetic products without significant evidence that they improve chronic changes of the skin caused by sunlight.

Actinic keratoses: There are several options, depending on the number and location of lesions:

- Cryotherapy or curettage with electrocautery
- Topical 5-FU
- Photodynamic therapy
- Topical imiquimod or ingenol mebutate

If only a few actinic keratoses are present, especially if large, cryotherapy (freezing with liquid nitrogen) or curettage with electrocautery are rapid and highly effective treatments.

If there are too many lesions for cryotherapy or curettage with electrocautery, topical 5-FU applied to the affected area nightly or twice daily for 2 to 6 wk often clears the majority of lesions. Several strengths and formulations of 5-FU are commercially available. Many patients tolerate 0.5% 5-FU cream applied once/day for 4 wk on the face better than stronger concentrations. Actinic keratoses on the arms may require stronger concentrations, such as 5% cream.

Topical 5-FU causes an inflammatory reaction, with redness, scaling, and burning, often affecting areas with no visible actinic keratoses. The intensity of this unsightly and uncomfortable reaction correlates with the effectiveness of treatment. However, if the reaction is too uncomfortable, application may be suspended for 1 to 3 days and, if necessary, can be suppressed with topical corticosteroids. Topical 5-FU has few significant adverse effects except for this reaction. 5-FU should not be used to treat basal cell carcinomas, except those shown by biopsy to be superficial.

Photodynamic therapy involves topical application of a systemic photosensitizer (eg, aminolevulinate or methyl aminolevulinate), followed by light of a specific wavelength that causes preferential damage of photodamaged skin vs normal skin. After treatment, the skin appears similar to how it would look after a mild to moderate sunburn. Significant benefits include the ability to treat multiple lesions at one time and a shorter downtime (when skin appears red, scaly, and irritated) compared to topical creams such as imiquimod and 5-FU.

The topical immunomodulator imiquimod is often used for treatment of actinic keratoses and superficial basal cell carcinomas. Imiquimod stimulates the immune system to recognize and destroy these precancerous skin lesions and early skin cancers. Duration of treatment for actinic keratoses is about 12 to 16 wk. A newer topical gel, ingenol mebutate, can be applied for 2 to 3 days to treat actinic keratoses and has the advantage of a short course of therapy. The skin reactions to imiquimod and ingenol mebutate are similar to those of 5-FU, with redness, scaling, and crusting occurring in most patients.

For treatment of skin cancers, see p. 1011.

PHOTOSENSITIVITY

Photosensitivity is a cutaneous overreaction to sunlight. It may be idiopathic or occur after exposure to certain toxic or allergenic drugs or chemicals, and it is sometimes a feature of systemic disorders (eg, SLE, porphyria, pellagra, xeroderma pigmentosum). Diagnosis is clinical. Treatment varies by type.

In addition to the acute and chronic effects of sunlight, a variety of less common reactions may occur after sun exposure. Unless the cause is obvious, patients with pronounced photosensitivity should be evaluated for systemic or cutaneous disorders associated with light sensitivity such as SLE and porphyria.

Solar urticaria: In certain patients, urticaria develops at a site of sun exposure within a few minutes. Rarely, if large areas are involved, syncope, dizziness, wheezing, and other systemic symptoms may develop. Etiology is unclear but may involve endogenous skin constituents functioning as photoallergens, leading to mast cell degranulation as in other types of urticaria. Solar urticaria can be distinguished from other types of urticaria in that wheals in solar urticaria occur only on exposed skin after UV light exposure.

Solar urticaria can be classified based on the component of the UV spectrum (UVA, UVB, and visible light) that causes them (and thus how such exposures could be subsequently prevented or minimized). If necessary, patients can be tested by exposing part of the skin to natural light or artificial light at particular wavelengths (phototesting).

Treatment can be difficult and may include H_1 blockers, antimalarial drugs, topical corticosteroids, sunscreens, psoralen plus ultraviolet A (PUVA) light, and/or narrow band UVB light. The wheals of solar urticaria usually last just minutes to hours, but the disorder is chronic and can wax and wane over years.

Chemical photosensitivity: Over 100 substances, ingested or applied topically, are known to predispose to cutaneous reactions after sun exposure. A limited number are responsible for most reactions (see Table 136–1). Reactions are divided

Table 136–1. SOME SUBSTANCES THAT CAUSE CUTANEOUS PHOTOSENSITIVITY

CATEGORY	SPECIFIC SUBSTANCE
Acne drugs	Isotretinoin
Analgesics	NSAIDs (especially piroxicam and ketoprofen)
Antibiotics	Quinolones
	Sulfonamides
	Tetracyclines
	Trimethoprim
Antidepressants	Tricyclics
Antifungals	Griseofulvin
Antihyperglycemics	Sulfonylureas
Antimalarials	Chloroquine
	Quinine
Antipsychotics	Phenothiazines
Anxiolytics	Alprazolam
	Chlordiazepoxide
Chemotherapy drugs	Dacarbazine
	Fluorouracil
	Methotrexate
	Vinblastine
Diuretics	Furosemide
	Thiazides
Heart drugs	Amiodarone
	Quinidine
Topical preparations*	Antibacterials (eg, chlorhexidine, hexachlorophene)
	Coal tar
	Fragrances
	Furocoumarin-containing plants (eg, limes, celery, parsley)
	Sunscreens

*There are many topical preparations. The specific substances listed are examples.

into phototoxicity and photoallergy. Phototesting can help confirm the diagnosis. Treatment for chemical photosensitivity is topical corticosteroids and avoidance of the causative substance.

In **phototoxicity,** light-absorbing compounds directly generate free radicals and inflammatory mediators, causing tissue damage manifesting as pain and erythema (like sunburn). This reaction does not require prior sun exposure and can appear in any person, although reaction is highly variable. Typical causes of phototoxic reactions include topical (eg, perfumes, coal tar, furocoumarin-containing plants [such as limes, celery, and parsley], drugs used for photodynamic therapy) or ingested (eg, tetracyclines, diuretics) agents. Phototoxic reactions do not generalize to non-sun-exposed skin.

Photoallergy is a type IV (cell-mediated) immune response. Light absorption causes structural changes in the drug or substance, allowing it to bind to tissue protein and function as a hapten, making the complex allergenic. Prior exposure to the allergen is required. The reaction is usually eczematous, with erythema, scaling, pruritus and sometimes vesicles. Typical causes of photoallergic reactions include aftershave lotions, sunscreens, and sulfonamides. Photoallergy occurs less often than phototoxicity, and the reaction may extend to non-sun-exposed skin.

Polymorphous light eruption: Polymorphous light eruption is a common photosensitive reaction to UV and sometimes visible light. It does not seem to be associated with systemic disease or drugs. A positive family history in some patients suggests a genetic risk factor.

Eruptions appear on sun-exposed areas, usually 30 min to several hours after exposure; however, sometimes eruptions do not appear for up to several days. Lesions are pruritic, erythematous, and often papular but may be papulovesicular or plaquelike. They are more common among women and people from northern climates when first exposed to spring or summer sun than among those exposed to sun year-round. Lesions often subside within several days to weeks.

Diagnosis is made by history, skin findings, and exclusion of other sun-sensitivity disorders. Diagnosis sometimes requires reproduction of the lesions with phototesting when the patient is not using any potentially photosensitizing drugs.

Often, lesions are self-limited and spontaneously improve as summer progresses. Preventive measures include using a broad-spectrum sunscreen and moderating sun exposure. More severely affected patients may benefit from desensitization in early spring by graduated exposure to UV light with low-dose psoralen plus ultraviolet A (PUVA—see p. 1072) or narrowband UVB (312 nm) phototherapy. Mild to moderate eruptions are treated with topical corticosteroids. Patients with disabling disease may require a course of oral immunosuppressive therapy such as prednisone, azathioprine, cyclosporine, or hydroxychloroquine.

SUNBURN

Sunburn is characterized by erythema and sometimes pain and blisters caused by overexposure to solar UV radiation. Treatment is similar to that for thermal burns, including cool compresses, NSAIDs, and, for severe cases, sterile dressings and topical antimicrobials. Prevention by sun avoidance and use of sunscreens is crucial.

Sunburn results from overexposure of the skin to UV radiation; wavelengths in the UVB spectrum (280 to 320 nm) cause the most pronounced effects.

Symptoms and Signs

Symptoms and signs appear in 1 to 24 h and, except in severe reactions, peak within 72 h (usually between 12 h and 24 h). Skin changes range from mild erythema, with subsequent superficial scaling, to pain, swelling, skin tenderness, and blisters. Constitutional symptoms (eg, fever, chills, weakness, shock), similar to a thermal burn, may develop if a large portion of the body surface is affected; these symptoms may be caused by the release of inflammatory cytokines such as IL-1. Very sunburned skin may exfoliate days later.

The most common complications are secondary infection, permanent blotchy pigmentation, and significantly increased risk of skin cancer. Exfoliated skin may be extremely vulnerable to sunlight for several weeks.

Treatment

- Cold compresses, NSAIDs

Further exposure should be avoided until sunburn has completely subsided. Cold tap-water compresses and oral NSAIDs help relieve symptoms, as may topical treatments (eg, aloe vera, petrolatum-based products such as petroleum jelly). Topical corticosteroids are no more effective than cool compresses. Blistered areas should be managed similarly to other partial-thickness burns (see p. 2957), with sterile dressings and silver sulfadiazine. Ointments or lotions containing local anesthetics (eg, benzocaine) or diphenhydramine typically should be avoided because of the risk of allergic contact dermatitis.

Early treatment of extensive, severe sunburn with a systemic corticosteroid (eg, prednisone 20 to 30 mg po bid for 4 days for adults or adolescents) may decrease the discomfort, but this use is controversial.

Prevention

Simple precautions (eg, avoiding the sun especially during midday; wearing tightly woven clothing, a hat, and sunglasses; applying sunscreens) significantly reduce the chances of sunburn.

137 Sweating Disorders

There are two types of sweat glands: apocrine and eccrine.

Apocrine glands are clustered in the axillae, areolae, genitals, and anus; modified apocrine glands are found in the external auditory meatus. Apocrine glands become active at puberty; their excretions are oily and viscid and are presumed to play a role in sexual olfactory messages. The most common disorder of apocrine glands is

- Bromhidrosis

Hidradenitis suppurativa also affects the apocrine glands and is discussed elsewhere.

Eccrine glands are sympathetically innervated, distributed over the entire body, and active from birth. Their secretions are watery and serve to cool the body in hot environments or during activity. Disorders of eccrine glands include

- Hyperhidrosis
- Hypohidrosis
- Miliaria

BROMHIDROSIS

Bromhidrosis is excessive or abnormal body odor caused by decomposition by bacteria and yeasts of sweat gland secretions and cellular debris.

Apocrine secretions are lipid-rich, sterile, and odorless but become odoriferous when decomposed by bacteria into volatile acids on the skin surface.

Eccrine sweat is generally not malodorous because it is nearly 100% water.

Eccrine bromhidrosis can occur when bacteria degrade keratin that has been softened by eccrine sweat. Eccrine bromhidrosis can also result from ingestion of foods (eg, curry, garlic, onion, alcohol) and drugs (eg, penicillin).

Recent studies suggest a strong correlation between bromhidrosis and wetness or stickiness of earwax (in association with a single nucleotide polymorphism of the *ABCC11*).[1]

In some people, a few days of washing with an antiseptic soap, which may be combined with use of antibacterial creams containing clindamycin or erythromycin, may be necessary. Shaving the hair in the armpits may also help control odor.

1. Nakano M, Miwa N, Hirano A, et al: A strong association of axillary osmidrosis with the wet earwax type determined by genotyping of the *ABCC11* gene. *BMC Genetics* 10:42, 2009. doi:10.1186/1471-2156-10-42.

HYPERHIDROSIS

Hyperhidrosis is excessive sweating, which can be focal or diffuse and has multiple causes. Sweating of the axillae, palms, and soles is most often a normal response due to stress, exercise, or environmental heat; diffuse sweating is usually idiopathic but, in patients with compatible findings, should raise suspicion for cancer, infection, and endocrine disease. Diagnosis is obvious, but tests for underlying causes may be indicated. Treatments include topical aluminum chloride, tap-water iontophoresis, botulinum toxin, oral glycopyrrolate, and, in extreme cases, surgery.

Etiology

Hyperhidrosis can be focal or generalized.

Focal sweating: Emotional causes are common, causing sweating on the palms, soles, axillae, and forehead at times of anxiety, excitement, anger, or fear. It may be due to a generalized stress-increased sympathetic outflow. Sweating is also common during exercise and in hot environments. Although such sweating is a normal response, patients with hyperhidrosis sweat excessively and under conditions that do not cause sweating in most people.

Gustatory sweating occurs around the lips and mouth when ingesting foods and beverages that are spicy or hot in temperature. There is no known cause in most cases, but gustatory sweating can be increased in diabetic neuropathy, facial herpes zoster, cervical sympathetic ganglion invasion, CNS injury or disease, or parotid gland injury. In the case of parotid gland injury, surgery, infection, or trauma may disrupt parotid gland innervation and lead to regrowth of parotid parasympathetic fibers into sympathetic fibers innervating local sweat glands in skin where the injury took place, usually over the parotid gland. This condition is called Frey syndrome. Asymmetric sweating can be caused by a neurologic abnormality.

Other causes of focal sweating include pretibial myxedema (shins), hypertrophic osteoarthropathy (palms), and blue rubber bleb nevus syndrome and glomus tumor (over lesions). Compensatory sweating is intense sweating after sympathectomy.

Generalized sweating: Generalized sweating involves most of the body. Although most cases are idiopathic, numerous conditions can be involved (see Table 137–1).

Symptoms and Signs

Sweating is often present during examination and sometimes is extreme. Clothing can be soaked, and palms or soles may become macerated and fissured. Hyperhidrosis can cause emotional distress to patients and may lead to social withdrawal. Palmar or plantar skin may appear pale.

Diagnosis

- History and examination
- Iodine and starch test
- Tests to identify a cause

Hyperhidrosis is diagnosed by history and examination but can be confirmed with the iodine and starch test. For this test, iodine solution is applied to the affected area and allowed to dry. Cornstarch is then dusted on the area, which makes areas of sweating appear dark. Testing is necessary only to confirm foci of sweating (as in Frey syndrome, or to locate the area needing surgical or botulinum toxin treatment) or in a semiquantitative way when following the course of treatment. Asymmetry in the pattern of sweating suggests a neurologic cause.

Table 137–1. SOME CAUSES OF GENERALIZED SWEATING

TYPE	EXAMPLES
Cancer*	Lymphoma, leukemia
CNS	Trauma, autonomic neuropathy, cervical sympathetic ganglion invasion
Drugs	Antidepressants, aspirin, NSAIDs, hypoglycemic agents, caffeine, theophylline; opioid withdrawal
Endocrine disorders	Hyperthyroidism, hypoglycemia, excessive secretion of sex hormones caused by GnRH agonists
Idiopathic	—
Infections*	TB, endocarditis, systemic fungal infections
Other	Carcinoid syndrome, pregnancy, menopause, anxiety

*Primarily nocturnal generalized sweating (night sweats).
GnRH = gonadotropin-releasing hormone.

Laboratory tests to identify a cause of hyperhidrosis are guided by the patient's other symptoms and might include, for example, CBC to detect leukemia, serum glucose to detect diabetes, and thyroid-stimulating hormone to screen for thyroid dysfunction.

Treatment

- Aluminum chloride hexahydrate solution
- Tap-water iontophoresis
- Botulinum toxin type A
- Oral anticholinergic drugs
- Surgery

Initial treatment of focal and generalized sweating is similar.

Aluminum chloride hexahydrate 6 to 20% solution in absolute ethyl alcohol is indicated for topical treatment of axillary, palmar, and plantar sweating; these preparations require a prescription. The solution precipitates salts, which block sweat ducts; it is most effective when applied nightly; it should be washed off in the morning. Sometimes an anticholinergic drug is taken before applying to prevent sweat from washing the aluminum chloride away. Initially, several applications weekly are needed to achieve control, then a maintenance schedule of once or twice weekly is followed. If treatment under occlusion is irritating, it should be tried without occlusion. This solution should not be applied to inflamed, broken, wet, or recently shaved skin. High-concentration, water-based aluminum chloride solutions may provide adequate relief in milder cases.

Tap-water iontophoresis, in which salt ions are introduced into the skin using electric current, is an option for patients unresponsive to topical treatments. The affected areas (typically palms or soles) are placed in tap-water basins each containing an electrode across which a 15- to 25-mA current is applied for 10 to 20 min. This routine is done daily for 1 wk and then repeated weekly or bimonthly. Iontophoresis may be made more effective by dissolving anticholinergic tablets (eg, glycopyrrolate) into the water of the iontophoresis basins. Although the treatments are usually effective, the technique is time-consuming and somewhat cumbersome, and some patients tire of the routine.

Botulinum toxin type A is a neurotoxin that decreases the release of acetylcholine from sympathetic nerves serving eccrine glands. Injected directly into the axillae, palms, or forehead, botulinum toxin inhibits sweating for about 5 mo depending on dose. Of note, botulinum toxin is FDA-approved only for axillary hyperhidrosis and may not be covered by insurance for other sites of hyperhidrosis. Complications include local muscle weakness and headache. Injections are effective but painful and expensive.

Oral anticholinergic drugs may help some patients. Glycopyrrolate or oxybutynin can be used until the degree of sweating becomes tolerable or anticholinergic adverse effects become intolerable. Potential side effects include dry mouth, dry skin, flushing, blurred vision, urinary retention, mydriasis, and cardiac arrhythmias.

Surgery is indicated if more conservative treatments fail. Patients with axillary sweating can be treated with surgical excision of axillary sweat glands through open dissection or by liposuction (the latter appears to have lower morbidity). Patients with palmar sweating can be treated with endoscopic transthoracic sympathectomy. The potential morbidity of surgery must be considered, especially in sympathectomy. Potential complications include phantom sweating (a sensation of sweating in the absence of sweating), compensatory hyperhidrosis (increased sweating in untreated parts of the body), gustatory sweating, neuralgia, and Horner syndrome. Compensatory hyperhidrosis is most common after endoscopic transthoracic sympathectomy, developing in up to 80% of patients, and can be disabling and far worse than the original problem.

KEY POINTS

- Asymmetric hyperhidrosis suggests a neurologic cause.
- Although diffuse sweating is usually normal, consider cancer, infection, and endocrine disorders as directed by patient symptoms.
- Obtain laboratory tests to determine systemic causes based on clinical findings.
- Treat using aluminum chloride solutions, tap-water iontophoresis, botulinum toxin, or oral glycopyrrolate.

HYPOHIDROSIS

Hypohidrosis is inadequate sweating.

Hypohidrosis due to skin abnormalities is rarely clinically significant. It is most commonly focal and caused by local skin injury (eg, due to trauma, radiation, infection [eg, leprosy], or inflammation) or by atrophy of glands resulting from connective tissue disease (eg, systemic sclerosis, systemic lupus erythematosus, Sjögren syndrome).

Hypohidrosis may be caused by drugs, especially those with anticholinergic properties. It is also caused by diabetic neuropathy and a variety of congenital syndromes. Heatstroke causes inadequate sweating but is a CNS rather than a skin disorder.

Diagnosis is by clinical observation of decreased sweating or by heat intolerance. Treatment is by cooling measures (eg, air-conditioning, wet garments).

MILIARIA

In miliaria, sweat flow is obstructed and trapped within the skin, causing skin lesions.

Miliaria most often occurs in warm humid weather but may occur in cool weather in an overdressed, hospitalized, or bedridden patient. Lesions vary depending on the depth of tissue at which the sweat duct is obstructed.

- **Miliaria crystallina** is ductal obstruction in the uppermost epidermis, with retention of sweat subcorneally. It causes clear, droplike vesicles that rupture with light pressure.
- **Miliaria rubra** (prickly heat) is ductal obstruction in the mid-epidermis with retention of sweat in the epidermis and dermis. It causes irritated, pruritic papules (prickling).
- **Miliaria pustulosa** is similar to miliaria rubra but manifests as pustules rather than papules.
- **Miliaria profunda** is ductal obstruction at the entrance of the duct into the dermal papillae at the dermo-epidermal junction, with retention of sweat in the dermis. It causes papules that are larger and more deeply seated than those of miliaria rubra. Papules are frequently painful.

Diagnosis is by clinical appearance in the context of a hot environment or skin occlusion (eg, hospitalized or bedridden patients who lie with their back against the hospital bed for prolonged periods).

Treatment is cooling and drying of the involved areas and avoidance of conditions that may induce sweating; an air-conditioned environment is ideal. Once the rash develops, corticosteroid creams or lotions can be used, sometimes with a bit of menthol added.

138 Viral Skin Diseases

MOLLUSCUM CONTAGIOSUM

Molluscum contagiosum is characterized by clusters of pink, dome-shaped, smooth, waxy, or pearly and umbilicated papules 2 to 5 mm in diameter caused by molluscum contagiosum virus, a poxvirus. Diagnosis is based on clinical appearance. Treatment aims to prevent spread or remove cosmetically unacceptable lesions and can include mechanical methods (eg, curettage, cryosurgery) and topical irritants (eg, imiquimod, cantharidin, tretinoin).

Molluscum contagiosum virus commonly causes a localized chronic infection. Transmission is by direct contact; spread occurs by autoinoculation and via fomites (eg, towels, bath sponges) and bath water. Molluscum contagiosum is common among children. Adults acquire the infection via close skin-to-skin contact with an infected person (eg, sexual contact, wrestling). Patients with immunocompromise (eg, due to HIV/AIDS, corticosteroid use, or chemotherapy) may develop a more widespread infection.

Symptoms and Signs

Molluscum contagiosum can appear anywhere on the skin except the palms and soles. Lesions consist of clusters of pink, dome-shaped, smooth, waxy, or pearly and umbilicated papules, usually 2 to 5 mm in diameter, which occur most commonly on the face, trunk, and extremities in children and on the pubis, penis, or vulva in adults. Lesions may grow to 10 to 15 mm in diameter, especially among patients with HIV infection and other immunodeficiencies.

Lesions are usually not pruritic or painful and may be discovered only coincidentally during a physical examination. However, the lesions can become inflamed and itchy as the body fights off the virus.

Diagnosis

- Clinical evaluation

Diagnosis of molluscum contagiosum is based on clinical appearance; skin biopsy or smear of expressed material shows characteristic inclusion bodies but is necessary only when diagnosis is uncertain.

Differential diagnosis includes folliculitis, milia, and warts (for lesions < 2 mm) and juvenile xanthogranuloma and Spitz nevus (for lesions > 2 mm).

Treatment

- Curettage, cryosurgery, laser therapy, or electrocautery
- Topical irritants (eg, trichloroacetic acid, cantharidin, tretinoin, tazarotene, podophyllotoxin)
- Sometimes combination therapies

Most lesions spontaneously regress in 1 to 2 yr, but they can remain for 2 to 3 yr. Treatment of molluscum contagiosum is indicated for cosmetic reasons or for prevention of spread. Options include curettage, cryosurgery, laser therapy, electrocautery, trichloroacetic acid (25 to 40% solution), cantharidin, podophyllotoxin (in adults), tretinoin, and tazarotene. Some clinicians use salicylic acid, but others consider it too irritating for many body areas where molluscum occurs. Similar concerns exist with use of potassium hydroxide (KOH). Imiquimod is usually not recommended.[1] Molluscum lesions within the orbital rim should be removed via gentle destruction by a skilled health care practitioner. Lesions may be gently squeezed with a forceps to remove the central core. Treatments that cause minimal pain (eg, tretinoin, tazarotene, cantharidin) are used first, especially in children.

Curettage or liquid nitrogen can be used 40 to 60 min after application of a topical anesthetic such as eutectic mixture of local anesthetics (EMLA) or 4% lidocaine cream under an occlusive dressing. EMLA cream must be applied judiciously because it can cause systemic toxicity, especially in children. In adults, curettage is very effective but painful if done without anesthetic. Dermatologists often use combination therapy such as liquid nitrogen or cantharidin in the office or a retinoid cream at home. This form of therapy is typically successful, but resolution often takes 1 to 2 mo in some patients.

Cantharidin is safe and effective but can cause blistering. Cantharidin is applied in 1 small drop directly to the molluscum lesion. Areas that patients (especially children) may rub are covered with a bandage because contact with the fingers should be avoided. Cantharidin should not be applied to the face or near the eyes because blistering is unpredictable. If cantharidin comes into contact with the cornea, it can cause scarring. Cantharidin should be washed off with soap and water in 6 h. Fewer than 15 lesions should be treated in one session because infection may occur after application of cantharidin. Parents should be warned about blistering if their children are prescribed this drug.

Children should not be excluded from school or day care. However, their lesions should be covered to reduce the risk of spread.

1. Katz KA: Dermatologists, imiquimod, and treatment of molluscum contagiosum in children: righting wrongs. *JAMA Dermatol* 151(2):125–126, 2015. doi: 10.1001/jamadermatol.2014.3335.

KEY POINTS

- Molluscum contagiosum, caused by a poxvirus, commonly spreads by direct contact (eg, sexual contact, wrestling), fomites, and bath water.
- Lesions tend to be asymptomatic clusters of 2- to 5-mm diameter papules that are pink, dome-shaped, smooth, waxy, or pearly and umbilicated.
- Diagnosis is based on clinical appearance.
- Treatment is for cosmetic reasons or prevention of spread.
- Treatments can include destructive methods (eg, curettage, cryosurgery, laser therapy, electrocautery) or topical irritants (eg, trichloroacetic acid, cantharidin, tretinoin, tazarotene, podophyllotoxin).

WARTS

(Verrucae Vulgaris)

Warts are common, benign, epidermal lesions caused by human papillomavirus infection. They can appear anywhere on the body in a variety of morphologies. Diagnosis is by examination. Warts are usually self-limited but may

Table 138–1. WART VARIANTS

CLINICAL FORM	HUMAN PAPILLOMAVIRUS TYPE	DESCRIPTION
Bowenoid papulosis*	16, 18, 33, 39	Flat, brown, verrucous papules on the vulva and penis (benign)
Buschke-Löwenstein tumor	6, 11	Large cauliflower-like tumors on the anogenital surface
Butcher's wart (meat handler's wart)	7	Common warts, usually benign, that occur on the hands of meat workers May appear more cauliflower-like than common warts
Epidermodysplasia verruciformis	1–5, 7–9, 10, 12, 14, 15, 17–20, 23–25, 36, 47, 50	Rare, inherited predisposition to develop widespread HPV infection and often skin cancer (such as squamous cell carcinoma) as early as a patient's 20s
Keratoacanthoma	77	Thought to be a well-differentiated squamous cell carcinoma
Oral focal epithelial hyperplasia (Heck disease)	13, 32	Multiple pale, flat-topped, cobblestoned papules in the lining of the mouth Benign
Warts in kidney transplant patients	75–77	Often multiple and difficult to treat

*Affected women and female partners of affected patients should be frequently evaluated for cervical cancer.
HPV = human papillomavirus.

be treated by destructive methods (eg, excision, cautery, cryotherapy, liquid nitrogen) and topical or injected agents.

Warts are almost universal in the population; they affect patients of all ages but are most common among children and are uncommon among the elderly.

Etiology

Warts are caused by human papillomavirus (HPV) infection; there are over 100 HPV subtypes. Trauma and maceration facilitate initial epidermal inoculation. Spread may then occur by autoinoculation. Local and systemic immune factors appear to influence spread; immunosuppressed patients (especially those with HIV infection or a kidney transplant) are at particular risk of developing generalized lesions that are difficult to treat. Humoral immunity provides resistance to HPV infection; cellular immunity helps established infection to regress.

Symptoms and Signs

Warts are named by their clinical appearance and location; different forms are linked to different HPV types (for unusual manifestations, see Table 138–1). Most types are usually asymptomatic. However, some warts are tender, so those on weight-bearing surfaces (eg, bottom of the feet) may cause mild pain.

Common warts: Common warts (verrucae vulgaris) are caused by HPV types 1, 2, 4, 27, and 29. They are usually asymptomatic but sometimes cause mild pain when they are located on a weight-bearing surface (eg, bottom of the feet). Common warts are sharply demarcated, rough, round or irregular, firm, and light gray, yellow, brown, or gray-black nodules 2 to 10 mm in diameter. They appear most often on sites subject to trauma (eg, fingers, elbows, knees, face) but may spread elsewhere. Variants of unusual shape (eg, pedunculated or resembling a cauliflower) appear most frequently on the head and neck, especially the scalp and beard area.

Filiform warts: These warts are long, narrow, frondlike growths, usually located on the eyelids, face, neck, or lips. They are usually asymptomatic. This morphologically distinct variant of the common wart is benign and easy to treat.

Flat warts: Flat warts, caused by HPV types 3, 10, 28, and 49, are smooth, flat-topped, yellow-brown, pink, or flesh-colored papules, most often located on the face and along scratch marks; they are more common among children and young adults and develop by autoinoculation. They generally cause no symptoms but are usually difficult to treat.

Palmar warts and plantar warts: These warts, caused by HPV type 1, occur on the palms and soles; they are flattened by pressure and surrounded by cornified epithelium (see Plate 63). They are often tender and can make walking and standing uncomfortable. They can be distinguished from corns and calluses by their tendency to pinpoint bleeding when the surface is pared away.

Mosaic warts: Mosaic warts are plaques formed by the coalescence of myriad smaller, closely set plantar warts. As with other plantar warts, they are often tender.

Periungual warts: These warts appear as thickened, fissured, cauliflower-like skin around the nail plate. They are usually asymptomatic, but the fissures cause pain as the warts enlarge. Patients frequently lose the cuticle and are susceptible to paronychia. Periungual warts are more common among patients who bite their nails or who have occupations where their hands are chronically wet such as dishwashers and bartenders.

Genital warts: Genital warts manifest as discrete flat to broad-based smooth to velvety papules to rough and pedunculated excrescences on the perineal, perirectal, labial, and penile areas (see Plate 78). Infection with high-risk HPV types (most notably types 16 and 18) is the main cause of cervical cancer. These warts are usually asymptomatic. Perirectal warts often itch.

Diagnosis

- Clinical evaluation
- Rarely biopsy

Diagnosis of warts is based on clinical appearance; biopsy is rarely needed. A cardinal sign of warts is the absence of skin lines crossing their surface and the presence of pinpoint

PEARLS & PITFALLS

- If necessary, confirm the diagnosis of a wart by shaving its surface to reveal thrombosed capillaries in the form of black dots.

black dots (thrombosed capillaries) or bleeding when warts are shaved.

Differential diagnosis of warts includes the following:

- Corns (clavi): May obscure skin lines but do not have thrombosed capillaries when shaved
- Lichen planus: May mimic flat warts but may be accompanied by lacy oral lesions and Wickham striae and may be symmetrically distributed
- Seborrheic keratosis: May appear more stuck on, be pigmented, and include keratin-filled horn cysts
- Skin tags (achrocordon): May be pedunculated and smoother and more flesh-colored than warts
- Squamous cell carcinoma: May be ulcerated, persistent, and grow irregularly

DNA typing of the virus is available in some medical centers but is generally not needed.

Prognosis

Many warts regress spontaneously (particularly common warts); others persist for years and recur at the same or different sites, even with treatment. Factors influencing recurrence appear to be related to the patient's overall immune status as well as local factors. Patients subject to local trauma (eg, athletes, mechanics, butchers) may have recalcitrant and recurrent HPV infection. Genital HPV infection has malignant potential, but malignant transformation is rare in HPV-induced skin warts, except among immunosuppressed patients.

Treatment

- Topical irritants (eg, salicylic acid, cantharidin, podophyllum resin)
- Destructive methods (eg, cryosurgery, electrocautery, curettage, excision, laser)

There are no firm indications for treatment of warts. Treatment should be considered for warts that are cosmetically unacceptable, in locations that interfere with function, or painful. Patients should be motivated to adhere to treatment, which may require a prolonged course and can be unsuccessful. Treatments are less successful in patients with impaired immune systems.

Mechanisms of many irritants include eliciting an immune response to HPV. Such irritants include salicylic acid (SCA), trichloroacetic acid, 5-fluorouracil, podophyllum resin, tretinoin, and cantharidin.

Topical imiquimod 5% cream induces skin cells to locally produce antiviral cytokines. Topical cidofovir, HPV vaccines, and contact immunotherapy (eg, squaric acid dibutyl ester and *Candida* allergen) have been used to treat warts. Warts can first be soaked in hot water at 113° F for 30 min ≥ 3 times/wk. After soaking, the skin is more permeable to topical drugs.

Oral treatments include cimetidine (which has questionable efficacy), isotretinoin, and zinc. IV cidofovir can also be used. In most instances, modalities should be combined to increase the likelihood of success. Direct antiviral effects can be achieved with intralesional injection of bleomycin and interferon alfa-2b, but these treatments are reserved for the most recalcitrant warts.

These drugs can be used in combination with a destructive method (eg, cryosurgery, electrocautery, curettage, excision, laser) because even though a wart may be physically removed by a destructive method, virus may remain in the tissues and cause recurrence.

Common warts: In immunocompetent patients, common warts usually spontaneously regress within 2 to 4 yr, but some linger for many years. Numerous treatments are available. Destructive methods include electrocautery, cryosurgery with liquid nitrogen, and laser surgery. SCA preparations are also commonly used.

Which method is used depends on the location and severity of involvement.

The most common topical agent to be used is SCA. SCA is available as a liquid or plaster or impregnated within tape. For example, 17% liquid SCA can be used on the fingers, and 40% plaster SCA can be used on the soles. Patients apply SCA to their warts at night and leave it on for 8 to 48 h depending on the site.

Cantharidin can be used alone or in combination (1%) with SCA (30%) and podophyllum (5%) in a collodion base. Cantharidin alone is removed with soap and water after 6 h; cantharidin with SCA or podophyllum is removed in 2 h. The longer these agents are left in contact with the skin, the more brisk the blistering response.

Cryosurgery is painful but extremely effective. Electrodesiccation with curettage, laser surgery, or both is effective and indicated for isolated lesions but may cause scarring. Recurrent or new warts occur in about 35% of patients within 1 yr; therefore, methods that scar should be avoided as much as possible so that multiple scars do not accumulate. When possible, scarring treatments are reserved for cosmetically unimportant areas and recalcitrant warts.

Filiform warts: Treatment of filiform warts is removal with scalpel, scissors, curettage, or liquid nitrogen. Liquid nitrogen should be applied so that up to 2 mm of skin surrounding the wart turns white. Damage to the skin occurs when the skin thaws, which usually takes 10 to 20 sec. Blisters can occur 24 to 48 h after treatment with liquid nitrogen. Care must be taken when treating cosmetically sensitive sites, such as the face and neck, because hypopigmentation or hyperpigmentation frequently occurs after treatment with liquid nitrogen. Patients with darkly pigmented skin can develop permanent depigmentation.

Flat warts: Treatment of flat warts is difficult, and flat warts are often longer-lasting than common warts, recalcitrant to treatments, and, in cosmetically important areas, make the most effective (destructive) methods less desirable. Usual first-line treatment is daily tretinoin (retinoic acid 0.05% cream). If peeling is not sufficient for wart removal, another irritant (eg, 5% benzoyl peroxide) or 5% SCA cream can be applied sequentially with tretinoin. Imiquimod 5% cream can be used alone or in combination with topical drugs or destructive measures. Topical 5-fluorouracil (1% or 5% cream) can also be used.

Plantar warts: Treatment of plantar warts is vigorous maceration with 40% SCA plaster kept in place for several days. The wart is then debrided while damp and soft, followed by destruction by freezing or using caustics (eg, 30 to 70% trichloroacetic acid). Other destructive treatments (eg, CO_2 laser, pulsed-dye laser, various acids) are often effective.

PEARLS & PITFALLS

- Take care when treating periungual and lateral finger warts because aggressive liquid nitrogen and cautery can cause permanent nail deformity and rarely nerve injury.

Periungual warts: Combination therapy with liquid nitrogen and imiquimod 5% cream, tretinoin, or SCA is effective and usually safer than liquid nitrogen or cautery.

Recalcitrant warts: Several methods whose long-term value and risks are not fully known are available for the treatment of recalcitrant warts. Intralesional injection of small amounts of a 0.1% solution of bleomycin in saline often cures stubborn plantar and periungual warts. However, Raynaud syndrome or vascular damage may develop in injected digits, especially when the drug is injected at the base of the digit, so caution is warranted. Interferon, especially interferon alfa, given intralesionally (3 times/wk for 3 to 5 wk) or IM, has also cleared recalcitrant skin and genital warts. Extensive warts sometimes abate or clear with oral isotretinoin or acitretin. HPV vaccine has been reported as useful for recalcitrant warts in children, but efficacy of this intervention is not proved.[1]

1. Abeck D, Fölster-Holst R: Quadrivalent human papillomavirus vaccination: a promising treatment for recalcitrant cutaneous warts in children. *Acta Derm Venereol* 95(8):1017–1019, 2015. doi: 10.2340/00015555-2111.

KEY POINTS

- Cutaneous warts are caused by HPVs, are very common, and have multiple forms.
- Spread is usually by autoinoculation and is facilitated by trauma and maceration.
- Most warts are asymptomatic but can be mildly painful with pressure.
- Most warts resolve spontaneously, particularly common warts.
- Treatments, when indicated, commonly include topical irritants (eg, SCA, cantharidin, podophyllum resin) and/or destructive methods (eg, cryosurgery, electrocautery, curettage, excision, laser).

ZOONOTIC DISEASES

Two viral skin diseases are rarely transmitted from animals to humans.

Contagious ecthyma: Contagious ecthyma (contagious pustular dermatitis) is caused by orf virus, a poxvirus that infects ruminants (most often sheep and goats). Farmers, veterinarians, zoo caretakers, and others with direct animal contact are at risk. The cutaneous findings pass through 6 stages that together last about 1 wk:

- Stage 1 (papular): A single red edematous papule on a finger (most commonly right index finder)
- Stage 2 (target): A larger nodule with a red center surrounded by a white ring with a red periphery
- Stage 3 (acute): A rapidly growing infected-looking tumor
- Stage 4 (regenerative): A nodule with black dots covered with a thin transparent crust
- Stage 5 (papillomatous): A nodule with a surface studded with small projections
- Stage 6 (regressive): A flattened nodule with a thick crust

Patients can develop regional adenopathy, lymphangitis, and fever.

Diagnosis of contagious ecthyma is by history of contact; differential diagnosis is extensive depending on the stage of the lesion. Acute lesions must be differentiated from milker's nodules, *Mycobacterium marinum* infection (see Cutaneous disease on p. 1661), and other bacterial infections; regressed lesions must be differentiated from cutaneous tumors, such as Bowen disease or squamous cell carcinoma.

Lesions spontaneously heal; no treatment is necessary.

Milker's nodules: These nodules are caused by paravaccinia virus, a parapoxvirus that causes udder lesions in cows. Infection requires direct contact and causes macules that progress to papules, vesicles, and nodules. This infection has 6 stages, which are similar to those of contagious ecthyma. Fever and lymphadenopathy are uncommon.

Diagnosis of milker's nodules is by history o.f contact and cutaneous findings. Differential diagnosis varies depending on morphology but can include primary inoculation TB (a chancre that can develop at the site of TB inoculation), sporotrichosis, anthrax, and tularemia.

- Lesions heal spontaneously; no treatment is necessary.

SECTION 12

Hematology and Oncology

139 Approach to the Patient with Anemia

RED BLOOD CELL PRODUCTION

Red blood cell (RBC) production (erythropoiesis) takes place in the bone marrow under the control of the hormone erythropoietin (EPO). Juxtaglomerular cells in the kidney produce EPO in response to decreased oxygen delivery (as in anemia and hypoxia) and increased levels of androgens. In addition to EPO, RBC production requires adequate supplies of substrates, mainly iron, vitamin B_{12}, and folate. Vitamin B_{12} and folate are discussed on p. 37; iron is discussed on p. 12 and iron deficiency anemia on p. 1095. Heme synthesis is discussed on p. 1330.

RBCs survive about 120 days. They then lose their cell membranes and are largely cleared from the circulation by the phagocytic cells of the spleen, liver, and bone marrow. Hemoglobin (Hb) is broken down in these cells and in hepatocytes primarily by the heme oxygenase system with conservation (and subsequent reutilization) of iron, degradation of heme to bilirubin through a series of enzymatic steps, and reutilization of protein. Maintenance of a steady number of RBCs requires daily renewal of 1/120 of the cells; immature RBCs (reticulocytes) are continually released and constitute 0.5 to 1.5% of the peripheral RBC population.

With aging, Hb and hematocrit (Hct) decrease slightly, but not below normal values. In women, other factors that frequently contribute to lower levels of RBCs include cumulative menstrual blood loss and increased demand for iron due to multiple pregnancies.

ETIOLOGY OF ANEMIA

Anemia is a decrease in the number of RBCs, Hct, or Hb content.

The RBC mass represents the balance between production and destruction or loss of RBCs. Thus, anemia can result from one or more of 3 basic mechanisms (see Table 139–1):

- Blood loss
- Deficient erythropoiesis
- Excessive hemolysis (RBC destruction)

Blood loss can be acute or chronic. Anemia does not develop until several hours after acute blood loss, when interstitial fluid diffuses into the intravascular space and dilutes the remaining RBC mass. During the first few hours, however, levels of polymorphonuclear granulocytes, platelets, and, in severe hemorrhage, immature WBCs and normoblasts may rise. Chronic blood loss results in anemia if loss is more rapid than can be replaced or, more commonly, if accelerated erythropoiesis depletes body iron stores (see p. 1095).

Deficient erythropoiesis has myriad causes. Complete cessation of erythropoiesis results in a decline in RBCs of about 7 to 10%/wk (1%/day). Impaired erythropoiesis, even if not sufficient to decrease the numbers of RBCs, often causes abnormal RBC size and shape.

Excessive hemolysis can be caused by intrinsic abnormalities of RBCs or by extrinsic factors, such as the presence of antibodies or complement on their surface, that lead to their early destruction. An enlarged spleen sequesters and destroys RBCs more rapidly than normal. Some causes of hemolysis deform as well as destroy RBCs. Hemolysis normally causes increased reticulocyte production unless iron or other essential nutrients are depleted.

EVALUATION OF ANEMIA

Anemia is a decrease in the number of RBCs, Hct, or Hb content. In men, anemia is Hb < 14 g/dL, Hct < 42%, or RBC < 4.5 million/μL. In women, Hb < 12 g/dL, Hct < 37%, or RBC < 4 million/μL is considered anemia. For infants, normal values vary with age, necessitating use of age-related tables.

Anemia is not a diagnosis; it is a manifestation of an underlying disorder (see Etiology of Anemia). Thus, even mild, asymptomatic anemia should be investigated so that the primary problem can be diagnosed and treated.

Anemia is usually suspected based on the history and physical examination. Common symptoms and signs of anemia include

- General fatigue
- Weakness
- Dyspnea on exertion
- Pallor

History and physical examination are followed by laboratory testing with a complete blood count and peripheral smear. The differential diagnosis (and cause of anemia) can then be further refined based on the results of testing.

Table 139–1. CLASSIFICATION OF ANEMIA BY CAUSE

MECHANISM	EXAMPLES
Blood loss	
Acute	Childbirth GI bleeding Injuries Surgery
Chronic	Bladder tumors Cancer or polyps in GI tract Heavy menstrual bleeding Kidney tumors Ulcers in the stomach or small intestine
Deficient erythropoiesis*	
Microcytic	Iron deficiency Iron reutilization defect (anemia of chronic inflammation, infection, cancer) Iron-transport deficiency (iron refractory iron deficiency anemia [IRIDA]) Iron utilization defect (inherited sideroblastic anemia) Thalassemias (also classified under excessive hemolysis due to intrinsic RBC defects)
Normochromic-normocytic	Anemia of chronic inflammation, infection, or cancer Kidney disease Endocrine failure (thyroid, pituitary) Malnutrition Myelodysplasia Myelophthisis Pure RBC aplasia
Macrocytic	Alcohol use disorder Copper deficiency Folate deficiency Liver disease Malabsorption (eg, tropical sprue) Myelodysplasia Vitamin B_{12} deficiency
Excessive hemolysis due to extrinsic RBC defects	
Reticuloendothelial hyperactivity with splenomegaly	Hypersplenism
Immunologic abnormalities	Cold agglutinin disease Drug-induced Paroxysmal cold hemoglobinuria Thrombotic thrombocytopenic purpura (TTP) and hemolytic uremic syndrome (HUS) Warm antibody hemolytic anemia
Infection	Clostridial infections Ebstein Barr virus (EBV) infection Malaria
Mechanical injury	Cardiac valvular disease Foot strike hemolysis
Drugs/toxins	Phenazopyridine Ribavirin Spider bites
Excessive hemolysis due to intrinsic RBC defects	
Membrane alterations, acquired	Hypophosphatemia Paroxysmal nocturnal hemoglobinuria Stomatocytosis
Membrane alterations, congenital	Hereditary elliptocytosis Hereditary spherocytosis

Table continues on the following page.

Table 139–1. CLASSIFICATION OF ANEMIA BY CAUSE (*Continued*)

MECHANISM	EXAMPLES
Metabolic disorders (inherited enzyme deficiencies)	Embden-Meyerhof pathway defects G6PD deficiency
Hemoglobinopathies	Hb C disease Hb E disease Hb S-C disease Hb S–beta-thalassemia disease Sickle cell disease (Hb S) Thalassemias (beta, beta-delta, and alpha)

*Classified according to RBC indices.

History

The history should address

- Risk factors for particular anemias
- Symptoms of anemia itself
- Symptoms that reflect the underlying disorder

Risk factors for anemia: Anemia has many risk factors. For example, a vegan diet predisposes to vitamin B_{12} deficiency anemia, whereas alcoholism increases the risk of folate deficiency anemia. A number of hemoglobinopathies are inherited, and certain drugs predispose to hemolysis. Cancer, rheumatic disorders, and chronic inflammatory disorders can suppress bone marrow activity or enlarge the spleen.

Symptoms of anemia: The symptoms of anemia are neither sensitive nor specific and do not help differentiate between types of anemias. Symptoms reflect compensatory responses to tissue hypoxia and usually develop when the Hb level falls well below the patient's individual baseline. Symptoms are generally more pronounced in patients with limited cardiopulmonary reserve or in whom the anemia developed very rapidly.

Symptoms such as weakness, fatigue, drowsiness, angina, syncope, and dyspnea on exertion can indicate anemia. Vertigo, headache, pulsatile tinnitus, amenorrhea, loss of libido, and GI complaints may also occur. Heart failure or shock can develop in patients with severe tissue hypoxia or hypovolemia.

Symptoms that suggest cause of anemia: Certain symptoms may suggest the cause of the anemia. For example, melena, epistaxis, hematochezia, hematemesis, or menorrhagia indicates bleeding. Jaundice and dark urine, in the absence of liver disease, suggest hemolysis. Weight loss may suggest cancer. Diffuse severe bone or chest pain may suggest sickle cell disease, and stocking-glove paresthesias may suggest vitamin B_{12} deficiency.

PEARLS & PITFALLS

- Anemia is not a diagnosis; it is a manifestation of an underlying disorder. Thus, even mild, asymptomatic anemia should be investigated so that the primary problem can be diagnosed and treated.

Physical Examination

Complete physical examination is necessary. Signs of anemia itself are neither sensitive nor specific; however, pallor is common with severe anemia.

Signs of underlying disorders are often more diagnostically accurate than are signs of anemia. Heme-positive stool identifies GI bleeding. Hemorrhagic shock (eg, hypotension, tachycardia, pallor, tachypnea, diaphoresis, confusion) may result from acute bleeding. Jaundice may suggest hemolysis. Splenomegaly may occur with hemolysis, hemoglobinopathy, connective tissue disease, myeloproliferative disorder, infection, or cancer. Peripheral neuropathy suggests vitamin B_{12} deficiency. Abdominal distention in a patient with blunt trauma suggests acute hemorrhage. Petechiae develop in thrombocytopenia or platelet dysfunction. Fever and heart murmurs suggest infective endocarditis, a possible cause of hemolysis. Rarely, high-output heart failure develops as a compensatory response to anemia-induced tissue hypoxia.

Testing

- CBC with WBC and platelets
- RBC indices and morphology
- Reticulocyte count
- Peripheral smear
- Sometimes bone marrow aspiration and biopsy

Laboratory evaluation begins with a CBC, including WBC and platelet counts, RBC indices and morphology (MCV, MCH, MCHC, RDW), and examination of the peripheral smear. The reticulocyte count demonstrates how well the bone marrow compensates for the anemia. Subsequent tests are selected on the basis of these results and on the clinical presentation. Recognition of general diagnostic patterns can expedite the diagnosis (see Table 139–2).

Complete blood count and RBC indices: The automated CBC directly measures Hb, RBC count, WBC count. and number of platelets, MCV (a measure of RBC volume). Hct (a measure of the percentage of blood made up of RBCs), mean corpuscular hemoglobin (MCH, a measure of the Hb content in individual RBCs), and mean corpuscular Hb concentration (a measure of the Hb concentration in individual RBCs) are calculated values.

The **diagnostic criterion for anemia** is

- For men: Hb < 14 g/dL, Hct < 42%, or RBC < 4.5 million/μL
- For women: Hb < 12 g/dL, Hct < 37%, or RBC < 4 million/μL

For infants, normal values vary with age, necessitating use of age-related tables. RBC populations are termed microcytic (small cells) if MCV is < 80 fL, and macrocytic (large cells) if MCV is > 100 fL. However, because reticulocytes are also larger than mature red cells, large numbers of reticulocytes can elevate the MCV and not represent an alteration of RBC production.

Automated techniques can also determine the degree of variation in RBC size, expressed as the RBC volume distribution width (RDW). A high RDW may be the only indication of simultaneous microcytic and macrocytic disorders (or simultaneous microcytosis and reticulocytosis); such a pattern may result in

Table 139–2. CHARACTERISTICS OF COMMON ANEMIAS

ETIOLOGY OR TYPE	MORPHOLOGIC CHANGES	SPECIAL FEATURES
Blood loss, acute	Normochromic-normocytic, with polychromatophilia	If severe, possible nucleated RBCs and left shift of WBCs Leukocytosis Thrombocytosis
Blood loss, chronic	Same as iron deficiency	Same as iron deficiency
Folate deficiency	Same as vitamin B_{12} deficiency	Serum folate < 5 ng/mL (< 11 nmol/L) RBC folate < 225 ng/mL RBCs (< 510 nmol/L) Nutritional deficiency and malabsorption (in sprue, pregnancy, infancy, or alcoholism)
Hereditary spherocytosis	Spheroidal microcytes Normoblastic erythroid hyperplasia	Increased mean RBC Hb level Increased RBC fragility Shortened survival of labeled RBCs
Hemolysis	Normochromic-normocytic Reticulocytosis Marrow erythroid hyperplasia	Increased serum bilirubin and lactate dehydrogenase Increased stool and urine urobilinogen Hemoglobinuria in fulminating cases Hemosiderinuria
Infection, cancer, or chronic inflammation	Normochromic-normocytic early, then microcytic Normoblastic marrow Normal iron stores	Decreased serum iron Decreased total iron-binding capacity Normal serum ferritin Normal marrow iron content
Iron deficiency	Microcytic, with anisocytosis and poikilocytosis Reticulocytopenia Hyperplastic marrow, with delayed hemoglobination	Possible achlorhydria, smooth tongue, and spoon nails Absent stainable marrow iron Low serum iron Increased total iron-binding capacity Low serum ferritin
Marrow failure	Normochromic-normocytic (may be macrocytic) Reticulocytopenia Failed marrow aspiration (often) or evident hypoplasia of erythroid series or of all elements	Idiopathic (> 50%) or secondary to exposure to toxic drugs or chemicals (eg, chloramphenicol, quinacrine, hydantoins, insecticides)
Marrow replacement (myelophthisis)	Anisocytosis and poikilocytosis Nucleated RBCs Early granulocyte precursors Marrow aspiration possibly failing or showing leukemia, myeloma, or metastatic cells	Marrow infiltration with infectious granulomas, tumors, fibrosis, or lipid histiocytosis Possible hepatomegaly and splenomegaly Possible bone changes
Cold agglutinin disease	Red cell agglutination	Follows exposure to cold Results from a cold agglutinin or hemolysin Sometimes postinfectious
Paroxysmal nocturnal hemoglobinuria	Leukopenia Thrombocytopenia	Dark morning urine Hemosiderinuria Thrombosis
Sickle cell disease	Anisocytosis and poikilocytosis Some sickle cells in peripheral smear Sickling of all RBCs in preparation with hypoxia or hyperosmolar exposure	Largely limited to blacks in the US Urinary isosthenuria Hb S detected during electrophoresis Possibly painful vaso-occlusive crises and leg ulcers Bone changes on x-ray
Sideroblastic anemia	Usually hypochromic but dimorphic with normocytes and macrocytes Hyperplastic marrow, with delayed hemoglobination Ringed sideroblasts	Inborn or acquired metabolic defect Stainable marrow iron (plentiful) Some congenital forms respond to vitamin B6 administration Can be part of myelodysplastic syndrome (MDS)
Thalassemia	Microcytic Target cells Basophilic stippling Anisocytosis and poikilocytosis Nucleated RBCs in homozygotes	Decreased RBC fragility Elevated Hb A_2 and Hb F (in beta-thalassemia) Mediterranean ancestry (common) In homozygotes, anemia from infancy Splenomegaly Bone changes on x-ray
Vitamin B_{12} deficiency	Oval macrocytes Anisocytosis Reticulocytopenia Hypersegmented WBCs Megaloblastic marrow	Serum B_{12} < 180 pg/mL (< 130 pmol/L) Frequent GI and CNS involvement Elevated serum bilirubin Increased LDH Antibodies to intrinsic factor in serum (pernicious anemia) Sometimes absent gastric intrinsic factor secretion

a normal MCV, which measures only the mean value. The term hypochromia refers to RBC populations in which MCH is < 27 pg/RBC or MCHC is < 30%. RBC populations with normal MCH and MCHC values are normochromic.

The RBC indices can help indicate the mechanism of anemia and narrow the number of possible causes. Microcytic indices occur with altered heme or globin synthesis. The most common causes are iron deficiency, thalassemia, and related Hb-synthesis defects. In some patients with anemia of chronic disease, the MCV is microcytic or borderline microcytic. Macrocytic indices occur with impaired DNA synthesis (eg, due to vitamin B_{12} or folate deficiencies or chemotherapeutic drugs such as hydroxyurea and antifolate agents) and in alcoholism because of abnormalities of the cell membrane. Acute bleeding may briefly produce macrocytic indices because of the release of large young reticulocytes. Normocytic indices occur in anemias resulting from deficient erythropoietin (EPO) or inadequate response to it (hypoproliferative anemias). Hemorrhage, before iron deficiency develops, usually results in normocytic and normochromic anemia unless the number of large reticulocytes is excessive.

Peripheral smear: The peripheral smear is highly sensitive for excessive RBC production and hemolysis. It is more accurate than automated technologies for recognition of altered RBC structure, thrombocytopenia, nucleated RBCs, or immature granulocytes and can detect other abnormalities (eg, malaria and other parasites, intracellular RBC or granulocyte inclusions) that can occur despite normal automated blood cell counts. RBC injury may be identified by finding RBC fragments, portions of disrupted cells (schistocytes), or evidence of significant membrane alterations from oval-shaped cells (ovalocytes) or spherocytic cells. Target cells (thin RBCs with a central dot of Hb) are RBCs with insufficient Hb or excess cell membrane (eg, due to hemoglobinopathies or liver disorders). The peripheral smear can also reveal variation in RBC shape (poikilocytosis) and size (anisocytosis).

Reticulocyte count: The reticulocyte count is expressed as the percentage of reticulocytes (normal range, 0.5 to 1.5%) or as the absolute reticulocyte count (normal range, 50,000 to 150,000/μL). Higher values indicate excessive production, or reticulocytosis; in the presence of anemia, reticulocytosis suggests excessive RBC destruction. Low numbers in the presence of anemia indicate decreased RBC production. The reticulocyte response can usually be estimated based on the number of blue-stained cells found when the peripheral smear is stained with a supravital stain.

Bone marrow aspiration and biopsy: Bone marrow aspiration and biopsy provide direct observation and assessment of RBC precursors. The presence of abnormal maturation (dyspoiesis) of blood cells and the amount, distribution, and cellular pattern of iron content can be assessed. Bone marrow aspiration and biopsy are usually not indicated in the evaluation of anemia and are only done when one of the following conditions is present:

- Unexplained anemia
- More than one cell lineage abnormality (ie, concurrent anemia and thrombocytopenia or leukopenia)
- Suspected primary bone marrow disorder (eg, leukemia, multiple myeloma, aplastic anemia, MDS, metastatic carcinoma, myelofibrosis)

Cytogenetic and molecular analyses can be done on aspirate material in hematopoietic or other tumors or in suspected congenital lesions of RBC precursors (eg, Fanconi anemia). Flow cytometry can be done in suspected lymphoproliferative or myeloproliferative states to define the immunophenotype. Bone marrow aspiration and biopsy are not technically difficult and do not pose significant risk of morbidity. These procedures are safe and helpful when hematologic disease is suspected. Both usually can be done as a single procedure. Because biopsy requires adequate bone depth, the sample is usually taken from the posterior (or, less commonly, anterior) iliac crest. If only aspiration is necessary, the sternum may be used.

Other tests for evaluation of anemia: Serum bilirubin and lactate dehydrogenase (LDH) can sometimes help differentiate between hemolysis and blood loss; both are elevated in hemolysis and normal in blood loss. Other tests, such as vitamin B_{12} and folate levels, iron and iron binding capacity, are done depending on the suspected cause of anemia. Other tests are discussed under specific anemias and bleeding disorders.

TREATMENT OF ANEMIA

When possible, the cause of the anemia is treated. When the Hb falls dangerously low (eg, < 7 g/dL for patients without cardiopulmonary insufficiency or higher for patients with it), RBC transfusion temporarily increases oxygen-carrying capacity. RBC transfusion should be reserved for patients

- With or at high risk of cardiopulmonary symptoms
- With active, uncontrollable blood loss
- With some form of hypoxic or ischemic end-organ failure (eg, neurologic ischemic symptoms, angina, tachycardia in patients with underlying heart failure or severe COPD)

Transfusion procedures and blood components are discussed elsewhere.

140 Anemias Caused by Deficient Erythropoiesis

Anemia (a decrease in the number of RBCs, Hb content, or Hct) can result from decreased RBC production (erythropoiesis), increased RBC destruction, blood loss, or a combination of these factors.

Anemias due to decreased erythropoiesis (termed hypoproliferative anemias) are recognized by reticulocytopenia, which is usually evident on the peripheral smear.

The RBC indices, mainly the mean corpuscular volume (MCV), can narrow the differential diagnosis of deficient erythropoiesis and help determine what further testing is necessary.

Microcytic anemias result from deficient or defective heme or globin synthesis. Microcytic anemias include iron deficiency anemias, iron-transport deficiency anemias, iron-utilization anemias (including some sideroblastic anemias and lead poisoning), and thalassemias (which also cause hemolysis). Patients with microcytic anemias typically require testing of iron stores.

Normocytic anemias are characterized by a normal RBC distribution width (RDW) and normochromic indices. The two most common causes are hypoproliferation due to a deficiency of or inadequate response to erythropoietin (EPO) and anemia of chronic disease. Acquired primary bone marrow disorders such as aplastic anemia, pure red cell aplasia, and myelodysplastic syndrome (MDS) can also present with a normocytic anemia.

Macrocytic anemias can be caused by impaired DNA synthesis leading to megaloblastosis, as occurs with deficiencies of vitamin B_{12} or folate (see p. 1101). Other causes include chronic alcohol intake (independent of vitamin deficiency), liver disease, MDS, and hemolysis. Some patients with hypothyroidism have macrocytic RBC indices, including some without anemia.

Many anemias have variable findings on the peripheral smear. Anemia of chronic disease may be microcytic or normocytic. Anemias due to MDSs may be normocytic or macrocytic. Anemias due to endocrine disorders (such as hypothyroidism) or elemental deficiencies (such as copper or zinc) can have variable manifestations, including a normocytic or macrocytic anemia.

Treatment of deficient RBC production depends on the cause.

IRON DEFICIENCY ANEMIA

(Anemia of Chronic Blood Loss; Chlorosis)

Iron deficiency is the most common cause of anemia and usually results from blood loss; malabsorption is a much less common cause. Symptoms are usually nonspecific. RBCs tend to be microcytic and hypochromic, and iron stores are low, as shown by low serum ferritin and low serum iron levels with high serum total iron-binding capacity. If the diagnosis is made, occult blood loss should be suspected until proven otherwise. Treatment involves iron replacement and treatment of the cause of blood loss.

Pathophysiology

Iron is distributed in active metabolic and storage pools. Total body iron is about 3.5 g in healthy men and 2.5 g in women; the difference relates to women's smaller body size and dearth of stored iron because of iron loss due to menses. The distribution of body iron is

- Hemoglobin 2 g (men), 1.5 g (women)
- Ferritin 1 g (men), 0.6 g (women)
- Hemosiderin, 300 mg
- Myoglobin, 200 mg
- Tissue enzymes (heme and nonheme), 150 mg
- Transport-iron compartment, 3 mg

Iron absorption: Iron is absorbed in the duodenum and upper jejunum. Absorption of iron is determined by the type of iron molecule and by what other substances are ingested. Iron absorption is best when food contains heme iron (meat). Dietary nonheme iron is usually in the ferric state and must be reduced to the ferrous state and released from food binders by gastric secretions. Nonheme iron absorption is reduced by other food items (eg, vegetable fiber phytates and polyphenols; tea tannates, including phosphoproteins; bran) and certain antibiotics (eg, tetracycline). Ascorbic acid is the only common food element known to increase nonheme iron absorption.

The average American diet, which contains 6 mg of elemental iron/1000 kcal of food, is adequate for iron homeostasis. Of about 15 mg/day of dietary iron, adults absorb only 1 mg, which is the approximate amount lost daily by cell desquamation from the skin and intestines. In iron depletion, absorption increases due to the suppression of hepcidin, a key regulator of iron metabolism; however, absorption rarely increases to > 6 mg/day unless supplemental iron is added.[1] Children have a greater need for iron and appear to absorb more to meet this need.

Iron transport and usage: Iron from intestinal mucosal cells is transferred to transferrin, an iron-transport protein synthesized in the liver; transferrin can transport iron from cells (intestinal, macrophages) to specific receptors on erythroblasts, placental cells, and liver cells. For heme synthesis, transferrin transports iron to the erythroblast mitochondria, which insert the iron into protoporphyrin for it to become heme. Transferrin (plasma half-life, 8 days) is extruded for reutilization. Synthesis of transferrin increases with iron deficiency but decreases with any type of chronic disease.

Iron storage and recycling: Iron not used for erythropoiesis is transferred by transferrin, an iron-transporting protein, to the storage pool; iron is stored in 2 forms, ferritin and hemosiderin. The most important is ferritin (a heterogeneous group of proteins surrounding an iron core), which is a soluble and active storage fraction located in the liver (in hepatocytes), bone marrow, and spleen (in macrophages); in RBCs; and in serum. Iron stored in ferritin is readily available for any body requirement. Circulating (serum) ferritin level parallels the size of the body stores (1 ng/mL = 8 mg of iron in the storage pool). The 2nd storage pool of iron is in hemosiderin, which is relatively insoluble and is stored primarily in the liver (in Kupffer cells) and in bone marrow (in macrophages).

Because iron absorption is so limited, the body recycles and conserves iron. Transferrin grasps and recycles available iron from aging RBCs undergoing phagocytosis by mononuclear phagocytes. This mechanism provides about 97% of the daily iron needed (about 25 mg of iron). With aging, iron stores tend to increase because iron elimination is slow.

Iron deficiency: Deficiency develops in stages. In the first stage, iron requirement exceeds intake, causing progressive depletion of bone marrow iron stores. As stores decrease, absorption of dietary iron increases in compensation. During later stages, deficiency impairs RBC synthesis, ultimately causing anemia.

Severe and prolonged iron deficiency also may cause dysfunction of iron-containing cellular enzymes.

1. Nemeth E, Tuttle MS, Powelson J, et al: Hepcidin regulates cellular iron efflux by binding to ferroportin and inducing its internalization. *Science* 306(5704): 2090–2093, 2004.

Etiology

Because iron is poorly absorbed, dietary iron barely meets the daily requirement for most people. Even so, people who eat a typical Western diet are unlikely to become iron deficient solely as a result of dietary deficiency. However, even modest losses, increased requirements, or decreased intake readily causes iron deficiency.

Blood loss is almost always the cause. In men and postmenopausal women, the most frequent cause is chronic occult bleeding, usually from the GI tract (eg, from peptic ulcer disease, malignancy, hemorrhoids). In premenopausal women, cumulative menstrual blood loss (mean, 0.5 mg iron/day) is a common cause. Intestinal bleeding due to hookworm infection is a common cause in developing countries. Less common causes include recurrent pulmonary hemorrhage (see Diffuse Alveolar Hemorrhage on p. 435) and chronic intravascular hemolysis when the amount of iron released during hemolysis exceeds the haptoglobin-binding capacity.

Increased iron requirement may contribute to iron deficiency. From birth to age 2 and during adolescence, when rapid growth requires a large iron intake, dietary iron often is inadequate. During pregnancy, the fetal iron requirement increases the maternal iron requirement (mean, 0.5 to 0.8 mg/day—see Anemia in Pregnancy on p. 2386) despite the absence of menses. Lactation also increases the iron requirement (mean, 0.4 mg/day).

Decreased iron absorption can result from gastrectomy or malabsorption syndromes such as celiac disease, atrophic gastritis, and achlorhydria. Rarely, absorption is decreased by dietary deprivation from undernutrition.

Symptoms and Signs

Most symptoms of iron deficiency are due to anemia. Such symptoms include fatigue, loss of stamina, shortness of breath, weakness, dizziness, and pallor.

In addition to the usual manifestations of anemia, some uncommon symptoms occur in severe iron deficiency. Patients may have pica, an abnormal craving to eat substances (eg, ice, dirt, paint). Other symptoms of severe deficiency include glossitis, cheilosis, and concave nails (koilonychia).

Diagnosis

- CBC, serum iron, iron-binding capacity, serum ferritin, transferrin saturation, reticulocyte count, red cell distribution width (RDW), and peripheral blood smear
- Rarely bone marrow examination

Iron deficiency anemia is suspected in patients with chronic blood loss or microcytic anemia, particularly if pica is present. In such patients, CBC, serum iron and iron-binding capacity, and serum ferritin and reticulocyte count are obtained.

Iron and iron-binding capacity (or transferrin) are measured because their relationship is important. Various tests exist; the range of normal values relates to the test used. In general, normal serum iron is 75 to 150 μg/dL (13 to 27 μmol/L) for men and 60 to 140 μg/dL (11 to 25 μmol/L) for women; total iron-binding capacity is 250 to 450 μg/dL (45 to 81 μmol/L). Serum iron level is low in iron deficiency and in many chronic diseases and is elevated in hemolytic disorders and in iron-overload syndromes. The iron-binding capacity increases in iron deficiency, while the transferrin saturation decreases.

Serum ferritin levels closely correlate with total body iron stores. The range of normal in most laboratories is 30 to 300 ng/mL, and the mean is 88 ng/mL in men and 49 ng/mL in women. Low levels (< 12 ng/mL) are specific for iron deficiency. However, ferritin is an acute-phase reactant, and levels increase in inflammatory and infectious disorders (eg, hepatitis), and neoplastic disorders (especially acute leukemia, Hodgkin lymphoma, and GI tract tumors). In these settings, a serum ferritin up to 100 ng/mL remains compatible with iron deficiency.

The **reticulocyte count** is low in iron deficiency. The peripheral smear generally reveals hypochromic red cells with significant anisopoikilocytosis, which is reflected in a high red cell distribution width (RDW).

The most sensitive and specific criterion for iron-deficient erythropoiesis is absent bone marrow stores of iron, although a bone marrow examination is rarely needed.

Stages of iron deficiency: Laboratory test results help stage iron deficiency anemia.

Stage 1 is characterized by decreased bone marrow iron stores; Hb and serum iron remain normal, but serum ferritin level falls to < 20 ng/mL. The compensatory increase in iron absorption causes an increase in iron-binding capacity (transferrin level).

During **stage 2,** erythropoiesis is impaired. Although the transferrin level is increased, the serum iron level decreases; transferrin saturation decreases. Erythropoiesis is impaired when serum iron falls to < 50 μg/dL (< 9 μmol/L) and transferrin saturation to < 16%. The serum transferrin receptor level rises (> 8.5 mg/L).

During **stage 3,** anemia with normal-appearing RBCs and indices develops.

During **stage 4,** microcytosis and then hypochromia develop.

During **stage 5,** iron deficiency affects tissues, resulting in symptoms and signs.

Diagnosis of iron deficiency anemia prompts consideration of its cause, usually bleeding. Patients with obvious blood loss (eg, women with menorrhagia) may require no further testing. Men and postmenopausal women without obvious blood loss should undergo evaluation of the GI tract, because anemia may be the only indication of an occult GI cancer. Rarely, chronic epistaxis or GU bleeding is underestimated by the patient and requires evaluation in patients with normal GI study results.

Other microcytic anemias: Iron deficiency anemia must be differentiated from other microcytic anemias (see Table 140–1). If tests exclude iron deficiency in patients with microcytic anemia, then anemia of chronic disease and structural Hb abnormalities (eg, hemoglobinopathies) are considered. Clinical features, Hb studies (eg, Hb electrophoresis and Hb A_2), and genetic testing (eg, for alpha-thalassemia) may help distinguish these entities.

Treatment

- Oral supplemental iron
- Rarely parenteral iron

Iron therapy without pursuit of the cause is poor practice; the bleeding site should be sought even in cases of mild anemia.

Iron can be provided by various iron salts (eg, ferrous sulfate, gluconate, fumarate) or saccharated iron po 30 min before meals (food or antacids may reduce absorption). A typical initial dose is 60 mg of elemental iron (eg, as 325 mg of ferrous sulfate) given once/day.[1] Larger doses are largely unabsorbed but increase adverse effects especially. Ascorbic acid either as a pill (500 mg) or as orange juice when taken with iron enhances iron absorption without increasing gastric distress.

Parenteral iron causes the same therapeutic response as oral iron but can cause adverse effects, such as anaphylactoid reactions, serum sickness, thrombophlebitis, and pain. It is reserved for patients who do not tolerate or who will not take oral iron or for patients who steadily lose large amounts of blood because of capillary or vascular disorders (eg, hereditary hemorrhagic telangiectasia). The dose of parenteral iron is determined by a hematologist. Oral or parenteral iron therapy should continue for ≥ 6 mo after correction of Hb levels to replenish tissue stores.

The response to treatment is assessed by serial Hb measurements until normal RBC values are achieved. Hb rises little for 2 wk but then rises 0.7 to 1 g/wk until near normal, at which time rate of increase tapers. Anemia should be corrected within 2 mo. A subnormal response suggests continued hemorrhage, underlying infection or cancer, insufficient iron intake, or malabsorption of oral iron.

Table 140–1. DIFFERENTIAL DIAGNOSIS OF MICROCYTIC ANEMIA DUE TO DECREASED RBC PRODUCTION

DIAGNOSTIC CRITERIA	IRON DEFICIENCY	IRON-TRANSPORT DEFICIENCY	SIDEROBLASTIC IRON UTILIZATION	CHRONIC DISEASE/ INFLAMMATION
Peripheral smear				
Microcytosis (M) vs hypochromia (H)	M > H	M > H	M > H, may be normocytic	Frequently normocytic
Polychromatophilic targeted cells	Absent	Absent	Present	Absent
Stippled RBCs	Absent	Absent	Present	Absent
RBCs				
RBC distribution width (RDW)	↑	↑	↑	Normal
Serum iron				
Serum iron	↓	↓	↑	Normal or decreased (↓)
Iron-binding capacity	↑	↓	Normal	Normal or decreased (↓)
% Saturation of transferrin	< 10	0	> 50	Normal or decreased (0–50)
Serum ferritin				
(Normal, 30–300 ng/mL)	< 12 ng/mL	Usually normal	> 400 ng/mL	30–400 ng/mL
Bone marrow				
RBC:granulocyte ratio (normal, 1:3–1:5)	1:1–1:2	1:1–1:2	1:1–5:1	1:1–1:2
Marrow iron	Absent	Present	↑	Present
Ringed sideroblasts	Absent	Absent	Present	Absent

> = more common than; ↑ = increased; ↓ = decreased.

1. Moretti D, Goede JS, Zeder C, et al: Oral iron supplements increase hepcidin and decrease iron absorption from daily or twice-daily doses in iron-depleted young women. *Blood* 126(17):1981–1989, 2015. doi: 10.1182/blood-2015-05-642223.

KEY POINTS

- Iron deficiency anemia is usually caused by blood loss (eg, GI, menstrual) but may be due to hemolysis, malabsorption or increased demand for iron (eg, in pregnancy, lactation, periods of rapid growth in children).
- Differentiate iron deficiency anemia from other microcytic anemias (eg, anemia of chronic disease, hemoglobinopathies).
- Measure serum iron, iron-binding capacity, and serum ferritin levels.
- Iron deficiency typically causes low serum iron, high iron-binding capacity, and low serum ferritin levels.
- Always seek a cause of iron deficiency, even when anemia is mild.
- Oral iron supplements are usually adequate; reserve use of parenteral iron for hematologists because of risks of adverse effects (eg, anaphylactoid reactions, serum sickness, thrombophlebitis).

SIDEROBLASTIC ANEMIAS

Sideroblastic anemias are a diverse group of anemias characterized by the presence of ringed sideroblasts (erythroblasts with perinuclear iron-engorged mitochondria). Sideroblastic anemias may be acquired or congenital. Acquired sideroblastic anemia is frequently associated with myelodysplastic syndrome (but may be produced by drugs or toxins) and causes a macrocytic anemia. Congenital sideroblastic anemia is caused by one of numerous X-linked or autosomal mutations and is usually a microcytic-hypochromic anemia with increased serum iron and ferritin and transferrin saturation.

Sideroblastic anemias are characterized by inadequate marrow utilization of iron for heme synthesis despite the presence of adequate or increased amounts of iron (iron-utilization anemias). Sideroblastic anemias are sometimes characterized by the presence of polychromatophilia and stippled RBCs (siderocytes).

In both acquired and congenital sideroblastic anemia, heme synthesis is impaired due to the inability to incorporate iron into protoporphyrin, leading to the formation of ringed sideroblasts.

Acquired sideroblastic anemia: Acquired sideroblastic anemias are often part of a

- Myelodysplastic syndrome

Less common causes include

- Drugs (eg, chloramphenicol, cycloserine, isoniazid, linezolid, pyrazinamide)
- Toxins (including ethanol and lead)
- Pyridoxine or copper deficiency

Deficient reticulocyte production, intramedullary death of RBCs, and bone marrow erythroid hyperplasia (and dysplasia) occur. Although hypochromic RBCs are produced, other RBCs may be large, producing normocytic or macrocytic indices; if so, variation in RBC size (dimorphism) usually produces a high RBC distribution width (RDW).

Congenital sideroblastic anemia: The most common congenital sideroblastic anemia is an X-linked form caused by heterozygous germline mutations in the ALAS2, a gene involved in heme biosynthesis. Pyridoxine (B_6) is an essential cofactor for this enzyme, thus patients may respond to pyridoxine supplementation. Numerous other X-linked, autosomal and mitochondrial forms have been identified with mutations in genes involved in heme synthesis. RBCs are usually microcytic and hypochromic, but this is not always the case.

Diagnosis

Sideroblastic anemia is suspected in patients with microcytic anemia or a high RDW anemia, particularly with increased serum iron, serum ferritin, and transferrin saturation (see p. 1095). The peripheral smear shows RBC dimorphism. RBCs may appear stippled. Bone marrow examination is necessary and reveals erythroid hyperplasia. Iron staining reveals the pathognomonic iron-engorged perinuclear mitochondria in developing RBCs (ringed sideroblasts). Other features of myelodysplasia, such as cytopenias and dysplasia, may be evident. Serum lead is measured if sideroblastic anemia has an unknown cause.

Treatment

Elimination of a toxin or drug (especially alcohol), or mineral/vitamin supplementation (copper or pyridoxine) can lead to recovery. Congenital cases may respond to pyridoxine 50 mg po tid, but usually incompletely.

ANEMIA OF CHRONIC DISEASE

(Anemia of Chronic Inflammation)

Anemia of chronic disease is a multifactorial anemia. Diagnosis generally requires the presence of a chronic inflammatory condition, such as infection, autoimmune disease, kidney disease, or cancer. It is characterized by a microcytic or normocytic anemia and low reticulocyte count. Values for serum iron transferrin are typically low to normal, while ferritin can be normal or elevated. Treatment is to reverse the underlying disorder and in some cases, to give erythropoietin.

Worldwide, anemia of chronic disease is the 2nd most common anemia. Early on, the RBCs are normocytic; with time they become microcytic. The major issue is that erythropoiesis is restricted due to inappropriate iron sequestration.

Etiology

This type of anemia occurs as part of a chronic inflammatory disorder, most often chronic infection, autoimmune disease (especially RA), kidney disease, or cancer; however, the same process appears to begin acutely during virtually any infection or inflammation, including trauma or post-surgery. (See also Anemia of Renal Disease on p. 1099.)

Three pathophysiologic mechanisms have been identified:

- Slightly shortened RBC survival, thought to be due to release of inflammatory cytokines, occurs in patients with cancer or chronic granulomatous infections.
- Erythropoiesis is impaired because of decreases in both erythropoietin (EPO) production and marrow responsiveness to EPO.
- Iron metabolism is altered due to an increase in hepcidin, which inhibits iron absorption and recycling, leading to iron sequestration.

Reticuloendothelial cells retain iron from senescent RBCs, making iron unavailable for Hb synthesis. There is thus a failure to compensate for the anemia with increased RBC production. Macrophage-derived cytokines (eg, IL-1-beta, tumor necrosis factor-alpha, interferon-beta) in patients with infections, inflammatory states, and cancer contribute to the decrease in EPO production and the impaired iron metabolism by increasing hepatic synthesis of hepcidin.

Diagnosis

- Symptoms and signs of underlying disorder
- CBC and serum iron, ferritin, transferrin, and reticulocyte count

Clinical findings are usually those of the underlying disorder (infection, inflammation, or cancer). Anemia of chronic disease should be suspected in patients with microcytic or normocytic anemia with chronic illness, infection, inflammation, or cancer. If anemia of chronic disease is suspected, serum iron, transferrin, reticulocyte count and serum ferritin are measured. Hb usually is > 8 g/dL unless an additional mechanism contributes to anemia, such as concomitant iron deficiency (see Table 140–1).

A serum ferritin level of < 100 ng/mL in the setting of inflammation (< 200 ng/mL in patients with renal failure) suggests that iron deficiency may be superimposed on anemia of chronic disease. However, serum ferritin may be falsely elevated as an acute-phase reactant.

Treatment

- Treatment of underlying disorder
- Sometimes recombinant erythropoietin (EPO) and iron supplements

Treating the underlying disorder is most important. Because the anemia is generally mild, transfusions usually are not required. Recombinant EPO has been shown to be most useful in the setting of chronic kidney disease. Because both reduced production of and marrow resistance to EPO occur, the EPO dose may need to be 150 to 300 units/kg sc 3 times/wk. A good response is likely if, after 2 wk of therapy, Hb has increased > 0.5 g/dL and serum ferritin is < 400 ng/mL. Iron supplements (see p. 1096) are required to ensure an adequate response to EPO. However, careful monitoring of Hb response is needed because adverse effects (eg, venous thromboembolism, MI, death) may occur when Hb rises to > 12 g/dL.

KEY POINTS

- Almost any chronic infection, inflammation, or cancer can cause anemia; Hb usually is > 8 g/dL unless an additional mechanism contributes.
- Multiple factors are involved, including shortened RBC survival, impaired erythropoiesis, and impaired iron metabolism.
- Anemia is initially normocytic and then can become microcytic.
- Serum iron and transferrin are typically decreased, while ferritin is normal to increased.
- Treat the underlying disorder and consider recombinant EPO.

ANEMIA OF RENAL DISEASE

Anemia of renal disease is a hypoproliferative anemia resulting primarily from deficient erythropoietin (EPO) or a diminished response to it; it tends to be normocytic and normochromic. Treatment includes measures to correct the underlying disorder and supplementation with EPO and sometimes iron.

Anemia in chronic renal disease is multifactorial.

The **most common mechanism** is

- Hypoproliferation due to decreased EPO production

Other factors include

- Uremia (in which mild hemolysis is common due to an increase in RBC deformity)
- Blood loss due to dysfunctional platelets, dialysis, and/or angiodysplasia
- Secondary hyperparathyroidism

Less common is RBC fragmentation (traumatic hemolytic anemia), which occurs when the renovascular endothelium is injured (eg, in malignant hypertension, membranoproliferative glomerulonephritis, polyarteritis nodosa, or acute cortical necrosis).

The deficiency in renal production of EPO and the severity of anemia do not always correlate with the extent of renal dysfunction; anemia occurs when creatinine clearance is < 45 mL/min. Renal glomerular lesions (eg, from amyloidosis, diabetic nephropathy) generally result in the most severe anemia for their degree of excretory failure.

Diagnosis is based on demonstration of renal insufficiency, normocytic anemia, and peripheral reticulocytopenia. Bone marrow may show erythroid hypoplasia. RBC fragmentation on the peripheral smear, particularly if there is thrombocytopenia, suggests simultaneous traumatic hemolysis.

Therapy is directed at improving renal function and increasing RBC production. If renal function returns to normal, anemia is slowly corrected. In patients receiving long-term dialysis, EPO, beginning with 50 to 100 units/kg IV or sc 3 times/wk with iron supplements, is the treatment of choice. In almost all cases, maximum increases in RBCs are reached by 8 to 12 wk. Reduced doses of EPO (about ½ the induction dose) can then be given 1 to 3 times/wk. Transfusions are rarely necessary. Careful monitoring of the response is needed to avoid adverse effects when Hb increases to > 12 g/dL.

APLASTIC ANEMIA

(Hypoplastic Anemia)

Aplastic anemia is a disorder of the hematopoietic stem cell that results in a loss of blood cell precursors, hypoplasia or aplasia of bone marrow, and cytopenias in two or more cell lines (RBCs, WBCs, and/or platelets). Symptoms result from anemia, thrombocytopenia (petechiae, bleeding), or leukopenia (infections). Diagnosis requires demonstration of peripheral pancytopenia and a bone marrow biopsy revealing a hypocellular marrow. Treatment usually involves immunosuppression with equine antithymocyte globulin (ATG) and cyclosporine, or bone marrow transplantation.

The term aplastic anemia commonly implies a panhypoplasia of the marrow with cytopenias in at least two hematopoietic lineages. In contrast, pure RBC aplasia is restricted to the erythroid cell line.

Etiology

True **aplastic anemia** (most common in adolescents and young adults) is idiopathic in about half of cases. Recognized causes are

- Chemicals (eg, benzene, inorganic arsenic)
- Radiation
- Drugs (eg, antineoplastic drugs, antibiotics, NSAIDs, anticonvulsants, acetazolamide, gold salts, penicillamine, quinacrine)
- Pregnancy
- Viruses (EBV and CMV)
- Hepatitis (seronegative for hepatitis viruses)

The precise mechanism remains unclear but appears to involve an immune attack on the hematopoietic stem cell.

Symptoms and Signs

The onset of aplastic anemia usually is insidious, often occurring over weeks or months after exposure to a toxin, though occasionally it can be acute.

In aplastic anemia, anemia may cause weakness and easy fatigability while severe thrombocytopenia may cause petechiae, ecchymosis, and bleeding from the gums, into the conjunctivae, or other tissues. Agranulocytosis commonly causes life-threatening infections. Splenomegaly is absent unless induced by transfusion hemosiderosis.

Diagnosis

- CBC, reticulocyte count
- Bone marrow examination

Aplastic anemia is suspected in patients, particularly young patients, with pancytopenia. Severe aplastic anemia is defined by the presence of 2 or more of the following:

- Bone marrow cellularity < 30%
- Absolute neutrophil count < 500/μL
- Absolute reticulocyte count < 60,000/μL
- Platelet count < 20,000/μL

Treatment

- Hematopoietic stem cell transplantation is first-line therapy.
- If transplantation is not an option, immunosuppression with equine ATG and cyclosporine is given.

In aplastic anemia, hematopoietic stem cell transplantation can be curative and is the treatment of choice, particularly in younger patients with a matched donor. At diagnosis, siblings are evaluated for HLA compatibility. Because transfusions pose a risk to subsequent transplantation, blood products are used only when essential.

In those patients unfit for transplant or lacking a donor, immunosuppressive treatment with equine ATG combined with cyclosporine produces overall response rates of approximately 60 to 80%. Allergic reactions and serum sickness may occur. In refractory cases, thrombopoietin agonists have shown some efficacy in clinical trials.

KEY POINTS

- Aplastic anemia involves panhypoplasia of the marrow with anemia, leukopenia, and thrombocytopenia.
- Many cases are idiopathic, but chemicals, drugs, or radiation may be involved.

- Bone marrow examination shows a variable degree of hypocellularity
- Treatment is with stem cell transplant or immunosuppression with ATG and cyclosporine.

PURE RED BLOOD CELL APLASIA

Acquired pure red blood cell aplasia is a disorder of erythroid precursors that results in an isolated normocytic anemia. White blood cells and platelets are not affected. Symptoms result from anemia and include fatigue, lethargy, decreased exercise tolerance and pallor. Diagnosis requires demonstration of peripheral normocytic anemia and a normocellular bone marrow biopsy with absence of erythroid maturation. Treatment usually involves treatment of underlying cause and in some cases thymectomy or immunosuppression.

Congenital pure red cell aplasia (Diamond-Blackfan anemia) is discussed on p. 2784.

Etiology

Pure RBC aplasia is most often due to an inappropriate immune response causing suppression of erythropoiesis. Well-known causes include

- Thymomas
- Drugs (eg, tranquilizers, anticonvulsants)
- Toxins (organic phosphates)
- Riboflavin deficiency
- Pregnancy
- HIV
- Lymphoproliferative diseases (chronic lymphocytic leukemia or large granular lymphocyte leukemia)
- ABO-mismatched bone marrow transplant
- Parvovirus B19, particularly in immunocompromised patients such as those with HIV infection (the parvovirus binds to the blood group P antigen on erythroid precursors and is directly cytotoxic to the cells)

Symptoms

Symptoms of pure RBC aplasia are generally mild and relate to the degree of the anemia or to the underlying disorder. The onset of pure red blood cell anemia usually is insidious, often occurring over weeks or months. Symptoms related to anemia include fatigue, lethargy, decreased exercise tolerance and pallor.

Diagnosis

- CBC, reticulocyte count
- Bone marrow examination

Pure RBC aplasia presents with a normocytic anemia but normal WBC and platelet counts. Reticulocytes are decreased. The bone marrow reveals normal cellularity with a maturation arrest at the proerythroblast stage. In parvovirus B19 infection, giant pronormoblasts may be present.

Treatment

- Immunosuppression
- Sometimes intravenous immunoglobulin (IV Ig) or thymectomy

Pure RBC aplasia has been successfully managed with immunosuppressants (prednisone, cyclosporine, or cyclophosphamide), especially when an autoimmune mechanism is suspected. Pure RBC aplasia secondary to parvovirus infection is treated with intravenous immunoglobulin. Because patients with thymoma-associated pure RBC aplasia improve after thymectomy but are not always cured, CT is used to seek the presence of such a lesion, and surgery is considered.

KEY POINTS

- Pure red cell aplasia involves pure erythroid hypoplasia.
- Immune-mediated suppression of the erythroid cell line is the most likely cause.
- Bone marrow cellularity is normal with an arrest of erythroid maturation causing a normocytic anemia.
- Direct treatment of underlying cause with thymectomy, IV immune globulin (IVIG), or immunosuppression.

MYELOPHTHISIC ANEMIA

Myelophthisic anemia is a normocytic-normochromic anemia that occurs when normal marrow space is infiltrated and replaced by nonhematopoietic or abnormal cells. Causes include tumors, granulomatous disorders, lipid storage diseases, and primary myelofibrosis. Bone marrow fibrosis often occurs as a secondary process as well. Splenomegaly may develop. Characteristic changes in peripheral blood include anisocytosis, poikilocytosis, and excessive numbers of RBC and WBC precursors. Diagnosis usually requires bone marrow biopsy. Treatment is supportive and includes measures directed at the underlying disorder.

Descriptive terms used in this anemia can be confusing. Myelofibrosis, which is replacement of marrow by fibrous tissue bands, may be idiopathic (primary) or secondary. Primary myelofibrosis is a stem cell defect in which the fibrosis is secondary to other hematopoietic intramedullary events. Myelosclerosis is new bone formation that sometimes accompanies myelofibrosis. Myeloid metaplasia refers to extramedullary hematopoiesis in the liver, spleen, or lymph nodes that may accompany myelophthisis due to any cause. An old term, agnogenic myeloid metaplasia, indicates primary myelofibrosis with or without myeloid metaplasia.

Etiology

The **most common cause** of myelophthisic anemia is

- Replacement of bone marrow by metastatic cancer

Cancers most often involved include breast or prostate; less often kidney, lung, adrenal, or thyroid. Extramedullary hematopoiesis tends to be modest.

Other causes include myeloproliferative disorders such as primary myelofibrosis or evolution from polycythemia vera or essential thrombocytosis, granulomatous diseases, and lipid storage diseases such as Gaucher disease or other causes of marrow fibrosis.

Decreased functional hematopoietic tissue due to bone marrow infiltration is the main cause of anemia.

Symptoms and Signs

Myeloid metaplasia may result in splenomegaly, particularly in patients with storage diseases. In severe cases, symptoms of anemia and of the underlying disorder may be present. Massive splenomegaly can cause abdominal pressure, early satiety, cachexia, portal hypertension, and left upper quadrant abdominal pain; hepatomegaly may be present. Hepatosplenomegaly is rare with myelofibrosis from malignant tumors.

Diagnosis

- CBC, RBC indices, reticulocyte count, and peripheral smear
- Bone marrow examination

Myelophthisic anemia is suspected in patients with normocytic anemia, particularly when splenomegaly or a potential underlying cancer is present. If it is suspected, a peripheral smear should be obtained, because a leukoerythroblastic pattern (immature myeloid cells and nucleated RBCs, such as normoblasts in the smear) suggests myelophthisic anemia. Extramedullary hematopoiesis or disruption of the marrow sinusoids causes release of immature myeloid cells and well as nucleated red cells into the periphery. Abnormally shaped RBCs, typically teardrop-shaped (dacrocytes), are also seen. Anemia, usually moderately severe, is characteristically normocytic but may be slightly macrocytic. RBC morphology may show extreme variation (anisocytosis and poikilocytosis) in size and shape. The WBC count may vary. The platelet count is often low, and platelets are often large and bizarre in shape.

Although examination of peripheral blood can be suggestive, diagnosis usually requires bone marrow examination. Indications include a leukoerythroblastic pattern and unexplained splenomegaly. The marrow may be difficult to aspirate; marrow trephine biopsy is usually required (see p. 1094). Findings vary according to the underlying disorder. Erythropoiesis is normal or increased in some cases. Hematopoiesis may be present in the spleen and liver.

X-rays, if obtained incidentally, may disclose bony lesions (myelosclerosis) characteristic of long-standing myelofibrosis or other osseous changes (ie, osteoblastic or lytic lesions of a tumor), suggesting the cause of anemia.

Treatment

- Treatment of underlying disorder
- Transfusions as needed

The underlying disorder is treated. Management is supportive with transfusions.

KEY POINTS

- Myelophthisic anemia is a normocytic-normochromic anemia that occurs when normal marrow space is infiltrated and replaced by nonhematopoietic or abnormal cells.
- The most common cause is replacement of bone marrow by metastatic cancer; other causes include myeloproliferative disorders, granulomatous diseases, and lipid storage diseases.
- Suspect myelophthisic anemia in patients with normocytic anemia and characteristic findings on peripheral smear, particularly in those with splenomegaly or a known causative disorder; confirm with bone marrow examination.
- Treat the cause and transfuse as needed.

MEGALOBLASTIC MACROCYTIC ANEMIAS

Megaloblastic anemias result most often from deficiencies of vitamin B_{12} and folate. Ineffective hematopoiesis affects all cell lines but particularly RBCs. Diagnosis is usually based on a CBC and peripheral smear, which usually shows a macrocytic anemia with anisocytosis and poikilocytosis, large oval RBCs (macro-ovalocytes), hypersegmented neutrophils, and reticulocytopenia. Treatment is directed at the underlying disorder.

Megaloblasts are large nucleated RBC precursors with noncondensed chromatin. Macrocytes are enlarged RBCs (ie, MCV > 100 fL/cell). Macrocytic RBCs occur in a variety of clinical circumstances, many unrelated to megaloblastosis.

Nonmegaloblastic macrocytosis: Most macrocytic (ie, MCV > 100 fL/cell) anemias are megaloblastic. Nonmegaloblastic macrocytosis occurs in various clinical states, not all of which are understood. Anemia commonly occurs in patients with macrocytosis but usually results from mechanisms independent of macrocytosis.

Macrocytosis due to excess RBC membrane occurs in patients with chronic liver disease when cholesterol esterification is defective. Macrocytosis with an MCV of about 100 to 105 fL/cell can occur with chronic alcohol use in the absence of folate deficiency. Mild macrocytosis can occur in aplastic anemia, especially as recovery occurs. Macrocytosis is also common in myelodysplasia. Because RBC membrane molding occurs in the spleen after cell release from the marrow, RBCs may be slightly macrocytic after splenectomy, although these changes are not associated with anemia. Reticulocytosis (in a hemolytic anemia, for example) can also cause macrocytosis.

Nonmegaloblastic macrocytosis is suspected in patients with macrocytic anemias when testing excludes vitamin B_{12}, folate deficiencies, and reticulocytosis. The macro-ovalocytes on peripheral smear and the increased RDW that are typical of classic megaloblastic anemia may be absent. If nonmegaloblastic macrocytosis is unexplained clinically (eg, by the presence of aplastic anemia, chronic liver disease, or alcohol use) or if myelodysplasia is suspected, bone marrow examination and cytogenetic analysis are done to exclude myelodysplasia. In nonmegaloblastic macrocytosis, the marrow is not megaloblastic, but in myelodysplasia and advanced liver disease there are megaloblastoid RBC precursors with dense nuclear chromatin that differ from the usual fine fibrillar pattern in megaloblastic anemias.

Etiology

The **most common causes** of megaloblastic states are

- Vitamin B_{12} deficiency
- Defective utilization of vitamin B_{12}
- Folate deficiency

The most common cause of B_{12} deficiency is pernicious anemia due to impaired intrinsic factor secretion (usually secondary to the presence of autoantibodies—see Autoimmune Metaplastic Atrophic Gastritis on p. 117). Other common causes are malabsorption due to gastritis, gastric bypass or tapeworm infection. Dietary deficiency is rare.

Common causes of folate deficiency include celiac disease and alcoholism.

Other causes of megaloblastosis include drugs (generally antineoplastics such as hydroxyurea, or immunosuppressants) that interfere with DNA synthesis and rare metabolic disorders (eg, hereditary orotic aciduria).

Pathophysiology

Megaloblastic states result from defective DNA synthesis. RNA synthesis continues, resulting in a large cell with a large nucleus. All cell lines have dyspoiesis, in which cytoplasmic maturity is greater than nuclear maturity; this dyspoiesis produces megaloblasts in the marrow before they appear in the peripheral blood. Dyspoiesis results in intramedullary cell death, making erythropoiesis ineffective. Because dyspoiesis affects all cell lines, reticulocytopenia and, during later stages leukopenia and thrombocytopenia develop. Large, oval RBCs (macro-ovalocytes) enter the circulation. Hypersegmentation of polymorphonuclear neutrophils is common.

Symptoms and Signs

Anemia develops insidiously and may not cause symptoms until it is severe. Gastrointestinal manifestations are common, including diarrhea, glossitis, and anorexia. Neurologic manifestations, including peripheral neuropathy, gait instability, and dementia, are unique to B_{12} deficiency and can be permanent if prolonged.

Diagnosis

- CBC, RBC indices, reticulocyte count, and peripheral smear
- B_{12} and folate levels

Megaloblastic anemia is suspected in anemic patients with macrocytic indices. Diagnosis is usually based on peripheral smear. When fully developed, the anemia is macrocytic, with MCV > 100 fL/cell in the absence of iron deficiency, thalassemia trait, or renal disease. The smear shows macro-ovalocytosis, anisocytosis, and poikilocytosis. The RDW is high. Howell-Jolly bodies (residual fragments of the nucleus) are common. Reticulocytopenia is present. Hypersegmentation of the granulocytes develops early; neutropenia develops later. Thrombocytopenia is often present in severe cases, and platelets may be bizarre in size and shape.

Serum B_{12} and folate levels should be measured. A B_{12} level < 200 pg/mL or folate level < 2 ng/mL is generally diagnostic of deficiency. B_{12} levels between 200 to 300 pg/mL are nondiagnostic, and in this case, both a methylmalonic acid (MMA) and homocysteine (HCY) level should be checked. Serum levels of MMA and HCY are both elevated in B_{12} deficiency, while only HCY is elevated in folate deficiency.

Treatment

- Appropriate vitamin supplementation

Supplementation with the proper vitamin is required. Always rule out B_{12} deficiency prior to supplementation with folate. Failure to do so can mask a concomitant B_{12} deficiency and lead to progression of neurologic complications.

For treatment of folate and vitamin B_{12} deficiencies, see pp. 38 and 46. Drugs causing megaloblastic states may need to be eliminated or given in reduced doses.

The etiology of any vitamin deficiency should also be investigated and treated.

KEY POINTS

- Megaloblasts are large nucleated RBC precursors with non-condensed chromatin.
- The most common causes of megaloblastic, macrocytic anemia are deficiency or defective utilization of vitamin B_{12} or folate.
- Do CBC, RBC indices, reticulocyte count, and peripheral smear.
- Measure vitamin B_{12} and folate levels and consider MMA and HCY testing.
- Treat the cause of B_{12} or folate deficiency.

MYELODYSPLASIA AND IRON-TRANSPORT DEFICIENCY ANEMIA

In MDS, anemia is commonly prominent. The anemia is usually normocytic or macrocytic with a dimorphic (large and small) population of circulating cells. Bone marrow examination shows decreased erythroid activity, megaloblastoid and dysplastic changes, and, sometimes, increased numbers of ringed sideroblasts. Treatment is directed at the malignancy, and growth factors are frequently used.

Iron-transport deficiency anemia (atransferrinemia) is exceedingly rare. It occurs when iron cannot move from storage sites (eg, mucosal cells, liver) to the erythropoietic precursors. One well-known form is iron-refractory iron-deficiency anemia (IRIDA), caused by germline mutations in the *TMPRSS6* gene. Patients have a microcytic anemia with very low transferrin saturation and are refractory to oral iron. TMPRSS6 encodes a transmembrane protein that regulates production of hepcidin. Patients have defective hepcidin regulation, with inappropriately elevated levels despite iron deficiency.

141 Anemias Caused by Hemolysis

At the end of their normal life span (about 120 days), RBCs are removed from the circulation. Hemolysis involves premature destruction and hence a shortened RBC life span (< 120 days). Anemia results when bone marrow production can no longer compensate for the shortened RBC survival; this condition is termed uncompensated hemolytic anemia. If the marrow can compensate, the condition is termed compensated hemolytic anemia.

Etiology

Hemolysis can be classified according to whether the hemolysis is

- Extrinsic: From a source outside the red cell; disorders extrinsic to the RBC are usually acquired.
- Intrinsic: Due to an defect within the red cell; intrinsic RBC abnormalities (see Table 141–1) are usually inherited.

Disorders extrinsic to the RBC: Causes of disorders extrinsic to the RBC include

- Reticuloendothelial hyperactivity (hypersplenism)
- Immunologic abnormalities (eg, autoimmune hemolytic anemia, thrombotic thrombocytopenic purpura)
- Mechanical injury (traumatic hemolytic anemia)
- Drugs (quinine, quinidine, penicillins, methyldopa, ticlopidine, clopidogrel)
- Toxins (lead, copper)
- Infections

Infectious organisms may cause hemolytic anemia through the direct action of toxins (eg, from *Clostridium perfringens*, α- or β-hemolytic streptococci, meningococci), by invasion and destruction of the RBC by the organism (eg, *Plasmodium* sp, *Bartonella* sp), or by antibody production (Epstein-Barr virus, mycoplasma).

Intrinsic RBC abnormalities: Defects intrinsic to the RBC that can cause hemolysis involve abnormalities of the RBC membrane, cell metabolism, or Hb structure. Abnormalities include hereditary and acquired cell membrane disorders (eg, spherocytosis), disorders of RBC metabolism (eg, G6PD deficiency), and hemoglobinopathies (eg, sickle cell diseases, thalassemias). Quantitative and functional abnormalities of certain RBC membrane proteins (α- and β-spectrin, protein 4.1, F-actin, ankyrin) cause hemolytic anemias.

Pathophysiology

Hemolysis may be acute, chronic, or episodic. Hemolysis can be extravascular, intravascular, or both.

Table 141–1. HEMOLYTIC ANEMIAS

MECHANISM	DISORDER OR AGENT
Disorders Extrinsic to the RBC	
Immunologic abnormalities	Autoimmune hemolytic anemias: • Cold antibody • Drug-induced • Epstein-Barr virus • Hemolytic uremic syndrome • Mycoplasma • Paroxysmal cold hemoglobinuria • Thrombotic thrombocytopenic purpura • Warm antibody
Infectious organisms	*Babesia* sp *Bartonella bacilliformis* *Plasmodium falciparum* *P. malariae* *P. vivax*
Mechanical trauma	March hemoglobinuria Valvular heart disorders
Reticuloendothelial hyperactivity	Hypersplenism
Toxin production by infectious organisms	*Clostridium perfringens* α- and β-hemolytic streptococci Meningococci
Toxins	Compounds with oxidant potential (eg, dapsone, phenazopyridine) Copper (Wilson disease) Lead Insect venom Snake venom
Intrinsic RBC abnormalities	
Acquired RBC membrane disorders	Hypophosphatemia Paroxysmal nocturnal hemoglobinuria Stomatocytosis
Congenital RBC membrane disorders	Hereditary elliptocytosis Hereditary spherocytosis Hereditary stomatocytosis
Disorders of Hb synthesis	Hb C disease Hb E disease Hb S-C disease Sickle cell disease Thalassemias
Disorders of RBC metabolism	Embden-Meyerhof pathway defects (eg, pyruvate kinase deficiency) Hexose monophosphate shunt defects (eg, G6PD deficiency)

Normal RBC processing: Senescent RBCs lose membrane and are cleared from the circulation largely by the phagocytic cells of the spleen, liver, bone marrow, and reticuloendothelial system. Hb is broken down in these cells primarily by the heme oxygenase system. The iron is conserved and reutilized, and heme is degraded to bilirubin, which is conjugated in the liver to bilirubin glucuronide and excreted in the bile.

Extravascular hemolysis: Most pathologic hemolysis is extravascular and occurs when damaged or abnormal RBCs are cleared from the circulation by the spleen and liver. The spleen usually contributes to hemolysis by destroying mildly abnormal RBCs or cells coated with warm antibodies. An enlarged spleen may sequester even normal RBCs. Severely abnormal RBCs or RBCs coated with cold antibodies or complement (C3) are destroyed within the circulation and in the liver, which (because of its large blood flow) can remove damaged cells efficiently. In extravascular hemolysis, the peripheral smear may show microspherocytes.

Intravascular hemolysis: Intravascular hemolysis is an important reason for premature RBC destruction and usually occurs when the cell membrane has been severely damaged by any of a number of different mechanisms, including autoimmune phenomena, direct trauma (eg, march hemoglobinuria), shear stress (eg, defective mechanical heart valves), and toxins (eg, clostridial toxins, venomous snake bite). The peripheral smear may show schistocytes or other fragmented red cells.

Intravascular hemolysis results in hemoglobinemia when the amount of Hb released into plasma exceeds the Hb-binding capacity of the plasma-binding protein haptoglobin, a protein normally present in concentrations of about 100 mg/dL (1.0 g/L) in plasma. Unbound plasma haptoglobin levels will be low. With hemoglobinemia, unbound Hb dimers are filtered into the urine and reabsorbed by renal tubular cells; hemoglobinuria results when reabsorptive capacity is exceeded. Iron is embedded in hemosiderin within the tubular cells; some of the iron is assimilated for reutilization and some reaches the urine when the tubular cells slough.

Consequences of hemolysis: Unconjugated (indirect) hyperbilirubinemia and jaundice occur when the conversion of Hb to bilirubin exceeds the liver's capacity to conjugate and excrete bilirubin (see p. 213). Bilirubin catabolism causes increased stercobilin in the stool and urobilinogen in the urine and sometimes cholelithiasis.

The bone marrow responds to the excess loss of RBCs by accelerating production and release of RBCs, resulting in a reticulocytosis.

Symptoms and Signs

Systemic manifestations resemble those of other anemias and include pallor, fatigue, dizziness, and possible hypotension. Scleral icterus and/or jaundice may occur, and the spleen may be enlarged.

Hemolytic crisis (acute, severe hemolysis) is uncommon; it may be accompanied by chills, fever, pain in the back and abdomen, prostration, and shock. Hemoglobinuria causes red or reddish-brown urine.

Diagnosis

- Peripheral smear and reticulocyte count
- Serum bilirubin, LDH, haptoglobin, and ALT
- Coombs test and/or hemoglobinopathy screen

Hemolysis is suspected in patients with anemia and reticulocytosis. If hemolysis is suspected, peripheral smear is examined and serum bilirubin, LDH, haptoglobin, and ALT are measured. The peripheral smear and reticulocyte count are the most important tests to diagnose hemolysis. Coombs testing or hemoglobinopathy screening (eg, HPLC) can help identify the cause of hemolysis.

Abnormalities of RBC morphology are seldom diagnostic but often suggest the presence and cause of hemolysis (see Table 141–2). Other suggestive findings include increased levels of serum LDH and indirect bilirubin with a normal ALT, and the presence of urinary urobilinogen.

Intravascular hemolysis is suggested by RBC fragments (schistocytes) on the peripheral smear and by decreased serum haptoglobin levels; however, haptoglobin levels can decrease because of hepatocellular dysfunction and can increase because of systemic inflammation. Intravascular hemolysis is also suggested by urinary hemosiderin. Urinary Hb, like hematuria and myoglobinuria, produces a positive benzidine reaction on dipstick testing; it can be differentiated from hematuria by the absence of RBCs on microscopic urine examination. Free Hb may make plasma reddish brown, noticeable often in centrifuged blood; myoglobin does not.

Once hemolysis has been identified, the etiology is sought. To narrow the differential diagnosis in hemolytic anemias

- Consider risk factors (eg, geographic location, genetics, underlying disorder)
- Examine the patient for splenomegaly
- Do a direct antiglobulin (direct Coombs) test

Most hemolytic anemias cause abnormalities in one of these variables that can direct further testing.

Other laboratory tests that can help discern the causes of hemolysis include the following:

- Quantitative Hb electrophoresis
- RBC enzyme assays
- Flow cytometry
- Cold agglutinins
- Osmotic fragility

Although some tests can help differentiate intravascular from extravascular hemolysis, making the distinction is sometimes difficult. During increased RBC destruction, both types are commonly involved, although to differing degrees.

Table 141–2. RBC MORPHOLOGIC CHANGES IN HEMOLYTIC ANEMIAS

RBC MORPHOLOGY	CAUSES
Spherocytes	Transfused blood Warm antibody hemolytic anemia Hereditary spherocytosis
Schistocytes	Microangiopathy Intravascular prostheses
Target cells	Hemoglobinopathies (sickle cell disease, Hb C disease, thalassemias) Liver dysfunction
Sickled cells	Sickle cell disease
Agglutinated cells	Cold agglutinin disease
Heinz bodies or bite cells	G6PD deficiency Oxidant stress Unstable Hb
Nucleated erythroblasts and basophilia	Thalassemia major
Acanthocytes	Liver disease Abetalipoproteinemia

Treatment

Treatment depends on the specific mechanism of hemolysis.

Corticosteroids are helpful in the initial treatment of warm antibody autoimmune hemolysis. Long-term transfusion therapy may cause excessive iron accumulation, necessitating chelation therapy. Splenectomy is beneficial in some situations, particularly when splenic sequestration is the major cause of RBC destruction. If possible, splenectomy is delayed until 2 wk after vaccination with pneumococcal, *Haemophilus influenzae*, and meningococcal vaccines. In cold agglutinin disease, avoidance of cold is recommended, and sometimes blood is warmed before transfusion. Folate replacement is needed for patients with ongoing long-term hemolysis.

AUTOIMMUNE HEMOLYTIC ANEMIA

Autoimmune hemolytic anemia (AIHA) is caused by autoantibodies that react with RBCs at temperatures ≥ 37° C (warm antibody hemolytic anemia) or < 37° C (cold agglutinin disease). Hemolysis is usually extravascular. The direct antiglobulin (direct Coombs) test establishes the diagnosis and may suggest the cause. Treatment depends on the cause and may include corticosteroids, splenectomy, IV immune globulin, immunosuppressants, avoidance of blood transfusions, and withdrawal of drugs.

Etiology

AIHA is caused by abnormalities extrinsic to the RBC.

Warm antibody hemolytic anemia: Warm antibody hemolytic anemia is the most common form of AIHA; it is more common among women. Autoantibodies in warm antibody hemolytic anemia generally react at temperatures ≥ 37° C. AIHA may be classified as

- Primary (idiopathic)
- Secondary (occurring in association with an underlying disorder such as SLE, lymphoma, chronic lymphocytic leukemia or after use of certain drugs)

Some drugs (eg, α-methyldopa, levodopa—see Table 141–3) stimulate production of autoantibodies against Rh antigens (α-methyldopa-type of AIHA). Other drugs stimulate production of autoantibodies against the antibiotic–RBC-membrane complex as part of a transient hapten mechanism; the hapten may be stable (eg, high-dose penicillin, cephalosporins) or unstable (eg, quinidine, sulfonamides).

In warm antibody hemolytic anemia, hemolysis occurs primarily in the spleen and is not due to direct lysis of RBCs. It is often severe and can be fatal. Most of the autoantibodies in warm antibody hemolytic anemia are IgG. Most are panagglutinins and have limited specificity.

Cold agglutinin disease: Cold agglutinin disease (cold antibody disease) is caused by autoantibodies that react at temperatures < 37° C. Causes include

- Infections (especially mycoplasmal pneumonias or infectious mononucleosis)
- Lymphoproliferative disorders (antibodies are usually directed against the I antigen)
- Idiopathic (usually associated with a clonal B-cell population)

Table 141–3. DRUGS THAT CAN CAUSE WARM ANTIBODY HEMOLYTIC ANEMIA

MECHANISM	DRUGS
Autoantibody to Rh antigens	Cephalosporins Diclofenac Ibuprofen Interferon alfa Levodopa Mefenamic acid α-methyldopa Procainamide Teniposide Thioridazine Tolmetin
Stable hapten	Cephalosporins Fluorescein sodium Penicillins Tetracycline Tolbutamide
Unstable hapten or unknown mechanism	*p*-Aminosalicylic acid Amphotericin B Antazoline Cephalosporins Chlorpropamide Diclofenac Diethylstilbestrol Doxepin Hydrochlorothiazide Isoniazid Probenecid Quinidine Quinine Rifampin Sulfonamides Thiopental Tolmetin

Infections tend to cause acute disease, whereas idiopathic disease (the common form in older adults) tends to be chronic. The hemolysis occurs largely in the extravascular mononuclear phagocyte system of the liver and spleen. The anemia is usually mild (Hb > 7.5 g/dL). Autoantibodies in cold agglutinin disease are usually IgM. The higher the temperature (ie, the closer to normal body temperature) at which these antibodies react with the RBC, the greater the hemolysis.

Paroxysmal cold hemoglobinuria: Paroxysmal cold hemoglobinuria (PCH; Donath-Landsteiner syndrome) is a rare type of cold agglutinin disease. PCH is more common in children. Hemolysis results from exposure to cold, which may even be localized (eg, from drinking cold water, from washing hands in cold water). An IgG antibody binds to the P antigen on RBCs at low temperatures and causes intravascular hemolysis after warming. It occurs most often after a nonspecific viral illness or in otherwise healthy patients, although it occurs in some patients with congenital or acquired syphilis. The severity and rapidity of development of the anemia varies and may be fulminant. In children, this disease is often self-resolving.

Symptoms and Signs

Symptoms of warm antibody hemolytic anemia tend to be due to the anemia. If the disorder is severe, fever, chest pain, syncope, or heart failure may occur. Mild splenomegaly is typical.

Cold agglutinin disease manifests as an acute or chronic hemolytic anemia. Other cryopathic symptoms or signs may be present (eg, acrocyanoses, Raynaud syndrome, cold-associated occlusive changes).

Symptoms of PCH may include severe pain in the back and legs, headache, vomiting, diarrhea, and passage of dark brown urine; hepatosplenomegaly may be present.

Diagnosis

- Peripheral smear, reticulocyte count, LDH
- Direct antiglobulin test

AIHA should be suspected in any patient with a hemolytic anemia (as suggested by the presence of anemia and reticulocytosis). The peripheral smear usually shows microspherocytes (and the reticulocyte count will be high). Laboratory tests typically suggest extravascular hemolysis (eg, hemosiderinuria is absent; haptoglobin levels are near normal, schistocytes are absent on smear) unless anemia is sudden and severe or PCH is the cause. Spherocytosis and a high mean corpuscular Hb concentration (MCHC) are typical.

AIHA is diagnosed by detection of autoantibodies with the direct antiglobulin (direct Coombs) test. Antiglobulin serum is added to washed RBCs from the patient; agglutination indicates the presence of immunoglobulin or complement (C) bound to the RBCs. Generally IgG is present in warm antibody hemolytic anemia, and C3 (C3b and C3d) in cold antibody disease. The test is ≤ 98% sensitive for AIHA; false-negative results can occur if antibody density is very low or if the autoantibodies are IgA or IgM. In most cases of warm AIHA, the antibody is an IgG identified only as a panagglutinin, meaning the antigen specificity of the antibody can not be determined. In cold AIHA, the antibody is usually an IgM directed against the I/i carbohydrate on the RBC surface. Antibody titers can usually be determined but do not always correlate with disease activity.

The indirect antiglobulin (indirect Coombs) test is a complementary test that consists of mixing the patient's plasma with normal RBCs to determine whether such antibodies are free in the plasma. A positive indirect antiglobulin test and a negative direct test generally indicate an alloantibody caused by pregnancy, prior transfusions, or lectin cross-reactivity rather than immune hemolysis. Even identification of a warm antibody does not define hemolysis, because 1/10,000 healthy blood donors has a positive test result.

Once AIHA has been identified by the antiglobulin test, testing should differentiate between warm antibody hemolytic anemia and cold agglutinin disease as well as the mechanism responsible for warm antibody hemolytic anemia. This determination can often be made by observing the pattern of the direct antiglobulin reaction. Three patterns are possible:

- The reaction is positive with anti-IgG and negative with anti-C3. This pattern is common in idiopathic AIHA and in the drug-associated or α-methyldopa-type of AIHA, usually warm antibody hemolytic anemia.
- The reaction is positive with anti-IgG and anti-C3. This pattern is common in patients with SLE and idiopathic AIHA, usually warm antibody hemolytic anemia, and is rare in drug-associated cases.
- The reaction is positive with anti-C3 but negative with anti-IgG. This pattern occurs in cold agglutinin disease (where the antibody is most commonly an IgM). It can also occur in warm antibody hemolytic anemia when the IgG antibody is of low affinity, in some drug-associated cases, and in PCH.

Other studies can suggest the cause of AIHA but are not definitive. In cold agglutinin disease, RBCs clump on the peripheral smear, and automated cell counts often reveal an increased MCV and spuriously low Hb due to such clumping; hand warming of the tube and recounting result in values significantly closer to normal. Warm antibody hemolytic anemia can often be differentiated from cold agglutinin disease by the temperature at which the direct antiglobulin test is positive; a test that is positive at temperatures ≥ 37° C indicates warm antibody hemolytic anemia, whereas a test that is positive at lower temperatures indicates cold agglutinin disease.

If PCH is suspected, the Donath-Landsteiner test, which is specific for PCH, should be done. In this test, the patient's serum is incubated with normal RBCs at 4° for 30 min to allow for fixation of complement and then warmed to body temperature. Hemolysis of the RBCs during this test is indicative of PCH. Because the PCH antibody fixes complement at low temperatures, the direct antiglobulin (direct Coombs) test is positive for C3 and negative for IgG. However, the antibody in PCH is an IgG against the P antigen.

Treatment

- Blood transfusion for severe, life-threatening anemia
- For drug-induced warm antibody hemolytic anemia, drug withdrawal and sometimes IV immune globulin
- For idiopathic warm antibody hemolytic anemia, corticosteroids and, in refractory cases, rituximab, IV immune globulin, or splenectomy
- For cold agglutinin disease, avoidance of cold and treatment of underlying disorder
- For PCH, avoidance of cold, immunosuppressants, and treatment of syphilis if present. In children, this disease is often self-resolving.

Blood transfusion is the most important treatment for symptomatic patients who rapidly develop severe, life-threatening anemia. In this situation, transfusion should never be withheld due to lack of "compatible" units. In general, patients who have not had a previous blood transfusion or been pregnant are at low risk for hemolysis of ABO-compatible blood. Even if transfused cells are hemolyzed, blood transfusion can be life-saving until more definitive therapy can be done.

Treatment depends on the specific mechanism of the hemolysis.

Warm antibody hemolytic anemias: In **drug-induced warm antibody hemolytic anemias,** drug withdrawal decreases the rate of hemolysis. With α-methyldopa-type AIHA, hemolysis usually ceases within 3 wk; however, a positive antiglobulin test may persist for > 1 yr. With hapten-mediated AIHA, hemolysis ceases when the drug is cleared from the plasma. Corticosteroids have only little effect in drug-induced hemolysis; infusions of immune globulin may be more effective.

In **idiopathic warm antibody AIHA,** corticosteroids (eg, prednisone 1 mg/kg po once/day) are the standard first-line treatment. When stable RBC values are achieved, corticosteroids are tapered slowly with laboratory monitoring of hemolysis (eg, by Hb and reticulocyte count). The goal is to wean the patient completely from corticosteroids or to maintain remission with the lowest possible corticosteroid dose. About two-thirds of patients respond to corticosteroid treatment. In patients who relapse after corticosteroid cessation or who are refractory to corticosteroids, rituximab is usually used as a second-line drug.

Other treatments include use of additional immunosuppressive drugs and/or splenectomy. About one-third to one-half of patients have a sustained response after splenectomy.

In cases of fulminant hemolysis, high-dose pulse corticosteroids can be used. For less severe but uncontrolled hemolysis, immune globulin infusions have provided temporary control.

Long-term management with immunosuppressants (including cyclosporine) has been effective in patients in whom corticosteroids and splenectomy have been ineffective.

The presence of panagglutinating antibodies in warm antibody hemolytic anemia makes cross-matching of donor blood difficult. In addition, transfusions often superimpose an alloantibody on the autoantibody, accelerating hemolysis. Thus, transfusions should be avoided when anemia is not life-threatening.

Cold agglutinin disease: In many cases, avoidance of cold environments and other triggers of hemolysis may be all that is needed to prevent symptomatic anemia.

In cases associated with a lymphoproliferative disease, treatment is directed at the underlying disorder. Rituximab is commonly used, and chemotherapy regimens used to treat B-cell cancers can be effective.

In severe cases, plasmapheresis is an effective temporary treatment. Transfusions should be given sparingly, with the blood warmed through an on-line warmer.

Splenectomy is usually of no value. and immunosuppressants have only modest effectiveness.

Paroxysmal cold hemoglobinuria: In PCH, therapy consists of strict avoidance of exposure to cold. Immunosuppressants have been effective, but use should be restricted to patients with progressive or idiopathic cases.

Splenectomy is of no value.

Treatment of concomitant syphilis may cure PCH.

KEY POINTS

- AIHA is divided into warm antibody hemolytic anemia and cold agglutinin disease based on the temperature at which the autoantibodies react with RBCs.
- Hemolysis tends to be more severe in warm antibody hemolytic anemia and can be fatal.
- Immunoglobulin and/or complement bound to the patient's RBCs is demonstrated by the occurrence of agglutination after antiglobulin serum is added to washed RBCs (positive direct antiglobulin test).
- The pattern of the direct antiglobulin reaction can help distinguish warm antibody hemolytic anemia from cold agglutinin disease and sometimes identify the mechanism responsible for warm antibody hemolytic anemia.
- Treatment is directed at the cause (including stopping drugs, avoiding cold, treating underlying disorder); IV immune globulin may be used for drug-induced AIHA, and immunosuppressants or splenectomy for idiopathic warm antibody hemolytic disease.

EMBDEN-MEYERHOF PATHWAY DEFECTS

Embden-Meyerhof pathway defects are autosomal recessive RBC metabolic disorders that cause hemolytic anemia.

The **most common** defect is

- Pyruvate kinase deficiency

Other defects that cause hemolytic anemia include deficiencies of

- Erythrocyte hexokinase
- Glucose phosphate isomerase
- Phosphofructokinase

In all of these pathway defects, hemolytic anemia occurs only in homozygotes. The exact mechanism of hemolysis is unknown. Symptoms are related to the degree of anemia and may include jaundice and splenomegaly. Spherocytes are absent, but small numbers of irregularly shaped spheres may be present.

In general, assays of ATP and diphosphoglycerate help identify any metabolic defect and localize the defective sites for further analysis.

Treatment

- Supportive care
- Sometimes splenectomy

There is no specific therapy for these hemolytic anemias. Most patients require no treatment other than supplemental folate 1 mg po once/day during acute hemolysis. In severe cases, patients may be transfusion dependent in which case, splenectomy may be done. Hemolysis and anemia persist after splenectomy, although some improvement may occur, particularly in patients with pyruvate kinase deficiency.

GLUCOSE-6-PHOSPHATE DEHYDROGENASE DEFICIENCY

Glucose-6-phosphate dehydrogenase (G6PD) deficiency is an X-linked enzymatic defect common in blacks that can result in hemolysis after acute illnesses or intake of oxidant drugs (including salicylates and sulfonamides). Diagnosis is based on assay for G6PD, although tests are often falsely negative during acute hemolysis. Treatment is supportive.

G6PD deficiency, a defect in the hexose monophosphate shunt pathway, is the most common disorder of RBC metabolism. The G6PD gene is located on the X chromosome and exhibits a high amount of variation (polymorphism) resulting in a range of G6PD activity from normal to severely deficient. Variants are classified I through V by the amount of activity of the G6PD enzyme. Because the gene is X-linked, males are more likely to present with clinically significant hemolysis, although females who are homozygous, or who are heterozygous with skewed X inactivation that results in a high proportion of affected X chromosomes (see Mosaicism on p. 3194), may also be affected.

This defect occurs in about 10% of black males and in < 10% of black females in the US and in lower frequencies among people with ancestors from the Mediterranean basin (eg, Italians, Greeks, Arabs, Sephardic Jews).

Pathophysiology

G6PD deficiency renders the RBC susceptible to oxidative stress, which shortens RBC survival. Hemolysis occurs following an oxidative challenge, commonly after fever, acute viral or bacterial infections, and diabetic acidosis. Hemolysis is episodic and self-limited, although rare patients have chronic, ongoing hemolysis in the absence of oxidative challenge.

Less commonly, hemolysis occurs after exposure to drugs or to other substances that produce peroxide and cause oxidation of Hb and RBC membranes. These drugs and substances include primaquine, salicylates, sulfonamides, nitrofurans, phenacetin, naphthalene, some vitamin K derivatives, dapsone, phenazopyridine, nalidixic acid, methylene blue, and, in some cases, fava beans. The amount of hemolysis depends on the degree of G6PD deficiency and the oxidant potential of the drug.

Symptoms and Signs

In most cases, hemolysis affects < 25% of RBC mass and causes transient jaundice and dark urine. Some patients have back and/or abdominal pain. However, when the deficiency is more severe, profound hemolysis may lead to hemoglobinuria and acute kidney injury.

Diagnosis

- Peripheral smear
- G6PD assay

The diagnosis is considered in patients with evidence of acute hemolysis, particularly males with a direct antiglobulin–negative hemolytic anemia. Anemia, jaundice, and reticulocytosis develop during hemolysis. The peripheral smear may reveal RBCs that appear to have had one or more bites (1-μm wide) taken from the cell periphery (bite or blister cells) and RBCs with inclusions termed Heinz bodies, which are particles of denatured Hb. These cells may be visible early during the hemolytic episode but do not persist in patients with an intact spleen because they are removed.

Testing for G6PD activity is available. However, during and immediately after a hemolytic episode, tests may yield false-negative results because of destruction of the older, more deficient RBCs and the presence of reticulocytes rich in G6PD. Thus, testing may need to be repeated several weeks after the acute event. Several screening tests are available, including point-of-care tests; positive results should be confirmed with a quantitative test.

Treatment

- Avoidance of triggers, removal of offending drug or agent, and supportive care

During acute hemolysis, treatment is supportive; transfusions are rarely needed. Patients are advised to avoid drugs or substances that initiate hemolysis.

Hb C DISEASE

Hb C disease is a hemoglobinopathy that causes symptoms of a hemolytic anemia.

The prevalence of Hb C in blacks in the US is about 2 to 3%. Heterozygotes are asymptomatic. Homozyotes have chronic hemolytic anemia and splenomegaly and symptoms consistent with anemia. Cholelithiasis is the most common complication, and splenic sequestration is possible.

Hb C disease is suspected in all patients with a family history and evidence of a hemolytic anemia, particularly in adults with splenomegaly. The anemia is usually mild but can be severe. The smear is normocytic, with frequent target cells, spherocytes, and, rarely, crystal-containing RBCs. Nucleated RBCs may be present. The RBCs do not sickle. On electrophoresis, the Hb is type C. In heterozygotes, the only laboratory abnormality is centrally targeted RBCs.

No specific treatment is recommended. Anemia usually is not severe enough to require blood transfusion.

Hb E DISEASE

Homozygous Hb E disease (a hemoglobinopathy) causes a mild hemolytic anemia, usually without splenomegaly.

Hb E is the 3rd most prevalent Hb worldwide (after Hb A and Hb S), primarily in Southeast Asian (> 15% incidence of homozygous disease) populations, although rarely in Chinese populations. Heterozygotes (Hb AE) are asymptomatic. Patients heterozygous for Hb E and β-thalassemia have a hemolytic disease more severe than S-thalassemia or homozygous Hb E disease and usually have splenomegaly.

In heterozygotes (Hb AE), a microcytosis is present without anemia, and target cells can be seen on peripheral blood smear. In homozygotes, a mild microcytic anemia with prominent target cells exists.

Diagnosis of Hb E disorders is by Hb electrophoresis.

Most patients do not require treatment. However, patients with severe disease may benefit from chronic transfusions or splenectomy.

Hb S-C DISEASE

Hb S-C disease is a hemoglobinopathy that causes symptoms similar to those of sickle cell disease, but usually less severe.

Because 10% of blacks carry the Hb S trait (which is responsible for sickle cell disease), the heterozygous S-C combination is more common than homozygous Hb C disease. The anemia in Hb S-C disease is milder than the anemia in sickle cell disease; some patients even have normal Hb levels.

Symptoms are similar to the symptoms of sickle cell disease, but are usually less frequent and less severe. However, gross hematuria, retinal hemorrhages, and aseptic necrosis of the femoral head are common. Splenomegaly may be present.

Hb S-C disease is suspected in patients whose clinical features suggest sickle cell disease or whose RBCs demonstrate sickling. Stained blood smears show target cells, spherocytes, and rarely sickle cells or oat-shaped cells. Sickling is identified in a sickling preparation, and Hb electrophoresis establishes the diagnosis.

Treatment can be similar to the treatment of sickle cell disease but is determined by severity of symptoms.

Hb S–β-THALASSEMIA DISEASE

Hb S–β-thalassemia disease is a hemoglobinopathy that causes symptoms similar to those of sickle cell disease, but milder.

Because of the increased frequency of both Hb S (the abnormal Hb that is responsible for sickle cell disease) and β-thalassemia genes in similar population groups, inheritance of both defects is relatively common. β-thalassemia results from decreased production of the β-polypeptide chains of Hb due to either mutations or deletions in the β globin gene, leading to impaired production of Hb A (see also Thalassemias on p. 1113).

Clinically, Hb S–β-thalassemia causes symptoms of moderate anemia and signs of sickle cell disease, which are usually less frequent and less severe than those of sickle cell disease. Mild to moderate microcytic anemia is usually present along with some sickled RBCs on stained blood smears.

Diagnosis requires quantitative Hb studies. The Hb A_2 is > 3%. Hb S predominates on electrophoresis, and Hb A is decreased or absent. Hb F increase is variable.

Treatment, if necessary, is the same as treatment of sickle cell disease.

HEREDITARY SPHEROCYTOSIS AND HEREDITARY ELLIPTOCYTOSIS

Hereditary spherocytosis and hereditary elliptocytosis are congenital RBC membrane disorders. Symptoms, generally milder in hereditary elliptocytosis, include variable degrees of anemia, jaundice, and splenomegaly. Diagnosis requires demonstration of increased RBC osmotic fragility and a negative direct antiglobulin test. Rarely, patients < 45 yr with symptomatic disease require splenectomy.

Hereditary spherocytosis (chronic familial icterus; congenital hemolytic jaundice; familial spherocytosis; spherocytic anemia) is an autosomal dominant disease with variable gene penetrance. It is characterized by hemolysis of spheroidal RBCs and anemia.

Hereditary elliptocytosis (ovalocytosis) is a rare autosomal dominant disorder in which RBCs are oval or elliptical. Hemolysis is usually absent or slight, with little or no anemia; splenomegaly is often present.

Pathophysiology

Alterations in membrane proteins cause the RBC abnormalities in both disorders.

- In **hereditary spherocytosis,** the cell membrane surface area is decreased disproportionately to the intracellular content. The decreased surface area of the cell impairs the flexibility needed for the cell to traverse the spleen's microcirculation, causing intrasplenic hemolysis.
- In **hereditary elliptocytosis,** genetic mutations result in weakness of the cytoskeleton of the cell, leading to deformation of the cell. The abnormally shaped RBCs are taken up and destroyed by the spleen.

Symptoms and Signs

In **hereditary spherocytosis,** symptoms and signs are usually mild. The anemia may be so well compensated that it is not recognized until an intercurrent viral illness, such as parvovirus infection, transiently decreases RBC production, causing an aplastic crisis. These episodes can be self-limited, resolving with resolution of the infection, while others require urgent treatment. Moderate jaundice and symptoms of anemia are present in severe cases. Splenomegaly is almost invariable but only rarely causes abdominal discomfort. Hepatomegaly may be present. Cholelithiasis (pigment stones) is common and may be the presenting symptom. Congenital skeletal abnormalities (eg, tower-shaped skull, polydactylism) occasionally occur. Although usually one or more family members have had symptoms, several generations may be skipped because of variations in the degree of gene penetrance.

In **hereditary elliptocytosis,** clinical features are similar to those of hereditary spherocytosis but tend to be milder.

Diagnosis

- Peripheral blood smear, RBC fragility assay, RBC autohemolysis assay, and direct antiglobulin (Coombs) test

Hereditary spherocytosis or hereditary elliptocytosis is suspected in patients with unexplained hemolysis (as suggested by the presence of anemia and reticulocytosis), particularly if splenomegaly, a family history of similar manifestations, or suggestive RBC indices are present.

In hereditary spherocytosis, because RBCs are spheroidal and the MCV is normal, the mean corpuscular diameter is below normal, and RBCs resemble microspherocytes. MCHC is increased. Reticulocytosis of 15 to 30% and leukocytosis are common. In hereditary elliptocytosis, the RBCs are typically elliptical or cigar-shaped; however, the clinical presentation is variable. Diagnosis is usually made by the presence of at least 60% elliptocytes on peripheral smear and a family history of similar disease.

If these disorders are suspected, the following tests are done:

- RBC osmotic fragility test, which mixes RBCs with varying concentrations of saline
- RBC autohemolysis test, which measures the amount of spontaneous hemolysis occurring after 48 h of sterile incubation
- Direct antiglobulin (direct Coombs) test, to rule out spherocytosis due to AIHA

RBC fragility is characteristically increased, but in mild cases, it may be normal unless sterile defibrinated blood is first incubated at 37° C for 24 h. RBC autohemolysis is increased and can be corrected by the addition of glucose. The direct antiglobulin test results are negative.

Treatment

- Sometimes splenectomy

Splenectomy, after appropriate vaccination, is the only specific treatment for hereditary spherocytosis or hereditary elliptocytosis but is rarely needed. It is indicated in patients with symptomatic hemolysis or complications such as biliary colic or persistent aplastic crisis. If the gallbladder has stones or other evidence of cholestasis, it should be removed during splenectomy. Although spherocytosis persists after splenectomy, the cells survive longer in the circulation. Usually, symptoms resolve and anemia and reticulocytosis decrease. However, RBC fragility remains high.

PAROXYSMAL NOCTURNAL HEMOGLOBINURIA

Paroxysmal nocturnal hemoglobinuria (PNH) is a rare acquired disorder characterized by intravascular hemolysis and hemoglobinuria. Leukopenia, thrombocytopenia, arterial and venous thromboses, and episodic crises are common. Diagnosis requires flow cytometry. Treatment is supportive and with eculizumab, a terminal complement inhibitor.

PNH is most common among men in their 20s, but it occurs in both sexes and at any age. Hemolysis occurs throughout the day not just at night-time.

Etiology

PNH is a clonal disorder caused by an acquired mutation in the *PIGA* gene of hematopoietic stem cells. *PIGA*, located on the X chromosome, encodes a protein that is integral for formation of the glycosylphosphatidylinositol (GPI) anchor for membrane proteins. Mutations in *PIGA* result in loss of all GPI-anchored proteins, including CD59, an important complement-regulating protein, on the surface of blood cells. As a consequence, cells are susceptible to complement activation, leading to ongoing intravascular hemolysis of RBCs.

Pathophysiology

Both arterial and venous thrombosis can occur, including thrombosis of less common sites such as portal veins and cerebral venous sinuses. Protracted urinary Hb loss may result in iron deficiency. PNH is associated with bone marrow dysfunction, often leading to leukopenia and thrombocytopenia. About 20% of patients with severe aplastic anemia, another clonal hematopoietic disorder, have a detectable PNH clone.

Symptoms

Crises are usually precipitated by a "trigger," such as infection, iron use, vaccination, or menstruation. Abdominal, chest, and lumbar pain and symptoms of severe anemia may occur; gross hemoglobinuria and splenomegaly are common. Manifestations of vascular thrombosis depend on the affected vessel and are discussed elsewhere in The Manual.

Diagnosis

- Flow cytometry

PNH is suspected in patients who have typical symptoms of anemia (eg, pallor, fatigue, dizziness, possible hypotension) or unexplained normocytic anemia with intravascular hemolysis, particularly if leukopenia or thrombocytopenia and/or thrombotic events are present.

Historically, if PNH was suspected, the acid hemolysis (Ham test) or sugar-water test was usually the first test done. These tests relied on activation of complement via acidification of serum or high-concentration sucrose solutions.

Currently, diagnosis of PNH is with flow cytometry, which is used to determine the absence of specific RBC or WBC cell surface proteins (CD59 and CD55). This test is highly sensitive and specific.

Bone marrow examination is not necessary but, if done to exclude other disorders, usually shows erythroid hyperplasia.

Gross hemoglobinuria is common during crises, and the urine may contain hemosiderin.

Treatment

- Supportive measures
- Eculizumab

Patients with small clones (ie, < 10% by flow cytometry) who are largely asymptomatic generally do not need treatment. Indications for treatment include

- Symptomatic hemolysis requiring transfusions
- Thrombosis
- Other cytopenias

Supportive measures include oral iron and folate supplementation and sometimes transfusions. Corticosteroids (eg, prednisone 20 to 40 mg po once/day) can control symptoms and stabilize RBC values in > 50% of patients and can be used when eculizumab is unavailable. However, due to the adverse effects of long-term use, corticosteroids should be avoided for chronic treatment. Generally, transfusions are reserved for crises. Transfusions containing plasma (and thus C3) should be avoided. Washing RBCs with saline before transfusion is no longer necessary. Heparin followed by warfarin or other anticoagulants may be required for thromboses but should be used cautiously.

Eculizumab, a monoclonal antibody that binds to C5 and acts as a terminal complement inhibitor, has remarkably changed the course of the disorder. It is given to all patients who require treatment. Eculizumab reduces transfusion requirements, thromboembolism risk, and symptoms and improves quality of life. However, eculizumab increases the risk of infection with *Neisseria meningitidis*, so patients should receive the meningococcal vaccine at least 14 d before starting eculizumab.

SICKLE CELL DISEASE

(Hb S Disease)

Sickle cell disease (a hemoglobinopathy—see Sidebar 141–1) causes a chronic hemolytic anemia occurring almost exclusively in blacks. It is caused by homozygous inheritance of Hb S. Sickle-shaped RBCs cause vaso-occlusion and are prone to hemolysis, leading to severe pain crises, organ ischemia, and other systemic complications. Acute exacerbations (crises) may develop frequently. Infection, bone marrow aplasia, or lung involvement (acute chest syndrome) can develop acutely and be fatal. Anemia is present, and sickle cells are usually evident on the peripheral smear. Diagnosis requires Hb electrophoresis. Painful crises are treated with analgesics and other supportive measures. Transfusions are occasionally required. Vaccines against bacterial infections, prophylactic antibiotics, and aggressive treatment of infections prolong survival. Hydroxyurea may decrease the frequency of crises and the acute chest syndrome.

Homozygotes (about 0.3% of blacks in the US) have sickle cell anemia; heterozygotes (8 to 13% of blacks) are typically not anemic but have an increased risk of other complications.

Pathophysiology

In Hb S, valine is substituted for glutamic acid in the 6th amino acid of the β chain. Oxygenated Hb S is much less soluble than oxygenated Hb A; it forms a semisolid gel that causes RBCs to deform into a sickle shape at sites of low PO_2. Distorted, inflexible RBCs adhere to vascular endothelium and plug small arterioles and capillaries, which leads to infarction. Vaso-occlusion also causes endothelial injury, which results in inflammation and can lead to thromboses. Because sickled RBCs are fragile, the mechanical trauma of circulation causes hemolysis. Chronic compensatory marrow hyperactivity deforms the bones.

Acute exacerbations: Acute exacerbations (crises) occur intermittently, often for no known reason. In some cases, crisis appears to be precipitated by

- Fever
- Viral infection
- Local trauma

Vaso-occlusive crisis (pain crisis) is the most common type; it is caused by ischemia, tissue hypoxia and infarction, typically of the bones, but also of the spleen, lungs, or kidneys.

Aplastic crisis occurs when marrow erythropoiesis slows during acute infection due to human parvovirus, during which an acute erythroblastopenia may occur.

Acute chest syndrome results from pulmonary microvascular occlusion and is a common cause of death, with mortality rates of up to 10%. It occurs in all age groups but is most common in childhood. Repeated episodes predispose to chronic pulmonary hypertension.

In children, acute sequestration of sickled cells in the spleen may occur, exacerbating anemia.

Priapism, a serious complication that can cause erectile dysfunction, is most common in young men.

Complications: Chronic spleen damage can lead to autoinfarction and increases susceptibility to infection, particularly pneumococcal and *Salmonella* infections (including *Salmonella* osteomyelitis). These infections are especially common in early childhood and can be fatal.

Recurrent ischemia and infarction can cause chronic dysfunction of multiple different organ systems. Complications include ischemic stroke, seizures, avascular necrosis of the hips, renal concentrating defects, renal failure, heart failure, pulmonary hypertension and fibrosis, and retinopathy.

Heterozygotes: Patients who are heterozygous (Hb AS) do not experience hemolysis or painful crises. However, they do have an increased risk of chronic kidney disease and pulmonary embolism. In addition, rhabdomyolysis and sudden death may occur during sustained, exhausting exercise. Impaired ability to concentrate urine (hyposthenuria) is common. Unilateral hematuria (by unknown mechanisms and usually from the left kidney) can occur but is self-limited. Typical renal papillary necrosis can occur but is less common than among homozygous patients, and there is an association with the extremely rare medullary carcinoma of the kidney.

Sidebar 141–1. Hemoglobinopathies

Hb molecules consist of polypeptide chains whose chemical structure is genetically controlled. The normal adult Hb molecule (Hb A) consists of 2 pairs of chains designated α and β. Normal blood also contains a ≤ 2.5% concentration of Hb A_2 (composed of α and δ chains). Fetal Hb (Hb F, which has γ chains in the place of β chains) gradually decreases, particularly in the first months of life, until it makes up < 2% of total Hb in adults (see p. 2387). Hb F concentration increases in certain disorders of Hb synthesis and in aplastic and myeloproliferative states.

Some hemoglobinopathies result in anemias that are severe in patients who are homozygous but mild in those who are heterozygous. Some patients are compound heterozygotes for 2 different hemoglobinopathies and have anemia of varying severity.

Different Hbs, as distinguished by electrophoretic mobility, are alphabetically designated in order of discovery (eg, A, B, C), although the first abnormal Hb, sickle cell Hb, was designated Hb S. Structurally different Hbs with the same electrophoretic mobility are named for the city or location in which they were discovered (eg, Hb S Memphis, Hb C Harlem). Standard description of a patient's Hb composition places the Hb of greatest concentration first (eg, AS in sickle cell trait).

In the US, important anemias are caused by genetic mutations resulting in Hb S or Hb C and the thalassemias, and immigration of Southeast Asians has made Hb E disease common.

Symptoms and Signs

Most symptoms occur only in patients who are homozygous and result from

- Anemia
- Vaso-occlusive events resulting in tissue ischemia and infarction

Anemia is usually severe but varies among patients and is usually compensated; mild jaundice and pallor are common.

Hepatosplenomegaly is common in children, but because of repeated infarctions and subsequent fibrosis (autosplenectomy), the spleen in adults is commonly atrophied. Cardiomegaly and systolic ejection (flow) murmurs are common. Cholelithiasis and chronic punched-out ulcers around the ankles are common.

Painful crisis causes severe pain in long bones, the hands and feet, back, and joints. Hip pain may result from avascular necrosis of the femoral head. Severe abdominal pain may develop with or without vomiting and is usually accompanied by back and joint pain.

Acute chest syndrome is characterized by sudden onset of fever, chest pain, and pulmonary infiltrates. It may follow bacterial pneumonia. Hypoxemia may develop rapidly, causing dyspnea.

Diagnosis

- DNA testing (prenatal diagnosis)
- Peripheral smear
- Solubility testing
- Hb electrophoresis (or thin-layer isoelectric focusing)

The type of testing done depends on the age of the patient. DNA testing can be used for prenatal diagnosis or to confirm a diagnosis of the sickle cell genotype. Screening of neonates is available in most US states and involves Hb electrophoresis. Screening and diagnosis in children and adults involve examination of the peripheral smear, Hb solubility testing, and Hb electrophoresis.

Prenatal screening: The sensitivity of prenatal diagnosis has been greatly improved with the availability of the PCR technique. It is recommended for families at risk for sickle cell (eg, couples with medical or family histories of anemia or of suggestive ethnic background). DNA samples can be obtained by chorionic villus sampling at 8 to 10 wk gestation. Amniotic fluid can also be tested at 14 to 16 wk. Diagnosis is important for genetic counseling.

Newborn screening: Universal testing is currently recommended and is frequently one of a battery of newborn screening tests. To distinguish between Hbs F, S, A, and C, the recommended tests are Hb electrophoresis using cellulose acetate or acid citrate agar, thin-layer isoelectric focusing, or Hb fractionation by high performance liquid chromatography (HPLC). Repeat testing at age 3 to 6 mo may be necessary for confirmation. Solubility testing for Hb S is unreliable during the first few months of life.

Screening and diagnosis of children and adults: Patients with a family history of sickle cell disease or trait should be screened with peripheral smear, Hb solubility testing, and Hb electrophoresis.

Patients with symptoms or signs suggesting the disorder or its complications (eg, poor growth, acute and unexplained bone pain, aseptic necrosis of the femoral head, unexplained hematuria), and black patients with normocytic anemia (particularly if hemolysis is present) require laboratory tests for hemolytic anemia, Hb electrophoresis, and examination of RBCs for sickling. If sickle cell disease is present, RBC count is usually between 2 and 3 million/μL with Hb reduced proportionately; cells are normocytic (microcytosis suggests a concomitant α-thalassemia). Nucleated RBCs frequently appear in the peripheral blood, and reticulocytosis ≥ 10% is common. Dry-stained smears may show sickled RBCs (crescent-shaped, often with elongated or pointed ends).

The homozygous state is differentiated from other sickle hemoglobinopathies by electrophoresis showing only Hb S with a variable amount of Hb F. The heterozygote is differentiated by the presence of more Hb A than Hb S on electrophoresis. Hb S must be distinguished from other Hb with a similar electrophoretic pattern by showing the pathognomonic RBC morphology.

Bone marrow examination is not used for diagnosis. If it is done to differentiate other anemias, it shows hyperplasia, with normoblasts predominating; bone marrow may become aplastic during sickling or severe infections. ESR, if done to exclude other disorders (eg, juvenile RA causing hand and foot pain), is low.

Incidental findings on skeletal x-rays may include widening of the diploic spaces of the skull and a sun-ray appearance of the diploic trabeculations. The long bones often show cortical thinning, irregular densities, and new bone formation within the medullary canal.

Unexplained hematuria, even among patients not suspected of having sickle cell disease, should prompt consideration of sickle cell trait.

Evaluation of exacerbations: If patients with known sickle cell disease have acute exacerbations, including pain, fever, or other symptoms of infection, aplastic crisis is considered and CBC and reticulocyte count are done. Reticulocyte count < 1% suggests aplastic crisis, particularly when Hb decreases below the patient's usual level. In a painful crisis without aplasia, WBC count rises, often with a shift to the left, particularly during bacterial infection. Platelet count usually increases. If measured, serum bilirubin is usually elevated (eg, 2 to 4 mg/dL [34 to 68 μmol/L]), and urine may contain urobilinogen.

In patients with chest pain or difficulty breathing, acute chest syndrome and pulmonary embolism are considered; chest x-ray and pulse oximetry are necessary. Because acute chest syndrome is the leading cause of death in sickle cell disease, early recognition and treatment are critical. Hypoxemia or pulmonary parenchymal infiltrates on chest x-ray suggest acute chest syndrome or pneumonia. Hypoxemia without pulmonary infiltrates suggests pulmonary embolism.

In patients with fever, infection and acute chest syndrome are considered; cultures, chest x-ray, and other appropriate diagnostic tests are done.

Prognosis

The life span of homozygous patients has steadily increased to > 50 yr. Common causes of death are acute chest syndrome, intercurrent infections, pulmonary emboli, infarction of a vital organ, and renal failure.

Treatment

- Broad-spectrum antibiotics (for infection)
- Analgesics and IV hydration (for vaso-occlusive pain crisis)
- Sometimes transfusions
- Immunizations, folate supplementation, and hydroxyurea (for health maintenance)

Treatment includes regular health maintenance measures as well as specific treatment of the complications as they arise. Complications are treated supportively. No effective in vivo anti-sickling drug is available. Splenectomy is valueless.

Hematopoietic stem cell transplantation remains the only curative treatment for sickle cell disease. Given the risks associated with this therapy, it is generally restricted to patients with advanced disease complications. However, this field is rapidly evolving and use of stem cell therapy may expand in the near future.

Gene therapy offers hope for a cure, but it is still under study.

Indications for hospitalization include suspected serious (including systemic) infection, aplastic crisis, acute chest syndrome, and, often, intractable pain or the need for transfusion. Fever alone may not be a reason to hospitalize. However, patients who appear acutely ill and have a temperature > 38° C should be admitted so that cultures can be obtained from multiple areas and IV antibiotics can be given.

Antibiotics: Patients with suspected serious bacterial infections or acute chest syndrome require broad-spectrum antibiotics immediately.

Analgesics: Painful crises are managed with liberal administration of analgesics, usually opioids. IV morphine (continuous or bolus) is effective and safe; meperidine is avoided. During crises, pain and fever may persist for as long as 5 days. Nonsteroidal anti-inflammatory drugs (NSAIDS) are often useful in reducing opioid requirements; however, they must be used cautiously in patients with renal disease.

Intravenous hydration: Although dehydration contributes to sickling and may precipitate crises, it is unclear whether vigorous hydration is helpful during crises. Nevertheless, maintaining normal intravascular volume has been a mainstay of therapy.

Transfusion: Transfusion is given in many situations in which its efficacy has not been demonstrated. However, chronic transfusion therapy is indicated for prevention of recurrent cerebral thrombosis, especially in children, in an effort to maintain the Hb S percentage less than 30%.

In the acute setting, specific indications include acute splenic sequestration, aplastic crises, cardiopulmonary symptoms or signs (eg, high-output heart failure, hypoxemia with PO_2 < 65 mm Hg), preoperative use, priapism, and life-threatening events that would benefit from improved oxygen delivery (eg, sepsis, severe infection, acute chest syndrome, stroke, acute organ ischemia). Transfusion is not helpful during an uncomplicated painful crisis. Transfusion may be needed during pregnancy.

Simple transfusion can be done when the goal is to correct anemia, such as during aplastic crisis or splenic sequestration. Exchange transfusion is done during other acute events in order to decrease the Hb S percent and prevent ischemia. It can be done with modern apheresis machines. If the initial Hb is low (< 7 g/dL), this process cannot be initiated before first transfusing red cells. Partial exchange transfusion minimizes iron accumulation and hyperviscosity.

Health maintenance: For long-term management the following interventions have reduced mortality, particularly during childhood:

- Pneumococcal, *Haemophilus influenzae*, influenza (inactivated, not live), and meningococcal vaccines
- Early identification and treatment of serious bacterial infections
- Prophylactic antibiotics, including continuous prophylaxis with oral penicillin from age 4 mo to 6 yr
- Use of hydroxyurea and folate supplementation

Supplemental folate, 1 mg po once/day, is usually prescribed.

Hydroxyurea, by increasing Hb F and thereby reducing sickling, decreases painful crises (by 50%) and decreases acute chest syndrome and transfusion requirements. It is indicated in patients with recurrent pain crises or other complications. The dose of hydroxyurea is variable and is adjusted based on blood counts and adverse effects. Hydroxyurea is a leukemogen and causes neutropenia and thrombocytopenia. It is also a teratogen and should not be given to females of child-bearing age.

Transcranial Doppler flow studies in children can help predict risk of stroke, and many experts recommend annual screening for children from age 2 to 16 yr. Children at high risk appear to benefit from prophylactic, chronic exchange transfusions to keep HbS at < 30% of total Hb; iron overload is common and must be screened for and treated.

KEY POINTS

- Patients homozygous for Hb S have an abnormal β chain, resulting in fragile, relatively inflexible RBCs that can plug capillaries, causing tissue infarction and that are prone to hemolysis, causing anemia.
- Patients have various acute exacerbations including painful crisis, sequestration crisis, aplastic crisis, and acute chest syndrome.
- Long term consequences include pulmonary hypertension, chronic kidney disease, stroke, aseptic necrosis, and increased risk of infection.
- Diagnose using Hb electrophoresis.
- For acute crises, give opioid analgesics for pain, check for worsening anemia (suggesting aplastic or sequestration crisis) and signs of acute chest syndrome or infection, restore normal intravascular volume using 0.9% saline and then give maintenance fluids.
- Prevent infection by using vaccinations and prophylactic antibiotics; limit painful crises and risk of acute chest syndrome by giving hydroxyurea.

STOMATOCYTOSIS AND ANEMIA CAUSED BY HYPOPHOSPHATEMIA

Stomatocytosis (RBCs with a transverse slit or stoma across the center) and hypophosphatemia cause RBC membrane abnormalities that can result in hemolytic anemia.

Stomatocytosis: Stomatocytosis is a rare condition of RBCs in which a mouthlike or slitlike pattern replaces the normal central zone of pallor. Stomatocytosis can be congenital or acquired; both may be asymptomatic or result in hemolysis. Symptoms, if present, result mainly from the anemia.

Congenital stomatocytosis, which shows autosomal dominant inheritance, is rare. It can cause a severe hemolytic anemia presenting very early in life. The RBC membrane is hyperpermeable to monovalent cations (sodium and potassium); movement of divalent cations and anions is normal. The percentage of stomatocytes varies and RBC fragility is increased, as is autohemolysis with inconstant correction with glucose. Splenectomy ameliorates anemia in some cases.

Acquired stomatocytosis with hemolytic anemia occurs primarily with recent excessive alcohol ingestion. Stomatocytes in the peripheral blood and hemolysis disappear within 2 wk of alcohol withdrawal.

Anemia caused by hypophosphatemia: RBC pliability varies according to intracellular ATP levels. Because the serum phosphate concentration affects RBC ATP levels, low serum phosphate level (< 0.5 mg/dL [< 0.16 mmol/L]) depletes ATP levels in RBCs. The complex metabolic sequelae of hypophosphatemia also include 2,3-diphosphoglyceric acid depletion, a shift to the left in the oxygen dissociation curve, decreased glucose utilization, and increased lactate production. The resultant rigid, nonyielding RBCs are susceptible to injury in the capillary circulatory bed, leading to hemolysis and small, sphere-shaped RBCs (microspherocytosis).

Severe hypophosphatemia may occur in

- Alcohol withdrawal
- Diabetes mellitus
- Refeeding after starvation
- The recovery (diuretic) phase after severe burns
- Hyperalimentation
- Severe respiratory alkalosis
- Uremic patients receiving dialysis who are taking antacids

Phosphate supplements prevent or reverse the anemia and are considered for patients at risk of or who have hypophosphatemia.

THALASSEMIAS

(Mediterranean Anemia; Thalassemia Major and Minor)

Thalassemias are a group of inherited microcytic, hemolytic anemias characterized by defective Hb synthesis. α-thalassemia is particularly common among people of African, Mediterranean, or Southeast Asian ancestry. β-thalassemia is more common in people of Mediterranean, Middle Eastern, Southeast Asian, or Indian ancestry. Symptoms and signs result from anemia, hemolysis, splenomegaly, bone marrow hyperplasia, and, if there have been multiple transfusions, iron overload. Diagnosis is based on genetic tests and quantitative Hb analysis. Treatment for severe forms may include transfusion, splenectomy, chelation, and stem cell transplantation.

Pathophysiology

Thalassemia is a hemoglobinopathy that is among the most common inherited disorders of Hb production. It results from unbalanced Hb synthesis caused by decreased production of at least one globin polypeptide chain (β, α, γ, δ).

α-thalassemia: α-thalassemia results from decreased production of α-polypeptide chains due to a deletion of one or more α genes. People normally have four α alleles (two on each of a pair of chromosomes) because the α gene is duplicated. Disease classification is based on the number and location of deletions:

- **α + thalassemia:** Loss of a single gene on one chromosome (α/--)
- **α 0 thalassemia:** Loss of both genes on the same chromosome (--/--)

β-thalassemia: β-thalassemia results from decreased production of β-polypeptide chains due to either mutations or deletions in the β globin gene, leading to impaired production of Hb A. Mutations or deletions may result in partial loss (β + allele) or complete loss (β 0 allele) of β globin function. There are two β globin genes, and patients may have heterozygous, homozygous, or compound heterozygous mutations. In addition, patients may be heterozygous or homozygous for abnormalities in 2 different globin genes (eg, β and δ).

β-δ-thalassemia is a less common form of β-thalassemia in which production of both the δ chain as well as the β chain is impaired. These mutations may be heterozygous or homozygous.

Symptoms and Signs

Clinical features of thalassemias are similar but vary in severity depending on the amount of normal Hb present.

α-thalassemia: Patients with a single α + allele are clinically normal (silent carriers).

Heterozygotes with defects in 2 of the 4 genes (either two α + alleles or one α 0 allele) tend to develop mild to moderate microcytic anemia but no symptoms. These patients have α thalassemia trait.

Defects in 3 of the 4 genes (coinheritance of both α + and α 0) severely impair α-chain production, resulting in the formation of tetramers of excess β-chains (Hb H) or, in infancy, γ-chains (Bart's Hb). Patients with Hb H disease often have symptomatic hemolytic anemia and splenomegaly.

Defects in all 4 genes (two α 0 alleles) is a lethal condition in utero (hydrops fetalis), because Hb that lacks α chains does not transport oxygen.

β-thalassemia: In β-thalassemia, clinical phenotypes are classified into 3 groups based on the degree to which β globin production is impaired:

- Minor (or trait)
- Intermedia
- Major

β-thalassemia minor (trait) occurs in heterozygotes, who are usually asymptomatic with mild to moderate microcytic anemia.

β-thalassemia intermedia causes a variable clinical picture that is intermediate between thalassemia major or minor.

β-thalassemia major (or Cooley anemia) occurs in homozygotes or compound heterozygotes (containing a β 0 allele) and results from severe β globin deficiency. These patients develop severe anemia and bone marrow hyperactivity. β-thalassemia major manifests by age 1 to 2 yr with symptoms of severe anemia and transfusional and absorptive iron overload. Patients are jaundiced, and leg ulcers and cholelithiasis occur (as in sickle cell disease). Splenomegaly, often massive, is common. Splenic sequestration may develop, accelerating destruction of transfused normal RBCs. Bone marrow hyperactivity causes thickening of the cranial bones and malar eminences. Long bone involvement predisposes to pathologic fractures and impairs growth, possibly delaying or preventing puberty.

With iron overload, iron deposits in heart muscle may cause heart failure. Hepatic siderosis is typical, leading to functional impairment and cirrhosis. Iron chelation is usually necessary.

Diagnosis

- Evaluation for hemolytic anemia if suspected
- Peripheral smear
- Hb electrophoresis
- DNA testing (prenatal diagnosis)

Thalassemia trait is commonly detected when routine peripheral blood smear and complete blood count show microcytic anemia and elevated red cell count. If desired, the diagnosis of β thalassemia trait can be confirmed with quantitative Hb studies. No intervention is needed.

More severe thalassemias are suspected in patients with a family history, suggestive symptoms or signs, or microcytic hemolytic anemia. If thalassemias are suspected, laboratory tests for microcytic and hemolytic anemias and quantitative Hb studies are done. Serum bilirubin, iron, and ferritin levels are increased.

In α-thalassemias, the percentages of Hb F and Hb A_2 are generally normal, and the diagnosis of single or double gene defect thalassemias may be carried out with newer genetic tests and often is one of exclusion of other causes of microcytic anemia.

In β-thalassemia major, anemia is severe, often with Hb ≤ 6 g/dL. RBC count is elevated relative to Hb because the cells are very microcytic. The blood smear is virtually diagnostic, with many nucleated erythroblasts; target cells; small, pale RBCs; and punctate and diffuse basophilia.

In quantitative Hb studies, elevation of Hb A_2 is diagnostic for β-thalassemia minor. In β-thalassemia major, Hb F is usually increased, sometimes to as much as 90%, and Hb A_2 is usually elevated to > 3%.

Hb H disease can be diagnosed by demonstrating the fast-migrating Hb H or Bart's fractions on Hb electrophoresis. The specific molecular defect can be characterized but does not alter the clinical approach.

Recombinant DNA approaches of gene mapping (particularly the PCR) have become standard for prenatal diagnosis and genetic counseling.

If bone marrow examination is done for anemia (eg, to exclude other causes), it shows marked erythroid hyperplasia. X-rays done for other reasons in patients with β-thalassemia major show changes due to chronic bone marrow hyperactivity. The skull may show cortical thinning, widened diploic space, a sun-ray appearance of the trabeculae, and a granular or ground-glass appearance. The long bones may show cortical thinning, marrow space widening, and areas of osteoporosis. The vertebral bodies may have a granular or ground-glass appearance. The phalanges may appear rectangular or biconvex.

Prognosis

Life expectancy is normal for people with β-thalassemia minor or α-thalassemia minor. The prognosis of Hb H disease and β-thalassemia intermedia varies.

Life expectancy is decreased in people with β-thalassemia major mostly due to complication from chronic transfusions.

Treatment

- Often RBC transfusion, with or without iron chelation therapy
- Splenectomy if splenomegaly is present
- Allogeneic stem cell transplantation if possible

α-thalassemia trait or β-thalassemia trait: No treatment.

Hb H disease: splenectomy may be helpful if anemia is severe or splenomegaly is present.

Patients with β-thalassemia intermedia should receive as few transfusions as possible to avoid iron overload. However, suppression of abnormal hematopoiesis by periodic RBC transfusion may be valuable in severely affected patients. In β thalassemia major, give transfusions as needed to maintain the Hb around 9 to 10 g/dL and avoid severe clinical manifestations. To prevent or delay complications due to iron overload, excess (transfusional) iron must be removed (eg, via chronic iron chelation therapy). Chelation therapy is generally initiated when serum ferritin levels are > 1000 ng/mL or after about 1 to 2 yr of scheduled transfusions. Splenectomy may help decrease transfusion requirements for patients with splenomegaly.

Allogeneic stem cell transplantation is the only curative option and should be considered in all patients.

KEY POINTS

- Thalassemias result from decreased production of at least one globin polypeptide chain (β, α, γ, δ); the resultant abnormal RBCs are microcytic, often abnormally shaped, and prone to hemolysis (causing anemia).
- Splenomegaly, often massive, is common and can result in splenic sequestration that accelerates destruction of RBCs (including transfused ones).
- Iron overload is common because of increased absorption (due to defective erythropoiesis) and frequent transfusions.
- Diagnose using Hb electrophoresis.
- Transfuse as needed, but monitor for iron overload and use chelation therapy.
- Splenectomy may help decrease transfusion requirements for patients with splenomegaly.
- Allogeneic stem cell transplantation is curative.

TRAUMATIC HEMOLYTIC ANEMIA

(Microangiopathic Hemolytic Anemia)

Traumatic hemolytic anemia is intravascular hemolysis caused by excessive shear or turbulence in the circulation.

Trauma causes fragmented RBCs (eg, triangles, helmet shapes) called schistocytes in the peripheral blood; their appearance on the peripheral smear is diagnostic. Small schistocytes cause low MCV and high RBC distribution width (the latter reflecting the anisocytosis).

When RBC fragmentation occurs in the setting of microvascular injury, the process is termed microangiopathic hemolytic anemia (MAHA). Causes of fragmentation hemolysis include

- Disseminated intravascular coagulation, a consumptive process secondary to other disorders such as sepsis, malignancy, pregnancy complications, trauma or surgery
- Stenotic or mechanical heart valves, or prosthetic valve dysfunction (ie, perivalvular leak)
- Thrombotic thrombocytopenic purpura
- Hemolytic uremic syndrome or related disorders such as the HELLP syndrome (hemolysis, elevated liver enzymes, and low platelet count), and systemic sclerosis renal crisis
- Rare cases of significant repetitive impact, such as foot strike hemolysis (march hemoglobinuria), karate strikes, or hand drumming

Treatment addresses the underlying process. Iron deficiency anemia occasionally is superimposed on the hemolysis as a result of chronic hemosiderinuria and, when present, responds to iron-replacement therapy.

142 Bleeding Due to Abnormal Blood Vessels

Bleeding may result from abnormalities in

- Platelets
- Coagulation factors
- Blood vessels

Vascular bleeding disorders result from defects in blood vessels, typically causing petechiae, purpura, and bruising but, except for hereditary hemorrhagic telangiectasia, seldom leading to serious blood loss. Bleeding may result from deficiencies of vascular and perivascular collagen in Ehlers-Danlos syndrome and in other rare hereditary connective tissue disorders (eg, pseudoxanthoma elasticum, osteogenesis imperfecta, Marfan syndrome). Hemorrhage may be a prominent feature of scurvy, or immunoglobulin A–associated vasculitis, a hypersensitivity vasculitis common during childhood.

In vascular bleeding disorders, tests of hemostasis are usually normal. For most disorders, diagnosis is clinical; specific tests are available for some.

AUTOERYTHROCYTE SENSITIZATION

(Gardner-Diamond Syndrome)

Autoerythrocyte sensitization is a rare and poorly understood disorder affecting mainly women. It is characterized by local pain and burning preceding unexplained painful ecchymoses that occur primarily on the extremities.

Autoerythrocyte sensitization typically occurs in white women who are experiencing emotional stress or who have concomitant psychiatric illness. Episodes of ecchymosis are painful and can occur spontaneously or after trauma or surgery. Bruising can occur on sites of the body distant from where trauma occurs. Ecchymoses virtually never occur on the back of the torso because this area is anatomically difficult to reach.

The etiology and pathophysiology of this syndrome are poorly understood. In some women with autoerythrocyte sensitization, intradermal injection of 0.1 mL of autologous RBCs or RBC stroma may result in pain, swelling, and induration at the injection site. This result suggests that escape of RBCs into the tissues is involved in the pathogenesis of the lesion. However, most patients also have associated severe psychiatric symptoms, and some patients self-induce purpura.

Diagnosis is by careful history, physical examination, and laboratory tests to rule out other potential bleeding disorders. Tests of the coagulation system are normal.

Treatment is psychiatric therapy.

DYSPROTEINEMIAS CAUSING VASCULAR PURPURA

Conditions that cause an abnormal protein content in the blood, typically in the form of immunoglobulins, can affect vascular fragility and lead to purpura.

Purpura refers to purplish cutaneous or mucosal lesions caused by hemorrhage. Small lesions (< 2 mm) are termed petechiae, and large lesions are termed ecchymoses or bruises.

Amyloidosis: Amyloidosis causes amyloid deposition within vessels in the skin and subcutaneous tissues, which may increase vascular fragility, causing purpura. Purpura typically occur on the upper extremities in contrast to immune thrombocytopenia, in which purpura occur mostly in the lower extremities. In some patients, coagulation factor X is adsorbed by amyloid and becomes deficient, but this deficiency is usually not the cause of bleeding. Periorbital purpura or a purpuric rash that develops in a nonthrombocytopenic patient after gentle stroking of the skin suggests amyloidosis. Some patients with amyloidosis have macroglossia (enlarged tongue).

Most patients have elevated levels of serum free light chains. The diagnosis is confirmed by tissue biopsy (eg, Congo red birefringence staining of fat pad aspirate).

Cryoglobulinemia: Cryoglobulinemia produces immunoglobulins that precipitate when plasma is cooled (ie, cryoglobulins) while flowing through the skin and subcutaneous tissues of the extremities. Monoclonal immunoglobulins formed in Waldenstrom macroglobulinemia (lymphoplasmacytic lymphoma) or in multiple myeloma occasionally behave as cryoglobulins, as may mixed IgM-IgG immune complexes formed in some chronic infectious diseases, most commonly hepatitis C. Cryoglobulinemia can also lead to small-vessel vasculitis, which can cause purpura. Cryoglobulins can be detected by laboratory testing.

Hypergammaglobulinemic purpura: Hypergammaglobulinemic purpura is a vasculitic purpura that primarily affects women. Recurrent crops of small, palpable purpuric lesions develop on the lower legs. These lesions leave small residual brown spots. Many patients have manifestations of an underlying immunologic disorder (eg, Sjögren syndrome, SLE). The diagnostic finding is a polyclonal increase in IgG.

Hyperviscosity syndrome: Hyperviscosity syndrome, usually resulting from a markedly elevated plasma IgM concentration, may also result in purpura and other forms of abnormal bleeding (eg, profuse epistaxis) in patients with macroglobulinemia. Marked elevations of other immunoglobulins (especially IgA and IgG_3) can also be associated with hyperviscosity syndrome.

HEREDITARY HEMORRHAGIC TELANGIECTASIA

(Osler-Weber-Rendu Syndrome)

Hereditary hemorrhagic telangiectasia is a hereditary disorder of vascular malformation transmitted as an autosomal dominant trait affecting men and women.

More than 80% of patients have mutations in the endoglin (*ENG*) gene, which encodes a receptor for transforming growth factor beta-1 (TGF-β1) and transforming growth factor beta-3 or in the *MADH4* gene, which encodes SMAD4, a protein active in the TGF beta signalling pathway.

Symptoms and Signs

The most characteristic lesions are small red-to-violet telangiectatic lesions on the face, lips, oral and nasal mucosa, and tips of the fingers and toes (see Plate 64). Similar lesions may be present throughout the mucosa of the GI tract, resulting in recurrent GI bleeding. Patients may experience recurrent, profuse nosebleeds. Some patients have pulmonary arteriovenous malformations (AVM). These fistulas may cause significant right-to-left shunts, which can result in dyspnea, fatigue, cyanosis, or polycythemia. However, the first sign of the presence of fistulas may be a brain abscess, transient ischemic attack, or stroke as a result of infected or noninfected emboli. Cerebral or spinal AVMs occur in some families and may cause subarachnoid hemorrhage, seizures, or paraplegia. Hepatic AVMs may lead to liver failure and high output heart failure.

Diagnosis

- Clinical evaluation
- Sometimes endoscopy or angiography
- Sometimes genetic testing

Diagnosis is based on the finding of characteristic AVMs on the face, mouth, nose, and digits. Endoscopy or angiography is sometimes needed. Laboratory findings are usually normal except for iron deficiency anemia in many patients.

Testing for the *ENG* and *MADH4* mutations may be helpful in some patients with atypical features or for screening asymptomatic family members.

Screening: If a family history of pulmonary, hepatic, or cerebral AVMs exists, screening at puberty and at the end of adolescence with pulmonary CT, hepatic CT, and cerebral MRI is recommended.

Treatment

- Sometimes laser ablation, surgical resection, or embolization of symptomatic AVMs
- Supplemental iron therapy
- Possibly blood transfusions
- Sometimes antifibrinolytic drugs (eg, aminocaproic acid, tranexamic acid)
- Sometimes angiogenesis inhibitors (eg, bevacizumab, pomalidomide, thalidomide)

Treatment for most patients is supportive, but accessible telangiectasias (eg, in the nose or GI tract via endoscopy) may be treated with laser ablation. Arteriovenous fistulas may be treated by surgical resection or embolization.

Repeated blood transfusions may be needed; therefore, immunization with hepatitis B vaccine is important.

Many patients require continuous iron therapy to replace iron lost in repeated mucosal bleeding (see Treatment of Iron Deficiency Anemia on p. 1096); many patients require parenteral iron and sometimes erythropoietin. Treatment with drugs that inhibit fibrinolysis, such as aminocaproic acid or tranexamic acid may be beneficial. Treatment with drugs that inhibit angiogenesis such as bevacizumab, pomalidomide, or thalidomide can reduce the number and density of abnormal vessel growth.

KEY POINTS

- Nasal and GI telangiectasias may cause significant external hemorrhage.
- Vascular malformations in the CNS, lungs, and liver may bleed; hepatic and pulmonary malformations may cause significant shunting.
- Accessible mucosal telangiectasias and AVMs may be treated with laser ablation; embolization or surgical resection may be needed for other vascular malformations.
- Many patients require parenteral iron supplements because of chronic blood loss.

PURPURA SIMPLEX

(Easy Bruising)

Purpura simplex is increased bruising that results from vascular fragility.

Purpura refers to purplish cutaneous or mucosal lesions caused by hemorrhage. Small lesions (< 2 mm) are termed petechiae, and large lesions are termed ecchymoses or bruises.

Purpura simplex is extremely common. The cause and mechanism are unknown. Purpura simplex may represent a heterogeneous group of disorders or merely a variation of normal.

The disorder usually affects women. Bruises develop on the thighs, buttocks, and upper arms in people without known trauma. The history usually reveals no other abnormal bleeding, but easy bruising may be present in family members. Serious bleeding does not occur.

The platelet count and tests of platelet function, blood coagulation, and fibrinolysis are normal.

No drug prevents the bruising; patients are often advised to avoid aspirin and aspirin-containing drugs, but there is no evidence that bruising is related to or worsened by their use. Patients should be reassured that the condition is not serious. All patients should be evaluated for the possibility of physical abuse.

SENILE PURPURA

Senile purpura causes ecchymoses and results from increased vessel fragility due to connective tissue damage to the dermis caused by chronic sun exposure, aging, and drugs.

Purpura refers to purplish cutaneous or mucosal lesions caused by hemorrhage. Small lesions (< 2 mm) are termed petechiae, and large lesions are termed ecchymoses or bruises.

Senile purpura typically affects elderly patients as their dermal tissues atrophy and blood vessels become more fragile. Patients develop persistent dark purple ecchymoses, which are characteristically confined to the extensor surfaces of the hands and forearms. New lesions appear without recognized trauma and then resolve over several days, leaving a brownish discoloration caused by deposits of hemosiderin. This discoloration may clear over weeks to months or may be permanent. The skin and subcutaneous tissue of the involved area often appear thinned and atrophic.

Drugs (eg, corticosteroids, warfarin, aspirin, clopidogrel) may exacerbate the ecchymoses.

No treatment hastens lesion resolution or is needed. Although cosmetically displeasing, the disorder has no health consequences and does not herald severe bleeding elsewhere.

143 Coagulation Disorders

Abnormal bleeding can result from disorders of the coagulation system, of platelets, or of blood vessels. Disorders of coagulation can be acquired or hereditary.

The **major causes of acquired coagulation disorders** are

- Vitamin K deficiency
- Liver disease
- Disseminated intravascular coagulation (DIC)
- Development of circulating anticoagulants

Severe liver disease (eg, cirrhosis, fulminant hepatitis, acute fatty liver of pregnancy) may disturb hemostasis by impairing clotting factor synthesis. Because all coagulation factors are made in the liver, both the prothrombin time (PT) and partial thromboplastin time (PTT) are elevated in severe liver disorders. (PT results are typically reported as INR.) Occasionally, decompensated liver disease also causes excessive fibrinolysis and bleeding due to decreased hepatic synthesis of alpha 2-antiplasmin.

The **most common hereditary disorder of hemostasis** is

- von Willebrand disease (VWD)

The **most common hereditary coagulation disorders** are

- The hemophilias

Testing

Patients in whom a coagulation disorder is suspected require laboratory evaluation beginning with PT and PTT. CBC with platelet count and a peripheral blood smear are also done. Results of these tests narrow the diagnostic possibilities and guide further testing.

Normal results on initial tests exclude many bleeding disorders. The main exceptions are VWD and hereditary hemorrhagic telangiectasia. VWD is a common entity in which the associated deficiency of factor VIII is frequently insufficient to prolong the PTT. Patients who have normal initial test results, along with symptoms or signs of bleeding and a positive family history, should be tested for VWD by measuring plasma von Willebrand factor (VWF) antigen, ristocetin cofactor activity (an indirect test for large VWF multimers), VWF multimer pattern, and factor VIII levels.

If **thrombocytopenia** is present, the peripheral blood smear often suggests the cause. If the smear is normal, patients should be tested for HIV infection. If the result of the HIV test is negative and the patient is not pregnant and has not taken a drug known to cause platelet destruction, then idiopathic thrombocytopenic purpura is likely. If there are signs of hemolysis (fragmented RBCs on smear, decreasing Hb level), thrombotic thrombocytopenic purpura (TTP) or hemolytic-uremic syndrome (HUS) is suspected, although sometimes other hemolytic disorders can cause these findings. HUS occurs in patients with hemorrhagic colitis. An "atypical" form of HUS occurs uncommonly in individuals with congenital abnormalities of the alternative complement pathway. The Coombs test is negative in TTP and HUS. If the CBC and peripheral blood smear demonstrate other cytopenias or abnormal WBCs, a hematologic abnormality affecting multiple cell types is suspected, and a bone marrow aspiration and biopsy are necessary for diagnosis.

Prolonged PTT with normal platelets and PT suggests hemophilia A or B. Factor VIII and IX assays are indicated. Inhibitors that specifically prolong the PTT include an autoantibody against factor VIII and antibodies against protein-phospholipid complexes (lupus anticoagulant). Clinicians suspect one of these inhibitors when a prolonged PTT does not correct after 1:1 mixing with normal plasma.

Prolonged PT with normal platelets and PTT suggests factor VII deficiency. Congenital factor VII deficiency is rare; however, the short half-life of factor VII in plasma causes factor VII to decrease to low levels more rapidly than other vitamin K–dependent coagulation factors in patients beginning warfarin anticoagulation or in patients with incipient liver disease.

Prolonged PT and PTT with thrombocytopenia suggest DIC, especially in association with obstetric complications, sepsis, cancer, or shock. Confirmation is by finding elevated levels of D-dimers (or fibrin degradation products) and decreasing plasma fibrinogen levels on serial testing.

Prolonged PT or PTT with normal platelet count occurs with liver disease or vitamin K deficiency or during anticoagulation with warfarin, unfractionated heparin, or the newer oral inhibitors of thrombin or factor Xa. Liver disease is suspected based on history and is confirmed by finding elevations of serum aminotransferases and bilirubin; hepatitis testing is recommended.

DISSEMINATED INTRAVASCULAR COAGULATION

(Consumption Coagulopathy; Defibrination Syndrome)

Disseminated intravascular coagulation (DIC) involves abnormal, excessive generation of thrombin and fibrin in the circulating blood. During the process, increased platelet aggregation and coagulation factor consumption occur. DIC that evolves slowly (over weeks or months) causes primarily venous thrombotic and embolic manifestations; DIC that evolves rapidly (over hours or days) causes primarily bleeding. Severe, rapidly evolving DIC is diagnosed by demonstrating thrombocytopenia, an elevated PTT and PT, increased levels of plasma D-dimer (or serum fibrin degradation products), and a decreasing plasma fibrinogen level. Treatment includes correction of the cause and replacement of platelets, coagulation factors (in fresh frozen plasma), and fibrinogen (in cryoprecipitate) to control severe bleeding. Heparin is used as therapy (or prophylaxis) in patients with slowly evolving DIC who have (or are at risk of) venous thromboembolism.

Etiology

DIC usually results from exposure of tissue factor to blood, initiating the coagulation cascade. In addition, DIC activates the fibrinolytic pathway (see Fig. 145–3 on p. 1131). Stimulation of endothelial cells by cytokines and perturbed microvascular blood flow causes the release of tissue plasminogen activator (tPA) from endothelial cells. Both tPA and plasminogen attach to fibrin polymers, and plasmin (generated by tPA cleavage of plasminogen) cleaves fibrin into D-dimers and other fibrin degradation products). DIC therefore causes both thrombosis and bleeding.

DIC occurs most often in the following clinical circumstances:

- Complications of obstetrics (eg, abruptio placentae, saline-induced therapeutic abortion, retained dead fetus or products of conception, amniotic fluid embolism): Placental tissue with tissue factor activity enters or is exposed to the maternal circulation.
- Infection, particularly with gram-negative organisms: Gram-negative endotoxin causes generation or exposure of tissue factor activity in phagocytic, endothelial, and tissue cells.
- Cancer, particularly mucin-secreting adenocarcinomas of the pancreas,adenocarcinomas of the prostate, and acute promyelocytic leukemia: Tumor cells express or release tissue factor.
- Shock due to any condition that causes ischemic tissue injury and release of tissue factor.

Less common causes of DIC include

- Severe tissue damage due to head trauma, burns, frostbite, or gunshot wounds
- Complications of prostate surgery that allow prostatic material with tissue factor activity (along with plasminogen activators) to enter the circulation
- Venomous snake bites in which enzymes enter the circulation, activate one or several coagulation factors, and either generate thrombin or directly convert fibrinogen to fibrin
- Profound intravascular hemolysis
- Aortic aneurysms or cavernous hemangiomas (Kasabach-Merritt syndrome) associated with vessel wall damage and areas of blood stasis

Slowly-evolving DIC typically results mainly from cancer, aneurysms or cavernous hemangiomas.

Pathophysiology

Slowly evolving DIC primarily causes venous thromboembolic manifestations (eg, deep venous thrombosis, pulmonary embolism), although occasionally cardiac valve vegetations occur; abnormal bleeding is uncommon.

Severe, rapidly evolving DIC, in contrast, causes thrombocytopenia and depletion of plasma coagulation factors and fibrinogen, which cause bleeding. Bleeding into organs, along with microvascular thromboses, may cause dysfunction and failure in multiple organs. Delayed dissolution of fibrin polymers by fibrinolysis may result in the mechanical disruption of RBCs, producing schistocytes and mild intravascular hemolysis.

Symptoms and Signs

In slowly evolving DIC, symptoms of venous thrombosis and/or symptoms of pulmonary embolism may be present.

In severe, rapidly evolving DIC, skin puncture sites (eg, IV or arterial punctures) bleed persistently, ecchymoses form at sites of parenteral injections, and serious GI bleeding may occur.

Diagnosis

- Platelet count, PT, PTT, plasma fibrinogen, plasma D-dimer

DIC is suspected in patients with unexplained bleeding or venous thromboembolism, especially if a predisposing condition exists. If DIC is suspected, platelet count, PT, PTT, plasma fibrinogen level, and plasma D-dimer level (an indication of in vivo fibrin deposition and degradation) are obtained.

Slowly evolving DIC produces mild thrombocytopenia, a normal to minimally prolonged PT (results are typically reported as INR) and PTT, a normal or moderately reduced fibrinogen level, and an increased plasma D-dimer level. Because various disorders stimulate increased synthesis of fibrinogen as an acute-phase reactant, a declining fibrinogen level on 2 consecutive measurements can help make the diagnosis of DIC. Initial PTT values in slowly evolving DIC may actually be shorter than normal, probably because of the presence of activated coagulation factors in the plasma.

Severe, rapidly evolving DIC results in more severe thrombocytopenia, more prolonged PT and PTT, a rapidly declining plasma fibrinogen level, and a high plasma D-dimer level.

A factor VIII level can sometimes be helpful if severe, acute DIC must be differentiated from massive hepatic necrosis, which can cause similar abnormalities in coagulation studies. The factor VIII level is elevated in hepatic necrosis because factor VIII is made in hepatic endothelial cells and released as they are destroyed; factor VIII is reduced in DIC because of the thrombin-induced generation of activated protein C, which proteolyses the activated form of factor VIII.

Treatment

- Treatment of cause
- Possibly replacement therapy (eg, platelets, cryoprecipitate, fresh frozen plasma))
- Sometimes heparin

Immediate correction of the cause is the priority (eg, broad-spectrum antibiotic treatment of suspected gram-negative sepsis, evacuation of the uterus in abruptio placentae). If treatment is effective, DIC should subside quickly.

Severe bleeding: If bleeding is severe or involves a critical location (eg, brain, GI tract), or if there is an urgent need for surgery, then adjunctive replacement therapy is indicated. Replacement may consist of

- Platelet concentrates to correct thrombocytopenia (in case of rapidly declining platelet count or platelets < 10,000 to 20,000/μL)
- Cryoprecipitate to replace fibrinogen (and factor VIII) if the fibrinogen level is declining rapidly or is < 100 mg/dL.
- Fresh frozen plasma to increase levels of other clotting factors and natural anticoagulants (antithrombin, proteins C, S, and Z)

The effectiveness of infusion of concentrates of antithrombin in severe, rapidly evolving DIC is unresolved. Volume resuscitation when hypotension is present is essential to arrest the DIC.

Slowly evolving DIC: Heparin is useful in the treatment of slowly evolving DIC with venous thrombosis or pulmonary embolism. Heparin usually is not indicated in rapidly evolving DIC with bleeding or bleeding risk, except in women with a retained dead fetus and evolving DIC with a progressive decrease in platelets, fibrinogen, and coagulation factors. In these patients, heparin is given for several days to control DIC, increase fibrinogen and platelet levels, and decrease excessive coagulation factor consumption. Heparin is then stopped and the uterus evacuated.

KEY POINTS

- In DIC, the coagulation cascade is activated when blood is exposed to tissue factor. In association with the coagulation system, the fibrinolytic pathway is also activated.
- DIC usually begins rapidly and causes bleeding and microvascular occlusion, leading to organ failure.
- DIC sometimes begins slowly and causes thromboembolic phenomena rather than bleeding.
- Severe, rapid-onset DIC causes severe thrombocytopenia, prolonged PT and PTT, a rapidly declining plasma fibrinogen level, and a high plasma D-dimer level.
- Immediate correction of the cause is the priority; severe bleeding may also require replacement therapy with platelet concentrate, cryoprecipitate, and fresh frozen plasma.
- Heparin is useful in slow-onset DIC, but rarely in DIC of rapid onset (mainly in women with a retained dead fetus).

HEMOPHILIA

Hemophilias are common hereditary bleeding disorders caused by deficiencies of either clotting factor VIII or IX. The extent of factor deficiency determines the probability and severity of bleeding. Bleeding into deep tissues or joints usually develops within hours of trauma. The diagnosis is suspected in a patient with an elevated PTT and normal PT and platelet count; it is confirmed by specific factor assays. Treatment includes replacement of the deficient factor if acute bleeding is suspected, confirmed, or likely to develop (eg, before surgery).

Hemophilia A (factor VIII deficiency), which affects about 80% of patients with hemophilia, and hemophilia B (factor IX deficiency) have identical clinical manifestations and screening test abnormalities. Both are X-linked genetic disorders. Specific factor assays are required to distinguish the two.

Etiology

Hemophilia is an inherited disorder that results from mutations, deletions, or inversions affecting the factor VIII or factor IX gene. Because these genes are located on the X chromosome, hemophilia affects males almost exclusively. Daughters of men with hemophilia are obligate carriers, but sons are normal. Each son of a carrier has a 50% chance of having hemophilia, and each daughter has a 50% chance of being a carrier.

Pathophysiology

Normal hemostasis requires > 30% of normal factor VIII and IX levels. Most patients with hemophilia have levels < 5%; some have extremely low levels (< 1%). The functional level (activity) of factor VIII or IX in hemophilia A and B, and thus bleeding severity, varies depending on the specific mutation in the factor VIII or IX gene.

Carriers usually have levels of about 50%; rarely, random inactivation of their normal X chromosome in early embryonic life results in a carrier having factor VIII or IX levels of < 30%.

Most patients with hemophilia who were treated in the early 1980s were infected with HIV due to contaminated factor concentrates. Occasional patients developed immune thrombocytopenia secondary to HIV infection, which exacerbated bleeding.

Symptoms and Signs

Patients with hemophilia bleed into tissues (eg, hemarthroses, muscle hematomas, retroperitoneal hemorrhage). The bleeding may be immediate or occur slowly, depending on the extent of trauma and plasma level of factor VIII or IX. Pain often occurs as bleeding commences, sometimes before other signs of bleeding develop. Chronic or recurrent hemarthroses can lead to synovitis and arthropathy. Even a trivial blow to the head can cause intracranial bleeding. Bleeding into the base of the tongue can cause life-threatening airway compression.

Severe hemophilia (factor VIII or IX level < 1% of normal) causes severe bleeding throughout life, usually beginning soon after birth (eg, scalp hematoma after delivery or excessive bleeding after circumcision). Moderate hemophilia (factor levels 1 to 5% of normal) usually causes bleeding after minimal trauma. In mild hemophilia (factor levels 5 to 25% of normal), excessive bleeding may occur after surgery or dental extraction.

Diagnosis

- Platelet count, PT, PTT, factor VIII and IX assays
- Sometimes VWF activity and antigen and multimer composition

Hemophilia is suspected in patients with recurrent bleeding, unexplained hemarthroses, or a prolongation of the PTT. If hemophilia is suspected, PTT, PT, platelet count, and factor VIII and IX assays are obtained. In hemophilia, the PTT is prolonged, but the PT and platelet count are normal. Factor VIII and IX assays determine the type and severity of the hemophilia. Because factor VIII levels may also be reduced in VWD, VWF activity, antigen, and multimer composition are measured in patients with newly diagnosed hemophilia A, particularly if the disorder is mild and a family history indicates that both male and female family members are affected. Determining if a female is a true carrier of hemophilia A is sometimes possible by measuring the factor VIII level. Similarly, measuring the factor IX level often identifies a carrier of hemophilia B. PCR analysis of DNA that comprises the factor VIII gene, available at specialized centers, can be used for diagnosis of the hemophilia A carrier state and for prenatal diagnosis of hemophilia A by chorionic villus sampling at 12 wk or amniocentesis at 16 wk. These procedures carry a 0.5 to 1% risk of miscarriage.

After repeated exposure to factor VIII replacement, about 15 to 35% of patients with hemophilia A develop factor VIII isoantibodies (alloantibodies) that inhibit the coagulant activity of any additional factor VIII infused. Patients should be screened for isoantibodies (eg, by measuring the degree of PTT shortening immediately after mixing the patient's plasma with an equal volume of normal plasma, and then by repeating the measurement after incubation for 1 h), especially before an elective procedure that requires replacement therapy. If isoantibodies are present, their titers can be measured by determining the extent of factor VIII inhibition by serial dilutions of patient plasma.

PEARLS & PITFALLS

- Because factor VIII levels may also be reduced in von Willebrand disease, measure von Willebrand factor (VWF) activity, antigen, and multimer composition in patients with newly diagnosed hemophilia A.

Prevention

Patients should avoid aspirin and NSAIDs (both inhibit platelet function). Regular dental care is essential so that tooth extractions and other dental surgery can be avoided. Drugs should be given orally or IV; IM injections can cause hematomas. Patients with hemophilia should be vaccinated against hepatitis B.

Treatment

- Replacement of deficient factor
- Sometimes antifibrinolytics

If symptoms suggest bleeding, treatment should begin immediately, even before diagnostic tests are completed. For example, treatment for headache that might indicate intracranial hemorrhage should begin before CT is completed.

Replacement of the deficient factor is the primary treatment. In hemophilia A, the factor VIII level should be raised transiently to

- About 30% of normal to prevent bleeding after dental extraction or to abort an incipient joint hemorrhage
- 50% of normal if severe joint or IM bleeding is already evident
- 100% of normal before major surgery or if bleeding is intracranial, intracardiac, or otherwise life threatening

Repeated infusions at 50% of the initial calculated dose should then be given every 8 to 12 h to keep trough levels > 50% for 7 to 10 days after major surgery or life-threatening hemorrhage. Each unit/kg of factor VIII increases the factor VIII level by about 2%. Thus, to increase the level from 0% to 50%, about 25 units/kg are required.

Factor VIII can be given as purified factor VIII concentrate, which is derived from multiple donors. It undergoes viral inactivation, but inactivation may not eliminate parvovirus or hepatitis A virus. Recombinant factor VIII is free of viruses and is usually preferred unless patients are already seropositive for HIV or for hepatitis B or C virus.

In hemophilia B, factor IX can be given as a purified or recombinant viral-inactivated product every 24 h. The target levels of factor correction are the same as in hemophilia A. However, to achieve these levels, the dose must be higher than in hemophilia A because factor IX is smaller than factor VIII and, in contrast to VIII, has an extensive extravascular distribution.

Fresh frozen plasma contains factors VIII and IX. However, unless plasma exchange is done, sufficient whole plasma usually cannot be given to patients with severe hemophilia to raise factor VIII or IX to levels that prevent or control bleeding.

Fresh frozen plasma should, therefore, be used only if rapid replacement therapy is necessary and factor concentrate is unavailable or the patient has a coagulopathy that is not yet defined precisely.

A recombinant factor VIII-Fc fusion protein,[1] as well as a recombinant factor IX-Fc fusion protein[2] and a pegylated recombinant factor IX,[3] with longer in vivo survival times have recently been reported to successfully control bleeding in hemophilia A and B.

In patients with hemophilia who develop a factor VIII inhibitor, treatment is best accomplished using recombinant activated factor VII (VIIa) in repeated high doses (eg, 90 mcg/kg).

Both VWF and factor VIII are stored in the Weibel-Palade bodies of endothelial cells, and secreted in response to endothelial cell stimulation.[4] Adjunctive therapy for hemophilia A thus includes in vivo stimulation of patient endothelial cells with the synthetic vasopressin analogue DDAVP (deamino-D-arginine vasopressin, also known as desmopressin). As described for VWD, desmopressin may temporarily raise factor VIII levels. The patient's response should be tested before desmopressin is used therapeutically. Its use after minor trauma or before elective dental surgery may obviate replacement therapy. Desmopressin should be used only for patients with mild hemophilia A (basal factor VIII levels ≥ 5%) who have demonstrated responsiveness.

An antifibrinolytic agent (aminocaproic acid 2.5 to 4 g po qid for 1 wk or tranexamic acid 1.0 to 1.5 g po tid or qid for 1 wk) may also be used as adjunctive therapy in hemophilia A or B to prevent late bleeding after dental extraction or other oropharyngeal mucosal trauma (eg, tongue laceration).

1. Mahlangu J, Powell JS, Ragni MV, et al: Phase 3 study of recombinant factor VIII Fc fusion protein in severe hemophilia A. *Blood* 123:317–325, 2014.
2. Powell JS, Pasi KJ, Ragni MV, et al: Phase 3 study of recombinant factor IX Fc fusion protein in hemophilia B. *N Engl J Med* 369:2313–2323, 2013.
3. Collins PW, Young G, Knobe K, et al: Recombinant long-acting glycoPEGylated factor IX in hemophilia B: A multinational randomized phase 3 trial. *Blood* 124:3880–3886, 2014.
4. Turner NA, Moake JL: Factor VIII is synthesized in human endothelial cells, packaged in Weibel-Palade bodies and secreted bound to ULVWF strings. *PLoS ONE* 10(10):e0140740, 2015.

KEY POINTS

- Hemophilias are X-linked recessive disorders of coagulation.
- Hemophilia A (about 80% of patients) involves factor VIII deficiency, and hemophilia B involves factor IX deficiency.
- Patients bleed into tissues (eg, hemarthroses, muscle hematomas, retroperitoneal hemorrhage) following minimal trauma; fatal intracranial hemorrhage may occur.
- The PTT is prolonged but the PT and platelet count are normal; factor VIII and IX assays determine the type and severity of the hemophilia.
- Patients with bleeding or in whom bleeding is anticipated (eg, before surgery or dental extraction) are given replacement factor, preferably using a recombinant product; dose depends on the circumstances.
- About 15 to 35% of patients with hemophilia A who require repeated factor VIII infusions develop antibodies to factor VIII.

COAGULATION DISORDERS CAUSED BY CIRCULATING ANTICOAGULANTS

Circulating anticoagulants are usually autoantibodies that neutralize specific clotting factors in vivo (eg, an autoantibody against factor VIII or factor V) or inhibit phospholipid-bound proteins in vitro (antiphospholipid antibodies). Occasionally, the latter type of autoantibody causes bleeding by binding in vivo to prothrombin-phospholipid complexes.

Circulating anticoagulants should be suspected in patients with excessive bleeding combined with either a prolonged PTT or PT that does not correct when the test is repeated with a 1:1 mixture of normal plasma and the patient's plasma.

Antiphospholipid antibodies typically cause thrombosis (the antiphospholipid antibody syndrome). However, in a subset of patients, the antibodies bind to prothrombin-phospholipid complexes and induce hypoprothrombinemia and bleeding.

Factor VIII Anticoagulants

Isoantibodies to factor VIII develop in about 15 to 35% of patients with severe hemophilia A as a complication of repeated exposure to normal factor VIII molecules during replacement therapy for hemophilia A. Factor VIII autoantibodies also arise occasionally in patients without hemophilia, eg, in postpartum women as a manifestation of an underlying systemic autoimmune disorder or of transiently disordered immune regulation; or in elderly patients without overt evidence of other underlying disorders. Patients with a factor VIII anticoagulant can develop life-threatening hemorrhage.

Plasma containing a factor VIII antibody has a prolonged PTT that does not correct when normal plasma or another source of factor VIII is added in a 1:1 mixture to the patient's plasma. Testing is done immediately after mixture and again after incubation.

Treatment

- In patients without hemophilia, cyclophosphamide, corticosteroids, or rituximab
- In patients with hemophilia, recombinant activated factor VII

Therapy with cyclophosphamide, corticosteroids, or rituximab (monoclonal antibody to CD20 on lymphocytes) may suppress autoantibody production in patients without hemophilia (eg, in postpartum women). The autoantibodies may disappear spontaneously.

Management of acute hemorrhage in patients with hemophilia who have factor VIII isoantibodies or autoantibodies is by recombinant activated factor VII.

UNCOMMON HEREDITARY COAGULATION DISORDERS

Most hereditary coagulation disorders other than hemophilia are rare autosomal recessive conditions that cause excessive bleeding only in homozygous people (see Table 143–1). The rare inherited coagulation disorders can involve factors II, V, VII, X, XI, and XIII. Of these, factor XI deficiency is the most common.

Factor XI deficiency: Factor XI deficiency is uncommon in the general population but common among descendants of European Jews (gene frequency about 5 to 9%). Bleeding

Table 143–1. SCREENING LABORATORY TEST RESULTS IN INHERITED DEFECTS IN BLOOD COAGULATION

SCREENING TEST RESULTS*	DEFECT	COMMENTS
PTT long PT normal	Factor XII, high molecular weight kininogen, or prekallikrein	Laboratory test abnormality without clinical bleeding Specific assays required to distinguish from factor XI deficiency, in which posttraumatic and perioperative bleeding may occur
PTT long PT normal	Factor XI	Autosomal recessive Increased frequency in Ashkenazi Jews Posttraumatic and perioperative bleeding Diagnosis by specific assay For bleeding: Fresh frozen plasma 5–20 mL/kg/day to keep factor XI level > 30% of normal
PTT long PT normal	Factor VIII or IX	Factor VIII deficiency (hemophilia A) Factor IX deficiency (hemophilia B) X-linked transmission Mild or severe bleeding in males, depending on factor VIII or IX level
PTT normal PT long	Factor VII	Autosomal recessive Rare If deficiency is severe (< 2% of normal values), serious bleeding If levels are > 5%, mild or no bleeding Therapy of choice: Recombinant activated factor VII
PTT long PT long	Factor X, V, or prothrombin	Autosomal recessive Rare Mild to severe bleeding Diagnosed by specific assays For bleeding episodes due to factor X or prothrombin deficiency: Fresh frozen plasma or prothrombin complex concentrate For treatment of factor V deficiency: Fresh frozen plasma with or without platelet concentrates (to supply platelet factor V)
In afibrinogenemia (fibrinogen < 10 mg/dL), no clotting in PTT or PT because machine end point is not triggered In hypofibrinogenemia (fibrinogen 70–100 mg/dL), PTT and PT often prolonged by several seconds and thrombin time long	Fibrinogen	Severe bleeding in afibrinogenemia (homozygous state) Posttraumatic and perioperative bleeding in hypofibrinogenemia (heterozygous state) For treatment: Cryoprecipitate (5–10 bags, with each containing about 250 mg fibrinogen)
PTT and PT long Thrombin time long	Dysfibrinogenemia	Various manifestations (no, or only mild, posttraumatic and perioperative bleeding, tendency for thrombosis, wound dehiscence) Fibrinogen low in clotting assay but normal in immunologic assay
PTT normal PT normal Thrombin time normal Clot lysis in 5M urea	Factor XIII	Autosomal recessive Rare Poor wound healing Spontaneous abortions in women Severe bleeding when levels are < 1% of normal For treatment: Fresh frozen plasma (1–2 units q 4–6 wk is effective because half-life of factor XIII is about 10 days)
PTT and PT normal Clot lysis times in 5M urea or saline accelerated	Alpha 2-antiplasmin deficiency	Severe bleeding in homozygotes Posttraumatic and perioperative bleeding in heterozygotes Specific assay required for confirmation of diagnosis

*PT results are typically reported as INR.

typically occurs after significant injuries, including trauma or surgery, in people who are homozygotes or compound heterozygotes.

Deficiency of alpha 2-antiplasmin: Severe deficiency of alpha 2-antiplasmin (levels 1 to 3% of normal), the major physiologic inhibitor of plasmin, can also cause bleeding as a result of poor control of plasmin-mediated proteolysis of fibrin polymers. Diagnosis is based on a specific alpha 2-antiplasmin assay. Aminocaproic acid or tranexamic acid is used to control or prevent acute bleeding by blocking plasminogen binding to fibrin polymers. Heterozygous people with alpha 2-antiplasmin levels of 40 to 60% of normal can occasionally experience excessive surgical bleeding if secondary fibrinolysis is extensive (eg, in patients who have released excessive amounts of urokinase-type plasminogen activator during open prostatectomy).

144 Eosinophilic Disorders

Eosinophils are granulocytes derived from the same progenitor cells as monocytes-macrophages, neutrophils, and basophils. They are a component of the innate immune system. Eosinophils have a variety of functions, including

- Defense against parasitic infections
- Defense against intracellular bacteria
- Modulation of immediate hypersensitivity reactions

Eosinophils are especially important in defense against parasitic infections. However, although eosinophilia commonly accompanies helminthic infections and eosinophils are toxic to helminths in vitro, there is no direct evidence that they kill parasites in vivo.

Although they are phagocytic, eosinophils are less efficient than neutrophils in killing intracellular bacteria.

Eosinophils may modulate immediate hypersensitivity reactions by degrading or inactivating mediators released by mast cells, such as histamine, leukotrienes (which may cause vasoconstriction and bronchoconstriction), lysophospholipids, and heparin.

Prolonged eosinophilia may result in tissue damage by mechanisms that are not fully understood.

Eosinophil production and function: Eosinophil production appears to be regulated by T cells through the secretion of the hematopoietic growth factors granulocyte-macrophage colony-stimulating factor (GM-CSF), interleukin-3 (IL-3), and interleukin-5 (IL-5). Although GM-CSF and IL-3 also increase the production of other myeloid cells, IL-5 increases eosinophil production exclusively.

Eosinophil granules contain major basic protein and eosinophil cationic protein; these proteins are toxic to several parasites and to mammalian cells. These proteins bind heparin and neutralize its anticoagulant activity. Eosinophil-derived neurotoxin can severely damage myelinated neurons. Eosinophil peroxidase, which differs significantly from peroxidase of other granulocytes, generates oxidizing radicals in the presence of hydrogen peroxide and a halide. Charcot-Leyden crystals are primarily composed of phospholipase B and are located in sputum, tissues, and stool in disorders in which there is eosinophilia (eg, asthma, eosinophilic pneumonia).

Eosinophil count: The normal peripheral blood eosinophil count varies, but it is generally accepted that a count > 500/μL is elevated. Peripheral eosinophilia is characterized as

- Mild: 500 to 1500/μL
- Moderate: 1500 to 5000/μL
- Severe: > 5000/μL

Diurnal levels vary inversely with plasma cortisol levels; the peak occurs at night and the trough in the morning.

The eosinophil count can decrease with stress, with the use of beta-blockers or corticosteroids, and sometimes during bacterial or viral infections.

The count can increase (eosinophilia) in allergic disorders, during certain infections (typically parasitic), and as a result of numerous other causes.

The circulating half-life of eosinophils is 6 to 12 h, with most eosinophils residing in tissues (eg, the upper respiratory tract, GI tract, skin, uterus).

EOSINOPHILIA

Eosinophilia is defined as a peripheral blood eosinophil count > 500/μL. Causes and associated disorders are myriad but often represent an allergic reaction or a parasitic infection. Diagnosis involves selective testing directed at clinically suspected causes. Treatment is directed at the cause.

Eosinophilia has features of an immune response: an agent such as *Trichinella spiralis* invokes a primary response with relatively low levels of eosinophils, whereas repeated exposures result in an augmented or secondary eosinophilic response. Several compounds released by mast cells and basophils induce IgE-mediated eosinophil production. Such substances include eosinophil chemotactic factor of anaphylaxis, leukotriene B4, complement complex (C5-C6-C7), and histamine (over a narrow range of concentration).

Peripheral eosinophilia is characterized as

- Mild: 500 to 1500/μL
- Moderate: 1500 to 5000/μL
- Severe: > 5000/μL

Mild eosinophilia itself does not cause symptoms, but levels ≥ 1500/μL may cause organ damage. Organ damage typically occurs because of tissue inflammation and reaction to the cytokines and chemokines released by the eosinophils as well as to immune cells which are recruited to the tissues. Although any organ may be involved, the heart, lungs, spleen, skin, and nervous system are typically affected (for manifestations see Table 144–3 on p. 1126). Occasionally, patients with very severe eosinophilia (eg, eosinophil counts of > 100,000/μL), usually with eosinophilic leukemia, develop complications when eosinophils form aggregates that occlude small blood vessels, causing tissue ischemia and microinfarctions. Manifestations typically include those of brain or lung hypoxia (eg, encephalopathy, dyspnea, respiratory failure).

Hypereosinophilic syndrome (HES) is a condition characterized by peripheral blood eosinophilia with manifestations of organ system involvement or dysfunction directly related to eosinophilia in patients who do not have parasitic, allergic, or other causes of eosinophilia.

Etiology

Eosinophilia may be

- Primary: A clonal proliferation of eosinophils associated with hematologic disorders such as leukemias and myeloproliferative disorders
- Secondary: Caused by or associated with nonhematologic disorders (see Table 144–1)
- Idiopathic: Causes cannot be identified

The **most common cause** in the US is

- Allergic or atopic disorders (typically respiratory or dermatologic)

Other common causes include

- Infections (typically parasitic)
- Certain tumors (hematologic or solid, benign or malignant)

Almost any parasitic invasion of tissues can elicit eosinophilia, but protozoa and noninvasive metazoa usually do not.

Table 144–1. IMPORTANT DISORDERS AND TREATMENTS ASSOCIATED WITH EOSINOPHILIA

CAUSE OR ASSOCIATED DISORDER	EXAMPLES
Allergic or atopic disorders	Asthma Allergic bronchopulmonary aspergillosis Allergic rhinitis Atopic dermatitis Drug reactions (eg, to antibiotics or NSAIDs) Episodic angioedema with eosinophilia Milk-protein allergy Occupational lung disease Urticaria
Connective tissue, vasculitic, or granulomatous disorders (especially those involving the lungs)	Eosinophilic fasciitis Idiopathic eosinophilic synovitis Inflammatory bowel disease Polyarteritis nodosa Post myocardial infarction syndrome (Dressler syndrome) Progressive systemic sclerosis (scleroderma) Rheumatoid arthritis Sarcoidosis Sjögren syndrome SLE
Endocrine disorders	Adrenal hypofunction
Immune disorders (often with eczema)	Congenital immunodeficiency syndrome (eg, IgA deficiency, hyper-IgE syndrome, Wiskott-Aldrich syndrome) Graft-vs-host disease
Myeloproliferative disorders	Acute or chronic eosinophilic leukemia Acute lymphocytic leukemia (certain types) Chronic myelogenous leukemia HES
Nonparasitic infections	Aspergillosis Brucellosis Cat-scratch disease Chlamydial pneumonia of infancy Coccidioidomycosis (acute) Infectious lymphocytosis Infectious mononucleosis Mycobacterial disease Scarlet fever
Parasitic infections (especially due to tissue-invasive metazoans)	Ascariasis Clonorchiasis Cysticercosis (caused by *Taenia solium*) Echinococcosis Fascioliasis Filariasis Hookworm infection Paragonimiasis *Pneumocystis jirovecii* infection Schistosomiasis Strongyloidiasis Toxocariasis Trichinosis Trichuriasis
Skin disorders	Dermatitis herpetiformis Exfoliative dermatitis Pemphigus Psoriasis
Syndromes of pulmonary infiltration with eosinophilia	Allergic bronchopulmonary aspergillosis Chronic eosinophilic pneumonia Eosinophilic granulomatosis with polyangiitis Löffler syndrome Tropical pulmonary eosinophilia

Table continues on the following page.

Table 144–1. IMPORTANT DISORDERS AND TREATMENTS ASSOCIATED WITH EOSINOPHILIA (*Continued*)

CAUSE OR ASSOCIATED DISORDER	EXAMPLES
Tumors	Angioimmunoblastic T-cell lymphoma (previously known as angioimmunoblastic lymphadenopathy with dysproteinemia or AILD) in association with systemic symptoms and autoimmune hemolytic anemia Carcinomas and sarcomas of the lung, pancreas, colon, cervix, or ovary Hodgkin lymphoma Non-Hodgkin lymphomas
Miscellaneous	Cirrhosis Familial eosinophilia Peritoneal dialysis Radiation therapy

Of hematologic tumors, Hodgkin lymphoma may elicit marked eosinophilia, whereas eosinophilia is less common in non-Hodgkin lymphoma, chronic myelogenous leukemia, and acute lymphocytic leukemia.

The pulmonary infiltrates with eosinophilic syndrome comprise a spectrum of clinical manifestations characterized by peripheral eosinophilia and eosinophilic pulmonary infiltrates but is usually of unknown cause.

Patients with eosinophilic drug reactions may be asymptomatic or have various syndromes, including interstitial nephritis, serum sickness, cholestatic jaundice, hypersensitivity vasculitis, and immunoblastic lymphadenopathy.

Eosinophilia-myalgia syndrome is rare; the cause is unknown. However, in 1989, several hundred patients were reported to have developed this syndrome after taking L-tryptophan for sedation or psychotropic support. This syndrome was probably caused by a contaminant rather than by L-tryptophan. The symptoms, including severe muscle pain, tenosynovitis, muscle edema, and rash, lasted weeks to months, and several deaths occurred.

Drug reaction with eosinophilia and systemic symptoms (DRESS) is a rare syndrome characterized by fever, rash, eosinophilia, atypical lymphocytosis, lymphadenopathy, and signs and symptoms related to end-organ involvement (typically, heart, lungs, spleen, skin, nervous system).

Evaluation

The number of possible causes and associated disorders is very large. Common causes (eg, allergic, infectious, or neoplastic disorders) should be considered first, but even they are often difficult to identify, so a thorough history and physical examination are always required.

History: The questions most likely to be helpful pertain to the following:

- Travel (suggesting possible parasite exposure)
- Allergies
- Drug use
- Use of herbal products and dietary supplements, including L-tryptophan
- Systemic symptoms (eg, fever, weight loss, myalgias, arthralgias, rashes, lymphadenopathy)

Systemic symptoms suggest that a minor allergic or drug cause is less likely, and a detailed evaluation for an infectious, neoplastic, connective tissue, or other systemic disorder should be done. Other important parts of the history include family history of blood dyscrasias and a complete review of systems, including symptoms of allergies and pulmonary, cardiac, GI, and neurologic dysfunction.

Physical examination: General physical examination should focus on the heart, skin, and neurologic and pulmonary systems. Certain physical findings may suggest causes or associated disorders. Examples include rash (allergic, dermatologic, or vasculitic disorders), abnormal lung findings (asthma, lung infections, or syndromes of pulmonary infiltration with eosinophilia), and generalized lymphadenopathy or splenomegaly (myeloproliferative disorders or cancer).

Testing: Eosinophilia is typically recognized when CBC is done for other reasons. Additional testing often includes the following:

- Stool ova and parasite testing
- Other tests to detect organ damage or for specific causes based on clinical findings

In general, if a drug or allergic cause is not suspected based on clinical findings, 3 stool specimens should be examined for ova and parasites; however, negative findings do not rule out a parasitic cause (eg, trichinosis requires a muscle biopsy; visceral larva migrans and filarial infections require other tissue biopsies; duodenal aspirates may be needed to exclude specific parasites, eg, *Strongyloides* sp).

Other specific diagnostic tests are determined by the clinical findings (particularly travel history) and may include chest x-ray, urinalysis, liver and kidney function tests, and serologic tests for parasitic and connective tissue disorders. If patients have generalized lymphadenopathy, splenomegaly, or systemic symptoms, blood tests are done. An elevated serum vitamin B_{12} level or abnormalities on the peripheral blood smear suggest an underlying myeloproliferative disorder, and a bone marrow aspirate and biopsy with cytogenetic studies may be helpful. Also, if routine evaluation does not reveal a cause, tests are done to detect organ damage. Testing can include some of the tests previously mentioned as well as LDH and liver function tests (suggesting liver damage or possibly a myeloproliferative disorder), echocardiography, and pulmonary function tests. Once a specific cause has been determined, additional testing may be needed.

Treatment

- Sometimes corticosteroids

For corticosteroid treatment of HES, see Immediate therapy on p. 1126.

Drugs known to be associated with eosinophilia are stopped. Other identified causes are treated.

If no cause is detected, the patient is followed for complications. A brief trial with low-dose corticosteroids may lower the eosinophil count if eosinophilia is secondary (eg, to allergy, connective tissue disorders, or parasitic infection) rather than primary. Such a trial is indicated if eosinophilia is persistent and progressive in the absence of a treatable cause.

HYPEREOSINOPHILIC SYNDROME

(Idiopathic Hypereosinophilic Syndrome)

Hypereosinophilic syndrome (HES) is a condition characterized by peripheral blood eosinophilia with manifestations of organ system involvement or dysfunction directly related to eosinophilia in the absence of parasitic, allergic, or other secondary causes of eosinophilia. Symptoms are myriad, depending on which organs are dysfunctional. Diagnosis involves excluding other causes of eosinophilia plus bone marrow and cytogenetic tests. Treatment usually begins with prednisone and, in one common subtype, includes imatinib.

HES is traditionally defined as peripheral blood eosinophilia > 1500/μL persisting ≥ 6 mo.

HES was previously considered to be idiopathic but is now known to result from various disorders, some of which have known causes. One limitation of the traditional definition is that it does not include those patients with some of the same abnormalities (eg, chromosomal defects) that are known causes of HES but who do not fulfill the traditional HES definition for degree or duration of eosinophilia. Another limitation is that some patients with eosinophilia and organ damage that characterize HES require treatment earlier than the 6 mo necessary to confirm the traditional diagnostic criteria.

HES is rare, has an unknown prevalence, and most often affects people age 20 through 50. Only some patients with prolonged eosinophilia develop organ dysfunction that characterizes hypereosinophilic syndrome. Although any organ may be involved, the heart, lungs, spleen, skin, and nervous system are typically affected. Cardiac involvement can cause significant morbidity and mortality.

Subtypes: There are two broad subtypes of HES (see Table 144–2):

- Myeloproliferative variant
- Lymphoproliferative variant

The **myeloproliferative variant** is often associated with a small interstitial deletion in chromosome 4 at the *CHIC2* site that causes the *FIP1L1/PDGFRA*-associated fusion gene (which has tyrosine kinase activity that can transform hematopoietic cells). Patients often have

- Splenomegaly
- Thrombocytopenia
- Anemia
- Elevated serum vitamin B_{12} levels
- Hypogranular or vacuolated eosinophils
- Myelofibrosis

Patients with this subtype often develop endomyocardial fibrosis and may rarely develop acute myeloid or lymphoblastic leukemia. Patients with the *FIP1L1/PDGFRA*-associated fusion gene are more often males and may be responsive to low-dose imatinib (a tyrosine kinase inhibitor).

A small proportion of patients with the myeloproliferative variant of HES have cytogenetic changes involving platelet derived growth factor receptor beta (PDGFRB) and may also be responsive to tyrosine kinase inhibitors such as imatinib.[1]

The **lymphoproliferative variant** is associated with a clonal population of T cells with aberrant phenotype. PCR shows a clonal T-cell receptor rearrangement. Patients more often have

- Angioedema, skin abnormalities, or both
- Hypergammaglobulinemia (especially IgE)
- Circulating immune complexes (sometimes with serum sickness)

They also more often respond favorably to corticosteroids and occasionally develop T-cell lymphoma.

Other HES variants include chronic eosinophilic leukemia, Gleich syndrome (cyclical eosinophilia and angioedema), familial HES mapped to 5q 31-33, and other organ-specific syndromes. Hyperleukocytosis may occur in patients with eosinophilic leukemia and very high eosinophil counts (eg, > 100,000 cells/μL). Eosinophils can form aggregates that occlude small blood vessels, causing tissue ischemia and microinfarctions. Common manifestations include brain or lung hypoxia (eg, encephalopathy, dyspnea or respiratory failure).

1. Apperley JF, Gardembas M, Melo JV, et al: Response to imatinib mesylate in patients with chronic myeloproliferative diseases with rearrangements of the platelet-derived growth factor receptor beta. *N Engl J Med* 347:481–487, 2002.

Symptoms and Signs

Symptoms are diverse and depend on which organs are dysfunctional (see Table 144–3).

Table 144–2. SUBTYPES OF HYPEREOSINOPHILIC SYNDROME

FEATURE	MYELOPROLIFERATIVE VARIANT	LYMPHOPROLIFERATIVE VARIANT
Genetics	Small interstitial deletion in chromosome 4 *FIP1L1/PDGFRA*-associated fusion gene	Clonal population of T cells with aberrant phenotype
Clinical manifestations and laboratory findings	Anemia Elevated serum vitamin B_{12} levels Endomyocardial fibrosis Hypogranular or vacuolated eosinophils Myelofibrosis Splenomegaly Thrombocytopenia	Angioedema Circulating immune complexes (sometimes with serum sickness) Hypergammaglobulinemia (especially IgE) Skin abnormalities
Increased risk of future disorder	Acute lymphoblastic leukemia Acute myeloid leukemia	T-cell lymphoma
Responsiveness to drugs	Imatinib and other tyrosine kinase inhibitors	Corticosteroids

Occasionally, patients with very severe eosinophilia (eg, eosinophil counts of > 100,000/μL) develop complications of hyperleukocytosis, such as manifestations of brain or lung hypoxia (eg, encephalopathy, dyspnea or respiratory failure).

Diagnosis

- Exclusion of secondary eosinophilia
- Tests to identify organ damage
- Bone marrow examination with cytogenetic testing

Evaluation for HES should be considered in patients who have peripheral blood eosinophilia > 1500/μL present on more than one occasion that is unexplained, particularly when there are manifestations of organ damage. Testing to exclude disorders causing eosinophilia should be done.

Evaluation for organ damage should include blood chemistries (including liver enzymes, creatine kinase, renal function, and troponin); ECG; echocardiography; pulmonary function tests; and CT of the chest, abdomen, and pelvis. Bone marrow aspirate and biopsy with flow cytometry, cytogenetic testing, and reverse transcriptase-PCR or fluorescence in situ hybridization (FISH) is done to identify the *FIP1L1/PDGFRA*-associated fusion gene and other possible causes of eosinophilia (eg, *BCR-ABL* abnormalities characteristic of chronic myelogenous leukemia).

Prognosis

Death usually results from organ, particularly heart, dysfunction. Cardiac involvement is not predicted by the degree or duration of eosinophilia. Prognosis varies depending on response to therapy. Response to imatinib improves the prognosis among patients with the *FIP1L1/PDGFRA*-associated fusion gene. Current therapy has improved prognosis.

Treatment

- Corticosteroids for hypereosinophilia and often for ongoing treatment of organ damage
- Imatinib for patients with the *FIP1L1/PDGFRA*-associated fusion gene
- Sometimes drugs to control eosinophil counts (eg, hydroxyurea, interferon alfa, etoposide, cladribine)
- Supportive care

Treatments include immediate therapy, definitive therapies (treatments directed at the disorder itself), and supportive therapies.[1]

Immediate therapy: For patients with very severe eosinophilia, complications of hyperleukocytosis, or both (usually patients with eosinophilic leukemia), high-dose IV corticosteroids (eg, prednisone 1 mg/kg or equivalent) should be initiated as soon as possible. If the eosinophil count is much lower (eg, by ≥ 50%) after 24 h, corticosteroid dose can be repeated daily; if not, an alternative treatment (eg, hydroxyurea) is begun. Once the eosinophil count begins to decline and is under better control, additional drugs may be started.

Definitive therapy: Patients with the *FIP1L1/PDGFRA*-associated fusion gene are usually treated with imatinib[2] and, particularly if heart damage is suspected, corticosteroids. If imatinib is ineffective or poorly tolerated, another tyrosine kinase inhibitor (eg, dasatinib, nilotinib, sorafenib) can be used, or allogeneic hematopoietic stem cell transplantation can be used.

Patients without the *FIP1L1/PDGFRA*-associated fusion gene, even if asymptomatic, are often given one dose of prednisone 60 mg (or 1 mg/kg) po to determine corticosteroid responsiveness (ie, a decrease in the eosinophil count). In patients with symptoms or organ damage, prednisone is continued at the same

Table 144–3. ABNORMALITIES IN PATIENTS WITH HYPEREOSINOPHILIC SYNDROME

SYSTEM	PREVALENCE	MANIFESTATIONS
Constitutional	≈ 50%	Anorexia Fatigue Fever Myalgias Weakness Weight loss
Cardiopulmonary	> 70%	Mural thrombi with emboli Restrictive or infiltrative cardiomyopathy or mitral or tricuspid regurgitation with cough, dyspnea, heart failure, arrhythmias, endomyocardial disease, pulmonary infiltrates, and pleural effusions
Dermatologic	> 50%	Angioedema Dermatographism Pruritus Rashes (including eczema and urticaria)
Hematologic	> 50%	Anemia Lymphadenopathy Splenomegaly Thromboembolic phenomena Thrombocytopenia
Neurologic	> 50%	Cerebral emboli with focal deficits Diffuse encephalopathy with altered behavior and cognitive function and spasticity Peripheral neuropathy
GI	> 40%	Abdominal cramps Diarrhea Nausea
Immunologic	≈ 40%	Circulating immune complexes with serum sickness Elevated levels of immunoglobulins (especially IgE)

dose for 2 wk, then tapered. Patients without symptoms and organ damage are monitored for at least 6 mo for these complications. If corticosteroids cannot be easily tapered, a corticosteroid-sparing drug (eg, hydroxyurea, interferon alfa) can be used. Mepolizumab, a fully human monoclonal antibody against interleukin-5 (a regulator of eosinophil production), is undergoing clinical trials.

Supportive care: Supportive drug therapy and surgery may be required for cardiac manifestations (eg, infiltrative cardiomyopathy, valvular lesions, heart failure). Thrombotic complications may require the use of antiplatelet drugs (eg, aspirin, clopidogrel, ticlopidine); anticoagulation is indicated if a left ventricular mural thrombus is present or if transient ischemic attacks persist despite use of aspirin.

1. Ogbogu PU, Bochener BS, Butterfield HJ, et al: Hypereosinophilic syndromes: A multicenter, retrospective analysis of clinical characteristics and response to therapy. *J Allergy Clin Immunol* 124:1319–1325, 2009.
2. Cortes J, Ault P, Koller C, et al: Efficacy of imatinib mesylate in the treatment of idiopathic hypereosinophilic syndrome. *Blood* 101:4714–4716, 2003.

KEY POINTS

- HES is peripheral blood eosinophilia (> 1500/μL) not caused by parasitic, allergic, or other secondary causes of eosinophilia, that has persisted ≥ 6 mo and caused organ damage or dysfunction.
- HES appears to be a manifestation of a number of hematopoietic disorders, some of which have a genetic cause.
- Any organ may be involved but the heart, lungs, spleen, skin, and nervous system are typically affected; cardiac involvement can cause significant morbidity and mortality.
- Do tests for organ involvement, including liver enzymes; creatine kinase, creatinine, and troponin levels; ECG and echocardiography; pulmonary function tests; and CT of the chest, abdomen, and pelvis.
- Do bone marrow examination with cytogenetic testing to identify a cause.
- Give corticosteroids for severe eosinophilia and/or organ damage. Tyrosine kinase inhibitors such as low-dose imatinib may be of benefit in subtypes associated with distinct chromosomal abnormalities.

145 Hemostasis

Hemostasis, the arrest of bleeding from an injured blood vessel, requires the combined activity of vascular, platelet, and plasma factors. Regulatory mechanisms counterbalance the tendency of clots to form. Hemostatic abnormalities can lead to excessive bleeding or thrombosis.

Vascular Factors

Vascular factors reduce blood loss due to trauma through local vasoconstriction (an immediate reaction to injury) and compression of injured vessels by extravasation of blood into surrounding tissues. Vessel wall injury triggers the attachment and activation of platelets and production of fibrin; platelets and fibrin combine to form a clot.

Platelet Factors

Various mechanisms, including endothelial cell nitric oxide and prostacyclin, promote blood fluidity by preventing platelet stasis and dilating intact blood vessels. These mediators are no longer produced when the vascular endothelium is disrupted. Under these conditions, platelets adhere to the damaged intima and form aggregates. Initial platelet adhesion is to von Willebrand factor (VWF), previously secreted by endothelial cells into the subendothelium. VWF binds to receptors on the platelet surface membrane (glycoprotein Ib/IX). Platelets anchored to the vessel wall undergo activation. During activation, platelets release mediators from storage granules, including adenosinediphosphate (ADP).

Other biochemical changes resulting from activation include hydrolysis of membrane phospholipids, inhibition of adenylate cyclase, mobilization of intracellular calcium, and phosphorylation of intracellular proteins. Arachidonic acid is converted to thromboxane A_2; this reaction requires cyclooxygenase and is inhibited irreversibly by aspirin and reversibly by many NSAIDs. ADP, thromboxane A_2, and other mediators induce activation and aggregation of additional platelets on the injured endothelium. Another receptor is assembled on the platelet surface membrane from glycoproteins IIb and IIIa. Fibrinogen binds to the glycoprotein IIb/IIIa complexes of adjacent platelets, connecting them into aggregates.

Platelets provide surfaces for the assembly and activation of coagulation complexes and the generation of thrombin. Thrombin converts fibrinogen to fibrin. Fibrin strands bind aggregated platelets to help secure the platelet-fibrin hemostatic plug.

Plasma Factors

Plasma coagulation factors interact to produce thrombin, which converts fibrinogen to fibrin. By radiating from and anchoring the hemostatic plug, fibrin strengthens the clot.

In the intrinsic pathway, factor XII, high molecular weight kininogen, prekallikrein, and activated factor XI (factor XIa) interact to produce factor IXa from factor IX. Factor IXa then combines with factor VIIIa and procoagulant phospholipid (present on the surface of activated platelets and tissue cells) to form a complex that activates factor X. In the extrinsic pathway, factor VIIa and tissue factor (TF) directly activate factor X (the factor VIIa/tissue factor complex also activates factor IX—see Fig. 145–1 and Table 145–1).

Activation of the intrinsic or extrinsic pathway activates the common pathway, resulting in formation of the fibrin clot. Three steps are involved in common pathway activation:

1. A prothrombin activator is produced on the surface of activated platelets and tissue cells. The activator is a complex of an enzyme, factor Xa, and 2 cofactors, factor Va and procoagulant phospholipid.
2. The prothrombin activator cleaves prothrombin into thrombin and another fragment.
3. Thrombin induces the generation of fibrin polymers from fibrinogen. Thrombin also activates factor XIII, an enzyme that catalyzes formation of stronger bonds between adjacent fibrin monomers, as well as activating factor VIII and factor XI.

Calcium ions are needed in most thrombin-generating reactions (calcium-chelating agents [eg, citrate, ethylenediaminetetraacetic acid] are used in vitro as anticoagulants).

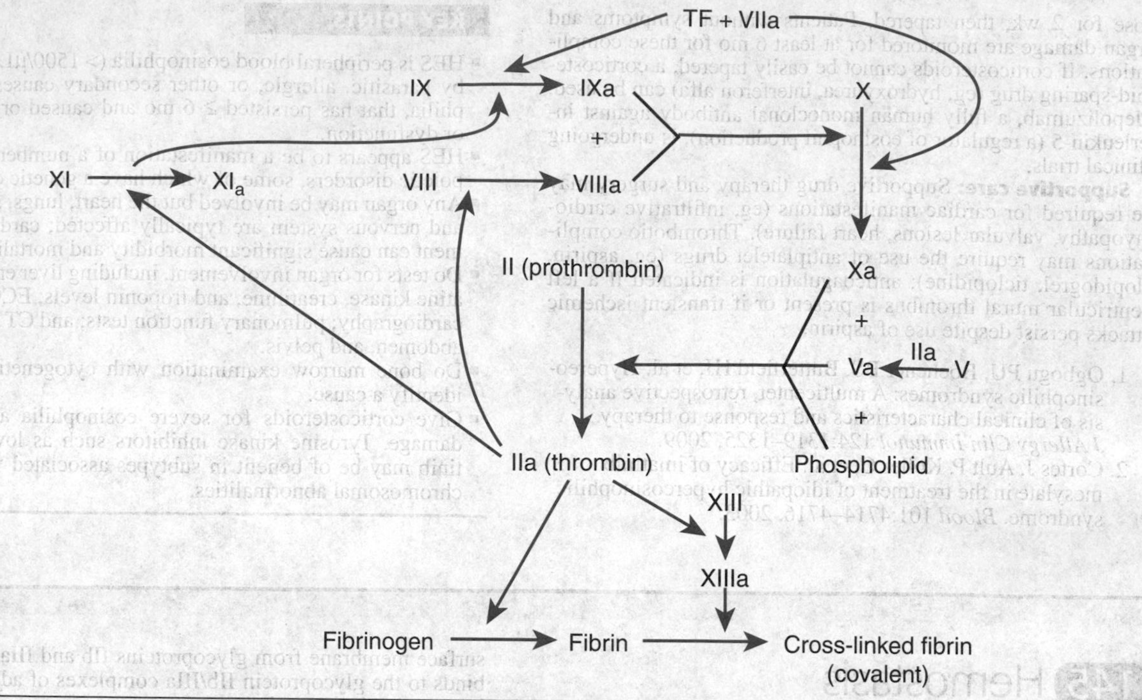

Fig. 145–1. Pathways in blood coagulation.

Table 145–1. COMPONENTS OF BLOOD COAGULATION REACTIONS

FACTOR NUMBER OR NAME	SYNONYM	PURPOSE
Plasma factors		
I	Fibrinogen	A precursor of fibrin
II	Prothrombin	A precursor of thrombin, which converts fibrinogen to fibrin; activates factors V, VIII, XI, and XIII; and binds to thrombomodulin to activate protein C Is vitamin K–dependent
V	Proaccelerin	Is activated to factor Va, a cofactor for the enzyme factor Xa in the factor Xa/Va/phospholipid complex, which cleaves prothrombin to thrombin Is present in alpha granules in platelets Factor Va inactivated by activated protein C in complex with free protein S
VII	Proconvertin	Binds to tissue factor and is then activated to form the enzymatic component of the factor VIIa/tissue factor complex, which activates factors IX and X Is vitamin K–dependent
VIII	Antihemophilic globulin	Is activated to factor VIIIa, a cofactor for the enzyme factor IXa in the factor IXa/VIIIa/phospholipid complex, which activates factor X Is a large cofactor protein (as is factor V) Circulates in plasma bound to von Willebrand factor multimers As factor VIIIa, is inactivated by activated protein C in complex with free protein S (as is factor Va)
IX	Christmas factor	Is activated to factor IXa, the enzyme of the factor IXa/VIIIa/phospholipid complex, which activates factor X Is vitamin K–dependent
X	Stuart-Prower factor	Is activated to factor Xa, the enzyme of the factor Xa/Va/phospholipid complex, which cleaves prothrombin to thrombin Is vitamin K–dependent
XI	Plasma thromboplastin antecedent	Is activated to factor XIa, which activates factor IX in a reaction requiring calcium ions

Table 145–1. COMPONENTS OF BLOOD COAGULATION REACTIONS (*Continued*)

FACTOR NUMBER OR NAME	SYNONYM	PURPOSE
Prekallikrein	Fletcher factor	Participates in a reciprocal reaction in which it is activated to kallikrein by factor XIIa As kallikrein, catalyzes further activation of factor XII to factor XIIa Circulates as a biomolecular complex with high molecular weight kininogen
High molecular weight kininogen	Fitzgerald factor	Circulates as a bimolecular complex with prekallikrein
XII	Hageman factor	When activated to factor XIIa by surface contact, kallikrein, or other factors, activates prekallikrein and factor XI, triggering the intrinsic coagulation pathway in vitro
XIII	Fibrin stabilizing factor	When activated by thrombin, catalyzes formation of peptide bonds between adjacent fibrin monomers, thus strengthening and stabilizing the fibrin clot
Protein C	—	Is activated by thrombin bound to thrombomodulin; then proteolyzes and inhibits (in the presence of free protein S and phospholipid) the cofactor activity of factors VIIIa and Va Is vitamin K–dependent
Protein S	—	Circulates in plasma as free protein S and as protein S bound to C4b-binding protein of the complement system Functions in its free form as a cofactor for activated protein C Is vitamin K–dependent
Cell surface factors		
Tissue factor	Tissue thromboplastin	Is a lipoprotein that is constitutively present on the membrane of certain tissue cells, including perivascular fibroblasts, boundary epithelial cells (eg, epithelial cells of the skin, amnion, and GI and GU tracts), and glial cells of the nervous system May also develop in pathologic states on activated monocytes and macrophages and on activated vascular endothelium Is present on some tumor cells Binds factor VIIa, which initiates the extrinsic coagulation pathway
Procoagulant phospholipid	—	Acidic phospholipid (primarily phosphatidyl serine) present on the surface of activated platelets and other tissue cells Is a component of the factor IXa/VIIIa/phospholipid complex which activates factor X and of the factor Xa/Va/phospholipid complex which activates prothrombin Functions as the lipid moiety of tissue factor
Thrombomodulin	—	Is an endothelial cell surface binding site for thrombin, which, when bound to thrombomodulin, activates protein C

Vitamin K–dependent clotting factors (factors II, VII, IX, and X) cannot bind normally to phospholipid surfaces through calcium bridges and function in blood coagulation when the factors are synthesized in the absence of vitamin K.

Although the coagulation pathways are helpful in understanding mechanisms and laboratory evaluation of coagulation disorders, in vivo coagulation is predominantly via the extrinsic pathway. People with hereditary deficiencies of factor XII, high molecular weight kininogen, or prekallikrein have no bleeding abnormality. People with hereditary factor XI deficiency have a mild to moderate bleeding disorder. In vivo, factor XI (an intrinsic pathway factor) is activated when a small amount of thrombin is generated. Factor IX can be activated both by factor XIa and factor VIIa/tissue factor complexes.

In vivo, initiation of the extrinsic pathway occurs when injury to blood vessels brings blood into contact with tissue factor on membranes of cells within and around the vessel walls. This contact with tissue factor generates factor VIIa/tissue factor complexes that activate factor X and factor IX. Factor IXa, combined with its cofactor, factor VIIIa, on phospholipid membrane surfaces generates additional factor Xa. Factor X activation by both factor VIIa/tissue factor and factor IXa/VIIIa complexes is required for normal hemostasis. This requirement for factors VIII and IX explains why hemophilia type A (deficiency of factor VIII) or type B (deficiency of factor IX) results in bleeding despite an intact extrinsic coagulation pathway initiated by factor VIIa/tissue factor complexes.

Regulatory Mechanisms

Several inhibitory mechanisms prevent activated coagulation reactions from amplifying uncontrollably, causing extensive local thrombosis or disseminated intravascular coagulation. These mechanisms include

- Inactivation of procoagulant enzymes
- Fibrinolysis
- Hepatic clearance of activated clotting factors

Inactivation of coagulation factors: Plasma protease inhibitors (antithrombin, tissue factor pathway inhibitor, α_2-macroglobulin, heparin cofactor II) inactivate coagulation enzymes. Antithrombin inhibits thrombin, factor Xa, factor XIa, and factor IXa.

Two vitamin K–dependent proteins, protein C and free protein S, form a complex that inactivates factors VIIIa and Va by

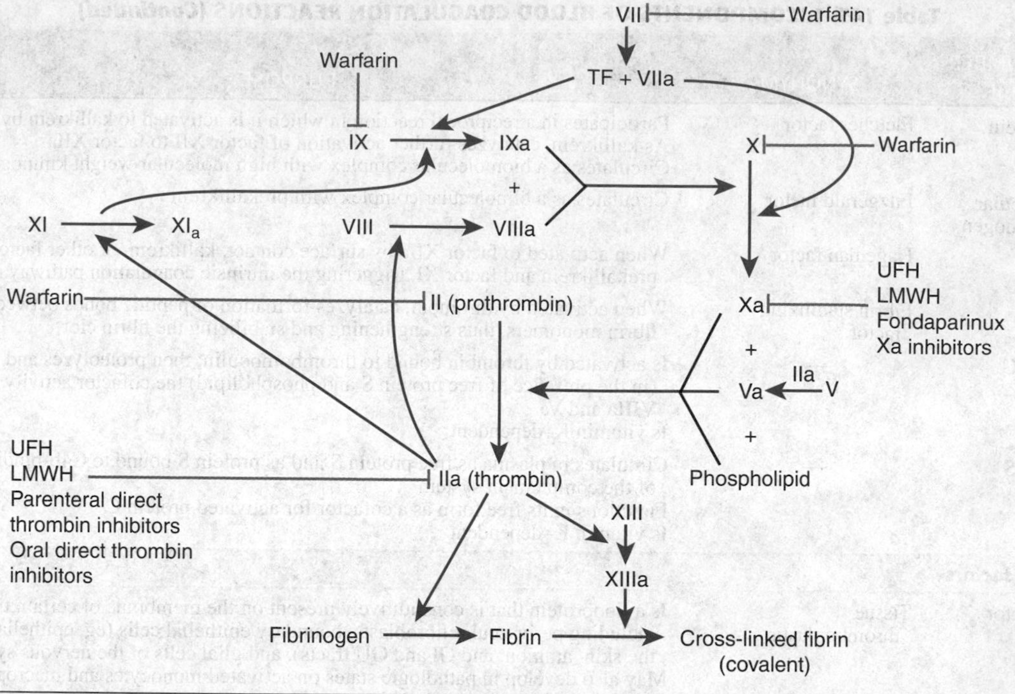

Fig. 145–2. Anticoagulants and their sites of action. LMWH = low molecular weight heparin; TF = tissue factor; UFH = unfractionated heparin.

proteolysis. Thrombin, when bound to a receptor on endothelial cells (thrombomodulin), activates protein C. Activated protein C, in combination with free protein S and phospholipid cofactors, proteolyzes and inactivates factors VIIIa and Va.

In addition to intrinsic inactivators, there are a number of anticoagulant drugs that potentiate the inactivation of coagulation factors (see Fig. 145–2).

Heparin enhances antithrombin activity. Warfarin is a vitamin K antagonist. It inhibits regeneration of the active form of vitamin K and, therefore, inhibits generation of functional forms of the vitamin K–dependent clotting factors II, VII, IX and X. Unfractionated heparin (UFH) and low molecular weight heparins (LMWH) enhance activity of antithrombin and inactivate factors IIa (thrombin) and Xa. LMWHs include enoxaparin, dalteparin, and tinzaparin. Fondaparinux is a small, synthetic molecule, containing the essential pentasaccharide portion of the heparin structure that enhances antithrombin inactivation of factor Xa (but not IIa). Parenteral direct thrombin inhibitors include argatroban and lepirudin. The newer oral anticoagulants include oral direct thrombin inhibitors (dabigatran) and oral direct factor Xa inhibitors (apixaban, rivaroxaban, edoxaban). The use of these drugs, including risks, benefits, and reversal agents, are discussed in the Manual sections on atrial fibrillation, deep venous thrombosis (DVT), and pulmonary embolism (PE).

Fibrinolysis: Fibrin deposition and lysis must be balanced to maintain temporarily, and subsequently remove, the hemostatic seal during repair of an injured vessel wall. The fibrinolytic system dissolves fibrin by means of plasmin, a proteolytic enzyme. Fibrinolysis is activated by plasminogen activators released from vascular endothelial cells. Plasminogen activators and plasminogen (from plasma) bind to fibrin, and plasminogen activators cleave plasminogen into plasmin (see Fig. 145–3). Plasmin then proteolyzes fibrin into soluble fibrin degradation products that are swept away in the circulation.

There are several plasminogen activators:

- **Tissue plasminogen activator** (tPA), from endothelial cells, is a poor activator when free in solution but an efficient activator when bound to fibrin in proximity to plasminogen.
- **Urokinase** exists in single-chain and double-chain forms with different functional properties. Single-chain urokinase cannot activate free plasminogen but, like tPA, can readily activate plasminogen bound to fibrin. A trace concentration of plasmin cleaves single-chain to double-chain urokinase, which activates plasminogen in solution as well as plasminogen bound to fibrin. Epithelial cells that line excretory passages (eg, renal tubules, mammary ducts) secrete urokinase, which is the physiologic activator of fibrinolysis in these channels.
- **Streptokinase,** a bacterial product not normally found in the body, is another potent plasminogen activator.

Streptokinase, urokinase, and recombinant tPA (alteplase) have all been used therapeutically to induce fibrinolysis in patients with acute thrombotic disorders.

Regulation of fibrinolysis: Fibrinolysis is regulated by plasminogen activator inhibitors (PAIs) and plasmin inhibitors that slow fibrinolysis. PAI-1, the most important PAI, inactivates tPA and urokinase and is released from vascular endothelial cells and activated platelets. The primary plasmin inhibitor is alpha$_2$-antiplasmin, which quickly inactivates any free plasmin escaping from clots. Some alpha$_2$-antiplasmin is also cross-linked to fibrin polymers by the action of factor XIIIa during clotting. This cross-linking may prevent excessive plasmin activity within clots.

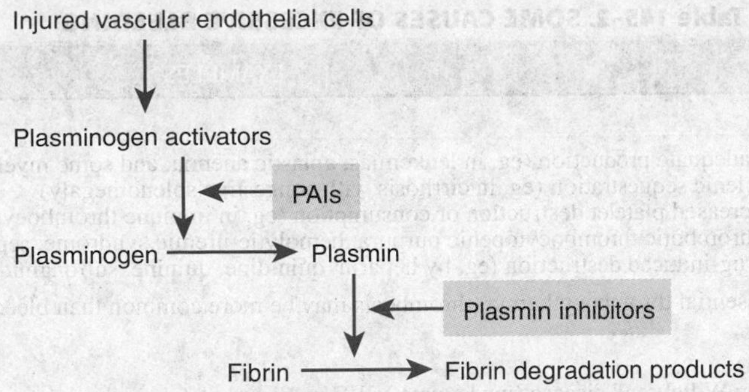

Fig. 145–3. Fibrinolytic pathway. Fibrin deposition and fibrinolysis must be balanced during repair of an injured blood vessel wall. Injured vascular endothelial cells release plasminogen activators (tissue plasminogen activator, urokinase), activating fibrinolysis. Plasminogen activators cleave plasminogen into plasmin, which dissolves clots. Fibrinolysis is controlled by plasminogen activator inhibitors (PAIs; eg, PAI-1) and plasmin inhibitors (eg, α_2-antiplasmin).

tPA and urokinase are rapidly cleared by the liver, which is another mechanism of preventing excessive fibrinolysis.

EXCESSIVE BLEEDING

Unusual or excessive bleeding may be indicated by several different signs and symptoms. Patients may present with unexplained nosebleeds (epistaxis), excessive or prolonged menstrual blood flow (menorrhagia), or prolonged bleeding after minor cuts, tooth brushing or flossing, or trauma. Other patients may have unexplained skin lesions, including petechiae (small intradermal or mucosal hemorrhages), purpura (areas of mucosal or skin hemorrhage larger than petechiae), ecchymoses (bruises), or telangiectasias (dilated small vessels visible on skin or mucosa). Some critically ill patients may suddenly bleed from vascular punctures or skin lesions and have severe hemorrhage from these sites or from the GI or GU tract. In some patients, the first sign is a laboratory test abnormality suggesting the susceptibility to excessive bleeding that is found incidentally.

Etiology

Excessive bleeding can result from several mechanisms (see Table 145–2), including the following:

- Platelet disorders
- Coagulation disorders
- Defects in blood vessels

Platelet disorders may involve an abnormal number of platelets (typically too few platelets, although an extremely elevated platelet count may be associated either with thrombosis or with excessive bleeding), defective platelet function, or both. Coagulation disorders may be acquired or hereditary.

Overall, the most common causes of excessive bleeding include

- Severe thrombocytopenia
- Excessive anticoagulation, as with warfarin or heparin
- Liver disease (inadequate production of coagulation factors)

Evaluation

History: History of present illness should determine the bleeding sites, the amount and duration of bleeding, and the relationship of bleeding to any possible precipitating events.

Review of systems should specifically query about bleeding from sites other than those volunteered (eg, patients complaining of easy bruising should be questioned about frequent nosebleeds, gum bleeding while tooth brushing, melena, hemoptysis, blood in stool or urine). Patients should be asked about symptoms of possible causes, including abdominal pain and diarrhea (GI illness); joint pain (connective tissue disorders); and amenorrhea and morning sickness (pregnancy).

Past medical history should seek known systemic conditions associated with defects in platelets or coagulation, particularly

- Severe infection, cancer, cirrhosis, HIV infection, pregnancy, SLE, or uremia
- Prior excessive or unusual bleeding or transfusions
- Family history of excessive bleeding

Drug history should be reviewed, particularly use of heparin, warfarin, newer oral inhibitors of thrombin or factor Xa, aspirin, and NSAIDs. Patients who are taking warfarin also should be questioned about intake of drugs and foods (including herbal supplements) that decrease the metabolism of warfarin and thus increase its anticoagulant effect.

Physical examination: Vital signs and general appearance can indicate hypovolemia (tachycardia, hypotension, pallor, diaphoresis) or infection (fever, tachycardia, hypotension with sepsis).

The skin and mucous membranes (nose, mouth, vagina) are examined for petechiae, purpura, and telangiectasias. GI bleeding can often be identified by digital rectal examination. Signs of bleeding in deeper tissues may include tenderness during movement and local swelling, muscle hematomas, and, for intracranial bleeding, confusion, stiff neck, focal neurologic abnormalities, or a combination of these findings.

Characteristic findings of alcohol abuse or liver disease are ascites, splenomegaly (secondary to portal hypertension), and jaundice.

Red flags: The following findings are of particular concern:

- Signs of hypovolemia or hemorrhagic shock
- Pregnancy or recent delivery
- Signs of infection or sepsis

Interpretation of findings: Bleeding in a patient taking warfarin is especially likely if there has been a recent increase in dose or the addition of a drug or food that may interfere with

Table 145–2. SOME CAUSES OF EXCESSIVE BLEEDING

CATEGORY	EXAMPLES
Platelet disorders	
Decreased number of platelets (quantitative disorder)	Inadequate production (eg, in leukemias, aplastic anemia, and some myelodysplastic syndromes) Splenic sequestration (eg, in cirrhosis with congestive splenomegaly) Increased platelet destruction or consumption (eg, in immune thrombocytopenia [ITP], DIC, thrombotic thrombocytopenic purpura, hemolytic-uremic syndrome, sepsis, and HIV infection) Drug-induced destruction (eg, by heparin, quinidine, quinine, sulfonamides, sulfonylureas, or rifampin)
Increased number of platelets (quantitative disorder)	Essential thrombocythemia (thrombosis may be more common than bleeding)
Inadequate platelet function (qualitative disorder)	von Willebrand disease (inadequate VWF-mediated platelet adhesion) Drug-induced dysfunction (eg, by aspirin or NSAIDs) Systemic disorders (uremia; occasionally, myeloproliferative or myelodysplastic syndromes, multiple myeloma)
Coagulation disorders	
Acquired	Vitamin K deficiency Liver disease Anticoagulation with warfarin, heparin or the direct oral inhibitors of thrombin or factor Xa DIC
Hereditary	Hemophilia A (factor VIII deficiency) Hemophilia B (factor IX deficiency)
Vascular disorders	
Acquired	Vitamin C deficiency Immunoglobulin A–associated vasculitis
Hereditary	Connective tissue disorders (eg, Ehlers-Danlos syndrome, osteogenesis imperfecta, Marfan syndrome) Hereditary hemorrhagic telangiectasia

DIC = disseminated intravascular coagulation; VWF = von Willebrand factor.

warfarin inactivation. Telangiectasias on the face, lips, oral or nasal mucosa, and tips of the fingers and toes in a patient with a positive family history of excessive bleeding is likely to indicate hereditary hemorrhagic telangiectasia.

Bleeding from superficial sites, including skin and mucous membranes, suggests a quantitative or qualitative defect in platelets or a defect in blood vessels (eg, amyloidosis).

Bleeding into deep tissues (eg, hemarthroses, muscle hematomas, retroperitoneal hemorrhage) suggests a defect in coagulation (coagulopathy).

A family history of excessive bleeding suggests an inherited coagulopathy (eg, hemophilia), a qualitative platelet disorder, a type of von Willebrand disease (VWD), or hereditary hemorrhagic telangiectasia. Absence of a known family history does not, however, exclude an inherited disorder of hemostasis.

Bleeding in a patient who is pregnant or has recently delivered, who is in shock, or who has a serious infection suggests disseminated intravascular coagulation (DIC).

Bloody diarrhea and thrombocytopenia in a patient with fever and GI symptoms suggest the hemolytic-uremic syndrome (HUS), which is often associated with infection by *Escherichia coli* O157:H7 (or other *Shiga*-like toxin-producing type of *E. coli*).

In a child, a palpable, purpuric rash on the extensor surfaces of the extremities suggests immunoglobulin A–associated vasculitis, particularly if accompanied by fever, polyarthralgia, or GI symptoms.

Patients with known alcohol abuse or liver disease may have coagulopathy, splenomegaly, or thrombocytopenia.

In patients with a history of IV drug abuse or possible sexual exposure, HIV infection should be considered.

Testing: Most patients require laboratory evaluation (see Table 145–3). The initial tests are

- CBC with platelet count
- Peripheral blood smear
- Prothrombin time (PT) and partial thromboplastin time (PTT)

Screening tests evaluate the components of hemostasis, including the number of circulating platelets and the plasma coagulation pathways. The most common screening tests for bleeding disorders are the platelet count, PT, and PTT. If results are abnormal, a specific test can usually pinpoint the defect. Determination of the level of fibrin degradation products measures in vivo activation of fibrinolysis (usually secondary to excessive coagulation in DIC).

Prothrombin time (PT) screens for abnormalities in the extrinsic and common pathways of coagulation (plasma factors VII, X, V, prothrombin, and fibrinogen). The PT is reported as the international normalized ratio (INR), which reflects the ratio of the patient's PT to the laboratory's control value; the INR controls for differences in reagents among different laboratories. Because commercial reagents and instrumentation vary widely, each laboratory determines its own normal range for PT and PTT; a typical normal range for the PT is between 10 and 13 sec. An INR > 1.5 or a PT ≥ 3 sec longer than a laboratory's normal control value is usually abnormal and requires further evaluation. The INR is valuable in screening for abnormal coagulation in various acquired conditions (eg, vitamin K

Table 145–3. LABORATORY TESTS OF HEMOSTASIS BY PHASE

TEST	PURPOSE
Formation of initial platelet plugs	
Platelet count	Quantifies platelet number
Platelet aggregation	Evaluates adequacy of platelet responsiveness to physiologic stimuli that activate platelets (eg, collagen, ADP, arachidonic acid) Detects abnormal patterns in hereditary or acquired platelet functional disorders
VWF antigen	Measures total concentration of plasma VWF protein
VWF multimer composition	Evaluates distribution of VWF multimers in plasma (eg, large multimers are missing in type 2 variants of VWD)
Ristocetin agglutination	Screens for large multimers of VWF in patient platelet-rich plasma (often done as part of routine laboratory evaluation for VWD)
Ristocetin cofactor activity	Quantifies large multimers of VWF in patient plasma using formalin-fixed test platelets
Formation of fibrin	
PT	Screens for the factors in extrinsic and common pathways (factors VII, X, and V; prothrombin; and fibrinogen)
PTT	Screens for the factors in intrinsic and common pathways (prekallikrein; high molecular weight kininogen; factors XII, XI, IX, VIII, X, and V; prothrombin; and fibrinogen)
Specific functional assays for coagulation factors	Determines activity of the specific coagulant factor tested as a percentage of normal
Thrombin time	Evaluates the last step of coagulation (thrombin cleavage of fibrinogen to fibrin) Is prolonged by heparin activation of antithrombin and in conditions resulting in qualitative fibrinogen abnormalities or hypofibrinogenemia
Reptilase time	If it is normal and thrombin time is prolonged, provides presumptive evidence that a plasma sample contains heparin (eg, residual heparin after extracorporeal bypass or in a sample drawn from an IV line kept open with heparin flushes) because reptilase time is not affected by heparin activation of antithrombin
Fibrinogen level	Quantifies plasma fibrinogen, which is increased in acute phase reactions and decreased in severe liver disease and severe DIC
Fibrinolysis	
Clot stability during 24-h incubation in saline and in 5M urea	Lysis of clots occurs in saline if fibrinolytic activity is excessive or in 5M urea if factor XIII is deficient Should be done in patients with defective wound healing or frequent miscarriages
Plasminogen activity	Quantifies plasma plasminogen, which is decreased in patients with congenital early-onset venous thromboembolism (rare)
Alpha$_2$-antiplasmin	Quantifies plasma level of this fibrinolysis inhibitor, which is reduced in patients with excessive bleeding due to increased fibrinolysis (rare)
Serum fibrinogen and fibrin degradation products	Screens for DIC Increased levels when plasmin has acted on fibrinogen or fibrin in vivo (eg, in DIC) Superseded by plasma D-dimer assay
Plasma D-dimer	Is measured with a monoclonal antibody latex agglutination test or with an ELISA If high, indicates that thrombin has been generated in vivo with resultant generation of fibrin, activation of the cross-linking enzyme factor XIII, and secondary fibrinolysis Has the practical advantage that it can be done on citrate-treated plasma and thus, unlike the test for serum fibrin degradation products, does not require blood clotting in a special tube to prepare serum free of residual fibrinogen Is useful in the diagnosis of DIC and in vivo thrombosis (eg, DVT, PE), especially the sensitive ELISA version

ADP = adenosinediphosphate; DIC = disseminated intravascular coagulation; ELISA = enzyme-linked immunosorbent assay; VWD = von Willebrand disease; VWF = von Willebrand factor.

deficiency, liver disease, DIC). It is also used to monitor therapy with the oral vitamin K antagonist, warfarin.

Partial thromboplastin time (PTT) screens plasma for abnormalities in factors of the intrinsic and common pathways (prekallikrein; high molecular weight kininogen; factors XII, XI, IX, VIII, X, and V; prothrombin; fibrinogen). The PTT tests for deficiencies of all clotting factors except factor VII (measured by the PT) and factor XIII. A typical normal range is 28 to 34 sec. A normal result indicates that at least 30% of all coagulation factors in the pathway are present in the plasma.

Heparin prolongs the PTT, and the PTT is often used to monitor heparin therapy. Inhibitors that prolong the PTT include an autoantibody against factor VIII (see pp. 1118 and 1120) and antibodies against protein-phospholipid complexes (lupus anticoagulant—see pp. 1120 and 1206).

Prolongation of PT or PTT may reflect

- Clotting factor deficiency
- Presence of an inhibitor of a component of the coagulation pathway (including the presence in circulation of a direct inhibitor of thrombin or factor Xa)

The PT and PTT do not become prolonged until one or more of the clotting factors tested are about 70% deficient. For determining whether prolongation reflects a deficiency of one or more clotting factor or the presence of an inhibitor, the test is repeated after mixing the patient's plasma with normal plasma in a 1:1 ratio. Because this mixture contains at least 50% of normal levels of all coagulation factors, failure of the mixture to correct almost completely the prolongation suggests the presence of an inhibitor in patient plasma.

The previously used bleeding time test is of doubtful reliability.

Normal results on initial tests exclude many bleeding disorders. The main exceptions are VWD and hereditary hemorrhagic telangiectasia. VWD is a common entity in which the associated deficiency of factor VIII is frequently insufficient to prolong the PTT. Patients who have normal initial test results, along with symptoms or signs of bleeding and a positive family history, should be tested for VWD by measuring plasma VWF antigen, ristocetin cofactor activity (an indirect test for large VWF multimers), VWF multimer pattern, and factor VIII levels.

If **thrombocytopenia** is present, the peripheral blood smear often suggests the cause (see Table 156–3 on p. 1200). If the smear is normal, patients should be tested for HIV infection. If the result of the HIV test is negative and the patient is not pregnant and has not taken a drug known to cause platelet destruction, then idiopathic thrombocytopenic purpura is likely. If there are signs of hemolysis (fragmented RBCs on smear, decreasing Hb level), thrombotic thrombocytopenic purpura (TTP) or hemolytic uremic syndrome (HUS) is suspected, although sometimes other hemolytic disorders can cause these findings. HUS occurs in patients with hemorrhagic colitis. The Coombs test is negative in TTP and HUS. If the CBC and peripheral blood smear demonstrate other cytopenias or abnormal WBCs, a hematologic abnormality affecting multiple cell types is suspected, and a bone marrow aspiration and biopsy are necessary for diagnosis.

Prolonged PTT with normal platelets and PT suggests hemophilia A or B. Factor VIII and IX assays are indicated. Inhibitors that specifically prolong the PTT include an autoantibody against factor VIII and antibodies against protein-phospholipid complexes (lupus anticoagulant). Clinicians suspect one of these inhibitors when a prolonged PTT does not correct after 1:1 mixing with normal plasma.

Prolonged PT with normal platelets and PTT suggests factor VII deficiency. Congenital factor VII deficiency is rare; however, the short half-life of factor VII in plasma causes factor VII to decrease to low levels more rapidly than other vitamin K–dependent coagulation factors in patients beginning warfarin anticoagulation or in patients with incipient liver disease.

Prolonged PT and PTT with thrombocytopenia suggest DIC, especially in association with obstetric complications, sepsis, cancer, or shock. Confirmation is by finding elevated levels of D-dimers (or fibrin degradation products) and decreasing plasma fibrinogen levels on serial testing.

Prolonged PT or PTT with normal platelet count occurs with liver disease or vitamin K deficiency or during anticoagulation with warfarin, UFH, or the newer oral inhibitors of thrombin or factor Xa. Liver disease is suspected based on history and is confirmed by finding elevations of serum aminotransferases and bilirubin; hepatitis testing is recommended.

Imaging tests are often required to detect occult bleeding in patients with bleeding disorders. For example, head CT should be done in patients with severe headaches, head injuries, or impairment of consciousness. Abdominal CT is needed in patients with abdominal pain or other findings compatible with intraperitoneal or retroperitoneal hemorrhage.

Treatment

- Treat underlying disorder

Treatment is directed at the underlying disorder and at any hypovolemia. For immediate treatment of bleeding due to a coagulopathy that has not yet been diagnosed, fresh frozen plasma, which contains all coagulation factors, should be infused pending definitive evaluation.

KEY POINTS

- DIC should be suspected in patients with sepsis, shock, or complications of pregnancy or delivery.
- Mild platelet dysfunction caused by aspirin or NSAIDs is common.
- Easy bruising with no other clinical manifestations and normal laboratory test results is probably benign.

146 Histiocytic Syndromes

The histiocytic syndromes are clinically heterogeneous disorders that result from an abnormal proliferation of histiocytes—either monocyte-macrophages (antigen-processing cells) or dendritic cells (antigen-presenting cells). Classifying these disorders is difficult (see Table 146–1) and has changed over time as an understanding of the biology of these cells has evolved. There are other rare histiocytic disorders such as Erdheim-Chester disease, juvenile xanthogranuloma, and others.

LANGERHANS CELL HISTIOCYTOSIS

Langerhans cell histiocytosis (LCH) is a proliferation of dendritic mononuclear cells with infiltration into organs locally or diffusely. Most cases occur in children. Manifestations may include lung infiltrates; bone lesions; rashes; and hepatic, hematopoietic, and endocrine dysfunction. Diagnosis is based on biopsy. Factors predicting a poor prognosis include age < 2 yr and dissemination, particularly involving the hematopoietic system, liver, spleen, or a combination. Treatments include supportive measures and

Table 146–1. SOME HISTIOCYTIC SYNDROMES

CATEGORY	USUAL DISORDERS*
Histiocytic disorders of varied biologic behavior	
Dendritic cell–related	Juvenile xanthrogranuloma Erdheim Chester disease Langerhans cell histiocytosis†
Macrophage-related	Primary hemophagocytic syndromes Secondary hemophagocytic syndromes Rosai-Dorfman disease‡
Malignant histiocytic disorders	
Leukemias	Acute monocytic and myelomonocytic leukemia Chronic myelomonocytic leukemia (CMML)

*Other, rare disorders exist in each category.

†Includes the disorders formerly called eosinophilic granuloma, Letterer-Siwe disease, and Hand-Schüller-Christian disease.

‡Also called sinus histiocytosis with massive lymphoadenopathy.

Adapted from Komp DM, Perry MC: Introduction: The histiocytic syndromes. *Seminars in Oncology* 18:1, 1991 and Favara BE, Feller AC, Pauli M, eds.: Contemporary classification of histiocytic disorders. *Medical and Pediatric Oncology* 29:157, 1997.

chemotherapy or local treatment with surgery or radiation therapy as indicated by the extent of disease.

LCH is a dendritic cell (antigen-presenting cell) disorder. It can cause distinct clinical syndromes that have been historically described as eosinophilic granuloma, Hand-Schüller-Christian disease, and Letterer-Siwe disease. Because these syndromes may be varied manifestations of the same underlying disorder and because most patients with LCH have manifestations of more than one of these syndromes, the designations of the separate syndromes (except for eosinophilic granuloma) are now mostly of historical significance. Estimates of the prevalence of LCH vary widely (eg, from about 1:50,000 to 1:200,000). Incidence is 5 to 8 cases/million children.

All patients with LCH have evidence of activation of the RAS-RAF-MEK-ERK signaling pathway. *BRAFV600E* mutations are identified in 50 to 60% of patients who have LCH. This mutation is monoallelic and acts like a dominant driving oncogene. About 10 to 15% of patients have MAP2K1 mutations. Because of these mutations, LCH is now considered an oncogene-driven cancer of myeloid lineage.

In LCH, abnormally proliferating dendritic cells infiltrate one or more organs. Bones, skin, teeth, gingival tissue, ears, endocrine organs, lungs, liver, spleen, lymph nodes, and bone marrow may be involved. Organs may be affected by infiltration, causing dysfunction, or by compression from adjacent enlarged structures. In about half of patients, more than one organ is involved.

Symptoms and Signs

Symptoms and signs vary considerably depending on which organs are infiltrated.

Patients are divided into 2 groups based on organ involvement:

- Single system
- Multisystem

Single system disease is unifocal or multifocal involvement of one of the following organs: bone, skin, lymph nodes, lungs, central nervous system, or other, rare locations (eg, thyroid, thymus). An example of single system disease is eosinophilic granuloma.

Multisystem disease is disease in two or more organ systems. Risk organs may or may not be affected. An example of multisystem disease without risk organ involvement is Hand-Schüller-Christian disease. An example of multisystem disease with risk organ involvement is Letterer-Siwe disease.

Involvement of the zygomatic, sphenoid, orbital, ethmoid, or temporal bones denotes a category of CNS risk lesions that imparts a higher risk of neurodegenerative disease in the skull and front of the face.

Involvement of risk organs implies a worse prognosis. Risk organs include the liver, spleen, and organs of the hematopoietic system.

Patients with single system disease (unifocal, multifocal, and CNS risk organs) and multisystem disease without risk organ involvement are considered low risk. Patients with multsystem disease and risk organ involvement are considered high risk.

Here, the syndromes are described by their historical designations, but few patients present with classic manifestations, and other than eosinophilic granuloma, these designations are no longer used.

Eosinophilic granuloma (single system disease): Unifocal or multifocal eosinophilic granuloma (60 to 80% of LCH cases) occurs predominantly in older children and young adults, usually by age 30; incidence peaks between ages 5 and 10 yr. Lesions most frequently involve bones, often with pain, the inability to bear weight, or both and with overlying tender (sometimes warm) swelling.

Hand-Schüller-Christian disease (multisystem disease without risk organ involvement): This syndrome (15 to 40% of LCH cases) occurs in children aged 2 to 5 yr and in some older children and adults. Classic findings in this systemic disorder include involvement of the flat bones of the skull, ribs, pelvis, scapula, or a combination. Long bones and lumbosacral vertebrae are less frequently involved; the wrists, hands, knees, feet, and cervical vertebrae are rarely involved. In classic cases, patients have proptosis caused by orbital tumor mass. Rarely, vision loss or strabismus is caused by optic nerve or orbital muscle involvement. Tooth loss caused by apical and gingival infiltration is common in older patients.

Chronic otitis media and otitis externa due to involvement of the mastoid and petrous portions of the temporal bone with partial obstruction of the auditory canal are fairly common. Diabetes insipidus, the last component of the classic triad that includes flat bone involvement and proptosis, affects 5 to 50% of patients, with higher percentages in children who have systemic disease and involvement of the orbit and skull. Up to 40% of children with systemic disease have short stature. Hyperprolactinemia and hypogonadism can result from hypothalamic infiltration.

Letterer-Siwe disease (multisystem disease with risk organ involvement): This syndrome (10% of LCH cases), a systemic disorder, is the most severe form of LCH. Typically, a child < 2 yr presents with a scaly seborrheic, eczematoid, sometimes purpuric rash involving the scalp, ear canals, abdomen, and intertriginous areas of the neck and face. Denuded skin may facilitate microbial invasion, leading to sepsis. Frequently, there is ear drainage, lymphadenopathy, hepatosplenomegaly, and, in severe cases, hepatic dysfunction with hypoproteinemia and diminished synthesis of clotting factors. Anorexia, irritability, failure to thrive, and pulmonary manifestations (eg, cough, tachypnea, pneumothorax) may also occur. Significant anemia and sometimes neutropenia occur; thrombocytopenia is of grave prognostic significance. Parents frequently report precocious eruption of teeth, when in fact the gums are receding to expose immature dentition. Patients may appear abused or neglected.

Diagnosis

- Biopsy

LCH is suspected in patients (particularly young patients) with unexplained pulmonary infiltrates, bone lesions, or ocular or craniofacial abnormalities; and in children < 2 yr with typical rashes or severe, unexplained multiorgan disease.

X-rays are often done because of presenting symptoms. Bone lesions are usually sharply marginated, and round or oval, with a beveled edge giving the appearance of depth. However, some lesions are radiographically indistinguishable from Ewing sarcoma, osteosarcoma, other benign and malignant conditions, or osteomyelitis.

Diagnosis is based on biopsy. Langerhans cells are usually prominent, except in older lesions. These cells are identified by a pathologist experienced in the diagnosis of LCH according to their immunohistochemical characteristics, which include cell surface CD 1a, CD207 (langerin), and S-100 (although not specific). Tumor tissue should be tested for *BRAFV600E* mutation and other mutations. Once the diagnosis is established, the extent of disease must be determined by appropriate imaging and laboratory studies.

Laboratory studies used to define the extent of disease include the following:

- Complete blood count with differential
- Comprehensive metabolic panel
- Coagulation studies
- Early morning urinalysis

Imaging studies include the following:

- Skeletal survey, including chest x-ray
- Ultrasonography of the abdomen
- MRI of the brain (to evaluate the pituitary gland)
- MRI of the spine
- MRI or CT of the skull (to look for temporal bone lesions)
- MRI or CT of the orbit (to look for facial bone lesions)
- CT of the chest (if the chest x-ray is abnormal)
- CT or MRI of the abdomen (if examination reveals hepatosplenomegaly or if liver function test results are abnormal)
- PET/CT if available (because it can identify bone lesions not seen on skeletal survey)

Prognosis

Prognosis is good for patients with both of the following:

- Disease restricted to skin, lymph nodes, or bones
- Age > 2 yr

With treatment, almost all such patients survive.

Morbidity and mortality are increased in patients with multisystem involvement, particularly those with

- Age < 2 yr
- Involvement of risk organs (the hematopoietic system, liver, or spleen)

With treatment, the overall survival rate for patients with multisystem disease without risk organ involvement is 100%, but event-free survival is about 70%. Death is more likely among at-risk patients who do not respond to initial therapy. Disease recurrence is common. A chronic remitting and exacerbating course may occur, particularly among adults.

Some evidence suggests that patients who have *BRAFV600E* mutations are more prone to relapses.

Treatment

- Supportive care
- Sometimes hormone replacement therapy for hypopituitarism, most commonly diabetes insipidus
- Chemotherapy for multisystem involvement, single system multifocal involvement, and involvement in certain sites such as skull based lesions
- Sometimes surgery, corticosteroid injection, or rarely, radiation therapy (usually for unifocal bone involvement)

Because these syndromes are rare and complex, patients are usually referred to institutions experienced in the treatment of LCH. The majority of patients should be treated using protocols developed by the Histiocyte Society (see the Histiocyte Society web site at https://www.histio.org).

General supportive care is essential and may include scrupulous hygiene to limit ear, cutaneous, and dental lesions. Debridement or resection of severely affected gingival tissue limits oral involvement. Seborrhea-like dermatitis of the scalp may diminish with use of a selenium-based shampoo twice/wk. If shampooing is ineffective, topical corticosteroids are used in small amounts and briefly in small areas.

Patients with systemic disease are monitored for potential chronic disabilities, such as cosmetic or functional orthopedic and cutaneous disorders and neurotoxicity as well as for psychologic problems that may require psychosocial support.

Many patients require hormone replacement for diabetes insipidus or other manifestations of hypopituitarism.

Chemotherapy is indicated for patients with multisystem involvement, single system multifocal involvement, and disease in certain sites, such as skull based lesions (including zygomatic, orbital, sphenoid, temporal, and ethmoid bones). Protocols sponsored by the Histiocyte Society are used; treatment protocols vary according to the risk category. Almost all patients with a good response to therapy can stop treatment. Protocols for poor responders with goals of early aggressive salvage are under study.

Local surgery, corticosteroid injection, curettage, or rarely, radiation therapy is used for disease involving a single bone. Surgery, corticosteroid injections, curettage, and radiation therapy should be done by specialists experienced in treating LCH. Easily accessible lesions in noncritical locations undergo surgical curettage. Surgery should be avoided when it may result in significant cosmetic deformities, orthopedic deformities, or loss of function.

Radiation therapy may be given to patients at risk of skeletal deformity, vision loss secondary to proptosis, pathologic fractures, vertebral collapse, and spinal cord injury or to patients with severe pain.

Patients with LCH that progresses despite standard therapy usually respond to more aggressive chemotherapy. Patients who do not respond to salvage chemotherapy may undergo reduced intensity hematopoietic stem cell transplantation, experimental chemotherapy, or immunosuppressive or other immunomodulatory therapy. Patients with *BRAFV600E* mutations who fail multiple lines of therapy may be candidates for RAS-RAF-MEK-ERK inhibitor therapy (eg, vemurafenib).

KEY POINTS

- Langerhans cell histiocytosis (LCH) involves a proliferation of dendritic mononuclear cells that infiltrate one or more organs.
- Manifestations vary significantly depending on the organ(s) affected.
- Bone lesions cause pain; lesions at the skull base may affect vision, hearing, and pituitary function (particularly causing diabetes insipidus).
- Liver, spleen, lymph nodes, and bone marrow may be affected, resulting in a worse prognosis.
- Use surgery, curettage with or without corticosteroid injection, or rarely, radiation therapy for only single bone lesions.
- Use chemotherapy for multisytem, multifocal, and skull-based site involvement.

HEMOPHAGOCYTIC LYMPHOHISTIOCYTOSIS

Hemophagocytic lymphohistiocytosis (HLH) is an uncommon disorder causing immune dysfunction in infants and young children. Many patients have an underlying immune disorder, although in some patients the underlying disorder is not known. Manifestations may include lymphadenopathy, hepatosplenomegaly, fever, and neurologic abnormalities. Diagnosis is by specific clinical and testing (genetic) criteria. Treatment is usually with chemotherapy and, in refractory cases or in cases with a genetic cause, hematopoietic stem cell transplantation.

HLH is uncommon. It affects mostly infants < 18 mo. It involves a defect in targeted killing and the inhibitory controls of natural killer and cytotoxic T cells, resulting in excessive cytokine production and accumulation of activated T cells and macrophages in various organs. Cells in the bone marrow and/or spleen may attack RBCs, WBCs, and/or platelets.

HLH can be:

- Familial (primary)
- Acquired (secondary)

HLH is diagnosed when patients fulfill at least 5 of the criteria described below or have a mutation in a known HLH-associated gene.

Acquired HLH can be associated with infections (eg, Epstein-Barr virus, cytomegalovirus, or others), cancer (eg, leukemias, lymphomas), and immune disorders (eg, SLE, RA, polyarteritis nodosa, sarcoidosis, progressive systemic sclerosis, Sjögren syndrome, Kawasaki disease) and can occur in kidney or liver transplant recipients.

In both forms, genetic abnormalities, clinical manifestations, and outcomes tend to be similar.

Symptoms and Signs

Common early manifestations include fever, hepatomegaly, splenomegaly, rash, lymphadenopathy, and neurologic abnormalities (eg, seizures, retinal hemorrhages, ataxia, altered consciousness or coma).

Diagnosis

- Clinical and testing criteria

HLH can be diagnosed if there is a mutation in a known causative gene or if at least 5 of 8 diagnostic criteria are met:

- Fever (peak temperature of > 38.5° C for > 7 days)
- Splenomegaly (spleen palpable > 3 cm below costal margin)
- Cytopenia involving > 2 cell lines (Hb < 9 g/dL, absolute neutrophil count < 100/μL, platelets < 100,000/μL)
- Hypertriglyceridemia (fasting triglycerides > 2.0 mmol/L or > 3 standard deviations [SD] more than normal value for age) or hypofibrinogenemia (fibrinogen < 1.5 g/L or > 3 SD less than normal value for age)
- Hemophagocytosis (in biopsy samples of bone marrow, spleen, or lymph nodes)
- Low or absent natural killer cell activity
- Serum ferritin > 500 μg/L
- Elevated soluble IL-2 (CD25) levels (> 2400 U/mL or very high for age)

Genetic mutations associated with HLH include PRF1, UNC13D, STX11, STXBP2, RAB27, and XLP.

Because some of these tests may not be widely available and HLH is uncommon, patients are usually referred to specialized centers for evaluation.

Treatment

- Chemotherapy, cytokine inhibitors, immune suppression, and sometimes hematopoietic stem cell transplantation

Treatment should be started if the disorder is suspected, even if not all diagnostic criteria are fulfilled. Patients are usually treated by a pediatric hematologist and in a referral center experienced in treating patients with HLH. Treatment depends on the presence of factors such as a family history of HLH, coexisting infections, and demonstrated immune system defects. Treatment for HLH may include cytokine inhibitors, immune therapy, chemotherapy, some combination of these, and possibly stem cell transplantation.

ROSAI-DORFMAN DISEASE

(Sinus Histiocytosis With Massive Lymphadenopathy)

Rosai-Dorfman disease is a rare disorder characterized by accumulation of histiocytes and massive lymphadenopathy, particularly in the neck and head.

Rosai-Dorfman disease is most common among patients < 20 yr, particularly blacks. Cause is unknown.

The most common presenting symptoms are fever and massive, painless cervical lymphadenopathy. Other nodal sites, including the mediastinum, retroperitoneum, axillae, and inguinal region, may be involved, as may the nasal cavity, salivary gland tissue, other regions of the head and neck, and CNS. Other manifestations may include lytic bone lesions, pulmonary nodules, and rash. The bone marrow and spleen are typically spared.

Laboratory testing usually shows leukocytosis, polyclonal hypergammaglobulinemia, hypochromic or normocytic anemia, and elevated ESR.

The disorder commonly resolves without treatment. In patients with progressive disease, chemotherapy has been tried.

147 Iron Overload

(Hemochromatosis; Hemosiderosis)

Typical adults lose about 1 mg iron (Fe) per day in shed epidermal and GI cells; menstruating females lose on average an additional 0.5 to 1 mg/day from menses. This iron loss is balanced by absorption of a portion of the 10 to 20 mg of iron in a typical US diet. Iron absorption is regulated based on the body's iron stores and is usually in balance with the body's needs. However, because there is no physiologic mechanism to remove iron from the body, iron absorbed in excess of bodily needs (or acquired through repeated transfusion) is deposited in tissues:

- **Hemosiderosis** is focal deposition of iron that does not cause tissue damage.
- **Hemochromatosis** (iron overload) is a typically systemic process in which iron deposition can cause tissue damage.

Iron overload may result from hereditary hemochromatosis (a genetic disorder of iron metabolism) or from secondary hemochromatosis, an acquired form of the disease that is due to excess oral intake or absorption of iron or to repeated blood transfusions.[1, 2] Morbidity is mainly due to iron accumulation in the endocrine organs (especially the pancreas, gonads, and pituitary), liver, and heart.

African iron overload occurs most often in sub-Saharan Africa among people who consume an iron-rich fermented drink. A genetic component is thought to contribute to the pathogenesis of African iron overload, but no gene has yet been identified.

1. Bacon BR, Adams PC, Kowdley KV, et al: Diagnosis and management of hemochromatosis: 2011 Practice Guideline by the AASLD. *Hepatology* 54(1): 328–343, 2011.
2. Fleming RE, Ponka P: Iron overload in human disease. *New Engl J Med* 366:348–359, 2012.

HEMOSIDEROSIS

Hemosiderosis is focal deposition of iron that does not cause tissue damage.

Focal hemosiderosis can result from hemorrhage within an organ. Iron liberated from extravasated RBCs is deposited within that organ, and significant hemosiderin deposits may eventually develop. Occasionally, iron loss due to tissue hemorrhage causes iron deficiency anemia because iron in tissues cannot be reused.

Usually the lungs are affected, and the cause usually is recurrent pulmonary hemorrhage, either idiopathic (eg, Goodpasture syndrome) or due to chronic pulmonary hypertension (eg, as a result of primary pulmonary hypertension, pulmonary fibrosis, severe mitral stenosis).

Another common site of accumulation is the kidneys, where hemosiderosis can result from extensive intravascular hemolysis. Free Hb is filtered at the glomerulus, resulting in iron deposition in the kidneys. The renal parenchyma is not damaged, but severe hemosiderinuria may result in iron deficiency.

HEREDITARY HEMOCHROMATOSIS

(Primary Hemochromatosis)

Hereditary hemochromatosis is a genetic disorder characterized by excessive iron (Fe) accumulation that results in tissue damage. Manifestations can include systemic symptoms, liver disorders, cardiomyopathy, diabetes, erectile dysfunction, and arthropathy. Diagnosis is by elevated serum ferritin, iron, and transferrin saturation levels and confirmed by a gene assay. Treatment is usually with serial phlebotomies.

Etiology

There are 4 types of hereditary hemochromatosis, types 1 through 4, depending on the gene that is mutated.

- Type 1: Mutations of the *HFE* gene
- Type 2 (juvenile hemochromatosis): Mutations in the *HJV* and *HAMP* genes
- Type 3: Mutations in the *TFR2* gene
- Type 4 (ferroportin disease): Mutations in the *SLC40A1* gene

Other much rarer genetic disorders can cause hepatic iron overload, but the clinical picture is usually dominated by symptoms and signs due to failure of other organs (eg, anemia in hypotransferrinemia or atransferrinemia, or neurologic defects in aceruloplasminemia).

Although these types vary markedly in age of onset, clinical consequences of iron overload are the same in all.[1]

Type 1 hereditary hemochromatosis: Type 1 is classic hereditary hemochromatosis, also termed *HFE*-related hemochromatosis. More than 80% of cases are caused by the homozygous *C282Y* or *C282Y/H63D* compound heterozygote mutation. The disorder is autosomal recessive, with a homozygous frequency of 1:200 and a heterozygous frequency of 1:8 in people of northern European ancestry. It is uncommon among blacks and rare among people of Asian ancestry. Of patients with clinical hemochromatosis, 83% are homozygous. However, for unknown reasons, phenotypic (clinical) disease is much less common than predicted by the frequency of the gene (ie, many homozygous people do not manifest the disorder).

Type 2 hereditary hemochromatosis: Type 2 hereditary hemochromatosis (juvenile hemochromatosis) is a rare autosomal recessive disorder caused by mutations in the *HJV* gene that affect the transcription protein hemojuvelin or mutations in the *HAMP* gene, which directly codes for hepcidin. It often manifests in adolescents.

Type 3 hereditary hemochromatosis: Mutations in transferrin receptor 2 (TFR2), a protein that appears to control saturation of transferrin, can cause a rare autosomal recessive form of hemochromatosis.

Type 4 hereditary hemochromatosis: Type 4 hereditary hemochromatosis (ferroportin disease) occurs largely in people of southern European ancestry. It results from an autosomal dominant mutation in the *SLC40A1* gene and affects the ability of ferroportin to bind hepcidin.

Transferrin and ceruloplasmin deficiency: In transferrin deficiency (hypotransferrinemia or atransferrinemia), absorbed iron that enters the portal system not bound to transferrin is deposited in the liver. Subsequent iron transfer to sites of RBC production is reduced because of transferrin deficiency.

In ceruloplasmin deficiency (aceruloplasminemia), lack of ferroxidase causes defective conversion of Fe^{2+} to Fe^{3+}; such conversion is necessary for binding to transferrin. Defective transferrin binding impairs the movement of iron from intracellular stores to plasma transport, resulting in accumulation of iron in tissues.

1. Pietrangelo A: Hereditary hemochromatosis: pathogenesis, diagnosis, and treatment. *Gastroenterology* 139:393–408, 2010.

Pathophysiology

Normal total body iron content is about 2.5 g in women and 3.5 g in men. Because symptoms may be delayed until iron accumulation is excessive (eg, > 10 to 20 g), hemochromatosis may not be recognized until later in life, even though it is an inherited abnormality. In women, clinical manifestations are uncommon before menopause because iron loss due to menses (and sometimes pregnancy and childbirth) tends to offset iron accumulation.

The mechanism for iron overload in both *HFE* and non-*HFE*-hemochromatosis is increased iron absorption from the GI tract, leading to chronic deposition of iron in the tissues. Hepcidin, a liver-derived peptide, is the critical control mechanism for iron absorption. Hepcidin is normally up-regulated when iron stores are elevated and, through its inhibitory effect on ferroportin (which participates in iron absorption), it prevents excessive iron absorption and storage in normal people. Hemochromatosis types 1 through 4 share the same pathogenic basis (eg, lack of hepcidin synthesis or activity) and key clinical features.

In general, tissue injury appears to result from reactive free hydroxyl radicals generated when iron deposition in tissues catalyzes their formation. Other mechanisms may affect particular organs (eg, skin hyperpigmentation can result from increased melanin as well as iron accumulation). In the liver, iron-associated lipid peroxidation induces hepatocyte apoptosis, which stimulates Kupffer cell activation and release of pro-inflammatory cytokines. These cytokines activate hepatic stellate cells to produce collagen, resulting in pathologic accumulation of liver fibrosis.

Symptoms and Signs

The clinical consequences of iron overload are the same regardless of the etiology and pathophysiology of the overload.

Historically, experts believed that symptoms did not develop until significant organ damage had occurred. However, organ damage is slow and subtle, and fatigue and nonspecific systemic symptoms and signs often occur early. For example, liver dysfunction can manifest insidiously with fatigue, right upper quadrant abdominal pain, and hepatomegaly. Laboratory abnormalities of iron overload and hepatitis usually precede symptoms.

In **type 1** hereditary (*HFE*) hemochromatosis, symptoms relate to the organs with the largest iron deposits (see Table 147–1). In men, the initial symptoms may be hypogonadism and erectile dysfunction caused by gonadal iron deposition. Glucose intolerance or diabetes mellitus is another common initial presentation. Some patients present with hypothyroidism.

Liver disease is the most common complication and may progress to cirrhosis; 20 to 30% of patients with cirrhosis develop hepatocellular carcinoma. Liver disease is the most common cause of death.

Cardiomyopathy with heart failure is the 2nd most common fatal complication. Hyperpigmentation (bronze diabetes) and porphyria cutanea tarda are common, as is symptomatic arthropathy.

In **type 2** disease, symptoms and signs include progressive hepatomegaly and hypogonadotropic hypogonadism.

In **type 3** disease, symptoms and signs are similar to type 1 hereditary (*HFE*) hemochromatosis.

Type 4 disease manifests in the first decade of life as increased serum ferritin levels with low or normal transferrin saturation; progressive saturation of transferrin occurs when patients are in their 20s and 30s. Clinical manifestations are milder than in type 1 disease, with modest liver disease and mild anemia.

Table 147–1. COMMON MANIFESTATIONS OF HEREDITARY HEMOCHROMATOSIS

MANIFESTATION	PREVALENCE (APPROXIMATE)
Systemic symptoms (eg, weakness, lethargy)	75%
Abnormal liver function test results	75%
Skin hyperpigmentation	70%
Diabetes mellitus	50%
Arthropathy	45%
Erectile dysfunction	45% (of men)
Cardiomyopathy	15%

Diagnosis

- Serum ferritin, fasting serum iron, and transferrin saturation
- Genetic testing
- Sometimes liver biopsy

Symptoms and signs may be nonspecific, subtle, and of gradual onset, so that index of suspicion should be high. Primary hemochromatosis should be suspected when typical manifestations, particularly combinations of such manifestations, remain unexplained after routine evaluation. Family history of hemochromatosis, cirrhosis, or hepatocellular carcinoma is a more specific clue. All patients with chronic liver disease should be evaluated for iron overload.

Serum ferritin measurement is the simplest and most direct initial test. Elevated levels (> 200 ng/mL in women or > 250 ng/mL in men) are usually present in hereditary hemochromatosis but can result from other abnormalities, such as inflammatory liver disorders (eg, chronic viral hepatitis, nonalcoholic steatohepatitis, alcoholic liver disease), cancer, certain systemic inflammatory disorders (eg, rheumatoid arthritis, hemophagocytic lymphohistiocytosis), or obesity. Further testing is done if ferritin level is abnormal; testing includes fasting serum iron (usually > 300 mg/dL) and iron binding capacity (transferrin saturation; levels usually > 50%). A transferrin saturation of < 45% has a negative predictive value of 97% for iron overload.

In type 2 disease, ferritin levels are > 1000 ng/mL, and transferrin saturation is > 90%.

In transferrin or ceruloplasmin deficiency, serum transferrin (ie, iron-binding capacity) and ceruloplasmin levels are profoundly low or undetectable.

Gene assay is diagnostic of hereditary hemochromatosis caused by *HFE* gene mutations. About 70% of patients with C282Y homozygous mutations of the *HFE* gene have an elevated ferritin level, but only about 10% of these patients have evidence of organ dysfunction. Clinically significant iron overload is even less common in patients with heterozygous mutations of the *HFE* gene (ie, C282Y/H63D). Hemochromatosis types 2 to 4 is suspected in the less common instances in which ferritin and iron blood tests indicate iron overload and genetic testing is negative for the *HFE* gene mutation, particularly in younger patients. Confirmation of these diagnoses is evolving.

Up to 80% of patients with cirrhosis and a homozygous C282Y mutation will have a ferritin of > 1000 ng/mL, elevated AST and ALT, and platelet count < 200 × 10^3/μL). Because the presence of cirrhosis affects prognosis, when the ferritin is > 1000 ng/mL, liver biopsy is commonly done and tissue iron content is measured (when available). Liver biopsy is also recommended in patients with serologic evidence of iron overload but negative genetic evaluation. MRI with noncontrast MR elastography (MRE), a noninvasive alternative for estimating hepatic iron content and hepatic fibrosis, is becoming increasingly accurate.

Screening is required for first-degree relatives of people with hereditary hemochromatosis by measuring serum ferritin levels and testing for the *C282Y* and *H63D* mutations in the *HFE* gene.

Treatment

- Phlebotomy

Treatment is indicated for patients with clinical manifestations, elevated serum ferritin levels (particularly levels > 1000 ng/mL), or elevated transferrin saturation. Asymptomatic patients need only periodic (eg, yearly) clinical evaluation and measurement of serum iron, ferritin, transferrin saturation, and liver enzymes.

Phlebotomy is the simplest and most effective method to remove excess iron. It delays progression of fibrosis to cirrhosis, sometimes even reversing cirrhotic changes, and prolongs survival, but it does not prevent hepatocellular carcinoma. About 500 mL of blood (about 250 mg of iron) is removed weekly or biweekly (every other week) until serum ferritin levels reach 50 to 100 ng/mL. Weekly or biweekly phlebotomy may be needed for many months (eg, if 250 mg of iron are removed per week, 40 wk will be required to remove 10 g of iron). When iron levels are normal, phlebotomies can be intermittent to maintain ferritin between 50 and 100 ng/mL.

Diabetes mellitus, cardiomyopathy, erectile dysfunction, and other secondary manifestations are treated as indicated. Patients with advanced fibrosis or cirrhosis due to iron overload should be screened for hepatocellular carcinoma every 6 months with a liver ultrasound.

Patients should follow a balanced diet; it is not necessary to restrict consumption of iron-containing foods (eg, red meat, liver). Alcohol should be consumed only in moderation because it can increase iron absorption and, in high amounts, increases the risk of cirrhosis. Vitamin C supplements should be avoided.

In patients with type 4 disease, tolerance to vigorous phlebotomy is poor; serial monitoring of Hb level and transferrin saturation is required.

Treatment of transferrin deficiency and ceruloplasmin deficiency is experimental; eg, iron chelators may be better tolerated than phlebotomy because patients typically have anemia.

KEY POINTS

- There are 4 types of hereditary hemochromatosis, which all involve mutations that impair the ability of the body to inhibit iron absorption when iron stores are excessive.
- The effects of iron overload are similar in all types and include liver disease (leading to cirrhosis), skin pigmentation, diabetes, arthropathy, erectile dysfunction, and sometimes heart failure.
- Diagnose by measuring serum ferritin level; if elevated, confirm by demonstrating elevated serum iron, transferrin saturation, and genetic testing.
- Once diagnosis is made, do liver biopsy to identify cirrhosis and determine prognosis; consider genetic testing and screening of first-degree relatives.
- Treat with phlebotomy and moderation of alcohol consumption.

SECONDARY IRON OVERLOAD

(Secondary Hemochromatosis)

Secondary iron overload results from excess absorption of iron, repeated blood transfusions, or excess oral intake, typically in patients with disorders of erythropoiesis. Consequences can include systemic symptoms, liver disorders, cardiomyopathy, diabetes, erectile dysfunction, and arthropathy. Diagnosis is by elevated serum ferritin, iron, and transferrin saturation levels. Treatment is usually by iron chelation.

Etiology

Secondary iron overload typically occurs in patients who have

- Hemoglobinopathies (eg, sickle cell disease, thalassemia, sideroblastic anemias)
- Congenital hemolytic anemias
- Myelodysplasia

Iron overload results from the following mechanisms:

- Increased iron absorption
- Exogenous iron given to treat anemia
- Repeated blood transfusions (each unit of blood provides about 250 mg of iron; tissue deposition becomes significant when more than about 40 units of blood are transfused)

Increased iron absorption in patients with ineffective erythropoiesis may be partly due to the secretion, by erythroid precursors, of erythroferrone (ERFE), which suppresses hepcidin (an inhibitor of iron absorption).

Patients with hemoglobinopathies and congenital hemolytic anemias now typically live into adulthood, so complications of iron overload are now common and clinically important. In such patients, iron overload involving the heart, the liver, and endocrine organs has become a common cause of death, but survival can be prolonged by iron removal.

Symptoms and Signs

The clinical consequences of iron overload are the same regardless of the etiology and pathophysiology of the overload.

Historically, experts believed that symptoms did not develop until significant organ damage had occurred. However, organ damage is slow and subtle, and fatigue and nonspecific systemic symptoms often occur early.

In men, the initial symptoms may be hypogonadism and erectile dysfunction caused by gonadal iron deposition. Glucose intolerance or diabetes mellitus is another common initial presentation. Some patients present with hypothyroidism.

Liver disease is the most common complication and may progress to cirrhosis. Patients who develop cirrhosis are at increased risk of hepatocellular carcinoma. The liver disease can present insidiously with nonspecific symptoms and signs, such as fatigue, and with right upper quadrant abdominal pain and hepatomegaly. Laboratory abnormalities of iron overload and hepatitis typically will be present well before clinical symptoms develop. Liver disease is the most common cause of death. Cardiomyopathy with heart failure is the 2nd most common fatal complication. Hyperpigmentation (bronze diabetes) and porphyria cutanea tarda are common, as is symptomatic arthropathy.

Diagnosis

- Measure serum ferritin, iron, and transferrin saturation

Patients with ineffective erythropoiesis should be evaluated for secondary iron overload, which is diagnosed by measuring serum ferritin, serum iron, and transferrin saturation. Serum ferritin measurement is the simplest and most direct initial test. Elevated levels (> 200 ng/mL in women or > 250 ng/mL in men) are usually present in secondary iron overload but can result from other abnormalities, such as hereditary hemochromatosis, inflammatory liver disorders (eg, chronic viral hepatitis, nonalcoholic steatohepatitis, alcoholic liver disease), cancer, certain systemic inflammatory disorders (eg, rheumatoid arthritis, hemophagocytic lymphohistiocytosis), or obesity. Further testing is done if ferritin level is abnormal; testing includes fasting serum iron (usually > 300 mg/dL) and iron binding capacity (transferrin saturation; levels usually > 50%). Hereditary hemochromatosis may be ruled out by history and genetic testing. A transferrin saturation < 45% has a negative predictive value of 97% for iron overload.

Treatment

- Usually iron chelation with deferasirox or deferoxamine, or sometimes deferiprone

Some patients can be treated with phlebotomy and given erythropoietin to maintain erythropoiesis. However, because it worsens anemia, phlebotomy is not recommended for many patients (eg, those with Hb level < 10 g/dL, those who are transfusion dependent, and those who develop symptoms of anemia after phlebotomy). Treatment in these patients is iron chelation. The goal of treatment is a transferrin saturation of < 50%.

Deferoxamine is the drug traditionally used for iron chelation therapy. It is given by a slow subcutaneous infusion overnight through a portable pump for 5 to 7 nights/wk or via 24-h IV infusion. Dose is 1 to 2 g in adults and 20 to 40 mg/kg in children. However, this therapy is complex to administer and requires an unusual time commitment from patients, resulting in a high rate of nonadherence. Important adverse effects include hypotension, GI disturbances, and anaphylaxis (acutely) and vision and hearing loss (with chronic use).

Deferasirox, an oral chelating agent, is an effective and increasingly used alternative to deferoxamine. Deferasirox reduces iron levels and prevents or delays onset of complications of iron overload. Initial dose is 20 mg/kg po once/day. Patients are monitored monthly with dose increases of up to 30 mg/kg once/day. Treatment can be interrupted when serum ferritin is < 500 ng/mL. Adverse effects (which occur in about 10% of patients) can include nausea, abdominal pain, diarrhea, and rash. Liver and kidney function may become abnormal; liver and kidney function tests should be done periodically (eg, monthly, sometimes more frequently for high-risk patients).

Deferiprone, another oral iron chelator, is indicated for the treatment of patients with transfusional iron overload due to thalassemia syndromes when chelation therapy with deferasirox or deferoxamine is inadequate. Initial dose is 25 mg/kg po tid. Maximum dose is 33 mg/kg po tid. Absolute neutrophil counts are obtained weekly to look for neutropenia (precedes agranulocytosis). Serum ferritin is measured every 2 to 3 mo; treatment is temporarily interrupted when levels are consistently < 500 ng/mL.

Diabetes mellitus, cardiomyopathy, erectile dysfunction, and other secondary manifestations are treated as indicated. Patients with advanced fibrosis or cirrhosis due to iron overload should be screened for hepatocellular carcinoma every 6 months with a liver ultrasound.

Patients should follow a balanced diet; it is not necessary to restrict consumption of iron-containing foods (eg, red meat, liver). Alcohol should be consumed only in moderation because it can increase iron absorption and, in high amounts, increases the risk of cirrhosis. Vitamin C supplements should be avoided.

KEY POINTS

- Secondary iron overload results from excess absorption of iron, repeated blood transfusions, or excess oral intake.
- The effects of secondary iron overload include liver disease (leading to cirrhosis), skin pigmentation, diabetes, arthropathy, erectile dysfunction, and sometimes heart failure.
- Diagnose by measuring serum ferritin level; if elevated, confirm by demonstrating elevated serum iron and transferrin saturation.
- Treat with chelation.

148 Leukemias

The leukemias are cancers of the WBCs involving bone marrow, circulating WBCs, and organs such as the spleen and lymph nodes.

Etiology

Risk of developing leukemia is increased in patients with

- History of exposure to ionizing radiation (eg, post–atom bomb in Nagasaki and Hiroshima) or to chemicals (eg, benzene)
- Prior treatment with certain antineoplastic drugs, particularly procarbazine, nitrosureas (cyclophosphamide, melphalan), and epipodophyllotoxins (etoposide, teniposide)
- Infection with a virus (eg, human T-lymphotropic virus 1 and 2, Epstein-Barr virus)
- Chromosomal translocations
- Preexisting conditions, including immunodeficiency disorders, chronic myeloproliferative disorders, and chromosomal disorders (eg, Fanconi anemia, Bloom syndrome, ataxia-telangiectasia, Down syndrome, infantile X-linked agammaglobulinemia)

Pathophysiology

Malignant transformation usually occurs at the pluripotent stem cell level, although it sometimes involves a committed stem cell with more limited capacity for self-renewal. Abnormal proliferation, clonal expansion, and diminished apoptosis (programmed cell death) lead to replacement of normal blood elements with malignant cells.

Manifestations of leukemia are due to

- Suppression of normal blood cell formation
- Organ infiltration by leukemic cells

Inhibitory factors produced by leukemic cells and replacement of marrow space may suppress normal hematopoiesis, with ensuing anemia, thrombocytopenia, and granulocytopenia.

Organ infiltration results in enlargement of the liver, spleen, and lymph nodes and, occasionally, in kidney and gonadal involvement. Meningeal infiltration results in clinical features associated with increasing intracranial pressure (eg, cranial nerve palsies).

Classification

Leukemias were originally termed acute or chronic based on life expectancy but now are classified according to cellular phenotype and degree of differentiation on initial presentation.

Acute leukemias: Acute leukemias consist of predominantly immature, poorly differentiated cells (usually blast forms). Acute leukemias are divided into ALL and acute myelogenous leukemia (AML), which may be further subdivided by the French-American-British (FAB) classification (see Table 148–1).

Chronic leukemias: Chronic leukemias have more mature cells than do acute leukemias. They usually manifest as abnormal leukocytosis with or without cytopenia in an otherwise asymptomatic person. Findings and management differ significantly between chronic lymphocytic leukemia (CLL) and chronic myelogenous leukemia (CML—see Table 148–2).

Myelodysplastic syndromes: Myelodysplastic syndromes involve progressive bone marrow failure but with an insufficient proportion of blast cells (< 30%) for making a definite diagnosis of AML; 40 to 60% of cases evolve into AML.

Table 148–1. FRENCH-AMERICAN-BRITISH (FAB) CLASSIFICATION OF ACUTE LEUKEMIAS

FAB CLASSIFICATION	DESCRIPTION
Acute lymphocytic leukemia	
L1	Lymphoblasts with uniform, round nuclei and scant cytoplasm
L2	More variability of lymphoblasts Sometimes irregular nuclei with more cytoplasm than L1
L3	Lymphoblasts with finer nuclear chromatin and blue to deep blue cytoplasm that contains vacuoles
Acute myelogenous leukemia	
M1	Undifferentiated myeloblastic No cytoplasmic granulation
M2	Differentiated myeloblastic Sparse granulation in few to many cells
M3	Promyelocytic Granulation typical of promyelocytic morphology
M4	Myelomonoblastic Mixed myeloblastic and monocytoid morphology
M5	Monoblastic Pure monoblastic morphology
M6	Erythroleukemic Predominantly immature erythroblastic morphology, sometimes megaloblastic appearance
M7	Megakaryoblastic Cells with shaggy borders that may show some budding

Leukemoid reaction: A leukemoid reaction is marked granulocytic leukocytosis (ie, WBC > 50,000/μL) produced by normal bone marrow in response to systemic infection or cancer. Although not a neoplastic disorder, a leukemoid reaction with a very high WBC count may require testing to distinguish it from CML.

ACUTE LEUKEMIA OVERVIEW

Acute leukemia occurs when a hematopoietic stem cell undergoes malignant transformation into a primitive, undifferentiated cell with abnormal longevity.

These lymphoid cells (ALL) or myeloid cells (acute myelogenous leukemia [AML]) proliferate, replacing normal marrow tissue and hematopoietic cells and inducing anemia, thrombocytopenia, and granulocytopenia. Because they are bloodborne, they can infiltrate various organs and sites, including the liver, spleen, lymph nodes, CNS, kidneys, and gonads.

Symptoms and Signs

Symptoms may be present for only days to weeks before diagnosis. Disrupted hematopoiesis leads to the most common presenting symptoms (anemia, infection, easy bruising and bleeding). Other presenting symptoms and signs are usually nonspecific (eg, pallor, fatigue, fever, malaise, weight loss, tachycardia, chest pain) and are attributable to anemia and a hypermetabolic state. The cause of fever often is not found, although granulocytopenia may lead to a rapidly progressing and potentially life-threatening bacterial infection.

Bleeding is usually manifested by petechiae, easy bruising, epistaxis, bleeding gums, or menstrual irregularity. Hematuria and GI bleeding are uncommon.

Bone marrow and periosteal infiltration may cause bone and joint pain, especially in children with ALL. Initial CNS involvement or leukemic meningitis (manifesting as headaches, vomiting, irritability, cranial nerve palsies, seizures, and papilledema) is uncommon. Extramedullary infiltration by leukemic cells may cause lymphadenopathy, splenomegaly, hepatomegaly, and leukemia cutis (a raised, nonpruritic rash). Gum hyperplasia may be prominent, particularly in acute monocytic leukemias.

Diagnosis

- CBC and peripheral blood smear
- Bone marrow examination
- Histochemical studies, cytogenetics, immunophenotyping, and molecular biology studies
- Imaging

CBC and peripheral smear are the first tests done; pancytopenia and peripheral blasts suggest acute leukemia. Blast cells in the peripheral smear may approach 90% of WBC count.

Bone marrow examination (aspiration or needle biopsy) is routinely done, although the diagnosis can usually be made from the peripheral smear. Blast cells in the bone marrow are classically between 25 and 95%. Aplastic anemia, viral infections such as infectious mononucleosis, and vitamin B_{12} and folate deficiencies should be considered in the differential diagnosis of severe pancytopenia. Leukemoid reactions to infectious disease (such as TB) can rarely manifest with high blast counts.

Histochemical studies, cytogenetics, immunophenotyping, and molecular biology studies help distinguish the blasts of ALL from those of AML or other disease processes. Specific B-cell, T-cell, and myeloid-antigen monoclonal antibodies, together with flow cytometry, are essential in classifying the acute leukemias, which is critical for treatment.

Other laboratory findings may include hyperuricemia, hyperphosphatemia, hyperkalemia or hypokalemia, hypocalcemia, elevated serum hepatic transaminases or LDH, hypoglycemia, and hypoxia.

CT of the head is done in patients with CNS symptoms. Chest x-ray should be done to detect mediastinal masses, especially before the patient is given anesthesia. CT, MRI, or abdominal ultrasonography may help assess splenomegaly or leukemic infiltration of other organs. Echocardiography is typically done to assess baseline cardiac function.

Prognosis

Cure is a realistic goal for both ALL and AML, especially in younger patients. Prognosis is worse in infants and the elderly and in those with hepatic or renal dysfunction, CNS involvement, testicular involvement, myelodysplasia, or a high WBC count (> 25,000/μL). Survival in untreated acute leukemia generally is 3 to 6 mo. Prognosis varies according to multiple variables including patient age, karyotype, response to therapy, and performance status.

Treatment

- Chemotherapy
- Supportive care

Table 148–2. FINDINGS AT DIAGNOSIS IN THE MOST COMMON LEUKEMIAS

FEATURE	ACUTE LYMPHOCYTIC	ACUTE MYELOGENOUS	CHRONIC LYMPHOCYTIC	CHRONIC MYELOGENOUS
Peak age of incidence	Childhood	Any age	Middle and old age	Young adulthood
WBC count	High in 50% Normal or low in 50%	High in 60% Normal or low in 40%	High in 98% Normal or low in 2%	High in 100%
Differential WBC count	Many lymphoblasts	Many myeloblasts	Small lymphocytes	Entire myeloid series
Anemia	Severe in > 90%	Severe in > 90%	Mild in about 50%	Mild in 80%
Platelets	Low in > 80%	Low in > 90%	Low in 20 to 30%	High in 60% Low in 10%
Lymphadenopathy	Common	Occasional	Common	Infrequent
Splenomegaly	In 60%	In 50%	Usual and moderate	Usual and severe
Other features	Without prophylaxis, CNS commonly involved	CNS rarely involved Sometimes Auer rods in myeloblasts	Occasionally hemolytic anemia and hypogammaglobulinemia	Low leukocyte alkaline phosphatase level Philadelphia chromosome–positive in > 90%

The goal of treatment is complete remission, including resolution of abnormal clinical features, restoration of normal blood counts and normal hematopoiesis with < 5% blast cells in the bone marrow, and elimination of the leukemic clone. Although basic principles in treating ALL and AML are similar, the drug regimens differ. The complex nature of patients' clinical situations and the available treatment protocols necessitate an experienced team. Whenever possible, patients should be treated at specialized medical centers, particularly during critical phases (eg, remission induction).

Supportive care: Supportive care is similar in the acute leukemias and may include

- Transfusions
- Antibiotics or antifungal drugs
- Hydration and urine alkalinization
- Psychologic support

Transfusions of platelets, RBCs, and granulocytes are administered as needed to patients with bleeding, anemia, and neutropenia, respectively. Prophylactic platelet transfusion is done when platelets fall to < 10,000/μL; a higher threshold (20,000/μL) is used for patients with the triad of fever, disseminated intravascular coagulation (DIC), and mucositis secondary to chemotherapy. Anemia (Hb < 8 g/dL) is treated with transfusions of packed RBCs. Granulocyte transfusions may help neutropenic patients with gram-negative or other serious infections but have no proven benefit as prophylaxis.

Antimicrobials are often needed because patients are neutropenic and immunosuppressed; in such patients, infections can progress quickly with little clinical prodrome. After appropriate studies and cultures have been done, febrile patients with neutrophil counts < 500/μL should begin treatment with a broad-spectrum bactericidal antibiotic that is effective against gram-positive and gram-negative organisms (eg, ceftazidime, imipenem, cilastatin). Fungal infections, especially pneumonias, are becoming more common; these are difficult to diagnose, so chest CT should be done early (ie, < 72 h, depending on degree of suspicion) to detect fungal pneumonia. Empiric antifungal therapy should be given if antibacterial therapy is not effective within 72 h. In patients with refractory pneumonitis, *Pneumocystis jirovecii* infection or a viral infection should be suspected and confirmed by bronchoscopy and bronchoalveolar lavage and treated appropriately. Empiric therapy with trimethoprim/sulfamethoxazole (TMP/SMX), amphotericin B, and acyclovir or other analogs, often with granulocyte transfusions, is often necessary. In patients with drug-induced immunosuppression at risk of opportunistic infections, TMP/SMX is given to prevent *P. jirovecii* pneumonia.

Hydration (twice the daily maintenance volume), urine alkalinization (pH 7 to 8), and electrolyte monitoring can prevent the hyperuricemia, hyperphosphatemia, hypocalcemia, and hyperkalemia (ie, tumor lysis syndrome) caused by the rapid lysis of leukemic cells during initial therapy (particularly in ALL). Hyperuricemia can be minimized by reducing the conversion of xanthine to uric acid by giving allopurinol (a xanthine oxidase inhibitor) or rasburicase (a recombinant urate-oxidase enzyme) before starting chemotherapy.

Psychologic support may help patients and their families weather the shock of illness and the rigors of treatment for a potentially life-threatening condition.

ACUTE LYMPHOCYTIC LEUKEMIA

(Acute Lymphoblastic Leukemia)

Acute lymphocytic leukemia (ALL) is the most common pediatric cancer; it also strikes adults of all ages. Malignant transformation and uncontrolled proliferation of an abnormally differentiated, long-lived hematopoietic progenitor cell results in a high circulating number of blasts, replacement of normal marrow by malignant cells, and the potential for leukemic infiltration of the CNS and abdominal organs. Symptoms include fatigue, pallor, infection, bone pain, and easy bruising and bleeding. Examination of peripheral blood smear and bone marrow is usually diagnostic. Treatment typically includes combination chemotherapy to achieve remission, intrathecal chemotherapy for CNS prophylaxis and/or cerebral irradiation for intracerebral leukemic infiltration, consolidation chemotherapy with or without stem cell transplantation, and maintenance chemotherapy for up to 3 yr to avoid relapse.

Two-thirds of all ALL cases occur in children, with a peak incidence at age 2 to 5 yr; ALL is the most common cancer in children and the 2nd most common cause of death in children < 15 yr. A second rise in incidence occurs after age 45.

Prognosis

Prognostic factors help determine treatment protocol and intensity.

Favorable prognostic factors are

- Age 3 to 9 yr
- WBC count < 25,000/μL (< 50,000/μL in children)
- French-American-British (FAB) L1 morphology
- Leukemic cell karyotype with > 50 chromosomes and t(12;21)
- No CNS disease at diagnosis

Unfavorable factors include

- A leukemic cell karyotype with chromosomes that are normal in number but abnormal in morphology (pseudodiploid)
- Presence of the Philadelphia (Ph) chromosome t(9;22)
- Increased age in adults
- B-cell immunophenotype with surface or cytoplasmic immunoglobulin
- Early precursor T-cell phenotype; BCR-ABL–like molecular signature
- Low chromosome number in the leukemia cells
- BCR/ABL-like molecular signature

Regardless of prognostic factors, the likelihood of initial remission is ≥ 95% in children and 70 to 90% in adults. Of children, 75% or more have continuous disease-free survival for 5 yr and appear cured. Of adults, 30 to 40% have continuous disease-free survival for 5 yr. Imatinib improves outcome in adults and children with Ph chromosome–positive ALL. Most investigatory protocols select patients with poor prognostic factors for more intense therapy, because the increased risk of and toxicity from treatment are outweighed by the greater risk of treatment failure leading to death.

Treatment

- Chemotherapy
- Sometimes stem cell transplantation or radiation therapy
- Antibody therapy

The **4 general phases of chemotherapy** for ALL include

- Remission induction
- CNS prophylaxis
- Postremission consolidation or intensification
- Maintenance

Induction therapy: The goal is to induce remission. Several regimens emphasize early introduction of an intensive multidrug regimen. Remission can be induced with daily oral prednisone and weekly IV vincristine with the addition of an anthracycline or asparaginase. Other drugs and combinations that may be introduced early in treatment are cytarabine and etoposide as well as cyclophosphamide. In some regimens, intermediate-dose or high-dose IV methotrexate is given with leucovorin rescue. The combinations and their dosages are modified according to the presence of risk factors. Imatinib can be added to the drug regimen in patients with Ph chromosome–positive ALL.

CNS prophylaxis: An important site of leukemic infiltration is the meninges; prophylaxis and treatment may include intrathecal methotrexate, cytarabine, and corticosteroids in combination or methotrexate and cytarabine singly. Cranial nerve or whole-brain irradiation may be necessary and is often used for patients at high risk of CNS disease (eg, high WBC count, high serum LDH, B-cell phenotype), but its use has been decreasing in recent years.

Consolidation therapy: The goal of consolidation is to prevent leukemic regrowth. Consolidation therapy usually lasts a few months and combines drugs that have different mechanisms of action than drugs used in induction regimens. Allogeneic stem cell transplantation is recommended as consolidation therapy for Ph chromosome–positive ALL in adults or for second or later relapses or remissions.

Maintenance therapy: Most regimens include maintenance therapy with methotrexate and mercaptopurine. Therapy duration is usually 2½ to 3 yr but may be shorter when regimens that are more intensive in earlier phases are used. Clinical testing of monoclonal antibodies directed against proteins on the leukemic cell surface are underway, with some new agents showing promise.

Therapy is usually short and intensive for Burkitt leukemia or ALL with mature B cells (FAB L3 morphology). For patients in continuous complete remission for 1 yr after therapy stops, the risk of relapse is small.

Relapse: Leukemic cells may reappear in the bone marrow, the CNS, the testes, or other sites. Bone marrow relapse is particularly ominous. Although a new round of chemotherapy may induce a second remission in 80 to 90% of children (30 to 40% of adults), subsequent remissions tend to be brief. Chemotherapy causes only a few patients with early bone marrow relapse to achieve long disease-free second remissions or cure.

New immunotherapy approaches show impressive early results in relapsed/refractory ALL. Antibodies, such as blinatumomab, that bring T cells in close proximity to leukemic blasts demonstrate activity in relapsed ALL. Chimeric antigen receptor T cells, generated from pheresed T-cells from the patient, induce remission in relapsed patients with remarkable efficacy, albeit with significant toxicity.[1]

If an HLA-matched sibling is available, stem cell transplantation offers the greatest hope of long-term remission or cure. Cells from other relatives or from matched, unrelated donors are sometimes used. Transplantation is rarely used for patients > 65 yr because it is much less likely to be successful and because adverse effects are much more likely to be fatal.

When **relapse involves the CNS,** treatment includes intrathecal methotrexate (with or without cytarabine or corticosteroids) twice weekly until all signs disappear. Most regimens include systemic reinduction chemotherapy because of the likelihood of systemic spread of blast cells. The role of continued intrathecal drug use or CNS irradiation is unclear.

Testicular relapse may be evidenced clinically by painless firm swelling of a testis or may be identified on biopsy. If unilateral testicular involvement is clinically evident, the apparently uninvolved testis should undergo biopsy. Treatment is radiation therapy of the involved testis and administration of systemic reinduction therapy as for isolated CNS relapse.

1. Lee DW, Kochenderfer JN, Stetler-Stevenson M, et al: T cells expressing CD19 chimeric antigen receptors for acute lymphoblastic leukaemia in children and young adults: a phase 1 dose-escalation trial. *Lancet* 385(9967):517–528, 2015.

KEY POINTS

- ALL is the most common cancer in children but also occurs in adults.
- CNS involvement is common; most patients receive intrathecal chemotherapy and corticosteroids and sometimes CNS radiation therapy.

- Response to treatment is good, with cure possible in about 75% of children and 30 to 40% of adults.
- Stem cell transplantation and new immunotherapies may be helpful for relapse.

ACUTE MYELOGENOUS LEUKEMIA

(Acute Myelocytic Leukemia; Acute Myeloid Leukemia)

In acute myelogenous leukemia (AML), malignant transformation and uncontrolled proliferation of an abnormally differentiated, long-lived myeloid progenitor cell results in high circulating numbers of immature blood forms and replacement of normal marrow by malignant cells. Symptoms include fatigue, pallor, easy bruising and bleeding, fever, and infection; symptoms of extramedullary leukemic infiltration are present in only about 5% of patients (often as skin manifestations). Examination of peripheral blood smear and bone marrow is diagnostic. Treatment includes induction chemotherapy to achieve remission and postremission chemotherapy (with or without stem cell transplantation) to avoid relapse.

The incidence of acute myelogenous leukemia increases with age; it is the more common acute leukemia in adults, with a median age of onset of 50 yr. AML may occur as a secondary cancer after chemotherapy or radiation therapy for a different type of cancer. Secondary AML is difficult to treat with chemotherapy alone.

AML has a number of subtypes that are distinguished from each other by morphology, immunophenotype, and cytochemistry. Five classes are described, based on predominant cell type, including

- Myeloid
- Myeloid-monocytic
- Monocytic
- Erythroid
- Megakaryocytic

Acute promyelocytic leukemia (APL) is a particularly important subtype, representing 10 to 15% of all cases of AML, striking a younger age group (median age 31 yr) and particular ethnicity (Hispanics), in which the patient commonly presents with a coagulation disorder.

Prognosis

Remission induction rates range from 50 to 85%. Long-term disease-free survival occurs in 20 to 40% of patients and increases to 40 to 50% in younger patients treated with intensive chemotherapy or stem cell transplantation.

Prognostic factors help determine treatment protocol and intensity; patients with strongly negative prognostic features are usually given more intense forms of therapy because the potential benefits are thought to justify the increased treatment toxicity.

The **leukemia cell karyotype** is an important prognostic factor. The specific chromosomal rearrangements of the different forms of AML affect the outcome. Three clinical groups have been identified: favorable, intermediate, and poor. Patients who have the cytogenetic findings of t(8;21), t(15;17), and inv(16) typically have a favorable response to therapy, durable remission, and improved survival. Patients with a normal karyotype have an intermediate prognosis, and patients with a poor prognosis are those with a deletion of chromosome 5 or 7, trisomy 8, or a karyotype with > 3 abnormalities.

Molecular genetic abnormalities are becoming more important in refining prognosis and therapy in AML. The large fraction of patients with cytogenetically normal blasts can now be further characterized. Patients with mutations in nucleophosmin (NPM1) or in CEBPA have a more favorable prognosis. Mutations in Flt3 kinase, on the other hand, have a poorer prognosis (including patients also having an otherwise favorable NPM1 mutation). Other negative factors include increasing age, a preceding myelodysplastic phase, secondary leukemia, high WBC count, and absence of Auer rods. Except in APL, the FAB or WHO classification alone does not predict response.

Treatment

- Chemotherapy (induction and consolidation)
- Sometimes stem cell transplantation

Induction therapy: Initial therapy attempts to induce remission and differs most from ALL in that AML responds to fewer drugs. The basic induction regimen includes cytarabine by continuous IV infusion or high doses for 5 to 7 days; daunorubicin or idarubicin is given IV for 3 days during this time. Some regimens include 6-thioguanine, etoposide, vincristine, and prednisone, but their contribution is unclear. Treatment usually results in significant myelosuppression, with infection or bleeding. There is significant latency before marrow recovery. During this time, meticulous preventive and supportive care is vital.

In APL and some other cases of AML, DIC may be present when leukemia is diagnosed and may worsen as leukemic cell lysis releases procoagulant. In APL with the translocation t(15;17), all-*trans* retinoic acid (tretinoin) corrects the DIC in 2 to 5 days; combined with daunorubicin or idarubicin, this regimen can induce remission in 80 to 90% of patients and bring about long-term survival in 65 to 70%. Arsenic trioxide is also very active in APL. Tretinoin and arsenic trioxide without conventional cytotoxic chemotherapy have been successful in APL, and this approach is undergoing further study in clinical trials. Molecular testing for mutations that might be targeted (eg, IDH, Flt3) is becoming standard at diagnosis.

Consolidation therapy: After remission, many regimens involve a phase of intensification with the same drugs used for induction or with other drugs. High-dose cytarabine regimens may lengthen remission duration, particularly when given for consolidation in patients < 60 yr. CNS prophylaxis usually is not given to adult patients because with better systemic disease control, CNS leukemia is a less frequent complication. In AML patients who have completed consolidation, maintenance therapy has no demonstrated role.

Relapse: Patients who have not responded to treatment and younger patients who are in remission but who are at high risk of relapse (generally identified by high-risk molecular or chromosomal abnormalities) may be given high-dose chemotherapy and stem cell transplantation. Extramedullary sites are infrequently involved in isolated relapse. When relapse occurs, additional chemotherapy for patients unable to undergo stem cell transplantation is less effective and often poorly tolerated. Another course of chemotherapy is most effective in younger patients and in patients whose initial remission lasted > 1 yr.

KEY POINTS

- AML is the most common acute leukemia in adults.
- There are a number of subtypes, typically involving very immature myeloid cells.
- Chromosomal and molecular genetic abnormalities are common and have implications for prognosis and treatment.
- Chemotherapy often prolongs survival.
- Stem cell transplantation may help patients who do not respond to treatment and younger patients.

CHRONIC LYMPHOCYTIC LEUKEMIA

(Chronic Lymphatic Leukemia)

The most common type of leukemia in the Western world, chronic lymphocytic leukemia (CLL) involves mature-appearing defective neoplastic lymphocytes (almost always B cells) with an abnormally long life span. The peripheral blood, bone marrow, spleen, and lymph nodes are infiltrated. Symptoms may be absent or may include lymphadenopathy, splenomegaly, hepatomegaly, and nonspecific symptoms attributable to anemia (fatigue, malaise) and immunosuppression (eg, fever). Diagnosis is by examination of peripheral blood smear and bone marrow aspirate. Treatment, delayed until symptoms develop, is aimed at lengthening life and decreasing symptoms and may involve chlorambucil or fludarabine, prednisone, and cyclophosphamide or doxorubicin or both. Monoclonal antibodies, such as alemtuzumab, rituximab, and obinutuzumab, are increasingly being used. Palliative radiation therapy is reserved for patients whose lymphadenopathy or splenomegaly interferes with other organs.

The incidence of CLL increases with age; 75% of cases are diagnosed in patients > 60 yr. CLL is twice as common in men. Although the cause is unknown, some cases appear to have a hereditary component. CLL is rare in Japan and China, and the incidence does not seem to be increased among Japanese expatriates in the US, suggesting the importance of genetic factors. CLL is more common among Jews of Eastern European descent.

Pathophysiology

In about 98% of cases, CD5+ B cells undergo malignant transformation, with lymphocytes initially accumulating in the bone marrow and then spreading to lymph nodes and other lymphoid tissues, eventually inducing splenomegaly and hepatomegaly. As CLL progresses, abnormal hematopoiesis results in anemia, neutropenia, thrombocytopenia, and decreased immunoglobulin production. Many patients develop hypogammaglobulinemia and impaired antibody response, perhaps related to increased T-suppressor cell activity. Patients have increased susceptibility to autoimmune disease characterized by immunohemolytic anemias (usually Coombs test–positive) or thrombocytopenia and a modest increase in risk of developing other cancers.

In 2 to 3% of cases, the clonal expansion is T cell in type, and even this group has a subtype (eg, large granular lymphocytes with cytopenias).

In addition, other chronic leukemic patterns have been categorized under CLL:

- Prolymphocytic leukemia
- Leukemic phase of cutaneous T-cell lymphoma (ie, Sézary syndrome)
- Hairy cell leukemia
- Lymphoma progressing to leukemia (ie, leukemic changes that occur in advanced stages of malignant lymphoma)

Differentiation of these subtypes from typical CLL is usually made by using light microscopy and phenotyping.

Diagnosis

- CBC and peripheral smear
- Bone marrow examination
- Immunophenotyping

CLL is confirmed by examining the peripheral smear and bone marrow; the hallmark is sustained, absolute peripheral lymphocytosis (> 5000/μL) and increased lymphocytes (> 30%) in the bone marrow. Differential diagnosis is simplified by immunophenotyping. Other findings at diagnosis may include hypogammaglobulinemia (< 15% of cases) and, rarely, elevated lactate dehydrogenase. About 10% of patients present with moderate anemia (sometimes immunohemolytic), thrombocytopenia, or both. A monoclonal serum immunoglobulin spike of the same type may be found on the leukemic cell surface in 2 to 4% of cases.

Clinical staging is useful for prognosis and treatment. Two common approaches are Rai and Binet staging, primarily based on hematologic changes and extent of disease (see Table 148–3).

Prognosis

The median survival of patients with B-cell CLL or its complications is about 7 to 10 yr. Patients in Rai stage 0 to II at diagnosis may survive for 5 to 20 yr without treatment. Patients in Rai stage III or IV are more likely to die within 3 to 4 yr of diagnosis. Progression to bone marrow failure is usually associated with short survival. Patients with CLL are more likely to develop a secondary cancer, especially skin cancer.

Treatment

- Symptom amelioration
- Supportive care
- Specific therapy

Although CLL is progressive, some patients may be asymptomatic for years; therapy is not indicated until progression

Table 148–3. CLINICAL STAGING OF CHRONIC LYMPHOCYTIC LEUKEMIA*

CLASSIFICATION AND STAGE	DESCRIPTION
Rai	
Stage 0	Absolute lymphocytosis of > 10,000/μL in blood and ≥ 30% lymphocytes in bone marrow
Stage I	Stage 0 plus enlarged lymph nodes
Stage II	Stage 0 plus hepatomegaly or splenomegaly
Stage III	Stage 0 plus anemia with Hb < 11 g/dL
Stage IV	Stage 0 plus thrombocytopenia with platelet counts < 100,000/μL
Binet	
Stage A	Absolute lymphocytosis of > 10,000/μL in blood and ≥ 30% lymphocytes in bone marrow Hb ≥ 10 g/dL Platelets ≥100,000/μL ≤ 2 involved sites*
Stage B	As for stage A, but 3–5 involved sites
Stage C	As for stage A or B, but Hb < 10 g/dL or platelets < 100,000/μL

*Sites considered: Cervical, axillary, and inguinal lymph nodes; liver; and spleen.

or symptoms occur. Cure usually is not possible, so treatment attempts to ameliorate symptoms and prolong life.

Supportive care includes

- Transfusion of packed RBCs or erythropoietin injections for anemia
- Platelet transfusions for bleeding associated with thrombocytopenia
- Antimicrobials for bacterial, fungal, or viral infections

Because neutropenia and agammaglobulinemia limit bacterial killing, antibiotic therapy should be bactericidal. Therapeutic infusions of gamma-globulin should be considered in patients with hypogammaglobulinemia and repeated or refractory infections or for prophylaxis when ≥ 2 severe infections occur within 6 mo.

Specific therapy includes

- Chemotherapy
- Corticosteroids
- Monoclonal antibody therapy
- Radiation therapy

These modalities may alleviate symptoms and prolong survival. *Overtreatment is more dangerous than undertreatment.*

Chemotherapy: Chemotherapy may be instituted when symptoms begin. Symptoms that prompt treatment include

- Constitutional symptoms (fever, night sweats, extreme fatigue, weight loss)
- Significant hepatomegaly, splenomegaly, or lymphadenopathy
- Lymphocytosis > 100,000/μL
- Infections accompanied by anemia, neutropenia, or thrombocytopenia

Alkylating drugs, especially chlorambucil, alone or with corticosteroids, have long been the usual therapy for B-cell CLL. However, fludarabine is more effective. Combination chemotherapy with fludarabine, cyclophosphamide, and rituximab more often induces complete remissions. It also lengthens remission duration and prolongs survival. Interferon alfa, deoxycoformycin, and 2-chlorodeoxyadenosine are highly effective for hairy cell leukemia. Patients with polymphocytic leukemia and lymphoma leukemia usually require multidrug chemotherapy and often respond only partially.

Ibrutinib is a novel, oral inhibitor of Bruton tyrosine kinase. Bruton tyrosine kinase is an enzyme essential for activation of several downstream B-cell mediated pathways that enhance survival of CLL cells. Ibrutinib appears to be highly active in CLL and has induced durable remissions in some patients with relapsed or refractory CLL. Its role as a single agent or as part of combination chemotherapy is evolving.

Corticosteroids: Immunohemolytic anemia and thrombocytopenia are indications for corticosteroids. Prednisone 1 mg/kg po once/day may occasionally result in striking, rapid improvement in patients with advanced CLL, although response is often brief. The metabolic complications and increasing rate and severity of infections warrant caution in its prolonged use. Prednisone used with fludarabine increases the risk of *Pneumocystis jirovecii* and *Listeria* infections.

Monoclonal antibody therapy: Rituximab is the first monoclonal antibody used in the successful treatment of lymphoid cancers. In previously untreated patients, the response rate is 75%, with 20% of patients achieving complete remission. Alemtuzumab has a 33% response rate in previously treated patients refractory to fludarabine and a 75 to 80% response rate in previously untreated patients. More problems with immunosuppression occur with alemtuzumab than with rituximab. Rituximab has been combined with fludarabine and with fludarabine and cyclophosphamide; these combinations have markedly improved the complete remission rate in both previously treated and untreated patients. Alemtuzumab is now being combined with rituximab and with chemotherapy to treat minimal residual disease and has effectively cleared bone marrow infiltration. Reactivation of cytomegalovirus and other opportunistic infections has occurred with alemtuzumab. Reactivation of hepatitis B infection may occur with rituximab.

Obinutuzumab is a newer monoclonal antibody that targets the same CLL cell surface protein as rituximab. The combination of obinutuzumab and chlorambucil was recently found to be superior to rituximab in prolonging progression-free survival and achieving a complete response to treatment.

Obinutuzumab plus chlorambucil has now been approved as frontline therapy for elderly patients or frail patients with comorbidities.[1] In the specific instance of CLL with a deletion of 17p, the Bruton tyrosine kinase inhibitor (TKI) ibrutinib has shown excellent activity. Single-agent ibrutinib is an approved frontline treatment for such patients. This is distinct from the group of CLL patients with deletion 11q abnormalities, who seem to benefit most from initial alkylator therapy. In patients with relapsed or refractory disease, new options include idelalisib (a phosphoinositide 3-kinase inhibitor) plus rituximab and monotherapy with ibrutinib.

In general, monoclonal antibodies are well tolerated, although they may cause allergic reactions and significant immunosuppression. This favorable toxicity profile allows these agents to be combined with conventional chemotherapy, often with excellent clinical efficacy.

Radiation therapy: Local irradiation for palliation may be given to areas of lymphadenopathy or for liver and spleen involvement that does not respond to chemotherapy. Total body irradiation in small doses is occasionally successful in temporarily ameliorating symptoms.

1. Goede V, Fischer K, Busch R, et al: Obinutuzumab plus chlorambucil in patients with CLL and coexisting conditions. *New Engl J Med* 370:1101–1111, 2014.

KEY POINTS

- CLL, a slowly progressing leukemia, involves mature appearing lymphocytes and is most common in older patients.
- Treatment is generally not curative and is usually not begun until symptoms develop.
- Chemotherapy with or without monoclonal antibody therapy decreases symptoms and improves survival.

CHRONIC MYELOGENOUS LEUKEMIA

(Chronic Granulocytic Leukemia; Chronic Myelocytic Leukemia; Chronic Myeloid Leukemia)

Chronic myelogenous leukemia (CML) occurs when a pluripotent stem cell undergoes malignant transformation and clonal myeloproliferation, leading to a striking overproduction of immature granulocytes. Initially asymptomatic, CML progression is insidious, with a nonspecific "benign" stage (malaise, anorexia, weight loss) eventually giving way to accelerated or blast phases with more ominous signs, such as splenomegaly, pallor, easy bruising and bleeding, fever, lymphadenopathy, and skin changes. Peripheral blood smear, bone marrow aspirate, and demonstration of Philadelphia chromosome are diagnostic. Treatment is with

imatinib, which significantly improves response and prolongs survival. The curative potential of imatinib is undefined. Myelosuppressive drugs (eg, hydroxyurea), stem cell transplantation, and interferon alfa are also used.

CML accounts for about 15% of all adult leukemias. CML can strike at any age, although it is uncommon before age 10, and the median age at diagnosis is 45 to 55. CML may occur in either sex.

Pathophysiology

Classical CML is induced by a translocation known as the Philadelphia (Ph) chromosome. It is a reciprocal translocation t(9;22) in which a piece of chromosome 9 containing the oncogene *c-abl* is translocated to chromosome 22 and fused to the gene *BCR*. The fusion gene *BCR-ABL* is essential in the pathogenesis and expression of CML and results in the production of a specific constitutively tyrosine kinase. CML ensues when an abnormal pluripotent hematopoietic progenitor cell initiates excessive production of granulocytes, primarily in the bone marrow but also in extramedullary sites (eg, spleen, liver). Although granulocyte production predominates, the neoplastic clone includes RBCs, megakaryocytes, monocytes, and even some T and B cells. Normal stem cells are retained and can emerge after drug suppression of the CML clone.

CML has 3 phases:

- **Chronic phase:** An initial indolent period that may last months to years
- **Accelerated phase:** Treatment failure, worsening anemia, progressive thrombocytopenia or thrombocytosis, persistent or worsening splenomegaly, clonal evolution, increasing blood basophils, and increasing marrow or blood blasts
- **Blast phase:** Accumulation of blasts in extramedullary sites (eg, bone, CNS, lymph nodes, skin), blasts in blood or marrow increased to > 20%

The blast phase leads to fulminant complications resembling those of acute leukemia, including sepsis and bleeding. Some patients progress directly from the chronic to the blast phase.

Symptoms and Signs

Patients are often asymptomatic early on, with insidious onset of nonspecific symptoms (eg, fatigue, weakness, anorexia, weight loss, fever, night sweats, a sense of abdominal fullness), which may prompt evaluation. Initially, pallor, bleeding, easy bruising, and lymphadenopathy are unusual, but moderate or occasionally extreme splenomegaly is common (60 to 70% of cases).

With disease progression, splenomegaly may increase, and pallor and bleeding occur. Fever, marked lymphadenopathy, and maculopapular skin involvement are ominous developments.

Diagnosis

- CBC and peripheral smear
- Bone marrow examination
- Cytogenetic studies (Ph chromosome)

CML is most frequently diagnosed by a CBC obtained incidentally or during evaluation of splenomegaly. Granulocyte count is elevated, usually < 50,000/μL in asymptomatic patients and 200,000/μL to 1,000,000/μL in symptomatic patients. The platelet count is normal or moderately increased. The Hb level is usually > 10 g/dL.

Peripheral smear may help differentiate CML from leukocytosis of other etiology. In CML, the peripheral smear frequently shows immature granulocytes as well as absolute eosinophilia and basophilia. However, in patients with WBC counts ≤ 50,000/μL and even some with higher WBC counts, immature granulocytes may not be seen, making the absence of immature granulocytes nondiagnostic. Leukocytosis in patients with myelofibrosis is usually associated with nucleated RBCs, teardrop-shaped RBCs, anemia, and thrombocytopenia. Leukemoid reaction, defined as a neutrophil count > 50,000/mL not caused by malignant transformation of a hematopoietic stem cell, can result from a variety of causes (eg, cancer, infection, inflammation, other stimuli such as hemorrhage, drugs or electrical shock). Usually the cause is apparent, but apparent benign neutrophilia can be mimicked by chronic neutrophilic leukemia or CML.

The leukocyte alkaline phosphatase score is usually low in CML and increased in leukemoid reactions. Bone marrow examination should be done to evaluate the karyotype as well as cellularity and extent of myelofibrosis.

Diagnosis is confirmed by finding the Ph chromosome in samples examined with cytogenetic or molecular studies. The classic Ph cytogenetic abnormality is absent in 5% of patients, but the use of fluorescence in situ hybridization (FISH) or reverse transcription polymerase chain reaction (RT-PCR) can confirm the diagnosis.

During the accelerated phase of disease, anemia and thrombocytopenia usually develop. Basophils may increase, and granulocyte maturation may be defective. The proportion of immature cells and the leukocyte alkaline phosphatase score may increase. In the bone marrow, myelofibrosis may develop and sideroblasts may be seen on microscopy. Evolution of the neoplastic clone may be associated with development of new abnormal karyotypes, often an extra chromosome 8 or isochromosome 17.

Further evolution may lead to a blast phase with myeloblasts (60% of patients), lymphoblasts (30%), and megakaryoblasts (10%). In 80% of these patients, additional chromosomal abnormalities occur.

Prognosis

With imatinib, survival is > 90% at 5 yr after diagnosis for chronic phase CML. Before imatinib was used, with treatment, 5 to 10% of patients died within 2 yr of diagnosis; 10 to 15% died each year thereafter. Median survival was 4 to 7 yr. Most (90%) deaths followed a blast phase or an accelerated phase of the disease. Median survival after blast crisis was about 3 to 6 mo or longer if remission was achieved.

Ph chromosome–negative CML, chronic neutrophilic leukemia, and chronic myelomonocytic leukemia have a worse prognosis than Ph chromosome–positive CML and are considered myelodysplastic syndromes.

Treatment

- A tyrosine kinase inhibitor (TKI), sometimes with chemotherapy
- Sometimes stem cell transplantation

Except when stem cell transplantation is successful, treatment is not known to be curative. However, when TKIs are used, survival is prolonged and maximum overall survival has not been reached. Some patients may be able to discontinue tyrosine kinase inhibitors and remain in remission. The durability of these remissions is as yet not known.

Imatinib and several newer drugs (dasatinib, nilotinib) inhibit the specific tyrosine kinase that results from the *BCR-ABL* gene product. TKIs are dramatically effective in achieving complete clinical and cytogenetic remissions of Ph chromosome–positive CML and are clearly superior to other regimens (eg, interferon with or without cytarabine). Imatinib also is superior to other treatments in the accelerated and blast phases. In the blast phase, combinations of chemotherapy with imatinib have a higher response rate than does therapy with either approach alone. Treatment tolerance is excellent. The high level of durable complete remissions associated with TKI therapy has led to the prospect of cure of the disease. However, the gene products of some *BCR-ABL* mutations, particularly the T315I mutation, are resistant to current TKIs and remain very difficult to control. Ponatinib has activity in patients with the T315I mutation.

Older chemotherapy regimens are reserved for *BCR-ABL*–negative patients, patients who relapse after receiving a TKI, and patients in the blast phase. The main agents are busulfan, hydroxyurea, and interferon.

Hydroxyurea is easiest to manage and has the fewest adverse effects. The starting dosage is generally 500 to 1000 mg po bid. Blood counts should be done every 1 to 2 wk and the dosage adjusted accordingly. Busulfan often causes unexpected general myelosuppression, and recombinant interferon causes a flu-like syndrome that frequently is unacceptable to patients; the pegylated form of interferon is better tolerated and more acceptable to patients.

The main benefit of hydroxyurea, busulfan, and interferon is reduction in distressing splenomegaly and adenopathy and control of the tumor burden to reduce the incidence of tumor lysis and gout. None of these therapies prolongs median survival > 1 yr compared with untreated patients; thus, reduction in symptoms is the major goal, and therapy is not continued when patients have significant toxic symptoms.

Allogeneic stem cell transplantation can be useful for patients refractory to therapy.

Although splenic radiation is rarely used, it may be helpful in refractory cases of CML or in patients with terminal disease and marked splenomegaly. Total dosage usually ranges from 6 to 10 Gy delivered in fractions of 0.25 to 2 Gy/day. Treatment should begin with very low doses and with careful evaluation of the WBC count. Response is usually disappointing.

Splenectomy may alleviate abdominal discomfort, lessen thrombocytopenia, and relieve transfusion requirements when splenomegaly cannot be controlled with chemotherapy or irradiation. Splenectomy does not play a significant role during the chronic phase of CML.

KEY POINTS

- CML involves a chromosomal translocation that creates the Philadelphia chromosome.
- Peripheral smear (typically showing immature granulocytes, basophilia, and eosinophilia) helps distinguish CML from leukocytosis of other etiologies (eg, leukocytosis due to cancer, infection, myelofibrosis).
- TKIs, such as imatinib, dasatinib or nilotinib, markedly prolong remission of CML and may even be curative.
- Chemotherapy may help in the blast phase.
- Stem cell transplantation may help patients who do not respond to drug therapy or who progress to accelerated or blast phase.

MYELODYSPLASTIC SYNDROME

The myelodysplastic syndrome (MDS) is group of disorders typified by peripheral cytopenia, dysplastic hematopoietic progenitors, a hypercellular bone marrow, and a high risk of conversion to acute myelogenous leukemia (AML). Symptoms are referable to the specific cell line most affected and may include fatigue, weakness, pallor (secondary to anemia), increased infections and fever (secondary to neutropenia), and increased bleeding and bruising (secondary to thrombocytopenia). Diagnosis is by blood count, peripheral smear, and bone marrow aspiration. Treatment with azacitidine may help; if AML supervenes, it is treated per the usual protocols.

Pathophysiology

MDS is a group of clonal hematopoietic stem cell disorders unified by the presence of distinct mutations of hematopoietic stem cells, most frequently in genes involved in RNA splicing. MDSs are characterized by ineffective and dysplastic hematopoiesis and include the following:

- Refractory anemia
- Sideroblastic anemia
- Philadelphia chromosome–negative CML
- Chronic myelomonocytic leukemia
- Chronic neutrophilic leukemia

Etiology is often unknown. Risk increases with age due to the acquisition of somatic mutations that can promote clonal expansion and dominance of a particular hematopoietic stem cell, and possibly due to exposure to environmental toxins such as benzene, radiation, and chemotherapeutic agents (particularly long or intense regimens and those involving alkylating agents and/or epipodophyllotoxins). Chromosomal abnormalities (eg, deletions, duplications, structural abnormalities) are often present.

The bone marrow can be hypocellular or hypercellular. The ineffective hematopoiesis causes anemia (most common), neutropenia, thrombocytopenia, or a combination of these, even to the point of marrow aplasia. Patients with significant anemia can develop iron overload from transfusions and/or increased iron absorption from the gut.

The disordered cell production is also associated with morphologic cellular abnormalities in bone marrow and blood. Extramedullary hematopoiesis may occur, leading to hepatomegaly and splenomegaly. Myelofibrosis may develop during the course of MDS. Classification is by blood and bone marrow findings (see Table 148–4) and also by karyotype and mutation. The MDS clone is unstable and tends to progress to acute myelogenous leukemia.

Symptoms and Signs

Symptoms tend to reflect the most affected cell line and may include pallor, weakness, and fatigue (anemia); fever and infections (neutropenia); and increased bruising, petechiae, epistaxis, and mucosal bleeding (thrombocytopenia). Splenomegaly and hepatomegaly are common.

Symptoms may also be referable to other underlying disorders; eg, in elderly patients with preexisting cardiovascular disorders, anemia from MDS may exacerbate anginal pain or heart failure.

Diagnosis

- CBC
- Peripheral smear
- Bone marrow examination

MDS is suspected in patients (especially the elderly) with refractory anemia, leukopenia, or thrombocytopenia. Cytopenias secondary to autoimmune disorders, vitamin deficiencies, idiopathic aplastic anemia, paroxysmal noctural hemoglobinuria, or drug effects must be ruled out. The diagnosis is suggested by

Table 148–4. MYELODYSPLASTIC SYNDROME BONE MARROW FINDINGS AND SURVIVAL

CLASSIFICATION	CRITERIA	MEDIAN SURVIVAL (YR)
Refractory anemia	Anemia with reticulocytopenia Normal or hypercellular marrow with erythroid hyperplasia and dyserythropoiesis Blasts ≤ 5% of nucleated marrow cells (NMC)	≥ 5
Refractory anemia with sideroblasts	Same as refractory anemia, but with ringed sideroblasts > 15% of NMC	≥ 5
Refractory anemia with excess blasts	Some cytopenia of ≥ 2 cell lines with morphologic abnormalities of blood cells Hypercellular marrow with dyserythropoiesis and dysgranulopoiesis Blasts 5–20% of NMC	1.5
Chronic myelomonocytic leukemia	Same as refractory anemia with excess blasts and absolute monocytosis in blood Significant increase in marrow monocyte precursors	1.5
Refractory anemia with excess blasts in transformation	Refractory anemia with excess blasts and ≥ 1 of the following: • ≥ 5% blasts in blood • 20–30% blasts in marrow • Auer rods in granulocyte precursors	0.5

NMC = nucleated marrow cells.

the finding of peripheral blood and bone marrow morphologic abnormalities in 10 to 20% of cells of a particular lineage but is established by demonstrating specific cytogenetic abnormalities and somatic mutations.

Anemia is the most common feature, associated usually with macrocytosis and anisocytosis. With automatic cell counters, these changes are indicated by an increased MCV and RBC distribution width.

Some degree of thrombocytopenia is usual; on peripheral smear, platelets vary in size, and some appear hypogranular.

The WBC count may be normal, increased, or decreased. Neutrophil cytoplasmic granularity is abnormal, with anisocytosis and variable numbers of granules. Eosinophils also may have abnormal granularity. Pseudo Pelger-Huët cells (hyposegmented neutrophils) may be seen.

Monocytosis is characteristic of the chronic myelomonocytic leukemia subgroup, and immature myeloid cells may occur in the less well differentiated subgroups. The cytogenetic pattern is usually abnormal, with one or more clonal cytogenetic abnormalities often involving chromosomes 5 or 7. The 5q- syndrome is a unique form of MDS, occurring primarily in women in whom macrocytic anemia and thrombocytosis are typically present; this form is very responsive to lenalidomide.

Prognosis

Prognosis depends greatly on classification and on any associated disorder. Patients with the 5q- syndrome, refractory anemia, or refractory anemia with ringed sideroblasts are less likely to progress to the more aggressive forms and may die of unrelated causes.

Treatment

- Symptom amelioration
- Supportive care
- Possibly stem cell transplantation

Azacitidine relieves symptoms, decreases the rate of transformation to leukemia and the need for transfusions, and improves survival. Other therapy is supportive, including RBC transfusions as indicated, platelet transfusions for bleeding, and antibiotic therapy for bacterial infection. Deoxyazacitidine, a hypomethylating agent, is sometimes effective, even in patients who do not respond to azacitidine.

Drugs that provide hematopoietic support can improve cytopenias in some patients but have not increased survival:

- Anemia: Erythropoietin, either alone or with granulocyte colony stimulating factor (effective only if the serum erythropoietin level is < 5 mU/mL
- Granulocytopenia (severe, symptomatic): Granulocyte colony-stimulating factor
- Thrombocytopenia (severe): A thrombopoietin mimetic

Thrombopoietin may also improve marrow function in general.

Combination therapy with azacitidine or decitabine plus an immune modulator such as lenalidomide is currently under investigation. Lenalidomide alone is particularly useful in patients with the 5q- syndrome and also appears to be effective in 25% of anemic MDS patients who do not have the 5q- syndrome. In patients with hypoplastic MDS, cyclosporine with or without antithymocyte globulin has been successful.

Allogeneic stem cell transplantation is the treatment of choice for young patients, and nonablative allogeneic bone marrow transplantations are now being studied for patients > 50 yr. Response of MDS to chemotherapy, typically regimens similar to those used for AML, is similar to that of AML after age and karyotype are considered.

KEY POINTS

- MDS is a disorder of hematopoietic cell production involving clonal proliferation of an abnormal hematopoietic stem cell.
- Patients usually present with a deficiency of red cells (most common), white cells, and/or platelets.
- Transformation to acute myelogenous leukemia is common.
- Azacitidine may ameliorate symptoms and decrease the rate of transformation to acute leukemia.
- Stem cell transplantation is the treatment of choice in young patients.

149 Leukopenias

Leukopenia is a reduction in the circulating WBC count to < 4000/μL. It is usually characterized by a reduced number of circulating neutrophils, although a reduced number of lymphocytes, monocytes, eosinophils, or basophils may also contribute. Thus, immune function is generally decreased.

Neutropenia is a reduction in blood neutrophil count to < 1500/μL in whites and < 1200/μL in blacks. It is sometimes accompanied by monocytopenia and lymphocytopenia, which cause additional immune deficits.

Lymphocytopenia, in which the total number of lymphocytes is < 1000/μL in adults, is not always recognized as a decrease in the total WBC count because lymphocytes account for only 20 to 40% of the total WBC count. The consequence of the lymphopenia can depend on the lymphocyte subpopulation(s) that are decreased.

Monocytopenia is a reduction in blood monocyte count to < 500/μL. Monocytes migrate into the tissues where they become macrophages, with characteristics depending on their tissue localization.

LYMPHOCYTOPENIA

Lymphocytopenia is a total lymphocyte count of < 1000/μL in adults or < 3000/μL in children < 2 yr. Sequelae include opportunistic infections and an increased risk of malignant and autoimmune disorders. If the CBC reveals lymphocytopenia, testing for immunodeficiency and analysis of lymphocyte subpopulations should follow. Treatment is directed at the underlying disorder.

The normal lymphocyte count in adults is 1000 to 4800/μL; in children < 2 yr, 3000 to 9500/μL. At age 6 yr, the lower limit of normal is 1500/μL.

Both B and T cells are present in the peripheral blood; about 75% of the lymphocytes are T cells and 25% B cells. Because lymphocytes account for only 20 to 40% of the total WBC count, lymphocytopenia may go unnoticed when WBC count is checked without a differential.

Almost 65% of blood T cells are CD4+ (helper) T cells. Most patients with lymphocytopenia have a reduced absolute number of T cells, particularly in the number of CD4+ T cells. The average number of CD4+ T cells in adult blood is 1100/μL (range, 300 to 1300/μL), and the average number of cells of the other major T-cell subgroup, CD8+ (suppressor) T cells, is 600/μL (range, 100 to 900/μL).

Etiology

Lymphocytopenia can be

- Acquired
- Inherited

Acquired lymphocytopenia: Acquired lymphocytopenia can occur with a number of other disorders (see Table 149–1). The most common causes include

- Protein-energy undernutrition
- AIDS and certain other viral infections

Protein-energy undernutrition is the most common cause worldwide.

AIDS is the most common infectious disease causing lymphocytopenia, which arises from destruction of CD4+ T cells infected with HIV. Lymphocytopenia may also reflect impaired lymphocyte production arising from destruction of thymic or lymphoid architecture. In acute viremia due to HIV or other viruses, lymphocytes may undergo accelerated destruction from active infections with the virus, may be trapped in the spleen or lymph nodes, or may migrate to the respiratory tract.

Iatrogenic lymphocytopenia is caused by cytotoxic chemotherapy, radiation therapy, or the administration of antilymphocyte globulin (or other lymphocyte antibodies). Long-term treatment for psoriasis using psoralen and ultraviolet A irradiation may destroy T cells. Glucocorticoids can induce lymphocyte destruction.

Lymphocytopenia may occur with lymphomas, autoimmune diseases such as SLE, rheumatoid arthritis, myasthenia gravis, and protein-losing enteropathy.

Inherited lymphocytopenia: Inherited lymphocytopenia (see Table 149–1) most commonly occurs in

- Severe combined immunodeficiency disorder
- Wiskott-Aldrich syndrome

It may occur with inherited immunodeficiency disorders and disorders that involve impaired lymphocyte production. Other inherited disorders, such as Wiskott-Aldrich syndrome, adenosine deaminase deficiency, and purine nucleoside phosphorylase deficiency, may involve accelerated T-cell destruction. In many disorders, antibody production is also deficient.

Symptoms and Signs

Lymphocytopenia per se generally causes no symptoms. However, findings of an associated disorder may include

- Absent or diminished tonsils or lymph nodes, indicative of cellular immunodeficiency
- Skin abnormalities (eg, alopecia, eczema, pyoderma, telangiectasia)
- Evidence of hematologic disease (eg, pallor, petechiae, jaundice, mouth ulcers)
- Generalized lymphadenopathy and splenomegaly, which may suggest HIV infection or Hodgkin lymphoma

Lymphocytopenic patients experience recurrent infections or develop infections with unusual organisms. Pneumocystis jirovecii, cytomegalovirus, rubeola, and varicella pneumonias often are fatal. Lymphocytopenia is also a risk factor for the development of cancers and for autoimmune disorders.

Diagnosis

- Clinical suspicion (repeated or unusual infections)
- CBC with differential
- Measurement of lymphocyte subpopulations and immunoglobulin levels

Lymphocytopenia is suspected in patients with recurrent viral, fungal, or parasitic infections but is usually detected incidentally on a CBC. *P. jirovecii*, cytomegalovirus, rubeola, or varicella pneumonias with lymphocytopenia suggest immunodeficiency. Lymphocyte subpopulations are measured in patients with lymphocytopenia. Measurement of immunoglobulin levels should also be done to evaluate antibody

Table 149–1. CAUSES OF LYMPHOCYTOPENIA

MECHANISM	EXAMPLES
Acquired	AIDS
	Other infectious disorders, including hepatitis, influenza, TB, typhoid fever, and sepsis
	Dietary deficiency in patients with ethanol abuse, protein-energy undernutrition, or zinc deficiency
	Protein losing enteropathy
	Iatrogenic after use of cytotoxic chemotherapy, glucocorticoids, high-dose psoralen and ultraviolet A radiation therapy, lymphocyte antibody therapy, immunosuppressants, radiation therapy, or thoracic duct drainage
	Systemic disorders with autoimmune features (eg, aplastic anemia, Hodgkin lymphoma, myasthenia gravis, protein-losing enteropathy, RA, chronic kidney disease, sarcoidosis, SLE, thermal injury)
Hereditary	Aplasia of lymphopoietic stem cells
	Ataxia-telangiectasia
	Cartilage-hair hypoplasia syndrome
	Idiopathic CD4+ T lymphocytopenia
	Immunodeficiency with thymoma
	Severe combined immunodeficiency associated with a defect in the IL-2 receptor gamma-chain, deficiency of ADA or PNP, or an unknown defect
	Wiskott-Aldrich syndrome

ADA = adenosine deaminase; PNP = purine nucleoside phosphorylase.

production. Patients with a history of recurrent infections undergo complete laboratory evaluation for immunodeficiency, even if initial screening tests are normal.

Treatment

- Treatment of associated infections
- Treatment of underlying disorder
- Sometimes IV immune globulin
- Possibly hematopoietic stem cell transplantation

In acquired lymphocytopenias, lymphocytopenia usually remits with removal of the underlying factor or successful treatment of the underlying disorder. IV immune globulin is indicated if patients have chronic IgG deficiency, lymphocytopenia, and recurrent infections. Hematopoietic stem cell transplantation can be considered for all patients with congenital immunodeficiencies and may be curative.

KEY POINTS

- Lymphocytopenia is most often due to AIDS or undernutrition, but it also may be inherited or caused by various infections, drugs, or autoimmune disorders.
- Patients have recurrent viral, fungal, or parasitic infections.
- Lymphocyte subpopulations and immunoglobulin levels should be measured.
- Treatment is usually directed at the cause, but occasionally, IV immune globulin or, in patients with congenital immunodeficiency, stem cell transplantation is helpful.

MONOCYTOPENIA

Monocytopenia is a reduction in blood monocyte count to < 500/μL. Risk of certain infections is increased. It is diagnosed by CBC with differential. Treatment with hematopoietic stem cell transplantation may be needed.

Monocytopenia frequently occurs with chemotherapy-induced myelosuppression. A severe deficiency or absence of monocytes can occur in patients with mutations of the hematopoietic transcription factor gene, *GATA2*. Dendritic cells are decreased, and there may also be lymphocytopenia (mainly natural killer and B cells).

Despite near-absence of circulating monocytes, tissue macrophages are usually preserved. Also, immunoglobulin levels are usually normal even when circulating B cells are depressed.

Bone marrow is hypocellular and can show fibrosis and multilineage dysplasia. Karyotypic abnormalities, including monosomy 7 and trisomy 8, may be present.

Infections with *Mycobacterium avian* complex (MAC) or other nontuberculous mycobacterial infections are common (MonoMAC syndrome). Fungal infections (ie, histoplasmosis, aspergillosis) also are typical. Infections with human papillomavirus (HPV) may occur with subsequent risk of progression to secondary cancers.

There is a high risk of progression to hematologic disorders (myelodysplasia, acute myelogenous leukemia, chronic myelomonocytic leukemia, lymphomas) with a resulting poor prognosis.

Unvaccinated patients should be given HPV vaccination. Any infections are treated with appropriate antimicrobials. Allogeneic hematopoietic stem cell transplantation should be considered for symptomatic patients.

NEUTROPENIA

(Agranulocytosis; Granulocytopenia)

Neutropenia is a reduction in the blood neutrophil count. If it is severe, the risk and severity of bacterial and fungal infections increase. Focal symptoms of infection may be muted, but fever is present during most serious infections. Diagnosis is by WBC count with differential, but evaluation requires identification of the cause. If fever is present, infection is presumed, and immediate, empiric broad-spectrum antibiotics are necessary, especially if the neutropenia is severe. Treatment with granulocyte-macrophage colony-stimulating factor or granulocyte colony-stimulating factor is sometimes helpful.

Neutrophils (granulocytes) are the body's main defense against bacterial infections and fungal infections. When neutropenia is present, the inflammatory response to such infections is ineffective.

Normal lower limit of the neutrophil count (total WBC × % neutrophils and bands) is 1500/μL in whites and is somewhat lower in blacks (about 1200/μL). Neutrophil counts are not as stable as other cell counts and may vary considerably over short periods, depending on many factors such as activity status, anxiety, infections, and drugs. Thus, several measurements may be needed when determining the severity of neutropenia.

Severity of neutropenia relates to the relative risk of infection and is classified as follows:

- Mild (1000 to 1500/μL)
- Moderate (500 to 1000/μL)
- Severe (< 500/μL)

When neutrophil counts fall to < 500/μL, endogenous microbial flora (eg, in the mouth or gut) can cause infections. If the count falls to < 200/μL, inflammatory response may be muted and the usual inflammatory findings of leukocytosis or WBCs in the urine or at the site of infection may not occur. Acute, severe neutropenia, particularly if another factor (eg, cancer) is present, significantly impairs the immune system and can lead to rapidly fatal infections. The integrity of the skin and mucous membranes, the vascular supply to tissue, and the nutritional status of the patient also influence the risk of infections.

The **most frequently occurring infections** in patients with profound neutropenia are

- Cellulitis
- Furunculosis
- Pneumonia
- Septicemia

Vascular catheters and other puncture sites confer extra risk of skin infections; the most common bacterial causes are coagulase-negative staphylococci and *Staphylococcus aureus*, but other gram-positive and gram-negative infections also occur. Stomatitis, gingivitis, perirectal inflammation, colitis, sinusitis, paronychia, and otitis media often occur. Patients with prolonged neutropenia after hematopoietic stem cell transplantation or chemotherapy and patients receiving high doses of corticosteroids are predisposed to fungal infections.

Etiology

Acute neutropenia (occurring over hours to a few days) can develop as a result of rapid neutrophil use or destruction or due to impaired production.

Chronic neutropenia (lasting months to years) usually arises as a result of reduced production or excessive splenic sequestration.

Neutropenia also may be classified as primary due to an intrinsic defect in marrow myeloid cells or as secondary (due to factors extrinsic to marrow myeloid cells—see Table 149–2).

Neutropenia caused by intrinsic defects in myeloid cells or their precursors: Neutropenia caused by intrinsic defects in myeloid cells or their precursors is uncommon, but when present, the **most common causes** include

- Chronic idiopathic neutropenia
- Congenital neutropenia

Chronic benign neutropenia is a type of chronic idiopathic neutropenia in which the rest of the immune system appears to remain intact; even with neutrophil counts < 200/μL, serious infections usually do not occur, probably because neutrophils are sometimes produced in adequate quantities in response to infection. It is most common in women.

Table 149–2. CLASSIFICATION OF NEUTROPENIAS

CLASSIFICATION	ETIOLOGY
Neutropenia due to intrinsic defects in myeloid cells or their precursors	Aplastic anemia Chronic idiopathic neutropenia, including benign neutropenia Cyclic neutropenia Myelodysplasia Neutropenia associated with dysgammaglobulinemia Paroxysmal nocturnal hemoglobinuria Severe congenital neutropenia (Kostmann syndrome) Syndrome-associated neutropenias (eg, cartilage-hair hypoplasia syndrome, dyskeratosis congenita, glycogen storage disease type IB, WHIM* syndrome, Shwachman-Diamond syndrome)
Secondary neutropenias	Alcoholism Autoimmune neutropenia, including chronic secondary neutropenia in AIDS Bone marrow replacement (eg, due to cancer, myelofibrosis, granuloma, or Gaucher cells) Cytotoxic chemotherapy or radiation therapy Drug-induced neutropenia Folate deficiency, vitamin B_{12} deficiency, or severe undernutrition Hypersplenism Infection T cell large granular lymphocyte disease

*WHIM = warts, hypogammaglobulinemia, infections, myelokathexis.

Severe congenital neutropenia (SCN, or Kostmann syndrome) is a heterogenous group of rare disorders that are characterized by an arrest in myeloid maturation at the promyelocyte stage in the bone marrow, resulting in an absolute neutrophil count of < 200/μL and significant infections starting in infancy. SCN can be autosomal dominant or recessive, X-linked, or sporadic. Several genetic abnormalities that cause SCN have been identified, including mutations affecting neutrophil elastase (*ELANE/ELA2*), HAX1, GFI1, and the G-CSF receptor (CSF3R). Most SCN patients will respond to chronic growth factor therapy, but bone marrow transplant may need to be considered for poor responders. SCN patients have an increased risk of developing myelodysplasia or acute myelogenous leukemia.

Cyclic neutropenia is a rare congenital granulocytopoietic disorder, usually transmitted in an autosomal dominant fashion and usually caused by a mutation in the gene for neutrophil elastase (*ELANE/ELA2*), resulting in abnormal apoptosis. It is characterized by regular, periodic oscillations in the number of peripheral neutrophils. The mean oscillatory period is 21 ± 3 days.

Benign ethnic neutropenia (BEN) occurs in members of some ethnic groups (eg, some people of African, Middle Eastern, and Jewish descent). They normally have lower neutrophil counts but do not have increased risk of infection. In some cases this finding has been linked to the Duffy RBC antigen; some experts think neutropenia in these populations is related to protection from malaria.

Neutropenia can also result from bone marrow failure due to rare congenital syndromes (eg, cartilage-hair hypoplasia syndrome, Chédiak-Higashi syndrome, dyskeratosis congenita, glycogen storage disease type IB, Shwachman-Diamond syndrome, WHIM syndrome). Neutropenia is also a feature of myelodysplasia, where it may be accompanied by megaloblastoid features in the bone marrow, and of aplastic anemia and can occur in dysgammaglobulinemia and paroxysmal nocturnal hemoglobinemia.

Secondary neutropenia: Secondary neutropenia can result from use of certain drugs, bone marrow infiltration or replacement, certain infections, or immune reactions.

The **most common causes** include

- Drugs
- Infections and immune reactions
- Marrow infiltrative processes

Drug-induced neutropenia is one of the most common causes of neutropenia. Drugs can decrease neutrophil production through toxic, idiosyncratic, or hypersensitivity mechanisms; or they can increase peripheral neutrophil destruction through immune mechanisms. Only the toxic mechanism (eg, with phenothiazines) causes dose-related neutropenia. Idiosyncratic reactions are unpredictable and occur with a wide variety of drugs, including alternative medicine preparations or extracts, and toxins.

Hypersensitivity reactions are rare and occasionally involve anticonvulsants (eg, phenytoin, phenobarbital). These reactions may last for only a few days or for months or years. Often, hepatitis, nephritis, pneumonitis, or aplastic anemia accompanies hypersensitivity-induced neutropenia.

Immune-mediated drug-induced neutropenia, thought to arise from drugs that act as haptens to stimulate antibody formation, usually persists for about 1 wk after the drug is stopped. It may result from aminopyrine, propylthiouracil, penicillin, or other antibiotics.

Severe dose-related neutropenia occurs predictably after cytotoxic cancer drugs or radiation therapy due to suppression of bone marrow production.

Neutropenia due to ineffective bone marrow production can occur in megaloblastic anemias caused by vitamin B_{12} or folate deficiency. Usually, macrocytic anemia and sometimes mild thrombocytopenia develop simultaneously. Ineffective production can also accompany myelodysplastic disorders.

Bone marrow infiltration by leukemia, myeloma, lymphoma, or metastatic solid tumors (eg, breast cancer, prostate cancer) can impair neutrophil production. Tumor-induced myelofibrosis may further exacerbate neutropenia. Myelofibrosis can also occur due to granulomatous infections, Gaucher disease, and radiation therapy.

Hypersplenism of any cause can lead to moderate neutropenia, thrombocytopenia, and anemia.

Infections can cause neutropenia by impairing neutrophil production or by inducing immune destruction or rapid use of neutrophils. Sepsis is a particularly serious cause. Neutropenia that occurs with common childhood viral diseases develops during the first 1 to 2 days of illness and may persist for 3 to 8 days. Transient neutropenia may also result from virus- or endotoxemia-induced redistribution of neutrophils from the circulating to the marginal pool. Alcohol may contribute to neutropenia by inhibiting the neutrophilic response of the marrow during some infections (eg, pneumococcal pneumonia).

Immune defects can cause neutropenia. Neonatal isoimmune neutropenia can occur with fetal/maternal neutrophil antigen incompatibility associated with transplacental transfer of IgG antibodies against the newborn's neutrophils (most commonly to HNA-1 antigens). Autoimmune neutropenia can occur at any age and may be operative in many cases of idiopathic chronic neutropenia. Testing for antineutrophil antibodies (immunofluorescence, agglutination, or flow cytometry) are not always available or reliable.

Chronic secondary neutropenia often accompanies HIV infection because of impaired production of neutrophils and accelerated destruction of neutrophils by antibodies. Autoimmune neutropenias may be acute, chronic, or episodic. They may involve antibodies directed against circulating neutrophils or neutrophil precursor cells. They may also involve cytokines (eg, gamma interferon, tumor necrosis factor) that can cause neutrophil apoptosis. Most patients with autoimmune neutropenia have an underlying autoimmune disorder or lymphoproliferative disorder (eg, SLE, Felty syndrome).

Symptoms and Signs

Neutropenia is asymptomatic until infection develops. Fever is often the only indication of infection. Typical signs of inflammation (erythema, swelling, pain, infiltrates, leukocytic reaction) may be muted or absent. Focal symptoms (eg, oral ulcers) may develop but are often subtle. Patients with drug-induced neutropenia due to hypersensitivity may have a fever, rash, and lymphadenopathy as a result of the hypersensitivity.

Some patients with chronic benign neutropenia and neutrophil counts < 200/μL do not experience many serious infections. Patients with cyclic neutropenia or severe congenital neutropenia tend to have episodes of oral ulcers, stomatitis, or pharyngitis and lymph node enlargement during severe neutropenia. Pneumonias and septicemia often occur.

Diagnosis

- Clinical suspicion (repeated or unusual infections)
- Confirmatory CBC with differential
- Evaluation for infection with cultures and imaging
- Identification of mechanism and cause of neutropenia

Neutropenia is suspected in patients with frequent, severe, or unusual infections or in patients at risk (eg, those receiving cytotoxic drugs or radiation therapy). Confirmation is by CBC with differential.

Evaluation for infection: The first priority is to determine whether an infection is present. Because infection may be subtle, **physical examination** systematically assesses the most common primary sites of infection: mucosal surfaces, such as the alimentary tract (gums, pharynx, anus); lungs; abdomen; urinary tract; skin and fingernails; venipuncture sites; and vascular catheters.

If neutropenia is acute or severe, laboratory evaluation must proceed rapidly.

Cultures are the mainstay of evaluation. At least 2 sets of bacterial and fungal blood cultures are obtained from all febrile patients; if an indwelling IV catheter is present, cultures are drawn from the catheter and from a separate peripheral vein. Persistent or chronic drainage material is also cultured for fungi and atypical mycobacteria. Mucosal ulcers are swabbed and cultured for herpes virus. Skin lesions are aspirated or biopsied for cytology and culture. Samples for urinalysis and urine cultures are obtained from all patients. If diarrhea is present, stool is evaluated for enteric bacterial pathogens and *Clostridium* *difficile* toxins. Sputum cultures are obtained to evaluate for pulmonary infections.

Imaging studies are helpful. Chest x-rays are done on all patients. A chest CT may also be necessary in immunosuppressed patients. CT of the paranasal sinuses may be helpful if symptoms or signs of sinusitis (eg, positional headache, upper tooth or maxillary pain, facial swelling, nasal discharge) are present. CT scan of the abdomen is usually done if symptoms (eg, pain) or history (eg, recent surgery) suggests an intra-abdominal infection.

Identification of cause: Next, mechanism and cause of neutropenia are determined. The **history** addresses all drugs, other preparations, and possible toxin exposure or ingestion. **Physical examination** addresses the presence of splenomegaly and signs of other underlying disorder (eg, arthritis, lymphadenopathy).

If no obvious cause is identified (eg, chemotherapy), the most important test is

- Bone marrow examination

Bone marrow examination determines whether neutropenia is due to decreased marrow production or is secondary to increased destruction or use of the cells (determined by normal or increased production of the myeloid cells). Bone marrow examination may also indicate the specific cause of the neutropenia (eg, aplastic anemia, myelofibrosis, leukemia). Additional marrow studies (eg, cytogenetic analysis; special stains and flow cytometry for detecting leukemia, other malignant disorders, and infections) are done.

Further testing for the cause of neutropenia may be necessary, depending on the diagnoses suspected. In patients at risk of nutritional deficiencies, levels of copper, folate, and vitamin B_{12} are determined. Testing for the presence of antineutrophil antibodies is done if immune neutropenia is suspected. Differentiation between neutropenia caused by certain antibiotics and infection can sometimes be difficult. The WBC count just before the start of antibiotic treatment usually reflects the change in blood count due to the infection.

Patients who have had chronic neutropenia since infancy and a history of recurrent fevers and chronic gingivitis have WBC counts with differential done 3 times/wk for 6 wk, so that periodicity suggestive of cyclic neutropenia can be evaluated. Platelet and reticulocyte counts are done simultaneously. In patients with cyclic neutropenia, eosinophils, reticulocytes, and platelets frequently cycle synchronously with the neutrophils, whereas monocytes and lymphocytes may cycle out of phase.

Treatment

- Treatment of associated conditions (eg, infections, stomatitis)
- Sometimes antibiotic prophylaxis
- Myeloid growth factors
- Discontinuation of suspected etiologic agent (eg, drug)
- Sometimes corticosteroids

Acute neutropenia: Suspected infections are always treated immediately. If fever or hypotension is present, serious infection is assumed, and empiric, high-dose, broad-spectrum antibiotics are given IV. Regimen selection is based on the most likely infecting organisms, the antimicrobial susceptibility of pathogens at that particular institution, and the regimen's potential toxicity. Because of the risk of creating resistant organisms, vancomycin is used only if gram-positive organisms resistant to other drugs are suspected.

Indwelling vascular catheters can usually remain in place even if bacteremia is suspected or documented, but removal is considered if infections involve *S. aureus* or *Bacillus* sp, *Corynebacterium* sp, or *Candida* sp or if blood cultures are persistently positive despite appropriate antibiotics. Infections caused by coagulase-negative staphylococci generally resolve with antimicrobial therapy alone. Indwelling Foley catheters can also predispose to infections in these patients, and change or removal of the catheter should be considered for persistent urinary infections.

If cultures are positive, antibiotic therapy is adjusted to the results of sensitivity tests. If a patient defervesces within 72 h, antibiotics are continued for at least 7 days and until the patient has no symptoms or signs of infection. When neutropenia is transient (such as that following myelosuppressive chemotherapy), antibiotic therapy is usually continued until the neutrophil count is > 500/μL; however, stopping antimicrobials can be considered in selected patients with persistent neutropenia, especially those in whom symptoms and signs of inflammation have resolved, if cultures remain negative.

Fever that persists > 72 h despite antibiotic therapy suggests a nonbacterial cause, infection with a resistant species, a superinfection with a 2nd bacterial species, inadequate serum or tissue levels of the antibiotics, or localized infection, such as an abscess. Neutropenic patients with persistent fever are reassessed every 2 to 4 days with physical examination, cultures, and chest x-ray. If the patient is well except for the presence of fever, the initial antibiotic regimen can be continued, and drug-induced fever should be considered. If the patient is deteriorating, alteration of the antimicrobial regimen is considered.

Fungal infections are the most likely cause of persistent fevers and deterioration. Antifungal therapy is added empirically if unexplained fever persists after 3 to 4 days of broad-spectrum antibiotic therapy. Selection of the specific antifungal drug (eg, fluconazole, caspofungin, voriconazole, posaconazole) depends on the type of risk (eg, duration and severity of neutropenia, past history of fungal infection, persistent fever despite use of narrower spectrum antifungal drug) and should be guided by an infectious disease specialist. If fever persists after 3 wk of empiric therapy (including 2 wk of antifungal therapy) and the neutropenia has resolved, then stopping all antimicrobials can be considered and the cause of fever reevaluated.

For **afebrile patients with neutropenia,** antibiotic prophylaxis with fluoroquinolones (levofloxacin, ciprofloxacin) is used in some centers for patients who receive chemotherapy regimens that commonly result in neutrophils ≤ 100/μL for > 7 days. Prophylaxis is usually started by the treating oncologist. Antibiotics are continued until the neutrophil count increases to > 1500/μL. Also, antifungal therapy can be given for afebrile neutropenic patients at higher risk of fungal infection (eg, after hematopoietic stem cell transplantation, intensive chemotherapy for acute myelogenous leukemia or a myelodysplastic disorder, prior fungal infections). Selection of the specific antifungal drug should be guided by an infectious disease specialist. Antibiotic and antifungal prophylaxis is not routinely recommended for afebrile neutropenic patients without risk factors who are anticipated to remain neutropenic for < 7 days on the basis of their specific chemotherapy regimen.

Myeloid growth factors (ie, granulocyte colony-stimulating factor [G-CSF]) are widely used to increase the neutrophil count and to prevent infections in patients with severe neutropenia (eg, after hematopoietic stem cell transplantation and intensive cancer chemotherapy). They are expensive. However, if the risk of febrile neutropenia is ≥ 30% (as assessed by neutrophil count < 500 μL, presence of infection during a previous cycle of chemotherapy, associated comorbid disease, or age > 75), growth factors are indicated. In general, most clinical benefit occurs when the growth factor is administered beginning about 24 h after completion of chemotherapy. Patients with neutropenia caused by an idiosyncratic drug reaction may also benefit from myeloid growth factors, particularly if a delayed recovery is anticipated. The dose for G-CSF (filgrastim) is 5 to 10 mcg/kg sc once/day, and the dose for pegylated G-CSF (pegfilgrastim) is 6 mg sc once per chemotherapy cycle.

Glucocorticoids, anabolic steroids, and vitamins do not stimulate neutrophil production but can affect distribution and destruction. If acute neutropenia is suspected to be drug- or toxin-induced, all potentially etiologic agents are stopped. If neutropenia develops during treatment with a drug known to induce low counts (eg, chloramphenicol), then switching to an alternative antibiotic may be helpful.

Saline or hydrogen peroxide gargles every few hours, liquid oral rinses (containing viscous lidocaine, diphenhydramine, and liquid antacid), anesthetic lozenges (benzocaine 15 mg q 3 or 4 h), or chlorhexidine mouth rinses (1% solution) bid or tid may relieve the discomfort of stomatitis with oropharyngeal ulcerations. Oral or esophageal candidiasis is treated with nystatin (400,000 to 600,000 units oral rinse qid; swallowed if esophagitis is present), clotrimazole troche (10 mg slowly dissolved in the mouth 5 times a day), or systemic antifungal drugs (eg, fluconazole). A semisolid or liquid diet may be necessary during acute stomatitis or esophagitis, and topical analgesics (eg,viscous lidocaine) may be needed to minimize discomfort.

Chronic neutropenia: Neutrophil production in congenital neutropenia, cyclic neutropenia, and idiopathic neutropenia can be increased with administration of G-CSF 1 to 10 mcg/kg sc once/day. Effectiveness can be maintained with daily or intermittent G-CSF for months or years. Long-term G-CSF has also been used in other patients with chronic neutropenia, including those with myelodysplasia, HIV, and autoimmune disorders. In general, neutrophil counts increase, although clinical benefits are less clear, especially for patients who do not have severe neutropenia. For patients with autoimmune disorders or who have had an organ transplant, cyclosporine can also be beneficial.

In some patients with accelerated neutrophil destruction caused by autoimmune disorders, corticosteroids (generally, prednisone 0.5 to 1.0 mg/kg po once/day) can increase blood neutrophils. This increase often can be maintained with alternate-day G-CSF therapy.

Splenectomy has been used in the past to increase the neutrophil count in some patients with splenomegaly and splenic sequestration of neutrophils (eg, Felty syndrome); however, because growth factors and other newer therapies are often effective, splenectomy should be avoided in most patients. However, splenectomy can be considered for patients with persistent painful splenomegaly or with severe neutropenia (ie, < 500/μL) and serious problems with infections in whom other treatments have failed. Patients should be vaccinated against infections caused by *Streptococcus pneumoniae*, *Neisseria meningitidis*, and *Haemophilus influenzae* before splenectomy because splenectomy predisposes patients to infection by encapsulated organisms.

KEY POINTS

- Neutropenia predisposes to bacterial and fungal infections.
- The risk of infection is proportional to the severity of neutropenia; patients with neutrophil counts < 500/μL are at greatest risk.
- Because the inflammatory response is limited, clinical findings may be muted, although fever is usually present.
- Febrile neutropenic patients are treated empirically with broad-spectrum antibiotics pending definitive identification of infection.
- Antibiotic prophylaxis is indicated in high-risk patients.

150 Lymphomas

Lymphomas are a heterogeneous group of tumors arising in the reticuloendothelial and lymphatic systems. The major types are Hodgkin lymphoma and non-Hodgkin lymphoma (NHL—Table 150–1).

Lymphomas were once thought to be absolutely distinct from leukemias. However, better understanding of cell markers and tools with which to evaluate those markers now show that the distinction between these 2 cancers is often vague. The notion that lymphoma is relatively restricted to the lymphatic system and leukemias to the bone marrow, at least in early stages, is also not always true.

HODGKIN LYMPHOMA

Hodgkin lymphoma is a localized or disseminated malignant proliferation of cells of the lymphoreticular system, primarily involving lymph node tissue, spleen, liver, and bone marrow. Symptoms include painless lymphadenopathy, sometimes with fever, night sweats, unintentional weight loss, pruritus, splenomegaly, and hepatomegaly. Diagnosis is based on lymph node biopsy. Treatment is curative in about 75% of cases and consists of chemotherapy with or without radiation therapy.

In the US, about 9000 new cases of Hodgkin lymphoma are diagnosed annually. The male:female ratio is 1.4:1. Hodgkin lymphoma is rare before age 10 and is most common between ages 15 and 40; a 2nd peak occurs in people > 50 to 60.

Pathophysiology

Hodgkin lymphoma results from the clonal transformation of cells of B-cell origin, giving rise to pathognomic binucleated Reed-Sternberg cells. The cause is unknown, but genetic susceptibility and environmental associations (eg, occupation, such as woodworking; history of treatment with phenytoin, radiation therapy, or chemotherapy; infection with Epstein-Barr virus, *Mycobacterium tuberculosis*, herpesvirus type 6, HIV) play a role. Risk is slightly increased in people with certain types of immunosuppression (eg, posttransplant patients taking immunosuppressants); in people with congenital immunodeficiency disorders (eg, ataxia-telangiectasia, Klinefelter syndrome, Chédiak-Higashi syndrome, Wiskott-Aldrich syndrome); and in people with certain autoimmune disorders (RA, celiac sprue, Sjögren syndrome, SLE).

Most patients also develop a slowly progressive defect in cell-mediated immunity (T-cell function) that, in advanced disease, contributes to common bacterial and unusual fungal,

Table 150–1. COMPARISON OF HODGKIN LYMPHOMA AND NON-HODGKIN LYMPHOMA

FEATURE	HODGKIN LYMPHOMA	NON-HODGKIN LYMPHOMA
Nodal involvement	Localized to a specific group of nodes	Usually disseminated among > 1 nodal group
Spread	Tends to spread in an orderly, contiguous fashion	Spreads noncontiguously
Effect on Waldeyer ring and mesenteric lymph nodes	Usually does not affect	Commonly affects mesenteric nodes May affect Waldeyer ring
Extranodal involvement	Infrequent	Frequent
Stage at diagnosis	Usually early	Usually advanced
Histologic classification in children	Usually one with a favorable prognosis	Usually high grade

viral, and protozoal infections. Humoral immunity (antibody production) is depressed in advanced disease. Death often results from sepsis.

Symptoms and Signs

Most patients present with painless cervical adenopathy. Although the mechanism is unclear, pain may occur in diseased areas immediately after drinking alcoholic beverages, thereby providing an early indication of the diagnosis.

Other manifestations develop as the disease spreads through the reticuloendothelial system, generally to contiguous sites. Intense pruritus may occur early. Constitutional symptoms include fever, night sweats, and unintentional weight loss (> 10% of body weight in previous 6 mo), which may signify involvement of internal lymph nodes (mediastinal or retroperitoneal), viscera (liver), or bone marrow. Splenomegaly is often present; hepatomegaly may be present. Pel-Ebstein fever (a few days of high fever regularly alternating with a few days to several weeks of normal or below-normal temperature) occasionally occurs. Cachexia is common as disease advances.

Bone involvement is often asymptomatic but may produce vertebral osteoblastic lesions (ivory vertebrae) and, rarely, pain with osteolytic lesions and compression fracture. Intracranial, gastric, and cutaneous lesions are rare and when present suggest HIV-associated Hodgkin lymphoma.

Local compression by tumor masses often causes symptoms, including

- Jaundice secondary to intrahepatic or extrahepatic bile duct obstruction
- Leg edema secondary to lymphatic obstruction in the pelvis or groin
- Severe dyspnea and wheezing secondary to tracheobronchial compression
- Lung cavitation or abscess secondary to infiltration of lung parenchyma, which may simulate lobar consolidation or bronchopneumonia

Epidural invasion that compresses the spinal cord may result in paraplegia. Horner syndrome and laryngeal paralysis may result when enlarged lymph nodes compress the cervical sympathetic and recurrent laryngeal nerves. Neuralgic pain follows nerve root compression.

Diagnosis

- Chest x-ray
- CT of chest, abdomen, and pelvis
- CBC, alkaline phosphatase, LDH, liver function tests, albumin, Ca, BUN, and creatinine
- Lymph node biopsy
- PET for staging and MRI if neurologic symptoms are present
- Sometimes bone marrow biopsy

Hodgkin lymphoma is usually suspected in patients with painless lymphadenopathy or mediastinal adenopathy detected on routine chest x-ray. Similar lymphadenopathy can result from infectious mononucleosis, toxoplasmosis, cytomegalovirus infection, non-Hodgkin lymphoma, or leukemia. Similar chest x-ray findings can result from lung cancer, sarcoidosis, or TB (for evaluation of a mediastinal mass, see p. 468).

A chest x-ray is obtained if not already done. X-ray is usually followed by lymph node biopsy if findings are confirmed with CT or PET scan of the chest. If only mediastinal nodes are enlarged, mediastinoscopy or Chamberlain procedure (a limited left anterior thoracostomy allowing biopsy of mediastinal lymph nodes inaccessible by cervical mediastinoscopy) may be indicated. CT-guided biopsy may also be considered, but results of fine-needle aspiration are often inaccurate, so node core biopsy is needed. CBC, alkaline phosphatase, and kidney and liver function tests are generally done. Other tests are done depending on findings (eg, MRI for symptoms of cord compression).

Biopsy reveals Reed-Sternberg cells (large, binucleated cells) in a characteristically heterogeneous cellular infiltrate, consisting of histiocytes, lymphocytes, monocytes, plasma cells, and eosinophils. Classic Hodgkin lymphoma has 4 histopathologic subtypes (see Table 150–2); there is also a lymphocyte-predominant type. Certain antigens on Reed-Sternberg cells may help differentiate Hodgkin lymphoma from non-Hodgkin lymphoma, and classic Hodgkin lymphoma from the lymphocyte-predominant type.

Other test results may be abnormal but are nondiagnostic. CBC may show slight polymorphonuclear leukocytosis. Lymphocytopenia may occur early and become pronounced with advanced disease. Eosinophilia is present in about 20% of patients, and thrombocytosis may be present. Anemia, often microcytic, usually develops with advanced disease. In advanced anemia, defective iron reutilization is characterized by low serum iron, low iron-binding capacity, and increased bone marrow iron. Pancytopenia is occasionally caused by bone marrow invasion, usually by the lymphocyte-depleted type. Hypersplenism (see p. 1197) may occur in patients with marked splenomegaly. Elevated serum alkaline phosphatase levels may be present, but elevations do not always indicate bone marrow or liver involvement. Increases in leukocyte alkaline phosphatase, serum haptoglobin, and other acute-phase reactants usually reflect active disease.

Staging: After diagnosis, stage is determined to guide therapy. The commonly used Ann Arbor staging system (see Table 150–3) incorporates symptoms; physical examination findings; results of imaging tests, preferably a combined FDG-PET/CT scan of the chest, abdomen, and pelvis, or, alternatively, a contrast-enhanced CT scan of those areas; and less frequently, unilateral bone marrow biopsy. Laparotomy is not required for staging. Other staging tests include cardiac

Table 150–2. HISTOPATHOLOGIC SUBTYPES OF HODGKIN LYMPHOMA (WHO CLASSIFICATION)

HISTOLOGIC TYPE	MORPHOLOGIC APPEARANCE	TUMOR CELL IMMUNOPHENOTYPE	INCIDENCE
Classic			
Nodular sclerosis	Dense fibrous tissue* surrounding nodules of Hodgkin tissue	CD15+, CD30+, CD20–	67%
Mixed cellularity	A moderate number of Reed-Sternberg cells with a mixed background infiltrate	CD15+, CD30+, CD20–	25%
Lymphocyte-rich	Few Reed-Sternberg cells Many B cells Fine sclerosis	CD15+, CD30+, CD20–	3%
Lymphocyte-depleted	Numerous Reed-Sternberg cells Extensive fibrosis	CD15+, CD30+, CD20–	Rare
Nodular lymphocyte-predominant			
	Few neoplastic cells (lymphocytic or histiocytic cells or both) Many small B cells Nodular pattern	CD15–, CD30–, CD20+, EMA+	3%

*Shows characteristic birefringence with polarized light.
EMA = epithelial membrane antigen.

and pulmonary function tests in anticipation of therapy. The Cotswold modifications of the Ann Arbor staging system incorporate the prognostic implications of tumor bulkiness and disease sites.

Designation of the letter A to any stage means that no systemic symptoms are being experienced. Designation of the letter B means that at least one systemic symptom is experienced. The presence of symptoms correlates with response to treatment.

Prognosis

In classic Hodgkin lymphoma, disease-free survival 5 yr after therapy is considered a cure. Relapse is very rare after 5 yr. Chemotherapy with or without radiation therapy achieves cure in 70 to 80% of patients. Increased potential for relapse depends on many factors, including male sex, age > 45 yr, involvement of multiple extranodal sites, and presence of constitutional symptoms at diagnosis. Patients who do not achieve complete remission or who relapse within 12 mo have a poor prognosis.

Table 150–3. COTSWOLD MODIFICATION OF ANN ARBOR STAGING OF HODGKIN LYMPHOMA AND NON-HODGKIN LYMPHOMA

STAGE*	CRITERIA
I	In 1 lymph region only
II	In ≥ 2 lymph regions on the same side of the diaphragm
III	In the lymph nodes, spleen, or both and on both sides of the diaphragm
IV	Extranodal involvement (eg, bone marrow, lungs, liver)

*Subclassification E indicates extranodal involvement adjacent to an involved lymph node (eg, disease of mediastinal nodes and hilar adenopathy with adjacent lung infiltration is classified as stage IIE). Stages can be further classified by A to indicate the absence or B to indicate the presence of systemic symptoms (weight loss, fever, or night sweats). Systemic symptoms usually occur in stages III and IV (20 to 30% of patients). The suffix X is used to denote bulky disease, which is > 10 cm in maximum dimension or involves more than one third of the chest diameter (seen on chest x-ray).

Treatment

- Chemotherapy
- Radiation therapy
- Surgery
- Sometimes hematopoietic stem cell transplantation

The choice of treatment modality is complex and depends on the precise stage of disease. Before treatment, men should be offered sperm banking, and women should discuss fertility options with their oncologists.

Stage IA, IIA, IB, or IIB disease is generally treated with an abbreviated chemotherapy regimen of doxorubicin (Adriamycin), bleomycin, vinblastine, and dacarbazine (ABVD) plus radiation therapy or with longer-course chemotherapy alone. Such treatment cures about 80% of patients. In patients with bulky mediastinal disease, chemotherapy may be of longer duration or of a different type, and radiation therapy is typically used.

Stage IIIA and IIIB disease is usually treated with ABVD combination chemotherapy alone. Cure rates of 75 to 80% have been achieved in patients with stage IIIA disease, and rates from 70 to 80% in patients with stage IIIB disease.

For stage IVA and IVB disease, ABVD combination chemotherapy is the standard regimen, producing complete remission in 70 to 80% of patients; > 50% remain disease-free at 5 yr. Other effective drugs include nitrosoureas, ifosfamide, procarbazine, cisplatin or carboplatin, and etoposide. Other drug combinations are bleomycin, etoposide, doxorubicin (Adriamycin), cyclophosphamide, vincristine (Oncovin), procarbazine, and prednisone (known as BEACOPP), and melchlorethamine, doxorubicin, vinblastine, vincristine, etoposide, bleomycin, and prednisone (known as Stanford V). Standford V incorporates involved field irradiation for consolidation.

Autologous transplantation using peripheral stem cell products should be considered for all physiologically eligible patients who fail induction therapy or who relapse and respond to salvage chemotherapy (eg, with newer agents such as brentuximab, nivolumab, or pembroizumab).

Complications of treatment: Chemotherapy, particularly with drugs such as mechlorethamine, vincristine, procarbazine, and prednisone, increases the risk of leukemia, which typically develops after > 3 yr. Both chemotherapy and radiation therapy increase the risk of malignant solid tumors (eg, breast, GI, lung, soft tissue). Mediastinal radiation increases the risk of coronary atherosclerosis. Breast cancer risk is increased in women beginning about 7 yr after they have received radiation treatment to adjacent nodal regions.

Posttreatment surveillance: Patients in remission should be monitored for relapse. Imaging with PET/CT or CT alone should be done mainly based on symptoms and signs rather than a calendar schedule as was previously recommended, although some clinicians scan asymptomatic patients at 1 and 2 yr post-therapy. For a schedule of posttreatment surveillance, see Table 150–4.

KEY POINTS

- Hodgkin lymphoma is of B-cell origin.
- Patients usually present with painless lymphadenopathy or with incidental mediastinal adenopathy discovered on chest x-ray.
- Biopsy shows pathognomic, binucleated Reed-Sternberg cells.
- Cure rate overall is 70 to 80% using combination chemotherapy and sometimes radiation therapy.

Table 150–4. HODGKIN LYMPHOMA POSTTREATMENT SURVEILLANCE

EVALUATION	SCHEDULE
History and physical examination, CBC, platelets, electrolytes, BUN, creatinine, liver function tests	First 2 yr, q 3–4 mo Yr 3–5, q 6 mo > 5 yr, q 12 mo
Chest x-ray at each visit	—
PET/CT	Any time symptoms develop; possibly at 1 and 2 yr post-therapy in asymptomatic patients
Thyroid-stimulating hormone levels	Every 6 mo after radiation to neck
Mammography	Annually beginning at yr 7 if radiation above the diaphragm began at age < 30 yr Annually beginning at age 37 if radiation above the diaphragm began at age ≥ 30 yr
Breast MRI	For high-risk patients (those who received radiation above the diaphragm before age 30 yr), alternating every 6 mo with mammography (one test every 6 mo)

NON-HODGKIN LYMPHOMAS

(Non-Hodgkin's Lymphoma)

Non-Hodgkin lymphomas (NHL) are a heterogeneous group of disorders involving malignant monoclonal proliferation of lymphoid cells in lymphoreticular sites, including lymph nodes, bone marrow, the spleen, the liver, and the GI tract. Presenting symptoms usually include peripheral lymphadenopathy. However, some patients present without lymphadenopathy but with abnormal lymphocytes in circulation. Compared with Hodgkin lymphoma, there is a greater likelihood of disseminated disease at the time of diagnosis. Diagnosis is usually based on lymph node or bone marrow biopsy or both. Treatment typically involves chemoimmunotherapy and sometimes also radiation therapy. Stem cell transplantation is usually reserved for salvage therapy after incomplete remission or relapse.

NHL is more common than Hodgkin lymphoma. It is the 6th most common cancer in the US; about 70,000 new cases are diagnosed annually in all age groups. However, NHL is not one disease but rather a category of lymphocyte cancers. Incidence increases with age (median age, 50 yr).

Etiology

The cause of NHL is unknown, although, as with the leukemias, substantial evidence suggests a viral cause (eg, human T-cell leukemia-lymphoma virus, Epstein-Barr virus, hepatitis C virus, HIV). Risk factors for NHL include immunodeficiency (secondary to posttransplant immunosuppression, AIDS, primary immune disorders, sicca syndrome, RA), *Helicobacter pylori* infection, certain chemical exposures, and previous treatment for Hodgkin lymphoma. NHL is the 2nd most common cancer in HIV-infected patients (see p. 1643), and some AIDS patients present with lymphoma. C-*myc* gene rearrangements are characteristic of some AIDS-associated lymphomas.

Pathophysiology

Most (80 to 85%) NHL arise from B cells; the remainder arise from T cells or natural killer cells. Either precursor or mature cells may be involved. Overlap exists between leukemia and NHL because both involve proliferation of lymphocytes or their precursors. A leukemia-like picture with peripheral lymphocytosis and bone marrow involvement may be present in up to 50% of children and in about 20% of adults with some types of NHL. Differentiation can be difficult, but generally patients with more extensive nodal involvement (especially mediastinal), fewer circulating abnormal cells, and fewer blast forms in the marrow (< 25%) are considered to have lymphoma. A prominent leukemic phase is less common in aggressive lymphomas, except Burkitt (see p. 1162) and lymphoblastic lymphomas.

Hypogammaglobulinemia caused by a progressive decrease in immunoglobulin production occurs in 15% of patients, primarily those with histology that resembles chronic lymphocytic leukemia, and may predispose to serious bacterial infection.

PEARLS & PITFALLS

- There is considerable overlap between non-Hodgkin lymphoma and leukemia; both may have peripheral lymphocytosis and bone marrow involvement.

Classification

Pathologic classification of NHL continues to evolve, reflecting new insights into the cells of origin and the biologic bases of these heterogeneous diseases. The WHO classification[1] classifies lymphomas as mature because it B-cell tumors or mature T-cell and NK cell tumors. There are numerous subtypes. This classification is valuable because it incorporates immunophenotype, genotype, and cytogenetics, but numerous other systems exist (eg, Lyon classification). Among the most important lymphomas newly recognized by the WHO system are mucosa-associated lymphoid tumors (MALT—see p. 123), mantle cell lymphoma (previously diffuse small cleaved cell lymphoma), and anaplastic large cell lymphoma. Anaplastic large cell lymphoma is a heterogeneous disorder with 75% of cases of T-cell origin, 15% of B-cell origin, and 10% unclassified. However, despite the plethora of entities, treatment is often similar except in certain T-cell lymphomas.

Lymphomas are commonly also categorized as indolent or aggressive. Indolent lymphomas are slowly progressive and responsive to therapy but are not curable with standard approaches. Aggressive lymphomas are rapidly progressive but responsive to therapy and often curable.

In children, NHL is almost always aggressive. Follicular and other indolent lymphomas are very rare. The treatment of these aggressive lymphomas (Burkitt, diffuse large B cell, and lymphoblastic lymphoma) presents special concerns, including GI tract involvement (particularly in the terminal ileum); meningeal spread (requiring CSF prophylaxis or treatment); and other sanctuary sites of involvement (eg, testes, brain). In addition, with these potentially curable lymphomas, treatment adverse effects as well as outcome must be considered, including late risks of secondary cancer, cardiorespiratory sequelae, fertility preservation, and developmental consequences. Current research is focused on these areas as well as on the molecular events and predictors of lymphoma in children.

1. Swerdlow SH, et al: The 2016 revision of the World Health Organization classification of lymphoid neoplasms. *Blood* i27:2375–2390, 2016.

Symptoms and Signs

Many patients present with asymptomatic peripheral lymphadenopathy. Enlarged lymph nodes are rubbery and discrete and later become matted. Disease is localized in some patients, but most patients have several areas of involvement. Mediastinal and retroperitoneal lymphadenopathy may cause pressure symptoms on various organs. Extranodal sites may dominate clinically (eg, gastric involvement can simulate GI carcinoma; intestinal lymphoma may cause a malabsorption syndrome; HIV patients who develop NHL often present with CNS involvement).

The skin and bones are initially involved in 15% of patients with aggressive lymphoma and in 7% of those with indolent lymphoma. Occasionally, patients with extensive abdominal or thoracic disease develop chylous ascites or pleural effusion because of lymphatic obstruction. Weight loss, fever, night sweats, and asthenia indicate disseminated disease. Patients may have hepatomegaly and splenomegaly as well.

Two problems are common in NHL but rare in Hodgkin lymphoma: Congestion and edema of the face and neck from pressure on the superior vena cava (superior vena cava or superior mediastinal syndrome) may occur. Also, ureters may be compressed by retroperitoneal or pelvic lymph nodes or both; this compression may interfere with urinary flow and cause secondary renal failure.

PEARLS & PITFALLS

- Superior vena cava syndrome and ureteral compression are common in non-Hodgkin lymphoma but rare in Hodgkin lymphoma.

Anemia is initially present in about 33% of patients and eventually develops in most. It may be caused by bleeding due to GI lymphoma, with or without low platelet levels; hemolysis due to hypersplenism or Coombs'-positive hemolytic anemia; bone marrow infiltration due to lymphoma; or marrow suppression due to chemotherapy or radiation therapy.

The acute illness of adult T-cell leukemia-lymphoma (ATLL, associated with human T-lymphotropic virus 1 [HTLV-1]) has a fulminating clinical course with skin infiltrates, lymphadenopathy, hepatosplenomegaly, and leukemia. The leukemic cells are malignant T cells, many with convoluted nuclei. Hypercalcemia often develops, related to humoral factors rather than to direct bone invasion.

Patients with anaplastic large cell lymphoma have rapidly progressive skin lesions, adenopathy, and visceral lesions. This disease may be mistaken for Hodgkin lymphoma or metastatic undifferentiated carcinoma.

Diagnosis

- Chest x-ray
- CT of chest, abdomen, and pelvis and/or PET–CT
- CBC, alkaline phosphatase, LDH, liver function tests, albumin, Ca, BUN, creatinine, electrolytes, and uric acid
- HIV, hepatitis B virus, and hepatitis C virus testing; testing for HTLV-1 if ATLL is found
- Lymph node and bone marrow biopsy
- MRI of spine if neurologic symptoms are present

As with Hodgkin lymphoma, NHL is usually suspected in patients with painless lymphadenopathy or when mediastinal adenopathy is detected on routine chest x-ray. Painless lymphadenopathy can also result from infectious mononucleosis, toxoplasmosis, cytomegalovirus infection, primary HIV infection, or leukemia. Similar chest x-ray findings can result from lung carcinoma, sarcoidosis, or TB. Less commonly, patients present after a finding of peripheral lymphocytosis on CBC done for nonspecific symptoms. In such cases, the differential diagnosis includes leukemia, Epstein-Barr virus infection, and Duncan syndrome (X-linked lymphoproliferative syndrome).

A lymph node biopsy is done if lymphadenopathy is confirmed on chest x-ray, CT, or PET. If only mediastinal nodes are enlarged, patients require CT-guided needle biopsy or mediastinoscopy. Usually, tests should include CBC, alkaline phosphatase, kidney and liver function tests, LDH, and uric acid. Other tests are done depending on findings (eg, MRI for symptoms of spinal cord compression or CNS abnormalities).

Histologic criteria on biopsy include destruction of normal lymph node architecture and invasion of the capsule and adjacent fat by characteristic neoplastic cells. Immunophenotyping studies to determine the cell of origin are of great value in identifying specific subtypes and helping define prognosis and management; these studies also can be done on peripheral cells. Demonstration of the leukocyte common antigen CD45 by immunoperoxidase rules out metastatic cancer, which is often in the differential diagnosis of "undifferentiated" cancers. The test for leukocyte common antigen, most surface marker studies, and gene rearrangement (to document B-cell or T-cell clonality) can be done on fixed tissues. Cytogenetics and flow cytometry require fresh tissue.

Staging: Although localized NHL does occur, the disease is typically disseminated when first recognized. Staging procedures include FDG-PET/CT scan of the chest, abdomen, and pelvis, or, alternately, a contrast-enhanced CT scan of those areas. The final staging of NHL (see Table 150–3) is similar to that of Hodgkin lymphoma and is based on clinical and pathologic findings.

Prognosis

Patients with peripheral T-cell or NK/T-cell lymphomas generally have a worse prognosis than do those with B-cell types, although newer intensive treatment regimens may lessen this difference. Prognosis for each NHL variant is related to differences in tumor cell biology.

Survival also varies with other factors. The International Prognostic Index (IPI) is frequently used in aggressive lymphomas. It considers 5 risk factors:

- Age > 60
- Poor performance status (can be measured using the Eastern Cooperative Oncology Group tool)
- Elevated LDH
- > 1 extranodal site
- Stage III or IV disease

Outcome is worse with an increasing number of risk factors. Survival, as determined by IPI factor, has improved with the addition of rituximab to the standard chemotherapeutic regimen. Patients in the highest risk groups (patients with 4 or 5 risk factors) now have a 50% 5-yr survival. Patients without any of the risk factors have a very high cure rate. A modified IPI (follicular lymphoma IPI [FLIPI]) is being used in follicular lymphomas and in diffuse large B-cell lymphoma (revised IPI [R-IPI]).

Treatment

- Chemotherapy, radiation therapy, or both
- Anti-CD20 monoclonal antibody, with or without chemotherapy
- Sometimes hematopoietic stem cell transplantation

Treatment varies considerably with cell type, which are too numerous to permit detailed discussion. Generalizations can be made regarding localized vs advanced disease and aggressive vs indolent forms. Burkitt lymphoma (see p. 1162) and mycosis fungoides (see p. 1162) are discussed separately.

Localized disease (stages I and II): Patients with indolent lymphomas rarely present with localized disease, but when they do, regional radiation therapy may offer long-term control. However, relapses may occur > 10 yr after radiation therapy.

About half of patients with aggressive lymphomas present with localized disease, for which combination chemotherapy, with or without regional radiation, is usually curative. Patients with lymphoblastic lymphomas or Burkitt lymphoma, even if apparently localized, must receive intensive combination chemotherapy with meningeal prophylaxis. Treatment may require maintenance chemotherapy, but cure is expected.

Advanced disease (stages III and IV): For indolent lymphomas, treatment varies considerably. A watch-and-wait approach or treatment with the B-cell specific monoclonal anti-CD20 antibody rituximab alone or combined with chemotherapy (single drug or 2- or 3-drug regimens) may be used. Criteria considered in selecting management options include age, general health, distribution of disease, tumor bulk, histology, and anticipated benefits of therapy. Radiolabeled-antibody therapy is also sometimes used.

In patients with the aggressive B-cell lymphomas (eg, diffuse large B cell), the standard drug combination is rituximab plus cyclophosphamide, hydroxydaunorubicin (doxorubicin), vincristine, and prednisone (R-CHOP). Complete disease regression is expected in ≥ 70% of patients, depending on the IPI category. More than 70% of complete responders are cured, and relapses > 2 yr after treatment ceases are rare.

Cure rates have improved with the use of R-CHOP, so autologous transplantation is reserved for patients with relapsed or refractory aggressive B-cell lymphomas, some younger patients with mantle cell lymphoma, and some patients with aggressive T-cell lymphomas.

Lymphoma relapse: The first relapse after initial chemotherapy is almost always treated with autologous stem cell transplantation. Patients usually should be ≤ 75 yr or in equivalent health and have responsive disease, good performance status, a source of uncontaminated stem cells, and an adequate number of CD34+ stem cells (harvested from peripheral blood or bone marrow). Consolidation myeloablative therapy may include chemotherapy with or without irradiation. Posttreatment immunotherapy (eg, rituximab, vaccination, IL-2) is being studied.

An allogeneic transplant is the donation of stem cells from a compatible donor (brother, sister, matched unrelated donor, or umbilical cord blood). The stem cells have a 2-fold effect: reconstituting normal blood counts and providing a possible graft-vs-tumor effect.

In aggressive lymphoma, a cure may be expected in 30 to 50% of eligible patients undergoing myeloablative therapy and transplantation.

In indolent lymphomas, cure with autologous stem cell transplantation remains uncertain, although remission may be superior to that with secondary palliative therapy alone. Reduced intensity allogenic transplantation is a potentially curative option in some patients with indolent lymphoma.

The mortality rate of patients undergoing myeloablative transplantation has decreased dramatically to 1 to 2% for most autologous procedures and to < 15% for most allogeneic procedures.

Complications of treatment: A late sequela of standard and high-dose chemotherapy is the occurrence of 2nd tumors, especially myelodysplasias and acute myelogenous leukemia. Chemotherapy combined with radiation therapy increases this risk, although its incidence is still only about 3%.

KEY POINTS

- Non-Hodgkin lymphomas are a group of related cancers involving lymphocytes; they vary significantly in their rate of growth and response to treatment.
- Non-Hodgkin lymphomas overlap considerably with leukemias.
- The disease is usually already disseminated at the time of diagnosis.
- Molecular and genetic tests are essential for diagnosis and management.

BURKITT LYMPHOMA

Burkitt lymphoma is a B-cell lymphoma occurring primarily in children. Endemic (African), sporadic (non-African), and immunodeficiency-related forms exist.

Burkitt lymphoma is endemic in central Africa and constitutes 30% of childhood lymphomas in the US. The form endemic to Africa often manifests as enlargement of the jaw or facial bones. In sporadic (non-African) Burkitt lymphoma, abdominal disease predominates, often arising in the region of the ileocecal valve or the mesentery. Tumor may cause bowel obstruction. The kidneys, ovaries, or breasts may also be involved. In adults, disease may be bulky and generalized, often with massive involvement of liver, spleen, and bone marrow. CNS involvement is often present at diagnosis or with relapsing lymphoma.

Burkitt lymphoma is the most rapidly growing human tumor, and pathology reveals a high mitotic rate, a monoclonal proliferation of B cells, and a "starry-sky" pattern of benign macrophages that have engulfed apoptotic malignant lymphocytes. There is a distinctive genetic translocation involving the *C-myc* gene on chromosome 8 and the immunoglobulin heavy chain of chromosome 14. The disease is closely associated with Epstein-Barr virus infection in endemic lymphoma; however, it is uncertain whether Epstein-Barr virus plays an etiologic role. Burkitt lymphoma occurs frequently in patients with AIDS and may be an AIDS-defining disease.

Diagnosis

Diagnosis is based on biopsy of lymph node or tissue from another suspected disease site. Rarely, laparotomy may be used for both diagnosis and treatment. Staging includes FDG-PET/CT scan of the chest, abdomen, and pelvis, or alternately, a contrast-enhanced CT scan of those areas, bone marrow biopsy, and CSF cytology. Staging studies must be expedited because of rapid tumor growth.

Treatment

- Intensive chemotherapy

Treatment must be initiated rapidly because tumors grow rapidly. An intensive alternating regimen of cyclophosphamide, vincristine, doxorubicin, methotrexate, ifosfamide, etoposide, and cytarabine (CODOX-M/IVAC) plus rituximab results in a cure rate of > 90% for children and adults. Other regimens such as rituximab plus etoposide, prednisone, vincristine (Oncovin), and doxorubicin (R-EPOCH) and rituximab plus cyclophosphamide, vincristine, doxorubicin (Adriamycin), and dexamethasone (R-Hyper CVAD) are also commonly used with success. Meningeal prophylaxis is essential. With treatment, tumor lysis syndrome (see p. 1195) is common, and patients must receive IV hydration, allopurinol often with rasburicase, alkalinization, and close attention to electrolytes (particularly K and Ca).

If the patient presents with bowel obstruction secondary to tumor but the tumor is completely resected at initial diagnostic-therapeutic laparotomy, then aggressive therapy is still indicated. Salvage therapy for treatment failures is generally unsuccessful, underscoring the importance of very aggressive initial therapy.

MYCOSIS FUNGOIDES

Mycosis fungoides is an uncommon chronic T-cell lymphoma primarily affecting the skin and occasionally the internal organs.

Mycosis fungoides is rare compared with Hodgkin lymphoma and non-Hodgkin lymphoma. Unlike most other lymphomas, it is insidious in onset, sometimes appearing as a chronic, pruritic rash that is difficult to diagnose. It begins focally but may spread to involve most of the skin. Lesions are plaquelike but may become nodular or ulcerated. Eventually, systemic involvement of lymph nodes, liver, spleen, and lungs occurs, resulting in the advent of symptoms, which include fever, night sweats, and unintentional weight loss.

Diagnosis

- Skin biopsy
- For staging, bone marrow biopsy and CT of chest, abdomen, and pelvis

Diagnosis is based on skin biopsy, but histology may be equivocal early in the course because of insufficient quantities of lymphoma cells. The malignant cells are mature T cells (T4+, T11+, T12+).

Characteristic Pautrier microabscesses are present in the epidermis. In some cases, a leukemic phase called Sézary syndrome is characterized by the appearance of malignant T cells with serpentine nuclei in the peripheral blood.

Once mycosis fungoides has been confirmed, the stage is commonly determined using the ISCL/EORTC (International Society of Cutaneous Lymphomas/European Organization of Research and Treatment of Cancer) staging system, which incorporates results of physical examination, histopathology, and imaging tests.

Prognosis

Most patients are > 50 yr at diagnosis; average life expectancy is 7 to 10 yr after diagnosis, even without treatment. However, survival rates vary markedly depending on stage at diagnosis. Patients who receive treatment for stage IA disease have a life expectancy analogous to that of similar people without mycosis fungoides. Patients who receive treatment for stage IIB disease survive for about 3 yr. Patients treated for stage III disease survive an average of 4 to 6 yr. Patients treated for stage IVA or IVB disease (extracutaneous disease) survive < 1.5 yr.

Treatment

- Radiation therapy, topical chemotherapy, phototherapy, or topical corticosteroids
- Sometimes systemic chemotherapy

Electron beam radiation therapy, in which most of the energy is absorbed in the first 5 to 10 mm of tissue, and topical nitrogen mustard have proved highly effective. Plaques may also be treated with sunlight and topical corticosteroids. Systemic treatment with alkylating drugs and folic acid antagonists produces transient tumor regression, but systemic treatment is primarily used when other therapies have failed, after relapse, or in patients with documented extranodal or extracutaneous disease. Extracorporeal phototherapy with a chemosensitive drug has shown modest success. New agents include histone deacetylase (HDAC) inhibitors, which may be given IV or orally.

151 Myeloproliferative Disorders

Myeloproliferative disorders are abnormal proliferations of bone marrow stem cells, which can manifest as increased platelets, RBCs, or WBCs in the circulation and sometimes as increased fibrosis in the bone marrow with consequent extramedullary hematopoiesis (cell production outside the marrow). Based on these abnormalities, they are classified as

- Essential thrombocythemia (increased platelets)
- Primary myelofibrosis (marrow fibrosis or scarring)
- Polycythemia vera (some combination of increased WBCs, RBCs, and/or platelets)
- Chronic myelogenous leukemia

Essential thrombocythemia (ET), primary myelofibrosis, and polycythemia vera are Philadelphia chromosome–negative myeloproliferative disorders. Myeloproliferative disorders sometimes lead to acute leukemia.

Less common myeloproliferative disorders include the hypereosinophilic syndromes and mastocytosis. There are also rare myeloproliferative disorders that overlap with myelodysplastic syndrome.

Each disorder is identified according to its predominant feature or site of proliferation (see Table 151–1). Despite overlap, each disorder has a somewhat typical constellation of clinical features, laboratory findings, and course. Although proliferation of one cell line may dominate the clinical picture, each disorder is typically caused by clonal proliferation of a pluripotent stem cell, causing varying degrees of abnormal proliferation of RBC, WBC, and platelet progenitors in the bone marrow. This abnormal clone does not, however, produce bone marrow fibroblasts, which can proliferate in a polyclonal reactive fashion.

Mutations of the Janus kinase 2 *(JAK2)* gene are responsible for polycythemia vera and a high proportion of cases of ET and primary myelofibrosis. JAK2 is a member of the tyrosine kinase family of enzymes and is involved in signal transduction for erythropoietin, thrombopoietin, and granulocyte colony-stimulating factor (G-CSF) among other entities. The thrombopoietin receptor gene (*MPL*), or the calreticulin (*CALR*) gene is mutated in a significant proportion of ET and primary myelofibrosis patients.

Table 151–1. CLASSIFICATION OF MYELOPROLIFERATIVE DISORDERS

DISORDER	PREDOMINANT FEATURE
Polycythemia vera	Erythrocytosis often with concurrent increased WBC and platelet count
Primary myelofibrosis	Bone marrow fibrosis with extramedullary hematopoiesis
ET	Thrombocytosis
Chronic myelogenous leukemia	Granulocytosis

ESSENTIAL THROMBOCYTHEMIA

(Essential Thrombocytosis; Primary Thrombocythemia)

Essential thrombocythemia (ET) is a myeloproliferative disorder characterized by an increased platelet count, megakaryocytic hyperplasia, and a hemorrhagic or thrombotic tendency. Symptoms and signs may include weakness, headaches, paresthesias, bleeding, splenomegaly, and erythromelalgia with digital ischemia. Diagnosis is based on a platelet count > 450,000/μL, normal RBC mass or normal Hct in the presence of adequate iron stores, and the absence of myelofibrosis, the Philadelphia chromosome (or *BCR-ABL* rearrangement), or any other disorder that could cause thrombocytosis. Treatment is controversial but may include aspirin. Patients > 60 yr and those with previous thromboses and transient ischemic attacks are at higher risk for subsequent thromboembolic events. Data suggest that risk of thrombosis is not proportional to platelet count.

Etiology

ET is a clonal hematopoietic stem cell disorder that causes increased platelet production. ET usually occurs with bimodal peaks of between ages 50 and 70 yr and a separate peak among young females.

A JAK2 enzyme mutation, *JAK2V617F*, is present in about 50% of patients; JAK2 is a member of the tyrosine kinase family of enzymes and is involved in signal transduction for erythropoietin, thrombopoietin, and G-CSF among other entities. Other patients have mutations in exon 9 of the calreticulin gene (*CALR*) and a few have acquired somatic thrombopoietin receptor gene mutations (*MPL*). Some myelodysplastic syndromes (refractory anemia with ringed sideroblasts and thrombocytosis [RARS-T] and the 5q- syndrome) may present with elevated platelet count.

Pathophysiology

Thrombocythemia may lead to

- Microvascular occlusions (usually reversible)
- Large vessel thrombosis
- Serious bleeding

Microvascular occlusions often involve small vessels of the distal extremities (causing erythromelalgia), the eye (causing ocular migraine), or the CNS (causing transient ischemic attack).

The risk of large vessel thrombosis causing deep venous thrombosis or pulmonary embolism is increased, but the risk does not increase proportional to the platelet count.

Bleeding is more likely with extreme thrombocytosis (ie, about 1.5 million platelets/μL); it is due to an acquired deficiency of von Willebrand factor caused because the platelets adsorb and proteolyze high molecular weight von Willebrand multimers.

Symptoms and Signs

Common symptoms are

- Weakness
- Bruising and bleeding
- Gout

- Ocular migraines
- Paresthesias of the hands and feet
- Thrombotic events

Thrombosis may cause symptoms in the affected site (eg, neurologic deficits with stroke or transient ischemic attack; leg pain, swelling or both with lower extremity thrombosis; chest pain and dyspnea with pulmonary embolism).

Bleeding is usually mild and manifests as epistaxis, easy bruisability, or GI bleeding. However, serious bleeding may occur in a small percentage of cases.

Erythromelalgia (burning pain in hands and feet, with warmth, erythema, and sometimes digital ischemia) may occur. Splenomegaly (usually not extending > 3 cm below the left costal margin) occurs in < 50% of patients. Hepatomegaly may rarely occur. Thrombosis may cause recurrent spontaneous abortions.

Diagnosis

- CBC and peripheral blood smear
- Exclusion of causes of secondary thrombocythemia
- Cytogenetic studies
- *JAK2* mutation by PCR, and, if negative, *CALR* or *MPL* mutation analysis
- Possibly bone marrow examination

ET is a diagnosis of exclusion and should be considered in patients in whom common reactive causes (see p. 1165) and other myeloproliferative disorders are excluded.

If ET is suspected, CBC, peripheral blood smear, iron studies and cytogenetic studies, including Philadelphia chromosome or BCR-ABL assay, should be done to distinguish ET from other myeloproliferative disorders that cause thrombocytosis. The diagnosis of ET requires a normal Hct, MCV, and iron studies; absence of the Philadelphia chromosome and *BCR-ABL* translocation; and absence of teardrop-shaped RBCs.

The platelet count can be > 1,000,000/μL but may be as low as 450,000/μL. Platelet count may decrease during pregnancy. The peripheral smear may show giant platelets and megakaryocyte fragments.

World Health Organization guidelines suggest that a bone marrow biopsy showing increased numbers of enlarged, mature megakaryocytes is required for a diagnosis of ET, so biopsy is recommended, if possible. Biopsy will also help rule out other myeloproliferative or myelodysplastic syndromes, such as primary myelofibrosis, which often initially manifests as isolated thrombocytosis. The bone marrow in ET shows megakaryocytic hyperplasia, with an abundance of platelets being released. Bone marrow iron is usually present.

Testing for the *JAK2V617F* mutation should be done; its presence helps distinguish ET from other causes of thrombocythemia. However, the *JAK2V617F* mutation also is present in many patients with polycythemia vera (PV). Thus, those few cases of PV that initially manifest with thrombocytosis can be confused with ET (thrombocytosis may predominate in PV either because of plasma volume expansion or because the other manifestations of polycythemia have not yet appeared.

If the *JAK2* mutation is not present, testing for *CALR* and *MPL* should be done.

Prognosis

Life expectancy is near normal. Although symptoms are common, the course of the disease is often benign. Serious arterial and venous thrombotic complications are rare but can be life-threatening. Leukemic transformation occurs in < 2% of patients but may increase after exposure to cytotoxic therapy, including hydroxyurea. Some patients develop secondary myelofibrosis, particularly men with the *JAK2V617F* or *CALR* type 1 mutations.

Treatment

- Aspirin
- Platelet-lowering drugs (eg, hydroxyurea, anagrelide)
- Rarely plateletpheresis
- Rarely cytotoxic agents
- Rarely interferon
- Rarely stem cell transplantation

For mild vasomotor symptoms (eg, headache, mild digital ischemia, erythromelalgia) and to decrease the risk of thrombosis in low-risk patients, aspirin 81 mg po once/day is usually sufficient but a higher dose may be used if necessary. Severe migraine may require platelet count reduction for control. The utility of aspirin during pregnancy is unproven.

Aminocaproic acid is effective in controlling hemorrhage due to acquired von Willebrand disease for minor procedures such as dental work. Major procedures may require optimization of platelet counts.

Allogeneic stem cell transplantation is rarely used in ET but can be effective in younger patients if other treatments are unsuccessful and a suitable donor is available.

Lowering platelet count: Because prognosis is usually good, potentially toxic drugs that lower the platelet count should not be used just to normalize the platelet count in asymptomatic patients. Generally agreed-upon indications for platelet-lowering therapy include

- Previous thromboses or transient ischemic attack
- Age > 60 yr
- Significant bleeding
- Need for a surgical procedure in patients with extreme thrombocytosis and low ristocetin cofactor activity
- Sometimes severe migraine

However, there are no data that prove cytotoxic therapy to reduce the platelet count lowers thrombotic risk, or improves survival.

Drugs used to lower platelet count include anagrelide, interferon alfa-2b, and hydroxyurea. Hydroxyurea is generally considered the drug of choice for short-term use. Because anagrelide and hydroxyurea cross the placenta, they are not used during pregnancy; interferon alfa-2b can be used in pregnant women when necessary. Interferon is the safest therapy for migraine.

Hydroxyurea should be prescribed only by specialists familiar with its use and monitoring. It is started at a dose of 500 to 1000 mg po once/day. Patients are monitored with a weekly CBC. If the WBC count falls to < 4000/μL, hydroxyurea is withheld and reinstituted at 50% of the dose when the value normalizes. When a steady state is achieved, the interval between CBCs is lengthened to 2 wk and then to 4 wk. There is no specific target platelet count; the aim of therapy is a platelet count that restores ristocetin cofactor activity if bleeding is the problem or that alleviates symptoms.

Platelet removal (plateletpheresis) has been used in rare patients with serious hemorrhage or recurrent thrombosis or before emergency surgery to immediately reduce the platelet count. However, plateletpheresis is rarely necessary and its effects are transient. Hydroxyurea or anagrelide do not provide an immediate effect but should be started at the same time as pheresis.

KEY POINTS

- ET is a clonal abnormality of a multipotent hematopoietic stem cell resulting in increased platelets.
- Patients are at risk of microvascular thrombosis, hemorrhage, and rarely macrovascular thrombosis.
- ET is a diagnosis of exclusion; in particular, other myeloproliferative disorders and reactive (secondary) thrombocytosis must be ruled out.
- Asymptomatic patients require no therapy. Aspirin is usually effective for microvascular events (ocular migraine, erythromelalgia and transient ischemic attacks).
- Some patients with extreme thrombocytosis require more aggressive treatment to control the platelet count; and such measures include hydroxyurea, anagrelide, interferon alfa-2b, or plateletpheresis.

REACTIVE THROMBOCYTOSIS

(Secondary Thrombocythemia)

Reactive thrombocytosis is an elevated platelet count (> 450,000/μL) that develops secondary to another disorder.

Some causes of reactive thrombocytosis include

- Chronic inflammatory disorders (eg, RA, inflammatory bowel disease, TB, sarcoidosis, granulomatosis with polyangiitis)
- Acute infection
- Hemorrhage
- Iron deficiency
- Hemolysis
- Cancer
- Splenectomy or hyposplenism

There are also congenital familial thrombocytoses such as those due to thrombopoietin and thrombopoietin receptor gene mutations. For thrombocytosis that is not secondary to another disorder, see p. 1163.

Platelet function is usually normal. Unlike in ET, reactive thrombocytosis does not increase the risk of thrombotic or hemorrhagic complications unless patients have severe arterial disease or prolonged immobility.

With secondary thrombocytosis, the platelet count is usually < 1,000,000/μL, and the cause may be obvious from the history and physical examination (perhaps with confirmatory testing). CBC and peripheral blood smear should help suggest iron deficiency or hemolysis.

If a cause of secondary thrombocythemia is not obvious, patients should be evaluated for a myeloproliferative disorder. Such evaluation may include cytogenetic studies, including Philadelphia chromosome or *BCR-ABL* assay, and possibly bone marrow examination, especially in patients with anemia, macrocytosis, leukopenia, and/or hepatosplenomegaly.

Treatment of the underlying disorder usually returns the platelet count to normal.

PRIMARY MYELOFIBROSIS

(Agnogenic Myeloid Metaplasia; Myelofibrosis with Myeloid Metaplasia)

Primary myelofibrosis (PMF) is a chronic myeloproliferative disorder characterized by bone marrow fibrosis, splenomegaly, and anemia with nucleated and teardrop-shaped RBCs. Diagnosis requires bone marrow examination and exclusion of other conditions that can cause myelofibrosis (secondary myelofibrosis). Treatment is often supportive, but JAK inhibitors such as ruxolitinib may decrease symptoms, and stem cell transplantation may be curative.

Pathophysiology

Myelofibrosis is a reactive, reversible increase in bone marrow collagen often with extramedullary hematopoiesis (primarily in the spleen). Myelofibrosis may be

- Primary (more common)
- Secondary to a number of hematologic, malignant, and nonmalignant conditions (see Table 151–2).

PMF results from neoplastic transformation of a multipotent bone marrow stem cell. These PMF progeny cells stimulate bone marrow fibroblasts (which are not part of the neoplastic transformation) to secrete excessive collagen. The peak incidence of PMF is between 50 and 70 yr and predominantly in males.

Mutations of the Janus kinase 2 (*JAK2*) gene are responsible a high proportion of cases of PMF. JAK2 is a member of the tyrosine kinase family of enzymes and is involved in signal transduction for erythropoietin, thrombopoietin, and G-CSF

Table 151–2. CONDITIONS ASSOCIATED WITH MYELOFIBROSIS

CONDITION	EXAMPLES
Malignancies	Cancer with bone marrow metastases Hodgkin lymphoma Leukemias (particularly chronic myelogenous leukemia and hairy cell leukemia) Multiple myeloma Non-Hodgkin lymphoma PV (15 to 30% of patients) ET
Hematologic disorders	ET PV
Infections	Osteomyelitis TB
Primary pulmonary hypertension	–
Toxins	Benzene Thorium dioxide X- or γ-radiation
Autoimmune disorders (rarely)	SLE Systemic sclerosis

among other entities. Mutations of the thrombopoietin receptor gene (*MPL*), or the calreticulin (*CALR*) gene also may be the cause of PMF.

In PMF, nucleated RBCs (normoblasts) and myelocytes are released into the circulation (leukoerythroblastosis) when there is extramedullary hematopoiesis (ie, non-marrow organs have taken over blood cell production because of the fibrosed marrow). Serum LDH level is often elevated. Bone marrow failure eventually occurs, with consequent anemia and thrombocytopenia. Rapidly progressive, chemotherapy-incurable acute leukemia develops in about 30% of patients.

Malignant or acute myelofibrosis, has a more rapidly progressive downhill course and is generally due to an acute leukemia.

Symptoms and Signs

In many patients, myelofibrosis is asymptomatic. Other patients have symptoms of anemia, splenomegaly, or, in later stages, general malaise, weight loss, fever, or splenic infarction. Hepatomegaly occurs in some patients. Lymphadenopathy is rare. Severe extramedullary hematopoiesis can disturb the function of organs in which it occurs, including the brain.

Diagnosis

- CBC and peripheral blood smear
- Bone marrow examination
- Testing for *JAK2*, *CALR*, and *MPL* mutations

PMF should be suspected in patients with splenomegaly, splenic infarction, and anemia. If the disorder is suspected, CBC should be done and peripheral blood morphology and a bone marrow biopsy should be examined. If myelofibrosis is present on bone marrow examination (as detected by reticulin staining or trichrome staining indicating excess collagen and osteosclerosis), other disorders associated with myelofibrosis (see Table 151–2) should be excluded by appropriate clinical and laboratory evaluation. The diagnosis of PMF is confirmed by detecting a mutation in *JAK2*, *CALR*, or *MPL*.

Anemia is typically present and usually increases over time. Blood cell morphology is variable. RBCs are poikilocytic. Reticulocytosis and polychromatophilia may be present; teardrop-shaped RBCs (dacryocytes) are characteristic morphologic features. Nucleated RBCs and neutrophil precursors are typically present in peripheral blood. WBC counts are usually increased but are highly variable. In advanced stages, myeloblasts may be present, even in the absence of acute leukemia. Platelet counts initially may be high, normal, or decreased; however, thrombocytopenia tends to supervene as the disorder progresses.

Prognosis

The median survival in PMF is 5 yr from onset, but variation is wide; some patients have a rapidly progressing disorder, including development of acute myelogenous leukemia, with short survival, but most have a more indolent course. Only allogeneic stem cell transplantation is curative.

Unfavorable prognostic markers include Hb < 10 g/dL, a history of transfusions, leukocytosis, and a platelet count < 100,000/μL. Patients in the least favorable risk group usually survive < 1 yr. Several prognostic scoring systems are available to predict survival.

Treatment

- Symptomatic therapy
- Sometimes allogeneic stem cell transplantation
- Sometimes ruxolitinib

Treatment is directed at symptoms and complications. Some patients can be observed without treatment.

In early PMF, interferon has been shown to reduce marrow fibrosis and spleen size.

Currently, for advanced PMF, the nonspecific JAK pathway inhibitor ruxolitinib is the therapy of choice. It can also be combined with thalidomide for maintaining the platelet count, which often falls with ruxolitinib. Ruxolitinib is effective whether or not a *JAK2* mutation or splenomegaly is present. Care must be taken when stopping ruxolitinib because a withdrawal syndrome may occur, with significant worsening of symptoms in part due to splenic enlargement and a rebound in inflammatory cytokines. Low-dose corticosteroids may be used short term for symptom control.

For younger patients with advanced disease, allogeneic stem cell transplantation may be beneficial. Nonmyeloablative allogeneic stem cell transplantation has been successfully used even in older patients.

Androgens, erythropoietin, splenectomy, chemotherapy, thalidomide, lenalidomide, and splenic embolization and radiation therapy have been tried for palliation. However, these are of limited effectiveness. Splenectomy should be avoided if possible; splenic irradiation has only a temporary effect and can cause severe neutropenia and infection.

KEY POINTS

- Myelofibrosis is excessive bone marrow fibrosis, often with loss of hematopoietic cells and consequent extramedullary hematopoiesis.
- Myelofibrosis is often primary but may occur secondary to a number of hematologic, malignant, and nonmalignant disorders, including PV and essential thrombocytosis.
- PMF is a clonal hematopoietic disorder and often involves *JAK2*, *CALR*, or *MPL* mutations.
- Diagnose with blood count, examination of peripheral blood smear and bone marrow, and molecular testing for *JAK2*, *MPL*, and/or *CALR* mutations.
- Some patients have an indolent course and do not require therapy immediately, but some patients have a rapidly progressive downhill course with short survival.
- Ruxolitinib is the therapy of choice for control of symptoms; allogeneic stem cell transplantation may be beneficial in selected cases.

POLYCYTHEMIA VERA

(Primary Polycythemia)

Polycythemia vera (PV) is a chronic myeloproliferative disorder characterized by an increase in morphologically normal red cells, white cells and platelets; erythrocytosis is typical. Ten to 30 % of patients eventually develop myelofibrosis and marrow failure; acute leukemia occurs spontaneously in 1.0 to 2.5 %. There is an increased risk of bleeding and arterial or venous thrombosis. Common manifestations include splenomegaly, microvascular events (eg, transient ischemic attacks, erythromelalgia, ocular

migraine), and aquagenic pruritus (itching triggered by exposure to hot water). Diagnosis is made by CBC, testing for *JAK2* or *CALR* mutations, and clinical criteria. Treatment involves phlebotomy, low-dose aspirin, ruxolitinib, interferon, and rarely stem cell transplantation.

PV is the most common of the myeloproliferative disorders; incidence in the US is estimated to be 1.9/100,000, with incidence increasing with age. The mean age at diagnosis is about 60 yr.

Pathophysiology

PV involves increased production of all cell lines, including RBCs, WBCs, and platelets. Thus, PV is a panmyelosis because of elevations of all 3 peripheral blood components. Increased production confined to the RBC line is termed erythrocytosis; isolated erythrocytosis may occur with PV but is more commonly due to other causes (secondary erythrocytosis). In PV, RBC production proceeds independently of erythropoietin.

Extramedullary hematopoiesis may occur in the spleen, liver, and other sites that have the potential for blood cell formation. In PV, in contrast to the secondary erythrocytoses, the red cell mass increase is often initially masked by an increase in the plasma volume that leaves the hematocrit in the normal range. This is particularly the case in women, who most commonly present with hepatic vein thrombosis and a normal Hct.

Iron deficiency may eventually occur because of the increased need for iron to produce RBCs. In the presence of iron deficiency of any kind, RBCs become increasingly smaller (microcytic erythrocytosis) because the red cell hemoglobin concentration (MCHC) is defended at the expense of red cell volume (MCV). Although patients with iron deficiency from other causes become anemic, patients with PV have increased RBC production and thus even when iron-deficient initially have a *normal* Hct level but microcytic RBC indices ; this combination of findings (iron-limited hematopoiesis) is a hallmark of PV.

Eventually, progression leads to a spent phase, with a phenotype indistinguishable from PMF.

Transformation to acute leukemia is rare, although the risk is increased with exposure to alkylating agents, such as chlorambucil, radioactive phosphorus (mostly of historic significance), and possibly hydroxyurea.

Genetic basis: PV is caused by clonal hematopoiesis due to a mutation in an hematopoietic stem cell.

Mutations of the Janus kinase 2 (*JAK2*) gene are responsible in a high proportion of cases of PV. *JAK2* is a member of the tyrosine kinase family of enzymes and is involved in signal transduction for erythropoietin, thrombopoietin, and G-CSF among other entities. Specifically, the *JAK2V617F* mutation or the *JAK2* exon12 mutation is present in most patients with PV. However, recently calreticulin (*CALR*) mutations have been found in PV patients lacking a *JAK2* mutation, and lymphocytic adaptor protein (*LNK*) mutations have been found in patients with isolated erythrocytosis. These mutations lead to sustained activation of the JAK2 kinase, which causes excess blood cell production independent of erythropoietin.

Complications: Complications of PV include

- Thrombosis
- Bleeding

In PV, blood volume expands and the increased number of RBCs can cause hyperviscosity. Hyperviscosity predisposes to macrovascular thrombosis, resulting in stroke, deep venous thrombosis, MI, retinal artery or vein occlusion, splenic infarction (often with a friction rub), or, particularly in women, the Budd-Chiari syndrome, Microvascular events (eg, transient ischemic attack, erythromelalgia, ocular migraine) also may occur. There is no evidence that the increase in other cell lines (leukocytosis, thrombocytosis) increases risk of thrombosis.

Platelets may function abnormally if the platelet count is about 1,500,000/μL due to acquired deficiency of von Willebrand factor because the platelets adsorb and proteolyze high molecular weight von Willebrand multimers. This acquired von Willebrand disease predisposes to increased bleeding.

Increased cell turnover may cause hyperuricemia, increasing the risk of gout and urate kidney stones. PV patients are prone to acid-peptic disease due to *H. pylori* infection.

Symptoms and Signs

PV itself is often asymptomatic, but eventually the increased red cell volume and viscosity cause weakness, headache, light-headedness, visual disturbances, fatigue, and dyspnea. Pruritus often occurs, particularly after a hot bath or shower (aquagenic pruritus) and may be the earliest symptom. The face may be red and the retinal veins engorged. The palms and feet may be red, warm, and painful, sometimes with digital ischemia (erythromelalgia). Over 30% of patients have splenomegaly (which may be massive).

Thrombosis may cause symptoms in the affected site (eg, neurologic deficits with stroke or transient ischemic attack, leg pain, swelling or both with lower extremity thrombosis, unilateral vision loss with retinal vascular occlusion).

Bleeding (typically GI) occurs in about 10% of patients.

Hypermetabolism can cause low-grade fevers and weight loss and suggests progression to secondary myelofibrosis, which is clinically indistinguishable from PMF but has a better prognosis.

Diagnosis

- CBC
- Testing for *JAK2*, *CALR*, or *LNK* mutations (done sequentially)
- Sometimes bone marrow examination and serum erythropoietinlevel
- Sometimes RBC mass determination

PV is often first suspected because of an abnormal CBC (eg, Hb > 18.5 g/dL in men or > 16.5 g/dL in women), but it must be considered in patients with suggestive symptoms or thrombotic events in unusual sites, particularly the Budd-Chiari syndrome (women) or portal vein thrombosis (men). Neutrophils and platelets are often, but not invariably, increased; in patients with only elevated Hct, PV may be present, but secondary erythrocytosis, a more common cause of elevated Hct, must be considered first. PV should also be considered in patients with a normal Hct level but microcytic erythrocytosis and evidence of iron deficiency; this combination of findings can occur with iron-limited hematopoiesis, which is a hallmark of PV.

The challenge in diagnosing PV is that several other myeloproliferative disorders can cause the same genetic mutations and bone marrow findings and because some patients with PV do not initially manifest an elevated Hb level. Thus, multiple findings must be integrated.

Patients suspected of having PV typically should have testing for *JAK2V617F* and *JAK2* exon12 mutations. If these are negative, do testing for *CALR* and *LNK* mutations. The presence of a known causative mutation in a patient with clear erythrocytosis is strongly suggestive of the diagnosis. If erythrocytosis is *not* clearly present, do a direct measure of red cell mass and plasma volume (eg, with chromium-labeled RBCs, although this test is usually available only at specialized centers) to help differentiate between true and relative polycythemia and between PV and other myeloproliferative disorders (which do not have increased red cell mass). If erythrocytosis is present but secondary causes have not been excluded, serum erythropoietin level may be done; patients with PV typically have low or low-normal serum erythropoietin levels; elevated levels suggest secondary erythrocytosis.

Bone marrow examination is not diagnostic of PV. When done, bone marrow examination typically shows panmyelosis, large and clumped megakaryocytes, and sometimes an increase in reticulin fibers. However, no bone marrow findings absolutely differentiate PV from other disorders of excessive erythrocytosis, such as congenital familial polycythemia, or from other myeloprolierative disorders, which is important because PV is the most common myeloproliferative neoplasm.

Acquired von Willebrand disease (as a cause of bleeding) may be diagnosed by showing decreased plasma von Willebrand factor antigen using the ristocetin cofactor test.

Nonspecific laboratory abnormalities that may occur in PV include elevated vitamin B_{12} and B_{12}-binding capacity, hyperuricemia and hyperuricosuria (present in ≥ 30% of patients), and decreased expression of C-mpl (the receptor for thrombopoietin) in megakaryocytes and platelets. These tests are not needed for diagnosis.

Prognosis

Generally, PV is associated with a shortened life span. In a recent retrospective study, median survival was 27 yr but this is anticipated to improve as new therapies become more widely used.

Thrombosis is the most common cause of morbidity and death, followed by the complications of myelofibrosis and development of leukemia. In the future, gene expression profiling or other characteristics may aid in the identification of prognostic subgroups.

Treatment

- Phlebotomy
- Possibly aspirin therapy
- Possibly targeted therapy with ruxolitinib or pegylated interferon. Currently, ruxolitinib is approved in the US only for patients who have not responded to or are intolerant of hydroxyurea.

Because PV is the only form of erythrocytosis for which myelosuppressive therapy may be indicated, accurate diagnosis is critical. Therapy must be individualized according to age, sex, medical status, clinical manifestations, and hematologic findings. However, previous criteria used to stratify treatment by high- or low-risk classification have not been prospectively validated and are not recommended.

Phlebotomy: Phlebotomy is the mainstay of therapy. The targets for phlebotomy are a Hct < 45% in men and < 42% in women. A randomized controlled trial published in 2013 showed that patients randomized to a Hct < 45% had a significantly lower rate of cardiovascular death and thrombosis than did those with a target Hct of 45 to 50%. Indeed, phlebotomy to a Hct < 45 % in men and < 42% in women eliminates the risk of thrombosis.

Initially, 300 to 500 mL of blood are removed every other day. Less blood is removed (ie, 200 to 300 mL twice/wk) from elderly patients and from patients with cardiac or cerebrovascular disorders. Once the Hct is below the target value, it is checked monthly and maintained at this level by additional phlebotomies as needed. If necessary, intravascular volume can be maintained with crystalloid or colloid solutions. Platelets may increase with phlebotomy, but this is transient, and a gradual increase in the platelet count as well as the leukocyte count is a feature of PV and requires no therapy in asymptomatic patients.

In some patients treated only with phlebotomy, the phlebotomy requirement may eventually markedly diminish. This is not a sign of marrow failure (ie, the so-called spent phase) but rather is due to an expansion of plasma volume.

Aspirin: Aspirin alleviates symptoms of microvascular events. Thus, patients with symptoms of erythromelalgia, ocular migraine, or transient ischemic attacks should be given aspirin 81 to 100 mg po once/day unless contraindicated (eg, because of acquired von Willebrand disease); higher doses may be required but clearly increase the risk of hemorrhage. Aspirin does not reduce the incidence of microvascular events and thus is not indicated in asymptomatic PV patients (in the absence of other indications).

Myelosuppressive therapy: Numerous studies have shown that many previously used myelosuppressive treatments, including hydroxyurea, radioactive phosphorus, and alkylating agents such as busulfan and chlorambucil, do not reduce incidence of thrombosis, and fail to improve survival over appropriate phlebotomy. The alkylating agents such as chlorambucil and hydroxyurea also increase the incidence of acute leukemia and solid tumors; these agents are no longer recommended.

If intervention other than phlebotomy is necessary (eg, because of symptoms or thrombotic events), interferon or ruxolitinib are preferred. Anagrelide has been used to control the platelet count but has both cardiac and renal toxicity and can cause anemia.

Interferon alfa-2b or alfa-2a specifically targets the affected cell and not normal stem cells in PV. Its pegylated versions are usually well tolerated and are effective in controlling pruritus and excessive blood production as well as reducing spleen size. About 20 % of patients achieve a complete molecular remission.

Ruxolitinib, a nonspecific JAK inhibitor, is approved for use in PV with inadequate response to or intolerance to hydroxyurea and in post-PV myelofibrosis. In PV, it is usually given at 10 mg po twice/day continued as long as response is occurring without undue toxicity.

Hydroxyurea is in widespread use in PV, but its role is evolving with the advent of JAK inhibitors such as ruxolitinib. Hydroxyurea should be prescribed only by specialists familiar with its use and monitoring. If JAK inhibitor drugs are not available and cytoreduction is needed, hydroxyurea is started at a dose of 500 to 1000 mg po once/day. Patients are monitored with a weekly CBC. If the WBC count falls to < 4000/μL or the platelet count is < 100,000/μL, hydroxyurea is withheld and reinstituted at 50% of the dose when the value normalizes. When a steady state is achieved, the interval between CBCs is lengthened to 2 wk and then to 4 wk.

Treatment of complications: Hyperuricemia should be treated with allopurinol 300 mg po once/day if it causes symptoms or if patients are receiving simultaneous myelosuppressive therapy.

Pruritus may be managed with antihistamines but is often difficult to control; ruxolitinib and interferon are effective. Cholestyramine, cyproheptadine, cimetidine, paroxetine, or PUVA light therapy may also be successful. After bathing, the skin should be dried gently.

KEY POINTS

- PV is a chronic myeloproliferative disorder that involves increased production of RBCs, WBCs, and platelets.
- PV is due to mutations involving *JAK2*, *CALR* or rarely, *LNK* in hematopoietic stem cells that lead to sustained activation of the JAK2 kinase, which causes excess blood cell production.
- Complications include thrombosis, bleeding, and hyperuricemia; some patients eventually develop myelofibrosis or rarely transformation to acute leukemia.
- PV is often first suspected because of an elevated Hb (> 18.5 g/dL in men, > 16.5 g/dL in women); neutrophils and platelets are often, but not invariably, increased.
- Test for *JAK2*, *CALR*, or *LNK* mutations and sometimes obtain bone marrow examination and serum erythropoietin level.
- Phlebotomy to target Hct < 45% in men or < 42% in women is essential; ruxolitinib and interferon are the preferred myelosuppressants. Cytotoxic agents should be avoided if possible and then used only temporarily.

SECONDARY ERYTHROCYTOSIS

(Secondary Polycythemia)

Secondary erythrocytosis is erythrocytosis that develops secondary to disorders that cause tissue hypoxia, inappropriately increase erythropoietin production, or increase sensitivity to erythropoietin.

In secondary erythrocytosis, only RBCs are increased, whereas in PV, RBCs, WBCs, and platelets may be increased. Any elevation of Hb or Hct above normal values for age and sex is considered erythrocytosis.

Common causes of secondary erythrocytosis include

- Smoking
- Chronic arterial hypoxemia
- Tumors (tumor-associated erythrocytosis)
- Use of androgenic steroids
- Surreptitious erythropoietin use

Less common causes include certain congenital disorders such as

- High oxygen-affinity hemoglobinopathies
- Erythropoietin receptor mutations
- Chuvash polycythemia (in which a mutation in the *VHL* gene affects the hypoxia-sensing pathway)
- Proline hydroxylase 2 and hypoxia-inducible factor 2 alpha (*HIF-2α*) mutations

Spurious erythrocytosis may occur with hemoconcentration (eg, due to burns, diarrhea, or diuretics).

In patients who smoke, reversible erythrocytosis results mainly from tissue hypoxia due to elevation of blood carboxyhemoglobin concentration; levels often normalize with smoking cessation.

Patients with chronic hypoxemia (arterial Hb oxygen concentration < 92%), typically due to lung disease, right-to-left intracardiac shunts, renal transplantation, prolonged exposure to high altitudes, or hypoventilation syndromes, often develop erythrocytosis. The primary treatment is to alleviate the underlying condition, but oxygen therapy may help, and phlebotomy may decrease viscosity and alleviate symptoms. Because in some cases the elevated Hct is physiologic, phlebotomy should be limited to the extent necessary to relieve symptoms (in contrast to PV, where the goal is to normalize the hematocrit).

Tumor-associated erythrocytosis can occur when renal tumors, cysts, hepatomas, cerebellar hemangioblastomas, or uterine leiomyomas secrete erythropoietin. Removal of the lesion is curative.

High oxygen–affinity hemoglobinopathies are very rare. This diagnosis is suggested by a family history of erythrocytosis; it is established by measuring the P_{50} (the partial pressure of oxygen at which Hb becomes 50% saturated) and, if possible, determining the complete oxyhemoglobin dissociation curve. Standard Hb electrophoresis may be normal and cannot reliably exclude this cause of erythrocytosis.

Evaluation: Tests done when isolated erythrocytosis is present include

- Arterial oxygen saturation
- Serum erythropoietin levels
- P_{50} to rule out a high oxygen-affinity hemoglobinopathy

A low or normal serum erythropoietin level is diagnostically nonspecific. If PV is suspected, the patient should be worked up as for PV and other causes for inappropriate erythropoietin production such as renal dysfunction should be sought.

Serum erythropoietin level is elevated in patients with hypoxia-induced erythrocytosis (or level is inappropriately normal for their elevated Hct) and patients with tumor-associated erythrocytosis. Patients with elevated erythropoietin levels (and no indication of hypoxia) or microscopic hematuria should undergo abdominal imaging, CNS imaging, or both to seek a renal lesion or other tumor sources of erythropoietin.

P_{50} measures the affinity of Hb for oxygen; a normal result excludes a high-affinity Hb (a familial abnormality) as the cause of erythrocytosis.

152 Overview of Cancer

Cancer is an unregulated proliferation of cells. Its prominent properties are a lack of differentiation of cells, local invasion of adjoining tissue, and, often, metastasis (spread to distant sites through the bloodstream or the lymphatic system). The immune system likely plays a significant role in eliminating early cancers or premalignant cells because immunodeficiency states are associated with an increased incidence of various kinds of cancer, particularly those associated with viral infection, and tumors arising in the lymphatic system and the skin.

The majority of cancers are now curable, particularly if detected at an early stage, and long-term remission is often possible in those detected at later stages. There is still uncertainty as to whether all cancers, particularly breast cancers detected at a very early stage by mammography or prostate cancers detected by prostate-specific antigen (PSA) testing, will progress and become life threatening, but it is certain that early detection of cancer enhances the potential for cure. When cure is not possible, as in many cases of advanced cancer, judicious treatment with radiation therapy, drugs, and/or surgery may improve quality of life and prolong survival. However, in other patients, particularly in the elderly and in those with comorbid conditions, such treatment may be poorly tolerated, and palliative care may be the best choice.

CELLULAR AND MOLECULAR BASIS OF CANCER

Cellular Kinetics

Generation time is the time required for a quiescent cell to complete a cycle in cell division (see see Fig. 152–1) and give rise to 2 daughter cells. Malignant cells, particularly those arising from the bone marrow or lymphatic system, may have a short generation time, and there usually are a smaller percentage of cells in G_0 (resting phase). Initial exponential tumor growth is followed by a plateau phase when cell death nearly equals the rate of formation of daughter cells. The slowing in growth rate may be related to exhaustion of the supply of nutrients and O_2 for the rapidly expanding tumor. Small tumors have a greater percentage of actively dividing cells than do large tumors.

A subpopulation within many tumors, identified by surface proteins, may have the properties of primitive "normal" stem cells, as found in the early embryo. Thus, these cells are capable of entering a proliferative state. They are less susceptible to injury by drugs or irradiation. They are believed to repopulate tumors after surgical, chemical, or radiation treatment.

Cellular kinetics of particular tumors is an important consideration in the design of antineoplastic drug regimens and may influence the dosing schedules and timing intervals of treatment. Many antineoplastic drugs, such as antimetabolites, are most effective if cells are actively dividing, and some drugs work only during a specific phase of the cell cycle and thus require prolonged administration to catch dividing cells during the phase of maximal sensitivity.

Tumor Growth and Metastasis

As a tumor grows, nutrients are provided by direct diffusion from the circulation. Local growth is facilitated by enzymes (eg, proteases) that destroy adjacent tissues. As tumor volume increases, tumor angiogenesis factors, such as vascular endothelial growth factor (VEGF), are produced by tumors to promote formation of the vascular supply required for further tumor growth.

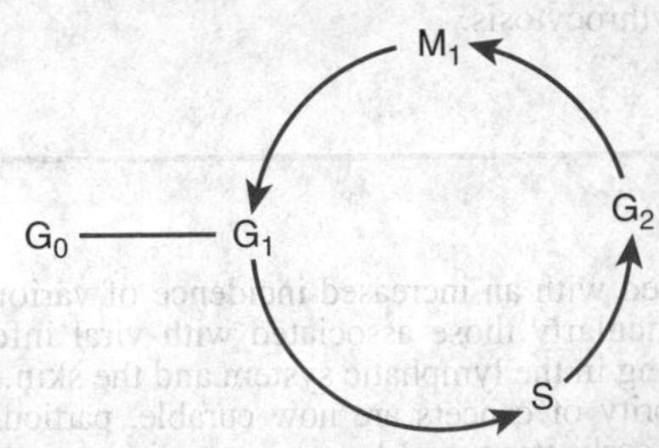

Fig. 152–1. The cell cycle. G_0 = resting phase (nonproliferation of cells); G_1 = variable pre-DNA synthetic phase (12 h to a few days); S = DNA synthesis (usually 2 to 4 h); G_2 = post-DNA synthesis (2 to 4 h)—a tetraploid quantity of DNA is found within cells; M_1 = mitosis (1 to 2 h).

Almost from inception, a tumor may shed cells into the circulation. From animal models, it is estimated that a 1-cm tumor sheds > 1 million cells/24 h into the venous circulation. Circulating tumor cells are present in many patients with advanced cancer and even in some with localized disease. Although most circulating tumor cells die in the intravascular space, an occasional cell may adhere to the vascular endothelium and penetrate into surrounding tissues, generating independent tumors (metastases) at distant sites. Metastatic tumors grow in much the same manner as primary tumors and may subsequently give rise to other metastases.

Experiments suggest that the ability to invade, migrate, and successfully implant and stimulate new blood vessel growth are all important properties of metastatic cells, which likely represent a subset of cells in the primary tumor.

Molecular Abnormalities

Genetic mutations are responsible for the generation of cancer cells and are thus present in all cancers. These mutations alter the quantity or function of protein products that regulate cell growth and division and DNA repair. Two major categories of mutated genes are oncogenes and tumor suppressor genes.

Oncogenes: These are abnormal forms of normal genes (proto-oncogenes) that regulate various aspects of cell growth. Mutation of these genes may result in direct and continuous stimulation of the pathways (eg, cell surface growth factor receptors, intracellular signal transduction pathways, transcription factors, secreted growth factors) that control cellular growth and division, DNA repair, angiogenesis, and other physiologic processes.

There are > 100 known oncogenes that may contribute to human neoplastic transformation. For example, the *RAS* gene encodes the ras protein, which carries signals from membrane bound receptors down the RAS-MAPKinase pathway to the cell nucleus, and thereby regulates cell division. Mutations may result in the inappropriate activation of the ras protein, leading to uncontrolled cell growth. In fact, the ras protein is abnormal in about 25% of human cancers. Other oncogenes have been implicated in specific cancers. These include

- *HER2-NEU* (amplified but not mutated in breast cancer)
- *BCR-ABL* (a translocation of 2 genes that underlies chronic myelocytic leukemia and some B-cell acute lymphocytic leukemias)
- *C-MYC* (Burkitt lymphoma)
- *N-MYC* (small cell lung cancer, neuroblastoma)
- Mutated *EGFR* (adenocarcinoma of the lung)
- *EML4-ALK* (a translocation that activates the ALK tyrosine kinase and causes a unique form of adenocarcinoma of the lung)

Specific oncogenes may have important implications for diagnosis, therapy, and prognosis (see individual discussions under the specific cancer type).

Oncogenes typically result from acquired somatic cell mutations secondary to point mutations (eg, from chemical carcinogens), gene amplification (eg, an increase in the number of copies of a normal gene), or translocations (in which pieces of different genes merge to form a unique sequence). These changes may either increase the activity of the gene product (protein) or change its function. Occasionally, mutation of genes results in inheritance of a cancer predisposition, as in the inherited cancer syndrome associated with mutation and loss of function of *BRCA1*, *BRCA2*, or *p53*.

Tumor suppressor genes: Genes such as the *p53* gene play a role in normal cell division and DNA repair and are critical for detecting inappropriate growth signals or DNA damage in cells. If these genes, as a result of inherited or acquired mutations, become unable to function, the system for monitoring DNA integration becomes inefficient, cells with spontaneous genetic mutations persist and proliferate, and tumors result.

As with most genes, 2 alleles are present that encode for each tumor suppressor gene. A defective copy of one gene may be inherited, leaving only one functional allele for the individual tumor suppressor gene. If a mutation is acquired in the other allele, the normal protective mechanism of the 2nd normal tumor suppressor gene is lost. For example, the retinoblastoma (*RB*) gene encodes for the protein Rb, which regulates the cell cycle by stopping DNA replication. Mutations in the *RB* gene family occur in many human cancers, allowing affected cells to divide continuously.

Another important regulatory protein, p53, prevents replication of damaged DNA in normal cells and promotes cell death (apoptosis) in cells with abnormal DNA. Inactive or altered p53 allows cells with abnormal DNA to survive and divide. Mutations are passed to daughter cells, conferring a high probability of replicating error-prone DNA, and neoplastic transformation results. The *p53* gene is defective in many human cancers. As with oncogenes, mutation of tumor suppressor genes such as *p53* or *RB* in germ cell lines may result in vertical transmission and a higher incidence of cancer in offspring.

Chromosomal abnormalities: Gross chromosomal abnormalities (see p. 2491) can occur through deletion, translocation, or duplication. If these alterations activate or inactivate genes that result in a proliferative advantage over normal cells, then a tumor may develop. Chromosomal abnormalities occur in most human cancers. In some congenital diseases (Bloom syndrome, Fanconi anemia, Down syndrome), DNA repair processes are defective and chromosomes breaks are frequent, putting children at high risk of developing acute leukemia and lymphomas.

Other influences: Most epithelial cancers likely result from a sequence of mutations that lead to neoplastic conversion. For example, the development of tumor in familial polyposis takes place through a sequence of genetic events: epithelium hyperproliferation (loss of a suppressor gene on chromosome 5), early adenoma (change in DNA methylation), intermediate adenoma (overactivity of the *RAS* oncogene), late adenoma (loss of a suppressor gene on chromosome 18), and finally, cancer (loss of a gene on chromosome 17). Further genetic changes may be required for metastasis.

Telomeres are nucleoprotein complexes that cap the ends of chromosomes and maintain their integrity. In normal tissue, telomere shortening (which occurs with aging) results in a finite limit in cell division. The enzyme telomerase, if activated in tumor cells, provides for new telomere synthesis and allows continuous proliferation of tumors.

Environmental Factors

Infections: Viruses contribute to the pathogenesis of human cancers (see Table 152–1). Pathogenesis may occur through the integration of viral genetic elements into the host DNA. These new genes are expressed by the host; they may affect cell growth or division or disrupt normal host genes required for control of cell growth and division. Alternatively, viral infection may result in immune dysfunction, leading to decreased immune surveillance for early tumors.

Bacteria may also cause cancer. *Helicobacter pylori* infection increases the risk of several kinds of cancer (gastric adenocarcinoma, gastric lymphoma, mucosa-associated lymphoid tissue [MALT] lymphoma).

Parasites of some types can lead to cancer. *Schistosoma haematobium* causes chronic inflammation and fibrosis of the bladder, which may lead to cancer. *Opisthorchis sinensis* has been linked to carcinoma of the pancreas and bile ducts.

Table 152–1. CANCER-ASSOCIATED VIRUSES

VIRUS	ASSOCIATED CANCER
Epstein-Barr virus	Burkitt lymphoma Nasopharyngeal carcinoma
Hepatitis B or hepatitis C virus	Hepatocellular carcinoma
Human herpesvirus 8	Kaposi sarcoma
Human papilloma viruses	Anal carcinoma Cervical carcinoma Head and neck carcinoma
Human T-lymphotropic virus	T-cell lymphomas

Radiation: Ultraviolet radiation may induce skin cancer (eg, basal and squamous cell carcinoma, melanoma) by damaging DNA. This DNA damage consists of formation of thymidine dimers, which may escape excision and resynthesis of a normal DNA strand because of inherent defects in DNA repair (eg, xeroderma pigmentosum) or through rare, random events.

Ionizing radiation is also carcinogenic. For example, survivors of the atomic bomb explosions in Hiroshima and Nagasaki have a higher-than-expected incidence of leukemia and other cancers. Similarly, exposure to therapeutic irradiation may lead to leukemia, breast cancer, and other solid tumors years after exposure. Use of x-rays in diagnostic imaging studies is thought to increase risk of cancer (see p. 3221). Industrial exposure (eg, to uranium by mine workers, to asbestos) is linked to development of lung cancer after a 15- to 20-yr latency. Long-term exposure to occupational irradiation or to internally deposited thorium dioxide predisposes people to angiosarcomas and acute nonlymphocytic leukemia.

Exposure to the radioactive gas radon, which is released from soil, increases the risk of lung cancer. Normally, radon disperses rapidly into the atmosphere and causes no harm. However, when a building is placed on soil with high radon content, radon can accumulate within the building, sometimes producing sufficiently high levels in the air to cause harm. In exposed people who also smoke, the risk of lung cancer is further increased.

Drugs and chemicals: Estrogen in oral contraceptives may slightly increase the risk of breast cancer, but this risk decreases over time. Estrogen and progestin used for hormone replacement therapy also increase the risk of breast cancer. Diethylstilbestrol (DES) increases the risk of breast cancer in women who took the drug and increases the risk of vaginal carcinoma in daughters of these women who were exposed before birth. Long-term use of anabolic steroids may increase the risk of liver cancer. Treatment of cancer with chemotherapy drugs alone or with radiation therapy increases the risk of developing a second cancer.

Chemical carcinogens can induce gene mutations and result in uncontrolled growth and tumor formation (see Table 152–2). Other substances, called co-carcinogens, have little or no inherent carcinogenic potency but enhance the carcinogenic effect of another agent when exposed simultaneously.

Dietary substances: Certain substances consumed in the diet can increase the risk of cancer. For instance, a diet high in fat and obesity itself have been linked to an increased risk of colon, breast, and possibly prostate cancer. People who drink large amounts of alcohol are at much higher risk of developing head and neck and esophageal cancer. A diet high in smoked

Table 152–2. COMMON CHEMICAL CARCINOGENS

CARCINOGENS	TYPE OF CANCER
Environmental and industrial	
Aromatic amines	Bladder cancer
Arsenic	Lung cancer Skin cancer
Asbestos	Lung cancer Mesothelioma
Benzene	Leukemia
Chromates	Lung cancer
Diesel exhaust	Lung cancer
Formaldehyde	Nasal cancer Nasopharyngeal cancer
Hair dyes	Bladder cancer
Ionizing radiation	Leukemia
Manufactured mineral fibers	Lung cancer
Nickel	Lung cancer Nasal sinus cancer
Painting materials	Lung cancer
Pesticides, nonarsenic	Lung cancer
Radon	Lung cancer
Radiation therapy	Leukemia
Ultraviolet radiation	Skin cancer
Vinyl chloride	Hepatic angiosarcoma
Lifestyle	
Betel nuts	Oropharyngeal cancer
Tobacco	Bladder cancer Cervical cancer Esophageal cancer Head and neck cancer Kidney cancer Lung cancer Pancreatic cancer Stomach cancer
Drugs*	
Alkylating drugs (cyclophosphamide, platinum analogs)	Leukemia
Diethylstilbestrol (DES)	Cervicovaginal cancer in women exposed in utero
Oxymetholone	Liver cancer
Topoisomerase inhibitors (anthracyclines, etoposide)	Leukemia

*Health care practitioners exposed to antineoplastic drugs are also at risk of adverse effects on reproduction.

and pickled foods or in meats cooked at a high temperature increases the risk of developing stomach cancer. People who are overweight or obese have a higher risk of cancer of the breast, endometrium, colon, kidney, and esophagus.

Physical factors: Chronic skin, lung, GI, or thyroid inflammation may predispose to development of cancer. For example, patients with long-standing inflammatory bowel disease (ulcerative colitis) have an increased risk of colorectal carcinoma. Sunlight and tanning light exposure increases the risk of skin cancers and melanoma.

Immunologic Disorders

Immune system dysfunction as a result of inherited genetic mutation, acquired disorders, aging, or immunosuppressants interferes with normal immune surveillance of early tumors and results in higher rates of cancer. Known cancer-associated immune disorders include

- Ataxia-telangiectasia (acute lymphocytic leukemia [ALL], brain tumors, gastric cancer)
- Wiskott-Aldrich syndrome (lymphoma, ALL)
- X-linked agammaglobulinemia (lymphoma, ALL)
- Immune deficiency secondary to immunosuppressants or HIV infection (large cell lymphoma, cervical cancer, head and neck cancer, Kaposi sarcoma)
- Rheumatologic conditions, such as SLE, RA, and Sjögren syndrome (B-cell lymphoma)
- Fanconi anemia (AML)

CANCER DIAGNOSIS

A diagnosis of cancer may be suspected based on history and physical examination but requires confirmation by tumor biopsy and histopathologic examination. Sometimes the first indication is an abnormal laboratory test result (eg, anemia resulting from colon cancer).

A complete history and physical examination may reveal unexpected clues to early cancer.

History

Physicians must be aware of predisposing factors and must specifically ask about familial cancer, environmental exposure (including smoking history), and prior or present illnesses (eg, autoimmune disorders, previous immunosuppressive therapy, hepatitis B or hepatitis C, HIV infection, abnormal Papanicolaou [Pap] test, human papillomavirus [HPV] infection). Symptoms suggesting occult cancer can include

- Fatigue
- Weight loss
- Fevers
- Night sweats
- Cough
- Hemoptysis
- Hematemesis
- Hematochezia
- Change in bowel habits
- Persistent pain

Physical examination

Particular attention should be paid to skin, lymph nodes, lungs, breasts, abdomen, and testes. Prostate, rectal, and vaginal examinations are also important. Findings help direct further testing, including x-rays and biopsies.

Testing

Tests include imaging tests, serum tumor markers, and biopsy; one or more may be indicated in patients with a suggestive history or physical or laboratory findings.

Imaging tests often include plain x-rays, ultrasonography, CT, PET, and MRI. These tests assist in identifying abnormalities, determining qualities of a mass (solid or cystic), providing dimensions, and establishing the relationship to surrounding structures, which may be important if surgery or biopsy is being considered.

Serum tumor markers may offer corroborating evidence in patients with findings suggestive of a specific cancer (see p. 1218). Most are not used as routine screening tests, except in high-risk patients. Useful examples include

- α-Fetoprotein (hepatocellular carcinoma, testicular carcinoma)
- Carcinoembryonic antigen (colon cancer)
- β-human chorionic gonadotropin (choriocarcinoma, testicular carcinoma)
- Serum immunoglobulins (multiple myeloma)
- DNA probes (eg, *BCR* probe to identify a chromosomal 9-22 translocation in chronic myelogenous leukemia)
- CA 125 (ovarian cancer)
- CA 27-29 (breast cancer)
- Prostate specific antigen (prostate cancer)

Some of these serum tumor markers may be most useful in monitoring the response to treatment rather than in tumor detection.

Biopsy to confirm the diagnosis and tissue of origin is almost always required when cancer is suspected or detected. The choice of biopsy site is usually determined by ease of access and degree of invasiveness. If lymphadenopathy is present, fine-needle or core biopsy may yield the tumor type; if nondiagnostic, open biopsy is indicated. Other biopsy routes include bronchoscopy for easily accessible mediastinal or central pulmonary tumors, percutaneous liver biopsy if liver lesions are present, and CT- or ultrasound-guided biopsy of lung or soft tissue masses. If these procedures are not suitable, open biopsy may be necessary.

Grading is a histologic measure of tumor aggressiveness and provides important prognostic information. It is determined by examining the biopsy specimen. Grade is based on the morphologic appearance of tumor cells, including the appearance of the nuclei, cytoplasm, and nucleoli; frequency of mitoses; and amount of necrosis. For many cancers, grading scales have been developed.

Molecular tests such as chromosomal analysis, fluorescent in situ hybridization (FISH), PCR, and cell surface antigens (eg, in lymphomas, leukemias, lung, and GI cancers) help delineate the origin of metastatic cancers, particularly for cancers of unknown primary origin, and may be helpful in selecting therapy.

Staging

Once a histologic diagnosis is made, staging (ie, determination of the extent of disease) helps in treatment decision-making and influences prognosis. Clinical staging uses data from the history, physical examination, imaging tests, laboratory tests, and biopsy of bone marrow, lymph nodes, or other sites of suspected disease. For staging of specific neoplasms, see details in the organ-relevant chapter.

Imaging tests: Imaging tests, especially CT, PET, and MRI, can detect metastases to brain, lungs, or abdominal viscera, including the adrenal glands, retroperitoneal lymph nodes, liver, and spleen. MRI (with gadolinium contrast) is the procedure of choice for recognition and evaluation of brain tumors, both primary and metastatic. PET scanning is increasingly being used to determine the metabolic activity of a suspect lymph node or mass. Integrated PET–CT can be valuable, especially in lung, head and neck, and breast cancer and in lymphoma.

Ultrasonography can be used to study breast, orbital, thyroid, cardiac, pericardial, hepatic, pancreatic, renal, testicular, and retroperitoneal masses. It may guide percutaneous biopsies and differentiate fluid-filled cysts from solid masses.

Nuclear scans can identify several types of metastases. Bone scans identify abnormal bone growth (ie, osteoblastic activity) before it is visible on plain x-ray. Thus, this technique is useless in neoplasms that are purely lytic (eg, multiple myeloma); routine bone x-rays are the study of choice in such diseases.

Laboratory tests: Serum chemistries and enzymes may help staging. Elevated liver enzyme (alkaline phosphatase, LDH, ALT) levels and elevated bilirubin levels suggest the presence of liver metastases. Elevated alkaline phosphatase and serum Ca may be the first evidence of bone metastases. Elevated BUN or creatinine levels may indicate an obstructive uropathy secondary to a pelvic mass, intrarenal obstruction from tubular precipitation of myeloma protein, or uric acid nephropathy from lymphoma or other cancers. Elevated uric acid levels often occur in patients with rapidly proliferating tumors and in those with myeloproliferative and lymphoproliferative disorders.

Invasive tests: Mediastinoscopy (see p. 386) is especially valuable in the staging of non–small cell lung cancer. When mediastinal lymph node involvement is found, patients may benefit from initial chemoradiation and subsequent tumor resection.

Bone marrow aspiration and biopsy are especially useful in detecting metastases from malignant lymphomas and small cell lung cancer. Bone marrow biopsy is positive at diagnosis in 50 to 70% of patients with malignant lymphoma (low and intermediate grade) and in 15 to 18% of patients with small cell lung cancer. Bone marrow biopsy should be done in patients with unexplained hematologic abnormalities (ie, anemia, thrombocytopenia, pancytopenia).

Biopsy of regional lymph nodes is part of the evaluation of many tumors, such as breast, lung, or colon cancers. Removal of a sentinel lymph node (as defined by uptake of dye or radioactivity injected into the tumor site) may allow limited but definitive lymph node sampling.

CANCER SCREENING

Cancer can sometimes be detected in asymptomatic patients via regular physical examinations and screening tests.

Physical examinations for cancers of the thyroid, oral cavity, skin, lymph nodes, testes, prostate, and ovaries should also be a part of routine medical care.

Screening tests are tests that are done in asymptomatic patients at risk (see also p. 3144). The rationale is that early diagnosis may decrease cancer mortality by detecting cancer at an early and curable stage. Early detection may allow for less radical therapy and reduce costs. Risks, however, include false-positive results, which necessitate confirmatory tests (eg, biopsy, endoscopy) that can lead to anxiety, significant morbidity, and significant costs; and false-negative results, which may give a mistaken sense of security, causing patients to ignore subsequent symptoms.

Screening for cancer should be done in the following circumstances:

- When distinct high-risk groups can be identified (eg, people who have a strong family history of breast or prostate cancer)
- When the disorder has an asymptomatic period during which treatment would alter outcome (breast cancer, colon cancer)
- When the morbidity of the disorder is significant if detection is delayed
- When a screening test is available that is sensitive, specific, and cost effective

Table 152–3. SCREENING PROCEDURES IN AVERAGE-RISK ASYMPTOMATIC PEOPLE AS RECOMMENDED BY THE AMERICAN CANCER SOCIETY*

TYPE OF CANCER	PROCEDURE	FREQUENCY
Breast cancer	Mammography	Yearly ages 45–54 and every other year ages ≥ 55. Women should have the opportunity to begin screening at age 40.
	MRI	Yearly (in addition to mammography), starting at age 40 only for certain women at high risk
Cervical cancer	Papanicolaou (Pap) test sometimes with the human papillomavirus (HPV) test	Pap test every 3 yr between ages 21 and 29 Pap test plus HPV test every 5 yr between ages 30 and 65 *or* Pap test every 3 yr After age 65, no testing if previous testing was done and results were normal
Uterine and ovarian cancers	Pelvic examination	Every 1 to 3 yr between ages 18 and 40, then yearly
Prostate cancer	Blood test for PSA	Because the benefit of screening is uncertain, patient and physician should discuss the risks and possible benefits of prostate cancer screening.
Rectal and colon cancer	Stool testing: Fecal occult blood, fecal immunochemical test, or stool DNA test *or*	Yearly, starting at age 50
	Flexible sigmoidoscopy *or*	Every 5 yr, starting at age 50
	Colonoscopy *or*	Every 10 yr, starting at age 50
	CT colonography	Every 5 yr, starting at age 50

*Examinations for cancers of the thyroid, oral cavity, skin, lymph nodes, testes, and ovaries should also be done during routine medical care.
Modified from the American Cancer Society Guidelines for the Early Detection of Cancer.

Recommended screening schedules are constantly evolving based on ongoing studies (see Table 152–3).

CLINICAL SEQUELAE OF CANCER

Cancer may lead to pain, weight loss fatigue or obstruction of visceral organs. Death typically occurs as a result of inanition and organ failure.

Pain in patients with metastatic cancer frequently results from bone metastases, nerve or plexus involvement, or pressure exerted by a tumor mass or effusion. Aggressive pain management is essential in the treatment of cancer and for maintenance of quality of life (see p. 1968).

Pleural effusions should be drained if symptomatic and monitored for reaccumulation. If the effusion reaccumulates rapidly, thoracostomy tube drainage (see p. 390) and sclerosing agents or repeated catheter drainage should be considered.

Spinal cord compression (see p. 2031) can result from cancer spread to the vertebrae and requires immediate surgery or radiation therapy. Symptoms may include back pain, lower extremity paresthesias, and bowel and bladder dysfunction. Diagnosis is confirmed by CT or MRI.

Clots in the veins of the lower extremities, leading to pulmonary emboli, are frequent in patients with pancreatic, lung, and other solid tumors and in patients with brain tumors. Tumors produce procoagulants, such as tissue factors, leading to excess clot formation, particularly after surgery. Anticoagulation may be necessary to prevent pulmonary emboli.

Metabolic and immune consequences of cancer can include hypercalcemia, hyperuricemia, increased ACTH production, antibodies that produce neurologic dysfunction, hemolytic anemia, and many other paraneoplastic complications (see p. 1175).

METASTATIC CARCINOMA OF UNKNOWN PRIMARY ORIGIN

A patient is considered to have carcinoma of unknown primary origin when a tumor is detected at one or more metastatic sites and routine evaluation fails to identify a primary tumor. Metastatic carcinoma of unknown primary origin constitutes up to 7% of all cancers and poses a therapeutic dilemma, because cancer treatment is typically determined by the specific primary tissue of origin.

The most common causative primary tumors are those of the testes, lungs, colon and rectum, and pancreas. Examination of these areas should be thorough.

Types of testing used to help specify the primary site include

- Laboratory testing
- Imaging tests
- Immunocytochemical and immunoperoxidase staining
- Tissue analysis

Laboratory tests should include a CBC, urinalysis, stool examination for occult blood, and serum chemistries (including PSA assays in males).

Imaging should be limited to a chest x-ray, abdominal CT, and mammography. Endoscopic examination of the upper and lower GI tract should be done if blood is present in the stool.

Increasing numbers of immunocytochemical stains can be used to test available cancerous tissue to help determine the primary tissue site and can potentially identify tumors arising from the lung, colon, or breast. In addition, immunoperoxidase staining for immunoglobulin, chromosomal studies, and immunophenotyping may help diagnose the various subtypes of malignant lymphomas, which may be difficult to recognize and differentiate from other tumors (even carcinomas) when they manifest outside lymph nodes. Immunoperoxidase staining of tumor cells for α-fetoprotein or β-human chorionic gonadotropin may suggest readily treatable germ cell tumors. Tissue analysis for estrogen and progesterone receptors helps identify breast cancer, and immunoperoxidase staining for PSA helps identify prostate cancer.

Even if a precise histologic diagnosis cannot be made, a constellation of findings may suggest an origin. Poorly differentiated carcinomas near or at midline regions of the mediastinum or retroperitoneum in young or middle-aged males should be considered germ cell neoplasms—even in the absence of a testicular mass. Patients with this type of carcinoma should be treated with a cisplatin-based regimen, because nearly 50% of such patients experience long disease-free intervals. For most other unknown primary cancers, the responses to this regimen and to other multidrug chemotherapy regimens are modest and of brief duration (eg, median survival < 1 yr).

PARANEOPLASTIC SYNDROMES

Paraneoplastic syndromes are symptoms that occur at sites distant from a tumor or its metastasis.

Although the pathogenesis remains unclear, these symptoms may be secondary to substances secreted by the tumor or may be a result of antibodies directed against tumors that cross-react with other tissue. Symptoms may occur in any organ or physiologic system. Up to 20% of cancer patients experience paraneoplastic syndromes, but often these syndromes are unrecognized.

The most common cancers associated with paraneoplastic syndromes include

- Lung carcinoma (most common)
- Renal carcinoma
- Hepatocellular carcinoma
- Leukemias
- Lymphomas
- Breast tumors
- Ovarian tumors
- Neural cancers
- Gastric cancers
- Pancreatic cancers

Successful treatment is best obtained by controlling the underlying cancer, but some symptoms can be controlled with specific drugs (eg, cyproheptadine or somatostatin analogs for carcinoid syndrome, bisphosphonates and corticosteroids for hypercalcemia).

General paraneoplastic symptoms: Patients with cancer often experience fever, night sweats, anorexia, and cachexia. These symptoms may arise from release of cytokines involved in the inflammatory or immune response or from mediators involved in tumor cell death, such as tumor necrosis factor-α. Alterations in liver function and steroidogenesis may also contribute.

Cutaneous paraneoplastic syndromes: Patients may experience many skin symptoms.

Itching is the most common cutaneous symptom experienced by patients with cancer (eg, leukemia, lymphomas) and may result from hypereosinophilia.

Flushing may also occur and is likely related to tumor-generated circulating vasoactive substances (eg, prostaglandins).

Pigmented skin lesions, or keratoses, may appear, including acanthosis nigricans (GI cancer), generalized dermic melanosis (lymphoma, melanoma, hepatocellular carcinoma), Bowen disease (lung, GI, GU cancer), and large multiple seborrheic keratoses, ie, Leser-Trélat signs (lymphoma, GI cancer).

Herpes zoster may result from reactivation of latent virus in patients with immune system depression or dysfunction.

Endocrine paraneoplastic syndromes: The endocrine system is often affected by paraneoplastic syndromes.

Cushing syndrome (cortisol excess, leading to hyperglycemia, hypokalemia, hypertension, central obesity, moon facies) may result from ectopic production of ACTH or ACTH-like molecules, most often with small cell cancer of the lung.

Abnormalities in water and electrolyte balance, including hyponatremia, may result from production of ADH and parathyroid hormone–like hormones from small cell and non–small cell lung cancer.

Hypoglycemia may result from production of insulin-like growth factors or insulin production by pancreatic islet cell tumors or hemangiopericytomas.

Refractory **hyperglycemia** may be due to glucagon-producing pancreatic tumors.

Hypertension may result from abnormal epinephrine and norepinephrine secretion (pheochromocytomas) or from cortisol excess (ACTH-secreting tumors).

Other ectopically produced hormones include parathyroid hormone-related peptide (PTHRP—from squamous cell lung cancer, head and neck cancer, bladder cancer), calcitonin (from breast cancer, small cell lung cancer, and medullary thyroid carcinoma), and thyroid-stimulating hormone (from gestational choriocarcinoma). PTHRP causes hypercalcemia and its associated symptoms (polyuria, dehydration, constipation, muscle weakness); calcitonin causes a fall in the serum Ca level, leading to muscle twitching and cardiac arrhythmias.

GI paraneoplastic syndromes: Watery diarrhea with subsequent dehydration and electrolyte imbalances may result from tumor-related secretion of prostaglandins or vasoactive intestinal peptide. Implicated tumors include pancreatic islet cell tumors and others. Carcinoid tumors produce serotonin degradation products that lead to flushing, diarrhea, and breathing difficulty. Protein-losing enteropathies may result from tumor mass inflammation, particularly with lymphomas.

Hematologic paraneoplastic syndromes: Patients with cancer may develop pure RBC aplasia, anemia of chronic disease, leukocytosis (leukemoid reaction), thrombocytosis, eosinophilia, basophilia, and disseminated intravascular coagulation. In addition, immune thrombocytopenia and a Coombs-positive hemolytic anemia can complicate the course of lymphoid cancers and Hodgkin lymphoma. Erythrocytosis may occur in various cancers, especially renal cancers and hepatomas, due to ectopic production of erythropoietin or erythropoietin-like substances, and monoclonal gammopathies may sometimes be present.

Demonstrated mechanisms of hematologic abnormalities include tumor-generated substances that mimic or block normal endocrine signals for hematologic line development and generation of antibodies that cross-react with receptors or cell lines.

Neurologic paraneoplastic syndromes: Several types of peripheral neuropathy are among the neurologic paraneoplastic syndromes. Cerebellar syndromes and other central neurologic paraneoplastic syndromes also occur.

Peripheral neuropathy is the most common neurologic paraneoplastic syndrome. It is usually a distal sensorimotor polyneuropathy that causes mild motor weakness, sensory loss, and absent distal reflexes. The syndrome is indistinguishable from that accompanying many chronic illnesses.

Subacute sensory neuropathy is a more specific but rare peripheral neuropathy. Dorsal root ganglia degeneration and progressive sensory loss with ataxia but little motor weakness develop; the disorder may be disabling. Anti-Hu, an autoantibody, is found in the serum of some patients with lung cancer. There is no treatment.

Guillain-Barré syndrome, another ascending peripheral neuropathy, is a rare finding in the general population and probably more common in patients with Hodgkin lymphoma.

Eaton-Lambert syndrome is an immune-mediated, myasthenia-like syndrome with weakness usually affecting the limbs and sparing ocular and bulbar muscles. It is presynaptic, resulting from impaired release of acetylcholine from nerve terminals. An IgG antibody is involved. The syndrome can precede, occur with, or develop after the diagnosis of cancer. It occurs most commonly in men with intrathoracic tumors (70% have small or oat cell lung carcinoma). Symptoms and signs include fatigability, weakness, pain in proximal limb muscles, peripheral paresthesias, dry mouth, erectile dysfunction, and ptosis. Deep tendon reflexes are reduced or lost. The diagnosis is confirmed by finding an incremental response to repetitive nerve stimulation: Amplitude of the compound muscle action potential increases > 200% at rates > 10 Hz. Treatment is first directed at the underlying cancer and sometimes induces remission. Guanidine (initially 125 mg po qid, gradually increased to a maximum of 35 mg/kg), which facilitates acetylcholine release, often lessens symptoms but may depress bone marrow and liver function. Corticosteroids and plasma exchange benefit some patients.

Subacute cerebellar degeneration causes progressive bilateral leg and arm ataxia, dysarthria, and sometimes vertigo and diplopia. Neurologic signs may include dementia with or without brain stem signs, ophthalmoplegia, nystagmus, and extensor plantar signs, with prominent dysarthria and arm involvement. Cerebellar degeneration usually progresses over weeks to months, often causing profound disability. Cerebellar degeneration may precede the discovery of the cancer by weeks to years. Anti-Yo, a circulating autoantibody, is found in the serum or CSF of some patients, especially women with breast or ovarian cancer. MRI or CT may show cerebellar atrophy, especially late in the disease. Characteristic pathologic changes include widespread loss of Purkinje cells and lymphocytic cuffing of deep blood vessels. CSF occasionally has mild lymphocytic pleocytosis. Treatment is nonspecific, but some improvement may follow successful cancer therapy.

Opsoclonus (spontaneous chaotic eye movements) is a rare cerebellar syndrome that may accompany childhood neuroblastoma. It is associated with cerebellar ataxia and myoclonus of the trunk and extremities. Anti-Ri, a circulating autoantibody, may be present. The syndrome often responds to corticosteroids and treatment of the cancer.

Subacute motor neuronopathy is a rare disorder causing painless lower motor neuron weakness of upper and lower extremities, usually in patients with Hodgkin lymphoma or other lymphomas. Anterior horn cells degenerate. Spontaneous improvement usually occurs.

Subacute necrotizing myelopathy is a rare syndrome in which rapid ascending sensory and motor loss occurs in gray and white matter of the spinal cord, leading to paraplegia. MRI helps rule out epidural compression from metastatic tumor—a much more common cause of rapidly progressive spinal cord dysfunction in patients with cancer. MRI may show necrosis in the spinal cord.

Encephalitis may occur as a paraneoplastic syndrome, taking several different forms, depending on the area of the brain involved. Global encephalitis has been proposed to explain the encephalopathy that occurs most commonly in small cell lung cancer. Limbic encephalitis is characterized by anxiety and depression, leading to memory loss, agitation, confusion, hallucinations, and behavioral abnormalities. Anti-Hu antibodies, directed against RNA binding proteins, may be present in the serum and spinal fluid. MRI may disclose areas of increased contrast uptake and edema.

Renal paraneoplastic syndrome: Membranous glomerulonephritis may occur in patients with colon cancer, ovarian cancer, and lymphoma as a result of circulating immune complexes.

Rheumatologic paraneoplastic syndromes: Rheumatologic disorders mediated by autoimmune reactions can also be a manifestation of paraneoplastic syndromes.

Arthropathies (rheumatic polyarthritis, polymyalgia) or systemic sclerosis may develop in patients with hematologic cancers or with cancers of the colon, pancreas, or prostate. Systemic sclerosis or SLE may also develop in patients with lung and gynecologic cancers.

Hypertrophic osteoarthropathy is prominent with certain lung cancers and manifests as painful swelling of the joints (knees, ankles, wrists, elbows, metacarpophalangeal joints) with effusion and sometimes fingertip clubbing.

Secondary amyloidosis may occur with myeloma, lymphomas, or renal cell carcinomas.

Dermatomyositis and, to a lesser degree, polymyositis (see p. 257) are thought to be more common in patients with cancer, especially in those > 50 yr. Typically, proximal muscle weakness is progressive with pathologically demonstrable muscle inflammation and necrosis. A dusky, erythematous butterfly rash with a heliotrope hue may develop on the cheeks with periorbital edema. Corticosteroids may be helpful.

153 Plasma Cell Disorders

(Dysproteinemias; Monoclonal Gammopathies; Paraproteinemias; Plasma Cell Dyscrasias)

Plasma cell disorders are a diverse group of disorders of unknown etiology characterized by

- Disproportionate proliferation of a single clone of B cells
- Presence of a structurally and electrophoretically homogeneous (monoclonal) immunoglobulin or polypeptide subunit in serum, urine, or both

Pathophysiology

After developing in the bone marrow, undifferentiated B cells enter peripheral lymphoid tissues, such as lymph nodes, spleen, and gut (eg, Peyer patches). Here, they begin to differentiate into cells, each of which can respond to a limited number of antigens. After encountering the appropriate antigen, some B cells undergo clonal proliferation into plasma cells. Each clonal plasma cell line is committed to synthesizing one specific immunoglobulin antibody that consists of 2 identical heavy chains (gamma [γ], mu [μ], alpha [α], delta [δ], or epsilon [ε]) and 2 identical light chains (kappa [κ] or lambda [λ]). A slight excess of light chains is normally produced, and urinary excretion of small amounts of free polyclonal light chains (≤ 40 mg/24 h) is normal.

Plasma cell disorders are of unknown etiology and are characterized by the disproportionate proliferation of one clone. The result is a corresponding increase in the serum level of its product, the monoclonal immunoglobulin protein (M-protein). M-proteins may consist of both heavy and light chains or of only one type of chain.

Complications of plasma cell proliferation and M-protein production include the following:

- Autoimmune damage of organs (particularly the kidneys): Some M-proteins show antibody activity
- Impaired immunity: Decreased production of other immunoglobulins
- Bleeding tendency: M-protein may coat platelets, inactivate clotting factors, increase blood viscosity, and cause bleeding by other mechanisms
- Secondary amyloidosis: M-protein can be deposited within organs
- Osteoporosis, hypercalcemia, anemia, or pancytopenia: Clonal cells can infiltrate bone matrix and/or marrow

Plasma cell disorders can vary from asymptomatic, stable conditions (in which only the protein is present) to progressive cancers (eg, multiple myeloma—for classification, see Table 153–1). Rarely, transient plasma cell disorders occur in patients with drug hypersensitivity (sulfonamide, phenytoin, and penicillin), with presumed viral infections, and after heart or transplant surgery.

Diagnosis

Plasma cell disorders may be suspected because of clinical manifestations, findings during evaluation of anemia, or an incidental finding of elevated serum protein or proteinuria that leads to further evaluation with serum or urine protein electrophoresis. Electrophoresis detects M-protein, which is further evaluated with immunofixation electrophoresis for identification of heavy and light chain classes.

HEAVY CHAIN DISEASES

Heavy chain diseases are neoplastic plasma cell disorders characterized by overproduction of monoclonal immunoglobulin heavy chains. Symptoms, diagnosis, and treatment vary according to the specific disorder.

Heavy chain diseases are plasma cell disorders that are typically malignant. In most plasma cell disorders, M-proteins are structurally similar to normal antibody molecules. In contrast, in heavy chain diseases, incomplete monoclonal immunoglobulins (true paraproteins) are produced. They consist of only heavy chain components (either alpha [α], gamma [γ], mu [μ],

Table 153–1. CLASSIFICATION OF PLASMA CELL DISORDERS

SYMPTOMS	DESCRIPTION	EXAMPLES
Monoclonal gammopathy of undetermined significance*		
Asymptomatic, usually nonprogressive	Associated with nonlymphoreticular tumors	Carcinomas of the breasts, biliary tree, GI tract, kidneys, and prostate
Occurring in apparently healthy people or in those with other conditions	Associated with chronic inflammatory and infectious conditions	Chronic cholecystitis, osteomyelitis, pyelonephritis, RA, TB
	Associated with various other disorders	Familial hypercholesterolemia, Gaucher disease, Kaposi sarcoma, lichen myxedematosus, liver disorders, myasthenia gravis, pernicious anemia, thyrotoxicosis
Malignant plasma cell disorders		
Asymptomatic, progressive	Usually light chains (Bence Jones) only, but occasionally intact immunoglobulin molecules (IgG, IgA, IgM, IgD)	Early multiple myeloma
Symptomatic, progressive	Excess production of IgM	Macroglobulinemia
	Most often IgG, IgA, or light chains (Bence Jones) only	Multiple myeloma
	Usually light chains (Bence Jones) only, but occasionally intact immunoglobulin molecules (IgG, IgA, IgM, IgD)	Nonhereditary primary systemic amyloidosis
	Heavy chain diseases	IgG heavy chain disease (sometimes benign) IgA heavy chain disease IgM heavy chain disease IgD heavy chain disease
Transient plasma cell disorders		
Not necessarily symptomatic	Associated with drug hypersensitivity, viral infections, and heart or transplant surgery	Hypersensitivity to sulfonamide, phenytoin, or penicillin

*Age-related incidence.

or delta [δ]) without light chains (epsilon [ε] heavy chain disease has not been described). Most heavy chain proteins are fragments of their normal counterparts with internal deletions of variable length; these deletions appear to result from structural mutations. The clinical picture is more like lymphoma than multiple myeloma. Heavy chain diseases are considered in patients with clinical manifestations suggesting lymphoproliferative disorders.

IgA Heavy Chain Disease (Alpha Chain Disease)

IgA heavy chain disease is the most common heavy chain disease and is similar to Mediterranean lymphoma (immunoproliferative small intestinal disease).

IgA heavy chain disease usually appears between ages 10 and 30 and is geographically concentrated in the Middle East. The cause may be an aberrant immune response to a parasite or other microorganism. Villous atrophy and plasma cell infiltration of the jejunal mucosa are usually present and, sometimes, infiltration of the mesenteric lymph nodes. The peripheral lymph nodes, bone marrow, liver, and spleen usually are not involved. A respiratory tract form of the disease has been reported rarely. Osteolytic lesions do not occur.

Almost all patients present with diffuse abdominal lymphoma and malabsorption. CBC may show anemia, leukopenia, thrombocytopenia, eosinophilia, and circulating atypical lymphocytes or plasma cells. Serum protein electrophoresis is normal in half of cases; often, there is an increased α_2 and β (beta) fraction or a decreased γ fraction. Diagnosis requires the detection of a monoclonal alpha chain on immunofixation electrophoresis. This chain is sometimes found in concentrated urine. If it cannot be found in serum or urine, biopsy is required. The abnormal protein can sometimes be detected in intestinal secretions. The intestinal cellular infiltrate may be pleomorphic and not overtly malignant. Bence Jones proteinuria is absent.

The course is highly variable: Some patients die in 1 to 2 yr, whereas others have remissions that last many years, particularly after treatment with corticosteroids, cytotoxic drugs, and broad-spectrum antibiotics.

IgG Heavy Chain Disease (Gamma Chain Disease)

IgG heavy chain disease is generally similar to an aggressive malignant lymphoma but is occasionally asymptomatic and benign.

IgG heavy chain disease occurs primarily in elderly men but can occur in children. Associated chronic disorders include RA, Sjögren syndrome, SLE, TB, myasthenia gravis, hypereosinophilic syndrome, autoimmune hemolytic anemia, and thyroiditis. Reductions in normal immunoglobulin levels occur. Lytic bone lesions are uncommon. Amyloidosis sometimes develops.

Common manifestations include lymphadenopathy and hepatosplenomegaly, fever, and recurring infections. Palatal edema occurs in about one quarter of patients.

The CBC may show anemia, leukopenia, thrombocytopenia, eosinophilia, and circulating atypical lymphocytes or plasma cells. Diagnosis requires demonstration by immunofixation of free monoclonal heavy chain fragments of IgG in serum and urine. Of affected patients, half have monoclonal serum components > 1 g/dL (often broad and heterogeneous), and half have proteinuria > 1 g/24 h. Although heavy chain proteins may involve any IgG subclass, the G3 subclass is especially common. Bone marrow or lymph node biopsy, done if other tests are not diagnostic, reveals variable histopathology.

The median survival with aggressive disease is about 1 yr. Death usually results from bacterial infection or progressive malignancy. Alkylating agents, vincristine, or corticosteroids, and radiation therapy may yield transient remissions.

IgM Heavy Chain Disease (Mu Chain Disease)

IgM heavy chain disease, which is rare, produces a clinical picture similar to chronic lymphocytic leukemia or other lymphoproliferative disorders.

IgM heavy chain disease most often affects adults > 50 yr. Visceral organ involvement (spleen, liver, abdominal lymph nodes) is common, but extensive peripheral lymphadenopathy is not. Pathologic fractures and amyloidosis may occur. Serum protein electrophoresis usually is normal or shows hypogammaglobulinemia. Bence Jones proteinuria (type κ) is present in 10 to 15% of patients. CBC may show anemia, leukopenia, thrombocytopenia, eosinophilia, and circulating atypical lymphocytes or plasma cells.

Diagnosis usually requires bone marrow examination; vacuolated plasma cells are present in two thirds of patients and, when present, are virtually pathognomonic. Death can occur in a few months or in many years. The usual cause of death is uncontrollable proliferation of chronic lymphocytic leukemia cells.

Treatment depends on the patient's condition but may consist of alkylating agents plus corticosteroids or may be similar to treatment of the lymphoproliferative disorder that it most closely resembles.

MACROGLOBULINEMIA

(Primary Macroglobulinemia; Waldenström Macroglobulinemia)

Macroglobulinemia is a malignant plasma cell disorder in which B cells produce excessive amounts of IgM M-proteins. Manifestations may include hyperviscosity, bleeding, recurring infections, and generalized adenopathy. Diagnosis requires bone marrow examination and demonstration of M-protein. Treatment includes plasma exchange as needed for hyperviscosity, and systemic therapy with alkylating drugs, corticosteroids, nucleoside analogs, or monoclonal antibodies.

Macroglobulinemia, an uncommon B-cell cancer, is clinically more similar to a lymphomatous disease than to myeloma and other plasma cell disorders. Cause is unknown. Men are affected more often than women; median age is 65.

After myeloma, macroglobulinemia is the 2nd most common malignant disorder associated with a monoclonal gammopathy. Excessive amounts of IgM M-proteins can also accumulate in other disorders, causing manifestations similar to macroglobulinemia. Small monoclonal IgM components are present in the sera of about 5% of patients with B-cell non-Hodgkin lymphoma; this circumstance is termed macroglobulinemic lymphoma. Additionally, IgM M-proteins are occasionally present in patients with chronic lymphocytic leukemia or other lymphoproliferative disorders.

Clinical manifestations of macroglobulinemia may be due to the large amount of high molecular weight monoclonal IgM proteins circulating in plasma, but most patients do not develop problems related to high IgM levels. Some of these proteins are antibodies directed toward autologous IgG (rheumatoid factors) or I antigens (cold agglutinins). About 10% are cryoglobulins. Secondary amyloidosis occurs in 5% of patients.

Symptoms and Signs

Most patients are asymptomatic, but many present with anemia or manifestations of hyperviscosity syndrome: fatigue, weakness, skin and mucosal bleeding, visual disturbances, headache, symptoms of peripheral neuropathy, and other changing neurologic manifestations. An increased plasma volume can precipitate heart failure. Cold sensitivity, Raynaud syndrome, or recurring bacterial infections may occur.

Examination may disclose lymphadenopathy, hepatosplenomegaly, and purpura (which rarely can be the first manifestation). Marked engorgement and localized narrowing of retinal veins, which resemble sausage links, suggests hyperviscosity syndrome. Retinal hemorrhages, exudates, microaneurysms, and papilledema occur in late stages.

PEARLS & PITFALLS

- Marked engorgement and localized narrowing of retinal veins, which resemble sausage links, suggests hyperviscosity syndrome.

Diagnosis

- CBC with platelets, RBC indices, and peripheral blood smear
- Serum protein electrophoresis followed by serum and urine immunofixation and quantitative immunoglobulin levels
- Serum viscosity assay
- Bone marrow examination
- Sometimes lymph node biopsy

Macroglobulinemia is suspected in patients with symptoms of hyperviscosity or other typical symptoms, particularly if anemia is present. However, it is often diagnosed incidentally when protein electrophoresis reveals an M-protein that proves to be IgM by immunofixation. Laboratory evaluation includes tests used to evaluate plasma cell disorders (see Multiple Myeloma on p. 1180) as well as measurement of cryoglobulins, rheumatoid factor, and cold agglutinins; coagulation studies; and direct Coombs test.

Moderate normocytic, normochromic anemia, marked rouleau formation, and a very high ESR are typical. Leukopenia, relative lymphocytosis, and thrombocytopenia occasionally occur. Cryoglobulins, rheumatoid factor, or cold agglutinins may be present. If cold agglutinins are present, the direct Coombs test usually is positive. Various coagulation and platelet function abnormalities may occur. Results of routine blood studies may be spurious if cryoglobulinemia or marked hyperviscosity is present. Normal immunoglobulins are decreased in half of patients.

Immunofixation electrophoresis of concentrated urine frequently shows a monoclonal light chain (usually kappa [κ]), but gross Bence Jones proteinuria is unusual. Bone marrow studies show a variable increase in plasma cells, lymphocytes, plasmacytoid lymphocytes, and mast cells. Periodic acid-Schiff–positive material may be present in lymphoid cells. Lymph node biopsy, done if bone marrow examination is normal, is frequently interpreted as diffuse well-differentiated or plasmacytic lymphocytic lymphoma. Serum viscosity is measured to confirm suspected hyperviscosity and when present is usually > 4.0 (normal, 1.4 to 1.8).

Treatment

- Plasma exchange (when hyperviscosity is present)
- Corticosteroids, alkylating drugs, nucleoside analogs, monoclonal antibodies (rituximab), or a combination
- Possibly a proteasome inhibitor (bortezomib or carfilzomib), an immunomodulatory agent (thalidomide, pomalidomide, or lenalidomide), ibrutinib, or idelalisib

The course is variable, with a median survival of 7 to 10 yr. Age > 60 yr, anemia, and cryoglobulinemia predict shorter survival.[1]

Often, patients require no treatment for many years.[1] If hyperviscosity is present, initial treatment is plasma exchange, which rapidly reverses bleeding as well as neurologic abnormalities. Plasma exchange often needs to be repeated.

Corticosteroids may be effective in reducing tumor load. Treatment with oral alkylating drugs may be indicated for palliation, but bone marrow toxicity can occur. Nucleoside analogs (fludarabine and 2-chlorodeoxyadenosine) produce responses in large numbers of newly diagnosed patients but have been associated with a high risk of myelodysplasia and myeloid leukemia. Rituximab can reduce tumor burden without suppressing normal hematopoiesis. However, during the first several months, IgM levels may increase, requiring plasma exchange. The proteasome inhibitors bortezomib or carfilzomib and the immunomodulating agents thalidomide, lenalidomide, and pomalidomide are also effective in this cancer. Ibrutinib, a Bruton tyrosine kinase inhibitor, and idelalisib, a PI3K inhibitor, are also effective in these patients.

1. Oza A, Rajkumar SV. Waldenstrom macroglobulinemia: prognosis and management. *Blood Cancer J* 5(3):e296, 2015. doi: 10.1038/bcj.2015.28.

KEY POINTS

- Macroglobulinemia is a malignant plasma cell disorder in which B cells produce excessive amounts of IgM M-proteins.
- Most patients are initially asymptomatic, but many present with anemia or hyperviscosity syndrome (fatigue, weakness, skin and mucosal bleeding, visual disturbances, headache, peripheral neuropathy and other neurologic manifestations).
- Do serum protein electrophoresis followed by serum and urine immunofixation, and quantitative immunoglobulin levels.
- Treat hyperviscosity using plasma exchange, which rapidly reverses bleeding as well as neurologic abnormalities.
- Corticosteroids, fludarabine, rituximab, proteasome inhibitors (bortezomib and carfilzomib), immunomodulatory agents (thalidomide, lenalidomide, and pomalidomide), ibrutimib, or idelalisib may be helpful; alkylating drugs can be used for palliation.

MONOCLONAL GAMMOPATHY OF UNDETERMINED SIGNIFICANCE

Monoclonal gammopathy of undetermined significance (MGUS) is the production of M-protein by noncancerous plasma cells in the absence of other manifestations typical of multiple myeloma.

The incidence of MGUS increases with age, from 1% of people aged 25 yr to > 5% of people > 70 yr. MGUS may occur in association with other disorders (see Table 153–1), in which case M-proteins may be antibodies produced in large amounts in response to protracted antigenic stimuli.

MGUS usually is asymptomatic, but peripheral neuropathy can occur, and patients are at higher risk of enhanced bone loss and fractures. Although most cases are initially benign, up to 25% (1%/yr) progress to myeloma or a related B-cell disorder, such as macroglobulinemia, amyloidosis, or lymphoma.

Diagnosis is usually suspected when M-protein is incidentally detected in blood or urine during a routine examination. On laboratory evaluation, M-protein is present in low levels in serum (< 3 g/dL) or urine (< 300 mg/24 h). MGUS is differentiated from other plasma cell disorders because M-protein levels remain relatively stable over time and lytic bone lesions, anemia, and renal dysfunction are absent. Because of fracture risk, baseline evaluation with a skeletal survey (ie, plain x-rays of skull, long bones, spine, pelvis, and ribs) and bone densitometry should be done. Bone marrow shows only mild plasmacytosis (< 10% of nucleated cells).

No antineoplastic treatment is recommended. However, recent studies suggest that MGUS patients with associated bone loss (osteopenia or osteoporosis) may benefit from treatment with bisphosphonates. Every 6 to 12 mo, patients should undergo clinical examination and serum and urine protein electrophoresis to evaluate for disease progression.

MULTIPLE MYELOMA

(Myelomatosis; Plasma Cell Myeloma)

Multiple myeloma is a cancer of plasma cells that produce monoclonal immunoglobulin and invade and destroy adjacent bone tissue. Common manifestations include bone pain, renal insufficiency, hypercalcemia, anemia, and recurrent infections. Diagnosis typically requires demonstration of M-protein (sometimes present in urine and not serum, and rarely absent entirely) and either lytic bone lesions, light-chain proteinuria, or excessive plasma cells in bone marrow. A bone marrow biopsy is usually needed. Specific treatment most often includes some combination of conventional chemotherapy, corticosteroids, and one or more of the newer agents such as bortezomib, carfilzomib, lenalidomide, thalidomide, pomalidomide, daratumumab, or elotuzumab. High-dose melphalan followed by autologous peripheral blood stem cell transplantation may also be used.

The incidence of multiple myeloma is 2 to 4/100,000. Male:female ratio is 1.6:1, and the median age is about 65 yr. Prevalence in blacks is twice that in whites. Etiology is unknown, although chromosomal and genetic factors, radiation, and chemicals have been suggested.

Pathophysiology

The M-protein produced by the malignant plasma cells is IgG in about 55% of myeloma patients and IgA in about 20%; of patients producing either IgG or IgA, 40% also have Bence Jones proteinuria, which is free monoclonal kappa (κ) or lambda (λ) light chains in the urine. In 15 to 20% of patients, plasma cells secrete only Bence Jones protein. IgD myeloma accounts for about 1% of cases. Rarely, patients have no M-protein in blood and urine, although a new serum free light chain assay now demonstrates monoclonal light chains in many of these patients.

Diffuse osteoporosis or discrete osteolytic lesions develop, usually in the pelvis, spine, ribs, and skull. Lesions are caused by bone replacement by expanding plasmacytomas or by cytokines that are secreted by malignant plasma cells that activate osteoclasts and suppress osteoblasts. The osteolytic lesions are usually multiple; occasionally, they are solitary intramedullary masses. Increased bone loss may also lead to hypercalcemia. Extraosseous solitary plasmacytomas are unusual but may occur in any tissue, especially in the upper respiratory tract.

In many patients, renal failure (myeloma kidney) is present at diagnosis or develops during the course of the disorder. Renal failure has many causes, most commonly, it results from deposition of light chains in the distal tubules or hypercalcemia. Patients also often develop anemia usually due to kidney disease or suppression of erythropoiesis by cancer cells but sometimes also due to iron deficiency.

Susceptibility to bacterial infection may occur in some patients. Viral infections, especially herpes zoster infections, are increasingly occurring as a result of newer treatment modalities, especially use of the proteasome inhibitors bortezomib and carfilzomib. Amyloidosis occurs in 10% of myeloma patients, most often in patients with 2λ-type M-proteins.

Variant expressions of multiple myeloma occur (see Table 153–2).

Symptoms and Signs

Persistent bone pain (especially in the back or thorax), renal failure, and recurring bacterial infections are the most common problems on presentation, but many patients are identified when routine laboratory tests show an elevated total protein level in the blood or show proteinuria. Pathologic fractures are common, and vertebral collapse may lead to spinal cord compression and paraplegia. Symptoms of anemia predominate or may be the sole reason for evaluation in some patients, and a few patients have manifestations of hyperviscosity syndrome (see p. 1179). Peripheral neuropathy, carpal tunnel syndrome, abnormal bleeding, and symptoms of hypercalcemia (eg, polydipsia, dehydration) are common. Patients may also present with renal failure. Lymphadenopathy and hepatosplenomegaly are unusual.

Diagnosis

- CBC with platelets, peripheral blood smear, ESR, and chemistry panel (BUN, creatinine, calcium, uric acid, LDH)

Table 153–2. VARIANT EXPRESSIONS OF MULTIPLE MYELOMA

FORM	CHARACTERISTICS
Extramedullary plasmacytoma	Plasmacytomas that occur outside of the medullary system
Solitary plasmacytoma of bone	Single bone plasmacytomas, which usually produce no M-protein
Osteosclerotic myeloma (POEMS syndrome)	Polyneuropathy (chronic inflammatory polyneuropathy) Organomegaly (hepatomegaly, splenomegaly, or lymphadenopathy) Endocrinopathy (eg, gynecomastia, testicular atrophy) M-protein Skin changes (eg, hyperpigmentation, excess hair)
Nonsecretory myeloma	Absence of M-protein in serum and urine Presence of M-protein in plasma cells

- Serum and urine protein electrophoresis followed by immunofixation; quantitative immunoglobulins; serum free light chains
- X-rays (skeletal survey)
- Bone marrow examination

Multiple myeloma is suspected in patients > 40 yr with persistent unexplained bone pain, particularly at night or at rest, other typical symptoms, or unexplained laboratory abnormalities, such as elevated blood protein or urinary protein, hypercalcemia, renal insufficiency, or anemia. Laboratory evaluation includes routine blood tests, protein electrophoresis, x-rays, and bone marrow examination.[1,2]

Routine blood tests include CBC, ESR, and chemistry panel. Anemia is present in 80% of patients, usually normocytic-normochromic anemia with formation of rouleau, which are clusters of 3 to 12 RBCs that occur in stacks. WBC and platelet counts are usually normal. ESR usually is > 100 mm/h; BUN, serum creatinine, LDH, and serum uric acid may be elevated. Anion gap is sometimes low. Hypercalcemia is present at diagnosis in about 10% of patients.

Protein electrophoresis is done on a serum sample and on a urine sample concentrated from a 24-h collection to quantify the amount of urinary M-protein. Serum electrophoresis identifies M-protein in about 80 to 90% of patients. The -remaining 10 to 20% are usually patients with only free monoclonal light chains (Bence Jones protein) or IgD. They almost always have M-protein detected by urine protein electrophoresis. Immunofixation electrophoresis can identify the immunoglobulin class of the M-protein (IgG, IgA, or uncommonly IgD, IgM, or IgE) and can often detect light-chain protein if serum immunoelectrophoresis is falsely negative; immunofixation electrophoresis is done even when the serum test is negative if multiple myeloma is strongly suspected. Serum free light-chain analysis with delineation of kappa and lambda ratios helps confirm the diagnosis and can also be used to monitor efficacy of therapy and provide prognostic data. Serum level of beta-2 microglobulin is measured if diagnosis is confirmed or very likely and along with serum albumin is used to stage patients as part of the international staging system (see Table 153–3).

X-rays include a skeletal survey (ie, plain x-rays of skull, long bones, spine, pelvis, and ribs). Punched-out lytic lesions or diffuse osteoporosis is present in 80% of cases. Radionuclide bone scans usually are not helpful. MRI can provide more detail and is obtained if specific sites of pain or neurologic symptoms are present. PET-CT may provide prognostic information and can help determine whether patients have solitary plasmacytoma or multiple myeloma.

Bone marrow aspiration and biopsy are done and reveal sheets or clusters of plasma cells; myeloma is diagnosed when

Table 153–3. INTERNATIONAL STAGING SYSTEM FOR MULTIPLE MYELOMA

STAGE	CRITERIA	MEDIAN SURVIVAL (mos)
I	Beta-2 microglobulin < 3.5 mcg/mL *and* Serum albumin ≥ 3.5 g/dL	62
II	Not stage I or III	44
III	Beta-2 microglobulin ≥ 5.5 mcg/mL	29

> 10% of the cells are of this type. However, bone marrow involvement is patchy; therefore, some samples from patients with myeloma may show < 10% plasma cells. Still, the number of plasma cells in bone marrow is rarely normal. Plasma cell morphology does not correlate with the class of immunoglobulin synthesized. Chromosomal studies on bone marrow (eg, using cytogenetic testing methods such as fluorescent in situ hybridization [FISH] and immunohistochemistry) may reveal specific karyotypic abnormalities in plasma cells associated with differences in survival.

Diagnosis and differentiation from other malignancies (eg, metastatic carcinoma, lymphoma, leukemia) and monoclonal gammopathy of undetermined significance typically requires multiple criteria

- Clonal bone marrow plasma cells or plasmacytoma
- M-protein in plasma and/or urine
- Organ impairment (hypercalcemia, renal insufficiency, anemia, or bony lesions)

In patients without serum M protein, myeloma is indicated by Bence Jones proteinuria > 300 mg/24 h or abnormal serum free light chains, osteolytic lesions (without evidence of metastatic cancer or granulomatous disease), and sheets or clusters of plasma cells in the bone marrow.

1. Rajkumar SV, Kumar S: Multiple myeloma: diagnosis and treatment. *Mayo Clinic Proc* 91(1):101–119, 2016. doi: 10.1016/j.mayocp.2015.11.007.
2. Rajkumar V: Myeloma today: disease definitions and treatment advances. *Am J Hematol* 91(1):90–100, 2016. doi: 10.1002/ajh.24392.

Prognosis

The disease is progressive and incurable, but median survival has recently improved to > 5 yr as a result of advances in treatment. Unfavorable prognostic signs at diagnosis are lower serum albumin and higher beta-2 microglobulin levels. Patients initially presenting with renal failure also do poorly unless kidney function improves with therapy (which typically happens with current treatment options). Certain cytogenetic abnormalities increase risk of poor outcome.

Because multiple myeloma is ultimately fatal, patients are likely to benefit from discussions of end-of-life care that involve their doctors and appropriate family and friends. Points for discussion may include advance directives, the use of feeding tubes, and pain relief.

Treatment

- Chemotherapy for symptomatic patients
- Thalidomide, lenalidomide, or pomalidomide, and/or bortezomib or carfilzomib, plus corticosteroids and/or conventional chemotherapy
- Monoclonal antibodies, including elotuzumab and daratumumab
- Possibly maintenance therapy with corticosteroids, thalidomide and/or lenalidomide
- Possibly autologous stem cell transplantation
- Possibly radiation therapy to specific symptomatic areas that do not respond to systemic therapy
- Treatment of complications (anemia, hypercalcemia, renal insufficiency, infections, skeletal lesions)

Treatment of myeloma has improved in the past decade, and long-term survival is a reasonable therapeutic target.[1-3] Therapy involves direct treatment of malignant cells in symptomatic patients or those with myeloma-related organ dysfunction (anemia, renal dysfunction, hypercalcemia, or bone disease). Asymptomatic patients probably do not benefit from treatment, which is usually withheld until symptoms or complications develop. Patients with evidence of lytic lesions or bone loss (osteopenia or osteoporosis) should be treated with monthly infusions of zoledronic acid or pamidronate to reduce the risk of skeletal complications.

1. Rajkumar SV, Kumar S: Multiple myeloma: diagnosis and treatment. *Mayo Clinic Proc* 91(1):101–119, 2016. doi: 10.1016/j.mayocp.2015.11.007.
2. Rajkumar V: Myeloma today: disease definitions and treatment advances. *Am J Hematol* 91(1):90–100, 2016. doi: 10.1002/ajh.24392.
3. Berenson J, Spektor T, Wang J: Advances in the management of multiple myeloma. 2016.

Treatment of malignant cells: Until recently, conventional chemotherapy consisted only of oral melphalan and prednisone given in cycles of 4 to 6 wk with monthly evaluation of response. Recent studies show superior outcome with the addition of either bortezomib or thalidomide. Other chemotherapeutic drugs, including cyclophosphamide, bendamustine, doxorubicin and its newer analog liposomal pegylated doxorubicin also are more effective when combined with an immunomodulatory drug (thalidomide, lenalidomide, or its newer analog pomalidomide) or a proteasome inhibitor (bortezomib, or a newer drug, carfilzomib). Many other patients are effectively treated with bortezomib, corticosteroids, and either thalidomide (or lenalidomide), chemotherapy, or both.

Chemotherapy response (see Table 154–1 on p. 1183) is indicated by reduction in bone pain and fatigue, decreases in serum and urine M-protein, decreases in levels of the involved serum free light chain, increases in RBCs, and improvement in renal function among patients presenting with renal failure.

Autologous peripheral blood stem cell transplantation may be considered for patients who have adequate cardiac, hepatic, pulmonary, and renal function, particularly those whose disease is stable or responsive after several cycles of initial therapy. However, recent studies suggest that the newer treatment options are highly effective and may make transplantation less often necessary. Allogeneic stem cell transplantation after nonmyeloablative chemotherapy (eg, low-dose cyclophosphamide and fludarabine) or low-dose radiation therapy can produce myeloma-free survival of 5 to 10 yr in some patients. However, allogeneic stem cell transplantation with myeloablative or nonmyeloablative chemotherapy remains experimental because of the high morbidity and mortality resulting from graft vs host disease.

In relapsed or refractory myeloma, combinations of bortezomib or carfilzomib, and thalidomide, lenalidomide, or pomalidomide, with chemotherapy or corticosteroids may be used. These drugs are usually combined with other effective drugs that the patient has not yet been treated with, although patients with prolonged remissions may respond to retreatment with the same regimen that led to the remission. Patients who fail to respond to a given combination of drugs may respond when another drug in the same class (eg, proteasome inhibitors, immunomodulatory agents, chemotherapeutic drugs) is substituted. Following disease progression, monoclonal antibodies may be effective, including daratumumab and elotuzumab, the latter when combined with lenalidomide and dexamethasone, and the new oral proteasome inhibitor ixazomib.

Maintenance therapy has been tried with nonchemotherapeutic drugs, including interferon alfa, which prolongs remission but does not improve survival and is associated with significant adverse effects. Following a response to corticosteroid-based regimens, corticosteroids alone are effective as a maintenance treatment. Thalidomide may also be effective as a maintenance treatment, and recent studies show that lenalidomide alone or with corticosteroids is also effective maintenance treatment. However, there is some recent concern about secondary malignancy among patients receiving long-term lenalidomide therapy, especially after autologous stem cell transplantation.

Treatment of complications: In addition to direct treatment of malignant cells, therapy must also be directed at complications, which include anemia, hypercalcemia, renal insufficiency, infections, and skeletal lesions.

Anemia can be treated with recombinant erythropoietin (40,000 units sc once/wk) in patients whose anemia is inadequately relieved by chemotherapy. If anemia causes cardiovascular or significant systemic symptoms, packed RBCs are transfused. Plasma exchange is indicated if hyperviscosity develops (see p. 1179). Often patients are iron deficient and require intravenous iron. Patients with anemia should have periodic measurement of serum iron, transferrin, and ferritin levels to monitor iron stores.

Hypercalcemia is treated with vigorous saluresis, IV bisphosphonates after rehydration, and sometimes with calcitonin or prednisone.

Hyperuricemia may occur in some patients with high tumor burden and underlying metabolic problems. However, most patients do not require allopurinol. Allopurinol is indicated for patients with high levels of serum uric acid or high tumor burden and a high risk of tumor lysis syndrome with treatment.

Renal compromise can be ameliorated with adequate hydration. Even patients with prolonged, massive Bence Jones proteinuria (≥ 10 to 30 g/day) may have intact renal function if they maintain urine output > 2000 mL/day. Dehydration combined with high-osmolar IV contrast may precipitate acute oliguric renal failure in patients with Bence Jones proteinuria. Plasma exchange may be effective in some cases.

Infection is more likely during chemotherapy-induced neutropenia. In addition, infections with the herpes zoster virus are occurring more frequently in patients treated with newer antimyeloma drugs, especially bortezomib or carfilzomib. Documented bacterial infections should be treated with antibiotics; however, prophylactic use of antibiotics is not routinely recommended. Prophylactic use of antiviral drugs (eg, acyclovir, valganciclovir, famciclovir) is indicated for patients receiving either bortezomib or carfilzomib. Prophylactic IV immune globulin may reduce the risk of infection but is generally reserved for patients with recurrent infections. Pneumococcal and influenza vaccines are indicated to prevent infection. However, use of live vaccines is not recommended in these immunocompromised patients.

Skeletal lesions require multiple supportive measures. Maintenance of ambulation and supplemental calcium and vitamin D help preserve bone density. Vitamin D levels should be measured at diagnosis and periodically and dosing of vitamin D adjusted accordingly. Analgesics and palliative doses of radiation therapy (18 to 24 Gy) can relieve bone pain. However, radiation therapy may cause significant toxicity and, because it suppresses bone marrow function, may impair the patient's ability to receive cytotoxic doses of systemic chemotherapy. Most patients, especially those with lytic lesions and generalized osteoporosis or osteopenia, should receive a monthly IV bisphosphonate (either pamidronate or zoledronic acid). Bisphosphonates reduce skeletal complications and lessen bone pain and may have an antitumor effect.

KEY POINTS

- Malignant plasma cells produce monoclonal immunoglobulin and invade and destroy bone.
- Expanding plasmacytomas and cytokine secretion cause multiple, discrete, osteolytic lesions (usually in the pelvis, spine, ribs, and skull) and diffuse osteoporosis; pain, fractures, and hypercalcemia are common.
- Anemia and renal failure are common.
- Amyloidosis develops in about 10%, typically patients who produce excess lambda light chains.
- Perform serum and urine protein electrophoresis followed by immunofixation, quantitative immunoglobulins, and measurement of serum free light chains.
- Symptomatic patients and those with organ dysfunction should be treated with drug therapy and, for certain patients, autologous stem cell transplantation.

154 Principles of Cancer Therapy

Curing cancer requires eliminating all cancer cells. The major modalities of therapy are

- Surgery (for local and local-regional disease)
- Radiation therapy (for local and local-regional disease)
- Chemotherapy (for systemic disease)

Other important methods include

- Hormonal therapy (for selected cancers, eg, prostate, breast, endometrium)
- Immunotherapy (monoclonal antibodies, interferons, and other biologic response modifiers and tumor vaccines—see p. 1218)
- Differentiating drugs such as retinoids
- Targeted drugs that exploit the growing knowledge of cellular and molecular biology

Overall treatment should be coordinated among a radiation oncologist, surgeon, and medical oncologist, where appropriate. Choice of modalities constantly evolves, and numerous controlled research trials continue. When available and appropriate, clinical trial participation should be considered and discussed with patients.

Various terms are used to describe the response to treatment (see Table 154–1). The disease-free interval often serves as an indicator of cure and varies with cancer type. For example, lung, colon, bladder, large cell lymphomas, and testicular cancers are usually cured if a 5-yr disease-free interval occurs. However, breast and prostate cancers may recur long after 5 yr, an event defining tumor dormancy (now a major area of research); thus, a 10-yr disease-free interval is more indicative of cure.

Treatment decisions should weigh the likelihood of adverse effects against the likelihood of benefit; these decisions require frank communication and possibly the involvement of a multidisciplinary cancer team. Patient preferences for how to live out the end of life should be established early in the course of cancer treatment despite the difficulties of discussing death at such a sensitive time (see p. 3212).

MODALITIES OF CANCER THERAPY

Treatment of cancer can involve any of several modalities:

- Surgery
- Radiation therapy
- Chemotherapy
- Hormonal therapy
- Immunotherapy

Often, modalities are combined to create a treatment program that is appropriate for the patient and is based on patient and tumor characteristics as well as patient preferences.

Survival rates with the different modalities, alone and in combination, are listed for selected cancers (see Table 154–2).

Surgery

Surgery is the oldest form of effective cancer therapy. It may be used alone or in combination with other modalities. The size, type, and location of the primary tumor may determine operability and outcome. The presence of metastases may preclude an aggressive surgical approach to the primary tumor.

Factors that increase operative risk in cancer patients include

- Age
- Comorbid conditions
- Debilitation due to cancer
- Paraneoplastic syndromes (less common—see p. 1175)

Cancer patients often have poor nutrition due to anorexia and the catabolic influences of tumor growth, and these factors may

Table 154–1. DEFINING RESPONSE TO CANCER TREATMENT

TERM	DEFINITION
Cure	Long-term absence of symptoms or signs of a disease, although patients who appear to be cured may still have viable tumor cells that eventually cause relapse
Complete remission (complete response)	Disappearance of clinical evidence of disease
Partial response	> 50% reduction in size of tumor mass or masses, sometimes leading to significant palliation and prolongation of life but with inevitable regrowth of the tumor
Stable disease	Neither improvement nor worsening
Disease-free survival (disease-free interval)	Interval between disappearance of the tumor and relapse
Progression-free survival	Time from initiation of treatment to time of overt progression in a surviving patient
Survival time	Time from diagnosis to death

Table 154–2. 5-YR DISEASE-FREE SURVIVAL RATES BY CANCER THERAPY

SITE OR TYPE	STAGE	5-YR DISEASE-FREE SURVIVAL RATE (%)
Surgery alone		
Bladder	0, A	81
	B_1	66
Cervix	I	94
Colon	I, II	81
Endometrium	I	74
Kidney	I, II	67
Larynx	I, II	76
Lung (non-small cell)	I	50–70
	II	37
Oral cavity	I, II	67–76
Ovary	I, II	72
Prostate	I	80
Testis (nonseminoma)	I	65
Radiation therapy alone		
Cervix	II, III	60
Esophagus	—	10
Hodgkin lymphoma	Pathologic stage IA	80
Larynx	I, II	76
Lung (non-small cell)	III M0 (excluding Pancoast tumor)	9
Nasal sinuses	I, II, III	35
Nasopharynx	I, II, III	35
Non-Hodgkin lymphoma	Pathologic stage I	60
Prostate	I, II	80
Testis (seminoma)	II, III	84
Chemotherapy (sometimes plus radiation)		
Burkitt lymphoma	I, II, III	60
Choriocarcinoma (in women)	All stages	95
Hodgkin lymphoma	IIIB,IVA, B	74
Leukemia (in children, ALL)	I, II, III	85
Leukemia (in children, ANLL)	—	50
Leukemia (in people ≤ 45 yr, ANLL)	—	40–50
Leukemia (in people 45–65 yr, ANLL)	—	25
Leukemia (in people > 65 yr, ANLL)	—	5
Lung (small cell)	Limited	25
Lymphoma (diffuse large cell)	II, III, IV	60
Testis (nonseminoma)	III	88
Surgery plus radiation		
Bladder	B_2, C	54
Endometrium	II	62
Hypopharynx	II, III	33
Lung (Pancoast tumor)	III M0	32
Oral cavity	III	36
Testis (seminoma)	I	94

Table 154–2. 5-YR DISEASE-FREE SURVIVAL RATES BY CANCER THERAPY (*Continued*)

SITE OR TYPE	STAGE	5-YR DISEASE-FREE SURVIVAL RATE (%)
Surgery plus chemotherapy		
Colon	III	70
Ovary (carcinoma)	III, IV	15
Radiation plus chemotherapy		
Anus (squamous cell carcinoma)	—	70
CNS (medulloblastoma)	—	70–80
Ewing sarcoma	All stages	70
Lung (small cell)	Limited	25
Surgery, radiation, plus chemotherapy		
Breast (with radiation therapy and/or hormonal therapy)	I, II	70–90
Embryonal rhabdomyosarcoma	All stages	80
Kidney (Wilms tumor)	All stages	80
Oral cavity or hypopharynx	III, IV	20–40
Rectum	II, III	50–70

ALL = acute lymphocytic leukemia; ANLL = acute nonlymphocytic leukemia.

inhibit or slow recovery from surgery. Patients may be neutropenic or thrombocytopenic or may have clotting disorders; these conditions increase the risk of sepsis and hemorrhage. Therefore, preoperative assessment is paramount (see p. 3128).

Primary tumor resection: If a primary tumor has not metastasized, surgery may be curative. Establishing a complete margin of normal tissue around the primary tumor (as in breast cancer surgery) is critical for the success of primary tumor resection and prevention of recurrence. Intraoperative examination of frozen tissue sections by a pathologist may be needed. Immediate resection of additional tissue is done if margins are positive for tumor cells. However, examination of frozen tissue is inferior to examination of processed and stained tissue. Later review of margin tissue may prove the need for wider resection.

Surgical resection for primary tumor with local spread may also require removal of involved regional lymph nodes, resection of an involved adjacent organ, or en bloc resection. Survival rates with surgery alone are listed for selected cancers (see Table 154–2).

When the primary tumor has spread into adjacent normal tissues extensively, surgery may be delayed so that other modalities (eg, chemotherapy, radiation therapy) can be used to reduce the size of the required resection.

Resection of metastases: When cancer has metastasized to regional lymph nodes, nonsurgical modalities may be the best initial treatments, as in locally advanced lung cancer or head and neck cancer. Single metastases, especially those in the lungs or liver, can sometimes be resected with a reasonable rate of cure.

Patients with a limited number of metastases, particularly to the liver, brain, or lungs, may benefit from surgical resection of both the primary and metastatic tumor. For example, in colon cancer with liver metastases, resection produces 5-yr survival rates of 30 to 40% if < 4 hepatic lesions exist and if adequate tumor margins can be obtained.

Cytoreduction: Cytoreduction (surgical resection to reduce tumor burden) is often an option when removal of all tumor tissue is impossible, as in most cases of ovarian cancer. Cytoreduction may increase the sensitivity of the remaining tissue to other treatment modalities through mechanisms that are not entirely clear. Primary renal cell carcinomas and ovarian cancers should be resected, if feasible, even in the presence of metastases. Cytoreduction also has yielded favorable results in pediatric solid tumors.

Palliative surgery: Surgery to relieve symptoms and preserve quality of life may be a reasonable alternative when cure is unlikely or when an attempt at cure produces adverse effects that are unacceptable to the patient. Tumor resection may be indicated to control pain, to reduce the risk of hemorrhage, or to relieve obstruction of a vital organ (eg, intestine, urinary tract). Nutritional supplementation with a feeding gastrostomy or jejunostomy tube may be necessary if proximal obstruction exists.

Reconstructive surgery: Reconstructive surgery may improve a patient's comfort or quality of life after tumor resection (eg, breast reconstruction after mastectomy).

Radiation Therapy

Radiation therapy can cure many cancers (see Table 154–2), particularly those that are localized or that can be completely encompassed within the radiation field. Radiation therapy plus surgery (for head and neck, laryngeal, or uterine cancer) or combined with chemotherapy and surgery (for sarcomas or breast, esophageal, lung, or rectal cancers) improves cure rates and allows for more limited surgery as compared with traditional surgical resection.

Radiation therapy can provide significant palliation when cure is not possible:

- For brain tumors: Prolongs patient functioning and prevents neurologic complications
- For cancers that compress the spinal cord: Prevents progression of neurologic deficits
- For superior vena cava syndromes: Relieves venous obstruction
- For painful bone lesions: Usually relieves symptoms

Radiation cannot destroy malignant cells without destroying some normal cells as well. Therefore, the risk to normal tissue must be weighed against the potential gain in treating the malignant cells. The final outcome of a dose of radiation depends on numerous factors, including

- Nature of the delivered radiation (mode, timing, volume, dose)
- Properties of the tumor (cell cycle phase, oxygenation, molecular properties, inherent sensitivity to radiation)

In general, cancer cells are selectively damaged because of their high metabolic and proliferative rates. Normal tissue repairs itself more effectively, resulting in greater net destruction of tumor.

Important considerations in the use of radiation therapy include the following:

- Treatment timing (critical)
- Dose fractionation (critical)
- Normal tissue within or adjacent to the proposed radiation field
- Target volume
- Configuration of radiation beams
- Dose distribution
- Modality and energy most suited to the patient's situation

Treatment is tailored to take advantage of the cellular kinetics of tumor growth, with the aim of maximizing damage to the tumor while minimizing damage to normal tissues.

Radiation therapy sessions begin with the precise positioning of the patient. Foam casts or plastic masks are often constructed to ensure exact repositioning for serial treatments. Laser-guided sensors are used. Typical courses consist of large daily doses given over 3 wk for palliative treatment or smaller doses given once/day 5 days/wk for 6 to 8 wk for curative treatment.

Types of radiation therapy: There are several different types of radiation therapy.

External beam radiation therapy can be done with photons (gamma radiation), electrons, or protons. Gamma radiation using a linear accelerator is the most common type of radiation therapy. The radiation dose to adjacent normal tissue can be limited by conformal technology, which reduces scatter at the field margins. Electron beam radiation therapy has little tissue penetration and is best for skin or superficial cancers. Different energies of electrons are used based on the desired depth of penetration and type of tumor. Proton therapy, although limited in availability, has advantages over gamma radiation therapy in that it deposits energy at a depth from the surface, whereas gamma radiation damages all tissues along the path of the beam. Proton beam therapy also can provide sharp margins that may result in less injury to immediately adjacent tissue and is thus particularly useful for tumors of the eye, the base of the brain, and the spine.

Stereotactic radiation therapy is radiosurgery with precise stereotactic localization of a tumor to deliver a single high dose or multiple fractionated doses to a small intracranial or other target. It is frequently used to treat metastatic tumors in the CNS. Advantages include complete tumor ablation where conventional surgery would not be possible and minimal adverse effects. Disadvantages include limitations involving the size of the area that can be treated and the potential danger to adjacent tissues because of the high dose of radiation. In addition, it cannot be used in all areas of the body. Patients must be immobilized and the area kept completely still.

Brachytherapy involves placement of radioactive seeds into the tumor bed itself (eg, in the prostate or cervix). Typically, placement is guided by CT or ultrasonography. Brachytherapy achieves higher effective radiation doses over a longer period than could be accomplished by use of fractionated, external beam radiation therapy.

Systemic radioactive isotopes can direct radiation to cancer in organs that have specific receptors for uptake of the isotope (ie, radioactive iodine for thyroid cancer) or when the radionuclide is attached to a monoclonal antibody (eg, iodine-131 plus tositumomab for non-Hodgkin lymphoma). Isotopes can also accomplish palliation of generalized bony metastases (ie, radiostrontium for prostate cancer).

Other agents or strategies, particularly chemotherapy, can sensitize tumor tissue to the delivered radiation and increase efficacy.

Adverse effects: Radiation can damage any intervening normal tissue.

Acute adverse effects depend on the area receiving radiation and may include

- Lethargy
- Fatigue
- Mucositis
- Dermatologic manifestations (erythema, pruritus, desquamation)
- Esophagitis
- Pneumonitis
- Hepatitis
- GI symptoms (nausea, vomiting, diarrhea, tenesmus)
- GU symptoms (frequency, urgency, dysuria)
- Cytopenias

Early detection and management of these adverse effects is important not only for the patient's comfort and quality of life but also to ensure continuous treatment; prolonged interruption can allow for tumor regrowth.

Late complications can include cataracts, keratitis, and retinal damage if the eye is in the treatment field. Additional late complications include hypopituitarism, xerostomia, hypothyroidism, pneumonitis, pericarditis, esophageal stricture, hepatitis, ulcers, gastritis, nephritis, sterility, and muscular contractures. Radiation that reaches normal tissue can lead to poor healing of the tissues if further procedures or surgery is necessary. For example, radiation to the head and neck impairs recovery from dental procedures (eg, restoration, extraction) and thus should be administered only after all necessary dental work has been done.

Radiation therapy can increase the risk of developing other cancers, particularly leukemias, sarcomas in the radiation pathway, and carcinomas of the thyroid or breast. Peak incidence occurs 5 to 20 yr after exposure and depends on the patient's age at the time of treatment. For example, chest radiation therapy for Hodgkin lymphoma in adolescent girls leads to a higher risk of breast cancer than does the same treatment for postadolescent women.

Chemotherapy

The ideal chemotherapeutic drug would target and destroy only cancer cells. Only a few such drugs exist. Common chemotherapeutic drugs and their adverse effects are described (see Table 154–3).

The most common routes of administration are IV for cytotoxic drugs and oral for targeted drugs. Frequent dosing for extended periods may necessitate subcutaneously implanted venous access devices (central or peripheral), multilumen external catheters, or peripherally inserted central catheters.

Table 154–3. COMMONLY USED ANTINEOPLASTIC DRUGS

DRUG	MECHANISM OF ACTION	COMMONLY RESPONSIVE TUMORS	TOXICITY AND COMMENTS
Antimetabolites: Folate antagonists			
Methotrexate	Binds to dihydrofolate reductase and interferes with thymidylate synthesis	Acute lymphocytic leukemia Choriocarcinoma (women) Head and neck cancer Malignant lymphoma Osteogenic sarcoma Ovarian cancer	Mucosal ulceration Bone marrow suppression Increased toxicity with impaired renal function or ascitic fluid (with pooling of drug) Reversal of toxicity with leucovorin rescue at 24 h (10–20 mg q 6 h for 10 doses)
Pemetrexed	Inhibits thymidylate synthase	Lung cancer Mesothelioma Ovarian cancer	Bone marrow suppression Mucosal ulceration
Antimetabolites: Purine antagonists			
Cladribine	Inhibits ribonucleotide reductase	Leukemia Lymphoma	Myelosuppression Immunosuppression
Clofarabine	Inhibits DNA synthesis	Acute lymphocytic leukemia refractory to at least 2 prior chemotherapy regimens	Myelosuppression Immunosuppression Nausea Diarrhea
Fludarabine	Terminates DNA synthesis and inhibits ribonucleotide reductase	Leukemia Lymphoma	Myelosuppression Immunosuppression Autoimmune reactions
6-Mercaptopurine	Blocks de novo purine synthesis	Acute leukemia	Myelosuppression Immunosuppression
Nelarabine	Inhibits DNA synthesis	Leukemia Lymphoma	Myelosuppression Immunosuppression
Pentostatin	Inhibits DNA synthesis	Leukemia	Myelosuppression Immunosuppression Nausea Vomiting
Antimetabolites: Pyrimidine antagonists			
Capecitabine	Inhibits thymidylate synthase	Breast cancer GI tumors	Mucositis Alopecia Myelosuppression Diarrhea Vomiting Hand or foot tenderness Ulceration
Cytarabine	Terminates chain when incorporated into DNA	Acute leukemia (especially nonlymphocytic) Lymphoma	Myelosuppression Nausea Vomiting Cerebellar toxicity (at high doses) Conjunctival toxicity (at high doses) Rash
5-Fluorouracil	Inhibits thymidylate synthase	Breast cancer GI tumors	Mucositis Alopecia Myelosuppression Diarrhea Vomiting
Gemcitabine	Terminates chain when incorporated into DNA and inhibits ribonucleotide reductase	Bladder cancer Lung cancer Pancreatic cancer	Myelosuppression Hemolytic-uremic syndrome
Hydroxyurea	Inhibits ribonucleotide reductase	Chronic myelocytic leukemia	Myelosuppression

Table continues on the following page.

Table 154–3. COMMONLY USED ANTINEOPLASTIC DRUGS (*Continued*)

DRUG	MECHANISM OF ACTION	COMMONLY RESPONSIVE TUMORS	TOXICITY AND COMMENTS
Biologic response modifiers			
Interferon alfa	Has antiproliferative effect	Chronic myelocytic leukemia Hairy cell leukemia Kaposi's sarcoma Lymphomas Melanoma Renal cell cancer	Fatigue Fever Myalgias Arthralgias Myelosuppression Nephrotic syndrome (rare)
Bleomycins			
Bleomycin	Causes DNA strands to break	Lymphoma Squamous cell cancer Testicular cancer	Anaphylaxis Chills and fever Rash Pulmonary fibrosis at dosage > 200 mg/m^2 Requires renal excretion
DNA alkylating agents: Nitrosoureas			
Carmustine	Alkylates DNA with restricted uncoiling and replication of strands	Brain tumors Lymphoma	Myelosuppression Pulmonary toxicity (fibrosis) Renal toxicity
Lomustine	Alkylates DNA with restricted uncoiling and replication of strands	Brain tumors (astrocytoma, glioblastoma)	Myelosuppression Pulmonary toxicity (delayed) Renal toxicity
DNA cross-linking drugs and alkylating agents			
Bendamustine Chlorambucil Cyclophosphamide Ifosfamide Mechlorethamine (nitrogen mustard) Melphalan	Form adducts with DNA, causing DNA strands to break	Breast cancer Chronic lymphocytic leukemia Gliomas Hodgkin lymphoma Lymphoma Multiple myeloma Small cell lung cancer Testicular cancer	Alopecia with high IV dosage Nausea Vomiting Myelosuppression Hemorrhagic cystitis (especially with cyclophosphamide and ifosfamide), which can be ameliorated with mesna Mutagenesis Secondary leukemias Aspermia Permanent sterility (possible)
Dacarbazine Temozolomide	Form adducts with DNA	Melanoma Malignant glioma	Neutropenia Nausea Vomiting Secondary leukemias
Procarbazine	Unclear	Hodgkin lymphoma	Neutropenia Nausea Vomiting Secondary leukemias
Enzymes			
Asparaginase	Depletes asparagine, on which leukemic cells depend	Acute lymphocytic leukemia	Acute anaphylaxis Hyperthermia Pancreatitis Hyperglycemia Hypofibrinogenemia
Hormones			
Bicalutamide Flutamide	Bind to androgen receptor	Prostate cancer	Decreased libido Hot flushes Gynecomastia

Table 154–3. COMMONLY USED ANTINEOPLASTIC DRUGS (*Continued*)

DRUG	MECHANISM OF ACTION	COMMONLY RESPONSIVE TUMORS	TOXICITY AND COMMENTS
Fulvestrant	Binds to estrogen receptor	Metastatic breast cancer	Nausea Vomiting Constipation Diarrhea Abdominal pain Headache Back pain Hot flushes Pharyngitis
Leuprolide acetate	Inhibits gonadotropin secretion	Prostate cancer	Hot flushes Decreased libido Irritation at injection site
Megestrol acetate	Progesterone agonist	Breast cancer Endometrial cancer	Weight gain Fluid retention
Tamoxifen	Binds to estrogen receptor	Breast cancer	Hot flushes Hypercalcemia Deep venous thrombosis
Hormones: Aromatase inhibitors			
Anastrozole Exemestane Letrozole	Block conversion of androgen to estrogen	Breast cancer	Osteoporosis Hot flushes
Monoclonal antibodies			
Alemtuzumab	Binds to B and T cells	Lymphomas	Immunosuppression
Bevacizumab	Binds to vascular endothelial growth factor	Colon cancer Renal cancer	Hypersensitivity Bleeding Hypertension
Brentuximab vedotin (linked to antimitotic agent auristatin E)	Binds to CD30 on lymphoma cells	Lymphomas	Progressive multifocal leukoencephalopathy Combining with bleomycin is contraindicated due to pulmonary toxicity
Gemtuzumab	Binds to CD33 on leukemic cells	Acute myelocytic leukemia	Myelosuppression
Ibritumomab tiuxetan	Binds to CD20 on lymphoid cells	Lymphomas	Delivers radiation to cancer cells
Ipilimumab	Anti-CTLA-4	Inoperable or advanced metastatic melanoma	Colitis Hepatitis Toxic epidermal necrolysis
Iodine-131 tositumomab	Bind to CD20 on lymphoid cells	Lymphomas	Myelosuppression Fever Rash
Ofatumumab	Binds to CD20 on lymphoid cells	CLL refractory to fludarabine and alemtuzumab	Myelosuppression
Rituximab	Binds to CD20 on B cells	B-cell lymphoma	Hypersensitivity Immunosuppression
Trastuzumab	Binds to HER2/neu receptor	Breast cancer	Hypersensitivity Cardiac toxicity
Other antibiotics			
Mitomycin	Inhibits DNA synthesis by acting as a bifunctional alkylator	Breast cancer Colon cancer Gastric adenocarcinoma Lung cancer Transitional cell cancer of the bladder	Local extravasation causing tissue necrosis Myelosuppression, with leukopenia and thrombocytopenia 4 to 6 wk after treatment Alopecia Lethargy Fever Hemolytic-uremic syndrome

Table continues on the following page.

Table 154–3. COMMONLY USED ANTINEOPLASTIC DRUGS (*Continued*)

DRUG	MECHANISM OF ACTION	COMMONLY RESPONSIVE TUMORS	TOXICITY AND COMMENTS
Platinum complexes			
Carboplatin	Establishes cross-links within and between DNA strands	Breast cancer Lung cancer Ovarian cancer	Myelosuppression Peripheral neuropathy
Cisplatin	Establishes cross-links within and between DNA strands	Bladder cancer Breast cancer Head and neck cancer Gastric cancer Lung cancer (especially small cell) Testicular cancer	Anemia Ototoxicity Nausea Vomiting Peripheral neuropathy Myelosuppression
Oxaliplatin	Establishes cross-links within and between DNA strands	Colon cancer	Myelosuppression Neuropathic throat pain Peripheral neuropathy
Proteosome inhibitors			
Bortezomib Carfilzomib	Inhibit proteosome functions	Multiple myeloma	Myelosuppression Diarrhea Nausea Constipation Peripheral neuropathy
Spindle poison (from plants): Taxanes			
Docetaxel	Promotes assembly of micro-tubules	Breast cancer Head and neck cancer Lung cancer Ovarian cancer	Myelosuppression Alopecia Rash Fluid retention
Carbezitaxel Paclitaxel (as solution or albumin-bound microspheres)	Promote assembly of micro-tubules	Bladder cancer Breast cancer Head and neck cancer Lung cancer Ovarian cancer	Myelosuppression Alopecia Myalgia Arthralgia Neuropathy
Spindle poison (from plants): Vincas			
Vinblastine	Arrests mitosis by inhibiting polymerization of micro-tubules	Breast cancer Ewing's sarcoma Leukemia Lymphomas Testicular cancer	Alopecia Myelosuppression Peripheral neuropathy
Vincristine	Arrests mitosis by inhibiting polymerization of micro-tubules	Acute leukemia Lymphoma	Peripheral neuropathy Ileus Syndrome of inappropriate antidiuretic hormone secretion
Vinorelbine	Arrests mitosis by inhibiting polymerization of microtubules	Breast cancer Lung cancer	Myelosuppression Neuropathy
Topoisomerase inhibitors: Anthracyclines			
Daunorubicin (daunomycin) Idarubicin	Inhibit topoisomerase II and causes DNA strands to break	Leukemia	Myelosuppression Cardiac toxicity at cumulative dosage > 1000 mg/m^2
Doxorubicin	Inhibits topoisomerase II and causes DNA strands to break	Acute leukemia Breast cancer Lung cancer Lymphoma	Nausea Vomiting Alopecia Myelosuppression Cardiac toxicity at cumulative dosage > 550 mg/m^2

Table 154–3. COMMONLY USED ANTINEOPLASTIC DRUGS (*Continued*)

DRUG	MECHANISM OF ACTION	COMMONLY RESPONSIVE TUMORS	TOXICITY AND COMMENTS
Epirubicin	Inhibits topoisomerase II and causes DNA strands to break	Acute myelocytic leukemia Breast cancer Gastric cancer	Myelosuppression Cardiac toxicity at cumulative dosage > 1000 mg/m^2
Topoisomerase inhibitors: Camptothecins			
Irinotecan	Inhibits topoisomerase I	Colon cancer Lung cancer Rectal cancer	Diarrhea Myelosuppression Alopecia
Topotecan	Inhibits topoisomerase I	Ovarian cancer Small cell lung cancer	Myelosuppression
Topoisomerase inhibitors: Podophyllotoxins			
Etoposide Teniposide	Inhibit topoisomerase II and cause DNA strands to break	Acute leukemia Hodgkin lymphoma Lymphoma Lung cancer (especially small cell) Testicular cancer	Nausea Vomiting Myelosuppression Peripheral neuropathy Increased toxicity in renal failure Neutropenia Cleared by liver and kidneys
Mitoxantrone	Inhibits topoisomerase II and causes DNA strands to break	Acute leukemia Lymphoma	Neutropenia Nausea Vomiting
Tyrosine kinase inhibitors			
Bosutinib Desatinib Imatinib Nilotinib Ponantinib	Inhibit BCR-ABL kinase and C-kit kinase	Chronic myelocytic leukemia GI stromal tumors	Leukopenia Hepatocellular toxicity Edema
Crizotinib	Inhibits the EML-4/ALK kinase	Non–small cell lung cancer	Diarrhea Hepatocellular toxicity
Erlotinib Gefitinib	Inhibit epidermal growth factor receptor	Non–small cell lung cancer	Acne Diarrhea Pneumonitis
Lapatinib	Inhibits *Her2/neu* activity Blocks epidermal growth factor receptor	Breast cancer	Diarrhea Nausea Rash Vomiting Fatigue
Pazopanib	Inhibits vascular endothelial growth factor	Sarcomas	Hypertension Proteinuria Hepatocellular toxicity QT prolongation
Sorafenib	Inhibits intracellular and cell surface kinases (eg, vascular endothelial growth factor receptor)	Hepatocellular cancer Renal cancer	Hypertension Proteinuria
Sunitinib	Inhibits receptor tyrosine kinases (C-kit) Blocks vascular endothelial growth factor receptor	GI stromal tumors Renal cancer	Hypertension Proteinuria Poor wound healing Intestinal perforations
Vandetanib	Blocks vascular endothelial growth factor receptor Epidermal growth factor receptor	Thyroid cancer	Torsades de pointes ventricular tachycardia
Vemurafenib	B-Raf tyrosine kinase	Melanoma	Diarrhea Hepatotoxicity

Drug resistance can occur to chemotherapy. Identified mechanisms include overexpression of target genes, mutation of target genes, development of alternative pathways, drug inactivation by tumor cells, defective apoptosis in tumor cells, and loss of receptors for hormonal agents. For cytotoxic drugs, one of the best characterized mechanisms is overexpression of the *MDR-1* gene, a cell membrane transporter that causes efflux of certain drugs (eg, vinca alkaloids, taxanes, anthracyclines). Attempts to alter *MDR-1* function and thus prevent drug resistance have been unsuccessful.

Cytotoxic drugs: Traditional cytotoxic chemotherapy, which damages cell DNA, kills many normal cells in addition to cancer cells. Antimetabolites, such as 5-fluorouracil and methotrexate, are cell cycle–specific and have no linear dose-response relationship. In contrast, other chemotherapeutic drugs (eg, DNA cross-linkers, also known as alkylating agents) have a linear dose-response relationship, producing more tumor killing as well as more toxicity at higher doses. At their highest doses, DNA cross-linkers may cause bone marrow aplasia, necessitating bone marrow/stem cell transplantation to restore bone marrow function.

Single-drug chemotherapy may cure selected cancers (eg, choriocarcinoma, hairy cell leukemia). More commonly, multidrug regimens incorporating drugs with different mechanisms of action and different toxicities are used to increase the tumor cell kill, reduce dose-related toxicity, and decrease the probability of drug resistance. These regimens can provide significant cure rates (eg, in acute leukemia, testicular cancer, Hodgkin lymphoma, non-Hodgkin lymphoma, and, less commonly, solid tumors such as small cell lung cancer and nasopharyngeal cancer). Multidrug regimens typically are given as repetitive cycles of a fixed combination of drugs. The interval between cycles should be the shortest one that allows for recovery of normal tissue. Continuous infusion may increase cell kill with some cell cycle–specific drugs (eg, 5-fluorouracil).

For each patient, the probability of significant toxicities should be weighed against the likelihood of benefit. End-organ function should be assessed before chemotherapeutic drugs with organ-specific toxicities are used (eg, echocardiography before doxorubicin use). Dose modification or exclusion of certain drugs may be necessary in patients with chronic lung disease (eg, bleomycin), renal failure (eg, methotrexate), or hepatic dysfunction (eg, taxanes).

Despite these precautions, adverse effects commonly result from cytotoxic chemotherapy. The normal tissues most commonly affected are those with the highest intrinsic turnover rate: bone marrow, hair follicles, and the GI epithelium.

Imaging (eg, CT, MRI, PET) is frequently done after 2 to 3 cycles of therapy to evaluate response to treatment. Therapy continues if there is a clear response. If the tumor progresses despite therapy, the regimen is often amended or stopped. If the disease remains stable with treatment and the patient can tolerate therapy, then a decision to continue is reasonable with the understanding that the disease will eventually progress.

Hormonal therapy: Hormonal therapy uses hormone agonists or antagonists to influence the course of cancer. It may be used alone or in combination with other treatment modalities.

Hormonal therapy is particularly useful in prostate cancer, which grows in response to androgens. Other cancers with hormone receptors on their cells (eg, breast, endometrium) can often be palliated by hormone antagonist therapy or hormone ablation. Hormonal agents may block the secretion of pituitary hormones (luteinizing hormone-releasing hormone agonists), block the androgen (bicalutamide, enzalutamide) or estrogen receptor (tamoxifen), suppress the conversion of androgens to estrogens by aromatase (letrozole), or inhibit the synthesis of adrenal androgens (abiraterone). All hormonal blockers cause symptoms related to hormone deficiency, such as hot flashes, and the androgen antagonists also induce a metabolic syndrome that increases the risk of diabetes and heart disease.

Use of prednisone, a glucocorticosteroid, is also considered hormonal therapy. It is frequently used to treat tumors derived from the immune system (lymphomas, lymphocytic leukemias, multiple myeloma).

Biologic response modifiers: Interferons are proteins synthesized by cells of the immune system as a physiologic immune protective response to foreign antigens (viruses, bacteria, other foreign cells). In pharmacologic amounts, they can palliate some cancers, including hairy cell leukemia, chronic myelocytic leukemia, locally advanced melanoma, metastatic renal cell cancer, and Kaposi sarcoma. Significant toxic effects of interferon include fatigue, depression, nausea, leukopenia, chills and fever, and myalgias.

Interleukins, primarily the lymphokine IL-2 produced by activated T cells, can be used in metastatic melanomas and can provide modest palliation in renal cell cancer.

Ipilimimab, which promotes autoimmune responses, activates the antitumor response to melanoma and other tumors.

Differentiating drugs: These drugs induce differentiation in cancer cells. All-*trans*-retinoic acid has been highly effective in treating acute promyelocytic leukemia. Other drugs in this class include arsenic compounds and the hypomethylating agents azacitidine and deoxyazacytidine. When used alone, these drugs have only transient effects, but their role in prevention and in combination with cytotoxic drugs is promising.

Antiangiogenesis drugs: Solid tumors produce growth factors that form new blood vessels necessary to support ongoing tumor growth. Several drugs that inhibit this process are available. Thalidomide is antiangiogenic, among its many effects. Bevacizumab, a monoclonal antibody to vascular endothelial growth factor (VEGF), is effective against renal cancers and colon cancer. VEGF receptor inhibitors, such as sorafenib and sunitinib, are also effective in renal cancer, hepatocellular cancers, and other tumors.

Signal transduction inhibitors: Many epithelial tumors possess mutations that activate signaling pathways that cause their continuous proliferation and failure to differentiate. These mutated pathways include growth factor receptors and the downstream proteins that transmit messages to the cell nucleus from growth factor receptors on the cell surface. Three such drugs, imatinib (an inhibitor of the BCR-ABL tyrosine kinase in chronic myelocytic leukemia) and erlotinib and gefitinib (inhibitors of the epidermal growth factor receptor), are now in routine clinical use. Other inhibitors of these signaling pathways are under study.

Monoclonal antibodies: Monoclonal antibodies directed against unique tumor antigens have some efficacy against neoplastic tissue (see also p. 1219). Trastuzumab, an antibody directed against a protein called HER-2 or ErbB-2, plus chemotherapy has shown benefit in metastatic breast cancer that expressed HER-2. Antibodies against CD antigens expressed on neoplastic cells, such as CD20 and CD33, are used to treat patients with non-Hodgkin lymphoma (rituximab, anti-CD20 antibody) and acute myelocytic leukemia (gemtuzumab, an antibody linked to a potent toxin).

The effectiveness of monoclonal antibodies may be increased by linking them to radioactive nuclide. One such drug, ibritumomab, is used to treat non-Hodgkin lymphoma.

Vaccines: Vaccines designed to trigger or enhance immune system response to cancer cells have been extensively studied and have typically provided little benefit. However, recently, sipuleucel-T, an autologous dendritic cell–derived immunotherapy, has demonstrated modest prolongation of life in patients with metastatic prostate cancer.

A new modality being studied modifies a patient's T cells to recognize and target tumor-associated antigens (eg, CD19). Initial reports show improvement in patients with chronic lymphocytic leukemia and certain types of acute leukemia that have become resistant to chemotherapy.

Multimodality and Adjuvant Chemotherapy

In some tumors with a high likelihood of relapse despite optimal initial surgery or radiation therapy, relapse may be prevented by addition of adjuvant chemotherapy. Increasingly, combined-modality therapy (eg, radiation therapy, chemotherapy, surgery) is used. It may permit organ-sparing procedures and preserve organ function.

Adjuvant therapy: Adjuvant therapy is systemic chemotherapy or radiation therapy given to eradicate residual occult tumor *after* initial surgery. Patients who have a high risk of recurrence may benefit from its use. General criteria are based on degree of local extension of the primary tumor, presence of positive lymph nodes, and certain morphologic or biologic characteristics of individual cancer cells. Adjuvant therapy has increased disease-free survival and cure rate in breast and in colorectal cancer.

Neoadjuvant therapy: Neoadjuvant therapy is chemotherapy, radiation therapy, or both given *before* surgical resection. This treatment may enhance resectability and preserve local organ function. For example, when neoadjuvant therapy is used in head and neck, esophageal, or rectal cancer, a smaller subsequent resection may be possible. Another advantage of neoadjuvant therapy is in assessing response to treatment; if the primary tumor does not respond, micrometastases are unlikely to be eradicated, and an alternate regimen should be considered. Neoadjuvant therapy may obscure the true pathologic stage of the cancer by altering tumor size and margins and converting histologically positive nodes to negative, complicating clinical staging. The use of neoadjuvant therapy has improved survival in inflammatory and locally advanced breast, stage IIIA lung, nasopharyngeal, and bladder cancers.

Bone Marrow/Stem Cell Transplantation

Bone marrow or stem cell transplantation is an important component of the treatment of otherwise refractory lymphomas, leukemias, and multiple myeloma (for an in-depth discussion of this topic, see p. 1413).

Gene Therapy

Genetic modulation is under intense investigation. Strategies include the use of antisense therapy, systemic viral vector transfection, DNA injection into tumors, genetic modulation of resected tumor cells to increase their immunogenicity, and alteration of immune cells to enhance their antitumor response.

MANAGEMENT OF ADVERSE EFFECTS OF CANCER THERAPY

Patients being treated for cancer frequently experience adverse effects. Managing these effects improves quality of life.

Nausea and Vomiting

Nausea and vomiting are commonly experienced by cancer patients and may result from the cancer itself (eg, paraneoplastic syndromes) or from its treatment (eg, chemotherapy, radiation therapy to the brain or abdomen). However, refractory nausea and vomiting should prompt further investigation, including basic laboratory testing (electrolytes, liver function tests, lipase) and x-rays to investigate possible bowel obstruction or intracranial metastases.

Serotonin-receptor antagonists are the most effective drugs but are also the most expensive. Virtually no toxicity occurs with granisetron and ondansetron aside from headache and orthostatic hypotension. A 0.15-mg/kg dose of ondansetron or a 10-mcg/kg dose of granisetron is given IV 30 min before chemotherapy. Doses of ondansetron can be repeated 4 and 8 h after the first dose. The efficacy against highly emetogenic drugs, such as the platinum complexes, can be improved with coadministration of dexamethasone 8 mg IV given 30 min before chemotherapy with repeat doses of 4 mg IV q 8 h.

A substance P/neurokinin-1 antagonist, aprepitant, can limit nausea and vomiting resulting from highly emetogenic chemotherapy. Dosage is 125 mg po 1 h before chemotherapy on day 1, then 80 mg po 1 h before chemotherapy on days 2 and 3.

Other traditional antiemetics, including phenothiazines (eg, prochlorperazine 10 mg IV q 8 h, promethazine 12.5 to 25 mg po or IV q 8 h) and metoclopramide 10 mg po or IV given 30 min before chemotherapy with repeated doses q 6 to 8 h, are alternatives restricted to patients with mild to moderate nausea and vomiting.

Dronabinol (Δ-9-tetrahydrocannabinol [THC]) is an alternative treatment for nausea and vomiting caused by chemotherapy. THC is the principal psychoactive component of marijuana. Its mechanism of antiemetic action is unknown, but cannabinoids bind to opioid receptors in the forebrain and may indirectly inhibit the vomiting center. Dronabinol is administered in doses of 5 mg/m^2 po 1 to 3 h before chemotherapy, with repeated doses q 2 to 4 h after the start of chemotherapy (maximum of 4 to 6 doses/day). However, it has variable oral bioavailability, is not effective for inhibiting the nausea and vomiting of platinum-based chemotherapy regimens, and has significant adverse effects (eg, drowsiness, orthostatic hypotension, dry mouth, mood changes, visual and time sense alterations). Smoking marijuana may be more effective. Marijuana for this purpose can be obtained legally in some states. It is used less commonly because of barriers to availability and because many patients cannot tolerate smoking.

Benzodiazepines, such as lorazepam 1 to 2 mg po or IV given 10 to 20 min before chemotherapy with repeated doses q 4 to 6 h prn, are sometimes helpful for refractory or anticipatory nausea and vomiting.

Cytopenias

Anemia, leukopenia, and thrombocytopenia may develop during chemotherapy or radiation therapy.

Anemia: Clinical symptoms and decreased efficacy of radiation therapy usually occur at Hct levels of < 30% or Hb levels < 10 g/dL, sooner in patients with coronary artery disease or peripheral vascular disease. Recombinant erythropoietin therapy may be started when Hb falls to < 10 mg/dL, depending on symptoms. In general, 150 to 300 units/kg sc 3 times/wk (a convenient adult dose is 10,000 units) is effective and reduces the need for transfusions. Longer-acting formulations of erythropoietin require less frequent dosing (darbepoetin alfa 2.25 to

4.5 mcg/kg sc q 1 to 2 wk). Unnecessary use of erythropoietin should be avoided because it increases the risk of cardiovascular thrombosis. Packed RBC transfusions may be needed to relieve acute cardiorespiratory symptoms but should generally not be given to asymptomatic anemic patients unless they have significant underlying cardiopulmonary disease.

Thrombocytopenia: A platelet count < 10,000/mL, especially with bleeding, requires transfusion of platelet concentrates. Small molecules that mimic thrombopoietin are available but are not commonly used in cancer treatment.

Leukocyte depletion of transfused blood products may prevent alloimmunization to platelets and should be used in patients who are expected to need platelet transfusions during multiple courses of chemotherapy or for candidates for stem cell transplantation. Leukocyte depletion also lowers the probability of cytomegalovirus being transferred to the patient through WBCs. Using gamma radiation of blood products to inactivate lymphocytes and prevent transfusion-induced graft-vs-host disease is also indicated in patients undergoing severely immunosuppressive chemotherapy.

Neutropenia: Neutropenia (see also p. 1152), usually defined by an absolute neutrophil count < 500/μL, predisposes to immediate life-threatening infection.

Afebrile patients with neutropenia require close outpatient follow-up for detection of fever and should be instructed to avoid contact with sick people or areas frequented by large numbers of people (eg, shopping malls, airports). Although most patients do not require antibiotics, patients with severe immunosuppression (ie, concomitant T-cell depletion or loss of function) *and* leukopenia are sometimes given trimethoprim/sulfamethoxazole (one double-strength tablet/day) as prophylaxis for *Pneumocystis jirovecii*. In transplant patients or others receiving high-dose chemotherapy, antiviral prophylaxis (acyclovir 800 mg po bid or 400 mg IV q 12 h) should be considered if serologic tests are positive for herpes simplex virus.

Fever > 38° C in a patient with neutropenia is an emergency. Evaluation should include immediate chest x-ray and cultures of blood, sputum, urine, stool, and any suspect skin lesions. Examination includes possible abscess sites (eg, skin, ears), skin and mucosa for presence of herpetic lesions, retina for vascular lesions suggestive of metastatic infection, and catheter sites. Rectal examination and use of a rectal thermometer are avoided if possible in neutropenic patients because of the risk of bacteremia.

Febrile neutropenic patients should receive broad-spectrum antibiotics chosen on the basis of the most likely organism. Typical regimens include cefepime or ceftazidime 2 g IV q 8 h immediately after samples for culture are obtained. If diffuse pulmonary infiltrates are present, sputum should be tested for *P. jirovecii*, and if positive, appropriate therapy should be started. If fever resolves within 72 h after starting empiric antibiotics, then antibiotics are continued until the absolute neutrophil count is > 500/μL. If fever continues for 120 h, antifungal drugs should be added to treat possible fungal causes. Reassessment for occult infection (often including CT of the chest and abdomen) should be undertaken at this time.

In selected patients with neutropenia related to chemotherapy, especially after high-dose chemotherapy, granulocyte colony-stimulating factor (G-CSF) or granulocyte-macrophage colony-stimulating factor (GM-CSF) may be started to shorten the leukopenic period. G-CSF 5 mcg/kg sc once/day up to 14 days and longer-acting forms (eg, pegfilgrastim 6 mg sc single dose once per chemotherapy cycle) may be used to accelerate WBC recovery. These drugs should not be administered in the first 24 h after chemotherapy, and for pegfilgrastim, at least 14 days should elapse until the next planned chemotherapy dose. These drugs are begun at the onset of fever or sepsis or, in afebrile high-risk patients, when neutrophil counts fall to < 500/μL.

Many centers use outpatient treatment with G-CSF in selected low-risk patients with fever and neutropenia. Candidates must not have hypotension, altered mental status, respiratory distress, uncontrolled pain, or serious comorbid illnesses, such as diabetes, heart disease, or hypercalcemia. The regimen in such cases requires daily follow-up and often involves visiting nurse services and home antibiotic infusion. Some regimens involve oral antibiotics, such as ciprofloxacin 750 mg po bid plus amoxicillin/clavulanate 875 mg po bid or 500 mg po tid. If no defined institutional program for follow-up and treatment of neutropenic fever is available in an outpatient setting, then hospitalization is required.

Gastrointestinal Effects

GI adverse effects are common among cancer patients.

Oral lesions: Oral lesions, such as ulcers, infections, and inflammation, are common.

Oral candidiasis can be treated with nystatin oral suspension 5 to 10 mL qid, clotrimazole troches 10 mg qid, or fluconazole 100 mg po once/day.

Mucositis due to radiation therapy can cause pain and preclude sufficient oral intake, leading to undernutrition and weight loss. Rinses with analgesics and topical anesthetics (2% viscous lidocaine 5 to 10 mL q 2 h or other commercially available mixtures) before meals, a bland diet without citrus food or juices, and avoidance of temperature extremes may allow patients to eat and maintain weight. If not, a feeding tube may be helpful if the small intestine is functional. For severe mucositis and diarrhea or an abnormally functioning intestine, parenteral alimentation may be needed.

Diarrhea: Diarrhea due to pelvic radiation therapy or chemotherapy can be alleviated with antidiarrheal drugs as needed (eg, kaolin/pectin suspension 60 to 120 mL regular strength, or 30 to 60 mL concentrate, po at first sign of diarrhea and after each loose stool or prn; loperamide 2 to 4 mg po after each loose stool; or diphenoxylate/atropine 1 to 2 tablets po q 6 h). Patients who underwent abdominal surgery or received broad-spectrum antibiotics within the preceding 3 mo should undergo stool testing for *Clostridium difficile*.

Constipation: Constipation may result from opioid use. A stimulant laxative such as senna 2 to 6 tablets po at bedtime or bisacodyl 10 mg po at bedtime should be initiated when repeated opioid use is anticipated. Established constipation can be treated with various drugs (eg, bisacodyl 5 to 10 mg po q 12 to 24 h, milk of magnesia 15 to 30 mL po at bedtime, lactulose 15 to 30 mL q 12 to 24 h, Mg citrate 250 to 500 mL po once). Enemas and suppositories should be avoided in patients with neutropenia or thrombocytopenia.

Anorexia: Appetite may decrease secondary to cancer treatment or to a paraneoplastic syndrome. Corticosteroids (eg, dexamethasone 4 mg po once/day, prednisone 5 to 10 mg po once/day) and megestrol acetate 400 to 800 mg once/day are most effective. However, the primary benefits are variably increased appetite and weight gain, not improved survival or quality of life.

Pain

Pain should be anticipated and aggressively treated (see also p. 1968). Use of multiple drug classes may provide better pain control with fewer or less severe adverse effects than use of a single drug class. NSAIDs should be avoided in patients with thrombocytopenia. Opioids are the mainstay of treatment, given around the clock in generally efficient doses, with supplemental doses given for occasional worse pain. If the oral route is unavailable, fentanyl is given transdermally. When opioids are given, antiemetics and prophylactic bowel regimens are often needed.

Neuropathic pain can be treated with gabapentin; the dose required is high (up to 1200 mg po tid) but must be started low (eg, 300 mg tid) and then increased over a few weeks. Alternatively, a tricyclic antidepressant (eg, nortriptyline 25 to 75 mg po at bedtime) may be tried.

Useful nondrug treatments for pain include focal radiation therapy, nerve blockade, and surgery.

Depression

Depression is often overlooked. It may occur in response to the disease (its symptoms and feared consequences), adverse effects of the treatments, or both. Patients receiving interferon can develop depression as an adverse effect. Also, alopecia as an adverse effect of radiation therapy or chemotherapy can contribute to depression. Frank discussion of a patient's fears can often relieve anxiety. Depression can often be treated effectively (see p. 1757).

Tumor Lysis Syndrome

Tumor lysis syndrome may occur secondary to release of intracellular components into the bloodstream as a result of tumor cell death after chemotherapy. It occurs mainly in acute leukemias and non-Hodgkin lymphomas but can also occur in other hematologic cancers and, uncommonly, after treatment of solid tumors. It should be suspected in patients with a large tumor burden who develop acute kidney injury after initial treatment. T-cell vaccines used to treat B-cell leukemias (see p. 1193) may precipitate life threatening tumor lysis and cytokine release days to weeks after vaccine administration.

The diagnosis is confirmed by some combination of the following findings:

- Renal failure
- Hypocalcemia (< 8 mg/dL)
- Hyperuricemia (> 15 mg/dL)
- Hyperphosphatemia (> 8 mg/dL)

Allopurinol 200 to 400 mg/m^2 once/day, maximum 600 mg/day and normal saline IV to achieve urine output > 2 L/day should be initiated with close laboratory and cardiac monitoring. Patients who have a cancer with rapid cell turnover should receive allopurinol for at least 2 days before and during chemotherapy; for patients with high cell burden, this regimen can be continued for 10 to 14 days after therapy. All such patients should receive vigorous IV hydration to establish a diuresis of at least 100 mL/h before treatment. Although some physicians advocate $NaHCO_3$ IV to alkalinize the urine and increase solubilization of uric acid, alkalinization may promote Ca phosphate deposition in patients with hyperphosphatemia, and a pH of about 7 should be avoided. Alternatively, rasburicase, an enzyme that oxidizes uric acid to allantoin (a more soluble molecule), may be used to prevent tumor lysis. The dose is 0.15 to 0.2 mg/kg IV over 30 min once/day for 5 to 7 days, typically initiated 4 to 24 h before the first chemotherapy treatment. Adverse effects may include anaphylaxis, hemolysis, hemoglobinuria, and methemoglobinemia.

CACHEXIA IN CANCER

Cachexia is wasting of both adipose tissue and skeletal muscle. It occurs in many conditions and is common with many cancers when remission or control fails. Some cancers, especially pancreatic and gastric cancers, cause profound cachexia. Affected patients may lose 10 to 20% of body weight. Men tend to experience worse cachexia as a result of cancer than do women. Neither tumor size nor the extent of metastatic disease predicts the degree of cachexia. Cachexia is associated with reduced response to chemotherapy, poor functional performance, and increased mortality.

The primary cause of cachexia is not anorexia or decreased caloric intake. Rather, this complex metabolic condition involves increased tissue catabolism; protein synthesis is decreased and degradation increased. Cachexia is mediated by certain cytokines, especially tumor necrosis factor-α, IL-1b, and IL-6, which are produced by tumor cells and host cells in the tissue mass. The ATP-ubiquitin-protease pathway plays a role as well.

Cachexia is easy to recognize, primarily by weight loss, which is most apparent with loss of temporalis muscle mass in the face. The loss of subcutaneous fat increases the risk of pressure ulcers over bony prominences.

Treatment

Treatment involves treatment of the cancer. If the cancer can be controlled or cured, regardless of modality, cachexia resolves.

Additional caloric supplementation does not relieve cachexia. Any weight gain is usually minimal and is likely to consist of adipose tissue rather than muscle. Neither function nor prognosis is improved. Thus, in most patients with cancer and cachexia, high-calorie supplementation is not recommended, and parenteral nutritional support is not indicated, except in situations where oral intake of adequate nutrition is impossible.

However, other treatments can mitigate cachexia and improve function. Corticosteroids increase appetite and may improve a sense of well-being but do little to increase body weight. Likewise, cannabinoids (marijuana, dronabinol) increase appetite but not weight. Progestogens, such as megestrol acetate 40 mg po bid or tid, may increase both appetite and body weight. Drugs to alter cytokine production and effects are being studied.

INCURABLE CANCER

Even in cases of incurable cancer, palliative or experimental therapy may improve quality and extent of life. But in many cases, physicians must resist the urge to administer a relatively ineffective chemotherapy drug. A better choice is to discuss the likely results of such treatments and to set realistic goals with the patient. A patient's decision to forgo cancer treatment must be respected. Another alternative is the clinical trial, the risks and benefits of which deserve discussion.

Regardless of prognosis, quality of life in cancer patients may improve with nutritional support, effective pain management, other symptomatic palliative care, and psychiatric and social support of the patient and family. Above all, patients must know that the clinical team will remain involved and accessible for supportive care, regardless of the prognosis. Hospice or other related end-of-life care programs are important parts of cancer treatment. For more information pertaining to patients with incurable disease, see p. 3175.

155 Spleen Disorders

By structure and function, the spleen is like 2 organs. The white pulp, consisting of periarterial lymphatic sheaths and germinal centers, acts as an immune organ. The red pulp, consisting of macrophages and granulocytes lining vascular spaces (the cords and sinusoids), acts as a phagocytic organ.

The **white pulp** is a site of production and maturation of B cells and T cells. B cells in the spleen generate protective humoral antibodies; in certain autoimmune disorders (eg, immune thrombocytopenia [ITP], Coombs-positive immune hemolytic anemias), inappropriate autoantibodies to circulating blood elements also may be synthesized.

The **red pulp** removes antibody-coated bacteria, senescent or defective RBCs, and antibody-coated blood cells (as may occur in immune cytopenias such as ITP, Coombs-positive hemolytic anemias, and some neutropenias). The red pulp also serves as a reservoir for blood elements, especially WBCs and platelets. During its culling and pitting of RBCs, the spleen removes inclusion bodies, such as Heinz bodies (precipitates of insoluble globin), Howell-Jolly bodies (nuclear fragments), and whole nuclei; thus, after splenectomy or in the functionally hyposplenic state, RBCs with these inclusions appear in the peripheral circulation. Hematopoiesis may occur if injury to bone marrow (eg, by fibrosis or tumors) allows hematopoietic stem cells to circulate and repopulate the adult spleen (see Myelodysplastic Syndrome on p. 1149 and Primary Myelofibrosis on p. 1165).

SPLENOMEGALY

Splenomegaly is almost always secondary to other disorders. Causes of splenomegaly are myriad, as are the many possible ways of classifying them (see Table 155–1). In temperate climates, the **most common causes** are

- Myeloproliferative disorders
- Lymphoproliferative disorders
- Storage diseases (eg, Gaucher disease)
- Connective tissue disorders

In the tropics, the most common causes are

- Infectious diseases (eg, malaria, kala-azar)

If splenomegaly is massive (spleen palpable 8 cm below the costal margin), the cause is usually chronic lymphocytic leukemia, non-Hodgkin lymphoma, chronic myelogenous leukemia, polycythemia vera, myelofibrosis with myeloid metaplasia, or hairy cell leukemia.

Splenomegaly can lead to cytopenias, a disorder called hypersplenism.

Evaluation

History: Most of the presenting symptoms result from the underlying disorder. However, splenomegaly itself may cause early satiety by encroachment of the enlarged spleen on the stomach. Fullness and left upper quadrant abdominal pain are also possible. Severe pain suggests splenic infarction. Recurrent infections, symptoms of anemia, or bleeding manifestations suggest cytopenia and possible hypersplenism.

Table 155–1. COMMON CAUSES OF SPLENOMEGALY

TYPE	EXAMPLES
Congestive	Cirrhosis External compression or thrombosis of portal or splenic veins Certain malformations of the portal venous vasculature
Infectious and inflammatory	Acute infections (eg, infectious mononucleosis, infectious hepatitis, subacute bacterial endocarditis, psittacosis) Chronic infections (eg, miliary TB, malaria, brucellosis, kala-azar, syphilis) Sarcoidosis Secondary amyloidosis Connective tissue disorder (eg, SLE, Felty syndrome)
Myeloproliferative and lymphoproliferative	Myelofibrosis with myeloid metaplasia Lymphomas, especially hairy cell leukemia Leukemias, especially chronic lymphocytic, large granular lymphocytic, and chronic myelocytic Polycythemia vera Primary thrombocythemia
Chronic hemolytic anemia	RBC shape abnormalities (eg, hereditary spherocytosis, hereditary elliptocytosis) Hemoglobinopathies, including thalassemias, sickle cell hemoglobin variants (eg, hemoglobin S-C disease), and congenital Heinz body hemolytic anemias RBC enzymopathies (eg, pyruvate kinase deficiency)
Storage diseases	Lipoid (eg, Gaucher disease, Niemann-Pick disease, Hand-Schüller-Christian disease, and Wolman disease) Nonlipoid (eg, Letterer-Siwe disease)
Structural	Splenic cysts, usually caused by resolution of previous intrasplenic hematoma

Adapted from Williams WJ, et al: *Hematology*. New York, McGraw-Hill Book Company, 1976.

Physical examination: The sensitivity for detection of ultrasound-documented splenic enlargement is 60 to 70% for palpation and 60 to 80% for percussion. Up to 3% of normal, thin, people have a palpable spleen. Also, a palpable left upper quadrant mass may indicate a problem other than an enlarged spleen such as a hypernephroma.

Other helpful signs include a splenic friction rub that suggests splenic infarction and epigastric and splenic bruits that suggest congestive splenomegaly. Generalized adenopathy may suggest a lymphoproliferative, infectious, or autoimmune disorder.

Testing: If confirmation of splenomegaly is necessary because the examination is equivocal, ultrasonography is the test of choice because of its accuracy and low cost. CT and MRI may provide more detail of the organ's consistency. MRI is especially useful in detecting portal or splenic vein thromboses. Nuclear scanning is accurate and can identify accessory splenic tissue but is expensive and cumbersome.

Specific causes suggested clinically should be confirmed by appropriate testing. If no cause is suggested, the highest priority is exclusion of occult infection, because early treatment affects the outcome of infection more than it does most other causes of splenomegaly. Testing should be thorough in areas of high geographic prevalence of infection or if the patient appears to be ill. CBC, blood cultures, and bone marrow examination and culture should be considered. If the patient is not ill, has no symptoms besides those due to splenomegaly, and has no risk factors for infection, the extent of testing is controversial but probably includes CBC, peripheral blood smear, liver function tests, and abdominal CT. Flow cytometry and immunochemical assays such as light chain measurements of peripheral blood and/or bone marrow sections is indicated if lymphoma is suspected.

Specific peripheral blood findings may suggest underlying disorders (eg, small-cell lymphocytosis in chronic lymphocytic leukemia, large granular lymphocytosis in T-cell granular lymphocyte [TGL] hyperplasia or TGL leukemia, atypical lymphocytes in hairy cell leukemia, and leukocytosis and immature forms in other leukemias). Excessive basophils, eosinophils, or nucleated or teardrop RBCs suggest myeloproliferative disorders. Cytopenias suggest hypersplenism. Spherocytosis suggests hypersplenism or hereditary spherocytosis. Liver function test results are diffusely abnormal in congestive splenomegaly with cirrhosis; an isolated elevation of serum alkaline phosphatase suggests hepatic infiltration, as in myeloproliferative and lymphoproliferative disorders and miliary TB.

Some other tests may be useful, even in asymptomatic patients. Serum protein electrophoresis identifying a monoclonal gammopathy or decreased immunoglobulins suggests lymphoproliferative disorders or amyloidosis; diffuse hypergammaglobulinemia suggests chronic infection (eg, malaria, kala-azar, brucellosis, TB) or cirrhosis with congestive splenomegaly, sarcoidosis, or connective tissue disorders. Elevation of serum uric acid suggests a myeloproliferative or lymphoproliferative disorder. Elevation of WBC alkaline phosphatase suggests a myeloproliferative disorder, whereas decreased levels suggest chronic myelocytic leukemia.

If testing reveals no abnormalities other than splenomegaly, the patient should be reevaluated at intervals of 6 to 12 mo or when new symptoms develop.

Treatment

- Treatment of underlying disorder

Treatment is directed at the underlying disorder. The enlarged spleen itself needs no treatment unless severe hypersplenism is present. Patients with palpable or very large spleens probably should avoid contact sports to decrease the risk of splenic rupture.

HYPERSPLENISM

Hypersplenism is cytopenia caused by splenomegaly.

Hypersplenism is a secondary process that can arise from splenomegaly of almost any cause (see Table 155–1). Splenomegaly increases the spleen's mechanical filtering and destruction of RBCs and often of WBCs and platelets. Compensatory bone marrow hyperplasia occurs in those cell lines that are reduced in the circulation.

Symptoms and Signs

Splenomegaly is the hallmark; spleen size correlates with the degree of cytopenia. Other clinical findings usually result from the underlying disorder.

Diagnosis

- Physical examination, sometimes ultrasonography
- CBC

Hypersplenism is suspected in patients with splenomegaly and anemia or cytopenias. Evaluation is similar to that of splenomegaly.

Unless other mechanisms coexist to compound their severity, anemia and other cytopenias are modest and asymptomatic (eg, platelet counts, 50,000 to 100,000/μL; WBC counts, 2500 to 4000/μL with normal WBC differential count). RBC morphology is generally normal except for occasional spherocytosis. Reticulocytosis is usual.

Treatment

- Possibly splenic ablation (splenectomy or radiation therapy)
- Vaccination for splenectomized patients

Treatment is directed at the underlying disorder. However, if hypersplenism is the only serious manifestation of the disorder (eg, Gaucher disease), splenic ablation by splenectomy or radiation therapy may be indicated. The indications for splenectomy or radiation therapy in hypersplenism are detailed below (see Table 155–2).

Table 155–2. INDICATIONS FOR SPLENECTOMY OR RADIATION THERAPY IN HYPERSPLENISM

INDICATION	EXAMPLES
Hemolytic syndromes in which splenomegaly further shortens the survival of intrinsically abnormal RBCs	Hereditary spherocytosis Thalassemia
Severe pancytopenia associated with massive splenomegaly	Hairy cell leukemia Lipid-storage diseases*
Vascular insults affecting the spleen	Recurrent infarctions Bleeding esophageal varices associated with excessive splenic venous return
Mechanical encroachment on other abdominal organs	Stomach with early satiety Calyceal obstruction in left kidney
Excessive bleeding	Hypersplenic thrombocytopenia

*The spleen may be up to 30 times larger than normal.

Because the intact spleen protects against serious infections with encapsulated bacteria, splenectomy should be avoided whenever possible, and patients undergoing splenectomy require vaccination against infections caused by *Streptococcus pneumoniae*, *Neisseria meningitidis*, and *Haemophilus influenzae*.

After splenectomy, patients are particularly susceptible to severe sepsis with encapsulated microorganisms and are often given daily prophylactic antibiotics such as penicillin or erythromycin. Patients who develop fever should receive empiric antibiotics.

156 Thrombocytopenia and Platelet Dysfunction

OVERVIEW OF PLATELET DISORDERS

Platelets are cell fragments that function in the clotting system. Thrombopoietin helps control the number of circulating platelets by stimulating the bone marrow to produce megakaryocytes, which in turn shed platelets from their cytoplasm. Thrombopoietin is produced in the liver at a constant rate and its circulating level is determined by the extent to which circulating platelets are cleared, and possibly by bone marrow megakaryocytes. Platelets circulate for 7 to 10 days. About one-third are always transiently sequestered in the spleen.

The platelet count is normally 140,000 to 440,000/μL. However, the count can vary slightly according to menstrual cycle phase, decrease during near-term pregnancy (gestational thrombocytopenia), and increase in response to inflammatory cytokines (secondary, or reactive, thrombocytosis). Platelets are eventually destroyed by apoptosis, a process independent of the spleen.

Platelet disorders include

- An abnormal increase in platelets (thrombocythemia and reactive thrombocytosis)
- A decrease in platelets (thrombocytopenia)
- Platelet dysfunction

Any of these conditions, even those in which platelets are increased, may cause defective formation of hemostatic plugs and bleeding.

The risk of bleeding is inversely proportional to the platelet count and platelet function (see Table 156–1). When platelet function is reduced (eg, as a result of uremia or aspirin use), the risk of bleeding increases.

Etiology

Thrombocythemia and thrombocytosis: Essential thrombocythemia is a myeloproliferative disorder involving overproduction of platelets because of a clonal abnormality of a hematopoietic stem cell. A markedly elevated platelet count is typically associated with thrombosis, but some patients with extreme thrombocytosis (ie, > 1,000,000/μL) develop bleeding due to loss of high molecular weight VWF multimers.

Reactive thrombocytosis is platelet overproduction in response to another disorder. There are many causes, including acute infection, chronic inflammatory disorders (eg, RA, inflammatory bowel disease, TB, sarcoidosis), iron deficiency, and certain cancers. Reactive thrombocytosis is not typically associated with an increased risk of thrombosis.

Thrombocytopenia: Causes of thrombocytopenia can be classified by mechanism (see Table 156–2) and include decreased platelet production, increased splenic sequestration of platelets with normal platelet survival, increased platelet destruction or consumption (both immunologic and nonimmunologic causes), dilution of platelets, and a combination of these mechanisms.

Increased splenic sequestration is suggested by splenomegaly.

A large number of drugs may cause thrombocytopenia (see p. 1203), typically by triggering immunologic destruction.

Overall, the **most common specific causes** of thrombocytopenia include

- Gestational thrombocytopenia
- Drug-induced thrombocytopenia due to immune-mediated platelet destruction (commonly, heparin, trimethoprim/sulfamethoxazole, rarely quinine)
- Drug-induced thrombocytopenia due to dose-dependent bone marrow suppression (eg, chemotherapeutic agents, ethanol)
- Thrombocytopenia accompanying systemic infection
- Immune thrombocytopenia (ITP, formerly called immune thrombocytopenic purpura)

Platelet dysfunction: Platelet dysfunction may stem from an intrinsic platelet defect or from an extrinsic factor that alters the function of normal platelets. Dysfunction may be hereditary or acquired. Hereditary disorders of platelet function consist of von Willebrand disease, the most common hereditary hemorrhagic disease, and hereditary intrinsic platelet disorders, which are much less common. Acquired disorders of platelet dysfunction are commonly due to diseases (eg, renal failure) as well as to aspirin and other drugs.

Table 156–1. PLATELET COUNT AND BLEEDING RISK

PLATELET COUNT	RISK OF BLEEDING*
≥ 50,000/μL	Minimal
20,000–50,000/μL	Minor bleeding after trauma
< 20,000/μL	Spontaneous bleeding
< 5000/μL	Severe, possibly life-threatening spontaneous bleeding

*Reduced platelet function (eg, due to uremia or aspirin use) adds to risk of bleeding in each platelet count range.

Symptoms and Signs

Platelet disorders result in a typical pattern of bleeding:

- Multiple petechiae in the skin (typically most evident on the lower legs)
- Scattered small ecchymoses at sites of minor trauma
- Mucosal bleeding (oropharyngeal, nasal, GI, GU)
- Excessive bleeding after surgery

Heavy GI bleeding and bleeding into the CNS may be life threatening. However, bleeding into tissues (eg, deep visceral hematomas or hemarthroses) rarely occurs with thrombocytopenia, which causes immediate, superficial bleeding following an injury. Bleeding into the tissues (often delayed

Table 156–2. CLASSIFICATION OF THROMBOCYTOPENIA

CAUSE	CONDITIONS
Diminished or absent megakaryocytes in bone marrow	Aplastic anemia Leukemia Myelosuppressive drugs (eg, hydroxyurea, interferon alfa-2b, chemotherapy drugs) Paroxysmal nocturnal hemoglobinuria (some patients)
Diminished platelet production despite the presence of megakaryocytes in bone marrow	Alcohol-induced thrombocytopenia Bortezomib use HIV-associated thrombocytopenia Myelodysplastic syndromes (some) Vitamin B_{12} or folate (folic acid) deficiency
Platelet sequestration in enlarged spleen	Cirrhosis with congestive splenomegaly Gaucher disease Myelofibrosis with myeloid metaplasia Sarcoidosis
Immunologic destruction	Antiphospholipid antibody syndrome Connective tissue disorders Drug-induced thrombocytopenia HIV-associated thrombocytopenia Immune thrombocytopenia Lymphoproliferative disorders Neonatal alloimmune thrombocytopenia Posttransfusion purpura Sarcoidosis
Nonimmunologic destruction	Certain systemic infections (eg, hepatitis, Epstein-Barr virus, cytomegalovirus, or dengue virus infection) Disseminated intravascular coagulation Pregnancy (gestational thrombocytopenia) Sepsis Thrombocytopenia in acute respiratory distress syndrome Thrombotic thrombocytopenic purpura–hemolytic-uremic syndrome
Dilution	Massive RBC replacement or exchange transfusion (most RBC transfusions use stored RBCs that do not contain many viable platelets)

for up to a day after trauma) suggests a coagulation disorder (eg, hemophilia).

Diagnosis

- Clinical presentation of petechiae and mucosal bleeding
- CBC with platelets, coagulation studies, peripheral blood smear
- Sometimes bone marrow aspiration
- Sometimes von Willebrand antigen and factor activity studies

Platelet disorders are suspected in patients with petechiae and mucosal bleeding. A CBC with platelet count, coagulation studies, and a peripheral blood smear are obtained. Excessive platelets and thrombocytopenia are diagnosed based on the platelet count; coagulation studies are normal unless there is a simultaneous coagulopathy. In patients with a normal CBC, platelet count, INR, and PTT, platelet dysfunction is suspected.

PEARLS & PITFALLS

- Suspect platelet or vessel wall dysfunction in patients with petechiae and/or hemorrhage but with normal platelet count and coagulation test results.

Thrombocytopenia: Peripheral smear examination is important in patients with thrombocytopenia because automated platelet counts sometimes show pseudothrombocytopenia due to platelet clumping caused by a reaction with the EDTA reagent present in some blood collection tubes. Also, schistocytes may be seen, which can indicate thrombotic thrombocytopenic purpura (TTP), hemolytic-uremic syndrome (HUS), or disseminated intravascular coagulation (DIC—see Table 156–3).

Bone marrow aspiration is indicated if the smear shows abnormalities other than thrombocytopenia, such as nucleated RBCs or abnormal or immature WBCs. Bone marrow aspiration reveals the number and appearance of megakaryocytes and is the definitive test for many disorders causing bone marrow failure. However, normal number and appearance of megakaryocytes does not always indicate normal platelet production. For example, in patients with ITP, platelet production may be decreased despite the normal appearance and increased number of megakaryocytes.

If the bone marrow is normal but the spleen is enlarged, increased splenic sequestration is the likely cause of thrombocytopenia. If the bone marrow is normal and the spleen is not enlarged, excess platelet destruction is the likely cause. Measurement of antiplatelet antibodies is not clinically useful. HIV testing is done in patients at risk of HIV infection. Bone marrow examination is rarely required in patients who present with typical features of ITP.

Suspected platelet dysfunction: In patients with platelet dysfunction, a drug cause is suspected if symptoms began only after the patient started taking a potentially causative drug (eg, clopidogrel, ticagrelor). Platelet dysfunction caused by drugs may be severe, but specialized tests are rarely needed.

A hereditary cause is suspected if there is a lifelong history of easy bruising; bleeding after tooth extractions, surgery,

Table 156–3. PERIPHERAL BLOOD FINDINGS IN THROMBOCYTOPENIC DISORDERS

FINDINGS	CONDITIONS
Normal RBCs and WBCs	Drug-induced thrombocytopenia Gestational thrombocytopenia HIV-related thrombocytopenia ITP Posttransfusion purpura
RBC fragmentation (schistocytes)	Metastatic cancer DIC Preeclampsia with DIC TTP and HUS
WBC abnormalities	Hypersegmented polymorphonuclear leukocytes in megaloblastic anemias Immature cells or increased mature lymphocytes in leukemia Markedly diminished granulocytes in aplastic anemia
Frequent giant platelets (approaching the size of RBCs)	Bernard-Soulier syndrome Disorders related to the myosin, heavy chain 9, non-muscle gene (*MYH9*) Other congenital thrombocytopenias
RBC abnormalities, nucleated RBCs, and immature granulocytes	Myelodysplasia
Platelet clumping	Pseudothrombocytopenia

DIC = disseminated intravascular coagulation.

childbirth, or circumcision; or heavy menstruation. In the case of a suspected hereditary cause, von Willebrand factor (VWF) antigen and VWF activity studies are routinely done. In some patients, platelet aggregation tests may identify a defect in how the platelet responds to various platelet agonists (adenosine diphosphate [ADP], collagen, thrombin) and thereby demonstrate the type of platelet defect.

Platelet dysfunction caused by systemic disorders is typically mild and of minor clinical importance. In these patients, the causative systemic disorder is the clinical concern, and hematologic tests are unnecessary.

Treatment

- Stopping drugs that impair platelet function
- Rarely platelet transfusions

In patients with thrombocytopenia or platelet dysfunction, drugs that further impair platelet function, particularly aspirin and other NSAIDs, should not be given. Patients who are already taking such drugs should consider alternative drugs, such as acetaminophen, or simply stop using them.

Patients may require platelet transfusion, but transfusions are given only in limited situations. Prophylactic transfusions are used sparingly because they may lose their effectiveness with repeated use due to the development of platelet alloantibodies. In platelet dysfunction or thrombocytopenia caused by decreased production, transfusions are reserved for patients with active bleeding, severe thrombocytopenia (eg, platelet count < 10,000/μL), or in need of invasive procedures. In thrombocytopenia caused by platelet destruction, transfusions are reserved for life-threatening or CNS bleeding.

ACQUIRED PLATELET DYSFUNCTION

Acquired platelet dysfunction, which is common, may result from aspirin, other NSAIDs, or systemic disorders.

Acquired abnormalities of platelet function are very common. Causes include

- Drugs
- Systemic disorders
- Cardiopulmonary bypass

Acquired platelet dysfunction is suspected and diagnosed when an isolated prolongation of bleeding is observed and other possible diagnoses have been eliminated. Platelet aggregation studies are unnecessary.

Drugs: Aspirin, other NSAIDs, inhibitors of the platelet P2Y12 ADP receptor (eg, clopidogrel, prasugrel, ticagrelor), and glycoprotein IIb/IIIa receptor inhibitors (eg, abciximab, eptifibatide, tirofiban) may induce platelet dysfunction. Sometimes this effect is incidental (eg, when the drugs are used to relieve pain and inflammation) and sometimes therapeutic (eg, when aspirin or the P2Y12 inhibitors are used for prevention of stroke or coronary thrombosis).

Aspirin and NSAIDs prevent cyclooxygenase-mediated production of thromboxane A_2. This effect can last 5 to 7 days. Aspirin modestly increases bleeding in healthy people but may markedly increase bleeding in patients with underlying platelet dysfunction or a severe coagulation disturbance (eg, patients receiving heparin, patients with severe hemophilia). Clopidogrel, prasugrel, and ticagrelor all can markedly reduce platelet function and increase bleeding.

A number of other drugs can also cause platelet dysfunction.[1]

Systemic disorders: Many disorders (eg, myeloproliferative and myelodysplastic disorders, uremia, macroglobulinemia, multiple myeloma, cirrhosis, SLE) can impair platelet function.

Uremia prolongs bleeding via unknown mechanisms. If bleeding is observed clinically, bleeding may be reduced with vigorous dialysis, cryoprecipitate administration, or desmopressin infusion. If necessary, increasing the hemoglobin concentration to > 10 g/dL by transfusion or by giving erythropoietin also reduces bleeding.

Cardiopulmonary bypass: As blood circulates through a pump oxygenator during cardiopulmonary bypass, platelets may become dysfunctional, prolonging bleeding. The mechanism appears to be activation of fibrinolysis on the platelet surface with resultant loss of the glycoprotein Ib/IX binding site for VWF. Regardless of platelet count, patients who bleed excessively after cardiopulmonary bypass are often transfused with platelets. Giving aprotinin (a protease inhibitor) during bypass may preserve platelet function and reduce the need for transfusion.

1. Scharf RE: Drugs that affect platelet function. *Semin Thromb Hemost* 38(8): 865–883, 2012. doi: 10.1055/s-0032-1328881. Epub 2012 Oct 30.

HEREDITARY INTRINSIC PLATELET DISORDERS

Hereditary intrinsic platelet disorders are rare and cause lifelong bleeding tendencies. Diagnosis is confirmed by platelet aggregation tests. Platelet transfusion is usually necessary to control serious bleeding.

Normal hemostasis requires platelet adhesion and activation.

Platelet adhesion (ie, of platelets to exposed vascular subendothelium) requires VWF and the platelet glycoprotein Ib/IX complex.

Platelet activation promotes platelet aggregation and fibrinogen binding and requires the platelet glycoprotein IIb/IIIa complex. Activation involves release of adenosine diphosphate (ADP) from platelet storage granules and conversion of arachidonic acid to thromboxane A_2 via a cyclooxygenase-mediated reaction. The released ADP acts on the P2Y12 receptor on other platelets, thereby activating them and recruiting them to the site of injury. Additionally, ADP (and thromboxane A_2) then promotes changes in the platelet glycoprotein IIb/IIIa complex, which in turn increases fibrinogen binding, thereby allowing platelets to aggregate.

Hereditary intrinsic platelet disorders can involve defects in any of these substrates and steps. These disorders are suspected in patients with lifelong bleeding disorders who have normal platelet counts and coagulation study results. Diagnosis usually is based on platelet aggregation tests; however, the results of platelet aggregation tests can be highly variable, and interpretation of results is often inconclusive (see Table 156–4). Platelet aggregation tests assess the ability of platelets to clump in response to the addition of various activators (eg, collagen, epinephrine, ADP, ristocetin). Platelet aggregometry studies are unreliable when platelet counts are < 100,000/µL.

Disorders of platelet adhesion: Bernard-Soulier syndrome is a rare autosomal recessive disorder. It impairs platelet adhesion via a defect in the glycoprotein Ib/IX complex that binds endothelial VWF. Bleeding may be severe. Platelets are unusually large. They do not aggregate with ristocetin but aggregate normally with ADP, collagen, and epinephrine.

Large platelets associated with functional abnormalities also occur in the May-Hegglin anomaly, a thrombocytopenic disorder with abnormal WBCs, and in the Chédiak-Higashi syndrome.

Platelet transfusion is necessary to control serious bleeding.

von Willebrand disease is due to a deficiency or defect in the VWF that is needed to permit platelet adhesion. It is often treated with desmopressin or VWF replacement with pasteurized intermediate-purity factor VIII concentrate or the newer recombinant VWF products.

Disorders of platelet activation: Disorders of amplification of platelet activation are the most common hereditary intrinsic platelet disorders and produce mild bleeding. They may result from decreased ADP in the platelet granules (storage pool deficiency), from an inability to generate thromboxane A_2 from arachidonic acid, or from an inability of platelets to aggregate in response to thromboxane A_2.

Platelet aggregation tests reveal impaired aggregation after exposure to collagen, epinephrine, and low levels of ADP and normal aggregation after exposure to high levels of ADP. The same pattern can result from use of NSAIDs or aspirin, the effect of which can persist for several days. Therefore, platelet aggregation tests should not be done in patients who have recently taken these drugs.

Thrombasthenia (Glanzmann disease) is a rare autosomal recessive disorder causing a defect in the platelet glycoprotein IIb/IIIa complex; platelets cannot aggregate. Patients may have severe mucosal bleeding (eg, nosebleeds that stop only after nasal packing and transfusions of platelet concentrates). The diagnosis is confirmed by the finding that platelets fail to aggregate after exposure to epinephrine, collagen, or even high levels of ADP but do aggregate transiently after exposure to ristocetin. Platelet transfusion is necessary to control serious bleeding.

IMMUNE THROMBOCYTOPENIA

(Idiopathic Thrombocytopenic Purpura; Immune Thrombocytopenic Purpura)

Immune thrombocytopenia (ITP) is a bleeding disorder caused by thrombocytopenia not associated with a systemic disease. Typically, it is chronic in adults, but it is usually acute and self-limited in children. Spleen size is normal in the absence of another underlying condition. Diagnosis requires that other disorders be excluded through selective tests. Treatment includes corticosteroids, splenectomy, immunosuppressants, and thrombopoietin receptor agonist drugs. For life-threatening bleeding, platelet transfusions, IV corticosteroids, IV anti-D immune globulin, or IV immune globulin (IVIG) may be used individually or in combination.

ITP usually results from development of an autoantibody directed against a structural platelet antigen. In childhood ITP, the autoantibody may be triggered by viral antigens. The trigger in adults is unknown, although in some countries (eg, Japan, Italy), ITP has been associated with *Helicobacter pylori* infection, and treatment of the infection has been followed by remission of the ITP. ITP tends to worsen during pregnancy and increases the risk of maternal morbidity (see p. 2388).

Symptoms and Signs

The symptoms and signs of ITP are

- Petechiae
- Purpura
- Mucosal bleeding

Gross GI bleeding and hematuria are less common. The spleen is of normal size unless it is enlarged by a coexisting viral infection or autoimmune hemolytic anemia (Evans syndrome). Like the other disorders of increased platelet destruction, ITP is also associated with an increased risk of thrombosis.

Table 156–4. RESULTS OF AGGREGATION TESTS IN HEREDITARY DISORDERS OF PLATELET FUNCTION

DISORDER	COLLAGEN, EPINEPHRINE, AND LOW-DOSE ADP	HIGH-DOSE ADP	RISTOCETIN
Disorders of amplification of platelet activation	Impaired	Normal	Normal
Thrombasthenia (eg, loss of the glycoprotein IIb/IIIa receptor)	Absent	Absent	Normal or impaired
Disorders of platelet adhesion (eg, Bernard-Soulier syndrome, von Willebrand disease)	Normal	Normal	Impaired

ADP = adenosinediphosphate.

Diagnosis

- CBC with platelets, peripheral blood smear
- Rarely bone marrow aspiration
- Exclusion of other thrombocytopenic disorders

ITP is suspected in patients with isolated thrombocytopenia (ie, otherwise normal CBC and peripheral blood smear). Because manifestations of ITP are nonspecific, other causes of isolated thrombocytopenia (eg, drugs, alcohol, lymphoproliferative disorders, other autoimmune diseases, viral infections) need to be excluded by clinical evaluation and appropriate testing. Typically, patients have coagulation studies, liver function tests, and tests for infection with hepatitis C and HIV. Testing for antiplatelet antibodies usually does not aid diagnosis or treatment.

Bone marrow examination is not required to make the diagnosis but is done if blood counts or blood smear reveals abnormalities in addition to thrombocytopenia, when clinical features are not typical, or if patients fail to respond to standard therapies. In patients with ITP, bone marrow examination reveals normal or possibly increased numbers of megakaryocytes in an otherwise normal bone marrow sample.

Prognosis

Children typically recover spontaneously, even from severe thrombocytopenia, in several weeks to months.

In adults, spontaneous remission may occur, but it is uncommon after the first year of disease. However, many patients have mild and stable disease (ie, platelet counts > 30,000/μL) with minimal or no bleeding; such cases may be more common than previously thought, many being discovered by the automated platelet counting now routinely done with CBC. Other patients have significant, symptomatic thrombocytopenia, although life-threatening bleeding and death are rare.

Treatment

- Oral corticosteroids
- IVIG
- IV anti-D immune globulin
- Splenectomy
- Thrombopoietin receptor agonist drugs
- Rituximab
- Other immunosuppressants
- For severe bleeding, IVIG, IV anti-D immune globulin, IV corticosteroids, and/or platelet transfusions

Adults with bleeding and a platelet count < 30,000/μL are usually given an oral corticosteroid (eg, prednisone 1 mg/kg po once/day) initially. An alternative, but probably less effective, corticosteroid regimen is dexamethasone 40 mg po once/day for 4 days. The majority of patients respond with a rise in platelet count within 2 to 5 days, but in some patients, it may take as long as 2 to 4 wk before a response occurs; however, when the corticosteroid is tapered after response, most adult patients relapse. Repeated corticosteroid treatments may be effective but increase the risk of adverse effects. Corticosteroids should not usually be continued beyond the first several months; other drugs may be tried in an attempt to avoid splenectomy.

Oral corticosteroids or IVIG or IV anti-D immune globulin may also be given when a transient increase of the platelet count is required for tooth extractions, childbirth, surgery, or other invasive procedures.

Splenectomy can achieve a complete remission in about two thirds of patients who relapse after initial corticosteroid therapy, but it is usually reserved for patients with severe thrombocytopenia, bleeding, or both. Splenectomy may not be appropriate for patients with mild disease. If thrombocytopenia can be controlled with medical therapies, splenectomy is often deferred for 6 to 12 mo to allow for the chance of spontaneous remission.[1] Splenectomy results in an increased risk of thrombosis and infection (particularly with encapsulated bacteria such as pneumococcus); patients require vaccination against *Streptococcus pneumoniae*, *Haemophilus influenzae*, and *Neisseria meningitidis* (ideally > 2 wk before the procedure).

Second-line medical therapies: **Second-line medical therapies** are available for patients

- Who are seeking to defer splenectomy in hope of a spontaneous remission
- Who are not candidates for or refuse splenectomy
- In whom splenectomy has not been effective

Such patients usually have platelet counts < 10,000 to 20,000/μL (and thus are at risk for bleeding). Second-line medical therapies include thrombopoietin receptor agonists, rituximab, and other immunosuppressive agents. Thrombopoietin receptor agonist drugs, such as romiplostim 1 to 10 mcg/kg sc once/wk and eltrombopag 25 to 75 mg po once/day, have response rates > 85%. However, thrombopoietin receptor agonists need to be administered continuously to maintain the platelet count > 50,000/μL. Rituximab (375 mg/m^2 IV once/wk for 4 wk) has a response rate of 57%, but only 21% of adult patients remain in remission after 5 yr.[2]

More intensive immunosuppression may be required with drugs such as cyclophosphamide and azathioprine in patients unresponsive to other drugs who have severe, symptomatic thrombocytopenia.

Life-threatening bleeding in ITP: In children or adults with ITP and life-threatening bleeding, rapid phagocytic blockade is attempted by giving IVIG 1 g/kg once/day for 1 to 2 days or, in Rh positive patients, a single dose of IV anti-D immune globulin 75 mcg/kg. IV anti-D immunoglobulin is only effective in patients who have not had a splenectomy and may be associated with severe complications such as severe hemolysis and DIC. This treatment usually causes the platelet count to rise within 2 to 4 days, but the count remains high for only 2 to 4 wk. High-dose methylprednisolone (1 g IV once/day for 3 days) is less expensive than IVIG or IV anti-D immune globulin and is easier to administer but may not be as effective. Patients with ITP and life-threatening bleeding are also given platelet transfusions. Platelet transfusions are not used prophylactically. Vincristine (1.4 mg/kg; maximum dose of 2 mg) has also been used in emergency situations.

Treatment of children with ITP: Treatment of children with ITP is usually supportive because most children spontaneously recover. Even after months or years of thrombocytopenia, most children have spontaneous remissions. If mucosal bleeding occurs, corticosteroids or IVIG may be given. Corticosteroid and IVIG use is controversial because the increased platelet count may not improve clinical outcome. Splenectomy is rarely done in children. However, if thrombocytopenia is severe and symptomatic for > 6 mo, then thrombopoietin receptor agonists (romiplostim, eltrombopag) or splenectomy is considered.

1. Neunert C, Lim W, Crowther M, et al: The American Society of Hematology 2011 evidence-based practice guideline for immune thrombocytopenia. *Blood* 117:4190–4207, 2011.
2. Patel VL, Mahevas M, Lee SY, et al: Outcomes 5 years after response to rituximab therapy in children and adults with immune thrombocytopenia. *Blood* 119:5989–5995, 2012.

KEY POINTS

- The immune system destroys platelets in the circulation and at the same time attacks bone marrow megakaryocytes, thereby reducing platelet production.
- Other causes of isolated thrombocytopenia (eg, drugs, alcohol, lymphoproliferative disorders, other autoimmune diseases, viral infections) need to be excluded.
- Children usually have spontaneous remission; in adults, spontaneous remission may occur during the first year but is uncommon thereafter.
- Corticosteroids (and sometimes IVIG or IV anti-D immune globulin) are first-line treatments for bleeding or severe thrombocytopenia.
- Splenectomy is often effective but is reserved for patients in whom medical therapy is ineffective or those whose disease persists after 12 mo.
- Platelet transfusion is given only for life-threatening bleeding.

THROMBOCYTOPENIA DUE TO SPLENIC SEQUESTRATION

Increased splenic platelet sequestration can occur in various disorders that cause splenomegaly However, thrombocytopenia that occurs in advanced cirrhosis is mostly due to reduced thrombopoietin production by the liver (and consequent reduced platelet production) rather than splenic sequestration.[1]

The platelet count usually is > 30,000/μL unless the disorder causing splenomegaly also impairs platelet production (eg, in myelofibrosis with myeloid metaplasia).

Sequestered platelets are released from the spleen at times of stress. Therefore, thrombocytopenia caused only by splenic sequestration rarely causes bleeding.

In patients with normal hepatic function, splenectomy corrects the thrombocytopenia; however, splenectomy is not indicated unless severe thrombocytopenia due to simultaneous bone marrow failure is present.

1. Peck-Radosavljevic M, Wichlas M, Zacherl J, et al: Thrombopoietin induces rapid resolution of thrombocytopenia after orthotopic liver transplantation through increased platelet production. *Blood* 95:795–801, 2009.

THROMBOCYTOPENIA: OTHER CAUSES

Platelet destruction can develop because of immunologic causes (viral infection, drugs, connective tissue or lymphoproliferative disorders, blood transfusions) or nonimmunologic causes (sepsis, acute respiratory distress syndrome). Manifestations are petechiae, purpura, and mucosal bleeding. Laboratory findings depend on the cause. The history may be the only suggestion of the diagnosis. Treatment is correction of the underlying disorder.

Acute respiratory distress syndrome: Patients with acute respiratory distress syndrome may develop nonimmunologic thrombocytopenia, possibly secondary to deposition of platelets in the pulmonary capillary bed.

Blood transfusions: Posttransfusion purpura causes immunologic platelet destruction indistinguishable from ITP, except for a history of a blood transfusion within the preceding 7 to 10 days. The patient, usually a woman, lacks a platelet antigen (PLA-1) present in most people. Transfusion with PLA-1–positive platelets stimulates formation of anti–PLA-1 antibodies, which (by an unknown mechanism) can react with the patient's PLA-1–negative platelets. Severe thrombocytopenia results, taking 2 to 6 wk to subside. Treatment with IVIG is usually successful.

Connective tissue and lymphoproliferative disorders: Connective tissue (eg, SLE) or lymphoproliferative disorders (eg, lymphoma, large granular lymphocytosis) can cause immunologic thrombocytopenia. Corticosteroids and the usual treatments for ITP are effective; treating the underlying disorder does not always lengthen remission.

Drug-induced immunologic destruction: Commonly used drugs that occasionally induce thrombocytopenia include

- Heparin
- Quinine
- Trimethoprim/sulfamethoxazole
- Glycoprotein IIb/IIIa inhibitors (eg, abciximab, eptifibatide, tirofiban)
- Hydrochlorothiazide
- Carbamazepine
- Acetaminophen
- Chlorpropamide
- Ranitidine
- Rifampin
- Vancomycin

Drug-induced thrombocytopenia occurs typically when a drug bound to the platelet creates a new and "foreign" antigen, causing an immune reaction. This disorder is indistinguishable from ITP except for the history of drug ingestion. When the drug is stopped, the platelet count typically begins to increase within 1 to 2 days and recovers to normal within 7 days.

Heparin-induced thrombocytopenia: Heparin-induced thrombocytopenia (HIT) occurs in up to 1% of patients receiving unfractionated heparin. HIT may occur even when very-low-dose heparin (eg, used in flushes to keep IV or arterial lines open) is used. The mechanism is usually immunologic. Bleeding rarely occurs, but more commonly platelets clump excessively, causing vessel obstruction, leading to paradoxical arterial and venous thromboses, which may be life threatening (eg, thromboembolic occlusion of limb arteries, stroke, acute MI).

Heparin should be stopped in any patient who becomes thrombocytopenic and develops a new thrombosis or whose platelet count decreases by more than 50%. All heparin preparations should be stopped immediately and presumptively, and tests are done to detect antibodies to heparin bound to platelet factor 4. Anticoagulation with nonheparin anticoagulants (eg, argatroban, bivalirudin, fondaparinux) is necessary at least until platelet recovery.

Low molecular weight heparin (LMWH) is less immunogenic than unfractionated heparin but cannot be used to anticoagulate patients with HIT because most HIT antibodies cross-react with LMWH. Warfarin should not be substituted for heparin in patients with HIT and, if long-term anticoagulation is required, should be started only after the platelet count has recovered.

Infections: **HIV infection** may cause immunologic thrombocytopenia indistinguishable from ITP except for the association with HIV. The platelet count may increase when glucocorticoids are given. However, glucocorticoids are often withheld unless the platelet count falls to < 20,000/μL because these drugs may further depress immune function. The platelet count also usually increases after treatment with antiviral drugs.

Hepatitis C infection is commonly associated with thrombocytopenia. Active infection can create a thrombocytopenia that is indistinguishable from ITP with platelets < 10,000/μL. Milder degrees of thrombocytopenia (platelet count 40,000 to 70,000/μL) may be due to liver damage that reduced production of thrombopoietin, the hematopoietic growth factor that regulates megakaryocyte growth and platelet production. Hepatitis C–induced thrombocytopenia responds to the same treatments as does ITP.

Other infections, such as systemic viral infections (eg, Epstein-Barr virus, cytomegalovirus), rickettsial infections (eg, Rocky Mountain spotted fever), and bacterial sepsis, are often associated with thrombocytopenia.

Pregnancy: Thrombocytopenia, typically asymptomatic, occurs late in gestation in about 5% of normal pregnancies (gestational thrombocytopenia); it is usually mild (platelet counts < 70,000/μL are rare), requires no treatment, and resolves after delivery. However, severe thrombocytopenia may develop in pregnant women with preeclampsia and the HELLP syndrome (hemolysis, elevated liver function tests, and low platelets; such women typically require immediate delivery, and platelet transfusion is considered if platelet count is < 20,000/μL (or < 50,000/μL if delivery is to be cesarean).

Sepsis: Sepsis often causes nonimmunologic thrombocytopenia that parallels the severity of the infection. The thrombocytopenia has multiple causes: DIC, formation of immune complexes that can associate with platelets, activation of complement, deposition of platelets on damaged endothelial surfaces, removal of the platelet surface glycoproteins resulting in increased platelet clearance by the Ashwell-Morell receptor in the liver, and platelet apoptosis.

THROMBOTIC THROMBOCYTOPENIC PURPURA AND HEMOLYTIC-UREMIC SYNDROME

Thrombotic thrombocytopenic purpura (TTP) and hemolytic-uremic syndrome (HUS) are acute, fulminant disorders characterized by thrombocytopenia and microangiopathic hemolytic anemia. Other manifestations may include alterations in level of consciousness and kidney failure. Diagnosis requires demonstrating characteristic laboratory test abnormalities, including direct antiglobulin test–negative hemolytic anemia. Treatment is plasma exchange and corticosteroids in adults and supportive care (sometimes including hemodialysis) in children; eculizumab is rarely indicated.

Pathophysiology

TTP and HUS involve nonimmunologic platelet destruction. Loose strands of platelets and fibrin are deposited in multiple small vessels and damage passing platelets and RBCs, causing significant thrombocytopenia and anemia. Platelets are also consumed within multiple small thrombi. Multiple organs develop bland platelet-VWF thrombi (without the vessel wall granulocytic infiltration characteristic of vasculitis) localized primarily to arteriocapillary junctions, described as thrombotic microangiopathy. The brain, heart, and kidneys are particularly likely to be affected.

TTP and HUS differ mainly in the relative degree of kidney failure. Typically, disorders in adults are described as TTP and are less likely to involve kidney failure. HUS is used to describe the disorder in children, which typically involves kidney failure.

Etiology

Children: Most cases follow acute hemorrhagic colitis resulting from *Shiga* toxin–producing bacteria (eg, *Escherichia coli* O157:H7, some strains of *Shigella dysenteriae*—see p. 1584).

Adults: Many cases are idiopathic. Known causes and associations include

- Immunosuppressants (eg, cyclosporine) and cancer chemotherapy drugs (eg, mitomycin C)
- Pregnancy (often indistinguishable from severe preeclampsia or eclampsia)
- Hemorrhagic colitis due to *Escherichia coli* O157:H7 or *E. coli* O104:H4

A predisposing factor in many patients is congenital or acquired deficiency of the plasma enzyme ADAMTS13, which cleaves VWF and thus eliminates abnormally large VWF multimers that can cause platelet thrombi.

Symptoms and Signs

Manifestations of ischemia develop with varying severity in multiple organs. These manifestations include weakness, confusion or coma, abdominal pain, nausea, vomiting, diarrhea, and arrhythmias caused by myocardial damage. Children usually have a prodrome of vomiting, abdominal pain, and diarrhea (frequently bloody). Fever does not usually occur in TTP or HUS. The symptoms and signs of TTP and HUS are indistinguishable, except that neurologic symptoms are less common with HUS.

Diagnosis

- CBC with platelets, peripheral blood smear, direct antiglobulin (Coombs) test, LDH, PT, PTT, fibrinogen
- ADAMTS 13 activity levels
- Exclusion of other thrombocytopenic disorders

TTP-HUS is suspected in patients with suggestive symptoms, thrombocytopenia, and anemia. If the disorder is suspected, urinalysis, peripheral blood smear, reticulocyte count, serum LDH, renal function tests, ADAMTS13 assay, serum bilirubin (direct and indirect), and direct antiglobulin test are done. The diagnosis is suggested by

- Thrombocytopenia and anemia
- Fragmented RBCs on the blood smear indicative of microangiopathic hemolysis (schistocytes: helmet cells, triangular RBCs, distorted-appearing RBCs)
- Evidence of hemolysis (falling Hb level, polychromasia, elevated reticulocyte count, elevated serum LDH and bilirubin, reduced haptoglobin)
- Negative direct antiglobulin test

Testing for ADAMTS13 activity is appropriate in patients with suspected TTP-HUS, except in children who have typical diarrhea-associated HUS. Although the results of ADAMTS13 testing do not usually affect initial treatment, results are important to guide subsequent treatment. ADAMTS13 levels < 10% with the presence of antibody against ADAMTS13 is characteristic of most adults with TTP, and these patients respond to plasma exchange and immunosuppression. Patients with higher levels of ADAMTS13 and no antibody against ADAMTS13 are unlikely to respond to such therapies and should be assessed for treatment with complement inhibition.

Otherwise unexplained thrombocytopenia and microangiopathic hemolytic anemia are sufficient evidence for a presumptive diagnosis.

Causes: Although causes (eg, cyclosporine) or associations (eg, pregnancy) are clear in some patients, in most patients

TTP-HUS appears suddenly and spontaneously without apparent cause. TTP-HUS is often indistinguishable, even with renal biopsy, from syndromes that cause identical thrombotic microangiopathies (eg, preeclampsia, systemic sclerosis, accelerated hypertension, acute renal allograft rejection).

Stool testing (*Shiga* toxin enzyme-linked immunosorbent assay or specific culture media for *E. coli* O157:H7) is done in children with diarrhea and also adults who had a prodrome of bloody diarrhea; however, the organism and toxin may have cleared by the time of presentation.

Treatment

- In children with HUS, supportive care, often including hemodialysis
- In adults with TTP, plasma exchange and corticosteroids
- In refractory atypical HUS, eculizumab

Typical diarrhea-associated HUS in children caused by enterohemorrhagic infection usually spontaneously remits and is treated with supportive care and not antibiotics or plasma exchange; over half of patients require renal dialysis.

Untreated TTP is almost always fatal. With plasma exchange, however, > 85% of patients recover completely. Plasma exchange is continued daily until evidence of disease activity has subsided, as indicated by a normal platelet count, which may require several days to many weeks. Adults with TTP are also given corticosteroids.

Most patients experience only a single episode of TTP. However, relapses occur in about 40% of patients who have a severe deficiency of ADAMTS13 activity caused by an autoantibody inhibitor. In patients with recurrence when plasma exchange is stopped or in patients with relapses, more intensive immunosuppression with rituximab may be effective. Patients must be evaluated quickly if symptoms suggestive of a relapse develop.

In patients with HUS refractory to plasma exchange and/or corticosteroids and worsening renal insufficiency, complement inhibition with eculizumab can sometimes reverse the renal insufficiency. Children with known or presumed hereditary deficiency in complement regulatory proteins such as factor H are particularly likely to respond to eculizumab.

KEY POINTS

- Platelets and RBCs are destroyed non-immunologically, leading to thrombocytopenia and anemia; renal failure is common in children.
- Cause in children is typically hemorrhagic colitis resulting from *Shiga* toxin–producing bacteria.
- Cause in adults is commonly associated with antibody against the ADAMTS13 protease but may also be due to certain drugs, pregnancy, and infectious colitis.
- Typical diarrhea-associated HUS in children usually spontaneously remits with supportive care, although over half of affected children require renal dialysis.
- Adults with TTP require plasma exchange and often corticosteroids.
- Rarely, worsening renal insufficiency in HUS refractory to other treatment may respond to eculizumab.

VON WILLEBRAND DISEASE

Von Willebrand disease (VWD) is a hereditary deficiency of von Willebrand factor (VWF), which causes platelet dysfunction. Bleeding tendency is usually mild. Screening tests show a normal platelet count and, possibly, a slightly prolonged PTT. Diagnosis is based on low levels of VWF antigen and abnormal ristocetin cofactor activity. Treatment involves control of bleeding with replacement therapy (virally inactivated, intermediate-purity factor VIII concentrate) or desmopressin.

VWF is synthesized and secreted by vascular endothelium to form part of the perivascular matrix. VWF promotes the platelet adhesion phase of hemostasis by binding with a receptor on the platelet surface membrane (glycoprotein Ib/IX), thus connecting the platelets to the vessel wall. VWF is also required to maintain normal plasma factor VIII levels. Levels of VWF can temporarily increase in response to stress, exercise, pregnancy, inflammation, or infection.

Von Willebrand disease is classified into 3 types:

- Type 1: A quantitative deficiency of VWF, which is the most common form and is an autosomal dominant disorder
- Type 2: A qualitative impairment in synthesis of VWF that can result from various genetic abnormalities and is an autosomal dominant disorder
- Type 3: A rare autosomal recessive disorder in which homozygotes have no detectable VWF

Although VWD, like hemophilia A, is a hereditary disorder that may, when severe, cause factor VIII deficiency, factor VIII deficiency is usually only moderate.

Symptoms and Signs

Bleeding manifestations are mild to moderate and include easy bruising, mucosal bleeding, bleeding from small skin cuts that may stop and start over hours, sometimes increased menstrual bleeding, and abnormal bleeding after surgical procedures (eg, tooth extraction, tonsillectomy). Platelets function well enough that petechiae and purpura rarely occur.

Diagnosis

- Total plasma VWF antigen, VWF function, and plasma factor VIII level

Von Willebrand disease is suspected in patients with unexplained bleeding, particularly those with a family history of a similar bleeding diathesis. Screening coagulation tests reveal a normal platelet count, normal INR, and sometimes a slightly prolonged PTT. Bleeding time testing is unreliable and no longer done.

Diagnosis requires measuring total plasma VWF antigen, VWF function as determined by the ability of plasma to support agglutination of normal platelets by ristocetin (ristocetin cofactor activity), and plasma factor VIII level. Stimuli that temporarily increase VWF levels can cause false-negative results in mild VWD; tests may need to be repeated.

In the common (type 1) form of VWD, results are concordant; ie, VWF antigen, VWF function, and plasma factor VIII level are equally depressed. The degree of depression varies from about 15 to 60% of normal and determines the severity of a patient's abnormal bleeding. Levels of VWF antigen can also be as low as 40% of normal in healthy people with type O blood.

Type 2 variants are suspected if test results are discordant, ie, VWF antigen is higher than expected for the degree of abnormality in ristocetin cofactor activity. VWF antigen is higher than expected because the VWF defect in type 2 is qualitative (loss of high molecular weight VWF multimers) not quantitative. Diagnosis is confirmed by demonstrating a reduced concentration of large VWF multimers on agarose gel electrophoresis. Four different type 2 variants are recognized, distinguished by different functional abnormalities of the VWF molecule.

Patients with type 3 VWD have no detectable VWF and a marked deficiency of factor VIII.

Treatment

- Desmopressin
- VWF replacement when necessary

Patients with Von Willebrand disease are treated only if they are actively bleeding or are undergoing an invasive procedure (eg, surgery, dental extraction).

Desmopressin is an analog of vasopressin (antidiuretic hormone) that stimulates release of VWF into the plasma and may increase levels of factor VIII. Desmopressin can be helpful for type 1 VWD but is usually of no value in other types and may even be harmful in some. To ensure adequate response to the drug, physicians give patients a test dose and measure the response of VWF antigen. Desmopressin 0.3 mcg/kg given in 50 mL of 0.9% saline solution IV over 15 to 30 min may enable patients to undergo minor procedures (eg, tooth extraction, minor surgery) without needing replacement therapy. If a replacement product is needed, desmopressin may reduce the required dose.

One dose of desmopressin is effective for about 8 to 10 h. About 48 h must elapse for new stores of VWF to accumulate, permitting a 2nd injection of desmopressin to be as effective as the initial dose. For many patients, intra-nasal desmopressin may be as effective as IV treatment.

For more significant procedures or for patients with types 2 or 3 VWD, treatment involves replacement of VWF by infusion of intermediate-purity factor VIII concentrates, which contain components of VWF. These concentrates are virally inactivated and therefore do not transmit HIV infection or hepatitis. Because they do not cause transfusion-transmitted infections, these concentrates are preferred to the previously used cryoprecipitate. High-purity factor VIII concentrates are prepared by immunoaffinity chromatography and contain no VWF and should not be used.

For women with heavy menstrual bleeding due to von Willebrand disease, a brief period of treatment with tranexamic acid by mouth may decrease bleeding.

KEY POINTS

- Patients have easy bruising and purpura, usually mucosal, and rarely joint bleeding.
- Screening tests reveal a normal platelet count, normal INR, and sometimes a slightly prolonged PTT.
- Confirming tests include total plasma VWF antigen, VWF function (VWF ristocetin cofactor assay), and plasma factor VIII level.
- Treatment, desmopressin or sometimes intermediate-purity factor VIII concentrate, is given for active bleeding and before an invasive procedure.

157 Thrombotic Disorders

In healthy people, homeostatic balance exists between procoagulant (clotting) forces and anticoagulant and fibrinolytic forces. Numerous genetic, acquired, and environmental factors can tip the balance in favor of coagulation, leading to the pathologic formation of thrombi in veins (eg, deep venous thrombosis [DVT]), arteries (eg, myocardial infarction, ischemic stroke), or cardiac chambers. Thrombi can obstruct blood flow at the site of formation or detach and embolize to block a distant blood vessel (eg, pulmonary embolism, embolic stroke).

Etiology

Genetic defects that increase the propensity for venous thromboembolism include

- Factor V Leiden mutation, which causes resistance to activated protein C (APC)
- Prothrombin 20210 gene mutation
- Deficiency of protein C
- Deficiency of protein S
- Deficiency of protein Z
- Antithrombin deficiency

Acquired defects also predispose to venous and arterial thrombosis (see Table 157–1).

Other disorders and environmental factors can increase the risk of thrombosis, especially if a genetic abnormality is also present.

Symptoms and Signs

Common manifestations of a thrombotic disorder include unexplained deep venous thrombosis and pulmonary embolism (PE). Superficial thrombophlebitis can also develop. Other consequences may include arterial thrombosis (eg, causing stroke or mesenteric ischemia). Symptoms depend on the location of the clot, as in the following examples:

- Chest pain and shortness of breath: Possible PE
- Leg warmth, redness, and swelling: DVT
- Weakness/numbness of one side of the body, problems speaking, and problems with balance and walking: Possible ischemic stroke
- Abdominal pain: Possible mesenteric ischemia

Women may have a history of multiple spontaneous abortions.

Diagnosis

Diagnoses are summarized elsewhere in THE MANUAL specific to the location of the thrombus (eg, deep venous thrombosis, pulmonary embolism, ischemic stroke).

Predisposing factors: Predisposing factors should always be considered. In some cases, the condition is clinically obvious (eg, recent surgery or trauma, prolonged immobilization, cancer, generalized atherosclerosis). If no predisposing factor is readily apparent, further evaluation should be conducted in patients with

- Family history of venous thrombosis
- More than one episode of venous thrombosis
- Venous or arterial thrombosis before age 50
- Unusual sites of venous thrombosis (eg, cavernous sinus, mesenteric veins)

Table 157–1. ACQUIRED CAUSES OF THROMBOEMBOLISM

CONDITION	COMMENTS
Antiphospholipid antibodies	Autoimmune disorder with increased risk of venous or arterial thrombi
Atherosclerosis	Increases risk of arterial thrombi Higher risk in patients with preexisting stenosis When atherosclerotic plaques rupture, they expose or release tissue factor, activate coagulation, initiate local platelet adhesion and aggregation, and cause thrombosis
Cancer (promyelocytic leukemia; lung, breast, prostate, pancreas, stomach, and colon tumors)	May activate coagulation by secreting a factor X–activating protease, by expressing/exposing tissue factor on exposed membrane surfaces, or both
Heparin-induced thrombocytopenia	Associated with platelet aggregation and increased risk of thrombosis
Hyperhomocysteinemia	Possible cause Due to folate, vitamin B_{12}, or vitamin B_6 deficiency
Infection, if severe (eg, sepsis)	Increases risk of venous thrombosis Increases expression/exposure of tissue factor by monocytes and macrophages
Oral contraceptives that contain estrogen	Low risk with low-dose regimens More frequent in patients who have a genetic abnormality that predisposes to venous thromboembolism and in women who smoke
Tissue injury	Due to trauma or surgery
Venous stasis	Due to surgery, orthopedic or paralytic immobilization, heart failure, pregnancy, or obesity

As many as half of all patients with spontaneous DVT have a genetic predisposition.

Testing for predisposing congenital factors includes specific assays that measure the quantity or activity of natural anticoagulant molecules in plasma, and screening for specific gene defects, as follows:

- Clotting assay for lupus anticoagulant
- Clotting assay for resistance to activated protein C
- Genetic test for factor V Leiden
- Genetic test for prothrombin gene mutation (G20210A)
- Functional assay of antithrombin
- Functional assay of protein C
- Functional assay of protein S
- Antigenic assays of total and free protein S.
- Measurement of plasma homocysteine levels
- Immunoassays for antiphospholipid antibodies

Treatment

Treatment is summarized elsewhere in The Manual specific to the location of the thrombus.

ANTIPHOSPHOLIPID ANTIBODY SYNDROME

(Anticardiolipin Antibody Syndrome; Lupus Anticoagulant Syndrome)

Antiphospholipid antibody syndrome (APS) is an autoimmune disorder in which patients have autoantibodies to phospholipid-bound proteins. Venous or arterial thrombi may occur. The pathophysiology is not precisely known. Diagnosis is with blood testing. Anticoagulation is used for prevention and treatment.

The APS is an autoimmune disorder that consists of thrombosis and (in pregnancy) fetal demise caused by various antibodies directed against one or more phospholipid-bound proteins (eg, $beta_2$-glycoprotein I, prothrombin, annexin A5). Annexin A5 may bind to phospholipid membrane constituents to prevent the cell membrane from initiating the activation of coagulation. The autoantibodies displace annexin A5 and, thus, produce procoagulant endothelial cell surfaces that can cause arterial or venous thromboses. The mechanism of thrombosis in patients with autoantibodies to phospholipid-bound $beta_2$-glycoprotein I (apolipoprotein H, a type of cardiolipin) or prothrombin is unknown.

Results of in vitro clotting tests may paradoxically be prolonged because the autoantibodies to phospholipid-bound proteins interfere with coagulation factor assembly and activation on the phospholipid components added to plasma to initiate the tests. The lupus anticoagulant is an autoantibody that binds to phospholipid-bound protein complexes. It was initially recognized in patients with systemic lupus erythematosis (SLE), but these patients now account for only a minority of people with the autoantibody.

Other symptoms of venous or arterial thrombosis may also develop. Patients with autoantibodies to phospholipid-bound prothrombin may have levels of circulating prothrombin that are low enough to increase risk of bleeding.

Diagnosis

- Laboratory testing, beginning with PTT

PTT testing is done in patients who are expected to undergo an invasive procedure or in those with unexplained bleeding or clotting. The lupus anticoagulant is suspected if the PTT is prolonged and does not correct immediately upon 1:1 mixing with normal plasma but does return to normal upon the addition of an excessive quantity of phospholipids (done in the clinical pathology laboratory). Antiphospholipid antibodies in patient plasma are then directly measured by immunoassays of IgG and IgM antibodies that bind to phospholipid/$beta_2$-glycoprotein I complexes on microtiter plates.

Treatment

- Anticoagulation

Heparin, warfarin (except in pregnant women), and aspirin have been used for prophylaxis and treatment.

It is not yet known if the newer oral anticoagulants that inhibit either thrombin (dabigatran) or factor Xa (eg, rivaroxaban, apixaban) can be used in place of heparin or warfarin for this disorder.

ANTITHROMBIN DEFICIENCY

Because antithrombin inhibits thrombin and factors Xa, IXa, and XIa, deficiency of antithrombin predisposes to venous thrombosis.

Antithrombin is a protein that inhibits thrombin and factors Xa, IXa, and XIa, thereby inhibiting thrombosis.

Heterozygous deficiency of plasma antithrombin has a prevalence of about 0.2 to 0.4%; about half of people affected develop venous thromboses. Homozygous deficiency is probably lethal to the fetus in utero.

Acquired deficiencies occur in patients with disseminated intravascular coagulation (DIC), liver disease, or nephrotic syndrome, or during heparin therapy. Heparin exerts its anticoagulant effect by activating antithrombin.

Laboratory testing is done for patients with an unexplained blood clot and involves quantification of the capacity of patient plasma to inhibit thrombin in the presence of heparin.

Treatment

- Warfarin to prevent venous thromboembolism

Oral warfarin is used for prophylaxis against venous thromboembolism.

It is not yet known if the newer oral anticoagulants that inhibit either thrombin (dabigatran) or factor Xa (eg, rivaroxaban, apixaban) can be used in place of warfarin in this disorder.

HYPERHOMOCYSTEINEMIA

Hyperhomocysteinemia may predispose to arterial and venous thrombosis.

Hyperhomocysteinemia may predispose to arterial thrombosis and venous thromboembolism, possibly because of injury to vascular endothelial cells. Some experts believe, however, that there is insufficient evidence definitively to link hyperhomocysteinemia to thrombosis.

Plasma homocysteine levels are elevated ≥ 10-fold in homozygous cystathionine beta-synthase deficiency. Milder elevations occur in heterozygous deficiency and in other abnormalities of folate metabolism, including methyltetrahydrofolate dehydrogenase deficiency. The most common causes of hyperhomocysteinemia are acquired deficiencies of

- Folate
- Vitamin B_{12}
- Vitamin B_6 (pyridoxine)

Folate deficiency is rare in the Western world due to folate fortification of wheat flour.

The abnormality is established by measuring plasma homocysteine levels.

Treatment

- Dietary supplementation

Plasma homocysteine levels may be normalized by dietary supplementation with folate, vitamin B_{12}, or vitamin B_6 alone or in combination; however, it is not been shown that this therapy reduces the risk of arterial or venous thrombosis.

FACTOR V RESISTANCE TO ACTIVATED PROTEIN C

Mutations of factor V make it resistant to its normal cleavage and inactivation by activated protein C and predispose to venous thrombosis.

Activated protein C (APC), in complex with protein S, degrades coagulation factors Va and VIIIa, thus inhibiting coagulation. Any of several mutations to factor V make it resistant to inactivation by APC, increasing the tendency for thrombosis.

Factor V Leiden is the most common of these mutations. Homozygous mutations increase the risk of thrombosis more than do heterozygous mutations.

Factor V Leiden as a single gene defect is present in about 5% of European populations, but it rarely occurs in native Asian or African populations. It is present in 20 to 60% of patients with spontaneous venous thrombosis.

Diagnosis

- Plasma coagulation assay

Diagnosis is based on a functional plasma coagulation assay (eg, the failure of patient's plasma PTT to become prolonged in the presence of snake venom–activated patient protein C) and on molecular analysis of the factor V gene.

Treatment

- Anticoagulation

Anticoagulation with parenteral heparin or low molecular weight heparin, followed by oral warfarin, is used for venous thrombosis or for prophylaxis for patients at increased thrombotic risk (eg, by immobilization, severe injury, surgery).

It is not yet known if the newer oral anticoagulants that inhibit either thrombin (dabigatran) or factor Xa (eg, rivaroxaban, apixaban) can be used in place of warfarin for this disorder.

PROTEIN C DEFICIENCY

Because activated protein C degrades coagulation factors Va and VIIIa, deficiency of protein C predisposes to venous thrombosis.

Protein C is a vitamin K–dependent protein, as are coagulation factors VII, IX, and X, prothrombin, and proteins S and Z. Because activated protein C (APC) degrades factors Va and VIIIa, APC is a natural plasma anticoagulant. Decreased protein C due to genetic or acquired causes promotes venous thrombosis.

Heterozygous deficiency of plasma protein C has a prevalence of 0.2 to 0.5%; about 75% of people with this defect experience a venous thromboembolism (50% by age 50).

Homozygous or doubly heterozygous deficiency causes neonatal purpura fulminans, ie, severe neonatal DIC.

Acquired decreases occur in patients with liver disease or DIC, and during warfarin therapy.

Diagnosis is based on antigenic and functional plasma assays.

Treatment

- Anticoagulation

Patients with symptomatic thrombosis require anticoagulation with heparin or low molecular weight heparin, followed by warfarin. Use of the vitamin K antagonist, warfarin, as initial therapy occasionally causes thrombotic skin infarction by lowering vitamin K–dependent protein C levels before a therapeutic decrease has occurred in most vitamin K–dependent coagulation factors.

It is not known whether the newer oral anticoagulants that inhibit either thrombin (dabigatran) or factor Xa (eg, rivaroxaban, apixaban) can be used in place of other anticoagulants for this disorder.

Neonatal purpura fulminans is fatal without replacement of protein C (using normal plasma or purified concentrate) and anticoagulation with heparin or low molecular weight heparin.

PROTEIN S DEFICIENCY

Because protein S binds and assists activated protein C in the degradation of coagulation factors Va and VIIIa, deficiency of protein S predisposes to venous thrombosis.

Protein S, a vitamin K–dependent protein, is a cofactor for activated protein C–mediated cleavage of factors Va and VIIIa.

Heterozygous deficiency of plasma protein S predisposes to venous thrombosis. Heterozygous protein S deficiency is similar to heterozygous protein C deficiency in genetic transmission, prevalence, laboratory testing, treatment, and precautions.

Homozygous deficiency of protein S can cause neonatal purpura fulminans that is clinically indistinguishable from that caused by homozygous deficiency of protein C.

Acquired deficiencies of protein C (and, soon thereafter, protein S) occur during DIC and warfarin therapy.

Diagnosis is based on antigenic assays of total or free plasma protein S (free protein S is the form unbound to the protein S carrier molecule, C4-binding protein).

Treatment

- Anticoagulation

The treatment of protein S deficiency associated with venous thrombosis is identical to the treatment of protein C deficiency, with one exception. Because there is no purified protein S concentrate available for transfusion, normal plasma is used to replace protein S during a thrombotic emergency.

It is not known if the newer oral anticoagulants that inhibit either thrombin (dabigatran) or factor Xa (eg, rivaroxaban, apixaban) can be used in place of other anticoagulants for this disorder.

PROTEIN Z DEFICIENCY

Because protein Z helps inactivate coagulation factor Xa, deficiency or dysfunction of protein Z predisposes to venous thrombosis (mainly in patients with other clotting abnormalities).

Protein Z, a vitamin K–dependent protein, functions as a cofactor to down-regulate coagulation by forming a complex with the plasma protein, Z-dependent protease inhibitor (ZPI). The complex predominantly inactivates factor Xa on phospholipid surfaces.

The consequence of protein Z or ZPI deficiency, or of autoantibodies to protein Z, in the pathophysiology of thrombosis and fetal loss is not completely clear; however, either defect may make thrombosis more likely if an affected patient also has another congenital coagulation abnormality (eg, factor V Leiden).

Quantification of protein Z, ZPI, and protein Z autoantibodies is done in specialized regional laboratories by plasma electrophoresis, immunoblotting, and enzyme-linked immunosorbent assay.

It is not yet known whether anticoagulant therapy or prophylaxis is indicated in protein Z or ZPI deficiency.

PROTHROMBIN (FACTOR II) 20210 GENE MUTATION

A genetic mutation causes increased serum levels of prothrombin (factor II), predisposing to venous thrombosis.

Prothrombin (factor II) is a vitamin K-dependent precursor of thrombin, the end-product of the coagulation cascade. A mutation of the prothrombin 20210 gene results in increased plasma prothrombin levels (with potentially increased thrombin generation) and increases the risk of venous thromboembolism. The prevalence of the mutation ranges from < 1% to 6.5%, depending on the population studied.

The diagnosis is made by genetic analysis of the prothrombin 20210 gene using blood samples.

Treatment

- Anticoagulation

Anticoagulation with heparin or low molecular weight heparin, followed by warfarin, is used for venous thrombosis, or for prophylaxis in patients at increased thrombotic risk (eg, by immobilization, severe injury, or surgery).

It is not known if the newer oral anticoagulants that inhibit either thrombin (dabigatran) or factor Xa (eg, rivaroxaban, apixaban) can be used in place of other anticoagulants for this disorder.

158 Transfusion Medicine

BLOOD COLLECTION

More than 25 million units of blood components are transfused yearly in the US, from about 9 million volunteer donors. Although transfusion is probably safer than ever, risk (and the public's perception of risk) mandates informed consent whenever practical.

In the US, the collection, storage, and transport of blood and its components are standardized and regulated by the FDA, the AABB (formerly known as the American Association of Blood Banks), and sometimes by state or local health authorities. Donor screening includes an extensive questionnaire and health interview; measurement of temperature, heart rate, and blood pressure; and Hb determination. Some potential donors are deferred either temporarily or permanently (see Table 158–1). Criteria for deferral protect prospective donors from possible ill effects of donation and recipients from disease.

Table 158–1. SOME REASONS FOR BLOOD DONATION DEFERRAL OR DENIAL

REASON	DONATION OUTCOME	COMMENT
AIDS or participation in certain high-risk activities[‡]	Denial	Includes any positive test for HIV, ever High-risk activity includes • IV drug use (ever) • Engaged in sex for compensation (ever)
Activities that increase risk of HIV infection[‡]	Deferral	The FDA has changed recommendations for certain high-risk activities from denial to deferral for 12 mo from last such activity. Activities include • Men who have sex with men (MSM) and women who have sex with MSM • Sexual contact with a person who ever had a positive HIV test, ever engaged in sex for compensation, or ever used IV drugs
Anemia	Deferral	Donation permitted after anemia resolves
Bovine insulin use (because of risk of variant Creutzfeldt-Jacob disease)	Denial	People who have used bovine insulin since 1980: Ineligible to donate
Cancer	Denial	Some people with mild, treatable forms (eg, small skin cancers): Possibly able to donate
Congenital bleeding disorder	Denial	—
Drugs (selected)	Deferral	Waiting period depends on drug: • Finasteride: Defer for 1 mo after last dose • Isotretinoin: Defer for 1 mo after last dose • Dutasteride: Defer for 6 mo after last dose • Acitretin: Defer for 3 yr after last dose • Etretinate: Defer indefinitely
Exposure to hepatitis	Deferral	Wait 12 mo after possible exposure
Hepatitis	Denial	Ineligible to donate if ever diagnosed with viral hepatitis
Hypertension	Deferral	Defer donation until BP is controlled
Malaria or exposure to malaria	Deferral	Wait 3 yr after treatment for malaria or living in an area in which malaria is endemic; wait 12 mo after visit to an area in which malaria is endemic
Military personnel residing on US bases in Europe at risk for variant Creutzfeldt-Jacob disease	Denial	UK, Germany, Belgium, Netherlands: ≥ 6 mo between 1980 and 1990 Elsewhere in Europe: ≥ 6 mo between 1980 and 1996
Pregnancy	Deferral	Wait 6 wk after giving birth
Severe asthma	Denial	—
Severe heart disease	Denial	—
Stay in UK or Europe for people at risk of variant Creutzfeldt-Jacob disease	Denial	UK: Cumulative stay of > 3 mo between 1980 and 1996 Europe (except France): Cumulative stay of ≥ 5 yr since 1980 France: Cumulative stay of > 5 yr since 1980
Tattoo	Deferral	Wait 12 mo
Transfusion that can increase risk of variant Creutzfeldt-Jacob disease	Deferral Denial	Wait 12 mo Recipients of any blood product since 1980 in the UK
Vaccinations (selected)	Deferral	Waiting period depends on vaccination: • Toxoids or synthetic or killed viral, bacterial, or rickettsial vaccines* in symptom-free and afebrile donors: No deferral • Measles, mumps, polio (Sabin), or typhoid (oral) vaccines[†]: Defer for 2 wk • Rubella or varicella vaccines[†]: Defer for 4 wk
Zika virus infection	Deferral	For recent Zika virus infection, the US FDA recommends a 120-day deferral from resolution of symptoms or the last positive test, whichever is longer The FDA no longer recommends screening donor for risk factors; instead all donor blood is to be tested for Zika

*These vaccines include anthrax, cholera, diphtheria, hepatitis A, hepatitis B, influenza, Lyme disease, paratyphoid, pertussis, plague, pneumococcal polysaccharide, polio (Salk), Rocky Mountain spotted fever, tetanus, and typhoid injection.

†Recipients of other live-attenuated viral or bacterial vaccines may be deferred 2 or 4 wk, depending on the vaccine.

‡Reflects FDA Dec 2015 Guidance document: Revised Recommendations for Reducing the Risk of Human Immunodeficiency Virus Transmission by Blood and Blood Products. (See also www.fda.gov/downloads/BiologicsBloodVaccines/GuidanceComplianceRegulatoryInformation/Guidances/Blood/UCM446580.pdf)

UK = United Kingdom.

Whole blood donations are limited to once every 56 days, whereas apheresis RBC donations (donations of twice the usual amount of RBCs in one sitting) are limited to once every 112 days. Apheresis platelet donations are limited to once every 72 h with a maximum of 24/yr. With rare exceptions, blood donors are unpaid. (See also the American Red Cross for information regarding donor eligibility.)

In standard blood donation, about 450 mL of whole blood is collected in a plastic bag containing an anticoagulant preservative. Whole blood or packed RBCs preserved with citrate-phosphate-dextrose-adenine may be stored for 35 days. Packed RBCs may be stored for 42 days if an adenine-dextrose-saline solution is added.

Autologous donation, which is use of the patient's own blood, is less preferred as a method of transfusion. When done before elective surgery, up to 3 or 4 units of whole blood or packed RBCs are collected in the 2 to 3 wk preceding surgery. The patient is then given iron supplements. Such elective autologous donation may be considered when matched blood is difficult to obtain because the patient has made antibodies to red cell antigens or has a rare blood type. Special blood salvage procedures are also available for collecting and autotransfusing blood shed after trauma and during surgery.

Pretransfusion Testing

Donor blood testing includes

- ABO and Rh_0(D) antigen typing
- Antibody screening,
- Testing for infectious disease markers (see Table 158–2)

Compatibility testing tests the recipient's RBCs for antigens A, B, and Rh_0(D); screens the recipient's plasma for antibodies against other RBC antigens; and includes a cross-match to ensure that the recipient's plasma is compatible with antigens on donor RBCs. Compatibility testing is done before a transfusion; however, in an emergency, testing is done after releasing blood from the blood bank. It can also help in diagnosing transfusion reactions.

Table 158–2. INFECTIOUS DISEASE TRANSMISSION TESTING

INFECTIOUS AGENT	TYPE OF TESTING
Chagas disease	Antibody testing
Hepatitis B core	Antibody testing
Hepatitis B surface	Antigen testing
Hepatitis C virus	Nucleic acid testing and antibody testing*
HIV	Nucleic acid testing
HIV-1 and HIV-2*	Antibody testing
Human T-cell lymphotropic viruses 1 and 2	Antibody testing
Treponema pallidum (syphilis)	Antigen testing
West Nile virus	Nucleic acid testing
Zika virus	Nucleic acid testing†

*If antibody test is positive, infection is confirmed by Western blot or recombinant immunoblotting assay.

†Test is available with FDA investigational new drug (IND) status in areas where there is a high risk of infection.

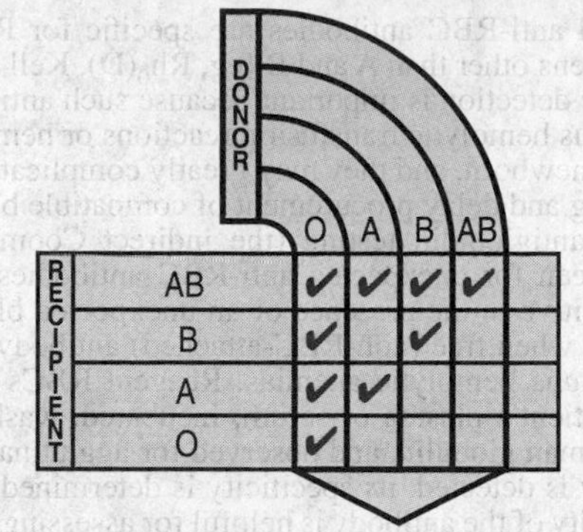

Fig. 158–1. Compatible RBC types.

The addition of a cross-match to ABO/Rh typing and antibody screening increases detection of incompatibility by only 0.01% (see Fig. 158-1). Therefore, many hospitals do computerized electronic cross-matches rather than physical cross-matches in a test tube in patients who have negative antibody screening. If the recipient has a clinically significant anti-RBC antibody, donor blood is restricted to RBC units negative for the corresponding antigen; further testing for compatibility is done by combining recipient plasma, donor RBCs, and antihuman globulin. In recipients without clinically significant anti-RBC antibodies, an immediate spin cross-match, which omits the antiglobulin phase, confirms ABO compatibility.

Emergency transfusion is done when not enough time (generally < 60 min) is available for thorough compatibility testing because the patient is in hemorrhagic shock. When time permits (about 10 min is needed), ABO/Rh type-specific blood may be given. In more urgent circumstances, type O RBCs are transfused if the ABO type is uncertain, and Rh-negative blood is given to females of child-bearing age if the Rh type is uncertain; otherwise, either Rh-negative or Rh-positive O blood can be used.

"Type and screen" may be requested in circumstances not likely to require transfusion, as in elective surgery. The patient's blood is typed for ABO/Rh antigens and screened for antibodies. If antibodies are absent and the patient needs blood, ABO/Rh type specific or compatible RBCs may be released without the antiglobulin phase of the cross-match. If an unexpected antibody is present, full testing is required.

ABO and Rh_0 typing: ABO typing of donor and recipient blood is done to prevent transfusion of incompatible RBCs (see Fig. 158–1). As a rule, blood for transfusion should be of the same ABO type as that of the recipient. In urgent situations or when the correct ABO type is in doubt or unknown, type O Rh-negative packed RBCs (not whole blood—see Acute Hemolytic Transfusion Reaction on p. 1213), which contains neither A nor B antigens, may be used for patients of any ABO type.

Rh typing determines whether the Rh factor Rh_0(D) is present on (Rh-positive) or absent from (Rh-negative) the RBCs. Rh-negative patients should always receive Rh-negative blood except in life-threatening emergencies when Rh-negative blood is unavailable. Rh-positive patients may receive Rh-positive or Rh-negative blood. Occasionally, RBCs from some Rh-positive people react weakly on standard Rh typing (weak D, or D^u, positive), but these people are still considered Rh-positive.

Antibody screening: Antibody screening for unexpected anti-RBC antibodies is routinely done on blood from prospective recipients and prenatally on maternal specimens.

Unexpected anti-RBC antibodies are specific for RBC blood group antigens other than A and B [eg, Rh_0(D), Kell (K), Duffy (Fy)]. Early detection is important because such antibodies can cause serious hemolytic transfusion reactions or hemolytic disease of the newborn, and they may greatly complicate compatibility testing and delay procurement of compatible blood.

Indirect antiglobulin testing (the indirect Coombs test) is used to screen for unexpected anti-RBC antibodies. This test may be positive in the presence of an unexpected blood group antibody or when free (non-RBC-attached) antibody is present in autoimmune hemolytic anemias. Reagent RBCs are mixed with the patient's plasma or serum, incubated, washed, tested with antihuman globulin, and observed for agglutination. Once an antibody is detected, its specificity is determined. Knowing the specificity of the antibody is helpful for assessing its clinical significance, selecting compatible blood, and managing hemolytic disease of the newborn.

Direct antiglobulin testing (the direct Coombs test) detects antibodies that have coated the patient's RBCs in vivo. It is used when immune-mediated hemolysis is suspected. Patients' RBCs are directly tested with antihuman globulin and observed for agglutination. A positive result, if correlated with clinical findings and laboratory indicators of hemolysis, suggests autoimmune hemolytic anemia, drug-induced hemolysis, a transfusion reaction, or hemolytic disease of the newborn.

Antibody titration is done when a clinically significant, unexpected anti-RBC antibody is identified in the plasma of a pregnant woman or in a patient with cold agglutinin disease. The maternal antibody titer correlates fairly well with the severity of hemolytic disease in the incompatible fetus and is often used to guide treatment in hemolytic disease of the newborn along with ultrasonography and amniotic fluid study.

Infectious disease testing: Donated blood products are tested for the presence of a number of infectious agents.

BLOOD PRODUCTS

Whole blood can provide improved oxygen-carrying capacity, volume expansion, and replacement of clotting factors and was previously recommended for rapid massive blood loss. However, because component therapy is equally effective and is a more efficient use of donated blood, whole blood is not generally available in the US.

RBCs: Packed RBCs are ordinarily the component of choice with which to increase Hb. Indications depend on the patient. Oxygen-carrying capacity may be adequate with Hb levels as low as 7 g/L in healthy patients, but transfusion may be indicated with higher Hb levels in patients with decreased cardiopulmonary reserve or ongoing bleeding. One unit of RBCs increases an average adult's Hb by about 1 g/dL (and the Hct by about 3%) above the pretransfusion value. When only volume expansion is required, other fluids can be used concurrently or separately. In patients with multiple blood group antibodies or with antibodies to high-frequency RBC antigens, rare frozen RBCs are used.

Washed RBCs are free of almost all traces of plasma, most WBCs, and platelets. They are generally given to patients who have severe reactions to plasma (eg, severe allergies, paroxysmal nocturnal hemoglobinuria, IgA immunization). In IgA-immunized patients, blood collected from IgA-deficient donors may be preferable for transfusion.

WBC-depleted RBCs are prepared with special filters that remove ≥ 99.99% of WBCs. They are indicated for patients who have experienced nonhemolytic febrile transfusion reactions, for exchange transfusions, for patients who require cytomegalovirus-negative blood that is unavailable, and possibly for the prevention of HLA alloimmunization to help prevent refractoriness to platelet transfusion (failure to achieve the target level of blood platelets after platelet transfusion).

Fresh frozen plasma: Fresh frozen plasma (FFP) is an unconcentrated source of all clotting factors without platelets. Indications include correction of bleeding secondary to factor deficiencies for which specific factor replacements are unavailable, multifactor deficiency states (eg, massive transfusion, disseminated intravascular coagulation [DIC], liver failure), and urgent warfarin reversal, although prothrombin complex concentrate (PCC) is the first choice if available. FFP can supplement RBCs when whole blood is unavailable for neonatal exchange transfusion. FFP should not be used simply for volume expansion or correction of mild to moderate coagulopathy before surgical procedures.

Cryoprecipitate: Cryoprecipitate is a concentrate prepared from FFP. Each concentrate usually contains about 80 units each of factor VIII and von Willebrand factor and about 250 mg of fibrinogen. It also contains ADAMTS13 (an enzyme that is deficient in congenital thrombotic thrombocytopenic purpura), fibronectin, and factor XIII. Although originally used for hemophilia and von Willebrand disease, cryoprecipitate is currently used as a source of fibrinogen in acute DIC with bleeding, treatment of uremic bleeding, cardiothoracic surgery (fibrin glue), obstetric emergencies such as abruptio placentae and HELLP syndrome (hemolysis, elevated liver enzymes, and low platelet count), and rare factor XIII deficiency when human coagulation factor XIII concentrate is unavailable. In general, it should not be used for other indications.

WBCs: Granulocytes may be transfused when sepsis occurs in a patient with profound persistent neutropenia (neutrophils < 500/μL) who is unresponsive to antibiotics. Granulocytes must be given within 24 h of harvest; however, testing for HIV, hepatitis, human T-cell lymphotropic virus, and syphilis may not be completed before infusion. Because of improved antibiotic therapy and drugs that stimulate granulocyte production during chemotherapy, granulocytes are seldom used.

Immune globulins: RhIg, given IM or IV, prevents development of maternal Rh antibodies that can result from fetomaternal hemorrhage. The standard dose of intramuscular RhIg (300 mcg) must be given to an Rh-negative mother immediately after abortion or delivery (live or stillborn) unless the infant is Rh_0(D) and D^u negative or the mother's serum already contains anti-Rh_0(D). If fetomaternal hemorrhage is > 30 mL, a larger dose is needed. If hemorrhage of this amount is suspected, testing of the volume of fetomaternal hemorrhage begins with the screening rosette test, which, if positive, is followed by a quantitative test (eg, Kleihauer-Betke test). RhIg is also used to treat immune thrombocytopenia (ITP), in which case it is given IV.

Other immune globulins are available for postexposure prophylaxis for patients exposed to a number of infectious diseases, including cytomegalovirus (CMV), hepatitis A and B, measles, rabies, respiratory syncytial virus, rubella, tetanus, smallpox, and varicella (for usage, see under specific disease).

Platelets: Platelet concentrates are used

- To prevent bleeding in asymptomatic severe thrombocytopenia (platelet count < 10,000/μL)
- For bleeding patients with less severe thrombocytopenia (platelet count < 50,000/μL)
- For bleeding patients with platelet dysfunction due to antiplatelet drugs but with normal platelet count
- For patients receiving massive transfusion that causes dilutional thrombocytopenia

Platelet concentrates are also sometimes used before invasive surgery, particularly with extracorporeal circulation for > 2 h (which often makes platelets dysfunctional). One platelet concentrate unit increases the platelet count by about 10,000/μL, and adequate hemostasis is achieved with a platelet count of about 10,000/μL in a patient without complicating conditions and about 50,000/μL for those undergoing surgery. Therefore, platelet concentrates derived from a pool of 4 to 5 units of whole blood are commonly used in adults.

Platelet concentrates are increasingly being prepared by automated devices that harvest the platelets (or other cells) and return unneeded components (eg, RBCs, plasma) to the donor. This procedure, called cytapheresis, provides enough platelets from a single donation (equivalent to 4 to 5 whole blood platelet units) for transfusion to an adult, which, because it minimizes infectious and immunogenic risks, is preferred to multiple donor transfusions in certain conditions.

Certain patients may not respond to platelet transfusions (called refractoriness), possibly because of splenic sequestration, platelet consumption due to DIC, or destruction due to HLA or platelet-specific antigen alloimmunization (and immune-mediated destruction). If patients are refractory to transfusion, they are tested for alloimmunization if possible. Patients with immune-mediated destruction may respond to pooled whole blood platelets (because of greater likelihood that some units are HLA compatible), platelets from family members, or ABO- or HLA-matched platelets. HLA alloimmunization may be mitigated by transfusing WBC-depleted RBCs and WBC-depleted platelet concentrates.

Other products: Irradiated blood products are used to prevent graft-vs-host disease (GVHD) in patients at risk. Many attempts have been made to develop blood substitutes using inert chemicals (eg, perfluorocarbons) or Hb solutions to carry and deliver oxygen to tissues. Although these Hb substitutes had promising ability to deliver oxygen to tissues during an emergency, several clinical trials have failed due to increased mortality and severe adverse cardiovascular toxicities (eg, hypotension). Currently, attempts to regenerate platelets and RBCs from various stem cell sources are underway.

Hematopoietic progenitor cells (stem cells) from autologous or allogenic donors can be transfused as a way of reconstituting hematopoietic function (particularly immune function) in patients undergoing myeloablative or myelotoxic therapy (see p. 1413).

TECHNIQUE OF TRANSFUSION

CAUTION: *Before transfusion is started, consent should be obtained, and the patient's wristband, blood unit label, and compatibility test report must be checked at the bedside to ensure that the blood component is the one intended for the recipient.*

Use of an 18-gauge (or larger) needle prevents mechanical damage to and hemolysis of RBCs. A standard filter should always be used for infusion of any blood component. Only 0.9% saline IV should be allowed into the blood bag or in the same tubing with blood. Hypotonic solutions lyse RBCs, and the calcium in Ringer's lactate can cause clotting.

Transfusion of 1 unit of blood or blood component should be completed by 4 h; longer duration increases the risk of bacterial growth. If transfusion must be given slowly because of heart failure or hypervolemia, units may be divided into smaller aliquots in the blood bank. For children, 1 unit of blood can be provided in small sterile aliquots used over several days, thereby minimizing exposure to multiple donors.

Close observation is important, particularly during the first 15 min, and includes recording temperature, blood pressure, pulse, and respiratory rate. Periodic observation continues throughout and after the transfusion, during which fluid status is assessed. The patient is kept covered and warm to prevent chills, which may be interpreted as a transfusion reaction. Elective transfusions at night are discouraged.

COMPLICATIONS OF TRANSFUSION

The **most common complications** of transfusion are

- Febrile nonhemolytic reactions
- Chill-rigor reactions

The **most serious complications,** which have very high mortality rates, are

- Transfusion-associated circulatory overload
- Transfusion-related acute lung injury
- Acute hemolytic reaction due to ABO incompatibility

Early recognition of symptoms suggestive of a transfusion reaction and prompt reporting to the blood bank are essential. The most common symptoms are chills, rigor, fever, dyspnea, light-headedness, urticaria, itching, and flank pain. If any of these symptoms (other than localized urticaria and itching) occur, the transfusion should be stopped immediately and the IV line kept open with normal saline. The remainder of the blood product and clotted and anticoagulated samples of the patient's blood should be sent to the blood bank for investigation. NOTE: *The unit in question should not be restarted, and transfusion of any previously issued unit should not be initiated.* Further transfusion should be delayed until the cause of the reaction is known, unless the need is urgent, in which case type O Rh negative RBCs should be used.

Hemolysis of donor or recipient RBCs (usually the former) during or after transfusion can result from ABO/Rh incompatibility, plasma antibodies, or hemolyzed or fragile RBCs (eg, by overwarming stored blood or contact with hypotonic IV solutions). Hemolysis is most common and most severe when incompatible donor RBCs are hemolyzed by antibodies in the recipient's plasma. Hemolytic reactions may be acute (within 24 h) or delayed (from 1 to 14 days).

Acute hemolytic transfusion reaction: About 20 people die yearly in the US as a result of acute hemolytic transfusion reaction (AHTR). AHTR usually results from recipient plasma antibodies to donor RBC antigens. ABO incompatibility is the most common cause of AHTR. Antibodies against blood group antigens other than ABO can also cause AHTR. Mislabeling the recipient's pretransfusion sample at collection and failing to match the intended recipient with the blood product immediately before transfusion are the usual causes.

Hemolysis is intravascular, causing hemoglobinuria with varying degrees of acute renal failure and possibly DIC. The severity of AHTR depends on the degree of incompatibility, the amount of blood given, the rate of administration, and the integrity of the kidneys, liver, and heart. An acute phase usually develops within 1 h of initiation of transfusion, but it may occur late during the transfusion or immediately afterward. Onset is usually abrupt. The patient may complain of discomfort and anxiety. Dyspnea, fever, chills, facial flushing, and severe pain may occur, especially in the lumbar area. Shock may develop, causing a rapid, feeble pulse; cold, clammy skin; low blood pressure; and nausea and vomiting. Jaundice may follow acute hemolysis.

If AHTR occurs while the patient is under general anesthesia, the only symptom may be hypotension, uncontrollable bleeding from incision sites and mucous membranes caused by an associated DIC, or dark urine that reflects hemoglobinuria.

If AHTR is suspected, one of the first steps is to recheck the sample and patient identifications. Diagnosis is confirmed by a positive direct antiglobulin test, measuring urinary Hb, serum LDH, bilirubin, and haptoglobin. Intravascular hemolysis produces free Hb in the plasma and urine; haptoglobin levels are very low. Hyperbilirubinemia may follow.

After the acute phase, the degree of acute kidney injury determines the prognosis. Diuresis and a decreasing BUN usually portend recovery. Permanent renal insufficiency is unusual. Prolonged oliguria and shock are poor prognostic signs.

If AHTR is suspected, the transfusion should be stopped and supportive treatment begun. The goal of initial therapy is to achieve and maintain adequate blood pressure and renal blood flow with IV 0.9% saline and furosemide. IV saline is given to maintain urine output of 100 mL/h for 24 h. The initial furosemide dose is 40 to 80 mg (1 to 2 mg/kg in children), with later doses adjusted to maintain urinary flow > 100 mL/h during the first day.

Drug treatment of hypotension must be done cautiously. Pressor drugs that decrease renal blood flow (eg, epinephrine, norepinephrine, high-dose dopamine) are contraindicated. If a pressor drug is necessary, dopamine 2 to 5 mcg/kg/min is usually used.

A nephrologist should be consulted as early as possible, particularly if no diuretic response occurs within about 2 to 3 h after initiating therapy, which may indicate acute tubular necrosis. Further fluid and diuretic therapy may be contraindicated, and early dialysis may be helpful.

Delayed hemolytic transfusion reaction: Occasionally, a patient who has been sensitized to an RBC antigen has very low antibody levels and negative pretransfusion tests. After transfusion with RBCs bearing this antigen, a primary or anamnestic response may result (usually in 1 to 4 wk) and cause a delayed hemolytic transfusion reaction. A delayed hemolytic transfusion reaction usually does not manifest as dramatically as AHTR. Patients may be asymptomatic or have a slight fever. Rarely, severe symptoms occur. Usually, only destruction of the transfused RBCs (with the antigen) occurs, resulting in a falling Hct and a slight rise in lactate dehydrogenase and bilirubin and a positive direct antiglobulin test. Because delayed hemolytic transfusion reaction is usually mild and self-limited, it is often unidentified, and the clinical clue may be an unexplained drop in Hb to the pretransfusion level occurring 1 to 2 wk posttransfusion. Severe reactions are treated similarly to acute reactions.

Febrile nonhemolytic transfusion reaction: Febrile reactions may occur without hemolysis. Antibodies directed against WBC HLA in otherwise compatible donor blood are one possible cause. This cause is most common in multitransfused or multiparous patients. Cytokines released from WBCs during storage, particularly in platelet concentrates, are another possible cause.

Clinically, febrile reactions consist of a temperature increase of ≥ 1° C, chills, and sometimes headache and back pain. Simultaneous symptoms of allergic reaction are common. Because fever and chills also herald a severe hemolytic transfusion reaction, all febrile reactions must be investigated as for AHTR, as with any transfusion reaction.

Most febrile reactions are treated successfully with acetaminophen and, if necessary, diphenhydramine. Patients should also be treated (eg, with acetaminophen) before future transfusions. If a recipient has experienced more than one febrile reaction, special leukoreduction filters are used during future transfusions; most hospitals use prestorage, leukoreduced blood components.

Allergic reactions: Allergic reactions to an unknown component in donor blood are common, usually due to allergens in donor plasma or, less often, to antibodies from an allergic donor. These reactions are usually mild and include urticaria, edema, occasional dizziness, and headache during or immediately after the transfusion. Simultaneous fever is common. Less frequently, dyspnea, wheezing, and incontinence may occur, indicating a generalized spasm of smooth muscle. Rarely, anaphylaxis occurs, particularly in IgA-deficient recipients.

In a patient with a history of allergies or an allergic transfusion reaction, an antihistamine may be given prophylactically just before or at the beginning of the transfusion (eg, diphenhydramine 50 mg po or IV). NOTE: *Drugs must never be mixed with the blood.* If an allergic reaction occurs, the transfusion is stopped. An antihistamine (eg, diphenhydramine 50 mg IV) usually controls mild urticaria and itching, and transfusion may be resumed. However, a moderate allergic reaction (generalized urticaria or mild bronchospasm) requires hydrocortisone (100 to 200 mg IV), and a severe anaphylactic reaction requires additional treatment with epinephrine 0.5 mL of 1:1000 solution sc and 0.9% saline IV (see p. 1378) along with investigation by the blood bank. Further transfusion should not occur until the investigation is completed. Patients with severe IgA deficiency require transfusion of washed RBCs, washed platelets, and plasma from an IgA-deficient donor.

Volume overload: Although volume overload is underrecognized and underreported, recently it has been recognized as the second most common cause of transfusion-related deaths (20%) reported to the FDA. The high osmotic load of blood products draws volume into the intravascular space over the course of hours, which can cause volume overload in susceptible patients (eg, those with cardiac or renal insufficiency). RBCs should be infused slowly. The patient should be observed and, if signs of heart failure (eg, dyspnea, crackles) occur, the transfusion should be stopped and treatment for heart failure begun.

Typical treatment is with a diuretic such as furosemide 20 to 40 mg IV. Occasionally, patients requiring a higher volume of plasma infusion to reverse a warfarin overdose may be given a low dose of furosemide simultaneously; however, PCC is the first choice for such patients. Patients at high risk of volume overload (eg, those with heart failure or severe renal insufficiency) are treated prophylactically with a diuretic (eg, furosemide 20 to 40 mg IV).

Acute lung injury: Transfusion-related acute lung injury is an infrequent complication caused by anti-HLA and/or antigranulocyte antibodies in donor plasma that agglutinate and degranulate recipient granulocytes within the lung. Acute respiratory symptoms develop, and chest x-ray has a characteristic pattern of noncardiogenic pulmonary edema. This complication is the most common cause of transfusion-related death (45% of deaths reported to the FDA). Incidence is 1 in 5,000 to one in 10,000, but many cases are mild. Mild to moderate transfusion-related acute lung injury probably is commonly missed. General supportive therapy typically leads to recovery without long-lasting sequelae. Diuretics should be avoided. Using blood donated by men reduces the risk of this reaction. Cases should be reported to the hospital transfusion medicine service or blood bank.

Altered oxygen affinity: Blood stored for > 7 days has decreased RBC 2,3-diphosphoglycerate (DPG), and the 2,3-DPG is absent after > 10 days. This absence results in an increased affinity for oxygen and slower release of oxygen to the tissues. There is little evidence that 2,3-DPG deficiency is clinically significant except in exchange transfusions in infants, in sickle cell patients with acute chest syndrome and stroke, and in some patients with severe heart failure. After transfusion of RBCs, 2,3-DPG regenerates within 12 to 24 h.

Graft-vs-host disease: Transfusion-associated GVHD (see also p. 1404) is usually caused by transfusion of products containing immunocompetent lymphocytes to an immunocompromised host. The donor lymphocytes attack host tissues. GVHD can occur occasionally in immunocompetent patients if they receive blood from a donor (usually a close relative) who is homozygous for an HLA haplotype for which they are heterozygous. Symptoms and signs include fever, rash (centrifugally spreading rash becoming erythroderma with bullae), vomiting, watery and bloody diarrhea, lymphadenopathy, and pancytopenia due to bone marrow aplasia. Jaundice and elevated liver enzyme levels are also common. GVHD occurs 4 to 30 days after transfusion and is diagnosed based on clinical suspicion and skin and bone marrow biopsies. GVHD has > 90% mortality because no specific treatment is available.

Prevention of GVHD is with irradiation (to damage DNA of the donor lymphocytes) of all transfused blood products. It is done

- If the recipient is immunocompromised (eg, patients with congenital immune deficiency syndromes, hematologic cancers, or hematopoietic stem cell transplants; neonates)
- If donor blood is obtained from a 1st-degree relative
- When HLA-matched components, excluding stem cells, are transfused

Treatment with corticosteroids and other immunosuppressants, including those used for solid organ transplantation, is not an indication for blood irradiation.

Complications of massive transfusion: Massive transfusion is transfusion of a volume of blood greater than or equal to one blood volume in 24 h (eg, 10 units in a 70-kg adult). When a patient receives standard resuscitation fluids of packed RBCs (colloid) plus crystalloid (Ringer's lactate or normal saline) in such large volume, the plasma clotting factors and platelets are diluted, causing a coagulopathy (dilutional coagulopathy). This coagulopathy worsens the consumptive coagulopathy due to major trauma itself (ie, as a result of extensive activation of the clotting cascade) and leads to a lethal triad of acidosis, hypothermia, and bleeding. Recently, protocols for massive transfusions have been developed in which FFP and platelets are given earlier in resuscitation *before* coagulopathy develops, rather than trying to "catch up." Such protocols have been shown to decrease mortality, although the ideal ratios of RBCs, plasma, and platelets are still being developed. A recent trial showed no significant mortality difference between giving one unit of plasma and one platelet concentrate for each 2 units of RBCs (1:1:2) versus giving one unit of plasma and one platelet concentrate for every 1 unit of RBCs (1:1:1).[1]

Hypothermia due to rapid transfusion of large amounts of cold blood can cause arrhythmias or cardiac arrest. Hypothermia is avoided by using an IV set with a heat-exchange device that gently warms blood. Other means of warming blood (eg, microwave ovens) are contraindicated because of potential RBC damage and hemolysis.

Citrate and potassium toxicities generally are not of concern even in massive transfusion; however, toxicities of both may be amplified in the presence of hypothermia. Patients with liver failure may have difficulty metabolizing citrate. Hypocalcemia can result but rarely necessitates treatment (which is 10 mL of a 10% solution of calcium gluconate IV diluted in 100 mL D_5W, given over 10 min). Patients with kidney failure may have elevated potassium if transfused with blood stored for > 1 wk (potassium accumulation is usually insignificant in blood stored for < 1 wk). Mechanical hemolysis during transfusion may increase potassium. Hypokalemia may occur about 24 h after transfusion of older RBCs (> 3 wk), which take up potassium.

Post-transfusion purpura: Post-transfusion purpura is a very rare complication in which the platelet count falls rapidly 4 to 14 days after an RBC transfusion, causing moderate to severe thrombocytopenia. Almost all patients are multiparous women who typically received RBC transfusion during a surgical procedure. The exact etiology is unclear. However, the most accepted hypothesis is that a patient who is negative for human platelet antigen 1a (HPA1a) develops alloantibodies due to exposure to HPA1a antigen from the fetus during pregnancy. Because stored RBCs contain platelet microparticles and because most (99%) donors are HPA1a positive, platelet microparticles from the donor blood may trigger an antibody response in previously sensitized patients (anamnestic response). Because these platelet microparticles attach to the recipient's platelets (and thus coat them with HPA1a antigen), the alloantibodies destroy the recipient's platelets, causing thrombocytopenia. The disorder resolves spontaneously as the antigen-coated platelets are destroyed.

Patients develop purpura along with moderate to severe bleeding—usually from the surgical site. Platelet and red cell transfusions make the condition worse.

The differential diagnosis usually includes heparin-induced thrombocytopenia (HIT), although HIT is not associated with bleeding. Diagnosis is made by documenting HPA1a antibodies in the patient's plasma and absence of corresponding antigen on the patient's platelets.

Treatment is high-dose IV immunoglobulins (1 to 2 g/kg) and avoidance of further transfusion of platelets or RBCs. Plasma exchange may be considered in severe cases and, for patients with severe bleeding, platelets donated by HPA1a-negative donors could be transfused if available.

Infectious complications: Bacterial contamination of packed RBCs occurs rarely, possibly due to inadequate aseptic technique during collection or to transient asymptomatic donor bacteremia. Refrigeration of RBCs usually limits bacterial growth except for cryophilic organisms such as *Yersinia* sp, which may produce dangerous levels of endotoxin. All RBC units are inspected before dispensing for bacterial growth, which is indicated by a color change. Because platelet concentrates are stored at room temperature, they have greater potential for bacterial growth and endotoxin production if contaminated. To minimize growth, storage is limited to 5 days. The risk of bacterial contamination of platelets is 1:2500. Therefore, platelets are routinely tested for bacteria.

Rarely, syphilis is transmitted in fresh blood or platelets. Storing blood for ≥ 96 h at 4 to 10° C kills the spirochete. Although federal regulations require a serologic test for syphilis on donor blood, infective donors are seronegative early in the disease. Recipients of infected units may develop the characteristic secondary rash.

Hepatitis may occur after transfusion of any blood product. The risk has been reduced by viral inactivation through heat treatment of serum albumin and plasma proteins and by the use of recombinant factor concentrates. Tests for hepatitis are required for all donor blood (see Table 158–2). The estimated risk of hepatitis B is 1:500,000; of hepatitis C, 1:2.6 million. Because its transient viremic phase and concomitant clinical illness likely preclude blood donation, hepatitis A (infectious hepatitis) is not a significant cause of transfusion-associated hepatitis.

HIV infection in the US is almost entirely HIV-1, although HIV-2 is also of concern. Testing for antibodies to both strains is required. Nucleic acid testing for HIV-1 antigen and HIV-1 p24 antigen testing are also required. Additionally, blood donors are asked about behaviors that may put them at high risk of HIV infection. HIV-0 has not been identified among blood donors. The estimated risk of HIV transmission due to transfusion is 1:2.6 million.

CMV can be transmitted by WBCs in transfused blood. It is not transmitted through FFP. Because CMV does not cause disease in immunocompetent recipients, routine antibody testing of donor blood is not required. However, CMV may cause serious or fatal disease in immunocompromised patients, who should receive CMV-negative blood products that have been provided by CMV antibody-negative donors or by blood depleted of WBCs by filtration.

Human T-cell lymphotropic virus 1 (HTLV-1), which can cause adult T-cell lymphoma/leukemia and HTLV-1–associated myelopathy/tropical spastic paraparesis, causes posttransfusion seroconversion in some recipients. All donor blood is tested for HTLV-1 and HTLV-2 antibodies. The estimated risk of false-negative results on testing of donor blood is 1:641,000.

Creutzfeldt-Jakob disease has never been reported to be transmitted by transfusion, but current practice precludes donation from a person who has received human-derived growth hormone or a dura mater transplant or who has a family member with Creutzfeldt-Jakob disease. New variant Creutzfeldt-Jakob disease (vCJD, or mad cow disease) has not been transmitted by blood transfusion. However, donors who have spent significant time in the United Kingdom and some other parts of Europe may be permanently deferred from donation (see Table 158–1).

Malaria is transmitted easily through infected RBCs. Many donors are unaware that they have malaria, which may be latent and transmissible for 10 to 15 yr. Storage does not render blood safe. Prospective donors must be asked about malaria or whether they have been in a region where it is prevalent. Donors who have had a diagnosis of malaria or who are immigrants, refugees, or citizens from countries in which malaria is considered endemic are deferred for 3 yr; travelers to endemic countries are deferred for 1 yr.

Babesiosis, Chagas disease, and West Nile virus have rarely been transmitted by transfusion.

Zika virus infection has been reported to be transmitted via blood products in Brazil. Therefore, the FDA has mandated testing for Zika virus in the US and its territories. In lieu of Zika testing, pathogen reduction technologies approved for platelets and plasma could also be used; however, their use is currently very limited, and this technology is still unavailable for red cells.

1. Holcomb JB, Tilley BC, Baraniuk S, et al: Transfusion of plasma, platelets, and red blood cells in a 1:1:1 vs a 1:1:2 ratio and mortality in patients with severe trauma: the PROPPR randomized clinical trial. *JAMA* 313(5):471–482, 2015. doi:10.1001/jama.2015.12.

THERAPEUTIC APHERESIS

Therapeutic apheresis includes plasma exchange and cytapheresis, which are generally tolerated by healthy donors. However, many minor and a few major risks exist. Insertion of the large IV catheters necessary for apheresis can cause complications (eg, bleeding, infection, pneumothorax). Citrate anticoagulant may decrease serum ionized calcium. Replacement of plasma with a noncolloidal solution (eg, saline) shifts fluid from the intravascular space. Colloidal replacement solutions do not replace IgG and coagulation factors.

Most complications can be managed with close attention to the patient and manipulation of the procedure, but some severe reactions and a few deaths have occurred.

Plasma exchange: Therapeutic plasma exchange removes plasma components from blood. A blood cell separator extracts the patient's plasma and returns RBCs and platelets in plasma or a plasma-replacing fluid; for this purpose, 5% albumin is preferred to FFP (except for patients with thrombotic thrombocytopenic purpura) because it causes fewer reactions and transmits no infections. Therapeutic plasma exchange resembles dialysis but, in addition, can remove protein-bound toxic substances. A one-volume exchange removes about 65% of such components.

To be of benefit, plasma exchange should be used for diseases in which the plasma contains a known pathogenic substance, and plasma exchange should remove this substance more rapidly than the body produces it. For example, in rapidly progressive autoimmune disorders, plasma exchange may be used to remove existing harmful plasma components (eg, cryoglobulins, antiglomerular basement membrane antibodies) while immunosuppressive or cytotoxic drugs suppress their future production.

There are numerous, complex indications. Clinicians typically follow Guidelines on the Use of Therapeutic Apheresis from the American Society for Apheresis.[1] The frequency of plasma exchange, the volume to be removed, the replacement fluid, and other variables are individualized. Low density lipoprotein cholesterol can be selectively removed from plasma by adsorption over a column (called LDL apheresis). In photopheresis, mononuclear cells are selectively removed by centrifugation and treated with photoactivatable drugs (eg, 8-methoxypsoralen) that are then activated with ultraviolet light; it is a form of immunomodulatory therapy. In immunoadsorption, an antibody or antigen is removed from plasma by combining with an antigen or antibody chosen to bind the target antibody or antigen over a column. Complications of plasma exchange are similar to those of therapeutic cytapheresis.

Cytapheresis: Therapeutic cytapheresis removes cellular components from blood, returning plasma. It is most often used to remove defective RBCs and substitute normal ones in patients with sickle cell disease who have the following conditions: acute chest syndrome, stroke, pregnancy, or frequent, severe sickle cell crises. RBC exchange achieves Hb S levels of < 30% without the risk of increased viscosity that can occur because of increased Hct with simple transfusion.

Therapeutic cytapheresis may also be used to reduce severe thrombocytosis or leukocytosis (cytoreduction) in acute leukemia or in accelerated or blast crisis phase of chronic myelogenous leukemia when there is risk of hemorrhage, thrombosis, or pulmonary or cerebral complications of extreme leukocytosis (leukostasis). Cytapheresis is effective in thrombocytosis because platelets are not replaced as rapidly as WBCs. One or two procedures may reduce platelet counts to safe levels. Therapeutic WBC removal (leukapheresis) can remove kilograms of buffy coat in a few procedures, and it often relieves leukostasis. However, the reduction in WBC count itself may be mild and only temporary.

Other uses of cytapheresis include collection of peripheral blood stem cells for autologous or allogeneic bone marrow reconstitution (an alternative to bone marrow transplantation) and collection of lymphocytes for use in immune modulation cancer therapy (adoptive immunotherapy).

1. Schwartz J, Padmanabhan A, Aqui N, et al: Guidelines on the Use of Therapeutic Apheresis in Clinical Practice–Evidence-Based Approach from the Writing Committee of the American Society for Apheresis: the Seventh Special Issue. *J Clin Apheresis* 31:149–338, 2016. doi:10.1002/jca.21470.

159 Tumor Immunology

TUMOR ANTIGENS

Many tumor cells produce antigens, which may be released in the bloodstream or remain on the cell surface. Antigens have been identified in most of the human cancers, including Burkitt lymphoma, neuroblastoma, malignant melanoma, osteosarcoma, renal cell carcinoma, breast carcinoma, prostate cancer, lung carcinomas, and colon cancer. A key role of the immune system is detection of these antigens to permit subsequent targeting for eradication. However, despite their foreign structure, the immune response to tumor antigens varies and is often insufficient to prevent tumor growth.

Tumor-associated antigens (TAAs) are relatively restricted to tumor cells, whereas tumor-specific antigens (TSAs) are unique to tumor cells. TSAs and TAAs typically are portions of intracellular molecules expressed on the cell surface as part of the major histocompatibility complex (MHC).

Suggested mechanisms of origin for tumor antigens include

- Introduction of new genetic information from a virus (eg, human papillomavirus E6 and E7 proteins in cervical cancer)
- Alteration of oncogenes or tumor suppressor genes by carcinogens, which result in formation of neoantigens (novel protein sequences or accumulation of proteins that are normally not expressed or are expressed at very low levels, such as *ras* or *p53*), either by generating the novel protein sequence directly or by inducing accumulation of these proteins
- Missense mutations in various genes not directly associated with tumor suppressor or oncogenes and that cause appearance of tumor-specific neoantigens on the cell surface
- Abnormally high levels of proteins that normally are present at substantially lower levels (eg, prostate-specific antigens, melanoma-associated antigens) or that are expressed only during embryonic development (carcinoembryonic antigens)
- Uncovering of antigens normally buried in the cell membrane because of defective membrane homeostasis in tumor cells
- Release of antigens normally sequestered within the cell or its organelles when tumor cells die

HOST RESPONSE TO TUMORS

The immune response to foreign antigens consists of

- Humoral mechanisms (eg, antibodies)
- Cellular mechanisms

Most humoral responses cannot prevent tumor growth. However, effector cells, such as T cells, macrophages, and natural killer (NK) cells, have relatively effective tumoricidal abilities. Effector cell activity is induced by cells that present TSAs or TAAs on their surface (these cells are called antigen-presenting cells) and is supported by cytokines (eg, interleukins, interferons). Despite the activity of effector cells, host immunoreactivity may fail to control tumor occurrence and growth.

Cellular Immunity

The **T cell** is the primary cell responsible for direct recognition and killing of tumor cells. T cells carry out immunologic surveillance, then proliferate and destroy newly transformed tumor cells after recognizing TAAs. The T-cell response to tumors is modulated by other cells of the immune system; some cells require the presence of humoral antibodies directed against the tumor cells (antibody-dependent cellular cytotoxicity) to initiate the interactions that lead to the death of tumor cells. In contrast, suppressor T cells inhibit the immune response against tumors.

Cytotoxic T lymphocytes (CTLs) recognize antigens on target cells and lyse these cells. These antigens may be cell surface proteins or may be intracellular proteins (eg, TAAs) that are expressed on the surface in combination with class I MHC molecules. Tumor-specific CTLs have been found with neuroblastomas; malignant melanomas; sarcomas; and carcinomas of the colon, breast, cervix, endometrium, ovary, testis, nasopharynx, and kidney.

NK cells are another population of effector cells with tumoricidal activity. In contrast to CTLs, NK cells lack the receptor for antigen detection but can still recognize normal cells infected with viruses or tumor cells. Their tumoricidal activity is termed natural because it is not induced by a specific antigen. The mechanism by which NK cells discriminate between normal and abnormal cells is under study. Evidence suggests that class I MHC molecules on the surface of normal cells inhibit NK cells and prevent lysis. Thus, the decreased level of class I molecule expression characteristic of many tumor cells may allow activation of NK cells and subsequent tumor lysis.

Macrophages can kill specific tumor cells when activated by a combination of factors, including lymphokines (soluble factors produced by T cells) and interferon. They are less effective than T-cell-mediated cytotoxic mechanisms. Under certain circumstances, macrophages may present TAAs to T cells and stimulate tumor-specific immune response. There are at least 2 classes of tumor-associated macrophages (TAM):

- TAM-1 (M1) cells facilitate T cell killing of tumors
- TAM-2 (M2) cells promote tumor tolerance

Dendritic cells are dedicated antigen-presenting cells present in barrier tissues (eg, skin, lymph nodes). They play a central role in initiation of tumor-specific immune response. These cells take up tumor-associated proteins, process them, and present TAAs to T cells to stimulate the CTL response against tumor. Several classes of dendritic cells can mediate tumor promotion or suppression.

Lymphokines produced by immune cells stimulate growth or induce activities of other immune cells. Such lymphokines include IL-2, also known as T-cell growth factor, and the interferons. IL-12 is produced by dendritic cells and specifically induces CTLs, thereby enhancing antitumor immune responses.

Regulatory T cells are normally present in the body and help prevent autoimmune reactions. They are produced during the active phase of immune responses to pathogens and limit the strong immune response that could damage the host. Accumulation of these cells in cancers inhibits antitumor immune responses.

Myeloid-derived suppressor cells consist of immature myeloid cells and their precursors. These cells accumulate in large numbers in cancers and potently suppress immune responses.

Humoral Immunity

In contrast to T-cell cytotoxic immunity, humoral antibodies do not appear to confer significant protection against tumor growth. Most antibodies cannot recognize TAAs. Regardless, humoral antibodies that react with tumor cells in vitro have been detected in the sera of patients with various tumors, including Burkitt lymphoma; malignant melanoma; osteosarcoma; neuroblastoma; and carcinomas of the lung, breast, and GI tract.

Cytotoxic antibodies are directed against surface antigens of tumor cells. These antibodies can exert anti-tumor effects through complement fixation or by serving as a flag for destruction of tumor cells by T cells (antibody-dependent cell-mediated cytotoxicity). Another population of humoral antibodies, called enhancing antibodies (blocking antibodies), may actually favor rather than inhibit tumor growth. The mechanisms and relative importance of such immunologic enhancement are not well understood.

Failure of Host Defenses

Although many tumors are eliminated by the immune system (and thus are never detected), others continue to grow despite the presence of TAAs. Several mechanisms have been proposed to explain this deficient host response to the TAA, including the following:

- Specific immunologic tolerance to TAAs in a process that involves antigen-presenting cells and suppressor T cells, possibly secondary to prenatal exposure to the antigen
- Suppression of immune response by chemical, physical, or viral agents (eg, helper T-cell destruction by HIV)
- Suppression of the immune response by cytotoxic drugs or radiation
- Suppression of the immune response by the tumor itself through various complex and largely uncharacterized mechanisms that cause various problems including decreased T, B, and antigen-presenting cell function, decreased IL-2 production, and increased circulating soluble IL-2 receptors (which bind and hence inactivate IL-2)
- Presence and activity of TAM-2 (M2) cells, promoting tumor tolerance

TUMOR IMMUNODIAGNOSIS

TAAs can help diagnose various tumors and sometimes determine the response to therapy or recurrence. An ideal tumor marker would be released only from tumor tissue, be specific for a given tumor type, be detectable at low levels of tumor cell burden, have a direct relationship to the tumor cell burden, and be present in all patients with the tumor. However, although most tumors release detectable antigenic macromolecules into the circulation, no tumor marker has all the requisite characteristics to provide enough specificity or sensitivity to be used in early diagnosis or mass cancer screening programs.

Carcinoembryonic antigen (CEA) is a protein-polysaccharide complex present in colon carcinomas and in normal fetal intestine, pancreas, and liver. Blood levels are elevated in patients with colon carcinoma, but the specificity is relatively low because positive results also occur in heavy cigarette smokers and in patients with cirrhosis, ulcerative colitis, and other cancers (eg, breast, pancreas, bladder, ovary, cervix). Monitoring CEA levels may be useful for detecting cancer recurrence after tumor excision if the patient initially had an elevated CEA and for refining estimates of prognosis by stage.

α-fetoprotein, a normal product of fetal liver cells, is also present in the sera of patients with primary hepatoma, nonseminomatous germ cell tumors, and, frequently, ovarian or testicular embryonal carcinoma. Levels are sometimes useful for estimating prognosis or, less often, for diagnosis.

β subunit of human chorionic gonadotropin (β-hCG), measured by immunoassay, is the major clinical marker in women with gestational trophoblastic neoplasia (GTN)—a disease spectrum that includes hydatidiform mole, nonmetastatic GTN, and metastatic GTN—and in about two-thirds of men with testicular embryonal carcinoma or choriocarcinoma. The β subunit is measured because it is specific for hCG. This marker is present in low levels in healthy people. Levels are elevated during pregnancy.

Prostate-specific antigen (PSA), a glycoprotein located in ductal epithelial cells of the prostate gland, can be detected in low concentrations in the sera of healthy men. Using an appropriate upper limit of normal, assays with monoclonal antibodies detect elevated serum levels of PSA in about 90% of patients with advanced prostate cancer, even in the absence of defined metastatic disease. It is more sensitive than prostatic acid phosphatase. However, because PSA is elevated in other conditions (eg, benign prostatic hypertrophy, prostatitis, recent GU tract instrumentation), it is less specific. PSA can be used to monitor recurrence after prostatic carcinoma has been diagnosed and treated.

CA 125 is clinically useful for screening, diagnosing, and monitoring therapy for ovarian cancer, although any peritoneal inflammatory process and some other cancers can increase levels.

β-2 microglobulin is often elevated in multiple myeloma and in some lymphomas. Its primary use is in prognosis.

CA 19-9 was originally developed to detect colorectal cancer but proved more sensitive for pancreatic cancer. It is primarily used to judge the response to treatment in patients with advanced pancreatic cancers. CA 19-9 can also be elevated in other GI cancers, particularly cancer of the bile ducts, and some benign bile duct and cholestatic disorders.

CA 15-3 and **CA 27-29** are elevated in most patients with metastatic breast cancer. Levels may also be elevated in other conditions. These markers are primarily used to monitor the response to therapy.

Chromogranin A is used as a marker for carcinoid and other neuroendocrine tumors. Sensitivity and specificity for neuroendocrine tumors can exceed 75%, and diagnostic accuracy is higher with diffuse than with localized tumors. Levels can be elevated in other cancers, such as lung and prostate, and some benign disorders (eg, primary hypertension, chronic kidney disease, chronic atrophic gastritis).

Thyroglobulin is produced by the thyroid and may be elevated with various thyroid disorders. It is primarily used after complete thyroidectomy to detect recurrent thyroid cancer and to monitor the response to treatment in metastatic thyroid cancer.

TA-90 is a highly immunogenic subunit of a urinary tumor–associated antigen that is present in 70% of melanomas; soft-tissue sarcomas; and carcinomas of the breast, colon, and lung. Some studies have shown that TA-90 levels can accurately predict survival and the presence of subclinical disease after surgery for melanoma.

IMMUNOTHERAPY OF CANCER

A number of immunologic interventions, both passive and active, can be directed against tumor cells.

Passive Cellular Immunotherapy

In passive cellular immunotherapy, specific effector cells are directly infused and are not induced or expanded within the patient.

Lymphokine-activated killer (LAK) cells are produced from the patient's endogenous T cells, which are extracted and grown in a cell culture system by exposing them to the lymphokine IL-2. The proliferated LAK cells are then returned to the patient's bloodstream. Animal studies have shown that LAK cells are more effective against cancer cells than are the original endogenous T cells, presumably because of their greater number. Clinical trials of LAK cells in humans are ongoing.

Tumor-infiltrating lymphocytes (TILs) may have greater tumoricidal activity than LAK cells. These cells are grown in culture in a manner similar to LAK cells. However, the progenitor cells consist of T cells that are isolated from resected tumor tissue. This process theoretically provides a line of T cells that has greater tumor specificity than those obtained from the bloodstream. Recent clinical studies have shown highly promising results.

Genetically modified T cells can express

- **T-cell receptors** (TCR) that recognize TAAs with high specificity to tumor cells. This approach is under study and may provide significant clinical benefit. Results of initial trials are encouraging.
- **Chimeric antigen receptors** (CAR) that recognize specific proteins on the surface of tumor cells. This approach has demonstrated great potential in first clinical trials in patients with B-cell leukemia.

In contrast to TCR T cells, CAR T cells recognize only relatively large proteins on the surface of tumor cells. Therefore CAR T cells and TCR T cells may represent complementary approaches to cancer therapy.

Concomitant use of interferon enhances the expression of MHC antigens and TAAs on tumor cells, thereby augmenting the killing of tumor cells by the infused effector cells.

Passive Humoral Immunotherapy

Administration of exogenous antibodies constitutes passive humoral immunotherapy. Antilymphocyte serum has been used in the treatment of chronic lymphocytic leukemia and in T-cell and B-cell lymphomas, resulting in temporary decreases in lymphocyte counts or lymph node size.

Monoclonal antitumor antibodies may also be conjugated with toxins (eg, ricin, diphtheria) or with radioisotopes so that the antibodies deliver these toxic agents specifically to the tumor cells. Another technique involves bispecific antibodies, or linkage of one antibody that reacts with the tumor cell to a second antibody that reacts with a cytotoxic effector cell. This technique brings the effector cell in close opposition to the tumor cell, resulting in increased tumoricidal activity. However, these techniques are in early stages of testing; thus, potential clinical benefits are uncertain.

Active Specific Immunotherapy

Inducing cellular immunity (involving cytotoxic T cells) in a host that failed to spontaneously develop an effective response generally involves methods to enhance presentation of tumor antigens to host effector cells. Cellular immunity can be induced to specific, very well-defined antigens. Several techniques can be used to stimulate a host response; these techniques may involve giving peptides, DNA, or tumor cells (from the host or another patient). Peptides and DNA are often given using antigen-presenting cells (dendritic cells). These dendritic cells can also be genetically modified to secrete additional immune-response stimulants (eg, granulocyte-macrophage colony-stimulating factor [GM-CSF]).

Peptide-based vaccines use peptides from defined TAAs. An increasing number of TAAs have been identified as the targets of T cells in cancer patients and are being tested in clinical trials. Recent data indicate that responses are most potent if TAAs are delivered using dendritic cells. These cells are obtained from the patient, loaded with the desired TAA, and then reintroduced intradermally; they stimulate endogenous T cells to respond to the TAA. The peptides also can be delivered by co-administration with immunogenic adjuvants.

DNA vaccines use recombinant DNA that encodes a specific (defined) antigenic protein. The DNA is incorporated into viruses that are injected directly into patients or, more often, introduced into dendritic cells obtained from the patients, which are then injected back into them. The DNA expresses the target antigen, which triggers or enhances patients' immune response.

Autochthonous tumor cells (cells taken from the patient) have been reintroduced to the patient after use of ex vivo techniques (eg, irradiation, neuraminidase treatment, hapten conjugation, hybridization with other cell lines) to reduce their malignant potential and increase their antigenic activity. Sometimes the tumor cells are genetically modified to produce immunostimulatory molecules (including cytokines such as GM-CSF or IL-2, costimulatory molecules such as B7-1, and allogeneic class I MHC molecules); this modification helps attract effector molecules and enhances systemic tumor targeting. Clinical trials with GM-CSF–modified tumor cells have produced encouraging preliminary results.

Allogeneic tumor cells (cells taken from other patients) have been used in patients with acute lymphocytic leukemia and acute myelogenous leukemia. Remission is induced by intensive chemotherapy and radiation therapy. Then, irradiated allogeneic tumor cells that have been modified either genetically or chemically to increase their immunogenic potential are injected into the patient. Sometimes patients are also given Bacille Calmette-Guérin (BCG) vaccine or other adjuvants to enhance the immune response against the tumor. Prolonged remissions or improved reinduction rates have been reported in some series but not in most.

A novel approach to cancer treatment combining immunotherapy and conventional chemotherapy has shown some success (vs historic controls) in nonrandomized phase I and phase II clinical trials involving various cancers, types of vaccines, and chemotherapy.

Immunotherapy and Targeting Inhibitors of Immune Responses

Immune checkpoint blockers are antibodies that target molecules involved in natural inhibition of immune responses. These target molecules include the following:

- Cytotoxic T lymphocyte-associated protein 4 (CTLA4)
- Programmed cell death protein 1 (PD1) and programmed cell death ligands 1 (PD-L1) and 2 (PD-L2)
- Others

Cytotoxic T-lymphocyte-associated protein 4 (CTLA-4) can downregulate the activation of CD4+ and CD8+ T cells that is triggered by antigen-presenting cells (APCs). The mechanism may be the higher affinity of CTL4 for CD80 and CD86 (costimulatory receptors) than the costimulatory receptor CD28 on APCs. CTLA-4 is upregulated by activation of T cell receptor and by cytokines such as interferon-gamma and interleukin-12. The CTLA-4 inhibitor ipilimumab prolongs survival in metastatic melanoma and can be used as an alternative to interferon as adjuvant treatment in high-risk melanoma.

Tremelimumab, another CTLA-4 inhibitor, is being studied in mesothelioma and other tumors.

PD-1 and PD ligand 1 and 2 inhibitors can counteract certain immune inhibitory effects triggered by the interaction of PD-1 and PD-L1 or PD-L2. PD-1 (expressed on T cells, B cells, natural killer (NK) cells, and some others (eg, monocytes, dendritic cells) binds to PD-L1 (expressed on many tumor cells, hematopoietic cells, and some other cells) and PD-L2 (expressed mainly on hematopoietic cells). This binding inhibits tumor cell apoptosis and facilitates T cell exhaustion and the conversion of T cell cytotoxic and helper T cells to regulatory T cells. PD-1 and PD-L1/2 are upregulated by cytokines such as interleukin-12 and interferon-gamma. Nivolumab and pembrolizumab are IgG4 PD-1 inhibitors that prolong survival in metastatic melanoma and non-small cell lung cancer. They are also in phase III clinical trials as treatment for other cancers (eg, lymphomas, head and neck cancer, renal cell carcinoma, certain colorectal carcinomas).

Others under study are generally in earlier stages of clinical development. These include, for example, B and T cell lymphocyte attenuator (BTLA, which decreases production of cytokines and CD4 cell proliferation), lymphocyte activator gene 3 (LAG3, which increases T cell regulator activity), T cell immunoglobulin and mucin domain 3 (TIM-3, which kills helper Th1 cells), and V-domain Ig suppressor of T cell activation (VISTA, inhibition of which increases T cell activity in tumors).

Nonspecific Immunotherapy

Interferons (IFN-α, -β, -γ) are glycoproteins that have antitumor and antiviral activity. Depending on dose, interferons may either enhance or decrease cellular immune function and humoral immune function. Interferons also inhibit division and certain synthetic processes in a variety of cells. Clinical trials have indicated that interferons have antitumor activity in various cancers, including hairy cell leukemia, chronic myelocytic leukemia, AIDS-associated Kaposi sarcoma, non-Hodgkin lymphoma, multiple myeloma, and ovarian carcinoma. However, interferons may have significant adverse effects, such as fever, malaise, leukopenia, alopecia, and myalgias.

Certain **bacterial adjuvants** (BCG and derivatives, killed suspensions of *Corynebacterium parvum*) have tumoricidal properties. They have been used with or without added tumor antigen to treat a variety of cancers, usually along with intensive chemotherapy or radiation therapy. For example, direct injection of BCG into cancerous tissues has resulted in regression of melanoma and prolongation of disease-free intervals in superficial bladder carcinomas and may help prolong drug-induced remission in acute myelogenous leukemia, ovarian carcinoma, and non-Hodgkin lymphoma.

SECTION 13

Endocrine and Metabolic Disorders

160 Principles of Endocrinology

The endocrine system coordinates functioning between different organs through hormones, which are chemicals released into the bloodstream from specific types of cells within endocrine (ductless) glands. Once in circulation, hormones affect function of the target tissues, which may be another endocrine gland or an end organ. Some hormones exert an effect on cells of the organ from which they were released (paracrine effect), some even on the same cell type (autocrine effect).

Hormones can be

- Peptides of various sizes
- Steroids (derived from cholesterol)
- Amino acid derivatives

Hormones bind selectively to receptors located inside or on the surface of target cells. Receptors inside cells interact with hormones that regulate gene function (eg, corticosteroids, vitamin D, thyroid hormone). Receptors on the cell surface bind with hormones that regulate enzyme activity or affect ion channels (eg, growth hormone, thyrotropin-releasing hormone).

Endocrine disorders result from disruptions of the endocrine glands and/or their target tissues.

Hypothalamic-Pituitary Relationships

Peripheral endocrine organ functions are controlled to varying degrees by pituitary hormones. Some functions (eg, secretion of insulin by the pancreas, primarily controlled by the blood glucose level) are controlled to a minimal extent, whereas many (eg, secretion of thyroid or gonadal hormones) are controlled to a great extent. Secretion of pituitary hormones is controlled by the hypothalamus.

The interaction between the hypothalamus and pituitary (hypothalamic-pituitary axis) is a feedback control system. The hypothalamus receives input from virtually all other areas of the CNS and uses it to provide input to the pituitary. In response, the pituitary releases various hormones that stimulate certain endocrine glands throughout the body. Changes in circulating levels of hormones produced by these endocrine glands are detected by the hypothalamus, which then increases or decreases its stimulation of the pituitary to maintain homeostasis.

The hypothalamus modulates the activities of the anterior and posterior lobes of the pituitary in different ways. Neurohormones synthesized in the hypothalamus reach the anterior pituitary (adenohypophysis) through a specialized portal vascular system and regulate synthesis and release of the 6 major peptide hormones of the anterior pituitary (see Fig.170–1 on p. 1318). These anterior pituitary hormones regulate peripheral endocrine glands (the thyroid, adrenals, and gonads) as well as growth and lactation. No direct neural connection exists between the hypothalamus and the anterior pituitary. In contrast, the posterior pituitary (neurohypophysis) comprises axons originating from neuronal cell bodies located in the hypothalamus. These axons serve as storage sites for 2 peptide hormones, vasopressin (antidiuretic hormone) and oxytocin, synthesized in the hypothalamus; these hormones act in the periphery to regulate water balance, milk ejection, and uterine contraction.

Virtually all hormones produced by the hypothalamus and the pituitary are released in a pulsatile fashion; periods of such release are interspersed with periods of inactivity. Some hormones (eg, adrenocorticotropic hormone [ACTH], growth hormone, prolactin) have definite circadian rhythms; others (eg, luteinizing hormone and follicle-stimulating hormone during the menstrual cycle) have month-long rhythms with superimposed circadian rhythms.

Hypothalamic Controls

Thus far, 7 physiologically important hypothalamic neurohormones have been identified (see Table 160–1). Except for the biogenic amine dopamine, all are small peptides. Several are produced in the periphery as well as in the hypothalamus and function in local paracrine systems, especially in the GI tract. Vasoactive intestinal peptide, which also stimulates the release of prolactin, is one.

Neurohormones may control the release of multiple pituitary hormones. Regulation of most anterior pituitary hormones depends on stimulatory signals from the hypothalamus; the exception is prolactin, which is regulated by inhibitory stimuli. If the pituitary stalk (which connects the pituitary to the hypothalamus) is severed, prolactin release increases, whereas release of all other anterior pituitary hormones decreases.

Many hypothalamic abnormalities (including tumors and encephalitis and other inflammatory lesions) can alter the release of hypothalamic neurohormones. Because neurohormones are synthesized in different centers within the hypothalamus, some disorders affect only one neuropeptide, whereas others affect several. The result can be undersecretion or oversecretion of neurohormones. Clinical syndromes that result from the ensuing pituitary hormone dysfunction (eg, diabetes insipidus,

Table 160–1. HYPOTHALAMIC NEUROHORMONES

NEUROHORMONE	ANTERIOR PITUITARY HORMONES AFFECTED	EFFECT
Corticotropin-releasing hormone	ACTH	Stimulate
Dopamine	Prolactin LH FSH TSH	Inhibit Inhibit Inhibit Inhibit
Gonadotropin-releasing hormone	LH FSH	Stimulate* Stimulate*
Growth hormone–releasing hormone	GH	Stimulate
Prolactin-releasing hormone	Prolactin	Stimulate
Somatostatin	GH TSH	Inhibit Inhibit
Thyrotropin-releasing hormone	TSH Prolactin	Stimulate Stimulate

*Under physiologic conditions and when administered exogenously in intermittent pulses. Continuous infusion inhibits the release of LH and FSH.

ACTH = adrenocorticotropic hormone (corticotropin); FSH = follicle-stimulating hormone; GH = growth hormone; LH = luteinizing hormone; TSH = thyroid-stimulating hormone.

acromegaly, and hypopituitarism) are discussed in Pituitary Disorders on p. 1317.

Anterior Pituitary Function

The cells of the anterior lobe (which constitutes 80% of the pituitary by weight) synthesize and release several hormones necessary for normal growth and development and also stimulate the activity of several target glands.

Adrenocorticotropic hormone (ACTH): ACTH is also known as corticotropin. Corticotropin-releasing hormone (CRH) is the primary stimulator of ACTH release, but vasopressin plays a role during stress. ACTH induces the adrenal cortex to release cortisol and several weak androgens, such as dehydroepiandrosterone (DHEA). Circulating cortisol and other corticosteroids (including exogenous corticosteroids) inhibit the release of CRH and ACTH. The CRH-ACTH-cortisol axis is a central component of the response to stress. Without ACTH, the adrenal cortex atrophies and cortisol release virtually ceases.

Thyroid-stimulating hormone (TSH): TSH regulates the structure and function of the thyroid gland and stimulates synthesis and release of thyroid hormones. TSH synthesis and release are stimulated by the hypothalamic hormone thyrotropin-releasing hormone (TRH) and suppressed (by negative feedback) by circulating thyroid hormones.

Luteinizing hormone (LH) and follicle-stimulating hormone (FSH): LH and FSH control the production of the sex hormones. Synthesis and release of LH and FSH are stimulated mainly by gonadotropin-releasing hormone (GnRH) and suppressed by estrogen and testosterone. One factor controlling GnRH release is kisspeptin, a hypothalamic peptide that is triggered by increased leptin levels at puberty. Two gonadal hormones, activin and inhibin, affect only FSH; activin is stimulative, and inhibin is inhibitory.

In women, LH and FSH stimulate ovarian follicular development and ovulation. In men, FSH acts on Sertoli cells and is essential for spermatogenesis; LH acts on Leydig cells of the testes to stimulate testosterone biosynthesis.

Growth hormone (GH): GH stimulates somatic growth and regulates metabolism. Growth hormone–releasing hormone (GHRH) is the major stimulator and somatostatin is the major inhibitor of the synthesis and release of GH. GH controls synthesis of insulin-like growth factor 1 (IGF-1, also called somatomedin-C), which largely controls growth. Although IGF-1 is produced by many tissues, the liver is the major source. A variant of IGF-1 occurs in muscle, where it plays a role in enhancing muscle strength. It is less under control of GH than is the liver variant.

The metabolic effects of GH are biphasic. GH initially exerts insulin-like effects, increasing glucose uptake in muscle and fat, stimulating amino acid uptake and protein synthesis in liver and muscle, and inhibiting lipolysis in adipose tissue. Several hours later, more profound anti–insulin-like metabolic effects occur. They include inhibition of glucose uptake and use, causing blood glucose and lipolysis to increase, which increases plasma free fatty acids. GH levels increase during fasting, maintaining blood glucose levels and mobilizing fat as an alternative metabolic fuel. Production of GH decreases with aging. Ghrelin, a hormone produced in the fundus of the stomach, promotes GH release from the pituitary, increases food intake, and improves memory.

Prolactin: Prolactin is produced in cells called lactotrophs that constitute about 30% of the cells of the anterior pituitary. The pituitary doubles in size during pregnancy, largely because of hyperplasia and hypertrophy of lactotrophs. In humans, the major function of prolactin is stimulating milk production. Also, prolactin release occurs during sexual activity and stress. Prolactin may be a sensitive indicator of pituitary dysfunction; prolactin is the hormone most frequently produced in excess by pituitary tumors, and it may be one of the hormones to become deficient from infiltrative disease or tumor compression of the pituitary.

Other hormones: Several other hormones are produced by the anterior pituitary. These include pro-opiomelanocortin (POMC, which gives rise to ACTH), alpha- and beta-melanocyte-stimulating hormone (MSH), beta-lipotropin (β-LPH), the enkephalins, and the endorphins. POMC and MSH can cause hyperpigmentation of the skin and are only significant clinically in disorders in which ACTH levels are markedly elevated (eg, Addison disease, Nelson syndrome). The function of β-LPH is unknown. Enkephalins and endorphins are endogenous opioids that bind to and activate opioid receptors throughout the CNS.

Posterior Pituitary Function

The posterior pituitary releases vasopressin (also called arginine vasopressin or antidiuretic hormone [ADH]) and oxytocin. Both hormones are released in response to neural impulses and have half-lives of about 10 min.

Vasopressin (antidiuretic hormone, ADH): Vasopressin acts primarily to promote water conservation by the kidneys by increasing the permeability of the distal tubular epithelium to water. At high concentrations, vasopressin also causes vasoconstriction. Like aldosterone, vasopressin plays an important role in maintaining fluid homeostasis and vascular and cellular hydration. The main stimulus for vasopressin release is increased osmotic pressure of water in the body, which is sensed by osmoreceptors in the hypothalamus. The other major stimulus is volume depletion, which is sensed by baroreceptors in the left atrium, pulmonary veins, carotid sinus, and aortic arch, and then transmitted to the CNS through the vagus and glossopharyngeal nerves. Other stimulants for vasopressin release include pain, stress, emesis, hypoxia, exercise, hypoglycemia, cholinergic agonists, beta-blockers, angiotensin, and prostaglandins. Inhibitors of vasopressin release include alcohol, alpha-blockers, and glucocorticoids.

A lack of vasopressin causes central diabetes insipidus. An inability of the kidneys to respond normally to vasopressin causes nephrogenic diabetes insipidus. Removal of the pituitary gland usually does not result in permanent diabetes insipidus because some of the remaining hypothalamic neurons produce small amounts of vasopressin.

Copeptin is coproduced with vasopressin in the posterior pituitary. Measuring it may be useful in distinguishing the cause of hyponatremia.

Oxytocin: Oxytocin has 2 major targets:

- Myoepithelial cells of the breast, which surround the alveoli of the mammary gland
- Smooth muscle cells of the uterus

Suckling stimulates the production of oxytocin, which causes the myoepithelial cells to contract. This contraction causes milk to move from the alveoli to large sinuses for ejection (ie, the milk letdown reflex of nursing mothers). Oxytocin stimulates contraction of uterine smooth muscle cells, and uterine sensitivity to oxytocin increases throughout pregnancy. However, plasma levels do not increase sharply during parturition, and the role of oxytocin in the initiation of labor is unclear.

There is no recognized stimulus for oxytocin release in men, although men have extremely low levels.

OVERVIEW OF ENDOCRINE DISORDERS

Endocrine disorders can result from

- Dysfunction originating in the peripheral endocrine gland itself (primary disorders)
- Understimulation by the pituitary (secondary disorders)
- Overstimulation by the pituitary (secondary disorders)

The disorders can result in hormone overproduction (hyperfunction) or underproduction (hypofunction). Rarely, endocrine disorders (usually hypofunction) occur because of abnormal tissue responses to hormones. Clinical manifestations of hypofunction disorders are often insidious and nonspecific.

Endocrine hyperfunction: Hyperfunction of endocrine glands may result from overstimulation by the pituitary but is most commonly due to hyperplasia or neoplasia of the gland itself. In some cases, cancers from other tissues can produce hormones (ectopic hormone production). Hormone excess also can result from exogenous hormone administration. In some cases, patients take hormones without telling the physician (factitious disease). Tissue hypersensitivity to hormones can occur. Antibodies can stimulate peripheral endocrine glands, as occurs in hyperthyroidism of Graves disease. Disruption of a peripheral endocrine gland can rapidly release stored hormone (eg, thyroid hormone release in subacute thyroiditis). Enzyme defects in the synthesis of a peripheral endocrine hormone can result in overproduction of hormones proximal to the block. Finally, overproduction of a hormone can occur as an appropriate response to a disease state.

Endocrine hypofunction: Hypofunction of an endocrine gland can result from understimulation by the pituitary. Hypofunction originating within the peripheral gland itself can result from congenital or acquired disorders (including autoimmune disorders, tumors, infections, vascular disorders, and toxins). Genetic disorders causing hypofunction can result from deletion of a gene or by production of an abnormal hormone. A decrease in hormone production by the peripheral endocrine gland with a resulting increase in production of pituitary regulating hormone can lead to peripheral endocrine gland hyperplasia. For example, if synthesis of thyroid hormone is defective, thyroid-stimulating hormone (TSH) is produced in excessive amounts, causing goiter.

Several hormones require conversion to an active form after secretion from the peripheral endocrine gland. Certain disorders can block this step (eg, renal disease can inhibit production of the active form of vitamin D). Antibodies to the circulating hormone or its receptor can block the ability of the hormone to bind to its receptor. Disease or drugs can cause increased rate of clearance of hormones. Circulating substances may also block the function of hormones. Abnormalities of the receptor or elsewhere in the peripheral endocrine tissue can also cause hypofunction.

Laboratory Testing for Endocrine Disorders

Because symptoms of endocrine disorders can begin insidiously and may be nonspecific, clinical recognition is often delayed for months or years. For this reason, biochemical diagnosis is usually essential; it typically requires measuring blood levels of the peripheral endocrine hormone, the pituitary hormone, or both.

Because most hormones have circadian rhythms, measurements need to be made at a prescribed time of day. Hormones that vary over short periods (eg, luteinizing hormone) necessitate obtaining 3 or 4 values over 1 or 2 h or using a pooled blood sample. Hormones with week-to-week variation (eg, testosterone) necessitate obtaining separate values a week apart.

Blood hormone measurements: Free or bioavailable hormone (ie, hormone not bound to a specific binding hormone) is generally believed to be the active form. Free or bioavailable hormones are measured using equilibrium dialysis, ultrafiltration, or a solvent-extraction method to separate the free and albumin-bound hormone from the binding globulin. These methods can be expensive and time-consuming. Analog and competitive free hormone assays, although often used commercially, are not always accurate and should not be used.

Blood hormone estimates: Free hormone levels can be estimated indirectly by assessing levels of the binding protein and using them to adjust levels of the total serum hormone. However, indirect methods are inaccurate if the binding capacity of the hormone-binding protein has been altered (eg, by a disorder).

In some cases, other indirect estimates are used. For example, because growth hormone (GH) has a short serum half-life and is difficult to detect in serum, serum insulin-like growth factor 1 (IGF-1), which is produced in response to GH, is often measured as an index of GH activity. Whether measurement of circulating hormone metabolites indicates the amount of bioavailable hormone is under investigation.

Sometimes, instead of blood levels, urine (eg, free cortisol when testing for Cushing disease) or salivary hormone levels may be used.

Dynamic tests: In many cases, a dynamic test is necessary. Thus, in the case of hypofunctioning organs, a stimulation test (eg, ACTH stimulation) can be used. In hyperfunction, a suppression test (eg, dexamethasone suppression) can be used.

Treatment

- Replacing deficient hormone
- Suppressing excessive hormone production

Hypofunction disorders are usually treated by replacement of the *peripheral* endocrine hormone regardless of whether the defect is primary or secondary (an exception is GH, a pituitary hormone replacement used for pituitary dwarfism). If resistance to the hormone exists, drugs that reduce resistance can be used (eg, metformin or thiazolidinediones for type 2 diabetes mellitus). Occasionally, a hormone-stimulating drug is used.

Radiation therapy, surgery, and drugs that suppress hormone production are used to treat hyperfunction disorders. In some cases, a receptor antagonist is used.

Aging and Endocrinology

Hormones undergo many changes as a person ages.

- Most hormone levels decrease.
- Some hormone levels remain normal, including TSH, ACTH (basal), thyroxine, cortisol (basal), 1,25-dihydroxycholecalciferol, insulin (sometimes increases), and estradiol (in men).
- Some hormone levels increase.

Hormones that increase, including ACTH (increased response to corticotropin-releasing hormone), follicle-stimulating hormone, sex-hormone binding globulin, activin (in men), gonadotropins (in women), epinephrine (in the oldest old), parathyroid hormone, norepinephrine, cholecystokinin, vasoactive intestinal peptide, vasopressin (also loss of circadian rhythm), and atrial natriuretic factor, are associated with either receptor defects or postreceptor defects, resulting in hypofunction.

Many age-related changes are similar to those in patients with hormone deficiency, leading to the hypothesis of a hormonal fountain of youth (ie, speculation that some changes associated with aging can be reversed by the replacement of one or more deficient hormones). Some evidence suggests that replacing certain hormones in the elderly can improve functional outcomes (eg, muscle strength, bone mineral density), but little evidence exists regarding effects on mortality. In some cases, replacing hormones may be harmful, as in estrogen replacement in most older women.

A competing theory is that the age-related decline in hormone levels represents a protective slowing down of cellular metabolism. This concept is based on the rate of living theory of aging (ie, the faster the metabolic rate of an organism, the quicker it dies). This concept is seemingly supported by studies on the effects of dietary restriction. Restriction decreases levels of hormones that stimulate metabolism, thereby slowing metabolic rate; restriction also prolongs life in rodents.

Specific age-related hormone decreases: DHEA and its sulfate levels decline dramatically with age. Despite optimism for the role of DHEA supplementation in older people, most controlled trials failed to show any major benefits.

Pregnenolone is the precursor of all known steroid hormones. As with DHEA, its levels decline with age. Studies in the 1940s showed its safety and benefits in people with arthritis, but additional studies failed to show any beneficial effects on memory and muscle strength.

Levels of GH and its peripheral endocrine hormone (IGF-1) decline with age. GH replacement in older people sometimes increases muscle mass but does not increase muscle strength (although it may in malnourished people). Adverse effects (eg, carpal tunnel syndrome, arthralgias, water retention) are very common. GH may have a role in the short-term treatment of some undernourished older patients, but in critically ill undernourished patients, GH increases mortality. Secretagogues that stimulate GH production in a more physiologic pattern may improve benefit and decrease risk.

Levels of melatonin, a hormone produced by the pineal gland, also decline with aging. This decline may play an important role in the loss of circadian rhythms with aging.

Estrogen replacement in older women is discussed on p. 2276. Testosterone replacement in older men is discussed on p. 2131.

161 Acid-Base Regulation and Disorders

Metabolic processes continually produce acid and, to a lesser degree, base. Hydrogen ion (H^+) is especially reactive; it can attach to negatively charged proteins and, in high concentrations, alter their overall charge, configuration, and function. To maintain cellular function, the body has elaborate mechanisms that maintain blood H^+ concentration within a narrow range—typically 37 to 43 nmol/L (pH 7.43 to 7.37, where pH = –log [H^+]) and ideally 40 nmol/L (pH = 7.40). Disturbances of these mechanisms can have serious clinical consequences.

Acid-base equilibrium is closely tied to fluid metabolism and electrolyte balance, and disturbances in one of these systems often affect another.

Acid-Base Physiology

Most acid comes from

- Carbohydrate and fat metabolism

Metabolism of carbohydrates and fats generates 15,000 to 20,000 mmol of carbon dioxide (CO_2) daily. CO_2 is not an acid itself, but in the presence of a member of the carbonic anhydrase family of enzymes, CO_2 combines with water (H_2O) in the blood to create carbonic acid (H_2CO_3), which dissociates into hydrogen ion (H^+) and bicarbonate (HCO_3^-). The H^+ binds with hemoglobin in RBCs and is released with oxygenation in the alveoli, at which time the reaction is reversed by another form of carbonic anhydrase, creating water (H_2O), which is excreted by the kidneys, and CO_2, which is exhaled in each breath.

Lesser amounts of organic acid derive from the following:

- Incomplete metabolism of glucose and fatty acids into lactic acid and ketoacids
- Metabolism of sulfur-containing amino acids (cysteine, methionine) into sulfuric acid
- Metabolism of cationic amino acids (arginine, lysine)
- Hydrolysis of dietary phosphate

This "fixed" or "metabolic" acid load cannot be exhaled and therefore must be neutralized or excreted by the kidneys.

Most base comes from metabolism of anionic amino acids (glutamate and aspartate) and from oxidation and consumption of organic anions such as lactate and citrate, which produce HCO_3^-.

Acid-Base Balance

Acid-base balance is maintained by chemical buffering and pulmonary and renal activity.

Chemical buffering: Chemical buffers are solutions that resist changes in pH. Intracellular and extracellular buffers provide an immediate response to acid-base disturbances. Bone also plays an important buffering role, especially of acid loads. A buffer is made up of a weak acid and its conjugate base. The conjugate base can accept H^+ and the weak acid can relinquish it, thereby minimizing changes in free H^+ concentration. A buffer system works best to minimize changes in pH near its equilibrium constant (pKa); so, although there are potentially many buffer pairs in the body, only some are physiologically relevant. The relationship between the pH of a buffer system and the concentration of its components is described by the Henderson-Hasselbalch equation:

$$pH = pKa + \log\left(\frac{[\text{anion}]}{[\text{weak acid}]}\right)$$

where pKa is the dissociation constant of the weak acid.

The most important extracellular buffer is the HCO_3^-/CO_2 system, described by the equation:

$$H^+ + HCO_3^- \Leftrightarrow H_2CO_3 \Leftrightarrow CO_2 + H_2O$$

An increase in H^+ drives the equation to the right and generates CO_2. This important buffer system is highly regulated; CO_2 concentrations can be finely controlled by alveolar ventilation, and H^+ and HCO_3^- concentrations can be finely regulated by renal excretion.

The relationship between pH, HCO_3^-, and CO_2 in the system as described by the Henderson-Hasselbalch equation is thus:

$$pH = 6.1 + \log\left(\frac{[HCO_3^-]}{[0.03 \times Pco_2]}\right)$$

Or similarly, by the Kassirer-Bleich equation, derived from the Henderson-Hasselbalch equation:

$$H^+ = 24 \times \frac{Pco_2}{HCO_3^-}$$

Note: to convert arterial pH to $[H^+]$ use:

$$pH = -\log[H^+]$$

or

$$[H^+] = 10\text{^}(-pH)$$

Both equations illustrate that acid-base balance depends on the ratio of Pco_2 and HCO_3^-, not on the absolute value of either one alone. With these formulas, any 2 variables can be used to calculate the third.

Other important physiologic buffers include intracellular organic and inorganic phosphates and proteins, including Hb in RBCs. Less important are extracellular phosphate and plasma proteins. Bone becomes an important buffer after consumption of an acid load. Bone initially releases sodium bicarbonate ($NaHCO_3$) and calcium bicarbonate ($Ca(HCO_3)_2$) in exchange for H^+. With prolonged acid loads, bone releases calcium carbonate ($CaCO_3$) and calcium phosphate ($CaPO_4$). Long-standing acidemia therefore contributes to bone demineralization and osteoporosis.

Pulmonary regulation: CO_2 concentration is finely regulated by changes in tidal volume and respiratory rate (minute ventilation). A decrease in pH is sensed by arterial chemoreceptors and leads to increases in tidal volume or respiratory rate; CO_2 is exhaled and blood pH increases. In contrast to chemical buffering, which is immediate, pulmonary regulation occurs over minutes to hours. It is about 50 to 75% effective and does not completely normalize pH.

Renal regulation: The kidneys control pH by adjusting the amount of HCO_3^- that is excreted or reabsorbed. Reabsorption of HCO_3^- is equivalent to excreting free H^+. Changes in renal acid-base handling occur hours to days after changes in acid-base status.

All of the HCO_3^- in serum is filtered as it passes through the glomerulus. HCO_3^- reabsorption occurs mostly in the proximal tubule and, to a lesser degree, in the collecting tubule. The H_2O within the distal tubular cell dissociates into H^+ and hydroxide (OH^-); in the presence of carbonic anhydrase, the OH^- combines with CO_2 to form HCO_3^-, which is transported back into the peritubular capillary, while the H^+ is secreted into the tubular lumen and joins with freely filtered HCO_3^- to form CO_2 and H_2O, which are also reabsorbed. Thus, the distally reabsorbed HCO_3^- ions are newly generated and not the same as those that were filtered. Decreases in effective circulating volume (such as occur with diuretic therapy) increase HCO_3^- reabsorption, while increases in parathyroid hormone in response to an acid load decrease HCO_3^- reabsorption. Also, increased Pco_2 leads to increased HCO_3^- reabsorption, while chloride (Cl^-) depletion (typically due to volume depletion) leads to increased sodium (Na^+) reabsorption and HCO_3^- generation by the proximal tubule.

Acid is actively excreted into the proximal and distal tubules where it combines with urinary buffers—primarily freely filtered phosphate (HPO_4^{-2}), creatinine, uric acid, and ammonia—to be transported outside the body. The ammonia buffering system is especially important because other buffers are filtered in fixed concentrations and can be depleted by high acid loads; by contrast, tubular cells actively regulate ammonia production in response to changes in acid load. Arterial pH is the main determinant of acid secretion, but excretion is also influenced by potassium (K^+), Cl^-, and aldosterone levels. Intracellular K^+ concentration and H^+ secretion are reciprocally related; K^+ depletion causes increased H^+ secretion and hence metabolic alkalosis.

ACID-BASE DISORDERS

Acid-base disorders are pathologic changes in arterial pH and CO_2 partial pressure (Pco_2), and in serum bicarbonate (HCO_3^-).

- Acidemia is serum pH < 7.35.
- Alkalemia is serum pH > 7.45.
- Acidosis refers to physiologic processes that cause acid accumulation or alkali loss.
- Alkalosis refers to physiologic processes that cause alkali accumulation or acid loss.

Actual changes in pH depend on the degree of physiologic compensation and whether multiple processes are present.

Classification

Primary acid-base disturbances are defined as metabolic or respiratory based on clinical context and whether the primary change in pH is due to an alteration in serum HCO_3^- or in P_{CO_2}.

Metabolic acidosis is serum $HCO_3^- < 24$ mEq/L. Causes are

- Increased acid production
- Acid ingestion
- Decreased renal acid excretion
- GI or renal HCO_3^- loss

Metabolic alkalosis is serum $HCO_3^- > 24$ mEq/L. Causes are

- Acid loss
- HCO_3^- retention

Respiratory acidosis is $P_{CO_2} > 40$ mm Hg (hypercapnia). Cause is

- Decrease in minute ventilation (hypoventilation)

Respiratory alkalosis is $P_{CO_2} < 40$ mm Hg (hypocapnia). Cause is

- Increase in minute ventilation (hyperventilation)

Whenever an acid-base disorder is present, compensatory mechanisms begin to correct the pH (see Table 161–1). Compensation cannot return pH completely to normal and never overshoots.

A **simple acid-base disorder** is a single acid-base disturbance with its accompanying compensatory response.

Mixed acid-base disorders comprise ≥ 2 primary disturbances.

PEARLS & PITFALLS

- Compensatory mechanisms for acid-base disturbances cannot return pH completely to normal and never overshoot.

Symptoms and Signs

Compensated or mild acid-base disorders cause few symptoms or signs. Severe, uncompensated disorders have multiple cardiovascular, respiratory, neurologic, and metabolic consequences (see Table 161–2 and Fig. 50–4 on p. 397).

Diagnosis

- ABG
- Serum electrolytes
- Anion gap calculated
- If metabolic acidosis is present, delta gap calculated and Winters formula applied
- Search for compensatory changes

Evaluation is with ABG and serum electrolytes. The ABG directly measures arterial pH and P_{CO_2}. HCO_3^- levels on ABG are calculated using the Henderson-Hasselbalch equation; HCO_3^- levels on serum chemistry panels are directly measured and are considered more accurate in cases of discrepancy. Acid-base balance is most accurately assessed with measurement of pH and P_{CO_2} on arterial blood. In cases of circulatory failure or during cardiopulmonary resuscitation, measurements on venous blood may more accurately reflect conditions at the tissue level and may be a more useful guide to bicarbonate administration and adequacy of ventilation.

The pH establishes the primary process (acidosis or alkalosis), although it moves toward the normal range with compensation. Changes in P_{CO_2} reflect the respiratory component, and changes in HCO_3^- reflect the metabolic component.

Complex or mixed acid-base disturbances involve more than one primary process. In these mixed disorders, values may be deceptively normal. Thus, it is important when evaluating acid-base disorders to determine whether changes in P_{CO_2} and HCO_3^- show the expected compensation (see Table 161–1). If not, then a second primary process causing the abnormal compensation should be suspected. Interpretation must also consider clinical conditions (eg, chronic lung disease, renal failure, drug overdose).

Table 161–1. PRIMARY CHANGES AND COMPENSATIONS IN SIMPLE ACID-BASE DISORDERS

PRIMARY DISTURBANCE	PH	BICARBONATE (HCO_3^-)	P_{CO_2}	EXPECTED COMPENSATION*
Metabolic acidosis	< 7.35	Primary decrease	Compensatory decrease	1.2 mm Hg decrease in P_{CO_2} for every 1 mmol/L decrease in HCO_3^- *or* $P_{CO_2} = (1.5 \cdot HCO_3^-) + 8\ (\pm 2)$ *or* $P_{CO_2} = HCO_3^- + 15$ *or* P_{CO_2} = last 2 digits of pH ·100
Metabolic alkalosis	> 7.45	Primary increase	Compensatory increase	0.6–0.75 mm Hg increase in P_{CO_2} for every 1 mmol/L increase in HCO_3^- (P_{CO_2} should not rise above 55 mm Hg in compensation)
Respiratory acidosis	< 7.35	Compensatory increase	Primary increase	**Acute:** 1–2 mmol/L increase in HCO_3^- for every 10 mm Hg increase in P_{CO_2} **Chronic:** 3–4 mmol/L increase in HCO_3^- for every 10 mm Hg increase in P_{CO_2}
Respiratory alkalosis	> 7.45	Compensatory decrease	Primary decrease	**Acute:** 1–2 mmol/L decrease in HCO_3^- for every 10 mm Hg decrease in P_{CO_2} **Chronic:** 4–5 mmol/L decrease in HCO_3^- for every 10 mm Hg decrease in P_{CO_2}

*Imprecise but convenient rules of thumb.

Table 161–2. CLINICAL CONSEQUENCES OF ACID-BASE DISORDERS

SYSTEM	ACIDEMIA	ALKALEMIA
Cardiovascular	Impaired cardiac contractility Arteriolar dilation Venoconstriction Centralization of blood volume Increased pulmonary vascular resistance Decreased cardiac output Decreased systemic BP Decreased hepatorenal blood flow Decreased threshold for cardiac arrhythmias Attenuation of responsiveness to catecholamines	Arteriolar constriction Reduced coronary blood flow Reduced anginal threshold Decreased threshold for cardiac arrhythmias
Metabolic	Insulin resistance Inhibition of anaerobic glycolysis Reduction in ATP synthesis Hyperkalemia Protein degradation Bone demineralization (chronic)	Stimulation of anaerobic glycolysis Formation of organic acids Decreased oxyhemoglobin dissociation Decreased ionized calcium Hypokalemia Hypomagnesemia Hypophosphatemia
Neurologic	Inhibition of metabolism and cell-volume regulation Obtundation and coma	Tetany Seizures Lethargy Delirium Stupor
Respiratory	Compensatory hyperventilation with possible respiratory muscle fatigue	Compensatory hypoventilation with hypercapnia and hypoxemia

The **anion gap** (see Sidebar 161–1) should always be calculated; elevation almost always indicates a metabolic acidosis. A normal anion gap with a low HCO_3^- (eg, < 24 mEq/L) and high serum chloride (Cl^-) indicates a non-anion gap (hyperchloremic) metabolic acidosis. If metabolic acidosis is present, a delta gap is calculated (see Sidebar 161–1) to identify concomitant metabolic alkalosis, and Winters formula is applied to determine whether respiratory compensation is appropriate or reflects a 2nd acid-base disorder (predicted $P_{CO_2} = 1.5\,[HCO_3^-] + 8 \pm 2$; if P_{CO_2} is higher, there is also a primary respiratory acidosis—if lower, respiratory alkalosis).

Respiratory acidosis is suggested by P_{CO_2} > 40 mm Hg; HCO_3^- should compensate acutely by increasing 3 to 4 mEq/L for each 10 mm Hg rise in P_{CO_2} sustained for 4 to 12 h (there may be no increase or only 1 to 2 mEq/L, which slowly increases to 3 to 4 mEq/L over days). Greater increase in HCO_3^- implies a primary metabolic alkalosis; lesser increase suggests no time for compensation or coexisting primary metabolic acidosis.

Metabolic alkalosis is suggested by $HCO_3^- > 28$ mEq/L. The P_{CO_2} should compensate by increasing about 0.6 to 0.75 mm Hg for each 1 mEq/L increase in HCO_3^- (up to about 55 mm Hg). Greater increase implies concomitant respiratory acidosis; lesser increase, respiratory alkalosis.

Respiratory alkalosis is suggested by P_{CO_2} < 38 mm Hg. The HCO_3^- should compensate over 4 to 12 h by decreasing 5 mEq/L for every 10 mm Hg decrease in P_{CO_2}. Lesser decrease means there has been no time for compensation or a primary metabolic alkalosis coexists. Greater decrease implies a primary metabolic acidosis.

Nomograms (acid-base maps) are an alternative way to diagnose mixed disorders, allowing for simultaneous plotting of pH, HCO_3^-, and P_{CO_2}.

KEY POINTS

- Acidosis and alkalosis refer to physiologic *processes* that cause accumulation or loss of acid and/or alkali; blood pH may or may not be abnormal.
- Acidemia and alkalemia refer to an abnormally acidic (pH < 7.35) or alkalotic (pH > 7.45) serum pH.
- Acid-base disorders are classified as *metabolic* if the change in pH is primarily due to an alteration in serum HCO_3^- and *respiratory* if the change is primarily due to a change in P_{CO_2} (increase or decrease in ventilation).
- The pH establishes the primary process (acidosis or alkalosis), changes in P_{CO_2} reflect the respiratory component, and changes in HCO_3^- reflect the metabolic component.
- All acid-base disturbances result in *compensation* that tends to normalize the pH. Metabolic acid-base disorders result in respiratory compensation (change in P_{CO_2}); respiratory acid-base disorders result in metabolic compensation (change in HCO_3^-).
- More than one primary acid-base disorder may be present simultaneously. It is important to identify and address each primary acid-base disorder.
- Initial laboratory evaluation of acid-base disorders includes ABG and serum electrolytes and calculation of the anion gap.
- Use one of several formulas, rules-of-thumb, or acid-base nomogram to determine if laboratory values are consistent with a single acid-base disorder (and compensation) or if a second primary acid-base disorder is also present.
- Treat each primary acid-base disorder.

Sidebar 161–1. The Anion Gap

The anion gap is defined as serum sodium (Na) concentration minus the sum of chloride (Cl^-) and bicarbonate (HCO_3^-) concentrations; $Na^+ - (Cl^- + HCO_3^-)$.

The term "gap" is misleading, because the law of electroneutrality requires the same number of positive and negative charges in an open system; the gap appears on laboratory testing because certain cations (+) and anions (–) are not measured on routine laboratory chemistry panels. Thus

$$Na^+ + \text{unmeasured cations (UC)} = Cl^- + HCO_3^- + \text{unmeasured anions (UA)}$$

and

$$\text{the anion gap, } Na^+ - (Cl^- + HCO_3^-) = UA - UC$$

The predominant "unmeasured" anions are phosphate (PO_4^{3-}), sulfate (SO_4^-), various negatively charged proteins, and some organic acids, accounting for 20 to 24 mEq/L. The predominant "unmeasured" extracellular cations are potassium (K^+), calcium (Ca^{++}), and magnesium (Mg^{++}) and account for about 11 mEq/L. Thus the typical anion gap is 23 − 11 = 12 mEq/L. The anion gap can be affected by increases or decreases in the UC or UA.

Increased anion gap is most commonly caused by metabolic acidosis in which negatively charged acids—mostly ketones, lactate, sulfates, or metabolites of methanol, ethylene glycol, or salicylate—consume (are buffered by) HCO_3^-. Other causes of increased anion gap include hyperalbuminemia and uremia (increased anions) and hypocalcemia or hypomagnesemia (decreased cations).

Decreased anion gap is unrelated to metabolic acidosis but is caused by hypoalbuminemia (decreased anions); hypercalcemia, hypermagnesemia, lithium intoxication, and hypergammaglobulinemia as occurs in myeloma (increased cations); or hyperviscosity or halide (bromide or iodide) intoxication. The effect of low albumin can be accounted for by adjusting the normal range for the anion gap 2.5 mEq/L downward for every 1-g/dL fall in albumin.

Negative anion gap occurs rarely as a laboratory artifact in severe cases of hypernatremia, hyperlipidemia, and bromide intoxication.

The delta gap: The difference between the patient's anion gap and the normal anion gap is termed the delta gap. This amount is considered an HCO_3^- equivalent, because for every unit rise in the anion gap, the HCO_3^- should lower by 1 (by buffering). Thus, if the delta gap is added to the measured HCO_3^-, the result should be in the normal range for HCO_3^-; elevation indicates the additional presence of a metabolic alkalosis.

Example: A vomiting, ill-appearing alcoholic patient has laboratory results showing

$$Na, 137; K, 3.8; Cl, 90; HCO_3^-, 22; \quad pH, 7.40; P_{CO_2}, 41; P_{O_2}, 85$$

At first glance, results appear unremarkable. However, calculations show elevation of the anion gap:

$$137 - (90 + 22) = 25 \text{ (normal, 10 to 12)}$$

indicating a metabolic acidosis. Respiratory compensation is evaluated by Winters formula:

$$\text{Predicted } P_{CO_2} = 1.5\,(22) + 8 \pm 2 = 41 \pm 2$$

Predicted = measured, so respiratory compensation is appropriate.

Because there is metabolic acidosis, the delta gap is calculated, and the result is added to measured HCO_3^-:

$$25 - 10 = 15$$
$$15 + 22 = 37$$

The resulting corrected HCO_3^- is above the normal range for HCO_3^-, indicating a primary metabolic alkalosis is also present. Thus, the patient has a mixed acid-base disorder. Using clinical information, one could theorize a metabolic acidosis arising from alcoholic ketoacidosis combined with a metabolic alkalosis from recurrent vomiting with loss of Cl^- and volume.

METABOLIC ACIDOSIS

Metabolic acidosis is primary reduction in bicarbonate (HCO_3^-), typically with compensatory reduction in CO_2 partial pressure (P_{CO_2}); pH may be markedly low or slightly subnormal. Metabolic acidoses are categorized as high or normal anion gap based on the presence or absence of unmeasured anions in serum. Causes include accumulation of ketones and lactic acid, renal failure, and drug or toxin ingestion (high anion gap) and GI or renal HCO_3^- loss (normal anion gap). Symptoms and signs in severe cases include nausea and vomiting, lethargy, and hyperpnea. Diagnosis is clinical and with ABG and serum electrolyte measurement. The cause is treated; IV sodium bicarbonate may be indicated when pH is very low.

Etiology

Metabolic acidosis is acid accumulation due to

- Increased acid production or acid ingestion
- Decreased acid excretion
- GI or renal HCO_3^- loss

Acidemia (arterial pH < 7.35) results when acid load overwhelms respiratory compensation. Causes are classified by their effect on the anion gap (see Sidebar 161–1 and Table 161–3).

High anion gap acidosis: The most common causes of a high anion gap metabolic acidosis are

- Ketoacidosis
- Lactic acidosis
- Renal failure
- Toxic ingestions

Ketoacidosis is a common complication of type 1 diabetes mellitus (see Diabetic Ketoacidosis on p. 1267), but it also occurs with chronic alcoholism (see alcoholic ketoacidosis), undernutrition, and, to a lesser degree, fasting. In these conditions, the body converts from glucose to free fatty acid (FFA) metabolism; FFAs are converted by the liver into ketoacids, acetoacetic acid, and beta-hydroxybutyrate (all unmeasured anions). Ketoacidosis is also a rare manifestation of congenital isovaleric and methylmalonic acidemia.

Lactic acidosis is the most common cause of metabolic acidosis in hospitalized patients. Lactate accumulation results from a combination of excess formation and decreased utilization of lactate. Excess lactate production occurs during states of anaerobic metabolism. The most serious form occurs

Table 161–3. CAUSES OF METABOLIC ACIDOSIS

CAUSE	EXAMPLES
High anion gap	
Ketoacidosis	Diabetes Chronic alcoholism Undernutrition Fasting
Lactic acidosis (due to physiologic processes)	Shock Primary hypoxia due to lung disorders Seizures Alcohol (chronic abuse)
Lactic acidosis (due to exogenous toxins)	Carbon monoxide Cyanide Iron Isoniazid Toluene (initially high gap; subsequent excretion of metabolites normalizes gap) HIV nucleoside reverse transcriptase inhibitors Biguanides (rare except with acute kidney injury) Propofol
D-Lactate generation	Bacterial overgrowth/short bowel syndrome
Renal failure	—
Toxins metabolized to acids	Methanol (formate) Ethylene glycol (oxalate) Paraldehyde (acetate, chloracetate) Salicylates
Rhabdomyolysis	—
Normal anion gap (hyperchloremic acidosis)	
GI bicarbonate (HCO_3^-) loss	Colostomy Diarrhea Enteric fistulas Ileostomy Use of ion-exchange resins Calcium chloride ($CaCl_2$) Magnesium sulfate ($MgSO_4$)
Urologic procedures	Ureterosigmoidostomy Ureteroileal conduit
Renal HCO_3^- loss	Tubulointerstitial renal disease Renal tubular acidosis, types 1, 2, and 4 Hyperparathyroidism Acetazolamide
Parenteral infusion	Arginine Lysine Ammonium chloride (NH_4Cl) Rapid sodium chloride (NaCl) infusion
Other	Hypoaldosteronism Hyperkalemia Toluene (late)

during the various types of shock. Decreased utilization generally occurs with hepatocellular dysfunction from decreased liver perfusion or as a part of generalized shock. Diseases and drugs that impair mitochondrial function can cause lactic acidosis.

Renal failure causes anion gap acidosis by decreased acid excretion and decreased HCO_3^- reabsorption. Accumulation of sulfates, phosphates, urate, and hippurate accounts for the high anion gap.

Toxins may have acidic metabolites or trigger lactic acidosis. Rhabdomyolysis is a rare cause of metabolic acidosis thought to be due to release of protons and anions directly from muscle.

Normal anion gap acidosis: The most common causes of normal anion gap acidosis are

- GI or renal HCO_3^- loss
- Impaired renal acid excretion

Normal anion gap metabolic acidosis is also called hyperchloremic acidosis because the kidneys reabsorb chloride (Cl^-) instead of reabsorbing HCO_3^-.

Many GI secretions are rich in HCO_3^- (eg, biliary, pancreatic, and intestinal fluids); loss due to diarrhea, tube drainage, or fistulas can cause acidosis. In ureterosigmoidostomy (insertion of ureters into the sigmoid colon after obstruction or cystectomy), the colon secretes and loses HCO_3^- in exchange for urinary Cl^- and absorbs urinary ammonium, which dissociates into ammonia (NH_3^+) and hydrogen ion (H^+). Ion-exchange resin uncommonly causes HCO_3^- loss by binding HCO_3^-.

The renal tubular acidoses either impair H^+ secretion (types 1 and 4) or HCO_3^- absorption (type 2). Impaired acid excretion and a normal anion gap also occur in early renal failure, tubulointerstitial renal disease, and when carbonic anhydrase inhibitors (eg, acetazolamide) are taken.

Symptoms and Signs

Symptoms and signs (see Table 161–2) are primarily those of the cause. Mild acidemia is itself asymptomatic. More severe acidemia (pH < 7.10) may cause nausea, vomiting, and malaise. Symptoms may appear at higher pH if acidosis develops rapidly.

The most characteristic sign is hyperpnea (long, deep breaths at a normal rate), reflecting a compensatory increase in alveolar ventilation; this hyperpnea is not accompanied by a feeling of dyspnea.

PEARLS & PITFALLS

- The hyperpnea triggered by metabolic acidosis does not cause a sensation of dyspnea.

Severe, acute acidemia predisposes to cardiac dysfunction with hypotension and shock, ventricular arrhythmias, and coma. Chronic acidemia causes bone demineralization disorders (eg, rickets, osteomalacia, osteopenia).

Diagnosis

- ABG and serum electrolytes
- Anion gap and delta gap calculated
- Winters formula for calculating compensatory changes
- Testing for cause

Recognition of metabolic acidosis and appropriate respiratory compensation are discussed on p. 1228. Determining the cause of metabolic acidosis begins with the anion gap.

The cause of an **elevated anion gap** may be clinically obvious (eg, hypovolemic shock, missed hemodialysis), but if not, blood testing should include glucose, BUN, creatinine, lactate, and tests for possible toxins. Salicylate levels can be measured in most laboratories, but methanol and ethylene glycol frequently cannot; their presence may be suggested by presence of an osmolar gap. Calculated serum osmolarity (2 [sodium] + [glucose]/18 + BUN/2.8 + blood alcohol/5) is subtracted from measured osmolarity. A difference > 10 implies the presence of an osmotically active substance, which in the case of a high anion gap acidosis is methanol or ethylene glycol. Although ingestion of ethanol may cause an osmolar gap and a mild acidosis, it should never be considered the cause of a significant metabolic acidosis.

If the **anion gap is normal** and no cause is obvious (eg, marked diarrhea), urinary electrolytes are measured and the urinary anion gap is calculated as [sodium] + [potassium] − [chloride]. A normal urinary anion gap (including in patients with GI losses) is 30 to 50 mEq/L; an elevation suggests renal HCO_3^- loss (for evaluation of renal tubular acidosis, see p. 2155).

In addition, when metabolic acidosis is present, a **delta gap** is calculated (see Sidebar 161–1) to identify concomitant metabolic alkalosis, and Winters formula (see p. 1228) is applied to see whether respiratory compensation is appropriate or reflects a 2nd acid-base disorder.

Treatment

- Cause treated
- Sodium bicarbonate ($NaHCO_3$) primarily for severe acidemia—give with caution

Treatment is directed at the underlying cause. Hemodialysis is required for renal failure and sometimes for ethylene glycol, methanol, and salicylate poisoning.

Treatment of acidemia with $NaHCO_3$ is clearly indicated only in certain circumstances and is probably deleterious in others. When metabolic acidosis results from loss of HCO_3^- or accumulation of inorganic acids (ie, normal anion gap acidosis), HCO_3^- therapy is generally safe and appropriate. However, when acidosis results from organic acid accumulation (ie, high anion gap acidosis), HCO_3^- therapy is controversial; it does not clearly decrease mortality in these conditions, and there are several possible risks.

With treatment of the underlying condition, lactate and ketoacids are metabolized back to HCO_3^-; exogenous HCO_3^- loading may therefore cause an "overshoot" metabolic alkalosis. In any condition, HCO_3^- may also cause sodium and volume overload, hypokalemia, and, by inhibiting respiratory drive, hypercapnia. Furthermore, because HCO_3^- does not diffuse across cell membranes, intracellular acidosis is not corrected and may paradoxically worsen because some of the added HCO_3^- is converted to CO_2, which does cross into the cell and is hydrolyzed to H^+ and HCO_3^-.

Despite these and other controversies, most experts still recommend HCO_3^- IV for severe metabolic acidosis (pH < 7.10).

Treatment requires 2 calculations. The first is the level to which HCO_3^- must be raised, calculated by the Kassirer-Bleich equation, using a value for [H^+] of 63 nmol/L, which corresponds to a pH of 7.20 (target for high anion gap acidosis is [H^+] of 79 nmol/L, pH < 7.10):

$$63 = 24 \times P_{CO_2}/HCO_3^-$$

or

$$\text{desired } HCO_3^- = 0.38 \times P_{CO_2}$$

The amount of HCO_3^- needed to achieve that level is

$$NaHCO_3 \text{ required (mEq)} = (\text{desired } [HCO_3^-] - \text{observed } [HCO_3^-]) \times 0.4 \times \text{body weight (kg)}$$

This amount of $NaHCO_3$ is given over several hours. Blood pH and HCO_3^- levels can be checked 30 min to 1 h after administration, which allows for equilibration with extravascular HCO_3^-.

Alternatives to $NaHCO_3$ include

- Tromethamine, an amino alcohol that buffers both metabolic (H^+) and respiratory (carbonic acid [H_2CO_3]) acid
- Carbicarb, an equimolar mixture of $NaHCO_3$ and carbonate (the latter consumes CO_2 and generates HCO_3^-)
- Dichloroacetate, which enhances oxidation of lactate

These alternatives are all of unproven benefit over $NaHCO_3$ alone and can cause complications of their own.

K^+ depletion, common in metabolic acidosis, should be identified through frequent serum K^+ monitoring and treated as needed with oral or parenteral potassium chloride.

KEY POINTS

- Metabolic acidosis can be caused by acid accumulation due to increased acid production or acid ingestion; decreased acid excretion; or GI or renal HCO_3^- loss.
- Metabolic acidoses are categorized based on whether the anion gap is high or normal.
- High anion gap acidoses are most often due to ketoacidosis, lactic acidosis, renal failure, or certain toxic ingestions.
- Normal anion gap acidoses are most often due to GI or renal HCO_3^- loss.
- Calculate delta gap to identify concomitant metabolic alkalosis, and apply Winters formula to see whether respiratory compensation is appropriate or reflects a 2nd acid-base disorder.
- Treat the underlying cause.
- $NaHCO_3$ is indicated when acidosis is due to a change in HCO_3^- (normal anion gap acidosis).
- Intravenous $NaHCO_3$ is controversial in high anion gap acidosis (but may be considered when pH < 7.00, with a target pH of ≤ 7.10).

Lactic Acidosis

Lactic acidosis is a high anion gap metabolic acidosis due to elevated blood lactate. Lactic acidosis results from overproduction of lactate, decreased metabolism of lactate, or both.

Lactate is a normal by-product of glucose and amino acid metabolism. There are 2 main types of lactic acidosis:

- Type A lactic acidosis
- Type B lactic acidosis

Type D-lactic acidosis is an unusual type.

Type A lactic acidosis: Type A lactic acidosis, the most serious form, occurs when lactic acid is overproduced in ischemic tissue to generate ATP during O_2 deficit. Overproduction typically occurs during tissue hypoperfusion in hypovolemic, cardiac, or septic shock and is worsened by decreased lactate metabolism in the poorly perfused liver. It may also occur with primary hypoxia due to lung disease and with various hemoglobinopathies.

Type B lactic acidosis: Type B lactic acidosis occurs in states of normal global tissue perfusion (and hence ATP production) and is less ominous. Lactate production may be increased from local relative hypoxia as with vigorous muscle use (eg, exertion, seizures, hypothermic shivering) and with cancer and ingestion of certain drugs or toxins (see Table 161–3). Drugs include the nucleoside reverse transcriptase inhibitors and the biguanides phenformin and, less so, metformin; although phenformin has been removed from the market in most of the world, it is still available from China (including as a component of some Chinese proprietary medicines). Metabolism may be decreased due to hepatic insufficiency or thiamin deficiency.

Type D-lactic acidosis: D-Lactic acidosis is an unusual form of lactic acidosis in which D-lactic acid, the product of bacterial carbohydrate metabolism in the colon of patients with jejunoileal bypass or intestinal resection, is systemically absorbed. It persists in circulation because human lactate dehydrogenase can metabolize only L-lactate.

Symptoms and Signs

Symptoms and signs are dominated by those of the underlying cause (eg, septic shock, toxin ingestion).

Diagnosis

- ABG and serum electrolytes
- Anion gap and delta gap calculated
- Blood lactate level

Findings in types A and B lactic acidosis are as for other metabolic acidoses. Diagnosis requires blood pH < 7.35 and lactate > 5 to 6 mmol/L. Less extreme lactate and pH changes are referred to as hyperlactatemia.

In D-lactic acidosis, the anion gap is lower than expected for the decrease in bicarbonate (HCO_3^-), and there may be a urinary osmolar gap (difference between calculated and measured urine osmolarity). Typical laboratory lactate assays are not sensitive to D-lactate. Specific D-lactate levels are available and sometimes needed to clarify the cause of acidosis in patients with multiple potential causes including bowel problems.

Treatment

- Treatment of cause

Treatment of types A and B lactic acidosis is similar to treatment of other metabolic acidoses. Treatment of the cause is paramount. Bicarbonate is potentially dangerous in high anion gap acidosis but may be considered when pH < 7.00, with a target pH of ≤ 7.10.

In D-lactic acidosis, treatment is IV fluids, restriction of carbohydrates, and sometimes oral antibiotics (eg, metronidazole).

METABOLIC ALKALOSIS

Metabolic alkalosis is primary increase in bicarbonate (HCO_3^-) with or without compensatory increase in CO_2 partial pressure (PCO_2); pH may be high or nearly normal. Common causes include prolonged vomiting, hypovolemia, diuretic use, and hypokalemia. Renal impairment of HCO_3^- excretion must be present to sustain alkalosis. Symptoms and signs in severe cases include headache, lethargy, and tetany. Diagnosis is clinical and with ABG and serum electrolyte measurement. The underlying condition is treated; oral or IV acetazolamide or hydrochloric acid is sometimes indicated.

Etiology

Metabolic alkalosis is bicarbonate HCO_3^- accumulation due to

- Acid loss
- Alkali administration
- Intracellular shift of hydrogen ion (H^+—as occurs in hypokalemia)
- HCO_3^- retention

Regardless of initial cause, persistence of metabolic alkalosis indicates that the kidneys have increased their HCO_3^- reabsorption, because HCO_3^- is normally freely filtered by the kidneys and hence excreted. Volume depletion and hypokalemia are the most common stimuli for increased HCO_3^- reabsorption, but any condition that elevates aldosterone or mineralocorticoids (which enhance sodium [Na] reabsorption and potassium [K] and H^+ excretion) can elevate HCO_3^-. Thus, hypokalemia is both a cause and a frequent consequence of metabolic alkalosis. Causes are listed; the most common are volume depletion (particularly when involving loss of gastric acid and chloride [Cl] due to recurrent vomiting or nasogastric suction) and diuretic use (see Table 161–4).

Metabolic alkalosis can be

- Chloride-responsive: Involves loss or excess secretion of Cl; it typically corrects with IV administration of NaCl-containing fluid.
- Chloride-unresponsive: Does not correct with NaCl-containing fluids, and typically involves severe magnesium and/or potassium deficiency or mineralocorticoid excess.

The 2 forms can coexist (eg, in patients with volume overload made hypokalemic by high-dose diuretics).

Symptoms and Signs

Symptoms and signs of mild alkalemia are usually related to the underlying disorder. More severe alkalemia increases protein binding of ionized calcium (Ca^{++}), leading to hypocalcemia and subsequent headache, lethargy, and neuromuscular excitability, sometimes with delirium, tetany, and seizures. Alkalemia also lowers threshold for anginal symptoms and arrhythmias. Concomitant hypokalemia may cause weakness.

Diagnosis

- ABG and serum electrolytes
- Diagnosis of cause usually clinical
- Sometimes measurement of urinary Cl^- and K^+

Recognition of metabolic alkalosis and appropriate respiratory compensation is discussed on p. 1228 and requires ABG and measurement of serum electrolytes (including Ca and Mg).

Common causes can often be determined by history and physical examination. If history is unrevealing and renal function is normal, urinary Cl^- and K^+ concentrations are measured (values are not diagnostic in renal insufficiency). Urinary Cl < 20 mEq/L indicates significant renal Cl^- reabsorption and hence a Cl-responsive cause (see Table 161–4). Urinary Cl > 20 mEq/L suggests a Cl-unresponsive form.

Urinary K and presence or absence of hypertension help differentiate Cl-unresponsive alkaloses. Urinary K < 30 mEq/day signifies hypokalemia or laxative misuse. Urinary K > 30 mEq/day without hypertension suggests diuretic abuse or Bartter or Gitelman syndrome. Urinary K > 30 mEq/day with hypertension requires evaluation for hyperaldosteronism, mineralocorticoid excess, and renovascular disease. Tests typically include plasma renin activity and aldosterone and cortisol levels (see pp. 1240 and 1243).

Treatment

- Cause treated
- IV 0.9% saline solution for Cl-responsive metabolic alkalosis

Underlying conditions are treated, with particular attention paid to correction of hypovolemia and hypokalemia.

Patients with Cl-responsive metabolic alkalosis are given 0.9% saline solution IV; infusion rate is typically 50 to 100 mL/h

Table 161–4. CAUSES OF METABOLIC ALKALOSIS

CAUSE	COMMENTS
GI acid loss*	
Gastric acid loss due to vomiting or nasogastric suction	Loss of HCl and acid coupled with contraction alkalosis due to release of aldosterone and subsequent resorption of HCO_3
Congenital chloridorrhea	Fecal Cl loss and HCO_3 retention
Villous adenoma	Probably secondary to K depletion
Renal acid loss	
Primary hyperaldosteronism†	Includes congenital adrenal hyperplasia
Secondary hyperaldosteronism†	Occurs with volume depletion, heart failure, cirrhosis with ascites, nephrotic syndrome, Cushing syndrome or disease, renal artery stenosis, or renin-secreting tumor
Use of glycyrrhizin-containing compounds† (eg, licorice, chewing tobacco, carbenoxolone, Lydia Pinkham's vegetable compound)	Glycyrrhizin inhibition of enzymatic conversion of cortisol to less active metabolites
Bartter syndrome†	Rare congenital disease causing hyperaldosteronism and hypokalemic metabolic alkalosis that manifests in early childhood with renal salt wasting and volume depletion
Gitelman syndrome†	Similar to Bartter syndrome Characterized in addition by hypomagnesemia and hypocalciuria Manifests in young adults
Diuretics (thiazide and loop)‡	Multiple mechanisms: Secondary hyperaldosteronism due to volume depletion, Cl depletion, or contraction alkalosis; may be Cl-unresponsive because of concomitant K depletion
Hypokalemia and hypomagnesemia†	Stimulate K and Mg reabsorption and H excretion; alkalosis unresponsive to NaCl and volume replacement until deficiencies corrected; low K causing H to shift into cells, raising extracellular pH
HCO_3 excess	
Posthypercapnic*	Persistent elevation of compensatory HCO_3 levels, often with volume, K, and Cl depletion
Postorganic acidosis	Conversion of lactic acid or ketoacid to HCO_3 worsened by HCO_3 therapy for acidosis
$NaHCO_3$ loading	Occurs with overzealous loading or with loading in patients who have hypokalemia; serum becomes more alkalotic as H shifts back into cells
Milk-alkali syndrome	Chronic ingestion of calcium carbonate antacids provides Ca and HCO_3 load; hypercalcemia lowers PTH, increasing HCO_3 reabsorption
Contraction alkalosis*	
Diuretics (all types) Sweat loss in cystic fibrosis	NaCl loss concentrates a fixed amount of HCO_3 in a smaller total body volume
Other	
Carbohydrate refeeding after starvation	Resolution of starvation ketosis or acidosis with improved cellular function
Laxative abuse*	Unclear mechanism
Some antibiotics (eg, carbenicillin, penicillin, ticarcillin)	Contain nonreabsorbable anion, which increases K and H excretion

*Chloride-responsive.
†Chloride-unresponsive.
‡May be either chloride-responsive or chloride-unresponsive.
Ca = calcium; Cl = chloride; H = hydrogen; HCl = hydrochloric acid; HCO_3 = bicarbonate; K = potassium; Mg = magnesium; NaCl = sodium chloride; $NaHCO_3$ = sodium bicarbonate.

greater than urinary and other sensible and insensible fluid losses until urinary Cl rises to > 25 mEq/L and urinary pH normalizes after an initial rise from bicarbonaturia. Patients with Cl-unresponsive metabolic alkalosis rarely benefit from rehydration alone.

Patients with severe metabolic alkalosis (eg, pH > 7.6) sometimes require more urgent correction of blood pH. Hemofiltration or hemodialysis is an option, particularly if volume overload and renal dysfunction are present. Acetazolamide 250 to 375 mg po or IV once/day or bid increases HCO_3^- excretion but may also accelerate urinary losses of K^+ and phosphate (PO_4^-); volume-overloaded patients with diuretic-induced metabolic alkalosis and those with posthypercapnic metabolic alkalosis may especially benefit.

In patients with severe metabolic alkalosis (pH > 7.6) and kidney failure who otherwise cannot or should not undergo dialysis, hydrochloric acid in a 0.1 to 0.2 normal solution IV is safe and effective but must be given through a central catheter because it is hyperosmotic and scleroses peripheral veins. Dosage is 0.1 to 0.2 mmol/kg/h. Frequent monitoring of ABG and electrolytes is needed.

KEY POINTS

- Metabolic alkalosis is HCO_3^- accumulation due to acid loss, alkali administration, intracellular shift of hydrogen ion, or HCO_3^- retention.
- The most common causes are volume depletion (particularly when involving loss of gastric acid and Cl from recurrent vomiting or nasogastric suction) and diuretic use.
- Metabolic alkalosis involving loss or excess secretion of Cl is termed Cl-responsive.
- Treat the cause and give patients with Cl-responsive metabolic alkalosis 0.9% saline IV.
- Cl-resistant metabolic alkalosis is due to increased aldosterone effect.
- Treatment of Cl-resistant metabolic alkalosis involves correction of hyperaldosteronism.

RESPIRATORY ACIDOSIS

Respiratory acidosis is primary increase in CO_2 partial pressure (Pco_2) with or without compensatory increase in bicarbonate (HCO_3^-); pH is usually low but may be near normal. Cause is a decrease in respiratory rate and/or volume (hypoventilation), typically due to CNS, pulmonary, or iatrogenic conditions. Respiratory acidosis can be acute or chronic; the chronic form is asymptomatic, but the acute, or worsening, form causes headache, confusion, and drowsiness. Signs include tremor, myoclonic jerks, and asterixis. Diagnosis is clinical and with ABG and serum electrolyte measurements. The cause is treated; oxygen (O_2) and mechanical ventilation are often required.

Respiratory acidosis is CO_2 accumulation (hypercapnia) due to a decrease in respiratory rate and/or respiratory volume (hypoventilation). Causes of hypoventilation (discussed under Ventilatory Failure on p. 566) include

- Conditions that impair CNS respiratory drive
- Conditions that impair neuromuscular transmission and other conditions that cause muscular weakness
- Obstructive, restrictive, and parenchymal pulmonary disorders

Hypoxia typically accompanies hypoventilation.

Respiratory acidosis may be acute or chronic. Distinction is based on the degree of metabolic compensation; CO_2 is initially buffered inefficiently, but over 3 to 5 days the kidneys increase HCO_3^- reabsorption significantly.

Symptoms and Signs

Symptoms and signs depend on the rate and degree of Pco_2 increase. CO_2 rapidly diffuses across the blood-brain barrier. Symptoms and signs are a result of high CO_2 concentrations (low CNS pH) in the CNS and any accompanying hypoxemia.

Acute (or acutely worsening chronic) respiratory acidosis causes headache, confusion, anxiety, drowsiness, and stupor (CO_2 narcosis). Slowly developing, stable respiratory acidosis (as in COPD) may be well tolerated, but patients may have memory loss, sleep disturbances, excessive daytime sleepiness, and personality changes. Signs include gait disturbance, tremor, blunted deep tendon reflexes, myoclonic jerks, asterixis, and papilledema.

Diagnosis

- ABG and serum electrolytes
- Diagnosis of cause usually clinical

Recognition of respiratory acidosis and appropriate renal compensation (see p. 1228) requires ABG and measurement of serum electrolytes. Causes are usually obvious from history and examination. Calculation of the alveolar-arterial (A-a) O_2 gradient (inspired Po_2 − [arterial Po_2 + $5/4$ arterial Pco_2]) can help distinguish pulmonary from extrapulmonary disease; a normal gradient essentially excludes pulmonary disorders.

Treatment

- Adequate ventilation
- $NaHCO_3$ almost always contraindicated

Treatment is provision of adequate ventilation by either endotracheal intubation or noninvasive positive pressure ventilation (for specific indications and procedures, see p. 559). Adequate ventilation is all that is needed to correct respiratory acidosis, although chronic hypercapnia generally must be corrected slowly (eg, over several hours or more), because too-rapid Pco_2 lowering can cause a posthypercapnic "overshoot" alkalosis when the underlying compensatory hyperbicarbonatemia becomes unmasked; the abrupt rise in CNS pH that results can lead to seizures and death. Any potassium and chloride deficits are corrected.

$NaHCO_3$ is almost always contraindicated, because of the potential for paradoxical acidosis within the CNS. One exception may be in cases of severe bronchospasm, in which HCO_3^- may improve responsiveness of bronchial smooth muscle to beta-agonists.

KEY POINTS

- Respiratory acidosis involves a decrease in respiratory rate and/or volume (hypoventilation).
- Common causes include impaired respiratory drive (eg, due to toxins, CNS disease), and airflow obstruction (eg, due to asthma, COPD, sleep apnea, airway edema).
- Recognize chronic hypoventilation by the presence of metabolic compensation (elevated HCO_3^-) and clinical signs of tolerance (less somnolence and confusion than expected for the degree of hypercarbia).
- Treat the cause and provide adequate ventilation, using tracheal intubation or noninvasive positive pressure ventilation as needed.

RESPIRATORY ALKALOSIS

Respiratory alkalosis is a primary decrease in Pco_2 with or without compensatory decrease in bicarbonate (HCO_3^-); pH may be high or near normal. Cause is an increase in respiratory rate or volume (hyperventilation) or both. Respiratory alkalosis can be acute or chronic. The chronic form is

asymptomatic, but the acute form causes light-headedness, confusion, paresthesias, cramps, and syncope. Signs include hyperpnea or tachypnea and carpopedal spasms. Diagnosis is clinical and with ABG and serum electrolyte measurements. Treatment is directed at the cause.

Etiology

Respiratory alkalosis is a primary decrease in Pco_2 (hypocapnia) due to an increase in respiratory rate and/or volume (hyperventilation). Ventilation increase occurs most often as a physiologic response to hypoxia (eg, at high altitude), metabolic acidosis, and increased metabolic demands (eg, fever) and, as such, is present in many serious conditions. In addition, pain and anxiety and some CNS disorders can increase respirations without a physiologic need.

Pathophysiology

Respiratory alkalosis can be

- Acute
- Chronic

Distinction is based on the degree of metabolic compensation. Excess HCO_3^- is buffered by extracellular hydrogen ion (H^+) within minutes, but more significant compensation occurs over 2 to 3 days as the kidneys decrease H^+ excretion.

Pseudorespiratory alkalosis: Pseudorespiratory alkalosis is low arterial Pco_2 and high pH in mechanically ventilated patients with severe metabolic acidosis due to poor systemic perfusion (eg, cardiogenic shock, during CPR). Pseudorespiratory alkalosis occurs when mechanical ventilation (often hyperventilation) eliminates larger-than-normal amounts of alveolar CO_2. Exhalation of large amounts of CO_2 causes respiratory alkalosis in arterial blood (hence on ABG measurements), but poor systemic perfusion and cellular ischemia cause cellular acidosis, leading to acidosis of venous blood. Diagnosis is by demonstration of marked differences in arterial and venous Pco_2 and pH and by elevated lactate levels in patients whose ABG shows respiratory alkalosis; treatment is improvement of systemic hemodynamics.

Symptoms and Signs

Symptoms and signs depend on the rate and degree of fall in Pco_2. Acute respiratory alkalosis causes light-headedness, confusion, peripheral and circumoral paresthesias, cramps, and syncope. Mechanism is thought to be change in cerebral blood flow and pH. Tachypnea or hyperpnea is often the only sign; carpopedal spasm may occur in severe cases due to decreased levels of ionized calcium in the blood (driven inside cells in exchange for hydrogen ion [H^+]).

Chronic respiratory alkalosis is usually asymptomatic and has no distinctive signs.

Diagnosis

- ABG and serum electrolytes
- If hypoxia present, cause vigorously pursued

Recognition of respiratory alkalosis and appropriate renal compensation (see p. 1228) requires ABG and serum electrolyte measurements. Minor hypophosphatemia and hypokalemia due to intracellular shifts and decreased ionized calcium (Ca^{++}) due to an increase in protein binding may be present.

Presence of hypoxia or an increased alveolar-arterial (A-a) O_2 gradient (inspired Po_2 – [arterial Po_2 + $^5/_4$ arterial Pco_2]) requires search for a cause. Other causes are often apparent on history and examination. However, because pulmonary embolism often manifests without hypoxia, embolism must be strongly considered in a hyperventilating patient before ascribing the cause to anxiety.

Treatment

- Treatment of underlying disorder

Treatment is directed at the underlying disorder. Respiratory alkalosis is not life threatening, so no interventions to lower pH are necessary. Increasing inspired CO_2 through rebreathing (such as from a paper bag) is common practice but may be dangerous in at least some patients with CNS disorders in whom CSF pH may already be below normal.

KEY POINTS

- Respiratory alkalosis involves an increase in respiratory rate and/or volume (hyperventilation).
- Hyperventilation occurs most often as a response to hypoxia, metabolic acidosis, increased metabolic demands (eg, fever), pain, or anxiety.
- Do not presume anxiety is the cause of hyperventilation until more serious disorders are excluded.
- Treat the cause; respiratory alkalosis is not life threatening, so interventions to lower pH are unnecessary.

162 Adrenal Disorders

The adrenal glands, located on the cephalad portion of each kidney (see Fig. 162–1), consist of a

- Cortex
- Medulla

The adrenal cortex and adrenal medulla each have separate endocrine functions.

Adrenal cortex: The adrenal cortex produces

- Glucocorticoids (primarily cortisol)
- Mineralocorticoids (primarily aldosterone)
- Androgens (primarily dehydroepiandrosterone and androstenedione)

Glucocorticoids promote and inhibit gene transcription in many cells and organ systems. Prominent effects include anti-inflammatory actions and increased hepatic gluconeogenesis.

Mineralocorticoids regulate electrolyte transport across epithelial surfaces, particularly renal conservation of sodium in exchange for K.

Adrenal androgens' chief physiologic activity occurs after conversion to testosteroneand dihydrotestosterone.

The physiology of the hypothalamic-pituitary-adrenocortical system is further discussed elsewhere.

Adrenal medulla: The adrenal medulla is composed of chromaffin cells, which synthesize and secrete catecholamines (mainly epinephrine and lesser amounts of norepinephrine). Chromaffin cells also produce bioactive amines and peptides (eg, histamine, serotonin, chromogranins, neuropeptide hormones). Epinephrine and norepinephrine, the major effector

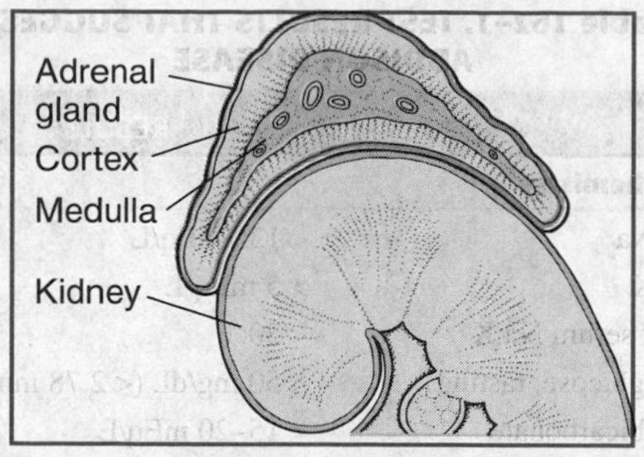

Fig. 162–1. Adrenal glands.

amines of the sympathetic nervous system, are responsible for the "flight or fight" response (ie, chronotropic and inotropic effects on the heart; bronchodilation; peripheral and splanchnic vasoconstriction with skeletal muscular vasodilation; metabolic effects including glycogenolysis, lipolysis, and renin release).

Clinical syndromes: Most **adrenal deficiency syndromes** affect output of all adrenocortical hormones. Hypofunction may be primary (malfunction of the adrenal gland itself, as in Addison disease) or secondary (due to lack of adrenal stimulation by the pituitary or hypothalamus, although some experts refer to hypothalamic malfunction as tertiary).

Adrenal hyperfunction causes distinct clinical syndromes depending on the hormone involved:

- Hypersecretion of androgens results in adrenal virilism.
- Hypersecretion of glucocorticoids results in Cushing syndrome.
- Hypersecretion of aldosterone results in hyperaldosteronism.
- Hypersecretion of epinephrine and norepinephrine results in pheochromocytoma.

These syndromes frequently have overlapping features.

Hyperfunction may be compensatory, as in congenital adrenal hyperplasia (CAH), or due to acquired hyperplasia, adenomas, or adenocarcinomas.

ADDISON DISEASE

(Primary or Chronic Adrenocortical Insufficiency)

Addison disease is an insidious, usually progressive hypofunctioning of the adrenal cortex. It causes various symptoms, including hypotension and hyperpigmentation, and can lead to adrenal crisis with cardiovascular collapse. Diagnosis is clinical and by finding elevated plasma adrenocorticotropic hormone (ACTH) with low plasma cortisol. Treatment depends on the cause but generally includes hydrocortisone and sometimes other hormones.

Addison disease develops in about 4/100,000 annually. It occurs in all age groups, about equally in each sex, and tends to become clinically apparent during metabolic stress or trauma.

Onset of severe symptoms (adrenal crisis) may be precipitated by acute infection (a common cause, especially with septicemia). Other causes include trauma, surgery, and Na loss due to excessive sweating. Even with treatment, Addison disease may cause a slight increase in mortality. It is not clear whether this increase is due to mistreated adrenal crises or long-term complications of inadvertent over-replacement.

Etiology

About 70% of cases in the US are due to idiopathic atrophy of the adrenal cortex, probably caused by autoimmune processes. The remainder result from destruction of the adrenal gland by granuloma (eg, TB, histoplasmosis), tumor, amyloidosis, hemorrhage, or inflammatory necrosis. Hypoadrenocorticism can also result from administration of drugs that block corticosteroid synthesis (eg, ketoconazole, the anesthetic etomidate).

Addison disease may coexist with diabetes mellitus or hypothyroidism in polyglandular deficiency syndrome. In children, the most common cause of primary adrenal insufficiency is CAH, but other genetic disorders are being increasingly recognized as causes.

Pathophysiology

Both mineralocorticoids and glucocorticoids are deficient.

Mineralocorticoid deficiency: Because mineralocorticoids stimulate Na reabsorption and K excretion, deficiency results in increased excretion of Na and decreased excretion of K, chiefly in urine but also in sweat, saliva, and the GI tract. A low serum concentration of Na and a high concentration of K result.

Urinary salt and water loss cause severe dehydration, plasma hypertonicity, acidosis, decreased circulatory volume, hypotension, and, eventually, circulatory collapse. However, when adrenal insufficiency is caused by inadequate ACTH production (secondary adrenal insufficiency), electrolyte levels are often normal or only mildly deranged, and the circulatory problems are less severe.

Glucocorticoid deficiency: Glucocorticoid deficiency contributes to hypotension and causes severe insulin sensitivity and disturbances in carbohydrate, fat, and protein metabolism. In the absence of cortisol, insufficient carbohydrate is formed from protein; hypoglycemia and decreased liver glycogen result. Weakness follows, due in part to deficient neuromuscular function. Resistance to infection, trauma, and other stress is decreased. Myocardial weakness and dehydration reduce cardiac output, and circulatory failure can occur.

Decreased blood cortisol results in increased pituitary ACTH production and increased blood beta-lipotropin, which has melanocyte-stimulating activity and, together with ACTH, causes the hyperpigmentation of skin and mucous membranes characteristic of Addison disease. Thus, adrenal insufficiency secondary to pituitary failure does not cause hyperpigmentation.

Symptoms and Signs

Weakness, fatigue, and orthostatic hypotension are early symptoms and signs of Addison disease.

Hyperpigmentation is characterized by diffuse tanning of exposed and, to a lesser extent, unexposed portions of the body, especially on pressure points (bony prominences), skin folds, scars, and extensor surfaces. Black freckles are common on the forehead, face, neck, and shoulders. Bluish black discolorations of the areolae and mucous membranes of the lips, mouth, rectum, and vagina occur.

Anorexia, nausea, vomiting, and diarrhea often occur. Decreased tolerance to cold, with hypometabolism, may be noted. Dizziness and syncope may occur.

The gradual onset and nonspecific nature of early symptoms often lead to an incorrect initial diagnosis of neurosis. Weight loss, dehydration, and hypotension are characteristic of the later stages of Addison disease.

Adrenal crisis: Adrenal crisis is characterized by

- Profound asthenia
- Severe pain in the abdomen, lower back, or legs
- Peripheral vascular collapse
- Renal shutdown with azotemia

Body temperature may be low, although severe fever often occurs, particularly when crisis is precipitated by acute infection.

A significant number of patients with partial loss of adrenal function (limited adrenocortical reserve) appear well but experience adrenal crisis when under physiologic stress (eg, surgery, infection, burns, critical illness). Shock and fever may be the only signs.

Diagnosis

- Electrolytes
- Serum cortisol
- Serum ACTH
- Sometimes ACTH stimulation testing

Clinical symptoms and signs suggest adrenal insufficiency. Sometimes the diagnosis is considered only on discovery of characteristic abnormalities of serum electrolytes, including low Na (< 135 mEq/L), high K (> 5 mEq/L), low bicarbonate (15 to 20 mEq/L), and high BUN (see Table 162–1).

Differential diagnosis: Hyperpigmentation can result from bronchogenic carcinoma, ingestion of heavy metals (eg, iron, silver), chronic skin conditions, or hemochromatosis. Peutz-Jeghers syndrome is characterized by pigmentation of the buccal and rectal mucosa. Frequently, hyperpigmentation occurs with vitiligo, which may indicate Addison disease, although other diseases can cause this association.

Weakness resulting from Addison disease subsides with rest, unlike neuropsychiatric weakness, which is often worse in the morning than after activity. Most myopathies that cause weakness can be differentiated by their distribution, lack of abnormal pigmentation, and characteristic laboratory findings.

Patients with adrenal insufficiency develop **hypoglycemia** after fasting because of decreased gluconeogenesis. In contrast, patients with hypoglycemia due to oversecretion of insulin can have attacks at any time, usually have increased appetite with weight gain, and have normal adrenal function.

Low serum sodium due to Addison disease must be differentiated from that of edematous patients with cardiac or liver disease (particularly those taking diuretics), the dilutional hyponatremia of the syndrome of inappropriate ADH secretion, and salt-losing nephritis. These patients are not likely to have hyperpigmentation, hyperkalemia, and increased BUN.

Testing: Laboratory tests, beginning with morning serum cortisol and ACTH levels, confirm adrenal insufficiency (see Table 162–2). Elevated ACTH (≥ 50 pg/mL) with low cortisol (< 5 μg/dL [< 138 nmol/L]) is diagnostic, particularly in patients who are severely stressed or in shock. Low ACTH (< 5 pg/mL) and cortisol suggest secondary adrenal insufficiency. It is important to note that ACTH levels within the normal range are inappropriate when cortisol levels are very low.

If ACTH and cortisol levels are borderline and adrenal insufficiency is clinically suspected—particularly in a patient who is about to undergo major surgery—provocative testing must be done. If time is too short (eg, emergency surgery), the patient is given hydrocortisone empirically (eg, 100 mg IV or IM), and provocative testing is done subsequently.

Provocative testing: Addison disease is diagnosed by showing failure of exogenous ACTH to increase serum cortisol. Secondary adrenal insufficiency is diagnosed by a prolonged ACTH stimulation test, insulin tolerance test, or glucagon test.

Table 162–1. TEST RESULTS THAT SUGGEST ADDISON DISEASE

TEST	RESULT
Blood chemistry	
Serum Na	< 135 mEq/L
Serum K	> 5 mEq/L
Ratio of serum Na:K	< 30:1
Plasma glucose, fasting	< 50 mg/dL (< 2.78 mmol/L)
Plasma bicarbonate	< 15–20 mEq/L
BUN	> 20 mg/dL (> 7.1 mmol/L)
Hematology	
Hct	Elevated
WBC count	Low
Lymphocytes	Relative lymphocytosis
Eosinophils	Increased
Imaging	
X-ray or CT	Evidence of • Calcification in adrenal area • Renal TB • Pulmonary TB

ACTH stimulation testing is done by injecting cosyntropin (synthetic ACTH) 250 mcg IV or IM followed by measurement of serum cortisol levels. Some authorities believe that in patients with suspected secondary adrenal insufficiency, a low-dose ACTH stimulation test using 1 mcg IV instead of the standard 250 mcg-dose should be done because such patients may react normally to the higher dose. Patients taking glucocorticoid supplements or spironolactone should not take them on the day of the test.

Normal preinjection serum cortisol levels vary somewhat depending on the laboratory assay in use but typically range from 5 to 25 μg/dL (138 to 690 nmol/L) and double in 30 to 90 min, reaching at least 20 μg/dL (552 nmol/L). Patients with Addison disease have low or low-normal preinjection values that do not rise above a peak value of 15 to 18 μg/dL at 30 min. However, the

Table 162–2. CONFIRMATORY SERUM TESTING FOR ADDISON DISEASE

TEST	RESULT
Serum ACTH	High (≥ 50 pg/mL)
Serum cortisol	Low (< 5 μg/dL [< 138 nmol/L])
ACTH stimulation test	Subnormal (ie, peak cortisol should be < 15-18 μg/dL, according to the assay)
Prolonged (24-h) ACTH stimulation test	Cortisol should be subnormal at 1 h and should not rise further at 24 h

ACTH = adrenocorticotropic hormone.

precise normal values depend on the specific cortisol assay used, and the normal range should be verified for each laboratory.

A normal response to cosyntropin may occur in secondary adrenal insufficiency. However, because pituitary failure may cause adrenal atrophy (and hence failure to respond to ACTH), the patient may need to be primed with long-acting ACTH 1 mg IM once/day for 3 days before the ACTH stimulation test if pituitary disease is suspected.

A **prolonged ACTH stimulation test** (sampling for 24 h) may be used to diagnose secondary (or tertiary, ie, hypothalamic) adrenal insufficiency. Cosyntropin 1 mg IM is given, and cortisol is measured at intervals for 24 h, typically at 1, 6, 12, and 24 h. Results for the first hour are similar for both the short (sampling stopped after 1 h) and prolonged tests, but in Addison disease there is no further rise beyond 60 min. In secondary and tertiary adrenal insufficiency, cortisol levels continue to rise for ≥ 24 h. Only in cases of prolonged adrenal atrophy is adrenal priming (with long-acting ACTH) necessary. The simple, short test is usually done initially, because a normal response obviates the need for further investigation.

If adrenal crisis is suspected, confirmation of Addison disease by ACTH stimulation testing is deferred until the patient has recovered. If ACTH stimulation testing is done, elevated ACTH levels together with low cortisol levels confirm the diagnosis.

Testing for etiology: In Western societies, the cause is usually assumed to be autoimmune, unless there is evidence otherwise. Adrenal autoantibodies can be assessed. A chest x-ray should be done for TB; if doubt exists, CT of the adrenals is helpful. In patients with autoimmune disease, the adrenals are atrophied, whereas in patients with TB or other granulomas, the adrenals are enlarged (initially) with frequent calcification. Bilateral adrenal hyperplasia, particularly in children and young adults, suggests a genetic enzyme defect.

Treatment

- Hydrocortisone or prednisone
- Fludrocortisone
- Dose increase during intercurrent illness

Normally, cortisol is secreted maximally in the early morning and minimally at night. Thus, hydrocortisone (identical to cortisol) is given in 2 or 3 divided doses with a typical total daily dose of 15 to 30 mg. One regimen gives half the total in the morning, and the remaining half split between lunchtime and early evening (eg, 10 mg, 5 mg, 5 mg). Others give two-thirds in the morning and one-third in the evening. Doses immediately before bed should generally be avoided because they may cause insomnia. Alternatively, prednisone 5 mg po in the morning and possibly an additional 2.5 mg po in the evening may be used. Additionally, fludrocortisone 0.1 to 0.2 mg po once/day is recommended to replace aldosterone. The easiest way to adjust the dosage is to ensure that the renin level is within the normal range.

Normal hydration and absence of orthostatic hypotension are evidence of adequate replacement therapy. In some patients, fludrocortisone causes hypertension, which is treated by reducing the dosage or starting a nondiuretic antihypertensive. Some clinicians tend to give too little fludrocortisone in an effort to avoid use of antihypertensives.

Intercurrent illnesses (eg, infections) are potentially serious and should be vigorously treated; the patient's hydrocortisone dose should be doubled during the illness. If nausea and vomiting preclude oral therapy, parenteral therapy is necessary. Patients should be instructed when to take supplemental prednisone or hydrocortisone and taught to self-administer parenteral hydrocortisone for urgent situations. A preloaded syringe with 100 mg hydrocortisone should be available to the patient. A bracelet or wallet card giving the diagnosis and corticosteroid dose may help in case of adrenal crisis that renders the patient unable to communicate.

When salt loss is severe, as in very hot climates, the dose of fludrocortisone may need to be increased.

In coexisting diabetes mellitus and Addison disease, the hydrocortisone dose usually should not be > 30 mg/day; otherwise, insulin requirements are increased.

Treatment of adrenal crisis: Therapy should be instituted immediately upon suspicion. (CAUTION: *In adrenal crisis, a delay in instituting corticosteroid therapy, particularly if there is hypoglycemia and hypotension, may be fatal.*) If the patient is acutely ill, confirmation by an ACTH stimulation test should be postponed until the patient has recovered.

Hydrocortisone 100 mg is injected IV over 30 sec and repeated q 6 to 8 h for the first 24 h. Immediate intravascular volume expansion is done by giving 1 L of a 5% dextrose in 0.9% saline solution over 1 to 2 h. Additional 0.9% saline is given IV until hypotension, dehydration, and hyponatremia have been corrected. Serum K may fall during rehydration, requiring replacement. Mineralocorticoids are not required when high-dose hydrocortisone is given. When illness is less acute, hydrocortisone 50 or 100 mg IM q 6 h can be given. Restoration of BP and general improvement should occur within 1 h after the initial dose of hydrocortisone. Inotropic agents may be needed until the effects of hydrocortisone are achieved.

A total dose of 150 mg hydrocortisone is usually given over the 2nd 24-h period if the patient has improved markedly, and 75 mg is given on the 3rd day. Maintenance oral doses of hydrocortisone (15 to 30 mg) and fludrocortisone (0.1 mg) are given daily thereafter, as described above. Recovery depends on treatment of the underlying cause (eg, infection, trauma, metabolic stress) and adequate hydrocortisone therapy.

For patients with some residual adrenal function who develop adrenal crisis when under stress, hydrocortisone treatment is the same, but fluid requirements may be much lower.

PEARLS & PITFALLS

- When adrenal crisis is suspected, give hydrocortisone treatment immediately; any delay, including for testing, may be fatal.

Treatment of complications: Fever > 40.6° C occasionally accompanies the rehydration process. Except in the presence of falling BP, antipyretics (eg, aspirin 650 mg) may be given po with caution. Complications of corticosteroid therapy may include psychotic reactions. If psychotic reactions occur after the first 12 h of therapy, the hydrocortisone dose should be reduced to the lowest level consistent with maintaining BP and good cardiovascular function. Antipsychotics may be temporarily required, but use should not be prolonged.

KEY POINTS

- Addison disease is primary adrenal insufficiency.
- Weakness, fatigue, and hyperpigmentation (generalized tanning or focal black spots involving skin and mucous membranes) are typical.
- Low serum Na, high serum K, and high BUN occur.
- Usually, serum ACTH is high and cortisol levels are low.
- Replacement doses of hydrocortisone and fludrocortisone are given; doses should be increased during intercurrent illness.

ADRENAL VIRILISM

(Adrenogenital Syndrome)

Adrenal virilism is a syndrome in which excessive adrenal androgens cause virilization. Diagnosis is clinical and confirmed by elevated androgen levels with and without dexamethasone suppression; determining the cause may involve adrenal imaging. Treatment depends on the cause.

Adrenal virilism is caused by

- Androgen-secreting adrenal tumors
- Adrenal hyperplasia

Malignant adrenal tumors may secrete excess androgens, cortisol, or mineralocorticoids (or all three), resulting in Cushing syndrome with suppression of ACTH secretion and atrophy of the contralateral adrenal as well as hypertension.

Adrenal hyperplasia is usually congenital; delayed virilizing adrenal hyperplasia is a variant of CAH. Both are caused by a defect in hydroxylation of cortisol precursors; cortisol precursors accumulate and are shunted into the production of androgens. The defect is only partial in delayed virilizing adrenal hyperplasia, so clinical disease may not develop until adulthood.

Symptoms and Signs

Effects depend on the patient's sex and age at onset and are more noticeable in women than in men.

Female infants with CAH may have fusion of the labioscrotal folds and clitoral hypertrophy resembling male external genitalia, thus presenting as a disorder of sexual differentiation.

In **prepubertal children,** growth may accelerate. If untreated, premature epiphyseal closure and short stature occur. Affected prepubertal males may experience premature sexual maturation.

Adult females may have amenorrhea, atrophy of the uterus, clitoral hypertrophy, decreased breast size, acne, hirsutism, deepening of the voice, baldness, increased libido, and increased muscularity.

In **adult males,** the excess adrenal androgens may suppress gonadal function and cause infertility. Ectopic adrenal tissue in the testes may enlarge and simulate tumors.

Diagnosis

- Testosterone
- Other adrenal androgens (dehydroepiandrosterone sulfate [DHEAS], androstenedione)
- Dexamethasone suppression test
- Adrenal imaging
- 17-hydroxyprogesterone

Adrenal virilism is suspected clinically, although mild hirsutism and virilization with hypomenorrhea and elevated plasma testosterone may also occur in polycystic ovary syndrome (Stein-Leventhal syndrome). Adrenal virilism is confirmed by showing elevated levels of adrenal androgens.

In adrenal hyperplasia, urinary dehydroepiandrosterone (DHEA) and its sulfate (DHEAS) are elevated, pregnanetriol excretion is often increased, and urinary free cortisol is normal or diminished. Plasma DHEA, DHEAS, 17-hydroxyprogesterone, testosterone, and androstenedione may be elevated. A 17-hydroxyprogesterone level of > 30 nmol/L (1000 ng/dL) 30 min after administration of cosyntropin (synthetic ACTH) 0.25 mg IM strongly suggests the most common form of adrenal hyperplasia.

Virilizing tumors are excluded if dexamethasone 0.5 mg po q 6 h for 48 h suppresses production of excess androgens. If excessive androgen excretion is not suppressed, CT or MRI of the adrenals and ultrasonography of the ovaries are done to search for a tumor.

Treatment

- Oral glucocorticoids for hyperplasia
- Removal of tumors

Glucocorticoids are used for adrenal hyperplasia, typically oral hydrocortisone 10 mg on arising, 5 mg at midday, and 5 mg in the late afternoon. Alternatively, dexamethasone 0.5 to 1 mg po may be given at bedtime, but even these small doses may cause signs of Cushing syndrome. Giving the dose at bedtime is most appropriate in terms of suppressing ACTH secretion but may cause insomnia. Cortisol 25 mg po once/day or prednisone 5 to 10 mg po once/day can be used instead. Although most symptoms and signs of virilism disappear, hirsutism and baldness disappear slowly, the voice may remain deep, and fertility may be impaired.

Tumors require adrenalectomy. For patients with cortisol-secreting tumors, hydrocortisone should be given preoperatively and postoperatively because their nontumorous adrenal cortex will be atrophic and suppressed.

KEY POINTS

- Adrenal virilism is due to an androgen-secreting adrenal tumor or to adrenal hyperplasia.
- Virilization is more noticeable in women; men may be infertile due to suppressed gonadal function.
- Urinary and plasma DHEA and its sulfate (DHEAS) and often plasma testosterone are elevated.
- ACTH stimulation testing and/or dexamethasone suppression testing may be done.
- Hyperplasia is treated with dexamethasone; tumors require adrenalectomy.

CUSHING SYNDROME

Cushing syndrome is a constellation of clinical abnormalities caused by chronic high blood levels of cortisol or related corticosteroids. Cushing disease is Cushing syndrome that results from excess pituitary production of adrenocorticotropic hormone (ACTH), generally secondary to a pituitary adenoma. Typical symptoms and signs include moon face and truncal obesity, easy bruising, and thin arms and legs. Diagnosis is by history of receiving corticosteroids or by finding elevated serum cortisol. Treatment depends on the cause.

Etiology

Hyperfunction of the adrenal cortex can be ACTH dependent or ACTH independent.

ACTH-dependent hyperfunction may result from

- Hypersecretion of ACTH by the pituitary gland (Cushing disease)
- Secretion of ACTH by a nonpituitary tumor, such as small cell carcinoma of the lung or a carcinoid tumor (ectopic ACTH syndrome)
- Administration of exogenous ACTH

ACTH-independent hyperfunction usually results from therapeutic administration of corticosteroids or from adrenal adenomas or carcinomas. Rare causes include primary pigmented nodular adrenal dysplasia (usually in adolescents) and macronodular dysplasia (in older patients).

Whereas the term Cushing syndrome denotes the clinical picture resulting from cortisol excess from any cause, Cushing disease refers to hyperfunction of the adrenal cortex from pituitary ACTH excess. Patients with Cushing disease usually have a small adenoma of the pituitary gland.

Symptoms and Signs

Clinical manifestations of Cushing syndrome include

- Moon face with a plethoric appearance (see Plate 66)
- Truncal obesity with prominent supraclavicular and dorsal cervical fat pads (buffalo hump)
- Usually, very slender distal extremities and fingers

Muscle wasting and weakness are present. The skin is thin and atrophic, with poor wound healing and easy bruising. Purple striae may appear on the abdomen. Hypertension, renal calculi, osteoporosis, glucose intolerance, reduced resistance to infection, and mental disturbances are common. Cessation of linear growth is characteristic in children.

Females usually have menstrual irregularities. In females with adrenal tumors, increased production of androgens may lead to hypertrichosis, temporal balding, and other signs of virilism.

Diagnosis

- Urinary free cortisol (UFC) level
- Dexamethasone suppression test
- Midnight serum or salivary cortisol levels
- Serum ACTH levels; if detectable, provocative testing

Diagnosis is usually suspected based on the characteristic symptoms and signs. Confirmation (and identification of the cause) generally requires hormonal and imaging tests.

Urinary free cortisol measurement: In some centers, testing begins with measurement of UFC, the best assay for urinary excretion (normal, 20 to 100 μg/24 h [55.2 to 276 nmol/24 h]). UFC is elevated > 120 μg/24 h (> 331 nmol/24 h) in almost all patients with Cushing syndrome. However, many patients with UFC elevations between 100 and 150 μg/24 h (276 and 414 nmol/24 h) have obesity, depression, or polycystic ovaries but not Cushing syndrome.

A patient with suspected Cushing syndrome with grossly elevated UFC (> 4 times the upper limit of normal) almost certainly has Cushing syndrome. Two to three normal collections usually excludes the diagnosis. Slightly elevated levels generally necessitate further investigation, as do normal levels when clinical suspicion is high.

A baseline morning (eg, 9 AM) serum cortisol measurement should also be done.

Dexamethasone suppression test: An alternative approach to investigation uses the dexamethasone suppression test, in which 1, 1.5, or 2 mg of dexamethasone is given po at 11 to 12 PM and serum cortisol is measured at 8 to 9 AM the next morning. In most normal patients, this drug suppresses morning serum cortisol to ≤ 1.8 μg/mL (≤ 50 nmol/L), whereas patients with Cushing syndrome virtually always have a higher level. A more specific but equally sensitive test is to give dexamethasone 0.5 mg po q 6 h for 2 days (low dose). In general, a clear failure to suppress cortisol levels in response to low-dose dexamethasone establishes the diagnosis.

Midnight cortisol measurements: If results of UFC measurements and the dexamethasone suppression test are indeterminate, the patient is hospitalized for measurement of serum cortisol at midnight, which is more likely to be conclusive. Alternatively, salivary cortisol samples may be collected and stored in the refrigerator at home. Cortisol normally ranges from 5 to 25 μg/dL (138 to 690 nmol/L) in the early morning (6 to 8 AM) and declines gradually to < 1.8 μg/dL (< 50 nmol/L) at midnight. Patients with Cushing syndrome occasionally have a normal morning cortisol level but lack normal diurnal decline in cortisol production, such that the midnight serum cortisol levels are above normal and the total 24-h cortisol production may be elevated.

Serum cortisol may be spuriously elevated in patients with congenital increases of corticosteroid-binding globulin or in those receiving estrogen therapy, but diurnal variation is normal in these patients.

Serum ACTH measurement: ACTH levels are measured to determine the cause of Cushing syndrome. Undetectable levels, both basally and particularly in response to corticotropin-releasing hormone (CRH), suggest a primary adrenal cause. High levels suggest a pituitary cause. If ACTH is detectable, provocative tests help differentiate Cushing disease from ectopic ACTH syndrome, which is rarer. In response to high-dose dexamethasone (2 mg po q 6 h for 48 h), the 9 AM serum cortisol falls by > 50% in most patients with Cushing disease but infrequently in those with ectopic ACTH syndrome. Conversely, ACTH rises by > 50% and cortisol rises by 20% in response to human or ovine-sequence CRH (100 mcg IV or 1 mcg/kg IV) in most patients with Cushing disease but very rarely in those with ectopic ACTH syndrome (see Table 162–3).

An alternative approach to localization, which is more accurate but more invasive, is to catheterize both petrosal veins (which drain the pituitary) and measure ACTH from these veins 5 min after a 100 mcg or 1 mcg/kg bolus of CRH (human or ovine). A central-to-peripheral ACTH ratio > 3 virtually excludes ectopic ACTH syndrome, whereas a ratio < 3 suggests a need to seek such a source.

Imaging: Pituitary imaging is done if ACTH levels and provocative tests suggest a pituitary cause; gadolinium-enhanced MRI is most accurate, but some microadenomas are visible on CT. If testing suggests a nonpituitary cause, imaging includes high-resolution CT of the chest, pancreas, and adrenals; scintiscanning or PET scanning with radiolabeled octreotide; and occasionally fluorodeoxyglucose (FDG)-PET scanning.

In children with Cushing disease, pituitary tumors are very small and usually cannot be detected with MRI. Petrosal sinus sampling is particularly useful in this situation. MRI is preferred to CT in pregnant women to avoid fetal exposure to radiation.

Treatment

- High protein intake, and K administration (or K-sparing agents such as spironolactone)
- Adrenal inhibitors such as metyrapone, mitotane, or ketoconazole
- Surgery or radiation therapy to remove pituitary, adrenal, or ectopic ACTH-producing tumors
- Sometimes somatostatin analogs, dopamine agonists, or mifepristone

Initially, the patient's general condition should be supported by high protein intake and appropriate administration of K. If clinical manifestations are severe, it may be reasonable to block corticosteroid secretion with metyrapone 250 mg to 1 g po tid or ketoconazole 400 mg po once/day, increasing to a maximum of 400 mg tid. Ketoconazole is probably slower in onset and sometimes hepatotoxic.

Table 162–3. DIAGNOSTIC TESTS IN CUSHING SYNDROME

DIAGNOSIS	SERUM CORTISOL, 9 AM	SALIVARY OR SERUM CORTISOL, MIDNIGHT	URINARY FREE CORTISOL	LOW-DOSE OR OVERNIGHT DEXAMETHASONE	HIGH-DOSE DEXAMETHASONE	CORTICOTROPIN-RELEASING HORMONE	ACTH LEVEL
Normal	N	N	N*	S	S	N	N
Cushing disease	N or ↑	↑	↑	NS	S	N or ↑	N or ↑
Ectopic ACTH	N or ↑	↑	↑	NS	NS	Flat	↑↑
Adrenal tumor	N or ↑	↑	↑	NS	NS	Flat	↓

*May be elevated in non-Cushing conditions.

Flat = no significant rise in ACTH or cortisol; N = normal; NS = nonsuppression; S = suppression; ↑↑ = greatly increased; ↑ = increased; ↓ = decreased.

Pituitary tumors that produce excessive ACTH are removed surgically or extirpated with radiation therapy. If no tumor is shown on imaging but a pituitary source is likely, total hypophysectomy may be attempted, particularly in older patients. Younger patients usually receive supervoltage irradiation of the pituitary, delivering 45 Gy. However, in children, irradiation may reduce secretion of growth hormone and occasionally cause precocious puberty. In special centers, heavy particle beam irradiation, providing about 100 Gy, is often successful, as is a single focused beam of radiation therapy given as a single dose (radiosurgery). Response to irradiation occasionally requires several years, but response is more rapid in children.

Studies suggest that mild cases of persistent or recurrent disease may benefit from the somatostatin analog pasireotide. However, hyperglycemia is a significant adverse effect. The dopamine agonist cabergoline may also occasionally be useful. Alternatively, the corticosteroid receptors can be blocked with mifepristone. Mifepristone increases serum cortisol but blocks the effects of the corticosteroid and may cause hypokalemia.

Bilateral adrenalectomy is reserved for patients with pituitary hyperadrenocorticism who do not respond to both pituitary exploration (with possible adenomectomy) and irradiation, or in patients in whom surgery was unsuccessful and radiotherapy is contraindicated. Adrenalectomy requires lifelong corticosteroid replacement.

Adrenocortical tumors are removed surgically. Patients must receive cortisol during the surgical and postoperative periods because their nontumorous adrenal cortex will be atrophic and suppressed. Benign adenomas can be removed laparoscopically. With multinodular adrenal hyperplasia, bilateral adrenalectomy may be necessary. Even after a presumed total adrenalectomy, functional regrowth occurs in a few patients.

Ectopic ACTH syndrome is treated by removing the nonpituitary tumor that is producing the ACTH. However, in some cases, the tumor is disseminated and cannot be excised. Adrenal inhibitors, such as metyrapone 500 mg po tid (and up to a total of 6 g/day) or mitotane 0.5 g po once/day, increasing to a maximum of 3 to 4 g/day, usually control severe metabolic disturbances (eg, hypokalemia). When mitotane is used, large doses of hydrocortisone or dexamethasone may be needed. Measures of cortisol production may be unreliable, and severe hypercholesterolemia may develop. Ketoconazole 400 to 1200 mg po once/day also blocks corticosteroid synthesis, although it may cause liver toxicity and can cause addisonian symptoms. Mifepristone also may be useful for treating ectopic ACTH syndrome.

Sometimes ACTH-secreting tumors respond to long-acting somatostatin analogs, although administration for > 2 yr requires close follow-up, because mild gastritis, gallstones, cholangitis, and malabsorption may develop.

Nelson syndrome: Nelson syndrome occurs when the pituitary gland continues to expand after bilateral adrenalectomy, causing a marked increase in the secretion of ACTH and its precursors, resulting in severe hyperpigmentation. It occurs in ≤ 50% of patients who undergo adrenalectomy. The risk is probably reduced if the patient undergoes pituitary radiation therapy.

Although irradiation may arrest continued pituitary growth, many patients also require hypophysectomy. The indications for hypophysectomy are the same as for any pituitary tumor: an increase in size such that the tumor encroaches on surrounding structures, causing visual field defects, pressure on the hypothalamus, or other complications.

Routine irradiation is often done after hypophysectomy if it was not done previously, especially when a tumor is clearly present. Radiation therapy may be delayed if there is no obvious lesion. Radiosurgery, or focused radiation therapy, can be given in a single fraction when standard external beam radiation therapy has already been done, as long as the lesion is at a reasonable distance from the optic nerve and chiasm.

KEY POINTS

- Diagnosis is usually made by elevated nocturnal serum or salivary cortisol levels, or 24-h urinary free cortisol, and a dexamethasone suppression test.
- Pituitary causes are distinguished from nonpituitary causes by ACTH levels.
- Imaging is then done to identify any causative tumor.
- Tumors are usually treated surgically or with radiation therapy.
- Metyrapone or ketoconazole may be given to suppress cortisol secretion prior to definitive treatment.

NONFUNCTIONAL ADRENAL MASSES

Nonfunctional adrenal masses are space-occupying lesions of the adrenal glands that have no hormonal activity. Symptoms, signs, and treatment depend on the nature and size of the mass.

The most common nonfunctioning adrenal mass in adults is an adenoma (50%), followed by carcinomas and metastatic tumors. Cysts and lipomas make up most of the remainder. However, the precise proportions depend on the clinical presentation. Masses discovered on incidental screening are usually adenomas. Less commonly, in neonates, spontaneous adrenal hemorrhage may cause large adrenal masses, simulating neuroblastoma or Wilms tumor. In adults, bilateral massive adrenal hemorrhage may result from thromboembolic disease or coagulopathy.

Benign cysts are observed in elderly patients and may be due to cystic degeneration, vascular accidents, lymphomas, bacterial infections, fungal infections (eg, histoplasmosis), or parasitic infestations (eg, due to *Echinococcus*). Hematogenous spread of TB organisms may cause adrenal masses. A nonfunctional adrenal carcinoma causes a diffuse and infiltrating retroperitoneal process. Hemorrhage can occur, causing adrenal hematomas.

Symptoms and Signs

Most patients are asymptomatic. With any adrenal mass, adrenal insufficiency is rare unless both glands are involved.

The major signs of bilateral massive adrenal hemorrhage are abdominal pain, falling Hct, signs of acute adrenal failure, and suprarenal masses on CT or MRI. TB of the adrenals may cause calcification and Addison disease. Nonfunctional adrenal carcinoma usually manifests as invasive or metastatic disease.

Diagnosis

- Adrenal hormone measurements
- Fine-needle biopsy

Nonfunctional adrenal masses are usually found incidentally during tests such as CT or MRI conducted for other reasons. Nonfunctionality is established clinically and confirmed by adrenal hormonal measurements. If metastatic disease is possible, fine-needle biopsy can be diagnostic but is contraindicated if adrenal carcinoma or pheochromocytoma is strongly suspected.

Treatment

- Sometimes excision, depending on size and/or imaging results
- Periodic monitoring

Although new imaging modalities (eg, in-phase and out-of-phase MRI) may be diagnostic, if the tumor is solid, of adrenal origin, and > 4 cm, it should usually be excised unless the imaging characteristics are quite clearly benign.

Tumors 2 to 4 cm in diameter are a particularly difficult clinical problem. If scanning does not suggest cancer and hormonal function does not seem altered (eg, normal electrolytes and metanephrines, no evidence of Cushing syndrome), it is reasonable to reevaluate periodically with imaging studies, usually for 1 to 2 yr. If no progression is seen by then, further follow-up is unnecessary. However, many of these tumors secrete cortisol in quantities too small to cause symptoms, and whether they would eventually cause symptoms and morbidity if untreated is unclear. Most clinicians merely observe patients with these tumors, but clinicians should consider removal of these tumors if there is significant cortisol secretion.

Adrenal adenomas < 2 cm require no special treatment but should be observed for growth or development of secretory function (such as by looking for clinical signs and periodically measuring electrolytes).

Nonfunctional adrenal carcinoma that has metastasized is not amenable to surgery, though mitotane plus corticosteroids may help control the disease.

PRIMARY ALDOSTERONISM

(Conn Syndrome)

Primary aldosteronism is aldosteronism caused by autonomous production of aldosterone by the adrenal cortex (due to hyperplasia, adenoma, or carcinoma). Symptoms and signs include episodic weakness, elevated BP, and hypokalemia. Diagnosis includes measurement of plasma aldosterone levels and plasma renin activity. Treatment depends on cause. A tumor is removed if possible; in hyperplasia, spironolactone or related drugs may normalize BP and eliminate other clinical features.

Aldosterone is the most potent mineralocorticoid produced by the adrenals. It causes Na retention and K loss. In the kidneys, aldosterone causes transfer of Na from the lumen of the distal tubule into the tubular cells in exchange for K and hydrogen. The same effect occurs in salivary glands, sweat glands, cells of the intestinal mucosa, and in exchanges between intracellular fluid (ICF) and extracellular fluid (ECF).

Aldosterone secretion is regulated by the renin-angiotensin system and, to a lesser extent, by ACTH. Renin, a proteolytic enzyme, is stored in the juxtaglomerular cells of the kidneys. Reduction in blood volume and flow in the afferent renal arterioles induces secretion of renin. Renin transforms angiotensinogen from the liver to angiotensin I, which is transformed by angiotensin-converting enzyme (ACE) to angiotensin II. Angiotensin II causes secretion of aldosterone and, to a much lesser extent, secretion of cortisol and deoxycorticosterone; it also has pressor activity. Na and water retention resulting from increased aldosterone secretion increases the blood volume and reduces renin secretion.

Primary aldosteronism is caused by an adenoma, usually unilateral, of the glomerulosa cells of the adrenal cortex or, more rarely, by adrenal carcinoma or hyperplasia. Adenomas are extremely rare in children, but the syndrome sometimes occurs in childhood adrenal carcinoma or hyperplasia. In adrenal hyperplasia, which is more common among older men, both adrenals are overactive, and no adenoma is present. The clinical picture can also occur with CAH from deficiency of 11 beta-hydroxylase and the dominantly inherited dexamethasone-suppressible hyperaldosteronism. Hyperplasia as a cause of hyperaldosteronism may be more common than previously recognized but remains an infrequent cause in the presence of hypokalemia.

Symptoms and Signs

Hypernatremia, hypervolemia, and a hypokalemic alkalosis may occur, causing episodic weakness, paresthesias, transient paralysis, and tetany. Diastolic hypertension and hypokalemic nephropathy with polyuria and polydipsia are common. In many cases, the only manifestation is mild to moderate hypertension. Edema is uncommon.

Diagnosis

- Electrolytes
- Plasma aldosterone
- Plasma renin activity (PRA)
- Adrenal imaging
- Bilateral adrenal vein catheterization (for cortisol and aldosterone levels)

Diagnosis is suspected in patients with hypertension and hypokalemia. Initial laboratory testing consists of plasma aldosterone levels and plasma renin activity. Ideally, the patient should not take any drugs that affect the renin-angiotensin system (eg, thiazide diuretics, ACE inhibitors, angiotensin antagonists, beta-blockers) for 4 to 6 wk before tests are done. Plasma renin activity is usually measured in the morning with the patient recumbent. Patients with primary aldosteronism typically have plasma aldosterone > 15 ng/dL (> 0.42 nmol/L) and low levels of PRA, with a ratio of plasma aldosterone (in ng/dL) to plasma renin activity (in ng/mL/h) > 20.

Low levels of both plasma renin activity and aldosterone suggest nonaldosterone mineralocorticoid excess (eg, due to licorice ingestion, Cushing syndrome, or Liddle syndrome). High levels of both plasma renin activity and aldosterone suggest secondary hyperaldosteronism. The principal differences between primary and secondary aldosteronism are shown in Table 162–4. In children, Bartter syndrome is distinguished from primary hyperaldosteronism by the absence of hypertension and marked elevation of PRA.

Patients with findings suggesting primary hyperaldosteronism should undergo CT or MRI to determine whether the cause is a tumor or hyperplasia. However, imaging tests are relatively insensitive, and most patients require bilateral catheterization of the adrenal veins to measure cortisol and aldosterone levels to confirm whether the aldosterone excess is unilateral (tumor) or bilateral (hyperplasia). It is possible that in the future PET-radionuclide imaging may be more helpful.

Treatment

- Surgical removal of tumors
- Spironolactone or eplerenone for hyperplasia

Tumors should be removed laparoscopically. After removal of an adenoma, serum K normalizes and BP decreases in all patients; complete normalization of the BP without the need for hypotensive therapy occurs in 50 to 70% of patients.

Among patients with adrenal hyperplasia, 70% remain hypertensive after bilateral adrenalectomy; thus, surgery is not recommended. Hyperaldosteronism in these patients can usually be controlled by a selective aldosterone blocker such as spironolactone, starting with 50 mg po once/day and increasing over 1 to 3 mo to a maintenance dose, usually around 100 mg once/day; or by amiloride 5 to 10 mg po once/day or another K-sparing diuretic. The more specific drug eplerenone 50 mg po once/day to 200 mg po bid may be used because, unlike spironolactone, it does not block the androgen receptor; it is the drug of choice for long-term treatment in men.

About half of patients with hyperplasia need additional antihypertensive treatment.

KEY POINTS

- Diagnosis should be suspected in hypertensive patients with hypokalemia in the absence of Cushing syndrome.
- Initial testing includes measurement of plasma aldosterone levels and plasma renin activity.
- Adrenal imaging tests are done, but usually bilateral adrenal vein catheterization is needed to distinguish tumor from hyperplasia.
- Tumors are removed and patients with adrenal hyperplasia are treated with aldosterone blockers such as spironolactone or eplerenone.

PHEOCHROMOCYTOMA

A pheochromocytoma is a catecholamine-secreting tumor of chromaffin cells typically located in the adrenals. It causes persistent or paroxysmal hypertension. Diagnosis is by measuring catecholamine products in blood or urine. Imaging tests, especially CT or MRI, help localize tumors. Treatment involves removal of the tumor when possible. Drug therapy for control of BP includes alpha-blockade, usually combined with beta-blockade.

The catecholamines secreted include norepinephrine, epinephrine, dopamine, and dopa in varying proportions. About 90% of pheochromocytomas are in the adrenal medulla, but they may also be located in other tissues derived from neural crest cells. Possible sites include the following:

- Paraganglia of the sympathetic chain
- Retroperitoneally along the course of the aorta
- Carotid body
- Organ of Zuckerkandl (at the aortic bifurcation)
- GU system
- Brain
- Pericardial sac
- Dermoid cysts

Pheochromocytomas in the adrenal medulla occur equally in both sexes, are bilateral in 10% of cases (20% in children), and are malignant in < 10%. Of extra-adrenal tumors, 30% are

Table 162–4. DIFFERENTIAL DIAGNOSIS OF ALDOSTERONISM

	PRIMARY ALDOSTERONISM		SECONDARY ALDOSTERONISM	
CLINICAL FINDING	Adenoma	Hyperplasia	Renovascular or Accelerated Hypertension	Edematous Disorders
BP	↑↑	↑	↑↑↑↑	N or ↑
Edema	Rare	Rare	Rare	Present
Serum Na	N or ↑	N or ↑	N or ↓	N or ↓
Serum K	↓	N or ↓	↓	N or ↓
Plasma renin activity*	↓↓	↓↓	↑↑	↑
Aldosterone	↑	↑	↑↑	↑

*When corrected for age; elderly patients have lower mean plasma renin activity.
↑↑↑↑ = very greatly increased; ↑↑ = greatly increased; ↑ = increased; ↓↓ = greatly decreased; ↓ = decreased; N = normal.

malignant. Although pheochromocytomas occur at any age, peak incidence is between the 20s and 40s. About 25 to 30% are now thought to be due to germline mutations.

Pheochromocytomas vary in size but average 5 to 6 cm in diameter. They weigh 50 to 200 g, but tumors weighing several kilograms have been reported. Rarely, they are large enough to be palpated or cause symptoms due to pressure or obstruction. Regardless of the histologic appearance, the tumor is considered benign if it has not invaded the capsule and no metastases are found, although exceptions occur. In general, larger tumors are more likely to be malignant.

Pheochromocytomas may be part of the syndrome of familial multiple endocrine neoplasia (MEN) types 2A and 2B, in which other endocrine tumors (parathyroid or medullary carcinoma of the thyroid) coexist or develop subsequently. Pheochromocytoma develops in 1% of patients with neurofibromatosis (von Recklinghausen disease) and may occur with hemangioblastomas and renal cell carcinoma, as in von Hippel-Lindau disease. Familial pheochromocytomas and carotid body tumors may be due to mutations of the enzyme succinate dehydrogenase as well as of the genes responsible for other more recently described signaling molecules.

Symptoms and Signs

Hypertension, which is paroxysmal in 45% of patients, is prominent. About 1/1000 hypertensive patients has a pheochromocytoma. Common symptoms and signs are

- Tachycardia
- Diaphoresis
- Postural hypotension
- Tachypnea
- Cold and clammy skin
- Severe headache
- Angina
- Palpitations
- Nausea and vomiting
- Epigastric pain
- Visual disturbances
- Dyspnea
- Paresthesias
- Constipation
- A sense of impending doom

Paroxysmal attacks may be provoked by palpation of the tumor, postural changes, abdominal compression or massage, induction of anesthesia, emotional trauma, unopposed beta-blockade (which paradoxically increases BP by blocking beta-mediated vasodilation), or micturition (if the tumor is in the bladder). In elderly patients, severe weight loss with persistent hypertension is suggestive of pheochromocytoma.

Physical examination, except for the presence of hypertension, is usually normal unless done during a paroxysmal attack. Retinopathy and cardiomegaly are often less severe than might be expected for the degree of hypertension, but a specific catecholamine cardiomyopathy can occur.

Diagnosis

- Plasma free metanephrines or urinary metanephrines
- Chest and abdomen imaging (CT or MRI) if catecholamine screen positive
- Possibly nuclear imaging with ^{123}I-metaiodobenzylguanidine (MIBG)

Pheochromocytoma is suspected in patients with typical symptoms or particularly sudden, severe, or intermittent unexplained hypertension. Diagnosis involves demonstrating high levels of catecholamine products in the serum or urine.

Blood tests: Plasma free metanephrine is up to 99% sensitive. This test has superior sensitivity to measurement of circulating epinephrine and norepinephrine because plasma metanephrines are elevated continuously, unlike epinephrine and norepinephrine, which are secreted intermittently. Grossly elevated plasma norepinephrine renders the diagnosis highly probable.

Urine tests: Urinary metanephrine is slightly less specific than plasma free metanephrine, but sensitivity is about 95%. Two or 3 normal results while the patient is hypertensive render the diagnosis extremely unlikely. Measurement of urinary norepinephrine and epinephrine is nearly as accurate. The principal urinary metabolic products of epinephrine and norepinephrine are the metanephrines, vanillylmandelic acid (VMA), and homovanillic acid (HVA). Healthy people excrete only very small amounts of these substances. Normal values for 24 h are as follows:

- Free epinephrine and norepinephrine < 100 μg (< 582 nmol)
- Total metanephrine < 1.3 mg (< 7.1 μmol)
- VMA < 10 mg (< 50 mmol)
- HVA < 15 mg (< 82.4 mmol)

In pheochromocytoma, increased urinary excretion of epinephrine and norepinephrine and their metabolic products is intermittent. Elevated excretion of these compounds may also occur in other disorders (eg, neuroblastoma, coma, dehydration, sleep apnea) or extreme stress; in patients being treated with rauwolfia alkaloids, methyldopa, or catecholamines; or after ingestion of foods containing large quantities of vanilla (especially if renal insufficiency is present).

Other tests: Blood volume is constricted and may falsely elevate Hb and Hct levels. Hyperglycemia, glycosuria, or overt diabetes mellitus may be present, with elevated fasting levels of plasma free fatty acid and glycerol. Plasma insulin level is inappropriately low for the plasma glucose. After removal of the pheochromocytoma, hypoglycemia may occur, especially in patients treated with oral antihyperglycemics.

Provocative tests with histamine or tyramine *are hazardous and should not be used.* Glucagon 0.5 to 1 mg injected rapidly IV provokes a rise in BP of > 35/25 mm Hg within 2 min in normotensive patients with pheochromocytoma but is now generally unnecessary. *Phentolamine mesylate must be available to terminate any hypertensive crisis.*

PEARLS & PITFALLS

- Provocative tests with histamine or tyramine are hazardous and should not be done.

Screening tests are preferred to provocative tests. The general approach is to measure plasma or urinary metanephrines as a screening test and to avoid provocative tests. In patients with elevated plasma catecholamines, a suppression test using oral clonidine or IV pentolinium can be used but is rarely necessary.

Imaging tests to localize tumors are usually done in patients with abnormal screening results. Tests should include CT and MRI of the chest and abdomen with and without contrast. With isotonic contrast media, no adrenoceptor blockade is necessary. FDG-PET has also been used successfully, especially in patients with succinate dehydrogenase mutations.

Repeated sampling of plasma catecholamine concentrations during catheterization of the vena cava with sampling at different locations, including the adrenal veins, can help localize the tumor: there will be a step up in norepinephrine level in a vein draining the tumor. Adrenal vein norepinephrine:epinephrine ratios may help in the hunt for a small adrenal source, but determining these ratios is now rarely necessary.

Radiopharmaceuticals with nuclear imaging techniques can also help localize pheochromocytomas. MIBG is the most used compound; 0.5 mCi ^{123}I-MIBG is injected IV, and the patient is scanned on days 1, 2, and 3. Normal adrenal tissue rarely picks up this isotope, but 85% of pheochromocytomas do. The imaging is usually positive only when the lesion is large enough to be obvious on CT or MRI, but it can help confirm that a mass is likely to be the source of the catecholamines. ^{131}I-MIBG is a less sensitive alternative.

Signs of an associated genetic disorder (eg, café-au-lait patches in neurofibromatosis) should be sought. Patients should be screened for MEN with a serum calcitonin measurement and any other tests as directed by clinical findings. Many centers routinely do genetic testing, especially when pheochromocytoma involves the sympathetic paraganglia.

Treatment

- Hypertension control with combination of alpha-blockers and beta-blockers
- Surgical removal of tumor with careful perioperative control of BP and volume status

Surgical removal is the treatment of choice. The operation is usually delayed until hypertension is controlled by a combination of alpha-blockers and beta-blockers (usually phenoxybenzamine 20 to 40 mg po tid and propranolol 20 to 40 mg po tid). Beta-blockers should not be used until adequate alpha-blockade has been achieved. Some alpha-blockers, such as doxazosin, may be equally effective but better tolerated.

PEARLS & PITFALLS

- Give alpha-blockers first before beta-blockers. Unopposed beta-blockade can cause paradoxical increase in blood pressure by blocking beta-mediated vasodilation.

The most effective and safest preoperative alpha-blockade is phenoxybenzamine 0.5 mg/kg IV in 0.9% saline over 2 h on each of the 3 days before the operation, but oral phenoxybenzamine is usually very effective as long as 7 to 14 days are available for volume equilibration. Nitroprusside can be infused for hypertensive crises preoperatively or intraoperatively. When bilateral tumors are documented or suspected (as in a patient with MEN), sufficient hydrocortisone (100 mg IV bid) given before and during surgery avoids acute glucocorticoid insufficiency due to bilateral adrenalectomy.

Most pheochromocytomas can be removed laparoscopically. BP must be continuously monitored via an intra-arterial catheter, and volume status is closely monitored. Anesthesia should be induced with a nonarrhythmogenic drug (eg, a thiobarbiturate) and continued with an inhaled drug (eg, enflurane, isoflurane). During surgery, paroxysms of hypertension should be controlled with injections of phentolamine 1 to 5 mg IV or nitroprusside infusion (2 to 4 mcg/kg/min), and tachyarrhythmias should be controlled with propranolol 0.5 to 2 mg IV. If a muscle relaxant is needed, drugs that do not release histamine are preferred. *Atropine should not be used preoperatively.*

Preoperative blood transfusion (1 to 2 units) may be given before the tumor is removed in anticipation of blood loss. If BP has been well controlled before surgery, a diet high in salt is recommended to increase blood volume. An infusion of norepinephrine 4 to 12 mg/L in a dextrose-containing solution may be considered if hypotension develops. Some patients whose hypotension responds poorly to norepinephrine may benefit from hydrocortisone 100 mg IV, but adequate fluid replacement is usually all that is required.

Malignant metastatic pheochromocytoma should be treated with alpha-blockers and beta-blockers. The tumor may be indolent and survival long-lasting. However, even with rapid tumor growth, BP can be controlled. ^{131}I-MIBG can help relieve symptoms in patients with residual disease. Metyrosine, a tyrosine hydroxylase inhibitor, may be used to decrease catecholamine production in patients whose BP is difficult to control. Radiation therapy may reduce bone pain. Chemotherapy is rarely effective, but the most common regimen tried is the combination of cyclophosphamide, vincristine, and dacarbazine. Recent data have shown some promising results with the chemotherapy agent temozolomide and targeted therapy with sunitinib.

KEY POINTS

- Hypertension may be constant or episodic.
- Diagnosis involves demonstrating high levels of catecholamine products (typically metanephrine) in the serum or urine.
- Tumors should be localized with imaging tests, sometimes using radiolabeled compounds.
- A combination of alpha-blockers and beta-blockers are given, pending tumor removal.

SECONDARY ADRENAL INSUFFICIENCY

Secondary adrenal insufficiency is adrenal hypofunction due to a lack of ACTH. Symptoms are the same as for Addison disease, but there is usually less hypovolemia. Diagnosis is clinical and by laboratory findings, including low plasma ACTH with low plasma cortisol. Treatment depends on the cause but generally includes hydrocortisone.

Secondary adrenal insufficiency may occur in panhypopituitarism, in isolated failure of ACTH production, in patients receiving corticosteroids (by any route, including high doses of inhaled, intra-articular, or topical corticosteroids), or after corticosteroids are stopped. Inadequate ACTH can also result from failure of the hypothalamus to stimulate pituitary ACTH production, which is sometimes called tertiary adrenal insufficiency.

Panhypopituitarism may occur secondary to pituitary tumors, various tumors, granulomas, and, rarely, infection or trauma that destroys pituitary tissue. In younger people, panhypopituitarism may occur secondary to a craniopharyngioma. Patients receiving corticosteroids for > 4 wk may have insufficient ACTH secretion during metabolic stress to stimulate the adrenals to produce adequate quantities of corticosteroids, or they may have atrophic adrenals that are unresponsive to ACTH. These problems may persist for up to 1 yr after corticosteroid treatment is stopped.

Symptoms and Signs

Symptoms and signs are similar to those of Addison disease and include fatigue, weakness, weight loss, nausea, vomiting, and diarrhea. Differentiating clinical or general laboratory features include the absence of hyperpigmentation and relatively normal electrolyte and BUN levels; hyponatremia, if it occurs, is usually dilutional.

Patients with panhypopituitarism have depressed thyroid and gonadal function and hypoglycemia. Coma may supervene when symptomatic secondary adrenal insufficiency occurs. Adrenal crisis is especially likely if a patient is treated for a single endocrine gland problem, particularly with thyroxine, without hydrocortisone replacement.

Diagnosis

- Serum cortisol
- Serum ACTH
- ACTH stimulation testing
- CNS imaging

Tests to differentiate primary and secondary adrenal insufficiency are discussed under Addison disease. Patients with confirmed secondary adrenal insufficiency (see Table 162–5) should have CT or MRI of the brain to rule out a pituitary tumor or pituitary atrophy.

Adequacy of the hypothalamic-pituitary-adrenal axis during tapering or after stopping long-term corticosteroid treatment can be determined by injecting cosyntropin 250 mcg IV or IM. After 30 min, serum cortisol should be > 20 μg/dL (> 552 nmol/L); specific levels vary somewhat depending on the laboratory assay in use. An insulin stress test to induce hypoglycemia and a rise in cortisol is the standard for testing integrity of the hypothalamic-pituitary-adrenal axis in many centers.

The corticotropin-releasing hormone (CRH) test can be used to distinguish between hypothalamic and pituitary causes but is rarely used in clinical practice. After administration of CRH 100 mcg (or 1 mcg/kg) IV, the normal response is a rise of serum ACTH of 30 to 40 pg/mL; patients with pituitary failure do not respond, whereas those with hypothalamic disease usually do.

Treatment

- Hydrocortisone or prednisone
- Fludrocortisone not indicated
- Dose increase during intercurrent illness

Glucocorticoid replacement is similar to that described for Addison disease. Each case varies regarding the type and degree of specific hormone deficiencies. Fludrocortisone is not required because the intact adrenals produce aldosterone. During acute febrile illness or after trauma, patients receiving corticosteroids for nonendocrine disorders may require supplemental doses to augment their endogenous hydrocortisone production. In panhypopituitarism, other pituitary deficiencies should be treated appropriately.

Table 162–5. CONFIRMATORY SERUM TESTING FOR SECONDARY ADRENAL INSUFFICIENCY

TEST	RESULT
ACTH	Low (< 5 pg/mL)
Cortisol	Low (< 5 μg/dL [138 nmol/L])
ACTH stimulation test	Normal or subnormal
Prolonged (24-h) ACTH stimulation test	Cortisol should continue to rise for 24 h

ACTH = adrenocorticotropic hormone.

KEY POINTS

- Secondary adrenal insufficiency involves ACTH deficiency due to pituitary or, less often, hypothalamic causes (including suppression by long-term corticosteroid use).
- Other endocrine deficiencies (eg, hypothyroidism, growth hormone deficiency) may coexist.
- Unlike in Addison disease, hyperpigmentation does not occur and serum Na and K levels are relatively normal.
- ACTH and cortisol levels both are low.
- Glucocorticoid replacement is required, but mineralocorticoids (eg, fludrocortisone) are not necessary.

SECONDARY ALDOSTERONISM

Secondary aldosteronism is increased adrenal production of aldosterone in response to nonpituitary, extra-adrenal stimuli such as renal hypoperfusion. Symptoms are similar to those of primary aldosteronism. Diagnosis includes measurement of plasma aldosterone levels and plasma renin activity. Treatment involves correcting the cause.

Secondary aldosteronism is caused by reduced renal blood flow, which stimulates the renin-angiotensin mechanism with resultant hypersecretion of aldosterone. Causes of reduced renal blood flow include obstructive renal artery disease (eg, atheroma, stenosis), renal vasoconstriction (as occurs in accelerated hypertension), and edematous disorders (eg, heart failure, cirrhosis with ascites, nephrotic syndrome). Secretion may be normal in heart failure, but hepatic blood flow and aldosterone metabolism are reduced, so circulating levels of the hormone are high.

Symptoms and Signs

Symptoms are similar to those of primary aldosteronism and include hypokalemic alkalosis that causes episodic weakness, paresthesias, transient paralysis, and tetany. In many cases, the only manifestation is hypertension. Peripheral edema may be present.

Diagnosis

- Serum electrolyte levels
- Plasma aldosterone
- Plasma renin activity (PRA)

Diagnosis is suspected in patients with hypertension and hypokalemia. Initial laboratory testing consists of plasma aldosterone levels and PRA. Ideally, the patient should not take any drugs that affect the renin-angiotensin system (eg, thiazide diuretics, ACE inhibitors, angiotensin antagonists, beta-blockers) for 4 to 6 wk before tests are done. Elevated aldosterone and plasma renin activity is indicative of secondary aldosteronism. The principal differences between primary and secondary aldosteronism are shown in Table 162–4.

Treatment

- Treament of cause
- Sometimes aldosterone antagonists

Treatment involves correcting the cause. Hypertension can usually be controlled with a selective aldosterone blocker such as spironolactone, starting with 50 mg po once/day and increasing over 1 to 3 mo to a maintenance dose, usually around 100 mg once/day or another K-sparing diuretic. The more specific drug eplerenone 50 mg po once/day to 200 mg po bid may be used because, unlike spironolactone, it does not block the androgen receptor; it is the drug of choice for long-term treatment in men.

KEY POINTS

- Diagnosis is suspected in hypertensive patients with hypokalemia.
- Initial testing includes measurement of plasma aldosterone and plasma renin activity.
- Unlike primary aldosteronism, plasma renin activity is elevated.
- Treatment includes correcting the cause. Hypertension may be controlled with aldosterone antagonists.

163 Amyloidosis

Amyloidosis is any of a group of disparate conditions characterized by extracellular deposition of insoluble fibrils composed of misaggregated proteins. These proteins may accumulate locally, causing relatively few symptoms, or widely, involving multiple organs and causing severe multiorgan failure. Amyloidosis can occur *de novo* or be secondary to various infectious, inflammatory, or malignant conditions. Diagnosis is by biopsy of affected tissue; the amyloidogenic protein is typed using a variety of immunohistologic and biochemical techniques. Treatment varies with the type of amyloidosis.

Amyloid deposits are composed of small (about 10 nm diameter), insoluble fibrils that form beta-pleated sheets that can be identified by x-ray diffraction. In addition to the fibrillar amyloid protein, the deposits also contain serum amyloid P component and glycosaminoglycans. Amyloid fibrils are made of misfolded proteins that aggregate into oligomers and then fibrils. A number of normal (wild-type) and mutant proteins are susceptible to such misfolding and aggregation (amyloidogenic proteins), thus accounting for the wide variety of causes and types of amyloidosis. For amyloidosis to develop, in addition to production of amyloidogenic proteins, there is probably also a failure of the normal clearance mechanisms for such misfolded proteins. The amyloid deposits themselves are metabolically inert but interfere physically with organ structure and function. However, some prefibrillar oligomers of amyloidogenic proteins have direct cellular toxicity, an important component of disease pathogenesis.

Amyloid deposits stain pink with hematoxylin and eosin, contain carbohydrate constituents that stain with periodic acid-Schiff dye or with Alcian blue, but most characteristically have apple-green birefringence under polarized light microscopy after Congo red staining. On autopsy inspection, affected organs may appear waxy.

Etiology

In **systemic amyloidosis,** circulating amyloidogenic proteins form deposits in a variety of organs. Major systemic types include

- AL (primary amyloidosis): Caused by acquired overexpression of clonal immunoglobulin light chains
- AF (familial amyloidosis): Caused by inheritance of a mutant gene encoding a protein prone to misfolding, most commonly transthyretin (*TTR*)
- ATTRwt (wild-type ATTR; previously termed senile systemic amyloidosis or SSA): Caused by misfolding and aggregation of wild-type *TTR (wild-type ATTR)*
- AA (secondary amyloidosis): Caused by aggregation of an acute phase reactant, serum amyloid A

Amyloidosis caused by aggregation of beta-2-microglobulin can occur in patients on long-term hemodialysis, but the incidence has declined with use of modern high-flow dialysis membranes.

Localized forms of amyloidosis appear to be caused by local production and deposition of an amyloidogenic protein (most often immunoglobulin light chains) within the affected organ rather than by deposition of circulating proteins. Frequently involved sites include the CNS (eg, in Alzheimer disease), skin, upper or lower airways, lung parenchyma, bladder, eyes, and breasts.

AL amyloidosis: AL is caused by overproduction of an amyloidogenic immunoglobulin light chain in patients with a monoclonal plasma cell or other B cell lymphoproliferative disorder. Light chains can also form nonfibrillar tissue deposits (ie, light chain deposition disease). Rarely, immunoglobulin heavy chains form amyloid fibrils (called AH amyloidosis). Common sites for amyloid deposition include the skin, nerves, heart, GI tract (including the tongue), kidneys, liver, spleen, and blood vessels. Usually, a low-grade plasmacytosis is present in the bone marrow, which is similar to that in multiple myeloma, although most patients do not have true multiple myeloma (with lytic bone lesions, hypercalcemia, renal tubular casts, and anemia). However, about 10 to 20% of patients with multiple myeloma develop AL amyloidosis.

AF amyloidosis: AF is caused by inheritance of a gene encoding a mutated aggregation-prone serum protein, usually a protein abundantly produced by the liver. Serum proteins that can cause AF include transthyretin (TTR), apolipoprotein A-I and A-II, lysozyme, fibrinogen, gelsolin, and cystatin C. A recently identified form that is speculated to be familial is caused by the serum protein leukocyte chemotactic factor 2 (LECT2); however, a specific inherited gene mutation for this latter type has not been clearly demonstrated.

Amyloidosis caused by TTR (ATTR) is the most common type of AF. More than 100 mutations of the *TTR* gene have been associated with amyloidosis. The most prevalent mutation, *V30M*, is common in Portugal, Sweden, Brazil, and Japan, and a *V122I* mutation is present in about 4% of American blacks. Disease penetrance and age of onset are highly variable but are consistent within families and ethnic groups. ATTR causes peripheral sensory and autonomic neuropathy and cardiomyopathy. Carpal tunnel syndrome commonly precedes other neurologic disease manifestations. Vitreous deposits may develop due to production of mutant TTR by the retinal epithelium, or leptomeningeal deposits may develop if the choroid plexus produces mutant TTR.

ATTRwt amyloidosis: ATTRwt is caused by aggregation and deposition of wild-type TTR, clinically targeting the heart. ATTRwt is increasingly recognized as a cause of infiltrative cardiomyopathy in older men. The genetic and epigenetic factors leading to ATTRwt are unknown. Because ATTRwt and AL amyloidosis both can cause cardiomyopathy, and because amyloidogenic monoclonal gammopathies may be present in patients in this age group, it is essential to accurately type the amyloid so that patients with ATTRwt are not inappropriately treated with chemotherapy (which is used for AL).

AA amyloidosis: This form can occur secondary to several infectious, inflammatory, and malignant conditions and is caused by aggregation of isoforms of the acute-phase reactant serum amyloid A. Common causative infections include TB, bronchiectasis, osteomyelitis, and leprosy. Predisposing inflammatory conditions include RA, juvenile idiopathic arthritis, Crohn disease, inherited periodic fever syndromes such as familial Mediterranean fever, and Castleman disease. Inflammatory cytokines (eg, IL-1, tumor necrosis factor, IL-6) that are produced in these disorders or ectopically by tumor cells cause increased hepatic synthesis of serum amyloid A.

AA shows a predilection for the spleen, liver, kidneys, adrenal glands, and lymph nodes. Involvement of the heart and peripheral or autonomic nerves occurs late in the disease course.

Localized amyloidosis: Localized amyloidosis outside the brain is most frequently caused by deposits of clonal immunoglobulin light chains and within the brain by amyloid beta protein. Localized amyloid deposits typically involve the airways and lung tissue, bladder and ureters, skin, breasts, and eyes. Rarely, other locally produced proteins cause amyloidosis, such as keratin isoforms that can form deposits locally in the skin.

Amyloid beta protein deposits in the brain contribute to Alzheimer disease or cerebrovascular amyloid angiopathy. Other proteins produced in the CNS can misfold, aggregate, and damage neurons, leading to neurodegenerative diseases (eg, Parkinson disease, Huntington disease). Clonal immunoglobulin light chains produced by mucosal-associated lymphoid tissue in the GI tract, airways, and bladder can lead to localized AL in those organs.

Symptoms and Signs

Symptoms and signs of systemic amyloidosis are nonspecific, often resulting in delays in diagnosis. Suspicion of amyloidosis should be increased in patients with a progressive multisystem disease process.

Renal amyloid deposits typically occur in the glomerular membrane leading to proteinuria, but in about 15% of cases the tubules are affected, causing azotemia with minimal proteinuria. These processes can progress to nephrotic syndrome with marked hypoalbuminemia, edema, and anasarca or to end-stage renal disease.

Hepatic involvement causes painless hepatomegaly, which may be massive. Liver function tests typically suggest intrahepatic cholestasis with elevation of alkaline phosphatase and later bilirubin, although jaundice is rare. Occasionally, portal hypertension develops, with resulting esophageal varices and ascites.

Airway involvement leads to dyspnea, wheezing, hemoptysis, or airway obstruction.

Infiltration of the myocardium causes a restrictive cardiomyopathy, eventually leading to diastolic dysfunction and heart failure; heart block or arrhythmia may occur. Hypotension is common.

Peripheral neuropathy with paresthesias of the toes and fingers is a common presenting manifestation in AL and ATTR amyloidoses. Autonomic neuropathy may cause orthostatic hypotension, erectile dysfunction, sweating abnormalities, and GI motility disturbances.

Cerebrovascular amyloid angiopathy most often causes spontaneous lobar cerebral hemorrhage but some patients have brief, transient neurologic symptoms.

GI amyloid may cause motility abnormalities of the esophagus and small and large intestines. Gastric atony, malabsorption, bleeding, or pseudo-obstruction may also occur. Macroglossia is common in AL amyloidosis.

Amyloidosis of the thyroid gland may cause a firm, symmetric, nontender goiter resembling that found in Hashimoto thyroiditis. Other endocrinopathies can also occur.

Lung involvement (mostly in AL amyloidosis) can be characterized by focal pulmonary nodules, tracheobronchial lesions, or diffuse alveolar deposits.

Amyloid vitreous opacities and bilateral scalloped pupillary margins develop in several hereditary amyloidoses.

Other manifestations include bruising, including bruising around the eyes (raccoon eyes), which is caused by amyloid deposits in blood vessels. Amyloid deposits cause weakening of the blood vessels, which may rupture after minor trauma, such as sneezing or coughing.

Diagnosis

- Biopsy
- Amyloid typing
- Testing for organ involvement

Diagnosis of amyloidosis is made by demonstration of fibrillar deposits in an involved organ. Aspiration of subcutaneous abdominal fat is positive in about 80% of patients with AL, 50% in AF, but only about 25% of patients with ATTRwt. If the fat biopsy result is negative, a clinically involved organ should be biopsied. Tissue sections are stained with Congo red dye and examined with a polarizing microscope for characteristic birefringence. Nonbranching 10-nm fibrils can also be recognized by electron microscopy on biopsy specimens from heart or kidneys.

Amyloid typing: After amyloidosis has been confirmed by biopsy, the type is determined using a variety of techniques. For some types of amyloidosis, immunohistochemistry or immunofluorescence may be diagnostic, but false-positive typing results occur. Other useful techniques include gene sequencing for AF, and biochemical identification by mass spectrometry.

If AL is suspected, patients should be evaluated for an underlying plasma cell disorder using quantitative measurement of serum free immunoglobulin light chains, qualitative detection of serum or urine monoclonal light chains using immunofixation electrophoresis (serum protein electrophoresis and urine protein electrophoresis are insensitive in patients with AL), and a bone marrow biopsy with flow cytometry or immunohistochemistry to establish plasma cell clonality. Patients with > 10% clonal plasma cells should be tested to see if they meet criteria for multiple myeloma, including screening for lytic bone lesions, anemia, renal insufficiency, and hypercalcemia.

Organ involvement: Patients are screened for organ involvement beginning with noninvasive testing:

- Kidneys: Urinalysis and measurement of serum BUN and creatinine
- Liver: Liver function tests

- Heart: ECG and measurement of brain (B-type) natriuretic peptide (BNP) or N-terminal-pro-BNP (NT-proBNP) and troponin
- Lungs: Chest x-ray, chest CT, and/or pulmonary function tests

Cardiac involvement can be suggested by low voltage on ECG (caused by a thickened ventricle), and/or dysrhythmias. If cardiac involvement is suspected because of symptoms, ECG, or cardiac biomarkers, echocardiography is done to measure diastolic relaxation and systolic function and to screen for biventricular hypertrophy. In ambiguous cases, cardiac MRI can be done to detect delayed subendocardial gadolinium enhancement, a characteristic finding. Technetium pyrophosphate nuclear imaging is a newly validated, highly sensitive and specific test for ATTR amyloid cardiomyopathy.

Prognosis

Prognosis depends on the type of amyloidosis and the organ system involved, but with appropriate disease-specific and supportive care, many patients have an excellent life expectancy.

AL complicated by severe cardiomyopathy still has the poorest prognosis, with median survival of < 1 yr. Untreated ATTR amyloidosis usually progresses to end-stage cardiac or neurologic disease within 5 to 15 yr. ATTRwt was once thought to have the slowest progression of any systemic amyloidosis involving the heart; however, patients with ATTRwt do progress to symptomatic heart failure and death within a few years of diagnosis.

Prognosis in AA amyloidosis depends largely upon the effectiveness of treatment of the underlying infectious, inflammatory, or malignant disorder.

Treatment

- Supportive care
- Type-specific treatment

Currently, there are specific treatments for most forms of amyloidosis, although some therapies are investigational. For all forms of systemic amyloidosis, supportive care measures can help relieve symptoms and improve quality of life.

Supportive care: Supportive care measures are directed at the affected organ system:

- **Renal:** Patients with nephrotic syndrome and edema should be treated with salt and fluid restriction, and loop diuretics; because of the ongoing protein loss, protein intake should not be restricted. Kidney transplantation is an option when the underlying disease process is controlled, and can provide long-term survival comparable to that in other renal diseases.
- **Cardiac:** Patients with cardiomyopathy should be treated with salt and fluid restriction and loop diuretics. Other drugs for heart failure, including digoxin, ACE inhibitors, calcium channel blockers, and beta-blockers are poorly tolerated and contraindicated. Heart transplantation has been successful in carefully selected patients with AL amyloidosis and severe cardiac involvement. To prevent recurrence in the transplanted heart, patients must be given aggressive chemotherapy directed at clonal plasma cell disorder.
- **GI:** Patients with diarrhea may benefit from loperamide. Those with early satiety and gastric retention may benefit from metoclopramide.
- **Nerves**: In patients with peripheral neuropathy, gabapentin or pregabalin may relieve pain.

Orthostatic hypotension often improves with high doses of midodrine; this drug can cause urinary retention in older males, but supine hypertension is rarely a problem in this population. Support stockings can also help, and fludrocortisone can be used in patients without peripheral edema, anasarca, or heart failure.

Type-specific treatment: For **AL amyloidosis**, prompt initiation of antiplasma cell therapy is essential to preserve organ function and prolong life. Most drugs used for multiple myeloma have been used in AL amyloidosis; choice of drug, dose, and schedule often must be modified when organ function is impaired. Chemotherapy using an alkylating agent (eg, melphalan, cyclophosphamide) combined with corticosteroids was the first regimen to show any benefit. High-dose IV melphalan, combined with autologous stem cell transplantation can be highly effective in selected patients.[1] Proteasome inhibitors (eg, bortezomib) and immunomodulators (eg, lenalidomide) also can be effective. Combination and sequential regimens are being investigated. Localized AL can be treated with low-dose external beam radiation therapy because plasma cells are highly radiosensitive.

For **ATTR amyloidosis,** liver transplantation—which removes the site of synthesis of the mutant protein—can be effective in certain *TTR* mutations with early neuropathy and no heart involvement. Recently, certain drugs have been shown to stabilize TTR in the plasma, preventing misfolding and fibril formation and inhibiting neurologic disease progression while preserving quality of life. These TTR stabilizers include diflunisal, which is widely available, and tafamidis, which is available in Europe, Brazil, and Japan.[2] *TTR* gene silencing using anti-sense RNA or RNA interference to block translation of mRNA into protein effectively reduces serum levels of TTR and is in clinical trials.[3]

For **ATTRwt amyloidosis,** TTR stabilization should also be effective but has not been tested; liver transplantation is not effective for patients with ATTRwt because the amyloidogenic protein is wild-type TTR.

For **AA amyloidosis** caused by familial Mediterranean fever, colchicine 0.6 mg po once/day or bid is effective. Colchicine is not effective in other disorders predisposing to AA amyloidosis. For other AA types, treatment is directed at the underlying infection, inflammatory disease, or cancer. Eprodisate, a sulfonated molecule that alters the stability of AA amyloid deposits, is a promising drug now under study.

1. Sanchorawala V, Sun F, Quillen K, et al: Long-term outcome of patients with AL amyloidosis treated with high-dose melphalan and stem cell transplantation: 20-year experience. *Blood* 126:2345–2347, 2015. doi: 10.1182/blood-2015-08-662726. Epub 2015 Oct 6.
2. Berk JL, Suhr OB, Obici L, et al: Repurposing diflunisal for familial amyloid polyneuropathy: a randomized clinical trial. *JAMA* 310:2658–2667, 2013. doi: 10.1001/jama.2013.283815.
3. Suhr OB, Coelho T, Buades J, et al: Efficacy and safety of patisiran for familial amyloidotic polyneuropathy: a phase II multi-dose study. *Orphanet J Rare Dis* 10:109, 2015. doi: 10.1186/s13023-015-0326-6.

KEY POINTS

- Amyloidosis is a group of disorders in which certain misfolded proteins aggregate into insoluble fibrils that are deposited within organs, causing dysfunction.
- Many different proteins are prone to misfold; some of these proteins are produced by a genetic defect or by certain disease states, while others are immunoglobulin light chains produced by monoclonal plasma cell or other B-cell lymphoproliferative disorders.
- The amyloidogenic protein determines the amyloid type and clinical course of disease, although the clinical manifestations of the different types may overlap.
- Many organs can be affected, but cardiac involvement carries a particularly poor prognosis; amyloid cardiomyopathy typically leads to diastolic dysfunction, heart failure, and heart block and/or arrhythmia.
- Diagnosis is by biopsy; type of amyloidosis is determined by a variety of immunologic, genetic, and biochemical tests.
- Appropriate supportive care will help relieve symptoms and improve quality of life; organ transplantation can help selected patients.
- Treat the underlying process; for AL amyloidosis due to plasma cell or lymphoproliferative disorders, chemotherapy can be highly effective; for secondary AA amyloidosis, anti-infectious and anti-inflammatory therapies can help; for some hereditary AF amyloidosis, small molecule therapies and gene-targeting therapies hold great promise.

164 Carcinoid Tumors

Carcinoid tumors develop from neuroendocrine cells in the GI tract (90%—see p. 58), pancreas, and pulmonary bronchi (see p. 526). More than 95% of all GI carcinoids originate in only 3 sites: the appendix, ileum, and rectum.

Although carcinoids are often benign or only locally invasive, those affecting the ileum and bronchus are frequently malignant.

Carcinoids can be

- Endocrinologically inert
- Endocrinologically active (produce hormones)

The most common endocrinologic syndrome is carcinoid syndrome; however, most patients with carcinoids do not develop carcinoid syndrome. The likelihood that a tumor will be endocrinologically active varies with its site of origin, being highest for tumors originating in the ileum and proximal colon (40 to 50%). The likelihood is lower with bronchial carcinoids, lower still with appendiceal carcinoids, and essentially zero with rectal carcinoids.

Endocrinologically inert carcinoids are suspected because of their symptoms and signs (eg, pain, luminal bleeding, GI obstruction). They can be detected by angiography, CT, or MRI. Small-bowel carcinoids may exhibit filling defects or other abnormalities on barium x-rays. Definitive diagnosis is made histologically after biopsy or resection.

Treatment of nonmetastatic carcinoid tumors is usually surgical resection. The type of surgery depends on the location in the GI tract and the size of the tumor.

Endocrinologically active carcinoids are diagnosed and treated as described for carcinoid syndrome.

CARCINOID SYNDROME

Carcinoid syndrome develops in some people with carcinoid tumors and is characterized by cutaneous flushing, abdominal cramps, and diarrhea. Right-sided valvular heart disease may develop after several years. The syndrome results from vasoactive substances (including serotonin, bradykinin, histamine, prostaglandins, polypeptide hormones) secreted by the tumor, which is typically a metastatic intestinal carcinoid. Diagnosis is clinical and by demonstrating increased urinary 5-hydroxyindoleacetic acid. Tumor localization may require a radionuclide scan or laparotomy. Treatment of symptoms is with the somatostatin analog, octreotide, but surgical removal is done where possible; chemotherapy may be used for malignant tumors.

Etiology

Endocrinologically active tumors of the diffuse peripheral endocrine or paracrine system produce various amines and polypeptides with corresponding symptoms and signs, including carcinoid syndrome. Carcinoid syndrome is usually due to endocrinologically active malignant tumors that develop from neuroendocrine cells (mostly in the ileum) and produce serotonin. It can, however, occur as a result of tumors elsewhere in the GI tract (particularly the appendix and rectum), pancreas, bronchi, or, rarely, the gonads. Rarely, certain highly malignant tumors (eg, oat cell carcinoma of the lung, pancreatic islet cell carcinoma, medullary thyroid carcinoma) are responsible.

An intestinal carcinoid does not usually cause the syndrome unless hepatic metastases have occurred because metabolic products released by the tumor are rapidly destroyed by blood and liver enzymes in the portal circulation (eg, serotonin by hepatic monoamine oxidase). Hepatic metastases, however, release metabolic products via the hepatic veins directly into the systemic circulation. Metabolic products released by primary pulmonary and ovarian carcinoids bypass the portal route and may similarly induce symptoms. Rare intestinal carcinoids with only intra-abdominal spread can drain directly into the systemic circulation or the lymphatics and cause symptoms.

Pathophysiology

Serotonin acts on smooth muscle to cause diarrhea, colic, and malabsorption. Histamine and bradykinin, through their vasodilator effects, cause flushing.

The role of prostaglandins and various polypeptide hormones, which may be produced by paracrine cells, awaits further investigation; elevated human chorionic gonadotropin and pancreatic polypeptide levels are occasionally present with carcinoids.

Some patients develop right-sided endocardial fibrosis, leading to pulmonary stenosis and tricuspid regurgitation. Left heart lesions, which have been reported with bronchial carcinoids, are rare because serotonin is destroyed during passage through the lungs.

Symptoms and Signs

The most common (and often earliest) sign is

- Uncomfortable flushing, typically of the head and neck

Flushing is often precipitated by emotional stress or the ingestion of food, hot beverages, or alcohol.

Striking skin color changes may occur, ranging from pallor or erythema to a violaceous hue. Abdominal cramps with recurrent diarrhea occur and are often the patient's major complaint. Malabsorption syndrome may occur. Patients with valvular lesions may have a heart murmur. A few patients have asthmatic wheezing, and some have decreased libido and erectile dysfunction. Pellagra develops rarely.

Diagnosis

- Urinary 5-hydroxyindoleacetic acid (5-HIAA)

Serotonin-secreting carcinoids are suspected based on their symptoms and signs. Diagnosis is confirmed by demonstrating increased urinary excretion of the serotonin metabolite 5-HIAA. To avoid false-positive results, clinicians do the test after the patient has abstained from serotonin-containing foods (eg, bananas, tomatoes, plums, avocados, pineapples, eggplant, walnuts) for 3 days. Certain drugs, including guaifenesin, methocarbamol, and phenothiazines, also interfere with the test and should be stopped temporarily before testing. On the 3rd day, a 24-h urine sample is collected for assay. Normal excretion of 5-HIAA is < 10 mg/day (< 52 μmol/day); in patients with carcinoid syndrome, excretion is usually > 50 mg/day (> 260 μmol/day).

In the past, provocative tests with calcium gluconate, catecholamines, pentagastrin, or alcohol have been used to induce flushing. Although these tests may be helpful when the diagnosis is in doubt, they are rarely used and must be done with care.

Tumor localization: Localization of the tumor involves angiography, CT, or MRI, the same techniques used to localize a nonfunctioning carcinoid. Localization may require extensive evaluation, sometimes including laparotomy. A scan with radionuclide-labeled somatostatin receptor ligand indium-111 pentetreotide or with iodine-123 metaiodobenzylguanidine may show metastases.

Exclusion of other causes of flushing: Other conditions that manifest with flushing and that could, therefore, be confused with carcinoid syndrome should be excluded. In patients in whom 5-HIAA excretion is not increased, disorders that involve systemic activation of mastocytes (eg, systemic mastocytosis with increased urinary levels of histamine metabolites and increased serum tryptase level) and idiopathic anaphylaxis may be responsible.

Additional causes of flushing include menopause, ethanol ingestion, drugs such as niacin, and certain tumors (eg, vipomas, renal cell carcinoma, medullary thyroid carcinoma).

Prognosis

Prognosis depends on primary site, grade, and stage. Despite metastatic disease, these tumors are slow growing, and survival of 10 to 15 yr is not unusual.

Treatment

- Surgical resection
- Octreotide for symptoms

Surgical resection: Resection of primary lung carcinoids is often curative.

For patients with hepatic metastases, surgical debulking, while not curative, may relieve symptoms and, in certain instances, increase survival. In addition, locoregional therapies for liver metastases could include transarterial chemoembolization (TACE), bland embolization, radioembolization with yttrium-90 microspheres, and radiofrequency ablation. Radiation therapy is unsuccessful, in part because of the poor tolerance of normal hepatic tissue to radiation. No effective chemotherapeutic regimen has been established, but streptozocin with 5-fluorouracil is most widely used, sometimes with doxorubicin.

Symptom relief: Certain symptoms, including flushing, have been relieved by octreotide (which inhibits release of most hormones) without lowering urinary 5-HIAA or gastrin. Numerous studies have suggested good results with octreotide, a long-acting analog of somatostatin. Octreotide is the drug of choice for controlling diarrhea and flushing. Case reports indicate that tamoxifen has been effective infrequently; leukocyte interferon (IFN-α) has temporarily relieved symptoms.

Flushing also can be treated with phenothiazines (eg, prochlorperazine 5 to 10 mg or chlorpromazine 25 to 50 mg po q 6 h). Histamine type 2 (H_2) blockers may also be used. Phentolamine (an alpha-blocker) 5 to 15 mg IV has prevented experimentally induced flushes. Corticosteroids (eg, prednisone 5 mg po q 6 h) may be useful for severe flushing caused by bronchial carcinoids.

Diarrhea may be controlled by codeine 15 mg po q 4 to 6 h, tincture of opium 0.6 mL po q 6 h, loperamide 4 mg po as a loading dose and 2 mg after each loose bowel to a maximum of 16 mg/day, diphenoxylate 5 mg po qid, or peripheral serotonin antagonists such as cyproheptadine 4 to 8 mg po q 6 h.

Niacin and adequate protein intake are needed to prevent pellagra because dietary tryptophan is diverted to serotonin by the tumor. Enzyme inhibitors that prevent the conversion of 5-hydroxytryptophan to serotonin include methyldopa 250 to 500 mg po q 6 h.

KEY POINTS

- Only some carcinoid tumors secrete the substances that cause carcinoid syndrome.
- The main causative substances are serotonin, which causes abdominal cramps and diarrhea, and histamine, which causes flushing.
- Diagnosis is made by detection of the serotonin metabolite 5-HIAA.
- Octreotide may help control symptoms.
- Surgical resection may be curative in the absence of metastases.
- Surgical debulking may help relieve symptoms and possibly prolong survival in patients with hepatic metastases.

165 Diabetes Mellitus and Disorders of Carbohydrate Metabolism

DIABETES MELLITUS

Diabetes mellitus (DM) is impaired insulin secretion and variable degrees of peripheral insulin resistance leading to hyperglycemia. Early symptoms are related to hyperglycemia and include polydipsia, polyphagia, polyuria, and blurred vision. Later complications include vascular disease, peripheral neuropathy, nephropathy, and predisposition to infection. Diagnosis is by measuring plasma glucose. Treatment is diet, exercise, and drugs that reduce glucose levels, including insulin and oral antihyperglycemic drugs. Complications can be delayed or prevented with adequate glycemic control; heart disease remains the leading cause of mortality in DM.

There are 2 main categories of DM—type 1 and type 2, which can be distinguished by a combination of features (see Table 165–1). Terms that describe the age of onset (juvenile or adult) or type of treatment (insulin- or non–insulin-dependent) are no longer accurate because of overlap in age groups and treatments between disease types.

Impaired glucose regulation (impaired glucose tolerance, or impaired fasting glucose—see Table 165–2) is an intermediate, possibly transitional, state between normal glucose metabolism and DM that becomes more common with aging. It is a significant risk factor for DM and may be present for many years before onset of DM. It is associated with an increased risk of cardiovascular disease, but typical diabetic microvascular complications are not very common (albuminuria and/or retinopathy develop in 6 to 10%).

Complications: Years of poorly controlled hyperglycemia lead to multiple, primarily vascular complications that affect small vessels (microvascular), large vessels (macrovascular), or both. (For additional detail, see p.1260.)

Microvascular disease underlies 3 common and devastating manifestations of DM:

- Retinopathy
- Nephropathy
- Neuropathy

Microvascular disease may also impair skin healing, so that even minor breaks in skin integrity can develop into deeper ulcers and easily become infected, particularly in the lower extremities. Intensive control of plasma glucose can prevent or delay many of these complications but may not reverse them once established.

Macrovascular disease involves atherosclerosis of large vessels, which can lead to

- Angina pectoris and myocardial infarction
- Transient ischemic attacks and strokes
- Peripheral arterial disease

Immune dysfunction is another major complication and develops from the direct effects of hyperglycemia on cellular immunity. Patients with DM are particularly susceptible to bacterial and fungal infections.

Table 165–1. GENERAL CHARACTERISTICS OF TYPES 1 AND 2 DIABETES MELLITUS

CHARACTERISTIC	TYPE 1	TYPE 2
Age at onset	Most commonly < 30 yr	Most commonly > 30 yr
Associated obesity	Uncommon	Very common
Propensity to ketoacidosis requiring insulin treatment for control	Yes	No
Plasma levels of endogenous insulin	Extremely low to undetectable	Variable; may be low, normal, or elevated depending on degree of insulin resistance and insulin secretory defect
Twin concordance	≤ 50%	> 90%
Associated with specific HLA-D antigens	Yes	No
Pancreatic autoantibodies at diagnosis	Yes, but may be absent	No
Islet pathology	Insulitis, selective loss of most beta cells	Smaller, normal-appearing islets; amyloid (amylin) deposition common
Prone to develop diabetic complications (retinopathy, nephropathy, neuropathy, atherosclerotic cardiovascular disease)	Yes	Yes
Hyperglycemia responds to oral antihyperglycemic drugs	No	Yes, initially in many patients

Table 165–2. DIAGNOSTIC CRITERIA FOR DIABETES MELLITUS AND IMPAIRED GLUCOSE REGULATION*

TEST	NORMAL	IMPAIRED GLUCOSE REGULATION	DIABETES
FPG (mg/dL [mmol/L])	< 100 (< 5.6)	100–125 (5.6–6.9)	≥ 126 (≥ 7.0)
OGTT (mg/dL [mmol/L])	< 140 (< 7.7)	140–199 (7.7–11.0)	≥ 200 (≥ 11.1)
HbA_{1C} (%)	< 5.7	5.7–6.4	≥ 6.5

*See also American Diabetes Association: Standards of Medical Care in Diabetes. *Diabetes Care* 39:Supplement 1:S1–S119, 2016.
FPG = fasting plasma glucose; HbA_{1C} = glycosylated Hb; OGTT = oral glucose tolerance test, 2-h glucose level.

Etiology

Type 1 diabetes:

- Insulin production absent because of autoimmune pancreatic beta-cell destruction

In type 1 DM (previously called juvenile-onset or insulin-dependent), insulin production is absent because of autoimmune pancreatic beta-cell destruction possibly triggered by an environmental exposure in genetically susceptible people. Destruction progresses subclinically over months or years until beta-cell mass decreases to the point that insulinconcentrations are no longer adequate to control plasma glucose levels. Type 1 DM generally develops in childhood or adolescence and until recently was the most common form diagnosed before age 30; however, it can also develop in adults (latent autoimmune diabetes of adulthood, which often initially appears to be type 2 DM). Some cases of type 1 DM, particularly in nonwhite populations, do not appear to be autoimmune in nature and are considered idiopathic. Type 1 accounts for < 10% of all cases of DM.

The pathogenesis of the autoimmune beta-cell destruction involves incompletely understood interactions between susceptibility genes, autoantigens, and environmental factors.

Susceptibility genes include those within the major histocompatibility complex (MHC)—especially HLA-DR3, DQB1*0201 and HLA-DR4,DQB1*0302, which are present in > 90% of patients with type 1 DM—and those outside the MHC, which seem to regulate insulinproduction and processing and confer risk of DM in concert with MHC genes. Susceptibility genes are more common among some populations than among others and explain the higher prevalence of type 1 DM in some ethnic groups (Scandinavians, Sardinians).

Autoantigens include glutamic acid decarboxylase, insulin, proinsulin, insulinoma-associated protein, zinc transporter ZnT8, and other proteins in beta cells. It is thought that these proteins are exposed or released during normal beta-cell turnover or beta-cell injury (eg, due to infection), activating primarily a T cell–mediated immune response resulting in beta-cell destruction (insulitis). Glucagon-secreting alpha cells remain unharmed. Antibodies to autoantigens, which can be detected in serum, seem to be a response to (not a cause of) beta-cell destruction.

Several **viruses** (including coxsackievirus, rubella virus, cytomegalovirus, Epstein-Barr virus, and retroviruses) have been linked to the onset of type 1 DM. Viruses may directly infect and destroy beta cells, or they may cause beta-cell destruction indirectly by exposing autoantigens, activating autoreactive lymphocytes, mimicking molecular sequences of autoantigens that stimulate an immune response (molecular mimicry), or other mechanisms.

Diet may also be a factor. Exposure of infants to dairy products (especially cow's milk and the milk protein beta casein), high nitrates in drinking water, and low vitamin D consumption have been linked to increased risk of type 1 DM. Early (< 4 mo) or late (> 7 mo) exposure to gluten and cereals increases islet cell autoantibody production. Mechanisms for these associations are unclear.

Type 2 diabetes:

- Resistance to insulin

In type 2 DM (previously called adult-onset or non-insulin-dependent), insulin secretion is inadequate because patients have developed resistance to insulin. Hepatic insulin resistance leads to an inability to suppress hepatic glucose production, and peripheral insulin resistance impairs peripheral glucose uptake. This combination gives rise to fasting and postprandial hyperglycemia. Often insulinlevels are very high, especially early in the disease. Later in the course of the disease, insulin production may fall, further exacerbating hyperglycemia.

The disease generally develops in adults and becomes more common with increasing age; up to one third of adults > age 65 have impaired glucose tolerance. In older adults, plasma glucose levels reach higher levels after eating than in younger adults, especially after meals with high carbohydrate loads. Glucose levels also take longer to return to normal, in part because of increased accumulation of visceral and abdominal fat and decreased muscle mass.

Type 2 DM is becoming increasingly common among children as childhood obesity has become epidemic. Over 90% of adults with DM have type 2 disease. There are clear genetic determinants, as evidenced by the high prevalence of the disease within ethnic groups (especially American Indians, Hispanics, and Asians) and in relatives of people with the disease. Although several genetic polymorphisms have been identified over the past several years, no single gene responsible for the most common forms of type 2 DM has been identified.

Pathogenesis is complex and incompletely understood. Hyperglycemia develops when insulin secretion can no longer compensate for insulin resistance. Although insulin resistance is characteristic in people with type 2 DM and those at risk of it, evidence also exists for beta-cell dysfunction and impaired insulin secretion, including impaired first-phase insulin secretion in response to IV glucose infusion, a loss of normally pulsatile insulin secretion, an increase in proinsulin secretion signaling impaired insulin processing, and an accumulation of islet amyloid polypeptide (a protein normally secreted with insulin). Hyperglycemia itself may impair insulin secretion, because high glucose levels desensitize beta cells, cause beta-cell dysfunction (glucose toxicity), or both. These changes typically take years to develop in the presence of insulin resistance.

Obesity and weight gain are important determinants of insulin resistance in type 2 DM. They have some genetic determinants but also reflect diet, exercise, and lifestyle. An inability to suppress lipolysis in adipose tissue increases plasma levels of free fatty acids that may impair insulin-stimulated glucose transport and muscle glycogen synthase activity. Adipose tissue also appears to function as an endocrine organ, releasing multiple factors (adipocytokines) that favorably (adiponectin) and adversely (tumor necrosis factor-alpha, IL-6, leptin, resistin) influence glucose metabolism. Intrauterine growth restriction and low birth weight have also been associated with insulin resistance in later life and may reflect adverse prenatal environmental influences on glucose metabolism.

Miscellaneous types of diabetes: Miscellaneous causes of DM that account for a small proportion of cases include genetic defects affecting beta-cell function, insulin action, and mitochondrial DNA (eg, maturity-onset diabetes of youth); pancreatic diseases (eg, cystic fibrosis, pancreatitis, hemochromatosis, pancreatectomy); endocrinopathies (eg, Cushing syndrome, acromegaly); toxins (eg, the rodenticide pyriminyl [Vacor]); and drug-induced diabetes, most notably due to glucocorticoids, beta-blockers, protease inhibitors, and therapeutic doses of niacin. Pregnancy causes some insulin resistance in all women, but only a few develop gestational diabetes.

Symptoms and Signs

The most common symptoms of DM are those of hyperglycemia. The mild hyperglycemia of early DM is often asymptomatic; therefore, diagnosis may be delayed for many years. More significant hyperglycemia causes glycosuria and thus an osmotic diuresis, leading to urinary frequency, polyuria, and polydipsia that may progress to orthostatic hypotension and dehydration. Severe dehydration causes weakness, fatigue, and mental status changes. Symptoms may come and go as plasma glucose levels fluctuate. Polyphagia may accompany symptoms of hyperglycemia but is not typically a primary patient concern. Hyperglycemia can also cause weight loss, nausea and vomiting, and blurred vision, and it may predispose to bacterial or fungal infections.

Patients with type 1 DM typically present with symptomatic hyperglycemia and sometimes with DKA. Some patients experience a long but transient phase of near-normal glucose levels after acute onset of the disease (honeymoon phase) due to partial recovery of insulin secretion.

Patients with type 2 DM may present with symptomatic hyperglycemia but are often asymptomatic, and their condition is detected only during routine testing. In some patients, initial symptoms are those of diabetic complications, suggesting that the disease has been present for some time. In some patients, hyperosmolar hyperglycemic state occurs initially, especially during a period of stress or when glucose metabolism is further impaired by drugs, such as corticosteroids.

Diagnosis

- Fasting plasma glucose (FPG) levels
- Glycosylated Hb (HbA_{1C})
- Sometimes oral glucose tolerance testing

DM is indicated by typical symptoms and signs and confirmed by measurement of plasma glucose.[1] Measurement after an 8- to 12-h fast (FPG) or 2 h after ingestion of a concentrated glucose solution (oral glucose tolerance testing [OGTT]) is best (see Table 165–2). OGTT is more sensitive for diagnosing DM and impaired glucose tolerance but is less convenient and reproducible than FPG. It is therefore rarely used routinely, except for diagnosing gestational diabetes and for research purposes.

In practice, DM or impaired fasting glucose regulation is often diagnosed using random measures of plasma glucose or of HbA_{1C}. A random glucose value > 200 mg/dL (> 11.1 mmol/L) may be diagnostic, but values can be affected by recent meals and must be confirmed by repeat testing; testing twice may not be necessary in the presence of symptoms of diabetes.

HbA_{1C} measurements reflect glucose levels over the preceding 3 mo. HbA_{1C} measurements are now included in the diagnostic criteria for DM:

- $HbA_{1C} \geq 6.5\%$ = DM
- HbA_{1C} 5.7 to 6.4% = prediabetes or at risk of DM

However, HbA_{1C} values may be falsely high or low (see Monitoring on p. 1257), and tests must be done in a certified clinical laboratory with an assay that is certified and standardized to a reference assay. Point-of-care HbA_{1C} measurements should not be used for diagnostic purposes, although they can be used for monitoring DM control.

Urine glucose measurement, once commonly used, is no longer used for diagnosis or monitoring because it is neither sensitive nor specific.

PEARLS & PITFALLS

- Point-of-care HbA_{1C} tests are not accurate enough to be used for initial diagnosis of diabetes.

Screening for disease: Screening for DM should be conducted for people at risk of the disease. Patients *with* DM are screened for complications.

People at high risk of type 1 DM (eg, siblings and children of people with type 1 DM) can be tested for the presence of islet cell or anti-glutamic acid decarboxylase antibodies, which precede onset of clinical disease. However, there are no proven preventive strategies for people at high risk, so such screening is usually reserved for research settings.

Risk factors for type 2 diabetes include

- Age ≥ 45
- Overweight or obesity
- Sedentary lifestyle
- Family history of DM
- History of impaired glucose regulation
- Gestational DM or delivery of a baby > 4.1 kg
- History of hypertension
- Dyslipidemia (HDL cholesterol < 35 mg/dL or triglyceride level > 250 mg/dL)
- History of cardiovascular disease
- Polycystic ovary syndrome
- Black, Hispanic, Asian American, or American Indian ethnicity

People ≥ age 45 and all adults with additional risk factors described above should be screened for DM with an FPG level, HbA_{1C}, or a 2-h value on a 75-g OGTT at least once every 3 yr as long as plasma glucose measurements are normal and at least annually if results reveal impaired fasting glucose levels (see Table 165–2).

Screening for complications: All patients with type 1 DM should begin screening for diabetic complications 5 yr after diagnosis. For patients with type 2 DM, screening begins at diagnosis. Typical screening for complications includes

- Foot examination
- Funduscopic examination
- Urine testing for albuminuria
- Measurement of serum creatinine and lipid profile

Foot examination should be done at least annually for impaired sense of pressure, vibration, pain, or temperature, which is characteristic of peripheral neuropathy. Pressure sense is best tested with a monofilament esthesiometer (see Fig. 165–1).

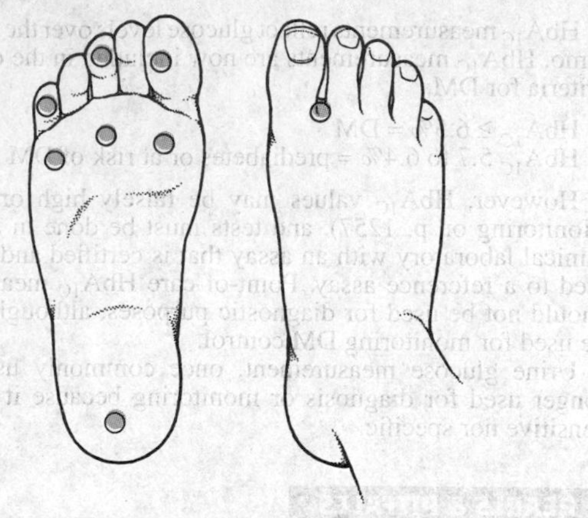

Fig. 165–1. Diabetic foot screening. A 10-g monofilament esthesiometer is touched to specific sites on each foot and is pushed until it bends. This test provides a constant, reproducible pressure stimulus (usually a 10-g force), which can be used to monitor change in sensation over time. Both feet are tested, and presence (+) or absence (–) of sensation at each site is recorded.

The entire foot, and especially skin beneath the metatarsal heads, should be examined for skin cracking and signs of ischemia, such as ulcerations, gangrene, fungal nail infections, deceased pulses, and hair loss.

Funduscopic examination should be done by an ophthalmologist; the screening interval is typically annually for patients with any retinopathy to every 2 yr for those without retinopathy on a prior examination. If retinopathy shows progression, more frequent evaluation may be needed.

Spot or 24-h urine testing is indicated annually to detect albuminuria, and serum creatinine should be measured annually to assess renal function.

Many physicians consider baseline ECG important given the risk of heart disease. Lipid profile should be checked at least annually and more often when abnormalities are present. Blood pressure should be measured at every examination.

1. American Diabetes Association: Standards of Medical Care in Diabetes. *Diabetes Care* 39:Supplement 1: S1–S119 , 2016.

Treatment

- Diet and exercise
- For type 1 DM, insulin
- For type 2 DM, oral antihyperglycemics, injectable glucagon-like peptide-1 (GLP-1) receptor agonists, insulin, or a combination
- To prevent complications, often renin-angiotensin-aldosterone system blockers (ACE inhibitors or angiotensin II receptor blockers), statins, and aspirin

Treatment of DM involves both lifestyle changes and drugs. Patients with type 1 diabetes require insulin. Some patients with type 2 diabetes may be able to avoid or cease drug treatment if they are able to maintain plasma glucose levels with diet and exercise alone. For detailed discussion, see Drug Treatment of Diabetes on p. 1261.

Goals and methods: Treatment involves control of hyperglycemia to relieve symptoms and prevent complications while minimizing hypoglycemic episodes.

Goals for glycemic control are

- Preprandial blood glucose between 80 and 130 mg/dL (4.4 and 7.2 mmol/L)
- Peak postprandial (1 to 2 h after beginning of the meal) blood glucose < 180 mg/dL (10 mmol/L)
- HbA_{1C} levels < 7%

Glucose levels are typically determined by home monitoring of capillary blood glucose (eg, from a fingerstick) and maintenance of HbA_{1C} levels < 7%. These goals may be adjusted for patients in whom strict glucose control may be inadvisable, such as the frail elderly; patients with a short life expectancy; patients who experience repeated bouts of hypoglycemia, especially with hypoglycemic unawareness; and patients who cannot communicate the presence of hypoglycemia symptoms (eg, young children, patients with dementia). Conversely, providers may recommend stricter HbA_{1C} goals (< 6.5%) in select patients if these goals can be achieved without hypoglycemia. Potential candidates for tighter glycemic control include patients not being treated with drugs that induce hypoglycemia, those who have short duration of DM, those who have a long life expectancy, and who have no cardiovascular disease.

Key elements for all patients are patient education, dietary and exercise counseling, and monitoring of glucose control.

All patients with type 1 DM require insulin therapy.

Patients with type 2 DM and mildly elevated plasma glucose should be prescribed a trial of diet and exercise, followed by an oral antihyperglycemic drug if lifestyle changes are insufficient, additional oral drugs and/or GLP-1 receptor agonist as needed (combination therapy), and insulin when combination therapy is ineffective for meeting recommended goals. Metformin is usually the first oral drug used, although no evidence supports the use of a particular drug or class of drugs; the decision often involves consideration of adverse effects, convenience, and patient preference.

Patients with type 2 DM and more significant glucose elevations at diagnosis are typically prescribed lifestyle changes and one or more antihyperglycemic drugs simultaneously.

Insulin is indicated as initial therapy for women with type 2 DM who are pregnant and for patients who present with acute metabolic decompensation, such as hyperosmolar hyperglycemic state (HHS) or DKA. Patients with severe hyperglycemia (plasma glucose > 400 mg/dL [22,2 mmol/L]) may respond better to therapy after glucose levels are normalized with a brief period of insulin treatment.

Patients with impaired glucose regulation should receive counseling addressing their risk of developing DM and the importance of lifestyle changes for preventing DM. They should be monitored closely for development of DM symptoms or elevated plasma glucose. Ideal follow-up intervals have not been determined, but annual or biannual checks are probably appropriate.

Patient education: Education about causes of DM, diet, exercise, drugs, self-monitoring with fingerstick testing, and the symptoms and signs of hypoglycemia, hyperglycemia, and diabetic complications is crucial to optimizing care. Most patients with type 1 DM can also be taught how to adjust their insulin doses. Education should be reinforced at every physician visit and hospitalization. Formal diabetes education programs, generally conducted by diabetes nurses, and nutrition specialists, are often very effective.

Diet: Adjusting diet to individual circumstances can help patients control fluctuations in their glucose level and, for patients with type 2 DM, lose weight.

In general, all patients with DM need to be educated about a diet that is low in saturated fat and cholesterol and contains moderate amounts of carbohydrate, preferably from whole grain sources with higher fiber content. Although dietary protein and fat contribute to caloric intake (and thus, weight gain or loss), only carbohydrates have a direct effect on blood glucose levels. A low-carbohydrate, high-fat diet improves glucose control for some patients and can be used for a short time, but its long-term safety is uncertain.

Patients with type 1 DM should use carbohydrate counting or the carbohydrate exchange system to match insulin dose to carbohydrate intake and facilitate physiologic insulin replacement. "Counting" the amount of carbohydrate in the meal is used to calculate the preprandial insulin dose. For example, if a carbohydrate-to-insulin ratio (CIR) of 15 gram:1 unit is used, a patient will require 1 unit of rapid-acting insulin for each 15 g of carbohydrate in a meal. These ratios can vary significantly between patients, depending on their degree of insulin sensitivity and must be tailored to the patient. This approach requires detailed patient education and is most successful when guided by a dietitian experienced in working with patients with diabetes. Some experts have advised use of the glycemic index (a measure of the impact of an ingested carbohydrate-containing food on the blood glucose level) to delineate between rapid and slowly metabolized carbohydrates, although there is little evidence to support this approach.

Patients with type 2 DM should restrict calories, eat regularly, increase fiber intake, and limit intake of refined carbohydrates and saturated fats. Nutrition consultation should complement physician counseling; the patient and the person who prepares the patient's meals should both be present.

Exercise: Physical activity should increase incrementally to whatever level a patient can tolerate. Both aerobic exercise and resistance exercise have been shown to improve glycemic control in type 2 diabetes, and several studies have shown a combination of resistance and aerobic exercise to be superior to either alone.

Patients who experience hypoglycemic symptoms during exercise should be advised to test their blood glucose and ingest carbohydrates or lower their insulin dose as needed to get their glucose slightly above normal just before exercise. Hypoglycemia during vigorous exercise may require carbohydrate ingestion during the workout period, typically 5 to 15 g of sucrose or another simple sugar.

Patients with known or suspected cardiovascular disease may benefit from exercise stress testing before beginning an exercise program. Activity goals may need to be modified for patients with complications of diabetes such as neuropathy and retinopathy.

Weight loss: Weight loss drugs, including orlistat, lorcaserin, phentermine/topiramate, and naltrexone/bupropion may be useful in selected patients as part of a comprehensive weight loss program, although lorcaserin may be used only short term. Orlistat, an intestinal lipase inhibitor, reduces dietary fat absorption; it reduces serum lipids and helps promote weight loss. Lorcaserin is a selective serotonin receptor agonist that causes satiety and thus reduces food intake. Phentermine/topiramate is a combination drug that reduces appetite through multiple mechanisms in the brain. Many of these drugs also have been shown to significantly decrease HbA_{1C} a.

Surgical treatment for obesity, such as gastric banding, sleeve gastrectomy, or gastric bypass, also leads to weight loss and improved glucose control (independent of weight loss) in patients who have DM and are unable to lose weight through other means.

Foot care: Regular professional podiatric care, including trimming of toenails and calluses, is important for patients with sensory loss or circulatory impairment. Such patients should be advised to inspect their feet daily for cracks, fissures, calluses, corns, and ulcers. Feet should be washed daily in lukewarm water, using mild soap, and dried gently and thoroughly. A lubricant (eg, lanolin) should be applied to dry, scaly skin. Nonmedicated foot powders should be applied to moist feet. Toenails should be cut, preferably by a podiatrist, straight across and not too close to the skin. Adhesive plasters and tape, harsh chemicals, corn cures, water bottles, and electric pads should not be used on skin. Patients should change stockings daily and not wear constricting clothing (eg, garters, socks or stockings with tight elastic tops).

Shoes should fit well, be wide-toed without open heels or toes, and be changed frequently. Special shoes should be prescribed to reduce trauma if the foot is deformed (eg, previous toe amputation, hammer toe, bunion). Walking barefoot should be avoided.

Patients with neuropathic foot ulcers should avoid weight bearing until ulcers heal. If they cannot, they should wear appropriate orthotic protection. Because most patients with these ulcers have little or no macrovascular occlusive disease, debridement and antibiotics frequently result in good healing and may prevent major surgery. After the ulcer has healed, appropriate inserts or special shoes should be prescribed. In refractory cases, especially if osteomyelitis is present, surgical removal of the metatarsal head (the source of pressure) or amputation of the involved toe or transmetatarsal amputation may be required. A neuropathic joint can often be satisfactorily managed with orthopedic devices (eg, short leg braces, molded shoes, sponge-rubber arch supports, crutches, prostheses).

Vaccination: All patients with DM should be vaccinated against *Streptococcus pneumoniae* (once) and influenza virus (annually).

Monitoring: DM control can be monitored by measuring blood levels of

- Glucose
- HbA_{1C}
- Fructosamine

Self-monitoring of whole blood glucose using fingertip blood, test strips, and a glucose meter is most important. It should be used to help patients adjust dietary intake and insulin dosing and to help physicians recommend adjustments in the timing and doses of drugs.

Many different monitoring devices are available. Nearly all require test strips and a means for pricking the skin and obtaining a blood sample. Most come with control solutions, which should be used periodically to verify proper meter calibration. Choice among devices is usually based on patient preferences for features such as time to results (usually 5 to 30 sec), size of display panel (large screens may benefit patients with poor eyesight), and need for calibration. Meters that allow for testing at sites less painful than fingertips (palm, forearm, upper arm, abdomen, thigh) are also available.

Continuous glucose monitoring systems using a subcutaneous catheter can provide real-time results, including an alarm to warn of hypoglycemia, hyperglycemia, or rapidly changing glucose levels. Such devices are expensive and do not eliminate the need for daily fingerstick glucose testing, but they may be useful for selected patients (eg, those with hypoglycemia unawareness or nocturnal hypoglycemia).

Patients with poor glucose control and those given a new drug or a new dose of a currently used drug may be asked to self-monitor 1 (usually morning fasting) to ≥ 5 times/day, depending on the patient's needs and abilities and the complexity of the treatment regimen. Most patients with type 1 DM benefit from testing at least 4 times/day.

HbA_{1C} levels reflect glucose control over the preceding 3 mo and hence assess control between physician visits. HbA_{1C} should be assessed quarterly in patients with type 1 DM and at least twice per year in patients with type 2 DM when plasma glucose appears stable and more frequently when control is uncertain. Home testing kits are useful for patients who are able to follow the testing instructions rigorously.

Control suggested by HbA_{1C} values sometimes appears to differ from that suggested by daily glucose readings because of falsely elevated or normal values. False elevations may occur with low RBC turnover (as occurs with iron, folate, or vitamin B_{12} deficiency anemia), high-dose aspirin, and high blood alcohol concentrations. Falsely normal values occur with increased RBC turnover, as occurs with hemolytic anemias and hemoglobinopathies (eg, HbS, HbC) or during treatment of deficiency anemias. In patients with chronic kidney disease stages 4 and 5, correlation between HbA_{1C} and glycemic levels is poor and HbA_{1C} can be falsely decreased in these populations.

Fructosamine, which is mostly glycosylated albumin but also comprises other glycosylated proteins, reflects glucose control in the previous 1 to 2 wk. Fructosamine monitoring may be used during intensive treatment of DM and for patients with Hb variants or high RBC turnover (which cause false HbA_{1C} results), but it is mainly used in research settings.

Urine glucose monitoring provides a crude indication of hyperglycemia and can be recommended only when blood glucose monitoring is impossible. By contrast, self-measurement of urine ketones is recommended for patients with type 1 DM if they experience symptoms, signs, or triggers of ketoacidosis, such as nausea or vomiting, abdominal pain, fever, cold or flu-like symptoms, or unusual sustained hyperglycemia (> 250 to 300 mg/dL [13.9 to 16.7 mmol/L]) during glucose self-monitoring.

Pancreas transplantation: Pancreas transplantation and transplantation of pancreatic islet cellsare alternative means of insulindelivery; both techniques effectively transplant insulin-producing beta-cells into insulin-deficient (type 1) patients. Indications, tissue sources, procedures, and limitations of both procedures are discussed elsewhere.

Special Populations and Settings

The term brittle diabetes has been used to refer to patients who have dramatic, recurrent swings in glucose levels, often for no apparent reason. However, this concept has no biologic basis and should not be used. Labile plasma glucose levels are more likely to occur in patients with type 1 DM because endogenous insulin production is completely absent, and in some patients, counter-regulatory response to hypoglycemia is impaired. Other causes include occult infection, gastroparesis (which leads to erratic absorption of dietary carbohydrates), and endocrinopathies (eg, Addison disease).

Patients with chronic difficulty maintaining acceptable glucose levels should be evaluated for situational factors that affect glucose control. Such factors include inadequate patient education or understanding that leads to errors in insulin administration, inappropriate food choices, and psychosocial stress that expresses itself in erratic patterns of drug use and food intake.

The initial approach is to thoroughly review self-care techniques, including insulin preparation and injection and glucose testing. Increased frequency of self-testing may reveal previously unrecognized patterns and provides the patient with helpful feedback. A thorough dietary history, including timing of meals, should be taken to identify potential contributions to poor control. Underlying disorders should be ruled out by physical examination and appropriate laboratory tests.

For some insulin-treated patients, changing to a more intensive regimen that allows for frequent dose adjustments (based on glucose testing) is helpful. In some cases, the frequency of hypoglycemic and hyperglycemic episodes diminishes over time even without specific treatment, suggesting life circumstances may contribute to causation.

Children: Diabetes in children is discussed in more detail elsewhere.

Children with type 1 DM require physiologic insulinreplacement as do adults, and similar treatment regimens, including insulin pumps, are used. However, the risk of hypoglycemia, because of unpredictable meal and activity patterns and limited ability to report hypoglycemic symptoms, may require modification of treatment goals. Most young children can be taught to actively participate in their own care, including glucose testing and insulininjections. School personnel and other caregivers must be informed about the disease and instructed about the detection and treatment of hypoglycemic episodes. Screening for microvascular complications can generally be deferred until after puberty.

Children with type 2 DM require the same attention to diet and weight control and recognition and management of dyslipidemia and hypertension as do adults. Most children with type 2 DM are obese, so lifestyle modification is the cornerstone of therapy. Children with mild hyperglycemia generally begin treatment with metformin unless they have ketosis, renal insufficiency, or another contraindication to metformin use. Dosage is 500 to 1000 mg bid. If response is insufficient, insulin may be added. Some pediatric specialists also consider using thiazolidinediones, sulfonylureas, GLP1 receptor agonists and dipeptidyl peptidase-4 inhibitors as part of combination therapy.

Adolescents: Diabetes in adolescents is discussed in more detail elsewhere. Glucose control typically deteriorates as children with DM enter adolescence. Multiple factors contribute, including pubertal and insulin-induced weight gain; hormonal changes that decrease insulinsensitivity; psychosocial factors that lead to insulin nonadherence (eg, mood and anxiety disorders); family conflict, rebellion, and peer pressure; eating disorders that lead to insulin omission as a means of controlling weight; and experimentation with cigarette, alcohol, and substance use. For these reasons, some adolescents experience recurrent episodes of hyperglycemia and DKA requiring emergency department visits and hospitalization.

Treatment often involves intensive medical supervision combined with psychosocial interventions (eg, mentoring or support groups), individual or family therapy, and psychopharmacology when indicated. Patient education is important so that adolescents can safely enjoy the freedoms of early adulthood. Rather than judging personal choices and behaviors, providers must continually reinforce the need for careful glycemic control, especially frequent blood sugar monitoring and use of frequent, low-dose, fast-acting insulins as needed.

Hospitalization: DM can be a primary reason for hospitalization or can accompany other illnesses that require inpatient care. All diabetic patients with DKA, HHS, or prolonged or severe hypoglycemia should be hospitalized. Patients with hypoglycemia induced by sulfonylureas, poorly controlled hyperglycemia, or acute worsening of diabetic complications may benefit from brief hospitalization. Children and adolescents with new-onset diabetes may also benefit from hospitalization. Control may worsen on discharge when insulin regimens developed in controlled inpatient settings prove inadequate to the uncontrolled conditions outside the hospital.

When other illnesses mandate hospitalization, some patients can continue on their home diabetes treatment regimens. However, glucose control often proves difficult, and it is often neglected when other diseases are more acute. Restricted physical activity and acute illness worsen hyperglycemia in some patients, whereas dietary restrictions and symptoms that accompany illness (eg, nausea, vomiting, diarrhea, anorexia) precipitate hypoglycemia in others—especially when antihyperglycemic drug doses remain unchanged. In addition, it may be difficult to control glucose adequately in hospitalized patients because usual routines (eg, timing of meals, drugs, and procedures) are inflexibly timed relative to diabetes treatment regimens.

In the inpatient setting, oral antihyperglycemic drugs often need to be stopped. Metformin can cause lactic acidosis in patients with renal insufficiency and has to be stopped if contrast agents need to be given and is, therefore, withheld in all but the most stable hospitalized patients. Sulfonylureas can cause hypoglycemia and should also be stopped. Most patients can be appropriately treated with basal insulin without or with supplemental short-acting insulin. Dipeptidyl peptidase-4 inhibitors are relatively safe, even in patients with kidney disease, and they may also be used for postprandial glucose lowering. Sliding-scale insulin should not be the only intervention to correct hyperglycemia; it is reactive rather than proactive, and no data suggest it leads to outcomes equivalent to or better than other approaches. Longer-acting insulins should be adjusted to prevent hyperglycemia rather than just using short-acting insulins to correct it.

Inpatient hyperglycemia worsens short-term prognosis for many acute conditions, most notably stroke and acute myocardial infarction, and often prolongs hospital stay. Critical illness causes insulin resistance and hyperglycemia even in patients without known DM. Insulin infusion to maintain plasma glucose between 140 and 180 mg/dL (7.8 and 8.3 mmol/L) prevents adverse outcomes such as organ failure, may enhance recovery from stroke, and leads to improved survival in patients requiring prolonged (> 5 days) critical care. Previously, glucose target levels were lower; however, it appears that the less stringent targets as described above may be sufficient to prevent adverse outcomes, particularly in patients who do not have heart disease. Severely ill patients, especially those receiving glucocorticoids or pressors, may need very high doses of insulin (> 5 to 10 units/h) because of insulin resistance. Insulin infusion should also be considered for patients receiving TPN and for patients with type 1 DM who cannot ingest anything orally.

Surgery: The physiologic stress of surgery can increase plasma glucose in patients with DM and induce DKA in those with type 1 DM. For shorter procedures, subcutaneous insulin can be used. In type 1 patients, one half to two thirds of the usual morning dose of intermediate-acting insulin or 70 to 80% of the dose of long-acting insulin (glargine or detemir) can be given the morning before surgery with an IV infusion of a 5% dextrose solution at a rate of 100 to 150 mL/h. During and after surgery, plasma glucose (and ketones if hyperglycemia suggests the need) should be measured at least every 2 h. Glucose infusion is continued, and regular or short-acting insulin is given sc q 4 to 6 h as needed to maintain the plasma glucose level between 100 and 200 mg/dL (5.55 and 11.01 mmol/L) until the patient can be switched to oral feedings and resume the usual insulin regimen. Additional doses of intermediate- or long-acting insulin should be given if there is a substantial delay (> 24 h) in resuming the usual regimen. This approach may also be used for insulin-treated patients with type 2 DM, but frequent measurement of ketones may be omitted.

Some physicians prefer to withhold sc or inhaled insulinon the day of surgery and to give insulin by IV infusion. For patients undergoing a long or major surgery, a continuous insulin infusion is preferable, especially since insulin requirements can increase with the stress of surgery. IV insulin infusion can be given at the same time as intravenous dextrose solution to maintain blood glucose. One approach is to combine glucose, insulin, and K in the same bag (GIK regimen), for example, by combining 10% dextrose with 10 mmol K, and 15 units of insulin in a 500-mL bag. The insulin doses are adjusted in 5-unit increments. This approach is not used at many institutions because of the frequent remixing and changing of bags needed to adjust to the patient's level of glycemia. A more common approach in the US is to infuse insulin and dextrose separately. Insulin can be infused at a rate of 1 to 2 U/h with 5% dextrose infusing at 75 to 150 mL/h. The insulin rate may need to be decreased for more insulin-sensitive type 1 diabetic patients and increased for more insulin-resistant type 2 diabetic patients. 10% dextrose may also be used. It is important, especially in type 1 diabetes not to stop insulin infusion, to avoid development of DKA Insulin adsorption onto IV tubing can lead to inconsistent effects, which can be minimized by preflushing the IV tubing with insulin solution. Insulininfusion is continued through recovery, with insulin adjusted based on the plasma glucose levels obtained in the recovery room and at 1- to 2-h intervals thereafter.

Most patients with type 2 DM who are treated with oral antihyperglycemic drugs maintain acceptable glucose levels when fasting and may not require insulin in the perioperative period. Most oral drugs, including sulfonylureas and metformin, should be withheld on the day of surgery, and plasma glucose levels should be measured preoperatively and postoperatively and every 6 h while patients receive IV fluids. Oral drugs may be resumed when patients are able to eat, but metformin should be withheld until normal renal function is confirmed 48 h after surgery.

Prevention

Type 1 diabetes: No treatments definitely prevent the onset or progression of type 1 DM. Azathioprine, corticosteroids, and cyclosporine induce remission of early type 1 DM in some patients, presumably through suppression of autoimmune beta-cell destruction. However, toxicity and the need for lifelong treatment limit their use. In a few patients, short-term treatment with anti-CD3 monoclonal antibodies reduces insulin requirements for at least the first year of recent-onset disease by suppressing autoimmune T-cell response.

Type 2 diabetes: Type 2 DM usually can be prevented with lifestyle modification. Weight loss of as little as 7% of baseline body weight, combined with moderate-intensity physical activity (eg, walking 30 min/day), may reduce the incidence of DM in high-risk people by > 50%. Metformin and acarbose have also been shown to reduce the risk of DM in patients with impaired glucose regulation. Thiazolidinediones may also be protective. However, further study is needed before thiazolidinediones can be recommended for routine preventive use.

Complications: Risk of complications of diabetes can be decreased by strict control of plasma glucose, defined as HbA_{1C} < 7%, and by control of hypertension and lipid levels. Specific measures for prevention of progression of complications once detected are described under Complications and Treatment on pp. 1256 and 1260.

KEY POINTS

- Type 1 diabetes is caused by an absence of insulin due to autoimmune-mediated inflammation in pancreatic beta cells.
- Type 2 diabetes is caused by hepatic insulin resistance (causing an inability to suppress hepatic glucose production), peripheral insulin resistance (which impairs peripheral glucose uptake) in combination with a beta-cell secretory defect.
- Microvascular complications include nephropathy, neuropathy, and retinopathy.
- Macrovascular complications involve atherosclerosis resulting in coronary artery disease, TIA/stroke, and peripheral arterial insufficiency.
- Diagnose by elevated fasting plasma glucose level and/or elevated HbA_{1C}, and/or 2-h value on OGTT.
- Do regular screening for complications.
- Treat with diet, exercise, and insulin, and/or oral antihyperglycemic drugs.
- Often, give ACE inhibitors, statins, and aspirin to prevent complications.

COMPLICATIONS OF DIABETES MELLITUS

In patients with DM, years of poorly controlled hyperglycemia lead to multiple, primarily vascular, complications that affect small vessels (microvascular), large vessels (macrovascular), or both.

The mechanisms by which vascular disease develops include

- Glycosylation of serum and tissue proteins with formation of advanced glycation end products
- Superoxide production
- Activation of protein kinase C, a signaling molecule that increases vascular permeability and causes endothelial dysfunction
- Accelerated hexosamine biosynthetic and polyol pathways leading to sorbitol accumulation within tissues
- Hypertension and dyslipidemias that commonly accompany DM
- Arterial microthromboses
- Proinflammatory and prothrombotic effects of hyperglycemia and hyperinsulinemia that impair vascular autoregulation

Immune dysfunction is another major complication and develops from the direct effects of hyperglycemia on cellular immunity.

Microvascular disease underlies 3 common and devastating manifestations of DM:

- Retinopathy
- Nephropathy
- Neuropathy

Microvascular disease may also impair skin healing, so that even minor breaks in skin integrity can develop into deeper ulcers and easily become infected, particularly in the lower extremities. Intensive control of plasma glucose can prevent or delay many of these complications but may not reverse them once established.

Macrovascular disease involves atherosclerosis of large vessels, which can lead to

- Angina pectoris and myocardial infarction
- Transient ischemic attacks and strokes
- Peripheral arterial disease

Immune dysfunction is another major complication and develops from the direct effects of hyperglycemia on cellular immunity. Diabetic patients are particularly susceptible to bacterial and fungal infections.

Diabetic Retinopathy

Diabetic retinopathy is the most common cause of adult blindness in the US. It is characterized initially by retinal capillary microaneurysms (background retinopathy) and later by neovascularization (proliferative retinopathy) and macular edema. There are no early symptoms or signs, but focal blurring, vitreous or retinal detachment, and partial or total vision loss eventually develop; rate of progression is highly variable.

Screening and diagnosis are by retinal examination, which should be done regularly (usually annually) in both type 1 and type 2 DM. Early detection and treatment are critical to preventing vision loss. Treatment for all patients includes intensive glycemic and blood pressure control. More advanced retinopathy may require panretinal laser photocoagulation or more rarely vitrectomy. Vascular endothelial growth factor (VEGF) inhibitors are promising new drugs for macular edema and as adjunctive therapy for proliferative retinopathy.

Diabetic Nephropathy

Diabetic nephropathy is a leading cause of chronic kidney disease in the US. It is characterized by thickening of the glomerular basement membrane, mesangial expansion, and glomerular sclerosis. These changes cause glomerular hypertension and progressive decline in GFR. Systemic hypertension may accelerate progression. The disease is usually asymptomatic until nephrotic syndrome or renal failure develops.

Diagnosis is by detection of urinary albumin. Once diabetes is diagnosed (and annually thereafter), urinary albumin level should be monitored so that nephropathy can be detected early. Monitoring can be done by measuring the albumin:creatinine ratio on a spot urine specimen or total urinary albumin in a 24-h collection. A ratio > 30 mg/g or an albumin excretion of 30 to 300 mg/24 h signifies moderately increased albuminuria (previously called microalbuminuria) and early diabetic nephropathy. An albumin excretion > 300 mg/day is considered severely increased albuminuria (previously called macroalbuminuria), or overt proteinuria, and signifies more advanced diabetic nephropathy. Typically a urine dipstick is positive only if the protein excretion exceeds 300 to 500 mg/day.

Treatment is rigorous glycemic control combined with blood pressure control. An ACE inhibitor or an angiotensin II receptor blocker should be used to treat hypertension and, at the earliest sign of albuminuria, to prevent progression of renal disease because these drugs lower intraglomerular blood pressure and thus have renoprotective effects. These drugs have not been shown to be beneficial for primary prevention (ie, in patients who do not have albuminuria).

Diabetic Neuropathy

Diabetic neuropathy is the result of nerve ischemia due to microvascular disease, direct effects of hyperglycemia on neurons, and intracellular metabolic changes that impair nerve function. There are multiple types, including

- Symmetric polyneuropathy (with small- and large-fiber variants)
- Autonomic neuropathy
- Radiculopathy
- Cranial neuropathy
- Mononeuropathy

Symmetric polyneuropathy is most common and affects the distal feet and hands (stocking-glove distribution); it manifests as paresthesias, dysesthesias, or a painless loss of sense of touch, vibration, proprioception, or temperature. In the lower extremities, these symptoms can lead to blunted perception of foot trauma due to ill-fitting shoes and abnormal weight bearing, which can in turn lead to foot ulceration and infection or to fractures, subluxation, and dislocation or destruction of normal foot architecture (Charcot joint). Small-fiber neuropathy is characterized by pain, numbness, and loss of temperature sensation with preserved vibration and position sense. Patients are prone to foot ulceration and neuropathic joint degeneration and have a high incidence of autonomic neuropathy. Predominant large-fiber neuropathy is characterized by muscle weakness, loss of vibration and position sense, and lack of deep tendon reflexes. Atrophy of intrinsic muscles of the feet and foot drop are common.

Autonomic neuropathy can cause orthostatic hypotension, exercise intolerance, resting tachycardia, dysphagia, nausea and vomiting (due to gastroparesis), constipation and diarrhea (including dumping syndrome), fecal incontinence, urinary retention and incontinence, erectile dysfunction and retrograde ejaculation, and decreased vaginal lubrication.

Radiculopathies most often affect the proximal L2 through L4 nerve roots, causing pain, weakness, and atrophy of the lower extremities (diabetic amyotrophy), or the proximal T4 through T12 nerve roots, causing abdominal pain (thoracic polyradiculopathy).

Cranial neuropathies cause diplopia, ptosis, and anisocoria when they affect the 3rd cranial nerve or motor palsies when they affect the 4th or 6th cranial nerve.

Mononeuropathies cause finger weakness and numbness (median nerve) or foot drop (peroneal nerve). Patients with DM are also prone to nerve compression disorders, such as carpal tunnel syndrome. Mononeuropathies can occur in several places simultaneously (mononeuritis multiplex). All tend to affect older patients predominantly and usually abate spontaneously over months; however, nerve compression disorders do not.

Diagnosis of symmetric polyneuropathy is by detection of sensory deficits and diminished ankle reflexes. Loss of ability to detect the light touch of a nylon monofilament identifies patients at highest risk of foot ulceration (see Fig. 165–1). Alternatively, a 128-Hz tuning fork can be used to assess vibratory sense on the dorsum of the first toe.

Electromyography and nerve conduction studies may be needed for all forms of neuropathy and are sometimes used to exclude other causes of neuropathic symptoms, such as nondiabetic radiculopathy and carpal tunnel syndrome.

Management of neuropathy involves a multidimensional approach including glycemic control, regular foot care, and management of pain. Strict glycemic control may lessen neuropathy. Treatments to relieve symptoms include topical capsaicin cream, tricyclic antidepressants (eg, amitriptyline), serotonin-norepinephrine reuptake inhibitors (eg, duloxetine), and anticonvulsants (eg, pregabalin, gabapentin). Patients with sensory loss should examine their feet daily to detect minor foot trauma and prevent it from progressing to limb-threatening infection.

Macrovascular Disease

Large-vessel atherosclerosis is a result of the hyperinsulinemia, dyslipidemias, and hyperglycemia characteristic of DM. Manifestations are

- Angina pectoris and myocardial infarction
- Transient ischemic attacks and strokes
- Peripheral arterial disease

Diagnosis is made by history and physical examination; the role of screening tests, such as coronary calcium score, is evolving. Treatment is rigorous control of atherosclerotic risk factors, including normalization of plasma glucose, lipids, and blood pressure, combined with smoking cessation and daily intake of aspirin and ACE inhibitors. A multifactorial approach that includes management of glycemic control, hypertension, and dyslipidemia may be effective in reducing the rate of cardiovascular events. In contrast with microvascular disease, intensive control of plasma glucose alone has been shown to reduce risk in type 1 diabetes but not in type 2.

Cardiomyopathy

Diabetic cardiomyopathy is thought to result from many factors, including epicardial atherosclerosis, hypertension and left ventricular hypertrophy, microvascular disease, endothelial and autonomic dysfunction, obesity, and metabolic disturbances. Patients develop heart failure due to impairment in left ventricular systolic and diastolic function and are more likely to develop heart failure after myocardial infarction.

Infection

Patients with poorly controlled DM are prone to bacterial and fungal infections because of adverse effects of hyperglycemia on granulocyte and T-cell function. In addition to an overall increase in risk for infectious diseases, individuals with diabetes have an increased susceptibility to mucocutaneous fungal infections (eg, oral and vaginal candidiasis) and bacterial foot infections (including osteomyelitis), which are typically exacerbated by lower extremity vascular insufficiency and diabetic neuropathy. Hyperglycemia is a well-established risk factor for surgical site infections.

Other Complications

Diabetic foot complications (skin changes, ulceration, infection, gangrene) are common and are attributable to vascular disease, neuropathy, and relative immunosuppression.

Patients with DM have an increased risk of developing some rheumatologic diseases, including muscle infarction, carpal tunnel syndrome, Dupuytren contracture, adhesive capsulitis, and sclerodactyly. They may also develop ophthalmologic disease unrelated to diabetic retinopathy (eg, cataracts, glaucoma, corneal abrasions, optic neuropathy); hepatobiliary diseases (eg, nonalcoholic fatty liver disease [steatosis and steatohepatitis], cirrhosis, gallstones); and dermatologic disease (eg, tinea infections, lower-extremity ulcers, diabetic dermopathy, necrobiosis lipoidica diabeticorum, diabetic systemic sclerosis, vitiligo, granuloma annulare, acanthosis nigricans [a sign of insulin resistance—see Plate 27]). Depression and dementia are also common.

DRUG TREATMENT OF DIABETES MELLITUS

General treatment for all patients with DM involves lifestyle changes, including diet and exercise. Regular monitoring of blood glucose levels is essential to prevent complications of diabetes.

Patients with type 1 DM are treated with insulin as well as diet and exercise.

Patients with type 2 DM are often initially treated with diet and exercise. If those measures are not sufficient for glycemic control, patients may be prescribed oral antihyperglycemic drugs, injectable glucagon-like peptide-1 (GLP-1) receptor agonists, insulin, or a combination of these drugs.

For some patients with diabetes, renin-angiotensin-aldosterone system (RAAS) blockers (ACE inhibitors or angiotensin II receptor blockers), statins, and aspirin often are given to prevent complications.

Insulin

Insulin is required for all patients with type 1 DM if they become ketoacidotic without it; it is also helpful for management of many patients with type 2 DM.

Insulin replacement in type 1 DM should ideally mimic beta-cell function using 2 insulin types to provide basal and prandial requirements (physiologic replacement); this approach requires close attention to diet and exercise as well as to insulin timing and dose.

When insulin is needed for patients with type 2 DM, glycemic control can often be achieved with basal insulin combined with non-insulin anti-hyperglycemic drugs, although prandial insulin may be needed in some patients.

Except for use of regular insulin, which is given IV in hospitalized patients, insulin is almost always administered subcutaneously. Recently, an inhaled insulin preparation has also become available.

Most insulin preparations are now recombinant human, practically eliminating the once-common allergic reactions to the drug when it was extracted from animal sources. A number of analogs are available. These analogs were created by modifying the human insulin molecule that alters absorption rates and duration and time to action.

Insulin types are commonly categorized by their time to onset and duration of action (see Table 165–3). However, these parameters vary within and among patients, depending on many factors (eg, site and technique of injection, amount of subcutaneous fat, blood flow at the injection site).

Rapid-acting insulins, including lispro and aspart, are rapidly absorbed because reversal of an amino acid pair prevents the insulin molecule from associating into dimers and polymers. They begin to reduce plasma glucose often within 15 min but have short duration of action (< 4 h). These insulins are best used at mealtime to control postprandial spikes in plasma glucose. Inhaled regular insulin is a newer rapid acting insulin that is taken with meals.

Regular insulin is slightly slower in onset (30 to 60 min) than lispro and aspart but lasts longer (6 to 8 h). It is the only insulin form for IV use.

Neutral protamine Hagedorn (NPH, or insulin isophane) is intermediate-acting; onset of action is about 2 h after injection, peak effect is 4 to 12 h after injection, and duration of action is 18 to 26 h. Concentrated regular insulin U-500 has a similar peak and duration of action (peak 4 to 8 h; duration 13 to 24 h) and can be dosed 2 to 3 times per day.

Long-acting insulins, insulin glargine, insulindetemir, and U-300 insulin glargine, unlike NPH, have no discernible peak of action and provide a steady basal effect over 24 h. Insulin degludec (another long-acting insulin) has an even longer duration of action of over 40 h. It is dosed daily, and although it requires 3 days to achieve steady state, the timing of dosing is less rigid.

Combinations of NPH and regular insulin and of insulin lispro and NPL (neutral protamine lispro or a form of lispro modified to act like NPH) are commercially available in premixed preparations (see Table 165–3). Other premixed formulations include NPA (neutral protamine aspart or a form of

Table 165–3. ONSET, PEAK, AND DURATION OF ACTION OF HUMAN INSULIN PREPARATIONS*

INSULIN PREPARATION	ONSET OF ACTION	PEAK ACTION	DURATION OF ACTION
Rapid-acting			
Lispro, aspart, glulisine†	5–15 min	45–75 min	3–5 h
Inhaled regular	< 15 min	50 min	2–3 h
Short-acting			
Regular†	30–60 min	2–4 h	6–8 h
Intermediate-acting			
NPH‡	About 2 h	4–12 h	18–26 h
U-500 regular	30 min	4–8 h	13–24 h
Long-acting			
Glargine	3–4 h	No peak	24 h
U-300 insulin glargine	6 h	No peak	24 h
Detemir	1–2 h	No peak	14–24 h
Degludec	1–2 h	No peak	> 40 h
Premixed			
70% NPH/30% regular	30–60 min	Dual (NPH & R)	10–16 h
50% NPL/50% lispro	30–60 min	Dual (NPL & lispro)	10–16 h
75% NPL/25% lispro	5–15 min	Dual (NPL & lispro)	10–16 h
70% NPA/30% aspart	5–15 min	Dual (NPA & aspart)	10–16 h
70% degludec/ 30% aspart	15 min	Dual (degludec/aspart)	> 40 h

*Times are approximate, assume subcutaneous administration, and may vary with injection technique and factors influencing absorption.
†Lispro and aspart are also available in premixed forms with intermediate-acting insulins.
‡NPH also exists in premixed form (NPH/regular).
NPA = neutral protamine aspart; NPH = neutral protamine Hagedorn; NPL = neutral protamine lispro.

aspart modified to act like NPH) with insulin aspart and a formulation of premixed degludec and aspart.

Different insulin types can be drawn into the same syringe for injection but should not be premixed in bottles except by a manufacturer. On occasion, mixing insulins may affect rates of insulin absorption, producing variability of effect and making glycemic control less predictable, especially if mixed > 1 h before use. Insulin glargine should never be mixed with any other insulin.

Many prefilled insulin pen devices are available as an alternative to the conventional vial and syringe method. Insulin pens may be more convenient for use away from home and may be preferable for patients with limited vision or manual dexterity. Spring-loaded self-injection devices (for use with a syringe) may be useful for the occasional patient who is fearful of injection, and syringe magnifiers are available for patients with low vision.

Lispro, aspart, or regular insulin can also be given continuously using an insulin pump. Continuous subcutaneous insulin infusion pumps can eliminate the need for multiple daily injections, provide maximal flexibility in the timing of meals, and substantially reduce variability in glucose levels. Disadvantages include cost, mechanical failures leading to interruptions in insulin supply, and the inconvenience of wearing an external device. Frequent and meticulous self-monitoring and close attention to pump function are necessary for safe and effective use of the insulin pump. The first hybrid, closed-loop insulin delivery system is now available. A closed loop system or "artificial pancreas" is one in which an algorithm is used to calculate and automatically deliver insulin doses through an insulin pump, based on input from a continuous glucose monitor. The approved system still requires input from the user for bolus doses.

Complications of insulin treatment: The **most common complication** is

- Hypoglycemia

Uncommon complications include

- Hypokalemia
- Local allergic reactions
- Generalized allergic reaction
- Local fat atrophy or hypertrophy
- Circulating anti-insulin antibodies

Hypoglycemia is the most common complication of insulin treatment, occurring more often as patients try to achieve strict glucose control and approach near-normoglycemia. Symptoms of mild or moderate hypoglycemia include headache, diaphoresis, palpitations, light-headedness, blurred vision, agitation, and confusion. Symptoms of more severe hypoglycemia include seizures and loss of consciousness. In older patients, hypoglycemia may cause strokelike symptoms of aphasia or hemiparesis and is more likely to precipitate stroke, myocardial infarction, and sudden death. Patients with type 1 DM of long duration may be unaware of hypoglycemic episodes because they no longer experience autonomic symptoms (hypoglycemia unawareness).

Patients should be taught to recognize symptoms of hypoglycemia, which usually respond rapidly to the ingestion of sugar, including candy, juice, and glucose tablets. Typically, 15 g of glucose or sucrose should be ingested. Patients should check their glucose levels 15 min after glucose or sucrose ingestion and ingest an additional 15 g if their glucose level is not > 80 mg/dL (4.4 mmol/L). For patients who are unconscious or unable to swallow, hypoglycemia can be treated immediately with glucagon 1 mg sc or IM or a 50% dextrose solution 50 mL IV (25 g) followed, if necessary, by IV infusion of a 5% or 10% dextrose solution to maintain adequate plasma glucose levels.

Hyperglycemia may follow hypoglycemia either because too much sugar was ingested or because hypoglycemia caused a surge in counter-regulatory hormones (glucagon, epinephrine, cortisol, growth hormone). Too high a bedtime insulin dose can drive glucose down and stimulate a counter-regulatory response, leading to morning hyperglycemia (Somogyi phenomenon). A more common cause of unexplained morning hyperglycemia, however, is a rise in early morning growth hormone (dawn phenomenon). In this case, the evening insulin dose should be increased, changed to a longer-acting preparation, or injected later.

Hypokalemia may be caused by intracellular shifts of K due to insulin-induced stimulation of the sodium-potassium pump, but it is uncommon. Hypokalemia more commonly occurs in acute care settings when body stores may be depleted and IV insulin is used.

Local allergic reactions at the site of insulin injections are rare, especially with the use of human insulins, but they may still occur in patients with latex allergy because of the natural rubber latex contained in vial stoppers. They can cause immediate pain or burning followed by erythema, pruritus, and induration—the latter sometimes persisting for days. Most reactions spontaneously disappear after weeks of continued injection and require no specific treatment, although antihistamines may provide symptomatic relief.

Generalized allergic reaction is extremely rare with human insulins but can occur when insulin is restarted after a lapse in treatment. Symptoms develop 30 min to 2 h after injection and include urticaria, angioedema, pruritus, bronchospasm, and anaphylaxis. Treatment with antihistamines often suffices, but epinephrine and IV glucocorticoids may be needed. If insulin treatment is needed after a generalized allergic reaction, skin testing with a panel of purified insulin preparations and desensitization should be done.

Local fat atrophy or hypertrophy at injection sites is relatively rare and is thought to result from an immune reaction to a component of the insulin preparation. Either may resolve by rotation of injection sites.

Circulating anti-insulin antibodies are a very rare cause of insulin resistance. This type of insulin resistance can sometimes be treated by changing insulin preparations (eg, from animal to human insulin) and by administering corticosteroids if necessary.

Insulin regimens for type 1 diabetes: Regimens range from twice/day split-mixed (eg, split doses of rapid- and intermediate-acting insulins) to more physiologic basal-bolus regimens using multiple daily injections (eg, single fixed [basal] dose of long-acting and variable prandial [bolus] doses of rapid-acting insulin) or an insulin pump. Intensive treatment, defined as glucose monitoring ≥ 4 times/day and ≥ 3 injections/day or continuous insulin infusion, is more effective than conventional treatment (1 to 2 insulin injections daily with or without monitoring) for preventing diabetic retinopathy, nephropathy, and neuropathy. However, intensive therapy may result in more frequent episodes of hypoglycemia and weight gain and is more effective in patients who are able and willing to take an active role in their self-care.

In general, most patients with type 1 DM can start with a total dose of 0.2 to 0.8 units of insulin/kg/day. Obese patients may require higher doses. Physiologic replacement involves giving 40 to 60% of the daily insulin dose as an intermediate- or long-acting preparation to cover basal needs, with the remainder given as a rapid- or short-acting preparation to cover postprandial increases. This approach is most effective when the dose of rapid- or short-acting insulin is adjusted for preprandial blood glucose level and anticipated meal content. A correction factor, also known as the insulin sensitivity factor, is the amount that 1 unit of insulin will lower a patient's blood glucose level over 2 to 4 hours; this factor is often calculated using the "1800 rule" when rapid-acting insulin is used for correction (1800/total daily dose of insulin). For regular insulin, a "1500 rule" can be used. A correction dose (current glucose level – target glucose level/correction factor) is the dose of insulin that will lower the blood glucose level into the target range. This correction dose can be added to the prandial insulin dose that is calculated for the number of carbohydrates in a meal, using the carbohydrate to insulin ration (CIR). The CIR is often calculated using the "500 rule" (500/total daily dose).

To illustrate calculation of a lunchtime dose, assume the following:

- Preprandial fingerstick glucose: 240 mg/dL
- Total daily dose of insulin: 30 units basal insulin + 10 units bolus insulin per meal = 60 units total, daily
- Correction factor (insulin sensitivity factor): 1800/60 = 30 mg/dL/unit
- Estimated carbohydrate content of upcoming meal: 50 g
- Carbohydrate:insulin ratio (CIR): 500/60 = 8:1
- Target glucose: 120 mg/dL

Prandial insulin dose = 50 g carbohydrate divided by 8 g/unit insulin = 6 units

Correction dose = (240 mg/dL – 120 mg/dL)/30 correction factor = 4 units

Total dose prior to this meal = prandial dose + correction dose = 6 + 4 = 10 units rapid-acting insulin

Such physiologic regimens allow greater freedom of lifestyle because patients can skip or time-shift meals and maintain normoglycemia. these recommendations are for initiation of therapy; thereafter, choice of regimens generally rests on physiologic response and patient and physician preferences. The carbohydrate to insulin ratio and sensitivity factors need to be fine-tuned and changed according to how the patient responds to insulin doses. This adjustment requires working closely with a diabetes specialist.

Insulin regimens for type 2 diabetes: Regimens for type 2 DM also vary. In many patients, glucose levels are adequately controlled with lifestyle changes and non-insulin antihyperglycemic drugs, but insulin should be added when glucose remains inadequately controlled by ≥ 3 drugs. Although uncommon, adult-onset type 1 DM may be the cause. Insulinshould replace non-insulin antihyperglycemic drugs in women who become pregnant. The rationale for combination therapy is strongest for use of insulin with oral biguanides and insulin sensitizers. Regimens vary from a single daily injection of long- or intermediate-acting insulin (usually at bedtime) to the multiple-injection regimen used by patients with type 1 DM. In general, the simplest effective regimen is preferred. Because of insulin resistance, some patients with type 2 DM require very large doses (> 2 units/kg/day). A common complication is weight gain, which is mostly attributable to reduction in loss of glucose in urine and improved metabolic efficiency.

Table 165–4. CHARACTERISTICS OF ORAL ANTIHYPERGLYCEMICS

GENERIC NAME	DAILY DOSAGE	DURATION OF ACTION	COMMENTS
Sulfonylureas			
Acetohexamide*	250 mg once/day–750 mg bid	12–24 h	No longer available in US
Chlorpropamide*	100 mg once/day–750 mg once/day	24–36 h	Chlorpropamide: May cause hyponatremia and flushing after alcohol ingestion
Tolbutamide*	250 mg once/day–1500 mg bid	12 h	—
Tolazamide*	100 mg once/day–500 mg bid	14–16 h	No longer available in US
Glyburide, regular-release†	1.25 mg once/day–10 mg bid	12–24 h	Glipizide and glyburide: No evidence of increased effectiveness of doses above 10 mg/day
Glyburide, micronized†	0.75 mg once/day–6 mg bid	12–24 h	
Glipizide, regular-release†	2.5 mg once/day–20 mg bid	12–24 h	
Glipizide, extended-release†	2.5–20 mg once/day	24 h	
Glimepiride†	1–8 mg once/day	24 h	—
Insulin secretagogues: Short-acting			
Nateglinide	60–120 mg tid with meals	3–4 h	Augment pancreatic beta-cell insulin secretion
Repaglinide	0.5–4 mg tid with meals	3–4 h	Can be used alone or in combination with other oral drugs and insulin
Insulin sensitizers: Biguanides			
Metformin, regular-release	500 mg once/day–1250 mg bid	6–10 h	Augment suppression of hepatic glucose production by insulin Can be used alone or in combination with other oral drugs and insulin Major adverse effects: Lactic acidosis (rare) Contraindicated in at-risk patients, including those with renal insufficiency, metabolic acidosis, hypoxia, alcoholism, or dehydration Does not cause hypoglycemia Other adverse effects: GI distress (diarrhea, nausea, pain), vitamin B_{12} malabsorption Potentiates weight loss
Metformin, extended-release	500 mg–2 g once/day	24 h	

Table 165–4. CHARACTERISTICS OF ORAL ANTIHYPERGLYCEMICS (*Continued*)

GENERIC NAME	DAILY DOSAGE	DURATION OF ACTION	COMMENTS
Insulin sensitizers: Thiazolidinediones			
Pioglitazone	15–45 mg once/day	24 h	Augment suppression of hepatic glucose production by insulin Can be used alone or in combination with other oral drugs and insulin Major adverse effects: Weight gain, fluid retention, anemia (mild) Hepatotoxicity rare, but liver function monitoring required Pioglitazone: May increase risk of bladder cancer, heart failure, and fractures
Rosiglitazone	2–8 mg once/day	24 h	Rosiglitazone: May increase low-density lipoprotein cholesterol and may increase risk of heart failure, angina, myocardial infarction, stroke, and fractures
Alpha-glucosidase inhibitors			
Acarbose	25–100 mg tid with meals	6–10 h	Intestinal enzyme inhibitors Used as monotherapy or combination therapy with other oral drugs or insulin to decrease postprandial plasma glucose levels Must be taken with the first bite of meal GI adverse effects (flatulence, diarrhea, bloating) common but may decrease over time Started with small dose (25 mg/day) and gradually titrated over several weeks
Miglitol	25–100 mg tid with meals	6–10 h	
Dipeptidyl peptidase-4 (DPP4) inhibitors			
Alogliptin	6.25–25 mg once/day	24 h	All DPP-4 inhibitors can be used in moderate to severe renal insufficiency. All, except linagliptin, require dose adjustment for eGFR. Well-tolerated but cause only modest improvements in hemoglobin A_{1C} A slight increase in risk of pancreatitis seen in several studies
Linagliptin	5 mg once/day	24 h	
Saxagliptin	2.5–5 mg once/day	24 h	
Sitagliptin	25–100 mg once/day	24 h	
Sodium-glucose co-transporter 2 (SGLT2) inhibitors			
Canagliflozin	100 or 300 mg once/ day	24 h	SGLT-2 inhibitors may cause weight loss, orthostatic hypotension, yeast infections, and UTIs Use cautiously in the elderly and in patients with renal impairment Possible increase in risk of DKA Empagliflozin may have cardiovascular benefits
Dapagliflozin	5–10 mg once/day	24 h	
Empagliflozin	10–25 mg daily	24 h	

*1st-generation sulfonylureas.
†2nd-generation sulfonylureas.

Oral Antihyperglycemic Drugs

Oral antihyperglycemic drugs (see Tables 165–4 and 165–5) are a mainstay of treatment for type 2 DM, along with glucagon-like peptide-1 (GLP-1) receptor agonists. Insulin is often added when ≥ 3 drugs fail to provide adequate glycemic control. Oral antihyperglycemic drugs may

- Enhance pancreatic insulin secretion (secretagogues)
- Sensitize peripheral tissues to insulin (sensitizers)
- Impair GI absorption of glucose
- Increase glycosuria

Drugs with different mechanisms of action may be synergistic.

Sulfonylureas: Sulfonylureas (SUs) are insulin secretagogues. They lower plasma glucose by stimulating pancreatic beta-cell insulin secretion and may secondarily improve peripheral and hepatic insulin sensitivity by reducing glucose toxicity. First-generation drugs (see Table 165–4) are more likely to cause adverse effects and are used infrequently. All SUs promote hyperinsulinemia and weight gain of 2 to 5 kg, which over time may potentiate insulin resistance and limit their usefulness. All also can cause hypoglycemia. Risk factors include age > 65, use of long-acting drugs (especially chlorpropamide, glyburide, or glipizide), erratic eating and exercise, and renal or hepatic insufficiency.

Hypoglycemia caused by long-acting drugs may last for days after treatment cessation, occasionally causes permanent neurologic disability, and can be fatal. For these reasons, some physicians hospitalize hypoglycemic patients, especially older ones. Chlorpropamide also causes the syndrome of inappropriate ADH secretion. Most patients taking SUs alone eventually require additional drugs to achieve normoglycemia, suggesting that SUs may exhaust beta-cell function. However, worsening of insulin secretion and insulin resistance is probably more a feature of DM itself than of drugs used to treat it.

Table 165–5. COMBINATION ORAL ANTIHYPERGLYCEMICS BY CLASS

DRUGS	AVAILABLE STRENGTHS (MG/MG)
Sulfonylurea/biguanide	
Glipizide/metformin	2.5/250, 2.5/500, 5/500
Glyburide/metformin	1.25/250, 2.5/500, 5/500
Repaglinide/metformin	1/500, 2/500
Thiazolidinedione/biguanide	
Pioglitazone/metformin	15/500, 15/850
Rosiglitazone/metformin	1/500, 2/500, 4/500, 2/1000, 4/1000
Thiazolidinedione/sulfonylurea	
Pioglitazone/glimepiride	30/2, 30/4
Rosiglitazone/glimepiride	4/1, 4/2, 4/4
Dipeptidyl peptidase-4 inhibitor/biguanide	
Linagliptin/metformin	2.5/500, 2.5/850, 2.5/1000
Saxagliptin/metformin, extended-release	5/1000, 5/500, 2.5/1000
Sitagliptin/metformin	50/500, 50/1000
Sitagliptin/metformin extended release	50/500, 50/1000, 100/1000
Metformin/SGLT-2 in inhibitor	
Canagliflozin/metformin	50/500, 50/1000, 150/500, 150/1000
Dapagliflozin/metformin, extended release	5/500, 5/1000, 10/500, 10/1000
DPP-4 inhibitor/SGLT-2 inhibitor	
Empagliflozin/linagliptin	10/5, 25/5

Short-acting insulin secretagogues: Short-acting insulin secretagogues (repaglinide, nateglinide) stimulate insulin secretion in a manner similar to SUs. They are faster acting, however, and may stimulate insulin secretion more during meals than at other times. Thus, they may be especially effective for reducing postprandial hyperglycemia and appear to have lower risk of hypoglycemia. There may be some weight gain, although apparently less than with SUs. Patients who have not responded to other oral drug classes (eg, SUs, metformin) are not likely to respond to these drugs.

Biguanides: Biguanides lower plasma glucose by decreasing hepatic glucose production (gluconeogenesis and glycogenolysis). They are considered peripheral insulin sensitizers, but their stimulation of peripheral glucose uptake may simply be a result of reductions in glucose from their hepatic effects. Biguanides also lower lipid levels and may also decrease GI nutrient absorption, increase beta-cell sensitivity to circulating glucose, and decrease levels of plasminogen activator inhibitor 1, thereby exerting an antithrombotic effect. Metformin is the only biguanide commercially available in the US. It is at least as effective as SUs in reducing plasma glucose, rarely causes hypoglycemia, and can be safely used with other drugs and insulin. In addition, metformin does not cause weight gain and may even promote weight loss by suppressing appetite. However, the drug commonly causes GI adverse effects (eg, dyspepsia, diarrhea), which for most people recede with time. Less commonly, metformin causes vitamin B_{12} malabsorption, but clinically significant anemia is rare.

Contribution of metformin to life-threatening lactic acidosis is very rare, but the drug is contraindicated in patients at risk of acidemia (including those with significant renal insufficiency, hypoxia or severe respiratory disease, alcoholism, other forms of metabolic acidosis, or dehydration). The drug should be withheld during surgery, administration of IV contrast, and any serious illness. Many people receiving metformin monotherapy eventually require an additional drug.

Thiazolidinediones: Thiazolidinediones (TZDs) decrease peripheral insulin resistance (insulin sensitizers), but their specific mechanisms of action are not well understood. The drugs bind a nuclear receptor primarily present in fat cells (peroxisome-proliferator-activated receptor-gamma [PPAR-γ]) that is involved in the transcription of genes that regulate glucose and lipid metabolism. TZDs also increase HDL levels, lower triglycerides, and may have anti-inflammatory and anti-atherosclerotic effects. TZDs are as effective as SUs and metformin in reducing HbA_{1C}. TZDs may be beneficial in treatment of non-alcoholic fatty liver disease (NAFLD).

Though one TZD (troglitazone) caused acute liver failure, currently available drugs have not proven hepatotoxic. Nevertheless, periodic monitoring of liver function is recommended. TZDs may cause peripheral edema, especially in patients taking insulin, and may worsen heart failure in susceptible patients. Weight gain, due to fluid retention and increased adipose tissue mass, is common and may be substantial (> 10 kg) in some patients. Rosiglitazone may increase risk of heart failure, angina, myocardial infarction, stroke, and fracture. Pioglitazone may increase the risk of bladder cancer (although data are conflicting), heart failure, and fractures.

Alpha-glucosidase inhibitors: Alpha-glucosidase inhibitors (AGIs) competitively inhibit intestinal enzymes that hydrolyze dietary carbohydrates; carbohydrates are digested and absorbed more slowly, thereby lowering postprandial plasma glucose. AGIs are less effective than other oral drugs in reducing plasma glucose, and patients often stop the drugs because they may cause dyspepsia, flatulence, and diarrhea. But the drugs are otherwise safe and can be used in combination with all other oral drugs and with insulin.

Dipeptidyl peptidase-4 inhibitors: Dipeptidyl peptidase-4 inhibitors (eg, alogliptin, linagliptin, saxagliptin, sitagliptin) prolong the action of endogenous glucagon-like peptide-1 (GLP-1) by inhibiting the enzyme dipeptidyl peptidase-4 (DPP-4), which is involved in the breakdown of GLP-1. There is a slight increase in risk for pancreatitis with DPP-4 inhibitors, but they are otherwise considered safe and well-tolerated. The HbA_{1C} decrease is modest with DPP-4 inhibitors.

Sodium-glucose co-transporter 2 inhibitors: Sodium-glucose co-transporter 2 (SGLT2) inhibitors (canagliflozin, dapagliflozin, empagliflozin) inhibit SGLT2 in the proximal tubule of the kidney, which blocks glucose reabsorption, thus causing glycosuria and lowering plasma glucose. SGLT2 inhibitors may also cause modest weight loss and lowering of blood pressure. Empagliflozin was shown to decrease cardiovascular events in diabetic patients at high risk for cardiovascular disease.

The most common side effects are genitourinary infections, especially mycotic infections. Orthostatic symptoms can also occur. There have been reports of DKA in patients with both type 1 DM and type 2 DM.

Dopamine agonist: Bromocriptine is a dopamine agonist that lowers HbA_{1C} about 0.5% by an unknown mechanism. Although approved for type 2 diabetes, it is not commonly used because of potential adverse effects.

Injectable Antihyperglycemic Drugs

Injectable antihyperglycemic drugs other than insulin are the glucagon-like peptide-1 (GLP-1) receptor agonists and the amylin analog, pramlintide (see Table 165–6). These drugs are used in combination with other antihyperglycemics.

Glucagon-like peptide-1 (GLP-1) receptor agonists: GLP-1 agonists (exenatide [an incretin hormone], liraglutide, dulaglutide, albiglutide) enhance glucose-dependent insulin secretion and slow gastric emptying. GLP-1 agonists may also reduce appetite and promote weight loss and stimulate beta-cell proliferation. Formulations are available for dosing twice/day, once/day, and weekly. The most common adverse effects of GLP-1 agonists are gastrointestinal, especially nausea and vomiting. GLP-1 agonists also cause a slight increase in the risk of pancreatitis. They are contraindicated in patients with a personal or family history of medullary thyroid cancer because an increased risk of this cancer has occurred in tested rodents.

Amylin analog: The amylin analog pramlintide mimics amylin, a pancreatic beta-cell hormone that helps regulate postprandial glucose levels. Pramlintide suppresses postprandial glucagon secretion, slows gastric emptying, and promotes satiety. It is given by injection and is used in combination with mealtime insulin. Patients with type 1 diabetes are given 30 to 60 mcg sc before meals, and those with type 2 diabetes are given 120 mcg.

Adjunctive Drug Therapy for Diabetes

Pharmacologic measures to prevent or treat complications of DM[1] are critical, including

- ACE inhibitors or angiotensin II receptor blockers
- Aspirin
- Statins

ACE inhibitors or angiotensin II receptor blockers are indicated for patients with evidence of early diabetic nephropathy (albuminuria), even in the absence of hypertension, and are a good choice for treating hypertension in patients who have DM and who have not yet shown renal impairment.

ACE inhibitors also help prevent cardiovascular events in patients with DM.

Aspirin 81 to 325 mg once/day provides cardiovascular protection and should be used by most adults with DM in the absence of a specific contraindication.

Statins are currently recommended by the American Heart Association/American College of Cardiology guidelines for all diabetic patients 40 to 75 yr of age. Moderate to high intensity treatment is used, and there are no target lipid levels. For patients < 40 or > 75, statins are given based upon individual assessment of the risk:benefit ratio and patient preference. Patients with type 2 DM tend to have high levels of triglycerides and small, dense low-density lipoproteins (LDL) and low levels of HDL; they should receive aggressive treatment with the same treatment goals as those of patients with known coronary artery disease (LDL < 100 mg/dL [< 2.6 mmol/L], HDL > 40 mg/dL [> 1.1 mmol/L], and triglycerides < 150 mg/dL [< 1.7 mmol/L]).

1. Fox CS, Golden SH, Anderson C, et al: AHA/ADA Scientific Statement: update on prevention of cardiovascular disease in adults with type 2 DM in light of recent evidence. *Circulation* 132:691–718, 2015.

DIABETIC KETOACIDOSIS

Diabetic ketoacidosis (DKA) is an acute metabolic complication of diabetes characterized by hyperglycemia, hyperketonemia, and metabolic acidosis. Hyperglycemia causes an osmotic diuresis with significant fluid and electrolyte loss. DKA occurs mostly in type 1 diabetes mellitus (DM). It causes nausea, vomiting, and abdominal pain and can progress to cerebral edema, coma, and death. DKA is diagnosed by detection of hyperketonemia and anion gap metabolic acidosis in the presence of hyperglycemia. Treatment involves volume expansion, insulin replacement, and prevention of hypokalemia.

Table 165–6. CHARACTERISTICS OF INJECTABLE NON-INSULIN ANTIHYPERGLYCEMIC DRUGS

GENERIC NAME	DAILY DOSAGE	DURATION OF ACTION	COMMENTS
Glucagon-like peptide-1 (GLP-1) agonists			
Albiglutide	30 mg or 50 mg sc once/wk	7 days	Low risk of hypoglycemia; may promote modest weight loss Increased risk of pancreatitis Thyroid C-cell tumors (medullary carcinoma) noted in rodents Weekly preparations may cause fewer GI adverse effects. When given once/day or bid, lowest starting dose may minimize nausea
Dulaglutide	0.75 mg or 1.5 mg sc once/wk	7 days	
Exenatide	5 mcg or 10 mcg sc bid before meals	4–6 h	
Exenatide, once/wk	2 mg sc once/wk	7 days	
Liraglutide	1.2–1.8 mg sc once/day	24 h	
Amylin analog			
Pramlintide	For type 1 DM: 30–60 mcg sc before meals For type 2 DM: 120 mcg sc before meals	2–4 h	For use in combination with insulin, but injected using a separate syringe May need to adjust insulin dose to avoid hypoglycemia Nausea common but declining with time May promote modest weight loss

DKA is most common among patients with type 1 DM and develops when insulin levels are insufficient to meet the body's basic metabolic requirements. DKA is the first manifestation of type 1 DM in a minority of patients. Insulin deficiency can be absolute (eg, during lapses in the administration of exogenous insulin) or relative (eg, when usual insulin doses do not meet metabolic needs during physiologic stress).

Common **physiologic stresses** that can trigger DKA include

- Acute infection (particularly pneumonia and UTI)
- Myocardial infarction
- Stroke
- Pancreatitis
- Trauma

Some **drugs** implicated in causing DKA include

- Corticosteroids
- Thiazide diuretics
- Sympathomimetics
- Sodium-glucose co-transporter 2 (SGLT-2) inhibitors

DKA is less common in type 2 DM, but it may occur in situations of unusual physiologic stress. Ketosis-prone type 2 diabetes is a variant of type 2 diabetes, which is sometimes seen in obese individuals, often of African (including African-American or Afro-Caribbean) origin. People with ketosis-prone diabetes (also referred to as Flatbush diabetes) can have significant impairment of beta cell function with hyperglycemia, and are therefore more likely to develop DKA in the setting of significant hyperglycemia. SGLT-2 inhibitors have been implicated in causing DKA in both type 1 and type 2 DM.

Pathophysiology

Insulin deficiency causes the body to metabolize triglycerides and amino acids instead of glucose for energy. Serum levels of glycerol and free fatty acids (FFAs) rise because of unrestrained lipolysis, as does alanine because of muscle catabolism. Glycerol and alanine provide substrate for hepatic gluconeogenesis, which is stimulated by the excess of glucagon that accompanies insulin deficiency.

Glucagon also stimulates mitochondrial conversion of FFAs into ketones. Insulinnormally blocks ketogenesis by inhibiting the transport of FFA derivatives into the mitochondrial matrix, but ketogenesis proceeds in the absence of insulin. The major ketoacids produced, acetoacetic acid and beta-hydroxybutyric acid, are strong organic acids that create metabolic acidosis. Acetone derived from the metabolism of acetoacetic acid accumulates in serum and is slowly disposed of by respiration.

Hyperglycemia due to insulin deficiency causes an osmotic diuresis that leads to marked urinary losses of water and electrolytes. Urinary excretion of ketones obligates additional losses of Na and K. Serum Na may fall due to natriuresis or rise due to excretion of large volumes of free water. K is also lost in large quantities, sometimes > 300 mEq/24 h. Despite a significant total body deficit of K, initial serum K is typically normal or elevated because of the extracellular migration of K in response to acidosis. K levels generally fall further during treatment as insulin therapy drives K into cells. If serum K is not monitored and replaced as needed, life-threatening hypokalemia may develop.

Symptoms and Signs

Symptoms and signs of DKA include symptoms of hyperglycemia with the addition of nausea, vomiting, and—particularly in children—abdominal pain. Lethargy and somnolence are symptoms of more severe decompensation. Patients may be hypotensive and tachycardic due to dehydration and acidosis; they may breathe rapidly and deeply to compensate for acidemia (Kussmaul respirations). They may also have fruity breath due to exhaled acetone. Fever is not a sign of DKA itself and, if present, signifies underlying infection. In the absence of timely treatment, DKA progresses to coma and death.

Acute cerebral edema, a complication in about 1% of DKA patients, occurs primarily in children and less often in adolescents and young adults. Headache and fluctuating level of consciousness herald this complication in some patients, but respiratory arrest is the initial manifestation in others. The cause is not well understood but may be related to too-rapid reductions in serum osmolality or to brain ischemia. It is most likely to occur in children < 5 yr when DKA is the initial manifestation of DM. Children with the highest BUN and lowest $Paco_2$ at presentation appear to be at greatest risk. Delays in correction of hyponatremia and the use of bicarbonate during DKA treatment are additional risk factors.

Diagnosis

- Arterial pH
- Serum ketones
- Calculation of anion gap

In patients suspected of having DKA, serum electrolytes, BUN and creatinine, glucose, ketones, and osmolarity should be measured. Urine should be tested for ketones. Patients who appear significantly ill and those with positive ketones should have arterial blood gas measurement.

DKA is diagnosed by an arterial pH < 7.30 with an anion gap > 12 (see Sidebar 161–1 on p. 1230) and serum ketones in the presence of hyperglycemia. A presumptive diagnosis can be made when urine glucose and ketones are strongly positive. Urine test strips and some assays for serum ketones may underestimate the degree of ketosis because they detect acetoacetic acid and not beta-hydroxybutyric acid, which is usually the predominant ketoacid.

Symptoms and signs of a triggering illness should be pursued with appropriate studies (eg, cultures, imaging studies). Adults should have an ECG to screen for acute myocardial infarction and to help determine the significance of abnormalities in serum K.

Other laboratory abnormalities include hyponatremia, elevated serum creatinine, and elevated plasma osmolality. Hyperglycemia may cause dilutional hyponatremia, so measured serum Na is corrected by adding 1.6 mEq/L for each 100 mg/dL elevation of serum glucose over 100 mg/dL. To illustrate, for a patient with serum Na of 124 mEq/L and glucose of 600 mg/dL, add 1.6 ([600 – 100]/100) = 8 mEq/L to 124 for a corrected serum Na of 132 mEq/L. As acidosis is corrected, serum K drops. An initial K level < 4.5 mEq/L indicates marked K depletion and requires immediate K supplementation.

Serum amylase and lipase are often elevated, even in the absence of pancreatitis (which may be present in patients with alcoholic ketoacidosis and in those with coexisting hypertriglyceridemia).

Prognosis

Overall mortality rates for DKA are < 1%; however, mortality is higher in the elderly and in patients with other life-threatening illnesses. Shock or coma on admission indicates a worse prognosis. Main causes of death are circulatory collapse, hypokalemia, and infection. Among children with cerebral edema, about 57% recover completely, 21% survive with neurologic sequelae, and 21% die.

Treatment

- IV 0.9% saline
- Correction of any hypokalemia
- IV insulin (as long as serum K is ≥ 3.3 mEq/L)
- Rarely IV Na bicarbonate (if pH < 7 after 1 h of treatment)

The most urgent goals for treating DKA are rapid intravascular volume repletion, correction of hyperglycemia and acidosis, and prevention of hypokalemia.[1] Identification of precipitating factors is also important. Treatment should occur in intensive care settings because clinical and laboratory assessments are initially needed every hour or every other hour with appropriate adjustments in treatment.

Volume repletion: Intravascular volume should be restored rapidly to raise blood pressure and ensure glomerular perfusion; once intravascular volume is restored, remaining total body water deficits are corrected more slowly, typically over about 24 h. Initial volume repletion in adults is typically achieved with rapid IV infusion of 1 to 3 L of 0.9% saline solution, followed by saline infusions at 1 L/h or faster as needed to raise blood pressure, correct hyperglycemia, and keep urine flow adequate. Adults with DKA typically need a minimum of 3 L of saline over the first 5 h. When blood pressure is stable and urine flow adequate, normal saline is replaced by 0.45% saline. When plasma glucose falls to < 200 mg/dL (11.1 mmol/L), IV fluid should be changed to 5% dextrose in 0.45% saline.

For children, fluid deficits are estimated at 60 to 100 mL/kg body weight. Pediatric maintenance fluids (for ongoing losses) must also be provided. Initial fluid therapy should be 0.9% saline (20 mL/kg) over 1 to 2 h, followed by 0.45% saline once blood pressure is stable and urine output adequate. The remaining fluid deficit should be replaced over 36 h, typically requiring a rate (including maintenance fluids) of about 2 to 4 mL/kg/h, depending on the degree of dehydration.

Correction of hyperglycemia and acidosis: Hyperglycemia is corrected by giving regular insulin 0.1 unit/kg IV bolus initially, followed by continuous IV infusion of 0.1 unit/kg/h in 0.9% saline solution. *Insulin should be withheld until serum K is ≥ 3.3 mEq/L* (see p. 1270). Insulin adsorption onto IV tubing can lead to inconsistent effects, which can be minimized by preflushing the IV tubing with insulin solution. If plasma glucose does not fall by 50 to 75 mg/dL (2.8 to 4.2 mmol/L) in the first hour, insulin doses should be doubled. Children should be given a continuous IV insulin infusion of 0.1 unit/kg/h or higher with or without a bolus.

Ketones should begin to clear within hours if insulin is given in sufficient doses. However, clearance of ketones may appear to lag because of conversion of beta-hydroxybutyrate to acetoacetate (which is the "ketone" measured in most hospital laboratories) as acidosis resolves. Serum pH and bicarbonate levels should also quickly improve, but restoration of a normal serum bicarbonate level may take 24 h. Rapid correction of pH by bicarbonate administration may be considered if pH remains < 7 after about an hour of initial fluid resuscitation, but bicarbonate is associated with development of acute cerebral edema (primarily in children) and should not be used routinely. If used, only modest pH elevation should be attempted (target pH of about 7.1), with doses of 50 to 100 mEq over 30 to 60 min, followed by repeat measurement of arterial pH and serum K.

When plasma glucose becomes < 200 mg/dL (< 11.1 mmol/L) in adults, 5% dextrose should be added to IV fluids to reduce the risk of hypoglycemia. Insulin dosage can then be reduced to 0.02 to 0.05 unit/kg/h, but the continuous IV infusion of regular insulin should be maintained until the anion gap has narrowed and blood and urine are consistently negative for ketones. Insulin replacement may then be switched to regular insulin 5 to 10 units sc q 4 to 6 h. When the patient is stable and able to eat, a typical split-mixed or basal-bolus insulin regimen is begun. IV insulin should be continued for 1 to 4 h after the initial dose of sc insulin is given. Children should continue to receive 0.05 unit/kg/h insulin infusion until sc insulin is initiated and pH is > 7.3.

Hypokalemia prevention: Hypokalemia prevention requires replacement of 20 to 30 mEq K in each liter of IV fluid to keep serum K between 4 and 5 mEq/L. If serum K is < 3.3 mEq/L, insulin should be withheld and K given at 40 mEq/h until serum K is ≥ 3.3 mEq/L; if serum K is > 5 mEq/L, K supplementation can be withheld.

Initially normal or elevated serum K measurements may reflect shifts from intracellular stores in response to acidemia and belie the true K deficits that almost all patients with DKA have. Insulinreplacement rapidly shifts K into cells, so levels should be checked hourly or every other hour in the initial stages of treatment.

Other measures: Hypophosphatemia often develops during treatment of DKA, but phosphate repletion is of unclear benefit in most cases. If indicated (eg, if rhabdomyolysis, hemolysis, or neurologic deterioration occurs), K phosphate 1 to 2 mmol/kg of phosphate, can be infused over 6 to 12 h. If K phosphate is given, the serum calcium level usually decreases and should be monitored.

Treatment of suspected cerebral edema is hyperventilation, corticosteroids, and mannitol, but these measures are often ineffective after the onset of respiratory arrest.

1. Kitabchi AE, Umpierrez GE, Miles JM, et al: Hyperglycemic crises in adult patients with diabetes. *Diabetes Care* 32:1335–1343, 2009.

KEY POINTS

- Acute physiologic stressors (eg, infections, myocardial infarction) can trigger acidosis, moderate glucose elevation, dehydration, and severe K loss in patients with type 1 diabetes.
- Acute cerebral edema is a rare (about 1%) but lethal complication, primarily in children and less often in adolescents and young adults.
- Diagnose by an arterial pH < 7.30, with an anion gap > 12 and serum ketones in the presence of hyperglycemia.
- Acidosis typically corrects with IV fluid and insulin; consider bicarbonate only if marked acidosis (pH < 7) persists after 1 hr of therapy.
- Withhold insulin until serum K is ≥ 3.3 mEq/L.

HYPEROSMOLAR HYPERGLYCEMIC STATE

Hyperosmolar hyperglycemic state is a metabolic complication of diabetes mellitus (DM) characterized by severe hyperglycemia, extreme dehydration, hyperosmolar plasma, and altered consciousness. It most often occurs in type 2 DM, often in the setting of physiologic stress. HHS is diagnosed by severe hyperglycemia and plasma hyperosmolality and absence of significant ketosis. Treatment is IV saline solution and insulin. Complications include coma, seizures, and death.

Hyperosmolar hyperglycemic state (HHS—previously referred to as hyperglycemic hyperosmolar nonketotic coma [HHNK] and nonketotic hyperosmolar syndrome) is a complication of type 2 DM and has an estimated mortality rate of up to

20%, which is significantly higher than the mortality for DKA (currently < 1%). It usually develops after a period of symptomatic hyperglycemia in which fluid intake is inadequate to prevent extreme dehydration due to the hyperglycemia-induced osmotic diuresis.

Precipitating factors include

- Acute infections and other medical conditions
- Drugs that impair glucose tolerance (glucocorticoids) or increase fluid loss (diuretics)
- Nonadherence to diabetes treatment

Serum ketones are not present because the amounts of insulin present in most patients with type 2 DM are adequate to suppress ketogenesis. Because symptoms of acidosis are not present, most patients endure a significantly longer period of osmotic dehydration before presentation, and thus plasma glucose (> 600 mg/dL [> 33.3 mmol/L]) and osmolality (> 320 mOsm/L) are typically much higher than in DKA.

Symptoms and Signs

The primary symptom of HHS is altered consciousness varying from confusion or disorientation to coma, usually as a result of extreme dehydration with or without prerenal azotemia, hyperglycemia, and hyperosmolality. In contrast to DKA, focal or generalized seizures and transient hemiplegia may occur.

Diagnosis

- Blood glucose level
- Serum osmolarity

Generally, hyperosmolar hyperglycemic state is initially suspected when a markedly elevated glucose level is found in a fingerstick specimen obtained in the course of a workup of altered mental status. If measurements have not already been obtained, measurement of serum electrolytes, BUN and creatinine, glucose, ketones, and plasma osmolality should be done. Urine should be tested for ketones. Serum K levels are usually normal, but Na may be low or high depending on volume deficits. Hyperglycemia may cause dilutional hyponatremia, so measured serum Na is corrected by adding 1.6 mEq/L for each 100 mg/dL elevation of serum glucose over 100 mg/dL. BUN and serum creatinine levels are markedly increased. Arterial pH is usually > 7.3, but occasionally mild metabolic acidosis develops due to lactate accumulation.

The fluid deficit can exceed 10 L, and acute circulatory collapse is a common cause of death. Widespread thrombosis is a frequent finding on autopsy, and in some cases bleeding may occur as a consequence of disseminated intravascular coagulation. Other complications include aspiration pneumonia, acute renal failure, and acute respiratory distress syndrome.

Treatment

- IV 0.9% saline
- Correction of any hypokalemia
- IV insulin (as long as serum K is ≥ 3.3 mEq/L)

Treatment consists of IV saline, correction of hypokalemia, and IV insulin.[1]

Treatment is 0.9% (isotonic) saline solution at a rate of 15 to 20 mL/kg/ h, for the first few hours. After that, the corrected Na should be calculated. If the corrected Na is < 135 mEq/L, then isotonic saline should be continued at a rate of 250 to 500 mL/h. If the corrected Na is normal or elevated, then 0.45% saline (half normal) should be used.

Dextrose should be added once the glucose level reaches 250 to 300mg/dL. The rate of infusion of IV fluids should be adjusted depending on BP, cardiac status, and the balance between fluid input and output.

Insulin is given at 0.1 unit/kg IV bolus followed by a 0.1 unit/kg/h infusion after the first liter of saline has been infused. Hydration alone can sometimes precipitously decrease plasma glucose, so insulin dose may need to be reduced. A too-quick reduction in osmolality can lead to cerebral edema. Occasional patients with insulin-resistant type 2 diabetes with HHS require larger insulin doses. Once plasma glucose reaches 300 mg/dL (16.7 mmol/L), insulin infusion should be reduced to basal levels (1 to 2 units/h) until rehydration is complete and the patient is able to eat.

Target plasma glucose is between 250 and 300 mg/dL (13.9 to 16.7 mmol/L) After recovery from the acute episode, patients are usually switched to adjusted doses of sc insulin.

K replacement is similar to that in DKA: 40 mEq/h for serum K < 3.3 mEq/L; 20 to 30 mEq/h for serum K between 3.3 and 4.9 mEq/L; and none for serum K ≥ 5 mEq/L.

1. Kitabchi AE, Umpierrez GE, Miles JM, et al: Hyperglycemic crises in adult patients with diabetes. *Diabetes Care* 32:1335–1343, 2009.

KEY POINTS

- Infections, nonadherence, and certain drugs can trigger marked glucose elevation, dehydration, and altered consciousness in patients with type 2 diabetes.
- Patients have adequate insulin present to prevent ketoacidosis.
- The fluid deficit can exceed 10 L; treatment is 0.9% saline solution IV plus insulin infusion.
- Target plasma glucose in acute treatment is between 250 and 300 mg/dL (13.9 to 16.7 mmol/L).
- Give K replacement depending on serum K levels.

ALCOHOLIC KETOACIDOSIS

Alcoholic ketoacidosis is a metabolic complication of alcohol use and starvation characterized by hyperketonemia and anion gap metabolic acidosis without significant hyperglycemia. Alcoholic ketoacidosis causes nausea, vomiting, and abdominal pain. Diagnosis is by history and findings of ketoacidosis without hyperglycemia. Treatment is IV saline solution and dextrose infusion.

Alcoholic ketoacidosis is attributed to the combined effects of alcohol and starvation on glucose metabolism.

Pathophysiology

Alcohol diminishes hepatic gluconeogenesis and leads to decreased insulin secretion, increased lipolysis, impaired fatty acid oxidation, and subsequent ketogenesis, causing an elevated anion gap metabolic acidosis. Counter-regulatory hormones are increased and may further inhibit insulin secretion. Plasma glucose levels are usually low or normal, but mild hyperglycemia sometimes occurs.

Symptoms and Signs

Typically, an alcohol binge leads to vomiting and the cessation of alcohol or food intake for ≥ 24 h. During this period of starvation, vomiting continues and abdominal pain develops, leading the patient to seek medical attention. Pancreatitis may occur.

Diagnosis

- Clinical evaluation
- Calculation of anion gap
- Exclusion of other disorders

Diagnosis requires a high index of suspicion; similar symptoms in an alcoholic patient may result from acute pancreatitis, methanol or ethylene glycol poisoning, or DKA. In patients suspected of having alcoholic ketoacidosis, serum electrolytes (including magnesium), BUN and creatinine, glucose, ketones, amylase, lipase, and plasma osmolality should be measured. Urine should be tested for ketones. Patients who appear significantly ill and those with positive ketones should have arterial blood gas and serum lactate measurement.

The absence of hyperglycemia makes DKA improbable. Those with mild hyperglycemia may have underlying DM, which may be recognized by elevated levels of glycosylated Hb (HbA_{1C}).

Typical laboratory findings include a high anion gap metabolic acidosis, ketonemia, and low levels of K, magnesium, and phosphorus. Detection of acidosis may be complicated by concurrent metabolic alkalosis due to vomiting, resulting in a relatively normal pH; the main clue is the elevated anion gap. If history does not rule out toxic alcohol ingestion as a cause of the elevated anion gap, serum methanol and ethylene glycol levels should be measured. Calcium oxalate crystals in the urine also suggests ethylene glycol poisoning. Lactic acid levels are often elevated because of hypoperfusion and the altered balance of reduction and oxidation reactions in the liver.

Treatment

- IV thiamin and other vitamins plus magnesium
- IV 5% dextrose in 0.9% saline

Patients are initially given thiamin 100 mg IV to prevent development of Wernicke encephalopathy or Korsakoff psychosis. Then an IV infusion of 5% dextrose in 0.9% saline solution is given. Initial IV fluids should contain added water-soluble vitamins and magnesium, with K replacement as required.

Ketoacidosis and GI symptoms usually respond rapidly. Use of insulin is appropriate only if there is any question of atypical DKA or if hyperglycemia > 300 mg/dL (16.7 mmol/L) develops.

HYPOGLYCEMIA

Hypoglycemia unrelated to exogenous insulin therapy is an uncommon clinical syndrome characterized by low plasma glucose level, symptomatic sympathetic nervous system stimulation, and central nervous system (CNS) dysfunction. Many drugs and disorders cause it. Diagnosis requires blood tests done at the time of symptoms or during a 72-h fast. Treatment is provision of glucose combined with treatment of the underlying disorder.

Most commonly, symptomatic hypoglycemia is a complication of drug treatment of DM. Oral antihyperglycemics or insulin may be involved.

Symptomatic hypoglycemia unrelated to treatment of DM is relatively rare, in part because the body has extensive counter-regulatory mechanisms to compensate for low blood glucose levels. Glucagon and epinephrine levels surge in response to acute hypoglycemia and appear to be the first line of defense. Cortisol and growth hormone levels also increase acutely and are important in the recovery from prolonged hypoglycemia. The threshold for release of these hormones is usually above that for hypoglycemic symptoms.

Etiology

Causes of physiologic hypoglycemia can be classified as

- Reactive (postprandial) or fasting
- Insulin-mediated or non-insulin-mediated
- Drug-induced or non-drug-induced

Insulin-mediated causes include exogenous administration of insulin or an insulinsecretagogue and insulin-secreting tumors (insulinomas).

A helpful practical classification is based on clinical status: whether hypoglycemia occurs in patients who appear healthy or ill. Within these categories, causes of hypoglycemia can be divided into drug-induced and other causes.

Non–islet cell tumor hypoglycemia (NICTH) is a rare cause of hypoglycemia in which excess insulin growth factor 2 (IGF-2) produced by the tumor is the cause of hypoglycemia.

Pseudohypoglycemia occurs when processing of blood specimens in untreated test tubes is delayed and cells, such as RBCs and leukocytes (especially if increased, as in leukemia or polycythemia), consume glucose. Factitious hypoglycemia is true hypoglycemia induced by nontherapeutic administration of sulfonylureas or insulin.

Symptoms and Signs

The surge in autonomic activity in response to low plasma glucose causes sweating, nausea, warmth, anxiety, tremulousness, palpitations, and possibly hunger and paresthesias. Insufficient glucose supply to the brain causes headache, blurred or double vision, confusion, difficulty speaking, seizures, and coma.

In controlled settings, autonomic symptoms begin at or beneath a plasma glucose level of about 60 mg/dL (3.3 mmol/L), whereas CNS symptoms occur at or below a glucose level of about 50 mg/dL (2.8 mmol/L). However, symptoms suggestive of hypoglycemia are far more common than the condition itself. Most people with glucose levels at these thresholds have no symptoms, and most people with symptoms suggestive of hypoglycemia have normal glucose concentrations.

Diagnosis

- Blood glucose level correlated with clinical findings
- Response to dextrose (or other sugar) administration
- Sometimes 48- or 72-h fast
- Sometimes insulin, C-peptide, and proinsulin levels

In principle, diagnosis requires verification that a low plasma glucose level (< 50 mg/dL [< 2.8 mmol/L]) exists at the time hypoglycemic symptoms occur and that the symptoms are responsive to dextrose administration. If a practitioner is present when symptoms occur, blood should be sent for glucose testing. If glucose is normal, hypoglycemia is ruled out and no further testing is needed. If glucose is abnormally low, serum insulin, C-peptide, and proinsulin measured from the same tube can distinguish insulin-mediated from non–insulin-mediated and factitious from physiologic hypoglycemia and can obviate the need for further testing.

In practice, however, it is unusual that practitioners are present when patients experience symptoms suggestive of hypoglycemia. Home glucose meters are unreliable for quantifying hypoglycemia, and there are no clear glycosylated Hb (HbA_{1C}) thresholds that distinguish long-term hypoglycemia from normoglycemia. So the need for more extensive diagnostic testing is based on the probability that an underlying disorder that could cause hypoglycemia exists given a patient's clinical appearance and coexisting illnesses.

A 72-h fast done in a controlled setting is the gold standard for diagnosis. However, in almost all patients with a hypoglycemic disorder, a 48-h fast is adequate to detect hypoglycemia and a full 72-h fast may not be necessary. Patients drink only noncaloric, noncaffeinated beverages, and plasma glucose is measured at baseline, whenever symptoms occur, and every 4 to 6 h or every 1 to 2 h if glucose falls below 60 mg/dL (3.3 mmol/L). Serum insulin, C-peptide, and proinsulin should be measured at times of hypoglycemia to distinguish endogenous from exogenous (factitious) hypoglycemia. The fast is terminated at 72 h if the patient has experienced no symptoms and glucose remains normal, sooner if glucose decreases to ≤ 45 mg/dL (≤ 2.5 mmol/L) in the presence of hypoglycemic symptoms.

End-of-fast measurements include beta-hydroxybutyrate (which should be low in insulinoma), serum sulfonylurea to detect drug-induced hypoglycemia, and plasma glucose after IV glucagon injection to detect an increase characteristic of insulinoma. Sensitivity, specificity, and predictive values for detecting hypoglycemia by this protocol have not been reported.

There is no definitive lower limit of glucose that unequivocally defines pathologic hypoglycemia during a monitored fast. Normal women tend to have lower fasting glucose levels than men and may have glucose levels as low as 30 mg/dL (1.7 mmol/L) without symptoms. If symptomatic hypoglycemia has not occurred by 48 to 72 h, the patient should exercise vigorously for about 30 min. If hypoglycemia still does not occur, insulinoma is essentially excluded and further testing is generally not indicated.

Treatment

- Oral sugar or IV dextrose
- Sometimes parenteral glucagon

Immediate treatment of hypoglycemia involves provision of glucose. Patients able to eat or drink can drink juices, sucrose water, or glucose solutions; eat candy or other foods; or chew on glucose tablets when symptoms occur. Infants and younger children may be given 10% dextrose solution 2 to 5 mL/kg IV bolus. Adults and older children unable to eat or drink can be given glucagon 0.5 (< 20 kg) or 1 mg (≥ 20 kg) sc or IM or 50% dextrose 50 to 100 mL IV bolus, with or without a continuous infusion of 5 to 10% dextrose solution sufficient to resolve symptoms. The efficacy of glucagon depends on the size of hepatic glycogen stores; glucagon has little effect on plasma glucose in patients who have been fasting or who are hypoglycemic for long periods.

Underlying disorders causing hypoglycemia must also be treated. Islet cell and non–islet cell tumors must first be localized, then removed by enucleation or partial pancreatectomy; about 6% recur within 10 yr. Diazoxide and octreotide can be used to control symptoms while the patient is awaiting surgery or when a patient refuses or is not a candidate for a procedure.

Islet cell hypertrophy is most often a diagnosis of exclusion after an islet cell tumor is sought but not identified.

Drugs that cause hypoglycemia, including alcohol, must be stopped.

Treatment of hereditary and endocrine disorders; liver failure, renal failure, heart failure; sepsis and shock are described elsewhere.

KEY POINTS

- Hypoglycemia is low plasma glucose level (< 50 mg/dL [< 2.8 mmol/L]) *plus* simultaneous hypoglycemic symptoms that reverse with dextrose administration.
- Most hypoglycemia is caused by drugs used to treat DM (including surreptitious use); insulin-secreting tumors are rare causes.
- If etiology is unclear, do a 48- or 72-h fast with measurement of plasma glucose at regular intervals and whenever symptoms occur.
- Measure serum insulin, C-peptide, and proinsulin at times of hypoglycemia to distinguish endogenous from exogenous (factitious) hypoglycemia.

166 Electrolyte Disorders

HYPONATREMIA

Hyponatremia is decrease in serum Na concentration < 136 mEq/L caused by an excess of water relative to solute. Common causes include diuretic use, diarrhea, heart failure, liver disease, renal disease, and the syndrome of inappropriate ADH secretion (SIADH). Clinical manifestations are primarily neurologic (due to an osmotic shift of water into brain cells causing edema), especially in acute hyponatremia, and include headache, confusion, and stupor; seizures and coma may occur. Diagnosis is by measuring serum Na. Serum and urine electrolytes and osmolality and assessment of volume status help determine the cause. Treatment involves restricting water intake and promoting water loss, replacing any Na deficit, and correcting the underlying disorder.

Etiology

Hyponatremia reflects an excess of total body water (TBW) relative to total body Na content. Because total body Na content is reflected by ECF volume status, hyponatremia must be considered along with status of the ECF volume: hypovolemia, euvolemia, and hypervolemia (see Table 166–1). Note that the ECF volume is not the same as effective plasma volume. For example, decreased effective plasma volume may occur with decreased ECF volume (as with diuretic use or hemorrhagic shock), but it may also occur with an increased ECF volume (eg, in heart failure, hypoalbuminemia, or capillary leak syndrome).

Sometimes, a low serum Na measurement is caused by an excess of certain substances (eg, glucose, lipid) in the blood (translocational hyponatremia, pseudohyponatremia) rather than by a water-Na imbalance.

Hypovolemic hyponatremia: Deficiencies in both TBW and total body Na exist, although proportionally more Na than water has been lost; the Na deficit causes hypovolemia. In hypovolemic hyponatremia, both serum osmolality and blood volume decrease. Vasopressin (antidiuretic hormone—ADH) secretion increases despite a decrease in osmolality to maintain blood

Table 166–1. PRINCIPAL CAUSES OF HYPONATREMIA

MECHANISM	CATEGORY	EXAMPLES
Hypovolemic hyponatremia		
Decreased TBW and Na, with a relatively greater decrease in Na	GI losses*	Diarrhea Vomiting
	3rd-space losses*	Burns Pancreatitis Peritonitis Rhabdomyolysis Small-bowel obstruction
	Renal losses	Diuretics Mineralocorticoid deficiency Osmotic diuresis (glucose, urea, mannitol) Salt-losing nephropathies (eg, interstitial nephritis, medullary cystic disease, partial urinary tract obstruction, polycystic kidney disease)
Euvolemic hyponatremia		
Increased TBW with near-normal total body Na	Drugs	Thiazide diuretics, barbiturates, carbamazepine, chlorpropamide, clofibrate, opioids, tolbutamide, vincristine 3,4-Methylenedioxymethamphetamine (MDMA [ecstasy]) Possibly cyclophosphamide, NSAIDs, oxytocin, SSRIs
	Disorders	Adrenal insufficiency as in Addison disease Hypothyroidism Syndrome of inappropriate ADH secretion
	Increased intake of fluids	Primary polydipsia
	States that increase nonosmotic release of vasopressin (ADH)	Emotional stress Nausea Pain Postoperative states
Hypervolemic hyponatremia		
Increased total body Na with a relatively greater increase in TBW	Extrarenal disorders	Cirrhosis Heart failure
	Renal disorders	Acute kidney injury Chronic kidney disease Nephrotic syndrome

*GI and 3rd-space losses cause hyponatremia if replacement fluids are hypotonic compared with losses.
TBW = total body water.

volume. The resulting water retention increases plasma dilution and hyponatremia.

Extrarenal fluid losses, such as those that occur with the losses of Na-containing fluids as in protracted vomiting, severe diarrhea, or sequestration of fluids in a 3rd space (see Table 166–2), can cause hyponatremia typically when losses are replaced by ingesting plain water or liquids low in Na (see Table 166–3) or by hypotonic IV fluid. Significant ECF fluid losses also cause release of vasopressin, causing water retention by the kidneys, which can maintain or worsen hyponatremia. In extrarenal causes of hypovolemia, because the normal renal response to volume loss is Na conservation, urine Na concentration is typically < 10 mEq/L.

Renal fluid losses resulting in hypovolemic hyponatremia may occur with mineralocorticoid deficiency, thiazide diuretic therapy, osmotic diuresis, or salt-losing nephropathy. Salt-losing nephropathy encompasses a loosely defined group of intrinsic renal disorders with primarily renal tubular dysfunction. This group includes interstitial nephritis, medullary cystic disease, partial urinary tract obstruction, and, occasionally, polycystic kidney disease. Renal causes of hypovolemic hyponatremia can usually be differentiated from extrarenal causes by the history. Patients with ongoing renal fluid losses can also be distinguished from patients with extrarenal fluid losses because the urine Na concentration is inappropriately high (> 20 mEq/L). Urine Na concentration may not help in differentiation when metabolic alkalosis (as occurs with protracted vomiting) is present and large amounts of HCO_3 are spilled in the urine, obligating the excretion of Na to maintain electrical neutrality. In metabolic alkalosis, urine chloride concentration frequently differentiates renal from extrarenal sources of volume depletion.

Diuretics may also cause hypovolemic hyponatremia. Thiazide diuretics, in particular, decrease the kidneys' diluting

Table 166–2. COMPOSITION OF BODY FLUIDS

FLUID SOURCE	SODIUM*	POTASSIUM*	CHLORIDE*
Gastric	20–80	5–20	100–150
Pancreatic	120–140	5–15	90–120
Small bowel	100–140	5–15	90–130
Bile	120–140	5–15	80–120
Ileostomy	45–135	3–15	20–115
Diarrhea	10–90	10–80	10–110
Sweat	10–30	3–10	10–35
Burns	140	5	110

*Unit is mEq/L.

Table 166–3. APPROXIMATE SODIUM CONTENT OF COMMON BEVERAGES

BEVERAGE	SODIUM (mEq/L)
Apple juice	1.3
Beer	2.2
Coffee	1
Cola	5–6.5
Diet cola	4.5–6.5
Light beer	1.3
Orange juice	3.7
Sports drink	8–33
Water (including tap water)	< 1

capacity and increase Na excretion. Once volume depletion occurs, the nonosmotic release of vasopressin causes water retention and worsens hyponatremia. Concomitant hypokalemia shifts Na intracellularly and enhances vasopressin release, thereby worsening hyponatremia. This effect of thiazides may last for up to 2 wk after cessation of therapy; however, hyponatremia usually responds to replacement of potassium and volume deficits along with judicious monitoring of water intake until the drug effect dissipates. Elderly patients may have increased Na diuresis and are especially susceptible to thiazide-induced hyponatremia, particularly when they have a preexisting defect in renal capacity to excrete free water. Rarely, such patients develop severe, life-threatening hyponatremia within a few weeks after the initiation of a thiazide diuretic. Loop diuretics much less commonly cause hyponatremia.

Euvolemic hyponatremia: In euvolemic (dilutional) hyponatremia, total body Na and thus ECF volume are normal or near-normal; however, TBW is increased.

Primary polydipsia can cause hyponatremia only when water intake overwhelms the kidneys' ability to excrete water. Because normal kidneys can excrete up to 25 L urine/day, hyponatremia due solely to polydipsia results only from the ingestion of large amounts of water or from defects in renal capacity to excrete free water. Patients affected include those with psychosis or more modest degrees of polydipsia plus renal insufficiency.

Euvolemic hyponatremia may also result from excessive water intake in the presence of Addison disease, hypothyroidism, or nonosmotic vasopressin release (eg, due to stress; postoperative states; use of drugs such as chlorpropamide, tolbutamide, opioids, barbiturates, vincristine, clofibrate, or carbamazepine). Postoperative hyponatremia most commonly occurs because of a combination of nonosmotic vasopressin release and excessive administration of hypotonic fluids after surgery. Certain drugs (eg, cyclophosphamide, NSAIDs, chlorpropamide) potentiate the renal effect of endogenous vasopressin, whereas others (eg, oxytocin) have a direct vasopressin-like effect on the kidneys. Intoxication with 3,4-methylenedioxymethamphetamine (MDMA [ecstasy]) causes hyponatremia by inducing excess water drinking and enhancing vasopressin secretion. A deficiency in water excretion is common in all these conditions. Diuretics can cause or contribute to euvolemic hyponatremia if another factor causes water retention or excessive water intake.

The syndrome of inappropriate ADH secretion (SIADH—see Sidebar 166–1) is another cause of euvolemic hyponatremia.

Hypervolemic hyponatremia: Hypervolemic hyponatremia is characterized by an increase in both total body Na (and thus ECF volume) and TBW with a relatively greater increase in TBW. Various edematous disorders, including heart failure and cirrhosis, cause hypervolemic hyponatremia. Rarely, hyponatremia occurs in nephrotic syndrome, although pseudohyponatremia may be due to interference with Na measurement by elevated lipids. In each of these disorders, a decrease in effective circulating volume results in the release of vasopressin and angiotensin II. The following factors contribute to hyponatremia:

- The antidiuretic effect of vasopressin on the kidneys
- Direct impairment of renal water excretion by angiotensin II
- Decreased GFR
- Stimulation of thirst by angiotensin II

Urine Na excretion is usually < 10 mEq/L, and urine osmolality is high relative to serum osmolality.

Hyponatremia in AIDS: Hyponatremia has been reported in > 50% of hospitalized patients with AIDS. Among the many potential contributing factors are

- Administration of hypotonic fluids
- Impaired renal function
- Nonosmotic vasopressinrelease due to intravascular volume depletion
- Administration of drugs that impair renal water excretion

In addition, adrenal insufficiency has become increasingly common among AIDS patients as the result of cytomegalovirus adrenalitis, mycobacterial infection, or interference with adrenal glucocorticoid and mineralocorticoid synthesis by

Sidebar 166–1. Syndrome of Inappropriate ADH Secretion

The syndrome of inappropriate ADH (vasopressin) secretion (SIADH) is attributed to excessive vasopressin release. It is defined as less-than-maximally-dilute urine in the presence of plasma hypo-osmolality (hyponatremia) without volume depletion or overload, emotional stress, pain, diuretics, or other drugs that stimulate vasopressin secretion (eg, chlorpropamide, carbamazepine, vincristine, clofibrate, antipsychotic drugs, aspirin, ibuprofen, vasopressin) in patients with normal cardiac, hepatic, renal, adrenal, and thyroid function. SIADH is associated with myriad disorders (see Table 166–4).

Table 166–4. DISORDERS ASSOCIATED WITH SYNDROME OF INAPPROPRIATE ADH SECRETION

DISORDER	EXAMPLES
Cancer	CNS Duodenum Lung (especially, small cell carcinoma) Lymphoma Pancreas
Neurologic disorders	Acute intermittent porphyria Acute psychosis Brain abscess Encephalitis Guillain-Barré syndrome Head trauma Meningitis Stroke Subdural or subarachnoid hemorrhage
Pulmonary disorders and treatments	Aspergillosis Lung abscess Pneumonia Positive-pressure breathing TB
Miscellaneous	Protein-energy undernutrition

ketoconazole. SIADH may be present because of coexistent pulmonary or CNS infections.

Symptoms and Signs

Symptoms mainly involve CNS dysfunction. However, when hyponatremia is accompanied by disturbances in total body Na content, signs of ECF volume depletion or volume overload also occur. In general, older chronically ill patients with hyponatremia develop more symptoms than younger otherwise healthy patients. Symptoms are also more severe with faster-onset hyponatremia. Symptoms generally occur when the effective plasma osmolality falls to < 240 mOsm/kg. Symptoms can be subtle and consist mainly of changes in mental status, including altered personality, lethargy, and confusion. As the serum Na falls to < 115 mEq/L, stupor, neuromuscular hyperexcitability, hyperreflexia, seizures, coma, and death can result.

Severe cerebral edema may occur in premenopausal women with acute hyponatremia, perhaps because estrogen and progesterone inhibit brain Na^+, K^+ -ATPase and decrease solute extrusion from brain cells. Sequelae include hypothalamic and posterior pituitary infarction and occasionally osmotic demyelination syndrome or brain stem herniation.

Diagnosis

- Serum and urine electrolytes and osmolality
- Clinical assessment of volume status

Hyponatremia is occasionally suspected in patients who have neurologic abnormalities and are at risk. However, because findings are nonspecific, hyponatremia is often recognized only after serum electrolyte measurement.

Exclusion of translocational hyponatremia and pseudohyponatremia: Serum Na may be low when severe hyperglycemia (or exogenously administered mannitol or glycerol) increases osmolality and water moves out of cells into the ECF. Serum Na concentration falls about 1.6 mEq/L for every 100-mg/dL (5.55-mmol/L) rise in the serum glucose concentration above normal. This condition is often called translocational hyponatremia because it is caused by translocation of water across cell membranes.

Pseudohyponatremia with normal serum osmolality may occur in hyperlipidemia or extreme hyperproteinemia, because the lipid or protein occupies space in the volume of serum taken for analysis; the concentration of Na in serum itself is not affected. Newer methods of measuring serum electrolytes with ion-selective electrodes circumvent this problem.

Identification of the cause: Identifying the cause of hyponatremia can be complex. The history sometimes suggests a cause (eg, significant fluid loss due to vomiting or diarrhea, renal disease, compulsive fluid ingestion, intake of drugs that stimulate vasopressin release or enhance vasopressin action).

The **volume status,** particularly the presence of obvious volume depletion or volume overload, suggests certain causes (see Table 167–1 on p. 1300).

- Overtly **hypovolemic** patients usually have an obvious source of fluid loss and typically have been treated with hypotonic fluid replacement.
- Overtly **hypervolemic** patients usually have a readily recognizable condition, such as heart failure or hepatic or renal disease.
- **Euvolemic** patients and patients with equivocal volume status require more laboratory testing to identify a cause.

Laboratory tests should include serum and urine osmolality and electrolytes. Euvolemic patients should also have thyroid and adrenal function tested. Hypo-osmolality in euvolemic patients should cause excretion of a large volume of dilute urine (eg, osmolality < 100 mOsm/kg and specific gravity < 1.003). Serum Na concentration and serum osmolality that are low and urine osmolality that is inappropriately high (120 to 150 mmol/L) with respect to the low serum osmolality suggest volume overload, volume contraction, or SIADH. Volume overload and volume contraction are differentiated clinically.

When neither volume overload or volume contraction appears likely, SIADH is considered. Patients with SIADH are usually euvolemic or slightly hypervolemic. BUN and creatinine values are normal, and serum uric acid is generally low. Urine Na concentration is usually > 30 mmol/L, and fractional excretion of Na is > 1% (for calculation, see p. 2052).

In patients with hypovolemia and normal renal function, Na reabsorption results in a urine Na of < 20 mmol/L. Urine Na > 20 mmol/L in hypovolemic patients suggests mineralocorticoid deficiency or salt-losing nephropathy. Hyperkalemia suggests adrenal insufficiency.

Treatment

- When hypovolemic, 0.9% saline
- When hypervolemic, fluid restriction, sometimes a diuretic, occasionally a vasopressin antagonist
- When euvolemic, treatment of cause
- In severe, rapid onset or highly symptomatic hyponatremia, partial rapid correction with hypertonic (3%) saline

Hyponatremia can be life threatening and requires prompt recognition and proper treatment. Too-rapid correction of hyponatremia risks neurologic complications, such as osmotic demyelination syndrome. Even with severe hyponatremia, serum Na concentration should not be increased by more than 8 mEq/L over the first 24 h. And, except during the first few hours of treatment of severe hyponatremia, Na should be corrected no faster than 0.5 mEq/L/h. The degree of hyponatremia, the duration and rate of onset, and the patient's symptoms are used to determine which treatment is most appropriate.

In patients with **hypovolemia** and normal adrenal function, administration of 0.9% saline usually corrects both hyponatremia and hypovolemia. When the serum Na is < 120 mEq/L, hyponatremia may not completely correct upon restoration of intravascular volume; restriction of free water ingestion to 500 to 1000 mL/24 h may be needed.

In **hypervolemic patients,** in whom hyponatremia is due to renal Na retention (eg, heart failure, cirrhosis, nephrotic syndrome) and dilution, water restriction combined with treatment of the underlying disorder is required. In patients with heart failure, an ACE inhibitor, in conjunction with a loop diuretic, can correct refractory hyponatremia. In other patients in whom simple fluid restriction is ineffective, a loop diuretic in escalating doses can be used, sometimes in conjunction with IV 0.9% normal saline. K and other electrolytes lost in the urine must be replaced. When hyponatremia is more severe and unresponsive to diuretics, intermittent or continuous hemofiltration may be needed to control ECF volume while hyponatremia is corrected with IV 0.9% normal saline. Severe or resistant hyponatremia generally occurs only when heart or liver disease is near end-stage.

In **euvolemia,** treatment is directed at the cause (eg, hypothyroidism, adrenal insufficiency, diuretic use). When SIADH is present, severe water restriction (eg, 250 to 500 mL/24 h) is generally required. Additionally, a loop diuretic may be combined with IV 0.9% saline as in hypervolemic hyponatremia. Lasting correction depends on successful treatment of the underlying disorder. When the underlying disorder is not correctable, as in metastatic cancer, and patients find severe water restriction unacceptable, demeclocycline 300 to 600 mg po q 12 h may be helpful by inducing a concentrating defect in the kidneys. However, demeclocycline is not widely used due to the possibility of drug-induced acute kidney injury. IV conivaptan, a vasopressin receptor antagonist, causes effective water diuresis without significant loss of electrolytes in the urine and can be used in hospitalized patients for treatment of resistant hyponatremia. Oral tolvaptan, is another vasopressin receptor antagonist with similar action to conivaptan. Tolvaptan use is limited to less than 30 days due to the potential for liver toxicity and it should not be used in patients with liver or kidney disease.

Mild to moderate hyponatremia: Mild to moderate, asymptomatic hyponatremia (ie, serum Na ≥ 121 and < 135 mEq/L) requires restraint because small adjustments are generally sufficient. In diuretic-induced hyponatremia, elimination of the diuretic may be enough; some patients need some Na or K replacement. Similarly, when mild hyponatremia results from inappropriate hypotonic parenteral fluid administration in patients with impaired water excretion, merely altering fluid therapy may suffice.

Severe hyponatremia: In **asymptomatic patients,** severe hyponatremia (serum Na < 121 mEq/L; effective osmolality < 240 mOsm/kg) can be treated safely with stringent restriction of water intake.

In **patients with neurologic symptoms** (eg, confusion, lethargy, seizures, coma), treatment is more controversial. The debate primarily concerns the rate and degree of hyponatremia correction. Many experts recommend that, in general, serum Na be raised no faster than 1 mEq/L/h. However, replacement rates of up to 2 mEq/L/h for the first 2 to 3 h have been suggested for patients with seizures or significantly altered sensorium. Regardless, the rise should be ≤ 8 mEq/L over the first 24 h. More vigorous correction risks precipitating osmotic demyelination syndrome.

Rapid-onset hyponatremia: Acute hyponatremia with known rapid onset (ie, within < 24 h) is a special case. Such rapid onset can occur with

- Acute psychogenic polydipsia
- Use of the recreational drug ecstasy (MDMA)
- Post op patients who received hypotonic fluid during surgery
- Marathon runners

Rapid-onset hyponatremia is problematic because the cells of the CNS have not had time to remove some of the intracellular osmolar compounds used to balance intracellular and extracellular osmolality. Thus, the intracellular environment becomes relatively hypertonic compared to the serum, causing intracellular fluid shifts that can rapidly cause cerebral edema, potentially progressing to brain stem herniation and death. In these patients, rapid correction with hypertonic saline is indicated even when neurologic symptoms are mild (eg, forgetfulness). If more severe neurologic symptoms, including seizures, are present, rapid correction of Na by 4 to 6 mEq/L using hypertonic saline is indicated. The patient should be monitored in an intensive care unit and serum Na levels monitored every 2 h. After Na level has increased by the initial target of 4 to 6 mEq/L, the rate of correction is slowed so that serum Na level does not rise by > 8 mEq/L in the first 24 h.

Hypertonic saline solution: Hypertonic (3%) saline (containing 513 mEq Na/L) use requires frequent (q 2) electrolyte determinations. In some situations, it may be used with a loop diuretic. A newer recommendation includes concurrent administration of desmopressin 1 to 2 mcg q 8 h. The desmopressin prevents an unpredictable water diuresis that can follow the abrupt normalization of endogenous vasopressin that can occur as the underlying disorder causing hyponatremia is corrected.

For patients with rapid-onset hyponatremia and neurologic symptoms, rapid correction is accomplished by giving 100 mL of hypertonic saline IV over 15 min. This dose can be repeated once if neurologic symptoms are still present.

For patients with seizures or coma but slower onset hyponatremia, ≤ 100 mL/h may be administered over 4 to 6 h in amounts sufficient to raise the serum Na 4 to 6 mEq/L. This amount (in mEq) may be calculated using the Na deficit formula as

$$(\text{Desired Change in Na}) \times \text{TBW}$$

where TBW is 0.6 × body weight in kg in men and 0.5 × body weight in kg in women.

For example, the amount of Na needed to raise the Na level from 106 to 112 mEq/L in a 70-kg man can be calculated as follows:

$$(112\ \text{mEq/L} - 106\ \text{mEq/L}) \times (0.6\ \text{L/kg} \times 70\ \text{kg}) = 252\ \text{mEq}$$

Because there is 513 mEq Na/L in hypertonic saline, roughly 0.5 L of hypertonic saline is needed to raise the Na level from 106 to 112 mEq/L. To result in a correction rate of 1 mEq/L/h, this 0.5 L volume would be infused over about 6 h.

Adjustments may be needed based on serum Na concentrations, which are monitored closely during the first few hours of treatment. Patients with seizures, coma, or altered mental status need supportive treatment, which may involve endotracheal intubation, mechanical ventilation, and benzodiazepines (eg, lorazepam 1 to 2 mg IV q 5 to 10 min prn) for seizures.

Selective vasopressin receptor antagonists: The selective vasopressin (V_2) receptor antagonists conivaptan (IV) and tolvaptan (oral) are relatively new treatment options for severe or resistant hyponatremia. These drugs are potentially dangerous because they may correct serum Na concentration too rapidly;

they are typically reserved for severe (< 121 mEq/L) and/or symptomatic hyponatremia that is resistant to correction with fluid restriction. The same pace of correction as for fluid restriction, ≤ 10 mEq/L over 24 h, is used. These drugs should not be used for hypovolemic hyponatremia or in patients with liver disease or advanced chronic kidney disease.

Conivaptan is indicated for treatment of hypervolemic and euvolemic hyponatremia. It requires close monitoring of patient status, fluid balance, and serum electrolytes and so its use is restricted to hospitalized patients. A loading dose is given followed by a continuous infusion over a maximum of 4 days. It is not recommended in patients with advanced chronic kidney disease (estimated GFR < 30 mL/min) and should not be used if anuria is present. Caution is advised in moderate to severe cirrhosis.

Tolvaptan is a once daily tablet indicated for hypervolemic and euvolemic hyponatremia. Close monitoring is recommended especially during initiation and dosage changes. Tolvaptan use is limited to 30 days because of the risk of liver toxicity. Tolvaptan is not recommended for patients with advanced chronic kidney disease or liver disease. Its effectiveness can be limited by increased thirst. Tolvaptan use is also limited by excessive cost.

Both of these drugs are strong inhibitors of CYP3A and as such have multiple drug interactions. Other strong CYP3A inhibitors (eg, ketoconazole, itraconazole, clarithromycin, retroviral protease inhibitors) should be avoided. Clinicians should review the other drugs the patient is taking for potentially dangerous interactions with V_2 receptor antagonists before initiating a treatment trial.

Osmotic demyelination syndrome: Osmotic demyelination syndrome (previously called central pontine myelinolysis) may follow too-rapid correction of hyponatremia. Demyelination classically affects the pons, but other areas of the brain can also be affected. Lesions are more common among patients with alcoholism, undernutrition, or other chronic debilitating illness. Flaccid paralysis, dysarthria, and dysphagia can evolve over a few days or weeks after a hyponatremic episode. The classic pontine lesion may extend dorsally to involve sensory tracts and leave patients with a "locked-in" syndrome (an awake and sentient state in which patients, because of generalized motor paralysis, cannot communicate, except by vertical eye movements controlled above the pons). Damage often is permanent. When Na is replaced too rapidly (eg, > 14 mEq/L/8 h) and neurologic symptoms start to develop, it is critical to prevent further serum Na increases by stopping hypertonic fluids. In such cases, inducing hyponatremia with hypotonic fluid may mitigate the development of permanent neurologic damage.

KEY POINTS

- Hyponatremia may occur with normal, increased, or decreased extracellular fluid volume.
- Common causes include diuretic use, diarrhea, heart failure, liver and renal disease.
- Hyponatremia is potentially life threatening. The degree, duration and symptoms of hyponatremia are used to determine how quickly to correct the serum Na.
- Treatment varies depending on fluid volume status, but in all cases serum Na level should be corrected slowly—by ≤ 8 mEq/L over 24 h, although fairly rapid correction by 4 to 6 mEq/L using hypertonic saline over the first several hours is frequently needed to reverse severe neurologic symptoms.
- Osmotic demyelination syndrome may follow too-rapid correction of hyponatremia.

HYPERNATREMIA

(For hypernatremia in neonates, see p. 2733.)

Hypernatremia is a serum Na concentration > 145 mEq/L. It implies a deficit of total body water (TBW) relative to total body Na, caused by water intake being less than water losses. A major symptom is thirst; other clinical manifestations are primarily neurologic (due to an osmotic shift of water out of brain cells), including confusion, neuromuscular excitability, seizures, and coma. Diagnosis requires measurement of serum Na and sometimes other laboratory tests. Treatment is usually controlled water replacement. When the response to treatment is poor, testing (eg, monitored water deprivation or administration of vasopressin) is directed at detecting causes other than decreased water intake.

Etiology

Hypernatremia reflects a deficit of TBW relative to total body Na content. Because total body Na content is reflected by ECF volume status, hypernatremia must be considered along with status of the ECF volume: hypovolemia, euvolemia, and hypervolemia. Note that the ECF volume is not the same as effective plasma volume. For example, decreased effective plasma volume may occur with decreased ECF volume (as with diuretic use or hemorrhagic shock), but it may also occur with an increased ECF volume (eg, in heart failure, hypoalbuminemia, or capillary leak syndrome).

Hypernatremia usually involves an impaired thirst mechanism or limited access to water, either as contributing factors or primary causes. The severity of the underlying disorder that results in an inability to drink in response to thirst and the effects of hyperosmolality on the brain are thought to be responsible for a high mortality rate in hospitalized adults with hypernatremia. There are several common causes of hypernatremia (see Table 166–5).

Hypovolemic hypernatremia: Hypernatremia associated with hypovolemia occurs with Na loss accompanied by a relatively greater loss of water from the body. Common extrarenal causes include most of those that cause hyponatremia and volume depletion. Either hypernatremia or hyponatremia can occur with severe volume loss, depending on the relative amounts of Na and water lost and the amount of water ingested before presentation.

Renal causes of hypernatremia and volume depletion include therapy with diuretics. Loop diuretics inhibit Na reabsorption in the concentrating portion of the nephrons and can increase water clearance. Osmotic diuresis can also impair renal concentrating capacity because of a hypertonic substance present in the tubular lumen of the distal nephron. Glycerol, mannitol, and occasionally urea can cause osmotic diuresis resulting in hypernatremia.

The most common cause of hypernatremia due to osmotic diuresis is hyperglycemia in patients with diabetes. Because glucose does not penetrate cells in the absence of insulin, hyperglycemia further dehydrates the ICF compartment. The degree of hyperosmolality in hyperglycemia may be obscured by the lowering of serum Na resulting from movement of water out of cells into the ECF (translational hyponatremia). Patients with renal disease can also be predisposed to hypernatremia when their kidneys are unable to maximally concentrate urine.

Euvolemic hypernatremia: Hypernatremia with euvolemia is a decrease in TBW with near-normal total body Na (pure water deficit). Extrarenal causes of water loss, such as excessive sweating, result in some Na loss, but because sweat

Table 166–5. PRINCIPAL CAUSES OF HYPERNATREMIA

DESCRIPTION	CATEGORY	EXAMPLES
Hypovolemic hypernatremia		
Decreased TBW and Na with a relatively greater decrease in TBW	GI losses	Diarrhea Vomiting
	Skin losses	Burns Excessive sweating
	Renal losses	Intrinsic renal disease Loop diuretics Osmotic diuresis (glucose, urea, mannitol)
Euvolemic hypernatremia		
Decreased TBW with near-normal total body Na	Extrarenal losses from the respiratory tract	Tachypnea
	Extrarenal losses from the skin	Excessive sweating Fever
	Renal losses	Central diabetes insipidus Nephrogenic diabetes insipidus
	Other	Inability to access water Primary hypodipsia Reset osmostat
Hypervolemic hypernatremia		
Increased Na with normal or increased TBW	Hypertonic fluid administration	Hypertonic saline $NaHCO_3$ TPN
	Mineralocorticoid excess	Adrenal tumors secreting deoxycorticosterone Congenital adrenal hyperplasia (caused by 11-hydroxylase defect)

TBW = total body water.

is hypotonic, hypernatremia can result before significant hypovolemia. A deficit of almost purely water also occurs in central diabetes insipidus and nephrogenic diabetes insipidus.

Essential hypernatremia (primary hypodipsia) occasionally occurs in children with brain damage and in chronically ill elderly adults. It is characterized by an impaired thirst mechanism (eg, caused by lesions of the brain's thirst center). Altered osmotic trigger for vasopressin release is another possible cause of euvolemic hypernatremia; some lesions cause both an impaired thirst mechanism and an altered osmotic trigger. The nonosmotic release of vasopressin appears intact, and these patients are generally euvolemic.

Hypervolemic hypernatremia: Hypernatremia in rare cases is associated with volume overload. In this case, hypernatremia results from a grossly elevated Na intake associated with limited access to water. One example is the excessive administration of hypertonic $NaHCO_3$ during treatment of lactic acidosis. Hypernatremia can also be caused by the administration of hypertonic saline or incorrectly formulated hyperalimentation.

Hypernatremia in the elderly: Hypernatremia is common among the elderly, particularly postoperative patients and those receiving tube feedings or parenteral nutrition. Other contributing factors may include the following:

- Dependence on others to obtain water
- Impaired thirst mechanism
- Impaired renal concentrating capacity (due to diuretics, impaired vasopressin release, or nephron loss accompanying aging or other renal disease)
- Impaired angiotensin II production (which may contribute directly to the impaired thirst mechanism)

Symptoms and Signs

The major symptom of hypernatremia is thirst. The absence of thirst in conscious patients with hypernatremia suggests an impaired thirst mechanism. Patients with difficulty communicating or ambulating may be unable to express thirst or obtain access to water. Sometimes patients with difficulty communicating express thirst by becoming agitated.

The major signs of hypernatremia result from CNS dysfunction due to brain cell shrinkage. Confusion, neuromuscular excitability, hyperreflexia, seizures, or coma may result. Cerebrovascular damage with subcortical or subarachnoid hemorrhage and venous thromboses have been described in children who died of severe hypernatremia.

In chronic hypernatremia, osmotically active substances are generated in CNS cells (idiogenic osmoles) and increase intracellular osmolality. Therefore, the degree of brain cell dehydration and resultant CNS symptoms are less severe in chronic than in acute hypernatremia.

When hypernatremia occurs with abnormal total body Na, the typical symptoms of volume depletion or volume overload are present. Patients with renal concentrating defects typically excrete a large volume of hypotonic urine. When losses are extrarenal, the route of water loss is often evident (eg, vomiting, diarrhea, excessive sweating), and the urinary Na concentration is low.

Diagnosis

- Serum Na

The diagnosis is clinical and by measuring serum Na. In patients who do not respond to simple rehydration or in whom hypernatremia recurs despite adequate access to water, further diagnostic testing is warranted. Determination of the underlying disorder requires assessment of urine volume and osmolality, particularly after water deprivation.

In patients with increased urine output, a water deprivation test is occasionally used to differentiate among several polyuric states, such as central diabetes insipidus and nephrogenic diabetes insipidus.

Treatment

- Replacement of intravascular volume and of free water

Replacement of intravascular volume and of free water is the main goal of treatment. Oral hydration is effective in conscious patients without significant GI dysfunction. In severe hypernatremia or in patients unable to drink because of continued vomiting or mental status changes, IV hydration is preferred. Hypernatremia that has occurred within the last 24 h should be corrected over the next 24 h. However, hypernatremia that is chronic or of unknown duration should be corrected over 48 h, and the serum osmolality should be lowered at a rate of no faster than 0.5 mOsm/L/h to avoid cerebral edema caused by excess brain solute. The amount of water (in liters) necessary to replace existing deficits may be estimated by the following formula:

$$\text{Free water deficit} = \text{TBW} \times \left[\left(\frac{\text{Serum Na}}{140}\right) - 1\right]$$

where TBW is in liters and is estimated by multiplying weight in kilograms by 0.6 for men and by 0.5 for women; serum Na is in mEq/L. This formula assumes constant total body Na content. In patients with hypernatremia and depletion of total body Na content (ie, who have volume depletion), the free water deficit is greater than that estimated by the formula.

In patients with hypernatremia and ECF volume overload (excess total body Na content), the free water deficit can be replaced with 5% D/W, which can be supplemented with a loop diuretic. However, too-rapid infusion of 5% D/W may cause glucosuria, thereby increasing salt-free water excretion and hypertonicity, especially in patients with diabetes mellitus. Other electrolytes, including serum K, should be monitored and should be replaced as needed.

In patients with hypernatremia and euvolemia, free water can be replaced using either 5% D/W or 0.45% saline.

Treatment of patients with central diabetes insipidus and acquired nephrogenic diabetes insipidus are discussed elsewhere.

In patients with hypernatremia and hypovolemia, particularly in patients with diabetes with nonketotic hyperglycemic coma, 0.45% saline can be given as an alternative to a combination of 0.9% normal saline and 5% D/W to replenish Na and free water. Alternatively, ECF volume and free water can be replaced separately, using the formula given previously to estimate the free water deficit. When severe acidosis (pH < 7.10) is present, $NaHCO_3$ solution can be added to 5% D/W or 0.45% saline, as long as the final solution remains hypotonic.

KEY POINTS

- Hypernatremia is usually caused by limited access to water or an impaired thirst mechanism, and less commonly by diabetes insipidus.
- Manifestations include confusion, neuromuscular excitability, hyperreflexia, seizures, and coma.
- Patients who do not respond to simple rehydration or in whom there is no obvious cause may need assessment of urine volume and osmolality, particularly after water deprivation.
- Replace intravascular volume and free water orally or intravenously at a rate dictated by how acutely (< 24 h) or chronically (> 24 h) the hypernatremia has developed, while watching other serum electrolyte levels (especially K and HCO_3) as well.

OVERVIEW OF DISORDERS OF POTASSIUM CONCENTRATION

K is the most abundant intracellular cation, but only about 2% of total body K is extracellular. Because most intracellular K is contained within muscle cells, total body K is roughly proportional to lean body mass. An average 70-kg adult has about 3500 mEq of K.

K is a major determinant of intracellular osmolality. The ratio between K concentration in the ICF and concentration in the ECF strongly influences cell membrane polarization, which in turn influences important cell processes, such as the conduction of nerve impulses and muscle (including myocardial) cell contraction. Thus, relatively small alterations in serum K concentration can have significant clinical manifestations. Total serum K concentration may be too high (hyperkalemia) or too low (hypokalemia). Clinical manifestations of disorders of K concentration can involve muscle weakness and cardiac arrhythmias.

In the absence of factors that shift K in or out of cells, the serum K concentration correlates closely with total body K content. Once intracellular and extracellular concentrations are stable, a decrease in serum K concentration of about 1 mEq/L indicates a total K deficit of about 200 to 400 mEq. Patients with stable K concentration < 3 mEq/L typically have a significant K deficit.

PEARLS & PITFALLS

- A decrease in serum K concentration of about 1 mEq/L indicates a total K deficit of about 200 to 400 mEq.

K shifts: Factors that shift K in or out of cells include the following:

- Insulin concentrations
- Beta-adrenergic activity
- Acid-base status

Insulin moves K into cells; high concentrations of insulin thus lower serum K concentration. Low concentrations of insulin, as in diabetic ketoacidosis, cause K to move out of cells, thus raising serum K, sometimes even in the presence of total body K deficiency.

Beta-adrenergic agonists, especially selective beta2-agonists, move K into cells, whereas beta-blockade and alpha-agonists promote movement of K out of cells.

Acute metabolic acidosis causes K to move out of cells, whereas acute metabolic alkalosis causes K to move into cells. However, changes in serum HCO_3 concentration may be more important than changes in pH; acidosis caused by accumulation of mineral acids (nonanion gap, hyperchloremic acidosis) is more likely to elevate serum K. In contrast, metabolic acidosis due to accumulation of organic acids (increased anion gap acidosis) does not cause hyperkalemia. Thus, the hyperkalemia common in diabetic ketoacidosis results more from insulin deficiency than from acidosis. Acute respiratory acidosis and alkalosis affect serum K concentration less than metabolic acidosis and alkalosis. Nonetheless, serum K concentration should always be interpreted in the context of the serum pH (and HCO_3 concentration).

Potassium metabolism: Dietary K intake normally varies between 40 and 150 mEq/day. In the steady state, fecal losses are usually close to 10% of intake. The remaining 90% is excreted in the urine so alternations in renal K secretion greatly affect K balance.

When K intake is > 150 mEq/day, about 50% of the excess K appears in the urine over the next several hours. Most of the remainder is transferred into the intracellular compartment, thus minimizing the rise in serum K. When elevated K intake continues, aldosterone secretion is stimulated and thus renal K excretion rises. In addition, K absorption from stool appears to be under some regulation and may fall by 50% in chronic K excess.

When K intake falls, intracellular K again serves to buffer wide swings in serum K concentration. Renal K conservation develops relatively slowly in response to decreases in dietary K and is far less efficient than the kidneys' ability to conserve Na. Thus, K depletion is a frequent clinical problem. Urinary K excretion of 10 mEq/day represents near-maximal renal K conservation and implies significant K depletion.

Acute acidosis impairs K excretion, whereas chronic acidosis and acute alkalosis can promote K excretion. Increased delivery of Na to the distal nephrons, as occurs with high Na intake or loop diuretic therapy, promotes K excretion.

False K concentrations: Pseudohypokalemia, or falsely low serum K, occasionally is found when blood specimens from patients with chronic myelogenous leukemia and a WBC count > 10^5/μL remain at room temperature before being processed because abnormal leukocytes in the sample take up serum K. It is prevented by prompt separation of plasma or serum in blood samples.

Pseudohyperkalemia, or falsely elevated serum K, is more common, typically occurring due to hemolysis and release of intracellular K. To prevent false results, phlebotomy personnel should not rapidly aspirate blood through a narrow-gauge needle or excessively agitate blood samples. Pseudohyperkalemia can also result from platelet count > 400,000/μL due to release of K from platelets during clotting; in these cases, the plasma K (unclotted blood), as opposed to serum K, is normal.

HYPOKALEMIA

Hypokalemia is serum K concentration < 3.5 mEq/L caused by a deficit in total body K stores or abnormal movement of K into cells. The most common causes are excess losses from the kidneys or GI tract. Clinical features include muscle weakness and polyuria; cardiac hyperexcitability may occur with severe hypokalemia. Diagnosis is by serum measurement. Treatment is giving K and managing the cause.

Etiology

Hypokalemia can be caused by decreased intake of K but is usually caused by excessive losses of K in the urine or from the GI tract .

GI tract losses: Abnormal GI K losses occur in all of the following:

- Chronic diarrhea, including chronic laxative abuse and bowel diversion
- Clay (bentonite) ingestion, which binds K and greatly decreases absorption
- Rarely, villous adenoma of the colon, which causes massive K secretion

Protracted vomiting or gastric suction (which removes volume and hydrochloric acid) causes renal K losses due to metabolic alkalosis and stimulation of aldosterone due to volume depletion; aldosterone and metabolic alkalosis both cause the kidneys to excrete K.

Intracellular shift: The transcellular shift of K into cells may also cause hypokalemia. This shift can occur in any of the following:

- Glycogenesis during TPN or enteral hyperalimentation (stimulating insulin release)
- After administration of insulin
- Stimulation of the sympathetic nervous system, particularly with beta2-agonists (eg, albuterol, terbutaline), which may increase cellular K uptake
- Thyrotoxicosis (occasionally) due to excessive beta-sympathetic stimulation (hypokalemic thyrotoxic periodic paralysis)
- Familial periodic paralysis

Familial periodic paralysis is a rare autosomal dominant disorder characterized by transient episodes of profound hypokalemia thought to be due to sudden abnormal shifts of K into cells. Episodes frequently involve varying degrees of paralysis. They are typically precipitated by a large carbohydrate meal or strenuous exercise.

Renal K losses: Various disorders can increase renal K excretion. Excess mineralocorticoid (ie, aldosterone) effect can directly increase K secretion by the distal nephrons and occurs in any of the following:

- Adrenal steroid excess that is due to Cushing syndrome, primary hyperaldosteronism, rare renin-secreting tumors, glucocorticoid-remediable aldosteronism (a rare inherited disorder involving abnormal aldosterone metabolism), and congenital adrenal hyperplasia.
- Ingestion of substances such as glycyrrhizin (present in natural licorice and used in the manufacture of chewing tobacco), which inhibits the enzyme 11 beta-hydroxysteroid dehydrogenase (11 β-HSDH), preventing the conversion of cortisol, which has some mineralocorticoid activity, to cortisone, which does not, resulting in high circulating concentrations of cortisol and renal K wasting.
- Bartter syndrome, an uncommon genetic disorder that is characterized by renal K and Na wasting, excessive production of renin and aldosterone, and normotension. Bartter syndrome is caused by mutations in a loop diuretic–sensitive ion transport mechanism in the loop of Henle.
- Gitelman syndrome is an uncommon genetic disorder characterized by renal K and Na wasting, excessive production of renin and aldosterone, and normotension. Gitelman syndrome is caused by loss of function mutations in a thiazide-sensitive ion transport mechanism in the distal nephron.

Liddle syndrome is a rare autosomal dominant disorder characterized by severe hypertension and hypokalemia. Liddle syndrome is caused by unrestrained Na reabsorption in the distal nephron due to one of several mutations found in genes encoding for epithelial Na channel subunits. Inappropriately high reabsorption of Na results in both hypertension and renal K wasting.

Renal K wasting can also be caused by numerous congenital and acquired renal tubular diseases, such as the renal tubular acidoses and Fanconi syndrome, an unusual syndrome resulting in renal wasting of K, glucose, PO_4, uric acid, and amino acids.

Hypomagnesemia is a common correlate of hypokalemia. Much of this correlation is attributable to common causes (ie, diuretics, diarrhea), but hypomagnesemia itself may also result in increased renal K losses.

Drugs: Diuretics are by far the most commonly used drugs that cause hypokalemia. K-wasting diuretics that block Na reabsorption proximal to the distal nephron include

- Thiazides
- Loop diuretics
- Osmotic diuretics

By inducing diarrhea, laxatives, especially when abused, can cause hypokalemia. Surreptitious diuretic or laxative use or both is a frequent cause of persistent hypokalemia, particularly among patients preoccupied with weight loss and among health care practitioners with access to prescription drugs.

Other drugs that can cause hypokalemia include

- Amphotericin B
- Antipseudomonal penicillins (eg, carbenicillin)
- Penicillin in high doses
- Theophylline (both acute and chronic intoxication)

Symptoms and Signs

Mild hypokalemia (serum K 3 to 3.5 mEq/L) rarely causes symptoms. Serum K < 3 mEq/L generally causes muscle weakness and may lead to paralysis and respiratory failure. Other muscular dysfunction includes cramping, fasciculations, paralytic ileus, hypoventilation, hypotension, tetany, and rhabdomyolysis. Persistent hypokalemia can impair renal concentrating ability, causing polyuria with secondary polydipsia.

Diagnosis

- Serum K measurement
- ECG
- When the mechanism not evident clinically, 24-h urinary K excretion and serum Mg concentration

Hypokalemia (serum K < 3.5 mEq/L) may be found during routine serum electrolyte measurement. It should be suspected in patients with typical changes on an ECG or who have muscular symptoms and risk factors and confirmed by blood testing.

ECG: ECG should be done on patients with hypokalemia. Cardiac effects of hypokalemia are usually minimal until serum K concentrations are < 3 mEq/L. Hypokalemia causes sagging of the ST segment, depression of the T wave, and elevation of the U wave. With marked hypokalemia, the T wave becomes progressively smaller and the U wave becomes increasingly larger. Sometimes, a flat or positive T wave merges with a positive U wave, which may be confused with QT prolongation (see Fig. 166–1). Hypokalemia may cause premature ventricular and atrial contractions, ventricular and atrial tachyarrhythmias, and 2nd- or 3rd-degree atrioventricular block. Such arrhythmias become more severe with increasingly severe hypokalemia; eventually, ventricular fibrillation may occur. Patients with significant preexisting heart disease and patients receiving digoxin are at risk of cardiac conduction abnormalities as a result of even mild hypokalemia.

Diagnosis of cause: The cause is usually apparent by history (particularly the drug history); when it is not, further investigation is warranted.

After acidosis and other causes of intracellular K shift (increased beta-adrenergic effect, hyperinsulinemia) have been eliminated, 24-h urinary K and serum Mg concentrations are measured. In hypokalemia, K secretion is normally < 15 mEq/L. Extrarenal (GI) K loss or decreased K ingestion is suspected in chronic unexplained hypokalemia when renal K secretion

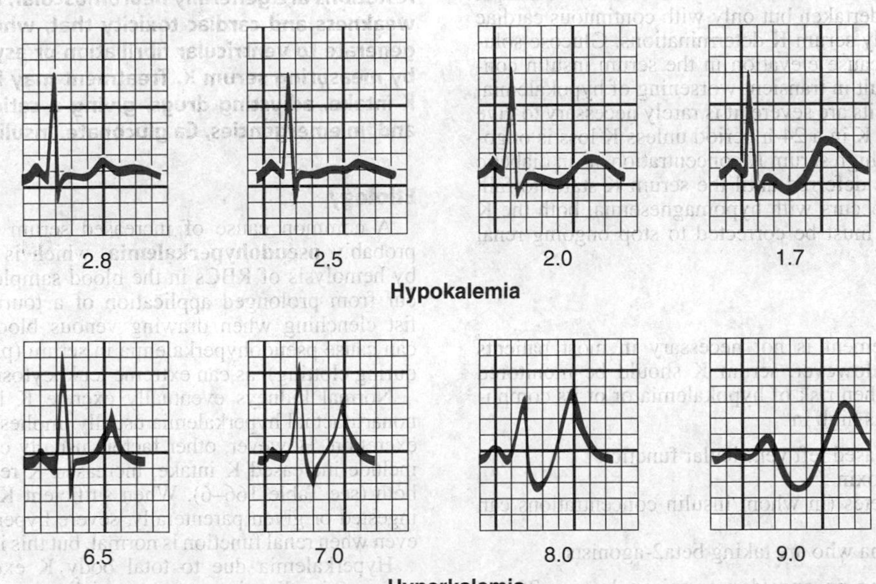

Fig. 166–1. ECG patterns in hypokalemia and hyperkalemia. (Serum K is in mEq/L.)

is < 15 mEq/L. Secretion of > 15 mEq/L suggests a renal cause for K loss. Unexplained hypokalemia with increased renal K secretion and hypertension suggests an aldosterone-secreting tumor or Liddle syndrome. Unexplained hypokalemia with increased renal K loss and normal BP suggests Bartter syndrome or Gitelman syndrome, but hypomagnesemia, surreptitious vomiting, and diuretic abuse are more common and should also be considered.

Treatment

- Oral K supplements
- IV K supplements for severe hypokalemia or ongoing K losses

Many oral potassium supplements are available. Because high single doses can cause GI irritation and occasional bleeding, deficits are usually replaced in divided doses. Liquid K chloride given orally elevates concentrations within 1 to 2 h but has a bitter taste and is tolerated particularly poorly in doses > 25 to 50 mEq. Wax-impregnated K chloride preparations are safe and better tolerated. GI bleeding may be even less common with microencapsulated K chloride preparations. Several of these preparations contain 8 or 10 mEq/capsule. Because a decrease in serum K of 1 mEq/L correlates with about a 200- to 400-mEq deficit in total body K stores, total deficit can be estimated and replaced over a number of days at 20 to 80 mEq/day.

When hypokalemia is severe (eg, with ECG changes or severe symptoms), is unresponsive to oral therapy, or occurs in hospitalized patients who are taking digoxin or who have significant heart disease or ongoing losses, K must be replaced IV. Because K solutions can irritate peripheral veins, the concentration should not exceed 40 mEq/L. The rate of correction of hypokalemia is limited because of the lag in K movement from the extracellular space into cells. *Routine infusion rates should not exceed 10 mEq/h.*

In hypokalemia-induced arrhythmia, IV K chloride must be given more rapidly, usually through a central vein or using multiple peripheral veins simultaneously. Infusion of 40 mEq K chloride/h can be undertaken but only with continuous cardiac monitoring and hourly serum K determinations. Glucose solutions are avoided because elevation in the serum insulin concentrations could result in transient worsening of hypokalemia.

Even when K deficits are severe, it is rarely necessary to give > 100 to 120 mEq of K in a 24-h period unless K loss is ongoing. In K deficit with high serum K concentration, as in diabetic ketoacidosis, IV K is deferred until the serum K starts to fall. When hypokalemia occurs with hypomagnesemia, both the K and Mg deficiencies must be corrected to stop ongoing renal K wasting.

Prevention

Routine K replacement is not necessary in most patients receiving diuretics. However, serum K should be monitored during diuretic use when risk of hypokalemia or of its complications is high. Risk is high in

- Patients with decreased left ventricular function
- Patients taking digoxin
- Patients with diabetes (in whom insulin concentrations can fluctuate)
- Patients with asthma who are taking beta2-agonists

Triamterene 100 mg po once/day or spironolactone 25 mg po qid does not increase K excretion and may be useful in patients who become hypokalemic but must use diuretics. When hypokalemia develops, K supplementation, usually with oral K chloride, is indicated.

KEY POINTS

- Hypokalemia can be caused by decreased intake of K or shift of extracellular K into cells, but it is usually caused by excessive losses of K in the urine or from the GI tract.
- Clinical signs include muscle weakness, cramping, fasciculations, paralytic ileus, and when hypokalemia is severe, hypoventilation, and hypotension.
- ECG changes typically occur when serum K is < 3 mEq/L, and include ST segment sagging, T wave depression, and U wave elevation. With marked hypokalemia, the T wave becomes progressively smaller and the U wave becomes increasingly larger.
- Hypokalemia may cause premature ventricular and atrial contractions, ventricular and atrial tachyarrhythmias, and 2nd- or 3rd-degree atrioventricular block; eventually, ventricular fibrillation may occur.
- Replace K orally, giving 20 to 80 mEq/day unless patients have ECG changes or severe symptoms.
- For hypokalemic arrhythmia, give IV K chloride through a central vein at a maximum of 40 mEq/h and only with continuous cardiac monitoring; routine IV infusion should be no more than 10 mEq/h.

HYPERKALEMIA

Hyperkalemia is a serum K concentration > 5.5 mEq/L, usually resulting from decreased renal K excretion or abnormal movement of K out of cells. There are usually several simultaneous contributing factors, including increased K intake, drugs that impair renal K excretion, and acute kidney injury or chronic kidney disease. Hyperkalemia can also occur in metabolic acidosis as in diabetic ketoacidosis. Clinical manifestations are generally neuromuscular, resulting in muscle weakness and cardiac toxicity that, when severe, can degenerate to ventricular fibrillation or asystole. Diagnosis is by measuring serum K. Treatment may involve decreasing K intake, adjusting drugs, giving a cation exchange resin and, in emergencies, Ca gluconate, insulin, and dialysis.

Etiology

A common cause of increased serum K concentration is probably **pseudohyperkalemia,** which is most often caused by hemolysis of RBCs in the blood sample. This can also occur from prolonged application of a tourniquet or excessive fist clenching when drawing venous blood. Thrombocytosis can cause pseudohyperkalemia in serum (platelet K is released during clotting), as can extreme leukocytosis.

Normal kidneys eventually excrete K loads, so sustained, nonartifactual hyperkalemia usually implies diminished renal K excretion. However, other factors usually contribute. They can include increased K intake, increased K release from cells, or both (see Table 166–6). When sufficient K chloride is rapidly ingested or given parenterally, severe hyperkalemia may result even when renal function is normal, but this is usually temporary.

Hyperkalemia due to total body K excess is particularly common in oliguric states (especially acute kidney injury) and with rhabdomyolysis, burns, bleeding into soft tissue or the GI tract, and adrenal insufficiency. In chronic kidney disease, hyperkalemia is uncommon until the GFR falls to < 10 to 15 mL/min unless dietary or IV K intake is excessive.

Symptoms and Signs

Although flaccid paralysis occasionally occurs, hyperkalemia is usually asymptomatic until cardiac arrhythmias develop.

In the rare disorder hyperkalemic familial periodic paralysis, weakness frequently develops during attacks and can progress to frank paralysis.

Diagnosis

- Serum K measurement
- ECG
- Review of drug use
- Assessment of renal function

Hyperkalemia (serum K > 5.5 mEq/L) may be found on routine serum electrolyte measurement. It should be suspected in patients with typical changes on an ECG or patients at high risk, such as those with renal failure, advanced heart failure, or urinary obstruction, or treated with ACE inhibitors and K-sparing diuretics.

Pseudohyperkalemia should be considered in patients without risk factors or ECG abnormalities. Hemolysis may be reported by the laboratory. When pseudohyperkalemia is suspected, K concentration should be repeated, taking measures to avoid hemolysis of the sample (such as avoiding small-gauge needles or tourniquet use and limited fist clenching) and blood should be promptly processed by the laboratory.

ECG: ECG should be done on patients with hyperkalemia. ECG changes (see Fig. 166–1) are frequently visible when serum K is > 5.5 mEq/L. Slowing of conduction characterized by an increased PR interval and shortening of the QT interval as well as tall, symmetric, peaked T waves are visible initially. K > 6.5 mEq/L causes further slowing of conduction with widening of the QRS interval, disappearance of the P wave, and nodal and escape ventricular arrhythmias. Finally, the QRS complex degenerates into a sine wave pattern, and ventricular fibrillation or asystole ensues.

Diagnosis of cause: Diagnosis of the cause of hyperkalemia requires a detailed history, including a review of drugs, a physical examination with emphasis on volume status, and measurement of electrolytes, BUN, and creatinine. In cases in which renal failure is present, additional tests, including renal ultrasonography to exclude obstruction, are needed.

Treatment

- Treatment of the cause
- For mild hyperkalemia, Na polystyrene sulfonate
- For moderate or severe hyperkalemia, IV insulin and glucose, an IV Ca solution, possibly an inhaled beta2-agonist, and usually hemodialysis

Mild hyperkalemia: Patients with serum K < 6 mEq/L and no ECG abnormalities may respond to diminished K intake or stopping K-elevating drugs. The addition of a loop diuretic enhances renal K excretion as long as volume depletion is not present.

Na polystyrene sulfonate in sorbitol can be given (15 to 30 g in 30 to 70 mL of 70% sorbitol po q 4 to 6 h). It acts as a cation exchange resin and removes K through the GI mucosa. Sorbitol is administered with the resin to ensure passage through the GI tract. Patients unable to take drugs orally because of nausea or other reasons may be given similar doses by enema. Enemas are not as effective at lowering K in patients with ileus. Enemas should not be used if acute abdomen is suspected. About 1 mEq of K is removed per gram of resin given. Resin therapy is slow and often fails to lower serum K significantly in hypercatabolic states. Because Na is exchanged for K when Na polystyrene sulfonate is used, Na overload may occur, particularly in oliguric patients with preexisting volume overload.

In patients with recurrent hyperkalemia, avoidance of drugs that can induce hyperkalemia (see Table 166–6) is generally all that is needed. In patients who need ACE inhibitors and angiotensin receptor blocking agents (eg, patients with chronic heart failure or diabetic nephropathy), newly available polymer resin patiromer can be taken daily to help decrease gut absorption of K and prevent hyperkalemia.

Table 166–6. FACTORS CONTRIBUTING TO HYPERKALEMIA

CATEGORY	EXAMPLES
Decreased potassium excretion	
Drugs	ACE inhibitors Angiotensin II receptor blockers Direct renin inhibitor (aliskiren) Cyclosporine Heparin K-sparing diuretics Lithium NSAIDs Tacrolimus Trimethoprim
Hypoaldosteronism	Adrenal insufficiency
Kidney disorders	Acute kidney injury Chronic kidney disease Obstruction Renal tubular acidosis type IV
Other	Decreased effective circulating volume
Increased K intake (usually iatrogenic)	
Oral	Dietary Oral K supplements
IV	Blood transfusions IV fluids with supplemental K K citrate solutions K-containing drugs (eg, penicillin G) TPN
Increased K movement out of cells	
Drugs	Beta-blockers Digoxin toxicity
Increased tissue catabolism	Acute tumor lysis Acute intravascular hemolysis Bleeding into soft tissues or GI tract Burns Rhabdomyolysis
Insulin deficiency	Diabetes mellitus Fasting
Disorders	Hyperkalemic familial periodic paralysis (rare)
Other	Exercise Metabolic acidosis

Moderate to severe hyperkalemia: Serum K between 6 and 6.5 mEq/L needs prompt attention, but the actual treatment depends on the clinical situation. If no ECG changes are present and renal function is intact, maneuvers as for mild hyperkalemia are usually effective. Follow-up serum K measurements are needed to ensure that the hyperkalemia has been successfully treated. If serum K is > 6.5 mEq/L, more aggressive therapy is required. Administration of regular insulin 5 to 10 units IV is followed immediately by or administered simultaneously with rapid infusion of 50 mL 50% glucose. Infusion of 10% D/W should follow at 50 mL/h to prevent hypoglycemia. The effect on serum K peaks in 1 h and lasts for several hours.

If ECG changes include the loss of P-wave or widening of the QRS complex, treatment with IV Ca as well as insulin and glucose is indicated; 10 to 20 mL 10% Ca gluconate (or 5 to 10 mL 22% Ca gluceptate) is given IV over 5 to 10 min. Ca antagonizes the effect of hyperkalemia on cardiac muscle. Ca should be given with caution to patients taking digoxin because of the risk of precipitating hypokalemia-related arrhythmias. If the ECG shows a sine wave pattern or asystole, Ca gluconate may be given more rapidly (5 to 10 mL IV over 2 min). Ca chloride can also be used but can be irritating to peripheral veins and cause tissue necrosis if extravasated. Ca chloride should be given only through a correctly positioned central venous catheter. The benefits of Ca occur within minutes but last only 20 to 30 min. Ca infusion is a temporizing measure while awaiting the effects of other treatments or initiation of hemodialysis and may need to be repeated.

A high-dose beta2-agonist, such as albuterol 10 to 20 mg inhaled over 10 min (5 mg/mL concentration), can lower serum K by 0.5 to 1.5 mEq/L and may be a helpful adjunct. The peak effect occurs in 90 min. However, beta2-agonists are contraindicated in patients with unstable angina or acute myocardial infarction.

Administration of IV $NaHCO_3$ is controversial. It may lower serum K over several hours. Reduction may result from alkalinization or the hypertonicity due to the concentrated Na in the preparation. The amount of Na that it contains may be harmful for dialysis patients who also may have volume overload. Another possible complication of IV $NaHCO_3$ is to acutely lower ionized Ca concentration which would further enhance the cardiotoxicity of hyperkalemia. When given, the typical dose is 3 ampules of 7.5% $NaHCO_3$ in one liter 5% D/W infused over 2 to 4 h. HCO_3 therapy has little effect when used by itself in patients with severe renal insufficiency unless acidemia is also present.

In addition to strategies for lowering K by shifting it into cells, maneuvers to remove K from the body should also be done early in the treatment of severe or symptomatic hyperkalemia. K can be removed via the GI tract by administration of Na polystyrene sulfonate (see p. 1283), but because the rate of K removal is somewhat unpredictable, close monitoring is needed. Patiromer is not recommended for use as an emergency treatment to acutely lower K because of its delayed onset of action.

Hemodialysis should be instituted promptly after emergency measures in patients with renal failure or when emergency treatment is ineffective. Dialysis should be considered early in patients with end-stage renal disease and hyperkalemia because they are at increased risk of progression to more severe hyperkalemia and serious cardiac arrhythmias. Peritoneal dialysis is relatively inefficient at removing K acutely.

KEY POINTS

- Common causes of hyperkalemia include K-retaining drugs, renal insufficiency, adrenal insufficiency, and disorders involving cellular breakdown (eg, rhabdomyolysis, burns, bleeding into soft tissue or the GI tract).
- Hyperkalemia is usually asymptomatic until cardiac toxicity develops, although some patients have weakness.
- ECG changes begin with an increased PR interval, shortening of the QT interval, and tall, symmetric, peaked T waves; with K > 6.5 mEq/L, QRS interval widens, and P wave disappears; ultimately, the QRS complex degenerates into a sine wave pattern, and ventricular fibrillation or asystole ensues.
- Give Na polystyrene sulfonate for mild hyperkalemia.
- Give IV insulin, glucose, and Ca, and possibly an inhaled beta2-agonist for moderate to severe hyperkalemia.
- Use hemodialysis for patients with chronic kidney disease and those with significant ECG changes.

OVERVIEW OF DISORDERS OF CALCIUM CONCENTRATION

Ca is required for the proper functioning of muscle contraction, nerve conduction, hormone release, and blood coagulation. In addition, proper Ca concentration is required for various other metabolic processes.

Maintenance of body Ca stores (to avoid hypocalcemia or hypercalcemia) depends on

- Dietary Ca intake
- Absorption of Ca from the GI tract
- Renal Ca excretion

In a balanced diet, roughly 1000 mg of Ca is ingested each day and about 200 mg/day is secreted into the GI tract in the bile and other GI secretions. Depending on the concentration of circulating parathyroid hormone (PTH) and active vitamin D, $1,25(OH)_2D$ (1,25-dihydroxycholecalciferol, calcitriol), roughly 200 to 400 mg of this Ca is absorbed from the intestine each day. The remaining 800 to 1000 mg appears in the stool. Ca balance is maintained through renal Ca excretion averaging 200 mg/day, which also depends on circulating PTH and calcitonin levels.

Both extracellular and intracellular Ca concentrations are tightly regulated by bidirectional Ca transport across the plasma membrane of cells and intracellular organelles, such as the endoplasmic reticulum, the sarcoplasmic reticulum of muscle cells, and the mitochondria.

Ionized Ca is the physiologically active form. Cytosolic ionized Ca is maintained within the micromolar range (< 1/1000 of the serum concentration). Ionized Ca acts as an intracellular 2nd messenger; it is involved in skeletal muscle contraction, excitation-contraction coupling in cardiac and smooth muscle, and activation of protein kinases and enzyme phosphorylation. Ca is also involved in the action of other intracellular messengers, such as cAMP and inositol 1,4,5-triphosphate, and thus mediates the cellular response to numerous hormones, including epinephrine, glucagon, vasopressin (ADH), secretin, and cholecystokinin.

Despite its important intracellular roles, about 99% of body Ca is in bone, mainly as hydroxyapatite crystals. About 1% of bone Ca is freely exchangeable with the ECF and, therefore, is available for buffering changes in Ca balance.

Normal **total serum Ca** concentration ranges from 8.8 to 10.4 mg/dL (2.20 to 2.60 mmol/L). About 40% of the total blood Ca is bound to plasma proteins, primarily albumin. The remaining 60% includes ionized Ca plus Ca complexed with PO_4 and citrate. Total Ca (ie, protein-bound, complexed, and ionized Ca) is usually what is determined by clinical laboratory measurement.

However, ideally, **ionized (or free) Ca** should be estimated or measured because it is the physiologically active form of Ca in plasma and because its blood level does not always correlate with total serum Ca.

- Ionized Ca is generally assumed to be about 50% of the total serum Ca.
- Ionized Ca can be estimated, based on total serum Ca and serum albumin levels (see Sidebar 166–2).
- Direct determination of ionized Ca, because of its technical difficulty, is usually restricted to patients in whom significant alteration of protein binding of serum Ca is suspected.

Normal ionized serum Ca concentration range varies somewhat between laboratories, but is typically 4.7 to 5.2 mg/dL (1.17 to 1.30 mmol/L).

Regulation of Ca Metabolism

The metabolism of Ca and of PO_4 (see p. 1294) is intimately related. The regulation of both Ca and PO_4 balance is greatly influenced by concentrations of circulating PTH, vitamin D, and, to a lesser extent, calcitonin. Ca and PO_4 concentrations are also linked by their ability to chemically react to form Ca PO_4. The product of concentrations of Ca and PO_4 (in mEq/L) is estimated to be < 60 normally; when the product exceeds 70, precipitation of Ca PO_4 crystals in soft tissue is much more likely. Calcification of vascular tissue accelerates arteriosclerotic vascular disease and may occur when the Ca and PO_4 product is even lower (> 55), especially in patients with chronic kidney disease.

PTH is secreted by the parathyroid glands. It has several actions, but perhaps the most important is to defend against hypocalcemia. Parathyroid cells sense decreases in serum Ca and, in response, release preformed PTH into the circulation. PTH increases serum Ca within minutes by increasing renal and intestinal absorption of Ca and by rapidly mobilizing Ca and PO_4 from bone (bone resorption). Renal Ca excretion generally parallels Na excretion and is influenced by many of the same factors that govern Na transport in the proximal tubule. However, PTH enhances distal tubular Ca reabsorption independently of Na.

Sidebar 166–2. Estimation of Ionized Calcium Concentration

Ionized Ca concentration can be estimated from routine laboratory tests, usually with reasonable accuracy.

In hypoalbuminemia, measured serum Ca is often low, mainly reflecting a low concentration of protein-bound Ca, while ionized Ca can be normal. Measured total serum Ca decreases or increases by about 0.8 mg/dL (0.2 mmol/L) for every 1 g/dL decrease or increase in albumin. Thus, an albumin concentration of 2.0 g/dL (normal, 4.0 g/dL) should itself reduce measured serum Ca by 1.6 mg/dL (0.4 mmol/L).

Similarly, increases in serum proteins, as occur in multiple myeloma, can raise total serum Ca. Acidosis increases ionized Ca by decreasing protein binding, whereas alkalosis decreases ionized Ca.

PTH also decreases renal PO_4 reabsorption and thus increases renal PO_4 losses. Renal PO_4 loss prevents the solubility product of Ca and PO_4 from being exceeded in plasma as Ca concentrations rise in response to PTH.

PTH also increases serum Ca by stimulating conversion of vitamin D to its most active form, calcitriol. This form of vitamin D increases the percentage of dietary Ca absorbed by the intestine. Despite increased Ca absorption, long-term increases in PTH secretion generally result in further bone resorption by inhibiting osteoblastic function and promoting osteoclastic activity. PTH and vitamin D both function as important regulators of bone growth and bone remodeling (see p. 50).

Radioimmunoassays for the intact PTH molecule are still the recommended way to test for PTH. Second-generation assays for intact PTH are available. These tests measure bioavailable PTH or complete PTH. They give values equal to 50 to 60% of those obtained with the older assay. Both types of assays can be used for diagnosing primary hyperparathyroidism or monitoring hyperparathyroidism secondary to renal disease, as long as normal ranges are noted.

PTH increases urinary cAMP. Sometimes total or nephrogenous cAMP excretion is measured in diagnosis of pseudohypoparathyroidism.

Calcitonin is secreted by the thyroid parafollicular cells (C cells). Calcitonin tends to lower serum Ca concentration by enhancing cellular uptake, renal excretion, and bone formation. The effects of calcitonin on bone metabolism are much weaker than those of either PTH or vitamin D.

HYPOCALCEMIA

Hypocalcemia is a total serum Ca concentration < 8.8 mg/dL (< 2.20 mmol/L) in the presence of normal plasma protein concentrations or a serum ionized Ca concentration < 4.7 mg/dL (< 1.17 mmol/L). Causes include hypoparathyroidism, vitamin D deficiency, and renal disease. Manifestations include paresthesias, tetany, and, when severe, seizures, encephalopathy, and heart failure. Diagnosis involves measurement of serum Ca with adjustment for serum albumin concentration. Treatment is administration of Ca, sometimes with vitamin D.

Etiology

Hypocalcemia has a number of causes, including

- Hypoparathyroidism
- Pseudohypoparathyroidism
- Vitamin D deficiency and dependency
- Renal disease

Hypoparathyroidism: Hypoparathyroidism is characterized by hypocalcemia and hyperphosphatemia and often causes chronic tetany. Hypoparathyroidism results from deficient parathyroid hormone (PTH), which can occur in autoimmune disorders or after the accidental removal of or damage to several parathyroid glands during thyroidectomy. Transient hypoparathyroidism is common after subtotal thyroidectomy, but permanent hypoparathyroidism occurs after < 3% of such thyroidectomies done by experienced surgeons. Manifestations of hypocalcemia usually begin about 24 to 48 h postoperatively but may occur after months or years. PTH deficiency is more common after radical thyroidectomy for cancer or as the result of surgery on the parathyroid glands (subtotal or total parathyroidectomy). Risk factors for severe hypocalcemia after subtotal parathyroidectomy include

- Severe preoperative hypercalcemia
- Removal of a large adenoma
- Elevated alkaline phosphatase
- Chronic kidney disease

Idiopathic hypoparathyroidism is an uncommon sporadic or inherited condition in which the parathyroid glands are absent or atrophied. It manifests in childhood. The parathyroid glands are occasionally absent and thymic aplasia and abnormalities of the arteries arising from the brachial arches (DiGeorge syndrome) are present. Other inherited forms include polyglandular autoimmune failure syndrome, autoimmune hypoparathyroidism associated with mucocutaneous candidiasis, and X-linked recessive idiopathic hypoparathyroidism.

Pseudohypoparathyroidism: Pseudohypoparathyroidism is an uncommon group of disorders characterized not by hormone deficiency but by target organ resistance to PTH. Complex genetic transmission of these disorders occurs.

Type Ia pseudohypoparathyroidism (Albright hereditary osteodystrophy) is caused by a mutation in the stimulatory Gs-alpha1 protein of the adenylyl cyclase complex (*GNAS1*). The result is failure of normal renal phosphaturic response or increase in urinary cAMP to PTH. Patients are usually hypocalcemic and hyperphosphatemic. Secondary hyperparathyroidism and hyperparathyroid bone disease can occur. Associated abnormalities include short stature, round facies, intellectual disability with calcification of the basal ganglia, shortened metacarpal and metatarsal bones, mild hypothyroidism, and other subtle endocrine abnormalities. Because only the maternal allele for *GNAS1* is expressed in the kidneys, patients whose abnormal gene is paternal, although they have many of the somatic features of the disease, do not have hypocalcemia, hyperphosphatemia, or secondary hyperparathyroidism; this condition is sometimes described as pseudopseudohypoparathyroidism.

Type Ib pseudohypoparathyroidism is less well known. Affected patients have hypocalcemia, hyperphosphatemia, and secondary hyperparathyroidism but do not have the other associated abnormalities.

Type II pseudohypoparathyroidism is even less common than type I. In affected patients, exogenous PTH raises the urinary cAMP normally but does not raise serum Ca or urinary PO_4. An intracellular resistance to cAMP has been proposed.

Vitamin D deficiency and dependency: Vitamin D deficiency and dependency are discussed in full elsewhere.

Vitamin D is ingested in foods naturally high in vitamin D or fortified with it. It is also formed in the skin in response to sunlight (UV light). Vitamin D deficiency may result from inadequate dietary intake or decreased absorption due to hepatobiliary disease or intestinal malabsorption. It can also result from alterations in vitamin D metabolism as occur with certain drugs (eg, phenytoin, phenobarbital, rifampin) or from decreased formation in the skin due to lack of exposure to sunlight. Aging also decreases skin synthetic capacity.

Decreased skin synthesis is an important cause of acquired vitamin D deficiency among people who spend a great deal of time indoors, who live in high northern or southern latitudes, and who wear clothing that covers them completely or frequently use sunblocking agents. Accordingly, subclinical vitamin D deficiency is fairly common, especially during winter months in temperate climates among the elderly. The institutionalized elderly are at particular risk because of decreased skin synthetic capacity, undernutrition, and lack of sun exposure. In fact, most people with deficiency have both decreased skin synthesis and dietary deficiency. However, most clinicians feel that the significant dangers of skin cancer outweigh the as yet unproven risk of moderately low vitamin D levels so increasing sun exposure or doing without sunblocks is not recommended; vitamin D supplements are readily available for patients with concerns.

Vitamin D–dependency results from the inability to convert vitamin D to its active form or decreased responsiveness of end-organs to adequate levels of active vitamin.

- Type I vitamin D–dependent rickets (pseudovitamin D–deficiency rickets) is an autosomal recessive disorder involving a mutation in the gene encoding the 1-alpha-hydroxylase enzyme. Normally expressed in the kidney, 1-alpha-hydroxylase is needed to convert inactive vitamin D to the active form calcitriol.
- In type II vitamin D–dependent rickets, target organs cannot respond to calcitriol. Vitamin D deficiency, hypocalcemia, and severe hypophosphatemia occur. Muscle weakness, pain, and typical bone deformities can occur.

Renal disease: Renal tubular disease, including acquired proximal renal tubular acidosis due to nephrotoxins (eg, heavy metals, cadmium in particular) and distal renal tubular acidosis, can cause severe hypocalcemia due to abnormal renal loss of Ca and decreased renal conversion of vitamin D to active $1,25(OH)_2D$.

Renal failure can result in diminished formation of $1,25(OH)_2D$ due to

- Direct renal cell damage
- Suppression of 1-alpha-hydroxylase (needed for the vitamin D conversion) by hyperphosphatemia

Other causes: Other causes of hypocalcemia include

- Mg depletion (can cause relative PTH deficiency and end-organ resistance to PTH action, usually when serum Mg concentrations are < 1.0 mg/dL [< 0.5 mmol/L]; Mg repletion increases PTH concentrations and improves renal Ca conservation)
- Acute pancreatitis (when lipolytic products released from the inflamed pancreas chelate Ca)
- Hypoproteinemia (reduces the protein-bound fraction of serum Ca; hypocalcemia due to diminished protein binding is asymptomatic—because ionized Ca is unchanged, this entity has been termed factitious hypocalcemia)
- Hungry bone syndrome (persistent hypocalcemia and hypophosphatemia occurring after surgical or medical correction of moderate to severe hyperparathyroidism in patients in whom serum Ca concentrations had been supported by high bone turnover induced by greatly elevated PTH—hungry bone syndrome has been described after parathyroidectomy, after renal transplantation, and rarely in patients with end-stage renal disease treated with calcimimetics)
- Septic shock (due to suppression of PTH release and decreased conversion of 25(OH)D to $1,25(OH)_2D$)
- Hyperphosphatemia (causes hypocalcemia by poorly understood mechanisms; patients with renal failure and subsequent PO_4 retention are particularly prone)
- Drugs including anticonvulsants (eg, phenytoin, phenobarbital) and rifampin, which alter vitamin D metabolism, and drugs generally used to treat hypercalcemia
- Transfusion of > 10 units of citrate-anticoagulated blood and use of radiocontrast agents containing the divalent ion-chelating agent ethylenediaminetetraacetate (EDTA—can decrease the concentration of bioavailable ionized Ca while total serum Ca concentrations remain unchanged)
- Infusion of gadolinium (may spuriously lower Ca concentration)

Although excessive secretion of calcitonin might be expected to cause hypocalcemia, calcitonin actually has only a minor effect on serum Ca. For example, low serum Ca concentrations rarely occur in patients with large amounts of circulating calcitonin due to medullary carcinoma of the thyroid.

Symptoms and Signs

Hypocalcemia is frequently asymptomatic. The presence of hypoparathyroidism is often suggested by the clinical manifestations of the underlying disorder (eg, short stature, round facies, intellectual disability, basal ganglia calcification in type 1a pseudohypoparathyroidism).

Major clinical manifestations of hypocalcemia are due to disturbances in cellular membrane potential, resulting in neuromuscular irritability.

Neurologic manifestations: Muscle cramps involving the back and legs are common.

Insidious hypocalcemia may cause mild, diffuse encephalopathy and should be suspected in patients with unexplained dementia, depression, or psychosis.

Papilledema occasionally occurs.

Severe hypocalcemia with serum Ca < 7 mg/dL (< 1.75 mmol/L) may cause hyperreflexia, tetany, laryngospasm, or generalized seizures.

Tetany characteristically results from severe hypocalcemia but can result from reduction in the ionized fraction of serum Ca without marked hypocalcemia, as occurs in severe alkalosis. Tetany is characterized by the following:

- Sensory symptoms consisting of paresthesias of the lips, tongue, fingers, and feet
- Carpopedal spasm, which may be prolonged and painful
- Generalized muscle aching
- Spasm of facial musculature

Tetany may be overt with spontaneous symptoms or latent and requiring provocative tests to elicit. Latent tetany generally occurs at less severely decreased serum Ca concentrations: 7 to 8 mg/dL (1.75 to 2.20 mmol/L).

Chvostek and Trousseau signs are easily elicited at the bedside to identify latent tetany.

Chvostek sign is an involuntary twitching of the facial muscles elicited by a light tapping of the facial nerve just anterior to the exterior auditory meatus. It is present in ≤ 10% of healthy people and in most people with acute hypocalcemia but is often absent in chronic hypocalcemia.

Trousseau sign is the precipitation of carpal spasm by reduction of the blood supply to the hand with a tourniquet or BP cuff inflated to 20 mm Hg above systolic BP applied to the forearm for 3 min. Trousseau sign also occurs in alkalosis, hypomagnesemia, hypokalemia, and hyperkalemia and in about 6% of people with no identifiable electrolyte disturbance.

Other manifestations: Many other abnormalities may occur with chronic hypocalcemia, such as dry and scaly skin, brittle nails, and coarse hair. *Candida* infections occasionally occur in hypocalcemia but most commonly occur in patients with idiopathic hypoparathyroidism. Cataracts occasionally occur with long-standing hypocalcemia and are not reversible by correction of serum Ca.

Diagnosis

- Estimation or measurement of ionized Ca (the physiologically active form of Ca)
- Sometimes further testing, including measurement of Mg, PTH, PO_4, alkaline phosphatase, and vitamin D concentrations in blood and cAMP and PO_4 concentrations in urine

Hypocalcemia may be suspected in patients with characteristic neurologic manifestations or cardiac arrhythmias but is often found incidentally. Hypocalcemia is diagnosed by a total serum Ca concentration < 8.8 mg/dL (< 2.20 mmol/L). However, because low plasma protein can lower total, but not ionized, serum Ca, ionized Ca should be estimated based on albumin concentration (see Sidebar 166–2).

Suspicion of low ionized Ca mandates its direct measurement, despite normal total serum Ca. A serum ionized Ca concentration < 4.7 mg/dL (< 1.17 mmol/L) is low.

Hypocalcemic patients should undergo measurement of renal function (eg, BUN, creatinine), serum PO_4, Mg, and alkaline phosphatase.

When no etiology (eg, alkalosis, renal failure, drugs, or massive blood transfusion) is obvious, further testing is needed (see Table 166–7). Additional testing begins with serum concentrations of Mg, PO_4, PTH, alkaline phosphatase, and occasionally vitamin D levels (25(OH)D, and $1,25(OH)_2D$). Urinary PO_4 and cAMP concentrations are measured when pseudohypoparathyroidism is suspected.

PTH concentration should be measured as an assay of the intact molecule. Because hypocalcemia is the major stimulus for PTH secretion, PTH normally should be elevated in response to hypocalcemia. Thus,

- Low or even low-normal PTH concentrations are inappropriate and suggest hypoparathyroidism.
- An undetectable PTH concentration suggests idiopathic hypoparathyroidism.
- A high PTH concentration suggests pseudohypoparathyroidism or an abnormality of vitamin D metabolism.

Hypoparathyroidism is further characterized by high serum PO_4 and normal alkaline phosphatase.

In type I pseudohypoparathyroidism, despite the presence of a high concentration of circulating PTH, urinary cAMP and urinary PO_4 are absent. Provocative testing by injection of parathyroid extract or recombinant human PTH fails to raise serum or urinary cAMP. Patients with type Ia pseudohypoparathyroidism frequently also have skeletal abnormalities, including short stature and shortened 1st, 4th, and 5th metacarpals. Patients with type Ib disease have renal manifestations without skeletal abnormalities.

In vitamin D deficiency, osteomalacia or rickets may be present, usually with typical skeletal abnormalities on x-ray. Diagnosis of vitamin D deficiency and dependency and measurement of vitamin D concentrations are discussed on p. 50.

Severe hypocalcemia can affect the ECG. It typically shows prolongation of the QTc and ST intervals. Changes in repolarization, such as T-wave peaking or inversion, also occur. ECG may show arrhythmia or heart block occasionally in patients with severe hypocalcemia. However, evaluation of isolated hypocalcemia does not mandate ECG testing.

Treatment

- IV Ca gluconate for tetany
- Oral Ca for postoperative hypoparathyroidism
- Oral Ca and vitamin D for chronic hypocalcemia

Tetany: For tetany, Ca gluconate 10 mL of 10% solution IV over 10 min is given. Response can be dramatic but may last for only a few hours. Repeated boluses or a continuous infusion with 20 to 30 mL of 10% Ca gluconate in 1 L of 5% D/W over the next 12 to 24 h may be needed. Infusions of Ca are hazardous in patients receiving digoxin and should be given slowly and with continuous ECG monitoring after checking for (and correcting) hypokalemia. When tetany is associated with

Table 166–7. TYPICAL LABORATORY TEST RESULTS IN SOME DISORDERS CAUSING HYPOCALCEMIA

DISORDER	FINDINGS
Surgical hypoparathyroidism	Low or low-normal PTH Normal or high serum PO_4 Low urinary PO_4 Normal serum alkaline phosphatase
Idiopathic hypoparathyroidism	Undetectable PTH High serum PO_4 Low urinary PO_4 Normal serum alkaline phosphatase
Type Ia pseudohypoparathyroidism (Albright hereditary osteodystrophy)	High PTH High serum PO_4 No urinary cAMP or increase in PO_4 excretion even after injection of parathyroid extract or PTH Skeletal and other abnormalities
Type Ib pseudohypoparathyroidism	High PTH High serum PO_4 No urinary cAMP or increase in PO_4 excretion even after injection of parathyroid extract or PTH No skeletal abnormalities
Type II pseudohypoparathyroidism	High PTH High serum PO_4 No urinary cAMP or PO_4 Injection of PTH increases urinary cAMP but not urinary PO_4 Normal or high vitamin D concentrations
Vitamin D deficiency	High PTH Low serum PO_4 High alkaline phosphatase Low 25(OH)D*
Type I hereditary vitamin D–dependent rickets	High PTH Low serum PO_4 High alkaline phosphatase X-ray evidence of rickets Normal serum 25(OH)D Low serum $1,25(OH)_2D$
Type II hereditary vitamin D–dependent rickets	High PTH Low serum PO_4 High alkaline phosphatase X-ray evidence of rickets Normal or high serum 25(OH)D Normal or high $1,25(OH)_2D$

*Measurement of serum 25(OH)D and $1,25(OH)_2D$ may help distinguish vitamin D deficiency from vitamin D–dependent states.
1,25(OH)2D = 1,25-dihydroxychoecalciferol or calcitriol; 25(OH)D = inactive vitamin D; PO_4 = phosphate; PTH = parathyroid hormone.

hypomagnesemia, it may respond transiently to Ca or K administration but is permanently relieved only by repletion of Mg, typically given as a 10% Mg sulfate solution (1 g/10 mL) IV, followed by oral Mg salts (eg, Mg gluconate 500 to 1000 mg po tid).

PEARLS & PITFALLS

- Infusions of Ca are hazardous in patients receiving digoxin and should be given slowly and with continuous ECG monitoring after checking for (and correcting) hypokalemia.

Transient hypoparathyroidism: In transient hypoparathyroidism after thyroidectomy or partial parathyroidectomy, supplemental oral Ca may be sufficient: 1 to 2 g of elemental Ca/day may be given as Ca gluconate (90 mg elemental Ca/1 g) or $CaCO_3$ (400 mg elemental Ca/1 g).

Hypocalcemia may be particularly severe and prolonged after subtotal parathyroidectomy, particularly in patients with chronic kidney disease or in patients from whom a large tumor was removed. Prolonged parenteral administration of Ca may be necessary postoperatively; supplementation with as much as 1 g/day of elemental Ca (eg, 111 mL of Ca gluconate, which contains 90 mg elemental Ca/10 mL) may be required for 5 to 10 days before oral Ca and vitamin D are sufficient. Elevated serum alkaline phosphatase in such patients may be a sign of rapid uptake of Ca into bone. The need for large amounts of parenteral Ca usually does not fall until the alkaline phosphatase concentration begins to decrease.

Chronic hypocalcemia: In chronic hypocalcemia, oral Ca and occasionally vitamin D supplements are usually sufficient: 1 to

2 g of elemental Ca/day may be given as Ca gluconate or Ca carbonate. In patients without renal failure, vitamin D is given as a standard oral supplement (eg, cholecalciferol 800 IU once/day). Vitamin D therapy is not effective unless adequate dietary or supplemental Ca and PO_4 (see p. 1295) are supplied.

For patients with renal failure, calcitriol or another $1,25(OH)_2D$ analog is used because these drugs require no renal metabolic alteration. Patients with hypoparathyroidism have difficulty converting cholecalciferol to its active form and also usually require calcitriol, usually 0.5 to 2 mcg po once/day. Pseudohypoparathyroidism can occasionally be managed with oral Ca supplementation alone. When used, calcitriol requires 1 to 3 mcg/day.

Vitamin D analogs include dihydrotachysterol (usually given orally at 0.8 to 2.4 once/day for a few days, followed by 0.2 to 1.0 mg once/day) and calcidiol (eg, 4000 to 6000 IU po once/wk). Use of vitamin D analogs, particularly the longer-acting calcidiol, can be complicated by vitamin D toxicity, with severe symptomatic hypercalcemia. Serum Ca concentration should be monitored weekly at first and then at 1- to 3-mo intervals after Ca concentrations have stabilized. The maintenance dose of calcitriol or its analog, dihydrotachysterol, usually decreases with time.

KEY POINTS

- Causes of hypocalcemia include hypoparathyroidism, pseudohypoparathyroidism, vitamin D deficiency, and renal failure.
- Mild hypocalcemia may be asymptomatic or cause muscle cramps.
- Severe hypocalcemia (serum Ca < 7 mg/dL [< 1.75 mmol/L]) may cause hyperreflexia, tetany (paresthesias of the lips, tongue, fingers, and feet, carpopedal and/or facial spasms, muscle aches), or generalized seizures.
- Diagnose by estimation or measurement of *ionized* (not total) serum Ca.
- Typically, measure serum concentrations of Mg, PO_4, PTH, alkaline phosphatase, and occasionally vitamin D levels.
- Give IV Ca gluconate to patients with tetany; treat others with oral Ca supplements.

HYPERCALCEMIA

Hypercalcemia is a total serum Ca concentration > 10.4 mg/dL (> 2.60 mmol/L) or ionized serum Ca > 5.2 mg/dL (> 1.30 mmol/L). Principal causes include hyperparathyroidism, vitamin D toxicity, and cancer. Clinical features include polyuria, constipation, muscle weakness, confusion, and coma. Diagnosis is by measuring serum ionized Ca and parathyroid hormone (PTH) concentrations. Treatment to increase Ca excretion and reduce bone resorption of Ca involves saline, Na diuresis, and drugs such as zoledronate.

Etiology

Hypercalcemia usually results from excessive bone resorption. There are many causes of hypercalcemia (see Table 166–8), but the most common are

- Hyperparathyroidism
- Cancer

Pathophysiology

Primary hyperparathyroidism: Primary hyperparathyroidism is a generalized disorder resulting from excessive secretion of PTH by one or more parathyroid glands. It probably is the most common cause of hypercalcemia, particularly among patients who are not hospitalized. Incidence increases with age and is higher in postmenopausal women. It also occurs in high frequency ≥ 3 decades after neck irradiation. Familial and sporadic forms exist.

Familial forms due to parathyroid adenoma occur in patients with other endocrine tumors (see p. 1313). Primary hyperparathyroidism causes hypophosphatemia and excessive bone resorption. Although asymptomatic hypercalcemia is the most frequent presentation, nephrolithiasis is also common, particularly when hypercalciuria occurs due to long-standing hypercalcemia. Histologic examination shows a parathyroid adenoma in about 85% of patients with primary hyperparathyroidism, although it is sometimes difficult to distinguish an adenoma from a normal gland. About 15% of cases are due to hyperplasia of ≥ 2 glands. Parathyroid cancer occurs in < 1% of cases.

Familial hypocalciuric hypercalcemia: The syndrome of familial hypocalciuric hypercalcemia (FHH) is transmitted as an autosomal dominant trait. Most cases involve an inactivating mutation of the Ca-sensing receptor gene, resulting in higher concentrations of serum Ca being needed to inhibit PTH secretion. Subsequent PTH secretion induces renal PO_4 excretion. Persistent hypercalcemia (usually asymptomatic) and often from an early age, normal to slightly elevated concentrations of PTH, hypocalciuria, and hypermagnesemia occur. Renal function is normal, and nephrolithiasis is unusual. However, severe pancreatitis occasionally occurs. This syndrome, which is associated with parathyroid hyperplasia, is not relieved by subtotal parathyroidectomy.

Secondary hyperparathyroidism: Secondary hyperparathyroidism occurs most commonly in advanced chronic kidney disease when decreased formation of active vitamin D in the kidneys and other factors lead to hypocalcemia and chronic stimulation of PTH secretion. Hyperphosphatemia that develops in response to chronic kidney disease also contributes. Once established, hypercalcemia or normocalcemia may occur. The sensitivity of the parathyroid to Ca may be diminished because of pronounced glandular hyperplasia and elevation of the Ca set point (ie, the amount of Ca necessary to reduce secretion of PTH).

Tertiary hyperparathyroidism: Tertiary hyperparathyroidism results in autonomous hypersecretion of PTH regardless of serum Ca concentration. Tertiary hyperparathyroidism generally occurs in patients with long-standing secondary hyperparathyroidism, as in patients with end-stage renal disease of several years' duration.

Cancer: Cancer is a common cause of hypercalcemia, usually in hospitalized patients. Although there are several mechanisms, elevated serum Ca ultimately occurs as a result of bone resorption.

Humoral hypercalcemia of cancer (ie, hypercalcemia with no or minimal bone metastases) occurs most commonly with squamous cell carcinoma, renal cell carcinoma, breast cancer, prostate cancer, and ovarian cancer. Many cases of humoral hypercalcemia of cancer were formerly attributed to ectopic production of PTH. However, some of these tumors secrete a PTH-related peptide that binds to PTH receptors in both bone and kidney and mimics many of the effects of the hormone, including osteoclastic bone resorption.

Osteolytic hypercalcemia can be caused by metastatic solid tumors (eg, breast, prostate, non-small cell lung cancers) or hematologic cancers, most often multiple myeloma, but also certain lymphomas and lymphosarcomas. Hypercalcemia may result from local elaboration of osteoclast-activating

Table 166–8. PRINCIPAL CAUSES OF HYPERCALCEMIA

MECHANISM	CATEGORY	EXAMPLES
Excessive bone resorption	Humoral hypercalcemia of cancer	Bladder Breast Leukemia Lymphoma Ovarian Renal cell Squamous cell (lung, head and neck)
	Osteolytic hypercalcemia of cancer, due to bone metastases or hematologic cancer	Leukemia Lymphoma Metastatic breast, prostate, non–small cell lung cancers Multiple myeloma
	Increased mobilization of Ca from bone	Immobilization (eg, orthopedic casting traction) Paget disease of bone Osteoporosis in the elderly Paraplegia or quadriplegia Rapid growth during childhood and adolescence Hyperthyroidism
	PTH excess	Familial hypocalciuric hypercalcemia Parathyroid carcinoma Primary hyperparathyroidism Secondary hyperparathyroidism Tertiary hyperparathyroidism
	Vitamin toxicity	Vitamin A toxicity Vitamin D toxicity
Excessive GI Ca absorption, intake, or both	Sarcoidosis and other granulomatous diseases	Berylliosis Coccidioidomycosis Histoplasmosis Leprosy Silicosis TB
	Other disorders	Milk-alkali syndrome Vitamin D toxicity
Elevated plasma protein concentration: Uncertain mechanism	Drugs	Lithium toxicity Theophylline toxicity Thiazide treatment
	Endocrine dysfunction	Addison disease Cushing disease, postoperative Myxedema
	Other disorders	Aluminum-induced osteomalacia Idiopathic infantile hypercalcemia Neuroleptic malignant syndrome
Artifactual	—	Exposure of blood to contaminated glassware Prolonged venous stasis as blood sample was obtained

cytokines or prostaglandins that stimulate osteoclasts to resorb bone, direct bone resorption by the tumor cells, or both. Diffuse osteopenia may also occur.

Vitamin D toxicity: Vitamin D toxicity can be caused by high concentrations of endogenous $1,25(OH)_2D$. Although serum concentrations are low in most patients with solid tumors, patients with lymphoma and T-cell leukemia sometimes have elevated concentrations due to dysregulation of the 1-alpha-hydroxylase enzyme present in tumor cells. Exogenous vitamin D in pharmacologic doses causes excessive bone resorption as well as increased intestinal Ca absorption, resulting in hypercalcemia and hypercalciuria.

Granulomatous disorders: Granulomatous disorders, such as sarcoidosis, TB, leprosy, berylliosis, histoplasmosis, and coccidioidomycosis, lead to hypercalcemia and hypercalciuria. In sarcoidosis, hypercalcemia and hypercalciuria appear to be due to unregulated conversion of 25(OH)D to $1,25(OH)_2D$, presumably due to expression of the 1-alpha-hydroxylase enzyme in mononuclear cells within sarcoid granulomas. Similarly, elevated serum concentrations of $1,25(OH)_2D$ have been reported in hypercalcemic patients with TB and silicosis. Other mechanisms must account for hypercalcemia in some instances, because depressed $1,25(OH)_2D$ concentrations occur in some patients with hypercalcemia and leprosy.

Immobilization: Immobilization, particularly complete prolonged bed rest in patients at risk (see Table 166–8), can result in hypercalcemia due to accelerated bone resorption. Hypercalcemia develops within days to weeks of onset of bed rest. Reversal of hypercalcemia occurs promptly on resumption of weight bearing. Young adults with several bone fractures and people with Paget disease of bone are particularly prone to hypercalcemia when at bed rest.

Idiopathic infantile hypercalcemia: Idiopathic infantile hypercalcemia (Williams syndrome—see Table 296–2 on p. 2492) is an extremely rare sporadic disorder with dysmorphic facial features, cardiovascular abnormalities, renovascular hypertension, and hypercalcemia. PTH and vitamin D metabolism are normal, but the response of calcitonin to Ca infusion may be abnormal.

Milk-alkali syndrome: In milk-alkali syndrome, excessive amounts of Ca and absorbable alkali are ingested, usually during self-treatment with Ca carbonate antacids for dyspepsia or to prevent osteoporosis, resulting in hypercalcemia, metabolic alkalosis, and renal insufficiency. The availability of effective drugs for peptic ulcer disease and osteoporosis has greatly reduced the incidence of this syndrome.

Symptoms and Signs

In mild hypercalcemia, many patients are asymptomatic. Clinical manifestations of hypercalcemia include constipation, anorexia, nausea and vomiting, abdominal pain, and ileus. Impairment of the renal concentrating mechanism leads to polyuria, nocturia, and polydipsia. Elevation of serum Ca > 12 mg/dL (> 3.00 mmol/L) can cause emotional lability, confusion, delirium, psychosis, stupor, and coma. Hypercalcemia may cause neuromuscular symptoms, including skeletal muscle weakness. Hypercalciuria with nephrolithiasis is common.

Less often, prolonged or severe hypercalcemia causes reversible acute renal failure or irreversible renal damage due to nephrocalcinosis (precipitation of Ca salts within the kidney parenchyma). Peptic ulcers and pancreatitis may occur in patients with hyperparathyroidism for reasons that are not related to hypercalcemia.

Severe hypercalcemia causes a shortened QT_c interval on ECG, and arrhythmias may occur, particularly in patients taking digoxin. Hypercalcemia > 18 mg/dL (> 4.50 mmol/L) may cause shock, renal failure, and death.

Diagnosis

- Total serum (and sometimes ionized) Ca concentration
- Chest x-ray; measurement of electrolytes, BUN, creatinine, ionized Ca, PO_4, PTH, alkaline phosphatase, and serum protein immunoelectrophoresis to determine the cause
- Sometimes PTH and urinary excretion of Ca with or without PO_4

Hypercalcemia is diagnosed by a serum Ca concentration > 10.4 mg/dL (> 2.60 mmol/L) or ionized serum Ca > 5.2 mg/dL (> 1.30 mmol/L). The condition is frequently discovered during routine laboratory screening.

Serum Ca can be artifactually elevated by high serum protein levels (see Table 166–9). True ionized hypercalcemia can also be masked by low serum protein. When protein and albumin are abnormal and when ionized hypercalcemia is suspected because of clinical findings (eg, because of symptoms of hypercalcemia), ionized serum Ca should be measured.

Initial evaluation: Initial evaluation should include

- Review of the history, particularly of past serum Ca concentration
- Physical examination
- Chest x-ray
- Laboratory studies, including electrolytes, BUN, creatinine, ionized Ca, PO_4, PTH, alkaline phosphatase, and serum protein immunoelectrophoresis

The cause is apparent from clinical data and results of these tests in ≥ 95% of patients. Patients without an obvious cause of hypercalcemia after this evaluation should undergo measurement of intact PTH and 24-h urinary Ca. When no cause is obvious, serum Ca < 11 mg/dL (< 2.75 mmol/L) suggests hyperparathyroidism or other nonmalignant causes, whereas serum Ca > 13 mg/dL (> 3.25 mmol/L) suggests cancer.

Asymptomatic hypercalcemia that has been present for years or is present in several family members raises the possibility of FHH. Primary hyperparathyroidism generally manifests late in life but can be present for several years before symptoms occur.

Measurement of intact PTH levels help differentiate PTH-mediated hypercalcemia (eg, caused by hyperparathyroidism or FHH), in which PTH levels are high or high-normal, from most other (PTH-independent) causes. In PTH-independent causes, levels are usually < 20 pg/mL.

The **chest x-ray** is particularly helpful, revealing most granulomatous disorders, such as TB, sarcoidosis, and silicosis, as well as primary lung cancer and lytic and Paget lesions in bones of the shoulder, ribs, and thoracic spine.

Chest and bone (eg, skull, extremity) x-rays can also show the effects on bone of secondary hyperparathyroidism, most commonly in long-term dialysis patients. In osteitis fibrosa cystica (often due to primary hyperparathyroidism), increased osteoclastic activity from overstimulation by PTH causes rarefaction of bone with fibrous degeneration and cyst and fibrous nodule formation. Because characteristic bone lesions occur only with relatively advanced disease, bone x-rays are recommended only for symptomatic patients. X-rays typically show bone cysts, a heterogeneous appearance of the skull, and subperiosteal resorption of bone in the phalanges and distal clavicles.

Hyperparathyroidism: In hyperparathyroidism, the serum Ca is rarely > 12 mg/dL (> 3.00 mmol/L), but the ionized serum Ca is almost always elevated. Low serum PO_4 concentration suggests hyperparathyroidism, especially when coupled with elevated PO_4 renal excretion. When hyperparathyroidism results in increased bone turnover, serum alkaline phosphatase is frequently increased. Increased intact PTH, particularly inappropriate elevation (ie, a high concentration in the absence of hypocalcemia) or an inappropriate high-normal concentration (ie, despite hypercalcemia), is diagnostic.

Urinary Ca excretion is usually normal or high in hyperparathyroidism. Chronic kidney disease suggests the presence of secondary hyperparathyroidism, but primary hyperparathyroidism can also be present. In patients with chronic kidney disease, high serum Ca and normal serum PO_4 suggest primary hyperparathyroidism, whereas elevated PO_4 suggests secondary hyperparathyroidism.

The need for localization of parathyroid tissue before surgery on the parathyroid(s) is controversial. High-resolution CT with or without CT-guided biopsy and immunoassay of thyroid venous drainage, MRI, high-resolution ultrasonography, digital subtraction angiography, and thallium-201–technetium-99 scanning all have been used and are highly accurate, but they have not improved the usually high cure rate of parathyroidectomy done by experienced surgeons. Technetium-99 sestamibi, a radionuclide agent for parathyroid imaging, is more sensitive and specific than older agents and may be useful for identifying solitary adenomas.

For residual or recurrent hyperparathyroidism after initial parathyroid surgery, imaging is necessary and may reveal abnormally functioning parathyroid glands in unusual locations

Table 166–9. LABORATORY AND CLINICAL FINDINGS IN SOME DISORDERS CAUSING HYPERCALCEMIA

CAUSE	FINDINGS
Primary hyperparathyroidism	Serum Ca elevated, but < 12 mg/dL Ionized serum Ca > 5.2 mg/dL Low serum PO_4 (particularly with high renal PO_4 excretion) High alkaline phosphatase (often) Inappropriately high PTH Normal or high urinary Ca excretion No family history of endocrine neoplasia, no neck irradiation during childhood, no other obvious cause of hyperparathyroidism (typically)
Secondary hyperparathyroidism	Serum Ca low, normal, or high, but < 12 mg/dL Ionized serum Ca > 5.2 mg/dL High serum PO_4 (particularly with high renal PO_4 excretion) High alkaline phosphatase (often) Inappropriately high PTH Normal or high urinary Ca excretion Chronic kidney disease (typically)
Humoral hypercalcemia of cancer	Serum Ca > 12 mg/dL Low PTH Normal or low PO_4 Possibly metabolic alkalosis, hypochloremia, and hypoalbuminemia
Familial hypocalciuric hypercalcemia	Ratio of Ca clearance to creatinine clearance of < 1% Hypermagnesemia (often) High or normal PTH Lifelong and asymptomatic hypercalcemia Hypercalcemia without hypercalciuria in patients and family members
Milk-alkali syndrome	No hypercalciuria Metabolic alkalosis Azotemia (occasionally) Low PTH (usually) Normalization of serum Ca when Ca and alkali ingestion stops High intake of Ca antacids (typically)

Ca = calcium; PO_4 = phosphate; PTH = parathyroid hormone.

throughout the neck and mediastinum. Technetium-99 sestamibi is probably the most sensitive imaging test. Use of several imaging studies (MRI, CT, or high-resolution ultrasonography in addition to technetium-99 sestamibi) before repeat parathyroidectomy is sometimes necessary.

Cancer: A serum Ca > 13 mg/dL (> 3.00 mmol/L) suggests some cause of hypercalcemia other than hyperparathyroidism. Urinary Ca excretion is usually normal or high in cancer. In humoral hypercalcemia of cancer, PTH is often decreased or undetectable; PO_4 is often decreased; and metabolic alkalosis, hypochloremia, and hypoalbuminemia are often present. Suppressed PTH differentiates humoral hypercalcemia of cancer from primary hyperparathyroidism. Humoral hypercalcemia of cancer can also be diagnosed by detection of PTH-related peptide in serum.

Multiple myeloma is suggested by simultaneous anemia, azotemia, and hypercalcemia or by the presence of a monoclonal gammopathy. Myeloma is confirmed by bone marrow examination.

Familial hypocalciuric hypercalcemia: FHH is very rare but should be considered in patients with hypercalcemia and elevated or high-normal intact PTH levels. FHH is distinguished from primary hyperparathyroidism by the early age of onset (it is a lifelong condition), absence of symptoms, frequent occurrence of hypermagnesemia, and presence of hypercalcemia without hypercalciuria in other family members. The fractional excretion of Ca (ratio of Ca clearance to creatinine clearance) is low (< 1%) in FHH; it is almost always elevated (1 to 4%) in primary hyperparathyroidism. Intact PTH can be elevated or normal, perhaps reflecting altered feedback regulation of the parathyroid glands.

Milk-alkali syndrome: In addition to a history of increased intake of Ca antacids, milk-alkali syndrome is recognized by the combination of hypercalcemia, metabolic alkalosis, and, occasionally, azotemia with hypocalciuria. The diagnosis can be confirmed when the serum Ca concentration rapidly returns to normal when Ca and alkali ingestion stops, although renal insufficiency can persist when nephrocalcinosis is present. Circulating PTH usually is suppressed.

Other causes: Vitamin D toxicity is characterized by elevated $1,25(OH)_2D$ concentration. In hypercalcemia due to sarcoidosis, other granulomatous disorders, and some lymphomas, serum concentration of $1,25(OH)_2D$ may be elevated. In other endocrine causes of hypercalcemia, such as thyrotoxicosis and Addison disease, typical laboratory findings of the underlying disorder help establish the diagnosis. When Paget disease is suspected, plain x-rays are done first and may show characteristic abnormalities.

Treatment

- Oral PO_4 for serum Ca < 11.5 mg/dL with mild symptoms and no kidney disease
- IV saline and furosemide for more rapid correction of elevated serum Ca < 18 mg/dL
- Bisphosphonates or other Ca-lowering drugs for serum Ca 11.5 – 18 mg/dL and/or moderate symptoms

- Hemodialysis for serum Ca > 18 mg/dL
- Surgical removal for moderate, progressive primary hyperparathyroidism and sometimes for mild disease
- Phosphate restriction and binders and sometimes calcitriol for secondary hyperparathyroidism

There are 4 main strategies for lowering serum Ca:

- Decrease intestinal Ca absorption
- Increase urinary Ca excretion
- Decrease bone resorption
- Remove excess Ca through dialysis

The treatment used depends on both the degree and the cause of hypercalcemia. Volume repletion with saline is an essential element of care.

Mild hypercalcemia: In mild hypercalcemia (serum Ca < 11.5 mg/dL [< 2.88 mmol/L]), in which symptoms are mild, treatment is deferred pending definitive diagnosis. After diagnosis, the underlying disorder is treated.

When symptoms are significant, treatment aimed at lowering serum Ca is necessary. Oral PO_4 can be used. When taken with meals, it binds some Ca, preventing its absorption. A starting dose is 250 mg of elemental PO_4 (as Na or K salt) qid. The dose can be increased to 500 mg qid prn unless diarrhea develops.

Another treatment is increasing urinary Ca excretion by giving isotonic saline plus a loop diuretic. Initially, 1 to 2 L of saline is given over 2 to 4 h unless significant heart failure is present because nearly all patients with significant hypercalcemia are hypovolemic. Furosemide 20 to 40 mg IV q 2 to 4 h is given as needed to maintain a urine output of roughly 250 mL/h (monitored hourly). Care must be taken to avoid volume depletion. K and Mg are monitored as often as every 4 h during treatment and replaced IV as needed to avoid hypokalemia and hypomagnesemia. Serum Ca begins to decrease in 2 to 4 h and falls to near-normal within 24 h.

Moderate hypercalcemia: Moderate hypercalcemia (serum Ca > 11.5 mg/dL [< 2.88 mmol/L] and < 18 mg/dL [< 4.51 mmol/L]) can be treated with isotonic saline and a loop diuretic as is done for mild hypercalcemia or, depending on its cause, drugs that decrease bone resorption (usually bisphosphonates, calcitonin, or infrequently plicamycin or gallium nitrate), corticosteroids, or chloroquine.

Bisphosphonates inhibit osteoclasts. They are usually the drugs of choice for cancer-associated hypercalcemia. Zoledronate can be given in doses of 4 to 8 mg IV and lowers serum Ca very effectively for an average of > 40 days.

Pamidronate can be given for cancer-associated hypercalcemia as a one-time dose of 30 to 90 mg IV, repeated only after 7 days. It lowers serum Ca for ≤ 2 wk.

Ibandronate 4 to 6 mg IV can be given for cancer-associated hypercalcemia; it is effective for about 14 days.

Etidronate 7.5 mg/kg IV once/day for 3 to 5 days is used to treat Paget disease and cancer-associated hypercalcemia. Maintenance dosage is 20 mg/kg po once/day, but the dose must be reduced when GFR is low.

Repetitive use of IV bisphosphonates to treat hypercalcemia associated with metastatic bone disease or myeloma has been associated with osteonecrosis of the jaw. Some reports suggest this finding may be more common with zoledronate. Renal toxicity has been reported in patients receiving zoledronate. Oral bisphosphonates (eg, alendronate or risedronate) can be given to maintain Ca in the normal range but are not generally used for treating hypercalcemia acutely.

Denosumab, 120 mg sc q 4 wk with additional doses on days 8 and 15 of the first month of treatment, is a monoclonal antibody inhibitor of osteoclastic activity that can be used for cancer-associated hypercalcemia that does not respond to bisphosphonates. Ca and vitamin D are given as needed to avert hypocalcemia.

Calcitonin (thyrocalcitonin) is a rapidly acting peptide hormone normally secreted in response to hypercalcemia by the C cells of the thyroid. Calcitonin appears to lower serum Ca by inhibiting osteoclastic activity. A dosage of 4 to 8 IU/kg sc q 12 h of salmon calcitonin is safe. Calcitonin can lower serum Ca levels by 1 to 2 mg/dL within a few hours. Its usefulness in the treatment of cancer-associated hypercalcemia is limited by its short duration of action with the development of tachyphylaxis (often after about 48 h) and by the lack of response in ≥ 40% of patients. However, the combination of salmon calcitonin and prednisone may control serum Ca for several months in some patients with cancer. If calcitonin stops working, it can be stopped for 2 days (while prednisone is continued) and then resumed.

Corticosteroids (eg, prednisone 20 to 40 mg po once/day) can help control hypercalcemia as adjunctive therapy by decreasing calcitriol production and thus intestinal Ca absorption in most patients with vitamin D toxicity, idiopathic hypercalcemia of infancy, and sarcoidosis. Some patients with myeloma, lymphoma, leukemia, or metastatic cancer require 40 to 60 mg of prednisone once/day. However, > 50% of such patients fail to respond to corticosteroids, and response, when it occurs, takes several days; thus, other treatment usually is necessary.

Chloroquine PO_4 500 mg po once/day inhibits $1,25(OH)_2D$ synthesis and reduces serum Ca concentration in patients with sarcoidosis. Routine ophthalmologic surveillance (eg, retinal examinations every 6 to 12 mo) is mandatory to detect dose-related retinal damage.

Plicamycin 25 mcg/kg IV once/day in 50 mL of 5% D/W over 4 to 6 h is effective in patients with hypercalcemia due to cancer but is rarely used because other treatments are safer.

Gallium nitrate is also effective in hypercalcemia due to cancer but is used infrequently because of renal toxicity and limited clinical experience.

Severe hypercalcemia: In severe hypercalcemia (serum Ca > 18 mg/dL [> 4.50 mmol/L] or with severe symptoms), hemodialysis with low-Ca dialysate may be needed in addition to other treatments. Although there is no completely satisfactory way to correct severe hypercalcemia in patients with renal failure, hemodialysis is probably the safest and most reliable short-term treatment.

IV PO_4 (disodium PO4 or monopotassium PO_4) should be used only when hypercalcemia is life threatening and unresponsive to other methods and when short-term hemodialysis is not possible. No more than 1 g should be given IV in 24 h; usually 1 or 2 doses over 2 days lower serum Ca for 10 to 15 days. Soft-tissue calcification and acute renal failure may result. (NOTE: IV infusion of Na sulfate is even more hazardous and less effective than PO_4 infusion and should not be used.)

Hyperparathyroidism: Treatment for hyperparathyroidism depends on severity.

Patients with **asymptomatic primary hyperparathyroidism** with no indications for surgery may be treated conservatively with methods to ensure that serum Ca concentrations remain low. Patients should remain active (ie, avoid immobilization that could exacerbate hypercalcemia), follow a low-Ca diet, drink plenty of fluids to minimize the chance of nephrolithiasis, and avoid drugs that can raise serum Ca, such as thiazide diuretics. Serum Ca and renal function are monitored every 6 mo. Bone density is monitored every 12 mo. However, subclinical bone disease, hypertension, and longevity are concerns. Osteoporosis is treated with bisphosphonates.

Surgery is indicated for patients with symptomatic or progressive hyperparathyroidism. The indications for surgery in patients with asymptomatic, primary hyperparathyroidism are controversial. Surgical parathyroidectomy increases bone density and may have modest effects on some quality of life symptoms, but most patients do not have progressive deterioration in biochemical abnormalities or bone density. Still, concerns about hypertension and longevity remain. Many experts recommend surgery in the following circumstances:

- Serum Ca 1 mg/dL (0.25 mmol/L) greater than the upper limits of normal
- Calciuria > 400 mg/day (> 10 mmol/day)
- Creatinine clearance less than 60 mL/min
- Peak bone density at the hip, lumbar spine, or radius 2.5 standard deviations below controls (T score = −2.5)
- Age < 50 yr
- The possibility of poor adherence with follow-up

Surgery consists of removal of adenomatous glands. PTH concentration can be measured before and after removal of the presumed abnormal gland using rapid assays. A fall of 50% or more 10 min after removal of the adenoma indicates successful treatment. In patients with disease of > 1 gland, several glands are removed, and often a small portion of a normal-appearing parathyroid gland is reimplanted in the belly of the sternocleidomastoid muscle or subcutaneously in the forearm to prevent hypoparathyroidism. Parathyroid tissue is also occasionally preserved using cryopreservation to allow for later autologous transplantation in case persistent hypoparathyroidism develops.

When hyperparathyroidism is mild, the serum Ca concentration drops to just below normal within 24 to 48 h after surgery; serum Ca must be monitored. In patients with severe osteitis fibrosa cystica, prolonged, symptomatic hypocalcemia may occur postoperatively unless 10 to 20 g elemental Ca is given in the days before surgery. Even with preoperative Ca administration, large doses of Ca and vitamin D may be required (see p. 1287) while bone Ca is repleted.

Hyperparathyroidism in renal failure is usually secondary. Measures used for treatment can also be used for prevention. One aim is to prevent hyperphosphatemia. Treatment combines dietary PO_4 restriction and PO_4 binding agents, such as Ca carbonate or sevelamer. Despite the use of PO_4 binders, dietary restriction of PO_4 is needed. Aluminum-containing compounds have been used to limit PO_4 concentration, but they should be avoided, especially in patients receiving long-term dialysis, to prevent aluminum accumulation in bone resulting in severe osteomalacia. Vitamin D administration is potentially hazardous in renal failure because it can increase PO_4 absorption and contribute to hypercalcemia; administration requires frequent monitoring of Ca and PO_4 levels. Treatment should be limited to patients with any of the following:

- Symptomatic osteomalacia (unrelated to aluminum)
- Secondary hyperparathyroidism
- Postparathyroidectomy hypocalcemia

Although oral calcitriol is often given along with oral Ca to suppress secondary hyperparathyroidism, the results are variable in patients with end-stage renal disease. The parenteral form of calcitriol, or vitamin D analogs such as paricalcitol, may better prevent secondary hyperparathyroidism in such patients, because the higher attained serum concentration of $1,25(OH)_2D$ directly suppresses PTH release. Simple osteomalacia may respond to calcitriol 0.25 to 0.5 mcg po once/day, whereas correction of postparathyroidectomy hypocalcemia may require prolonged administration of as much as 2 mcg of calcitriol po once/day and ≥ 2 g of elemental Ca/day.

The calcimimetic, cinacalcet, modulates the set point of the Ca-sensing receptor on parathyroid cells and decreases PTH concentration in dialysis patients without increasing serum Ca. In patients with osteomalacia caused by having taken large amounts of aluminum-containing PO_4 binders, removal of aluminum with deferoxamine is necessary before calcitriol administration reduces bone lesions.

Familial hypocalciuric hypercalcemia: Although FHH results from histologically abnormal parathyroid tissue, the response to subtotal parathyroidectomy is unsatisfactory. Because overt clinical manifestations are rare, drug therapy is not routinely indicated.

KEY POINTS

- The most common causes of hypercalcemia are hyperparathyroidism and cancer.
- Clinical features include polyuria, constipation, anorexia, and hypercalciuria with renal stones; patients with high Ca concentrations may have muscle weakness, confusion, and coma.
- Do chest x-ray; measure electrolytes, BUN, creatinine, ionized Ca, PO_4, PTH, and alkaline phosphatase, and do serum protein immunoelectrophoresis.
- In addition to treating the cause, treat mild hypercalcemia (serum Ca < 11.5 mg/dL [< 2.88 mmol/L]) with oral PO_4 or isotonic saline plus a loop diuretic.
- For moderate hypercalcemia (serum Ca > 11.5 mg/dL [< 2.88 mmol/L] and < 18 mg/dL [< 4.51 mmol/L]), add a bisphosphonate, corticosteroids and sometimes calcitonin.
- For severe hypercalcemia, hemodialysis may be needed.

OVERVIEW OF DISORDERS OF PHOSPHATE CONCENTRATION

Phosphorus is one of the most abundant elements in the human body. Most phosphorus in the body is complexed with oxygen as PO_4.

About 85% of the about 500 to 700 g of PO_4 in the body is contained in bone, where it is an important constituent of crystalline hydroxyapatite. In soft tissues, PO_4 is mainly found in the intracellular compartment as an integral component of several organic compounds, including nucleic acids and cell membrane phospholipids.

Phosphate is also involved in aerobic and anaerobic energy metabolism. RBC 2,3-diphosphoglycerate (2,3-DPG) plays a crucial role in oxygen delivery to tissue. Adenosinediphosphate (ADP) and ATP contain PO_4 and use chemical bonds between PO_4 groups to store energy.

Phosphate is a major intracellular anion but is also present in plasma.

The normal serum PO_4 concentration in adults ranges from 2.5 to 4.5 mg/dL (0.81 to 1.45 mmol/L). PO_4 concentration is 50% higher in infants and 30% higher in children, possibly because of the important roles the PO_4-dependent processes play in growth.

Phosphate concentration can become

- Too high (hyperphosphatemia), usually as a result of chronic kidney disease, hypoparathyroidism, and metabolic or respiratory acidosis
- Too low (hypophosphatemia), usually as a result of alcoholism, burns, starvation, or diuretic use

The typical American diet contains about 800 to 1500 mg of PO_4. The amount in stool varies depending on the amount of

PO_4-binding compounds (mainly Ca) in the diet. Also, like Ca, GI PO_4 absorption is enhanced by vitamin D. Renal PO_4 excretion roughly equals GI absorption to maintain PO_4 balance. PO_4 depletion can occur in various disorders and normally results in conservation of PO_4 by the kidneys. PO_4 in bone serves as a reservoir, which can buffer changes in plasma and intracellular PO_4.

HYPOPHOSPHATEMIA

Hypophosphatemia is a serum PO_4 concentration < 2.5 mg/dL (0.81 mmol/L). Causes include alcoholism, burns, starvation, and diuretic use. Clinical features include muscle weakness, respiratory failure, and heart failure; seizures and coma can occur. Diagnosis is by serum PO_4 concentration. Treatment consists of PO_4 supplementation.

Hypophosphatemia occurs in 2% of hospitalized patients but is more prevalent in certain populations (eg, it occurs in up to 10% of hospitalized patients with alcoholism).

Etiology

Hypophosphatemia has numerous causes but clinically significant acute hypophosphatemia occurs in relatively few clinical settings, including the following:

- The recovery phase of diabetic ketoacidosis
- Acute alcoholism
- Severe burns
- When receiving TPN
- Refeeding after prolonged undernutrition
- Severe respiratory alkalosis

Acute severe hypophosphatemia with serum PO_4 < 1 mg/dL (< 0.32 mmol/L) is most often caused by transcellular shifts of PO_4 often superimposed on chronic PO_4 depletion.

Chronic hypophosphatemia usually is the result of decreased renal PO_4 reabsorption. Causes include the following:

- Increased PTH levels, as in primary and secondary hyperparathyroidism
- Other hormonal disturbances, such as Cushing syndrome and hypothyroidism
- Vitamin D deficiency
- Electrolyte disorders, such as hypomagnesemia and hypokalemia
- Theophylline intoxication
- Long-term diuretic use

Severe chronic hypophosphatemia usually results from a prolonged negative PO_4 balance. Causes include

- Chronic starvation or malabsorption, often in patients with alcoholism, especially when combined with vomiting or copious diarrhea
- Long-term ingestion of large amounts of PO_4-binding aluminum, usually in the form of antacids

Patients with advanced chronic kidney disease (especially those on dialysis), often take PO_4 binders with meals to reduce absorption of dietary PO_4. The prolonged use of these binders can cause hypophosphatemia in, particularly when combined with greatly decreased dietary intake of PO_4.

Symptoms and Signs

Although hypophosphatemia usually is asymptomatic, anorexia, muscle weakness, and osteomalacia can occur in severe chronic depletion. Serious neuromuscular disturbances may occur, including progressive encephalopathy, seizures, coma, and death. The muscle weakness of profound hypophosphatemia may be accompanied by rhabdomyolysis, especially in acute alcoholism. Hematologic disturbances of profound hypophosphatemia include hemolytic anemia, decreased release of oxygen from Hb, and impaired leukocyte and platelet function.

Diagnosis

- Serum PO_4 levels

Hypophosphatemia is diagnosed by a serum PO_4 concentration < 2.5 mg/dL (< 0.81 mmol/L). Most causes of hypophosphatemia (eg, diabetic ketoacidosis, burns, refeeding) are readily apparent. Testing to diagnose the cause is done when clinically indicated (eg, suggestive liver function test results or signs of cirrhosis in patients with suspected alcoholism).

Treatment

- Treat underlying disorder
- Oral PO_4 replacement
- IV PO_4 when serum PO_4 is < 1 mg/dL (< 0.32 mmol/L) or symptoms are severe

Oral treatment: Treatment of the underlying disorder and oral PO_4 replacement are usually adequate in asymptomatic patients, even when the serum concentration is very low. PO_4 can be given in doses up to about 1 g po tid in tablets containing Na PO_4 or K PO_4. Oral Na PO_4 or K PO_4 may be poorly tolerated because of diarrhea. Ingestion of 1 L of low-fat or skim milk provides 1 g of PO_4 and may be more acceptable. Removal of the cause of hypophosphatemia may include stopping PO_4-binding antacids or diuretics or correcting hypomagnesemia.

Parenteral treatment: Parenteral PO_4 is usually given IV. It should be administered in any of the following circumstances:

- When serum PO_4 is < 1 mg/dL (< 0.32 mmol/L)
- Rhabdomyolysis, hemolysis, or CNS symptoms are present
- Oral replacement is not feasible due to underlying disorder

IV administration of K PO_4 (as buffered mix of K_2HPO_4 and KH_2PO_4) is relatively safe when renal function is well preserved. Parenteral K PO_4 contains 93 mg (3 mmol) phosphorus and 170 mg (4.4 mEq) K per mL. The usual dose is 0.5 mmol phosphorus/kg (0.17 mL/kg) IV over 6 h. Patients with alcoholism may require ≥ 1 g/day during TPN; supplemental PO_4 is stopped when oral intake is resumed. If patients have impaired renal function or serum K > 4 mEq/L, Na PO_4 preparations generally should be used; these preparations also contain 3 mmol/mL of phosphorus and are thus given at the same dose.

Serum Ca and PO_4 concentrations should be monitored during therapy, particularly when PO_4 is given IV or to patients with impaired renal function. In most cases, no more than 7 mg/kg (about 500 mg for a 70-kg adult) of PO_4 should be given over 6 h. Close monitoring is done and more rapid rates of PO_4 administration should be avoided to prevent hypocalcemia, hyperphosphatemia, and metastatic calcification due to excessive Ca PO_4 product.

KEY POINTS

- Acute hypophosphatemia most often occurs in the setting of alcoholism, burns, or starvation.
- Acute severe hypophosphatemia can cause serious neuromuscular disturbances, rhabdomyolysis, seizures, coma, and death.

- Chronic hypophosphatemia may be due to hormonal disorders (eg, hyperparathyroidism, Cushing syndrome, hypothyroidism), chronic diuretic use, or use of aluminum-containing antacids by patients with chronic kidney disease.
- Hypophosphatemia is usually asymptomatic, but severe depletion can cause anorexia, muscle weakness, and osteomalacia.
- Treat the underlying disorder, but some patients require oral, or rarely, IV PO_4 replacement.

HYPERPHOSPHATEMIA

Hyperphosphatemia is a serum PO_4 concentration > 4.5 mg/dL (> 1.46 mmol/L). Causes include chronic kidney disease, hypoparathyroidism, and metabolic or respiratory acidosis. Clinical features may be due to accompanying hypocalcemia and include tetany. Diagnosis is by serum PO_4 measurement. Treatment includes restriction of PO_4 intake and administration of PO_4-binding antacids, such as Ca carbonate.

Etiology

The **usual cause of hyperphosphatemia** is

- Decrease in renal excretion of PO_4

Advanced renal insufficiency (GFR < 30 mL/min) reduces excretion sufficiently to increase serum PO_4. Defects in renal excretion of PO_4 in the absence of renal failure also occur in pseudohypoparathyroidism, hypoparathyroidism and parathyroid suppression (as from hypercalcemia due to vitamin A or D excess or granulomatous disease).

Hyperphosphatemia occasionally results from a transcellular shift of PO_4 into the extracellular space that is so large that the renal excretory capacity is overwhelmed. This transcellular shift occurs most frequently in diabetic ketoacidosis (despite total body PO_4 depletion), crush injuries, and nontraumatic rhabdomyolysis as well as in overwhelming systemic infections and tumor lysis syndrome. Hyperphosphatemia can also occur with excessive oral PO_4 administration and occasionally with overzealous use of enemas containing PO_4.

Hyperphosphatemia can be spurious in cases of hyperproteinemia (multiple myeloma or macroglobulinemia), hyperlipidemia, hemolysis, or hyperbilirubinemia.

Pathophysiology

Hyperphosphatemia plays a critical role in the development of secondary hyperparathyroidism and renal osteodystrophy in patients with advanced chronic kidney disease as well as in patients on dialysis.

Hyperphosphatemia can lead to Ca precipitation into soft tissues, especially when the serum Ca × PO_4 product is chronically > 55 in patients with chronic kidney disease. Soft-tissue calcification in the skin is one cause of excessive pruritis in patients with end-stage renal disease on chronic dialysis. Vascular calcification also occurs in dialysis patients with a chronically elevated Ca × PO_4 product; this vascular calcification is a major risk factor for cardiovascular morbidity including stroke, myocardial infarction, and claudication.

Symptoms and Signs

Most patients with hyperphosphatemia are asymptomatic, although symptoms of hypocalcemia, including tetany, can occur when concomitant hypocalcemia is present. Soft-tissue calcifications are common among patients with chronic kidney disease; they manifest as easily palpable, hard subcutaneous nodules often with overlying scratches. Imaging studies frequently show vascular calcifications lining major arteries.

Diagnosis

- Phosphate concentration > 4.5 mg/dL (> 1.46 mmol/L)

Hyperphosphatemia is diagnosed by PO_4 concentration. When the etiology is not obvious (eg, rhabdomyolysis, tumor lysis syndrome, renal failure, overingestion of PO_4-containing laxatives), additional evaluation is warranted to exclude hypoparathyroidism or pseudohypoparathyroidism, which is end-organ resistance to PTH. False elevation of serum PO_4 also should be excluded by measuring serum protein, lipid, and bilirubin concentrations.

Treatment

- Phosphate restriction
- Phosphate binders
- Sometimes saline diuresis or hemodialysis

The mainstay of treatment in patients with advanced chronic kidney disease is reduction of PO_4 intake, which is usually accomplished with avoidance of foods containing high amounts of PO_4 and with use of PO_4-binding drugs taken with meals. Although quite effective, aluminum-containing antacids should not be used as PO_4 binding agents in patients with end-stage renal disease because of the possibility of aluminum-related dementia and osteomalacia, Ca carbonate and Ca acetate are frequently used as PO_4 binders. But require close monitoring because of the possibility of excessive Ca × PO_4 product causing vascular calcification in dialysis patients taking Ca-containing binders. A PO_4-binding resin without Ca, sevelamer, is widely used in dialysis patients in doses of 800 to 2400 mg po tid with meals. Lanthanum carbonate is another PO_4 binder that lacks Ca used in dialysis patients. It is given in doses of 500 to 1000 mg po tid with meals. Sucroferric oxyhydroxide combines the need many dialysis patients have for elemental iron with PO_4 binding. It is given in doses of 500 mg po tid with meals. Hemodialysis does remove some PO_4, but not enough to allow most end-stage renal disease patients to avoid significant hyperphosphatemia without the dietary interventions listed above.

Saline diuresis can be used to enhance PO_4 elimination in cases of acute hyperphosphatemia with intact kidney function. Hemodialysis can lower PO_4 levels in cases of severe acute hyperphosphatemia.

KEY POINTS

- The usual cause of hyperphosphatemia is advanced renal insufficiency; hypoparathyroidism and pseudohypoparathyroidism are less common causes.
- Most patients are asymptomatic, but those who also are hypocalcemic may have tetany.
- Treat by restricting dietary PO_4 and sometimes with PO_4 binders.
- Saline diuresis or hemodialysis may be needed.

OVERVIEW OF DISORDERS OF MAGNESIUM CONCENTRATION

Mg is the 4th most plentiful cation in the body. A 70-kg adult has about 2000 mEq of Mg. About 50% is sequestered in bone and is not readily exchangeable with Mg in other compartments. The ECF contains only about 1% of total body Mg. The remainder resides in the intracellular compartment. Normal serum Mg concentration ranges from 1.8 to 2.6 mg/dL (0.74 to 1.07 mmol/L).

The maintenance of serum Mg concentration is largely a function of dietary intake and effective renal and intestinal conservation. Within 7 days of initiation of a Mg-deficient diet, renal and stool Mg excretion each fall to about 12.5 mg/day (0.5 mmol/day).

About 70% of serum Mg is filtered by the kidney; the remainder is bound to protein. Protein binding of Mg is pH dependent. Serum Mg concentration is not closely related to either total body Mg or intracellular Mg content. However, severe serum hypomagnesemia may reflect diminished total body Mg. Hypermagnesemia is most often caused by renal failure.

Many enzymes are activated by or are dependent on Mg. Mg is required by all enzymatic processes involving ATP and by many of the enzymes involved in nucleic acid metabolism. Mg is required for thiamine pyrophosphate cofactor activity and appears to stabilize the structure of macromolecules such as DNA and RNA. Mg is also related to Ca and K metabolism in an intimate but poorly understood way.

HYPOMAGNESEMIA

Hypomagnesemia is serum magnesium concentration < 1.8 mg/dL (< 0.70 mmol/L). Causes include inadequate Mg intake and absorption or increased excretion due to hypercalcemia or drugs such as furosemide. Clinical features are often due to accompanying hypokalemia and hypocalcemia and include lethargy, tremor, tetany, seizures, and arrhythmias. Treatment is with Mg replacement.

Serum Mg concentration, even when free Mg ion is measured, may be normal even with decreased intracellular or bone Mg stores.

Etiology

Mg depletion usually results from inadequate intake plus impairment of renal conservation or GI absorption. There are numerous causes of clinically significant Mg deficiency (see Table 166–10). Hypomagnesemia is common among hospitalized patients and frequently occurs with other electrolyte disorders, including hypokalemia and hypocalcemia. Hypomagnesemia is related to decreased intake in patients with malnutrition or long-term chronic alcoholism. Decreased oral intake is frequently compounded by increased urinary excretion exacerbated by diuretic use which increase urinary excretion of Mg.

Drugs can cause hypomagnesemia. Examples include chronic (> 1 yr) use of a protein pump inhibitor and concomitant use of diuretics. Amphotericin B can cause hypomagnesemia, hypokalemia, and acute kidney injury. The risk of each of these is increased with duration of therapy with amphotericin B and concomitant use of another nephrotoxic agent. Liposomal amphotericin B is less likely to cause either kidney injury or hypomagnesemia. Hypomagnesemia generally resolves with cessation of therapy. Cisplatin can cause increased Mg losses by the kidney as well as generalized decrease in kidney function. Mg loses can be severe and persist despite discontinuation of cisplatin. Discontinuation of cisplatin is still recommended if signs of renal toxicity occur during therapy.

Table 166–10. CAUSES OF HYPOMAGNESEMIA

CAUSE	COMMENT
Alcoholism	Due to inadequate intake and excessive renal excretion
GI losses	Chronic diarrhea Steatorrhea Small-bowel bypass Chronic protein pump inhibitor use
Pregnancy-related	Pregnancy (especially 3rd trimester; excessive renal excretion, other factors; usually physiologic) Lactation (increased Mg requirements)
Primary renal losses	Rare disorders that cause inappropriately high Mg excretion (eg, Gitelman syndrome)
Secondary renal losses	Loop and thiazide diuretics Hypercalcemia After removal of parathyroid tumor Diabetic ketoacidosis Hypersecretion of aldosterone, thyroid hormones, or vasopressin Nephrotoxins (eg, amphotericin B, cisplastin, cyclosporine, aminoglycosides)

Symptoms and Signs

Clinical manifestations are anorexia, nausea, vomiting, lethargy, weakness, personality change, tetany (eg, positive Trousseau or Chvostek sign or spontaneous carpopedal spasm, hyperreflexia), and tremor and muscle fasciculations. The neurologic signs, particularly tetany, correlate with development of concomitant hypocalcemia, hypokalemia, or both. Myopathic potentials are found on electromyography but are also compatible with hypocalcemia or hypokalemia. Severe hypomagnesemia may cause generalized tonic-clonic seizures, especially in children.

Diagnosis

- Considered in patients with risk factors and with unexplained hypocalcemia or hypokalemia
- Serum Mg concentration < 1.8 mg/dL (< 0.70 mmol/L)

Hypomagnesemia is diagnosed by a serum Mg concentration. Severe hypomagnesemia usually results in concentrations of < 1.25 mg/dL (< 0.50 mmol/L). Associated hypocalcemia and hypocalciuria are common. Hypokalemia with increased urinary K excretion and metabolic alkalosis may be present. Mg deficiency should be suspected even when serum Mg concentration is normal in patients with unexplained hypocalcemia or refractory hypokalemia. Mg deficiency should also be suspected in patients with unexplained neurologic symptoms and alcoholism, with chronic diarrhea, or after cyclosporine use, cisplatinum-based chemotherapy, or prolonged therapy with amphotericin B or aminoglycosides.

Treatment

- Oral Mg salts
- IV or IM Mg sulfate for severe hypomagnesemia or inability to tolerate or adhere to oral therapy

Treatment with Mg salts is indicated when Mg deficiency is symptomatic or persistently < 1.25 mg/dL (< 0.50 mmol/L). Patients with alcoholism are treated empirically. In such cases, deficits approaching 12 to 24 mg/kg are possible. About twice the amount of the estimated deficit should be given in patients with intact renal function, because about 50% of the administered Mg is excreted in urine. Oral Mg salts (eg, Mg gluconate 500 to 1000 mg po tid) are given for 3 to 4 days. Oral treatment is limited by the onset of diarrhea.

Parenteral administration is reserved for patients with severe, symptomatic hypomagnesemia who cannot tolerate oral drugs. Sometimes a single injection is given in patients with alcoholism who are unlikely to adhere to ongoing oral therapy. When Mg must be replaced parenterally, a 10% Mg sulfate solution (1 g/10 mL) is available for IV use and a 50% solution (1 g/2 mL) is available for IM use. The serum Mg concentration should be monitored frequently during Mg therapy, particularly when Mg is given to patients with renal insufficiency or in repeated parenteral doses. In these patients, treatment is continued until a normal serum Mg concentration is achieved.

In severe, symptomatic hypomagnesemia (eg, Mg < 1.25 mg/dL [< 0.5 mmol/L] with seizures or other severe symptoms), 2 to 4 g of Mg sulfate IV is given over 5 to 10 min. When seizures persist, the dose may be repeated up to a total of 10 g over the next 6 h. In patients in whom seizures stop, 10 g in 1 L of 5% D/W can be infused over 24 h, followed by up to 2.5 g q 12 h to replace the deficit in total Mg stores and prevent further drops in serum Mg. When serum Mg is ≤ 1.25 mg/dL (< 0.5 mmol/L) but symptoms are less severe, Mg sulfate may be given IV in 5% D/W at a rate of 1 g/h as slow infusion for up to 10 h. In less severe cases of hypomagnesemia, gradual repletion may be achieved by administration of smaller parenteral doses over 3 to 5 days until the serum Mg concentration is normal.

Concurrent hypokalemia or hypocalcemia should be specifically addressed in addition to hypomagnesemia. These electrolyte disturbances are difficult to correct until Mg has been repleted. Additionally, hypocalcemia can be worsened by isolated treatment of hypomagnesemia with intravenous Mg sulfate because sulfate binds ionized Ca.

KEY POINTS

- Hypomagnesemia may occur in alcoholics, in patients with uncontrolled diabetes, and with hypercalcemia or use of loop diuretics.
- Symptoms include anorexia, nausea, vomiting, lethargy, weakness, personality change, tetany (eg, positive Trousseau or Chvostek sign, spontaneous carpopedal spasm, hyperreflexia), tremor, and muscle fasciculations.
- Treat with Mg salts when Mg deficiency is symptomatic or persistently < 1.25 mg/dL (< 0.50 mmol/L).
- Give oral Mg salts unless patients have seizures or other severe symptoms, in which case, give 2 to 4 g of Mg sulfate IV over 5 to 10 min.

HYPERMAGNESEMIA

Hypermagnesemia is a serum Mg concentration > 2.6 mg/dL (> 1.05 mmol/L). The major cause is renal failure. Symptoms include hypotension, respiratory depression, and cardiac arrest. Diagnosis is by serum Mg concentration. Treatment includes IV administration of Ca gluconate and possibly furosemide; hemodialysis can be helpful in severe cases.

Symptomatic hypermagnesemia is fairly uncommon. It occurs most commonly in patients with renal failure after ingestion of Mg-containing drugs, such as antacids or purgatives.

Symptoms and signs include hyporeflexia, hypotension, respiratory depression, and cardiac arrest.

Diagnosis

- Serum Mg concentrations > 2.6 mg/dL (> 1.05 mmol/L)

At serum Mg concentrations of 6 to 12 mg/dL (2.5 to 5 mmol/L), the ECG shows prolongation of the PR interval, widening of the QRS complex, and increased T-wave amplitude. Deep tendon reflexes disappear as the serum Mg concentration approaches 12 mg/dL (5.0 mmol/L); hypotension, respiratory depression, and narcosis develop with increasing hypermagnesemia. Cardiac arrest may occur when blood Mg concentration is > 15 mg/dL (6.0 to 7.5 mmol/L).

Treatment

- Ca gluconate
- Diuresis or dialysis

Treatment of severe Mg toxicity consists of circulatory and respiratory support with administration of 10% Ca gluconate 10 to 20 mL IV. Ca gluconate may reverse many of the Mg-induced changes, including respiratory depression.

Administration of IV furosemide can increase Mg excretion when renal function is adequate; volume status should be maintained. Hemodialysis may be valuable in severe hypermagnesemia, because a relatively large fraction (about 70%) of blood Mg is not protein bound and thus is removable with hemodialysis. When hemodynamic compromise occurs and hemodialysis is impractical, peritoneal dialysis is an option.

167 Fluid Metabolism

WATER AND SODIUM BALANCE

Body fluid volume and electrolyte concentration are normally maintained within very narrow limits despite wide variations in dietary intake, metabolic activity, and environmental stresses. Homeostasis of body fluids is preserved primarily by the kidneys.

Water and sodium balance are closely interdependent. Total body water (TBW) is about 60% of body weight in men (ranging from about 50% in obese people to 70% in lean people) and about 50% in women. Almost two-thirds of TBW is in the intracellular compartment (intracellular fluid, or ICF); the other one third is extracellular (extracellular fluid, or ECF). Normally, about 25% of the ECF is in the intravascular compartment; the other 75% is interstitial fluid (see Fig. 167–1).

The major intracellular cation is potassium. The major extracellular cation is Na. Concentrations of intracellular and extracellular cations are as follows:

- Intracellular potassium concentration averages 140 mEq/L.
- Extracellular potassium concentration is 3.5 to 5 mEq/L.
- Intracellular Na concentration is 12 mEq/L.
- Extracellular Na concentration averages 140 mEq/L.

Osmotic forces: The concentration of combined solutes in water is osmolarity (amount of solute per L of solution), which, in body fluids, is similar to osmolality (amount of solute per kg

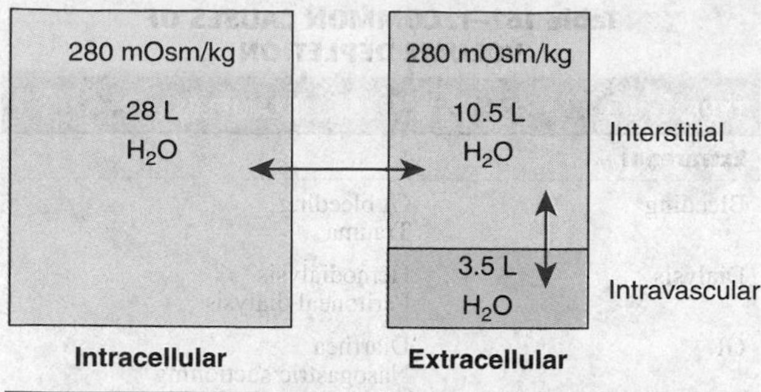

Fig. 167–1. Fluid compartments in an average 70-kg man. Total body water = 70 kg · 0.60 = 42 L.

of solution). Plasma osmolality can be measured in the laboratory or estimated according to the formula

Plasma osmolality (mOsm/kg) =

$$2\,[\text{Serum Na}] + \frac{[\text{Glucose}]}{18} + \frac{[\text{BUN}]}{2.8}$$

where serum Na is expressed in mEq/L, and glucose and BUN are expressed in mg/dL. Osmolality of body fluids is normally between 275 and 290 mOsm/kg. Na is the major determinant of plasma osmolality. Apparent changes in calculated osmolality may result from errors in the measurement of Na (which can occur in patients with hyperlipidemia or extreme hyperproteinemia because the lipid or protein occupies space in the volume of serum taken for analysis; the concentration of Na in serum itself is not affected. Newer methods of measuring serum electrolytes with direct ion-selective electrodes circumvent this problem. An osmolar gap is present when measured osmolality exceeds estimated osmolality by ≥ 10 mOsm/kg. It is caused by unmeasured osmotically active substances present in the plasma. The most common are alcohols (ethanol, methanol, isopropanol, ethylene glycol), mannitol, and glycine.

Water crosses cell membranes freely from areas of low solute concentration to areas of high solute concentration. Thus, osmolality tends to equalize across the various body fluid compartments, resulting primarily from movement of water, not solutes. Solutes such as urea that freely diffuse across cell membranes have little or no effect on water shifts (little or no osmotic activity), whereas solutes that are restricted primarily to one fluid compartment, such as Na and potassium, have the greatest osmotic activity.

Tonicity, or effective osmolality, reflects osmotic activity and determines the force drawing water across fluid compartments (the osmotic force). Osmotic force can be opposed by other forces. For example, plasma proteins have a small osmotic effect that tends to draw water into the plasma; this osmotic effect is normally counteracted by vascular hydrostatic forces that drive water out of the plasma.

Water intake and excretion: The average daily fluid intake is about 2.5 L. The amount needed to replace losses from the urine and other sources is about 1 to 1.5 L/day in healthy adults. However, on a short-term basis, an average young adult with normal kidney function may ingest as little as 200 mL of water each day to excrete the nitrogenous and other wastes generated by cellular metabolism. More is needed in people with any loss of renal concentrating capacity. Renal concentrating capacity is lost in

- The elderly
- People with diabetes insipidus, certain renal disorders, hypercalcemia, severe salt restriction, chronic overhydration, or hyperkalemia
- People who ingest ethanol, phenytoin, lithium, demeclocycline, or amphotericin B
- People with osmotic diuresis (eg, due to high-protein diets or hyperglycemia)

Other obligatory water losses are mostly insensible losses from the lungs and skin, averaging about 0.4 to 0.5 mL/kg/h or about 650 to 850 mL/day in a 70-kg adult. With fever, another 50 to 75 mL/day may be lost for each degree C of temperature elevation above normal. GI losses are usually negligible, except when marked vomiting, diarrhea, or both occur. Sweat losses can be significant during environmental heat exposure or excessive exercise.

Water intake is regulated by thirst. Thirst is triggered by receptors in the anterolateral hypothalamus that respond to increased plasma osmolality (as little as 2%) or decreased body fluid volume. Rarely hypothalamic dysfunction decreases the capacity for thirst.

Water excretion by the kidneys is regulated primarily by vasopressin (ADH). Vasopressin is released by the posterior pituitary and results in increased water reabsorption in the distal nephron. Vasopressin release is stimulated by any of the following:

- Increased plasma osmolality
- Decreased blood volume
- Decreased BP
- Stress

Vasopressin release may be impaired by certain substances (eg, ethanol, phenytoin), by tumors or infiltrative disorders affecting the posterior pituitary, and by trauma to the brain. In many cases a specific cause cannot be identified.

Water intake decreases plasma osmolality. Low plasma osmolality inhibits vasopressin secretion, allowing the kidneys to produce dilute urine. The diluting capacity of healthy kidneys in young adults is such that maximum daily fluid intake can be as much as 25 L; greater amounts quickly lower plasma osmolality.

OVERVIEW OF DISORDERS OF FLUID VOLUME

Because Na is the major osmotically active ion in the ECF, total body Na content determines ECF volume. Deficiency or excess of total body Na content causes ECF volume depletion or volume overload. Serum Na concentration does not necessarily reflect total body Na.

Dietary intake and renal excretion regulate total body Na content. When total Na content and ECF volume are low, the kidneys increase Na conservation. When total Na content and ECF volume are high, Na excretion (natriuresis) increases so that volume decreases.

Renal Na excretion can be adjusted widely to match Na intake. Renal Na excretion requires delivery of Na to the kidneys and so depends on renal blood flow and GFR. Thus, inadequate Na excretion may be secondary to decreased renal blood flow, as in chronic kidney disease or heart failure.

Renin-angiotensin-aldosterone axis: The renin-angiotensin-aldosterone axis is the main regulatory mechanism of renal Na excretion. In volume-depleted states, GFR and Na delivery to the distal nephrons decreases, causing release of renin. Renin cleaves angiotensinogen (renin substrate) to form angiotensin I. ACE then cleaves angiotensin I to angiotensin II. Angiotensin II does the following:

- Increases Na retention by decreasing the filtered load of Na and enhancing proximal tubular Na reabsorption
- Increases BP (has pressor activity)
- Increases thirst
- Directly impairs water excretion
- Stimulates the adrenal cortex to secrete aldosterone, which increases Na reabsorption via multiple renal mechanisms

Angiotensin I can also be transformed to angiotensin III, which stimulates aldosterone release as much as angiotensin II but has much less pressor activity. Aldosterone release is also stimulated by hyperkalemia.

Other natriuretic factors: Several other natriuretic factors have been identified, including atrial natriuretic peptide (ANP), brain natriuretic peptide (BNP), and a C-type natriuretic peptide (CNP).

ANP is secreted by cardiac atrial tissue. Concentration increases in response to ECF volume overload (eg, heart failure, chronic kidney disease, cirrhosis with ascites) and primary aldosteronism and in some patients with primary hypertension. Decreases have occurred in the subset of patients with nephrotic syndrome who have presumed ECF volume contraction. High concentrations increase Na excretion and increase GFR even when BP is low.

BNP is synthesized mainly in the atria and left ventricle and has similar triggers and effects to ANP. BNP assays are readily available. High BNP concentration is used to diagnose volume overload.

CNP, in contrast to ANP and BNP, is primarily vasodilatory.

Sodium depletion and excess: Na depletion requires inadequate Na intake plus abnormal losses from the skin, GI tract, or kidneys (defective renal Na conservation). Defective renal Na conservation may be caused by primary renal disease, adrenal insufficiency, or diuretic therapy.

Na overload requires higher Na intake than excretion; however, because normal kidneys can excrete large amounts of Na, Na overload generally reflects defective regulation of renal blood flow and Na excretion (eg, as occurs in heart failure, cirrhosis, or chronic kidney disease).

VOLUME DEPLETION

Volume depletion, or ECF volume contraction, occurs as a result of loss of total body Na. Causes include vomiting, excessive sweating, diarrhea, burns, diuretic use, and kidney failure. Clinical features include diminished skin turgor, dry mucous membranes, tachycardia, and orthostatic hypotension. Diagnosis is clinical. Treatment involves administration of Na and water.

Because water crosses plasma membranes in the body via passive osmosis, loss of the major extracellular cation (Na) quickly results in water loss from the ECF space as well. In this way, Na loss always causes water loss. However, depending on many factors, serum Na concentration can be high, low, or normal in volume-depleted patients (despite the decreased total body Na content). ECF volume is related to effective circulating volume. A decrease in ECF (hypovolemia) generally causes a decrease in effective circulating volume, which in turn causes decreased organ perfusion and leads to clinical sequelae. Common causes of volume depletion are listed in Table 167–1.

Table 167–1. COMMON CAUSES OF VOLUME DEPLETION

TYPE	EXAMPLES
Extrarenal	
Bleeding	GI bleeding Trauma
Dialysis	Hemodialysis Peritoneal dialysis
GI	Diarrhea Nasogastric suctioning Vomiting
Skin	Burns Excessive sweating Exfoliation
3rd-space losses	Intestinal lumen Intraperitoneal Retroperitoneal
Renal, adrenal, and pituitary	
Acute renal failure	Diuretic phase of recovery
Adrenal disorders	Adrenal insufficiency (causing adrenal steroid deficiency), including Addison disease Hypoaldosteronism
Genetic disorders causing renal Na and potassium wasting	Bartter syndrome Gitelman syndrome
Hypothalamic or pituitary disorders causing vasopressin ADH deficiency	Central diabetes insipidus (eg, due to trauma, tumor, infection)
Osmotic diuresis	Diabetes mellitus with extreme glucosuria
Diuretics	Loop diuretics Thiazide diuretics
Salt-wasting renal disease	Interstitial nephritis Medullary cystic disease Myeloma (occasionally) Pyelonephritis (occasionally)

Symptoms and Signs

When **fluid loss is < 5% of ECF** (mild volume depletion), the only sign may be diminished skin turgor (best assessed at the upper torso). Skin turgor may be low in elderly patients regardless of volume status. Patients may complain of thirst. Dry mucous membranes do not always correlate with volume depletion, especially in the elderly and in mouth-breathers. Oliguria is typical.

When **ECF volume has diminished by 5 to 10%** (moderate volume depletion), orthostatic tachycardia, hypotension, or both are usually, but not always, present. Also, orthostatic changes can occur in patients without ECF volume depletion, particularly patients deconditioned or bedridden. Skin turgor may decrease further.

When **fluid loss exceeds 10% of ECF volume** (severe volume depletion), signs of shock (eg, tachypnea, tachycardia, hypotension, confusion, poor capillary refill) can occur.

Diagnosis

- Clinical findings
- Sometimes serum electrolytes, BUN, and creatinine
- Rarely plasma osmolality and urine chemistries

Volume depletion is suspected in patients at risk, most often in patients with a history of inadequate fluid intake (especially in comatose or disoriented patients), increased fluid losses, diuretic therapy, and renal or adrenal disorders.

Diagnosis is usually clinical. When the cause is obvious and easily correctable (eg, acute gastroenteritis in otherwise healthy patients), laboratory testing is unnecessary; otherwise, serum electrolytes, BUN, and creatinine are measured. Plasma osmolality and urine Na, creatinine, and osmolality are measured when there is suspicion of clinically meaningful electrolyte abnormality that is not clear from results of serum tests and for patients with cardiac or renal disease. When metabolic alkalosis is present, urine chloride is also measured.

Central venous pressure and pulmonary artery occlusion pressure are decreased in volume depletion, but measurement is rarely required. Measurement, which requires an invasive procedure, is occasionally necessary for patients for whom even small amounts of added volume may be detrimental, such as those with unstable heart failure or advanced chronic kidney disease.

The following concepts are helpful when interpreting urine electrolyte and osmolality values:

- During volume depletion, normally functioning kidneys conserve Na. Thus, the urine Na concentration is usually < 15 mEq/L; the fractional excretion of Na (urine Na/serum Na divided by urine creatinine/serum creatinine) is usually < 1%; also, urine osmolality is often > 450 mOsm/kg.
- When metabolic alkalosis is combined with volume depletion, urine Na concentration may be high because large amounts of bicarbonate are spilled in the urine, obligating the excretion of Na to maintain electrical neutrality. In this instance, a urine chloride concentration of < 10 mEq/L more reliably indicates volume depletion.
- Misleadingly high urinary Na (generally > 20 mEq/L) or low urine osmolality can also occur due to renal Na losses resulting from renal disease, diuretics, or adrenal insufficiency.

Volume depletion frequently increases the BUN and serum creatinine concentrations; the ratio of BUN to creatinine is often > 20:1. Values such as Hct often increase in volume depletion but are difficult to interpret unless baseline values are known.

Treatment

- Replacement of Na and water

The cause of volume depletion is corrected and fluids are given to replace existing volume deficits as well as any ongoing fluid losses and to provide daily fluid requirements. Mild-to-moderate volume deficits may be replaced by increased oral intake of Na and water when patients are conscious and not vomiting. When volume deficits are severe or when oral fluid replacement is impractical, IV 0.9% saline is given. For typical IV regimens, see p. 576; for oral regimens, see p. 2557.

VOLUME OVERLOAD

Volume overload generally refers to expansion of the ECF volume. ECF volume expansion typically occurs in heart failure, kidney failure, nephrotic syndrome, and cirrhosis. Renal Na retention leads to increased total body Na content. This increase results in varying degrees of volume overload. Serum Na concentration can be high, low, or normal in volume-overloaded patients (despite the increased total body Na content). Treatment involves removal of excess fluid with diuretics or mechanical fluid removal via methods such as dialysis and paracentesis.

An increase in total body Na is the key pathophysiologic event. It increases osmolality, which triggers compensatory mechanisms that cause water retention. When sufficient fluid accumulates in the ECF (usually > 2.5 L), edema develops.

Among the most common causes of ECF volume overload are the following:

- Heart failure
- Cirrhosis
- Kidney failure
- Nephrotic syndrome
- Premenstrual edema
- Pregnancy

Diagnosis

- Clinical evaluation

Diagnosis is mainly clinical. Clinical features include weight gain and edema. The location and amount of edema are dependent on many factors, including whether the patient has been sitting, lying, or standing recently. Clinical findings vary significantly depending on the cause and are discussed in detail elsewhere in The Manual.

Serum Na concentration can be high, low, or normal in volume-overloaded patients (despite the increased total body Na content). Urinary Na may help differentiate acute kidney failure from other (non-renal related) acute causes of volume overload. In renal failure, the urinary Na is > 20mEq/L as compared to < 10 mEq/L in heart failure, cirrhosis and nephrotic syndrome.

Treatment

- Treatment of cause

Treatment aims to correct the cause. Treatment of heart failure, cirrhosis, kidney failure, and nephrotic syndrome are addressed elsewhere in the Manual, but in general treatment includes diuretics and sometimes mechanical fluid removal via methods such as dialysis and paracentesis.

Dietary Na intake is restricted. Diuretics are given in heart failure, cirrhosis, renal insufficiency, and nephrotic syndrome. Daily weights are the best way to follow the progress of therapy for ECF volume overload. The speed of correction of ECF volume overload should be limited to 0.25 to 0.5 kg body weight/day, depending on the degree of volume overload (faster with a copious excess, slower with less excess) and the patient's other medical problems (slower with hypotension and renal insufficiency).

Outpatients should be monitored closely when undergoing active diuresis. When there is more severe organ system dysfunction or multiple organ systems are involved or little progress is being made with oral diuretics, inpatient treatment and monitoring are needed.

168 Lipid Disorders

Lipids are fats that are either absorbed from food or synthesized by the liver. Triglycerides (TGs) and cholesterol contribute most to disease, although all lipids are physiologically important. The primary function of TGs is to store energy in adipocytes and muscle cells; cholesterol is a ubiquitous constituent of cell membranes, steroids, bile acids, and signaling molecules.

All lipids are hydrophobic and mostly insoluble in blood, so they require transport within hydrophilic, spherical structures called lipoproteins, which possess surface proteins (apoproteins, or apolipoproteins) that are cofactors and ligands for lipid-processing enzymes (see Table 168–1). Lipoproteins are classified by size and density (defined as the ratio of lipid to protein) and are important because high levels of low-density lipoproteins (LDL) and low levels of high-density lipoproteins (HDL) are major risk factors for atherosclerotic heart disease.

Physiology

Pathway defects in lipoprotein synthesis, processing, and clearance can lead to accumulation of atherogenic lipids in plasma and endothelium.

Exogenous (dietary) lipid metabolism: Over 95% of dietary lipids are TGs; the rest are phospholipids, free fatty acids (FFAs), cholesterol (present in foods as esterified cholesterol), and fat-soluble vitamins. Dietary TGs are digested in the stomach and duodenum into monoglycerides (MGs) and FFAs by gastric lipase, emulsification from vigorous stomach peristalsis, and pancreatic lipase. Dietary cholesterol esters are de-esterified into free cholesterol by these same mechanisms. MGs, FFAs, and free cholesterol are then solubilized in the intestine by bile acid micelles, which shuttle them to intestinal villi for absorption. Once absorbed into enterocytes, they are reassembled into TGs and packaged with cholesterol into chylomicrons, the largest lipoproteins.

Chylomicrons transport dietary TGs and cholesterol from within enterocytes through lymphatics into the circulation. In the capillaries of adipose and muscle tissue, apoprotein C-II (apo C-II) on the chylomicron activates endothelial lipoprotein lipase (LPL) to convert 90% of chylomicron TG to fatty acids and glycerol, which are taken up by adipocytes and muscle cells for energy use or storage. Cholesterol-rich chylomicron remnants then circulate back to the liver, where they are cleared in a process mediated by apoprotein E (apo E).

Endogenous lipid metabolism: Lipoproteins synthesized by the liver transport endogenous TGs and cholesterol. Lipoproteins circulate through the blood continuously until the TGs they contain are taken up by peripheral tissues or the lipoproteins themselves are cleared by the liver. Factors that stimulate hepatic lipoprotein synthesis generally lead to elevated plasma cholesterol and TG levels.

Very-low-density lipoproteins (VLDL) contain apoprotein B-100 (apo B), are synthesized in the liver, and transport TGs and cholesterol to peripheral tissues. VLDL is the way the liver exports excess TGs derived from plasma FFA and chylomicron remnants; VLDL synthesis increases with increases in intrahepatic FFA, such as occur with high-fat diets and when excess adipose tissue releases FFAs directly into the circulation (eg, in obesity, uncontrolled diabetes mellitus). Apo C-II on the VLDL

Table 168–1. MAJOR APOPROTEINS AND ENZYMES IMPORTANT TO LIPID METABOLISM

COMPONENT	LOCATION	FUNCTION
Apoproteins		
Apo A-I	HDL	Major component of HDL particle
Apo A-II	HDL	Component of HDL particle
Apo B-100	VLDL, IDL, LDL, Lp(a)	LDL receptor ligand
Apo B-48	Chylomicrons	Major component of chylomicron
Apo C-II	Chylomicrons, VLDL, HDL	LPL cofactor
Apo C-III	Chylomicrons, VLDL, HDL	Inhibits LPL
Apo E	Chylomicrons, remnants, VLDL, HDL	LDL receptor ligand
Apo(a)	Lp(a)	Component of Lp(a) and links to LDL particle
Enzymes		
ABCA1	Within cells	Contributes to intracellular cholesterol transport to membrane
CETP	HDL	Mediates transfer of cholesteryl esters from HDL to VLDL
LPL	Endothelium	Hydrolyzes TGs of chylomicrons and VLDL to release free fatty acids
LCAT	HDL	Esterifies free cholesterol for transport within HDL

ABCA1 = ATP-binding cassette transporter A1; apo = apoprotein; CETP = cholesteryl ester transfer protein; HDL = high-density lipoprotein; IDL = intermediate-density lipoprotein; LCAT = lecithin-cholesterol acyltransferase; LDL = low-density lipoprotein; LPL = lipoprotein lipase; Lp(a) = lipoprotein (a); VLDL = very-low-density lipoprotein.

surface activates endothelial LPL to break down TGs into FFAs and glycerol, which are taken up by cells.

Intermediate-density lipoproteins (IDL) are the product of LPL processing of VLDL and chylomicrons. IDL are cholesterol-rich VLDL and chylomicron remnants that are either cleared by the liver or metabolized by hepatic lipase into LDL, which retains apo B.

Low-density lipoproteins (LDL), the products of VLDL and IDL metabolism, are the most cholesterol-rich of all lipoproteins. About 40 to 60% of all LDL are cleared by the liver in a process mediated by apo B and hepatic LDL receptors. The rest are taken up by either hepatic LDL or nonhepatic non-LDL (scavenger) receptors. Hepatic LDL receptors are down-regulated by delivery of cholesterol to the liver by chylomicrons and by increased dietary saturated fat; they can be up-regulated by decreased dietary fat and cholesterol. Nonhepatic scavenger receptors, most notably on macrophages, take up excess oxidized circulating LDL not processed by hepatic receptors.

Monocytes rich in oxidized LDL migrate into the subendothelial space and become macrophages; these macrophages then take up more oxidized LDL and form foam cells within atherosclerotic plaques (see p. 653). The size of LDL particles varies from large and buoyant to small and dense. Small, dense LDL is especially rich in cholesterol esters, is associated with metabolic disturbances such as hypertriglyceridemia and insulin resistance, and is especially atherogenic. The increased atherogenicity of small, dense LDL derives from less efficient hepatic LDL receptor binding, leading to prolonged circulation and exposure to endothelium and increased oxidation.

High-density lipoproteins (HDL) are initially cholesterol-free lipoproteins that are synthesized in both enterocytes and the liver. HDL metabolism is complex, but one role of HDL is to obtain cholesterol from peripheral tissues and other lipoproteins and transport it to where it is needed most—other cells, other lipoproteins (using cholesteryl ester transfer protein [CETP]), and the liver (for clearance). Its overall effect is antiatherogenic. Efflux of free cholesterol from cells is mediated by ATP-binding cassette transporter A1 (ABCA1), which combines with apoprotein A-I (apo A-I) to produce nascent HDL. Free cholesterol in nascent HDL is then esterified by the enzyme lecithin-cholesterol acyl transferase (LCAT), producing mature HDL. Blood HDL levels may not completely represent reverse cholesterol transport.

Lipoprotein (a) [Lp(a)] is LDL that contains apoprotein (a), characterized by 5 cysteine-rich regions called kringles. One of these regions is homologous with plasminogen and is thought to competitively inhibit fibrinolysis and thus predispose to thrombus. The Lp(a) may also directly promote atherosclerosis. The metabolic pathways of Lp(a) production and clearance are not well characterized, but levels increase in patients with diabetic nephropathy.

DYSLIPIDEMIA

(Hyperlipidemia)

Dyslipidemia is *elevation* of plasma cholesterol, triglycerides (TGs), or both, or a low high-density lipoprotein level that contributes to the development of atherosclerosis. Causes may be primary (genetic) or secondary. Diagnosis is by measuring plasma levels of total cholesterol (TC), TGs, and individual lipoproteins. Treatment involves dietary changes, exercise, and lipid-lowering drugs.

There is no natural cutoff between normal and abnormal lipid levels because lipid measurements are continuous. A linear relation probably exists between lipid levels and cardiovascular risk, so many people with "normal" cholesterol levels benefit from achieving still lower levels. Consequently, there are no numeric definitions of dyslipidemia; the term is applied to lipid levels for which treatment has proven beneficial. Proof of benefit is strongest for lowering elevated low density lipoprotein (LDL) levels. In the overall population, evidence is less strong for a benefit from lowering elevated TG and increasing low high-density lipoprotein (HDL) levels.

HDL levels do not always predict cardiovascular risk. For example, high HDL levels caused by some genetic disorders may not protect against cardiovascular disorders, and low HDL levels caused by some genetic disorders may not increase the risk of cardiovascular disorders. Although HDL levels predict cardiovascular risk in the overall population, the increased risk may be caused by other factors, such as accompanying lipid and metabolic abnormalities, rather than the HDL level itself.

Classification

Dyslipidemias were traditionally classified by patterns of elevation in lipids and lipoproteins (Fredrickson phenotype—see Table 168–2). A more practical system categorizes dyslipidemias as primary or secondary and characterizes them by

- Increases in cholesterol only (pure or isolated hypercholesterolemia)
- Increases in TGs only (pure or isolated hypertriglyceridemia),
- Increases in both cholesterol and TGs (mixed or combined hyperlipidemias)

This system does not take into account specific lipoprotein abnormalities (eg, low HDL or high LDL) that may contribute to disease despite normal cholesterol and TG levels.

Etiology

Primary (genetic) causes and secondary (lifestyle and other) causes contribute to dyslipidemias in varying degrees. For example, in familial combined hyperlipidemia, expression may occur only in the presence of significant secondary causes.

Primary causes: Primary causes are single or multiple gene mutations that result in either overproduction or defective clearance of TG and LDL cholesterol, or in underproduction or excessive clearance of HDL (see Table 168–3). The names of

Table 168–2. LIPOPROTEIN PATTERNS (FREDRICKSON PHENOTYPES)

PHENOTYPE	ELEVATED LIPOPROTEIN(S)	ELEVATED LIPIDS
I	Chylomicrons	TGs
IIa	LDL	Cholesterol
IIb	LDL and VLDL	TGs and cholesterol
III	VLDL and chylomicron remnants	TGs and cholesterol
IV	VLDL	TGs
V	Chylomicrons and VLDL	TGs and cholesterol

LDL = low-density lipoprotein; TGs = triglycerides; VLDL = very-low-density lipoprotein.

Table 168–3. GENETIC (PRIMARY) DYSLIPIDEMIAS

DISORDER	GENETIC DEFECT/ MECHANISM	INHERITANCE	PREVALENCE	CLINICAL FEATURES	TREATMENT
Familial hypercholesterolemia	LDL receptor defect Diminished LDL clearance	Codominant or complex with multiple genes	Present worldwide but increased among French Canadian, Christian Lebanese, and South African populations	—	Diet Lipid-lowering drugs LDL apheresis (for homozygotes and heterozygotes with severe disease) Liver transplantation (for homozygotes)
			Heterozygotes: 1/200 to 1/500	Tendon xanthomas, arcus corneae, premature CAD (ages 30–50), responsible for about 5% of MIs in people < 60 yr TC: 250–500 mg/dL (7–13 mmol/L)	
			Homozygotes: 1/1 million (increased among French Canadian, Christian Lebanese, and South African populations)	Planar and tendon xanthomas and tuberous xanthomas, premature CAD (before age 18) TC > 500 mg/dL (> 13 mmol/L)	
Familial defective apo B-100	Apo B (LDL receptor–binding region defect) Diminished LDL clearance	Dominant	1/700	Xanthomas, arcus corneae, premature CAD TC: 250–500 mg/dL (7–13 mmol/L)	Diet Lipid-lowering drugs
PCSK9 gain of function mutations	Increased degradation of LDL receptors	Dominant	Unknown	Similar to familial hypercholesterolemia	Diet Lipid-lowering drugs
Polygenic hypercholesterolemia	Unknown, possibly multiple defects and mechanisms	Variable	Common	Premature CAD TC: 250–350 mg/dL (6.5–9.0 mmol/L)	Diet Lipid-lowering drugs
LPL deficiency	Endothelial LPL defect Diminished chylomicron clearance	Recessive	Rare but present worldwide	Failure to thrive (in infants), eruptive xanthomas, hepatosplenomegaly, pancreatitis TG: > 750 mg/dL (> 8.5 mmol/L)	Diet: Total fat restriction with fat-soluble vitamin supplementation and medium-chain TG supplementation Gene therapy (approved in European Union)
Apo C-II deficiency	Apo C-II (causing functional LPL deficiency)	Recessive	< 1/1 million	Pancreatitis (in some adults), metabolic syndrome (often present) TG: > 750 mg/dL (> 8.5 mmol/L)	Diet: Total fat restriction with fat-soluble vitamin supplementation and medium-chain TG supplementation

Table 168–3. GENETIC (PRIMARY) DYSLIPIDEMIAS (*Continued*)

DISORDER	GENETIC DEFECT/ MECHANISM	INHERITANCE	PREVALENCE	CLINICAL FEATURES	TREATMENT
Familial hypertriglyceridemia	Unknown, possibly multiple defects and mechanisms	Dominant	1/100	Usually no symptoms or findings; occasionally hyperuricemia, sometimes early atherosclerosis TG: 200–500 mg/dL (2.3–5.7 mmol/L), possibly higher depending on diet and alcohol use	Diet Weight loss Lipid-lowering drugs
Familial combined hyperlipidemia	Unknown, possibly multiple defects and mechanisms	Dominant	1/50 to 1/100	Premature CAD, responsible for about 15% of MIs in people < 60 yr Apo B: Disproportionately elevated TC: 250–500 mg/dL (6.5–13.0 mmol/L) TG: 250–750 mg/dL (2.8–8.5 mmol/L)	Diet Weight loss Lipid-lowering drugs
Familial dysbetalipoproteinemia	Apo E (usually e2/e2 homozygotes) Diminished chylomicron and VLDL clearance	Recessive (more common) or dominant (less common)	1/5000 Present worldwide	Xanthomas (especially tuberous and palmar), yellow palmar creases, premature CAD TC: 250–500 mg/dL (6.5–13.0 mmol/L) TG: 250–500 mg/dL (2.8–5.6 mmol/L)	Diet Lipid-lowering drugs
Primary hypoalphalipoproteinemia (familial or nonfamilial)	Unknown, possibly apo A-I, C-III, or A-IV	Dominant	About 5%	Premature CAD HDL: 15–35 mg/dL	Exercise LDL-lowering drugs
Familial apo A/apo C-III deficiency/mutations	Apo A or apo C-III Increased HDL catabolism	Unknown	Rare	Corneal opacities, xanthomas, premature CAD (in some people) HDL: 15–30 mg/dL	Nonspecific
Familial LCAT deficiency	*LCAT* gene	Recessive	Extremely rare	Corneal opacities, anemia, renal failure HDL: < 10 mg/dL	Fat restriction Renal transplantation
Fisheye disease (partial LCAT deficiency)	*LCAT* gene	Recessive	Extremely rare	Corneal opacities HDL: < 10 mg/dL	Nonspecific
Tangier disease	*ABCA1* gene	Recessive	Rare	Premature CAD (in some people), peripheral neuropathy, hemolytic anemia, corneal opacities, hepatosplenomegaly, orange tonsils HDL: < 5 mg/dL	Low-fat diet
Familial HDL deficiency	*ABCA1* gene	Dominant	Rare	Premature CAD	Low-fat diet
Hepatic lipase deficiency	Hepatic lipase	Recessive	Extremely rare	Premature CAD TC: 250–1500 mg/dL TG: 395–8200 mg/dL HDL: Variable	Empiric: Diet, lipid-lowering drugs

Table continues on the following page.

Table 168–3. GENETIC (PRIMARY) DYSLIPIDEMIAS (*Continued*)

DISORDER	GENETIC DEFECT/ MECHANISM	INHERITANCE	PREVALENCE	CLINICAL FEATURES	TREATMENT
Cerebrotendinous xanthomatosis	Hepatic mitochondrial 27-hydroxylase defect Blockage of bile acid synthesis and conversion of cholesterol to cholestanol, which accumulates	Recessive	Rare	Cataracts, premature CAD, neuropathy, ataxia	Chenodeoxycholic acid
Sitosterolemia	*ABCG5* and *ABCG8* genes	Recessive	Rare	Tendon xanthomas, premature CAD	Fat restriction Bile acid sequestrants Ezetimibe
Cholesteryl ester storage disease and Wolman disease	Lysosomal esterase deficiency	Recessive	Rare	Premature CAD Accumulation of cholesteryl esters and TG in lysosomes in the liver, spleen, and lymph nodes Cirrhosis	Possibly statins Enzyme replacement

ABCA1 = ATP-binding cassette transporter A1; ABCG5 and 8 = ATP-binding cassette subfamily G members 5 and 8; apo = apoprotein; CAD = coronary artery disease; HDL = high-density lipoprotein; LCAT = lecithin-cholesterol acyltransferase; LDL = low-density lipoprotein; LPL = lipoprotein lipase; MI = myocardial infarction; PCSK9 = proprotein convertase subtilisin-like/kexin type 9; TC = total cholesterol; TG = triglyceride; VLDL = very-low-density lipoprotein.

many primary disorders reflect an old nomenclature in which lipoproteins were detected and distinguished by how they separated into alpha (HDL) and beta (LDL) bands on electrophoretic gels.

Secondary causes: Secondary causes contribute to many cases of dyslipidemia in adults. The **most important** secondary cause in developed countries is

- A sedentary lifestyle with excessive dietary intake of saturated fat, cholesterol, and trans fats

Trans fats are polyunsaturated or monounsaturated fatty acids to which hydrogen atoms have been added; they are used in some processed foods and are as atherogenic as saturated fat. Other common secondary causes include

- Diabetes mellitus
- Alcohol overuse
- Chronic kidney disease
- Hypothyroidism
- Primary biliary cirrhosis and other cholestatic liver diseases
- Drugs, such as thiazides, β-blockers, retinoids, highly active antiretroviral agents, cyclosporine, tacrolimus, estrogen and progestins, and glucocorticoids

Secondary causes of low levels of HDL cholesterol include cigarette smoking, anabolic steroids, HIV infection, and nephrotic syndrome.

Diabetes is an especially significant secondary cause because patients tend to have an atherogenic combination of high TGs; high small, dense LDL fractions; and low HDL (diabetic dyslipidemia, hypertriglyceridemic hyperapo B). Patients with type 2 diabetes are especially at risk. The combination may be a consequence of obesity, poor control of diabetes, or both, which may increase circulating FFAs, leading to increased hepatic very-low-density lipoprotein (VLDL) production. TG-rich VLDL then transfers TG and cholesterol to LDL and HDL, promoting formation of TG-rich, small, dense LDL and clearance of TG-rich HDL. Diabetic dyslipidemia is often exacerbated by the increased caloric intake and physical inactivity that characterize the lifestyles of some patients with type 2 diabetes. Women with diabetes may be at special risk of cardiac disease from this form.

Symptoms and Signs

Dyslipidemia itself usually causes no symptoms but can lead to symptomatic vascular disease, including coronary artery disease (CAD), stroke, and peripheral arterial disease. High levels of TGs (> 1000 mg/dL [> 11.3 mmol/L]) can cause acute pancreatitis. High levels of LDL can cause arcus corneae and tendinous xanthomas at the Achilles, elbow, and knee tendons and over metacarpophalangeal joints.

Patients with the homozygous form of familial hypercholesterolemia may have the above findings plus planar or tuberous xanthomas. Planar xanthomas are flat or slightly raised yellowish patches. Tuberous xanthomas are painless, firm nodules typically located over extensor surfaces of joints. Patients with severe elevations of TGs can have eruptive xanthomas over the trunk, back, elbows, buttocks, knees, hands, and feet. Patients with the rare dysbetalipoproteinemia can have palmar and tuberous xanthomas.

Severe hypertriglyceridemia (> 2000 mg/dL [> 22.6 mmol/L]) can give retinal arteries and veins a creamy white appearance (lipemia retinalis). Extremely high lipid levels also give a lactescent (milky) appearance to blood plasma. Symptoms can include paresthesias, dypsnea, and confusion.

Diagnosis

- Serum lipid profile (measured TC, TG, and HDL cholesterol and calculated LDL cholesterol and VLDL)

Dyslipidemia is suspected in patients with characteristic physical findings or complications of dyslipidemia (eg, atherosclerotic disease). Primary lipid disorders are suspected when patients have physical signs of dyslipidemia, onset of premature atherosclerotic disease (at < 60 yr), a family history of atherosclerotic disease, or serum cholesterol > 240 mg/dL (> 6.2 mmol/L). Dyslipidemia is diagnosed by measuring serum lipids. Routine measurements (lipid profile) include TC, TGs, HDL cholesterol, and LDL cholesterol.

Lipid profile measurement: TC, TGs, and HDL cholesterol are measured directly. TC and TG values reflect cholesterol and TGs in all circulating lipoproteins, including chylomicrons, VLDL, IDL, LDL, and HDL. TC values can vary by 10% and TGs by up to 25% day-to-day even in the absence of a disorder. TC and HDL cholesterol can be measured in the nonfasting state, but most patients should have all lipids measured while fasting (usually for 12 h) for maximum accuracy and consistency.

Testing should be postponed until after resolution of acute illness because TG and lipoprotein(a) levels increase and cholesterol levels decrease in inflammatory states. Lipid profiles can vary for about 30 days after an acute MI; however, results obtained within 24 h after MI are usually reliable enough to guide initial lipid-lowering therapy.

LDL cholesterol values are most often calculated as the amount of cholesterol not contained in HDL and VLDL. VLDL is estimated by TG ÷ 5 because the cholesterol concentration in VLDL particles is usually one fifth of the total lipid in the particle. Thus,

$$\text{LDL cholesterol} = \text{Total cholesterol} - \left[\text{HDL cholesterol} + \left(\frac{\text{Triglycerides}}{5}\right)\right]$$

This calculation is valid only when TGs are < 400 mg/dL and patients are fasting, because eating increases TGs. The calculated LDL cholesterol value incorporates measures of all non-HDL, nonchylomicron cholesterol, including that in IDL and lipoprotein (a) [Lp(a)].

LDL can also be measured directly using plasma ultracentrifugation, which separates chylomicrons and VLDL fractions from HDL and LDL, and by an immunoassay method. Direct measurement may be useful in some patients with elevated TGs, but these direct measurements are not routinely necessary. The role of apo B testing is under study because values reflect all non-HDL cholesterol (in VLDL, VLDL remnants, IDL, and LDL) and may be more predictive of CAD risk than LDL cholesterol. Non-HDL cholesterol (TC − HDL cholesterol) may also be more predictive of CAD risk than LDL cholesterol.

Other tests: Patients with premature atherosclerotic cardiovascular disease (ASCVD), cardiovascular disease with normal or near-normal lipid levels, or high LDL levels refractory to drug therapy should probably have Lp(a) levels measured. Lp(a) levels may also be directly measured in patients with borderline high LDL cholesterol levels to determine whether drug therapy is warranted. C-reactive protein may be considered in the same populations. Measurements of LDL particle number or apoprotein B-100 (apo B) may be useful in patients with elevated TGs and the metabolic syndrome. Apo B provides similar information to LDL particle number because there is one apo B molecule for each LDL particle. Apo B measurement includes all atherogenic particles, including remnants and Lp(a).

Secondary causes: Tests for secondary causes of dyslipidemia—including measurements of fasting glucose, liver enzymes, creatinine, thyroid-stimulating hormone (TSH), and urinary protein—should be done in most patients with newly diagnosed dyslipidemia and when a component of the lipid profile has inexplicably changed for the worse.

Screening: Universal screening using a fasting lipid profile (TC, TGs, HDL cholesterol, and calculated LDL cholesterol) should be done in all children between age 9 and 11 (or at age 2 if children have a family history of severe hyperlipidemia or premature CAD). Adults are screened at age 20 yr and every 5 yr thereafter. Lipid measurement should be accompanied by assessment of other cardiovascular risk factors, defined as

- Diabetes mellitus
- Cigarette use
- Hypertension
- Family history of CAD in a male 1st-degree relative before age 55 or a female 1st-degree relative before age 65

A definite age after which patients no longer require screening has not been established, but evidence supports screening of patients into their 80s, especially in the presence of ASCVD.

Patients with an extensive family history of heart disease should also be screened by measuring Lp(a) levels.

Treatment

- Risk assessment by explicit criteria
- Lifestyle changes (eg, exercise, dietary modification)
- For high LDL cholesterol, statins, sometimes bile acid sequestrants, ezetimibe, niacin, and other measures
- For high TG, niacin, fibrates, omega-3 fatty acids, and sometimes other measures

General principles: The main indication for dyslipidemia treatment is prevention of ASCVD, including acute coronary syndromes, stroke, transient ischemic attack, or peripheral arterial disease presumed caused by atherosclerosis. Treatment is indicated for all patients with ASCVD (secondary prevention) and for some without (primary prevention).

Treatment of children is controversial; dietary changes may be difficult to implement, and no data suggest that lowering lipid levels in childhood effectively prevents heart disease in adulthood. Moreover, the safety and effectiveness of long-term lipid-lowering treatment are questionable. Nevertheless, the American Academy of Pediatrics (AAP) recommends treatment for some children who have elevated LDL cholesterol levels. Children with heterozygous familial hypercholesterolemia should be treated beginning at age 10. Children with homozygous familial hypercholesterolemia require diet, medications, and often LDL apheresis to prevent premature death; treatment is begun when diagnosis is made.

Treatment options depend on the specific lipid abnormality, although different lipid abnormalities often coexist. In some patients, a single abnormality may require several therapies; in others, a single treatment may be adequate for several abnormalities. Treatment should always include treatment of hypertension and diabetes, smoking cessation, and in patients with a 10-yr risk of MI or death from CAD of ≥ 20% (as determined from the NHLBI Cardiac Risk Calculator), low-dose daily aspirin. In general, treatment options for men and women are the same.

Elevated LDL cholesterol treatment: Treatment options to lower LDL cholesterol in all age groups include lifestyle changes (diet and exercise), drugs, dietary supplements, procedural interventions, and experimental therapies. Many of these options are also effective for treating other lipid abnormalities.

Dietary changes include decreasing intake of saturated fats and cholesterol; increasing the proportion of dietary fiber, and complex carbohydrates; and maintaining ideal body weight. Referral to a dietitian is often useful, especially for older people. Exercise lowers LDL cholesterol in some people and also helps maintain ideal body weight. Dietary changes and exercise should be used whenever feasible but AHA/ACC guidelines recommend also using drug treatment for certain groups of patients after discussion of the risks and benefits of statin therapy.

For **drug treatment in adults,** AHA/ACC recommends treatment with a statin for 4 groups of patients, comprised of those with any of the following:

- Clinical ASCVD
- LDL cholesterol ≥ 190 mg/dL
- Age 40 to 75, with diabetes and LDL cholesterol 70 to 189 mg/dL
- Age 40 to 75, LDL cholesterol 70 to 189 mg/dL, and estimated 10-yr risk of ASCVD ≥ 7.5%

Risk of ASCVD is estimated using the pooled cohort risk assessment equations (see Downloadable AHA/ACC Risk Calculator), which replace previous risk calculation tools. This new risk calculator is based on sex, age, race, total and HDL cholesterol, systolic BP (and whether BP is being treated), diabetes, and smoking status. When considering whether to give a statin, clinicians may also take into account other factors, including LDL cholesterol ≥ 160 mg/dL, family history of premature ASCVD (ie, age of onset < 55 in male 1st degree relative, or < 65 in female 1st degree relative), high-sensitivity C-reactive protein ≥ 2 mg/L, coronary artery calcium score ≥ 300 Agatston units (or ≥ 75th percentile for the patient's demographic), ankle-brachial BP index < 0.9, and increased lifetime risk. Increased lifetime risk (identified using the ACC/AHA risk calculator) is relevant because 10-year risk may be low in younger patients, in whom longer-term risk should be taken into account.

Statins are the treatment of choice for LDL cholesterol reduction because they demonstrably reduce cardiovascular morbidity and mortality. Other classes of lipid-lowering drugs are not the first choice because they have not demonstrated equivalent efficacy for decreasing ASCVD. Statin treatment is classified as high, moderate, or low intensity and is given based on treatment group and age (see Table 168–4). The choice of statin may depend on the patient's co-morbidities, other medications, risk factors for adverse events, statin intolerance, cost, and patient preference. Statins inhibit hydroxymethylglutaryl CoA reductase, a key enzyme in cholesterol synthesis, leading to up-regulation of LDL receptors and increased LDL clearance. They reduce LDL cholesterol by up to 60% and produce small increases in HDL and modest decreases in TGs. Statins also appear to decrease intra-arterial inflammation, systemic inflammation, or both by stimulating production of endothelial nitric oxide and may have other beneficial effects.

Adverse effects are uncommon but include liver enzyme elevations and myositis or rhabdomyolysis. Liver enzyme elevations are uncommon, and serious liver toxicity is extremely rare. Muscle problems occur in up to 10% of patients taking statins and may be dose-dependent in many patients. Muscle symptoms can occur without enzyme elevation. Adverse effects are more common among older patients, patients with several disorders, and patients taking several drugs. In some patients, changing from one statin to another or lowering the dose relieves the problem. Muscle toxicity seems to be most common when some of the statins are used with drugs that inhibit cytochrome P3A4 (eg, macrolide antibiotics, azole antifungals, cyclosporine) and with fibrates, especially gemfibrozil. Statins are contraindicated during pregnancy and lactation.

Previous guidelines recommended using specific target LDL cholesterol levels to guide drug treatment. However, evidence suggests that using such targets does not improve ASCVD prevention but does increase risk of adverse effects. Instead, response to therapy is determined by whether LDL cholesterol levels decrease as expected based on therapy intensity (ie, patients receiving high-intensity therapy should have a ≥ 50% decrease in LDL cholesterol). If response is less than anticipated, the first intervention is to reinforce the importance of adherence to the drug regimen and lifestyle changes, and assess for drug side effects and secondary causes of hyperlipidemia (eg, hypothyroidism, nephrotic syndrome).

Table 168–4. STATINS FOR ATHEROSCLEROTIC CARDIOVASCULAR DISEASE PREVENTION

CLASSIFICATION	EFFECTS*	RECOMMENDED FOR	EXAMPLES†
High-intensity	Lowers LDL-C ≥ 50%	Clinical ASCVD, age ≤ 75 LDL-C ≥ 190 mg/dL Diabetes, age 40 to 75, and 10-yr ASCVD risk ≥ 7.5% Age 40 to 75, 10-yr ASCVD risk ≥ 7.5% Consider additional risk factors	Atorvastatin 40–80 mg Rosuvastatin 20–40 mg
Moderate-intensity	Lowers LDL-C 30 to < 50%	Clinical ASCVD, age > 75 Diabetes, age 40 to 75, and 10-yr ASCVD risk < 7.5% Age 40 to 75, 10-yr ASCVD risk ≥ 7.5%	Atorvastatin 10–20 mg Fluvastatin XL 80 mg Lovastatin 40 mg Pitavastatin 2–4 mg Pravastatin 40–80 mg Rosuvastatin 5–10 mg Simvastatin 20–40 mg
Low-intensity	Lowers LDL-C < 30%	Patients who cannot tolerate high or moderate intensity treatment	Fluvastatin 20–40 mg Lovastatin 20 mg Pitavastatin 1 mg Pravastatin 10–20 mg

*Individual response may vary.

†All doses oral and once/day.

If response remains less than expected after this, then the statin can be changed or dosage increased. If response continues to be less than expected after patients are on the maximum tolerated intensity of statin therapy, then a non-statin lipid-lowering drug(s) (see Table 168–5) can be added if the ASCVD risk reduction benefit appears to outweigh the potential for adverse effects, particularly for secondary prevention and in patients with genetic dyslipidemias such as familial hypercholesterolemia.

Bile acid sequestrants block intestinal bile acid reabsorption, forcing up-regulation of hepatic LDL receptors to recruit circulating cholesterol for bile synthesis. They are proved to reduce cardiovascular mortality. Bile acid sequestrants are usually used with statins or with nicotinic acid to augment LDL cholesterol reduction and are the drugs of choice for women who are or are planning to become pregnant. Bile acid sequestrants are safe, but their use is limited by adverse effects of bloating, nausea, cramping, and constipation. They may also increase TGs, so their use is contraindicated in patients with hypertriglyceridemia. Cholestyramine and colestipol, but not usually colesevelam, interfere with absorption of other drugs—notably thiazides, beta-blockers, warfarin, digoxin, and thyroxine—an effect that can be decreased by administration at least 4 h before or 1 h after other drugs. Bile acid sequestrants should be given with meals to increase their efficacy.

Cholesterol absorption inhibitors, such as ezetimibe, inhibit intestinal absorption of cholesterol and phytosterol. Ezetimibe usually lowers LDL cholesterol by 15 to 20% and causes small increases in HDL and a mild decrease in TGs. Ezetimibe can be used as monotherapy in patients intolerant to statins or added to statins for patients on maximum doses with persistent LDL cholesterol elevation. Adverse effects are infrequent.

PCSK9 monoclonal antibodies are available as subcutaneous injections given once or twice per month. These drugs keep PCSK9 from attaching to LDL receptors, leading to improved function of these receptors. LDL cholesterol is lowered by 40 to 70%. A cardiovascular outcomes trial with evolocumab showed a decrease in cardiovascular events in patients with prior atherosclerotic cardiovacular disease.

Dietary supplements that lower LDL cholesterol levels include fiber supplements and commercially available margarines and other products containing plant sterols (sitosterol and campesterol) or stanols. The latter reduce LDL cholesterol by up to 10% without affecting HDL or TGs by competitively displacing cholesterol from intestinal micelles.

Drugs for homozygous familial hypercholesterolemia include mipomersen and lomitapide. Mipomersen is an apo B antisense oligonucleotide that decreases synthesis of apo B in liver cells and decreases levels of LDL, apo B, and Lp(a). It is given by subcutaneous injection and can cause injection site reactions, flu-like symptoms, and increased hepatic fat and liver enzyme elevations. Lomitapide is an inhibitor of microsomal TG transfer protein inhibitor that interferes with the secretion of TG-rich lipoproteins in the liver and intestine. Dose is begun low and gradually titrated up about every 2 wk. Patients must follow a diet with less than 20% of calories from fat. Lomitapide can cause GI adverse effects (eg, diarrhea, increased hepatic fat, elevated liver enzymes).

Procedural approaches are reserved for patients with severe hyperlipidemia (LDL cholesterol > 300 mg/dL (> 7.74 mmol/L) in patients without vascular disease, and for LDL apheresis, LDL cholesterol > 200 mg/dL (> 5.16 mmol/L) in patients with vascular disease) that is refractory to conventional therapy, such as occurs with familial hypercholesterolemia. Options include LDL apheresis (in which LDL is removed by extracorporeal plasma exchange) and, rarely, ileal bypass (to block reabsorption of bile acids), liver transplantation (which transplants LDL receptors), and portocaval shunting (which decreases LDL production by unknown mechanisms). LDL apheresis is the procedure of choice in most instances when maximally tolerated therapy fails to lower LDL adequately. Apheresis is also the usual therapy in patients with the homozygous form of familial hypercholesterolemia who have limited or no response to drug therapy.

Future therapies to reduce LDL include peroxisome proliferator–activated receptor agonists that have thiazolidinedione-like and fibrate-like properties, LDL-receptor activators, LPL activators, and recombinant apo E. Cholesterol vaccination (to induce anti-LDL antibodies and hasten LDL clearance from serum) and gene transfer are conceptually appealing therapies that are under study but years away from being available for use.

Elevated LDL cholesterol in children: Childhood risk factors besides family history and diabetes include cigarette smoking, hypertension, low HDL cholesterol (< 35 mg/dL), obesity, and physical inactivity.

For children, the AAP recommends dietary treatment for children with LDL cholesterol > 110 mg/dL (> 2.8 mmol/L). Drug therapy is recommended for children > 8 yr and with either of the following:

- Poor response to dietary therapy, LDL cholesterol ≥ 190 mg/dL (≥ 4.9 mmol/L), and no family history of premature cardiovascular disease
- LDL cholesterol ≥ 160 mg/dL (> 4.13 mmol/L) and a family history of premature cardiovascular disease or ≥ 2 risk factors for premature cardiovascular disease

Drugs used in children include many of the statins. Children with familial hypercholesterolemia may require a second drug to achieve LDL cholesterol reduction of at least 50%.

Elevated TGs: Although it is unclear whether elevated TGs independently contribute to cardiovascular disease, they are associated with multiple metabolic abnormalities that contribute to CAD (eg, diabetes, metabolic syndrome). Consensus is emerging that lowering elevated TGs is beneficial. No target goals exist, but levels < 150 mg/dL (< 1.7 mmol/L) are generally considered desirable. No guidelines specifically address treatment of elevated TGs in children.

The **overall treatment strategy** is to first implement lifestyle changes, including exercise, weight loss, and avoidance of concentrated dietary sugar and alcohol. Intake of 2 to 4 servings/wk of marine fish high in omega-3 fatty acids may be effective, but the amount of omega-3 fatty acids is often lower than needed; supplements may be helpful. In patients with diabetes, glucose levels should be tightly controlled. If these measures are ineffective, lipid-lowering drugs should be considered. Patients with very high TGs may need to begin drug therapy at diagnosis to more quickly reduce the risk of acute pancreatitis.

Fibrates reduce TGs by about 50%. They appear to stimulate endothelial LPL, leading to increased fatty acid oxidation in the liver and muscle and decreased hepatic VLDL synthesis. They also increase HDL by up to 20%. Fibrates can cause GI adverse effects, including dyspepsia, abdominal pain, and elevated liver enzymes. They uncommonly cause cholelithiasis. Fibrates may potentiate muscle toxicity when used with statins and potentiate the effects of warfarin.

Statins can be used in patients with TGs < 500 mg/dL (< 5.65 mmol/L) if LDL cholesterol elevations are also present; statins may reduce both LDL cholesterol and TGs through reduction of VLDL. If only TGs are elevated, fibrates are the drug of choice.

Omega-3 fatty acids in high doses (1 to 6 g/day of eicosapentaenoic acid [EPA] and docosahexaenoic acid [DHA]) can be effective in reducing TGs. The omega-3 fatty acids EPA and DHA are the active ingredients in marine fish oil or omega-3 capsules. Adverse effects include eructation and diarrhea. These

Table 168–5. NON-STATIN LIPID-LOWERING DRUGS

DRUGS	ADULT DOSES	COMMENTS
Bile acid sequestrants		Lower LDL-C (primary), slightly increase HDL (secondary), may increase TGs
Cholestyramine	4–8 g po 1–3 times/day with meals	—
Colesevelam	2.4–4.4 g po once/day with a meal	—
Colestipol	5–30 g po once/day with a meal or divided with two or more meals	—
Cholesterol absorption inhibitor		Lowers LDL-C (primary), minimally increases HDL-C
Ezetimibe	10 mg po once/day	—
Drugs for homozygous familial hypercholesteremia		
Lomitapide	5–60 mg po once/day	Risk of hepatotoxicity Increase dose gradually (about every 2 wk) Measure transaminase levels before increasing dosage
Mipomersen	200 mg sc once/wk	Used as an adjunct to diet and other lipid-lowering drugs in patients with familial hypercholesteremia Can cause hepatotoxicity
Fibrates		Lower TGs and VLDL, increase HDL, may increase LDL-C (in patients with high TGs)
Bezafibrate	200 mg po tid or 400 mg po once/day	Decreased dose required in renal insufficiency Not available in US
Ciprofibrate	100–200 mg po once/day	Not available in US
Fenofibrate	34–201 mg po once/day	Decreased dose required in renal insufficiency May be safest fibrate for use with statins
Gemfibrozil	600 mg po bid	Decreased dose required in renal insufficiency
Nicotinic acid (niacin)	Immediate-release: 500 mg bid–1000 mg po tid Extended-release: 500–2000 mg po once/day at bedtime	Increases HDL; lowers TGs (low doses), LDL-C (higher doses), and Lp(a) (secondary) Frequent adverse effects: Flushing, impaired glucose tolerance, increased uric acid Aspirin and administration with food minimize flushing
PCSK9 monoclonal antibodies		
Alirocumab	75–150 mg sc q 2 wk	For patients with familial hypercholesterolemia and for other high-risk patients
Evolocumab	Primary or mixed dyslipidemia: 140 mg sc q 2 wk or 420 mg sc once/month* Familial hypercholesterolemia: 420 mg sc once/ month or 420 mg sc q 2 wk*	For patients with familial hypercholesterolemia and for other high-risk patients
Prescription omega-3 fatty acids		
Omega-3 acid ethyl esters	3–4 g po once/day (4 capsules)	Lower TGs only
Combination products		Combined effects of the 2 drugs
Ezetimibe + atorvastatin	Ezetimibe 10 mg + atorvastatin 10, 20, 40, 80 mg po once/day	Not recommended as initial therapy. Simvastatin 80 mg should not be used unless patients have already taken it for > 1 yr without adverse effects
Ezetimibe + simvastatin	Ezetimibe 10 mg + simvastatin 10, 20, 40, or 80 mg po once/day	
Niacin extended release + lovastatin	Niacin 500 mg + lovastatin 20 mg po once/day Niacin 2000 mg + lovastatin 40 mg po once/day	
Niacin extended release + simvastatin	Niacin 500 mg + simvastatin 20 mg po once/day at bedtime (starting dose) or niacin 750 or 1000 mg + simvastatin 20 mg po once/day at bedtime	

*Proposed dosages, pending FDA approval.

HDL = high-density lipoprotein; HDL-C = HDL cholesterol; LDL = low-density lipoprotein; LDL-C = LDL cholesterol; Lp(a) = lipoprotein (a); TG = triglyceride.

effects may be decreased by giving the fish oil capsules with meals in divided doses (eg, bid or tid). Omega-3 fatty acids can be a useful adjunct to other therapies. Prescription omega-3 fatty acid preparations are indicated for TG levels > 500 mg/dL (> 5.65 mmol/L).

Low HDL: Although higher HDL levels are associated with lower cardiovascular risk, it is not clear whether treatments to increase HDL cholesterol levels decrease risk of death. ATPIII guidelines define low HDL cholesterol as < 40 mg/dL [< 1.04 mmol/L]; the guidelines do not specify an HDL cholesterol target level and recommend interventions to raise HDL cholesterol only after LDL cholesterol targets have been reached. Treatments for LDL cholesterol and TG reduction often increase HDL cholesterol, and the 3 objectives can sometimes be achieved simultaneously. No guidelines specifically address treatment of low HDL cholesterol in children.

PEARLS & PITFALLS

- Although higher HDL levels are associated with lower cardiovascular risk, it is not clear whether treatments to increase HDL cholesterol levels decrease risk of death.

Treatment includes **lifestyle changes** such as an increase in exercise and weight loss. Alcohol raises HDL cholesterol but is not routinely recommended as a therapy because of its many other adverse effects. Drugs may be successful in raising levels when lifestyle changes alone are insufficient, but it is uncertain whether raising HDL levels reduces mortality.

Nicotinic acid (niacin) is the most effective drug for increasing HDL. Its mechanism of action is unknown, but it appears to both increase HDL production and inhibit HDL clearance; it may also mobilize cholesterol from macrophages. Niacin also decreases TGs and, in doses of 1500 to 2000 mg/day, reduces LDL cholesterol. Niacin causes flushing, pruritus, and nausea; premedication with low-dose aspirin may prevent these adverse effects. Extended-release preparations cause flushing less often. However, most OTC slow-release preparations are not recommended; an exception is polygel controlled-release niacin. Niacin can cause liver enzyme elevations and occasionally liver failure, insulin resistance, and hyperuricemia and gout. It may also increase homocysteine levels. The combination of high doses of niacin with statins may increase the risk of myopathy. In patients with average LDL cholesterol and below-average HDL cholesterol levels, niacin combined with statin treatment may be effective in preventing cardiovascular disorders. In patients treated with statins to lower LDL cholesterol to < 70 mg/dL (< 1.8 mmol/L), niacin does not appear to have added benefit.

Fibrates increase HDL. Fibrates may decrease cardiovascular risk in patients with TGs > 200 mg/dL (< 2.26 mmol/L) and HDL cholesterol < 40 mg/dL (< 1.04 mmol/L).

Cholesterol ester transport protein (CETP) inhibitors raise HDL levels by inhibiting CETP. Several have not shown a benefit, but anacetrapib may be beneficial.

Elevated Lp(a): The upper limit of normal for Lp(a) is about 30 mg/dL (0.8 mmol/L), but values in African Americans run higher. Few data exist to guide the treatment of elevated Lp(a) or to establish treatment efficacy. Niacin is the only drug that directly decreases Lp(a); it can lower Lp(a) by > 20% at higher doses. The usual approach in patients with elevated Lp(a) is to lower LDL cholesterol aggressively. LDL apheresis has been used to lower Lp(a) in patients with high Lp(a) levels and progressive vascular disease.

Secondary causes: Treatment of diabetic dyslipidemia should always involve lifestyle changes and statins to reduce LDL cholesterol. To decrease the risk of pancreatitis, fibrates can be used to decrease TGs when levels are > 500 mg/dL (> 5.65 mmol/L). Metformin lowers TGs, which may be a reason to choose it over other oral antihyperglycemic drugs when treating diabetes. Some thiazolidinediones (TZDs) increase both HDL cholesterol and LDL cholesterol. Some TZDs also decrease TGs. These antihyperglycemic drugs should not be chosen over lipid-lowering drugs to treat lipid abnormalities in diabetic patients but may be useful adjuncts. Patients with very high TG levels and less than optimally controlled diabetes may have better response to insulin than to oral antihyperglycemic drugs.

Treatment of dyslipidemia in patients with hypothyroidism, renal disease, liver disease, or a combination of these disorders involves treating the underlying disorders primarily and lipid abnormalities secondarily. Abnormal lipid levels in patients with low-normal thyroid function (high-normal TSH levels) improve with hormone replacement. Reducing the dosage of or stopping drugs that cause lipid abnormalities should be considered.

Monitoring treatment: Lipid levels should be monitored periodically after starting treatment. No data support specific monitoring intervals, but measuring lipid levels 2 to 3 mo after starting or changing therapies and once or twice yearly after lipid levels are stabilized is common practice.

Despite the low incidence of liver and severe muscle toxicity with statin use (0.5 to 2% of all users), current recommendations are for baseline measurements of liver and muscle enzyme levels at the beginning of treatment. Routine monitoring of liver enzyme levels is not necessary, and routine measurement of CK is not useful to predict the onset of rhabdomyolysis. Muscle enzyme levels need not be checked regularly unless patients develop myalgias or other muscle symptoms. If statin-induced muscle damage is suspected, statin use is stopped and CK may be measured. When muscle symptoms subside, a lower dose or a different statin can be tried. If symptoms do not subside within 1 to 2 wk of stopping the statin, another cause should be sought for the muscle symptoms (eg, polymyalgia rheumatica).

KEY POINTS

- Elevated lipid levels are a risk factor for atherosclerosis and thus can lead to symptomatic CAD and peripheral arterial disease.
- Causes of dyslipidemia include a sedentary lifestyle with excessive dietary intake of saturated fat, cholesterol, and trans fats and/or genetic (familial) abnormalities of lipid metabolism.
- Diagnose using serum lipid profile (measured TC, TG, and HDL cholesterol and calculated LDL cholesterol and VLDL).
- Screening tests should be done at age 9 to 11 years (age 2 if there is a strong family history of severe hyperlipidemia or premature CAD) and again at age 17 to 21 yr; adults are screened every 5 yr beginning at age 20.
- Treatment with a statin is indicated to reduce risk of ASCVD for all patients in 4 major risk groups as defined by the AHA and for those without who have certain other combinations of risk factors and elevated lipid levels.
- Optimize adherence, lifestyle changes, and statin usage before adding a non-statin drug (eg, bile acid sequestrants, ezetimibe, and/or niacin).
- Other treatment depends on the specific lipid abnormality but should always include lifestyle changes, treatment of hypertension and diabetes, smoking cessation, and in patients with increased risk of MI or death from CAD, daily low-dose aspirin.

ELEVATED HIGH-DENSITY LIPOPROTEIN LEVELS

Elevated high-density lipoprotein (HDL) level is HDL cholesterol > 80 mg/dL (> 2.1 mmol/L).

Elevated HDL cholesterol levels usually correlate with decreased cardiovascular risk; however, high HDL cholesterol levels caused by some genetic disorders may not protect against cardiovascular disease, probably because of accompanying lipid and metabolic abnormalities.

Primary causes of elevated HDL levels are single or multiple genetic mutations that result in overproduction or decreased clearance of HDL. **Secondary causes** of high HDL cholesterol include all of the following:

- Chronic alcoholism without cirrhosis
- Primary biliary cirrhosis
- Hyperthyroidism
- Drugs (eg, corticosteroids, insulin, phenytoin)

The unexpected finding of high HDL cholesterol in patients not taking lipid-lowering drugs should prompt a diagnostic evaluation for a secondary cause with measurements of AST, ALT, and TSH; a negative evaluation suggests a possible primary cause.

Cholesteryl ester transfer protein (CETP) deficiency is a rare autosomal recessive disorder caused by a *CETP* gene mutation. CETP facilitates transfer of cholesterol esters from HDL to other lipoproteins, and CETP deficiency affects LDL cholesterol and slows HDL clearance. Affected patients display no symptoms or signs but have HDL cholesterol > 150 mg/dL (> 3.9 mmol/L). Protection from cardiovascular disorders has not been proved. No treatment is necessary.

Familial hyperalphalipoproteinemia is an autosomal dominant condition caused by various unidentified and known genetic mutations, including those that cause apoprotein A-I overproduction and apoprotein C-III variants. The disorder is usually diagnosed incidentally when plasma HDL cholesterol levels are > 80 mg/dL. Affected patients have no other symptoms or signs. No treatment is necessary.

HYPOLIPIDEMIA

Hypolipidemia is a decrease in plasma lipoprotein caused by primary (genetic) or secondary factors. It is usually asymptomatic and diagnosed incidentally on routine lipid screening. Treatment of secondary hypolipidemia involves treating underlying disorders. Treatment of primary hypolipidemia is often unnecessary, but patients with some genetic disorders require high-dose vitamin E and dietary supplementation of fats and other fat-soluble vitamins.

Etiology

Hypolipidemia is defined as a TC < 120 mg/dL (< 3.1 mmol/L) or LDL cholesterol < 50 mg/dL (< 1.3 mmol/L). Secondary causes are far more common than primary causes and include all of the following:

- Hyperthyroidism
- Chronic infections (including hepatitis C infection) and other inflammatory states
- Hematologic and other cancers
- Undernutrition (including that accompanying chronic alcohol use)
- Malabsorption

The unexpected finding of low cholesterol or low LDL cholesterol in a patient not taking a lipid-lowering drug should prompt a diagnostic evaluation, including measurements of AST, ALT, and TSH; a negative evaluation suggests a possible primary cause.

There are 3 primary disorders in which single or multiple genetic mutations result in underproduction or increased clearance of LDL.

Abetalipoproteinemia (Bassen-Kornzweig syndrome): This autosomal recessive condition is caused by mutations in the gene for microsomal TG transfer protein, a protein critical to chylomicron and VLDL formation. Dietary fat cannot be absorbed, and lipoproteins in both metabolic pathways are virtually absent from serum; TC is typically < 45 mg/dL (< 1.16 mmol/L), TGs are < 20 mg/dL (< 0.23 mmol/L), and LDL is undetectable.

The condition is often first noticed in infants with fat malabsorption, steatorrhea, and failure to thrive. Intellectual disability may result. Because vitamin E is distributed to peripheral tissues via VLDL and LDL, most affected people eventually develop severe vitamin E deficiency. Symptoms and signs include visual changes from slow retinal degeneration, sensory neuropathy, posterior column signs, and cerebellar signs of dysmetria, ataxia, and spasticity, which can eventually lead to death. RBC acanthocytosis is a distinguishing feature on blood smear.

Diagnosis is made by the absence of apoprotein B (apo B) in plasma; intestinal biopsies show lack of microsomal transfer protein.

Treatment is with high doses (100 to 300 mg/kg once/day) of vitamin E with supplementation of dietary fat and other fat-soluble vitamins. The prognosis is poor.

Hypobetalipoproteinemia: Hypobetalipoproteinemia is an autosomal dominant or codominant condition caused by mutations in the gene coding for apo B. Heterozygous patients have truncated apo B, leading to rapid LDL clearance. Heterozygous patients manifest no symptoms or signs except for TC < 120 mg/dL (< 3.1 mmol/L) and LDL cholesterol < 80 mg/dL (< 2.1 mmol/L). TGs are normal. Homozygous patients have either shorter truncations, leading to lower lipid levels (TC < 80 mg/dL [< 2.1 mmol/L], LDL cholesterol < 20 mg/dL [< 0.52 mmol/L]), or absent apo B synthesis, leading to symptoms and signs of abetalipoproteinemia.

Diagnosis is by finding low levels of LDL cholesterol and apo B; hypobetalipoproteinemia and abetalipoproteinemia are distinguished from one another by family history. People who are heterozygous and people who are homozygous with low but detectable LDL cholesterol require no treatment. Treatment of people who are homozygous with no LDL is the same as for abetalipoproteinemia.

Loss of function mutations of *PCSK9* are another cause of low LDL levels. There are no adverse consequences and no treatment.

Chylomicron retention disease: Chylomicron retention disease is a very rare autosomal recessive condition caused by an unknown mutation leading to deficient apo B secretion from enterocytes. Chylomicron synthesis is absent, but VLDL synthesis remains intact. Affected infants have fat malabsorption, steatorrhea, and failure to thrive and may develop neurologic disorders similar to those in abetalipoproteinemia. Diagnosis is by intestinal biopsy of patients with low cholesterol levels and absence of postprandial chylomicrons. Treatment is supplementation of fat and fat-soluble vitamins.

169 Multiple Endocrine Neoplasia Syndromes

(Familial Endocrine Adenomatosis; Multiple Endocrine Adenomatosis)

The multiple endocrine neoplasias (MEN) syndromes comprise 3 genetically distinct familial diseases involving adenomatous hyperplasia and malignant tumors in several endocrine glands.

- MEN 1 involves primarily hyperplasia or sometimes adenomas of the parathyroid glands (with resultant hyperparathyroidism) and tumors of the pancreatic islet cells and/or pituitary gland.
- MEN 2A involves primarily medullary thyroid carcinoma (MTC), pheochromocytoma, hyperplasia or sometimes adenomas of the parathyroid glands (with resultant hyperparathyroidism), and occasionally cutaneous lichen amyloidosis.
- MEN 2B involves primarily MTC, pheochromocytoma, multiple mucosal and intestinal neuromas, and marfanoid habitus.

Clinical features depend on the glandular elements involved. Each syndrome is inherited as an autosomal dominant trait with a high degree of penetrance, variable expressivity, and production of seemingly unrelated effects by a single mutant gene. The specific mutation is not always known.

Symptoms and signs develop at any age. Proper management includes early identification of affected individuals within a kindred and surgical removal of the tumors when possible. Although these syndromes are genetically and clinically distinct, significant overlap exists (see Table 169–1).

MULTIPLE ENDOCRINE NEOPLASIA, TYPE 1

(Multiple Endocrine Adenomatosis, Type I; Wermer Syndrome)

Multiple endocrine neoplasia, type 1 (MEN 1) is a hereditary syndrome characterized by hyperplasia or sometimes adenomas of the parathyroid glands and tumors of the pancreatic islet cells and/or pituitary gland. Duodenal gastrinomas, carcinoid tumors of the foregut, benign adrenal adenomas, and lipomas also occur. Clinical features most commonly include hyperparathyroidism and asymptomatic hypercalcemia. Genetic screening is used to detect carriers. Diagnosis is by hormonal and imaging tests. Tumors are surgically removed when possible.

MEN 1 is caused by an inactivating mutation of the gene that encodes the nuclear protein menin; > 500 mutations of this gene have been identified. The exact function of menin is unknown, but it appears to have tumor suppressing effects.

About 40% of MEN 1 cases involve tumors of all 3 affected glands:

- Parathyroids
- Pancreas
- Pituitary

Almost any combination of the tumors and symptom complexes outlined below is possible. A patient with a MEN 1 gene mutation and one of the MEN 1 tumors is at risk of developing any of the other tumors later on. Age at onset ranges from 4 to 81 yr, but peak incidence occurs in the 20s to 40s. Men and women are equally affected.

Symptoms and Signs

The clinical features depend on the glandular elements affected (see Table 169–1).

Parathyroid: Hyperparathyroidism is present in ≥ 95% of patients. Asymptomatic hypercalcemia is the most common manifestation, but about 25% of patients have evidence of nephrolithiasis or nephrocalcinosis. In contrast to sporadic cases of hyperparathyroidism, diffuse hyperplasia, which is often asymmetric, is typical.

Pancreas: Pancreatic islet cell tumors occur in 30 to 90% of patients. Tumors are usually multicentric and sometimes synthesize several hormones. Multiple adenomas or diffuse islet cell hyperplasia commonly occurs; such tumors may arise from the small bowel rather than the pancreas. About 30% of tumors are malignant and have local or distant metastases. Malignant islet cell tumors due to MEN 1 syndrome often have a more benign course than do sporadically occurring malignant islet cell tumors.

The most common functional enteropancreatic tumor in MEN 1 is the gastrinoma, which can arise from the pancreas

Table 169–1. CONDITIONS ASSOCIATED WITH MEN SYNDROMES

CONDITION	MEN 1	MEN 2A	MEN 2B
Hyperparathyroidism	≥ 95%	10–20%	—
Enteropancreatic tumors	30–80%	—	—
Pituitary adenomas	15–42%	—	—
Medullary thyroid cancer	—	> 95%	> 95%
Pheochromocytomas	—	40–50%	50%
Mucosal neuromas	—	—	≈ 100%
Marfanoid habitus	—	—	≈ 100%

MEN = multiple endocrine neoplasia.

or the duodenum. Up to 80% of patients with MEN 1 have either multiple peptic ulcers due to gastrin-stimulated increased gastric acid secretion or asymptomatic elevated gastrin levels.

Insulinomas are the second most common functional pancreatic tumor and can cause fasting hypoglycemia. The tumors are often small and multiple. Age of onset is often < 40.

Nonfunctioning enteropancreatic tumors occur in about one third of MEN 1 patients. Most islet cell tumors, including nonfunctioning tumors, secrete pancreatic polypeptide. Although the clinical significance is unknown, pancreatic polypeptide may be helpful for screening. The size of the nonfunctioning tumor correlates with risk of metastasis and death.

Less commonly, other functional enteropancreatic tumors can occur in MEN 1. A severe secretory diarrhea can develop and cause fluid and electrolyte depletion with non-beta-cell tumors. This complex, referred to as the watery diarrhea, hypokalemia, and achlorhydria syndrome (WDHA, or pancreatic cholera), has been ascribed to vasoactive intestinal polypeptide, although other intestinal hormones or secretagogues (including prostaglandins) may contribute. Hypersecretion of glucagon, somatostatin, chromogranin, or calcitonin, ectopic secretion of ACTH or corticotropin-releasing hormone (causing Cushing syndrome), and hypersecretion of growth hormone–releasing hormone (causing acromegaly) sometimes occur in non-beta-cell tumors.

Pituitary: Pituitary tumors occur in 15 to 42% of MEN 1 patients. From 25 to 90% are prolactinomas. About 25% of pituitary tumors secrete growth hormone or growth hormone and prolactin. Excess prolactin may cause galactorrhea in affected women, and excess growth hormone causes acromegaly clinically indistinguishable from sporadically occurring acromegaly. About 3% of tumors secrete ACTH, causing Cushing disease. Most of the remainder are nonfunctional.

Local tumor expansion may cause visual disturbance, headache, and hypopituitarism.

Pituitary tumors in patients with MEN 1 may be larger and behave more aggressively and may occur at an earlier age than sporadic pituitary tumors; however, a recent long-term cohort study found MEN 1–associated pituitary tumors were more indolent, similar to sporadic pituitary tumors.[1]

Other manifestations: Carcinoid tumors, particularly those derived from the embryologic foregut (thymus, lungs, stomach), occur in 5 to 15% of MEN 1 patients. Thymic carcinoids are more common in affected males. Adrenal adenomas occur in 10 to 20% of patients and may be bilateral. Adenomatous hyperplasia of the thyroid occurs occasionally in MEN 1 patients. Hormone secretion is rarely altered as a result, and the significance of this abnormality is uncertain. Multiple subcutaneous and visceral lipomas, angiofibromas, meningiomas, ependymomas, and collagenomas may also occur.

1. de Laat JM, Dekkers OM, Pieterman CR, et al: Long-term natural course of pituitary tumors in patients with MEN1: results from the DutchMEN1 Study Group (DMSG). *J Clin Endocrinol Metab* 100(9):3288–3296, 2015.

Diagnosis

- Genetic testing
- Clinical evaluation for other tumors of the triad
- Serum calcium, parathyroid hormone (PTH), gastrin, and prolactin levels
- Tumor localization with MRI, CT, or ultrasonography

MEN 1 syndrome should be considered in patients with tumors of the parathyroids, pancreas, or pituitary, particularly those with a family history of endocrinopathy. Screening should also be considered in individuals diagnosed with hyperparathyroidism diagnosed prior to age 30.[1] At risk individuals should undergo genetic testing with direct DNA sequencing of the MEN 1 gene and clinical screening for other tumors of MEN 1, including the following:

- Asking about symptoms of peptic ulcer disease, diarrhea, nephrolithiasis, hypoglycemia, and hypopituitarism
- Examining for visual field defects, galactorrhea in women, and features of acromegaly and subcutaneous lipomas
- Measuring levels of serum calcium, intact PTH, gastrin, and prolactin

Additional laboratory or radiologic tests should be done if these screening tests suggest an endocrine abnormality related to MEN 1.

A gastrin-secreting non-beta-cell tumor of the pancreas or duodenum is diagnosed by elevated basal plasma gastrin levels, an exaggerated gastrin response to infused calcium, and a paradoxical rise in gastrin level after infusion of secretin. An insulin-secreting beta-cell tumor of the pancreas is diagnosed by detecting fasting hypoglycemia with an elevated plasma insulin level. An elevated basal level of pancreatic polypeptide or gastrin or an exaggerated response of these hormones to a standard meal may be the earliest sign of pancreatic involvement.

Ultrasonography or CT can help localize tumors. Because these tumors are often small and difficult to localize, other imaging tests (eg, helical [spiral] CT, angiography, endoscopic ultrasonography, intraoperative ultrasonography) may be necessary.

Acromegaly is diagnosed by elevated growth hormone levels that are not suppressed by glucose administration and by elevated levels of serum insulin-like growth factor 1 (somatomedin C).

Screening: When an index case is identified, 1st-degree relatives should be given the option of genetic screening. Although early presymptomatic screening of family members of patients with MEN 1 has not been shown to reduce morbidity or mortality, a recent large cohort study reported a clinically relevant lag time between diagnosis of the index case and diagnosis in the rest of the family.[2]

Some clinicians monitor gene carriers by doing pancreatic and pituitary imaging every 3 to 5 yr, although such screening has not been shown to improve outcomes.

1. Thakker RV, Newey PJ, Walls GV, et al: Clinical practice guidelines for multiple endocrine neoplasia type 1 (MEN1). *J Clin Endocrinol Metab* 97(9):2990–3011, 2012.
2. van Leeuwaarde RS, van Nesselrooij BP, Hermus AR, et al. Impact of delay in diagnosis in outcomes in MEN1: results from the Dutch MEN1 Study Group. *J Clin Endocrinol Metab* 101(3):1159–1165, 2016.

Treatment

- Surgical excision when possible
- Drug management of hormone excess

Treatment of **hyperparathyroidism** is primarily surgical, with subtotal parathyroidectomy; however, the hyperparathyroidism frequently recurs. Octreotide and cinacalcet may help control recurrent or persistent postoperative hypercalcemia.

Prolactinoma is usually managed with dopamine agonists; other pituitary tumors are treated surgically.

Islet cell tumors are more difficult to manage because the lesions are often small and difficult to find, multiple lesions are common, and surgery often is not curative.

The treatment of **gastrin-secreting non-beta-cell tumors** is complex. When possible, the tumor is located and removed, although it is unclear whether surgery decreases the likelihood of late metastatic disease. If localization is impossible, a proton pump inhibitor frequently provides long-term control of symptomatic peptic ulcer disease.

If a single tumor cannot be found in patients with insulinomas, distal subtotal pancreatectomy with enucleation of any palpable tumors in the head of the pancreas is recommended. Diazoxide or a somatostatin analogue (octreotide, lanreotide) may help treat hypoglycemia. Streptozocin and other cytotoxic drugs may relieve symptoms by reducing tumor burden.

Somatostatin analogs also can block hormone secretion from other non-gastrin-secreting pancreatic tumors and are well tolerated. Palliative treatments for metastatic pancreatic tumors include hepatic debulking surgery and hepatic artery chemoembolization. Streptozocin, doxorubicin, and other cytotoxic drugs may relieve symptoms by reducing tumor burden.

KEY POINTS

- Consider MEN 1 in patients with tumors of the parathyroids, pancreas, or pituitary.
- The main clinical manifestations are those of hormone excess, particularly hypercalcemia due to hyperparathyroidism.
- Patients should have genetic testing of the MEN 1 gene and clinical evaluation for other tumors of the syndrome.
- Tumors are excised when possible, but lesions are often multiple and/or difficult to find.
- Sometimes hormone excess can be managed by drugs.

MULTIPLE ENDOCRINE NEOPLASIA, TYPE 2A

(MEN 2; Multiple Endocrine Adenomatosis, Type 2; Sipple Syndrome)

Multiple endocrine neoplasia, type 2A (MEN 2A) is a hereditary syndrome characterized by medullary carcinoma of the thyroid (MTC), pheochromocytoma, parathyroid hyperplasia or adenomas (causing hyperparathyroidism), and occasionally cutaneous lichen amyloidosis. Clinical features depend on the glandular elements affected. Familial MTC is a distinct variant of MEN 2A. Diagnosis involves genetic testing. Hormonal and imaging tests help locate the tumors, which are removed surgically when possible.

Mutations in the *RET* proto-oncogene on chromosome 10 have been identified in MEN 2A, MEN 2B, and familial MTC. The RET protein is a receptor tyrosine kinase; MEN 2A and familial MTC mutations result in activation of certain intracellular pathways.

Symptoms and Signs

Clinical features depend on the type of tumor present (see Table 169–1).

Thyroid: Almost all patients have MTC. The tumor usually develops during childhood and begins with thyroid parafollicular C-cell hyperplasia. Tumors are frequently multicentric.

Adrenal: Pheochromocytoma usually originates in the adrenal glands. Pheochromocytoma occurs in 40 to 50% of patients within a MEN 2A kindred, and in some kindreds pheochromocytoma accounts for 30% of deaths. In contrast to sporadic pheochromocytoma, the familial variety within MEN 2A begins with adrenal medullary hyperplasia and is multicentric and bilateral in > 50% of cases. Extra-adrenal pheochromocytomas are rare. Pheochromocytomas are almost always benign, but some tend to recur locally.

Pheochromocytomas that occur with MEN 2A (and MEN 2B) usually produce epinephrine disproportionately to norepinephrine, in contrast to sporadic cases.

Hypertensive crisis secondary to pheochromocytoma is a common manifestation. Hypertension in MEN 2A patients with pheochromocytoma is more often paroxysmal than sustained, in contrast to the usual sporadic case. Patients with pheochromocytomas may have paroxysmal palpitations, anxiety, headaches, or sweating; many are asymptomatic.

Parathyroid: Ten to 20% of patients have evidence of hyperparathyroidism (which may be long-standing), with hypercalcemia, nephrolithiasis, nephrocalcinosis, or renal failure. Hyperparathyroidism frequently involves multiple glands as either diffuse hyperplasia or multiple adenomas, and mild abnormalities in parathyroid function may also be present in MEN 2A.

Other manifestations: Cutaneous lichen amyloidosis, a pruritic, scaly, papular skin lesion, located in the interscapular region or on extensor surfaces, occurs in some MEN 2A kindreds. Hirschsprung disease is present in 2 to 5% of MEN 2A patients.

Diagnosis

- Clinical suspicion
- Genetic testing
- Serum calcium and PTH, plasma free metanephrines, and urinary catecholamine levels
- Pheochromocytoma localization with MRI or CT

Many cases are identified during screening of family members of known cases. MEN 2A should also be suspected in patients with bilateral pheochromocytoma or at least 2 of its characteristic endocrine manifestations. The diagnosis can be confirmed with genetic testing. Although only 25% of MTC cases are familial, genetic testing of people with apparent sporadic MTC should be considered if patients are < 35 yr, tumors are bilateral or multicentric, or a family history is suspected; some experts recommend genetic testing for *RET* germline mutations in all patients with newly diagnosed MTC.[1]

Because pheochromocytoma may be asymptomatic, its exclusion may be difficult. The most sensitive tests are measurement of plasma free metanephrines and fractionated urinary catecholamines (particularly epinephrine).

CT or MRI is useful in localizing the pheochromocytoma or establishing the presence of bilateral lesions.

Hyperparathyroidism is diagnosed by finding hypercalcemia, hypophosphatemia, and increased PTH level.

Screening: Genetic screening of family members of MEN 2A patients is now the diagnostic test of choice; the availability of such testing has made biochemical screening for early MTC largely obsolete. The specific *RET* mutation also predicts phenotypic characteristics such as age of onset, aggressiveness of MCT, and presence of other endocrinopathies, so is important in clinical management. Preimplantation genetic diagnosis and prenatal chorionic villus sampling or amniocentesis have been used for antenatal diagnosis.

Among affected family members, annual screening for hyperparathyroidism and pheochromocytoma should begin in early childhood and continue indefinitely. Screening for hyperparathyroidism entails measurement of serum calcium levels.

Screening for pheochromocytoma includes questions about symptoms, measurement of pulse rate and BP, and laboratory testing.

1. Kloos RT, Eng C, Evans D, et al: Medullary thyroid cancer: management guidelines of the American Thyroid Association. *Thyroid* 19:565–612, 2009.

Treatment

- Surgical excision of identified tumors
- Prophylactic thyroidectomy

In patients presenting with pheochromocytoma and either MTC or hyperparathyroidism, the pheochromocytoma should be removed first, even if asymptomatic because it greatly increases risk during other surgeries. Laparoscopic adrenalectomy, which has lower morbidity, is preferred to open laparotomy. Because bilateral pheochromocytomas are common, adrenal-sparing surgery may be appropriate in some patients.[1]

Surgery for MTC should include total thyroidectomy and central compartment lymph node dissection, with additional lymph node dissection if indicated based on preoperative imaging. Postsurgical assessment for residual or recurrent disease should include measurement of serum calcitonin and imaging with neck ultrasonography and, when indicated, CT or MRI of neck and chest, bone scan, or PET scan.

Once MTC has metastasized, tyrosine kinase inhibitors, including newly available cabozantinib and vandetanib, can lengthen progression-free survival. Clinical trials of other tyrosine kinase inhibitors for metastatic MTC are ongoing. Cytotoxic chemotherapy and radiation therapy are largely ineffective in lengthening survival but may slow disease progression. Postoperative adjuvant external beam radiation should be considered in patients at high risk of local recurrence and those at risk for airway obstruction. Some studies have shown lengthened survival with immunotherapy (eg, tumor-derived vaccines or tumor cell transfectants) and radioimmunotherapy (eg, radioisotope-coupled monoclonal antibodies).

Once genetic testing identifies a child as having a *RET* mutation, prophylactic thyroidectomy is recommended. Depending on the particular mutation, prophylactic thyroidectomy as early as the first months of life may be indicated. MTC can be cured or prevented by early thyroidectomy.

1. Castinetti F, Qi XP, Walz AL, et al: Outcomes of adrenal-sparing surgery or total adrenalectomy in phaeochromoctyoma associated with multiple endocrine neoplasia type 2: an international retrospective population-based study. *Lancet Oncol* 15(6):648–655, 2014.

KEY POINTS

- Most patients have MTC, typically beginning in childhood.
- Other manifestations are those of hormone excess, particularly hypertension due to pheochromocytoma and hypercalcemia due to hyperparathyroidism.
- Patients should have genetic testing for *RET* proto-oncogene mutations and clinical evaluation for other tumors of the syndrome.
- Tumors are excised when possible, beginning with any pheochromocytoma.
- Prophylactic thyroidectomy is recommended.

MULTIPLE ENDOCRINE NEOPLASIA, TYPE 2B

(Mucosal Neuroma Syndrome; Multiple Endocrine Adenomatosis, Type 2B)

Multiple endocrine neoplasia, type 2B (MEN 2B) is an autosomal dominant syndrome characterized by medullary thyroid cancer (MTC), pheochromocytoma, multiple mucosal neuromas and intestinal ganglioneuromas, and often a marfanoid habitus and other skeletal abnormalities. Symptoms depend on the glandular elements present. Diagnosis and treatment are the same as for MEN 2A.

Ninety-five percent of MEN 2B cases result from a single amino acid substitution in the RET protein. As in MEN 2A and familial MTC, this mutation results in activation of *RET* proto-oncogene-mediated cellular processes. More than 50% are de novo mutations and thus may be sporadic rather than familial.

Symptoms and Signs

Symptoms and signs reflect the glandular abnormalities present (see Table 169–1). About 50% of patients have the complete syndrome with mucosal neuromas, pheochromocytomas, and MTC. Fewer than 10% have neuromas and pheochromocytomas alone, whereas the remaining patients have neuromas and MTC without pheochromocytoma.

Often, mucosal neuromas are the earliest sign, and they occur in most or all patients. Neuromas appear as small glistening bumps on the lips, tongue, and buccal mucosae.

The eyelids, conjunctivae, and corneas also commonly develop neuromas; infants are often unable to make tears. Thickened eyelids and everted, diffusely hypertrophied lips are characteristic.

GI abnormalities related to altered motility (constipation, diarrhea, and, occasionally, megacolon) are common and thought to result from diffuse intestinal ganglioneuromatosis.

Patients almost always have a marfanoid habitus. Skeletal abnormalities are common, including deformities of the spine (lordosis, kyphosis, scoliosis), slipped capital femoral epiphyses, dolichocephaly (hull-shaped skull, also called scaphocephaly), pes cavus, and talipes equinovarus.

MTC and pheochromocytoma resemble the corresponding disorders in MEN 2A syndrome; both tend to be bilateral and multicentric. MTC, however, tends to be particularly aggressive in MEN 2B and may be present in very young children.

Although the neuromas, facial characteristics, and GI disorders are present at an early age, the syndrome may not be recognized until MTC or pheochromocytoma manifests in later life.

Diagnosis

- Clinical suspicion
- Genetic testing
- Plasma free metanephrines and urinary catecholamine levels
- Pheochromocytoma localization with MRI or CT

MEN 2B is suspected in patients with a family history of MEN 2B, pheochromocytoma, multiple mucosal neuromas, or MTC. Genetic testing is highly accurate and is done to confirm the disorder. Genetic testing also is done to screen 1st-degree relatives and any symptomatic family members of patients with MEN 2B as in MEN 2A.

Pheochromocytoma may be suspected clinically and is confirmed by measuring plasma free metanephrines and urinary catecholamines. Laboratory testing for MTC may be done. MRI or CT is used to search for pheochromocytomas and MTC.

Treatment

- Surgical excision of identified tumors
- Prophylactic thyroidectomy

Affected patients should have total thyroidectomy as soon as the diagnosis is established. Pheochromocytoma, if present, should be removed before thyroidectomy is done.

Gene carriers should undergo prophylactic thyroidectomy before age 1 yr.

KEY POINTS

- MEN 2B has a mutation of the same gene as in MEN 2A and manifests similarly except for the absence of hyperparathyroidism, the presence of more aggressive MTC, and the presence of multiple mucosal neuromas and a marfanoid habitus.
- Patients should have genetic testing for *RET* proto-oncogene mutations and blood or urine tests for pheochromocytoma.
- Pheochromocytoma is excised and prophylactic thyroidectomy is done.

170 Pituitary Disorders

The pituitary gland controls the functions of peripheral endocrine glands (see Fig. 170–1). Pituitary structure and function and relationships between the hypothalamus and the pituitary gland are discussed in Ch. 160.

Specific pituitary disorders include

- Pituitary lesions
- Generalized hypopituitarism
- Selective disorders of pituitary hormone deficiencies (including central diabetes insipidus)
- Pituitary hormone excesses, including gigantism, acromegaly, galactorrhea, syndrome of inappropriate ADH secretion, and Cushing disease

CENTRAL DIABETES INSIPIDUS

(Vasopressin-Sensitive Diabetes Insipidus)

Diabetes insipidus (DI) results from a deficiency of vasopressin (ADH) due to a hypothalamic-pituitary disorder (central DI [CDI]) or from resistance of the kidneys to vasopressin (nephrogenic DI [NDI]). Polyuria and polydipsia develop. Diagnosis is by water deprivation test showing failure to maximally concentrate urine; vasopressin levels and response to exogenous vasopressin help distinguish CDI from NDI. Treatment is with intranasal desmopressin or lypressin. Nonhormonal treatment includes use of diuretics (mainly thiazides) and vasopressin-releasing drugs, such as chlorpropamide.

(See also Sidebar 166–1 on p. 1274 and Nephrogenic Diabetes Insipidus on p. 2152.)

Pathophysiology

The posterior lobe of the pituitary is the primary site of vasopressin storage and release, but vasopressin is synthesized within the hypothalamus. Newly synthesized hormone can still be released into the circulation as long as the hypothalamic nuclei and part of the neurohypophyseal tract are intact. Only about 10% of neurosecretory neurons must remain intact to avoid CDI. The pathology of CDI thus always involves the supraoptic and paraventricular nuclei of the hypothalamus or a major portion of the pituitary stalk.

CDI may be complete (absence of vasopressin) or partial (insufficient amounts of vasopressin). CDI may be primary, in which there is a marked decrease in the hypothalamic nuclei of the neurohypophyseal system.

Etiology

Primary CDI: Genetic abnormalities of the vasopressin gene on chromosome 20 are responsible for autosomal dominant forms of primary CDI, but many cases are idiopathic.

Secondary CDI: CDI may also be secondary (acquired), caused by various lesions, including hypophysectomy, cranial injuries (particularly basal skull fractures), suprasellar and intrasellar tumors (primary or metastatic), Langerhans cell histiocytosis (Hand-Schüller-Christian disease), lymphocytic hypophysitis, granulomas (sarcoidosis or TB), vascular lesions (aneurysm, thrombosis), and infections (encephalitis, meningitis).

Symptoms and Signs

Onset may be insidious or abrupt, occurring at any age. The only symptoms in primary CDI are polydipsia and polyuria. In secondary CDI, symptoms and signs of the associated lesions are also present. Enormous quantities of fluid may be ingested, and large volumes (3 to 30 L/day) of very dilute urine (specific gravity usually < 1.005 and osmolality < 200 mOsm/L) are excreted. Nocturia almost always occurs. Dehydration and hypovolemia may develop rapidly if urinary losses are not continuously replaced.

Polyuria may result from

- Diabetes mellitus (most common)
- CDI (a deficiency of vasopressin)
- NDI (renal resistance to vasopressin)
- Compulsive or habitual water drinking (psychogenic polydipsia)

Diagnosis

- Water deprivation test
- Sometimes vasopressin levels

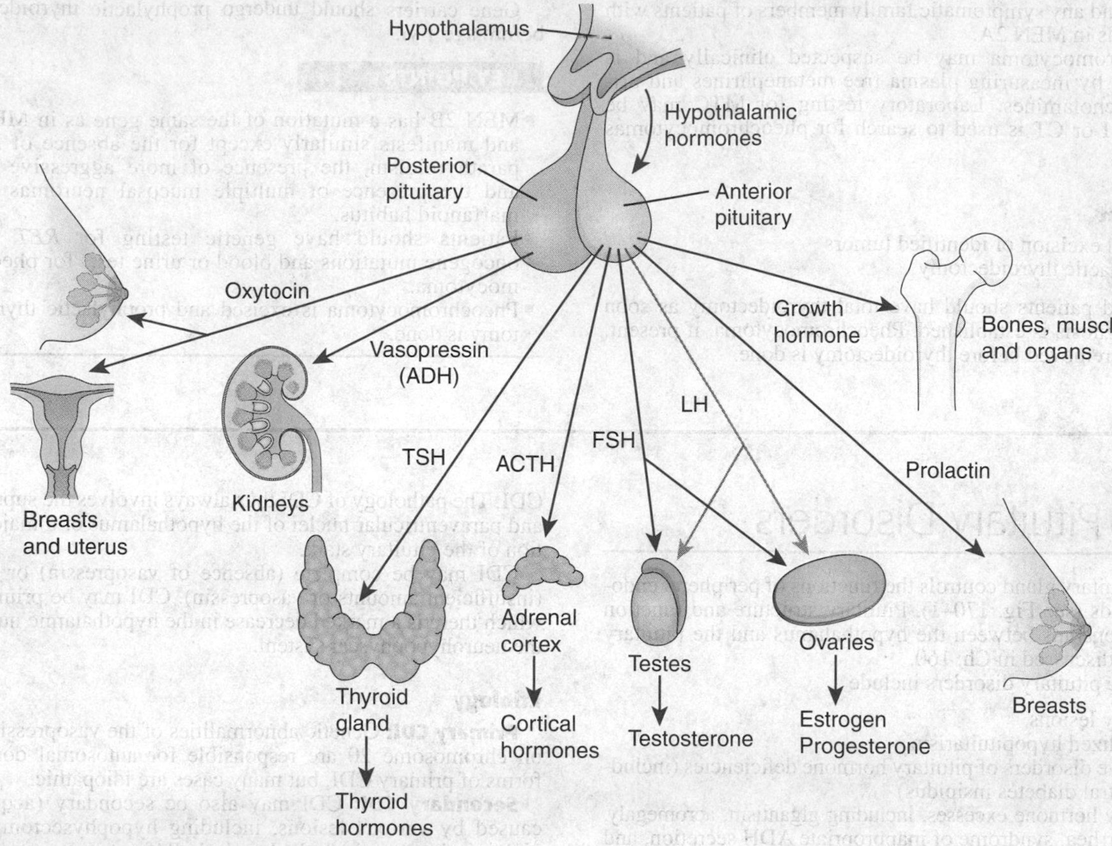

Fig. 170–1. The pituitary and its target organs.

CDI must be differentiated from other causes of polyuria, particularly psychogenic polydipsia (see Table 170–1) and NDI. All tests for CDI (and for NDI) are based on the principle that increasing the plasma osmolality in normal people will lead to decreased excretion of urine with increased urine osmolality.

The **water deprivation test** is the simplest and most reliable method for diagnosing CDI but *should be done only while the patient is under constant supervision. Serious dehydration may result.* Additionally, if psychogenic polydipsia is suspected, the patient must be observed to prevent surreptitious drinking. The test is started in the morning by weighing the patient, obtaining venous blood to determine electrolyte concentrations and osmolality, and measuring urinary osmolality. Voided urine is collected hourly, and its specific gravity or, preferably, osmolality is measured. Dehydration is continued until orthostatic hypotension and postural tachycardia appear, ≥ 5% of the initial body weight has been lost, or the urinary concentration does not increase > 0.001 specific gravity or > 30 mOsm/L in sequentially voided specimens. Serum electrolytes and osmolality are again determined. Exogenous vasopressin is then given (5 units of aqueous vasopressin sc, 10 mcg desmopressin [DDAVP] intranasally, or 4 mcg IM or IV). Urine for specific gravity or osmolality measurement is collected one final time 60 min post-injection, and the test is terminated.

A normal response produces maximum urine osmolality after dehydration (often > 1.020 specific gravity or > 700 mOsm/L), exceeding the plasma osmolality; osmolality does not increase more than an additional 5% after injection of vasopressin. Patients with CDI are generally unable to concentrate urine to greater than the plasma osmolality but are able to increase their urine osmolality by > 50 to > 100% after exogenous vasopressin administration. Patients with partial CDI are often able to concentrate urine to above the plasma osmolality but show a rise in urine osmolality of 15 to 50% after vasopressin administration. Patients with NDI are unable to concentrate urine to greater than the plasma osmolality and show no additional response to vasopressin administration (see Table 170–2).

Measurement of circulating vasopressin is the most direct method of diagnosing CDI; levels at the end of the water deprivation test (before the vasopressin injection) are low in CDI and appropriately elevated in NDI. However, vasopressin levels are difficult to measure, and the test is not routinely available. In addition, water deprivation is so accurate that direct measurement of vasopressin is unnecessary. Plasma vasopressin levels are diagnostic after either dehydration or infusion of hypertonic saline.

Psychogenic polydipsia: Psychogenic polydipsia may present a difficult problem in differential diagnosis. Patients may

Table 170–1. COMMON CAUSES OF POLYURIA

MECHANISM	EXAMPLE
Vasopressin-sensitive polyuria	
Decreased synthesis of vasopressin	Primary diabetes insipidus, hereditary (usually autosomal dominant) Primary diabetes insipidus, hereditary associated with diabetes mellitus, optic nerve atrophy, nerve deafness, and atonia of bladder and ureters Acquired (secondary) diabetes insipidus (causes outlined in text)
Decreased release of vasopressin	Psychogenic polydipsia (dipsogenic diabetes insipidus)
Vasopressin-resistant polyuria	
Renal resistance to vasopressin	Congenital nephrogenic diabetes insipidus (usually X-linked recessive trait) Acquired nephrogenic diabetes insipidus: Chronic kidney disease, systemic or metabolic disease (eg, myeloma, amyloidosis, hypercalcemic or hypokalemic nephropathy, sickle cell disease), certain drugs (eg, lithium, demeclocycline)
Osmotic diuresis	Hyperglycemia (in diabetes mellitus) Poorly resorbed solutes (mannitol, sorbitol, urea)

ingest and excrete up to 6 L of fluid/day and are often emotionally disturbed. Unlike patients with CDI and NDI, they usually do not have nocturia, nor does their thirst wake them at night. Continued ingestion of large volumes of water in this situation can lead to life-threatening hyponatremia.

Patients with acute psychogenic water drinking are able to concentrate their urine during water deprivation. However, because chronic water intake diminishes medullary tonicity in the kidney, patients with long-standing polydipsia are not able to concentrate their urine to maximal levels during water deprivation, a response similar to that of patients with partial CDI. However, unlike CDI, patients with psychogenic polydipsia show no response to exogenous vasopressin after water deprivation. This response resembles NDI, except that basal vasopressin levels are low compared with the elevated levels present in NDI. After prolonged restriction of fluid intake to ≤ 2 L/day, normal concentrating ability returns within several weeks.

Treatment

- Hormonal drugs, eg, desmopressin
- Nonhormonal drugs, eg, diuretics

CDI can be treated with hormone replacement and treatment of any correctable cause. In the absence of appropriate management, permanent renal damage can result.

Restricting salt intake may also help because it reduces urine output by reducing solute load.

Hormonal drugs: Desmopressin, a synthetic analog of vasopressin with minimal vasoconstrictive properties, has prolonged antidiuretic activity lasting for 12 to 24 h in most patients and may be administered intranasally, sc, IV, or orally. Desmopressin is the preparation of choice for both adults and children and is available as an intranasal solution in 2 forms. A dropper bottle with a calibrated nasal catheter has the advantage of delivering incremental doses from 5 to 20 mcg but is awkward to use. A spray bottle that delivers 10 mcg of desmopressin in 0.1 mL of fluid is easier to use but delivers a fixed quantity. For each patient, the duration of action of a given dose must be established, because variation among individuals is great. The duration of action can be established by following timed urine volumes and osmolality. The nightly dose is the lowest dose required to prevent nocturia. The morning and evening doses should be adjusted separately. The usual dosage range in adults is 10 to 40 mcg, with most adults requiring 10 mcg bid. For children age 3 mo to 12 yr, the usual dosage range is 2.5 to 10 mcg bid.

Overdosage can lead to fluid retention and decreased plasma osmolality, possibly resulting in seizures in small children. In such instances, furosemide can be given to induce diuresis. Headache may be a troublesome adverse effect but generally disappears if the dosage is reduced. Infrequently, desmopressin causes a slight increase in BP. Absorption from the nasal mucosa may be erratic, especially when URI or allergic rhinitis occurs. When intranasal delivery of desmopressin is inappropriate, it may be administered sc using about one-tenth of the intranasal dose. Desmopressin may be used IV if a rapid effect is necessary (eg, for hypovolemia). With oral desmopressin, dose equivalence with the intranasal formulation is unpredictable, so individual dose titration is needed. The initial dose is 0.1 mg po tid, and the maintenance dose is usually 0.1 to 0.2 mg tid.

Table 170–2. WATER DEPRIVATION TEST RESULTS

PARAMETER	NORMAL	COMPLETE CDI	PARTIAL CDI	COMPLETE NDI	PARTIAL NDI	PSYCHOGENIC POLYDIPSIA
U_{osm} after dehydration (step 1)	Very high (> 700–800 mOsm/kg)	Very low (less than plasma osmolality)	Low (≥ 300 mOsm/kg)	Very low (less than plasma osmolality)	Very low (less than plasma osmolality)	High (500–600 mOsm/kg)
U_{osm} increase after vasopressin (step 2)	Minimal (< 5%)	50 to > 100%	15–50%	< 50 mOsm/kg	Up to 45%	No change

U_{osm} = urine osmolality.

PEARLS & PITFALLS

- The duration of action of a given dose of desmopressin varies greatly among individuals and must be established for each patient.

Lypressin (lysine-8-vasopressin), a synthetic agent, is given by nasal spray at doses of 2 to 4 units (7.5 to 15 mcg) q 3 to 8 h but, because of its short duration of action, has been largely replaced by desmopressin.

Aqueous vasopressin 5 to 10 units sc or IM can be given to provide an antidiuretic response that usually lasts ≤ 6 h. Thus, this drug has little use in long-term treatment but can be used in the initial therapy of unconscious patients and in patients with CDI who are undergoing surgery. Synthetic vasopressin can also be administered bid to qid as a nasal spray, with the dosage and interval tailored to each patient. Vasopressin tannate in oil 0.3 to 1 mL (1.5 to 5 units) IM may control symptoms for up to 96 h.

Nonhormonal drugs: At least 3 groups of nonhormonal drugs are useful in reducing polyuria:

- Diuretics, primarily thiazides
- Vasopressin-releasing drugs (eg, chlorpropamide, carbamazepine, clofibrate)
- Prostaglandin inhibitors

These drugs have been particularly useful in partial CDI and do not cause the adverse effects of exogenous vasopressin.

Thiazide diuretics paradoxically reduce urine volume in partial and complete CDI (and NDI), primarily as a consequence of reducing ECF volume and increasing proximal tubular resorption. Urine volumes may fall by 25 to 50% with 15 to 25 mg/kg of chlorothiazide.

Chlorpropamide, carbamazepine, and clofibrate can reduce or eliminate the need for vasopressin in some patients with partial CDI. None are effective in NDI. Chlorpropamide 3 to 5 mg/kg po once/day or bid causes some release of vasopressin and also potentiates the action of vasopressin on the kidney. Clofibrate 500 to 1000 mg po bid or carbamazepine 100 to 400 mg po bid is recommended for adults only. These drugs may be used synergistically with a diuretic. However, significant hypoglycemia may result from chlorpropamide.

Prostaglandin inhibitors (eg, indomethacin 0.5 to 1.0 mg/kg po tid, although most NSAIDs are effective) are modestly effective. They may reduce urine volume, but generally by no more than 10 to 25%, perhaps by decreasing renal blood flow and GFR. Together with indomethacin, restriction of sodium intake and a thiazide diuretic help further reduce urine volume in NDI.

KEY POINTS

- Central diabetes insipidus (CDI) is caused by a deficiency of vasopressin, which decreases the kidneys' ability to reabsorb water, resulting in massive polyuria (3 to 30 L/day).
- The cause may be a primary genetic disorder or various tumors, infiltrative lesions, injuries, or infections that affect the hypothalamic-pituitary system.
- Diagnosis using a water deprivation test; patients cannot maximally concentrate urine following dehydration but can concentrate urine after receiving exogenous vasopressin.
- Low vasopressin levels are diagnostic, but vasopressin levels are difficult to measure and the test is not routinely available.
- Address any treatable causes and give desmopressin, a synthetic analog of vasopressin.

GALACTORRHEA

Galactorrhea is lactation in men or in women who are not breastfeeding. It is generally due to a prolactin-secreting pituitary adenoma. Diagnosis is by measurement of prolactin levels and imaging tests. Treatment involves tumor inhibition with dopamine agonist drugs and sometimes removal or destruction of the adenoma.

Galactorrhea involves secretion of breast milk. A discussion of nipple discharge in general is provided elsewhere.

Etiology

Galactorrhea is generally due to a prolactin-secreting pituitary adenoma (prolactinoma). Most tumors in women are microadenomas (< 10 mm in diameter), but a small percentage are macroadenomas (> 10 mm) when diagnosed. The frequency of microadenomas is much lower in men, perhaps because of later recognition. Nonfunctioning pituitary mass lesions also can increase prolactin levels by compressing the pituitary stalk and thus reducing the action of dopamine, a prolactin inhibitor.

Hyperprolactinemia and galactorrhea also may be caused by ingestion of certain drugs, including phenothiazines, other antipsychotics, certain antihypertensives (especially alpha-methyldopa), and opioids. Primary hypothyroidism can cause hyperprolactinemia and galactorrhea, because increased levels of thyroid-releasing hormone increase secretion of prolactin as well as thyroid-stimulating hormone (TSH). It is unclear why hyperprolactinemia is associated with hypogonadotropism and hypogonadism (see Table 170–3).

Symptoms and Signs

Abnormal lactation is not defined quantitatively; it is milk release that is inappropriate, persistent, or worrisome to the patient. Spontaneous lactation is more unusual than milk released in response to manual expression. The milk is white. Women with galactorrhea commonly also have amenorrhea or oligomenorrhea. Women with galactorrhea and amenorrhea may also have symptoms and signs of estrogen deficiency, including dyspareunia, due to inhibition of pulsatile luteinizing hormone and follicle-stimulating hormone release by high prolactin levels. However, estrogen production may be normal, and signs of androgen excess have been observed in some women with hyperprolactinemia. Hyperprolactinemia may occur with other menstrual cycle disturbances besides amenorrhea, including infrequent ovulation and corpus luteum dysfunction.

Men with prolactin-secreting pituitary tumors typically have headaches or visual difficulties. About two-thirds of affected men have loss of libido and erectile dysfunction.

Diagnosis

- Prolactin levels
- Thyroxine (T_4) and TSH levels
- CT or MRI

Diagnosis of galactorrhea due to a prolactin-secreting pituitary adenoma is based on elevated prolactin levels (typically > 5 times normal, sometimes much higher) and decrease in lesion size in response to drug treatment. In general, prolactin levels correlate with the size of a pituitary tumor and can be used to follow patients over time. With a nonfunctioning pituitary mass, prolactin levels are not usually elevated > 3 to 4 times normal.

Table 170–3. CAUSES OF HYPERPROLACTINEMIA

CAUSE	EXAMPLE
Physiologic	Nipple stimulation in women Pregnancy Postpartum period Stress Food ingestion Sexual intercourse in some women Sleep Hypoglycemia Early infancy (up to 3 mo)
Hypothalamic disorders	Hypothalamic tumors Nontumerous hypothalamic infiltration: Sarcoidosis, TB, Langerhans cell histiocytosis (Hand-Schüller-Christian disease) Postencephalitis Idiopathic galactorrhea (presumed abnormality in dopamine secretion) Head trauma
Pituitary disorders	Prolactin-secreting pituitary tumors Tumors causing pituitary stalk compression Surgical pituitary stalk section and other stalk lesions Empty sella syndrome
Other endocrine disorders	Acromegaly Cushing disease Primary hypothyroidism
Disorders of other systems	Chronic renal failure Liver disease Ectopic production of prolactin: Bronchogenic carcinoma (not squamous cell; mostly small cell undifferentiated) Hypernephroma
Chest wall lesions	Surgical scars Trauma Tumors Herpes zoster
Pharmacologic	Antihypertensive drugs: Resperine, alpha-methyldopa, labetalol, atenolol, verapamil, clonidine H_2-antagonists (eg, ranitidine) Oral contraceptives and estrogens Opioids Psychoactive drugs, eg, phenothiazines, tricyclic and some other antidepressants, butyrphenones (haloperidol), benzamides (metoclopramide, sulpiride) Thyrotropin-releasing hormone

Data from Rebar RW: Practical evaluation of hormonal status. In *Reproductive Endocrinology: Physiology, Pathophysiology and Clinical Management*, edited by SSC Yen and RB Jaffe. Philadelphia, WB Saunders Company, 1978, p. 493.

A trial of dopamine agonist therapy can help distinguish between prolactin-secreting and nonfunctioning lesions; in both types of lesion, prolactin levels decrease after treatment, but prolactin-secreting lesions decrease in size, whereas nonfunctioning lesions do not.

Serum gonadotropin and estradiol levels are either low or in the normal range in women with hyperprolactinemia. Primary hypothyroidism is easily ruled out by absence of elevated TSH.

High-resolution CT or MRI is the method of choice in identifying microadenomas. Visual field examination is indicated in all patients with macroadenomas and in any patient who elects drug therapy or surveillance only.

Treatment

- Depends on sex, cause, symptoms, and other factors

The treatment of microprolactinomas is controversial. Asymptomatic patients who have prolactin levels < 100 ng/mL and normal CT or MRI results or who have only microadenomas can probably be observed; serum prolactin often normalizes within years. Patients with hyperprolactinemia should be monitored with quarterly measurement of prolactin levels and undergo sellar CT or MRI annually for at least an additional 2 yr. The frequency of sellar imaging can then be reduced if prolactin levels do not increase.

In women, indications for treatment include

- Desire for pregnancy
- Amenorrhea or significant oligomenorrhea (because of the risk of osteoporosis)
- Hirsutism
- Low libido
- Troublesome galactorrhea

In men, galactorrhea itself is rarely troublesome enough to require treatment; indications for treatment include

- Hypogonadism (because of the risk of osteoporosis)
- Erectile dysfunction
- Low libido
- Troublesome infertility

The initial treatment is usually a dopamine agonist such as bromocriptine 1.25 to 5 mg po bid or the longer-acting cabergoline 0.25 to 1.0 mg po once/wk or twice/wk, which lower prolactin levels. Cabergoline is the treatment of choice because it appears to be more easily tolerated and more potent than bromocriptine. Women trying to become pregnant should switch to bromocriptine at least 1 mo before planned conception and stop bromocriptine use at the time of a positive pregnancy test result; long-term safety data are better established for bromocriptine than for cabergoline, although evidence for the safety of cabergoline is increasing. Exogenous estrogen can be given to women with a microadenoma who are clinically hypoestrogenic or have low estradiol levels. Exogenous estrogen is unlikely to cause tumor expansion. Quinagolide, a nonergot-derived dopamine agonist, is also an option for hyperprolactinemia. It is started at 25 mcg po once/day and titrated over 7 days up to the usual maintenance dose of 75 mcg once/day (maximum dose 600 mcg once/day).

Patients with macroadenomas generally should be treated with dopamine agonists or surgically but only after thorough testing of pituitary function and evaluation for radiation therapy. Dopamine agonists are usually the initial treatment of choice and usually shrink a prolactin-secreting tumor but will not shrink a nonfunctioning tumor causing pituitary stalk compression, although prolactin levels will decrease. If prolactin levels fall and symptoms and signs of compression by the tumor abate, no other therapy may be necessary. However, typically, larger, nonfunctioning lesions need additional treatment, usually surgery. Surgery or radiation therapy may be easier to do or yield better results after tumor shrinkage induced by a dopamine agonist. Although dopamine agonist treatment usually needs to be continued long-term, prolactin-secreting tumors sometimes remit, either spontaneously or perhaps aided by the drug therapy. Sometimes, therefore, dopamine agonists can be stopped without a recurrence of the tumor or a rise in prolactin levels; remission is more likely with microadenomas than macroadenomas. Remission is also more likely after pregnancy.

High doses of dopamine agonists, particularly cabergoline and pergolide, are thought to have caused valvular heart disease in some patients with Parkinson disease. It is not clear whether the lower doses of dopamine agonists used for hyperprolactinemia similarly increase the risk of valvular heart disease, but the possibility should be discussed with patients, and echocardiographic surveillance should be considered. The risk may be less with bromocriptine or quinagolide. Dopamine agonists in the doses used for hyperprolactinemia also sometimes cause behavioral and psychiatric changes, characterized by increased impulsivity and occasionally psychosis, and this limits their use in some patients.

Radiation therapy should be used only in patients with progressive disease who do not respond to other forms of therapy. With irradiation, hypopituitarism often develops several years after therapy. Monitoring endocrine function and sellar imaging are indicated yearly for life.

KEY POINTS

- Galactorrhea is milk release that is inappropriate, persistent, or worrisome to the patient.
- The most common cause is a pituitary tumor, but many drugs, and endocrine, hypothalamic, or other disorders may be responsible.
- Measure prolactin levels and do CNS imaging to detect a causative tumor.
- For microprolactinomas, give a dopamine agonist if certain troublesome symptoms are present.
- For macroadenomas, give a dopamine agonist and consider surgical ablation or sometimes radiation therapy.

GENERALIZED HYPOPITUITARISM

Generalized hypopituitarism refers to endocrine deficiency syndromes due to partial or complete loss of anterior lobe pituitary function. Various clinical features occur depending on the specific hormones that are deficient. Diagnosis involves imaging tests and measurement of pituitary hormone levels basally and after various provocative stimuli. Treatment depends on cause but generally includes removal of any tumor and administration of replacement hormones.

Hypopituitarism is divided into

- Primary: Caused by disorders that affect the pituitary gland
- Secondary: Caused by disorders of the hypothalamus

The different causes of primary and secondary hypopituitarism are listed in the table below (see Table 170–4).

Symptoms and Signs

Symptoms and signs relate to the underlying disorder and to the specific pituitary hormones that are deficient or absent. Onset is usually insidious and may not be recognized by the patient; occasionally, onset is sudden or dramatic.

Most commonly, growth hormone (GH) is lost first, then gonadotropins, and finally thyroid-stimulating hormone (TSH) and ACTH. Vasopressin deficiency is rare in primary pituitary disorders but is common with lesions of the pituitary stalk and hypothalamus. Function of all target glands decreases when all hormones are deficient (panhypopituitarism).

Lack of luteinizing hormone (LH) and follicle-stimulating hormone (FSH) in children leads to delayed puberty. Premenopausal women develop amenorrhea, reduced libido, regression of secondary sexual characteristics, and infertility. Men develop erectile dysfunction, testicular atrophy, reduced libido, regression of secondary sexual characteristics, and decreased spermatogenesis with consequent infertility.

GH deficiency may contribute to decreased energy but is usually asymptomatic and clinically undetectable in adults. Suggestions that GH deficiency accelerates atherosclerosis are unproved. Effects of GH deficiency in children are discussed elsewhere.

TSH deficiency leads to hypothyroidism, with such symptoms as facial puffiness, hoarse voice, bradycardia, and cold intolerance.

ACTH deficiency results in hypoadrenalism with attendant fatigue, hypotension, and intolerance to stress and infection. ACTH deficiency does not result in the hyperpigmentation characteristic of primary adrenal failure.

Table 170–4. CAUSES OF HYPOPITUITARISM

CAUSE	EXAMPLES
Causes primarily affecting the pituitary gland (primary hypopituitarism)	
Pituitary tumors	Adenoma Craniopharyngioma
Infarction or ischemic necrosis	Hemorrhagic infarction (pituitary apoplexy) Shock, especially postpartum (Sheehan syndrome), or in diabetes mellitus or sickle cell anemia Vascular thrombosis or aneurysm, especially of the internal carotid artery
Inflammatory processes	Meningitis (tubercular, other bacterial, fungal, malarial) Pituitary abscess Sarcoidosis
Infiltrative disorders	Hemochromatosis Langerhans cell histiocytosis
Idiopathic isolated or multiple pituitary hormone deficiencies	—
Iatrogenic	Drugs (eg, hypophysitis due to antimelanoma monoclonal antibodies) Irradiation Surgical extirpation
Autoimmune dysfunction	Lymphocytic hypophysitis
Causes primarily affecting the hypothalamus (secondary hypopituitarism)	
Hypothalamic tumors	Craniopharyngioma Ependymoma Meningioma Metastatic tumor Pinealoma
Inflammatory processes	Sarcoidosis
Neurohormone deficiencies of the hypothalamus	Isolated Multiple
Iatrogenic	Surgical transection of the pituitary stalk
Trauma	Basal skull fracture

Hypothalamic lesions, which can result in hypopituitarism, can also disturb the centers that control appetite, causing a syndrome resembling anorexia nervosa, or sometimes hyperphagia with massive obesity.

Sheehan syndrome, which affects postpartum women, is pituitary necrosis due to hypovolemia and shock occurring in the immediate peripartum period. Lactation does not start after childbirth, and the patient may complain of fatigue and loss of pubic and axillary hair.

Pituitary apoplexy is a symptom complex caused by hemorrhagic infarction of either a normal pituitary gland or, more commonly, a pituitary tumor. Acute symptoms include severe headache, stiff neck, fever, visual field defects, and oculomotor palsies. The resulting edema may compress the hypothalamus, resulting in somnolence or coma. Varying degrees of hypopituitarism may develop suddenly, and the patient may present with vascular collapse because of deficient ACTH and cortisol. The CSF often contains blood, and MRI documents hemorrhage.

Diagnosis

- MRI or CT
- Free thyroxine (T_4), TSH, prolactin, LH, FSH, and testosterone (in men) or estradiol (in women) levels
- Cortisol levels plus provocative testing of pituitary-adrenal axis
- Sometimes other provocative testing

Clinical features are often nonspecific, and the diagnosis must be established with certainty before committing the patient to a lifetime of hormone replacement therapy. Pituitary dysfunction must be distinguished from anorexia nervosa, chronic liver disease, myotonia dystrophica, polyglandular autoimmune disease (see Table 170–5), and disorders of the other endocrine glands. The clinical picture may be particularly confusing when the function of more than one gland decreases at the same time. Evidence of structural pituitary abnormalities and of hormonal deficiencies should be sought with imaging and laboratory tests.

Imaging tests: Patients should undergo high-resolution CT or MRI, with contrast media as required (to rule out structural abnormalities, such as pituitary adenomas). PET is a research tool used in a few specialized centers and therefore is rarely done. When no modern neuroradiologic facilities are available, a simple cone-down lateral x-ray of the sella turcica can identify pituitary macroadenomas with a diameter > 10 mm. Cerebral angiography is indicated only when other imaging tests suggest perisellar vascular anomalies or aneurysms.

Laboratory testing: Initial evaluation should include testing for TSH and ACTH deficiencies, because both conditions are potentially life threatening. Testing for deficiencies of other hormones is also discussed elsewhere.

Free T_4 and TSH levels should be determined. Levels of both are usually low in generalized hypopituitarism; a pattern of normal TSH level with low free T_4 may also occur. In contrast, elevated TSH levels with low free T_4 indicate a primary abnormality of the thyroid gland.

Synthetic thyrotropin-releasing hormone (TRH), 200 to 500 mcg IV given over 15 to 30 sec, may help identify patients with hypothalamic as opposed to pituitary dysfunction, although this test is not often done. Serum TSH levels are generally measured at 0, 20, and 60 min after injection. If pituitary function is intact, TSH should rise by > 5 mU/L, peaking by 30 min after injection. A delayed rise in serum TSH levels may occur in patients with hypothalamic disease. However, some patients with primary pituitary disease also show a delayed rise.

Serum cortisol levels alone are not reliable indicators of ACTH-adrenal axis function, although a very low morning serum cortisol level (< 3.5 mg/dL between 7:30 and 9:00 AM) almost certainly indicates cortisol deficiency. One of several provocative tests should be done. The **short ACTH stimulation test** is a safer and less labor-intensive test for cortisol deficiency than the insulin tolerance test. In the short ACTH stimulation test, synthetic ACTH 250 mcg IV or IM (standard-dose test) or 1 mcg IV (low-dose test) is given, and the blood cortisol level is measured immediately before and 30 and 60 min after administration of synthetic ACTH. Cortisol should rise significantly; a peak of < 20 mg/dL is abnormal. However, the short ACTH

Table 170–5. DIFFERENTIATION OF GENERALIZED HYPOPITUITARISM FROM OTHER SELECTED DISORDERS

DISORDER	DIFFERENTIATING FEATURES
Anorexia nervosa	Female predominance; cachexia; abnormal ideation regarding food and body image; maintenance of secondary sexual characteristics despite amenorrhea; increased levels of basal growth hormone and cortisol
Alcoholic liver disease or hemochromatosis*	Evidence of liver disease; laboratory testing
Myotonia dystrophica	Progressive weakness; premature balding; cataracts; facial features of accelerated aging; laboratory testing
Polyglandular autoimmune disease†	Pituitary hormone levels

*May cause hypogonadism and general debility.
†If the affected glands are target glands of the pituitary.

stimulation test is abnormal in secondary cortisol deficiency only when the test done at least 2 to 4 wk after onset of the deficiency; before this time, the adrenal glands have not atrophied and remain responsive to exogenous ACTH.

The **insulin tolerance test** is considered the most accurate way of evaluating ACTH (as well as GH and prolactin) reserve, but because of its demands, it is probably best reserved for patients who fail the short ACTH stimulation test (if confirmation is needed) or when a test must be done within 2 to 4 wk of a possible pituitary injury. Regular insulin at a dosage of 0.1 units/kg body weight IV is given over 15 to 30 sec, and venous blood samples are obtained to determine GH, cortisol, and glucose levels at baseline (before insulin administration) and 20, 30, 45, 60, and 90 min later. If glucose drops to < 40 mg/dL (< 2.22 mmol/L) or symptoms of hypoglycemia develop, cortisol should increase by > 7 µg/dL or to > 20 µg/dL. (CAUTION: *This test is hazardous in patients with severe documented panhypopituitarism or diabetes mellitus and in the elderly and is contraindicated in patients with coronary artery disease or epilepsy. A health care practitioner should be present during the test.*) Usually, only transient perspiration, tachycardia, and nervousness occur. If the patient complains of palpitations, loses consciousness, or has a seizure, the test should be stopped promptly by giving 50 mL of 50% glucose solution IV.

Neither the short ACTH stimulation test nor the insulin tolerance test alone will differentiate between primary (Addison disease) and secondary (hypopituitary) adrenal insufficiency. Tests to make this distinction and to evaluate the hypothalamic-pituitary-adrenal axis are described under Addison disease.

The **corticotropin-releasing hormone** (CRH) test is done to distinguish between primary, secondary (pituitary), and tertiary (hypothalamic) causes of adrenal insufficiency. CRH 1 mcg/kg IV is given by rapid injection. Serum ACTH and cortisol levels are measured 15 min before, then at baseline, and 15, 30, 60, 90, and 120 min after the injection. Adverse effects include temporary flushing, a metallic taste in the mouth, and slight and transient hypotension.

Prolactin levels are routinely measured. These levels are often elevated up to 5 times normal values when a large pituitary tumor is present, even if it does not produce prolactin. The tumor compresses the pituitary stalk, preventing dopamine, which inhibits pituitary prolactin production and release, from reaching the pituitary. Patients with such hyperprolactinemia often have hypogonadotropism and secondary hypogonadism.

Measurement of basal levels of LH and FSH is most helpful in evaluating hypopituitarism in postmenopausal women not taking exogenous estrogens in whom circulating gonadotropin concentrations are normally high (> 30 mIU/mL). Although gonadotropin levels tend to be low in other patients with panhypopituitarism, overlap exists with the normal range. Levels of both hormones should increase in response to synthetic gonadotropin-releasing hormone (GnRH) at a dose of 100 mcg IV, with LH peaking about 30 min and FSH peaking 40 min after GnRH administration. However, normal, diminished, or absent responses to GnRH may occur in hypothalamic-pituitary dysfunction. Normal increases in LH and FSH in response to GnRH vary. Administration of exogenous GnRH is not helpful in distinguishing primary hypothalamic disorders from primary pituitary disorders.

Screening for GH deficiency in adults is not recommended unless GH treatment is contemplated (eg, for unexplained reduced energy and quality of life in patients with hypopituitarism in which other hormones have been fully replaced). GH deficiency is suspected if ≥ 2 other pituitary hormones are deficient. Because GH levels vary by time of day and other factors and are difficult to interpret, levels of insulin-like growth factor 1 (IGF-1), which reflect GH, are used; low levels suggest GH deficiency, but normal levels do not rule it out. A provocative test of GH release (see p. 2567) may be necessary.

Although the usefulness of provocative testing of pituitary function using releasing hormones remains to be established, if such testing is elected, it is most efficient to evaluate multiple hormones simultaneously. Growth hormone–releasing hormone (1 mcg/kg), CRH (1 mcg/kg), TRH (200 mcg), and GnRH (100 mcg) are given together IV over 15 to 30 sec. Glucose, cortisol, GH, TSH, prolactin, LH, FSH, and ACTH are measured at frequent intervals for the ensuing 180 min. The normal responses are the same as those delineated earlier for individual testing.

Treatment

- Hormone replacement
- Treatment of cause (eg, tumor)

Treatment is replacement of the hormones of the hypofunctioning target glands, as discussed in the pertinent chapters in this section and elsewhere in THE MANUAL. Adults ≤ 50 yr deficient in GH are now sometimes treated with GH doses of 0.002 to 0.012 mg/kg sc once/day. Benefits of treatment include improved energy and quality of life, increased body muscle mass, and decreased body fat mass. Suggestions that GH replacement can prevent an acceleration of atherosclerosis induced by GH deficiency are unproved.

In pituitary apoplexy, immediate surgery is warranted if visual field disturbances or oculomotor palsies develop suddenly or if somnolence progresses to coma because of hypothalamic compression. Although management with high-dose corticosteroids and general support may suffice in a few cases, transsphenoidal decompression of the tumor should generally be undertaken promptly.

Surgery and radiation therapy may be followed by the loss of other pituitary hormone functions. Irradiated patients may lose endocrine function slowly over years. Therefore, posttreatment hormonal status should be evaluated frequently, preferably at 3 and 6 mo and yearly thereafter for at least 10 yr and preferably up to 15 yr after radiation therapy. Such evaluation should include at least assessment of thyroid and adrenal function. Patients may also develop visual difficulties related to fibrosis of the optic chiasm. Sellar imaging and visual field assessment should be done at least every 2 yr initially for about 10 yr, particularly if residual tumor tissue is present.

GIGANTISM AND ACROMEGALY

Gigantism and acromegaly are syndromes of excessive secretion of growth hormone (hypersomatotropism) that are nearly always due to a pituitary adenoma. Before closure of the epiphyses, the result is gigantism. Later, the result is acromegaly, which causes distinctive facial and other features. Diagnosis is clinical and by skull and hand x-rays and measurement of growth hormone levels. Treatment involves removal or destruction of the responsible adenoma.

Many growth hormone (GH)–secreting adenomas contain a mutant form of the G_s protein, which is a stimulatory regulator of adenylate cyclase. Cells with the mutant form of G_s protein secrete GH even in the absence of growth hormone–releasing hormone (GHRH). A few cases of ectopic GHRH-producing tumors, especially of the pancreas and lung, also have been described.

Symptoms and Signs

Pituitary gigantism: This rare condition occurs if GH hypersecretion begins in childhood, before closure of the epiphyses. Skeletal growth velocity and ultimate stature are increased, but little bony deformity occurs. However, soft-tissue swelling occurs, and the peripheral nerves are enlarged. Delayed puberty or hypogonadotropic hypogonadism is also frequently present, resulting in a eunuchoid habitus.

Acromegaly: In acromegaly, GH hypersecretion usually starts between the 20s and 40s. When GH hypersecretion begins after epiphyseal closure, the earliest clinical manifestations are coarsening of the facial features (see Plate 65) and soft-tissue swelling of the hands and feet. Appearance changes, and larger rings, gloves, and shoes are needed. Photographs of the patient are important in delineating the course of the disease.

In adults with acromegaly, coarse body hair increases and the skin thickens and frequently darkens. The size and function of sebaceous and sweat glands increase, such that patients frequently complain of excessive perspiration and offensive body odor. Overgrowth of the mandible leads to protrusion of the jaw (prognathism) and malocclusion of teeth. Cartilaginous proliferation of the larynx leads to a deep, husky voice. The tongue is frequently enlarged and furrowed. In long-standing acromegaly, costal cartilage growth leads to a barrel chest. Articular cartilaginous proliferation occurs early in response to GH excess, with the articular cartilage possibly undergoing necrosis and erosion. Joint symptoms are common, and crippling degenerative arthritis may occur.

Peripheral neuropathies occur commonly because of compression of nerves by adjacent fibrous tissue and endoneural fibrous proliferation. Headaches are common because of the pituitary tumor. Bitemporal hemianopia may develop if suprasellar extension compresses the optic chiasm. The heart, liver, kidneys, spleen, thyroid gland, parathyroid glands, and pancreas are larger than normal. Cardiac disease (eg, coronary artery disease, cardiomegaly, sometimes cardiomyopathy) occurs in perhaps one third of patients, with a doubling in the risk of death from cardiac disease. Hypertension occurs in up to one third of patients. The risk of cancer, particularly of the GI tract, increases 2-fold to 3-fold. GH increases tubular reabsorption of phosphate and leads to mild hyperphosphatemia. Impaired glucose tolerance occurs in nearly half the patients with acromegaly and in gigantism, but clinically significant diabetes mellitus occurs in only about 10% of patients.

Galactorrhea occurs in some women with acromegaly, usually in association with hyperprolactinemia. However, galactorrhea may occur with GH excess alone, because GH itself stimulates lactation. Decreased gonadotropin secretion often occurs with GH-secreting tumors. About one-third of men with acromegaly develop erectile dysfunction, and nearly all women develop menstrual irregularities or amenorrhea.

Diagnosis

- CT or MRI
- Insulin-like growth factor 1 (IGF-1) levels
- Usually GH levels

Diagnosis can be made from the characteristic clinical findings. CT, MRI, or skull x-rays disclose cortical thickening, enlargement of the frontal sinuses, and enlargement and erosion of the sella turcica. X-rays of the hands show tufting of the terminal phalanges and soft-tissue thickening.

Serum IGF-1 should be measured in patients with suspected acromegaly; IGF-1 levels are typically substantially elevated (3-fold to 10-fold), and because IGF-1 levels do not fluctuate like GH levels do, they are the simplest way to assess GH hypersecretion. IGF-1 levels also can be used to monitor response to therapy.

Plasma GH levels measured by radioimmunoassay are typically elevated. Blood should be taken before the patient eats breakfast (basal state); in normal people, basal GH levels are < 5 ng/mL. Transient elevations of GH are normal and must be distinguished from pathologic hypersecretion. The degree of GH suppression after a glucose load remains the standard and thus should be measured in patients with elevated plasma GH; however, the results are assay-dependent, and the cutoff for normal suppression is controversial. Secretion in normal people is suppressed to < 2 ng/mL (a cutoff of < 1 ng/mL is often used) within 90 min of administration of glucose 75 g po. Most patients with acromegaly have substantially higher values. Basal plasma GH levels are also important in monitoring response to therapy.

CT or **MRI** of the head should be done to look for a tumor. If a tumor is not visible, excessive secretion of pituitary GH may be due to a non-CNS tumor producing excessive amounts of ectopic GHRH. Demonstration of elevated levels of plasma GHRH can confirm the diagnosis. Lungs and pancreas may be first evaluated in searching for the sites of ectopic production.

Screening for complications, including diabetes, heart disease, and GI cancer, should be done at the time of diagnosis. Fasting plasma glucose levels, glycosylated Hb (HbA_{1C}), or an oral glucose tolerance test can be done to test for diabetes. ECG and, preferably, echocardiography are done to detect heart disease. Colonoscopy is done to detect colon cancer. Follow-up screening depends on the results of the initial testing and the patient's response to treatment.

Treatment

- Surgery or radiation therapy
- Sometimes pharmacologic suppression of GH secretion or activity

Ablative therapy: Ablative therapy with surgery or radiation is generally indicated. Transsphenoidal resection is preferred, but choices vary at different institutions. Stereotactic supervoltage radiation, delivering about 5000 cGy to the pituitary, is used, but GH levels may not fall to normal for several years. Treatment with accelerated protons (heavy particle radiation) permits delivery of larger doses of radiation (equivalent to 10,000 cGy) to the pituitary; such therapy poses higher risk of cranial nerve and hypothalamic damage and is available only in a few centers. Development of hypopituitarism several years after irradiation is common. Because radiation damage is cumulative, proton beam therapy should *not* be used after conventional gamma-irradiation. A combined approach with both surgery and radiation therapy is indicated for patients with progressive extrasellar involvement by a pituitary tumor and for patients whose entire tumor cannot be resected, which is often the case.

Surgical removal of the tumor is likely to have been curative if GH levels measured after a glucose load and IGF-1 levels reach normal values. If one or both values are abnormal, further therapy is usually needed. If GH excess is poorly controlled, hypertension, heart failure, and a doubling in the death rate occur. If GH levels are < 5 ng/mL, however, mortality does not increase.

Drug therapy: In general, drug therapy is indicated if surgery and radiation therapy are contraindicated, if they have not been curative, or if radiation therapy is being given time to work. In such instances, a somatostatin analog, octreotide, is given at 0.05 to 0.15 mg sc q 8 to 12 h; it suppresses GH secretion effectively. Longer-acting somatostatin analogs, such as mannitol-modified release octreotide (octreotide LAR) given 10 to 30 mg IM q 4 to 6 wk and lanreotide given 30 mg IM q 10 to 14 days, are more convenient. Bromocriptine mesylate (1.25 to 5 mg po bid) may effectively lower GH levels in a small percentage of patients but is less effective than somatostatin analogs.

Pegvisomant, a GH receptor blocker, has been shown to reduce the effects of GH and lower IGF-1 levels in people with acromegaly, without apparent increase in pituitary tumor size. This drug may find a place in treating patients who are partially or totally unresponsive to somatostatin analogs.

KEY POINTS

- Gigantism and acromegaly are usually caused by a pituitary adenoma that secretes excessive amounts of GH; rarely, they are caused by non-pituitary tumors that secrete GHRH.
- Gigantism occurs if GH hypersecretion begins in childhood, before closure of the epiphyses.
- Acromegaly involves GH hypersecretion beginning in adulthood; a variety of bony and soft tissue abnormalities develop.
- Diagnose by measuring IGF-1 and GH levels; do CNS imaging to detect a pituitary tumor.
- Remove pituitary tumors surgically or using radiation therapy.
- If tumors cannot be removed, give octreotide or lanreotide to suppress GH secretion.

PITUITARY LESIONS

Patients with hypothalamic-pituitary lesions generally present with some combination of

- Symptoms and signs of a mass lesion: headaches, altered appetite, thirst, visual field defects—particularly bitemporal hemianopia or the hemifield slide phenomenon (images drifting apart)
- Imaging evidence of a mass lesion as an incidental finding
- Hypersecretion or hyposecretion of one or more pituitary hormones

The most common cause of hypopituitary or hyperpituitary secretion is a pituitary or hypothalamic tumor. A pituitary tumor tends to produce an enlarged sella (sella turcica). Alternatively, an enlarged sella may represent empty sella syndrome.

Empty sella syndrome: In this disorder, the sella appears empty because it is filled with CSF, which flattens the pituitary gland against the wall of the sella. The syndrome may be

- Congenital
- Primary
- Secondary to injury (eg, ischemia after childbirth, surgery, head trauma, radiation therapy)

The typical patient is female (> 80%), obese (about 75%), and hypertensive (30%) and may have idiopathic intracranial hypertension (10%) or spinal fluid rhinorrhea (10%).

Pituitary function in patients with empty sella syndrome is frequently normal. However, hypopituitarism may occur, as may headaches and visual field defects. Occasionally, patients have small coexisting pituitary tumors that secrete growth hormone (GH), prolactin, or ACTH.

Diagnosis can be confirmed by CT or MRI.

No specific therapy is needed for an empty sella alone.

Anterior lobe lesions: Hypersecretion of anterior lobe hormones (hyperpituitarism) is almost always selective, although occasionally a tumor hypersecretes both growth hormone and prolactin. The anterior pituitary hormones most commonly secreted in excess are GH (as in acromegaly, gigantism), prolactin (as in galactorrhea), and ACTH (resulting in Cushing disease).

Hyposecretion of anterior lobe hormones (hypopituitarism) may be generalized, usually due to a pituitary tumor, or is idiopathic or may involve the selective loss of one or a few pituitary hormones.

Posterior lobe lesions: The 2 posterior lobe hormones are

- Oxytocin
- Vasopressin (ADH)

In women, oxytocin causes myoepithelial cells of the breast and myometrial cells of the uterus to contract. Oxytocin is present in men but has no proven function.

Deficiency of vasopressin results in central diabetes insipidus. Excess vasopressin secretion results in the syndrome of inappropriate ADH secretion (SIADH).

SELECTIVE PITUITARY HORMONE DEFICIENCIES

Selective deficiencies of pituitary hormones may represent an early stage in the development of more generalized hypopituitarism. Patients must be observed for signs of other pituitary hormone deficiencies, and sellar imaging should be done at intervals to check for signs of a pituitary tumor.

Isolated growth hormone (GH) deficiency is responsible for many cases of pituitary short stature. Although one autosomal dominant form of complete GH deficiency is associated with a deletion of the GH structural gene, such gene defects probably account for a minority of cases. Treatment of GH deficiency in adults < 50 yr is discussed elsewhere (see Generalized Hypopituitarism—p. 1322).

Isolated gonadotropin deficiency occurs in both sexes and must be distinguished from primary hypogonadism; men have low serum testosterone levels and infertility, and women have amenorrhea, low serum estrogen levels, and infertility. A eunuchoid habitus is generally present. However, patients with primary hypogonadism have elevated levels of luteinizing hormone (LH) and follicle-stimulating hormone (FSH), whereas those with gonadotropin deficiency, either secondary (pituitary) or tertiary (hypothalamic), have low-normal, low, or unmeasurable levels of LH and FSH. Although most cases of hypogonadotropic hypogonadism involve deficiencies of both LH and FSH, in rare cases the secretion of only one is impaired. Isolated gonadotropin deficiency must also be distinguished from hypogonadotropic amenorrhea secondary to exercise, diet, or mental stress. Although the history may be helpful, differential diagnosis may be impossible.

In **Kallmann syndrome,** the specific lack of gonadotropin-releasing hormone (GnRH) is associated with midline facial defects, including anosmia and cleft lip or palate, and with color blindness. Embryologic studies have shown that GnRH neurons originally develop in the epithelium of the olfactory placode and migrate into the septal-preoptic region of the hypothalamus early in development. In at least some cases, gene defects, localized to the X chromosome in the X-linked form of the disorder and termed the *KALIG-1* (Kallmann syndrome interval gene 1) gene, have been found in the adhesion proteins facilitating this neuronal migration. Administration of GnRH is not indicated.

Isolated ACTH deficiency is rare. Weakness, hypoglycemia, weight loss, and decreased axillary and pubic hair suggest the diagnosis. Blood and urinary steroid levels are low and rise to normal after ACTH replacement. Clinical and laboratory evidence of other hormonal deficiencies is absent. Treatment is with cortisol replacement, as for Addison disease; mineralocorticoid replacement is not required.

Isolated thyroid-stimulating hormone deficiency is likely when clinical features of hypothyroidism exist, serum TSH levels are low or not elevated, and no other pituitary hormone deficiencies exist. Serum TSH levels, as measured by immunoassay, are not always lower than normal, suggesting that the TSH secreted is biologically inactive. Administration of recombinant human TSH increases thyroid hormone levels.

Isolated prolactin deficiency has been noted rarely in women who fail to lactate after delivery. Basal prolactin levels are low and do not increase in response to provocative stimuli, such as thyroid-releasing hormone. Administration of prolactin is not indicated.

171 Polyglandular Deficiency Syndromes

POLYGLANDULAR DEFICIENCY SYNDROMES

(Autoimmune Polyglandular Syndromes; Polyendocrine Deficiency Syndromes)

Polyglandular deficiency syndromes (PDS) are characterized by sequential or simultaneous deficiencies in the function of several endocrine glands that have a common cause. Etiology is most often autoimmune. Categorization depends on the combination of deficiencies, which fall within 1 of 3 types. Diagnosis requires measurement of hormone levels and autoantibodies against affected endocrine glands. Treatment includes replacement of missing or deficient hormones and sometimes immunosuppressants.

Etiology

The etiology is most often autoimmune. Risk factors for development of autoimmunity include

- Genetic factors
- Environmental triggers

Genetic factors include the *AIRE* gene mutation, which is causative of type 1, and certain HLA subtypes, which are important in the development of types 2 and 3. Environmental triggers include viral infections, dietary factors, and other as yet unknown exposures.

Pathophysiology

The underlying autoimmune reaction involves autoantibodies against endocrine tissues, cell-mediated autoimmunity, or both and leads to inflammation, lymphocytic infiltration, and partial or complete gland destruction. More than one endocrine gland is involved, although clinical manifestations are not always simultaneous. The autoimmune reaction and associated immune system dysfunction can also damage nonendocrine tissues.

Classification

Three patterns of autoimmune failure have been described (see Table 171–1), which likely reflect different autoimmune abnormalities. Some experts combine type 2 and type 3 into a single group.

Type 1: Type 1 usually begins in childhood. It is defined by the presence of ≥ 2 of the following:

- Chronic mucocutaneous candidiasis
- Hypoparathyroidism
- Adrenal insufficiency (Addison disease)

Candidiasis is usually the initial clinical manifestation, most often occurring in patients < 5 yr. Hypoparathyroidism occurs next, usually in patients < 10 yr. Lastly, adrenal insufficiency occurs in patients < 15 yr. Accompanying endocrine and nonendocrine disorders (see Table 171–1) continue to appear at least until patients are about age 40.

Type 2 (Schmidt syndrome): Type 2 usually occurs in adults; peak incidence is age 30. It occurs 3 times more often in women. It typically manifests with the following:

- Adrenal insufficiency
- Hypothyroidism or hyperthyroidism
- Type 1 diabetes (autoimmune etiology)

More rare features may also be present (see Table 171–1).

Table 171–1. CHARACTERISTICS OF TYPES 1, 2, AND 3 POLYGLANDULAR DEFICIENCY SYNDROMES

CHARACTERISTIC	TYPE 1	TYPE 2	TYPE 3
Demographics			
Age at onset	Childhood (3–5 yr)	Adulthood (peak 30 yr)	Adulthood (particularly middle-aged women)
Female:male	4:3	3:1	N/A
Genetics			
HLA types	May influence the development of specific components of the disorder	Primarily, B8, DW3, DR3, DR4 Others in specific disorders	DR3, DR4
Inheritance	Autosomal recessive mutation of the *AIRE* gene	Polygenic	Polygenic
Glands affected			
Common	Parathyroid Adrenals Gonads	Adrenals Thyroid Pancreas	Thyroid Pancreas
Less common	Pancreas Thyroid	Gonads	Variable
Clinical			
Adrenal insufficiency (Addison disease)	73–100%	100%	Not seen
Alopecia	26–32%	Not seen	*
Celiac disease	Rare	Incidence uncertain	*
Chronic active hepatitis	20%	Not seen	N/A
Chronic mucocutaneous candidiasis	73–97%	Not seen	N/A
Diabetes mellitus (type 1)	2–30%	52%	*
Gonadal failure	In men, 15–25% In women, 60%	3.5%	*
Hypoparathyroidism	76–99%	Not seen	Not seen
Malabsorption	22–24%	Not seen	N/A
Myasthenia gravis	Not seen	Incidence uncertain	*
Pernicious anemia	13–30%	< 1%	*
Sarcoidosis	Not seen	Not seen	*
Thyroid disorders†	10–11%	69%	100%
Vitiligo	4–30%	5–50%	N/A

*Associated; incidence uncertain.
†Usually chronic lymphocytic thyroiditis but also includes Graves disease.
N/A = data not available.
Data from Husebye ES, Perheentupa J, Rautemaa R, Kampe O: Clinical manifestations and management of patients with autoimmune polyendocrine syndrome type 1. *Journal of Internal Medicine* 265:519–529, 2009; Trence DL, Morley JE, Handwerger BS: Polyglandular autoimmune syndromes. *American Journal of Medicine* 77(1):107–116, 1984; Leshin M: Polyglandular autoimmune syndromes. *American Journal of Medical Sciences* 290(2):77–88, 1985; Dittmar M, Kahaly GJ: Polyglandular autoimmune syndromes: immunogenetics and long-term follow-up. *Journal of Clinical Endocrinology and Metabolism* 88:2983–2992, 2003; and Eisenbarth GS, Gottlieb PA. Autoimmune polyendocrine syndromes. *New England Journal of Medicine* 350:2068–2079, 2004.

Type 3: Type 3 is characterized by

- Glandular failure occurring in adults, particularly middle-aged women
- Hypothyroidism
- At least one of a variety of other disorders (see Table 171–1)

Type 3 does not involve the adrenal cortex.

Symptoms and Signs

The clinical appearance of patients with PDS is the sum of the individual endocrine deficiencies and associated nonendocrine disorders; their symptoms and signs are discussed elsewhere in THE MANUAL. The deficiencies do not always appear at the same time and may require a period of years to manifest; in such cases they do not follow a particular sequence.

Diagnosis

- Measurement of hormone levels
- Sometimes autoantibody titers

Diagnosis is suggested clinically and confirmed by detecting deficient hormone levels. Other causes of multiple endocrine deficiencies include hypothalamic-pituitary dysfunction and coincidental endocrine dysfunction due to separate causes (eg, tuberculous hypoadrenalism and nonautoimmune hypothyroidism in the same patient). Detecting autoantibodies to each affected glandular tissue can help differentiate PDS from the other causes, and elevated levels of pituitary tropic hormones (eg, thyroid-stimulating hormone) suggest the hypothalamic-pituitary axis is intact (although some patients with type 2 PDS have hypothalamic-pituitary insufficiency).

Because decades may pass before the appearance of all manifestations, lifelong follow-up is prudent; unrecognized hypoparathyroidism or adrenal insufficiency can be life threatening.

Relatives should be made aware of the diagnosis and screened when appropriate. Trials following relatives of patients with type 1 diabetes for development of autoimmunity are currently enrolling.

Treatment

- Hormone replacement

Treatment of the various individual glandular deficiencies is discussed elsewhere in The Manual; the treatment of multiple deficiencies can be more complex than treatment of an isolated endocrine deficiency. For example, treatment of hypothyroidism with thyroid hormone replacement can precipitate an adrenal crisis in patients with undiagnosed adrenal insufficiency.

Chronic mucocutaneous candidiasis usually requires lifelong antifungal therapy (eg, oral fluconazole or ketoconazole).

Clinical trials of interventions to slow the autoimmune process in type 1 diabetes have shown some promise in delaying the complete destruction of insulin-producing beta-cells. Treatments that have been evaluated include immunotherapy and umbilical cord blood transplantation. Treatments are still experimental. [1, 2]

1. Cai J, Wu Z, Xu X, et al: Umbilical cord mesenchymal stromal cell with autologous bone marrow cell transplantation in established type 1 diabetes: A pilot randomized controlled open-label clinical study to assess safety and impact on insulin secretion. *Diabetes Care* 39(1): 149–157, 2016.
2. Haller MJ, Gitelman SE, Gottlieb PA, et al: Anti-thymocyte globulin/G-CSF treatment preserves β cell function in patients with established type 1 diabetes. *J Clin Invest* 125(1):448–455, 2015.

KEY POINTS

- PDS involve deficiencies in the function of several endocrine glands, which may occur simultaneously or sequentially.
- Nonendocrine organs also may be affected.
- Most cases are autoimmune; triggers are often unknown but may involve viruses or dietary substances.
- PDS are distinguished by the glands affected.

IPEX SYNDROME

IPEX (immune dysregulation, polyendocrinopathy, enteropathy, X-linked) is a recessive syndrome involving aggressive autoimmunity.

This rare disorder results from mutation of the transcriptional activator, FoxP3, which causes regulatory T-cell dysfunction and a subsequent autoimmune disorder.

IPEX syndrome manifests as severe enlargement of the secondary lymphoid organs, type 1 diabetes mellitus, eczema, food allergies, and infections. Secondary enteropathy leads to persistent diarrhea.

Diagnosis is suggested by clinical features and confirmed by genetic analysis.

Treatment

- Hematopoietic stem cell transplantation

Untreated, IPEX syndrome is usually fatal in the first year of life. Hematopoietic stem cell transplantation has been shown to be effective. Long-term follow-up of patients with IPEX treated with hematopoietic stem cell transplantation continues.[1]

1. Nademi Z, Slatter M, Gambineri E, et al. Single centre experience of haematopoietic SCT for patients with immunodysregulation, polyendocrinopathy, enteropathy, X-linked syndrome. *Bone Marrow Transplant* 49(2):310–312, 2014.

POEMS SYNDROME

(Crow-Fukase Syndrome; PEP Syndrome; Takatsuki Disease)

POEMS (polyneuropathy, organomegaly, endocrinopathy, monoclonal gammopathy, skin changes) is a nonautoimmune polyglandular deficiency syndrome.

POEMS syndrome is probably caused by circulating immunoglobulins caused by a plasma cell dyscrasia. Circulating cytokines (IL-1-β, IL-6), vascular endothelial growth factor, and tumor necrosis factor-alpha are also increased.

Patients may have the following:

- Hepatomegaly
- Lymphadenopathy
- Hypogonadism
- Diabetes mellitus type 2
- Primary hypothyroidism
- Hyperparathyroidism
- Adrenal insufficiency (Addison disease)
- Excess production of monoclonal IgA and IgG due to plasmacytomas
- Skin abnormalities (eg, hyperpigmentation, dermal thickening, hirsutism, angiomas, hypertrichosis)

Other symptoms and signs may include edema, ascites, pleural effusion, papilledema, and fever.

Like other syndromes of undefined pathophysiology, POEMS syndrome is diagnosed based on the constellation of symptoms and signs. Criteria include the presence of polyneuropathy and monoclonal paraproteinemia plus any 2 of the other manifestations of the disorder.

Treatment

- Radiation therapy
- Chemotherapy with or without hematopoietic stem cell transplantation

Treatment consists of radiation therapy or chemotherapy sometimes followed by autologous hematopoietic stem cell transplantation. Five-year survival is about 60%.

172 Porphyrias

Porphyrias result from genetic or acquired deficiencies of enzymes of the heme biosynthetic pathway. These deficiencies allow heme precursors to accumulate, causing toxicity. Porphyrias are defined by the specific enzyme deficiency. Two major clinical manifestations occur: neurovisceral abnormalities (the acute porphyrias) and cutaneous photosensitivity (the cutaneous porphyrias).

Heme, an iron-containing pigment, is an essential cofactor of numerous hemoproteins. Virtually all cells of the human body require and synthesize heme. However, most heme is synthesized in the bone marrow (by erythroblasts and reticulocytes) and is incorporated into hemoglobin. The liver is the second most active site of heme synthesis, most of which is incorporated into cytochrome P-450 enzymes. Heme synthesis requires 8 enzymes (see Table 172–1). These enzymes produce and transform molecular species called porphyrins (and their precursors); accumulation of these substances causes the clinical manifestations of the porphyrias.

Table 172–1. SUBSTRATES AND ENZYMES OF THE HEME BIOSYNTHETIC PATHWAY AND THE DISEASES ASSOCIATED WITH THEIR DEFICIENCY

SUBSTRATE/*ENZYME**	PORPHYRIA	NEUROVISCERAL SYMPTOMS	CUTANEOUS SYMPTOMS	INHERITANCE
Glycine + succinyl CoA *Erythroid specific delta-aminolevulinic acid synthase-2 (ALAS 2)*[†]	X-linked protoporphyria (due to *increased* enzyme activity)[†]	No	Phenotypically similar to EPP	X-linked
Delta-aminolevulinic acid *Delta-aminolevulinic acid dehydratase (ALAD)*	ALAD-deficient porphyria	Yes	No	Autosomal recessive
Porphobilinogen *Porphobilinogen deaminase*	Acute intermittent porphyria	Yes	No	Autosomal dominant
Hydroxymethylbilane *Uroporphyrinogen III cosynthase*	Congenital erythropoietic porphyria	No	Severe, mutilating skin disease	Autosomal recessive
Uroporphyrinogen III *Uroporphyrinogen decarboxylase*	Porphyria cutanea tarda	No	Fragile skin, blisters	Two variants: • Autosomal dominant (20–25% of cases) • Without known genetic correlate (sporadic, 75–80%)
	Hepatoerythropoietic porphyria	No	Severe blistering	Autosomal recessive
Coproporphyrinogen III *Coproporphyrinogen oxidase*	Hereditary coproporphyria	Yes	Fragile skin, blisters	Autosomal dominant
Protoporphyrinogen IX *Protoporphyrinogen oxidase*	Variegate porphyria	Yes	Fragile skin, blisters	Autosomal dominant
Protoporphyrin IX[†] *Ferrochelatase*	Erythropoietic protoporphyria (EPP)	No, except in patients with severe hepatobiliary pathology	Skin pain, lichenification and other minor skin changes, but no blistering	Autosomal recessive
Heme (final product incorporated in various heme proteins)	—	—	—	—

*Listed are successive intermediates in the heme biosynthetic pathway, beginning with glycine and succinyl CoA and ending with heme. Deficiency of an enzyme causes buildup of precursor compounds.

[†]XLPP results from gain-of-function mutations that *increase* the activity of ALAS 2, causing accumulation of protoporphyrin. *Decreased* activity of ALAS 2 causes a sideroblastic anemia.

Etiology

With the exception of the sporadic type of porphyria cutanea tarda (PCT), the porphyrias are inherited diseases. Autosomal dominant (AD) inheritance is most common.

In the AD porphyrias, homozygous or compound heterozygous states (ie, 2 separate heterozygous mutations, one in each allele of the same gene in the same patient) may be incompatible with life, typically causing fetal death. Disease penetrance in heterozygotes varies; thus, clinically expressed disease is less common than genetic prevalence. The 2 most common porphyrias, PCT and acute intermittent porphyria (AIP), are AD (20% of PCT is AD). The prevalence of PCT is about 1/10,000. The prevalence of the causative genetic mutation for AIP is about 1/1500, but because penetrance is low, the prevalence of clinical disease is also about 1/10,000. Prevalence of both PCT and AIP varies widely among regions and ethnic groups.

In the autosomal recessive porphyrias, only homozygous or compound heterozygous states cause disease. Erythropoietic protoporphyria (EPP), the 3rd most common porphyria, is autosomal recessive.

X-linked inheritance occurs in one of the porphyrias, X-linked protoporphyria (XLPP).

Pathophysiology

Porphyrias result from a deficiency of any of the last 7 enzymes of the heme biosynthetic pathway or from *increased* activity of the first enzyme in the pathway, ALAS 2. (*Deficiency* of ALAS 2 causes sideroblastic anemia rather than porphyria.) Single genes encode each enzyme; any of numerous possible mutations can alter the levels and/or the activity of the enzyme encoded by that gene. When an enzyme of heme synthesis is deficient or defective, its substrate and any other heme precursors normally modified by that enzyme may accumulate in bone marrow, liver, skin, or other tissues and have toxic effects. These precursors may appear in excess in the blood and be excreted in urine, bile, or stool.

Although porphyrias are most precisely defined according to the deficient enzyme, classification by major clinical features (phenotype) is often useful. Thus, porphyrias are usually divided into 2 classes:

- Acute
- Cutaneous

Acute porphyrias manifest as intermittent attacks of abdominal, mental, and neurologic symptoms. They are typically triggered by drugs, cyclic hormonal activity in young women, and other exogenous factors. Cutaneous porphyrias tend to cause continuous or intermittent symptoms involving cutaneous photosensitivity. Some acute porphyrias (hereditary coproporphyria, variegate porphyria) may also have cutaneous manifestations. Because of variable penetrance in heterozygous porphyrias, clinically expressed disease is less common than genetic prevalence (see Table 172–2).

Urine discoloration (red or reddish brown) may occur in the symptomatic phase of all porphyrias except EPP and ALAD-deficiency porphyria. Discoloration results from oxidation of the porphyrinogens, the porphyrin precursor porphobilinogen (PBG), or both. Sometimes the color develops after the urine has stood in light for about 30 min, allowing time for non-enzymatic oxidation. In the acute porphyrias, except in ALAD-deficiency porphyria, about 1 in 3 heterozygotes (more frequently in females than males) also have increased urinary excretion of PBG (and urine discoloration) during the latent phase.

Diagnosis

- Blood or urine testing

Patients with symptoms suggesting porphyria are screened by blood or urine tests for porphyrins or the porphyrin precursors PBG and ALA (see Table 172–3). Abnormal results on screening are confirmed by further testing.

Asymptomatic patients, including suspected carriers and people who are between attacks, are evaluated similarly. However, the tests are less sensitive in these circumstances; measurement of RBC or WBC enzyme activity is considerably more sensitive. Genetic analysis is highly accurate and preferentially used within families when the mutation is known. Prenatal testing (involving amniocentesis or chorionic villus sampling) is possible but rarely indicated.

Secondary Porphyrinuria

Several diseases unrelated to porphyrias may involve increased urinary excretion of porphyrins; this phenomenon is described as secondary porphyrinuria.

Hematologic disorders, hepatobiliary diseases, and toxins (eg, alcohol, benzene, lead) can cause elevated urinary coproporphyrin excretion. Elevated coproporphyrin excretion in the

Table 172–2. MAJOR FEATURES OF THE TWO MOST COMMON PORPHYRIAS

PORPHYRIA	PRESENTING SYMPTOMS	EXACERBATING FACTORS	MOST IMPORTANT SCREENING TESTS*	TREATMENT
Acute intermittent porphyria	Neurovisceral (intermittent, acute)	Drugs (mostly cytochrome P-450 inducers) Fasting Alcohol ingestion Organic solvents Infections Stress	Urinary PBG	Glucose Heme
Porphyria cutanea tarda	Blistering skin lesions (chronic)	Iron Alcohol ingestion Estrogens Hepatitis C virus Halogenated hydrocarbons	Urinary or plasma porphyrins	Phlebotomy Low-dose chloroquine or hydroxychloroquine

*In symptomatic phase.
PBG = porphobilinogen.

Table 172–3. SCREENING FOR PORPHYRIAS

TESTING	IN PATIENTS WITH ACUTE NEUROVISCERAL SYMPTOMS	IN PATIENTS WITH PHOTOSENSITIVITY
Screening	Urinary PBG (semiquantitative, random urine sample)	Plasma porphyrins*
Confirmation (when screening test results are significantly abnormal)	Urinary ALA and PBG† (quantitative‡) Fecal and urinary porphyrins† RBC PBG deaminase Plasma porphyrins*	RBC porphyrins Urinary ALA, PBG, and porphyrins (quantitative) Fecal porphyrins† Plasma porphyrins*

*The preferred method is by direct fluorescent spectrophotometry.
†Urinary and fecal porphyrins are fractionated only if the total is increased.
‡Results are corrected according to urine creatinine level.
ALA = delta-aminolevulinic acid; PBG =porphobilinogen.

urine can occur in any hepatobiliary disorder because bile is one the routes of porphyrin excretion. Uroporphyrin may also be elevated in patients with hepatobiliary disorders. Protoporphyrin is not excreted in urine because it is water insoluble.

Some patients present with abdominal pain and neurologic symptoms mimicking acute porphyrias. Urinary ALA and PBG are typically not elevated in these diseases, and normal levels help distinguish secondary porphyrinuria from acute porphyrias. However, some patients with lead poisoning can have elevated urinary ALA levels. Blood lead levels should be measured in such patients. If urinary ALA and PBG are normal or only slightly increased, measurement of urinary total porphyrins and high-performance liquid chromatography profiles of these porphyrins are helpful for differential diagnosis of acute porphyric syndromes.

ACUTE PORPHYRIAS

Acute porphyrias result from deficiency of certain enzymes in the heme biosynthetic pathway, resulting in accumulation of heme precursors that cause intermittent attacks of abdominal pain and neurologic symptoms. Attacks are precipitated by certain drugs and other factors. Diagnosis is based on elevated levels of the porphyrin precursors delta-aminolevulinic acid (ALA) and porphobilinogen in the urine during attacks. Attacks are treated with glucose or, if more severe, IV heme. Symptomatic treatment, including analgesia, is given as necessary.

Acute porphyrias include, in order of prevalence:

- Acute intermittent porphyria (AIP)
- Variegate porphyria (VP)
- Hereditary coproporphyria (HCP)
- Delta-aminolevulinic acid dehydratase (ALAD)–deficiency porphyria (exceedingly rare)

Patients with VP and HCP, with or without neurovisceral symptoms, may develop bullous eruptions especially on the hands, forearms, face, neck, or other areas of the skin exposed to sunlight.

Among heterozygotes, acute porphyrias are rarely expressed clinically before puberty; after puberty, they are expressed in only about 2 to 4%. Among homozygotes and compound heterozygotes, onset typically is in childhood, and symptoms are often severe.

Precipitating Factors

Many precipitating factors exist, typically accelerating heme biosynthesis above the catalytic capacity of the defective enzyme. Accumulation of the porphyrin precursors porphobilinogen (PBG) and ALA, or in the case of ALAD-deficiency porphyria, ALA alone, results.

Attacks probably result from several, sometimes unidentifiable, factors. Identified precipitating factors include

- Hormonal changes in women
- Drugs
- Low-calorie, low-carbohydrate diets
- Alcohol
- Exposure to organic solvents
- Infections and other illnesses
- Surgery
- Emotional stress

Hormonal factors are important. Women are more prone to attacks than men, particularly during periods of hormonal change (eg, luteal phase of the menstrual cycle, during oral contraceptive use, during early weeks of gestation, in the immediate postpartum period). Nevertheless, pregnancy is not contraindicated.

Other factors include drugs (including barbiturates, hydantoins, other antiepileptic drugs, and sulfonamide antibiotics—see Table 172–4) and reproductive hormones (progesterone and related steroids), particularly those that induce hepatic ALA synthase and cytochrome P-450 enzymes. Attacks usually occur within 24 h after exposure to a precipitating drug.

Exposure to sunlight precipitates cutaneous symptoms in variegate porphyria and hereditary coproporphyria.

Symptoms and Signs

Symptoms and signs of acute porphyrias involve the nervous system, abdomen, or both (neurovisceral). Attacks develop over hours or days and can last up to several weeks. Most gene carriers experience no, or only a few, attacks during their lifetime. Others experience recurrent symptoms. In women, recurrent attacks often coincide with the luteal phase of the menstrual cycle.

The acute porphyric attack: Constipation, fatigue, irritability, and insomnia typically precede an acute attack. The most common symptoms of an attack are abdominal pain and vomiting. The pain may be excruciating and is disproportionate to abdominal tenderness or other physical signs. Abdominal manifestations may result from effects on visceral nerves or from local vasoconstrictive ischemia. Because there is no

Table 172–4. DRUGS AND PORPHYRIA*

CATEGORY/DISORDER TREATED	UNSAFE	SAFE	PROBABLY SAFE
Analgesic	Dextropropoxyphene[†] Diclofenac Meprobamate Propoxyphene[†] Tramadol	Aspirin Buprenorphine Caffeine Codeine Morphine Propofol	Atropine Dexibuprofen[†] Fentanyl Hydromorphone Ketobemidone[†] Ketoprofen Naproxen
Anesthetic (local)	Lidocaine	Bupivacaine	Articaine
Anesthetic (premedication, induction, or maintenance)	Barbiturates	Atropine Morphine Propofol	Alfentanil Desflurane Droperidol Fentanyl Isoflurane- Remifentanil Scopolamine Sufentanil
Antidepressant	—	Lithium	Fluoxetine
Antidiarrheal	—	Active carbon Loperamide	—
Antiemetic	—	Chlorpromazine	Granisetron Ondansetron Scopolamine Tropisetron[†]
Anticonvulsant	Barbiturates Carbamazepine Diones (paramethadione[†], trimethadione) Felbamate Lamotrigine Mephenytoin[†] Phenytoin Primidone Succinimides (ethosuximide, methsuximide) Valproate	—	Clonazepam Diazepam (active seizure) Gabapentin Levetiracetam Topiramate Vigabatrin
Antihyperglycemic	Sulfonylureas	Acarbose Insulin Metformin	—
Anti-infective	Chloramphenicol Clindamycin Erythromycin Indinavir Ketoconazole Mecillinam[†] Nitrofurantoin Pivampicillin[†] Pivmecillinam[†] Rifampin Ritonavir Sulfonamides Trimethoprim	Acyclovir Amikacin Amoxicillin Amoxicillin with a beta-lactamase inhibitor Ampicillin Cloxacillin[†] Dicloxacillin Fusidic acid[†] Ganciclovir Gentamicin Immune globulin Immune sera Methenamine hippurate Netilmicin[†] Oseltamivir Penicillin G Penicillin V Piperacillin Teicoplanin[†] Tobramycin Vaccines Valacyclovir Vancomycin Zanamivir	Amphotericin B Azithromycin Bacampicillin[†] Cephalosporins Ciprofloxacin Didanosine Ethambutol Ertapenem Famciclovir Flucytosine Foscarnet Fosfomycin Imipenem/cilastatin Levofloxacin Meropenem Moxifloxacin Norfloxacin[†] Ofloxacin Piperacillin with tazobactam Ribavirin

Table continues on the following page.

Table 172–4. DRUGS AND PORPHYRIA* (*Continued*)

CATEGORY/DISORDER TREATED	UNSAFE	SAFE	PROBABLY SAFE
Anti-inflammatory or antirheumatic	—	Hyaluronic acid Penicillamine Salicylates	Abacavir Dexibuprofen† Ibuprofen Ketoprofen Lamivudine Lornoxicam† Naproxen Piroxicam Tenofovir disoproxil fumarate Tenoxicam† Zalcitabine†
Anxiolytic, sedative-hypnotic, or antipsychotic	Ethchlorvynol† Glutethimide† Hydroxyzine Meprobamate	Chlorpromazine Droperidol Fluoxetine Fluphenazine Haloperidol Levomepromazine† Prochlorperazine Propiomazine†	Alprazolam Clozapine Dixyrazine† Eszopiclone Lorazepam Olanzapine Oxazepam Perphenazine Triazolam
Cardiovascular disorders	Dihydralazine† Ergoloid mesylates Hydralazine Lidocaine Methyldopa Nifedipine Spironolactone	Amiloride Beta-blockers Cholestyramine Colestipol Digoxin Diltiazem Enalapril Epinephrine Heparins Lisinopril Losartan Niacin Organic nitrates	Adenosine Amrinone Bendroflumethiazide Bezafibrate† Bumetanide Digitalis glycosides Dobutamine Dopamine Dopexamine† Doxazosin Ethacrynic acid Etilefrine† Fenofibrate Furosemide Hydrochlorothiazide Milrinone Phenylephrine Prostaglandins Quinidine
Hormones	Danazol Progesterone Synthetic progestins	Nonreproductive hormones, including glucocorticoids	Natural estrogens
Laxatives	—	Bisacodyl Cascara sagrada Dietary fiber Lactitol† Lactulose Lauryl sulfate Psyllium seed Senna glycosides Sodium docusate Sodium picosulfate† Sorbitol	—
Migraines	Ergots	—	—
Muscle relaxants	Carisoprodol Orphenadrine	Atracurium Cisatracurium Mivacurium† Pancuronium Rocuronium Succinylcholine (suxamethonium) Vecuronium	Baclofen

Table 172–4. DRUGS AND PORPHYRIA* (*Continued*)

CATEGORY/DISORDER TREATED	UNSAFE	SAFE	PROBABLY SAFE
Osteoporosis	—	Bisphosphonates Calcium supplements	—
Peptic ulcers	—	Alginic acid Calcium-containing antacids Cimetidine Magnesium-containing antacids Sucralfate	Famotidine Misoprostol Nizatidine Ranitidine
Respiratory disorders	Clemastine Dimenhydrinate	Albuterol (salbutamol) Alimemazine† Codeine Corticosteroids Dipalmitoyl phosphatidylcholine Dornase alfa Ephedrine Ethylmorphine Ipratropium Phenylpropanolamine† Phospholipid surfactant	Bambuterol† Cromolyn Desloratadine Fenoterol† Fexofenadine Formoterol Levocabastine† Lidocaine (solution for gargling) Loratadine Mizolastine† Oxymetazoline Salmeterol Terbutaline Tiotropium

*The classification of the drugs in the list is based on a combination of clinical observations, case reports in the literature, and theoretical considerations derived from the structure and metabolism of the substances. However, clinical observations may in many cases be unreliable. Also, the biochemical and molecular-biologic models for the activation of the disease are incomplete. This list is meant as guidance only and is neither complete nor applicable to all patients. Drugs must always be used cautiously in people who carry genes for acute porphyria. For questions about specific drugs, physicians can consult www.drugs-porphyria.org.

†Not available in the US.

inflammation, the abdomen is not tender and there are no peritoneal signs. Temperature and WBC count are normal or only slightly increased. Bowel distention may develop as a result of paralytic ileus. The urine is red or reddish brown and positive for PBG during an attack.

All components of the peripheral nervous system and the CNS may be involved. Motor neuropathy is common with severe and prolonged attacks. Muscle weakness usually begins in the extremities but can involve any motor neuron or cranial nerve and proceed to tetraplegia. Bulbar involvement can cause respiratory failure.

CNS involvement may cause seizures or mental disturbances (eg, apathy, depression, agitation, frank psychosis, hallucinations). Seizures, psychotic behavior, and hallucinations may be due to or exacerbated by hyponatremia or hypomagnesemia, which can also contribute to cardiac arrhythmias. Hyponatremia may occur during an acute attack due to excessive vasopressin (antidiuretic hormone [ADH]) release and/or administration of hypotonic IV solutions (5% or 10% dextrose in water), a standard therapy for acute attacks.

Excess catecholamines generally cause restlessness and tachycardia. Rarely, catecholamine-induced arrhythmias cause sudden death. Labile hypertension with transiently high BP may cause vascular changes progressing to irreversible hypertension if untreated. Renal failure in acute porphyria is multifactorial; acute hypertension (possibly leading to chronic hypertension) is likely a main precipitating factor.

Subacute or subchronic symptoms: Some patients have prolonged symptoms of lesser intensity (eg, obstipation, fatigue, headache, back or thigh pain, paresthesia, tachycardia, dyspnea, insomnia, depression, anxiety or other disturbances of mood, seizures).

Skin symptoms in variegate porphyria and hereditary coproporphyria: Fragile skin and bullous eruptions may develop on sun-exposed areas, even in the absence of neurovisceral symptoms. Often patients are not aware of the connection to sun exposure. Cutaneous manifestations are identical to those of PCT; lesions typically occur on the dorsal aspects of the hands and forearms, the face, ears, and neck.

Late manifestations of acute porphyrias: Motor involvement during acute attacks may lead to persistent muscle weakness and muscle atrophy between attacks. Cirrhosis, hepatocellular carcinoma, systemic arterial hypertension, and renal impairment become more common after middle age in AIP and possibly also in VP and HCP, especially in patients with previous porphyric attacks.

Diagnosis

- Urine screen for PBG
- If urine results are positive, quantitative ALA and PBG determination
- For confirmation of AIP, measurement of PBG deaminase activity in erythrocytes
- Genetic analysis if type is to be identified

Acute attack: Misdiagnosis is common because the acute attack is confused with other causes of acute abdomen (sometimes leading to unnecessary surgery) or with a primary neurologic or mental disorder. However, in patients previously diagnosed as gene carriers or who have a positive family history, porphyria should be suspected. Still, even in known gene carriers, other causes must be considered.

Red or reddish brown urine, not present before onset of symptoms, is a cardinal sign and is present during full-blown attacks. A urine specimen should be examined in patients with abdominal pain of unknown cause, especially if severe constipation, vomiting, tachycardia, muscle weakness, bulbar involvement, or mental symptoms occur.

If porphyria is suspected, the urine is analyzed for PBG using a rapid qualitative or semiquantitative determination. A positive result or high clinical suspicion necessitates quantitative ALA and PBG measurements preferentially obtained from the same specimen. PBG and ALA levels > 5 times normal indicate an acute porphyric attack unless patients are gene carriers in whom porphyrin precursor excretion occurs at similar levels even during the latent phase of the disorder.

If urinary PBG and ALA levels are normal, an alternative diagnosis must be considered. Measurement of urinary total porphyrins and high-performance liquid chromatography profiles of these porphyrins are helpful. Elevated urinary ALA and coproporphyrin with normal or slightly increased PBG suggests lead poisoning, ALAD-deficiency porphyria, or hereditary tyrosinemia type 1. Analysis of a 24-h urine specimen is not necessary. Instead, a random urine specimen is used, and PBG and ALA levels are corrected for dilution by relating to the creatinine level of the sample.

Electrolytes including magnesium should be measured. Hyponatremia may be present because of excessive vomiting or diarrhea after hypotonic fluid replacement or because of the syndrome of inappropriate antidiuretic hormone secretion (SIADH).

Determination of acute porphyria type: Because treatment does not depend on the type of acute porphyria, identification of the specific type is valuable mainly for finding gene carriers among relatives. When the type and mutation are already known from previous testing of relatives, the diagnosis is clear but may be confirmed by gene analysis.

Activity of the enzymes ALAD and PBGD in the red blood cells is readily measurable and can be helpful for establishing the diagnosis in ALAD-deficiency porphyria and AIP, respectively. RBC PBG deaminase levels that are about 50% of normal suggest AIP.

If there is no family history to guide the diagnosis, the different forms of acute porphyria are distinguished by characteristic patterns of porphyrin (and precursor) accumulation and excretion in plasma, urine, and stool. When urinalysis reveals increased levels of ALA and PBG, fecal porphyrins may be measured. Fecal porphyrins are usually normal or minimally increased in AIP but elevated in HCP and VP. Often, these markers are not present in the quiescent phase of the disorder. Plasma fluorescence emission after excitation with Soret band of light (~410 nm) can be used to differentiate HCP and VP, which have different peak emissions.

Family studies in acute porphyrias: Children of a gene carrier for an AD form of acute porphyria (AIP, HCP, VP) have a 50% risk of inheriting the disorder. In contrast, children of patients with ALAD-deficiency porphyria (autosomal recessive inheritance) are obligate carriers but are very unlikely to develop clinical disease. Because early diagnosis followed by counseling reduces the risk of morbidity, children in affected families should be tested before the onset of puberty. Genetic testing is used if the mutation has been identified in the index case. If not, pertinent RBC or WBC enzyme levels are measured. Gene analysis can be used for in utero diagnosis (using amniocentesis or chorionic villus sampling) but is seldom indicated because of the favorable outlook for most gene carriers.

Prognosis

Advances in medical care and self-care have improved the prognosis of acute porphyrias for symptomatic patients. Still, some patients develop recurrent crises or progressive disease with permanent paralysis or renal failure. Also, frequent need for opioids analgesics may give rise to opioid dependence.

Treatment

- Triggers eliminated if possible
- Dextrose (oral or IV)
- IV heme

Treatment of the acute attack is identical for all the acute porphyrias. Possible triggers (eg, excessive alcohol use, drugs) are identified and eliminated. Unless the attack is mild, patients are hospitalized in a darkened, quiet, private room. Heart rate, BP, and fluid and electrolyte balance are monitored. Neurologic status, bladder function, muscle and tendon function, respiratory function, and oxygen saturation are continuously monitored. Symptoms (eg, pain, vomiting) are treated with nonporphyrinogenic drugs as needed (see Table 172–4).

Dextrose 300 to 500 g daily down-regulates hepatic ALA synthase (ALAS 1) and relieves symptoms. Dextrose can be given by mouth if patients are not vomiting; otherwise, it is given IV. The usual regimen is 3 L of 10% dextrose solution, given by a central venous catheter over 24 h (125 mL/h). However, to avoid overhydration with consequent hyponatremia, 1 L of 50% dextrose solution can be used instead.

IV heme is more effective than dextrose and should be given immediately in severe attacks, electrolyte imbalance, or muscle weakness. Heme usually resolves symptoms in 3 to 4 days. If heme therapy is delayed, nerve damage is more severe and recovery is slower and possibly incomplete. Heme is available in the US as lyophilized hematin to be reconstituted in a glass vial with sterile water. The dose is 3 to 4 mg/kg IV once/day for 4 days. An alternative is heme arginate, which is given at the same dose, except that it is diluted in 5% dextrose or half-normal or quarter-normal saline. Hematin and heme arginate may cause venous thrombosis and/or thrombophlebitis. Risk of these adverse events appears to be lower if the heme is administered bound to human serum albumin. Such binding also decreases the rate of development of hematin aggregates. Thus, most authorities recommend administration of hematin or heme arginate with human serum albumin.

Recurrent attacks: In patients with severe recurrent attacks, who are at risk of renal damage or permanent neurologic damage, liver transplantation is an option. Successful liver transplantation leads to permanent cure of AIP. The deficiency in hepatic PBG deaminase is corrected with liver transplantation, resulting in biochemical (normal levels of PBG and ALA) and symptomatic resolution.[1] Clinical experience with liver transplantation for AIP has been limited to 14 described cases, with survival rates similar to transplantation for other indications; survival at 3 mo was 93%, and at 5 yr, survival was 77%. Liver transplantation has not been described in hereditary coproporphyria. One child with ALAD underwent liver transplantation with a decrease in hospitalizations but no improvement in biochemical markers.[2]

Although not recognized in the latest American Association for the Study of Liver Disease (AASLD) as a distinct indication for liver transplantation, the hepatic porphyrias would accurately be included within the liver-based metabolic conditions with systemic manifestations. In the absence of standardized Model for End-Stage Liver Disease (MELD) exception points, liver transplantation for AIP would rely upon petition to the regional review board within the transplant center's United Network for Organ Sharing (UNOS) region.

Patients with acute porphyrias should not serve as liver donors even though their liver may appear structurally normal (ie, no cirrhosis) because recipients have developed acute porphyric syndromes; such an outcome helped establish that the acute porphyrias are hepatic disorders. Kidney transplantation, with or without simultaneous liver exchange, should be considered in patients with active disease and terminal renal failure because there is considerable risk that nerve damage will progress at the start of dialysis.

1. Dowman JK, Gunson BK, Mirza DF, et al: Liver transplant for acute intermittent porphyria is complicated by a high rate of hepatic artery thrombosis. *Liver Transpl* 18: 195–200, 2012. doi: 10.1002/lt.22345.
2. Thunell S, Henrichson A, Floderus Y, et al: Liver transplantation in a boy with acute porphyria due to aminolaevulinate dehydratase deficiency. *Eur J Clin Chem Clin Biochem* 30:599–606, 1992.

Prevention

Carriers of acute porphyria should avoid the following:

- Potentially harmful drugs (see Table 172–4)
- Heavy alcohol use
- Physical or emotional stress or exhaustion
- Exposure to organic solvents (eg, in painting or dry cleaning)
- Crash diets
- Periods of starvation

Diets for obesity should provide gradual weight loss and be adopted only during periods of remission. Carriers of VP or HCP should minimize sun exposure; sunscreens that block only ultraviolet B light are ineffective, but opaque zinc oxide or titanium dioxide preparations are beneficial. Support associations, such as the American Porphyria Foundation and the European Porphyria Network, can provide written information and direct counseling.

Patients should be identified prominently in the medical record as carriers and should carry a card verifying the carrier state and precautions to be observed.

A high-carbohydrate diet may decrease the risk of acute attacks. Some patients can sometimes treat mild acute attacks by increasing their intake of dextrose or glucose. Prolonged use should be avoided in order to decrease risk of obesity and dental caries.

Patients who experience recurrent and predictable attacks (typically women with attacks related to the menstrual cycle) may benefit from prophylactic heme therapy given shortly before the expected onset. There is no standardized regimen; a specialist should be consulted. Frequent premenstrual attacks in some women are aborted by administration of a gonadotropin-releasing hormone agonist plus low-dose estrogen. Low-dose oral contraceptives are sometimes used successfully, but the progestin component is likely to exacerbate the porphyria.

To prevent renal damage, chronic hypertension should be treated aggressively (using safe drugs). Patients with evidence of impaired renal function are referred to a nephrologist. Recent anecdotal experience indicates that tolvaptan, a vasopressin receptor blocker, is helpful in the management of hyponatremia during acute attacks.

The incidence of hepatocellular cancer is high among carriers of acute porphyria, especially in patients with active disease. Patients who are > 50 should undergo yearly or twice yearly surveillance, including liver screening with ultrasonography. Early intervention can be curative and increases life expectancy.

KEY POINTS

- Acute porphyrias cause intermittent attacks of abdominal pain and neurologic symptoms; some types also have cutaneous manifestations that are triggered by sun exposure.
- Attacks have many triggers, including hormones, drugs, low-calorie and low-carbohydrate diets, and alcohol ingestion.
- Attacks typically involve severe abdominal pain (with a non-tender abdomen) and vomiting; any component of the peripheral and central nervous system may be affected but muscle weakness is common.
- Urine is often reddish-brown during an attack.
- Do a qualitative urine test for porphobilinogen (PBG) and confirm a positive result with quantitative ALA and PBG measurements.
- Treat acute attacks with oral or IV dextrose and, for severe attacks, IV heme.

OVERVIEW OF CUTANEOUS PORPHYRIAS

Cutaneous porphyrias result from deficiency (and in one case, excess) of certain enzymes in the heme biosynthetic pathway (see Table 172–1), resulting in a relatively steady production of phototoxic porphyrins in the liver or bone marrow. These porphyrins accumulate in the skin and, on sunlight exposure (visible light, including near-ultraviolet [UV]), generate cytotoxic radicals that cause recurrent or unremitting cutaneous manifestations.

Cutaneous porphyrias include

- Porphyria cutanea tarda (PCT)
- Erythropoietic protoporphyria (EPP)
- Congenital erythropoietic porphyria (CEP—see Table 172–5)
- XLPP, sometimes regarded as a clinical variant of EPP
- Hepatoerythropoietic porphyria (HEP—see Table 172–5), sometimes regarded as a type of PCT (extremely rare)

The acute porphyrias variegate porphyria (VP) and hereditary coproporphyria (HCP) also have cutaneous manifestations. For porphyria etiology and pathophysiology, see p. 1330.

In all cutaneous porphyrias except EPP and XLPP, cutaneous photosensitivity manifests as fragile skin and bullous eruptions. Skin changes generally occur on sun-exposed areas (eg, face, neck, dorsal aspects of hands and forearms) or traumatized skin. The cutaneous reaction is insidious, and often patients are unaware of the connection to sun exposure. In contrast, the photosensitivity in EPP and XLPP occurs within minutes or hours after sun exposure, manifesting as a burning pain that persists for hours, without any blistering and often without any objective signs on the skin. However, swelling and erythema may occur. Chronic liver disorders are common in cutaneous porphyrias.

The cutaneous porphyrias are all accompanied by elevated total plasma porphyrins, and are specifically diagnosed by measurements of porphyrins in RBCs, plasma, urine, and stool, as well as by genetic or enzyme analysis. Treatment involves avoidance of sunlight, measures to protect the skin, and sometimes other treatments directed according to the specific diagnosis.

Table 172–5. SOME LESS COMMON PORPHYRIAS

DESCRIPTION	SYMPTOMS AND SIGNS	DIAGNOSIS	TREATMENT
Congenital erythropoietic porphyria (Günther disease)			
Severe deficiency of uroporphyrinogen III cosynthase (UROS)	In utero or shortly after birth: Severe cases manifesting as nonimmune hydrops Soon after birth: Skin blistering, hemolytic anemia, hyperbilirubinemia, red urine, dark diapers that show a red fluorescence under UV light Phototherapy for hyperbilirubinemia leads to severe skin blistering. In adulthood: Facial disfiguration, increased hair growth, corneal scarring (possibly severe), hemolytic anemia, splenomegaly, erythrodontia, deposition of porphyrins in bone, bone demineralization (possibly substantial)	Porphyrins in plasma, urine, and stool elevated to levels higher than those in other porphyrias, with uroporphyrin I and coproporphyrin I the predominant porphyrins in urine and stool Urinary ALA and PBG virtually normal Can be confirmed by low RBC UROS activity (< 10%), but test not readily available Genetic analysis of UROS gene, which reveals homozygous or compound heterozygous mutations on chromosome 10 (most common mutation is C73R) For in utero diagnosis: Measurement of amniotic porphyrins or genetic analysis	Avoidance of sunlight (including lights for treating neonatal hyperbilirubinemia) Use of sun-protective clothing Avoidance of skin trauma Prompt treatment of secondary bacterial infections to help prevent scarring Splenectomy possibly beneficial for patients with hemolytic anemia Repeated RBC transfusions and hydroxyurea to keep bone marrow porphyrin production low; deferoxamine for transfusion-related iron overload Hematopoietic stem cell transplantation potentially curative
Hepatoerythropoietic porphyria			
Severe deficiency of uroporphyrinogen decarboxylase (UROD)	Skin blistering Red urine Anemia	Elevated isocoproporphyrin in stool and urine Elevated zinc protoporphyrin in RBCs (to differentiate from PCT) Confirmed by very low RBC UROD activity Genetic analysis of UROD gene, which reveals homozygous or compound heterozygous mutations	Avoidance of sunlight Phlebotomy possibly beneficial to patients with milder cases Treatment of severe disease similar to that of congenital erythropoietic porphyria
Dual porphyria			
Disorders resulting from deficiencies of > 1 enzyme of the heme biosynthetic pathway	Clinical and biochemical manifestations of both disorders In acute porphyrias: Neurovisceral symptoms triggered by porphyrogenic agents In cutaneous porphyrias: Hypersensitivity to sunlight with blistering and fragile skin	Porphyrin and porphyrin precursor excretion patterns Confirmed by family history and enzyme analyses	In acute porphyrias: Avoidance of triggering agents In cutaneous porphyrias: Skin protection and avoidance of sunlight

ALA = delta-aminolevulinic acid; PBG = porphobilinogen; PCT = porphyria cutanea tarda; UV = ultraviolet.

PORPHYRIA CUTANEA TARDA

Porphyria cutanea tarda (PCT) is a comparatively common hepatic porphyria affecting mainly the skin. Liver disease is also common. PCT is due to an acquired or inherited deficiency in the activity of hepatic UROD, an enzyme in the heme biosynthetic pathway (see Table 172–1). Porphyrins accumulate, particularly when there is increased oxidative stress in the hepatocytes, which is usually due to increased hepatic iron, but which may also be due to alcohol, smoking, estrogens, or hepatitis C or HIV infection. Symptoms include fragile, easily blistered skin, mainly on sun-exposed areas. Diagnosis is by porphyrin analysis of urine and stool. Differentiation from the acute, cutaneous porphyrias hereditary coproporphyria and variegate porphyria is important. Treatment includes iron depletion by phlebotomy and enhancing porphyrin excretion by treatment with low dose chloroquine or hydroxychloroquine. Prevention is by

avoidance of sunlight, alcohol, smoking, estrogens, and iron-containing drugs and successful treatment of any concomitant hepatitis C and HIV infections.

Pathophysiology

PCT results from hepatic deficiency of UPGD (see Table 172–1). Porphyrins accumulate in the liver and are transported to the skin, where they cause photosensitivity.

The partial (~50%) deficiency in UROD activity in heterozygous patients itself is not sufficient to cause biochemical or clinical features of PCT; additional factors (eg, elevated hepatic iron, alcohol use, halogenated hydrocarbon exposure, hepatitis C virus or HIV infection) are required to cause the > 75% decrease in hepatic UROD activity needed for features of PCT to manifest. These factors increase the oxidation of uroporphyrinogens and other porphyrinogens to the corresponding porphyrins and also help form inhibitors of UROD. The drugs that commonly trigger acute porphyria (see Table 172–4) do not trigger PCT.

Liver disease is common in PCT and may be due partly to porphyrin accumulation, chronic hepatitis C infection, concomitant hemosiderosis, or excess alcohol ingestion. Cirrhosis occurs in ≤ 35% of patients, and hepatocellular carcinoma occurs in 7 to 24% (more common among middle-aged men).

There are two main types of PCT:

- Type 1: Acquired or sporadic
- Type 2: Hereditary or familial

Type 1 accounts for 75 to 80% of cases, and type 2 for 20 to 25%.

In **type 1 PCT,** decarboxylase deficiency is restricted to the liver and no genetic predisposition is present. It usually manifests in middle age or later.

In **type 2 PCT,** decarboxylase deficiency is inherited in an AD fashion with limited penetrance. Deficiency occurs in all cells, including RBCs. It may develop earlier than type 1, occasionally in childhood. The partial (~50%) deficiency in UROD activity in heterozygous patients itself is not sufficient to cause biochemical or clinical features of PCT; additional factors (eg, elevated hepatic iron, alcohol use, halogenated hydrocarbon exposure, hepatitis C virus or HIV infection) are required to cause the > 75% decrease in hepatic UROD activity needed for features of PCT to manifest. These factors increase the oxidation of uroporphyrinogens and other porphyrinogens to the corresponding porphyrins and also help form inhibitors of UROD.

Hepatoerythropoietic porphyria (HEP—see Table 172–5), which features profound UROD deficiency, is very rare and is often regarded as an autosomal recessive form of type 2 PCT.

Type 3 PCT, which is very rare, is hereditary but without any defect in the *UROD* gene; a defect in another, unidentified gene appears to be the cause. Type 3 accounts for < 1% of cases.

Types 1 and 2 are the major forms of the disease. They have the same precipitants, symptoms, and treatment. Overall prevalence may be on the order of 1/10,000 but is probably higher in people exposed to halogenated aromatic hydrocarbons or other precipitants of the disease.

Pseudoporphyria: Renal failure, ultraviolet radiation (UVA) and certain drugs can cause PCT-like symptoms without elevated porphyrin levels (pseudoporphyria). Commonly implicated drugs are furosemide, tetracyclines, sulfonamides, and naproxen and other NSAIDs.

Because porphyrins are poorly dialyzed, some patients receiving long-term hemodialysis develop a skin condition that resembles PCT; this condition is termed pseudoporphyria of end-stage renal disease.

Symptoms and Signs

Patients with PCT present with fragile skin, mainly on sun-exposed areas. Phototoxicity is delayed: patients do not always connect sun exposure with symptoms.

Spontaneously or after minor trauma, tense bullae develop. Some bullae are hemorrhagic. Accompanying erosions and ulcers may develop secondary infection; they heal slowly, leaving atrophic scars. Sun exposure occasionally leads to erythema, edema, or itching.

Hyperemic conjunctivitis may develop, but other mucosal sites are not affected.

Areas of hypopigmentation or hyperpigmentation may develop, as may facial hypertrichosis and pseudosclerodermoid changes.

Diagnosis

- Elevated levels of plasma porphyrins, urinary uroporphyrin and heptacarboxyl porphyrin, and fecal isocoproporphyrin

In otherwise healthy patients, fragile skin and blister formation suggest PCT. Differentiation from acute porphyrias with cutaneous symptoms (variegate porphyria [VP] and hereditary coproporphyria [HCP]) is important because in patients with VP and HCP, the erroneous prescription of porphyrogenic drugs may trigger the severe neurovisceral symptoms of the acute porphyrias. Previous unexplained neurologic symptoms or abdominal pain may suggest an acute porphyria. A history of exposure to chemicals that can cause pseudoporphyria should be sought.

Although all porphyrias that cause skin lesions are accompanied by elevated plasma porphyrins, elevated urinary uroporphyrin and heptacarboxyl porphyrin and fecal isocoproporphyrin indicate PCT. Urine levels of PBG is normal in PCT. Urinary ALA may be slightly increased (< 3 times the upper limit of normal). RBC activity of UROD is normal in type 1 and type 3 PCT but decreased (by ~50%) in type 2.

All patients with PCT should be tested for hepatitis C and HIV infections. They should also be tested for iron overload with serum iron and ferritin levels, and total iron-binding capacity; if results suggest iron overload, genetic testing for hereditary hemochromatosis is done.

Treatment

Two different therapeutic strategies are available:

- Reduction of body iron stores
- Increase in porphyrin excretion

These strategies can be combined for more rapid remission. The treatment is monitored by determinations of serum ferritin (if iron reduction therapy is used) and urinary porphyrin excretion every other or every 3rd month until full remission.

Iron removal by therapeutic phlebotomy is usually effective. A unit of blood is removed every week or two. When serum ferritin falls slightly below normal, phlebotomy is stopped. Usually, 6 to 10 sessions are needed. Urine and plasma porphyrins fall gradually with treatment, lagging behind but paralleling the fall in ferritin. The skin eventually becomes normal. After remission, further phlebotomy is needed only if there is a recurrence.

Low-dose chloroquine or hydroxychloroquine 100 to 125 mg po twice/wk removes excess porphyrins from the liver and perhaps other tissues by increasing the excretion rate. Higher doses can cause transient liver damage and worsening of porphyria. When remission is achieved, the regimen is stopped.

Chloroquine and hydroxychloroquine are not effective in advanced renal disease, and phlebotomy is usually contraindicated because of underlying anemia. However, recombinant erythropoietin mobilizes excess iron and resolves the anemia enough to permit phlebotomy. In end-stage renal disease, deferoxamine is an adjunct to phlebotomy for reduction of hepatic iron, the complexed iron being removed during dialysis. Dialyzers with ultrapermeable membranes and extra high blood flow rates are needed.

Patients with overt PCT and hepatitis C infection should be evaluated for treatment with pegylated interferon alfa-2a, ribavirin, and an antiviral drug (telaprevir, boceprevir). Previous iron depletion augments the response to antiviral therapy.

Children with symptomatic PCT are treated with small-volume phlebotomies or oral chloroquine; dosage is determined by body weight.

Skin symptoms occurring during pregnancy are treated with phlebotomy. In refractory cases, low-dose chloroquine can be added; no teratogenic effects have been recognized. Depending on degree of hemodilution and iron depletion, the skin symptoms usually abate as pregnancy advances.

Postmenopausal estrogen supplementation is interrupted during treatment for PCT. Stopping estrogens often induces remission.

Prevention

Patients should avoid sun exposure; hats and clothing protect best, as do zinc or titanium oxide sunscreens. Typical sunscreens that block UV light are ineffective, but UVA-absorbing sunscreens, such as those containing dibenzylmethanes, may help somewhat. Alcohol ingestion should be avoided permanently, but estrogen supplementation can usually be resumed safely after a disease remission.

KEY POINTS

- PCT is usually acquired but may be hereditary.
- Triggers include elevated hepatic iron, alcohol use, halogenated hydrocarbon exposure, and hepatitis C virus or HIV infection.
- Drugs that commonly trigger acute porphyria do not trigger PCT.
- Measure urinary uroporphyrin and heptacarboxyl porphyrin, and fecal isocoproporphyrin.
- Test for iron overload with serum iron and ferritin levels and total iron-binding capacity.
- Reduce elevated iron stores by phlebotomy.
- Remove excess porphyrins by giving low-dose chloroquine or hydroxychloroquine.

ERYTHROPOIETIC PROTOPORPHYRIA AND X-LINKED PROTOPORPHYRIA

Erythropoietic protoporphyria (EPP) is due to an inherited deficiency in the activity of the enzyme ferrochelatase, and X-linked protoporphyria (XLPP) is due to an inherited increase in the activity of ALAS 2; both enzymes are in the heme biosynthetic pathway (see Table 172–1). EPP and XLPP are nearly identical clinically. They typically manifest in infancy with itching or burning skin pain after even short exposure to sunlight. Gallstones are common later in life, and chronic liver disease occurs in about 10%. Diagnosis is based on symptoms and increased levels of protoporphyrin in RBCs and plasma. Prevention is by avoidance of triggers (eg, sunlight, alcohol, fasting) and perhaps use of oral beta-carotene. Acute skin symptoms can be alleviated by cold baths or wet towels, analgesics, and topical and/or oral corticosteroids. Patients with liver failure may need liver transplantation, but liver transplantation is not curative because the predominant source of excess protoporphyrin production is the bone marrow.

Because XLPP is so similar to EPP, it is sometimes regarded as a variant of EPP. For porphyria etiology and pathophysiology, see p. 1330.

Etiology

EPP, which comprises about 90% of EPP phenotypic presentations results from inherited deficiency of the enzyme ferrochelatase (FECH). The inheritance pattern is autosomal recessive; thus, clinical manifestations occur only in people with 2 defective FECH alleles, or more commonly, one defective and one low-expressing wild-type allele.

XLPP, which comprises the remaining 10% of cases, results from gain-of-function mutations that increase the activity of erythroid-specific delta-aminolevulinate synthase (ALAS 2) in the bone marrow; the inheritance is X-linked. The phenotype of heterozygous females can vary from asymptomatic that of affected males.

Prevalence of EPP phenotype is about 1/75,000. Protoporphyrin accumulates in bone marrow and RBCs, enters the plasma, and is deposited in the skin or excreted by the liver into bile. About 10% of patients develop chronic liver disease; a few of these patients develop cirrhosis, which may progress to liver failure. A more common complication is pigment gallstones due to heavy protoporphyrin excretion.

Symptoms and Signs

Symptom severity in erythropoietic protoporphyria and XLPP varies greatly, even among patients within a single family. Most patients develop symptoms in early childhood. Brief exposure to sunlight can cause severe pain, burning, erythema, and edema of the exposed skin. Usually, an infant or young child cries for hours after even short exposure to sun. Sometimes skin swelling and erythema may be subtle or absent, and EPP and XLPP may go undiagnosed longer than any other of the porphyrias.

Crusting may develop around the lips and on the back of the hands after prolonged sun exposure. However, blistering and scarring, as are typical in PCT, hereditary coproporphyria, and congenital erythropoietic porphyria (see Table 172–5), do not occur.

If skin protection is chronically neglected, rough, thickened, and leathery skin (lichenification) may develop, especially over the knuckles. Linear perioral furrows (carp mouth) may develop. Patients with XLPP tend to have more severe photosensitivity and liver disease than those with EPP.

If unrecognized, EPP and XLPP may cause psychosocial problems because children inexplicably refuse to go outdoors.

The fear or anticipation of pain may be so distressing that children become nervous, tense, aggressive, or even develop feelings of detachment from the surroundings or suicidal thoughts.

Diagnosis

- RBC and plasma protoporphyrin measurement
- Genetic testing for *FECH* or *ALAS 2* gene mutations

EPP or XLPP should be suspected in children and adults with painful cutaneous photosensitivity who experience no blisters or scarring. Gallstones in children should prompt testing for EPP and XLPP. Family history is usually negative.

The diagnosis is confirmed by finding increased RBC and plasma protoporphyrin levels. RBC protoporphyrin should also be fractionated to determine the proportions of metal-free and zinc protoporphyrin. In EPP, the proportion of RBC protoporphyrin that is metal-free is almost always > 85%. The presence of > 15% zinc protoporphyrin suggests XLPP.

If measured, plasma coproporphyrin and urinary porphyrin levels are normal. Stool protoporphyrin may be elevated, but coproporphyrin level is normal.

Potential carriers among relatives can be identified by showing increased RBC protoporphyrin and by genetic testing if a mutation has been identified in the index case.

Treatment

- Avoidance of sun exposure through use of protective clothing and opaque sunscreens
- Symptomatic treatment for skin burning with cold compresses, NSAIDs, and topical and/or oral corticosteroids
- Sometimes oral beta-carotene for prevention
- Management of hepatobiliary complications
- Afamelanotide for prevention of phototoxic events and relief of symptoms

Patients with erythropoietic protoporphyria or XLPP should avoid sun exposure; protective clothing, hats, and light-opaque titanium dioxide or zinc oxide containing sunscreens should be used.

Oral beta-carotene, an antioxidant, reduces photosensitivity. However, patient adherence with beta-carotene is often poor because it is not very effective in controlling symptoms and also causes orange skin pigmentation. Beta-carotene dose depends on patient's age (see Table 172–6).

Other drugs that also may decrease photosensitivity include cysteine, an antioxidant, and afamelanotide, a synthetic analog of melanocyte stimulating hormone. Afamelanotide is currently available in parts of the European Union. In two multicenter randomized, double-blind, placebo-controlled trials (United States and European Union) in patients with erythropoietic protoporphyria, afamelanotide decreased the number of phototoxic events, decreased recovery time from phototoxic events, and improved quality of life with an acceptable adverse effect profile.[1]

Drugs that trigger acute porphyrias need not be avoided (see Table 172–4).

Acute skin symptoms can be alleviated by cold baths or wet towels, analgesics, and topical and/or oral corticosteroids. Symptoms can take up to a week to resolve. If these measures are ineffective (eg, patients have increasing photosensitivity, rising porphyrin levels, progressive jaundice), giving hematin and/or RBC hypertransfusion (ie, to above-normal Hb levels) may reduce protoporphyrin overproduction. Administration of bile acids may facilitate biliary excretion of protoporphyrin. Oral cholestyramine or charcoal have been used to interrupt the enterohepatic circulation of protoporphyrin and increase fecal excretion.

Patients who develop decompensated end-stage liver disease require liver transplantation. As with AIP, patients with EPP are not eligible for standardized Model for End-Stage Liver Disease (MELD)–exception points. However, liver transplantation does not correct the underlying metabolic defect and EPP hepatopathy often develops in the transplanted liver.

Hematopoietic stem cell transplantation is curative for EPP but is not routinely done because the risk typically outweighs the benefits. The strategy of hematopoietic stem cell transplantation after liver transplantation cures EPP and prevents recurrent EPP from damaging the allograft, but the optimal timing of this strategy has not been established. Patients should be protected from operating lights during liver transplantation or other prolonged surgery to avoid serious phototoxic injury to internal organs. Light sources should be covered with commercially available filters that block wavelengths ~380 to 420 nm. Endoscopy, laparoscopy, and brief (< 1.5 h) abdominal surgery do not usually cause phototoxic damage.

PEARLS & PITFALLS

- Operating room lights can cause phototoxic injury to internal organs in patients with erythropoietic protoporphyria.

Regular physician-patient consultations that provide information, discussion, and opportunities for genetic counseling together with physical checkups are important. Liver function and RBC and plasma protoporphyrin levels should be checked annually. Patients with abnormal liver function test results should be evaluated by a hepatologist; a liver biopsy may be needed to stage the degree of fibrosis. Patients with known chronic liver disease should undergo screening ultrasonography every 6 mo to check for hepatocellular carcinoma.

Vitamin D levels should be checked because deficiency is common (patients tend to avoid sun exposure); supplements are given if levels are low.

All patients with EPP should receive hepatitis A vaccine and hepatitis B vaccine and be advised to avoid alcohol.

1. Langendonk JG, Balwani M, Anderson KE, et al: Afamelanotide for erythropoietic protoporphyria. *N Engl J Med* 373:48–59, 2015. doi: 10.1056/NEJMoa1411481.

Table 172–6. DOSES OF BETA-CAROTENE IN ERYTHROPOIETIC PROTOPORPHYRIA

PATIENT AGE (YR)	DOSE (ORAL)
1–4	60–90 mg once/day
5–8	90–120 mg once/day
9–12	120–150 mg once/day
13–16	150–180 mg once/day
> 16	Up to 300 mg once/day*

*To maintain serum levels of 11–15 μmol/L.

KEY POINTS

- EPP causes burning pain with exposure to sunlight; symptoms are not brought on by drugs that trigger other porphyrias.
- Cirrhosis develops in about 10%, sometimes progressing to liver failure.
- Brief exposure to sunlight can cause severe pain, burning, erythema, and edema of exposed skin.
- Measure RBC and plasma protoporphyrin levels.
- Prevent symptoms by avoiding sun exposure and sometimes using drugs (eg, beta-carotene, cysteine).
- Hematin and/or RBC hypertransfusion may reduce protoporphyrin overproduction.
- XLPP is clinically similar to EPP, but photosensitivity and liver disease are more severe than in EPP.
- A useful clue for XLPP is a high proportion of RBC protoporphyrin that is zinc protoporphyrin.

173 Thyroid Disorders

The thyroid gland, located in the anterior neck just below the cricoid cartilage, consists of 2 lobes connected by an isthmus. Follicular cells in the gland produce the 2 main thyroid hormones:

- Tetraiodothyronine (thyroxine, T_4)
- Triiodothyronine (T_3)

These hormones act on cells in virtually every body tissue by combining with nuclear receptors and altering expression of a wide range of gene products. Thyroid hormone is required for normal brain and somatic tissue development in the fetus and neonate, and, in people of all ages, regulates protein, carbohydrate, and fat metabolism.

T_3 is the most active form in binding to the nuclear receptor; T_4 has only minimal hormonal activity. However, T_4 is much longer lasting and can be converted to T_3 (in most tissues) and thus serves as a reservoir for T_3. A 3rd form of thyroid hormone, reverse T_3 (rT_3), has no metabolic activity; levels of rT_3 increase in certain diseases.

Additionally, C cells secrete the hormone calcitonin, which is released in response to hypercalcemia and lowers serum Ca levels (see p. 1285).

Synthesis and Release of Thyroid Hormones

Synthesis of thyroid hormones requires iodine (see Fig. 173–1). Iodine, ingested in food and water as iodide, is actively

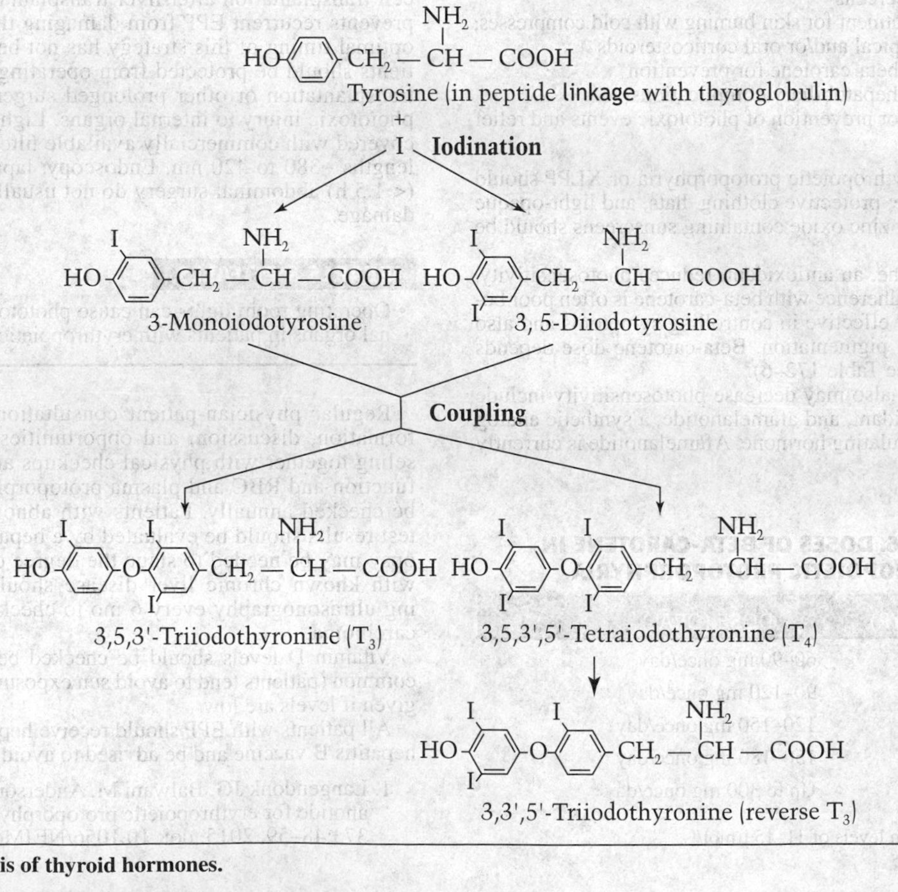

Tyrosine (in peptide linkage with thyroglobulin)
\+ I Iodination
3-Monoiodotyrosine
3, 5-Diiodotyrosine
Coupling
3,5,3'-Triiodothyronine (T_3)
3,5,3',5'-Tetraiodothyronine (T_4)
3,3',5'-Triiodothyronine (reverse T_3)

Fig. 173–1. Synthesis of thyroid hormones.

concentrated by the thyroid and converted to organic iodine (organification) within follicular cells by thyroid peroxidase. The follicular cells surround a space filled with colloid, which consists of thyroglobulin, a glycoprotein containing tyrosine within its matrix. Tyrosine in contact with the membrane of the follicular cells is iodinated at 1 (monoiodotyrosine) or 2 (diiodotyrosine) sites and then coupled to produce the 2 forms of thyroid hormone (diiodotyrosine + diiodotyrosine → T_4; diiodotyrosine + monoiodotyrosine → T_3).

T_3 and T_4 remain incorporated in thyroglobulin within the follicle until the follicular cells take up thyroglobulin as colloid droplets. Once inside the thyroid follicular cells, T_3 and T_4 are cleaved from thyroglobulin. Free T_3 and T_4 are then released into the bloodstream, where they are bound to serum proteins for transport, the major one being thyroxine-binding globulin (TBG), which has high affinity but low capacity for T_3 and T_4. TBG normally carries about 75% of bound thyroid hormones. The other binding proteins are T_4-binding prealbumin (transthyretin), which has high affinity but low capacity for T_4, and albumin, which has low affinity but high capacity for T_3 and T_4. About 0.3% of total serum T_3 and 0.03% of total serum T_4 are free and in equilibrium with bound hormones. Only free T_3 and free T_4 are available to act on the peripheral tissues.

All reactions necessary for the formation and release of T_3 and T_4 are controlled by thyroid-stimulating hormone (TSH), which is secreted by pituitary thyrotropic cells. TSH secretion is controlled by a negative feedback mechanism in the pituitary: Increased levels of free T_4 and T_3 inhibit TSH synthesis and secretion, whereas decreased levels increase TSH secretion. TSH secretion is also influenced by thyrotropin-releasing hormone (TRH), which is synthesized in the hypothalamus. The precise mechanisms regulating TRH synthesis and release are unclear, although negative feedback from thyroid hormones inhibits TRH synthesis.

Most circulating T_3 is produced outside the thyroid by monodeiodination of T_4. Only one-fifth of circulating T_3 is secreted directly by the thyroid.

Laboratory Testing of Thyroid Function

TSH measurement: TSH measurement is the best means of determining thyroid dysfunction (see Table 173–1). Normal results essentially rule out hyperthyroidism or hypothyroidism, except in patients with central hypothyroidism due to disease in the hypothalamus or pituitary gland or in rare patients with pituitary resistance to thyroid hormone. Serum TSH can be falsely low in very sick people.

The serum TSH level also defines the syndromes of subclinical hyperthyroidism (low serum TSH) and subclinical hypothyroidism (elevated serum TSH), both of which are characterized by normal serum T_4, free T_4, serum T_3, and free T_3 levels.

T_4 measurement: Total serum T_4 is a measure of bound and free hormone. Changes in levels of thyroid hormone–binding serum proteins produce corresponding changes in total T_4, even though levels of physiologically active free T_4 are unchanged. Thus, a patient may be physiologically normal but have an abnormal total serum T_4 level. Free T_4 in the serum can be measured directly, avoiding the pitfalls of interpreting total T_4 levels.

Free T_4 index is a calculated value that corrects total T_4 for the effects of varying amounts of thyroid hormone–binding serum proteins and thus gives an estimate of free T_4 when total T_4 is measured. The thyroid hormone–binding ratio or T_3 resin uptake is used to estimate protein binding. Free T_4 index is readily available and compares well with direct measurement of free T_4.

T_3 measurement: Total serum T_3 and free T_3 can also be measured. Because T_3 is tightly bound to TBG (although 10 times less so than T_4), total serum T_3 levels are influenced by alterations in serum TBG level and by drugs that affect binding to TBG. Free T_3levels in the serum are measured by the same direct and indirect methods (free T_3 index) described for T_4 and are used mainly for evaluating thyrotoxicosis.

T_4-binding globulin: TBG can be measured. It is increased in pregnancy, by estrogen therapy or oral contraceptive use, and in the acute phase of infectious hepatitis. TBG may also be increased by an X-linked abnormality. It is most commonly

Table 173–1. RESULTS OF THYROID FUNCTION TESTS IN VARIOUS CLINICAL SITUATIONS

PHYSIOLOGIC STATE	SERUM TSH	SERUM FREE T_4	SERUM T_3	24-H RADIOIODINE UPTAKE
Hyperthyroidism				
Untreated	Low*	High	High	High
T_3 toxicosis	Low	Normal	High	Normal or high
Hypothyroidism				
Primary, untreated	High	Low	Low or normal	Low or normal
Secondary to pituitary disease	Low or normal	Low	Low or normal	Low or normal
Euthyroidism				
Patient taking iodine	Normal	Normal	Normal	Low
Patient taking exogenous thyroid hormone	Normal	Normal in patient taking T_4, low in patient taking T_3	High in patient taking T_3, normal in patient taking T_4	Low
Patient taking estrogen	Normal	Normal	High	Normal
Euthyroid sick syndrome	Normal, low, or high	Normal or low	Low	Normal

*TSH is low in patients with hyperthyroidism except in the rare instance when the etiology is a TSH-secreting pituitary adenoma or pituitary resistance to the normal inhibition by thyroid hormone.

T_3 = triiodothyronine; T_4 = thyroxine; TSH = thyroid-stimulating hormone.

decreased by illnesses that reduce hepatic protein synthesis, use of anabolic steroids, and excessive corticosteroid use. Large doses of certain drugs, such as phenytoin and aspirin and their derivatives, displace T_4 from its binding sites on TBG, which spuriously lowers total serum T_4 levels.

Autoantibodies to thyroid peroxidase: Autoantibodies to thyroid peroxidase are present in almost all patients with Hashimoto thyroiditis (some of whom also have autoantibodies to thyroglobulin) and in most patients with Graves disease. These autoantibodies are markers of autoimmune disease but probably do not cause disease. However, an autoantibody directed against the TSH receptor on the thyroid follicular cell is responsible for the hyperthyroidism in Graves disease. Antibodies against T_4 and T_3 may be found in patients with autoimmune thyroid disease and may affect T_4 and T_3 measurements but are rarely clinically significant.

Thyroglobulin: The thyroid is the only source of thyroglobulin, which is readily detectable in the serum of healthy people and is usually elevated in patients with nontoxic or toxic goiter. The principal use of serum thyroglobulin measurement is in evaluating patients after near-total or total thyroidectomy (with or without ^{131}I ablation) for differentiated thyroid cancer. Normal or elevated serum thyroglobulin values indicate the presence of residual normal or cancerous thyroid tissue in patients receiving TSH-suppressive doses of L-thyroxine or after withdrawal of L-thyroxine. However, thyroglobulin antibodies interfere with thyroglobulin measurement.

Screening for thyroid dysfunction: Screening every 5 yr by measuring serum TSH is recommended for all men ≥ 65 and for all women ≥ 35. Screening is also recommended for all newborns and for pregnant women. For those with risk factors for thyroid disease, the serum TSH should be checked more often. Screening for hypothyroidism is as cost effective as screening for hypertension, hypercholesterolemia, and breast cancer. This single test is highly sensitive and specific in diagnosing or excluding two prevalent and serious disorders (hypothyroidism and hyperthyroidism), both of which can be treated effectively. Because of the high incidence of hypothyroidism in the elderly, screening on an annual basis is reasonable for those > age 70.

Radionuclide Imaging

Radioactive iodine uptake can be measured. A trace amount of radioiodine is given orally or IV; a scanner then detects the amount of radioiodine taken up by the thyroid. The preferred radioiodine isotope is ^{123}I, which exposes the patient to minimal radiation (much less than ^{131}I). Thyroid ^{123}I uptake varies widely with iodine ingestion and is low in patients exposed to excess iodine.

The test is valuable in the differential diagnosis of hyperthyroidism (high uptake in Graves disease, low uptake in thyroiditis—see p. 1347). It may also help in the calculation of the dose of ^{131}I needed for treatment of hyperthyroidism.

Imaging using a scintillation camera can be done after radioisotope administration (radioiodine or technetium 99m pertechnetate) to produce a graphic representation of isotope uptake. Focal areas of increased (hot) or decreased (cold) uptake help distinguish areas of possible cancer (thyroid cancers exist in < 1% of hot nodules compared with 10 to 20% of cold nodules).

APPROACH TO THE PATIENT WITH A THYROID NODULE

Thyroid nodules are common, increasingly so with increasing age. The reported incidence varies with the method of assessment. In middle-aged and elderly patients, palpation reveals nodules in about 5%. Results of ultrasonography and autopsy studies suggest that nodules are present in about 50% of older adults. Many nodules are found incidentally on thyroid imaging studies done for other disorders.

Etiology

Most nodules are benign. Benign causes include

- Hyperplastic colloid goiter
- Thyroid cysts
- Thyroiditis
- Thyroid adenomas

Malignant causes include thyroid cancers.

Evaluation

History: Pain suggests thyroiditis or hemorrhage into a cyst. An asymptomatic nodule may be malignant but is usually benign. Symptoms of hyperthyroidism suggest a hyperfunctioning adenoma or thyroiditis, whereas symptoms of hypothyroidism suggest Hashimoto thyroiditis. Risk factors for thyroid cancer include

- History of thyroid irradiation, especially in infancy or childhood
- Age < 20 yr
- Male sex
- Family history of thyroid cancer or multiple endocrine neoplasia type 2
- A solitary nodule
- Dysphagia
- Dysphonia
- Increasing size (particularly rapid growth or growth while receiving thyroid suppression treatment)

Physical examination: Signs that suggest thyroid cancer include stony, hard consistency or fixation to surrounding structures, cervical lymphadenopathy, and hoarseness due to recurrent laryngeal nerve paralysis.

Testing: Initial evaluation of a thyroid nodule consists of measurement of thyroid hormones, specifically

- Thyroid-stimulating hormone (TSH)
- Antithyroid peroxidase antibodies

If TSH is suppressed, radioiodine scanning is done. Nodules with increased radionuclide uptake (hot) are seldom malignant. If thyroid function tests do not indicate hyperthyroidism or Hashimoto thyroiditis, fine-needle aspiration biopsy is done to distinguish benign from malignant nodules. Early use of fine-needle aspiration biopsy is a more economic approach than routine use of radioiodine scans.

Ultrasonography is useful in determining the size of the nodule; fine-needle aspiration biopsy is not routinely indicated for nodules < 1 cm on ultrasonography or nodules that are entirely cystic. Ultrasonography is rarely diagnostic of cancer, although cancer is suggested by certain ultrasonographic or x-ray findings:

- Fine, stippled, psammomatous calcification (papillary thyroid carcinoma)
- Hypoechogenicity, irregular borders, increased intranodular vascularity, height greater than width on transverse section, irregular macrocalcifications, or rarely dense, homogeneous calcification (medullary thyroid carcinoma)

Treatment

- Treatment of underlying disorder

Treatment is directed at the underlying disorder. T_4 suppression of TSH to shrink smaller benign nodules is effective in no more than half the cases and is seldom done.

EUTHYROID SICK SYNDROME

Euthyroid sick syndrome is low serum levels of thyroid hormones in clinically euthyroid patients with nonthyroidal systemic illness. Diagnosis is based on excluding hypothyroidism. Treatment is of the underlying illness; thyroid hormone replacement is not indicated.

Patients with various acute or chronic nonthyroid disorders may have abnormal thyroid function test results. Such disorders include acute and chronic illness, particularly fasting, starvation, protein-energy undernutrition, severe trauma, myocardial infarction, chronic kidney disease, diabetic ketoacidosis, anorexia nervosa, cirrhosis, thermal injury, and sepsis.

Decreased triiodothyronine (T_3) levels are most common. Patients with more severe or prolonged illness also have decreased T_4 levels. Serum reverse T_3(rT_3) is increased. Patients are clinically euthyroid and do not have elevated TSH levels.

Pathogenesis is unknown but may include decreased peripheral conversion of T_4 to T_3, decreased clearance of rT_3 generated from T_4, and decreased binding of thyroid hormones to T_4-binding globulin (TBG). Proinflammatory cytokines (eg, tumor necrosis factor-alpha, IL-1) may be responsible for some changes.

Interpretation of abnormal thyroid function test results in ill patients is complicated by the effects of various drugs, including the iodine-rich contrast agents and amiodarone, which impairs the peripheral conversion of T_4 to T_3, and by drugs such as dopamine and corticosteroids, which decrease pituitary secretion of TSH, resulting in low serum TSH levels and subsequent decreased T_4 secretion.

PEARLS & PITFALLS

- Thyroid function tests should not be ordered for ICU patients unless thyroid dysfunction is highly suspected.

Diagnosis

- TSH
- Serum cortisol
- Clinical judgment

The diagnostic dilemma is whether the patient has hypothyroidism or euthyroid sick syndrome. The best test is measurement of TSH, which in euthyroid sick syndrome is low, normal, or slightly elevated but not as high as it would be in hypothyroidism. Serum rT_3 is elevated, although this measurement is rarely done. Serum cortisol is often elevated in euthyroid sick syndrome and low or low-normal in hypothyroidism due to pituitary-hypothalamic disease. Because tests are nonspecific, clinical judgment is required to interpret abnormal thyroid function tests in the acutely or chronically ill patient. Unless thyroid dysfunction is highly suspected, thyroid function tests should not be ordered for patients in the ICU.

Treatment

- Treatment of underlying disorder

Treatment with thyroid hormone replacement is not appropriate. When the underlying disorder is treated, results of thyroid tests normalize.

KEY POINTS

- Many seriously ill patients have low levels of thyroid hormones but are not clinically hypothyroid and do not require thyroid hormone supplementation.
- Patients with euthyroid sick syndrome have low, normal, or only slightly elevated TSH levels, unlike the marked TSH elevations present in true hypothyroidism.

HASHIMOTO THYROIDITIS

(Autoimmune Thyroiditis; Chronic Lymphocytic Thyroiditis)

Hashimoto thyroiditis is chronic autoimmune inflammation of the thyroid with lymphocytic infiltration. Findings include painless thyroid enlargement and symptoms of hypothyroidism. Diagnosis involves demonstration of high titers of thyroid peroxidase antibodies. Lifelong L-thyroxine replacement is typically required.

Hashimoto thyroiditis is believed to be the most common cause of primary hypothyroidism in North America. It is several times more prevalent among women. Incidence increases with age and in patients with chromosomal disorders, including Down syndrome, Turner syndrome, and Klinefelter syndrome. A family history of thyroid disorders is common.

Hashimoto thyroiditis, like Graves disease, is sometimes associated with other autoimmune disorders, including Addison disease (adrenal insufficiency), type 1 diabetes mellitus, hypoparathyroidism, vitiligo, premature graying of hair, pernicious anemia, connective tissue disorders (eg, RA, SLE, Sjögren syndrome), celiac disease, and Schmidt syndrome (Addison disease, diabetes, and hypothyroidism secondary to Hashimoto thyroiditis). There may be an increased incidence of thyroid tumors, rarely thyroid lymphoma. Pathologically, there is extensive infiltration of lymphocytes with lymphoid follicles and scarring.

Symptoms and Signs

Patients complain of painless enlargement of the thyroid or fullness in the throat. Examination reveals a nontender goiter that is smooth or nodular, firm, and more rubbery than the normal thyroid. Many patients present with symptoms of hypothyroidism, but some present with hyperthyroidism.

Diagnosis

- Thyroxine (T_4)
- Thyroid-stimulating hormone (TSH)
- Thyroid autoantibodies

Testing consists of measuring T_4, TSH, and thyroid autoantibodies. Early in the disease, T_4 and TSH levels are normal and there are high levels of thyroid peroxidase antibodies and, less commonly, of antithyroglobulin antibodies.

Thyroid radioactive iodine uptake may be increased, perhaps because of defective iodide organification together with a gland that continues to trap iodine. Patients later develop hypothyroidism with decreased T_4, decreased thyroid radioactive iodine uptake, and increased TSH.

Testing for other autoimmune disorders is warranted only when clinical manifestations are present.

Treatment

- Thyroid hormone replacement

Occasionally, hypothyroidism is transient, but most patients require lifelong thyroid hormone replacement, typically L-thyroxine 75 to 150 mcg po once/day.

KEY POINTS

- Hashimoto thyroiditis is autoimmune inflammation of the thyroid.
- Patients sometimes have other autoimmune disorders.
- T_4 and TSH levels initially are normal, but later, T_4 declines and TSH rises, and patients become clinically hypothyroid.
- There are high levels of thyroid peroxidase antibodies and, less commonly, of antithyroglobulin antibodies.
- Lifelong thyroid hormone replacement is typically needed.

HYPERTHYROIDISM

(Thyrotoxicosis)

Hyperthyroidism is characterized by hypermetabolism and elevated serum levels of free thyroid hormones. Symptoms are many and include tachycardia, fatigue, weight loss, nervousness, and tremor. Diagnosis is clinical and with thyroid function tests. Treatment depends on cause.

Hyperthyroidism can be classified on the basis of thyroid radioactive iodine uptake and the presence or absence of circulating thyroid stimulators (see Table 173–1).

Etiology

Hyperthyroidism may result from increased synthesis and secretion of thyroid hormones (thyroxine [T_4] and triiodothyronine [T_3]) from the thyroid, caused by thyroid stimulators in the blood or by autonomous thyroid hyperfunction. It can also result from excessive release of thyroid hormone from the thyroid without increased synthesis. Such release is commonly caused by the destructive changes of various types of thyroiditis. Various clinical syndromes also cause hyperthyroidism.

The **most common causes** overall include

- Graves disease
- Thyroiditis
- Multinodular goiter
- Single, autonomous, hyperfunctioning "hot" nodule

Graves disease (toxic diffuse goiter), the most common cause of hyperthyroidism, is characterized by hyperthyroidism and one or more of the following:

- Goiter
- Exophthalmos
- Infiltrative dermopathy

Graves disease is caused by an autoantibody against the thyroid receptor for TSH; unlike most autoantibodies, which are inhibitory, this autoantibody is stimulatory, thus causing continuous synthesis and secretion of excess T_4 and T_3. Graves disease (like Hashimoto thyroiditis) sometimes occurs with other autoimmune disorders, including type 1 diabetes mellitus, vitiligo, premature graying of hair, pernicious anemia, connective tissue disorders, and polyglandular deficiency syndrome. Heredity increases risk of Graves disease, although the genes involved are still unknown.

The pathogenesis of infiltrative ophthalmopathy (responsible for the exophthalmos in Graves disease) is poorly understood but may result from immunoglobulins directed to the TSH receptors in the orbital fibroblasts and fat that result in release of proinflammatory cytokines, inflammation, and accumulation of glycosaminoglycans. Ophthalmopathy may also occur before the onset of hyperthyroidism or as late as 20 yr afterward and frequently worsens or abates independently of the clinical course of hyperthyroidism. Typical ophthalmopathy in the presence of normal thyroid function is called euthyroid Graves disease.

Inappropriate TSH secretion is a rare cause. Patients with hyperthyroidism have essentially undetectable TSH except for those with a TSH-secreting anterior pituitary adenoma or pituitary resistance to thyroid hormone. TSH levels are high, and the TSH produced in both disorders is biologically more active than normal TSH. An increase in the alpha-subunit of TSH in the blood (helpful in differential diagnosis) occurs in patients with a TSH-secreting pituitary adenoma.

Molar pregnancy, choriocarcinoma, and hyperemesis gravidarum produce high levels of serum human chorionic gonadotropin (hCG), a weak thyroid stimulator. Levels of hCG are highest during the 1st trimester of pregnancy and result in the decrease in serum TSH and mild increase in serum free T_4 sometimes observed at that time. The increased thyroid stimulation may be caused by increased levels of partially desialated hCG, an hCG variant that appears to be a more potent thyroid stimulator than more sialated hCG. Hyperthyroidism in molar pregnancy, choriocarcinoma, and hyperemesis gravidarum is transient; normal thyroid function resumes when the molar pregnancy is evacuated, the choriocarcinoma is appropriately treated, or the hyperemesis gravidarum abates.

Nonautoimmune autosomal dominant hyperthyroidism manifests during infancy. It results from mutations in the TSH receptor gene that produce continuous thyroid stimulation.

Toxic solitary or multinodular goiter (Plummer disease) sometimes results from TSH receptor gene mutations causing continuous thyroid activation. Patients with toxic nodular goiter have none of the autoimmune manifestations or circulating antibodies observed in patients with Graves disease. Also, in contrast to Graves disease, toxic solitary and multinodular goiters usually do not remit.

Inflammatory thyroid disease (thyroiditis) includes subacute granulomatous thyroiditis, Hashimoto thyroiditis, and silent lymphocytic thyroiditis, a variant of Hashimoto thyroiditis. Hyperthyroidism results from destructive changes in the gland and release of stored hormone, not from increased synthesis. Hypothyroidism may follow.

Drug-induced hyperthyroidism can result from amiodarone and interferon-alfa, which may induce thyroiditis with hyperthyroidism and other thyroid disorders. Although more commonly causing hypothyroidism, lithium can rarely cause hyperthyroidism. Patients receiving these drugs should be closely monitored.

Thyrotoxicosis factitia is hyperthyroidism resulting from conscious or accidental overingestion of thyroid hormone.

Excess iodine ingestion causes hyperthyroidism with a low thyroid radioactive iodine uptake. It most often occurs in patients with underlying nontoxic nodular goiter (especially elderly patients) who are given drugs that contain iodine (eg, amiodarone, iodine-containing expectorants) or who undergo radiologic studies using iodine-rich contrast agents. The etiology may be that the excess iodine provides substrate for functionally autonomous (ie, not under TSH regulation) areas of the thyroid to produce hormone. Hyperthyroidism usually persists as long as excess iodine remains in the circulation.

Metastatic thyroid cancer is a possible cause. Overproduction of thyroid hormone occurs rarely from functioning metastatic follicular carcinoma, especially in pulmonary metastases.

Struma ovarii develops when ovarian teratomas contain enough thyroid tissue to cause true hyperthyroidism. Radioactive iodine uptake occurs in the pelvis, and uptake by the thyroid is usually suppressed.

Pathophysiology

In hyperthyroidism, serum T_3 usually increases more than does T_4, probably because of increased secretion of T_3 as well as conversion of T_4 to T_3 in peripheral tissues. In some patients, only T_3 is elevated (T_3 toxicosis). T_3 toxicosis may occur in any of the usual disorders that cause hyperthyroidism, including Graves disease, multinodular goiter, and the autonomously functioning solitary thyroid nodule. If T_3 toxicosis is untreated, the patient usually also develops laboratory abnormalities typical of hyperthyroidism (ie, elevated T_4 and ^{123}I uptake). The various forms of thyroiditis commonly have a hyperthyroid phase followed by a hypothyroid phase.

Symptoms and Signs

Most symptoms and signs are the same regardless of the cause. Exceptions include infiltrative ophthalmopathy and dermopathy, which occur only in Graves disease.

PEARLS & PITFALLS

- Elderly patients may have symptoms more akin to depression or dementia.

The clinical presentation may be dramatic or subtle. A goiter or nodule may be present. Many common symptoms of hyperthyroidism are similar to those of adrenergic excess, such as nervousness, palpitations, hyperactivity, increased sweating, heat hypersensitivity, fatigue, increased appetite, weight loss, insomnia, weakness, and frequent bowel movements (occasionally diarrhea). Hypomenorrhea may be present. Signs may include warm, moist skin; tremor; tachycardia; widened pulse pressure and atrial fibrillation.

Elderly patients, particularly those with toxic nodular goiter, may present atypically (apathetic or masked hyperthyroidism) with symptoms more akin to depression or dementia. Most do not have exophthalmos or tremor. Atrial fibrillation, syncope, altered sensorium, heart failure, and weakness are more likely. Symptoms and signs may involve only a single organ system.

Eye signs include stare, eyelid lag, eyelid retraction, and mild conjunctival injection and are largely due to excessive adrenergic stimulation. They usually remit with successful treatment. Infiltrative ophthalmopathy, a more serious development, is specific to Graves disease and can occur years before or after hyperthyroidism. It is characterized by orbital pain, lacrimation, irritation, photophobia, increased retro-orbital tissue, exophthalmos (see Plate 67), and lymphocytic infiltration of the extraocular muscles, causing ocular muscle weakness that frequently leads to double vision.

Infiltrative dermopathy, also called pretibial myxedema (a confusing term, because myxedema suggests hypothyroidism), is characterized by nonpitting infiltration by proteinaceous ground substance, usually in the pretibial area (see Plate 68). It rarely occurs in the absence of Graves ophthalmopathy. The lesion is often pruritic and erythematous in its early stages and subsequently becomes brawny. Infiltrative dermopathy may appear years before or after hyperthyroidism.

Thyroid storm: Thyroid storm is an acute form of hyperthyroidism that results from untreated or inadequately treated severe hyperthyroidism. It is rare, occurring in patients with Graves disease or toxic multinodular goiter (a solitary toxic nodule is a less common cause and generally causes less severe manifestations). It may be precipitated by infection, trauma, surgery, embolism, diabetic ketoacidosis, or preeclampsia.

Thyroid storm causes abrupt florid symptoms of hyperthyroidism with one or more of the following: fever, marked weakness and muscle wasting, extreme restlessness with wide emotional swings, confusion, psychosis, coma, nausea, vomiting, diarrhea, and hepatomegaly with mild jaundice. The patient may present with cardiovascular collapse and shock. *Thyroid storm is a life-threatening emergency requiring prompt treatment.*

Diagnosis

- TSH
- Free T_4, plus either free T_3 or total T_3
- Sometimes radioactive iodine uptake

Diagnosis is based on history, physical examination, and thyroid function tests. Serum TSH measurement is the best test because TSH is suppressed in hyperthyroid patients except in the rare instance when the etiology is a TSH-secreting pituitary adenoma or pituitary resistance to the normal inhibition by thyroid hormone.

Screening selected populations for TSH level is warranted. Free T_4 is increased in hyperthyroidism. However, T_4 can be falsely normal in true hyperthyroidism in patients with a severe systemic illness (similar to the falsely low levels that occur in euthyroid sick syndrome) and in T_3 toxicosis. If free T_4 level is normal and TSH is low in a patient with subtle symptoms and signs of hyperthyroidism, then serum T_3 should be measured to detect T_3 toxicosis; an elevated level confirms that diagnosis.

The cause can often be diagnosed clinically (eg, exposure to a drug, the presence of signs specific to Graves disease). If not, radioactive iodine uptake by the thyroid may be measured by using ^{123}I. When hyperthyroidism is due to hormone overproduction, radioactive iodine uptake by the thyroid is usually elevated. When hyperthyroidism is due to thyroiditis, iodine ingestion, or ectopic hormone production, radioactive iodine uptake is low.

TSH receptor antibodies can be measured to detect Graves disease, but measurement is rarely necessary except during the 3rd trimester of pregnancy to assess the risk of neonatal Graves disease; TSH receptor antibodies readily cross the placenta to stimulate the fetal thyroid. Most patients with Graves disease have circulating antithyroid peroxidase antibodies, and fewer have antithyroglobulin antibodies.

Inappropriate TSH secretion is uncommon. The diagnosis is confirmed when hyperthyroidism occurs with elevated circulating free T_4 and T_3 concentrations and normal or elevated serum TSH.

If thyrotoxicosis factitia is suspected, serum thyroglobulin can be measured; it is usually low or low-normal—unlike in all other causes of hyperthyroidism.

Treatment

Treatment depends on cause but may include

- Methimazole or propylthiouracil
- Beta-blockers
- Iodine
- Radioactive iodine
- Surgery

Methimazole and propylthiouracil: These antithyroid drugs block thyroid peroxidase, decreasing the organification of iodide, and impair the coupling reaction. Propylthiouracil in high doses also inhibits the peripheral conversion of T_4 to T_3. About 20 to 50% of patients with Graves disease remain in remission after a 1- to 2-yr course of either drug. The return to normal or a marked decrease in gland size, the restoration of a normal serum TSH level, and less severe hyperthyroidism before therapy are good prognostic signs of long-term remission. The concomitant use of antithyroid drug therapy and L-thyroxine does not improve the remission rate in patients with Graves disease. Because toxic nodular goiter rarely goes into remission, antithyroid drug therapy is given only in preparation for surgical treatment or ^{131}I therapy.

Because of severe hepatic failure in some patients < 40, especially children, propylthiouracil is now recommended only in special situations (eg, in the 1st trimester of pregnancy, in thyroid storm). Methimazole is the preferred drug. The usual starting dosage of methimazole is 5 to 20 mg po tid and of propylthiouracil is 100 to 150 mg po q 8 h. When T_4 and T_3 levels normalize, the dosage is decreased to the lowest effective amount, usually methimazole 5 to 15 mg once/day or propylthiouracil 50 mg bid or tid. Usually, control is achieved in 2 to 3 mo. More rapid control can be achieved by increasing the dosage of propylthiouracil to 150 to 200 mg q 8 h. Such dosages or higher ones (up to 400 mg q 8 h) are generally reserved for severely ill patients, including those with thyroid storm, to block the conversion of T_4 to T_3. Maintenance doses of methimazole can be continued for one or many years depending on the clinical circumstances. Carbimazole, which is used widely in Europe, is rapidly converted to methimazole. The usual starting dose is similar to that of methimazole; maintenance dosage is 5 to 20 mg po once/day, 2.5 to 10 mg bid, or 1.7 to 6.7 mg tid.

Adverse effects include rash, allergic reactions, abnormal liver function (including hepatic failure with propylthiouracil), and, in about 0.1% of patients, reversible agranulocytosis. Patients allergic to one drug can be switched to the other, but cross-sensitivity may occur. If agranulocytosis occurs, the patient cannot be switched to the other drug; other therapy (eg, radioiodine, surgery) should be used.

PEARLS & PITFALLS

- If agranulocytosis occurs with one of the antithyroid peroxidase drugs, avoid using another drug in the same class; use another therapy (eg, radioiodine, surgery) instead.

Each drug has advantages and disadvantages. Methimazole need only be given once/day, which improves adherence. Furthermore, when methimazole is used in dosages of < 20 mg/day, agranulocytosis is less common; with propylthiouracil, agranulocytosis may occur at any dosage. Methimazole has been used successfully in pregnant and nursing women without fetal or infant complications, but rarely methimazole has been associated with scalp and GI defects in neonates and with a rare embryopathy. Because of these complications, propylthiouracil is used in the 1st trimester of pregnancy. Propylthiouracil is preferred for the treatment of thyroid storm, because the dosages used (800 to 1200 mg/day) partially block the peripheral conversion of T_4 to T_3.

The combination of high-dose propylthiouracil and dexamethasone, also a potent inhibitor of T_4 to T_3 conversion, can relieve symptoms of severe hyperthyroidism and restore the serum T_3 level to normal within a week.

Beta-blockers: Symptoms and signs of hyperthyroidism due to adrenergic stimulation may respond to beta-blockers; propranolol has had the greatest use, but atenolol or metoprolol may be preferable.

Other manifestations typically do not respond.

- Manifestations typically responding to beta-blockers: Tachycardia, tremor, mental symptoms, eyelid lag; occasionally heat intolerance and sweating, diarrhea, proximal myopathy
- Manifestations typically not responding to beta-blockers: Oxygen consumption, exophthalmos, goiter, bruit, circulating T_4 levels, weight loss

Propranolol is indicated in thyroid storm (see Table 173–2). It rapidly decreases heart rate, usually within 2 to 3 h when given orally and within minutes when given IV. Esmolol may be used in the ICU because it requires careful titration and monitoring. Propranolol is also indicated for tachycardia with hyperthyroidism, especially in elderly patients, because antithyroid drugs usually take several weeks to become fully effective. Calcium channel blockers may control tachyarrhythmias in patients in whom beta-blockers are contraindicated.

Iodine: Iodine in pharmacologic doses inhibits the release of T_3 and T_4 within hours and inhibits the organification of iodine, a transitory effect lasting from a few days to a week, after which inhibition usually ceases. Iodine is used for emergency management of thyroid storm, for hyperthyroid patients undergoing emergency nonthyroid surgery, and (because it also decreases the vascularity of the thyroid) for preoperative preparation of hyperthyroid patients undergoing thyroidectomy. Iodine generally is not used for routine treatment of hyperthyroidism. The usual dosage is 2 to 3 drops (100 to 150 mg) of a saturated potassium iodide solution po tid or qid or sodium iodide in 1 L 0.9% saline solution 0.5 to 1 g IV given slowly once/day.

Complications of iodine therapy include inflammation of the salivary glands, conjunctivitis, and rash.

Radioactive sodium iodine (^{131}I, radioiodine): In the US, ^{131}I is the most common treatment for hyperthyroidism. Radioiodine is often recommended as the treatment of choice for

Table 173–2. TREATMENT OF THYROID STORM

Propylthiouracil: 600 mg po given before iodine, then 400 mg q 6 h
Iodine: 5 drops saturated solution of potassium iodide po tid *or* 10 drops Lugol solution po tid *or* 1g sodium iodide slowly by IV drip over 24 h
Propranolol: 40 mg po qid *or* 1 mg slowly IV q 4 h (not to exceed 1 mg/min) under close monitoring A repeat 1-mg dose given after 2 min, if needed, or esmolol
IV dextrose solutions
Correction of dehydration and electrolyte imbalance
Cooling blanket for hyperthermia
Antiarrhythmics (eg, calcium channel blockers, adenosine, beta-blockers) if necessary for atrial fibrillation
Treatment of underlying disorder, such as infection
Corticosteroids: Hydrocortisone 100 mg IV q 8 h *or* Dexamethasone 8 mg IV once/day
Definitive therapy after control of the crisis via ablation of the thyroid with ^{131}I or surgical treatment

Graves disease and toxic nodular goiter in all patients, including children. Dosage of ^{131}I is difficult to adjust because the response of the gland cannot be predicted; some physicians give a standard dose of 8 to 15 mCi. Others adjust the dose based on estimated thyroid size and the 24-h uptake to provide a dose of 80 to 120 microCi/g thyroid tissue.

When sufficient ^{131}I is given to cause euthyroidism, about 25 to 50% of patients become hypothyroid 1 yr later, and the incidence continues to increase yearly. Thus, most patients eventually become hypothyroid. However, if smaller doses are used, incidence of recurrence is higher. Larger doses, such as 10 to 15 mCi, often cause hypothyroidism within 6 mo.

Radioactive iodine is not used during lactation because it can enter breast milk and cause hypothyroidism in the infant. It is not used during pregnancy because it crosses the placenta and can cause severe fetal hypothyroidism. There is no proof that radioiodine increases the incidence of tumors, leukemia, thyroid cancer, or birth defects in children born to previously hyperthyroid women who become pregnant later in life.

Surgery: Surgery is indicated for patients with Graves disease whose hyperthyroidism has recurred after courses of antithyroid drugs and who refuse ^{131}I therapy, patients who cannot tolerate antithyroid drugs, patients with very large goiters, and in some younger patients with toxic adenoma and multinodular goiter. Surgery may be done in elderly patients with giant nodular goiters.

Surgery usually restores normal function. Postoperative recurrences vary between 2 and 16%; risk of hypothyroidism is directly related to the extent of surgery. Vocal cord paralysis and hypoparathyroidism are uncommon complications. Saturated solution of potassium iodide 3 drops (about 100 to 150 mg) po tid should be given for 10 days before surgery to reduce the vascularity of the gland. Methimazole must also be given because the patient should be euthyroid before iodide is given. Dexamethasone can be added to rapidly restore euthyroidism. Surgical procedures are more difficult in patients who previously underwent thyroidectomy or radioiodine therapy.

Treatment of thyroid storm: A treatment regimen for thyroid storm is shown in Table 173–2.

Treatment of infiltrative dermopathy and ophthalmopathy: In infiltrative dermopathy (in Graves disease), topical corticosteroids or corticosteroid injections into the lesions may decrease the dermopathy. Dermopathy sometimes remits spontaneously after months or years. Ophthalmopathy should be treated jointly by the endocrinologist and ophthalmologist and may require selenium, corticosteroids, orbital radiation, and surgery. Surgical thyroidectomy may help resolve or prevent progression of ophthalmopathy. Radioiodine therapy may accelerate progression of ophthalmopathy when ophthalmopathy is active, and is thus contraindicated in this active phase.

Subclinical hyperthyroidism: Subclinical hyperthyroidism is low serum TSH in patients with normal serum free T_4 and T_3 and absent or minimal symptoms of hyperthyroidism.

Subclinical hyperthyroidism is far less common than subclinical hypothyroidism.

Many patients with subclinical hyperthyroidism are taking L-thyroxine. The other causes of subclinical hyperthyroidism are the same as those for clinically apparent hyperthyroidism.

Patients with serum TSH < 0.1 mU/L have an increased incidence of atrial fibrillation (particularly elderly patients), reduced bone mineral density, increased fractures, and increased mortality. Patients with serum TSH that is only slightly below normal are less likely to have these features.

In patients with subclinical hyperthyroidism who are taking L-thyroxine, reduction of the dose is the most appropriate management unless therapy is aimed at maintaining suppressed TSH levels in patients with thyroid cancer.

Therapy is indicated for patients with endogenous subclinical hyperthyroidism (serum TSH < 0.1 mU/L), especially those with atrial fibrillation or reduced bone mineral density. The usual treatment is ^{131}I, but low doses of methimazole are also effective.

KEY POINTS

- Hyperthyroidism has many causes; these may involve excessive stimulation of a normal thyroid gland (eg, by TSH, hCG, ingestion of iodine or iodine-containing drugs), excessive hormone synthesis by an abnormal thyroid (eg, Graves disease, some thyroid cancers), or excessive release of thyroid hormones (eg, due to thyroiditis).
- Symptoms and signs are many but include tachycardia, fatigue, weight loss, nervousness, and tremor; patients with Graves disease may also have exophthalmos and infiltrative dermopathy.
- Free T_4, and/or free or total T_3 are elevated, and TSH is suppressed (except in rarer cases of pituitary causes of hyperthyroidism).
- Thyroid storm—resulting from untreated or inadequately treated severe hyperthyroidism—is a life-threatening emergency.
- Hormone synthesis can be suppressed with methimazole (or in certain cases, propylthiouracil) and adrenergic symptoms relieved with beta-blockers; long-term treatment may require thyroid ablation with radioactive iodine or surgery.

HYPOTHYROIDISM

(Myxedema)

Hypothyroidism is thyroid hormone deficiency. It is diagnosed by clinical features such as a typical facial appearance, hoarse slow speech, and dry skin and by low levels of thyroid hormones. Management includes treatment of the cause and administration of thyroxine.

Hypothyroidism occurs at any age but is particularly common among the elderly, where it may present subtly and be difficult to recognize. Hypothyroidism may be

- Primary: Caused by disease in the thyroid
- Secondary: Caused by disease in the hypothalamus or pituitary

Primary hypothyroidism: Primary hypothyroidism is due to disease in the thyroid; TSH is increased. The most common cause is autoimmune. It usually results from Hashimoto thyroiditis and is often associated with a firm goiter or, later in the disease process, with a shrunken fibrotic thyroid with little or no function. The 2nd most common cause is post-therapeutic hypothyroidism, especially after radioactive iodine therapy or surgery for hyperthyroidism or goiter. Hypothyroidism during overtreatment with propylthiouracil, methimazole, and iodide abates after therapy is stopped.

Most patients with non-Hashimoto goiters are euthyroid or have hyperthyroidism, but goitrous hypothyroidism may occur in endemic goiter. Iodine deficiency decreases thyroid hormonogenesis. In response, TSH is released, which causes the thyroid to enlarge and trap iodine avidly; thus, goiter results. If iodine deficiency is severe, the patient becomes hypothyroid, a rare occurrence in the US since the advent of iodized salt.

Iodine deficiency can cause congenital hypothyroidism. In severely iodine-deficient regions worldwide, congenital hypothyroidism (previously termed endemic cretinism) is a major cause of intellectual disability.

Rare inherited enzymatic defects can alter the synthesis of thyroid hormone and cause goitrous hypothyroidism (see p. 2560).

Hypothyroidism may occur in patients taking lithium, perhaps because lithium inhibits hormone release by the thyroid. Hypothyroidism may also occur in patients taking amiodarone or other iodine-containing drugs, in patients taking interferon-alfa, and in patients taking checkpoint inhibitors or some tyrosine kinase inhibitors for cancer.

Hypothyroidism can result from radiation therapy for cancer of the larynx or Hodgkin lymphoma (Hodgkin disease). The incidence of permanent hypothyroidism after radiation therapy is high, and thyroid function (through measurement of serum TSH) should be evaluated at 6- to 12-mo intervals.

Secondary hypothyroidism: Secondary hypothyroidism occurs when the hypothalamus produces insufficient thyrotropin-releasing hormone (TRH) or the pituitary produces insufficient TSH. Sometimes, deficient TSH secretion due to deficient TRH secretion is termed tertiary hypothyroidism.

Subclinical hypothyroidism: Subclinical hypothyroidism is elevated serum TSH in patients with absent or minimal symptoms of hypothyroidism and normal serum levels of free T_4.

Subclinical thyroid dysfunction is relatively common; it occurs in more than 15% of elderly women and 10% of elderly men, particularly in those with underlying Hashimoto thyroiditis.

In patients with serum TSH > 10 mU/L, there is a high likelihood of progression to overt hypothyroidism with low serum levels of free T_4 in the next 10 yr. These patients are also more likely to have hypercholesterolemia and atherosclerosis. They should be treated with L-thyroxine, even if they are asymptomatic.

For patients with TSH levels between 4.5 and 10 mU/L, a trial of L-thyroxine is reasonable if symptoms of early hypothyroidism (eg, fatigue, depression) are present.

L-thyroxine therapy is also indicated in pregnant women and in women who plan to become pregnant to avoid deleterious effects of hypothyroidism on the pregnancy and fetal development. Patients should have annual measurement of serum TSH and free T_4 to assess progress of the condition if untreated or to adjust the L-thyroxine dosage.

Symptoms and Signs

Symptoms and signs of primary hypothyroidism are often subtle and insidious. Various organ systems may be affected.

- Metabolic manifestations: Cold intolerance, modest weight gain (due to fluid retention and decreased metabolism), hypothermia
- Neurologic manifestations: Forgetfulness, paresthesias of the hands and feet (often due to carpal tunnel syndrome caused by deposition of proteinaceous ground substance in the ligaments around the wrist and ankle); slowing of the relaxation phase of deep tendon reflexes
- Psychiatric manifestations: Personality changes, dull facial expression, dementia or frank psychosis (myxedema madness)
- Dermatologic manifestations: Facial puffiness; myxedema; sparse, coarse and dry hair; coarse, dry, scaly and thick skin; carotenemia, particularly notable on the palms and soles (caused by deposition of carotene in the lipid-rich epidermal layers); macroglossia due to deposition of proteinaceous ground substance in the tongue
- Ocular manifestations: Periorbital swelling due to infiltration with the mucopolysaccharides hyaluronic acid and chondroitin sulfate), droopy eyelids because of decreased adrenergic drive
- Gastrointestinal manifestations: Constipation
- Gynecologic manifestations: Menorrhagia or secondary amenorrhea
- Cardiovascular manifestations: Slow heart rate (a decrease in both thyroid hormone and adrenergic stimulation causes bradycardia), enlarged heart on examination and imaging (partly because of dilation but chiefly because of pericardial effusion; pericardial effusions develop slowly and only rarely cause hemodynamic distress)
- Other manifestations: Pleural or abdominal effusions (pleural effusions develop slowly and only rarely cause respiratory or hemodynamic distress), hoarse voice, and slow speech

Symptoms can differ significantly in elderly patients.

Although secondary hypothyroidism is uncommon, its causes often affect other endocrine organs controlled by the hypothalamic-pituitary axis. In a woman with hypothyroidism, indications of secondary hypothyroidism are a history of amenorrhea rather than menorrhagia and some suggestive differences on physical examination. Secondary hypothyroidism is characterized by skin and hair that are dry but not very coarse, skin depigmentation, only minimal macroglossia, atrophic breasts, and low BP. Also, the heart is small, and serous pericardial effusions do not occur. Hypoglycemia is common because of concomitant adrenal insufficiency or growth hormone deficiency.

Myxedema coma: Myxedema coma is a life-threatening complication of hypothyroidism, usually occurring in patients with a long history of hypothyroidism. Its characteristics include coma with extreme hypothermia (temperature 24° to 32.2° C), areflexia, seizures, and respiratory depression with carbon dioxide retention. Severe hypothermia may be missed unless low-reading thermometers are used. Rapid diagnosis based on clinical judgment, history, and physical examination is imperative, because death is likely without rapid treatment. Precipitating factors include illness, infection, trauma, drugs that suppress the CNS, and exposure to cold.

Diagnosis

- TSH
- Free T_4

Serum TSH is the most sensitive test, and screening of selected populations is warranted. In primary hypothyroidism, there is no feedback inhibition of the intact pituitary, and serum TSH is always elevated, whereas serum free T_4 is low. In secondary hypothyroidism, free T_4 and serum TSH are low (sometimes TSH is normal but with decreased bioactivity).

Many patients with primary hypothyroidism have normal circulating levels of T_3, probably caused by sustained TSH stimulation of the failing thyroid, resulting in preferential synthesis and secretion of biologically active T_3. Therefore, serum T_3 is not sensitive for hypothyroidism.

Anemia is often present, usually normocytic-normochromic and of unknown etiology, but it may be hypochromic because of menorrhagia and sometimes macrocytic because of associated pernicious anemia or decreased absorption of folate. Anemia is rarely severe (Hb usually > 9 g/dL). As the hypometabolic state is corrected, anemia subsides, sometimes requiring 6 to 9 mo.

Serum cholesterol is usually high in primary hypothyroidism but less so in secondary hypothyroidism.

In addition to primary and secondary hypothyroidism, other conditions may cause decreased levels of total T_4, such as serum T_4-binding globulin (TBG) deficiency, some drugs, Hashimoto thyroiditis, and euthyroid sick syndrome.

Treatment

- L-thyroxine, adjusted until TSH levels are in midnormal range

Various thyroid hormone preparations are available for replacement therapy, including synthetic preparations of T_4 (L-thyroxine), T_3 (liothyronine), combinations of the 2 synthetic hormones, and desiccated animal thyroid extract. L-thyroxine is preferred; the usual maintenance dose is 75 to 150 mcg po once/day, depending on age, body mass index, and absorption (for pediatric doses, see p. 2571). The starting dose in young or middle-aged patients who are otherwise healthy can be 100 mcg or 1.7 mcg/kg po once/day.

However, in patients with heart disease, therapy is begun with low doses, usually 25 mcg once/day. The dose is adjusted every 6 wk until maintenance dose is achieved. The maintenance dose may need to be increased in pregnant women. Dose may also need to be increased if drugs that decrease T_4 absorption or increase its biliary excretion are administered concomitantly. The dose used should be the lowest that restores serum TSH levels to the midnormal range (though this criterion cannot be used in patients with secondary hypothyroidism). In secondary hypothyroidism the dose of L-thyroxine should achieve a free T_4 in the midnormal range.

Liothyronine should not be used alone for long-term replacement because of its short half-life and the large peaks in serum T_3 levels it produces. The administration of standard replacement amounts (25 to 37.5 mcg bid) results in rapidly increasing serum T_3 to between 300 and 1000 ng/dL (4.62 to 15.4 nmol/L) within 4 h due to its almost complete absorption; these levels return to normal by 24 h. Additionally, patients receiving liothyronine are chemically hyperthyroid for at least several hours a day, potentially increasing cardiac risks.

Similar patterns of serum T_3 occur when mixtures of T_3 and T_4 are taken po, although peak T_3 is lower because less T_3 is given. Replacement regimens with synthetic T_4 preparations reflect a different pattern in serum T_3 response. Increases in serum T_3 occur gradually, and normal levels are maintained when adequate doses of T_4 are given. Desiccated animal thyroid preparations contain variable amounts of T_3 and T_4 and should not be prescribed unless the patient is already taking the preparation and has normal serum TSH.

In patients with secondary hypothyroidism, L-thyroxine should not be given until there is evidence of adequate cortisol secretion (or cortisol therapy is given), because L-thyroxine could precipitate adrenal crisis.

Myxedema coma: Myxedema coma is treated as follows:

- T_4 given IV
- Corticosteroids
- Supportive care as needed
- Conversion to oral T_4 when patient is stable

Patients require a large initial dose of T_4 (300 to 500 mcg IV) or T_3 (25 to 50 mcg IV). The IV maintenance dose of T_4 is 75 to 100 mcg once/day and of T_3, 10 to 20 mcg bid until T_4 can be given orally. Corticosteroids are also given because the possibility of central hypothyroidism usually cannot be initially ruled out. The patient should not be rewarmed rapidly, which may precipitate hypotension or arrhythmias. Hypoxemia is common, so Pa_{O_2} should be monitored. If ventilation is compromised, immediate mechanical ventilatory assistance is required. The precipitating factor should be rapidly and appropriately treated and fluid replacement given carefully, because hypothyroid patients do not excrete water appropriately. Finally, all drugs should be given cautiously because they are metabolized more slowly than in healthy people.

Geriatrics Essentials

Hypothyroidism is particularly common among the elderly. It occurs in close to 10% of women and 6% of men > 65. Although typically easy to diagnose in younger adults, hypothyroidism may be subtle and manifest atypically in the elderly.

Elderly patients have significantly fewer symptoms than do younger adults, and complaints are often subtle and vague. Many elderly patients with hypothyroidism present with nonspecific geriatric syndromes—confusion, anorexia, weight loss, falling, incontinence, and decreased mobility. Musculoskeletal symptoms (especially arthralgias) occur often, but arthritis is rare. Muscular aches and weakness, often mimicking polymyalgia rheumatica or polymyositis, and an elevated CK level may occur. In the elderly, hypothyroidism may mimic dementia or parkinsonism.

In the elderly, L-thyroxine therapy is begun with low doses, usually 25 mcg once/day. Maintenance doses may also need to be lower in elderly patients.

KEY POINTS

- Primary hypothyroidism is most common; it is due to disease in the thyroid, and TSH levels are high.
- Secondary hypothyroidism is less common; it is due to pituitary or hypothalamic disease, and TSH levels are low.
- Symptoms develop insidiously and typically include cold intolerance, constipation, and cognitive and/or personality changes; later, the face becomes puffy and the facial expression dull.
- Myxedema coma is a life-threatening complication that requires rapid diagnosis and treatment.
- Free thyroxine (T_4) level is always low, but T_3 may remain normal early in some disorders.
- Serum TSH is the best diagnostic test, and screening is warranted in select populations (eg, the elderly) because the disease is so subtle and insidious.
- Oral T_4 (L-thyroxine) is the preferred treatment and is given in the lowest dose that restores serum TSH levels to the midnormal range.

SILENT LYMPHOCYTIC THYROIDITIS

Silent lymphocytic thyroiditis is a self-limited, subacute disorder occurring most commonly in women during the postpartum period. Symptoms are initially of hyperthyroidism, then hypothyroidism, and then generally recovery to the euthyroid state. Treatment of the hyperthyroid phase is with a beta-blocker. If hypothyroidism is permanent, lifelong T_4 supplementation is needed.

The term "silent" refers to the absence of thyroid tenderness in contrast with subacute thyroiditis, which usually causes thyroid tenderness. Silent lymphocytic thyroiditis causes most cases of postpartum thyroid dysfunction. It occurs in about 5 to 10% of postpartum women.

Thyroid biopsy reveals lymphocytic infiltration as in Hashimoto thyroiditis but without lymphoid follicles and scarring. Thyroid peroxidase autoantibodies and, less commonly, antithyroglobulin antibodies are almost always positive during pregnancy and the postpartum period in these patients. Thus, this disorder would appear to be a variant of Hashimoto thyroiditis.

Symptoms and Signs

The condition begins in the postpartum period, usually within 12 to 16 wk. Silent lymphocytic thyroiditis is characterized by a variable degree of painless thyroid enlargement with a hyperthyroid phase of several weeks, often followed by transient hypothyroidism due to depleted thyroid hormone stores but usually eventual recovery to the euthyroid state (as noted for painful subacute thyroiditis). The hyperthyroid phase is self-limited and may be brief or overlooked. Many women with this disorder are diagnosed when they become hypothyroid, which occasionally is permanent.

Diagnosis

- Clinical evaluation
- Serum T_4, T_3, and TSH levels

Silent lymphocytic thyroiditis is frequently undiagnosed. Suspicion of the diagnosis generally depends on clinical findings, typically once hypothyroidism has occurred. Eye signs and pretibial myxedema do not occur.

Thyroid function test results vary depending on the phase of illness. Initially, serum T_4 and T_3 are elevated and TSH is suppressed. In the hypothyroid phase, these findings are reversed. WBC count and ESR are normal. Needle biopsy provides definitive diagnosis but is usually unnecessary.

PEARLS & PITFALLS

- Screen even asymptomatic pregnant women for silent lymphocytic thyroiditis if they have had it in previous pregnancies.

Treatment

- Usually a beta-blocker
- Sometimes thyroid hormone replacement

Because silent lymphocytic thyroiditis lasts only a few months, treatment is conservative, usually requiring only a beta-blocker (eg, propranolol) during the hyperthyroid phase. Antithyroid drugs, surgery, and radioiodine therapy are contraindicated.

Thyroid hormone replacement may be required during the hypothyroid phase. Most patients recover normal thyroid function, although some remain permanently hypothyroid. Therefore, thyroid function should be reevaluated after 9 to 12 mo of thyroxine therapy; replacement is stopped for 5 wk, and TSH is remeasured. This disorder usually recurs after subsequent pregnancies.

KEY POINTS

- This disorder affects mostly women in the postpartum period.
- Most patients go through a transient hyperthyroid phase, followed by a longer hypothyroid phase; most but not all recover spontaneously.
- The disorder often goes undiagnosed.
- A beta-blocker is often needed in the hyperthyroid phase, and thyroid hormone replacement is typically needed in the hypothyroid phase.

SUBACUTE THYROIDITIS

(de Quervain Thyroiditis; Giant Cell Thyroiditis; Granulomatous Thyroiditis)

Subacute thyroiditis is an acute inflammatory disease of the thyroid probably caused by a virus. Symptoms include fever and thyroid tenderness. Initial hyperthyroidism is common, sometimes followed by a transient period of hypothyroidism. Diagnosis is clinical and with thyroid function tests. Treatment is with high doses of NSAIDs or with corticosteroids. The disease usually resolves spontaneously within months.

History of an antecedent viral URI is common. Histologic studies show less lymphocytic infiltration of the thyroid than in Hashimoto thyroiditis or silent lymphocytic thyroiditis, but there is characteristic giant cell infiltration, polymorphonuclear lymphocytes, and follicular disruption.

Symptoms and Signs

There is pain in the anterior neck and fever of 37.8° to 38.3° C. Neck pain characteristically shifts from side to side and may settle in one area, frequently radiating to the jaw and ears. It is often confused with dental pain, pharyngitis, or otitis and is aggravated by swallowing or turning of the head. Symptoms of hyperthyroidism are common early in the disease because of hormone release from the disrupted follicles. There is more lassitude and prostration than in other thyroid disorders. On physical examination, the thyroid is asymmetrically enlarged, firm, and tender.

Diagnosis

- Clinical findings
- Free thyroxine (T_4) and thyroid-stimulating hormone (TSH) levels
- ESR
- Radioactive iodine uptake

Diagnosis is primarily clinical, based on finding an enlarged, tender thyroid in patients with the appropriate clinical history. Thyroid testing with TSH and at least a free T_4 measurement is usually also done. Radioactive iodine uptake should be measured to confirm the diagnosis. When the diagnosis is uncertain, fine-needle aspiration biopsy is useful. Thyroid ultrasonography with color Doppler shows multiple irregular sonolucent areas and reduced blood flow in contrast with the increased flow of Graves disease.

Laboratory findings early in the disease include an increase in free T_4 and T_3, a marked decrease in TSH and thyroid radioactive iodine uptake (often 0), and a high ESR. After several weeks, the thyroid is depleted of T_4 and T_3 stores, and transient hypothyroidism develops accompanied by a decrease in free T_4 and T_3, a rise in TSH, and recovery of thyroid radioactive iodine uptake. Weakly positive thyroid antibodies may be present. Measurement of free T_4, T_3, and TSH at 2- to 4-wk intervals identifies the stages of the disease.

Prognosis

Subacute thyroiditis is self-limited, generally subsiding in a few months; occasionally, it recurs and may result in permanent hypothyroidism when follicular destruction is extensive.

Treatment

- NSAIDs
- Sometimes corticosteroids, a beta-blocker, or both

Discomfort is treated with high doses of aspirin or NSAIDs. In severe and protracted cases, corticosteroids (eg, prednisone 15 to 30 mg po once/day, gradually decreasing the dose over 3 to 4 wk) eradicate all symptoms within 48 h.

Bothersome hyperthyroid symptoms may be treated with a short course of a beta-blocker. If hypothyroidism is pronounced or persists, thyroid hormone replacement therapy may be required, rarely permanently.

KEY POINTS

- Manifestations are usually fever, neck pain, and an enlarged, tender thyroid.
- Patients are initially hyperthyroid, with low TSH and elevated free T_4; they sometimes then become transiently hypothyroid, with high TSH and low free T_4.
- Treatment is with NSAIDs plus sometimes corticosteroids and/or a beta-blocker.

SIMPLE NONTOXIC GOITER

(Euthyroid Goiter)

Simple nontoxic goiter, which may be diffuse or nodular, is noncancerous hypertrophy of the thyroid without hyperthyroidism, hypothyroidism, or inflammation. Except in severe iodine deficiency, thyroid function is normal and patients are asymptomatic except for an obviously enlarged, nontender thyroid. Diagnosis is clinical and with determination of normal thyroid function. Treatment is directed at the cause, but partial surgical removal may be required for very large goiters.

Simple nontoxic goiter, the most common type of thyroid enlargement, is frequently noted at puberty, during pregnancy, and at menopause. The cause at these times is usually unclear. Known causes include

- Intrinsic thyroid hormone production defects
- Ingestion of foods that contain substances that inhibit thyroid hormone synthesis (goitrogens, eg, cassava, broccoli, cauliflower, cabbage), as may occur in countries in which iodine deficiency is common
- Drugs that can decrease the synthesis of thyroid hormone (eg, amiodarone or other iodine-containing compounds, lithium)

Iodine deficiency is rare in North America but remains the most common cause of goiter worldwide (termed endemic goiter). Compensatory small elevations in TSH occur, preventing hypothyroidism, but the TSH stimulation results in goiter formation. Recurrent cycles of stimulation and involution may result in nontoxic nodular goiters. However, the true etiology of most nontoxic goiters in iodine-sufficient areas is unknown.

Symptoms and Signs

The patient may have a history of low iodine intake or overingestion of food goitrogens, but these phenomena are rare in North America. In the early stages, the goiter is typically soft, symmetric, and smooth. Later, multiple nodules and cysts may develop.

Diagnosis

- Thyroidal radioactive iodine uptake
- Thyroid scan
- Thyroid ultrasonography
- T_4, T_3, and TSH levels

In the early stages, thyroidal radioactive iodine uptake may be normal or high with normal thyroid scans. Thyroid function test results are usually normal. Thyroid antibodies are measured to rule out Hashimoto thyroiditis.

In endemic goiter, serum TSH may be slightly elevated, and serum T_4 may be low-normal or slightly low, but serum T_3 is usually normal or slightly elevated.

Thyroid ultrasonography is done to determine whether there are nodules that are suggestive of cancer.

Treatment

- Depends on cause

In iodine-deficient areas, iodine supplementation of salt; oral or IM administration of iodized oil yearly; and iodination of water, crops, or animal fodder eliminates iodine-deficiency goiter. Goitrogens being ingested should be stopped.

In other instances, suppression of the hypothalamic-pituitary axis with thyroid hormone blocks TSH production (and hence stimulation of the thyroid). Full TSH-suppressive doses of L-thyroxine (100 to 150 mcg/day po depending on the serum TSH) are useful in younger patients.

L-thyroxine is contraindicated in older patients with nontoxic nodular goiter, because these goiters rarely shrink and may harbor areas of autonomy so that L-thyroxine therapy can result in hyperthyroidism.

Large goiters occasionally require surgery or ^{131}I to shrink the gland enough to prevent interference with respiration or swallowing or to correct cosmetic problems.

KEY POINTS

- Thyroid function is usually normal.
- When the cause is iodine deficiency, iodine supplementation is effective treatment.
- Blocking TSH production by giving L-thyroxine is useful in younger patients to halt stimulation of the thyroid and shrink the goiter.
- Surgery or ^{131}I may be needed for large goiters.

THYROID CANCERS

There are 4 general types of thyroid cancer. Most thyroid cancers manifest as asymptomatic nodules. Rarely, lymph node, lung, or bone metastases cause the presenting symptoms of small thyroid cancers. Diagnosis is often by fine-needle aspiration biopsy but may involve other tests. Treatment is surgical removal, usually followed by ablation of residual tissue with radioactive iodine.

There are 4 general types of thyroid cancer:

- Papillary
- Follicular
- Medullary
- Anaplastic

Papillary and follicular carcinoma together are called differentiated thyroid cancer because of their histologic resemblance to normal thyroid tissue and because differentiated function (eg, thyroglobulin secretion) is preserved.

Except for anaplastic and metastatic medullary carcinoma, most thyroid cancers are not highly malignant and are seldom fatal.

Most thyroid cancers manifest as asymptomatic nodules. Rarely, lymph node, lung, or bone metastases cause the presenting symptoms of small thyroid cancers. Diagnosis is often by fine-needle aspiration biopsy but may involve other tests.

Treatment is surgical removal, usually followed by ablation of residual tissue with radioactive iodine.

Papillary Thyroid Carcinoma

Papillary carcinoma accounts for 80 to 90% of all thyroid cancers. The female:male ratio is 3:1. It may be familial in up to 5% of patients. Most patients present between ages 30 and 60.

The tumor is often more aggressive in elderly patients. Many papillary carcinomas contain follicular elements. One variant is called noninvasive follicular thyroid neoplasm with papillary-like nuclear features (previously known as noninvasive encapsulated follicular variant of papillary thyroid carcinoma).[1]

The tumor spreads via lymphatics to regional lymph nodes in one third of patients and may metastasize to the lungs. Patients < 45 yr with small tumors confined to the thyroid have an excellent prognosis.

Tumors > 4 cm or that are diffusely spreading require total or near-total thyroidectomy with postoperative radioiodine ablation of residual thyroid tissue with appropriately large doses of ^{131}I administered when the patient is hypothyroid or after recombinant TSH injections. Treatment may be repeated every 6 to 12 mo to ablate any remaining thyroid tissue. TSH-suppressive doses of L-thyroxine are given after treatment, and serum thyroglobulin levels help detect recurrent or persistent disease. Neck ultrasonography will detect recurrence in lymph nodes. About 20 to 30% of patients, mainly elderly patients, have recurrent or persistent disease.

Treatment for encapsulated tumors < 1.5 cm localized to one lobe is usually near-total thyroidectomy, although some experts recommend only lobectomy and isthmusectomy; surgery is almost always curative. Thyroid hormone in TSH-suppressive doses is given to minimize chances of regrowth and cause regression of any microscopic remnants of papillary carcinoma.

1. Nikiforov YE, Seethala RR, Tallini G, et al: Nomenclature revision for encapsulated follicular variant of papillary thyroid carcinoma: a paradigm shift to reduce overtreatment of indolent tumors. *JAMA Oncol* Published online April 14, 2016. doi: 10.1001/jamaoncol.2016.0386.

Follicular Thyroid Carcinoma

Follicular carcinoma, including the Hürthle cell variant, accounts for about 10% of thyroid cancers. It is more common among elderly patients and in regions of iodine deficiency. It is more malignant than papillary carcinoma, spreading hematogenously with distant metastases.

Treatment requires near-total thyroidectomy with postoperative radioiodine ablation of residual thyroid tissue as in treatment for papillary carcinoma. Metastases are more responsive to radioiodine therapy than are those of papillary carcinoma. TSH-suppressive doses of L-thyroxine are given after treatment. Serum thyroglobulin and neck ultrasongraphy should be monitored to detect recurrent or persistent disease.

Medullary Thyroid Carcinoma

Medullary carcinoma constitutes about 3% of thyroid cancers and is composed of C cells that produce calcitonin. It may be sporadic (usually unilateral); however, it is often familial, caused by a mutation of the *ret* proto-oncogene. The familial form may occur in isolation or as a component of multiple endocrine neoplasia (MEN) syndrome type 2A and MEN 2B. Although calcitonin can lower serum calcium and phosphate levels, serum calcium is normal because the high level of calcitonin ultimately down-regulates its receptors. Characteristic amyloid deposits that stain with Congo red are also present.

Metastases spread via the lymphatic system to cervical and mediastinal nodes and sometimes to liver, lungs, and bone.

Patients typically present with an asymptomatic thyroid nodule, although many cases are now diagnosed during routine screening of affected kindreds with MEN 2A or MEN 2B before a palpable tumor develops.

Medullary carcinoma may have a dramatic biochemical presentation when associated with ectopic production of other hormones or peptides (eg, ACTH, vasoactive intestinal polypeptide, prostaglandins, kallikreins, serotonin).

The best test is measurement of serum calcitonin, which is greatly elevated. A challenge with calcium (15 mg/kg IV over 4 h) provokes excessive secretion of calcitonin.

X-rays may show a dense, homogenous, conglomerate calcification.

All patients with medullary carcinoma should have genetic testing; relatives of those with mutations should have genetic testing and measurement of basal and stimulated calcitonin levels.

Total thyroidectomy is indicated even if bilateral involvement is not obvious. Lymph nodes are also dissected. If hyperparathyroidism is present, removal of hyperplastic or adenomatous parathyroids is required.

Pheochromocytoma, if present, is usually bilateral. Pheochromocytomas should be identified and removed before thyroidectomy because of the danger of provoking hypertensive crisis during the operation. Long-term survival is common in patients with medullary carcinoma and MEN 2A; more than two-thirds of affected patients are alive at 10 yr. Medullary carcinoma of the sporadic type has a worse prognosis.

Relatives with an elevated calcitonin level without a palpable thyroid abnormality should undergo thyroidectomy because there is a greater chance of cure at this stage. Some experts recommend surgery in relatives who have normal basal and stimulated serum calcitonin levels but who have the *ret* proto-oncogene mutation.

Anaplastic Thyroid Carcinoma

Anaplastic carcinoma is an undifferentiated cancer that accounts for about 2% of thyroid cancers. It occurs mostly in elderly patients and slightly more often in women. The tumor is characterized by rapid, painful enlargement. Rapid enlargement of the thyroid may also suggest thyroid lymphoma, particularly if found in association with Hashimoto thyroiditis.

No effective therapy exists, and the disease is generally fatal. About 80% of patients die within 1 yr of diagnosis. In a few patients with smaller tumors, thyroidectomy followed by external beam radiation therapy has been curative. Chemotherapy is mainly experimental.

Radiation-Induced Thyroid Cancer

Thyroid tumors develop in people whose thyroid is exposed to large amounts of environmental radiation, as occurs as a result of atomic bomb blasts, nuclear reactor accidents, or incidental thyroid irradiation due to radiation therapy. Tumors may be detected 10 yr after exposure, but risk remains increased for 30 to 40 yr. Such tumors are usually benign; however, about 10% are papillary thyroid carcinoma. The tumors are frequently multicentric or diffuse.

Patients who had thyroid irradiation should undergo yearly thyroid palpation, ultrasonography, and measurement of thyroid autoantibodies (to exclude Hashimoto thyroiditis). A thyroid scan does not always reflect areas of involvement.

If ultrasonography reveals a nodule, fine-needle aspiration biopsy should be done. In the absence of suspicious or malignant lesions, many physicians recommend lifelong TSH-lowering doses of thyroid hormone to suppress thyroid function and thyrotropin secretion and possibly decrease the chance of developing a thyroid tumor.

Surgery is required if fine-needle aspiration biopsy suggests cancer. Near-total or total thyroidectomy is the treatment of choice, to be followed by radioiodine ablation of any residual thyroid tissue if a cancer is found (depending on the size, histology, and invasiveness).

SECTION 14

Immunology; Allergic Disorders

174 Biology of the Immune System

The immune system distinguishes self from nonself and eliminates potentially harmful nonself molecules and cells from the body. The immune system also has the capacity to recognize and destroy abnormal cells that derive from host tissues. Any molecule capable of being recognized by the immune system is considered an antigen (Ag).

The skin, cornea, and mucosa of the respiratory, GI, and GU tracts form a physical barrier that is the body's first line of defense. Some of these barriers also have active immune functions:

- Outer, keratinized epidermis: Keratinocytes in the skin secrete antimicrobial peptides (defensins), and sebaceous and sweat glands secrete microbe-inhibiting substances (eg, lactic acid, fatty acids). Also, many immune cells (eg, mast cells, intraepithelial lymphocytes, Ag-sampling Langerhans cells) reside in the skin.
- Mucosa of the respiratory, GI, and GU tracts: The mucus contains antimicrobial substances, such as lysozyme, lactoferrin, and secretory IgA antibody (SIgA).

Breaching of anatomic barriers can trigger 2 types of immune response:

- Innate
- Acquired

Many molecular components (eg, complement, cytokines, acute phase proteins) participate in both innate and acquired immunity.

Innate immunity: Innate (natural) immunity does not require prior exposure to an Ag (ie, immunologic memory) to be effective. Thus, it can respond immediately to an invader. It recognizes mainly Ag molecules that are broadly distributed rather than specific to one organism or cell.

Components include

- Phagocytic cells
- Innate lymphoid cells (eg, natural killer [NK] cells)
- Polymorphonuclear leukocytes

Phagocytic cells (neutrophils in blood and tissues, monocytes in blood, macrophages in tissues) ingest and destroy invading Ags. Attack by phagocytic cells can be facilitated when Ags are coated with antibody (Ab), which is produced as part of acquired immunity, or when complement proteins opsonize Ags.

NK cells kill virus-infected cells and some tumor cells.

Polymorphonuclear leukocytes (neutrophils, eosinophils, basophils) and **mononuclear cells** (monocytes, macrophages, mast cells) release inflammatory mediators.

Acquired immunity: Acquired (adaptive) immunity requires prior exposure to an Ag and thus takes time to develop after the initial encounter with a new invader. Thereafter, response is quick. The system remembers past exposures and is Ag-specific.

Components include

- T cells
- B cells

Acquired immunity includes

- **Cell-mediated:** Derived from certain T-cell responses
- **Humoral immunity:** Derived from B-cell responses (B cells secrete soluble Ag-specific Ab)

B cells and T cells work together to destroy invaders. Antigen-presenting cells are needed to present Ags to T cells.

Immune Response

Successful immune defense requires activation, regulation, and resolution of the immune response.

Activation: The immune system is activated when a foreign antigen (Ag) is recognized by circulating antibodies (Abs) or cell surface receptors. These receptors may be

- Highly specific (Ab expressed on B cells or T-cell receptors)
- Broadly specific (eg, pattern-recognition receptors such as Toll-like, mannose, and scavenger receptors on dendritic and other cells)

Broadly specific receptors recognize common microbial pathogen-associated molecular patterns in ligands, such as gram-negative lipopolysaccharide, gram-positive peptidoglycans, bacterial flagellin, unmethylated cytosine-guanosine dinucleotides (CpG motifs), and viral double-stranded RNA. These receptors can also recognize molecules that are produced by stressed or infected human cells (called damage-associated molecular patterns).

Activation may also occur when Ab-Ag and complement-microorganism complexes bind to surface receptors for the crystallizable fragment (Fc) region of IgG (Fc-gamma R) and for C3b and iC3b.

Once recognized, an Ag, Ag-Ab complex, or complement-microorganism complex is phagocytosed. Most microorganisms are killed after they are phagocytosed, but others inhibit the phagocyte's intracellular killing ability (eg, mycobacteria that have been engulfed by a macrophage inhibit that cell's killing ability). In such cases, T cell–derived cytokines, particularly interferon-gamma (IFN-gamma), stimulate the phagocyte to produce more lytic enzymes and other microbicidal products and thus enhance its ability to kill or sequester the microorganism.

Unless Ag is rapidly phagocytosed and entirely degraded (an uncommon event), the acquired immune response is recruited. This response begins in

- The spleen for circulating Ag
- Regional lymph nodes for tissue Ag
- Mucosa-associated lymphoid tissues (eg, tonsils, adenoids, Peyer patches) for mucosal Ag

For example, Langerhans dendritic cells in the skin phagocytose Ag and migrate to local lymph nodes; there, peptides derived from the Ag are expressed on the cell surface within class II major histocompatibility complex (MHC) molecules, which present the peptide to CD4 helper T (T_H) cells. When the T_H cell engages the MHC-peptide complex and receives various costimulatory signals, it is activated to express receptors for the cytokine IL-2 and secretes several cytokines. Each subset of T_H cells secretes different combinations of substances and thus effect different immune responses.

Class II MHC molecules typically present peptides derived from extracellular (exogenous) Ag (eg, from many bacteria) to CD4 T_H cells; in contrast, class I MHC molecules typically present peptides derived from intracellular (endogenous) Ag (eg, from viruses) to CD8 cytotoxic T cells. The activated cytotoxic T cell then kills the infected cell.

Regulation: The immune response must be regulated to prevent overwhelming damage to the host (eg, anaphylaxis, widespread tissue destruction). Regulatory T cells (most of which express Foxp3 transcription factor) help control the immune response via secretion of immunosuppressive cytokines, such as IL-10 and transforming growth factor-beta (TGF-beta), or via a poorly defined cell contact mechanism.

These regulatory cells help prevent autoimmune responses and probably help resolve ongoing responses to nonself Ag.

Resolution: The immune response resolves when Ag is sequestered or eliminated from the body. Without stimulation by Ag, cytokine secretion ceases, and activated cytotoxic T cells undergo apoptosis. Apoptosis tags a cell for immediate phagocytosis, which prevents spillage of the cellular contents and development of subsequent inflammation. T and B cells that have differentiated into memory cells are spared this fate.

Geriatrics Essentials

With aging, the immune system becomes less effective in the following ways:

- The immune system becomes less able to distinguish self from nonself, making autoimmune disorders more common.
- Macrophages destroy bacteria, cancer cells, and other antigens (Ag) more slowly, possibly contributing to the increased incidence of cancer among the elderly.
- T cells respond less quickly to Ag.
- There are fewer lymphocytes that can respond to new Ag.
- The aging body produces less complement in response to bacterial infections.
- Although overall antibody (Ab) concentration does not decline significantly, the binding affinity of Ab to Ag is decreased, possibly contributing to the increased incidence of pneumonia, influenza, infectious endocarditis, and tetanus and the increased risk of death due to these disorders among the elderly. These changes may also partly explain why vaccines are less effective in the elderly.

CELLULAR COMPONENTS OF THE IMMUNE SYSTEM

The immune system consists of cellular components and molecular components that work together to destroy antigens.

Antigen-Presenting Cells

Although some antigens (Ags) can stimulate the immune response directly, T cell–dependent acquired immune responses typically require antigen-presenting cells (APCs) to present Ag-derived peptides within major histocompatibility complex (MHC) molecules.

Intracellular antigens (eg, viruses) can be processed and presented to CD8 cytotoxic T cells by any nucleated cell because all nucleated cells express class I MHC molecules. By encoding proteins that interfere with this process, some viruses (eg, cytomegalovirus) can evade elimination.

Extracellular antigens (eg, from many bacteria) must be processed into peptides and complexed with surface class II MHC molecules on professional APCs to be recognized by CD4 helper T (T_H) cells. The following cells constitutively express class II MHC molecules and therefore act as professional APCs:

- B cells
- Monocytes
- Macrophages
- Dendritic cells

Monocytes in the circulation are precursors to tissue macrophages. Monocytes migrate into tissues, where over about 8 h, they develop into macrophages under the influence of macrophage colony-stimulating factor (M-CSF), secreted by various cell types (eg, endothelial cells, fibroblasts). At infection sites, activated T cells secrete cytokines (eg, interferon-gamma [IFN-gamma]) that induce production of macrophage migration inhibitory factor, preventing macrophages from leaving.

Macrophages are activated by IFN-gamma and granulocyte-macrophage colony-stimulating factor (GM-CSF). Activated macrophages kill intracellular organisms and secrete IL-1 and tumor necrosis factor-alpha (TNF-alpha). These cytokines potentiate the secretion of IFN-gamma and GM-CSF and increase the expression of adhesion molecules on endothelial cells, facilitating leukocyte influx and destruction of pathogens. Based on different gene expression profiles, subtypes of macrophages (eg, M1, M2) have been identified (see Table 174–1).

Dendritic cells are present in the skin (as Langerhans cells), lymph nodes, and tissues throughout the body. Dendritic cells in the skin act as sentinel APCs, taking up Ag, then traveling to local lymph nodes where they can activate T cells. Follicular dendritic cells are a distinct lineage, do not express class II MHC molecules, and therefore do not present Ag to T_H cells. They are not phagocytic; they have receptors for the crystallizable fragment (Fc) region of IgG and for complement, which enable them to bind with immune complexes and present the complex to B cells in germinal centers of secondary lymphoid organs.

Lymphocytes

The 2 main types of lymphocytes are

- B cells (which mature in bone marrow)
- T cells (which mature in the thymus)

They are morphologically indistinguishable but have different immune functions. They can be distinguished by Ag-specific surface receptors and molecules called clusters of differentiation (CDs), whose presence and absence define some subsets. More than 300 CDs have been identified. Each lymphocyte recognizes a specific Ag via surface receptors.

Table 174–1. MACROPHAGE SUBTYPES

CHARACTERISTICS	M1	M2
Activation agent	Stimulation of Toll-like receptors IFN-gamma (a cytokine produced by T_H1 cells)	IL-4 and IL-13 (cytokines produced by T_H2 cells)
Cytokines produced	Proinflammatory cytokines (eg, TNF-alpha)	Immunosuppressive cytokines (eg, IL-10)
Other functions	Promote T_H1 responses Are strongly microbicidal	Promote tissue remodelling

IFN = interferon; IL = interleukin; T_H1 cells = type 1 helper T cells; T_H2 cells = type 2 helper T cells; TNF = tumor necrosis factor.

B cells: About 5 to 15% of lymphocytes in the blood are B cells; they are also present in the bone marrow, spleen, lymph nodes, and mucosa-associated lymphoid tissues.

B cells can present antigen (Ag) to T cells and release cytokines, but their primary function is to develop into plasma cells, which manufacture and secrete antibodies (Abs).

Patients with B-cell immunodeficiencies (eg, X-linked agammaglobulinemia—see p. 1406) are especially susceptible to recurrent bacterial infections.

After random rearrangement of the genes that encode immunoglobulin (Ig), B cells collectively have the potential to recognize an almost limitless number of unique Ags. Gene rearrangement occurs in programmed steps in the bone marrow during B-cell development. The process starts with a committed stem cell, continues through pro-B and pre-B cell stages, and results in an immature B cell. At this point, any cells that interact with self Ag (autoimmune cells) are removed from the immature B cell population via inactivation or apoptosis (immune tolerance). Cells that are not removed (ie, those that recognize nonself Ag) continue to develop into mature naive B cells, leave the marrow, and enter peripheral lymphoid organs, where they may encounter Ag.

Their response to Ag has 2 stages:

- **Primary immune response:** When mature naive B cells first encounter Ag, they become lymphoblasts, undergo clonal proliferation, and differentiate into memory cells, which can respond to the same Ag in the future, or into mature Ab-secreting plasma cells. After first exposure, there is a latent period of days before Ab is produced. Then, only IgM is produced. After that, with the help of T cells, B cells can further rearrange their Ig genes and switch to production of IgG, IgA, or IgE. Thus, after first exposure, the response is slow and provides limited protective immunity.
- **Secondary (anamnestic or booster) immune response:** When memory B and T_H cells are reexposed to the Ag, the memory B cells rapidly proliferate, differentiate into mature plasma cells, and promptly produce large amounts of Ab (chiefly IgG because of a T cell–induced isotype switch). The Ab is released into the blood and other tissues, where it can react with Ag. Thus, after reexposure, the immune response is faster and more effective.

T cells: T cells develop from bone marrow stem cells that travel to the thymus, where they go through rigorous selection. There are 3 main types of T cells:

- Helper
- Regulatory (suppressor)
- Cytotoxic

In selection, T cells that react to self antigen (Ag) presented by self MHC molecules or to self MHC molecules (regardless of the Ag presented) are eliminated by apoptosis. Only T cells that can recognize nonself Ag complexed to self MHC molecules survive; they leave the thymus for peripheral blood and lymphoid tissues.

Most mature T cells express either CD4 or CD8 and have an Ag-binding, Ig-like surface receptor called the T-cell receptor (TCR). There are 2 types of TCR:

- Alpha-beta (αβ) TCR: Composed of TCR alpha and beta chains; present on the most T cells
- Gamma-delta (γδ) TCR: Composed of TCR gamma and delta chains; present on a small population of T cells

Genes that encode the TCR, like Ig genes, are rearranged, resulting in defined specificity and affinity for Ag. Most T cells (those with an alpha-beta TCR) recognise Ag-derived peptide displayed in the MHC molecule of an APC. Gamma-delta T cells recognize protein Ag directly or recognize lipid Ag displayed by an MHC-like molecule called CD1. As for B cells, the number of T-cell specificities is almost limitless.

For alpha-beta T cells to be activated, the TCR must engage with Ag-MHC. Costimulatory accessory molecules must also interact; otherwise, the T cell becomes anergic or dies by apoptosis. Some accessory molecules (eg, CTLA-4) inhibit previously activated T cells and thus dampen the immune response. Polymorphisms in the CTLA-4 gene are associated with certain autoimmune disorders, including Graves disease (see p. 1346) and type I diabetes (see p. 1254).

Helper T (T_H) cells are usually CD4 but may be CD8. They differentiate from T_H0 cells into one of the following:

- T_H1 cells: In general, T_H1 cells promote cell-mediated immunity via cytotoxic T cells and macrophages and are thus particularly involved in defense against intracellular pathogens (eg, viruses). They can also promote the production of some Ab classes.
- T_H2 cells: T_H2 cells are particularly adept at promoting Ab production by B cells (humoral immunity) and thus are particularly involved in directing responses aimed at extracellular pathogens (eg, bacteria, parasites).
- T_H17 cells: T_H17 cells promote tissue inflammation.

Each cell type secretes several cytokines (see Table 174–2). Different patterns of cytokine production identify other T_H-cell functional phenotypes. Depending on the stimulating pathogen, T_H1 and T_H2 cells can, to a certain extent, downregulate each other's activity, leading to dominance of a T_H1 or a T_H2 response.

The distinction between the different T_H cells is clinically relevant. For example, a T_H1 response dominates in tuberculoid

Table 174–2. FUNCTIONS OF T CELLS

TYPE	SUBSTANCES PRODUCED	PRIMARY FUNCTION
T_H1	IFN-gamma IL-2 Lymphotoxin	Facilitate macrophage and cytotoxic T-cell responses
T_H2	IL-4 IL-5 IL-6 IL-10 IL-13	Stimulate antibody production by B cells
T_H17	IL-17 IL-21 IL-22	Promote inflammatory responses
Regulatory	TGF-beta IL-10 IL-35	Suppress immune responses
T_C	Perforin Granzymes FasL Cytokines	Kill infected cells
Activated NKT cells	IL-4 IFN-gamma	May help regulate immune responses

FasL = Fas ligand; IFN = interferon; IL = interleukin; NK = natural killer; T_C = cytotoxic T cell; TGF = transforming growth factor; T_H = helper T cell.

leprosy, and a T_H2 response dominates in lepromatous leprosy. A T_H1 response is characteristic of certain autoimmune disorders (eg, type 1 diabetes, multiple sclerosis), and a T_H2 response promotes IgE production and development of allergic disorders, as well as helps B cells produce autoantibodies in some autoimmune disorders (eg, Graves disease, myasthenia gravis). T_H17 cells, via their role in inflammation, may also contribute to autoimmune disorders such as psoriasis and RA. Patients with immunodeficiencies characterized by defective T_H17 cells (eg, hyper-IgE [Job] syndrome) are especially susceptible to infection with *Candida albicans* and *Staphylococcus aureus*.

Regulatory (suppressor) T cells mediate suppression of immune responses and usually express the Foxp3 transcription factor. The process involves functional subsets of CD4 or CD8 T cells that either secrete cytokines with immunosuppressive properties or suppress the immune response by poorly defined mechanisms that require cell-to-cell contact. Patients with functional mutations in Foxp3 develop the autoimmune disorder IPEX (immunodysregulation, polyendocrinopathy, enteropathy, X-linked) syndrome.

Cytotoxic T (T_C) cells are usually CD8 but may be CD4; they are vital for eliminating intracellular pathogens, especially viruses. T_C cells play a role in organ transplant rejection.

T_C-cell development involves 3 phases:

- A precursor cell that, when appropriately stimulated, can differentiate into a T_C cell
- An effector cell that has differentiated and can kill its appropriate target
- A memory cell that is quiescent (no longer stimulated) but is ready to become an effector when restimulated by the original Ag-MHC combination

Fully activated T_C cells, like NK cells, can kill an infected target cell by inducing apoptosis.

T_C cells can secrete cytokines and, like T_H cells, have been divided into types T_C1 and T_C2 based on their patterns of cytokine production.

T_C cells may be

- Syngeneic: Generated in response to self (autologous) cells modified by viral infection or other foreign proteins
- Allogeneic: Generated in response to cells that express foreign MHC products (eg, in organ transplantation when the donor's MHC molecules differ from the recipient's)

Some T_C cells can directly recognize foreign MHC (direct pathway); others may recognize fragments of foreign MHC presented by self MHC molecules of the transplant recipient (indirect pathway).

Natural killer T (NKT) cells are a distinct subset of T cells. Activated NKT cells secrete IL-4 and IFN-gamma and may help regulate immune responses. NKT cells differ from NK cells in phenotype and certain functions.

Mast Cells

Mast cells are tissue-based and functionally similar to basophils circulating in the blood.

Mucosal mast cell granules contain tryptase and chondroitin sulfate; connective tissue mast cell granules contain tryptase, chymase, and heparin. By releasing these mediators, mast cells play a key role in generating protective acute inflammatory responses; basophils and mast cells are the source of type I hypersensitivity reactions associated with atopic allergy. Degranulation can be triggered by cross-linking of IgE receptors or by the anaphylatoxin complement fragments C3a and C5a.

NK Cells

Typical NK cells belong to a category of cells collectively referred to as innate lymphoid cells (which also includes ILC1, ILC2, and ILC3). NK cells constitute 5 to 15% of peripheral blood mononuclear cells and have a round nucleus and granular cytoplasm. They induce apoptosis in infected or abnormal cells by a number of pathways. Like other innate lymphoid cells, they lack antigen-specific receptors; however, recent evidence suggests that some NK cells have a form of immunologic memory.

NK cells are best characterized by CD2+, CD3–, CD4–, CD8+, CD16+ (a receptor for IgG-Fc), and CD56+ surface markers.

Typical NK cells are thought to be important for tumor surveillance. NK cells express both activating and inhibitory receptors. The activating receptors on NK cells can recognize numerous ligands on target cells (eg, MHC class I–related chain A [MICA] and chain B [MICB]); the inhibitory receptors on NK cells recognize MHC class I molecules. NK cells can kill their target only when there is no strong signal from inhibitory receptors. The presence of MHC class I molecules (normally expressed on nucleated cells) on cells therefore prevents destruction of cells; their absence indicates that the cell is infected with certain viruses that inhibit MHC expression or has lost MHC expression because cancer has changed the cell.

NK cells can also secrete several cytokines (eg, IFN-gamma, IL-1, TNF-alpha); they are a major source of IFN-gamma. By secreting IFN-gamma, NK cells can influence the acquired immune system by promoting differentiation of type 1 helper T (T_H1) cells and inhibiting that of type 2 (T_H2) cells.

Patients with NK-cell deficiencies (eg, some types of severe combined immunodeficiency) are especially susceptible to herpes and human papillomavirus infections.

Polymorphonuclear Leukocytes

Polymorphonuclear (PMN) leukocytes, also called granulocytes because their cytoplasm contains granules, include

- Neutrophils
- Eosinophils
- Basophils

PMNs occur in the circulation and have multilobed nuclei.

Neutrophils: Neutrophils constitute 40 to 70% of total circulating WBCs; they are a first line of defense against infection. Mature neutrophils have a half-life of about 2 to 3 days.

During acute inflammatory responses (eg, to infection), neutrophils, drawn by chemotactic factors and alerted by the expression of adhesion molecules on blood vessel endothelium, leave the circulation and enter tissues. Their purpose is to phagocytose and digest pathogens. Microorganisms are killed when phagocytosis generates lytic enzymes and reactive O_2 compounds (eg, superoxide, hypochlorous acid) and triggers release of granule contents (eg, defensins, proteases, bactericidal permeability-increasing protein, lactoferrin, lysozymes). DNA and histones are also released, and they, with granule contents such as elastase, generate fibrous structures called neutrophil extracellular traps (NETs) in the surrounding tissues; these structures facilitate killing by trapping bacteria and focusing enzyme activity.

Patients with immunodeficiencies that affect the phagocytes' ability to kill pathogens (eg, chronic granulomatous disease) are especially susceptible to chronic bacterial and fungal infections.

Eosinophils: Eosinophils constitute up to 5% of circulating WBCs.

They target organisms too large to be engulfed; they kill by secreting toxic substances (eg, reactive O_2 compounds similar to those produced in neutrophils), major basic protein (which is toxic to parasites), eosinophil cationic protein, and several enzymes.

Eosinophils are also a major source of inflammatory mediators (eg, prostaglandins, leukotrienes, platelet-activating factor, many cytokines).

Basophils: Basophils constitute < 5% of circulating WBCs and share several characteristics with mast cells, although the 2 cell types have distinct lineages. Both have high-affinity receptors for IgE called Fc-epsilon RI (FcεRI). When these cells encounter certain Ags, the bivalent IgE molecules bound to the receptors become cross-linked, triggering cell degranulation with release of preformed inflammatory mediators (eg, histamine, platelet-activating factor) and generation of newly synthesized mediators (eg, leukotrienes, prostaglandins, thromboxanes).

MOLECULAR COMPONENTS OF THE IMMUNE SYSTEM

The immune system consists of cellular components and molecular components that work together to destroy antigens (Ags).

Acute Phase Reactants

Acute phase reactants are plasma proteins whose levels dramatically increase (called positive acute phase reactants) or, in some cases, decrease (called negative acute phase reactants) in response to the elevated circulating levels of IL-1 and IL-6 that occur when infection or tissue damage occurs. Most dramatically increased are C-reactive protein (CRP) and mannose-binding lectin (which fix complement and act as opsonins), the transport protein alpha-1 acid glycoprotein, and serum amyloid P component. CRP and ESR are often measured; elevated levels are a nonspecific indicator suggesting infection or inflammation. Increased fibrinogen is the main reason ESR is elevated.

Many acute phase reactants are made in the liver. Collectively, they may help limit tissue injury, enhance host resistance to infection, and promote tissue repair and resolution of inflammation.

Antibodies

Antibodies (Abs) act as the antigen (Ag) receptor on the surface of B cells and, in response to Ag, are subsequently secreted by plasma cells. Abs recognize specific configurations (epitopes, or antigenic determinants) on the surfaces of Ags (eg, proteins, polysaccharides, nucleic acids). Abs and Ags fit tightly together because their shape and other surface properties (eg, charge) are complementary. The same Ab molecule can cross-react with related Ags if their epitopes are similar enough to those of the original Ag.

Antibody structure: Abs consist of 4 polypeptide chains (2 identical heavy chains and 2 identical light chains) joined by disulfide bonds to produce a Y configuration (see Fig. 174–1). The heavy and light chains are divided into a variable (V) region and a constant (C) region.

V regions are located at the amino-terminal ends of the Y arms; they are called variable because the amino acids they contain are different in different Abs. Within the V regions, hypervariable regions determine the specificity of the Ig. They also function as antigens (idiotypic determinants) to which certain natural (anti-idiotype) Abs can bind; this binding may help regulate B-cell responses.

The **C region** of the heavy chains contains a relatively constant sequence of amino acids (isotype) that is distinctive for each Ig class. A B cell can change the isotype it produces and thus switch the class of Ig it produces. Because the Ig retains the variable part of the heavy chain V region and the entire light chain, it retains its antigenic specificity.

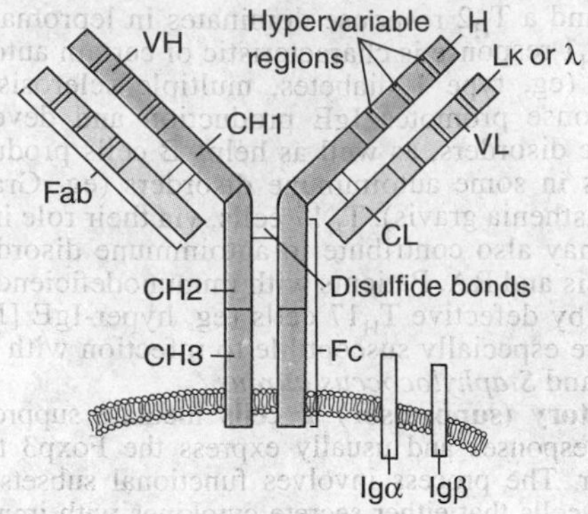

Fig. 174–1. B-cell receptor. The B-cell receptor consists of an Ig molecule anchored to the cell's surface. CH = heavy chain constant region; CL = light chain constant region; Fab = antigen-binding fragment; Fc = crystallizable fragment; Ig = immunoglobulin; L-kappa (κ) or lambda (λ) = 2 types of light chains; VH = heavy chain variable region; VL = light chain variable region.

The amino-terminal (variable) end of the Ab binds to Ag to form an Ab-Ag complex. The Ag-binding (Fab) portion of Ig consists of a light chain and part of a heavy chain and contains the V region of the Ig molecule (ie, the combining sites). The crystallizable fragment (Fc) contains most of the C region of the heavy chains; Fc is responsible for complement activation and binds to Fc receptors on cells.

Antibody classes: Antibodies are divided into 5 classes:

- IgM
- IgG
- IgA
- IgD
- IgE

The classes are defined by their type of heavy chain: mu (μ) for IgM, gamma (γ) for IgG, alpha (α) for IgA, epsilon (ε) for IgE, and delta (δ) for IgD. There are also 2 types of light chains: kappa (κ) and lambda (λ). Each of the 5 Ig classes can bear either kappa or lambda light chains.

IgM is the first Ab formed after exposure to new Ag. It has 5 Y-shaped molecules (10 heavy chains and 10 light chains), linked by a single joining (J) chain. IgM circulates primarily in the intravascular space; it complexes with and agglutinates Ag and can activate complement, thereby facilitating phagocytosis. Isohemagglutinins are predominantly IgM. Monomeric IgM acts as a surface Ag receptor on B cells. Patients with hyper-IgM syndrome have a defect in the genes involved in antibody class switching (eg, genes that encode CD40, CD154 [also known as CD40L], or NEMO [nuclear factor–kappa-B essential modulator]); therefore, IgA, IgG, and IgE levels are low or absent, and levels of circulating IgM are often high.

IgG is the most prevalent Ig isotype in serum and is also present in intravascular and extravascular spaces. It coats Ag to activate complement and facilitate phagocytosis by neutrophils and macrophages. IgG is the primary circulating Ig produced after reexposure to Ag (secondary immune response) and is the predominant isotype contained in commercial gamma-globulin products. IgG protects against bacteria, viruses, and toxins;

it is the only Ig isotype that crosses the placenta. Therefore, this class of antibody is important for protecting neonates, but pathogenic IgG antibodies (eg, anti-Rh_0[D] antibodies, stimulatory anti-TSH receptor autoantibodies), if present in the mother, can potentially cause significant disease in the fetus.

There are 4 subclasses of IgG: IgG1, IgG2, IgG3, and IgG4. They are numbered in descending order of serum concentration. IgG subclasses differ functionally mainly in their ability to activate complement; IgG1 and IgG3 are most efficient, IgG2 is less efficient, and IgG4 is inefficient. IgG1 and IgG3 are efficient mediators of Ab-dependent cellular cytotoxicity; IgG4 and IgG2 are less so.

IgA occurs at mucosal surfaces, in serum, and in secretions (saliva; tears; respiratory, GU, and GI tract secretions; colostrum), where it provides an early antibacterial and antiviral defense. J chain links IgA into a dimer to form secretory IgA. Secretory IgA is synthesized by plasma cells in the subepithelial regions of the GI and respiratory tracts. Selective IgA deficiency is relatively common but often has little clinical impact because there is cross-functionality with other classes of antibody.

IgD is coexpressed with IgM on the surface of naive B cells. Whether these 2 classes function differently on the surface of the B cell and, if so, how differently are unclear. They may simply be an example of molecular degeneracy. Serum IgD levels are very low, and the function of circulating IgD is unknown.

IgE is present in low levels in serum and in respiratory and GI mucous secretions. IgE binds with high affinity to receptors present in high levels on mast cells and basophils and to a lesser extent on several other hematopoietic cells, including dendritic cells. If Ag bridges 2 IgE molecules bound to the mast cell or basophil surface, the cells degranulate, releasing chemical mediators that cause an inflammatory response. IgE levels are elevated in atopic disorders (eg, allergic or extrinsic asthma, hay fever, atopic dermatitis) and parasitic infections.

Cytokines

Cytokines are polypeptides secreted by immune and other cells when the cell interacts with a specific Ag, with pathogen-associated molecules such as endotoxin, or with other cytokines. Main categories include

- Chemokines
- Hematopoietic CSFs
- Interleukins
- Interferons (IFN-alpha, IFN-beta, IFN-gamma)
- TGFs
- Tumor necrosis factors (TNF-alpha, lymphotoxin-alpha, lymphotoxin-beta)

Although lymphocyte interaction with a specific Ag triggers cytokine secretion, cytokines themselves are not Ag-specific; thus, they bridge innate and acquired immunity and generally influence the magnitude of inflammatory or immune responses. They act sequentially, synergistically, or antagonistically. They may act in an autocrine or paracrine manner.

Cytokines deliver their signals via cell surface receptors. For example, the IL-2 receptor consists of 3 chains: alpha (α), beta (β), and gamma (γ). The receptor's affinity for IL-2 is

- High if all 3 chains are expressed
- Intermediate if only the beta and gamma chains are expressed
- Low if only the alpha chain is expressed

Mutations or deletion of the gamma chain is the basis for X-linked severe combined immunodeficiency.

Chemokines: Chemokines induce chemotaxis and migration of leukocytes. There are 4 subsets (C, CC, CXC, CX3C), defined by the number and spacing of their amino terminal cysteine residues. Chemokine receptors (CCR5 on memory T cells, monocytes/macrophages, and dendritic cells; CXCR4 on resting T cells) act as coreceptors for entry of HIV into cells.

CSF: G-CSF is produced by endothelial cells and fibroblasts. The main effect of G-CSF is

- Stimulation of neutrophil precursors growth

Clinical uses of G-CSF include

- Reversal of neutropenia after chemotherapy, radiation therapy, or both

GM-CSF is produced by endothelial cells, fibroblasts, macrophages, mast cells, and T_H cells.

The main effects of GM-CSF are

- Stimulation of growth of monocyte, neutrophil, eosinophil, and basophil precursors
- Activation of macrophages

Clinical uses of GM-CSF include

- Reversal of neutropenia after chemotherapy, radiation therapy, or both

M-CSF is produced by endothelial cells, epithelial cells, and fibroblasts.

The main effect of M-CSF is

- Stimulation of monocyte precursor growth

Clinical uses of M-CSF include

- Therapeutic potential for stimulating tissue repair

SCF is produced by bone marrow stromal cells.
The main effect of SCF is

- Stimulation of stem cell division

Clinical uses of SCF include

- Therapeutic potential for stimulating tissue repair

Interferons: IFN-alpha is produced by leukocytes.
The main effects of IFN-alpha are

- Inhibition of viral replication
- Augmentation of class I MHC expression

Clinical uses of IFN-alpha include

- Treatment of chronic hepatitis C, AIDS-related Kaposi sarcoma, hairy cell leukemia, chronic myelogenous leukemia, and metastatic melanoma

IFN-beta is produced by fibroblasts.
The main effects of IFN-beta are

- Inhibition of viral replication
- Augmentation of class I MHC expression

Clinical uses of IFN-beta include

- Reduction of the number of flare-ups in relapsing multiple sclerosis

IFN-gamma is produced by NK cells, T_C1 cells, and T_H1 cells.
The main effects of IFN-gamma are

- Inhibition of viral replication
- Augmentation of classes I and II MHC expression
- Activation of macrophages
- Antagonism of several actions of IL-4
- Inhibition of T_H2 cell proliferation

Clinical uses of IFN-gamma include

- Control of infection in chronic granulomatous disease
- Delay of progression in severe malignant osteopetrosis

Interleukins: IL-1 (alpha and beta) is produced by B cells, dendritic cells, endothelium, macrophages, monocytes, and NK cells.

The main effects of IL-1 are

- Costimulation of T-cell activation by enhancing production of cytokines (eg, IL-2 and its receptor)
- Enhancement of B-cell proliferation and maturation
- Enhancement of NK-cell cytotoxicity
- Induction of IL-1, IL-6, IL-8, TNF, GM-CSF, and prostaglandin E_2 production by macrophages
- Proinflammatory activity by inducing chemokines, ICAM-1, and VCAM-1 on endothelium
- Induction of sleep, anorexia, release of tissue factor, acute phase reactants, and bone resorption by osteoclasts
- Endogenous pyrogenic activity

Clinical relevance of IL-1 includes

- For **anti–IL-1 beta mAb,** treatment of cryopyrin-associated periodic syndromes and juvenile idiopathic arthritis
- For **IL-1 receptor antagonist (IL-1RA),** treatment of adults with moderate to severe RA and patients with neonatal-onset multisystem inflammatory disease (NOMID)

IL-2 is produced by T_H1 cells.

The main effects of IL-2 are

- Induction of activated T- and B-cell proliferation
- Enhancement of NK-cell cytotoxicity and killing of tumor cells and bacteria by monocytes and macrophages

Clinical relevance of IL-2 includes

- For **IL-2,** treatment of metastatic renal cell carcinoma and metastatic melanoma
- For **anti-IL-2 receptor mAb,** help with prevention of acute kidney rejection

IL-4 is produced by mast cells, NK cells, NKT cells, gamma-delta T cells, T_C2 cells, and T_H2 cells.

The main effects of IL-4 are

- Induction of T_H2 cells
- Stimulation of activated B-, T-, and mast cell proliferation
- Upregulation of class II MHC molecules on B cells and on macrophages and CD23 on B cells
- Downregulation of IL-12 production, thereby inhibiting T_H1 cell-differentiation
- Augmentation of macrophage phagocytosis
- Induction of switch to IgG1 and IgE

Clinical relevance of IL-4 includes

- Involvement of IL-4 (with IL-13) in the production of IgE in atopic allergy

IL-5 is produced by mast cells and T_H2 cells.

The main effects of IL-5 are

- Induction of eosinophil and activated B-cell proliferation
- Induction of switch to IgA

Clinical relevance of IL-5 includes

- For **anti–IL-5 mAb,** efficacy in the treatment of patients with severe eosinophilic asthma

IL-6 is produced by dendritic cells, fibroblasts, macrophages, monocytes, and T_H2 cells.

The main effects of IL-6 are

- Induction of differentiation of B cells into plasma cells and differentiation of myeloid stem cells
- Induction of acute phase reactants
- Enhancement of T-cell proliferation
- Induction of T_C-cell differentiation
- Pyrogenic activity

Clinical relevance of IL-6 includes

- For **anti–IL-6 mAb,** treatment of multicentric Castleman disease in patients who are negative for HIV and human herpesvirus 8 (HHV-8)
- For **anti–IL-6 receptor mAb,** treatment of RA when the response to TNF-antagonists is inadequate and treatment of juvenile idiopathic arthritis

IL-7 is produced by bone marrow and thymus stromal cells.

The main effects of IL-7 are

- Induction of differentiation of lymphoid stem cells into T- and B-cell precursors
- Activation of mature T cells

The role of IL-7 in T-cell differentiation has led to clinical trials of IL-7 as a potential immunostimulatory agent in the treatment of viral infections and cancer.

IL-8 (chemokine) is produced by endothelial cells, macrophages, and monocytes.

The main effect of IL-8 is

- Mediation of chemotaxis and activation of neutrophils

Clinical relevance of IL-8 includes

- For **IL-8 antagonists,** potential for the treatment of chronic inflammatory disorders

IL-9 is produced by T_H cells.

The main effects of IL-9 are

- Induction of thymocyte proliferation
- Enhancement of mast cell growth
- Synergistic action with IL-4 to induce switch to IgG1 and IgE

Clinical trials of anti-IL-9 mAb in asthma have generally failed to demonstrate efficacy.

IL-10 is produced by B cells, macrophages, monocytes, T_C cells, T_H2 cells, and regulatory T cells.

The main effects of IL-10 are

- Inhibition of IL-2 secretion by human T_H1 cells
- Downregulation of production of class II MHC molecules and cytokines (eg, IL-12) by monocytes, macrophages, and dendritic cells, thereby inhibiting T_H1-cell differentiation
- Inhibition of T-cell proliferation
- Enhancement of B-cell differentiation

Clinical uses of IL-10 include

- Possible suppression of pathogenic immune response in allergy and autoimmune disorders

IL-12 is produced by B cells, dendritic cells, macrophages, and monocytes.

The main effects of IL-12 are

- A critical role in T_H1 differentiation
- Induction of proliferation of T_H1 cells, CD8 T cells, gamma-delta T cells, and NK cells and their production of IFN-gamma
- Enhancement of NK and CD8 T-cell cytotoxicity

Clinical relevance of IL-12 includes

- For **anti–IL-12 mAb,** treatment of plaque psoriasis and psoriatic arthritis

IL-13 is produced by mast cells and T_H2 cells.

The main effects of IL-13 are

- Inhibition of activation and cytokine secretion by macrophages
- Coactivation of B-cell proliferation
- Upregulation of class II MHC molecules and CD23 on B cells and monocytes
- Induction of switch to IgG1 and IgE
- Induction of VCAM-1 on endothelium

Clinical relevance of IL-13 includes

- Involvement of IL-13 (with IL-4) in the production of IgE in atopic allergy

IL-15 is produced by B cells, dendritic cells, macrophages, monocytes, NK cells, and T cells.
The main effects of IL-15 are

- Induction of proliferation of T, NK, and activated B cells
- Induction of cytokine production and cytotoxicity of NK cells and CD8 T cells
- Chemotactic activity for T cells
- Stimulation of intestinal epithelium growth

Clinical uses of IL-15 include

- Potential as an immunostimulatory agent in the treatment of cancer

IL-17 (A and F) is produced by T_H17 cells, gamma-delta T cells, NKT cells, and macrophages
The main effects of IL-17 are

- Proinflammatory action
- Stimulation of production of cytokines (eg, TNF, IL-1 beta, IL-6, IL-8, G-CSF)

Clinical relevance of IL-17 includes

- For **anti-IL-17A mAb,** treatment of adults with active ankylosing spondylitis, active psoriatic arthritis, or moderate to severe plaque psoriasis

IL-18 is produced by monocytes, macrophages, and dendritic cells.
The main effects of IL-18 are

- Induction of IFN-gamma production by T cells
- Enhancement of NK-cell cytotoxicity

IL-18 has been investigated as an immunotherapeutic agent in cancer, but efficacy has not been established.
IL-21 is produced by NKT cells and T_H cells.
The main effects of IL-21 are

- Stimulation of B-cell proliferation after CD40 cross-linking
- Stimulation of NK cells
- Costimulation of T cells
- Stimulation of bone marrow precursor cell proliferation

Clinical relevance of IL-21 includes

- In clinical trials, stimulation of cytotoxic T cells and NK cells in cancer
- For **IL-21 antagonists,** potential in the treatment of autoimmune disorders

IL-22 is produced by NK cells, T_H17 cells, and gamma-delta cells.
The main effects of IL-22 are

- Proinflammatory activity
- Induction of acute phase reactant synthesis

Clinical relevance of IL-22 includes

- For **IL-22 antagonists,** potential in the treatment of autoimmune disorders

IL-23 is produced by dendritic cells and macrophages.
The main effect of IL-23 is

- Induction of T_H-cell proliferation

Clinical relevance of IL-23 includes

- For **anti–IL-23 mAb,** treatment of plaque psoriasis and psoriatic arthritis

IL-24 is produced by B cells, macrophages, monocytes, and T cells.
The main effects of IL-24 are

- Suppression of tumor cell growth
- Induction of apoptosis in tumor cells

Clinical uses of IL-24 include

- Potential in the treatment of cancer

IL-27 is produced by dendritic cells, monocytes, and macrophages.
The main effect of IL-27 is

- Induction of T_H1 cells

Clinical uses of IL-27 include

- Potential in the treatment of cancer

IL-32 is produced by NK cells and T cells.
The main effects of IL-32 are

- Proinflammatory activity
- Participation in activation-induced T cell apoptosis

Clinical uses of IL-32 include

- Potential in the treatment of autoimmune disorders

IL-33 is produced by endothelial cells, stromal cells, and dendritic cells.
The main effects of IL-33 are

- Induction of T_H2 cytokines
- Promotion of eosinophilia

Clinical relevance of IL-33 includes

- For **IL-33 antagonists,** potential in the treatment of asthma

IL-35 is produced by regulatory T cells, macrophages, and dendritic cells.
The main effect of IL-35 is

- Suppression of inflammation (eg, by inducing regulatory T and B cells and inhibiting T_H17 cells)

Clinical uses of IL-35 include

- Potential to suppress pathogenic immune responses in allergy and autoimmune disorders

TGF: TGF-beta is produced by B cells, macrophages, mast cells, and T_H3 cells.
The main effects of TGF-beta are

- Proinflammatory activity (eg, by chemoattraction of monocytes and macrophages) but also anti-inflammatory activity (eg, by inhibiting lymphocyte proliferation)
- Induction of switch to IgA
- Promotion of tissue repair

Clinical trials of **TGF-beta antagonists** (eg, antisense oligonucleotides) in cancer are ongoing.

TNFs: TNF-alpha (cachectin) is produced by B cells, dendritic cells, macrophages, mast cells, monocytes, NK cells, and T_H cells.

The main effects of TNF-alpha include

- Cytotoxicity to tumor cells
- Cachexia
- Induction of secretion of several cytokines (eg, IL-1, GM-CSF, IFN-gamma)
- Induction of E-selectin on endothelium
- Activation of macrophages
- Antiviral activity

Clinical relevance of TNF-alpha includes

- For **TNF-alpha antagonists** (mAb or soluble receptor), treatment of RA, plaque psoriasis, Crohn disease refractory to standard treatments, ulcerative colitis, hidradenitis suppurativa, ankylosing spondylitis, psoriatic arthritis, and polyarticular juvenile idiopathic arthritis.

TNF-beta (lymphotoxin) is produced by T_C cells, and T_H1 cells.

The main effects of TNF-beta include

- Cytotoxicity to tumor cells
- Antiviral activity
- Enhancement of phagocytosis by neutrophils and macrophages
- Involvement in lymphoid organ development

Clinical relevance of TNF-beta includes

- For **TNF-beta antagonists**, similar effects to well-established TNF-alpha antagonists but have not been shown to be superior

HUMAN LEUKOCYTE ANTIGEN SYSTEM

The human leukocyte antigen (HLA) system, the major histocompatibility complex (MHC) in humans, is controlled by genes located on chromosome 6. It encodes cell surface molecules specialized to present antigenic peptides to the T-cell receptor (TCR) on T cells. MHC molecules that present antigen (Ag) are divided into 2 main classes:

- Class I MHC molecules
- Class II MHC molecules

Class I MHC molecules are present as transmembrane glycoproteins on the surface of all nucleated cells. Intact class I molecules consist of an alpha heavy chain bound to a beta-2 microglobulin molecule. The heavy chain consists of 2 peptide-binding domains, an Ig-like domain, and a transmembrane region with a cytoplasmic tail. The heavy chain of the class I molecule is encoded by genes at HLA-A, HLA-B, and HLA-C loci. Lymphocytes that express CD8 molecules react with class I MHC molecules. These lymphocytes often have a cytotoxic function, requiring them to be capable of recognizing any infected cell. Because every nucleated cell expresses class I MHC molecules, all infected cells can act as antigen-presenting cells for CD8 T cells (CD8 binds to the nonpolymorphic part of the class I heavy chain). Some class I MHC genes encode nonclassical MHC molecules, such as HLA-G (which may play a role in protecting the fetus from the maternal immune response) and HLA-E (which presents peptides to certain receptors on NK cells).

Class II MHC molecules are usually present only on professional Ag-presenting cells (B cells, macrophages, dendritic cells, Langerhans cells), thymic epithelium, and activated (but not resting) T cells; most nucleated cells can be induced to express class II MHC molecules by interferon (IFN)-gamma. Class II MHC molecules consist of 2 polypeptide (alpha [α] and beta [β]) chains; each chain has a peptide-binding domain, an Ig-like domain, and a transmembrane region with a cytoplasmic tail. Both polypeptide chains are encoded by genes in the HLA-DP, -DQ, or -DR region of chromosome 6. Lymphocytes reactive to class II molecules express CD4 and are often helper T cells.

The **MHC class III region** of the genome encodes several molecules important in inflammation; they include complement components C2, C4, and factor B; TNF-alpha; lymphotoxin; and three heat shock proteins.

Individual serologically defined antigens encoded by the class I and II gene loci in the HLA system are given standard designations (eg, HLA-A1, -B5, -C1, -DR1). Alleles defined by DNA sequencing are named to identify the gene, followed by an asterisk, numbers representing the allele group (often corresponding to the serologic antigen encoded by that allele), a colon, and numbers representing the specific allele (eg, A*02:01, DRB1*01:03, DQA1*01:02). Sometimes additional numbers are added after a colon to identify allelic variants that encode identical proteins, and after another colon, other numbers are added to denote polymorphisms in introns or in 5' or 3' untranslated regions (eg, A*02:101:01:02, DRB1*03:01:01:02).

The MHC class I and II molecules are the most immunogenic antigens that are recognized during rejection of an allogeneic transplant. The strongest determinant is HLA-DR, followed by HLA-B and -A. These 3 loci are therefore the most important for matching donor and recipient.

Some autoimmune disorders are linked to specific HLA alleles—for example,

- Psoriasis to HLA-C*06:02
- Ankylosing spondylitis and reactive arthritis to HLA-B27
- Narcolepsy to HLA-DR2 and HLA–DQB1*06:02
- Type 1 diabetes mellitus to HLA-DQ2 and HLA-DQ8
- Multiple sclerosis to HLA-DR2
- RA to HLA-DR4

COMPLEMENT SYSTEM

The complement system is an enzyme cascade that helps defend against infection. Many complement proteins occur in serum as inactive enzyme precursors (zymogens); others reside on cell surfaces. The complement system bridges innate and acquired immunity by

- Augmenting antibody (Ab) responses and immunologic memory
- Lysing foreign cells
- Clearing immune complexes and apoptotic cells

Complement components have many biologic functions (eg, stimulation of chemotaxis, triggering of mast cell degranulation independent of IgE).

Complement activation: There are 3 pathways of complement activation (see Fig. 174–2):

- Classical
- Lectin
- Alternative

Classical pathway components are labeled with a C and a number (eg, C1, C3), based on the order in which they were identified. Alternative pathway components are often lettered (eg, factor B, factor D) or named (eg, properdin).

Classical pathway activation is either

- Ab-dependent, occurring when C1 interacts with Ag-IgM or aggregated Ag-IgG complexes

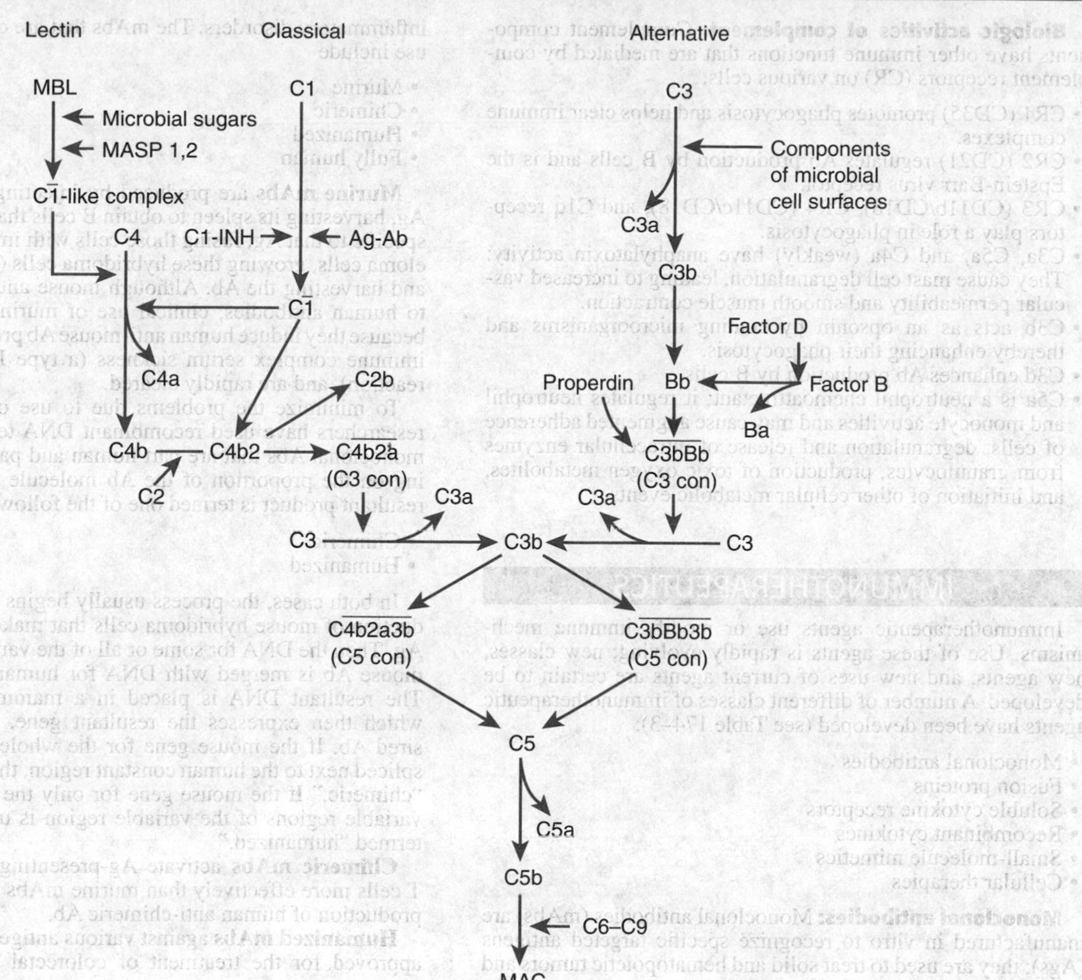

Fig. 174–2. Complement activation pathways. The classical, lectin, and alternative pathways converge into a final common pathway when C3 convertase (C3 con) cleaves C3 into C3a and C3b. Ab = antibody; Ag = antigen; C1-INH = C1 inhibitor; MAC = membrane attack complex; MASP = MBL-associated serine protease; MBL = mannose-binding lectin. Overbar indicates activation.

- Ab-independent, occurring when polyanions (eg, heparin, protamine, DNA and RNA from apoptotic cells), gram-negative bacteria, or bound C-reactive protein reacts directly with C1

This pathway is regulated by C1 inhibitor (C1-INH). Hereditary angioedema is due to a genetic deficiency of C1-INH.

Lectin pathway activation is Ab-independent; it occurs when mannose-binding lectin (MBL), a serum protein, binds to mannose, fuctose, or *N*-acetylglucosamine groups on bacterial cell walls, yeast walls, or viruses. This pathway otherwise resembles the classical pathway structurally and functionally.

Alternate pathway activation occurs when components of microbial cell surfaces (eg, yeast walls, bacterial cell wall lipopolysaccharide [endotoxin]) or Ig (eg, nephritic factor, aggregated IgA) cleave small amounts of C3. This pathway is regulated by properdin, factor H, and decay-accelerating factor (CD55).

The 3 activation pathways converge into a final common pathway when C3 convertase cleaves C3 into C3a and C3b (see Fig. 174–2). C3 cleavage may result in formation of the membrane attack complex (MAC), the cytotoxic component of the complement system. MAC causes lysis of foreign cells.

Factor I, with cofactors including membrane cofactor protein (CD46), inactivates C3b and C4b.

Complement deficiencies and defects: Deficiencies or defects in specific complement components have been linked to specific disorders; the following are examples:

- Deficiency in C1, C2, C3, MBL, MASP-2, factor H, factor I, or complement receptor 2 (CR2): Susceptibility to recurrent bacterial infections
- Deficiency of C5, C9, factor B, factor D, or properdin: Susceptibility to neisserial infections
- Defects in C1, C4, and C5: SLE
- Defects in CR2: Common variable immunodeficiency
- Defects of CR3: Leukocyte adhesion deficiency type 1
- Mutations in the genes for factor B, factor H, factor I, membrane cofactor protein (CD46), or C3: Development of the atypical variant of hemolytic uremic syndrome

Biologic activities of complement: Complement components have other immune functions that are mediated by complement receptors (CR) on various cells.

- CR1 (CD35) promotes phagocytosis and helps clear immune complexes.
- CR2 (CD21) regulates Ab production by B cells and is the Epstein-Barr virus receptor.
- CR3 (CD11b/CD18), CR4 (CD11c/CD18), and C1q receptors play a role in phagocytosis.
- C3a, C5a, and C4a (weakly) have anaphylatoxin activity: They cause mast cell degranulation, leading to increased vascular permeability and smooth muscle contraction.
- C3b acts as an opsonin by coating microorganisms and thereby enhancing their phagocytosis.
- C3d enhances Ab production by B cells.
- C5a is a neutrophil chemoattractant; it regulates neutrophil and monocyte activities and may cause augmented adherence of cells, degranulation and release of intracellular enzymes from granulocytes, production of toxic oxygen metabolites, and initiation of other cellular metabolic events.

IMMUNOTHERAPEUTICS

Immunotherapeutic agents use or modify immune mechanisms. Use of these agents is rapidly evolving; new classes, new agents, and new uses of current agents are certain to be developed. A number of different classes of immunotherapeutic agents have been developed (see Table 174–3):

- Monoclonal antibodies
- Fusion proteins
- Soluble cytokine receptors
- Recombinant cytokines
- Small-molecule mimetics
- Cellular therapies

Monoclonal antibodies: Monoclonal antibodies (mAbs) are manufactured in vitro to recognize specific targeted antigens (Ags); they are used to treat solid and hematopoietic tumors and inflammatory disorders. The mAbs that are currently in clinical use include

- Murine
- Chimeric
- Humanized
- Fully human

Murine mAbs are produced by injecting a mouse with an Ag, harvesting its spleen to obtain B cells that are producing Ab specific to that Ag, fusing those cells with immortal mouse myeloma cells, growing these hybridoma cells (eg, in cell culture), and harvesting the Ab. Although mouse antibodies are similar to human antibodies, clinical use of murine mAbs is limited because they induce human anti-mouse Ab production, can cause immune complex serum sickness (a type III hypersensitivity reaction), and are rapidly cleared.

To minimize the problems due to use of pure mouse Ab, researchers have used recombinant DNA techniques to create monoclonal Abs that are part human and part mouse. Depending on the proportion of the Ab molecule that is human, the resultant product is termed one of the following:

- Chimeric
- Humanized

In both cases, the process usually begins as above with production of mouse hybridoma cells that make Ab to the desired Ag. Then the DNA for some or all of the variable portion of the mouse Ab is merged with DNA for human immunoglobulin. The resultant DNA is placed in a mammalian cell culture, which then expresses the resultant gene, producing the desired Ab. If the mouse gene for the whole variable region is spliced next to the human constant region, the product is termed "chimeric." If the mouse gene for only the Ag-binding hypervariable regions of the variable region is used, the product is termed "humanized."

Chimeric mAbs activate Ag-presenting cells (APCs) and T cells more effectively than murine mAbs but can still induce production of human anti-chimeric Ab.

Humanized mAbs against various antigens (Ags) have been approved for the treatment of colorectal and breast cancer,

Table 174–3. SOME IMMUNOTHERAPEUTIC AGENTS IN CLINICAL USE

AGENT	EFFECTS	INDICATIONS
Monoclonal antibodies*		
Adalimumab	Anti–TNF-alpha	Moderate to severe RA Plaque psoriasis Moderate to severe Crohn disease refractory to standard treatments Ulcerative colitis Ankylosing spondylitis Psoriatic arthritis Moderate to severe polyarticular juvenile idiopathic arthritis Hidradenitis suppurativa
Alemtuzumab	Anti–B cell (CD52)	B-cell chronic lymphocytic leukemia refractory to standard treatments
Atezolizumab	Anti–PD-L1	Locally advanced or metastatic transitional cell urothelial carcinoma if it progresses during or after platinum-based chemotherapy
Basiliximab	Anti–IL-2 receptor	Prevention of acute kidney rejection
Belimumab	Anti–B-lymphocyte stimulator protein (anti-BLyS)	Autoantibody-positive SLE in adults receiving standard treatment

Table 174–3. SOME IMMUNOTHERAPEUTIC AGENTS IN CLINICAL USE (*Continued*)

AGENT	EFFECTS	INDICATIONS
Bevacizumab	Anti–VEGF-A	Metastatic colorectal cancer (used with IV 5-fluorouracil–based chemotherapy as 1st- or 2nd-line treatment) Metastatic colorectal cancer (used with fluoropyrimidine-, irinotecan-, or fluoropyrimidine-oxaliplatin–based chemotherapy as 2nd-line treatment) if the cancer progressed during treatment with a 1st-line regimen that contains bevacizumab Unresectable, locally advanced, recurrent, or metastatic nonsquamous non–small cell lung cancer (used with carboplatin and paclitaxel as 1st-line treatment) Glioblastoma in adults if the disorder progresses after other treatments have been tried Metastatic renal cell carcinoma (used with IFN-alpha) Persistent, recurrent, or metastatic cervical cancer (used with paclitaxel and cisplatin or paclitaxel and topotecan) Platinum-resistant, recurrent epithelial ovarian cancer, fallopian tube cancer, or primary peritoneal cancer (used with paclitaxel, pegylated liposomal doxorubicin, or topotecan)
Blinatumomab	Bispecific: Anti-CD19 and anti-CD3	Philadelphia chromosome–negative relapsed or refractory B-cell precursor ALL
Brentuximab vedotin	Anti-CD30 (linked to the antimitotic agent monomethyl auristatin E)	Hodgkin lymphoma after failure of autologous stem cell transplantation (ASCT) or of at least 2 multidrug chemotherapy regimens in patients who are not candidates for ASCT Systemic anaplastic large cell lymphoma after failure of at least one multidrug chemotherapy regimen
Canakinumab	Anti–IL-1 beta	Cryopyrin-associated periodic syndromes (cryopyrinopathies) in patients ≥ 4 yr Juvenile idiopathic arthritis in patients ≥ 2 yr
Certolizumab (pegylated Fab' fragment)	Anti–TNF-alpha	Moderate to severe RA in adults Moderate to severe Crohn disease if response to conventional treatments is inadequate Psoriatic arthritis Ankylosing spondylitis
Cetuximab	Anti-EGFR	Locally or regionally advanced squamous cell carcinoma of the head and neck (used with radiation therapy) Recurrent locoregional or metastatic squamous cell carcinoma of the head and neck (used with platinum-based therapy and 5-fluorouracil) Recurrent or metastatic squamous cell carcinoma of the head and neck if it progresses after platinum-based therapy Wild-type *KRAS*, EGFR-expressing, metastatic colorectal cancer, given as follows: • With FOLFIRI as first-line treatment • With irinotecan if the cancer is refractory to irinotecan-based chemotherapy • As a single agent if oxaliplatin- and irinotecan-based chemotherapy is ineffective or patients cannot tolerate irinotecan
Daclizumab	Anti–IL-2 receptor	Prevention of acute kidney rejection
Daratumumab	Anti-CD 38	Multiple myeloma if • Patients have received ≥ 3 prior drug regimens that included a proteasome inhibitor and an immunomodulatory drug. *or* • The cancer is refractory to both a proteasome inhibitor and an immunomodulatory drug.

Table continues on the following page.

Table 174–3. SOME IMMUNOTHERAPEUTIC AGENTS IN CLINICAL USE (*Continued*)

AGENT	EFFECTS	INDICATIONS
Denosumab	Anti-RANKL	Prevention of skeletal-related events (eg, fractures, bone pain) in patients with bone metastases from solid tumors Treatment of adults and skeletally mature adolescents with a giant cell tumor of bone if the tumor is unresectable or if surgical resection is likely to result in severe morbidity Treatment of hypercalcemia of malignancy refractory to bisphosphonate therapy
Dinutuximab	Anti-GD2 glycolipid	High-risk pediatric neuroblastoma that has at least partially responded to prior first-line multidrug, multimodality therapy (used with GM-CSF, IL-2, and isotretinoin [13-*cis*-retinoic acid])
Eculizumab	Anti–complement component C5	Paroxysmal nocturnal hemoglobinuria Atypical hemolytic-uremic syndrome
Efalizumab[†]	Anti-CD11a	Chronic moderate to severe plaque psoriasis
Elotuzumab	Anti-SLAMF7	Multiple myeloma in patients who have received 1 to 3 prior therapies (used with lenalidomide and dexamethasone)
Golimumab	Anti–TNF-alpha	Moderate to severe RA (used with methotrexate) Psoriatic arthritis Ankylosing spondylitis Moderate to severe ulcerative colitis if • Patients have an inadequate response to or are intolerant of prior treatments. *or* • They require continuous corticosteroid therapy.
Ibritumomab	Anti–B cell (CD20; linked to the radioactive agent yttrium 90)	Relapsed or refractory low-grade follicular or transformed B-cell non-Hodgkin lymphoma
Infliximab	Anti–TNF-alpha	Moderate to severe Crohn disease or ulcerative colitis if response to conventional treatments is inadequate Moderate to severe RA (used with methotrexate) Active ankylosing spondylitis Active psoriatic arthritis Chronic severe plaque psoriasis when other treatments are less appropriate
Ipilimumab	Anti–CTLA-4	Inoperable or metastatic advanced melanoma Melanoma with pathologic involvement of regional lymph nodes of > 1 mm in patients who have had complete resection, including total lymphadenectomy
Natalizumab	Anti–alpha-4 integrin subunit	Relapsing multiple sclerosis or Crohn disease when other treatments are inadequate
Necitumumab	EGFR1	Metastatic squamous non–small cell lung cancer as 1st-line treatment (used with gemcitabine and cisplatin)
Nivolumab	Anti–PD-1	Unresectable or metastatic melanoma (used with ipilimumab and, if the melanoma is *BRAF* V600 mutation–positive, with a BRAF inhibitor) Metastatic non–small cell lung cancer if it progresses during or after platinum-based chemotherapy Advanced renal cell cancer in patients who have received prior antiangiogenesis therapy Hodgkin lymphoma that recurs or progresses after autologous hematopoietic stem cell transplantation and post-transplantation treatment with brentuximab vedotin
Obinutuzumab	Anti-CD20	Follicular lymphoma that recurred after or is refractory to a regimen that contains rituximab (used first with bendamustine, then given as monotherapy) Previously untreated CLL (used with chlorambucil)

Table 174–3. SOME IMMUNOTHERAPEUTIC AGENTS IN CLINICAL USE (*Continued*)

AGENT	EFFECTS	INDICATIONS
Ofatumumab	Anti-B cell (CD20)	Extended treatment of CLL in patients with complete or partial response after ≥ 2-drug regimens for recurrent or progressive disease CLL refractory to fludarabine and alemtuzumab
Omalizumab	Anti-IgE	Moderate to severe asthma in patients > 12 yr with documented allergic disorders inadequately controlled by inhaled corticosteroids Chronic idiopathic urticaria in patients ≥ 12 yr who remain symptomatic despite H_1 antihistamine treatment
Panitumumab	Anti-EGFR	Wild-type *KRAS* metastatic colorectal cancer as first-line treatment (used with FOLFOX or as monotherapy) if cancer progresses after prior treatment with fluoropyrimidine, oxaliplatin, and irinotecan
Pembrolizumab	Anti–PD-1	Inoperable or metastatic advanced melanoma PD-L1+ non–small lung cell carcinoma if it progresses during or after platinum-based chemotherapy
Pertuzumab	Anti-HER2	HER2+ metastatic breast cancer in patients who have not received prior anti-HER2 therapy or chemotherapy for metastatic cancer (used with trastuzumab and docetaxel) HER2+, locally advanced, inflammatory, or early-stage breast cancer (either > 2 cm in diameter or node-positive) for neoadjuvant treatment (used with trastuzumab and docetaxel) as part of a complete treatment regimen for early breast cancer
Ramucirumab	Anti–VEGFR-2	Metastatic colorectal cancer that has progressed during or after a first-line drug regimen that contains bevacizumab, oxaliplatin, and a fluoropyrimidine (used with FOLFIRI) Metastatic non–small cell lung cancer that progressed during or after platinum-based chemotherapy (used with docetaxel) Advanced or metastatic gastric or gastroesophageal junction adenocarcinoma if it progresses during or after prior chemotherapy that contains a fluoropyrimidine or platinum-based drug
Ranibizumab	Anti-VEGF	Neovascular (wet) age-related macular degeneration Macular edema after retinal vein occlusion Diabetic macular edema Diabetic retinopathy in patients with diabetic macular edema
Rituximab	Anti–B cell (CD20)	Relapsed or refractory CD20+, low-grade or follicular B-cell non-Hodgkin lymphoma CD20+ CLL (used with fludarabine and cyclophosphamide) Moderate to severe RA (used with methotrexate) when response to TNF-antagonists is inadequate Granulomatosis with polyangiitis (Wegener granulomatosis) Microscopic polyangiitis
Secukinumab	Anti–IL-17A	Ankylosing spondylitis Psoriatic arthritis Moderate to severe plaque psoriasis
Siltuximab	Anti–IL-6	Multicentric Castleman disease in patients who are HIV- and HHV-8–negative
Tocilizumab	Anti–IL-6 receptor (anti–IL-6R)	Moderate to severe RA when response to TNF-antagonists is inadequate Polyarticular or systemic juvenile idiopathic arthritis in patients ≥ 2 yr
Tositumomab	Anti–B cell (CD20; linked to radioactive iodine [^{131}I])	Refractory and relapsed CD20+ low-grade follicular or transformed non-Hodgkin lymphoma

Table continues on the following page.

Table 174–3. SOME IMMUNOTHERAPEUTIC AGENTS IN CLINICAL USE (*Continued*)

AGENT	EFFECTS	INDICATIONS
Trastuzumab	Anti–HER2	HER2+ breast cancer HER2+ metastatic gastric or gastroesophageal junction adenocarcinoma
Ustekinumab	Anti–IL-12 and –IL-23	Moderate to severe plaque psoriasis Psoriatic arthritis
Vedolizumab	Anti–alpha-4 beta-7 integrin	Moderate to severe active ulcerative colitis if response to conventional therapy or TNF-antagonists is inadequate Moderate to severe Crohn disease if response to conventional therapy or TNF-antagonists is inadequate
Fusion proteins		
Abatacept (CTLA-4 extracellular domain fused to the Fc region of IgG1)	Inhibition of T-cell activation	Moderate to severe RA
Denileukin diftitox (fusion of IL-2 to diphtheria toxin)	Delivery of toxin to CD25 component of IL-2 receptor	CD25+ cutaneous T-cell lymphoma
Etanercept (fusion of 2 CD120b TNF-alpha receptors to Fc region of IgG1)	Decrease in TNF levels	RA Polyarticular juvenile idiopathic arthritis in patients ≥ 2 yr Psoriatic arthritis Ankylosing spondylitis Plaque psoriasis
Soluble cytokine receptor		
Anakinra (IL-1 receptor antagonist, sometimes pegylated for longer half-life)	Competitive inhibition of IL-1 alpha and IL-1 beta activities	In patients ≥ 18 yr: Moderate to severe RA, cryopyrin-associated periodic syndromes
Cytokines		
IFN-alpha	Antiproliferative and antiviral	In patients ≥ 18 yr: Chronic hepatitis C, AIDS-related Kaposi sarcoma, hairy cell leukemia, chronic myelogenous leukemia, metastatic melanoma
IFN-beta	Antiproliferative and antiviral	Reduction of number of flare-ups in relapsing multiple sclerosis
IFN-gamma	Immunostimulatory and antiviral	Control of infection in chronic granulomatous disease, delay of progression in severe malignant osteopetrosis
IL-2	Immunostimulatory	Metastatic renal cell carcinoma and metastatic melanoma
IL-11	Thrombopoietic growth factor	Prevention of thrombocytopenia after myelosuppressive chemotherapy
G-CSF	Stimulation of granulocyte production	Reversal of neutropenia after chemotherapy, radiation therapy, or both
GM-CSF	Stimulation of granulocyte and monocyte/macrophage production	Reversal of neutropenia after chemotherapy, radiation therapy, or both
Cellular therapy		
Sipuleucel-T	Autologous circulating ICAM-1+ peripheral blood mononuclear cells activated with prostatic acid phosphatase and GM-CSF	Asymptomatic or minimally symptomatic metastatic prostate cancer refractory to castration (hormone therapy)

*mAbs used for diagnostic testing and radiologic imaging are not included.

†Efalizumab is not available in the US.

ALL = acute lymphocytic leukemia; ANCA = antineutrophil cytoplasmic antibodies; CD = cluster of differentiation; CLL = chronic lymphocytic leukemia; CTLA = cytotoxic T-lymphocyte antigen; EGFR = epidermal growth factor receptor; Fc = crystallizable fragment; FOLFIRI = leucovorin (folinic acid), fluorouracil, plus irinotecan; FOLFOX = leucovorin (folinic acid), fluorouracil, plus oxaliplatin; G-CSF = granulocyte colony-stimulating factor; GM-CSF = granulocyte-macrophage colony-stimulating factor; HER2 = human epidermal growth factor receptor 2; HHV-8 = human herpesvirus 8; ICAM = intercellular adhesion molecule; IFN = interferon; mAb = monoclonal antibody; PD-L1 = programmed death–ligand 1; RANKL = receptor activator of nuclear factor kappa beta ligand; SLAMF7 = signaling lymphocyte activation molecule family member 7; TNF = tumor necrosis factor; VEGF-A = vascular endothelial growth factor A; VEGFR = VEGF receptor.

leukemia, allergy, autoimmune disease, transplant rejection, and respiratory syncytial virus infection.

Fully human mAbs are produced using transgenic mice that contain human immunoglobulin genes or using phage display (ie, a bacteriophage-based cloning method) of immunoglobulin genes isolated from human B cells. Fully human mAbs have decreased immunogenicity and therefore may have fewer adverse effects in patients.

Fusion proteins: These hybrid proteins are created by linking together the gene sequences encoding all or part of 2 different proteins to generate a chimeric polypeptide that incorporates desirable attributes from the parent molecules (eg, a cell-targeting component combined with a cell toxin). The circulating half-life of therapeutic proteins can also often be improved by fusing them to another protein that naturally has a longer serum half-life (eg, the Fc region of IgG).

Soluble cytokine receptors: Soluble versions of cytokine receptors are used as therapeutic reagents. They can block the action of cytokines by binding with them before they attach to their normal cell surface receptor.

Etanercept, a fusion protein, consists of 2 identical chains from the CD120b receptor for TNF-alpha. This agent thus blocks TNF-alpha and is used to treat RA refractory to other treatments, ankylosing spondylitis, psoriatic arthritis, and plaque psoriasis.

Soluble IL receptors (eg, those for IL-1, IL-2, IL-4, IL-5, and IL-6) are being developed for treatment of inflammatory and allergic disorders and cancer.

Recombinant cytokines: CSF, such as erythropoietin, G-CSF, and GM-CSF, are used in patients undergoing chemotherapy or transplantation for hematologic disorders and cancers (see Table 174–3 on p. 1366). Interferon-alpha (IFN-alpha) and IFN-gamma are used to treat cancer, immunodeficiency disorders, and viral infections; IFN-beta is used to treat relapsing multiple sclerosis. Many other cytokines are being studied.

Anakinra, used to treat RA, is a recombinant, slightly modified form of the naturally occurring IL-1R antagonist; this drug attaches to the IL-1 receptor and thus prevents binding of IL-1, but unlike IL-1, it does not activate the receptor.

Cells expressing cytokine receptors can be targeted by modified versions of the relevant cytokine (eg, denileukin diftitox, which is a fusion protein containing sequences from IL-2 and from diphtheria toxin). Denileukin is used in cutaneous T-cell lymphoma to target the toxin to cells expressing the CD25 component of the IL-2 receptor.

Small-molecule mimetics: Small linear peptides, cyclicized peptides, and small organic molecules are being developed as agonists or antagonists for various applications. Screening libraries of peptides and organic compounds can identify potential mimetics (eg, agonists for receptors for erythropoietin, thrombopoietin, and G-CSF).

Cellular therapies: Immune system cells are harvested (eg, by leukapheresis) and activated in vitro before they are returned to the patient. The aim is to amplify the normally inadequate natural immune response to cancer. Methods of activating immune cells include using cytokines to stimulate and increase numbers of antitumor cytotoxic T cells and using pulsed exposure to antigen-presenting cells such as dendritic cells with tumor antigens.

175 Allergic, Autoimmune, and Other Hypersensitivity Disorders

OVERVIEW OF ALLERGIC AND ATOPIC DISORDERS

Allergic (including atopic) and other hypersensitivity disorders are inappropriate or exaggerated immune reactions to foreign antigens. Inappropriate immune reactions include those that are misdirected against intrinsic body components, leading to autoimmune disorders.

Classification of Hypersensitivity Reactions

Hypersensitivity reactions are divided into 4 types by the Gell and Coombs classification. Hypersensitivity disorders often involve more than 1 type.

Type I: Type I reactions (immediate hypersensitivity) are IgE-mediated. Antigen binds to IgE that is bound to tissue mast cells and blood basophils, triggering release of preformed mediators (eg, histamine, proteases, chemotactic factors) and synthesis of other mediators (eg, prostaglandins, leukotrienes, platelet-activating factor, cytokines). These mediators cause vasodilation, increased capillary permeability, mucus hypersecretion, smooth muscle spasm, and tissue infiltration with eosinophils, type 2 helper T (T_H2) cells, and other inflammatory cells.

Type I reactions develop < 1 h after exposure to antigen.

Type I hypersensitivity reactions underlie all atopic disorders (eg, allergic asthma, rhinitis, conjunctivitis) and many allergic disorders (eg, anaphylaxis, some cases of angioedema, urticaria, latex and some food allergies). The terms atopy and allergy are often used interchangeably but are different:

- **Atopy** is an exaggerated IgE-mediated immune response; all atopic disorders are type I hypersensitivity disorders.
- **Allergy** is any exaggerated immune response to a foreign antigen regardless of mechanism.

Thus, all atopic disorders are considered allergic, but many allergic disorders (eg, hypersensitivity pneumonitis) are not atopic. Allergic disorders are the most common disorders among people.

Atopic disorders most commonly affect the nose, eyes, skin, and lungs. These disorders include conjunctivitis, extrinsic atopic dermatitis, immune-mediated urticaria, immune-mediated angioedema, acute latex allergy, some allergic lung disorders (eg, allergic asthma, IgE-mediated components of allergic bronchopulmonary aspergillosis), allergic rhinitis, and allergic reactions to venomous stings.

Type II: Type II reactions (antibody-dependent cytotoxic hypersensitivity) result when antibody binds to cell surface antigens or to a molecule coupled to a cell surface. The antigen-antibody complex activates cells that participate in antibody-dependent cell-mediated cytotoxicity (eg, natural killer cells, eosinophils, macrophages), complement, or both. The result is cell and tissue damage.

Disorders involving type II reactions include hyperacute graft rejection of an organ transplant, Coombs-positive hemolytic

Sidebar 175–1. Latex Sensitivity

Latex sensitivity is an exaggerated immune response to water-soluble proteins in latex products (eg, rubber gloves, dental dams, condoms, tubing for respiratory equipment, catheters, enema tips with inflatable latex cuffs).

Beginning in the late 1980s, incidence increased among health care workers when emphasis on universal precautions resulted in routine use of latex gloves.

Reactions to latex may be

- Acute (IgE-mediated)
- Delayed (cell-mediated)

Acute reactions cause urticaria and anaphylaxis; delayed reactions cause dermatitis.

After health care workers wear latex gloves, the skin often becomes irritated and crusted, but this reaction is usually chemical irritation, not latex allergy.

Diagnosis of latex sensitivity is based primarily on history. Skin testing and assays for detecting IgE antilatex antibodies are available.

Treatment is avoidance of latex. Health care institutions should have latex-free gloves and equipment available.

anemias, Hashimoto thyroiditis, and anti–glomerular basement membrane disease (eg, Goodpasture syndrome).

Type III: Type III reactions (immune complex disease) cause inflammation in response to circulating antigen-antibody immune complexes deposited in vessels or tissue. These complexes can activate the complement system or bind to and activate certain immune cells, resulting in release of inflammatory mediators. Consequences of immune complex formation depend in part on the relative proportions of antigen and antibody in the immune complex. Early, there is excess antigen with small antigen-antibody complexes, which do not activate complement. Later, when antigen and antibody are more balanced, immune complexes are larger and tend to be deposited in various tissues (eg, glomeruli, blood vessels), causing systemic reactions. The isotype of induced antibodies changes, and glycosylation, size, and charge of the complex's components contribute to the clinical response.

Type III disorders include serum sickness, SLE, RA, leukocytoclastic vasculitis, cryoglobulinemia, acute hypersensitivity pneumonitis, and several types of glomerulonephritis.

Type III reactions develop 4 to 10 days after exposure to antigen and, if exposure to the antigen continues, can become chronic.

Type IV: Type IV reactions (delayed hypersensitivity) are T cell–mediated.

T cells, sensitized after contact with a specific antigen, are activated by reexposure to the antigen; they damage tissue by direct toxic effects or through release of cytokines, which activate eosinophils, monocytes and macrophages, neutrophils, or natural killer cells.

Disorders involving type IV reactions include contact dermatitis (eg, poison ivy), subacute and chronic hypersensitivity pneumonitis, allograft rejection, the immune response to TB, and many forms of drug hypersensitivity.

Etiology

Complex genetic, environmental, and site-specific factors contribute to development of allergies.

Genetic factors may be involved, as suggested by familial inheritance of disease, association between atopy and specific HLA loci, and polymorphisms of several genes, including those for the high-affinity IgE receptor beta-chain, IL-4 receptor alpha-chain, IL-4, IL-13, CD14, dipeptidyl-peptidase 10 (DPP10), and a disintegrin and metalloprotease domain 33 (*ADAM33*).

Environmental factors interact with genetic factors to maintain type 2 helper T (T_H2) cell–directed immune responses. T_H2 cells activate eosinophils, promote IgE production, and are proallergic. Early childhood exposure to bacterial and viral infections and endotoxins (eg, lipopolysaccharide) may normally shift native T_H2-cell responses to type 1 helper T (T_H1)–cell responses, which suppress T_H2 cells and therefore discourage allergic responses. Regulatory T (CD4+CD25+Foxp3+; T_{reg}) cells (which are capable of suppressing T_H2-cell responses) and IL-12–secreting dendritic cells (which drive T_H1-cell responses) are perhaps also involved. But trends in developed countries toward smaller families with fewer children, cleaner indoor environments, and early use of antibiotics may limit children's exposure to the infectious agents that drive a predominantly T_H1-cell response; such trends may explain the increased prevalence of some allergic disorders. Other factors thought to contribute to allergy development include chronic allergen exposure and sensitization, diet, and environmental pollutants.

Site-specific factors include adhesion molecules in bronchial epithelium and skin and molecules in the GI tract that direct T_H2 cells to target tissues.

Allergens: By definition, an allergen induces type I IgE-mediated or type IV T cell–mediated immune responses. Allergic triggers are almost always low molecular weight proteins; many of them can become attached to airborne particles.

Allergens that most commonly cause acute and chronic allergic reactions include

- House dust mite feces
- Animal dander
- Pollens (tree, grass, weed)
- Molds

Pathophysiology

When allergen binds to IgE-sensitized mast cells and basophils, histamine is released from their intracellular granules. Mast cells are widely distributed but are most concentrated in skin, lungs, and GI mucosa; histamine facilitates inflammation and is the primary mediator of clinical atopy. Physical disruption of tissue and various substances (eg, tissue irritants, opiates, surface-active agents, complement components C3a and C5a) can trigger histamine release directly, independent of IgE.

Histamine causes the following:

- Local vasodilation (causing erythema)
- Increased capillary permeability and edema (producing a wheal)
- Vasodilation of surrounding arterioles mediated by neuronal reflex mechanisms (causing flare—the redness around a wheal)
- Stimulation of sensory nerves (causing itching)
- Smooth muscle contraction in the airways (bronchoconstriction) and in the GI tract (increasing GI motility)
- Increased nasal, salivary, and bronchial gland secretions

When released systemically, histamine is a potent arteriolar dilator and can cause extensive peripheral pooling of blood and hypotension; cerebral vasodilation may be a factor in vascular headache. Histamine increases capillary permeability; the resulting loss of plasma and plasma proteins from the vascular space can worsen circulatory shock. This loss triggers a compensatory catecholamine surge from adrenal chromaffin cells.

Symptoms and Signs

Common symptoms of allergic disorders include

- Rhinorrhea, sneezing, and nasal congestion (upper respiratory tract)
- Wheezing and dyspnea (lower respiratory tract)
- Itching (eyes, nose, skin)

Signs may include nasal turbinate edema, sinus pain during palpation, wheezing, conjunctival hyperemia and edema, urticaria, angioedema, dermatitis, and skin lichenification. Stridor, wheezing, and hypotension are life-threatening signs of anaphylaxis.

Diagnosis

- Clinical evaluation
- Sometimes CBC and occasionally serum IgE levels (nonspecific tests)
- Often skin testing and allergen-specific serum IgE testing (specific tests)
- Rarely provocative testing

A thorough history is generally more reliable than testing or screening. History should include

- Questions about frequency and duration of attacks and changes over time
- Triggering factors if identifiable
- Relation to seasonal or situational settings (eg, predictably occurring during pollen seasons; after exposure to animals, hay, or dust; during exercise; or in particular places)
- Family history of similar symptoms or of atopic disorders
- Responses to attempted treatments

Age at onset may be important in asthma because childhood asthma is likely to be atopic and asthma beginning after age 30 is not.

Health care workers may be unaware that exposure to latex products could be causing their allergic reaction.

Nonspecific tests: Certain tests can suggest but not confirm an allergic origin of symptoms.

CBC may be done to detect eosinophilia if patients are not taking corticosteroids, which reduce the eosinophil count. However, CBC is of limited value because although eosinophils may be increased in atopy or other conditions (eg, drug hypersensitivity, cancer, some autoimmune disorders, parasitic infection), a normal eosinophil count does not exclude allergy. Total WBC is usually normal. Anemia and thrombocytosis are not typical of allergic responses and should prompt consideration of a systemic inflammatory disorder.

Conjunctival or nasal secretions or sputum can be examined for leukocytes; finding any eosinophils suggests that T_H2-mediated inflammation is likely.

Serum IgE levels are elevated in atopic disorders but are of little help in diagnosis because they may also be elevated in parasitic infections, infectious mononucleosis, autoimmune disorders, drug reactions, immunodeficiency disorders (hyper-IgE syndrome and Wiskott-Aldrich syndrome), and in some forms of multiple myeloma. IgE levels are probably most helpful for following response to therapy in allergic bronchopulmonary aspergillosis.

Specific tests: Skin testing uses standardized concentrations of antigen introduced directly into skin and is indicated when a detailed history and physical examination do not identify the cause and triggers for persistent or severe symptoms. Skin testing has higher positive predictive values for diagnosing allergic rhinitis and conjunctivitis than for diagnosing allergic asthma or food allergy; negative predictive value for food allergy is high.

The most commonly used antigens are pollens (tree, grass, weed), molds, house dust mite feces, animal danders and sera, insect venom, foods, and beta-lactam antibiotics. Choice of antigens to include is based on patient history and geographic prevalence.

Two skin test techniques can be used:

- Percutaneous (prick)
- Intradermal

The prick test can detect most common allergies. The intradermal test is more sensitive but less specific; it can be used to evaluate sensitivity to allergens when prick test results are negative or equivocal.

For the **prick test**, a drop of antigen extract is placed on the skin, which is then tented up and pricked or punctured through the extract with the tip of a 27-gauge needle held at a 20° angle or with a commercially available prick device.

For the **intradermal test**, just enough extract to produce a 1- or 2-mm bleb (typically 0.02 mL) is injected intradermally with a 0.5- or 1-mL syringe and a 27-gauge short-bevel needle.

Prick and intradermal skin testing should include the diluent alone as a negative control and histamine (10 mg/mL for prick tests, 0.01 mL of a 1:1000 solution for intradermal tests) as a positive control. For patients who have had a recent (< 1 yr) generalized reaction to the test antigen, testing begins with the standard reagent diluted 100-fold, then 10-fold, and then the standard concentration. A test is considered positive if a wheal and flare reaction occurs and wheal diameter is 3 to 5 mm greater than that of the negative control after 15 to 20 min. False positives occur in dermatographism (a wheal and flare reaction provoked by stroking or scraping the skin). False negatives occur when allergen extracts have been stored incorrectly or are outdated. Certain drugs can also interfere with results and should be stopped a few days to a week before testing. These drugs include OTC and prescription antihistamines, tricyclic antidepressants, and monoamine oxidase inhibitors. Some clinicians suggest that testing should be avoided in patients taking beta-blockers because these patients are more likely to have risk factors for severe reactions. These risk factors tend to predict limited cardiopulmonary reserve and include coronary artery disease, arrhythmias, and older age. Also, beta-blockers can interfere with treatment of severe reactions by blocking response to beta-adrenergic agonists such as epinephrine.

Allergen-specific serum IgE tests use an enzyme-labeled anti-IgE antibody to detect binding of serum IgE to a known allergen. They are done when skin testing might be ineffective or risky—for example, when drugs that interfere with test results cannot be temporarily stopped before testing or when a skin disorder such as eczema or psoriasis would make skin testing difficult. For allergen-specific serum IgE tests, the allergen is immobilized on a synthetic surface. After incubation with patient serum and enzyme-labeled anti-IgE antibody, a substrate for the enzyme is added; the substrate provides colorimetric fluorescent or chemiluminescent detection of binding. Allergen-specific IgE tests have replaced radioallergosorbent testing (RAST), which used ^{125}I-labeled anti-IgE antibody. Although the allergen-specific serum IgE tests are not radioactive, they are still sometimes referred to as RAST.

Provocative testing involves direct exposure of the mucosae to allergen and is indicated for patients who must document their reaction (eg, for occupational or disability claims) and sometimes for diagnosis of food allergy. For example, patients may be asked to exercise to diagnose exercise-induced asthma, or an ice cube may be placed on the skin for 4 min to diagnose cold-induced urticaria.

Ophthalmic testing has no advantage over skin testing and is rarely used.

Nasal and bronchial challenge are primarily research tools, but bronchial challenge is sometimes used when the clinical significance of a positive skin test is unclear or when no antigen extracts are available (eg, for occupation-related asthma).

Treatment

- Emergency treatment
- Removal or avoidance of allergic triggers
- H_1 blockers
- Mast cell stabilizers
- Anti-inflammatory corticosteroids and leukotriene inhibitors
- Immunotherapy (desensitization)

Emergency treatment: Severe allergic reactions (eg, anaphylaxis) require prompt emergency treatment.

If the airways are affected (eg, in angioedema), securing an airway is the highest priority. Treatment may include epinephrine and/or endotracheal intubation.

Patients who have severe allergic reactions should be advised to always carry a prefilled, self-injecting syringe of epinephrine and oral antihistamines and, if a severe reaction occurs, to use these treatments as quickly as possible and then go to the emergency department. There, patients can be closely monitored and treatment can be repeated or adjusted as needed.

Environmental control: Removal or avoidance of allergic triggers is the primary treatment for allergy, as well as the primary preventive strategy.

H_1 blockers: Antihistamines block receptors; they do not affect histamine production or metabolism.

H_1 blockers are a mainstay of treatment for allergic disorders. H_2 blockers are used primarily for gastric acid suppression and have limited usefulness for allergic reactions; they may be indicated as adjunctive therapy for certain atopic disorders, especially chronic urticaria.

Oral H_1 blockers (see Table 175–1) relieve symptoms in various atopic and allergic disorders (eg, seasonal hay fever, allergic rhinitis, conjunctivitis, urticaria, other dermatoses, minor reactions to blood transfusion incompatibilities); they are less effective for allergic bronchoconstriction and systemic vasodilation. Onset of action is usually 15 to 30 min, with peak effects in 1 h; duration of action is usually 3 to 6 h.

Products that contain an oral H_1 blocker and a sympathomimetic (eg, pseudoephedrine) are widely available OTC for use in adults and children ≥ 12 yr. These products are particularly useful when both an antihistamine and a nasal decongestant are needed; however, they are sometimes contraindicated (eg, if patients are taking an MAOI).

Oral H_1 blockers are classified as

- Sedating
- Nonsedating (better thought of as less sedating)

Sedating antihistamines are widely available without prescription. All have significant sedative and anticholinergic properties; they pose particular problems for the elderly and for patients with glaucoma, benign prostatic hyperplasia, constipation, orthostatic hypotension, delirium, or dementia.

Nonsedating (nonanticholinergic) antihistamines are preferred except when sedative effects may be therapeutic (eg, for nighttime relief of allergy, for short-term treatment of insomnia in adults or nausea in younger patients). Anticholinergic effects may also partially justify use of sedating antihistamines to relieve rhinorrhea in URIs.

Antihistamine solutions may be

- Intranasal (azelastine or olopatadine to treat rhinitis)
- Ocular (azelastine, emedastine, ketotifen, levocabastine, olopatadine, or pemirolast to treat conjunctivitis)

Topical diphenhydramine is available but should not be used; its efficacy is unproved, drug sensitization (ie, allergy) may occur, and anticholinergic toxicity can develop in young children who are simultaneously taking oral H_1 blockers.

Mast cell stabilizers: These drugs block the release of mediators from mast cells.

Mast cell stabilizers are used when other drugs (eg, antihistamines, topical corticosteroids) are ineffective or not well-tolerated. These drugs may be given

- Orally (cromolyn)
- Intranasally (eg, azelastine, cromolyn)
- Ocularly (eg, azelastine, cromolyn, lodoxamide, ketotifen, nedocromil, olopatadine, pemirolast)

Several ocular and nasal drugs are dual-acting mast cell stabilizers/antihistamines (see above).

Anti-inflammatory drugs: Corticosteroids can be given intranasally (see Tables 175–2 and 175–3) or orally.

Oral corticosteroids are indicated for the following:

- Allergic disorders that are severe but self-limited and not easily treated with topical corticosteroids (eg, acute asthma exacerbations, severe widespread contact dermatitis)
- Disorders refractory to other measures

Ocular corticosteroids are used only when an ophthalmologist is involved because infection is a risk.

NSAIDs are typically not useful, with the exception of topical forms used to relieve conjunctival injection and itching due to allergic conjunctivitis.

Other drugs: Leukotriene modifiers are indicated for treatment of the following:

- Mild persistent asthma
- Seasonal allergic rhinitis

Anti-IgE antibody (omalizumab) is indicated for the following:

- Moderately persistent or severe asthma refractory to standard treatment
- Chronic idiopathic urticaria refractory to antihistamine therapy

Immunotherapy: Exposure to allergen in gradually increasing doses (hyposensitization or desensitization) via injection or in high doses sublingually can induce tolerance and is indicated when allergen exposure cannot be avoided and drug treatment is inadequate.

Mechanism is unknown but may involve induction of the following:

- IgG antibodies, which compete with IgE for allergen or block IgE from binding with mast cell IgE receptors
- Interferon-gamma, IL-12, and cytokines secreted by T_H1 cells
- Regulatory T cells

For full effect, injections are initially given once or twice/wk. Dose typically starts at 0.1 to 1.0 biologically active units (BAU), depending on initial sensitivity, and is increased weekly or every 2 wk by ≤ 2 times with each injection until the maximum tolerated dose (the dose that begins to elicit moderate adverse effects) is established; *patients should be observed for about 30 min postinjection during dose escalation because anaphylaxis may occur after injection*. Subsequently, injections of the maximum tolerated dose should be given q 2 to 4 wk year-round; year-round treatment is better than preseasonal or coseasonal treatment, even for seasonal allergies.

Allergens used are those that typically cannot be avoided: pollens, house dust mite feces, molds, and venom of stinging insects. Insect venoms are standardized by weight; a typical

Table 175–1. ORAL H_1 BLOCKERS

DRUG	USUAL ADULT DOSAGE	USUAL PEDIATRIC DOSAGE	AVAILABLE PREPARATIONS
Sedating*			
Brompheniramine	4 mg q 4–6 h or 8 mg q 8–12 h	**< 2 yr:** Contraindicated **2–6 yr:** 0.125 mg/kg q 6 h (maximum dose 6–8 mg/day) **6–11 yr:** 2–4 mg q 6–8 h (maximum dose 12–16 mg/day) **≥ 12 yr:** Adult dose	4-, 8-, and 12-mg tablets 2 mg/5 mL elixir 8- and 12-mg tablets (sustained-release)
Chlorpheniramine	2–4 mg q 4–6 h	**< 2 yr:** Contraindicated **2–6 yr:** Not recommended **6–11 yr:** 2 mg q 4–6 h (maximum dose 12 mg/day) **≥ 12 yr:** Adult dose	2-mg chewable tablets 4-, 8-, and 12-mg tablets 2 mg/5 mL syrup 8- and 12-mg tablets or capsules (timed-release)
Clemastine	1.34 mg (1.0 mg of base) bid to 2.68 mg tid	**< 1 yr:** Contraindicated **1–3 yr:** 0.33–0.67 mg q 12 h **3–5 yr:** 0.67 mg q 12 h **6–11 yr:** 0.67–1.34 mg q 12 h **≥ 12 yr:** Adult dose	1.34- and 2.68-mg tablets 0.67 mg/5 mL syrup
Cyproheptadine	4 mg tid or qid (maximum 0.5 mg/kg/day)	**< 2 yr:** Contraindicated **2–6 yr:** 2 mg bid to tid (maximum 12 mg/day) **7–14 yr:** 4 mg bid to tid (maximum 16 mg/day)	4-mg tablets† 2 mg/5 mL syrup
Dexchlorpheniramine	2 mg q 4–6 h	**< 2 yr:** Contraindicated **2–5 yr:** 0.5 mg q 4–6 h (maximum dose 3 mg/day) **6–11 yr:** 1 mg q 4–6 h (maximum dose 6 mg/day) **≥ 12 yr:** Adult dose	2-mg tablets 2 mg/5 mL syrup 4- and 6-mg tablets (extended-release)
Diphenhydramine	25–50 mg q 4–6 h	**< 2 yr:** Contraindicated **2–11 yr:** 1.25 mg/kg q 6 h (maximum dose 300 mg/day) **≥ 12 yr:** Adult dose	25- and 50-mg capsules or tablets 12.5 mg/mL syrup 12.5 mg/5 mL elixir
Hydroxyzine	25–50 mg tid or qid	**< 2 yr:** Not recommended **2–11 yr:** 0.7 mg/kg tid **≥ 12 yr:** Adult dose	25-, 50-, and 100-mg capsules 10-, 25-, 50-, and 100-mg tablets 10 mg/5 mL syrup 25 mg/5 mL oral suspension
Promethazine	12.5–25 mg bid	**< 2 yr:** Contraindicated **≥ 2 yr:** 6.25–12.5 mg bid or tid	12.5-, 25-, and 50-mg tablets† 6.25 mg/5 mL and 25 mg/5 mL syrup
Nonsedating			
Acrivastine/pseudoephedrine	8/60 mg bid or tid	**< 12 yr:** Not recommended **≥ 12 yr:** Adult dose	8-mg acrivastine plus 60-mg pseudoephedrine capsules
Cetirizine	5–10 mg once/day	**6–11 mo:** 2.5 mg once/day **12–23 mo:** 2.5 mg bid **2–5 yr:** 5 mg once/day **≥ 6 yr:** Adult dose	5- and 10-mg tablets 1 mg/mL syrup
Desloratadine	5 mg once/day	**6–11 mo:** 1 mg/day **1–5 yr:** 1.25 mg/day **6–11 yr:** 2.5 mg once/day **≥ 12 yr:** Adult dose	5-mg tablets 0.5 mg/mL syrup
Fexofenadine	60 mg bid or 180 mg once/day	**6–23 mo:** 15 mg bid **2–11 yr:** 30 mg bid **≥ 12 yr:** Adult dose	30-, 60-, and 180-mg tablets 6 mg/mL oral suspension
Levocetirizine	5 mg once/day	**< 6 yr:** Contraindicated **6–11 yr:** 2.5 mg once/day **≥ 12 yr:** Adult dose	5-mg tablets 0.5 mg/mL oral suspension
Loratadine	10 mg once/day	**2–5 yr:** 5 mg once/day **≥ 6 yr:** Adult dose	10-mg tablets 1 mg/mL syrup
Mizolastine	10 mg once/day	**< 12 yr:** Not recommended **≥ 12 yr:** Adult dose	10-mg tablets

*All sedating antihistamines have strong anticholinergic properties. Generally, they should not be used in the elderly or in patients with glaucoma, benign prostatic hyperplasia, constipation, delirium, dementia, or orthostatic hypotension. These drugs commonly cause dry mouth, blurred vision, urinary retention, constipation, and orthostatic hypotension.

†Dosing frequency in children should not be increased.

Table 175–2. INHALED NASAL CORTICOSTEROIDS

DRUG	DOSE PER SPRAY	INITIAL DOSE (SPRAYS PER NOSTRIL)
Beclomethasone	42 mcg	**6–12 yr:** 1 spray bid **> 12 yr:** 1 spray bid to qid
Budesonide	32 mcg	**≥ 6 yr:** 1 spray once/day
Flunisolide	29 mcg	**6–14 yr:** 1 spray tid or 2 sprays bid **Adults:** 2 sprays bid
Fluticasone	50 mcg	**4–12 yr:** 1 spray once/day **> 12 yr:** 2 sprays once/day
Mometasone	50 mcg	**2–11 yr:** 1 spray once/day **≥ 12 yr:** 2 sprays once/day
Triamcinolone	55 mcg	**> 6–12 yr:** 1 spray once/day **> 12 yr:** 2 sprays once/day

starting dose is 0.01 mcg, and usual maintenance dose is 100 to 200 mcg. Animal dander desensitization is ordinarily limited to patients who cannot avoid exposure (eg, veterinarians, laboratory workers), but there is little evidence that it is useful. Desensitization for food allergens is under study. Desensitization for penicillin and certain other drugs and for foreign (xenogeneic) serum can be done.

Adverse effects are most commonly related to overdose, occasionally via inadvertent IM or IV injection of a dose that is too high, and range from mild cough or sneezing to generalized urticaria, severe asthma, anaphylactic shock, and, rarely, death. Adverse effects can be prevented by the following:

- Increasing the dose in small increments
- Repeating or decreasing the dose if local reaction to the previous injection is large (≥ 2.5 cm in diameter)
- Reducing the dose when a fresh extract is used

Reducing the dose of pollen extract during pollen season is recommended. Epinephrine, O_2, and resuscitation equipment should be immediately available for prompt treatment of anaphylaxis.

Sublingual immunotherapy can be used for allergic rhinitis.

Allergy treatment during pregnancy and breastfeeding: For pregnant women with allergies, avoidance of the allergen is the best way to control symptoms. If symptoms are severe, an antihistamine nasal spray is recommended. An oral antihistamine should be used only if antihistamine nasal sprays are inadequate.

During breastfeeding, antihistamines should not be used if possible. But if antihistamines are necessary, antihistamine nasal sprays are preferred to oral antihistamines. If oral antihistamines are essential for controlling symptoms, they should be taken immediately after breastfeeding.

Prevention

Allergic triggers should be removed or avoided. Strategies include the following:

- Using synthetic fiber pillows and impermeable mattress covers
- Frequently washing bed sheets, pillowcases, and blankets in hot water
- Removing upholstered furniture, soft toys, and carpets
- Exterminating cockroaches to eliminate exposure
- Using dehumidifiers in basements and other poorly aerated, damp rooms
- Treating homes with heat-steam
- Using high-efficiency particulate air (HEPA) vacuums and filters
- Avoiding food triggers
- Limiting pets to certain rooms or keeping them out of the house
- Frequently cleaning the house

Adjunctive nonallergenic triggers (eg, cigarette smoke, strong odors, irritating fumes, air pollution, cold temperatures, high humidity) should also be avoided or controlled when possible.

KEY POINTS

- Atopic reactions (commonly caused by mite feces, animal dander, pollen, or mold) are IgE-mediated allergic reactions that trigger histamine release.
- Take a thorough history, including a detailed description of the frequency and duration of attacks, relationship of symptoms to seasons or situations, family history, possible triggers, and responses to attempted treatments, because history is more reliable than testing.
- When the history and examination do not identify the cause, skin tests or an allergen-specific serum IgE test may help identify the allergen.
- Eliminating or avoiding the allergen is key to treatment and prevention; to relieve symptoms, use H_1 blockers, topical corticosteroids, and/or mast cell stabilizers.
- If the allergen cannot be avoided and other treatments are ineffective, immunotherapy may be needed.

ALLERGIC RHINITIS

Allergic rhinitis is seasonal or perennial itching, sneezing, rhinorrhea, nasal congestion, and sometimes conjunctivitis, caused by exposure to pollens or other allergens. Diagnosis is by history and occasionally skin testing. First-line treatment is with a nasal corticosteroid (with or without an oral or a nasal antihistamine) or with an oral antihistamine plus an oral decongestant.

Allergic rhinitis may occur seasonally or throughout the year (as a form of perennial rhinitis). Seasonal rhinitis is usually allergic. At least 25% of perennial rhinitis is nonallergic.

Table 175–3. INHALED NASAL MAST CELL STABILIZERS

DRUG	DOSE PER SPRAY	INITIAL DOSE (SPRAYS PER NOSTRIL)
Azelastine	137 mcg	**5–11 yr:** 1 spray bid **> 12 yr:** 1–2 sprays bid
Cromolyn	5.2 mg	**≥ 6 yr:** 1 spray tid or qid
Olopatadine	665 mcg	**6–11 yr:** 1 spray bid **> 12 yr:** 2 sprays bid

Seasonal allergic rhinitis (hay fever) is most often caused by plant allergens, which vary by season. Common plant allergens include

- **Spring:** Tree pollens (eg, oak, elm, maple, alder, birch, juniper, olive)
- **Summer:** Grass pollens (eg, Bermuda, timothy, sweet vernal, orchard, Johnson) and weed pollens (eg, Russian thistle, English plantain)
- **Fall:** Other weed pollens (eg, ragweed)

Causes also differ by region, and seasonal allergic rhinitis is occasionally caused by airborne fungal (mold) spores.

Perennial rhinitis is caused by year-round exposure to indoor inhaled allergens (eg, dust mite feces, cockroaches, animal dander) or by strong reactivity to plant pollens in sequential seasons.

Allergic rhinitis and asthma frequently coexist; whether rhinitis and asthma result from the same allergic process (one-airway hypothesis) or rhinitis is a discrete asthma trigger is unclear.

The numerous nonallergic forms of perennial rhinitis include infectious, vasomotor, drug-induced (eg, aspirin- or NSAID-induced), and atrophic rhinitis.

Symptoms and Signs

Patients have itching (in the nose, eyes, or mouth), sneezing, rhinorrhea, and nasal and sinus obstruction. Sinus obstruction may cause frontal headaches; sinusitis is a frequent complication. Coughing and wheezing may also occur, especially if asthma is also present.

The most prominent feature of perennial rhinitis is chronic nasal obstruction, which, in children, can lead to chronic otitis media; symptoms vary in severity throughout the year. Itching is less prominent than in seasonal rhinitis. Chronic sinusitis and nasal polyps may develop.

Signs include edematous, bluish red nasal turbinates, and, in some cases of seasonal allergic rhinitis, conjunctival injection and eyelid edema.

Diagnosis

- Clinical evaluation
- Occasionally skin testing, allergen-specific serum IgE tests, or both

Allergic rhinitis can almost always be diagnosed based on history alone. Diagnostic testing is not routinely needed unless patients do not improve when treated empirically; for such patients, skin tests are done to identify a reaction to pollens (seasonal) or to dust mite feces, cockroaches, animal dander, mold, or other antigens (perennial), which can be used to guide additional treatment. Occasionally, skin test results are equivocal, or testing cannot be done (eg, because patients are taking drugs that interfere with results); then, an allergen-specific serum IgE test is done.

Eosinophilia detected on nasal smear plus negative skin tests suggests aspirin sensitivity or nonallergic rhinitis with eosinophilia (NARES).

Nonallergic perennial rhinitis is usually also diagnosed based on history. Lack of a clinical response to treatment for assumed allergic rhinitis and negative results on skin tests and/or an allergen-specific serum IgE test also suggest a nonallergic cause; disorders to consider include nasal tumors, enlarged adenoids, hypertrophic nasal turbinates, granulomatosis with polyangiitis (Wegener granulomatosis), and sarcoidosis.

Treatment

- Antihistamines
- Decongestants
- Nasal corticosteroids
- For seasonal or severe refractory rhinitis, sometimes desensitization

Treatment of seasonal and perennial allergic rhinitis is generally the same, although attempts at removal or avoidance of allergens (eg, eliminating dust mites and cockroaches) are recommended for perennial rhinitis. For seasonal or severe refractory rhinitis, desensitization immunotherapy may help.

The most effective first-line drug treatments are

- Nasal corticosteroids with or without oral or nasal antihistamines (see Table 175–2)
- Oral antihistamines plus oral decongestants

Less effective alternatives include nasal mast cell stabilizers (eg, cromolyn) given tid to qid, the nasal H_1 blocker azelastine 1 to 2 puffs twice/day, and nasal ipratropium 0.03% 2 puffs q 4 to 6 h, which relieves rhinorrhea. Nasal drugs are often preferred to oral drugs because less of the drug is absorbed systemically.

Intranasal saline, often forgotten, helps mobilize thick nasal secretions and hydrate nasal mucous membranes; various saline solution kits and irrigation devices (eg, squeeze bottles, bulb syringes) are available OTC, or patients can make their own solutions.

Desensitization immunotherapy may be more effective for seasonal than for perennial allergic rhinitis; it is indicated when

- Symptoms are severe.
- Allergen cannot be avoided.
- Drug treatment is inadequate.

First attempts at desensitization should begin soon after the pollen season ends to prepare for the next season; adverse reactions increase when desensitization is started during the pollen season because the person's allergic immunity is already maximally stimulated.

Sublingual immunotherapy using 5–grass pollen sublingual tablets (an extract of 5 grass pollens) can be used to treat grass pollen-induced allergic rhinitis. Dosage is

- For adults: One 300-IR (index of reactivity) tablet daily
- For patients aged 10 to 17 yr: One 100-IR tablet on day 1, two 100-IR tablets simultaneously on day 2, then the adult dose from day 3 onward

The first dose is given in a health care setting and *patients should be observed for 30 min after administration because anaphylaxis may occur*. If the first dose is tolerated, patients can take subsequent doses at home. Treatment is initiated 4 mo before the onset of each grass pollen season and maintained throughout the season.

Patients with allergic rhinitis should carry a prefilled, self-injecting epinephrine syringe.

Montelukast, a leukotriene blocker, relieves allergic rhinitis symptoms, but its role relative to other treatments is uncertain.

Omalizumab, an anti-IgE antibody, is under study for treatment of allergic rhinitis but will probably have a limited role because less expensive, effective alternatives are available.

Treatment of NARES is nasal corticosteroids.

Treatment of aspirin sensitivity is avoidance of aspirin and nonselective NSAIDs (which can cross-react with aspirin), plus desensitization and leukotriene blockers as needed.

Prevention

For perennial allergies, triggers should be removed or avoided if possible. Strategies include the following:

- Using synthetic fiber pillows and impermeable mattress covers
- Frequently washing bed sheets, pillowcases, and blankets in hot water

- Removing upholstered furniture, soft toys, and carpets
- Exterminating cockroaches to eliminate exposure
- Using dehumidifiers in basements and other poorly aerated, damp rooms
- Treating homes with heat-steam
- Using high-efficiency particulate air (HEPA) vacuums and filters
- Avoiding food triggers
- Limiting pets to certain rooms or keeping them out of the house
- Frequently cleaning the house

Adjunctive nonallergenic triggers (eg, cigarette smoke, strong odors, irritating fumes, air pollution, cold temperatures, high humidity) should also be avoided or controlled when possible.

KEY POINTS

- Seasonal rhinitis is usually an allergic reaction to pollens.
- Patients with allergic rhinitis may have cough, wheezing, frontal headache, sinusitis, or, particularly in children with perennial rhinitis, otitis media.
- Diagnosis of allergic rhinitis is usually based on the history; skin tests and sometimes an allergen-specific serum IgE test are needed only when patients do not respond to empiric treatment.
- Try nasal corticosteroids first because they are the most effective treatment and have few systemic effects.

ANAPHYLAXIS

Anaphylaxis is an acute, potentially life-threatening, IgE-mediated allergic reaction that occurs in previously sensitized people when they are reexposed to the sensitizing antigen. Symptoms can include stridor, dyspnea, wheezing, and hypotension. Diagnosis is clinical. Treatment is with epinephrine. Bronchospasm and upper airway edema may require inhaled or injected beta-agonists and sometimes endotracheal intubation. Persistent hypotension requires IV fluids and sometimes vasopressors.

Etiology

Anaphylaxis is typically triggered by

- Drugs (eg, beta-lactam antibiotics, insulin, streptokinase, allergen extracts)
- Foods (eg, nuts, eggs, seafood)
- Proteins (eg, tetanus antitoxin, blood transfusions)
- Animal venoms
- Latex

Peanut and latex allergens may be airborne. Occasionally, exercise or cold exposure (eg, in patients with cryoglobulinemia) can trigger or contribute to an anaphylactic reaction.

History of atopy does not increase risk of anaphylaxis but increases risk of death when anaphylaxis occurs.

Pathophysiology

Interaction of antigen with IgE on basophils and mast cells triggers release of histamine, leukotrienes, and other mediators that cause diffuse smooth muscle contraction (eg, resulting in bronchoconstriction, vomiting, or diarrhea) and vasodilation with plasma leakage (eg, resulting in urticaria or angioedema).

Anaphylactoid reactions: These reactions are clinically indistinguishable from anaphylaxis but do not involve IgE and do not require prior sensitization. They occur via direct stimulation of mast cells or via immune complexes that activate complement.

The most common triggers of anaphylactoid reactions are

- Iodinated radiopaque contrast agents
- Aspirin and other NSAIDs
- Opioids
- Ig
- Exercise

Symptoms and Signs

Symptoms of anaphylaxis typically begin within 15 min of exposure and involve the skin, upper or lower airways, cardiovascular system, or GI tract. One or more areas may be affected, and symptoms do not necessarily progress from mild (eg, urticaria) to severe (eg, airway obstruction, refractory shock), although each patient typically manifests the same reaction to subsequent exposure.

Symptoms range from mild to severe and include flushing, pruritus, urticaria, sneezing, rhinorrhea, nausea, abdominal cramps, diarrhea, a sense of choking or dyspnea, palpitations, and dizziness.

Signs of anaphylaxis include hypotension, tachycardia, urticaria, angioedema, wheezing, stridor, cyanosis, and syncope. Shock can develop within minutes, and patients may have seizures, become unresponsive, and die. Cardiovascular collapse can occur without respiratory or other symptoms.

Late-phase reactions may occur 4 to 8 h after the exposure or later. Symptoms and signs are usually less severe than they were initially and may be limited to urticaria; however, they may be more severe or fatal.

Diagnosis

- Clinical evaluation
- Sometimes measurement of 24-h urinary levels of *N*-methylhistamine or serum levels of tryptase

Diagnosis of anaphylaxis is clinical. Anaphylaxis should be suspected if any of the following suddenly occur without explanation:

- Shock
- Respiratory symptoms (eg, dyspnea, stridor, wheezing)
- Two or more other manifestations of possible anaphylaxis (eg, angioedema, rhinorrhea, GI symptoms)

Risk of rapid progression to shock leaves no time for testing, although mild equivocal cases can be confirmed by measuring 24-h urinary levels of *N*-methylhistamine or serum levels of tryptase.

The cause is usually easily recognized based on history. If health care workers have unexplained anaphylactic symptoms, latex allergy should be considered.

PEARLS & PITFALLS

- Consider latex allergy in health care workers with unexplained anaphylactic symptoms.

Treatment

- Epinephrine given immediately
- Sometimes intubation
- IV fluids and sometimes vasopressors for persistent hypotension
- Antihistamines
- Inhaled beta-agonists for bronchoconstriction

Epinephrine: Epinephrine is the cornerstone of treatment for anaphylaxis; it may help relieve all symptoms and signs and should be given immediately.

Epinephrine can be given sc or IM (usual dose is 0.3 to 0.5 mL of a 1:1000 [0.1%] solution in adults or 0.01 mL/kg in children, repeated every 10 to 30 min). Maximal absorption occurs when the drug is given IM in the lateral thigh.

Patients with cardiovascular collapse or severe airway obstruction may be given epinephrine IV in a single dose (3 to 5 mL of a 1:10,000 [0.01%] solution over 5 min) or by continuous drip (1 mg in 250 mL 5% D/W for a concentration of 4 mcg/mL, starting at 1 mcg/min and titrated up to 4 mcg/min [15 to 60 mL/h]). Epinephrine may also be given by sublingual injection (0.5 mL of 1:1000 solution) or through an endotracheal tube (3 to 5 mL of a 1:10,000 solution diluted to 10 mL with saline). A second injection of epinephrine sc may be needed.

Glucagon 1-mg bolus (20 to 30 mcg/kg in children) followed by 1-mg/h infusion should be used in patients taking oral beta-blockers, which attenuate the effect of epinephrine.

Other treatments: Patients who have stridor and wheezing unresponsive to epinephrine should be given O_2 and be intubated. Early intubation is recommended because waiting for a response to epinephrine may allow upper airway edema to progress sufficiently to prevent endotracheal intubation and require cricothyrotomy.

Hypotension often resolves after epinephrine is given. Persistent hypotension can usually be treated with 1 to 2 L (20 to 40 mL/kg in children) of isotonic IV fluids (eg, 0.9% saline). Hypotension refractory to fluids and IV epinephrine may require vasopressors (eg, dopamine 5 mcg/kg/min).

Antihistamines—both H_1 blockers (eg, diphenhydramine 50 to 100 mg IV) and H_2 blockers (eg, cimetidine 300 mg IV)—should be given q 6 h until symptoms resolve.

Inhaled beta-agonists are useful for managing bronchoconstriction that persists after treatment with epinephrine; albuterol 5 to 10 mg by continuous nebulization can be given.

Corticosteroids have no proven role but may help prevent a late-phase reaction; methylprednisolone 125 mg IV initially is adequate.

Prevention

Primary prevention is avoidance of known triggers. Desensitization is used for allergen triggers that cannot reliably be avoided (eg, insect stings).

Patients with past reactions to a radiopaque contrast agent should not be reexposed. When exposure is absolutely necessary, patients are given 3 doses of prednisone 50 mg po q 6 h, starting 18 h before the procedure, and diphenhydramine 50 mg po 1 h before the procedure; however, evidence to support the efficacy of this approach is limited.

Patients with an anaphylactic reaction to insect stings, foods, or other known substances should wear an alert bracelet and carry a prefilled, self-injecting epinephrine syringe (containing 0.3 mg for adults and 0.15 mg for children) and oral antihistamines for prompt self-treatment after exposure.

KEY POINTS

- Common triggers of anaphylaxis include drugs (eg, beta-lactam antibiotics, allergen extracts), foods (eg, nuts, seafood), proteins (eg, tetanus antitoxin, blood transfusions), animal venoms, and latex.
- Non–IgE-mediated reactions that have anaphylactic-like manifestations (anaphylactoid reactions) can be caused by iodinated radiopaque dye, aspirin, other NSAIDs, opioids, blood transfusions, Ig, and exercise.
- Consider anaphylaxis if patients have unexplained hypotension, respiratory symptoms, or ≥ 2 anaphylactic manifestations (eg, angioedema, rhinorrhea, GI symptoms).
- Give epinephrine immediately because anaphylactic symptoms may rapidly progress to airway occlusion or shock; epinephrine can help relieve all symptoms.

ANGIOEDEMA

Angioedema is edema of the deep dermis and subcutaneous tissues. It is usually an acute mast cell–mediated reaction caused by exposure to drug, venom, dietary, pollen, or animal dander allergens. Angioedema can also be an acute reaction to ACE inhibitors, a chronic reaction, or a hereditary or an acquired disorder characterized by an abnormal complement response. The main symptom is swelling, which can be severe. Diagnosis is by examination. Treatment is with airway management as needed, elimination or avoidance of the allergen, and drugs to minimize swelling (eg, H_1 blockers).

Angioedema is swelling (usually localized) of the subcutaneous tissues due to increased vascular permeability and extravasation of intravascular fluid. Known mediators of increased vascular permeability include the following:

- Mast cell–derived mediators (eg, histamine, leukotrienes, prostaglandins)
- Bradykinin and complement-derived mediators

Mast cell–derived mediators tend to also affect layers superficial to subcutaneous tissue, including the dermal-epidermal junction. There, these mediators cause urticaria and pruritus, which thus usually accompany mast cell–mediated angioedema.

In bradykinin-mediated angioedema, the dermis is usually spared, so urticaria and pruritus are absent.

In some cases, the mechanism and cause of angioedema are unknown. Several causes (eg, calcium channel blockers, fibrinolytic drugs) have no identified mechanism; sometimes a cause (eg, muscle relaxants) with a known mechanism is overlooked clinically.

Angioedema can be acute or chronic (> 6 wk). There are hereditary and acquired forms.

Acute angioedema: Acute angioedema is mast cell–mediated in > 90% of cases. Mast cell–mediated mechanisms include acute allergic, typically IgE-mediated reactions. IgE-mediated angioedema is usually accompanied by acute urticaria (local wheals and erythema in the skin). It may often be caused by the same allergens (eg, drug, venom, dietary, extracted allergens) that are responsible for acute IgE-mediated urticaria.

Acute angioedema can also result from agents that directly stimulate mast cells without involving IgE. Causes can include opiates, radiopaque contrast agents, aspirin, and NSAIDs.

ACE inhibitors cause up to 30% of cases of acute angioedema seen in emergency departments. ACE inhibitors can directly increase levels of bradykinin. The face and upper airways are most commonly affected, but the intestine may be affected. Urticaria does not occur. Angioedema may occur soon or years after therapy begins.

Chronic angioedema: The cause of chronic (> 6 wk) angioedema is usually unknown. IgE-mediated mechanisms are rare, but chronic ingestion of an unsuspected drug or chemical (eg, penicillin in milk, a nonprescription drug, preservatives, other food additives) is sometimes the cause. A few cases are due to hereditary or acquired C1 inhibitor deficiency.

Idiopathic angioedema is angioedema that occurs without urticaria, is chronic and recurrent, and has no identifiable cause.

Hereditary and acquired angioedema: Hereditary angioedema and acquired angioedema are disorders that are characterized by abnormal complement responses and caused by deficiency or dysfunction of C1 inhibitor. Symptoms are those of bradykinin-mediated angioedema.

Symptoms and Signs

In angioedema, edema is often asymmetric and mildly painful. It often involves the face, lips (see Plate 69), and/or tongue and may also occur on the back of hands or feet or on the genitals. Edema of the upper airways may cause respiratory distress and stridor; the stridor may be mistaken for asthma. The airways may be completely obstructed. Edema of the intestines may cause nausea, vomiting, colicky abdominal pain, and/or diarrhea.

Other manifestations depend on the mediator.

Mast cell–mediated angioedema

- Tends to develop over minutes to several hours
- May be accompanied by other manifestations of acute allergic reactions (eg, pruritus, urticaria, flushing, bronchospasm, anaphylactic shock)

Bradykinin-mediated angioedema

- Tends to develop over hours to a few days
- Is not accompanied by other manifestations of allergic reactions

Diagnosis

- Clinical evaluation

For diagnosis of urticaria, see p. 981.

Patients with localized swelling but no urticaria are asked specifically about use of ACE inhibitors.

The cause of angioedema is often obvious, and diagnostic tests are seldom required because most reactions are self-limited and do not recur. When angioedema is acute, no test is particularly useful. When it is chronic, thorough drug and dietary evaluation are warranted; if no cause is obvious or if family members have it, testing for C1 inhibitor deficiency should be considered to check for hereditary or acquired angioedema.

Erythropoietic protoporphyria may mimic allergic forms of angioedema; both can cause edema and erythema after exposure to sunlight. The two can be distinguished by measuring blood and fecal porphyrins.

PEARLS & PITFALLS

- If angioedema is not accompanied by urticaria and recurs without clear cause or is present in family members, consider hereditary or acquired angioedema.

Treatment

- Airway management
- For mast cell-mediated angioedema, an antihistamine and sometimes a systemic corticosteroid and epinephrine
- For ACE inhibitor–related angioedema, occasionally fresh frozen plasma and C1 inhibitor concentrate
- For recurrent idiopathic angioedema, an oral antihistamine given bid

Securing an airway is the highest priority. In mast cell–mediated angioedema, treatment usually rapidly reduces airway edema; however, in bradykinin-mediated angioedema, edema usually takes > 30 min to decrease after treatment begins. Thus, endotracheal intubation is more likely to be needed in bradykinin-mediated angioedema. If angioedema involves the airways, epinephrine sc or IM is given as for anaphylaxis unless the mechanism is obviously bradykinin-mediated (eg, due to use of an ACE inhibitor or to known hereditary or acquired angioedema).

Treatment of angioedema also includes removing or avoiding the allergen and using drugs that relieve symptoms. If a cause is not obvious, all nonessential drugs should be stopped.

For **mast cell–mediated angioedema**, drugs that may relieve symptoms include H_1 blockers. Prednisone 30 to 40 mg po once/day is indicated for more severe reactions. Topical corticosteroids are useless. If symptoms are severe, a corticosteroid and antihistamine can be given IV (eg, methylprednisolone 125 mg and diphenhydramine 50 mg). Long-term treatment may involve H_1 and H_2 blockers and occasionally corticosteroids.

For **bradykinin-mediated angioedema**, epinephrine, corticosteroids, and antihistamines have not been shown to be effective. Angioedema due to ACE inhibitor use usually resolves about 24 to 48 h after stopping the drug. If symptoms are severe, progressing, or refractory, treatments used for hereditary or acquired angioedema can be tried. They include fresh frozen plasma, C1 inhibitor concentrate, and possibly ecallantide (which inhibits plasma kallikrein, required for the generation of bradykinin) and icatibant (which blocks bradykinin).

For **idiopathic angioedema,** a high dose of a nonsedating oral antihistamine can be tried.

Patients who have severe mast-cell mediated reactions should be advised to always carry a prefilled, self-injecting syringe of epinephrine and oral antihistamines and, if a severe reaction occurs, to use these treatments as quickly as possible and then go to the emergency department. There, they can be closely monitored and treatment can be repeated or adjusted as needed.

KEY POINTS

- In the emergency department, up to 30% of cases of acute angioedema are caused by ACE inhibitors (bradykinin-mediated), although overall, > 90% of cases are mast cell–mediated.
- The cause of chronic angioedema is usually unknown.
- Swelling always develops; bradykinin-mediated angioedema tends to develop more slowly and to cause fewer symptoms of an acute allergic reaction (eg, pruritus, urticaria, anaphylactic shock) than does mast cell–mediated angioedema.
- For chronic angioedema, take a thorough drug and dietary history, and possibly test for C1 inhibitor deficiency; testing is rarely necessary for acute angioedema.
- First, make sure the airway is secure; if the airway is affected, give epinephrine sc or IM unless the cause is obviously bradykinin-mediated angioedema, which is more likely to require endotracheal intubation.
- Eliminating or avoiding the allergen is key.
- For symptomatic and adjunctive treatment, an antihistamine (eg, H_1 blocker) and a systemic corticosteroid can relieve symptoms of mast cell–mediated angioedema; frozen plasma, C1 inhibitor concentrate, and/or ecallantide or icatibant may be tried if bradykinin-mediated angioedema is severe or refractory.

HEREDITARY AND ACQUIRED ANGIOEDEMA

(Acquired C1 Inhibitor Deficiency)

Hereditary angioedema and acquired angioedema (acquired C1 inhibitor deficiency) are caused by deficiency or dysfunction of C1 inhibitor, a protein that regulates the classical complement activation pathway. Diagnosis is by measurement of complement levels. C1 inhibitor is used to treat acute attacks. Prophylaxis is with attenuated androgens, which increase C1 inhibitor levels.

C1 inhibitor deficiency or dysfunction results in increased levels of bradykinin because C1 inhibitor inhibits activated kallikrein (required for the generation of bradykinin) in the kinin system pathway.

Hereditary angioedema: Hereditary angioedema has 2 types:

- Type 1 (85%): Characterized by C1 inhibitor deficiency
- Type 2 (15%): Characterized by C1 inhibitor dysfunction

Inheritance is autosomal dominant. Clinical presentation is usually during childhood or adolescence.

Acquired C1 inhibitor deficiency: C1 inhibitor deficiency may be acquired when

- Complement is consumed in neoplastic disorders (eg, B-cell lymphoma) or immune complex disorders.
- C1 inhibitor autoantibody is produced in monoclonal gammopathy.
- Rarely, C1 inhibitor autoantibody is produced in autoimmune disorders (eg, SLE, dermatomyositis).

Clinical presentation is usually at an older age, when patients have an associated disorder.

Triggers: In all forms of hereditary and acquired angioedema, attacks can be precipitated by mild trauma (eg, dental work, tongue piercing), viral illness, cold exposure, pregnancy, or ingestion of certain foods; angioedema may be aggravated by emotional stress.

Symptoms and Signs

Symptoms and signs are similar to those of other forms of bradykinin-mediated angioedema, with asymmetric and mildly painful swelling that often involves the face, lips, and/or tongue. Swelling may also occur on the back of hands or feet or on the genitals.

The GI tract is often involved, with manifestations that suggest intestinal obstruction, including nausea, vomiting, and colicky discomfort.

Pruritus, urticaria, and bronchospasm do not occur, but laryngeal edema may be present, causing stridor (and sometimes death).

Swelling resolves within about 1 to 3 days of onset. In hereditary angioedema, symptoms resolve as complement components are consumed.

Diagnosis

- Measurement of complement levels

Levels of C4, C1 inhibitor, and C1q (a component of C1) are measured. Hereditary angioedema or acquired C1 inhibitor deficiency is confirmed by

- Low levels of C4 (and C2, if measured)
- Decreased C1 inhibitor function

Other findings include

- Type 1 hereditary angioedema: Low C1 inhibitor levels and normal levels of C1q
- Type 2 hereditary angioedema: Normal or increased C1 inhibitor levels and normal C1q levels
- Acquired C1 inhibitor deficiency: Low C1q levels

If angioedema is not accompanied by urticaria and recurs without any clear cause, clinicians should suspect hereditary angioedema or acquired C1 inhibitor deficiency. If family members have it, they should suspect hereditary angioedema.

Treatment

- For acute attacks, C1 inhibitor, ecallantide, or icatibant
- For prophylaxis, attenuated androgens

Acute attacks are treated with purified human C1 inhibitor, ecallantide, or icatibant. If none of these drugs is available, fresh frozen plasma or, in the European Union, tranexamic acid has been used. A recombinant form of C1 inhibitor (recombinant human C1 esterase inhibitor [rhC1INH], or conestat alfa) is available in Europe.

If the airways are affected, securing an airway is the highest priority. Epinephrine may provide transient benefit in acute attacks when airways are involved. However, the benefit may not be sufficient or may be temporary; then endotracheal intubation may be necessary. Corticosteroids and antihistamines are not effective.

Analgesics, antiemetics, and fluid replacement can be used to relieve symptoms.

PEARLS & PITFALLS

- Antihistamines and corticosteroids are not effective for hereditary or acquired angioedema.

For **long-term prophylaxis,** attenuated androgens (eg, stanozolol 2 mg po tid, danazol 200 mg po tid) are used to stimulate hepatic C1 inhibitor synthesis. This treatment may be less effective for the acquired form. C1 inhibitor is effective but expensive.

Short-term prophylaxis is indicated before high-risk procedures (eg, dental or airway procedures) if C1 inhibitor is not available to treat an acute attack. Patients are usually given attenuated androgens 5 days before the procedure until 2 days afterward. If C1 inhibitor is available, some experts advocate giving it 1 h before high-risk procedures rather than attenuated androgens for short-term prophylaxis.

KEY POINTS

- Onset is usually during childhood or adolescence (hereditary) or during later adulthood (acquired), often in patients with a neoplastic or an autoimmune disorder.
- Mild trauma, viral illness, cold exposure, pregnancy, or ingestion of certain foods may trigger attacks; emotional stress may aggravate them.
- Measure complement levels; low levels of C4 and decreased C1 inhibitor function indicate hereditary angioedema or acquired C1 inhibitor deficiency.
- For acute attacks, use purified human C1 inhibitor, ecallantide, or icatibant, and for symptom relief, use analgesics, antiemetics, and fluids; antihistamines and corticosteroids are ineffective.

- For prophylaxis (long-term and short-term—eg, before dental or airway procedures), consider attenuated androgens (eg, stanozolol, danazol); a C1 inhibitor can also be considered for short-term prophylaxis.

AUTOIMMUNE DISORDERS

In autoimmune disorders, the immune system produces antibodies to an endogenous antigen (autoantigen). The following hypersensitivity reactions may be involved:

- **Type II:** Antibody-coated cells, like any similarly coated foreign particle, activate the complement system, resulting in tissue injury.
- **Type III:** The mechanism of injury involves deposition of antibody-antigen complexes.
- **Type IV:** Injury is T cell-mediated.

For specific autoimmune disorders, see elsewhere in THE MANUAL.

Women are affected more often than men.

Etiology

Mechanisms: Several mechanisms may account for the body's attack on itself:

- Autoantigens may become immunogenic if they are altered in some way.
- Antibodies to a foreign antigen may cross-react with an unaltered antigen (eg, antibodies to streptococcal M protein may cross-react with human heart muscle).
- Antigens normally sequestered from the immune system can become exposed and cause an autoimmune reaction (eg, systemic release of melanin-containing uveal cells after eye trauma triggers sympathetic ophthalmia).

Autoantigens may be altered chemically, physically, or biologically:

- Chemical: Certain chemicals can bind with body proteins, making them immunogenic, as occurs in drug-induced hemolytic anemia.
- Physical: For example, ultraviolet light induces keratinocyte apoptosis and subsequent altered immunogenicity of autoantigens, resulting in photosensitivity, as can occur in cutaneous lupus erythematosus.
- Biologic: For example, in animal models, persistent infection with an RNA virus that combines with host tissues alters autoantigens biologically, resulting in an autoimmune disorder resembling SLE.

Genetic factors: Relatives of patients with autoimmune disorders often also have autoantibodies. The specificity of autoantibodies in patients and in their relatives is frequently, but not always, similar. The incidence of autoimmune disorders is higher in identical twins than in fraternal twins.

Most autoimmune disorders have a polygenic etiology, and allelic variants within the HLA-gene locus nearly always contribute.

Defense mechanisms: Normally, potentially pathologic autoimmune reactions are avoided because of the immunologic tolerance mechanisms of clonal deletion and clonal anergy. Any autoreactive lymphocytes not controlled by these mechanisms are usually restrained by Foxp3+ regulatory T cells. A regulatory T-cell defect may interfere with any of these protective mechanisms, resulting in autoimmunity. Anti-idiotype antibodies (antibodies to the antigen-combining site of other antibodies) may interfere with regulation of antibody activity.

DRUG HYPERSENSITIVITY

Drug hypersensitivity is an immune-mediated reaction to a drug. Symptoms range from mild to severe and include rash, anaphylaxis, and serum sickness. Diagnosis is clinical; skin testing is occasionally useful. Treatment is drug discontinuation, supportive treatment (eg, with antihistamines), and sometimes desensitization.

Drug hypersensitivity differs from toxic and adverse effects that may be expected from the drug and from problems due to drug interactions.

Pathophysiology

Some protein and large polypeptide drugs (eg, insulin, therapeutic antibodies) can directly stimulate antibody production. However, most drugs act as haptens, binding covalently to serum or cell-bound proteins, including peptides embedded in major histocompatibility complex (MHC) molecules. The binding makes the protein immunogenic, stimulating antidrug antibody production, T-cell responses against the drug, or both. Haptens may also bind directly to the MHC II molecule, directly activating T cells. Some drugs act as prohaptens. When metabolized, prohaptens become haptens; eg, penicillin itself is not antigenic, but its main degradation product, benzylpenicilloic acid, can combine with tissue proteins to form benzylpenicilloyl (BPO), a major antigenic determinant. Some drugs bind and stimulate T-cell receptors (TCR) directly; the clinical significance of nonhapten TCR binding is being determined.

How primary sensitization occurs and how the immune system is initially involved is unclear, but once a drug stimulates an immune response, cross-reactions with other drugs within and between drug classes can occur. For example, penicillin-sensitive patients are highly likely to react to semisynthetic penicillins (eg, amoxicillin, carbenicillin, ticarcillin). In early, poorly designed studies, about 10% of patients who had a vague history of penicillin sensitivity reacted to cephalosporins, which have a similar beta-lactam structure; this finding has been cited as evidence of cross-reactivity between these drug classes. However, in recent, better-designed studies, only about 2% of patients with a penicillin allergy detected during skin testing react to cephalosporins; about the same percentage of patients react to structurally unrelated antibiotics (eg, sulfa drugs). Sometimes this and other apparent cross-reactions (eg, between sulfonamide antibiotics and nonantibiotics) are due to a predisposition to allergic reactions rather than to specific immune cross-reactivity. Also, not every apparent reaction is allergic; for example, amoxicillin causes a rash that is not immune-mediated and does not preclude future use of the drug.

PEARLS & PITFALLS

- Penicillin allergy does not always rule out use of cephalosporins.

Symptoms and Signs

Symptoms and signs of drug allergies vary by patient and drug, and a single drug may cause different reactions in different patients. The most serious is anaphylaxis; exanthema (eg, morbilliform eruption), urticaria, and fever are common. Fixed drug reactions—reactions that recur at the same body site each time a patient is exposed to the same drug—are uncommon.

Some distinct clinical syndromes exist:

- **Serum sickness:** This reaction typically occurs 7 to 10 days after exposure and causes fever, arthralgias, and rash. Mechanism involves drug-antibody complexes and complement activation. Some patients have frank arthritis, edema, or GI symptoms. Symptoms are self-limited, lasting 1 to 2 wk. Beta-lactam and sulfonamide antibiotics, iron-dextran, and carbamazepine are most commonly implicated.
- **Hemolytic anemia:** This disorder may develop when an antibody-drug-RBC interaction occurs or when a drug (eg, methyldopa) alters the RBC membrane, uncovering an antigen that induces autoantibody production.
- **DRESS (drug rash with eosinophilia and systemic symptoms):** This reaction, also called drug-induced hypersensitivity syndrome (DHS), can start up to 12 wk after initiation of drug treatment and can occur after a dose increase. Symptoms may persist or recur for several weeks after stopping drug treatment. Patients have prominent eosinophilia and often develop hepatitis, exanthema, facial swelling, generalized edema, and lymphadenopathy. Carbamazepine, phenytoin, allopurinol, and lamotrigine are frequently implicated.
- **Pulmonary effects:** Some drugs induce respiratory symptoms (distinct from the wheezing that may occur with type I hypersensitivity), deterioration in pulmonary function, and other pulmonary changes (see p. 450).
- **Renal effects:** Tubulointerstitial nephritis is the most common allergic renal reaction; methicillin, antimicrobials, and cimetidine are commonly implicated.
- **Other autoimmune phenomena:** Hydralazine, propylthiouracil, and procainamide can cause an SLE-like syndrome. The syndrome may be mild (with arthralgias, fever, and rash) or fairly dramatic (with serositis, high fevers, and malaise), but it tends to spare the kidneys and CNS. The antinuclear antibody test is positive. Penicillamine can cause SLE and other autoimmune disorders (eg, myasthenia gravis). Some drugs can cause perinuclear antineutrophil cytoplasmic autoantibodies (p-ANCA)–associated vasculitis. These autoantibodies are directed against myeloperoxidase (MPO).

Diagnosis

- Patient's report of a reaction soon after taking a drug
- Skin testing
- Sometimes drug provocation testing
- Sometimes direct and indirect antiglobulin assays

The following can help differentiate drug hypersensitivity from toxic and adverse drug effects and from problems due to drug interactions:

- Time of onset
- Known effects of a drug
- Results of a repeat drug challenge

For example, a dose-related reaction is often drug toxicity, not drug hypersensitivity.

Drug hypersensitivity is suggested when a reaction occurs within minutes to hours after drug administration. However, many patients report a past reaction of uncertain nature. In such cases, if there is no equivalent substitute (eg, when penicillin is needed to treat syphilis), testing should be considered.

Skin testing: Tests for immediate-type (IgE-mediated) hypersensitivity help identify reactions to beta-lactam antibiotics, foreign (xenogeneic) serum, and some vaccines and polypeptide hormones. However, typically, only 10 to 20% of patients who report a penicillin allergy have a positive reaction on skin tests. Also, for most drugs (including cephalosporins), skin tests are unreliable and, because they detect only IgE-mediated reactions, do not predict the occurrence of morbilliform eruptions, hemolytic anemia, or nephritis.

Penicillin skin testing is needed if patients with a history of an immediate hypersensitivity reaction must take a penicillin. BPO-polylysine conjugate and penicillin G are used with histamine and saline as controls. The prick test is used first. If patients have a history of a severe explosive reaction, reagents should be diluted 100-fold for initial testing. If prick tests are negative, intradermal testing may follow. If skin tests are positive, treating patients with penicillin may induce an anaphylactic reaction. If tests are negative, a serious reaction is less likely but not excluded. Although the penicillin skin test has not induced de novo sensitivity in patients, patients should usually be tested only immediately before essential penicillin therapy is begun.

For **xenogeneic serum skin testing**, patients who are not atopic and who have not previously received xenogeneic (eg, horse) serum should first be given a prick test with a 1:10 dilution; if this test is negative, 0.02 mL of a 1:1000 dilution is injected intradermally. A wheal > 0.5 cm in diameter develops within 15 min in sensitive patients. Initially, for all patients who may have previously received serum—whether or not they reacted—and for those with a suspected allergic history, a prick test should be done using a 1:1000 dilution; if results are negative, 1:100 is used, and if results are again negative, 1:10 is used as above. A negative result rules out the possibility of anaphylaxis but does not predict incidence of subsequent serum sickness.

Other testing: For drug provocation testing, a drug suspected of causing a hypersensitivity reaction is given in escalating doses to precipitate the reaction (see Table 175–4). This test is usually safe and effective if done in a controlled setting.

Because drug hypersensitivity is associated with certain HLA class I haplotypes, genotyping of patients from particular ethnic groups can identify those at higher risk of hypersensitivity reactions.

Tests for hematologic drug reactions include direct and indirect antiglobulin tests. Tests for other specific drug hypersensitivity (eg, allergen-specific serum IgE testing, histamine release, basophil or mast cell degranulation, lymphocyte transformation) are unreliable or experimental.

Prognosis

Hypersensitivity decreases with time. IgE antibodies are present in 90% of patients 1 yr after an allergic reaction but in only about 20 to 30% after 10 yr. Patients who have anaphylactic reactions are more likely to retain antibodies to the causative drug longer.

Table 175–4. SOME HLA-BASED RISK FACTORS FOR DRUG HYPERSENSITIVITY

DRUG	ETHNICITY	HLA HAPLOTYPE
Abacavir	Caucasians	HLA-B*5701
Allopurinol	Han Chinese, Japanese, Koreans, Thai Less often, Europeans	HLA-B*5801
Carbamazepine	Caucasians, Japanese	HLA-A*3101
Carbamazepine	Asians	HLA-B*1502
Fosphenytoin Phenytoin	Asians	HLA-B*1502
Lamotrigine	Asians	HLA-B*1502

People with drug allergies should be taught about avoiding the drug and should carry identification or an alert bracelet. Charts should always be appropriately marked.

Treatment

- Drug discontinuation
- Supportive treatment (eg, antihistamines, corticosteroids, epinephrine)
- Sometimes desensitization

Treatment of drug allergies is stopping the implicated drug; most symptoms and signs clear within a few days after the drug is stopped.

Symptomatic and supportive treatment for acute reactions may include

- Antihistamines for pruritus
- NSAIDs for arthralgias
- Corticosteroids for severe reactions (eg, exfoliative dermatitis, bronchospasm)
- Epinephrine for anaphylaxis

Conditions such as drug fever, a nonpruritic rash, or mild organ system reactions require no treatment (for treatment of specific clinical reactions, see elsewhere in THE MANUAL).

Desensitization: Rapid desensitization may be necessary if sensitivity has been established and if treatment is essential and no alternative exists. Rapid desensitization reduces sensitivity only temporarily. If possible, desensitization should be done in collaboration with an allergist. The procedure should not be attempted in patients who have had Stevens-Johnson syndrome. Whenever desensitization is used, O_2, epinephrine, and resuscitation equipment must be available for prompt treatment of anaphylaxis.

Desensitization is based on incremental dosing of the antigen every 15 to 20 min, beginning with a minute dose to induce subclinical anaphylaxis before exposure to therapeutic doses. This procedure depends on constant presence of drug in the serum and so must not be interrupted; desensitization is immediately followed by full therapeutic doses. Hypersensitivity typically returns 24 to 48 h after treatment is stopped. Minor reactions (eg, itching, rash) are common during desensitization.

For **penicillin,** oral or IV regimens can be used; sc or IM regimens are not recommended. If only the intradermal skin test is positive, 100 units (mcg)/mL IV in a 50-mL bag (5000 units total) should be given very slowly (eg, < 1 mL/min) at first. If no symptoms appear after 20 to 30 min, flow rate can be increased gradually until the bag is empty. The procedure is then repeated with concentrations of 1,000 units/mL and 10,000 units/mL, followed by the full therapeutic dose. If any allergic symptoms develop, flow rate should be slowed, and patients are given appropriate drug treatment (see above). If the prick test for penicillin was positive or patients have had a severe anaphylactic reaction, the starting dose should be lower.

Oral penicillin desensitization begins with 100 units (mcg); doses are doubled every 15 min up to 400,000 units (dose 13). Then, the therapeutic dose of the drug is given parenterally to treat the infection, and if symptoms of drug hypersensitivity occur, appropriate antianaphylactic drugs are used.

For allergies to trimethoprim-sulfamethoxazole and vancomycin, regimens similar to those for penicillin can be used.

If a skin test to xenogeneic serum is positive, risk of anaphylaxis is high. If serum treatment is essential, desensitization must precede it.

KEY POINTS

- Diagnosis can usually be based on history (mainly the patient's report of a reaction soon after taking the drug), but known adverse and toxic effects of the drug and drug-drug interactions must be excluded.
- If the diagnosis is unclear, usually skin tests but occasionally drug provocation testing or other specific tests can identify some drugs as the cause.
- A negative skin test result rules out the possibility of anaphylaxis but does not predict incidence of subsequent serum sickness.
- Hypersensitivity tends to decrease over time.
- Treat acute reactions supportively with antihistamines for pruritus, NSAIDs for arthralgias, corticosteroids for severe reactions (eg, exfoliative dermatitis, bronchospasm), and epinephrine for anaphylaxis.
- If the causative drug must be used, try rapid desensitization, in collaboration with an allergist if possible, to temporarily reduce drug sensitivity.

FOOD ALLERGY

Food allergy is an exaggerated immune response to dietary components, usually proteins. Manifestations vary widely and can include atopic dermatitis, GI or respiratory symptoms, and anaphylaxis. Diagnosis is by history and sometimes allergen-specific serum IgE testing, skin testing, and/or elimination diets. Treatment is with elimination of the food that triggers the reaction and sometimes oral cromolyn.

Food allergy should be distinguished from nonimmune reactions to food (eg, lactose intolerance, irritable bowel syndrome, infectious gastroenteritis) and reactions to additives (eg, monosodium glutamate, metabisulfite, tartrazine) or food contaminants (eg, latex dust in food handled by workers wearing latex gloves), which cause most food reactions. Prevalence of true food allergy ranges from < 1 to 3% and varies by geography and method of ascertainment; patients tend to confuse intolerance with allergy.

Etiology

Almost any food or food additive can cause an allergic reaction, but the most common triggers include

- **In infants and young children:** Milk, soy, eggs, peanuts, and wheat
- **In older children and adults:** Nuts and seafood

Cross-reactivity between food and nonfood allergens exists, and sensitization may occur nonenterally. For example, patients with oral allergies (typically, pruritus, erythema, and edema of the mouth when fruits and vegetables are eaten) may have been sensitized by exposure to pollens that are antigenically similar to food antigens; children with peanut allergy may have been sensitized by topical creams containing peanut oil used to treat rashes. Many patients who are allergic to latex are also allergic to bananas, kiwis, avocados, or a combination.

In general, food allergy is mediated by IgE, T cells, or both. IgE-mediated allergy (eg, urticaria, asthma, anaphylaxis) is acute in onset, usually develops during infancy, and occurs most often in people with a strong family history of atopy. T cell–mediated allergy (eg, dietary protein gastroenteropathies, celiac disease) manifests gradually and is chronic; it is most common among infants and children. Allergies mediated by both IgE and

T cells (eg, atopic dermatitis, eosinophilic gastroenteropathy) tend to be delayed in onset or chronic.

Eosinophilic gastroenteropathy: This unusual disorder causes pain, cramps, and diarrhea with blood eosinophilia, eosinophilic infiltrates in the gut, and protein-losing enteropathy; patients have a history of atopic disorders.

Eosinophilic esophagitis sometimes accompanies eosinophilic gastroenteropathy and may cause dysphagia, nonacid-related dyspepsia, and dysmotility or, in children, feeding intolerance and abdominal pain.

Symptoms and Signs

Symptoms and signs of food allergies vary by allergen, mechanism, and patient age. The most common manifestation in infants is atopic dermatitis alone or with GI symptoms (eg, nausea, vomiting, diarrhea). Children usually outgrow these manifestations and react increasingly to inhaled allergens, with symptoms of asthma and rhinitis; this progression is called atopic march. By age 10 yr, patients rarely have respiratory symptoms after the allergenic food is eaten, even though skin tests remain positive. If atopic dermatitis persists or appears in older children or adults, its activity seems largely independent of IgE-mediated allergy, even though atopic patients with extensive dermatitis have much higher serum IgE levels than atopic patients who are free of dermatitis.

When food allergy persists in older children and adults, the reactions tend to be more severe (eg, explosive urticaria, angioedema, even anaphylaxis). In a few patients, food (especially wheat and shrimp) triggers anaphylaxis only if they exercise soon afterward; mechanism is unknown. Food may also trigger nonspecific symptoms (eg, light-headedness, syncope). Occasionally, cheilitis, aphthous ulcers, pylorospasm, spastic constipation, pruritus ani, and perianal eczema are attributed to food allergy.

T cell–mediated reactions tend to involve the GI tract, causing symptoms such as subacute or chronic abdominal pain, nausea, cramping, and diarrhea.

PEARLS & PITFALLS

- Consider food allergy if patients have cryptogenic subacute or chronic abdominal pain, nausea, vomiting, cramping, or diarrhea.

Diagnosis

- Allergen-specific serum IgE testing
- Skin testing
- Trial elimination diet (alone or after skin testing or allergen-specific serum IgE testing)

Severe food allergy is usually obvious in adults. When it is not or when it occurs in children (the most commonly affected age group), diagnosis may be difficult, and the disorder must be differentiated from functional GI problems. For diagnosis of celiac disease, see p. 151.

Testing (eg, allergen-specific serum IgE testing, skin testing) and elimination diets are most useful in diagnosing IgE-mediated reactions.

If a food reaction is suspected, the relationship of symptoms to foods is assessed by one of the following:

- An allergen-specific serum IgE test
- Skin testing

In either case, a positive test does not confirm a clinically relevant allergy. Both tests can have false-positive or false-negative results. Skin testing is generally more sensitive than the allergen-specific serum IgE test but is more likely to have to false-positive results. The skin test provides a result within 15 to 20 min, much more quickly than the allergen-specific serum IgE test. If either test is positive, the tested food is eliminated from the diet; if eliminating the food relieves symptoms, the patient is reexposed to the food (preferably in a double-blind test) to see whether symptoms recur. (See also the National Institute of Allergy and Infectious Diseases [NIAID] medical position statement: Guidelines for the diagnosis and management of food allergy in the United States [http://www.jacionline.org].)

Alternatives to skin testing include one or both of the following:

- Eliminating foods the patient suspects of causing symptoms
- Prescribing a diet that consists of relatively nonallergenic foods and that eliminates common food allergens (see Table 175–5)

For the latter diet, no foods or fluids may be consumed other than those specified. Pure products must always be used. Many commercially prepared products and meals contain an undesired food in large amounts (eg, commercial rye bread contains wheat flour) or in traces as flavoring or thickeners, and determining whether an undesired food is present may be difficult.

If no improvement occurs after 1 wk, another diet should be tried; however, T cell–mediated reactions may take weeks to resolve. If symptoms are relieved, one new food is added and eaten in large amounts for > 24 h or until symptoms recur. Alternatively, small amounts of the food to be tested are eaten in the clinician's presence, and the patient's reactions observed. Aggravation or recrudescence of symptoms after addition of a new food is the best evidence of allergy.

Treatment

- Food elimination diet
- Sometimes oral cromolyn
- Sometimes corticosteroids for eosinophilic enteropathy

Treatment of food allergies consists of eliminating the food that triggers the allergic reaction. Thus, diagnosis and treatment overlap. When assessing an elimination diet's effect, clinicians must consider that food sensitivities may disappear spontaneously.

Oral desensitization (by first eliminating the allergenic food for a time, then giving small amounts and increasing them daily) and immunotherapy using sublingual drops of food extracts are under study.

Oral cromolyn has been used to decrease the allergic reaction with apparent success. Antihistamines are of little value except in acute general reactions with urticaria and angioedema. Prolonged corticosteroid treatment is helpful for symptomatic eosinophilic enteropathy.

Patients with severe food allergies should be advised to carry antihistamines to take immediately if a reaction starts and a prefilled, self-injecting syringe of epinephrine to use when needed for severe reactions.

Prevention

For many years, avoiding feeding young infants allergenic foods (eg, peanuts) has been recommended as a way to prevent food allergies. However, a recent study showed that early introduction and regular consumption of food that contains peanuts can prevent peanut allergy in infants at high risk of developing this allergy (eg, infants with egg allergy or eczema).

Table 175–5. ALLOWABLE FOODS IN ELIMINATION DIETS*

FOOD	DIET NO. 1 (NO BEEF, PORK, FOWL, MILK, RYE, OR CORN)	DIET NO. 2 (NO BEEF, LAMB, MILK, OR RICE)	DIET NO. 3 (NO LAMB, FOWL, RYE, RICE, CORN, OR MILK)
Cereal	Rice products	Corn products	None
Vegetables	Artichokes, beets, carrots, lettuce, spinach	Asparagus, corn, peas, squash, string beans, tomatoes	Beets, lima beans, potatoes (white and sweet), string beans, tomatoes
Meats	Lamb	Bacon, chicken	Bacon, beef
Flour (bread or biscuits)	Rice	Corn, 100% rye (ordinary rye bread contains wheat)	Lima bean, potato, soybean
Fruits	Grapefruit, lemons, pears	Apricots, peaches, pineapple, prunes	Apricots, grapefruit, lemons, peaches
Fat	Cottonseed oil, olive oil	Corn oil, cottonseed oil	Cottonseed oil, olive oil
Beverages	Coffee (black), lemonade, tea	Coffee (black), lemonade, tea	Coffee (black), lemonade, juice from approved fruit, tea
Miscellaneous	Cane sugar, gelatin, maple sugar, olives, salt, tapioca pudding	Cane sugar, corn syrup, gelatin, salt	Cane sugar, gelatin, maple sugar, olives, salt, tapioca pudding

*Diet No. 4: If symptoms persist when patients are following any of the above 3 elimination diets and diet is still suspected, daily diet may be restricted to an elemental diet (using extensively hydrolyzed or amino acid–based formulas).

KEY POINTS

- Food allergy is commonly mediated by IgE (typically resulting in acute systemic allergic reactions) or T cells (typically resulting in chronic GI symptoms).
- Food allergy should be distinguished from nonimmune reactions to food (eg, lactose intolerance, irritable bowel syndrome, infectious gastroenteritis) and reactions to additives (eg, monosodium glutamate, metabisulfite, tartrazine) or food contaminants.
- If the diagnosis is not clinically obvious in adults or if children are being evaluated, skin tests, an allergen-specific serum IgE test, or an elimination diet may be used.
- Make sure patients understand that in an elimination diet, they can eat only foods on the list and only pure foods (which excludes many commercially prepared foods).

MASTOCYTOSIS

Mastocytosis is mast cell infiltration of skin or other tissues and organs. Symptoms result mainly from mediator release and include pruritus, flushing, and dyspepsia due to gastric hypersecretion. Diagnosis is by skin or bone marrow biopsy or both. Treatment is with antihistamines and control of any underlying disorder.

Mastocytosis is a group of disorders characterized by proliferation of mast cells and infiltration of the skin, other organs, or both. Pathology results mainly from release of mast cell mediators, including histamine, heparin, leukotrienes, and various inflammatory cytokines. Histamine causes many symptoms, including gastric symptoms, but other mediators also contribute. Significant organ infiltration may cause organ dysfunction. Mediator release may be triggered by physical touch, exercise, alcohol, NSAIDs, opioids, insect stings, or foods.

Etiology in many patients involves an activating mutation (D816V) in the gene coding for the stem cell factor receptor c-kit, which is present on mast cells. The result is autophosphorylation of the receptor, which causes uncontrolled mast cell proliferation.

Classification

Mastocytosis may be cutaneous or systemic.

Cutaneous mastocytosis: This type typically occurs in children. Most patients present with urticaria pigmentosa, a local or diffusely distributed salmon or brown maculopapular rash caused by multiple small mast cell collections. Less common are diffuse cutaneous mastocytosis, which is skin infiltration without discrete lesions, and mastocytoma, which is a large (1 to 5 cm) solitary collection of mast cells.

Systemic mastocytosis: This type most commonly occurs in adults and is characterized by multifocal bone marrow lesions; it often involves other organs, most commonly skin, lymph nodes, liver, spleen, or GI tract.

Systemic mastocytosis is classified as

- Indolent mastocytosis, with no organ dysfunction and a good prognosis
- Mastocytosis associated with other hematologic disorders (eg, myeloproliferative disorders, myelodysplasia, lymphoma)
- Aggressive mastocytosis, characterized by impaired organ function
- Mast cell leukemia, with > 20% mast cells in bone marrow, no skin lesions, multiorgan failure, and a poor prognosis

Symptoms and Signs

Skin involvement is often pruritic. Changes in temperature, contact with clothing or other materials, or use of some drugs (including NSAIDs) may worsen itching, as may consuming hot beverages, spicy foods, or alcohol or exercising. Stroking or rubbing skin lesions causes urticaria and erythema around the lesion (Darier sign); this reaction differs from dermatographism, which involves normal skin.

Systemic symptoms can occur with any form. The most common is flushing; the most dramatic are anaphylactoid and anaphylactic reactions with syncope and shock. Other symptoms include epigastric pain due to peptic ulcer disease, nausea, vomiting, chronic diarrhea, arthralgias, bone pain, and neuropsychiatric changes (eg, irritability, depression, mood lability). Hepatic and splenic infiltration may cause portal hypertension with resultant ascites.

Diagnosis

- Clinical evaluation
- Skin lesion biopsy and sometimes bone marrow biopsy

Diagnosis of mastocytosis is suggested by clinical presentation. Diagnosis is confirmed by biopsy of skin lesions and sometimes of bone marrow. Multifocal, dense infiltrates of mast cells are present.

Tests may be done to rule out disorders that cause similar symptoms (eg, anaphylaxis, pheochromocytoma, carcinoid syndrome, Zollinger-Ellison syndrome); these tests include the following:

- Serum gastrin level to rule out Zollinger-Ellison syndrome in patients with ulcer symptoms
- Urinary excretion of 5-hydroxyindoleacetic acid (5-HIAA) to rule out carcinoid syndrome in patients with flushing
- Measurement of plasma-free metanephrines or urinary metanephrines to help rule out pheochromocytoma

PEARLS & PITFALLS

- Rule out disorders that cause symptoms similar to those of mastocytosis (eg, anaphylaxis, carcinoid syndrome, pheochromocytoma, Zollinger-Ellison syndrome).

If the diagnosis is uncertain, levels of mast cell mediators and their metabolites (eg, urinary *N*-methylhistamine, *N*-methylimidazole acetic acid) may be measured in plasma and urine; elevated levels support the diagnosis of mastocytosis. The level of tryptase (a marker of mast cell degranulation) is elevated in systemic mastocytosis but is typically normal in cutaneous mastocytosis. A bone scan, GI workup, and identification of the D816V *c-kit* mutation can also be helpful in cases where the diagnosis requires confirmation.

Treatment

- For cutaneous mastocytosis, H_1 blockers and possibly psoralen plus ultraviolet light or topical corticosteroids
- For systemic mastocytosis, H_1 and H_2 blockers and sometimes cromolyn
- For aggressive forms, interferon alfa-2b, corticosteroids, or splenectomy

Cutaneous mastocytosis: H_1 blockers are effective for symptoms. Children with cutaneous forms require no additional treatment because most cases resolve spontaneously. Adults with cutaneous forms may be treated with psoralen plus ultraviolet light or with topical corticosteroids once/day or bid. Mastocytoma usually involutes spontaneously and requires no treatment.

Cutaneous forms rarely progress to systemic disease in children but may do so in adults.

Systemic mastocytosis: All patients should be treated with H_1 and H_2 blockers and should carry a prefilled, self-injecting epinephrine syringe. Aspirin controls flushing but may enhance leukotriene production, thereby contributing to mast cell–related symptoms; it should not be given to children because Reye syndrome is a risk.

Cromolyn 200 mg po qid (100 mg qid for children 2 to 12 yr; not to exceed 40 mg/kg/day) may help by preventing mast cell degranulation. Ketotifen 2 to 4 mg po bid is inconsistently effective. No treatment can reduce the number of tissue mast cells.

In patients with an aggressive form, interferon alfa-2b 4 million units sc once/wk to a maximum of 3 million units/day induces regression of bone lesions. Corticosteroids (eg, prednisone 40 to 60 mg po once/day for 2 to 3 wk) may be required. Splenectomy may improve survival.

Cytotoxic drugs (eg, daunomycin, etoposide, 6-mercaptopurine) may be indicated for treatment of mast cell leukemia, but efficacy is unproved. Imatinib (a tyrosine kinase receptor inhibitor) may be useful in some patients but is ineffective in patients with the D816V *c-kit* mutation. Midostaurin (a 2nd-generation tyrosine kinase receptor inhibitor) is under study in such patients.

KEY POINTS

- Patients with cutaneous mastocytosis, usually children, typically present with a diffuse salmon or brown, often pruritic maculopapular rash.
- Systemic mastocytosis causes multifocal bone marrow lesions, usually in adults, but often affects other organs.
- All types can cause systemic symptoms (most commonly, flushing but sometimes anaphylactoid reactions).
- For cutaneous mastocytosis, use H_1 blockers to relieve symptoms, and in adults, consider treatment with psoralen plus ultraviolet light or topical corticosteroids.
- For systemic mastocytosis, use H_1 and H_2 blockers and sometimes cromolyn, and for aggressive mastocytosis, consider interferon alfa-2b, systemic corticosteroids, or splenectomy.
- Make sure all patients with mastocytosis carry a prefilled, self-injecting epinephrine syringe.

176 Immunodeficiency Disorders

Immunodeficiency disorders are associated with or predispose affected patients to various complications, including infections, autoimmune disorders, and lymphomas and other cancers. Primary immunodeficiencies are hereditary; secondary immunodeficiencies are acquired. Secondary immunodeficiencies are much more common.

Evaluation of immunodeficiency includes history, physical examination, and immune function testing. Testing varies based on the following:

- Whether a primary or secondary immunodeficiency is suspected
- For primary immunodeficiency, which component of the immune system is thought to be deficient

Table 176–1. CAUSES OF SECONDARY IMMUNODEFICIENCY

CATEGORY	EXAMPLES
Endocrine	Diabetes mellitus
GI	Hepatic insufficiency, hepatitis, intestinal lymphangiectasia, protein-losing enteropathy
Hematologic	Aplastic anemia, cancers (eg, chronic lymphocytic leukemia, multiple myeloma, Hodgkin lymphoma), graft-vs-host disease, sickle cell disease, splenectomy
Iatrogenic	Certain drugs (see Table 176–2), such as chemotherapeutic drugs, immunosuppressants, corticosteroids; radiation therapy; splenectomy
Infectious	Viral infections (eg, cytomegalovirus, Epstein-Barr virus, HIV, measles virus, varicella-zoster virus), bacterial infections, rare bacterial infections with superantigens (antigens that can activate large numbers of T cells, resulting in massive cytokine production, most notably from *Staphylococcus aureus*), mycobacterial infections
Nutritional	Alcoholism, undernutrition
Physiologic	Physiologic immunodeficiency in infants due to immaturity of the immune system, pregnancy
Renal	Nephrotic syndrome, renal insufficiency, uremia
Rheumatologic	SLE
Other	Burns, cancers, chromosomal abnormalities (eg, Down syndrome), congenital asplenia, critical and chronic illness, histiocytosis, sarcoidosis

Secondary Immunodeficiencies

Causes (see Table 176–1) include

- Systemic disorders (eg, diabetes, undernutrition, HIV infection)
- Immunosuppressive treatments (eg, cytotoxic chemotherapy, bone marrow ablation before transplantation, radiation therapy)
- Prolonged serious illness

Secondary immunodeficiency also occurs among critically ill, older, or hospitalized patients. Prolonged serious illness may impair immune responses; impairment is often reversible if the underlying illness resolves.

Immunodeficiency can result from loss of serum proteins (particularly IgG and albumin) through the following:

- The kidneys in nephrotic syndrome
- The skin in severe burns or dermatitis
- The GI tract in enteropathy

Enteropathy may also lead to lymphocyte loss, resulting in lymphopenia. All of these disorders can mimic B- and T-cell defects. Treatment focuses on the underlying disorder; a diet high in medium-chain triglycerides may decrease loss of immunoglobulins (Igs) and lymphocytes from the GI tract and be remarkably beneficial.

If a specific secondary immunodeficiency disorder is suspected clinically, testing should focus on that disorder (eg, diabetes, HIV infection, cystic fibrosis, primary ciliary dyskinesia).

Primary Immunodeficiencies

These disorders are genetically determined; they may occur alone or as part of a syndrome. More than 100 of these disorders have been described, and heterogeneity within each disorder may be considerable. The molecular basis for about 80% is known.

Primary immunodeficiencies typically manifest during infancy and childhood as abnormally frequent (recurrent) or unusual infections. About 70% of patients are < 20 yr at onset; because transmission is often X-linked, 60% are male. Overall incidence of symptomatic disease is about 1/280 people.

Primary immunodeficiencies are classified by the main component of the immune system that is deficient, absent, or defective:

- Humoral immunity
- Cellular immunity
- Combined humoral and cellular immunity
- Phagocytic cells
- Complement proteins

As more molecular defects are defined, classifying immunodeficiencies by their molecular defects will become more appropriate.

Primary immunodeficiency syndromes are genetically determined immunodeficiencies with immune and nonimmune defects. Nonimmune manifestations are often more easily recognized than those of the immunodeficiency. Examples are ataxia-telangiectasia, cartilage-hair hypoplasia, DiGeorge syndrome, hyper-IgE syndrome, and Wiskott-Aldrich syndrome.

Immunodeficiency typically manifests as recurrent infections. The age at which recurrent infections began provides a clue as to which component of the immune system is affected. Other characteristic findings tentatively suggest a clinical diagnosis (see Table 176–9 on p. 1394). However, tests are needed

Table 176–2. SOME DRUGS THAT CAUSE IMMUNOSUPPRESSION

CLASS	EXAMPLES
Anticonvulsants	Lamotrigine, phenytoin, valproate
Disease-modifying anti-rheumatic drugs (DMARDs)	IL-1 inhibitors (eg, anakinra) IL-6 inhibitors (eg, tocilizumab) IL-17 inhibitors (eg, brodalumab) TNF inhibitors (eg, adalimumab, etanercept, infliximab) T-cell activation inhibitors (eg, abatacept, basiliximab) CD20 inhibitors (eg, rituximab) CD3 inhibitors (eg, muromonab-CD3) Janus kinase (JAK) inhibitors (eg, ruxolitinib)
Calcineurin inhibitors	Cyclosporine, tacrolimus
Corticosteroids	Methylprednisolone, prednisone
Cytotoxic chemotherapy drugs	Multiple (see Table 154–3 on p. 1187)
Purine metabolism inhibitors	Azathioprine, mycophenolate mofetil
Rapamycins	Everolimus, sirolimus
Immunosuppressive immunoglobulins	Antilymphocyte globulin, antithymocyte globulin

to confirm a diagnosis of immunodeficiency (see Table 176–10 on p. 1395). If clinical findings or initial tests suggest a specific disorder of immune cell or complement function, additional tests are indicated (see Table 176–11 on p. 1396).

The prognosis in primary immunodeficiency disorders depends on the specific disorder.

Humoral immunity deficiencies: Humoral immunity deficiencies (B-cell defects) that cause antibody deficiencies account for 50 to 60% of primary immunodeficiencies (see Table 176–3). Serum antibody titers decrease, predisposing to bacterial infections.

The most common B-cell disorder is

- Selective IgA deficiency

For diagnostic evaluation of humoral immunity deficiencies, see Approach to the Patient With Suspected Immunodeficiency on p. 1392 and Table 176–11 on p. 1396.

Cellular immunity deficiencies: Cellular immunity deficiencies (T-cell defects) account for about 5 to 10% of primary immunodeficiencies and predispose to infection by viruses, *Pneumocystis jirovecii*, fungi, other opportunistic organisms, and many common pathogens (see Table 176–4). T-cell disorders also cause Ig deficiencies because the B- and T-cell immune systems are interdependent.

The most common T-cell disorders are

- DiGeorge syndrome
- ZAP-70 deficiency
- X-linked lymphoproliferative syndrome
- Chronic mucocutaneous candidiasis

Primary natural killer (NK) cell defects, which are very rare, may predispose to viral infections and tumors. Secondary NK cell defects can occur in patients who have various other primary or secondary immunodeficiencies.

For diagnostic evaluation of cellular immunity deficiencies, see Tables 176–10 and 176–11 on pp. 1395 and 1396.

Combined humoral and cellular immunity deficiencies: Combined humoral and cellular immunity deficiencies (B- and

Table 176–3. HUMORAL IMMUNITY DEFICIENCIES

DISORDER	INHERITANCE	GENE AFFECTED	CLINICAL FINDINGS
Common variable immunodeficiency	Variable	*TACI, ICOS, BAFFR*	Recurrent sinopulmonary infections, autoimmune disorders (eg, immune thrombocytopenia, autoimmune hemolytic anemia), malabsorption, giardiasis, granulomatous interstitial lung disease, nodular lymphoid hyperplasia of GI tract, bronchiectasis, lymphoid interstitial pneumonia, splenomegaly; in 10%, gastric carcinoma and lymphoma Usually diagnosed in patients aged 20–40 yr
Hyper-IgM syndrome with AID or UNG deficiencies	Autosomal recessive	*AID, UNG*	Similar to X-linked hyper-IgM syndrome but with lymphoid hyperplasia No leukopenia
Hyper-IgM syndrome with CD40 deficiency	Autosomal recessive	*CD40*	Similar to X-linked hyper-IgM syndrome Lymphoid hypoplasia, neutropenia
Hyper-IgM syndrome with CD40 ligand deficiency	X-linked	CD40 ligand (CD40L)	Similar to X-linked agammaglobulinemia (eg, recurrent pyogenic bacterial sinopulmonary infections) but greater frequency of *Pneumocystis jirovecii* pneumonia, cryptosporidiosis, severe neutropenia, and lymphoid hypoplasia
Selective antibody deficiency with normal immunoglobulins	Unknown	—	Recurrent sinopulmonary infections Sometimes atopic manifestations (eg, atopic dermatitis, asthma, chronic rhinitis) Can occur in mild, moderate, severe, and memory phenotypes
Selective IgA deficiency	Unknown	In some cases, *TACI*	Most often asymptomatic Recurrent sinopulmonary infections, diarrhea, allergies (including anaphylactic transfusion reactions [rare]), autoimmune disorders (eg, celiac disease, inflammatory bowel disease, SLE, chronic active hepatitis)
Transient hypogammaglobulinemia of infancy	Unknown	—	Usually asymptomatic Sometimes recurrent sinopulmonary or GI infections, candidiasis, meningitis
X-linked agammaglobulinemia	X-linked	*BTK*	Recurrent sinopulmonary and skin infections during infancy, transient neutropenia, lymphoid hypoplasia Persistent CNS infections resulting from live-attenuated oral polio vaccine, echoviruses, or coxsackieviruses Increased risk of infectious arthritis, bronchiectasis, and certain cancers

AID = activation-dependent (induced) cytidine deaminase; *BAFFR* = B-cell activating factor receptor; *BTK* = Bruton tyrosine kinase; CAML = calcium-modulator and cyclophilin ligand; CD = clusters of differentiation; *ICOS* = inducible T-cell co-stimulator; *TACI* = transmembrane activator and CAML interactor; *UNG* = uracil DNA glycosylase.

Table 176–4. CELLULAR IMMUNITY DEFICIENCIES

DISORDER	INHERITANCE	GENE AFFECTED	CLINICAL FINDINGS
Chronic mucocutaneous candidiasis	Autosomal dominant or recessive	*STAT1* (dominant) *AIRE* (recessive)	Persistent or recurrent candidal infections, onychomycosis, autosomal recessive autoimmune polyendocrinopathy–candidosis-ectodermal dystrophy (with hypoparathyroidism and adrenal insufficiency)
DiGeorge syndrome	Autosomal	Genes at chromosomal region 22q11.2 Genes at chromosome 10p13	Unusual facies with low-set ears, a congenital heart disorder (eg, aortic arch abnormalities), thymic hypoplasia or aplasia, hypoparathyroidism with hypocalcemic tetany, recurrent infections, developmental delay
X-linked lymphoproliferative syndrome	X-linked	*SH2D1A* (type 1) *XIAP* (type 2)	Asymptomatic until onset of Epstein-Barr virus infection, then fulminant or fatal infectious mononucleosis with liver failure, B-cell lymphomas, splenomegaly, aplastic anemia
Zeta-associated protein 70 (ZAP-70) deficiency	Autosomal recessive	—	Common and opportunistic infections No CD8 cells

AIRE = autoimmune regulator; CD = clusters of differentiation; *SH2D1A* = SH2 domain containing 1A; *STAT* = signal transducer and activator of transcription; *XIAP* = X-linked inhibitor of apoptosis.

T-cell defects) account for about 20% of primary immunodeficiencies (see Table 176–5).

The most important form is

- Severe combined immunodeficiency (SCID)

In some forms of combined immunodeficiency (eg, purine nucleoside phosphorylase deficiency), Ig levels are normal or elevated, but because of inadequate T-cell function, antibody formation is impaired.

For diagnostic evaluation of combined humoral and cellular immunodeficiencies, see Table 176–11 on p. 1396.

Phagocytic cell defects: Phagocytic cell defects account for 10 to 15% of primary immunodeficiencies; the ability of phagocytic cells (eg, monocytes, macrophages, granulocytes such as

Table 176–5. COMBINED HUMORAL AND CELLULAR IMMUNITY DEFICIENCIES

DISORDER	INHERITANCE	GENE AFFECTED	CLINICAL FINDINGS
Ataxia-telangiectasia	Autosomal recessive	*ATM*	Ataxia, telangiectasias, recurrent sinopulmonary infections, endocrine abnormalities (eg, gonadal dysgenesis, testicular atrophy, diabetes mellitus), increased risk of cancer
Cartilage-hair hypoplasia	Autosomal recessive	—	Short-limbed dwarfism, common and opportunistic infections
Combined immunodeficiency with inadequate but not absent T-cell function and normal or elevated immunoglobulins	Autosomal recessive or X-linked	*NEMO*	Common and opportunistic infections, lymphopenia, lymphadenopathy, hepatosplenomegaly, skin lesions resembling those of Langerhans cell histiocytosis in some patients
Hyper-IgE syndrome	Autosomal dominant or recessive	*STAT3* (dominant) *TYK2*, *DOCK8* (recessive)	Sinopulmonary infections; staphylococcal abscesses of skin, lungs, joints, and viscera; pulmonary pneumatoceles; pruritic dermatitis; coarse facial features; delayed shedding of baby teeth; osteopenia; recurrent fractures; tissue and blood eosinophilia
MHC antigen deficiencies	Autosomal recessive	—	Common and opportunistic infections
Severe combined immunodeficiency	Autosomal recessive or X-linked	*JAK3*, PTPRC (*CD45*), *RAG1*, *RAG2* (autosomal recessive) *IL-2RG* (X-linked)	Oral candidiasis, *Pneumocystis jirovecii* pneumonia, diarrhea before 6 mo, failure to thrive, graft vs host disease, absent thymic shadow, lymphopenia, bone abnormalities (in ADA deficiency), exfoliative dermatitis as part of Omenn syndrome
Wiskott-Aldrich syndrome	X-linked recessive	*WASP*	Typically, pyogenic and opportunistic infections, eczema, thrombocytopenia Possibly GI bleeding (eg, bloody diarrhea), recurrent respiratory infections, cancer (in 10% of patients > 10 yr), varicella-zoster virus infection, herpesvirus infection

ADA = adenosine deaminase; *ATM* = ataxia telangiectasia–mutated; *DOCK* = dedicator of cytokinesis; *IL-2RG* = IL-2 receptor gamma; *JAK* = Janus kinase; MHC = major histocompatibility complex; *NEMO* = nuclear factor–kappa-B essential modulator; PTPRC = protein tyrosine phosphatase, receptor type, C; *RAG* = recombination activating gene; *STAT* = signal transducer and activator of transcription; *TYK* = tyrosine kinase; *WASP* = Wiskott-Aldrich syndrome protein.

Table 176–6. PHAGOCYTIC CELL DEFECTS

DISORDER	INHERITANCE	GENE AFFECTED	CLINICAL FINDINGS
Chédiak-Higashi syndrome	Autosomal recessive	*LYST* (CHS1)	Oculocutaneous albinism, recurrent infections, fever, jaundice, hepatosplenomegaly, lymphadenopathy, neuropathy, pancytopenia, bleeding diathesis
Chronic granulomatous disease	X-linked or autosomal recessive	gp91phox (*CYBB*; X-linked) p22phox, p47phox, p67phox (autosomal recessive)	Granulomatous lesions in the lungs, liver, lymph nodes, and GI and GU tract (causing obstruction); lymphadenitis; hepatosplenomegaly; skin, lymph node, lung, liver, and perianal abscesses; osteomyelitis; pneumonia; staphylococcal, gram-negative, and aspergillus infections
Leukocyte adhesion deficiency	Autosomal recessive	*ITGB2* gene, encoding CD18 of beta-2 integrins (type 1) GDP-fucose transporter gene (type 2)	Soft-tissue infections, periodontitis, poor wound healing, delayed umbilical cord detachment, leukocytosis, no formation of pus Developmental delay (type 2)
Mendelian susceptibility to mycobacterial disease (MSMD)	Autosomal dominant or recessive	Defects in genes encoding the IFN-gamma receptor, IL-12, or the IL-12 receptor	Mycobacterial infections Varying clinical severity based on genetic defect
Cyclic neutropenia	Autosomal dominant	*ELA2*	Pyogenic bacterial infections during recurrent episodes of neutropenia (eg, every 14 to 35 days)

CD = clusters of differentiation; CHS = Chédiak-Higashi syndrome; *CYBB* = cytochrome b-245, beta polypeptide; *ELA* = elastase; gp = glycoprotein; IFN = interferon; *ITGB2* = integrin beta-2; *LYST* = lysosomal transporter.

neutrophils and eosinophils) to kill pathogens is impaired (see Table 176–6). Cutaneous staphylococcal and gram-negative infections are characteristic.

The most common (although still rare) phagocytic cell defects are

- Chronic granulomatous disease
- Leukocyte adhesion deficiency (types 1 and 2)
- Cyclic neutropenia
- Chédiak-Higashi syndrome

For diagnostic evaluation of phagocytic cell defects, see Tables 176–10 and 176–11 on pp. 1395 and 1396.

Complement deficiencies: Complement deficiencies are rare (≤ 2%); they include isolated deficiencies of complement components or inhibitors and may be hereditary or acquired (see Table 176–7). Hereditary deficiencies are autosomal recessive except for deficiencies of C1 inhibitor, which is autosomal dominant, and properdin, which is X-linked. The deficiencies result in defective opsonization, phagocytosis, and lysis of pathogens and in defective clearance of antigen-antibody complexes.

The most serious consequences are

- Recurrent infection, which is due to defective opsonization
- Autoimmune disorders (eg, SLE, glomerulonephritis), which is due to defective clearance of antigen-antibody complexes

A deficiency in a complement regulatory protein causes hereditary angioedema.

Complement deficiencies can affect the classical and/or alternate pathways (see p. 1364). The alternate pathway shares C3 and C5 through C9 with the classical pathway but has additional components: factor D, factor B, properdin (P), and regulatory factors H and I.

For diagnostic evaluation of complement deficiencies, see Tables 176–10 and 176–11 on pp. 1395 and 1396.

Geriatrics Essentials

Some decrease in immunity occurs with aging. For example, in the elderly, the thymus tends to produce fewer naive T cells; thus, fewer T cells are available to respond to new antigens. The number of T cells does not decrease (because of oligoclonality), but these cells can recognize only a limited number of antigens.

Signal transduction (transmission of antigen-binding signal across the cell membrane into the cell) is impaired, making T cells less likely to respond to antigens. Also, helper T cells may be less likely to signal B cells to produce antibodies.

The number of neutrophils does not decrease, but these cells become less effective in phagocytosis and microbicidal action.

Undernutrition, common among the elderly, impairs immune responses. Calcium, zinc, and vitamin E are particularly important to immunity. Risk of calcium deficiency is increased in the elderly, partly because with aging, the intestine becomes less able to absorb calcium. Also, the elderly may not ingest enough calcium in their diet. Zinc deficiency is very common among the institutionalized elderly and homebound patients.

Certain disorders (eg, diabetes, chronic kidney disease, undernutrition), which are more common among the elderly, and certain therapies (eg, immunosuppressants, immunomodulatory drugs and treatments), which the elderly are more likely to use, can also impair immunity.

KEY POINTS

- Secondary (acquired) immunodeficiencies are much more common than primary (hereditary) immunodeficiencies.
- Primary immunodeficiencies can affect humoral immunity (most commonly), cellular immunity, both humoral and cellular immunity, phagocytic cells, or the complement system.
- Patients who have primary immunodeficiencies may have nonimmune manifestations that can be recognized more easily than the immunodeficiencies.
- Immunity tends to decrease with aging partly because of age-related changes; also, conditions that impair immunity (eg, certain disorders, use of certain drugs) are more common among the elderly.

Table 176–7. COMPLEMENT DEFICIENCIES

DISORDER	INHERITANCE	CLINICAL FINDINGS
C1	Autosomal recessive	SLE
C2	Autosomal recessive	SLE, recurrent pyogenic infections with encapsulated bacteria (especially pneumococcal) that start in early childhood, other autoimmune disorders (eg, glomerulonephritis, polymyositis, vasculitis, Henoch-Schönlein purpura, Hodgkin lymphoma)
C3	Autosomal recessive	Recurrent pyogenic infections with encapsulated bacteria that start at birth, glomerulonephritis, other antigen-antibody complex disorders, sepsis
C4	Autosomal recessive	SLE, other autoimmune disorders (eg, IgA nephropathy, progressive systemic sclerosis, Henoch-Schönlein purpura, type 1 diabetes mellitus, autoimmune hepatitis)
C5, C6, C7, C8, C9 (membrane attack complex)	Autosomal recessive	Recurrent *Neisseria meningitidis* and disseminated *N. gonorrhoeae* infections
Complement deficiencies in the MBL pathway		
MBL	Autosomal recessive	Recurrent pyogenic infections with encapsulated bacteria that start at birth; unexplained sepsis; increased severity of infection in secondary immunodeficiencies due to corticosteroid use, cystic fibrosis, or chronic lung disorders
MASP-2	Unknown	Autoimmune disorders (eg, inflammatory bowel disease, erythema multiforme), recurrent pyogenic infections with encapsulated bacteria (eg, *Streptococcus pneumoniae*)
Complement deficiencies in the alternative pathway		
Factor B	Autosomal recessive	Pyogenic infections
Factor D	Autosomal	Pyogenic infections
Properdin	X-linked	Increased risk of fulminant neisserial infection
Complement regulatory protein deficiencies		
C1 inhibitor	Autosomal dominant	Angioedema
Factor I	Autosomal codominant	Same as C3 deficiency
Factor H	Autosomal codominant	Same as C3 deficiency Hemolytic-uremic syndrome
Decay accelerating factor	Autosomal recessive	Paroxysmal nocturnal hemoglobinuria
Complement receptor (CR) deficiencies		
CR1	Acquired	Secondary finding in immune (antigen-antibody) complex–mediated disease
CR3	Autosomal recessive	Leukocyte adhesion deficiency syndrome (recurrent *Staphylococcus aureus* and *Pseudomonas aeruginosa* infections)

C = complement; MASP = mannose-binding lectin-associated serine protease; MBL = mannose-binding lectin.

APPROACH TO THE PATIENT WITH SUSPECTED IMMUNODEFICIENCY

Immunodeficiency can be

- Primary: Genetically determined, typically manifesting during infancy or childhood
- Secondary: Acquired

There are many causes of secondary immunodeficiency, but most immunodeficiencies result from one or more of the following:

- Systemic disorders (eg, diabetes, undernutrition, HIV infection)
- Immunosuppressive treatments (eg, cytotoxic chemotherapy, bone marrow ablation before transplantation, radiation therapy)
- Prolonged serious illness (particularly in critically ill, older, and/or hospitalized patients)

Primary immunodeficiencies are classified by the main component of the immune system that is deficient, absent, or defective:

- Humoral immunity
- Cellular immunity
- Combined humoral and cellular immunity
- Phagocytic cells
- Complement proteins

Immunodeficiency typically manifests as recurrent infections. However, more likely causes of recurrent infections in children are repeated exposures to infection at day care or school (infants and children may normally have up to 10 respiratory infections/yr), and more likely causes in children and adults are inadequate duration of antibiotic treatment, resistant organisms, and other disorders that predispose to infection (eg, congenital heart defects, allergic rhinitis, ureteral or urethral stenosis, immotile cilia syndrome, asthma, cystic fibrosis, severe dermatitis).

Immunodeficiency should be suspected when recurrent infections are the following:

- Severe
- Complicated
- In multiple locations
- Resistant to treatment
- Caused by unusual organisms
- Present in family members

Initially, infections due to immunodeficiency are typically upper and lower respiratory tract infections (eg, sinusitis, bronchitis, pneumonia) and gastroenteritis, but they may be serious bacterial infections (eg, meningitis, sepsis).

Immunodeficiency should also be suspected in infants or young children with chronic diarrhea and failure to thrive, especially when the diarrhea is caused by unusual viruses (eg, adenovirus) or fungi (eg, *Cryptosporidium* sp). Other signs include skin lesions (eg, eczema, warts, abscesses, pyoderma, alopecia), oral or esophageal thrush, oral ulcers, and periodontitis.

Less common manifestations include severe viral infection with herpes simplex or varicella zoster virus and CNS problems (eg, chronic encephalitis, delayed development, seizure disorder). Frequent use of antibiotics may mask many of the common symptoms and signs. Immunodeficiency should be considered particularly in patients with infections and an autoimmune disorder (eg, hemolytic anemia, thrombocytopenia).

Evaluation

History and physical examination are helpful but must be supplemented by immune function testing. Prenatal testing is available for many disorders and is indicated if there is a family history of immunodeficiency and the mutation has been identified in family members.

History: Clinicians should determine whether patients have risk factors for infection or a history of symptoms of secondary immunodeficiency disorders and/or risk factors for them. Family history is very important.

Age when recurrent infections began is important.

- Onset before age 6 mo suggests a T-cell defect because maternal antibodies are usually protective for the first 6 to 9 mo.
- Onset between the age of 6 and 12 mo may suggest combined B- and T-cell defects or a B-cell defect, which becomes evident when maternal antibodies are disappearing (at about age 6 mo).
- Onset much later than 12 mo usually suggests a B-cell defect or secondary immunodeficiency.

In general, the earlier the age at onset in children, the more severe the immunodeficiency. Often, certain other primary immunodeficiencies (eg, common variable immunodeficiency [CVID]) do not manifest until adulthood.

Certain infections suggest certain immunodeficiency disorders (see Table 176–8); however, no infection is specific to any one disorder, and certain common infections (eg, respiratory viral or bacterial infections) occur in many.

Physical examination: Patients with immunodeficiency may or may not appear chronically ill. Macular rashes, vesicles, pyoderma, eczema, petechiae, alopecia, or telangiectasia may be evident.

Cervical lymph nodes and adenoid and tonsillar tissue are typically very small or absent in X-linked agammaglobulinemia, X-linked hyper-IgM syndrome, SCID, and other T-cell immunodeficiencies despite a history of recurrent infections. In certain other immunodeficiencies (eg, chronic granulomatous

Table 176–8. SOME CLUES IN PATIENT HISTORY TO TYPE OF IMMUNODEFICIENCY

FINDING	IMMUNODEFICIENCY
Recurrent *Streptococcus pneumoniae* and *Haemophilus influenzae* infections	Ig, C2, or IRAK-4 deficiency
Recurrent *Giardia intestinalis (lamblia)* infection	Antibody deficiency syndromes
Familial clustering of autoimmune disorders (eg, SLE, pernicious anemia)	Common variable immunodeficiency or selective IgA deficiency
Pneumocystis infections, cryptosporidiosis, or toxoplasmosis	T-cell disorders or occasionally Ig deficiency
Viral, fungal, or mycobacterial (opportunistic) infections	T-cell disorders
Clinical infection due to live-attenuated vaccines (eg, varicella, polio, BCG)	T-cell disorders
Graft-vs-host disease due to blood transfusions	T-cell disorders
Staphylococcal infections, infections with gram-negative organisms (eg, *Serratia* or *Klebsiella* sp), or fungal infections (eg, aspergillosis)	Phagocytic cell defects or hyper-IgE syndrome
Skin infections	Neutrophil defect or Ig deficiency
Recurrent gingivitis	Neutrophil defect
Recurrent neisserial infections	Certain complement deficiencies
Recurrent sepsis	Certain complement deficiencies, hyposplenism, or IgG deficiency
Family history of childhood death or of infections in a maternal uncle that are similar to those in the patient	X-linked disorders (eg, severe combined immunodeficiency, X-linked agammaglobulinemia, Wiskott-Aldrich syndrome, hyper-IgM syndrome)

BCG = bacille Calmette-Guérin; Ig = immunoglobulin; IRAK = IL-1R-associated kinase; SLE = systemic lupus erythematosus.

disease), lymph nodes of the head and neck may be enlarged and suppurative.

Tympanic membranes may be scarred or perforated. The nostrils may be crusted, indicating purulent nasal discharge. Chronic cough is common, as are lung crackles, especially in adults with CVID.

The liver and spleen are often enlarged in patients with CVID or chronic granulomatous disease. Muscle mass and fat deposits of the buttocks are decreased.

In infants, skin around the anus may break down because of chronic diarrhea. Neurologic examination may detect delayed developmental milestones or ataxia.

Other characteristic findings tentatively suggest a clinical diagnosis (see Table 176–9).

Initial testing: If a specific secondary immunodeficiency disorder is suspected clinically, testing should focus on that disorder (eg, diabetes, HIV infection, cystic fibrosis, primary ciliary dyskinesia).

Tests are needed to confirm a diagnosis of immunodeficiency (see Table 176–10). Initial screening tests should include

- CBC with manual differential
- Quantitative immunoglobulin (Ig) measurements
- Antibody titers
- Skin testing for delayed hypersensitivity

If results are normal, immunodeficiency (especially Ig deficiency) can be excluded. If results are abnormal, further tests in specialized laboratories are needed to identify specific

Table 176–9. CHARACTERISTIC CLINICAL FINDINGS IN SOME PRIMARY IMMUNODEFICIENCY DISORDERS

AGE GROUP	FINDINGS*	DISORDER
< 6 mo	Diarrhea, failure to thrive	Severe combined immunodeficiency
	Life-threatening infections (eg, pneumonia, sepsis, meningitis)	
	Maculopapular rash, splenomegaly	Severe combined immunodeficiency when accompanied by graft-vs-host disease (eg, caused by transplacentally transferred T cells)
	Hypocalcemic tetany, a congenital heart disorder, unusual facies with low-set ears, developmental delay	DiGeorge syndrome
	Recurrent pyogenic infections, sepsis	C3 deficiency
	Oculocutaneous albinism, neurologic changes, lymphadenopathy	Chédiak-Higashi syndrome
	Cyanosis, a congenital heart disorder, midline liver	Congenital asplenia
	Delayed umbilical cord detachment, leukocytosis, periodontitis, poor wound healing	Leukocyte adhesion deficiency
	Abscesses, lymphadenopathy, antral obstruction, pneumonia, osteomyelitis	Chronic granulomatous disease
	Recurrent staphylococcal abscesses of the skin, lungs, joints, and viscera; pneumatoceles; coarse facial features; pruritic dermatitis	Hyper-IgE syndrome
	Chronic gingivitis, recurrent aphthous ulcers and skin infections, severe neutropenia	Severe congenital neutropenia
	GI bleeding (eg, bloody diarrhea), eczema	Wiskott-Aldrich syndrome
6 mo to 5 yr	Paralysis after oral polio immunization	X-linked agammaglobulinemia
	Severe progressive infectious mononucleosis	X-linked lymphoproliferative syndrome
	Persistent oral candidiasis, nail dystrophy, endocrine disorders (eg, hypoparathyroidism, Addison disease)	Chronic mucocutaneous candidiasis
> 5 yr (including adults)	Ataxia, recurrent sinopulmonary infections, neurologic deterioration, telangiectasias	Ataxia-telangiectasia
	Recurrent *Neisseria* meningitis	C5, C6, C7, or C8 deficiency
	Recurrent sinopulmonary infections, malabsorption, splenomegaly, autoimmune disorders, nodular lymphoid hyperplasia of the GI tract, giardiasis, lymphoid interstitial pneumonia, bronchiectasis	Common variable immunodeficiency
	Progressive dermatomyositis with chronic echovirus encephalitis	X-linked agammaglobulinemia

*In addition to infection.

Adapted from Stiehm, ER, Conley ME: Immunodeficiency diseases: general considerations, in *Immunodeficiency Disease in Infants and Children,* ed 4, edited by ER Stiehm. Philadelphia, WB Saunders Company, 1996, p. 212.

Table 176–10. INITIAL AND ADDITIONAL LABORATORY TESTS FOR IMMUNODEFICIENCY

TYPE	INITIAL TESTS	ADDITIONAL TESTS
Humoral immunity deficiency	IgG, IgM, IgA, and IgE levels Isohemagglutinin titers Antibody response to vaccine antigens (eg, *Haemophilus influenzae* type b, tetanus, diphtheria, conjugated and nonconjugated pneumococcal, and meningococcal antigens)	B-cell phenotyping and count using flow cytometry and monoclonal antibodies to B cells Flow cytometry for CD40 and CD40 ligand Evaluation for mutations in genes that encode BTK and NEMO Sweat test
Cellular immunity deficiency	Absolute lymphocyte count Delayed hypersensitivity skin tests (eg, using *Candida*) HIV testing Chest x-ray for size of thymus in infants only	T-cell phenotyping and count using flow cytometry and monoclonal antibodies to T cells and subsets T-cell proliferative response to mitogens TREC test (a genetic test that identifies infants with abnormal T cells or a low T-cell count due to SCID or other disorders)
Phagocytic cell defects	Phagocytic cell count and morphology	Flow cytometric oxidative burst measurement using dihydrorhodamine 123 (DHR) or nitroblue tetrazolium (NBT) Flow cytometry for CD18 and CD15 Neutrophil chemotaxis
Complement deficiency	C3 level C4 level CH50 activity (for total activity of the classical pathway) and AH50 activity (for total activity of the alternate complement pathways) C1 inhibitor level and function	Specific component assays

BTK = Bruton tyrosine kinase; C = complement; CH = hemolytic complement; NEMO = nuclear factor–kappa-B essential modulator; SCID = severe combined immunodeficiency; TREC = T-cell receptor excision circle.

deficiencies. If chronic infections are objectively documented, initial and specific tests may be done simultaneously. If clinicians suspect that immunodeficiency may be still developing, tests may need to be repeated, with monitoring over time, before a definitive diagnosis is made.

CBC can detect abnormalities in one or more cell types (eg, WBCs, platelets) characteristic of specific disorders, as in the following:

- **Neutropenia** (absolute neutrophil count < 1200 cells/μL) may be congenital or cyclic or may occur in aplastic anemia.
- **Lymphopenia** (lymphocytes < 2000/μL at birth, < 4500/μL at age 9 mo, or < 1000/μL in older children or adults) suggests a T-cell disorder because 70% of circulating lymphocytes are T cells.
- **Leukocytosis** that persists between infections may occur in leukocyte adhesion deficiency.
- **Thrombocytopenia** in male infants suggests Wiskott-Aldrich syndrome.
- **Anemia** may suggest anemia of chronic disease or autoimmune hemolytic anemia, which may occur in CVID and other immunodeficiencies.

However, many abnormalities are transient manifestations of infection, drug use, or other factors; thus, abnormalities should be confirmed and followed.

Peripheral blood smear should be examined for Howell-Jolly bodies and other unusual RBC forms, which suggest primary asplenia or impaired splenic function. Granulocytes may have morphologic abnormalities (eg, giant granules in Chédiak-Higashi syndrome).

Quantitative serum Ig levels are measured. Low serum levels of IgG, IgM, or IgA suggest antibody deficiency, but results must be compared with those of age-matched controls. An IgG level < 200 mg/dL usually indicates significant antibody deficiency, although such levels may occur in protein-losing enteropathies or nephrotic syndrome.

IgM antibodies can be assessed by measuring isohemagglutinin titers (anti-A, anti-B). All patients except infants < 6 mo and people with blood type AB have natural antibodies at a titer of ≥ 1:8 (anti-A) or ≥ 1:4 (anti-B). Antibodies to blood groups A and B and to some bacterial polysaccharides are selectively deficient in certain disorders (eg, Wiskott-Aldrich syndrome, complete IgG2 deficiency).

IgG antibody titers can be assessed in immunized patients by measuring antibody titers before and after administration of vaccine antigens (*Haemophilus influenzae* type B, tetanus, diphtheria, conjugated or nonconjugated pneumococcal, and meningococcal antigens); a less-than-twofold increase in titer at 2 to 3 wk suggests antibody deficiency regardless of Ig levels. Natural antibodies (eg, antistreptolysin O, heterophil antibodies) may also be measured.

With **skin testing,** most immunocompetent adults, infants, and children react to 0.1 mL of *Candida albicans* extract (1:100 for infants and 1:1000 for older children and adults) injected intradermally. Positive reactivity, defined as erythema and induration > 5 mm at 24, 48, and 72 h, excludes a T-cell disorder. Lack of response does not confirm immunodeficiency in patients with no previous exposure to *Candida*.

Chest x-ray may be useful in some infants; an absent thymic shadow suggests a T-cell disorder, especially if the x-ray is obtained before onset of infection or other stresses that may shrink the thymus. Lateral pharyngeal x-ray may show absence of adenoidal tissue.

Additional testing: If clinical findings or initial tests suggest a specific disorder of immune cell or complement function, other tests are indicated.

If patients have recurrent infections and lymphopenia, lymphocyte phenotyping using flow cytometry and monoclonal antibodies to T, B, and NK cells is indicated to check for lymphocyte deficiency.

If cellular immunity deficiency is suspected, the T-cell receptor excision circle (TREC) test can be done to identify infants with low T-cell counts. If tests show that T cells are low in number or absent, in vitro mitogen stimulation studies are done to assess T-cell function. If MHC antigen deficiency is suspected, serologic (not molecular) HLA typing is indicated. Some experts recommend screening all neonates with a TREC test; testing is done routinely in some US states.

If humoral immunity deficiency is suspected, patients may be tested for specific mutations—for example, in the genes that encode for Bruton tyrosine kinase (BTK), CD40 and CD40 ligand, and nuclear factor-kappa-B essential modulator (NEMO). A sweat test is typically done during the evaluation to rule out cystic fibrosis.

If combined cellular and humoral immunity is impaired and SCID is suspected, patients can be tested for certain typical mutations (eg, in the IL-2 receptor gamma [*IL-2RG*, or *IL-2Rγ*] gene).

If phagocytic cell defects are suspected, CD15 and CD18 are measured by flow cytometry and neutrophil chemotaxis is tested. A flow cytometric oxidative (respiratory) burst assay (measured by dihydrorhodamine 123 [DHR] or nitroblue tetrazolium [NBT]) can detect whether O_2 radicals are produced during phagocytosis; no production is characteristic of chronic granulomatous disease.

If the type or pattern of infections suggests complement deficiency, the serum dilution required to lyse 50% of antibody-coated RBCs is measured. This test (called CH50) detects complement component deficiencies in the classical complement pathway but does not indicate which component is abnormal. A similar test (AH50) can be done to detect complement deficiencies in the alternative pathway.

If examination or screening tests detect abnormalities suggesting lymphocyte or phagocytic cell defects, other tests can more precisely characterize specific disorders (see Table 176–11).

Prenatal and neonatal diagnosis: An increasing number of primary immunodeficiency disorders can be diagnosed prenatally using chorionic villus sampling, cultured amniotic cells, or fetal blood sampling, but these tests are used only when a mutation in family members has already been identified.

X-linked agammaglobulinemia, Wiskott-Aldrich syndrome, ataxia-telangiectasia, X-linked lymphoproliferative syndrome, all forms of SCID (using the TREC test), and all forms of chronic granulomatous disease can be detected.

Sex determination by ultrasonography can be used to exclude X-linked disorders.

Prognosis

Prognosis depends on the primary immunodeficiency disorder.

Most patients with an Ig or a complement deficiency have a good prognosis with a near-normal life expectancy if they are diagnosed early, are treated appropriately, and have no coexisting chronic disorders (eg, pulmonary disorders such as bronchiectasis).

Other immunodeficient patients (eg, those with a phagocytic cell defect or combined immunodeficiencies, such as Wiskott-Aldrich syndrome or ataxia-telangiectasia) have a guarded prognosis; most require intensive and frequent treatment.

Some immunodeficient patients (eg, those with SCID) die during infancy unless immunity is provided through transplantation. All forms of SCID could be diagnosed at birth if a WBC count and manual differential of cord or peripheral blood were routinely done in neonates. Suspicion for SCID, a true pediatric emergency, must be high because prompt diagnosis is essential for survival. If SCID is diagnosed before patients reach age 3 mo, transplantation of stem cells from a matched or half-matched (haploidentical) relative is lifesaving in 95%.

PEARLS & PITFALLS

- To prevent early death, strongly consider screening all neonates for SCID using a T-cell receptor excision circle (TREC) test.

Treatment

- Vaccines and avoidance of exposure to infection
- Antibiotics and sometimes surgery
- Replacement of missing immune components

Treatment of immunodeficiency disorders generally involves preventing infection, managing acute infection, and replacing missing immune components when possible.

Infection prevention: Infection can be prevented by advising patients to avoid environmental exposures and not giving them live-virus vaccines (eg, varicella, rotavirus, measles, mumps, rubella, herpes zoster, yellow fever, oral polio, intranasal influenza vaccines) or BCG.

Patients at risk of serious infections (eg, those with SCID, chronic granulomatous disease, Wiskott-Aldrich syndrome, or asplenia) or of specific infections (eg, with *Pneumocystis jirovecii*

Table 176–11. SPECIFIC AND ADVANCED LABORATORY TESTS FOR IMMUNODEFICIENCY*

TEST	INDICATIONS	INTERPRETATION
Humoral immunity deficiency		
IgE level measurement	Abscesses	Levels are high in patients with abscesses and pneumatoceles hyper-IgE syndrome, partial T-cell deficiencies, allergic disorders, or parasitic infections. Levels may be high or low in patients with incomplete B-cell defects or deficiencies. Isolated deficiency is not clinically significant.
B-cell quantification via flow cytometry	Low Ig levels	< 1% B cells suggests X-linked agammaglobulinemia. B cells are absent in Omenn syndrome.
Lymph node biopsy	For some patients with lymphadenopathy, to determine whether germinal centers are normal and to exclude cancer and infection	Interpretation varies by histology.

Table 176–11. SPECIFIC AND ADVANCED LABORATORY TESTS FOR IMMUNODEFICIENCY* (*Continued*)

TEST	INDICATIONS	INTERPRETATION
Genetic testing (genetic sequencing or mutation analysis)	B cells < 1% (detected by flow cytometry) Suspicion of a disorder with one or more characteristic mutations	Abnormalities in genes suggest or confirm a diagnosis, as in the following: • *BTK*: X-linked agammaglobulinemia • *SAP*[†]: X-linked lymphoproliferative syndrome • *NEMO*: A combined immunodeficiency Results can also provide prognostic information.
T-cell deficiency		
T-cell enumeration using flow cytometry and monoclonal antibodies[‡]	Lymphopenia, suspected SCID or complete DiGeorge syndrome	Interpretation varies by molecular type of SCID.
T-cell proliferation assays to mitogens, antigens, or irradiated allogeneic WBCs	Low percentage of T cells, lymphopenia, suspected SCID, or complete DiGeorge syndrome	Low or absent uptake of radioactive thymidine during cell division indicates a T-cell or combined defect.
Detection of antigens (eg, class II MHC molecules) using monoclonal antibodies or serologic HLA typing	Suspected MHC deficiency, absence of MHC stimulation by cells	Absence of class I or class II HLA antigens by serologic HLA typing is diagnostic for MHC antigen deficiency.
RBC adenosinedeaminase assay	Severe lymphopenia	Levels are low in a specific form of SCID.
Purine nucleoside phosphorylase assay	Severe persistent lymphopenia	Levels are low in combined immunodeficiency with normal or elevated Ig levels.
T-cell receptor and signal transduction assays	Phenotypically normal T cells that do not proliferate normally in response to mitogen antigen	Interpretation varies by test.
T-cell receptor excision circle (TREC) test	Screening for SCID and other T-cell disorders	Low numbers suggest a defect that disrupts development or maturation of T cells or that causes apoptosis of T cells.
Combined humoral and cellular immunity deficiencies		
Genetic testing	A suspected combined immunodeficiency disorder	Abnormalities in genes suggest or confirm certain disorders; for example, abnormalities in *NEMO* suggest combined immunodeficiency with defects of NF–kappa-B regulation, and abnormalities in *IL-2RG* suggest SCID.
Phagocytic cell defects		
Assays for oxidant products (hydrogen peroxide, superoxide) or proteins (CR3 [CD11] adhesive glycoproteins, NADPH oxidase components)	History of staphylococcal abscesses or certain gram-negative or fungal infections (eg, *Serratia marcescens* aspergillosis)	Abnormalities confirm phagocytic cell defects or deficiencies.
Phosphorylation assays for signal transducer and activator of transcription (STAT), including STAT1 and STAT4	Recurrent mycobacterial infections	This test is the first one done to check for mendelian susceptibility to mycobacterial disease (MSMD).
Complement deficiency		
Measurement of levels of specific complement components	Suspicion of a complement disorder	Interpretation varies by test.

*Some of these tests may be used for screening or initial testing.

[†]SAP is also called SH2 domain protein 1A [SH2D1A], or DSHP.

[‡]Test uses anti-CD3 for all T cells, anti-CD4 for helper T cells, anti-CD8 for cytotoxic T cells, anti-CD45RO or anti-CD45RA for activated and naive T cells, anti-CD25 for regulatory T cells, and anti-CD16 and anti-CD56 for natural killer cells.

BTK = Bruton tyrosine kinase; CH = hemolytic complement; Ig = immunoglobulin; IL-2RG = IL-2 receptor gamma; MHC = major histocompatibility complex; NADPH = nicotinamide adenine dinucleotide phosphate; NEMO = NF–kappa-B essential modifier; NF–kappa-B = nuclear factor-kappa-B; SAP = SLAM-associated protein; SCID = severe combined immunodeficiency; SLAM = signaling lymphocyte activation molecule.

in patients with T-cell disorders) can be given prophylactic antibiotics (eg, 5 mg/kg trimethoprim/sulfamethoxazole po bid).

To prevent graft-vs-host disease after transfusions, clinicians should use blood products from cytomegalovirus-negative donors; the products should be filtered to remove WBCs and irradiated (15 to 30 Gy).

Management of acute infection: After appropriate cultures are obtained, antibiotics that target likely causes should be given promptly. Sometimes surgery (eg, to drain abscesses) is needed.

Usually, self-limited viral infections cause severe persistent disease in immunocompromised patients. Antivirals (eg, amantadine, rimantadine, oseltamivir, or zanamivir for influenza; acyclovir for herpes simplex and varicella-zoster infections; ribavirin for respiratory syncytial virus or parainfluenza 3 infections) may be lifesaving.

Replacement of missing immune components: Such replacement helps prevent infection. Therapies used in more than one primary immunodeficiency disorder include the following:

- **IV immune globulin (IVIG)** is effective replacement therapy in most forms of antibody deficiency. The usual dose is 400 mg/kg once/mo; treatment is begun at a low infusion rate. Some patients need higher or more frequent doses. IVIG 800 mg/kg once/mo helps some antibody-deficient patients who do not respond well to conventional doses, particularly those with a chronic lung disorder. High-dose IVIG aims to keep IgG trough levels in the normal range (> 600 mg/dL).
- **Subcutaneous immune globulin (SCIG)** can be given instead of IVIG. SCIG can be given at home, usually by patients themselves. The usual dose is 100 to 150 mg/kg once/wk. Because SCIG and IVIG differ in bioavailability, the dose of SCIG may need to be adjusted if patients are switched from IVIG. With SCIG, local site reactions are a risk, but SCIG seems to have fewer systemic adverse effects.
- **Hematopoietic stem cell transplantation** using bone marrow, cord blood, or adult peripheral blood stem cells is effective for lethal T cell and other immunodeficiencies. Pretransplantation chemotherapy is unnecessary in patients without T cells (eg, those with SCID). However, patients with intact T-cell function or partial T-cell deficiencies (eg, Wiskott-Aldrich syndrome, combined immunodeficiency with inadequate but not absent T-cell function) require pretransplantation chemotherapy to ensure graft acceptance. When a matched sibling donor is unavailable, haploidentical bone marrow from a parent can be used. In such cases, mature T cells that cause graft-vs-host disease must be rigorously depleted from parental marrow before it is given. Umbilical cord blood from an HLA-matched sibling can also be used as a source of stem cells. In some cases, bone marrow or umbilical cord blood from a matched unrelated donor can be used, but after transplantation, immunosuppressants are required to prevent graft-vs-host disease, and their use delays restoration of immunity.

Retroviral vector gene therapy has been successful in a few patients with X-linked and ADA-deficient SCID, but this treatment is not widely used because some patients with X-linked SCID developed leukemia.

KEY POINTS

- Consider a primary immunodeficiency if infections are unusually frequent or severe, particularly if they occur in family members, or if patients have thrush, oral ulcers, periodontitis, or certain skin lesions.
- Do a complete physical examination, including the skin, all mucous membranes, lymph nodes, spleen, and rectum.
- Begin testing with CBC (with manual differential), quantitative Ig levels, antibody titers, and skin testing for delayed hypersensitivity.
- Select additional tests based on what type of immune defect is suspected (humoral, cellular, phagocytic cell, or complement).
- Test the fetus (eg, using fetal blood, chorionic villus sampling, or cultured amniotic cells) if family members are known to have an immunodeficiency disorder.
- Teach patients how to avoid infections, give indicated vaccines, and prescribe prophylactic antibiotics for patients with certain disorders.
- Consider immune globulin replacement for antibody deficiencies and hematopoietic stem cell transplantation for severe immunodeficiencies, particularly T-cell immunodeficiencies.

ATAXIA-TELANGIECTASIA

Ataxia-telangiectasia results from a DNA repair defect that frequently results in humoral and cellular deficiency; it causes progressive cerebellar ataxia, oculocutaneous telangiectasias, and recurrent sinopulmonary infections.

Ataxia-telangiectasia is an autosomal-recessive primary immunodeficiency disorder that involves combined humoral and cellular deficiencies. Estimated incidence is 1 in 20,000 to 100,000 births. Ataxia-telangiectasia is caused by mutations in the gene that encodes ataxia-telangiectasia–mutated (ATM) protein. ATM is involved in detection of DNA damage and helps control the rate of cell growth and division.

Patients often lack IgA and IgE and have a progressive T-cell defect.

Symptoms and Signs

Age at onset of neurologic symptoms and evidence of immunodeficiency vary.

Ataxia is frequently the first symptom and usually develops when children begin to walk. Progression of neurologic symptoms leads to severe disability. Speech becomes slurred, choreoathetoid movements and nystagmus develop, and muscle weakness usually progresses to muscle atrophy.

Telangiectasias may not appear until age 4 to 6 yr; they are most prominent on the bulbar conjunctivae, ears, antecubital and popliteal fossae, and sides of the neck.

Recurrent sinopulmonary infections lead to recurrent pneumonia, bronchiectasis, and chronic restrictive pulmonary disease.

Certain endocrine abnormalities (eg, gonadal dysgenesis, testicular atrophy, diabetes mellitus) may occur.

Frequency of cancer (especially leukemia, lymphoma, brain tumors, and gastric cancer) is high. Cancer typically occurs after age 10 and at a rate of about 1%/yr but is a lifelong risk and can occur at any age.

Diagnosis

- IgA and serum alpha-1 fetoprotein levels
- Genetic testing

The following clinical findings suggest the diagnosis of ataxia-telangiectasia:

- Cerebellar ataxia (particularly when telangiectasias are present)
- Low levels of IgA (present in 80% of patients with this disorder)
- High levels of serum alpha-1 fetoprotein

If karyotype analysis is done, chromosome breaks, consistent with a defect in DNA repair, are often seen.

Diagnosis of ataxia-telangiectasia is confirmed by identifying mutations on both alleles of the gene for ATM protein. Because carriers of an ataxia-telangiectasia mutation usually remain asymptomatic, testing siblings for a carrier state can help predict their chance of having an affected child.

Testing for endocrine abnormalities and cancers is done based on clinical presentation.

Treatment

- Supportive care using prophylactic antibiotics or immune globulin (IgG) replacement therapy

Treatment with prophylactic antibiotics or immune globulin may help patients with ataxia-telangiectasia.

In one small study, treatment with amantadine resulted in minimal improvement in motor function, but there is no effective treatment for the progressive neurologic deterioration, which causes death, usually by age 30.

Chemotherapy is often indicated for treatment of associated cancers.

CHÉDIAK-HIGASHI SYNDROME

Chédiak-Higashi syndrome is a rare, autosomal recessive syndrome characterized by impaired lysis of phagocytized bacteria, resulting in recurrent bacterial respiratory and other infections and oculocutaneous albinism.

Chédiak-Higashi syndrome is a rare, autosomal recessive primary immunodeficiency disorder that involves phagocytic cell defects. The syndrome is caused by a mutation in the *LYST* (lysosomal trafficking regulator; *CHS1*) gene. Giant lysosomal granules develop in neutrophils and other cells (eg, melanocytes, neural Schwann cells). The abnormal lysosomes cannot fuse with phagosomes, so ingested bacteria cannot be lysed normally.

Symptoms and Signs

Clinical findings of Chédiak-Higashi syndrome include oculocutaneous albinism and susceptibility to recurrent respiratory and other infections.

In about 80% of patients, an accelerated phase occurs, causing fever, jaundice, hepatosplenomegaly, lymphadenopathy, pancytopenia, bleeding diathesis, and neurologic changes. Once the accelerated phase occurs, the syndrome is usually fatal within 30 mo.

Diagnosis

- Genetic testing

Neutropenia, decreased NK–cell cytotoxicity, and hypergammaglobulinemia are common. A peripheral blood smear is examined for giant granules in neutrophils and other cells; a bone marrow smear is examined for giant inclusion bodies in leukocyte precursor cells.

The diagnosis of Chédiak-Higashi syndrome can be confirmed with genetic testing for *LYST* mutations.

Because this disorder is extremely rare, there is no need to screen relatives unless clinical suspicion is high.

Treatment

- Supportive care using antibiotics, interferon gamma and sometimes corticosteroids
- Hematopoietic stem cell transplantation

Prophylactic antibiotics can help prevent infections, and interferon gamma can help restore some immune system function. Pulse doses of corticosteroids and splenectomy sometimes induce transient remission.

However, unless hematopoietic stem cell transplantation is done, most patients die of infections by age 7 yr. Transplantation of unfractionated HLA-identical bone marrow after pretransplantation cytoreductive chemotherapy may be curative. Five-yr posttransplantation survival rate is about 60%.

CHRONIC GRANULOMATOUS DISEASE

Chronic granulomatous disease (CGD) is characterized by WBCs that cannot produce activated O_2 compounds and by defects in phagocytic cell microbicidal function. Manifestations include recurrent infections; multiple granulomatous lesions of the lungs, liver, lymph nodes, and GI and GU tract; abscesses; lymphadenitis; hypergammaglobulinemia; elevated ESR; and anemia. Diagnosis is by assessing O_2 radical production in WBCs via a flow cytometric oxidative burst assay. Treatment is with antibiotics, antifungal drugs, and interferon gamma; granulocyte transfusions may be needed.

CGD is a primary immunodeficiency disorder that involves phagocytic cell defects. More than 50% of cases of CGD are inherited as an X-linked recessive trait and thus occur only in males; in the rest, inheritance is autosomal recessive. Common mutations responsible for CGD affect the gp91phox (X-linked form), p22phox, p47phox, and p67phox genes.

In CGD, WBCs do not produce hydrogen peroxide, superoxide, and other activated O_2 compounds because nicotinamide adenine dinucleotide phosphate oxidase activity is deficient. Phagocytic cell microbicidal function is defective; thus, bacteria and fungi are not killed despite normal phagocytosis.

Symptoms and Signs

CGD usually begins with recurrent abscesses during early childhood, but in a few patients, onset is delayed until the early teens. Typical pathogens are catalase-producing organisms (eg, *Staphylococcus aureus*; *Escherichia coli*; *Serratia*, *Klebsiella*, and *Pseudomonas* sp; fungi). *Aspergillus* infections are the leading cause of death.

Multiple granulomatous lesions occur in the lungs, liver, lymph nodes, and GI and GU tract (causing obstruction). Suppurative lymphadenitis, hepatosplenomegaly, pneumonia, and hematologic evidence of chronic infection are common. Skin, lymph node, lung, liver, and perianal abscesses; stomatitis; and osteomyelitis also occur.

Growth may be delayed.

Diagnosis

- Flow cytometric oxidative (respiratory) burst assay

Diagnosis of CGD is by a flow cytometric oxidative (respiratory) burst assay to detect O_2 radical production using dihydrorhodamine 123 (DHR) or nitroblue tetrazolium (NBT). This test can also identify female carriers of the X-linked form and recessive forms.

Genetic testing is done only in research settings and is not required to make the diagnosis. Siblings are usually screened using DHR shortly after the diagnosis.

Hypergammaglobulinemia and anemia can occur; ESR is elevated.

Treatment

- Prophylactic antibiotics and usually antifungals
- Usually interferon gamma
- For severe infections, granulocyte transfusions
- Hematopoietic stem cell transplantation

Treatment of CGD is continuous prophylactic antibiotics, particularly trimethoprim/sulfamethoxazole 160/800 mg po bid. Oral antifungals are given as primary prophylaxis or are added if fungal infections occur even once; most useful are

- Itraconazole po q 12 h (100 mg for patients < 13 yr, 200 mg for those ≥ 13 yr or weighing > 50 kg)
- Voriconazole po q 12 h (100 mg for those weighing < 40 kg; 200 mg for those weighing ≥ 40 kg)
- Posaconazole (400 mg bid)

Interferon gamma may reduce severity and frequency of infections and is usually included in the treatment regimen. Usual dose is 50 mcg/m^2 sc 3 times/wk.

Granulocyte transfusions can be lifesaving when infections are severe.

When preceded by pretransplantation chemotherapy, HLA-identical sibling hematopoietic stem cell transplantation is usually successful.

Gene therapy is under study.

KEY POINTS

- Suspect CGD if patients have recurrent abscesses during childhood (sometimes not until the early teens), particularly if the pathogen is a catalase-producing organism (eg, *Staphylococcus aureus*; *Escherichia coli*; *Serratia*, *Klebsiella*, or *Pseudomonas* sp; fungi).
- Use the flow cytometric oxidative burst assay to diagnose CGD and identify carriers.
- Treat most patients with prophylactic antibiotics, antifungals, and interferon gamma.
- For severe infections, give granulocyte transfusions.
- Consider hematopoietic stem cell transplantation.

CHRONIC MUCOCUTANEOUS CANDIDIASIS

Chronic mucocutaneous candidiasis is persistent or recurrent candidal infection due to inherited T-cell defects.

Chronic mucocutaneous candidiasis is a primary immunodeficiency disorder that involves T-cell defects. Inheritance may be

- Autosomal dominant: Involving a mutation in the signal transducer and activator of transcription 1 gene (*STAT1*)
- Autosomal recessive: Involving a mutation in the autoimmune regulator gene (*AIRE*)

In the **recessive form** (autoimmune polyendocrinopathy–candidosis-ectodermal dystrophy), autoimmune manifestations typically develop; they include endocrine disorders (eg, hypoparathyroidism, adrenal insufficiency, hypogonadism, thyroid disorders, diabetes), alopecia areata, pernicious anemia, and hepatitis. Mutations may also occur in genes that encode various proteins involved in the innate immune response to fungi—notably, the following:

- *PTPN22* (protein tyrosine phosphatase, non-receptor type 22 [*also called LYP*, or lymphoid tyrosine phosphatase], which is involved in T cell–receptor signalling)
- Dectin-1 (an innate pattern recognition receptor essential for the control of fungal infections)
- CARD9 (caspase recruitment domain-containing protein 9, which is an adaptor molecule important in the production of IL-17 and for protection against fungal invasion)

Patients have cutaneous anergy to *Candida*, absent proliferative responses to *Candida* antigen (but normal proliferative responses to mitogens), and intact antibody response to *Candida* and other antigens. Candidiasis recurs or persists, usually beginning during infancy but sometimes during early adulthood. Life span is not affected. Some patients also have deficient humoral immunity (sometimes called antibody deficiency), characterized by abnormal antibody responses to polysaccharide antigens despite normal immunoglobulin levels.

Symptoms and Signs

Thrush is common, as are infections of the scalp, skin, nails, and GI and vaginal mucosa. Severity varies. Nails may be thickened, cracked, and discolored, with edema and erythema of the surrounding periungual tissue, resembling clubbing. Skin lesions are crusted, pustular, erythematous, and hyperkeratotic. Scalp lesions may result in scarring alopecia.

Infants often present with refractory thrush, candidal diaper rash, or both.

Diagnosis

- Clinical evaluation

Candidal lesions are confirmed by standard tests (eg, potassium hydroxide wet mount of scrapings).

Diagnosis of chronic mucocutaneous candidiasis is based on the presence of recurrent candidal skin or mucosal lesions when no other known causes of candidal infection (eg, diabetes, antibiotic use) are present.

Patients are screened for endocrine disorders based on clinical suspicion.

If an AIRE mutation is detected, screening can be offered to the patient's siblings and children.

Treatment

- Antifungal drugs
- Treatment of endocrine and autoimmune manifestations

Usually, the infections can be controlled with a topical antifungal, If patients have a poor response to topical antifungals, long-term treatment with a systemic antifungal drug (eg, amphotericin B, fluconazole, ketoconazole) may be needed. Immune globulin should be considered if patients have antibody deficiency.

Autoimmune (including endocrine) manifestations are treated aggressively.

Hematopoietic stem cell transplantation was successful in 2 cases and could be considered as last-line treatment in severe cases.

KEY POINTS

- Inheritance of chronic mucocutaneous candidiasis is autosomal dominant or recessive.
- Patients with the recessive form can have autoimmune (including endocrine) manifestations.
- Diagnose the disorder by confirming mucocutaneous candidiasis and excluding other causes.
- Treat candidiasis with antifungal drugs (using a systemic drug if needed), and treat autoimmune manifestations.

COMMON VARIABLE IMMUNODEFICIENCY

Common variable immunodeficiency (CVID—acquired or adult-onset hypogammaglobulinemia) is characterized by low immunoglobulin (Ig) levels with phenotypically normal B cells that can proliferate but do not develop into Ig-producing cells.

CVID is a primary immunodeficiency disorder that involves humoral immunity deficiencies. It includes several different molecular defects, but in most patients, the molecular defect is unknown. Mutations are sporadic in > 90% of cases. CVID is clinically similar to X-linked agammaglobulinemia in the types of infections that develop, but onset tends to be later (typically between ages 20 and 40). T-cell immunity may be impaired in some patients.

Symptoms and Signs

Patients with CVID have recurrent sinopulmonary infections.

Autoimmune disorders (eg, autoimmune thrombocytopenia, autoimmune hemolytic or pernicious anemia, SLE, Addison disease, thyroiditis, RA, alopecia areata) can occur, as can malabsorption, nodular lymphoid hyperplasia of the GI tract, granuloma formation, lymphoid interstitial pneumonia, splenomegaly, and bronchiectasis. Gastric carcinoma and lymphoma occur in 10% of patients.

Diagnosis

- Measurement of serum Ig and antibody titers
- Flow cytometry for T-cell and B-cell subsets
- Serum protein electrophoresis

Diagnosis of CVID is suggested by recurrent sinopulmonary infections and requires all of the following:

- Low (at least 2 standard deviations below the mean) levels of IgG
- Low levels of IgA, IgM, or both
- Impaired response to immunizations (usually both protein and polysaccharide vaccines)
- Exclusion of other immunodeficiency disorders

Antibody levels should not be measured if patients have been treated with IV immune globulin (IVIG) within the previous 6 mo because any detected antibodies are from the IVIG.

B-cell and T-cell quantification by flow cytometry is done to exclude other immunodeficiency disorders and to distinguish CVID from X-linked agammaglobulinemia, multiple myeloma, and chronic lymphocytic leukemia; findings may include low numbers of class-switched memory B cells or CD21+ cells. Serum protein electrophoresis is done to screen for monoclonal gammopathies (eg, myeloma), which may be associated with reduced levels of other Ig isotypes.

Spirometry, CBC, liver function tests, and a basic metabolic panel are recommended yearly to check for associated disorders. If lung function changes, CT should be done.

Because mutations are usually sporadic, screening relatives is not recommended unless there is a significant family history of CVID.

Treatment

- Prophylactic immune globulin (IgG) replacement therapy
- Antibiotics for infections

Treatment of CVID consists of immune globulin and antibiotics as needed to treat infection.

Rituximab, TNF-alpha inhibitors (eg, etanercept, infliximab), corticosteroids, and/or other treatments may be required to treat complications such as autoimmune disorders, lymphoid interstitial pneumonia, and granuloma formation.

DIGEORGE SYNDROME

DiGeorge syndrome is thymic and parathyroid hypoplasia or aplasia leading to T-cell immunodeficiency and hypoparathyroidism.

DiGeorge syndrome is a primary immunodeficiency disorder that involves T cell defects. It results from gene deletions in the DiGeorge chromosomal region at 22q11, mutations in genes at chromosome 10p13, and mutations in other unknown genes, which cause dysembryogenesis of structures that develop from pharyngeal pouches during the 8th wk of gestation. Most cases are sporadic; boys and girls are equally affected.

DiGeorge syndrome may be partial (some T-cell function exists) or complete (T-cell function is absent).

Symptoms and Signs

Infants have low-set ears, midline facial clefts, a small receding mandible, hypertelorism, a shortened philtrum, developmental delay, and congenital heart disorders (eg, interrupted aortic arch, truncus arteriosus, tetralogy of Fallot, atrial or ventricular septal defects). They also have thymic and parathyroid hypoplasia or aplasia, causing T-cell deficiency and hypoparathyroidism.

Recurrent infections begin soon after birth, but the degree of immunodeficiency varies considerably, and T-cell function may improve spontaneously. Hypocalcemic tetany appears within 24 to 48 h of birth.

Prognosis often depends on severity of the heart disorder.

Diagnosis

- Immune function assessment with immunoglobulin (Ig) levels, vaccine titers, and lymphocyte subset counts
- Parathyroid function assessment
- Chromosome analysis

Diagnosis of DiGeorge syndrome is based on clinical findings.

An absolute lymphocyte count is done, followed by B- and T-cell counts and lymphocyte subsets if leukopenia is detected; blood tests to evaluate T-cell and parathyroid function are done. Ig levels and vaccine titers are measured. If complete DiGeorge syndrome is suspected, the T-cell receptor excision circle (TREC) test should also be done.

A lateral chest x-ray may help evaluate thymic shadow.

Fluorescent in situ hybridization (FISH) testing can detect the chromosomal deletion in the 22q11 region; standard chromosomal tests to check for other abnormalities may also be done.

If DiGeorge syndrome is suspected, echocardiography is done. Cardiac catheterization may be necessary if patients present with cyanosis.

Because most cases are sporadic, screening of relatives is not necessary.

Treatment

- Partial syndrome: Calcium and vitamin D supplementation
- Complete syndrome: Transplantation of cultured thymus tissue or hematopoietic stem cells

In partial DiGeorge syndrome, hypoparathyroidism is treated with calcium and vitamin D supplementation; long-term survival is not affected.

Complete DiGeorge syndrome is fatal without treatment, which is transplantation of cultured thymus tissue or hematopoietic stem cell transplantation.

HYPER-IgE SYNDROME

(Hyperimmunoglobulinemia E Syndrome; Buckley Syndrome)

Hyper-IgE syndrome is a hereditary combined B- and T-cell immunodeficiency characterized by recurrent staphylococcal abscesses of the skin, sinopulmonary infections, and severe pruritic eosinophilic dermatitis.

Hyper-IgE syndrome is a primary immunodeficiency disorder that involves combined humoral and cellular immunity deficiencies. Inheritance can be

- Autosomal dominant: Caused by mutations in the *STAT3* (signal transducer and activator of transcription 3) gene
- Autosomal recessive: Appears to be caused by homozygous null mutations in *TYK2* (tyrosine kinase 2) or *DOCK8* (dedicator of cytokinesis 8) genes

Hyper-IgE syndrome starts during infancy.

Symptoms and Signs

Hyper-IgE syndrome typically causes recurrent staphylococcal abscesses of the skin, lungs, joints, and viscera; sinopulmonary infections; pulmonary pneumatoceles; and a severe pruritic eosinophilic dermatitis.

Patients have coarse facial features, delayed shedding of baby teeth, osteopenia, and recurrent fractures. All have tissue and blood eosinophilia and very high IgE levels (> 2000 IU/mL).

Diagnosis

- Serum IgE levels

Diagnosis of hyper-IgE syndrome is suspected based on symptoms and confirmed by measurement of serum IgE levels.

Genetic testing can identify the gene mutations and is done mainly to confirm the diagnosis or to help predict inheritance patterns.

Treatment

- Prophylactic antistaphylococcal antibiotics
- Sometimes interferon gamma for severe infection

Treatment of hyper-IgE syndrome consists of lifelong prophylactic antistaphylococcal antibiotics (usually trimethoprim/sulfamethoxazole).

Dermatitis is treated with skin hydration, emollient creams, antihistamines. and, if infections are suspected, antibiotics. Pulmonary complications are treated early and aggressively with antibiotics.

Interferon gamma has been used successfully for life-threatening infections.

HYPER-IgM SYNDROME

Hyper-IgM syndrome is an immunoglobulin (Ig) deficiency characterized by normal or elevated serum IgM levels and decreased levels or absence of other serum immunoglobulins, resulting in susceptibility to bacterial infections.

Hyper-IgM syndrome is a primary immunodeficiency disorder that involves combined humoral and cellular immunity deficiencies. It may be X-linked or autosomal. Manifestations vary depending on the mutation and its location.

X-linked hyper-IgM syndrome: Most cases are X-linked and caused by mutations in a gene on the X chromosome that encodes a protein (CD154, or CD40 ligand) on the surfaces of activated helper T cells. In the presence of cytokines, normal CD40 ligand interacts with B cells and thus signals them to switch from producing IgM to producing IgA, IgG, or IgE. In X-linked hyper-IgM syndrome, T cells lack functional CD40 ligand and cannot signal B cells to switch. Thus, B cells produce only IgM; IgM levels may be normal or elevated.

Patients with this form may have severe neutropenia and often present during infancy with *Pneumocystis jirovecii* pneumonia. Lymphoid tissue is very small because deficient CD 40 ligand signaling does not activate B cells. Otherwise, clinical presentation is similar to that of X-linked agammaglobulinemia and includes recurrent pyogenic bacterial sinopulmonary infections during the first 2 yr of life. Susceptibility to *Cryptosporidium* infections may be increased. Many patients die before puberty, and those who live longer often develop cirrhosis or B-cell lymphomas.

Autosomal recessive hyper-IgM syndrome: In autosomal recessive hyper-IgM syndrome with CD40 mutation, manifestations are similar to those of the X-linked form.

At least 4 autosomal recessive forms involve a B-cell defect. In 2 of these forms (deficiency of activation-induced cytidine deaminase [AID] or uracil DNA glycosylase [UNG]), serum IgM levels are much higher than in the X-linked form; lymphoid hyperplasia (including lymphadenopathy, splenomegaly, and tonsillar hypertrophy) is present, and autoimmune disorders may be present. Leukopenia is absent.

Diagnosis

- CD40 ligand expression and genetic testing

Diagnosis of hyper-IgM syndrome is suspected based on clinical criteria. Serum Ig levels are measured; normal or elevated serum IgM levels and low levels or absence of other immunoglobulins support the diagnosis. Flow cytometry testing of CD40 ligand expression on T-cell surfaces should be done. When possible, the diagnosis is confirmed by genetic testing. Prenatal genetic testing can be offered to women considering pregnancy if they have a family history of CD40 ligand deficiency. Genetic testing of other relatives is not routinely done.

Other laboratory findings include a reduced number of memory B cells (CD27) and absence of class-switched memory B cells (IgD-CD27).

Treatment

- Prophylactic immune globulin (IgG) replacement therapy and sometimes trimethoprim/sulfamethoxazole
- Hematopoietic stem cell transplantation when possible

Treatment of hyper-IgM syndrome usually includes immune globulin replacement therapy.

Patients with the X-linked form or CD40 mutations are given trimethoprim/sulfamethoxazole to prevent *P. jirovecii* infection, and environmental precautions are taken to reduce the risk of *Cryptosporidium* infection (see p. 127). However, because the prognosis is poor, hematopoietic stem cell transplantation is preferred if an HLA-identical sibling donor is available.

SELECTIVE IgA DEFICIENCY

Selective IgA deficiency is an IgA level < 7 mg/dL with normal IgG and IgM levels. It is the most common primary immunodeficiency. Many patients are asymptomatic, but some develop recurrent infections and autoimmune disorders. Some patients develop common variable immunodeficiency over time, and some remit spontaneously. Diagnosis is by measuring serum immunoglobulins. Treatment is antibiotics as needed (sometimes prophylactically) and usually avoidance of blood products that contain IgA.

IgA deficiency involves B cell defects. Prevalence ranges from 1/100 to 1/1000.

The inheritance pattern is unknown, but having a family member with selective IgA deficiency increases the risk by about 50 times.

Some patients have mutations in the *TACI* (transmembrane activator and calcium-modulator and cyclophilin ligand interactor) gene. Selective IgA deficiency is also commonly associated with certain HLA haplotypes; rare alleles or deletions of genes in the major histocompatibility complex (MHC) class III region are common.

Drugs such as phenytoin, sulfasalazine, gold, and D-penicillamine may lead to IgA deficiency in some patients.

Symptoms and Signs

Most patients are asymptomatic; others have recurrent sinopulmonary infections, diarrhea, allergies (eg, asthma, associated nasal polyps), or autoimmune disorders (eg, celiac or inflammatory bowel disease, SLE, chronic active hepatitis).

Anti-IgA antibodies may develop after exposure to IgA in transfusions, immune globulin (IVIG), or other blood products; rarely, if reexposed to these products, patients may have anaphylactic reactions.

Diagnosis

- Clinical evaluation
- Measurement of serum Ig levels
- Measurement of antibody response to vaccine antigens

Diagnosis of selective IgA deficiency is suspected in patients who have recurrent infections (including giardiasis), anaphylactic transfusion reactions, or a family history of CVID, IgA deficiency, or autoimmune disorders or who are taking drugs that lead to IgA deficiency.

Diagnosis is confirmed by a serum IgA level < 7 mg/dL with normal IgG and IgM levels and normal antibody titers in response to vaccine antigens.

Testing of family members is not recommended because most patients with low IgA have no clinically significant manifestations.

Prognosis

A few IgA-deficient patients develop CVID over time; others improve spontaneously. Prognosis is worse if an autoimmune disorder develops.

Treatment

- Antibiotics as needed for treatment and, in severe cases, for prophylaxis
- Avoidance of blood products that contain IgA

Allergic manifestations are treated. Antibiotics are given as needed for bacterial infections of the ears, sinuses, lungs, or GI or GU tract and, in severe cases, are given prophylactically.

Blood products that contain IgA are avoided because even trace amounts can elicit an anti-IgA–mediated anaphylactic reaction. If RBC transfusion is needed, only washed packed RBCs can be used.

Because immune globulin replacement therapy contains mostly IgG, patients with IgA deficiency do not benefit from it; also, anaphylactic reactions are a risk because patients may have developed anti-IgA antibodies. Rarely, if patients have no antibody response to vaccines and if prophylactic antibiotics are ineffective, specially formulated immune globulin preparations that contain extremely low levels of IgA can be tried and may be somewhat effective.

Patients are advised to wear an identification bracelet to prevent inadvertent plasma or immune globulin administration, which could lead to anaphylaxis.

KEY POINTS

- Selective IgA deficiency is the most common primary immunodeficiency.
- Patients may be asymptomatic or have recurrent infections or autoimmune disorders; some develop CVID over time, but in others, selective IgA deficiency spontaneously resolves.
- Suspect selective IgA deficiency if patients have anaphylactic reactions to transfusions, take drugs that lead to IgA deficiency, or have recurrent infections or a suggestive family history.
- Confirm the diagnosis by measuring Ig levels and antibody titers after vaccines are given; an IgA level < 7mg/dL and normal IgG and IgM levels and antibody titers are diagnostic.
- Give antibiotics as needed and, in severe cases, prophylactically.
- Avoid giving patients blood products that contain IgA.

LEUKOCYTE ADHESION DEFICIENCY

Leukocyte adhesion deficiency (LAD) results from an adhesion molecule defect that causes granulocyte and lymphocyte dysfunction and recurrent soft-tissue infections.

LAD is a primary immunodeficiency disorder that involves phagocytic cell defects. Inheritance is autosomal recessive.

LAD is caused by deficiency of adhesive glycoproteins on the surfaces of WBCs; these glycoproteins facilitate cellular interactions, cell attachment to blood vessel walls, cell movement, and interaction with complement fragments. Deficiencies impair the ability of granulocytes (and lymphocytes) to migrate out of the intravascular compartment, to engage in cytotoxic reactions, and to phagocytose bacteria. Severity of disease correlates with degree of deficiency.

Three different types of syndromes have been identified:

- LAD 1 (deficient or defective beta-2 integrin family)
- LAD 2 (absent fucosylated carbohydrate ligands for selectins)
- LAD 3 (defective activation of all beta integrins [1, 2, and 3])

Type 1 results from mutations in the integrin beta-2 gene (*ITGB2*), encoding CD18 of beta-2 integrins. Type 2 results from mutations in the glucose diphosphate (GDP)-fucose transporter gene.

Symptoms and Signs

Symptoms usually begin in infancy.

Severely affected infants have recurrent or progressive necrotic soft-tissue infections with staphylococcal and gram-negative bacteria, periodontitis, poor wound healing, no pus formation, leukocytosis, and delayed (> 3 wk) umbilical cord detachment. WBC counts remain high even between infections. Infections become increasingly difficult to control.

Less severely affected infants have few serious infections and mild alterations in blood counts.

Developmental delay is common in type 2.

Diagnosis

- Testing for adhesive glycoproteins on the surface of WBCs

Diagnosis of LAD is by detecting absence or severe deficiency of adhesive glycoproteins on the surface of WBCs using monoclonal antibodies (eg, anti-CD11, anti-CD18) and flow cytometry. Leukocytosis on CBC is common but nonspecific.

Genetic testing is recommended for siblings.

Treatment

- Supportive care using prophylactic antibiotics and granulocyte transfusions
- Hematopoietic stem cell transplantation

Treatment of LAD is with prophylactic antibiotics, often given continuously (usually trimethoprim/sulfamethoxazole). Granulocyte transfusions can also help.

Hematopoietic stem cell transplantation is the only effective treatment to date and can be curative. Gene therapy, which is under study, appears promising.

For patients with type II, correcting the underlying defect with fucose supplementation should be tried.

Patients with mild or moderate disease can survive into young adulthood. Most patients with severe disease die by age 5 unless treated successfully with hematopoietic stem cell transplantation.

SELECTIVE ANTIBODY DEFICIENCY WITH NORMAL IMMUNOGLOBULINS

Selective antibody deficiency with normal immunoglobulins (SADNI) is characterized by deficient specific antibody response to polysaccharide antigens but not to protein antigens, despite normal or near normal serum levels of immunoglobulins, including IgG subclasses.

SADNI is a primary immunodeficiency disorder. It is one of the most common immunodeficiencies that manifests with recurrent sinopulmonary infections. Selective antibody deficiencies can occur in other disorders, but SADNI is a primary disorder in which deficient response to polysaccharide antigens is the only abnormality (see Table 176–3 on p. 1389). The inheritance and pathophysiology have not been elucidated, but some evidence suggests that the cause may be inherited molecular abnormalities.

A subset of patients with SADNI initially have an appropriate response to polysaccharide antigen but lose antibody titers within 6 to 8 mo (called SADNI memory phenotype).

Patients have recurrent sinopulmonary infections and sometimes manifestations that suggest atopy (eg, chronic rhinitis, atopic dermatitis, asthma). Severity of the disorder varies.

Young children may have a form of SADNI that resolves spontaneously over time.

Diagnosis

- Immunoglobulin levels (IgG, IgA, IgM, and IgG subclasses)
- Responses to polysaccharide vaccines

Because healthy children < 2 yr can have recurrent sinopulmonary infections and weak responses to polysaccharide vaccines, testing for SADNI is not done unless patients are > 2 yr. Then, levels of IgG, IgA, IgM, and IgG subclasses and responses to vaccines are measured. The only abnormality in laboratory testing is a deficient response to polysaccharide vaccines (eg, pneumococcal vaccine). Responses to protein vaccines are normal.

Treatment

- Pneumococcal conjugate vaccine
- Sometimes prophylactic antibiotics and sometimes immune globulin replacement therapy

Patients should be vaccinated with the pneumococcal conjugate (eg, 13-valent) vaccine.

Sinopulmonary infections and atopic manifestations are treated aggressively. Uncommonly, when infections continue to recur, prophylactic antibiotics (eg, amoxicillin, trimethoprim/sulfamethoxazole) can be given.

Rarely, when infections recur frequently despite prophylactic antibiotics, immune globulin replacement therapy can be given.

SEVERE COMBINED IMMUNODEFICIENCY

Severe combined immunodeficiency (SCID) is characterized by low to absent T cells and a low, high, or normal number of B cells and NK cells. Most infants develop opportunistic infections within the first 3 mo of life. Diagnosis is by detecting lymphopenia, absence or a very low number of T cells, and impaired lymphocyte proliferative responses to mitogens. Patients must be kept in a protected environment; definitive treatment is hematopoietic stem cell transplantation.

SCID is a primary immunodeficiency disorder that involves combined humoral and cellular immunity deficiencies. It is caused by mutations in any one of many different genes (eg, for autosomal recessive forms, Janus kinase 3 [*JAK3*], protein tyrosine phosphatase, receptor type, C [*PTPRC*, or *CD45*], recombination activating genes 1 [*RAG1*] and 2 [*RAG2*]). Most types are autosomal recessive defects, so for the infant to be affected with SCID, the same gene must be mutated on both chromosomes.

There are 4 different abnormal lymphocyte phenotypes. In all forms of SCID, T cells are absent (T-); the number of B cells and/or NK cells may be low or none (B-; NK-) or high or normal (B+; NK+), depending on the form of SCID. However, B cells, even when normal in number, cannot function because T cells are absent. Natural killer cell function is usually impaired.

The most common form is X-linked. It affects the IL-2 receptor common gamma chain (a component of at least 6 cytokine receptors) and thus causes severe disease; phenotype is T- B+ NK-. It results from a mutation in the IL-2 receptor gamma gene (*IL-2RG*).

The 2nd most common form results from adenosine deaminase (ADA) deficiency, which leads to apoptosis of precursors for B, T, and NK cells; phenotype is T- B- NK-.

The next most common form results from IL-7 receptor alpha-chain deficiency; phenotype is T- B+ NK+.

Symptoms and Signs

By age 6 mo, most infants with SCID develop candidiasis, persistent viral infections, *Pneumocystis jirovecii* pneumonia, and diarrhea, leading to failure to thrive. Some have graft-vs-host disease due to maternal lymphocytes or blood transfusions. Other infants present at age 6 to 12 mo. Exfoliative dermatitis may develop as part of Omenn syndrome, one form of SCID. ADA deficiency may cause bone abnormalities. In all forms, the thymus is extremely small, and lymphoid tissue may be decreased or absent.

All forms of SCID are fatal during infancy unless they are diagnosed and treated early.

Diagnosis

- Routine neonatal screening using the T-cell receptor excision circle (TREC) test
- History of persistent infections
- WBC count
- Mitogen and vaccine antigen stimulation assays

Screening all neonates using the TREC test is often recommended and is done routinely in many US states.

SCID is suspected in infants with a history of persistent infections or other characteristic manifestations. CBC, including absolute WBC count and differential, is done; immunoglobulin levels are measured. Responses to mitogens and to standard vaccine antigens are determined to evaluate WBC and antibody function.

The disorder is diagnosed in patients with the following:

- Lymphopenia
- A low number of or no T cells
- Absent lymphocyte proliferative responses to mitogens

Other tests are done to determine the type of SCID; they include flow cytometry to determine T, B, and NK cell counts. ADA and purine nucleoside phosphorylase levels in WBCs, RBCs, and fibroblasts are measured. X-inactivation tests may be done to determine whether SCID is X-linked. To help determine severity and prognosis, clinicians often test patients for common mutations that are characteristic of SCID (eg, *IL-2RG*, *RAG1* and *RAG2*, *JAK3*, *Artemis* [*DCLRE1C*]).

Genetic testing of relatives is not recommended, except for siblings born after the diagnosis is made.

Treatment

- Reverse isolation
- Supportive care using immune globulin replacement therapy, antibiotics, and antifungals
- Hematopoietic stem cell transplantation
- Enzyme replacement for ADA deficiency
- Gene therapy for ADA-deficient SCID

Patients must be kept in reverse isolation.

Treatment with immune globulin replacement therapy, antibiotics (including *P. jirovecii* prophylaxis), and antifungals can help prevent infections but is not curative.

In 90 to 100% of infants with SCID or its variants, hematopoietic stem cell transplantation from an HLA-identical, mixed leukocyte culture–matched sibling restores immunity. When an HLA-identical sibling is not available, haploidentical hematopoietic stem cells from a parent that is rigorously depleted of T cells can be used. If SCID is diagnosed by age 3 mo, the survival rate after transplantation with either type of hematopoietic stem cells is 96%. Pretransplantation chemotherapy is unnecessary because patients do not have T cells and therefore cannot reject a graft.

Patients with ADA deficiency who do not receive a bone marrow graft may be treated with injections of polyethylene glycol–modified bovine ADA once or twice/wk.

Gene therapy has been successful in ADA-deficient SCID, and no posttreatment leukemias or lymphomas have been reported. Gene therapy has also been successful in X-linked SCID but has caused T-cell leukemias, precluding its use. Gene therapy for other forms of SCID is under study.

KEY POINTS

- Suspect SCID if infants have recurrent infections, graft-vs-host disease, or exfoliative dermatitis.
- The diagnosis is confirmed if patients have lymphopenia, deficient numbers of T cells, and no lymphocyte proliferative responses to mitogens.
- Determine T, B, and NK cell counts to identify the type of SCID.
- Give prophylactic immune globulin and antimicrobials.
- Do hematopoietic stem cell transplantation early whenever possible.
- If patients with ADA-deficient SCID do not receive a bone marrow graft, use ADA replacement and sometimes gene therapy.

TRANSIENT HYPOGAMMAGLOBULINEMIA OF INFANCY

Transient hypogammaglobulinemia of infancy is a temporary decrease in serum IgG and sometimes IgA and other Ig isotypes to levels below age-appropriate normal values.

Transient hypogammaglobulinemia of infancy is a primary immunodeficiency disorder that involves humoral immunity deficiencies. In this disorder, IgG levels continue to be low after the physiologic fall in maternal IgG at about age 3 to 6 mo. The cause and inheritance patterns are unknown.

The condition rarely leads to significant infections and is not thought to be a true immunodeficiency. The condition is usually asymptomatic. However, a few patients develop sinopulmonary or GI infections, candidiasis, and/or meningitis.

Diagnosis of transient hypogammaglobulinemia is based on low serum Ig levels (at least 2 standard deviations below the mean for age) and tests showing that antibody production in response to vaccine antigens (eg, tetanus, diphtheria) is normal. Thus, this condition can be distinguished from permanent forms of hypogammaglobulinemia, in which specific antibodies to vaccine antigens are not produced.

Patients with recurrent infections can be temporarily treated with prophylactic antibiotics. Immune globulin is usually unnecessary.

This condition may persist for months to a few years but usually resolves.

WISKOTT-ALDRICH SYNDROME

Wiskott-Aldrich syndrome results from a combined B- and T-cell defect and is characterized by recurrent infection, eczema, and thrombocytopenia.

Wiskott-Aldrich syndrome is a primary immunodeficiency disorder that involves combined humoral and cellular immunity deficiencies.

Inheritance is X-linked recessive. Wiskott-Aldrich syndrome is caused by mutations in the gene that encodes the Wiskott-Aldrich syndrome protein (WASP), a cytoplasmic protein necessary for normal B- and T-cell signaling.

Because B- and T-cell functions are impaired, infections with pyogenic bacteria and opportunistic organisms, particularly viruses and *Pneumocystis jirovecii*, develop. Infections with varicella zoster virus and herpesvirus are common.

Symptoms and Signs

The first manifestations are often hemorrhagic (usually bloody diarrhea), followed by recurrent respiratory infections, eczema, and thrombocytopenia.

Cancers, especially Epstein-Barr virus lymphomas and acute lymphoblastic leukemia, develop in about 10% of patients > 10 yr.

Diagnosis

- Immunoglobulin levels
- Platelet count and volume assessment
- WBC function tests (eg, neutrophil chemotaxis, T-cell function)

Diagnosis of Wiskott-Aldrich syndrome is based on the following:

- Decreased T-cell count and function
- Elevated IgE and IgA levels
- Low IgM levels
- Low or normal IgG levels
- Decreased NK cell cytotoxicity
- Impaired neutrophil chemotaxis

Antibodies to polysaccharide antigens (eg, blood group antigens A and B) may be selectively deficient. Platelets are small and defective, and splenic destruction of platelets is increased, causing thrombocytopenia. Mutation analysis may be used to confirm the diagnosis.

Genetic testing is recommended for 1st-degree relatives.

Because risk of lymphoma and leukemia is increased, a CBC with differential is usually done every 6 mo. Acute changes in symptoms related to B-cell dysfunction require more in-depth evaluations.

Treatment

- Supportive care using prophylactic immune globulin, antibiotics, and acyclovir
- For symptomatic thrombocytopenia, platelet transfusion and rarely splenectomy
- Hematopoietic stem cell transplantation

Treatment is prophylactic antibiotics and immune globulin to prevent recurrent bacterial infections, acyclovir to prevent severe herpes simplex virus infections, and platelet transfusions to treat hemorrhage. If thrombocytopenia is severe, splenectomy can be done, but it is usually avoided because it increases risk of septicemia.

The only established cure is hematopoietic stem cell transplantation, but gene therapy is under study.

Without transplantation, most patients die by age 15; however, some patients survive into adulthood.

X-LINKED AGAMMAGLOBULINEMIA

(Bruton Disease)

X-linked agammaglobulinemia is characterized by low levels or absence of immunoglobulins and absence of B cells, leading to recurrent infections with encapsulated bacteria.

X-linked agammaglobulinemia is a primary immunodeficiency disorder that involves humoral immunity deficiencies. It results from mutations in a gene on the X chromosome that encodes Bruton tyrosine kinase (BTK). BTK is essential for B-cell development and maturation; without it, maturation stops before the B-cell stage resulting in no mature B cells and hence no antibodies.

As a result, male infants have very small tonsils and do not develop lymph nodes; they have recurrent pyogenic lung, sinus, and skin infections with encapsulated bacteria (eg, *Streptococcus pneumoniae*, *Haemophilus influenzae*). Patients are also susceptible to persistent CNS infections resulting from live-attenuated oral polio vaccine and from echoviruses and coxsackieviruses; these infections can also manifest as progressive dermatomyositis with or without encephalitis. Risk of infectious arthritis, bronchiectasis, and certain cancers is also increased.

With early diagnosis and appropriate treatment, prognosis is good unless CNS viral infections develop.

Diagnosis

- Low immunoglobulin levels and absent B cells
- Genetic testing

Diagnosis of X-linked agammaglobulinemia is by detecting low (at least 2 standard deviations below the mean) levels of immunoglobulins (IgG, IgA, IgM) and absent B cells (< 1% of all lymphocytes are CD19+ cells, detected by flow cytometry). Transient neutropenia may also be present.

Genetic testing can be used to confirm a diagnosis but is not required. It is usually recommended for 1st-degree relatives. If the mutation has been identified in family members, mutational analysis of chorionic villus, amniocentesis, or percutaneous umbilical cord blood samples can provide prenatal diagnosis.

Treatment

- Immune globulin replacement therapy

Treatment is immune globulin replacement therapy.

Prompt use of adequate antibiotics for each infection is crucial; bronchiectasis may require frequent rotation of antibiotics. Live-virus vaccines are contraindicated.

X-LINKED LYMPHOPROLIFERATIVE SYNDROME

(Duncan Syndrome)

X-linked lymphoproliferative syndrome (XLP) results from a T-cell and NK-cell defect and is characterized by an abnormal response to Epstein-Barr virus infection, leading to liver failure, immunodeficiency, lymphoma, fatal lymphoproliferative disease, or bone marrow aplasia.

XLP is a primary immunodeficiency disorder that involves cellular immunity deficiencies. It is caused by mutations in genes on the X chromosome. It is a recessive disorder and thus manifests only in males.

XLP type 1 is the most common type (about 60% of cases). It is caused by a mutation in the gene that encodes the signaling lymphocyte activation molecule (SLAM)–associated protein (SAP, also called the SH2 domain protein 1A [SH2D1A] or DSHP). Without SAP, lymphocytes proliferate unchecked in response to Epstein-Barr virus (EBV) infection, and NK cells do not function.

XLP type 2 is clinically similar to type 1 and predisposes to hemophagocytic lymphohistiocytosis (HLH), an uncommon disorder that causes immunodeficiency in infants and young children. XLP2 is caused by mutations in a gene that encodes the X-linked inhibitor of apoptosis protein (XIAP).

Symptoms and Signs

The syndrome is usually asymptomatic until EBV infection develops. Then, most patients develop fulminating or fatal infectious mononucleosis with liver failure (caused by cytotoxic T cells that react to EBV-infected B or other tissue cells). Survivors of initial infection develop B-cell lymphomas, aplastic anemia, hypogammaglobulinemia (resembling that in common variable immunodeficiency), splenomegaly, or a combination.

Diagnosis

- Genetic testing

The diagnosis of XLP should be considered in young males who have severe EBV infection, HLH, a suggestive family history, or other common manifestations.

Genetic testing is the gold standard test for confirming the diagnosis (before and after EBV infection and symptoms develop) as well as the carrier state. However, genetic testing can take weeks to complete, so other testing is done if the diagnosis must be made earlier (eg, flow cytometry to assess SH2D1A protein expression).

Suggestive findings include

- Decreased antibody responses to antigens (particularly to EBV nuclear antigen)
- Impaired T-cell proliferative responses to mitogens
- Decreased NK-cell function
- An inverted CD4:CD8 ratio

These findings are typical before and after EBV infection. A bone marrow biopsy can help confirm HLH.

In survivors, laboratory and imaging tests are done yearly to check for lymphoma and anemia.

Genetic testing is done in relatives when a case or carrier is identified in a family. Prenatal screening is recommended for people if a mutation that causes XLP has been identified in their family.

Treatment

- Hematopoietic stem cell transplantation

About 75% of patients die by age 10, and all die by age 40 unless hematopoietic stem cell transplantation is done. About 80% of patients who receive a transplant survive. Transplantation is curative if done before EBV infection or other disorders become irreversible.

Rituximab can help prevent severe EBV infection before transplantation.

ZAP-70 DEFICIENCY

ZAP-70 (zeta-associated protein 70) deficiency is impaired T-cell activation caused by a signaling defect.

ZAP-70 deficiency is a primary immunodeficiency disorder that involves cellular immunity deficiencies. Inheritance is autosomal recessive.

ZAP-70 is important in T-cell signaling and in T-cell selection in the thymus. ZAP-70 deficiency causes T-cell activation defects.

Patients who have ZAP-70 deficiency present during infancy or early childhood with recurrent infections similar to those in SCID; however, they live longer, and the deficiency may not be diagnosed until they are several years old. Patients have normal, low, or elevated serum immunoglobulin levels and normal or elevated numbers of circulating CD4 T cells but essentially no CD8 T cells. Their CD4 T cells do not respond to mitogens or allogeneic cells in vitro and do not produce cytotoxic T cells. In contrast, NK cell activity is normal.

Diagnosis of ZAP-70 deficiency is similar to that for SCID.

The disorder is fatal unless treated by hematopoietic stem cell transplantation.

177 Transplantation

Transplants may be

- The patient's own tissue (autografts; eg, bone, bone marrow, and skin grafts)
- Genetically identical (syngeneic [between monozygotic twins]) donor tissue (isografts)
- Genetically dissimilar donor tissue (allografts, or homografts)
- Rarely, grafts from a different species (xenografts, or heterografts)

Transplanted tissue may be

- Cells (as for hematopoietic stem cell [HSC], lymphocyte, and pancreatic islet cell transplants)
- Parts or segments of an organ (as for hepatic or pulmonary lobar transplants and skin grafts)
- Entire organs (as for heart or kidney transplants)
- Tissues (eg, composite tissue grafts)

Tissues may be grafted to an anatomically normal site (orthotopic; eg, heart transplants) or abnormal site (heterotopic; eg, a kidney transplanted into the iliac fossa).

Almost always, transplantation is done to improve patient survival. However, some procedures (eg, hand, larynx, tongue, and facial transplantation) enhance the quality of life but do not improve survival and have significant risks related to surgery and immunosuppression. These procedures are in an early experimental phase (see p. 1422).

With rare exceptions, clinical transplantation uses allografts from living related, living unrelated, or deceased donors. Living donors are often used for kidney and HSC transplants and less frequently for segmental liver, pancreas, and lung transplants. Use of deceased-donor organs (from heart-beating or non–heart-beating donors) has helped reduce the disparity between organ demand and supply; however, demand still far exceeds supply, and the number of patients waiting for organ transplants continues to grow.

Graft rejection and graft-vs-host disease: All allograft recipients are at risk of graft rejection; the recipient's immune system recognizes the graft as foreign and seeks to destroy it. Recipients of grafts containing immune cells (particularly bone marrow, intestine, and liver) are at risk of graft-vs-host disease. Risk of these complications is minimized by pretransplantation screening and immunosuppressive therapy during and after transplantation.

Organ allocation: Allocation depends on disease severity for some organs (liver, heart) and on disease severity, time on the waiting list, or both for others (kidney, lung, bowel).

In the US and Puerto Rico, organs are allocated first among 12 geographic regions, then among local Organ Procurement Organizations. If no recipient in the first region is suitable, organs are reallocated to recipients in other regions.

Pretransplantation Screening

Before the risk and expense of transplantation are undertaken and scarce donor organs are committed, medical teams screen potential recipients for medical and nonmedical factors that may affect the likelihood of success.

Tissue compatibility: In pretransplantation screening, **recipients and donors** are tested for

- Human leukocyte antigens (HLAs; also called the major histocompatibility complex [MHC])
- ABO antigens

Recipients are tested for

- Presensitization to donor antigens

HLA tissue typing is most important for the following:

- Kidney transplantation
- The most common types of HSC transplantation

Transplantation of the following typically occurs urgently, often before HLA tissue typing can be completed, so the role of matching for these organs is less well-established.

- Heart
- Liver
- Pancreas
- Lung

HLA tissue typing of peripheral blood or lymph node lymphocytes is used to match the most important known determinants of histocompatibility in the donor and recipient. More than 1250 alleles determine 6 HLA antigens (HLA-A, -B, -C, -DP, -DQ, -DR), so matching is a challenge; eg, in the US, only 2 of 6 antigens on average are matched in kidney donors and recipients. Matching of as many HLA antigens as possible significantly improves functional survival of grafts from living related kidney and HSC donors; HLA matching of grafts from unrelated donors also improves survival, although much less so because of multiple undetected histocompatibility differences. Better immunosuppressive therapy has expanded eligibility for transplantation; HLA mismatches no longer automatically disqualify patients for transplantation because immunosuppressive therapy has become more effective.

ABO compatibility and HLA compatibility are important for graft survival. ABO mismatches can precipitate hyperacute rejection of vascularized grafts (eg, kidney, heart), which have ABO antigens on the endothelial surfaces. Presensitization to HLA and ABO antigens results from prior blood transfusions, transplantations, or pregnancies and can be detected with serologic tests or, more commonly, with a lymphocytotoxic test using the recipient's serum and donor's lymphocytes in the presence of complement. A positive cross-match indicates that the recipient's serum contains antibodies directed against ABO or class I HLA antigens in the donor; it is an absolute contraindication to transplantation, except possibly in infants (up to age 14 mo) who have not yet produced isohemagglutinins.

High-dose IV immune globulin and plasma exchange have been used to suppress HLA antibodies and facilitate transplantation when a more compatible graft is not available. Costs are high, but midterm outcomes are encouraging and appear similar to those in unsensitized patients.

Even a negative cross-match does not guarantee safety; when ABO antigens are compatible but not identical (eg, donor O and recipient A, B, or AB), hemolysis is a potential complication due to antibody production by transplanted (passenger) donor lymphocytes.

Although matching for HLA and ABO antigens generally improves graft survival, nonwhite patients are disadvantaged because

- Organ donation is less common among nonwhites and thus, the number of potential nonwhite donors is limited.
- End-stage renal disease is more common among blacks, and thus, the need for organs is greater.
- Nonwhite patients may have different HLA polymorphisms from white donors, a higher rate of presensitization to HLA antigens, and a higher incidence of blood types O and B.

Infection: Donor and recipient exposure to common infectious pathogens and active as well as latent infections must be detected before transplantation to minimize risk of transmitting infection from the donor and risk of worsening or reactivating existing infection in the recipient (due to use of immunosuppressants).

This screening usually includes the history and tests for cytomegalovirus (CMV), Epstein-Barr virus (EBV), herpes simplex virus (HSV), varicella-zoster virus (VZV), hepatitis B and C viruses, HIV, West Nile virus (if exposure is suspected), and *Mycobacterium tuberculosis* (for TB). Positive findings may require posttransplantation antiviral treatment (eg, for CMV infection or hepatitis B) or contraindicate transplantation until the infection is controlled (eg, if HIV with AIDS is detected).

Contraindications to transplantation: Absolute contraindications to transplantation include the following:

- Active infection, except possibly infection in the recipient if it is confined to the organ being replaced (eg, liver abscesses)
- Cancer (except hepatocellular carcinoma confined to the liver and certain neuroendocrine tumors in the recipient)
- A positive cross-match identified by lymphocytotoxic testing

Relative contraindications include the following:

- Age > 65
- Poor functional or nutritional status (including severe obesity)
- HIV infection
- Multiorgan insufficiency

Psychologic and social factors also play an important role in success of transplantation. For example, people who abuse drugs or who are psychologically unstable are less likely to firmly adhere to the necessary lifelong regimen of treatments and follow-up visits.

Eligibility decisions for patients with relative contraindications differ by medical center. Immunosuppressants are well-tolerated by and effective in HIV-positive transplant recipients.

Posttransplantation Immunosuppression

Immunosuppressants control graft rejection and are primarily responsible for the success of transplantation. However, they suppress all immune responses and contribute to many posttransplantation complications, including development of cancer, acceleration of cardiovascular disease, and even death due to overwhelming infection.

Immunosuppressants must usually be continued long after transplantation, but initially high doses can be reduced a few weeks after the procedure, and low doses can be continued indefinitely unless rejection occurs. Further reduction of immunosuppressant doses long after transplantation and protocols for inducing tolerance of donor organs are under study.

Corticosteroids: A high dose is usually given at the time of transplantation, then is reduced gradually to a maintenance dose, which is given indefinitely. Several months after transplantation, corticosteroids can be given on alternate days; this regimen helps prevent growth restriction in children. If rejection occurs, high doses are reinstituted.

Regimens that reduce the need for corticosteroids (steroid-sparing regimens) are being developed.

Calcineurin inhibitors (CNIs): These drugs (cyclosporine, tacrolimus) block T-cell transcription processes required for production of cytokines, thereby selectively inhibiting T-cell proliferation and activation.

Cyclosporine is the most commonly used drug in heart and lung transplantation. It can be given alone but is usually given with other drugs (eg, azathioprine, prednisone), so that lower, less toxic doses can be used. The initial dose is reduced to a maintenance dose soon after transplantation. The drug is metabolized by the cytochrome P-450 3A enzyme, and blood levels are affected by many other drugs.

The most serious dose-dependent adverse effect of cyclosporine is nephrotoxicity; cyclosporine causes vasoconstriction of afferent (preglomerular) arterioles, leading to glomerular apparatus damage, refractory glomerular hypoperfusion, and, eventually, chronic renal failure. Also, B-cell lymphomas and polyclonal B-cell lymphoproliferation occur more often in patients receiving high doses of cyclosporine or combinations of cyclosporine and other immunosuppressants directed at T cells, possibly because of an association with EBV. Other adverse effects include diabetes, hepatotoxicity, tophaceous gout, refractory hypertension, neurotoxicity (including tremor), increased incidence of other tumors, and less serious effects (eg, gum hypertrophy, hirsutism, hypertrichosis). Serum cyclosporine levels do not correlate with effectiveness or toxicity.

Tacrolimus is the most commonly used drug in kidney, liver, pancreas, and small-bowel transplantation. Tacrolimus may be started at the time of transplantation or days after the procedure. Dosing should be guided by blood levels, which are influenced by the same drug interactions as for cyclosporine. Tacrolimus may be useful when cyclosporine is ineffective or has intolerable adverse effects.

Adverse effects of tacrolimus are similar to those of cyclosporine except tacrolimus is more prone to induce diabetes; gum hypertrophy and hirsutism are less common. In patients taking tacrolimus, lymphoproliferative disorders seem to occur more often, even just weeks after transplantation, and may resolve partly or completely when the drug is stopped. If lymphoproliferative disorders occur, tacrolimus should be stopped, and cyclosporine or another immunosuppressive drug should be substituted.

Purine metabolism inhibitors: Examples are azathioprine and mycophenolate mofetil.

Azathioprine, an antimetabolite, is usually started at the time of transplantation. Most patients tolerate it indefinitely. The most serious adverse effects are bone marrow depression and, rarely, hepatitis. Systemic hypersensitivity reactions occur in > 5% of patients. Azathioprine is often used with low doses of calcineurin inhibitors.

Mycophenolate mofetil (MMF), a prodrug metabolized to mycophenolic acid, reversibly inhibits inosine monophosphate dehydrogenase, an enzyme in the guanine nucleotide pathway that is rate-limiting in lymphocyte proliferation. MMF is given with cyclosporine (or tacrolimus) and corticosteroids to patients with a kidney, heart, or liver transplant. The most common adverse effects are leukopenia, nausea, vomiting, and diarrhea.

Rapamycins: These drugs (sirolimus, everolimus) block a key regulatory kinase (mammalian target of rapamycin [mTOR]) in lymphocytes, resulting in arrest of the cell cycle and in inhibition of lymphocyte response to cytokine stimulation.

Sirolimus is typically given with cyclosporine and corticosteroids and may be useful for patients with renal insufficiency. Adverse effects include hyperlipidemia, interstitial pneumonitis, leg edema, impaired wound healing, and bone marrow depression with leukopenia, thrombocytopenia, and anemia.

Everolimus is used to prevent kidney and liver transplant rejection. Adverse effects are similar to those of sirolimus.

Immunosuppressive immunoglobulins: Examples are

- Antilymphocyte globulin (ALG)
- Antithymocyte globulin (ATG)

Both are fractions of animal antisera directed against human cells: lymphocytes (ALG) and thymus cells (ATG). ALG and ATG suppress cellular immunity while preserving humoral immunity. They are used with other immunosuppressants to allow those drugs to be used in lower, less toxic doses. Use of ALG or ATG to control acute episodes of rejection improves graft survival rates; use at the time of transplantation may decrease rejection incidence and allow CNIs to be started later, thereby reducing toxicity.

Use of highly purified serum fractions has greatly reduced incidence of adverse effects (eg, anaphylaxis, serum sickness, antigen-antibody–induced glomerulonephritis).

Monoclonal antibodies (mAbs): mAbs directed against T cells provide a higher concentration of anti-T-cell antibodies and fewer irrelevant serum proteins than do ALG and ATG.

OKT3 (a mouse antibody) inhibits T-cell receptor (TCR)–antigen binding, resulting in immunosuppression. OKT3 was used primarily to control episodes of acute rejection; it was also used at the time of transplantation to reduce incidence or delay onset of rejection episodes. However, the drug is no longer available.

Anti–IL-2 receptor monoclonal antibodies inhibit T-cell proliferation by blocking the effect of IL-2, secreted by activated T cells. Basiliximab, which is a humanized anti–IL-2 receptor antibody, is used to treat acute rejection of kidney, liver, and small-bowel transplants; it is also used as adjunct immunosuppressive therapy at the time of transplantation. The only adverse effect reported is anaphylaxis, but an increased risk of lymphoproliferative disorders cannot be excluded.

Irradiation: Irradiation of a graft, local recipient tissues, or both can be used to treat kidney transplant rejection when other treatment (eg, corticosteroids and ATG) has been ineffective. Total lymphatic irradiation is experimental but appears to safely suppress cellular immunity, at first by stimulation of suppressor T cells and later possibly by clonal deletion of specific antigen-reactive cells. However, because immunosuppressants are now so effective, the need for irradiation is extremely rare.

Future therapies: Protocols and agents to induce graft antigen-specific tolerance without suppressing other immune responses are being sought (see Table 177–1). Two strategies are promising:

- Blockade of T-cell costimulatory pathways using a cytotoxic T lymphocyte–associated antigen 4 (CTLA-4)-IgG1 fusion protein
- Induction of chimerism (coexistence of donor and recipient immune cells in which graft tissue is recognized as self) using nonmyeloablative pretransplantation treatment (eg, with cyclophosphamide, thymic irradiation, ATG, and cyclosporine) to induce transient T-cell depletion, engraftment of donor HSCs, and subsequent tolerance of solid organ transplants from the same donor (under study)

Table 177–1. IMMUNOSUPPRESSANTS USED TO TREAT TRANSPLANT REJECTION

IMMUNOSUPPRESSANT	MECHANISM OF ACTION	INDICATION	MAIN ADVERSE EFFECTS
Antilymphocyte globulin (ALG) Antithymocyte globulin (ATG)	Inhibition of lymphocytes (ALG) or thymus cells (ATG)	Induction, maintenance, and treatment of acute rejection	Anaphylaxis, serum sickness, antigen-antibody–induced glomerulonephritis
Azathioprine	Purine metabolism inhibitor	Maintenance	Myelosuppression, hepatitis
Basiliximab	Inhibition of T-cell proliferation by blocking the effect of IL-2	Mostly induction	Infection, anaphylaxis, myeloproliferative disorders
Belatacept	Antibody that inhibits T-cell costimulatory pathways	Maintenance	Progressive mutifocal leukoencephalopathy, other viral infections
Corticosteroids	Anti-inflammatory	Induction, maintenance, and adjunctive treatment of acute rejection	Diabetes, hypertension, osteoporosis, atherosclerosis
Cyclosporine	Calcineurin inhibition (blocking T-cell transcription)	Induction (rarely), maintenance, and treatment of acute and chronic rejection	Nephrotoxicity, neurotoxicity, hyperlipidemia, hirsutism, hypertrichosis, diabetes, hepatotoxicity, tophaceous gout, refractory hypertension, increased incidence of other tumors, gum hypertrophy
Everolimus Sirolimus	Inhibition of mTOR, inhibiting lymphocyte response to cytokine stimulation	Maintenance	Interstitial pneumonitis, leg edema, hyperlipidemia, impaired wound healing, bone marrow depression
Mycophenolate mofetil	Purine metabolism inhibitor	Maintenance	Myelosuppression, nausea, vomiting, diarrhea
Tacrolimus	Calcineurin inhibition (blocking T-cell transcription)	Induction, maintenance, and treatment of acute and chronic rejection	Nephrotoxicity, neurotoxicity, hyperlipidemia, alopecia, hypertension

mTOR = mammalian target of rapamycin.

Belatacept, another antibody that inhibits T-cell costimulatory pathways, can be used in kidney transplant recipients. However, incidence of progressive multifocal leukoencephalopathy, a deadly CNS disorder, appears to be increased, and incidence of viral infections is increased. Posttransplant lymphoproliferative disorder is another concern.

Posttransplantation Complications

Complications include the following:

- Rejection
- Infection
- Renal insufficiency
- Cancer
- Atherosclerosis

Rejection: Rejection of solid organs may be hyperacute, accelerated, acute, or chronic (late). These categories can be distinguished histopathologically and approximately by the time of onset. Symptoms vary by organ (see Table 177–2).

Hyperacute rejection has the following characteristics:

- Occurs within 48 h of transplantation
- Is caused by preexisting complement-fixing antibodies to graft antigens (presensitization)
- Is characterized by small-vessel thrombosis and graft infarction

It has become rare (1%) as pretransplantation screening has improved. No treatment is effective except graft removal.

Accelerated rejection has the following characteristics:

- Occurs 3 to 5 days after transplantation
- Is caused by preexisting non-complement-fixing antibodies to graft antigens
- Is characterized histopathologically by cellular infiltrate with or without vascular changes

Accelerated rejection is also rare. Treatment is with high-dose pulse corticosteroids or, if vascular changes occur, antilymphocyte preparations. Plasma exchange, which may clear circulating antibodies more rapidly, has been used with some success.

Acute rejection is graft destruction after transplantation and has the following characteristics:

- Occurs later, about 5 days after transplantation (because unlike hyperacute and accelerated rejection, acute rejection is mediated by a de novo anti-graft T-cell response, not by preexisting antibodies)
- Is caused by a T cell–mediated delayed hypersensitivity reaction to allograft histocompatibility antigens
- Is characterized by mononuclear cellular infiltration, with varying degrees of hemorrhage, edema, and necrosis but with vascular integrity usually maintained (although vascular endothelium appears to be a primary target)

Acute rejection accounts for about half of all rejection episodes that occur within 10 yr. Acute rejection is often reversed

Table 177–2. MANIFESTATIONS OF TRANSPLANT REJECTION BY CATEGORY

ORGAN	HYPERACUTE	ACCELERATED	ACUTE	CHRONIC
Kidney	Fever, anuria	Fever, oliguria, graft swelling and tenderness	Fever, increased serum creatinine, hypertension, weight gain, graft swelling, tenderness Appearance of protein, lymphocytes, and renal tubular cells in urine sediment	Proteinuria with or without hypertension, nephrotic syndrome
Liver	Fever, very elevated liver function test results (AST, bilirubin), coagulopathy	Fever, coagulopathy, very elevated liver function test results (AST, bilirubin), ascites	Anorexia, pain, fever, jaundice, light- (clay-) colored stools, dark urine, elevated liver function test results (AST, bilirubin)	Jaundice, vanishing bile duct syndrome (with elevated bilirubin, alkaline phosphatase, and GGT), slightly elevated liver function test results (AST, bilirubin), ascites
Heart*	Cardiogenic shock	Atrial arrhythmia, cardiogenic shock	Heart failure, atrial arrhythmia	Dyspnea during exertion, low stress tolerance
Lung	Poor oxygenation, fever, cough, dyspnea, decreased FEV_1	Poor oxygenation, fever, cough, dyspnea, infiltrate seen on chest x-ray, decreased FEV_1	Same as those for accelerated Interstitial perivascular infiltrate (detected by transbronchial biopsy)	Obliterative bronchiolitis, cough, dyspnea
Pancreas	Pancreatic necrosis, fever, hyperglycemia	Pancreatitis, hyperglycemia, elevated amylase and lipase	Same as those for accelerated	Hyperglycemia, mildly elevated amylase and lipase
Small bowel	Fever, very elevated lactic acid	Fever, diarrhea, elevated lactic acid	Fever, diarrhea, malabsorption, mildly elevated lactic acid	Diarrhea, malabsorption

*Most patients with heart transplant rejection are asymptomatic.
FEV_1 = forced expiratory volume in 1 sec; GGT = gamma-glutamyl transpeptidase.

by intensifying immunosuppressive therapy (eg, with pulse corticosteroids, ALG, or both). After rejection reversal, severely damaged parts of the graft heal by fibrosis, the remainder of the graft functions normally, immunosuppressant doses can be reduced to very low levels, and the allograft can survive for long periods.

Chronic rejection is graft dysfunction, often without fever. It has the following characteristics:

- Typically occurs months to years after transplantation but sometimes within weeks
- Has multiple causes, including early antibody-mediated rejection, periprocedural ischemia and reperfusion injury, drug toxicity, infection, and vascular factors (eg, hypertension, hyperlipidemia)
- Is characterized pathologically by proliferation of neointima consisting of smooth muscle cells and extracellular matrix (transplantation atherosclerosis), which gradually and eventually occludes vessel lumina, resulting in patchy ischemia and fibrosis of the graft

Chronic rejection accounts for most of the other half of all rejection episodes. Chronic rejection progresses insidiously despite immunosuppressive therapy; no established treatments exist. Tacrolimus has been reported to control chronic liver rejection in a few patients.

Infection: Transplant patients become vulnerable to infections because of

- Use of immunosuppressants
- Secondary immunodeficiencies that accompany organ failure
- Surgery

Rarely, a transplanted organ is the source of infection (eg, CMV).

The most common sign is fever, often without localizing signs. Fever can also be a symptom of acute rejection but is usually accompanied by signs of graft dysfunction. If these signs are absent, the approach is similar to that for other FUO; timing of symptoms and signs after transplantation helps narrow the differential diagnosis.

In the first month after transplantation, most infections are caused by the same hospital-acquired bacteria and fungi that infect other surgical patients (eg, *Pseudomonas* sp causing pneumonia, gram-positive bacteria causing wound infections). The greatest concern with early infection is that organisms can infect a graft or its vascular supply at suture sites, causing mycotic aneurysms or dehiscence.

Opportunistic infections occur 1 to 6 mo after transplantation (for treatment, see elsewhere in THE MANUAL). Infections may be bacterial (eg, listeriosis, nocardiosis), viral (eg, due to CMV, EBV, VZV, or hepatitis B or C virus), fungal (eg, aspergillosis, cryptococcosis, *Pneumocystis jirovecii* infection), or parasitic (eg, strongyloidiasis, toxoplasmosis, trypanosomiasis, leishmaniasis). Historically, many of these infections were associated with the use of high-dose corticosteroids.

Risk of infection returns to baseline in about 80% of patients after 6 mo. About 10% develop complications of early infections, such as viral infection of the graft, metastatic infection (eg, CMV retinitis, colitis), or virus-induced cancers (eg, hepatitis and subsequent hepatocellular carcinoma, human papillomavirus and subsequent basal cell carcinoma). Others develop chronic rejection, require high doses of immunosuppressants (5 to 10%), and remain at high risk of opportunistic infections indefinitely. Risk of infection varies depending on the graft received and is lowest for recipients of kidney allografts and highest for recipients of liver and lung transplants.

After transplantation, most patients are given antimicrobials to reduce risk of infection. Choice of drug depends on individual risk and type of transplantation; regimens include trimethoprim/sulfamethoxazole 80/400 mg po once/day for 4 to 12 mo to prevent *P. jirovecii* infection or to prevent UTIs in kidney transplant patients. Neutropenic patients are sometimes given quinolone antibiotics (eg, levofloxacin 500 mg po or IV once/day) to prevent infection with gram-negative organisms. Often, patients are treated prophylactically with ganciclovir or acyclovir because CMV and other viral infections occur more frequently in the first months after transplantation, when doses of immunosuppressants are highest. The doses given depend on patients' renal function.

Inactivated vaccines can be safely given posttransplantation. Risks due to live-attenuated vaccines must be balanced against their potential benefits because clinically evident infection and exacerbation of rejection are possible in immunosuppressed patients, even if blood levels of immunosuppressants are low.

Renal disorders: GFR decreases 30 to 50% during the first 6 mo after solid organ transplantation in 15 to 20% of patients. These patients usually also develop hypertension. Incidence is highest for recipients of small-bowel transplants (21%) because high blood levels of immunosuppressants (usually CNIs) are needed to maintain the graft. Incidence is lowest for recipients of heart-lung transplants (7%). Nephrotoxic and diabetogenic effects of CNIs are the most important contributor, but periprocedural renal damage, pretransplantation renal insufficiency, and use of other nephrotoxic drugs also contribute.

After the initial decrease, GFR typically stabilizes or decreases more slowly; nonetheless, mortality risk quadruples in patients progressing to end-stage renal disease requiring dialysis unless subsequent kidney transplantation is done. Renal insufficiency after transplantation may be prevented by early weaning from CNIs, but a safe minimum dose has not been determined.

Cancer: Long-term immunosuppression increases incidence of virus-induced cancer, especially squamous and basal cell carcinoma, lymphoproliferative disorders (mainly B-cell non-Hodgkin lymphoma), anogenital (including cervical) and oropharyngeal cancer, and Kaposi sarcoma.

Treatment is similar to that of cancer in nonimmunosuppressed patients; reduction or interruption of immunosuppression is not usually required for low-grade tumors but is recommended for more aggressive tumors and lymphomas. In particular, purine metabolism antagonists (azathioprine, mycophenolate mofetil) are stopped, and tacrolimus is stopped if a lymphoproliferative disorder develops.

Other complications: Osteoporosis can develop in patients who are at risk of osteoporosis before transplantation (eg, because of reduced physical activity, use of tobacco and/or alcohol, or a preexisting renal disorder) because immunosuppressants (especially corticosteroids and CNIs) increase bone resorption. Although not routine, use of vitamin D, bisphosphonates, or other antiresorptive drugs after transplantation may play a role in prevention.

Failure to grow, primarily as a consequence of chronic corticosteroid use, is a concern in children. Growth failure can be mitigated by tapering corticosteroids to the minimum dose that does not lead to graft rejection.

Atherosclerosis can result from hyperlipidemia due to use of CNIs, rapamycins (sirolimus, everolimus), or corticosteroids; it typically occurs in kidney transplant recipients > 15 yr posttransplantation.

Graft vs host disease (GVHD) occurs when donor T cells react against recipient's self-antigens. GVHD primarily affects hematopoietic stem cell recipients but may also affect liver and small-bowel transplant recipients. It can include inflammatory damage to tissues, especially the liver, intestine, and skin, as well as blood dyscrasia.

HEART TRANSPLANTATION

Heart transplantation is an option for patients who have any of the following and who remain at risk of death and have intolerable symptoms despite optimal use of drugs and medical devices:

- End-stage heart failure
- Coronary artery disease (CAD)
- Arrhythmias
- Hypertrophic cardiomyopathy
- Congenital heart disease

Transplantation may also be indicated for patients who

- Cannot be weaned from temporary cardiac-assist devices after MI or nontransplant cardiac surgery
- Have cardiac sequelae of a lung disorder requiring lung transplantation

The **only absolute contraindication** for heart transplantation is

- Pulmonary hypertension that does not respond to preoperative treatments

Relative contraindications include organ insufficiency (eg, pulmonary, renal, hepatic) and local or systemic infiltrative disorders (eg, cardiac sarcoma, amyloidosis).

All donated hearts come from brain-dead donors, who are usually required to be < 60 and have normal cardiac and pulmonary function and no history of CAD or other heart disorders. Donor and recipient must have compatible ABO blood type and heart size. About 25% of eligible recipients die before a donor organ becomes available. Left ventricular assist devices and artificial hearts provide interim hemodynamic support for patients waiting for a transplant. However, these devices carry a risk of sepsis, device failure, and thromboembolism.

Bridge and destination ventricular assist devices: In recent years, implantable ventricular assist devices have greatly improved, and these devices are being used to treat some patients who previously would have needed heart transplantation and patients for whom transplantation is contraindicated. These devices are usually used to assist the left ventricle as interim (bridge-to-transplantation) or long-term (destination) treatment. Infection, which may originate at the skin insertion site of the drivelines, is a concern. However, there are now patients who have survived alive and have been well for several years after these devices were implanted.

Procedure

Donor hearts are preserved by hypothermic storage. They must be transplanted within 4 to 6 h. The recipient is placed on a bypass pump, and the recipient heart is removed, preserving the posterior right atrial wall in situ. The donor heart is then transplanted orthotopically (in its normal position) with aortic, pulmonary artery, and pulmonary vein anastomoses; a single anastomosis joins the retained posterior atrial wall to that of the donor organ. Use of an in vitro pump system that modifies cell metabolism in the donor heart and thus may prolong transplant viability > 4 to 6 h is under study.

Immunosuppressive regimens vary but are similar to those for kidney or liver transplantation (eg, anti-IL-2 receptor monoclonal antibodies, a calcineurin inhibitor, corticosteroids—see Table 177–1).

Complications

Rejection: About 50 to 80% of patients have at least 1 episode of rejection (average 2 to 3); most patients are asymptomatic, but about 5% develop left ventricle dysfunction or atrial arrhythmias. Incidence of acute rejection peaks at 1 mo, decreases over the next 5 mo, and levels off by 1 yr.

Risk factors for rejection include

- Younger age
- Female recipient
- Female or black donor
- HLA mismatching
- Possibly cytomegalovirus (CMV) infection

Because graft damage can be irreversible and catastrophic, surveillance endomyocardial biopsy is usually done once/yr; degree and distribution of mononuclear cell infiltrate and presence of myocyte injury in specimens are determined. Differential diagnosis includes perioperative ischemia, CMV infection, and idiopathic B-cell infiltration (Quilty lesions).

Mild rejection (grade 1) without detectable clinical sequelae requires no treatment; moderate or severe rejection (grades 2 to 4) or mild rejection with clinical sequelae is treated with corticosteroid pulses (500 mg or 1 g daily for several days) and antithymocyte globulin as needed (see Table 177–3).

Cardiac allograft vasculopathy: The main complication of heart transplantation is cardiac allograft vasculopathy, a form of atherosclerosis that diffusely narrows or obliterates vessel lumina (in 25% of patients). Its cause is probably multifactorial and relates to donor age, cold and reperfusion ischemia, dyslipidemia, immunosuppressants, chronic rejection, and viral infection (adenovirus in children, CMV in adults).

For early detection, surveillance stress testing or coronary angiography with or without intravascular ultrasonography is often done at the time of endomyocardial biopsy.

Treatment is aggressive lipid lowering and diltiazem.

Prognosis

Survival rates at 1 yr after heart transplantation are 85 to 90%, and annual mortality thereafter is about 4%.

Pretransplantation predictors of 1-yr mortality include

- Need for preoperative ventilation or left ventricular assist devices
- Cachexia
- Female recipient or donor
- Diagnoses other than heart failure or CAD

Table 177–3. MANIFESTATIONS OF HEART TRANSPLANT REJECTION BY CATEGORY*

REJECTION CATEGORY	MANIFESTATIONS
Hyperacute	Cardiogenic shock
Accelerated	Atrial arrhythmia, cardiogenic shock
Acute	Heart failure, atrial arrhythmia
Chronic	Dyspnea during exertion, low stress tolerance

*Most patients with heart transplant rejection are asymptomatic.

Posttransplantation predictors include

- Elevated C-reactive protein and troponin levels

Most often, death within 1 yr results from acute rejection or infection; after 1 yr, death most often results from cardiac allograft vasculopathy or a lymphoproliferative disorder.

Functional status of heart transplant recipients alive at > 1 yr is excellent; exercise capacity remains below normal but is sufficient for daily activities and may increase over time with sympathetic reinnervation. More than 95% of patients reach New York Heart Association class I cardiac status, and > 70% return to full-time employment.

HEMATOPOIETIC STEM CELL TRANSPLANTATION

Hematopoietic stem cell (HSC) transplantation is a rapidly evolving technique that offers a potential cure for hematologic cancers (leukemias, lymphomas, myeloma) and other hematologic disorders (eg, primary immunodeficiency, aplastic anemia, myelodysplasia). HSC transplantation is also sometimes used for solid tumors (eg, some germ cell tumors) that respond to chemotherapy.

HSC transplantation contributes to a cure by

- Restoring bone marrow after myeloablative cancer-eradicating treatments
- Replacing abnormal bone marrow with normal bone marrow in nonmalignant hematologic disorders

HSC transplantation may be autologous or allogeneic. Stem cells may be harvested from

- Bone marrow
- Peripheral blood
- Umbilical cord blood

Peripheral blood has largely replaced bone marrow as a source of stem cells, especially in autologous HSC transplantation, because stem cell harvest is easier and neutrophil and platelet counts recover faster. Umbilical cord HSC transplantation has been restricted mainly to children because there are too few stem cells in umbilical cord blood for an adult. A potential future source of stem cells is induced pluripotent stem cells (certain cells taken from adults and reprogrammed to act like stem cells).

There are no contraindications to autologous HSC transplantation.

Contraindications to allogeneic HSC transplantation are relative and include age > 50, previous HSC transplantation, and significant comorbidities.

Allogeneic HSC transplantation is limited mainly by lack of histocompatible donors. An HLA-identical sibling donor is ideal, followed by an HLA-matched sibling donor. Because only one fourth of patients have such a sibling donor, mismatched related or matched unrelated donors (identified through international registries) are often used. However, long-term disease-free survival rates may be lower than those with HLA-identical sibling donors.

The technique for umbilical cord HSC transplantation is still being defined, but HLA-matching is probably unimportant.

Procedure

For **bone marrow stem cell harvest,** 700 to 1500 mL (maximum 15 mL/kg) of marrow is aspirated from the donor's posterior iliac crests; a local or general anesthetic is used.

For **peripheral blood harvest,** the donor is treated with recombinant growth factors (granulocyte colony-stimulating factor or granulocyte-macrophage colony-stimulating factor) to stimulate proliferation and mobilization of stem cells; standard apheresis is done 4 to 6 days afterward. Fluorescence-activated cell sorting is used to identify and separate stem cells from other cells.

Stem cells are then infused over 1 to 2 h through a large-bore central venous catheter.

Conditioning regimens: Before allogeneic HSC transplantation for cancer, the recipient first is given a conditioning regimen (eg, a myeloablative regimen such as cyclophosphamide 60 mg/kg IV once/day for 2 days with full-dose total body irradiation or busulfan 1 mg/kg po qid for 4 days plus cyclophosphamide without total body irradiation) to induce remission and suppress the immune system so that the graft can be accepted.

Similar conditioning regimens are used before allogeneic HSC transplantation, even when cancer is not the indication, to reduce incidence of rejection and relapse.

Such conditioning regimens are not used before autologous HSC transplantation for cancer; cancer-specific drugs are used instead.

Nonmyeloablative conditioning regimens (eg, with cyclophosphamide, thymic irradiation, antithymocyte globulin [ATG], and/or cyclosporine) may reduce morbidity and mortality risks and may be useful for elderly patients, patients with comorbidities, and patients susceptible to a graft-vs-tumor effect (eg, those with multiple myeloma).

Posttransplantation: After transplantation, recipients are given colony-stimulating factors to shorten duration of posttransplantation leukopenia, prophylactic anti-infective drugs, and, after allogeneic HSC transplantation, up to 6 mo of prophylactic immunosuppressants (typically methotrexate and cyclosporine) to prevent donor T cells from reacting against recipient HLA molecules (graft-vs-host disease [GVHD]). Broad-spectrum antibiotics are usually withheld unless fever develops.

Engraftment typically occurs 10 to 20 days after HSC transplantation (earlier with peripheral blood stem cells) and is defined by an absolute neutrophil count > 500 $\times 10^6$/L.

Complications

Complications of stem cell transplantation can occur early (< 100 days after transplantation) or later. After allogeneic HSC transplantation, risk of infections is increased.

Early complications: Major early complications include

- Failure to engraft
- Rejection
- Acute GVHD

Failure to engraft and **rejection** affect < 5% of patients and manifest as persistent pancytopenia or irreversible decline in blood counts. Treatment is corticosteroids for several weeks.

Acute GVHD occurs in recipients of allogeneic HSC transplants (in 40% of HLA-matched sibling graft recipients and 80% of unrelated donor graft recipients). It causes fever, rash, hepatitis with hyperbilirubinemia, vomiting, diarrhea, abdominal pain (which may progress to ileus), and weight loss.

Risk factors for acute GVHD include

- HLA and sex mismatching
- Unrelated donor
- Older age of recipient, donor, or both
- Donor presensitization
- Inadequate GVHD prophylaxis

Diagnosis of acute GVHD is obvious based on history, physical examination, and liver function test results. Treatment is methylprednisolone 2 mg/kg IV once/day, increased to 10 mg/kg if there is no response within 5 days.

Later complications: Major later complications include

- Chronic GVHD
- Disease relapse

Chronic GVHD may occur by itself, develop from acute GVHD, or occur after resolution of acute GVHD. It typically occurs 4 to 7 mo after HSC transplantation (range 2 mo to 2 yr). Chronic GVHD occurs in recipients of allogeneic HSC transplants (in about 35 to 50% of HLA-matched sibling graft recipients and 60 to 70% of unrelated donor graft recipients).

Chronic GVHD affects primarily the skin (eg, lichenoid rash, scleroderma) and mucous membranes (eg, keratoconjunctivitis sicca, periodontitis, orogenital lichenoid reactions), but it also affects the GI tract and liver. Immunodeficiency is a primary feature; bronchiolitis obliterans similar to that after lung transplantation can also develop. Ultimately, GVHD causes death in 20 to 40% of patients who have it.

Treatment may not be necessary for GVHD that affects the skin and mucous membrane; treatment of more extensive disease is similar to that of acute GVHD. T-cell depletion of allogeneic donor grafts using monoclonal antibodies or mechanical separation reduces incidence and severity of GVHD but also eliminates the graft-vs-tumor effect that may enhance stem cell proliferation and engraftment and reduce disease relapse rates. Relapse rates with autologous HSC transplantation are higher because there is no graft-vs-tumor effect and because circulating tumor cells may be transplanted. Ex vivo tumor cell purging before autologous transplantation is under study.

In patients without chronic GVHD, all immunosuppression can be stopped 6 mo after HSC transplantation; thus, late complications are rare in these patients.

Prognosis

Prognosis after HSC transplantation varies by indication and procedure.

Overall, disease relapse occurs in

- 40 to 75% of recipients of autologous HSC transplants
- 10 to 40% of recipients of allogeneic HSC transplants

Success (cancer-free bone marrow) rates are

- 30 to 40% for patients with relapsed, chemotherapy-sensitive lymphoma
- 20 to 50% for patients with acute leukemia in remission

Compared with chemotherapy alone, HSC transplantation improves survival of patients with multiple myeloma. Success rates are low for patients with more advanced disease or with responsive solid cancers (eg, germ cell tumors). Relapse rates are reduced in patients with GVHD, but overall mortality rates are increased if GVHD is severe.

Intensive conditioning regimens, effective GVHD prophylaxis, cyclosporine-based regimens, and improved supportive care (eg, antibiotics as needed, herpesvirus and cytomegalovirus prophylaxis) have increased long-term disease-free survival after HSC transplantation.

KIDNEY TRANSPLANTATION

Kidney transplantation is the most common type of solid organ transplantation.

The **primary indication** for kidney transplantation is

- End-stage renal failure

Absolute contraindications include

- Comorbidities that could compromise graft survival (eg, severe heart disorders, cancer), which can be detected via thorough screening

Relative contraindications include

- Poorly controlled diabetes, which can lead to renal failure
- Certain viral infections (eg, hepatitis C with end-stage liver disease), which could be worsened by the immunosuppression required by transplantation

Patients in their 70s and sometimes 80s may be candidates for transplants if they are otherwise healthy and functionally independent with good social support, if they have a reasonably long life expectancy, and if transplantation is likely to substantially improve function and quality of life beyond simply freeing them from dialysis. Patients with type 1 diabetes may be candidates for simultaneous pancreas-kidney or pancreas-after-kidney transplantation.

Kidney donors: More than one half of donated kidneys come from previously healthy, brain-dead people. About one third of these kidneys are marginal, with physiologic or procedure-related damage, but are used because demand is so great.

More kidneys from non-heart-beating donors (called donation-after-cardiac-death [DCD] grafts) are being used. These kidneys may have been damaged by ischemia before the donor's death, and their function is often impaired because of acute tubular necrosis; however, over the long term, they seem to function as well as kidneys from donors that meet standard criteria (called standard criteria donors [SCD]).

The remaining donated kidneys (about another 40%) come from living donors; because of limited supply, allografts from carefully selected living unrelated donors are being increasingly used. Living donors relinquish reserve renal capacity, may put themselves at risk of procedural and long-term morbidity, and may have psychologic conflicts about donation; therefore, they are evaluated for normal bilateral renal function, absence of systemic disease, histocompatibility, emotional stability, and ability to give informed consent. Hypertension, diabetes, and cancer (except possibly CNS tumors) in prospective living donors usually preclude kidney donation.

Use of kidneys from unrelated living donors has been increasing; kidney exchange programs often match a prospective donor and recipient who are incompatible with other similar incompatible pairs. When many such pairs are identified, chain exchanges are possible, greatly increasing the potential for a good match between recipient and donor.

If ABO matching is not feasible, sometimes ABO-incompatible transplantation can be done; with careful selection of donors and recipients and with pretransplant treatment (plasma exchange and/or IV immune globulins [IVIG]), outcomes can be comparable to those of ABO-compatible transplantation.

Procedure

The **donor kidney** is removed during a laparoscopic (or rarely, an open) procedure, perfused with cooling solutions containing relatively large concentrations of poorly permeating substances (eg, mannitol, hetastarch) and electrolyte concentrations approximating intracellular levels, then stored in an iced solution. Kidneys preserved this way usually function well if transplanted within 24 h. Although not commonly used, continuous pulsatile hypothermic perfusion with an oxygenated, plasma-based perfusate can extend ex vivo viability up to 48 h.

For **recipients,** dialysis may be required before transplantation to ensure a relatively normal metabolic state, but living-donor allografts appear to survive slightly better in recipients who have not begun long-term dialysis before transplantation.

Recipient nephrectomy is usually not required unless native kidneys are infected.

Whether transfusions are useful for anemic patients anticipating an allograft is unclear; transfusions can sensitize patients to alloantigens, but allografts may survive better in recipients who receive transfusions but do not become sensitized, possibly because transfusions induce some form of tolerance.

The transplanted kidney is usually placed in the iliac fossa. Renal vessels are anastomosed to the iliac vessels, and the donor ureter is implanted into the bladder or anastomosed to the recipient ureter. Vesicoureteral reflux occurs in about 30% of recipients, but usually without adverse effects.

Immunosuppressive regimens vary (see Table 177–1). Commonly, calcineurin inhibitors are begun immediately after transplantation in doses titrated to minimize toxicity and rejection while maintaining trough blood levels high enough to prevent rejection. On the day of transplantation, IV or oral corticosteroids are also given; dose is tapered over the following weeks depending on the protocol used.

Complications

Rejection: Despite use of immunosuppressants, about 20% of kidney transplant recipients have one or more rejection episodes within the first year after transplantation. Most episodes are easily treated with a corticosteroid bolus; however, they contribute to long-term insufficiency, graft failure, or both. Signs of rejection vary by type of rejection (see Table 177–4).

Rejection can be diagnosed by percutaneous needle biopsy if the diagnosis is unclear clinically. Biopsy may also help distinguish antibody-mediated from T cell–mediated rejection and identify other common causes of graft insufficiency or failure (eg, calcineurin inhibitor toxicity, diabetic or hypertensive nephropathy, polyomavirus type 1 infection). Advanced tests that may improve accuracy of rejection diagnosis include measurement of urinary mRNA-encoding mediators of rejection and gene expression profiling of biopsy samples using DNA microarrays.

Intensified immunosuppressive therapy (eg, with high-dose pulse corticosteroids or antilymphocyte globulin) usually reverses accelerated or acute rejection. If immunosuppressants are ineffective, dose is tapered and hemodialysis is resumed until a subsequent transplant is available.

Table 177–4. MANIFESTATIONS OF KIDNEY TRANSPLANT REJECTION BY CATEGORY

REJECTION CATEGORY	MANIFESTATIONS
Hyperacute	Fever, anuria
Accelerated	Fever, oliguria, graft swelling and tenderness
Acute	Fever, increased serum creatinine, hypertension, weight gain, graft swelling, tenderness Appearance of protein, lymphocytes, and renal tubular cells in urine sediment
Chronic	Proteinuria with or without hypertension, nephrotic syndrome

Nephrectomy of the transplanted kidney is necessary if hematuria, graft tenderness, or fever develops after immunosuppressants are stopped.

Chronic allograft nephropathy: Chronic allograft nephropathy refers to graft insufficiency or failure ≥ 3 mo after transplantation. Most cases are attributable to one or more of the above causes. Some experts believe the term should be reserved to describe graft insufficiency or failure when biopsy shows chronic interstitial fibrosis and tubular atrophy not attributable to any other cause.

Cancer: Compared with the general population, kidney transplant recipients are about 10 to 15 times more likely to develop cancer, probably because the modulated immune system's response to cancer as well as infections is weakened. Cancer of the lymphatic system (lymphoma) is 30 times more common among kidney transplant recipients than the general population, but lymphoma is still uncommon. Skin cancer becomes common among kidney transplant recipients after many years of immunosuppression.

Prognosis

Most rejection episodes and other complications occur within 3 to 4 mo after transplantation; most patients then return to more normal health and activity but must take maintenance doses of immunosuppressants indefinitely.

At 1 yr after kidney transplantation, survival rates are

- Living-donor grafts: 98% (patients) and 94% (grafts)
- Deceased-donor grafts: 95% (patients) and 88% (grafts)

Subsequent annual graft loss rates are 3 to 5% with a living-donor graft and 5 to 8% with a deceased-donor graft.

Among patients whose graft survives the first year, half die of other causes with the graft functioning normally; half develop chronic allograft nephropathy with the graft malfunctioning in 1 to 5 yr. Rates of late failure are higher for blacks than for whites.

Doppler ultrasonographic measurement of peak systolic and minimal end-diastolic flow in renal segmental arteries ≥ 3 mo after transplantation may help assess prognosis.

The **best clinical predictor** remains

- Serial determination of serum creatinine

In a specific patient, the most recently obtained creatinine levels should be compared with previous levels; a sudden increase in creatinine indicates the need to consider rejection or another problem (eg, vascular compromise, obstruction of the ureter). Ideally, serum creatinine should be normal in all post-transplant patients 4 to 6 wk after kidney transplantation.

LIVER TRANSPLANTATION

Liver transplantation is the second most common type of solid organ transplantation.

Indications for liver transplantation include

- Cirrhosis (70% of transplantations in the US; 60 to 70% of these cases are attributed to hepatitis C)
- Fulminant hepatic necrosis (about 8%)
- Hepatocellular carcinoma (about 7%)
- Biliary atresia and metabolic disorders, primarily in children (about 3% each)
- Other cholestatic (eg, primary sclerosing cholangitis) and non-cholestatic (eg, autoimmune hepatitis) disorders (about 8%)

For patients with hepatocellular carcinoma, transplantation is indicated for 1 tumor < 5 cm or up to 3 tumors < 3 cm (Milan criteria) and for some fibrolamellar types. For patients with liver metastases, transplantation is indicated only for neuroendocrine tumors without extrahepatic growth after removal of the primary tumor.

Absolute contraindications to liver transplantation are

- Elevated intracranial pressure (> 40 mm Hg) or low cerebral perfusion pressure (< 60 mm Hg) in patients with fulminant hepatic necrosis
- Severe pulmonary hypertension (mean pulmonary arterial pressure > 50 mm Hg)
- Sepsis
- Advanced or metastatic hepatocellular carcinoma

All of these conditions lead to poor outcomes during or after transplantation.

Liver donors: Nearly all donated livers come from size- and ABO-matched brain-dead (deceased), heart-beating donors. Prospective tissue typing and HLA matching are not always required. ABO-incompatible liver transplants have been transplanted successfully in children < 2 yr; in older children and adults, these transplants are not used because there is a high risk of rejection and bile duct damage (ductopenia) with cholestasis, which requires retransplantation.

Annually, about 250 transplants come from living donors, who can live without their right lobe (in adult-to-adult transplantation) or the lateral segment of their left lobe (in adult-to-child transplantation). Advantages of living donation for the recipient include shorter waiting times and shorter cold ischemic times for explanted organs, largely because transplantation can be scheduled to optimize the patient's condition. Disadvantages to the donor include mortality risk of 1/600 to 700 (compared with 1/3300 in living-donor kidney transplantation) and complications (especially bile leakage) in up to one fourth. Clinicians must make every effort to prevent psychologic coercion of donors.

A few livers come from deceased, non-heart-beating donors (called donation-after-cardiac-death [DCD] donors), but in such cases, bile duct complications develop in up to one-third of recipients because the liver had been damaged by ischemia before donation.

Donor (deceased or living) risk factors for graft failure in the recipient include

- Age > 50
- Hepatic steatosis
- Elevated liver enzymes, bilirubin, or both
- Prolonged stay in ICU
- Hypotension requiring vasopressors
- Hypernatremia
- Possibly transplantation from female donors to male recipients

But because imbalance between supply and demand is greatest for liver transplants (and is growing because prevalence of hepatitis-induced cirrhosis is increasing), livers from donors > 50, livers with longer cold ischemia times, those with fatty infiltration, and those with viral hepatitis (for transplantation into recipients with viral hepatitis-induced cirrhosis) are increasingly being used.

Additional techniques to increase supply include

- **Split liver transplantation:** Deceased-donor livers are divided into right and left lobes or right lobe and left lateral segment (done in or ex situ) and given to 2 recipients
- **Domino transplantation:** Occasionally, a deceased-donor liver is given to a recipient with an infiltrative disease (eg, amyloidosis), and the explanted diseased liver is given to an

elderly recipient who can benefit from the diseased liver but is not expected to live long enough to experience adverse effects of transplant dysfunction.

Despite these innovations, many patients die waiting for transplants. Liver-assist devices (extracorporeal perfusion of cultured hepatocyte suspensions or immortalized hepatoma cell lines) are used in some centers to keep patients alive until a liver is available or acute dysfunction resolves.

Organ distribution: For distribution of available organs, patients on the national waitlist are given a prognostic score derived from creatinine, bilirubin, and INR measurements (using the Model for End-Stage Liver Disease [MELD] for adults) or from age and serum albumin, bilirubin, INR, and growth failure measurements (using the model for Pediatric End-Stage Liver Disease [PELD] for children). MELD and PELD are formulas that are used to calculate the probability of a patient dying of liver disease while waiting for a liver transplantation. Patients more likely to die are given higher priority for organs from matched donors. For patients with hepatocellular carcinoma, a score is assigned to reflect mortality risk based on tumor size and wait time.

Procedure

Deceased-donor livers are removed after exploratory laparotomy confirms absence of intra-abdominal disease that would preclude transplantation. Living donors undergo lobar or segmental resection.

Explanted livers are perfused and stored in a cold preservation solution for up to 18 h before transplantation; incidence of graft nonfunction and ischemic-type biliary injury increases with prolonged storage.

Recipient hepatectomy is the most demanding part of the procedure because it is often done in patients with portal hypertension and coagulation defects. Intraoperative blood loss can total > 100 units in rare cases, but use of a cell saver machine and autotransfusion devices reduces allogeneic transfusion requirements to an average of 5 to 10 units. After hepatectomy, the suprahepatic vena cava of the donor graft is anastomosed to the recipient's vena cava in an end-to-side fashion (piggy-back technique). Donor and recipient portal veins, hepatic arteries, and bile ducts are then anastomosed. With this technique, a bypass pump is not needed to carry portal venous blood to the systemic venous circuit. Heterotopic placement of the liver (not in its normal location) provides an auxiliary liver and obviates several technical difficulties, but outcomes have been discouraging, and this technique is still experimental.

Immunosuppressive regimens vary (see Table 177–1). Commonly, anti-IL-2 receptor monoclonal antibodies are given on the day of transplantation, with a calcineurin inhibitor (cyclosporine or tacrolimus), mycophenolate mofetil, and corticosteroids. Except in patients with autoimmune hepatitis, corticosteroids can be tapered within weeks and often stopped after 3 to 4 mo. Compared with other solid organ transplantation, liver transplantation requires the lowest doses of immunosuppressants.

Complications

Rejection: Liver allografts are less aggressively rejected than other organ allografts for unknown reasons; hyperacute rejection occurs less frequently than expected in patients presensitized to HLA or ABO antigens, and immunosuppressants can often be tapered relatively quickly and eventually stopped. Most episodes of acute rejection are mild and self-limited, occur in the first 3 to 6 mo, and do not affect graft survival.

Risk factors for rejection include

- Younger recipient age
- Older donor age
- Greater HLA mismatching
- Longer cold ischemia times
- Autoimmune disorders

Worse nutritional status (eg, in alcoholism) appears protective.

Symptoms and signs of rejection depend on the type of rejection (see Table 177–5). Symptoms of acute rejection occur in about 50% of patients; symptoms of chronic rejection occur in < 2%.

Differential diagnosis of acute rejection includes viral hepatitis (eg, cytomegalovirus or Epstein-Barr virus infection; recurrent hepatitis B, C, or both), calcineurin inhibitor toxicity, and cholestasis. Rejection can be diagnosed by percutaneous needle biopsy if the diagnosis is unclear clinically.

Suspected rejection is treated with IV corticosteroids; antithymocyte globulin is an option when corticosteroids are ineffective (in 10 to 20%). Retransplantation is tried when rejection is refractory to immunosuppressants.

Hepatitis recurrence after transplantation: Immunosuppression contributes to recurrence of viral hepatitis in patients who had viral hepatitis-induced cirrhosis before transplantation. Hepatitis C recurs in nearly all patients; usually, viremia and infection are clinically silent but may cause active hepatitis and cirrhosis.

Risk factors for clinically significant reinfection may be related to the

- Recipient: Eg, older age, HLA type, and hepatocellular carcinoma
- Donor: Eg, older age, fatty infiltration, prolonged ischemic time, and living donor
- Virus: High viral load, genotype 1B, failure to respond to interferon
- Postprocedural events: Immunosuppressant doses, acute rejection treated with corticosteroids and cytomegalovirus infection

Standard treatment of hepatitis C is only marginally effective, although there is hope that newer antiviral drugs (eg, telaprevir)

Table 177–5. MANIFESTATIONS OF LIVER TRANSPLANT REJECTION BY CATEGORY

REJECTION CATEGORY	MANIFESTATIONS
Hyperacute	Fever, very elevated liver function test results (AST, bilirubin), coagulopathy
Accelerated	Fever, coagulopathy, very elevated liver function test results (AST, bilirubin), ascites
Acute	Anorexia, pain, fever, jaundice, light- (clay-) stools, dark urine, elevated liver function test results (AST, bilirubin)
Chronic	Jaundice, vanishing bile duct syndrome (with elevated bilirubin, alkaline phosphatase, and GGT), slightly elevated liver function test results (AST, bilirubin), ascites

GGT = gamma-glutamyl transpeptidase.

will improve outcomes of patients with recurrent hepatitis C. Hepatitis B recurs in all but has been successfully managed with antiviral drugs; coinfection with hepatitis D appears protective against recurrence.

Other complications: **Early complications** (within 2 mo) of liver transplantation include

- Primary nonfunction in 1 to 5%
- Biliary dysfunction (eg, ischemic anastomotic strictures, bile leakage, ductal obstructions, leakage around T-tube site) in 15 to 20%
- Portal vein thrombosis in < 5%
- Hepatic artery thrombosis in 3 to 5% (especially in small children or recipients of split grafts)
- Hepatic artery mycotic aneurysm or pseudoaneurysm and hepatic artery rupture

Typically, symptoms and signs of early complications include fever, hypotension, and abnormal liver function test results.

The **most common late complications** are

- Intrahepatic or anastomotic bile duct strictures, which cause symptoms of cholestasis and cholangitis

After liver transplantation with DCD grafts, strictures are particularly common, occurring in about one fourth to one third of recipients. Strictures can sometimes be treated endoscopically or using percutaneous transhepatic cholangiographic dilation, stenting, or both, but they often ultimately require retransplantation.

Prognosis

At 1 yr after liver transplantation, survival rates are

- Living-donor grafts: 90% (patients) and 82% (grafts)
- Deceased-donor grafts: 86% (patients) and 82% (grafts)

Overall survival rates are

- At 3 yr: 79% (patients) and 72% (grafts)
- At 5 yr: 73% (patients) and 65% (grafts)

Survival is better for chronic than for acute liver failure. Death after 1 yr is usually attributable to a recurrent disorder (eg, cancer, hepatitis) rather than to posttransplantation complications.

Recurrent hepatitis C leads to cirrhosis in 15 to 30% of patients by 5 yr. Hepatic disorders with an autoimmune component (eg, primary biliary cirrhosis, primary sclerosing cholangitis, autoimmune hepatitis) recur in 20 to 30% by 5 yr.

LUNG AND HEART-LUNG TRANSPLANTATION

Lung or heart-lung transplantation is an option for patients who have respiratory insufficiency or failure and who remain at risk of death despite optimal medical treatment.

The **most common indications for lung transplantation** are

- COPD
- Idiopathic pulmonary fibrosis
- Cystic fibrosis
- Alpha-1 antitrypsin deficiency
- Primary pulmonary hypertension

Less common indications include interstitial lung disorders (eg, sarcoidosis), bronchiectasis, and congenital heart disease.

Single and double lung procedures are equally appropriate for most lung disorders without cardiac involvement; the exception is chronic diffuse infection (eg, bronchiectasis), for which double lung transplantation is best.

Indications for heart-lung transplantation are

- Eisenmenger syndrome
- Any lung disorder with severe ventricular dysfunction likely to be irreversible

Cor pulmonale often reverses after lung transplantation alone and is therefore rarely an indication for heart-lung transplantation; however, sometimes a heart-lung transplantation is necessary.

Relative contraindications include age (single lung recipients must be < 65; double lung recipients, < 60; and heart-lung recipients, < 55), current cigarette smoking, previous thoracic surgery, and, for some cystic fibrosis patients and at some medical centers, lung infection with resistant strains of *Burkholderia cepacia*, which greatly increases mortality risk.

Single and double lung procedures are about equally common and are at least 8 times more common than heart-lung transplantation.

Lung donors: Nearly all donated lungs are from brain-dead (deceased), heart-beating donors.

Grafts from non–heart-beating donors, called donation-after-cardiac-death (DCD) donors, are being increasingly used because lungs from more suitable donors are lacking.

Rarely, living adult (usually parent-to-child) lobar transplantation is done when deceased-donor organs are unavailable.

Donors must be < 65 and never-smokers and have no active lung disorder as evidenced by

- **Oxygenation:** Pao_2/Fio_2 (fractional inspired O_2) > 250 to 300, with Pao_2 in mm Hg and Fio_2 in decimal fraction (eg, 0.5)
- **Lung compliance:** Peak inspiratory pressure < 30 cm H_2O at tidal volume (V_T) 15 mL/kg and positive end-expiratory pressure = 5 cm H_2O
- **Gross appearance:** Using bronchoscopy

Donor and recipients must be size-matched anatomically (by chest x-ray), physiologically (by total lung capacity), or both.

Timing of transplantation referral: Timing of referral for transplantation should be determined by factors such as

- Degree of obstructive defect: Forced expiratory volume in 1 sec (FEV_1) < 25 to 30% predicted in patients with COPD, alpha-1 antitrypsin deficiency, or cystic fibrosis
- $Paco_2$ < 55 mm Hg
- $Paco_2$ > 50 mm Hg
- Right atrial pressure > 10 mm Hg and peak systolic pressure > 50 mm Hg for patients with primary pulmonary hypertension
- Progression rate of clinical, radiographic, or physiologic disease

Procedure

The donor is anticoagulated, and a cold crystalloid preservation solution containing prostaglandins is flushed through the pulmonary arteries into the lungs. Donor organs are cooled with iced saline slush in situ or via cardiopulmonary bypass, then removed. Prophylactic antibiotics are often given.

Single lung transplantation: Single lung transplantation requires posterolateral thoracotomy. The native lung is removed, and the bronchus, pulmonary artery, and pulmonary veins of the donor lung are anastomosed to their respective cuffs. The bronchial anastomosis requires intussusception or wrapping with omentum or pericardium to facilitate adequate healing.

Advantages of single lung transplantation include a simpler operation, avoidance of cardiopulmonary bypass and systemic anticoagulation (usually), more flexibility concerning size matching, and availability of the contralateral lung from the same donor for another recipient.

Disadvantages include the possibility of ventilation/perfusion mismatch between the native and transplant lungs and the possibility of poor healing of the single bronchial anastomosis.

Double lung transplantation: Double lung transplantation requires sternotomy or anterior transverse thoracotomy; the procedure is similar to 2 sequential single transplants.

The **primary advantage** is definitive removal of all diseased lung tissue in the recipient.

The **disadvantage** is poor healing of the tracheal anastomosis.

Heart-lung transplantation: Heart-lung transplantation requires median sternotomy with cardiopulmonary bypass. Aortic, right atrial, and tracheal anastomoses are required; the trachea is anastomosed immediately above the bifurcation.

The **primary advantages** are improved graft function and more dependable healing of the tracheal anastomosis because of coronary-bronchial collaterals within the heart-lung block.

Disadvantages include long operative time with the need for cardiopulmonary bypass, the need for close size matching, and use of 3 donor organs by one recipient.

Immunosuppression: A common 3-drug immunosuppressive regimen combines

- A calcineurin inhibitor (cyclosporine or tacrolimus)
- A purine metabolism inhibitor (azathioprine or mycophenolate mofetil)
- Methylprednisolone or another corticosteroid

First, patients are given high doses perioperatively; methylprednisolone IV is often given intraoperatively before reperfusion of the transplanted lung. Lower doses are given for maintenance thereafter (see Table 177–1).

Antithymocyte globulin (ATG) or alemtuzumab is often given as induction therapy. These drugs can also minimize immunosuppressive therapy posttransplantation. Often, tacrolimus monotherapy is sufficient if induction therapy is given.

Corticosteroids may be omitted to facilitate healing of the bronchial anastomosis; higher doses of other drugs (eg, cyclosporine, azathioprine) are then used instead. Immunosuppressants are continued indefinitely.

Complications

Rejection: Rejection develops in most patients despite immunosuppressive therapy. Symptoms and signs are similar in hyperacute, acute, and chronic forms and include fever, dyspnea, cough, decreased SaO_2 (arterial O_2 saturation), and a decrease in FEV_1 by > 10 to 15% (see Table 177–6).

Hyperacute rejection must be distinguished from early graft dysfunction caused by ischemic injury during the transplantation procedure, and acute rejection must be differentiated from infection. Interstitial infiltrate, seen on chest x-rays, is typical in patients with accelerated or acute rejection. Rejection is usually diagnosed by bronchoscopy, including bronchoscopic transbronchial biopsy. If rejection has occurred, biopsy shows perivascular lymphocytic infiltration in small vessels; polymorphonuclear leukocytes in alveolar infiltrates and infectious pathogens suggest infection. IV corticosteroids are usually effective for hyperacute, accelerated, or acute rejection. Treatment of recurrent or resistant cases varies and includes higher corticosteroid doses, aerosolized cyclosporine, and ATG.

Table 177–6. MANIFESTATIONS OF LUNG TRANSPLANT REJECTION BY CATEGORY

REJECTION CATEGORY	MANIFESTATIONS
Hyperacute	Poor oxygenation, fever, cough, dyspnea, decreased FEV_1
Accelerated	Poor oxygenation, fever, cough, dyspnea, infiltrate seen on chest x-ray, decreased FEV_1
Acute	Same as those for accelerated Interstitial perivascular infiltrate (detected by transbronchial biopsy)
Chronic	Obliterative bronchiolitis, cough, dyspnea

FEV_1 = forced expiratory volume in 1 sec.

Chronic rejection develops after > 1 yr in up to 50% of patients; it manifests as obliterative bronchiolitis or, less commonly, as atherosclerosis. Acute rejection may increase risk of chronic rejection. Patients with obliterative bronchiolitis present with cough, dyspnea, and decreased $FEF_{25-75\%}$ or FEV_1, with or without physical and radiographic evidence of an airway process. Differential diagnosis includes pneumonia. Diagnosis is usually by bronchoscopy with biopsy. No treatment has proved effective, but options include corticosteroids, ATG, inhaled cyclosporine, and retransplantation.

Surgical complications: The most common surgical complications are

- Poor healing of the bronchial or tracheal anastomosis (diagnosed when mediastinal air or pneumothorax is detected)
- Infection

Up to 20% of single-lung recipients develop bronchial stenosis that causes wheezing and airway obstruction; it can be treated with dilation or stent placement.

Other surgical complications include hoarseness and diaphragmatic paralysis, caused by damage to the recurrent laryngeal or phrenic nerves; GI dysmotility, caused by damage to the thoracic vagus nerve; and pneumothorax. Supraventricular arrhythmias develop in some patients, probably because of conduction changes caused by pulmonary vein-atrial suturing.

Prognosis

Patient survival rates are

- At 1 yr: 84% with living-donor grafts and 83% with deceased-donor grafts
- At 5 yr: 34% with living-donor grafts and 46% with deceased-donor grafts

Mortality rate is higher for patients with primary pulmonary hypertension, idiopathic pulmonary fibrosis, or sarcoidosis and lower for those with COPD or alpha-1 antitrypsin deficiency. Mortality rate is higher for single lung transplantation than for double.

Most common causes of death are

- Within 1 mo: Primary graft failure, ischemia and reperfusion injury, and infection (eg, pneumonia) excluding cytomegalovirus
- Between 1 mo and 1 yr: Infection
- After 1 yr: Obliterative bronchiolitis

Mortality risk factors include cytomegalovirus mismatching (donor positive, recipient negative), human leukocyte antigen (HLA-DR) mismatching, diabetes, and prior need for mechanical ventilation or inotropic support.

Uncommonly, the original disorder, particularly some interstitial lung disorders, recurs. Exercise capacity is slightly limited because of a hyperventilatory response.

With **heart-lung transplantation,** overall survival rate at 1 yr is 60% for patients and grafts.

PANCREAS TRANSPLANTATION

Pancreas transplantation is a form of pancreatic beta-cell replacement that can restore normoglycemia in diabetic patients.

Because the recipient exchanges risks of insulin injection for risks of immunosuppression, eligibility is limited mostly to

- Patients who have type 1 diabetes with renal failure and who are thus candidates for kidney transplantation

More than 90% of pancreas transplantations include transplantation of a kidney.

At many centers, repeated failure to control glycemia with standard treatment and episodes of hypoglycemic unawareness are also eligibility criteria.

Relative contraindications include age > 55 and significant atherosclerotic cardiovascular disease, defined as a previous MI, coronary artery bypass graft surgery, percutaneous coronary intervention, or a positive stress test; these factors dramatically increase perioperative risk.

Options include

- Simultaneous pancreas-kidney (SPK) transplantation
- Pancreas-after-kidney (PAK) transplantation
- Pancreas-alone transplantation

The **advantages of simultaneous pancreas-kidney transplantation** are one-time exposure to induction immunosuppression, potential protection of the newly transplanted kidney from adverse effects of hyperglycemia, and the ability to monitor rejection in the kidney; the kidney is more prone to rejection than the pancreas, where rejection is difficult to detect.

The **advantage of pancreas-after-kidney transplantation** is the ability to optimize HLA matching and timing of kidney transplantation using a living donor.

Pancreas-alone transplantation offers an advantage to patients who do not have end-stage renal disease but have other severe diabetic complications, including labile glucose control.

Pancreas donors: Donors are usually recently deceased patients who are aged 10 to 55 and have no history of glucose intolerance or alcohol abuse.

For simultaneous pancreas-kidney transplantation, the pancreas and kidney come from the same donor, and the same restrictions for kidney donation apply.

A few (< 1%) segmental transplantations from living donors have been done, but this procedure has substantial risks for the donor (eg, splenic infarction, abscess, pancreatitis, pancreatic leak and pseudocyst, secondary diabetes), which limit its widespread use.

Procedure

The donor is anticoagulated, and a cold preservation solution is flushed into the celiac artery. The pancreas is cooled in situ with iced saline slush, then removed en bloc with the liver (for transplantation into a different recipient) and the 2nd portion of the duodenum containing the ampulla of Vater. The iliac artery is also removed.

The donor pancreas is positioned intraperitoneally and laterally in the lower abdomen.

In simultaneous pancreas-kidney transplantation, the pancreas is placed into the right lower quadrant of the recipient's abdomen and the kidney into the left lower quadrant. The native pancreas is left in place. The donor iliac artery is used for reconstruction on the back table to reconstruct the splenic artery and superior mesenteric artery of the pancreas graft. This technique results in one artery for connection to the recipient blood vessels. The final anastomoses are made between the donor iliac artery and one of the recipient's iliac arteries and between the donor portal vein and recipient iliac vein. Thus, endocrine secretions drain systemically, causing hyperinsulinemia; sometimes the donor pancreatic venous system is anastomosed to a portal vein tributary to re-create physiologic conditions, although this procedure is more demanding and its benefits are unclear. The duodenum is sewn to the bladder dome or to the jejunum for drainage of exocrine secretions.

Immunosuppression regimens vary but typically include immunosuppressive Igs, a calcineurin inhibitor, a purine synthesis inhibitor, and corticosteroids, which can be slowly tapered over 12 mo (see Table 177–1 on p. 1410).

Complications

Rejection: Despite adequate immunosuppression, acute rejection develops in 40 to 60% of patients, primarily affecting exocrine, not endocrine, components.

Compared with kidney transplantation alone, simultaneous pancreas-kidney transplantation has a greater risk of rejection, and rejection episodes tend to occur later, to recur more often, and to be corticosteroid-resistant. Symptoms and signs are nonspecific (see Table 177–7 on p. 1410).

After simultaneous pancreas-kidney transplantation and pancreas-after-kidney transplantation, pancreas rejection is best detected by an increase in serum creatinine because pancreas rejection almost always accompanies kidney rejection. After pancreas-alone transplantation, a stable urinary amylase concentration in patients with urinary drainage excludes rejection; a decrease suggests some form of graft dysfunction but is not specific to rejection. Early detection is therefore difficult.

Diagnosis is confirmed by ultrasound-guided percutaneous or cystoscopic transduodenal biopsy.

Treatment is with antithymocyte globulin.

Other complications: Early complications affect 10 to 15% of patients and include wound infection and dehiscence, gross hematuria, intra-abdominal urinary leak, reflux pancreatitis, recurrent UTI, small-bowel obstruction, abdominal abscess, and graft thrombosis.

Late complications relate to urinary loss of pancreatic sodium bicarbonate ($NaHCO_3^-$), causing volume depletion and

Table 177–7. MANIFESTATIONS OF PANCREAS TRANSPLANT REJECTION BY CATEGORY

REJECTION CATEGORY	MANIFESTATIONS
Hyperacute	Pancreatic necrosis, fever, hyperglycemia
Accelerated	Pancreatitis, hyperglycemia, elevated amylase and lipase
Acute	Same as those for accelerated
Chronic	Hyperglycemia, mildly elevated amylase and lipase

non-anion gap metabolic acidosis. Hyperinsulinemia does not appear to adversely affect glucose or lipid metabolism.

Prognosis

Overall, 1-yr survival rates are

- Patients: > 90%
- Grafts: 78%

Whether survival is higher than that of patients without transplantation is unclear; however, the primary benefits of the procedure are freedom from insulin therapy and stabilization or some amelioration of many diabetic complications (eg, nephropathy, neuropathy).

Graft survival is

- Simultaneous pancreas-kidney transplantation: 95%
- Pancreas-after-kidney transplantation: 74%
- Pancreas-alone transplantation: 76%

The rate of immunologic graft loss for pancreas-after-kidney transplantation and pancreas-alone transplants is higher, possibly because such a transplanted pancreas lacks a reliable monitor of rejection; in contrast, rejection after simultaneous pancreas-kidney transplantation can be monitored using established indicators of rejection for the transplanted kidney.

PANCREATIC ISLET CELL TRANSPLANTATION

Islet cell transplantation (into the recipient's liver) has theoretical advantages over pancreas transplantation; the most important is that the procedure is less invasive. A secondary advantage is that islet cell transplantation appears to help maintain normoglycemia in patients who require total pancreatectomy for pain due to chronic pancreatitis. Nevertheless, the procedure remains developmental, although steady improvements appear to be occurring.

Its disadvantages are that transplanted glucagon-secreting alpha cells are nonfunctional (possibly complicating hypoglycemia) and several pancreata are usually required for a single islet cell recipient (exacerbating disparities between graft supply and demand and limiting use of the procedure).

Indications are the same as those for pancreas transplantation. Simultaneous islet cell–kidney transplantation may be desirable after the technique is improved.

Procedure

A pancreas is removed from a brain-dead donor; collagenase is infused into the pancreatic duct to separate islets from pancreatic tissue. A purified islet cell fraction is infused percutaneously into the portal vein by direct puncture of that vein or via a branch of the mesenteric vein. Islet cells travel into hepatic sinusoids, where they lodge and secrete insulin.

Results are best when 2 cadavers are used, with each supplying 2 or 3 infusions of islet cells, followed by an immunosuppressive regimen consisting of an anti-IL-2 receptor antibody (basiliximab), tacrolimus, and sirolimus (Edmonton protocol); corticosteroids are used sparingly because they cause hyperglycemia. Immunosuppression must be continued lifelong or until islet cell function ceases.

Complications

Rejection is poorly defined but can be detected by deterioration in blood glucose control and an increase in glycosylated hemoglobin (HbA_{1c}); treatment of rejection is not established.

Procedural complications include percutaneous hepatic puncture with bleeding, portal vein thrombosis, and portal hypertension.

Prognosis

Successful islet cell transplantation maintains short-term normoglycemia, but long-term outcomes are unknown; additional injections of islet preparations may be necessary to obtain longer-lasting insulin independence.

SMALL-BOWEL TRANSPLANTATION

Small-bowel transplantation is done infrequently (eg, about 106 transplants in the US in 2012). It is being done less frequently because there are new treatments for secondary cholestatic liver disease (eg, Omegaven®, a nutritional supplement rich in omega fatty acids) and safer TPN line placement techniques.

Small-bowel transplantation is indicated for patients who

- Are at risk of death because of intestinal failure secondary to intestinal disorders (eg, gastroschisis, Hirschsprung disease, autoimmune enteritis, congenital enteropathies such as microvillus inclusion disease) or intestinal resection (eg, for mesenteric thromboembolism or extensive Crohn disease)
- Develop complications of TPN used to treat intestinal failure (eg, liver failure secondary to cholestatic liver disease, recurrent sepsis, total loss of venous access)
- Have locally invasive tumors that cause obstruction, abscesses, fistulas, ischemia, or hemorrhage (usually desmoid tumors associated with familial polyposis)

Procedure

Procurement from a brain-dead, beating-heart donor is complex, partly because the small bowel can be transplanted alone, with a liver, or with a stomach, liver, duodenum, and pancreas. The role of living-related donation for small-bowel allografts has yet to be defined.

Procedures vary by medical center; immunosuppressive regimens also vary, but a typical regimen includes antilymphocyte globulin for induction, followed by high-dose tacrolimus and mycophenolate mofetil for maintenance.

Complications

Rejection: Weekly endoscopy is indicated to check for rejection. About 30 to 50% of recipients have one or more bouts of rejection within the first year after transplantation.

Symptoms and signs of rejection include diarrhea, fever, and abdominal cramping. Endoscopic findings include mucosal erythema, friability, ulceration, and exfoliation; changes are distributed unevenly, may be difficult to detect, and can be differentiated from cytomegalovirus enteritis by viral inclusion bodies. Biopsy findings include blunted villi and inflammatory infiltrates in the lamina propria (see Table 177–8).

Treatment of acute rejection is high-dose corticosteroids, antithymocyte globulin, or both.

Other complications: Surgical complications affect 50% of patients and include anastomotic leaks, biliary leaks and strictures, hepatic artery thrombosis, and chylous ascites.

Nonsurgical complications include graft ischemia and graft-vs-host disease caused by transplantation of gut-associated lymphoid tissue.

Table 177–8. MANIFESTATIONS OF SMALL-BOWEL TRANSPLANT REJECTION BY CATEGORY

REJECTION CATEGORY	MANIFESTATIONS
Hyperacute	Fever, very elevated lactic acid
Accelerated	Fever, diarrhea, elevated lactic acid
Acute	Fever, diarrhea, malabsorption, mildly elevated lactic acid
Chronic	Diarrhea, malabsorption

Prognosis

At 3 yr, survival rates after small-bowel transplantation alone are

- Patients: 65%
- Grafts: > 50%

Infections commonly contribute to death.

With liver and small-bowel transplantation, survival rates are lower because the procedure is more extensive and the recipient's condition is more serious. However, after the perioperative phase, graft and patient survival rates are higher than those after small-bowel transplantation alone, presumably because the transplanted liver has a protective effect, preventing rejection by absorbing and neutralizing antibodies.

TISSUE TRANSPLANTATION

Composite Transplantation (Hand, Extremity, Face)

Composite transplants involve multiple tissues, usually including skin and soft tissues and sometimes musculoskeletal structures. Many of these procedures are now possible because of advances in immunosuppressive therapy. However, the procedures are ethically controversial because they typically do not extend life, are very expensive and resource-intensive, and can potentially cause morbidity and mortality due to infections.

The first successful composite transplants were hand transplants. Since then, perhaps as many as 10 different structures have been replaced in about 150 patients, with varying functional success rates.

The first hand transplantation was done in 1998. Since then, double hand and upper-extremity transplantations have been done. Recovery of the hand function varies widely; some recipients regain enough function and sensitivity to do daily activities.

The first face transplantation was done in 2005. As of 2011, 17 such procedures have been done. To date, no graft failure has been reported, but the recipient of the first face transplant died in 2016. Ethical questions about face transplantation are even more prominent than those about extremity transplantation because the surgical procedure is extremely demanding and the immunosuppression required puts the recipient at considerable risk of opportunistic infections.

Immunosuppression usually consists of induction therapy (antithymocyte globulin [ATG] or IL-2 receptor blocker), followed by triple maintenance immunosuppression with a corticosteroid, an antiproliferative drug (eg, basiliximab), and a calcineurin inhibitor (see Table 177–1 on p. 1410). Sometimes topical creams containing calcineurin inhibitors or corticosteroids are used.

Skin Grafts

Skin grafts may be

- Autografts
- Allografts

Skin autografts: Skin autografts use the patient's own intact skin as the source.

Split-thickness grafts are usually used; for these grafts, a thin layer of epidermis and some dermis are excised and placed on the recipient site. Such grafts are typically used for burns but may also be used to accelerate healing of small wounds. Because a significant amount of dermal elements remain at the donor site, the site eventually heals and can be harvested again.

Full-thickness grafts are composed of epidermis and dermis and provide better appearance and function than split-thickness grafts. However, because the donor site will not heal primarily, it must be a loose area of redundant skin (eg, abdominal or thoracic wall, sometimes scalp) so that the site can be sutured closed. Thus, full-thickness grafting is usually reserved for cosmetically sensitive areas (eg, face) or areas requiring a thicker, more protective skin layer (eg, hands). Because full-thickness grafts are thicker and more vascular, they do not have quite as high a survival rate as split-thickness grafts.

The patient's own skin cells may be grown in culture, then returned to a burned patient to help cover extensive burns. Alternatively, artificial skin, composed of cultured cells or a thin, split-thickness skin graft placed on a synthetic underlayer, may also be used.

Skin allografts: Skin allografts use donor skin (typically from cadavers). Skin allografts are used for patients with extensive burns or other conditions causing such massive skin loss that the patient does not have enough undamaged skin to provide the graft. Allografts can be used to cover broad denuded areas and thus reduce fluid and protein losses and discourage invasive infection.

Unlike solid organ transplants, skin allografts are ultimately rejected, but the resulting denuded areas develop well-vascularized granulations onto which autografts from the patient's healed sites take readily.

Cartilage Transplantation

Cartilage transplantation is used for children with congenital nasal or ear defects and adults with severe injuries or joint destruction (eg, severe osteoarthritis). Chondrocytes are more resistant to rejection, possibly because the sparse population of cells in hyaline cartilage is protected from cellular attack by the cartilaginous matrix around them. Immunosuppression is therefore not indicated.

Bone Transplantation

Bone transplantation is used for reconstruction of large bony defects (eg, after massive resection of bone cancer). No viable donor bone cells survive in the recipient, but dead matrix from allografts can stimulate recipient osteoblasts to recolonize the matrix and lay down new bone. This matrix acts as scaffolding for bridging and stabilizing defects until new bone is formed.

Cadaveric allografts are preserved by freezing to decrease immunogenicity of the bone (which is dead at the time of implantation) and by glycerolization to maintain chondrocyte viability.

No postimplantation immunosuppressive therapy is used. Although patients develop anti-HLA antibodies, early follow-up detects no evidence of cartilage degradation.

Adrenal Autografting

Adrenal autografting by stereotactically placing medullary tissue within the CNS has been reported to alleviate symptoms in patients with Parkinson disease.

Allografts of adrenal tissue, especially from fetal donors, have also been proposed. Fetal ventral mesencephalic tissue stereotactically implanted in the putamen of patients with Parkinson disease has been reported to reduce rigidity and bradykinesia. However, with the ethical and political debates about the propriety of using human fetal tissue, a controlled trial large enough to adequately assess fetal neural transplantation appears unlikely.

Xenografts of endocrinologically active cells from porcine donors are being tested.

Fetal Thymus Implants

Fetal thymus implants obtained from stillborn infants may restore immunologic responsiveness in children with thymic aplasia and resulting abnormal development of the lymphoid system (DiGeorge syndrome).

Because the recipient is immunologically unresponsive, immunosuppression is not required; however, severe graft-vs-host disease may occur.

SECTION 15

Infectious Diseases

178 Biology of Infectious Disease

A healthy person lives in harmony with the microbial flora that helps protect its host from invasion by pathogens, usually defined as microorganisms that have the capacity to cause disease. The microbial flora is mostly bacteria and fungi and includes normal resident flora, which is present consistently and which promptly reestablishes itself if disturbed, and transient flora, which may colonize the host for hours to weeks but does not permanently establish itself. Organisms that are normal flora can occasionally cause disease, especially when defenses are disrupted.

Tropisms (attractions to certain tissues) determine which body sites microorganisms colonize. Normal flora is influenced by tropisms and many other factors (eg, diet, hygiene, sanitary conditions, air pollution). For example, lactobacilli are common in the intestines of people with a high intake of dairy products; *Haemophilus influenzae* colonizes the tracheobronchial tree in patients with COPD. As a result, different body habitats contain microbial communities, forming microbiomes that differ by microbial composition and function.

HOST DEFENSE MECHANISMS AGAINST INFECTION

Host defenses that protect against infection include

- Natural barriers (eg, skin, mucous membranes)
- Nonspecific immune responses (eg, phagocytic cells [neutrophils, macrophages] and their products)
- Specific immune responses (eg, antibodies, lymphocytes)

Natural Barriers

Skin: The skin usually bars invading microorganisms unless it is physically disrupted (eg, by injury, IV catheter, or surgical incision). Exceptions include the following:

- Human papillomavirus, which can invade normal skin, causing warts
- Some parasites (eg, *Schistosoma mansoni*, *Strongyloides stercoralis*)

Mucous membranes: Many mucous membranes are bathed in secretions that have antimicrobial properties (eg, cervical mucus, prostatic fluid, and tears containing lysozyme, which splits the muramic acid linkage in bacterial cell walls, especially in gram-positive organisms). Local secretions also contain immunoglobulins, principally IgG and secretory IgA, which prevent microorganisms from attaching to host cells.

Respiratory tract: The respiratory tract has upper airway filters. If invading organisms reach the tracheobronchial tree, the mucociliary epithelium transports them away from the lung. Coughing also helps remove organisms. If the organisms reach the alveoli, alveolar macrophages and tissue histiocytes engulf them. However, these defenses can be overcome by large numbers of organisms or by compromised effectiveness resulting from air pollutants (eg, cigarette smoke) or interference with protective mechanisms (eg, endotracheal intubation, tracheostomy).

GI tract: GI tract barriers include the acid pH of the stomach and the antibacterial activity of pancreatic enzymes, bile, and intestinal secretions.

Peristalsis and the normal loss of epithelial cells remove microorganisms. If peristalsis is slowed (eg, because of drugs such as belladonna or opium alkaloids), this removal is delayed and prolongs some infections, such as symptomatic shigellosis.

Compromised GI defense mechanisms may predispose patients to particular infections (eg, achlorhydria predisposes to salmonellosis).

Normal bowel flora can inhibit pathogens; alteration of this flora with antibiotics can allow overgrowth of inherently pathogenic microorganisms (eg, *Salmonella* Typhimurium) or superinfection with ordinarily commensal organisms (eg, *Candida albicans*).

GU tract: GU tract barriers include the length of the urethra (20 cm) in men, the acid pH of the vagina in women, and the hypertonic state of the kidney medulla.

The kidneys also produce and excrete large amounts of Tamm-Horsfall mucoprotein, which binds certain bacteria, facilitating their harmless removal.

Nonspecific Immune Responses

Cytokines (including IL-1, IL-6, tumor necrosis factor-alpha, and interferon-gamma) are produced principally by macrophages and activated lymphocytes and mediate an acute-phase response that develops regardless of the inciting microorganism. The response involves fever and increased production of neutrophils by the bone marrow. Endothelial cells also produce large amounts of IL-8, which attracts neutrophils.

The inflammatory response directs immune system components to injury or infection sites and is manifested by increased blood supply and vascular permeability, which allows chemotactic peptides, neutrophils, and mononuclear cells to leave the intravascular compartment.

Microbial spread is limited by engulfment of microorganisms by phagocytes (eg, neutrophils, macrophages). Phagocytes are drawn to microbes via chemotaxis and engulf them, releasing phagocytic lysosomal contents that help destroy microbes. Oxidative products such as hydrogen peroxide are generated by the phagocytes and kill ingested microbes. When quantitative or qualitative defects in neutrophils result in infection, the infection is usually prolonged and recurrent and responds slowly to antimicrobial drugs. Staphylococci, gram-negative organisms, and fungi are the pathogens usually responsible.

Specific Immune Responses

After infection, the host can produce a variety of antibodies (complex glycoproteins known as immunoglobulins) that bind to specific microbial antigenic targets. Antibodies can help eradicate the infecting organism by attracting the host's WBCs and activating the complement system.

The complement system destroys cell walls of infecting organisms, usually through the classical pathway. Complement can also be activated on the surface of some microorganisms via the alternative pathway.

Antibodies can also promote the deposition of substances known as opsonins (eg, the complement protein C3b) on the surface of microorganisms, which helps promote phagocytosis. Opsonization is important for eradication of encapsulated organisms such as pneumococci and meningococci.

Host Genetic Factors

For many pathogens, the host's genetic makeup influences the host's susceptibility and the resulting morbidity and mortality. For example, patients who have deficiencies of the terminal complement components (C5 through C8, perhaps C9) have an increased susceptibility to infections caused by neisserial species.

FACTORS FACILITATING MICROBIAL INVASION

Microbial invasion can be facilitated by the following:

- Virulence factors
- Microbial adherence
- Resistance to antimicrobials
- Defects in host defense mechanisms

Virulence Factors

Virulence factors assist pathogens in invasion and resistance of host defenses; these factors include

- Capsule
- Enzymes
- Toxins

Capsule: Some organisms (eg, certain strains of pneumococci, meningococci, type B *Haemophilus influenzae*) have a capsule that blocks phagocytosis, making these organisms more virulent than nonencapsulated strains. However, capsule-specific opsonic antibodies can bind to the bacterial capsule and facilitate phagocytosis.

Enzymes: Bacterial proteins with enzymatic activity (eg, protease, hyaluronidase, neuraminidase, elastase, collagenase) facilitate local tissue spread. Invasive organisms (eg, *Shigella flexneri*, *Yersinia enterocolitica*) can penetrate and traverse intact eukaryotic cells, facilitating entry from mucosal surfaces.

Some bacteria (eg, *Neisseria gonorrhoeae*, *H. influenzae*, *Proteus mirabilis*, clostridial species, *Streptococcus pneumoniae*) produce IgA-specific proteases that cleave and inactivate secretory IgA on mucosal surfaces.

Toxins: Organisms may release toxins (called exotoxins), which are protein molecules that may cause disease (eg, diphtheria, cholera, tetanus, botulism) or increase the severity of the disease. Most toxins bind to specific target cell receptors. With the exception of preformed toxins responsible for some food-borne illnesses (eg, botulism, staphylococcal or *Bacillus cereus* food poisoning), toxins are produced by organisms during the course of infection.

Endotoxin is a lipopolysaccharide produced by gram-negative bacteria and is part of the cell wall. Endotoxin triggers humoral enzymatic mechanisms involving the complement, clotting, fibrinolytic, and kinin pathways and causes much of the morbidity in gram-negative sepsis.

Other factors: Some microorganisms are more virulent because they do the following:

- Impair antibody production
- Resist the lytic effects of serum complement
- Resist the oxidative steps in phagocytosis
- Produce superantigens

Many microorganisms have mechanisms that impair antibody production by inducing suppressor cells, blocking antigen processing, and inhibiting lymphocyte mitogenesis.

Resistance to the lytic effects of serum complement confers virulence. Among species of *N. gonorrhoeae*, resistance predisposes to disseminated rather than localized infection.

Some organisms resist the oxidative steps in phagocytosis. For example, *Legionella* and *Listeria* either do not elicit or actively suppress the oxidative step, whereas other organisms produce enzymes (eg, catalase, glutathione reductase, superoxide dismutase) that mitigate the oxidative products.

Some viruses and bacteria produce superantigens that bypass the immune system, cause nonspecific activation of inordinate numbers of naive T cells, and thus cause excessive and potentially destructive inflammation mediated by massive release of proinflammatory cytokines.

Microbial Adherence

Adherence to surfaces helps microorganisms establish a base from which to penetrate tissues. Among the factors that determine adherence are adhesins (microbial molecules that mediate attachment to a cell) and host receptors to which the adhesins bind. Host receptors include cell surface sugar residues and cell surface proteins (eg, fibronectin) that enhance binding of certain gram-positive organisms (eg, staphylococci).

Other determinants of adherence include fine structures on certain bacterial cells (eg, streptococci) called fibrillae, by which some bacteria bind to human epithelial cells. Other bacteria, such as Enterobacteriaceae (eg, *Escherichia coli*), have specific adhesive organelles called fimbriae or pili. Fimbriae enable the organism to attach to almost all human cells, including neutrophils and epithelial cells in the GU tract, mouth, and intestine.

Biofilm: Biofilm is a slime layer that can form around certain bacteria and confer resistance to phagocytosis and antibiotics. It develops around *Pseudomonas aeruginosa* in the lungs of patients with cystic fibrosis and around coagulase-negative staphylococci on synthetic medical devices, such as IV catheters, prosthetic vascular grafts, and suture material.

Factors that affect the likelihood of biofilm developing on such medical devices include the material's roughness, chemical composition, and hydrophobicity.

Antimicrobial Resistance

Genetic variability among microbes is inevitable. Use of antimicrobial drugs eventually selects for survival of strains that are capable of resisting them.

Emergence of antimicrobial resistance may be due to spontaneous mutation of chromosomal genes. In many cases, resistant bacterial strains have acquired mobile genetic elements from other microorganisms. These elements are encoded on plasmids or transposons and enable the microorganisms to synthesize enzymes that

- Modify or inactivate the antimicrobial agent
- Change the bacterial cell's ability to accumulate the antimicrobial agent
- Resist inhibition by the antimicrobial agent

Minimizing inappropriate use of antibiotics is important for public health.

For further discussion, see Antibiotic Resistance on p. 1506.

Defects in Host Defense Mechanisms

Two types of immune deficiency states affect the host's ability to fight infection:

- Primary immune deficiency
- Secondary (acquired) immune deficiency

Primary immune deficiencies are genetic in origin; > 100 primary immune deficiency states have been described. Most primary immune deficiencies are recognized during infancy; however, up to 40% are recognized during adolescence or adulthood.

Acquired immune deficiencies are caused by another disease (eg, cancer, HIV infection, chronic disease) or by exposure to a chemical or drug that is toxic to the immune system.

Mechanisms: Defects in immune responses may involve

- Cellular immunity
- Humoral immunity
- Phagocytic system
- Complement system

Cellular deficiencies are typically T-cell or combined immune defects. T cells contribute to the killing of intracellular organisms; thus, patients with T-cell defects can present with opportunistic infections such as *Pneumocystis jirovecii* or cryptococcal infections. Chronicity of these infections can lead to failure to thrive, chronic diarrhea, and persistent oral candidiasis.

Humoral deficiencies are typically caused by the failure of B cells to make functioning immunoglobulins. Patients with this type of defect usually have infections involving encapsulated organisms (eg, *H. influenzae*, streptococci). Patients can present with poor growth, diarrhea, and recurrent sinopulmonary infections.

A defect in the phagocytic system affects the immediate immune response to bacterial infection and can result in development of recurrent abscesses or severe pneumonias.

Primary complement system defects are particularly rare. Patients with this type of defect may present with recurrent infections with pyogenic bacteria (eg, encapsulated bacteria, *Neisseria* sp) and have an increased risk of autoimmune disorders (eg, SLE).

MANIFESTATIONS OF INFECTION

Manifestations may be local (eg, cellulitis, abscess) or systemic (most often fever). Manifestations may develop in multiple organ systems. Severe, generalized infections may have life-threatening manifestations (eg, sepsis, septic shock). Most manifestations resolve with successful treatment of the underlying infection.

Clinical: Most infections increase the pulse rate and body temperature, but others (eg, typhoid fever, tularemia, brucellosis, dengue) may not elevate the pulse rate commensurate with the degree of fever. Hypotension can result from hypovolemia, septic shock, or toxic shock. Hyperventilation and respiratory alkalosis are common.

Alterations in sensorium (encephalopathy) may occur in severe infection regardless of whether CNS infection is present. Encephalopathy is most common and serious in the elderly and may cause anxiety, confusion, delirium, stupor, seizures, and coma.

Hematologic: Infectious diseases commonly increase the numbers of mature and immature circulating neutrophils. Mechanisms include demargination and release of immature granulocytes from bone marrow, IL-1- and IL-6-mediated release of neutrophils from bone marrow, and colony-stimulating factors elaborated by macrophages, lymphocytes, and other tissues. Exaggeration of these phenomena (eg, in trauma, inflammation, and similar stresses) can result in release of excessive numbers of immature leukocytes into the circulation (leukemoid reaction), with leukocyte counts up to 25 to 30×10^9/L.

Conversely, some infections (eg, typhoid fever, brucellosis) commonly cause leukopenia. In overwhelming, severe infections, profound leukopenia is often a poor prognostic sign.

Characteristic morphologic changes in the neutrophils of septic patients include Döhle bodies, toxic granulations, and vacuolization.

Anemia can develop despite adequate tissue iron stores. If anemia is chronic, plasma iron and total iron-binding capacity may be decreased. Serious infection may cause thrombocytopenia and disseminated intravascular coagulation (DIC).

Other organ systems: Pulmonary compliance may decrease, progressing to acute respiratory distress syndrome (ARDS) and respiratory muscle failure.

Renal manifestations range from minimal proteinuria to acute renal failure, which can result from shock and acute tubular necrosis, glomerulonephritis, or tubulointerstitial disease.

Hepatic dysfunction, including cholestatic jaundice (often a poor prognostic sign) or hepatocellular dysfunction, occurs with many infections, even though the infection does not localize to the liver. Upper GI bleeding due to stress ulceration may occur during sepsis.

Endocrinologic dysfunctions include

- Increased production of thyroid-stimulating hormone, vasopressin, insulin, and glucagon
- Breakdown of skeletal muscle proteins and muscle wasting secondary to increased metabolic demands
- Bone demineralization

Hypoglycemia occurs infrequently in sepsis, but adrenal insufficiency should be considered in patients with hypoglycemia and sepsis. Hyperglycemia may be an early sign of infection in diabetics.

FEVER

Fever is elevated body temperature (> 37.8° C orally or > 38.2° C rectally) or an elevation above a person's known normal daily value. Fever occurs when the body's thermostat (located in the hypothalamus) resets at a higher temperature, primarily in response to an infection. Elevated body temperature that is not caused by a resetting of the temperature set point is called hyperthermia.

Many patients use "fever" very loosely, often meaning that they feel too warm, too cold, or sweaty, but they have not actually measured their temperature.

Symptoms are due mainly to the condition causing the fever, although fever itself can cause chills, sweats, and discomfort and make patients feel flushed and warm.

Pathophysiology

During a 24-h period, temperature varies from lowest levels in the early morning to highest in late afternoon. Maximum variation is about 0.6° C.

Body temperature is determined by the balance between heat production by tissues, particularly the liver and muscles, and heat loss from the periphery. Normally, the hypothalamic thermoregulatory center maintains the internal temperature between 37° and 38° C. Fever results when something raises the hypothalamic set point, triggering vasoconstriction and shunting of blood from the periphery to decrease heat loss; sometimes shivering, which increases heat production, is induced. These processes continue until the temperature of the blood bathing the hypothalamus reaches the new set point. Resetting the hypothalamic set point downward (eg, with antipyretic drugs) initiates heat loss through sweating and vasodilation.

The capacity to generate a fever is reduced in certain patients (eg, alcoholics, the very old, the very young).

Pyrogens are substances that cause fever. Exogenous pyrogens are usually microbes or their products. The best studied are the lipopolysaccharides of gram-negative bacteria (commonly called endotoxins) and *Staphylococcus aureus* toxin, which causes toxic shock syndrome. Fever is the result of exogenous pyrogens that induce release of endogenous pyrogens, such as interleukin-1 (IL-1), tumor necrosis factor-alpha (TNF-alpha), IL-6 and other cytokines, which then trigger cytokine receptors, or of exogenous pyrogens that directly trigger Toll-like receptors.

Prostaglandin E_2 synthesis appears to play a critical role.

Consequences of fever: Although many patients worry that fever itself can cause harm, the modest transient core temperature elevations (ie, 38 to 40°) caused by most acute illnesses are well tolerated by healthy adults.

However, extreme temperature elevation (typically > 41° C) may be damaging. Such elevation is more typical of severe environmental hyperthermia but sometimes results from exposure to illicit drugs (eg, cocaine, phencyclidine), anesthetics, or antipsychotic drugs. At this temperature, protein denaturation occurs, and inflammatory cytokines that activate the inflammatory cascade are released. As a result, cellular dysfunction occurs, leading to malfunction and ultimately failure of most organs; the coagulation cascade is also activated, leading to DIC.

Because fever can increase the BMR by about 10 to 12% for every 1° C increase over 37° C, fever may physiologically stress adults with preexisting cardiac or pulmonary insufficiency. Fever can also worsen mental status in patients with dementia.

Fever in healthy children can cause febrile seizures.

Etiology

Many disorders can cause fever. They are broadly categorized as

- Infectious (most common)
- Neoplastic
- Inflammatory (including rheumatic, nonrheumatic, and drug-related)

The cause of an acute (ie, duration ≤ 4 days) fever in adults is highly likely to be infectious. When patients present with fever due to a noninfectious cause, the fever is almost always chronic or recurrent. Also, an isolated, acute febrile event in patients with a known inflammatory or neoplastic disorder is still most likely to be infectious. In healthy people, an acute febrile event is unlikely to be the initial manifestation of a chronic illness.

Infectious causes: Virtually all infectious illnesses can cause fever. But overall, the most likely causes are

- Upper and lower respiratory tract infections
- GI infections
- UTIs
- Skin infections

Most acute respiratory tract and GI infections are viral.

Specific patient and external factors also influence which causes are most likely.

Patient factors include health status, age, occupation, and risk factors (eg, hospitalization, recent invasive procedures, presence of IV or urinary catheters, use of mechanical ventilation).

External factors are those that expose patients to specific diseases—eg, through infected contacts, local outbreaks, disease vectors (eg, mosquitoes, ticks), a common vehicle (eg, food, water), or geographic location (eg, residence in or recent travel to an endemic area).

Some causes appear to predominate based on these factors (see Table 178–1).

Table 178–1. SOME CAUSES OF ACUTE FEVER

PREDISPOSING FACTOR	CAUSE
None (healthy)	Upper or lower respiratory tract infection GI infection UTI Skin infection
Hospitalization	IV catheter infection UTI (particularly in patients with an indwelling catheter) Pneumonia (particularly in patients using a ventilator) Atelectasis Surgical site infection (postoperatively) Deep venous thrombosis or pulmonary embolism Diarrhea (*Clostridium difficile*–induced) Drugs Hematoma Transfusion reaction Decubitus ulcers
Travel to endemic areas	Coccidioidomycosis Dengue fever (less common) Diarrheal disorders Hantavirus Histoplasmosis Legionnaires' disease Malaria Multidrug resistant bacteria Plague Tularemia Typhoid fever Viral hepatitis Zika virus infection
Vector exposure (in US)	Ticks: Rickettsiosis, ehrlichiosis, anaplasmosis, Lyme disease, babesiosis, tularemia Mosquitoes: Arboviral encephalitis Wild animals: Tularemia, rabies, hantavirus infection Fleas: Plague Domestic animals: Brucellosis, cat-scratch disease, Q fever, toxoplasmosis Birds: Psittacosis Reptiles: *Salmonella* infection Bats: Rabies, histoplasmosis
Immunocompromise	**Viruses:** Varicella-zoster virus or cytomegalovirus infection **Bacteria:** Infection due to encapsulated organisms (eg, pneumococci, meningococci), *Staphylococcus aureus*, gram-negative bacteria (eg, *Pseudomonas aeruginosa*), *Nocardia* sp, or *Mycobacteria* sp **Fungi:** Infection due to *Candida*, *Aspergillus*, *Histoplasma*, or *Coccidioides* sp; *Pneumocystis jirovecii*; or fungi that cause mucormycosis **Parasites:** Infection due to *Toxoplasma gondii*, *Strongyloides stercoralis*, *Cryptosporidium* sp, microsporidia, or *Cystoisospora* (previously *Isospora*) *belli*
Drugs that can increase heat production	Amphetamines Cocaine Methylenedioxymethamphetamine (MDMA, or Ecstasy) Antipsychotics Anesthetics
Drugs that can trigger fever	Beta-lactam antibiotics Sulfa drugs Phenytoin Carbamazepine Procainamide Quinidine Amphotericin B Interferons

Evaluation

Two general issues are important in the initial evaluation of acute fever:

- Identifying any localizing symptoms (eg, headache, cough): These symptoms help narrow the range of possible causes. The localizing symptom may be part of the patient's chief complaint or identified only by specific questioning.
- Determining whether the patient is seriously or chronically ill (particularly if such illness is unrecognized): Many causes of fever in healthy people are self-limited, and many of the possible viral infections are difficult to diagnose specifically. Limiting testing to the seriously or chronically ill can help avoid many expensive, unnecessary, and often fruitless searches.

History: **History of present illness** should cover magnitude and duration of fever and method used to take the temperature. True rigors (severe, shaking, teeth-chattering chills—not simply feeling cold) suggest fever due to infection but are not otherwise specific. Pain is an important clue to the possible source; the patient should be asked about pain in the ears, head, neck, teeth, throat, chest, abdomen, flank, rectum, muscles, and joints.

Other localizing symptoms include nasal congestion and/or discharge, cough, diarrhea, and urinary symptoms (frequency, urgency, dysuria). Presence of rash (including nature, location, and time of onset in relation to other symptoms) and lymphadenopathy may help.

Infected contacts and their diagnosis should be identified.

Review of systems should identify symptoms of chronic illness, including recurrent fevers, night sweats, and weight loss.

Past medical history should particularly cover the following:

- Recent surgery
- Known conditions that predispose to infection (eg, HIV infection, diabetes, cancer, organ transplantation, sickle cell disease, valvular heart disorders—particularly if an artificial valve is present)
- Other known disorders that predispose to fever (eg, rheumatologic disorders, SLE, gout, sarcoidosis, hyperthyroidism, cancer)

Questions to ask about recent travel include location, time since return, locale (eg, in back country, only in cities), vaccinations received before travel, and any use of prophylactic antimalarial drugs (if required).

All patients should be asked about possible exposures (eg, via unsafe food or water, insect bites, animal contact, or unprotected sex).

Vaccination history, particularly against hepatitis A and B and against organisms that cause meningitis, influenza, or pneumococcal infection, should be noted.

Drug history should include specific questions about the following:

- Drugs known to cause fever (see Table 178–1)
- Drugs that predispose to increased risk of infection (eg, corticosteroids, anti-TNF drugs, chemotherapeutic and antirejection drugs, other immunosuppressants)
- Illicit use of injection drugs (predisposing to endocarditis, hepatitis, septic pulmonary emboli, and skin and soft-tissue infections)

Physical examination: Physical examination begins with confirmation of fever. Fever is most accurately diagnosed by measuring rectal temperature. Oral temperatures are normally about 0.6° C lower and may be falsely even lower for many reasons, such as recent ingestion of a cold drink, mouth breathing, hyperventilation, and inadequate measurement time (up to several minutes are required with mercury thermometers). Measurement of tympanic membrane temperature by infrared sensor is less accurate than rectal temperature. Monitoring skin temperature using temperature-sensitive crystals incorporated into plastic strips placed on the forehead is insensitive for detecting elevations in the core temperature.

Other vital signs are reviewed for presence of tachypnea, tachycardia, or hypotension.

For patients with localizing symptoms, examination proceeds as discussed elsewhere in The Manual. For febrile patients without localizing symptoms, a complete examination is necessary because clues to the diagnosis may be in any organ system.

The patient's general appearance, including any weakness, lethargy, confusion, cachexia, and distress, should be noted.

All of the skin should be inspected for rash, particularly petechial or hemorrhagic rash and any lesions or areas of erythema or blistering suggesting skin or soft-tissue infection. Neck, axillae, and epitrochlear and inguinal areas should be examined for adenopathy.

In hospitalized patients, presence of any IVs, NGTs, urinary catheters, and any other tubes or lines inserted into the body should be noted. If patients have had recent surgery, surgical sites should be thoroughly inspected.

For the head and neck examination, the following should be done:

- Tympanic membranes: Examined for infection
- Sinuses (frontal and maxillary): Percussed
- Temporal arteries: Palpated for tenderness
- Nose: Inspected for congestion and discharge (clear or purulent)
- Eyes: Inspected for conjunctivitis or icterus
- Fundi: Inspected for Roth spots (suggesting endocarditis)
- Oropharynx and gingiva: Inspected for inflammation or ulceration (including any lesions of candidiasis, which suggests immunocompromise)
- Neck: Flexed to detect discomfort, stiffness, or both, indicating meningismus, and palpated for adenopathy

The lungs are examined for crackles or signs of consolidation, and the heart is auscultated for murmurs (suggesting possible endocarditis).

The abdomen is palpated for hepatosplenomegaly and tenderness (suggesting infection).

The flanks are percussed for tenderness over the kidneys (suggesting pyelonephritis).

A pelvic examination is done in women to check for cervical motion or adnexal tenderness; a genital examination is done in men to check for urethral discharge and local tenderness.

The rectum is examined for tenderness and swelling, suggesting perirectal abscess (which may be occult in immunosuppressed patients).

All major joints are examined for swelling, erythema, and tenderness (suggesting a joint infection or rheumatologic disorder). The hands and feet are inspected for signs of endocarditis, including splinter hemorrhages under the nails, painful erythematous subcutaneous nodules on the tips of digits (Osler nodes), and nontender hemorrhagic macules on the palms or soles (Janeway lesions).

The spine is percussed for focal tenderness.

Neurologic examination is done to detect focal deficits.

Red flags: The following findings are of particular concern:

- Altered mental status
- Headache, stiff neck, or both
- Petechial rash
- Hypotension
- Dyspnea
- Significant tachycardia or tachypnea

- Temperature > 40° C or < 35° C
- Recent travel to an area where serious diseases (eg, malaria) are endemic
- Recent use of immunosuppressants

Interpretation of findings: The degree of elevation in temperature usually does not predict the likelihood or cause of infection. Fever pattern, once thought to be significant, is not.

Likelihood of serious illness is considered. If serious illness is suspected, immediate and aggressive testing and often hospital admission are needed.

Red flag findings strongly suggest a serious disorder, as in the following:

- Headache, stiff neck, and petechial or purpuric rash suggest meningitis.
- Tachycardia (beyond the modest elevation normally present with fever) and tachypnea, with or without hypotension or mental status changes, suggest sepsis.
- Malaria should be suspected in patients who have recently traveled to an endemic area.

Immunocompromise, whether caused by a known disorder or use of immunosuppressants or suggested by examination findings (eg, weight loss, oral candidiasis), is also of concern, as are other known chronic illnesses, injection drug use, and heart murmur.

The elderly, particularly those in nursing homes, are at particular risk of serious bacterial infection (see p. 1437).

Localizing findings identified by history or physical examination are evaluated and interpreted (see elsewhere in THE MANUAL). Other suggestive findings include generalized adenopathy and rash.

Generalized adenopathy may occur in older children and younger adults who have acute mononucleosis; it is usually accompanied by significant pharyngitis, malaise, and hepatosplenomegaly. Primary HIV infection or secondary syphilis should be suspected in patients with generalized adenopathy, sometimes accompanied by arthralgias, rash, or both. HIV infection develops 2 to 6 wk after exposure (although patients may not always report unprotected sexual contact or other risk factors). Secondary syphilis is usually preceded by a chancre, with systemic symptoms developing 4 to 10 wk later. However, patients may not notice a chancre because it is painless and may be located out of sight in the rectum, vagina, or oral cavity.

Fever and rash have many infectious and drug causes. Petechial or purpuric rash is of particular concern; it suggests possible meningococcemia, Rocky Mountain spotted fever (particularly if the palms or soles are involved), or, less commonly, some viral infections (eg, dengue fever, hemorrhagic fevers). Other suggestive skin lesions include the classic erythema migrans rash of Lyme disease, target lesions of Stevens-Johnson syndrome, and the painful, tender erythema of cellulitis and other bacterial soft-tissue infections. The possibility of delayed drug hypersensitivity (even after long periods of use) should be kept in mind.

If no localizing findings are present, healthy people with acute fever and only nonspecific findings (eg, malaise, generalized aches) most likely have a self-limited viral illness, unless a history of exposure to infected contacts (including a new, unprotected sexual contact), to disease vectors, or in an endemic area (including recent travel) suggests otherwise.

Patients with significant underlying disorders are more likely to have an occult bacterial or parasitic infection. Injection drug users and patients with a prosthetic heart valve may have endocarditis. Immunocompromised patients are predisposed to infection caused by certain microorganisms (see Table 178–1).

Drug fever (with or without rash) is a diagnosis of exclusion, often requiring a trial of stopping the drug. One difficulty is that if antibiotics are the cause, the illness being treated may also cause fever. Sometimes a clue is that the fever and rash begin after clinical improvement from the initial infection and without worsening or reappearance of the original symptoms (eg, in a patient being treated for pneumonia, fever reappears without cough, dyspnea, or hypoxia).

Testing: Testing depends on whether localized findings are present.

If localizing findings are present, testing is guided by clinical suspicion and findings (see also elsewhere in THE MANUAL), as for the following:

- Mononucleosis or HIV infection: Serologic testing
- Rocky Mountain spotted fever: Biopsy of skin lesions to confirm the diagnosis (acute serologic testing is unhelpful)
- Bacterial or fungal infection: Blood cultures to detect possible bloodstream infections
- Meningitis: Immediate lumbar puncture and IV dexamethasone and antibiotics (head CT should be done before lumbar puncture if patients are at risk of brain herniation; IV dexamethasone and antibiotics must be given immediately after blood cultures are obtained and before head CT is done)
- Specific disorders based on exposure (eg, to contacts, to vectors, or in endemic areas): Testing for those disorders, particularly a peripheral blood smear for malaria

If no localizing findings are present in otherwise healthy patients and serious illness is not suspected, patients can usually be observed at home without testing. In most, symptoms resolve quickly; the few who develop worrisome or localizing symptoms should be reevaluated and tested based on the new findings.

If serious illness is suspected in patients who have no localizing findings, testing is needed. Patients with red flag findings suggesting sepsis require cultures (urine and blood), chest x-ray, and evaluation for metabolic abnormalities with measurement of serum electrolytes, glucose, BUN, creatinine, lactate, and liver enzymes. CBC is typically done, but sensitivity and specificity for diagnosing serious bacterial infection are low. However, WBC count is important prognostically for patients who may be immunosuppressed (ie, a low WBC count may be associated with a poor prognosis).

Patients with certain underlying disorders may need testing even if they have no localizing findings and do not appear seriously ill. Because of the risk and devastating consequences of endocarditis, febrile injection drug users are usually admitted to the hospital for serial blood cultures and often echocardiography. Patients taking immunosuppressants require CBC; if neutropenia is present, testing is initiated and chest x-ray is done, as are cultures of blood, sputum, urine, stool, and any suspicious skin lesions. Because bacteremia and sepsis are frequent causes of fever in patients with neutropenia, empiric broad-spectrum IV antibiotics should be given promptly, without waiting for culture results.

Febrile elderly patients often require testing (see p. 1437).

Treatment

Specific causes of fever are treated with anti-infective therapy; empiric anti-infective therapy is required when suspicion of serious infection is high.

Whether fever due to infection should be treated with antipyretics is controversial. Experimental evidence, but not clinical studies, suggests that fever enhances host defenses.

Fever should probably be treated in certain patients at particular risk, including adults with cardiac or pulmonary insufficiency or with dementia.

Drugs that inhibit brain cyclooxygenase effectively reduce fever:

- Acetaminophen 650 to 1000 mg po q 6 h
- Ibuprofen 400 to 600 mg po q 6 h

The daily dose of acetaminophen should not exceed 4 g to avoid toxicity; patients should be warned not to simultaneously take nonprescription cold or flu remedies that contain acetaminophen. Other NSAIDs (eg, aspirin, naproxen) are also effective antipyretics. Salicylates should not be used to treat fever in children with viral illnesses because use has been associated with Reye syndrome.

If temperature is ≥ 41° C, other cooling measures (eg, evaporative cooling with tepid water mist, cooling blankets) should also be started.

Geriatrics Essentials: Fever

In the frail elderly, infection is less likely to cause fever, and even when elevated by infection, temperature may be lower than the standard definition of fever. Similarly, other inflammatory symptoms, such as focal pain, may be less prominent. Frequently, alteration of mental status or decline in daily functioning may be the only other initial manifestations of pneumonia or UTI.

In spite of their less severe manifestations of illness, the febrile elderly are significantly more likely to have a serious bacterial illness than are febrile younger adults. As in younger adults, the cause is commonly a respiratory infection or UTI, but in the elderly, skin and soft-tissue infections are among the top causes.

Focal findings are evaluated as for younger patients. But unlike younger patients, elderly patients probably require urinalysis, urine culture, and chest x-ray. Blood cultures should be done to exclude septicemia; if septicemia is suspected or vital signs are abnormal, patients should be admitted to the hospital.

KEY POINTS

- Most fevers in healthy people are due to viral respiratory tract or GI infections.
- Localizing symptoms guide evaluation.
- Consider underlying chronic disorders, particularly those impairing the immune system.

FEVER OF UNKNOWN ORIGIN

Fever of unknown origin (FUO) is body temperature ≥ 38.3° C (101° F) rectally that does not result from transient and self-limited illness, rapidly fatal illness, or disorders with clear-cut localizing symptoms or signs or with abnormalities on common tests such as chest x-ray, urinalysis, or blood cultures.

FUO is currently classified into 4 distinct categories:

- **Classic FUO:** Fever for > 3 wk with no identified cause after 3 days of hospital evaluation or ≥ 3 outpatient visits
- **Health care–associated FUO:** Fever in hospitalized patients receiving acute care and with no infection present or incubating at admission if the diagnosis remains uncertain after 3 days of appropriate evaluation
- **Immune-deficient FUO:** Fever in patients with immunodeficiencies if the diagnosis remains uncertain after 3 days of appropriate evaluation, including negative cultures after 48 h
- **HIV-related FUO:** Fever for > 3 wk in outpatients with confirmed HIV infection or > 3 days in inpatients with confirmed HIV infection if the diagnosis remains uncertain after appropriate evaluation

Etiology

Causes of FUO are usually divided into 4 categories (see Table 178–2):

- Infections (25 to 50%)
- Connective tissue disorders (10 to 20%)
- Neoplasms (5 to 35%)
- Miscellaneous (15 to 25%)

Infections are the most common cause of FUO. In patients with HIV infection, opportunistic infections (eg, TB; infection by atypical mycobacteria, disseminated fungi, or cytomegalovirus) should be sought.

Common connective tissue disorders include SLE, RA, giant cell arteritis, vasculitis, and juvenile RA of adults (adult Still disease).

The **most common neoplastic causes** are lymphoma, leukemia, renal cell carcinoma, hepatocellular carcinoma, and metastatic carcinomas. However, the incidence of neoplastic causes of FUO has been decreasing, probably because they are being detected by ultrasonography and CT, which are now widely used during initial evaluation.

Important miscellaneous causes include drug reactions, deep venous thrombosis, recurrent pulmonary emboli, sarcoidosis, inflammatory bowel disease, and factitious fever.

No cause of FUO is identified in about 10% of adults.

Evaluation

In puzzling cases, such as FUO, assuming that all information was gathered or was gathered accurately by previous clinicians is usually a mistake. Clinicians should be aware of what patients previously reported (to resolve discrepancies) but should not simply copy details of previously recorded history (eg, family history, social history). Initial errors of omission have been perpetuated through many clinicians over many days of hospitalization, causing much unnecessary testing. Even when initial evaluation was thorough, patients often remember new details when questioning is repeated.

Conversely, clinicians should not ignore previous test results and should not repeat tests without considering how likely results are to be different (eg, because the patient's condition has changed, because a disorder develops slowly).

History: History aims to uncover focal symptoms and facts (eg, travel, occupation, family history, exposure to animal vectors, dietary history) that suggest a cause.

History of present illness should cover duration and pattern (eg, intermittent, constant) of fever. Fever patterns usually have little or no significance in the diagnosis of FUO, although a fever that occurs every other day (tertian) or every 3rd day (quartan) may suggest malaria in patients with risk factors. Focal pain often indicates the location (although not the cause) of the underlying disorder. Clinicians should ask generally, then specifically, about discomfort in each body part.

Review of systems should include nonspecific symptoms, such as weight loss, anorexia, fatigue, night sweats, and headaches. Also, symptoms of connective tissue disorders (eg, myalgias, arthralgias, rashes) and GI disorders (eg, diarrhea, steatorrhea, abdominal discomfort) should be sought.

Past medical history should include disorders known to cause fever, such as cancer, TB, connective tissue disorders, alcoholic cirrhosis, inflammatory bowel disease, rheumatic fever,

Table 178–2. SOME CAUSES OF FEVER OF UNKNOWN ORIGIN

CAUSE	SUGGESTIVE FINDINGS	DIAGNOSTIC APPROACH*
Infectious		
Abscesses (abdominal, pelvic, dental)	Abdominal or pelvic discomfort, usually tenderness Sometimes history of surgery, trauma, diverticulosis, peritonitis, or gynecologic procedure	CT or MRI
Cat-scratch disease	History of being scratched or licked by a cat Regional adenopathy, Parinaud oculoglandular syndrome, headache	Culture (sometimes of lymph node aspirate), antibody titers, PCR testing
CMV infection	History of blood transfusion from CMV-positive donor Syndrome that resembles mononucleosis (fatigue, mild hepatitis, splenomegaly, adenopathy), chorioretinitis	CMV IgM antibody titers Possibly PCR testing
EBV infection	Sore throat, adenopathy, right upper quadrant tenderness, splenomegaly, fatigue Usually occurring in adolescents and young adults In older patients, typical findings possibly absent	Serologic testing
HIV infection	History of high-risk behaviors (eg, unprotected sex, sharing needles) Weight loss, night sweats, fatigue, adenopathy, opportunistic infections	Testing for HIV antibodies (ie, ELISA, Western blot) Sometimes testing for HIV RNA (for acute HIV infection)
Infective endocarditis	Often history of risk factors (eg, structural heart disease, prosthetic heart valve, periodontal disease, IV catheter, injection drug use) Usually a heart murmur, sometimes extracardiac manifestations (eg, splinter hemorrhages, petechiae, Roth spots, Osler nodes, Janeway lesions, joint pain or effusion, splenomegaly)	Serial blood cultures, echocardiography
Lyme disease	Visiting or living in an endemic area Erythema migrans rash, headache, fatigue, Bell palsy, meningitis, radiculopathy, heart block, joint pain and swelling	Serologic testing
Osteomyelitis	Localized pain, swelling, erythema	X-rays Sometimes MRI (most accurate test), radionuclide scanning with indium-111, bone scanning
Sinusitis	Prolonged congestion, headache, facial pain	CT of sinuses
TB (pulmonary and disseminated)	History of high-risk exposure Cough, weight loss, fatigue Use of immunosuppressants History of HIV infection	Chest x-ray, PPD, interferon-gamma release assay Sputum smear for acid-fast bacilli, nucleic acid amplification testing (NAAT), culture of body fluids (eg, gastric aspirates, sputum, CSF)
Uncommon infections (eg, brucellosis, malaria, Q fever, toxoplasmosis, trichinosis, typhoid fever)	History of travel to endemic areas Exposure to or ingestion of certain animal products	Serologic testing for individual causes Peripheral blood smear for malaria
Connective tissue		
Adult Still disease	Evanescent salmon-pink rash, arthralgias, arthritis, myalgias, cervical adenopathy, sore throat, cough, chest pain	ANA, RF, serum ferritin concentration, x-rays of affected joints
Giant cell (temporal) arteritis	Unilateral headache, visual disturbances Often symptoms of polymyalgia rheumatica, sometimes jaw claudication Tenderness of temporal artery when palpated	ESR, temporal artery biopsy
Polyarteritis nodosa	Fever, weight loss, myalgias, arthralgias, purpura, hematuria, abdominal pain, testicular pain, angina, livedo reticularis, new-onset hypertension	Biopsy of involved tissues or angiography

Table 178–2. SOME CAUSES OF FEVER OF UNKNOWN ORIGIN (*Continued*)

CAUSE	SUGGESTIVE FINDINGS	DIAGNOSTIC APPROACH*
Polymyalgia rheumatica	History of morning stiffness in shoulders, hips, and neck Malaise, fatigue, anorexia Possibly synovitis, bursitis, pitting edema of extremities	Creatinine kinase, ANA, RF, ESR Possibly MRI of extremities
Reactive arthritis	Sometimes recent history of infection with *Chlamydia*, *Salmonella*, *Yersinia*, *Campylobacter*, or *Shigella* Asymmetric oligoarthritis, urethritis, conjunctivitis, genital ulcerations	ANA, RF, serologic testing for causative pathogens
Rheumatoid arthritis	Symmetric peripheral polyarthritis, prolonged morning stiffness, subcutaneous rheumatoid nodules in pressure sites (extensor surface of ulna, sacrum, back of head, Achilles tendon)	ANA, RF, citrullinated peptide antibody (anti-CCP), x-rays (to identify bone erosions)
SLE	Fatigue, arthralgia, pleuritic chest pain, malar rash, tender swollen joints, mild peripheral edema, Raynaud syndrome, serositis, nephritis, alopecia	Clinical criteria, ANA, antibodies to double-stranded DNA
Neoplastic		
Colon carcinoma	Abdominal pain, change in bowel habits, hematochezia, weakness, nausea, vomiting, weight loss, fatigue	Colonoscopy, biopsy
Hepatoma	History of chronic liver disease, abdominal pain, weight loss, early satiety, palpable mass in right upper quadrant	Abdominal ultrasonography and CT, liver biopsy
Leukemia	Sometimes history of myelodysplastic disorder Fatigue, weight loss, bleeding, pallor, petechiae, ecchymoses, anorexia, splenomegaly, bone pain	CBC, bone marrow examination
Lymphoma	Painless adenopathy, weight loss, malaise, night sweats, splenomegaly, hepatomegaly	Lymph node biopsy
Metastatic cancer	Symptoms dependent on the site of metastasis (eg, cough and shortness of breath for lung metastasis, headache and dizziness for brain metastasis) Often asymptomatic, discovered during a routine medical evaluation	Biopsy of suspicious mass or node, imaging tests appropriate for area of concern
Myeloproliferative disorders	Frequently asymptomatic, abnormal indices incidentally detected during screening CBC	Testing based on the suspected disorder
Renal cell carcinoma	Weight loss, night sweats, flank pain, hematuria, palpable flank mass, hypertension	Serum calcium (to check for hypercalcemia), urinalysis, CT of kidneys
Miscellaneous		
Alcoholic cirrhosis	Long history of alcohol use Sometimes ascites, jaundice, small or enlarged liver, gynecomastia, Dupuytren contracture, testicular atrophy	PT/PTT, alkaline phosphatase, transaminases, albumin, bilirubin Sometimes abdominal ultrasonography and CT
Deep venous thrombosis	Pain, swelling, sometimes redness of leg	Ultrasonography Sometimes D-dimer assay
Drug fever	Fever coincident with administration of a drug (usually within 7–10 days) Sometimes a rash	Withdrawal of drug
Factitious fever	Dramatic, atypical presentation, vague and inconsistent details, knowledge of textbook descriptions, compulsive or habitual lying (pseudologia fantastica)	Diagnosis of exclusion
Inflammatory bowel disease	Abdominal pain, diarrhea (sometimes bloody), weight loss, guaiac-positive stools Sometimes fistulas, perianal and oral ulcerations, arthralgias	Upper GI endoscopy with small-bowel follow-through or CT enterography (Crohn disease) Colonoscopy (ulcerative colitis or Crohn colitis)

*Patients with FUO may lack typical findings, but such findings should be sought.

ANA = antinuclear antibodies; ANCA = antineutrophil cytoplasmic antibody; CMV = cytomegalovirus; EBV = Epstein-Barr virus; ELISA = enzyme-linked immunosorbent assay; RF = rheumatoid factor.

and hyperthyroidism. Clinicians should note disorders or factors that predispose to infection, such as immunocompromise (eg, due to disorders such as HIV infection, cancer, diabetes, or use of immunosuppressants), structural heart disorders, urinary tract abnormalities, operations, and insertion of devices (eg, IV lines, pacemakers, joint prostheses).

Drug history should include questions about specific drugs known to cause fever.

Social history should include questions about risk factors for infection such as injection drug use, high-risk sexual practices (eg, unprotected sex, multiple partners), infected contacts (eg, with TB), travel, and possible exposure to animal or insect vectors. Risk factors for cancer, including smoking, alcohol use, and occupational exposure to chemicals, should also be identified.

Family history should include questions about inherited causes of fever (eg, familial Mediterranean fever).

Medical records are checked for previous test results, particularly those that effectively rule out certain disorders.

Physical examination: The general appearance, particularly for cachexia, jaundice, and pallor, is noted.

The skin is thoroughly inspected for focal erythema (suggesting a site of infection) and rash (eg, malar rash of SLE); inspection should include the perineum and feet, particularly in diabetics, who are prone to infections in these areas. Clinicians should also check for cutaneous findings of endocarditis, including painful erythematous subcutaneous nodules on the tips of digits (Osler nodes), nontender hemorrhagic macules on the palms or soles (Janeway lesions), petechiae, and splinter hemorrhages under the nails.

The entire body (particularly over the spine, bones, joints, abdomen, and thyroid) is palpated for areas of tenderness, swelling, or organomegaly; digital rectal examination and pelvic examination are included. The teeth are percussed for tenderness (suggesting apical abscess). During palpation, any regional or systemic adenopathy is noted; eg, regional adenopathy is characteristic of cat-scratch disease in contrast to the diffuse adenopathy of lymphoma.

The heart is auscultated for murmurs (suggesting bacterial endocarditis) and rubs (suggesting pericarditis due to a rheumatologic or infectious disorder).

Sometimes key physical abnormalities in patients with FUO are or seem so subtle that repeated physical examinations may be necessary to suggest causes (eg, by detecting new adenopathy, heart murmurs, rash, or nodularity and weak pulsations in the temporal artery).

Red flags: The following are of particular concern:

- Immunocompromise
- Heart murmur
- Presence of inserted devices (eg, IV lines, pacemakers, joint prostheses)
- Recent travel to endemic areas

Interpretation of findings: After a thorough history and physical examination, the following scenarios are typical:

- Localizing symptoms or signs that were not present, not detected, or not managed during previous examinations are discovered. These findings are interpreted and investigated as indicated (see Table 178–2).
- More commonly, evaluation detects only nonspecific findings that occur in many different causes of FUO, but it identifies risk factors that can help guide testing (eg, travel to an endemic area, exposure to animal vectors). Sometimes risk factors are less specific but may suggest a class of illness; eg, weight loss without anorexia is more consistent with infection than cancer, which usually causes anorexia. Possible causes should be investigated further.
- In the most difficult scenario, patients have only nonspecific findings and no or multiple risk factors, making a logical, sequential approach to testing essential. Initial testing is used to narrow the diagnostic possibilities and guide subsequent testing.

Testing: Previous test results, particularly for cultures, are reviewed. Cultures for some organisms may require a long time to become positive.

As much as possible, clinical information is used to focus testing (see Table 178–2). For example, housebound elderly patients with headache would not be tested for tick-borne infections or malaria, but those disorders should be considered in younger travelers who have hiked in an endemic area. Elderly patients require evaluation for giant cell arteritis; younger patients do not.

In addition to specific testing, the following should usually be done:

- CBC with differential
- ESR
- Liver function tests
- Serial blood cultures (ideally before antimicrobial therapy)
- HIV antibody test, RNA concentration assays, and PCR assay
- Tuberculin skin test or interferon-gamma release assay

Even if done earlier, these tests may suggest a helpful trend.

Urinalysis, urine culture, and chest x-ray, usually already done, are repeated only if findings indicate that they should be.

Any available fluid or material from abnormal areas identified during the evaluation is cultured (eg, for bacteria, mycobacteria, fungi, viruses, or specific fastidious bacteria as indicated). Organism-specific tests, such as PCR and serologic titers (acute and convalescent), are helpful mainly when guided by clinical suspicion, not done in a shotgun approach.

Serologic tests, such as antinuclear antibody (ANA) and rheumatoid factor, are done to screen for rheumatologic disorders.

Imaging tests are guided by symptoms and signs. Typically, areas of discomfort should be imaged—eg, in patients with back pain, MRI of the spine (to check for infection or tumor); in patients with abdominal pain, CT of the abdomen. However, CT of the chest, abdomen, and pelvis should be considered to check for adenopathy and occult abscesses even when patients do not have localizing symptoms or signs.

If blood cultures are positive or heart murmurs or peripheral signs suggest endocarditis, echocardiography is done.

In general, CT is useful for delineating abnormalities localized to the abdomen or chest.

MRI is more sensitive than CT for detecting most causes of FUO involving the CNS and should be done if a CNS cause is being considered.

Venous duplex imaging may be useful for identifying cases of deep venous thrombosis.

Radionuclide scanning with indium-111-labeled granulocytes may help localize some infectious or inflammatory processes. This technique has generally fallen out of favor because it is thought to contribute very little to diagnosis, but some reports suggest that it provides a higher diagnostic yield than CT.

PET may also be useful in detecting the focus of fever.

Biopsy may be required if an abnormality is suspected in tissue that can be biopsied (eg, liver, bone marrow, skin, pleura, lymph nodes, intestine, muscle). Biopsy specimens should be evaluated by histopathologic examination and cultured for bacteria, fungi, viruses, and mycobacteria or sent for molecular (PCR) diagnostic testing. Muscle biopsy or skin biopsy of rashes may confirm vasculitis. Bilateral temporal artery biopsy may confirm giant cell arteritis in elderly patients with unexplained ESR elevation.

Treatment

Treatment of FUO focuses on the causative disorder. Antipyretics should be used judiciously, considering the duration of fever.

Geriatrics Essentials: FUO

Causes of FUO in the elderly are usually similar to those in the general population, but connective tissue disorders are identified more often. The most common causes are

- Giant cell arteritis
- Lymphomas
- Abscesses
- TB

KEY POINTS

- Classic FUO is body temperature ≥ 38.0° C rectally for > 3 wk with no identified cause after 3 days of hospital investigation or ≥ 3 outpatient visits.
- Identified causes can be categorized as infectious, connective tissue, neoplastic, or miscellaneous.
- Evaluation should be based on synthesis of history and physical examination, with particular consideration of risk factors and likely causes based on individual circumstances.

ABSCESSES

Abscesses are collections of pus in confined tissue spaces, usually caused by bacterial infection. Symptoms include local pain, tenderness, warmth, and swelling (if abscesses are near the skin layer) or constitutional symptoms (if abscesses are deep). Imaging is often necessary for diagnosis of deep abscesses. Treatment is surgical drainage and often antibiotics.

Etiology

Numerous organisms can cause abscesses, but the most common is

- *Staphylococcus aureus*

Organisms may enter the tissue by

- Direct implantation (eg, penetrating trauma with a contaminated object)
- Spread from an established, contiguous infection
- Dissemination via lymphatic or hematogenous routes from a distant site
- Migration from a location where there are resident flora into an adjacent, normally sterile area because natural barriers are disrupted (eg, by perforation of an abdominal viscus causing an intra-abdominal abscess)

Abscesses may begin in an area of cellulitis or in compromised tissue where leukocytes accumulate. Progressive dissection by pus or necrosis of surrounding cells expands the abscess. Highly vascularized connective tissue may then surround the necrotic tissue, leukocytes, and debris to wall off the abscess and limit further spread.

Predisposing factors to abscess formation include the following:

- Impaired host defense mechanisms (eg, impaired leukocyte defenses)
- The presence of foreign bodies
- Obstruction to normal drainage (eg, in the urinary, biliary, or respiratory tracts)
- Tissue ischemia or necrosis
- Hematoma or excessive fluid accumulation in tissue
- Trauma

Symptoms and Signs

The symptoms and signs of cutaneous and subcutaneous abscesses are pain, heat, swelling, tenderness, and redness.

If superficial abscesses are ready to spontaneously rupture, the skin over the center of the abscess may thin, sometimes appearing white or yellow because of the underlying pus (termed pointing). Fever may occur, especially with surrounding cellulitis.

For deep abscesses, local pain and tenderness and systemic symptoms, especially fever, as well as anorexia, weight loss, and fatigue are typical.

The predominant manifestation of some abscesses is abnormal organ function (eg, hemiplegia due to a brain abscess).

Complications of abscesses include

- Bacteremic spread
- Rupture into adjacent tissue
- Bleeding from vessels eroded by inflammation
- Impaired function of a vital organ
- Inanition due to anorexia and increased metabolic needs

Diagnosis

- Clinical evaluation
- Sometimes ultrasonography, CT, or MRI

Diagnosis of cutaneous and subcutaneous abscesses is by physical examination.

Diagnosis of deep abscesses often requires imaging. Ultrasonography is noninvasive and detects many soft-tissue abscesses; CT is accurate for most, although MRI is usually more sensitive.

Treatment

- Surgical drainage
- Sometimes antibiotics

Superficial abscesses may resolve with heat and oral antibiotics. However, healing usually requires drainage.

Minor cutaneous abscesses may require only incision and drainage. All pus, necrotic tissue, and debris should be removed. Eliminating open (dead) space by packing with gauze or by placing drains may be necessary to prevent reformation of the abscess. Predisposing conditions, such as obstruction of natural drainage or the presence of a foreign body, require correction.

Deep abscesses can sometimes be adequately drained by percutaneous needle aspiration (typically guided by ultrasonography or CT); this method often avoids the need for open surgical drainage.

Spontaneous rupture and drainage may occur, sometimes leading to the formation of chronic draining sinuses. Without drainage, an abscess occasionally resolves slowly after proteolytic digestion of the pus produces a thin, sterile fluid that is resorbed into the bloodstream. Incomplete resorption may leave a cystic loculation within a fibrous wall that may become calcified.

Systemic antimicrobial drugs are indicated as adjunctive therapy as follows:

- If the abscess is deep (eg, intra-abdominal)
- If abscesses are multiple
- If there is significant surrounding cellulitis
- Perhaps if size is > 2 cm

Antimicrobial drugs are usually ineffective without drainage. Empiric antimicrobial therapy is based on location and likely infecting pathogen. Gram stain, culture, and susceptibility results guide further antimicrobial therapy.

KEY POINTS

- Cutaneous and subcutaneous abscesses are diagnosed clinically; deeper abscesses often require imaging.
- Usually, drain the abscess by incision or sometimes by needle aspiration.
- Use antibiotics when abscesses are deep or surrounded by significant cellulitis.

BACTEREMIA

Bacteremia is the presence of bacteria in the bloodstream. It can occur spontaneously, during certain tissue infections, with use of indwelling GU or IV catheters, or after dental, GI, GU, wound-care, or other procedures. Bacteremia may cause metastatic infections, including endocarditis, especially in patients with valvular heart abnormalities. Transient bacteremia is often asymptomatic but may cause fever. Development of other symptoms usually suggests more serious infection, such as sepsis or septic shock.

Bacteremia may be transient and cause no sequelae, or it may have metastatic or systemic consequences. Systemic consequences include

- Systemic inflammatory response syndrome
- Septic shock

Etiology

Bacteremia has many possible causes, including

- Catheterization of an infected lower urinary tract
- Surgical treatment of an abscess or infected wound
- Colonization of indwelling devices, especially IV and intracardiac catheters, urethral catheters, and ostomy devices and tubes

Gram-negative bacteremia secondary to infection usually originates in the GU or GI tract or in the skin of patients with decubitus ulcers. Chronically ill and immunocompromised patients have an increased risk of gram-negative bacteremia. They may also develop bacteremia with gram-positive cocci and anaerobes, and are at risk of fungemia. Staphylococcal bacteremia is common among injection drug users and patients with IV catheters. *Bacteroides* bacteremia may develop in patients with infections of the abdomen and the pelvis, particularly the female genital tract. If an infection in the abdomen causes bacteremia, the organism is most likely a gram-negative bacillus. If an infection above the diaphragm causes bacteremia, the organism is most likely gram-positive.

Pathophysiology

Transient or sustained bacteremia can cause metastatic infection of the meninges or serous cavities, such as the pericardium or larger joints. Metastatic abscesses may occur almost anywhere. Multiple abscess formation is especially common with staphylococcal bacteremia.

Bacteremia may cause endocarditis, most commonly with enterococcal, streptococcal, or staphylococcal bacteremia and less commonly with gram-negative bacteremia or fungemia. Patients with structural heart disease (eg, valvular disease, certain congenital anomalies), prosthetic heart valves, or other intravascular prostheses are predisposed to endocarditis. Staphylococci can cause bacterial endocarditis, particularly in injection drug users, and usually involving the tricuspid valve.

Symptoms and Signs

Some patients are asymptomatic or have only mild fever.

Development of symptoms such as tachypnea, shaking chills, persistent fever, altered sensorium, hypotension, and GI symptoms (abdominal pain, nausea, vomiting, diarrhea) suggests sepsis or septic shock. Septic shock develops in 25 to 40% of patients with significant bacteremia. Sustained bacteremia may cause metastatic focal infection or sepsis.

Diagnosis

- Cultures

If bacteremia, sepsis, or septic shock is suspected, cultures of blood and any other appropriate specimens are obtained.

Treatment

- Antibiotics

In patients with suspected bacteremia, empiric antibiotics are given after appropriate cultures are obtained. Early treatment of bacteremia with an appropriate antimicrobial regimen appears to improve survival.

Continuing therapy involves adjusting antibiotics according to the results of culture and susceptibility testing, surgically draining any abscesses, and usually removing any internal devices that are the suspected source of bacteria.

KEY POINTS

- Bacteremia is often transient and of no consequence, but sustained bacteremia may cause metastatic focal infection or sepsis.
- Bacteremia is more common after invasive procedures, particularly those involving indwelling devices or material.
- If bacteremia is suspected, give empiric antibiotics after cultures of potential sources and blood are obtained.

179 Laboratory Diagnosis of Infectious Disease

Laboratory tests may identify organisms directly (eg, visually, using a microscope, growing the organism in culture) or indirectly (eg, identifying antibodies to the organism). General types of tests include

- Microscopy
- Culture
- Immunologic tests (agglutination tests such as latex agglutination, enzyme immunoassays, Western blot, precipitation tests, and complement fixation tests)
- Nucleic acid–based identification methods
- Non-nucleic acid–based identification methods

Culture is normally the gold standard for identification of organisms, but results may not be available for days or weeks, and not all pathogens can be cultured, making alternative tests useful. When a pathogen is cultured and identified, the laboratory can also assess its susceptibility to antimicrobial drugs. Sometimes molecular methods can be used to detect specific resistance genes.

Some tests (eg, Gram stain, routine aerobic culture) can detect a large variety of pathogens and are commonly done for many suspected infectious illnesses. However, because some pathogens are missed on these tests, clinicians must be aware of the limitations of each test for each suspected pathogen. In such cases, clinicians should request tests specific for the suspected pathogen (eg, special stains or culture media) or advise the laboratory to select more specific tests.

MICROSCOPY

Microscopy can be done quickly, but accuracy depends on the experience of the microscopist and quality of equipment. Regulations often limit physicians' use of microscopy for diagnostic purposes outside a certified laboratory. Microscopic examination of tissue may be required to distinguish invasive disease from surface colonization—a distinction not easily achieved by culture methods.

Most specimens are treated with stains that color pathogens, causing them to stand out from the background, although wet mounts of unstained samples can be used to detect fungi, parasites (including helminth eggs and larvae), vaginal clue cells, motile organisms (eg, *Trichomonas*), and syphilis (*Treponema* spirochetes, via darkfield microscopy). Visibility of fungi can be increased by applying 10% potassium hydroxide (KOH) to dissolve surrounding tissues and nonfungal organisms.

The clinician orders a stain based on the likely pathogens, but no stain is 100% specific. Most samples are treated with Gram stain and, if mycobacteria are suspected, with an acid-fast stain. However, some pathogens are not easily visible using these stains; if these pathogens are suspected, different stains or other identification methods are required. Because microscopic detection usually requires a microbe concentration of at least about $1 \times 10^{4\text{-}5}$/mL, most body fluid specimens (eg, CSF) are concentrated (eg, by centrifugation) before examination.

Gram stain: The Gram stain does the following:

- Classifies bacteria according to whether they retain crystal violet stain (gram-positive—blue) or not (gram-negative—red)
- Highlights cell morphology (eg, bacilli, cocci) and cell arrangement (eg, clumps, chains, diploids)

Such characteristics can direct antibiotic therapy pending definitive identification. Finding a mixture of microorganisms with multiple morphologies and staining characteristics on Gram stain suggests a contaminated specimen or a polymicrobial bacterial infection.

To do a Gram stain, technicians heat-fix specimen material to a slide and stain it by sequential exposure to Gram crystal violet, iodine, decolorizer, and counterstain (typically safranin).

Acid-fast and modified acid-fast stains: These stains are used to identify the following:

- Acid-fast organisms (*Mycobacterium* sp)
- Moderately acid-fast organisms (primarily *Nocardia* sp)
- *Rhodococcus* and related genera
- Oocysts of some parasites (eg, *Cryptosporidium*, *Cystoisospora [Isospora] belli*)

Although detection of mycobacteria in sputum requires at least 10,000 organisms/mL, mycobacteria are often present in lower levels, so sensitivity is limited. Usually, several mL of sputum are decontaminated with sodium hydroxide and concentrated by centrifugation for acid-fast staining. Specificity is better, although some moderately acid-fast organisms are difficult to distinguish from mycobacteria.

Fluorescent stains: These stains allow detection at lower concentrations ($< 1 \times 10^4$ cells/mL). Examples are

- Acridine orange (bacteria and fungi)
- Auramine-rhodamine and auramine O (mycobacteria)
- Calcofluor white (fungi, especially dermatophytes)

Coupling a fluorescent dye to an antibody directed at a pathogen (direct or indirect immunofluorescence) should theoretically increase sensitivity and specificity. However, these tests are difficult to read and interpret, and few (eg, *Pneumocystis* and *Legionella* direct fluorescent antibody tests) are commercially available and commonly used.

India ink (colloidal carbon) stain: This stain is used to detect mainly *Cryptococcus neoformans* and other encapsulated fungi in a cell suspension (eg, CSF sediment). The background field, rather than the organism itself, is stained, making any capsule around the organism visible as a halo. In CSF, the test is not as sensitive as cryptococcal antigen. Specificity is also limited; leukocytes may appear encapsulated.

Warthin-Starry stain and Dieterle stain: These silver stains are used to visualize bacteria such as

- Spirochetes
- *Helicobacter pylori*
- Microsporidia
- *Bartonella henselae* (the cause of cat-scratch disease)

Wright stain and Giemsa stain: These stains are used for detection of the following:

- Parasites in blood
- *Histoplasma capsulatum* in phagocytes and tissue cells
- Intracellular inclusions formed by viruses and chlamydia
- Trophozoites of *Pneumocystis jirovecii*
- Some intracellular bacteria

Trichrome stain (Gomori-Wheatley stain) and iron hematoxylin stain: These stains are used to detect intestinal protozoa.

The **Gomori-Wheatley stain** is used to detect microsporidia. It may miss helminth eggs and larvae and does not reliably identify *Cryptosporidium*. Fungi and human cells take up the stain.

The **iron hematoxylin stain** differentially stains cells, cell inclusions, and nuclei. Helminth eggs may stain too dark to permit identification.

CULTURE

Culture is microbial growth on or in a nutritional solid or liquid medium; increased numbers of organisms simplify identification. Culture also facilitates testing of antimicrobial susceptibility.

Communication with the laboratory is essential. Although most specimens are placed on general purpose media (eg, blood or chocolate agar), some pathogens require inclusion of specific nutrients and inhibitors or other special conditions (see Table 179–1); if one of these pathogens is suspected or if the patient has been taking antimicrobials, the laboratory should be advised. The specimen's source is reported so that the laboratory can differentiate pathogens from site-specific normal flora.

Specimen collection: Specimen collection is important. For diagnosis of infectious disease, the rule of thumb is sample where the infection is. For lesions, the leading edge, not the center, should be sampled.

Use of swabs is discouraged. However, if a swab is used, a flocked swab is preferred because it can recover more specimen. Swabs used for molecular assays (see p. 1447) must be compatible for the specific molecular assay for which they are intended. The wrong type of swab can produce false-negative results. Wooden-shafted swabs are toxic to some viruses. Cotton-tipped swabs are toxic for some bacteria, including chlamydiae.

Blood cultures require decontamination and disinfection of the skin (eg, povidone iodine swab, allowed to dry, removed with 70% alcohol). Multiple samples, each from a different site are generally used; they are taken nearly simultaneously with fever spikes if possible. Normal flora of skin and mucous membranes that grows in only a single blood sample is usually interpreted as contamination. If a blood specimen is obtained from a central line, a peripheral blood specimen should also be obtained to help differentiate systemic bacteremia from catheter infection. Cultures from infected catheters generally turn positive more quickly and contain more organisms than simultaneously drawn peripheral blood cultures. Some fungi, particularly molds (eg, *Aspergillus* spp), usually cannot be cultured from blood.

The specimen must be transported rapidly, in the correct medium, and in conditions that limit growth of any potentially contaminating normal flora. For accurate quantification of the pathogen, additional pathogen growth must be prevented; specimens should be transported to the laboratory immediately or, if transport is delayed, refrigerated (in most cases).

Special considerations for culture: Certain cultures have special considerations.

Anaerobic bacteria should not be cultured from sites where they are normal flora because differentiation of pathogens from normal flora may be impossible. Specimens must be shielded from air, which can be difficult. For swab specimens, anaerobic

Table 179–1. SELECTIVE MEDIA FOR ISOLATION OF COMMON BACTERIA

ORGANISM	PREFERRED MEDIUM
Bacteroides sp	Kanamycin-vancomycin laked blood agar
Bacteroides fragilis	*Bacteroides* bile-esculin (with gentamicin and bile)
Bordetella pertussis	Bordet-Gengou agar plus methicillin or cephalexin Regan-Lowe cephalexin agar Horse blood–charcoal agar
Burkholderia cepacia	*Pseudomonas cepacia* agar
Campylobacter jejuni or *C. coli*	*Campylobacter*-selective agars (eg, cefoperazone-vancomycin agar)
Corynebacterium diphtheriae	Tinsdale agar Cystine-tellurite blood agar Löffler coagulated serum medium
Escherichia coli or enterohemorrhagic pathogens (Shiga toxin producers, including O157-H7)	MacConkey-sorbitol agar
Francisella tularensis	Blood- or chocolate-cystine agar
Legionella sp	Buffered charcoal yeast extract agar
Leptospira sp	Fletcher or Stuart medium with rabbit serum or *Leptospira* medium with bovine serum albumin-Tween 80
Neisseria gonorrhoeae or *N. meningitidis*	Modified Thayer-Martin agar New York City agar
Salmonella and *Shigella* sp	May grow on standard MacConkey or eosin-methylene blue Alternative: Hektoen or xylose-lysine-desoxycholate, *Salmonella-Shigella* agar, gram-negative or selenite enrichment broth
Vibrio sp	Thiosulfate-citrate-bile salts–sucrose agar
Yersinia sp	Cefsulodin-Irgasan-novobiocin agar

transport media are available. However, fluid specimens (eg, abscess contents) are superior to swab specimens for recovery of anaerobic bacteria. Fluid specimens should be collected with a syringe from which all air was expressed (to minimize contact of the specimen with oxygen) and sent to a laboratory in the syringe (capped without the needle) or transferred to an anaerobic transport vial.

Mycobacteria are difficult to culture. Specimens containing normal flora (eg, sputum) must first be decontaminated and concentrated. *Mycobacterium tuberculosis* and some other mycobacteria grow slowly. Growth of *M. tuberculosis* is typically faster in liquid than in solid media; routine use of automated systems with liquid media can result in growth within 2 wk vs ≥ 4 wk on solid media such as Lowenstein-Jensen agar. In addition, few organisms may be present in a specimen. Multiple specimens from the same site may help maximize yield. Specimens should be allowed to grow for 8 wk before being discarded. If an atypical mycobacterium is suspected, the laboratory should be notified.

Viruses are generally cultured from swabs and tissue specimens usually transported in media that contain antibacterial and antifungal agents. Specimens are inoculated onto tissue cultures that support the suspected virus and inhibit all other microbes. Viruses that are highly labile (eg, varicella zoster) should be inoculated onto tissue cultures within 1 h of collection. Standard tissue cultures are most sensitive. Rapid tissue cultures (shell vials) may provide more rapid results. Some common viruses cannot be detected using routine culture methods and require alternative methods for diagnosis (see Table 179–2), as for the following:

- Enzyme immunoassay for Epstein-Barr virus, hepatitis B and E viruses, HIV, and human T-lymphotropic virus
- Serologic tests for hepatitis A and D viruses
- Nucleic acid–based methods for HIV

Fungi specimens obtained from nonsterile sites must be inoculated onto media containing antibacterial agents. Specimens should be allowed to grow for 3 to 4 wk before being discarded.

SUSCEPTIBILITY TESTING

Susceptibility tests determine a microbe's vulnerability to antimicrobial drugs by exposing a standardized concentration of organism to specific concentrations of antimicrobial drugs. Susceptibility testing can be done for bacteria, fungi, and viruses. For some organisms, results obtained with one drug predict results with similar drugs. Thus, not all potentially useful drugs are tested.

Susceptibility testing occurs in vitro and may not account for many in vivo factors (eg, pharmacodynamics and pharmacokinetics, site-specific drug concentrations, host immune status, site-specific host defenses) that influence treatment success. Thus, susceptibility test results do not always predict treatment outcome.

TABLE 179–2. DIAGNOSTIC TESTS FOR COMMON VIRUSES THAT DO NOT GROW IN ROUTINE VIRAL CULTURES

COMMON CONDITIONS	VIRUS	DIAGNOSTIC TESTS
Acute febrile illness, meningoencephalitis	Alphavirus, flaviviruses, bunyaviruses (eg, St. Louis encephalitis virus, La Crosse encephalitis virus)	EIA, nucleic acid–based methods
Diarrhea	Rotaviruses, caliciviruses (noroviruses), astroviruses	EM or IEM, nucleic acid–based methods
Infectious mononucleosis	Epstein-Barr virus	EIA, nucleic acid–based methods
Hemorrhagic fevers, lymphocytic choriomeningitis	Filoviruses, arenaviruses (eg, Lassa fever, Ebola virus)	EM, nucleic acid–based methods
Hepatitis	Hepatitis A, hepatitis D	Serologic testing, nucleic acid–based methods
	Hepatitis B, hepatitis E	EIA, nucleic acid–based methods
	Hepatitis C, hepatitis G	Nucleic acid–based methods, EIA
Roseola, Kaposi sarcoma, disseminated infections	Herpesviruses 6, 7, 8	Nucleic acid–based methods, EIA
AIDS	HIV	Nucleic acid–based methods, EIA, Western blot
Condylomata acuminata, genital skin cancer	Human papillomaviruses	Nucleic-acid–based methods, EIA
Fifth disease	Human parvovirus B19	Nucleic acid–based methods, EIA
Adult T-cell leukemia	Human T-lymphotropic virus	EIA, nucleic acid–based methods
Progressive multifocal leukoencephalopathy, kidney infection	Polyoma viruses (JC and BK)	Nucleic acid–based methods
Smallpox, monkeypox, vaccinia, molluscum contagiosum	Poxviruses	Nucleic acid–based methods, EM, culture depending on virus
Rabies	Rabies virus	EM, IFA, nucleic acid–based methods
Rubella	Rubella virus	EIA, IFA, nucleic acid–based methods

EIA = enzyme immunoassay; EM = electron microscopy; IEM = immunoelectron microscopy; IFA = immunofluorescence assay.

Susceptibility testing can be done qualitatively, semiquantitatively, or using nucleic acid–based methods. Testing can also determine the effect of combining different antimicrobials (synergy testing).

Qualitative methods: Qualitative methods are less precise than semiquantitative. Results are usually reported as one of the following:

- Susceptible (S)
- Intermediate (I)
- Resistant (R)

Some strains that do not have established criteria for resistance may be reported only as susceptible or nonsusceptible. Establishment of which specific drug concentrations represent S, I, and R is based on multiple factors, particularly pharmacokinetic, pharmacodynamic, clinical, and microbiologic data.

The commonly used **disk diffusion method** (also known as the Kirby-Bauer test) is appropriate for rapidly growing organisms. It places antibiotic-impregnated disks on agar plates inoculated with the test organism. After incubation (typically 16 to 18 h), the diameter of the zone of inhibition around each disk is measured. Each organism-antibiotic combination has different diameters signifying S, I, or R.

Other methods that require less rigid adherence to test parameters can be used to rapidly screen for resistance of a single organism to a single drug or drug class or to specific antimicrobial combinations (eg, oxacillin resistance of methicillin-resistant *Staphylococcus aureus*, β-lactamase production).

Semiquantitative methods: Semiquantitative methods determine the minimal concentration of a drug that inhibits growth of a particular organism in vitro. This minimum inhibitory concentration (MIC) is reported as a numerical value that may then be translated to 1 of 4 groupings: S (sensitive), I (intermediate), R (resistant), or sometimes nonsusceptible. MIC determination is used primarily for isolates of bacteria, including mycobacteria and anaerobes, and sometimes for fungi, especially *Candida* sp.

Minimal killing (bactericidal) concentration (MBC) can also be determined but is technically difficult, and standards for interpretation have not been agreed on. The value of MBC testing is that it indicates whether a drug may be bacteriostatic or bactericidal.

The antibiotic can be diluted in agar or broth, which is then inoculated with the organism. Broth dilution is the gold standard but is labor intensive because only one drug concentration can be tested per tube. A more efficient method uses a strip of polyester film impregnated with antibiotic in a concentration gradient along its length. The strip is laid on an agar plate containing the inoculum, and the MIC is determined by the location on the strip where inhibition begins; multiple antibiotics can be tested on one plate.

The MIC allows correlation between drug susceptibility of the organism and the achievable tissue concentration of free drug (ie, drug not bound to protein). If the tissue concentration of free drug is higher than the MIC, successful treatment is likely. Designations of S, I, and R derived from the MIC study usually correlate with achievable serum, plasma, or urine concentrations of free drug.

Nucleic acid–based methods: These tests incorporate nucleic acid techniques similar to those used for organism identification but modified to detect known resistance genes or mutations. An example is *mecA*, a gene for oxacillin resistance in *S. aureus*; if this gene is present, the organism is considered resistant to most beta-lactam drugs regardless of apparent susceptibility results. However, although a number of such genes are known, their presence does not uniformly confer in vivo resistance. Also, because new mutations or other resistance genes may be present, their absence does not guarantee drug susceptibility. For these reasons, routine, phenotypic susceptibility testing methods remain the standard approach for assessing susceptibility of bacteria and fungi to antimicrobial drugs. However, nucleic acid methods are preferred for rapid diagnosis of multidrug resistant TB in at-risk groups and for rapid detection of possible resistance in organisms directly obtained from positive blood cultures.

IMMUNOLOGIC TESTS FOR INFECTIOUS DISEASE

Immunologic tests use one of the following:

- **Antigen** to detect antibodies to a pathogen in the patient's specimen
- **Antibody** to detect an antigen of the pathogen in the patient's specimen

Specimen handling varies, but if testing is to be delayed, the specimen should typically be refrigerated or frozen to prevent overgrowth of bacterial contaminants.

Agglutination tests: In agglutination tests (eg, latex agglutination, coaggregation), a particle (latex bead, gelatin particles, bacterium) is coupled to a reagent antigen or antibody. The resulting particle complex is mixed with the specimen (eg, CSF, serum); if the target antibody or antigen is present in the specimen, it cross-links the particles, producing measurable agglutination.

If results are positive, the body fluid is serially diluted and tested. Agglutination with more dilute solutions indicates higher concentrations of the target antigen or antibody. The titer is correctly reported as the reciprocal of the most dilute solution yielding agglutination (eg, 32 indicates that agglutination occurred in a solution diluted to 1/32 of the starting concentration).

Usually, agglutination tests are rapid but less sensitive than many other methods. They can also determine serotypes of some bacteria.

Complement fixation: This test measures complement-consuming (complement-fixing) antibody in serum or CSF. The test is used for diagnosis of some viral and fungal infections, particularly coccidioidomycosis.

The specimen is incubated with known quantities of complement and the antigen that is the target of the antibody being measured. The degree of complement fixation indicates the relative quantity of the antibody in the specimen.

The test can measure IgM and IgG antibody titers or can be modified to detect certain antigens. It is accurate but has limited applications, is labor intensive, and requires numerous controls.

Enzyme immunoassays: These tests use antibodies linked to enzymes to detect antigens and to detect and quantify antibodies. The enzyme immunoassay (EIA) and enzyme-linked immunosorbent assay (ELISA) are examples.

Because sensitivities of most enzyme immunoassays are high, they are usually used for screening. Titers can be determined by serially diluting the specimen as for agglutination tests.

Test sensitivities, although usually high, can vary, sometimes according to patient age, microbial serotype, specimen type, or stage of clinical disease.

Precipitation tests: These tests measure an antigen or antibody in body fluids by the degree of visible precipitation of antigen-antibody complexes within a gel (agarose) or in solution. There are many types of precipitation tests (eg, Ouchterlony double diffusion, counterimmunoelectrophoresis), but their applications are limited.

Usually, a blood specimen is mixed with test antigen to detect patient antibodies, most often in suspected fungal infection or pyogenic meningitis. Because a positive result requires a large amount of antibody or antigen, sensitivity is low.

Western blot test: This test detects antimicrobial antibodies in the patient's sample (eg, serum, other body fluid) by their reaction with target antigens (eg, viral components) that have been immobilized onto a membrane by blotting.

The Western blot typically has good sensitivity, although often less than that of screening tests such as ELISA, but generally is highly specific. Thus, it is usually used to confirm a positive result obtained with a screening test.

Technical modifications of the Western blot are

- The line immunoassay (LIA)
- The recombinant immunoblot assay (RIBA), which uses synthetic or recombinant-produced antigens
- Immunochromatographic assays, which can rapidly screen specimens for specific microbial antigens or patient antibodies

Of the three, the immunochromatographic assay is easiest to do and the most commonly used—eg, to detect Shiga toxin–producing microorganisms, *Cryptococcus neoformans* capsular antigen, and influenza virus.

NON-NUCLEIC ACID–BASED IDENTIFICATION METHODS FOR INFECTIOUS DISEASE

Once an organism has been isolated by culture, it must be identified. Non-nucleic acid–based identification methods use phenotypic (functional or morphologic) characteristics of organisms rather than genetic identification.

Characteristics of an organism's growth on culture media, such as colony size, color, and shape, provide clues to species identification and, combined with Gram stain, direct further testing.

Numerous biochemical tests are available; each is restricted to organisms of a certain type (eg, aerobic or anaerobic bacteria). Some assess an organism's ability to use different substrates for growth. Others assess presence or activity of key enzymes (eg, coagulase, catalase). Tests are done sequentially, with previous results determining the next test to be used. The sequences of tests are myriad and differ somewhat among laboratories.

Non-nucleic acid–based identification tests may involve manual methods, automated systems, or chromatographic methods. Some commercially available kits contain a battery of individual tests that may be done simultaneously using a single inoculum of a microorganism and may be useful for a wider range of organisms. Multiple test systems can be highly accurate but may require several days to yield results.

Chromatographic methods: Microbial components or products are separated and identified using high-performance liquid chromatography (HPLC) or gas chromatography. Usually, identification is by comparison of an organism's fatty acids to a database.

Chromatographic methods can be used to identify aerobic and anaerobic bacteria, mycobacteria, and fungi. Test accuracy depends on the conditions used to culture the specimen and the quality of the database, which may be inaccurate or incomplete.

Mass spectroscopy: Mass spectrometry can detect various proteins of different masses in a specimen. Specific pathogens have unique proteins, and the relative mass and abundance of each protein can sometimes be used to identify a microorganism. Mass spectroscopy is one of a number of innovative technologies that are being or have been developed for detection and identification of biological warfare and bioterrorism agents. However, this method is limited because it, unlike some nucleic acid–based methods, is not readily deployable in the field.

Currently, a form of mass spectrometry called matrix-assisted laser desorption ionization–time of flight (MALDI-TOF) is being used to identify bacteria (including mycobacteria), yeasts, molds, and potentially viruses. The advantage of this method is that microorganisms can be identified in < 1 h; traditional methods may require 24 to 48 h.

NUCLEIC ACID–BASED IDENTIFICATION METHODS FOR INFECTIOUS DISEASE

Nucleic acid–based (molecular) identification has become commonplace in clinical settings; the resulting rapid identification allows the patient to be placed on specific antimicrobial therapy and avoid prolonged management on empiric, potentially inappropriate drugs.

Nucleic acid–based methods detect organism-specific DNA or RNA sequences extracted from the microorganism. Sequences may or may not be amplified in vitro.

Nucleic acid–based methods are generally specific and highly sensitive and can be used for all categories of microbes. Results can be provided rapidly. Because each test typically is specific to a single organism, the clinician must know the diagnostic possibilities and request tests accordingly. For example, if a patient has symptoms suggesting influenza but the influenza season is over, doing a more general viral diagnostic test (eg, viral culture) rather than a specific flu test is better because another virus (eg, parainfluenza, adenovirus) may be the cause.

Recent advances have led to the development of multiplex assays, in which a single nucleic acid–based test can detect and differentiate between ≥ 2 causative microorganisms. Multiplex assays are usually less sensitive than single-target, qualitative assays. Multiplex assays are currently available for detecting biological warfare agents.

Nucleic acid–based tests are qualitative, but quantification methods exist for a limited but increasing number of infections (eg, HIV, cytomegalovirus, human T-cell lymphotropic virus); these methods can be useful for diagnosis and for monitoring response to treatment.

Unamplified testing: Techniques that target nucleic acid sequences but do not require amplification of those sequences are usually restricted to situations in which the organism has been first cultured or is present in high concentration in the specimen (eg, in pharyngitis caused by group A *Streptococcus*, in genital infections caused by *Chlamydia trachomatis* or *Neisseria gonorrhoeae*).

Amplification: Nucleic acid amplification techniques take tiny amounts of DNA or RNA, replicate them many times, and thus can detect minute traces of an organism in a specimen, avoiding the need for culture. These techniques are particularly useful for organisms that are difficult to culture or identify using other methods (eg, viruses, obligate intracellular pathogens, fungi, mycobacteria, some other bacteria) or that are present in low numbers.

These tests may involve

- Target amplification (eg, PCR, reverse transcriptase–PCR [RT-PCR], strand displacement amplification, transcription amplification)
- Signal amplification (eg, branched DNA assays, hybrid capture)
- Probe amplification (eg, ligase chain reaction, cleavase-invader, cycling probes)
- Postamplification analysis (eg, sequencing of the amplified product, microarray analysis, and melting curve analysis, as is done in real-time PCR).

Appropriate specimen collection and storage before arrival at the molecular diagnostic laboratory are critical. Because amplification methods are so sensitive, false-positive results from trace contamination of the specimen or equipment can easily occur.

Despite high sensitivity, false-negative results sometimes occur even when a patient is symptomatic (eg, in West Nile virus infection). False-negative results can be minimized by the following:

- Avoiding use of swabs with wooden shafts or cotton tips (the swab that has been validated for the amplification assay must be used)
- Transporting specimens rapidly
- Freezing or refrigerating specimens if transport is likely to take > 2 h

Freezing is the typical storage method for nucleic acid amplification assays. However, specimens should be refrigerated rather than frozen if labile viruses (eg, varicella-zoster virus, influenza virus, HIV-2) are suspected or if viral cultures are also to be done (frozen specimens may not be usable for standard cultures).

180 Immunization

Immunity can be achieved

- Actively by using antigens (eg, vaccines, toxoids)
- Passively by using antibodies (eg, immune globulins, antitoxins)

A **toxoid** is a bacterial toxin that has been modified to be nontoxic but that can still stimulate antibody formation.

A **vaccine** is a suspension of whole (live or inactivated) or fractionated bacteria or viruses rendered nonpathogenic. For vaccines available in the US, see Table 180–1.

The most current recommendations for immunization are available on the Centers for Disease Control and Prevention (CDC) web site (www.cdc.gov) and free mobile app. See also Table 180–2 and Tables 291–2 and 291–3 on pp. 2462 and 2467 (CDC's Childhood Immunization Schedule). For the contents of each vaccine (including additives), see that vaccine's package insert.

Vaccination has been extremely effective in preventing serious disease and in improving health worldwide. Because of vaccines, infections that were once very common and/or fatal (eg, smallpox, polio, measles, diphtheria) are now rare or have been eliminated. However, these infections still occur in parts of the developing world.

Effective vaccines are not yet available for many important infections, including

- Most sexually transmitted diseases (eg, HIV, herpes, syphilis, gonorrhea, chlamydial infections)
- Tick-borne infections (eg, Lyme disease, ehrlichiosis and anaplasmosis, babesiosis)
- Many tropical diseases (eg, malaria, Chikungunya disease, dengue)
- Emerging diseases (eg, Ebola hemorrhagic fever, West Nile virus infection)

Certain vaccines are recommended routinely for all adults at certain ages who have not previously been vaccinated or have no evidence of previous infection. Other vaccines (eg, rabies, BCG, typhoid, yellow fever) are not routinely given but are recommended only for specific people and circumstances (see the Centers for Disease Control and Prevention's [CDC's] Recommended Adult Immunization Schedule and under the specific disorder, elsewhere in THE MANUAL).

Some adults do not get the vaccines recommended for them. For example, only 55.1% of those > 65 were given a tetanus vaccine within a 10-yr period. Also, vaccination rates tend to be lower in blacks, Asians, and Hispanics than in whites.

Vaccine Administration

Vaccines should be given exactly as recommended on the package insert; however, for most vaccines, the interval between a series of doses may be lengthened without losing efficacy.

Injection vaccines are usually given IM into the midlateral thigh (in infants and toddlers) or into the deltoid muscle (in school-aged children and adults). Some vaccines are given sc. For details on vaccine administration, see the CDC's Vaccination Administration Recommendations and Guidelines at www.cdc.gov and the Immunization Action Coalition's Administering Vaccines to Adults at www.immunize.org.

Clinicians should have a process in place to ensure that patient vaccination status is reviewed at each visit so that vaccines are given as per recommendations. Patients (or caregivers) should be encouraged to keep a history (written or electronic) of their vaccinations and share this information with new health care practitioners and institutions to make sure that vaccinations are up to date.

PEARLS & PITFALLS

- If a vaccine series is interrupted, practitioners should give the next recommended dose the next time the patient presents, provided that the recommended interval between doses has passed; they should not restart the series (ie, with dose 1).

If a vaccine series (eg, for hepatitis B or human papillomavirus) is interrupted, practitioners should give the next recommended dose the next time the patient presents, provided that the recommended interval between doses has passed. They should not restart the series (ie, with dose 1).

Simultaneous administration of different vaccines: With rare exceptions, simultaneous administration is safe, effective, and convenient (see p. 2466); it is particularly recommended when children may be unavailable for future vaccination or when adults require multiple simultaneous vaccines (eg, before international travel). An exception is simultaneous administration of pneumococcal conjugate vaccine (PCV13) and the meningococcal conjugate vaccine MenACWY-D (Menactra®) to children with functional or anatomic asplenia; these vaccinations should not be given during the same visit but should be separated by ≥ 4 wk.

Simultaneous administration may involve combination vaccines (see Table 180–1) or use of ≥ 1 single-antigen vaccines. More than one vaccine may be given at the same time using different injection sites and syringes.

If live-virus vaccines (varicella and MMR) are not given at the same time, they should be given ≥ 4 wk apart.

Restrictions, Precautions, and High-Risk Groups

Restrictions and **precautions** are conditions that increase the risk of an adverse reaction to a vaccine or that compromise the ability of a vaccine to produce immunity. These conditions are usually temporary, meaning the vaccine can be given later.

Table 180–1. VACCINES AVAILABLE IN THE US

VACCINE	TYPE	ROUTE
Anthrax	Inactivated bacteria	sc
BCG (for tuberculosis)	Live *Mycobacteria bovis*	Intradermal or sc
Cholera	Live-attenuated vaccine	Oral
Diphtheria-tetanus-acellular pertussis (DTaP or Tdap)	Toxoids and inactivated bacterial components	IM
DTaP plus *Haemophilus influenzae* type b conjugate (DTaP-Hib)	Toxoids, inactivated whole bacteria, and bacterial polysaccharide conjugated to protein	IM
DTaP-hepatitis B-polio (DTaP-HepB-IPV)	Toxoids, recombinant viral antigen, and inactivated poliovirus	IM
DTaP-IPV	Toxoids, inactivated bacteria, and inactivated poliovirus	IM
DTaP-IPV-Hib	Toxoids, inactivated bacteria, inactivated poliovirus, and bacterial polysaccharide conjugated to protein	IM
Haemophilus influenzae type b conjugate (Hib)	Bacterial polysaccharide conjugated to protein	IM
Hepatitis A (HepA)	Inactivated virus	IM
Hepatitis B (HepB)	Recombinant viral antigen	IM
Hepatitis A and hepatitis B	Inactivated virus plus recombinant viral antigens	IM
HbCV plus Hep B	Bacterial polysaccharide conjugate plus inactivated viral antigen	IM
Human papillomavirus (HPV)	Noninfectious viruslike particles	IM
Influenza	Live influenza A and B virus	Intranasal
Influenza, types A and B	Inactivated virus or viral components	IM or intradermal
Japanese encephalitis	Inactivated virus	sc
Measles-mumps-rubella (MMR)	Live viruses	sc
Measles-mumps-rubella-varicella (MMRV)	Live viruses	sc
Meningococcal, polysaccharide (MPSV4)	Bacterial polysaccharides of serogroups A/C/Y/W-135	sc
Meningococcal, conjugate (MenACWY)	Bacterial polysaccharides of serogroups A, C, Y, and W-135 conjugated to diphtheria toxoid protein	IM
Meningococcal group B (MenB)	Recombinant vaccine composed of two LP2086 antigens (factor H–binding proteins)	IM
Pneumococcal, polysaccharide (PPSV23)	Bacterial polysaccharides of 23 pneumococcal types	IM or sc
Pneumococcal, conjugate (PCV13)	Polysaccharides of 13 types, conjugated to diphtheria toxin	IM
Poliovirus (IPV)	Inactivated viruses of all 3 serotypes	IM
Rabies	Inactivated virus	Intradermal* or sc
Rotavirus	Live virus	Oral
Smallpox	Live vaccinia virus	Intradermal via multiple puncture device
Tetanus	Inactivated toxin (toxoid)	IM†
Tetanus and diphtheria toxoids adsorbed (Td)‡ or diphtheria-tetanus (DT)	Inactivated toxins (toxoids)	IM†
Tuberculosis (see BCG)	—	
Typhoid	Capsular polysaccharide	IM
Typhoid	Live-attenuated vaccine	Oral
Varicella	Live virus	sc
Zoster (shingles)	Live virus	sc
Yellow fever	Live virus	sc

*Intradermal dose is lower and used only for preexposure vaccination.
†Preparations with adjuvants should be given IM.
‡Td contains the same amount of tetanus toxoid as DTP or DT but a reduced dose of diphtheria toxoid.
Modified from the Vaccine Recommendations of the Advisory Committee for Immunization Practices (ACIP). Accessed 12/11/14.

Table 180–2. VACCINE ADMINISTRATION GUIDELINES FOR ADULTS

PARAMETER	NEEDLE SIZE	COMMENTS
By route		
sc	23–25 gauge 5/8" long	The needle should be inserted into fatty tissue over the triceps.
IM	23–25 gauge for injection into the deltoid	Needle length is determined by sex and weight (see below).
By sex and weight for IM injection		
Male or female, < 60 kg	5/8–1" long	A 5/8" needle may be used for IM injection in the deltoid muscle only if subcutaneous tissue is not bunched and injection is made at a 90° angle.
Females, 60–90 kg	1–1.5" long	—
Males, 60–118 kg	1–1.5" long	—
Females, > 90 kg	1.5" long	—
Males, > 118 kg	1.5" long	—

Sometimes vaccination is indicated when a precaution exists because the protective effects of the vaccine outweigh the risk of an adverse reaction to the vaccine.

Contraindications are conditions that increases the risk of a serious adverse reaction. A vaccine should not be given when a contraindication is present.

Allergy: For many vaccines, the only contraindication is a serious allergic reaction (eg, anaphylactic reaction) to the vaccine or to one of its components.

Egg allergy is common in the US. Some vaccines produced in cell culture systems, including most influenza vaccines (see p. 1455), contain trace amounts of egg antigens; thus, there is concern about using such vaccines in patients who are allergic to eggs. CDC guidelines for the influenza vaccine state that although mild reactions may occur, serious allergic reactions (ie, anaphylaxis) are unlikely, and vaccination with inactivated influenza vaccine (IIV) is contraindicated only in patients who have had anaphylaxis after a previous dose of any influenza vaccine or to a vaccine component, including egg protein. Live influenza vaccine is not recommended for patients with a history of any egg allergy. Patients with a history of less severe reactions to eggs (eg, hives) may be given an egg-prepared, IIV provided the clinician has experience managing allergic reactions and observes the patient for 30 min after vaccination.

Asplenia: Asplenic patients are predisposed to overwhelming bacteremic infection, primarily due to encapsulated organisms such as *Streptococcus pneumoniae*, *Neisseria meningitidis*, or *Haemophilus influenzae* type b (Hib). Asplenic adults should be given the following vaccines (before splenectomy if possible):

- Hib conjugate vaccine (HbCV): A single dose and no booster
- Meningococcal conjugate vaccine (MenACY—see p. 1452): 2 doses 8 to 12 wk apart and boosters every 5 yr
- Pneumococcal conjugate (PCV13) and polysaccharide vaccines (PPSV23): PCV13 if patients did not receive a full series previously as a routine vaccination, then PPSV23 8 wk later (≥ 2 wk before or after splenectomy) with a single PPSV23 booster after 5 yr and a routine booster dose at age 65 (see p. 1457)

Additional doses may be given based on clinical judgment.

Blood product use: Live-microbial vaccines should not be given simultaneously with blood or plasma transfusions or immune globulin; these products can interfere with development of desired antibodies. Ideally, live-microbial vaccines should be given 2 wk before or 6 to 12 wk after the immune globulins.

Fever or other acute illness: A significant fever (temperature of > 39° C) or severe illness without fever requires delaying vaccination, but minor infections, such as the common cold (even with low-grade fever), do not. This precaution prevents confusion between manifestations of the underlying illness and possible adverse effects of the vaccine and prevents superimposition of adverse effects of the vaccine on the underlying illness. Vaccination is postponed until the illness resolves, if possible.

Guillain-Barré syndrome: Patients who developed Guillain-Barré syndrome (GBS) within 6 wk after a previous influenza or DTaP vaccination may be given the vaccine if the benefits of vaccination are thought to outweigh the risks. For example, for patients who developed the syndrome after a dose of DTaP, clinicians may consider giving them a dose of the vaccine if a pertussis outbreak occurs; however, such decisions should be made in consultation with an infectious disease specialist.

The Advisory Committee on Immunization Practices (ACIP) no longer considers a history of GBS to be a precaution for use of the MenACY, although it remains listed as a precaution in the package insert.

Immunocompromise: Immunocompromised patients should, in general, not receive live-virus vaccines, which could provoke severe or fatal infections. If immunocompromise is caused by immunosuppressive therapy (eg, high-dose corticosteroids [≥ 20 mg prednisone or equivalent for ≥ 2 wk], antimetabolites, immune modulators, alkylating compounds, radiation), live-virus vaccines should be withheld until the immune system recovers after treatment (the interval of time varies depending on the therapy used). For patients receiving long-term immunosuppressive therapy, clinicians should discuss risks and benefits of vaccination and/or revaccination with an infectious disease specialist.

Patients with HIV infection should generally receive inactivated vaccines (eg, diphtheria-tetanus-acellular pertussis [Tdap], polio [IPV], Hib) according to routine recommendations. Despite the general caution against giving a live-virus vaccine, patients who have CD4 counts ≥ 200/μL (ie, are not severely immunocompromised) can be given certain live-virus vaccines, including measles-mumps-rubella (MMR). Patients with HIV infection should receive both pneumococcal conjugate and polysaccharide vaccines (and be revaccinated after 5 yr).

Live-virus vaccines: Live-microbial vaccines .should not be given simultaneously with blood, plasma, or immune globulin, which can interfere with development of desired antibodies; ideally, such vaccines should be given 2 wk before or 6 to 12 wk after the immune globulins.

Pregnancy: Pregnancy is a contraindication to vaccination with MMR, intranasal (live) influenza vaccine, varicella, and other live-virus vaccines. Vaccination with HPV vaccine is not recommended (see p. 1449).

Transplantation: Before solid organ transplantation, patients should receive all appropriate vaccines. Patients who have had allogeneic or autogeneic hematopoietic stem cell transplantation should be considered unimmunized and should receive repeat doses of all appropriate vaccines. Care of these patients is complex, and vaccination decisions for these patients should involve consultation with the patient's hematologist-oncologist and an infectious disease specialist.

Vaccine Safety

In the US, the safety of vaccines is ensured through several surveillance systems; selected events that occur after routine vaccination must be reported by mail, by fax, or electronically to the CDC's Vaccine Adverse Event Reporting System (VAERS) Vaccine Safety Datalink (VSD—see p. 2460). For additional information about the safety of individual vaccines, see Vaccine Safety at the CDC web site (www.cdc.gov).

Nonetheless, many parents remain concerned about the safety and possible adverse effects (particularly autism) of childhood vaccines. These concerns, perpetuated on the Internet, have led some parents to not allow their children to be given some or all of the recommended vaccines (see p. 2461). As a result, outbreaks of diseases made uncommon by vaccination (eg, measles, pertussis) are becoming more common among unvaccinated children in North America and Europe.

One of the main parental concerns is that vaccines may increase the risk of autism. Reasons cited include

- Use of the combination MMR vaccine (see p. 2461)
- Thimerosal, a mercury-based preservative used in some vaccines (see p. 2466)
- Use of multiple, simultaneous vaccines, given as recommended (see p. 2466)

In 1998, Andrew Wakefield and colleagues published a brief report in *The Lancet* (see p. 2461). In it, Wakefield postulated a link between the measles virus in the MMR vaccine and autism. This report received significant media attention worldwide, and many parents began to doubt the safety of the MMR vaccine. However, since then, *The Lancet* has retracted the report because it contained serious scientific flaws; many subsequent, large studies have failed to show any link between the vaccine and autism.

Gerbner and Offit reviewed epidemiologic and biologic studies concerning this issue and found no evidence to support an association between use of vaccines and risk of autism.[1] The US Institute of Medicine Immunization Safety Review Committee reviewed epidemiologic studies (published and unpublished) to determine whether the MMR vaccine and vaccines containing thimerosal cause autism and to identify possible biologic mechanisms for such an effect; based on the evidence, this group rejected a causal relationship between these vaccines and autism.[2]

At this time, virtually every vaccine given to children is thimerosal-free. Small amounts of thimerosal continue to be used in multidose vials of influenza vaccine and in several other vaccines intended for use in adults. For information about vaccines that contain low levels of mercury or thimerosal, see the FDA's web site (www.fda.gov) and Thimerosal Content in Some US Licensed Vaccines (www.vaccinesafety.edu). Thimerosal is also used in many vaccines produced in developing countries.

As with any treatment, clinicians should talk to their patients about the relative risks and benefits of recommended vaccines. In particular, clinicians must make sure that the parents of their patients are aware of the possible serious effects (including death) of vaccine-preventable childhood diseases such as measles, Hib infection, and pertussis, and clinicians discuss any concerns parents may have about vaccinating their children; resources for these discussions are available at the CDC web site (www.cdc.gov): Provider Resources for Vaccine Conversations with Parents (see also Talking with Parents about Vaccines for Infants and Some Common Misconceptions About Vaccination and How to Respond to Them).

1. Gerber JS, Offit PA: Vaccines and autism: a tale of shifting hypotheses. *Clin Infect Dis* 48(4):456–461, 2009.
2. Institute of Medicine: Immunization safety review: Vaccines and autism. Washington DC, National Academies Press, 2004.

Immunization for Travelers

Immunizations may be required for travel to areas where infectious diseases are endemic (see Table 383–3 on p. 3208). The CDC can provide this information; a telephone service (1-800-232-4636 [CDC-INFO]) and web site (www.cdc.gov) are available 24 h/day.

DIPHTHERIA-TETANUS-PERTUSSIS VACCINE

For more information, see DTaP ACIP (Advisory Committee on Immunization Practices) Vaccine Recommendations at www.cdc.gov.

Preparations

Diphtheria (D) vaccines contain toxoids prepared from *Corynebacterium diphtheriae*. Tetanus (T) vaccines contain toxoids prepared from *Clostridium tetani*. Acellular (a) pertussis (P) vaccines contain semipurified or purified components of *Bordetella pertussis*. Whole-cell pertussis vaccine is no longer available in the US because of concerns about adverse effects, but it is still available in other parts of the world. There are 2 preparations of the acellular vaccine:

- DTaP for children < 7 yr
- Tdap for adolescents and adults

Tdap contains lower doses of diphtheria and pertussis components (indicated by the lower case d and p).

Indications

DTaP is a routine childhood vaccination (see Table 291–2 on p. 2462).

Tdap is routinely given as a single lifetime dose to children at age 11 or 12 yr and to people ≥ 13 yr who have never received Tdap (regardless of the interval since the last tetanus-diphtheria [Td] vaccine—see p. 1452) or whose vaccine status is unknown.

Additional boosters of Tdap are also recommended for

- Pregnant women during *each* pregnancy (preferably at 27 to 36 wk gestation), regardless of the interval since any previous dose of Tdap
- Postpartum women who have never received Tdap and who were not vaccinated during pregnancy

Adults who require a tetanus toxoid-containing vaccine as part of wound management and who have not previously received Tdap are given Tdap instead of Td.

People who have had pertussis should still receive a pertussis-containing vaccine as per routine recommendations.

Contraindications and Precautions

Contraindications for DTaP and Tdap are

- A severe allergic reaction (eg, anaphylaxis) after a previous dose or to a vaccine component
- For the pertussis component: Encephalopathy (eg, coma, decreased level of consciousness, prolonged seizures) that occurred within 7 days of a previous dose of DTaP or Tdap and that is not attributable to another identifiable cause

Because tetanus vaccination is important, people who have had an anaphylactic reaction to components in DTaP or Tdap should be referred to an allergist to determine whether they are allergic to tetanus toxoid (TT). If not, they can be vaccinated with TT vaccine. Adults with a history of encephalopathy can be vaccinated with Td, and children can be given diphtheria-tetanus (DT) instead of Tdap.

Precautions vary depending on the formulation.

For DTaP and Tdap, they include

- Moderate or severe acute illness with or without fever (vaccination is postponed until illness resolves if possible)
- Guillain-Barré syndrome within 6 wk after a previous dose to a vaccine containing TT
- For the pertussis component only: A progressive or unstable neurologic disorder, uncontrolled seizures, or progressive encephalopathy (vaccination is postponed until a treatment regimen is established and the disorder is stabilized)

For DTaP only, precautions include

- A seizure, with or without fever, within 3 days after a previous dose of DTaP
- ≥ 3 h of persistent, severe, inconsolable screaming or crying within 48 h after a previous dose of DTaP
- Collapse or shock-like state (hypotonic hyporesponsive episode) within 48 h after a previous dose of DTaP
- Temperature of ≥ 40.5° C, unexplained by another cause, within 48 h after a previous dose of DTaP

For Tdap only, precautions include

- History of type III hypersensitivity reactions after a previous dose of a vaccine containing tetanus or diphtheria toxoid (vaccination is postponed ≥ 10 yr since the last dose of TT-containing vaccine)

Dose and Administration

The dose for DTaP or Tdap is 0.5 mL IM.

The DTaP vaccine is given as 5 primary and 1 booster IM injections during childhood as follows: at age 2 mo, 4 mo, 6 mo, 15 to 18 mo, and 4 to 6 yr (before school entry). The 5th dose is not necessary if the 4th dose was given at age ≥ 4 yr.

A single booster of Tdap is given, except for pregnant women, who should have a dose during each pregnancy.

Adverse Effects

Adverse effects are rare and are mostly attributable to the pertussis component. They include encephalopathy within 7 days; a seizure, with or without fever, within 3 days; ≥ 3 h of persistent, severe, inconsolable screaming or crying within 48 h; collapse or shock within 48 h; temperature of ≥ 40.5° C, unexplained by another cause, within 48 h; and immediate severe or anaphylactic reaction to the vaccine.

If the pertussis vaccine is contraindicated, a combined diphtheria and tetanus vaccine is available without the pertussis component (see below).

Mild adverse effects include redness, swelling, and soreness at the injection site.

TETANUS-DIPHTHERIA VACCINE

Preparations

The most widely used preparations combine tetanus toxoid (TT) with diphtheria toxoid (Td for adults; DT, which contains a higher dose of diphtheria toxoid, for children); a preparation with only TT is also available but is not recommended because periodic boosting is needed for both antigens. Tdap is an adult preparation that contains a pertussis component (see p. 1451).

Indications

Td boosters are given routinely every 10 yr after the Tdap booster is given at age 11 to 12 yr. Patients who have not received or completed a primary vaccination series of at least 3 doses of tetanus and diphtheria vaccine should begin or complete the series.

Patients who have a wound that poses an increased risk of tetanus (see Table 181–2 on p. 1472) should be given a Td booster if ≥ 5 yr have elapsed since the previous dose. One dose of Tdap should be substituted for a Td booster if adults have never received Tdap.

Contraindications and Precautions

The **main contraindication is**

- A severe allergic reaction (eg, anaphylaxis) after a previous dose or to a vaccine component

Precautions include

- Guillain-Barré syndrome within 6 wk after a previous dose of a vaccine that contains TT
- Moderate or severe acute illness with or without fever
- History of type III hypersensitivity reactions after a previous dose of a vaccine that contains tetanus or diphtheria toxoid (vaccination is postponed until ≥ 10 yr since the last dose of a vaccine that contains TT)

Dose and Administration

Td 0.5 mL IM is injected into the deltoid with a 22- to 25-gauge needle. Booster vaccinations are given every 10 yr.

Adverse Effects

Adverse effects are very rare. They include anaphylactic reactions and brachial neuritis. Mild effects include erythema, swelling, and soreness at the injection site.

MENINGOCOCCAL VACCINE

For more information, see Meningococcal ACIP (Advisory Committee for Immunization Practices) Vaccine Recommendations and Infant Meningococcal Vaccination update at www.cdc.gov.

The meningococcal serogroups that most often cause disease in the US are serogroups B, C, and Y. Serogroups A and W cause disease outside the US. Current vaccines are directed against some but not all of these serogroups.

For serogroups ACWY (quadrivalent):

- Meningococcal conjugate vaccines (MCV4): MenACWY-D (Menactra®) or MenACWY-CRM (Menveo®)
- Meningococcal polysaccharide vaccine (MPSV4 [Menomune®])

For serogroups CY (bivalent):

- A Hib-MenCY-TT (MenHibrix®), in which tetanus toxoid and *Haemophilus influenzae* type b capsular polysaccharide are conjugated with meningococcal serogroup C and Y polysaccharides

For serogroup B (monovalent):

- MenB-4C (Bexsero®) and MenB-FHbp (Trumenba®)

Indications

The meningococcal vaccine is a routine childhood vaccination given to adolescents, preferably at age 11 or 12 yr, with a booster dose at age 16 yr (see Table 291–3 on p. 2467). It is also recommended for younger children who are at high risk of infection (see Table 291–2 on p. 2462).

MenACWY conjugate vaccines are recommended for adults who have conditions that increase risk of meningococcal infection, such as

- Anatomic or functional asplenia
- Persistent complement component deficiencies
- Research in a microbiology laboratory involving routine exposure to isolates of *N. meningitidis*
- Military recruitment
- Travel to or residence in endemic areas
- First year of residence in a college dormitory if students are ≤ 21 yr and have not already received a dose on or after their 16th birthday
- Exposure to an outbreak attributable to a vaccine serogroup

If 1st-yr college students aged ≤ 21 yr received only 1 dose of vaccine before their 16th birthday, they should be given a booster dose before enrollment.

MenACWY is recommended for all adolescents (aged 11 to 18 yr), including those with HIV infection. But otherwise, it is indicated only when people with HIV infection are at increased risk for other reasons.

MenACWY is preferred for people aged 11 to 55 yr and for those > 55 yr who were vaccinated previously with MenACWY and require revaccination or who may require multiple doses of vaccine.

Revaccination with MenACWY every 5 yr is recommended for adults who were previously vaccinated with MenACWY or MPSV4 and who remain at increased risk of infection (eg, adults with anatomic or functional asplenia or persistent complement component deficiencies, microbiologists).

MPSV4 is preferred for people > 55 yr who have not received MenACWY previously and who require only a single dose (eg, travelers).

MenB-4C or MenB-FHpb is indicated for people 10 yr or older with certain high-risk conditions (including functional asplenia, complement deficiencies).

Contraindications and Precautions

The **main contraindication** is

- A severe allergic reaction (eg, anaphylaxis) after previous dose or to a vaccine component

The **main precaution** is

- Moderate or severe illness with or without a fever (vaccination is postponed until illness resolves if possible)

Dose and Administration

The dose is 0.5 mL IM for MenACWY and 0.5 mL sc for MPSV4.

Two doses of MenACWY, given ≥ 2 mo apart and followed by a booster every 5 yr, are required for adults with anatomic or functional asplenia or persistent complement component deficiencies. Adolescents (aged 11 to 18 yr) with HIV infection are routinely vaccinated with a 2-dose primary series, given 8 wk apart.

A single dose of meningococcal vaccine is given to microbiologists who are routinely exposed to isolates of *N. meningitidis*, military recruits, people at risk during an outbreak attributable to a vaccine serogroup, and those who travel to or live in endemic areas. If risk continues (eg, for microbiologists who continue working with *N. meningitidis*), booster doses are needed.

Two doses of MenB-4C are given at least 1 mo apart or 3-dose series of MenB-FHbp is given with second dose at least 1 to 2 mo after the first and the third dose at least 6 mo after the first. The same MenB must be used for all doses.

Adverse Effects

Adverse effects are usually mild. They include pain and redness at the injection site, fever, headache, and fatigue.

HAEMOPHILUS INFLUENZAE TYPE B VACCINE

For more information, see Hib ACIP Vaccine Recommendations at www.cdc.gov.

Preparations

These vaccines are prepared from the purified capsule of *Haemophilus influenzae* type b (Hib). All Hib vaccines use polyribosylribitol phosphate (PRP) as the polysaccharide, but 4 different protein carriers are used in the 4 different Hib conjugate vaccines available:

- Diphtheria toxoid (PRP-D)
- *Neisseria meningitidis* outer membrane protein (PRP-OMP)
- Tetanus toxoid (PRP-T)
- Diphtheria mutant carrier protein CRM_{197} (HbOC)

PRP-D and HbOC vaccines are no longer available in the US.

Combination vaccines that contain Hib conjugate vaccine include DTaP-IPV/Hib (Pentacel®), Hib-HepB (COMVAX®), and Hib-MenCY (MenHibrix®).

Some Hib vaccines—PRP-T (ActHIB®, Pentacel®, or MenHibrix®) and PRP-OMP (PedvaxHIB® or COMVAX®)—can be used in infants as young as 6 wk. Another Hib vaccine (Hiberix®) can be used only for the last dose of the Hib schedule in children ≥ 12 mo.

Indications

The Hib vaccine is a routine childhood vaccination (see Table 291–2 on p. 2462).

This vaccine is also recommended for

- Adults with anatomic or functional asplenia and those scheduled for elective splenectomy if they are unimmunized (ie, if they have not previously received a primary series plus booster dose or ≥ 1 dose of Hib vaccine after age 14 mo), although some experts suggest giving a dose before elective splenectomy regardless of vaccination history
- Immunocompromised adults (eg, because of cancer chemotherapy or HIV infection) if they are unimmunized
- People who have had a hematopoietic stem cell transplantation regardless of their vaccination history

Contraindications and Precautions

The **main contraindication** is

- A severe allergic reaction (eg, anaphylaxis) after previous dose or to a vaccine component

The **main precaution** is

- Moderate or severe illness with or without a fever (vaccination is postponed until the illness resolves)

Dose and Administration

Hib vaccine 0.5 mL is given IM. A primary childhood series is given in 3 doses at age 2, 4, and 6 mo or in 2 doses at age 2 and 4 mo, depending on the formulation. In either case, a booster is recommended at age 12 to 15 mo.

One dose is given to older children, adolescents, and adults who have asplenia or who are scheduled for an elective splenectomy if they are unimmunized. Some experts suggest giving a dose before elective splenectomy regardless of vaccination history. The dose is given ≥ 14 days before elective splenectomy if possible.

A 3-dose regimen is given 6 to 12 mo after hematopoietic stem cell transplantation; doses are separated by ≥ 4 wk.

Adverse Effects

Adverse effects are rare. They can include pain, redness, and swelling at the injection site and, in children, fever, crying, and irritability.

HEPATITIS A VACCINE

Preparations

Hepatitis A (HepA) vaccines are prepared from formalin-inactivated, cell culture–derived hepatitis A virus. There are 2 hepatitis A vaccines (Havrix® and Vaqta®); both are available in pediatric and adult formulations.

A vaccine that combines hepatitis A and hepatitis B vaccine (Twinrix®) is also available.

Indications

The HepA vaccine is a routine childhood vaccination (see Table 291–2 on p. 2462).

HepA vaccine is indicated when any of the following is present:

- A desire for protection from hepatitis A in people not previously vaccinated
- Travel to or work in endemic areas
- Occupational exposure (eg, working with primates infected with hepatitis A virus [HAV] or HAV in a research laboratory)
- Sex between men
- Use of illicit drugs (injected or not), such as methamphetamine
- Treatment with clotting factor concentrates
- A chronic liver disorder
- Anticipated close personal contact (eg, as members of the household or as regular babysitters) with an adopted child during the first 60 days after the child's arrival in the US from an endemic area

The combination HepA and HepB vaccine can be used in people ≥ 18 yr who have indications for either hepatitis A or hepatitis B vaccine and who have not been previously vaccinated with one of the vaccine components.

Contraindications and Precautions

The **main contraindication** is

- A severe allergic reaction (eg, anaphylaxis) after previous dose or to a vaccine component

The **main precaution** is

- Moderate or severe illness with or without a fever (vaccination is postponed until the illness resolves)

Dose and Administration

The dose is 0.5 mL IM up to age 18 yr or 1 mL IM for adults (age ≥ 19 yr).

Children are given a 2-dose series typically at age 12 to 23 mo and 6 to 18 mo after the 1st dose.

Adults are given the vaccine in a 2-dose series at either 0 and 6 to 12 mo (Havrix®) or 0 and 6 to 18 mo (Vaqta®).

Or adults may be given the combination HepA and HepB vaccine on a 3-dose schedule: at 0, 1, and 6 mo. The 1st and 2nd doses should be separated by ≥ 4 wk, and the 2nd and 3rd doses should be separated by ≥ 5 mo. Alternatively, the vaccine may be given on a 4-dose schedule: on days 0, 7, and 21 to 30, followed by a booster 12 mo after the 1st dose.

As soon as an adoption of a child from an endemic area is planned, close contacts should be given the 1st dose of the 2-dose HepA vaccine series, ideally ≥ 2 wk before the adopted child arrives.

Adverse Effects

No serious adverse effects have been reported.

Mild effects include pain, erythema, swelling, and occasionally induration at the injection site.

HEPATITIS B VACCINE

For more information, see Hepatitis B ACIP Vaccine Recommendations at www.cdc.gov.

Preparations

Hepatitis B (HepB) vaccine is produced using recombinant DNA technology. A plasmid containing the gene for HBsAg is inserted into common baker's yeast, which then produces HBsAg. The HBsAg is harvested and purified. This vaccine cannot cause HBV infection because no potentially infectious viral DNA or complete viral particles are produced during this process.

Single-antigen and a combination formulation that combines hepatitis A and hepatitis B vaccines (Twinrix®), are available.

Indications

HepB vaccine is a routine childhood vaccination (see Table 291–2 on p. 2462).

HepB vaccine is indicated for people who have not been previously vaccinated when any of the following is present:

- A desire for protection from hepatitis B in people who have not been previously vaccinated
- A sexually active lifestyle in people who are not in a long-term, mutually monogamous relationship (eg, > 1 sex partner during the previous 6 mo)
- Need for evaluation or treatment of a sexually transmitted disease (STD)
- Current or recent use of illicit injection drugs
- Sex between men
- Employment in which workers may be exposed to blood or other potentially infectious body fluids (eg, as health care, custodial, or public safety workers)
- Diabetes in people < 60 yr (as soon as feasible after diagnosis) and sometimes in those ≥ 60 yr (based on their risk of becoming infected, having severe consequences if infected, and having an adequate immune response to vaccination)
- End-stage renal disease (eg, being treated with hemodialysis)
- HIV infection
- A chronic liver disorder

- Household contact and/or sexual contact with people who are positive for hepatitis B surface antigen (HBsAg)
- Travel to endemic areas
- Time spent (as patients, residents, or employees) in correctional facilities or in facilities that provide STD treatment, HIV testing and treatment, drug abuse treatment and prevention services, services to injection-drug users or men who have sex with men, or care for patients with developmental disabilities or with end-stage renal disease (including those receiving long-term hemodialysis)

The combination HepA and HepB vaccine can be used in people ≥ 18 yr who have indications for either hepatitis A or hepatitis B vaccine and who have not been previously vaccinated with one of the vaccine components.

Contraindications and Precautions

The **main contraindication** is

- A severe allergic reaction (eg, anaphylaxis) after previous dose or to baker's yeast or any vaccine component

The **main precaution** is

- Moderate or severe illness with or without a fever (vaccination is postponed until the illness resolves)

Dose and Administration

The dose is 0.5 mL IM up to age 20 yr or 1 mL IM for adults (≥ 20 yr).

The vaccine is typically given to children in a 3-dose series at age 0 mo, at 1 to 2 mo, and at 6 to 18 mo.

All children not previously vaccinated with HepB vaccine should be vaccinated at age 11 or 12 yr. A 3-dose schedule is used; the 1st and 2nd doses are separated by ≥ 4 wk, and the 3rd dose is given 4 to 6 mo after the 2nd dose. However, a 2-dose schedule using Recombivax HB® can be used; the 2nd dose is given 4 to 6 mo after the first.

The usual schedule for adults is 2 doses separated by ≥ 4 wk, and a 3rd dose 4 to 6 mo after the 2nd dose.

Unvaccinated adults who are being treated with hemodialysis or who are immunocompromised should be given 1 dose of Recombivax HB® 40 mcg/mL in a 3-dose schedule at 0, 1, and 6 mo or 2 doses of Engerix-B® 20 mcg/mL given simultaneously in a 4-dose schedule at 0, 1, 2, and 6 mo.

If people are not vaccinated or not completely vaccinated, the missing doses should be given to complete the 3-dose HepB series. The 2nd dose is given 1 mo after the 1st dose; the 3rd dose is given ≥ 2 mo after the 2nd dose (and ≥ 4 mo after the 1st dose). If the combined hepatitis A and hepatitis B vaccine (Twinrix®) is used, 3 doses are given at 0, 1, and 6 mo, or 4 doses are given on days 0, 7, and 21 to 30, followed by a booster dose at 12 mo. If a person was lost to follow-up before the series was completed, the series does not need to be restarted.

Adverse Effects

Serious adverse effects are very rare and include anaphylaxis. Mild effects include pain at the injection site and occasionally an increase in temperature to about 38° C.

HUMAN PAPILLOMAVIRUS VACCINE

Preparations

Three vaccines protect against HPV:

- A 9-valent vaccine that protects against HPV types 6 and 11 (which cause > 90% of visible genital warts), types 16 and 18 (which cause most cervical cancers), and types 31, 33, 45, 52, and 58
- A quadrivalent vaccine (HPV4) that protects against types 6, 11, 16, and 18
- A bivalent vaccine (HPV2) that protects against types 16 and 18

Only the 9-valent vaccine is now available in the US.

Recombinant DNA technology is used to prepare HPV vaccines from the major capsid (L1) protein of HPV. The L1 proteins self-assemble into noninfectious, nononcogenic virus-like particles (VLPs).

Indications

The HPV vaccine is a routine childhood vaccination (see Table 291–3 on p. 2467).

HPV4 or HPV2 is recommended for females at age 11 or 12 yr and for females up through age 26 yr if they were not previously vaccinated.

HPV4 is recommended for males at age 11 or 12 yr and previously unvaccinated males through age 26 yr; HPV4 is recommended for all men who are in this age group and who have sex with men.

Vaccination is recommended for all people who are immunocompromised, including HIV patients, through age 26 if they were not vaccinated at a younger age.

Contraindications and Precautions

Contraindications include

- A severe allergic reaction (eg, anaphylaxis) after previous dose or to a vaccine component
- Pregnancy

Although HPV vaccines are not recommended for pregnant women, pregnancy testing is not needed before vaccination. If pregnancy is diagnosed after the vaccination series has been started, no intervention is needed, but the remaining doses of the series should be delayed until pregnancy is completed.

The **main precaution** is

- Moderate or severe acute illness with or without fever (vaccination is postponed until the illness resolves)

Dose and Administration

The dose is 0.5 mL IM, given in a 3-dose series at 0 mo, at 2 mo, and at 6 mo.

Adverse Effects

No serious adverse effects have been reported. Mild effects include pain, redness, swelling, and tenderness at the injection site.

INFLUENZA VACCINE

For more information, see Influenza ACIP Vaccine Recommendations and Provider Vaccine Information Statements (VIS) Supplements at www.cdc.gov.

Based on recommendations by the WHO and US Centers for Disease Control and Prevention (CDC), vaccines are modified annually to include the most prevalent strains (usually 2 strains of influenza A and 1 or 2 strains of influenza B). Sometimes slightly different vaccines are used in the northern and southern hemispheres.

Preparations

There are 2 basic types of vaccine:

- Inactivated influenza vaccine (IIV)
- Live-attenuated influenza vaccine (LAIV)

Trivalent vaccines are gradually being superseded by quadrivalent vaccines that cover an additional B virus strain. A trivalent recombinant influenza vaccine (RIV3) and a cell culture–based vaccine (ccIIV3) that do not contain egg protein are available. A high-dose trivalent vaccine is available for patients ≥ 65 yr.

Indications

Annual vaccination against influenza is recommended for

- All people ≥ 6 mo

IIV can be given to all people ≥ 6 mo, including pregnant women.

An age-appropriate formulation should be used.

Adults ≥ 65 yr should be given high-dose IIV. The high dose is recommended only for those ≥ 65 yr.

RIV3 can be used in people aged 18 to 49 yr.

LAIV can be given to healthy people aged 2 to 49 yr who are not pregnant and who do not have immunocompromising conditions. Safety of LAIV has not been established in people with disorders that predispose them to complications from influenza, including advanced lung disease or asthma.

Health care workers who care for immunocompromised people (ie, those who require care in a protected environment) should be given IIV or RIV3 rather than LAIV (or they should avoid contact with the immunocompromised people for 7 days after getting the vaccine).

Contraindications and Precautions

The **main contraindication for IIV** is

- A severe allergic reaction (eg, anaphylaxis) after previous dose of IIV

Precautions with IIV include

- Moderate or severe acute illness with or without fever (vaccination is postponed until illness resolves)
- Guillain-Barré syndrome (GBS) within 6 wk after a previous dose of an influenza vaccine

Contraindications for LAIV include

- A severe allergic reaction (eg, anaphylaxis) after previous dose of LAIV
- Immunocompromise (eg, due to disorders, including HIV infection, or use of immunosuppressants)
- Certain chronic disorders (eg, asthma; reactive airway disease; diabetes; hemoglobinopathy; lung, heart, or kidney disorders)
- For children and adolescents, long-term treatment with aspirin or other salicylates
- Pregnancy
- Age < 2 yr or ≥ 50 yr
- Age < 5 yr if reactive airway disease (eg, known asthma, recurrent or recent wheezing episodes) is present

Precautions for LAIV include

- Moderate or severe acute illness with or without fever (vaccination is postponed until illness resolves)
- GBS within 6 wk after a previous dose of an influenza vaccine
- Use of specific antiviral drugs: ie, amantadine, rimantadine, zanamivir, oseltamivir (these drugs are stopped 48 h before vaccination and are not resumed for 14 days after vaccination)

The **main contraindication for RIV3** is

- A severe allergic reaction (eg, anaphylaxis) after a previous dose of RIV3

Precautions for RIV3 include:

- Moderate or severe acute illness with or without fever (vaccination is postponed until illness resolves)
- GBS within 6 wk after a previous dose of an influenza vaccine

Precautions for patients with suspected egg allergy: Patients with a history of egg allergy who have experienced only hives after exposure to egg should receive influenza vaccine. Any influenza vaccine that is otherwise recommended based on the recipient's age and health status can be used.

Patients who report reactions to egg involving symptoms other than hives, such as angioedema, respiratory distress, lightheadedness, or recurrent emesis, or who required epinephrine or another emergency medical intervention, may similarly receive any influenza vaccine that is otherwise recommended based on the recipient's age and health status. The vaccine should be given in an inpatient or outpatient medical setting and supervised by a health care practitioner capable of recognizing and managing severe allergic conditions.

Dose and Administration

The influenza vaccine is given yearly.

For IIV, the dose is

- 0.25 mL IM for children aged 6 to 35 mo
- 0.5 mL IM for people ≥ 3 yr
- 0.1 mL for people aged 18 to 64 yr, given intradermally

The smaller, intradermal dose can be used to conserve vaccine in times of shortage.

For LAIV, the dose is 0.1 mL, sprayed into each nostril (total dose is 0.2 mL).

For RIV3, the dose is 0.5 mL, given IM.

Adverse Effects

For IIV, adverse effects are usually limited to mild pain at the injection site. Fever, myalgia, and other systemic effects are relatively uncommon; however, people who have been vaccinated may mistakenly think that the vaccine is causing influenza. Such reactions do not contraindicate future vaccination, which should be encouraged.

Multidose vials contain thimerosal, a mercury-based preservative. Public concerns about a possible link between thimerosal and autism have proved unfounded (see p. 2466); however single-dose vials, which are thimerosal-free, are available.

For LAIV, adverse effects are mild; rhinorrhea is the most common, and mild wheezing may occur.

MEASLES, MUMPS, AND RUBELLA VACCINE

For more information, see MMR ACIP Vaccine Recommendations (Measles, Mumps and Rubella) at www.cdc.gov.

Preparations

The measles, mumps, and rubella (MMR) vaccine contains live-attenuated measles and mumps viruses, prepared in chicken embryo cell cultures. It also contains live-attenuated rubella virus, prepared in human diploid lung fibroblasts.

MMR vaccine and varicella vaccine are available as a combined vaccine (MMRV vaccine).

Indications

The MMR vaccine is a routine childhood vaccination (see Table 291–2 on p. 2462).

All adults who were born in 1957 or later should be given 1 dose of the vaccine unless they have one of the following:

- Documentation of vaccination with one or more doses of MMR
- Laboratory evidence that indicates immunity to the 3 diseases
- A contraindication to the vaccine

Documented diagnosis of disease by a physician is not considered acceptable evidence of immunity for measles, mumps, or rubella.

A 2nd dose of MMR vaccine is recommended for adults who are likely to be exposed:

- Students in colleges or other post–high school educational institutions
- Health care workers
- International travelers

Because rubella during pregnancy can have dire consequences for the fetus (eg, miscarriage, multiple birth defects), all women of childbearing age, regardless of birth year, should be screened for rubella immunity. If there is no evidence of immunity, women who are not pregnant should be vaccinated. Pregnant women who do not have evidence of immunity should be vaccinated when pregnancy is completed and before they are discharged from the health care facility.

People who were vaccinated with inactivated (killed) measles vaccine or measles vaccine of unknown type during 1963 to 1967 should be revaccinated with 2 doses of MMR vaccine.

People who were vaccinated before 1979 with killed mumps vaccine or mumps vaccine of unknown type and who are at high risk of mumps exposure should be offered revaccination with 2 doses of MMR vaccine.

Contraindications and Precautions

Contraindications include

- A severe allergic reaction (eg, anaphylaxis) after a previous dose or to a vaccine component, including neomycin
- Known severe primary or acquired immunodeficiency (eg, due to leukemia, lymphomas, solid tumors, tumors that affect bone marrow or the lymphatic system, AIDS, severe HIV infection, treatment with chemotherapy, or long-term use of immunosuppressants)
- Pregnancy (vaccination is postponed until pregnancy is completed)

HIV infection is a contraindication only if immunocompromise is severe (CDC immunologic category 3 with CD4 < 15% or CD4 count < 200 cells/μL—see Table 312–2 on p. 2602); if immunocompromise is not severe, risks of wild measles outweigh risk of acquiring measles from the live vaccine.

Women who have been vaccinated should avoid becoming pregnant for ≥ 28 days afterward. The vaccine virus may be capable of infecting a fetus during early pregnancy. The vaccine does not cause congenital rubella syndrome, but risk of fetal damage is estimated at ≤ 3%.

Precautions include

- Moderate or severe acute illness with or without fever (vaccination is postponed until illness resolves)
- Recent (within 11 mo) treatment with blood products that contain antibody (specific interval depends on the product)
- History of thrombocytopenia or thrombocytopenic purpura

If a person is infected with *Mycobacterium tuberculosis*, MMR and possibly MMRV vaccine may temporarily suppress the response to tuberculin testing. Thus, if needed, this test can be done before or at the same time as vaccination. If people have already been vaccinated, testing should be postponed for 4 to 6 wk after vaccination.

Dose and Administration

Dose is 0.5 mL, given sc. The MMR vaccine is routinely given to children in 2 doses: one at age 12 to 15 mo and one at age 4 to 6 yr.

Adverse Effects

The vaccine causes a mild or inapparent, noncommunicable infection. Symptoms include fever > 38° C, sometimes followed by a rash. CNS reactions are very rare; the vaccine does not cause autism (see MMR vaccine and autism on p. 2461 and Vaccine Safety on p. 1451).

Occasionally, the rubella component causes painful joint swelling in adults, usually in women.

PNEUMOCOCCAL VACCINE

For more information, see Pneumococcal ACIP Vaccine Recommendations at www.cdc.gov.

Certain medical conditions (eg, chronic disorders, immunocompromising conditions, CSF leaks, cochlear implants) increase the risk of pneumococcal disease.

Preparations

The 13-valent pneumococcal conjugate vaccine (PCV13, Prevnar®) contains 13 purified capsular polysaccharides of *Streptococcus pneumoniae*; each is coupled to a nontoxic variant of diphtheria toxin. This vaccine has replaced the 7-valent vaccine (PCV7); PCV13 contains the 7 serotypes in PCV7 plus 6 additional serotypes. The 23-valent pneumococcal polysaccharide vaccine (PPSV23, Pneumovax®) contains antigens from the 23 most virulent of the 83 subtypes of *S. pneumococcus*. Unlike the older PPSV23, PCV13 can stimulate antibody responses in infants. It also seems to confer greater protection against invasive pneumococcal disorders than PPSV23. PPSV23 reduces bacteremia by 56 to 81% in adults overall but is less effective in debilitated elderly people. It reduces pneumonia incidence.

Indications

PCV13: PCV13 is recommended for

- All children (routine childhood vaccine—see Table 291–2 on p. 2462)
- All adults ≥ 65 yr

PCV13 is also recommended for people aged 6 to 64 yr with any of the following high-risk conditions:

- A cochlear implant
- CSF leak
- Sickle cell disease or other hemoglobinopathy
- Congenital or acquired asplenia
- Immunocompromising conditions (eg, congenital immunodeficiency, chronic renal failure, nephrotic syndrome, HIV infection, leukemia, lymphomas, generalized cancer, use of immunosuppressants, solid organ transplant)

PPSV23: PPSV23 is recommended for

- All adults ≥ 65 yr

PPSV23 is also recommended for people aged 6 to 64 yr with the high-risk conditions listed above. Additional criteria for adults aged 19 to 64 yr include the following:

- A chronic lung disorder (including asthma)
- Chronic cardiovascular disorders (excluding hypertension)

- Diabetes mellitus
- A chronic liver disorder
- Chronic alcoholism
- Cigarette smoking

PPSV23 is no longer recommended for routine use in American Indians and Alaska natives < 65 yr unless they have a medical condition or other indication for PPSV23. However, American Indians and Alaskan natives aged 50 to 64 yr may be given PPSV23 if they live in areas where risk of invasive pneumococcal disease is increased.

Contraindications and Precautions

The **main contraindication for PCV13** is

- A severe allergic reaction (eg, anaphylaxis) after a previous dose of PCV7 or PCV13, to a vaccine component, or to any vaccine containing diphtheria toxoid

The **main contraindication for PPSV23** is

- A severe allergic reaction after a previous dose of the vaccine or to a vaccine component

Precautions include

- Moderate or severe acute illness with or without fever (vaccination is postponed until illness resolves)

Administration

The usual dose is 0.5 mL IM for PCV13 and 0.5 mL IM or sc for PCSV23.

PCV13 is recommended as a 4-dose IM series for infants at age 2, 4, 6, and 12 to 15 mo. Children aged 7 to 59 mo who have not been vaccinated with PCV7 or PCV13 previously should be given 1 to 3 doses of PCV13, depending on their age at the initiation of the vaccination series and the presence of medical conditions. Children aged 24 to 71 mo with chronic medical conditions that increase their risk of pneumococcal disease should be given 2 doses of PCV13 at least 8 wk apart if unvaccinated. Interruption of the vaccination schedule does not require starting the entire series over or giving extra doses.

Children at high risk of pneumococcal disease (eg, children with sickle cell disease, asplenia, or a chronic disorder) should be given a dose of PPSV23 at age 24 mo at least 8 wk after the most recent dose of PCV13.

Children aged 14 to 59 mo who have received a complete age-appropriate series of PCV7 should be given a single supplemental dose of PCV13.

If children aged 6 to 18 yr with an immunocompromising condition, a cochlear implant, or a CSF leak have not been vaccinated with PCV13 or PPSV23, they should be given 1 dose of PCV13, followed by 1 dose of PPSV23 ≥ 8 wk later. If they have been vaccinated with PPSV23 but not PCV13, they are given 1 dose of PCV13 ≥ 8 wk after the last dose of PPSV23. Children with an immunocompromising condition should be revaccinated once with PPSV23 5 yr after the first dose. They should not be given > 2 doses of PPSV23.

If people need both vaccines, PCV13 should be given first, followed by PPSV23 at least 8 wk later. If people have already been vaccinated with PPSV23, administer PCV13 at least 8 wk after the most recent dose of PPSV23.

Adults aged ≥ 19 yr with immunocompromising conditions (eg, functional or anatomic asplenia, HIV infection), CSF leaks, or cochlear implants should be vaccinated with PCV13 and PSV23. If they have not previously been given PCV13 or PPSV23, they should be vaccinated with a dose of PCV13, followed by a dose of PPSV23 ≥ 8 wk later. If they have been given PPSV23 but not PCV13, they are given a dose of PCV13 ≥ 1 yr after the last dose of PPSV23.

People with asymptomatic or symptomatic HIV infection should be vaccinated as soon as possible after their diagnosis.

Adults aged 19 to 64 yr at highest risk of pneumococcal disease (eg, with functional or anatomic asplenia, chronic kidney disease, or another immunocompromising condition, including cancer and use of corticosteroids) should be given a 2nd dose of PPSV23 5 yr after the first PPSV23 dose.

All people should be vaccinated with PPSV23 at age 65. If people were given 1 or 2 doses of PPSV23 before age 65 for any indication and ≥ 5 yr have elapsed since their previous PPSV23 dose, they should be given another dose of the vaccine at age 65 or later. The 2nd dose is given 5 yr after the first (eg, at age 69 if the previous dose was given at age 64). Those who are given PPSV23 at or after age 65 should be given only 1 dose.

If elective splenectomy is planned, PCV13 should be given ≥ 12 wk before surgery, followed by a dose of PPSV23 ≥ 8 wk after PCV13 is given. PPSV23 should be given at least 2 wk before elective splenectomy. If splenectomy must be done immediately, PCV13 should be given, followed by PPSV23 ≥ 8 wk later. If patients have already received PCV13, PPSV23 should not be given until ≥ 2 wk after splenectomy.

When cancer chemotherapy or other immunosuppressive therapy is being considered, the interval between vaccination and initiation of immunosuppressive therapy should be ≥ 2 wk. People should be not be vaccinated during chemotherapy or radiation therapy.

Adverse Effects

Adverse effects are usually mild and include fever, irritability, drowsiness, anorexia, vomiting, and local pain and erythema.

POLIOMYELITIS VACCINE

Preparations

Inactivated poliovirus vaccine (IPV) contains a mixture of formalin-inactivated poliovirus types 1, 2, and 3. IPV may contain trace amounts of streptomycin, neomycin, and polymyxin B. The live-attenuated oral formulation is no longer available in the US because it causes polio in about 1 of every 2.4 million people who are given the vaccine.

Combination vaccines with IPV, DTaP, and sometimes also hepatitis B or Hib are also available.

Indications

IPV is a routine childhood vaccine (see Table 291–2 on p. 2462).

Routine primary poliovirus vaccination of adults living in the US is not recommended. Unimmunized or incompletely immunized adults who may be exposed to wild poliovirus (eg, travelers to endemic areas, laboratory workers who handle specimens that may contain poliovirus) should be vaccinated with IPV. Completely vaccinated adults who are at an increased risk of exposure to poliovirus can be given a booster dose of IPV. For current information about which countries are considered at high risk for polio, see the CDC Travel Destinations List and Polio: Traveler Information at www.cdc.gov.

Contraindications and Precautions

The **main contraindication** is

- A severe allergic reaction (eg, anaphylaxis) after a previous dose of the vaccine or to a vaccine component

The **main precaution** is

- Moderate or severe acute febrile illness (vaccination is postponed until the illness resolves)

Administration

The dose is 0.5 mL IM or sc.

A 4-dose IM series is given at age 2 mo, 4 mo, 6 to 18 mo, and 4 to 6 yr. Typically, a combination vaccine is used for the first 3 vaccinations and a single-antigen vaccine for the last dose. If children miss an IPV dose at age 4 to 6 yr, they should be given a booster dose as soon as possible.

When DTaP-IPV/Hib (Pentacel®) is used for the 4-dose schedule (at ages 2, 4, 6, and 15 to 18 mo), an additional booster dose of IPV-containing vaccine (IPV or DTaP-IPV [Kinrix®]) should be given at age 4 to 6 yr, resulting in a 5-dose schedule; however, DTaP-IPV/Hib should not be used for the booster dose at age 4 to 6 yr. The minimum interval between doses 4 and 5 should be ≥ 6 mo to optimize the booster response.

A primary series of IPV is recommended for unvaccinated adults at increased risk of exposure to poliovirus. The recommended interval between doses 1 and 2 is 1 to 2 mo; the 3rd dose is given 6 to 12 mo later. If protection is needed in 2 to 3 mo, 3 doses are given ≥ 1 mo apart. If it is needed in 1 to 2 mo, 2 doses are given ≥ 1 mo apart, and if it is needed in < 1 mo, 1 dose is given.

Adverse Effects

No adverse effects have been associated with IPV. Because it may contain trace amounts of neomycin, streptomycin, and polymyxin B, people who are sensitive to any of these drugs may have an allergic reaction to the vaccine.

VARICELLA VACCINE

Preparations

The vaccine contains an attenuated wild strain of varicella and trace amounts of gelatin and neomycin. It is available as a single-antigen vaccine or as a combination vaccine with MMR (MMRV).

Indications

Varicella vaccine is a routine childhood vaccine (see Table 291–2 on p. 2462).

Single-antigen varicella vaccine is recommended for

- All people ≥ 13 yr who do not have evidence of immunity to varicella

Evidence of immunity consists of one of the following:

- Documentation of 2 doses of varicella vaccine given ≥ 4 wk apart
- History of varicella or herpes zoster verified by a physician
- Laboratory confirmation of protective levels of varicella antibodies
- Birth in the US before 1980, except for health care workers, pregnant women, and people with immunocompromising conditions

The vaccine is recommended particularly for people who do not have evidence of immunity and are likely to be exposed or transmit varicella, including the following:

- Health care workers
- Household contacts of immunocompromised people
- People who live or work in places where exposure or transmission is likely (eg, teachers, students, child care workers, residents and employes of institutional settings, inmates and employees of correctional institutions, military personnel)
- Women of childbearing age who are not pregnant
- Adolescents and adults living in households with children
- International travelers

Postexposure vaccination with the single-antigen varicella vaccine is recommended for children with no evidence of immunity and should be offered to adults with no evidence of immunity. The vaccine is effective in preventing or ameliorating disease if it is given within 3 days and possibly up to 5 days after exposure. The vaccine should be given as soon as possible. If exposure to varicella does not cause infection, postexposure vaccination should induce protection against subsequent exposures, even if the vaccine is given > 5 days postexposure.

Varicella-zoster immune globulin (see Table 180–3) is recommended for postexposure prophylaxis in people who have no evidence of immunity, are at increased risk of severe varicella, and/or have contraindications to the varicella vaccine. These people include

- Immunocompromised people without evidence of immunity
- Pregnant women without evidence of immunity
- Neonates whose mothers developed varicella within 5 days before to 2 days after delivery
- Hospitalized premature infants who were born at ≥ 28 wk gestation and whose mothers do not have evidence of immunity to varicella
- Hospitalized premature infants who were born at < 28 wk gestation or who weigh ≤ 1000 g at birth, regardless of their mother's evidence of immunity to varicella

Contraindications and Precautions

Contraindications include

- A severe allergic reaction (eg, anaphylaxis) after a previous dose of the vaccine or to a vaccine component
- Known severe primary or acquired immunodeficiency (eg, due to leukemia, lymphomas, solid tumors, tumors that affect bone marrow or the lymphatic system, AIDS, severe HIV infection, treatment with chemotherapy, or long-term use of immunosuppressants)
- Unless people are known to be immunocompetent, 1st-degree relatives who have congenital hereditary immunodeficiency
- Confirmed or suspected pregnancy

The single-antigen varicella vaccine may be given to children aged 1 to 8 yr who have HIV infection if their CD4 percentage is ≥ 15%; it may be given to those > 8 yr if their CD4 count is ≥ 200 μL.

Precautions include

- Moderate or severe acute illness with or without fever (vaccination is postponed until illness resolves)
- Recent (within 11 mo) treatment with blood products that contain antibody (specific interval depends on the product)
- Use of specific antiviral drugs: acyclovir, famciclovir, or valacyclovir (if possible, these drugs are stopped 24 h before vaccination and are not resumed for 14 days after vaccination)

Breastfeeding is not a contraindication to vaccination. Women who are breastfeeding and do not have evidence of immunity can be vaccinated postpartum and continue breastfeeding.

Dose and Administration

The dose is 0.5 mL given sc in 2 doses: at age 12 to 15 mo and at age 4 to 6 yr. If children, adolescents, or adults have been given only 1 dose, a catch-up dose is recommended. The recommended minimum interval between the 1st dose and the catch-up 2nd dose is 3 mo for children aged ≤ 12 yr and 4 wk for people aged ≥ 13 yr; the 2nd dose may be given at any interval longer than the minimum.

If adults think that they have not had varicella or are likely to be exposed to or to transmit varicella, levels of protective antibodies should be measured to check for evidence of immunity and thus determine the need for vaccination.

No immune globulins, particularly varicella-zoster immune globulin, should be given within 5 mo before or 2 mo after vaccination because immune globulins may prevent development of protective antibodies.

Eligible children with HIV infection are given 2 doses of single-antigen varicella vaccine 3 mo apart. Because impaired cellular immunity increases the risk of complications after vaccination with a live vaccine, these children should be encouraged to return for evaluation if a varicella-like rash develops after vaccination.

Prenatal assessment of women for evidence of varicella immunity is indicated. Birth before 1980 is not considered evidence of immunity for pregnant women. After completion or termination of pregnancy, women who do not have evidence of immunity should be given the 1st dose of vaccine before discharge and the 2nd dose 4 to 8 wk later, usually at the postpartum visit. Women should be advised to avoid becoming pregnant for 1 mo after each dose.

Adverse Effects

Most adverse effects are minimal and include transient pain, tenderness, and redness at the injection site. Occasionally, within 1 mo of vaccination, a mild maculopapular or varicella-like rash develops in 1 to 3% of people who are vaccinated. Vaccine recipients who develop this rash should diligently avoid contact with immunocompromised people until it resolves. Spread of the virus from vaccine recipients to susceptible people is rare but can result in severe problems, including pneumonia, hepatitis, severe rash, and shingles with meningitis. However, such problems rarely develop.

Because Reye syndrome can develop, recipients < 16 yr should avoid salicylates for 6 wk after the vaccine is given.

HERPES ZOSTER VACCINE

For more information, see Zoster (Shingles) ACIP Vaccine Recommendations at www.cdc.gov.

Preparations

The vaccine contains an attenuated wild strain of varicella, similar to the varicella vaccine but with a higher amount of the attenuated virus.

Indications

The zoster vaccine is recommended for adults ≥ 60 yr whether they have had herpes zoster or not. It is not routinely recommended for people aged 50 to 59 yr but can be used in this age group.

Contraindications and Precautions

Contraindications include

- A severe allergic reaction (eg, anaphylaxis) to a vaccine component
- Known severe primary or acquired immunodeficiency (eg, due to leukemia, lymphomas, solid tumors, tumors that affect bone marrow or the lymphatic system, AIDS, severe HIV infection, treatment with chemotherapy, or long-term use of immunosuppressants)
- Pregnancy

Precautions include

- Moderate or severe acute illness with or without fever (vaccination is postponed until illness resolves)
- Use of specific antiviral drugs: acyclovir, famciclovir, or valacyclovir (if possible, vaccination is postponed until 24 h after use of these drugs, and the drugs are not resumed for 14 days after vaccination)

Dose and Administration

The vaccine is given as a single 0.65-mL dose sc in the deltoid region of the upper arm.

Zoster vaccine should be given ≥ 14 days before immunosuppressive therapy is begun; some experts prefer waiting 1 mo after zoster vaccination to begin immunosuppressive therapy if possible.

This vaccine must be kept frozen between –50° C (–58° F) and –15° C (5° F) and must be reconstituted immediately after removal from the freezer.

Adverse Effects

No serious adverse effects have been reported. Soreness at the site of the injection may occur.

PASSIVE IMMUNIZATION

Passive immunization is provided in the following circumstances:

- When people cannot synthesize antibody
- When people have been exposed to a disease that they are not immune to or that is likely to cause complications
- When people have a disease and the effects of the toxin must be ameliorated

For immune globulins and antitoxins available in the US, see Table 180–3.

Human immune globulin (IG): IG is a concentrated antibody-containing solution prepared from plasma obtained from normal donors. It consists primarily of IgG, although trace amounts of IgA, IgM, and other serum proteins may be present. IG very rarely contains transmissible viruses (eg, hepatitis B or C, HIV) and is stable for many months if stored at 4° C. IG is given IM.

Because maximal serum antibody levels may not occur until about 48 h after IM injection, IG must be given as soon after exposure as possible. Half-life of IG in the circulation is about 3 wk.

IG may be used for prophylaxis in

- Hepatitis A
- Measles
- Immunoglobulin deficiency
- Varicella (in immunocompromised patients when varicella-zoster IG is unavailable)
- Rubella exposure during the 1st trimester of pregnancy

IG provides only temporary protection; the antibody content against specific agents varies by as much as 10-fold among preparations. Administration is painful, and anaphylaxis can occur.

IV immune globulin (IVIG) was developed to provide larger and repeated doses of human immune globulin. IVIG is used to treat or prevent severe bacterial and viral infections,

Table 180–3. IMMUNE GLOBULINS AND ANTITOXINS* AVAILABLE IN THE US

IMMUNOBIOLOGIC AGENT	TYPE	INDICATIONS
Botulinum antitoxin	Specific equine antibodies	Treatment of botulism
Botulinum antitoxin (BIG)	Specific human antibodies	Treatment of botulism in infants
Cytomegalovirus immune globulin, IV (CMV-IGIV)	Specific human antibodies	Prophylaxis in hematopoietic stem cell and kidney transplant recipients
Diphtheria antitoxin	Specific equine antibodies	Treatment of respiratory diphtheria
Hepatitis B immune globulin (HBIG)	Specific human antibodies	Prophylaxis for hepatitis B postexposure
Immune globulin (IG)	Pooled human antibodies	Prophylaxis for hepatitis A preexposure and postexposure, measles postexposure, immunoglobulin deficiency, rubella during the 1st trimester of pregnancy, varicella (if varicella zoster immune globulin is unavailable)
Immune globulin, intravenous (IVIG)	Pooled human antibodies	Prophylaxis for and treatment of severe bacterial and viral infections (eg, HIV infection in children), primary immunodeficiency disorders, autoimmune thrombocytopenic purpura, chronic B-cell lymphocytic leukemia, Kawasaki disease, autoimmune disorders (eg, myasthenia gravis, Guillain-Barré syndrome, polymyositis/dermatomyositis) Prophylaxis for graft-vs-host disease
Immune globulin, sc (SCIG)	Pooled human antibodies	Treatment of primary immunodeficiency disorders
Rabies immune globulin (HRIG)†	Specific human antibodies	Management of rabies postexposure in people not previously immunized with rabies vaccine (see on p. 1853)
Respiratory syncytial virus murine monoclonal antibody (RSV-mAb)	Murine monoclonal antibody (palivizumab)	Prevention of RSV in high-risk infants (see p. 2764)
Tetanus immune globulin (TIG)	Specific human antibodies	Treatment of tetanus Postexposure prophylaxis in people not adequately immunized with tetanus toxoid
Vaccinia immune globulin (VIG)	Specific human antibodies	Treatment of eczema vaccinatum, vaccinia necrosum, and ocular vaccinia
Varicella-zoster immune globulin (VariZIG)	Specific human antibodies	Postexposure prophylaxis in people who have no evidence of immunity, are at increased risk of severe varicella, and have contraindications to the varicella vaccine (see p. 1460)

*Immune globulin preparations and antitoxins are given IM unless otherwise indicated.
†HRIG is administered around wounds as well as IM.
From General Recommendations on Immunization. Recommendations of the Advisory Committee on Immunization Practices (ACIP). *Morbidity and Mortality Weekly Report* 43:1, January 28, 1994. Updated through the Center for Biologics Evaluation and Research of the U.S. Food and Drug Administration, 2008.

autoimmune disorders, and immunodeficiency disorders, particularly the following:

- Kawasaki disease
- HIV infection in children
- Chronic B-cell lymphocytic leukemia
- Primary immunodeficiencies
- Immune thrombocytopenia
- Prevention of graft-vs-host disease

Adverse effects are uncommon, although fever, chills, headache, faintness, nausea, vomiting, hypersensitivity, anaphylactic reactions, coughing, and volume overload have occurred.

Subcutaneous immune globulin (SCIG) is also prepared from pooled human plasma; SCIG is intended for home use in patients with a primary immunodeficiency.

Injection site reactions are common, but systemic adverse effects (eg, fever, chills) are much less common than with IVIG.

Hyperimmune globulin: Hyperimmune globulin is prepared from the plasma of people with high titers of antibody against a specific organism or antigen. It is derived from people convalescing from natural infections or donors artificially immunized.

Hyperimmune globulins are available for hepatitis B, infant botulism, rabies, tetanus, cytomegalovirus, vaccinia, and varicella-zoster. Administration is painful, and anaphylaxis may occur.

Monoclonal antibodies: Specific monoclonal antibodies active against infectious agents are of great theoretical interest, and a number are currently being studied. However, only one product, palivizumab, is currently available; it is active against respiratory syncytial virus (RSV) and is used for prevention of RSV infection in certain high-risk children (see p. 2764).

181 Anaerobic Bacteria

Bacteria can be classified by their need and tolerance for O_2:

- Facultative: Grow aerobically or anaerobically in the presence or absence of O_2
- Microaerophilic: Require a low O_2 concentration (eg, 5%) and, for many, a high CO_2 concentration (eg, 10%); grow very poorly anaerobically
- Obligate anaerobic: Are incapable of aerobic metabolism but are variably tolerant of O_2

Obligate anaerobes replicate at sites with low oxidation-reduction potential (eg, necrotic, devascularized tissue). Oxygen is toxic to them. Obligate anaerobes have been categorized based on their O_2 tolerance:

- Strict: Tolerate only $\leq 0.5\%$ O_2
- Moderate: Tolerate 2 to 8% O_2
- Aerotolerant anaerobes: Tolerate atmospheric O_2 for a limited time

The obligate anaerobes that commonly cause infection can tolerate atmospheric O_2 for at least 8 h and frequently for up to 72 h.

Obligate anaerobes are major components of the normal microflora on mucous membranes, especially of the mouth, lower GI tract, and vagina; these anaerobes cause disease when normal mucosal barriers break down.

Gram-negative anaerobes and some of the infections they cause include

- *Bacteroides* (most common): Intra-abdominal infections
- *Fusobacterium*: Abscesses, wound infections, and pulmonary and intracranial infections
- *Porphyromonas*: Aspiration pneumonia and periodontitis
- *Prevotella*: Intra-abdominal and soft-tissue infections

Gram-positive anaerobes and some of the infections they cause include

- *Actinomyces*: Head, neck, abdominal, and pelvic infections and aspiration pneumonia (actinomycosis)
- Clostridia: Intra-abdominal infections (eg, clostridial necrotizing enteritis), soft-tissue infections, and gas gangrene due to *C. perfringens*; food poisoning due to *C. perfringens type A*; botulism and infant botulism due to *C. botulinum*; tetanus due to *C. tetani*; and *C. difficile*–induced diarrhea (pseudomembranous colitis)
- *Peptostreptococcus*: Oral, respiratory, and intra-abdominal infections
- *Propionibacterium:* Foreign body infections (eg, in a cerebrospinal fluid shunt, prosthetic joint, or cardiac device)

Anaerobic infections are typically suppurative, causing abscess formation and tissue necrosis and sometimes septic thrombophlebitis, gas formation, or both. Many anaerobes produce tissue-destructive enzymes, as well as some of the most potent paralytic toxins known.

Usually, multiple species of anaerobes are present in infected tissues; aerobes are frequently also present (mixed anaerobic infections).

Clues to anaerobic infection include

- Polymicrobial results on Gram stain or culture
- Gas in pus or infected tissues
- Foul odor of pus or infected tissues
- Necrotic infected tissues
- Site of infection near mucosa where anaerobic microflora normally reside

Testing: Specimens for anaerobic culture should be obtained by aspiration or biopsy from normally sterile sites. Delivery to the laboratory should be prompt, and transport devices should provide an O_2-free atmosphere of carbon dioxide, hydrogen, and nitrogen. Swabs are best transported in an anaerobically sterilized, semisolid medium such as Cary-Blair transport medium.

ACTINOMYCOSIS

Actinomycosis is a chronic localized or hematogenous anaerobic infection caused by Actinomyces israelii. Findings are a local abscess with multiple draining sinuses, a TB-like pneumonitis, and low-grade septicemia. Diagnosis is by the typical appearance plus laboratory identification. Treatment is with a long course of antibiotics and surgery.

The causative organisms, *Actinomyces* sp (most commonly *A. israelii*), are often present commensally on the gums, tonsils, and teeth. However, many, if not most, infections are polymicrobial, with other bacteria (oral anaerobes, staphylococci, streptococci, *Aggregatibacter* [previously *Actinobacillus*] *actinomycetemcomitans,* Enterobacteriaceae) frequently cultured from lesions.

Actinomycosis most often occurs in adult males and takes several forms:

- **Cervicofacial (lumpy jaw):** The most common portal of entry is decayed teeth.
- **Thoracic:** Pulmonary disease results from aspiration of oral secretions.
- **Abdominal:** Disease presumably results from a break in the mucosa of a diverticulum or the appendix or from trauma.
- **Uterine:** This localized pelvic form is a complication of certain types of intrauterine device (IUD).
- **Generalized:** Rarely, the infection spreads from primary sites, presumably by hematogenous seeding.

Symptoms and Signs

The characteristic lesion is an indurated area of multiple, small, communicating abscesses surrounded by granulation tissue. Lesions tend to form sinus tracts that communicate to the skin and drain a purulent discharge containing "sulfur" granules (rounded or spherical, usually yellowish, and ≤ 1 mm in diameter). Infection spreads to contiguous tissues, but only rarely hematogenously.

The **cervicofacial form** usually begins as a small, flat, hard swelling, with or without pain, under the oral mucosa or the skin of the neck or as a subperiosteal swelling of the jaw. Subsequently, areas of softening appear and develop into sinuses and fistulas that discharge the characteristic sulfur granules. The cheek, tongue, pharynx, salivary glands, cranial bones, meninges, or brain may be affected, usually by direct extension.

In the **abdominal form**, the intestines (usually the cecum and appendix) and the peritoneum are infected. Pain, fever, vomiting, diarrhea or constipation, and emaciation are characteristic. One or more abdominal masses develop and cause signs of partial intestinal obstruction. Draining sinuses and intestinal fistulas may develop and extend to the external abdominal wall.

In the **localized pelvic form**, patients who use an IUD have vaginal discharge and pelvic or lower abdominal pain.

In the **thoracic form**, lung involvement resembles TB. Extensive invasion may occur before chest pain, fever, and productive cough appear. Perforation of the chest wall, with chronic draining sinuses, may result.

In the **generalized form**, infection spreads hematogenously to multiple areas, including the skin, vertebral bodies, brain, liver, kidneys, ureters, and, in women, pelvic organs. Diverse symptoms (eg, back pain, headache, abdominal pain) related to these sites may occur.

Diagnosis

- Microscopy
- Culture

Diagnosis is suspected clinically and confirmed by identification of *A. israelii* using microscopy and culture of sputum (ideally obtained endoscopically), pus, or a biopsy specimen. Imaging tests (eg, chest x-ray, abdominal or thoracic CT) are often done depending on findings.

In pus or tissue, the microorganism appears as the distinctive sulfur granules or as tangled masses of branched and unbranched wavy bacterial filaments, pus cells, and debris, surrounded by an outer zone of radiating, club-shaped, hyaline, and refractive filaments that take hematoxylin-eosin stain in tissue but are positive on Gram stain.

Lesions in any location may simulate malignant growths. Lung lesions must be distinguished from those of TB and cancer. Most abdominal lesions occur in the ileocecal region and are difficult to diagnose, except during laparotomy or when draining sinuses appear in the abdominal wall. Aspiration liver biopsy should be avoided because it can cause a persistent sinus.

Prognosis

The disease is slowly progressive. Prognosis relates directly to early diagnosis and is most favorable in the cervicofacial form and progressively worse in the thoracic, abdominal, and generalized forms, especially if the CNS is involved.

Treatment

- High-dose penicillin

Most patients respond to antibiotics, although response is usually slow because of extensive tissue induration and the relatively avascular nature of the lesions. Therefore, treatment must be continued for at least 8 wk and occasionally for ≥ 1 yr, until symptoms and signs have resolved.

High doses of penicillin G (eg, 3 to 5 million units IV q 6 h) are usually effective. Penicillin V 1 g po qid may be substituted after about 2 to 6 wk. Tetracycline 500 mg po q 6 h or doxycycline 100 mg q 12 h may be given instead of penicillin. Minocycline, clindamycin, and erythromycin have also been successful. Antibiotic regimens may be broadened to cover other pathogens cultured from lesions.

Anecdotal reports suggest that hyperbaric O_2 therapy is helpful. Extensive and repeated surgical procedures may be required. Sometimes small abscesses can be aspirated; large ones are drained, and fistulas are excised surgically.

KEY POINTS

- Actinomycosis usually involves multiple small, communicating abscesses with sinus tracts that drain a purulent discharge.
- Infection typically involves the neck and face, lungs, or abdominal and pelvic organs.
- Microscopically, *Actinomyces* appears as distinctive "sulfur" granules (rounded or spherical particles, usually yellowish, and ≤ 1 mm in diameter) or as tangled masses of branched and unbranched wavy bacterial filaments.
- Drain abscesses and excise fistulas.
- High-dose penicillin is usually effective but must be given long-term (8 wk to 1 yr).

OVERVIEW OF CLOSTRIDIAL INFECTIONS

Clostridia are spore-forming, gram-positive bacilli present widely in dust, soil, and vegetation and as normal flora in mammalian GI tracts.

Nearly 100 *Clostridium* sp have been identified, but only 25 to 30 commonly cause human or animal disease.

Pathophysiology

The pathogenic species produce tissue-destructive and neural exotoxins that are responsible for disease manifestations. Clostridia may become pathogenic when tissue O_2 tension and pH are low. Such an anaerobic environment may develop in ischemic or devitalized tissue, as occurs in primary arterial insufficiency or after severe penetrating or crushing injuries. The deeper and more severe the wound, the more prone the patient is to clostridial infection, especially if there is even minimal contamination by foreign matter.

Clostridial disease can also occur after injection of street drugs.

Serious noninfectious disease can occur after ingestion of home-canned foods in which clostridia have produced toxins.

Diseases Caused by Clostridia

Diseases caused by clostridia (see Table 181–1) include

- Botulism (due to *C. botulinum*)
- *C. difficile*–induced colitis
- Gastroenteritis
- Soft-tissue infections
- Tetanus (due to *C. tetani*)
- Clostridial necrotizing enteritis (due to *C. perfringens* type C)
- Neutropenic enterocolitis (due to *C. septicum*)

The most frequent clostridial infection is minor, self-limited gastroenteritis, typically due to *C. perfringens type A*. Serious clostridial diseases are relatively rare but can be fatal.

Abdominal disorders, such as cholecystitis, peritonitis, ruptured appendix, and bowel perforation can involve *C. perfringens, C. ramosum*, and many others.

Muscle necrosis and soft-tissue infection, which is characterized by crepitant cellulitis, myositis, and clostridial myonecrosis, can be caused by *C. perfringens*.

Skin and tissue necrosis can be caused by bloodborne *C. septicum* from the colon.

Clostridia also appear as components of mixed flora in common mild wound infections; their role in such infections is unclear.

Table 181–1. SELECTED CONDITIONS ASSOCIATED WITH CLOSTRIDIAL INFECTIONS

CONDITION	AGENT	TOXIN
Soft-tissue infection		
Crepitant cellulitis, myositis, clostridial myonecrosis, hemolysis	*C. perfringens*	α-Toxin (phospholipase C), θ-toxin, others
Gas gangrene, tissue necrosis, hemolysis	*C. septicum*	α-Toxin, β-toxin, hyaluronidase γ-toxin, septicolysin δ-toxin
Enteric diseases		
Food poisoning	*C. perfringens* type A	Enterotoxin
Enteritis necroticans	*C. perfringens* type C	β-Toxin
Antibiotic-associated colitis	*C. difficile*	Toxin A or B or *C. difficile* binary toxin (CDT)
Neutropenic enterocolitis	*C. septicum,* others	Unknown, possibly β-toxin
Colorectal cancer	*C. septicum*	—
Abdominal infections: Cholecystitis, peritonitis, ruptured appendix, bowel perforation	*C. perfringens, C. ramosum,* many others	β-Toxin*
Neurologic syndromes		
Tetanus	*C. tetani*	Tetanospasmin
Botulism	*C. botulinum*	Botulinal toxins A–H

*β-Toxin is produced by *C. perfringens* type C, but most of these infections are caused by *C. perfringens* type A, which does not produce β-toxin.

Hospital-acquired clostridial infection is increasing, particularly in postoperative and immunocompromised patients. Severe clostridial sepsis may complicate intestinal perforation and obstruction.

BOTULISM

Botulism is poisoning that is due to *Clostridium botulinum* toxin and that affects the peripheral nerves. Botulism may occur without infection if toxin is ingested, injected, or inhaled. Symptoms are symmetric cranial nerve palsies accompanied by a symmetric descending weakness and flaccid paralysis without sensory deficits. Diagnosis is clinical and by laboratory identification of toxin. Treatment is with support and antitoxin.

C. botulinum is one of several species of clostridia that cause human disease. Botulism is a rare, life-threatening disorder that occurs when botulinum toxin spreads hematogenously and interferes with release of acetylcholine at peripheral nerve endings. Botulism is a medical emergency and sometimes a public health emergency.

C. botulinum elaborates 8 types of antigenically distinct neurotoxins (types A through H). Five of the toxins (types A, B, E, and rarely F and H) affect humans. Types A and B are highly poisonous proteins resistant to digestion by GI enzymes. About 50% of food-borne outbreaks in the US are caused by type A toxin, followed by types B and E. Type A toxin occurs predominantly west of the Mississippi River, type B in the eastern states, and type E in Alaska and the Great Lakes area (type E is frequently associated with ingestion of fish products). Type H is the most potent toxin known.

Botulism can occur when neurotoxin is elaborated in vivo by *C. botulinum* or when it is acquired.

In vivo elaboration causes the following forms:

- Wound botulism
- Infant botulism (the most common form)
- Adult enteric botulism (rare)

In **wound botulism**, neurotoxin is elaborated in infected tissue.

In **infant botulism** and in **adult enteric botulism**, spores are ingested, and neurotoxin is elaborated in the GI tract. Adult enteric botulism usually occurs only in adults with impaired resistance.

Acquisition of preformed neurotoxin causes the following forms:

- Food-borne botulism
- Iatrogenic botulism
- Inhalation botulism

In **food-borne botulism**, neurotoxin produced in contaminated food is eaten.

In **iatrogenic botulism**, type A toxin is injected therapeutically to relieve excess muscle activity; rarely, botulism has occurred after cosmetic injections.

In **inhalation botulism**, toxins becomes aerosolized either accidentally or when intentionally used as a bioweapon; aerosolized toxins do not occur in nature.

C. botulinum spores are highly heat-resistant and may survive boiling for several hours at 100° C. However, exposure to moist heat at 120° C for 30 min kills the spores. Toxins, on the other hand, are readily destroyed by heat, and cooking food at 80° C for 30 min safeguards against botulism. Toxin production (especially type E) can occur at temperatures as low as 3° C (ie, inside a refrigerator) and does not require strict anaerobic conditions.

PEARLS & PITFALLS

- *C. botulinum* can produce toxin at temperatures as low as 3° C, so if food is contaminated, refrigeration is not protective.

Sources of toxin: Home-canned foods, particularly low-acid foods (ie, pH > 4.5), are the most common sources of ingested toxin, but commercially prepared foods have been implicated in about 10% of outbreaks. Vegetables (but usually not tomatoes), fish, fruits, and condiments are the most common vehicles, but beef, milk products, pork, poultry, and other foods have been involved. Of outbreaks caused by seafood, type E causes about 50%; types A and B cause the rest. In recent years, foods that are not canned (eg, foil-wrapped baked potatoes, chopped garlic in oil, patty melt sandwiches) have caused restaurant-associated outbreaks.

Sometimes the toxin is absorbed through the eyes or a break in the skin and, in such cases, may cause serious disease.

C. botulinum spores are common in the environment; most cases of infant botulism are caused by ingestion of spores.

Spores can also enter the body when drugs are injected with unsterilized needles; wound botulism may result. Injecting contaminated heroin into a muscle or under the skin (skin popping) is riskiest; it can cause gas gangrene.

If botulinum toxins enter the bloodstream, botulism results, regardless of how the toxins are acquired.

Symptoms and Signs

Common botulism symptoms and signs include

- Dry mouth
- Blurred or double vision
- Drooping eyelids
- Slurred speech
- Dysphagia

Pupillary light reflex is diminished or totally lost. Dysphagia can lead to aspiration pneumonia. These neurologic symptoms are characteristically bilateral and symmetric, beginning with the cranial nerves and followed by descending weakness or paralysis.

There are no sensory disturbances, and the sensorium usually remains clear.

Muscles of respiration and of the extremities and trunk progressively weaken in a descending pattern. Fever is absent, and the pulse remains normal or slow unless intercurrent infection develops. Constipation is common after neurologic impairment appears.

Major complications include

- Respiratory failure caused by diaphragmatic paralysis
- Pulmonary and other nosocomial infections

Food-borne botulism: Symptoms begin abruptly, usually 18 to 36 h after toxin ingestion, although the incubation period may vary from 4 h to 8 days. Nausea, vomiting, abdominal cramps, and diarrhea frequently precede neurologic symptoms.

Wound botulism: Neurologic symptoms appear, as in food-borne botulism, but there are no GI symptoms or evidence implicating food as a cause. A history of a traumatic injury or a deep puncture wound (particularly if due to injection of illicit drugs) in the preceding 2 wk may suggest the diagnosis.

A thorough search should be made for breaks in the skin and for skin abscesses caused by self-injection of illegal drugs.

Diagnosis

- Toxin assays
- Sometimes electromyography

Botulism may be confused with Guillain-Barré syndrome, poliomyelitis, stroke, myasthenia gravis, tick paralysis, and poisoning caused by curare or belladonna alkaloids. Electromyography shows characteristic augmented response to rapid repetitive stimulation in most cases.

In **food-borne botulism**, the pattern of neuromuscular disturbances and ingestion of a likely food source are important diagnostic clues. The simultaneous presentation of at least 2 patients who ate the same food simplifies diagnosis, which is confirmed by demonstrating *C. botulinum* toxin in serum or stool or by isolating the organism from stool. Finding *C. botulinum* toxin in suspect food identifies the source.

In **wound botulism**, finding toxin in serum or isolating *C. botulinum* organisms on anaerobic culture of the wound confirms the diagnosis.

Toxin assays are done only by certain laboratories, which may be located through local health authorities or the Centers for Disease Control and Prevention (CDC).

Treatment

- Supportive care
- Equine heptavalent antitoxin

Anyone known or thought to have been exposed to contaminated food must be carefully observed. Administration of activated charcoal may be helpful. Patients with significant symptoms often have impaired airway reflexes, so if charcoal is used, it should be given via gastric tube, and the airway should be protected by a cuffed endotracheal tube.

The greatest threat to life is

- Respiratory impairment and its complications

Patients should be hospitalized and closely monitored with serial measurements of vital capacity. Progressive paralysis prevents patients from showing signs of respiratory distress as their vital capacity decreases. Respiratory impairment requires management in an ICU, where intubation and mechanical ventilation are readily available. Improvements in such supportive care have reduced the mortality rate to < 10%.

Nasogastric intubation is the preferred method of alimentation because it

- Simplifies management of calories and fluids
- Stimulates intestinal peristalsis (which eliminates *C. botulinum* from the gut)
- Allows the use of breast milk in infants
- Avoids the potential infectious and vascular complications inherent in IV alimentation

Patients with wound botulism require wound debridement and parenteral antibiotics such as penicillin or metronidazole.

Antitoxin: A new heptavalent equine antitoxin (A to G) is now also available in the US; it replaces the older trivalent antitoxin. Antitoxin does not inactivate toxin that is already bound at the neuromuscular junction; therefore, preexisting neurologic impairment cannot be reversed rapidly. (Ultimate recovery depends on regeneration of nerve endings, which may take weeks or months.) However, antitoxin may slow or halt further progression. In patients with wound botulism, antitoxin can reduce complications and mortality rate.

Antitoxin should be given as soon as possible after clinical diagnosis and not delayed to await culture results. Antitoxin is less likely to be of benefit if given > 72 h after symptom onset.

One 20- or 50-mL vial of the heptavalent antitoxin, diluted 1:10, is given to adults as a slow infusion; dose and infusion rate are adjusted for infants and children. All patients who require the antitoxin must be reported to state health authorities, who then request the antitoxin from the CDC, which is the only source; practitioners cannot obtain antitoxin directly from the CDC. Because antitoxin is derived from horse serum, there is a risk of anaphylaxis or serum sickness. (For precautions, see p. 1382; for treatment, see p. 1378).

Prevention

Because even minute amounts of *C. botulinum* toxin can cause serious illness, all materials suspected of containing toxin require special handling. Toxoids are available for active immunization of people working with *C. botulinum* or its toxins. Details regarding specimen collection and handling can be obtained from state health departments or the CDC.

Correct canning and adequate heating of home-canned food before serving are essential. Canned foods showing evidence of spoilage and swollen or leaking cans should be discarded.

KEY POINTS

- Botulism may develop from ingestion of food-borne toxin, from elaboration of toxin from a clostridial wound infection, or, in infants, from ingestion and enteric colonization by *C. botulinum* spores.
- Botulism may result from man-made botulism toxin that is injected therapeutically or for cosmetic reasons or is inhaled (in an aerosolized form).
- Botulinum toxins block release of acetylcholine at peripheral nerve endings and cause bilateral, symmetric, descending weakness, beginning with the cranial nerves.
- Sensation and mental status are unaffected.
- Cooking destroys botulinum toxin but not the spores.
- For diagnosis, use toxin assays.
- Give equine antitoxin obtained from CDC via the state department of health.

INFANT BOTULISM

Infant botulism results from ingestion of *Clostridium botulinum* spores, their colonization of the large intestine, and toxin production in vivo.

Infant botulism occurs most often in infants < 6 mo. The youngest reported patient was 2 wk, and the oldest was 12 mo. Unlike food-borne botulism, infant botulism is not caused by ingestion of a preformed toxin. Most cases are idiopathic, although some have been traced to ingestion of honey, which may contain *C. botulinum* spores; thus, infants < 12 mo should not be fed honey.

Most cases involve type A or B toxin.

Symptoms and Signs

Constipation is present initially in 90% of cases and is followed by neuromuscular paralysis, beginning with the cranial nerves and proceeding to peripheral and respiratory musculature. Cranial nerve deficits typically include ptosis, extraocular muscle palsies, weak cry, poor suck, decreased gag reflex, pooling of oral secretions, poor muscle tone (floppy baby syndrome), and an expressionless face.

Severity varies from mild lethargy and slowed feeding to severe hypotonia and respiratory insufficiency.

Diagnosis

- Stool tests

Initially, botulism should be suspected based on clinical findings. Treatment should not be delayed pending test results.

Infant botulism may be confused with sepsis, congenital muscular dystrophy, spinal muscular atrophy, hypothyroidism, and benign congenital hypotonia.

Finding *C. botulinum* toxin or organisms in the stool establishes the diagnosis.

Treatment

- Human botulism immune globulin

Infants are hospitalized, and supportive care (eg, ventilatory support) is given as needed. Because the organism and toxin are excreted in the stool for weeks to months after symptom onset, appropriate contact precautions must be followed.

Specific treatment of botulism is with human botulism immune globulin, which is available from the Infant Botulism Treatment and Prevention Program (IBTPP—[510] 231-7600; see also the IBTPP web site). This antitoxin is derived from pooled human donors who have high titers of antibodies to A and/or B toxin.

Treatment is started as soon as the diagnosis is suspected; waiting for confirmatory test results, which may take days, is dangerous. The dose is 75 mg/kg IV once, given slowly.

The horse serum heptavalent antitoxin used in adults is not recommended for infants.

Antibiotics are not given because they may lyse *C. botulinum* in the gut and increase toxin availability.

CLOSTRIDIUM DIFFICILE–INDUCED DIARRHEA

(Pseudomembranous Colitis)

Toxins produced by *Clostridium difficile* strains in the GI tract cause pseudomembranous colitis, typically after antibiotic use. Symptoms are diarrhea, sometimes bloody, rarely progressing to sepsis and acute abdomen. Diagnosis is by identifying *C. difficile* toxin in stool. Treatment is with oral metronidazole or vancomycin.

C. difficile is the most common cause of antibiotic-associated colitis and is typically hospital-acquired, but community-acquired cases are increasing. *C. difficile*–induced diarrhea occurs in up to 8% of hospitalized patients and is responsible for 20 to 30% of cases of hospital-acquired diarrhea.

Risk factors for *C. difficile*–induced diarrhea include

- Extremes of age
- Severe underlying disease
- Prolonged hospital stay
- Living in a nursing home

C. difficile is carried asymptomatically by 15 to 70% of neonates, 3 to 8% of healthy adults, and perhaps 20% of hospitalized adults (more in long-term care facilities) and is common in the environment (eg, soil, water, household pets). Disease may follow overgrowth of intrinsic intestinal organisms or infection from an external source. Health care workers are frequently the source of transmission.

Recently, a more virulent strain, BI/NAP1/027 (North American pulsed-field type 1 [NAP1]/ribotype 027), has become prominent in hospital outbreaks. This strain produces substantially more toxin, causes more severe illness with greater chance of relapse, is more transmissible, and responds less well to antibiotic treatment.

Pathophysiology

Antibiotic-induced changes in GI flora are the dominant predisposing factor. Although most antibiotics have been implicated, cephalosporins (particularly 3rd-generation), penicillins (particularly ampicillin and amoxicillin), clindamycin, and fluoroquinolones pose the highest risk. *C. difficile*–induced colitis may also follow use of certain antineoplastic drugs.

The organism secretes both a cytotoxin and an enterotoxin. The main effect is on the colon, which secretes fluid and develops characteristic pseudomembranes—discrete yellow-white plaques that are easily dislodged. Plaques may coalesce in severe cases.

Toxic megacolon, which rarely develops, is somewhat more likely after use of antimotility drugs. Limited tissue dissemination occurs very rarely, as do sepsis and acute abdomen. Reactive arthritis has occurred after *C. difficile*–induced diarrhea.

Symptoms and Signs

Symptoms typically begin 5 to 10 days after starting antibiotics but may occur on the first day or up to 2 mo later. Diarrhea may be mild and semiformed or frequent and watery. Cramping or pain is common, but nausea and vomiting are rare. The abdomen may be slightly tender.

Patients with significant colitis or toxic megacolon have more pain and appear very ill, with tachycardia and abdominal distention and tenderness. Peritoneal signs are present in those with perforation.

Diagnosis

- Stool assay for toxin
- Sometimes sigmoidoscopy

Diagnosis should be suspected in any patient who develops diarrhea within 2 mo of antibiotic use or 72 h of hospital admission. Diagnosis is confirmed by stool (sample, not swab) assay for *C. difficile* toxin. A new real-time PCR test for the toxin gene *tcdB* may be superior to current assays. A single sample is usually adequate, but repeat samples should be submitted when suspicion is high and the first sample is negative. Fecal leukocytes are often present but not specific.

Sigmoidoscopy, which can confirm the presence of pseudomembranes, should be done if patients have ileus or if toxin assays are nondiagnostic. Abdominal x-rays, CT, or both are usually done if fulminant colitis, perforation, or megacolon is suspected.

Treatment

- Oral or IV metronidazole or oral vancomycin

The therapy of choice is

- Metronidazole 500 mg po q 8 h for 10 days

Alternatively, vancomycin 125 to 500 mg po q 6 h for 10 days may be given when severe illness is present (WBC count > 15,000 and/or creatinine > 1.5 times baseline). Metronidazole 500 mg IV q 8 h may be used when patients cannot tolerate oral drugs, or it may be given with oral vancomycin for very severe disease. In exceptional cases, vancomycin can be given by enema; dosage is similar to that of oral vancomycin. Fidaxomicin 200 mg po q 12 h, which is relatively new, is another alternative. Some patients require bacitracin 500 mg po q 6 h for 10 days, cholestyramine resin, or *Saccharomyces boulardii* yeast. Nitazoxanide 500 mg po q 12 h appears to be comparable to oral vancomycin 125 mg but is not commonly used in the US.

A few patients require total colectomy for cure.

Treatment of recurrences: Disease recurs in 15 to 20% of patients, typically within a few weeks of stopping treatment. Recurrence often results from reinfection (with the same or different strain), but some cases may involve persistent spores from the initial infection. For recurrences, vancomycin is given at a higher dose (250 to 500 mg po q 6 h) than is used for initial treatment.

Infusion of donor feces (fecal transplant) increases the likelihood of resolution in patients who have frequent, severe recurrences; presumably, the mechanism is restoration of normal fecal microbiota. About 200 to 300 mL of donor feces are used; donors are tested for enteric and systemic pathogens. Feces can be infused using a nasal-duodenal tube, colonoscope, or enema; the optimal method has not been determined.

Prevention of spread: Infection control measures are vital to reduce the spread of *C. difficile* among patients and health care workers.

KEY POINTS

- Antibiotic therapy can cause intestinal overgrowth of toxin-secreting *Clostridium difficile*, resulting in a pseudomembranous colitis that can be severe and difficult to cure.
- Cephalosporins (particularly 3rd-generation), penicillins, clindamycin, and fluoroquinolones pose the highest risk.
- Diagnose using a stool assay for *C. difficile* toxin.
- Treat severe disease with oral metronidazole and sometimes vancomycin or fidaxomicin.
- Recurrence is common; re-treat with a higher dose of vancomycin (250 to 500 mg po q 6 h), and consider fecal transplantation for refractory and severe recurrences.

CLOSTRIDIAL INTRA-ABDOMINAL AND PELVIC INFECTIONS

Clostridia, primarily *Clostridium perfringens*, are common in mixed intra-abdominal infections due to a ruptured viscus or pelvic inflammatory disease.

Clostridial infections of the abdomen and pelvis are serious and sometimes fatal.

Clostridium sp are common residents of the GI tract and are present in many abdominal infections, generally mixed with other enteric organisms. Clostridia are often the primary agents in the following:

- Emphysematous cholecystitis
- Gas gangrene of the uterus (which may occur after delivery and was previously common in patients who had a septic abortion)
- Certain other female genital tract infections (tubo-ovarian, pelvic, and uterine abscesses)
- Infection after perforation in colon carcinoma

The primary organisms are *C. perfringens* and, in the case of colon carcinoma, *C. septicum*. The organism produces exotoxins (lecithinases, hemolysins, collagenases, proteases, lipases) that can cause suppuration. Gas formation is common. Clostridial septicemia may cause hemolytic anemia because lecithinase (α-toxin) disrupts RBC membranes. With severe hemolysis and coexisting toxicity, acute renal failure can occur.

Symptoms and Signs

Symptoms are similar to those of other abdominal infections (eg, pain, fever, abdominal tenderness, a toxic appearance). Patients with a uterine infection may have a foul-smelling, bloody vaginal discharge, and gas sometimes escape through the cervix. Rarely, acute tubular necrosis develops.

Sepsis: Sepsis may be a complication of intra-abdominal or uterine clostridial infections. Initial symptoms can include fever, chills, vomiting, diarrhea, abdominal pain, hypotension, tachycardia, jaundice, cyanosis, and oliguria.

In 7 to 15% of patients with sepsis due to *C. perfringens*, acute massive intravascular hemolysis occurs. These patients have jaundice and red-tinged serum and urine. Spherocytes, ghost cells, and sometimes *C. perfringens* can be seen in a stained blood smear. Blood cultures are positive for *C. perfringens*.

Clostridial sepsis may result in multiorgan failure, which is frequently fatal, often within 24 h of hospital admission.

Diagnosis

- Gram stain and culture

Early diagnosis requires a high index of suspicion. Early and repeated Gram stains and cultures of the site, pus, lochia, and blood are indicated. Because *C. perfringens* can occasionally be isolated from healthy vagina and lochia, cultures are not specific.

X-rays may show local gas production (eg, in the biliary tree, gallbladder wall, or uterus).

Treatment

- Surgical debridement
- High-dose penicillin

Treatment is surgical debridement and penicillin G 5 million units IV q 6 h for at least 1 wk. Organ removal (eg, hysterectomy) may be necessary and can be lifesaving if debridement is insufficient.

If acute tubular necrosis develops, dialysis is needed.

The usefulness of hyperbaric O_2 has not been established.

CLOSTRIDIAL NECROTIZING ENTERITIS

(Darmbrand; Enteritis Necroticans; Pigbel)

Clostridial necrotizing enteritis is necrotizing inflammation of the jejunum and ileum caused by *Clostridium perfringens*.

Clostridial necrotizing enteritis is a mild to severe clostridial infection, which can be fatal if not treated promptly.

C. perfringens type C occasionally causes severe inflammatory disease in the small bowel (primarily, the jejunum). Disease is caused by clostridial β-toxin, which is very sensitive to proteolytic enzymes and is inactivated by normal cooking. Inflammation is segmental, involving small or large patches with varying degrees of hemorrhage and necrosis. Perforation may occur.

Disease occurs primarily in populations with multiple risk factors, including the following:

- Protein deprivation (causing inadequate synthesis of protease enzymes)
- Poor food hygiene
- Episodic meat feasting
- Staple diets containing trypsin inhibitors (eg, sweet potatoes)
- *Ascaris* infestation (these parasites secrete a trypsin inhibitor)

These factors are typically present collectively only in the hinterlands of New Guinea and parts of Africa, Central and South America, and Asia. In New Guinea, the disease is known as pigbel and is usually spread through contaminated pork, other meats, and perhaps peanuts.

Severity varies from mild diarrhea to a fulminant course of severe abdominal pain, vomiting, bloody stool, septic shock, and sometimes death within 24 h.

Diagnosis of clostridial necrotizing enteritis is based on clinical presentation plus toxin in stool.

Treatment of clostridial necrotizing enteritis is with antibiotics (penicillin G, metronidazole). Perhaps 50% of seriously ill patients require surgery for perforation, persistent intestinal obstruction, or failure to respond to antibiotics. An experimental toxoid vaccine has been used successfully in endemic areas but is not available commercially.

Neutropenic enterocolitis (typhlitis): This similar life-threatening syndrome develops in the cecum of neutropenic patients (eg, those with leukemia or receiving cancer chemotherapy). It may be associated with sepsis due to *C. septicum*.

Symptoms are fever, abdominal pain, GI bleeding, and diarrhea.

Diagnosis of neutropenic enterocolitis is based on symptoms, the presence of severe neutropenia, and results of abdominal CT and blood and stool cultures and toxin tests.

Neutropenic enterocolitis must be distinguished from *C. difficile*–induced diarrhea, graft-vs-host disease, and colitis due to cytomegalovirus.

Treatment of neutropenic enterocolitis is with antibiotics, but surgery may be necessary.

Neonatal necrotizing enterocolitis: Neonatal necrotizing enterocolitis, which occurs in neonatal ICUs, may be caused by *C. perfringens, C. butyricum,* or *C. difficile,* although the role of these organisms needs further study.

CLOSTRIDIUM PERFRINGENS FOOD POISONING

***Clostridium perfringens* food poisoning is acute gastroenteritis caused by ingestion of contaminated food.**

C. perfringens food poisoning is usually a mild clostridial infection.

C. perfringens is widely distributed in feces, soil, air, and water. Contaminated meat has caused many outbreaks. Because *C. perfringens* spores sometimes survive cooking, they can germinate and produce toxin when cooked meat that is contaminated with *C. perfringens* is left at room temperature or even up to 60° C (140° F, as on a warming table) for a period of time. Outbreaks typically occur in commercial establishments and rarely at home.

Once inside the GI tract, *C. perfringens* produces an enterotoxin that acts on the small bowel. Only *C. perfringens* type A has been definitively linked to this food poisoning syndrome. The enterotoxin produced is sensitive to heat (> 75° C).

Mild gastroenteritis is most common, with onset of symptoms 6 to 24 h after ingestion of contaminated food. The most common symptoms are watery diarrhea and abdominal cramps. Vomiting and fever are unusual. Symptoms typically resolve within 24 h; severe or fatal cases rarely occur.

Diagnosis of *C. perfringens* food poisoning is based on epidemiologic evidence and isolation of large numbers of organisms from contaminated food or from stools of affected people or on direct identification of enterotoxin in stool samples.

To prevent disease, people should promptly refrigerate leftover cooked meat and reheat it thoroughly (internal temperature, 75° C) before serving.

Treatment of *C. perfringens* food poisoning is supportive; antibiotics are not given.

CLOSTRIDIAL SOFT-TISSUE INFECTIONS

(Clostridial Myonecrosis; Gas Gangrene)

Clostridial soft-tissue infections include cellulitis, myositis, and clostridial myonecrosis. They usually occur after trauma. Symptoms may include edema, pain, gas with crepitation, foul-smelling exudates, intense coloration of the site, and progression to shock, renal failure, and sometimes death. Diagnosis is by inspection and smell, confirmed by culture. Treatment is with penicillin and surgical debridement. Hyperbaric O_2 is sometimes beneficial.

Clostridial infections of soft tissues may occur after an injury or spontaneously. Infection typically results in gas in soft tissues.

Clostridium perfringens is the most common species involved.

Clostridial soft-tissue infections usually develop hours or days after an extremity is injured by severe crushing or penetrating trauma that devitalizes tissue, creating anaerobic conditions. The presence of foreign material (even if sterile) markedly increases risk of clostridial infection. Infection may also occur in operative wounds, particularly in patients with underlying occlusive vascular disease.

Rarely, spontaneous cases occur, usually caused by *C. septicum* bacteremia originating from occult colon perforation in patients with colon cancer, diverticulitis, or bowel ischemia. Because *C. septicum* is aerotolerant, infection can spread widely to normal skin and soft tissues. Concurrent neutropenia, regardless of cause, predisposes to *C. septicum* bacteremia, which results in a poor prognosis; the prognosis is worse if intravascular hemolysis occurs.

In suitable conditions (low oxidation-reduction potential, low pH), as occur in devitalized tissue, infection progresses rapidly, from initial injury through shock, toxic delirium, and death within as little as 1 day.

Symptoms and Signs

Clostridial cellulitis occurs as a localized infection in a superficial wound, usually ≥ 3 days after injury. Infection may spread extensively along fascial planes, often with evident crepitation and abundant gas bubbling, but toxicity is much less severe than with extensive myonecrosis, and pain is minimal. Bullae are frequently evident, with foul-smelling, serous, brown exudate. Discoloration and gross edema of the extremity are rare. Clostridial skin infections associated with primary vascular occlusion of an extremity rarely progress to severe toxic myonecrosis or extend beyond the line of demarcation.

Clostridial myositis (suppurative infection of muscle without necrosis) is most common among parenteral drug users. It resembles staphylococcal pyomyositis and lacks the systemic symptoms of clostridial myonecrosis. Edema, pain, and frequently gas in the tissues occur. The infection spreads rapidly and may progress to myonecrosis.

In **clostridial myonecrosis** (gas gangrene), initial severe pain is common, sometimes even before other findings. The wound site may be pale initially, but it becomes red or bronze, often with blebs or bullae, and finally turns blackish green. The area is tensely edematous and tender to palpation. Crepitation is less obvious early than it is in clostridial cellulitis but is ultimately palpable in about 80%. Wounds and drainage have a particularly foul odor.

With progression, patients appear toxic, with tachycardia, pallor, and hypotension. Shock and renal failure occur, although patients often remain alert until the terminal stage. Bacteremia, sometimes with overt hemolysis, occurs in about 15% of patients with traumatic gas gangrene. Whenever massive hemolysis occurs, mortality of 70 to 100%, due to acute renal failure and septicemia, can be expected.

Diagnosis

- Clinical evaluation
- Gram stain and culture

Early suspicion and intervention are essential; clostridial cellulitis responds well to treatment, but myonecrosis has a mortality rate of ≥ 40% with treatment and 100% without treatment.

Although localized cellulitis, myositis, and spreading myonecrosis may be clinically distinct, differentiation often requires surgical exploration. In myonecrosis, muscle tissue is visibly necrotic; the affected muscle is a lusterless pink, then deep red, and finally gray-green or mottled purple and does not contract with stimulation. X-rays may show local gas production, and CT and MRI delineate the extent of gas and necrosis.

Wound exudate should be cultured for anaerobic and aerobic organisms. Because clostridia double in number every 7 min, anaerobic cultures of *Clostridia* may be positive in as little as 6 h. However, other anaerobic and aerobic bacteria, including members of the Enterobacteriaceae family and *Bacteroides, Streptococcus,* and *Staphylococcus* spp, alone or mixed, can cause severe clostridia like cellulitis, extensive fasciitis, or myonecrosis (see p. 999). Also, many wounds, particularly if open, are contaminated with both pathogenic and nonpathogenic clostridia that are not responsible for the infection.

The presence of clostridia is significant when

- Gram stain shows them in large numbers.
- Few PMNs are found in the exudates.
- Free fat globules are demonstrated with Sudan stain.

However, if PMNs are abundant and the smear shows many chains of cocci, an anaerobic streptococcal or staphylococcal infection should be suspected. Abundant gram-negative bacilli may indicate infection with one of the Enterobacteriaceae or a *Bacteroides* sp (see p. 1472). Detection of clostridial toxins in the wound or blood is useful only in the rare case of wound botulism.

Treatment

- Drainage and debridement
- Penicillin plus clindamycin

When clinical signs of clostridial infection (eg, gas, myonecrosis) are present, rapid, aggressive intervention is mandatory. Thorough drainage and debridement are as important as antibiotics; both should be instituted rapidly.

Penicillin G 3 to 4 million units IV q 4 to 6 h and clindamycin 600 to 900 mg IV q 6 to 8 h should be given immediately for severe cellulitis and myonecrosis. If gram-negative organisms are seen or suspected, a broad-spectrum antibiotic (eg, ticarcillin plus clavulanate, ampicillin plus sulbactam, piperacillin plus tazobactam) should be added. If penicillin-allergic patients have a life-threatening infection, clindamycin, with or without metronidazole 500 mg IV q 6 h, may be used.

Hyperbaric O_2 therapy may be helpful in extensive myonecrosis, particularly in the extremities, as a supplement to antibiotics and surgery. Hyperbaric O_2 therapy may salvage tissue and lessen mortality and morbidity if it is started early, *but it should not delay surgical debridement.*

KEY POINTS

- Rapidly progressing infection develops hours or days after an injury, particularly when crushing or penetrating trauma devitalizes tissue, creating an anaerobic environment.
- Clostridial cellulitis often causes minimal pain, but typically, myositis and myonecrosis are painful; crepitance due to gas in tissues is common in all forms.
- Drain and debride wounds quickly and thoroughly.
- Give penicillin plus clindamycin.
- For extensive myonecrosis, consider hyperbaric O_2 therapy, but do not let it delay surgical treatment.

TETANUS

(Lockjaw)

Tetanus is acute poisoning from a neurotoxin produced by *Clostridium tetani*. Symptoms are intermittent tonic spasms of voluntary muscles. Spasm of the masseters accounts for the name lockjaw. Diagnosis is clinical. Treatment is with human tetanus immune globulin and intensive support.

Tetanus bacilli form durable spores that occur in soil and animal feces and remain viable for years. Worldwide, tetanus is estimated to cause over half a million deaths annually, mostly in neonates and young children, but the disease is so rarely reported that all figures are only rough estimates. In the US, an average of 29 cases/yr were reported from 2001 through 2008.

Disease incidence is directly related to the immunization level in a population, attesting to the effectiveness of preventive efforts. In the US, well over half of elderly patients have inadequate antibody levels and account for one third to one half of cases. Most of the rest occur in inadequately immunized patients aged 20 to 59 yr. Patients < 20 yr account for < 10%.

Patients with burns, surgical wounds, or a history of injection drug abuse are especially prone to developing tetanus. However, tetanus may follow trivial or even inapparent wounds. Infection may also develop postpartum in the uterus (maternal tetanus) and in a neonate's umbilicus (tetanus neonatorum).

Pathophysiology

C. tetani spores usually enter through contaminated wounds. Manifestations of tetanus are caused by an exotoxin (tetanospasmin) produced when bacteria lyse. The toxin enters peripheral nerve endings, binds there irreversibly, then travels retrograde along the axons and synapses, and ultimately enters the CNS. As a result, release of inhibitory transmitters from nerve terminals is blocked, thereby causing unopposed muscle stimulation by acetylcholine and generalized tonic spasticity, usually with superimposed intermittent tonic seizures. Disinhibition of autonomic neurons and loss of control of adrenal catecholamine release cause autonomic instability and a hypersympathetic state. Once bound, the toxin cannot be neutralized.

Most often, tetanus is generalized, affecting skeletal muscles throughout the body. However, tetanus is sometimes localized to muscles near an entry wound.

PEARLS & PITFALLS

- Tetanus toxin binds irreversibly to nerve terminals, and once bound, it cannot be neutralized.

Symptoms and Signs

The incubation period ranges from 2 to 50 days (average, 5 to 10 days). Symptoms include

- Jaw stiffness (most frequent)
- Difficulty swallowing
- Restlessness
- Irritability
- Stiff neck, arms, or legs
- Headache
- Sore throat
- Tonic spasms

Later, patients have difficulty opening their jaw (trismus).

Spasms: Facial muscle spasm produces a characteristic expression with a fixed smile and elevated eyebrows (risus sardonicus). Rigidity or spasm of abdominal, neck, and back muscles and sometimes opisthotonos—generalized rigidity of the body with arching of the back and neck—may occur. Sphincter spasm causes urinary retention or constipation. Dysphagia may interfere with nutrition.

Characteristic painful, generalized tonic spasms with profuse sweating are precipitated by minor disturbances such as a draft, noise, or movement. Mental status is usually clear, but coma may follow repeated spasms. During generalized spasms, patients are unable to speak or cry out because of chest wall rigidity or glottal spasm. Rarely, fractures result from sustained spasms.

Spasms also interfere with respiration, causing cyanosis or fatal asphyxia.

Autonomic instability: Temperature is only moderately elevated unless a complicating infection, such as pneumonia, is present. Respiratory and pulse rates are increased. Reflexes are often exaggerated. Protracted tetanus may manifest as a very labile and overactive sympathetic nervous system, including periods of hypertension, tachycardia, and myocardial irritability.

Causes of death: Respiratory failure is the most common cause of death. Laryngeal spasm and rigidity and spasms of the abdominal wall, diaphragm, and chest wall muscles cause asphyxiation. Hypoxemia can also induce cardiac arrest, and pharyngeal spasm leads to aspiration of oral secretions with subsequent pneumonia, contributing to a hypoxemic death. Pulmonary embolism is also possible. However, the immediate cause of death may not be apparent.

Localized tetanus: In localized tetanus, there is spasticity of muscles near the entry wound but no trismus; spasticity may persist for weeks.

Cephalic tetanus is a form of localized tetanus that affects the cranial nerves. It is more common among children; in them, it may occur with chronic otitis media or may follow a head wound. Incidence is highest in Africa and India. All cranial nerves can be involved, especially the 7th. Cephalic tetanus may become generalized.

Tetanus neonatorum: Tetanus in neonates is usually generalized and frequently fatal. It often begins in an inadequately cleansed umbilical stump in children born of inadequately immunized mothers. Onset during the first 2 wk of life is characterized by rigidity, spasms, and poor feeding. Bilateral deafness may occur in surviving children.

Diagnosis

- Clinical evaluation

A history of a recent wound in a patient with muscle stiffness or spasms is a clue.

Tetanus can be confused with meningoencephalitis of bacterial or viral origin, but the following combination suggests tetanus:

- An intact sensorium
- Normal CSF
- Muscle spasms

Trismus must be distinguished from peritonsillar or retropharyngeal abscess or another local cause. Phenothiazines can induce tetanus-like rigidity (eg, dystonic reaction, neuroleptic malignant syndrome).

C. tetani can sometimes be cultured from the wound, but culture is not sensitive; only 30% of patients with tetanus have positive cultures. Also, false-positive cultures can occur in patients without tetanus.

Prognosis

Tetanus has a mortality rate of

- Worldwide: 50%
- In untreated adults: 15 to 60%
- In neonates, even if treated: 80 to 90%

Mortality is highest at the extremes of age and in drug abusers.

The prognosis is poorer if the incubation period is short and symptoms progress rapidly or if treatment is delayed. The course tends to be milder when there is no demonstrable focus of infection.

Treatment

- Supportive care, particularly respiratory support
- Wound debridement
- Tetanus antitoxin
- Benzodiazepines for muscle spasms
- Metronidazole or penicillin
- Sometimes drugs for autonomic dysfunction

Therapy requires maintaining adequate ventilation. Additional interventions include early and adequate use of human immune globulin to neutralize nonfixed toxin; prevention of further toxin production; sedation; control of muscle spasm, hypertonicity, fluid balance, and intercurrent infection; and continuous nursing care.

General principles: The patient should be kept in a quiet room. Three principles should guide all therapeutic interventions:

- Prevent further toxin release by debriding the wound and giving an antibiotic
- Neutralize unbound toxin outside the CNS with human tetanus immune globulin and tetanus toxoid (TT), taking care to inject into different body sites and thus avoid neutralizing the antitoxin
- Minimize the effect of toxin already in the CNS

Wound care: Because dirt and dead tissue promote *C. tetani* growth, prompt, thorough debridement, especially of deep puncture wounds, is essential. Antibiotics are not substitutes for adequate debridement and immunization.

Antitoxin: The benefit of human-derived antitoxin depends on how much tetanospasmin is already bound to the synaptic membranes—only free toxin is neutralized. For adults, human tetanus immune globulin 3000 to 6000 units IM is given once; this large volume may be split and given at separate sites around the wound. Dose can range from 500 to 6000 units, depending on wound severity, but some authorities feel that 500 units are adequate.

Antitoxin of animal origin is far less preferable because it does not maintain the patient's serum antitoxin level well and risk of serum sickness is considerable. If horse serum must be used, the usual dose is 50,000 units IM or IV (CAUTION: see Skin Testing on p. 1383).

If necessary, immune globulin or antitoxin can be injected directly into the wound, but this injection is not as important as good wound care.

Management of muscle spasm: Drugs are used to manage spasms.

Benzodiazepines are the standard of care to control rigidity and spasms. They block reuptake of an endogenous inhibiting neurotransmitter, γ-aminobutyric acid (GABA), at the $GABA_A$ receptor.

Diazepam can help control seizures, counter muscle rigidity, and induce sedation. Dosage varies and requires meticulous titration and close observation. The most severe cases may require 10 to 20 mg IV q 3 h (not exceeding 5 mg/kg). Less severe cases can be controlled with 5 to 10 mg po q 2 to 4 h. Dosage varies by age:

- Infants > 30 days: 1 to 2 mg IV given slowly, repeated q 3 to 4 h as necessary
- Young children: 0.1 to 0.8 mg/kg/day up to 0.1 to 0.3 mg/kg IV q 4 to 8 h
- Children > 5 yr: 5 to 10 mg IV q 3 to 4 h
- Adults: 5 to 10 mg po q 4 to 6 h or up to 40 mg/h IV drip

Diazepam has been used most extensively, but midazolam (adults, 0.1 to 0.3 mg/kg/h IV infusion; children, 0.06 to 0.15 mg/kg/h IV infusion) is water soluble and preferred for prolonged therapy. Midazolam reduces risk of lactic acidosis due to propylene glycol solvent, which is required for diazepam and lorazepam, and reduces risk of long-acting metabolites accumulating and causing coma.

Benzodiazepines may not prevent reflex spasms, and effective respiration may require neuromuscular blockade with vecuronium 0.1 mg/kg IV or other paralytic drugs and mechanical ventilation. Pancuronium has been used but may worsen autonomic instability. Vecuronium is free of adverse cardiovascular effects but is short-acting. Longer-acting drugs (eg, pipecuronium, rocuronium) also work, but no randomized clinical comparative trials have been done.

Intrathecal baclofen (a $GABA_A$ agonist) is effective but has no clear advantage over benzodiazepines. It is given by continuous infusion; effective doses range between 20 and 2000 mcg/day. A test dose of 50 mcg is given first; if response is inadequate, 75 mcg may be given 24 h later, and 100 mcg 24 h after that. Patients who do not respond to 100 mcg are not candidates for chronic infusion. Coma and respiratory depression requiring ventilatory support are potential adverse effects.

Dantrolene (loading dose 1.0 to 1.5 mg/kg IV, followed by infusion of 0.5 to 1.0 mg/kg q 4 to 6 h for ≤ 25 days) relieves muscle spasticity. Dantrolene given orally can be used in place of infusion therapy for up to 60 days. Hepatotoxicity and expense limit its use.

Management of autonomic dysfunction: Morphine may be given q 4 to 6 h to control autonomic dysfunction, especially cardiovascular; total daily dose is 20 to 180 mg.

β-Blockade with long-acting drugs such as propranolol is not recommended. Sudden cardiac death is a feature of tetanus, and β-blockade can increase risk; however, esmolol, a short-acting β-blocker, has been used successfully. Atropine at high doses has been used; blockade of the parasympathetic nervous system markedly reduces excessive sweating and secretions. Lower mortality has been reported in clonidine-treated patients than in those treated with conventional therapy.

Mg sulfate at doses that maintain serum levels between 4 to 8 mEq/L (eg, 4 g bolus followed by 2 to 3 g/h) has a stabilizing effect, eliminating catecholamine stimulation. Patellar tendon reflex is used to assess overdosage. Tidal volume may be impaired, so ventilatory support must be available.

Pyridoxine (100 mg once/day) lowers mortality in neonates. Other drugs that may prove useful include Na valproate (which blocks GABA-aminotransferase, inhibiting GABA catabolism), ACE inhibitors (which inhibit angiotensin II and reduce norepinephrine release from nerve endings), dexmedetomidine (a potent α-2 adrenergic agonist), and adenosine (which reduces presynaptic norepinephrine release and antagonizes the inotropic effect of catecholamines). Corticosteroids are of unproven benefit; their use is not recommended.

Antibiotics: The role of antibiotic therapy is minor compared with wound debridement and general support. Typical antibiotics include penicillin G 6 million units IV q 6 h, doxycycline 100 mg po bid, and metronidazole 500 mg po q 6 to 8 h.

Supportive care: In moderate or severe cases, patients should be intubated. Mechanical ventilation is essential when neuromuscular blockade is required to control muscle spasms that impair respirations.

IV hyperalimentation avoids the hazard of aspiration secondary to gastric tube feeding. Because constipation is usual, stools should be kept soft. A rectal tube may control distention. Bladder catheterization is required if urinary retention occurs.

Chest physiotherapy, frequent turning, and forced coughing are essential to prevent pneumonia. Analgesia with opioids is often needed.

Prevention

A primary series of vaccinations followed by regular boosters is required. Children < 7 yr require 5 primary vaccinations, and unimmunized patients > 7 yr require 3. The vaccine may be TT alone, but toxoid is typically combined with diphtheria and/or pertussis. Children's vaccines have higher doses of the diphtheria and pertussis components (DTaP, DT) than adult's vaccines (Tdap, Td).

Children are given DTaP at ages 2 mo, 4 mo, 6 mo, 15 to 18 mo, and 4 to 6 yr; they should get a Tdap booster at age 11 to 12 yr, and Td every 10 yr thereafter (see Tables 291–2 on p. 2462 and 291–3 on p. 2467).

Unimmunized adults are given Tdap initially, then Td 4 wk and 6 to 12 mo later, and Td every 10 yr thereafter. Adults who have not had a vaccine that contains pertussis should be given a single dose of Tdap instead of one of the Td boosters. Adults ≥ 65 who anticipate close contact with an infant < 12 mo and who have not previously received Tdap should be given a single dose of Tdap. Pregnant women should be given Tdap at 27 to 36 wk gestation regardless of when they were last vaccinated; the fetus can develop passive immunity from vaccines given at this time.

For routine diphtheria, tetanus, and pertussis immunization and booster recommendations, see pp. 1451 and 1452.

After injury, tetanus vaccination is given depending on wound type and vaccination history; tetanus immune globulin may also be indicated (see Table 181–2). Patients not previously vaccinated are given a 2nd and 3rd dose of toxoid at monthly intervals.

Because tetanus infection does not confer immunity, patients who have recovered from clinical tetanus should be vaccinated.

KEY POINTS

- Tetanus is caused by a toxin produced by *Clostridium tetani* in contaminated wounds.
- Tetanus toxin blocks release of inhibitory neurotransmitters, causing generalized muscle stiffness with intermittent spasms; seizures and autonomic instability may occur.
- Mortality is 15 to 60% in untreated adults and 80 to 90% in neonates even if treated.
- Prevent further toxin release by debriding the wound and giving an antibiotic (eg, penicillin, doxycycline), and neutralize unbound toxin with human tetanus immune globulin.
- Give IV benzodiazepines for muscle spasm, and neuromuscular blockade and mechanical ventilation as needed for respiratory insufficiency due to muscle spasm.
- Prevent tetanus by following routine immunization recommendations.

MIXED ANAEROBIC INFECTIONS

Anaerobes can infect normal hosts and hosts with compromised resistance or damaged tissues. Mixed anaerobic infections can include both single anaerobic species or multiple anaerobic species with any number of nonanaerobic isolates. Symptoms depend on site of infection. Diagnosis is

Table 181–2. TETANUS PROPHYLAXIS IN ROUTINE WOUND MANAGEMENT

HISTORY OF ADSORBED TETANUS TOXOID	CLEAN, MINOR WOUNDS		ALL OTHER WOUNDS*	
	Td†	TIG‡	Td†	TIG‡
Unknown or < 3 doses	Yes	No	Yes	Yes
≥ 3 doses	Yes if > 10 yr since last dose	No	Yes if > 5 yr since last dose	No

*Such as (but not limited to) wounds contaminated with dirt, feces, soil, or saliva; puncture wounds; crush injuries; avulsions; and wounds resulting from missiles, burns, or frostbite.

†For patients ≥ 10 yr who have not previously received a dose of Tdap, a single dose of Tdap should be given instead of one Td booster. Children < 7 yr should be given DTaP or, if pertussis vaccine is contraindicated, DT. Children aged 7–9 yr should be given Td.

‡TIG 250–500 units IM.

DT = diphtheria and tetanus toxoids (for children); DTaP = diphtheria and tetanus toxoids, acellular pertussis (for children); Td = tetanus and diphtheria toxoids adsorbed (for adults); Tdap = tetanus and diphtheria toxoids, acellular pertussis (for adults); TIG = tetanus immune globulin (human).

clinical combined with Gram stain and anaerobic cultures. Treatment is with antibiotics and surgical drainage and debridement.

Hundreds of species of nonsporulating anaerobes are part of the normal flora of the skin, mouth, GI tract, and vagina. If this commensal relationship is disrupted (eg, by surgery, other trauma, poor blood supply, or tissue necrosis), a few of these species together can cause infections with high morbidity and mortality. After becoming established in a primary site, infection can spread locally and hematogenously to distant sites.

Because aerobic and anaerobic bacteria are frequently present in the same infected site, appropriate procedures for isolation and culture are necessary to keep from overlooking the anaerobes.

Anaerobes can be the main cause of infection in the following:

- The pleural spaces and lungs
- Intra-abdominal, gynecologic, CNS, upper respiratory tract, and cutaneous diseases
- Bacteremia

Etiology

The principal anaerobic gram-positive cocci involved in mixed anaerobic infections are

- Peptococci
- Peptostreptococci

These anaerobes are part of the normal flora of the mouth, upper respiratory tract, and large intestine.

The principal anaerobic gram-negative bacilli involved in mixed anaerobic infections include

- *Bacteroides fragilis*
- *Prevotella melaninogenica*
- *Fusobacterium* sp

The *B. fragilis* group is part of the normal bowel flora and includes the anaerobic pathogens most frequently isolated from intra-abdominal and pelvic infections. Organisms in the *Prevotella* group and *Fusobacterium* sp are part of the normal oral and large-bowel flora.

Pathophysiology

Mixed anaerobic infections can usually be characterized as follows:

- They tend to occur as localized collections of pus or abscesses.
- The reduced O_2 tension and low oxidation-reduction potential that prevail in avascular and necrotic tissues are critical for their survival.
- When bacteremia occurs, it usually does not lead to disseminated intravascular coagulation (DIC) and purpura.

Clostridial infections can lead to septic shock, but most other anaerobic infections do not.

Some anaerobic bacteria possess distinct virulence factors. The virulence factors of *B. fragilis* probably account for its frequent isolation from clinical specimens despite its relative rarity in normal flora compared with other *Bacteroides* sp. This organism has a polysaccharide capsule that apparently stimulates abscess formation. An experimental model of intra-abdominal sepsis has shown that *B. fragilis* alone can cause abscesses, whereas other *Bacteroides* sp require the synergistic effect of another organism. Another virulence factor, a potent endotoxin, is implicated in septic shock associated with severe *Fusobacterium* pharyngitis.

Morbidity and mortality rates for anaerobic and mixed bacterial sepsis are as high as those for sepsis caused by a single aerobic organism. Anaerobic infections are often complicated by deep-seated tissue necrosis. The overall mortality rate for severe intra-abdominal sepsis and mixed anaerobic pneumonias tends to be high. *B. fragilis* bacteremia has a high mortality rate, especially in the elderly and in patients with cancer.

Symptoms and Signs

Patients usually have fever, rigors, and critical illness; shock is usually absent. DIC may occur in *Fusobacterium* sepsis.

For specific infections (and symptoms) caused by mixed anaerobic organisms, see elsewhere in The Manual and Table 181–3.

Anaerobes are rare in UTI, septic arthritis, and infective endocarditis.

Diagnosis

- Clinical suspicion
- Gram stain and culture

Table 181–3. DISORDERS OFTEN CAUSED BY MIXED* ANAEROBIC ORGANISMS

Anaerobic cellulitis
Aspiration pneumonia
Bartholin gland infections
Brain abscesses
Chronic otitis media
Chronic sinusitis
Decubitus or ischemic ulcer infections
Dental abscesses
Endometritis
Epidural and subdural empyema
Human bite infections
Intra-abdominal abscess
Liver abscess
Ludwig angina
Lung abscess
Mandibular osteomyelitis
Necrotizing gingivitis
Necrotizing ulcerative mucositis (cancrum oris)
Nongonococcal tubo-ovarian abscess
Parametrial abscess
Pelvic peritonitis
Periodontitis
Peritonitis
Septic thrombophlebitis
Skene glands infection
Vincent angina

*With aerobes or other anaerobes.

Clinical clues to the presence of anaerobic organisms include

- Infection adjacent to mucosal surfaces that bear anaerobic flora
- Ischemia, tumor, penetrating trauma, foreign body, or perforated viscus
- Spreading gangrene involving skin, subcutaneous tissue, fascia, and muscle
- Feculent odor in pus or infected tissues
- Abscess formation
- Gas in tissues
- Septic thrombophlebitis
- Failure to respond to antibiotics that do not have significant anaerobic activity

Anaerobic infection should be suspected when any wound smells foul or when a Gram stain of pus from an infected site shows mixed pleomorphic bacteria but aerobic cultures show no growth. Only specimens from normally sterile sites should be cultured because commensal contaminants may easily be mistaken for pathogens.

Gram stains and aerobic cultures should be obtained for all specimens. Gram stain, particularly in *Bacteroides* infection, and cultures for anaerobes may be falsely negative. Antibiotic susceptibility testing of anaerobes is exacting, and data may not be available for ≥ 1 wk after initial culture. However, if the species is known, susceptibility patterns can usually be predicted. Therefore, many laboratories do not routinely test anaerobic organisms for susceptibility.

Treatment

- Drainage and debridement
- Antibiotic choice varying by site of infection

In established infection, pus is drained, and devitalized tissue, foreign bodies, and necrotic tissue are removed. Organ perforations must be treated by closure or drainage. Whenever possible, blood supply should be reestablished. Septic thrombophlebitis may require vein ligation as well as antibiotics.

Because anaerobic culture results may not be available for 3 to 5 days, antibiotics are started. Antibiotics sometimes work even when some of the bacterial species in a mixed infection are resistant to the antibiotic, especially if surgical debridement and drainage are adequate. Antibiotics are chosen based on infection site and thus likely organisms.

Oropharyngeal anaerobic infections and lung abscesses: Oropharyngeal anaerobic infections may not respond to penicillin and thus require a drug effective against penicillin-resistant anaerobes (see below).

Oropharyngeal infections and lung abscesses should be treated with clindamycin or a β-lactam/β-lactamase inhibitor combination such as amoxicillin/clavulanate. In patients allergic to penicillin, clindamycin or metronidazole (plus a drug active against aerobes and microaerophiles) is useful.

GI or female pelvic anaerobic infections: GI or female pelvic anaerobic infections are likely to contain obligate anaerobic gram-negative bacilli such as *B. fragilis* plus facultative gram-negative bacilli such as *Escherichia coli;* antibiotic regimens must be active against both. Resistance of *B. fragilis* and other obligate anaerobic gram-negative bacilli to penicillins and 3rd- and 4th-generation cephalosporins occurs. However, the following drugs have excellent in vitro activity against *B. fragilis* and are effective:

- Metronidazole
- Carbapenems (eg, imipenem/cilastatin, meropenem, ertapenem)
- β-lactam/β-lactamase combinations (eg, piperacillin/tazobactam, ampicillin/sulbactam, amoxicillin/clavulanate, ticarcillin/clavulanate)
- Tigecycline
- Moxifloxacin

No single regimen appears to be superior. Drugs that are less predictably active in vitro against *B. fragilis* include clindamycin, cefoxitin, and cefotetan. All except clindamycin and metronidazole can be used as monotherapy because these drugs also have good activity against facultative anaerobic gram-negative bacilli.

Metronidazole is active against clindamycin-resistant *B. fragilis,* has unique anaerobic bactericidal activity, and usually avoids the pseudomembranous colitis sometimes associated with clindamycin. Concerns about metronidazole's potential mutagenicity have not been of clinical consequence.

Because many regimens currently used to treat GI or female pelvic anaerobic infections are also effective against facultative gram-negative bacilli, use of a potentially nephrotoxic aminoglycoside (to cover enteric facultative gram-negative bacilli) plus an antibiotic active against *B. fragilis* is no longer warranted.

Prevention

Before elective colorectal surgery, patients should have bowel preparation consisting of

- Cathartics
- Enemas
- Antibiotics

Most surgeons give both oral and parenteral antibiotics. For emergency colorectal surgery, parenteral antibiotics are used alone. Examples of oral regimens are neomycin (or kanamycin) plus erythromycin or metronidazole; these drugs are given no more than 18 to 24 h before the procedure. Examples of parenteral preoperative regimens are cefotetan, cefoxitin, cefazolin plus metronidazole, and ertapenem; these drugs are given within 1 h before the procedure. Preoperative parenteral antibiotics control bacteremia, reduce secondary or metastatic suppurative complications, and prevent local spread of infection around the surgical site.

During lengthy procedures, intraoperative antibiotics may be given every 1 to 2 half-lives of the antibiotic. Typically, postoperative antibiotics are not continued beyond 24 h after surgery.

For patients with confirmed allergy or adverse reaction to β-lactams, one of the following regimens is recommended:

- Clindamycin plus gentamicin, aztreonam, or ciprofloxacin
- Metronidazole plus gentamicin or ciprofloxacin

KEY POINTS

- Mixed anaerobic infections occur when the normal commensal relationship among the normal flora of mucosal surfaces (eg, skin, mouth, GI tract, vagina) is disrupted (eg, by surgery, injury, ischemia, or tissue necrosis).
- Infections tend to occur as localized collections of pus or abscesses.
- Base clinical suspicion on the clinical setting and the presence of gangrene, pus, abscess, tissue gas, and/or feculent odor.
- Draining and debride the infected area, and give antibiotics selected based on the infection location (and thus likely organisms).

182 Approach to Parasitic Infections

Human parasites are organisms that live on or in a person and derive nutrients from that person (its host). There are 3 types of parasites:

- Single-cell protozoa
- Multicellular helminths (worms)
- Ectoparasites such as scabies and lice

Parasitic infections due to protozoa and helminths are responsible for substantial morbidity and mortality worldwide. They are prevalent in Central and South America, Africa, and Asia. They are much less common in Australia, Canada, Europe, Japan, New Zealand, and the US. By far, the greatest impact is on residents of impoverished tropical areas with poor sanitation, but parasitic infections are encountered in developed countries among immigrants and travelers returning from endemic regions and, on occasion, even among residents who have not traveled, particularly those with AIDS or other conditions that cause immunodeficiency.

Many parasitic infections are spread through fecal contamination of food or water. They are most frequent in areas where sanitation and hygiene are poor. Some parasites, such as the hookworm, can enter the skin during contact with contaminated dirt or, in the case of schistosomes, with freshwater. Others, such as malaria, are transmitted by arthropod vectors. Rarely, parasites are transmitted via blood transfusions or shared needles or congenitally from mother to fetus.

Some parasites are endemic in the US and other developed countries. Examples are the pinworm *Enterobius vermicularis*, *Trichomonas vaginalis*, *Toxoplasma gondii*, and enteric parasites such as *Giardia intestinalis* (also known as *G. duodenalis* or *G. lamblia*) and *Cryptosporidium* spp.

The characteristics of protozoan and helminthic infections vary in important ways.

Protozoa: Protozoa are single-celled organisms that multiply by simple binary division (see pp. 1542 and 1644). Protozoa can multiply in their human hosts, increasing in number to cause overwhelming infection. With rare exceptions, protozoan infections do not cause eosinophilia.

Helminths: Helminths are multicellular and have complex organ systems. Helminths can be further divided into

- Roundworms (nematodes—see p. 1667)
- Flatworms (platyhelminthes), which include tapeworms (cestodes—see p. 1529) and flukes (trematodes— see p. 1720)

Some parasites have adapted to living in the lumen of the intestine where conditions are anaerobic; others reside in blood or tissues in aerobic conditions.

In contrast to protozoa, helminths do not multiply in humans but can elicit eosinophilic responses when they migrate through tissue. Most helminths have complex life cycles that involve substantial time outside their human hosts. A few, including *Strongyloides stercoralis*, *Capillaria philippinensis*, and *Hymenolepis nana*, can increase in number because of autoinfection (offspring reinfect the same host rather than being shed to infect another host). In strongyloidiasis, autoinfection can result in life-threatening, disseminated hyperinfections in immunosuppressed people, particularly those taking corticosteroids.

The severity of helminthic infections usually correlates with the worm burden, but there are exceptions as when a single ascaris causes life-threatening pancreatitis by migrating into and obstructing the pancreatic duct. The worm burden depends on the degree of environmental exposure, parasite factors, and the host's genetically determined immune responses. If a person moves from an endemic area, the number of adult worms diminishes over time. Although a few parasites (eg, *Clonorchis sinensis*) can survive for decades, many species have life spans of only a few years or less.

Nematodes are nonsegmented cylindric worms ranging from 1 mm to 1 m in length. Nematodes have a body cavity, distinguishing them from tapeworms and flukes. Depending on the species, different stages in the life cycle are infectious to humans. Hundreds of millions of humans are infected with nematodes; the most common are *Ascaris* (ascariasis), hookworms, and *Trichuris* (trichuriasis).

Cestodes (tapeworms) as adults are multisegmented flatworms that lack a digestive tract and absorb nutrients directly from the host's small bowel. In the host's digestive tract, adult tapeworms can become large, up to 40 m for one species. Tapeworms that infect humans include the fish tapeworm (*Diphyllobothrium latum*), beef tapeworm (*Taenia saginata*), and pork tapeworm (*Taenia solium*).

Trematodes (flukes) are nonsegmented flatworms that infect the blood vessels, GI tract, lungs, or liver. They are usually no more than a few centimeters in length; however, some are only 1 mm, and some are as large as 7 cm. In humans, most fluke infections are caused by *Schistosoma* sp (schistosomiasis), *Paragonimus westermani* (paragonimiasis), and *Clonorchis sinensis* (clonorchiasis).

Microsporidia: Microsporidia are intracellular spore-forming organisms that used to be classified as protozoa, but genetic analysis indicates that they are fungi or closely related to them. Human disease is mainly limited to people who have AIDS or another severe immunocompromising conditions. The clinical manifestations include gastroenteritis, focal involvement of the eyes, and disseminated infection.

Diagnosis

- Microscopic examination
- Antigen and DNA tests

Methods used to diagnose specific parasitic diseases are summarized in Table 182–1 (see also specific infections elsewhere in THE MANUAL).

Parasitic infections should be considered in the differential diagnosis of clinical syndromes in residents of or travelers to areas where sanitation and hygiene are poor or where vector-borne diseases are endemic. For example, fever in the returning traveler suggests the possibility of malaria. Experience indicates that people who have immigrated from endemic areas to developed countries and who return home to visit friends and relatives are at particular risk. They frequently do not seek or cannot afford pretravel advice on disease prevention and are more likely to enter high-risk settings than tourists who stay at resort facilities.

Although less frequent, the possibility of an endemic or imported parasitic infection must also be considered in residents of developed countries who present with suggestive clinical syndromes, even if they have not traveled.

Historical information, physical findings, and laboratory data may also suggest specific parasitic infections. For example, eosinophilia is common when helminths migrate through tissue and suggests a parasitic infection in an immigrant or returning traveler.

Table 182–1. COLLECTING AND HANDLING SPECIMENS FOR MICROSCOPIC DIAGNOSIS OF PARASITIC INFECTIONS*

PARASITE	OPTIMAL SPECIMEN	COLLECTION DETAILS	COMMENTS
Blood			
Plasmodium sp	Thick and thin smears of capillary blood (ie, finger or earlobe, using a disposable lancet) or 5–10 mL of fresh anticoagulated blood (preferably in collection tubes that contain EDTA)	Collect multiple samples during acute illness. Prepare smears from capillary or anticoagulated blood within 3 h after collection.	Use Wright or Giemsa stain. Ensure that glass slides are clean.
Babesia sp	Thick and thin smears as for *Plasmodium* sp	Collect as for *Plasmodium* sp.	Use Wright or Giemsa stain. Morphology is similar to *Plasmodium* sp ring forms but without pigment and gametocytes. Tetrads are diagnostic of *Babesia* sp but are infrequent.
Trypanosoma sp	Thin smears of capillary blood or 5–6 mL of anticoagulated blood	Collect capillary or anticoagulated blood. Smear on glass slides.	Various concentration techniques are used to enhance sensitivity. Motile trypanosomes are seen in wet preparations; Giemsa (or Field) stain is used to identify them in fixed preparations.
Filarial worms	Thick and thin smears from 1 mL of anticoagulated blood; if first specimen is negative, 5–10 mL, concentrated by centrifugation or filtration	Microfilariae of *Wuchereria bancrofti* and *Brugia malayi*: Draw blood between 10 PM and 2 AM. *Loa loa, Dipetalonema perstans*, and *Mansonella ozzardi*: Draw blood between 10 AM and 6 PM.	Use Giemsa or hematoxylin-eosin stain directly or, for greater sensitivity, after concentration in 2% formalin (Knott technique) or after filtration through a Nucleopore® membrane.
Bone marrow, other reticuloendothelial tissue, or CSF			
Leishmania sp	Aspirates of bone marrow, spleen, liver, or lymph nodes or smears from the buffy coat	Smear on glass slides.	Use Giemsa, Wright-Giemsa, or hematoxylin-eosin stain.
Naegleria *Acanthamoeba* *Balamuthia*	Fresh spinal fluid	Use aseptic collection technique. Examine specimen as soon as possible.	Examine using light or phase-contrast microscopy. Parasites may be detected by their movements; they can be fixed and stained with Giemsa or cultured.
Trypanosoma brucei gambiense and *rhodesiense*	Aspirates of lymph nodes or chancre Fresh spinal fluid	Use aseptic collection technique.	Use wet mount to identify motile parasites, or fix and stain with Giemsa or Field stain before or after concentration by centrifugation.
Duodenal aspirate or jejunal biopsy			
Giardia sp *Cryptosporidium* sp *Cystoisospora* sp *Cyclospora* sp Microsporidia *Strongyloides* sp	Duodenal aspirate or jejunal biopsy specimen	Examine aspirates immediately, or fix and stain them. Do histopathologic examination of biopsy specimens.	Use a wet mount of aspirate to identify ova or *Strongyloides* larvae. Multiple stains may be used for diagnosis (see Feces below for details). Transmission electron microscopy is the gold standard for detection of microsporidia.
Rectal biopsy			
Schistosoma mansoni *Schistosoma japonicum*	Rectal biopsy specimen from level of dorsal fold (Houston valve), about 9 cm from anus	Fix for histopathologic examination, and crush a segment between slides for increased sensitivity.	Speciation is based on the morphology of ova.

Table 182–1. COLLECTING AND HANDLING SPECIMENS FOR MICROSCOPIC DIAGNOSIS OF PARASITIC INFECTIONS* (*Continued*)

PARASITE	OPTIMAL SPECIMEN	COLLECTION DETAILS	COMMENTS
Sigmoidoscopy (proctoscopy)			
Entamoeba histolytica	Fresh scrapings with a curet or Volkmann spoon, a piece of mucosa snipped off with a surgical instrument, or aspirate from a lesion via a 1-mL serologic pipette with a rubber bulb (cotton-tipped swabs are not satisfactory)	Examine specimen immediately or after fixation and staining.	Use wet mounts or fixed stained slides (eg, with Trichrome stain) to detect trophozoites and cysts. Stool should be assayed for *E. histolytica* antigen; this test is more sensitive and can differentiate *E. histolytica* from nonpathogenic ameba.
Feces			
Entamoeba histolytica *Entamoeba dispar* *Entamoeba moshkovski* Other amebas	Multiple freshly passed stools (≥ 3) collected in AM	Examine unformed or diarrheal specimens within 15 min. Keep formed stools refrigerated until examination. Preserve in formalin or another fixative.	Use wet mounts and permanent stained slides (eg, Trichrome stain) and concentration techniques for cysts. Stool should be assayed for specific *E. histolytica* antigen, which is more sensitive and can differentiate *E. histolytica* from the nonpathologic *E. dispar*, *E. moshkovski*, and other nonpathogenic organisms.
Giardia sp	Multiple freshly passed stools (≥ 3) collected in AM every other day	Examine fresh, or preserve in formalin or another fixative. Trophozoites can also be detected in duodenal aspirates.	Examine direct and concentrated specimens. Cysts are usually seen in wet mounts and trophozoites are seen in fixed, Trichrome-stained slides. Assays for fecal antigens are more sensitive.
Cryptosporidium sp	Multiple freshly passed stools (≥ 3) collected daily or every other day	Refrigerate and examine fresh samples, or preserve in formalin or another fixative. Handle with care; fresh and dichromate-preserved stools are infectious. Duodenal aspirate or biopsy can be diagnostic.	Examine wet mounts by conventional light, differential interference contrast, and immunofluorescence microscopy. Stain specimens with modified acid-fast or modified safranin. Assays for fecal antigens are more sensitive.
Cystoisospora sp	Multiple freshly passed stools collected daily or every other day	Examine fresh, or preserve in formalin or other fixative. Concentration techniques enhance sensitivity.	Oocysts can be visualized in wet mounts by bright field differential interference contrast or epifluorescence microscopy. Stain fixed specimens with modified acid-fast stain. When stools are negative, examination of duodenal aspirate or a biopsy specimen can be diagnostic.
Cyclospora spp	Multiple freshly passed stools collected daily or every other day	Specimens should be refrigerated and examined fresh or frozen, or preserved in 10% formalin and 2.5% potassium dichromate. Different laboratory tests require different preservation techniques. Concentration techniques increase sensitivity.	Examine wet mounts by conventional light, bright-field differential interference contrast, and UV fluorescence microscopy. Oocysts are autofluorescent under UV light. Fixed specimens can be stained with modified acid-fast stain or modified safranin. A sporulation assay can differentiate *Cyclospora* from blue-green algae.
Microsporidia	Multiple stools collected daily or every other day	Small-bowel biopsies may be necessary if stools are negative.	Specimens stained by chromotropic methods are most widely used. Chemofluorescent agents such as calcofluor white can also be used for quick identification. Electron microscopy is the most sensitive method and used for speciation.

Table continues on the following page.

Table 182–1. COLLECTING AND HANDLING SPECIMENS FOR MICROSCOPIC DIAGNOSIS OF PARASITIC INFECTIONS* (*Continued*)

PARASITE	OPTIMAL SPECIMEN	COLLECTION DETAILS	COMMENTS
Trichuris sp *Ascaris* sp Hookworms *Strongyloides* sp Tapeworms Flukes	Multiple stools collected daily (up to 7 needed for *Strongyloides*)	Refrigerate specimen, and examine fresh, or fix in 10% formalin and concentrate using formalin–ethyl acetate sedimentation.	Active larvae are seen with *Strongyloides*; ova are seen with other intestinal helminths. For *Strongyloides*, the agar plate assay is more sensitive than ova and parasite examination. If stool is held at ambient temperature, *Strongyloides* larvae may appear similar to hatched hookworm larvae.
Enterobius sp	Ova collected from area around the anus on cellophane tape and placed on glass slide	Collect from area around the anus in the AM before a bowel movement or bath.	*Enterobius* ova are occasionally seen in a stool specimen or in vaginal contents obtained during a Papanicolaou test. Adult worms may be observed on the perianal region or in the vagina.
Sputum or aspirate from respiratory tract			
Paragonimus sp	Fresh sputum	Examine specimen as soon as possible, or preserve for later examination.	Concentration techniques may be necessary. Occasionally, ova are present in pleural fluid.
Strongyloides sp (hyperinfection)	Sputum, any aspirated material, fluid obtained by BAL or drainage material	Examine specimen as soon as possible, or preserve it for later examination.	Active larvae may be seen in wet mounts or can be fixed and stained with Giemsa.
Lung biopsy			
Paragonimus sp	Open lung biopsy or percutaneous biopsy guided by fluoroscopy or CT	Collect and place in sterile container with sterile saline. Fix and stain with Giemsa or hematoxylin-eosin.	Ova and adult flukes can be identified.
Skin			
Onchocerca volvulus	For patients infected in Africa, skin snips from the thigh, buttocks, or iliac crest For patients infected in Latin America, skin snips from the head, scapula, or buttocks	For skin snips, disinfect the skin with alcohol, insert a 25-gauge needle just under the epidermis, raise it, and slice off small piece of tissue with a scalpel or razor blade, or use a sclerocorneal punch biopsy tool. Bleeding should not occur. Examine fresh, or fix in methanol and stain with Giemsa or hematoxylin-eosin.	Examine the specimen suspended in saline for motile microfilaria migrating from the skin snip. Microfilariae may be seen in tissue sections.
Leishmania sp	Biopsy of a nonulcerated area of the lesion and touch preparations or slip smear scrapings	Look for amastigotes in Giemsa-stained touch preparations or smears and in hematoxylin-eosin-stained biopsy specimens.	*Leishmania* amastigotes are morphologically indistinguishable from those of *Trypanosoma cruzi*. *Leishmania* can be cultured from skin biopsies, but growth in vitro may take weeks. Molecular assays for leishmania DNA are available.
Urogenital secretions or biopsy			
Trichomonas sp	Sterile swabs of vaginal, urethral, or prostatic secretions placed in a tube with a small amount of sterile saline	Tell female patients not to douche for 3–4 days before collecting the specimen. Send specimen to the laboratory as soon as possible.	Identification of motile organisms by wet mount is the most rapid. Direct fluorescent antibody for parasites is more sensitive; culture is most sensitive but takes 3–7 days.
Schistosoma haematobium, occasionally *S. japonicum*	Fresh urine or biopsy from the area around the trigone	Recommended time for urine collection is between noon and 3 PM. Centrifugation increases detection.	Ova can be seen in wet mounts of urine or in biopsy specimens from the bladder.

BAL = bronchoalveolar lavage; EDTA = ethylene diamine tetraacetic acid; UV = ultraviolet.
Based on the CDC: Laboratory Identification of Parasitic Diseases of Public Health Concern, which provides detailed instructions.

The diagnosis of parasitic infections was once based on the identification of ova, larvae, or adult parasites in stool, blood, tissue or other samples or the presence of antibodies in serum, but diagnosis is being increasingly based on identification of parasite antigens or molecular tests for parasite DNA.

Physicians with expertise in parasitic infections and tropical medicine are available for consultation at many major medical centers, travel clinics, and public health facilities.

For detailed descriptions of diagnostic methods, see the CDC's Laboratory Identification of Parasites of Public Health Concern at www.cdc.gov.

GI tract parasites: Various stages of protozoa and helminths that infect the GI tract are typically shed in the stool. Routine detection requires examination of stool specimens, preferably 3 collected on different days, because shedding can vary. Sensitivity of stool examination for ova and parasites is low enough that when clinical suspicion is strong, empirical treatment should be considered. Sensitive and specific assays are now available to detect antigens of *G. intestinalis*, *Cryptosporidium* spp, and *Entamoeba histolytica* in stool. Although expensive, molecular tests for *G. intestinalis*, *Cryptosporidium* spp, *E. histolytica*, and *Cyclospora* are included in PCR-based screens for enteric bacterial, viral, and parasitic pathogens in stool samples (see Table 182–2).

Freshly passed stools uncontaminated with urine, water, dirt, or disinfectants should be sent to the laboratory within 1 h; unformed or watery stools are most likely to contain motile

Table 182–2. SEROLOGIC AND MOLECULAR TESTS FOR PARASITIC INFECTIONS

INFECTION	ANTIBODY	ANTIGEN OR DNA/RNA
Protozoans		
African trypanosomiasis (West)	CATT	—
Amebiasis	EIA, IHA	**Stool:** Antigen (EIA), PCR
Babesiosis	IFA	**Blood:** PCR
Chagas disease	IFA, EIA, RIPA	**Blood, tissue, or CSF:** PCR
Cryptosporidiosis	—	**Stool:** Antigen (EIA), PCR
Cyclosporiasis	—	PCR
Giardiasis	—	**Stool:** Antigen (EIA), DFA, PCR
Leishmaniasis	IFA or EIA (for visceral but not cutaneous leishmaniasis)	**Blood or tissue:** PCR
Malaria	IFA	**Blood:** ICG for antigen (rapid diagnostic test), PCR
Microsporidiosis	—	**Stool or intestinal tissue:** IFA, IIF, TEM, PCR
Toxoplasmosis	IFA, EIA (IgG and IgM)	**Tissue or blood:** PCR
Roundworms		
Filariasis	—	**Blood:** Antigen (ICG; not available in the US)
Strongyloidiasis	EIA, IFA, IHA	—
Trichinellosis	EIA	—
Toxocariasis	EIA	—
Flukes		
Paragonimiasis	CF, IB, EIA	—
Schistosomiasis	FAST-ELISA, IB	—
Tapeworms		
Cysticercosis	IB (serum or CSF), EIA	**Serum or CSF:** Antigen (used to assess responses to therapy; not sensitive enough for diagnosis) **CSF:** PCR
Echinococcosis	EIA, IHA, IFA, IB	—

CATT = card agglutination trypanosomiasis test for *Trypanosoma brucei gambiense*; CDC = Centers for Disease Control and Prevention; CF = complement fixation; DFA = direct fluorescent antibody; EIA = enzyme immunoassay; FAST-ELISA = Falcon assay screening test–enzyme-linked immunosorbent assay; IB = immunoblot; ICG = immunochromatographic assay; IFA = indirect fluorescent antibody test; IHA = indirect hemagglutination assay; IIF = immunofluorescence assay; PCR = polymerase chain reaction; RIPA = radioimmunoprecipitation assay; TEM = transmission electronic microscopy.

NOTE: Some antigen and parasite detection kits are available commercially. Others are available at the CDC or other reference laboratories. Molecular tests (eg, PCR) for DNA are available to detect enteric protozoa in stool samples, but they are expensive. Molecular tests for a number of other parasites are available in reference or research laboratories.

Based on CDC's Laboratory Identification of Parasites of Public Health Concern.

trophozoites. If not examined immediately, stools should be refrigerated, but not frozen. Portions of fresh stools should also be emulsified in fixative to preserve GI protozoa. Concentration techniques can be used to improve sensitivity. Anal cellophane tape or swabs may collect pinworm or tapeworm eggs. If strongyloidiasis is suspected, fresh stool should be smeared on an agar plate and incubated to identify the tracks of migrating larvae. Antibiotics, x-ray contrast material, purgatives, and antacids can hinder detection of ova and parasites for several weeks.

Sigmoidoscopy or colonoscopy should be considered when routine stool examinations are negative and amebiasis is suspected in patients with persistent GI symptoms. Sigmoidoscopic specimens should be collected with a curet or spoon (cotton swabs are not suitable) and processed immediately for microscopy. Duodenal aspirates or small-bowel biopsy specimens may be necessary for diagnosis of such infections as cryptosporidiosis and microsporidiosis.

Serologic testing for parasitic infections: Some parasites can be detected by serologic tests (see Table 182–2).

Treatment

- Various treatments, depending on the specific infection

Advice for treating parasitic infections is available from experts at major medical and public health centers and travel clinics, at the CDC web site (www.cdc.gov), in textbooks of infectious diseases and tropical medicine, and in summary form from *The Medical Letter on Drugs and Therapeutics*.

Drugs for unusual parasitic infections can often be obtained from the CDC Drug Service or the manufacturer.

Prevention

Despite substantial investment and research, no vaccines are yet available for prevention of human parasitic infections. Prevention is based on avoidance strategies.

Transmission of most intestinal parasites can be prevented by

- Sanitary disposal of feces
- Adequate cooking of food
- Provision of purified water

For the international traveler, the best advice is "cook it, boil it, peel it, or forget it." When followed, these measures reduce but do not eliminate the risk of intestinal parasitic infections as well as the risk of bacterial and viral gastroenteritis. Meat, particularly pork, and fish, particularly freshwater varieties, should be thoroughly cooked before ingestion. Other safety measures include removing cat litter boxes from areas where food is prepared to prevent toxoplasmosis. People should not swim in freshwater lakes, streams, or rivers in areas where schistosomiasis is endemic or walk barefoot or sit bare-bottom in areas where hookworms are found.

Prevention of malaria and many other vector-borne diseases involves

- Wearing long-sleeved shirts and pants
- Applying diethyltoluamide (DEET)-containing insect repellants to exposed skin and permethrin to clothing
- Using window screens, air-conditioning, and mosquito nets impregnated with permethrin or other insecticides
- For residents of nonendemic areas who travel in regions where malaria is transmitted, taking prophylactic antimalarial drugs

Travelers to rural Latin America should not sleep in adobe dwellings where reduviid bugs can transmit Chagas disease (see p. 1546). In Africa, travelers should avoid bright-colored clothing and wear long-sleeved shirts and pants to avoid tsetse flies in regions where African sleeping sickness occurs (see p. 1543).

Country-specific recommendations for travel are available from the CDC (www.cdc.gov).

183 Arboviruses, Arenaviridae, and Filoviridae

Arbovirus (arthropod-borne virus) applies to any virus that is transmitted to humans and/or other vertebrates by certain species of blood-feeding arthropods, chiefly insects (flies and mosquitoes) and arachnids (ticks). Arbovirus is not part of the current viral classification system, which is based on the nature and structure of the viral genome. Families in the current classification system that have *some* arbovirus members include

- Bunyaviridae (comprising the bunyaviruses, phleboviruses, nairoviruses, and hantaviruses)
- Flaviviridae (comprising only the flaviviruses)
- Reoviridae (comprising the coltiviruses and orbiviruses)
- Togaviridae (comprising the alphaviruses)

PEARLS & PITFALLS

- Arbovirus is not a family of viruses; the term indicates only that a virus is transmitted by certain species of arthropods—*ar*thropod-*bo*rne *virus*).
- Members of many different viral families may be arboviruses.

Most viruses associated with hemorrhagic fevers are classified in the families Arenaviridae and Filoviridae. However, some flaviviruses (yellow fever, dengue viruses) and some Bunyaviridae (Rift Valley fever virus, Crimean-Congo hemorrhagic fever virus, and the hantaviruses) may be associated with hemorrhagic symptoms.

Arboviruses number > 250 and are distributed worldwide; at least 80 cause human disease. Birds are often reservoirs for arboviruses, which are transmitted by mosquitoes to horses, other domestic animals, and humans. Other reservoirs for arboviruses include arthropods and vertebrates (often rodents, monkeys, and humans). These viruses may spread to humans directly from nonhuman reservoirs, but human-to-human transmission may also occur. Most arboviral diseases are not transmissible by humans, perhaps because the typical viremia is inadequate to infect the arthropod vector; exceptions include dengue fever, yellow fever, Zika virus (ZV) infection, and chikungunya disease, which can be transmitted from person to person via mosquitoes. Also, ZV can be transmitted during sexual activity from infected symptomatic or asymptomatic men to their sex partners (male or female) or from infected women to their sex partner.

Some infections (eg, West Nile virus infection, Colorado tick fever, dengue; theoretically, ZV) have been spread by blood transfusion or organ donation.

The Arenaviridae includes lymphocytic choriomeningitis virus, Lassa fever virus, Mopeia virus, Tacaribe virus, Junin virus, Lujo virus, and Guaroa virus; all are transmitted by rodents and thus are not arboviruses. Lassa fever can be transmitted from person to person.

The Filoviridae consists of 2 genera: Ebola virus (consisting of 5 species) and Marburg virus (consisting of 2 species). The specific vectors of these viruses have not been confirmed, but fruit bats are the prime candidates; thus, Filoviridae are not arboviruses. Human-to-human transmission of Ebola virus and Marburg virus occurs readily.

Many of these infections are asymptomatic. When symptomatic, they generally begin with a minor nonspecific flu-like illness that may evolve to one of a few syndromes (see Table 183–1). These syndromes include lymphadenopathy, rashes, aseptic meningitis, encephalitis, arthralgias, arthritis, and noncardiogenic pulmonary edema. Many cause fever and bleeding tendencies (hemorrhagic fever). Decreased synthesis of vitamin K–dependent coagulation factors, disseminated intravascular coagulation, and altered platelet function contribute to bleeding.

Laboratory diagnosis often involves viral cultures, PCR, electron microscopy, and antigen and antibody detection methods where available.

Treatment

- Supportive care
- Sometimes ribavirin

Treatment for most of these infections is supportive.

In hemorrhagic fevers, bleeding may require phytonadione (vitamin K_1). Transfusion of packed RBCs or fresh frozen plasma may also be necessary. Aspirin and other NSAIDs are contraindicated because of antiplatelet activity.

The following is recommended for hemorrhagic fever caused by arenaviruses or bunyaviruses including Lassa fever, Rift Valley fever, and Crimean-Congo hemorrhagic fever:

- Ribavirin 30 mg/kg IV (maximum, 2 g) loading dose followed by 16 mg/kg IV (maximum, 1 g/dose) q 6 h for 4 days, then 8 mg/kg IV (maximum, 500 mg/dose) q 8 h for 6 days

For dosage in hemorrhagic fever with renal syndrome (HFRS), see p. 1485.

Antiviral treatment for other syndromes has not been adequately studied. Ribavirin has not been effective in animal models of filovirus and flavivirus infections.

Prevention

- Vector control
- Sometimes vaccination

The abundance and diversity of arboviruses means that it is often easier and cheaper to control arbovirus infections by destroying their arthropod vectors, preventing bites, and eliminating their breeding habitats than by developing specific vaccines or drug treatments.

Vector control: Diseases transmitted by mosquitoes or ticks can often be prevented by the following:

- Wearing clothing that covers as much of the body as possible
- Using insect repellants (eg, DEET [diethyltoluamide])
- Minimizing the likelihood of exposure to the insect (eg, for mosquitoes, limiting time outdoors in wet areas; for ticks, see Sidebar 201–1 on p. 1696)

Diseases transmitted by rodent excreta can be prevented by the following:

- Sealing sites of potential rodent entry into homes and nearby buildings
- Preventing rodent access to food
- Eliminating potential nesting sites around the home

Guidelines for cleaning up after rodents and working in areas with potential rodent excreta are available through the Centers for Disease Control and Prevention (CDC).

Because transmission of the filoviruses Ebola virus and Marburg virus is predominantly from person to person, prevention of spread requires strict quarantine and isolation measures.

Vaccination: At present, there are effective vaccines only for Yellow fever virus and Japanese encephalitis virus. Vaccines for tick-borne encephalitis are available in Europe, Russia and China. A vaccine for dengue is approved in several countries outside the US, but efficacy is only moderate and varies by serotype and patient age; studies are ongoing.

DENGUE

(Breakbone Fever; Dandy Fever)

Dengue is a mosquito-borne disease caused by a flavivirus. Dengue fever usually results in abrupt onset of high fever, headache, myalgias, arthralgias, and generalized lymphadenopathy, followed by a rash that appears with a 2nd temperature rise after an afebrile period. Respiratory symptoms, such as cough, sore throat, and rhinorrhea, can occur. Dengue can also cause potentially fatal hemorrhagic fever with a bleeding tendency and shock. Diagnosis involves serologic testing and PCR. Treatment is symptomatic and, for dengue hemorrhagic fever (DHF), includes meticulously adjusted intravascular volume replacement.

Dengue is endemic to the tropical regions of the world in latitudes from about 35° north to 35° south. Outbreaks are most prevalent in Southeast Asia but also occur in the Caribbean, including Puerto Rico and the US Virgin Islands, Oceania, and the Indian subcontinent; more recently, dengue incidence has increased in Central and South America. Each year, only about 100 to 200 cases are imported to the US by returning tourists, but an estimated 50 to 100 million cases occur worldwide, with about 20,000 deaths.

The causative agent, a flavivirus with 4 serogroups, is transmitted by the bite of *Aedes* mosquitoes. The virus circulates in the blood of infected humans for 2 to 7 days; *Aedes* mosquitoes may acquire the virus when they feed on humans during this period.

Symptoms and Signs

After an incubation period of 3 to 15 days, fever, chills, headache, retro-orbital pain with eye movement, lumbar backache, and severe prostration begin abruptly. Extreme aching in the legs and joints occurs during the first hours, accounting for the traditional name of breakbone fever. The temperature rises rapidly to up to 40° C, with relative bradycardia. Bulbar and palpebral conjunctival injection and a transient flushing or pale pink macular rash (particularly of the face) may occur. Cervical, epitrochlear, and inguinal lymph nodes are often enlarged.

Fever and other symptoms persist 48 to 96 h, followed by rapid defervescence with profuse sweating. Patients then feel well for about 24 h, after which fever may occur again (saddleback pattern), typically with a lower peak temperature than the first. Simultaneously, a blanching maculopapular rash spreads from the trunk to the extremities and face.

Sore throat, GI symptoms (eg, nausea, vomiting), and hemorrhagic symptoms can occur. Some patients develop DHF. Neurologic symptoms are uncommon and can include encephalopathy and seizures; some patients develop Guillain-Barré syndrome (GBS).

Table 183–1. ARBOVIRUS, ARENAVIRUS, AND FILOVIRUS DISEASES

DISTINGUISHING SYMPTOMS	VIRAL AGENT OR DISEASE	FAMILY	VECTOR	MAJOR DISTRIBUTION*
Fever, malaise, headaches, myalgias				
Additional features: none	Colorado tick fever	Reoviridae (Coltivirus)	Ticks *Dermacentor* sp	Western US, western Canada
	Phlebotomus fever	Bunyaviridae (Phlebovirus)	Sand flies *Phlebotomus* sp	Mediterranean basin, Balkans, Middle East, Pakistan, India, China, eastern Africa, Panama, Brazil
	Venezuelan equine encephalitis	Togaviridae (Alphavirus)	Mosquitoes *Culex* sp	Argentina, Brazil, northern South America, Panama, Mexico, Florida
	Rift Valley fever†	Bunyaviridae (Phlebovirus)	Mosquitoes Several species	South Africa, eastern Africa, Egypt
Rash	Dengue fever	Flaviviridae	Mosquitoes *Aedes* sp	Southeast Asia, West Africa, Oceania, Australia, South America, Mexico, Caribbean, US
	Zika virus	Flaviviridae	Mosquitoes *Aedes* sp	Central and South America, Caribbean
	West Nile fever‡	Flaviviridae	Mosquitoes *Culex* sp	Africa, Middle East, southern France, Russia, India, Indonesia, US
Arthralgia, rash	Chikungunya disease	Togaviridae (Alphavirus)	Mosquitoes *Aedes* sp	Africa, India, Guam, Southeast Asia, New Guinea, limited areas of Europe
	Mayaro virus	Togaviridae (Alphavirus)	Mosquitoes *Haemagogus* sp	Brazil, Bolivia, Trinidad
	Ross River virus	Togaviridae (Alphavirus)	Mosquitoes *Aedes* sp	Australia, New Guinea, Solomon Islands, Samoa, Cook Islands
	Barmah Forest virus	Togaviridae (Alphavirus)	Mosquitoes *Aedes* sp	Australia
	Sindbis virus disease (Ockelbo disease, Karelian fever)	Togaviridae (Alphavirus)	Mosquitoes *Culex* sp	Africa, Australia, former Soviet Union, Finland, Sweden
Hemorrhagic signs§	Yellow fever	Flaviviridae	Mosquitoes *Aedes* spp	Central and South America, Africa
	Dengue hemorrhagic fever	Flaviviridae	Mosquitoes *Aedes* sp	Southeast Asia, West Africa, Oceania, Caribbean
	Kyasanur Forest disease	Flaviviridae	Ticks *Haemaphysalis* sp	India
	Omsk hemorrhagic fever	Flaviviridae	Ticks *Dermacentor* spp	Russia
	Crimean-Congo hemorrhagic fever	Bunyaviridae (Nairovirus)	Ticks *Hyalomma* sp	Africa, southern and eastern Europe, India, China, Middle East, former Soviet Union
	Hantaan virus	Bunyaviridae (Hantavirus)	Rodent	Korea, Japan, China, Southeast Asia, Europe
	Seoul virus	Bunyaviridae (Hantavirus)	Rodent	Korea, Japan, Europe
	Puumala virus (nephropathia epidemica)	Bunyaviridae (Hantavirus)	Rodent	Scandinavia, former Soviet Union
	Machupo virus	Arenaviridae	Rodent	Bolivia
	Junin virus	Arenaviridae	Rodent	Argentina

Table 183–1. ARBOVIRUS, ARENAVIRUS, AND FILOVIRUS DISEASES (*Continued*)

DISTINGUISHING SYMPTOMS	VIRAL AGENT OR DISEASE	FAMILY	VECTOR	MAJOR DISTRIBUTION*
	Guanarito virus	Arenaviridae	Rodent	Venezuela
	Lassa fever virus	Arenaviridae	Rodent *Mastomys* sp	West Africa
	Lujo virus	Arenaviridae	Unknown	Zambia
	Marburg virus	Filoviridae	Human to human Monkey Bat	Zimbabwe, Kenya, Uganda, Democratic Republic of Congo, South Africa
	Ebola virus	Filoviridae	Human to human Monkey Bat	Zaire, Sudan Guinea, Liberia, Sierra Leone, Democratic Republic of Congo, Gabon, Côte d'Ivoire, Uganda
Noncardiogenic pulmonary edema	Hantavirus: Sin Nombre, Black Creek Canal, Bayou, New York-1, Rio Mamore	Bunyaviridae (Hantavirus)	Rodent	US (west of Mississippi River), Canada, Brazil, Bolivia, Paraguay, Argentina
Severe fever with thrombocytopenia syndrome (SFTS)	SFTS virus	Bunyaviridae	Ticks	China, Korea, Japan
Fever and CNS involvement				
	Eastern equine encephalitis	Togaviridae (Alphavirus)	Mosquitoes *Culex* sp	Atlantic and Gulf coasts of US, Caribbean, upper New York, western Michigan
	Western equine encephalitis	Togaviridae (Alphavirus)	Mosquito	US, Canada, Central and South America
	West Nile virus	Flaviviridae	Mosquitoes *Culex* sp	Africa, Middle East, southern France, former Soviet Union, India, Indonesia, US
	St. Louis encephalitis	Flaviviridae	Mosquitoes *Culex* sp	US, Caribbean
	Venezuelan equine encephalitis	Togaviridae (Alphavirus)	Mosquitoes *Culex* sp	Argentina, Brazil, northern South America, Panama, Mexico, Florida
	La Crosse encephalitis	Bunyaviridae	Mosquitoes *Aedes* spp.	North Central States, New York
	Japanese encephalitis	Flaviviridae	Mosquitoes *Culex* sp	Japan, Korea, China, India, Philippines, Southeast Asia, Russia
	Powassan virus	Flaviviridae	Tick	Eastern Canada, New York
	Murray Valley encephalitis	Flaviviridae	Mosquitoes *Culex* sp	Australia, New Guinea
	Kyasanur Forest disease	Flaviviridae	Ticks	India
	Tick-borne encephalitis	Flaviviridae	Ticks *Haemaphysalis* sp	Europe, Balkans, Russia
Lymphocytic choriomeningitis	Rodents	Arenaviridae	Organ transplantation	US, Argentina, Germany, Balkans

*Changes in climatic conditions can affect the geographic range of arboviruses by extending or contracting the habitats of their vectors.
†Rift Valley fever also causes hemorrhage, meningoencephalitis, and ocular disorders.
‡West Nile virus also causes encephalitis.
§The Seoul, Puumala, Dobrava, and Hantaan hantaviruses cause hemorrhagic fever with renal syndrome.

Mild cases of dengue, usually lacking lymphadenopathy, remit in < 72 h. In more severe disease, asthenia may last several weeks. Death is rare. Immunity to the infecting strain is long-lasting, whereas broader immunity to other strains lasts only 2 to 12 mo.

Diagnosis

- Acute and convalescent serologic testing

Dengue fever is suspected in patients who live in or have traveled to endemic areas if they develop sudden fever, severe retro-orbital headache, myalgias, and adenopathy, particularly with the characteristic rash or recurrent fever. Evaluation should rule out alternative diagnoses, especially malaria and leptospirosis.

Diagnostic studies include acute and convalescent serologic testing, antigen detection, and PCR of blood. Serologic testing involves hemagglutination inhibiting or complement fixation tests using paired sera, but cross-reactions with other flavivirus antibodies are possible. Antigen detection is available in some parts of the world (not in the US), and PCR is usually done only in laboratories with special expertise.

Although rarely done and difficult, cultures can be done using mosquitoes or specialized cell lines in specialized laboratories.

CBC may show leukopenia by the 2nd day of fever; by the 4th or 5th day, the WBC count may be 2000 to 4000/μL with only 20 to 40% granulocytes. Urinalysis may show moderate albuminuria and a few casts. Thrombocytopenia may also be present.

Treatment

- Supportive care

Treatment of dengue is symptomatic. Acetaminophen can be used, but NSAIDs, including aspirin, should be avoided because bleeding is a risk. Aspirin increases the risk of Reye syndrome in children and should be avoided for that reason.

Prevention

People in endemic areas should try to prevent mosquito bites. To prevent further transmission by mosquitoes, patients with dengue should be kept under mosquito netting until the 2nd bout of fever has resolved.

Several vaccine candidates are being evaluated. One vaccine was licensed in Mexico in December 2015 for use in people aged 9 to 45 yr living in endemic areas.

KEY POINTS

- The dengue virus is transmitted by the bite of *Aedes* mosquitoes.
- Dengue fever typically causes sudden fever, severe retro-orbital headache, myalgias, adenopathy, a characteristic rash, and extreme aching in the legs and joints during the first hours.
- Dengue fever can cause a potentially fatal hemorrhagic fever with a bleeding tendency and shock (DHF).
- Suspect dengue fever if patients who live in or have traveled to endemic areas if they have typical symptoms; diagnose using serologic tests, antigen tests, or PCR of blood.

Dengue Hemorrhagic Fever

(Dengue Shock Syndrome; Philippine, Thai, or Southeast Asian Hemorrhagic Fever)

Dengue hemorrhagic fever (DHF) is a variant presentation that occurs primarily in children < 10 yr living in areas where dengue is endemic. DHF requires prior infection with the dengue virus.

DHF is an immunopathologic disease; dengue virus–antibody immune complexes trigger release of vasoactive mediators by macrophages. The mediators increase vascular permeability, causing vascular leakage, hemorrhagic manifestations, hemoconcentration, and serous effusions, which lead to circulatory collapse (ie, dengue shock syndrome).

Symptoms and Signs

DHF often begins with abrupt fever and headache and is initially indistinguishable from classic dengue. Warning signs that predict possible progression to severe dengue include

- Severe abdominal pain and tenderness
- Persistent vomiting
- Hematemesis
- Epistaxis or bleeding from the gums
- Black, tarry stools (melena)
- Edema
- Lethargy, confusion. or restlessness
- Hepatomegaly, pleural effusion, or ascites
- Marked change in temperature (from fever to hypothermia)

Shock and increasing illness may develop rapidly 2 to 6 days after onset.

Bleeding tendencies manifest as follows:

- Usually as purpura, petechiae, or ecchymoses at injection sites
- Sometimes as hematemesis, melena, or epistaxis
- Occasionally as subarachnoid hemorrhage

Bronchopneumonia with or without bilateral pleural effusions is common. Myocarditis can occur.

Mortality is usually < 1% in experienced centers but otherwise can range to up 30%.

Diagnosis

- Clinical and laboratory criteria

DHF is suspected in children with WHO-defined clinical criteria for the diagnosis:

- Sudden fever that stays high for 2 to 7 days
- Hemorrhagic manifestations
- Hepatomegaly

Hemorrhagic manifestations include at least a positive tourniquet test and petechiae, purpura, ecchymoses, bleeding gums, hematemesis, or melena. The tourniquet test is done by inflating a BP cuff to midway between the systolic and diastolic BP for 15 min. The number of petechiae that form within a 2.5-cm diameter circle are counted; > 20 petechiae suggests capillary fragility.

CBC, coagulation tests, urinalysis, liver function tests, and dengue serologic tests should be done. Coagulation abnormalities include

- Thrombocytopenia (≤ 100,000 platelets/μL)
- A prolonged PT
- Prolonged activated partial thromboplastin time
- Decreased fibrinogen
- Increased amount of fibrin split products

There may be hypoproteinemia, mild proteinuria, and increases in AST levels. Complement fixation antibody titers against flaviviruses are usually high (demonstration of a 4-fold or greater change in reciprocal IgG or IgM antibody titers to ≥ 1 dengue virus antigens in paired serum samples).

Patients with WHO-defined clinical criteria plus thrombocytopenia (≤ 100,000/μL) or hemoconcentration (Hct increased by ≥ 20%) are presumed to have the disease (see the CDC's Dengue Virus: Clinical Guidance at www.cdc.gov).

Treatment

- Supportive care

Patients with DHF require intensive treatment to maintain euvolemia. Both hypovolemia (which can cause shock) and overhydration (which can cause acute respiratory distress syndrome) should be avoided. Urine output and the degree of hemoconcentration can be used to monitor intravascular volume.

No antivirals have been shown to improve outcome.

KEY POINTS

- DHF occurs primarily in children < 10 yr living in areas where dengue is endemic and requires prior infection with the dengue virus.
- DHF may initially resemble dengue, but certain findings (eg, severe abdominal pain and tenderness, persistent vomiting, hematemesis, epistaxis, melena) indicate possible progression to severe dengue.
- Diagnose based on specific clinical and laboratory criteria.
- Maintaining euvolemia is crucial.

HANTAVIRUS INFECTION

Bunyaviridae contain the genus Hantavirus, which consists of at least 4 serogroups with 9 viruses causing 2 major, sometimes overlapping, clinical syndromes:

- Hemorrhagic fever with renal syndrome (HFRS)
- Hantavirus pulmonary syndrome (HPS)

Viruses causing HFRS are Hantaan, Seoul, Dobrava (Belgrade), and Puumala. Those causing HPS are Sin Nombre, Black Creek Canal, Bayou, and New York-1.

Hantaviruses occur throughout the world in wild rodents, which shed the virus throughout life in urine and feces. Transmission occurs between rodents. Transmission to humans is through inhalation of aerosols of rodent excreta. Recent evidence suggests human-to-human transmission may occur rarely. Naturally and laboratory-acquired infections are becoming more common.

Laboratory diagnosis of hantavirus infection is established by serologic tests and reverse transcriptase–PCR (RT-PCR). Serologic tests include enzyme-linked immunosorbent assay (ELISA) and Western and strip immunoblot assays. Growth of the virus is technically difficult and requires a biosafety level 3 laboratory.

Hemorrhagic Fever With Renal Syndrome

(Epidemic Nephrosonephritis; Korean Hemorrhagic Fever; Nephropathia Epidemica)

Hemorrhagic fever with renal syndrome (HFRS) begins as a flu-like illness and may progress to shock, bleeding, and renal failure. Diagnosis is with serologic tests and PCR. Mortality is 6 to 15%. Treatment includes IV ribavirin.

Some forms of HFRS are mild (eg, nephropathia epidemica, caused by Puumala virus, as occur in Scandinavia, the western part of the former Soviet Union, and Europe). Others are severe (eg, those caused by Hantaan and Dobrava viruses, as occur in Korea or the Balkans).

Infection is transmitted to humans via inhalation of rodent excreta.

Symptoms and Signs

Incubation is about 2 wk. In mild forms, infection is often asymptomatic.

When symptoms occur, onset is sudden, with high fever, headache, backache, and abdominal pain. On the 3rd or 4th day, subconjunctival hemorrhages, palatal petechiae, and a truncal petechial rash may appear. Diffuse reddening of the face that resembles sunburn, with dermatographism, occurs in > 90% of patients.

Relative bradycardia is present, and transient mild hypotension occurs in about half of patients, with shock in a minority. After the 4th day, renal failure develops.

About 20% of patients become obtunded. Seizures or severe focal neurologic symptoms occur in 1%. The rash subsides; patients develop polyuria and recover over several weeks. Proteinuria, hematuria, and pyuria may develop. Renal failure may occur.

Diagnosis

- Serologic testing or PCR

HFRS is suspected in patients with possible exposure if they have fever, a bleeding tendency, and renal failure.

CBC, electrolyte levels, renal function tests, coagulation tests, and urinalysis are then done. During the hypotensive phase, Hct increases and leukocytosis and thrombocytopenia develop. Albuminuria, hematuria, and RBC and WBC casts may develop, usually between the 2nd and 5th day. During the diuretic phase, electrolyte abnormalities are common.

Diagnosis of HFRS is ultimately based on serologic testing or PCR.

Prognosis

Death can occur during the diuretic phase, secondary to volume depletion, electrolyte disturbances, or secondary infections. Recovery usually takes 3 to 6 wk but may take up to 6 mo. Overall, mortality is 6 to 15%, almost always occurring in patients with the more severe forms. Residual renal dysfunction is uncommon except in the severe form that occurs in the Balkans.

Treatment

- Ribavirin
- Sometimes renal dialysis

Treatment is with IV ribavirin: loading dose 33 mg/kg (maximum, 2.64 g), followed by 16 mg/kg q 6 h (maximum, 1.28 g q 6 h) for 4 days, then 8 mg/kg q 8 h (maximum, 0.64 g q 8 h) for 3 days.

Supportive care, which may include renal dialysis, is critical, particularly during the diuretic phase.

Hantavirus Pulmonary Syndrome

Hantavirus pulmonary syndrome (HPS) occurs in the US primarily in the southwestern states. It begins as a flu-like illness and, within days, causes noncardiogenic pulmonary edema. Diagnosis is with serologic tests and reverse transcriptase–PCR. Mortality is 50 to 75%. Treatment is supportive.

Most cases of HPS are caused by

- The Sin Nombre hantavirus (Four Corners virus, Muerto Canyon virus)

Others are caused by

- The Black Creek Canal virus or Bayou virus in the southeastern US
- The New York virus on the East Coast of the US
- The Andes virus or Laguna Negra virus in South America

Infection is transmitted to humans via inhalation of excreta of sigmodontine rodents (especially the deer mouse). Most cases occur west of the Mississippi River in spring or summer, typically after heavy rains.

Symptoms and Signs

HPS begins as a nonspecific flu-like illness, with acute fever, myalgia, headache, and GI symptoms. Two to 15 days later (median 4 days), patients rapidly develop noncardiogenic pulmonary edema and hypotension. Several patients have had a combination of HFRS and HPS. Mild cases of HPS can occur.

Diagnosis

- Serologic testing or PCR

HPS is suspected in patients with possible exposure if they have unexplained clinical or radiographic pulmonary edema. Chest x-ray may show increased vascular markings, Kerley B lines, bilateral infiltrates, or pleural effusions.

If HPS is suspected, echocardiography should be done to exclude cardiogenic pulmonary edema.

CBC, liver function tests, and urinalysis are also usually done. HPS causes mild neutrophilic leukocytosis, hemoconcentration, and thrombocytopenia. Modest elevation of LDH, AST, and ALT, with decreased serum albumin, is typical. Urinalysis shows minimal abnormalities.

Diagnosis is with serologic testing or reverse transcriptase–PCR.

Prognosis

Patients who survive the first few days improve rapidly and recover completely over 2 to 3 wk, often without sequelae. Mortality averages 36%.

Treatment

- Supportive care

Treatment is supportive. Mechanical ventilation, meticulous volume control, and vasopressors may be required. For severe cardiopulmonary insufficiency, extracorporeal mechanical oxygenation may be lifesaving.

IV ribavirin is ineffective.

LASSA FEVER

Lassa fever is an often fatal arenavirus infection that occurs mostly in West Africa. It may involve multiple organ systems. Diagnosis is with serologic tests and PCR. Treatment includes IV ribavirin.

Lassa fever outbreaks have occurred in Nigeria, Liberia, and Sierra Leone. Cases have been imported to the US and the United Kingdom.

The reservoir is *Mastomys natalensis*, a rat that commonly inhabits houses in Africa. Most human cases probably result from contamination of food with rodent urine or feces, but human-to-human transmission can occur via urine, feces, saliva, vomitus, or blood.

Based on serologic data, indigenous people in endemic areas have a very high rate of infection—much higher than their rate of hospitalization for Lassa fever—suggesting that many infections are mild and self-limited. However, some observational studies of missionaries sent to endemic areas show they have a much higher rate of severe illness and mortality. The Centers for Disease Control and Prevention (CDC) estimates that about 80% of infected people have mild disease and about 20% have severe, multisystem disease.

Symptoms and Signs

The incubation period is 5 to 16 days.

Symptoms of Lassa fever begin with gradually progressive fever, weakness, malaise, and GI symptoms (eg, nausea, vomiting, diarrhea, dysphagia, stomach ache); symptoms and signs of hepatitis may occur. Over the subsequent 4 to 5 days, symptoms progress to prostration with sore throat, cough, chest pain, and vomiting. The sore throat becomes more severe during the first week; patches of white or yellow exudate may appear on the tonsils, often coalescing into a pseudomembrane.

In 60 to 80% of patients, systolic BP is < 90 mm Hg with pulse pressures of < 20 mm Hg, and relative bradycardia is possible. Facial and neck swelling and conjunctival edema occur in 10 to 30%. Occasionally, patients have tinnitus, epistaxis, bleeding from the gums and venipuncture sites, maculopapular rash, cough, and dizziness. Sensorineural hearing loss develops in 20%; it is often permanent.

Patients who recover defervesce in 4 to 7 days. Progression to severe illness results in shock, delirium, rales, pleural effusion, and, occasionally, generalized seizures. Pericarditis occasionally occurs. Degree of fever and aminotransferase levels correlate with disease severity.

Late sequelae include alopecia, iridocyclitis, and transient blindness.

Diagnosis

- PCR or serologic testing

Lassa fever is suspected in patients with possible exposure if they have a viral prodrome followed by unexplained disease of any organ system.

Liver function tests, urinalysis, serologic tests, and possibly CBC should then be done. Proteinuria is common and may be massive. AST and ALT levels rise (to 10 times normal), as do LDH levels.

The most rapid diagnostic test is PCR, but demonstrating either Lassa IgM antibodies or a 4-fold rise in IgG antibody titer using an indirect fluorescent antibody technique is also diagnostic.

Although the virus can be grown in cell culture, cultures are not routine. Because infection is a risk, particularly in patients with hemorrhagic fever, cultures must be handled only in a biosafety level 4 laboratory.

Chest x-rays, obtained if lung involvement is suspected, may show basilar pneumonitis and pleural effusions.

Prognosis

Recovery or death usually occurs 7 to 31 days (average 12 to 15 days) after symptoms begin. In patients with severe, multisystem disease, mortality is 16 to 45%.

Disease is severe during pregnancy. Mortality is 50 to 92% in women who are pregnant or who have delivered within 1 mo. Most pregnant women lose the fetus.

Treatment

- Ribavirin

Ribavirin, if begun within the first 6 days, may reduce mortality up to 10-fold. Treatment with ribavirin is 30 mg/kg IV (maximum, 2 g) loading dose followed by 16 mg/kg IV (maximum, 1 g/dose) q 6 h for 4 days, then 8 mg/kg IV (maximum, 500 mg/dose) q 8 h for 6 days. Anti-Lassa fever plasma has been tried in very ill patients but has not been shown to be beneficial and is not currently recommended.

Supportive treatment, including correction of fluid and electrolyte imbalances, is imperative.

For infected pregnant women, particularly during the 3rd trimester, uterine evacuation appears to reduce maternal mortality.

Prevention

Universal precautions, airborne isolation (including use of goggles, high-efficiency masks, a negative-pressure room, and positive-pressure filtered air respirators), and surveillance of contacts are recommended.

No vaccine is available.

KEY POINTS

- Lassa fever is usually transmitted by consuming food contaminated with rodent excreta, but human-to-human transmission can occur via urine, feces, saliva, vomitus, or blood.
- Symptoms may progress from fever, weakness, malaise, and GI symptoms to prostration with sore throat, cough, chest pain, and vomiting; sometimes to shock, delirium, rales, and pleural effusion; and occasionally to severe illness and shock.
- For the most rapid diagnosis, use PCR, but antibody tests can also be used.
- Lassa fever is severe during pregnancy; most infected pregnant women lose the fetus.
- Ribavirin, if begun within the first 6 days, may reduce mortality up to 10-fold; supportive treatment, including correction of fluid and electrolyte imbalances, is imperative.

LYMPHOCYTIC CHORIOMENINGITIS

Lymphocytic choriomeningitis is caused by an arenavirus. It usually causes a flu-like illness or aseptic meningitis, sometimes with rash, arthritis, orchitis, parotitis, or encephalitis. Diagnosis is by viral isolation, PCR, or indirect immunofluorescence. Treatment is supportive.

Lymphocytic choriomeningitis is endemic in rodents. Human infection results most commonly from exposure to dust or food contaminated by the gray house mouse or hamsters, which harbor the virus and excrete it in urine, feces, semen, and nasal secretions. When transmitted by mice, the disease occurs primarily in adults during autumn and winter.

Symptoms and Signs

The incubation period for lymphocytic choriomeningitis is 1 to 2 wk.

Most patients have no or minimal symptoms. Some develop a flu-like illness. Fever, usually 38.5 to 40° C, with rigors is accompanied by malaise, weakness, myalgia (especially lumbar), retro-orbital headache, photophobia, anorexia, nausea, and light-headedness. Sore throat and dysesthesia occur less often.

After 5 days to 3 wk, patients may improve for 1 or 2 days. Many relapse with recurrent fever, headache, rashes, swelling of metacarpophalangeal and proximal interphalangeal joints, meningeal signs, orchitis, parotitis, or alopecia of the scalp.

Aseptic meningitis occurs in a minority of patients. Rarely, frank encephalitis, ascending paralysis, bulbar paralysis, transverse myelitis, or acute Parkinson disease can occur. Neurologic sequelae are rare in meningitis but occur in up to 33% of patients with encephalitis.

Infection during pregnancy may cause fetal abnormalities, including hydrocephalus, chorioretinitis, and intellectual disability. Infections that occur during the 1st trimester may result in fetal death.

Diagnosis

- PCR, CSF analysis, antibody detection, and viral culture

Lymphocytic choriomeningitis is suspected in patients with exposure to rodents and an acute illness, particularly aseptic meningitis or encephalitis. Aseptic meningitis may lower CSF glucose mildly but occasionally to as low as 15 mg/dL. CSF WBCs range from a few hundred to a few thousand cells, usually with > 80% lymphocytes. WBC counts of 2000 to 3000/μL and platelet counts of 50,000 to 100,000/μL typically occur during the first week of illness.

Diagnosis can be made by

- PCR or by isolation of the virus from the blood or CSF during the acute stage of illness
- Indirect immunofluorescence assays of inoculated cell cultures, although these tests are most likely to be used in research laboratories
- Tests that detect seroconversion of antibody to the virus

Treatment

- Supportive care

Treatment of lymphocytic choriomeningitis is supportive. Measures needed depend on the severity of the illness. If aseptic meningitis, encephalitis, or meningoencephalitis develops, patients should be hospitalized, and treatment with ribavirin can be considered.

Anti-inflammatory drugs (eg, corticosteroids) may be considered in certain circumstances.

KEY POINTS

- In humans, lymphocytic choriomeningitis is usually acquired via exposure to dust or consumption of food contaminated by mouse or hamster excreta.
- Most patients have no or minimal symptoms, but some develop a flu-like illness, and a few develop aseptic meningitis.
- Infection during pregnancy may cause fetal abnormalities; if infection occurs during the 1st trimester, the fetus may die.

MARBURG AND EBOLA VIRUS INFECTIONS

Marburg and Ebola are filoviruses that cause hemorrhage, multiple organ failure, and high mortality rates. Diagnosis is with ELISA, PCR, or electron microscopy. Treatment is supportive. Strict isolation and quarantine measures are necessary to contain outbreaks.

Marburg and Ebola viruses are filamentous filoviruses that are distinct from each other but that cause clinically similar diseases characterized by hemorrhagic fevers and capillary leakage. Ebola virus infection is slightly more virulent than Marburg virus infection.

Ebola virus isolates have been differentiated into 5 species:

- Zaire Ebola virus
- Sudan Ebola virus
- Tai Forest Ebola virus (formerly, Côte d'Ivoire Ebola virus [the Tai forest is located in Côte D'Ivoire])
- Bundibugyo Ebola virus
- Reston Ebola virus (which is present in Asia but does not cause disease in humans)

Most previous outbreaks of Marburg and Ebola virus infections have originated in sub-Saharan Central and West Africa. Past outbreaks have been rare and sporadic; they have been contained partly because they have occurred in isolated areas. Spread to other areas, when it occurs, has usually resulted from travelers returning from Africa. However, in 1967, a small Marburg hemorrhagic fever outbreak occurred in Germany and Yugoslavia among laboratory workers who had been exposed to tissues from imported green monkeys.

In December 2013, a large Ebola virus outbreak began in rural Guinea (West Africa), then spread to densely populated urban regions in Guinea and to neighboring Liberia and Sierra Leone. It was first recognized in March 2014. It has so far involved thousands of people and has a mortality rate of about 59%. Infected travelers have spread Ebola virus to Europe and North America. Cases of Ebola continued to occur in the first few months of 2016; Sierra Leone was finally declared Ebola-free in March 2016, Guinea, in May 2016, and Liberia, in June 2016.

Transmission: Most index cases involve exposure to nonhuman primates in sub-Saharan Africa. The vector and reservoir are not known precisely, although the Marburg virus has been identified in bats, and cases have occurred in people exposed to bats (eg, in mines or caves). Ebola virus outbreaks have been linked to consumption of meat from wild animals in affected areas (bush meat) or soup made from bats. Ebola and Marburg virus infections have also occurred after handling tissues from infected animals.

Filoviruses are highly contagious. Human-to-human transmission occurs via skin and mucous membrane contact with body fluids (saliva, blood, vomit, urine, stool, sweat, breast milk, semen) of an infected symptomatic person or rarely a nonhuman primate. Humans are not infectious until they develop symptoms. Symptoms and signs persist in surviving patients for as long as it takes to develop an effective immune response. Typically, surviving patients eliminate the virus entirely and no longer transmit the virus; however, Ebola virus may survive in certain immune-privileged sites (eye, brain, testes). The virus may re-emerge from these sites and cause late sequelae or relapse. Semen can transmit Ebola and Marburg virus infection for up to 7 mo in contrast to other body fluids.

Aerosol transmission has been postulated; however, if it occurs, it is probably rare.

Real-world transmission is mainly human-to-human, resulting from close contact with the blood, secretions, other body fluids, or organs of infected people. Burial ceremonies in which mourners have direct contact with the deceased have played an important role in transmission of infection.

Symptoms and Signs

Symptoms of Marburg and Ebola virus infection are very similar.

After an incubation period of 2 to 20 days, fever, myalgia, and headache occur, often with abdominal pain, nausea, and upper respiratory symptoms (cough, chest pain, pharyngitis). Photophobia, conjunctival injection, jaundice, and lymphadenopathy also occur. Vomiting and diarrhea may soon follow. Delirium, stupor, and coma may occur, indicating CNS involvement.

Hemorrhagic symptoms begin within the first few days and include petechiae, ecchymoses, and frank bleeding around puncture sites and mucous membranes. A maculopapular rash, primarily on the trunk, begins around day 5.

Severe hypovolemia can develop, resulting from

- Extensive fluid loss due to diarrhea and vomiting
- Capillary leakage, resulting in hypoalbuminemia and loss of fluid from the intravascular space

Loss of electrolytes can cause severe hyponatremia, hypokalemia, and hypocalcemia. Cardiac arrhythmias can result.

During the 2nd wk of symptoms, either defervescence occurs and patients begin recovery, or patients develop fatal multiple organ failure. Recovery is prolonged and may be complicated by recurrent hepatitis, uveitis, transverse myelitis, and orchitis. Mortality ranges from 25 to 90%.

Diagnosis

- Evaluation and testing per the Centers for Disease Control and Prevention (CDC) guidelines at www.cdc.gov
- Enzyme-linked immunosorbent blood assay (ELISA) and reverse transcriptase (RT)-PCR

Marburg or Ebola virus infection is suspected in patients with bleeding tendencies, fever, other symptoms consistent with early filovirus infection, and travel from endemic areas. The CDC has issued an algorithm and guidelines for evaluating travelers returning from endemic areas. A similar approach can be used if Marburg virus is suspected.

The WHO has also issued guidelines regarding the 2014 Ebola outbreak in West Africa.

Cases should be discussed with public health authorities, who can assist in all facets of management, including

- Deciding whether to pursue the diagnosis
- Arranging transport of samples for testing
- Treatment, including transport to selected centers and, when indicated, use of novel therapies
- Tracking contacts

Testing includes CBC, routine blood chemistries, liver function and coagulation tests, and urinalysis. Diagnostic tests include ELISA and RT-PCR. The gold standard is detection of characteristic virions with electron microscopy of infected tissue (especially liver) or blood.

Treatment

- Supportive care

No effective antiviral therapy exists. Treatment is supportive and includes the following:

- Maintenance of blood volume and electrolyte balance
- Replacement of depleted coagulation factors
- Minimization of invasive procedures
- Treatment of symptoms, including use of analgesics

Drugs are being tested, some under expedited procedures, but none have yet been proved effective and safe.

Prevention

Several vaccines and antiviral drugs are currently in development but are unlikely to be available imminently.

To prevent spread, symptomatic patients with possible Ebola or Marburg virus infection must be isolated in dedicated containment facilities. Standard intensive care units (ICUs) in public hospitals are not suitable. Special containment facilities provide for total control of fluid effluent and respiratory products.

Staff members in contact with patients must be completely covered in protective suits with internal containment of respiratory gases. Trained staff members must be available to help those in contact with patients remove the protective clothing. Protocols for donning and removing mask, goggles or face shields, gown, and gloves must be followed (see the CDC's Sequence for Donning Personal Protective Equipment at www.cdc.gov).

Thorough equipment sterilization, hospital closures, and community education have shortened previous epidemics.

All suspected cases, including the cadavers, require strict isolation and special handling.

For more information, see the WHO's interim recommendations for infection prevention and control (http://apps.who.int).

KEY POINTS

- Ebola and Marburg viruses, although distinct, cause similar hemorrhagic fevers; outbreaks are perpetuated mainly by human-to-human transmission via contact with infected body fluids.
- Transmission in the 2013–2014 Ebola virus outbreak was predominantly human to human, resulting from close contact with blood, secretions, other body fluids, or organs of infected people or cadavers.
- Suspect Marburg or Ebola virus infection in patients with bleeding tendencies, fever, other compatible symptoms, and travel from endemic areas.
- Isolate patients with possible infection, and use strict procedures to protect workers who care for these patients.
- Plan diagnosis, management, and prevention of transmission with public health authorities.

YELLOW FEVER

Yellow fever is a mosquito-borne flavivirus infection endemic in tropical South America and sub-Saharan Africa. Symptoms may include sudden onset of fever, relative bradycardia, headache, and, if severe, jaundice, hemorrhage, and multiple organ failure. Diagnosis is with viral culture, reverse transcription PCR, and serologic tests. Treatment is supportive. Prevention involves vaccination and mosquito control.

In urban yellow fever, the virus is transmitted by the bite of an *Aedes aegypti* mosquito infected about 2 wk previously by feeding on a person with viremia. In jungle (sylvatic) yellow fever, the virus is transmitted by *Haemagogus* and other forest canopy mosquitoes that acquire the virus from wild primates. Incidence is highest during months of peak rainfall, humidity, and temperature in South America and during the late rainy and early dry seasons in Africa.

Symptoms and Signs

Infection ranges from asymptomatic (in 5 to 50% of cases) to a hemorrhagic fever with 50% mortality. Incubation lasts 3 to 6 days. Onset is sudden, with fever of 39 to 40° C, chills, headache, dizziness, and myalgias. The pulse is usually rapid initially but, by the 2nd day, becomes slow for the degree of fever (Faget sign). The face is flushed, and the eyes are injected. Nausea, vomiting, constipation, severe prostration, restlessness, and irritability are common.

Mild disease may resolve after 1 to 3 days. However, in moderate or severe cases, the fever falls suddenly 2 to 5 days after onset, and a remission of several hours or days ensues. The fever recurs, but the pulse remains slow. Jaundice, extreme albuminuria, and epigastric tenderness with hematemesis often occur together after 5 days of illness. There may be oliguria, petechiae, mucosal hemorrhages, confusion, and apathy.

Disease may last > 1 wk with rapid recovery and no sequelae. In the most severe form (called malignant yellow fever), delirium, intractable hiccups, seizures, coma, and multiple organ failure may occur terminally. During recovery, bacterial superinfections, particularly pneumonia, can occur.

Diagnosis

- Viral culture, reverse transcription PCR (RT-PCR), or serologic testing

Yellow fever is suspected in patients in endemic areas if they develop sudden fever with relative bradycardia and jaundice; mild disease often escapes diagnosis.

CBC, urinalysis, liver function tests, coagulation tests, viral blood culture, and serologic tests should be done. Leukopenia with relative neutropenia is common, as are thrombocytopenia, prolonged clotting, and increased PT. Bilirubin and aminotransferase levels may be elevated acutely and for several months. Albuminuria, which occurs in 90% of patients, may reach 20 g/L; it helps differentiate yellow fever from hepatitis. In malignant yellow fever, hypoglycemia and hyperkalemia may occur terminally.

Diagnosis is confirmed by culture, serologic tests, RT-PCR, or identification of characteristic midzonal hepatocyte necrosis at autopsy.

Needle biopsy of the liver during illness is contraindicated because hemorrhage is a risk.

Treatment

- Supportive care

Up to 10% of patients with disease severe enough to be diagnosed die.

Treatment is mainly supportive. Bleeding may be treated with vitamin K. An H_2 blocker or a proton pump inhibitor and sucralfate can be helpful as prophylaxis for GI bleeding and can be used in all patients ill enough to require hospitalization.

Suspected or confirmed cases must be quarantined.

Prevention

Preventive measures include

- Mosquito avoidance
- Vaccination

The most effective way to prevent outbreaks is to reduce the number of mosquitoes and limit mosquito bites by using diethyltoluamide (DEET), mosquito netting, and protective attire. During jungle outbreaks, people should evacuate the area until they are immunized and mosquitoes are controlled. Prompt mass yellow fever vaccination of the population is used to control an ongoing yellow fever outbreak through immunization. A single dose of vaccine can provide life-long immunity against yellow fever.

For people traveling to endemic areas, active immunization with the 17D strain of live-attenuated yellow fever vaccine (0.5 mL sc q 10 yr) is indicated and is effective in 95%. Although a single dose of yellow fever vaccine provides long-lasting protection and the WHO and the CDC's Advisory Committee on Immunization Practices no longer recommend a booster dose every 10 yr for most travelers, not all points of entry into countries may be aware that this requirement has been suspended; thus, it is probably safer to get the booster and not risk being denied entry. In the US, the vaccine is given only at US Public Health Service–authorized Yellow Fever Vaccination Centers.

The vaccine is contraindicated in the following:

- Pregnant women
- Infants < 6 mo
- People with compromised immunity

If infants aged 6 to 8 mo cannot avoid travel to an endemic area, parents should discuss vaccination with their physician since the vaccine is typically not offered until age 9 mo.

To prevent further mosquito transmission, infected patients should be isolated in rooms that are well screened and sprayed with insecticides.

ZIKA VIRUS INFECTIONS

The zika virus (ZV) is a flavivirus that is similar to the viruses that cause dengue, yellow fever, and West Nile fever. ZV infection is typically asymptomatic but can cause fever, rash, joint pain, or conjunctivitis; ZV infection during pregnancy can cause microcephaly (a serious birth defect) and eye abnormalities. Diagnosis is with ELISA or reverse transcriptase–PCR. Treatment is supportive. Prevention involves avoiding mosquito bites, avoiding unprotected sex with a partner at risk of having ZV infection, and, for pregnant women, avoiding travel to areas with ongoing transmission.

ZV, like the viruses that cause dengue, yellow fever, and chikungunya disease, is transmitted by *Aedes* mosquitoes, which breed in areas of stagnant water. These mosquitoes prefer to bite people and live near people, indoors and outdoors; they bite aggressively during the day. They also bite at night.

The main vectors are *A. aegypti* and *A. albopictus*. In the US, *A. aegypti* is restricted to the deep South, but *A. albopictus*, which better adapted to colder climates, is present across a large part of the southeast. *A. aegypti* is considered to be the main vector for epidemic ZV infection; *A. albopictus* is thought to be a significant vector of epidemic ZV infection in the tropics, but whether it would do so in the more temperate climate of the US is unclear.

Epidemiology

In 1947, the ZV was first isolated from monkeys in the Zika Forest of Uganda but was not considered an important human pathogen until the first large-scale outbreaks in the South Pacific islands in 2007. In May 2015, local transmission was first reported in South America, then in Central America and in the Caribbean, reaching Mexico by late November 2015.

Currently, ongoing local transmission of ZV has been reported in the following regions:

- South America
- Central America
- Caribbean Islands
- Pacific Islands
- Cape Verde (a nation of islands off the northwest coast of Africa)
- Southeast Asia (sporadic cases)

The US CDC has issued travel alerts for many countries in these regions.

As of October 2016, cases of locally transmitted ZV infection have been reported in Miami-Dade County in southeastern Florida. ZV infection has also been reported in travelers returning to the US after travel to countries where the virus is transmitted locally.

Predicting where the ZV will spread is difficult. However, because the same mosquito that transmits Zika also transmits dengue and chikungunya, local transmission of ZV can be expected wherever dengue or chikungunya has been transmitted. Dengue has been locally acquired in Texas, Florida, and Hawaii; chikungunya has been locally acquired in Florida. Similarly, in areas of the US where dengue is now endemic (Puerto Rico and the US Virgin Islands in the Caribbean; American Samoa, Guam, and the Northern Mariana Islands in the Pacific Ocean), ZV infection may also become endemic.

Transmission

During the first week of infection, the ZV is present in blood. Mosquitoes can acquire the virus when they bite infected people; the mosquitoes can then transmit the virus to other people through bites. Travelers from areas of ongoing ZV transmission may have ZV in their blood when they return home, and if mosquito vectors are present locally, local transmission of ZV is possible. However, because contact between *Aedes*mosquitoes and people is infrequent in most of the continental US and Hawaii (because of mosquito control and people living and working in air-conditioned environments), local transmission of ZV is expected to be rare and limited.

Although the ZV is transmitted primarily by mosquitoes, other modes of transmission are possible. They include

- Sexual transmission
- Transmission through blood transfusion
- Transmission through organ or tissue transplantation (theoretically)
- Intrauterine transmission from mother to fetus, resulting in congenital infection

ZV is present in semen and can be transmitted by men to their sex partners through sexual intercourse, including vaginal and anal sex and probably oral sex (fellatio). Both male to female and male to male transmission during unprotected sexual activity (no condoms) has occurred (see also the CDC: Clinical Guidance for Healthcare Providers for Prevention of Sexual Transmission of ZV at www.cdc.gov).

ZV also persists in vaginal secretions after it disappears from blood and urine; female-to-male sexual transmission of ZV infection has recently been reported.[1]

Transmission by blood transfusion has been reported in Brazil; however, at present, no cases of transmission by blood transfusion have been confirmed in the US (see also the CDC: About ZV Disease at www.cdc.gov).

The ZV, like the viruses that cause dengue, chikungunya disease, West Nile fever, and yellow fever, can be transmitted from mother to child during pregnancy. The viruses that cause dengue and West Nile fever can be transmitted in breast milk. At present, there have been no reports of ZV transmission via breastfeeding, and because breastfeeding has many benefits, the CDC encourages mothers to breastfeed even in areas where ZV transmission is ongoing.

1. CDC media statement: First female-to-male sexual transmission of ZV infection reported in New York City. July 2016.

Symptoms and Signs

Most people who become infected have no symptoms.

Symptoms of ZV infection include fever, maculopapular rash, conjunctivitis (pinkeye), joint pain, retro-orbital pain, headache, and muscle pain. Symptoms last 4 to 7 days. Most infections are mild. Severe infection requiring hospitalization is uncommon. Death due to ZV infection is rare.

Very uncommonly, Guillain-Barré syndrome (GBS) develops after a ZV infection. GBS is an acute, usually rapidly progressive but self-limited inflammatory polyneuropathy thought to be caused by an autoimmune reaction. GBS has also developed after dengue and chikungunya disease.

Microcephaly: ZV infection during pregnancy can cause microcephaly (a congenital disorder involving incomplete brain development and small head size) and other severe fetal brain defects (see also the CDC: Clinical Guidance for Healthcare Providers Caring for Infants and Children at www.cdc.gov).

In the US, several cases of microcephaly have been linked to the ZV; the mothers of these infants probably contracted the infection through travel to a country with endemic infection. The CDC is monitoring a number of pregnant women who have ZV infection and who live on the US mainland or in Puerto Rico or other US territories; these women contracted the virus through travel or an infected partner.

Diagnosis

- Serologic testing
- Reverse transcriptase-PCR (RT-PCR) testing

(See also the CDC's Revised diagnostic testing for Zika, chikungunya, and dengue viruses at www.cdc.gov)

Clinicians are required to notify the CDC if they identify a case of ZV infection.

ZV infection is suspected based on symptoms and on places and dates of travel. However, clinical manifestations of ZV infection resemble those of many febrile tropical diseases (eg, malaria, leptospirosis, other arbovirus infections), and its geographic distribution resembles that of other arboviruses. Thus, diagnosis of ZV infection requires laboratory confirmation by one of the following:

- Serologic testing (ELISA for IgM, the plaque reduction neutralization test [PRNT] for ZV antibodies)
- RT-PCR to detect viral RNA in serum

Virus-specific IgM and neutralizing antibodies typically develop toward the end of the first week of illness, but cross-reaction with related flaviviruses (eg, dengue and yellow fever viruses) is common.

The PRNT measures virus-specific neutralizing antibodies and helps distinguish cross-reacting antibodies from closely related flaviviruses.

During the first week after symptom onset, the ZV can often be detected using RT-PCR on serum; urine samples should be collected < 14 days after symptom onset for RT-PCR testing.

In the US, emergency use authorization for the following diagnostic tests for ZV has been issued:

- Zika MAC-ELISA
- Trioplex Real-Time RT-PCR Assay

These tests are being distributed to laboratories that are certified to perform high-complexity tests in the US (for more information about these tests, see the CDC's ZV: Diagnostic Testing and ZV: Information for State and Local Public Health Laboratories at www.cdc.gov).

To aid in the diagnosis and treatment of ZV infection, the CDC has issued interim guidelines for pregnant women and interim guidelines for infants born to mothers who traveled to or live in an area with ongoing ZV transmission during pregnancy.

Currently, testing men to assess risk of sexual transmission is not recommended (see also the CDC: Clinical Guidance for Healthcare Providers for Prevention of Sexual Transmission of ZV at www.cdc.gov). Men who reside in or have traveled to an area of active ZV transmission and who have a pregnant partner should abstain from sexual activity or consistently and correctly use condoms during sex (ie, vaginal intercourse, anal intercourse, fellatio) for the duration of the pregnancy.

Maternal testing: For **pregnant travelers returning from areas with ongoing ZV transmission,** the CDC guidelines recommend serologic testing for all pregnant women, whether they have symptoms of ZV infection or not. In addition, if pregnant women may have been exposed to ZV, ultrasonography to assess fetal anatomy is recommended (see also the ZV: Clinical Guidance for Healthcare Providers Caring for Pregnant Women at www.cdc.gov).

- For asymptomatic pregnant women: Testing should be done 2 to 12 wk after pregnant women return from traveling.
- For symptomatic pregnant women: Testing should be done while they are symptomatic.

For **pregnant women who live in areas with ongoing ZV transmission,** ZV infection is a risk throughout pregnancy. If pregnant women develop symptoms suggesting ZV infection, testing should be done during the first week of illness. For asymptomatic pregnant women who live in areas with ongoing ZV transmission, the CDC recommends testing at the first prenatal visit and, if the results are negative, during the middle of the 2nd trimester; fetal ultrasonography should be done at 18 to 20 wk gestation.

Compared with pregnant travelers, pregnant women living in areas with ongoing ZV transmission are more likely to have a false-positive IgM result because they are more likely to have been exposed to a related flavivirus.

Infant testing and follow-up: If infants have possible congenital Zika virus infection and their mother traveled to or lived in an area affected by ZV infection during pregnancy, testing should be guided by what the mother's ZV test results are and whether the infant has microcephaly, intracranial calcifications, or eye abnormalities.

- If mothers have negative ZV test results or were not tested for ZV and their infant does not have microcephaly or intracranial calcifications, the infant should be given routine care.
- If mothers have positive or inconclusive ZV test results and their infant has microcephaly or intracranial calcifications, the CDC's Interim Guidelines for the Evaluation and Testing of Infants with Possible Congenital ZV Infection should be followed.

Treatment

- Supportive care

No specific antiviral treatment is available for ZV infection. Treatment is supportive; it includes the following:

- Rest
- Fluids to prevent dehydration
- Acetaminophen to relieve fever and pain
- Avoidance of aspirin and other NSAIDs

Aspirin and other NSAIDs are not typically used during pregnancy and should specifically be avoided in all patients treated for ZV infection until dengue can be ruled out because hemorrhage is a risk. Also, death and severe infection due to ZV has been related to immune thrombocytopenia and bleeding.[1,2]

If pregnant women have laboratory evidence of ZV in serum or amniotic fluid, serial ultrasonography every 3 to 4 wk should be considered to monitor fetal anatomy and growth. Referral to a maternal-fetal medicine or infectious disease specialist with expertise in pregnancy management is recommended.

1. Sharp TM, Muñoz-Jordán J, Perez-Padilla J, et al: Zika virus infection associated with severe thrombocytopenia. *Clin Infect Dis* 2016.
2. Karimi O, Goorhuis A, Schinkel J, et al: Thrombocytopenia and subcutaneous bleedings in a patient with Zika virus infection. *The Lancet* 387 (10022):939–940. 2016.

Prevention

Until more is known, the CDC has recommended that pregnant women consider postponing travel to areas with ongoing ZV transmission (see also CDC: For Pregnant Women at www.cdc.gov). If women decide to go, they should talk with their physician about risks of ZV infection and precautions to be taken to avoid mosquito bites during the trip.

There is currently no vaccine to prevent ZV infection.

Prevention of transmission via mosquitoes: Prevention of ZV infection depends on control of *Aedes* mosquitoes and prevention of mosquito bites when traveling to countries with ongoing ZV transmission.

To prevent mosquito bites, the following precautions should be taken:

- Wear long-sleeved shirts and long pants.
- Stay in places that have air conditioning or that use window and door screens to keep mosquitoes out.
- Sleep under a mosquito bed net in places that are not adequately screened or air-conditioned.
- Use Environmental Protection Agency–registered insect repellents with ingredients such as DEET (diethyltoluamide) or other approved active ingredients on exposed skin surfaces.
- Treat clothing and gear with permethrin insecticide (do not apply directly to the skin).

For children, the following precautions are recommended:

- Do not use insect repellent on infants < 2 mo.
- Do not use products containing oil of lemon eucalyptus (para-menthane-diol) on children < 3 yr.
- For older children, adults should spray repellent on their hands and then apply it to the children's skin.
- Dress children in clothing that covers their arms and legs, or cover the crib, stroller, or baby carrier with mosquito netting.
- Do not apply insect repellent to the hands, eyes, mouth, or cut or irritated skin of children.

Prevention of transmission via blood transfusion: Even though the risk of ZV transmission through blood transfusions is considered extremely low, the FDA has recommended that blood donors wait 28 days if they are at risk of ZV infection for any of the following reasons:

- Travel to or residence in an area with ongoing ZV transmission
- History of ZV infection (waiting for 4 wk after symptoms resolve before donating)
- Symptoms of ZV infection within 2 wk of travel to an area with ongoing ZV transmission
- Sexual contact with a man who has been diagnosed with ZV infection
- Sexual contact with a man who traveled to or lived in an area with ongoing ZV transmission in the 3 mo before the sexual contact

If donors give blood and subsequently develop symptoms of ZV infection, the Red Cross asks to be notified so that it can quarantine possibly affected donations.

Prevention of sexual transmission: Because ZV can be transmitted via semen, men who live in or have traveled to an area of ongoing ZV transmission should abstain from sexual activity or consistently and correctly use condoms during sex (vaginal intercourse, anal intercourse, fellatio) while their partner is pregnant. This recommendation applies whether men have symptoms or not because most ZV infections are asymptomatic, and when symptoms do develop, they are usually mild.

RNA of the ZV has been detected in semen up to 62 days after the onset of symptoms. The CDC has therefore made the following specific recommendations:

For men who have been diagnosed with ZV infection or who have or have had symptoms:

- They should consider using condoms or not having sex for ≥ 6 mo.

For couples with a male partner who has traveled to an area with ongoing ZV transmission:

- If the male partner has been diagnosed with ZV infection or has (or had) symptoms, the couple should consider using condoms or not having sex for ≥ 6 mo after symptom onset.
- If the male partner does not develop symptoms, the couple should consider using condoms or not having sex for ≥ 8 wk after the man returns.

For couples with a male partner living in an area with ongoing ZV transmission:

- If the male partner has been diagnosed with ZV infection or has (or had) symptoms, the couple should consider using condoms or not having sex for ≥ 6 mo after symptom onset.
- If the male partner has never developed symptoms, the couple should consider using condoms or not having sex as long as Zika is in the area.

There has been one case of female-to-male sexual transmission. Although no cases of woman-to-woman sexual transmission have been reported, the CDC now recommends that all pregnant women who have a sex partner (male or female) who has traveled to or resides in an area with Zika use barrier methods every time they have sex or they should not have sex during the pregnancy.[1] The CDC is continuing to update their recommendations for sexually active people.

If a female partner is not pregnant and lives in or has traveled to an area with ongoing ZV transmission, the couple can consider using condoms or not having sex (see also CDC: Zika and Sexual Transmission at www.cdc.gov).

1. CDC media statement: First female-to-male sexual transmission of Zika virus infection reported in New York City. July 2016.

KEY POINTS

- The ZV is transmitted primarily by *Aedes* mosquitoes.
- Most ZV infections are asymptomatic; symptomatic infections are usually mild, causing fever, a maculopapular rash, conjunctivitis, joint pain, retro-orbital pain, headache, and muscle pain (myalgia).
- ZV infection during pregnancy can cause a serious birth defect called microcephaly.
- Test pregnant women for ZV if they have traveled to or live in areas of ongoing ZV transmission using serologic testing (ELISA for IgM, the PRNT) or reverse transcriptase–PCR.

- Treat supportively; treat fever with acetaminophen and avoid using aspirin or NSAIDs until dengue has been excluded.
- Pregnant women should be advised to consider postponing travel to areas with ongoing ZV transmission.
- Prevention of ZV infection depends on controlling *Aedes* mosquitoes and avoiding mosquito bites.
- Because ZV can be transmitted sexually, men and women who live in or have traveled to an area of ongoing ZV transmission should abstain from sexual activity or consistently and correctly use barrier methods during sex while their partner is pregnant.

OTHER ARBOVIRUS INFECTIONS

Chikungunya disease: This disease is an acute febrile illness followed by more chronic polyarthritis. It is transmitted by *Aedes* mosquitoes and is common in Africa, India, Guam, Southeast Asia, New Guinea, China, Mexico, Central America, islands in the Caribbean, Indian Ocean and Pacific, and limited areas of Europe. Local transmission has been identified in Florida, Puerto Rico, and the US Virgin Islands.

Prevention of chikungunya disease involves avoiding mosquito bites.

Mayaro disease: This dengue-like disease is transmitted by mosquitoes. It is common in Brazil, Bolivia, and Trinidad.

Prevention of Mayaro disease involves avoiding mosquito bites.

Tick-borne encephalitis: In northern Asia, Russia, and Europe, this infection is caused by 3 subtypes of flaviviruses: a far-eastern subtype, a Siberian subtype, and a European subtype. In the US, tick-borne encephalitis is caused by Powassan virus, a flavivirus.

Initially, a mild flu-like illness occurs, accompanied by leukocytopenia and thrombocytopenia, which clears up within a few days. About 30% of patients develop more severe symptoms (eg, meningitis, meningoencephalitis).

A vaccine is available in Europe and Russia.

California encephalitis: The California encephalitis virus belongs to the *Bunyaviridae* family. This encephalitis and related infections are transmitted by mosquitoes and occur in the US Midwest and probably worldwide.

California encephalitis causes symptoms (eg, fever, somnolence, obtundation, focal neurologic findings, seizures) primarily in children. Temporal lobe involvement may mimic herpes encephalitis; 20% of patients develop behavioral problems or recurrent seizures. Mortality rate is < 1%.

No treatment is available.

Omsk hemorrhagic fever and Kyasanur Forest disease: These infections are transmitted by ticks or by direct contact with an infected animal (eg, rodent, monkey). Omsk hemorrhagic fever is caused by a flavivirus; it occurs in Russia, including Siberia; Kyasanur Forest disease, also caused by a flavivirus, occurs in India.

Omsk hemorrhagic fever and Kyasanur Forest disease are acute febrile illnesses accompanied by bleeding diathesis, low BP, leukopenia, and thrombocytopenia; some patients develop encephalitis in the 3rd wk. Mortality rate is < 3% for Omsk hemorrhagic fever and 3 to 5% for Kyasanur Forest disease.

Prevention involves avoiding tick bites and infected animals.

Rift Valley fever: This infection, caused by a phlebovirus, is spread by mosquitoes and can be transmitted by the following:

- Direct or indirect contact with the blood or organs of infected animals (eg, during slaughtering, butchering, or veterinary procedures)
- Inhalation of infected aerosols
- Ingestion of raw milk from infected animals

Rift Valley fever occurs in South Africa, East and West Africa, Arabia, and Egypt.

Rarely, Rift Valley fever progresses to ocular disorders, meningoencephalitis, or a hemorrhagic form (which has a 50% mortality rate).

A vaccine for livestock is available, and a human vaccine is under investigation.

184 Bacteria and Antibacterial Drugs

Bacteria are microorganisms that have circular double-stranded DNA and (except for mycoplasmas) cell walls. Most bacteria live extracellularly. Some bacteria (eg, *Salmonella typhi*; *Neisseria gonorrhoeae*; *Legionella*, *Mycobacterium*, *Rickettsia*, *Chlamydia*, and *Chlamydophila* spp) preferentially reside and replicate intracellularly. Some bacteria such as chlamydiae, *Chlamydophila* sp, and rickettsiae are obligate intracellular pathogens (ie, able to grow, reproduce, and cause disease only within the cells of the host). Others (eg, *Salmonella typhi*, *Brucella* sp, *Francisella tularensis*, *N. gonorrhoeae*, *N. meningitidis*, *Legionella* and *Listeria* spp, *Mycobacterium tuberculosis*) are facultative intracellular pathogens.

Many bacteria are present in humans as normal flora, often in large numbers and in many areas (eg, in the GI tract). Only a few bacterial species are human pathogens.

Bacteria are classified by the following criteria (see Table 184–1).

Morphology: Bacteria may be

- Cylindric (bacilli)
- Spherical (cocci)
- Spiral (spirochetes)

A few coccal, many bacillary, and most spirochetal species are motile.

Staining: The most common stain for general bacterial identification is Gram stain. Gram-positive bacteria retain crystal violet dye (appearing dark blue) after iodine fixation, alcohol decolorization, and counterstaining with safranin; gram-negative bacteria, which do not retain crystal violet, appear red. Gram-negative bacteria have an additional outer membrane containing lipopolysaccharide (endotoxin), increasing the virulence of these bacteria. (For other factors that enhance bacterial pathogenicity, see Factors Facilitating Microbial Invasion on p. 1431.)

Ziehl-Neelsen and Kinyoun stains are acid-fast stains used to identify mainly mycobacteria, particularly *M. tuberculosis*. They also can identify *Nocardia* and *Cryptosporidia* spp. Carbolfuchsin is applied, followed by decolorization with hydrochloric acid and ethanol and then counterstaining with methylene blue. Fluorochrome stains (eg, auramine-rhodamine) also identify acid-fast organisms, but a special fluorescent microscope is required.

Table 184–1. CLASSIFICATION OF COMMON PATHOGENIC BACTERIA

TYPE	BACTERIA
Obligate aerobic	
Gram-negative cocci	*Moraxella catarrhalis*, *Neisseria gonorrhoeae*, *N. meningitidis*
Gram-positive bacilli	*Corynebacterium jeikeium*
Acid-fast bacilli	*Mycobacterium avium* complex, *M. kansasii*, *M. leprae*, *M. tuberculosis*, *Nocardia* sp
Nonfermentative, non-Enterobacteriaceae	*Acinetobacter calcoaceticus*, *Elizabethkingia meningoseptica* (previously *Flavobacterium meningosepticum*), *Pseudomonas aeruginosa*, *P. alcaligenes*, other *Pseudomonas* sp, *Stenotrophomonas maltophilia*
Fastidious gram-negative coccobacilli and bacilli	*Brucella*, *Bordetella*, *Francisella*, and *Legionella* spp
Treponemataceae (spiral bacteria)	*Leptospira* sp
Obligate anaerobic	
Gram-negative bacilli	*Bacteroides fragilis*, other *Bacteroides* sp, *Fusobacterium* sp, *Prevotella* sp
Gram-negative cocci	*Veillonella* sp
Gram-positive cocci	*Peptococcus niger*, *Peptostreptococcus* sp
Non-spore-forming gram-positive bacilli	*Actinomyces*, *Bifidobacterium*, *Eubacterium*, and *Propionibacterium* spp
Endospore-forming gram-positive bacilli	*Clostridium botulinum*, *C. perfringens*, *C. tetani*, other *Clostridium* sp
Facultative anaerobic	
Gram-positive cocci, catalase-positive	*Staphylococcus aureus* (coagulase-positive), *S. epidermidis* (coagulase-negative), other coagulase-negative staphylococci
Gram-positive cocci, catalase-negative	*Enterococcus faecalis*, *E. faecium*, *Streptococcus agalactiae* (group B streptococcus), *S. bovis*, *S. pneumoniae*, *S. pyogenes* (group A streptococcus), viridans group streptococci (*S. mutans*, *S. mitis*, *S. salivarius*, *S. sanguis*), *S. anginosus* group (*S. anginosus*, *S. milleri*, *S. constellatus*), *Gemella morbillorum*
Gram-positive bacilli	*Bacillus anthracis*, *Erysipelothrix rhusiopathiae*, *Gardnerella vaginalis* (gram-variable)
Gram-negative bacilli	Enterobacteriaceae (*Citrobacter* sp, *Enterobacter aerogenes*, *Escherichia coli*, *Klebsiella* sp, *Morganella morganii*, *Proteus* sp, *Plesiomonas shigelloides*, *Providencia rettgeri*, *Salmonella typhi*, other *Salmonella* sp, *Serratia marcescens*, *Shigella* sp, *Yersinia enterocolitica*, *Y. pestis*)
Fermentative, non-Enterobacteriaceae	*Aeromonas hydrophila*, *Chromobacterium violaceum*, *Pasteurella multocida*
Fastidious gram-negative coccobacilli and bacilli	*Actinobacillus actinomycetemcomitans*, *Bartonella bacilliformis*, *B. henselae*, *B. quintana*, *Eikenella corrodens*, *Haemophilus influenzae*, other *Haemophilus* sp
Mycoplasma	*Mycoplasma pneumoniae*
Treponemataceae (spiral bacteria)	*Borrelia burgdorferi*, *Treponema pallidum*
Microaerophilic	
Curved bacilli	*Campylobacter jejuni*, *Helicobacter pylori*, *Vibrio cholerae*, *V. vulnificus*
Obligate intracellular parasitic	
Chlamydiaceae	*Chlamydia trachomatis*, *Chlamydophila pneumoniae*, *C. psittaci*
Coxiellaceae	*Coxiella burnetii*
Rickettsiales	*Rickettsia prowazekii*, *R. rickettsii*, *R. typhi*, *R. tsutsugamushi*, *Ehrlichia chaffeensis*, *Anaplasma phagocytophilum*

Encapsulation: Some bacteria are enclosed in capsules; for some encapsulated bacteria (eg, *Streptococcus pneumoniae*, *Haemophilus influenzae*), the capsule helps protect them from ingestion by phagocytes. Encapsulation increases bacterial virulence.

Oxygen requirements: Aerobic bacteria (obligate aerobes) require O_2 to produce energy and to grow in culture. They produce energy using aerobic cellular respiration.

Anaerobic bacteria (obligate anaerobes—see also p. 1462) do not require O_2 and do not grow in culture if air is present. They produce energy using fermentation or anaerobic respiration. Anaerobic bacteria are common in the GI tract, vagina, dental crevices, and wounds when blood supply is impaired.

Facultative bacteria can grow with or without O_2. They produce energy by fermentation or anaerobic respiration when O_2 is absent and by aerobic cellular respiration when O_2 is present. Microaerophilic bacteria prefer a reduced O_2 tension (eg, 2 to 10%).

Chlamydiae are obligate intracellular parasites that acquire energy from the host cell and do not produce it themselves.

OVERVIEW OF ANTIBACTERIAL DRUGS

Antibacterial drugs are derived from bacteria or molds or are synthesized de novo. Technically, "antibiotic" refers only to antimicrobials derived from bacteria or molds but is often (including in The Manual) used synonymously with "antibacterial drug."

Antibiotics have many mechanisms of action, including inhibiting cell wall synthesis, l, increasing cell membrane permeability, and interfering with protein synthesis, nucleic acid metabolism, and other metabolic processes (eg, folic acid synthesis).

Antibiotics sometimes interact with other drugs, raising or lowering serum levels of other drugs by increasing or decreasing their metabolism or by various other mechanisms (see Table 184–2). The most clinically important interactions involve drugs with a low therapeutic ratio (ie, toxic levels are close to therapeutic levels). Also, other drugs can increase or decrease levels of antibiotics.

Many antibiotics are chemically related and are thus grouped into classes. Although drugs within each class share structural and functional similarities, they often have different pharmacology and spectra of activity.

Selection and Use of Antibiotics

Antibiotics should be used only if clinical or laboratory evidence suggests bacterial infection. Use for viral illness or undifferentiated fever is inappropriate in most cases; it exposes patients to drug complications without any benefit and contributes to bacterial resistance.

Certain bacterial infections (eg, abscesses, infections with foreign bodies) require surgical intervention and do not respond to antibiotics alone.

Spectrum of activity: Cultures and antibiotic sensitivity testing are essential for selecting a drug for serious infections. However, treatment must often begin before culture results are available, necessitating selection according to the most likely pathogens (empiric antibiotic selection).

Whether chosen according to culture results or not, drugs with the narrowest spectrum of activity that can control the infection should be used. For empiric treatment of serious infections that may involve any one of several pathogens (eg, fever in neutropenic patients) or that may be due to multiple pathogens (eg, polymicrobial anaerobic infection), a broad spectrum of activity is desirable. The most likely pathogens and their susceptibility to antibiotics vary according to geographic location (within cities or even within a hospital) and can change from month to month.

For serious infections, combinations of antibiotics are often necessary because multiple species of bacteria may be present or because combinations act synergistically against a single species of bacteria. Synergism is usually defined as a more rapid and complete bactericidal action from a combination of antibiotics than occurs with either antibiotic alone. A common example is a cell wall–active antibiotic (eg, a β-lactam, vancomycin) plus an aminoglycoside.

Effectiveness: In vivo antibiotic effectiveness involves many factors, including

- Pharmacology (eg, absorption, distribution, concentration in fluids and tissues, protein binding, rate of metabolism or excretion)
- Pharmacodynamics (ie, the time course of antibacterial effects exerted by drug levels in blood and at the site of infection)
- Drug interactions or inhibiting substances
- Host defense mechanisms

Bactericidal drugs kill bacteria. Bacteriostatic drugs slow or stop in vitro bacterial growth. These definitions are not absolute; bacteriostatic drugs may kill some susceptible bacterial species, and bactericidal drugs may only inhibit growth of some susceptible bacterial species. Bactericidal antibiotics may be preferred for patients who have infections that impair host defenses locally (eg, meningitis, endocarditis) or who are immunocompromised (eg, neutropenic). More precise quantitative methods identify the minimum in vitro concentration at which an antibiotic can inhibit growth (minimum inhibitory concentration, or MIC) or kill (minimum bactericidal concentration, or MBC). An antibiotic with bactericidal activity is important if host defenses are impaired locally at the site of infection (eg, in meningitis or endocarditis) or systemically (eg, in patients who are neutropenic or immunocompromised in other ways).

The predominant determinant of bacteriologic response to antibiotics is either the

- Time that blood levels of the antibiotic exceed the MIC (time-dependence)
- Peak blood level relative to MIC (concentration-dependence)

β-Lactams and vancomycin exhibit time-dependent bactericidal activity. Increasing their concentration above the MIC does not increase their bactericidal activity, and their in vivo killing is generally slow. In addition, because there is no or very brief residual inhibition of bacterial growth after concentrations fall below the MIC (postantibiotic effect, or PAE), β-lactams are most often effective when serum levels of free drug (drug not bound to serum protein) exceed the MIC for ≥ 50% of the time. Because ceftriaxone has a long serum half-life, free serum levels exceed the MIC of very susceptible pathogens for the entire 24-h dosing interval. However, for β-lactams that have serum half-lives of ≤ 2 h, frequent dosing or continuous infusion is required. For vancomycin, trough levels should be maintained at least at 15 to 20 μg/mL.

Aminoglycosides, fluoroquinolones, and daptomycin exhibit concentration-dependent bactericidal activity. Increasing their concentrations from levels slightly above the MIC to levels far above the MIC increases their rate of bactericidal activity and decreases the bacterial load. In addition, if concentrations exceed the MIC even briefly, aminoglycosides and fluoroquinolones have a PAE on residual bacteria; duration of PAE is also concentration-dependent. If PAEs are long, drug levels can be below the MIC for extended periods without loss of efficacy, allowing less frequent dosing. Consequently, aminoglycosides and fluoroquinolones are usually most effective as intermittent

Table 184–2. COMMON EFFECTS OF ANTIBIOTICS ON OTHER DRUGS

DRUG	TOXICITY ENHANCED BY	NO CHANGE WITH
Digoxin	All macrolides (eg, azithromycin, clarithromycin, erythromycin) Doxycycline Tetracycline Trimethoprim	Aminoglycosides Cephalosporins Clindamycin Fluoroquinolones Ketoconazole Linezolid Metronidazole Penicillins Quinulpristine/dalfopristin Sulfonamides Vancomycin
Phenytoin	Chloramphenicol Ciprofloxacin Isoniazid Some macrolides (erythromycin, clarithromycin, telithromycin) Rifampin (decreased phenytoin levels) Sulfonamides	Azithromycin Aminoglycosides Cephalosporins Clindamycin Doxycycline Fluoroquinolones except ciprofloxacin Linezolid Metronidazole Penicillins Quinulpristine/dalfopristin Tetracycline Trimethoprim Vancomycin
Theophylline	Ciprofloxacin Clarithromycin Erythromycin Rifampin (decreased theophylline levels)	Aminoglycosides Azithromycin Cephalosporins Clindamycin Doxycycline Linezolid Metronidazole Penicillins Quinulpristine/dalfopristin Sulfonamides Tetracycline Trimethoprim Vancomycin
Warfarin	Cefoperazon* Cefotetan* Chloramphenicol Clarithromycin Doxycycline Erythromycin Certain fluoroquinolones (ciprofloxacin, levofloxacin, moxifloxacin, ofloxacin) Metronidazole Rifampin (decreased PT) Sulfonamides	Aminoglycosides (IV) Azithromycin Cephalosporins (some) Clindamycin Doxycycline Linezolid Penicillins Quinulpristine/dalfopristin Tetracycline Trimethoprim Vancomycin

*These drugs interfere with vitamin K–dependent clotting factors and, when used with antiplatelet drugs and thrombolytics, may increase risk of bleeding.

boluses that reach peak free serum levels ≥ 10 times the MIC of the bacteria; usually, trough levels are not important.

Route: For many antibiotics, oral administration results in therapeutic blood levels nearly as rapidly as IV administration. However, IV administration is preferred in the following circumstances:

- Oral antibiotics cannot be tolerated (eg, because of vomiting).
- Oral antibiotics cannot be absorbed (eg, because of malabsorption after intestinal surgery).
- Intestinal motility is impaired (eg, because of opioid use).
- No oral formulation is available (eg, for aminoglycosides).
- Patients are critically ill, possibly impairing GI tract perfusion or making even the brief delay with oral administration detrimental.

Special populations: Doses and scheduling of antibiotics may need to be adjusted for the following:

- Infants
- The elderly
- Patients with renal failure (see Table 184–3)
- Patients with hepatic insufficiency (most commonly for cefoperazone, chloramphenicol, metronidazole, rifabutin, and rifampin)

Table 184–3. USUAL DOSES OF COMMONLY PRESCRIBED ANTIBIOTICS

DRUG	ADULT DOSE			PEDIATRIC (AGE > 1 MO) DOSE		DOSE IN RENAL FAILURE[a] (CrCl < 10 mL/min)
	ORAL	PARENTERAL	SERIOUS INFECTIONS	ORAL	PARENTERAL	
Aminoglycosides						
Amikacin	N/A	15 mg/kg IV once/day *or* 7.5 mg/kg q 12 h	15 mg/kg IV once/day *or* 7.5 mg/kg IV q 12 h	N/A	5–7.5 mg/kg IV q 12 h	1.5–2.5 mg/kg IV q 24–48 h
Gentamicin	N/A	5–7 mg/kg IV once/day *or* 1.7 mg/kg IV q 8 h	5–7 mg/kg IV once/day	N/A	1–2.5 mg/kg IV q 8 h	0.34–0.51 mg/kg IV q 24–48 h
For synergy with a cell wall–active antibiotic to treat enterococcal endocarditis caused by strains susceptible to gentamicin	N/A	1 mg/kg IV q 8 h	N/A	N/A	1 mg/kg IV q 8 h	Infectious disease consultation required for dosage Dosage adjusted to achieve peak serum concentration of 3–4 μg/mL and trough concentration of < 1 μg/mL
For streptococcal or *Staphylococcus aureus* endocarditis	—	1 mg/kg IV q 8 h *or* 3 mg/kg IV once/day	N/A	N/A	1 mg/kg IV q 8 h *or* 3 mg/kg IV once/day	N/A
Neomycin						
For preoperative gut antisepsis (with erythromycin and mechanical cleansing)	1 g for 3 doses (eg, at 1, 2, and 11 pm on the day before surgery)	N/A	N/A	15 mg/kg q 4 h for 2 days *or* 25 mg/kg at 1, 2, and 11 pm on the day before surgery	N/A	N/A
For hepatic coma	1–3 g qid	N/A	N/A	0.6–1.75 g/m^2 q 6 h *or* 0.4–1.2 g/m^2 q 4 h	N/A	N/A
Streptomycin						
For TB	N/A	15 mg/kg IM q 24 h (maximum: 1.0 g/day) initially, then 1.0 g 2–3 times/wk	N/A	N/A	20–40 mg/kg IM once/day	7.5 mg/kg IM q 72–96 h (maximum: 1 g)
For synergy with a cell wall–active antibiotic to treat enterococcal endocarditis	N/A	7.5 mg/kg IM q 12 h	N/A	N/A	N/A	N/A

Table continues on the following page.

Table 184–3. USUAL DOSES OF COMMONLY PRESCRIBED ANTIBIOTICS (*Continued*)

DRUG	ADULT DOSE: ORAL	ADULT DOSE: PARENTERAL	ADULT DOSE: SERIOUS INFECTIONS	PEDIATRIC (AGE > 1 MO) DOSE: ORAL	PEDIATRIC (AGE > 1 MO) DOSE: PARENTERAL	DOSE IN RENAL FAILURE[a] (CrCl < 10 mL/min)
Tobramycin	N/A	5–7 mg/kg IV once/day *or* 1.7 mg/kg IV q 8 h	5–7 mg/kg IV once/day *or* 1.7 mg/kg IV q 8 h	N/A	1–2.5 mg/kg IV q 8 h	0.34–0.51 mg/kg IV q 24–48 h
β-Lactams: Cephalosporins (1st generation)						
Cefadroxil	0.5–1 g q 12 h	N/A	N/A	15 mg/kg q 12 h	N/A	0.5 g po q 36 h
Cefazolin	N/A	1–2 g IV q 8 h	2 g IV q 8 h	N/A	16.6–33.3 mg/kg IV q 8 h	1–2 g IV q 24–48 h
Cephalexin	0.25–0.5 g q 6 h	N/A	N/A	6.25–12.5 mg/kg q 6 h *or* 8.0–16 mg/kg q 8 h	N/A	0.25–0.5 g po q 24–48 h
β-Lactams: Cephalosporins (2nd generation)						
Cefaclor[b]	0.25–0.5 g q 8 h	N/A	N/A	10–20 mg/kg q 12 h *or* 6.6–13.3 mg/kg q 8 h	N/A	0.5 g po q 12 h
Cefotetan	N/A	1–3 g IV q 12 h	2–3 g IV q 12 h	N/A	20–40 mg/kg IV q 12 h	1–3 g IV q 48 h
Cefoxitin	N/A	1 g IV q 8 h to 2 g IV q 4 h	2 g IV q 4 h *or* 3 g IV q 6 h	N/A	27–33 mg/kg IV q 8 h or, for severe infections, 25–40 mg/kg q 6 h	0.5–1.0 g IV q 24–48 h
Cefprozil	0.25 g q 12 h *or* 0.5 g q 12–24 h	N/A	N/A	15 mg/kg q 12 h for otitis media	N/A	0.25 g po q 12–24 h
Cefuroxime	0.125–0.5 g q 12 h	0.75–1.5 g IV q 6–8 h	1.5 g IV q 6 h	10–15 mg/kg suspension q 12 h For older children: 125–250 mg tablets q 12 h	25–50 mg/kg IV q 8 h	0.25–0.5 g po q 24 h *or* 0.75 g IV q 24 h
For meningitis	—	—	3 g IV q 8 h	—	50–60 mg/kg IV q 6 h	—
β-Lactams: Cephalosporins (3rd generation)						
Cefotaxime	N/A	1 g q 12 h to 2 g IV q 4 h	2 g IV q 4 h	N/A	8.3–33.3 mg/kg IV q 4 h *or* 16.6–66.6 mg/kg q 6 h	1–2 g IV q 24 h
Cefpodoxime[c]	0.1–0.4 g q 12 h	N/A	N/A	5 mg/kg q 12 h	N/A	0.1–0.4 g po q 24 h
Ceftazidime	N/A	1 g IV q 12 h to 2 g q 8 h	2 g IV q 8 h	N/A	25–50 mg/kg IV q 8 h	0.5 g IV q 24–48 h

Table 184–3. USUAL DOSES OF COMMONLY PRESCRIBED ANTIBIOTICS (*Continued*)

DRUG	ADULT DOSE			PEDIATRIC (AGE > 1 MO) DOSE		DOSE IN RENAL FAILURE[a] (CrCl < 10 mL/min)
	ORAL	PARENTERAL	SERIOUS INFECTIONS	ORAL	PARENTERAL	
Ceftibuten[b]	0.4 g q 24 h	N/A	N/A	9 mg/kg once/day	N/A	0.1 g po q 24 h
Ceftriaxone	N/A	1–2 g IV q 24 h	2 g IV q 24 h	N/A	50–75 mg/kg IV q 24 h *or* 25–37.5 mg/kg q 12 h	Same as adult dose
For meningitis	N/A	2 g IV q 12 h	2 g IV q 12 h	N/A	50 mg/kg IV q 12 h or 100 mg/kg q 24 h (not to exceed 4 g/day) Possibly a loading dose of 100 mg/kg IV (not to exceed 4 g) at the start of therapy	2 g IV q 12 h
β-Lactams: Cephalosporin (4th generation)						
Cefepime	N/A	1–2 g IV q 8–12 h	2 g IV q 8 h	N/A	50 mg/kg IV q 8–12 h	0.25–1 g IV q 24 h
β-Lactams: Cephalosporin (5th generation)						
Ceftaroline	N/A	0.6 g IV q 12 h	0.6 g IV q 12 h	N/A	N/A	0.2 g IV q 12 h
β-Lactams: Penicillins						
Amoxicillin	0.25–0.5 g q 8 h *or* 0.875 g q 12 h	N/A	N/A	12.5–25 mg/kg q 12 h *or* 7–13 mg/kg q 8 h	N/A	0.25–0.5 g po q 24 h
For endocarditis prophylaxis	2 g for 1 dose	N/A	N/A	50 mg/kg 1 h before procedure	N/A	2 g po for 1 dose
Amoxicillin/ clavulanate	0.25–0.5 g q 8 h *or* 0.875 g q 12 h	N/A	N/A	If > 40 kg: Adult dose	N/A	0.25–0.5 g po q 24 h
Amoxicillin/ clavulanate, ES-600	N/A	N/A	N/A	45 mg/kg q 12 h	N/A	N/A
Amoxicillin/ clavulanate, extended-release	2 g q 12 h	N/A	N/A	N/A	N/A	N/A
Ampicillin	N/A	0.5–2.0 g IV q 4–6 h	2 g IV q 4 h	N/A	25–50 mg/kg IV q 6 h	0.5–2.0 g IV q 12–24 h
For meningitis	N/A	2 g IV q 4 h	2 g IV q 4 h	N/A	50–100 mg/kg IV q 6 h	2 g IV q 12 h
Ampicillin/ sulbactam (3 g = 2 g ampicillin + 1 g sulbactam)	N/A	1.5–3.0 g IV q 6 h	3 g IV q 6 h	N/A	25–50 mg/kg IV q 6 h	1.5–3.0 g IV q 24 h
Dicloxacillin[b]	0.125–0.5 g q 6 h	N/A	N/A	3.125–6.25 mg/kg q 6 h	N/A	0.125–0.5 g po q 6 h

Table continues on the following page.

Table 184–3. USUAL DOSES OF COMMONLY PRESCRIBED ANTIBIOTICS (*Continued*)

DRUG	ADULT DOSE			PEDIATRIC (AGE > 1 MO) DOSE		DOSE IN RENAL FAILURE[a] (CrCl < 10 mL/min)
	ORAL	PARENTERAL	SERIOUS INFECTIONS	ORAL	PARENTERAL	
Nafcillin	Rarely used	1–2 g IV q 4 h	2 g IV q 4 h	N/A	12.5–25 mg/kg IV q 6 h *or* 8.3–33.3 mg/kg q 4 h	1–2 g IV q 4 h
Oxacillin	Rarely used	1–2 g IV q 4 h	2 g IV q 4 h	N/A	12.5–25 mg/kg IV q 6 h *or* 8.3–33.3 mg/kg IV q 4 h	1–2 g IV q 4 h
Penicillin G[b]	0.25–0.5 g q 6–12 h (penicillin V)	1–4 million units IV q 4–6 h	4 million units IV q 4 h	Penicillin VK 6.25–12.5 mg/kg q 8 h	6,250–100,000 units/kg IV q 6 h *or* 4,166.6–66,666 units/kg IV q 4 h	0.5–2 million units IV q 4–6 h (maximum total daily dose: 6 million units/day)
Penicillin G benzathine (Bicillin© L-A)						
For streptococcal pharyngitis	N/A	1.2 million units IM for 1 dose	N/A	N/A	25,000–50,000 units/kg IM as a single dose *or* If < 27 kg: 300,000–600,000 units as a single dose *or* If ≥ 27 kg: 0.9 million units as a single dose	1.2 million units IM for 1 dose
Prophylaxis for rheumatic fever	N/A	1.2 million units IM q 3–4 wk	N/A	N/A	25,000–50,000 units/kg IM q 3–4 wk	1.2 million units IM q 3–4 wk
For early syphilis	N/A	2.4 million units IM for 1 dose	N/A	N/A	50,000 units/kg IM for 1 dose	2.4 million units IM for 1 dose
For late syphilis (excluding neurosyphilis)	N/A	2.4 million units IM/wk for 3 wk	N/A	N/A	50,000 units/kg IM in 3 doses 1 wk apart	2.4 million units IM for 1 dose
Penicillin G procaine (IM only)	N/A	0.3–0.6 million units IM q 12 h	N/A	N/A	25,000–50,000 units/kg IM q 24 h *or* 12,500–25,000 units/kg IM q 12 h	0.3 to 0.6 million units IM q 12 h
Piperacillin (1.9 mEq Na/g)	N/A	3 g IV q 4–6 h	3 g IV q 4 h	N/A	50–75 mg/kg IV q 6 h *or* 33.3–50 mg/kg IV q 4 h	3–4 g IV q 12 h
Piperacillin/ tazobactam (2.25 g = 2.0 g piperacillin + 0.25 g tazobactam)	N/A	3.375 g IV q 4–6 h	3.375 g IV q 4 h	N/A	80 mg/kg IV q 8 h	2.25 g IV q 8 h to 4.5 g IV q 12 h

Table 184–3. USUAL DOSES OF COMMONLY PRESCRIBED ANTIBIOTICS (*Continued*)

DRUG	ADULT DOSE			PEDIATRIC (AGE > 1 MO) DOSE		DOSE IN RENAL FAILURE[a] (CrCl < 10 mL/min)
	ORAL	PARENTERAL	SERIOUS INFECTIONS	ORAL	PARENTERAL	
Ticarcillin (5.2 mEq Na/g)	N/A	3 g IV q 4–6 h	3 g IV q 4 h	N/A	If < 60 kg: 50 mg/kg IV q 4–6 h	1–2 g IV q 12 h
Ticarcillin/clavulanate (3.1 g = 3 g ticarcillin + 0.1 g clavulanic acid)	N/A	3.1 g IV q 4–6 h	3.1 g IV q 4 h	N/A	If < 60 kg: 50 mg/kg IV (based on ticarcillin component) q 4–6 h	2 g IV q 12 h
β-Lactams: Monobactams						
Aztreonam	N/A	1–2 g IV q 6–12 h	2 g IV q 6 h	N/A	30–40 mg/kg IV q 6–8 h	0.5 g IV q 8 h
β-Lactams: Carbapenems						
Ertapenem	N/A	1 g IV q 24 h	1 g IV q 24 h	N/A	N/A	0.5 g IV q 24 h
Imipenem	N/A	0.5–1.0 g IV q 6 h	1 g IV q 6 h	N/A	For infants 4 wk to 3 mo: 25 mg/kg IV q 6 h For children >3 mo: 15–25 mg/kg IV q 6 h	0.125–0.25 g IV q 12 h (may increase risk of seizures)
Meropenem	N/A	1 g IV q 8 h	2 g IV q 8 h	N/A	20–40 mg/kg IV q 8 h	0.5 g IV q 24 h
Doripenem	N/A	0.5 g IV q 8 h	0.5 g IV q 8 h	N/A	N/A	0.25 g IV q 24 h
For meningitis	—	40 mg/kg IV q 8 h	40 mg/kg IV q 8 h	N/A	—	20 mg/kg IV q 24 h
Fluoroquinolones[d]						
Ciprofloxacin	0.5–0.75 g q 12 h	0.2–0.4 g IV q 8–12 h	0.4 g IV q 8 h	10–15 mg/kg IV q 12 h (in select circumstances)	10–15 mg/kg IV q 12 h (in select circumstances)	0.5–0.75 g po q 24 h *or* 0.2–0.4 g IV q 24 h
Extended-release for uncomplicated cystitis	0.5 g q 24 h for 3 days	N/A	N/A	N/A	N/A	N/A
Gemifloxacin	320 mg q 24 h	N/A	N/A	N/A	N/A	160 mg po q 24 h
Levofloxacin	0.25–0.75 g q 24 h	0.25–0.75 IV g q 24 h	0.75 g IV q 24 h	N/A	N/A	0.25–0.5 g po or IV q 48 h
Moxifloxacin	0.4 g q 24 h	0.4 g IV q 24 h	0.4 g IV q 24 h	N/A	N/A	0.4 g q 24 h po or IV
Norfloxacin[b]	0.4 g q 12 h	N/A	N/A	N/A	N/A	0.4 g po q 24 h
Ofloxacin	0.2–0.4 g q 12 h	0.4 g IV q 12 h	0.2–0.4 g IV q 12 h	N/A	N/A	0.1–0.2 g po or IV q 24 h
Macrolides						
Azithromycin	0.5 g on day 1, then 0.25 g q 24 h for 4 days	0.5 g IV q 24 h	0.5 g IV q 24 h	—	N/A	0.5 g po on day 1, then 0.25 g po q 24 h for 4 days or 0.5 g IV q 24 h

Table continues on the following page.

Table 184–3. USUAL DOSES OF COMMONLY PRESCRIBED ANTIBIOTICS (*Continued*)

DRUG	ADULT DOSE			PEDIATRIC (AGE > 1 MO) DOSE		DOSE IN RENAL FAILURE[a] (CrCl < 10 mL/min)
	ORAL	PARENTERAL	SERIOUS INFECTIONS	ORAL	PARENTERAL	
For nongonococcal cervicitis and urethritis	1 g for 1 dose	N/A	N/A	N/A	N/A	N/A
For traveler's diarrhea	1 g for 1dose	N/A	N/A	5–10 mg/kg for 1 dose	N/A	N/A
For tonsillitis or pharyngitis	N/A	N/A	N/A	12 mg/kg for 5 days	N/A	N/A
For otitis media or community-acquired pneumonia	N/A	N/A	N/A	10 mg/kg on day 1, then 5 mg/kg once/day on days 2–5	N/A	N/A
Clarithromycin	0.25–0.5 g q 12 h Extended-release: 1 g q 24 h	N/A	N/A	7.5 mg/kg q 12 h	N/A	0.25–0.5 g po q 24 h
Erythromycin base[b]	0.25–0.5 g q 6 h	N/A	N/A	10–16.6 mg/kg q 8 h *or* 7.5–12.5 mg/kg q 6 h	N/A	0.25 g po q 6 h
Fidaxomicin	0.2 g q 12 h	N/A	N/A	N/A	N/A	0.2 g po q 12 h
Lactobionate	N/A	0.5–1 g IV q 6 h	1 g IV q 6 h	N/A	3.75–5.0 mg/kg IV q 6 h	0.5 g IV q 6 h
Gluceptate	N/A	0.5–1 g IV q 6 h	1 g IV q 6 h	N/A	3.75–5.0 mg/kg IV q 6 h	0.5 g IV q 6 h
For GI preoperative bowel preparation	1 g for 3 doses	N/A	N/A	20 mg/kg for 3 doses	N/A	N/A
Telithromycin	800 mg q 24 h	N/A	N/A	N/A	N/A	800 mg po q 24 h
Sulfonamides and trimethoprim						
Sulfisoxazole	1.0 g q 6 h	25 mg/kg IV q 6 h (not available in US)	N/A	30–37.5 mg/kg q 6 h *or* 20–25 mg/kg q 4 h	N/A	1 g po q 12–24 h
Sulfamethizole	0.5–1 g q 6–8 h	N/A	N/A	7.5–11.25 mg/kg q 6 h	N/A	N/A
Sulfamethoxazole	1 g q 8–12 h	N/A	N/A	25–30 mg/kg q 12 h	N/A	1 g po q 24 h
Trimethoprim	0.1 g q 12 h *or* 0.2 g q 24 h	N/A	N/A	2 mg/kg q 12 h for 10 days for UTI	N/A	0.1 g po q 24 h
Trimethoprim/ sulfamethoxazole[e]	0.16/0.8 g q 12 h	3–5 mg TMP/kg IV q 6–8 h	5 mg TMP/kg IV q 6 h	3–6 mg TMP/kg q 12 h	3–6 mg TMP/kg IV q 12 h	(Not recommended if other alternatives are available)

Table 184–3. USUAL DOSES OF COMMONLY PRESCRIBED ANTIBIOTICS (*Continued*)

DRUG	ADULT DOSE			PEDIATRIC (AGE > 1 MO) DOSE		DOSE IN RENAL FAILURE[a] (CrCl < 10 mL/min)
	ORAL	PARENTERAL	SERIOUS INFECTIONS	ORAL	PARENTERAL	
For *Pneumocystis jirovecii* pneumonia[e]	0.32/1.6 g q 8 h for 21 days	5 mg TMP/kg IV q 8 h for 21 days	5 mg TMP/kg IV q 6–8 h	5–6.6 mg TMP/kg q 8 h *or* 3.75–5 mg TMP/kg q 6 h	5–6.6 mg TMP/kg IV q 8 h *or* 3.75–5 mg TMP/kg IV q 6 h	If essential, 5 mg TMP/kg IV q 24 h *or* 1.25 mg TMP/kg IV q 6 h
Tetracyclines						
Doxycycline	0.1 g q 12 h	0.1 g IV q 12 h	0.1 mg IV q 12 h	Age > 8 yr: 2–4 mg/kg q 24 h *or* 1–2 mg/kg q 12 h	Age > 8 yr: 2–4 mg/kg IV q 24 h *or* 1–2 mg/kg IV q 12 h	0.1 g IV or po q 12 h
Minocycline	0.1 g q 12 h	0.1 g IV q 12 h	0.1 g IV q 12 h	N/A	N/A	0.1 g IV or po q 12 h
Tetracycline[b]	0.25–0.5 g q 6 h	N/A	N/A	Age > 8 yr: 6.25–12.5 mg/kg q 6 h	N/A	Doxycycline used instead
Tigecycline	N/A	100 mg, then 50 mg (25 mg for severe hepatic dysfunction) IV q 12 hr	Same as adult dose[f]	N/A	N/A	Same as adult dose
Others						
Clindamycin	0.15–0.45 g q 6 h	0.6 g IV q 6 h to 0.9 IV g q 8 h	0.9 g IV q 8 h	2.6–6.6 mg/kg q 8 h *or* 2–5 mg/kg q 6 h	6.6–13.2 mg/kg IV q 8 h *or* 5–10 mg/kg IV q 6 h	0.15–0.45 g po q 6 h *or* 0.6–0.9 g IV q 6–8 h
Chloramphenicol	0.25–1 g q 6 h	0.25–1.0 g IV q 6 h	1 g IV q 6 h	N/A	12.5–18.75 mg/kg IV q 6 h	0.25–1.0 g IV q 6 h
For meningitis	N/A	12.5 mg/kg q 6 h (maximum: 4 g/day)	12.5 mg/kg IV q 6 h (maximum: 4 g/day)	N/A	18.75–25 mg/kg IV q 6 h	12.5 mg/kg IV q 6 h (maximum: 4 g/day)
Colistin (polymyxin E)	N/A	2.5–5 mg/kg/day IV in 2–4 doses	2.5–5 mg/kg/day IV in 2–4 doses[f]	N/A	N/A	1.5 mg/kg q 36 h
Dalbavancin	N/A	1000 mg as a single dose, followed by a 500-mg dose 1 wk later	1000 mg as a single dose, followed by 500-mg dose 1 wk later	N/A	N/A	1000 mg as a single dose, followed by a 500-mg dose 1 wk later
Daptomycin	N/A	4–6 mg/kg IV q 24 h	8–10 mg/kg IV q 24 h[f]	N/A	N/A	4–6 mg/kg IV q 48 h
Fosfomycin	A single dose of 3 g in 3–4 oz of water	N/A in US	N/A	N/A	N/A	A single dose of 3 g in 3–4 oz of water
Linezolid	0.6 g q 12 h	0.6 g IV q 12 h	0.6 g IV q 12 h	10 mg/kg q 8 h	10 mg/kg IV q 8 h	0.6 g IV or po q 12 h
Metronidazole						

Table continues on the following page.

Table 184–3. USUAL DOSES OF COMMONLY PRESCRIBED ANTIBIOTICS (*Continued*)

DRUG	ADULT DOSE			PEDIATRIC (AGE > 1 MO) DOSE		DOSE IN RENAL FAILURE[a] (CrCl < 10 mL/min)
	ORAL	PARENTERAL	SERIOUS INFECTIONS	ORAL	PARENTERAL	
For anaerobic infection	7.5 mg/kg q 6 h (not to exceed 4 g/day)	7.5 mg/kg IV q 6 h (not to exceed 4 g/day)	7.5 mg/kg IV q 6 h (not to exceed 4 g/day)	7.5 mg/kg q 6 h	7.5 mg/kg IV q 6 h	3.75 mg/kg IV or po q 6 h (not to exceed 2 g/day)
For trichomoniasis	2 g for 1 dose *or* 0.5 g q 12 h for 7 days	N/A	N/A	N/A	N/A	N/A
For *Clostridium difficile*–induced diarrhea (pseudomembranous colitis)	0.5 g q 6–8 h for 10–14 days	500 mg IV q 6–8 h	500 mg IV q 6 h	7.5 mg/kg q 8 h	7.5 mg/kg IV q 6 h	250 mg po or IV q 8 h
For amebiasis	0.5–0.75 g q 8 h for 10 days followed by paromomycin po 0.5 g q 8 h for 7 days	0.75 g IV q 8 h for 10 days followed by paromomycin po 0.5 g q 8 h for 7 days	0.75 g IV q 8 h for 10 days followed by paromomycin po 0.5 g q 8 h for 7 days	11.6–16.6 mg/kg q 8 h for 7–10 days	11.6–16.6 mg/kg IV q 8 h for 7–10 days	N/A
For giardiasis	0.25 g q 6–8 h for 5–7 days	N/A	N/A	5 mg/kg q 6–8 h for 5 days	N/A	N/A
Nitrofurantoin macrocrystals	50–100 mg q 6 h	N/A	N/A	1.25–1.75 mg/kg q 6 h	N/A	Not recommended
Nitrofurantoin monohydrate/ macrocrystals	100 mg q 12 h	N/A	N/A	N/A	N/A	N/A
Oritavancin	N/A	1200 mg as a single dose	1200 mg as a single dose	N/A	N/A	1200 mg as a single dose
Quinupristin/ dalfopristin	N/A	7.5 mg/kg IV q 8–12 h	7.5 mg/kg IV q 8 h	N/A	7.5 mg/kg IV q 12 h for complicated skin or skin structure infection *or* 7.5 mg/kg q 8 h for serious infections	7.5 mg/kg IV q 8–12 h
Rifampin[b]						
For TB	0.6 g q 24 h	0.6 g IV q 24 h	N/A	5–10 mg/kg q 12 h *or* 10–20 mg/kg q 24 h	10–20 mg/kg IV q 24 h	0.3–0.6 g IV or po q 24 h
For meningococcal exposure	0.6 g q 12 h for 4 doses	N/A	N/A	Age ≥ 1 mo: 10 mg/kg q 12 h for 2 days; Age < 1 mo: 5 mg/kg q 12 h for 2 days	N/A	0.6 g po q 12 h for 4 doses

Table 184–3. USUAL DOSES OF COMMONLY PRESCRIBED ANTIBIOTICS (*Continued*)

DRUG	ADULT DOSE			PEDIATRIC (AGE > 1 MO) DOSE		DOSE IN RENAL FAILURE[a] (CrCl < 10 mL/min)
	ORAL	PARENTERAL	SERIOUS INFECTIONS	ORAL	PARENTERAL	
For *Haemophilus influenzae* exposure	20 mg/kg q 24 h for 4 days (not to exceed 600 mg q 24 h)	N/A	N/A	20 mg/kg q 24 h for 4 days Age < 1 mo: 10 mg/kg q 24 h for 4 days	N/A	20 mg/kg q 24 h for 4 days (not to exceed 600 mg q 24 h)
For staphylococcal infections (used with a penicillin, cephalosporin, or vancomycin)	0.3 g q 8 h *or* 0.6–0.9 g q 24 h	0.3 g IV q 8 h *or* 0.6–0.9 g IV q 24 h	0.3 g IV q 8 h *or* 0.6–0.9 g IV q 24 h	—	—	0.3 g IV or po q 8 h *or* 0.6–0.9 g IV or po q 24 h
Rifapentine						
For pulmonary TB (as part of a 3- or 4- drug regimen)	Initial phase (2 mo): 0.6 g twice/wk Continuation phase (4 mo): 0.6 g once/wk	N/A	N/A	N/A	N/A	N/A
For latent TB (in combination with isoniazid)	0.9 g once/wk (3 mo)	N/A	N/A	N/A	N/A	N/A
Tedizolid	200 mg q 24 h	200 mg IV q 24 h	200 mg IV q 24 h	N/A	N/A	200 mg po or IV q 24 h
Telavancin	N/A	10 mg/kg IV q 24 h	10 mg/kg IV q 24 h	N/A	N/A	N/A
Vancomycin	125 mg q 6 h (only effective for *C. difficile*–induced diarrhea	15 mg/kg IV q 12 h (often 1 g q 12)	15 mg/kg IV q 12 h	N/A	13 mg/kg IV q 8 h *or* 10 mg/kg IV q 6 h	0.5–1.0 g IV q wk
For meningitis	N/A	1 g IV q 8 h *or* 1.5 g IV q 12 h[g]	1 g IV q 8 h *or* 1.5 g IV q 12 h	N/A	15 mg/kg IV q 6 h	15 mg/kg IV q wk

[a]Initial loading dose should be equivalent to the usual dose for patients with normal renal function, followed by a dose adjusted for renal failure. Dosing adjustments of aminoglycosides should be assisted by measuring peak (drawn 1 h after the start of a 30-min IV infusion) and trough (drawn 30 min before next dose) serum levels.
[b]Rate or extent of absorption is decreased when the drug is taken with food.
[c]Dosage should not exceed that for adults.
[d]These drugs are generally avoided in children.
[e]Dose is based on TMP.
[f]The standard of care for dosing of this antibiotic for serious infections is complex and rapidly evolving (see discussion of individual drug for a more information).
[g]In addition, intrathecal or intraventricular vancomycin 10–20 mg/day may be necessary, and dose may need to be adjusted to achieve trough CSF levels of 10–20 µg/mL.
N/A = not applicable; TMP = trimethoprim.

Pregnancy and breastfeeding affect choice of antibiotic. Penicillins, cephalosporins, and erythromycin are among the safest antibiotics during pregnancy; tetracyclines are contraindicated. Most antibiotics reach sufficient concentrations in breast milk to affect a breastfed baby, sometimes contraindicating their use in women who are breastfeeding.

Duration: Antibiotics should be continued until objective evidence of systemic infection (eg, fever, symptoms, abnormal laboratory findings) is absent for several days. For some infections (eg, endocarditis, TB, osteomyelitis), antibiotics are continued for weeks or months to prevent relapse.

Complications: Complications of antibiotic therapy include superinfection by nonsusceptible bacteria or fungi and cutaneous, renal, hematologic, and GI adverse effects.

Adverse effects frequently require stopping the causative drug and substituting another antibiotic to which the bacteria are susceptible; sometimes, no alternatives exist.

Antibiotic Resistance

Resistance to an antibiotic may be inherent in a particular bacterial species or may be acquired through mutations or acquisition of genes for antibiotic resistance that are obtained from another organism. Different mechanisms for resistance are encoded by these genes (see Table 184–4). Resistance genes can be transmitted between 2 bacterial cells by the following mechanisms:

- Transformation (uptake of naked DNA from another organism)
- Transduction (infection by a bacteriophage)
- Conjugation (exchange of genetic material in the form of either plasmids, which are pieces of independently replicating extrachromosomal DNA, or transposons, which are movable pieces of chromosomal DNA)

Plasmids and transposons can rapidly disseminate resistance genes.

Antibiotic use preferentially eliminates nonresistant bacteria, increasing the proportion of resistant bacteria that remain. Antibiotic use has this effect not only on pathogenic bacteria but also on normal flora; resistant normal flora can become a reservoir for resistance genes that can spread to pathogens.

AMINOGLYCOSIDES

Aminoglycosides (see Table 184–5) have concentration-dependent bactericidal activity. They bind to the 30S ribosome, thereby inhibiting bacterial protein synthesis. Spectinomycin is a bacteriostatic antibiotic chemically related to the aminoglycosides (see p. 1508).

Pharmacology

Aminoglycosides are poorly absorbed orally but are well absorbed from the peritoneum, pleural cavity, and joints (and should never be instilled in these body cavities) and from denuded skin. Aminoglycosides are usually given IV. Aminoglycosides are distributed well into ECF except for vitreous humor, CSF, respiratory secretions, and bile (particularly in patients with biliary obstruction). Intravitreous injection is required to treat endophthalmitis. Intraventricular injection is often required to reach intraventricular levels high enough to treat meningitis.

Aminoglycosides are excreted by glomerular filtration and have a serum half-life of 2 to 3 h; the half-life increases exponentially as the GFR falls (eg, in renal insufficiency, in the elderly).

Indications

Aminoglycosides are used for

- Serious gram-negative bacillary infections (especially those due to *Pseudomonas aeruginosa*)

Aminoglycosides are active against most gram-negative aerobic and facultative anaerobic bacilli but lack activity against anaerobes and most gram-positive bacteria, except for most staphylococci; however, some gram-negative bacilli and methicillin-resistant staphylococci are resistant.

Aminoglycosides that are active against *P. aeruginosa* include tobramycin (particularly), gentamicin, and amikacin. Streptomycin, neomycin, and kanamycin are not active against *P. aeruginosa*. Gentamicin and tobramycin have similar antimicrobial spectra against gram-negative bacilli, but tobramycin is more active against *P. aeruginosa*, and gentamicin is more

Table 184–4. COMMON MECHANISMS OF ANTIBIOTIC RESISTANCE

MECHANISM	EXAMPLE
Decreased cell wall permeability	Loss of outer membrane D2 porin in imipenem-resistant *Pseudomonas aeruginosa*
Enzymatic inactivation	Production of β-lactamases that inactivate penicillins in penicillin-resistant *Staphylococcus aureus*, *Haemophilus influenzae*, and *Escherichia coli* Production of aminoglycoside-inactivating enzymes in gentamicin-resistant enterococci
Changes in target	Decreased affinity of penicillin-binding proteins for β-lactam antibiotics (eg, in *Streptococcus pneumoniae* with reduced penicillin sensitivity) Decreased affinity of methylated ribosomal RNA target for macrolides, clindamycin, and quinupristin in MLSB-resistant *S. aureus* Decreased affinity of altered cell wall precursor for vancomycin (eg, in *Enterococcus faecium*) Decreased affinity of DNA gyrase for fluoroquinolones in fluoroquinolone-resistant *S. aureus*
Increased antibiotic efflux pump	Increased efflux of tetracycline, macrolides, clindamycin, or fluoroquinolones (eg, in *S. aureus*)
Bypass of antibiotic inhibition	Development of bacterial mutants that can subsist on products (eg, thymidine) present in the environment, not just products synthesized within the bacteria (eg, in certain bacteria exposed to trimethoprim/sulfamethoxazole)

MLSB = macrolide, lincoside, streptogramin B.

Table 184–5. AMINOGLYCOSIDES

Amikacin
Gentamicin
Kanamycin*
Neomycin*
Streptomycin
Tobramycin

*Should be used topically or orally only.

active against *Serratia marcescens*. Amikacin is frequently active against gentamicin- and tobramycin-resistant pathogens.

Aminoglycosides are infrequently used alone, except when used for plague and tularemia. They are usually used with a broad-spectrum β-lactam for severe infection suspected to be due to a gram-negative bacillary species. However, because of increasing aminoglycoside resistance, a fluoroquinolone can be substituted for the aminoglycoside in initial empiric regimens, or if the pathogen is found to be susceptible to the accompanying antibiotic, the aminoglycoside can be stopped after 2 to 3 days unless an aminoglycoside-sensitive *P. aeruginosa* is identified.

Gentamicin or, less commonly, streptomycin may be used with other antibiotics to treat endocarditis due to streptococci or enterococci. Enterococcal resistance to aminoglycosides has become a common problem. Because treatment of enterococcal endocarditis requires prolonged use of a potentially nephrotoxic and ototoxic aminoglycoside plus a bacterial cell wall–active drug (eg, penicillin, vancomycin) to achieve bactericidal synergy, the choice of aminoglycoside must be based on special in vitro susceptibility testing. Susceptibility only to high levels of aminoglycosides in vitro predicts synergy when low-dose aminoglycoside therapy is combined with a cell wall–active drug. If the strain is susceptible to high levels of gentamicin and streptomycin, gentamicin is preferred because serum levels can be readily determined and toxicity is less. High-level enterococcal resistance to gentamicin in vitro does not rule out susceptibility of these strains to high levels of streptomycin; in such cases, streptomycin should be used.

Few therapeutic options are available for endocarditis due to enterococci that are resistant to high levels of gentamicin and streptomycin; no synergistic cell wall–active drug/aminoglycoside combination exists for endocarditis due to such strains, but the combination of the cell wall–active drugs ampicillin and ceftriaxone has recently been shown to be effective and minimizes the risk of nephrotoxicity.

Streptomycin has limited uses because of resistance and toxicity. It is used to treat tularemia and plague and, with other antibiotics, to treat TB.

Because of toxicity, neomycin and kanamycin are limited to topical use in small amounts. Neomycin is available for eye, ear, oral, and rectal use and as a bladder irrigant. Oral neomycin is used topically against intestinal flora to prepare the bowel before surgery and to treat hepatic coma.

Contraindications

Aminoglycosides are contraindicated in patients who are allergic to them.

Use During Pregnancy and Breastfeeding

Aminoglycosides are in pregnancy category D (there is evidence of human risk, but clinical benefits may outweigh risk).

Aminoglycosides enter breast milk but are not well absorbed orally. Thus, they are considered compatible with use during breastfeeding.

Adverse Effects

All aminoglycosides cause

- Renal toxicity (often reversible)
- Vestibular and auditory toxicity (often irreversible)
- Prolongation of effects of neuromuscular blockers

Symptoms and signs of vestibular damage are vertigo and ataxia.

Risk factors for renal, vestibular, and auditory toxicity are

- Frequent or very high doses
- Very high blood levels of the drug
- Long duration of therapy (particularly > 3 days)
- Older age
- A preexisting renal disorder
- Coadministration of vancomycin, cyclosporine, or amphotericin B
- For renal toxicity, coadministration of contrast agents
- For auditory toxicity, a genetic predisposition, preexisting hearing problems, and coadministration of loop diuretics

High doses given over a long period of time typically cause more concern about renal toxicity, but even low doses given for a short time can worsen renal function.

Patients receiving aminoglycosides for > 2 wk and those at risk of vestibular and auditory toxicity should be monitored with serial audiography. At the first sign of toxicity, the drug should be stopped (if possible), or dosing should be adjusted.

Aminoglycosides can prolong the effect of neuromuscular blockers (eg, succinylcholine, curare-like drugs) and worsen weakness in disorders affecting neuromuscular transmission (eg, myasthenia gravis). These effects are particularly likely when the drug is given too rapidly or serum levels are excessively high. The effects sometimes resolve more rapidly if patients are given neostigmine or IV Ca. Other neurologic effects include paresthesias and peripheral neuropathy.

Hypersensitivity reactions are uncommon except for contact dermatitis due to topical neomycin. High oral doses of neomycin can cause malabsorption.

Dosing Considerations

Because toxicity depends more on duration of therapeutic levels than on peak levels and because efficacy is concentration-dependent rather than time-dependent (see p. 1495), frequent doses are avoided. Once/day IV dosing is preferred for most indications except enterococcal endocarditis. IV aminoglycosides are given slowly (30 min for divided daily dosing or 30 to 45 min for once/day dosing).

In patients with normal renal function, once/day dosing of gentamicin or tobramycin is 5 mg/kg (7 mg/kg if patients are critically ill) q 24 h, and once/day dosing for amikacin is 15 mg/kg q 24 h. If patients respond to the 7-mg/kg dose of gentamicin clinically and renal function continues to be normal, the once/day dose can be reduced to 5 mg/kg after the first few days of treatment.

In critically ill patients, peak serum levels should be determined after the first dose. In all patients, peak and trough levels are measured after the 2nd or 3rd dose (when the daily dose is divided) or when therapy lasts > 3 days, as well as after the dose is changed. Serum creatinine is measured every 2 to 3 days, and if it is stable, serum aminoglycoside levels need not be measured again. Peak concentration is the level 60 min after an IM injection or 30 min after the end of a 30-min IV infusion. Trough levels are measured during the 30 min before the next dose.

Peak levels in serum of at least 10 times the MIC are desirable. Dosing is adjusted to ensure a therapeutic peak serum level (to facilitate concentration-dependent activity) and nontoxic trough levels (see Table 184–6). In critically ill patients, who are likely to have expanded volumes of distribution and who are given higher initial doses, target peak serum levels are 16 to 24 μg/mL for gentamicin and tobramycin and 56 to 64 μg/mL for amikacin. For gentamicin and tobramycin, trough levels should be < 1 μg/mL at 18 to 24 h after the first dose with once/day dosing and between 1 and 2 μg/mL with divided daily dosing.

For patients with renal insufficiency, the loading dose is the same as that for patients with normal renal function; usually, the dosing interval is increased rather than the dose decreased. Guidelines for maintenance doses based on serum creatinine or creatinine clearance values are available (see Table 184–6), but they are not precise, and measurement of blood levels is preferred.

If patients are taking a high dose of a β-lactam (eg, piperacillin, ticarcillin) and an aminoglycoside, the high serum levels of the β-lactam can inactivate the aminoglycoside in vitro in serum specimens obtained to determine drug levels unless the specimen is assayed immediately or frozen. If patients with renal failure are concurrently taking an aminoglycoside and a high-dose β-lactam, the serum aminoglycoside level may be lower because interaction in vivo is prolonged.

SPECTINOMYCIN

Spectinomycin is a bacteriostatic antibiotic chemically related to the aminoglycosides (see p. 1506). Spectinomycin binds to the 30S subunit of the ribosome, thus inhibiting bacterial protein synthesis. Its activity is restricted to gonococci. Spectinomycin is excreted by glomerular filtration.

Indications include

- Gonococcal urethritis
- Cervicitis
- Proctitis

Spectinomycin is not effective for gonococcal pharyngitis. It is not available in the US, and where available, it is reserved for patients who cannot be treated with ceftriaxone or cefixime plus azithromycin or doxycycline.

Adverse effects, including hypersensitivity reactions and fever, are rare.

Table 184–6. DOSING FOR AMINOGLYCOSIDES IN ADULTS

1. Choose loading dose in mg/kg for peak serum levels in the range listed below for the aminoglycoside being used. If the patient's actual weight is > 20% higher than ideal weight* because of obesity, the weight used for dosing equals ideal weight plus 40% of excess body weight (actual weight minus ideal weight). If actual weight exceeds ideal weight because of ascites or edema, the weight used for dosing is the actual weight.

AMINOGLYCOSIDE	USUAL LOADING DOSES	EXPECTED PEAK SERUM LEVELS	TARGET SERUM TROUGH LEVELS
Gentamicin Tobramycin	1.5–2.0 mg/kg	4–10 μg/mL	1–2 μg/mL
Amikacin	5.0–7.5 mg/kg	15–30 μg/mL	5–10 μg/mL

2. Choose maintenance dose (as percentage of chosen loading dose) to maintain peak serum levels indicated above based on the selected dosing interval and the patient's corrected creatinine clearance†:

	PERCENTAGE OF LOADING DOSE REQUIRED FOR DOSAGE INTERVAL SELECTED		
CrCl (mL/min)‡	**8 h (%)**	**12 h (%)**	**24 h (%)**
90	84	—	—
70	76	88	—
50	65	79	—
30	48	63	86
20	37	50	75
15	31	42	67
10	24	34	56
5	16	23	41
0	8	11	21

*Ideal body weight = 50 kg (men) or 45.5 kg (women) at a height of 152 cm; 0.9 kg is subtracted for each cm of height < 152 cm or is added for each cm > 152 cm.

†CrCl(c) for men = (140 – age)wt in kg/70 × serum creatinine.
CrCl(c) for women = 0.85 × CrCl(c) for men.

‡If CrCl(c) is ≤ 90 mL/min, serum levels should be measured to help determine dosing.
CrCl = creatinine clearance; CrCl(c) = corrected CrCl.

Modified from Sarubbi FA Jr, Hull JH: Amikacin serum concentrations: prediction of levels and dosage guidelines. *Annals of Internal Medicine* 89:612–618, 1978.

β-LACTAMS

β-Lactams are antibiotics that have a β-lactam ring nucleus. Subclasses include

- Cephalosporins and cephamycins (cephems)
- Carbacephems
- Clavams
- Carbapenems
- Monobactams
- Penicillins

All β-lactams bind to and inactivate enzymes required for bacterial cell wall synthesis.

CARBAPENEMS

Carbapenems (imipenem, meropenem, doripenem, and ertapenem) are parenteral bactericidal β-lactam antibiotics that have an extremely broad spectrum. They are active against

- *Haemophilus influenzae*
- Anaerobes
- Most Enterobacteriaceae (including those that produce ampC β-lactamase and extended-spectrum β-lactamase [ESBL], although *P. mirabilis* tends to have higher imipenem minimum inhibitory concentration [MICs])
- Methicillin-sensitive staphylococci and streptococci, including *S. pneumoniae* (except possibly strains with reduced penicillin sensitivity)

Most *Enterococcus faecalis* and many *P. aeruginosa* strains, including those resistant to broad-spectrum penicillins and cephalosporins, are susceptible to imipenem, meropenem, and doripenem but are resistant to ertapenem. However, meropenem and doripenem are less active against *E. faecalis* than imipenem. Carbapenems are active synergistically with aminoglycosides against *P. aeruginosa*. *E. faecium, Stenotrophomonas maltophilia,* and methicillin-resistant staphylococci are resistant.

Many multidrug-resistant hospital-acquired bacteria are sensitive only to carbapenems. However, expanded use of carbapenems has resulted in some carbapenem resistance.

Imipenem and meropenem penetrate into CSF when meninges are inflamed. Meropenem is used for gram-negative bacillary meningitis; imipenem is not used in meningitis because it may cause seizures. Most seizures occur in patients who have CNS abnormalities or renal insufficiency and who are given inappropriately high doses.

Doripenem has a black box warning stating that when used to treat patients with ventilator-associated bacterial pneumonia, it has an increased risk of death compared with imipenem. Also, clinical response rates were lower with doripenem. Doripenem is not approved for the treatment of pneumonia.

CEPHALOSPORINS

Cephalosporins are bactericidal β-lactam antibiotics. They inhibit enzymes in the cell wall of susceptible bacteria, disrupting cell synthesis. There are 5 generations of cephalosporins (see Table 184–7).

Pharmacology

Cephalosporins penetrate well into most body fluids and the ECF of most tissues, especially when inflammation (which enhances diffusion) is present. However, the only cephalosporins that reach CSF levels high enough to treat meningitis are

- Ceftriaxone
- Cefotaxime
- Ceftazidime
- Cefepime

All cephalosporins penetrate poorly into ICF and the vitreous humor.

Most cephalosporins are excreted primarily in urine, so their doses must be adjusted in patients with renal insufficiency. Cefoperazone and ceftriaxone, which have significant biliary excretion, do not require such dose adjustment.

Indications

Cephalosporins are bactericidal for most of the following:

- Gram-positive bacteria
- Gram-negative bacteria

Cephalosporins are classified in generations (see Table 184–8). The 1st-generation drugs are effective mainly against gram-positive organisms. Higher generations generally have expanded spectra against aerobic gram-negative bacilli. The 5th-generation cephalosporin ceftaroline is active against

Table 184–7. CEPHALOSPORINS

DRUG	ROUTE
1st Generation	
Cefadroxil	Oral
Cefazolin	Parenteral
Cephalexin	Oral
Cephradine	Oral
2nd Generation	
Cefaclor	Oral
Cefotetan	Parenteral
Cefoxitin	Parenteral
Cefprozil	Oral
Cefuroxime	Parenteral or oral
3rd Generation	
Cefdinir	Oral
Cefditoren	Oral
Cefixime	Oral
Cefotaxime	Parenteral
Cefpodoxime	Oral
Ceftazidime	Parenteral
Ceftibuten	Oral
Ceftriaxone	Parenteral
4th Generation	
Cefepime	Parenteral
5th Generation	
Ceftaroline	Parenteral

Table 184–8. SOME CLINICAL USES OF 3RD- AND 4TH-GENERATION CEPHALOSPORINS

DRUG	INDICATIONS	COMMENTS
3rd- and 4th-generation cephalosporins	Polymicrobial infections involving gram-negative bacilli and gram-positive cocci (eg, intra-abdominal sepsis, decubitus ulcers, diabetic foot infections)	When necessary, used with other drugs to cover anaerobes or enterococci
Ceftriaxone and some other 3rd-generation drugs	Community-acquired pneumonia	Used with a macrolide to cover atypical pathogens (mycoplasmas, *Chlamydophila* sp, *Legionella* sp)
Cefotaxime Ceftriaxone	Acute meningitis suspected to be due to *Streptococcus pneumoniae*, *Haemophilus influenzae*, or *Neisseria meningitides*	Used with ampicillin to cover *Listeria monocytogenes* and with vancomycin to cover *S. pneumoniae* with reduced penicillin sensitivity (pending MIC results*)
Cefpodoxime (oral)	Uncomplicated skin and soft-tissue infections due to staphylococci or streptococci	Not used if methicillin-resistant *Staphylococcus aureus* is suspected
Ceftazidime	Empiric therapy for postneurosurgical meningitis to cover *Pseudomonas aeruginosa*	Used with vancomycin to cover methicillin-resistant *S. aureus*
Ceftriaxone	Endocarditis caused by HACEK organisms	—
	Endocarditis due to penicillin-sensitive streptococci	—
	Lyme disease with neurologic complications (except isolated Bell palsy), carditis, or arthritis	
	Uncomplicated gonococcal infections, chancroid, or both	Single IM dose

* Pneumococcal strains that are resistant to ceftriaxone and cefotaxime have been reported, and guidelines suggest that if CSF strains have MICs of ≥ 1.0 μg/mL, they should be considered nonsusceptible to 3rd-generation cephalosporins.

HACEK = *Haemophilus*, *Actinobacillus*, *Cardiobacterium*, *Eikenella*, and *Kingella* spp; MICs = minimum inhibitory concentrations.

methicillin-resistant *Staphylococcus aureus*. Cephalosporins have the following limitations:

- Lack of activity against enterococci (except for ceftaroline, which is active against *Enterococcus faecalis,* not *E. faecium*)
- Lack of activity against methicillin-resistant staphylococci (except for ceftaroline)
- Lack of activity against anaerobic gram-negative bacilli (except for cefotetan and cefoxitin)

First-generation cephalosporins: These drugs have excellent activity against

- Gram-positive cocci

Oral 1st-generation cephalosporins are commonly used for uncomplicated skin and soft-tissue infections, which are usually due to staphylococci and streptococci.

Parenteral cefazolin is frequently used for endocarditis due to methicillin-sensitive *S. aureus* and for prophylaxis before cardiothoracic, orthopedic, abdominal, and pelvic surgery.

Second-generation cephalosporins and cephamycins: Second-generation cephalosporins are active against

- Gram-positive cocci
- Certain gram-negative bacilli

Cephamycins are active against

- *Bacteroides* sp, including *B. fragilis*

These drugs may be slightly less active against gram-positive cocci than 1st-generation cephalosporins. Second-generation cephalosporins and cephamycins are often used for polymicrobial infections that include gram-negative bacilli and gram-positive cocci. Because cephamycins are active against *Bacteroides* sp, they can be used when anaerobes are suspected (eg, in intra-abdominal sepsis, decubitus ulcers, and diabetic foot infections). However, in some medical centers, these bacilli are no longer reliably susceptible to cephamycins.

Third-generation cephalosporins: These drugs are active against

- *Haemophilus influenzae* and some Enterobacteriaceae (eg, *Escherichia coli*, *Klebsiella pneumoniae*, *Proteus mirabilis*) that do not produce ampC β-lactamase or ESBL

Ceftazidime is also active against

- *Pseudomonas aeruginosa*

Some 3rd-generation cephalosporins have relatively poor activity against gram-positive cocci. Oral cefixime and ceftibuten have little activity against *S. aureus* and, if used for skin and soft-tissue infections, should be restricted to uncomplicated infections due to streptococci. These cephalosporins have many clinical uses, as does the 4th-generation cephalosporin (see Table 184–8).

Fourth-generation cephalosporin: The 4th-generation cephalosporin cefepime has activity against

- Gram-positive cocci (similar to cefotaxime)
- Gram-negative bacilli (enhanced activity), including *P. aeruginosa* (similar to ceftazidime), ESBL-producing *K. pneumoniae* and *E. coli*, and ampC β-lactamase–producing Enterobacteriaceae, such as *Enterobacter* sp

Fifth-generation cephalosporin: The 5th-generation cephalosporin ceftaroline is active against

- Methicillin-resistant *S. aureus* (MRSA) and *E. faecalis*

Its activity against other gram-positive cocci and gram-negative bacilli is similar to that of 3rd-generation cephalosporins. It is not active against *Pseudomonas* sp.

Contraindications

Cephalosporins are contraindicated in patients who are allergic to them or who have had an anaphylactic reaction to penicillins.

Ceftriaxone is contraindicated as follows:

- Ceftriaxone IV must not be coadministered with Ca-containing IV solutions (including continuous Ca-containing infusions such as parenteral nutrition) in neonates ≤ 28 days because precipitation of ceftriaxone-Ca salt is a risk. Fatal reactions with ceftriaxone-Ca precipitates in the lungs and kidneys of neonates have been reported. In some cases, different infusion lines were used, and ceftriaxone and Ca-containing solutions were given at different times. To date, no intravascular or pulmonary precipitates have been reported in patients other than neonates who are treated with ceftriaxone and Ca-containing IV solutions. However, because an interaction between ceftriaxone and IV Ca-containing solutions is theoretically possible in patients other than neonates, ceftriaxone and Ca-containing solutions should not be mixed or given within 48 h of each other (based on 5 half-lives of ceftriaxone)—even via different infusion lines at different sites—to any patient regardless of age. No data on potential interaction between ceftriaxone and oral Ca-containing products or on interaction between IM ceftriaxone and Ca-containing products (IV or oral) are available.
- Ceftriaxone should not be given to hyperbilirubinemic and preterm neonates because in vitro, ceftriaxone can displace bilirubin from serum albumin, potentially triggering kernicterus.

Use During Pregnancy and Breastfeeding

Cephalosporins are in pregnancy category B (animal studies show no risk and human evidence is incomplete, or animal studies show risk but human studies do not).

Cephalosporins enter breast milk and may alter bowel flora of the infant. Thus, use during breastfeeding is often discouraged.

Adverse Effects

Significant adverse effects include

- Hypersensitivity reactions (most common)
- *Clostridium difficile*–induced diarrhea (pseudomembranous colitis—see p. 1466)
- Leukopenia
- Thrombocytopenia
- Positive Coombs test (although hemolytic anemia is very uncommon)

Hypersensitivity reactions are the most common systemic adverse effects; rash is common, but immediate IgE-mediated urticaria and anaphylaxis are rare.

Cross-sensitivity between cephalosporins and penicillins is uncommon; cephalosporins can be given cautiously to patients with a history of delayed hypersensitivity to penicillin if necessary. However, cephalosporins should not be used in patients who have had an anaphylactic reaction to penicillin. Pain at the IM injection site and thrombophlebitis after IV use may occur.

Cefotetan may have a disulfiram-like effect when ethanol is ingested, causing nausea and vomiting. Cefotetan may also elevate the PT/INR and PTT, an effect that is reversible with vitamin K.

MONOBACTAMS

Monobactams are parenteral β-lactam bactericidal antibiotics.

Aztreonam is currently the only available monobactam. Aztreonam is as active as ceftazidime against

- Enterobacteriaceae that do not produce ampC β-lactamase or ESBL
- *Pseudomonas aeruginosa*

Aztreonam is not active against anaerobes. Gram-positive bacteria are resistant to aztreonam (in contrast to cephalosporins). Aztreonam acts synergistically with aminoglycosides.

Because the metabolic products of aztreonam differ from those of other β-lactams, cross-hypersensitivity is unlikely. Thus, aztreonam is used mainly for

- Severe aerobic gram-negative bacillary infections, including meningitis, in patients who have a serious β-lactam allergy but who nevertheless require β-lactam therapy

Other antibiotics are added to cover any suspected gram-positive cocci and anaerobes.

The dose is reduced in renal failure.

PENICILLINS

Penicillins (see Table 184–9) are β-lactam antibiotics that are bactericidal by unknown mechanisms but perhaps by activating autolytic enzymes that destroy the cell wall in some bacteria.

Resistance: Some bacteria produce β-lactamases, which inactivate β-lactam antibiotics; this effect can be blocked

Table 184–9. PENICILLINS

DRUG	ROUTE
Penicillin G–like drugs	
Penicillin G	Oral or parenteral
Penicillin G benzathine	Parenteral
Penicillin G procaine	Parenteral
Penicillin V	Oral
Ampicillin-like drugs	
Ampicillin	Oral or parenteral
Ampicillin plus sulbactam	Parenteral
Amoxicillin	Oral
Amoxicillin plus clavulanate	Oral
Penicillinase-resistant penicillins	
Dicloxacillin	Oral
Nafcillin	Oral or parenteral
Oxacillin	Oral or parenteral
Broad-spectrum (antipseudomonal) penicillins	
Carbenicillin	Oral
Piperacillin	Parenteral
Piperacillin plus tazobactam	Parenteral
Ticarcillin	Parenteral
Ticarcillin plus clavulanate	Parenteral

by adding a β-lactamase inhibitor (clavulanate, sulbactam, or tazobactam). However, available β-lactamase inhibitors do not inhibit ampC β-lactamases, commonly produced by *Enterobacter*, *Serratia*, *Citrobacter*, *Providencia*, and *Morganella* spp or by *Pseudomonas aeruginosa*, and these drugs may only partially inhibit ESBL produced by some *Klebsiella pneumoniae*, *Escherichia coli*, and other Enterobacteriaceae.

Carbapenemases, which can inactivate all β-lactam antibiotics, have become increasingly common in *Klebsiella* sp, other Enterobacteriaceae, *P. aeruginosa*, and *Acinetobacter* sp. Currently, there are no carbapenemase inhibitors available, although some are being developed.

Pharmacology

Food does not interfere with absorption of amoxicillin, but penicillin G should be given 1 h before or 2 h after a meal. Amoxicillin has generally replaced ampicillin for oral use because amoxicillin is absorbed better, has fewer GI effects, and can be given less frequently.

Penicillins are distributed rapidly in the ECF of most tissues, particularly when inflammation is present.

All penicillins except nafcillin are excreted in urine and reach high levels in urine. Parenteral penicillin G is rapidly excreted (serum half-life 0.5 h), except for repository forms (the benzathine or procaine salt of penicillin G); these forms are intended for deep IM injection only and provide a tissue depot from which absorption takes place over several hours to several days. Benzathine penicillin reaches its peak level more slowly and is generally longer-acting than procaine penicillin.

Indications

Penicillin G–like drugs: Penicillin G–like drugs (including penicillin V) are primarily used against

- Gram-positive bacteria
- Some gram-negative cocci (eg, meningococci)

A minority of gram-negative bacilli are also susceptible to large parenteral doses of penicillin G. Most staphylococci, most *Neisseria gonorrhoeae*, many anaerobic gram-negative bacilli, and about 30% of *Haemophilus influenzae* are resistant.

Penicillin G is the drug of choice for syphilis, for certain clostridial infections, and, with gentamicin, for endocarditis due to susceptible enterococci.

Benzathine penicillin G is available as pure benzathine penicillin, a mixture of equal amounts of benzathine and procaine penicillin G, and a mixture of 0.9 million units benzathine and 0.3 million units procaine penicillin G. Of the 3 products, only pure benzathine penicillin is recommended for treating syphilis and preventing rheumatic fever. Whether the mixture of equal amounts is effective in treating syphilis is unknown. Pure benzathine penicillin and the mixture of equal amounts are indicated for treating URIs and skin and soft-tissue infections caused by susceptible streptococci.

Amoxicillin and ampicillin: These drugs are more active against

- Enterococci
- Certain gram-negative bacilli, such as non-β-lactamase–producing *H. influenzae*, *E. coli*, and *Proteus mirabilis*; *Salmonella* sp; and *Shigella* sp

The addition of a β-lactamase inhibitor allows use against methicillin-sensitive staphylococci, *H. influenzae*, *Moraxella catarrhalis*, *Bacteroides* sp, *E. coli*, and *K. pneumoniae*.

Ampicillin is indicated primarily for infections typically caused by susceptible gram-negative bacteria:

- UTIs
- Meningococcal meningitis
- Biliary sepsis
- Respiratory infections
- *Listeria* meningitis
- Enterococcal infections
- Some typhoid fever and typhoid carriers

Penicillinase-resistant penicillins: These drugs are used primarily for

- Penicillinase-producing methicillin-sensitive *Staphylococcus aureus*

These drugs are also used to treat some *Streptococcus pneumoniae*, group A streptococcal, and methicillin-sensitive coagulase-negative staphylococcal infections.

Broad-spectrum (antipseudomonal) penicillin: These drugs have activity against

- Bacteria susceptible to ampicillin
- Some strains of *Enterobacter* and *Serratia* spp
- Many strains of *P. aeruginosa*

Ticarcillin is less active against enterococci than piperacillin. The addition of a β-lactamase inhibitor enhances activity against β-lactamase–producing methicillin-sensitive *S. aureus*, *E. coli*, *K. pneumoniae*, *H. influenzae*, and gram-negative anaerobic bacilli, but not against gram-negative bacilli that produce ampC β-lactamase, and may only partially inhibit ESBL produced by some *K. pneumoniae*, *E. coli*, and other Enterobacteriaceae. Broad-spectrum penicillins exhibit synergy with aminoglycosides and are usually used with this class to treat *P. aeruginosa* infections.

Contraindications

Penicillins are contraindicated in patients who have had serious allergic reactions to them.

Use During Pregnancy and Breastfeeding

Penicillins are in pregnancy category B (animal studies show no risk and human evidence is incomplete, or animal studies show risk but human studies do not).

Penicillins enter breast milk in small amounts. Their use is usually considered compatible with breastfeeding.

Adverse Effects

Adverse effects include

- Hypersensitivity reactions, including rashes (most common)

Other adverse effects occur less commonly.

Hypersensitivity: Most adverse effects are hypersensitivity reactions:

- Immediate reactions: Anaphylaxis (which can cause death within minutes), urticaria and angioneurotic edema (in 1 to 5/10,000 injections), and death (in about 0.3/10,000 injections)
- Delayed reactions (in up to 8% of patients): Serum sickness, rashes (eg, macular, papular, morbilliform), and exfoliative dermatitis (which usually appears after 7 to 10 days of therapy)

Most patients who report an allergic reaction to penicillin do not react to subsequent exposure to penicillin. Although small, risk of an allergic reaction is about 10 times higher for patients who have had a previous allergic reaction. Many patients report adverse reactions to penicillin that are not truly allergic (eg, GI adverse effects, nonspecific symptoms). If patients have a vague or inconsistent history of penicillin allergy and taking alternative antibiotics is not effective or convenient, skin testing may be done (see p. 1383). Desensitization may be attempted in patients with a positive skin test if there is no alternative to a penicillin-type drug. However, patients with a history of anaphylaxis to penicillin should not be given any β-lactam again (including for skin testing), except in very rare circumstances when no substitute can be found. In such cases, special precautions and desensitization regimens are required (see p. 1384).

Rashes: Rashes occur more often with ampicillin and amoxicillin than with other penicillins. Patients with infectious mononucleosis often develop a nonallergic rash, typically maculopapular, usually beginning between days 4 and 7 of treatment.

Other adverse effects: Penicillins can also cause

- CNS toxicity (eg, seizures) if doses are high, especially in patients with renal insufficiency
- Nephritis
- *C. difficile*–induced diarrhea (pseudomembranous colitis—see p. 1466)
- Coombs-positive hemolytic anemia
- Leukopenia
- Thrombocytopenia

Leukopenia seems to occur most often with nafcillin. Any penicillin used in very high IV doses can interfere with platelet function and cause bleeding, but ticarcillin is the most common cause, especially in patients with renal insufficiency.

Other adverse effects include pain at the IM injection site, thrombophlebitis when the same site is used repeatedly for IV injection, and, with oral formulations, GI disturbances. Rarely, black tongue, due to irritation of the glossal surface and keratinization of the superficial layers, occurs, usually when oral formulations are used.

Ticarcillin in high doses may cause Na overload because ticarcillin is a disodium salt. Ticarcillin can also cause hypokalemic metabolic alkalosis because the large amount of nonabsorbable anion presented to the distal tubules alters H^+ ion excretion and secondarily results in K^+ loss.

Dosing Considerations

Because penicillins, except nafcillin, reach high levels in urine, doses must be reduced in patients with severe renal insufficiency. Probenecid inhibits renal tubular secretion of many penicillins, increasing blood levels. It is sometimes given concurrently to maintain high blood levels.

CHLORAMPHENICOL

Chloramphenicol is primarily bacteriostatic. It binds to the 50S subunit of the ribosome, thereby inhibiting bacterial protein synthesis.

Pharmacology

Chloramphenicol is well absorbed orally. Parenteral therapy should be IV.

Chloramphenicol is distributed widely in body fluids, including CSF, and is excreted in urine. Because of hepatic metabolism, active chloramphenicol does not accumulate when renal insufficiency is present.

Indications

Chloramphenicol has a wide spectrum of activity against

- Gram-positive and gram-negative cocci and bacilli (including anaerobes)
- *Rickettsia*, *Mycoplasma*, *Chlamydia*, and *Chlamydophila* spp

Because of bone marrow toxicity, the availability of alternative antibiotics, and the emergence of resistance, chloramphenicol is no longer a drug of choice for any infection, except for

- Serious infections due to a few multidrug-resistant bacteria that remain susceptible to this antibiotic

However, when chloramphenicol has been used to treat meningitis caused by relatively penicillin-resistant pneumococci, outcomes have been discouraging, probably because chloramphenicol has poor bactericidal activity against these strains.

Contraindications

Chloramphenicol is contraindicated if another drug can be used instead.

Use During Pregnancy and Breastfeeding

Use of chloramphenicol during pregnancy results in fetal drug levels almost as high as maternal levels. Gray baby syndrome is a theoretical concern, particularly near term, but there is no clear evidence of fetal risk.

Chloramphenicol enters breast milk. Safety during breastfeeding has not been determined.

Adverse Effects

Adverse effects include

- Bone marrow depression (most serious)
- Nausea, vomiting, and diarrhea
- Gray baby syndrome (in neonates)

There are 2 types of bone marrow depression:

- Reversible dose-related interference with iron metabolism: This effect is most likely with high doses or prolonged treatment or in patients with a severe liver disorder.
- Irreversible idiosyncratic aplastic anemia: This anemia occurs in < 1/25,000 treated patients. It may not develop until after therapy is stopped. Chloramphenicol should not be used topically because small amounts may be absorbed and, rarely, cause aplastic anemia.

Hypersensitivity reactions are uncommon. Optic and peripheral neuritis may occur with prolonged use.

The neonatal gray baby syndrome, which involves hypothermia, cyanosis, flaccidity, and circulatory collapse, is often fatal. The cause is high blood levels, which occur because the immature liver cannot metabolize and excrete chloramphenicol. To avoid the syndrome, clinicians should not give infants ≤ 1 mo > 25 mg/kg/day initially, and doses should be adjusted based on blood levels of the drug.

DAPTOMYCIN

Daptomycin is a cyclic lipopeptide antibiotic that has a unique mechanism of action. It binds to the bacterial cell membranes, causing rapid depolarization of the membrane due to K efflux and associated disruption of DNA, RNA, and protein synthesis; the result is rapid concentration-dependent bacterial death (see p. 1495).

Indications

Daptomycin has activity against the following:

- Gram-positive bacteria (broad-spectrum activity)
- Multidrug-resistant gram-positive bacteria (because cross-resistance with other classes of antibiotics does not occur)

Daptomycin is used mainly for infections caused by

- Vancomycin- and methicillin-resistant *Staphylococcus aureus*
- Vancomycin-resistant enterococci (VRE)
- Pneumococci with reduced penicillin sensitivity

However, MRSA and VRE may become resistant during daptomycin therapy, resulting in relapsing or persistent infection.

Daptomycin is inferior to ceftriaxone for pneumonia, presumably because daptomycin can bind to pulmonary surfactant, reducing daptomycin's activity in the alveolar epithelial lining fluid.

Contraindications

Daptomycin is contraindicated in patients who have had an allergic reaction to it.

Use During Pregnancy and Breastfeeding

Daptomycin is in pregnancy category B (animal studies show no risk and human evidence is incomplete).

Daptomycin enters breast milk, but oral availability is low; effects on breastfeeding infants are unknown.

Adverse Effects

Adverse effects include

- Eosinophilic pneumonia
- Myopathy

Chronic use may cause reversible organizing pneumonia with eosinophilic pulmonary infiltrates, presumably because daptomycin binds to pulmonary surfactant and thus accumulates in the alveolar spaces.

Skeletal myopathy due to daptomycin is reversible but seldom occurs with once/day dosing.

Dosing Considerations

Daptomycin is given parenterally once/day. Over 90% is bound to serum protein.

Dosing is adjusted for renal failure.

Because daptomycin can cause reversible skeletal myopathy, patients should be monitored for muscle pain or weakness, and serum creatine kinase levels should be checked weekly.

FLUOROQUINOLONES

Fluoroquinolones (see Table 184–10) exhibit concentration-dependent bactericidal activity (see p. 1495) by inhibiting the activity of DNA gyrase and topoisomerase, enzymes essential for bacterial DNA replication.

Fluoroquinolones are divided into 2 groups, based on antimicrobial spectrum and pharmacology:

- Older group: Ciprofloxacin, norfloxacin, and ofloxacin
- Newer group: Gemifloxacin, levofloxacin, and moxifloxacin

Many newer fluoroquinolones have been withdrawn because of toxicity; they include trovafloxacin (because of severe hepatic toxicity), gatifloxacin (because of hypoglycemia and hyperglycemia), grepafloxacin (because of cardiac toxicity), temafloxacin (because of acute renal failure, hepatotoxicity, hemolytic anemia, coagulopathy, and hypoglycemia), and lomefloxacin, sparfloxacin, and enoxacin.

Table 184–10. FLUOROQUINOLONES

DRUG	ROUTE*
Ciprofloxacin	Oral or parenteral
Gemifloxacin	Oral
Levofloxacin	Oral or parenteral
Moxifloxacin	Oral or parenteral
Norfloxacin	Oral
Ofloxacin	Oral or parenteral

*Several fluoroquinolones are also available as otic and ophthalmic formulations.

Pharmacology

Oral absorption is diminished by coadministration of cations (aluminum, Mg, Ca, zinc, and iron preparations). After oral and parenteral administration, fluoroquinolones are widely distributed in most extracellular and intracellular fluids and are concentrated in the prostate, lungs, and bile.

Most fluoroquinolones are metabolized in the liver and excreted in urine, reaching high levels in urine. Moxifloxacin is eliminated primarily in bile.

Indications

Fluoroquinolones are active against the following:

- *Haemophilus influenzae*
- *Moraxella catarrhalis*
- *Mycoplasma* sp
- *Chlamydia* sp
- *Chlamydophila* sp
- *Legionella* sp
- Enterobacteriaceae
- *Pseudomonas aeruginosa* (particularly ciprofloxacin)
- *Mycobacterium tuberculosis*
- Some atypical mycobacteria
- Methicillin-sensitive staphylococci

Nosocomial methicillin-resistant staphylococci are usually resistant. Older fluoroquinolones have poor activity against streptococci and anaerobes. Newer fluoroquinolones have reliable activity against streptococci (including *Streptococcus pneumoniae* with reduced penicillin sensitivity) and some anaerobes; moxifloxacin in particular is active against most clinically significant obligates anaerobes. As use has increased, resistance, particularly to older fluoroquinolones, is developing among Enterobacteriaceae, *P. aeruginosa*, *S. pneumoniae*, and *Neisseria* sp. Nonetheless, fluoroquinolones have many clinical uses (see Table 184–11).

Fluoroquinolones are no longer recommended for treatment of gonorrhea in the US because of increasing resistance.

Contraindications

Contraindications include

- Previous allergic reaction to the drugs
- Certain disorders that predispose to arrhythmias (eg, QT-interval prolongation, uncorrected hypokalemia or hypomagnesemia, significant bradycardia)

Table 184–11. SOME CLINICAL USES OF FLUOROQUINOLONES

DRUG	USE	COMMENTS
Fluoroquinolones except moxifloxacin	UTIs when *Escherichia coli* resistance to trimethoprim/sulfamethoxazole is > 15%	Drugs of choice; however, increasing resistance of *E. coli* in some communities
Fluoroquinolones	Bacterial prostatitis	—
	Salmonella bacteremia	—
	Typhoid fever	Usually effective
	Infectious diarrhea	Effective against most bacterial causes (*Campylobacter* sp, salmonellae, shigellae, vibrios, *Yersinia enterocolitica*); however, increasing resistance of *C. jejuni* in some regions Not used for *E. coli* 0157:H7 or other enterohemorrhagic *E. coli* Not effective against *Clostridium difficile*
Ofloxacin	*Chlamydia trachomatis* infections	7-day course
Newer fluoroquinolones	Community-acquired pneumonia	Other drugs preferred if patients have taken fluoroquinolones recently
	Legionella pneumonia	Drugs of choice (or azithromycin)
Ciprofloxacin	Hospital-acquired pneumonia	Used empirically because it is effective against *Pseudomonas aeruginosa* Usually used with another antipseudomonal drug
	Long-term oral treatment of gram-negative bacillary or *Staphylococcus aureus* osteomyelitis	—
	Meningococcal prophylaxis	—
	Anthrax prophylaxis	Used extensively during 2001 after bioterrorist attack in US

- Use of drugs known to prolong the QT interval or to cause bradycardia (eg, metoclopramide, cisapride, erythromycin, clarithromycin, classes Ia and III antiarrhythmics, tricyclic antidepressants)

Fluoroquinolones have traditionally been considered to be contraindicated in children because they may cause cartilage lesions if growth plates are open. However, some experts, who challenge this view because evidence is weak, have recommended prescribing fluoroquinolones as a 2nd-line antibiotic and restricting use to a few specific situations, including *P. aeruginosa* infections in patients with cystic fibrosis, prophylaxis and treatment of bacterial infections in immunocompromised patients, life-threatening multiresistant bacterial infections in neonates and infants, and *Salmonella* or *Shigella* GI tract infections.

Use During Pregnancy and Breastfeeding

Fluoroquinolones are in pregnancy category C (animal studies show some risk, evidence in human and animal studies is inadequate, but clinical benefit sometimes exceeds risk).

Fluoroquinolones enter breast milk. Use during breastfeeding is not recommended.

Adverse Effects

Serious adverse effects are uncommon; main concerns include the following:

- Upper GI adverse effects occur in about 5% of patients because of direct GI irritation and CNS effects.
- CNS adverse effects (eg, mild headache, drowsiness, insomnia, dizziness, mood alteration) occur in < 5%. NSAIDs may enhance the CNS stimulatory effects of fluoroquinolones. Seizures are rare, but fluoroquinolones should not be used in patients with CNS disorders.
- Peripheral neuropathy may occur soon after taking the drug and may be permanent. If symptoms occur (eg, pain, burning, tingling, numbness, weakness, change in sensation), use of the fluoroquinolone should be stopped to prevent irreversible damage.
- Tendinopathy, including rupture of the Achilles tendon, may occur even after short-term use of fluoroquinolones.
- QT-interval prolongation can occur, potentially leading to ventricular arrhythmias and sudden cardiac death.
- Fluoroquinolone use has been strongly associated with *Clostridium difficile*–associated diarrhea (pseudomembranous colitis), especially that due to the hypervirulent *C. difficile* ribotype 027.

Diarrhea, leukopenia, anemia, and photosensitivity are uncommon. Rash is uncommon unless gemifloxacin is used for > 1 wk and is more likely to develop in women < 40. Nephrotoxicity is rare.

Dosing Considerations

Dose reduction, except for moxifloxacin, is required for patients with renal insufficiency. Older fluoroquinolones are normally given twice/day; newer ones and an extended-release form of ciprofloxacin are given once/day.

Ciprofloxacin raises theophylline levels, sometimes resulting in theophylline-related adverse effects (see p. 429).

FOSFOMYCIN

Fosfomycin is a novel class of antibacterial with a chemical structure unrelated to other known antibiotics. It is a bactericidal drug that disrupts cell wall synthesis by inhibiting phosphoenolpyruvate synthetase and thus interferes with the production of peptidoglycan.

In the US, it is available only as a powder formulation of fosfomycin tromethamine, which can be dissolved in liquid and taken orally. Outside the US, IV formulations are available.

Pharmacology

Fosfomycin is well absorbed orally and penetrates well into tissues, including sequestered sites such as the prostate and CSF.

Oral bioavailability of the fosfomycin tromethamine salt is low (about 40%), and consequently, serum levels are low relative to the minimum inhibitory concentrations (MICs). For this reason, the drug is used to treat uncomplicated lower UTIs, not pyelonephritis.

Fosfomycin is excreted in urine mainly by glomerular filtration without biotransformation. After oral dosing, urinary levels exceed the MICs of susceptible pathogens for over 24 h.

Indications

Fosfomycin has a broad spectrum of activity against both gram-positive and gram-negative organisms, including many antibiotic-resistant organisms such as

- *Staphylococcus aureus*, including MRSA
- *Enterococcus* sp, including VRE
- Enterobacteriaceae, including ESBL–producing *K. pneumoniae* and *Escherichia coli*
- *Pseudomonas aeruginosa*, which has variable rates of intrinsic resistance

Fosfomycin is used mainly for uncomplicated (ie, lower) UTIs caused by *E. coli* or *E. faecalis*. However, because it has a broad spectrum of activity, fosfomycin is sometimes used to treat infections with multidrug-resistant organisms at other anatomic sites.

Contraindications

There are no significant contraindications to its use other than known hypersensitivity to fosfomycin or to any component of the formulation.

Adverse Effects

Fosfomycin is generally well-tolerated and has a low rate of adverse effects, which include mainly GI symptoms (eg, nausea, diarrhea).

Dosing Considerations

For uncomplicated UTIs, a single oral dose of fosfomycin tromethamine 5.61 g (equivalent to 3 g of fosfomycin) dissolved in liquid is used.[1] A longer treatment course is probably necessary for infections at other sites (eg, prostate).

1. Falagas ME, Giannopoulou KP, Kokolakis GN, Rafailidis PI: Fosfomycin: use beyond urinary tract and gastrointestinal infections. *Clin Infect Dis* 46(7):1069–1077, 2008.

LINCOSAMIDES, OXAZOLIDINONES, AND STREPTOGRAMINS

Lincosamides (clindamycin—see below), oxazolidinones (linezolid, tedizolid—see p. 1517), and streptogramins (dalfopristin [streptogramin A] and quinupristin [streptogramin B]—see p. 1518) are grouped together because they have a similar mode of antibacterial action and similar antibacterial spectra. Macrolides (see p. 1518) and the ketolide telithromycin (see p. 1519) may be included with this group for similar reasons. All inhibit protein synthesis by binding to the 50S ribosomal subunit.

Cross-resistance occurs among the following antibiotics because they bind to the same target:

- Macrolides
- Clindamycin
- Quinupristin
- Telithromycin (to some extent)

However, cross-resistance does not occur between these antibiotics and dalfopristin and linezolid, which bind to different targets on the 50S ribosomal subunit.

CLINDAMYCIN

Clindamycin is a lincosamide antibiotic that is primarily bacteriostatic. It binds to the 50S subunit of the ribosome, thus inhibiting bacterial protein synthesis.

Pharmacology

Clindamycin is absorbed well orally and can be given parenterally. Clindamycin diffuses well into body fluids except CSF; it is concentrated in phagocytes. Most of the drug is metabolized; metabolites are excreted in bile and urine.

Indications

The spectrum of activity for clindamycin is similar to that of the macrolide erythromycin (see Table 184–13 on p. 1519) except that clindamycin is

- Effective for infections due to anaerobes (particularly *Bacteroides* sp, including *B. fragilis*), community-acquired methicillin-resistant *Staphylococcus aureus*, and macrolide-resistant, clindamycin-susceptible *Streptococcus pneumoniae*
- Not reliably active against mycoplasmas, chlamydiae, *Chlamydophila* sp, and legionellae

Aerobic gram-negative bacilli and enterococci are resistant.

Clindamycin is usually used for anaerobic infections; however, clindamycin resistance has emerged among these organisms in some regions. Because these infections often also involve aerobic gram-negative bacilli, additional antibiotics are also used. Clindamycin is part of combination therapy for the following:

- Infections caused by toxigenic streptococci (because clindamycin decreases the bacteria's toxin production)
- Cerebral toxoplasmosis
- Babesiosis
- Falciparum malaria
- *Pneumocystis jirovecii* pneumonia

Clindamycin can be used for infections (eg, skin and soft-tissue infections) in communities where community-associated methicillin-resistant *Staphylococcus aureus* (CA-MRSA) is common; whether clindamycin is useful depends on local resistance patterns.

Clindamycin can be used for infections due to clindamycin-and erythromycin-susceptible strains. However, some CA-MRSA strains are clindamycin-susceptible and erythromycin-resistant; erythromycin resistance in these strains may be due to an active efflux mechanism or to erythromycin-inducible modification of the ribosomal target. If the infecting strain of clindamycin-susceptible CA-MRSA is resistant to erythromycin because of the efflux mechanism, patients can be expected to respond to clindamycin. However, if the strain is erythromycin-resistant because of erythromycin-inducible ribosomal target modification, patients may not respond clinically to clindamycin because certain mutants can emerge during clindamycin therapy; these mutants are resistant to clindamycin and erythromycin because of constitutive modification of the ribosomal target. (Constitutive means that resistance is always present regardless of whether an inducer, such as erythromycin, is present.)

Erythromycin resistance due to efflux can be differentiated from that due to inducible ribosomal target modification with a commonly used double disk diffusion assay (D test). A clindamycin disk is placed at a standard distance from an erythromycin disk on an agar plate streaked with a standard inoculum of the CA-MRSA strain in question. Zone of growth inhibition (shaped like the letter "D") around the clindamycin disk, with a flattened zone nearest the erythromycin disk indicates inducible ribosomal resistance. Patients who have moderate to severe infection with an inducible ribosomal-resistant CA-MRSA strain and a positive D test should not be treated with clindamycin.

Clindamycin cannot be used for CNS infections (other than cerebral toxoplasmosis) because penetration into the brain and CSF is poor.

Topical clindamycin is used for acne.

Contraindications

Clindamycin is contraindicated in patients who have had an allergic reaction to it, and it should be used with caution in those who have a history of regional enteritis, ulcerative colitis, or antibiotic-associated colitis.

Use During Pregnancy and Breastfeeding

Clindamycin is in pregnancy category B (animal studies show no risk but human evidence is inadequate, or animal studies show risk and human studies do not).

Clindamycin enters breast milk. Use during breastfeeding is not recommended.

Adverse Effects

The main adverse effect is

- *Clostridium difficile*–associated diarrhea (pseudomembranous colitis—see p. 1466)

Clindamycin, penicillins, cephalosporins, and, most recently, fluoroquinolones have been associated with *C. difficile*–associated diarrhea. Clindamycin has been associated with *C. difficile*–associated diarrhea in up to 10% of patients regardless of route, including topical.

Hypersensitivity reactions may occur. If not swallowed with water, clindamycin may cause esophagitis.

Dosing Considerations

Dose adjustments are not required for renal failure. Clindamycin is given q 6 to 8 h.

LINEZOLID AND TEDIZOLID

Linezolid

Linezolid is an oxazolidinone antibiotic that has activity against the following:

- Streptococci
- Enterococci (*Enterococcus faecalis* and *E. faecium*)
- Staphylococci, including strains resistant to other classes of antibiotics
- Mycobacteria
- Anaerobes, such as *Fusobacterium*, *Prevotella*, *Porphyromonas*, and *Bacteroides* spp and peptostreptococci

Contraindications

Linezolid is contraindicated in patients with a prior allergic reaction to it.

Other contraindications include having risk factors for serotonin syndrome or hypertension.

Serotonin syndrome: Linezolid is a reversible, nonselective monamine oxidase inhibitor (MAOI); MAO inhibition causes levels of the neurotransmitter serotonin to increase. Thus, linezolid has the potential for causing serotonin syndrome (a hyperserotonergic state characterized by mental status changes, neurologic abnormalities, and autonomic instability—see p. 3019) when it is used in patients with either of the following:

- Endocrinologically active carcinoid tumors (see p. 1251)
- Use of drugs with serotonergic activity

Such drugs include SSRIs, MAOIs (eg, phenelzine, isocarboxazid), tricyclic antidepressants, serotonin 1B,1D receptor agonists (triptans), meperidine, bupropion, and buspirone. Patients who are taking such drugs and urgently need linezolid may be treated if the benefit is thought to outweigh the risk and if they

- Promptly stop the proserotonergic drug
- Are carefully monitored for manifestations of serotonin syndrome for 2 wk after stopping the drug (for fluoxetine, 5 wk) or for 24 h after the last linezolid dose

Linezolid is not been studied in patients with carcinoid syndrome; it should be used only if patients are closely monitored for symptoms and signs of serotonin syndrome.

Hypertension: Linezolid should not be given to the following patients unless they are monitored for potential increases in BP:

- Those taking any of the following: sympathomimetic drugs (eg, pseudoephedrine), vasopressors (eg, epinephrine, norepinephrine), or dopaminergic drugs (eg, dopamine, dobutamine)
- Those with uncontrolled hypertension
- Those with thyrotoxicosis
- Those with a pheochromocytoma

Use During Pregnancy and Breastfeeding

Linezolid is in pregnancy category C (animal studies show some risk, evidence in human studies is inadequate, but clinical benefit sometimes exceeds risk).

Whether linezolid is excreted in breast milk or is safe to use during breastfeeding is unknown.

Adverse Effects

Adverse effects include

- Reversible myelosuppression
- Irreversible peripheral neuropathy
- Reversible optic neuropathy
- Serotonin syndrome

Reversible myelosuppression, including thrombocytopenia, leukopenia, and anemia, occurs in about 3% of patients, usually when therapy is used > 2 wk. Consequently, CBC is monitored weekly, especially when therapy lasts > 2 wk.

Peripheral and optic neuropathy may occur with prolonged use, and patients taking long-term linezolid therapy should be closely monitored for these disorders.

Tedizolid

Tedizolid is an oxazolidinone antibiotic with a spectrum of activity similar to that of linezolid, although it may have activity against some linezolid-resistant gram-positive cocci.

In clinical trials, risk of serotonin syndrome and thrombocytopenia was lower with tedizolid than with linezolid. Tedizolid can cause significant neutropenia and its use is not recommended in patients with neutrophil counts of < 1000 cell/mm^3.

QUINUPRISTIN AND DALFOPRISTIN

Quinupristin and dalfopristin are lincosamide antibiotics (see p. 1516) that are semisynthetic derivatives of pristinamycin, a naturally occurring streptogramin. Quinupristin/dalfopristin (Q/D) is given together in a fixed 30/70 combination; this combination has synergistic bactericidal activity against the following:

- Streptococci and staphylococci, including strains resistant to other antibiotic classes
- Some gram-negative anaerobic bacilli
- *Clostridium perfringens*
- *Peptostreptococcus* sp
- Atypical respiratory pathogens (*Mycoplasma pneumoniae*, *Chlamydophila pneumoniae*, *Legionella pneumophila*)

Q/D inhibits *Enterococcus faecium*, including vancomycin-resistant strains. *E. faecalis* is resistant.

Q/D is given via a central IV catheter because phlebitis frequently occurs when Q/D is given via a peripheral vein. Up to 30% of patients develop significant myalgias.

Dosage reduction is required for severe hepatic insufficiency but not for renal insufficiency.

Q/D may inhibit the metabolism of drugs that are metabolized by the cytochrome P-450 (CYP450) 3A4 isoenzyme system.

MACROLIDES

Macrolides (see Table 184–12) are antibiotics that are primarily bacteriostatic; by binding to the 50S subunit of the ribosome, they inhibit bacterial protein synthesis.

Pharmacology

Except for telithromycin (see p. 1519), macrolides are relatively poorly absorbed orally. Fidaxomicin is minimally absorbed and active only locally in the GI tract. Food has the following effects on macrolide absorption:

- For extended-release clarithromycin, increased absorption
- For immediate-release clarithromycin tablet or suspension, no effect

Table 184–12. MACROLIDES

DRUG	ROUTE
Azithromycin	Oral or parenteral
Clarithromycin	Oral
Erythromycin	Oral or parenteral
Fidaxomicin	Oral
Telithromycin	Oral

- For azithromycin capsules and erythromycin (including base and stearate formulations), decreased absorption
- For fidaxomicin, minimal effects

Once absorbed macrolides diffuse well into body fluids, except CSF, and are concentrated in phagocytes. Excretion is mainly in bile.

Indications

Macrolides are active against

- Aerobic and anaerobic gram-positive cocci, except for most enterococci, many *Staphylococcus aureus* strains (especially methicillin-resistant strains), and some *Streptococcus pneumoniae* and *S. pyogenes* strains
- *Mycoplasma pneumoniae*
- *Chlamydia trachomatis*
- *Chlamydophila pneumoniae*
- *Legionella* sp
- *Corynebacterium diphtheriae*
- *Campylobacter* sp
- *Treponema pallidum*
- *Propionibacterium acnes*
- *Borrelia burgdorferi*

Bacteroides fragilis is resistant. Clarithromycin and azithromycin have enhanced activity against *Haemophilus influenzae* and activity against *Mycobacterium avium* complex.

Macrolides have been considered the drug of choice for group A streptococcal and pneumococcal infections when penicillin cannot be used. However, pneumococci with reduced penicillin sensitivity are often resistant to macrolides, and in some communities, up to 20% of *S. pyogenes* are macrolide-resistant. Because they are active against atypical respiratory pathogens, they are often used empirically for lower respiratory tract infections, but another drug is often necessary to cover macrolide-resistant pneumococci. Macrolides have other clinical uses (see Table 184–13). Macrolides are not used to treat meningitis.

Fidaxomicin has minimal to no activity against gram-negative bacteria but is bactericidal against *Clostridium difficile*.

Contraindications

Macrolides are contraindicated in patients who have had an allergic reaction to them.

Concomitant administration of macrolides with astemizole, cisapride, pimozide, or terfenadine is contraindicated because potentially fatal cardiac arrhythmias (QT prolongation, ventricular tachycardia, ventricular fibrillation, torsades de pointes) may occur when clarithromycin or erythromycin is given with these drugs. This effect is most likely due to inhibition of metabolism of these drugs by erythromycin and clarithromycin.

Table 184–13. SOME CLINICAL USES OF MACROLIDES

DRUG	INDICATION	COMMENTS
Macrolides	Infection due to *Mycoplasma pneumoniae*, *Legionella* sp, or *Bordetella pertussis*	Drugs of choice
	Eradication of *Corynebacterium diphtheriae* in carriers	
	Symptomatic cat-scratch disease (*Bartonella henselae*)	—
	Bacillary angiomatosis and peliosis hepatis in patients with AIDS (involving *B. henselae* or *B. quintana*)	—
Azithromycin	Cerebral toxoplasmosis	Used with other drugs
	Babesiosis	Used with other drugs
	Chlamydia trachomatis urethritis and cervicitis	—
Clarithromycin and azithromycin	*Mycobacterium avium* complex	Part of a multidrug regimen
Erythromycin	Uncomplicated skin infections	—
	Acne	Topical use
	Bowel preparation before GI tract surgery	Taken orally and used with an oral aminoglycoside
Fidaxomicin	*Clostridium difficile*	—

Use During Pregnancy and Breastfeeding

Erythromycin and azithromycin are in pregnancy category B (animal studies show no risk and human evidence is incomplete, or animal studies show risk but human studies do not). Erythromycin is considered safer because clinical use has been much more extensive.

Clarithromycin is in category C (animal studies show some risk, evidence in human studies is inadequate, but clinical benefit sometimes outweighs risk).

Erythromycin is considered compatible with breastfeeding. Safety of other macrolides during breastfeeding is unknown.

Adverse Effects

Main concerns include

- GI disturbances (mainly with erythromycin)
- QT-interval prolongation by erythromycin
- Inhibition of hepatic metabolism, leading to numerous drug interactions

Erythromycin commonly causes dose-related GI disturbances, including nausea, vomiting, abdominal cramps, and diarrhea; disturbances are less common with clarithromycin and azithromycin. Taking the drug with food may help decrease GI disturbances. Erythromycin may cause dose-related tinnitus, dizziness, and reversible hearing loss. Cholestatic jaundice occurs most commonly with erythromycin estolate. Jaundice usually appears after 10 days of use, primarily in adults but can occur earlier if the drug has been given previously. Erythromycin is not given IM because it causes severe pain; when given IV, it may cause phlebitis or pain. Hypersensitivity reactions are rare.

Erythromycin causes QT-interval prolongation and predisposes to ventricular tachyarrhythmia, especially in women, in patients who have QT-interval prolongation or electrolyte abnormalities, and in patients taking another drug that may prolong the QT interval.

Dosing Considerations

For azithromycin, no dosage adjustment is required for renal insufficiency.

Erythromycin and, to some extent, clarithromycin interact with numerous drugs because they inhibit hepatic metabolism via the cytochrome P-450 (CYP450) system. Azithromycin is the least likely to interact with other drugs. Interactions may occur when erythromycin or clarithromycin is taken with the following:

- Warfarin: Further elevation of the PT/INR
- Lovastatin and simvastatin: Rhabdomyolysis
- Midazolam and triazolam: Somnolence
- Theophylline: Nausea, vomiting, and seizures
- Tacrolimus, cyclosporine, and ergot alkaloids: Elevated serum levels of these drugs

TELITHROMYCIN

Telithromycin is a ketolide antibiotic. Ketolides are chemically related to macrolides (see p. 1518) and inhibit bacterial ribosomal protein synthesis without inducing resistance to macrolides, clindamycin, or streptogramins. Telithromycin can have serious adverse effects and typically should not be selected if other, less toxic alternatives are available.

Telithromycin is rapidly absorbed orally with or without food and is metabolized primarily in the liver.

Indications

Telithromycin is active against erythromycin-susceptible staphylococci and streptococci and multidrug-resistant *Streptococcus pneumoniae*. Telithromycin is also active against erythromycin-susceptible enterococci, *Bordetella pertussis*, *Haemophilus influenzae*, *Helicobacter pylori*, *Moraxella catarrhalis*, *Mycoplasma pneumoniae*, *Chlamydophila pneumoniae*, and *Legionella*, *Prevotella*, and *Peptostreptococcus* spp.

Because of safety concerns, telithromycin is recommended only for the treatment of adults ≥ 18 yr with community-acquired mild to moderate pneumonia due to the following:

- *S. pneumoniae* (including multidrug-resistant strains, ie, penicillin-resistant *S. pneumoniae*; isolates resistant to ≥ 2 of the following: penicillin, 2nd-generation cephalosporins [eg, cefuroxime], macrolides, tetracyclines, trimethoprim/sulfamethoxazole)

- *H. influenzae*
- *M. catarrhalis*
- *C. pneumoniae*
- *M. pneumoniae*

Contraindications

Contraindications include

- Myasthenia gravis because telithromycin may exacerbate symptoms and fatal respiratory failure has occurred in patients with this disorder
- Previous allergic reaction to telithromycin or any macrolide
- Previous hepatitis or jaundice after taking telithromycin or a macrolide
- Concurrent use of pimozide or cisapride because of cardiac arrhythmias (QT prolongation, ventricular tachycardia, ventricular fibrillation, torsades de pointes)
- Concurrent use of colchicine in patients with renal or hepatic impairment

Use During Pregnancy and Breastfeeding

Telithromycin is in pregnancy category C because animal studies show some risk, evidence in human studies is inadequate, but clinical benefit sometimes outweighs risk.

Safety of telithromycin during breastfeeding is unknown.

Adverse Effects

Adverse effects include

- GI disturbances
- QT-interval prolongation
- Severe hepatitis

Diarrhea, nausea, vomiting, and dizziness are the most common adverse effects.

Prolongation of the QT interval, hyperbilirubinemia, elevation of liver enzymes, transient loss of consciousness (sometimes associated with vagal syndrome), and visual disturbances (particularly a slowed ability to accommodate and to release accommodation) are less common. Because loss of consciousness or visual disturbance is a risk, patients should try to avoid potentially hazardous activities (eg, driving, operating dangerous equipment). Severe hepatotoxicity, which may require liver transplantation and which may be fatal, may occur.

Cross-sensitivity with macrolides can occur.

Dosing Considerations

Telithromycin inhibits cytochrome P-450 (CYP450) 3A4, increasing levels of the following drugs:

- Digoxin: Digoxin adverse effects or serum levels should be monitored.
- Ergot alkaloids: Concomitant use should be avoided.
- Benzodiazepines: Concomitant use requires caution.
- Metoprolol: Concomitant use in patients with heart failure requires caution.
- Statins: Concomitant use of simvastatin, lovastatin, or atorvastatin (but not pravastatin or fluvastatin) should be avoided.
- Cisapride: Concomitant use is contraindicated.
- Pimozide: Concomitant use is contraindicated.
- Sirolimus
- Tacrolimus

CYP3A4 inducers such as rifampin, phenytoin, carbamazepine, and phenobarbital decrease levels of telithromycin; the CYP3A4 inhibitors itraconazole and ketoconazole increase levels of telithromycin. Telithromycin decreases absorption of sotalol.

METRONIDAZOLE

Metronidazole is bactericidal. It enters bacterial cell walls and disrupts DNA and inhibits DNA synthesis in certain microorganisms.

Pharmacology

Oral metronidazole is absorbed well. It is usually given IV only if patients cannot be treated orally. It is distributed widely in body fluids and penetrates into CSF, resulting in high concentrations.

Metronidazole is metabolized presumably in the liver and excreted mainly in urine, but elimination is not decreased in patients with renal insufficiency.

Indications

Metronidazole is active against

- All obligate anaerobic bacteria (it is inactive against facultative anaerobic and aerobic bacteria)
- Certain protozoan parasites (eg, *Trichomonas vaginalis*, *Entamoeba histolytica*, *Giardia intestinalis [lamblia]*)

Metronidazole is used primarily for infections caused by obligate anaerobes, often with other antimicrobials. Metronidazole is the drug of choice for bacterial vaginosis. The drug has other clinical uses (see Table 184–14).

Contraindications

Metronidazole is contraindicated in patients who have had an allergic reaction to it.

Table 184–14. SOME CLINICAL USES OF METRONIDAZOLE

INDICATION	COMMENTS
Infections due to obligate anaerobes (eg, intra-abdominal, pelvic, soft-tissue, periodontal, and odontogenic infections; lung abscess)	Often used with other antimicrobials
Bacterial vaginosis	Drug of choice
Crohn disease	—
CNS infections (meningitis, brain abscess)	—
Endocarditis	—
Septicemia	—
Prophylaxis before intestinal surgery	—
Clostridium difficile–induced diarrhea (pseudomembranous colitis)	Oral use preferable
Peptic ulcers due to *Helicobacter pylori*	For treatment and prevention of relapses Used with other drugs
Acne rosacea	Topical or oral use

Use During Pregnancy and Breastfeeding

Metronidazole is in pregnancy category B (animal studies show no risk and human evidence is incomplete, or animal studies show risk but human studies do not). Nonetheless, metronidazole should be avoided during the 1st trimester because mutagenicity is a concern.

Metronidazole enters breast milk; use during breastfeeding is not recommended.

Adverse Effects

Adverse effects include

- GI disturbances
- CNS effects and peripheral neuropathy
- Disulfiram-like reaction

Nausea, vomiting, headache, seizures, syncope, other CNS effects, and peripheral neuropathy can occur; rash, fever, and reversible neutropenia have been reported. Metronidazole can cause a metallic taste and dark urine. A disulfiram-like reaction may occur if alcohol is ingested within 7 days of use.

Dosing Considerations

Metronidazole doses are not decreased in patients with renal failure but are usually decreased 50% in patients with significant liver disease.

Metronidazole inhibits metabolism of warfarin and may increase its anticoagulant effect.

MUPIROCIN

Mupirocin inhibits bacterial RNA and protein synthesis. It is available only as a 2% topical preparation, which is bactericidal against staphylococci and β-hemolytic streptococci. Systemic absorption of topical mupirocin is negligible.

Mupirocin is used for

- Impetigo (see p. 998)
- Minor superficial secondarily infected skin lesions
- Eradication of *Staphylococcus aureus* nasal carriage, although relapse rates may be high

Chronic therapy leads to mupirocin-resistant staphylococci.

Mupirocin is nontoxic but, when applied to denuded skin or mucous membranes, may cause itching and burning.

NITROFURANTOIN

Nitrofurantoin is bactericidal; the exact mechanism is unknown.

Nitrofurantoin is available only for oral use.

Pharmacology

After a single dose, serum drug levels are very low, but urine drug levels are therapeutic.

Indications

Nitrofurantoin is active against common uropathogens, such as

- *Escherichia coli*
- *Staphylococcus saprophyticus*
- *Enterococcus faecalis*

E. faecium, including vancomycin-resistant strains, and *Klebsiella* and *Enterobacter* sp are less susceptible. Most strains of *Proteus*, *Providencia*, *Morganella*, *Serratia*, *Acinetobacter*, and *Pseudomonas* spp are resistant. There is no cross-resistance with other antibiotic classes.

Nitrofurantoin is used only for

- Treatment or prophylaxis of uncomplicated UTI

In women with recurrent UTIs, it may decrease the number of episodes.

Contraindications

Contraindications to nitrofurantoin use include

- Previous allergic reaction to it
- Renal insufficiency (creatinine clearance < 60 L/min)
- Age < 1 mo

Use During Pregnancy and Breastfeeding

Nitrofurantoin is in pregnancy category B (animal studies show no risk and human evidence is incomplete, or animal studies show risk but human studies do not). Nonetheless, nitrofurantoin is contraindicated at term and during labor or delivery because it interferes with immature enzyme systems in RBCs of neonates, damaging the cells and resulting in hemolytic anemia.

Nitrofurantoin enters breast milk and is contraindicated during the first month of breastfeeding.

Adverse Effects

Adverse effects include

- GI disturbances
- Pulmonary toxicity
- Peripheral neuropathy
- Hemolytic anemia
- Hepatic toxicity

Common adverse effects are nausea and vomiting, which are less likely with the macrocrystalline form. Fever, rash, acute hypersensitivity pneumonitis (accompanied by fever and eosinophilia), and chronic progressive pulmonary interstitial fibrosis may occur. Paresthesias may result and may be followed by a severe ascending motor and sensory polyneuropathy if the drug is continued, especially in patients with renal failure. Leukopenia and hepatic toxicity (acute cholestatic or chronic active hepatitis) have been reported, and hemolytic anemia can occur in patients with G6PD deficiency and in infants < 1 mo. Chronic pulmonary and hepatic reactions occur when the drug is used for > 6 mo.

POLYPEPTIDE ANTIBIOTICS: BACITRACIN, COLISTIN, POLYMYXIN B

Polypeptide antibiotics disrupt bacterial cell walls (see Table 184–15).

Bacitracin is a polypeptide antibiotic that inhibits cell wall synthesis and is active against gram-positive bacteria.

Colistin (polymyxin E) and **polymyxin B** are cationic polypeptide antibiotics that disrupt the outer bacterial cell

Table 184–15. POLYPEPTIDES

Drug
Bacitracin
Colistin
Polymyxin B

membrane by binding to the anionic outer membrane and thereby neutralizing the bacteria's toxicity and causing bacterial cell death.

Colistin methane sulfonate (colistimethate sodium [CMS]) is a parenteral preparation of a prodrug that is transformed in blood and urine to colistin. CMS is less toxic than colistin.

Polypeptides other than colistin are usually used topically; systemic absorption is negligible.

Indications

Polypeptides are used for several types of infections (see Table 184–16).

Bacitracin is used mainly as a topical treatment for

- Superficial skin infections caused by *Staphylococcus aureus*

Polymyxin B and colistin have rapid concentration-dependent bactericidal activity (see p. 1495) against

- Most facultative and aerobic gram-negative bacilli, including *Pseudomonas aeruginosa* and *Acinetobacter* sp

These drugs are not active against *Proteus*, *Providencia*, *Burkholderia, and Serratia* spp and some obligate anaerobes, including *Bacteroides fragilis* and gram-positive bacteria. Development of resistance is uncommon.

The increasing prevalence of extensively drug-resistant gram-negative bacilli in hospitals has led to a resurgence of the use of IV colistin for serious systemic infections (eg, ventilator-associated pneumonia, bacteremia). However, IV polymyxin B and colistin should typically be used only when there are no less toxic options.

Table 184–16. SOME CLINICAL USES OF POLYPEPTIDES

PREPARATION	USES	COMMENTS
Combination treatments		
Ointment containing bacitracin plus neomycin, polymyxin B, or both	Wound infection	No confirmation of clinical efficacy
Spray containing neomycin, bacitracin, and polymyxin	Prevention of postoperative wound infections	Appears to help
Polymyxin B ophthalmic ointments and solutions with other antimicrobials (eg, bacitracin, neomycin, trimethoprim/sulfamethoxazole) and corticosteroids	Ophthalmic use	Significantly improved rates of early clinical remission (although acute bacterial conjunctivitis is frequently self-limited)
Otic suspension with polymyxin B, neomycin, and hydrocortisone or with colistin, neomycin, and hydrocortisone	Otitis externa (commonly due to *Pseudomonas aeruginosa*)	Clinically effective, but may be no more effective than 2% acetic acid with hydrocortisone In patients with a tympanostomy tube or known perforation of the tympanic membrane, must use a nonototoxic topical preparation (no aminoglycoside or alcohol)
Bacitracin		
Topical	Eradication of *Staphylococcus aureus* nasal carriage Impetigo	Less effective than other treatments
Oral	*Clostridium difficile*–induced diarrhea (pseudomembranous colitis)	Less effective and less palatable than oral vancomycin or metronidazole
Colistin		
Aerosolized colistin methane sulfonate (colistimethate sodium [CMS])	Cystic fibrosis Occasionally hospital-acquired pneumonia caused by multidrug-resistant gram-negative bacilli	Associated with fewer adverse effects (eg, chest tightness, throat irritation, cough) than colistin sulfate
Aerosolized colistin sulfate	Same as for aerosolized colistin methane sulfonate	May be beneficial for patients with cystic fibrosis or nosocomial pneumonia (ventilator-associated or not) due to multidrug-resistant gram-negative bacteria
Parenteral CMS	Severe infections due to multidrug-resistant gram-negative bacilli such as *P. aeruginosa* or *Acinetobacter* sp	Reduced dose in patients with renal insufficiency
Polymyxin B		
Solutions	GU irrigation	—

Contraindications

All polypeptides are contraindicated in patients who have had an allergic reaction to them.

CMS and polymyxin B should not be given simultaneously with drugs that block neuromuscular transmission or are nephrotoxic (eg, aminoglycosides, curare-like drugs).

Use During Pregnancy and Breastfeeding

Bacitracin may pose minimal risk during pregnancy and breastfeeding because systemic absorption is minimal; however, safety has not been established.

Polymyxin B is in pregnancy category B (animal studies show no risk and human evidence is incomplete, or animal studies show risk but human studies do not).

Colistin is in pregnancy category C (animal studies show some risk, evidence in human studies is inadequate, but clinical benefit sometimes outweighs risk); this drug crosses the placenta. Whether use during breastfeeding is safe is unknown.

Adverse Effects

Adverse effects include

- Nephrotoxicity
- Central and peripheral neurotoxicity

Polymyxins are nephrotoxic. CMS and polymyxin B may cause circumoral and extremity paresthesias, vertigo, slurred speech, and muscle weakness and respiratory difficulty due to neuromuscular blockade, especially in patients with renal insufficiency.

Dosing Considerations

Because colistin was released before the advent of modern pharmacokinetic/pharmacodynamic analysis, appropriate dosing has not been studied as rigorously as for many modern antibiotics. In addition, manufacturers do not use a uniform method of describing drug amount; some use international units, and others use mg of colistin base activity or mg of actual colistimethate.

Whatever units are used,[1] many experts believe that the manufacturer-recommended dose of 2.5 to 5 mg/kg of colistin base activity per day divided into 2 to 4 doses is too low and recommend higher dosing regimens, including the use of a loading dose. However, nephrotoxicity is dose-dependent and becomes a greater concern with higher doses. Dosing should be discussed with an expert.

1. Garonzik SM, et al: Population pharmacokinetics of colistin methanesulfonate and formed colistin in critically ill patients from a multicenter study provide dosing suggestions for various categories of patients. *Antimicrob Agents Chemother* 55(7):3284–3294, 2011.

RIFAMYCINS

The rifamycins are bactericidal and inhibit bacterial DNA-dependent RNA polymerase, suppressing RNA synthesis (see Table 184–17).

Table 184–17. RIFAMYCINS

Rifabutin
Rifaximin
Rifampin
Rifapentine

Rifampin, Rifabutin, and Rifapentine

Rifampin, rifabutin, and rifapentine have similar pharmacology, antimicrobial spectra, and adverse effects.

Pharmacology

Oral absorption is good, producing wide distribution in body tissues and fluids, including CSF.

Rifampin is concentrated in polymorphonuclear granulocytes and macrophages, facilitating clearance of bacteria from abscesses. It is metabolized in the liver and eliminated in bile and, to a much lesser extent, in urine.

Indications

Rifampin is active against

- Most gram-positive and some gram-negative bacteria
- *Mycobacterium* sp

Resistance develops rapidly, so rifampin is rarely used alone. Rifampin is used with other antibiotics for

- TB (see p. 1654)
- Atypical mycobacterial infection (rifampin is active against many nontuberculous mycobacteria, but rapidly growing mycobacteria, such as *Mycobacterium fortuitum*, *M. chelonae*, or *M. abscessus*, are naturally resistant)
- Leprosy (with dapsone with or without clofazimine)
- Staphylococcal infections, including osteomyelitis, prosthetic valve endocarditis, and infections involving foreign bodies such as a prosthetic joint (with other antistaphylococcal antibiotics)
- *Legionella* infections (older data suggest better outcomes for rifampin when used with erythromycin; use of rifampin with azithromycin or a fluoroquinolone offers no advantage)
- Pneumococcal meningitis when organisms are susceptible to rifampin (with vancomycin with or without ceftriaxone or cefotaxime for ceftriaxone- or cefotaxime-resistant organisms [MIC > 4 μg/mL]) or when expected clinical or microbiologic response is delayed

Rifampin can be used alone for prophylaxis of close contacts of patients with meningococcal or *Haemophilus influenzae* type b meningitis.

Rifabutin and rifampin are equally efficacious in regimens for TB in HIV-positive and HIV-negative patients.

Rifabutin is more active than rifampin against *M. avium* complex and is used preferentially in multidrug regimens for these infections, but otherwise, rifampin is preferred.

Rifapentine is used to treat pulmonary TB and latent TB.

Contraindications

Rifampin and rifabutin are contraindicated in patients who have had an allergic reaction to them.

Use During Pregnancy and Breastfeeding

Rifabutin is in pregnancy category B (animal studies show no risk and human evidence is incomplete, or animal studies show risk but human studies do not). Safety during breastfeeding is unknown.

Rifampin and rifapentine are in pregnancy category C (animal studies show some risk [in this case, teratogenicity], evidence in human studies is inadequate, but clinical benefit sometimes outweighs risk). The drug crosses the placenta. Still, if risk of maternal TB is moderate or high, treatment is thought to be less harmful for the fetus than untreated maternal TB and is thus recommended.

Because of potential tumorigenicity shown in animal studies, the manufacturer does not recommend use of rifampin during breastfeeding. However, the Centers for Disease Control and Prevention (CDC) does not consider rifampin a contraindication to breastfeeding; a decision to stop breastfeeding or to stop the drug should be made depending on the importance of the drug to the mother.

Adverse Effects

Adverse effects include

- Hepatitis (most serious)
- GI disturbances
- CNS effects
- Myelosuppression

Hepatitis occurs much more often when isoniazid or pyrazinamide is used concurrently with rifampin. During the first week of therapy, rifampin may cause a transient rise in unconjugated serum bilirubin, which results from competition between rifampin and bilirubin for excretion and which is not in itself an indication for interrupting treatment.

CNS effects may include headache, drowsiness, ataxia, and confusion. Rash, fever, leukopenia, hemolytic anemia, thrombocytopenia, interstitial nephritis, acute tubular necrosis, renal insufficiency, and interstitial nephritis are generally considered to be hypersensitivity reactions and occur when therapy is intermittent or when treatment is resumed after interruption of a daily dosage regimen; they are reversed when rifampin is stopped.

Less serious adverse effects are common; they include heartburn, nausea, vomiting, and diarrhea. Rifampin colors urine, saliva, sweat, sputum, and tears red-orange.

Dosing Considerations

If patients have a liver disorder, liver function tests should be done before rifampin therapy is started and every 2 to 4 wk during therapy, or an alternate drug should be used. Dose adjustments are unnecessary for renal insufficiency.

Rifampin interacts with many drugs because it is a potent inducer of hepatic cytochrome P-450 (CYP450) microsomal enzymes. Rifampin accelerates elimination and thereby may decrease the effectiveness of the following drugs: ACE inhibitors, atovaquone, barbiturates, β-blockers, Ca channel blockers, chloramphenicol, clarithromycin, oral and systemic hormone contraceptives, corticosteroids, cyclosporine, dapsone, digoxin, doxycycline, fluconazole, haloperidol, itraconazole, ketoconazole, the nonnucleoside reverse transcriptase inhibitors delavirdine and nevirapine, opioid analgesics, phenytoin, protease inhibitors, quinidine, sulfonylureas, tacrolimus, theophylline, thyroxine, tocainide, tricyclic antidepressants, voriconazole, warfarin, and zidovudine. To maintain optimum therapeutic effect of these drugs, clinicians may have to adjust the dosage when rifampin is started or stopped.

Conversely, protease inhibitors, as well as other drugs (eg, azoles, the macrolide clarithromycin, nonnucleoside reverse transcriptase inhibitors) inhibit CYP450 enzymes and increase levels of rifamycins and thus potentially increase the frequency of toxic reactions. For example, uveitis occurs more commonly when rifabutin is used with clarithromycin or azoles.

Rifaximin

Rifaximin is a derivative of rifamycin that is poorly absorbed after oral administration; 97% is recovered primarily unchanged in feces.

Rifaximin can be used for empiric treatment of traveler's diarrhea, which is caused primarily by enterotoxigenic and enteroaggregative *Escherichia coli*. Rifaximin is not known to be effective for diarrhea due to enteric pathogens other than *E. coli*. Because rifaximin is not systemically absorbed, it should not be used to treat infectious diarrhea caused by invasive enteric bacterial pathogens (eg, salmonellae, *Campylobacter* sp).

The dose is 200 mg po q 8 h for 3 days in adults and children > 12 yr.

Adverse effects include nausea, vomiting, abdominal pain, and flatulence.

SULFONAMIDES

Sulfonamides (see Table 184–18) are synthetic bacteriostatic antibiotics that competitively inhibit conversion of *p*-aminobenzoic acid to dihydropteroate, which bacteria need for folate synthesis and ultimately purine and DNA synthesis. Humans do not synthesize folate but acquire it in their diet, so their DNA synthesis is less affected.

Two sulfonamides, sulfisoxazole and sulfamethizole, are available as single drugs for oral use. Sulfamethoxazole is coformulated with trimethoprim (as TMP/SMX—see Trimethoprim and Sulfamethoxazole on p. 1525).

Sulfonamides available for topical use include silver sulfadiazine, vaginal cream and suppositories containing sulfanilamide, and ophthalmic sulfacetamide.

Pharmacology

Most sulfonamides are readily absorbed orally and, when applied to burns, topically. Sulfonamides are distributed throughout the body. They are metabolized mainly by the liver and excreted by the kidneys. Sulfonamides compete for bilirubin-binding sites on albumin.

Indications

Sulfonamides are active against

- A broad spectrum of gram-positive and many gram-negative bacteria
- *Plasmodium* and *Toxoplasma* spp

However, resistance is widespread, and resistance to one sulfonamide indicates resistance to all.

Sulfasalazine can be used orally for inflammatory bowel disease.

Sulfonamides are most commonly used with other drugs (eg, for nocardiosis, UTI, and chloroquine-resistant falciparum malaria).

Topical sulfonamides can be used to treat the following:

- Burns: Silver sulfadiazine and mafenide acetate
- Vaginitis: Vaginal cream and suppositories with sulfanilamide
- Superficial ocular infections: Ophthalmic sulfacetamide

Table 184–18. SULFONAMIDES

Sulfacetamide
Sulfadiazine
Sulfadoxine
Sulfamethizole
Sulfamethoxazole
Sulfanilamide
Sulfasalazine
Sulfisoxazole

Contraindications

Sulfonamides are contraindicated in patients who have had an allergic reaction to them or who have porphyria.

Sulfonamides do not eradicate group A streptococci in patients with pharyngitis and should not be used to treat group A streptococcal pharyngitis.

Use During Pregnancy and Breastfeeding

Most sulfonamides are in pregnancy category B (animal studies show no risk and human evidence is incomplete, or animal studies show risk but human studies do not). However, use near term and in breastfeeding mothers is contraindicated, as is use in patients < 2 mo (except as adjunctive therapy with pyrimethamine to treat congenital toxoplasmosis). If used during pregnancy or in neonates, these drugs increase blood levels of unconjugated bilirubin and increase risk of kernicterus in the fetus or neonate.

Sulfonamides enter breast milk.

Adverse Effects

Adverse effects can result from oral and sometimes topical sulfonamides; effects include

- Hypersensitivity reactions, such as rashes, Stevens-Johnson syndrome (see p. 1050), vasculitis, serum sickness, drug fever, anaphylaxis, and angioedema
- Crystalluria, oliguria, and anuria
- Hematologic reactions, such as agranulocytosis, thrombocytopenia, and, in patients with G6PD deficiency, hemolytic anemia
- Kernicterus in neonates
- Photosensitivity
- Neurologic effects, such as insomnia, and headache

Hypothyroidism, hepatitis, and activation of quiescent SLE may occur in patients taking sulfonamides. These drugs can exacerbate porphyrias.

Incidence of adverse effects is different for the various sulfonamides, but cross-sensitivity is common.

Sulfasalazine can reduce intestinal absorption of folate (folic acid). Thus, use of this drug may trigger folate deficiency in patients with inflammatory bowel disease, which also reduces absorption, especially if dietary intake is also inadequate.

Mafenide may cause metabolic acidosis by inhibiting carbonic anhydrase.

Dosing Considerations

To avoid crystalluria, clinicians should hydrate patients well (eg, to produce a urinary output of 1200 to 1500 mL/day). Sulfonamides can be used in patients with renal insufficiency, but peak plasma levels should be measured and sulfamethoxazole levels should not exceed 120 μg/mL.

Sulfonamides can potentiate sulfonylureas (with consequent hypoglycemia), phenytoin (with increased adverse effects), and coumarin anticoagulants.

TRIMETHOPRIM AND SULFAMETHOXAZOLE

Trimethoprim is available as a single drug or in combination with sulfamethoxazole (a sulfonamide antibiotic—see Sulfonamides on p. 1524). The drugs act synergistically to block sequential steps in bacterial folate metabolism:

- Trimethoprim prevents reduction of dihydrofolate to tetrahydrofolate.
- Sulfamethoxazole inhibits conversion of *p*-aminobenzoic acid to dihydropteroate.

This synergy results in maximal antibacterial activity, which is often bactericidal.

Trimethoprim/sulfamethoxazole (TMP/SMX) is available as a fixed combination consisting of a 1:5 ratio (80 mg TMP plus 400 mg SMX or a double-strength tablet of 160 mg TMP plus 800 mg SMX).

Pharmacology

Both drugs are well absorbed orally and are excreted in the urine. They have a serum half-life of about 11 h in plasma and penetrate well into tissues and body fluids, including CSF. TMP is concentrated in prostatic tissue.

Indications

TMP and TMP/SMX (see Table 184–19) are active against

- A broad spectrum of gram-positive bacteria (including some methicillin-resistant *Staphylococcus aureus*)
- A broad spectrum of gram-negative bacteria
- Protozoans *Cystoisospora* and *Cyclospora* spp
- The fungus *Pneumocystis jirovecii*

The **combination** is inactive against

- Anaerobes
- *Treponema pallidum*
- *Mycobacterium tuberculosis*
- *Mycoplasma* sp
- *Pseudomonas aeruginosa*

Enterococci, many Enterobacteriaceae, and *Streptococcus pneumoniae* strains are resistant. TMP/SMX is not clinically effective for group A streptococcal pharyngitis.

TMP alone is especially useful for

- Chronic bacterial prostatitis
- Prophylaxis and treatment of UTI in patients allergic to sulfonamides

Contraindications

TMP/SMX is contraindicated in patients who have had an allergic reaction to either drug.

Relative contraindications include folate deficiency, liver dysfunction, and renal insufficiency.

Use During Pregnancy and Breastfeeding

TMP/SMX is in pregnancy category C (animal studies show some risk, evidence in human studies is inadequate, but clinical benefit sometimes outweighs risk). However, use near term is contraindicated; if used during pregnancy or in neonates, TMP/SMX increases blood levels of unconjugated bilirubin and increases risk of kernicterus in the fetus or neonate.

Sulfonamides enter breast milk and use during breastfeeding is usually discouraged.

Adverse Effects

Adverse effects include

- Those associated with sulfonamide (see p. 1524)
- Folate deficiency
- Hyperkalemia (TMP can decrease renal tubular K excretion, leading to hyperkalemia)
- Renal insufficiency

Renal failure in patients with underlying renal insufficiency is probably secondary to interstitial nephritis or tubular necrosis. Also, TMP competitively inhibits renal tubular creatinine secretion and may cause an artificial increase in serum

Table 184–19. SOME INDICATIONS FOR TMP/SMX

INDICATION	COMMENTS
Chronic bacterial prostatitis	One of the few effective drugs, but cures < 1/2 of patients, even after 12 wk
Uncomplicated cystitis in women	As effective as fluoroquinolones for empiric short-course (3-day) therapy if the rate of TMP/SMX resistance is < 15%
Prophylaxis for recurrent UTI in women and children	Use of 1/2 to 1 double-strength tablet every night or every other night or, for women with previous recurrences after coitus, after coitus
Treatment of *Pneumocystis jirovecii* pneumonia and prophylaxis of this infection in patients with AIDS or cancer	Drug of choice
Intestinal infections due to various bacteria (eg, *Shigella* sp, *Vibrio* sp, *Escherichia coli*) and the protozoans *Cystoisospora* and *Cyclospora* spp	Usefulness limited by increasing prevalence of resistance
Nocardia and *Listeria monocytogenes* infections	—
Acute exacerbations of chronic bronchitis	—
Methicillin-resistant *Staphylococcus aureus* infections	Used if patients cannot tolerate vancomycin

TMP/SMX =trimethoprim/sulfamethoxazole.

creatinine, although GFR remains unchanged. Increases in serum creatinine are more likely in patients with preexisting renal insufficiency and especially in those with diabetes mellitus.

Most adverse effects are the same as for sulfonamides. TMP has adverse effects identical to those of SMX, but they are less common. Nausea, vomiting, and rash occur most often. AIDS patients have a high incidence of adverse effects, especially fever, rash, and neutropenia.

Folate deficiency (resulting in macrocytic anemia) can also occur. Use of folinic acid can prevent or treat macrocytic anemia, leukopenia, and thrombocytopenia, which sometimes occur with prolonged TMP/SMX use.

Rarely, severe hepatic necrosis occurs. The drug may also cause a syndrome resembling aseptic meningitis.

Dosing Considerations

TMP/SMX may increase warfarin activity and levels of phenytoin, methotrexate, and rifampin. SMX can increase the hypoglycemic effects of sulfonylureas.

TELAVANCIN

Telavancin is a semisynthetic lipoglycopeptide derivative of vancomycin that has bactericidal activity exclusively against gram-positive bacteria. Telavancin inhibits cell wall synthesis and disrupts cell membrane integrity.

Pharmacology

Parenteral telavancin penetrates well into pulmonary epithelial lining fluid and skin blisters.

Telavancin has a half-life of 7 to 9 h and a postantibiotic effect of about 4 h.

Telavancin is excreted by the kidneys so the dose must be adjusted in patients with renal insufficiency.

Indications

Telavancin is active against gram-positive bacteria such as

- Streptococci
- *Enterococcus faecalis*
- *E. faecium*
- *Staphylococcus aureus*, including *S. aureus* that is methicillin-resistant or vancomycin–intermediate-resistant

Telavancin is used for complicated skin and skin structure infections as well as for hospital-acquired and ventilator-acquired bacterial pneumonia caused by sensitive isolates of *S. aureus*. Outcome may be worse for patients with baseline moderate to severe renal insufficiency.

Contraindications

Telavancin is contraindicated in patients who are allergic to it. It should be used with care in patients who are allergic to vancomycin because cross-reactivity is possible.

Use During Pregnancy and Breastfeeding

Telavancin has had adverse effects on fetal development in animals, and there are no safety data in pregnant women to generate category C labeling.

There are no data regarding excretion in breast milk.

Adverse Effects

Common adverse effects include

- Nausea and vomiting
- Taste disturbance
- Foamy urine

Telavancin also interferes with certain coagulation and urine protein assays.

Significant adverse effects include

- A histamine-mediated pruritus and flushing of the face, neck, and shoulders, similar to the red-person syndrome that can occur with vancomycin
- Nephrotoxicity, which may occur slightly more often with telavancin than with vancomycin
- QTc prolongation

Pruritus and flushing can be prevented by infusing the drug over ≥ 60 min.

QTc prolongation occurred in healthy subjects in the clinical trials of telavancin; thus, telavancin should be used with caution or not be used in patients taking drugs that prolong the QT interval. Telavancin should not be used in patients with congenital long QT syndrome, known QTc prolongation, uncompensated heart failure, or severe left ventricular hypertrophy (patients with these disorders were excluded from the clinical trials).

Dosing Considerations

Telavancin dosing is based on creatinine clearance:

- Creatinine clearance > 50 mL/min: 10 mg/kg IV q 24 h
- Creatinine clearance 30 to 50 mL/min: 7.5 mg/kg q 24 h
- Creatinine clearance 10 to < 30 mL/min: 10 mg/kg q 48 h
- Creatinine clearance < 10 mL/min: Data limited, no recommendations available

TETRACYCLINES

Tetracyclines (see Table 184–20) are bacteriostatic antibiotics that bind to the 30S subunit of the ribosome, thus inhibiting bacterial protein synthesis.

Pharmacology

About 60 to 80% of tetracycline and ≥ 90% of doxycycline and minocycline are absorbed after oral use. However, absorption is decreased by metallic cations (eg, aluminum, Ca, Mg, iron); thus, tetracyclines cannot be taken with preparations containing these substances (eg, antacids, many vitamin and mineral supplements). Food decreases absorption of tetracycline but not of doxycycline or minocycline.

Tetracyclines penetrate into most body tissues and fluids. All are concentrated in unobstructed bile. However, CSF levels are not reliably therapeutic. Minocycline is the only tetracycline that reaches high concentrations in tears and saliva.

Tetracycline and minocycline are excreted primarily in urine. Doxycycline is excreted primarily in the intestinal tract.

Indications

Tetracyclines are active against infections caused by the following:

- Rickettsiae
- Spirochetes (eg, *Treponema pallidum*, *Borrelia burgdorferi*)
- *Helicobacter pylori*
- *Vibrio* sp
- *Yersinia pestis*
- *Francisella tularensis*
- *Brucella* sp
- *Bacillus anthracis*
- *Plasmodium vivax*
- *Plasmodium falciparum*
- *Mycoplasma* sp
- *Chlamydia* and *Chlamydophila* sp
- Some methicillin-resistant *Staphylococcus aureus*

About 5 to 10% of pneumococcal strains and many group A β-hemolytic streptococci, many gram-negative bacillary uropathogens, and penicillinase-producing gonococci are resistant.

Table 184–20. TETRACYCLINES

Doxycycline
Minocycline
Tetracycline

Tetracyclines are interchangeable for most indications, although minocycline has been most studied for MRSA infections.

Doxycycline is usually preferred for all of the following because it is better tolerated and can be given twice/day:

- Infections caused by rickettsiae or *Anaplasma, Chlamydia, Chlamydophila, Ehrlichia, Mycoplasma*, or *Vibrio* spp
- Acute exacerbations of chronic bronchitis
- Lyme disease
- Brucellosis
- Anthrax
- Plague
- Tularemia
- Granuloma inguinale
- Syphilis
- Prophylaxis of malaria caused by chloroquine-resistant *P. falciparum*

Because of its high concentration in tears and saliva, minocycline is the only tetracycline that can eradicate meningococci in carriers and is an alternate to rifampin for this indication.

Contraindications

Tetracyclines are contraindicated in patients who have had an allergic reaction to them, patients with renal insufficiency (except for doxycycline, which has no dosage adjustment for renal insufficiency), and children < 8 yr (except sometimes for inhalational anthrax or other severe illnesses when the benefit outweighs the potential risk of tooth staining).

Use During Pregnancy and Breastfeeding

Tetracyclines are in pregnancy category D (there is evidence of human risk, but clinical benefits may outweigh risk). Tetracyclines cross the placenta, enter fetal circulation, accumulate in fetal bones, and, if used during the 2nd or 3rd trimester, may cause permanent discoloration of teeth.

Hepatotoxicity may occur in pregnant women, particularly after IV administration and in those with azotemia or pyelonephritis. Taking high doses during pregnancy can lead to fatty degeneration of the liver, which may be fatal.

Tetracyclines enter breast milk, but usually in small amounts (particularly tetracycline). Use during breastfeeding is usually discouraged.

Adverse Effects

Adverse effects include

- GI disturbances
- *Clostridium difficile*–induced diarrhea (pseudomembranous colitis—see p. 1466)
- Candidiasis
- Photosensitivity
- Bone and dental effects in children
- Fatty liver
- Vestibular dysfunction (with minocycline)

All oral tetracyclines cause nausea, vomiting, and diarrhea and can cause *C. difficile*–induced diarrhea (pseudomembranous colitis) and candidal superinfections. If not swallowed with water, tetracyclines can cause esophageal erosions. Photosensitivity due to tetracyclines may manifest as an exaggerated sunburn reaction. Bone and dental effects include staining of teeth, hypoplasia of dental enamel, and abnormal bone growth in children < 8 yr and in fetuses. In infants, tetracyclines may cause idiopathic intracranial hypertension and bulging fontanelles.

Excessive blood levels due to use of high doses or renal insufficiency may lead to fatal acute fatty degeneration of the liver, especially during pregnancy.

Minocycline commonly causes vestibular dysfunction, limiting its use. Use of minocycline has been associated with development of autoimmune disorders such as SLE and polyarteritis nodosa, which may be reversible. Minocycline may also cause drug reaction with eosinophilia and systemic symptoms (DRESS), which is characterized by fever, rash, lymphadenopathy, hepatitis, atypical lymphocytosis, eosinophilia, and thrombocytopenia.

Tetracycline can exacerbate azotemia in patients with renal insufficiency.

Expired tetracycline pills can degenerate and, if ingested, cause Fanconi syndrome. Patients should be instructed to discard the drugs when they expire.

Dosing Considerations

Doxycycline, excreted primarily in the intestinal tract, requires no dose reduction in renal insufficiency.

Tetracyclines may decrease the effectiveness of oral contraceptives and potentiate the effects of oral anticoagulants.

TIGECYCLINE

Tigecycline, a derivative of the tetracycline minocycline, is the first available glycylcycline. Tigecycline inhibits protein synthesis by binding to the 30S ribosomal subunit. It is bacteriostatic.

Pharmacology

Tigecycline is given IV. Tigecycline has a large volume of distribution (> 12 L/kg), penetrating well into bone, lung, liver, and kidney tissues. However, because of its extensive distribution into tissue, high blood levels are not maintained, so tigecycline is probably not a good choice for patients with bacteremia.

A half-life of 36 h facilitates once/day dosing.

Most of the drug is excreted in bile and feces.

Indications

Tigecycline is effective against many resistant bacteria, including those with resistance to tetracyclines. Tigecycline is active against

- Many gram-positive bacteria, including methicillin-susceptible and methicillin-resistant *Staphylococcus aureus*, *Streptococcus pneumoniae* with reduced penicillin sensitivity, vancomycin-sensitive *Enterococcus faecalis*, vancomycin-resistant *E. faecium*, and *Listeria* sp
- Many gram-negative bacteria, such as multidrug-resistant *Acinetobacter baumannii*, *Stenotrophomonas maltophilia*, *Haemophilus influenzae*, and most Enterobacteriaceae (including some strains that produce ESBLs and other strains that were carbapenem-resistant based on production of a carbapenemase or metallo-β-lactamase)
- Many atypical respiratory pathogens (chlamydiae, *Mycoplasma* sp), *Mycobacterium abscessus*, *M. fortuitum*, and anaerobes, including *Bacteroides fragilis*, *Clostridium perfringens*, and *C. difficile*

It is not effective against *Pseudomonas aeruginosa*, *Providencia* sp, *Morganella morganii*, or *Proteus* sp.

Tigecycline is indicated for

- Complicated skin and soft-tissue infections
- Complicated intra-abdominal infections
- Community-acquired pneumonia

However, a recent meta-analysis showed that patients treated with tigecycline (particularly those treated for ventilator-associated pneumonia) had a higher mortality than those given other antibiotics, resulting in a black box warning from the FDA. In general, tigecycline should be reserved for infections with multidrug-resistant (MDR) organisms when other treatment options are more toxic or less effective. Because of its parenteral activity against *C. difficile,* tigecycline may be a useful antibiotic when a patient requires concurrent treatment of an MDR infection and a *C. difficile* infection.

Contraindications

Tigecycline is contraindicated in patients who have had an allergic reaction to it and in children < 8 yr.

Use During Pregnancy and Breastfeeding

Tigecycline is in pregnancy category D (there is evidence of human risk, but clinical benefits may outweigh risk); it, like tetracyclines, can affect fetal bones and teeth.

Whether tigecycline enters breast milk and is safe to use during breastfeeding is unknown; however, it has limited oral bioavailability.

Adverse Effects

Adverse effects include

- Nausea, vomiting, and diarrhea
- Photosensitivity
- Hepatotoxicity

Nausea and vomiting are common. Increases in serum amylase, total bilirubin concentration, PT, and transaminases can occur in patients treated with tigecycline. Isolated cases of significant hepatic dysfunction and hepatic failure have been reported in patients being treated with tigecycline. Many of tigecycline's adverse effects are similar to those of tetracyclines (eg, photosensitivity).

Dosing Considerations

Dose is adjusted in patients with hepatic dysfunction but not in those with renal dysfunction.

Serum levels of warfarin may increase, but INR does not appear to increase.

VANCOMYCIN

Vancomycin is a time-dependent bactericidal antibiotic that inhibits cell wall synthesis.

Pharmacology

Vancomycin is not appreciably absorbed from a normal GI tract after oral administration. Given parenterally, it penetrates into bile and pleural, pericardial, synovial, and ascitic fluids. However, penetration into even inflamed CSF is low and erratic.

Vancomycin is excreted unchanged by glomerular filtration.

Indications

Vancomycin is active against

- Most gram-positive cocci and bacilli, including almost all *Staphylococcus aureus* and coagulase-negative staphylococcal strains that are resistant to penicillins and cephalosporins
- Many strains of enterococci (via a bacteriostatic mechanism)

However, many strains of enterococci and some strains of *S. aureus* are resistant.

Vancomycin is a drug of choice for serious infection and endocarditis caused by the following (except for vancomycin-resistant strains):

- MRSA
- Methicillin-resistant coagulase-negative staphylococci
- Certain β-lactam– and multidrug-resistant *Streptococcus pneumoniae*
- β-Hemolytic streptococci (when β-lactams cannot be used because of drug allergy or resistance)
- *Corynebacterium* group JK
- Viridans streptococci (when β-lactams cannot be used because of drug allergy or resistance)
- Enterococci (when β-lactams cannot be used because of drug allergy or resistance)

However, vancomycin is less effective than antistaphylococcal β-lactams for *S. aureus* endocarditis. Vancomycin is used with other antibiotics when treating methicillin-resistant coagulase-negative staphylococcal prosthetic valve endocarditis or enterococcal endocarditis. Vancomycin has also been used as an alternative drug for pneumococcal meningitis caused by strains with reduced penicillin sensitivity; however, the erratic penetration of vancomycin into CSF (especially during concomitant use of dexamethasone) and reports of clinical failures make it less than optimal when used alone to treat pneumococcal meningitis.

Oral vancomycin is used to treat *Clostridium difficile*–induced diarrhea (pseudomembranous colitis—see p. 1466). It is preferred over metronidazole for patients who have severe *C. difficile* infection and is preferred for patients who do not respond to metronidazole.

Contraindications

Vancomycin is contraindicated in patients who have had an allergic reaction to it.

Use During Pregnancy and Breastfeeding

Vancomycin has not had adverse effects in animals, and evidence in human studies is inadequate. Oral vancomycin tablets are in pregnancy category B (animal studies show no risk and human evidence is incomplete, or animal studies show risk but human studies do not). Oral-solution vancomycin and IV vancomycin are in category C (animal studies show some risk, evidence in human and animal studies is inadequate, but clinical benefit sometimes exceeds risk).

Vancomycin enters breast milk, and so its use during breastfeeding is discouraged; however, because oral absorption is poor from a normal GI tract, adverse effects in infants are usually considered unlikely.

Adverse Effects

The main concern is

- Hypersensitivity (allergic or due to direct mast-cell degranulation)

Vancomycin should be infused over ≥ 60 min to avoid red-person syndrome (a histamine-mediated reaction that can cause pruritus and flushing on the face, neck, and shoulders). Other hypersensitivity reactions (eg, rash, fever) may occur, especially when therapy lasts for > 2 wk.

Other adverse effects include reversible neutropenia and thrombocytopenia. Nephrotoxicity is rare unless high doses are used or an aminoglycoside is given concomitantly. Phlebitis occurs uncommonly during IV infusion.

Dose-related ototoxicity is unusual with current formulations; incidence is increased when vancomycin is given concurrently with other ototoxic drugs.

Dosing Considerations

Doses used for meningitis must be higher than usual.

Dose reduction is required in renal insufficiency.

In critically ill patients, serum trough levels should be measured after the 2nd or 3rd dose and kept between 15 and 20 μg/mL.

Vancomycin MICs for many pathogens have been increasing during the past decade. Sensitivity for *S. aureus* based on vancomycin MIC is as follows:

- ≤ 2 μg/mL: Sensitive
- 4 to 8 μg/mL: Intermediate
- > 8 μg/mL: Resistant

However, infections due to *S. aureus* with a vancomycin MIC of 2 to 8 μg/mL may respond suboptimally to standard dosing and require higher doses with trough levels between 15 to 20 μg/mL, but this approach may be complicated by increased rates of nephrotoxicity.

185 Cestodes (Tapeworms)

All tapeworms cycle through 3 stages—eggs, larvae, and adults. Adults inhabit the intestines of definitive hosts, mammalian carnivores. Several of the adult tapeworms that infect humans are named after their intermediate host:

- The fish tapeworm (*Diphyllobothrium latum*)
- The beef tapeworm (*Taenia saginata*)
- The pork tapeworm (*Taenia solium*)

An exception is the Asian tapeworm (see Fig. 185–1; *Taenia asiatica*) which is similar to *T. saginata* in many respects, but it is acquired by eating pork in Asia.

Eggs laid by adult tapeworms living in the intestines of definitive hosts are excreted with feces into the environment and ingested by an intermediate host (typically another species), in which larvae develop, enter the circulation, and encyst in the musculature or other organs. When the intermediate host is eaten, the parasites are released from the ingested cysts in the intestines and develop into adult tapeworms in the definitive host, restarting the cycle. With some cestode species (eg, *T. solium*), the definitive host can also serve as an intermediate host; that is, if eggs rather than tissue cysts are ingested, the eggs develop into larvae, which enter the circulation and encyst in various tissues.

Adult tapeworms are multisegmented flat worms that lack a digestive tract and absorb nutrients directly from the host's small bowel. In the host's digestive tract, adult tapeworms can become large; the longest parasite in the world is the 40-m whale tapeworm, *Polygonoporus* sp.

Tapeworms have 3 recognizable portions:

- The scolex (head) functions as an anchoring organ that attaches to intestinal mucosa.
- The neck is an unsegmented region with high regenerative capacity. If treatment does not eliminate the neck and scolex, the entire worm may regenerate.
- The rest of the worm consists of numerous proglottids (segments). Proglottids closest to the neck are undifferentiated. As proglottids move caudally, each develops hermaphroditic sex organs. Distal proglottids are gravid and contain eggs in a uterus.

Symptoms and Signs

Adult tapeworms are so well-adapted to their host's GI tract that they usually cause minimal symptoms. There are some exceptions. Heavy infections with *Hymenolepis nana* can cause abdominal discomfort, diarrhea, and weight loss; *Diphyllobothrium latum* can cause vitamin B_{12} deficiency and megaloblastic anemia.

In contrast to adult tapeworms, larvae can cause severe and even lethal disease when they develop in extraintestinal sites, most importantly in the brain, but also in the liver, lungs, eyes, muscles, and subcutaneous tissues. In humans, *T. solium* causes cysticercosis, and *Echinococcus granulosus* and *E. multilocularis* cause hydatid disease. Larvae of *Spirometra* spp, *Sparganum proliferum*, *T. multiceps*, and *T. serialis* can also infect humans.

Diagnosis

- For adult tapeworm infections, microscopic examination of stool
- For larval disease, imaging

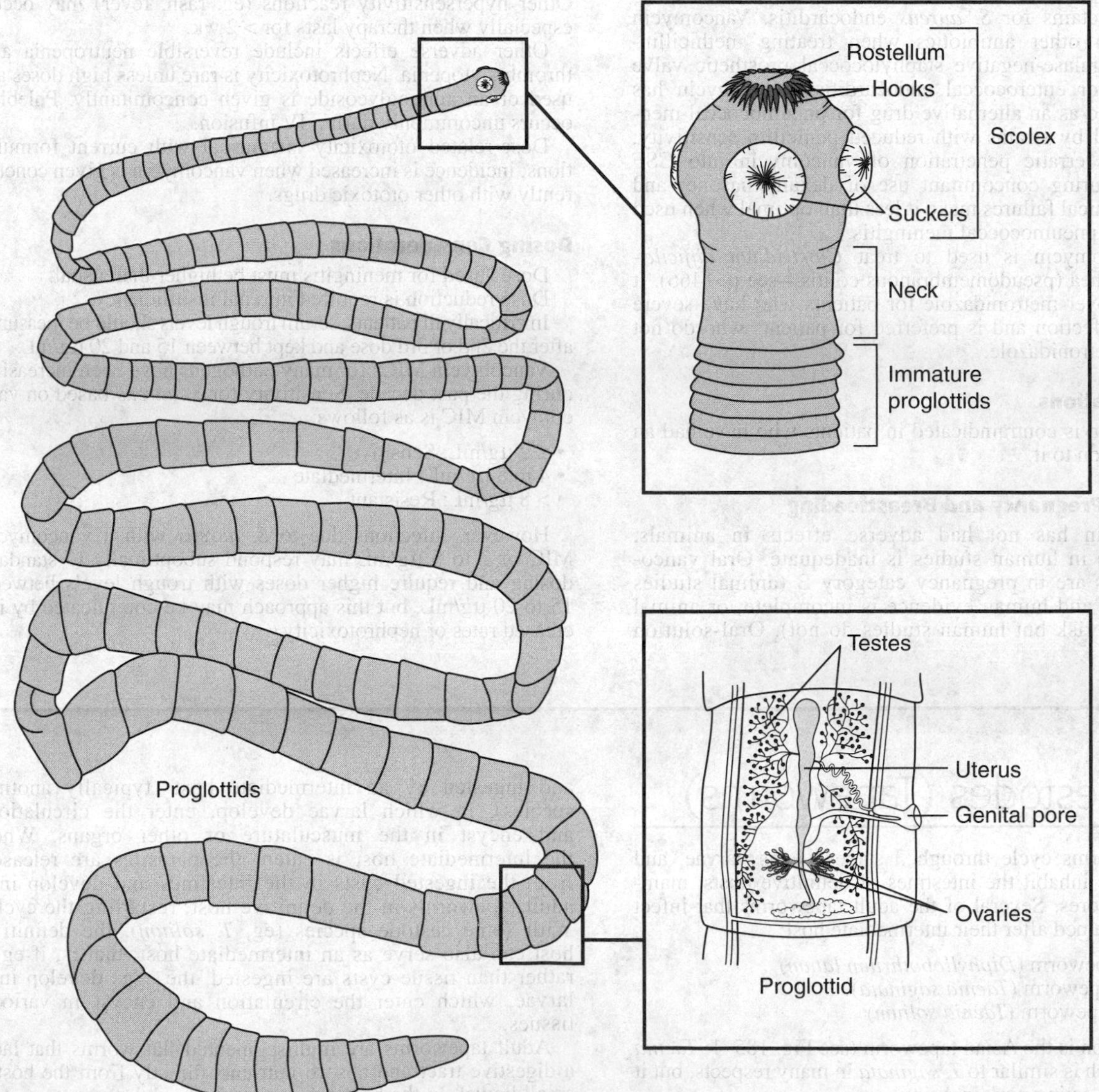

Fig. 185–1. Representative structure of a tapeworm, based on *Taenia solium*. Size and morphology vary depending on species and maturity.

Adult tapeworm infections are diagnosed by identifying eggs or gravid proglottid segments in stool. Larval disease is best identified by imaging (eg, brain CT and/or MRI). Serologic tests may also be helpful.

Treatment

- Anthelmintic drugs

The anthelmintic drug praziquantel is effective for intestinal tapeworm infections. Niclosamide is an alternative that is not available in the US. Nitazoxanide can be used for *H. nana* infections.

Some extraintestinal infections respond to anthelmintic treatment with albendazole and/or praziquantel; others require surgical intervention.

Prevention

Prevention and control involve the following:

- Thorough cooking (to a temperature > 57° C [> 135° F]) of pork, beef, lamb, game meat, and fish
- Prolonged freezing of meat for some tapeworms (eg, fish tapeworm)
- Regular deworming of dogs and cats
- Prevention of recycling through hosts (eg, dogs eating dead game or livestock)
- Reduction and avoidance of intermediate hosts such as rodents, fleas, and grain beetles
- Meat inspection
- Sanitary treatment of human waste

Smoking and drying meat are ineffective in preventing infection.

DIPHYLLOBOTHRIASIS

(Fish Tapeworm Infection)

Diphyllobothriasis is infection with the intestinal tapeworm, *Diphyllobothrium latum*, a parasite of freshwater fish. Treatment is with praziquantel.

D. latum is the largest parasite of humans (up to 10 m in length). *D. latum* and the cestodes that cause sparganosis are the only human tapeworms with aquatic life cycles. In freshwater, eggs of *D. latum* from human feces hatch into free-swimming larvae, which are ingested by microcrustaceans. The microcrustaceans are ingested by fish, in which the larvae become infective.

Diphyllobothriasis occurs worldwide, especially where cool lakes are contaminated by sewage. Infections in the US and northern Europe occur in people who eat raw freshwater fish. Infection is less common with current sewage treatment.

Infection is usually asymptomatic, but mild GI symptoms may be noted. Fish tapeworms take up dietary vitamin B_{12}, occasionally resulting in vitamin B_{12} deficiency and megaloblastic anemia.

Diagnosis of diphyllobothriasis is by identification of characteristic operculated eggs or broad proglottids (tapeworm segments) in stool. CBC is done to check for anemia.

Treatment

- Praziquantel
- Sometimes niclosamide (outside of the US)

Treatment of diphyllobothriasis is with a single oral dose of praziquantel 5 to 10 mg/kg. Alternatively, a single 2-g dose of niclosamide (unavailable in the US) is given as 4 tablets (500 mg each) that are chewed one at a time and swallowed. For children, the dose is 50 mg/kg (maximum 2 g) once.

Vitamin B_{12} may be needed to correct megaloblastic anemia if present.

Thoroughly cooking freshwater fish or freezing it at recommended temperatures can kill fish tapeworms. For freezing, recommendations include the following:

- Freezing at -20° C (-4° F) or below for 7 days (total time)
- Freezing at -35° C (-31° F) or below until solid and storing at -35° C (-31° F) or below for 15 h
- Freezing at -35° C (-31° F) or below until solid and storing at -20° C (-4° F) or below for 24 h

DIPYLIDIUM CANINUM INFECTION

***Dipylidium caninum* is a tapeworm that can cause intestinal infection, which is typically asymptomatic.**

D. caninum, the double-pored tapeworm, is present in dogs and cats. Fleas are the intermediate host. Ingestion of an infected flea, usually by a young child, causes an asymptomatic, self-limited infection, but proglottids (tapeworm segments) may be seen in stool.

Treatment is with a single oral dose of praziquantel 5 to 10 mg/kg. Alternatively, a single 2-g dose of niclosamide (unavailable in the US) is given as 4 tablets (500 mg each) that are chewed one at a time and swallowed. For children, the dose is 50 mg/kg (maximum 2 g) once.

ECHINOCOCCOSIS

(Hydatid Disease)

Echinococcosis is infection with larvae of the tapeworms *Echinococcus granulosus* or *E. multilocularis* (alveolar hydatid disease). Symptoms depend on the organ involved—eg, jaundice and abdominal discomfort with liver cysts or cough, chest pain, and hemoptysis with lung cysts. Cyst rupture can cause fever, urticaria, and serious anaphylactic reactions. Diagnosis is with imaging, examination of cyst fluid, or serologic tests. Treatment is with albendazole, surgery, or both or with cyst aspiration and instillation of a scolicidal agent.

E. granulosus is common in sheep-raising areas of the Mediterranean, Middle East, Australia, New Zealand, South Africa, and South America. Canines are definitive hosts, and herbivores (eg, sheep, horses, deer) or humans are intermediate hosts. Foci also exist in regions of Canada, Alaska, and California.

E. multilocularis worms are present in foxes, and the hydatid larvae occur in small wild rodents. Infected dogs and other canines are the main link to occasional human infection. *E. multilocularis* occurs mainly in Central Europe, Alaska, Canada, and Siberia. Its range of natural infection in the continental US extends from Wyoming and the Dakotas to the upper Midwest.

Rarely, *E. vogelii* or *E. oligarthus* causes polycystic hydatid disease in humans, primarily in the liver. These species occur in Central and South America.

Pathophysiology

Ingested eggs from animal feces (which may be present on the fur of dogs or other animals) hatch in the gut and release oncospheres (immature forms of the parasite enclosed in an embryonic envelope). Oncospheres penetrate the intestinal wall, migrate via the circulation, and lodge in the liver or lungs or, less frequently, in the brain, bone, or other organs. No adult worms are present in the GI tract of humans.

In tissue, *E. granulosus* oncospheres develop into cysts, which grow slowly (usually over many years) into large unilocular, fluid-filled lesions—hydatid cysts. Brood capsules containing numerous small infective protoscolices form within these cysts. Large cysts may contain > 1 L of highly antigenic hydatid fluid as well as millions of protoscolices. Daughter cysts sometimes form in or outside primary cysts. If a cyst in the liver leaks or ruptures, infection can spread to the peritoneum.

E. multilocularis produces spongy masses that are locally invasive and difficult or impossible to treat surgically. Cysts occur primarily in the liver but can occur in the lungs, or other tissues. The cysts are not large, but they invade and destroy surrounding tissue and can cause liver failure and death.

Symptoms and Signs

Although many infections are acquired during childhood, clinical signs may not appear for years, except when cysts are in vital organs. Symptoms and signs may resemble those of a space-occupying tumor.

Liver cysts eventually cause abdominal pain or a palpable mass. Jaundice may occur if the bile duct is obstructed. Rupture into the bile duct, peritoneal cavity, or lung may cause fever, urticaria, or a serious anaphylactic reaction.

Pulmonary cysts can rupture, causing cough, chest pain, and hemoptysis.

Diagnosis

- Imaging
- Serologic testing
- Examination of cyst fluid

Pulmonary cysts are usually discovered on routine chest x-ray as round, often irregular pulmonary masses.

CT, MRI, and ultrasound findings may be pathognomonic if daughter cysts and hydatid sand (protoscolices and debris) are present, but simple hydatid cysts may be difficult to differentiate from benign cysts, abscesses, or benign or malignant tumors. The presence of hydatid sand in aspirated cyst fluid is diagnostic.

Serologic tests (enzyme immunoassay, immunofluorescent assay, indirect hemagglutination assay) are variably sensitive but are useful if positive and should be done. CBC may detect eosinophilia.

Treatment

- Surgical removal or percutaneous aspiration followed by instillation of a scolicidal agent and reaspiration
- Sometimes albendazole

Treatment of echinococcosis varies depending on the type, location, and size of the cyst and on complications.

Surgery, sometimes via laparoscopy, can be curative. Albendazole is often given before surgery to prevent metastatic infections that can occur if cyst contents spill during the procedure. In some centers, percutaneous aspiration under CT guidance is done, followed by instillation of a scolicidal agent (eg, hypertonic saline) and reaspiration (PAIR [percutaneous aspiration-injection-reaspiration]).

PEARLS & PITFALLS

- Take care to avoid leakage of cyst contents during aspiration or surgery because metastatic infection can occur.

For *E. granulosis*, albendazole 400 mg po bid for 1 to 6 mo (7.5 mg/kg bid in children up to a maximum of 400 mg bid) is curative in 30 to 40% of patients.

Prognosis for patients with *E. multilocularis* infection is poor unless the entire larval mass can be removed. Surgery is indicated if it is feasible, which depends on the size, location, and manifestations of the lesion.

Albendazole in the above doses can suppress growth of inoperable lesions.

Liver transplantation has been lifesaving in a few patients.

KEY POINTS

- Echinococcosis occurs when ingested tapeworm eggs hatch, releasing oncospheres, which migrate into the liver or lungs or, less frequently, to the brain, bone, or other organs and develop into cysts; no adult worms are present in the GI tract of humans.
- The cysts develop slowly (usually over many years) into large (up to 1 L), fluid-filled cysts (hydatid cysts), which contain numerous infective protoscolices.
- Feces from infected dogs (and other canines) are the main source of human infection.
- Liver cysts cause pain and sometimes jaundice; lung cysts can cause pain, cough, and hemoptysis.
- *E. multilocularis* does not produce large cysts but invades and destroys surrounding tissue and can result in liver failure and death.
- Diagnose by analysis of cyst fluid and serologic testing.
- Treatment varies depending on the organism, cyst size and location, and complications; it may include surgery, cyst aspiration and instillation of a scolicidal agent, and/or prolonged treatment with albendazole.

HYMENOLEPIS DIMINUTA INFECTION

***Hymenolepis diminuta* is a tapeworm that can cause intestinal infection.**

H. diminuta, the rat tapeworm, has a life cycle similar to the indirect cycle of *H. nana*, involving grain insects. *H. diminuta* rarely infects humans but can cause mild diarrhea.

Diagnosis is by finding characteristic eggs in stool.

Treatment

- Praziquantel
- Alternatively, nitazoxanide or, outside the US, niclosamide

H. diminuta infection is effectively treated with

- Praziquantel 25 mg/kg po once

Alternatives include nitazoxanide and niclosamide (not available in the US).

For nitazoxanide, dosage is

- For patients > 11 yr: 500 mg po bid for 3 days
- For children aged 4 to 11 yr: 200 mg po bid for 3 days
- For children aged 1 to 4 yr: 100 mg po bid for 3 days

For niclosamide, dosage is

- For adults: 2 g po once/day for 7 days
- For children > 34 kg: 1.5 g in a single dose on day 1, then 1 g once/day for 6 days
- For children 11 to 34 kg: 1 g in a single dose on day 1, then 500 mg once/day for 6 days

HYMENOLEPIS NANA INFECTION

(Dwarf Tapeworm)

***Hymenolepis nana*, a tiny intestinal tapeworm, is the most common human cestode; infection is treated with praziquantel.**

H. nana is only 15 to 40 mm long. It requires only one host but can also cycle through two. Its larvae migrate only within the gut wall, and its life span is relatively short (4 to 6 wk).

H. nana is more frequent in populations living in conditions of poverty and poor hygiene, particularly when fleas are present.

H. nana has 3 modes of infection:

- Indirect 2 host cycle: Rodents are the primary definitive hosts, and grain beetles, fleas, or other insects feed on contaminated rodent droppings as intermediate hosts; humans can become infected by ingesting parasitized insects.
- Human-to-human oral-anal cycle: Eggs are passed from one human to another or recycle externally in a single host.
- Internal autoinfection: Eggs hatch within the gut and initiate a 2nd generation without ever exiting the host. Autoinfection can result in massive numbers of worms, which can cause nausea, vomiting, diarrhea, abdominal pain, weight loss, and nonspecific systemic symptoms.

Infections are often asymptomatic, but heavy infections may cause crampy abdominal pain, diarrhea, anorexia, weight loss and pruritis ani.

Diagnosis is made by finding eggs in stool samples.

Treatment

- Praziquantel
- Alternatively, nitazoxanide or, outside the US, niclosamide

The treatment of choice for *H. nana* infection is

- Praziquantel 25 mg/kg po once

Alternatives include nitazoxanide and niclosamide (not available in the US).

For nitazoxanide, dosage is

- For patients > 11 yr: 500 mg po bid for 3 days
- For children aged 4 to 11 yr: 200 mg po bid for 3 days
- For children aged 1 to 4 yr: 100 mg po bid for 3 days

For niclosamide, dosage is

- For adults: 2 g po once/day for 7 days
- For children > 34 kg: 1.5 g in a single dose on day 1, then 1 g once/day for 6 days
- For children 11 to 34 kg: 1 g in a single dose on day 1, then 500 mg once/day for 6 days

SPARGANOSIS

Sparganosis is infection with larvae of *Spirometra* spp or *Sparganum proliferum* tapeworms.

Adult *Spirometra* spp and *Sparganum proliferum* tapeworms infect dogs, cats, and other carnivores. Eggs are passed into freshwater where they are ingested by copepods (eg, *Cyclops*). Fish, reptiles, and amphibians (including frogs) ingest them and serve as intermediate hosts.

Humans and other mammals become infected by

- Accidental ingestion of copepods from water contaminated by cat or dog feces
- Ingestion of inadequately cooked flesh from another intermediate host
- Contact with poultices containing flesh from these sources

In humans, larvae typically migrate to subcutaneous tissue or muscle and form slowly growing masses. Other sites, including the CNS, may be involved but are much less common. Symptoms are caused by mass effect.

Diagnosis of sparganosis is typically made after surgical removal, although it may be suggested when imaging detects a mass.

Surgery is also the primary treatment and is typically done for symptomatic, space-occupying lesions. Generally, treatment with anthelmintics has not been effective.

COENUROSIS

(*Taenia multiceps, T. serialis*, or *T. brauni* Infection)

The tapeworms *Taenia multiceps*, *T. serialis*, and T. brauni are rare causes of human infection, which is acquired by accidental ingestion of eggs from dog feces.

Canines are the definitive hosts for adult *T. multiceps*, *T. seralis,* and *T. brauni* tapeworms; sheep and other herbivorous animals are intermediate hosts. Unwitting ingestion of material contaminated by dog feces causes human disease. In humans, the larvae invade and form a cyst (coenurus) in the CNS, subcutaneous tissues, muscles, or eyes.

Symptoms require several years to develop and depend on the organ infected. Involvement of the brain can cause increased intracranial pressure, seizures, loss of consciousness, and focal neurologic deficits. A coenurus in subcutaneous tissue or muscle may manifest as a fluctuant, tender nodule. If the eyes are involved, vision may be impaired.

Diagnosis of coenurosis is typically made after surgical removal, which is also the primary treatment. Surgery is typically done for symptomatic, space-occupying lesions.

Praziquantel can be effective. Some patients are treated with a combination of surgery and anthelmintics. But praziquantel is not used in patients with intraocular coenurosis because dying parasites can trigger severe inflammation, resulting in loss of vision.

TAENIA ASIATICA INFECTION

(Asian Tapeworm)

Infection with the Asian tapeworm, *Taenia asiatica*, is limited to Asia. It is very similar to infection with *T. saginata*, but the primary animal reservoir is pigs rather than cattle.

The morphology, clinical manifestations, diagnosis, and management of intestinal infection with the adult *T. asiatica* tapeworm are similar to those for infections with *T. saginata* (beef tapeworm), but infection is acquired by eating pork, not beef.

Infection with *T. asiatica* is limited to Asia and occurs mostly in China, Taiwan, Indonesia, Thailand, South Korea, India, and adjacent countries.

Pigs are the intermediate hosts for *T. asiatica*. Humans are infected by eating cysticerci (larvae) in raw or undercooked pork. After ingestion, the cysticerci mature into adult worms in the small intestine of humans.

Whether *T. asiatica* can cause cysticercosis in humans is not clear. Cysticercosis is infection with larvae, which develops after ingestion of ova excreted in human feces.

Symptoms

T. asiatica causes intestinal infection. Humans infected with adult *T. asiatica* worms are asymptomatic or have mild GI symptoms. They may see proglottids (tapeworm segments) in their stool.

Diagnosis

- Microscopic examination of stool for ova and proglottids

The stool should be examined for proglottids and ova; ova may also be present on anal swabs. Ova of *T. asiatica* are morphologically indistinguishable from those of *T. saginata* and *T. solium*. Molecular tests for parasite DNA can differentiate *T. asiatica* from *T. saginata*.

Treatment

- Praziquantel
- Alternatively, niclosamide (outside the US)

Treatment of *T. asiatica* infection is with a single oral dose of praziquantel 5 or 10 mg/kg.

Alternatively, a single 2-g dose of niclosamide (not available in the US) is given as 4 tablets (500 mg each) that are chewed one at a time and swallowed with a small amount of water. For children, the dose of niclosamide is 50 mg/kg (maximum dose 2 g) once.

TAENIA SAGINATA INFECTION

(Beef Tapeworm)

Infection with the beef tapeworm, *Taenia saginata*, may cause mild GI upset or passage of a motile segment in the stool. It is treated with praziquantel.

Cattle are intermediate hosts for *T. saginata*. Humans are infected by

- Eating cysticerci (larval form) in raw or undercooked beef

The larvae mature in about 2 mo to adult worms that can live for several years; usually, only 1 or 2 adult worms are present.

Infection occurs worldwide but especially in cattle-raising regions of the tropics and subtropics in Africa, the Middle East, Eastern Europe, Mexico, and South America. Infection is uncommon in US cattle and is monitored by federal inspection.

Patients may be asymptomatic or have mild digestive symptoms. Passage of a motile segment (proglottid) often brings an otherwise asymptomatic patient to medical attention.

Diagnosis

- Microscopic examination of stool for ova and proglottids

The stool should be examined for proglottids and ova; ova may also be present on anal swabs. The ova of *T. saginata* are indistinguishable from those of *T. solium* (pork tapeworm) and *T. asiatica*, as are the clinical features and management of intestinal infections due to these 3 tapeworms.

Treatment

- Praziquantel
- Alternatively, niclosamide (outside the US)

Treatment of *T. saginata* infection is with a single oral dose of praziquantel 5 or 10 mg/kg.

Alternatively, a single 2-g dose of niclosamide (not available in the US) is given as 4 tablets (500 mg each) that are chewed one at a time and swallowed with a small amount of water. For children, the dose of niclosamide is 50 mg/kg (maximum dose 2 g) once.

Treatment can be considered successful when no proglottids are passed for 4 mo.

TAENIA SOLIUM INFECTION AND CYSTICERCOSIS

(Pork Tapeworm)

***Taenia solium* infection (taeniasis) is an intestinal infection with adult tapeworms that follows ingestion of contaminated pork. Cysticercosis is infection with larvae of *T. solium*, which develops after ingestion of ova excreted in human feces. Adult worms may cause mild GI symptoms or passage of a motile segment in the stool. Cysticercosis is usually asymptomatic unless larvae invade the CNS, resulting in neurocysticercosis, which can cause seizures and various other neurologic signs. Neurocysticercosis may be recognized on brain imaging studies. Fewer than half of patients with neurocysticercosis have adult *T. solium* in their intestines and thus eggs or proglottids in their stool. Adult worms can be eradicated with praziquantel. Treatment of symptomatic neurocysticercosis is with corticosteroids, anticonvulsants, and, in some situations, albendazole or praziquantel. Surgery may be required.**

Presentation, diagnosis, and management of intestinal infection with the adult *T. solium* tapeworm are similar to those of T. saginata (beef tapeworm) infection.

However, humans may also act as intermediate hosts for *T. solium* larvae if they ingest *T. solium* eggs from human excreta

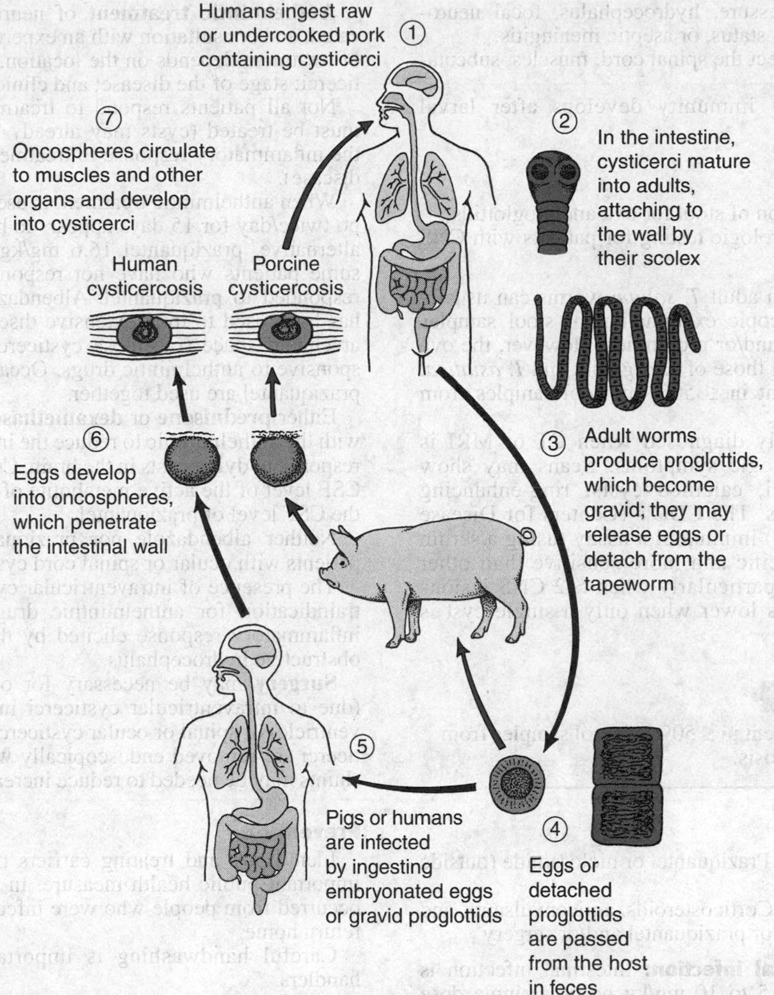

Humans ingest raw or undercooked pork containing cysticerci
1
In the intestine, cysticerci mature into adults, attaching to the wall by their scolex
2
Adult worms produce proglottids, which become gravid; they may release eggs or detach from the tapeworm
3
Eggs or detached proglottids are passed from the host in feces
4
Pigs or humans are infected by ingesting embryonated eggs or gravid proglottids
5
Eggs develop into oncospheres, which penetrate the intestinal wall
6
Human cysticercosis
Porcine cysticercosis
Oncospheres circulate to muscles and other organs and develop into cysticerci
7

Fig. 185–2. ***Taenia solium*** **life cycle.** Humans develop intestinal infection with adult worms after ingestion of contaminated pork or may develop cysticercosis after ingestion of *T. solium* eggs (making humans intermediate hosts).

(see Fig. 185–2). Some experts postulate that if an adult tapeworm is present in the intestine, gravid proglottids (tapeworm segments) may be passed retrograde from the intestine to the stomach, where oncospheres (immature form of the parasite enclosed in an embryonic envelope) may hatch and migrate to subcutaneous tissue, muscle, viscera, and the CNS.

Adult tapeworms may reside in the small bowel for years. They reach 2 to 7 m in length and produce up to 1000 proglottids; each contains about 50,000 eggs.

Taeniasis and cysticercosis occur worldwide. Cysticercosis is prevalent, and neurocysticercosis is a major cause of seizure disorders in Latin America. Cysticercosis is rare in Muslim countries. Infection in the US is most common among immigrants, but North Americans who have not traveled abroad have been infected by ingesting ova from immigrants harboring adult *T. solium.*

Rarely, zoonotic *Taenia* spp other than *T. solium* cause neurocysticercosis.

Symptoms and Signs

Intestinal infection: Humans infected with adult *T. solium* worms are asymptomatic or have mild GI complaints. They may see proglottids in their stool.

Cysticercosis: Viable cysticerci (larval form) in most organs cause minimal or no tissue reaction, but death of the cysts in the CNS can elicit an intense tissue response. Thus, symptoms often do not appear for years after infection.

Infection in the brain (cerebral cysticercosis) may result in severe symptoms due to mass effect and inflammation induced by degeneration of cysticerci and release of antigens.

Depending on the location and number of cysticerci, patients with neurocysticercosis may present with seizures, signs of increased intracranial pressure, hydrocephalus, focal neurologic signs, altered mental status, or aseptic meningitis.

Cysticerci may also infect the spinal cord, muscles, subcutaneous tissues, and eyes.

Substantial secondary immunity develops after larval infection.

Diagnosis

- Microscopic examination of stool for ova and proglottids
- CT and/or MRI and serologic testing for patients with CNS symptoms

Intestinal infection with adult *T. solium* worms can usually be diagnosed by microscopic examination of stool samples and identification of ova and/or proglottids. However, the ova are indistinguishable from those of *T. saginata* and *T. asiatica*. *T. solium* eggs are present in ≤ 50% of stool samples from patients with cysticercosis.

Cysticercosis is usually diagnosed when CT or MRI is done to evaluate neurologic symptoms. Scans may show solid nodules, cysticerci, calcified cysts, ring-enhancing lesions, or hydrocephalus. The CDC's (Centers for Disease Control and Prevention's) immunoblot assay (using a serum specimen) is highly specific and more sensitive than other enzyme immunoassays (particularly when > 2 CNS lesions are present; sensitivity is lower when only a single cyst is present).

PEARLS & PITFALLS

- *T. solium* eggs are present in ≤ 50% of stool samples from patients with cysticercosis.

Treatment

- For intestinal infection: Praziquantel or niclosamide (outside the US)
- For neurocysticercosis: Corticosteroids, anticonvulsants, and sometimes albendazole or praziquantel and/or surgery

Treatment of intestinal infection: Intestinal infection is treated with praziquantel 5 to 10 mg/kg po as a single dose to eliminate adult worms. Praziquantel should be used with caution in patients who also have neurocysticercosis because by killing cysts, praziquantel may trigger an inflammatory response associated with seizures or other symptoms.

Alternatively, a single 2-g dose of niclosamide (not available in the US) is given as 4 tablets (500 mg each) that are chewed one at a time and swallowed with a small amount of water. For children, the dose is 50 mg/kg (maximum 2 g) once.

Treatment of neurocysticercosis: The initial treatment goals for symptomatic neurocysticercosis are

- To reduce inflammation associated with degenerating cysticerci documented by MRI
- To prevent seizures if present or if risk is high
- To relieve increased intracranial pressure if present

Corticosteroids (prednisone 60 mg po once/day or dexamethasone 6 mg po once/day) are used to reduce inflammation and increased intracranial pressure.

Conventional anticonvulsants are given to patients who have seizures. These drugs can be used prophylactically in patients at high risk of seizures, particularly those who have multiple degenerating lesions with associated inflammation.

Neurosurgical intervention may be necessary for patients with increased intracranial pressure or intraventricular cysticerci.

Anthelmintic treatment of neurocysticercosis is complicated, and consultation with an expert is recommended. Choice of treatment depends on the location, number, and size of cysticerci; stage of the disease; and clinical manifestations.

Not all patients respond to treatment, and not all patients must be treated (cysts may already be dead and calcified, or the inflammatory response to treatment may be worse than the disease).

When anthelmintic treatment is used, albendazole 7.5 mg/kg po twice/day for 15 days appears to be more effective than the alternative, praziquantel 16.6 mg/kg po tid for 15 days, but some patients who have not responded to albendazole *have* responded to praziquantel. Albendazole given for ≥ 30 days has been used to treat extensive disease and cysts in the subarachnoid space (racemose cysticercosis), which are less responsive to anthelmintic drugs. Occasionally, albendazole and praziquantel are used together.

Either **prednisone** or **dexamethasone** is given concurrently with the anthelminthic to reduce the inflammation that occurs in response to dying cysts in the brain. Corticosteroids increase the CSF level of the active metabolite of albendazole but decrease the CSF level of praziquantel.

Neither albendazole nor praziquantel should be used in patients with ocular or spinal cord cysticerci.

The presence of intraventricular cysticerci is a relative contraindication for anthelminthic drugs because the resulting inflammatory response elicited by the dying cysts can cause obstructive hydrocephalus.

Surgery may be necessary for obstructive hydrocephalus (due to intraventricular cysticerci including those in the 4th ventricle) or spinal or ocular cysticercosis. Intraventricular cysticerci are removed endoscopically when possible. Ventricular shunts may be needed to reduce increased intracranial pressure.

Prevention

Identifying and treating carriers of adult tapeworms is an important public health measure. In the US, transmission has occurred from people who were infected in endemic areas and return home.

Careful handwashing is important, especially for food handlers.

When traveling to endemic areas with poor sanitation, people should be careful to avoid foods that might be contaminated by human feces.

KEY POINTS

- Ingestion of *T. solium* cysts may cause intestinal infection; ingestion of eggs may result in tissue cysts (cysticercosis), which are particularly problematic when in the brain.
- Patients with neurocysticercosis may have seizures, signs of increased intracranial pressure, altered mental status, focal neurologic signs, or aseptic meningitis.
- Diagnose infection with adult worms by microscopic examination of stool.
- Diagnose neurocysticercosis by neuroimaging and serologic testing.
- Give praziquantel for intestinal infection.
- Consult an expert for neurocysticercosis; typically corticosteroids are given with anticonvulsants to patients who have associated seizures or are thought to be at high risk of seizures.
- Use of anthelmintics and/or surgery for neurocysticercosis depends on the location, number, and size of cysticerci; stage of the disease; and clinical manifestations.

186 Chlamydia and Mycoplasmas

CHLAMYDIA

Three species of *Chlamydia* cause human disease, including sexually transmitted diseases (STDs) and respiratory infections. Most are susceptible to macrolides (eg, azithromycin), tetracyclines (eg, doxycycline), and fluoroquinolones.

Chlamydiae are nonmotile, obligate intracellular bacteria. They contain DNA, RNA, and ribosomes and make their own proteins and nucleic acids. However, they depend on the host cell for 3 of their 4 nucleoside triphosphates and use host adenosine triphosphate (ATP) to synthesize chlamydial protein.

The genus *Chlamydia* contains 9 species; 3 of them cause human disease:

- *Chlamydia trachomatis*
- *Chlamydia pneumoniae*
- *Chlamydia psittaci*

Chlamydial species can cause persistent infection, which is often subclinical.

C. trachomatis: *C. trachomatis* has 18 immunologically defined serovars:

- A, B, Ba, and C cause trachoma.
- D through K cause STDs localized to mucosal surfaces.
- L1, L2, and L3 cause STDs that lead to invasive lymph node disease (lymphogranuloma venereum).

In the US, *C. trachomatis* is the most common bacterial cause of STDs, including nongonococcal urethritis and epididymitis in men; cervicitis, urethritis, and pelvic inflammatory disease in women; and proctitis, lymphogranuloma venereum, and reactive arthritis (Reiter syndrome) in both sexes.

Maternal transmission of *C. trachomatis* causes neonatal conjunctivitis and pneumonia. Universal prenatal screening and treatment of pregnant women have greatly reduced the incidence of infant *C. trachomatis* infection in the US.

The organism can be isolated from the rectum and throat in adults (usually in men who have sex with men [MSM]). Rectal infection with L2 strains can cause severe proctocolitis that can mimic acute inflammatory bowel disease in HIV-positive MSM.

C. pneumoniae: *C. pneumoniae* can cause pneumonia (especially in children and young adults) that may be clinically indistinguishable from pneumonia caused by *Mycoplasma pneumoniae*. In some patients with *C. pneumoniae*, pneumonia, hoarseness, and sore throat may precede coughing, which may be persistent and complicated by bronchospasm.

From 6 to 19% of community-acquired pneumonia cases are due to *C. pneumoniae*; outbreaks of *C. pneumoniae* pneumonia pose a particular risk for people in closed populations (eg, nursing homes, schools, military installations, prisons). No seasonal variations in occurrence have been observed.

C. pneumoniae has also been implicated as an infectious trigger of reactive airway disease.

C. psittaci: *C. psittaci* causes psittacosis. Strains causing human disease are usually acquired from psittacine birds (eg, parrots), causing a disseminated disease characterized by pneumonitis. Outbreaks have occurred among workers that handle turkeys and ducks in poultry processing plants.

Diagnosis

- Nucleic acid–based testing

C. trachomatis is best identified in genital samples using nucleic acid amplification tests (NAATs) because these tests, although not currently FDA-approved for this use, are more sensitive than cell culture and have less stringent sample handling requirements. NAATs for genital infection can be done using noninvasively obtained samples, such as urine or vaginal swabs obtained by the patient or clinician. Serologic tests are of limited value except for diagnosing lymphogranuloma venereum and psittacosis.

C. pneumoniae is diagnosed by culture of respiratory tract specimens or by NAAT testing. There is one commercially available FDA-approved NAAT for *C. pneumoniae*, available as part of a panel that simultaneously tests for multiple respiratory pathogens.

A primary clue to diagnosis of *C. psittaci* infection is close contact with birds, typically parrots or parakeets. Diagnosis is confirmed by serologic tests. Culture is not generally available. There are no FDA-approved NAATs for *C. psittaci*.

Screening: Because chlamydial genital infection is so common and often asymptomatic or causes only mild or nonspecific symptoms (particularly in women), routine screening of asymptomatic people at high risk of STDs is recommended by the CDC (see 2015 Sexually Transmitted Diseases Treatment Guidelines at www.cdc.gov).

People who should be screened include the following.

Nonpregnant women (including women who have sex with women) are screened annually if they

- Are sexually active and ≤ 25
- Have a history of a prior STD
- Engage in high-risk sexual behavior (eg, have a new sex partner or multiple sex partners, engage in sex work, use condoms inconsistently)
- Have a partner who has an STD or engages in high-risk behavior

Women < 35 are screened when admitted to a correctional facility.

Pregnant women are screened during their initial prenatal visit; those ≤ 25 yr or with risk factors are screened again during the 3rd trimester.

Heterosexually active men are not screened except in settings with a high prevalence of chlamydial infection, including adolescent or STD clinics or at admission into correctional facilities.

MSM are screened if they have been sexually active within the previous year:

- For insertive anal intercourse: Urine screen
- For receptive anal intercourse: Rectal swab
- For oral intercourse: Pharyngeal swab

Treatment

- Azithromycin or doxycycline

Uncomplicated lower genital tract infection is typically treated with a single dose of azithromycin (1 g po) or with a 7-day regimen of doxycycline (100 mg po bid) or some fluoroquinolones (eg, levofloxacin 500 mg po once/day). Treatment of presumed chlamydial infection is routine when gonorrhea is present. Pelvic inflammatory disease, lymphogranuloma venereum, or epididymitis is usually treated with doxycycline for 10 days.

Specific infections are discussed elsewhere in THE MANUAL: Psittacosis and C. pneumoniae pneumonia, lymphogranuloma venereum and urethritis, epididymitis, reactive arthritis, neonatal conjunctivitis and neonatal pneumonia, trachoma, and inclusion conjunctivitis.

KEY POINTS

- *C. trachomatis* causes trachoma or STDs; maternal transmission can cause neonatal conjunctivitis and/or pneumonia.
- *C. pneumoniae* can cause pneumonia (especially in children and young adults and in enclosed populations).
- *C. psittaci* is a rare cause of pneumonia (psittacosis) that is usually acquired from psittacine birds (eg, parrots).
- Diagnose *C. trachomatis* and *C. pneumoniae* infections using NAATs.
- Screen high-risk, asymptomatic patients for sexually transmitted chlamydial infection.
- Treat with azithromycin or doxycycline.

MYCOPLASMAS

Mycoplasmas are ubiquitous bacteria that differ from other prokaryotes in that they lack a cell wall.

Mycoplasma pneumoniae is a common cause of pneumonia, particularly community-acquired pneumonia.

Increasing evidence suggests that *M. genitalium* and *Ureaplasma urealyticum* cause some cases of nongonococcal urethritis. They (and *M. hominis*) are often present in patients with other urogenital infections (eg, vaginitis, cervicitis, pyelonephritis, pelvic inflammatory disease) and some nonurogenital infections, but whether they cause these infections is not clear.

Mycoplasmas are not visible with light microscopy. Culture is technically difficult and often unavailable, but laboratory diagnosis is sometimes possible with NAATs or by detection of antibodies; frequently, diagnosis must be by exclusion. One NAAT for *M. pneumoniae* is part of a commercially available panel that tests for multiple respiratory pathogens.

Macrolides are usually the antimicrobials of choice. Most species are also sensitive to fluoroquinolones and tetracyclines. Macrolide-resistant infections have been reported; therefore, fluoroquinolones or tetracyclines should be considered in patients with refractory disease, especially in areas with significant macrolide resistance.

187 Enteroviruses

Enteroviruses include

- Coxsackieviruses A1 to A21, A24, and B1 to 6
- Echoviruses (enteric cytopathic human orphan viruses) 1 to 7, 9, 11 to 21, 24 to 27, and 29 to 33
- Enteroviruses 68 to 71, 73 to 91, and 100 to 101
- Polioviruses types 1 to 3

Enteroviruses, along with rhinoviruses (see p. 1685) and human parechoviruses, are picornaviruses (*pico*, or small, RNA viruses). Human parechoviruses types 1 and 2 were previously named echovirus 22 and 23 but have now been reclassified. All enteroviruses are antigenically heterogeneous and have wide geographic distribution.

Enteroviruses are shed in respiratory secretions and stool and sometimes are present in the blood and CSF of infected patients. Infection is usually transmitted by direct contact with respiratory secretions or stool but can be transmitted by contaminated environmental sources (eg, water).

Enteroviral diseases or epidemics in the US occur in summer and fall.

Infection transmitted by a mother during delivery can cause severe disseminated neonatal infection, which may include hepatitis or hepatic necrosis, meningoencephalitis, myocarditis, or a combination.

Intact humoral immunity and B-cell function are required for control of enteroviral disease. Severe enteroviral infections (often manifesting as a slowly progressive meningoencephalitis) occur in patients with agammaglobulinemia but usually not in those with other immune deficiencies.

Diseases Caused by Enteroviruses

Enteroviruses cause various syndromes (see Table 187–1). The following are caused almost exclusively by enteroviruses:

- Epidemic pleurodynia
- Hand-foot-and-mouth disease
- Herpangina
- Poliomyelitis

Other disorders (eg, aseptic meningitis, myopericarditis) may be caused by enteroviruses or other organisms.

Aseptic meningitis: Aseptic meningitis is most common among infants and children. In infants and young children, the cause is frequently one of the following:

- A group A or B coxsackievirus
- An echovirus
- A human parechovirus

In older children and adults, other enteroviruses as well as other viruses may cause aseptic meningitis.

The course is usually benign. A rash may accompany enteroviral aseptic meningitis. Rarely, encephalitis, which may be severe, also occurs.

Enterovirus D68: Enterovirus D68 (EV-D68) causes a respiratory illness, primarily in children; symptoms usually resemble those of a cold (eg, rhinorrhea, cough, malaise, fever in a few children). Some children, particularly those with asthma, have more serious symptoms involving the lower respiratory tract (eg, wheezing, respiratory distress).

Healthy adults can be infected, but they tend to have few or no symptoms. Immunocompromised adults may have severe respiratory disease.

Every year, respiratory infections caused by EV-D68 have been identified in a few children. However, in the late summer

Table 187–1. SYNDROMES CAUSED BY ENTEROVIRUSES

SYNDROME	SEROTYPES MOST OFTEN IMPLICATED
Aseptic meningitis	Coxsackieviruses A2, 4, 7, 9, and others and B2–5 Poliovirus types 1–3 Echoviruses 4, 6, 7, 9, 11, 30, and others Human parechoviruses 1–4
Aseptic meningitis with rash	Coxsackieviruses A9 and B4 Echoviruses 4 and 16 Enterovirus 71
Conjunctivitis (hemorrhagic)	Enterovirus 70 Coxsackievirus A24
Epidemic pleurodynia (Bornholm disease)	Coxsackieviruses B1–6
Hand-foot-and-mouth disease	Coxsackieviruses A6, 9, 16, and others Coxsackieviruses B2–5 Enterovirus 71
Herpangina	Coxsackieviruses A2, 4–6, 8, and 10 Probably coxsackieviruses B3 and others
Myopericarditis	Coxsackieviruses A4 and 16 and B1–5 Echoviruses 9 and human parechovirus 1
Paralysis	Polioviruses 1–3 Coxsackieviruses A7 and others Echoviruses 4, 6, 9, and others Enterovirus 71
Rash	Coxsackieviruses A9 and B1, 3, 4, and 5 (also implicated: A4–6 and 16) Echoviruses 9 and 16 (also implicated: 2, 4, 11, 14, 19, and 25)
Respiratory disease	Echoviruses 4, 8, 9, 11, 20, and others Coxsackieviruses A21 and 24 and B1 and 3–5 Enterovirus D68

and fall of 2014, over 1000 cases were confirmed in a large outbreak across the US. Severe respiratory distress developed in a significant number of children, and EV-D68 was detected in specimens from a few children who died. In addition, a few children developed focal limb weakness or paralysis with spinal cord lesions (seen on MRI) after a respiratory illness; EV-D68 was identified in respiratory specimens in about half of these cases. It is unclear whether EV-D68 infection was the main cause of death or paralysis or whether the virus happened to be present in children who also had other disorders. Investigation to determine the cause of death and neurologic symptoms is ongoing.

Hemorrhagic conjunctivitis: Rarely, hemorrhagic conjunctivitis occurs in epidemics in the US. Importation of the virus from Africa, Asia, Mexico, and the Caribbean may make outbreaks more common.

The eyelids rapidly swell. Hemorrhagic conjunctivitis, unlike uncomplicated conjunctivitis, often leads to subconjunctival hemorrhages or keratitis, causing pain, tearing, and photophobia. Systemic illness is uncommon. However, when hemorrhagic conjunctivitis is due to enterovirus 70, transient lumbosacral radiculomyelopathy or poliomyelitis-like illness (with paralysis) can occur but is rare. Recovery is usually complete within 1 to 2 wk of onset.

Coxsackievirus A24 also causes hemorrhagic conjunctivitis, but subconjunctival hemorrhage is less frequent, and neurologic complications have not been described. Most patients recover in 1 to 2 wk.

Myopericarditis: Cardiac infection may occur at any age, but most patients are 20 to 39 yr old. Patients may present with chest pain, arrhythmias, heart failure, or sudden death. Recovery is usually complete, but some patients develop dilated cardiomyopathy. Diagnosis may require reverse transcriptase (RT)–PCR of myocardial tissue.

Myocarditis neonatorum (cardiac infection at birth) is caused by group B coxsackieviruses, some echoviruses, and human parechoviruses. It causes fever and heart failure and has a high mortality rate.

Neonatal infection: Usually, several days after birth, the neonate suddenly develops a syndrome resembling sepsis with fever, lethargy, disseminated intravascular coagulation, bleeding, and multiple organ (including heart) failure. CNS, hepatic, myocardial, pancreatic, or adrenal lesions may occur simultaneously.

Recovery may occur within a few weeks, but death may result from circulatory collapse or, if the liver is involved, liver failure.

Rashes: Certain coxsackieviruses, echoviruses, and human parechoviruses may cause rashes, often during epidemics. Rashes are usually nonpruritic, do not desquamate, and occur on the face, neck, chest, and extremities. They are sometimes maculopapular or morbilliform but occasionally hemorrhagic, petechial, or vesicular. Fever is common. Aseptic meningitis may develop simultaneously.

The course is usually benign.

Respiratory infections: These infections may result from enteroviruses. Symptoms include fever, coryza, pharyngitis, and, in some infants and children, vomiting and diarrhea. Bronchitis and interstitial pneumonia occasionally occur in adults and children.

The course is usually mild.

Diagnosis

- Clinical evaluation
- Sometimes culture or reverse transcriptase–PCR (RT-PCR)

Diagnosis of enteroviral diseases is clinical.

Laboratory diagnosis is usually unnecessary but can often be made by

- Culturing the virus
- Detecting viral RNA using RT-PCR
- Less commonly, demonstrating seroconversion

Enteroviruses that cause aseptic meningitis can be detected in a sample from the throat, stool, blood, or CSF with RT-PCR tests done on blood and CSF. However, human parechoviruses are not identified by most standard enterovirus RT-PCR tests; specific parechovirus RT-PCR testing is required.

Treatment

- Supportive

Treatment of enteroviral disease is supportive.

Patients with agammaglobulinemia are treated with IV immune globulins with variable success.

EPIDEMIC PLEURODYNIA

(Bornholm Disease)

Epidemic pleurodynia is a febrile disorder caused most commonly by a group B coxsackievirus. Infection causes severe pleuritic chest or abdominal pain.

Epidemic pleurodynia may occur at any age but is most common among children.

Symptoms

Severe, frequently intermittent, often pleuritic pain begins suddenly in the epigastrium, abdomen, or lower anterior chest, with fever and often headache, sore throat, and malaise. The involved truncal muscles may become swollen and tender. Symptoms usually subside in 2 to 4 days but may recur within a few days and persist or recur for several weeks.

Cases are infrequently complicated by aseptic meningitis, orchitis, and, less commonly, myopericarditis. After recovery, subsequent infection with another group B coxsackievirus is possible.

Diagnosis

- Clinical evaluation

Diagnosis may be obvious in a child who has unexplained severe pleuritic or abdominal pain during an epidemic. However, in other situations, symptoms may be hard to distinguish from those due to other conditions that cause chest or abdominal pain.

Laboratory diagnosis is not routinely necessary; it consists of detecting the virus in a throat or stool sample or, less commonly, demonstrating seroconversion.

Treatment

- Symptom relief, including NSAIDs

Treatment includes NSAIDs and other symptomatic measures.

HAND-FOOT-AND-MOUTH DISEASE

Hand-foot-and-mouth disease is a febrile disorder usually caused by coxsackievirus A16, enterovirus 71, or other enteroviruses. Infection causes a vesicular eruption on the hands, feet (see Plate 81), and oral mucosa. Atypical hand-foot-and-mouth disease due to coxsackievirus A6 often causes high fever with papulovesicular lesions progressing to vesicobullous lesions and bullae that are widely distributed on the body.

The disease is most common among young children. The course is similar to that of herpangina.

Large outbreaks of disease due to enterovirus 71 (EV-71) have occurred in the Asia-Pacific region since 1997. Disease due to EV-71 is more serious than that due to other enteroviruses.

Children have a sore throat or mouth pain and may refuse to eat. Fever is common. Vesicles are distributed over the buccal mucosa and tongue, the palms of the hands and soles of the feet, and, occasionally, the buttocks or genitals; usually, the vesicles of typical HFMD are benign and short-lived.

Atypical HFMD has 4 distinct presentations:

- Widespread vesiculobullous lesions
- Eczema coxsackium with lesions concentrated in areas of eczematous skin
- Gianotti-Crosti type rash (multiple discrete, erythematous flat-topped papules symmetrically distributed on the face, buttocks, and extensor surface of the extremities)
- Purpuric lesions

Onychomadesis (painless nail shedding) is common during convalescence. Aseptic meningitis may complicate atypical HFMD, but most patients recover uneventfully.

Infection with EV-71 may be accompanied by severe neurologic manifestations (eg, meningitis, encephalitis, polio-like paralysis). Morbidity and mortality are significantly higher with EV-71 than with coxsackievirus A16 or other enteroviruses.

The **diagnosis** of HFMD is usually made clinically.

Treatment of HFMD is symptomatic. It includes meticulous oral hygiene (using a soft toothbrush and salt-water rinses), a soft diet that does not include acidic or salty foods, and topical measures (see p. 871).

Three inactivated EV-71 vaccines are currently under development; they appear safe and efficacious in preventing HFMD due to EV-71.

HERPANGINA

Herpangina is a febrile disorder caused by numerous group A coxsackieviruses and occasionally other enteroviruses. Infection causes oropharyngeal mucosal vesicular and ulcerative lesions.

Herpangina tends to occur in epidemics, most commonly in infants and children.

Symptoms

Herpangina is characterized by sudden onset of fever with sore throat, headache, anorexia, and frequently neck pain. Infants may vomit.

Within 2 days after onset, up to 20 (mean, 4 to 5) 1- to 2-mm diameter grayish papules develop and become vesicles with erythematous areolae. They occur most frequently on the tonsillar pillars but also on the soft palate, tonsils, uvula, or tongue. During the next 24 h, the lesions become shallow ulcers, seldom > 5 mm in diameter, and heal in 1 to 7 days.

Complications are unusual.

Lasting immunity to the infecting strain follows, but repeated episodes caused by other group A coxsackieviruses or other enteroviruses are possible.

Diagnosis

- Clinical evaluation

Diagnosis of herpangina is based on symptoms and characteristic oral lesions.

Confirmatory testing is not usually required but can be done by

- Isolating the virus from the lesions
- Detecting virus by reverse transcriptase–PCR
- Demonstrating a rise in specific antibody titer

Recurrent aphthous ulcers may appear similar. Rarely, Bednar aphthous ulcers occur in the pharynx but usually without systemic symptoms. Herpetic stomatitis occurs sporadically and causes larger, more persistent, and more numerous ulcers throughout the oropharynx than herpangina. Coxsackievirus

A10 causes lymphonodular pharyngitis, which is similar except that the papules become 2- to 3-mm whitish to yellowish nodules instead of vesicles and ulcers.

Treatment

- Symptom relief

Treatment of herpangina is symptomatic. It includes meticulous oral hygiene (using a soft toothbrush and salt-water rinses), a soft diet that does not include acidic or salty foods, and topical measures (see p. 871).

POLIOMYELITIS

(Acute Anterior Poliomyelitis; Infantile Paralysis; Polio)

Poliomyelitis is an acute infection caused by a poliovirus (an enterovirus). Manifestations include a nonspecific minor illness (abortive poliomyelitis), sometimes aseptic meningitis without paralysis (nonparalytic poliomyelitis), and, less often, flaccid weakness of various muscle groups (paralytic poliomyelitis). Diagnosis is clinical, although laboratory diagnosis is possible. Treatment is supportive.

Polioviruses have 3 serotypes. Type 1 is the most paralytogenic and used to be the most common cause of epidemics. Humans are the only natural host. Infection is highly transmittable via direct contact. Asymptomatic and minor infections (abortive poliomyelitis) are more common than nonparalytic or paralytic infections by ≥ 60:1 and are the main source of spread.

Extensive vaccination has almost eradicated the disease worldwide. However, cases still occur in regions with incomplete immunization, such as sub-Saharan Africa and southern Asia.

Pathophysiology

The virus enters via the fecal-oral or respiratory route, then enters the lymphoid tissues of the GI tract. A primary (minor) viremia follows with spread of virus to the reticuloendothelial system. Infection may be contained at this point, or the virus may further multiply and cause several days of secondary viremia, culminating in the development of symptoms and antibodies.

In **paralytic infections,** poliovirus enters the CNS—whether via secondary viremia or via migration up peripheral nerves is unclear. Significant damage occurs in only the spinal cord and brain, particularly in the nerves controlling motor and autonomic function. Inflammation compounds the damage produced by primary viral invasion. Factors predisposing to serious neurologic damage include

- Increasing age (throughout life)
- Recent tonsillectomy or intramuscular injection
- Pregnancy
- Impairment of B-cell function
- Physical exertion concurrent with onset of the CNS phase

Poliovirus is present in the throat and feces during incubation and, after symptom onset, persists 1 to 2 wk in the throat and ≥ 3 to 6 wk in feces; the fecal-oral and respiratory routes are the usual method of transmission.

PEARLS & PITFALLS

- Most poliovirus infections do not involve the CNS or cause paralysis.

Symptoms and Signs

Most (70 to 75%) infections cause no symptoms. Symptomatic disease is classified as

- Abortive poliomyelitis
- Paralytic or nonparalytic poliomyelitis

Abortive: Most symptomatic infections, particularly in young children, are minor, with 1 to 3 days of slight fever, malaise, headache, sore throat, and vomiting, which develop 3 to 5 days after exposure. There are no neurologic symptoms or signs, and physical examination is unremarkable except for the presence of fever.

Paralytic and nonparalytic: Paralytic poliomyelitis occurs in < 1% of all infections. It may develop without a preceding minor illness, particularly in older children and adults. Incubation is usually 7 to 21 days.

Common manifestations include aseptic meningitis, deep muscle pain, hyperesthesias, paresthesias, and, during active myelitis, urinary retention and muscle spasms. Asymmetric flaccid paralysis may develop and progress over 2 to 3 days. Encephalitic signs occasionally predominate.

Dysphagia, nasal regurgitation, and nasal voice are usually the earliest signs of bulbar involvement, but some patients have pharyngeal paralysis and cannot control oral secretions. As with skeletal muscle paralysis, bulbar involvement may worsen over 2 to 3 days and, in some patients, affects the respiratory and circulatory centers of the brain stem, leading to respiratory compromise. Infrequently, respiratory failure develops when the diaphragm or intercostal muscles are affected.

Some patients develop postpoliomyelitis syndrome years or decades after paralytic poliomyelitis. This syndrome is characterized by muscle fatigue and decreased endurance, often with weakness, fasciculations, and atrophy.

Diagnosis

- Lumbar puncture
- Viral culture (stool, throat, and CSF)
- Reverse transcriptase–PCR of blood or CSF
- Serologic testing for poliovirus serotypes, enteroviruses, and West Nile virus

When there are no CNS manifestations, symptomatic polio resembles other systemic viral infections and is typically not considered or diagnosed except during an epidemic.

Nonparalytic poliomyelitis resembles other viral meningitides. In such patients, lumbar puncture is usually done; typical CSF findings are normal glucose, mildly elevated protein, and a cell count of 10 to 500/μL (predominantly lymphocytes). Detection of the virus in a throat swab, feces, or CSF or demonstration of a rise in specific antibody titer confirms infection with poliovirus but is usually not needed in patients with uncomplicated aseptic meningitis.

Paralytic poliomyelitis may be suspected in nonimmunized children or young adults who have asymmetric flaccid limb paralysis or bulbar palsies without sensory loss during an acute febrile illness. However, certain group A and B coxsackieviruses (especially A7), several echoviruses, and enterovirus type 71 may produce similar findings. Also, cases of focal limb weakness or paralysis have been identified after infection with enterovirus D68. West Nile virus infection can also cause an acute flaccid paralysis that is clinically indistinguishable from paralytic poliomyelitis due to polioviruses. Guillain-Barré syndrome causes flaccid paralysis but can be distinguished because of the following:

- It usually causes no fever.
- Muscle weakness is symmetric.
- Sensory deficits occur in 70% of patients
- CSF protein is usually elevated and CSF cell count is normal.

Epidemiologic clues (eg, immunization history, recent travel, age, season) can help suggest the cause. Because identification of poliovirus or another enterovirus as the cause of acute flaccid paralysis is important for public health reasons, viral culture of throat swabs, stool, and CSF and reverse transcriptase–PCR of CSF and blood should be done in all cases. Specific serologic testing for polioviruses, other enteroviruses, and West Nile virus should also be done.

Prognosis

In **nonparalytic poliomyelitis,** recovery is complete.

In **paralytic poliomyelitis,** about two thirds of patients have residual permanent weakness. Bulbar paralysis is more likely to resolve than peripheral paralysis. Mortality is 4 to 6% but increases to 10 to 20% in adults and in patients with bulbar disease.

Treatment

- Supportive care

Standard treatment of poliomyelitis is supportive and includes rest, analgesics, and antipyretics as needed. Specific antiviral therapy is not available.

During active myelitis, precautions to avoid complications of bed rest (eg, deep venous thrombosis, atelectasis, UTI) and prolonged immobility (eg, contractures) may be necessary. Respiratory failure may require mechanical ventilation. Mechanical ventilation or bulbar paralysis requires intensive pulmonary toilet measures.

Prevention

All infants and children should be immunized with poliomyelitis vaccine. The American Academy of Pediatrics recommends vaccination at ages 2 mo, 4 mo, and 6 to 18 mo and a booster dose at age 4 to 6 yr (see Table 291–2 on p. 2462). Childhood vaccination produces immunity in > 95% of recipients.

Salk inactivated poliovirus vaccine (IPV) is preferred to Sabin live-attenuated oral polio vaccine (OPV), which causes paralytic poliomyelitis in about 1 case per 2,400,000 doses and is thus no longer available in the US. Serious adverse effects have not been associated with IPV. As part of the Global Polio Eradication Initiative, all countries were to implement routine IPV vaccination programs by the end of 2016.

Adults are not routinely vaccinated. Nonimmunized adults traveling to endemic or epidemic areas should receive primary vaccination with IPV, including 2 doses given 4 to 8 wk apart and a 3rd dose given 6 to 12 mo later. At least 1 dose is given before travel. Immunized adults traveling to endemic or epidemic areas should be given 1 dose of IPV. Immunocompromised patients and their household contacts should not be given OPV.

KEY POINTS

- Most poliovirus infections are asymptomatic or cause nonspecific minor illness or aseptic meningitis without paralysis; < 1% of patients develop the classic syndrome of flaccid weakness (paralytic poliomyelitis).
- Asymmetric flaccid limb paralysis or bulbar palsies without sensory loss during an acute febrile illness in a nonimmunized child or young adult may indicate paralytic poliomyelitis.
- Viral culture of throat swabs, stool, and CSF and reverse transcriptase–PCR of CSF and blood should be done.
- In paralytic poliomyelitis, about two thirds of patients have residual permanent weakness.
- All infants and children should be immunized, but adults are not routinely vaccinated unless they are at increased risk (eg, because of travel or occupation).

POSTPOLIOMYELITIS SYNDROME

(Postpolio Syndrome)

Postpoliomyelitis syndrome is a group of symptoms that develops years or decades after paralytic poliomyelitis and usually affects the same muscle groups as the initial infection.

In patients who have had paralytic poliomyelitis, muscle fatigue and decreased endurance, often accompanied by weakness, fasciculations, and atrophy, may develop years or decades later, particularly in older patients and in patients who are severely affected initially. Damage usually occurs in previously affected muscle groups. However, postpoliomyelitis syndrome rarely increases disability substantially.

The cause may be related to further loss of anterior horn cells due to aging in a population of neurons already depleted by earlier poliovirus infection.

Treatment of postpoliomyelitis syndrome is supportive.

188 Extraintestinal Protozoa

AFRICAN TRYPANOSOMIASIS

(African Sleeping Sickness)

African trypanosomiasis is infection with protozoa of the genus Trypanosoma, transmitted by the bite of a tsetse fly. Symptoms include characteristic skin lesions, intermittent fever, headache, rigors, transient edema, generalized lymphadenopathy, and often fatal meningoencephalitis. Diagnosis is by identification of the organism in blood, lymph node aspirate, or CSF or sometimes by serologic tests. Treatment is with suramin, pentamidine, melarsoprol, or eflornithine, depending on the infecting subspecies, clinical stage, and drug availability.

African trypanosomiasis is caused by *Trypanosoma brucei gambiense* in West and Central Africa and by *T. brucei rhodesiense* in East Africa; both species are endemic in Uganda.

The organisms are transmitted by tsetse flies and can be transmitted prenatally from mother to fetus. Rarely, the infection is transmitted through blood transfusions; theoretically, it could be transmitted through organ transplantation.

Pathophysiology

Metacyclic trypomastigotes inoculated by flies transform into bloodstream trypomastigotes, which multiply by binary fission and spread through the lymphatics and bloodstream after inoculation. Bloodstream trypomastigotes multiply until specific antibodies produced by the host sharply reduce parasite levels. However, a subset of parasites escape immune destruction by a change in their variant surface glycoprotein and start a new multiplication cycle. The cycle of multiplication and lysis repeats.

Late in the course of infection, trypanosomes appear in the interstitial fluid of many organs, including the myocardium and eventually the CNS. The cycle is continued when a tsetse fly bites an infected human or animal.

Humans are the main reservoir of *T. b. gambiense*, but this species may also reside in animals. Wild game animals are the main reservoir of *T. b. rhodesiense*.

Symptoms and Signs

Trypanosomiasis has 3 stages:

- Cutaneous
- Hemolymphatic
- CNS

Cutaneous: A papule may develop at the site of the tsetse fly bite within a few days to 2 wk. It evolves into a dusky red, painful, indurated nodule (trypanosomal chancre). A chancre is present in about half of Caucasians with *T.b. rhodesiense* but is less common in Africans with *T. b. rhodesiense* and seldom occurs with *T. b. gambiense*.

Hemolymphatic: Over several months in *T. b. gambiense* infection but a period of weeks with *T. b. rhodesiense*, intermittent fever, headaches, rigors, muscle and joint pain, and transient facial swelling develop. An evanescent, circinate erythematous rash may develop. It is most readily visible in light-skinned patients. Generalized lymphadenopathy often occurs.

Winterbottom sign (enlarged lymph nodes in the posterior cervical triangle) is characteristic with *T. b. gambiense* sleeping sickness.

CNS: In the Gambian form, CNS involvement occurs months to several years after onset of acute disease. In the Rhodesian form, disease is more fulminant, and CNS invasion often occurs within a few weeks.

CNS involvement causes persistent headache, inability to concentrate, personality changes (eg, progressive lassitude and indifference), daytime somnolence, tremor, ataxia, and terminal coma.

Without treatment, death occurs within months of disease onset with *T. b. rhodesiense* and during the 2nd or 3rd yr with *T. b. gambiense*. Untreated patients die in coma of undernutrition or secondary infections.

Diagnosis

- Light microscopy of blood (thin or thick smears) or other fluid sample

Diagnosis of trypanosomiasis is made by identifying trypanosomes in fluid from a chancre, lymph node aspirate, blood, bone marrow aspirate, or, during the late stage of infection, CSF. Preferred sources are blood smears for *T. b. rhodesiense* and fluid aspirated from an enlarged lymph node for *T. b. gambiense*. Wet preparations should be examined for motile trypanosomes, and smears should be fixed, stained with Giemsa (or Field) stain, and examined. The concentration of trypanosomes in blood is often low, and concentration techniques (eg, centrifugation, miniature anion-exchange centrifugation, quantitative buffy coat technique) enhance sensitivity.

Antibody detection assays are not very useful clinically because seroconversion occurs after the onset of symptoms. However, a card agglutination test for *T. b. gambiense* is useful in mass screening programs to identify candidates for microscopic examination.

A lumbar puncture should be done in all patients with African trypanosomiasis. When CSF is involved, opening pressure may be increased, and CSF has elevated levels of lymphocytes (≥ 5 cells/μL), total protein, and IgM. In addition to trypanosomes, characteristic Mott cells (plasma cells with cytoplasmic vacuoles that contain immunoglobulin [Russell bodies]) may be present.

Other, nonspecific laboratory findings include anemia, monocytosis, and markedly elevated serum levels of polyclonal IgM.

Treatment

- Without CNS involvement, pentamidine or eflornithine for *T. b. gambiense*; suramin for *T. b. rhodesiense*
- With CNS involvement, eflornithine or melarsoprol for *T. b. gambiense*; melarsoprol for *T. b. rhodesiense*

Without CNS involvement: Suramin and pentamidine are effective against bloodstream stages of both *T. brucei* subspecies but do not cross the blood-brain barrier and are not useful for CNS infection. Pentamidine is preferred for *T. b. gambiense*, and suramin is preferred for the hemolymphatic stage of *T. b. rhodesiense*. The dosage of pentamidine is 4 mg/kg IM or IV once/day for 7 to 10 days. An initial test dose of suramin 100 mg IV (to exclude hypersensitivity) is followed by 20 mg/kg (up to 1 g) IV on days 1, 3, 7, 14, and 21.

Eflornithine (obtainable from the WHO or, in the US, from the CDC; availability limited) is effective against all stages of *T. b. gambiense* (but not *T. b. rhodesiense*) trypanosomiasis. Dosage is 100 mg/kg IV qid for 14 days. When available, it is the drug of choice for *T. b. gambiense*.

With CNS involvement: When available, eflornithine 100 mg/kg IV qid for 14 days should be used for CNS disease due to *T. b. gambiense* (eflornithine is ineffective for *T. b. rhodesiense*). In the US, eflornithine can be obtained from the CDC.

Melarsoprol, an organic arsenical, is often used in African countries because of the limited availability of eflornithine, even though adverse effects can be severe and life threatening. Melarsoprol dosage is as follows:

- For *T. b. gambiense*: 2.2 mg/kg IV once/day for 10 days
- For *T. b. rhodesiense*: 2 to 3.6 mg/kg IV once/day for 3 days; after 7 days, 3.6 mg/kg once/day for 3 days, followed 7 days later by another 3-day course at this dose

Alternative regimens have been proposed for debilitated patients with severe CNS involvement. Serial follow-up examinations, including CSF analysis, are recommended every 6 mo (sooner if symptoms return) for 2 yr.

Serious adverse effects of melarsoprol include encephalopathic reactions, exfoliative dermatitis, cardiovascular toxicity (hypertension, arrhythmia, heart failure), and the GI and renal toxicity of arsenicals.

Corticosteroids have been used to decrease the risk of encephalopathic reactions.

Prevention

Prevention includes avoiding endemic areas and protecting against tsetse flies. Visitors to game parks should wear substantial wrist- and ankle-length clothing (tsetse flies bite through thin clothes) in neutral colors that blend with the background and should use insect repellents, although efficacy of repellents against tsetse flies may be limited.

Pentamidine can help prevent *T. b. gambiense* infection, but it may damage pancreatic beta cells, resulting in insulin release and hypoglycemia followed later by diabetes; thus, it is seldom used for prophylaxis.

KEY POINTS

- African trypanosomiasis is caused by *Trypanosoma brucei gambiense* in West and Central Africa and by *T. b. rhodesiense* in East Africa; tsetse flies are the main vector.
- There are 3 stages of disease: cutaneous, hemolymphatic, and CNS (sleeping sickness).
- Diagnose using light microscopy of blood (thin or thick smears) or another fluid sample.
- Treatment varies by species and stage of disease.
- Without CNS involvement, use pentamidine or eflornithine for *T. b. gambiense* and suramin for *T. b. rhodesiense*.
- With CNS involvement, use eflornithine or melarsoprol for *T. b. gambiense* and melarsoprol for *T. b. rhodesiense*.

BABESIOSIS

Babesiosis is infection with *Babesia* protozoa. Infections can be asymptomatic or cause a malaria-like illness with fever and hemolytic anemia. Disease is most severe in asplenic patients, the elderly, and patients with AIDS. Diagnosis is by identification of *Babesia* in a peripheral blood smear, serologic test, or PCR. Treatment, when needed, is with azithromycin plus atovaquone or with quinine plus clindamycin.

Endemic areas in the US include the islands and the mainland bordering Nantucket Sound in Massachusetts, Rhode Island, eastern Long Island and Shelter Island in New York, coastal Connecticut, and New Jersey, as well as foci in Wisconsin and Minnesota in the upper Midwest. *Babesia duncani* has been isolated from patients in Washington and California. A currently unnamed strain designated MO-1 has been reported in patients in Missouri. Other *Babesia* sp transmitted by different ticks infect humans in areas of Europe. In Europe, *B. divergens* is the principle cause of babesiosis in patients who have had a splenectomy.

Etiology

In the US, *Babesia microti* is the most common cause of babesiosis in humans. Rodents are the principal natural reservoir, and deer ticks of the family Ixodidae are the usual vectors. Larval ticks become infected while feeding on an infected rodent, then transform into nymphs that transmit the parasite to another animal or to a human. Adult ticks ordinarily feed on deer but may also transmit the parasite to humans. *Babesia* enter RBCs, mature, and then divide asexually. Infected erythrocytes eventually rupture and release organisms that invade other RBCs; thus, *Babesia* can also be transmitted by blood transfusion, possibly by organ transplantation, and congenitally. Currently, no tests to screen for *Babesia* in blood donors are available.

Ixodes ticks infected with *Babesia* are sometimes coinfected with *Borrelia burgdorferi* (which causes Lyme disease), *Anaplasma phagocytophilum* (which causes human granulocytic anaplasmosis [HGA]), or *Borrelia miyamotoi* (which causes an HGA-like illness).

Symptoms and Signs

Asymptomatic infection may persist for months to years and remain subclinical throughout its course in otherwise healthy people, especially those < 40 yr.

When symptomatic, the illness usually starts after a 1- to 2-wk incubation period with malaise, fatigue, chills, fever, headache, myalgia, and arthralgia, which may last for weeks. Hepatosplenomegaly with jaundice, mild to moderately severe hemolytic anemia, mild neutropenia, and thrombocytopenia may occur.

Babesiosis is sometimes fatal, particularly in the elderly, asplenic patients, and patients with AIDS. In such patients, babesiosis may resemble falciparum malaria, with high fever, hemolytic anemia, hemoglobinuria, jaundice, and renal failure. Splenectomy may cause previously acquired asymptomatic parasitemia to become symptomatic.

Diagnosis

- Light microscopy of blood smears
- Serologic and PCR-based tests

Most patients do not remember a tick bite, but they may reside in or report a history of travel to an endemic region.

Babesiosis is usually diagnosed by finding *Babesia* in blood smears, but differentiation from *Plasmodium* species can be difficult. Tetrad forms (the so-called Maltese cross formation), although not common, are unique to *Babesia* and helpful diagnostically.

Serologic and PCR-based tests are available. Antibody detection by indirect fluorescent antibody (IFA) testing using *B. microti* antigens can be helpful in patients with low-level parasitemia but may be falsely negative in those infected with other *Babesia* sp.

Treatment

- Atovaquone plus azithromycin
- Quinine plus clindamycin

Asymptomatic patients require no treatment, but therapy is indicated for patients with persistent high fever, rapidly increasing parasitemia, and falling Hct.

The combination of atovaquone and azithromycin given for 7 to 10 d has fewer adverse effects than traditional therapy with quinine plus clindamycin. Adult dosage is atovaquone 750 mg po q 12 h and azithromycin 500 to 1000 mg po the first day followed by a daily dose of 250 to 1000 mg. In children > 5 kg, dosage is atovaquone 20 mg/kg po bid plus azithromycin 10 mg/kg po once, then 5 mg/kg/day for 7 to 10 days.

Quinine 650 mg po tid plus clindamycin 600 mg po tid or 300 to 600 mg IV 4 times a day for 7 to 10 days can also be used. Pediatric dosage is quinine 10 mg/kg po tid plus clindamycin 7 to 14 mg/kg po tid. Quinine plus clindamycin is considered the standard of care for severely ill patients.

Exchange transfusion has been used in hypotensive patients with high parasitemia.

Prevention

Standard tick precautions (see Sidebar 201–1 on p. 1696) should be taken by all people in endemic areas. Asplenic patients and patients with AIDS should be particularly cautious.

KEY POINTS

- Endemic areas of babesiosis in the US include the coast and islands of southern New England and New Jersey as well as parts of the upper Midwest.
- Babesiosis ranges from a mild, asymptomatic infection to a severe, life-threatening illness (mainly in the elderly and asplenic or immunosuppressed patients).

- Symptoms resemble those of malaria, with prolonged fever, headache, myalgias, and sometimes jaundice.
- Diagnose using light microscopy of blood smears and sometimes PCR-based tests.
- Treat symptomatic patients with atovaquone plus azithromycin or, if symptoms are severe, quinine plus clindamycin.

CHAGAS DISEASE

(American Trypanosomiasis)

Chagas disease is infection with *Trypanosoma cruzi*, transmitted by Triatominae bug bites or, less commonly, via ingestion of sugar cane juice or foods contaminated with infected Triatominae bugs or their feces, transplacentally from an infected mother to her fetus, or via blood transfusion or an organ transplant from an infected donor. Symptoms after a Triatominae bite typically begin with a skin lesion or unilateral periorbital edema, then progress to fever, malaise, generalized lymphadenopathy, and hepatosplenomegaly; years later, some patients develop chronic cardiomyopathy, megaesophagus, or megacolon. Many who are infected never develop disease. In patients with AIDS, the skin or brain may be affected. Diagnosis is by detecting trypanosomes in peripheral blood or aspirates from infected organs. Antibody tests are sensitive and can be helpful. Treatment is with nifurtimox or benznidazole.

T. cruzi is transmitted by Triatominae (reduviid, kissing, or assassin) bugs in South and Central America, Mexico, and very rarely in the US. Nonhuman reservoirs include domestic dogs, opossums, armadillos, rats, raccoons, and many other animals. Less commonly, *T. cruzi* is transmitted via ingestion of sugar cane juice or food contaminated with infected Triatominae bugs or their feces, transplacentally from an infected mother to her fetus, or via blood transfusion or an organ transplant from an infected donor.

Worldwide, an estimated 8 million people are chronically infected with *T. cruzi*. Most reside in Latin America, but about 300,000 of those infected in Latin America now live in the US; others live in Europe or elsewhere. The incidence of *T. cruzi* infection has been decreasing in Latin America because of improved housing, screening of blood and organ donors, and other control measures.

Pathophysiology

Chagas disease is spread when a kissing bug bites an infected person or animal, then bites another person. While biting, infected bugs deposit feces containing metacyclic trypomastigotes on the skin. These infective forms enter through the bite wound or penetrate the conjunctivae or mucous membranes. The parasites invade macrophages at the site of entry and transform into amastigotes that multiply by binary fission; the amastigotes develop into trypomastigotes, enter the bloodstream and tissue spaces, and infect other cells. Cells of the reticuloendothelial system, myocardium, muscles, and nervous system are most commonly involved.

Symptoms and Signs

Chagas disease can occur in 3 stages:

- Acute
- Latent (indeterminate)
- Chronic

Acute infection is followed by a latent (indeterminate) period, which may remain asymptomatic or progress to chronic disease. Immunosuppression may reactivate latent infection, with high parasitemia and a 2nd acute stage, skin lesions, or brain abscesses.

About 1 to 5% of infected pregnant women transmit the infection transplacentally, resulting in abortion, stillbirth, or chronic neonatal disease with high mortality.

Acute: Acute infection in endemic areas usually occurs in childhood and can be asymptomatic. When present, symptoms start 1 to 2 wk after exposure. An indurated, erythematous skin lesion (a chagoma) appears at the site of parasite entry. When the inoculation site is the conjunctiva, unilateral periocular and palpebral edema with conjunctivitis and preauricular lymphadenopathy are collectively called the Romaña sign.

Acute Chagas disease is fatal in a small percentage of patients; death results from acute myocarditis with heart failure or meningoencephalitis. In the remainder, symptoms subside without treatment.

Primary acute Chagas disease in immunocompromised patients, such as those with AIDS, may be severe and atypical, with skin lesions and, rarely, brain abscesses.

Indeterminate: Patients with indeterminate infection have parasitologic and/or serologic evidence of *T. cruzi* infection but have neither symptoms, abnormal physical findings, nor evidence of cardiac or GI involvement as assessed by ECG and rhythm strip, cardiac ultrasonography, chest x-ray, or other studies.

Many infected patients are identified by screening enzyme-linked immunosorbent blood assay (ELISA) and confirmatory radioimmunoprecipitation assay (RIPA) when they donate blood.

Chronic: Chronic disease develops in 20 to 40% after a latent phase that may last years or decades. The main effects are

- Cardiac
- GI

Chronic cardiomyopathy leads to flaccid enlargement of all chambers, apical aneurysms, and localized degenerative lesions in the conduction system. Patients may present with heart failure, syncope, sudden death due to heart block or ventricular arrhythmia, or thromboembolism. ECG may show right bundle branch or complete heart block.

GI disease causes symptoms resembling achalasia or Hirschsprung disease. Chagas megaesophagus manifests as dysphagia and may lead to pulmonary infections caused by aspiration or to severe undernutrition. Megacolon may result in long periods of obstipation and intestinal volvulus.

Diagnosis

- Light microscopy of blood smears (thin or thick) or tissue (acute Chagas disease)
- Screening serologic test confirmed by a second test
- PCR-based tests

The number of trypanosomes in peripheral blood is large during the acute phase of Chagas disease and can be readily detected by examining thin or thick smears. In contrast, few parasites are present in blood during latent infection or chronic disease. Definitive diagnosis of acute-stage Chagas disease may also be made by examining tissue from lymph nodes or heart.

In immunocompetent patients with chronic Chagas disease, serologic tests, such as indirect fluorescent antibody (IFA), enzyme immunoassays (EIA), or enzyme-linked immunosorbent assay (ELISA), are often done to detect antibodies to *T. cruzi*. Serologic tests are sensitive but may yield false-positive results in patients with leishmaniasis or other diseases. Thus, an initial positive test is followed by one or more different tests (typically, radioimmunoprecipitation assay [RIPA] in the US) or sometimes light microscopy of blood smears or a tissue sample to confirm the diagnosis. Serologic tests are also used to screen blood donors for *T. cruzi* in endemic areas and the US.

PCR-based tests are used when the level of parasitemia is likely to be high, as occurs in acute Chagas disease, in transplacentally transmitted (congenital) Chagas disease, or after transmission via blood transfusion, transplantation, or laboratory exposure. In endemic areas, xenodiagnosis has been used; it involves examining the intestinal contents of Triatominae bugs raised in a laboratory after they took a blood meal from a person thought to have Chagas disease.

Ancillary testing in patients with chronic Chagas disease: After Chagas disease is diagnosed, the following tests should be done, depending on findings:

- No symptoms but documented *T. cruzi* infection: A screening ECG and rhythm strip and a chest x-ray
- Potential cardiac abnormalities on a screening test or symptoms suggesting heart disease: Echocardiography
- Dysphagia or other GI symptoms or findings: GI contrast studies and/or endoscopy.

Treatment

- Benznidazole or nifurtimox
- Supportive care

Treatment of acute-stage Chagas disease with antiparasitic drugs does the following:

- Rapidly reduces parasitemia
- Shortens the clinical illness
- Reduces risk of mortality
- Decreases the likelihood of chronic disease

Treatment is indicated for all cases of acute, congenital, or reactivated Chagas disease and for indeterminate infection in children up to age 18 yr. The younger the patient and the earlier treatment is started, the more likely that treatment will result in parasitologic cure.

For indeterminate infections, treatment of adults up to age 50 yr has been recommended. For patients > 50 yr, treatment is individualized based on potential risks and benefits.

Once signs of cardiac or GI manifestations of chronic Chagas disease appear, antiparasitic drugs are not thought to be helpful.

Supportive measures include treatment for heart failure, pacemakers for heart block, antiarrhythmic drugs, cardiac transplantation, esophageal dilation, botulinum toxin injection into the lower esophageal sphincter, and GI tract surgery for megacolon.

The only effective drugs are

- **Benznidazole:** For adults and children > 12 yr, 2.5 to 3.5 mg/kg po bid for 60 days. For children ≤ 12 yr, 2.5 to 3.75 mg/kg bid for 60 days
- **Nifurtimox:** For patients ≥ 17 yr, 2 to 2.5 mg/kg po qid for 90 days. For children aged 11 to 16 yr, 3 to 3.75 mg/kg qid for 90 days. For children aged 1 to 10 yr, 4 to 5 mg/kg qid for 90 days

Both drugs are available through the CDC. They have substantial toxicity, which increases with age. Contraindications for treatment include severe liver or kidney disease.

Common adverse effects of benznidazole include allergic dermatitis, peripheral neuropathy, anorexia, weight loss, and insomnia.

Common adverse effects of nifurtimox are anorexia, weight loss, polyneuropathy, nausea, vomiting, headache, dizziness, vertigo.

It is recommended that these drugs not be used in pregnant women or in breastfeeding mothers.

Prevention

Plastering walls and replacing thatched roofs or repeated spraying of houses with residual insecticides (those that have prolonged duration of action) can control Triatominae bugs. Infection in travelers is rare and can be avoided by not sleeping in adobe dwellings or by using bed nets if sleeping in such dwellings is unavoidable.

Blood and organ donors are screened in many endemic areas and, since 2006, in the US to prevent transfusion- and organ transplant–related Chagas disease.

KEY POINTS

- Chagas disease is caused by *Trypanosoma cruzi*, which is transmitted by Triatominae (reduviid, kissing, or assassin) bugs.
- Infection is endemic in South and Central America and Mexico; an estimated 8 million people worldwide, including an estimated 300,000 people in the US (primarily immigrants), are infected.
- Acute infection is followed by a latent (indeterminate) period, which may remain asymptomatic, but in 20 to 40%, it progresses to chronic disease, which particularly affects the heart and GI tract.
- Diagnose acute Chagas using light microscopy of blood smears (thin or thick) or a tissue sample.
- Diagnose chronic *T. cruzi* infection by screening enzyme-linked immunosorbent blood assay (ELISA) with confirmatory radioimmunoprecipitation assay (RIPA) or other assay for antibodies.
- Use PCR-based tests to evaluate cases potentially transmitted transplacentally or via transfusion, transplantation, or laboratory exposure.
- To detect chronic Chagas disease, do echocardiography if patients have symptoms suggesting heart disease or potential cardiac abnormalities on a chest x-ray, ECG, or rhythm strip; do GI contrast studies or endoscopy if they have dysphagia or other GI symptoms.
- Treat patients in the acute stage and many in the indeterminate stage with benznidazole or nifurtimox.
- Antiparasitic drugs are not effective in chronic Chagas disease, but supportive measures (eg, treatment of heart failure, pacemakers for heart block, antiarrhythmic drugs, cardiac transplantation, esophageal dilation, botulinum toxin injection into the lower esophageal sphincter, GI tract surgery) are often helpful.

FREE-LIVING AMEBAS

Free-living amebas are protozoa that live independently in soil or water and do not require a human or animal host. They rarely cause disease, in contrast to the parasitic ameba *Entamoeba histolytica*, which is a common cause of intestinal infection (amebiasis). Pathogenic free-living amebas are of the genera *Naegleria, Acanthamoeba*, *Balamuthia*, and *Sappinia*.

Three major syndromes occur:

- Primary amebic meningoencephalitis
- Granulomatous amebic encephalitis
- Amebic keratitis

Acanthamoeba and *Balamuthia* can also cause skin lesions or disseminated disease in immunocompromised people; *Acanthamoeba* can also cause infection of the sinuses or lungs.

Primary Amebic Meningoencephalitis

Primary amebic meningoencephalitis is a generally fatal, acute CNS infection caused by *Naegleria fowleri*.

Naegleria fowleri inhabit bodies of warm fresh water worldwide. Swimming in contaminated water exposes nasal mucosa to the organism, which can enter the CNS via olfactory neuroepithelium and the cribriform plate. Most patients are healthy children or young adults.

Symptoms and Signs

Symptoms of primary amebic meningoencephalitis begin within 1 to 2 wk of exposure, sometimes with alteration of smell and taste. Fulminant meningoencephalitis ensues, with headache, meningismus, and mental status change, progressing to death within 10 days, usually due to cerebral herniation. Only a few patients have survived.

Diagnosis

- CSF examination

Primary amebic meningoencephalitis is suspected based on history of swimming in fresh water, but confirmation is difficult because CT and routine CSF tests, although necessary to exclude other causes, are nonspecific.

Wet mount of CSF should be done; it may demonstrate motile amebic trophozoites (which can be seen in Giemsa-stained specimens but are destroyed by Gram stain techniques).

Immunohistochemistry, amebic culture, PCR of CSF, and/or brain biopsy are available in specialized reference laboratories.

Treatment

- Various treatment regimens
- Multiple drugs, including miltefosine plus antifungal drugs and antibiotics

Optimal treatment is unclear.

A reasonable regimen would include miltefosine, an antileishmanial drug, which has been used to successfully treat granulomatous amebic encephalitis. Miltefosine is available through consultation from the CDC (see CDC information on Naegleria at www.cdc.gov).

Other drugs that have been used in combination treatment regimens for *Naegleria* include

- Amphotericin B
- Rifampin
- An azole (fluconazole, voriconazole, or ketoconazole)
- Azithromycin

Anticonvulsants and dexamethasone are often needed to control seizures and cerebral edema.

KEY POINTS

- Primary amebic meningoencephalitis is usually fatal.
- The infection is acquired when swimming in contaminated fresh water; *Naegleria fowleri* enters the CNS via olfactory neuroepithelium and the cribriform plate.
- Diagnostic tests should include a wet mount and Giemsa-stained specimen of CSF.
- Treat the infection with appropriate antimicrobial drugs; if needed, treat seizures and cerebral edema with anticonvulsants and dexamethasone.

Granulomatous Amebic Encephalitis

Granulomatous amebic encephalitis is a generally fatal subacute CNS infection caused by Acanthamoeba sp in immunocompromised or debilitated hosts or by *Balamuthia mandrillaris*.

Acanthamoeba sp and *Balamuthia mandrillaris* are present worldwide in water, soil, and dust. Human exposure is common, but infection is rare. *Acanthamoeba* infection of the CNS occurs almost entirely in immunocompromised or otherwise debilitated patients, but *B. mandrillaris* may also infect healthy hosts. *Sappinia pedata* was implicated in one case of amebic encephalitis in Texas.

The life cycle of *Acanthamoeba* involves only 2 stages: cysts and trophozoites (the infective form). The trophozoites form double-walled cysts, which resist eradication. The entry portal is thought to be the skin or lower respiratory tract, with subsequent hematogenous dissemination to the CNS. In infected patients, cysts and trophozoites may be found in tissues.

Symptoms

Onset is insidious, often with focal neurologic manifestations. Mental status change, seizures, and headache are common.

Acanthamoeba sp *and B. mandrillaris* may also cause skin lesions; patients can present with ulcerative skin lesions and later develop neurologic symptoms and signs. In a few patients with AIDS, disseminated *Acanthamoeba* infection affects only the skin.

Survival is uncommon; death usually occurs between 7 and 120 days after onset.

Diagnosis

- CT with contrast and MRI
- CSF analysis
- Biopsy of skin lesions

Diagnosis of granulomatous amebic encephalitis is often postmortem.

Diagnosis of *Acanthamoeba* infections: In patients with *Acanthamoeba* infections, CT with contrast and MRI may show single or multiple space-occupying lesions with ring enhancement, most commonly in the temporal and parietal lobes. In CSF, WBC count (predominantly lymphocytes) is elevated, but trophozoites are rarely seen. These tests help exclude other possible causes but usually cannot confirm the diagnosis.

Visible skin lesions often contain amebas and should be biopsied; if detected, amebas may be cultured and tested for drug sensitivity. Brain biopsy is often positive.

PCR-based assays are available in specialized reference laboratories.

Diagnosis of *B. mandrillaris* infections: In patients with *B. mandrillaris* infection, CT and MRI typically show multiple nodular, ring-enhancing lesions. Intralesional hemorrhage is an important radiologic clue.

Treatment

- A combination of drugs, usually including miltefosine
- Consultation with the CDC

Optimal treatment of *Acanthamoeba* encephalitis is unclear. Multiple drugs (often > 5) are typically used in combination. Although the number of patients treated with a regimen containing miltefosine is small, miltefosine appears to offer a survival advantage. Miltefosine is available directly from the CDC.

Other drugs that have been used in combination to treat *Acanthamoeba* encephalitis include pentamidine, sulfadiazine or trimethoprim/sulfamethoxazole, flucytosine, an azole (fluconazole, itraconazole, or voriconazole), rifampin and amphotericin B.

For *B. mandrillaris* encephalitis, miltefosine in combination with other drugs such as flucytosine, pentamidine, fluconazole, and/or sulfadiazine plus either azithromycin or clarithromycin plus surgical resection have been used.

A case of *Sappinia pedata* encephalitis was successfully treated with a combination of azithromycin, pentamidine, itraconazole, and flucytosine plus surgical resection of the CNS lesion. Adding miltefosine to this regimen should be considered.

For all cases of amebic encephalitis, immediate consultation with the CDC is recommended (call the CDC Emergency Operations Center at 770-488-7100).

Skin infections caused by *Acanthamoeba* sp or *B. mandrillaris* are usually treated with the same drugs plus surgical debridement.

KEY POINTS

- Granulomatous amebic encephalitis is a rare, usually fatal CNS infection.
- *Acanthamoeba* encephalitis occurs almost entirely in immunocompromised or otherwise debilitated patients, but *B. mandrillaris* may infect healthy hosts.
- Do CT with contrast, MRI, and CSF tests to exclude other causes, and biopsy any skin lesions to check for amebas.
- Consult with the CDC about optimal treatment.
- Treat with miltefosine plus other drugs (eg, pentamidine, sulfadiazine, flucytosine, an azole).

Amebic Keratitis

Amebic keratitis is corneal infection with *Acanthamoeba* sp, typically occurring in contact lens wearers.

Acanthamoeba spp can cause chronic and progressively destructive keratitis in normal hosts. The main risk factor (85% of cases) is contact lens use, particularly if lenses are worn while swimming or if unsterile lens cleaning solution is used. Some infections follow corneal abrasion.

Acanthamoeba are present worldwide in water, soil, and dust. The life cycle of *Acanthamoeba* involves only 2 stages: cysts and trophozoites (the infective form). The trophozoites form double-walled cysts, which resist eradication. Both forms can enter the body through various means (eg, eyes, nasal mucous membranes, broken skin). When *Acanthamoeba* enter the eye, they can cause severe keratitis. In infected patients, cysts and trophozoites may be found in tissues.

Symptoms and Signs

Lesions are typically very painful and produce a foreign body sensation. Initially, lesions have a dendriform appearance resembling herpes simplex keratitis. Later, there are patchy stromal infiltrates and sometimes a characteristic ring-shaped lesion. Anterior uveitis is usually also present. Vision is diminished.

Diagnosis

- Examination and culture of corneal scrapings

Consultation with an ophthalmologist is important for diagnosis and treatment.

Diagnosis of amebic keratitis is confirmed by examination of Giemsa- or trichrome-stained corneal scrapings and by culture on special media. Viral culture is done if herpes is considered.

Treatment

- Corneal debridement
- Topical chlorhexidine, polyhexamethylene biguanide, or both
- In severe cases, systemic itraconazole or ketoconazole

Early, superficial infection responds better to treatment. The encysted stage of the life cycle appears to cause most problems.

Epithelial lesions are debrided, and intensive drug therapy is applied. The initial choice is

- Topical chlorhexidine 0.02%
- Topical polyhexamethylene biguanide 0.02%
- Both drugs

For the first 3 days, drugs are given every 1 to 2 h. Other topical drugs used as adjunct therapy include propamidine and hexamidine diisethionate.

Systemic treatment with itraconazole or ketoconazole has been used in conjunction with topical therapy, particularly in patients with anterior uveitis or involvement of the sclera. Systemic ketoconazole can cause severe liver injury and adrenal gland problems and should be used only when alternative antifungal drugs are not available or not tolerated.

Early recognition and treatment have eliminated the need for therapeutic keratoplasty in most instances, but keratoplasty remains an option when pharmacologic therapy fails. Intensive treatment is required for the first month; it is tapered per clinical response but often continued for 6 to 12 mo. Recurrence is common if treatment is stopped prematurely

Prevention

Contact lens solution should be kept clean. Nonsterile homemade contact lens solutions should not be used. Wearing contact lenses while swimming or showering should be avoided.

KEY POINTS

- *Acanthamoeba* spp can cause chronic and progressively destructive keratitis in otherwise healthy hosts, mainly in contact lens users.
- Consult with an ophthalmologist about management.
- Diagnose by examining Giemsa- or trichrome-stained corneal scrapings and by culturing the sample using special media.
- Herpes simplex keratitis can cause similar lesions; if it seems a possible diagnosis, do viral culture.
- Debride corneal lesions, and treat with topical chlorhexidine, polyhexamethylene biguanide, or both.
- For severe infections, consider treatment with systemic itraconazole, or if itraconazole is ineffective or not tolerated, consider ketoconazole.

LEISHMANIASIS

Leishmaniasis is caused by species of *Leishmania*. Manifestations include cutaneous, mucosal, and visceral syndromes. Cutaneous leishmaniasis causes painless chronic skin lesions

ranging from nodules to large ulcers that can persist for months to years but eventually heal. Mucosal leishmaniasis affects nasopharyngeal tissues and can cause gross mutilation of the nose and palate. Visceral leishmaniasis causes irregular fever, hepatosplenomegaly, pancytopenia, and polyclonal hypergammaglobulinemia with high mortality in untreated patients. Diagnosis is by demonstrating parasites in smears or cultures and increasingly by PCR-based assays at reference centers. Serologic testing can be helpful in diagnosing visceral but not cutaneous leishmaniasis. Treatment of visceral leishmaniasis is with liposomal amphotericin B. Alternatives include amphotericin B deoxycholate, pentavalent antimony compounds (sodium stibogluconate, meglumine antimonate), and miltefosine. A variety of topical and systemic treatments are available for cutaneous leishmaniasis depending on the causative species and clinical manifestations.

Leishmaniasis is present in scattered areas worldwide. Human infection is caused by 20 *Leishmania* sp that are morphologically indistinguishable but can be differentiated by laboratory analysis.

Etiology

Leishmania promastigotes are transmitted by sand flies (*Phlebotomus* sp, *Lutzomyia* sp) to vertebrate hosts. Vector sand flies are infected by biting infected humans or other animals. Animal reservoirs vary with the *Leishmania* sp and geographic location and include dogs, other canines, rodents, and other animals. In the Indian subcontinent, humans are the reservoir for *L. donovani*.

Rarely, infection is spread by blood transfusion, shared needles, congenitally, or sexually.

Pathophysiology

After inoculation by a sand fly, promastigotes are phagocytized by host macrophages; inside these cells, they transform into amastigotes.

The parasites may remain localized in the skin or spread to the mucosa of the nasopharynx or disseminate to bone marrow, the spleen, the liver, and occasionally other organs, resulting in 3 major clinical forms of leishmaniasis:

- Cutaneous
- Mucosal
- Visceral

Cutaneous leishmaniasis is also known as oriental or tropical sore, Delhi or Aleppo boil, uta or chiclero ulcer, or forest yaws. The causative agents are

- *L. major* and *L. tropica* in southern Europe, Asia, and Africa
- *L. mexicana* and related species in Mexico and Central and South America
- *L. braziliensis* and related species in Central and South America

Cases have occurred among US military personnel serving in Iraq and Afghanistan and among travelers to endemic areas in Central and South America, Israel, and elsewhere. Uncommonly, *L. braziliensis* spreads widely in the skin causing disseminated cutaneous leishmaniasis.

Mucosal leishmaniasis (espundia) is caused mainly by *L. braziliensis* but occasionally by other *Leishmania* sp. The parasites are thought to spread from the initial skin lesion through the lymphatics and blood to nasopharyngeal tissues. Symptoms and signs of mucosal leishmaniasis typically develop months to years after the appearance of the skin lesion.

Visceral leishmaniasis (kala-azar, Dumdum fever) is typically caused by *L. donovani* or *L. infantum* (previously called *L. chagasi* in Latin America) and occurs in India, Africa (particularly the Sudan), Central Asia, the Mediterranean basin, South and Central America, and infrequently China. Most cases occur in northeastern India. Parasites disseminate from the site of the sand fly bite in the skin to regional lymph nodes, the spleen, the liver, and bone marrow and cause symptoms. Subclinical infections are common; only a minority of infected patients develop progressive visceral disease. Symptomatic infection with *L. infantum* is more common among children than adults. Visceral leishmaniasis is an opportunistic infection in patients with AIDS or other immunocompromising conditions.

Symptoms and Signs

In **cutaneous leishmaniasis,** a well-demarcated skin lesion develops at the site of a sand fly bite, usually within several weeks to months. Multiple lesions may occur after multiple infective bites or with metastatic spread. Their appearance varies. The initial lesion is often a papule that slowly enlarges, ulcerates centrally, and develops a raised, erythematous border where intracellular parasites are concentrated. Ulcers are typically painless and cause no systemic symptoms unless secondarily infected. Lesions usually heal spontaneously after several months but may persist for years. They leave a depressed, burn-like scar. The course depends on the infecting *Leishmania* sp and the host's immune status.

Diffuse cutaneous leishmaniasis, a rare syndrome,results in widespread nodular skin lesions resembling those of lepromatous leprosy. It results from cell-mediated anergy to the organism.

Mucosal leishmaniasis starts with a primary cutaneous ulcer. This lesion heals spontaneously; progressive mucosal lesions may not become apparent for months to years. Typically, patients have nasal stuffiness, discharge, and pain. Over time, the infection may progress, resulting in gross mutilation of the nose, palate, or face.

In **visceral leishmaniasis,** the clinical manifestations usually develop gradually over weeks to months after inoculation of the parasite but can be acute. Irregular fever, hepatosplenomegaly, pancytopenia, and polyclonal hypergammaglobulinemia with a reversed albumin:globulin ratio occur. In some patients, there are twice-daily temperature spikes. Cutaneous skin lesions rarely occur. Emaciation and death occur within months to years in patients with progressive infections. Those with asymptomatic, self-resolving infections and survivors (after successful treatment) are resistant to further attacks unless cell-mediated immunity is impaired (eg, by AIDS). Relapse may occur years after initial infection.

Post kala-azar dermal leishmaniasis (PKDL) may develop after treatment for visceral leishmaniasis in patients in the Sudan and India. It is characterized by flat or nodular cutaneous lesions that contain many parasites. In patients in the Sudan, these lesions develop at the end of or within 6 mo of therapy and persist for a few months to a year after therapy. In patients in India and adjacent countries, the lesions develop 1 to 2 yr after therapy ends and can last for many years. PKDL lesions are thought to be a reservoir for the spread of infection in these areas.

Diagnosis

- Light microscopy of tissue samples, touch preparations, or aspirates; when available, PCR-based assays
- For visceral leishmaniasis, antibody titers

- For cutaneous and mucosal leishmaniasis, skin testing (not available in the US)
- Culture (special media required)

A definite diagnosis of leishmaniasis is made by any of the following:

- Demonstrating organisms in Giemsa-stained smears
- Isolating *Leishmania* in cultures
- PCR-based assays of aspirates from bone marrow, the spleen, or lymph nodes in patients with visceral leishmaniasis or of biopsy, aspirates, or touch preparations from a skin lesion

Parasites are usually difficult to find or isolate in culture from biopsies of mucosal lesions.

Organisms causing simple cutaneous leishmaniasis can be differentiated from those capable of causing mucosal leishmaniasis based on the site of acquisition, specific DNA probes, or analysis of cultured parasites.

Serologic tests can help diagnose visceral leishmaniasis; high titers of antibodies to a recombinant leishmanial antigen (rk39) are present in most immunocompetent patients with visceral leishmaniasis. But antibodies may be absent in patients with AIDS or other immunocompromising conditions. Serologic tests for antileishmanial antibodies are not helpful in the diagnosis of cutaneous leishmaniasis.

The leishmanin skin test is not available in the US. It is typically positive in patients with cutaneous and mucosal leishmaniasis but negative in those with active visceral leishmaniasis.

Treatment

- Various drugs depending on the clinical syndrome and other factors
- For topical treatment, sodium stibogluconate injection or topical paromomycin outside the US or heat therapy or cryotherapy
- For systemic treatment, liposomal amphotericin IV, amphotericin B deoxycholate IV, or miltefosine po
- Alternatively, pentavalent antimonials (sodium stibogluconate, meglumine antimoniate) only if the infecting *Leishmania* sp is likely to be susceptible

Treatment of leishmaniasis is complicated; which drugs are used depends on the following:

- Clinical syndrome
- Infecting *Leishmania* sp
- Geographic location of acquisition
- Organism's likelihood of susceptibility to treatment
- Immune status of the host

Detailed recommendations for treatment are available.[1,2]

Cutaneous leishmaniasis: Treatment of cutaneous leishmaniasis may be topical or systemic, depending on the lesion and organism.

If a lesion is small, spontaneously healing, and not caused by a *Leishmania* sp associated with mucosal leishmaniasis, it can be closely followed, rather than treated.

Topical treatment is an option for small, uncomplicated lesions. Intralesional injection of sodium stibogluconate has been used for many years for simple cutaneous leishmaniasis in Europe and Asia; it is not currently available in the US for intralesional use. Other topical options include heat therapy, which requires a specialized system for administration, and cryotherapy; both can be painful and are practical only when used to treat small lesions. In addition, topical paromomycin is used outside the US as an ointment that contains 15% paromomycin and 12% methylbenzethonium chloride in soft white paraffin.

Systemic therapy is used in patients who have the following:

- Infection by *L. braziliensis* or related organisms associated with mucosal leishmaniasis
- Complex cutaneous leishmaniasis with multiple, large, widespread, or disfiguring lesions
- Compromised cell-mediated immunity

In the US, systemic options include miltefosine, liposomal amphotericin B, amphotericin B deoxycholate, and sodium stibogluconate (only if infection was acquired in areas where resistance to them is not prevalent). Liposomal amphotericin B and amphotericin B deoxycholate are typically given in the regimens used for visceral leishmaniasis.

Miltefosine 2.5 mg/kg (maximum, 150 mg/day) po once/day for 28 days can be effective for cutaneous leishmaniasis. Adverse effects include nausea, vomiting, transient elevations in aminotransferases, and dizziness. Miltefosine is contraindicated during pregnancy; women of childbearing age who are taking this drug must use effective birth control measures.

Pentavalent antimonials (sodium stibogluconate, meglumine antimoniate) should be used only if the infecting *Leishmania* sp is likely to be susceptible. Sodium stibogluconate is available from the CDC (call the Emergency Operations Center at 770-488-7100). Meglumine antimoniate (a pentavalent antimonial) is used in Latin America. Doses of both are based on their pentavalent antimony content—20 mg/kg IV (slow infusion required) or IM once/day for 20 days. Adverse effects include nausea, vomiting, malaise, elevated amylase and/or liver enzymes, and cardiotoxicity (arrhythmias, myocardial depression, heart failure, ECG changes, cardiac arrest). The incidence of adverse effects increases with age. The drug is stopped if patients develop cardiotoxicity.

Alternatives include azoles (eg, fluconazole, itraconazole). Fluconazole 200 mg po once/day for 6 wk is commonly ineffective, sometimes leading to the use of higher daily doses.

Diffuse cutaneous leishmaniasis is relatively resistant to treatment.

Mucosal leishmaniasis: The optimal treatment is uncertain. Historically, pentavalent antimonials have been used.

Another option is amphotericin B deoxycholate 0.5 to 1.0 mg/kg once/day or every other day for a total daily dose of about 20 to 45 mg/kg. Recent studies suggest that liposomal amphotericin B with a cumulative dose ranging from 20 to 60 mg/kg or miltefosine 2.5 mg/kg (maximum, 150 mg/day) po once/day for 28 days is effective, but data are limited.

Reconstructive surgery may be required if mucosal leishmaniasis grossly distorts the nose or palate, but surgery should be delayed for 12 mo after successful chemotherapy to avoid losing grafts because of relapses.

Visceral leishmaniasis: Liposomal amphotericin B and miltefosine are approved by the FDA for treatment of visceral leishmaniasis; other lipid-associated amphotericin preparations may be effective but have been less well-studied.

Dosage of liposomal amphotericin B is

- For immunocompetent patients: 3 mg/kg IV once/day for 5 days and then once/day on days 14 and 21 (total dose of 21 mg/kg)
- For patients with AIDS or other immunocompromising conditions:s 4 mg/kg IV once/day on days 1 to 5, 10, 17, 24, 31, and 38 (total dose of 40 mg/kg)

Miltefosine 2.5 mg/kg po once/day (maximum 150 mg/day) for 28 days can be used to treat immunocompetent patients who acquired *L. donovani* in India or adjacent areas of South Asia, who are > 12 yr of age, who weigh > 30 kg, and who are not pregnant or breastfeeding.

Pentavalent antimonials can be used to treat visceral leishmaniasis acquired in Latin America or other areas of the world where the infection is not resistant to these drugs; they may be used in the US after consultation with the CDC. Dosage is 20 mg/kg (based on the antimony content) IV or IM once/day for 28 days.

An alternative is amphotericin B deoxycholate 1 mg/kg IV once/day for 15 to 20 days or every other day for up to 8 wk.

Relapses are common among patients with AIDS or other immunocompromising conditions. Antiretroviral drugs can help restore immune function, reducing the likelihood of relapse. Secondary prophylaxis with an antileishmanial drug may help prevent relapses in AIDS patients with CD4 counts < 200/μL.

Supportive measures (eg, adequate nutrition, transfusions, antibiotics for secondary bacterial infection) are often necessary for patients with visceral leishmaniasis.

1. Aronson N, Herwaldt BL, Libman M, et al: Diagnosis and treatment of leishmaniasis: clinical Practice Guidelines by the Infectious Diseases Society of America (IDSA) and the American Society of Tropical Medicine and Hygiene (ASTMH). *Clin Infect Dis* 63 (12):e202-e264, 2016. doi: 10.1093/cid/ciw670.
2. CDC: Resources for Health Professionals: Treatment.

Prevention

For prevention, the following may help:

- Treatment of leishmaniasis in a geographic area where humans are a reservoir
- Reduction of the vector population by spraying residual insecticide (one that has prolonged duration of action) in sites of domestic transmission
- Control of nonhuman reservoirs

Travelers to endemic areas should use insect repellents containing DEET. Insect screens, bed nets, and clothing are more effective if treated with permethrin or pyrethrum because the small sand flies can penetrate mechanical barriers.

Vaccines are not currently available.

KEY POINTS

- Leishmaniasis is present in scattered areas worldwide and is transmitted by bites of sand flies.
- The parasites may remain localized in the skin (cutaneous leishmaniasis), spread to the mucosa (mucosal leishmaniasis), or disseminate to the liver, the spleen, and bone marrow (visceral leishmaniasis).
- Diagnose using Giemsa-stained smears, cultures, or PCR-based assays; serologic tests can help diagnose visceral leishmaniasis in immunocompetent patients but are not helpful in patients with AIDS or with cutaneous or mucosal leishmaniasis.
- Treat small, uncomplicated skin lesions with locally applied heat or cryotherapy or, outside the US, with topical paromomycin or intralesional sodium stibogluconate.
- Systemic treatment options for complex cutaneous leishmaniasis, mucosal leishmaniasis, and visceral leishmaniasis includes liposomal amphotericin B, amphotericin B deoxycholate, and miltefosine; sodium stibogluconate is an alternative if infection is acquired in areas where *Leishmania* spp are likely to be susceptible.
- Drug resistance to antimonials is an increasing problem, particularly in India.

MALARIA

Malaria is infection with *Plasmodium* sp. Symptoms and signs include fever (which may be periodic), chills, sweating, hemolytic anemia, and splenomegaly. Diagnosis is by seeing *Plasmodium* in a peripheral blood smear and rapid diagnostic tests. Treatment and prophylaxis depend on the species and drug sensitivity and include artemisinin-based combination therapy, the fixed combination of atovaquone and proguanil, and regimens that contain chloroquine, quinine, or mefloquine. Patients infected with *P. vivax*and *P. ovale* also receive primaquine to prevent relapse.

About half of the world's population remains at risk of malaria. Malaria is endemic in Africa, India and other areas of South Asia, Southeast Asia, North and South Korea, Mexico, Central America, Haiti, the Dominican Republic, South America (including northern parts of Argentina), the Middle East (including Turkey, Syria, Iran, and Iraq), and Central Asia. The CDC provides information about specific countries where malaria is transmitted, types of malaria, resistance patterns, and recommended prophylaxis (see CDC: Malaria at www.cdc.gov).

In 2015, there were an estimated 214 million cases of malaria worldwide, with 438,000 deaths, mostly in children < 5 yr in Africa. Since 2000, deaths due to malaria have decreased by 60% through the efforts of the Roll Back Malaria Program, which has > 500 partners (including endemic countries and various organizations and institutions).

Malaria once was endemic in the US. Currently, about 1500 cases occur in the US each year. Nearly all are acquired abroad, but a small number result from blood transfusions or rarely from transmission by local mosquitoes that feed on infected immigrants or returning travelers.

Pathophysiology

The *Plasmodium* species that infect humans are

- *P. falciparum*
- *P. vivax*
- *P. ovale*
- *P. malariae*
- *P. knowlesi (rarely)*

Concurrent infection with more than one *Plasmodium* species is uncommon.

Also, simian malaria has been reported in humans; *P. knowlesi* is an emerging pathogen in Southeast Asia. The degree to which *P. knowlesi* is transmitted from human to human via the mosquito, without the natural intermediate monkey host, is under study.

The basic elements of the life cycle are the same for all *Plasmodium* sp (see Fig. 188–1). Transmission begins when a female *Anopheles* mosquito feeds on a person with malaria and ingests blood containing gametocytes.

During the following 1 to 2 wk, gametocytes inside the mosquito reproduce sexually and produce infective sporozoites. When the mosquito feeds on another human, sporozoites are inoculated and quickly reach the liver and infect hepatocytes.

The parasites mature into tissue schizonts within hepatocytes. Each schizont produces 10,000 to 30,000 merozoites, which are released into the bloodstream 1 to 3 wk later when the hepatocyte ruptures. Each merozoite can invade an RBC and there transform into a trophozoite.

Trophozoites grow, and most develop into erythrocyte schizonts; schizonts produce further merozoites, which 48 to 72 h later rupture the RBC and are released in plasma. These

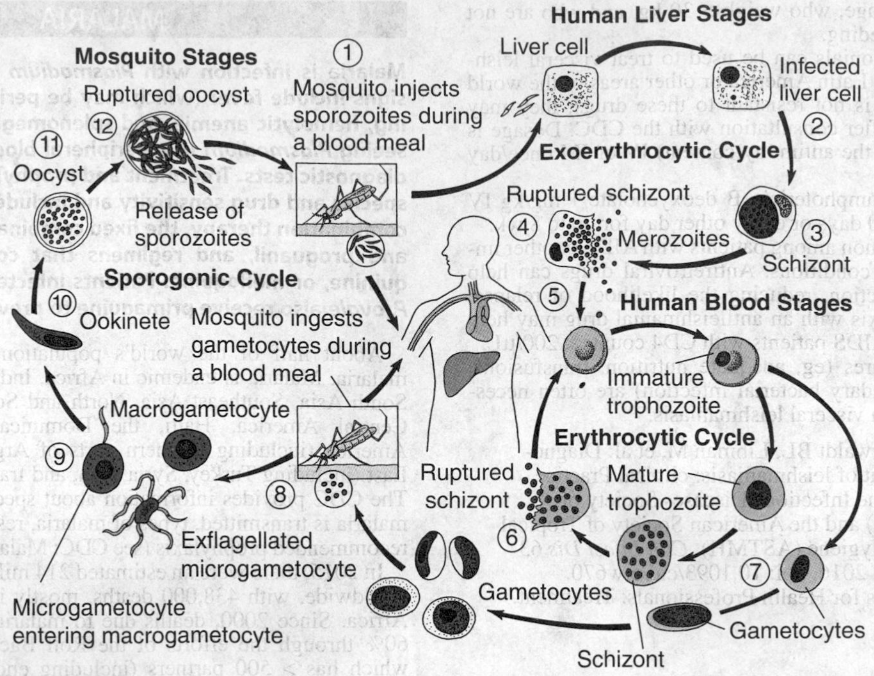

Fig. 188–1. ***Plasmodium* life cycle.** 1. The malaria parasite life cycle involves 2 hosts. During a blood meal, a malaria-infected female *Anopheles* mosquito inoculates sporozoites into the human host. 2. Sporozoites infect liver cells. 3. There, the sporozoites mature into schizonts. 4. The schizonts rupture and release merozoites. This initial replication in the liver is called the exoerythrocytic cycle. 5. Merozoites infect RBCs. There, the parasite multiples asexually (called the erythrocytic cycle). The merozites develop into ring-stage trophozoites. Some then mature into schizonts. 6. The schizonts rupture, releasing merozoites. 7. Some trophozoites differentiate into gametocytes. 8. During a blood meal, an *Anopheles* mosquito ingests the male (microgametocytes) and female (macrogametocytes) gametocytes, beginning the sporogonic cycle. 9. In the mosquito's stomach, the microgametes penetrate the macrogametes, producing zygotes. 10. The zygotes become motile and elongated, developing into ookinetes. 11. The ookinetes invade the midgut wall of the mosquito where they develop into oocysts. 12. The oocysts grow, rupture, and release sporozoites, which travel to the mosquito's salivary glands. Inoculation of the sporozoites into a new human host perpetuates the malaria life cycle.

merozoites then rapidly invade new RBCs, repeating the cycle. Some trophozoites develop into gametocytes, which are ingested by an *Anopheles* mosquito. They undergo sexual union in the gut of the mosquito, develop into oocysts, and release infective sporozoites, which migrate to the salivary glands.

With *P. vivax* and *P. ovale* (but not *P. falciparum* or *P. malariae*), tissue schizonts may persist as hypnozoites in the liver for years. Relapse of *P. ovale* has occurred as late as 6 yr after an episode of symptomatic malaria, and the infection was transmitted by blood transfusion from a person who was exposed 7 yr before donating blood. These dormant forms serve as time-release capsules, which cause relapses and complicate chemotherapy because they are not killed by most antimalarial drugs, which typically act on bloodstream parasites.

The pre-erythrocytic (hepatic) stage of the malarial life cycle is bypassed when infection is transmitted by blood transfusions, by sharing of contaminated needles, or congenitally. Therefore, these modes of transmission do not cause latent disease or delayed recurrences.

Rupture of RBCs during release of merozoites is associated with the clinical symptoms. If severe, hemolysis causes anemia and jaundice, which are worsened by phagocytosis of infected RBCs in the spleen. Anemia may be severe in *P. falciparum* or chronic *P. vivax* infection but tends to be mild in *P. malariae* infection.

Falciparum malaria: Unlike other forms of malaria, *P. falciparum* causes microvascular obstruction because infected RBCs adhere to vascular endothelial cells. Ischemia can develop with resultant tissue hypoxia, particularly in the brain, kidneys, lungs, and GI tract. Hypoglycemia and lactic acidosis are other potential complications.

Resistance to infection: Most West Africans have complete resistance to *P. vivax* because their RBCs lack the Duffy blood group, which is required for the attachment of *P. vivax* to RBCs; many African Americans also have such resistance. The development of *Plasmodium* in RBCs is retarded in patients with hemoglobin S, hemoglobin C, thalassemia, G6PD deficiency, or elliptocytosis.

Previous infections provide partial immunity. Once residents of hyperendemic areas leave, acquired immunity wanes over time (months to years), and symptomatic malaria may develop if they return home and become reinfected.

Symptoms and Signs

The incubation period is usually

- 12 to 17 days for *P. vivax*
- 9 to 14 days for *P. falciparum*
- 16 to 18 days or longer for *P. ovale*
- About 1 mo (18 to 40 days) or longer (years) for *P. malariae*

However, some strains of *P. vivax* in temperate climates may not cause clinical illness for months to > 1 yr after infection.

Manifestations common to all forms of malaria include

- Fever and rigors—the malarial paroxysm
- Anemia
- Jaundice
- Splenomegaly
- Hepatomegaly

The malarial paroxysm coincides with release of merozoites from ruptured RBCs. The classic paroxysm starts with malaise, abrupt chills and fever rising to 39 to 41° C, rapid and thready pulse, polyuria, headache, myalgia, and nausea. After 2 to 6 h, fever falls, and profuse sweating occurs for 2 to 3 h, followed by extreme fatigue. Fever is often hectic at the start of infection. In established infections, malarial paroxysms typically occur every 2 to 3 days depending on the species; intervals are not rigid.

Splenomegaly usually becomes palpable by the end of the first week of clinical disease but may not occur with *P. falciparum*. The enlarged spleen is soft and prone to traumatic rupture. Splenomegaly may decrease with recurrent attacks of malaria as functional immunity develops. After many bouts, the spleen may become fibrotic and firm or, in some patients, becomes massively enlarged (tropical splenomegaly). Hepatomegaly usually accompanies splenomegaly.

***P. falciparum* manifestations:** *P. falciparum* causes the most severe disease because of its microvascular effects. It is the only species likely to cause fatal disease if untreated; nonimmune patients may die within days of their initial symptoms. Temperature spikes and accompanying symptoms typically occur in an irregular pattern but can become synchronous, occurring in a tertian pattern (temperature spikes at 48-h intervals), particularly in residents of endemic areas who are partially immune.

Patients with cerebral malaria may develop symptoms ranging from irritability to seizures and coma. Acute respiratory distress syndrome (ARDS), diarrhea, icterus, epigastric tenderness, retinal hemorrhages, algid malaria (a shocklike syndrome), and severe thrombocytopenia may also occur.

Renal insufficiency may result from volume depletion, vascular obstruction by parasitized erythrocytes, or immune complex deposition. Hemoglobinemia and hemoglobinuria resulting from intravascular hemolysis may progress to blackwater fever (so named based on the dark color of the urine), either spontaneously or after treatment with quinine.

Hypoglycemia is common and may be aggravated by quinine treatment and associated hyperinsulinemia.

Placental involvement may lead to low birth weight, spontaneous abortion, stillbirth, or congenital infection.

***P. vivax, P. ovale,* and *P. malariae* manifestations:** *P. vivax, P. ovale*, and *P. malariae* typically do not compromise vital organs. Mortality is rare and is mostly due to splenic rupture or uncontrolled hyperparasitemia in asplenic patients.

The clinical course with *P. ovale* is similar to that of *P. vivax*. In established infections, temperature spikes occur at 48-h intervals—a tertian pattern.

P. malariae infections may cause no acute symptoms, but low-level parasitemia may persist for decades and lead to immune complex–mediated nephritis or nephrosis or tropical splenomegaly; when symptomatic, fever tends to occur at 72-h intervals—a quartan pattern.

Manifestations in patients taking chemoprophylaxis: In patients who have been taking chemoprophylaxis (see Table 188–4 on p. 1558), malaria may be atypical. The incubation period may extend weeks to months after the drug is stopped. Those infected may develop headache, backache, and irregular fever, but parasites may initially be difficult to find in blood samples.

Diagnosis

- Light microscopy of blood (thin and thick smears)
- Rapid diagnostic tests that detect *Plasmodium* antigens or enzymes in blood

Fever and chills in an immigrant or traveler returning from an endemic region should prompt immediate assessment for malaria. Symptoms usually appear in the first 6 mo after infection, but onset may take up to 2 yr or, rarely, longer.

Malaria can be diagnosed by finding parasites on microscopic examination of thick or thin blood smears. The infecting species (which determines therapy and prognosis) is identified by characteristic features on smears (see Table 188–1). Blood smears should be repeated at 4- to 6-h intervals if the initial smear is negative.

Thin blood smears stained with Wright-Giemsa stain allow assessment of parasite morphology within RBCs, often speciation, and determination of percentage parasitemia. Thick smears are more sensitive but more difficult to prepare and interpret as

Table 188–1. DIAGNOSTIC FEATURES OF *PLASMODIUM* SPECIES IN BLOOD SMEARS

CHARACTERISTIC	*PLASMODIUM VIVAX**	*PLASMODIUM FALCIPARUM*	*PLASMODIUM MALARIAE*†
Infected RBCs enlarged	Yes	No	No
Schüffner dots‡	Yes	No	No
Maurer dots or clefts	No	Yes§	No
Multiple infections in RBCs	Rare	Yes	No
Rings with 2 chromatin dots	Rare	Frequent	No
Crescentic gametocytes	No	Yes	No
Bayonet or band trophozoites	No	No	Yes
Schizonts present in peripheral blood	Yes	Rare	Yes
Number of merozoites per schizont (mean [range])	16 (12–24)	12 (8–24)¶	8 (6–12)

*RBCs infected with *P. ovale* are fimbriated, oval, and slightly enlarged; the parasites otherwise resemble *P. vivax*.
†*P. knowlesi* is morphologically similar to *P. malaria* and has been confused with it.
‡Schüffner dots are best seen when the blood smear is stained with Giemsa stain.
§This feature is not always visible.
¶Schizonts are trapped in viscera and usually are not present in peripheral blood.

the RBCs are lysed before staining. Sensitivity and accuracy of the results depend on the examiner's experience.

Commercial rapid diagnostic tests for malaria are based on the presence of certain plasmodium antigens or enzymatic activities. Assays may involve detection of a histidine-rich protein 2 (HRP-2) associated with malaria parasites (especially *P. falciparum*) and detection of plasmodium-associated lactate dehydrogenase (pLDH). The rapid diagnostic tests are generally comparable in sensitivity to microscopy in detecting low levels of parasitemia, but they do not differentiate single infection from concurrent infection with more than one *Plasmodium* sp or allow speciation except for *P. falciparum*.

Light microscopy and rapid diagnostic tests are complementary tests, and both should be done when available. They have similar sensitivity. Negative results in both does not exclude malaria in a patient with low parasitemia.

PCR and species-specific DNA probes can be used but are not widely available at the point of care. They can help identify the infecting *Plasmodium* sp after malaria is diagnosed. Because serologic tests may reflect prior exposure, they are not useful in the diagnosis of acute malaria.

Treatment

- Antimalarial drugs

Antimalarial drugs are chosen based on the following:

- Clinical manifestations
- Infecting *Plasmodium* sp
- Known resistance patterns of strains in the area of acquisition
- Efficacy and adverse effects of drugs available

Artemisinin-based combination therapy (ACT), such as artemether/lumefantrine, is the most rapidly active treatment, and in many situations, it is the drug of choice. Resistance to artemisinins has been reported but is not yet common.

In some endemic areas, a significant proportion of locally available antimalarial drugs are counterfeit. Thus, some clinicians advise travelers to remote, high-risk areas to take along a full course of an appropriate treatment regimen to be used if medically confirmed malaria is acquired despite prophylaxis; this strategy also avoids depleting limited drug resources in the destination country.

Malaria is particularly dangerous in children < 5 yr (mortality is highest in those < 2 yr), pregnant women, and previously unexposed visitors to endemic areas.

If *P. falciparum* is suspected, therapy should be initiated immediately, even if the initial smear is negative. *P. falciparum* and, more recently, *P. vivax* have become increasingly resistant to antimalarial drugs.

For recommended drugs and doses for treatment and prevention of malaria, see Tables 188–2 and 188–4. Common adverse effects and contraindications are listed in Table 188–3. See also the CDC web site at www.cdc.gov, or for emergency consultation about management, call the CDC Malaria Hotline at 770-488-7788 or 855-856-4713 toll-free Monday-Friday 9 AM to 5 PM EST (after hours, weekends, or holidays, call 770-488-7100).

In case of a febrile illness during travel in an endemic region, prompt professional medical evaluation is essential. When prompt evaluation is not possible (eg, because the region is very remote), self-medication with artemether/lumefantrine or atovaquone/proguanil can be considered pending evaluation. If travelers present with fever after returning from an endemic region and no other diagnosis is made, clinicians should consider giving empiric treatment for uncomplicated malaria even when malaria smears and/or rapid diagnostic tests are negative.

1. Aldámiz-Echevarría LT, López-Polín A, Norman FF et al: Delayed haemolysis secondary to treatment of severe malaria with intravenous artesunate: report on the experience of a referral centre for tropical infections in Spain. *Travel Med Infect Dis* 2016. pii: S1477–8939(16)30166-1. doi: 10.1016/j.tmaid.2016.10.013.

Table 188–2. TREATMENT OF MALARIA

PREFERENCES	DRUG[a]	ADULT DOSAGE	PEDIATRIC DOSAGE[b]
Uncomplicated malaria due to *P. falciparum* or unidentified species acquired in all malarious regions except those specified as chloroquine-sensitive—Oral drugs			
Drugs of choice	Atovaquone/proguanil[c]	4 adult tablets once/day for 3 days	< 5 kg: Not indicated 5–8 kg: 2 pediatric tablets once/day for 3 days 9–10 kg: 3 pediatric tablets once/day for 3 days 11–20 kg: 1 adult tablet once/day for 3 days 21–30 kg: 2 adult tablets once/day for 3 days 31–40 kg: 3 adult tablets once/day for 3 days > 40 kg: 4 adult tablets once/day for 3 days
	or		
	Artemether/lumefantrine[d]	6 doses (1 dose = 4 tablets) over 3 days (at 0, 8, 24, 36, 48, and 60 h)	6 doses at intervals as for the adults; dose = 5– < 15 kg: 1 tablet 15– < 25 kg: 2 tablets 25– < 35 kg: 3 tablets ≥ 35 kg: 4 tablets
	or		
	Quinine sulfate ***plus one of the following:***	650 mg salt tid for 3 or 7 days[e]	10 mg salt/kg q 8 h for 3 or 7 days[e]
	• Doxycycline[f]	100 mg bid for 7 days	2.2 mg/kg bid for 7 days
	• Tetracycline[f]	250 mg qid for 7 days	6.25 mg/kg qid for 7 days
	• Clindamycin[g]	7 mg/kg tid for 7 days	7 mg/kg tid for 7 days
Alternative (if other options cannot be used)	Mefloquine[h]	750 mg salt, then 500 mg salt 6–12 h later	15 mg salt/kg, then 10 mg salt/kg 6–12 h later

Table 188–2. TREATMENT OF MALARIA (*Continued*)

PREFERENCES	DRUG[a]	ADULT DOSAGE	PEDIATRIC DOSAGE[b]
Uncomplicated malaria due to *P. falciparum* and unidentified species acquired in chloroquine-sensitive areas (Central America west of Panama Canal, Haiti, Dominican Republic, most of the Middle East) and *P. malariae* and *P. knowlesi* in all regions—Oral drugs			
Drugs of choice	Chloroquine phosphate[i,j]	1 g salt (600 mg base), then 500 mg salt (300 mg base) at 6, 24, and 48 h	10 mg base/kg (up to 600 mg base), then 5 mg base/kg (up to 300 mg) at 6, 24, and 48 h
	or		
	Hydroxychloroquine[j]	800 mg salt (620 mg base), then 400 mg salt (310 mg base) at 6, 24, and 48 h	10 mg base/kg (up to 620 mg), then 5 mg/kg (up to 310 mg) at 6, 24, and 48 h
Uncomplicated malaria due to *P. vivax* (unless from chloroquine-resistant areas including Papua New Guinea and Indonesia) or *P. ovale*—Oral drugs			
Drugs of choice	Chloroquine phosphate[i,j] or hydroxychloroquine[j] dosed as above		
	plus		
	Primaquine[k]	30 mg base once/day for 14 days	0.5 mg base/kg (maximum 30 mg) once/day for 14 days
Uncomplicated malaria due to *P. vivax* acquired in areas known to harbor chloroquine-resistant *P. vivax*[l] (Papua New Guinea, Indonesia)—Oral drugs			
Drugs of choice	A. Quinine sulfate ***plus one of the following:***	650 mg salt tid for 3 or 7 days[e]	10 mg salt/kg tid for 3 or 7 days[e]
	• Doxycycline[f]	100 mg bid for 7 days	2.2 mg/kg bid for 7 days
	• Tetracycline[f]	250 mg qid for 7 days	6.25 mg/kg qid for 7 days
	or		
	B. Atovaquone/ proguanil[c]	4 adult tablets once/day for 3 days	< 5 kg: Not indicated 5–8 kg: 2 pediatric tablets once/day for 3 days 9–10 kg: 3 pediatric tablets once/day for 3 days 11–20 kg: 1 adult tablet once/day for 3 days 21–30 kg: 2 adult tablets once/day for 3 days 31–40 kg: 3 adult tablets once/day for 3 days > 40 kg: 4 adult tablets once/day for 3 days
	or		
	C. Mefloquine[h]	750 mg salt, then 500 mg 6–12 h later	15 mg salt/kg, then 10 mg/kg 6–12 h later
	For *P. vivax or P. ovale*: Regimen A, B, or C plus		
	Primaquine[k]	30 mg base once/day for 14 days	0.5 mg base/kg (maximum 30 mg) once/day for 14 days
Severe malaria, all *Plasmodium*—Parenteral drugs			
Drugs of choice	Quinidine gluconate[m] ***plus one of the following dosed as above:***	10 mg salt/kg loading dose in normal saline over 1–2 h, then continuous infusion of 0.02 mg salt/kg/min for at least 24 h	Same as for adults (except doxycycline and tetracycline are not used in children < 8 yr)
		or	
	• Doxycycline[f,n] • Tetracycline[f] • Clindamycin[g,o]	24 mg salt/kg loading dose over 4 h, then 12 mg salt/kg infused over 4 h q 8 h, starting 8 h after the loading dose Once parasite density is < 1% and patient can take oral drugs, complete treatment with oral quinine dosed as above	
	or (investigational)		
	Artesunate[p,q] ***followed by one of the following dosed as above:***	As per investigational new drug protocol (contact CDC for drug and dosing information)	Same as for adults (except doxycycline is not used in children)
	• Atovaquone-proguanil[c] • Doxycycline[f,n] • Clindamycin[g,o] • Mefloquine[h]		

Table continues on the following page.

Table 188–2. TREATMENT OF MALARIA (*Continued*)

PREFERENCES	DRUG[a]	ADULT DOSAGE	PEDIATRIC DOSAGE[b]
Prevention of relapses: *P. vivax* and *P. ovale* only			
Drug of choice	Primaquine	30 mg base po once/day for 14 days after leaving the endemic area	0.5 mg base/kg po once/day (maximum 30 mg) for 14 days after leaving the endemic area

[a]See Table 188–3 for adverse reactions and contraindications. If malaria develops during prophylactic drug therapy, that drug should not be used as part of the treatment regimen.

[b]The pediatric dose should not exceed the adult dose.

[c]Atovaquone/proguanil is available as a fixed-dose combination tablet: adult tablets (250 mg atovaquone/100 mg proguanil) and pediatric tablets (62.5 mg atovaquone/25 mg proguanil). To enhance absorption, patients should take it with food or a milky drink. This combination is contraindicated in patients with creatinine clearance < 30 mL/min. Generally, this combination is not recommended for pregnant women, particularly during the 1st trimester, because safety data are insufficient; it may be used if other options are unavailable or are not tolerated and benefits outweigh risks. Twice/day dosing reduces nausea and vomiting as does taking it with food or milk. If patients vomit within 30 min of taking a dose, the dose should be repeated.

[d]Artemether/lumefantrine is available as a fixed-dose combination tablet of 20 mg/120 mg. Generally, this combination is not recommended for use in pregnant women, particularly during the 1st trimester, because safety data are insufficient; it may be used if other options are unavailable or are not tolerated and benefits outweigh risks. Patients should take the drug with food or whole milk. If patients vomit within 30 min of taking a dose, the dose should be repeated.

[e]In the US, quinine sulfate capsules contain 324 mg, so 2 capsules are sufficient for adults. For children, dosing may be more difficult because noncapsule forms of quinine are not available. In Southeast Asia, relative resistance to quinine has increased, and treatment should be continued for 7 days. In other regions, treatment is continued for only 3 days. To reduce risk of GI adverse effects, patients should take quinine with food. Quinine plus doxycycline or tetracycline is generally preferred to quinine plus clindamycin because there is more data on efficacy.

[f]Use of tetracyclines is contraindicated during pregnancy and in children < 8 yr. In children < 8 yr with chloroquine-resistant *P. vivax*, mefloquine is recommended. If these drugs are not available or are not tolerated and if the benefits of treatment outweigh the risks, atovaquone/proguanil or artemether/lumefantrine can be used instead.

[g]Clindamycin is to be used during pregnancy and in children < 8 yr.

[h]Mefloquine is not recommended unless other options cannot be used because the rate of severe neuropsychiatric reactions is higher with mefloquine than with other options. Mefloquine is contraindicated in patients who have active depression, a recent history of depression, generalized anxiety disorder, psychosis, schizophrenia, other major psychiatric disorders, or seizures. Mefloquine is not recommended for infections acquired in Southeast Asia because resistance to mefloquine has been reported in some areas (eg, the Myanmar borders with Thailand, China, and Laos; Thailand-Cambodia border; southern Vietnam).

[i]To reduce risk of GI effects, patients should take chloroquine phosphate with food.

[j]Chloroquine or hydroxychloroquine is recommended for chloroquine-sensitive infections; however, regimens used to treat chloroquine-resistant infections may be used if they are more convenient or preferred or if chloroquine is unavailable.

[k]Primaquine is used to eradicate any hypnozoites that may remain dormant in the liver and thus prevent relapses in *P. vivax* and *P. ovale* infections. Because primaquine can cause hemolytic anemia in patients with G6PD deficiency, G6PD screening must occur before starting treatment with primaquine. For patients with borderline G6PD deficiency or as an alternate to the above regimen, primaquine 45 mg po once/wk may be given for 8 wk; clinicians should consult with an expert in infectious disease and/or tropical medicine if this alternative regimen is being considered for G6PD-deficient patients. Primaquine should not be used during pregnancy.

[l]If patients acquire *P. vivax* infection in regions not known to harbor chloroquine-resistant *P. vivax* infection, treatment should start with chloroquine. If they do not respond, treatment should be changed to a chloroquine-resistant *P. vivax* regimen, and clinicians should call the CDC Malaria Hotline at 770-488-7788 or 855-856-4713 toll-free Monday-Friday 9 AM to 5 PM EST (after hours, weekends, or holidays, 770-488-7100).

[m]The CDC recommends that patients with severe malaria be treated aggressively with parenteral (IV) quinidine started immediately with a loading dose. If patients have received > 40 mg/kg of quinine in the preceding 48 h or mefloquine within 12 h, the quinidine loading dose should be omitted. Consultation with a cardiologist and a physician with expertise in treating severe malaria is advised. BP monitoring for hypotension, cardiac monitoring for widening of the QRS complex or lengthening of the QTc interval, and blood glucose monitoring for hypoglycemia are necessary. Malaria is considered to be severe when patients have ≥ 1 of the following: impaired consciousness, coma or seizure, severe normocytic anemia, renal failure, pulmonary edema, acute respiratory distress syndrome, shock, disseminated intravascular coagulation, spontaneous bleeding, acidosis, hemoglobinuria, jaundice, or parasitemia > 5%. Severe malaria is most often caused by *P. falciparum*.

[n]If patients cannot take oral doxycycline, 100 mg is given IV q 12 h, then switched to oral administration as soon as patients are able. Rapid IV administration should be avoided. Treatment course is 7 days.

[o]If patients cannot take oral clindamycin, a loading dose of 10 mg base/kg is given IV, followed by 5 mg base/kg q 8 h, then switched to oral administration as soon as patients are able. Rapid IV administration should be avoided. Treatment course is 7 days.

[p]In the US, artesunate for IV administration is available only as an investigational new drug (obtained through the CDC by calling the CDC Malaria Hotline [770-488-7788 or 855-856-4713 or, after hours and on weekends and holidays, 770-488-7100]).

[q]One of the following (using oral treatment doses) should be given with artesunate:

- In adults: Atovaquone/proguanil, doxycycline, clindamycin (in pregnant women), or mefloquine
- In children: Atovaquone/proguanil, clindamycin, or mefloquine

G6PD = glucose-6-phosphate dehydrogenase.

Adapted from the Centers for Disease Control and Prevention: Malaria diagnosis and treatment in the United States.

Table 188–3. ADVERSE REACTIONS AND CONTRAINDICATIONS OF ANTIMALARIAL DRUGS

DRUG	SOME ADVERSE REACTIONS	CONTRAINDICATIONS
Artemether/lumefantrine	Headache, anorexia, dizziness, asthenia (usually mild) With lumefantrine, prolonged QT interval	During pregnancy, used only if potential benefit justifies potential risk to fetus Use of mefloquine prophylaxis
Artesunate	As with artemether Delayed hemolysis[1]	As with artemether
Atovaquone/proguanil	GI disturbances, headache, dizziness, rash, pruritus	During pregnancy, used only if there are no alternatives and potential benefit justifies potential risk to fetus Hypersensitivity, breastfeeding*, severe renal impairment (creatinine clearance < 30 mL/min)
Chloroquine phosphate Chloroquine hydrochloride Hydroxychloroquine sulfate	GI disturbances, headaches, dizziness, blurred vision, rashes or pruritus, exacerbation of psoriasis, blood dyscrasias, alopecia, ECG changes, retinopathy, psychosis (rare)	Hypersensitivity, retinal or visual field changes
Clindamycin	Hypotension, bone marrow toxicity, renal dysfunction, rashes, jaundice, tinnitus, *Clostridium difficile* infection (pseudomembranous colitis)	Hypersensitivity
Doxycycline	GI upset, photosensitivity, vaginal candidiasis, *C. difficile* infection (pseudomembranous colitis), erosive esophagitis	Pregnancy, children < 8 yr
Halofantrine	Prolongation of PR and QT intervals, cardiac arrhythmia, hypotension, GI disturbances, dizziness, mental changes, seizures, sudden death	During pregnancy, used only if potential benefit justifies potential risk to fetus Cardiac conduction defects, familial QT prolongation, use of drugs that affect QT interval, hypersensitivity
Mefloquine	Bad dreams, neuropsychiatric symptoms, dizziness, vertigo, confusion, psychosis, seizures, sinus bradycardia, GI disturbances	Hypersensitivity, history of seizures or psychiatric disorders, cardiac conduction disturbances or arrhythmia, coadministration of drugs that may prolong cardiac conduction (eg, beta-blockers, calcium channel blockers, quinine, quinidine, halofantrine), occupations that require fine coordination and spatial discrimination and in which vertigo may be life threatening, 1st trimester of pregnancy
Quinine sulfate Quinine dihydrochloride	GI disturbances, tinnitus, visual disturbances, allergic reactions, mental changes, arrhythmias, cardiotoxicity	Hypersensitivity, G6PD deficiency, optic neuritis, tinnitus, pregnancy (relative contraindication), past adverse quinine reaction (continuous ECG, BP [when drug is given IV], and glucose monitoring recommended)
Quinidine gluconate	Arrhythmias, widened QRS complex, prolonged QTc interval, hypotension, hypoglycemia	Hypersensitivity, thrombocytopenia (continuous ECG, BP, and glucose monitoring recommended) No loading dose in patients receiving > 40 mg/kg of quinine in the preceding 48 h or a dose of mefloquine in preceding 12 h
Primaquine phosphate	Severe intravascular hemolysis in people with G6PD deficiency, GI disturbances, leukopenia, methemoglobinuria	Concomitant use of quinacrine or potentially hemolytic or bone marrow suppressing agents, G6PD deficiency, pregnancy (because G6PD status of the fetus is unknown)
Pyrimethamine/sulfadoxine	Erythema multiforme, Stevens-Johnson syndrome, toxic epidermal neurolysis, urticaria, exfoliative dermatitis, serum sickness, hepatitis, seizures, mental changes, GI disturbances, stomatitis, pancreatitis, bone marrow toxicity, hemolysis, fever, nephrosis	Hypersensitivity, folate deficiency anemia, infants ≤ 2 mo, pregnancy, breastfeeding

*Proguanil is excreted in human milk; whether atovaquone is excreted in human milk is unknown. Safety and effectiveness of these drugs have not been established in children who weigh < 5 kg.

G6PD =glucose-6-phosphate dehydrogenase.

Table 188–4. PREVENTION OF MALARIA

DRUG[a]	USE	ADULT DOSAGE	PEDIATRIC DOSAGE	COMMENTS
Atovaquone/proguanil[b]	In all areas	1 adult tablet once/day	5–8 kg: one-half pediatric tablet once/day > 8–10 kg: three-fourths pediatric tablet once/day > 10–20 kg: 1 pediatric tablet once/day > 20–30 kg: 2 pediatric tablets once/day > 30–40 kg: 3 pediatric tablets once/day > 40 kg: 1 adult tablet once/day	Begun 1 to 2 days before travel and continued daily during the stay and for 7 days after leaving
Chloroquine phosphate	Only in areas with chloroquine-sensitive *Plasmodium*	500 mg salt (300 mg base) po once/wk	8.3 mg salt/ kg (5 mg base/kg), up to maximum 500 mg salt (300 mg base) po once/wk	Begun 1–2 wk before travel and continued weekly during the stay and for 4 wk after leaving
Doxycycline[c]	In all areas	100 mg po once/day	≥ 8 yr: 2.2 mg/kg (up to 100 mg) po once/day	Begun 1–2 days before travel and continued during the stay and for 4 wk after leaving
Hydroxychloroquine[d]	An alternative to chloroquine only in areas with chloroquine-sensitive *Plasmodium*	400 mg salt (310 mg base) po once/wk	6.5 mg salt/kg (5 mg base/kg), up to 400 mg salt (310 mg base) po once/wk	Begun 1–2 wk before travel and continued during the stay and for 4 wk after leaving
Mefloquine[e]	In areas with mefloquine-sensitive *Plasmodium*	250 mg salt (228 mg base) po once/wk	≤ 9 kg: 5 mg salt (4.6 mg/kg base) once/wk > 9–19 kg: one-fourth tablet once/wk > 19–30 kg: one-half tablet once/wk > 30–45 kg: three-fourths tablet once/wk > 45 kg: 1 tablet once/wk	Begun ≥ 2 wk before travel and continued during the stay and for 4 wk after leaving Contraindicated in patients with a history of depression, other psychologic problems, or seizures; not recommended for patients with cardiac conduction abnormalities
Primaquine[f]	For prophylaxis for brief travel in areas known to harbor mainly *P. vivax*	30 mg base (52.6 mg salt) po once/day	0.5 mg base/kg (0.8 mg salt /kg) up to adult dose po once/day	Begun 1 to 2 days before travel and continued daily during the stay and for 7 days after departure Document that the G6PD level is normal before use Contraindicated in people with G6PD deficiency and in pregnant and breastfeeding women unless the breastfed infant has a normal G6PD level
	For terminal prophylaxis to prevent relapse of infection in people with prolonged exposure to or prior infection with *P. vivax* or *P. ovale*	Dosed as above	Dosed as above	Given daily for 14 days after departure from endemic area. Document that the G6PD level is normal before use Contraindications as above

[a]See Table 188–3 for adverse reactions and contraindications.

[b]Atovaquone/proguanil is available as a fixed-dose combination tablet: adult tablets (250 mg atovaquone/100 mg proguanil) and pediatric tablets (62.5 mg atovaquone/25 mg proguanil). To enhance absorption, patients should take the drug with food or a milky drink. Atovaquone/proguanil is contraindicated in patients with a creatinine clearance < 30 mL/min. This combination is not recommended for children weighing < 5 kg or for pregnant or breastfeeding women.

[c]Use of tetracyclines is contraindicated during pregnancy and in children < 8 yr.

[d]Physicians should review the prescribing information for hydroxychloroquine before using it.

[e]Mefloquine has not been approved for use during pregnancy. The drug is contraindicated in patients who have active depression, a recent history of depression, generalized anxiety disorder, psychosis, schizophrenia, other major psychiatric disorders, or seizures; if patients have psychiatric disturbances or a previous history of depression, the drug should be used cautiously. The drug is not recommended for patients with cardiac conduction abnormalities.

[f]Primaquine is used as terminal prophylaxis to reduce risk of relapse in people who have taken chloroquine or a drug active against chloroquine-resistant malaria and have had prolonged exposure to *P. vivax* and/or *P. ovale*. Primaquine alone can also be used for primary prophylaxis in people at risk of malaria, particularly that due to *P. vivax*. It is contraindicated in people with G6PD deficiency and in pregnant or breastfeeding women (unless the breastfed infant has a normal G6PD level).

G6PD = glucose-6-phosphate dehydrogenase.

Adapted from the CDC's *Yellow Book*: Infectious diseases related to travel: Malaria.

Prevention of Relapses of *P. vivax* or *P. ovale* Malaria

Hypnozoites must be eliminated from the liver with primaquine to prevent relapses of *P. vivax* or *P. ovale*. Primaquine may be given simultaneously with chloroquine or afterward. Some *P. vivax* strains are less sensitive, and relapse may occur, requiring repeated treatment. Primaquine is not necessary for *P. falciparum* or *P. malariae* because these species do not have a persistent hepatic phase. If exposure to *P. vivax* or *P. ovale* is intense or prolonged or if travelers are asplenic, a 14-day prophylactic course of primaquine phosphate starting when travelers return reduces the risk of recurrence. The main adverse effect is hemolysis in people with glucose-6-phosphate dehydrogenase (G6PD) deficiency. G6PD levels should be determined before primaquine is given.

Primaquine is contraindicated during pregnancy and breastfeeding, unless the infant has been shown not to be G6PD deficient. In pregnant women, chemoprophylaxis with weekly chloroquine can be given for the remainder of pregnancy, and after delivery, women can be given primaquine, provided they are not G6PD deficient.

Prevention

Travelers to endemic regions should be given chemoprophylaxis (see Table 188–4). Information about countries where malaria is endemic is available from the CDC (www.cdc.gov); the information includes types of malaria, resistance patterns, geographic distribution, and recommended prophylaxis.

Malaria during pregnancy poses a serious threat to both mother and fetus. Chloroquine can be used during pregnancy in areas where *Plasmodium* sp are susceptible, but there is no other safe and effective prophylactic regimen, so pregnant women should avoid travel to chloroquine-resistant areas whenever possible. The safety of mefloquine during pregnancy has not been documented, but limited experience suggests that it may be used when the benefits are judged to outweigh the risks. Doxycycline, atovaquone/proguanil, and primaquine should not be used during pregnancy.

Artemisinins have a short half-life and are not useful for prophylaxis.

Prophylactic measures against mosquitoes include

- Using permethrin- or pyrethrum-containing residual insecticide sprays (which have prolonged duration of action)
- Placing screens on doors and windows
- Using mosquito netting (preferably impregnated with permethrin or pyrethrum) around beds
- Treating clothing and gear (eg, boots, pants, socks, tents) with products containing 0.5% permethrin, which remain protective through several washings (pretreated clothing is available and may protect longer)
- Applying mosquito repellents such as DEET 25 to 35% to exposed skin
- Wearing protective long-sleeved shirts and pants, especially between dusk and dawn, when *Anopheles* mosquitoes are active

People who plan to use repellents that contain DEET should be instructed to

- Apply repellents only to exposed skin as directed on the label and use them sparingly around ears (they should not be applied to or sprayed in the eyes or mouth).
- Wash hands after application.
- Not allow children to handle repellents (adults should apply the repellent to their hands first, then gently spread it on the child's skin).
- Apply just enough repellent to cover the exposed area.
- Wash the repellant off after returning indoors.
- Wash clothing before wearing again unless indicated otherwise by the product label.

Most repellents can be used on infants and children < 2 mo. The Environmental Protection Agency does not recommend additional precautions for using registered repellents on children or on pregnant or breastfeeding women.

Malaria vaccines are under development. A multicenter clinical trial of the RTS,S recombinant vaccine based on the *P. falciparum* circumsporozoite protein showed short-term partial efficacy, resulting in 46% fewer cases of clinical malaria in young children living in endemic regions of Africa, but not long-term protection. It is unclear when a vaccine is likely to become available.

KEY POINTS

- In 2015, there were an estimated 214 million people with malaria worldwide, and about 438,000 deaths occurred, mostly in children < 5 yr in Africa; since 2000, deaths due to malaria have decreased by about 60%.
- *P. falciparum* causes microvascular obstruction and tissue ischemia, particularly in the brain, kidneys, lungs, and GI tract of nonimmune infants and adults; patients may die within days of their initial symptoms.
- *P. vivax, P. ovale*, and *P. malariae* typically do not compromise vital organs; mortality is rare.
- Manifestations include recurrent fever and rigor, headache, myalgia, and nausea; hemolytic anemia and splenomegaly are common.
- Diagnose using light microscopy of blood (thin and thick smears) and rapid diagnostic blood tests.
- Treat with antimalarial drugs based on the species (if known) and drug resistance patterns in the area in which infection was acquired.
- Artemisinin-based combination therapy (eg, artemether/lumefantrine) is the most rapidly active therapy and is available worldwide; atovaquone plus proguanil is an alternative for patients with uncomplicated malaria.
- Use primaquine for confirmed or suspected infections with *P. vivax* and *P. ovale* to prevent relapse unless patients are pregnant or have G6PD deficiency.
- Give chemoprophylaxis to travelers to endemic areas, and teach them ways to prevent mosquito bites.

TOXOPLASMOSIS

Toxoplasmosis is infection with *Toxoplasma gondii*. Symptoms range from none to benign lymphadenopathy (a mononucleosis-like illness) to life-threatening CNS disease or involvement of other organs in immunocompromised people. Encephalitis can develop in patients with AIDS and low CD4 counts. Retinochoroiditis, seizures, and intellectual disability occur in congenital infection. Diagnosis is by serologic tests, histopathology, or PCR. Treatment is most often with pyrimethamine plus either sulfadiazine or clindamycin. Corticosteroids are given concurrently for retinochoroiditis.

Human exposure to toxoplasmosis is common wherever cats are found; an estimated 15% of residents in the US are seropositive, which indicates that they have been infected. The risk of developing disease is very low except for a fetus infected in utero and people who are or become immunocompromised.

Pathophysiology

T. gondii is ubiquitous in birds and mammals. This obligate intracellular parasite invades and multiplies asexually as tachyzoites within the cytoplasm of any nucleated cell (see Fig. 188–2). When host immunity develops, multiplication of tachyzoites ceases and tissue cysts form; cysts persist in a dormant state for years, especially in brain, eyes, and muscle. The dormant *Toxoplasma* forms within the cysts are called bradyzoites.

Sexual reproduction of *T. gondii* occurs only in the intestinal tract of cats; the resultant oocysts passed in the feces remain infectious in moist soil for months.

Infection can occur by

- Ingestion of oocysts
- Ingestion of tissue cysts
- Transplacental transmission
- Blood transfusion or organ transplantation

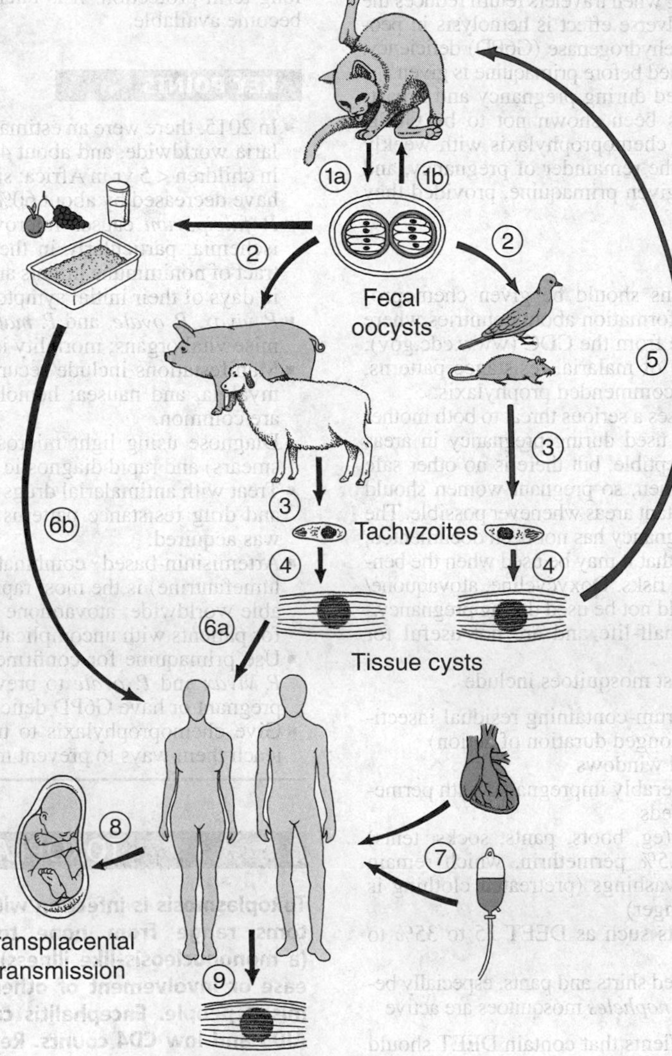

Fig. 188–2. *Toxoplasma gondii* life cycle. The only known definitive hosts for *T. gondii* are members of family Felidae (domestic cats and their relatives). 1a. Oocysts are shed in the cat's feces. Large numbers are shed, but usually only for 1–2 wk. Oocysts take 1–5 days to become infective. 1b. Cats become reinfected by ingesting sporulated oocysts. 2. Soil, water, plant material, or cat litter becomes contaminated with oocysts. Intermediate hosts in nature (eg, birds, rodents, wild game, animals bred for human consumption) become infected after ingesting infected materials. 3. Oocysts develop into tachyzoites shortly after ingestion. 4. Tachyzoites spread throughout the body and form tissue cysts in neural and muscle tissue. 5. Cats become infected after consuming intermediate hosts containing tissue cysts. 6a. Humans can become infected by ingesting undercooked meat containing tissue cysts. 6b. Humans can become infected by ingesting food or water contaminated with cat feces or other feces-contaminated materials (eg, soil) or contact with a pet cat's litter. 7. Rarely, human infection results from blood transfusion or organ transplantation. 8. Rarely, transplacental transmission from mother to fetus occurs. 9. In the human host, parasites form tissue cysts, most commonly in skeletal muscle, myocardium, the brain, and the eyes; these cysts may remain throughout the life of the host and can reactivate if the host becomes immunocompromised.

Ingestion of oocysts in food or water contaminated with cat feces is the most common mode of oral infection. Infection can also occur by eating raw or undercooked meat containing tissue cysts, most commonly lamb, pork, or rarely beef.

After ingestion of oocysts or tissue cysts, tachyzoites are released and spread throughout the body. This acute infection is followed by the development of protective immune responses and the formation of tissue cysts in many organs. The cysts can reactivate, primarily in immunocompromised patients. Toxoplasmosis reactivates in 30 to 40% of AIDS patients who are not taking antibiotic prophylaxis, but the widespread use of trimethoprim/sulfamethoxazole for *Pneumocystis* prophylaxis has dramatically reduced the incidence.

Toxoplasmosis can be transmitted transplacentally if the mother becomes infected during pregnancy or if immunosuppression reactivates a prior infection. Transmission of *Toxoplasma* to a fetus is extraordinarily rare in immunocompetent mothers who have had toxoplasmosis earlier in life.

Transmission may occur via transfusion of whole blood or WBCs or via transplantation of an organ from a seropositive donor.

In otherwise healthy people, congenital or acquired infection can reactivate. Past infection confers resistance to reinfection.

Symptoms and Signs

Infections may manifest in several ways:

- Acute toxoplasmosis
- CNS toxoplasmosis
- Congenital toxoplasmosis
- Ocular toxoplasmosis
- Disseminated or non-CNS disease in immunocompromised patients

Acute toxoplasmosis: Acute infection is usually asymptomatic, but 10 to 20% of patients develop bilateral, nontender cervical or axillary lymphadenopathy. A few of these also have a mild flu-like syndrome of fever, malaise, myalgia, hepatosplenomegaly, and less commonly, pharyngitis, which can mimic infectious mononucleosis and include lymphadenitis. Atypical lymphocytosis, mild anemia, leukopenia, and slightly elevated liver enzymes are common. The syndrome may persist for weeks but is almost always self-limited.

CNS toxoplasmosis: Most patients with AIDS or other immunocompromised patients who develop toxoplasmosis present with encephalitis and ring-enhancing intracranial mass lesions seen on CT scan with contrast. Risk is greatest among those with CD4 counts of < 50/μL; toxoplasmic encephalitis is rare when CD4 counts are > 200/μL. These patients typically have headache, altered mental status, seizures, coma, fever, and sometimes focal neurologic deficits, such as motor or sensory loss, cranial nerve palsies, visual abnormalities, and focal seizures.

Congenital toxoplasmosis: This type results from a primary, often asymptomatic infection acquired by the mother during pregnancy. Women infected before conception ordinarily do not transmit toxoplasmosis to the fetus unless the infection is reactivated during pregnancy by immunosuppression. Spontaneous abortion, stillbirth, or birth defects may occur. The percentage of surviving fetuses born with toxoplasmosis depends on when maternal infection is acquired; it increases from 15% during the 1st trimester to 30% during the 2nd to 60% during the 3rd.

Disease in neonates may be severe, particularly if acquired early in pregnancy; symptoms include jaundice, rash, hepatosplenomegaly, and the characteristic tetrad of abnormalities:

- Bilateral retinochoroiditis
- Cerebral calcifications
- Hydrocephalus or microcephaly
- Psychomotor retardation

Prognosis is poor.

Many children with less severe infections and most infants born to mothers infected during the 3rd trimester appear healthy at birth but are at high risk of seizures, intellectual disability, retinochoroiditis, or other symptoms developing months or even years later.

Ocular toxoplasmosis: This type usually results from congenital infection that is reactivated, often during the teens and 20s, but rarely, it occurs with acquired infections. Focal necrotizing retinitis and a secondary granulomatous inflammation of the choroid occur and may cause ocular pain, blurred vision, and sometimes blindness. Relapses are common.

Disseminated infection and non-CNS involvement: Disease outside the eye and CNS is much less common and occurs primarily in severely immunocompromised patients. They may present with pneumonitis, myocarditis, polymyositis, diffuse maculopapular rash, high fevers, chills, and prostration.

In toxoplasmic pneumonitis, diffuse interstitial infiltrates may progress rapidly to consolidation and cause respiratory failure, whereas endarteritis may lead to infarction of small lung segments. Myocarditis, in which conduction defects are common but often asymptomatic, may rapidly lead to heart failure.

Untreated disseminated infections are usually fatal.

Diagnosis

- Serologic testing
- For CNS involvement, CT or MRI and lumbar puncture
- Histopathologic evaluation of biopsies
- PCR-based assays of blood, CSF, tissue, or, during pregnancy, amniotic fluid

Toxoplasmosis is usually diagnosed serologically using an indirect fluorescent antibody (IFA) test or enzyme immunoassay (EIA) for IgG and IgM antibodies (see Table 188–5). Specific IgM antibodies appear during the first 2 wk of acute illness, peak within 4 to 8 wk, and eventually become undetectable, but they may be present for as long as 18 mo after acute infection. IgG antibodies arise more slowly, peak in 1 to 2 mo, and may remain high and stable for months to years. Assays for toxoplasma IgM lack specificity.

The diagnosis of acute toxoplasmosis during pregnancy and in the fetus or neonate can be difficult, and consultation with an expert is recommended. If the patient is pregnant and IgG and IgM are positive, an IgG avidity test should be done. High avidity antibodies in the first 12 to 16 wk of pregnancy essentially rules out an infection acquired during gestation. But a low IgG avidity result cannot be interpreted as indicating recent infection because some patients have persistent low IgG avidity for many months after infection. Suspected recent infection in a pregnant woman should be confirmed before intervention by having samples tested at a toxoplasmosis reference laboratory. If the patient has clinical illness compatible with toxoplasmosis but the IgG titer is low, a follow-up titer 2 to 3 wk later should show an increase in antibody titer if the illness is due to acute toxoplasmosis, unless the host is severely immunocompromised.

In general, detection of specific IgM antibody in neonates suggests congenital infection. Maternal IgG crosses the placenta, but IgM does not. Detection of *Toxoplasma*-specific IgA antibodies is more sensitive than IgM in congenitally infected infants, but it is available only at special reference facilities (eg, Palo Alto Medical Foundation [telephone 650-853-4828]). An expert should be consulted when fetal or congenital infection is suspected.

Table 188–5. INTERPRETATION OF *TOXOPLASMA* SEROLOGIC TESTING*

IgG	IgM	INTERPRETATION†
Negative	Negative	No evidence of infection
Negative	Equivocal	Possibly early infection or false-positive IgM result
Negative	Positive	Possibly acute infection or false-positive IgM result
Equivocal	Negative	Indeterminate
Equivocal	Equivocal	Indeterminate
Equivocal	Positive	Possibly acute infection
Positive	Negative	Infection for ≥ 6 mo
Positive	Equivocal	Infection for probably > 1 yr or false-positive IgM result
Positive	Positive	Possibly recent infection in the last 12 mo or false-positive IgM result

*Except in infants.

†If results are equivocal or interpretation is uncertain, testing additional samples at a reference laboratory or testing samples taken at a later time may provide useful information.

Adapted from the CDC: Toxoplasmosis: Laboratory Diagnosis.

Toxoplasma are occasionally demonstrated histologically. Tachyzoites, which are present during acute infection, take up Giemsa or Wright stain but may be difficult to find in routine tissue sections. Tissue cysts do not distinguish acute from chronic infection. *Toxoplasma* must be distinguished from other intracellular organisms, such as Histoplasma, Trypanosoma cruzi, and Leishmania. PCR tests for parasite DNA in blood, CSF, or amniotic fluid are available at several reference laboratories. PCR-based analysis of amniotic fluid is the preferred method to diagnose toxoplasmosis during pregnancy.

If CNS toxoplasmosis is suspected, patients should have head MRI, CT with contrast agent, or both plus a lumbar puncture if there are no signs of increased intracranial pressure. MRI is more sensitive than CT. MRI and CT with contrast typically show single or multiple rounded, ring-enhancing lesions. Although these lesions are not pathognomonic, their presence in patients with AIDS and CNS symptoms warrants a trial of chemotherapy for *T. gondii*. CSF may be positive for lymphocytic pleocytosis, and the protein level may be elevated.

Acute infection should be suspected in immunocompromised patients if the IgG is positive. However, IgG antibody levels in AIDS patients with *Toxoplasma* encephalitis are usually low to moderate, and IgG antibodies are sometimes absent; IgM antibodies are not present.

If the suspected diagnosis of toxoplasmosis is correct, clinical and radiographic improvement should become evident within 7 to 14 days. If symptoms worsen over the 1st wk or do not lessen by the end of the 2nd wk, a brain biopsy should be considered.

Ocular disease is diagnosed based on the appearance of the lesions in the eye, symptoms, course of disease, and results of serologic testing.

Treatment

- Pyrimethamine and sulfadiazine plus leucovorin (to prevent bone marrow suppression)
- Clindamycin or atovaquone plus pyrimethamine when the patient is allergic to sulfonamides or does not tolerate sulfadiazine

Treatment of toxoplasmosis is not indicated for immunocompetent patients who are asymptomatic or have mild, uncomplicated acute infection; treatment is required only when visceral disease is present or symptoms are severe or persist.

However, specific treatment is indicated for acute toxoplasmosis in the following:

- Neonates
- Pregnant women with acute toxoplasmosis
- Immunocompromised patients

PEARLS & PITFALLS

- No treatment is required for immunocompetent patients who are asymptomatic or have mild, uncomplicated acute toxoplasmosis.

Treatment of immunocompetent patients: The most effective regimen in immunocompetent patients is pyrimethamine plus sulfadiazine. Dosage is

- Pyrimethamine: 100 mg on day 1, then 25 to 50 mg once/day for 2 to 4 wk in adults (2 mg/kg po for 2 days, then 1 mg/kg once/day in children; maximum 25 mg/day).
- Sulfadiazine: 1 g po qid for 2 to 4 wk in adults (25 to 50 mg/kg qid in children)

Leucovorin is given concurrently to help protect against bone marrow suppression.

In patients who have or develop sulfonamide hypersensitivity, clindamycin 600 to 800 mg po tid is given with pyrimethamine instead of sulfonamides. Another option is atovaquone 1500 mg q 12 h plus pyrimethamine.

Treatment of immunocompromised patients: Higher doses of pyrimethamine are used in HIV-infected patients with CNS toxoplasmosis. A loading dose of pyrimethamine 200 mg is given the first day, then 50 to 100 mg/day plus sulfadiazine for at least 6 wk. Pyrimethamine bone marrow suppression can be minimized with leucovorin (also called folinic acid; not folate, which blocks the therapeutic effect). Dosage is 10 to 25 mg po once/day (7.5 mg once/day in children). Even when leucovorin is given, the CBC should be monitored weekly.

Antiretroviral therapy should be optimized in patients with concurrent HIV/AIDS or other immunocompromising infections. Relapses of toxoplasmosis are common in patients with AIDS, and suppressive treatment should continue indefinitely unless the CD4 count increases and remains > 200/μL and patients remain symptom-free for > 3 mo.

Treatment of ocular toxoplasmosis: Treatment of ocular toxoplasmosis is based on results of a complete ophthalmologic evaluation (degree of inflammation; visual acuity; size, location, and persistence of lesion). Dosages used for pyrimethamine, sulfadiazine, and leucovorin are similar to those of immunocompetent patients. The CDC (www.cdc.gov) recommends that therapy for ocular toxoplasmosis be continued for 4 to 6 wk, followed by reevaluation of the patient's condition.

Patients with ocular toxoplasmosis are also frequently given corticosteroids to reduce inflammation.

Treatment of pregnant patients: Treatment of pregnant women with acute toxoplasmosis can decrease the incidence of fetal infection.

Spiramycin 1 g po tid or qid has been used safely to reduce transmission in pregnant women during the 1st trimester (available from the FDA [telephone 301-827-2335]), but spiramycin is less active than pyrimethamine plus sulfonamide and does not cross the placenta. Spiramycin is continued until fetal infection is documented or excluded at the end of the 1st trimester.

Amniotic fluid is obtained at 18 wk gestational age and is tested using a PCR-based assay to determine whether a fetus is infected. If no transmission has occurred, spiramycin can be continued to term. If the fetus is infected, pyrimethamine plus sulfadiazine plus leucovorin is used during the 2nd and 3rd trimesters. Pyrimethamine is a potent teratogen and should not be used during the 1st trimester.

Consultation with an infectious diseases expert is recommended.

Treatment of infants with congenital toxoplasmosis: Congenitally infected infants should be treated with pyrimethamine every 2 to 3 days and with sulfadiazine once/day for 1 yr. Infants should also receive leucovorin while receiving pyrimethamine and for 1 wk after pyrimethamine is stopped to prevent bone marrow suppression.

Prevention

Washing hands thoroughly after handling raw meat, soil, or cat litter is essential. Food possibly contaminated with cat feces should be avoided. Meat should be cooked to 165 to 170° F (73.9 to 76.7° C).

Pregnant women are advised to avoid contact with cats. If contact is unavoidable, pregnant women should at least avoid cleaning cat litter boxes or wear gloves when doing so.

Chemoprophylaxis is recommended for patients with HIV and a positive IgG *T. gondii* serologic test once CD4 cell counts are < 100/μL. One double-strength tablet of trimethoprim/sulfamethoxazole once/day, which also is prophylactic against *Pneumocystis jirovecii*, is recommended. If this dosage is not tolerated, alternatives are one double-strength tablet 3 times/wk or one single-strength tablet daily. If patients cannot tolerate trimethoprim-sulfamethoxazole, dapsone plus pyrimethamine and leucovorin can be used. Atovaquone with or without pyrimethamine and leucovorin is another option. Chemoprophylaxis is continued until CD4 cell counts are > 200/μL for ≥ 3 mo.

KEY POINTS

- *T. gondii* reproduces sexually in the intestinal tract of cats; most human infections result from direct or indirect contact with cat feces but can be acquired transplacentally or by ingestion of poorly cooked meat that contains cysts.
- About 15% of the US population have been infected with *T. gondii*, but symptomatic disease is rare and occurs mainly in fetuses who are infected when the mother acquires acute infection during pregnancy and transmits the infection transplacentally or in people who are immunocompromised.
- Acute infection is usually asymptomatic, but 10 to 20% of patients have manifestations, similar to those of mononucleosis, including lymphadenitis.
- Immunocompromised patients typically present with encephalitis and have ring-enhancing intracranial mass lesions, seen on MRI or CT with contrast.
- To diagnose, use serologic tests (for IgG and IgM antibodies), histopathology, or PCR.
- Treatment is indicated mainly for congenitally infected neonates, pregnant women with acute infection, and immunocompromised patients.
- Use pyrimethamine and sulfadiazine plus leucovorin or, if the patient is allergic to sulfonamides or sulfadiazine is not tolerated, pyrimethamine and clindamycin.
- Pyrimethamine is a potent teratogen and should not be used during the 1st trimester.
- Antiretroviral therapy is optimized in patients with AIDS; suppressive treatment is continued until patients are asymptomatic and CD4 cell counts are > 200/uL for > 3 mo.

189 Fungi

Fungal infections are often classified as opportunistic or primary. Opportunistic infections are those that develop mainly in immunocompromised hosts; primary infections can develop in immunocompetent hosts. Fungal infections can be systemic or local. Local fungal infections typically involve the skin (see p. 1031), mouth (see p. 869), and/or vagina (see p. 2314) and may occur in normal or immunocompromised hosts.

Opportunistic fungal infections: Many fungi are opportunists and are usually not pathogenic except in an immunocompromised host. Causes of immunocompromise include AIDS, azotemia, diabetes mellitus, lymphoma, leukemia, other hematologic cancers, burns, and therapy with corticosteroids, immunosuppressants, or antimetabolites. Patients who spend more than several days in an ICU can become compromised because of medical procedures, underlying disorders, and/or undernutrition.

Typical opportunistic systemic fungal infections (mycoses) include

- Candidiasis
- Aspergillosis
- Mucormycosis (zygomycosis)
- Fusariosis

Systemic mycoses affecting severely immunocompromised patients often manifest acutely with rapidly progressive pneumonia, fungemia, or manifestations of extrapulmonary dissemination.

Primary fungal infections: These infections usually result from inhalation of fungal spores, which can cause a localized pneumonia as the primary manifestation of infection. In immunocompetent patients, systemic mycoses typically have a chronic course; disseminated mycoses with pneumonia and septicemia are rare and, if lung lesions develop, usually progress slowly. Months may elapse before medical attention is sought or a diagnosis is made. Symptoms are rarely intense in such chronic mycoses, but fever, chills, night sweats, anorexia, weight loss, malaise, and depression may occur. Various organs may be infected, causing symptoms and dysfunction.

Primary fungal infections may have a characteristic geographic distribution, which is especially true for the endemic mycoses caused by certain dimorphic fungi. For example,

- Coccidioidomycosis: Confined primarily to the southwestern US and northern Mexico
- Histoplasmosis: Occurring primarily in the eastern and Midwestern US
- Blastomycosis: Confined to North America and Africa
- Paracoccidioidomycosis (formerly, South American blastomycosis): Confined to that continent

However, travelers can manifest disease any time after returning from endemic areas.

When fungi disseminate from a primary focus in the lung, the manifestations may be characteristic, as for the following:

- Cryptococcosis: Usually, chronic meningitis
- Progressive disseminated histoplasmosis: Generalized involvement of the reticuloendothelial system (liver, spleen, bone marrow)
- Blastomycosis: Single or multiple skin lesions or involvement of the prostate
- Coccidioidomycosis: Bone and joint infections, skin lesions, and meningitis

Diagnosis

- Cultures and stains
- Serologic tests (mainly for *Aspergillus*, *Blastomyces*, *Candida*, *Coccidioides*, *Cryptococcus,* and *Histoplasma*)
- Histopathology

If clinicians suspect an acute or a chronic primary fungal infection, they should obtain a detailed travel and residential history to determine whether patients may have been exposed to certain endemic mycoses, perhaps years previously.

Pulmonary fungal infections must be distinguished from tumors and chronic pneumonias caused by nonfungal organisms such as mycobacteria (including TB). Specimens are obtained for fungal and mycobacterial culture and histopathology. Sputum samples may be adequate, but occasionally bronchoalveolar lavage, transthoracic needle biopsy, or even surgery may be required to obtain an acceptable specimen.

Fungi that cause primary systemic infections are readily recognized by their histopathologic appearance. However, identifying the specific fungus may be difficult and usually requires fungal culture. The clinical significance of positive sputum cultures may be unclear if they show commensal organisms (eg, *Candida albicans*) or fungi ubiquitous in the environment (eg, *Aspergillus* sp). Therefore, other evidence (eg, host factors such as immunosuppression, serologic evidence, tissue invasion) may be required to help establish a diagnosis.

Serologic tests may be used to check for many systemic mycoses if culture and histopathology are unavailable or unrevealing, although few provide definitive diagnoses. Particularly useful tests include the following:

- Measurement of organism-specific antigens, most notably from *Cryptococcus neoformans*, *Histoplasma capsulatum*, and *Aspergillus* sp (occasional cross-reactivity with other fungi has been noted with each of these serologic tests)
- Serum β-glucan, which is often positive in invasive candidiasis as well as *Pneumocystis jirovecii* infections
- Complement fixation assays and newer enzyme immunoassays for anticoccidioidal antibodies, which are satisfactorily specific and do not require proof of rising levels (high titers confirm the diagnosis and indicate high risk of extrapulmonary dissemination)

Most other tests for antifungal antibodies have low sensitivity, specificity, or both and, because measurement of acute and convalescent titers is required, cannot be used to guide initial therapy.

ANTIFUNGAL DRUGS

Drugs for systemic antifungal treatment include amphotericin B (and its lipid formulations), various azole derivatives, echinocandins, and flucytosine (see Table 189–1). Amphotericin B, an effective but relatively toxic drug, has long been the mainstay of antifungal therapy for invasive and serious mycoses. However, newer potent and less toxic triazoles and echinocandins are now often recommended as first-line drugs for many invasive fungal infections. These drugs have markedly changed the approach to antifungal therapy, sometimes even allowing oral treatment of chronic mycoses.

Amphotericin B

Amphotericin B has been the mainstay of antifungal therapy for invasive and serious mycoses, but other antifungals (eg, fluconazole, voriconazole, posaconazole, the echinocandins) are now considered first-line drugs for many of these infections. Although amphotericin B does not have good CSF penetration, it is still effective for certain mycoses such as cryptococcal meningitis.

For **chronic mycoses**, amphotericin B deoxycholate is usually started at ≥ 0.3 mg/kg IV once/day, increased as tolerated to the desired dose (0.4 to 1.0 mg/kg; generally not > 50 mg/day); many patients tolerate the target dose on the first day.

For **acute, life-threatening mycoses**, amphotericin B deoxycholate may be started at 0.6 to 1.0 mg/kg IV once/day.

Formulations: There are 2 formulations of amphotericin:

- Deoxycholate (standard)
- Lipid-based

The **standard formulation**, amphotericin B deoxycholate, must always be given in 5% D/W because salts can precipitate the drug. It is usually given over 2 to 3 h, although more rapid infusions over 20 to 60 min can be used in selected patients. However, more rapid infusions usually have no advantage. Many patients experience chills, fever, nausea, vomiting, anorexia, headache, and, occasionally, hypotension during and for several hours after an infusion. Amphotericin B may also cause chemical thrombophlebitis when given via peripheral veins; a central venous catheter may be preferable. Pretreatment with acetaminophen or NSAIDs is often used; if these drugs are ineffective, hydrocortisone 25 to 50 mg or diphenhydramine 25 mg is sometimes added to the infusion or given as a separate IV bolus. Often, hydrocortisone can be tapered and omitted during extended therapy. Severe chills and rigors can be relieved or prevented by meperidine 50 to 75 mg IV.

Several **lipid vehicles** reduce the toxicity of amphotericin B (particularly nephrotoxicity and infusion-related symptoms). Two preparations are available:

- Amphotericin B lipid complex
- Liposomal amphotericin B

Lipid formulations are preferred over conventional amphotericin B because they cause fewer infusion-related symptoms and less nephrotoxicity.

Adverse effects: The main adverse effects are

- Nephrotoxicity (most common)
- Hypokalemia
- Hypomagnesemia
- Bone marrow suppression

Renal impairment is the major toxic risk of amphotericin B therapy. Serum creatinine and BUN should be monitored before treatment and at regular intervals during treatment: several times/wk for the first 2 to 3 wk, then 1 to 4 times/mo as clinically indicated. Amphotericin B is unique among nephrotoxic antimicrobial drugs because it is not eliminated

Table 189–1. SOME DRUGS FOR SYSTEMIC FUNGAL INFECTIONS

DRUG	USES	DOSE	SOME ADVERSE EFFECTS
Amphotericin B	Most fungal infections (Not for *Pseudallescheria* sp)	Conventional (deoxycholate) formulation: 0.5–1.0 mg/kg IV once/day	Conventional formulation: Acute infusion reactions, neuropathy, GI upset, renal failure, anemia, thrombophlebitis, hearing loss, rash, hypokalemia, hypomagnesemia
		Various lipid formulations: 3–5 mg/kg IV once/day	Lipid formulations: Infusion reactions*, renal failure*
Anidulafungin	Candidiasis, including candidemia	200 mg IV on day 1, then 100 mg IV once/day For esophageal candidiasis, half of this dose	Hepatitis, diarrhea, hypokalemia, infusion reactions
Caspofungin	Aspergillosis Candidiasis, including candidemia	70 mg IV on day 1, then 50 mg IV once/day	Phlebitis, headache, GI upset, rash,
Fluconazole	Mucosal and systemic candidiasis Cryptococcal meningitis Coccidioidal meningitis	100–800 mg po or IV once/day (loading dose may be given) Children: 3–12 mg/kg po or IV once/day	GI upset, hepatitis, QT prolongation
Flucytosine	Candidiasis (systemic) Cryptococcosis	12.5–37.5 mg/kg po qid	Pancytopenia due to bone marrow toxicity, neuropathy, nausea, vomiting, hepatic and renal injury, colitis
Isavuconazole†	Aspergillosis Mucormycosis	372 mg po or IV q 8 h (6 doses) initially, then 372 mg po or IV once/day for maintenance	Nausea, vomiting, hepatitis
Itraconazole	Dermatomycosis Histoplasmosis, blastomycosis, coccidioidomycosis, sporotrichosis	100 mg po once/day to 200 mg po bid	Hepatitis, GI upset, rash, headache, dizziness, hypokalemia, hypertension, edema, QT prolongation
Micafungin	Candidiasis, including candidemia	100 mg IV once/day (dose 150 mg for esophageal candidiasis)	Phlebitis, hepatitis, rash, headache, nausea
Posaconazole	Prophylaxis for invasive aspergillosis and candidiasis	200 mg po tid	Hepatitis, GI upset, rash, QT prolongation
	Oral candidiasis	100 mg po bid on day 1, then 100 mg once/day for 13 days	
	Oral candidiasis refractory to itraconazole	400 mg po bid	
Voriconazole	Invasive aspergillosis Fusariosis Scedosporiosis	6 mg/kg IV for 2 loading doses, then 200 mg po q 12 h *or* 3 to 6 mg/kg IV q 12 h	GI upset, transient visual disturbances, peripheral edema, rash, hepatitis, QT prolongation

*This adverse effect is less common with lipid formulations than with the conventional formulation.

†Isavuconazole is given as the prodrug isavuconazonium; 372 mg of isavuconazonium is equivalent to 200 mg of isavuconazole.

appreciably via the kidneys and does not accumulate as renal failure worsens. Nevertheless, dosages should be lowered, or a lipid formulation should be used instead if serum creatinine rises to > 2.0 to 2.5 mg/dL (> 177 to 221 μmol/L) or BUN rises to > 50 mg/dL (> 18 mmol urea/L). Acute nephrotoxicity can be reduced by aggressive IV hydration with saline before amphotericin B infusion; at least 1 L of normal saline should be given before amphotericin infusion. Mild to moderate renal function abnormalities induced by amphotericin B usually resolve gradually after therapy is completed. Permanent damage occurs primarily after prolonged treatment; after > 4 g total dose, about 75% of patients have persistent renal insufficiency.

Amphotericin B also frequently suppresses bone marrow function, manifested primarily by anemia. Hepatotoxicity or other untoward effects are unusual.

Azole Antifungals

Azoles block the synthesis of ergosterol, an important component of the fungal cell membrane. They can be given orally to treat chronic mycoses. The first such oral drug, ketoconazole, has been supplanted by more effective, less toxic triazole derivatives, such as fluconazole, itraconazole, posaconazole, and voriconazole. Drug interactions can occur with all azoles but are less likely with fluconazole. The drug interactions mentioned below are not intended as a complete listing; clinicians should refer to a specific drug interaction reference before using azole antifungal drugs.

PEARLS & PITFALLS

- Drug and food interactions are common with azole antifungals; review all concurrent drug use before prescribing them.

Fluconazole: This water-soluble drug is absorbed almost completely after an oral dose. It is excreted largely unchanged in urine and has a half-life of > 24 h, allowing single daily doses. It has high penetration into CSF (≥ 70% of serum levels) and has been especially useful in treating cryptococcal and coccidioidal meningitis. It is also one of the first-line drugs for treatment of candidemia in nonneutropenic patients. Doses range from 200 to 400 mg po once/day to as high as 800 mg once/day in some seriously ill patients and in patients infected with *Candida glabrata* or other *Candida* sp (not *C. albicans* or *C. krusei*); daily doses of ≥ 1000 mg have been given and had acceptable toxicity.

Adverse effects that occur most commonly are GI discomfort and rash. More severe toxicity is unusual, but the following have occurred: hepatic necrosis, Stevens-Johnson syndrome, anaphylaxis, alopecia, and, when taken for long periods of time during the 1st trimester of pregnancy, congenital fetal anomalies.

Drug interactions occur less often with fluconazole than with other azoles. However, fluconazole sometimes elevates serum levels of Ca channel blockers, cyclosporine, rifabutin, phenytoin, tacrolimus, warfarin-type oral anticoagulants, sulfonylurea drugs (eg, tolbutamide), and zidovudine. Rifampin may lower fluconazole blood levels.

Isavuconazole: This is the latest broad spectrum triazole approved for the treatment of aspergillosis and the first oral treatment approved for treatment of mucormycosis. It is available as an IV formulation as well as an oral capsule. Drug level monitoring is not required.

Adverse effects that occur most commonly are GI upset and hepatitis, although QT interval may actually decrease.

Drug interactions occur with many drugs, although they may be less severe compared with other azoles.

Itraconazole: This drug has become the standard treatment for lymphocutaneous sporotrichosis as well as for mild or moderately severe histoplasmosis, blastomycosis, and paracoccidioidomycosis. It is also effective in mild cases of invasive aspergillosis, some cases of coccidioidomycosis, and certain types of chromoblastomycosis. Despite poor CSF penetration, itraconazole can be used to treat some types of fungal meningitis, but it is not the drug of choice. Because of its high lipid solubility and protein binding, itraconazole blood levels tend to be low, but tissue levels are typically high. Drug levels are negligible in urine and CSF. Use of itraconazole has declined as use of voriconazole and posaconazole has increased.

Adverse effects with doses of up to 400 mg/day most commonly are GI, but a few men have reported erectile dysfunction, and higher doses may cause hypokalemia, hypertension, and edema. Other reported adverse effects include allergic rash, hepatitis, and hallucinations. An FDA black box warning for heart failure has been issued, particularly with a total daily dose of 400 mg.

Drug and food interactions can be significant. When the capsule form is used, acidic drinks (eg, cola, acidic fruit juices) or foods (especially high-fat foods) improve absorption of itraconazole from the GI tract. However, absorption may be reduced if itraconazole is taken with prescription or OTC drugs used to lower gastric acidity. Several drugs, including rifampin, rifabutin, didanosine, phenytoin, and carbamazepine, may decrease serum itraconazole levels. Itraconazole also inhibits metabolic degradation of other drugs, elevating blood levels with potentially serious consequences. Serious, even fatal cardiac arrhythmias may occur if itraconazole is used with cisapride (not available in the US) or some antihistamines (eg, terfenadine, astemizole, perhaps loratadine). Rhabdomyolysis has been associated with itraconazole-induced elevations in blood levels of cyclosporine or statins. Blood levels of some drugs (eg, digoxin, tacrolimus, oral anticoagulants, sulfonylureas) may increase when these drugs are used with itraconazole.

Posaconazole: The triazole posaconazole is available as an oral suspension and a tablet. An IV formulation will probably be available soon. This drug is highly active against yeasts and molds and effectively treats various opportunistic mold infections, such as those due to dematiaceous (dark-walled) fungi (eg, *Cladophialophora* sp). It is effective against many of the species that cause mucormycosis. Posaconazole can also be used as fungal prophylaxis in neutropenic patients with various cancers and in bone marrow transplant recipients.

Adverse effects for posaconazole, as for other triazoles, include a prolonged QT interval and hepatitis.

Drug interactions occur with many drugs, including rifabutin, rifampin, statins, various immunosuppressants, and barbiturates.

Voriconazole: This broad-spectrum triazole is available as a tablet and an IV formulation. It is considered the treatment of choice for *Aspergillus* infections in immunocompetent and immunocompromised hosts. Voriconazole can also be used to treat *Scedosporium apiospermum* and *Fusarium* infections. Additionally, the drug is effective in candidal esophagitis and invasive candidiasis, although it is not usually considered a first-line treatment; it has activity against a broader spectrum of *Candida* sp than does fluconazole.

Adverse effects that must be monitored for include hepatotoxicity, visual disturbances (common), hallucinations, and dermatologic reactions. This drug can prolong the QT interval.

Drug interactions are numerous, notably with certain immunosuppressants used after organ transplantation.

Echinocandins

Echinocandins are water-soluble lipopeptides that inhibit glucan synthase. They are available only for IV administration. Their mechanism of action is unique among antifungal drugs; echinocandins target the fungal cell wall, making them attractive because they lack cross-resistance with other drugs and their target is fungal and has no mammalian counterpart. Drug levels in urine and CSF are not significant. Echinocandins available in the US are anidulafungin, caspofungin, and micafungin. There is little evidence to suggest that one is better than the other, but anidulafungin appears to interact with fewer drugs than the other two.

These drugs are potently fungicidal against most clinically important *Candida* sp but are considered fungistatic against *Aspergillus*.

Adverse effects include hepatitis and rash.

Flucytosine

Flucytosine, a nucleic acid analog, is water soluble and well-absorbed after oral administration. Preexisting or emerging resistance is common, so it is almost always used with another antifungal, usually amphotericin B. Flucytosine plus amphotericin B is used primarily to treat cryptococcosis but is also valuable for some cases of disseminated candidiasis (including endocarditis), other yeast infections, and severe invasive aspergillosis. Flucytosine plus antifungal azoles may be beneficial in treating cryptococcal meningitis and some other mycoses.

The usual dose (12.5 to 37.5 mg/kg po qid) leads to high drug levels in serum, urine, and CSF.

Major adverse effects are bone marrow suppression (thrombocytopenia and leukopenia), hepatotoxicity, and enterocolitis; only degree of bone marrow suppression is proportional to serum levels.

Because flucytosine is cleared primarily by the kidneys, blood levels rise if nephrotoxicity develops during concomitant use with amphotericin B, particularly when amphotericin B is used in doses > 0.4 mg/kg/day. Flucytosine serum levels should be monitored, and the dosage should be adjusted to keep levels between 40 and 90 μg/mL. CBC and renal and liver function tests should be done twice/wk. If blood levels are unavailable, therapy is begun at 25 mg/kg qid, and dosage is decreased if renal function deteriorates.

ASPERGILLOSIS

Aspergillosis is an opportunistic infection caused by inhaling spores of the mold *Aspergillus*, commonly present in the environment; the spores invade blood vessels, causing hemorrhagic necrosis and infarction. Symptoms may be those of asthma, pneumonia, sinusitis, or rapidly progressing systemic illness. Diagnosis is primarily clinical but may be aided by imaging, histopathology, and specimen staining and culture. Treatment is with voriconazole, amphotericin B (or its lipid formulations), caspofungin, or itraconazole. Fungus balls may require surgical resection.

(See also the Infectious Diseases Society of America's Practice Guidelines for Diseases Caused by Aspergillus at www.academic.oup.com.)

Pathophysiology

Invasive infections are usually acquired by inhalation of spores or, occasionally, by direct invasion through damaged skin.

Major risk factors include

- Neutropenia when prolonged (typically > 7 days)
- Long-term high-dose corticosteroid therapy
- Organ transplantation (especially bone marrow transplantation with graft-vs-host disease [GVHD])
- Hereditary disorders of neutrophil function (eg, chronic granulomatous disease)

Aspergillus sp tends to infect open spaces, such as pulmonary cavities caused by previous lung disorders (eg, bronchiectasis, tumor, TB), the sinuses, or ear canals (otomycosis). Such infections tend to be locally invasive and destructive, although systemic spread sometimes occurs, particularly in immunocompromised patients. However, aspergillosis is unusual in those with HIV infection.

A. fumigatus is the most common cause of invasive pulmonary disease; *A. flavus* most often causes invasive extrapulmonary disease, probably because these patients are more severely immunosuppressed than patients infected with *A. fumigatus*.

Focal infections, typically in the lung, sometimes form a fungus ball (aspergilloma), a characteristic growth of tangled masses of hyphae, with fibrin exudate and few inflammatory cells, typically encapsulated by fibrous tissue. Occasionally, there is some local invasion of tissue at the periphery of the cavity, but usually the fungus just resides within the cavity with no appreciable local invasion.

A chronic form of invasive aspergillosis occasionally occurs, particularly in patients taking corticosteroids long-term and those with chronic granulomatous disease, which is characterized by a hereditary phagocytic cell defect.

Aspergillus sp can also cause endophthalmitis after trauma or surgery to the eye or by hematogenous seeding and can infect intravascular and intracardiac prostheses.

Primary superficial aspergillosis is uncommon but may occur in burns; beneath occlusive dressings; after corneal trauma (keratitis); or in the sinuses, mouth, nose, or ear canal.

Allergic bronchopulmonary aspergillosis is a hypersensitivity reaction to *A. fumigatus* that results in lung inflammation unrelated to fungal invasion of tissues (see p. 416).

Symptoms and Signs

Acute invasive pulmonary aspergillosis usually causes cough, often with hemoptysis, pleuritic chest pain, and shortness of breath. If untreated, invasive pulmonary aspergillosis may lead to rapidly progressive, ultimately fatal respiratory failure.

Chronic pulmonary aspergillosis may manifest with mild, indolent symptoms despite significant disease.

In severely immunocompromised patients, extrapulmonary invasive aspergillosis begins with skin lesions, sinusitis, or pneumonia and may involve the liver, kidneys, brain, and other tissues; it is often rapidly fatal.

Aspergillosis in the sinuses can form an aspergilloma or cause allergic fungal sinusitis or a chronic, slowly invasive granulomatous inflammation with fever, rhinitis, and headache. Patients may have necrosing cutaneous lesions overlying the nose or sinuses, palatal or gingival ulcerations, signs of cavernous sinus thrombosis, or pulmonary or disseminated lesions.

Diagnosis

- Usually fungal culture and histopathology of tissue samples
- Galactomannan antigen test on serum and bronchoalveolar lavage fluid

Because *Aspergillus* sp are common in the environment, positive sputum cultures may be due to environmental contamination or noninvasive colonization in patients with chronic lung disease; positive cultures are significant mainly when sputum is obtained from patients with increased susceptibility due to immunosuppression or when there is high suspicion due to typical imaging findings. Conversely, sputum cultures from patients with aspergillomas or invasive pulmonary aspergillosis are often negative because cavities are often walled off from airways and because invasive disease progresses mainly by vascular invasion and tissue infarction.

Chest x-rays are taken; however, chest CT is far more sensitive and should be done if patients are at high risk (ie, neutropenic). CT of sinuses is done if sinus infection is suspected. A movable fungus ball within a cavitary lesion is characteristic on both, although most lesions are focal and solid. Sometimes imaging detects a halo sign (a hazy shadow surrounding a nodule) or cavitation within a necrotic lesion. Diffuse, generalized pulmonary infiltrates are seen in some patients.

Culture and histopathology of a tissue sample are usually necessary for confirmation; histopathology helps distinguish invasive infection from colonization. The sample is typically taken from the lungs via bronchoscopy or percutaneous needle biopsy and from the sinuses via anterior rhinoscopy. Because cultures take time and histopathology results may be false-negative, most decisions to treat are based on strong presumptive clinical evidence. In aspergillus endocarditis, large vegetations often release sizable emboli that may occlude blood vessels and provide specimens for diagnosis.

Detection of antigens such as galactomannan can be specific but, in serum, is often not sufficiently sensitive to identify most cases in their early stages. In invasive pulmonary aspergillosis, the galactomannan test on bronchoalveolar lavage fluid is much more sensitive than that on serum and is often the only option for patients with thrombocytopenia, for whom biopsy is contraindicated. Blood cultures are almost always negative, even in rare cases of endocarditis.

Treatment

- Voriconazole or isovuconazole
- Amphotericin B (including lipid formulations)
- Echinocandins as salvage therapy
- Sometimes surgery for aspergillomas

Invasive infections usually require aggressive treatment with voriconazole (considered the first-choice drug) or isavuconazole, which has equal efficacy and fewer side effects. Amphotericin B (particularly lipid formulations) is also effective, although more toxic. Oral posaconazole or itraconazole (but not fluconazole) can be effective in some cases. Caspofungin or other echinocandins may be used as salvage therapy. Combination therapy with voriconazole and echinocandins may be effective in certain patients.

Usually, complete cure requires reversal of immunosuppression (eg, resolution of neutropenia, discontinuation of corticosteroids). Recrudescence is common if neutropenia recurs.

Aspergillomas neither require nor respond to systemic antifungal therapy but may require resection because of local effects, especially hemoptysis.

Prophylaxis with posaconazole or itraconazole can be considered for high-risk patients (those with GVHD or neutropenia due to acute myelocytic leukemia).

KEY POINTS

- Inhaling spores of the mold *Aspergillus* can cause localized or invasive pulmonary disease and, rarely, disseminated infection (eg, to the brain) in severely immunocompromised patients.
- Aspergillosis is more common among immunocompromised patients, although it is unusual in those with HIV infection.
- Focal infections, typically in the lung or sinuses, sometimes form a fungus ball (aspergilloma).
- Culture and histopathology of a tissue sample are usually necessary, but the galactomannan test on bronchoalveolar lavage fluid can help diagnose pulmonary infection.
- Voriconazole or isavuconazole is the drug of choice; amphotericin B is an alternative.
- Aspergillomas neither require nor respond to antifungal drugs but may need surgical resection if they cause bleeding or other symptoms.

BLASTOMYCOSIS

(Gilchrist Disease; North American Blastomycosis)

Blastomycosis is a pulmonary disease caused by inhaling spores of the dimorphic fungus *Blastomyces dermatitidis*; occasionally, the fungi spread hematogenously, causing extrapulmonary disease. Symptoms result from pneumonia or from dissemination to multiple organs, most commonly the skin. Diagnosis is clinical, by chest x-ray, or both and is confirmed by laboratory identification of the fungi. Treatment is with itraconazole, fluconazole, or amphotericin B.

(See also the Infectious Diseases Society of America's Practice guidelines for the management of patients with blastomycosis at www.academic.oup.com.)

In North America, the endemic area for blastomycosis includes

- Ohio–Mississippi River valleys (extending into the middle Atlantic and southeastern states)
- Northern Midwest
- Upstate New York
- Southern Canada

Rarely, the infection occurs in the Middle East and Africa.

Immunocompetent people can contract this infection. Although blastomycosis may be more common and more severe in immunocompromised patients, it is a less common opportunistic infection than histoplasmosis or coccidioidomycosis.

B. dermatitidis grows as a mold at room temperature in soil enriched with animal excreta and in moist, decaying, acidic organic material, often near rivers. In the lungs, inhaled spores convert into large (15 to 20 μm) invasive yeasts, which form characteristic broad-based buds.

Once in the lungs, infection may

- Remain localized in the lungs
- Disseminate hematogenously

Hematogenous dissemination can cause focal infection in numerous organs, including the skin, prostate, epididymides, testes, kidneys, vertebrae, ends of long bones, subcutaneous tissues, brain, oral or nasal mucosa, thyroid, lymph nodes, and bone marrow.

Symptoms and Signs

Pulmonary: Pulmonary blastomycosis may be asymptomatic or cause an acute, self-limited disease that often goes unrecognized. It can also begin insidiously and develop into a chronic, progressive infection. Symptoms include a productive or dry hacking cough, chest pain, dyspnea, fever, chills, and drenching sweats.

Pleural effusion occurs occasionally. Some patients have rapidly progressive infections, and acute respiratory distress syndrome may develop.

Extrapulmonary: In extrapulmonary disseminated blastomycosis, symptoms depend on the organ involved.

Skin lesions are by far the most common; they may be single or multiple and may occur with or without clinically apparent pulmonary involvement. Papules or papulopustules usually appear on exposed surfaces and spread slowly. Painless miliary abscesses, varying from pinpoint to 1 mm in diameter, develop on the advancing borders. Irregular, wartlike papillae may form on surfaces. Sometimes bullae develop. As lesions enlarge, the centers heal, forming atrophic scars. When fully developed, an individual lesion appears as an elevated verrucous patch, usually ≥ 2 cm wide with an abruptly sloping, purplish red, abscess-studded border. Ulceration may occur if bacterial superinfection is present.

If bone lesions develop, overlying areas are sometimes swollen, warm, and tender.

Genital lesions cause painful epididymal swelling, deep perineal discomfort, or prostatic tenderness detected during rectal examination.

CNS involvement can manifest as brain abscess, epidural abscess, or meningitis.

Diagnosis

- Fungal cultures and smear
- *Blastomyces* urine antigen

A chest x-ray should be taken. Focal or diffuse infiltrates may be present, sometimes as patchy bronchopneumonia fanning out from the hilum. These findings must be distinguished from other causes of pneumonia (eg, other mycoses, TB, tumors). Skin lesions can be mistaken for sporotrichosis, TB, iodism, or basal cell carcinoma. Genital involvement may mimic TB.

Cultures of infected material are done; they are definitive when positive. Because culturing *Blastomyces* can pose a severe biohazard to laboratory personnel, the laboratory should be notified of the suspected diagnosis. The organism's characteristic appearance, seen during microscopic examination of tissues or sputum, is also frequently diagnostic. Serologic testing is not sensitive but is useful if positive.

A urine antigen test is useful, but cross-reactivity with *Histoplasma* is high.

Treatment

- For mild to moderate disease, itraconazole
- For severe, life-threatening infection, amphotericin B

Untreated blastomycosis is usually slowly progressive and is rarely ultimately fatal.

Treatment depends on severity of the infection. For mild to moderate disease, itraconazole 200 mg po tid for 3 days, followed by 200 mg po once/day or bid for 6 to 12 mo is used. Fluconazole appears less effective, but 400 to 800 mg po once/day may be tried in itraconazole-intolerant patients with mild disease. For severe, life-threatening infections, IV amphotericin B is usually effective; therapy is changed to itraconazole once patients improve.

Voriconazole and posaconazole are highly active against *B. dermatitidis*, but their role has not yet been defined.

KEY POINTS

- Inhaling spores of the dimorphic fungus *Blastomyces* can cause pulmonary disease and, less commonly, disseminated infection (particularly to the skin).
- In North America, blastomycosis is endemic in the regions around the Great Lakes and in the mid-Atlantic and Southeast.
- Diagnose using cultures of infected material; serologic testing is specific but not very sensitive.
- For mild to moderate disease, use itraconazole.
- For severe disease, use amphotericin B.

CANDIDIASIS (INVASIVE)

(Candidosis; Moniliasis)

Candidiasis is infection by *Candida* sp (most often *C. albicans*), manifested by mucocutaneous lesions, fungemia, and sometimes focal infection of multiple sites. Symptoms depend on the site of infection and include dysphagia, skin and mucosal lesions, blindness, vaginal symptoms (itching, burning, discharge), fever, shock, oliguria, renal shutdown, and disseminated intravascular coagulation. Diagnosis is confirmed by histopathology and cultures from normally sterile sites. Treatment is with amphotericin B, fluconazole, echinocandins, voriconazole, or posaconazole.

(See also the Infectious Diseases Society of America's Guidelines for treatment of candidiasis at http://www.idsociety.org.)

Candida sp are commensal organisms that inhabit the GI tract and sometimes the skin (see p. 1031). Unlike other systemic mycoses, candidiasis results from endogenous organisms. Most infections are caused by *C. albicans*; however, *C. glabrata* (formerly *Torulopsis glabrata*) and other non-albicans species are increasingly involved in fungemia, UTIs, and, occasionally, other focal disease. *C. glabrata* is frequently less susceptible to fluconazole than other species; *C. krusei* is inherently resistant.

Candida sp account for about 80% of major systemic fungal infections and are the most common cause of fungal infections in immunocompromised patients. Candidal infections are one of the most common hospital-acquired infections.

Candidiasis involving the mouth (see Plate 72) and esophagus (see Plate 71) is a defining opportunistic infection in AIDS. Although mucocutaneous candidiasis is frequently present in HIV-infected patients, hematogenous dissemination is unusual unless other specific risk factors are present (see below). Neutropenic patients (eg, those receiving cancer chemotherapy) are at high risk of developing life-threatening disseminated candidiasis.

Candidemia may occur in nonneutropenic patients during prolonged hospitalization. This bloodstream infection is often related to one or more of the following:

- Central venous catheters
- Major surgery
- Broad-spectrum antibacterial therapy
- IV hyperalimentation

IV lines and the GI tract are the usual portals of entry. Candidemia often prolongs hospitalization and increases mortality due to concurrent disorders. Prolonged or untreated candidemia may lead to endocarditis or meningitis as well as to focal involvement of skin, subcutaneous tissues, bones, joints, liver, spleen, kidneys, eyes, and other tissues. Endocarditis is commonly related to IV drug abuse, valve replacement, or intravascular trauma induced by indwelling IV catheters.

All forms of disseminated candidiasis should be considered serious, progressive, and potentially fatal.

Symptoms and Signs

Esophageal candidiasis is most often manifested by dysphagia.

Candidemia usually causes fever, but no symptoms are specific. Some patients develop a syndrome resembling bacterial sepsis, with a fulminating course that may include shock, oliguria, renal shutdown, and disseminated intravascular coagulation.

Candidal endophthalmitis starts as white retinal lesions that are initially asymptomatic but can progress, opacifying the vitreous and causing potentially irreversible scarring and blindness. In neutropenic patients, retinal hemorrhages occasionally also occur, but actual infection of the eye is rare.

Papulonodular skin lesions may also develop, especially in neutropenic patients, in whom they indicate widespread hematogenous dissemination to other organs. Symptoms of other focal infection depend on the organ involved.

Diagnosis

- Histopathology and fungal cultures
- Blood cultures
- Serum β-glucan testing

Because *Candida* spp are commensal, their culture from sputum, the mouth, the vagina, urine, stool, or skin does not necessarily signify an invasive, progressive infection. A characteristic clinical lesion must also be present, histopathologic evidence of tissue invasion (eg, yeasts, pseudohyphae, or hyphae in tissue specimens) must be documented, and other etiologies must be excluded. Positive cultures of specimens taken from normally sterile sites, such as blood, CSF, pericardium, pericardial fluid, or biopsied tissue, provide definitive evidence that systemic therapy is needed.

Serum β-glucan is often positive in patients with invasive candidiasis; conversely, a negative result indicates low likelihood of systemic infection.

Ophthalmologic examination to check for endophthalmitis is recommended for all patients with candidemia.

Treatment

- An echinocandin if patients are severely or critically ill or if infection with *C. glabrata* or *C. krusei* is suspected
- Fluconazole if patients are clinically stable or if infection with *C. albicans* or *C. parapsilosis* is suspected
- Alternatively, voriconazole or amphotericin B

In patients with invasive candidiasis, predisposing conditions (eg, neutropenia, immunosuppression, use of broad-spectrum antibacterial antibiotics, hyperalimentation, presence of indwelling lines) should be reversed or controlled if possible. In nonneutropenic patients, IV catheters should be removed.

When an echinocandin is indicated (if patients are moderately severely ill or critically ill [most neutropenic patients] or if *C. glabrata* or *C. krusei* is suspected), one of the following drugs can be used: caspofungin, loading dose 70 mg IV, then 50 mg IV once/day; micafungin 100 mg IV once/day; or anidulafungin, loading dose 200 mg IV, then 100 mg IV once/day.

If fluconazole is indicated (if patients are clinically stable or if *C. albicans* or *C. parapsilosis* is suspected), loading dose is 800 mg (12 mg/kg) po or IV once, followed by 400 mg (6 mg/kg) once/day.

Treatment is continued for 14 days after the last negative blood culture.

Esophageal candidiasis is treated with fluconazole 200 to 400 mg po or IV once/day or itraconazole 200 mg po once/day. If these drugs are ineffective or if infection is severe, voriconazole 4 mg/kg po or IV bid, posaconazole 400 mg po bid, or one of the echinocandins may be used. Treatment is continued for 14 to 21 days.

KEY POINTS

- Unlike other fungal infections, invasive candidiasis is usually due to endogenous organisms.
- Invasive infection typically occurs in immunocompromised and/or hospitalized patients, particularly those who have had surgery or been given broad-spectrum antibiotics.
- Positive cultures of specimens taken from normally sterile sites (eg, blood, CSF, tissue biopsy specimens) are needed to distinguish invasive infection from normal colonization; serum β-glucan is often positive in patients with invasive candidiasis.
- Use an echinocandin if patients are severely or critically ill or if infection with *C. glabrata* or *C. krusei* is suspected.
- Use fluconazole if patients are clinically stable or if infection with *C. albicans* or *C. parapsilosis* is suspected.

CHROMOBLASTOMYCOSIS

Chromoblastomycosis is a specific type of cutaneous infection caused by dematiaceous (pigmented) fungi. Symptoms are ulcerating nodules on exposed body parts. Diagnosis is by appearance, histopathology, and culture. Treatment is with itraconazole, another azole, or flucytosine and surgical excision.

Chromoblastomycosis is a cutaneous infection affecting normal, immunocompetent people mostly in tropical or subtropical areas; it is characterized by formation of papillomatous nodules that tend to ulcerate.

Symptoms and Signs

Most infections begin on the foot or leg, but other exposed body parts may be infected, especially where the skin is broken. Early small, itchy, enlarging papules may resemble dermatophytosis (ringworm). These papules extend to form dull red or violaceous, sharply demarcated patches with indurated bases. Several weeks or months later, new lesions, projecting 1 to 2 mm above the skin, may appear along paths of lymphatic drainage. Hard, dull red or grayish cauliflower-shaped nodular projections may develop in the center of patches and, if the infection is untreated, gradually extend to cover extremities over the course of many years. Lymphatics may be obstructed, itching may persist, and secondary bacterial superinfections may develop, causing ulcerations and occasionally septicemia.

Diagnosis

- Histopathology
- Culture

Late chromoblastomycosis lesions have a characteristic appearance, but early lesions may be mistaken for dermatophytoses.

Fontana-Masson staining for melanin helps confirm the presence of the sclerotic bodies (Medlar bodies), which are pathognomonic. Culture is needed to identify the causative species.

Treatment

- Itraconazole, sometimes with flucytosine
- Often surgery or cryotherapy.

Itraconazole is the most effective drug, although not all patients respond. Flucytosine is sometimes added to prevent relapse. Amphotericin B is ineffective. Anecdotal reports suggest that posaconazole, voriconazole, or terbinafine may also be effective. Adjunctive therapies such as cryotherapy are often helpful, although response is slow.

For localized lesions, surgical excision may be curative.

COCCIDIOIDOMYCOSIS

(San Joaquin Fever; Valley Fever)

Coccidioidomycosis is a pulmonary or hematogenously spread disseminated disease caused by the fungi *Coccidioides immitis* and *C. posadasii*; it usually occurs as an acute benign asymptomatic or self-limited respiratory infection. The organism occasionally disseminates to cause focal lesions in other tissues. Symptoms, if present, are those of lower respiratory infection or low-grade nonspecific disseminated disease. Diagnosis is suspected based on clinical and epidemiologic characteristics and confirmed by chest x-ray, culture, and serologic testing. Treatment, if needed, is usually with fluconazole, itraconazole, newer triazoles, or amphotericin B.

(See also the Infectious Diseases Society of America's Coccidioidomycosis at www.academic.oup.com.)

In North America, the endemic area for coccidioidomycosis includes

- The southwestern US
- Northern Mexico

The affected areas of the southwestern US include Arizona, the central valley of California, parts of New Mexico, and Texas west of El Paso. The area extends into northern Mexico, and foci occur in parts of Central America and Argentina. About 30 to 60% of people who live in an endemic region are exposed to the fungus at some point during their life. In the US, about 150,000 infections develop annually; over half of them are subclinical.

Pathophysiology

Infections are acquired by inhaling spore-laden dust. Thus, certain occupations (eg, farming, construction) and outdoor recreational activities increase risk. Epidemics can occur when heavy rains, which promote the growth of mycelia, are followed by drought and winds. Because of travel and delayed onset of clinical manifestations, infections can become evident outside endemic areas.

Once inhaled, *C. immitis* spores convert to large tissue-invasive spherules. As spherules enlarge and then rupture, each releases thousands of small endospores, which may form new spherules. Pulmonary disease is characterized by an acute, subacute, or chronic granulomatous reaction with varying degrees of fibrosis. Lesions may cavitate or form nodular-like coin lesions.

Sometimes disease progresses, with widespread lung involvement, systemic dissemination, or both; focal lesions may form in almost any tissue, most commonly in skin, subcutaneous tissues, bones (osteomyelitis), and meninges (meningitis).

Progressive coccidioidomycosis is uncommon in otherwise healthy people and more likely to occur in the following contexts:

- HIV infection
- Use of immunosuppressants
- Advanced age
- 2nd half of pregnancy or postpartum
- Certain ethnic backgrounds (Filipino, African American, Native American, Hispanic, and Asian, in decreasing order of relative risk)

Symptoms and Signs

Primary coccidioidomycosis: Most patients are asymptomatic, but nonspecific respiratory symptoms resembling those of influenza, acute bronchitis, or, less often, acute pneumonia or pleural effusion sometimes occur. Symptoms, in decreasing order of frequency, include fever, cough, chest pain, chills, sputum production, sore throat, and hemoptysis.

Physical signs may be absent or limited to scattered rales with or without areas of dullness to percussion over lung fields. Some patients develop hypersensitivity to the localized respiratory infection, manifested by arthritis, conjunctivitis, erythema nodosum, or erythema multiforme.

Primary pulmonary lesions sometimes leave nodular coin lesions that must be distinguished from tumors, TB, and other granulomatous infections. Sometimes residual cavitary lesions develop; they may vary in size over time and often appear thin-walled. A small percentage of these cavities fail to close spontaneously. Hemoptysis or the threat of rupture into the pleural space occasionally necessitates surgery.

Progressive coccidioidomycosis: Nonspecific symptoms develop a few weeks, months, or occasionally years after primary infection; they include low-grade fever, anorexia, weight loss, and weakness.

Extensive pulmonary involvement is uncommon in otherwise healthy people and occurs mainly in those who are immunocompromised. It may cause progressive cyanosis, dyspnea, and mucopurulent or bloody sputum.

Symptoms of extrapulmonary lesions depend on the site. Draining sinus tracts sometimes connect deeper lesions to the skin. Localized extrapulmonary lesions often become chronic and recur frequently, sometimes long after completion of seemingly successful antifungal therapy.

Untreated disseminated coccidioidomycosis is usually fatal and, if meningitis is present, is uniformly fatal without prolonged and possibly lifelong treatment. Mortality rates in patients with advanced HIV infection exceed 70% within 1 mo of diagnosis; whether treatment can alter mortality rates is unclear.

Diagnosis

- Cultures (routine or fungal)
- Microscopic examination of specimens to check for *C. immitis* spherules
- Serologic testing

Eosinophilia may be an important clue in identifying coccidioidomycosis. The diagnosis is suspected based on history and typical physical findings, when apparent; chest x-ray findings can help confirm the diagnosis, which can be established by fungal culture or by visualization of *C. immitis* spherules in sputum, pleural fluid, CSF, exudate from draining lesions, or biopsy specimens. Intact spherules are usually 20 to 80 μm in diameter, thick-walled, and filled with small (2 to 4 μm) endospores. Endospores released into tissues from ruptured spherules may be mistaken for nonbudding yeasts. Because culturing *Coccidioides* can pose a severe biohazard to laboratory personnel, the laboratory should be notified of the suspected diagnosis.

Serologic testing for anticoccidioidal antibodies using an immunodiffusion kit (for IgG and IgM antibodies) and complement fixation (for IgG antibodies) are the most useful tests. Titers ≥ 1:4 in serum are consistent with current or recent infection, and high titers (≥ 1:32) signify an increased likelihood of extrapulmonary dissemination. However, immunocompromised patients may have low titers. Titers should decline during successful therapy. The presence of complement-fixing antibodies in CSF is diagnostic of coccidioidal meningitis and is important because CSF cultures are rarely positive. A urine antigen test that may be useful in cases of pneumonia and disseminated infection has been developed.

Delayed cutaneous hypersensitivity to coccidioidin or spherulin usually develops within 10 to 21 days after acute infections in immunocompetent patients but is characteristically absent in progressive disease. Because this test is positive in most people in endemic areas, its primary value is for epidemiologic studies rather than for diagnosis.

Treatment

- For mild to moderate disease, fluconazole or itraconazole
- For severe disease, amphotericin B

Patients with primary coccidioidomycosis and risk factors for severe or progressive disease should be treated. Treatment for primary coccidioidomycosis is controversial in low-risk patients. Some experts give fluconazole because its toxicity is low and because even in low-risk patients, there is a small risk of hematogenous seeding, especially to bone or brain. In addition, symptoms resolve more quickly in treated patients than in those who are not treated with an antifungal. Others think that fluconazole may blunt the immune response and that risk of hematogenous seeding in primary infection is too low to warrant use of fluconazole. High complement fixation titers indicate spread and the need for treatment.

Mild to moderate nonmeningeal extrapulmonary involvement should be treated with fluconazole ≥ 400 mg po once/day or itraconazole 200 mg po bid. Voriconazole 200 mg po or IV bid or posaconazole 400 mg po bid are alternatives but have not been well-studied. For severe illness, amphotericin B 0.5 to 1.0 mg/kg IV over 2 to 6 h once/day is given for 4 to 12 wk until total dose reaches 1 to 3 g, depending on degree of infection. Lipid formulations of amphotericin B are preferred over conventional amphotericin B. Patients can usually be switched to an oral azole once they have been stabilized, usually within several weeks.

Patients with HIV- or AIDS-associated coccidioidomycosis require maintenance therapy to prevent relapse; fluconazole 200 mg po once/day or itraconazole 200 mg po bid usually is sufficient, given until the CD4 cell count is > 250/μL.

For meningeal coccidioidomycosis, fluconazole is used. The optimal dose is unclear; oral doses of 800 to 1200 mg once/day may be more effective than 400 mg once/day. Treatment for meningeal coccidioidomycosis should be given lifelong. Surgical removal of involved bone may be necessary to cure osteomyelitis.

KEY POINTS

- Coccidioidomycosis is a common fungal infection acquired by inhaling spore-laden dust.
- It is endemic to the southwestern US and northern Mexico; disease also occurs in certain parts of Central and South America.
- Most patients have an asymptomatic or mild pulmonary infection, but those who are immunocompromised or have other risk factors may develop severe, progressive pulmonary disease or disseminated infection (typically to skin, bone, or meninges).
- Diagnose using culture, staining, and/or serologic testing.
- For mild to moderate disease, use fluconazole or itraconazole.
- For severe disease, use a lipid formulation of amphotericin B.

CRYPTOCOCCOSIS

(European Blastomycosis; Torulosis)

Cryptococcosis is a pulmonary or disseminated infection acquired by inhalation of soil contaminated with the encapsulated yeast *Cryptococcus neoformans* or *C. gattii*. Symptoms are those of pneumonia, meningitis, or involvement of skin, bones, or viscera. Diagnosis is clinical and microscopic, confirmed by culture or fixed-tissue staining. Treatment, when necessary, is with azoles or amphotericin B, with or without flucytosine.

(See also the Infectious Diseases Society of America's Practice Guidelines for the Management of Cryptococcal Disease at www.academic.oup.com.)

Distribution of *C. neoformans* is worldwide; it is present in soil contaminated with bird droppings, particularly those of pigeons. Cryptococcosis is a defining opportunistic infection for AIDS (typically associated with CD4 counts < 100/μL), although patients with Hodgkin lymphoma, other lymphomas, or sarcoidosis and those taking long-term corticosteroid therapy are also at increased risk, as are recipients of a solid organ transplant.

C. gattii is primarily associated with trees, especially the eucalyptus and, unlike *C. neoformans*, is not associated with birds and is more likely to cause disease in immunocompetent hosts. Outbreaks have occurred in the Pacific Northwest and in Papua New Guinea and northern Australia.

Pathophysiology

Cryptococcosis is acquired by inhalation and thus typically affects the lungs. Many patients present with asymptomatic, self-limited primary lung lesions. In immunocompetent patients, the isolated pulmonary lesions usually heal spontaneously without disseminating, even without antifungal therapy.

After inhalation, *Cryptococcus* may disseminate, frequently to the brain and meninges, typically manifesting as microscopic multifocal intracerebral lesions. Meningeal granulomas and larger focal brain lesions may be evident. Although pulmonary involvement is rarely dangerous, meningitis is life threatening and requires aggressive therapy.

Focal sites of dissemination may also occur in skin, the ends of long bones, joints, liver, spleen, kidneys, prostate, and other tissues. Except for those in the skin, these lesions usually cause few or no symptoms. Rarely, pyelonephritis occurs with renal papillary necrosis.

Involved tissues typically contain cystic masses of yeasts that appear gelatinous because of accumulated cryptococcal capsular polysaccharide, but acute inflammatory changes are minimal or absent.

Symptoms and Signs

Manifestations depend on the affected area.

CNS: Because inflammation is not extensive, fever is usually low grade or absent, and meningismus is uncommon. In patients with AIDS, cryptococcal meningitis may cause minimal or no symptoms, but headache frequently occurs and sometimes slowly progressive altered mental status. Because most symptoms of cryptococcal meningitis result from cerebral edema, they are usually nonspecific (eg, headache, blurred vision, confusion, depression, agitation, other behavioral changes). Except for ocular or facial palsies, focal signs are rare until relatively late in the course. Blindness may develop because of cerebral edema or direct involvement of the optic tracts.

Lungs: Many patients are asymptomatic. Those with pneumonia usually have cough and other nonspecific respiratory symptoms. However, AIDS-associated cryptococcal pulmonary infection may manifest as severe, progressive pneumonia with acute dyspnea and an x-ray pattern suggesting *Pneumocystis* infection.

Skin: Dermatologic spread can manifest as pustular, papular, nodular, or ulcerated lesions, which sometimes resemble acne, molluscum contagiosum, or basal cell carcinoma.

Diagnosis

- Culture of CSF, sputum, urine, and blood
- Fixed-tissue specimen staining
- Serum and CSF testing for cryptococcal antigen

Clinical diagnosis is suggested by symptoms of an indolent infection in immunocompetent patients and a more severe, progressive infection in immunocompromised patients. Chest x-ray, urine collection, and lumbar puncture are done first.

Culture of *C. neoformans* is definitive. CSF, sputum, and urine yield organisms most often, and blood cultures may be positive, particularly in patients with AIDS. In disseminated cryptococcosis with meningitis, *C. neoformans* is frequently cultured from urine (prostatic foci of infection sometimes persist despite successful clearance of organisms from the CNS). Diagnosis is strongly suggested if experienced observers identify encapsulated budding yeasts in smears of body fluids, secretions, exudates, or other specimens. In fixed tissue specimens, encapsulated yeasts may also be identified and confirmed as *C. neoformans* by positive mucicarmine or Masson-Fontana staining.

Elevated CSF protein and a mononuclear cell pleocytosis are usual in cryptococcal meningitis. Glucose is frequently low, and encapsulated yeasts forming narrow-based buds can be seen on India ink smears in most patients, especially in those who have AIDS (who typically have a higher fungal burden than those without HIV infection). In some patients with AIDS, CSF parameters are normal, except for the presence of numerous yeasts on India ink preparation. The latex test for cryptococcal capsular antigen is positive in CSF or blood specimens or both in > 90% of patients with meningitis and is generally specific, although false-positive results may occur, usually with titers ≤ 1:8, especially if rheumatoid factor is also present.

Treatment

- For meningitis, amphotericin B with or without flucytosine, followed by fluconazole
- For nonmeningeal disease, fluconazole (which is usually effective)

Patients without AIDS: Patients may need no treatment for localized, asymptomatic pulmonary involvement, confirmed by normal CSF parameters, negative cultures of CSF and urine, and no evidence of cutaneous, bone, or other extrapulmonary lesions. Some experts give a course of fluconazole to prevent hematogenous dissemination and to shorten the course of the illness. Patients with pulmonary symptoms should be treated with fluconazole 200 to 400 mg po once/day for 6 to 12 mo.

In patients without meningitis, localized lesions in skin, bone, or other sites require systemic antifungal therapy, typically fluconazole 400 mg po once/day for 6 to 12 mo. For more severe disease, amphotericin B 0.5 to 1.0 mg/kg IV once/day with flucytosine 25 mg/kg po q 6 h is given for several weeks.

For meningitis, the standard regimen is induction with amphotericin B 0.7 mg/kg IV once/day plus flucytosine 25 mg/kg po q 6 h for 2 to 4 wk, followed by consolidation therapy with fluconazole 400 mg po once/day for 8 wk, then maintenance therapy with fluconazole 200 mg po once/day for 6 to 12 mo. Repeated lumbar puncture is important to manage elevated opening pressures.

Patients with AIDS: All patients require treatment. For meningitis or severe pulmonary disease, the standard regimen is amphotericin B 0.7 mg/kg IV once/day plus flucytosine 25 mg po q 6 h for the first 2 wk of treatment (longer induction therapy may be needed if clinical response is slow or cultures remain positive), followed by fluconazole 400 mg po once/day for 10 wk total. Once induction therapy is completed, long-term suppressive (maintenance) therapy is required. Repeated lumbar puncture is important to manage elevated opening pressures. Patients with mild to moderate symptoms of localized pulmonary involvement (confirmed by normal CSF parameters, negative cultures of CSF and urine, and no evidence of cutaneous, bone, or other extrapulmonary lesions) may be treated with fluconazole 400 mg po once/day for 6 to 12 mo.

Nearly all AIDS patients need maintenance therapy until CD4 cell counts are > 150. Fluconazole 200 mg po once/day is preferred, but itraconazole at the same dose is acceptable; however, itraconazole serum levels should be measured to make sure that patients are absorbing the drug.

KEY POINTS

- *C. neoformans* is present worldwide; it is acquired by inhaling dust from soil contaminated with bird droppings, particularly those of pigeons.
- In immunocompetent patients, infection is typically asymptomatic and self-limited.
- In immunocompromised patients, *Cryptococcus* may disseminate to many sites, commonly to the brain and meninges, and to the skin.
- Diagnose using culture, staining, and/or serum and CSF testing for cryptococcal antigen.
- For localized pulmonary disease, use fluconazole.
- For meningitis or other severe infection, use amphotericin B with or without flucytosine, followed by fluconazole.

HISTOPLASMOSIS

Histoplasmosis is a pulmonary and hematogenous disease caused by *Histoplasma capsulatum*; it is often chronic and usually follows an asymptomatic primary infection. Symptoms are those of pneumonia or of nonspecific chronic illness. Diagnosis is by identification of the organism in sputum or tissue or use of specific serum and urine antigen. Treatment, when necessary, is with amphotericin B or an azole.

(See also the Infectious Diseases Society of America's Practice Guidelines for the Management of Patients with Histoplasmosis at www.academic.oup.com.)

Histoplasmosis occurs worldwide.

In the US, the endemic area for histoplasmosis includes

- The Ohio–Mississippi River valleys extending into parts of northern Maryland, southern Pennsylvania, central New York, and Texas

Microfoci have been noted in other states, such as Florida, and along the St. Lawrence and Rio Grande rivers.

H. capsulatum grows as a mold in nature or in culture at room temperature but converts to a small (1 to 5 μm in diameter) yeast cell at 37° C and during invasion of host cells. Infection follows inhalation of conidia (spores produced by the mycelial form of the fungus) in soil or dust contaminated with bird or bat droppings. Severe disease is more common after heavy, prolonged exposure and in men, infants, or people with compromised T cell–mediated immunity.

Initial infection occurs in the lungs and usually remains there but may spread hematogenously to other organs if it is not controlled by normal cell-mediated host defenses. Progressive disseminated histoplasmosis is one of the defining opportunistic infections for AIDS.

Symptoms and Signs

Most histoplasmosis infections are asymptomatic or so mild that patients do not seek medical attention. The disease has 3 main forms.

Acute primary histoplasmosis is a syndrome with fever, cough, myalgias, chest pain, and malaise of varying severity. Acute pneumonia (evident on physical examination and chest x-ray) sometimes develops.

Chronic cavitary histoplasmosis is characterized by pulmonary lesions that are often apical and resemble cavitary

TB. Manifestations are worsening cough and dyspnea, progressing eventually to disabling respiratory dysfunction. Dissemination does not occur.

Progressive disseminated histoplasmosis characteristically includes generalized involvement of the reticuloendothelial system, with hepatosplenomegaly, lymphadenopathy, bone marrow involvement, and sometimes oral or GI ulcerations. The course is usually subacute or chronic, with only nonspecific, often subtle symptoms (eg, fever, fatigue, weight loss, weakness, malaise); the condition of HIV-positive patients may inexplicably worsen. The CNS may become involved, causing meningitis or focal brain lesions. Adrenal infection is rare but may result in Addison disease. Severe pneumonia is rare, but patients with AIDS may develop severe acute pneumonia with hypoxia suggesting *Pneumocystis jirovecii* infection, as well as hypotension, mental status changes, coagulopathy, or rhabdomyolysis.

Fibrosing mediastinitis, a chronic but rare form, ultimately causes circulatory compromise.

Patients with histoplasmosis may lose vision, but organisms are not present in ocular lesions, antifungal chemotherapy is not helpful, and the link to *H. capsulatum* infection is unclear.

Diagnosis

- Histopathology and cultures
- Antigen testing

The index of suspicion must be high because symptoms are nonspecific. Chest x-rays should be done and may show the following:

- In acute infection: Normal or a diffuse nodular or miliary pattern
- In chronic pulmonary histoplasmosis: Cavitary lesions in most patients
- In progressive disease: Hilar adenopathy with diffuse nodular infiltrates in about 50% of patients

Bronchoalveolar lavage or tissue biopsy may be necessary to obtain histology specimens; serologic testing and culture of urine, blood, and sputum specimens are also done. Because culturing *Histoplasma* can pose a severe biohazard to laboratory personnel, the laboratory should be notified of the suspected diagnosis.

Microscopic histopathology can strongly suggest the diagnosis, particularly in patients with AIDS and extensive infections; in such patients, intracellular yeasts may be seen in Wright- or Giemsa-stained peripheral blood or buffy coat specimens. Fungal culture confirms the diagnosis. Lysis-centrifugation or culture of buffy coat improves the yield from blood specimens.

A test for *H. capsulatum* antigen is sensitive and specific, particularly when simultaneous serum and urine specimens are tested; however, cross-reactivity with other fungi (*Coccidioides immitis*, *Blastomyces dermatitidis*, *Paracoccidioides brasiliensis*, *Penicillium marneffei*) has been noted.

Prognosis

The acute primary form is almost always self-limited, although very rarely, death occurs after massive infection. Chronic cavitary histoplasmosis can cause death due to severe respiratory insufficiency. Untreated progressive disseminated histoplasmosis has a mortality rate of > 90%.

Treatment

- Sometimes no treatment
- For mild to moderate infection, itraconazole
- For severe infection, amphotericin B

Acute primary histoplasmosis requires no antifungal therapy unless there is no spontaneous improvement after 1 mo; itraconazole 200 mg po is given tid for 3 days, then once/day for 6 to 12 wk. Fluconazole is less effective, and other azoles are not well-studied but have been used successfully. Severe pneumonia requires more aggressive therapy with amphotericin B.

For **chronic cavitary histoplasmosis**, itraconazole 200 mg po is given tid for 3 days, then once/day or bid for 12 to 24 mo. Other azoles or amphotericin B is used if patients are seriously ill or do not respond to or tolerate itraconazole.

For **severe disseminated histoplasmosis**, liposomal amphotericin B 3 mg/kg IV once/day (preferred) or amphotericin B 0.5 to 1.0 mg/kg IV once/day for 2 wk or until the patient is clinically stable is the treatment of choice. Patients can then be switched to itraconazole 200 mg po tid for 3 days, then twice/day continued for 12 mo after they become afebrile and require no ventilatory or BP support. For mild disseminated disease, itraconazole 200 mg po tid for 3 days, then twice/day for 12 mo can be used. In patients with AIDS, itraconazole is given indefinitely to prevent relapse or until CD4 cell counts are > 150. Blood levels of itraconazole and *Histoplasma* antigen levels should be monitored during therapy. Fluconazole may be less effective, but voriconazole and posaconazole are very active against *H. capsulatum* and may be effective in the treatment of patients with histoplasmosis. Further data and experience are required to determine which drug is the best in each clinical situation.

KEY POINTS

- Histoplasmosis is a common fungal infection acquired by inhaling spores.
- It is endemic to the Ohio–Mississippi River valleys, extending into parts of northern Maryland, southern Pennsylvania, central New York, and Texas.
- It may cause an acute primary pulmonary infection, a chronic cavitary pulmonary infection, or progressive disseminated infection.
- Diagnose using histopathology, cultures, and/or antigen testing.
- Acute primary infection is almost always self-limited.
- Untreated progressive disseminated histoplasmosis has a mortality rate of > 90%.
- For mild to moderate infection, use itraconazole.
- For severe infection, use liposomal amphotericin B, followed by itraconazole.

MUCORMYCOSIS

(Zygomycosis)

Mucormycosis refers to infection caused by diverse fungal species, including *Rhizopus*, *Rhizomucor*, and *Mucor*. Symptoms most frequently result from invasive necrotic lesions in the nose and palate, causing pain, fever, orbital cellulitis, proptosis, and purulent nasal discharge. CNS symptoms may follow. Pulmonary symptoms are severe and include productive cough, high fever, and dyspnea. Disseminated infection may occur in severely immunocompromised patients. Diagnosis is primarily clinical, requires a high index of suspicion, and is confirmed by histopathology and culture. Treatment is with IV amphotericin B and surgery to remove necrotic tissue. Even with aggressive treatment, mortality rates are high.

Infection is most common among immunocompromised people, in patients with poorly controlled diabetes (particularly those with ketoacidosis), and in patients receiving the iron-chelating drug deferoxamine.

The **most common form** of mucormycosis is

- Rhinocerebral

However, primary cutaneous, pulmonary, or GI lesions sometimes develop, and hematogenous dissemination to other sites can occur. Cutaneous *Rhizopus* infections have developed under occlusive dressings but more often result from trauma when the injured areas are contaminated with soil.

Symptoms and Signs

Rhinocerebral infections are usually severe and frequently fatal unless diagnosed early and treated aggressively.

Necrotic lesions appear on the nasal mucosa or sometimes the palate. Vascular invasion by hyphae leads to progressive tissue necrosis that may involve the nasal septum, palate, and bones surrounding the orbit or sinuses. Manifestations may include pain, fever, orbital cellulitis, proptosis, purulent nasal discharge, and mucosal necrosis.

Progressive extension of necrosis to the brain can cause signs of cavernous sinus thrombosis, seizures, aphasia, or hemiplegia.

Pulmonary infections resemble invasive aspergillosis. Pulmonary symptoms (eg, productive cough, high fever, dyspnea) are severe.

Diagnosis

- Examination of tissue samples for broad, ribbon-like, nonseptate hyphae
- Culture

Diagnosis requires a high index of suspicion and painstaking examination of tissue samples for large nonseptate hyphae with irregular diameters and right-angle branching patterns; the examination must be thorough because much of the necrotic debris contains no organisms. For unclear reasons, cultures may be negative, even when hyphae are clearly visible in tissues.

CTs and x-rays often underestimate or miss significant bone destruction.

Treatment

- Control of underlying condition
- Lipid amphotericin B formulations
- Surgical debridement

Effective therapy requires that diabetes be controlled or, if at all possible, immunosuppression be reversed or deferoxamine be stopped.

A high-dose lipid amphotericin B formulation (7.5 to 10 mg/kg IV once/day) is recommended as initial therapy, although isavuconazole was recently FDA approved as primary therapy. However, there is relatively limited clinical experience, and in severely ill patients, amphotericin B would likely remain the drug of choice. Posaconazole may also be effective, especially as consolidation therapy. Posaconazole has not been studied as primary therapy.

Complete surgical debridement of necrotic tissue is critical.

MYCETOMA

(Maduromycosis; Madura Foot)

Mycetoma is a chronic, progressive local infection caused by fungi or bacteria and involving the feet, upper extremities, or back. Symptoms include tumefaction and formation of sinus tracts. Diagnosis is clinical, confirmed by microscopic examination of exudates and culture. Treatment includes antimicrobials, surgical debridement, and sometimes amputation.

Bacteria, primarily *Nocardia* sp and other actinomycetes, cause more than half the cases. The remainder are caused by about 20 different fungal species. When caused by fungi, the lesions are sometimes called eumycetoma.

Mycetoma occurs mainly in tropical or subtropical areas, including the southern US, and is acquired when organisms enter through sites of local trauma on bare skin of the feet or on the extremities or backs of workers carrying contaminated vegetation or other objects. Men aged 20 to 40 are most often affected, presumably because of trauma incurred while working outdoors.

Infections spread through contiguous subcutaneous areas, resulting in tumefaction and formation of multiple draining sinuses that exude characteristic grains of clumped organisms. Microscopic tissue reactions may be primarily suppurative or granulomatous depending on the specific causative agent. As the infection progresses, bacterial superinfections can develop.

Symptoms and Signs

The initial lesion may be a papule, a fixed subcutaneous nodule, a vesicle with an indurated base, or a subcutaneous abscess that ruptures to form a fistula to the skin surface. Fibrosis is common in and around early lesions. Tenderness is minimal or absent unless acute suppurative bacterial superinfection is present.

Infection progresses slowly over months or years, gradually extending to and destroying contiguous muscles, tendons, fascia, and bones. Neither systemic dissemination nor symptoms and signs suggesting generalized infection occur. Eventually, muscle wasting, deformity, and tissue destruction prevent use of affected limbs. In advanced infections, involved extremities appear grotesquely swollen, forming a club-shaped mass of cystic areas. The multiple draining and intercommunicating sinus tracts and fistulas in these areas discharge thick or serosanguineous exudates containing characteristic grains, which may be white or black.

Diagnosis

- Examination and culture of exudates

Causative agents can be identified presumptively by gross and microscopic examination of grains from exudates, which contain irregularly shaped, variably colored, 0.5- to 2-mm granules. Crushing and culture of these granules provides definitive identification. Exudate specimens may yield multiple bacteria and fungi, some of which are potential causes of superinfections.

Treatment

- Antibacterial or antifungal drugs
- Sometimes surgery

Treatment may be required for > 10 yr. Death may result from bacterial superinfection and sepsis if treatment is neglected.

In infections caused by *Nocardia* (see p. 1615), sulfonamides and certain other antibacterial drugs, sometimes in combination, are used.

In infections caused by fungi, certain potential causative organisms may be at least partially sensitive to amphotericin B, itraconazole, or ketoconazole, but some are resistant to all antifungal drugs. Relapses occur after antifungal therapy in most patients, and many patients do not improve or even worsen during treatment, indicating the often refractory nature of the infection.

Surgical debridement is necessary, and limb amputation may be needed to prevent potentially fatal severe secondary bacterial infections.

PARACOCCIDIOIDOMYCOSIS

(South American Blastomycosis)

Paracoccidioidomycosis is progressive mycosis of the lungs, skin, mucous membranes, lymph nodes, and internal organs caused by *Paracoccidioides brasiliensis*. Symptoms are skin ulcers, adenitis, and pain due to abdominal organ involvement. Diagnosis is clinical and microscopic, confirmed by culture. Treatment is with azoles (eg, itraconazole), amphotericin B, or sulfonamides.

Infections occur only in discrete foci in South and Central America, most often in men aged 20 to 50, especially coffee growers of Colombia, Venezuela, and Brazil. An estimated 10 million people in South America are infected. Although a relatively unusual opportunistic infection, paracoccidioidomycosis sometimes occurs in immunocompromised patients, including those with AIDS. Although specific natural sites for *Paracoccidioides brasiliensis* remain undefined, it is presumed to exist in soil as a mold, with infection due to inhalation of conidia (spores produced by the mycelial form of the fungus). Conidia convert to invasive yeasts in the lungs and are assumed to spread to other sites via blood and lymphatics.

Symptoms and Signs

Most people who inhale conidia of *P. brasiliensis* do not become ill; illness, if it occurs, usually manifests as acute pneumonia, which may spontaneously resolve. Clinically apparent infections can become chronic and progressive but are not usually fatal. There are 3 patterns:

- **Mucocutaneous:** Infections most often involve the face, especially at the nasal and oral mucocutaneous borders. Yeasts are usually abundantly present within pinpoint lesions throughout granular bases of slowly expanding ulcers. Regional lymph nodes enlarge, become necrotic, and discharge necrotic material through the skin.
- **Lymphatic:** Cervical, supraclavicular, or axillary nodes enlarge but are painless.
- **Visceral:** Typically, focal lesions cause enlargement mainly of the liver, spleen, and abdominal lymph nodes, sometimes causing abdominal pain.

Infections may be mixed, involving combinations of all 3 patterns.

Diagnosis

- Culture and/or histopathology

Clinical findings suggest the diagnosis. Culture is diagnostic, although observation of large (often > 15 µm) yeasts that form characteristic multiple buds (pilot wheel) in specimens provides strong presumptive evidence. Because culturing *P. brasiliensis* can pose a severe biohazard to laboratory personnel, the laboratory should be notified of the suspected diagnosis.

Treatment

- Itraconazole

Azoles are highly effective. Oral itraconazole is generally considered the drug of choice, primarily because it costs less than other azoles that are available in endemic areas. IV amphotericin B can also eliminate the infection and is often used in very severe cases. Sulfonamides, which are widely used in some countries because they are inexpensive, can suppress growth of *Paracoccidioides* and cause lesions to regress but are not curative and must be given for up to 5 yr.

PHAEOHYPHOMYCOSIS

Phaeohyphomycosis refers to infections caused by many kinds of dark, melanin-pigmented dematiaceous fungi. It is distinguished from chromoblastomycosis and mycetoma by the absence of specific histopathologic findings.

Pigmented fungi have been increasingly recognized as opportunists, causing phaeohyphomycosis in immunocompetent and immunosuppressed patients. Phaeohyphomycosis can be caused by many species of dark, melanin-pigmented dematiaceous fungi including *Bipolaris*, *Cladophialophora*, *Cladosporium*, *Exophiala*, *Fonsecaea*, *Phialophora*, *Ochronosis*, *Rhinocladiella*, and *Wangiella*.

Dematiaceous fungi only rarely cause fatal infections in patients who have intact host defense mechanisms, although they may cause brain abscess in immunocompetent patients.

Clinical syndromes include invasive sinusitis, sometimes with bone necrosis, as well as subcutaneous nodules or abscesses, keratitis, lung masses, osteomyelitis, mycotic arthritis, endocarditis, brain abscess, and disseminated infection.

Diagnosis

- Examination using Masson-Fontana staining
- Culture to identify causative species

Dematiaceous fungi can frequently be discerned in tissue specimens stained with conventional hematoxylin and eosin; they appear as septate, brownish hyphae or yeast-like cells, reflecting their high melanin content. Masson-Fontana staining for melanin confirms their presence. Phaeohyphomycosis is distinguished from chromoblastomycosis and mycetoma by the absence of specific histopathologic findings such as sclerotic bodies or grains in tissue.

Culture is needed to identify the causative species.

Treatment

There is no standard therapy; treatment depends on the clinical syndrome and status of the patient.

For subcutaneous nodules, surgery alone may be curative. Itraconazole has excellent activity and has been used the most clinically, although voriconazole and posaconazole are being increasingly used with good results. Duration of therapy varies but may range from 6 wk to > 12 mo. Amphotericin B is often ineffective.

Combination therapy (eg, with 2 or 3 drugs, at least one of which is an azole) for brain abscess and disseminated infections is often used, although clinical outcomes are generally poor regardless of treatment.

SPOROTRICHOSIS

Sporotrichosis is a cutaneous infection caused by the saprophytic mold *Sporothrix schenckii*. Pulmonary and hematogenous involvement is uncommon. Symptoms are cutaneous nodules that spread via lymphatics and break down into abscesses and ulcers. Diagnosis is by culture. Treatment is with itraconazole or amphotericin B.

(See also the Infectious Diseases Society of America's Practice Guidelines for the Management of Sporotrichosis at www.academic.oup.com.)

Sporothrix schenckii resides on rose or barberry bushes, in sphagnum moss, and in other mulches. Horticulturists, gardeners, farm laborers, and timber workers are most often infected, typically after minor trauma involving contaminated material. In contrast to the other dimorphic fungi, *S. schenckii* is not usually inhaled but enters the body through small cuts and abrasions in the skin.

Symptoms and Signs

Lymphocutaneous infections are most common. They characteristically involve one hand and arm, although they can occur anywhere on the body; primary lesions may occur on exposed surfaces of the feet or face.

A primary lesion may appear as a small, nontender papule or, occasionally, as a slowly expanding subcutaneous nodule that eventually becomes necrotic and sometimes ulcerates. Typically, a few days or weeks later, a chain of lymph nodes that drain the affected area begins to enlarge slowly but progressively, forming movable subcutaneous nodules. Without treatment, overlying skin reddens and may later necrose, sometimes causing an abscess, ulceration, and bacterial superinfection. Systemic symptoms and signs of infection are notably absent.

Lymphocutaneous sporotrichosis is chronic and indolent; it is potentially fatal only if bacterial superinfections cause sepsis.

Rarely, in patients without primary lymphocutaneous lesions, hematogenous spread leads to indolent infections of multiple peripheral joints, sometimes bones, and, less often, genitals, liver, spleen, kidneys, or meninges. Equally rare is chronic pneumonia caused by inhaling spores and manifested by localized infiltrates or cavities, most often in patients with preexisting chronic lung disease.

Diagnosis

- Culture

The illness must be differentiated from local infections caused by *Mycobacterium tuberculosis*, atypical mycobacteria, *Nocardia*, or other organisms. During the early, nondisseminated stage, the primary lesion is sometimes misdiagnosed as a spider bite. Culture of tissue from the active infection site provides the definitive diagnosis. *S. schenckii* yeasts can be seen only rarely in fixed-tissue specimens, even with special staining. Serologic tests are not available.

Treatment

- Itraconazole

Oral itraconazole 200 mg po once/day given until 2 to 4 wk after all lesions have resolved (typically 3 to 6 mo) is the treatment of choice. Severe infection requires a lipid formulation of amphotericin B (3 to 5 mg/kg IV once/day); after a favorable response, treatment is switched to oral itraconazole for a total of 12 mo of treatment. AIDS patients may require lifelong maintenance therapy with itraconazole for meningeal and disseminated infection. Posaconazole may have a role.

MISCELLANEOUS OPPORTUNISTIC FUNGI

Many yeasts and molds can cause opportunistic, even life-threatening infections in immunocompromised patients. These infections only rarely affect immunocompetent people. Yeasts tend to cause fungemia as well as focal involvement of skin and other sites.

Blastoschizomyces capitatus and *Trichosporon* sp (including *T. ovoides*, *T. inkin*, *T. asahii*, *T. mucoides*, *T. asteroides*, and *T. cutaneum*) affect neutropenic patients in particular. Among *Trichosporon*, *T. asahii* is the most common cause of disseminated disease. The name *T. beigelii*, now obsolete, was formerly used for all or any of these *Trichosporon* sp.

Malassezia furfur fungemia typically affects infants and debilitated adults receiving lipid-containing IV hyperalimentation infusions.

Penicillium marneffei was recognized as an opportunistic invader in Southeast Asian patients with AIDS, and cases have been recognized in the US. *P. marneffei* skin lesions may resemble molluscum contagiosum.

Especially in neutropenic patients, various environmental molds, including species of *Fusarium* and *Scedosporium*, both of which are becoming more frequent, can cause focal vasculitic lesions mimicking invasive aspergillosis. *Fusarium* in particular may grow in routine blood cultures from patients with disseminated infection.

Specific diagnosis requires culture and species identification and is crucial because not all of these organisms respond to any single antifungal drug. For example, *Scedosporium* sp are typically resistant to amphotericin B. Optimal regimens of antifungal therapy for each member of this group of fungal opportunists must be defined.

190 Gram-Negative Bacilli

Gram-negative bacilli are responsible for numerous diseases. Some are commensal organisms present among normal intestinal flora. These commensal organisms plus others from animal or environmental reservoirs may cause disease.

UTIs, diarrhea, peritonitis, and bloodstream infections are commonly caused by gram-negative bacilli.

Gram-negative bacteria cause plague, cholera, and typhoid fever. These infections are rare in the US but are more common in areas of the world that are affected by poverty or war or have poor sanitation and/or an unsafe water and food supply. These infections can be serious.

OVERVIEW OF *BARTONELLA* INFECTIONS

Bartonella sp are gram-negative bacteria previously classified as Rickettsiae. They are facultative intracellular organisms that typically live within RBCs and endothelial cells. They cause several uncommon diseases:

- Cat-scratch disease
- An acute febrile anemia (Oroya fever)
- A chronic cutaneous eruption (bacillary angiomatosis)
- Disseminated disease (trench fever)

Risk is higher in immunocompromised hosts (see Table 190–1).

Bartonella infection (bartonellosis) is usually acquired by humans via an insect vector.

Table 190–1. SOME *BARTONELLA* INFECTIONS

SPECIES	MANIFESTATIONS*	AT RISK	INSECT VECTOR	TREATMENT
Bacillary angiomatosis				
B. henselae, B. quintana	Verrucous, fleshy skin lesions Disseminated visceral disease Lymphadenopathy Hepatosplenomegaly	Immunocompromised patients	Lice, fleas	Doxycycline†, azithromycin, erythromycin
Trench fever				
B. quintana	Prolonged or recurrent fever Bacteremia Endocarditis	People living in conditions of crowding or poor hygiene Immunocompromised patients at risk of disseminated infection	Body louse	‡Doxycycline†, erythromycin, rifampin
Cat-scratch disease				
B. henselae	Lymphadenopathy Fever Endocarditis in patients who have had a valvular heart disorder	Owners of cats Immunocompromised patients at risk of disseminated infection	Possibly cat fleas (which also transmit the organism among cats)	‡Doxycycline†, erythromycin, rifampin
Oroya fever, verruga peruana, Carrión disease				
B. bacilliformis	Acute febrile hemolytic anemia, skin lesions similar to those in bacillary angiomatosis Secondary infections	Residents of the Andes Mountains at elevations of 600–2400 m	*Phlebotomus* sandfly	Doxycycline†, chloramphenicol, rifampin, fluoroquinolones, streptomycin

*In normal host.
†Doxycycline is generally the preferred drug.
‡Treatment is not usually required in patients with normal immune systems; however, *Bartonella* bacteremia may be complicated by endocarditis.

CAT-SCRATCH DISEASE

(Cat-Scratch Fever)

Cat-scratch disease is infection caused by *Bartonella henselae*. Symptoms are a local papule and regional lymphadenitis. Diagnosis is clinical and confirmed by biopsy or serologic tests. Treatment is with local heat application, analgesics, and sometimes antibiotics.

The domestic cat, particularly kittens, is a major reservoir for *B. henselae*. The prevalence of *B. henselae* antibodies in US cats is 14 to 50%. About 99% of patients report contact with cats, most of which are healthy. The specific location of the organism in the cat is unclear; however, periods of asymptomatic bacteremia occur in cycles. Infection is spread to humans via a bite or scratch. The cat flea transmits infection among cats and may be the cause of disease in humans who have not had contact with cats, although this theory is unproved. Children are most often affected.

Symptoms and Signs

Within 3 to 10 days after a bite or scratch, most patients develop an erythematous, crusted papule (rarely, a pustule) at the scratch site. Regional lymphadenopathy develops within 2 wk. The nodes are initially firm and tender, later becoming fluctuant, and may drain with fistula formation. Fever, malaise, headache, and anorexia may accompany lymphadenopathy.

Unusual manifestations occur in 5 to 14% of patients:

- Parinaud oculoglandular syndrome (conjunctivitis associated with palpable preauricular nodes) in 6%
- Neurologic manifestations (encephalopathy, seizures, neuroretinitis, myelitis, paraplegia, cerebral arteritis) in 2%
- Hepatosplenic granulomatous disease in < 1%

Patients may also present with an FUO. *B. henselae* is one of the most common causes of culture-negative endocarditis, usually in patients with prior valvular heart disease. Severe disseminated illness may occur in patients with AIDS.

Lymphadenopathy subsides spontaneously within 2 to 5 mo. Complete recovery is usual, except in severe neurologic or hepatosplenic disease, which may be fatal or have residual effects.

Diagnosis

- Acute and convalescent serologic testing or PCR testing
- Sometimes lymph node biopsy

Diagnosis of cat-scratch disease is typically confirmed by positive serum Ab titers (testing acute and convalescent sera 6 wk apart is recommended) or PCR testing of samples from lymph node aspirates.

Because similar lymphadenopathy may be caused by other infections (eg, tularemia, mycobacterial infection, brucellosis, fungal infection, lymphogranuloma venereum), testing for those organisms may be done if the diagnosis is not clearly cat-scratch disease.

Lymph node biopsy may be done if cancer is suspected or if the diagnosis of cat-scratch disease needs to be confirmed. Diagnosis is suggested by characteristic histopathologic findings (eg, suppurative granulomas) or detection of organisms by immunofluorescence.

Immunocompromised patients and patients with systemic symptoms should also have blood cultures. Lymph node aspirates are rarely culture-positive. However, *Bartonella* sp can be isolated from cultures of lymph node biopsy specimens.

Treatment

- Local heat and analgesics
- Sometimes antibiotics for immunocompromised patients

Treatment of cat-scratch disease in immunocompetent patients is local heat application and analgesics for this typically self-limited disease. If a lymph node is fluctuant, needle aspiration usually relieves the pain.

Antibiotic treatment is not clearly beneficial and generally should not be given for localized infection in immunocompetent patients. However, azithromycin, erythromycin, or doxycycline is often given to reduce adenopathy and perhaps decrease the risk of systemic spread. A fluoroquinolone, rifampin, gentamicin, or doxycycline may be used for bacteremia in AIDS patients. Prolonged therapy (eg, weeks to months) is usually necessary for bacteremia to clear. In vitro antibiotic susceptibilities often do not correlate with clinical results.

OROYA FEVER AND VERRUGA PERUANA

(Carrión Disease)

Oroya fever and verruga peruana are infections caused by *Bartonella bacilliformis*. Oroya fever occurs after initial exposure; verruga peruana occurs after recovery from the primary infection.

Endemic only to the Andes Mountains in Colombia, Ecuador, and Peru, both Oroya fever and verruga peruana are passed from human to human by the *Phlebotomus* sandfly.

Oroya fever: Symptoms of Oroya fever include fever and profound anemia, which may be sudden or indolent in onset. The anemia is primarily hemolytic, but myelosuppression also occurs. Muscle and joint pain, severe headache, and often delirium and coma may occur. Superimposed bacteremia caused by *Salmonella* or other coliform organisms may occur. Mortality rates may exceed 50% in untreated patients.

Diagnosis of Oroya fever is confirmed by blood cultures.

Because Oroya fever is often complicated by *Salmonella* bacteremia, chloramphenicol 500 to 1000 mg po q 6 h for 7 days is the treatment of choice; some clinicians add another antibiotic, typically doxycycline or a beta-lactam, but trimethoprim/sulfamethoxazole (TMP/SMX), macrolides, and fluoroquinolones have also been used successfully.

Verruga peruana: Verruga peruana manifests as multiple skin lesions that strongly resemble bacillary angiomatosis; these raised, reddish purple skin nodules usually occur on the limbs and face. The lesions may persist for months to years and may be accompanied by pain and fever.

Verruga peruana is diagnosed by its appearance and sometimes by biopsy showing dermal angiogenesis.

Treatment with most antibiotics produces remission, but relapse is common and requires prolonged therapy.

Typical treatment is rifampin 10 mg/kg po once/day for 10 to 14 days or streptomycin 15 to 20 mg/kg IM once/day for 10 days. Ciprofloxacin 500 mg po bid for 7 to 10 days has been used successfully, as has azithromycin, doxycycline, and trimethoprim-sulfamethoxazole.

BACILLARY ANGIOMATOSIS

(Epithelioid Angiomatosis)

Bacillary angiomatosis is skin infection caused by *Bartonella henselae* or *B. quintana*.

Bacillary angiomatosis almost always occurs in immunocompromised people and is characterized by protuberant, reddish, berrylike lesions on the skin, often surrounded by a collar of scale. Lesions bleed profusely if traumatized. They may resemble Kaposi sarcoma or pyogenic granulomas.

Infection with *B. quintana* is spread by lice; infection with *B. henselae* is probably spread by fleas from household cats. Disease may spread throughout the reticuloendothelial system, causing bacillary peliosis (peliosis hepatis due to *Bartonella* bacteria), particularly in AIDS patients.

Diagnosis of bacillary angiomatosis relies on histopathology of the skin lesions, cultures, and PCR analysis. The laboratory should be notified that *Bartonella* is suspected because special stains and prolonged culture growth are necessary.

Treatment of bacillary angiomatosis is with erythromycin 500 mg po q 6 h or doxycycline 100 mg po q 12 h, continued for at least 3 mo. Fluoroquinolones and azithromycin are alternatives.

TRENCH FEVER

(Wolhynia, Shin Bone, or Quintan Fever)

Trench fever is a louse-borne disease caused by *Bartonella quintana* and observed originally in military populations during World Wars I and II. Symptoms are an acute, recurring febrile illness, occasionally with a rash. Diagnosis is by blood culture. Treatment is with a macrolide or doxycycline.

Humans are the only reservoir of this *Bartonella* infection. *B. quintana* is transmitted to humans when feces from infected lice are rubbed into abraded skin or the conjunctiva. Trench fever is endemic in Mexico, Tunisia, Eritrea, Poland, and the former Soviet Union and is reappearing in the homeless population in the US.

Symptoms and Signs

After a 14- to 30-day incubation period, onset of trench fever is sudden, with fever, weakness, dizziness, headache (with pain behind the eyes), conjunctival injection, and severe back and leg (shin) pains.

Fever may reach 40.5° C and persist for 5 to 6 days. In about half the cases, fever recurs 1 to 8 times at 5- to 6-day intervals.

A transient macular or papular rash and, occasionally, hepatomegaly and splenomegaly occur. Endocarditis may complicate some cases.

Relapses are common and have occurred up to 10 yr after the initial attack.

Diagnosis

- Blood cultures
- Serologic tests and PCR

Trench fever should be suspected in people living where louse infestation is heavy. Leptospirosis, typhus, relapsing fever, and malaria must be considered.

The organism is identified by blood culture, although growth may take 1 to 4 wk. The disease is marked by persistent bacteremia during the initial attack, during relapses, throughout the asymptomatic periods between relapses, and in patients with endocarditis.

Serologic testing is available and can provide support for the diagnosis. High titers of IgG antibodies should trigger evaluation for endocarditis. PCR testing of blood or tissue samples can be done.

Treatment

- Doxycycline, a macrolide, or ceftriaxone

Although recovery is usually complete in 1 to 2 mo and mortality is negligible, bacteremia may persist for months after clinical recovery, and prolonged (> 1 mo) doxycycline or macrolide treatment may be needed. Patients are given doxycycline 100 mg po bid for 4 to 6 wk plus, if endocarditis is suspected, gentamicin 3 mg/kg/day IV for the initial 2 wk.

Body lice must be controlled.

Patients with chronic bacteremia should be monitored for signs of endocarditis.

BRUCELLOSIS

(Undulant, Malta, Mediterranean, or Gibraltar Fever)

Brucellosis is caused by *Brucella* sp. Symptoms begin as an acute febrile illness with few or no localized signs and may progress to a chronic stage with relapses of fever, weakness, sweats, and vague aches and pains. Diagnosis is by culture, usually from the blood. Optimal treatment usually requires 2 antibiotics—doxycycline or trimethoprim/sulfamethoxazole plus gentamicin, streptomycin, or rifampin.

The causative organisms of human brucellosis are *B. abortus* (from cattle), *B. melitensis* (from sheep and goats), and *B. suis* (from hogs). *B. canis* (from dogs) has caused sporadic infections. Generally, *B. melitensis* and *B. suis* are more pathogenic than other *Brucella* sp.

The most common sources of infection are farm animals and raw dairy products. Deer, bison, horses, moose, caribou, hares, chickens, and desert rats may also be infected; humans can acquire the infection from these animals as well.

Brucellosis is acquired by

- Direct contact with secretions and excretions of infected animals
- Ingesting undercooked meat, raw milk, or milk products containing viable organisms
- Inhaling aerosolized infectious material
- Rarely, person-to-person transmission

Most prevalent in rural areas, brucellosis is an occupational disease of meatpackers, veterinarians, hunters, farmers, livestock producers, and microbiology laboratory technicians. Brucellosis is rare in the US, Europe, and Canada, but cases occur in the Middle East, Mediterranean regions, Mexico, and Central America.

Because very few organisms (perhaps as few as 10 to 100) may cause infection via aerosol exposure, *Brucella* sp are potential agents of biological terrorism.

Patients with acute, uncomplicated brucellosis usually recover in 2 to 3 wk, even without treatment. Some go on to subacute, intermittent, or chronic disease.

Complications: Complications of brucellosis are rare but include subacute bacterial endocarditis, meningitis, encephalitis, neuritis, orchitis, cholecystitis, hepatic suppuration, and osteomyelitis (particularly sacroiliac or vertebral).

Symptoms and Signs

The incubation period for brucellosis varies from 5 days to several months and averages 2 wk. Onset may be sudden, with chills and fever, severe headache, joint and low back pain, malaise, and occasionally diarrhea. Or onset may be insidious, with mild prodromal malaise, muscular pain, headache, and pain in the back of the neck, followed by a rise in evening temperature. As the disease progresses, temperature increases to 40 to 41° C, then subsides gradually to normal or near-normal with profuse sweating in the morning.

Typically, intermittent fever persists for 1 to 5 wk, followed by a 2- to 14-day remission when symptoms are greatly diminished or absent. In some patients, fever may be transient. In others, the febrile phase recurs once or repeatedly in waves (undulations) and remissions over months or years and may manifest as FUO.

After the initial febrile phase, anorexia, weight loss, abdominal and joint pain, headache, backache, weakness, irritability, insomnia, depression, and emotional instability may occur. Constipation is usually pronounced. Splenomegaly appears, and lymph nodes may be slightly or moderately enlarged. Up to 50% of patients have hepatomegaly.

Brucellosis is fatal in < 5% of patients, usually as a result of endocarditis or severe CNS complications.

Diagnosis

- Blood cultures
- Acute and convalescent serologic testing

Blood cultures should be obtained; growth may take > 7 days, and subcultures using special media may need to be held for up to 3 to 4 wk, so the laboratory should be notified of the suspicion of brucellosis.

Acute and convalescent sera should be obtained 3 wk apart. A 4-fold increase or an acute titer of 1:160 or higher is considered diagnostic, particularly if a history of exposure and characteristic clinical findings are present. The WBC count is normal or reduced with relative or absolute lymphocytosis during the acute phase.

Treatment

- Doxycycline plus either rifampin, an aminoglycoside (streptomycin or gentamicin), or ciprofloxacin

Activity should be restricted in acute cases, with bed rest recommended during febrile episodes. Severe musculoskeletal pains, especially over the spine, may require analgesia. *Brucella* endocarditis often requires surgery in addition to antibiotic therapy.

If antibiotics are given, combination therapy is preferred because relapse rates with monotherapy are high. Doxycycline 100 mg po bid for 6 wk plus streptomycin 1 g IM q 12 to 24 h (or gentamicin 3 mg/kg IV once/day) for 14 days lowers the rate of relapse. For uncomplicated cases, rifampin 600 to 900 mg po bid for 6 wk can be used instead of an aminoglycoside.

Regimens using ciprofloxacin 500 mg po bid for 14 to 42 days plus rifampin or doxycycline instead of an aminoglycoside have been shown to be equally effective. In children < 8 yr, trimethoprim/sulfamethoxazole (TMP/SMX) and oral rifampin for 4 to 6 wk have been used.

Even with antibiotic treatment, about 5 to 15% of patients relapse, so all should be followed clinically and with repeat serologic titers for 1 yr.

Prevention

Pasteurization of milk helps prevent brucellosis. Cheese that is made from unpasteurized milk and is aged < 3 mo may be contaminated.

People handling animals or carcasses likely to be infected should wear goggles and rubber gloves and protect skin breaks from exposure. Programs to detect infection in animals, eliminate infected animals, and vaccinate young seronegative cattle and swine are required in the US and in several other countries.

There is no human vaccine; use of the animal vaccine (a live-attenuated preparation) in humans can cause infection. Immunity after human infection is short-lived, lasting about 2 yr.

Postexposure antibiotic prophylaxis is recommended for high-risk patients (eg, those who have unprotected exposure to infected animals or laboratory samples or who received animal vaccine). Regimens include doxycycline 100 mg po bid plus rifampin 600 mg po once/day for 3 wk; rifampin is not used for exposure to the *B. abortus* (strain RB51) vaccine, which is resistant to rifampin.

KEY POINTS

- Brucellosis is acquired by direct contact with secretions and excretions of infected animals.
- Infection typically causes fever and constitutional symptoms, but specific organs (eg, brain, meninges, heart, liver, bones) are rarely affected.
- Most patients recover in 2 to 3 wk, even without treatment, but some develop subacute, intermittent, or chronic disease.
- Diagnose using blood cultures and acute and convalescent serologic testing.
- Treat most patients with 2 antibiotics, typically doxycycline plus either rifampin, an aminoglycoside, or ciprofloxacin; monitor patients up to 1 yr for relapse.

CAMPYLOBACTER AND RELATED INFECTIONS

***Campylobacter* infections commonly cause diarrhea and occasionally bacteremia, with consequent endocarditis, osteomyelitis, or septic arthritis.**

Campylobacter sp are motile, curved, microaerophilic, gram-negative bacilli that normally inhabit the GI tract of many domestic animals and fowl.

Several species are human pathogens. The major pathogens are *C. jejuni* and *C. fetus*. *C. jejuni* causes diarrhea in all age groups, although peak incidence appears to be from age 1 to 5 yr. *C. jejuni* accounts for more cases of diarrhea in the US than *Salmonella* and *Shigella* combined. *C. fetus* and several others typically cause bacteremia and systemic manifestations in adults, more often when underlying predisposing diseases, such as diabetes, cirrhosis, cancer, or HIV/AIDS, are present. In patients with immunoglobulin deficiencies, these organisms may cause difficult-to-treat, relapsing infections. *C. jejuni* can cause meningitis in infants.

The following have been implicated in outbreaks

- Contact with infected animals (eg, puppies)
- Contact with contaminated food or water (eg, handling food)
- Ingestion of contaminated food (especially undercooked poultry) or water

Person-to-person transmission through fecal-oral and sexual contact may also occur. However, in sporadic cases, the source of the infecting organism is frequently obscure.

Complications: *C. jejuni* diarrheal illness is associated with subsequent development of Guillain-Barré syndrome (GBS) because of cross-reaction between *C. jejuni* antibodies and surface components of peripheral nerves. Although only 1 case of GBS is estimated to occur per 2000 *C. jejuni* infections, about 25 to 40% of patients who develop GBS have had a prior *C. jejuni* infection.

Postinfectious (reactive) arthritis may occur in HLA-B27–positive patients a few days to several weeks after an episode of *C. jejuni* diarrhea. Other postinfectious complications include uveitis, hemolytic anemia, hemolytic-uremic syndrome, myopericarditis, immunoproliferative small intestinal disease, septic abortion, and encephalopathy.

Focal extraintestinal infections (eg, endocarditis, meningitis, septic arthritis) occur rarely with *C. jejuni* but are more common with *C. fetus*.

Symptoms and Signs

The most common manifestation of *Campylobacter* infection is watery and sometimes bloody diarrhea. Fever (38 to 40° C), which follows a relapsing or intermittent course, is the only constant feature of systemic *Campylobacter* infection, although abdominal pain (typically in the right lower quadrant), headache, and myalgias are frequent.

Patients can also present with subacute bacterial endocarditis (more often due to *C. fetus*), reactive arthritis, meningitis, or an indolent FUO rather than with diarrheal illness. Joint involvement with reactive arthritis is usually monoarticular, affecting the knees; symptoms resolve spontaneously over 1 wk to several months.

Diagnosis

- Stool culture
- Sometimes blood cultures

Diagnosis, particularly to differentiate *Campylobacter* infection from ulcerative colitis, requires microbiologic evaluation. Stool culture should be obtained plus blood cultures for patients with signs of focal infection or serious systemic illness. WBCs are present in stained smears of stool.

Treatment

- Sometimes erythromycin

Most enteric infections resolve spontaneously; if they do not, erythromycin 500 mg po q 6 h for 5 days may be helpful. Azithromycin 500 mg po once/day for 3 days is an alternative. Because resistance to ciprofloxacin is increasing, this drug should be used judiciously.

For patients with extraintestinal infections, antibiotics (eg, imipenem, gentamicin, ampicillin, a 3rd-generation cephalosporin, erythromycin) should be given for 2 to 4 wk to prevent relapses.

CHOLERA

Cholera is an acute infection of the small bowel by *Vibrio cholerae*, which secretes a toxin that causes copious watery diarrhea, leading to dehydration, oliguria, and circulatory collapse. Infection is typically through contaminated water or seafood. Diagnosis is by culture or serology. Treatment is vigorous rehydration and electrolyte replacement plus doxycycline.

The causative organism, *V. cholerae,* serogroups 01 and 0139, is a short, curved, motile, aerobic bacillus that produces enterotoxin, a protein that induces hypersecretion of an isotonic electrolyte solution by the small-bowel mucosa. These organisms do not invade the intestinal wall; thus, few or no WBCs are found in stool.

Both the El Tor and classic biotypes of *V. cholerae* 01 can cause severe disease. However, mild or asymptomatic infection is much more common with the currently predominant El Tor biotype and with non-01, non-0139 serogroups of *V. cholerae*.

Cholera is spread by ingestion of water, seafood, or other foods contaminated by the excrement of people with symptomatic or asymptomatic infection. Household contacts of patients with cholera are at high risk of infection that probably occurs through shared sources of contaminated food and water. Person-to-person transmission is less likely to occur because a large inoculum of organism is needed to transmit the infection.

Cholera is endemic in portions of Asia, the Middle East, Africa, South and Central America, and the Gulf Coast of the US. Cases transported into Europe, Japan, and Australia have caused localized outbreaks. In endemic areas, outbreaks usually occur during warm months. The incidence is highest in children. In newly affected areas, epidemics may occur during any season, and all ages are equally susceptible.

A milder form of gastroenteritis is caused by noncholera vibrios.

Susceptibility to infection varies and is greater for people with blood type O. Because vibrios are sensitive to gastric acid, hypochlorhydria and achlorhydria are predisposing factors.

People living in endemic areas gradually acquire a natural immunity.

Symptoms and Signs

The incubation period for cholera is 1 to 3 days. Cholera can be subclinical, a mild and uncomplicated episode of diarrhea, or a fulminant, potentially lethal disease.

Abrupt, painless, watery diarrhea and vomiting are usually the initial symptoms. Significant nausea is typically absent. Stool loss in adults may exceed 1 L/h but is usually much less. Often, stools consist of white liquid void of fecal material (rice-water stool). The resultant severe water and electrolyte depletion leads to intense thirst, oliguria, muscle cramps, weakness, and marked loss of tissue turgor, with sunken eyes and wrinkling of skin on the fingers. Hypovolemia, hemoconcentration, oliguria and anuria, and severe metabolic acidosis with K+ depletion (but normal serum Na+ concentration) occur. If cholera is untreated, circulatory collapse with cyanosis and stupor may follow. Prolonged hypovolemia can cause renal tubular necrosis.

Most patients are free of *V. cholerae* within 2 wk after cessation of diarrhea; chronic biliary tract carriers are rare.

Diagnosis

- Stool culture and serotyping

Diagnosis of cholera is confirmed by stool culture (use of selective media is recommended) plus subsequent serotyping. Tests for *V. cholerae* are available in reference laboratories; PCR testing is also an option. Rapid dipstick testing for cholera is available for public health use in areas with limited access to laboratory testing.

Cholera should be distinguished from clinically similar disease caused by enterotoxin-producing strains of *Escherichia coli* and occasionally by *Salmonella* and *Shigella.*

Serum electrolytes, BUN, and creatinine should be measured.

Treatment

- Fluid replacement
- Doxycycline, azithromycin, furazolidone, trimethoprim/sulfamethoxazole (TMP/SMX), or ciprofloxacin, depending on results of susceptibility testing

Fluid replacement: Replacement of fluid loss is essential. Mild cases can be treated with standard oral rehydration formulas. Rapid correction of severe hypovolemia is lifesaving. Prevention or correction of metabolic acidosis and hypokalemia is important. For hypovolemic and severely dehydrated patients, IV replacement with isotonic fluids should be used (for details on fluid resuscitation, see pp. 576 and 2557). Water should also be given freely by mouth. To replace potassium losses, KCl 10 to 15 mEq/L can be added to the IV solution, or $KHCO_3$ 1 mL/kg po of a 100-g/L solution can be given qid. Potassium replacement is especially important for children, who tolerate hypokalemia poorly.

Once intravascular volume is restored (rehydration phase), amounts for replacement of continuing losses should equal measured stool volume (maintenance phase). Adequacy of hydration is confirmed by frequent clinical evaluation (pulse rate and strength, skin turgor, urine output). Plasma, plasma volume expanders, and vasopressors should *not* be used in place of water and electrolytes.

Oral glucose-electrolyte solution is effective in replacing stool losses and may be used after initial IV rehydration, and it may be the only means of rehydration in epidemic areas where supplies of parenteral fluids are limited. Patients who have mild or moderate dehydration and who can drink may be rehydrated with the oral solution (about 75 mL/kg in 4 h). Those with more severe dehydration need more and may need to receive the fluid by nasogastric tube.

The oral rehydration solution (ORS) recommended by the WHO contains 13.5 g glucose, 2.6 g NaCl, 2.9 g trisodium citrate dihydrate (or 2.5 g $NaHCO_3$), and 1.5 g KCl per liter of drinking water. This solution is best prepared using widely available, premeasured, sealed packets of glucose and salts; one packet is mixed with 1 L of clean water. Using such prepared ORS packets minimizes the possibility of error when untrained people mix the solution. If ORS packets are not available, a reasonable substitute can be made by mixing half a small spoon of salt and 6 small spoons of sugar in 1 L of clean water. The ORS should be continued ad libitum after rehydration in amounts at least equal to continuing stool and vomitus losses. Solid food should be given only after vomiting stops and appetite returns.

Antimicrobials: Early treatment with an effective oral antimicrobial eradicates vibrios, reduces stool volume by 50%, and stops diarrhea within 48 h. The choice of antimicrobial should be based on the susceptibility of *V. cholerae* isolated from the community.

Drugs effective for susceptible strains include

- Doxycycline: For adults, a single dose of 300 mg po or 100 mg bid on day 1, then 100 mg once/day on days 2 and 3; or a single dose of azithromycin 1 g po (recommended for pregnant women) or 20 mg/kg for children
- Furazolidone (not available in the US): For adults, 100 mg po qid for 72 h; for children, 1.5 mg/kg qid for 72 h

- TMP/SMX: For adults, one double-strength tablet bid; for children, 5 mg/kg (of the TMP component) bid for 72 h
- Ciprofloxacin: For adults, a single dose of 1 g po or 250 mg po once/day for 3 days

Prevention

For control of cholera, human excrement must be correctly disposed of, and water supplies purified. In endemic regions, drinking water should be boiled or chlorinated, and vegetables and fish cooked thoroughly.

Vaxchora® is a live-attenuated **oral vaccine** that has been approved for use in the US for prevention of *V. cholerae* O1 in adults 18 to 64 yr of age traveling to cholera-affected areas.

Two killed whole-cell oral vaccines are currently available for use in children and adults internationally but not in the US:

- Dukoral®: This monovalent vaccine contains only *V. cholerae* 01 and El Tor bacteria plus a small amount of nontoxic b subunit cholera toxin; it must be taken with a large amount of buffer fluid (buffer packet is dissolved in 5 oz of cool water) at the time of vaccine administration.
- Shanchol®: This newer bivalent vaccine contains both 01 and 0139 strains of *V. cholerae* and has no added components, eliminating the requirement for excessive fluid ingestion at the time of vaccination.

Both vaccines provide 60 to 85% protection for up to 5 yr. Both require 2 doses, and booster doses are recommended after 2 yr for people with ongoing risk of cholera.

Injectable vaccines provide less protection for shorter periods of time with more adverse effects and are not recommended when an oral vaccine is available.

Antibiotic prophylaxis for household contacts of patients with cholera is not recommended because data supporting this measure are lacking.

KEY POINTS

- *V. cholerae* serogroups 01 and 0139 secrete an enterotoxin that can cause severe, sometimes fatal diarrheal illness that often occurs in large outbreaks caused by mass exposure to contaminated water or food.
- Other *V. cholerae* serogroups can cause milder, nonepidemic disease.
- Diagnose using stool culture and serotyping; a rapid dipstick test is helpful in identifying outbreaks in remote areas.
- Rehydration is critical; oral rehydration solution is adequate for most cases, but patients with severe volume depletion require IV fluids.
- Give infected adults doxycycline or azithromycin (TMP/SMX for children) pending results of susceptibility testing.

NONCHOLERA *VIBRIO* INFECTIONS

Noncholera vibrios include *Vibrio parahaemolyticus, V. mimicus, V. alginolyticus, V. hollisae*, and *V. vulnificus*; they may cause diarrhea, wound infection, or septicemia.

Noncholera vibrios are sometimes called nonagglutinable vibrios (ie, they do not agglutinate with serum from cholera patients). They typically inhabit warm salt water or mixed salt and fresh water (eg, in estuaries).

V. parahaemolyticus, V. mimicus, and *V. hollisae* usually cause food-borne outbreaks of diarrhea, typically involving inadequately cooked seafood (usually shellfish). *V. parahaemolyticus* infections typically occur in Japan and in coastal areas of the US. The organisms damage intestinal mucosa but do not produce enterotoxin or invade the bloodstream. Also, wound infection may develop when contaminated warm seawater enters a minor wound.

V. alginolyticus and *V. vulnificus* can cause serious wound infection; neither causes enteritis. *V. vulnificus*, when ingested by a compromised host (often someone with chronic liver disease or immunodeficiency), can cross the intestinal mucosa without causing enteritis and cause septicemia with a high mortality rate; occasionally, otherwise healthy people develop such infections.

Symptoms and Signs

Enteric illness begins suddenly after a 15- to 24-h incubation period; manifestations include cramping abdominal pain, large amounts of watery diarrhea (stools may be bloody and contain PMNs), tenesmus, weakness, and sometimes nausea, vomiting, and low-grade fever. Symptoms subside spontaneously in 24 to 48 h.

Cellulitis can rapidly develop in contaminated wounds in some cases (typically those involving *V. vulnificus*) and progress to necrotizing fasciitis with typical hemorrhagic, bullous lesions.

***V. vulnificus* septicemia** causes shock, bullous skin lesions, and often manifestations of disseminated intravascular coagulation (eg, thrombocytopenia, hemorrhage); mortality rate is high.

Diagnosis

- Cultures

Wound and bloodstream infections are readily diagnosed with routine cultures. When enteric infection is suspected, *Vibrio* organisms can be cultured from stool on thiosulfate citrate bile salts sucrose medium. Contaminated seafood also yields positive cultures.

Treatment

- Ciprofloxacin or doxycycline for enteric infection
- Antibiotics and often debridement for wound infection

Noncholera *Vibrio* enteric infections can be treated with a single dose of ciprofloxacin 1 g po or doxycycline 300 mg po. However, generally, such treatment is not necessary because the infection is self-limited, although treatment may be considered in severe cases.

If diarrhea is present, close attention to volume repletion and replacement of lost electrolytes are needed.

For wound infections, antibiotics are used—typically, doxycycline 100 mg po q 12 h, with or without a 3rd-generation cephalosporin for severe wound infection or septicemia. Ciprofloxacin is an acceptable alternative.

Patients with necrotizing fasciitis require surgical debridement.

KEY POINTS

- Noncholera vibrios may cause diarrhea, wound infection, or septicemia, depending on the species and mode of exposure.
- Diagnose using cultures of stool, wound, or blood as appropriate.
- Treat severe enteric infections with a single dose ciprofloxacin or doxycycline.
- Treat wound infections with doxycycline; for severe infection, add a 3rd-generation cephalosporin.

ESCHERICHIA COLI INFECTIONS

Escherichia coli **are the most numerous aerobic commensal inhabitants of the large intestine. Certain strains cause diarrhea, and all can cause infection when they invade sterile sites (eg, the urinary tract). Diagnosis is by standard culture techniques. Toxin assays may help identify the cause of diarrhea. Treatment with antibiotics is guided by susceptibility testing.**

Diseases caused by *E. coli*:

- UTI (most common)
- Enteric infection (certain strains)
- Invasive infection (rare, except in neonates)
- Infection at other sites

Most commonly, *E. coli* cause UTIs, which usually represent ascending infection (ie, from the perineum via the urethra). *E. coli* may also cause prostatitis and pelvic inflammatory disease (PID).

E. coli normally inhabit the GI tract; however, some strains have acquired genes that enable them to cause intestinal infection. When ingested, the following strains can cause diarrhea:

- **Enterohemorrhagic:** These strains (including serotype O157:H7 and others) produce several cytotoxins, neurotoxins, and enterotoxins, including Shiga toxin (verotoxin), and cause bloody diarrhea; hemolytic-uremic syndrome develops in 2 to 7% of cases. Such strains have most often been acquired from undercooked ground beef but may also be acquired from infected people by the fecal-oral route when hygiene is inadequate.
- **Enterotoxigenic:** These strains can cause watery diarrhea, particularly in infants and travelers (traveler's diarrhea).
- **Enteroinvasive:** These strains can cause inflammatory diarrhea.
- **Enteropathogenic:** These strains can cause watery diarrhea, particularly in infants.
- **Enteroaggregative:** Some strains are emerging as potentially important causes of persistent diarrhea in patients with AIDS and in children in tropical areas.

Other strains are capable of causing extraintestinal infection if normal intestinal anatomic barriers are disrupted (eg, by ischemia, inflammatory bowel disease, or trauma), in which case the organism may spread to adjacent structures or invade the bloodstream. Hepatobiliary, peritoneal, cutaneous, and pulmonary infections also occur. *E. coli* bacteremia may also occur without an evident portal of entry.

In neonates, particularly preterm infants, *E. coli* bacteremia and meningitis (caused by strains with the K1 capsule, a marker for neuroinvasiveness) are common.

Diagnosis

- Culture

Samples of blood, stool, or other clinical material are sent for culture. If an enterohemorrhagic strain is suspected, the laboratory must be notified because special culture media are required.

Treatment

- Various antibiotics depending on site of infection and susceptibility testing

Treatment of *E. coli* infections must be started empirically based on the site and severity of infection (eg, mild bladder infection, urosepsis) and then modified based on antibiotic susceptibility testing. Many strains are resistant to ampicillin and tetracyclines, so other drugs should be used; they include ticarcillin, piperacillin, cephalosporins, aminoglycosides, trimethoprim/sulfamethoxazole (TMP/SMX), and fluoroquinolones.

Surgery may be required to control the source of infection (eg, to drain pus, debride necrotic lesions, or remove foreign bodies).

Drug resistance: Besides being resistant to ampicillin and tetracycline, *E. coli* have become increasingly resistant to TMP/SMX and fluoroquinolones. Also, multidrug-resistant strains that produce extended-spectrum beta-lactamases (ESBLs) have emerged as an important cause of community-acquired UTI and sepsis. ESBLs can hydrolyze most beta-lactams, including penicillins and broad-spectrum cephalosporins and monobactams, but not carbapenems (imipenem, meropenem, doripenem, ertapenem); carbapenems should be used for ESBL-producing *E. coli*.

INFECTION BY *ESCHERICHIA COLI* O157:H7 AND OTHER ENTEROHEMORRHAGIC *E. COLI*

E. coli **O157:H7 and other enterohemorrhagic *E. coli* (EHEC) typically cause acute bloody diarrhea, which may lead to hemolytic-uremic syndrome. Symptoms are abdominal cramps and diarrhea that may be grossly bloody. Fever is not prominent. Diagnosis is by stool culture and toxin assay. Treatment is supportive; antibiotic use is not recommended.**

Epidemiology

EHEC include > 100 serotypes that produce Shiga and Shiga-like toxins (Shiga toxin–producing E. coli [STEC]; also known as verotoxin-producing *E. coli* [VTEC]).

E. coli O157:H7 is the most common STEC in North America. However, non-O157 STEC serotypes (particularly O26, O45, O91, O103, O111, O113, O121, O128, and O145) may also cause enterohemorrhagic illness, particularly outside the US. In 2011, serotype O104:H4 caused a significant, multinational outbreak in Europe.

In some parts of the US and Canada, *E. coli* O157:H7 infection may be a more common cause of bloody diarrhea than shigellosis or salmonellosis. *E. coli* O157:H7 infection can occur in people of all ages, although severe infection is most common among children and the elderly.

E. coli O157:H7 and other STEC have a bovine reservoir. Infection can be transmitted via food or water contaminated with cow manure, as in the outbreaks and sporadic cases that typically occur after ingestion of undercooked beef (especially ground beef) or unpasteurized milk. In the 2011 European O104:H4 outbreak, infection was transmitted by contaminated raw bean sprouts. The organism can also be transmitted by the fecal-oral route, especially among infants in diapers (eg, via inadequately chlorinated children's wading pools).

Pathophysiology

After ingestion, *E. coli* O157:H7 and similar STEC serotypes produce high levels of various toxins in the large intestine; these toxins are closely related to the potent cytotoxins produced by *Shigella dysenteriae* type 1. These toxins appear to directly damage mucosal cells and vascular endothelial cells in the gut wall. If absorbed, they exert toxic effects on other vascular endothelia (eg, renal).

About 5% of cases (mostly children < 5 yr and adults > 60 yr) are complicated by hemolytic-uremic syndrome, which typically develops in the 2nd wk of illness. Death may occur, especially in the elderly, with or without this complication.

Symptoms and Signs

EHEC infection typically begins acutely with severe abdominal cramps and watery diarrhea that may become grossly bloody within 24 h. Some patients report diarrhea as being "all blood and no stool," which has given rise to the term hemorrhagic colitis. Fever, usually absent or low grade, occasionally reaches 39° C. Diarrhea may last 1 to 8 days in uncomplicated infections.

Diagnosis

- Stool cultures
- Rapid stool assay for Shiga toxin

E. coli O157:H7 and other STEC infections should be distinguished from other infectious diarrheas by isolating the organism from stool cultures. Identifying the specific serotype helps identify the origin of an outbreak. Often, the clinician must specifically ask the laboratory to test for the organism.

Because bloody diarrhea and severe abdominal pain without fever suggest various noninfectious etiologies, *E. coli* O157:H7 infection should be considered in suspected cases of ischemic colitis, intussusception, and inflammatory bowel disease. Characteristically, no inflammatory cells are found in the stool fluid. A rapid stool assay for Shiga toxin or, when available, a test for the gene that encodes the toxin may help.

Patients at risk of noninfectious diarrheas may need sigmoidoscopy. If done, sigmoidoscopy may reveal erythema and edema; barium enema typically shows evidence of edema with thumbprinting.

Treatment

- Supportive care

The mainstay of treatment is supportive. Although *E. coli* is sensitive to most commonly used antibiotics, antibiotics have not been shown to alleviate symptoms, reduce carriage of the organism, or prevent hemolytic-uremic syndrome. Fluoroquinolones are suspected of increasing release of enterotoxins.

In the week after infection, patients at high risk of developing hemolytic-uremic syndrome (eg, children < 5 yr, the elderly) should be observed for early signs, such as proteinuria, hematuria, red cell casts, and rising serum creatinine. Edema and hypertension develop later. Patients who develop complications are likely to require intensive care, including dialysis and other specific therapies, at a tertiary medical center.

Prevention

Improved meat processing procedures in the US have helped reduce the rate of meat contamination.

Correct disposal of the stool of infected people, good hygiene, and careful hand washing with soap limit spread of infection.

Preventive measures that may be effective in the day care setting include grouping children known to be infected with STEC or requiring 2 negative stool cultures before allowing infected children to attend.

Pasteurization of milk and thorough cooking of beef prevent food-borne transmission.

Reporting outbreaks of bloody diarrhea to public health authorities is important because intervention can prevent additional infections.

KEY POINTS

- EHEC produce Shiga toxin, which causes severe, bloody diarrhea and sometimes hemolytic-uremic syndrome.
- There are > 100 serotypes of EHEC; O157:H7 is the best-known, but many others cause similar illness.
- EHEC have a bovine reservoir, so outbreaks often result from ingestion of undercooked beef, but many other foods (eg, fresh produce, raw milk) and sources (eg, direct exposure to animals) may be involved.
- Use stool tests to identify Shiga toxin and cultures to identify EHEC.
- Provide supportive care; antibiotics are not helpful.
- Monitor at-risk patients (eg, children < 5 yr, the elderly) for signs of hemolytic-uremic syndrome for a week or two after onset of illness.

HAEMOPHILUS INFECTIONS

***Haemophilus* sp cause numerous mild and serious infections, including bacteremia, meningitis, pneumonia, sinusitis, otitis media, cellulitis, and epiglottitis. Diagnosis is by culture and serotyping. Treatment is with antibiotics.**

Many *Haemophilus* sp are normal flora in the upper respiratory tract and rarely cause illness. Pathogenic strains enter the upper respiratory tract through droplet inhalation or direct contact. Spread is rapid in nonimmune populations. Children, particularly males, blacks, and Native Americans, are at highest risk of serious infection. Overcrowded living conditions and day care center attendance predispose to infection, as do immunodeficiency states, asplenia, and sickle cell disease.

There are several pathogenic species of *Haemophilus*; the most common is *H. influenzae*, which has 6 distinct encapsulated serotypes (a through f) and numerous nonencapsulated, nontypeable strains. Before the use of *H. influenzae* type b (Hib) conjugate vaccine, most cases of serious, invasive disease were caused by type b.

Diseases caused by *Haemophilus* sp: *H. influenzae* causes many childhood infections, including meningitis, bacteremia, septic arthritis, pneumonia, tracheobronchitis, otitis media, conjunctivitis, sinusitis, and acute epiglottitis. These infections, as well as endocarditis and UTIs, may occur in adults, although far less commonly. These illnesses are discussed elsewhere in THE MANUAL.

Nontypeable *H. influenzae* strains cause mainly mucosal infections (eg, otitis media, sinusitis, conjunctivitis, bronchitis). Occasionally, nonencapsulated strains cause invasive infections in children, but they may cause up to half of serious *H. influenzae* infections in adults.

H. influenzae biogroup aegyptius (formerly called *H. aegyptius*) may cause mucopurulent conjunctivitis and bacteremic Brazilian purpuric fever. *H. ducreyi* causes chancroid. *H. parainfluenzae* and *H. aphrophilus* are rare causes of bacteremia, endocarditis, and brain abscess.

Diagnosis

- Cultures
- Sometimes serotyping

Diagnosis of *Haemophilus* infections is by culture of blood and body fluids. Strains involved in invasive illness should be serotyped.

Treatment

- Various antibiotics depending on site and severity of infection

Treatment of *Haemophilus* infections depends on nature and location of the infection, but doxycycline, fluoroquinolones, 2nd- and 3rd-generation cephalosporins, and carbapenems are used for invasive disease. The Hib vaccine has markedly reduced the rate of bacteremia.

Children with serious illness are hospitalized with contact and respiratory isolation for 24 h after starting antibiotics.

Antibiotic choices depend strongly on the site of infection and require susceptibility testing; many isolates in the US produce beta-lactamase (eg, > 50% are resistant to ampicillin).

For invasive illness, including meningitis, cefotaxime or ceftriaxone is recommended. For less serious infections, oral cephalosporins (except cephalexin), macrolides, and amoxicillin/clavulanate are generally effective. (See individual disease entries for specific recommendations.)

Cefotaxime and ceftriaxone eliminate respiratory carriage of *H. influenzae,* but other antibiotics used for systemic infection do not do so reliably. Thus, children with systemic infection who were not treated with cefotaxime or ceftriaxone should be given rifampin immediately after completing treatment and before resuming contact with other children.

Prevention

Hib conjugate vaccines are available for children ≥ 2 mo of age and have reduced invasive infections (eg, meningitis, epiglottitis, bacteremia) by 99%. A primary series is given at age 2, 4, and 6 mo or at age 2 and 4 mo, depending on the vaccine product. A booster at age 12 to 15 mo is indicated.

Contacts within the household may have asymptomatic *H. influenzae* carriage. Unimmunized or incompletely immunized household contacts < 4 yr are at risk of illness and should receive a dose of vaccine. In addition, all household members (except pregnant women) should receive prophylaxis with rifampin 600 mg (20 mg/kg for children ≥ 1 mo; 10 mg/kg for children < 1 mo) po once/day for 4 days. Nursery or day care contacts should receive prophylaxis if ≥ 2 cases of invasive disease occurred in 60 days. The benefit of prophylaxis if only one case occurred has not been established.

KEY POINTS

- Several species of *Haemophilus* are pathogenic; the most common is *H. influenzae*.
- *H. influenzae* causes many types of mucosal and, less commonly, invasive infection, primarily in children.
- Antibiotic choices depend strongly on the site of infection and require susceptibility testing.
- Hib conjugate vaccines, given as part of routine childhood immunization to children ≥ 2 mo, have reduced invasive infections by 99%.
- Close contacts may be asymptomatic *H. influenzae* carriers and typically are given prophylaxis with rifampin.

HACEK INFECTIONS

The HACEK group includes weakly virulent, gram-negative organisms that primarily cause endocarditis.

The HACEK group of nonmotile, gram-negative bacilli or coccobacilli contains a number of minimally pathogenic, slow-growing, fastidious genera. Their primary pathology is endocarditis in susceptible people; about 5% of endocarditis cases are due to this group, making them the most common causes of gram-negative bacilli endocarditis. The group consists of

- *Haemophilus* sp (*H. parainfluenza*, *H. aphrophilus*, and *H. paraphrophilus*), which may cause respiratory infections or, less commonly, endocarditis
- *Aggregatibacter* (formerly *Actinobacillus*) *actinomycetemcomitans*, which usually occurs with *A. israelii* in actinomycosis
- *Cardiobacterium hominis*
- *Eikenella corrodens*, which usually occurs in human bite wounds, endocarditis (often in IV drug users), brain and visceral abscesses, osteomyelitis, respiratory infections (including empyemas), uterine infections related to intrauterine devices, and mixed soft-tissue infections
- *Kingella kingae*

Antibiotic sensitivities differ among species, so treatment should be directed by susceptibility testing. However, increasing beta-lactam resistance has made ceftriaxone and ampicillin/sulbactam the current antibiotics of choice.

KLEBSIELLA, *ENTEROBACTER*, AND *SERRATIA* INFECTIONS

***Klebsiella*, *Enterobacter*, and *Serratia* are closely related normal intestinal flora that rarely cause disease in normal hosts.**

Infections with *Klebsiella*, *Enterobacter*, and *Serratia* are often hospital-acquired and occur mainly in patients with diminished resistance. Usually, *Klebsiella*, *Enterobacter*, and *Serratia* cause a wide variety of infections, including bacteremia, surgical site infections, intravascular catheter infections, and respiratory or urinary tract infections that manifest as pneumonia, cystitis, or pyelonephritis and that may progress to lung abscess, empyema, bacteremia, and sepsis, as in the following:

- *Klebsiella* pneumonia, a rare and severe disease with dark brown or red currant–jelly sputum, lung abscess formation, and empyema, is most common among diabetics and alcoholics.
- *Serratia*, particularly *S. marcescens*, has greater affinity for the urinary tract.
- *Enterobacter* most often cause nosocomial infections but can cause otitis media, cellulitis, and neonatal sepsis.

Treatment

- Antibiotics based on results of susceptibility testing

Treatment is with 3rd-generation cephalosporins, cefepime, carbapenems, fluoroquinolones, piperacillin/tazobactam, or aminoglycosides. However, because some isolates are resistant to multiple antibiotics, susceptibility testing is essential.

Klebsiella strains that produce extended-spectrum beta-lactamase (ESBL) may develop resistance to cephalosporins during treatment, particularly with ceftazidime; these ESBL strains are inhibited to a variable extent by beta-lactamase inhibitors (eg, sulbactam, tazobactam, clavulanate). Carbapenemase-producing species of *K. pneumoniae* (KPC) have been isolated internationally as well as in the US, making treatment of some infections very problematic. Ceftazidime/avibactam (a new beta-lactamase inhibitor) has activity against KPC isolates.

Enterobacter strains may become resistant to most beta-lactam antibiotics, including 3rd-generation cephalosporins; the beta-lactamase enzyme they produce (AmpC beta-lactamase) is not inhibited by the usual beta-lactamase inhibitors (clavulanate, tazobactam, sulbactam). However, these *Enterobacter* strains may be susceptible to carbapenems (eg, imipenem, meropenem, ertapenem). Carbapenemase-resistant Enterobacteriaceae have also been detected. In certain cases, ceftazidime/avibactam, tigecycline, and perhaps colistin may be the only available active antibiotics.

LEGIONELLA INFECTIONS

***Legionella pneumophila* most often causes pneumonia with extrapulmonary features. Diagnosis requires specific growth media, serologic testing, or PCR analysis. Treatment is with macrolides fluoroquinolones or doxycycline.**

This organism was first recognized in 1976 after an outbreak at a convention of the American Legion in Philadelphia, Pennsylvania—thus, the name legionnaires' disease. This disease is the pneumonic form of an infection usually caused by *Legionella pneumophila* serogroup 1. Nonpneumonic infection is called Pontiac fever, which manifests as a febrile, viral-like illness.

The organisms are often present in soil and freshwater. Amebas present in freshwater are a natural reservoir for these bacteria. A building's water supply is often the source of a *Legionella* outbreak. *Legionella* organisms are embedded in a biofilm that forms on the inside of water pipes and containers. The infection is usually acquired by inhaling aerosols (or less often aspiration) of contaminated water (eg, as generated by shower heads, misters, whirlpool baths, or water cooling towers for air-conditioning). Nosocomial infection usually involves a contaminated hot water supply. The infection is not transmitted from person to person.

Diseases caused by *Legionella* sp: *Legionella* infection is more frequent and more severe in the following:

- Patients < 1 yr
- The elderly
- Patients with diabetes or COPD
- Cigarette smokers
- Immunocompromised patients (typically with diminished cell-mediated immunity)

The lungs are the most common site of infection; community- and hospital-acquired pneumonia may occur.

Extrapulmonary legionellosis is rare; manifestations include sinusitis, hip wound infection, myocarditis, pericarditis, and prosthetic valve endocarditis, frequently in the absence of pneumonia.

Symptoms and Signs

Legionnaires' disease is a flu-like syndrome with acute fever, chills, malaise, myalgias, headache, or confusion. Nausea, loose stools or watery diarrhea, abdominal pain, cough, and arthralgias also frequently occur. Pneumonic manifestations may include dyspnea, pleuritic pain, and hemoptysis. Bradycardia relative to fever may occur, especially in severe cases.

Overall mortality is low (about 5%) but can reach 40% in patients with hospital-acquired infections, the elderly, and immunocompromised patients.

Diagnosis

- Direct fluorescent antibody staining
- Sputum culture
- Rapid urinary antigen test (for serogroup 1 only)

Direct fluorescent antibody staining of sputum or lavage fluid is occasionally used but requires expertise. In addition, PCR with DNA probing is available and may help identify transmission pathways. A urinary antigen test is 60 to 95% sensitive and > 99% specific 3 days after symptom onset but detects only *L. pneumophila* (serogroup 1) and not non-*pneumophila Legionella*. Paired acute and convalescent antibody assays may yield a delayed diagnosis. A 4-fold increase or an acute titer of ≥ 1:128 is considered diagnostic.

Diagnosis of legionnaires' disease is by culture of sputum or bronchoalveolar lavage fluid; blood cultures are unreliable. Slow growth on laboratory media may delay identification for 3 to 5 days.

Chest x-ray should be done; it usually shows patchy and rapidly asymmetrically progressive infiltrates (even when effective antibiotic therapy is used), with or without small pleural effusions.

Laboratory abnormalities often include hyponatremia, hypophosphatemia, and elevated aminotransferase levels.

Treatment

- Fluoroquinolones
- Macrolides (preferably azithromycin)
- Sometimes doxycycline

A fluoroquinolone given IV or po for 7 to 14 days and, for severely immunocompromised patients, sometimes up to 3 wk is the preferred regimen. Azithromycin (for 5 to 10 days) is effective, but erythromycin may be less effective. Erythromycin should be used only for mild pneumonia in patients who are not immunocompromised. Doxycycline is an alternative for immunocompetent patients with mild pneumonia. The addition of rifampin is no longer recommended because benefit has not been proved and there is potential for harm.

KEY POINTS

- *L. pneumophila* usually causes pulmonary infection; it rarely causes extrapulmonary infections (most often involving the heart).
- *L. pneumophila* infection is typically acquired by inhaling aerosols (or less often by aspiration) of contaminated water; it is not transmitted from person to person.
- Diagnose using direct fluorescent antibody staining or PCR testing; sputum cultures are accurate but may take 3 to 5 days.
- Treat using a fluoroquinolone or azithromycin; doxycycline is an alternative.

MELIOIDOSIS

(Whitmore Disease)

Melioidosis is an infection caused by *Burkholderia* (formerly *Pseudomonas*) *pseudomallei*. Manifestations include pneumonia, septicemia, and localized infection in various organs. Diagnosis is by staining or culture. Treatment with antibiotics, such as ceftazidime, is prolonged.

The organism can be isolated from soil and water and is endemic in Southeast Asia; Australia; Central, West, and East Africa; India; the Middle East; and China.

Humans may contract melioidosis by contamination of skin abrasions or burns, ingestion, or inhalation but not directly from infected animals or other humans.

In endemic areas, melioidosis is likely to occur in patients with

- Diabetes
- Alcoholism
- Chronic renal disease
- Immunocompromise including AIDS

Melioidosis is also a potential agent of bioterrorism.

Symptoms and Signs

Infection may manifest acutely or remain latent for years after an inapparent primary infection. Mortality is < 10%, except in acute septicemic melioidosis, which is frequently fatal.

Acute pulmonary infection is the most common form. It varies from mild to overwhelming necrotizing pneumonia. Onset may be abrupt or gradual, with headache, anorexia, pleuritic or dull aching chest pain, and generalized myalgia. Fever is usually > 39° C. Cough, tachypnea, and rales are characteristic. Sputum may be blood-tinged. Chest x-rays usually show upper lobe consolidation, frequently cavitating and resembling TB. Nodular lesions, thin-walled cysts, and pleural effusion may also occur. The WBC count ranges from normal to 20,000/μL.

Acute septicemic infection begins abruptly, with septic shock and multiple organ involvement manifested by disorientation, extreme dyspnea, severe headache, pharyngitis, upper abdominal colic, diarrhea, and pustular skin lesions. High fever, hypotension, tachypnea, a bright erythematous flush, and cyanosis are present. Muscle tenderness may be striking. Signs of arthritis or meningitis sometimes occur. Pulmonary signs may be absent or may include rales, rhonchi, and pleural rubs.

Localized suppurative infection can occur in almost any organ but is most common at the site of inoculation in the skin (or lungs) and associated lymph nodes. Typical metastatic sites of infection include the liver, spleen, kidneys, prostate, bone, and skeletal muscle. Acute suppurative parotiditis is common among children in Thailand. Patients may be afebrile.

Diagnosis

- Staining and culture

B. pseudomallei can be identified in exudates by methylene blue or Gram stain and by culture. Blood cultures often remain negative except when there is marked bacteremia (eg, in septicemia). Serologic assays are often unreliable in endemic areas because positive results may be due to previous infection.

Chest x-rays usually show irregular, nodular (4 to 10 mm) densities but may also show lobar infiltrates, bilateral bronchopneumonia, or cavitary lesions.

Ultrasonography or CT of the abdomen and pelvis should probably be done to detect abscesses, which may be present regardless of the clinical presentation. The liver and spleen may be palpable. Liver function tests, AST, and bilirubin are often abnormal. Renal insufficiency and coagulopathy may be present in severe cases. The WBC count is normal or slightly increased.

Treatment

- Sometimes ceftazidime, followed by trimethoprim/sulfamethoxazole (TMP/SMX)

Asymptomatic infection needs no treatment. Symptomatic patients are given ceftazidime 30 mg/kg IV q 6 h for 2 to 4 wk (imipenem, meropenem, and piperacillin are acceptable substitutes), then oral antibiotics (one double-strength tablet of TMP/SMX bid or doxycycline 100 mg bid) for 3 to 6 mo. In children < 8 yr and pregnant women, amoxicillin/clavulanate 25/5 mg/kg tid is used instead of doxycycline.

KEY POINTS

- Melioidosis is acquired by skin contact, ingestion, or inhalation; it is not acquired directly from infected animals or people.
- The most common manifestation is an acute pulmonary infection (occasionally severe), but suppurative lesions may occur in the skin and/or many other organs; septicemia, which has high mortality, may result.
- Diagnose using staining and culture; blood cultures are done but often are negative except in severe septicemia.
- Treat symptomatic patients with IV ceftazidime followed by a prolonged course of oral TMP/SMX and either doxycycline or, in children < 8 yr and pregnant women, amoxicillin/clavulanate.

PERTUSSIS

(Whooping Cough)

Pertussis is a highly communicable disease occurring mostly in children and adolescents and caused by *Bordetella pertussis*. Symptoms are initially those of nonspecific URI followed by paroxysmal or spasmodic coughing that usually ends in a prolonged, high-pitched, crowing inspiration (the whoop). Diagnosis is by nasopharyngeal culture, PCR, and serologic assays. Treatment is with macrolide antibiotics.

Pertussis is endemic throughout the world. Its incidence in the US cycles every 3 to 5 yr. Pertussis occurs only in humans; there are no animal reservoirs.

Transmission is mainly via aerosols of *B. pertussis* (a small, nonmotile, gram-negative coccobacillus) from infected patients, particularly during the catarrhal and early paroxysmal stages. The infection is highly contagious and causes disease in ≥ 80% of close contacts. Transmission by contact with contaminated articles is rare. Patients are usually not infectious after the 3rd wk of the paroxysmal phase.

Pertussis is the only vaccine-preventable childhood disease that is increasing in incidence. In the US, the case rate in the 1980s was at an all-time low of about 1/100,000 population, which, by 2014, increased to about 10/100,000. The increase is due to immunity waning in previously vaccinated adolescents and adults and to parents refusing to vaccinate their children (see p. 2461). Such unprotected patients may become ill; furthermore, unprotected adolescents and adults are an important reservoir for *B. pertussis* and are thus often the source of infection for unprotected infants < 1 yr (who have had the highest increase in annual incidence and the highest case fatality rate.)[1]

In the US, there were 32,971 pertussis cases and 13 deaths in 2014.[2] Deaths occurred in all age groups, but the incidence was highest in infants < 6 mo and most deaths (8 of 13) occurred in infants < 3 mo. Most deaths are caused by bronchopneumonia and cerebral complications. Pertussis is also serious in the elderly (see Table 190–2).

One attack does not confer lifelong natural immunity, but secondary attacks and infections in previously vaccinated adolescents and adults whose immunity has waned are usually mild and often unrecognized.

Table 190–2. PERTUSSIS INCIDENCE BY AGE, 2014

AGE	NUMBER OF CASES (%)	INCIDENCE PER 100,000
< 6 mo	3,330 (10.1)	169
6–11 mo	875 (2.7)	44.4
1–6 yr	6,082 (18.5)	25.1
7–10 yr	5,576 (16.9)	34
11–19 yr	11,159 (33.8)	29.6
≥ 20 yr	5,839 (17.7)	2.2
Unknown	110 (0.3)	N/A

Based on National Center for Immunization and Respiratory Diseases Division of Bacterial Diseases: 2014 Final Pertussis Surveillance Report. Centers for Disease Control and Prevention, 2015.

Diseases caused by pertussis: Respiratory complications, including asphyxia in infants, are most common. Otitis media occurs frequently. Bronchopneumonia (common among the elderly) may be fatal at any age.

Seizures are common among infants but rare in older children.

Hemorrhage into the brain, eyes, skin, and mucous membranes can result from severe paroxysms and consequent anoxia. Cerebral hemorrhage, cerebral edema, and toxic encephalitis may result in spastic paralysis, intellectual disability (mental retardation), or other neurologic disorders.

Umbilical herniation and rectal prolapse occasionally occur.

Parapertussis: This disease, caused by *B. parapertussis,* may be clinically indistinguishable from pertussis but is usually milder and less often fatal.

1. Centers for Disease Control and Prevention: *The Pink Book: Pertussis.* 2015.
2. National Center for Immunization and Respiratory Diseases Division of Bacterial Diseases: *2014 Final Pertussis Surveillance Report.* Centers for Disease Control and Prevention, 2015.

Symptoms and Signs

The incubation period averages 7 to 14 days (maximum 3 wk). *B. pertussis* invades respiratory mucosa, increasing the secretion of mucus, which is initially thin and later viscid and tenacious. Uncomplicated disease lasts about 6 to 10 wk and consists of 3 stages:

- Catarrhal
- Paroxysmal
- Convalescent

The **catarrhal stage** begins insidiously, generally with sneezing, lacrimation, or other signs of coryza; anorexia; listlessness; and a troublesome, hacking nocturnal cough that gradually becomes diurnal. Hoarseness may occur. Fever is rare.

After 10 to 14 days, the **paroxysmal stage** begins with an increase in the severity and frequency of the cough. Repeated bouts of ≥ 5 rapidly consecutive forceful coughs occur during a single expiration and are followed by the whoop—a hurried, deep inspiration. Copious viscid mucus may be expelled or bubble from the nares during or after the paroxysms. Vomiting is characteristic. In infants, choking spells (with or without cyanosis) may be more common than whoops.

Symptoms diminish as the **convalescent stage** begins, usually within 4 wk of onset. Average duration of illness is about 7 wk (range 3 wk to 3 mo or more). Paroxysmal coughing may recur for months, usually induced in the still sensitive respiratory tract by irritation from a URI.

Diagnosis

- Nasopharyngeal cultures and PCR testing

The catarrhal stage is often difficult to distinguish from bronchitis or influenza. Adenovirus infections and TB should also be considered.

Cultures of nasopharyngeal specimens are positive for *B. pertussis* in 80 to 90% of cases in the catarrhal and early paroxysmal stages. Because special media and prolonged incubation are required, the laboratory should be notified that pertussis is suspected. Specific fluorescent antibody testing of nasopharyngeal smears accurately diagnoses pertussis but is not as sensitive as culture. PCR testing of nasopharyngeal samples is the most sensitive and preferred test. The WBC count is usually between 15,000 and 20,000/μL but may be normal or as high as 60,000/μL, usually with 60 to 80% small lymphocytes.

Parapertussis is differentiated by culture or the fluorescent antibody technique.

Treatment

- Supportive care
- Erythromycin or azithromycin

Hospitalization with respiratory isolation is recommended for seriously ill infants. Isolation is continued until antibiotics have been given for 5 days.

In infants, suction to remove excess mucus from the throat may be lifesaving. O_2 and tracheostomy or nasotracheal intubation is occasionally needed. Expectorants, cough suppressants, and mild sedation are of little value. Because any disturbance can precipitate serious paroxysmal coughing with anoxia, seriously ill infants should be kept in a darkened, quiet room and disturbed as little as possible. Patients treated at home should be isolated, particularly from susceptible infants, for at least 4 wk from disease onset and until symptoms have subsided.

Antibiotics given during the catarrhal stage may ameliorate the disease. After paroxysms are established, antibiotics usually have no clinical effect but are recommended to limit spread. Preferred drugs are erythromycin 10 to 12.5 mg/kg po q 6 h (maximum 2 g/day) for 14 days or azithromycin 10 to 12 mg/kg po once/day for 5 days. Trimethoprim/sulfamethoxazole may be substituted in patients ≥ 2 mo who are intolerant of or hypersensitive to macrolide antibiotics. Antibiotics should also be used for bacterial complications (eg, bronchopneumonia, otitis media).

Prevention

Active immunization against pertussis is part of standard childhood vaccination. Five doses of acellular pertussis vaccine are given (usually combined with diphtheria and tetanus [DTaP]) at age 2, 4, and 6 mo; boosters are given at 15 to 18 mo and 4 to 6 yr.

Significant adverse effects from the pertussis component of the vaccine include

- Encephalopathy within 7 days
- Seizure, with or without fever, within 3 days
- Persistent, severe, inconsolable screaming or crying for ≥ 3 h
- Collapse or shock within 48 h
- Fever ≥ 40.5° C within 48 h
- Immediate severe or anaphylactic reaction

These reactions contraindicate further use of pertussis vaccine; combined diphtheria and tetanus vaccine (DT) is available without the pertussis component. The acellular vaccine is better tolerated than the previously used vaccine that contains numerous cell components and is the currently available preparation. Neither vaccination nor natural disease confers lifelong protective immunity against pertussis or reinfection. Immunity tends to wane 5 to 10 yr after the last vaccine dose is given.

A single booster with Tdap (containing lower doses of the diphtheria and pertussis components than the childhood DTaP) instead of Td is recommended for all adults after age 19 yr (including those > 65 yr) as well as before pregnancy; it should be given during each pregnancy after 20 wk gestation (preferably at 27 to 36 wk gestation). These newer recommendations are intended to decrease risk of spread of pertussis from susceptible adolescents and adults to unprotected infants.

Immunity after natural infection lasts about 20 yr. Passive immunization is unreliable and is not recommended.

Close contacts < 7 yr who have had < 4 doses of vaccine should be vaccinated. Contacts of all ages, whether vaccinated or not, should receive a 10-day course of erythromycin 500 mg po qid or 10 to 12.5 mg/kg po qid.

KEY POINTS

- Pertussis is a respiratory infection that can occur at any age but is most common and most likely to be fatal in young children, particularly infants < 6 mo.
- A catarrhal stage with URI symptoms is followed by a paroxysmal stage with repeated bouts of rapid, consecutive coughs followed by a hurried, deep inspiration (the whoop).
- The illness lasts about 7 wk, but cough may continue for months.
- Diagnose using PCR testing or nasopharyngeal cultures; special media are required.
- Treat with a macrolide antibiotic to ameliorate disease (during the catarrhal stage) or minimize transmission (during the paroxysmal stage and later).
- Prevent the disease using acellular pertussis vaccine as part of scheduled immunizations (including a booster for adults), and treat close contacts with erythromycin.
- Neither having the disease nor being vaccinated provides lifelong protection, although any subsequent disease tends to be milder.

PLAGUE AND OTHER *YERSINIA* INFECTIONS

(Black Death; Bubonic Plague; Pestis)

Plague is caused by *Yersinia pestis*. Symptoms are either severe pneumonia or massive lymphadenopathy with high fever, often progressing to septicemia. Diagnosis is epidemiologic and clinical, confirmed by culture and serologic testing. Treatment is with streptomycin or gentamicin; alternatives are a fluoroquinolone or doxycycline.

Yersinia (formerly *Pasteurella*) *pestis* is a short bacillus that often shows bipolar staining (especially with Giemsa stain) and may resemble a safety pin.

Plague occurs primarily in wild rodents (eg, rats, mice, squirrels, prairie dogs) and is transmitted from rodent to human by the bite of an infected rat flea vector. Plague may also be spread through contact with fluid or tissue from an infected animal. Human-to-human transmission occurs by inhaling droplets from patients with pulmonary infection (primary pneumonic plague), which is highly contagious. In endemic areas in the US, several cases may have been caused by household pets, especially cats (infected by eating infected rodents). Transmission from cats can be by bite of an infected flea or, if the cat has pneumonic plague, by inhalation of infected respiratory droplets. Pneumonic plague can also be transmitted via exposure in a laboratory or intentional aerosol spread as an act of bioterrorism.

Massive human epidemics (eg, the Black Death of the Middle Ages, an epidemic in Manchuria in 1911) have occurred. More recently, plague has occurred sporadically or in limited outbreaks. The last urban outbreak of rat-associated plague in the US occurred in Los Angeles in 1924 to 1925. Since that time, > 90% of human plague in the US has occurred in rural or semirural areas of the Southwest, especially New Mexico, Arizona, California, and Colorado.

Symptoms and Signs

There are several distinct clinical manifestations:

- Bubonic plague (most common)
- Pneumonic plague (primary or secondary)
- Septicemic plague
- Pestis minor

In **bubonic plague,** the most common form, the incubation period is usually 2 to 5 days but varies from a few hours to 12 days. Onset of fever of 39.5 to 41° C is abrupt, often with chills. The pulse may be rapid and thready; hypotension may occur. Lymph nodes that drain the site of inoculation by the bacteria become enlarged and tender (buboes) and appear shortly after the fever. The femoral or inguinal lymph nodes are most commonly involved, followed by axillary, cervical, or multiple nodes. Typically, the nodes are extremely tender and firm, surrounded by considerable edema. They may suppurate in the 2nd wk. The overlying skin is smooth and reddened but often not warm. A primary cutaneous lesion, varying from a small vesicle with slight local lymphangitis to an eschar, occasionally appears at the flea bite. The patient may be restless, delirious, confused, and uncoordinated. The liver and spleen may be enlarged. Because the bacteria can spread through the bloodstream to other parts of the body, bubonic plague may be complicated by hematogenous (secondary) pneumonic plague.

Primary pneumonic plague has a 2- to 3-day incubation period, followed by abrupt onset of high fever, chills, tachycardia, chest pain, and headache, often severe. Cough, not prominent initially, develops within 24 h. Sputum is mucoid at first, rapidly develops blood specks, and then becomes uniformly pink or bright red (resembling raspberry syrup) and foamy. Tachypnea and dyspnea are present, but pleuritic chest pain is not. Signs of consolidation are rare, and rales may be absent.

Secondary pneumonic plague is more common than primary and results from hematogenous dissemination of organisms from a bubo or other foci of infection.

Septicemic plague may occur with the bubonic form or without the bubonic form (called primary septicemic plague) as an acute, fulminant illness. Abdominal pain, presumably due to mesenteric lymphadenopathy, occurs in 40% of patients. Disseminated intravascular coagulopathy, gangrene of the extremities (hence, the name Black Death), and multiorgan failure eventually develop.

Pestis minor, a more benign form of bubonic plague, usually occurs only in endemic areas. Lymphadenitis, fever, headache, and prostration subside within a week.

Pharyngeal plague and **plague meningitis** are less common forms.

The mortality rate for untreated patients with bubonic plague is about 60%; most deaths result from septicemia in 3 to 5 days. Most untreated patients with pneumonic plague die within 48 h of symptom onset. Septicemic plague may be fatal before bubonic or pulmonary manifestations predominate.

Diagnosis

- Staining, cultures, and serologic testing

Rapid diagnosis is important because mortality increases significantly the longer treatment is delayed.

Diagnosis is made by stain and culture of the organism, typically by needle aspiration of a bubo (surgical drainage may disseminate the organism); blood and sputum cultures should also be obtained. Other tests include immunofluorescent staining and serology; a titer of > 1:16 or a 4-fold rise between acute and convalescent titers is positive. PCR testing, if available, is diagnostic.

Prior vaccination does not exclude plague; clinical illness may occur in vaccinated people.

Patients with pulmonary symptoms or signs should have a chest x-ray, which shows a rapidly progressing pneumonia in pneumonic plague. The WBC count is usually 10,000 to 20,000/μL with numerous immature neutrophils.

Treatment

- Streptomycin or gentamicin
- Alternatively, doxycycline, ciprofloxacin, levofloxacin, or chloramphenicol

Immediate treatment reduces mortality to < 5%.

In septicemic or pneumonic plague, treatment must begin within 24 h with streptomycin 15 mg/kg (up to 1 g) IM bid or gentamicin 5 mg/kg IM or IV once/day (or 2 mg/kg loading dose followed by 1.7 mg/kg q 8 h) if renal function is normal; the drug is given for 10 days or until 3 days after temperature has returned to normal. Doxycycline 100 mg IV or po q 12 h is an alternative. Ciprofloxacin, levofloxacin, and chloramphenicol are also effective.

Chloramphenicol is preferred for patients with infection of tissue spaces into which other drugs pass poorly (eg, plague meningitis, endophthalmitis). Chloramphenicol should be given in a loading dose of 25 mg/kg IV, followed by 12.5 mg/kg IV or po q 6 h.

Routine isolation precautions are adequate for patients with bubonic plague. Those with primary or secondary pneumonic plague require strict respiratory isolation and droplet precautions (see the Centers for Disease Control and Prevention's Resources for Clinicians at www.cdc.gov).

Prevention

All pneumonic plague contacts should be under medical surveillance. Temperature should be taken q 4 h for 6 days. They and others in close contact with patients who have plague pneumonia or in direct contact with infected body fluids or tissues should receive prophylaxis for 7 days with

- Doxycycline 100 mg po q 12 h
- Ciprofloxacin 500 mg po q 12 h
- For children < 8 yr, trimethoprim/sulfamethoxazole [TMP/SMX] 20 mg/kg [of the SMX component] q 12 h

Levofloxacin taken for 7 days is an alternative.

Travelers should be given prophylaxis with doxycycline 100 mg po q 12 h during exposure periods.

Plague vaccine is no longer available in the US.

Rodents should be controlled and repellents used to minimize flea bites.

KEY POINTS

- Plague is a highly contagious, life-threatening infection now present in the US mainly in rural or semirural areas of the Southwest.
- Plague may cause massive, often suppurative lymphadenopathy (buboes), severe pulmonary infection, and/or septicemia.
- Rapid diagnosis using stain and culture of the organism is important because mortality increases significantly the longer treatment is delayed.
- Place patients with pneumonic plague in strict respiratory isolation; routine isolation is adequate for those with other forms.
- Treat with streptomycin or gentamicin; acceptable alternatives include doxycycline, ciprofloxacin, levofloxacin, and chloramphenicol.
- Monitor close contacts carefully, and treat them prophylactically with doxycycline, ciprofloxacin, or levofloxacin, and treat children with TMP/SMX; plague vaccine is no longer available in the US.

Other *Yersinia* Infections

Yersinia enterocolitica and *Y. pseudotuberculosis* are zoonoses acquired by ingestion of contaminated food or water; they occur worldwide.

Y. enterocolitica is a common cause of diarrheal disease and mesenteric adenitis that clinically mimics appendicitis. *Y. pseudotuberculosis* most commonly causes mesenteric adenitis and has been suspected in cases of interstitial nephritis, hemolytic-uremic syndrome, and a scarlet fever–like illness. Both species can cause pharyngitis, septicemia, focal infections in multiple organs, and postinfectious erythema nodosum and reactive arthritis. In patients with chronic liver disease or iron overload, mortality from septicemia may be as high as 50%, even with treatment.

The organisms can be identified in standard cultures from normally sterile sites. Selective culture methods are required for nonsterile specimens. Serologic assays are available but difficult and not standardized. Diagnosis, particularly of reactive arthritis, requires a high index of suspicion and close communication with the clinical laboratory.

Treatment of diarrhea is supportive because the disease is self-limited. Septic complications require beta-lactamase–resistant antibiotics guided by susceptibility testing. Third-generation cephalosporins, fluoroquinolones, and TMP/SMX are preferred.

Prevention focuses on food handling and preparation, household pets, and epidemiology of suspected outbreaks.

PROTEEAE INFECTIONS

The Proteeae are normal fecal flora that often cause infection in patients whose normal flora have been disturbed by antibiotic therapy.

The Proteeae constitute at least 3 genera of gram-negative organisms:

- *Proteus: P. mirabilis, P. vulgaris,* and *P. myxofaciens*
- *Morganella: M. morganii*
- *Providencia: P. rettgeri, P. alcalifaciens,* and *P. stuartii*

However, *P. mirabilis* causes most human infections. These organisms are normal fecal flora and are present in soil and water. They are often present in superficial wounds, draining ears, and sputum, particularly in patients whose normal flora has been eradicated by antibiotic therapy. They may cause bacteremia and deep-seated infections, particularly in the ears and mastoid sinuses, peritoneal cavity, and urinary tract of patients with chronic UTIs or with renal or bladder stones; *Proteus* organisms produce urease, which hydrolyzes urea, leading to alkaline urine and the formation of struvite (magnesium ammonium phosphate) stones.

P. mirabilis is often sensitive to ampicillin, carbenicillin, ticarcillin, piperacillin, cephalosporins, fluoroquinolones, and aminoglycosides and resistant to tetracyclines. Multidrug-resistant *P. mirabilis* is an emerging problem.

Indole-positive species (*P. vulgaris, M. morganii, P. rettgeri*) tend to be more resistant but generally are sensitive to fluoroquinolones, carbapenems, piperacillin/tazobactam, 3rd-generation cephalosporins, and cefixime.

PSEUDOMONAS AND RELATED INFECTIONS

Pseudomonas aeruginosa **and other members of this group of gram-negative bacilli are opportunistic pathogens that frequently cause hospital-acquired infections, particularly in ventilator patients, burn patients, and patients with chronic debility. Many sites can be infected, and infection is usually severe. Diagnosis is by culture. Antibiotic choice varies with the pathogen and must be guided by susceptibility testing because resistance is common.**

Epidemiology

Pseudomonas is ubiquitous and favors moist environments. In humans, *P. aeruginosa* is the most common pathogen, but infection may result from *P. paucimobilis, P. putida, P. fluorescens*, or *P. acidovorans*. Other important hospital-acquired pathogens formerly classified as *Pseudomonas* include *Burkholderia cepacia* and *Stenotrophomonas maltophilia. B. pseudomallei* causes a distinct disease known as melioidosis that is limited mostly to the Asian tropics.

P. aeruginosa is present occasionally in the axilla and anogenital areas of normal skin but rarely in stool unless antibiotics are being given. In hospitals, the organism is frequently present in sinks, antiseptic solutions, and urine receptacles. Transmission to patients by health care practitioners may occur, especially in burn and neonatal ICUs, unless infection control practices are meticulously followed.

Diseases Caused by *Pseudomonas*

Most *P. aeruginosa* infections occur in hospitalized patients, particularly those who are debilitated or immunocompromised. *P. aeruginosa* is a common cause of infections in ICUs. HIV-infected patients, particularly those in advanced stages, and patients with cystic fibrosis are at risk of community-acquired *P. aeruginosa* infections.

Pseudomonas infections can develop in many anatomic sites, including skin, subcutaneous tissue, bone, ears, eyes, urinary tract, lungs, and heart valves. The site varies with the portal of entry and the patient's vulnerability. In hospitalized patients, the first sign may be overwhelming gram-negative sepsis.

Skin and soft-tissue infections: In burns, the region below the eschar can become heavily infiltrated with organisms, serving as a focus for subsequent bacteremia—an often lethal complication.

Deep puncture wounds of the foot are often infected by *P. aeruginosa*. Draining sinuses, cellulitis, and osteomyelitis may result. Drainage from puncture wounds often has a sweet, fruity smell.

Folliculitis acquired in hot tubs is often caused by *P. aeruginosa*.

External otitis, common in tropical climates, is the most common form of *Pseudomonas* infection involving the ear. A more severe form, referred to as malignant external otitis, can develop in diabetic patients. It is manifested by severe ear pain, often with unilateral cranial nerve palsies, and requires parenteral therapy.

Ecthyma gangrenosum is a skin lesion that occurs in neutropenic patients and is usually caused by *P. aeruginosa*. It is characterized by erythematous, centrally ulcerated, purple-black areas about 1 cm in diameter occurring most often in the axillary, inguinal, or anogenital areas. Ecthyma gangrenosum typically occurs in patients with *P. aeruginosa* bacteremia.

Respiratory tract infections: *P. aeruginosa* is a frequent cause of ventilator-associated pneumonia. In HIV-infected patients, *Pseudomonas* most commonly causes pneumonia or sinusitis. *Pseudomonas* bronchitis is common late in the course of cystic fibrosis. Isolates from patients with cystic fibrosis have a characteristic mucoid colonial morphology and result in a worse prognosis than nonmucoid *Pseudomonas*.

Other infections: *Pseudomonas* is a common cause of nosocomial UTI, especially in patients who have had urologic manipulation or obstructive uropathy. *Pseudomonas* commonly colonizes the urinary tract in catheterized patients, especially those who have received broad-spectrum antibiotics.

Ocular involvement generally manifests as corneal ulceration, most often after trauma, but contamination of contact lenses or lens fluid has been implicated in some cases.

Rarely, *Pseudomonas* causes acute bacterial endocarditis, usually on prosthetic valves in patients who have had open-heart surgery or on natural valves in IV drug abusers.

Bacteremia: Many *Pseudomonas* infections can cause bacteremia. In nonintubated patients without a detectable urinary focus, especially if infection is due to a species other than *P. aeruginosa*, bacteremia suggests contaminated IV fluids, drugs, or antiseptics used in placing the IV catheter.

Diagnosis

- Culture

Diagnosis depends on culturing the organism from the site of infection: blood, skin lesions, drainage fluid, urine, CSF, or eye.

Localized infection may produce a fruity smell, and pus may be greenish.

Treatment

- Various antibiotics depending on site and severity of infection and susceptibility testing

Localized infection: Hot-tub folliculitis resolves spontaneously and does not require antibiotic therapy.

External otitis is treated with 1% acetic acid irrigations or topical drugs such as polymyxin B or colistin. More severe infection is treated with fluoroquinolones.

Focal soft-tissue infection may require early surgical debridement of necrotic tissue and drainage of abscesses in addition to antibiotics.

Small corneal ulcers are treated with ciprofloxacin 0.3% or levofloxacin 0.5%. Fortified (higher than stock concentration) antibiotic drops, such as tobramycin 15 mg/mL, are used for more significant ulcers. Frequent dosing (eg, q 1 h around the clock) is necessary initially. Eye patching is contraindicated because it produces a dark warm environment that favors bacterial growth and prevents administration of topical drugs.

Asymptomatic bacteriuria is not treated with antibiotics, except during pregnancy and before urologic manipulation. Patients with symptomatic UTIs can often be treated with levofloxacin 500 mg po once/day or ciprofloxacin 500 mg po bid.

Systemic infection: Parenteral therapy is required. Recently, single drug therapy with an active antipseudomonal beta-lactam (eg, ceftazidime) or a fluoroquinolone has been shown to produce outcomes equivalent to those of previously recommended combination therapy with an aminoglycoside plus an antipseudomonal beta-lactam, an antipseudomonal cephalosporin (eg, ceftazidime, cefepime, cefoperazone), a monobactam (eg, aztreonam), or a carbapenem (meropenem, imipenem, doripenem). Such single-drug therapy is also satisfactory for patients with neutropenia.

Right-sided endocarditis can be treated with antibiotics, but usually the infected valve must be removed to cure an infection involving the mitral, aortic, or prosthetic valve.

P. aeruginosa resistance may occur among patients treated with ceftazidime, cefepime, ciprofloxacin, gentamicin, meropenem, imipenem, or doripenem. Older antibiotics (eg, colistin) may be required to treat infections involving multidrug-resistant *Pseudomonas* sp. Ceftolozane/tazobactam maintains activity against many multidrug-resistant strains of *P. aeruginosa*.

KEY POINTS

- Most *P. aeruginosa* infections occur in hospitalized patients, particularly those who are debilitated or immunocompromised, but patients with cystic fibrosis or advanced HIV may acquire the infection in the community.
- Infection can develop in many sites, varying with the portal of entry (eg, skin in burn patients, lungs in patients on a ventilator, urinary tract in patients who have had urologic manipulation or obstructive uropathy); overwhelming gram-negative sepsis may occur.
- Surface infections (eg, folliculitis, external otitis, keratitis) may develop in healthy people.
- Diagnose using cultures.
- Treat systemic infection with parenteral therapy using a single drug (eg, an antipseudomonal beta-lactam, a fluoroquinolone).

OVERVIEW OF *SALMONELLA* INFECTIONS

The genus *Salmonella* is divided into 2 species, *S. enterica* and *S. bongori*, which include > 2400 known serotypes. Some of these serotypes are named. In such cases, common usage sometimes shortens the scientific name to include only the genus and serotype; for example, *S. enterica*, subspecies *enterica*, serotype Typhi is shortened to *Salmonella* Typhi.

Salmonella may also be divided into 3 groups based on how well the organism is adapted to human hosts:

- Those highly adapted to humans and having no nonhuman hosts: This group includes *S.* Typhi and *S.* Paratyphi types A, B (also called *S.* Schottmülleri), and C (also called *S.* Hirschfeldii), which are pathogenic only in humans and commonly cause enteric (typhoid) fever.
- Those adapted to nonhuman hosts or causing disease almost exclusively in animals. Some strains within this group—*S.* Dublin (cattle), *S.* Arizonae (reptiles), and *S.* Choleraesuis (swine)—also cause disease in humans.
- Those with a broad host range: This group includes > 2000 serotypes (eg, *S.* Enteritidis, *S.* Typhimurium) that cause gastroenteritis and account for 85% of all *Salmonella* infections in the US.

TYPHOID FEVER

Typhoid fever is a systemic disease caused by *Salmonella* serotype Typhi (*S.* Typhi—see above). Symptoms are high fever, prostration, abdominal pain, and a rose-colored rash. Diagnosis is clinical and confirmed by culture. Treatment is with ceftriaxone, ciprofloxacin, or azithromycin.

Epidemiology

About 400 to 500 cases of typhoid fever are reported annually in the US, mainly among US travelers returning from endemic regions.

Humans are the only natural host and reservoir. Typhoid bacilli are shed in stool of asymptomatic carriers or in stool or urine of people with active disease. The infection is transmitted by ingestion of food or water contaminated with feces. Inadequate hygiene after defecation may spread *S.* Typhi to community food or water supplies. In endemic areas where sanitary measures are generally inadequate, *S.* Typhi is transmitted more frequently by water than by food. In developed countries, transmission is chiefly by food that has been contaminated during preparation by healthy carriers. Flies may spread the organism from feces to food.

Occasional transmission by direct contact (fecal-oral route) may occur in children during play and in adults during sexual practices. Rarely, hospital personnel who have not taken adequate enteric precautions have acquired the disease when changing soiled bedclothes.

The organism enters the body via the GI tract and gains access to the bloodstream via the lymphatic channels. Intestinal ulceration, hemorrhage, and perforation may occur in severe cases.

Carrier state: About 3% of untreated patients, referred to as chronic enteric carriers, harbor organisms in their gallbladder and shed them in stool for > 1 yr. Some carriers have no history of clinical illness. Most of the estimated 2000 carriers in the US are elderly women with chronic biliary disease. Obstructive uropathy related to schistosomiasis or nephrolithiasis may predispose certain typhoid patients to urinary carriage.

Epidemiologic data indicate that typhoid carriers are more likely than the general population to develop hepatobiliary cancer.

Symptoms and Signs

The incubation period (usually 8 to 14 days) is inversely related to the number of organisms ingested. Onset is usually gradual, with fever, headache, arthralgia, pharyngitis, constipation, anorexia, and abdominal pain and tenderness. Less common symptoms include dysuria, nonproductive cough, and epistaxis.

Without treatment, the temperature rises in steps over 2 to 3 days, remains elevated (usually 39.4 to 40° C) for another 10 to 14 days, begins to fall gradually at the end of the 3rd wk, and reaches normal levels during the 4th wk. Prolonged fever is often accompanied by relative bradycardia and prostration. CNS symptoms such as delirium, stupor, or coma occur in severe cases. In about 10 to 20% of patients, discrete pink, blanching lesions (rose spots) appear in crops on the chest and abdomen during the 2nd wk and resolve in 2 to 5 days.

Splenomegaly, leukopenia, anemia, liver function abnormalities, proteinuria, and a mild consumption coagulopathy are common. Acute cholecystitis and hepatitis may occur.

Late in the disease, when intestinal lesions are most prominent, florid diarrhea may occur, and the stool may contain blood (occult in 20% of patients, gross in 10%). In about 2% of patients, severe bleeding occurs during the 3rd wk, with a mortality rate of about 25%. An acute abdomen and leukocytosis during the 3rd wk may suggest intestinal perforation, which usually involves the distal ileum and occurs in 1 to 2% of patients.

Pneumonia may develop during the 2nd or 3rd wk and may be due to secondary pneumococcal infection, although *S.* Typhi itself can also cause pneumonia. Bacteremia occasionally leads to focal infections such as osteomyelitis, endocarditis, meningitis, soft-tissue abscesses, glomerulitis, or GU tract involvement.

Atypical presentations, such as pneumonitis, fever only, or, very rarely, symptoms consistent with UTI, may delay diagnosis.

Convalescence may last several months.

In 8 to 10% of untreated patients, symptoms and signs similar to the initial clinical syndrome recur about 2 wk after defervescence. For unclear reasons, antibiotic therapy during the initial illness increases the incidence of febrile relapse to 15 to 20%. If antibiotics are restarted at the time of relapse, the fever abates rapidly, unlike the slow defervescence that occurs during the primary illness. Occasionally, a 2nd relapse occurs.

Diagnosis

- Cultures

Other infections causing a similar presentation include other *Salmonella* infections, the major rickettsioses, leptospirosis, disseminated TB, malaria, brucellosis, tularemia, infectious hepatitis, psittacosis, *Yersinia enterocolitica* infection, and lymphoma.

Cultures of blood, stool, and urine should be obtained. Because drug resistance is common, standard susceptibility testing is essential. The nalidixic acid susceptibility screening test is no longer recommended because it no longer reliably predicts susceptibility to ciprofloxacin. Blood cultures are usually positive only during the first 2 wk of illness, but stool cultures are usually positive during the 3rd to 5th wk. If these cultures are negative and typhoid fever is strongly suspected, culture from a bone marrow biopsy specimen may reveal the organism.

Typhoid bacilli contain antigens (O and H) that stimulate the host to form corresponding antibodies. A 4-fold rise in O and H antibody titers in paired specimens obtained 2 wk apart suggests *S.* Typhi infection. However, this test is only moderately (70%) sensitive and lacks specificity; many nontyphoidal *Salmonella* strains cross-react, and liver cirrhosis causes false-positives.

Prognosis

Without antibiotics, the mortality rate is about 12%. With prompt therapy, the mortality rate is 1%. Most deaths occur in malnourished people, infants, and the elderly.

Stupor, coma, or shock reflects severe disease and a poor prognosis.

Complications occur mainly in patients who are untreated or in whom treatment is delayed.

Treatment

- Ceftriaxone
- Sometimes a fluoroquinolone or azithromycin

Antibiotic resistance is common and increasing, particularly in endemic areas, so susceptibility testing should guide drug selection.

In general, preferred antibiotics include

- Ceftriaxone 1 g IM or IV q 12 h (25 to 37.5 mg/kg in children) for 14 days
- Various fluoroquinolones (eg, ciprofloxacin 500 mg po bid for 10 to 14 days, levofloxacin 500 mg po or IV once/day for 14 days, moxifloxacin 400 mg po or IV once/day for 14 days)

Chloramphenicol 500 mg po or IV q 6 h is still widely used, but resistance is increasing. Fluoroquinolones may be used in children, but caution is required. For fluoroquinolone-resistant strains, azithromycin 1 g po on day 1, then 500 mg once/day for 6 days can be tried. Resistance rates to alternative therapies (eg, amoxicillin, trimethoprim/sulfamethoxazole [TMP/SMX]) are high, so use of these drugs depends on in vitro sensitivity.

Corticosteroids may be added to antibiotics to treat severe toxicity. Defervescence and clinical improvement usually follow. Prednisone 20 to 40 mg once/day po (or equivalent) for the first 3 days of treatment usually suffices. Higher doses of corticosteroids (dexamethasone 3 mg/kg IV initially, followed by 1 mg/kg q 6 h for 48 h total), are used in patients with marked delirium, coma, or shock.

Nutrition should be maintained with frequent feedings. While febrile, patients are usually kept on bed rest. Salicylates (which may cause hypothermia and hypotension), as well as laxatives and enemas, should be avoided. Diarrhea may be minimized with a clear liquid diet; parenteral nutrition may be needed temporarily. Fluid and electrolyte therapy and blood replacement may be needed.

Intestinal perforation and associated peritonitis call for surgical intervention and broader gram-negative and anti–*Bacteroides fragilis* coverage.

Relapses are treated the same as the initial illness, although duration of antibiotic therapy seldom needs to be > 5 days.

Patients must be reported to the local health department and prohibited from handling food until proven free of the organism. Typhoid bacilli may be isolated for as long as 3 to12 mo after the acute illness in people who do not become carriers. Thereafter, 3 stool cultures at monthly intervals must be negative to exclude a carrier state.

Carriers: Carriers with normal biliary tracts should be given antibiotics. The cure rate is about 80% with amoxicillin, TMP-SMX, or ciprofloxacin given for 4 to 6 wk.

In some carriers with gallbladder disease, eradication has been achieved with TMP/SMX and rifampin. In other cases, cholecystectomy with 1 to 2 days of preoperative antibiotics and 2 to 3 days of postoperative antibiotics is effective. However, cholecystectomy does not ensure elimination of the carrier state, probably because of residual foci of infection elsewhere in the hepatobiliary tree.

Prevention

Drinking water should be purified, and sewage should be disposed of effectively. Chronic carriers should avoid handling food and should not provide care for patients or young children until they are proved free of the organism; adequate patient isolation precautions should be implemented. Special attention to enteric precautions is important.

Travelers in endemic areas should avoid ingesting raw leafy vegetables, other foods stored or served at room temperature, and untreated water (including ice cubes). Unless water is known to be safe, it should be boiled or chlorinated before drinking.

A live-attenuated oral typhoid vaccine is available (Ty21a strain); it is used for travelers to endemic regions and is about 70% effective. It may also be considered for household or other close contacts of carriers. It is given every other day for a total of 4 doses, which should be completed ≥ 1 wk before travel. A booster is required after 5 yr for people who remain at risk. The vaccine should be delayed for > 72 h after patients have taken any antibiotic and should not be used with the antimalarial drug mefloquine. Because the vaccine contains living *S.* Typhi organisms, it is contraindicated in patients who are immunosuppressed. In the US, the Ty21a vaccine is not used in children < 6 yr.

An alternative is the single-dose, IM VI polysaccharide vaccine, which is 64 to 72% effective and is well-tolerated, but it is not used in children < 2 yr. For people who remain at risk, a booster is required after 2 to 3 yr.

KEY POINTS

- Typhoid fever is spread enterically and causes fever and other constitutional symptoms (eg, headache, arthralgia, anorexia, abdominal pain and tenderness); later in the disease, some patients develop severe, sometimes bloody diarrhea and/or a characteristic rash (rose spots).
- Bacteremia occasionally causes focal infections (eg, osteomyelitis, endocarditis, meningitis, soft-tissue abscesses, glomerulitis).
- A chronic carrier state develops in about 3% of untreated patients; they harbor organisms in their gallbladder and shed them in stool for > 1 yr.
- Diagnose using blood and stool cultures; because drug resistance is common, susceptibility testing is essential.
- Treat with ceftriaxone, a fluoroquinolone, or azithromycin, guided by susceptibility testing; corticosteroids may be given to decrease severe symptoms.
- Give carriers a prolonged course of antibiotics; sometimes cholecystectomy is necessary.
- Patients must be reported to the local health department and prohibited from handling food until they are proved free of the organism.
- Vaccination may be appropriate for certain travelers to endemic regions.

NONTYPHOIDAL *SALMONELLA* INFECTIONS

Nontyphoidal *salmonellae* primarily cause gastroenteritis, bacteremia, and focal infection. Symptoms may be diarrhea, high fever with prostration, or symptoms of focal infection. Diagnosis is by cultures of blood, stool, or site specimens. Treatment, when indicated, is with trimethoprim/sulfamethoxazole, ciprofloxacin, azithromycin, or ceftriaxone with surgery for abscesses, vascular lesions, and bone and joint infections.

Nontyphoidal *Salmonella* infections are common and remain a significant public health problem in the US. Many serotypes of *Salmonella* have been given names and are referred to informally as if they were separate species even though they are not (see p. 1593). Most nontyphoidal *Salmonella* infections are caused by *S. enterica* subspecies *enterica* serotype Enteritidis, *S.* Typhimurium, *S.* Newport, *S.* Heidelberg, and *S.* Javiana.

Human disease occurs by direct and indirect contact with numerous species of infected animals, the foodstuffs derived from them, and their excreta. Contaminated meat, poultry, raw milk, eggs, egg products, and water are common sources of *Salmonella*. Other reported sources include infected pet turtles and reptiles, carmine red dye, and contaminated marijuana.

Risk factors: Subtotal gastrectomy, achlorhydria (or ingestion of antacids), hemolytic conditions (eg. sickle cell anemia, Oroya fever, malaria), bartonellosis, splenectomy, louse-borne relapsing fever, cirrhosis, leukemia, lymphoma, and HIV infection are all risk factors for *Salmonella* infection.

Diseases caused by nontyphoidal *Salmonella* sp: Each *Salmonella* serotype can cause any or all of the clinical syndromes described below, although given serotypes tend to produce specific syndromes. Enteric fever, for instance, is caused by *S.* Paratyphi types A, B, and C.

An asymptomatic carrier state may also occur. However, carriers are rare and do not appear to play a major role in large outbreaks of nontyphoidal gastroenteritis. Persistent shedding of organisms in the stool for ≥ 1 yr occurs in only 0.2 to 0.6% of patients with nontyphoidal *Salmonella* infections.

Symptoms and Signs

Salmonella infection may manifest as

- Gastroenteritis
- Enteric fever
- Bacteremia
- Focal disease

Gastroenteritis usually starts 12 to 48 h after ingestion of organisms, with nausea and cramping abdominal pain followed by diarrhea, fever, and sometimes vomiting. Usually, the stool is watery but may be a pastelike semisolid. Rarely, mucus or blood is present. The disease is usually mild, lasting 1 to 4 days. Occasionally, a more severe, protracted illness occurs. About 10 to 30% of adults develop reactive arthritis weeks to months after diarrhea stops. This disorder causes pain and swelling, usually in the hips, knees, and Achilles tendon.

Enteric fever is a less severe form than typhoid; it is characterized by fever, prostration, and septicemia.

Bacteremia is relatively uncommon in patients with gastroenteritis, except in infants and the elderly. However, *S.* Choleraesuis, *S.* Typhimurium, and *S.* Heidelberg, among others, can cause a sustained and frequently lethal bacteremic syndrome lasting ≥ 1 wk, with prolonged fever, headache, malaise, and chills but rarely diarrhea. Patients may have recurrent episodes of bacteremia or other invasive infections (eg, septic arthritis) due to *Salmonella*. Multiple *Salmonella* infections in a patient without other risk factors should prompt HIV testing.

Focal *Salmonella* infection can occur with or without sustained bacteremia, causing pain in or referred from the involved organ—the GI tract (liver, gallbladder, appendix), endothelial surfaces (eg, atherosclerotic plaques, ileofemoral or aortic aneurysms, heart valves), pericardium, meninges, lungs, joints, bones, GU tract, or soft tissues. Preexisting solid tumors are occasionally seeded and develop abscesses that may, in turn, become a source of *Salmonella* bacteremia. *S.* Choleraesuis and *S.* Typhimurium are the most common causes of focal infection.

Diagnosis

- Cultures

Diagnosis of nontyphoidal *Salmonella* infections is by isolating the organism from stool or another infected site. In bacteremic and focal forms, blood cultures are positive, but stool cultures are generally negative.

Antibiotic resistance is more common with nontyphoidal *Salmonella* than with *S.* Typhi, and antimicrobial susceptibility testing is important.

In patients with gastroenteritis, stool specimens stained with methylene blue often show WBCs, indicating inflammatory colitis.

Treatment

- Supportive care
- Ciprofloxacin, azithromycin, ceftriaxone, or trimethoprim/sulfamethoxazole (TMP/SMX) only for high-risk patients and patients with systemic or focal infections

Gastroenteritis due to nontyphoidal *Salmonella* infections is treated symptomatically with oral or IV fluids (see p. 127).

Antibiotics do not hasten resolution, may prolong excretion of the organism, and are unwarranted in uncomplicated cases. However, in elderly nursing home residents, infants, and patients with HIV infection, increased mortality dictates treatment with antibiotics. Acceptable antibiotic regimens include the following:

- TMP/SMX 5 mg/kg (of the TMP component) po q 12 h for children
- Ciprofloxacin 500 mg po q 12 h for adults
- Azithromycin 500 mg po on day 1 followed by 250 mg po once/day for 4 days
- Ceftriaxone 2 g IV once/day for 7 to 10 days.

Nonimmunocompromised patients should be treated for 3 to 5 days; patients with AIDS may require prolonged suppression to prevent relapses.

Systemic or focal disease should be treated with antibiotic doses as for typhoid fever. Sustained bacteremia is generally treated for 4 to 6 wk.

Abscesses should be drained surgically. At least 4 wk of antibiotic therapy should follow surgery.

Infected aneurysms and heart valves and bone or joint infections usually require surgical intervention and prolonged courses of antibiotics.

The prognosis is usually good, unless severe underlying disease is present.

Carriers: Asymptomatic carriage is usually self-limited, and antibiotic treatment is rarely required. In unusual cases (eg, in food handlers or health care workers), eradication may be attempted with ciprofloxacin 500 mg po q 12 h for 1 mo. Follow-up stool cultures should be obtained in the weeks after drug administration to document elimination of *Salmonella*.

Prevention

Preventing contamination of foodstuffs by infected animals and humans is paramount. Preventive measures for travelers also apply to most other enteric infections.

Case reporting is essential.

KEY POINTS

- Nontyphoidal *Salmonella* infections are common and result from direct and indirect contact with numerous species of infected animals, the foodstuffs derived from them, and their excreta.
- Clinical syndromes include gastroenteritis, enteric fever, and focal infections; bacteremia occasionally occurs.
- Diagnose using cultures.
- In uncomplicated cases, antibiotics are unnecessary; they do not hasten resolution and may prolong excretion of the organism.
- Treat high-risk patients (eg, elderly nursing home residents, infants, patients with HIV infection) with antibiotics, such as ciprofloxacin, azithromycin, ceftriaxone, or TMP/SMX.
- An asymptomatic carrier state may occur, but carriers do not play a major role in outbreaks, and treatment with antibiotics is rarely indicated.

SHIGELLOSIS

(Bacillary Dysentery)

Shigellosis is an acute infection of the intestine caused by *Shigella* sp. Symptoms include fever, nausea, vomiting, tenesmus, and diarrhea that is usually bloody. Diagnosis is clinical and confirmed by stool culture. Treatment of mild infection is supportive, mostly with rehydration; antibiotics (eg, ciprofloxacin, azithromycin, ceftriaxone) are given to moderate to severely ill and high-risk patients with bloody diarrhea or immunocompromise and may shorten the duration of illness and decrease contagiousness.

The genus *Shigella* is distributed worldwide and is the typical cause of inflammatory dysentery, responsible for 5 to 10% of diarrheal illness in many areas. *Shigella* is divided into 4 major subgroups:

- A (*S. dysenteriae*)
- B (*S. flexneri*)
- C (*S. boydii*)
- D (*S. sonnei*)

Each subgroup is further subdivided into serologically determined types. *S. flexneri* and *S. sonnei* are more widespread than *S. boydii* and the particularly virulent *S. dysenteriae. S. sonnei* is the most common isolate in the US.

The source of infection is the feces of infected people or convalescent carriers; humans are the only natural reservoir for *Shigella*. Direct spread is by the fecal-oral route. Indirect spread is by contaminated food and fomites. Flies serve as vectors.

Because *Shigella* are relatively resistant to gastric acid, ingestion of as few as 10 to 100 organisms can cause disease. Epidemics occur most frequently in overcrowded populations with inadequate sanitation. Shigellosis is particularly common among younger children living in endemic areas. Adults usually have less severe disease.

Convalescents and subclinical carriers may be significant sources of infection, but true long-term carriers are rare. Infection imparts little or no immunity.

Shigella organisms penetrate the mucosa of the colon, causing mucus secretion, hyperemia, leukocytic infiltration, edema, and often superficial mucosal ulcerations. *Shigella dysenteriae* type 1 (not commonly present in the US, except in travelers returning from endemic areas) produces Shiga toxin, which causes marked watery diarrhea and sometimes hemolytic-uremic syndrome.

Symptoms and Signs

The incubation period for *Shigella* is 1 to 4 days. The most common presentation, watery diarrhea, is indistinguishable from other bacterial, viral, and protozoan infections that induce secretory activity of intestinal epithelial cells.

In **adults,** initial symptoms of shigellosis may be

- Episodes of gripping abdominal pain
- Urgency to defecate (tenesmus)
- Passage of formed feces that temporarily relieves the pain

These episodes recur with increasing severity and frequency. Diarrhea becomes marked, with soft or liquid stools containing mucus, pus, and often blood. Rectal prolapse and consequent fecal incontinence may result from severe tenesmus. However, adults may present without fever, with nonbloody and nonmucoid diarrhea, and with little or no tenesmus.

The disease usually resolves spontaneously in adults—mild cases in 4 to 8 days, severe cases in 3 to 6 wk. Significant dehydration and electrolyte loss with circulatory collapse and death occur mainly in debilitated adults and children < 2 yr.

Rarely, shigellosis starts suddenly with rice-water or serous (occasionally bloody) stools. The patient may vomit and rapidly become dehydrated. Infection may manifest as delirium, seizures, and coma but with little or no diarrhea. Death may occur in 12 to 24 h.

In **young children,** onset is sudden, with fever, irritability or drowsiness, anorexia, nausea or vomiting, diarrhea, abdominal pain and distention, and tenesmus. Within 3 days, blood, pus, and mucus appear in the stools. The number of stools may increase to ≥ 20/day, and weight loss and dehydration become severe. If untreated, children may die in the first 12 days. If children survive, acute symptoms subside by the 2nd wk.

Complications: The hemolytic-uremic syndrome may complicate shigellosis due to *S. dysenteriae* type 1 in children. Secondary bacterial infections may occur, especially in debilitated and dehydrated patients. Severe mucosal ulcerations may cause significant acute blood loss. Patients (particularly those with the HLA-B27 genotype) may develop reactive arthritis (arthritis, conjunctivitis, urethritis) after shigellosis (and other enteritides).

Other complications are uncommon but include seizures in children, myocarditis, and, rarely, intestinal perforation.

Infection does not become chronic and is not an etiologic factor in ulcerative colitis.

Diagnosis

- Stool cultures

Diagnosis of shigellosis is facilitated by a high index of suspicion during outbreaks and in endemic areas and by the presence of fecal leukocytes on smears stained with methylene blue or Wright stain. Stool cultures are diagnostic and should be obtained; for severely ill or at-risk patients, antimicrobial sensitivity testing is done.

In patients with symptoms of dysentery (bloody and mucoid stools), the differential diagnosis should include invasive *Escherichia coli, Salmonella, Yersinia,* and *Campylobacter* infections; amebiasis; *Clostridium difficile* infection, and viral diarrheas.

The mucosal surface, as seen through a proctoscope, is diffusely erythematous with numerous small ulcers. Although leukopenia or marked leukocytosis may be present, WBC count averages 13,000/μL. Hemoconcentration is common, as is diarrhea-induced metabolic acidosis.

Treatment

- Supportive care
- For severely ill or at-risk patients, a fluoroquinolone, azithromycin, or a 3rd-generation cephalosporin

Fluid loss due to shigellosis is treated symptomatically with oral or IV fluids.

Antidiarrheal drugs (eg, loperamide) may prolong illness and should not be used.

Antibiotics can reduce the symptoms and shedding of *Shigella* but are not necessary for healthy adults with mild illness. However, certain patients, including the following, should usually be treated:

- Children
- The elderly
- Debilitated patients
- Patients with moderate to severe disease

For adults, the following antibiotic regimens may be used:

- A fluoroquinolone (such as ciprofloxacin 500 mg po q 12 h for 3 to 5 days)
- Azithromycin 500 mg po on day 1 and 250 mg once/day for 4 days
- Ceftriaxone 2 g/day IV for 5 days

Many *Shigella* isolates are likely to be resistant to ampicillin, trimethoprim/sulfamethoxazole (TMP/SMX), and tetracyclines, but patterns of resistance vary by geographic region.

Prevention

Hands should be washed thoroughly before handling food, and soiled garments and bedclothes should be immersed in covered buckets of soap and water until they can be boiled. Appropriate isolation techniques (especially stool isolation) should be used with patients and carriers.

A live oral vaccine is being developed, and field trials in endemic areas hold promise. However, immunity is generally type specific.

KEY POINTS

- *Shigella* sp are a highly contagious cause of dysentery; humans are the only reservoir.
- Watery diarrhea may be accompanied by abdominal pain and marked urgency to defecate; stools may contain mucus, pus, and often blood.
- *S. dysenteriae* type 1 (not common in the US, except in returning travelers) produces Shiga toxin, which may cause hemolytic-uremic syndrome.
- Significant dehydration and electrolyte loss with circulatory collapse and death occur mainly in debilitated adults and children < 2 yr.
- Supportive care is usually adequate, but give antibiotics (a fluoroquinolone, azithromycin, ceftriaxone) to young children and to elderly, debilitated, or severely ill patients; resistance to ampicillin, TMP/SMX, and tetracyclines is common.

TULAREMIA

(Deer Fly Fever; Rabbit Fever)

Tularemia is a febrile disease caused by *Francisella tularensis*; it may resemble typhoid fever. Symptoms are a primary local ulcerative lesion, regional lymphadenopathy, profound systemic symptoms, and, occasionally, atypical pneumonia. Diagnosis is primarily epidemiologic and clinical and supported by serologic tests. Treatment is with streptomycin, gentamicin, chloramphenicol, ciprofloxacin, or doxycycline.

There are 7 clinical syndromes associated with tularemia (see Table 190–3); clinical manifestations vary by the type of exposure to the organism.

The causative organism, *F. tularensis*, is a small, pleomorphic, nonmotile, nonsporulating aerobic bacillus that enters the body by

- Ingestion of contaminated food or water
- Bite of an infected arthropod vector (ticks, deer flies, fleas)
- Inhalation
- Direct contact with infected tissues or material

Tularemia does not spread from person to person.

The organism can penetrate apparently unbroken skin but may actually enter through microlesions.

Table 190–3. TYPES OF TULAREMIA

TYPE	FREQUENCY	COMMENTS
Ulceroglandular	Most common	Primary lesions on the hands or fingers with regional lymphadenitis
Typhoidal†	Common	Systemic illness without indication of the site of inoculation or localized infection
Oculoglandular	Uncommon	Conjunctivitis with inflammation of ipsilateral preauricular, submandibular, or cervical lymph nodes, probably caused by inoculation of an eye from an infected finger or hand
Glandular	Rare	Regional lymphadenitis but no primary lesion and often cervical adenopathy, suggesting oral ingestion of bacteria
Pneumonic*	Uncommon	Infiltrates with asymmetric hilar adenopathy, with or without bloody pleural effusion
Oropharyngeal	Rare	Sore throat and cervical adenopathy due to ingestion of contaminated food or water
Septicemic†	Rare	Severe systemic illness with hypotension, acute respiratory distress syndrome (ARDS), disseminated intravascular coagulation, and multiorgan dysfunction

*Tularemic pneumonia may be primary or may complicate any form of tularemia.
†Hematogenous spread to various organs (eg, lungs, bone, pericardium, peritoneum, heart valves, meninges) may also occur.

There are 2 types of *F. tularensis*:

- **Type A:** This type is a more virulent serotype for humans; it usually occurs in rabbits and rodents in the US and Canada.
- **Type B:** This type usually causes a mild ulceroglandular infection and occurs in water and aquatic animals in Europe and Asia.

Hunters, butchers, farmers, and fur handlers are most commonly infected. In winter months, most cases result from contact (especially during skinning) with infected wild rabbits. In summer months, infection usually follows handling of other infected animals or birds or bites of infected ticks or other arthropods. Rarely, cases result from eating undercooked infected meat, drinking contaminated water, or mowing fields in endemic areas. In the Western states, ticks, deer flies, horse flies, and direct contact with infected animals are other sources of infection. Human-to-human transmission has not been reported. Laboratory workers are at particular risk because infection is readily acquired during normal handling of infected specimens.

Tularemia is considered a possible agent of bioterrorism.

In disseminated cases, characteristic focal necrotic lesions in various stages of evolution are scattered throughout the body. They are 1 mm to 8 cm and whitish yellow; they are seen externally as the primary lesions on the fingers, eyes, or mouth and commonly occur in lymph nodes, spleen, liver, kidneys, and lungs. In pneumonia, necrotic foci occur in the lungs. Although severe systemic toxicity may occur, no toxins have been demonstrated.

Symptoms and Signs

Onset of tularemia is sudden, occurring 1 to 10 (usually 2 to 4) days after exposure, with headache, chills, nausea, vomiting, fever of 39.5° to 40° C, and severe prostration. Extreme weakness, recurring chills, and drenching sweats develop. Clinical manifestations depend to some extent on the type of exposure (see Table 190–3).

Within 24 to 48 h, an inflamed papule appears at the site of exposure (finger, arm, eye, roof of the mouth), except in glandular or typhoidal tularemia. The papule rapidly becomes pustular and ulcerates, producing a clean ulcer crater with a scanty, thin, colorless exudate. Ulcers are usually single on the extremities but multiple in the mouth or eyes. Usually, only one eye is affected. Regional lymph nodes enlarge and may suppurate and drain profusely. A typhoid-like state frequently develops by the 5th day, and the patient may develop atypical pneumonia, sometimes accompanied by delirium.

Pneumonic tularemia can occur after inhalation or by hematogenous spread from another type of tularemia; it develops in 10 to 15% of ulceroglandular tularemia cases and in about 50% of typhoidal tularemia cases. Although signs of consolidation are frequently present, reduced breath sounds and occasional rales may be the only physical findings in tularemic pneumonia. A dry, nonproductive cough is associated with a retrosternal burning sensation. A nonspecific roseola-like rash may appear at any stage of the disease. Splenomegaly and perisplenitis may occur. In untreated cases, temperature remains elevated for 3 to 4 wk and resolves gradually. Mediastinitis, lung abscess, and meningitis are rare complications.

Mortality is almost nil in treated cases and about 6% in untreated cases of ulceroglandular tularemia. Mortality rates are higher for type A infection and for typhoidal, septicemic, and pneumonic tularemia; they are as high as 33% for untreated cases. Death usually results from overwhelming infection, pneumonia, meningitis, or peritonitis. Relapses can occur in inadequately treated cases. One attack confers immunity.

Diagnosis

- Cultures
- Acute and convalescent serologic testing

Diagnosis of tularemia is suspected based on a history of contact with rabbits or wild rodents or exposure to arthropod vectors, the sudden onset of symptoms, and the characteristic primary lesion.

Patients should have cultures of blood and relevant clinical material (eg, sputum, lesions); routine cultures may be negative, and the laboratory should be notified that tularemia is suspected so that appropriate media can be used (and appropriate safety precautions ensured). Acute and convalescent antibody titers should be done 2 wk apart. A 4-fold rise or a single titer > 1:128 is diagnostic. The serum of patients with brucellosis may cross-react to *F. tularensis* antigens but usually in much lower titers. Fluorescent antibody or immunohistochemical staining is used by some laboratories. Leukocytosis is common, but the WBC count may be normal with an increase only in the proportion of PMNs.

Because this organism is highly infectious, samples and culture media from patients suspected of having tularemia should be handled with extreme caution and, if possible, processed by a high-level biosafety containment-equipped laboratory with a level 3 rating.

Treatment

- Streptomycin (plus chloramphenicol for meningitis)

The **preferred drug** is

- Streptomycin 1 g IM q 12 h for adults and 15 mg/kg IM q 12 h for children for 7 to 10 days for moderate to severe disease

Chloramphenicol 12.5 to 25 mg/kg IV q 6 h or doxycycline 100 mg twice/day for 14 to 21 days is added if there is evidence of meningitis.

Alternatives to streptomycin include the following:

- Gentamicin 1 to 2 mg/kg IM or IV q 8 h (for moderate to severe disease)
- Doxycycline 100 mg po q 12 h (for mild disease)
- Chloramphenicol 12.5 to 25 mg/kg IV q 6 h (used only for meningitis because there are more effective and safer alternatives; oral form not available in US)
- Ciprofloxacin 500 mg po q 12 h (for mild disease)

In a mass casualty setting if parenteral treatment is not feasible, oral doxycycline or ciprofloxacin may be used for adults and children. However, relapses occasionally occur with all of these drugs, and they may not prevent node suppuration.

Continuous wet saline dressings are beneficial for primary skin lesions and may diminish the severity of lymphangitis and lymphadenitis. Surgical drainage of large abscesses is rarely necessary unless therapy is delayed.

In **ocular tularemia,** applying warm saline compresses and using dark glasses give some relief. In severe cases, 2% homatropine 1 to 2 drops q 4 h may relieve symptoms.

Intense headache usually responds to oral opioids (eg, oxycodone or hydrocodone with acetaminophen).

Prevention

When entering endemic areas, people should use tick-proof clothing and repellents. A thorough search for ticks should be done after leaving tick-infested areas. Ticks should be removed at once (see Sidebar 201–1 on p. 1696).

When handling rabbits and rodents, especially in endemic areas, people should wear protective clothing, including rubber gloves and face masks, because organisms may be present in the animal and in tick feces on the animal's fur. Wild birds and game must be thoroughly cooked before eating.

Water that may be contaminated must be disinfected before use.

No vaccine is currently available, although one is currently under review by the FDA. Antibiotic prophylaxis with 14 days of oral doxycycline or ciprofloxacin is recommended after high-risk exposure (eg, a laboratory accident).

KEY POINTS

- *F. tularensis* is a highly infectious organism; in the US and Canada, the main reservoir is wild rabbits and rodents.
- Tularemia can be acquired in many ways, including direct contact with infected animals (particularly rabbits) or birds, bites of infected arthropods or insects, inadvertent contact with laboratory specimens, or, rarely, inhalation of an infectious aerosol or ingestion of contaminated meat or water.
- Patients have a fever of 39.5 to 40° C and other constitutional symptoms (eg, headache, chills, nausea, vomiting, severe prostration) along with specific manifestations related to the organ affected; skin lesions and/or lymphadenitis are most common, and pneumonia may occur.
- Diagnose using cultures of blood and relevant clinical material; acute and convalescent antibody titers and certain staining techniques may also be helpful.
- Treat with streptomycin (plus chloramphenicol for meningitis).
- Take appropriate precautions in endemic areas, including tick avoidance strategies, use of protective gear while handling rabbits and rodents, and thorough cooking of wild birds and game.

191 Gram-Positive Cocci

ENTEROCOCCAL INFECTIONS

Enterococci are gram-positive aerobic organisms. *Enterococcus faecalis* and *E. faecium* cause a variety of infections, including endocarditis, UTI, prostatitis, intra-abdominal infection, cellulitis, and wound infection as well as concurrent bacteremia.

Enterococci are part of the normal intestinal flora. They used to be classified as group D streptococci but are now considered a separate genus. There are > 17 species, but *E. faecalis* and *E. faecium* most commonly cause infections in humans.

Enterococci typically cause

- UTI
- Bacteremia
- Endocarditis
- Intra-abdominal and pelvic infections
- Wound infections

Treatment

- Varies by site of infection and susceptibility testing

(See also the American Heart Association's Infective Endocarditis: Diagnosis, Antimicrobial Therapy, and Management of Complications at http://circ.ahajournals.org.)

Enterococci associated with endocarditis are difficult to eradicate unless a combination of certain cell wall–active drugs (eg, penicillin, ampicillin, amoxicillin, piperacillin, vancomycin) plus an aminoglycoside (eg, gentamicin, streptomycin) is used to achieve bactericidal activity. However, some cell wall-active drugs have limited or no activity against enterococci; they include nafcillin, oxacillin, ticarcillin, meropenem, ertapenem, most cephalosporins, and aztreonam. *E. faecium* are more resistant to penicillin than *E. faecalis*. Imipenem is active against *E. faecalis*.

For complicated skin infections due to vancomycin-susceptible enterococci, daptomycin, linezolid tedizolid, and tigecycline are effective treatment options. Piperacillin-tazobactam and imipenem are recommended for complicated intra-abdominal infections when enterococci are known or presumed to be involved.

UTIs do not require bactericidal therapy and, if the causative organism is sensitive, are usually treated with a single antibiotic such as ampicillin. Nitrofurantoin and fosfomycin are often effective against vancomycin-resistant enterococcal UTI.

Resistance: In the past several decades, resistance to multiple antimicrobial drugs has increased rapidly, especially among *E. faecium*.

Resistance to aminoglycosides (eg, gentamicin, streptomycin), particularly with *E. faecium*, continues to emerge.

Vancomycin-resistant enterococci (VRE) may also be resistant to other glycopeptides (eg, teicoplanin), aminoglycosides, and cell wall–active β-lactams (eg, penicillin G, ampicillin). When identified, infected patients are strictly isolated. Recommended treatment includes streptogramins (quinupristin/dalfopristin for *E. faecium* only) and oxazolidinones (linezolid, tedizolid). Daptomycin and tigecycline have in vitro activity against VRE and may be off-label treatment options.

β-Lactamase–producing enterococci are occasionally encountered, particularly when large numbers of organisms are present (eg, in endocarditis vegetation). Resistance may be present clinically even though the organism appears susceptible based on standard testing. Vancomycin or combination β-lactam/β-lactamase inhibitor antibiotics (eg, piperacillin/tazobactam, ampicillin/sulbactam) can be used.

PNEUMOCOCCAL INFECTIONS

Streptococcus pneumoniae **(pneumococci) are gram-positive, α-hemolytic, aerobic, encapsulated diplococci. In the US, pneumococcal infection annually causes about 7 million cases of otitis media, 500,000 cases of pneumonia, 50,000 cases of sepsis, 3,000 cases of meningitis, and 40,000 deaths. Diagnosis is by Gram stain and culture. Treatment depends on the resistance profile and includes a β-lactam, a macrolide, a respiratory fluoroquinolone, and sometimes vancomycin.**

Pneumococci are fastidious microorganisms that require catalase to grow on agar plates. In the laboratory, pneumococci are identified by

- α-Hemolysis on blood agar
- Sensitivity to optochin
- Lysis by bile salts

Pneumococci commonly colonize the human respiratory tract, particularly in winter and early spring. Spread is via airborne droplets.

True epidemics of pneumococcal infections are rare; however, some serotypes seem to be associated with outbreaks in certain (eg, military, institutional) populations.

Serotypes: The pneumococcus capsule consists of a complex polysaccharide that determines serologic type and contributes to virulence and pathogenicity. Virulence varies somewhat within serologic types because of genetic diversity.

Currently, > 90 different serotypes have been identified. Most serious infections are caused by a small number of serotypes (4, 6B, 9V, 14, 18C, 19F, and 23F) that are included in the 13-valent pneumococcal conjugate vaccine. These serotypes cause about 90% of invasive infections in children and 60% in adults. However, these patterns are slowly changing, in part because of the widespread use of polyvalent vaccine. Serotype 19A, which is highly virulent and multidrug-resistant, has emerged as an important cause of respiratory tract infection and invasive disease; it is thus now included in the 13-valent pneumococcal conjugate vaccine.

Risk factors: Patients most susceptible to serious and invasive pneumococcal infections are

- Those with chronic illness (eg, chronic cardiorespiratory disease, diabetes, liver disease, alcoholism)
- Those with immunosuppression (eg, HIV)
- Those with functional or anatomic asplenia
- Those with sickle cell disease
- Residents of long-term care facilities
- Smokers
- Aborigines, Alaskan natives, and certain American Indian populations

The elderly, even those without other disease, tend to have a poor prognosis with pneumococcal infections.

Damage to the respiratory epithelium by chronic bronchitis or common respiratory viral infections, notably influenza, may predispose to pneumococcal invasion.

Diseases Caused by Pneumococci

Pneumococcal diseases include

- Otitis media
- Pneumonia
- Sinusitis
- Meningitis
- Endocarditis
- Septic arthritis
- Peritonitis (rare)

Primary infection usually involves the middle ear or lungs.

The diseases listed below are further discussed elsewhere in THE MANUAL.

Pneumococcal bacteremia: Pneumococcal bacteremia can occur in immunocompetent and immunosuppressed patients; patients who have had splenectomy are at particular risk.

Bacteremia may be the primary infection, or it may accompany the acute phase of any focal pneumococcal infection. When bacteremia is present, secondary seeding of distant sites may cause infections such as septic arthritis, meningitis, and endocarditis.

Despite treatment, the overall mortality rate for bacteremia is 15 to 20% in children (mainly in those who have meningitis, who are immunocompromised, and/or who have had splenectomy and have severe bacteremia) and in adults and is 30 to 40% in the elderly; risk of death is highest during the first 3 days.

Pneumococcal pneumonia: Pneumonia is the most frequent serious infection caused by pneumococci; it may manifest as lobar pneumonia or, less commonly, as bronchopneumonia. About 4 million cases of community-acquired pneumonia occur each year in the US; when community-acquired pneumonia requires hospitalization, pneumococci are the most common etiologic agent in patients of all ages.

Pleural effusion occurs in up to 40% of patients, but most effusions resolve during drug treatment; only about 2% of patients develop empyema, which may become loculated, thick, and fibrinopurulent. Lung abscess formation is rare.

Pneumococcal acute otitis media: Acute otitis media in infants (after the neonatal period) and children is caused by pneumococci in about 30 to 40% of cases. More than one third of children in most populations develop acute pneumococcal otitis media during the first 2 yr of life, and pneumococcal otitis commonly recurs. Relatively few serotypes of *S. pneumoniae* are responsible for most cases. After universal immunization of infants in the US beginning in 2000, nonvaccine serotypes of *S. pneumoniae* (particularly serotype 19A) have become the most common pneumococcal cause of acute otitis media.

Complications include

- Mild conductive hearing loss
- Vestibular balance dysfunction
- Tympanic membrane perforation
- Mastoiditis
- Petrositis
- Labyrinthitis

Intracranial complications are rare in developed countries but may include meningitis, epidural abscess, brain abscess, lateral venous sinus thrombosis, cavernous sinus thrombosis, subdural empyema, and carotid artery thrombosis.

Pneumococcal paranasal sinusitis: Paranasal sinusitis may be caused by pneumococci and may become chronic and polymicrobic.

Most commonly, the maxillary and ethmoid sinuses are affected. Infection of the sinuses causes pain and purulent discharge and may extend into the cranium, causing the following complications:

- Cavernous sinus thrombosis
- Brain, epidural, or subdural abscesses
- Septic cortical thrombophlebitis
- Meningitis

Pneumococcal meningitis: Acute purulent meningitis is frequently caused by pneumococci and may be secondary to bacteremia from other foci (notably pneumonia); direct extension from infection of the ear, mastoid process, or paranasal sinuses; or basilar fracture of the skull involving one of these sites or the cribriform plate (usually with cerebrospinal fluid leakage), thus giving bacteria in the paranasal sinuses, nasopharynx, or middle ear access to the CNS.

Typical meningitis symptoms (eg, headache, stiff neck, fever) occur.

Complications after pneumococcal meningitis include

- Hearing loss (in up to 50% of patients)
- Seizures
- Learning disabilities
- Mental dysfunction
- Palsies

Pneumococcal endocarditis: Acute bacterial endocarditis may result from pneumococcal bacteremia, even in patients without valvular heart disease, but is rare.

Pneumococcal endocarditis may produce a corrosive valvular lesion, with sudden rupture or fenestration, leading to rapidly progressive heart failure.

Pneumococcal septic arthritis: Septic arthritis, similar to septic arthritis caused by other gram-positive cocci, is usually a complication of pneumococcal bacteremia from another site.

Spontaneous pneumococcal peritonitis: Spontaneous pneumococcal peritonitis occurs most often in patients with cirrhosis and ascites, with no features to distinguish it from spontaneous bacterial peritonitis of other causes.

Diagnosis

- Gram stain and culture

Pneumococci are readily identified by their typical appearance on Gram stain as lancet-shaped diplococci.

The characteristic capsule can be best detected using the Quellung test. In this test, application of antiserum followed by staining with India ink causes the capsule to appear like a halo around the organism. The capsule is also visible in smears stained with methylene blue.

Culture confirms identification; antimicrobial susceptibility testing should be done. Serotyping and genotyping of isolates can be helpful for epidemiologic reasons (eg, to follow the spread of specific clones and antimicrobial resistance patterns). Differences in virulence within a serotype may be distinguished by techniques such as pulsed-field gel electrophoresis and multilocus sequence typing.

Treatment

- A β-lactam, macrolide, or a respiratory fluoroquinolone (eg, levofloxacin, moxifloxacin, gemifloxacin)

If pneumococcal infection is suspected, initial therapy pending susceptibility studies should be determined by local resistance patterns.

Although preferred treatment for pneumococcal infections is a β-lactam or macrolide antibiotic, treatment has become more challenging because resistant strains have emerged. Strains highly resistant to penicillin, ampicillin, and other β-lactams are common worldwide. The most common predisposing factor to β-lactam resistance is use of these drugs within the past several months. Resistance to macrolide antibiotics has also increased significantly; these drugs are no longer recommended as monotherapy for hospitalized patients with community-acquired pneumonia.

Intermediately resistant organisms may be treated with usual or high doses of penicillin G or another β-lactam.

Seriously ill patients with nonmeningeal infections caused by organisms that are highly resistant to penicillin can often be treated with ceftriaxone, cefotaxime, or ceftaroline. Very high doses of parenteral penicillin G (20 to 40 million units/day IV for adults) also work, unless the minimum inhibitory concentration of the isolate is very high. Fluoroquinolones (eg, moxifloxacin, levofloxacin, gemifloxacin) are effective for respiratory infections with highly penicillin-resistant pneumococci in adults. Evidence suggests that the mortality rate for bacteremic pneumococcal pneumonia is lower when combination therapy (eg, macrolide plus β-lactam) is used.

All penicillin-resistant isolates have been susceptible to vancomycin so far, but parenteral vancomycin does not always produce concentrations in CSF adequate for treatment of meningitis (especially if corticosteroids are also being used). Therefore, in patients with meningitis, ceftriaxone or cefotaxime, rifampin, or both are commonly used with vancomycin.

Prevention

Infection produces type-specific immunity that does not generalize to other serotypes. Otherwise, prevention involves

- Vaccination
- Prophylactic antibiotics

Pneumococcal vaccines: Two pneumococcal vaccines are available:

- A conjugated vaccine against 13 serotypes (PCV13)
- A polyvalent polysaccharide vaccine directed against the 23 serotypes (PPSV23) that account for > 90% of serious pneumococcal infections in adults and children

The vaccine schedules vary depending on age and medical conditions present in the patient.

Pneumococcal conjugated vaccine (PCV13) is recommended for the following:

- All children aged 2 mo to 6 yr (see Table 291–2 on p. 2462)
- Adults ≥ 65 yr
- Patients aged 6 to 64 yr with conditions that put them at high risk of pneumococcal infections

Conditions that put patients at high risk of pneumococcal infections include the following:

- A cochlear implant
- CSF leak
- Sickle cell disease or another hemoglobinopathy
- Congenital or acquired asplenia
- Immunocompromising conditions (eg, congenital immunodeficiency, chronic renal failure, nephrotic syndrome, HIV infection, leukemia, lymphomas, generalized cancer, use of immunosuppressants, solid organ transplant)

Pneumococcal polysaccharide vaccine (PPSV23) is recommended for the following:

- Adults ≥ 65 yr
- Patients aged 2 to 64 yr who have high-risk conditions, including the high-risk conditions listed above.

Additional vaccine criteria for adults aged 19 to 64 yr include the following:

- A chronic lung disorder (including asthma)
- Chronic cardiovascular disorders (excluding hypertension)
- Diabetes mellitus
- A chronic liver disorder
- Chronic alcoholism
- Cigarette smoking

(See also the the CDC's Recommended Immunization Schedule for Persons Aged 0 Through 18 Years and Recommended Adult Immunization Schedule, by Vaccine and Age Group [www.cdc.gov].)

Prophylactic antibiotics: For functional or anatomic asplenic children < 5 yr, prophylactic penicillin V 125 mg po bid is recommended. The duration for chemoprophylaxis is empiric, but some experts continue prophylaxis throughout childhood and into adulthood for high-risk patients with asplenia. Penicillin 250 mg po bid is recommended for older children or adolescents for at least 1 yr after splenectomy.

KEY POINTS

- Pneumococci cause many cases of otitis media and pneumonia and can also cause meningitis, sinusitis, and septic arthritis.
- Patients with chronic respiratory tract disease or asplenia are at high risk of serious and invasive pneumococcal infections, as are immunocompromised patients.
- Treat uncomplicated or mild infection with a β-lactam or macrolide antibiotic.
- Because resistance to β-lactam and macrolide antibiotics is increasing, seriously ill patients may be treated with an advanced-generation cephalosporin (eg, ceftriaxone, cefotaxime, ceftaroline) and/or a respiratory fluoroquinolone (eg, moxifloxacin, levofloxacin, gemifloxacin).
- Routine vaccination is recommended for all children aged 6 wk through 59 mo, all adults ≥ 65 yr, and people of other ages with certain risk factors.

STAPHYLOCOCCAL INFECTIONS

Staphylococci are gram-positive aerobic organisms. *Staphylococcus aureus* is the most pathogenic; it typically causes skin infections and sometimes pneumonia, endocarditis, and osteomyelitis. It commonly leads to abscess formation. Some strains elaborate toxins that cause gastroenteritis, scalded skin syndrome, and toxic shock syndrome. Diagnosis is by Gram stain and culture. Treatment is usually with penicillinase-resistant β-lactams, but because antibiotic resistance is common, vancomycin or other newer antibiotics may be required. Some strains are partially or totally resistant to all but the newest antibiotics, which include linezolid, tedizolid, quinupristin/dalfopristin, daptomycin, telavancin, dalbavancin, oritavancin, tigecycline, ceftobiprole (not available in the US), and ceftaroline.

The ability to clot blood by producing coagulase distinguishes the virulent pathogen, *Staphylococcus aureus*, from the less virulent coagulase-negative staphylococcal species. Coagulase-positive *S. aureus* is among the most ubiquitous and dangerous human pathogens, for both its virulence and its ability to develop antibiotic resistance.

Coagulase-negative species such as *S. epidermidis* are increasingly associated with hospital-acquired infections; *S. saprophyticus* causes urinary infections. *S. lugdunensis*, a coagulase-negative species, can cause invasive disease with virulence similar to that of *S. aureus*. Unlike most coagulase-negative staphylococcal species, *S. lugdunensis*, often remains sensitive to penicillinase-resistant β-lactam antibiotics.

Pathogenic staphylococci are ubiquitous. They are carried, usually transiently, in the anterior nares of about 30% of healthy adults and on the skin of about 20%; from these locations, staphylococci can cause infection in the host and others. Rates are higher in hospital patients and personnel.

Risk factors: People who are predisposed to staphylococcal infections include

- Neonates and breastfeeding mothers
- Patients with influenza, chronic bronchopulmonary disorders (eg, cystic fibrosis, emphysema), leukemia, tumors, chronic skin disorders, diabetes mellitus, or burns
- Patients with a transplant, an implanted prosthesis, other foreign bodies, or an indwelling intravascular plastic catheter surgical incisions
- Patients receiving adrenal steroids, irradiation, immunosuppressants, or antitumor chemotherapy
- Injection drug users

Predisposed patients may acquire antibiotic-resistant staphylococci from other patients, health care personnel, or inanimate objects in health care settings. Transmission via the hands of personnel is the most common means of spread, but airborne spread can also occur.

Diseases Caused by Staphylococci

Staphylococci cause disease by

- Direct tissue invasion
- Sometimes exotoxin production

Direct tissue invasion is the most common mechanism for staphylococcal disease, including the following:

- Skin infections
- Pneumonia
- Endocarditis
- Osteomyelitis
- Septic arthritis

Multiple **exotoxins** are sometimes produced by staphylococci. Some have local effects; others trigger cytokine release from certain T cells, causing serious systemic effects (eg, skin lesions, shock, organ failure, death). Panton-Valentine leukocidin (PVL) is a toxin produced by strains infected with a certain bacteriophage. PVL is typically present in strains of CA-MRSA and has been thought to mediate the ability to necrotize; however, this effect has not been verified.

Toxin-mediated staphylococcal diseases include the following:

- Toxic shock syndrome
- Staphylococcal scalded skin syndrome
- Staphylococcal food poisoning

The diseases listed below are further discussed elsewhere in THE MANUAL.

Staphylococcal bacteremia: Staphylococcal bacteremia, which frequently causes metastatic foci of infection, may occur with any localized staphylococcal infection but is particularly common with infection related to intravascular catheters or other foreign bodies. It may also occur without any obvious primary site. *S. epidermidis* and other coagulase-negative staphylococci increasingly cause hospital-acquired bacteremia associated with intravascular catheters and other foreign bodies because they can form biofilms on these materials. They are important causes of morbidity (especially prolongation of hospitalization) and mortality in debilitated patients.

Staphylococcal skin infections: Skin infections are the most common form of staphylococcal disease. Superficial infections may be diffuse, with vesicular pustules and crusting (impetigo) or sometimes cellulitis or with focal and nodular abscesses (furuncles and carbuncles). Deeper cutaneous abscesses are common. Severe necrotizing skin infections may occur.

Staphylococci are commonly implicated in wound and burn infections, postoperative incision infections, and mastitis or breast abscess in breastfeeding mothers.

Staphylococcal neonatal infections: Neonatal infections usually appear within 6 wk after birth and include

- Skin lesions with or without exfoliation
- Bacteremia
- Meningitis
- Pneumonia

Staphylococcal pneumonia: Pneumonia that occurs in a community setting is not common but may develop in patients who have influenza, who are receiving corticosteroids or immunosuppressants, or who have chronic bronchopulmonary or other high-risk diseases. Staphylococcal pneumonia may be a primary infection or result from hematogenous spread of *S. aureus* infection elsewhere in the body (eg, IV catheter infection, endocarditis, soft-tissue infection) or from injection drug use. However, *S. aureus* is a common cause of hospital-acquired pneumonia.

Staphylococcal pneumonia is occasionally characterized by formation of lung abscesses followed by rapid development of pneumatoceles and empyema. Community-associated methicillin-resistant *S. aureus* (CA-MRSA) often causes severe necrotizing pneumonia.

Staphylococcal endocarditis: Endocarditis (see p. 707) can develop, particularly in IV drug abusers and patients with prosthetic heart valves. Because intravascular catheter use and implantation of cardiac devices have increased, *S. aureus* has become a leading cause of bacterial endocarditis.

S. aureus endocarditis is an acute febrile illness often accompanied by visceral abscesses, embolic phenomena, pericarditis, subungual petechiae, subconjunctival hemorrhage, purpuric lesions, heart murmurs, and heart failure secondary to cardiac valve damage.

Staphylococcal osteomyelitis: Osteomyelitis (see p. 298) occurs more commonly in children, causing chills, fever, and pain over the involved bone. Subsequently, the overlying soft tissue becomes red and swollen. Articular infection may occur; it frequently results in effusion, suggesting septic arthritis rather than osteomyelitis. Most infections of the vertebrae and intervertebral disks in adults involve *S. aureus*.

Staphylococcal toxic shock syndrome: Staphylococcal toxic shock syndrome (TSS—see p. 1608) may result from use of vaginal tampons or complicate any type of *S. aureus* infection (eg, postoperative wound infection, infection of a burn, skin infection). Although most cases have been due to methicillin-susceptible *S. aureus* (MSSA), cases due to MRSA are becoming more frequent.

Staphylococcal scalded skin syndrome: Staphylococcal scalded skin syndrome, which is caused by several toxins termed exfoliatins, is an exfoliative dermatitis of childhood characterized by large bullae and peeling of the upper layer of skin (see p. 1000 and Plate 52). Eventually, exfoliation occurs. Scalded skin syndrome most commonly occurs in infants and children < 5 yr.

Staphylococcal food poisoning: Staphylococcal food poisoning is caused by ingesting a preformed heat-stable staphylococcal enterotoxin. Food can be contaminated by staphylococcal carriers or people with active skin infections. In food that is incompletely cooked or left at room temperature, staphylococci reproduce and elaborate enterotoxin. Many foods can serve as growth media, and despite contamination, they have a normal taste and odor. Severe nausea and vomiting begin 2 to 8 h after ingestion, typically followed by abdominal cramps and diarrhea. The attack is brief, often lasting < 12 h.

Diagnosis

- Gram stain and culture

Diagnosis is by Gram stain and culture of infected material.

Susceptibility tests should be done because methicillin-resistant organisms are now common and require alternative therapy.

When **staphylococcal scalded skin syndrome** is suspected, cultures should be obtained from blood, urine, the nasopharynx, the umbilicus, abnormal skin, or any suspected focus of infection; the intact bullae are sterile. Although the diagnosis is usually clinical, a biopsy of the affected skin may help confirm the diagnosis.

Staphylococcal food poisoning is usually suspected because of case clustering (eg, within a family, attendees of a social gathering, or customers of a restaurant). Confirmation (typically by the health department) entails isolating staphylococci from suspect food and sometimes testing for enterotoxins.

In **osteomyelitis,** x-ray changes may not be apparent for 10 to 14 days, and bone rarefaction and periosteal reaction may not be detected for even longer. Abnormalities in MRI, CT, or radionuclide bone scans are often apparent earlier. Bone biopsy (open or percutaneous) should be done for pathogen identification and susceptibility testing.

Screening: Some institutions that have a high incidence of MRSA nosocomial infections routinely screen admitted patients for MRSA (active surveillance) by using rapid laboratory techniques to evaluate nasal swab specimens. Some institutions screen only high-risk patients (eg, those who are admitted to the ICU, who have had previous MRSA infection, or who are about to undergo vascular, orthopedic, or cardiac surgery).

Quick identification of MRSA does the following:

- Allows carriers to be placed in contact isolation and, when preoperative antibiotic prophylaxis against skin organisms is required, to be given vancomycin as part of their drug regimen
- Decreases the spread of MRSA
- May decrease the incidence of nosocomial infections with MRSA

However, decolonization treatments (eg, giving topical nasal mupirocin), although sometimes done, are not yet proved effective, and mupirocin resistance is emerging. Bathing ICU patients with chlorhexidine daily decreases the incidence of MRSA infections.

Treatment

- Local measures (eg, debridement, removal of catheters)
- Antibiotics selected based on severity of infection and local resistance patterns

Management includes abscess drainage, debridement of necrotic tissue, removal of foreign bodies (including intravascular catheters), and use of antibiotics (see Table 191–1).

Initial choice and dosage of antibiotics depend on

- Infection site
- Illness severity
- Probability that resistant strains are involved

Thus, it is essential to know local resistance patterns for initial therapy (and ultimately, to know actual drug susceptibility).

Treatment of **toxin-mediated staphylococcal disease** (the most serious of which is toxic shock syndrome) involves decontamination of the toxin-producing area (exploration of surgical wounds, irrigation, debridement), intensive support (including IV fluids, vasopressors, and respiratory assistance), electrolyte balancing, and antimicrobials. In vitro evidence supports a preference for protein synthesis inhibitors (eg, clindamycin 900 mg IV q 8 h, linezolid 600 mg IV q 12 h) over other classes of antibiotics. IV immune globulin has been beneficial in severe cases.

Antibiotic resistance: Many staphylococcal strains produce penicillinase, an enzyme that inactivates several β-lactam antibiotics; these strains are resistant to penicillin G, ampicillin, and antipseudomonal penicillins.

Community-acquired strains are often susceptible to penicillinase-resistant penicillins (eg, methicillin, oxacillin, nafcillin, cloxacillin, dicloxacillin), cephalosporins, carbapenems (eg, imipenem, meropenem, ertapenem, doripenem), tetracyclines, macrolides, fluoroquinolones, trimethoprim/sulfamethoxazole (TMP/SMX), gentamicin, vancomycin, and teicoplanin.

MRSA isolates have become common, especially in hospitals. In addition, CA-MRSA has emerged over the past several years in most geographic regions. CA-MRSA tends to be less resistant to multiple drugs than hospital-acquired MRSA. These strains, although resistant to most β-lactams, are usually susceptible to TMP/SMX and tetracyclines (minocycline, doxycycline) and are often susceptible to clindamycin, but there is the potential for emergence of clindamycin resistance by strains inducibly resistant to erythromycin (laboratories may report these strains as D-test positive). Vancomycin is effective against most MRSA, sometimes with rifampin and an aminoglycoside added for some serious infections (ie, osteomyelitis, prosthetic joint infections, prosthetic valve endocarditis). An alternative drug (daptomycin, linezolid, tedizolid, dalbavancin, oritavancin, tigecycline, quinupristin/dalfopristin, TMP-SMX, possibly ceftaroline) should be considered when treating MRSA strains with a vancomycin MIC of > 1.5 mcg/mL.

Vancomycin-resistant *S. aureus* (**VRSA**; MIC > 16 mcg/mL) and vancomycin-intermediate-susceptible *S. aureus* (VISA; MIC 4 to 8 mcg/mL) strains have appeared in the US. These organisms require linezolid, tedizolid, quinupristin/dalfopristin, daptomycin, TMP/SMX, or ceftaroline.

Because incidence of MRSA has increased, initial empiric treatment for serious staphylococcal infections (particularly those that occur in a health care setting) should include a drug with reliable activity against MRSA. Thus, appropriate drugs include the following:

- For proven or suspected bloodstream infections, vancomycin or daptomycin
- For pneumonia, vancomycin, telavancin, or linezolid (because daptomycin is not reliably active in the lungs)

Table 191–1 summarizes treatment options.

Table 191–1. ANTIBIOTIC TREATMENT OF STAPHYLOCOCCAL INFECTIONS IN ADULTS

INFECTION	DRUGS
Community-acquired cutaneous infections (non-MRSA)	Dicloxacillin or cephalexin 250–500 mg po q 6 h for 7–10 days
Penicillin-allergic patients	Erythromycin 250–500 mg po q 6 h; clarithromycin 500 mg po q 12 h; azithromycin 500 mg po on the first day, then 250 mg po q 24 h; or clindamycin 300 mg po q 6 h
Community-acquired cutaneous infections likely to be due to MRSA	Trimethoprim/sulfamethoxazole 160/800 mg po q 8–12 h, clindamycin 300 mg po q 6 h or 600 mg po q 8 h, linezolid 600 mg po q 12 h, or tedizolid 200 mg po q 24 h
Sulfa-allergic patients	Clindamycin 600 mg po q 8 h or doxycycline 100 mg po q 12 h
Serious infections unlikely to be due to MRSA	Nafcillin or oxacillin 1–2 g IV q 4–6 h or cefazolin 1 g IV q 8 h
Penicillin-allergic patients	Clindamycin 600 mg IV q 8 h or vancomycin 15 mg/kg q 12 h
Serious infection highly likely to be due to MRSA	Vancomycin 15 mg/kg IV q 12 h, linezolid 600 mg IV q 12 h, tedizolid 200 mg IV q 24 h, daptomycin 4–6 mg/kg q 24 h (not for pulmonary infections), ceftobiprole 500 mg IV q 8 h, or ceftaroline 600 mg IV q 12 h
Documented MRSA	By reported sensitivities
Vancomycin-resistant staphylococci*	Linezolid 600 mg IV q 12 h, quinupristin/dalfopristin 7.5 mg/kg q 8 h, daptomycin 4–6 mg/kg q 24 h, dalbavancin 1000 mg IV followed by 500 mg IV a week later, oritavancin 1200 mg IV once, ceftobiprole 500 mg IV q 8 h, or ceftaroline 600 mg IV q 12 h

*No clinical data are available, but listed drugs appear to be active in vitro; doses have not been established.
MRSA = methicillin-resistant *Staphylococcus aureus*.

Prevention

Aseptic precautions (eg, thoroughly washing hands between patient examinations, sterilizing shared equipment) help decrease spread in institutions. Strict isolation procedures should be used for patients harboring resistant microbes until their infections have been cured. An asymptomatic nasal carrier need not be isolated unless the strain is MRSA or is the suspected source of an outbreak.

The organism recurs in up to 50% of carriers and frequently becomes resistant. For certain MRSA carriers (eg, preorthopedic, vascular and cardiovascular surgical patients), some experts recommend nasal decolonization with mupirocin ointment twice/day for 5 to 10 days and topical body decolonization regimens with a skin antiseptic solution (eg, chlorhexidine) or dilute bleach baths (about 5 mL/L) for 5 to 14 days. Oral antimicrobial therapy is recommended only for treatment of active infection. However, if infections recur despite topical treatments, clinicians should consider using rifampin plus either cloxacillin, dicloxacillin, TMP/SMX, or ciprofloxacin, depending on susceptibility. If MRSA is identified via nasal culture, vancomycin should be used.

Staphylococcal food poisoning can be prevented by appropriate food preparation. Patients with staphylococcal skin infections should not handle food, and food should be consumed immediately or refrigerated and not kept at room temperature.

KEY POINTS

- Coagulase-positive *Staphylococcus aureus* is the most dangerous staphylococcal species.
- Most staphylococcal diseases involve direct tissue invasion and cause skin and soft-tissue infections, pneumonia, endocarditis, or osteomyelitis.
- Some strains produce a toxin that can cause toxic shock syndrome, scalded skin syndrome, or food poisoning.
- Methicillin-resistant strains are common, and vancomycin resistance is appearing in the US.
- Drug choice depends on source and location of infection and community or institutional resistance patterns.

STREPTOCOCCAL INFECTIONS

Streptococci are gram-positive aerobic organisms that cause many disorders, including pharyngitis, pneumonia, wound and skin infections, sepsis, and endocarditis. Symptoms vary with the organ infected. Sequelae include rheumatic fever and glomerulonephritis. Most strains are sensitive to penicillin, although macrolide-resistant strains have recently emerged.

Classification of streptococci: Three different types of streptococci are initially differentiated by their appearance when they are grown on sheep blood agar:

- β-Hemolytic streptococci produce zones of clear hemolysis around each colony.
- α-Hemolytic streptococci (commonly called viridans streptococci) are surrounded by green discoloration resulting from incomplete hemolysis.
- γ-Hemolytic streptococci are nonhemolytic.

Subsequent classification, based on carbohydrates in the cell wall, divides streptococci into Lancefield groups A through H and K through T (see Table 191–2). Viridans streptococci form a separate group that is difficult to classify. In the Lancefield classification, enterococci were initially included among the group D streptococci. More recently, enterococci have been classified as a separate genus.

Virulence factors: Many streptococci elaborate virulence factors, including streptolysins, DNAases, and hyaluronidase, which contribute to tissue destruction and spread of infection. A few strains release exotoxins that activate certain T cells, triggering release of cytokines, including tumor necrosis factor-α, interleukins, and other immunomodulators. These cytokines activate the complement, coagulation, and fibrinolytic systems, leading to shock, organ failure, and death.

Diseases Caused by Streptococci

The most significant streptococcal pathogen is *S. pyogenes*, which is β-hemolytic and in Lancefield group A and is thus denoted as group A β-hemolytic streptococci (GABHS).

The **most common acute diseases due to GABHS** are

- Pharyngitis
- Skin infections

In addition, delayed, nonsuppurative complications (rheumatic fever, acute glomerulonephritis) sometimes occur ≥ 2 wk after infection.

Disease caused by other streptococcal species is less prevalent and usually involves soft-tissue infection or endocarditis (see Table 191–2). Some non-GABHS infections occur predominantly in certain populations (eg, group B streptococci in neonates and postpartum women).

Infections can spread through the affected tissues and along lymphatic channels to regional lymph nodes. They can also cause local suppurative complications, such as peritonsillar abscess, otitis media, sinusitis, and bacteremia. Suppuration depends on the severity of infection and the susceptibility of tissue.

Other serious streptococcal infections include septicemia, puerperal sepsis, endocarditis, and pneumonia.

Streptococcal pharyngitis: Streptococcal pharyngitis is usually caused by GABHS. About 20% of patients present with sore throat, fever, a beefy red pharynx, and a purulent tonsillar exudate. The remainder have less prominent symptoms, and the examination resembles that of viral pharyngitis. The cervical and submaxillary nodes may enlarge and become tender. Streptococcal pharyngitis can lead to peritonsillar abscess. Cough, laryngitis, and stuffy nose are not characteristic of streptococcal pharyngeal infection; their presence suggests another cause (usually viral or allergic).

An asymptomatic carrier state may exist in as many as 20%.

Scarlet fever: Scarlet fever is uncommon today, but outbreaks still occur. Transmission is enhanced in environments that result in close contact among people (eg, in schools or day-care centers).

Scarlet fever, a predominantly childhood disease, usually follows a pharyngeal streptococcal infection; less commonly, it follows streptococcal infections at other sites (eg, the skin). Scarlet fever is caused by group A streptococcal strains that produce an erythrogenic toxin, leading to a diffuse pink-red cutaneous flush that blanches with pressure.

The rash is seen best on the abdomen or lateral chest and as dark red lines in skinfolds (Pastia lines) or as circumoral pallor. The rash consists of characteristic numerous small (1- to 2-mm) papular elevations, giving a sandpaper quality to the skin. The upper layer of the previously reddened skin often desquamates after fever subsides. The rash usually lasts 2 to 5 days.

A strawberry tongue (inflamed papillae protruding through a bright red coating) also occurs and must be differentiated from that seen in TSS and Kawasaki disease.

Table 191–2. CLASSIFICATION OF STREPTOCOCCI

LANCEFIELD GROUP	SPECIES	HEMOLYSIS	ASSOCIATED DISEASES	TREATMENT
A	*S. pyogenes*	β	Pharyngitis, tonsillitis, wound and skin infections, septicemia, scarlet fever, pneumonia, rheumatic fever, glomerulonephritis	Penicillin, erythromycin, clindamycin
			Necrotizing fasciitis	Expeditious surgical management β-Lactam (usually broad spectrum until etiology is identified; if GABHS is confirmed, penicillin or cefazolin can be used) plus clindamycin
B	*S. agalactiae*	β	Sepsis, postpartum or neonatal sepsis, meningitis, skin infections, endocarditis, septic arthritis, UTIs	Penicillin or ampicillin, cephalosporin, vancomycin
C and G	*S. equi, S. canis*	β	Pharyngitis, pneumonia, cellulitis, pyoderma, erysipelas, impetigo, wound infections, puerperal sepsis, neonatal sepsis, endocarditis, septic arthritis	Penicillin, vancomycin, cephalosporins, macrolides (variable susceptibility)
D	Enterococcal: *Enterococcus faecalis, E. faecium* Nonenterococcal: *S. bovis, S. equinus*	α or γ	Endocarditis, UTI, intra-abdominal infection, cellulitis, wound infection as well as concurrent bacteremia	Penicillin, ampicillin, vancomycin (plus an aminoglycoside for serious infection) Vancomycin-resistant enterococci: Streptogramins (quinupristin/dalfopristin), oxazolidinones (linezolid), lipopeptide (daptomycin)
	S. gallolyticus (formerly *S. bovis* biotype I)		Colonic adenomas or carcinomas	
Viridans*	*S. mutans, S. sanguis, S. salivarius, S. mitior, S. milleri*	α or γ	Endocarditis, bacteremia, meningitis, localized infection, abscesses (particularly *S. milleri*)	Penicillin, ampicillin, vancomycin (plus an aminoglycoside for serious infection), other antibiotics based on in vitro susceptibility
	S. suis		Meningitis, sometimes toxic shock syndrome	
	S. iniae		Cellulitis, invasive infections from fish	Penicillin

*Do not conform to specific serogroups.
GABHS = group A β-hemolytic streptococci.

Other symptoms are similar to those in streptococcal pharyngitis, and the course and management of scarlet fever are the same as those of other group A infections.

Streptococcal skin infections: Skin infections include

- Impetigo
- Erysipelas
- Cellulitis

Impetigo is a superficial skin infection that causes crusting or bullae (see p. 998).

Erysipelas is a superficial cellulitis that also involves the lymphatics (see p. 995). Patients have shiny, red, raised, indurated lesions with distinct margins (see Plate 36). It is most often caused by GABHS, but other streptococcal and non-streptococcal organisms are sometimes involved.

Cellulitis involves the deeper layers of skin and may spread rapidly because of the numerous lytic enzymes and toxins produced mainly by group A streptococci (see p. 994).

Necrotizing fasciitis: Necrotizing fasciitis (see also p. 999) due to *S. pyogenes* is a severe dermal (and sometimes muscle) infection that spreads along fascial planes. Inoculation originates through the skin or bowel, and the defect may be surgical, trivial, distant from the disease site, or occult, as with colonic diverticula or an appendiceal abscess.

Necrotizing fasciitis is prevalent among IV drug abusers.

Formerly known as streptococcal gangrene and popularized as the flesh-eating bacteria, the same syndrome may also be polymicrobial, involving a host of aerobic and anaerobic flora, including *Clostridium perfringens*.

Symptoms of necrotizing fasciitis begin with fever and exquisite localized pain; pain increases rapidly over time and is often the first (and sometimes only) manifestation. Diffuse or local erythema may be present. Thrombosis of the microvasculature causes ischemic necrosis, leading to rapid spread and disproportionally severe toxicity. In 20 to 40% of patients, adjacent muscles are invaded. Shock and renal dysfunction are common. Mortality is high, even with treatment.

When necrotizing fasciitis occurs in the perineum, it is called Fournier gangrene (see Plate 75). Comorbid conditions, such as impaired immunity, diabetes, and alcoholism, are common.

Streptococcal toxic shock syndrome: Streptococcal toxic shock syndrome, similar to that caused by *S. aureus*, may result from toxin-producing strains of GABHS and occasionally from other streptococci (see p. 1608). Patients are usually otherwise healthy children or adults with skin and soft-tissue infections.

Delayed complications of streptococcal infection: The mechanism by which certain strains of GABHS cause delayed complications is unclear but may involve cross-reactivity of streptococcal antibodies against host tissue.

Rheumatic fever, an inflammatory disorder (see p. 2745), occurs in < 3% of patients in the weeks after untreated GABHS pharyngitis. It has become much less common in developed countries but is still common in developing countries. Diagnosis of a first episode is based on a combination of arthritis, carditis, chorea, specific cutaneous manifestations, and laboratory test results (Jones criteria—see Table 321–4 on p. 2747).

One of the most important reasons for treating strep throat is to prevent rheumatic fever.

Poststreptococcal acute glomerulonephritis is an acute nephritic syndrome following pharyngitis or skin infection due to a certain limited number of nephritogenic strains of GABHS (eg, M protein serotypes 12 and 49). After a throat or skin infection with one of these strains, about 10 to 15% of patients develop acute glomerulonephritis. It is most common among children, occurring 1 to 3 wk after infection. Nearly all children, but somewhat fewer adults, recover without permanent renal damage. Antibiotic treatment of GABHS infection has little effect on development of glomerulonephritis.

PANDAS syndrome (pediatric autoimmune neuropsychiatric disorder associated with group A streptococci) refers to a subset of obsessive disorders or tic disorders in children thought to be exacerbated by GABHS infection.

Certain forms of **psoriasis** (eg, guttate) may also be related to β-hemolytic streptococcal infections.

Diagnosis

- Culture
- Sometimes rapid antigen tests or antibody titers

Streptococci are readily identified by culture on a sheep blood agar plate.

Rapid antigen-detection tests that can detect GABHS directly from throat swabs are available (ie, for point-of-care use). Many tests use enzyme immunoassay, but more recently, tests using optical immunoassay have become available. These rapid tests have high specificity (> 95%) but vary considerably in sensitivity (55% to 80 to 90% for the newer optical immunoassay test). Thus, positive results can establish the diagnosis, but negative results, at least in children, should be confirmed by culture. Because streptococcal pharyngitis is less common among adults and adults are unlikely to have poststreptococcal complications, many clinicians do not confirm a negative rapid screening result in adults by culture unless use of a macrolide is being considered; in such cases, susceptibility testing to detect macrolide resistance should be done.

Demonstrating **antistreptococcal antibodies** in serum during convalescence provides only indirect evidence of infection. Antibodies are most useful in diagnosis of poststreptococcal diseases, such as rheumatic fever and glomerulonephritis.

Confirmation requires that sequential specimens show a rise in titer because a single value may be high because of a long antecedent infection. Serum specimens need not be taken more often than every 2 wk and may be taken every 2 mo. To be considered significant, a rise (or fall) in titer should span at least 2 serial dilutions. The antistreptolysin O (ASO) titer rises in only 75 to 80% of infections. For completeness in difficult cases, any one of the other tests (antihyaluronidase, antideoxyribonuclease B, antinicotinamide adenine dinucleotidase, antistreptokinase) can also be used. Penicillin given within the first 5 days for symptomatic streptococcal pharyngitis may delay the appearance and decrease the magnitude of the ASO response. Patients with streptococcal pyoderma usually do not have a significant ASO response but may have a response to other antigens (ie, anti-DNAase, antihyaluronidase).

Treatment

- Usually penicillin

Pharyngitis: (See also the Infectious Diseases Society of America's Practice Guidelines for the Diagnosis and Management of Group A Streptococcal Pharyngitis at https://academic.oup.com and The American Heart Association's Preventing Rheumatic Fever at http://www.jwatch.org.)

Ordinarily, pharyngeal GABHS infections, including scarlet fever, are self-limited. Antibiotics shorten the course in young children, especially those with scarlet fever, but have only modest effect on symptoms in adolescents and adults. However, antibiotics help prevent local suppurative complications (eg, peritonsillar abscess), otitis media, and rheumatic fever.

Penicillin is the drug of choice. No isolate of GABHS has demonstrated penicillin resistance clinically. However, some streptococcal strains appear to have in vitro tolerance to penicillin; the clinical significance of such strains is unclear.

A single injection of benzathine penicillin G, 600,000 units IM for small children (< 27 kg) or 1.2 million units IM for children weighing ≥ 27 kg, adolescents, and adults usually suffices.

Oral drugs may be used if the patient can be trusted to maintain the regimen for the required 10 days. Choices include

- Penicillin V 500 mg (250 mg for children < 27 kg) po q 12 h
- Amoxicillin 50 mg/kg (maximum 1 g) once/day for 10 days (which is an effective substitute for penicillin V)

Oral narrow-spectrum cephalosporins (eg, cephalexin, cefadroxil) are also effective and can be used unless patients have an anaphylactic reaction to penicillin. Azithromycin can be used for a 5-day course of therapy, although macrolides are inactive against *Fusobacterium necrophorum*, a common cause of pharyngitis in adolescents and adults. Delaying treatment 1 to 2 days until laboratory confirmation increases neither the duration of disease nor the incidence of complications.

When penicillin and a β-lactam are contraindicated, choices include

- Clindamycin 600 mg (6.7 mg/kg for children) po q 8 h
- Erythromycin or clarithromycin 250 mg (7.5 mg/kg for children) po q 12 h for 10 days
- Azithromycin 500 mg (15 mg/kg for children) once/day for 5 days

Because resistance of GABHS to macrolides has been detected, some authorities recommend in vitro confirmation of susceptibility if a macrolide is to be used and there is macrolide resistance in the community. Clindamycin 6.7 mg/kg po q 8 h is preferred in children who have relapses of chronic tonsillitis, possibly because it has good activity against penicillinase-producing staphylococci or anaerobes coinfecting the tonsillar crypts and inactivating penicillin G and because it appears to halt exotoxin production more rapidly than other drugs. Amoxicillin/clavulanate is also effective. Trimethoprim/sulfamethoxazole (TMP/SMX), some of the fluoroquinolones, and tetracyclines are unreliable for treating GABHS.

Sore throat, headache, and fever can be treated with analgesics or antipyretics. Aspirin should be avoided in children. Bed rest and isolation are unnecessary. Close contacts who are symptomatic or have a history of poststreptococcal complications should be examined for streptococci.

Skin infection: Cellulitis is often treated without doing a culture because isolating organisms can be difficult. Thus, regimens effective against both streptococci and staphylococci are used (eg, dicloxacillin or cephalexin if methicillin-resistant *Staphylococcus aureus* [MRSA] is not likely or TMP/SMX, linezolid, minocycline, or clindamycin if MRSA is suspected—see p. 995).

Necrotizing fasciitis should be treated in an ICU. Extensive (sometimes repeated) surgical debridement is required. A recommended initial antibiotic regimen is a β-lactam (often a broad-spectrum drug until etiology is confirmed by culture) plus clindamycin. Although streptococci remain susceptible to β-lactam antibiotics, animal studies show that penicillin is not always effective against a large bacterial inoculum because the streptococci are not rapidly growing and lack penicillin-binding proteins, which are the target of penicillin activity.

Other streptococcal infections: For treating **group B, C, and G infections,** drugs of choice are

- Penicillin
- Ampicillin
- Vancomycin

Cephalosporins or macrolides are usually effective, but susceptibility tests must guide therapy, especially in very ill, immunocompromised, or debilitated people and in people with foreign bodies at the infection site. Surgical wound drainage and debridement as adjuncts to antimicrobial therapy may be lifesaving.

S. bovis (including *S. gallolyticus*) is relatively susceptible to antibiotics. Although vancomycin-resistant *S. bovis* isolates have been reported, the organism remains susceptible to penicillin and aminoglycosides.

Most **viridans streptococci** are often susceptible to penicillin G and other β-lactams. Resistance is growing, and therapy for such strains should be dictated by results of in vitro susceptibility tests.

KEY POINTS

- The most significant streptococcal pathogen is *S. pyogenes*, which is denoted as GABHS.
- The 2 most common acute diseases due to GABHS are pharyngitis and skin infections.
- Delayed nonsuppurative complications, including rheumatic fever and poststreptococcal glomerulonephritis, can occur.
- Rapid antigen tests (ie, for point-of-care use) are very specific but not highly sensitive; confirm negative results using culture, at least in children.
- A penicillin or cephalosporin is preferred for pharyngitis; because macrolide resistance is increasing, susceptibility testing is recommended if that class of drugs is used.

TOXIC SHOCK SYNDROME

Toxic shock syndrome (TSS) is caused by staphylococcal or streptococcal exotoxins. Symptoms include high fever, hypotension, diffuse erythematous rash, and multiple organ dysfunction, which may rapidly progress to severe and intractable shock. Diagnosis is made clinically and by isolating the organism. Treatment includes antibiotics, intensive support, and immune globulin.

TSS is caused by exotoxin-producing cocci. Strains of phage-group 1 *Staphylococcus aureus* elaborate the TSS toxin-1 (TSST-1) or related exotoxins; certain strains of *Streptococcus pyogenes* produce at least 2 exotoxins.

Staphylococcal toxic shock: At highest risk of staphylococcal TSS are

- Women who have preexisting staphylococcal colonization of the vagina and who leave tampons or other devices (eg, contraceptive sponges, diaphragms) in the vagina

Mechanical or chemical factors related to tampon use probably enhance production of the exotoxin or facilitate its entry into the bloodstream through a mucosal break or via the uterus. Estimates made from small series suggest about 3 cases/100,000 menstruating women still occur, and cases are still reported in women who do not use tampons and in women who have infection after childbirth, abortion, or surgery. About 15% of cases occur postpartum or as a complication of postoperative staphylococcal wound infections, which frequently appear insignificant. Cases have also been reported in both men and women with any type of *S. aureus* infection.

Mortality from staphylococcal TSS is < 3%. Recurrences are common among women who continue to use tampons during the first 4 mo after an episode.

Streptococcal toxic shock: The syndrome is similar to that caused by *S. aureus*, but mortality is higher (20 to 60%) despite aggressive therapy. In addition, about 50% of patients have *S. pyogenes* bacteremia, and 50% have necrotizing fasciitis (neither is common with staphylococcal TSS). Patients are usually otherwise healthy children or adults. Primary infections in skin and soft tissue are more common than in other sites. In contrast to staphylococcal TSS, streptococcal TSS is more likely to cause acute respiratory distress syndrome (ARDS) and less likely to cause a typical cutaneous reaction.

S. pyogenes TSS is defined as any GABHS infection associated with shock and organ failure.

Risk factors for GABHS TSS include

- Minor trauma
- Surgical procedures
- Viral infections (eg, varicella)
- Use of NSAIDs

Symptoms and Signs

Onset is sudden, with fever (39 to 40.5° C, which remains elevated), hypotension (which can be refractory), a diffuse macular erythroderma, and involvement of at least 2 other organ systems.

Staphylococcal TSS is likely to cause vomiting, diarrhea, myalgia, elevated CK, mucositis, hepatic damage, thrombocytopenia, and confusion. The staphylococcal TSS rash is more likely to desquamate, particularly on the palms and soles, between 3 and 7 days after onset.

Streptococcal TSS commonly causes ARDS (in about 55% of patients), coagulopathy, and hepatic damage and is more likely to cause fever, malaise, and severe pain at the site of a soft-tissue infection.

Renal impairment is frequent and common to both. The syndrome may progress within 48 h to syncope, shock, and death. Less severe cases of staphylococcal TSS are fairly common.

Diagnosis

- Clinical evaluation
- Cultures

Diagnosis is made clinically and by isolating the organism from blood cultures (for *Streptococcus*) or from the local site.

TSS resembles Kawasaki disease, but Kawasaki disease usually occurs in children < 5 yr of age and does not cause shock, azotemia, or thrombocytopenia; the rash is maculopapular. Other disorders to be considered are scarlet fever, Reye syndrome, staphylococcal scalded skin syndrome, meningococcemia, Rocky Mountain spotted fever, leptospirosis, and viral exanthematous diseases. These disorders are ruled out by specific clinical differences, cultures, and serologic tests.

Specimens for culture should be taken from any lesions, the nose (for staphylococci), throat (for streptococci), vagina (for both), and blood. MRI or CT of soft tissue is helpful in localizing sites of infection. Continuous monitoring of renal, hepatic, bone marrow, and cardiopulmonary function is necessary.

Treatment

- Local measures (eg, decontamination, debridement)
- Fluid resuscitation and circulatory support
- Empiric antibiotic therapy (eg, clindamycin plus vancomycin or daptomycin) pending culture results

Patients suspected of having TSS should be hospitalized immediately and treated intensively. Tampons, diaphragms, and other foreign bodies should be removed at once. Suspected primary sites should be decontaminated thoroughly. Decontamination includes

- Reinspection and irrigation of surgical wounds, even if they appear healthy
- Repeated debridement of devitalized tissues
- Irrigation of potential naturally colonized sites (sinuses, vagina)

Fluids and electrolytes are replaced to prevent or treat hypovolemia, hypotension, and shock. Because fluid loss into tissues can occur throughout the body (because of systemic capillary leak syndrome and hypoalbuminemia), shock may be profound and resistant. Aggressive fluid resuscitation and circulatory, ventilatory, and/or hemodialysis support are sometimes required.

Obvious infections should be treated with antibiotics (for indications and doses, see Table 191–1). Pending culture results, clindamycin or linezolid (to suppress toxin production) plus vancomycin, daptomycin, linezolid, or ceftaroline—empiric choices that cover the most likely etiologic organisms—should be used. If a pathogen is isolated on culture, the antibiotic regimen is adjusted as needed, as for the following:

- For group A streptococci: Clindamycin plus a β-lactam
- For methicillin-susceptible *S. aureus* (MSSA): Clindamycin plus oxacillin or nafcillin
- For methicillin-resistant *Staphylococcus aureus* [MRSA]: Vancomycin or daptomycin plus clindamycin or linezolid, depending on the susceptibility

Antibiotics given during the acute illness may eradicate pathogen foci and prevent recurrences. Passive immunization to TSS toxins with IV immune globulin (2 g/kg, followed by 0.4 g/kg daily for up to 5 days) has been helpful in severe cases of both types of TSS and lasts for weeks, but the disease may not induce active immunity, so recurrences are possible.

If a test for seroconversion of the serum antibody responses to TSST-1 in acute- and convalescent-phase paired sera is negative, women who have had staphylococcal TSS should probably refrain from using tampons and cervical caps, plugs, and diaphragms. Advising all women, regardless of TSST-1 antibody status, to change tampons frequently or use napkins instead and to avoid hyperabsorbent tampons seems prudent.

KEY POINTS

- TSS is caused by exotoxin-producing strains of *Staphylococcus aureus* and *Streptococcus pyogenes*.
- Although classically described as occurring with tampon use, TSS may follow many staphylococcal or streptococcal soft-tissue infections.
- Onset of symptoms is sudden; symptoms include high fever, hypotension (which can be refractory), diffuse erythematous rash, and multiple organ dysfunction.
- Provide aggressive supportive care, and decontaminate and/or debride the source site.
- Give antibiotics (eg, clindamycin plus vancomycin or daptomycin) pending culture and susceptibility testing.
- Give IV immune globulin if TSS is severe.

192 Gram-Positive Bacilli

ANTHRAX

Anthrax is caused by *Bacillus anthracis*, toxin-producing, encapsulated, facultative anaerobic organisms. Anthrax, an often fatal disease of animals, is transmitted to humans by contact with infected animals or their products. In humans, infection is typically acquired through the skin. Inhalation infection is less common; oropharyngeal, meningeal, and GI infections are rare. For inhalation and GI infections, nonspecific local symptoms are typically followed in several days by severe systemic illness, shock, and often death. Empiric treatment is with ciprofloxacin or doxycycline. A vaccine is available.

(See also the Centers for Disease Control and Prevention's Emergency Preparedness regarding anthrax at www.cdc.gov.)

Etiology

Anthrax is an important domestic animal disease, occurring in goats, cattle, sheep, and horses. Anthrax also occurs in wildlife, such as hippos, elephants, and Cape buffalo. It is rare in humans and occurs mainly in countries that do not prevent industrial or agricultural exposure to infected animals or their products (eg, hides, carcasses, hair). The incidence of natural infection has decreased, particularly in the developed world.

However, the potential use of anthrax as a biological weapon has increased fear of this pathogen. Spores have been prepared in very finely powdered form (weaponized) to be used as agents of warfare and bioterrorism; in anthrax bioattacks of 2001, spores were spread in envelopes delivered via the United States Postal Service.

Pathophysiology

Bacillus anthracis readily form spores when they dry—an environmental condition unfavorable for growth. Spores resist destruction and can remain viable in soil, wool, and animal hair and hides for decades. Spores germinate and begin multiplying rapidly when they enter an environment rich in amino acids and glucose (eg, tissue, blood).

Human infection can be acquired by

- Cutaneous contact (most common)
- Ingestion
- Inhalation

Cutaneous infection is usually acquired by contact with infected animals or spore-contaminated animal products. Open wounds or abrasions increase susceptibility, but infection may occur when skin is intact. Skin infection may be transmitted from person to person by direct contact or fomites.

GI (including oropharyngeal) infection may occur after ingestion of inadequately cooked meat containing the vegetative forms of the organism, usually when a break in the pharyngeal or intestinal mucosa facilitates invasion. Ingested anthrax spores can cause lesions from the oral cavity to the cecum. Released toxin causes hemorrhagic necrotic ulcers and mesenteric lymphadenitis, which may lead to intestinal hemorrhage, obstruction, or perforation.

Pulmonary infection (inhalation anthrax), caused by inhaling spores, is almost always due to occupational exposure to contaminated animal products (eg, hides) and is often fatal.

GI and inhalation anthrax are not transmitted from person to person.

After entering the body, spores germinate inside macrophages, which migrate to regional lymph nodes where the bacteria multiply. In inhalation anthrax, spores are deposited in alveolar spaces, where they are ingested by macrophages, which migrate to mediastinal lymph nodes, usually causing a hemorrhagic mediastinitis.

Bacteremia may occur in any form of anthrax and occurs in nearly all fatal cases; meningeal involvement is common.

Virulence factors: The virulence of *B. anthracis* is due to its

- Antiphagocytic capsule
- Toxins (factors)
- Rapid replication capability

The predominant toxins are edema toxin and lethal toxin. A cell-binding protein, called protective antigen (PA), binds to target cells and facilitates cellular entry of edema toxin and lethal toxin. Edema toxin causes massive local edema. Lethal toxin triggers a massive release of cytokines from macrophages, which is responsible for the sudden death common in anthrax infections.

Symptoms and Signs

Most patients present within 1 to 6 days of exposure, but for inhalation anthrax, the incubation period can be > 6 wk.

Cutaneous anthrax begins as a painless, pruritic, red-brown papule 1 to 10 days after exposure to infective spores. The papule enlarges with a surrounding zone of brawny erythema and marked edema (see Plate 70). Vesiculation and induration are present. Central ulceration follows, with serosanguineous exudation and formation of a black eschar (the malignant pustule). Local lymphadenopathy is common, occasionally with malaise, myalgia, headache, fever, nausea, and vomiting. It may take several weeks for the wound to heal and the edema to resolve.

GI anthrax ranges from asymptomatic to fatal. Fever, nausea, vomiting, abdominal pain, and bloody diarrhea are common. Ascites may be present. Intestinal necrosis and septicemia with potentially lethal toxicity ensue.

Oropharyngeal anthrax manifests as edematous lesions with central necrotic ulcers on the tonsils, posterior pharyngeal wall, or hard palate. Soft-tissue swelling in the neck is marked, and cervical lymph nodes are enlarged. Symptoms include hoarseness, sore throat, fever, and dysphagia. Airway obstruction may occur.

Inhalation anthrax begins insidiously as a flu-like illness. Within a few days, fever worsens, and chest pain and severe respiratory distress develop, followed by cyanosis, shock, and coma. Severe hemorrhagic necrotizing lymphadenitis develops and spreads to adjacent mediastinal structures. Serosanguineous transudation, pulmonary edema, and bloody pleural effusion occur. Typical bronchopneumonia does not occur. Hemorrhagic meningoencephalitis or GI anthrax may develop.

Diagnosis

- Gram stain and culture

Occupational and exposure history is important.

Cultures and Gram stain of samples from clinically identified sites, including cutaneous or mucosal lesions, pleural fluid, CSF, ascites, or stool, should be done. Sputum examination and Gram stain are unlikely to identify inhalation anthrax because airspace disease is frequently absent. A PCR test and immunohistochemical methods can help.

Nasal swab testing for spores in people potentially exposed to inhalation anthrax is not recommended because the predictive value is unknown.

PEARLS & PITFALLS

- Sputum examination and Gram stain are unlikely to identify inhalation anthrax because airspace disease is frequently absent.

Chest x-ray (or CT) should be done if pulmonary symptoms are present. It typically shows widening of the mediastinum (because of enlarged hemorrhagic lymph nodes) and pleural effusion. Pneumonic infiltrates are uncommon.

Lumbar puncture should be done if patients have meningeal signs or a change in mental status.

An enzyme-linked immunosorbent assay (ELISA) is available, but confirmation requires a 4-fold change in antibody titer from acute to convalescent specimens.

Prognosis

Mortality in untreated anthrax varies depending on infection type:

- Inhalation and meningeal anthrax: 100%
- Cutaneous anthrax: 10 to 20%
- GI anthrax: About 50%
- Oropharyngeal anthrax: 12 to 50%

Treatment

- Antibiotics

With early diagnosis, treatment, and intensive support, including mechanical ventilation, fluids, and vasopressors, mortality may be reduced to less than the rate in previously documented cases (45% in the US 2001 anthrax attacks and 90% in cases before these attacks). If treatment is delayed (usually because the diagnosis is missed), death is likely.

Antibiotics: Cutaneous anthrax without significant edema or systemic symptoms is treated with one of the following antibiotics:

- Ciprofloxacin 500 mg (10 to 15 mg/kg for children) po q 12 h
- Levofloxacin 500 mg po q 24 h
- Doxycycline 100 mg (2.5 mg/kg for children) po q 12 h

Amoxicillin 500 mg q 8 h may still be used if the infection is thought to have been naturally acquired.

Cutaneous anthrax without significant edema, systemic symptoms, or risk of inhalation exposure is treated with antibiotics for 7 to 10 days. Treatment is extended to 60 days if concomitant inhalation exposure was possible.

Children and pregnant or breastfeeding women, who typically should not be given ciprofloxacin or doxycycline, should nonetheless be given one of these drugs; however, if prolonged treatment is needed, they may be switched to amoxicillin 500 mg (15 to 30 mg/kg for children) tid after 14 to 21 days if the organism is shown to be susceptible to penicillin. Mortality is rare with treatment, but the lesion will progress through the eschar phase.

Inhalation and other forms of anthrax, including cutaneous anthrax with significant edema or systemic symptoms, require therapy with 2 or 3 antibiotics. Antibiotic therapy should include ≥ 1 antibiotic with bactericidal activity, and ≥ 1 should be a protein synthesis inhibitor, which may block toxin production (eg, ciprofloxacin plus clindamycin).

Antibiotics with bactericidal activity include

- Ciprofloxacin 400 mg (10 to 15 mg/kg for children) IV q 12 h
- Levofloxacin 750 mg IV q 24 h
- Moxifloxacin 400 mg IV q 24 h
- Meropenem 2 g IV q 8 h
- Imipenem 1 g IV q 6 h
- Vancomycin IV dosing to maintain serum trough concentration of 15 to 20 mcg/mL
- Penicillin G 4 million units IV q 4 h (for penicillin-susceptible strains)
- Ampicillin 3 g IV q 4 h (for penicillin-susceptible stains)

Antibiotics that inhibit protein synthesis include

- Linezolid 600 mg IV q 12 h
- Clindamycin 900 mg IV q 8 h
- Doxycycline 200 mg IV initially, then 100 mg q 12 h
- Chloramphenicol 1 g IV q 6 to 8 h

Linezolid should be used with caution in patients with myelosuppression; it cannot be used for long periods because of its neurologic side effects.

Chloramphenicol has good CNS penetration and has been used to successfully treat anthrax.[1]

Rifampin, although not a protein synthesis inhibitor, may be used in this capacity because it has a synergistic effect with the primary antibiotic.

If meningitis is suspected, meropenem should be used with other antibiotics because it has good CNS penetration. If meropenem is not available, imipenem/cilastatin is an equivalent alternative. The initial IV combination therapy should be given for ≥ 2 wk or until patients are clinically stable, whichever is longer. If patients have been exposed to aerosolized spores, treatment should be continued for 60 days to prevent relapse due to any ungerminated spores that may have survived in their lungs after the initial exposure.

Once IV combination therapy is completed, therapy should be switched to a single oral antibiotic.

1. Hendricks KA, Wright ME, Shadomy SV, et al: Centers for Disease Control and Prevention Expert Panel meetings on prevention and treatment of anthrax in adults. *Emerg Infect Dis* 20(2), 2014.

Other drugs: Corticosteroids may be useful for meningitis and severe mediastinal edema but have not been evaluated adequately.

Ca channel blockers and ACE inhibitors may be considered.

Raxibacumab is a monoclonal antibody that can be used to treat effects of toxins already present and can be combined with antibacterial therapy. Raxibacumab has shown efficacy in animal models of inhalation anthrax, particularly when given early.

Drug resistance: Drug resistance is a theoretical concern. Although normally sensitive to penicillin, *B. anthracis* manifests inducible β-lactamases, so single-drug therapy with a penicillin or a cephalosporin is not recommended. Biological warfare researchers may have created strains of anthrax that are resistant to multiple antibiotics, but these strains have not yet been encountered in a clinical situation.

Prevention

An anthrax vaccine, composed of a cell-free culture filtrate, is available for people at high risk (eg, military personnel, veterinarians, laboratory technicians, employees of textile mills processing imported goat hair). A separate veterinary vaccine is also available. Repeated vaccination is required to ensure protection. Local reactions from vaccine can occur.

Limited data suggest that cutaneous anthrax does not result in acquired immunity, particularly if early effective antimicrobial therapy was used. Inhalation anthrax may provide some immunity in patients who survive, but data are very limited.

Postexposure prophylaxis: Postexposure measures include

- Antibiotics
- Vaccination

Asymptomatic people (including pregnant women and children) exposed to inhaled anthrax require prophylaxis with one of the following oral antibiotics, given for 60 days:

- Ciprofloxacin 500 mg (10 to 15 mg/kg for children) q 12 h
- Doxycycline 100 mg (2.5 mg/kg for children) q 12 h
- Levofloxacin 750 mg q 24 h
- Moxifloxacin 400 mg q 24 h

If the organism has been shown to be susceptible to penicillin, amoxicillin 500 mg (25 to 30 mg/kg for children) tid is an option when ciprofloxacin and doxycycline are contraindicated.

Viable spores have been detected in the lungs for ≥ 60 days after aerosol exposure. Because people exposed to aerosolized *B. anthracis* spores are presumed to be at risk of inhalation anthrax due to ungerminated spores remaining in their lungs after the initial exposure, antibiotic therapy is continued for 60 days to clear germinating organisms.

The Centers for Disease Control and Prevention (CDC) recommends that the anthrax vaccine be administered with antibiotic prophylaxis to patients exposed to anthrax spores. Postexposure antibiotic treatment is extended to 100 days in patients who are vaccinated.

KEY POINTS

- Anthrax is typically acquired from infected animals but has been used as a biological weapon.
- Potent toxins, including edema toxin and lethal toxin, are responsible for the most severe manifestations.
- The main clinical forms of anthrax are cutaneous (most common), oropharyngeal, GI, and inhalation (most lethal).
- GI and inhalation anthrax are not transmitted from person to person.
- Treat with ciprofloxacin or doxycycline plus an additional drug for inhalation anthrax.
- Give postexposure prophylaxis with ciprofloxacin, levofloxacin, or doxycycline and anthrax vaccine to people exposed to inhaled anthrax.

DIPHTHERIA

Diphtheria is an acute pharyngeal or cutaneous infection caused mainly by toxigenic strains of *Corynebacterium diphtheriae* and rarely by other, less common *Corynebacterium* sp. Symptoms are either nonspecific skin infections or pseudomembranous pharyngitis followed by myocardial and neural tissue damage secondary to the exotoxin. An asymptomatic carrier state also exists. Diagnosis is clinical and confirmed by culture. Treatment is with antitoxin and penicillin or erythromycin. Childhood vaccination should be routine.

Corynebacterium diphtheriae usually infect the nasopharynx (respiratory diphtheria) or skin.

Diphtheria toxin: Diphtheria strains infected by a β-phage, which carries a toxin-encoding gene, produce a potent toxin. This toxin first causes inflammation and necrosis of local tissues and then can damage the heart, nerves, and sometimes the kidneys.

Nontoxigenic strains of *C. diphtheriae* can also cause nasopharyngeal infection and sometimes systemic disease (eg, endocarditis, septic arthritis).

Epidemiology and transmission: Humans are the only known reservoir for *C. diphtheriae*. The organism is spread by

- Respiratory droplets
- Contact with nasopharyngeal secretions
- Contact with infected skin lesions
- Fomites (rare)

A carrier state is common in endemic regions but not in developed countries. Immunity derived from vaccination or active infection may not prevent patients from becoming carriers; however, most patients who are adequately treated do not become carriers. Patients with clinical illness or asymptomatic carriers may transmit the infection.

Poor personal and community hygiene contributes to the spread of cutaneous diphtheria. In the US, the highest incidence rates in the past were reported in states with substantial populations of Native Americans. However, currently there is no geographic concentration of cases in the US.

Diphtheria is endemic in many countries in Africa, South America, South and Southeast Asia, and the Middle East and in Haiti and the Dominican Republic (travel information about diphtheria is available at the Centers for Disease Control and Prevention [CDC] web site at www.cdc.gov).

Diphtheria is now rare in developed countries because childhood immunization is widespread. However, after the breakup of the former Soviet Union, vaccination rates in its constituent countries fell, followed by a marked rise in diphtheria cases. Susceptibility has also increased because booster immunization rates in adults are declining.

Symptoms and Signs

Symptoms vary depending on

- Where the infection is
- Whether the strain produces toxin

Most respiratory infections are caused by toxigenic strains. Cutaneous infections are caused by toxigenic and nontoxigenic strains. Toxin is poorly absorbed from the skin; thus, toxin complications are rare in cutaneous diphtheria.

Pharyngeal infection: After an incubation period, which averages 5 days, and a prodromal period of between 12 and 24 h, patients develop mild sore throat, dysphagia, low-grade fever, and tachycardia. Nausea, emesis, chills, headache, and fever are more common among children.

If a toxigenic strain is involved, the characteristic membrane appears in the tonsillar area. It may initially appear as a white, glossy exudate but typically becomes dirty gray, tough, fibrinous, and adherent so that removal causes bleeding. Local edema may cause a visibly swollen neck (bull neck), hoarseness, stridor, and dyspnea. The membrane may extend to the larynx, trachea, and bronchi and may partially obstruct the airway or suddenly detach, causing complete obstruction.

If a large amount of toxin is absorbed, severe prostration, pallor, tachycardia, stupor, and coma may occur; toxemia may cause death within 6 to 10 days.

Mild disease with a serosanguineous or purulent discharge and irritation of the external nares and upper lip occurs in patients who have only nasal diphtheria.

Skin infection: Skin lesions usually occur on the extremities and are varied in appearance, often indistinguishable from chronic skin conditions (eg, eczema, psoriasis, impetigo). A few patients have nonhealing, punched-out ulcers, occasionally with a grayish membrane. Pain, tenderness, erythema, and exudate are typical. If exotoxin is produced, lesions may be numb. Concomitant nasopharyngeal infection occurs in 20 to 40% by direct or indirect inoculation with the organism, often from preexisting chronic skin lesions.

Complications: The main complications are cardiac and neurologic.

Myocarditis is usually evident by the 10th to 14th day but can appear any time during the 1st to 6th wk, even while local respiratory symptoms are subsiding; risk of cardiac toxicity is related to degree of local infection. Insignificant ECG changes occur in 20 to 30% of patients, but atrioventricular dissociation, complete heart block, and ventricular arrhythmias may occur and are associated with a high mortality rate. Heart failure may develop.

Nervous system toxicity is uncommon (about 5%) and limited to patients with severe respiratory diphtheria. The toxin causes a demyelinating polyneuropathy that affects cranial and peripheral nerves. The toxic effects usually begin during the 1st wk of illness with loss of ocular accommodation and bulbar palsy, causing dysphagia and nasal regurgitation. Peripheral neuropathy appears during the 3rd to 6th wk. It is both motor and sensory, although motor symptoms predominate. Resolution occurs over many weeks.

Overall mortality is 3%; it is higher in those with delayed presentation or myocarditis, in children < 15 yr, and in adults > 40 yr.

Diagnosis

- Gram stain and culture

Diphtheria needs to be considered in patients with nonspecific findings of pharyngitis, cervical adenopathy, and low-grade fever if they also have systemic toxicity plus hoarseness, palatal paralysis, or stridor. The appearance of the characteristic membrane suggests the diagnosis.

Gram stain of the membrane may reveal gram-positive bacilli with metachromatic (beaded) staining in typical Chinese-character configuration. Material for culture should be obtained from below the membrane, or a portion of membrane itself should be submitted. The laboratory should be notified that *C. diphtheriae* is suspected, so that special culture media (Loeffler or Tindale) can be used. In vitro testing for toxin production (modified Elek test) is done to differentiate toxigenic from nontoxigenic strains. PCR testing for the diphtheria toxin gene can be done.

Cutaneous diphtheria should be considered when a patient develops skin lesions during an outbreak of respiratory diphtheria. Swab or biopsy specimens should be cultured. Patients with cutaneous diphtheria may be coinfected with group A streptococci or *Staphylococcus aureus*.

ECG should be done to look for ST-T wave changes, QTc prolongation, and/or 1st-degree heart block related to myocarditis, which often becomes evident as the respiratory symptoms resolve.

Treatment

- Diphtheria antitoxin
- Penicillin or erythromycin

Symptomatic patients with respiratory diphtheria should be hospitalized in an ICU to monitor for respiratory and cardiac complications. Isolation with respiratory-droplet and contact precautions is required and must continue until 2 cultures, taken 24 and 48 h after antibiotics are stopped, are negative.

Diphtheria antitoxin: Diphtheria antitoxin must be given without waiting for culture confirmation because the antitoxin neutralizes only toxin not yet bound to cells. The use of antitoxin for cutaneous disease, without evidence of respiratory disease, is of questionable value because toxic sequelae have rarely been reported in cutaneous diphtheria; however, some experts recommend it. In the US, antitoxin must be obtained from the CDC through the CDC's Emergency Operations Center at 770-488-7100 (see also the CDC's notice regarding availability of antitoxin).

CAUTION: Diphtheria antitoxin is derived from horses; therefore, a skin (or conjunctival) test to rule out sensitivity should always precede administration (see p. 1373). The dose of antitoxin, ranging from 20,000 to 100,000 units IM or IV, is determined by the following:

- Site and severity of symptoms
- Duration of the disease
- Complications

If an allergic reaction occurs, 0.3 to 1 mL epinephrine 1:1000 (0.01 mL/kg) should immediately be injected sc, IM, or slowly IV. In highly sensitive patients, IV administration of antitoxin is contraindicated.

Antibiotics: Antibiotics are required to eradicate the organism and prevent spread; they are not substitutes for antitoxin.

Adults may be given either of the following:

- Erythromycin 40 mg/kg/day (maximum, 2 g/day) po or by injection q 6 h for 14 days
- Procaine penicillin G IM daily (300,000 units/day for those weighing ≤ 10 kg and 600,000 units/day for those weighing > 10 kg) for 14 days

When patients are able to tolerate oral drugs, they should be switched to penicillin 250 mg po qid or erythromycin 500 mg po q 6 h for a total of 14 days treatment.

Children should be given procaine penicillin G 12,500 to 25,000 units/kg IM q 12 h or erythromycin 10 to 15 mg/kg (maximum, 2 g/day) IV q 6 h, with a similar switch to oral drugs when tolerated.

Vancomycin or linezolid can be used if antibiotic resistance is detected. Organism elimination should be documented by 2 consecutive negative throat and/or nasopharyngeal cultures done 1 to 2 days and 2 wk after completion of antibiotic treatment.

Other treatments: For **cutaneous diphtheria,** thorough cleansing of the lesion with soap and water and administration of systemic antibiotics for 10 days are recommended.

Vaccination is required after recovery for patients who had diphtheria because infection does not guarantee immunity.

Recovery from severe diphtheria is slow, and patients must be advised against resuming activities too soon. Even normal physical exertion may harm patients recovering from myocarditis.

Prevention

Prevention consists of

- Infection control measures (respiratory droplet isolation until 2 cultures at least 24 h apart are negative)
- Vaccination (primary and postexposure)
- Antibiotics

Vaccination: The vaccine for diphtheria contains diphtheria toxoid; it is available only in combination with other vaccines.

Everyone should be vaccinated at prescribed intervals using the following:

- Children: Diphtheria-tetanus–acellular pertussis (DTaP) vaccine
- Adolescents and adults: Tetanus-diphtheria (Td) or tetanus toxoid, reduced diphtheria toxoid, and acellular pertussis (Tdap)

(See also the CDC's National Immunization Program Childhood and Adolescent Immunization Schedule and their Adult Immunization Recommendations at www.cdc.gov.)

After exposure, diphtheria immunization should be updated in all contacts (including hospital personnel) who have not completed a primary series or who have gone > 5 yr since their last booster dose. The vaccine should also be given if immunization status is unknown. An age-appropriate diphtheria toxoid-containing vaccine is used.

Postexposure antibiotics: All close contacts should be examined; surveillance for evidence of disease is maintained for 7 days. Nasopharyngeal and throat cultures for *C. diphtheriae* should be done regardless of immunization status.

Asymptomatic contacts should be treated with erythromycin 500 mg (10 to 15 mg/kg for children) po q 6 h for 7 days or, if adherence is uncertain, a single dose of penicillin G benzathine (600,000 units IM for patients < 30 kg and 1.2 million units IM for those > 30 kg).

If cultures are positive, an additional 10-day course of erythromycin should be given; carriers should not be given antitoxin. After 3 days of treatment, carriers can safely resume work while continuing to take antibiotics. Cultures should be repeated; 24 h after the completion of antimicrobial therapy, 2 consecutive culture sets of the nose and throat should be collected 24 h apart. If results are positive, another course of antibiotics is given and cultures are done again.

KEY POINTS

- Usually, diphtheria is a cutaneous or nasopharyngeal infection, but a potent toxin produced by phage-infected organisms can damage the heart, nerves, and sometimes the kidneys.
- Diphtheria is rare in developed countries because of widespread vaccination but is endemic in many developing countries; rates are increasing slightly in developed countries because rates of vaccination and revaccination are declining.
- Pharyngeal infection causes a characteristic membrane in the tonsillar area; it may initially appear as a white, glossy exudate but typically becomes dirty gray, tough, fibrinous, and adherent.
- Treat with diphtheria antitoxin and penicillin or erythromycin; document cure by culture.

- Vaccinate patients after recovery, and vaccinate close contacts who have not completed a primary series or who have gone > 5 yr since their last booster.
- Do nasopharyngeal and throat cultures of close contacts regardless of their immunization status.
- Give antibiotics to close contacts; duration of treatment depends on culture results.

ERYSIPELOTHRICOSIS

Erysipelothricosis is infection caused by *Erysipelothrix rhusiopathiae*. The most common symptom is erysipeloid, an acute but slowly evolving localized cellulitis. Diagnosis is by culture of a biopsy specimen or occasionally PCR testing. Treatment is with antibiotics.

Erysipelothrix rhusiopathiae (formerly *E. insidiosa*) are thin, gram-positive capsulated, nonsporulating, nonmotile, microaerophilic bacilli with worldwide distribution; they are primarily saprophytes.

E. rhusiopathiae may infect a variety of animals, including insects, shellfish, fish, birds, and mammals (especially swine). In humans, infection is chiefly occupational and typically follows a penetrating wound in people who handle edible or nonedible animal matter (eg, infected carcasses, rendered products [grease, fertilizer], bones, shells). Most commonly, patients handle fish or work in slaughterhouses. Infection can also result from cat or dog bites. Nondermal infection is rare, usually occurring as arthritis or endocarditis.

Symptoms and Signs

Within 1 wk of injury, a characteristic raised, purplish red, nonvesiculated, indurated, maculopapular rash appears, accompanied by itching and burning. Local swelling, although sharply demarcated, may inhibit use of the hand, the usual site of infection. The lesion's border may slowly extend outward, causing discomfort and disability that may persist for 3 wk. The disease is usually self-limited.

Regional lymphadenopathy occurs in about one-third of cases. Erysipelothricosis rarely becomes generalized cutaneous disease, which is characterized by purple skin lesions that expand as the lesion's center clears, plus bullous lesions at the primary or distant sites.

Bacteremia is rare and is more often a primary infection than dissemination from cutaneous lesions. It may result in septic arthritis or infective endocarditis, even in people without known valvular heart disease. Endocarditis tends to involve the aortic valve, and the mortality rate and percentage of patients needing cardiac valve replacement are unusually high. Rarely, CNS, intra-abdominal, and bone infections occur.

Diagnosis

- Culture

Culture of a full-thickness biopsy specimen is superior to needle aspiration of the advancing edge of a lesion because organisms are located only in deeper parts of the skin. Culture of exudate obtained by abrading a florid papule may be diagnostic. Isolation from synovial fluid or blood is necessary for diagnosis of erysipelothrical arthritis or endocarditis. *E. rhusiopathiae* may be misidentified as lactobacilli.

PCR amplification may aid rapid diagnosis. Rapid diagnosis is particularly important if endocarditis suspected because treatment of endocarditis due to *E. rhusiopathiae* is often different from the usual empiric treatment of treatment of gram-positive bacillary endocarditis (eg, *E. rhusiopathiae* is resistant to vancomycin, which is typically used).

Treatment

- Penicillin, cephalosporins, fluoroquinolones, or clindamycin

For **localized cutaneous disease**, usual treatment is one of the following, given for 7 days:

- Penicillin V or ampicillin (500 mg po q 6 h)
- Ciprofloxacin (250 mg po q 12 h)
- Clindamycin (300 mg po q 8 h)

Cephalosporins are also effective. Daptomycin and linezolid are active in vitro and may be considered if patients are very allergic to β-lactams. Tetracyclines and macrolides may no longer be dependable.

E. rhusiopathiae are resistant to sulfonamides, aminoglycosides, and vancomycin.

Severe diffuse cutaneous or systemic infection is best treated with one of the following:

- IV penicillin G (2 to 3 million units q 4 h)
- Ceftriaxone (2 g IV once/day)
- A fluoroquinolone (eg, ciprofloxacin 400 mg IV q 12 h, levofloxacin 500 mg IV once/day)

Endocarditis is treated with penicillin G for 4 to 6 wk. Cephalosporins and fluoroquinolones are alternatives. Vancomycin is often used empirically for the treatment of gram-positive bacillary endocarditis; however, *E. rhusiopathiae* is resistant to vancomycin. Thus, rapid differentiation of *E. rhusiopathiae* from other gram-positive organisms is critical.

The same drugs and doses are appropriate for arthritis (given for at least 1 wk after defervescence or cessation of effusion), but repeated needle aspiration drainage of the infected joint is also necessary.

KEY POINTS

- Infection typically results from a penetrating wound in people who handle edible or nonedible animal matter (eg, in a slaughterhouse) or who work with fish or shellfish.
- Within 1 wk after the injury, a raised, purplish red, nonvesiculated, indurated, maculopapular rash appears, accompanied by itching and burning; about one third of patients have regional lymphadenopathy.
- Bacteremia is rare but may result in septic arthritis or infective endocarditis.
- Diagnose by culturing a full-thickness biopsy specimen or an exudate obtained by abrading a florid papule.
- If endocarditis due to *E. rhusiopathiae* is suspected, rapid identification of the pathogen is critical because treatment is often different; *E. rhusiopathiae* is resistant to vancomycin, which is typically used to treat gram-positive bacillary endocarditis.
- Treat with antibiotics (eg, penicillin, ciprofloxacin) based on extent and location of infection.

LISTERIOSIS

Listeriosis is bacteremia, meningitis, cerebritis, dermatitis, an oculoglandular syndrome, intrauterine and neonatal infections, or rarely endocarditis caused by *Listeria* sp. Symptoms vary with the organ system affected.

Intrauterine infection may cause fetal death. Diagnosis is by laboratory isolation. Treatment includes penicillin, ampicillin (often with aminoglycosides), and trimethoprim/sulfamethoxazole.

Listeria are small, non–acid-fast, noncapsulated, nonsporulating, β-hemolytic, aerobic, and facultative anaerobic gram-positive bacilli that have characteristic tumbling motility. They are present worldwide in the environment and in the gut of humans, nonhuman mammals, birds, arachnids, and crustaceans. There are several species of *Listeria*, but *L. monocytogenes* is the only pathogen in humans.

In the US, the average annual incidence of listeriosis in 2013 was 2.6/million, peaking in the summer; attack rates are highest in neonates and in adults ≥ 60 yr.

Transmission: Because *L. monocytogenes* is ubiquitous in the environment, opportunities for contamination are numerous during the food production process. Nearly all types of food can harbor and transmit *L. monocytogenes*, but infection usually occurs via ingestion of contaminated dairy products, raw vegetables, or meats and is favored by the ability of *L. monocytogenes* to survive and grow at refrigerator temperatures.

Infection may also occur by direct contact and during slaughter of infected animals.

PEARLS & PITFALLS

- *Listeria monocytogenes* can reproduce at refrigerator temperatures, so lightly contaminated refrigerated food can become heavily contaminated.

Risk factors: Because *L. monocytogenes* multiplies intracellularly, control of listeriosis requires cell-mediated immunity; thus, the following people are at high risk:

- Immunocompromised patients
- Neonates
- Elderly

Pregnant women are also at increased risk of developing listerial infection, which can spread antepartum and intrapartum from mother to child and can cause abortion or early infant death.

Listeria are a common cause of neonatal bacterial meningitis.

Symptoms and Signs

Primary listerial bacteremia is rare and causes high fever without localizing symptoms and signs. Endocarditis, peritonitis, osteomyelitis, septic arthritis, cholecystitis, and pleuropneumonia may occur. Febrile gastroenteritis may occur after ingestion of contaminated food. Listerial bacteremia during pregnancy can cause intrauterine infection, chorioamnionitis, premature labor, fetal death, or neonatal infections.

Meningitis is due to *Listeria* in about 20% of cases in neonates and in patients > 60 yr. Twenty percent of cases progress to cerebritis, either diffuse encephalitis or, rarely, rhombencephalitis and abscesses; rhombencephalitis manifests as altered consciousness, cranial nerve palsies, cerebellar signs, and motor or sensory loss.

Oculoglandular listeriosis can cause ophthalmitis and regional lymph node enlargement (Parinaud syndrome). It may follow conjunctival inoculation and, if untreated, may progress to bacteremia and meningitis.

Diagnosis

- Culture

Listerial infections are diagnosed by culture of blood or CSF. The laboratory must be informed when *L. monocytogenes* is suspected because the organism is easily confused with diphtheroids.

In all listerial infections, IgG agglutinin titers peak 2 to 4 wk after onset.

Treatment

- Ampicillin or penicillin G, usually with an aminoglycoside

Listerial meningitis is best treated with ampicillin 2 g IV q 4 h. Most authorities recommend adding gentamicin (1 mg/kg IV q 8 h) based on synergy in vitro. Cephalosporins are not effective. For treatment of neonatal meningitis, see p. 2635.

Endocarditis and primary listerial bacteremia are treated with ampicillin 2 g IV q 4 h plus gentamicin (for synergy) given for 6 wk (for endocarditis) or 2 wk (for bacteremia) beyond defervescence. Oculoglandular listeriosis and listerial dermatitis should respond to erythromycin 10 mg/kg po q 6 h, continued until 1 wk after defervescence. Cephalosporins have no in vitro activity and should not be used; failures with vancomycin have been reported. Trimethoprim/sulfamethoxazole 5/25 mg/kg IV q 8 h is an alternative. Linezolid is active in vitro, but clinical experience is lacking.

Prevention

Because food contamination is common and because *L. monocytogenes* can reproduce at refrigerator temperatures, lightly contaminated food can become heavily contaminated during refrigeration. This problem is of particular concern when foods (eg, refrigerated ready-to-eat foods) are eaten without further cooking. Thus, appropriate food hygiene is important, particularly for at-risk people (eg, immunocompromised patients, pregnant women, the elderly). Those at risk should avoid eating the following:

- Soft cheeses (eg, feta, Brie, Camembert)
- Refrigerated ready-to-eat foods (eg, hot dogs, deli meats, pâtés, meat spreads), unless they are heated to an internal temperature of 73.9° C (165° F) or until steaming hot just before serving
- Refrigerated smoked seafood (eg, nova-style, lox, kippered, smoked, jerky), unless it has been cooked
- Raw (unpasteurized) milk

KEY POINTS

- *L. monocytogenes* is very common in the environment but causes infection in only about 2.6 people/million annually, typically via contaminated food products.
- Attack rates are highest in neonates, adults ≥ 60 yr, and immunocompromised patients.
- Various organ systems can be affected; maternal infection during pregnancy may cause fetal death.
- Give ampicillin, usually plus gentamicin.
- Advise patients to prevent disease by promptly eating foods at risk of contamination and/or cooking them appropriately (or, for high-risk patients, to avoid such food).

NOCARDIOSIS

Nocardiosis is an acute or chronic, often disseminated, suppurative or granulomatous infection caused by various aerobic soil saprophytes of the genus *Nocardia*. Pneumonia is

typical, but skin and CNS infections are common. Diagnosis is by culture and special stains. Treatment is usually with sulfonamides.

Nocardia are obligate aerobic, partially acid-fast, beaded, branching, gram-positive bacilli. Several *Nocardia* sp, in the family Actinomycetaceae, cause human disease.

N. asteroides is the most common human pathogen; it usually causes pulmonary and disseminated infection.

N. brasiliensis most commonly causes skin infection, particularly in tropical climates. Infection is via inhalation or by direct inoculation of the skin.

Other *Nocardia* sp sometimes cause localized or, occasionally, systemic infections.

Nocardiosis occurs worldwide in all age groups, but incidence is higher in older adults, especially men, and immunocompromised patients. Person-to-person spread is rare.

Risk factors: Predisposing factors include

- Lymphoreticular cancers
- Organ transplantation
- High-dose corticosteroid or other immunosuppressive therapy
- Underlying pulmonary disease

However, about one half of patients have no preexisting disease or condition.

Nocardiosis is also an opportunistic infection in patients with advanced HIV infection.

Symptoms and Signs

Nocardiosis usually begins as a subacute pulmonary infection that resembles actinomycosis, but *Nocardia* are more likely to disseminate locally or hematogenously. Dissemination with abscess formation may involve any organ but most commonly affects the brain, skin, kidneys, bone, or muscle.

The most common symptoms of pulmonary involvement—cough, fever, chills, chest pain, weakness, anorexia, and weight loss—are nonspecific and may resemble those of TB or suppurative pneumonia. Pleural effusion may also occur. Metastatic brain abscesses, occurring in 30 to 50% of cases, usually cause severe headaches and focal neurologic abnormalities. Infection may be acute, subacute, or chronic.

Skin or subcutaneous abscesses occur frequently, sometimes as a primary local inoculation. They may appear as

- Firm cellulitis
- Lymphocutaneous syndrome
- An actinomycetoma

The lymphocutaneous syndrome consists of a primary pyoderma lesion and lymphatic nodules resembling sporotrichosis.

An actinomycetoma begins as a nodule, suppurates, spreads along fascial planes, and drains through chronic fistulas.

Diagnosis

- Microscopic examination or culture

Diagnosis is by identification of *Nocardia* sp in tissue or in culture of samples from localized lesions identified by physical examination, x-ray, or other imaging studies. Clumps of beaded, branching filaments of gram-positive bacteria (which may be weakly acid-fast) are often seen.

Prognosis

Without treatment, pulmonary nocardiosis and disseminated nocardiosis are usually fatal. Among patients who are treated with appropriate antibiotics, the mortality rate is highest (> 50%) in immunocompromised patients with disseminated infections and is about 10% in immunocompetent patients with lesions restricted to the lungs.

Cure rates for patients with skin infection are usually > 95%.

Treatment

- Trimethoprim/sulfamethoxazole (TMP/SMX)

TMP/SMX 15 mg/kg/day (of the TMP component) po q 6 to 12 h or high doses of a sulfonamide alone (eg, sulfadiazine 1 g po q 4 to 6 h) are used. Because most cases respond slowly, a dose that maintains a sulfonamide blood concentration of 12 to 15 mg/dL 2 h after the last dose must be continued for ≥ 6 mo. In immunocompromised patients and patients with disseminated disease, TMP/SMX should be used with amikacin, imipenem, or meropenem pending species identification and susceptibility testing results.

When sulfonamide hypersensitivity or refractory infection is present, amikacin, a tetracycline (particularly minocycline), imipenem/cilastatin, meropenem, ceftriaxone, cefotaxime, extended-spectrum fluoroquinolones (eg, moxifloxacin), dapsone, or cycloserine can be used. Linezolid and tigecycline may be effective alternatives. In vitro susceptibility data should guide the choice of alternative drugs.

KEY POINTS

- Immunosuppression and chronic pulmonary disease are predisposing factors, but about half of patients have no preexisting disease.
- Pneumonia is typical, but skin and CNS infections are common; hematogenous spread can involve almost any organ.
- Treat with trimethoprim/sulfamethoxazole (or one of the numerous alternatives) for several months.

193 Herpesviruses

Eight types of herpesviruses infect humans (see Table 193–1). After initial infection, all herpesviruses remain latent within specific host cells and may subsequently reactivate. Herpesviruses do not survive long outside a host; thus, transmission usually requires intimate contact. In people with latent infection, the virus can reactivate without causing symptoms; in such cases, asymptomatic shedding occurs and people can transmit infection.

Epstein-Barr virus (EBV) and human herpesvirus type 8 (HHV-8), also known as Kaposi sarcoma–associated herpesvirus (KSHV), can cause certain cancers. Roseola infantum is a childhood disease caused by herpesvirus 6 (and sometimes 7).

Drug Treatment of Herpesviruses

Drugs that have activity against herpesviruses include acyclovir, cidofovir, famciclovir, fomivirsen, foscarnet, ganciclovir, idoxuridine, penciclovir, trifluridine, valacyclovir, valganciclovir, and vidarabine (see Table 193–2).

Table 193–1. HERPESVIRUSES THAT INFECT HUMANS

COMMON NAME	OTHER NAME	TYPICAL MANIFESTATIONS
Herpes simplex virus type 1	Human herpesvirus 1	Gingivostomatitis, keratoconjunctivitis, cutaneous herpes, genital herpes, encephalitis, herpes labialis, viral meningitis, esophagitis*, pneumonia*, hepatitis*,†
Herpes simplex virus type 2	Human herpesvirus 2	Genital herpes, cutaneous herpes, gingivostomatitis, neonatal herpes, viral meningitis, disseminated infection*, hepatitis*,†
Varicella-zoster virus	Human herpesvirus 3	Chickenpox, herpes zoster, disseminated herpes zoster*
Epstein-Barr virus	Human herpesvirus 4	Infectious mononucleosis, hepatitis, encephalitis, nasopharyngeal carcinoma, Hodgkin lymphoma, Burkitt lymphoma, lymphoproliferative syndromes*, oral hairy leukoplakia*
Cytomegalovirus	Human herpesvirus 5	CMV mononucleosis, hepatitis, congenital cytomegalic inclusion disease, hepatitis*, retinitis*, pneumonia*, colitis*
Human herpesvirus 6	—	Roseola infantum, otitis media with fever; encephalitis
Human herpesvirus 7	—	Roseola infantum
Kaposi sarcoma–associated herpesvirus	Human herpesvirus 8	Not a known cause of acute illness but has a causative role in Kaposi sarcoma* and AIDS-related non-Hodgkin lymphomas that grow primarily in the pleural, pericardial, or abdominal cavities as lymphomatous effusions Also linked with multicentric Castleman disease

*In immunocompromised hosts.

†Uncommonly causes fulminant hepatitis without cutaneous lesions in immunocompetent hosts.

CHICKENPOX

(Varicella)

Chickenpox is an acute, systemic, usually childhood infection caused by the varicella-zoster virus (human herpesvirus type 3). It usually begins with mild constitutional symptoms that are followed shortly by skin lesions appearing in crops and characterized by macules, papules, vesicles, and crusting. Patients at risk of severe neurologic or other systemic complications (eg, pneumonia) include adults, neonates, and patients who are immunocompromised or have certain underlying medical conditions. Diagnosis is clinical. Those at risk of severe complications receive postexposure prophylaxis with immune globulin and, if disease develops, are treated with antiviral drugs (eg, valacyclovir, famciclovir, acyclovir). Vaccination provides effective prevention in immunocompetent patients.

Chickenpox is caused by the varicella-zoster virus (human herpesvirus type 3); chickenpox is the acute invasive phase of the infection, and herpes zoster (shingles) represents reactivation of the latent phase.

Chickenpox, which is extremely contagious, is spread by

- Mucosal (usually nasopharyngeal) inoculation via infected airborne droplets or aerosolized particles
- Direct contact with the virus (eg, via skin lesions)

Chickenpox is most communicable during the prodrome and early stages of the eruption. It is communicable from 48 h before the first skin lesions appear until the final lesions have crusted. Indirect transmission (by carriers who are immune) does not occur.

Table 193–2. DRUGS USED TO TREAT HERPESVIRUS INFECTIONS

DRUG	ACTIVITY	USES	ADVERSE EFFECTS
Acyclovir	Active against (in order of potency) HSV type 1 (HSV-1), HSV-2, VZV, and EBV Minimal activity against CMV	**Oral or IV** (IV indicated when a higher serum drug level is required, as for herpes simplex encephalitis)	**Oral:** Infrequent **IV:** Rarely, renal toxicity due to precipitation of acyclovir crystals; in immunocompromised patients, TTP/HUS
Cidofovir	In vitro inhibition of a broad spectrum of viruses, including HSV-1, HSV-2, VZV, CMV, EBV, KSHV, adenovirus, HPV, and human polyomavirus (JC and BK viruses)	**IV:** Generally used for CMV, but use limited by renal toxicity	Significant renal toxicity

Table continues on the following page.

Table 193–2. DRUGS USED TO TREAT HERPESVIRUS INFECTIONS (*Continued*)

DRUG	ACTIVITY	USES	ADVERSE EFFECTS
Famciclovir (prodrug of penciclovir)	Antiviral spectrum similar to acyclovir (strains resistant to acyclovir also resistant to famciclovir)	**Oral:** As effective as acyclovir for genital herpes and herpes zoster and more bioavailable than acyclovir after oral administration (which is theoretically important for VZV infection)	Infrequent
Fomivirsen	Potent activity against CMV (antisense oligonucleotide inhibits CMV protein synthesis)	**Intravitreal injection:** For patients with HIV infection and CMV retinitis that is resistant to other therapies	Increased intraocular pressure, corticosteroid-responsive uveitis
Foscarnet	Active against EBV, KSHV, human herpesvirus 6, acyclovir-resistant (and acyclovir-susceptible) HSV and VZV, and ganciclovir-resistant (and ganciclovir-susceptible) CMV Some anti-HIV activity	**IV:** Efficacy similar to that of ganciclovir for treating and delaying progression of CMV retinitis	Renal toxicity in up to one-third of patients if foscarnet is given without adequate hydration, electrolyte imbalances
Ganciclovir	In vitro activity against all herpesviruses, including CMV, but HSV strains that are resistant to acyclovir also cross-resistant to ganciclovir Typically drug of choice for CMV Used in patients with both HIV and CMV retinitis	**IV form:** Most common **Oral:** Only 6 to 9% bioavailable; requires 12 capsules/day for a standard dose (1 g tid), limiting its usefulness	Primarily, bone marrow suppression, particularly neutropenia, which sometimes requires treatment*
Idoxuridine	Active against HSV-1, HSV-2, VZV, vaccinia, and CMV	**Topical:** Because of its high systemic toxicity, limited to topical ophthalmic treatment of herpes simplex keratoconjunctivitis	Irritation, pain, photophobia, pruritus, inflammation or edema of the eyelids Rarely, allergic reactions
Penciclovir	Active against HSV-1, HSV-2, VZV, CMV, and EBV	**Topical (cream):** Used to treat recurrent herpes labialis in adults	Erythema
Trifluridine (trifluorothymidine)	Active against HSV-1 and HSV-2	**Topical:** Ophthalmic treatment of primary keratoconjunctivitis and recurrent keratitis or ulceration caused by HSV-1 and HSV-2 (Systemic use precluded by bone marrow suppression)	Ocular stinging, palpebral edema Less commonly, punctate keratitis, allergic reactions
Valacyclovir (prodrug of acyclovir)	Antiviral spectrum similar to that of acyclovir	**Oral:** 3–5 times more bioavailable than acyclovir	Similar to those of acyclovir TTP/HUS in some patients with advanced HIV and in transplant recipients who received valacyclovir in higher doses than currently recommended†
Valganciclovir (prodrug of ganciclovir)	Similar to ganciclovir	**Oral:** Taken as two 450-mg tablets once/day or q 12 h (more bioavailable than oral ganciclovir)	Similar to ganciclovir
Vidarabine (adenine arabinoside, ara-A)	For HSV infections	**IV form** not used anymore because of neurotoxicity **Ophthalmic preparations:** Effective for acute keratoconjunctivitis and recurrent superficial keratitis caused by HSV-1 and HSV-2	Superficial punctate keratitis with tearing, irritation, pain, and photophobia

*Severe neutropenia (< 500 neutrophils/μL) may require one of the following:

- Bone marrow stimulation with granulocyte colony-stimulating factor or granulocyte-macrophage colony-stimulating factor
- Discontinuation of ganciclovir
- Reduction of the dose

†Valacyclovir should be used with caution in patients with advanced HIV and in transplant recipients.

CMV = cytomegalovirus; EBV = Epstein-Barr virus; HPV = human papillomavirus; HSV = herpes simplex virus; KSHV = Kaposi sarcoma–associated herpesvirus; TTP/HUS = thrombotic thrombocytopenic purpura and hemolytic-uremic syndrome; VZV = varicella-zoster virus.

Epidemics occur in winter and early spring in 3- to 4-yr cycles. Some infants may have partial immunity, probably acquired transplacentally, until age 6 mo.

Symptoms and Signs

In immunocompetent children, chickenpox is rarely severe. In adults and immunocompromised children, infection can be serious.

Mild headache, moderate fever, and malaise may occur 10 to 21 days after exposure, about 24 to 36 h before lesions appear. This prodrome is more likely in patients > 10 yr and is usually more severe in adults.

Initial rash: The initial rash, a macular eruption, may be accompanied by an evanescent flush. Within a few hours, lesions progress to papules and then characteristic, sometimes pathognomonic teardrop vesicles, often intensely itchy, on red bases. The lesions become pustular and then crust.

Lesions initially develop on the face and trunk and erupt in successive crops; some macules appear just as earlier crops begin to crust. The eruption may be generalized (in severe cases) or more limited but almost always involves the upper trunk.

Ulcerated lesions may develop on the mucous membranes, including the oropharynx and upper respiratory tract, palpebral conjunctiva, and rectal and vaginal mucosa.

In the mouth, vesicles rupture immediately, are indistinguishable from those of herpetic gingivostomatitis, and often cause pain during swallowing.

Scalp lesions may result in tender, enlarged suboccipital and posterior cervical lymph nodes.

New lesions usually cease to appear by the 5th day, and the majority are crusted by the 6th day; most crusts disappear < 20 days after onset.

Breakthrough varicella: Sometimes vaccinated children develop varicella (called breakthrough varicella); in these cases, the rash is typically milder, fever is less common, and the illness is shorter; the lesions are infectious.

Complications: Secondary bacterial infection (typically streptococcal or staphylococcal) of the vesicles may occur, causing cellulitis or rarely necrotizing fasciitis or streptococcal toxic shock.

Pneumonia may complicate severe chickenpox in adults, neonates, and immunocompromised patients of all ages but usually not in immunocompetent young children.

Myocarditis, hepatitis, and hemorrhagic complications may also occur.

Acute postinfectious cerebellar ataxia is one of the most common neurologic complications; it occurs in 1/4000 cases in children.

Transverse myelitis may also occur.

Reye syndrome, a rare but severe childhood complication, may begin 3 to 8 days after onset of the rash; aspirin increases the risk.

In adults, encephalitis, which can be life threatening, occurs in 1 to 2/1000 cases of chickenpox.

Diagnosis

- Clinical evaluation

Chickenpox is suspected in patients with the characteristic rash, which is usually the basis for diagnosis. The rash may be confused with that of other viral skin infections.

If the diagnosis is in doubt, laboratory confirmation can be done; it requires one of the following:

- PCR for viral DNA
- Immunofluorescent detection of viral antigen in lesions or culture
- Serologic tests

In serologic tests, detection of IgM antibodies to varicella-zoster virus (VZV) or seroconversion from negative to positive for antibodies to VZV indicate acute infection.

Samples are generally obtained with scraping and transported to the laboratory in viral media.

Prognosis

Chickenpox in children is rarely severe. Severe or fatal disease is more likely in the following:

- Adults
- Patients with depressed T-cell immunity (eg, lymphoreticular cancer)
- Those receiving corticosteroids or chemotherapy

Treatment

- Symptomatic treatment
- Valacyclovir or famciclovir for patients ≥ 12 yr
- IV acyclovir for immunocompromised patients and others at risk of severe disease

Mild cases in children require only symptomatic treatment. Relief of itching and prevention of scratching, which predisposes to secondary bacterial infection, may be difficult. Wet compresses or, for severe itching, systemic antihistamines and colloidal oatmeal baths may help. Simultaneous use of large doses of systemic and topical antihistamines can cause encephalopathy and should be avoided.

To prevent secondary bacterial infection, patients should bathe regularly and keep their underclothing and hands clean and their nails clipped. Antiseptics should not be applied unless lesions become infected; bacterial superinfection is treated with antibiotics.

Oral antivirals, when given to immunocompetent patients within 24 h of the rash's onset, slightly decrease symptom duration and severity. However, because the disease is generally benign in children, antiviral treatment is not routinely recommended.

Oral valacyclovir, famciclovir, or acyclovir should be given to healthy people at risk of moderate to severe disease, including all patients ≥ 12 yr and those with skin disorders (particularly eczema) or chronic lung disease. The dose is famciclovir 500 mg tid or valacyclovir 1 g tid. Acyclovir is a less desirable choice because it has poorer oral bioavailability, but it can be given at 20 mg/kg qid with a maximum daily dose of 3200 mg.

Immunocompromised children > 1 yr should be given acyclovir 500 mg/m^2 q 8 h IV. Immunocompromised adults should be treated with acyclovir 10 to 12 mg/kg IV q 8 h.

Patients should not return to school or work until the final lesions have crusted.

Prevention

Infection provides lifelong protection.

Potentially susceptible people should take strict precautions to avoid people capable of transmitting the infection.

Vaccination: Three live-attenuated varicella vaccines are available in the US:

- Varicella vaccine
- Combination measles-mumps-rubella-varicella (MMRV) vaccine
- Herpes zoster vaccine

All healthy children and susceptible adults should receive 2 doses of live-attenuated varicella vaccine (see Tables 291–2 on p. 2462 and 291–3 on p. 2467). Vaccination is particularly important for women of child-bearing age and adults with underlying chronic medical conditions. Serologic testing to determine immune status before vaccination in adults is usually not required. Although the vaccine may cause chickenpox in immunocompetent patients, disease is usually mild (< 10 papules or vesicles) and brief and causes few systemic symptoms.

People ≥ 13 yr should not be given the MMRV vaccine.

The herpes zoster vaccine is recommended for people ≥ 60 yr. It is not routinely recommended for people aged 50 to 59 yr but can be given to them.

Vaccination of health care workers who do not have evidence of varicella immunity is recommended. Susceptible health care workers who have been exposed to varicella should be vaccinated as soon as possible and kept off duty for 21 days.

Vaccination is contraindicated in

- Patients with moderate to severe acute concurrent illness (vaccination is postponed until illness resolves)
- Immunocompromised patients
- Pregnant women and those who intend to become pregnant within 1 mo of vaccination (based on Advisory Committee on Immunization Practices recommendations) or within 3 mo of vaccination (based on vaccine labeling)
- Patients taking high doses of systemic corticosteroids
- Children using salicylates

Postexposure prophylaxis: After exposure, chickenpox can be prevented or attenuated by IM administration of varicella-zoster immune globulin. Candidates for postexposure prophylaxis include

- People with leukemia, immunodeficiencies, or other severe debilitating illness
- Susceptible pregnant women
- Neonates whose mother developed chickenpox within 5 days before or 2 days after delivery
- Neonates born at < 28 wk and exposed to a nonmaternal source even if their mother has evidence of immunity (neonates born at ≥ 28 wk and exposed to a nonmaternal source do not need immune globulin if their mother has evidence of immunity)

The immune globulin should be given as soon as possible (and within 10 days of exposure) and may modify or prevent varicella.

Vaccination should be given as soon as possible to susceptible healthy patients eligible for vaccination (eg, age ≥ 1 yr). Vaccination can be effective in preventing or ameliorating disease within 3 days and possibly up to 5 days after exposure.

To prevent nosocomial transmission, the Centers for Disease Control and Prevention (CDC) recommends postexposure prophylaxis with vaccination or varicella-zoster immunoglobulin, depending on immune status, for exposed health care workers and patients without evidence of immunity.

KEY POINTS

- Chickenpox causes pustular, crusting lesions on the skin (often including scalp) and may cause ulcerated lesions on mucous membranes.
- Complications include secondary bacterial infection of skin lesions, pneumonia, and cerebellar ataxia.
- Give oral valacyclovir or famciclovir to patients ≥ 12 yr and to those with skin disorders (particularly eczema) or chronic lung disease.
- Give IV acyclovir to immunocompromised patients and to other patients at risk of severe disease.
- Vaccinate all healthy children and susceptible adults.
- Give postexposure prophylaxis with varicella-zoster immune globulin to immunocompromised patients, susceptible pregnant women, and neonates whose mother developed chickenpox within 5 days before or 2 days after delivery.
- Give postexposure prophylaxis with varicella vaccine to immunocompetent patients ≥ 1 yr who are eligible for vaccination.

CYTOMEGALOVIRUS INFECTION

(Cytomegalic Inclusion Disease)

Cytomegalovirus (CMV) can cause infections that have a wide range of severity. A syndrome that is similar to infectious mononucleosis but lacks severe pharyngitis is common. Severe focal disease, including retinitis, can develop in HIV-infected patients and, rarely, in organ transplant recipients and other immunocompromised patients. Severe systemic disease can develop in neonates and immunocompromised patients. Laboratory diagnosis, helpful for severe disease, may involve culture, serologic testing, biopsy, or antigen or nucleic acid detection. Ganciclovir and other antiviral drugs are used to treat severe disease, particularly retinitis.

CMV (human herpesvirus type 5) is transmitted through blood, body fluids, or transplanted organs. Infection may be acquired transplacentally or during birth.

Prevalence increases with age; 60 to 90% of adults have CMV infection (resulting in lifelong latent infection). Lower socioeconomic groups tend to have a higher prevalence.

Congenital CMV infection may be asymptomatic or may cause abortion, stillbirth, or postnatal death. Complications include extensive hepatic and CNS damage.

Acquired infections are often asymptomatic.

An acute febrile illness, termed CMV mononucleosis, may cause chemical hepatitis with elevated aminotransferases, and atypical lymphocytosis similar to infectious mononucleosis due to EBV.

Postperfusion/posttransfusion syndrome can develop 2 to 4 wk after transfusion with blood products containing CMV. It causes fever lasting 2 to 3 wk and the same manifestations as CMV mononucleosis.

In immunocompromised patients, CMV is a major cause of morbidity and mortality. Disease often results from reactivation of latent virus. The lungs, GI tract, or CNS may be involved. In the terminal phase of AIDS, CMV infection causes retinitis in up to 40% of patients and causes funduscopically visible retinal abnormalities. Ulcerative disease of the colon (with abdominal pain and GI bleeding) or of the esophagus (with odynophagia) may occur.

Diagnosis

- Usually clinical evaluation
- Detection of CMV antigen or DNA
- Urine culture in infants
- Often biopsy in immunocompromised patients
- Serologic testing

CMV infection is suspected in

- Healthy people with mononucleosis-like syndromes
- Immunocompromised patients with GI, CNS, or retinal symptoms
- Neonates with systemic disease

CMV mononucleosis can sometimes be differentiated from infectious (EBV) mononucleosis by the absence of pharyngitis, a negative heterophile antibody test, and serologic testing. CMV infection can be differentiated from viral hepatitis by hepatitis serologic testing. Laboratory confirmation of primary CMV infection is necessary only to differentiate it from other, particularly treatable, conditions or serious disease.

Seroconversion can be demonstrated by development of CMV antibodies and indicates new CMV infection.However, much CMV disease results from reactivation of latent disease in the immunocompromised host. Reactivation of CMV can result in virus in the urine, other body fluids, or tissues, but the presence of CMV in body fluids and tissues does not always indicate disease and may merely represent shedding. Therefore, biopsy showing CMV-induced abnormalities is often necessary to demonstrate invasive disease. Quantitative detection of CMV antigen or DNA in the peripheral blood can also be very helpful because elevated or rising CMV titers are often highly suggestive of invasive disease.

Diagnosis in infants can be made by urine culture.

Treatment

- For serious disease, antivirals (eg, ganciclovir, valganciclovir, foscarnet, cidofovir)

CMV retinitis, which occurs mostly in AIDS patients, is treated with systemic antivirals.

Anti-CMV drugs are used to treat severe disease other than retinitis but are less consistently effective than in retinitis.

CMV retinitis: Drugs used to treat CMV retinitis in induction and maintenance regimens include

- Ganciclovir or valganciclovir
- Foscarnet, with or without ganciclovir
- Cidofovir

Most patients receive induction therapy with either ganciclovir 5 mg/kg IV q 12 h for 2 to 3 wk or valganciclovir 900 mg po q 12 h for 21 days. If induction fails more than once, another drug should be used. After induction, patients receive maintenance or suppressive therapy with valganciclovir 900 mg po once/day to delay progression. Maintenance therapy with ganciclovir 5 mg/kg IV once/day can also be used to prevent recurrence.

Alternatively, foscarnet can be given with or without ganciclovir. Foscarnet 60 mg/kg IV q 8 h for 2 to 3 wk is used for induction, followed by 90 to 120 mg/kg IV once/day for maintenance therapy. Adverse effects of IV foscarnet are significant and include nephrotoxicity, symptomatic hypocalcemia, hypomagnesemia, hyperphosphatemia, hypokalemia, and CNS effects. Combination therapy with ganciclovir and foscarnet increases efficacy as well as adverse effects.

Cidofovir therapy consists of 5 mg/kg IV once/wk (induction) for 2 wk, followed by a similar dose every other week for maintenance. Efficacy is similar to ganciclovir or foscarnet. Significant adverse effects, including renal failure, limit its use. Cidofovir may cause iritis or ocular hypotony (intraocular pressure ≤ 5 mm Hg). The potential for nephrotoxicity can be reduced by giving probenecid and prehydration with each dose. However, the adverse effects of probenecid, including rash, headache, and fever, may be significant enough to prevent its use.

Even patients receiving ocular injections need systemic therapy to prevent CMV in the contralateral eye and extraocular tissues. Ultimately, improvement of CD4+ count to > 100 cells/μL with systemic antiretroviral therapy should prevent the need for ocular implants and chemoprophylaxis.

Prevention

Prophylaxis or preemptive treatment (actively monitoring patients by viral load and giving antiviral drugs to those with evidence of infection) is effective for preventing CMV disease in solid organ or hematopoietic cell transplant recipients infected with CMV and at risk of CMV disease. Drugs used include ganciclovir, valganciclovir, and foscarnet.

KEY POINTS

- Sixty to 90% of adults have latent CMV infection.
- Healthy children and adults usually have mild, nonspecific symptoms or sometimes a mononucleosis-like syndrome.
- Congenital infection may cause stillbirth or severe, sometimes fatal postnatal complications including extensive hepatic or CNS damage.
- Severely immunocompromised patients may have severe disease involving the retina, lungs, GI tract, or CNS.
- Antiviral drugs may help treat retinitis but are less effective when other organs are affected.
- Transplant patients at risk of CMV infection require prophylactic antivirals or close monitoring for early indications of infection.

HERPES SIMPLEX VIRUS INFECTIONS

(Herpes Labialis; Herpetic Gingivostomatitis)

Herpes simplex viruses (human herpesviruses types 1 and 2) commonly cause recurrent infection affecting the skin, mouth, lips, eyes, and genitals. Common severe infections include encephalitis, meningitis, neonatal herpes, and, in immunocompromised patients, disseminated infection. Mucocutaneous infections cause clusters of small painful vesicles on an erythematous base. Diagnosis is clinical; laboratory confirmation by culture, PCR, direct immunofluorescence, or serologic testing can be done. Treatment is symptomatic; antiviral therapy with acyclovir, valacyclovir, or famciclovir is helpful for severe infections and, if begun early, for recurrent or primary infections.

Both types of herpes simplex virus (HSV), HSV-1 and HSV-2, can cause oral or genital infection. Most often, HSV-1 causes gingivostomatitis, herpes labialis, and herpes keratitis. HSV-2 usually causes genital lesions.

Transmission of HSV results from close contact with a person who is actively shedding virus. Viral shedding occurs from lesions but can occur even when lesions are not apparent.

After the initial infection, HSV remains dormant in nerve ganglia, from which it can periodically emerge, causing symptoms. Recurrent herpetic eruptions are precipitated by

- Overexposure to sunlight
- Febrile illnesses
- Physical or emotional stress
- Immunosuppression
- Unknown stimuli

Generally, recurrent eruptions are less severe and occur less frequently over time.

Diseases Caused by HSV

Diseases include

- Mucocutaneous infection (most common), including genital herpes
- Ocular infection (herpes keratitis)
- CNS infection
- Neonatal herpes

HSV rarely causes fulminant hepatitis in the absence of cutaneous lesions.

In patients with HIV infection, herpetic infections can be particularly severe. Progressive and persistent esophagitis, colitis, perianal ulcers, pneumonia, encephalitis, and meningitis may occur.

HSV outbreaks may be followed by erythema multiforme, possibly caused by an immune reaction to the virus. Eczema herpeticum is a complication of HSV infection in which severe herpetic disease develops in skin regions with eczema.

Mucocutaneous HSV infection: Lesions may appear anywhere on the skin or mucosa but are most frequent in the following locations:

- Mouth or lips (perioral infection)
- Genitals
- Conjunctiva and cornea

Generally, after a prodromal period (typically < 6 h in recurrent HSV-1) of tingling discomfort or itching, clusters of small, tense vesicles appear on an erythematous base. Clusters vary in size from 0.5 to 1.5 cm but may coalesce. Lesions on the nose, ears, eyes, fingers, or genitals may be particularly painful.

Vesicles typically persist for a few days, then rupture and dry, forming a thin, yellowish crust.

Healing generally occurs within 10 to 19 days after onset in primary infection or within 5 to 10 days in recurrent infection. Lesions usually heal completely, but recurrent lesions at the same site may cause atrophy and scarring. Skin lesions can develop secondary bacterial infection. In patients with depressed cell-mediated immunity due to HIV infection or other conditions, prolonged or progressive lesions may persist for weeks or longer. Localized infections can disseminate, particularly—and often dramatically—in immunocompromised patients.

Acute herpetic gingivostomatitis usually results from primary infection with HSV-1, typically in children. Herpetic pharyngitis can occur in adults as well as children. Occasionally, through oral-genital contact, the cause is HSV-2. Intraoral and gingival vesicles rupture, usually within several hours to 1 or 2 days, to form ulcers. Fever and pain often occur. Difficulty eating and drinking may lead to dehydration. After resolution, the virus resides dormant in the semilunar ganglion.

Herpes labialis is usually a recurrence of HSV. It develops as ulcers (cold sores) on the vermilion border of the lip or, much less commonly, as ulcerations of the mucosa of the hard palate.

Genital herpes is the most common ulcerative sexually transmitted disease in developed countries (see p. 1623). Genital HSV can be caused by HSV-1 or HSV-2.

Herpes simplex keratitis: Herpes simplex keratitis (HSV infection of the corneal epithelium—see also p. 925) causes pain, tearing, photophobia, and corneal ulcers that often have a branching pattern.

Herpetic whitlow: Herpetic whitlow, a swollen, painful, erythematous lesion of the distal phalanx, results from inoculation of HSV through the skin and is most common among health care practitioners (see also p. 291).

Neonatal herpes simplex: Neonatal HSV infection develops in neonates, including those whose mothers have no suggestion of current or past herpes infection (see also p. 2631). It is most commonly transmitted during birth through contact with vaginal secretions containing HSV and usually involves HSV-2.

Neonatal HSV infection usually develops between the 1st and 4th wk of life, often causing mucocutaneous vesicles or CNS involvement. It causes major morbidity and mortality.

CNS infection: Herpes encephalitis occurs sporadically and may be severe. Multiple early seizures are characteristic.

Viral meningitis may result from HSV-2. It is usually self-limited and may involve lumbosacral myeloradiculitis, which may cause urinary retention or obstipation.

Diagnosis

- Clinical evaluation
- Sometimes laboratory confirmation
- PCR of CSF and MRI for HSV encephalitis

Diagnosis is often clinical based on characteristic lesions.

Laboratory confirmation can be helpful, especially if infection is severe, the patient is immunocompromised or pregnant, or lesions are atypical. A Tzanck test (a superficial scraping from the base of a freshly ruptured vesicle stained with Wright-Giemsa stain) often reveals multinucleate giant cells in HSV or varicella-zoster virus infection.

Definitive diagnosis is with culture, seroconversion involving the appropriate serotype (in primary infections), PCR, and antigen detection. Fluid and material for culture should be obtained from the base of a vesicle or of a freshly ulcerated lesion. HSV can sometimes be identified using direct immunofluorescence assay of scrapings of lesions. PCR of CSF and MRI are used to diagnose HSV encephalitis.

HSV should be distinguished from herpes zoster, which rarely recurs and usually causes more severe pain and larger groups of lesions that are distributed along a dermatome.

Clusters of vesicles or ulcers on an erythematous base are unusual in genital ulcers other than those due to HSV infection.

If herpes infections recur frequently, do not resolve, or do not respond to antiviral drugs as expected, immunocompromise, possibly due to HIV infection, should be suspected.

Treatment

- Usually acyclovir, valacyclovir, or famciclovir
- For keratitis, topical trifluridine

Mucocutaneous infection: Isolated infections often go untreated without consequence.

Acyclovir, valacyclovir, or famciclovir can be used to treat infection, especially when it is primary. Infection with acyclovir-resistant HSV is rare and occurs almost exclusively in immunocompromised patients. Foscarnet may be effective for acyclovir-resistant infections.

Secondary bacterial infections are treated with topical antibiotics (eg, mupirocin or neomycin-bacitracin) or, if severe, with systemic antibiotics (eg, penicillinase-resistant β-lactams). Systemic analgesics may help.

Gingivostomatitis and **pharyngitis** may require symptom relief with topical anesthetics (eg, dyclonine, benzocaine, viscous lidocaine). (NOTE: Lidocaine must not be swallowed because it anesthetizes the oropharynx, the hypopharynx, and possibly the epiglottis. Children must be watched for signs of aspiration.) Severe cases can be treated with acyclovir, valacyclovir, or famciclovir.

Herpes labialis responds to oral and topical acyclovir. The duration of a recurrent eruption may be decreased by about a day by applying penciclovir 1% cream q 2 h while awake for 4 days, beginning during the prodrome or when the first lesion appears. Toxicity appears to be minimal. Famciclovir 1500 mg as one dose or valacyclovir 2 g po q 12 h for 1 day can be used to treat recurrent herpes labialis. Acyclovir-resistant strains are resistant to penciclovir, famciclovir, and valacyclovir. Docosanol 10% cream may be effective when used 5 times/day.

Herpetic whitlow heals in 2 to 3 wk without treatment. Topical acyclovir has not been shown to be effective. Oral or IV acyclovir can be used in immunosuppressed patients and those with severe infection.

PEARLS & PITFALLS

- Treating primary herpes infection with drugs, even if done early, does not prevent recurrence.

Herpes simplex keratitis: Treatment of herpes simplex keratitis involves topical antivirals, such as trifluridine, and should be supervised by an ophthalmologist.

Neonatal herpes simplex: Acyclovir 20 mg/kg IV q 8 h for 14 to 21 days should be used if renal function is normal. A dose of 20 mg/kg IV q 8 h for at least 21 days is indicated for CNS and disseminated HSV disease.

CNS infection: Encephalitis is treated with acyclovir 10 mg/kg IV q 8 h for 14 to 21 days if renal function is normal. Treatment for 14 to 21 days is preferred to prevent potential relapse. Higher doses up to 20 mg/kg IV q 8 h are used in children.

Viral meningitis is usually treated with IV acyclovir. Acyclovir is generally very well-tolerated. However, adverse effects can include phlebitis, renal dysfunction, and, rarely, neurotoxicity (lethargy, confusion, seizures, coma).

KEY POINTS

- HSV usually causes mucocutaneous infection but sometimes causes keratitis, and serious CNS infection can occur in neonates and in adults.
- After initial infection, HSV remains dormant in nerve ganglia, from which it can periodically emerge, causing symptoms.
- Diagnose mucocutaneous infections clinically, but do viral culture, PCR, or antigen detection if patients are neonates, immunocompromised, or pregnant or have a CNS infection or severe disease.
- Give IV acyclovir to patients with serious infections.
- For mucocutaneous infections, consider oral acyclovir, valacyclovir, or famciclovir; for herpes labialis, an alternative is topical penciclovir or docosanol.

GENITAL HERPES

Genital herpes is a sexually transmitted disease caused by human herpesvirus 1 or 2. It causes ulcerative genital lesions. Diagnosis is clinical with laboratory confirmation by culture, PCR, or serologic testing. Treatment is with antiviral drugs.

Genital herpes is the most common ulcerative sexually transmitted disease in developed countries. It is caused by human herpesviruses 1 (HSV-1) or 2 (HSV-2).

After the initial infection, HSV remains dormant in nerve ganglia, from which it can periodically emerge. When the virus emerges, it may or may not cause symptoms (ie, genital lesions). Transmission may occur through contact with the lesions or, more often, via skin-to-skin contact with sex partners when lesions are not apparent (called asymptomatic shedding).

Pregnant women with genital herpes can transmit HSV (usually HSV-2) to the fetus or neonate, Typically, HSV is transmitted during delivery via contact with vaginal secretions containing HSV. The virus is rarely transmitted transplacentally. Mothers of neonates with HSV infection tend to have newly acquired genital infection; many do not have symptoms at the time of delivery. Neonatal HSV infection is a serious, potentially fatal infection.

Symptoms and Signs

Most cases of primary genital herpes do not cause noticeable symptoms; many people infected with HSV-2 do not know that they have genital herpes.

Primary genital lesions develop 4 to 7 days after contact. The vesicles usually erode to form ulcers that may coalesce. Lesions may occur in the following locations:

- On the prepuce, glans penis, and penile shaft in men
- On the labia, clitoris, perineum, vagina, and cervix in women
- Around the anus and in the rectum in men (see Plate 76) or women who engage in receptive rectal intercourse

Urinary hesitancy, dysuria, urinary retention, constipation, or severe sacral neuralgia may occur.

Scarring may follow healing. The lesions recur in 80% of patients with HSV-2 and in 50% of those with HSV-1.

Primary genital lesions are usually more painful, prolonged, and widespread and are more likely to be bilateral and involve regional adenopathy and constitutional symptoms than recurrent genital lesions. Recurrent lesions may have severe prodromal symptoms and may involve the buttock, groin, or thigh.

Diagnosis

- Clinical evaluation
- Culture and PCR
- Serologic testing

Diagnosis of genital herpes is often clinical based on characteristic lesions; clusters of vesicles or ulcers on an erythematous base are unusual in genital ulcers other than those due to HSV. However, these lesions are absent in many patients.

Tests for HSV should be done to confirm the diagnosis if it is not clear.

Testing is usually done using a sample of fluid from the base of a vesicle or of a newly ulcerated lesion, if present. Absence of HSV in culture, especially in patients without active lesions, does not rule out HSV infection because viral shedding is intermittent. Also, culture has limited sensitivity; PCR is more sensitive and is being used increasingly.

Direct immunofluorescence with fluorescein-labeled monoclonal antibodies is sometimes available; it is specific but not sensitive.

Serologic tests can accurately detect HSV-1 and HSV-2 antibodies, which develop during the first several weeks after infection and then persist. Thus, if genital herpes is thought to be recently acquired, tests may have to be repeated.

HSV serologic testing should be considered for the following;

- To evaluate patients who have no suspicious genital lesions but who require or request evaluation (eg, because of past genital lesions or high-risk behaviors)
- To help determine risk of recurrence

- To identify pregnant women who do not have genital lesions but are at risk of transmitting herpes to the neonate during delivery
- To determine whether a person is susceptible to infection from a sex partner with genital herpes

Treatment

- Acyclovir, valacyclovir, or famciclovir

Genital herpes is treated with antiviral drugs.

Primary eruptions can be treated with one of the following:

- Acyclovir 400 mg po tid for 7 to 10 days
- Valacyclovir 1 g po q 12 h for 7 to 10 days
- Famciclovir 250 mg po tid for 7 to 10 days

These drugs reduce viral shedding and symptoms in severe primary infections. However, even early treatment of primary infections does not prevent recurrences.

In **recurrent eruptions,** symptom duration and severity can be reduced marginally by antiviral treatment, particularly during the prodromal phase. Recurrent eruptions can be treated with one of the following:

- Acyclovir 400 mg po tid for 5 days
- Valacyclovir 500 mg po q 12 h for 3 days
- Famciclovir 1000 mg po q 12 h for 1 day

For **frequent eruptions** (eg, > 6 eruptions/yr), suppressive antiviral therapy with one of the following may be used:

- Acyclovir 400 mg po q 12 h
- Valacyclovir 500 to 1000 mg po once/day
- Famciclovir 250 mg po q 12 h

Doses should be adjusted for renal insufficiency. Adverse effects are infrequent with oral administration but may include nausea, vomiting, diarrhea, headache, and rash.

Topical antiviral drugs have only little value, and their use is discouraged.

Evaluation of sex partners of patients with genital herpes is important.

Prevention

The best ways to avoid genital herpes are

- Abstaining from sexual contact (vaginal, anal, and oral sex)
- Being in a long-term mutually monogamous relationship with a partner who has been tested and is not infected

Risk of genital herpes can by reduced by

- Using latex condoms correctly and consistently

However, condoms do not cover all areas that can be affected and thus do not fully protect against genital herpes.

Patients with genital herpes should abstain from sexual activity when they have lesions or other herpes symptoms. Patients should be reminded that they can transmit the infection even when they do not have any symptoms.

Preventing neonatal HSV infection: Efforts to prevent neonatal transmission have not been very effective. Universal screening has not been recommended or shown to be effective.

Clinicians should ask all pregnant women whether they have had genital herpes and should emphasize the importance of not contracting herpes during pregnancy.

If women have herpes symptoms (eg, active genital lesions) when labor begins, cesarean delivery is recommended to prevent transmission to the neonate. Pregnant women with genital herpes can be given acyclovir starting at 36 wk gestation to reduce the risk of a recurrence and thus the need for cesarean delivery.

Fetal scalp monitors should not be used during labor on infants whose mothers have suspected active genital herpes.

KEY POINTS

- After the initial infection, HSV remains dormant in nerve ganglia, from which it can periodically emerge.
- Transmission may occur through contact with the lesions, but viral shedding and transmission can also occur when lesions are not apparent (asymptomatic shedding).
- Most initial infections do not cause symptoms, but primary genital lesions are usually more painful, prolonged, and widespread than recurrent genital lesions.
- Diagnose based on characteristic genital lesions in patients with lesions and confirm by culture, PCR, and/or serologic tests for HSV.
- Treat primary and recurrent eruptions with acyclovir, valacyclovir, or famciclovir.
- If pregnant women have genital herpes, consider giving acyclovir starting at 36 wk gestation to reduce the risk of a recurrence and transmission to the neonate during delivery.

HERPES ZOSTER

(Acute Posterior Ganglionitis; Shingles)

Herpes zoster is infection that results when varicella-zoster virus reactivates from its latent state in a posterior dorsal root ganglion. Symptoms usually begin with pain along the affected dermatome, followed in 2 to 3 days by a vesicular eruption that is usually diagnostic. Treatment is antiviral drugs given within 72 h after skin lesions appear.

Chickenpox and herpes zoster are caused by the varicella-zoster virus (human herpesvirus type 3); chickenpox is the acute invasive phase of the virus, and herpes zoster (shingles) represents reactivation of the latent phase.

Herpes zoster inflames the sensory root ganglia, the skin of the associated dermatome, and sometimes the posterior and anterior horns of the gray matter, meninges, and dorsal and ventral roots. Herpes zoster frequently occurs in elderly and HIV-infected patients and is more severe in immunocompromised patients because cell-mediated immunity in these patients is decreased. There are no clear-cut precipitants.

Symptoms and Signs

Lancinating, dysesthetic, or other pain develops in the involved site, followed in 2 to 3 days by a rash, usually crops of vesicles on an erythematous base. The site is usually one or more adjacent dermatomes in the thoracic (see Plate 82) or lumbar region, although a few satellite lesions may also appear. Lesions are typically unilateral. The site is usually hyperesthetic, and pain may be severe. Lesions usually continue to form for about 3 to 5 days.

Herpes zoster may disseminate to other regions of the skin and to visceral organs, especially in immunocompromised patients.

Geniculate zoster (Ramsay Hunt syndrome, herpes zoster oticus) results from involvement of the geniculate ganglion. Ear pain, facial paralysis, and sometimes vertigo occur. Vesicles erupt in the external auditory canal, and taste may be lost in the anterior two thirds of the tongue.

Ophthalmic herpes zoster results from involvement of the gasserian ganglion, with pain and vesicular eruption around the eye and on the forehead, in the distribution of the ophthalmic division of the 5th cranial nerve. Ocular disease can be severe. Vesicles on the tip of the nose (Hutchinson sign) indicate involvement of the nasociliary branch and a higher risk of severe ocular disease. However, the eye may be involved in the absence of lesions on the tip of the nose.

Intraoral zoster is uncommon but may produce a sharp unilateral distribution of lesions. No intraoral prodromal symptoms occur.

Postherpetic neuralgia: Fewer than 4% of patients with herpes zoster experience another outbreak. However, many patients, particularly the elderly, have persistent or recurrent pain in the involved distribution (postherpetic neuralgia), which may persist for months or years or permanently. Infection in the trigeminal nerve is particularly likely to lead to severe, persistent pain.

The pain of postherpetic neuralgia may be sharp and intermittent or constant and may be debilitating.

Diagnosis

- Clinical evaluation

Herpes zoster is suspected in patients with the characteristic rash and sometimes in patients with typical pain in a dermatomal distribution. Diagnosis is usually based on the virtually pathognomonic rash.

If the diagnosis is equivocal, detecting multinucleate giant cells with a Tzanck test can confirm infection, but the Tzanck test is positive with herpes zoster or herpes simplex. HSV may cause nearly identical lesions, but unlike herpes zoster, HSV tends to recur and is not dermatomal. Viruses can be differentiated by culture or PCR. Antigen detection from a biopsy sample can be useful.

Treatment

- Symptomatic treatment
- Antivirals (acyclovir, famciclovir, valacyclovir), especially for immunocompromised patients

Wet compresses are soothing, but systemic analgesics are often necessary.

For treatment of ophthalmic herpes zoster, an ophthalmologist should be consulted. For treatment of otic herpes zoster, an otolaryngologist should be consulted.

Antiviral therapy: Treatment with oral antivirals decreases the severity and duration of the acute eruption and the rate of serious complications in immunocompromised patients; it may decrease the incidence of postherpetic neuralgia.

Treatment should start as soon as possible, ideally during the prodrome, and is likely to be ineffective if given > 72 h after skin lesions appear. Famciclovir 500 mg po tid for 7 days and valacyclovir 1 g po tid for 7 days have better bioavailability with oral dosing than acyclovir, and therefore for herpes zoster, they are generally preferred to oral acyclovir 800 mg 5 times/day for 7 to 10 days. Corticosteroids do not decrease the incidence of postherpetic neuralgia.

For less severely immunocompromised patients, oral famciclovir, valacyclovir, or acyclovir (see above) is a reasonable option; famciclovir and valacyclovir are preferred. For severely immunocompromised patients, acyclovir is recommended at a dosage of 10 mg/kg IV q 8 h for 7 to 14 days for adults and 20 mg/kg IV q 8 h for 7 days for children < 12 yr.

Although data concerning the safety of acyclovir and valacyclovir during pregnancy are reassuring, the safety of antiviral therapy during pregnancy is not firmly established. Because congenital varicella can result from maternal varicella but rarely results from maternal zoster, the potential benefit of treatment of pregnant patients should outweigh possible risks to the fetus. Pregnant patients with severe rash, severe acute pain, or ophthalmic zoster can be treated with valacyclovir or acyclovir, especially in later stages of pregnancy.

Management of postherpetic neuralgia: Management of postherpetic neuralgia can be particularly difficult. Treatments include gabapentin, cyclic antidepressants, and topical capsaicin or lidocaine ointment. Opioid analgesics may be necessary. Intrathecal methylprednisolone may be of benefit.

A recent study suggests that injecting the entire affected area with botulinum toxin A (40 injections in a chessboard pattern) can reduce pain.

Prevention

Adults ≥ 60 yr should have a single dose of zoster vaccine (a more potent preparation of varicella vaccine) whether they have had herpes zoster or not. This vaccine has been shown to decrease the incidence of zoster.

KEY POINTS

- Herpes zoster is caused by reactivation of the varicella-zoster virus (the cause of chickenpox) from its latent phase.
- A painful rash, usually crops of vesicles on an erythematous base, develops on one or more adjacent dermatomes.
- Fewer than 4% of patients have another outbreak of zoster, but many, particularly the elderly, have persistent or recurrent pain for months or years (postherpetic neuralgia).
- Antivirals (acyclovir, famciclovir, valacyclovir) are beneficial, especially for immunocompromised patients.
- Analgesics are often necessary.
- Give adults ≥ 60 yr a single dose of zoster vaccine whether they have had herpes zoster or not.

INFECTIOUS MONONUCLEOSIS

Infectious mononucleosis is caused by Epstein-Barr virus (EBV—human herpesvirus type 4) and is characterized by fatigue, fever, pharyngitis, and lymphadenopathy. Fatigue may persist weeks or months. Severe complications, including airway obstruction, splenic rupture, and neurologic syndromes, occasionally occur. Diagnosis is clinical or with EBV serologic testing. Treatment is supportive.

EBV is a herpesvirus that infects 50% of children before age 5. Over 90% of adults are seropositive for EBV. Its host is humans.

EBV infection is usually asymptomatic.

Pathophysiology

After initial replication in the nasopharynx, the virus infects B cells. Morphologically abnormal (atypical) lymphocytes develop, mainly from CD8+ T cells that respond to the infection.

After primary infection, EBV remains within the host, primarily in B cells, for life and undergoes intermittent asymptomatic shedding from the oropharynx. The virus is detectable in oropharyngeal secretions of 15 to 25% of healthy EBV-seropositive adults. Shedding increases in frequency and titer in immunocompromised patients (eg, organ allograft recipients, HIV-infected people).

EBV has not been recovered from environmental sources and is not very contagious.

Transmission: Transmission may occur via transfusion of blood products but much more frequently occurs via kissing between an uninfected and an EBV-seropositive person who is shedding the virus asymptomatically. Only about 5% of patients acquire EBV from someone who has acute infection.

Early childhood transmission occurs more frequently among lower socioeconomic groups and in crowded conditions.

Associated disorders: EBV is statistically associated with and likely has a causal role in

- Burkitt lymphoma
- Certain B-cell tumors in immunocompromised patients
- Nasopharyngeal carcinoma

EBV does not cause chronic fatigue syndrome. However, it may occasionally cause a syndrome of fever, interstitial pneumonitis, pancytopenia, and uveitis (ie, chronic active EBV).

Symptoms and Signs

In most young children, primary EBV infection is asymptomatic. Symptoms of infectious mononucleosis develop most often in older children and adults.

The incubation period is about 30 to 50 days. Fatigue can last for months but is usually maximal during the first 2 to 3 wk.

Most patients have the triad of

- Fever
- Pharyngitis
- Adenopathy

Fever usually peaks in the afternoon or early evening, with a temperature around 39.5° C, although it may reach 40.5° C.

Pharyngitis may be severe, painful, and exudative and may resemble streptococcal pharyngitis.

Adenopathy is usually symmetric and may involve any group of nodes, particularly the anterior and posterior cervical chains. Adenopathy may be the only manifestation.

Other symptoms include

- Splenomegaly
- Mild hepatomegaly and hepatic percussion tenderness
- Periorbital edema and palatal petechiae
- Less frequently maculopapular eruptions
- Rarely jaundice

Splenomegaly, which occurs in about 50% of cases, is maximal during the 2nd and 3rd wk and usually results in only a barely palpable splenic tip.

Complications: Although recovery is usually complete, complications may be dramatic.

Neurologic complications are rare but may include encephalitis, seizures, Guillain-Barré syndrome, peripheral neuropathy, viral meningitis, myelitis, cranial nerve palsies, and psychosis. Encephalitis may manifest with cerebellar dysfunction, or it may be global and rapidly progressive, similar to herpes simplex encephalitis, but is usually self-limited.

Hematologic complications are usually self-limited. They include

- Granulocytopenia
- Thrombocytopenia
- Hemolytic anemia

Transient mild granulocytopenia or thrombocytopenia occurs in about 50% of patients; severe cases, associated with bacterial infection or bleeding, occur less frequently. Hemolytic anemia is often due to anti-i-specific cold-agglutinin antibodies.

Splenic rupture can have severe consequences. It can result from splenic enlargement and capsular swelling, which are maximal 10 to 21 days after presentation. A history of trauma is present only about half of the time. Rupture is usually painful but occasionally causes painless hypotension. For treatment, see p. 2937.

Respiratory complications include, rarely, upper airway obstruction due to pharyngeal or paratracheal lymphadenopathy; respiratory complications may respond to corticosteroids. Clinically silent interstitial pulmonary infiltrates occur mostly in children and are usually visible on x-rays.

Hepatic complications include elevated aminotransferase levels (about 2 to 3 times normal, returning to baseline over 3 to 4 wk); they occur in about 95% of patients. If jaundice or more severe enzyme elevations occur, other causes of hepatitis should be investigated.

Overwhelming infection with EBV occurs sporadically but may cluster in families, particularly those with X-linked lymphoproliferative syndrome. Survivors of overwhelming primary EBV infection are at risk of developing agammaglobulinemia or lymphoma.

Diagnosis

- Heterophile antibody test
- Sometimes EBV serologic testing

Infectious mononucleosis should be suspected in patients with typical symptoms and signs. Exudative pharyngitis, anterior cervical lymphadenopathy, and fever may be clinically indistinguishable from those caused by group A β-hemolytic streptococci. However, posterior cervical or generalized adenopathy or hepatosplenomegaly suggests infectious mononucleosis. Moreover, detection of streptococci in the oropharynx does not exclude infectious mononucleosis.

Differential diagnosis: Primary HIV infection can produce a clinical picture resembling acute EBV infection. If patients have risk factors for HIV infection, the following should be done:

- Quantitative HIV RNA viral blood count
- Combination antibody immunoassay and p24 antigen assay

HIV enzyme-linked immunosorbent assay (ELISA)/Western blot is usually negative during the acute infection and thus should not be used alone to diagnose early primary HIV infection. Quantitative HIV RNA and p24 antigen detection are more sensitive for diagnosing acute HIV infection because HIV RNA and p24 antigen are present in blood before HIV antibodies develop

PEARLS & PITFALLS

- Primary HIV infection can resemble acute EBV infection; patients with risk factors for HIV infection should be tested using quantitative HIV RNA viral count and combination antibody immunoassay and p24 antigen testing.

CMV may cause a syndrome similar to infectious mononucleosis, with atypical lymphocytosis as well as hepatosplenomegaly and hepatitis but usually not with severe pharyngitis.

Toxoplasmosis, hepatitis B, rubella, or atypical lymphocytes associated with adverse drug reactions can also cause infectious mononucleosis–like syndromes. These syndromes can usually be distinguished by their other clinical features or by specific testing.

Laboratory tests: Laboratory diagnosis usually involves a CBC and EBV serologic testing. Lymphocytes that are morphologically atypical account for up to 30% of the WBCs. Although individual lymphocytes may resemble leukemic lymphocytes, lymphocytes are heterogeneous, which is unlikely in leukemia.

Atypical lymphocytes may also be present in HIV or CMV infection, hepatitis B, influenza B, rubella, or other viral illnesses, so diagnosis requires serologic testing. However, very high atypical lymphocyte counts are typically seen only in primary EBV and CMV infection.

Two serologic tests are used to diagnose acute EBV infection:

- Heterophile antibody testing
- Specific EBV antibody testing

Heterophile antibodies are measured using various agglutination card (monospot) tests. However, heterophile antibodies are present in only 50% of patients < 5 yr and in about 80 to 90% of adolescents and adults with infectious mononucleosis. Importantly, the heterophile antibody test may be false-positive in some patients with acute HIV infection. The titer and prevalence of heterophile antibodies rise during the 2nd and 3rd wk of illness. Thus, if the diagnosis is strongly suspected but the heterophile antibody test is negative, repeating the test after 7 to 10 days of symptoms is reasonable.

If the test remains negative, antibodies to EBV should be measured. The presence of IgM antibodies to the EBV viral capsid antigen (VCA) indicates primary EBV infection (these antibodies disappear within 3 mo after infection). IgG VCA (EBV VCA-IgG) also develops early in primary EBV infection, but these antibodies persist for life. EBV nuclear antigen (EBNA-IgG) antibodies develop later (perhaps after 8 wk) in acute EBV infection and also persist for life. If EBV antibody titers are negative or indicate remote infection (ie, positive for IgG antibodies and negative for IgM antibodies), other diagnoses (eg, acute HIV infection, CMV infection) should be considered.

Prognosis

Infectious mononucleosis is usually self-limited. Duration of illness varies; the acute phase lasts about 2 wk. Generally, 20% of patients can return to school or work within 1 wk, and 50% within 2 wk. Fatigue may persist for several more weeks or, in 1 to 2% of cases, for months.

Death occurs in < 1%, mostly resulting from complications (eg, encephalitis, splenic rupture, airway obstruction).

Treatment

- Supportive care
- Corticosteroids possibly helpful for severe disease

Treatment is supportive. Patients are encouraged to rest during the acute phase but can resume activity when fever, pharyngitis, and malaise abate. To prevent splenic rupture, patients should avoid heavy lifting and contact sports for 1 mo after presentation and until splenomegaly (which can be monitored by ultrasonography) resolves.

Although corticosteroids hasten defervescence and relieve pharyngitis, they generally should not be used in uncomplicated disease. Corticosteroids can be helpful for complications such as impending airway obstruction, severe thrombocytopenia, and hemolytic anemia. Although oral or IV acyclovir decreases oropharyngeal shedding of EBV, there is no convincing evidence to warrant its clinical use.

KEY POINTS

- EBV infection is very common; the virus remains within the host for life and is intermittently and asymptomatically shed from the oropharynx.
- Only about 5% of patients acquire EBV from someone who has acute infection.
- Typical manifestations include fatigue (sometimes persisting weeks or rarely months), fever, pharyngitis, splenomegaly, and lymphadenopathy.
- Uncommon severe complications include encephalitis and other neurologic manifestations, splenic rupture, airway obstruction due to tonsillar enlargement, hemolytic anemia, thrombocytopenia, and jaundice.
- Do heterophile antibody testing and sometimes specific EBV antibody testing.
- Provide supportive care and recommend avoidance of heavy lifting and contact sports; antivirals are not indicated.
- Consider corticosteroids for complications such as impending airway obstruction, severe thrombocytopenia, and hemolytic anemia.

194 Human Immunodeficiency Virus

Human immunodeficiency virus (HIV) infection results from 1 of 2 similar retroviruses (HIV-1 and HIV-2) that destroy CD4+ lymphocytes and impair cell-mediated immunity, increasing risk of certain infections and cancers. Initial infection may cause nonspecific febrile illness. Risk of subsequent manifestations—related to immunodeficiency—is proportional to the level of CD4+ lymphocytes. HIV can directly damage the brain, gonads, kidneys, and heart, causing cognitive impairment, hypogonadism, renal insufficiency, and cardiomyopathy. Manifestations range from asymptomatic carriage to AIDS, which is defined by serious opportunistic infections or cancers or a CD4 count of < 200/μL. HIV infection can be diagnosed by antibody, nucleic acid (HIV RNA), or antigen (p24) testing. Screening should be routinely offered to all adults and adolescents. Treatment aims to suppress HIV replication by using combinations of ≥ 3 drugs that inhibit HIV enzymes; treatment can restore immune function in most patients if suppression of replication is sustained.

(See also p. 2599, the National Institute's of Health AIDSInfo web site [www.aidsinfo.nih.gov], and the recommendations of the HIV Medicine Association of the Infectious Diseases Society of America: Primary Care Guidelines for the Management of Persons Infected with HIV [https://academic.oup.com].)

Retroviruses are enveloped RNA viruses defined by their mechanism of replication via reverse transcription to produce DNA copies that integrate in the host cell genome. Several retroviruses, including 2 types of HIV and 2 types of human T-lymphotropic virus (HTLV—see Sidebar 194–1), cause serious disorders in people.

HIV-1 causes most HIV infections worldwide, but HIV-2 causes a substantial proportion of infections in parts of West Africa. In some areas of West Africa, both viruses are prevalent and may coinfect patients. HIV-2 appears to be less virulent than HIV-1.

HIV-1 originated in Central Africa in the first half of the 20th century, when a closely related chimpanzee virus first infected

Sidebar 194–1. HTLV Infections

Infection with human T-lymphotropic virus (HTLV) 1 or 2 can cause T-cell leukemias and lymphomas, lymphadenopathy, hepatosplenomegaly, skin lesions, and immunocompromise. Some HTLV-infected patients develop infections similar to those that occur in HIV-infected patients. HTLV-1 can also cause myelopathy (see on p. 2033).

Most cases are transmitted from mother to child by breast-feeding, but HTLV-1 can be transmitted sexually, through blood, and, rarely, via transplantation of organs from HTLV-1 seropositive donors.

humans. Epidemic global spread began in the late 1970s, and AIDS was recognized in 1981.

In 2016, about 36.7 million people, including 2.1 million children < 15 yr, were living with HIV worldwide, according to the World Health Organization (WHO)[1]. Almost half do not know they are infected. In 2016, 1 million died, and 1.8 million were newly infected. Most new infections (95%) occur in the developing world, and > 1/2 are in women. In many sub-Saharan African countries, incidence is declining markedly from the very high rates of a decade before.

In the US in 2014, 1,107,700 people aged ≥ 13 yr were estimated to be living with HIV infection; HIV was undiagnosed in about 15% of them. About 50,000 new cases are estimated to occur each year in the US. In 2015, there were 39,513 new cases. Over two thirds of new infections occurred in gay and bisexual men; black/African American gay and bisexual men accounted for the largest number of HIV diagnoses (10,315), followed by white and bisexual men (7,570[2]).

AIDS: AIDS is defined as one or more of the following:

- HIV infection that leads to any of the certain illnesses (see Sidebar 194–2)[3]
- A CD4+ T lymphocyte (helper cell) count of < 200/μL
- A CD4+ cell percentage of ≤ 14%

AIDS-defining illnesses are

- Serious opportunistic infections
- Certain cancers (eg, Kaposi sarcoma, non-Hodgkin lymphoma) to which defective cell-mediated immunity predisposes
- Neurologic dysfunction

1. UNAIDS. Fact sheet: Latest statistics on the status of the AIDS epidemic at www.unaids.org/en/resources/fact-sheet
2. CDC: HIV in the United States: At A Glance at www.cdc.gov/hiv/statistics/overview/ataglance.html
3. Selik RM, Mokotoff ED, Branson, B, et al: Revised Surveillance Case Definition for HIV Infection—United States, 2014. *MMWR* 63(RR03):1–10, 2014.

Transmission

Transmission of HIV requires contact with body fluids—specifically blood, semen, vaginal secretions, breast milk, saliva, or exudates from wounds or skin and mucosal lesions—that contain free HIV virions or infected cells. Transmission is more likely with the high levels of virions that are typical during primary infection, even when such infections are asymptomatic. Transmission by saliva or droplets produced by coughing or sneezing, although conceivable, is extremely unlikely. HIV is not transmitted by casual nonsexual contact as may occur at work, school, or home.

Transmission is usually

- Sexual: Direct transfer of genital, rectal or oral fluids through sexual intercourse
- Needle- or instrument-related: Sharing of blood-contaminated needles or exposure to contaminated instruments
- Maternal: Childbirth or breastfeeding
- Transfusion- or transplant-related

Sexual transmission: Sexual practices such as fellatio and cunnilingus appear to be relatively low risk but not absolutely safe (see Table 194–1). Risk does not increase significantly if semen or vaginal secretions are swallowed. However, open sores in the mouth may increase risk.

The sexual practices with the highest risks are those that cause mucosal trauma, typically intercourse. Anal-receptive intercourse poses the highest risk. Mucous membrane inflammation facilitates HIV transmission; sexually transmitted diseases, such as gonorrhea, chlamydial infection, trichomoniasis, and especially those that cause ulceration (eg, chancroid, herpes, syphilis), increase the risk severalfold.

In heterosexuals, the estimated risk per coital act is about 1/1000; however, risk is increased in the following:

- Early and advanced stages of HIV infection when HIV concentrations in plasma and genital fluids are higher
- Younger people
- People with ulcerative genital diseases

Sidebar 194–2. AIDS-Defining Illnesses

- Bacterial infections, multiple or recurrent
- Candidiasis of bronchi, trachea, or lungs
- Candidiasis of esophagus
- Cervical cancer, invasive
- Coccidioidomycosis, disseminated or extrapulmonary
- Cryptococcosis, extrapulmonary
- Cryptosporidiosis, chronic intestinal (lasting > 1 mo)
- Cytomegalovirus disease (other than liver, spleen, or lymph nodes), onset at age > 1 mo
- Cytomegalovirus retinitis (with loss of vision)
- Encephalopathy attributed to HIV
- Herpes simplex: chronic ulcers (lasting > 1 mo) or bronchitis, pneumonitis, or esophagitis (onset at age > 1 mo)
- Histoplasmosis, disseminated or extrapulmonary
- Isosporiasis, chronic intestinal (lasting > 1 mo)
- Kaposi sarcoma
- Lymphoma, Burkitt (or equivalent term)
- Lymphoma, immunoblastic (or equivalent term)
- Lymphoma, primary, of brain
- *Mycobacterium avium* complex or *Mycobacterium kansasii*, disseminated or extrapulmonary
- *Mycobacterium tuberculosis* of any site, pulmonary, disseminated, or extrapulmonary
- *Mycobacterium*, other species or unidentified species, disseminated or extrapulmonary
- *Pneumocystis jirovecii* (previously known as *Pneumocystis carinii*) pneumonia
- Pneumonia, recurrent
- Progressive multifocal leukoencephalopathy
- *Salmonella* septicemia, recurrent
- Toxoplasmosis of brain, onset at age > 1 mo
- Wasting syndrome attributed to HIV

See also Revised Surveillance Case Definition for HIV Infection.

Table 194–1. HIV TRANSMISSION RISK FOR SEVERAL SEXUAL ACTIVITIES

RISK	ACTIVITY
None (unless sores are present)	Dry kissing Body-to-body rubbing and massage Using unshared inserted sexual devices Genital stimulation by a partner but no contact with semen or vaginal fluids Bathing or showering together Contact with feces or urine if skin is intact
Theoretical (extremely low risk unless sores are present)	Wet kissing Fellatio (oral sex done to a male) without ejaculation if a condom is used Cunnilingus (oral sex done to a female) if a barrier is used Oral-anal contact Digital vaginal or anal penetration, with or without a glove Use of shared but disinfected inserted sexual devices
Low	Fellatio without a condom and with ejaculation Cunnilingus if no barrier is used Vaginal or anal intercourse if a condom is used correctly Use of shared but not disinfected inserted sexual devices
High	Vaginal or anal intercourse with or without ejaculation if a condom is not used or is not used correctly

Circumcision seems to reduce the risk of males acquiring HIV infection by about 50% by removing the penile mucosa (underside of foreskin), which is more susceptible to HIV infection than the keratinized, stratified squamous epithelium that covers the rest of the penis.

Needle- and instrument-related transmission: Risk of HIV transmission after skin penetration with a medical instrument contaminated with infected blood is on average about 1/300 without postexposure antiretroviral prophylaxis. Immediate prophylaxis probably reduces risk to < 1/1500. Risk appears to be higher if the wound is deep or if blood is inoculated (eg, with a contaminated hollow-bore needle). Risk is also increased with hollow-bore needles and with punctures of arteries of veins compared with solid needles or other penetrating objects coated with blood because larger volumes of blood may be transferred. Thus, sharing needles that have entered the veins of other injection drug users is a very high risk activity.

Risk of transmission from infected health care practitioners who take appropriate precautions is unclear but appears minimal. In the 1980s, one dentist transmitted HIV to ≥ 6 of his patients by unknown means. However, extensive investigations of patients cared for by other HIV-infected physicians, including surgeons, have uncovered few other cases.

Maternal transmission: HIV can be transmitted from mother to offspring

- Transplacentally
- Perinatally
- Via breast milk

Without treatment, risk of transmission at birth is about 25 to 35%.

HIV is excreted in breast milk, and breastfeeding by untreated HIV-infected mothers may transmit HIV to about 10 to 15% of infants who had previously escaped infection. These rates can be reduced dramatically by treating HIV-positive mothers with antiretroviral drugs while they are pregnant, in labor, and breastfeeding.

Because many HIV-positive pregnant women are treated or take prophylactic drugs, the incidence of AIDS in children is decreasing in many countries (see p. 2599).

Transfusion- and transplant-related transmission: Screening of blood donors with tests for both antibody to HIV and HIV RNA has minimized risk of transmission via transfusion. Current risk of transmitting HIV via blood transfusion is probably < 1/2,000,000 per unit transfused in the US. However, in many developing countries, where blood and blood products are not screened for HIV, the risk of transfusion-transmitted HIV infection remains high.

Rarely, HIV has been transmitted via transplantation of organs from HIV-seropositive donors. Infection has developed in recipients of kidney, liver, heart, pancreas, bone, and skin—all of which contain blood—but screening for HIV greatly reduces risk of transmission. HIV transmission is even more unlikely from transplantation of cornea, ethanol-treated and lyophilized bone, fresh-frozen bone without marrow, lyophilized tendon or fascia, or lyophilized and irradiated dura mater.

HIV transmission is possible via artificial insemination using sperm from HIV-positive donors. Some cases of infection occurred in the early 1980s, before safeguards were introduced. In the US, sperm washing is considered an effective method of reducing the risk of partner insemination from a known HIV-positive sperm donor.

Epidemiology

HIV has spread in 2 epidemiologically distinct patterns:

- Male homosexual intercourse or contact with infected blood (eg, through sharing needles in injection drug users; before effective screening of donors, through transfusions)
- Heterosexual intercourse (affecting men and women about equally)

In most countries, both patterns occur, but the first pattern usually predominates in developed countries; the second pattern predominates in Africa, South America, and southern Asia.

In areas where heterosexual transmission is dominant, HIV infection follows routes of trade, transportation, and economic migration to cities and spreads secondarily to rural areas. In Africa, particularly southern Africa, the HIV epidemic has killed tens of millions of young adults, creating millions of orphans. Factors that perpetuate spread include

- Poverty
- Poor education
- Deficient systems of medical care that do not provide access to HIV testing and antiretroviral drugs

However, as of 2016, through international efforts, an estimated 19.5 million people living with HIV infection were accessing antiretroviral drugs, dramatically reducing deaths and transmission in many countries.

Many opportunistic infections that complicate HIV are reactivations of latent infections. Thus, epidemiologic factors that determine the prevalence of latent infections also influence risk of specific opportunistic infections. In many developing countries, prevalence of latent TB and toxoplasmosis in the general population is higher than in developed countries. Dramatic increases in reactivated TB and toxoplasmic encephalitis have followed the epidemic of HIV-induced immunosuppression in these countries.

Similarly in the US, incidence of coccidioidomycosis, common in the Southwest, and histoplasmosis, common in the Midwest, has increased because of HIV infection.

Human herpesvirus 8 infection, which causes Kaposi sarcoma, is common among homosexual and bisexual men but uncommon among other HIV patients in the US and Europe. Thus, in the US, > 90% of AIDS patients who have developed Kaposi sarcoma are homosexual or bisexual men.

Pathophysiology

HIV attaches to and penetrates host T cells via CD4+ molecules and chemokine receptors (see Fig. 194–1). After attachment, HIV RNA and several HIV-encoded enzymes are released into the host cell.

Viral replication requires that reverse transcriptase (an RNA-dependent DNA polymerase) copy HIV RNA, producing proviral DNA; this copying mechanism is prone to errors, resulting in frequent mutations. These mutations facilitate the generation of HIV that can resist control by the host's immune system and by antiretroviral drugs.

Proviral DNA enters the host cell's nucleus and is integrated into the host DNA in a process that involves integrase, another HIV enzyme. With each cell division, the integrated proviral DNA is duplicated along with the host DNA. Subsequently, the proviral HIV DNA can be transcribed to HIV RNA and translated to HIV proteins, such as the envelope glycoproteins 41 and 120. These HIV proteins are assembled into HIV virions at the host cell inner membrane and budded from the cell surface within an envelope of modified human cell membrane. Each host cell may produce thousands of virions.

After budding, protease, another HIV enzyme, cleaves viral proteins, converting the immature virion into a mature, infectious virion.

Infected CD4+ lymphocytes produce > 98% of plasma HIV virions. A subset of infected CD4+ lymphocytes constitutes a reservoir of HIV that can reactivate (eg, if antiviral treatment is stopped).

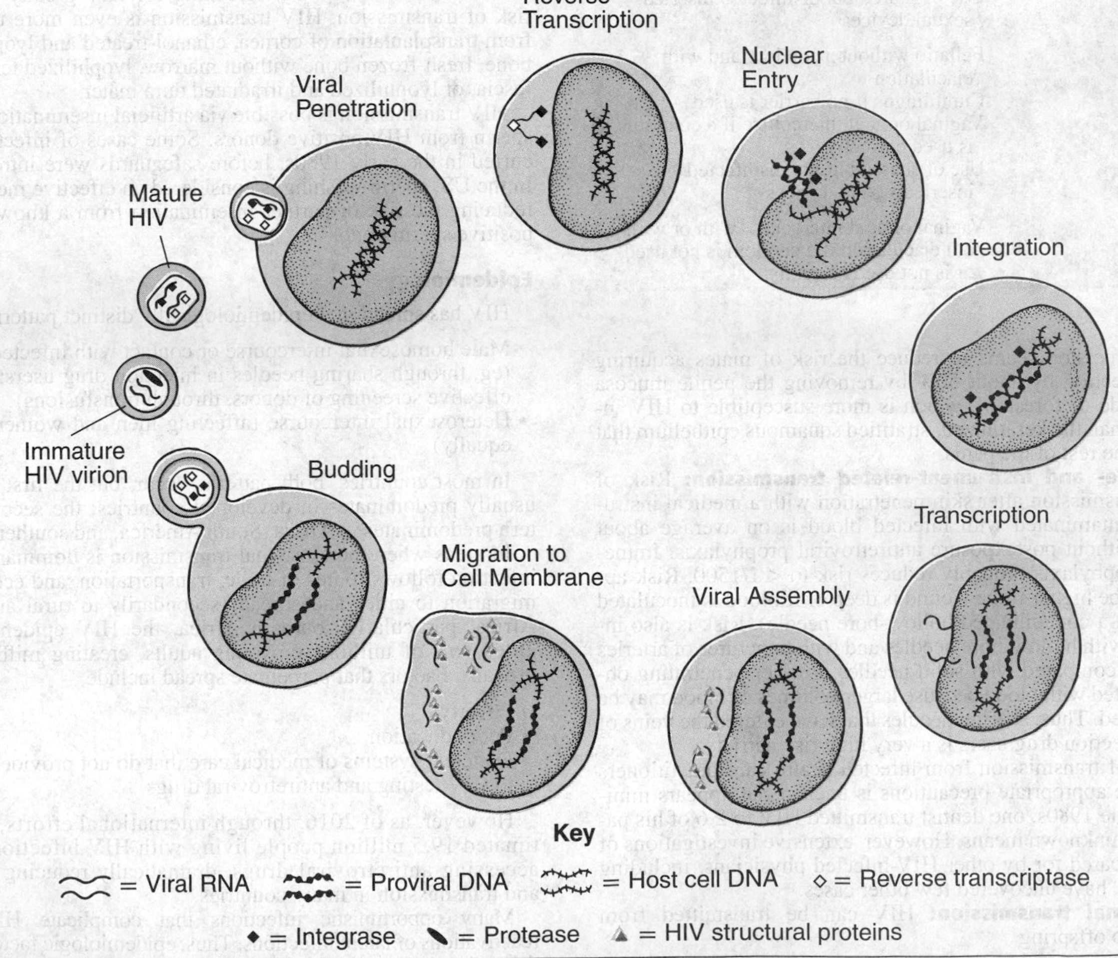

Fig. 194–1. Simplified HIV life cycle. HIV attaches to and penetrates host T cells, then releases HIV RNA and enzymes into the host cell. HIV reverse transcriptase copies viral RNA as proviral DNA. Proviral DNA enters the host cell's nucleus, and HIV integrase facilitates the proviral DNA's integration into the host's DNA. The host cell then produces HIV RNA and HIV proteins. HIV proteins are assembled into HIV virions and budded from the cell surface. HIV protease cleaves viral proteins, converting the immature virion to a mature, infectious virion.

Virions have a plasma half-life of about 6 h. In moderate to heavy HIV infection, about 10^8 to 10^9 virions are created and removed daily. The high volume of HIV replication and high frequency of transcription errors by HIV reverse transcriptase result in many mutations, increasing the chance of producing strains resistant to host immunity and drugs.

Immune system: Two main consequences of HIV infection are

- Damage to the immune system, specifically depletion of CD4+ lymphocytes
- Immune activation

CD4+ lymphocytes are involved in cell-mediated and, to a lesser extent, humoral immunity. CD4+ depletion may result from the following:

- Direct cytotoxic effects of HIV replication
- Cell-mediated immune cytotoxicity
- Thymic damage that impairs lymphocyte production

Infected CD4+ lymphocytes have a half-life of about 2 days, which is much shorter than that of uninfected CD4+ cells. Rates of CD4+ lymphocyte destruction correlate with plasma HIV level. Typically, during the initial or primary infection, HIV levels are highest (> 10^6 copies/mL), and the CD4 count drops rapidly.

The normal CD4 count is about 750/μL, and immunity is minimally affected if the count is > 350/μL. If the count drops below about 200/μL, loss of cell-mediated immunity allows a variety of opportunistic pathogens to reactivate from latent states and cause clinical disease.

The humoral immune system is also affected. Hyperplasia of B cells in lymph nodes causes lymphadenopathy, and secretion of antibodies to previously encountered antigens increases, often leading to hyperglobulinemia. Total antibody levels (especially IgG and IgA) and titers against previously encountered antigens may be unusually high. However, antibody response to new antigens (eg, in vaccines) decreases as the CD4 count decreases.

Abnormal elevation of immune activation may be caused in part by absorption of components of bowel bacteria. Immune activation contributes to CD4+ depletion and immunosupression by mechanisms that remain unclear.

Other tissues: HIV also infects nonlymphoid monocytic cells (eg, dendritic cells in the skin, macrophages, brain microglia) and cells of the brain, genital tract, heart, and kidneys, causing disease in the corresponding organ systems.

HIV strains in several compartments, such as the nervous system (brain and CSF) and genital tract (semen), can be genetically distinct from those in plasma, suggesting that they have been selected by or have adapted to these anatomic compartments. Thus, HIV levels and resistance patterns in these compartments may vary independently from those in plasma.

Disease progression: During the first few weeks of primary infection, there are humoral and cellular immune responses:

- **Humoral:** Antibodies to HIV are usually measurable within a few weeks after primary infection; however, antibodies cannot fully control HIV infection because mutated forms of HIV that are not controlled by the patient's current anti-HIV antibodies are generated.
- **Cellular:** Cell-mediated immunity is a more important means of controlling the high levels of viremia (usually over 10^6 copies/mL) at first. But rapid mutation of viral antigens that are targeted by lymphocyte-mediated cytotoxicity subvert control of HIV in all but a small percentage of patients.

Plasma HIV virion levels, expressed as number of HIV RNA copies/mL, stabilize after about 6 mo at a level (set point) that varies widely among patients but averages 30,000 to 100,000/mL (4.2 to 5 $\log_{10}$/mL). The higher this set point, the more quickly the CD4 count decreases to a level that seriously impairs immunity (< 200/μL) and results in the opportunistic infections and cancers that define AIDS.

Risk and severity of opportunistic infections, AIDS, and AIDS-related cancers are determined by 2 factors:

- CD4 count
- Exposure to potentially opportunistic pathogens

Risk of specific opportunistic infections increases below threshold CD4 counts of about 200/μL for some infections and 50/μL for others, as in the following:

- CD4 count < 200/μL: Increased risk of *Pneumocystis jirovecii* pneumonia, toxoplasmic encephalitis, and cryptococcal meningitis
- CD4 count < 50/μL: Increased risk of cytomegalovirus (CMV) and *Mycobacterium avium* complex (MAC) infections

For every 3-fold (0.5 $\log_{10}$) increase in plasma HIV RNA in untreated patients, risk of progression to AIDS or death over the next 2 to 3 yr increases about 50%.

Without treatment, risk of progression to AIDS is about 1 to 2%/yr in the first 2 to 3 yr of infection and about 5 to 6%/yr thereafter. Eventually, AIDS almost invariably develops in untreated patients.

Symptoms and Signs

Initial HIV infection: Initially, primary HIV infection may be asymptomatic or cause transient nonspecific symptoms (acute retroviral syndrome).

Acute retroviral syndrome usually begins within 1 to 4 wk of infection and usually lasts 3 to 14 days. Symptoms and signs are often mistaken for infectious mononucleosis or benign, nonspecific viral syndromes and may include fever, malaise, fatigue, several types of dermatitis, sore throat, arthralgias, generalized lymphadenopathy, and septic meningitis.

After the first symptoms disappear, most patients, even without treatment, have no symptoms or only a few mild, intermittent, nonspecific symptoms for a highly variable time period (2 to 15 yr).

Symptoms during this relatively asymptomatic period may result from HIV directly or from opportunistic infections. The following are most common:

- Lymphadenopathy
- White plaques due to oral candidiasis
- Herpes zoster
- Diarrhea
- Fatigue
- Fever with intermittent sweats

Asymptomatic, mild-to-moderate cytopenias (eg, leukopenia, anemia, thrombocytopenia) are also common. Some patients experience progressive wasting (which may be related to anorexia and increased catabolism due to infections) and low-grade fevers or diarrhea.

Worsening HIV infection: When the CD4 count drops to < 200/μL, nonspecific symptoms may worsen and a succession of AIDS-defining illnesses develop (see Sidebar 194–2).

Evaluation may detect infections that do not typically occur in the general population, such as *Mycobacterium* sp, *P. jirovecii*, *Cryptococcus neoformans*, or other fungal infections.

Infections that also occur in the general population but suggest AIDS if they are unusually severe or frequently recur include herpes zoster, herpes simplex, vaginal candidiasis, and *Salmonella* septicemia.

In patients with HIV infection, certain syndromes are common and may require different considerations (see Table 194–2). Some patients present with cancers (eg, Kaposi sarcoma, B-cell lymphomas) that occur more frequently, are unusually severe, or have unique features in patients with HIV infection (see p. 1643). In other patients, neurologic dysfunction may occur.

Diagnosis

- HIV antibody testing
- Nucleic acid amplification assays to determine HIV RNA level (viral load)

HIV infection is suspected in patients with persistent, unexplained, generalized adenopathy or any of the AIDS-defining illnesses (see Sidebar 194–2). It may also be suspected in high-risk patients with symptoms that could represent acute primary HIV infection.

Diagnostic tests: Detection of antibodies to HIV is sensitive and specific except during the first few weeks after infection. Enzyme-linked immunosorbent assay (ELISA) to detect HIV antibodies is highly sensitive, but rarely, results are false-positive. Positive ELISA results are therefore confirmed with a more specific test such as Western blot. However, these tests have drawbacks:

- ELISA requires complex equipment.
- Western blot requires well-trained technicians and is expensive.
- The full testing sequence takes at least a day.

Newer point-of-care tests using blood or saliva (eg, particle agglutination, immunoconcentration, immunochromatography) can be done quickly (in 15 min) and simply, allowing testing in a variety of settings and immediate reporting to patients. Positive results of these rapid tests should be confirmed by standard blood tests (eg, ELISA with or without Western blot) in developed countries and repetition with one or more other rapid tests in developing countries. Negative tests need not be confirmed.

If HIV infection is suspected despite negative antibody test results (eg, during the first few weeks after infection), the plasma HIV RNA level may be measured. The nucleic acid amplification assays used are highly sensitive and specific. HIV RNA assays require advanced technology, such as reverse transcription–PCR (RT-PCR), which is sensitive to extremely low HIV RNA levels. Measuring p24 HIV antigen (p24 is a core protein of the virus) by ELISA is less sensitive and less specific than directly detecting HIV RNA in blood.

Monitoring: When HIV is diagnosed, the following should be determined:

- CD4 count
- Plasma HIV RNA level

Both are useful for determining prognosis and monitoring treatment.

The CD4 count is calculated as the product of the following:

- WBC count (eg, 4000 cells/mL)
- Percentage of WBCs that are lymphocytes (eg, 30%)
- Percentage of lymphocytes that are CD4+ (eg, 20%)

Using the numbers above, the CD4 count (4000 x 0.3 x 0.2) is 240 cells/mL, or about 1/3 of the normal CD4 count in adults, which is about 750 ± 250/μL.

Plasma HIV RNA level (viral load) reflects HIV replication rates. The higher the set point (the relatively stable virus levels that occur after primary infection), the more quickly the CD4 count decreases and the greater the risk of opportunistic infection, even in patients without symptoms.

Staging: HIV infection can be staged based on the CD4 count. In patients ≥ 6 yr, stages are as follows:

- Stage 1: ≥ 500 cells/μL
- Stage 2: 200 to 499 cells/μL
- Stage 3: < 200 cells/μL

The CD4 count after 1 to 2 yr of treatment provides an indication of ultimate immune recovery; CD4 counts may not return to the normal range despite prolonged suppression of HIV.

HIV-related conditions: Diagnosis of the various opportunistic infections, cancers, and other syndromes that occur in HIV-infected patients is discussed elsewhere in THE MANUAL. Many have aspects unique to HIV infection.

Hematologic disorders (eg, cytopenias, lymphomas, cancers) are common and may be usefully evaluated with bone marrow aspiration and biopsy. This procedure can also help diagnose disseminated infections with MAC, *M. tuberculosis, Cryptococcus, Histoplasma*, human parvovirus B19, *P. jirovecii*, and *Leishmania*. Most patients have normocellular or hypercellular marrow despite peripheral cytopenia, reflecting peripheral destruction. Iron stores are usually normal or increased, reflecting anemia of chronic disease (an iron-reutilization defect). Mild to moderate plasmacytosis, lymphoid aggregates, increased numbers of histiocytes, and dysplastic changes in hematopoietic cells are common.

HIV-associated neurologic syndromes can be differentiated via lumbar puncture with CSF analysis and contrast-enhanced CT or MRI (see Table 194–2 and elsewhere in THE MANUAL).

Screening for HIV: Screening antibody tests should be offered routinely to adults and adolescents, particularly pregnant women, regardless of their perceived risk. For people at highest risk, especially sexually active people who have multiple partners and who do not practice safe sex, testing should be repeated every 6 to 12 mo. Such testing is confidential and available, often free of charge, in many public and private facilities throughout the world.

Prognosis

Risk of AIDS, death, or both is predicted by the

- CD4 count in the short term
- Plasma HIV RNA level in the longer term

For every 3-fold (0.5 $\log_{10}$) increase in viral load, mortality over the next 2 to 3 yr increases about 50%. HIV-associated morbidity and mortality vary by the CD4 count, with the most deaths from HIV-related causes occurring at counts of < 50/μL. However, with effective treatment, the HIV RNA level decreases to undetectable levels, CD4 counts often increase dramatically, and risk of illness and death falls but remains higher than that for age-matched populations not infected with HIV.

Another less well-understood prognostic factor is the level of immune activation as determined by evaluating the expression of activation markers on CD4 and CD8 lymphocytes. Activation, which may be caused by leakage of bacteria across the HIV-damaged colonic mucosa, is a strong prognostic predictor but is not used clinically because this test is not widely available and antiretroviral therapy changes the prognosis, making this test less important.

Table 194–2. COMMON MANIFESTATIONS OF HIV INFECTION BY ORGAN SYSTEM

SYNDROME	CAUSE	DIAGNOSTIC EVALUATION	TREATMENT	SYMPTOMS/ COMMENTS
Cardiac				
Cardiomyopathy	Direct viral damage to cardiac myocytes	Echocardiography	Antiretroviral drugs	Symptoms of heart failure
GI				
Esophagitis	Candidiasis, CMV, or herpes simplex virus	Esophagoscopy with biopsy of ulcers	Treatment of cause	Dysphagia, anorexia
Gastroenteritis or colitis	Intestinal *Salmonella*, MAC, *Cryptosporidium*, *Cyclospora*, CMV, microsporidia, *Cystoisospora (Isospora) belli* (cystoisosporiasis), or *Clostridium difficile*	Cultures and stains of stools or biopsy, but determination of cause possibly difficult	For all, supportive treatment for symptoms, treatment of cause, and prompt initiation of antiretroviral drugs, as for the following: • Antibiotics for *Salmonella*, MAC, and *C. difficile* • Prompt use of antiretroviral drugs for *Cryptosporidium*, *Cyclospora*, and microsporidia • TMP/SMX for *Cyclospora*, *Cystoisospora*, and microsporidia • Antiviral drugs for CMV	Diarrhea, weight loss, abdominal cramping
Cholecystitis or cholangitis	CMV, *Cryptosporidium*, *Cyclospora*, or microsporidia	Ultrasonography or endoscopy	Treatment of CMV Antiretroviral drugs for *Cryptosporidium, Cyclospora*, and microsporidia	Possibly pain or obstruction
Anal, rectal, and perirectal lesions	Herpes simplex virus, human papillomavirus, or anal cancer Possibly multiple causes	Examination Gram staining and culture Biopsy	Treatment of cause	High incidence in homosexual men who are infected with human papillomavirus via anal receptive sexual intercourse
Hepatocellular damage due to hepatitis viruses, opportunistic infections, or antiviral drug toxicity	TB, MAC, CMV, or peliosis (bartonellosis) Chronic hepatitis B or C, which may be worsened by HIV	Differentiation from hepatitis due to antiretroviral or other drugs Liver biopsy sometimes necessary	Treatment of cause	Symptoms of hepatitis (eg, anorexia, nausea, vomiting, jaundice)
Gynecologic				
Vaginal candidiasis	*Candida*	See p. 2314	See p. 2314	Possibly increased in severity or recurrent
Pelvic inflammatory disease	*Neisseria gonorrhoeae, Chlamydia trachomatis*, or other usual pathogens	See p. 2316	See p. 2316	Possibly increased in severity, atypical, and difficult to treat
Hematologic				
Anemia	Multifactorial: HIV-induced bone marrow suppression Immune-mediated peripheral destruction Anemia of chronic disease Infections, particularly human parvovirus B-19, disseminated MAC, or histoplasmosis Cancers	See p. 1090 For parvovirus B19 infection, bone marrow examination (to check for multinucleated erythroblasts) or serum or bone marrow PCR	Treatment of cause Transfusion as needed Erythropoietin for anemia due to antineoplastic drugs or zidovudine if severity warrants transfusion and erythropoietin level is < 500 mU/L IVIG for parvovirus	With parvovirus, sometimes acute severe anemia

Table continues on the following page.

Table 194–2. COMMON MANIFESTATIONS OF HIV INFECTION BY ORGAN SYSTEM (*Continued*)

SYNDROME	CAUSE	DIAGNOSTIC EVALUATION	TREATMENT	SYMPTOMS/ COMMENTS
Thrombocytopenia	Immune thrombocytopenia, drug toxicity, HIV-induced marrow suppression, immune-mediated peripheral destruction, infections, or cancer	CBC, clotting tests, PTT, peripheral smear, bone marrow biopsy, or von Willebrand factor measurement	Antiretroviral drugs IVIG for bleeding or preoperatively Possibly anti-Rho (D) IgG, vincristine, danazol, or interferon If severe and intractable, splenectomy	Often asymptomatic and may occur in otherwise asymptomatic HIV infection
Neutropenia	HIV-induced bone marrow suppression, immune-mediated peripheral destruction, infections, cancer, or drug toxicity	See p. 1154	For severe neutropenia (< 500/µL) plus fever, immediate broad-spectrum antibiotics If drug-induced, granulocyte or granulocyte-macrophage colony-stimulating factors	—
Neurologic				
Mild to severe cognitive impairment with or without motor deficits	Direct virus-induced brain damage	HIV RNA level in CSF CT or MRI to check for brain atrophy (nonspecific)	Antiretroviral drugs, which may reverse damage and improve function, although low levels of cognitive dysfunction commonly persist, even in treated patients	Progression to dementia uncommon in treated patients
Ascending paralysis	Guillain-Barré syndrome or CMV polyradiculopathy	Spinal cord MRI CSF testing	Treatment of CMV polyradiculopathy Supportive care for Guillain-Barré syndrome	Neutrophilic pleocytosis in patients with CMV polyradiculopathy, possibly simulating bacterial meningitis
Acute or subacute focal encephalitis	*Toxoplasma gondii* (toxoplasmosis)	CT or MRI to check for ring-enhancing lesions, especially near basal ganglia Antibody testing of CSF (sensitive but not specific) PCR testing to check for *T. gondii* DNA in CSF Brain biopsy (rarely indicated)	Pyrimethamine, folinic acid, sulfadiazine, and possibly trimethoprim/sulfamethoxazole (clindamycin if allergic to sulfa—see p. 1562) Often lifelong maintenance therapy	Primary prophylaxis with clindamycin and pyrimethamine or trimethoprim/ sulfamethoxazole (as for *Pneumocystis* pneumonia) indicated for patients with a CD4 count of < 100/µL and previous toxoplasmosis or positive antibodies; can be stopped if CD4 counts increase to > 200/µL for ≥ 3 mo in response to antiretroviral therapy
Subacute encephalitis	CMV Less often, herpes simplex virus or varicella-zoster virus	CSF PCR Response to treatment	Antiviral drugs	With CMV, often delirium, cranial nerve palsies, myoclonus, seizures, and progressively impaired consciousness at presentation Often responds rapidly to treatment
Myelitis or polyradiculopathy	CMV	Spinal cord MRI CSF PCR	Antiviral drugs	Simulates Guillain-Barré syndrome
Progressive encephalitis of white matter only	Progressive multifocal leukoencephalopathy due to reactivation of latent JC virus infection	Brain MRI CSF testing	Antiretroviral drugs to reverse the immunodeficiency (no drugs are effective for JC virus)	Usually fatal within a few months May respond to antiretroviral drugs
	HIV			

Table 194–2. COMMON MANIFESTATIONS OF HIV INFECTION BY ORGAN SYSTEM (*Continued*)

SYNDROME	CAUSE	DIAGNOSTIC EVALUATION	TREATMENT	SYMPTOMS/ COMMENTS
Subacute meningitis	*Cryptococcus*, *Histoplasma*, *Coccidioidomycosis*, or *Mycobacterium tuberculosis*	CT or MRI CSF stains, antigen tests, and cultures	Treatment of cause	Outcomes improved by early treatment
Peripheral neuropathy	Direct effects of HIV or CMV or antiviral drug toxicity	History Sensory and motor testing	Treatment of cause or withdrawal of toxic drugs	Very common Not quickly reversible
Ophthalmologic				
Retinitis	CMV	Direct retinoscopy	Specific anti-CMV drugs	Requires examination by specialist
Oral				
Oral candidiasis	Immunosuppression by HIV	Examination	Systemic antifungals	Possibly painless in early stages
Intraoral ulcers	Herpes simplex virus or aphthous stomatitis	Examination	For aphthous ulcers, intralesional or systemic corticosteroids and systemic montelukast and thalidomide For herpes, acyclovir	May be severe and result in undernutrition
Periodontal disease	Mixed oral bacterial flora	Examination	Improved hygiene and nutrition Antibiotics	May be severe, with bleeding, swelling, and tooth loss
Painless intraoral mass	Kaposi sarcoma, lymphoma, or human papillomavirus-related tumors	Biopsy	Treatment of neoplasm	—
Painless white filiform patches on the sides of the tongue (oral hairy leukoplakia)	Epstein-Barr virus	Examination	Acyclovir	Usually asymptomatic
Pulmonary				
Subacute (occasionally acute) pneumonia	Mycobacteria, fungi such as *P. jirovecii*, *C. neoformans*, *H. capsulatum*, *Coccidioides immitis*, or *Aspergillus*	Pulse oximetry Chest x-ray Skin tests (sometimes false-negative because of anergy) Bronchoscopy with special stains and cultures of bronchial lavage specimens sometimes necessary	Treatment of cause	Possibly cough, tachypnea, and chest discomfort at presentation Mild hypoxia or increased alveolar-arterial O_2 gradient possibly occurring before evidence of pneumonia on x-ray
Acute (occasionally subacute) pneumonia	Typical bacterial pathogens or *Haemophilus*, *Pseudomonas*, *Nocardia*, or *Rhodococcus*	In patients with known or suspected HIV and pneumonia, exclusion of opportunistic or unusual pathogens	Treatment of cause	Possibly cough, tachypnea, and chest discomfort at presentation
Tracheobronchitis	*Candida* or herpes simplex virus	—	Treatment of cause	Possibly cough, tachypnea, and chest discomfort at presentation
Subacute or chronic pneumonia or mediastinal adenopathy	Kaposi sarcoma or B-cell lymphoma	Chest CT Bronchoscopy	Treatment of cause	Possibly cough, tachypnea, and chest discomfort at presentation
Renal				
Nephrotic syndrome or renal insufficiency	Direct viral damage, resulting in focal glomerulosclerosis	Renal biopsy	Antiretroviral drugs or ACE inhibitors possibly useful	Increased incidence in African Americans and patients with a low CD4 count

Table continues on the following page.

Table 194–2. COMMON MANIFESTATIONS OF HIV INFECTION BY ORGAN SYSTEM (*Continued*)

SYNDROME	CAUSE	DIAGNOSTIC EVALUATION	TREATMENT	SYMPTOMS/ COMMENTS
Tubular dysfunction (glucosuria, proteinuria)	Some antiviral drugs	Urinalysis and/or blood tests	Dose reduction or discontinuation of the antiviral drug	—
Skin				
Herpes zoster	Varicella-zoster virus	Clinical evaluation	Acyclovir or related drugs	Common Possible prodrome of mild to severe pain or tingling before skin lesions
Herpes simplex ulcers	Herpes simplex virus	Usually clinical evaluation	Antiviral drugs if lesions are severe, extensive, persistent, or disseminated	Atypical lesions of herpes simplex that are extensive, severe, or persistent
Scabies	*Sarcoptes scabiei*	See p. 1060	See p. 1060	Possibly severe hyperkeratotic lesions
Violaceous or red papules or nodules	Kaposi sarcoma or bartonellosis	Biopsy	Antiretroviral drugs and treatment of cause	—
Centrally umbilicated skin lesions	Cryptococcosis or molluscum contagiosum	See pp. 1082 and 1572	See pp. 1082 and 1573	May be the presenting sign of cryptococcemia
Systemic				
Sepsis and septic shock due to nosocomial gram-negative bacillary and staphylococcal infections, disseminated opportunistic infections	Gram-negative bacilli, *Staphylococcus aureus, Candida, Salmonella, M. tuberculosis*, MAC, or *H. capsulatum*	Blood cultures Bone marrow examination	Treatment of cause	—
Wasting syndrome (substantial weight loss)	Multifactorial, including AIDS, AIDS-related opportunistic infections, AIDS-related cancers, and/or AIDS-induced hypogonadism	Defined as weight loss of > 10% of body weight	Antiretroviral drugs (the primary treatment for this syndrome) Treatment of underlying infections; treatment of AIDS-induced hypogonadism when indicated Measures to improve appetite and caloric intake	—

CMV = cytomegalovirus; IVIG = IV immune globulin; MAC = *Mycobacterium avium* complex; TMP/SMX = trimethoprim/sulfamethoxazole.

A subgroup of HIV-infected people (termed long-term nonprogressors) remains asymptomatic with high CD4 counts and low HIV levels in the blood without antiretroviral treatment. These people usually have vigorous cellular and humoral immune responses to their infecting HIV strain as measured by assays in vitro. The specificity of this effective response is shown by the following: When these people acquire a superinfection with a second strain of HIV to which their immune response is not as effective, they convert to a more typical pattern of progression. Thus, their unusually effective response to the first strain does not apply to the second strain. These cases provide a rationale for counseling HIV-infected people that they still need to avoid exposure to possible HIV superinfection through unsafe sex or needle sharing.

Cure of HIV infection has not been thought possible, and thus lifelong drug treatment is considered necessary. However, several recent cases of HIV-infected infants who were treated briefly with antiretroviral therapy after diagnosis and who have remained HIV-negative for many months after stopping treatment suggests that cure is possible in this setting.

Treatment

- Combinations of antiretroviral drugs (antiretroviral therapy [ART], sometimes called highly active ART [HAART] or combined ART [cART])
- Chemoprophylaxis for opportunistic infections in patients at high risk

Because disease-related complications can occur in untreated patients with high CD4 counts and because less toxic drugs have been developed, treatment with ART is now recommended for nearly all patients. A few exceptional patients can control their HIV strain without treatment, maintaining very low blood levels of HIV and normal CD4 counts for long periods. These patients may not require ART, but studies to determine whether treating them is helpful have not been done and would be difficult because there are few of these patients and they would likely do well not taking ART for long periods.

Antiretroviral therapy: General principles: ART aims to

- Reduce the plasma HIV RNA level to undetectable (ie, < 20 to 50 copies/mL)
- Restore the CD4 count to a normal level (immune restoration or reconstitution)

A poor CD4 count response is more likely if the CD4 count at initiation of treatment is low (especially if < 50/μL) and/or the HIV RNA level is high. However, marked improvement is likely even in patients with advanced immunosuppression. An increased CD4 count correlates with markedly decreased risk of opportunistic infections, other complications, and death. With immune restoration, patients, even those with complications that have no specific treatment (eg, HIV-induced cognitive dysfunction) or that were previously considered untreatable (eg, progressive multifocal leukoencephalopathy), may improve. Outcomes are also improved for patients with cancers (eg, lymphoma, Kaposi sarcoma) and most opportunistic infections.

ART can usually achieve its goals if patients take their drugs > 95% of the time. However, maintaining this degree of adherence is difficult. Partial suppression (failure to lower plasma levels to undetectable levels) may select for single or multiple accumulated mutations in HIV that make viruses partially or completely resistant to a single drug or entire classes of drugs. Unless subsequent treatment uses drugs of other classes to which HIV remains sensitive, treatment is more likely to fail.

Patients with most acute opportunistic infections benefit from early ART (initiated during the management of the opportunistic infection). However, for some opportunistic infections, such as tuberculous meningitis or cryptococcal meningitis, the evidence suggests that ART should be delayed until the first phase of antimicrobial therapy for these infections is finished.

The success of ART is assessed by measuring plasma HIV RNA levels every 8 to 12 wk for the first 4 to 6 mo or until HIV levels are undetectable and every 3 to 6 mo thereafter. Increasing HIV levels are the earliest evidence of treatment failure and may precede a decreasing CD4 count by months. Maintaining patients on failing drug regimens selects for HIV mutants that are more drug-resistant. However, compared with wild-type HIV, these mutants appear less able to reduce the CD4 count, and failing drug regimens are often continued when no fully suppressive regimen can be found.

If treatment fails, drug susceptibility (resistance) assays can determine the susceptibility of the dominant HIV strain to all available drugs. Genotypic and phenotypic assays are available and can help clinicians select a new regimen that should contain at least 2 and preferably 3 drugs to which the HIV strain is more susceptible. The dominant HIV strain in the blood of patients who are taken off antiretroviral therapy may revert over months to years to the wild-type (ie, susceptible) strain because the resistant mutants replicate more slowly and are replaced by the wild type. Thus, if patients have not been treated recently, the full extent of resistance may not be apparent through resistance testing, but when treatment resumes, strains with resistance mutations often reemerge from latency and again replace the wild-type HIV strain.

Classes of antiretrovirals: Multiple classes of antiretrovirals are used in ART (see Table 194–3). One class inhibits HIV entry, and the others inhibit one of the 3 HIV enzymes needed to replicate inside human cells; 3 classes inhibit reverse transcriptase by blocking its RNA-dependent and DNA-dependent DNA polymerase activity.

- **Nucleoside reverse transcriptase inhibitors (NRTIs)** are phosphorylated to active metabolites that compete for incorporation into viral DNA. They inhibit the HIV reverse transcriptase enzyme competitively and terminate synthesis of DNA chains.
- **Nucleotide reverse transcriptase inhibitors (nRTIs)** competitively inhibit the HIV reverse transcriptase enzyme, as do NRTIs, but do not require initial phosphorylation.
- **Non-nucleoside reverse transcriptase inhibitors (NNRTIs)** bind directly to the reverse transcriptase enzyme.
- **Protease inhibitors (PIs)** inhibit the viral protease enzyme that is crucial to maturation of immature HIV virions after they bud from host cells.
- **Entry inhibitors (EIs),** sometimes called fusion inhibitors, interfere with the binding of HIV to CD4+ receptors and chemokine co-receptors; this binding is required for HIV to enter cells. For example, CCR-5 inhibitors block the CCR-5 receptor.
- **Integrase inhibitors** prevent HIV DNA from being integrated into human DNA.

Antiretroviral regimens: Combinations of 3 or 4 drugs from different classes are usually necessary to fully suppress replication of wild-type HIV. The specific drugs are chosen based on the following:

- Anticipated adverse effects
- Simplicity of regimen
- Concomitant conditions (eg, hepatic or renal dysfunction)
- Other drugs being taken (to avoid drug interactions)

To maximize adherence, clinicians should choose an affordable, well-tolerated regimen that uses once/day (preferable) or bid dosing. Guidelines from expert panels for initiating, selecting, switching, and interrupting therapy and special issues concerning treatment of women and children change regularly.

Tablets containing fixed combinations of ≥ 2 drugs are now widely used to simplify regimens and improve adherence. Common combination tablets include

- Stribild: Elvitegravir 150 mg, cobicistat 150 mg, emtricitabine 200 mg, plus tenofovir disoproxil fumarate 300 mg, taken po once/day with food
- Atripla: Efavirenz 600 mg, tenofovir disoproxil fumarate 300 mg, plus emtricitabine 200 mg, taken po once/day on an empty stomach, preferably at bedtime
- Complera: Rilpivirine 25 mg, emtricitabine 200 mg, plus tenofovir disoproxil fumarate 300 mg, taken po once/day with food
- Truvada: Emtricitabine 200 mg plus tenofovir disoproxil fumarate 300 mg, taken once/day po with or without food
- Triumeq: Dolutegravir 50 mg, lamivudine 300 mg, plus abacavir 600 mg, taken po once/day with or without food

Tablets containing fixed combinations of one drug with a pharmacokinetic enhancer devoid of anti-HIV activity to increase the amount of medicine with HIV activity in the blood can be used. These combinations include

- Evotaz: Atazanavir 300 mg plus cobicistat 150 mg, taken po once/day with food
- Prezcobix: Darunavir 800 mg plus cobicistat 150 mg, taken po once/day with food

Adverse effects with combination tablets are the same as those for the individual drugs included.

Table 194–3. ANTIRETROVIRAL DRUGS

GENERIC NAME	ABBREVIATION	USUAL ADULT DOSE[a]	SOME ADVERSE EFFECTS[b]
Entry (fusion) inhibitors			
Enfuvirtide	T-20	90 mg sc bid	Hypersensitivity reactions, local injection site reactions, peripheral neuropathy, risk of bacterial pneumonia, insomnia, loss of appetite
Maraviroc (CCR5 inhibitor)	—	150–600 mg bid, depending on other drugs used	Myocardial ischemia or infarction
Integrase inhibitors			
Dolutegravir	—	50 mg once/day	Headache, insomnia
Elvitegravir	—	150 mg once/day	Nausea, diarrhea
Raltegravir	—	400 mg bid	Asymptomatic elevated creatinine phospokinase levels, myositis
Non-nucleoside reverse transcriptase inhibitors			Rash (occasionally severe or life threatening), liver dysfunction
Efavirenz	EFV	600 mg at bedtime	CNS symptoms, false-positive cannabinoid test results, excessive blood levels if the drug is taken after fatty meals
Etravirine	—	200 mg bid	Severe, potentially life-threatening rashes
Nevirapine	NVP	200 mg once/day for 2 wk, then 200 mg bid	Severe, potentially life-threatening hepatotoxicity and rashes, especially during the first 18 wk of treatment Increased cytochrome P-450, reducing levels of protease inhibitors, and other drugs (eg, efavirenz, clarithromycin, ethinyl estradiol, ketoconazole, itraconazole, methadone, certain antiarrhythmics, anticonvulsants, Ca channel blockers, immunosuppressants, cyclophosphamide, ergot alkaloids, fentanyl, cisapride, warfarin)
Rilpivirine	—	25 mg once/day	Fewer CNS adverse effects than efavirenz
Nucleoside reverse transcriptase inhibitors			Lactic acidosis (which can be life threatening), steatohepatitis
Abacavir	ABC	300 mg bid	Severe, potentially fatal hypersensitivity reactions with fever, rashes, nausea, vomiting, diarrhea, pharyngitis, dyspnea, and/or cough (risk is 100-fold higher in patients with HLA-B*57:01, which can be detected by genetic testing) Anorexia, nausea, vomiting Rechallenge contraindicated
Didanosine	ddI	400 mg once/day or 200 mg bid if ≥ 60 kg 250 mg once/day or 125 mg bid if < 60 kg	Peripheral neuropathy[c], Possibly life-threatening pancreatitis[d], severe hepatomegaly with steatosis, diarrhea
Emtricitabine	FTC	200 mg once/day	Minimal; skin hyperpigmentation
Lamivudine	3TC	150 mg bid or 300 mg once/day	Peripheral neuropathy, rarely pancreatitis
Stavudine	d4T	40 mg bid if ≥ 60 kg 30 mg bid if < 60 kg	Peripheral neuropathy, possibly life-threatening pancreatitis (rare), hepatic steatosis, fat redistribution with lipoatrophy of face and extremities
Zalcitabine	ddC	0.75 mg tid	Peripheral neuropathy, possibly life-threatening pancreatitis[d], oral ulcers
Zidovudine	ZDV, AZT	300 mg bid	Anemia and leukopenia[e], rarely pancreatitis, hepatic steatosis, myopathy, myositis
Nucleotide reverse transcriptase inhibitor			
Tenofovir disoproxil fumarate	TDF	300 mg once/day	Mild renal insufficiency (uncommon), other serious renal diseases (rare) Increased levels of ddI; otherwise minimal
Tenofovir alafenamide	TAF	10 mg/day	Less effect on renal factors and bone mineral density than TDF

Table 194–3. ANTIRETROVIRAL DRUGS (*Continued*)

GENERIC NAME	ABBREVIATION	USUAL ADULT DOSE[a]	SOME ADVERSE EFFECTS[b]
Protease inhibitors[f]			Nausea, vomiting, diarrhea, abdominal discomfort, increased serum glucose and hypercholesterolemia (common), increased abdominal fat, liver dysfunction, bleeding tendency (particularly in hemophiliacs)
Amprenavir	APV	1200 mg bid with food	Rash
Atazanavir	ATV	400 mg once/day	Rash, hyperbilirubinemia
Darunavir	—	800 mg once/day, taken with ritonavir 100 mg, or 600 mg bid, taken with ritonavir 100 mg bid and with food	Severe rash, hypersensitivity, fever
Fosamprenavir	None	1400 mg bid	Rash
Indinavir	IND	800 mg tid on an empty stomach (600 mg for patients taking DLV; should not be given with ddI because concurrent use reduces levels of indinavir)	Kidney stones, occasionally obstructive (patients should ingest 1300 mL of fluid daily) Cross-resistance with other protease inhibitors, especially ritonavir
Lopinavir	LPV	400 mg bid (in a fixed combination with 100 mg ritonavir) with food	Altered taste, circumoral paresthesias
Nelfinavir	NLF	1250 mg bid with food	Diarrhea
Ritonavir	RIT	600 mg bid with food	Altered taste, circumoral paresthesias Possibly decreased incidence and severity of adverse effects with dose reduction
Saquinavir	SQV	1200 mg tid, within 2 h of a meal (trough levels and efficacy possibly increased when used with ritonavir)	—
Tipranavir	TPV	500 mg with ritonavir 200 mg bid	Possibly life-threatening hepatitis and intracranial hemorrhage

[a]Doses are given orally, unless otherwise specified.
[b]All classes of antiretroviral drugs may contribute to chronic metabolic adverse effects, which include elevated cholesterol and triglycerides, insulin resistance, and centripetal redistribution of body fat. Adverse effects listed for drug class can occur when any drug in that class is used.
[c]Peripheral neuropathy may be reversible when the drug is stopped, and symptomatic treatment provides partial relief.
[d]If symptoms of pancreatitis (eg, nausea, vomiting, back and abdominal pain) occur, ddI or ddC must be immediately stopped until pancreatitis is confirmed or excluded.
[e]Anemia can be treated with transfusions or other drugs such as erythropoietin; leukopenia can be treated with colony-stimulating factor (granulocyte colony-stimulating factor or granulocyte-macrophage colony-stimulating factor).
[f]All are metabolized by the cytochrome P-450 system, creating potential for many drug interactions.

Drug interactions: Interactions between antiretrovirals may increase or decrease efficacy.

For example, efficacy can be increased by combining a subtherapeutic dose of ritonavir (100 mg once/day) with another PI (eg, lopinavir, amprenavir, indinavir, atazanavir, tipranavir). Ritonavir inhibits the hepatic enzyme that metabolizes the other PI. By slowing clearance of the therapeutically dosed PI, ritonavir increases the other drug's levels, maintains the increased levels longer, decreases the dosing interval, and increases efficacy. Another example is lamivudine (3TC) plus zidovudine (ZDV). Use of either drug as monotherapy quickly results in resistance, but the mutation that produces resistance in response to 3TC increases the susceptibility of HIV to ZDV. Thus, when used together, they are synergistic.

Conversely, interactions between antiretrovirals may decrease the efficacy of each drug. One drug may increase elimination of another drug (eg, by inducing hepatic cytochrome P-450 enzymes responsible for elimination). Another, poorly understood effect of some NRTI combinations (eg, ZDV plus stavudine [d4T]) results in decreased antiretroviral activity without increasing drug elimination.

Combining drugs often increases the risk that either drug will have an adverse effect. Possible mechanisms include the following:

- Hepatic metabolism of PIs by cytochrome P-450: The result is decreased metabolism (and increased levels) of other drugs.
- Additive toxicities: For example, combining NRTIs, such as d4T and didanosine (ddI), increases the chance of adverse metabolic effects and peripheral neuropathy.

Many drugs may interfere with antiretrovirals (see Guidelines for the Use of Antiretroviral Agents in HIV-1-Infected

Adults and Adolescents: Drug Interactions at https://aidsinfo.nih.gov); thus, interactions should always be checked before any new drug is started.

In addition to drug interactions, the following influence activity of some antiretroviral drugs and should be avoided:

- Grapefruit juice, which inhibits an enzyme in the GI tract that degrades the PI saquinavir and thus increases bioavailability of saquinavir
- St. John's wort, which can enhance metabolism of PIs and NNRTIs and thus decrease plasma PI and NNRTI levels

Adverse effects of antiretrovirals: Antiretrovirals can have serious adverse effects (see Table 194–3). Some of these effects, notably anemia, hepatitis, renal insufficiency, pancreatitis, and glucose intolerance, can be detected by blood tests before they cause symptoms. Patients should be screened regularly, both clinically and with appropriate laboratory testing (CBC; blood tests for hyperglycemia, hyperlidemia, hepatic and pancreatic damage, and renal function; urinalysis), especially after new drugs are started or unexplained symptoms develop.

Metabolic effects consist of interrelated syndromes of fat redistribution, hyperlipidemia, and insulin resistance. Subcutaneous fat is commonly redistributed from the face and extremities to the trunk, neck, breasts, and abdomen—a cosmetic effect that can stigmatize and distress patients. Treating the resulting deep facial grooves with injected collagen or polylactic acid can be beneficial.

Central obesity, hyperlipidemia, and insulin resistance, which together constitute the metabolic syndrome, increase the risk of MI, stroke, and dementia.

Antivirals from all classes appear to contribute to these metabolic effects, but PIs are the most clearly involved. Some drugs, such as ritonavir or d4T, commonly have metabolic effects. Others, such as tenofovir disoproxil fumarate, etravirine, atazanavir or darunavir (even when combined with low-dose ritonavir), raltegravir, and maraviroc, appear to have small to minimal effects on lipid levels.

Mechanisms for metabolic effects appear to be multiple; one is mitochondrial toxicity. Risk of metabolic effects (highest with PIs) and mitochondrial toxicity (highest with NRTIs) varies by drug class and within drug classes (eg, among NRTIs, highest with d4T).

Metabolic effects are dose-dependent and often begin in the first 1 to 2 yr of treatment. Lactic acidosis is uncommon but can be lethal. Nonalcoholic steatohepatitis is a risk. Long-term effects and optimal management of metabolic effects are unclear. Lipid-lowering drugs (statins) and insulin-sensitizing drugs (glitazones) may help. (See also the recommendations of the HIV Medicine Association of the Infectious Diseases Society of America and the Adult AIDS Clinical Trials Group: Guidelines for the evaluation and management of dyslipidemia in HIV-infected adults receiving antiretroviral therapy at https://academic.oup.com.)

Bone complications of ART include asymptomatic osteopenia and osteoporosis, which are common. Uncommonly, osteonecrosis of large joints such as the hip and shoulder causes severe joint pain and dysfunction. Mechanisms of bone complications are poorly understood.

Immune reconstitution inflammatory syndrome (IRIS): Patients beginning ART sometimes deteriorate clinically, even though HIV levels in their blood are suppressed and their CD4 count increases, because of an immune reaction to subclinical opportunistic infections or to residual microbial antigens after successful treatment of opportunistic infections. IRIS usually occurs in the first months of treatment but is occasionally delayed. IRIS can complicate virtually any opportunistic infection and even tumors (eg, Kaposi sarcoma) but is usually self-limited or responds to brief regimens of corticosteroids.

Determining whether clinical deterioration is caused by treatment failure, IRIS, or both requires assessment of the persistence of active infections with cultures and can be difficult.

Interruption of antiretroviral therapy: Interruption of ART is usually safe if all drugs are stopped simultaneously, but levels of slowly metabolized drugs (eg, nevirapine) may remain high and thus increase the risk of resistance. Interruption may be necessary if intervening illnesses require treatment or if drug toxicity is intolerable or needs to be evaluated. After interruption to determine which drug is responsible for toxicity, clinicians can safely restart most drugs as monotherapy for up to a few days. Note: The most important exception is abacavir; patients who had fever or rash during previous exposure to abacavir may develop severe, potentially fatal hypersensitivity reactions with reexposure.

PEARLS & PITFALLS

- If patients who had an adverse reaction to abacavir are reexposed to the drug, they may have a severe, potentially fatal hypersensitivity reaction, so they should not be given the drug again.
- Risk of an adverse reaction to abacavir is 100-fold higher in patients with HLA-B*57:01, which can be detected by genetic testing.

End-of-life care: Although antiretroviral therapy has dramatically increased life expectancy for patients with AIDS, many patients still deteriorate and die. Death may result from the following:

- Inability to take ART consistently, resulting in progressive immunosuppression
- Occurrence of untreatable opportunistic infections and cancers
- Liver failure due to hepatitis B or C
- Accelerated aging and age-related disorders

Death is rarely sudden; thus, patients usually have time to make plans. Nonetheless, patients should record their plans for health care early, with clear instructions for end-of-life care. Other legal documents, including powers of attorney and wills, should be in place. These documents are particularly important for homosexual patients because protection of assets and rights (including visitation and decision-making) for their partners may be problems.

As patients near the end of life, clinicians may need to prescribe drugs to relieve pain, anorexia, agitation, and other distressing symptoms. The profound weight loss in many people during the last stages of AIDS makes good skin care difficult. The comprehensive support provided by hospice programs helps many patients because hospice providers are unusually skilled at symptom management, and they support caregivers and patient autonomy.

Prevention

Vaccines against HIV have been difficult to develop because HIV surface proteins mutate easily, resulting in an enormous diversity of antigenic types. Nonetheless, various vaccine candidates are under study, and a few have shown promise in clinical trials. At the present time, there is no effective AIDS vaccine.

Prevention of transmission: Vaginal microbicides (including antiretroviral drugs) inserted before sexual contact have thus far proved ineffective, and some appear to increase risk for women, perhaps by damaging natural barriers to HIV.

Effective measures include the following:

- **Public education:** Education is effective and appears to have decreased rates of infection in some countries, notably Thailand and Uganda. Because sexual contact accounts for most cases, teaching people to avoid unsafe sex practices is the most relevant measure (see Table 194–1).
- **Safe sex practices:** Unless both partners are known to be free of HIV and remain monogamous, safe sex practices are essential. Safe sex practices are also advised when both partners are HIV-positive; unprotected sex between HIV-infected people may expose a person to resistant or more virulent strains of HIV and to other viruses (eg, cytomegalovirus, Epstein-Barr virus, herpes simplex virus, hepatitis B virus) that cause severe disease in AIDS patients, as well as to syphilis and other sexually transmitted diseases (STDs). Condoms offer the best protection. Oil-based lubricants should not be used because they may dissolve latex, increasing the risk of condom failure. (See also the recommendations of the Centers for Disease Control and Prevention (CDC), the Health Resources and Services Administration, the National Institutes of Health, and the HIV Medicine Association of the Infectious Diseases Society of America: Incorporating HIV Prevention into the Medical Care of Persons Living with HIV at www.cdc.gov.)
- **Counseling for parenteral drug users:** Counseling about the risk of sharing needles is important but is probably more effective if combined with provision of sterile needles, treatment of drug dependence, and rehabilitation.
- **Confidential testing for HIV infection:** Testing should be offered routinely to adolescents and adults in virtually all health care settings. To facilitate routine testing, some states no longer require written consent or extensive pre-test counseling.
- **Counseling for pregnant women:** Mother-to-child transmission has been virtually eliminated by HIV testing, treatment with ART, and, in developed countries, use of breast milk substitutes. If pregnant women test positive for HIV, risk of mother-to-child transmission should be explained. Pregnant women who do not accept immediate treatment for their HIV infection should be encouraged to accept therapy to protect the unborn baby, typically beginning at about 14 wk gestation. Combination therapy is typically used because it is more effective than monotherapy and less likely to result in drug resistance. Some drugs can be toxic to the fetus or woman and should be avoided. If women meet criteria for ART, they should begin a regimen tailored to their history and stage of pregnancy and continue it throughout pregnancy. Cesarean delivery can also reduce risk of transmission. Regardless of the antepartum regimen used or mode of delivery, all HIV-infected women should be given IV zidovudine during labor, and after birth, neonates should be given oral zidovudine, which is continued for 6 wk after delivery (see also Prevention of Perinatal Transmission on p. 2611). Some women choose to terminate their pregnancy because HIV can be transmitted in utero to the fetus or for other reasons.
- **Screening of blood and organs:** Transmission by blood transfusion is still remotely possible in the US because antibody results may be false-negative during early infection. Currently, screening blood for antibody and p24 antigen is mandated in the US and probably further reduces risk of transmission. Risk is reduced further by asking people with risk factors for HIV infection, even those with recent negative HIV antibody test results, not to donate blood or organs for transplantation. The FDA has issued draft guidance for deferral of blood donation, including deferral for 12 mo after the most recent sexual contact for men who have had sex with another man and for women who have had sex with a man who has had sex with another man (see Revised Recommendations for Reducing the Risk of HIV Transmission by Blood and Blood Products at www.fda.gov). However, use of sensitive HIV screening tests and deferral of donors of organs, blood, and blood products have not been implemented consistently in developing countries.
- **Preexposure prophylaxis with antiretrovirals (PrEP):** In PrEP, people who are not infected with HIV but are at high risk (eg, by having an HIV-infected sexual partner) take an antiretroviral drug daily to reduce their risk of infection. The combination of tenofovir disoproxil fumarate plus emtricitabine (TDF/FTC) can be used. Use of PrEP does not eliminate the need to use other methods of reducing risk of HIV infection, including using condoms and avoiding high-risk behaviors (eg, needle sharing). Data concerning infants of HIV-negative mothers taking TDF/FTC PrEP during pregnancy are incomplete, but currently, no adverse effects have been reported in children born to HIV-infected women treated with TDF/FTC. Use of PrEP to reduce the risk of HIV infection in injection drug users is being studied. For the current CDC recommendations, see Pre-Exposure Prophylaxis (PrEP) at www.cdc.gov.
- **Circumcision of men:** In young African men, circumcision has been shown to reduce their risk of acquiring HIV infection from female partners during vaginal sex by about 50%; male circumcision is probably similarly effective elsewhere. Whether male circumcision reduces HIV transmission from HIV-positive men to women or reduces the risk of acquiring HIV from an infected male partner is unknown.
- **Universal precautions:** Medical and dental health care practitioners should wear gloves in situations that may involve contact with any patient's mucous membranes or body fluids and should be taught how to avoid needlestick accidents. Home caregivers of patients with HIV infection should wear gloves if their hands may be exposed to body fluids. Surfaces or instruments contaminated by blood or other body fluids should be cleaned and disinfected. Effective disinfectants include heat, peroxide, alcohols, phenolics, and hypochlorite (bleach). Isolation of HIV-infected patients is unnecessary unless indicated by an opportunistic infection (eg, TB). Guidelines to prevent transmission from infected practitioners to patients have not been established. See also the CDC's Recommendations for Preventing Transmission of Human Immunodeficiency Virus and Hepatitis B Virus to Patients During Exposure-Prone Invasive Procedures at www.cdc.gov.
- **Treatment of HIV infection:** Treatment with ART lowers the risk of transmission

Postexposure prophylaxis (PEP): Potential consequences of exposure to HIV have prompted the development of policies and procedures, particularly preventive treatment, to decrease risk of infection to health care workers.

Preventive treatment is indicated after

- Penetrating injuries involving HIV-infected blood (usually needlesticks)
- Heavy exposure of mucous membranes (eye or mouth) to infected body fluids such as semen, vaginal fluids, or other body fluids containing blood (eg, amniotic fluid)

Body fluids such as saliva, urine, tears, nasal secretions, vomitus, or sweat are not considered potentially infectious unless they are visibly bloody.

After initial exposure to blood, the exposed area is immediately cleaned with soap and water for skin exposures and with antiseptic for puncture wounds. If mucous membranes are exposed, the area is flushed with large amounts of water.

The following are documented:

- Type of exposure
- Time elapsed since exposure
- Clinical information (including risk factors and serologic tests for HIV) about the source patient for the exposure and the person exposed

Type of exposure is defined by

- Which body fluid was involved
- Whether exposure involved a penetrating injury (eg, needlestick, cut with sharp object) and how deep the injury was
- Whether the fluid had contact with nonintact skin (eg, abraded or chapped skin) or mucous membrane

Risk of infection is about 0.3% (1:300) after a typical percutaneous exposure and about 0.09% (1:1100) after mucous membrane exposure. These risks vary, reflecting the amount of HIV transferred to the person with the injury; the amount of HIV transferred is affected by multiple factors, including viral load of the source and type of needle (eg, hollow or solid). However, these factors are no longer taken into account in PEP recommendations.

The source is qualified by whether it is known or unknown. If the source is unknown (eg, a needle on the street or in a sharps disposal container), risk should be assessed based on the circumstances of the exposure (eg, whether the exposure occurred in an area where injection drug use is prevalent, whether a needle discarded in a drug-treatment facility was used). If the source is known but HIV status is not, the source is assessed for HIV risk factors, and prophylaxis is considered (see Table 194–4).

The goal is to start PEP as soon after exposure as possible if prophylaxis is warranted. CDC recommends providing PEP within 24 to 36 h after exposure; a longer interval after exposure requires the advice of an expert.

Use of PEP is determined by risk of infection; guidelines recommend antiretroviral therapy with ≥ 3 antiretroviral drugs. The drugs should be carefully selected to minimize adverse effects and provide a convenient dosing schedule and thus encourage PEP completion. Preferred regimens include combination of 2 NRTIs and the addition of one or more drugs (eg, 2 NRTIs plus an integrase inhibitor, a PI, or an NNRTI); drugs are given for 28 days. Nevirapine is avoided because of the rare possibility of severe hepatitis. Although evidence is not conclusive, ZDV alone probably reduces risk of transmission after needlestick injuries by about 80%. For detailed recommendations, see the CDC's Guidelines for the Management of Occupational Exposures to HBV, HCV, and HIV and Recommendations for Postexposure Prophylaxis at www.cdc.gov or the University of California, Post-Exposure Prophylaxis (PEP) at http://nccc.ucsf.edu.

If the source's virus is known or suspected to be resistant to ≥ 1 drug, an expert in antiretroviral therapy and HIV transmission should be consulted. However, clinicians should not delay PEP pending expert consultation or drug susceptibility testing. Also, clinicians should provide immediate evaluation and face-to-face counseling and not delay follow-up care.

Prevention of opportunistic infections: (See also the US Public Health Service and the HIV Medicine Association of the Infectious Diseases Society of America's Guidelines for Prevention and Treatment of Opportunistic Infections in HIV-Infected Adults and Adolescents at www.cdc.com.)

Effective chemoprophylaxis is available for many opportunistic infections and reduces rates of disease due to *P. jirovecii*, *Candida*, *Cryptococcus*, and MAC. If therapy restores CD4 counts to above threshold values for > 3 mo, chemoprophylaxis can be stopped.

Primary prophylaxis depends on the CD4 count:

- CD4 count < 200/μL or oropharyngeal candidiasis (active or previous): Prophylaxis against *P. jirovecii* pneumonia is recommended. Double-strength trimethoprim/sulfamethoxazole (TMP/SMX) tablets given once/day or 3 times/wk are effective. Some adverse effects can be minimized with the 3 times/wk dose or by gradual dose escalation. Some patients who cannot tolerate TMP/SMX can tolerate dapsone (100 mg once/day). For the few patients who cannot tolerate either drug because of a troublesome adverse effect (eg, fever, neutropenia, rash), aerosolized pentamidine 300 mg once/day or atovaquone 1500 mg once/day can be used.
- CD4 count < 50/μL: Prophylaxis against disseminated MAC consists of azithromycin or clarithromycin; if neither of these drugs is tolerated, rifabutin can be used. Azithromycin can be given weekly as two 600-mg tablets; it provides protection (70%) similar to daily clarithromycin and does not interact with other drugs.

If latent TB is suspected (based on tuberculin skin tests, interferon-gamma release assays, high-risk exposure, personal history of active TB, or residence in a region with high TB

Table 194–4. POSTEXPOSURE PROPHYLAXIS RECOMMENDATIONS

INFECTION STATUS OF SOURCE	PROPHYLAXIS
HIV-positive (symptomatic or asymptomatic HIV infection, AIDS, acute seroconversion, known or unknown viral load)	PEP with ≥ 3 antiretroviral drugs
Unknown HIV status of source or unknown source	Generally, no PEP warranted*; however, consideration of PEP if source has HIV risk factors or if setting is likely to involve exposure to HIV-infected people
HIV-negative (based on antibody tests or nucleic acid amplification assays)	No PEP warranted

*PEP is optional and should be based on an individualized decision by the exposed person and the treating clinician. If PEP is offered and taken and the source is later determined to be HIV-negative, PEP should be stopped.

PEP = postexposure prophylaxis.

Adapted from the World Health Organization: Guidelines on postexposure prophylaxis for HIV and the use of co-trimoxazole prophylaxis for HIV-related infections among adults, adolescents and children: Recommendations for a public health approach—December 2014 supplement to the 2013 consolidated guidelines on the use of antiretroviral drugs for treating and preventing HIV infection.

prevalence), regardless of CD4 count, patients should be given isoniazid 5 mg/kg (up to 300 mg) po once/day plus pyridoxine (vitamin B_6) 10 to 25 mg po once/day for 9 mo to prevent reactivation.

For primary prophylaxis against some fungal infections (eg, esophageal candidiasis, cryptococcal meningitis or pneumonia), oral fluconazole 100 to 200 mg once/day or 400 mg weekly is successful but is infrequently used because the cost per infection prevented is high and diagnosis and treatment of these infections are usually successful.

Secondary prophylaxis (after control of the initial infection) is indicated if patients have had the following:

- Recurrent oral, vaginal, or esophageal candidiasis, coccidioidomycosis, or cryptococcal infections: Fluconazole is used.
- Histoplasmosis: Itraconazole is used.
- Latent toxoplasmosis: This asymptomatic condition is indicated by serum antibodies (IgG) to *Toxoplasma gondii*. TMP/SMX (in doses used to prevent *P. jirovecii* pneumonia) is used to prevent reactivation and consequent toxoplasmic encephalitis. Latent infection is less common (about 15% of adults) in the US than in Europe and most developing countries (up to 70 to 80% of adults).
- *P. jirovecii* pneumonia
- Herpes simplex infection
- Aspergillosis (possibly)

Detailed guidelines for prophylaxis of fungal (including *Pneumocystis*), viral, mycobacterial, and toxoplasmic infections are available at www.aidsinfo.nih.gov.

Immunization: The CDC 2015 recommendations for vaccination of HIV-infected patients include the following:

- Patients who have not received the conjugate pneumococcal vaccine (PCV13) or polysaccharide pneumococcal vaccine (PPSV23) should be given PCV13 followed by PPSV23 ≥ 8 wk after PCV13.
- All patients should be given the influenza vaccine annually.
- All patients should be given the hepatitis B vaccine.
- Patients at risk of hepatitis A or desiring protection from it should be given the hepatitis A vaccine.
- At the appropriate age, males and females should be given the human papillomavirus (HPV) vaccine to prevent HPV-related cervical and anal cancers.

Generally, inactivated vaccines should be used. These vaccines are effective less often in patients who are HIV-positive than in those who are HIV-negative.

Use of the herpes zoster vaccine (for boosting immunity to prevent reactivation as zoster) could be useful in HIV-infected adults but is contraindicated if the CD4 count is < 200/μL.

Because live-virus vaccines are potentially dangerous for patients with severe immunosuppression, expert opinion should be sought when dealing with patients at risk of primary varicella; recommendations vary (see p. 2611 and Table 312–6 on p. 2612).

KEY POINTS

- HIV infects CD4+ lymphocytes and thus interferes with cell-mediated and, to a lesser extent, humoral immunity.
- HIV is spread mainly by sexual contact, parenteral exposure to contaminated blood, and prenatal and perinatal maternal transmission.
- Frequent viral mutations combined with immune system damage significantly impair the body's ability to clear the HIV infection.
- Various opportunistic infections and cancers can develop and are the usual cause of death in untreated patients.
- Diagnose using antibody tests, and monitor by measuring viral load and CD4 count.
- Treat with a combination of antiretroviral drugs, which can restore immune function to nearly normal in most patients if they take the drugs consistently.
- Use postexposure and preexposure antiretroviral prophylaxis when indicated.
- Give primary prophylaxis against opportunistic infections based on the CD4 count.

CANCERS COMMON IN HIV-INFECTED PATIENTS

AIDS-defining cancers in HIV-infected patients are

- Kaposi sarcoma
- Lymphoma, Burkitt (or equivalent term)
- Lymphoma, immunoblastic (or equivalent term)
- Lymphoma, primary, of CNS
- Cervical cancer, invasive

Other cancers that appear to be dramatically increased in incidence or severity include

- Hodgkin lymphoma (especially the mixed cellularity and lymphocyte-depleted subtypes)
- Anal cancer
- Testicular cancer
- Melanoma
- Other skin and superficial eye cancers

Leiomyosarcoma is a rare complication of HIV infection in children. Also, the rates of other common cancers (eg, lung, head and neck, and cervical carcinomas; hepatomas) are several times higher in HIV-infected patients than in the general population. This finding may reflect, at least in part, greater exposure to the viruses or toxins that cause these cancers: hepatitis B and C for hepatoma, HPV for cervical and anal carcinoma, and alcohol and tobacco for lung and head and neck carcinomas.

Non-Hodgkin lymphoma: Incidence of non-Hodgkin lymphoma is 50 to 200 times higher in HIV-infected patients. Most cases are B-cell, aggressive, high-grade histologic subtype lymphomas. At diagnosis, extranodal sites are usually involved; they include bone marrow, GI tract, and other sites that are unusual in non–HIV-associated non-Hodgkin lymphoma, such as the CNS and body cavities (eg, pleural, pericardial, peritoneal).

Common presentations include rapidly enlarging lymph nodes or extranodal masses and systemic symptoms (eg, weight loss, night sweats, fevers).

Diagnosis is by biopsy with histopathologic and immunochemical analysis of tumor cells. Abnormal circulating lymphocytes or unexpected cytopenias suggest involvement of the bone marrow, mandating bone marrow biopsy. Tumor staging may require CSF examination and CT or MRI of the chest, abdomen, and other areas where tumors are suspected.

Poor **prognosis** is predicted by the following:

- CD4 count of < 100/μL
- Age > 35 yr
- Poor functional status
- Bone marrow involvement
- History of opportunistic infections
- High-grade histologic subtype

Treatment of non-Hodgkin lymphoma is with various regimens of systemic, multidrug chemotherapy that includes cyclophosphamide, doxorubicin, vincristine, prednisone, and etoposide. These drugs are combined with IV rituximab and an anti-CD20 monoclonal antibody and supplemented with antiretroviral therapy (ART), prophylactic antibiotics and antifungals, and hematologic growth factors. Therapy may be limited by severe myelosuppression, particularly when combinations of myelosuppressive antitumor or antiretroviral drugs are used. Radiation therapy may debulk large tumors and control pain or bleeding.

Primary CNS lymphoma: Incidence of primary CNS lymphoma is markedly increased in HIV-infected patients with very low CD4 counts.

These lymphomas consist of intermediate- or high-grade malignant B cells, originating in CNS tissue. These lymphomas do not spread systemically, but the prognosis is poor; median survival is < 6 mo.

Presenting symptoms include headache, seizures, neurologic deficits (eg, cranial nerve palsies), and mental status changes.

Acute treatment requires control of cerebral edema using corticosteroids. Although whole-brain radiation therapy and antitumor chemotherapy with high-dose methotrexate alone or combined with other chemotherapy drugs or rituximab are commonly used, none of these regimens has been rigorously evaluated. In observational studies of ART and in a single clinical trial of rituximab, survival appeared improved.

Cervical cancer: In HIV-infected women, prevalence of human papillomavirus (HPV) infection is increased, oncogenic subtypes (types 16, 18, 31, 33, 35, and 39) persist, and the incidence of cervical intraepithelial dysplasia (CIN) is up to 60%, but increased incidence of cervical cancer has not been proved. However, cervical cancers, if they occur, are more extensive, are more difficult to cure, and have higher recurrence rates after treatment.

Confirmed risk factors for cervical cancer in HIV-infected women include the following:

- Infection with HPV subtype 16 or 18
- CD4 count of < 200/μL
- Age > 34 yr

Management of CIN or cervical cancer is not changed by HIV infection. Frequent Papanicolaou tests are important to monitor for progression. ART may result in resolution of HPV infection and regression of CIN but has no clear effects on cancer.

Squamous cell cancer of the anus and vulva: Squamous cell cancers of the anus (see p. 58) and vulva (see p. 2267) are caused by the same oncogenic types of HPV as cervical cancers and occur more commonly in HIV-infected patients. The increased incidence of anal intraepithelial neoplasia and cancers in these patients appears to be caused by both high-risk behaviors (eg, anal-receptive intercourse) and immunosupression by HIV; ART may decrease risk of progression. Anal dysplasia is common, and squamous cell cancers can be very aggressive.

Treatments include surgical extirpation, radiation therapy, and combined chemotherapy with mitomycin or cisplatin and 5-fluorouracil.

195 Intestinal Protozoa and Microsporidia

The most important intestinal protozoan pathogens are

- *Entamoeba histolytica*
- *Giardia duodenalis* (*G. lamblia*, *G. intestinalis*)
- Intestinal coccidia: *Cryptosporidium* sp, *Cystoisospora (Isospora) belli*, and *Cyclospora cayetanensis*

Members of the phylum Microsporidia used to be classified as protozoa but are now, based on DNA studies, thought to be fungi or closely related to them.

Multiple pathogenic parasites and nonpathogenic commensal organisms may be present in the intestine at the same time. Nonintestinal protozoan infections are covered in other chapters.

Systemic protozoal diseases include malaria, babesiosis, leishmaniasis, toxoplasmosis, and trypanosomiasis.

Intestinal protozoa are spread by the fecal-oral route, so infections are widespread in areas with inadequate sanitation and water treatment. They are also common in the US in settings where fecal incontinence and poor hygiene prevail, as may occur in mental institutions and day care centers. Occasionally, large waterborne outbreaks of intestinal protozoan infection have occurred in the US (eg, the massive waterborne *Cryptosporidium* outbreak in Milwaukee in 1993). Some GI protozoa are spread sexually, especially with practices involving oral-anal contact, and several protozoan species cause severe opportunistic infections in patients with AIDS.

Diagnosis

Making a diagnosis based on symptoms and physical findings is difficult; stool testing for parasite antigens or microscopic examination of stool for cysts or organisms is necessary.

Fecal antigen tests that are sensitive and specific are available for

- *G. intestinalis*
- *Cryptosporidium* sp
- *E. histolytica*

Microscopic diagnosis may require several samples, concentration methods, and special stains; thus, the laboratory should be notified which pathogen or pathogens are suspected. Some patients require semi-invasive diagnostic techniques such as endoscopic biopsy (see Table 182–1 on p. 1476).

Molecular diagnosis using PCR-based assays is available for some enteric protozoa and holds promise for the future.

AMEBIASIS

(Entamebiasis)

Amebiasis is infection with *Entamoeba histolytica*. It is commonly asymptomatic, but symptoms ranging from mild diarrhea to severe dysentery may occur. Extraintestinal infections include liver abscesses. Diagnosis is by identifying *E. histolytica* in stool specimens or by serologic tests. Treatment for symptomatic disease is with metronidazole or tinidazole followed by paromomycin or other drugs active against cysts in the lumen.

Three species of *Entamoeba* are morphologically indistinguishable, but molecular techniques show that they are different species:

- *E. histolytica* (pathogenic)
- *E. dispar* (harmless colonizer, more common)
- *E. moshkovskii* (uncertain pathogenicity)

Amebiasis is caused by *E. histolytica* and tends to occur in regions with poor socioeconomic conditions and poor sanitation. Most infections occur in Central America, western South America, western and southern Africa, and the Indian subcontinent. In developed countries (eg, US), most cases occur among recent immigrants and travelers returning from endemic regions.

Worldwide each year, an estimated 40 to 50 million people develop amebic colitis or extraintestinal disease, and about 40,000 to 70,000 die.

Pathophysiology

Entamoeba spp exist in 2 forms:

- Trophozoite
- Cyst

The motile trophozoites feed on bacteria and tissue, reproduce, colonize the lumen and the mucosa of the large intestine, and sometimes invade tissues and organs. Trophozoites predominate in liquid stools but rapidly die outside the body and, if ingested, would be killed by gastric acids. Some trophozoites in the colonic lumen become cysts that are excreted with stool.

E. histolytica trophozoites can adhere to and kill colonic epithelial cells and polymorphonuclear leukocytes (PMNs) and can cause dysentery with blood and mucus but with few PMNs in stool. Trophozoites also secrete proteases that degrade the extracellular matrix and permit invasion into the intestinal wall and beyond. Trophozoites can spread via the portal circulation and cause necrotic liver abscesses. Infection may spread by direct extension from the liver to the right lung and pleural space or, rarely, through the bloodstream to the brain and other organs.

Cysts predominate in formed stools and resist destruction in the external environment. They may spread directly from person to person or indirectly via food or water. Amebiasis can also be sexually transmitted by oral-anal contact.

Symptoms and Signs

Most infected people are asymptomatic but chronically pass cysts in stools. Symptoms that occur with tissue invasion include

- Intermittent diarrhea and constipation
- Flatulence
- Cramping abdominal pain

Tenderness over the liver or ascending colon may occur, and stools may contain mucus and blood.

Amebic dysentery: This form, common in the tropics, manifests with episodes of frequent semiliquid stools that often contain blood, mucus, and live trophozoites. Abdominal findings range from mild tenderness to frank abdominal pain, with high fevers and toxic systemic symptoms. Abdominal tenderness frequently accompanies amebic colitis.

Between relapses, symptoms diminish to recurrent cramps and loose or very soft stools, but emaciation and anemia may develop. Symptoms suggesting appendicitis may occur. Surgery in such cases may result in peritoneal spread of amebas.

Chronic amebic infection: Chronic amebic infection can mimic inflammatory bowel disease and manifests as intermittent nondysenteric diarrhea with abdominal pain, mucus, flatulence, and weight loss. Chronic infection may also manifest as tender, palpable masses or annular lesions (amebomas) in the cecum and ascending colon.

Extraintestinal amebic disease: Extraintestinal amebic disease originates from infection in the colon and can involve any organ, but a liver abscess is the most common.

Liver abscess is usually single and in the right lobe. It can manifest in patients who have had no prior symptoms, is more common among men than among women (7:1 to 9:1), and may develop insidiously. Symptoms include pain or discomfort over the liver, which is occasionally referred to the right shoulder, as well as intermittent fever, sweats, chills, nausea, vomiting, weakness, and weight loss. Jaundice is unusual and low grade when present. The abscess may perforate into the subphrenic space, right pleural cavity, right lung, or other adjacent organs (eg, pericardium).

Skin lesions are occasionally observed, especially around the perineum and buttocks in chronic infection, and may also occur in traumatic or operative wounds.

Diagnosis

- Intestinal infection: Microscopic examination, enzyme immunoassay (EIA) of stool, and/or serologic testing
- Extraintestinal infection: Imaging and serologic testing or a therapeutic trial

Nondysenteric amebiasis may be misdiagnosed as irritable bowel syndrome, regional enteritis, or diverticulitis. A right-sided colonic mass may also be mistaken for cancer, tuberculosis, actinomycosis, or lymphoma.

Amebic dysentery may be confused with shigellosis, salmonellosis, schistosomiasis, or ulcerative colitis. In amebic dysentery, stools are usually less frequent and less watery than those in bacillary dysentery. They characteristically contain tenacious mucus and flecks of blood. Unlike stools in shigellosis, salmonellosis, and ulcerative colitis, amebic stools do not contain large numbers of WBCs because trophozoites lyse them.

Hepatic amebiasis and amebic abscess must be differentiated from other hepatic infections and tumors.

Diagnosis of amebiasis is supported by finding amebic trophozoites, cysts, or both in stool or tissues; however, pathogenic *E. histolytica* are morphologically indistinguishable from nonpathogenic *E. dispar* and *E. moshkovskii*. Immunoassays that detect *E. histolytica* antigens in stool are sensitive and specific and are done to confirm the diagnosis. Specific DNA detection assays for *E. histolytica* are available at diagnostic reference laboratories.

Serologic tests are positive in

- About 95% of patients with an amebic liver abscess
- > 70% of those with active intestinal infection
- 10% of asymptomatic carriers

EIA is the most widely used serologic test. Antibody titers can confirm *E. histolytica* infection but may persist for months or years, making it impossible to differentiate acute from past infection in residents from areas with a high prevalence of infection. Thus, serologic tests are helpful when previous infection is considered less likely (eg, in travelers to endemic areas).

Amebic intestinal infection: Identification of intestinal amebas may require examination of 3 to 6 stool specimens and concentration methods (see Table 182–1 on p. 1476). Antibiotics, antacids, antidiarrheals, enemas, and intestinal radiocontrast agents can interfere with recovery of the parasite and should not be given until the stool has been examined. *E. histolytica* has to be distinguished from *E. dispar* and *E. moshkovskii* as well as from other nonpathogenic amebas, including *E. coli*, *E. hartmanni*, *Endolimax nana*, and *Iodamoeba bütschlii*. Molecular analysis using PCR-based assays and EIA for fecal antigens are more sensitive and differentiate *E. histolytica* from nonpathogens.

In symptomatic patients, proctoscopy often shows characteristic flask-shaped mucosal lesions, which should be aspirated, and the aspirate should be examined for trophozoites. Biopsy specimens from rectosigmoid lesions may also show trophozoites.

Amebic extraintestinal infection: Amebic extraintestinal infection is more difficult to diagnose. Stool examination is usually negative, and recovery of trophozoites from aspirated pus is uncommon. If a liver abscess is suspected, ultrasonography, CT, or MRI should be done. They have similar sensitivity; however, no technique can differentiate amebic from pyogenic abscess with certainty.

Needle aspiration is reserved for the following:

- Lesions of uncertain etiology
- Those in which rupture seems imminent
- Those that respond poorly to drug therapy

Abscesses contain thick, semifluid material ranging from yellow to chocolate-brown. A needle biopsy may show necrotic tissue, but motile amebas are difficult to find in abscess material, and amebic cysts are not present.

A therapeutic trial of an amebicide is often the most helpful diagnostic tool for an amebic liver abscess.

PEARLS & PITFALLS

- Microscopic examination of stool is usually negative in patients with extraintestinal amebiasis.

Treatment

- Metronidazole or tinidazole initially
- Iodoquinol, paromomycin, or diloxanide furoate subsequently for cyst eradication

For **GI symptoms and extraintestinal amebiasis**, one of the following is used:

- Oral metronidazole 500 to 750 mg tid in adults (12 to 17 mg/kg tid in children) for 7 to 10 days
- Tinidazole 2 g po once/day in adults (50 mg/kg [maximum 2 g] po once/day in children > 3 yr) for 3 days for mild to moderate GI symptoms, 5 days for severe GI symptoms, and 3 to 5 days for amebic liver abscess

Metronidazole and tinidizole should not be given to pregnant women. Alcohol must be avoided because these drugs have a disulfiram-like effect. In terms of GI adverse effects, tinidazole is generally better tolerated than metronidazole.

Therapy for patients with significant GI symptoms should include rehydration with fluid and electrolytes and other supportive measures.

Although metronidazole and tinidazole have some activity against *E. histolytica* cysts, they are not sufficient to eradicate cysts. Consequently, a 2nd oral drug is used to eradicate residual cysts in the intestine.

Options for cyst eradication are

- Iodoquinol 650 mg po tid after meals in adults (10 to 13 mg/kg [maximum of 2 g/day] po tid in children) for 20 days
- Paromomycin 8 to 11 mg/kg po tid with meals for 7 days
- Diloxanide furoate 500 mg po tid in adults (7 mg/kg po tid in children) for 10 days

Diloxanide furoate is not available commercially in the US.

Asymptomatic people who pass *E. histolytica* cysts should be treated with paromomycin, iodoquinol, or diloxanide furoate (see above for doses) to prevent development of invasive disease and spreading elsewhere in the body and to others.

Treatment is not necessary for *E. dispar* or *E. moshkovskii* infections. However, if fecal antigen or PCR-based assays to differentiate them from *E. histolytica* are not available, the decision to treat is made clinically (eg, by the likelihood of exposure to *E. histolytica*).

Prevention

Contamination of food and water with human feces must be prevented—a problem complicated by the high incidence of asymptomatic carriers. Uncooked foods, including salads and vegetables, and potentially contaminated water and ice should be avoided in developing areas. Boiling water kills *E. histolytica* cysts. The effectiveness of chemical disinfection with iodine- or chlorine-containing compounds depends on the temperature of the water and amount of organic debris in it. Portable filters provide various degrees of protection.

Work continues on the development of a vaccine, but none is available yet.

KEY POINTS

- *E. histolytica* usually causes dysentery but sometimes causes liver abscesses.
- Diagnose amebic intestinal infection using stool antigen tests or microscopy.
- Diagnose amebic extraintestinal infection using serologic tests, which are most helpful when previous infection is considered unlikely (eg, in travelers to endemic areas), or a therapeutic trial of an amebicide.
- Treat with metronidazole or tinidazole to eliminate amebas, followed by iodoquinol or paromomycin to kill cysts in the intestine.

CRYPTOSPORIDIOSIS

Cryptosporidiosis is infection with *Cryptosporidium*. The primary symptom is watery diarrhea, often with other signs of GI distress. Illness is typically self-limited in immunocompetent patients but can be persistent and severe in patients with AIDS. Diagnosis is by identification of the organism or antigen in stool. Treatment of immunocompetent people, when necessary, is with nitazoxanide. For patients with AIDS, highly active antiretroviral therapy (ART) and supportive care are used.

Pathophysiology

Cryptosporidia are obligate, intracellular coccidian protozoa that replicate in small-bowel epithelial cells of a vertebrate host.

After *Cryptosporidium* oocysts are ingested, they excyst in the GI tract and release sporozoites, which parasitize GI epithelial cells. In these cells, the sporozoites transform into trophozoites, replicate, and produce oocysts.

Two types of oocysts are produced:

- Thick-walled oocysts, which are commonly excreted from the host
- Thin-walled oocysts, which are primarily involved in autoinfection

The thick-walled infective oocysts are shed into the lumen and passed in stool by the infected host; they are immediately infective and can be transmitted directly from person to person by the fecal-oral route. Very few oocysts (eg, < 100) are required to cause disease, thus increasing risk of person-to-person transmission.

When the infective oocysts are ingested by humans or another vertebrate host, the cycle begins again.

Oocysts are resistant to harsh conditions, including chlorine at levels usually used in public water treatment systems and swimming pools despite adherence to recommended residual chlorine levels.

Epidemiology

Cryptosporidium parvum (bovine genotype) and *C. hominis* (human genotype) are responsible for most human cases of cryptosporidiosis. Infections result from the following:

- Ingestion of fecally contaminated food or water (often water in public and residential pools, hot tubs, water parks, lakes, or streams)
- Direct person-to-person contact
- Zoonotic spread

The disease occurs worldwide. Cryptosporidiosis is responsible for 0.6 to 7.3% of diarrheal illness in developed countries and an even higher percentage in areas with poor sanitation. It has been the cause of large waterborne diarrhea outbreaks in the US.[1] In Milwaukee, Wisconsin, >400,000 people were affected during a waterborne outbreak in 1993, when the city's water supply was contaminated by sewage during spring rains and the filtration system was not working correctly.

Children, travelers to foreign countries, immunocompromised patients, and medical personnel caring for patients with cryptosporidiosis are at increased risk. Outbreaks have occurred in day care centers. The small number of oocysts required to cause infection, the prolonged excretion of oocysts, the resistance of oocysts to chlorination, and their small size raise concern about swimming pools used by diapered children.

Severe, chronic diarrhea due to cryptosporidiosis is a problem in patients with AIDS.

1. Painter JE, Gargano JW, Yoder JS, et al: Evolving epidemiology of reported cryptosporidiosis cases in the United States, 1995–2012. *Epidemiol Infect* 144(8):1792–1802, 2016. doi: 10.1017/S0950268815003131.

Symptoms and Signs

The incubation period is about 1 wk, and clinical illness occurs in > 80% of infected people. Onset is abrupt, with profuse watery diarrhea, abdominal cramping, and, less commonly, nausea, anorexia, fever, and malaise. Symptoms usually persist 1 to 2 wk, rarely ≥ 1 mo, and then abate. Fecal excretion of oocysts may continue for several weeks after symptoms have subsided. Asymptomatic shedding of oocysts is common among older children in developing countries.

In the immunocompromised host, onset may be more gradual, but diarrhea can be more severe. Unless the underlying immune defect is corrected, infection can persist, causing profuse intractable diarrhea for life. Fluid losses of > 5 to 10 L/day have been reported in some AIDS patients. The intestine is the most common site of infection in immunocompromised hosts; however, other organs (eg, biliary tract, pancreas, respiratory tract) may be involved.

Diagnosis

- EIA for fecal antigen
- Microscopic examination of stool (special techniques required)

Identifying the acid-fast oocysts in stool confirms the diagnosis, but conventional methods of stool examination (ie, routine "stool for ova and parasites" testing) are unreliable. Oocyst excretion is intermittent, and multiple stool samples may be needed. Several concentration techniques increase the yield. *Cryptosporidium* oocysts can be identified by phase-contrast microscopy or by staining with modified Ziehl-Neelsen or Kinyoun techniques. Immunofluorescence microscopy with fluorescein-labeled monoclonal antibodies allows for greater sensitivity and specificity.

EIA for fecal *Cryptosporidium* antigen is more sensitive than microscopic examination for oocysts. DNA-based assays for detection and speciation of *C. parvum* and *C. hominis* have been developed. They are being increasingly used in reference diagnostic laboratories.

Intestinal biopsy can demonstrate *Cryptosporidium* within epithelial cells.

Treatment

- Nitazoxanide in patients without AIDS and with persistent infection
- ART in patients with AIDS plus high-dose nitazoxanide

In immunocompetent people, cryptosporidiosis is self-limited. For persistent infections, oral nitazoxanide can be used; the recommended doses, given for 3 days, are as follows:

- Age 1 to 3 yr: 100 mg bid
- Age 4 to 11 yr: 200 mg bid
- Age ≥ 12 yr: 500 mg bid

In patients with AIDS, immune reconstitution with ART is key. High-dose nitazoxanide (500 to 1000 mg bid) for 14 days has been effective in adults with a CD4 count > 50/μL. Symptoms have abated after effective ART in some patients.

Supportive measures, oral and parenteral rehydration, and hyperalimentation are indicated for immunocompromised patients.

Prevention

Stools of patients with cryptosporidiosis are highly infectious; strict stool precautions should be observed. Special biosafety guidelines have been developed for handling clinical specimens. Boiling water for 1 min (3 min at altitudes > 2000 m [6562 ft]) is the most reliable decontamination method; only filters with pore sizes ≤ 1 μm (specified as "absolute 1 micron" or certified under NSF International Standard No. 53 or No. 58) remove *Cryptosporidium* cysts.

KEY POINTS

- Cryptosporidiosis spreads easily because fecal excretion of oocysts persists for weeks after symptoms resolve, a very small number of oocysts are required for infection, and oocysts are difficult to remove by conventional water filtration and are resistant to chlorination.
- Profuse, watery diarrhea with cramping is usually self-limited but can be severe and lifelong in patients with AIDS.
- Diagnose using EIA for fecal *Cryptosporidium* antigen; microscopic stool examination is less accurate and requires specialized techniques (eg, phase-contrast microscopy, acid-fast staining).
- For people without AIDS, use nitazoxanide if symptoms persist.
- Treat people with AIDS with ART and high doses of nitazoxanide; symptoms may abate when the immune system improves with ART.

CYCLOSPORIASIS AND CYSTOISOSPORIASIS

Cyclosporiasis is infection with *Cyclospora cayetanensis*; cystoisosporiasis is infection with *Cystoisospora (Isospora) belli*. Symptoms include watery diarrhea with GI and systemic symptoms. Diagnosis is by detection of characteristic oocysts in stool or intestinal biopsy specimens. Treatment is usually with trimethoprim/sulfamethoxazole.

Cyclosporiasis and cystoisosporiasis are obligate intracellular coccidian protozoa. They are most common in tropical and subtropical climates. Transmission is by the fecal-oral route via contaminated food or drink.

The life cycles of *C. cayetanensis* and *C. belli* are similar to that of Cryptosporidium, except that oocysts passed in stool are not sporulated. Thus, when freshly passed in stools, the oocysts are not infective, and direct fecal-oral transmission cannot occur. The oocysts require days to weeks in the environment to sporulate. The sporulated oocysts are ingested in contaminated food or water and excyst in the GI tract, releasing sporozoites. The sporozoites invade the epithelial cells of the small intestine, replicate, and mature into oocysts, which are shed in stool.

In the 1990s, outbreaks of *C. cayetanensis* in North America were caused by ingestion of raspberries imported from Guatemala. In the summer of 2013, a multistate outbreak involving hundreds of people in the US was attributed to ingestion of prewashed salad mixes.[1]

1. Abanyie F, Harvey RR, Harris JR, et al: 2013 multistate outbreaks of *Cyclospora cayetanensis* infections associated with fresh produce: focus on the Texas investigations. *Epidemiol Infect* 143(16):3451–3458, 2015. doi: 10.1017/S0950268815000370.

Symptoms and Signs

The primary symptom is sudden, nonbloody, watery diarrhea, with fever, abdominal cramps, nausea, anorexia, malaise, and weight loss. In immunocompetent patients, the illness usually resolves spontaneously but can last weeks.

In hosts with depressed cell-mediated immunity as occurs in AIDS, cyclosporiasis and cystoisosporiasis may cause severe, intractable, voluminous diarrhea resembling cryptosporidiosis. Extraintestinal disease in patients with AIDS may include cholecystitis and disseminated infection.

Diagnosis

- Microscopic examination of stool

Diagnosis of cyclosporiasis and cystoisosporiasis is by detection of oocysts via microscopic examination of the stool. A modified Ziehl-Neelsen or Kinyoun acid-fast staining technique can help identify *Cyclospora* and *Cystoisospora* oocysts. Oocysts of both *Cyclospora* and *Cystoisospora* are autofluorescent. *Cyclospora* oocysts are spherical and similar in morphology to but larger than *Cryptosporidium* oocysts. *Cystoisospora* oocysts are even larger and are ellipsoidal.

Multiple (≥ 3) stool specimens may be needed because cyst secretion may be intermittent. Molecular tests for parasite DNA are being developed.

Diagnosis is sometimes made only when intracellular parasite stages are detected in biopsies of intestinal tissue.

In cystoisosporiasis, the stool may contain Charcot-Leyden crystals (hexagonal, double-pointed, and often needlelike crystals) derived from eosinophils.

Unlike other protozoan infections, cystoisosporiasis may result in peripheral blood eosinophilia.

Treatment

- Trimethoprim/sulfamethoxazole

Treatment of choice for both cyclosporiasis and cystoisosporiasis is double-strength trimethoprim/sulfamethoxazole (TMP/SMX): 160 mg TMP and 800 mg SMX po bid for 7 to 10 days for cyclosporiasis or for 10 days for cystoisosporiasis. Children are given 5 mg/kg TMP and 25 mg/kg SMX po bid for the same number of days.

In patients with AIDS, higher doses and longer duration may be needed, and treatment of acute infection is usually followed by long-term suppressive therapy. Institution or optimization of ART is important.

For cyclosporiasis, an alternative to TMP/SMX has yet to be identified.

Ciprofloxacin 500 mg po bid for 7 days has been used to treat cystoisosporiasis, but it is less effective than TMP/SMX.

Prevention is as for amebiasis.

GIARDIASIS

Giardiasis is infection with the flagellated protozoan *Giardia duodenalis* (*G. lamblia*, *G. intestinalis*). Infection can be asymptomatic or cause symptoms ranging from intermittent flatulence to chronic malabsorption. Diagnosis is by identifying the organism in fresh stool or duodenal contents or by assays of *Giardia* antigen in stool. Treatment is with metronidazole, tinidazole, or nitazoxanide or, during pregnancy, paromomycin.

Giardia trophozoites firmly attach to the duodenal and proximal jejunal mucosa and multiply by binary fission. Some organisms transform into environmentally resistant cysts that are spread by the fecal-oral route.

Giardiasis is the most common intestinal parasitic disease in the US. Waterborne transmission is the major source of infection.[1] Transmission can also occur by ingestion of contaminated food and by direct person-to-person contact, especially in mental institutions and day care centers or between sex partners.

Giardia cysts remain viable in surface water and are resistant to routine levels of chlorination. Wild animals may also serve as reservoirs. Thus, mountain streams as well as chlorinated but poorly filtered municipal water supply systems have been implicated in waterborne epidemics.

There are 8 genetic groups (assemblages) of *G. duodenalis*. Two infect humans and animals; the others infect only animals. The clinical manifestations appear to vary with genotype.

1. Schnell K, Collier S, Derado G, et al: Giardiasis in the United States—an epidemiologic and geospatial analysis of county-level drinking water and sanitation data, 1993–2010. *J Water Health* 14(2):267–279, 2016. doi: 10.2166/wh.2015.283.

Symptoms and Signs

Many cases of giardiasis are asymptomatic. However, asymptomatic people can pass infective cysts.

Symptoms of acute giardiasis usually appear 1 to 14 days (average 7 days) after infection. They are usually mild and include watery malodorous diarrhea, abdominal cramps and distention, flatulence, eructation, intermittent nausea, epigastric discomfort, and sometimes low-grade malaise and anorexia.

Acute giardiasis usually lasts 1 to 3 wk. Malabsorption of fat and sugars can lead to significant weight loss in severe cases. Neither blood nor WBCs are present in stool.

A subset of infected patients develop chronic diarrhea with foul stools, abdominal distention, and malodorous flatus. Substantial weight loss may occur. Chronic giardiasis occasionally causes failure to thrive in children.

Diagnosis

- EIA for antigen in stool
- Microscopic examination of stool

EIA to detect parasite antigen in stool is more sensitive than microscopic examination. Characteristic trophozoites or cysts in stool are diagnostic, but parasite excretion is intermittent and at low levels during chronic infections. Thus, microscopic diagnosis may require repeated stool examinations.

Sampling of the upper intestinal contents can also yield trophozoites but is seldom necessary.

Specific DNA probes exist. Testing is available at the CDC and is likely to become increasingly available at reference laboratories.

Treatment

- Tinidazole, metronidazole, or nitazoxanide

For symptomatic infections, metronidazole, tinidazole, or nitazoxanide may be used.

Metronidazole is given as follows:

- Adults: 250 mg po tid for 5 to 7 days
- Children: 5 mg/kg po tid for 5 to 7 days

Tinidazole is as effective as metronidazole and is given as follows:

- Adults: 2 g po once
- Children: 50 mg/kg [maximum 2 g] po once

Adverse effects of metronidazole include nausea and headaches. Metronidazole and tinidizole should not be given to pregnant women. Alcohol must be avoided because these drugs have a disulfiram-like effect. In terms of GI adverse effects, tinidazole is generally better tolerated than metronidazole.

Nitazoxanide is given orally for 3 days as follows:

- Age 1 to 3 yr: 100 mg bid
- Age 4 to 11 yr: 200 mg bid
- Age > 12 yr (including adults): 500 mg bid

Nitazoxanide is available in liquid form for children. Resistance has been reported.

Metronidazole and tinidazole should not be given to pregnant women. The safety of nitazoxanide during pregnancy has not been assessed. If therapy cannot be delayed because of symptoms, the nonabsorbable aminoglycoside paromomycin (8 to 11 mg/kg po tid for 5 to 10 days) is an option.

Furazolidone and quinacrine are effective but are now rarely used because of potential toxicity.

Prevention

Prevention requires

- Appropriate public water treatment
- Hygienic food preparation
- Appropriate fecal-oral hygiene

Water can be decontaminated by boiling. *Giardia* cysts resist routine levels of chlorination. Disinfection with iodine-containing compounds is variably effective and depends on the turbidity and temperature of the water and duration of treatment. Some handheld filtration devices can remove *Giardia* cysts from contaminated water, but the efficacy of various filter systems has not been fully assessed.

Treatment of asymptomatic cyst passers can theoretically reduce the spread of infection, but whether it is cost-effective remains unclear.

KEY POINTS

- The major source of giardiasis is waterborne transmission, including via fresh-appearing mountain streams and poorly filtered municipal water supplies.
- *Giardia* cysts resist routine levels of chlorination, and disinfection with iodine-containing compounds is variably effective.
- EIA to detect parasite antigen in stool is preferred because it is more sensitive than microscopic examination.
- For symptomatic patients, use tinidazole, metronidazole, or nitazoxanide.

MICROSPORIDIOSIS

Microsporidiosis is infection with microsporidia. Symptomatic disease develops predominantly in patients with AIDS and includes chronic diarrhea, disseminated infection, and corneal disease. Diagnosis is by demonstrating organisms in biopsy specimens, stool, urine, other secretions, or corneal scrapings. Treatment is with albendazole or fumagillin (depending on the infecting species and clinical syndrome) or with topical fumagillin added for eye disease.

Microsporidia are obligate intracellular spore-forming parasitic fungi, which used to be classified as protozoa.

At least 15 of the > 1200 species of microsporidia are associated with human disease. Spores of the organisms are acquired by the following:

- Ingestion
- Inhalation
- Direct contact with the conjunctiva
- Animal contact
- Person-to-person transmission

Inside the host, they harpoon a host cell with their polar tubule or filament and inoculate it with an infective sporoplasm. Intracellularly, the sporoplasm divides and multiplies, producing sporoblasts that mature into spores; the spores can disseminate throughout the body or pass into the environment via respiratory aerosols, stool, or urine. An inflammatory response develops when spores are liberated from host cells.

Little is known about routes of transmission to humans or possible animal reservoirs.

Microsporidia probably are a common cause of subclinical or mild self-limited illness in otherwise healthy people, but only a few cases of human infection were reported in the pre-AIDS era—perhaps because overall awareness of microsporidial infection was less. Recently, microsporidial keratoconjunctivitis has become increasingly reported in immunocompetent people.

Microsporidia have emerged as opportunistic pathogens in patients with AIDS and, to a lesser degree, in those with other immunocompromising conditions. *Encephalitozoon bieneusi* and *E.* (formerly *Septata*) *intestinalis* can cause chronic diarrhea in patients with AIDS and CD4 cell counts of < 100/μL. Microsporidian species can also infect the liver, biliary tract, cornea, sinuses, muscles, respiratory tract, GU system, and, occasionally, the CNS.

The incidence of microsporidiosis has decreased substantially with the widespread use of effective ART and immune reconstitution.

Symptoms and Signs

Clinical illness caused by microsporidia varies with

- The parasite species
- The immune status of the host

In patients with AIDS, various species cause chronic diarrhea, malabsorption, wasting, cholangitis, punctate keratoconjunctivitis, peritonitis, hepatitis, myositis, or sinusitis. Infections of kidneys and the gallbladder have occurred. *Vittaforma (Nosema) corneum* and several other species can cause ocular infections ranging from punctuate keratopathy with redness and irritation to severe, vision-threatening stromal keratitis.

Diagnosis

- Light or electron microscopy with special stains
- Sometimes immunofluorescence or PCR-based assays

Infecting organisms can be demonstrated in specimens of affected tissue obtained by biopsy or in stool, urine, CSF, sputum, or corneal scrapings. Microsporidia are best seen with special staining techniques. Fluorescence brighteners (fluorochromes) are used to detect spores in tissues and smears. The quick-hot Gram chromotrope technique is the fastest.

Immunofluorescence assays (IFA) and PCR-based assays are available in specialized laboratories.

Transmission electron microscopy is currently the most sensitive test and is used for speciation.

Treatment

- For patients with AIDS, initiation or optimization of ART
- For GI, skin, muscle, or disseminated microsporidiosis, oral albendazole or fumagillin (where available), depending on the infecting species
- For keratoconjunctivitis, oral albendazole and topical fumagillin

For **GI microsporidiosis**, albendazole (400 mg po bid for weeks in adults) may be effective in controlling diarrhea due to *E. intestinalis*. The drug reduces the number of organisms in small-bowel biopsies but does not eliminate infection. Albendazole 400 mg po bid for weeks has been used to treat skin, muscle, or disseminated microsporidiosis due to *E. intestinalis* and many other microsporidial species.

Albendazole 400 mg po bid in combination with itraconazole 400 mg po daily has been used for *Trachipleistophora* and *Anncaliia* infections. Albendazole is not active against *E. bieneusi* and *V. corneum*.

In patients with AIDS, initiation or optimization of ART is important. Duration of albendazole therapy and outcome depend on the level of immune reconstitution with ART.

Oral fumagillin 20 mg tid for 14 days has been used for intestinal *E. bieneusi* infection, but it has potentially serious adverse effects, including severe reversible thrombocytopenia in up to half of patients. Oral fumagillin is not available in the US.

Ocular microsporidial keratoconjunctivitis can be treated with albendazole 400 mg po bid plus fumagillin eye drops 3 mg/mL (2 drops q 2 h for 4 days, then 2 drops qid). Topical fluoroquinolones, as well as topical voriconazole, have been effective in some patients. When topical and systemic therapy are ineffective, keratoplasty may be useful. Outcome is typically very good in immunocompetent patients; in patients with AIDS, it depends on the level of immune reconstitution with ART.

KEY POINTS

- Microsporidiosis occurs mainly in immunocompromised patients, predominantly those with AIDS, but keratoconjunctivitis is being increasingly reported in otherwise healthy people.
- Microsporidia spores can be acquired by ingestion, inhalation, direct contact with the conjunctiva, animal contact, or person-to-person transmission.
- Manifestations vary widely depending on the organism and the patient's immune status, but chronic diarrhea, malabsorption, wasting, cholangitis, punctate keratoconjunctivitis, peritonitis, hepatitis, myositis, or sinusitis may occur.
- Diagnose using light or electron microscopy with special stains; immunofluorescence assays and PCR-based assays are available in specialized laboratories.
- For patients with AIDS, initiation or optimization of ART is of primary importance.
- Albendazole and oral or topical fumagillin may be useful, depending on the infecting species and organs involved; oral fumagillin is not available in the US.

196 Mycobacteria

Mycobacteria are small, slow-growing, aerobic bacilli. They are distinguished by a complex, lipid-rich cell envelope responsible for their characterization as acid-fast (ie, resistant to decolorization by acid after staining with carbolfuchsin) and their relative resistance to Gram stain. The most common mycobacterial infection is tuberculosis (TB); others include leprosy and various diseases caused by *Mycobacterium avium* complex.

TUBERCULOSIS

TB is a chronic, progressive infection, often with a period of latency following initial infection. TB most commonly affects the lungs. Symptoms include productive cough, fever, weight loss, and malaise. Diagnosis is most often by sputum smear and culture and, increasingly, by rapid molecular-based diagnostic tests. Treatment is with multiple antimicrobial drugs given for at least 6 mo.

TB is a leading infectious cause of morbidity and mortality in adults worldwide, killing about 1.8 million people in 2015, most of them in low- and middle-income countries. HIV/AIDS is the most important factor predisposing to TB infection and mortality in parts of the world where both infections are prevalent.

Etiology

TB properly refers only to disease caused by *Mycobacterium tuberculosis* (for which humans are the main reservoir). Similar disease occasionally results from the closely related mycobacteria, *M. bovis*, *M. africanum*, and *M. microti*—together known as the *Mycobacterium tuberculosis* complex.

TB results almost exclusively from inhalation of airborne particles (droplet nuclei) containing *M. tuberculosis*. They disperse primarily through coughing, singing, and other forced respiratory maneuvers by people who have active pulmonary TB and whose sputum contains a significant number of organisms (typically enough to render the smear positive). People with pulmonary cavitary lesions are especially infectious because of the high number of bacteria contained within a lesion. Droplet nuclei (particles < 5 μ in diameter) containing tubercle bacilli may remain suspended in room air currents for several hours, increasing the chance of spread. However, once these droplets land on a surface, it is difficult to resuspend the organisms (eg, by sweeping the floor, shaking out bed linens) as respirable particles. Although such actions can resuspend dust particles containing tubercle bacilli, these particles are far too large to reach the alveolar surfaces necessary to initiate infection. Contact with fomites (eg, contaminated surfaces, food, and personal respirators) do not appear to facilitate spread.

How contagious patients with untreated active pulmonary TB are varies widely. Certain strains of *M. tuberculosis* are more contagious, and patients with positive sputum smears are more contagious than those with positive results only on culture. Patients with cavitary disease (which is closely associated with mycobacterial burden in sputum) are more contagious than those without. Environmental factors also are important. Transmission is enhanced by frequent or prolonged exposure to untreated patients who are dispersing large numbers of tubercle bacilli in overcrowded, poorly ventilated enclosed spaces; consequently, people living in poverty or in institutions are at particular risk. Health care practitioners who have close contact with active cases have increased risk. Thus, estimates of contagiousness vary widely; some studies suggest that only 1 in 3 patients with untreated pulmonary TB infect any close contacts; the WHO estimates that each untreated patient may infect 10 to 15 people per year. However, most of those who are infected do not develop active disease. Contagiousness decreases rapidly once effective treatment begins; organisms are less infectious even if they persist in sputum, and cough decreases. Studies of household contacts indicate that transmissibility ends within 2 wk of patients starting effective treatment.

Much less commonly, contagion results from aerosolization of organisms after irrigation of infected wounds, in mycobacteriology laboratories, or in autopsy rooms. TB of the tonsils, lymph nodes, abdominal organs, bones, and joints was once commonly caused by ingestion of milk or milk products (eg, cheese) contaminated with *M. bovis*, but this transmission route has been largely eradicated in developed countries by slaughter of cows that test positive on a tuberculin skin test (TB) and by pasteurization of milk. TB due to *M. bovis* still occurs in developing countries and in immigrants from developing countries where bovine TB is endemic (eg, some Latin American countries). The increasing popularity of cheese made from unpasteurized milk raises new concerns if the cheeses come from countries with a bovine TB problem (eg, Mexico, the United Kingdom).

Epidemiology

About one third of the world's population is infected (based on TST surveys). In 2015, an estimated 10.4 million new TB cases occurred worldwide. Six countries accounted for 60% of the new cases: India, Indonesia, China, Nigeria, Pakistan, and South Africa (listed in descending order of their number of cases). Worldwide, the rate of decline in TB incidence remained at only 1.5% from 2014 to 2015. There were an estimated 1.8 million deaths resulting from TB in 2015, which is a decrease of 22% from 2000. In 2015, there were an estimated 480,000 new cases of multidrug-resistant TB (MDR-TB); almost half of these occurred in India, China, and the Russian Federation.

In the US, in 2015, there were 9,557 TB cases reported (a rate of 3 cases per 100,000 persons). Although the number of TB cases declined yearly from 1993 to 2014, the incidence rate has remained relatively stable since 2013. In 2015, 66.4% of reported TB cases in the US occurred among foreign-born persons. The TB incidence rate among foreign-born persons (15.1/100,000) was about 13 times the rate among US-born persons (1.2/100,000). The majority of these foreign-born cases are among persons who have been in the US ≥ 5 yr. In the US, Asians, native Hawaiians, and other Pacific Islanders had the highest incidence rate (18.2/100,000), followed by American Indians or Alaska natives (6.1/100,000), blacks or African Americans (5.0/100,000), and Hispanics or Latinos (4.8/100,000).

A resurgence of TB occurred in parts of the US and other developed countries between 1985 and 1992; it was associated with several factors, including HIV coinfection, homelessness, a deteriorated public health infrastructure, and the appearance of multidrug-resistant TB (MDR-TB). Although substantially controlled in the US by effective public health and institutional infection control measures, the problem of MDR-TB, including extensively drug-resistant TB (XDR-TB), appears to be growing around the world, fueled by inadequate resources, including diagnostic and treatment delivery systems. In most parts of the world, drug-resistant TB cannot be rapidly diagnosed and promptly treated with effective regimens, including effective management of adverse effects of 2nd-line drugs. This situation results in ongoing transmission, low cure rates, and amplified resistance. Treatment of XDR-TB has even less favorable outcomes; the mortality rate is extremely high in patients coinfected with HIV, even when they are being treated with antiretroviral drugs. Effective treatment and adverse effect management, community outreach, and social support have resulted in more favorable downward epidemiologic trends for drug-resistant TB in a few areas (eg, Peru, the Tomsk region of Russia). India and China are just beginning to implement countrywide MDR-TB programs, and the future of MDR-TB may be greatly influenced by the success or failure of these programs.

Pathophysiology

M. tuberculosis bacilli initially cause a primary infection, which uncommonly causes acute illness. Most (about 95%) primary infections are asymptomatic and followed by a latent (dormant) phase. A variable percentage of latent infections subsequently reactivate with symptoms and signs of disease. Infection is usually not transmissible in the primary stage and is never contagious in the latent stage.

Primary infection: Infection requires inhalation of particles small enough to traverse the upper respiratory defenses and deposit deep in the lung, usually in the subpleural airspaces of the middle or lower lobes. Larger droplets tend to lodge in the more proximal airways and typically do not result in infection. Infection usually begins from a single droplet nucleus, which typically carries few organisms. Perhaps only a single organism may suffice to cause infection in susceptible people, but less susceptible people may require repeated exposure to develop infection.

To initiate infection, *M. tuberculosis* bacilli must be ingested by alveolar macrophages. Bacilli that are not killed by the macrophages actually replicate inside them, ultimately killing the host macrophage (with the help of CD8 lymphocytes); inflammatory cells are attracted to the area, causing a focal pneumonitis that coalesces into the characteristic tubercles seen histologically. In the early weeks of infection, some infected macrophages migrate to regional lymph nodes (eg, hilar, mediastinal), where they access the bloodstream. Organisms may then spread hematogenously to any part of the body, particularly the apical-posterior portion of the lungs, epiphyses of the long bones, kidneys, vertebral bodies, and meninges. Hematogenous dissemination is less likely in patients with partial immunity due to vaccination or to prior natural infection with *M. tuberculosis* or environmental mycobacteria.

In 95% of cases, after about 3 wk of uninhibited growth, the immune system suppresses bacillary replication, usually before symptoms or signs develop. Foci of bacilli in the lung or other sites resolve into epithelioid cell granulomas, which may have caseous and necrotic centers. Tubercle bacilli can survive in this material for years; the balance between the host's resistance and microbial virulence determines whether the infection ultimately resolves without treatment, remains dormant, or becomes active. Infectious foci may leave fibronodular scars in the apices of one or both lungs (Simon foci, which usually result from hematogenous seeding from another site of infection) or small areas of consolidation (Ghon foci). A Ghon focus with lymph node involvement is a Ghon complex, which, if calcified, is called a Ranke complex. The TST (see p. 1653) and interferon-gamma release blood assays (IGRA) become positive during the latent stage of infection. Sites of latent infection are dynamic processes, not entirely dormant as once believed.

Less often, the primary focus progresses immediately, causing acute illness with pneumonia (sometimes cavitary), pleural effusion, and marked mediastinal or hilar lymph node enlargement (which, in children, may compress bronchi). Small pleural effusions are predominantly lymphocytic, typically contain few organisms, and clear within a few weeks. This sequence may be more common among young children and recently infected or reinfected immunosuppressed patients. Extrapulmonary TB at any site can sometimes manifest without evidence of lung involvement. TB lymphadenopathy is the most common extrapulmonary presentation; however, meningitis is the most feared because of its high mortality in the very young and very old.

Active disease: Healthy people who are infected with TB have about a 5 to 10% lifetime risk of developing active disease, although the percentage varies significantly by age and other risk factors. In 50 to 80% of those who develop active disease, TB reactivates within the first 2 yr, but it can also occur decades later. Any organ initially seeded may become a site of reactivation, but reactivation occurs most often in the lung apices, presumably because of favorable local conditions such as high O_2 tension. Ghon foci and affected hilar lymph nodes are much less likely to be sites of reactivation.

Conditions that impair cellular immunity (which is essential for defense against TB) significantly facilitate reactivation. Thus, patients coinfected with HIV have about a 10% annual risk of developing active disease. Other conditions that facilitate reactivation, but to a lesser extent than HIV infection, include diabetes, head and neck cancer, gastrectomy, jejunoileal bypass surgery, dialysis-dependent chronic kidney disease, and significant weight loss. Drugs that suppress the immune system also facilitate development of active TB. Patients who require immunosuppression after solid organ transplantation are at the highest risk, but other immunosuppressants such as corticosteroids and TNF inhibitors also commonly cause reactivation. Tobacco use also is a risk factor.

In some patients, active disease develops when they are reinfected rather than when latent disease reactivates. Reinfection is more likely to be the mechanism in areas where TB is prevalent and patients are exposed to a large inoculum of bacilli. Reactivation of latent infection predominates in low-prevalence areas. In a given patient, it is difficult to determine whether active disease resulted from reinfection or reactivation.

TB damages tissues through delayed-type hypersensitivity (DTH—see p. 1372), typically producing granulomatous necrosis with a caseous histologic appearance. Lung lesions are characteristically but not invariably cavitary, especially in immunosuppressed patients with impaired DTH. Pleural effusion is less common than in progressive primary TB but may result from direct extension or hematogenous spread. Rupture of a large tuberculous lesion into the pleural space may cause empyema with or without bronchopleural fistula and sometimes causes pneumothorax. In the prechemotherapy era, TB empyema sometimes complicated medically induced pneumothorax therapy and was usually rapidly fatal, as was sudden massive hemoptysis due to erosion of a pulmonary artery by an enlarging cavity.

The course of disease varies greatly, depending on the virulence of the organism and the state of host defenses. The course may be rapid in members of isolated populations (eg, native Americans) who, unlike many Europeans and their American descendents, have not experienced centuries of selective pressure to develop innate or natural immunity to the disease. The course is often more indolent in these European and American populations.

Acute respiratory distress syndrome (ARDS), which appears to be due to hypersensitivity to TB antigens, develops rarely after diffuse hematogenous spread or rupture of a large cavity with spillage into the lungs.

Symptoms and Signs

In active pulmonary TB, even moderate or severe disease, patients may have no symptoms, except "not feeling well," anorexia, fatigue, and weight loss, which develop gradually over several weeks, or they may have more specific symptoms. Cough is most common. At first, it may be minimally productive of yellow or green sputum, usually when awakening in the morning, but cough may become more productive as the disease progresses. Hemoptysis occurs only with cavitary TB (due to granulomatous damage to vessels but sometimes due to fungal growth in a cavity). Low-grade fever is common but not invariable. Drenching night sweats are a classic symptom but are neither common in nor specific for TB. Dyspnea may result from lung parenchymal damage, spontaneous pneumothorax, or pleural TB with effusion.

With HIV coinfection, the clinical presentation is often atypical because DTH is impaired; patients are more likely to have symptoms of extrapulmonary or disseminated disease.

Extrapulmonary TB causes various systemic and localized manifestations depending on the affected organs (see p. 1659).

Diagnosis

- Chest x-ray
- Acid-fast stain and culture
- TST or IGRA
- When available, nucleic acid–based testing

Pulmonary TB is often suspected based on chest x-rays taken while evaluating respiratory symptoms (cough > 3 wk, hemoptysis, chest pain, dyspnea), an unexplained illness, FUO, or a positive TST (see p. 1653) or IGRA done as a screening test or during contact investigation. Suspicion for TB is higher in patients who have fever, cough lasting > 2 to 3 wk, night sweats, weight loss, and/or lymphadenopathy and in patients with possible TB exposure (eg, via infected family members, friends, or other contacts; institutional exposure; travel to TB-endemic areas).

Initial tests are chest x-ray and sputum examination and culture. If the diagnosis of active TB is still unclear after chest imaging and sputum examination, TST or IGRA may be done. Nucleic acid–based tests (eg, PCR) can be diagnostic.

Once TB is diagnosed, patients should be tested for HIV infection, and those with risk factors for hepatitis B or C should be tested for those viruses. Baseline tests of hepatic and renal function should typically be done.

Chest x-ray: In adults, a multinodular infiltrate above or behind the clavicle is most characteristic of active TB; it suggests reactivation of disease. It is best visualized in an apical-lordotic view or with chest CT. Middle and lower lung infiltrates are nonspecific but should prompt suspicion of primary TB in patients (usually young) whose symptoms or exposure history suggests recent infection, particularly if there is pleural effusion. Calcified hilar nodes may be present; they may result from primary TB infection but may also result from histoplasmosis in areas where histoplasmosis is endemic (eg, the Ohio River Valley).

Sputum examination and culture: Sputum testing is the mainstay for diagnosis of pulmonary TB. If patients cannot produce sputum spontaneously, aerosolized hypertonic saline can be used to induce it. If induction is unsuccessful, bronchial washings, which are particularly sensitive, can be obtained by fiberoptic bronchoscopy. Because induction of sputum and bronchoscopy entail some risk of infection for medical staff, these procedures should be done as a last resort in selected cases. Appropriate precautions (eg, negative-pressure room, N-95 or other fitted respirators) should be used.

The first step is typically microscopic examination to check for acid-fast bacilli (AFB). Tubercle bacilli are nominally gram-positive but take up Gram stain inconsistently; samples are best prepared with Ziehl-Neelsen or Kinyoun stains for conventional light microscopy or fluorochrome stains for fluorescent microscopy. Smear microscopy can detect about 10,000 bacilli/mL of sputum, making it insensitive when fewer bacilli are present, as occurs in early reactivation or in patients with HIV coinfection.

Although finding AFB in a sputum smear is strong presumptive evidence of TB, definitive diagnosis requires a positive mycobacterial culture or nucleic acid amplification test (NAAT). Culture is also required to isolate bacteria for drug-susceptibility testing and genotyping. Culture can detect as few as 10 bacilli/mL of sputum and can be done using solid or liquid media. However, it can take up to 3 mo for final confirmation of culture results. Liquid media are more sensitive and faster that solid media, with results available in 2 to 3 wk.

NAAT for TB can shorten the time to diagnosis from 1 to 2 wk to 1 to 2 days; some commercially available NAATs can provide results (including identification of rifampin [RIF] resistance) in 2 h. However, in low-prevalence situations, NAATs are usually done only on smear-positive specimens. They are approved for smear-negative specimens and are indicated when suspicion is high and a rapid diagnosis is essential for medical or public health reasons. Some NAATs are more sensitive than sputum smear and about as sensitive as culture for diagnosing TB.

If AFB smear results and confirmatory NAAT are positive, patients are presumed to have TB, and treatment can be started. If the NAAT result is positive and the AFB smear result is negative, an additional specimen is tested using NAAT; patients can be presumed to have TB if ≥ 2 specimens are NAAT-positive. If NAAT and AFB smear results are negative, clinical judgment is used to determine whether to begin anti-TB treatment while awaiting results of culture.

Drug susceptibility tests (DSTs) should be done on initial isolates from all patients to identify an effective anti-TB regimen. These tests should be repeated if patients continue to produce culture-positive sputum after 3 mo of treatment or if cultures become positive after a period of negative cultures. Results of DSTs may take up to 8 wk if conventional bacteriologic methods are used, but several new molecular DSTs can detect drug resistance to RIF or to RIF and isoniazid (INH) in a sputum sample within hours.

Tests of other specimens: Transbronchial biopsies can be done on infiltrative lesions, and samples are submitted for culture, histologic evaluation, and molecular testing. Gastric washings, which are culture-positive in a minority of samples, are no longer commonly used except in small children, who usually cannot produce a good sputum specimen. However, sputum induction is being used in young children who are able to cooperate. Ideally, biopsied samples of other tissue should be cultured fresh, but NAAT can be used for fixed tissues (eg, for biopsied lymph node if histologic examination unexpectedly detects granulomatous changes). The latter use of NAAT has not been approved but can be extremely useful, although positive and negative predictive values have not been established.

Skin testing: Multiple-puncture devices (tine test) are no longer recommended. The TST (Mantoux or PPD—purified protein derivative) is usually done, although it is a test of infection, latent or active, and is not diagnostic of active disease. The standard dose in the US of 5 tuberculin units (TU) of PPD in 0.1 mL of solution is injected on the volar forearm. It is critical to give the injection intradermally, not subcutaneously. A well-demarcated bleb or wheal should result immediately. The diameter of induration (not erythema) transverse to the long axis of the arm is measured 48 to 72 h after injection. Recommended cutoff points for a positive reaction depend on the clinical setting:

- **5 mm:** Patients at high risk of developing active TB if infected, such as those who have chest x-ray evidence of past TB, who are immunosuppressed because of HIV infection or drugs (eg, TNF-α inhibitors, corticosteroid use equivalent to prednisone 15 mg/day for > 1 mo), or who are close contacts of patients with infectious TB
- **10 mm:** Patients with some risk factors, such as injection drug users, recent immigrants from high-prevalence areas, residents of high-risk settings (eg, prisons, homeless shelters), patients with certain disorders (eg, silicosis, renal insufficiency, diabetes, head or neck cancer), and those who have had gastrectomy or jejunoileal bypass surgery
- **15 mm:** Patients with no risk factors (who typically should not be tested)

Results can be falsely negative, most often in patients who are febrile, elderly, HIV-infected (especially if CD4 count is < 200 cells/μL), or very ill, many of whom show no reaction to any skin test (anergy). Anergy probably occurs because inhibiting antibodies are present or because so many T cells have been mobilized to the disease site that too few remain to produce a significant skin reaction. False-positive results may occur if patients have nontuberculous mycobacterial infections or have received the BCG vaccine. However, the effect of BCG vaccination on TST wanes after several years; after this time, a positive test is likely to be due to TB infection.

IGRAs: The IGRA is a blood test based on the release of interferon-γ by lymphocytes exposed in vitro to TB-specific antigens. Although results of IGRAs are not always concordant with TST, these tests appear to be as sensitive as and more specific than TST in contact investigations. Importantly, they are often negative in patients with remote TB infection. Long-term studies are being done to see whether TST-positive, IGRA-negative patients (particularly those with immunosuppression) are at low risk of reactivation.

Prognosis

In immunocompetent patients with drug-susceptible pulmonary TB, even severe disease with large cavities, appropriate therapy is usually curative if it is instituted and completed. Still, TB causes or contributes to death in about 10% of cases, often in patients who are debilitated for other reasons. Disseminated TB and TB meningitis may be fatal in up to 25% of cases despite optimal treatment.

TB is much more aggressive in immunocompromised patients and, if not appropriately and aggressively treated, may be fatal in as little as 2 mo from a patient's initial presentation, especially with MDR-TB. However, with effective antiretroviral therapy (and appropriate anti-TB treatment), the prognosis for immunocompromised patients, even with MDR-TB, may approach that of immunocompetent patients. Poorer outcomes should be expected for patients with XDR-TB because there are so few effective drugs.

Treatment

Most patients with uncomplicated TB and all patients with complicating illnesses (eg, AIDS, hepatitis, diabetes), adverse drug reactions, or drug resistance should be referred to a TB specialist. (See also the Joint Statement from the American Thoracic Society, Centers for Disease Control and Prevention, and the Infectious Diseases Society of America: Treatment of Tuberculosis at www.cdc.com.) Most patients with TB can be treated as outpatients, with instructions on how to prevent transmission usually including

- Staying at home
- Avoiding visitors (except for previously exposed family members),
- Covering coughs with a tissue or elbow

Surgical face masks for TB patients are stigmatizing and are typically not recommended for cooperative patients. Precautions are needed until drug treatment has made patients sufficiently noncontagious. For patients with proven drug-susceptible or MDR-TB, precautions are maintained until there is a clinical response to therapy (typically, 1 to 2 wk). However, for XDR-TB, response to treatment may be slower, and the consequences of transmission even greater; thus, a more convincing response to therapy (eg, smear or culture conversion) is required to end precautions.

Hospitalization: The main indications for hospitalization are

- Serious concomitant illness
- Need for diagnostic procedures
- Social issues (eg, homelessness)
- Need for respiratory isolation, as for people living in congregate settings where previously unexposed people would be regularly encountered (important primarily if effective treatment cannot be ensured)

Initially, all hospitalized patients should be in respiratory isolation, ideally in a negative-pressure room with 6 to 12 air changes/h. Anyone entering the room should wear a respirator (not a surgical mask) that has been appropriately fitted and that meets National Institute for Occupational Safety and Health certification (N-95 or greater). Because risk of exposing other hospitalized patients is high, even though patients receiving effective treatment become noncontagious before sputum smears become negative, release from respiratory isolation usually requires 3 negative sputum smears over 2 days, including at least one early-morning negative specimen.

PEARLS & PITFALLS

- In hospitals and clinics, the highest risk of TB transmission is from patients who have undiagnosed TB or unidentified drug resistance and are receiving inadequate treatment, not from known TB patients who are receiving effective treatment.

Public health considerations: To improve treatment adherence, ensure cure, and limit transmission and the development of drug-resistant strains, public health programs closely monitor treatment, even if patients are being treated by a private physician. In most states, TB care (including skin testing, chest x-rays, and drugs) is available free through public health clinics to reduce barriers to treatment.

Increasingly, optimal patient case management includes supervision by public health personnel of the ingestion of every dose of drug, a strategy known as directly observed therapy (DOT). DOT increases the likelihood that the full treatment course will be completed from 61% to 86% (91% with enhanced DOT, in which incentives and enablers such as transportation vouchers, child care, outreach workers, and meals are provided). DOT is particularly important

- For children and adolescents
- For patients with HIV infection, psychiatric illness, or substance abuse
- After treatment failure, relapse, or development of drug resistance

In some programs, selective self-administered treatment (SAT) is an option for patients who are committed to treatment; ideally, fixed-dose combination drug preparations are used to avoid the possibility of monotherapy, which can lead to drug resistance. Mechanical drug monitoring devices have been advocated to improve adherence with SAT.

Public health departments usually visit homes to evaluate potential barriers to treatment (eg, extreme poverty, unstable housing, child care problems, alcoholism, mental illness), to check for other active cases, and to assess close contacts. Close contacts are people who share the same breathing space for prolonged periods, typically household residents, but often include people at work, school, and places of recreation. The precise duration and degree of contact that constitutes risk vary because TB patients vary greatly in contagiousness. For patients who are highly contagious as evidenced by multiple family members with disease or positive skin tests, even relatively casual contacts (eg, passengers on the bus they ride) should be referred for skin testing and evaluation for latent infection (see p. 1657); patients who do not infect any household contacts are less likely to infect casual contacts.

First-line drugs: The first-line drugs INH, RIF, pyrazinamide (PZA), and ethambutol (EMB) are used together in initial treatment (for regimens and doses, see p. 1657 and Table 196–1).

Table 196–1. DOSING OF ORAL FIRST-LINE ANTI-TB DRUGS*

DRUG	ADULTS OR CHILDREN	DAILY†	ONCE/WK	2 TIMES/WK	3 TIMES/WK
Isoniazid	Adults (maximum)	5 mg/kg (300 mg)	15 mg/kg (900 mg)	15 mg/kg (900 mg)	15 mg/kg (900 mg)
	Children (maximum)	10–20 mg/kg (300 mg)	N/A	20–40 mg/kg (900 mg)	N/A
Rifampin	Adults (maximum)	10 mg/kg (600 mg)	N/A	10 mg/kg (600 mg)	10 mg/kg (600 mg)
	Children (maximum)	10–20 mg/kg (600 mg)	N/A	10–20 mg/kg (600 mg)	N/A
Rifabutin	Adults (maximum)	5 mg/kg (300 mg)	N/A	5 mg/kg (300 mg)	5 mg/kg (300 mg)
	Children	10–20 mg/kg (300 mg)	N/A	10–20 mg/kg (300 mg)	10–20 mg/kg (600 mg)
Rifapentine‡	Adults	N/A	10 mg/kg (600 mg)	N/A	N/A
	Children	N/A	N/A	N/A	N/A
Pyrazinamide	Adults (whole tablets):				
	40–55 kg	1 g	N/A	2 g	1.5 g
	56–75 kg	1.5 g	N/A	3 g	2.5 g
	≥ 76 kg§	2 g	N/A	4 g	3 g
	Children (maximum)	15–30 mg/kg (2 g)	N/A	50 mg/kg (2 g)	N/A
Ethambutol	Adults (whole tablets):				
	40–55 kg	800 mg	N/A	2000 mg	1200 mg
	56–75 kg	1200 mg	N/A	2800 mg	2000 mg
	≥ 76 kg§	1600 mg	N/A	4000 mg	2400 mg
	Children (maximum)	15–20 mg/kg (1 g)	N/A	50 mg/kg (2.5 g)	N/A

*Specific regimens are discussed in text.
†Daily is considered either 5 or 7 days/wk. All dosing < 7 days/wk must be given as directly observed therapy.
‡Continuation phase only.
§Maximum dose.
N/A = not applicable.

INH is given orally once/day, has good tissue penetration (including CSF), and is highly bactericidal. It remains the single most useful and least expensive drug for TB treatment. Decades of uncontrolled use—often as monotherapy—in many countries (especially in East Asia) have greatly increased the percentage of resistant strains. In the US, about 10% of isolates are INH-resistant.

Adverse reactions include rash, fever, and, rarely, anemia and agranulocytosis. INH causes asymptomatic, transient aminotransferase elevations in up to 20% of patients and clinical (usually reversible) hepatitis in about 1/1000. Clinical hepatitis occurs more often in patients > 35 yr, alcoholics, postpartum women, and patients with chronic liver disease. Monthly liver function testing is not recommended unless patients have risk factors for liver disease. Patients with unexplained fatigue, anorexia, nausea, vomiting, or jaundice may have hepatic toxicity; treatment is suspended and liver function tests are done. Those with symptoms and any significant aminotransferase elevation (or asymptomatic elevation > 5 times normal) by definition have hepatic toxicity, and INH is stopped. After recovery from mild aminotransferase elevations and symptoms, patients can be safely challenged with a half-dose for 2 to 3 days. If this dose is tolerated (typically in about half of patients), the full dose may be restarted with close monitoring for recurrence of symptoms and deterioration of liver function. If patients are receiving INH, RIF, and PZA, all drugs must be stopped, and the challenge done with each drug separately. INH or PZA, rather than RIF, is the more likely cause of hepatotoxicity. Peripheral neuropathy can result from INH-induced pyridoxine (vitamin B_6) deficiency, most likely in pregnant or breastfeeding women, undernourished patients, patients with diabetes mellitus or HIV infection, alcoholics, patients with cancer or uremia, and the elderly. A daily dose of pyridoxine 25 to 50 mg can prevent this complication, although pyridoxine is usually not needed in children and healthy young adults. INH delays hepatic metabolism of phenytoin, requiring dose reduction. It can also cause a violent reaction to disulfiram, a drug occasionally used for alcoholism. INH is safe during pregnancy.

RIF, given orally, is bactericidal, is well-absorbed, penetrates well into cells and CSF, and acts rapidly. It also eliminates dormant organisms in macrophages or caseous lesions that can cause late relapse. Thus, RIF should be used throughout the course of therapy. Adverse effects include cholestatic jaundice (rare), fever, thrombocytopenia, and renal failure. RIF has a lower rate of hepatotoxicity than INH. Drug interactions must be considered when using RIF. It accelerates metabolism of anticoagulants, oral contraceptives, corticosteroids, digitoxin, oral antihyperglycemic drugs, methadone, and many other drugs. The interactions of rifamycins and many antiretroviral drugs are particularly complex; combined use requires specialized expertise. RIF is safe during pregnancy.

The following newer rifamycins are available for special situations:

- **Rifabutin** is used for patients taking drugs (particularly antiretroviral drugs) that have unacceptable interactions with RIF. Its action is similar to RIF, but it affects the metabolism of other drugs less. When used with clarithromycin or fluconazole, rifabutin has been associated with uveitis.

- **Rifapentine** is used in one dose/wk regimens (see Table 196–1) but is not used in children or patients with HIV (because of unacceptable treatment failure rates) or extrapulmonary TB. It is also used in a 12-dose, once/wk DOT regimen with INH for TB prophylaxis. This prophylactic combination is not recommended for children < 2 yr, HIV-infected patients receiving antiretroviral treatment, pregnant women, or women expecting to become pregnant during treatment because safety in these groups is unknown.

PZA is an oral bactericidal drug. When used during the intensive initial 2 mo of treatment, it shortens the duration of therapy to 6 mo and prevents development of resistance to RIF.

Its major adverse effects are GI upset and hepatitis. It often causes hyperuricemia, which is generally mild and only rarely induces gout. PZA is commonly used during pregnancy, but its safety has not been confirmed.

EMB is given orally and is the best tolerated of the first-line drugs. Its main toxicity is optic neuritis, which is more common at higher doses (eg, 25 mg/kg) and in patients with impaired renal function. Patients with optic neuritis present initially with an inability to distinguish blue from green, followed by impairment of visual acuity. Because both symptoms are reversible if detected early, patients should have a baseline test of visual acuity and color vision and should be questioned monthly regarding their vision. Patients taking EMB for > 2 mo or at doses higher than those listed in the table above should have monthly visual acuity and color vision testing. Caution is warranted if communication is limited by language and cultural barriers. For similar reasons, EMB is usually avoided in young children who cannot read eye charts but can be used if needed because of drug resistance or drug intolerance. Another drug is substituted for EMB if optic neuritis occurs. EMB can be used safely during pregnancy. Resistance to EMB is less common than that to the other first-line drugs.

Second-line drugs: Other antibiotics are active against TB and are used primarily when patients have drug-resistant TB (DR-TB) or do not tolerate one of the first-line drugs. The 2 most important classes are aminoglycosides (and the closely related polypeptide drug, capreomycin) and fluoroquinolones; aminoglycosides are available only for parenteral use.

Streptomycin, once the most commonly used aminoglycoside, is very effective and bactericidal. Resistance is still relatively uncommon in the US but is more common globally. CSF penetration is poor, and intrathecal administration should not be used if other effective drugs are available.

Dose-related adverse effects include renal tubular damage, vestibular damage, and ototoxicity. The dose is about 15 mg/kg IM. The maximum is usually 1 g for adults, reduced to 0.75 g [10 mg/kg] for those ≥ 60 yr. To limit dose-related adverse effects, clinicians give the drug only 5 days/wk for up to 2 mo. Then it may be given twice/wk for another 2 mo if necessary. In patients with renal insufficiency, dosing frequency should be reduced (eg, 12 to 15 mg/kg/ dose 2 or 3 times/wk). Patients should be monitored with appropriate testing of balance, hearing, and serum creatinine levels. Adverse effects include rash, fever, agranulocytosis, and serum sickness. Flushing and tingling around the mouth commonly accompany injection but subside quickly. Streptomycin is contraindicated during pregnancy because it may cause vestibular toxicity and ototoxicity in the fetus.

Kanamycin and **amikacin** may remain effective even if streptomycin resistance has developed. Their renal and neural toxicities are similar to those of streptomycin. Kanamycin is the most widely used injectable for MDR-TB.

Capreomycin, a related nonaminoglycoside parenteral bactericidal drug, has dosage, effectiveness, and adverse effects similar to those of aminoglycosides. It is an important drug for MDR-TB because isolates resistant to streptomycin are often susceptible to capreomycin, and it is somewhat better tolerated than aminoglycosides when prolonged administration is required.

Some **fluoroquinolones** (levofloxacin, moxifloxacin) are the most active and safest TB drugs after INH and RIF, but they are not first-line drugs for TB susceptible to INH and RIF. Moxifloxacin appears to be as active as INH when used with RIF.

Other 2nd-line drugs include ethionamide, cycloserine, and para-aminosalicylic acid (PAS). These drugs are less effective and more toxic than the first-line drugs but are essential in treatment of MDR-TB.

Bedaquiline, delamanid, and sutezolid are new anti-TB drugs that are typically reserved for highly resistant TB (precise indications are not yet fully defined) or for patients who cannot tolerate other 2nd-line drugs.

Drug resistance: Drug resistance develops through spontaneous genetic mutation. Incomplete, erratic, or single-drug therapy selects for these resistant organisms. Once a drug-resistant strain has developed and proliferates, it may acquire resistance to additional drugs through the same process. In this way, the organism can become resistant to multiple antibiotics in steps.

MDR-TB is resistant to INH and RIF, with or without resistance to other drugs. Numerous outbreaks of MDR-TB have been reported, and the global burden is increasing. The WHO estimates that 480,000 new cases occurred worldwide in 2015. In parts of the world where resistance testing is inadequate or unavailable, many patients who do not respond to first-line therapy probably have unrecognized MDR-TB. Multidrug resistance has major negative implications for TB control; alternative treatments require a longer treatment course with less effective, more toxic, and more expensive 2nd-line drugs.

Pre-XDR-TB is MDR-TB plus resistance to either a fluoroquinolone or an injectable drug but not both.

XDR-TB extends the resistance profile of MDR-TB to include fluoroquinolones and at least one injectable drug (eg, streptomycin, amikacin, kanamycin, capreomycin). This additional resistance has dire therapeutic implications. Although some patients with XDR-TB can be cured, mortality is higher, and the outcome depends on the number of effective drugs that remain as well as the extent of lung destruction caused by the bacilli. Surgery to remove localized areas of necrotic lung tissue is important in the treatment of advanced cases of MDR-TB or XDR-TB but is not widely available in high-burden areas.

Resistant strains can be transmitted from person to person. A person who is infected with a drug-resistant strain from another person is said to have primary drug resistance. Slightly more than half of all MDR-TB cases have not previously been treated, probably because of transmission of (often reinfection with) MDR or XDR strains. Uninhibited transmission of drug-resistant strains in congregate settings, such as hospitals, clinics, prisons, shelters, and refugee camps, is a major barrier to global control.

Several new anti-TB drugs that may be active against resistant strains are in preclinical or clinical development but will not be available for several more years. Furthermore, unless treatment programs are strengthened (eg, by full supervision of each dose and improved access to culture and susceptibility testing), stepwise resistance to new drugs is likely.

Successful treatment of DR-TB depends on the use of multiple active drugs simultaneously, so that any resistance to one drug is countered by the killing effects of a 2nd, 3rd or 4th drug. Furthermore, all drugs in the regimen must be taken scrupulously for an extended period. Any lapses in adherence may lead to further drug resistance and/or treatment failure.

The new anti-TB drugs bedaquiline, delamanid, and sutezolid are active against resistant strains and may help control the epidemic of DR-TB. However, success will continue to depend on strong global efforts to diagnose TB early, give patients appropriate therapy, and provide supervision of ingestion of each dose (DOT).

Treatment regimens: Treatment of all patients with new, previously untreated TB should consist of a

- 2-mo initial intensive phase
- 4- to 7-mo continuation phase

Initial intensive–phase therapy is with 4 antibiotics: INH, RIF, PZA, and EMB (see Table 196–1 for dosing). These drugs can be given daily throughout this phase or daily for 2 wk, followed by doses 2 or 3 times/week for 6 wk. Intermittent administration (usually with higher doses) is usually satisfactory because of the slow growth of tubercle bacilli and the residual postantibiotic effect on growth (bacterial growth is often delayed well after antibiotics are below the minimal inhibitory concentration). However, daily therapy is recommended for patients with MDR-TB or HIV coinfection. Regimens involving less than daily dosing must be carried out as DOT because each dose becomes more important.

After 2 mo of intensive 4-drug treatment, PZA and usually EMB are stopped, depending on the drug susceptibility pattern of the original isolate.

Continuation-phase treatment depends on results of drug susceptibility testing of initial isolates (where available), the presence or absence of a cavitary lesion on the initial chest x-ray, and results of cultures taken at 2 mo. If positive, 2-mo cultures indicate the need for a longer course of treatment. If both culture and smear are negative, regardless of the chest x-ray, or if the culture or smear is positive but x-ray showed no cavitation, INH and RIF are continued for 4 more mo (6 mo total). If the x-ray showed cavitation and the culture or smear is positive, INH and RIF are continued for 7 more mo (9 mo total). In either regimen, EMB is usually stopped if the initial culture shows no resistance to any drug. Continuation-phase drugs can be given daily or, if patients are not HIV-positive, 2 or 3 times/wk. Patients who have negative culture and smears at 2 mo and no cavitation on chest x-ray and who are HIV-negative may receive once/wk INH plus rifapentine. Patients who have positive cultures after 2 mo of treatment should be evaluated to determine the cause. Evaluation for MDR-TB, a common cause, should be thorough. Clinicians should also check for other common causes (eg, nonadherence, extensive cavitary disease, drug resistance, malabsorption of drugs).

For both initial and continuation phases, the total number of doses (calculated by doses/wk times number of weeks) should be given; thus if any doses are missed, treatment is extended and not stopped at the end of the time period.

Management of drug-resistant TB varies with the pattern of drug resistance. Generally, MDR-TB requires treatment for 18 to 24 mo using a regimen that contains 4 or 5 active drugs. Presumed activity is based on drug susceptibility test results, a known source case, prior exposure to anti-TB drugs, or drug susceptibility patterns in the community. The regimen should include all remaining active first-line drugs (including PZA, if the strain is susceptible) plus a 2nd-line injectable, a fluoroquinolone, and other 2nd-line drugs as needed to build a 4- or 5-drug regimen. Designing a treatment regimen for XDR-TB becomes even more challenging, often requiring the use of unproven and highly toxic drugs such as clofazimine and linezolid.

Managing adverse effects of these long, complex regimens is challenging. A TB specialist experienced with DR-TB should be consulted for assistance in managing these cases. DOT is essential to avoid development of additional drug resistance through nonadherance.

Other treatments: Surgical resection of a persistent TB cavity or a region of necrotic lung tissue is occasionally necessary. The main indication for resection is persistent, culture-positive MDR-TB or XDR-TB in patients with a region of necrotic lung tissue into which antibiotics cannot penetrate. Other indications include uncontrollable hemoptysis and bronchial stenosis.

Corticosteroids are sometimes used to treat TB when inflammation is a major cause of morbidity and are indicated for patients with acute respiratory distress syndrome or closed-space infections, such as meningitis and pericarditis. Dexamethasone 12 mg po or IV q 6 h is given to adults and children > 25 kg; children < 25 kg are given 8 mg. Treatment is continued for 2 to 3 wk. Corticosteroids that are needed for other indications pose no danger to patients who have active TB and who are receiving an effective TB regimen.

Screening

Screening for latent TB infection (LTBI) is done with TST or IGRA. Indications for testing include

- Close contact with a person who has active pulmonary TB
- Chest x-ray evidence of past TB infection
- Risk factors for exposure to TB (eg, people who have immigrated within 5 yr from high-risk areas, indigent patients, IV drug users, selected US health care practitioners such as respiratory therapists and practitioners working with high-risk populations)
- Risk factors for development of active TB (eg, HIV infection or other impaired immunity, gastrectomy, jejunoileal bypass surgery, silicosis, renal insufficiency, diabetes, head or neck cancer, age > 70 yr)
- Therapeutic immunosuppression with corticosteroids, TNF inhibitors, or cancer chemotherapy

In the US, most children and other people without specific TB risk factors should not be tested to avoid false-positive reactions.

A positive TST or IGRA test result (see p. 1653 for criteria) suggests LTBI. Patients with a positive TST or IGRA result are evaluated for other clinical and epidemiologic risk factors and have a chest x-ray. Those with x-ray abnormalities suggesting TB require evaluation for active TB as above, including sputum examination by microscopy and culture. Updated guidelines for testing and treatment of LTBI are available at the Centers for Disease Control and Prevention (CDC) web site (www.cdc.gov).

Booster reaction: Some patients with remote TB exposure, BCG vaccination, or infection with nontuberculous mycobacteria may have a negative TST or IGRA; however, the TST itself may serve as an immune booster so that a subsequent test done as little as 1 wk or as much as several years later may be positive (booster reaction). Thus, in people who are tested regularly (eg, health care workers), the 2nd routine test will be positive, giving the false appearance of recent infection (and hence mandating further testing and treatment). If recurrent testing for LTBI is indicated, a 2nd TST should be done 1 to 4 wk after the first to identify a booster reaction (because conversion in that brief interval is highly unlikely). Subsequent TST is done and interpreted normally.

The new IGRAs for LTBI do not involve injection of antigens and thus do not cause boosting. They also are not influenced by preexisting hypersensitivity from BCG vaccination or infection with environmental mycobacteria other than *M. kansasii*, *M. szulgai*, and *M. marinum*.

Treatment of LTBI: Treatment is indicated principally for

- People whose TST converted from negative to positive within the previous 2 yr
- People with x-ray changes consistent with old TB but no evidence of active TB

Other indications for preventive treatment include

- People who, if infected, are at high risk of developing active TB (eg, HIV-infected people, people with drug-induced immunosuppression)
- Any child < 5 yr who is a close contact of a person with smear-positive TB, regardless of whether there was TST conversion

Other people with an incidental positive TST or IGRA but without these risk factors are often treated for LTBI, but physicians should balance individual risks of drug toxicity against the benefits of treatment.

Treatment generally consists of INH unless resistance is suspected (eg, in exposure to a known INH-resistant case). The dose is 300 mg once/day for 9 mo for most adults and 10 mg/kg for 9 mo for children. An alternative for patients resistant to or intolerant of INH is RIF 600 mg once/day for 4 mo. DOT with INH plus rifapentine taken once/wk for 3 mo is also effective.

The main limitations of treatment of LTBI are hepatotoxicity and poor adherence. When used for LTBI, INH causes clinical hepatitis in 1/1000 cases; hepatitis usually reverses if INH is stopped promptly. Patients being treated for LTBI should be instructed to stop the drug if they experience any new symptoms, especially unexplained fatigue, loss of appetite, or nausea. Hepatitis due to RIF is less common than with INH, but drug interactions are frequent. Only about 50% of patients complete the recommended 9-mo course of INH. Adherence is better with 4 mo of RIF. Monthly visits to monitor symptoms and to encourage treatment completion are standard good clinical and public health practice.

Prevention

Vaccination: The BCG vaccine, made from an attenuated strain of *M. bovis* is given to > 80% of the world's children, primarily in high-burden countries. Overall average efficacy is probably only 50%. BCG clearly reduces the rate of extrathoracic TB in children, especially TB meningitis, and may prevent TB infection. Thus, it is considered worthwhile in high-burden regions. Immunization with BCG has few indications in the US, except unavoidable exposure of a child to an infectious TB case that cannot be effectively treated (ie, pre-XDR or XDR-TB) and possibly previously uninfected health care workers exposed to MDR-TB or XDR-TB on a regular basis.

Although BCG vaccination often converts the TST, the reaction is usually smaller than the response to natural TB infection, and it usually wanes more quickly. The TST reaction due to BCG is rarely > 15 mm, and 15 yr after BCG administration, it is rarely > 10 mm. The CDC recommends that all TST reactions in children who have had BCG be attributed to TB infection (and treated accordingly) because untreated latent infection can have serious complications. IGRAs are not influenced by BCG vaccination and should ideally be used in patients who have received BCG to be sure that the TST response is due to infection with *M. tuberculosis*.

Special Populations

Children: Children infected with TB are more likely than adults to develop active disease, which commonly manifests as extrapulmonary disease. Lymphadenitis (scrofula) is the most common extrapulmonary manifestation, but TB may also affect the vertebrae (Pott disease), the highly vascular epiphyses of long bones, or the CNS and meninges. Clinical presentation of active TB in children varies, making the diagnosis challenging. Most children have few symptoms other than a brassy cough.

Obtaining a sample for culture often requires gastric aspiration, sputum induction, or a more invasive procedure such as bronchoalveolar lavage. The most common sign on chest x-ray is hilar lymphadenopathy, but segmental atelectasis is possible. Adenopathy may progress, even after chemotherapy is started, and may cause lobar atelectasis, which usually clears during treatment. Cavitary disease is less common than in adults, and most children harbor far fewer organisms and are not contagious. Treatment strategies are similar to those for adults except that drugs must be dosed strictly based on the child's weight (see Table 196–1).

The elderly: Reactivated disease can involve any organ, but particularly the lungs, brain, kidneys, long bones, vertebrae, or lymph nodes. Reactivation may cause few symptoms and can be overlooked for weeks or months, delaying appropriate evaluation. The frequent presence of other disorders in old age further complicates the diagnosis. Regardless of their age, nursing home residents who were previously TST negative are at risk of disease due to recent transmission, which may cause apical, middle-lobe, or lower-lobe pneumonia as well as pleural effusion. The pneumonia may not be recognized as TB and may persist and spread to other people while it is being erroneously treated with ineffective broad-spectrum antibiotics. In the US, miliary TB and TB meningitis, commonly thought to affect mainly young children, are more common among the elderly.

Risks and benefits of preventive treatment should be carefully assessed before the elderly are treated. INH causes hepatotoxicity in up to 4 to 5% of patients > 65 yr (compared with < 1% of patients < 65 yr). As a result, chemoprophylaxis is usually given to the elderly only if the induration after TST increases ≥ 15 mm from a previously negative reaction. Close contacts of an active case and others at high risk and with a negative TST or IGRA should also be considered for preventive treatment unless contraindicated.

HIV-infected patients: TST sensitivity is generally poor in immunocompromised patients, who may be anergic. In some studies, IGRAs appear to perform better than the TST in immunocompromised patients, although this advantage has not yet been established.

In HIV-infected patients with LTBI, active TB develops in about 5 to 10%/yr, whereas in people who are not immunocompromised, it develops in about the same percentage over a lifetime. In the early 1990s, half of HIV-infected TB patients who were untreated or infected with an MDR strain died, with median survival of only 60 days. Now, outcomes are somewhat better in developed countries because of earlier TB diagnosis and antiretroviral therapy, but TB in HIV patients remains a serious concern. In developing countries, mortality continues to be high among patients coinfected with HIV and MDR-TB or XDR-TB.

Dissemination of bacilli during primary infection is usually much more extensive in patients with HIV infection. Consequently, a larger proportion of TB is extrapulmonary. Tuberculomas (mass lesions in the lungs or CNS due to TB) are more common and more destructive. HIV infection reduces both inflammatory reaction and cavitation of pulmonary lesions. As a result, a chest x-ray may show a nonspecific pneumonia or even be normal. Smear-negative TB is more common when HIV coinfection is present. Because smear-negative TB is common, HIV-TB coinfection is often considered a paucibacillary disease state.

TB may develop early in AIDS and may be its presenting manifestation. Hematogenous dissemination of TB in patients with HIV infection causes a serious, often baffling illness with symptoms of both infections. In AIDS patients, a mycobacterial illness that develops while the CD4 count is ≥ 200/μL is almost always TB. By contrast, depending on the probability of TB exposure, a mycobacterial infection that develops while the CD4 count is < 50/μL is usually due to *M. avium* complex (MAC—see p. 1660). Infection with MAC is not contagious and, in HIV-infected patients, affects primarily the blood and bone marrow, not the lungs.

HIV-infected patients who were not diagnosed before presenting with TB should receive 2 wk of antimycobacterial treatment before starting antiretroviral therapy to decrease the risk of developing the immune reconstitution inflammatory syndrome (IRIS). TB in HIV-infected patients generally responds well to usual regimens when in vitro testing shows drug susceptibility. However, for MDR-TB strains, outcomes are not as favorable because the drugs are more toxic and less effective. Therapy for susceptible TB should be continued for 6 to 9 mo after conversion of sputum cultures to negative but may be shortened to 6 mo if 3 separate pretreatment sputum smears are negative, suggesting a low burden of organisms. Current recommendations suggest that if the sputum culture is positive after 2 mo of therapy, treatment is prolonged to 9 mo. HIV-infected patients whose tuberculin reactions are ≥ 5 mm (or with a positive IGRA) should receive chemoprophylaxis. Current CDC TB treatment guidelines should be consulted at www.cdc.gov.

KEY POINTS

- TB causes a primary, often asymptomatic infection followed by latent infection and, in a few patients, an active disease phase.
- About one third of the world's population is infected with TB, and about 15 million have active disease at a given time.
- Active disease is much more likely in patients with impaired immunity, particularly those with HIV infection.
- Suspect the diagnosis based on symptoms, risk factors, TST, and IGRA; confirm by sputum testing (microscopic examination and culture) and/or NAATs.
- Treat with multiple drugs for several months.
- Drug resistance is a major concern and is increased by poor adherence, use of inappropriate drug regimens, and inadequate susceptibility testing.

EXTRAPULMONARY TUBERCULOSIS

Tuberculosis (TB) outside the lung usually results from hematogenous dissemination. Sometimes infection directly extends from an adjacent organ. Symptoms vary by site but generally include fever, malaise, and weight loss. Diagnosis is most often by sputum smear and culture and, increasingly, by rapid molecular-based diagnostic tests. Treatment is with multiple antimicrobial drugs given for at least 6 mo.

Miliary TB: Also known as generalized hematogenous TB, miliary TB occurs when a tuberculous lesion erodes into a blood vessel, disseminating millions of tubercle bacilli into the bloodstream and throughout the body. Uncontrolled massive dissemination can occur during primary infection or after reactivation of a latent focus. The lungs and bone marrow are most often affected, but any site may be involved. Miliary TB is most common among children < 4 yr, immunocompromised people, and the elderly.

Symptoms include fever, chills, weakness, malaise, and often progressive dyspnea. Intermittent dissemination of tubercle bacilli may lead to a prolonged FUO. Bone marrow involvement may cause anemia, thrombocytopenia, or a leukemoid reaction.

Genitourinary TB: Infection of the kidneys may manifest as pyelonephritis (eg, fever, back pain, pyuria) without the usual urinary pathogens on routine culture (sterile pyuria). Infection commonly spreads to the bladder and, in men, to the prostate, seminal vesicles, or epididymis, causing an enlarging scrotal mass. Infection may spread to the perinephric space and down the psoas muscle, sometimes causing an abscess on the anterior thigh.

Salpingo-oophoritis can occur after menarche, when the fallopian tubes become vascular. Symptoms include chronic pelvic pain and sterility or ectopic pregnancy due to tubal scarring.

TB meningitis: Meningitis often occurs in the absence of infection at other extrapulmonary sites. In the US, it is most common among the elderly and immunocompromised, but in areas where TB is common among children, TB meningitis usually occurs between birth and 5 yr. At any age, meningitis is the most serious form of TB and has high morbidity and mortality. It is the one form of TB believed to be prevented in childhood by vaccination with BCG.

Symptoms are low-grade fever, unremitting headache, nausea, and drowsiness, which may progress to stupor and coma. Kernig and Brudzinski signs may be positive. Stages are

1. Clear sensorium with abnormal CSF
2. Drowsiness or stupor with focal neurologic signs
3. Coma

Stroke may result from thrombosis of a major cerebral vessel. Focal neurologic symptoms suggest a tuberculoma.

TB peritonitis: Peritoneal infection represents seeding from abdominal lymph nodes or from salpingo-oophoritis. Peritonitis is particularly common among alcoholics with cirrhosis.

Symptoms may be mild, with fatigue, abdominal pain, and tenderness, or severe enough to mimic acute abdomen.

TB pericarditis: Pericardial infection may develop from foci in mediastinal lymph nodes or from pleural TB. In some high-incidence parts of the world, TB pericarditis is a common cause of heart failure.

Patients may have a pericardial friction rub, pleuritic and positional chest pain, or fever. Pericardial tamponade may occur, causing dyspnea, neck vein distention, paradoxical pulse, muffled heart sounds, and possibly hypotension.

TB lymphadenitis: Tuberculous lymphadenitis (scrofula) typically involves the lymph nodes in the posterior cervical and supraclavicular chains. Infection in these areas is thought to be due to contiguous spread from intrathoracic lymphatics. Mediastinal lymph nodes are also commonly enlarged as a part of primary pulmonary disease.

Cervical tuberculous lymphadenitis is characterized by progressive swelling of the affected nodes. In advanced cases, nodes may become inflamed and tender; the overlying skin may break down, resulting in a draining fistula.

TB of bones and joints: Weight-bearing joints are most commonly involved, but bones of the wrist, hand, and elbow may also be affected, especially after injury.

Pott disease is spinal infection, which begins in a vertebral body and often spreads to adjacent vertebrae, with narrowing of the disk space between them. Untreated, the vertebrae may collapse, possibly impinging on the spinal cord. Symptoms include progressive or constant pain in involved bones and chronic or subacute arthritis (usually monoarticular). In Pott disease, spinal cord compression produces neurologic deficits, including paraplegia; paravertebral swelling may result from an abscess.

Gastrointestinal TB: Because the entire GI mucosa resists TB invasion, infection requires prolonged exposure and enormous inocula. It is very unusual in developed countries where bovine TB is rare.

Ulcers of the mouth and oropharynx may develop from eating *M. bovis*–contaminated dairy products; primary lesions may also occur in the small bowel. Intestinal invasion generally causes hyperplasia and an inflammatory bowel syndrome with pain, diarrhea, obstruction, and hematochezia. It may also mimic appendicitis. Ulceration and fistulas are possible.

TB of the liver: Liver infection is common in patients with advanced pulmonary TB and widely disseminated or miliary TB. However, the liver generally heals without sequelae when the principal infection is treated. TB in the liver occasionally spreads to the gallbladder, leading to obstructive jaundice.

Other sites: Rarely, TB develops on abraded skin in patients with cavitary pulmonary TB. TB may infect the wall of a blood vessel and has even ruptured the aorta. Adrenal involvement, leading to Addison disease, formerly was common but now is rare. Tubercle bacilli may spread to tendon sheaths (tuberculous tenosynovitis) by direct extension from adjacent lesions in bone or hematogenously from any infected organ.

Diagnosis

- Acid-fast staining, microscopic analysis, and mycobacterial culture of fluid and tissue samples, and, when available, nucleic acid–based testing
- Chest x-ray
- TST or IGRA

Testing is similar to that for pulmonary TB (see p. 1652), including chest x-ray, TST or IGRA, and microscopic analysis (with appropriate staining) and mycobacterial cultures of affected body fluids (CSF, urine, or pleural, pericardial, or joint fluid) and tissue for mycobacteria. Nucleic acid–based testing can be done on fresh fluid or biopsy samples and on fixed tissue (eg, if TB was not suspected during a surgical procedure and cultures were not done). Blood culture results are positive in about 50% of patients with disseminated TB; such patients are often immunocompromised, often by HIV infection. However, cultures and smears of body fluids and tissues are often negative because few organisms are present; in this case, NAATs may be helpful.

Typically, lymphocytosis is present in body fluids. A very suggestive finding in the CSF is a glucose level < 50% of that in serum and an elevated protein level.

If all tests are negative and miliary TB is still a concern, biopsies of the bone marrow and the liver are done. If TB is highly suspected based on other features (eg, granuloma seen on biopsy, positive TST or IGRA plus unexplained lymphocytosis in pleural fluid or CSF), treatment should usually proceed despite inability to demonstrate TB organisms.

Chest x-ray and other imaging, TST, and IGRA can also provide helpful diagnostic information. Chest x-ray may show signs of primary or active TB; in miliary TB, it shows thousands of 2- to 3-mm interstitial nodules evenly distributed through both lungs. Other imaging tests are done based on clinical findings. Abdominal or GU involvement usually requires CT or ultrasonography; renal lesions are often visible. Bone and joint involvement requires CT or MRI; MRI is preferable for spinal disease. TST and IGRA may initially be negative, but a repeat test in a few weeks is likely to be positive. If it is not, the diagnosis of TB should be questioned or causes of anergy sought.

Treatment

Drug treatment is the most important modality and follows standard regimens and principles (see p. 1654). Six to 9 mo of therapy is probably adequate for most sites except the meninges, which require treatment for 9 to 12 mo. Corticosteroids may help in pericarditis and meningitis (for dosing, see p. 1657).

Drug resistance is a major concern; it is increased by poor adherence, use of too few drugs, and inadequate susceptibility testing.

Surgery is required for the following:

- To drain empyema, cardiac tamponade, and CNS abscess
- To close bronchopleural fistulas
- To resect infected bowel
- To decompress spinal cord encroachment

Surgical debridement is sometimes needed in Pott disease to correct spinal deformities or to relieve cord compression if there are neurologic deficits or pain persists; fixation of the vertebral column by bone graft is required in only the most advanced cases. Surgery is usually not necessary for TB lymphadenitis except for diagnostic purposes.

KEY POINTS

- TB can spread from the lungs through the bloodstream to many sites.
- Symptoms depend on the affected organ but typically include fever, malaise, and weight loss.
- Diagnose based identification of bacilli in infected fluid or tissue by microscopic examination and culture and/or NAATs.
- Treat with multiple drugs for several months and sometimes with surgery.
- Drug resistance is a major concern and is increased by poor adherence, use of too few drugs, and inadequate susceptibility testing.

OTHER MYCOBACTERIAL INFECTIONS RESEMBLING TUBERCULOSIS

Mycobacteria other than the tubercle bacillus sometimes infect humans. These organisms are commonly present in soil and water and are much less virulent in humans than is *M. tuberculosis*. Infections with these organisms have been called atypical, environmental, and nontuberculous mycobacterial infections. Most exposures and infections by these organisms do not cause disease, which usually requires a defect in local or systemic host defenses; the frail elderly and immunocompromised people are at the highest risk. *M. avium* complex (MAC)—the closely related species of *M. avium* and *M. intracellulare*—accounts for most diseases. Other causative species are *M. kansasii*, *M. xenopi*, *M. marinum*, *M. ulcerans*, and the *M. fortuitum* complex (*M. fortuitum*, *M. abscessus*, and *M. chelonae*). Person-to-person transmission has not been documented.

The lungs are the most common site of disease; most lung infections involve MAC but may be due to *M. kansasii*, *M. xenopi*, or *M. abscessus*. Occasional cases involve lymph nodes, bones and joints, the skin, and wounds. However, incidence of disseminated MAC disease is increasing in HIV-infected patients, and resistance to anti-TB drugs is the rule (except for *M. kansasii* and *M. xenopi*).

Diagnosis of nontuberculous mycobacterial infections is typically made via acid-fast stain and culture of samples.

Nontuberculous mycobacterial infections are best managed by a specialist with particular expertise in that area. The American Thoracic Society publishes updated diagnostic and therapeutic guidelines on the diagnosis and management of these challenging infections.

Pulmonary disease: The typical patient is a middle-aged and elderly women with bronchiectasis, scoliosis, pectus excavatum, or mitral valve prolapse but without known underlying lung abnormalities. MAC also causes pulmonary disease in middle-aged or older white men with previous lung problems such as chronic bronchitis, emphysema, healed TB, bronchiectasis, or silicosis. Whether MAC causes bronchiectasis or bronchiectasis leads to MAC is not always clear. In older, thin women with chronic nonproductive cough, this syndrome is often called Lady Windermere syndrome; it appears to be increasing in frequency for unknown reasons.

Cough and expectoration are common, often associated with fatigue, weight loss, and low-grade fever. The course may be slowly progressive or stable for long periods. Respiratory insufficiency and persistent hemoptysis may develop. Fibronodular infiltrates on chest x-ray resemble those of pulmonary TB, but cavitation tends to be thin-walled, and pleural effusion is rare. So-called tree-and-bud infiltrates, seen on chest CT, are also characteristic of MAC disease.

Determination of drug susceptibility may be helpful for certain organism/drug combinations but can be done only in highly specialized laboratories. For MAC, susceptibility to clarithromycin is a predictor of therapeutic response.

For moderately symptomatic disease due to MAC with positive sputum smears and cultures, clarithromycin 500 mg po bid or azithromycin 600 mg po once/day, RIF 600 mg po once/day, and EMB 15 to 25 mg/kg po once/day should be used for 12 to 18 mo or until cultures are negative for 12 mo. For progressive cases unresponsive to standard drugs, combinations of 4 to 6 drugs that include clarithromycin 500 mg po bid or azithromycin 600 mg po once/day, rifabutin 300 mg po once/day, ciprofloxacin 250 to 500 mg po or IV bid, clofazimine 100 to 200 mg po once/day, and amikacin 10 to 15 mg/kg IV once/day may be tried. Resection surgery is recommended in exceptional cases involving well-localized disease in young, otherwise healthy patients.

M. kansasii and *M. xenopi* infections respond to INH, rifabutin, and EMB, with or without streptomycin or clarithromycin, given for 18 to 24 mo. *M. abscessus* infections are treated with 3 drugs: amikacin, cefoxitin or imipenem, and an oral macrolide. All nontuberculous mycobacteria are resistant to PZA.

Lymphadenitis: In children 1 to 5 yr, chronic submaxillary and submandibular cervical lymphadenitis is commonly due to MAC or *M. scrofulaceum*. It is presumably acquired by oral ingestion of soil organisms.

Diagnosis is usually by excisional biopsy. Usually, excision is adequate treatment and chemotherapy is not required.

Cutaneous disease: Swimming pool granuloma is a protracted but self-limited superficial granulomatous ulcerating disease usually caused by *M. marinum* contracted from swimming in contaminated pools or from cleaning a home aquarium. *M. ulcerans* and *M. kansasii* are occasionally involved. Lesions, reddish bumps, enlarging and turning purple, most frequently occur on the upper extremities or knees. Healing may occur spontaneously, but minocycline or doxycycline 100 to 200 mg po once/day, clarithromycin 500 mg po bid, or RIF plus EMB for 3 to 6 mo have been effective against *M. marinum*.

Buruli ulcer, caused by *M. ulcerans*, occurs in rural areas of > 30 tropical and subtropical countries. It starts as a painless subcutaneous nodule, a large painless area of induration, or a diffuse painless swelling of the legs, arms, or face. The infection progresses to cause extensive destruction of the skin and soft tissue; large ulcers may form on the legs or arms. Healing may result in a severe contracture, scarring, and deformity. For diagnosis, PCR should be used. The WHO recommends 8 wk of once/day combination therapy with rifampicin 10 mg/kg po plus either streptomycin 15 mg/kg IM, clarithromycin 7.5 mg/kg po (preferred during pregnancy), or moxifloxacin 400 mg po.

Wounds and foreign body infections: *M. fortuitum* complex has caused serious infections of penetrating wounds in the eyes and skin (especially feet), in tattoos, and in patients receiving contaminated materials (eg, porcine heart valves, breast implants, bone wax).

Treatment usually requires extensive debridement and removal of the foreign material. Useful drugs include imipenem 1 g IV q 6 h, levofloxacin 500 mg IV or po once/day, clarithromycin 500 mg po bid, trimethoprim/sulfamethoxazole 1 double-strength tablet po bid, doxycycline 100 to 200 mg po once/day, cefoxitin 2 g IV q 6 to 8 h, and amikacin 10 to 15 mg/kg IV once/day, for 3 to 6 mo. Combination therapy with at least 2 drugs that have in vitro activity is recommended. Infections caused by *M. abscessus* and *M. chelonae* are usually resistant to most antibiotics, have proved extremely difficult or impossible to cure, and should be referred to an experienced specialist.

Disseminated disease: MAC causes disseminated disease commonly in patients with advanced AIDS and occasionally in those with other immunocompromised states, including organ transplantation and hairy cell leukemia. In AIDS patients, disseminated MAC usually develops late (unlike TB, which develops early), occurring simultaneously with other opportunistic infections.

Disseminated MAC disease causes fever, anemia, thrombocytopenia, diarrhea, and abdominal pain (features similar to Whipple disease). Diagnosis can be confirmed by cultures of blood or bone marrow or by biopsy (eg, percutaneous fine-needle biopsy of liver or necrotic lymph nodes). Organisms may be identified in stool and respiratory specimens, but organisms from these specimens may represent colonization rather than true disease.

Combination therapy to clear bacteremia and alleviate symptoms usually requires 2 or 3 drugs; one is clarithromycin 500 mg po bid or azithromycin 600 mg po once/day, plus EMB 15 to 25 mg/kg once/day. Sometimes rifabutin 300 mg once/day is also given. After successful treatment, chronic suppression with clarithromycin or azithromycin plus EMB is necessary to prevent relapse. HIV-infected patients who were not diagnosed before presenting with disseminated MAC should receive 2 wk of antimycobacterial treatment before starting antiretroviral therapy to decrease the risk of developing the IRIS.

HIV-infected patients with a CD4 count < 100 cells/μL require prophylaxis for disseminated MAC with azithromycin 1.2 g po once/week or clarithromycin 500 mg po bid.

LEPROSY

(Hansen Disease)

Leprosy is a chronic infection usually caused by the acid-fast bacilli *Mycobacterium leprae*, which has a unique tropism for peripheral nerves, skin, and mucous membranes of the upper respiratory tract. Symptoms are myriad and include anesthetic polymorphic skin lesions and peripheral neuropathy. Diagnosis is clinical and confirmed by biopsy. Treatment is typically with dapsone plus other antimycobacterial drugs. Patients rapidly become noncontagious after starting therapy.

M. leprae was the only known cause of leprosy until 2008, when a second species, *M. lepromatosis* was identified in Mexico.

Although leprosy is not highly contagious, rarely causes death, and can be effectively treated with antibiotics, it continues to be associated with considerable social stigma. Misunderstanding about the disease probably exists because leprosy was incurable before the advent of effective antibiotic therapy in the 1940s. People with the disease would become disfigured and often have significant disability, causing them to be feared and shunned by others. Because of this social stigma, the psychologic impact of leprosy is often significant.

Epidemiology

Globally, the number of leprosy cases is declining. During 2015, about 212,000 new cases were reported. About 80% of these cases occurred in India, Brazil, and Indonesia. In the US, about 150 to 250 people are infected each year. Most cases of leprosy in the US involve people who emigrated from developing countries.

Leprosy can develop at any age but appears most often in people aged 5 to 15 yr or > 30.

Pathophysiology

Humans are the main natural reservoir for *M. leprae*. Armadillos are the only confirmed source other than humans, although other animal and environmental sources may exist.

Leprosy is thought to be spread by passage from person to person through nasal droplets and secretions. Casual contact (eg, simply touching someone with the disease) and short-term contact does not seem to spread the disease. About half of people with leprosy probably contracted it through close, long-term contact with an infected person. Even after contact with the bacteria, most people do not contract leprosy; health care workers often work for many years with people who have leprosy without contracting the disease. Most (95%) immunocompetent people who are infected with *M. leprae* do not develop leprosy because of effective immunity. People who do develop leprosy probably have a poorly defined genetic predisposition.

M. leprae grow slowly (doubling in 2 wk). The usual incubation period ranges from 6 mo to 10 yr. Once infection develops, hematogenous dissemination can occur.

Classification: Leprosy can be categorized by type and number of skin areas affected:

- Paucibacillary: ≤ 5 skin lesions with no bacteria detected on samples from those areas
- Multibacillary: ≥ 6 skin lesions, bacteria detected on samples from skin lesions, or both

Leprosy can also be classified by cellular response and clinical findings:

- Tuberculoid
- Lepromatous
- Borderline

People with tuberculoid leprosy typically have a strong cell-mediated response, which limits disease to a few skin lesions (paucibacillary), and the disease is milder, less common, and less contagious. People with lepromatous or borderline leprosy typically have poor cell-mediated immunity to *M. leprae* and have more severe, systemic infection with widespread bacterial infiltration of skin, nerves, and other organs (eg, nose, testes, kidneys). They have more skin lesions (multibacillary), and the disease is more contagious.

In both classifications, the type of leprosy dictates long-term prognosis, likely complications, and duration of antibiotic treatment.

Symptoms and Signs

Symptoms usually do not begin until > 1 yr after infection (average 5 to 7 yr). Once symptoms begin, they progress slowly.

Leprosy affects mainly the skin and peripheral nerves. Nerve involvement causes numbness and weakness in areas controlled by the affected nerves.

- **Tuberculoid leprosy:** Skin lesions consist of one or a few hypoesthetic, centrally hypopigmented macules with sharp, raised borders. The rash, as in all forms of leprosy, is nonpruritic. Areas affected by this rash are numb because of damage to the underlying peripheral nerves, which may be palpably enlarged.
- **Lepromatous leprosy:** Much of the skin and many areas of the body, including the kidneys, nose, and testes, may be affected. Patients have skin macules, papules, nodules, or plaques, which are often symmetric. Peripheral neuropathy is more severe than in tuberculoid leprosy, with more areas of numbness; certain muscle groups may be weak. Patients may develop gynecomastia or lose eyelashes and eyebrows.
- **Borderline leprosy:** Features of both tuberculoid and lepromatous leprosy are present. Without treatment, borderline leprosy may become less severe and more like the tuberculoid form, or it may worsen and become more like the lepromatous form.

Complications: The most severe complications result from the peripheral neuropathy, which causes deterioration of the sense of touch and a corresponding inability to feel pain and temperature. Patients may unknowingly burn, cut, or otherwise harm themselves. Repeated damage may lead to loss of digits. Muscle weakness can result in deformities (eg, clawing of the 4th and 5th fingers caused by ulnar nerve involvement, foot drop caused by peroneal nerve involvement).

Papules and nodules can be particularly disfiguring on the face.

Other areas of the body may be affected:

- **Feet:** Plantar ulcers with secondary infection are a major cause of morbidity, making walking painful.
- **Nose:** Damage to the nasal mucosa can result in chronic nasal congestion and nosebleeds and, if untreated, erosion and collapse of the nasal septum.
- **Eyes:** Iritis may lead to glaucoma, and corneal insensitivity may lead to scarring and blindness.
- **Sexual function:** Men with lepromatous leprosy may have erectile dysfunction and infertility. The infection can reduce testosterone and sperm production by the testes.
- **Kidneys:** Amyloidosis and consequent renal failure occasionally occur in lepromatous leprosy.

Leprosy reactions: During the course of untreated or even treated leprosy, the immune system may produce inflammatory reactions. There are 2 types.

Type 1 reactions result from a spontaneous increase in cell-mediated immunity. These reactions can cause fever and inflammation of the preexisting skin and peripheral nerve lesions, resulting in skin edema, erythema, and tenderness and worsening nerve function. These reactions, particularly if not treated early, contribute significantly to nerve damage. Because the immune response is increased, these reactions are termed reversal reactions, despite the apparent clinical worsening.

Type 2 reactions (erythema nodosum leprosum, or ENL) are systemic inflammatory reactions that appear to be a vasculitis or panniculitis and probably involve circulating immune complex deposition or increased T-helper cell function. They have become less common since clofazimine was added to the drug regimen. Patients may develop erythematous and painful papules or nodules that may pustulate and ulcerate and cause fever, neuritis, lymphadenitis, orchitis, arthritis (particularly in large joints, usually knees), and glomerulonephritis. Hemolysis or bone marrow suppression may cause anemia, and hepatic inflammation may cause mild abnormalities in liver function tests.

Diagnosis

- Microscopic examination of skin biopsy specimen

Diagnosis is often delayed in the US because clinicians are unfamiliar with the clinical manifestations. The disease is suggested by the presence of skin lesions and peripheral neuropathy and confirmed by microscopic examination of biopsy specimens. The organism does not grow on artificial culture media. Biopsy specimens should be taken from the advancing edge of tuberculoid lesions or, in lepromatous leprosy, from nodules or plaques.

Serum IgM antibodies to *M. leprae* are specific but insensitive (present in only two thirds of patients with tuberculoid leprosy). Diagnostic usefulness is further limited in endemic areas because such antibodies may be present in asymptomatic infection.

Treatment

- Long-term, multidrug regimens with dapsone, RIF, and sometimes clofazimine
- Sometimes lifelong maintenance antibiotics

Antibiotics can stop the progression of leprosy but do not reverse any nerve damage or deformity. Thus, early detection and treatment are vitally important. Because of antibiotic resistance, multidrug regimens are used. The drugs chosen depend on the type of leprosy; multibacillary leprosy requires more intensive regimens and a longer duration than paucibacillary does. Advice about diagnosis and treatment is available from the National Hansen's Disease Program in Baton Rouge, LA (1-800-642-2477) or the US Health Resources and Services Administration. Standard regimens recommended by the WHO differ somewhat from those used in the US.

Multibacillary: The standard WHO regimen includes dapsone, RIF, and clofazimine. WHO provides these drugs free for all leprosy patients throughout the world. Patients take RIF 600 mg po and clofazimine 300 mg po once/mo under a health care practitioner's supervision and dapsone 100 mg po plus clofazimine 50 mg po once/day without supervision. This regimen is continued for 12 mo.

In the US, the regimen is RIF 600 mg po once/day, dapsone 100 mg po once/day, and clofazimine 100 mg po once/day for 24 mo. Dapsone is continued indefinitely for lepromatous leprosy and for 10 yr for borderline leprosy.

Paucibacillary: In the standard WHO regimen, patients take RIF 600 mg po once/mo with supervision and dapsone 100 mg po once/day without supervision for 6 mo. People who have only a single skin lesion are given a one-time oral dose of RIF 600 mg, ofloxacin 400 mg, and minocycline 100 mg.

In the US, the regimen is RIF 600 mg po once/day and dapsone 100 mg po once/day for 12 mo. Dapsone is continued for 3 yr for indeterminate and tuberculoid leprosy and for 5 yr for borderline tuberculoid.

Drugs for leprosy: Dapsone is relatively inexpensive and generally safe to use. Adverse effects include hemolysis and anemia (which are usually mild) and allergic dermatoses (which can be severe); rarely, dapsone syndrome (exfoliative dermatitis, high fever, mononucleosis-like WBC differential) occurs.

RIF, is primarily bactericidal for *M. leprae* and is even more effective than dapsone. However, if given at the recommended US dosage of 600 mg po once/day, it is too expensive for many developing countries. Adverse effects include hepatotoxicity, flu-like syndromes, and, rarely, thrombocytopenia and renal failure.

Clofazimine is extremely safe. The main side effect is reversible skin pigmentation, but discoloration may take months to resolve. Clofazimine can be obtained in the US only from the Department of Health and Human Services as an investigational new drug (contact number for the case officer is 225-756-3709).

Leprosy reactions: Patients with type 1 reactions (except minor skin inflammation) are given prednisone 40 to 60 mg po once/day initially, followed by low maintenance doses (often as low as 10 to 15 mg once/day) for a few months. Minor skin inflammation should not be treated.

First and 2nd episodes of ENL may be treated, if mild, with aspirin or, if significant, with 1 wk of prednisone 40 to 60 mg po once/day plus antimicrobials. For recurrent cases, thalidomide 100 to 300 mg po once/day is the drug of choice (in the US, available through the National Hansen's Disease Program). However, because of its teratogenicity, thalidomide should not be given to women who may become pregnant. Adverse effects are mild constipation, mild leukopenia, and sedation.

Prevention

Because leprosy is not very contagious, risk of spread is low. Only the untreated lepromatous form is contagious, but even then, the infection is not easily spread. However, household contacts (particularly children) of patients with leprosy should be monitored for development of symptoms and signs of leprosy. Once treatment has begun, leprosy cannot be spread. Avoiding contact with bodily fluids from and the rash on infected people is the best prevention.

The BCG vaccine, used to prevent TB, provides some protection against leprosy but is not often used for that purpose. There is no role for chemoprophylaxis.

KEY POINTS

- Leprosy is a chronic infection usually caused by the acid-fast bacilli *Mycobacterium leprae*.
- Leprosy is not very contagious in untreated patients and not at all contagious once treatment starts.
- Leprosy affects mainly the skin and peripheral nerves.
- The most severe complications result from loss of the sense of touch, pain, and temperature; muscle weakness that can result in deformities; and disfiguring lesions of the skin and nasal mucosa.
- Inflammatory reactions called leprosy reactions can occur and require treatment with corticosteroids.
- Diagnose based on biopsy; *M. leprae* cannot be grown in culture.
- Treatment depends on the form of leprosy but involves multidrug regimens typically using dapsone, RIF, and sometimes clofazimine.

197 Neisseriaceae

All pathogenic aerobic gram-negative cocci belong to the Neisseriaceae family, which is composed of 5 genera:

- Acinetobacter
- Kingella
- Moraxella (previously *Branhamella*)
- Neisseria
- Oligella

Of these, *Neisseria* includes the most important human pathogens:

- *N. meningitidis*
- *N. gonorrhoeae*

Numerous saprophytic Neisseriaceae commonly inhabit the oropharynx, vagina, or colon but rarely cause human disease.

Moraxella catarrhalis causes otitis media in children, sinusitis in people of all ages, and exacerbations of COPD, sometimes community-acquired pneumonia in adults, and infrequently bacteremia. Over half a dozen other *Moraxella* sp and the related *Kingella kingae* cause infections in the CNS, respiratory tract, urinary tract, endocardium, bones, and joints.

Humans are the only reservoir of *Neisseria*, and person-to-person spread is the prime mode of transmission. Both *N. meningitidis* (meningococcus) and *N. gonorrhoeae* (which causes gonorrhea), can exist in an asymptomatic carrier state. Carrier states are particularly important with meningococcus because of its association with epidemics.

ACINETOBACTER INFECTIONS

***Acinetobacter* sp can cause suppurative infections in any organ system; these bacteria are often opportunists in hospitalized patients.**

Acinetobacter are gram-negative aerobic bacilli that belong to the family Neisseriaceae. They are ubiquitous and can survive on dry surfaces for up to a month and are commonly carried on the skin of health care workers, increasing the likelihood of patients being colonized and medical equipment being contaminated. There are many species of *Acinetobacter*; all can cause human disease, but *A. baumannii* (AB) accounts for about 80% of infections.

Diseases Caused by *Acinetobacter*

The most common manifestations of *Acinetobacter* disease are

- Respiratory infections

AB infections typically occur in critically ill, hospitalized patients. Community-acquired infections (mostly pneumonia) are more common in tropical climates. Crude death rates associated with AB infection are 19 to 54%.

The most common site for infection is the respiratory system. *Acinetobacter* easily colonize tracheostomy sites and can cause community-acquired bronchiolitis and tracheobronchitis in healthy children and tracheobronchitis in immunocompromised adults. Hospital-acquired *Acinetobacter* pneumonias are frequently multilobar and complicated. Secondary bacteremia and septic shock are associated with a poor prognosis.

Acinetobacter sp can also cause suppurative infections (eg, abscesses) in any organ system, including the lungs, urinary tract, skin, and soft tissues; bacteremia may occur.

Rarely, these organisms cause meningitis (primarily after neurosurgical procedures), cellulitis, or phlebitis in patients with an indwelling venous catheter; ocular infections; native or prosthetic valve endocarditis; osteomyelitis; septic arthritis; or pancreatic and liver abscesses.

The significance of isolates from clinical specimens, such as respiratory secretions from intubated patients or specimens from open wounds, is difficult to determine because they often represent colonization.

Risk factors: Risk factors for *Acinetobacter* infection depend on the type of infection (hospital-acquired, community-acquired, multidrug resistant—see Table 197–1).

Drug resistance: Recently, multidrug resistant (MDR) AB has emerged, particularly in ICUs in immunosuppressed patients, patients with serious underlying disorders, and patients treated with broad-spectrum antibiotics after an invasive procedure. Spread in ICUs has been attributed to colonized health care practitioners, contaminated common equipment, and contaminated parenteral nutrition solutions.

Treatment

- Typically empiric multidrug therapy for serious infections

In patients with localized cellulitis or phlebitis associated with a foreign body (eg, IV catheter, suture), removal of the foreign body plus local care is usually sufficient. Tracheobronchitis

Table 197–1. RISK FACTORS FOR *ACINETOBACTER* INFECTION

TYPE OF INFECTION	RISK FACTORS
Hospital-acquired	Fecal colonization with *Acinetobacter* ICU stay Indwelling devices Length of hospital stay Mechanical ventilation Parenteral nutrition Previous infection Surgery Treatment with broad-spectrum antibiotics Wounds
Community-acquired	Alcoholism Cigarette smoking Chronic lung disease Diabetes mellitus Residence in a tropical developing country
Multidrug-resistant	Exposure to colonized or infected patients Invasive procedures Mechanical ventilation, particularly if prolonged Prolonged hospitalization (particularly in the ICU) Receipt of blood products Use of broad-spectrum antibiotics (eg, 3rd-generation cephalosporins, carbapenems, fluoroquinolones)

after endotracheal intubation may resolve with pulmonary toilet alone. Patients with more extensive infections should be treated with antibiotics and with debridement if necessary.

AB has long had intrinsic resistance to many antimicrobials. MDR-AB are defined as strains that are resistant to ≥ 3 classes of antimicrobials; some isolates are resistant to all. Before susceptibility results are available, possible initial options include a carbapenem (eg, meropenem, imipenem, doripenem), colistin, or a fluoroquinolone plus an aminoglycoside, rifampin, or both. Sulbactam (a beta-lactamase inhibitor) has intrinsic bactericidal activity against many MDR-AB strains. Tigecycline, a glycylcycline antibiotic, is also effective; however, borderline activity and emergence of resistance during therapy have been reported. Minocycline has in vitro activity.

Mild to moderate infections may respond to monotherapy. Traumatic wound infections can be treated with minocycline. Serious infections are treated with combination therapy—typically, imipenem, or ampicillin/sulbactam plus an aminoglycoside.

To prevent spread, health care practitioners should use contact precautions (hand washing, barrier precautions) and appropriate ventilator care and cleaning for patients colonized or infected with MDR-AB.

KEY POINTS

- *A. baumannii* (AB) accounts for about 80% of infections and tends to occur in critically ill, hospitalized patients.
- The most common site for infection is the respiratory system, but *Acinetobacter* sp can also cause suppurative infections in any organ system.
- Multidrug-resistant AB has become a problem; use multidrug treatment chosen based on susceptibility testing.

KINGELLA INFECTIONS

***Kingella* organisms colonize the human respiratory tract. They cause skeletal infections, endocarditis, and bacteremia and, rarely, pneumonia, epiglottitis, meningitis, abscesses, and ocular infections.**

Kingella, which belong to the family Neisseriaceae, are short, nonmotile, gram-negative coccobacilli that occur in pairs or short chains. The organisms are slow-growing and fastidious. *Kingella* are recovered from the human respiratory tract and are a rare cause of human disease.

Among *Kingella* species, *K. kingae* is the most frequent human pathogen; these organisms frequently colonize the respiratory mucous membranes. Children aged 6 mo to 4 yr have the highest rates of colonization and invasive disease from this respiratory tract pathogen. *K. kingae* is transmitted from child to child through close personal contact (eg, at day care centers). Infection has a seasonal distribution, with more cases in fall and winter.

Diseases Caused by *Kingella*

The most common manifestations of *K. kingae* disease are

- Skeletal infections (septic arthritis, osteomyelitis)
- Endocarditis
- Bacteremia

Rare manifestations include pneumonia, epiglottitis, meningitis, abscesses, and ocular infections.

The most common skeletal infection is septic arthritis, which most frequently affects large, weight-bearing joints, especially the knee and ankle. Osteomyelitis most frequently involves bones of the lower extremities. Onset is insidious, and diagnosis is often delayed. Hematogenous invasion of intervertebral disks can occur, most commonly in the lumbar intervertebral spaces.

Kingella endocarditis has been reported in all age groups. Endocarditis may involve native or prosthetic valves. *Kingella* is a component of the so-called HACEK group (*Haemophilus aphrophilus* and *H. parainfluenzae*, *Aggregatibacter*, *Cardiobacterium*, *Eikenella*, *Kingella*), which includes fastidious gram-negative bacteria capable of causing endocarditis.

Diagnosis of *Kingella* infections requires laboratory isolation from fluids or tissues thought to be infected.

Treatment

- A penicillin or cephalosporin

Kingella organisms are generally susceptible to various penicillins and cephalosporins. However, antimicrobial susceptibility testing is needed to guide therapy. Other useful drugs include aminoglycosides, trimethoprim/sulfamethoxazole, tetracyclines, erythromycin, and fluoroquinolones.

MENINGOCOCCAL DISEASES

Meningococci (*Neisseria meningitidis*) cause meningitis and meningococcemia. Symptoms, usually severe, include headache, nausea, vomiting, photophobia, lethargy, rash, multiple organ failure, shock, and disseminated intravascular coagulation. Diagnosis is clinical, confirmed by culture. Treatment is penicillin or a 3rd-generation cephalosporin.

Meningococci are gram-negative aerobic cocci that belong to the family Neisseriaceae. There are 13 serogroups; 5 (serogroups A, B, C, W135, and Y) cause most human disease.

Worldwide, the incidence of endemic meningococcal disease is 0.5 to 5/100,000, with an increased number of cases during winter and spring in temperate climates. Local outbreaks occur most frequently in sub-Saharan Africa between Senegal and Ethiopia, an area known as the meningitis belt. In major African epidemics (which were often caused by serogroup A), attack rates ranged from 100 to 800/100,000. After widespread use of the meningococcal A vaccine in the African meningitis belt, serogroup A has been replaced by other meningococcal serogroups and by *Streptococcus pneumoniae*.

In the US, the annual incidence ranges from 0.5 to 1.1/100,000. Over the past 20 yr, incidence of meningococcal disease has declined annually. Most cases are sporadic, typically in children < 2 yr; < 2% occur in outbreaks. Outbreaks tend to occur in semiclosed communities (eg, military recruit camps, college dormitories, schools, day-care centers) and often involve patients aged 5 to 19 yr. Serogroups B, C, and Y are the most frequent causes of disease in the US; each serogroup accounts for about one-third of reported cases. Serogroup A is rare in the US.

Diseases Caused by Meningococci

Over 90% of meningococcal infections involve

- Meningitis
- Meningococcemia

Infections of lungs, joints, respiratory passageways, GU organs, eyes, endocardium, and pericardium are less common.

Pathophysiology

Meningococci can colonize the nasopharynx of asymptomatic carriers. A combination of factors is probably responsible for transition from carrier state to invasive disease. Despite documented high rates of colonization (10 to 40% of healthy people), transition to invasive disease is rare and occurs primarily in previously uninfected patients. Transmission usually occurs via direct contact with respiratory secretions from a nasopharyngeal carrier. Nasopharyngeal carriage rates are highest in adolescents and young adults, who serve as reservoirs for transmission of *N. meningitidis*. Carrier rates rise dramatically during epidemics.

After invading the body, *N. meningitidis* causes meningitis and severe bacteremia in children and adults, resulting in profound vascular effects. Infection can rapidly become fulminant. The case-fatality rate is 4 to 6% for meningitis alone, compared with up to 40% for meningococcemia with septic shock. Of patients who recover, 10 to 15% have serious sequelae, such as permanent hearing loss, intellectual disability, or loss of phalanges or limbs.

Risk factors: The most frequently infected are

- Children aged 6 mo to 3 yr

Other high-risk groups include

- Adolescents
- Military recruits
- College freshmen living in dormitories
- Travelers to places where meningococcal disease is common (eg, certain countries in Africa and in Saudi Arabia during the Hajj)
- People with functional or anatomic asplenia or complement deficiencies
- Microbiologists working with *N. meningitidis* isolates

Infection or vaccination confers serogroup-specific immunity.

Incidence of meningococcal disease is higher in people with AIDS than in the general adult population. Antecedent viral infection, household crowding, chronic underlying illness, and both active and passive smoking are associated with increased risk of meningococcal disease.[1]

1. Advisory Committee on Immunization Practices: Prevention and control of meningococcal disease recommendations of the Advisory Committee on Immunization Practices (ACIP). *MMWR* 62(2):1–28, 2013.

Symptoms and Signs

Patients with meningitis frequently report fever, headache, and stiff neck (see p. 1918). Other symptoms include nausea, vomiting, photophobia, and lethargy. A maculopapular or hemorrhagic petechial rash often appears soon after disease onset. Meningeal signs are often apparent during physical examination.

Fulminant meningococcemia syndromes include Waterhouse-Friderichsen syndrome (septicemia, profound shock, cutaneous purpura, adrenal hemorrhage), sepsis with multiple organ failure, shock, and disseminated intravascular coagulation. A rare, chronic meningococcemia causes recurrent mild symptoms (mostly joint and cutaneous).

Diagnosis

- Gram stain and culture

Neisseria are small, gram-negative cocci readily identified with Gram stain and by other standard bacteriologic identification methods. Serologic methods, such as latex agglutination and coagglutination tests, allow rapid presumptive diagnosis of *N. meningitides* in blood, CSF, synovial fluid, and urine. However, both positive and negative results should be confirmed by culture. PCR testing of CSF, blood, and other normally sterile sites for *N. meningitidis* is more sensitive and specific than culture and may be useful when prior antibiotic administration interferes with isolating the organism.

Treatment

- Ceftriaxone
- Dexamethasone

While awaiting definitive identification of the causal organism, immunocompetent adults suspected of having meningococcal infection are given a 3rd-generation cephalosporin (eg, cefotaxime 2 g IV q 6 h, ceftriaxone 2 g IV q 12 h) plus vancomycin 30 to 60 mg/kg IV q 8 to 12 h. In immunocompromised patients and patients > 50 yr, coverage for *Listeria monocytogenes* should be considered by adding ampicillin 2 g IV q 4 h.

Once *N. meningitidis* has been definitively identified, the preferred treatment is ceftriaxone 2 g IV q 12 h or penicillin 4 million units IV q 4 h.

Corticosteroids decrease the incidence of neurologic complications in children and adults. When corticosteroids are used, they should be given with or before the first dose of antibiotics. Dexamethasone 0.15 mg/kg IV q 6 h in children (10 mg q 6 h in adults) is given for 4 days.

Prevention

Antibiotic prophylaxis: Close contacts of people with meningococcal disease are at increased risk of acquiring disease and should receive a prophylactic antibiotic. Options include

- Rifampin 600 mg (for children > 1 mo, 10 mg/kg; for children < 1 mo, 5 mg/kg) po q 12 h for 4 doses
- Ceftriaxone 250 mg (for children < 15 yr, 125 mg) IM for 1 dose
- In adults, a fluoroquinolone (ciprofloxacin or levofloxacin 500 mg or ofloxacin 400 mg) po for 1 dose

Azithromycin is not routinely recommended, but a recent study showed that a single 500-mg dose was equivalent to rifampin for chemoprophylaxis and so could be an alternative for patients with contraindications to recommended drugs.

Ciprofloxacin-resistant meningococcal disease has been reported in several countries (Greece, England, Wales, Australia, Spain, Argentina, France, India). More recently, 2 US states (North Dakota, Minnesota) reported ciprofloxacin-resistant meningococci and so recommended that ciprofloxacin chemoprophylaxis not be used as preventive treatment for people who have had close contact with someone diagnosed with meningococcal disease.

Vaccination: Several meningococcal vaccines are available in the US (see Meningococcal Disease: Recommendations of the Advisory Committee on Immunization Practices at www.cdc.gov). Available vaccines include

- 2 quadrivalent conjugate vaccines (MenACWY-D and MenACWY-CRM) that protect against 4 of the 5 common pathogenic serogroups of meningococcus (all but B)
- A bivalent conjugate vaccine that protects against serogroups C and Y and that is available only in combination with a *Haemophilus influenzae* type b vaccine (Hib-MenCY)
- A quadrivalent polysaccharide vaccine (MPSV4) for use in patients ≥ 56 yr
- 2 recombinant vaccines against serogroup B (MenB)

All children should receive MenACWY-D or MenACWY-CRM at age 11 to 12 yr, with a booster dose at age 16 yr. Vaccination is also recommended for people who are aged 19 to 55 and at risk, including military recruits, college freshmen living in a dormitory, travelers to hyperendemic or epidemic areas (a booster dose is given to those whose last vaccination was ≥ 5 yr before), and people with laboratory or industrial exposure to *N. meningitidis* aerosols. Adults with functional asplenia or persistent complement component deficiencies and patients with HIV infection (not a routine vaccination unless other risk factors are present) should receive 2 doses of MenACWY-D or MenACWY-CRM at least 2 mo apart.

At-risk people ≥ 56 yr should receive the MPSV4 polysaccharide vaccine. However, in this age group, MenACWY is preferred for the following people:

- Those who were vaccinated previously with MenACWY and are recommended for revaccination
- Those who are expected to need multiple doses (eg, people with asplenia, microbiologists)

MenB (2-dose series at least 1 mo apart or 3-dose vaccine at 0, 2, and 6 mo) is recommended for people ≥ 10 yr who are at increased risk of serogroup B meningococcal disease.

Children < 11 yr are not routinely vaccinated, but those at high risk should receive Hib-MenCY, MenACWY-D, or MenACWY-CRM. Vaccine selection varies with age and risk factors (see CDC Vaccination Schedule Birth Through 18 Yr at www.cdc.gov).

KEY POINTS

- Over 90% of meningococcal infections involve meningitis or septicemia.
- An asymptomatic nasopharyngeal carrier state is common; transmission usually occurs via direct contact with respiratory secretions from a carrier.
- Most cases are sporadic, typically in children < 2 yr, but outbreaks can occur, primarily in semiclosed communities (eg, military recruit camps, dormitories, day-care centers) and often involve patients aged 5 to 19 yr.
- Treat with ceftriaxone or penicillin; add dexamethasone for patients with meningitis.
- Give close contacts a prophylactic antibiotic; options include rifampin, ceftriaxone, and a fluoroquinolone.
- Vaccinate all children starting at age 11 to 12 yr, and selectively vaccinate high-risk younger children and other high-risk people.

MORAXELLA CATARRHALIS INFECTION

***Moraxella catarrhalis* causes ear and upper and lower respiratory infections.**

Previously classified as *Micrococcus*, then *Neisseria*, and also known as *Branhamella catarrhalis*, this organism is a frequent cause of otitis media in children, acute and chronic sinusitis at all ages, and lower respiratory infection in adults with chronic lung disease. It is the 2nd most common bacterial cause of COPD exacerbations after nontypeable *Haemophilus influenzae*. *M. catarrhalis* pneumonia resembles pneumococcal pneumonia. Although bacteremia is rare, half of patients die within 3 mo because of intercurrent diseases.

The prevalence of *M. catarrhalis* colonization depends on age. About 1 to 5% of healthy adults have upper respiratory tract colonization. Nasopharyngeal colonization with *M. catarrhalis* is common throughout infancy, may be increased during winter months, and is a risk factor for acute otitis media; early colonization is a risk factor for recurrent otitis media. Substantial regional differences in colonization rates occur. Living conditions, hygiene, environmental factors (eg, household smoking), genetic characteristics of the populations, host factors, and other factors may contribute to these differences.

The organism appears to spread contiguously from its colonizing position in the respiratory tract to the infection site.

There is no pathognomonic feature of *M. catarrhalis* otitis media, acute or chronic sinusitis, or pneumonia. In lower respiratory disease, patients experience increased cough, purulent sputum production, and increased dyspnea.

These gram-negative cocci resemble *Neisseria* sp but can be readily distinguished by routine biochemical tests after culture isolation from infected fluids or tissues.

All strains now produce beta-lactamase. The organism is generally susceptible to beta-lactam/beta-lactamase inhibitors, sulfamethoxazole, tetracyclines, extended-spectrum oral cephalosporins, aminoglycosides, macrolides, and fluoroquinolones.

OLIGELLA INFECTIONS

***Oligella* sp causes infection primarily of the GU tract.**

The genus *Oligella* contains 2 species, *Oligella urethralis* and *O. ureolytica*.

O. urethralis is a commensal of the GU tract, and most clinical isolates are from the urine, predominantly from men. Although symptomatic infections are rare, bacteremia, septic arthritis that mimics gonococcal arthritis, and peritonitis have been reported.

O. ureolytica also occurs primarily in the urine, usually from patients with long-term urinary catheters or other urinary drainage systems. These patients have a propensity to develop urinary stones, possibly because the organism hydrolyzes urea and alkalinizes the urine, leading to precipitation of phosphates. Bacteremia has occurred in a patient with obstructive uropathy.

Diagnosis of *Oligella* infections is by culture.

Because these organisms are rarely isolated, antimicrobial susceptibility data are limited; most are sensitive to beta-lactam antibiotics. However, a beta-lactamase–producing strain and strains resistant to ciprofloxacin have been identified.

198 Nematodes (Roundworms)

ANGIOSTRONGYLIASIS

Angiostrongyliasis is infection with larvae of worms of the genus *Angiostrongylus*; intestinal symptoms or eosinophilic meningitis occurs depending on the infecting species.

Angiostrongylus are parasites of rats (rat lung worms). Excreted larvae are taken up by intermediate hosts (snails and slugs) and paratenic or transport hosts (hosts that are not required for the parasite's development but that can transmit infection to humans). Human infection is acquired by ingestion of raw or undercooked snails or slugs or transport hosts (certain crabs and freshwater shrimp); it is unclear whether larval contamination of vegetables (eg, in slime from snails or slugs that crawl on the food) can cause infection.

A. cantonensis infection occurs predominantly in Southeast Asia and the Pacific Basin, although infection has been reported elsewhere, including the Caribbean, Hawaii, and

Louisiana. The larvae migrate from the GI tract to the meninges, where they cause eosinophilic meningitis, with fever, headache, and meningismus. Occasionally, ocular invasion occurs.

A. costaricensis infection occurs in the Americas, predominantly in Latin America and the Caribbean. Adult worms reside in arterioles of the ileocecal area, and eggs can be released into the intestinal tissues, resulting in local inflammation with abdominal pain, vomiting, and fever; this infection can mimic appendicitis. Also, abdominal angiostrongyliasis is often accompanied by eosinophilia, and a painful right lower quadrant mass may develop.

Diagnosis

- If meningitis signs are present, CSF analysis (for *A. cantonensis*)
- Sometimes identification of eggs and larvae during abdominal surgery (for *A. costaricensis*)

Angiostrongyliasis is suspected based on a history of ingesting potentially contaminated material.

Patients with meningeal findings require lumbar puncture; CSF shows eosinophilia, but *A. cantonensis* parasites are rarely visible.

Diagnosis of GI infection due to *A. costaricensis* is difficult because larvae and eggs are not present in stool; however, if surgery is done (eg, for suspected appendicitis), eggs and larvae can be identified in tissues removed during surgery.

Immunoassays are not widely available.

Treatment

- For meningitis, analgesics, corticosteroids, and removal of CSF

A. cantonensis meningitis is treated with analgesics, corticosteroids, and removal of CSF at frequent intervals to reduce CNS pressure. Anthelmintic therapy may increase the inflammatory response because it results in the release of parasite antigens. Most patients have a self-limited course and recover completely.

There is no specific treatment for *A. costaricensis* infection; most infections resolve spontaneously. Anthelmintics do not appear to be effective and may lead to additional migration of worms and worsening symptoms.

Prevention

People who live in or travel to areas with *A. cantonensis* should avoid eating raw or undercooked snails, slugs, freshwater shrimp, land crabs, frogs, and lizards, as well as potentially contaminated vegetables and vegetable juices.

People who live in or travel to areas with *A. costaricensis* should avoid eating raw or undercooked slugs and potentially contaminated vegetables or juices.

KEY POINTS

- Humans acquire *Angiostrongylus* when they consume raw or undercooked snails or slugs or the organisms' transport hosts (land crabs and freshwater shrimp).
- *A. cantonensis* larvae migrate from the GI tract to the meninges, where they cause eosinophilic meningitis; *A. costaricensis* eggs can be released into the intestinal tissues, causing abdominal pain, vomiting, and fever.
- Treat *A. cantonensis* meningitis with analgesics, corticosteroids, and, if intracranial pressure is elevated, removal of CSF at frequent intervals.
- Treating *A. costaricensis* infection with anthelmintics does not appear to be effective and may lead to additional migration of worms and worsening symptoms; most of these infections resolve spontaneously.

ANISAKIASIS

Anisakiasis is infection with larvae of worms of the genus *Anisakis* and related genera such as *Pseudoterranova*. Infection is acquired by eating raw or poorly cooked saltwater fish; larvae burrow into the mucosa of the GI tract, causing discomfort.

Anisakis is a parasite that resides in the GI tract of marine mammals. Excreted eggs hatch into free-swimming larvae, which are ingested by fish and squid; human infection is acquired by ingestion of these intermediate hosts in a raw or undercooked state. Thus, infection is particularly common in locations such as Japan and cultures in which raw fish is traditionally consumed. Larvae burrow into the stomach and small bowel of humans.

Symptoms and Signs

Symptoms of anisakiasis typically include abdominal pain, nausea, and vomiting within hours of ingesting the larvae. In the small intestine, the infection may result in an inflammatory mass, and symptoms resembling Crohn disease may develop 1 to 2 wk later.

Anisakiasis typically resolves spontaneously after several weeks; rarely, it persists for months.

Diagnosis

- Upper endoscopy

Anisakiasis is usually diagnosed by upper endoscopy; stool examination is unhelpful, but a serologic test is available in some countries.

Treatment

- Endoscopic removal of the larvae
- Albendazole

Endoscopic removal of the larvae is curative.

Treatment of anisakiasis with albendazole 400 mg po bid for 3 to 5 days may be effective, but data are limited.

Prevention

Larvae are destroyed by

- Cooking to > 63° C (> 145° F)
- Freezing at -20° C (-4° F) or below for 7 days
- Freezing at -35° C (-31° F) or below until solid, then storing at that temperature for ≥ 15 h, or at -20° C (-4° F) for 24 h

Larvae may resist pickling, salting, and smoking.

KEY POINTS

- Humans acquire *Anisakis* when they consume the intermediate hosts (fish or squid) that are raw or undercooked; thus, anisakiasis is common in Japan and other cultures where raw fish is traditionally consumed.
- Anisakiasis typically causes abdominal pain, nausea, and vomiting within hours of ingesting the larvae; an inflammatory mass may form in the small intestine and symptoms may resemble Crohn disease.

- Anisakiasis typically resolves spontaneously after several weeks.
- Do upper endoscopy to diagnose anisakiasis.
- Endoscopic removal of the larvae is curative.

ASCARIASIS

Ascariasis is infection with *Ascaris lumbricoides* or occasionally *Ascaris suum* (a closely related parasite of pigs). Light infections may be asymptomatic. Early symptoms are pulmonary (cough, wheezing); later symptoms are GI, with cramps or abdominal pain due to obstruction of GI lumina (intestines or biliary or pancreatic ducts) by adult worms. Chronically infected children may develop undernutrition. Diagnosis is by identifying eggs or adult worms in stool, adult worms that migrate from the nose or mouth, or larvae in sputum during the pulmonary migration phase. Treatment is with albendazole, mebendazole, or ivermectin.

Ascariasis occurs worldwide. It is concentrated in tropical and subtropical areas with poor sanitation. Ascariasis is the most common intestinal helminth infection in the world. Prevalence is highest in children aged 2 to 10 yr and decreases in older age groups. Current estimates suggest that about 800 million people are infected, and as many as 2,000 infected people (mostly children) may die each year of bowel or biliary obstruction.

In the US, most cases occur in refugees, immigrants, or travelers to endemic tropical areas.

Humans are infected with *A. lumbricoides* when they ingest its eggs, often in food contaminated by human feces. Infection can also occur when hands or fingers with contaminated dirt on them are put in the mouth.

Humans can also be infected with *A. suum*, a closely related roundworm of pigs, after cysts are ingested in food contaminated with feces or larvae are ingested in raw or undercooked pork.

Pathophysiology

Ingested *A. lumbricoides* eggs hatch in the duodenum, and the resulting larvae penetrate the wall of the small bowel and migrate via the portal circulation through the liver to the heart and lungs. Larvae lodge in the alveolar capillaries, penetrate alveolar walls, and ascend the bronchial tree into the oropharynx. They are swallowed and return to the small bowel, where they develop into adult worms, which mate and release eggs into the stool. The life cycle is completed in about 2 to 3 mo; adult worms live 1 to 2 yr.

A tangled mass of worms resulting from heavy infection can obstruct the bowel, particularly in children. Aberrantly migrating individual adult worms occasionally obstruct the biliary or pancreatic ducts, causing cholecystitis or pancreatitis; cholangitis, liver abscess, and peritonitis are less common. Fever due to other illnesses or certain drugs (eg, albendazole, mebendazole, tetrachloroethylene) may trigger aberrant migration.

Symptoms and Signs

Ascaris larvae migrating through the lungs may cause cough, wheezing, and occasionally hemoptysis or other respiratory symptoms in people without prior exposure to *Ascaris*.

Adult worms in small numbers usually do not cause GI symptoms, although passage of an adult worm by mouth or rectum may bring an otherwise asymptomatic patient to medical attention. Bowel or biliary obstruction causes cramping abdominal pain, nausea, and vomiting. Jaundice is uncommon.

Even moderate infections can lead to undernutrition in children. The pathophysiology is unclear and may include competition for nutrients, impairment of absorption, and depression of appetite.

Diagnosis

- Microscopic examination of stool
- Identification of adult worms in stool or emerging from the nose, mouth, or rectum

Diagnosis of ascariasis is by microscopic detection of eggs in stool or observation of adult worms emerging from the nose or mouth. Occasionally, larvae can be found in sputum during the pulmonary phase.

Eosinophilia can be marked while larvae migrate though the lungs but usually subsides later when adult worms reside in the intestine. Chest x-ray during the pulmonary phase may show infiltrates (Löffler syndrome).

Treatment

- Albendazole, mebendazole, or ivermectin

All intestinal infections should be treated.

Albendazole 400 mg po once, mebendazole 100 mg po bid for 3 days or 500 mg po once, or ivermectin 150 to 200 mcg/kg po once is effective. Albendazole, mebendazole, and ivermectin may harm the fetus, and risk of treatment in pregnant women infected with *Ascaris* must be balanced with risk of untreated disease.

Nitazoxanide is effective for mild *Ascaris* infections but less effective for heavy infections. Piperazine, once widely used, has been replaced by less toxic alternatives.

Obstructive complications may be effectively treated with anthelmintic drugs or require surgical or endoscopic extraction of adult worms.

When the lungs are affected, treatment is symptomatic; it includes bronchodilators and corticosteroids. Anthelmintic drugs are typically not used.

Prevention

Prevention of ascariasis requires adequate sanitation. Preventive strategies include

- Washing the hands thoroughly with soap and water before handling food
- Washing, peeling, and/or cooking all raw vegetables and fruits before eating
- Not eating uncooked or unwashed vegetables in areas where human feces is used as fertilizer
- Not defecating outdoors

KEY POINTS

- Ascariasis is the most prevalent intestinal helminth infection in the world.
- Eggs hatch in the intestines, and larvae migrate first to the lungs and then to the intestines, where they mature.
- Larvae in the lungs may cause cough and wheezing; adult worms may obstruct the intestines.
- Diagnose by microscopic examination of the stool; occasionally, adult worms are seen.
- Treat with albendazole, mebendazole, or ivermectin; obstructions may require surgical or endoscopic extraction of the worms.

BAYLISASCARIASIS

Baylisascariasis is a rare infection with the raccoon ascarid, *Baylisascaris procyonis*, which may cause fatal CNS infection in humans.

Infection usually occurs in children who play in dirt or with articles contaminated with raccoon feces. Most cases have been reported in the Middle Atlantic, Midwest, and Northeast of the US. Although baylisascariasis is rare in people, it is of concern because a large number of raccoons live near humans and the infection rate of *B. procyonis* in these animals is high.

Infected raccoons shed millions of eggs daily in their feces; the eggs can survive in the environment for years. Humans become infected by ingesting infective eggs.

After ingestion by humans, the eggs hatch into larvae. The larvae migrate through a wide variety of tissues (liver, heart, lungs, brain, eyes), resulting in visceral larva migrans (VLM) and ocular larva migrans (OLM), similar to those due to toxocariasis. However, in contrast to *Toxocara* larvae, *Baylisascaris* larvae continue to grow to a large size (up to 24 cm for females and 12 cm for males) within the CNS. Larvae in the CNS can cause inflammatory reactions and eosinophilic meningoencephalitis, damage tissue, and become encapsulated in granulomas.

The severity of neurologic disease in humans varies depending on the

- Number of eggs ingested
- Number of larvae migrating in the CNS

Tissue damage and symptoms and signs of baylisascariasis are often severe because *Baylisascaris* larvae tend to wander widely and do not readily die.

Diagnosis

- MRI
- Antibody tests

Baylisascaris encephalitis should be considered in patients with sudden onset of eosinophilic encephalitis and a history of possible exposure to raccoons and/or to areas where racoons defecate (eg, possibly resulting in ingestion of raccoon feces or contaminated soil).

Characteristic findings include CSF eosinophilic pleocytosis, peripheral eosinophilia, and deep, especially periventricular, white matter abnormalities seen on an MRI scan.

Diagnosis of baylisascariasis is difficult because serologic tests are not commercially available, but CSF or serum can be tested for antibodies at the CDC if the index of suspicion is high.

Viewing a larva during ocular examination is also a clue.

Treatment

- Albendazole

When suspicion of infection is high, immediate treatment with albendazole 25 to 50 mg/kg po once/day for 10 to 20 days may be effective.

KEY POINTS

- Baylisascariasis, a raccoon infection, is rare in people, but it is a concern because a large number of raccoons live near humans and the infection rate of *B. procyonis* in raccoons is high.
- Baylisascariasis usually occurs in children who play in dirt or with articles contaminated with raccoon feces.
- Tissue damage and manifestations are often severe because *Baylisascaris* larvae tend to wander widely and do not readily die.
- Diagnosis is difficult because serologic tests are not commercially available, but CSF or serum can be tested for antibodies at the CDC.
- When suspicion of baylisascariasis is high, immediate treatment with albendazole may be effective.

DRACUNCULIASIS

(Fiery Serpent; Guinea Worm Disease)

Dracunculiasis is infection with *Dracunculus medinensis*. Symptoms are a painful, inflamed skin lesion, which contains an adult worm, and debilitating arthritis. Diagnosis is by inspection. Treatment is slow removal of the adult worm. Dracunculiasis is close to being eradicated.

In the mid-1980s, 3.5 million people had dracunculiasis, but by 2015, thanks to international efforts to interrupt transmission, only 22 cases were reported. They occurred within a narrow belt of African countries—South Sudan, Chad, Mali, and Ethiopia.

The guinea worm is likely to be the first human parasite to be eradicated.[1]

1. Editorial: Guinea worm disease nears eradication. *The Lancet Infectious Diseases* 16(2):131, 2016. doi: http://dx.doi.org/10.1016/S1473-3099(16)00020-7.

Pathophysiology

Humans become infected by drinking water containing infected microcrustaceans (copepods). The larvae are released, penetrate the bowel wall, and mature in the abdominal cavity into adult worms in about 1 yr.

After mating, the male dies, and the gravid female migrates through subcutaneous tissues, usually to the distal lower extremities. The cephalic end of the worm produces an indurated papule that vesiculates and eventually ulcerates. On contact with water (eg, when a person attempts to relieve the severe discomfort by immersing the affected limb), a loop of the worm's uterus prolapses through the skin and discharges motile larvae. Worms that do not reach the skin die and disintegrate or become calcified. Larvae are ingested by copepods.

In most endemic areas, transmission is seasonal and each infectious episode lasts about 1 yr.

Symptoms and Signs

Dracunculiasis is typically asymptomatic for the first year. Symptoms typically develop when the worm erupts through the skin. Local symptoms include intense itching and a burning pain at the site of the skin lesion. Urticaria, erythema, dyspnea, vomiting, and pruritus are thought to reflect allergic reactions to worm antigens. If the worm is broken during expulsion or extraction, a severe inflammatory reaction ensues, causing disabling pain. Symptoms subside and the ulcer heals once the adult worm is expelled. In about 50% of cases, secondary bacterial infections occur along the track of the emerging worm.

The chronic stage of infection is associated with inflammation and pain in the joints and other signs of arthritis. Sequelae include fibrous ankylosis of joints and contraction of tendons.

Diagnosis

- Clinical evaluation

Diagnosis of dracunculiasis is obvious once the white, filamentous adult worm appears at the cutaneous ulcer. Calcified worms can be localized with x-ray examination; they have been found in Egyptian mummies.

No serodiagnostic tests are available.

Treatment

- Manual removal

Treatment of dracunculiasis consists of slow removal of the adult worm (which may be up to 80 cm long) over days to weeks by rolling it on a stick. Surgical removal under local anesthesia is an option but is seldom available in endemic areas.

There are no effective anthelmintic drugs for this disease; the beneficial effect of metronidazole (250 mg po tid for 10 days) has been ascribed to the drug's anti-inflammatory and antibacterial properties.

Prevention

Filtering drinking water through a piece of fine-mesh cloth, chlorination, or boiling effectively protects against dracunculiasis. Infected people should be instructed not to enter drinking water sources to avoid contaminating them.

KEY POINTS

- The guinea worm has almost been eradicated.
- When an infected person immerses the affected extremity in water to relieve the intense discomfort caused by eruption of the female worm through the skin, larvae are released and ingested by microcrustaceans; humans are infected when they ingest water contaminated with the microcrustaceans.
- If a worm is broken during expulsion or extraction, a severe inflammatory reaction ensues, causing disabling pain.
- Diagnose based on observation of a white, filamentous adult worm at a cutaneous ulcer.
- Treat dracunculiasis by slowly removing the adult worm over days to weeks by rolling it on a stick or sometimes by surgically removing it.
- Filtering drinking water through a piece of fine-mesh cloth, chlorination, or boiling effectively protects against dracunculiasis.

OVERVIEW OF FILARIAL NEMATODE INFECTIONS

Threadlike adult filarial worms reside in lymphatic or subcutaneous tissues. Gravid females produce live offspring (microfilariae) that circulate in blood or migrate through tissues. When ingested by a suitable bloodsucking insect (mosquitoes or flies), microfilariae develop into infective larvae that are inoculated or deposited in the skin of the next host during the insect bite. Life cycles of all filarial worms are similar except for the site of infection. Only a few filarial species infect humans. They can be grouped based on the location of adult worms.

Subcutaneous filariasis includes

- Loiasis caused by *Loa loa* (the African eye worm)
- Onchocerciasis (river blindness) caused by *Onchocerca volvulus*

Lymphatic filariasis includes

- Bancroftian and Brugian lymphatic filariasis caused by *Wuchereria bancrofti*, *Brugia malayi*, and *B. timori*

Rarely, *Dirofilaria immitis*, the dog heartworm, causes infection in humans (dirofilariasis).

Some specialty laboratories have a general screening serologic test for filarial infection (including *Wuchereria*, *Brugia*, *Onchocerca*, and *Mansonella* infections). The test is highly sensitive but cannot identify the specific filarial infection and cannot distinguish active from remote infection. This distinction is less important in symptomatic travelers, but limits the usefulness of the test in people from endemic areas.

DIROFILARIASIS

(Dog Heartworm Infection)

Dirofilariasis is a filarial nematode infection with *Dirofilaria immitis*, the dog heartworm, or other *Dirofilaria* spp, which are transmitted to humans by infected mosquitoes.

Symptomatic human infection is very rare, but larvae may become encapsulated in infarcted lung tissue and produce well-defined pulmonary nodules; rarely, larvae form nodules in the eyes, brain, and testes.

Patients may have chest pain, cough, and occasionally hemoptysis. Many patients remain asymptomatic, and a pulmonary nodule, which may suggest a tumor, is discovered during routine chest x-ray.

Dirofilariasis is diagnosed by histologic examination of a surgical specimen.

No anthelmintic treatment is indicated in humans; infection is self-limited.

LOIASIS

Loiasis is a filarial nematode infection with *Loa loa*. Symptoms include localized angioedema (Calabar swellings) and subconjunctival migration of adult worms. Diagnosis is by detecting microfilariae in peripheral blood or seeing worms migrating across the eye. Treatment is with diethylcarbamazine.

Loiasis is confined to the rain forest belt of western and central Africa. Humans are the only known natural reservoir for this parasite.

Loa loa microfilariae are transmitted by day-biting tabanid flies (*Chrysops* [deer fly or horse fly]). Microfilariae mature to adult worms in the subcutaneous tissues of the human host; females are 40 to 70 mm long, and males are 30 to 34 mm long. The adults produce microfilariae. Adults migrate in subcutaneous tissues and under the conjunctiva of the eye, and microfilariae circulate in blood. Flies become infected when they ingest blood from a human host during the day (when microfilaremia levels are the highest).

Occasionally, infection causes cardiomyopathy, nephropathy, or encephalitis. Eosinophilia is common but nonspecific.

Symptoms and Signs

Most infected people are asymptomatic, but eosinophilia is common. Infection produces areas of angioedema (Calabar swellings) that develop anywhere on the body but predominantly on the extremities; they are presumed to reflect hypersensitivity reactions to allergens released by migrating adult worms. In native residents, swellings usually last 1 to 3 days but are more frequent and severe in visitors. Worms may also migrate subconjunctivally across the eyes. This migration may be unsettling, but residual eye damage is uncommon.

Nephropathy generally manifests as proteinuria with or without mild hematuria and is believed to be due to immune complex deposition.

Encephalopathy is usually mild, with vague CNS symptoms.

Diagnosis

- Observation of an adult worm subconjunctivally crossing the eye
- Identification of an adult worm removed from the eye or skin
- Identification and quantification of microfilariae in blood by microscopy or quantitative PCR

Loiasis should be suspected in immigrants or travelers who have a history of exposure in an endemic area and who present with eye worms, Calabar swellings, or unexplained peripheral eosinophilia.

Occasionally, the diagnosis of loiasis is confirmed by observing an adult worm migrating under the conjunctiva or by identifying a worm after it is removed from the eye or skin.

Microscopic detection of microfilariae in peripheral blood establishes the diagnosis. Blood samples should be drawn between 10 am and 2 pm, when microfilaremia levels are the highest.

Many serologic tests for antibodies do not differentiate *Loa loa* from other filarial nematode infections. *Loa*-specific antibody tests have been developed, but they are not widely available in the US. A quantitative real-time PCR (qPCR) to confirm the diagnosis and determine the microfilarial burden is available at the Laboratory of Parasitic Diseases, National Institutes of Health.

People from endemic regions of Africa should be checked for *Loa loa* before they are treated with diethylcarbamazine or ivermectin for other disorders because these drugs can have substantial side effects in people with loiasis. If treated with diethylcarbamazine or ivermectin, people with > 8000 *Loa loa* microfilariae mL/blood are at risk of potentially fatal encephalopathy, caused by the release of antigens from dying microfilariae.

Treatment

- Diethylcarbamazine (DEC)
- For heavy infections, initial treatment with albendazole and/or apheresis

Treatment of loiasis is complicated. DEC is the only drug that kills microfilariae and adult worms. In the US, it is available only from the CDC after laboratory confirmation of loiasis; clinicians should seek expert advice before they initiate treatment, and they should do the following before initiating treatment with DEC:

- Measure the number of microfilariae in the blood because using DEC to treat heavy infections (> 8000 microfilariae/mL/blood) can result in potentially fatal encephalopathy
- Exclude coinfection with onchocerciasis because DEC can worsen eye disease in patients with onchocerciasis

Clinicians should seek expert assistance when measuring the number of microfilariae and thus determining the severity of the infection.

Treatment of light infection: Patients with symptomatic loiasis and < 8000 microfilariae/mL blood are given DEC as follows:

- 50 mg po on day 1
- 50 mg po tid on day 2
- 100 mg po tid on day 3
- Then 2.7 to 3.3 mg/kg tid on days 4 to 21

Treatment of heavy infection: In heavily infected patients, filarial antigens (released by the microfilariae as DEC kills them) may trigger encephalopathy, leading to coma and death. Patients with > 8000 microfilariae/mL blood are at risk of this effect and may benefit from apheresis or initial treatment with albendazole 200 mg po bid for 21 days; the goal is to reduce the microfilarial load to < 8000/mL before DEC is initiated. Multiple courses of DEC may be necessary.

Patients who have failed ≥ 2 rounds of treatment with DEC may be given albendazole 200 mg po bid for 21 days.

Ivermectin has also been used to reduce microfilaremia, but albendazole is preferred because its onset of action is slower and risk of precipitating encephalopathy is lower.

Prevention

DEC 300 mg po once/wk can be used to prevent loiasis.

Using insect repellents (including permethrin-impregnated clothing) and wearing long-sleeved and long-legged clothing may reduce the number of bites by infected flies. Because the flies are day-biting, mosquito (bed) nets do not help.

KEY POINTS

- Humans are the only known natural reservoir for *Loa loa,* which is transmitted by day-biting tabanid flies.
- Most infected people are asymptomatic, but some have areas of angioedema (Calabar swellings), which occur mainly on the extremities.
- Diagnose by microscopic examination of peripheral blood drawn between 10 am and 2 pm, when microfilaremia levels are the highest, and confirm by quantitative PCR.
- Occasionally, diagnosis of loiasis is confirmed by observing an adult worm migrating under the conjunctiva or by identifying a worm after it is removed from the eye or skin.
- DEC is the only drug that kills microfilariae and adult worms; in the US, it is available only from the CDC.
- Seek expert assistance in measuring the number of microfilariae and determining the severity of the infection, and seek expert advice before initiating treatment.
- In patients with heavy infection, pretreatment with apheresis or albendazole is recommended because in these patients, the filarial antigens released as diethylcarbamazine kills microfilariae may trigger encephalopathy, leading to coma and death.

BANCROFTIAN AND BRUGIAN LYMPHATIC FILARIASIS

Lymphatic filariasis is infection with any of 3 species of *Filarioidea*. Acute symptoms include fever, lymphadenitis, lymphangitis, funiculitis, and epididymitis. Chronic symptoms include abscesses, hyperkeratosis, polyarthritis, hydroceles, lymphedema, and elephantiasis. Tropical pulmonary eosinophilia (TPE) with bronchospasm, fever, and pulmonary infiltrates is another manifestation of infection. Diagnosis is by detection of microfilariae in blood, ultrasound visualization of adult worms, or serologic testing. Treatment is with diethylcarbamazine; antibiotics are used for complicating bacterial cellulitis.

Bancroftian filariasis is present in tropical and subtropical areas of Africa, Asia, the Pacific, and the Americas, including Haiti. Brugian filariasis is endemic in South and Southeast Asia.

Mass treatment programs have reduced the prevalence in many areas. Current estimates suggest that about 120 million people are infected worldwide.

Lymphatic filariasis is caused by *Wuchereria bancrofti*, *Brugia malayi*, or *B. timori*. Transmission is by mosquitoes. Infective larvae from the mosquito migrate to the lymphatics, where they develop into threadlike adult worms within 6 to 12 mo. Females are 80 to 100 mm long; males are about 40 mm long. Gravid adult females produce microfilariae that circulate in blood.

Symptoms and Signs

Infection can result in microfilaremia without overt clinical manifestations. Symptoms and signs are caused primarily by adult worms. Microfilaremia gradually disappears after people leave the endemic area.

Acute inflammatory filariasis consists of 4- to 7-day episodes (often recurrent) of fever and inflammation of lymph nodes with lymphangitis (termed acute adenolymphangitis [ADL]) or acute epididymitis and spermatic cord inflammation. Localized involvement of a limb may cause an abscess that drains externally and leaves a scar. ADL is often associated with secondary bacterial infections. ADL episodes usually precede onset of chronic disease by ≥ 2 decades. Acute filariasis is more severe in previously unexposed immigrants to endemic areas than in native residents.

Chronic filarial disease develops insidiously after many years. In most patients, asymptomatic lymphatic dilation occurs, but chronic inflammatory responses to adult worms and secondary bacterial infections may result in chronic lymphedema of the affected body area. Increased local susceptibility to bacterial and fungal infections further contributes to its development. Chronic pitting lymphedema of a lower extremity can progress to elephantiasis (chronic lymphatic obstruction). *W. bancrofti* can cause hydrocele and scrotal elephantiasis. Other forms of chronic filarial disease are caused by disruption of lymphatic vessels or aberrant drainage of lymph fluid, leading to chyluria and chyloceles.

Extralymphatic signs include chronic microscopic hematuria and proteinuria and mild polyarthritis, all presumed to result from immune complex deposition.

TPE is an uncommon manifestation with recurrent bronchospasm, transitory lung infiltrates, low-grade fever, and marked eosinophilia. It is most likely due to hypersensitivity reactions to microfilariae. Chronic TPE can lead to pulmonary fibrosis.

Diagnosis

- Microscopic examination of blood samples
- Antigen test for *W. bancrofti*
- Antibody tests

Microscopic detection of microfilariae in blood establishes the diagnosis of lymphatic filariasis. Filtered or centrifuged concentrates of blood are more sensitive than thick blood films. Blood samples must be obtained when microfilaremia peaks—at night in most endemic areas, but during the day in many Pacific islands. Viable adult worms can be visualized in dilated lymphatics by ultrasonography; their movement has been called the filarial dance.

Several blood tests are available:

- **Antigen detection:** A rapid-format immunochromatographic test for *W. bancrofti* antigens
- **Molecular diagnosis:** Polymerase chain reaction assays for *W. bancrofti* and *B. malayi*
- **Antibody detection:** Alternatively, enzyme immunoassay (EIA) tests for antifilarial IgG1 and IgG4

Patients with active filarial infection typically have elevated levels of antifilarial IgG4 in the blood. However, there is substantial antigenic cross-reactivity between filariae and other helminths, and a positive serologic test does not distinguish between past and current infection.

Treatment

- DEC

DEC kills microfilariae and a variable proportion of adult worms. In the US, DEC is available only from the CDC after laboratory confirmation of filariasis.

PEARLS & PITFALLS

- Before treatment with DEC, assess patients for coinfection with *Loa loa* and *Onchocerca volvulus* because DEC can cause serious reactions in patients with those infections.

Treatment of acute lymphatic filariasis: DEC 2 mg/kg po tid for 12 days has traditionally been used; 6 mg/kg po once is an alternative. Generally, the 1-day regimen seems to be as effective as the 12-day regimen.

Adverse effects with DEC are usually limited and depend on the number of microfilariae in the blood. The most common are dizziness, nausea, fever, headache, and pain in muscles or joints, which are thought to be related to release of filarial antigens.

Before treatment with DEC, patients should be assessed for coinfection with *Loa loa* (loiasis) and *Onchocerca volvulus* (onchocerciasis) because DEC can cause serious reactions in patients with those infections. A single dose of albendazole 400 mg po plus ivermectin (200 mcg/kg po) in areas where onchocerciasis is co-endemic or DEC (6 mg/kg) in areas without onchocerciasis and loiasis rapidly reduces microfilaremia levels, but ivermectin does not kill adult worms.

A number of drug combinations and regimens have been used in mass treatment programs.

Also, doxycycline has been given long-term (eg, 100 mg po bid for 4 to 8 wk). Doxycycline kills *Wolbachia* endosymbiont bacteria within filaria, leading to death of adult filarial worms. It can be given with DEC or used alone.

Acute attacks of ADL usually resolve spontaneously, although antibiotics may be required to control secondary bacterial infections.

Treatment of chronic lymphedema: Chronic lymphedema requires meticulous skin care, including use of systemic antibiotics to treat secondary bacterial infections; these antibiotics may slow or prevent progression to elephantiasis.

Whether DEC therapy prevents or lessens chronic lymphedema remains controversial.

Conservative measures such as elastic bandaging of the affected limb reduce swelling.

Surgical decompression using nodal-venous shunts to improve lymphatic drainage offers some long-term benefit in extreme cases of elephantiasis. Massive hydroceles can also be managed surgically.

Treatment of tropical pulmonary eosinophilia: TPE responds to DEC 2 mg/kg po tid for 14 to 21 days, but relapses occur in up to 25% of patients and require additional courses of therapy.

Prevention

Avoiding mosquito bites in endemic areas is the best protection (eg, by using diethyltoluamide [DEET] on exposed skin, permethrin-impregnated clothing, and bed nets).

Chemoprophylaxis with DEC or combinations of antifilarial drugs (ivermectin/albendazole or ivermectin/DEC) can suppress microfilaremia and thereby reduce transmission of the parasite by mosquitoes in endemic communities. DEC has even been used as an additive to table salt in some endemic areas.

KEY POINTS

- Lymphatic filariasis is transmitted by mosquitoes; infective larvae migrate to the lymphatics, where they develop into adult worms.
- Adult worms inside the lymphatics can cause inflammation resulting in acute ADL or epididymitis or in chronic lymphatic obstruction, which, in some patients, leads to elephantiasis or hydrocele.
- Diagnose based on microscopic detection of microfilariae in filtered or centrifuged concentrates of blood that is drawn at the time of day when microfilaremia peaks (varies by species).
- Tests for antigen, antibodies, and parasite DNA are alternatives to diagnosis by microscopy.
- Treat with diethylcarbamazine after checking for coinfection with *Loa loa*and *Onchocerca volvulus*.

ONCHOCERCIASIS

(River Blindness)

Onchocerciasis is a filarial nematode infection with *Onchocerca volvulus*. Symptoms are subcutaneous nodules, pruritus, dermatitis, adenopathy, lymphatic obstruction, and eye lesions that may lead to blindness. Diagnosis is by finding microfilariae in skin snips, the cornea, or the anterior chamber of the eye; identifying adult worms in subcutaneous nodules; or using PCR or DNA probes. Treatment is with ivermectin.

About 18 million people are infected; about 270,000 are blind, and an additional 750,000 are visually impaired. Onchocerciasis is the 2nd leading cause of blindness worldwide (after trachoma).

Onchocerciasis is most common in tropical and sub-Saharan regions of Africa. Small foci exist in Yemen, southern Mexico, Guatemala, Ecuador, Colombia, Venezuela, and the Brazilian Amazon. Blindness due to onchocerciasis is fairly rare in the Americas.

Pathophysiology

Onchocerciasis is spread by blackflies (*Simulium* sp) that breed in swiftly flowing streams (hence, the term river blindness).

Infective larvae inoculated into the skin during the bite of a blackfly develop into adult worms in 12 to 18 mo. Adult female worms may live up to 15 yr in subcutaneous nodules. Females are 33 to 50 cm long; males are 19 to 42 mm long. Mature female worms produce microfilariae that migrate mainly through the skin and invade the eyes.

Symptoms and Signs

Onchocerciasis typically affects

- Skin (nodules, dermatitis)
- Eyes

Nodules: The subcutaneous (or deeper) nodules (onchocercoma) that contain adult worms may be visible or palpable but are otherwise asymptomatic. They are composed of inflammatory cells and fibrotic tissue in various proportions. Old nodules may caseate or calcify.

Dermatitis: Onchocercal dermatitis is caused by the microfilarial stage of the parasite. Intense pruritus may be the only symptom in lightly infected people.

Skin lesions usually consist of a nondescript maculopapular rash with secondary excoriations, scaling ulcerations and lichenification, and mild to moderate lymphadenopathy. Premature wrinkling, skin atrophy, enlargement of inguinal or femoral nodes, lymphatic obstruction, patchy hypopigmentation, and transitory localized areas of edema and erythema can occur.

Onchocercal dermatitis is generalized in most patients, but a localized and sharply delineated form of eczematous dermatitis with hyperkeratosis, scaling, and pigment changes (Sowdah) is common in Yemen and Sudan.

Eye disease: Ocular involvement ranges from mild visual impairment to complete blindness. Lesions of the anterior portion of the eye include

- Punctate (snowflake) keratitis (an acute inflammatory infiltrate surrounding dying microfilariae that resolves without causing permanent damage)
- Sclerosing keratitis (an ingrowth of fibrovascular scar tissue that may cause subluxation of the lens and blindness)
- Anterior uveitis or iridocyclitis (which may deform the pupil)

Chorioretinitis, optic neuritis, and optic atrophy may also occur.

Diagnosis

- Microscopic examination of a skin sample
- Slit-lamp examination of the cornea and anterior chamber of the eye
- PCR of the skin

Demonstration of microfilariae in skin snips is the traditional diagnostic method; multiple samples are usually taken (see Table 182–1 on p. 1476). PCR-based methods to detect parasite DNA in skin snips are more sensitive than standard techniques but are available only in research settings.

Microfilariae may also be visible in the cornea and anterior chamber of the eye during slit-lamp examination.

Antibody detection is of limited value; there is substantial antigenic cross-reactivity among filaria and other helminths, and a positive serologic test does not distinguish between past and current infection.

Palpable nodules (or deep nodules detected by ultrasonography or MRI) can be excised and examined for adult worms, but this procedure is rarely necessary.

Treatment

- Ivermectin

Ivermectin is given as a single oral dose of 150 mcg/kg, repeated q 6 to 12 mo. Ivermectin reduces microfilariae in the skin and eyes and decreases production of microfilariae for many months. It does not kill adult female worms, but cumulative doses decrease their fertility. The optimal duration of therapy is uncertain. Although annual treatment could theoretically be continued for the life span of female worms (10 to 14 yr), it is often stopped after several years if pruritis has resolved and no evidence of microfilariae is detected by skin biopsy or eye examination.

Adverse effects of ivermectin are qualitatively similar to those of diethylcarbamazine (DEC) but are much less common and less severe. DEC is not used for onchocerciasis because it can cause a severe hypersensitivity (Mazzotti) reaction, which can further damage skin and eyes and lead to cardiovascular collapse.

Before treatment with ivermectin, patients should be assessed for coinfection with *Loa loa*, another filarial parasite, if they have been in areas of central Africa where both parasites are transmitted because ivermectin can cause severe reactions in patients coinfected with *Loa loa*.

PEARLS & PITFALLS

- Before treating onchocerciasis with ivermectin, exclude coinfection with *Loa loa* if patients have been exposed to this parasite in central Africa.

Doxycycline can kill the endosymbiont bacteria *Wolbachia*, which *O. volvulus* requires for survival and embryogenesis. Doxycycline kills > 60% of adult female worms and sterilizes or decreases the fertility of those that survive. A newer regimen includes one dose of ivermectin 150 mcg/kg, followed in 1 wk by doxycycline 100 mg po once/day or bid for 6 wk; ivermectin is then continued at yearly intervals as above.

Surgical removal of accessible onchocercomas can reduce skin microfilaria counts, but it has been replaced by ivermectin therapy.

Prevention

No drug has been shown to protect against infection with *O. volvulus*. However, annual or semiannual administration of ivermectin effectively controls disease and may decrease transmission.

Simulium bites can be minimized by avoiding fly-infested areas, by wearing protective clothing, and possibly by liberally applying insect repellents.

KEY POINTS

- Onchocerciasis is a filarial infection that causes skin lesions, rash, and, more importantly, eye disease, leading to visual impairment and sometimes blindness.
- Diagnose by slit-lamp examination of the eye and microscopic examination of a skin snip; where available, PCR testing may be helpful.
- Treat with ivermectin to kill microfilaria and reduce the fertility of female worms; ivermectin does not kill adult worms.
- Before treatment with ivermectin, patients should be assessed for coinfection with *Loa loa* if they have been in areas of central Africa where both parasites are transmitted.
- Consider adding a 6-wk course of doxycycline to kill and/or sterilize adult female worms.

HOOKWORM INFECTION

(Ancylostomiasis)

Ancylostomiasis is infection with the hookworm *Ancylostoma duodenale* or *Necator americanus*. Symptoms include rash at the site of larval entry and sometimes abdominal pain or other GI symptoms during early infection. Later, iron deficiency may develop because of chronic blood loss. Hookworms are a major cause of iron deficiency anemia in endemic regions. Diagnosis is by finding eggs in stool. Treatment is with albendazole or mebendazole.

The estimated prevalence of hookworm infection is 576 to 740 million, mostly in developing areas. Both *A. duodenale* and *N. americanus* occur in Africa, Asia, and the Americas. Only *A. duodenale* occurs in the Middle East, North Africa, and southern Europe. *N. americanus* predominates in the Americas and Australia; it was once widely distributed in the southern US and is still endemic on islands of the Caribbean and in Central and South America.

Pathophysiology

Both hookworm species have similar life cycles. Eggs passed in the stool hatch in 1 to 2 days (if they are deposited in a warm, moist place on loose soil) and release rhabditiform larvae, which molt once to become slender filariform larvae in 5 to 10 days. The larvae can survive 3 to 4 wk if environmental conditions are favorable. Filariform larvae penetrate human skin when people walk barefoot on or otherwise come into direct contact with infested soil.

The larvae reach the lungs via blood vessels, penetrate into pulmonary alveoli, ascend the bronchial tree to the epiglottis, and are swallowed. The larvae develop into adults in the small bowel; there, they attach to the wall, feeding on blood. Adult worms may live ≥ 2 yr.

Chronic blood loss leads to iron deficiency anemia. Development of anemia depends on worm burden and the amount of absorbable iron in the diet.

Zoonotic (animal) hookworm infections: Zoonotic hookworms infections include

- Cutaneous larva migrans
- Eosinophilic enterocolitis

A. braziliense and *A. caninum* are hookworms that have cats and dogs as the primary hosts. These hookworms cannot complete their life cycle in humans. If their larvae penetrate human skin, they typically wander in the skin, causing cutaneous larva migrans, rather than migrate to the intestine.

Rarely, *A. caninum* larvae migrate to the intestine, where they may cause eosinophilic enterocolitis. However, they do not cause significant blood loss and anemia, and because they do not mature to full adulthood, they do not lay eggs (making diagnosis difficult). Such intestinal infection may be asymptomatic or cause acute abdominal pain and eosinophilia.

Symptoms and Signs

Hookworm infection is often asymptomatic. However, a pruritic papulovesicular rash (ground itch) may develop at the site of larval penetration, usually on the feet. Migration of large numbers of larvae through the lungs occasionally causes Löffler syndrome, with cough, wheezing, eosinophilia, and sometimes hemoptysis. During the acute phase, adult worms in the intestine may cause colicky epigastric pain, anorexia, flatulence, diarrhea, and weight loss.

Chronic, heavy infection can lead to iron deficiency anemia, causing pallor, dyspnea, weakness, tachycardia, lassitude, and peripheral edema. A low-grade eosinophilia is often present. In children, chronic blood loss may lead to severe anemia, heart failure, and anasarca and, in pregnant women, to growth retardation in the fetus.

Cutaneous larva migrans can occur when animal hookworms infect humans. It is caused by the larvae as they migrate through the skin and is characterized by itchy, erythematous, serpiginous skin lesions.

Diagnosis

- Microscopic examination of stool

A. duodenale and *N. americanus* produce thin-shelled oval eggs that are readily detected in fresh stool. Concentration procedures are needed to diagnose light infections. If the stool is not kept cold and examined within several hours, the eggs may hatch and release larvae that may be confused with those of *Strongyloides stercoralis*.

Nutritional status, anemia, and iron stores should be evaluated.

Diagnosis of cutaneous larva migrans is based on the clinical manifestations. Ova are not present in the stool.

Treatment

- Albendazole, mebendazole, or pyrantel pamoate

One of the following drugs may be used:

- Albendazole 400 mg po as a single dose
- Mebendazole 100 mg po bid for 3 days or 500 mg as a single dose
- Pyrantel pamoate 11 mg/kg (maximum dose of 1 g) po once/day for 3 days

These drugs should only be used during pregnancy if benefits outweigh risks. Ivermectin is not effective.

General support and correction of iron deficiency anemia are needed if infection is heavy.

Cutaneous larva migrans is a self-limited infection, but symptoms can last 5 to 6 wk. Treatment with albendazole 400 mg once/day po for 3 or 7 days or ivermectin 200 mcg/kg as a single dose is curative.

Prevention

Preventing unhygienic defecation and avoiding direct skin contact with the soil (eg, wearing shoes, using barriers when seated on the ground) are effective in preventing infection but difficult to implement in many endemic areas. Periodic mass treatment of susceptible populations at 3- to 4-mo intervals has been used in high-risk areas.

Risk of developing cutaneous larva migrans can be reduced by the following:

- Avoiding direct skin contact with potentially infested beach sand or other soil
- Treating cats and dogs for hookworm

KEY POINTS

- Hookworm larvae penetrate the skin when people walk barefoot on or otherwise come into direct contact with infested soil.
- In humans, larvae of the hookworms *Ancylostoma duodenale* or *Necator americanus* travel through the bloodstream to the lungs, penetrate the alveoli, ascend to the epiglottis, are swallowed, and then mature in the intestines.
- Infection may be asymptomatic, but a pruritic rash may appear at the site of larval penetration, and pulmonary involvement may cause cough and wheezing.
- Intestinal involvement may cause iron deficiency anemia.
- Diagnose by microscopic examination of stool.
- Treat with albendazole, mebendazole, or pyrantel pamoate.

PINWORM INFESTATION

(Enterobiasis; Oxyuriasis)

Enterobiasis is an intestinal infestation by the pinworm *Enterobius vermicularis*, usually in children. Its major symptom is perianal itching. Diagnosis is by visual inspection for threadlike worms in the perianal area or the cellophane tape test for ova. Treatment is with mebendazole or albendazole.

Pinworm infestation is the most common helminthic infection in the US. Most cases occur in school-aged children, adults who care for children, or family members of an infected child.

Pathophysiology

Pinworm infestation usually results from transfer of ova from the perianal area to fomites (clothing, bedding, furniture, rugs, toys, toilet seats), from which the ova are picked up by the new host, transmitted to the mouth, and swallowed. Thumb sucking is a risk factor. Reinfestation (autoinfestation) easily occurs through finger transfer of ova from the perianal area to the mouth. Pinworm infections have also been attributed to anilingus among adults.

Pinworms reach maturity in the lower GI tract within 2 to 6 wk. The female worm migrates out of the anus to the perianal region (usually at night) to deposit ova. The sticky, gelatinous substance in which the ova are deposited and the movements of the female worm cause perianal pruritus. The ova can survive on fomites as long as 3 wk at normal room temperature.

Symptoms and Signs

Most infected people have no symptoms or signs, but some experience perianal pruritus and develop perianal excoriations from scratching. Rarely, migrating female worms ascend the human female genital tract, causing vaginitis and, even less commonly, peritoneal lesions.

Many other conditions (eg, abdominal pain, insomnia, seizures) have been attributed to pinworm infestation, but a causal relationship is unlikely. Pinworms have been found obstructing the appendiceal lumen in cases of appendicitis, but the presence of the parasites may be coincidental.

Diagnosis

- Examination of the perianal region for worms, ova, or both

Pinworm infestation can be diagnosed by finding the female worm, which is 8 to 13 mm long (males are 2 to 5 mm), in the perianal region 1 or 2 h after a child goes to bed at night or in the morning or by using a low-power microscope to identify ova on cellophane tape. The ova are obtained in the early morning before the child arises by patting the perianal skinfolds with a strip of cellophane tape, which is then placed sticky side down on a glass slide and viewed microscopically. The 50 by 30 μm ova are oval with a thin shell that contains a curled-up larva. A drop of toluene placed between tape and slide dissolves the adhesive and eliminates air bubbles under the tape, which can hamper identification of the ova. This procedure should be repeated on 3 successive mornings if necessary.

Eggs may also be encountered, but less frequently, in stool, urine, or vaginal smears.

Treatment

- Mebendazole, albendazole, or pyrantel pamoate

Because pinworm infestation is seldom harmful, prevalence is high, and reinfestation is common, treatment is indicated only for symptomatic infections. However, most parents actively seek treatment when their children have pinworms.

A single dose of any of the following, repeated in 2 wk, is effective in eradicating pinworms (but not ova) in > 90% of cases:

- Mebendazole 100 mg po (regardless of age)
- Albendazole 400 mg po
- Pyrantel pamoate 11 mg/kg (maximum dose of 1 g) po

Carbolated petrolatum (ie, containing carbolic acid) or other antipruritic creams or ointments applied to the perianal region may relieve itching.

Prevention

Pinworm reinfestation is common because viable ova may be excreted for 1 wk after therapy, and ova deposited in the environment before therapy can survive 3 wk. Multiple infestations within the household are common, and treatment of the entire family may be necessary.

The following can help prevent the spread of pinworm:

- Washing the hands with soap and warm water after using the toilet, after changing diapers, and before handling food (the most successful way)
- Frequently washing clothing, bedding, and toys
- If people are infected, showering every morning to help remove eggs on the skin
- Vacuuming he environment to try to eliminate eggs

KEY POINTS

- Pinworm infestation is the most common helminthic infection in the US; most cases occur in school-aged children, in adults who care for children, or in family members of an infected child.
- Pinworm infestation is seldom harmful, and reinfestation is common.
- Ova deposited in the environment can survive 3 wk.
- Pinworm eggs may be ingested when people touch their mouth after they scratch their perianal area or after they handle contaminated clothes or other objects (eg, bed linens).
- Most infected people have no symptoms or signs, but some experience perianal pruritus.
- Diagnose pinworm infestation by collecting ova in the morning on cellophane tape and using a low-power microscope to identify them; diagnosis can also be made by finding the female worm in the perianal region 1 or 2 h after a child goes to bed at night.
- If patients have symptomatic infections, treat with mebendazole, albendazole, or pyrantel pamoate.

STRONGYLOIDIASIS

(Threadworm Infection)

Strongyloidiasis is infection with *Strongyloides stercoralis*. Findings include rash and pulmonary symptoms (including cough and wheezing), eosinophilia, and abdominal pain with diarrhea. Diagnosis is by finding larvae in stool or small-bowel contents or occasionally in sputum or by detection of antibodies in blood. Treatment is with ivermectin or albendazole.

Strongyloidiasis is endemic throughout the tropics and subtropics, including rural areas of the southern US, at sites where bare skin is exposed to contaminated soil and conditions are unsanitary.

Serious *S. stercoralis* infections have occurred in recipients of solid organ transplants from asymptomatic donors who had lived in endemic areas.[1]

Strongyloides fülleborni, which infects chimpanzees and baboons, can cause limited infections in humans.

1. Abanyie FA, Gray EB, Delli Carpini KW, et al: Donor-derived *Strongyloides stercoralis* infection in solid organ transplant recipients in the United States, 2009–2013. *Am J Transplant* 15(5):1369–1375, 2015. doi: 10.1111/ajt.13137.

Pathophysiology

Strongyloides adult worms live in the mucosa and submucosa of the duodenum and jejunum. Released eggs hatch in the bowel lumen, liberating rhabditiform larvae. Most of the larvae are excreted in the stool. After a few days in soil, they develop into infectious filariform larvae. Like hookworms, *Strongyloides* larvae penetrate human skin, migrate via the bloodstream to the lungs, break through pulmonary capillaries, ascend the respiratory tract, are swallowed, and reach the intestine, where they mature in about 2 wk. In the soil, larvae that do not contact humans may develop into free-living adult worms that can reproduce for several generations before their larvae reenter a human host.

Some rhabditiform larvae convert within the intestine to infectious filariform larvae that immediately reenter the bowel wall, short-circuiting the life cycle (internal autoinfection). Sometimes filariform larvae are passed in stool and reenter through the skin of the buttocks and thighs (external autoinfection). Autoinfection explains why strongyloidiasis can persist for many decades and helps account for the extremely high worm burden in the hyperinfection syndrome.

Hyperinfection syndrome: Hyperinfection syndrome may result from a newly acquired *Strongyloides* infection or from activation of a previously asymptomatic one. In either case, it can result in disseminated disease involving organs not usually part of the parasite's normal life cycle (eg, CNS, skin, liver, heart). Hyperinfection syndrome usually occurs in patients who are taking corticosteroids or who have impaired T_H2 type cell-mediated immunity, particularly those infected with the human T-lymphotropic virus 1 (HTLV-1). However, hyperinfection and disseminated strongyloidiasis are less common than might be predicted among patients with HIV/AIDS, even those living in areas where *Strongyloides* is highly endemic.

Symptoms and Signs

Strongyloidiasis may be asymptomatic.

Larva currens (creeping infection) is a form of cutaneous larva migrans specific to *Strongyloides* infection; it results from autoinfection. The eruption usually begins in the perianal region and is accompanied by intense pruritus. Typically, larva currens is a linear or serpiginous, rapidly migrating, erythematous, urticarial skin lesion. Nonspecific maculopapular or urticarial eruptions may also occur.

Pulmonary symptoms are uncommon, although heavy infections may cause Löffler syndrome, with cough, wheezing, and eosinophilia. GI symptoms include anorexia, epigastric pain and tenderness, diarrhea, nausea, and vomiting. In heavy infections, malabsorption and protein-losing enteropathy may result in weight loss and cachexia.

Hyperinfection syndrome: GI and pulmonary symptoms are often prominent. Bacteremia may develop when the larvae invade the bowel or lungs. Ileus, obstruction, massive GI bleeding, severe malabsorption, and peritonitis may occur.

Pulmonary symptoms include dyspnea, hemoptysis, and respiratory failure. Infiltrates may be seen on chest x-ray.

Other symptoms depend on the organs involved. CNS involvement includes parasitic meningitis, brain abscess, and diffuse invasion of the brain. Secondary gram-negative meningitis and bacteremia, which occurs with high frequency, probably reflect disruption of bowel mucosa, carriage of bacteria on migrating larvae, or both. Liver infection may result in cholestatic and granulomatous hepatitis.

Infection may be fatal in immunocompromised patients, even with treatment.

Diagnosis

- Identification of larvae by microscopic examination of stool or the agar plate method
- EIA for antibodies

Microscopic examination of a single stool sample detects larvae in about 25% of uncomplicated *Strongyloides* infections. Repeated examination of concentrated stool samples raises the sensitivity; a minimum of 3 stool samples is recommended. The agar plate method has a sensitivity of > 85%. If the specimen stands at room temperature for several hours, rhabditiform larvae may transform into longer filariform larvae, leading to erroneous diagnosis of hyperinfection.

Sampling of the proximal small bowel by aspiration may be positive in low-level infections and should be done endoscopically to permit biopsy of suspicious duodenal and jejunal lesions in patients with findings that suggest strongyloidiasis (eg, eosinophilia).

In hyperinfection syndrome, filariform larvae may be found in stool, duodenal contents, sputum, and bronchial washings and, uncommonly, in CSF, urine, or pleural or ascitic fluid. Chest x-rays may show diffuse interstitial infiltrates, consolidation, or abscess.

Several immunodiagnostic tests are available for strongyloidiasis. EIA is recommended because of its greater sensitivity (> 90%). IgG antibodies can usually be detected even in immunocompromised patients with disseminated strongyloidiasis, but the absence of detectable antibodies does not exclude infection. Cross-reactions in patients with filariasis or other nematode infections may result in false-positive tests. Antibody test results cannot be used to differentiate current from past infection. A positive test warrants continuing efforts to establish a parasitologic diagnosis.

Serologic monitoring may be useful in follow-up because antibody levels decrease within 6 mo of successful chemotherapy.

PCR-based methods for the diagnosis of *S. stercoralis* are being developed.

Eosinophilia is often present but can be suppressed by drugs such as corticosteroids or cytotoxic chemotherapeutic drugs.

Treatment

- Ivermectin
- Alternatively, albendazole

All patients with strongyloidiasis should be treated. The cure rate is higher with ivermectin than albendazole.[1]

Ivermectin 200 mcg/kg po once/day for 2 days is used for uncomplicated infection and is generally well-tolerated. Before treatment with ivermectin, patients should be assessed for coinfection with *Loa loa* if they have traveled to areas of central Africa where *Loa loa* is endemic. Ivermectin can cause severe reactions in patients with loiasis. Albendazole 400 mg po bid for 7 days is an alternative.

In immunocompromised patients, prolonged therapy or repeated courses may be needed. In severely ill patients who are unable to take oral drugs, rectal preparations of ivermectin or sometimes the veterinary subcutaneous formulation of ivermectin has been used.

PEARLS & PITFALLS

- Before treating uncomplicated strongyloidiasis with ivermectin, assess patients for coinfection with *Loa loa*.

Hyperinfection syndrome in patients with strongyloidiasis is a life-threatening medical emergency. Ivermectin 200 mcg/kg po once/day is continued until sputum and stool examinations for rhabditiform and filariform larvae are negative for 2 wk. Broad-spectrum antibiotics are used to treat concurrent polymicrobial bacterial infections associated with larval invasion from the bowel.

After treatment of strongyloidiasis, cure should be documented by repeated stool examinations 2 to 4 wk later. If the stool remains positive, retreatment is indicated.

1. Henriquez-Camacho C, Gotuzzo E, Echevarria J, et al: Ivermectin versus albendazole or thiabendazole for *Strongyloides stercoralis* infection. *Cochrane Database Syst Rev* 18(1):CD007745, 2016. doi: 10.1002/14651858.CD007745.pub3.

Prevention

Prevention of primary *Strongyloides* infections is the same as for hookworms. It involves

- Preventing unhygienic defecation (eg, by using latrines or toilets)
- Avoiding direct skin contact with the soil (eg, by wearing shoes and using barriers when seated on the ground)

Prevention of hyperinfection syndrome: If patients are about to begin treatment with corticosteroids or other immunosuppressants, are infected with HTLV-1, or have impaired cell-mediated immunity for other reasons, they may be tested for *Strongyloides* infection. Several stool examinations and serologic testing should be done if patients have any of the following:

- Possible exposure to *Strongyloides* (history of travel to or residence in endemic areas, recently or even in the distant past)
- Unexplained eosinophilia
- Symptoms that suggest strongyloidiasis

Potential organ transplant recipients and donors from endemic regions should also be tested.

Such testing can help prevent potentially fatal hyperinfection syndrome.

If patients have strongyloidiasis, treatment should be instituted and parasitologic cure should be documented before immunosuppression. Immunosuppressed people who have recurrent strongyloidiasis require additional courses of treatment until cured.

KEY POINTS

- *Strongyloides* larvae penetrate human skin when people walk barefoot on infested soil.
- Larvae travel through the bloodstream to the lungs, penetrate the alveoli, ascend the respiratory tract, are swallowed, and

then mature in the intestines; adult worms produce ova that hatch in the intestines, releasing larvae; they can develop into infective filariform larvae, which may cause external or internal autoinfection, perpetuating the cycle.
- Patients who are coinfected with HTLV-1, who are taking corticosteroids, or who have impaired cell-mediated immunity for other reasons may develop potentially fatal hyperinfection syndrome—disseminated disease involving the lungs, intestines, skin, and other organs that are not part of the parasite's normal life cycle (eg, CNS, liver, heart).
- Symptoms include rash, pulmonary symptoms (including cough and wheezing), and abdominal pain with diarrhea.
- Diagnose by microscopic examination of multiple stool samples, the agar plate method, or duodenal aspirate; larvae may be identified in sputum in patients with hyperinfection.
- Treat uncomplicated infections with ivermectin for 2 days; albendazole for 7 days is an alternative.
- Hyperinfection syndrome requires prolonged ivermectin treatment.
- For all *Strongyloides* infections, document cure by repeated stool examinations.

TOXOCARIASIS

(Visceral or Ocular Larva Migrans)

Toxocariasis is human infection with nematode ascarid larvae that ordinarily infect animals. Symptoms are fever, anorexia, hepatosplenomegaly, rash, pneumonitis, asthma, or visual impairment. Diagnosis is by enzyme immunoassay (EIA). Treatment is with albendazole or mebendazole. Corticosteroids may be added for severe symptoms or eye involvement.

Pathophysiology

The eggs of *Toxocara canis, T. cati*, and other animal ascarid helminths mature in soil and infect dogs, cats, and other animals. Humans may accidentally ingest eggs in soil contaminated by stool from infected animals or may ingest undercooked infected transfer hosts (eg, rabbits). The eggs hatch in the human intestine. Larvae penetrate the bowel wall and may migrate through the liver, lungs, CNS, eyes, or other tissues. Tissue damage is caused by focal eosinophilic granulomatous reactions to the migrating larvae.

The larvae usually do not complete their development in the human body but can remain alive for many months.

Symptoms and Signs

Visceral larva migrans (VLM): VLM consists of fever, anorexia, hepatosplenomegaly, rash, pneumonitis, and asthmatic symptoms, depending on the affected organs. Larvae of other helminths including *Baylisascaris procyonis*, *Strongyloides* spp, and *Paragonimus* spp can cause similar symptoms and signs when they migrate through tissue.

VLM occurs mostly in 2- to 5-yr-old children with a history of geophagia or in adults who ingest clay.

The syndrome is self-limiting in 6 to 18 mo if egg intake ceases. Deaths due to invasion of the brain or heart occur rarely.

Ocular larva migrans (OLM): OLM, also called ocular toxocariasis, is usually unilateral and has no or very mild systemic manifestations. OLM lesions consist mostly of granulomatous inflammatory reactions to a larva, resulting in uveitis and/or chorioretinitis. As a result, vision can be impaired or lost.

OLM occurs in older children and less commonly in young adults. The lesion may be confused with retinoblastoma or other intraocular tumors.

Diagnosis

- EIA plus clinical findings

Diagnosis of toxocariasis is based on clinical, epidemiologic, and serologic findings.

EIA for *Toxocara* antigens is recommended to confirm the diagnosis. However, serum antibody titers may be low or undetectable in patients with OLM. Isoagglutinins may be elevated, but the finding is nonspecific. CT or MRI can show multiple, ill-defined, 1.0- to 1.5-cm oval lesions scattered in the liver or poorly defined subpleural nodules in the chest.

Hyperglobulinemia, leukocytosis, and marked eosinophilia are common in VLM.

Biopsies of the liver or other affected organs may show eosinophilic granulomatous reactions, but larvae are difficult to find in tissue sections and biopsies are low yield. Stool examinations are worthless.

OLM should be distinguished from retinoblastoma to prevent unnecessary surgical enucleation of the eye.

Treatment

- Albendazole or mebendazole
- Symptomatic treatment

Asymptomatic patients and patients with mild symptoms do not require anthelmintic therapy because infection is usually self-limited.

For patients with moderate to severe symptoms, albendazole 400 mg po bid for 5 days or mebendazole 100 to 200 mg po bid for 5 days is used, but the optimal duration of therapy has not been determined.

Antihistamines may suffice for mild symptoms. Corticosteroids (prednisone 20 to 40 mg po once/day) are indicated for patients with severe symptoms. Corticosteroids, both local and oral, are also indicated for acute OLM to reduce inflammation within the eye.

Laser photocoagulation has been used to kill larvae in the retina.

Prevention

Infection with *T. canis* in puppies is common in the US; infection with *T. cati* in cats is less common. Both animals should be dewormed regularly. Contact with dirt or sand contaminated with animal feces should be minimized. Sandboxes should be covered.

KEY POINTS

- The *Toxocara canis* life cycle normally involves dogs; humans are infected only accidentally, when they ingest eggs in soil contaminated by stool from infected animals or ingest undercooked infected transfer hosts (eg, rabbits).
- In humans, toxocariasis causes 2 main syndromes: VLM (which causes various symptoms depending on the organ infected) and OLM (which usually causes no or mild symptoms but can result in impaired or lost vision).
- Diagnose based on clinical evaluation and EIA for *Toxocara* antigens.
- Most cases of toxocariasis are self-limited and do not require treatment, but if needed, the following can be used: albendazole or mebendazole for moderate to severe symptoms, possibly antihistamines for mild symptoms, and corticosteroids for severe symptoms.
- Deworming dogs and cats can help prevent toxocariasis.

TRICHINOSIS

(Trichiniasis)

Trichinosis is infection with *Trichinella spiralis* or related *Trichinella* species. Symptoms include initial GI irritation followed by periorbital edema, muscle pain, fever, and eosinophilia. Diagnosis is clinical and with serologic tests. Muscle biopsy may be diagnostic but is seldom necessary. Treatment is with mebendazole or albendazole and, if symptoms are severe, with prednisone.

Trichinosis occurs worldwide. In addition to the classic agent *Trichinella spiralis*, trichinosis can be caused by *T. pseudospiralis, T. nativa, T. nelsoni*, and *T. britovi* in different geographic locations.

Pathophysiology

The *Trichinella* life cycle is maintained by animals that are fed (eg, pigs, horses) or eat (eg, bears, foxes, boars) other animals whose striated muscles contain encysted infective larvae (eg, rodents). Humans become infected by eating raw, undercooked, or underprocessed meat from infected animals, most commonly pigs, wild boar, or bear. Larvae excyst in the small bowel, penetrate the mucosa, and become adults in 6 to 8 days. Females are about 2.2 mm long, and males are about 1.2 mm long.

Mature females release living larvae for 4 to 6 wk and then die or are expelled. Newborn larvae migrate through the bloodstream and lymphatics but ultimately survive only within striated skeletal muscle cells. Larvae fully encyst in 1 to 2 mo and remain viable for several years as intracellular parasites. Dead larvae eventually are resorbed or calcify. The cycle continues only if encysted larvae are ingested by another carnivore.

Symptoms and Signs

Many *Trichinella* infections are asymptomatic or mild.

During the 1st wk, nausea, abdominal cramps, and diarrhea may occur.

One to 2 wk after infection, systemic symptoms and signs begin: facial or periorbital edema, myalgia, persistent fever, headache, and subconjunctival hemorrhages and petechiae. Eye pain and photophobia often precede myalgia.

Symptoms due to muscle invasion may mimic polymyositis. The muscles of respiration, speech, mastication, and swallowing may be painful. Severe dyspnea may occur in heavy infections.

Fever is generally remittent, rising to 39° C or higher, remaining elevated for several days, and then falling gradually. Eosinophilia usually begins when newborn larvae invade tissues, peaks 2 to 4 wk after infection, and gradually declines as the larvae encyst.

In heavy infections, the inflammation may cause complications: cardiac (myocarditis, heart failure, arrhythmia), neurologic (encephalitis, meningitis, visual or auditory disorders, seizures), or pulmonary (pneumonitis, pleurisy). Death may result from myocarditis or encephalitis.

Symptoms and signs gradually resolve, and most disappear by about the 3rd mo, when the larvae have become fully encysted in muscle cells and eliminated from other organs and tissues. Vague muscular pains and fatigue may persist for months.

Recurrent infections with *T. nativa* in northern latitudes can cause chronic diarrhea.

Diagnosis

- Enzyme immunoassay (EIA)
- Rarely muscle biopsy

No specific tests to diagnose the intestinal stage are available. After the 2nd wk of infection, a muscle biopsy may detect larvae and cysts but is seldom necessary. Diffuse inflammation in muscle tissue indicates recent infection.

A number of serologic tests have been used, but EIA using *T. spiralis* excretory-secretory (ES) antigen seems to be the quickest way to detect the infection and is used in the US. Antibodies are often not detectable for the first 3 to 5 wk of infection, so tests should be repeated at weekly intervals if results are initially negative. Because antibodies may persist for years, serologic tests are of most value if they are initially negative and then positive. Serologic tests and muscle biopsy are complementary tests; either one can be negative in a given patient with trichinosis. Skin testing with larval antigens is unreliable.

Muscle enzymes (creatine kinase and LDH) are elevated in 50% of patients and correlate with abnormal electromyograms.

Trichinosis must be differentiated from

- Acute rheumatic fever, acute arthritis, angioedema, and myositis
- Febrile illnesses such as TB, typhoid fever, sepsis, and undulant fever
- Pneumonitis
- Neurologic manifestations of meningitis, encephalitis, and poliomyelitis
- Eosinophilia due to Hodgkin lymphoma, eosinophilic leukemia, polyarteritis nodosa, or disease caused by other migrating nematodes

Treatment

- Symptomatic treatment
- Albendazole or mebendazole to eliminate adult worms

Anthelmintics eliminate adult worms from the GI tract but probably have little effect on encysted larvae.

Albendazole 400 mg po bid for 8 to 14 days or mebendazole 200 to 400 mg po tid for 3 days, followed by 400 to 500 mg tid for 10 days can be used.

Analgesics may help relieve muscle pains. For severe allergic manifestations or myocardial or CNS involvement, prednisone 20 to 60 mg po once/day is given for 3 or 4 days, then tapered over 10 to 14 days.

Prevention

Trichinosis is prevented by cooking pork or meat from wild animals until brown (> 71° C [> 160° F] throughout). Larvae can be killed in pork < 6 inches thick by freezing the pork at -15° C (-5° F) for 20 days. Freezing is not recommended for meat from wild animals because they may be infected with *Trichinella* spp that are resistant to low temperatures.

Smoking, microwave cooking, or salting meat does not reliably kill larvae.

Meat grinders and other items used to prepare raw meat should be thoroughly cleaned. Handwashing with soap and water is also important.

Domestic swine should not be fed uncooked meat.

KEY POINTS

- Humans become infected with *Trichinella* by eating raw, undercooked, or underprocessed meat from infected animals—most commonly pigs, wild boar, or bear.
- Larvae excyst in the small bowel, penetrate the mucosa, and become adults that release living larvae; the larvae migrate through the bloodstream and lymphatics and encyst within striated skeletal muscle cells.

- Symptoms begin with GI irritation followed by periorbital edema, muscle pain, fever, and eosinophilia.
- Manifestations gradually resolve by about the 3rd mo, when the larvae have become fully encysted, although vague muscular pains and fatigue may persist for months.
- Diagnose using EIA.
- Treat symptoms (eg, with analgesics for pain and prednisone for allergic manifestations or CNS or myocardial involvement); anthelmintics kill adult worms but have little effect on encysted larvae.
- Thoroughly cooking meat from pigs and wild animals can prevent trichinosis.

TRICHURIASIS

(Trichocephaliasis; Whipworm Infection)

Trichuriasis is infection with *Trichuris trichiura*. Symptoms may include abdominal pain, diarrhea, and, in heavy infections, anemia and undernutrition. Diagnosis is by finding eggs in stool. Treatment is with mebendazole, albendazole, or ivermectin.

Trichuriasis is the 3rd most common roundworm infection. An estimated 604 to 795 million people are infected worldwide. *Trichuris trichiura* occurs principally in developing tropical or subtropical areas where human feces is used as fertilizer or where people defecate onto soil, but infections also occur in the southern US. Children are most affected.

Infection is spread via the fecal-oral route. Ingested eggs hatch and enter the crypts of the small bowel as larvae. After maturing for 1 to 3 mo, the worms migrate to the cecum and ascending colon, where they attach to the superficial epithelium, mate, and lay eggs.

Adult worms are estimated to live 1 to 2 yr, although some may live longer.

Symptoms and Signs

Light *Trichuris* infections are often asymptomatic.

Patients with heavy infections may have abdominal pain, anorexia, and diarrhea; weight loss, anemia, and rectal prolapse may result, particularly in children.

Diagnosis

- Microscopic examination of stool

Diagnosis of trichuriasis is made by microscopic examination of stool; the characteristic lemon-shaped eggs with clear opercula at both ends are readily apparent. When anoscopy, proctoscopy, or colonoscopy is done for other indications, wiggling adult worms may be seen protruding into the bowel lumen.

CBC is done to check for anemia.

Treatment

- Mebendazole, albendazole, or ivermectin

Mebendazole 100 mg po bid for 3 days is recommended. A single dose of mebendazole 500 mg has been used in mass treatment programs. Alternatives are albendazole 400 mg po once/day for 3 days or ivermectin 200 mcg/kg po once/day for 3 days. These drugs should usually not be used during pregnancy.

If treatment with ivermectin is planned, patients should be assessed for coinfection with *Loa loa* if they have been in areas of central Africa where it is transmitted; ivermectin can induce severe reactions in patients with *Loa loa* infection.

Prevention of trichinosis is possible through good sanitation, handwashing, and good personal hygiene.

KEY POINTS

- Trichuriasis occurs principally in developing tropical or subtropical areas where human feces is used as fertilizer or where people defecate onto soil, but infections also occur in the southern US, mainly in children.
- Infection is spread via the fecal-oral route.
- Light infections are often asymptomatic; heavy infections may cause abdominal pain, anorexia, diarrhea, and, in children, weight loss, anemia, and rectal prolapse.
- To diagnose trichuriasis, examine a stool sample for the characteristic lemon-shaped eggs with clear opercula at both ends.
- Treat with mebendazole (recommended); albendazole and ivermectin are alternatives.
- If treatment with ivermectin is planned, assess patients for coinfection with *Loa loa* if they have been in areas of central Africa where it is transmitted; ivermectin can induce severe reactions in patients with *Loa loa* infections.

199 Pox Viruses

MONKEYPOX

Monkeypox virus is structurally related to the smallpox virus and causes similar, but usually milder illness.

Monkeypox, like smallpox, is a member of the Orthopoxvirus group. Although the reservoir is unknown, the leading candidates are small rodents and squirrels in the rain forests of Africa, mostly in western and central Africa. Human disease occurs in Africa sporadically and in occasional epidemics. Most reported cases have been in the Democratic Republic of the Congo; a recent 20-fold increase in incidence is thought to be due to the cessation of smallpox vaccination in 1980.

In the US, an outbreak of monkeypox occurred in 2003, when infected rodents imported as pets from Africa spread the virus to pet prairie dogs, which then infected people in the Midwest. The outbreak involved 35 confirmed, 13 probable, and 22 suspected cases in 6 states, but there were no deaths.

Monkeypox is probably transmitted from animals via wounds or mucous membranes. Person-to-person transmission occurs inefficiently, with an attack rate of 8 to 9%. Most patients are children. People who have received smallpox vaccine are at reduced risk. In Africa, mortality rate ranges from 4 to 22%.

Clinically, monkeypox is similar to smallpox; however, skin lesions occur more often in crops, and lymphadenopathy is more common. Secondary bacterial infection of the skin and lungs may occur.

Clinical differentiation of monkeypox from smallpox and chickenpox (a herpesvirus, not a pox virus—see Chickenpox on p. 1617) may be impossible. Diagnosis is by culture,

PCR, immunohistochemistry, or electron microscopy, depending on which tests are available.

Treatment is supportive. Potentially useful drugs include the antiviral drug cidofovir and the investigational drugs brincidofovir (CMX001) and tecovirimat (ST-246); all have activity against monkeypox in vitro and in experimental models. However, none of these drugs has been studied or used in endemic areas to treat monkeypox.

Cases are reported to public health authorities.

SMALLPOX

(Variola)

Smallpox is a highly contagious disease caused by the smallpox virus, an orthopoxvirus. It causes death in up to 30%. Indigenous infection has been eradicated. The main concern for outbreaks is from bioterrorism. Severe constitutional symptoms and a characteristic pustular rash develop. Treatment is supportive. Prevention involves vaccination, which, because of its risks, is done selectively.

No cases of smallpox have occurred in the world since 1977 because of worldwide vaccination. In 1980, the World Health Organization (WHO) recommended discontinuation of routine smallpox vaccination. Routine vaccination in the US ended in 1972. Because humans are the only natural host of the smallpox virus and because the virus cannot survive > 2 days in the environment, WHO has declared natural infection eradicated. Concerns about bioterrorism using smallpox virus from retained research stores or even from synthetically created virus raise the possibility of a recurrence (see p. 3045 and CDC: Smallpox: Emergency Preparedness and Response at www.cdc.gov).

Pathophysiology

There are at least 2 strains of smallpox virus:

- Variola major (classic smallpox), the more virulent strain
- Variola minor (alastrim), the less virulent strain

Smallpox is transmitted from person to person by inhalation or, less efficiently, by direct contact. Contaminated clothing or bed linens can also transmit infection. The infection is most communicable for the first 7 to 10 days after the rash appears. Once crusts form on the skin lesions, infectivity declines.

The attack rate is as high as 85% in unvaccinated people, and infection may lead to as many as 4 to 10 secondary cases from each primary case. However, infection tends to spread slowly and mainly among close contacts.

The virus invades the oropharyngeal or respiratory mucosa and multiplies in regional lymph nodes, causing subsequent viremia. It eventually localizes in small blood vessels of the dermis and the oropharyngeal mucosa. Other organs are seldom clinically involved, except for occasionally the CNS, with encephalitis. Secondary bacterial infection of the skin, lungs, and bones may develop.

Symptoms and Signs

Variola major has a 10- to 12-day incubation period (range 7 to 17 days), followed by a 2- to 3-day prodrome of fever, headache, backache, and extreme malaise. Sometimes severe abdominal pain and vomiting occur. After the prodrome, maculopapular lesions develop on the oropharyngeal mucosa, face, and arms, spreading shortly thereafter to the trunk and legs. The oropharyngeal lesions quickly ulcerate. After 1 or 2 days, the cutaneous lesions become vesicular, then pustular. Pustules are denser on the face and extremities than on the trunk, and they may appear on the palms. The pustules are round and tense and appear deeply embedded. Skin lesions of smallpox, unlike those of chickenpox, are all at the same stage of development on a given body part. After 8 or 9 days, the pustules become crusted. Severe residual scarring is typical. Mortality rate is about 30%. Death results from a massive inflammatory response causing shock and multiple organ failure and usually occurs during the 2nd wk of illness.

About 5 to 10% of people with variola major develop either a hemorrhagic or a malignant (flat) variant. The hemorrhagic form is rarer and has a shorter, more intense prodrome, followed by generalized erythema and cutaneous and mucosal hemorrhage. It is uniformly fatal within 5 or 6 days. The malignant form has a similar, severe prodrome, followed by development of confluent, flat, nonpustular skin lesions. In survivors, the epidermis frequently desquamates.

Variola minor results in symptoms that are similar but much less severe, with a less extensive rash. Mortality rate is < 1%.

Diagnosis

- PCR
- Electron microscopy

Unless laboratory exposure is documented or an outbreak (due to bioterrorism) is suspected, only patients that fit the clinical case definition for smallpox should be tested because of the risk that test results may be falsely positive. An algorithm for evaluating the risk of smallpox in patients with fever and rash is available on the CDC web site at www.cdc.gov (CDC Algorithm Poster for Evaluation of Suspected Smallpox), as is a worksheet that can be printed and sent to the CDC to aid in evaluation.

Diagnosis is confirmed by documenting the presence of variola DNA by PCR of vesicular or pustular samples. Or the virus can be identified by electron microscopy or viral culture of material scraped from skin lesions and subsequently confirmed by PCR. Suspected smallpox must be reported immediately to local public health agencies or the CDC at 770-488-7100. These agencies then arrange for testing in a laboratory with high-level containment capability (biosafety level 4).

Treatment

- Supportive care
- Isolation
- Possibly cidofovir, brincidofovir (CMX 001), or tecovirimat (ST-246)

Treatment is generally supportive, with antibiotics for secondary bacterial infections. The antiviral drug cidofovir may be considered. Brincidofovir (CMX001), and tecovirimat (ST-246) are investigational drugs but have been used to treat severe vaccine-related complications (vaccinia) and may also be useful for treatment. Currently, there is no licensed drug for the treatment of smallpox.

Isolation of people with smallpox is essential. In limited outbreaks, patients may be isolated in a hospital in a negative-pressure room equipped with high-efficiency particulate (HEPA) filters. In mass outbreaks, home isolation may be required. Contacts should be placed under surveillance, typically with daily temperature measurement; if they develop a temperature of > 38° C or other sign of illness, they should be isolated at home.

Prevention

Licensed smallpox vaccine in the US consists of live vaccinia virus (ACAM2000), which is related to smallpox and provides cross-immunity. Vaccine is administered with a bifurcated needle dipped in reconstituted vaccine. The needle is rapidly jabbed 15 times in an area about 5 mm in diameter and with sufficient force to draw a trace of blood. The vaccine site is covered with a dressing to prevent spread of the vaccine virus to other body sites or to close contacts. Fever, malaise, and myalgias are common the week after vaccination. Successful vaccination is indicated by development of a pustule by about the 7th day. Revaccination may cause only a papule surrounded by erythema, which peaks between 3 and 7 days. People without such signs of successful vaccination should be given another dose of vaccine. Two live-attenuated vaccines (modified vaccinia Ankara [MVA] and LC16m8) have been developed; MVA is licensed in Europe, and LC16m8 is licensed in Japan.

After a single vaccination, immunity begins to fade after 5 yr and is probably negligible after 20 yr. If people have been successfully revaccinated one or more times, some residual immunity may persist for ≥ 30 yr.

Until an outbreak in the population occurs, preexposure vaccination remains recommended only for people at high risk of exposure to the virus (eg, laboratory technicians).

Vaccine complications: Risk factors for complications include extensive skin disorders (particularly eczema), immunosuppressive diseases or therapies, ocular inflammation, and pregnancy. Widespread vaccination is not recommended because of the risk.

Serious complications occur in about 1 of 10,000 patients after their first (primary) vaccination and include

- Postvaccinial encephalitis
- Progressive vaccinia
- Eczema vaccinatum
- Generalized vaccinia
- Myocarditis and/or pericarditis
- Vaccinia virus keratitis
- Noninfectious rashes

Postvaccinial encephalitis occurs in about 1 of 300,000 recipients of primary vaccination, typically 8 to 15 days postvaccination.

Progressive vaccinia (vaccinia necrosum) results in a nonhealing vaccinial (vesicular) skin lesion that spreads to adjacent skin and ultimately other skin areas, bones, and viscera. Progressive vaccinia may occur after primary vaccination or revaccination but occurs almost exclusively in patients with an underlying defect in cell-mediated immunity; it can be fatal.

Eczema vaccinatum results in vaccinial skin lesions appearing on areas of active or even healed eczema.

Generalized vaccinia results from hematogenous dissemination of the vaccinia virus and causes vaccinia lesions at multiple body locations; it is usually benign.

Vaccinia virus keratitis occurs rarely, when vaccinia virus is inadvertently implanted in the eye.

Some serious vaccine complications are treated with vaccinia immune globulin (VIG); one case of eczema vaccinatum apparently treated successfully with VIG, cidofovir, and tecovirimat has been reported. In the past, high-risk patients who required vaccination because of viral exposure were simultaneously given VIG to try to prevent complications. The efficacy of this practice is unknown, and it is not recommended by the CDC. VIG is available only from the CDC.

Postexposure prophylaxis: Postexposure vaccination can prevent or significantly limit the severity of illness and is indicated for family members and close personal contacts of smallpox patients. Early administration is most effective, but some benefit is realized up to 4 days postexposure.

KEY POINTS

- No cases of smallpox have occurred since 1977, but concerns about possible use for bioterrorism remain.
- Diagnosis is made by PCR.
- Treatment is mainly supportive, but cidofovir may be considered; brincidofovir (CMX001) and tecovirimat (ST-246) are investigational drugs but may also be useful.
- Vaccination is highly protective, but rare complications (about 1:10,000) can be serious.
- Immunity fades over decades.

200 Respiratory Viruses

Viral infections commonly affect the upper or lower respiratory tract. Although these infections can be classified by the causative virus (eg, influenza), they are generally classified clinically according to syndrome (eg, the common cold, bronchiolitis, croup). Although specific pathogens commonly cause characteristic clinical manifestations (eg, rhinovirus typically causes the common cold, respiratory syncytial virus [RSV] typically causes bronchiolitis), each can cause many of the viral respiratory syndromes (see Table 200–1).

Severity of viral respiratory illness varies widely; severe disease is more likely in the elderly and infants. Morbidity may result directly from viral infection or may be indirect, due to exacerbation of underlying cardiopulmonary conditions or bacterial superinfection of the lung, paranasal sinuses, or middle ear.

Diagnosis

Detection of viral pathogens by PCR, cell culture, or serologic tests is generally too slow to be useful for patient care but is useful for epidemiologic surveillance (ie, identifying and determining the cause of an outbreak). More rapid diagnostic tests are available for influenza and RSV, but the utility of these tests for routine care is not clear; they should be reserved for situations in which pathogen-specific diagnosis affects clinical management. Management decisions are usually based on clinical data and epidemiology.

Treatment

Treatment of viral respiratory infections is usually supportive. Antibacterial drugs are ineffective against viral pathogens, and prophylaxis against secondary bacterial infections is not recommended. Antibiotics should be given only when secondary bacterial infections develop. In patients with chronic lung disease, antibiotics may be given with less restriction.

Aspirin should not be used in patients who are ≤ 18 yr and have respiratory infections because Reye syndrome is a risk.

Some patients continue to cough for weeks after resolution of an URI; these symptoms may lessen with use of an inhaled bronchodilator or corticosteroids.

Table 200–1. CAUSES OF COMMON VIRAL RESPIRATORY SYNDROMES

SYNDROME	COMMON CAUSES	LESS COMMON CAUSES
Bronchiolitis	RSV	Influenza viruses Parainfluenza viruses Adenoviruses Rhinoviruses
Common cold	Rhinoviruses Coronaviruses	Influenza viruses Parainfluenza viruses Enteroviruses Adenoviruses Human metapneumoviruses RSV
Croup	Parainfluenza viruses	Influenza viruses RSV
Influenza-like illness	Influenza viruses	Parainfluenza viruses Adenoviruses
Pneumonia	Influenza viruses RSV Adenoviruses	Parainfluenza viruses Enteroviruses Rhinoviruses Human metapneumoviruses Coronaviruses

RSV = respiratory syncytial virus.

In some cases, antiviral drugs are useful. Amantadine, rimantadine, oseltamivir, and zanamivir are effective for influenza. Ribavirin, a guanosine analog that inhibits replication of many RNA and DNA viruses, may be considered for severely immunocompromised patients with lower respiratory tract infection due to RSV. Palivizumab, a monoclonal antibody to RSV fusion protein, is being used to prevent RSV infection in certain high-risk infants.

ADENOVIRUS INFECTIONS

Infection with one of the many adenoviruses may be asymptomatic or result in specific syndromes, including mild respiratory infections, keratoconjunctivitis, gastroenteritis, cystitis, and primary pneumonia. Diagnosis is clinical. Treatment is supportive.

Adenoviruses are DNA viruses classified according to 3 major capsid antigens (hexon, penton, and fiber). Adenoviruses are commonly acquired by contact with secretions (including those on fingers of infected people) from an infected person or by contact with a contaminated object (eg, towel, instrument). Infection may be airborne or waterborne (eg, acquired while swimming). Asymptomatic respiratory or GI viral shedding may continue for months, or even years.

Symptoms and Signs

In immunocompetent hosts, most adenovirus infections are asymptomatic; when infections are symptomatic, a broad spectrum of clinical manifestations is possible. The most common syndrome, especially in children, involves fever that tends to be > 39° C and to last > 5 days. Sore throat, cough, rhinorrhea, or other respiratory symptoms may occur. A separate syndrome involves conjunctivitis, pharyngitis, and fever (pharyngoconjunctival fever). Rare adenoviral syndromes in infants include severe bronchiolitis (see p. 2825) and pneumonia. In closed populations of young adults (eg, military recruits), outbreaks of respiratory illness may occur; symptoms include fever and lower respiratory tract symptoms, usually tracheobronchitis but occasionally pneumonia.

Epidemic keratoconjunctivitis (see p. 941) is sometimes severe and occurs sporadically and in epidemics. Conjunctivitis is frequently bilateral. Preauricular adenopathy may develop. Chemosis, pain, and punctate corneal lesions that are visible with fluorescein staining may be present. Systemic symptoms and signs are mild or absent. Epidemic keratoconjunctivitis usually resolves within 3 to 4 wk, although corneal lesions may persist much longer.

Nonrespiratory adenoviral syndromes include hemorrhagic cystitis, diarrhea in infants, and meningoencephalitis.

Most patients recover fully. Even severe primary adenoviral pneumonia is not fatal except for rare fulminant cases, predominantly in infants, military recruits, and immunocompromised patients.

Diagnosis

- Clinical evaluation

Laboratory diagnosis of adenovirus infection rarely affects management. During the acute illness, virus can be isolated from respiratory and ocular secretions and frequently from stool and urine. A 4-fold rise in the serum antibody titer indicates recent adenoviral infection.

Treatment

- Symptomatic treatment

Treatment is symptomatic and supportive. Ribavirin and cidofovir have been used in immunocompromised patients; results varied.

To minimize transmission, heath care practitioners should change gloves and wash hands after examining infected patients, sterilize instruments adequately, and avoid using ophthalmologic instruments in multiple patients.

Prevention

Vaccines containing live adenovirus types 4 and 7, given orally in an enteric-coated capsule, can reduce lower respiratory disease. The vaccine was unavailable for a number of years but was reintroduced in 2011. However, it is available only for military personnel. It may be given to patients aged 17 through 50 yr and should not be given to women who are pregnant or breastfeeding.

COMMON COLD

(Coryza; Upper Respiratory Infection)

The common cold is an acute, usually afebrile, self-limited viral infection causing upper respiratory symptoms, such as rhinorrhea, cough, and sore throat. Diagnosis is clinical. Handwashing helps prevent its spread. Treatment is supportive.

About 50% of all colds are caused by one of the > 100 serotypes of rhinoviruses. Coronaviruses cause some outbreaks, and infections caused by influenza and parainfluenza viruses, enterovirus, adenovirus, respiratory syncytial viruses, and metapneumoviruses may also manifest as the common cold, particularly in patients who are experiencing reinfection.

Rhinovirus infections are most common during fall and spring and are less common during winter. Rhinoviruses are most efficiently spread by direct person-to-person contact, although spread may also occur via large-particle aerosols.

The most potent deterrent to infection is the presence of specific neutralizing antibodies in the serum and secretions, induced by previous exposure to the same or a closely related virus. Susceptibility to colds is not affected by exposure to cold temperature, host health and nutrition, or upper respiratory tract abnormalities (eg, enlarged tonsils or adenoids).

Symptoms and Signs

After an incubation period of 24 to 72 h, symptoms begin with a scratchy or sore throat, followed by sneezing, rhinorrhea, nasal obstruction, and malaise. Temperature is usually normal, particularly when the pathogen is a rhinovirus or coronavirus. Nasal secretions are watery and profuse during the first days but then become more mucoid and purulent. Mucopurulent secretions do not indicate a bacterial superinfection. Cough is usually mild but often lasts into the 2nd wk. Most symptoms due to uncomplicated colds resolve within 10 days. Colds may exacerbate asthma and chronic bronchitis.

Purulent sputum or significant lower respiratory tract symptoms are unusual with rhinovirus infection. Purulent sinusitis and otitis media may result from the viral infection itself or from secondary bacterial infection.

Diagnosis

- Clinical evaluation

Diagnosis is generally made clinically and presumptively, without diagnostic tests. Allergic rhinitis is the most important consideration in differential diagnosis.

Treatment

- Symptomatic treatment

No specific treatment exists. Antipyretics and analgesics may relieve fever and sore throat. Nasal decongestants may reduce nasal obstruction. Topical nasal decongestants are more effective than oral decongestants, but the use of topical drugs for > 3 to 5 days may result in rebound congestion. Rhinorrhea may be relieved with 1st-generation antihistamines (eg, chlorpheniramine) or intranasal ipratropium bromide (2 sprays of a 0.03% solution bid or tid); however, these drugs should be avoided in the elderly and people with benign prostatic hypertrophy or glaucoma. First-generation antihistamines frequently cause sedation, but 2nd-generation (nonsedating) antihistamines are ineffective for treating the common cold. Antihistamines and decongestants are not recommended for children < 4 yr.

Zinc, echinacea, and vitamin C have all been evaluated as common cold therapies, but none has been clearly shown to be beneficial.

Prevention

There are no vaccines. Polyvalent bacterial vaccines, citrus fruits, vitamins, ultraviolet light, glycol aerosols, and other folk remedies do not prevent the common cold. Handwashing and use of surface disinfectant in a contaminated environment may reduce spread of infection.

Antibiotics should not be given unless there is clear evidence of secondary bacterial infection. In patients with chronic lung disease, antibiotics may be given with less restriction.

INFLUENZA

(Flu; Grip; Grippe)

Influenza is a viral respiratory infection causing fever, coryza, cough, headache, and malaise. Mortality is possible during seasonal epidemics, particularly among high-risk patients (eg, those who are institutionalized, at the extremes of age, have cardiopulmonary insufficiency, or are in late pregnancy); during pandemics, even healthy, young patients may die. Diagnosis is usually clinical and depends on local epidemiologic patterns. Everyone aged ≥ 6 mo should receive annual influenza vaccination. Antiviral treatment reduces the duration of illness by about 1 day and should be specifically considered for high-risk patients.

Influenza refers to illness caused by the influenza viruses, but the term is commonly and incorrectly used to refer to similar illnesses caused by other viral respiratory pathogens. Influenza viruses are classified as type A, B, or C by their nucleoproteins and matrix proteins. Influenza C virus infection does not cause typical influenza illness and is not discussed here.

Influenza antigens: Hemagglutinin (H) is a glycoprotein on the influenza viral surface that allows the virus to bind to cellular sialic acid and fuse with the host cell membrane. Neuraminidase (NA), another surface glycoprotein, enzymatically removes sialic acid, promoting viral release from the infected host cell. There are 18 H types and 11 NA types, giving 198 possible combinations, but only a few are human pathogens.

Antigenic drift refers to relatively minor, progressive mutations in preexisting combinations of H and NA antigens, resulting in the frequent emergence of new viral strains. These new strains may cause seasonal epidemics because protection by antibody generated to the previous strain is decreased.

Antigenic shift refers to the relatively rare development of new combinations of H and/or NA antigens, which result from reassortment of subunits of the viral genome. Pandemics can result from antigenic shift because antibodies against other strains (resulting from vaccination or native infection) provide little or no protection against the new strain.

Epidemiology

Influenza causes widespread sporadic illness yearly during fall and winter in temperate climates (seasonal epidemics). Seasonal epidemics are caused by both influenza A and B viruses and often occur in 2 waves—the first in schoolchildren and their household contacts (generally younger people) and the 2nd mostly in housebound or institutionalized people, particularly the elderly. Influenza B viruses may cause milder disease but often cause epidemics with moderate or severe disease, usually in 3- to 5-yr cycles. Most influenza epidemics are caused by a predominant serotype, but different influenza viruses may appear sequentially in one location or may appear simultaneously, with one virus predominating in one location and another virus predominating elsewhere.

Pandemics are much less common. As of 2013, there have been 6 major pandemics, typically named after the presumed location of origin:

- 1889: Russian influenza (H2N2)
- 1900: Old Hong Kong influenza (H3N8)
- 1918: Spanish influenza (H1N1)
- 1957: Asian influenza (H2N2)
- 1968: Hong Kong influenza (H3N2)
- 2009: Swine influenza (influenza A [H1N1]pdm09)

Influenza viruses can be spread by airborne droplets, person-to-person contact, or contact with contaminated items. Airborne spread appears to be the most important mechanism.

At-risk groups: Certain patients are at high risk of complications from influenza:

- Children < 4 yr
- Adults > 65 yr
- People with chronic medical disorders (eg, cardiopulmonary disease, diabetes mellitus, renal or hepatic insufficiency, hemoglobinopathies, immuodeficiency)
- Women in the 2nd or 3rd trimester of pregnancy
- Patients with disorders that impair handling of respiratory secretions (eg, cognitive dysfunction, neuromuscular disorders, stroke, seizure disorders)
- Patients ≤ 18 yr taking aspirin (because Reye syndrome is a risk)

Morbidity and mortality in these patients may be due to exacerbation of underlying illness, acute respiratory distress syndrome, primary influenza pneumonia, or secondary bacterial pneumonia.

Symptoms and Signs

The incubation period ranges from 1 to 4 days with an average of about 48 h. In mild cases, many symptoms are like those of a common cold (eg, sore throat, rhinorrhea); mild conjunctivitis may also occur. Typical influenza in adults is characterized by sudden onset of chills, fever, prostration, cough, and generalized aches and pains (especially in the back and legs). Headache is prominent, often with photophobia and retrobulbar aching. Respiratory symptoms may be mild at first, with scratchy sore throat, substernal burning, nonproductive cough, and sometimes coryza. Later, lower respiratory tract illness becomes dominant; cough can be persistent, raspy, and productive. GI symptoms may occur and appear to be more common with the 2009 pandemic H1N1 strain. Children may have prominent nausea, vomiting, or abdominal pain, and infants may present with a sepsis-like syndrome.

After 2 to 3 days, acute symptoms rapidly subside, although fever may last up to 5 days. Cough, weakness, sweating, and fatigue may persist for several days or occasionally for weeks.

Complications: Pneumonia is suggested by a worsening cough, bloody sputum, dyspnea, and rales. Secondary bacterial pneumonia is suggested by persistence or recurrence of fever and cough after the primary illness appears to be resolving.

Encephalitis, myocarditis, and myoglobinuria, sometimes with renal failure, develop infrequently after influenza A or B infection. Reye syndrome (see p. 2756)—characterized by encephalopathy; fatty liver; elevation of liver enzymes, ammonia, or both; hypoglycemia; and lipidemia—often occurs during epidemics of influenza B, particularly in children who have ingested aspirin.

Diagnosis

- Clinical evaluation
- Sometimes rapid diagnostic testing
- Pulse oximetry and chest x-ray for patients with severe respiratory symptoms

The diagnosis is generally made clinically in patients with a typical syndrome when influenza is known to be present in the community. Although many rapid diagnostic tests are available and most have good specificity, their sensitivities vary widely, and they usually add little to patient management. Diagnostic tests should be done when results will affect clinical decisions. Reverse transcriptase–PCR (RT-PCR) assays are sensitive and specific and can differentiate influenza types and subtypes. If this assay is quickly available, results may be used to select appropriate antiviral therapy. These tests are also useful to determine whether outbreaks of respiratory disease are due to influenza. Cell culture of nasopharyngeal swabs or aspirates takes several days and is not useful for patient management decisions.

If patients have lower respiratory tract symptoms and signs (eg, dyspnea, rales noted during lung examination), pulse oximetry to detect hypoxemia and a chest x-ray to detect pneumonia should be done. Primary influenza pneumonia appears as focal or diffuse interstitial infiltrates or as acute respiratory distress syndrome. Secondary bacterial pneumonia is more likely to be lobar or segmental.

Prognosis

Most patients recover fully, although full recovery often takes 1 to 2 wk. However, influenza and influenza-related pneumonia are important causes of increased morbidity or mortality in high-risk patients. Use of antiviral treatment in these patients appears to reduce the incidence of lower respiratory disease and hospitalization. Appropriate antibacterial therapy decreases the mortality rate due to secondary bacterial pneumonia.

Treatment

- Symptomatic treatment
- Sometimes antiviral drugs

Treatment for most patients is symptomatic, including rest, hydration, and antipyretics as needed, but aspirin is avoided in patients ≤ 18 yr. Complicating bacterial infections require appropriate antibiotics.

Drugs for influenza: Antiviral drugs given within 1 to 2 days of symptom onset decrease the duration of fever, severity of symptoms, and time to return to normal activity. Treatment with antiviral drugs is recommended for high-risk patients who develop influenza-like symptoms; this recommendation is based on data suggesting that early treatment may prevent complications in these patients.

Drugs for influenza include the following:

- Oseltamivir and zanamivir (neuraminidase inhibitors)
- Amantadine and rimantadine (adamantanes)

Neuraminidase inhibitors interfere with release of influenza virus from infected cells and thus halt spread of infection.

Adamantanes block the M2 ion channel and thus interfere with viral uncoating inside the cell. They are effective only against influenza A viruses (influenza B viruses lack the M2 protein).

Choice of antiviral drug is complicated by resistance of different influenza types and subtypes to different drugs (see Table 200–2). If RT-PCR testing is rapidly available, results can be used to direct treatment. If RT-PCR is not available, patients may be treated with zanamivir alone or with rimantadine plus oseltamivir.

Zanamivir is given by an inhaler, 2 puffs (10 mg) bid; it can be used in adults and children ≥ 7 yr. Zanamivir sometimes causes bronchospasm and should not be given to patients with reactive airway disease; some people cannot use the inhalation device.

Oseltamivir 75 mg po bid is given to patients > 12 yr; lower doses may be used in children as young as 1 yr. Oseltamivir may cause occasional nausea and vomiting. In children, oseltamivir may decrease the incidence of otitis media; however, no other data clearly show that treatment of influenza prevents complications.

Rimantadine is the preferred adamantane because it has fewer side effects and is better tolerated. Treatment is stopped 1 to 2 days after symptoms resolve or after 3 to 5 days. For rimantadine or amantadine, 100 mg po bid can be used in adults ≤ 65, and 100 mg po once/day can be used in those > 65. To avoid adverse effects due to drug accumulation, clinicians reduce the dose for children (2.5 mg/kg bid to a maximum of 150 mg/day for children < 10 yr or 200 mg/day for children ≥ 10 yr). In patients with impaired renal function, dose is adjusted according to creatinine clearance. The dose of rimantadine should not exceed 100 mg/day if patients have hepatic dysfunction. Dose-related nervousness, insomnia, or other CNS effects occur in about 10% of people receiving amantadine and in about 2% of people receiving rimantadine. These effects usually occur within 48 h after starting the drug, are more prominent in the elderly and in patients with CNS diseases or impaired renal function, and often resolve during continued use. Anorexia, nausea, and constipation may also occur.

Prevention

Influenza infections can largely be prevented by

- Annual vaccination
- Sometimes chemoprophylaxis (ie, with antiviral drugs)

Current commercially available vaccines protect only against seasonal influenza. A vaccine for H5N1 avian influenza has been approved for people > 18 yr at high risk of H5N1 exposure but is available only through public health officials. No vaccines are currently available for the other avian influenza viruses rarely associated with human disease (H7N7, H9N2, H7N3, and H7N9).

Prevention is indicated for all patients but is especially important for high-risk patients and health care practitioners.

Vaccines: Based on recommendations by the WHO and US Centers for Disease Control and Prevention (CDC), vaccines are modified annually to include the most prevalent strains (usually 2 strains of influenza A and 1 or 2 strains of influenza B). Sometimes slightly different vaccines are used in the northern and southern hemisphere. When the vaccine contains the same HA and NA as the strains in the community, vaccination decreases infections by 70 to 90% in healthy adults. In the institutionalized elderly, vaccines are less effective for prevention but decrease the rate of pneumonia and death by 60 to 80%. Vaccine-induced immunity is decreased by antigenic drift and is absent if there is antigenic shift.

There are 2 basic types of vaccine:

- Multivalent inactivated influenza vaccine (MIV)
- Live-attenuated influenza vaccine (LAIV)

MIV is given by IM injection. Trivalent vaccines are gradually being superseded by quadrivalent vaccines that cover an additional B virus strain. An egg protein–free vaccine (RIV3) is available for patients who are aged 18 through 49 yr and have any degree of egg allergy. A high-dose trivalent vaccine is available for patients ≥ 65 yr, but efficacy is still being studied. For all MIVs, patients aged 6 mo to 35 mo are given 0.25 mL, and those ≥ 3 yr are given 0.5 mL. Adverse effects are usually limited to mild pain at the injection site; it lasts no more than a few days. Fever, myalgia, and other systemic effects are uncommon. Multidose vials contain thimerosal, a mercury-based preservative. Public concerns about a possible link between thimerosal and autism have proved unfounded (see p. 2466); however single-dose vials, which are thimerosal-free, are available.

LAIV is given intranasally at a dose of 0.25 mL in each nostril. It may be used for healthy people aged 2 to 49 yr. This vaccine is not recommended for high-risk patients, pregnant women, household contacts of patients with severe immunodeficiency (eg, with hematopoietic stem cell transplants), or children who are receiving long-term aspirin therapy. Also, it should not be given until 48 h after stopping drug treatment of influenza. Adverse effects associated with the vaccine are mild; rhinorrhea is the most common, and mild wheezing may occur. LAIV should not be given to children who are < 5 yr and have reactive airway disease (eg, known asthma, recurrent or recent wheezing episodes).

For both types of vaccines, children who are < 8 yr and have not been vaccinated should be given a primary dose and a booster dose 1 mo apart.

Table 200–2. DRUG SENSITIVITIES OF VARIOUS INFLUENZA STRAINS

VIRUS	AMANTADINE OR RIMANTADINE	OSELTAMIVIR	ZANAMIVIR
Influenza A viruses			
Seasonal H3N2	Resistant	Sensitive	Sensitive
Seasonal H1N1	Sensitive	Resistant	Sensitive
Pandemic H1N1	Resistant	Sensitive	Sensitive
Avian H5N1	Resistant	Sensitive	Sensitive
Influenza B viruses			
All	Resistant	Sensitive	Sensitive

A complete list of vaccines for the 2016–2017 season, is available from the CDC (see CDC Influenza Vaccines at www.cdc.com).

Vaccination recommendations: Annual vaccination is recommended for everyone ≥ 6 mo.

Influenza vaccine is given annually to maintain antibody titers and allow vaccine modification to compensate for antigenic drift. Vaccine is best given in the fall, so that antibody titers will be high during the winter influenza season (between November and March in the US).

Vaccination (both MIV and LAIV) should be avoided in people who

- Have a severe egg allergy (if the only allergic manifestation is urticaria, an egg-protein free vaccine can be used in patients aged 18 through 49 yr, or a standard vaccine can be used if appropriate precautions are taken to manage a possible allergic reaction)
- Previously had a severe reaction to influenza vaccine
- Developed Guillain-Barré syndrome (GBS) within 6 wk of a previous influenza vaccination (it is not known whether influenza vaccination increases risk of recurrent GBS in patients who have previously had GBS that was not related to influenza vaccination)
- Have had GBS in the previous 6 wk, regardless of cause
- Are < 6 mo old

Antiviral drugs: Although vaccination is the preferred method of prevention, antiviral drugs are also effective. Prophylactic antiviral drugs are indicated when influenza is circulating in the community for patients

- Who have been vaccinated only within the previous 2 wk
- For whom vaccination is contraindicated
- Who are immunocompromised and thus may not respond to vaccination

Antiviral drugs do not impair development of immunity from inactivated vaccine. They can be stopped 2 wk after vaccination. If vaccine cannot be given, antiviral drugs are continued for the duration of the epidemic.

If the circulating influenza types or subtypes are unknown, patients may be treated with either zanamivir alone (in patients for whom it is not contraindicated) or with a combination of rimantadine and oseltamivir.

KEY POINTS

- Minor antigenic drift in H and/or NA antigens produces strains that cause seasonal epidemics; rare antigenic shifts resulting in new combinations of H and NA antigens can cause a pandemic with significant mortality.
- Influenza itself may cause pneumonia, or patients with influenza may develop secondary bacterial pneumonia.
- Diagnosis is usually clinical, but sensitve and specific RT-PCR assays can differentiate influenza types and subtypes and thus help select antiviral therapy and determine whether outbreaks of respiratory disease are due to influenza.
- Treat most patients symptomatically.
- Antiviral drugs given early can slightly decrease duration and severity of symptoms but are typically used only in high-risk patients; different influenza types and subtypes are resistant to different drugs.
- Vaccinate everyone ≥ 6 mo annually; antiviral drugs can be used for prevention in immunocompromised patients (who may not respond to vaccination) and patients with contraindications to vaccination.

AVIAN INFLUENZA

(Bird Flu)

Avian influenza is caused by strains of influenza A that normally infect only wild birds and domestic poultry (and sometimes pigs). Infections due to these strains have recently been detected in humans.

Most cases of avian influenza in humans have been caused by strains of avian influenza type A H5N1 and, most recently, by type A H7N9, but types H7N7, H7N3, H9N2, and H10N8 have also caused some human infections. Infections with these strains are asymptomatic in wild birds but may cause highly lethal illness in domestic poultry.

The first human cases of H5N1 were discovered in Hong Kong in 1997. Spread to humans was contained by culling domestic bird populations. However, in 2003 and 2004, H5N1 infections in humans reappeared, and occasional cases continue to be reported, primarily in Asia and the Middle East. Human infections with other avian influenza strains have also been reported in Asia (H9N2), Canada (H7N3), the Netherlands (H7N7), and China (H10N8). At the end of 2013, the first 2 human cases of avian H10N8 influenza infection were diagnosed in southeastern China. One patient, an elderly woman with a compromised immune system, died. All her contacts remained asymptomatic. Although most cases of avian influenza occurred through exposure to infected birds, some person-to-person transmission probably occurred in the Netherlands and in Asia.

In early 2013, an extensive outbreak of H7N9 avian influenza occurred in several provinces of southeastern China. About one third of cases were fatal, but significant illness typically occurred only in the elderly. Sustained human-to-human transmission did not occur, although there is some evidence of limited human-to-human transmission. Human infection appeared to result from direct exposure to infected birds in live (wet) poultry markets, where birds are purchased for subsequent consumption at home. The outbreak peaked in late spring of 2013, subsided (partly because the markets were closed down), but then reappeared in early autumn. China is currently experiencing its 5th epidemic of Asian H7N9 avian influenza in humans; as of August 2017, 759 people have been infected in this epidemic, bringing the total cumulative number of people with Asian lineage H7N9 avian influenza to 1557. Some cases of Asian H7N9 avian influenza have been reported outside of mainland China, but most occurred in people who had traveled to mainland China before becoming ill.

It is likely that avian influenza viruses of any antigenic specificity can cause influenza in humans whenever the virus acquires mutations enabling it to attach to human-specific receptor sites in the respiratory tract. Because all influenza viruses are capable of rapid genetic change, there is a possibility that avian strains could acquire the ability to spread more easily from person to person via direct mutation or via reassortment of genome subunits with human strains during replication in a human, animal or, avian host. Many experts are concerned that if these strains acquire the ability to spread efficiently from person to person, an influenza pandemic could result.

Human infection with avian influenza H5N1 strains can cause severe respiratory symptoms. Mortality was 33% in the 1997 outbreak and has been > 60% in subsequent infections. Infection with the H7 strains most commonly causes conjunctivitis, although in the Netherlands outbreak, a few patients had flu-like symptoms and one patient (of 83) died.

Diagnosis

- Reverse transcriptase–PCR (RT-PCR)

An appropriate clinical syndrome in a patient exposed to a person known to be infected or to birds in an area with an ongoing avian influenza outbreak should prompt consideration of this infection. History of recent travel to regions with ongoing transmission of virus from domestic poultry to humans (eg, for H5N1, Egypt, Indonesia, and Vietnam) plus exposure to birds or infected people should prompt testing for influenza A by RT–PCR. Culture of the organism should not be attempted.

Suspected and confirmed cases are reported to the Centers for Disease Control and Prevention (CDC).

Treatment

- A neuraminidase inhibitor

Treatment with oseltamivir or zanamivir at usual doses is indicated. The H5N1 virus is resistant to amantadine and rimantadine; resistance to oseltamivir has also been reported.

PANDEMIC 2009 H1N1 INFLUENZA

(Swine Flu)

Pandemic 2009 H1N1 influenza is caused by a new strain of H1N1 influenza A virus, which genetically is a combination of swine, avian, and human influenza viruses.

Most often, pigs have been infected by strains of influenza that are slightly different from those that infect people. These strains very rarely spread to people, and when they do, they very rarely then spread from person to person. The H1N1 swine flu virus is a combination of swine, avian, and human influenza viruses that spreads easily from person to person. The infection is not acquired through ingestion of pork and is acquired very rarely by contact with infected pigs.

In June 2009, the World Health Organization declared H1N1 swine flu a pandemic; it spread to > 70 countries and to all 50 US states. The majority of the deaths initially occurred in Mexico. The attack rate and mortality for H1N1 swine flu are higher in young and middle-aged adults and lower in the elderly than they are for seasonal flu. The pandemic entered the post-pandemic period in August 2010. Subsequently, the virus name was standardized to influenza A(H1N1)pdm09 to denote the pandemic and distinguish the virus from seasonal H1N1 strains and the 1918 pandemic H1N1 strain.

Human cases of H3N2 virus infection have occurred sporadically in several US states where children and adults have had contact with apparently healthy domestic pigs at agricultural fairs. There have also been cases of possible human-to-human transmission. The H3N2 virus has genes from avian, swine, and human viruses and the matrix (M) gene from the A(H1N1)pdm09 virus.

Symptoms and Signs

Symptoms, signs, and complications resemble those of ordinary influenza (see p. 1686), although nausea, vomiting, and diarrhea may be more common. Symptoms are usually mild, but they can become severe, leading to pneumonia or respiratory failure. Currently circulating isolates appear to have lost some of their initial virulence.

Diagnosis

- Sometimes PCR testing of respiratory samples

Because A(H1N1)pdm09 swine flu is the predominant strain of influenza currently circulating worldwide, this diagnosis should be considered in any patient with influenza-like symptoms.

A PCR test can detect the A(H1N1)pdm09 virus in respiratory tract samples (eg, nasopharyngeal swabs, nasal washings, tracheal aspirates). Mildly ill patients do not require testing other than for epidemiologic or surveillance purposes; however, local hospital and public health requirements may vary. Rapid antigen detection tests have decreased sensitivity and generally are clinically useful in diagnosis only if results are positive.

Treatment

- Sometimes a neuraminidase inhibitor

Treatment focuses mainly on symptom relief (eg, acetaminophen or ibuprofen for fever and aches). Antiviral drugs may be used, particularly for high-risk patients (see p. 1686) and those who are seriously ill. Oseltamivir and zanamivir appear to be effective; they are most effective when started within 48 h after symptom onset. In the US, the FDA has issued Emergency Use Authorizations for the use of oseltamivir in patients < 1 yr old and for the emergency use of peramivir, an IV neuraminidase inhibitor, in severely ill hospitalized patients.

Most patients recover fully without taking these drugs.

Prevention

The current seasonal influenza vaccines are effective against the A(H1N1)pdm09 virus.

Common sense steps (eg, staying home if influenza-like symptoms develop; thorough, frequent handwashing with soap and water or an alcohol-based hand sanitizer) are recommended to reduce the spread of infection.

PARAINFLUENZA VIRUS INFECTIONS

Parainfluenza viruses include several closely related viruses that cause many respiratory illnesses varying from the common cold to an influenza-like syndrome or pneumonia; croup is the most common severe manifestation. Diagnosis is usually clinical. Treatment is supportive.

The parainfluenza viruses are paramyxoviruses types 1, 2, 3, and 4. They share antigenic cross-reactivity but tend to cause diseases of different severity. Type 4 has antigenic cross-reactivity with the mumps virus and appears to be an uncommon cause of respiratory disease.

Childhood outbreaks of parainfluenza virus infections can occur in nurseries, pediatric wards, and schools. Types 1 and 2 tend to cause epidemics in the autumn, with each serotype occurring in alternate years. Type 3 disease is endemic and infects most children < 1 yr; incidence is increased in the spring.

Parainfluenza viruses can cause repeated infections, but reinfection generally causes milder illness. Thus, in immunocompetent adults, most infections are asymptomatic or mild.

The most common illness in children is an upper respiratory illness with no or low-grade fever.

Parainfluenza type 1 probably causes croup (laryngotracheobronchitis—see p. 2826), primarily in infants aged 6 to 36 mo. Croup begins with common cold symptoms. Later, fever, a barking cough, hoarseness, and stridor develop. Respiratory failure due to upper airway obstruction is a rare, but potentially fatal complication.

Parainfluenza virus type 3 may cause pneumonia and bronchiolitis in young infants (see p. 2825). These illnesses are generally indistinguishable from disease caused by respiratory syncytial virus (see below) but are often less severe.

A specific viral diagnosis is unnecessary. Treatment is symptomatic.

CORONAVIRUSES AND ACUTE RESPIRATORY SYNDROMES (MERS AND SARS)

Coronaviruses are enveloped RNA viruses. Coronavirus infections in humans most frequently cause symptoms of the common cold. Coronaviruses 229E and OC43 cause the common cold; the serotypes NL63 and HUK1 have also been associated with this syndrome.

Two coronaviruses, MERS-CoV and SARS-CoV, cause much more severe respiratory infections in humans than other coronaviruses. In 2012, the coronavirus MERS-CoV was identified as the cause of Middle East respiratory syndrome (MERS). In late 2002, SARS-CoV was identified as the cause of an outbreak of severe acute respiratory syndrome (SARS).

MERS

MERS is a severe acute respiratory illness caused by the newly identified MERS coronavirus (MERS-CoV).

MERS-CoV infection was first reported in September 2012 in Saudi Arabia, but an outbreak in April 2012 in Jordan was confirmed retrospectively. Between April 2012 and September 2013, 130 cases were laboratory-confirmed; most of them occurred in Saudi Arabia, where new cases continue to appear. As of 2017, worldwide, 2066 cases of MERS-CoV infection (with at least 720 related deaths) have been reported; all cases of MERS have been linked through travel to or residence in countries in and near the Arabian Peninsula. The largest known outbreak of MERS outside the Arabian Peninsula occurred in the Republic of Korea in 2015. The outbreak was associated with a traveler returning from the Arabian Peninsula. Cases have also been confirmed in France, Germany, Italy, Tunisia, and the United Kingdom in patients who were either transferred there for care or became ill after returning from the Middle East.

Person-to-person transmission has been established by the development of infection in people whose only risk was close contact with people who had MERS. Most reported cases have involved severe respiratory illness requiring hospitalization, but at least 21% or patients had mild or no symptoms.

The reservoir of MERS-CoV is unknown; however, many coronavirus species are present in bats, and bats are the most probable source although MERS-CoV has not previously been identified in bats. Anti-MERS-CoV antibodies have been detected in a few camels, which are the only other currently suspected hosts.

The incubation period is about 5 days. More than half of cases have been fatal. Median patient age is 56 yr, and the male:female ratio is about 1.6:1. Infection tends to be more severe in elderly patients and in patients with a preexisting disorder such as diabetes, a chronic heart disorder, or a chronic renal disorder.

Fever, chills, myalgia, and cough are common. GI symptoms (eg, diarrhea, vomiting, abdominal pain) occur in about one third of patients. Cases may require ICU confinement, but recently, the proportion of such cases has declined sharply.

In all patients, chest imaging detects abnormalities, which may be subtle or extensive, unilateral or bilateral. In some patients, levels of LDH and AST are elevated and/or levels of platelets and lymphocytes are low. A few patients have acute kidney injury. Disseminated intravascular coagulation and hemolysis may develop.

Preliminary seroprevalence studies indicate that the infection is not widespread in Saudi Arabia.

The WHO considers the risk of contracting MERS-CoV infection to be very low for pilgrims traveling to Saudi Arabia for Umrah and Hajj; last year's Hajj did not result in an increase of patients with MERS-CoV infection. For additional information about pilgrimages to the Middle East, see World-travel advice on MERS-CoV for pilgrimages (available at www.who.int).

Diagnosis

- Real-time reverse-transcriptase PCR (RT-PCR) testing of lower respiratory secretions

MERS should be suspected in patients who have an unexplained acute lower respiratory infection and either

- Travel to or residence in an area where MERS has recently been reported or where transmission could have occurred
- Within 10 days before symptom onset, close contact with a patient who was ill with suspected MERS

The most recent recommendations are available from the WHO (Interim surveillance recommendations for human infection with novel coronavirus) and, in the US, the Centers for Disease Control and Prevention (Interim Guidelines for Investigation for MERS).

Testing should include real-time RT-PCR testing of lower respiratory secretions, ideally taken from different sites and at different times. Serum should be obtained from patients and from all, even asymptomatic close contacts, including health care workers (to help identify mild or asymptomatic MERS). Serum is obtained immediately after MERS is suspected or after contacts are exposed (acute serum) and 3 to 4 wk later (convalescent serum).

Treatment

- Supportive

Treatment is supportive. To help prevent spread from suspected cases, health care practitioners should use standard, contact, and airborne precautions.

There is no vaccine.

SARS

SARS is a severe, acute respiratory illness caused by the SARS coronavirus (SARS-CoV).

SARS is much more severe than other coronavirus infections. SARS is an influenza-like illness that occasionally leads to progressively severe respiratory insufficiency. SARS-CoV was first detected in the Guangdong province of China in November 2002 and subsequently spread to > 30 countries. In this outbreak, > 8000 cases were reported worldwide, with > 774 deaths (about 10% case mortality rate). This outbreak subsided, and no new cases have been identified since 2004. The immediate source was presumed to be civet cats, which had been infected through contact with a bat before being sold in a live meat market. Bats are frequent carriers hosts of coronaviruses.

Diagnosis is made clinically, and treatment is supportive. Eradication depends on rigidly maintained isolation.

SARS-CoV is the only human virus, besides the smallpox virus, to have been completely eradicated globally. It was eradicated largely because superspreaders (patients who infect an unusually large number of contacts) were quickly identified and isolated from the general population, thus interrupting transmission of the virus.

201 Rickettsiae and Related Organisms

Rickettsial diseases (rickettsioses) and related diseases (anaplasmosis, ehrlichiosis, Q fever, scrub typhus) are caused by a group of gram-negative, obligately intracellular coccobacilli. All, except for *Coxiella burnetii*, have an arthropod vector. Symptoms usually include sudden-onset fever with severe headache, malaise, prostration, and, in most cases, a characteristic rash. Diagnosis is clinical, confirmed by immunofluorescence assay or PCR. Treatment is with tetracyclines or, except for anaplasmosis and ehrlichiosis, chloramphenicol.

Rickettsia, *Orientia*, *Ehrlichia*, *Anaplasma*, and *Coxiella* spp were once thought to belong to the same family but now, based on genetic analysis, are considered distinct entities. Although this group of organisms require living cells for growth, they are true bacteria because they have metabolic enzymes and cell walls, use oxygen, and are susceptible to antibiotics.

These organisms typically have an animal reservoir and an arthropod vector; exceptions are *R. prowazekii,* for which humans are the primary reservoir, and *C. burnetii*, which does not require an arthropod vector. Specific vectors, reservoirs, and endemic regions differ widely (see Table 201–1).

There are many rickettsial species, but 3 cause most human rickettsial infections:

- *R. rickettsii*
- *R. prowazekii*
- *R. typhi*

Symptoms and Signs

Rickettsiae multiply at the site of arthropod attachment and often produce a local lesion (eschar). They penetrate the skin or mucous membranes; some (*R. rickettsii*) multiply in the endothelial cells of small blood vessels, causing vasculitis, and others replicate in WBCs (*Ehrlichia* sp in monocytes, *Anaplasma* sp in granulocytes).

Regional lymphadenopathy is common with infection by *Orientia* sp or members of the spotted fever group (except for *R. rickettsii*).

The endovasculitis of *R. rickettsii* causes a petechial rash (due to focal areas of hemorrhage), encephalitic signs, and gangrene of skin and tissues.

Patients seriously ill with a rickettsial disease of the typhus or spotted fever group may have ecchymotic skin necrosis, edema (due to increased vascular permeability), digital gangrene, circulatory collapse, shock, oliguria, anuria, azotemia, anemia, hyponatremia, hypochloremia, delirium, and coma.

Diagnosis

- Clinical features
- Biopsy of rash with fluorescent antibody staining to detect organisms
- Acute and convalescent serologic testing (serologic testing not useful acutely)
- PCR

Differentiating rickettsial from other infections: Rickettsial and related diseases must be differentiated from other acute infections, primarily meningococcemia, rubeola, and rubella. A history of louse or flea contact, tick bite, or presence in a known endemic area is helpful, but such history is often absent. Clinicians should specifically ask about travel to an endemic region within the incubation period of the disease.

Clinical features may help distinguish diseases:

- **Meningococcemia:** The rash may be pink, macular, maculopapular, or petechial in the subacute form and petechially confluent or ecchymotic in the fulminant form. The rash develops rapidly in acute meningococcal disease and, when ecchymotic, is usually tender when palpated.
- **Rubeola:** The rash begins on the face, spreads to the trunk and arms, and soon becomes confluent (see Plate 84).
- **Rubella:** The rash usually remains discrete (see Plate 83). Postauricular lymph node enlargement and lack of toxicity suggest rubella.

Differentiating among rickettsial diseases: Rickettsial diseases must also be differentiated from each other. Clinical features allow some differentiation, but overlap is considerable:

- **Rocky Mountain spotted fever (RMSF):** The rash usually appears on about the 4th febrile day as blanching macules on the extremities and gradually becomes petechial as it spreads to the trunk, palms, and soles over several days. Some patients with RMSF never develop a rash. Vasculitis often develops; it may affect the skin, subcutaneous tissues, CNS, lungs, heart, kidneys, liver, or spleen.
- **Epidemic typhus:** The rash usually appears initially in the axillary folds and on the trunk. Later, it spreads peripherally, rarely involving the palms, soles, and face. Severe physiologic and pathologic abnormalities similar to those of RMSF occur.
- **Murine typhus:** The rash is nonpurpuric, nonconfluent, and less extensive, and renal and vascular complications are uncommon.
- **Scrub typhus:** Manifestations are similar to those of RMSF and epidemic typhus. However, scrub typhus occurs in different geographic areas, and frequently, an eschar develops with satellite adenopathy.
- **Rickettsialpox:** This disease is mild, and the rash, in the form of vesicles with surrounding erythema, is sparse and may resemble varicella.
- **African tick bite fever** (due to *R. africae*): Symptoms are similar to those of other rickettsial diseases. The rash is characterized by multiple black eschars on the distal extremities with regional adenopathy.

Testing: Knowledge of residence and recent travel often helps in diagnosis because many rickettsiae are localized to certain geographic areas. However, testing is usually required.

The most useful tests for *R. rickettsii* are indirect immunofluorescence assay (IFA) and PCR of a biopsy specimen of the rash. Culture is difficult and not clinically useful. For *Ehrlichia* sp, PCR of blood is the best test. Serologic tests are not useful for acute diagnosis because they usually become positive only during convalescence.

Treatment

- Tetracyclines

Because diagnostic tests can take time and may be insensitive, antibiotics are usually begun presumptively to prevent significant deterioration, death, and prolonged recovery.

Table 201–1. DISEASES CAUSED BY *RICKETTSIA, ORIENTIA, EHRLICHIA, ANAPLASMA,* AND *COXIELLA* SPP

DISEASE	ORGANISM	RASH OR ESCHAR	VECTOR	ENDEMIC REGION
Typhus				
Epidemic typhus, Brill-Zinsser disease	*Rickettsia prowazekii*	Trunk to extremities May be absent in Brill-Zinsser disease No eschar	Body lice	Worldwide
Murine (endemic) typhus	*R. typhi, R. felis*	Trunk to extremities No eschar	Rat flea, cat flea	Worldwide
Scrub typhus				
Scrub typhus (tsutsugamushi disease)	*Orientia tsutsugamushi* (formerly *R. tsutsugamushi*)	Trunk to extremities Eschar present	Trombiculid mite larvae (chiggers)	Asia-Pacific area bounded by Japan, Korea, China, India, and northern Australia
Spotted fever				
Rocky Mountain spotted fever	*R. rickettsii*	Extremities to trunk No eschar	Ixodid (hard) ticks, including *Dermacentor andersoni* (wood tick), principally in the western US, and *D. variabilis* (dog tick), principally in the eastern and southern US	Western Hemisphere, including most of the US (except Maine, Hawaii, and Alaska); Central and South America
North Asian tick-borne rickettsiosis	*R. sibirica*	Trunk, extremities, face Multiple eschars present	Ixodid ticks	Armenia, central Asia, Siberia, Mongolia, China
Queensland tick typhus	*R. australis*	Trunk, extremities, face Eschar present	Ixodid ticks	Australia
African tick bite fever	*R. africae*	Multiple eschars on extremities at the sites of the tick bites	Ixodid ticks	Sub-Saharan Africa, West Indies
Mediterranean spotted fever (boutonneuse fever)*	*R. conorii*	Trunk, extremities, face Eschar present	*Rhipicephalus sanguineus* (brown dog tick)	Africa; India; southern Europe; the Middle East adjacent to the Mediterranean, Black, and Caspian Seas
Rickettsialpox	*R. akari*	Trunk, extremities, face Eschar present	Mites	US, Russia, Korea, Africa
R. parkeri rickettsiosis	*R. parkeri*	Eschar present	Gulf Coast tick (*Amblyomma maculatum*)	Southern US, South America
Ehrlichiosis and anaplasmosis				
Monocytic ehrlichiosis	*Ehrlichia chaffeensis*	Uncommon, but more common among children No eschar	Ticks (*A. americanum*, also known as the lone star tick)	Southeastern and south central US
Granulocytic anaplasmosis	*Anaplasma phagocytophilum*	None No eschar	Ticks (*Ixodes scapularis* in the eastern and Midwest US, *I. pacificus* in the western US, possibly *I. ricinus* in Europe)	In the US, the Northeast, mid-Atlantic, upper Midwest, and West Coast; Europe
Q Fever				
Q fever	*Coxiella burnetii*	Rare, but more common among children No eschar	No vector needed	Worldwide

*Often known by the area in which it occurs (eg, Indian tick typhus, Marseilles fever).

Tetracyclines are first-line treatment: doxycycline 200 mg po once followed by 100 mg bid until the patient improves, has been afebrile for 24 to 48 h, and has received treatment for at least 7 days. IV preparations are used in patients too ill to take oral drugs. Although tetracyclines can cause tooth staining in children, experts think that a course of doxycycline is warranted.

Chloramphenicol 500 mg po or IV qid for 7 days is 2nd-line treatment.

Both drugs are rickettsiostatic, not rickettsicidal.

Ciprofloxacin and other fluoroquinolones are effective against certain rickettsiae, but extensive clinical experience is lacking.

Because severely ill patients with RMSF or epidemic typhus may have a marked increase in capillary permeability in later stages, IV fluids should be given cautiously to maintain BP while avoiding worsening pulmonary and cerebral edema.

Heparin is not recommended in patients who develop disseminated intravascular coagulation.

KEY POINTS

- Rickettsial diseases and related diseases (anaplasmosis, ehrlichiosis, Q fever, scrub typhus) are caused by a group of gram-negative, obligately intracellular coccobacilli; all, except for *Coxiella burnetii*, have an arthropod vector.
- Rickettsial diseases cause fever and, depending on the disease, sometimes a local lesion (eschar), petechial rash, regional lymphadenopathy, encephalitic signs, vasculitis, gangrene of skin and tissues, organ dysfunction, and vascular collapse.
- Distinguish rickettsial and related diseases from other acute infections and from each others based on history, clinical features, and results of tests (eg, biopsy with indirect immunofluorescence assay, serologic tests, PCR).
- Treat with antibiotics presumptively, without waiting for diagnostic test results, to prevent significant deterioration, death, and prolonged recovery.
- First-line treatment is tetracyclines.

EHRLICHIOSIS AND ANAPLASMOSIS

Ehrlichiosis and anaplasmosis are caused by rickettsial-like bacteria. Ehrlichiosis is caused mainly by *Ehrlichia* chaffeensis; anaplasmosis is caused by *Anaplasma phagocytophilum*. Both are transmitted to humans by ticks. Symptoms resemble those of Rocky Mountain spotted fever (RMSF) except that a rash is much less common. Onset of illness, with fever, chills, headache, and malaise, is abrupt.

Ehrlichiosis and anaplasmosis are related to rickettsial diseases.

E. chaffeensis causes human monocytic ehrlichiosis. Most cases of monocytic ehrlichiosis have been identified in the southeastern and south central US, where its arthropod vector (the lone star tick) is endemic.

Anaplasma phagocytophilum (formerly *E. phagocytophila*) causes human granulocytic anaplasmosis, which occurs in the Northeast, mid-Atlantic, upper Midwest and West Coast of the US, where its arthropod vector (ixodid ticks) are endemic. Lyme disease and babesiosis have the same tick vector and endemic area, and occasionally patients acquire coinfections after being bitten by a tick infected with more than one type of organism. Several cases of anaplasmosis have been reported after blood transfusions from asymptomatic or acutely infected donors.

PEARLS & PITFALLS

- Because Lyme disease and babesiosis have the same tick vector and endemic area as anaplasmosis, ticks (and thus the people they bite) may be infected with more than one type of organism at the same time.

The difference in the primary target cell (monocytes for ehrlichiosis and granulocytes for anaplasmosis) results in only minor differences in clinical manifestations.

Symptoms and Signs

Clinical features of ehrlichiosis and anaplasmosis are similar. Although some infections are asymptomatic, most cause abrupt onset of an influenza-like illness with nonspecific symptoms such as fever, chills, myalgias, weakness, nausea, vomiting, cough. headache, and malaise, usually beginning about 12 days after the tick bite.

Rash is uncommon in anaplasmosis. Some patients infected with *E. chaffeensis* develop a maculopapular or petechial rash on the trunk and extremities.

Ehrlichiosis and anaplasmosis may result in disseminated intravascular coagulation, multiorgan failure, seizures, and coma.

Both infections appear to be more severe and have a higher mortality rate in patients with compromised immunity caused by immunosuppressants (eg, corticosteroids, cancer chemotherapy, long-term treatment with immunosuppressants after organ transplantation), HIV infection, or splenectomy.

Diagnosis

- PCR testing of a blood sample

Diagnostic serologic tests are available for ehrlichiosis and anaplasmosis, but PCR of blood is more sensitive and specific and can result in an early diagnosis because serologic tests require comparison of serial titers. Cytoplasmic inclusions in monocytes (ehrlichiosis) or in neutrophils (anaplasmosis) may be detected, but cytoplasmic inclusions are more commonly seen in anaplasmosis.

Blood and liver functions tests may detect hematologic and hepatic abnormalities, such as leukopenia, thrombocytopenia, and elevated aminotransferase levels.

Treatment

- Doxycycline

Treatment of ehrlichiosis and anaplasmosis is best started before laboratory results return. When treatment is started early, patients generally respond rapidly and well. A delay in treatment may lead to serious complications, including viral and fungal superinfections and death in 2 to 5%.

Primary treatment is doxycycline 200 mg po once followed by 100 mg bid until the patient improves and has been afebrile for 24 to 48 h but is continued for at least 7 days. Chloramphenicol is no longer effective.

Some patients continue to experience headache, weakness, and malaise for weeks after adequate treatment.

Measures can be taken to prevent tick bites (see Sidebar 201–1).

KEY POINTS

- Ehrlichiosis and anaplasmosis are related to rickettsial diseases.
- The lone star tick, endemic in the southeastern and south central US, is the vector for both.
- Clinical features of ehrlichiosis and anaplasmosis are similar, usually with abrupt onset of an influenza-like illness; rash is uncommon in anaplasmosis.
- Ehrlichiosis and anaplasmosis may result in disseminated intravascular coagulation, multiorgan failure, seizures, and coma.
- Do PCR testing of blood, which is more sensitive and specific than serologic tests and can result in an early diagnosis.
- Treat with doxycycline, best started before laboratory results return.

EPIDEMIC TYPHUS

(European, Classic, or Louse-Borne Typhus; Jail Fever)

Epidemic typhus is caused by *Rickettsia prowazekii*. Symptoms are prolonged high fever, intractable headache, and a maculopapular rash.

Epidemic typhus is a rickettsial disease.

Humans are the natural reservoir for *R. prowazekii*, which is prevalent worldwide and transmitted by body lice when louse feces are scratched or rubbed into bite or other wounds (or sometimes the mucous membranes of the eyes or mouth). In the US, humans occasionally contract epidemic typhus after contact with flying squirrels.

Fatalities are rare in children < 10 yr, but mortality increases with age and may reach 60% in untreated patients > 50 yr.

Symptoms and Signs

After an incubation period of 7 to 14 days, fever, headache, and prostration suddenly occur. Temperature reaches 40° C in several days and remains high, with slight morning remission, for about 2 wk. Headache is generalized and intense. Small, pink macules, which appear on the 4th to 6th day, rapidly cover the body, usually in the axillae and on the upper trunk and not on the palms, soles, and face. Later, the rash becomes dark and maculopapular. In severe cases, the rash becomes petechial and hemorrhagic.

Splenomegaly sometimes occurs. Hypotension occurs in most seriously ill patients. Vascular collapse, renal insufficiency, encephalitic signs, ecchymosis with gangrene, and pneumonia are poor prognostic signs.

Brill-Zinsser disease, a mild recrudescence of epidemic typhus, can occur years after the initial infection if host defenses falter.

Diagnosis

- Clinical features
- Biopsy of rash with fluorescent antibody staining to detect organisms
- Acute and convalescent serologic testing (serologic testing not useful acutely)
- PCR

Louse infestation is usually obvious and strongly suggests typhus, if history (eg, living in or visiting an endemic area) suggests possible exposure.

For details of diagnosis, see p. 1691.

Treatment

- Doxycycline

Primary treatment of epidemic typhus is doxycycline 200 mg po once followed by 100 mg bid until the patient improves, has been afebrile for 24 to 48 h, and has received treatment for at least 7 days.

Chloramphenicol 500 mg po or IV qid for 7 days is 2nd-line treatment.

Severely ill patients with epidemic typhus may have a marked increase in capillary permeability in later stages; thus, IV fluids should be given cautiously to maintain BP while avoiding worsening pulmonary and cerebral edema.

Prevention

Immunization and louse control are highly effective for prevention. However, vaccines are not available in the US. Lice may be eliminated by dusting infested people with malathion or lindane.

KEY POINTS

- Epidemic typhus is prevalent worldwide; humans are the natural reservoir.
- Infection is transmitted among humans by body lice when louse feces are scratched or rubbed into louse bites, wounds, or mucous membranes.
- Small, pink macules rapidly cover the body, later, becoming dark and maculopapular.
- Mortality increases with age and may reach 60% in untreated patients > 50 yr; vascular collapse, renal insufficiency, encephalitic signs, ecchymosis with gangrene, and pneumonia are poor prognostic signs.
- Suspect epidemic typhus based on clinical manifestations and signs of louse infestation; confirm with fluorescent antibody staining of skin biopsy.
- Treat with doxycycline or chloramphenicol.
- Brill-Zinsser disease, a mild recrudescence of epidemic typhus, can occur years after the initial infection if host defenses falter.

Brill-Zinsser Disease

Brill-Zinsser disease is a recrudescence of epidemic typhus, occurring years after an initial attack.

Patients with Brill-Zinsser disease acquired epidemic typhus earlier or lived in an endemic area. Apparently, when host defenses falter, viable organisms retained in the body are activated, causing recurrent typhus; thus, disease is sporadic, occurring at any season or geographic area, and in the absence of infected lice. Lice that feed on patients may acquire and transmit the agent.

Symptoms and signs of Brill-Zinsser disease are almost always mild and resemble those of epidemic typhus, with similar circulatory disturbances and hepatic, renal, and CNS changes. The remittent febrile course lasts about 7 to 10 days. The rash is often evanescent or absent. Mortality is nil.

For diagnosis and treatment, see above.

MURINE (ENDEMIC) TYPHUS

(Rat-Flea Typhus; Urban Typhus of Malaya)

Murine typhus is caused by *Rickettsia typhi* and *R. felis*, which are transmitted to humans by fleas; it is clinically

similar to, but milder than, epidemic typhus, causing chills, headache, fever, and rash.

Murine typhus is a rickettsial disease.

Animal reservoirs include wild rats, mice, and other rodents. Rat fleas and probably cat fleas transmit organisms to humans through bites. Fleas are also natural reservoirs for *R. typhi*; infected female fleas can transmit organisms to their progeny. Distribution is sporadic but worldwide; the incidence is low but higher in rat-infested areas.

Symptoms and Signs

After an incubation of 6 to 18 days (mean 10 days), a shaking chill accompanies headache and fever. The fever lasts about 12 days; then temperature gradually returns to normal.

The rash and other manifestations are similar to those of epidemic typhus but are much less severe. The early rash is sparse and discrete.

Mortality is low but is higher in elderly patients.

Diagnosis

- Clinical features
- Biopsy of rash with fluorescent antibody staining to detect organisms
- Acute and convalescent serologic testing (serologic testing not useful acutely)
- PCR

For details of diagnosis, see p. 1694.

Treatment

- Doxycycline

Primary treatment is doxycycline 200 mg po once followed by 100 mg bid until the patient improves, has been afebrile for 48 h, and has received treatment for at least 7 days. Chloramphenicol 500 mg po or IV qid for 7 days is 2nd line treatment.

For details of treatment, see p. 1691.

Incidence has been decreased by reducing rat and rat flea populations. No effective vaccine exists.

KEY POINTS

- Murine typhus is transmitted to humans by fleas.
- Symptoms begin with a shaking chill, headache, and fever; the rash and other manifestations are similar to those of epidemic typhus but are much less severe.
- Treat with doxycycline or chloramphenicol.

OTHER SPOTTED FEVER RICKETTSIOSES

Various rickettsiae transmitted by ixodid ticks cause spotted fever rickettsioses similar to but milder than Rocky Mountain spotted fever (RMSF). Symptoms are an initial skin lesion, satellite adenopathy, and an erythematous maculopapular rash.

Spotted fever rickettsioses include North Asian tick-borne rickettsiosis, Queensland tick typhus, African tick typhus, Mediterranean spotted fever (boutonneuse fever), and *Rickettsia parkeri* rickettsiosis (transmitted by the Gulf Coast tick [*Amblyomma maculatum*]—see Table 201–1). The causative agents belong to the spotted fever group of rickettsiae.

The epidemiology of these tick-borne rickettsioses resembles that of RMSF in the Western Hemisphere. Ixodid ticks and wild animals maintain the rickettsiae in nature. If humans intrude accidentally into the cycle, they become infected. In certain areas, the cycle of boutonneuse fever involves domiciliary environments, with the brown dog tick, *Rhipicephalus sanguineus*, as the dominant vector.

Symptoms and Signs

The symptoms and signs are similar for all spotted fever rickettsioses and generally milder than with RMSF.

After an incubation period of 5 to 7 days, fever, malaise, headache, and conjunctival injection develop. With the onset of fever, a small buttonlike ulcer 2 to 5 mm in diameter with a black center appears (an eschar or, in boutonneuse fever, tache noire). Usually, the regional or satellite lymph nodes are enlarged. On about the 4th day of fever, a red maculopapular rash appears on the forearms and extends to most of the body, including the palms and soles. Fever lasts into the 2nd wk.

Complications and death are rare except among elderly or debilitated patients. However, the disease should not be ignored; a fulminant form of vasculitis can occur.

Diagnosis

- Clinical features
- Biopsy of rash with fluorescent antibody staining to detect organisms
- Acute and convalescent serologic testing (serologic testing is not useful acutely)
- PCR

For details on diagnosis, see p. 1691.

Treatment

- Doxycycline or ciprofloxacin

Treatment of spotted fever rickettsioses is one of the following:

- Doxycycline 100 mg po bid for 5 days
- Ciprofloxacin 500 to 750 mg po bid for 5 days

Measures can be taken to prevent tick bites (see Sidebar 201–1).

Q FEVER

Q fever is an acute or chronic disease caused by the rickettsial-like bacillus *Coxiella burnetii*. Acute disease causes sudden onset of fever, headache, malaise, and interstitial pneumonitis. Chronic disease manifestations reflect the organ system affected. Diagnosis is confirmed by several serologic techniques, isolation of the organism, or PCR. Treatment is with doxycycline or chloramphenicol.

Coxiella burnetii is a small, intracellular, pleomorphic bacillus that is no longer classified as *Rickettsia*. Molecular studies have reclassified it as Proteobacteria in the same group as Legionella sp.

Q fever can be

- Acute
- Chronic

Acute disease causes a febrile illness that often affects the respiratory system, although sometimes the liver is involved. Women infected during pregnancy have an increased risk of spontaneous abortion and preterm delivery.

Chronic Q fever occurs in < 5% of patients. It usually manifests as endocarditis or hepatitis; osteomyelitis may occur.

Sidebar 201–1. Tick Bite Prevention

Preventing tick access to skin includes

- Staying on paths and trails
- Tucking trousers into boots or socks
- Wearing long-sleeved shirts
- Applying repellents with diethyltoluamide (DEET) to skin surfaces

DEET should be used cautiously in very young children because toxic reactions have been reported. Permethrin on clothing effectively kills ticks. Frequent searches for ticks, particularly in hairy areas and on children, are essential in endemic areas.

Engorged ticks should be removed with care and not crushed between the fingers because crushing the tick may result in disease transmission. The tick's body should not be grasped or squeezed. Gradual traction on the head with a small forceps dislodges the tick. The point of attachment should be swabbed with alcohol. Petroleum jelly, alcohol, lit matches, and other irritants are not effective ways to remove ticks and should not be used.

No practical means are available to rid entire areas of ticks, but tick populations may be reduced in endemic areas by controlling small-animal populations.

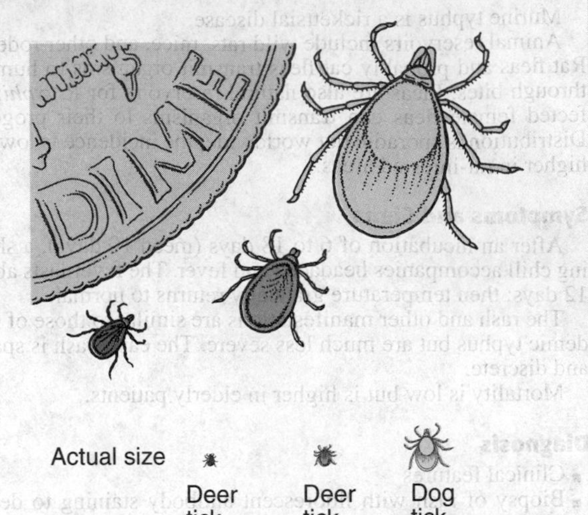

Worldwide in its distribution, Q fever is maintained as an inapparent infection in domestic or farm animals. Sheep, cattle, and goats are the principal reservoirs for human infection. *C. burnetii* persists in stool, urine, milk, and tissues (especially the placenta), so that fomites and infective aerosols form easily. *C. burnetii* is also maintained in nature through an animal-tick cycle, but arthropods are not involved in human infection.

Etiology

Cases of Q fever occur among workers whose occupations bring them in close contact with farm animals or their products. Transmission is usually by inhalation of infected aerosols, but the disease can also be contracted by ingesting infective raw milk.

C. burnetii is very virulent, resists inactivation, and remains viable in dust and stool for months; even a single organism can cause infection. Because of these characteristics, *C. burnetii* is a potential biological warfare agent.

Very rarely, the disease is transmitted from person to person.

Symptoms and Signs

The incubation period averages 18 to 21 days (range 9 to 28 days). Acute Q fever is often asymptomatic; in other patients, it begins abruptly with influenza-like symptoms: fever, severe headache, chills, severe malaise, myalgia, anorexia, and sweats. Fever may rise to 40° C and persist 1 to > 3 wk.

Rarely, acute Q fever manifests as encephalitis or meningoencephalitis.

Respiratory symptoms (a dry nonproductive cough, pleuritic chest pain) appear 4 to 5 days after onset of illness. These symptoms may be particularly severe in elderly or debilitated patients. During examination, lung crackles are commonly noted, and findings suggesting consolidation may be present. Unlike rickettsial diseases, acute Q fever does not cause a rash.

Acute hepatic involvement, occurring in some patients, resembles viral hepatitis, with fever, malaise, hepatomegaly with right upper abdominal pain, and possibly jaundice. Headache and respiratory signs are frequently absent.

Chronic Q fever may manifest within a few weeks to many years after the initial infection. Hepatitis may manifest as fever of unknown origin. Liver biopsy may show granulomas, which should be differentiated from other causes of liver granulomas (eg, TB, sarcoidosis, histoplasmosis, brucellosis, tularemia, syphilis).

Endocarditis resembles viridans group subacute bacterial endocarditis; the aortic valve is most commonly affected, but vegetations may occur on any valve. Marked finger clubbing, arterial emboli, hepatomegaly, splenomegaly, and a purpuric rash may occur.

The case-fatality rate is only about 1% in untreated patients but is higher in those with endocarditis. Some patients with neurologic involvement have residual impairment.

Diagnosis

- Immunofluorescence assay or PCR of infected tissue
- Sometimes acute and convalescent serologic tests

Symptoms do not readily suggest the diagnosis of Q fever. Early on, Q fever resembles many infections (eg, influenza, other viral infections, salmonellosis, malaria, hepatitis, brucellosis). Later, it resembles many forms of bacterial, viral, and mycoplasmal and other atypical pneumonias. Contact with animals or animal products is an important clue.

Immunofluorescence assay (IFA) of infected tissue is the diagnostic method of choice; alternatively, enzyme-linked immunosorbent assay (ELISA) may be done. Acute and convalescent serum specimens (typically complement fixation) may be used. Antibodies to phase II antigen are used to diagnose acute disease, and antibodies to both phase I and phase II antigens are used to diagnose chronic disease.

PCR can identify the organism in biopsy specimens, but negative results do not rule out the diagnosis.

C. burnetii may be isolated from clinical specimens, but only by special research laboratories; routine blood and sputum cultures are negative.

Patients with respiratory symptoms or signs require chest x-ray; findings may include atelectasis, pleural-based opacities, pleural effusion, and lobar consolidation. The gross appearance of the lungs may resemble bacterial pneumonia but, histologically, more closely resembles psittacosis and some viral pneumonias.

In acute Q fever, CBC may be normal, but about 30% of patients have an elevated WBC count. Alkaline phosphatase, AST, and ALT levels are mildly elevated to 2 to 3 times the normal level in typical cases. If obtained, liver biopsy specimens often show diffuse granulomatous changes.

Treatment

- Doxycycline

For **acute Q fever**, primary treatment is doxycycline 200 mg po once followed by 100 mg po bid until the patient improves, has been afebrile for about 5 days, and has received treatment for at least 7 days; typically, 2 to 3 wk of treatment is required. Tetracycline resistance has not been documented.

For **endocarditis**, treatment needs to be prolonged (months to years to lifelong), typically for at least 18 mo. Doxycycline 100 mg po bid plus hydroxychloroquine 200 mg po q 8 h is currently recommended. Clinical signs, ESR, blood count, and antibody titers should be monitored to help determine when to stop treatment. Consultation with an infectious disease specialist may help with managing the complexities of the disease and its treatment. Frequently, antibiotic treatment is only partially effective, and damaged valves must be replaced surgically, although some cures have occurred without surgery.

For **chronic granulomatous hepatitis**, the optimal regimen has not been determined.

Prevention

Vaccines are effective, and in Australia, where a Q fever vaccine is commercially available, vaccination is recommended to protect people with occupational risk (eg, slaughterhouse and dairy workers, rendering-plant workers, herders, woolsorters, farmers).

Prevaccination screening with skin and blood tests should be done to identify preexisting immunity to Q fever because vaccinating people who already have immunity can cause severe local reactions.

KEY POINTS

- Sheep, cattle, and goats are the principal reservoirs for human Q fever infection, which occurs worldwide.
- Transmission to humans is usually by inhalation of infected aerosols; arthropods are not involved.
- Acute symptoms resemble influenza; respiratory symptoms may be particularly severe in elderly or debilitated patients.
- Chronic Q fever occurs in < 5% of patients and usually manifests as endocarditis or hepatitis.
- Diagnose using immunofluorescence assay or PCR testing of infected tissue.
- Treat acute Q fever with doxycycline, typically for 2 to 3 wk; endocarditis requires prolonged treatment (months to years to lifelong).
- A vaccine to prevent Q fever is commercially available but only in Australia.

RICKETTSIALPOX

(Vesicular Rickettsiosis)

Rickettsialpox is caused by *Rickettsia akari*. Symptoms are an initial local lesion and a generalized papulovesicular rash.

Rickettsialpox, a rickettsial disease, occurs in many areas of the US and in Russia, Korea, and Africa. The vector, a small, colorless mite, is widely distributed. It infects the house mouse and some species of wild mice. Humans may be infected by chigger (mite larvae) or adult mite bites.

An eschar appears about 1 wk before onset of fever as a small papule 1 to 1.5 cm in diameter, then develops into a small ulcer with a dark crust that leaves a scar when it heals. Regional lymphadenopathy is present. An intermittent fever lasts about 1 wk, with chills, profuse sweating, headache, photophobia, and muscle pains. Early in the febrile course, a generalized maculopapular rash with intraepidermal vesicles appears, sparing the palms and soles.

The disease is mild; no deaths have been reported.

For details of diagnosis, see p. 1691.

Treatment is doxycycline 100 mg po bid for 5 days or ciprofloxacin 750 mg po bid for 5 days.

For prophylaxis, mouse harborages must be destroyed, and the vector controlled by residual insecticides.

ROCKY MOUNTAIN SPOTTED FEVER

(Spotted Fever; Tick Fever; Tick Typhus)

Rocky Mountain spotted fever (RMSF) is caused by *Rickettsia rickettsii* and transmitted by ixodid ticks. Symptoms are high fever, severe headache, and rash.

RMSF is a rickettsial disease.

Epidemiology

RMSF is limited to the Western Hemisphere. Initially recognized in the Rocky Mountain states, it occurs in practically all of the US and throughout Central and South America. In humans, infection occurs mainly from March to September, when adult ticks are active and people are most likely to be in tick-infested areas. In southern states, sporadic cases occur throughout the year. The incidence is highest in children < 15 yr and in people who frequent tick-infested areas for work or recreation.

Hard-shelled ticks (family Ixodidae) harbor *R. rickettsii*, and infected females transmit the agent to their progeny. These ticks are the natural reservoirs. *Dermacentor andersoni* (wood tick) is the principal vector in the western US. *D. variabilis* (dog tick) is the vector in the eastern and southern US.

RMSF is probably not transmitted directly from person to person.

Pathophysiology

Small blood vessels are the sites of the characteristic pathologic lesions. Rickettsiae propagate within damaged endothelial cells, and vessels may become blocked by thrombi, producing vasculitis in the skin, subcutaneous tissues, CNS, lungs, heart, kidneys, liver, and spleen. Disseminated intravascular coagulation often occurs in severely ill patients.

Symptoms and Signs

The incubation period for RMSF averages 7 days but varies from 3 to 12 days; the shorter the incubation period, the more severe the infection.

Onset is abrupt, with severe headache, chills, prostration, and muscular pains. Fever reaches 39.5 to 40° C within several days and remains high (for 15 to 20 days in severe cases), although morning remissions may occur.

Between the 1st and 6th day of fever, most patients with RMSF develop a rash on the wrists, ankles, palms, soles, and forearms that rapidly extends to the neck, face, axillae, buttocks, and trunk. Initially macular and pink, it becomes maculopapular and darker. In about 4 days, the lesions become petechial and may coalesce to form large hemorrhagic areas that later ulcerate.

Neurologic symptoms include headache, restlessness, insomnia, delirium, and coma, all indicative of encephalitis.

Hypotension develops in severe cases. Hepatomegaly may be present, but jaundice is infrequent. Nausea and vomiting are common. Localized pneumonitis may occur. Untreated patients may develop pneumonia, tissue necrosis, and circulatory failure, sometimes with brain and heart damage. Cardiac arrest with sudden death occasionally occurs in fulminant cases.

Diagnosis

- Clinical features
- Biopsy of rash with fluorescent antibody staining to detect organisms
- Acute and convalescent serologic testing (serologic testing not useful acutely)
- PCR

Clinicians should suspect RMSF in any seriously ill patient who lives in or near a wooded area anywhere in the Western Hemisphere and has unexplained fever, headache, and prostration, with or without a history of tick contact. A history of tick bite is elicited in about 70% of patients.

Testing is usually required to confirm RMSF but because of the limitations of currently available tests, clinicians typically must make treatment decisions before receiving results of confirmatory testing.

If patients have a rash, a skin biopsy should be taken from the rash site. PCR or immunohistochemical staining, which can provide fairly rapid results, is used. Sensitivity of these tests is about 70% when tissue specimens are collected during the acute illness and before antibiotic treatment is started. However, a negative test result does not justify withholding treatment when clinical manifestations suggest RMSF.

Culture of *R. rickettsii* is available only at specialized laboratories.

PEARLS & PITFALLS

- Negative test results for RMSF do not justify withholding treatment when clinical manifestations suggest RMSF.

Serologic tests are not useful for acute diagnosis because they usually become positive only during convalescence. Indirect immunofluorescence assay using 2 paired samples is usually done.

For additional specifics of diagnosis, see p. 1691.

Treatment

- Doxycycline

Starting antibiotics early significantly reduces mortality, from about 20 to 5%, and prevents most complications. If patients who have been in an endemic area have a tick bite but no clinical symptoms or signs, antibiotics should not be given immediately.

If fever, headache, and malaise occur with or without a rash, antibiotics should be started promptly.

Primary treatment is doxycycline 200 mg po once followed by 100 mg bid until the patient improves, has been afebrile for 24 to 48 h, and has received treatment for at least 7 days.

Chloramphenicol 500 mg po or IV qid for 7 days is 2nd-line treatment.

Severely ill patients with RMSF may have a marked increase in capillary permeability in later stages; thus, IV fluids should be given cautiously to maintain BP while avoiding worsening pulmonary and cerebral edema.

No effective vaccine is available. Measures can be taken to prevent tick bites (see Sidebar 201–1).

KEY POINTS

- Despite its name, RMSF occurs in practically all of the US and throughout Central and South America.
- Small-vessel vasculitis can cause serious illness affecting the CNS, lungs, heart, kidneys, liver, and spleen; untreated mortality is about 20%.
- Symptoms (severe headache, chills, prostration, muscle pain) begin abruptly, followed by fever and usually a rash.
- Neurologic symptoms (headache, restlessness, insomnia, delirium, coma) may develop, indicating encephalitis.
- Suspect RMSF in any seriously ill patient who lives in or near a wooded area anywhere in the Western Hemisphere and has unexplained fever, headache, and prostration, with or without a history of tick contact.
- Test during acute illness with PCR or immunohistology of a skin biopsy specimen, but because sensitivity is only about 70%, a negative result should not affect the decision to begin antibiotics.
- Treat with doxycycline and provide supportive care as needed for hypovolemia and/or organ involvement.

SCRUB TYPHUS

(Mite-Borne Typhus; Tropical Typhus; Tsutsugamushi Disease)

Scrub typhus is a mite-borne disease caused by *Orientia tsutsugamushi* (formerly *Rickettsia tsutsugamushi*). Symptoms are fever, a primary lesion, a macular rash, and lymphadenopathy.

Scrub typhus is related to rickettsial diseases.

O. tsutsugamushi is transmitted by trombiculid mite larvae (chiggers), which feed on forest and rural rodents, including rats, voles, and field mice. Human infection also follows a chigger bite. The mites are both the vector and the natural reservoir for *O. tsutsugamushi*.

Scrub typhus is endemic in an area of Asia-Pacific bounded by Japan, Korea, China, India, and northern Australia.

Symptoms and Signs

After an incubation period of 6 to 21 days (mean 10 to 12 days), fever, chills, headache, and generalized lymphadenopathy start suddenly. At onset of fever, an eschar often develops at the site of the chigger bite. The typical lesion of scrub typhus, common in whites but rare in Asians, begins as a red, indurated lesion about 1 cm in diameter; it eventually vesiculates, ruptures, and becomes covered with a black scab. Regional lymph nodes enlarge.

Fever rises during the 1st wk, often to 40 to 40.5° C. Headache is severe and common, as is conjunctival injection. A macular rash develops on the trunk during the 5th to 8th day of fever, often extending to the arms and legs. It may disappear rapidly or become maculopapular and intensely colored. Cough is present during the 1st wk of fever, and pneumonitis may develop during the 2nd wk.

In severe cases, pulse rate increases; BP drops; and delirium, stupor, and muscular twitching develop. Splenomegaly may be present, and interstitial myocarditis is more common than in other rickettsial diseases. In untreated patients, high fever may persist ≥ 2 wk, then falls gradually over several days. With therapy, defervescence usually begins within 36 h. Recovery is prompt and uneventful.

Diagnosis

- Clinical features
- Biopsy of rash with fluorescent antibody staining to detect organisms
- Acute and convalescent serologic testing (serologic testing not useful acutely)
- PCR

For details of diagnosis, see p. 1691.

Treatment

- Doxycycline

Primary treatment is doxycycline 200 mg po once followed by 100 mg bid until the patient improves, has been afebrile for 48 h, and has received treatment for at least 7 days.

Chloramphenicol 500 mg po or IV qid for 7 days is 2nd-line treatment.

Clearing brush and spraying infested areas with residual insecticides eliminate or decrease mite populations. Insect repellents (eg, diethyltoluamide [DEET]) should be used when exposure is likely.

KEY POINTS

- Scrub typhus, endemic in Asia-Pacific, is transmitted by the bite of chiggers (mite larvae).
- Fever (often accompanied by an eschar at the bite site), chills, severe headache, and generalized lymphadenopathy start suddenly; a rash develops and spreads.
- Treat with doxycycline, which results in rapid improvement even in severe cases.

202 Sexually Transmitted Diseases

Sexually transmitted diseases (STDs), also termed sexually transmitted infections (STIs), can be caused by a number of microorganisms that vary widely in size, life cycle, symptoms, and susceptibility to available treatments.

Bacterial STDs include

- Syphilis
- Gonorrhea
- Chancroid
- Lymphogranuloma venereum
- Granuloma inguinale
- Chlamydial, mycoplasmal, and ureaplasmal infections

Viral STDs include

- Genital and anorectal warts
- Genital herpes
- Molluscum contagiosum
- HIV infection

Parasitic infections that can be sexually transmitted include

- Trichomoniasis (caused by protozoa)
- Scabies (caused by mites)
- Pediculosis pubis (caused by lice)

Many other infections not considered primarily to be STDs—including salmonellosis, shigellosis, campylobacteriosis, amebiasis, giardiasis, hepatitis (A, B, and C), and cytomegalovirus infection—can be transmitted sexually.

Because sexual activity includes close contact with skin and mucous membranes of the genitals, mouth, and rectum, many organisms are efficiently spread between people. Some STDs cause inflammation (eg, in gonorrhea or chlamydial infection) or ulceration (eg, in herpes simplex, syphilis, or chancroid), which predispose to transmission of other infections (eg, HIV).

STD prevalence rates remain high in most of the world, despite diagnostic and therapeutic advances that can rapidly render patients with many STDs noninfectious. In the US, an estimated 20 million new cases of STDs occur each year; about half occur in people aged 15 to 24 yr.

Factors impeding control of STDs include

- Unprotected sexual activity with multiple partners
- Difficulty talking about sexual issues for both physicians and patients
- Inadequate funding for implementing existing diagnostic tests and treatments and for developing new tests and treatments
- Susceptibility to reinfection if both partners are not treated simultaneously
- Incomplete treatment, which can lead to development of drug-resistant organisms
- International travel, which facilitates rapid global dissemination of STDs

Symptoms and Signs

Symptoms and signs vary depending on the infection. Many STDs cause genital lesions (see Table 202–1).

Diagnosis

- Often clinical evaluation
- Gram staining and culture
- Laboratory tests

STDs are diagnosed and treated in a variety of settings; for many, diagnostic tests are limited or unavailable or patient follow-up is uncertain. Thus, identification of the causative organism is often not pursued. Often, diagnosis is based only on clinical findings.

Table 202–1. DIFFERENTIATING COMMON SEXUALLY TRANSMITTED GENITAL LESIONS

FINDING	OTHER FEATURES	CAUSE*
Solitary painless ulcer	Indurated, nontender or only slightly tender Relatively nontender adenopathy	Syphilitic chancre
Clusters of small, painful superficial ulcers on an erythematous base	Sometimes with vesicles Inguinal adenopathy	Herpes simplex virus infection
Shallow painful ulcer	Nonindurated, tender ulcers with ragged, undermined edges and a red border, varying in size and often coalescing Regional adenopathy	Chancroid
Small papule or ulcer, often asymptomatic or unnoticed	Severely tender and painful adenopathy, sometimes with distal lymphedema or drainage to the skin Sometimes fever	Lymphogranuloma venereum
Multiple, shallow ulcers	Characteristic extragenital lesions and burrows	Excoriated scabies
Multiple, shallow lesions Visible lice, or egg sacs (nits) attached to hair shafts	—	Pediculosis pubis with excoriation
Elevated lesion	Velvety, malodorous, granulating lesions No inguinal adenopathy	Granuloma inguinale

*Other causes of ulcers include mucous patches of secondary syphilis, erosive balanitis, gummatous ulceration of tertiary syphilis, Behçet syndrome, epithelioma, and trauma.

Diagnostic testing may include Gram staining and culture or laboratory tests such as nucleic acid amplification tests (NAATs). Diagnostic testing is done more often in the following situations:

- The diagnosis is unclear.
- The infection is severe.
- Initial treatment is ineffective.
- Other reasons (eg, public health surveillance, psychosocial reasons, including extreme mental distress and depression) are compelling.

Treatment

- Syndromic treatment
- Sometimes antimicrobials
- Simultaneous treatment of sex partners

Because diagnostic tests are often limited or unavailable and/or patient follow-up is uncertain, initial treatment is often syndromic—ie, directed at the organisms most likely to cause the presenting syndrome (eg, urethritis, cervicitis, genital ulcers, pelvic inflammatory disease [PID]).

Most STDs can be effectively treated with drugs. However, drug resistance is an increasing problem.

Patients who are being treated for a bacterial STD should abstain from sexual intercourse until the infection has been eliminated from them and their sex partners. Sex partners should be evaluated and treated simultaneously.

Viral STDs, especially herpes and HIV infection, usually persist for life. Antiviral drugs can control but not yet cure all of these infections.

Prevention

STD control depends on

- Adequate facilities and trained personnel for diagnosis and treatment
- Public health programs for locating and treating recent sex partners of patients
- Follow-up for treated patients to ensure that they have been cured
- Education of health care practitioners and the public
- Avoidance of high-risk behaviors by patients

Condoms and vaginal dams, if used correctly, greatly decrease risk of some STDs.

Vaccines are unavailable for most STDs, except for hepatitis A and B and human papillomavirus infection.

CHANCROID

Chancroid is infection of the genital skin or mucous membranes caused by *Haemophilus ducreyi* and characterized by papules, painful ulcers, and enlargement of the inguinal lymph nodes leading to suppuration. Diagnosis is usually clinical because culturing the organism is difficult. Treatment is with a macrolide (azithromycin or erythromycin), ceftriaxone, or ciprofloxacin.

H. ducreyi is a short, slender, gram-negative bacillus with rounded ends.

Chancroid occurs in rare outbreaks in developed countries but is a common cause of genital ulcers throughout much of the developing world and often acquired by men from prostitutes. Like other STD causing genital ulcers, chancroid increases risk of HIV transmission.

Symptoms and Signs

After an incubation period of 3 to 7 days, small, painful papules appear and rapidly break down into shallow, soft, painful ulcers with ragged, undermined edges (ie, with overhanging tissue) and a red border. Ulcers vary in size and often coalesce. Deeper erosion occasionally leads to marked tissue destruction.

The inguinal lymph nodes become tender, enlarged, and matted together, forming a pus-filled abscess (bubo). The skin over the abscess may become red and shiny and may break down to form a sinus. The infection may spread to other areas of skin, resulting in new lesions. Phimosis, urethral stricture, and urethral fistula may result from chancroid.

Diagnosis

- Clinical evaluation
- Sometimes culture or PCR

Chancroid is suspected in patients who have unexplained genital ulcers or buboes (which may be mistaken for abscesses) and who have been in endemic areas. Genital ulcers with other causes (see Table 202–1) may resemble chancroid.

If available, a sample of pus from a bubo or exudate from the edge of an ulcer should be sent to a laboratory that can identify *H. ducreyi*. However, diagnosis is usually based on clinical findings alone because culture of the bacteria is difficult and microscopic identification is confounded by the mixed flora in ulcers. PCR testing is not commercially available, but several institutions have certified tests that are highly sensitive (98.4%) and specific (99.6%) for *H. ducreyi*. Clinical diagnosis has a lower sensitivity (53 to 95%) and specificity (41 to 75%).

Serologic testing for syphilis and HIV and cultures for herpes should be done to exclude other causes of genital ulcers. However, interpretation of test results is complicated by the fact that genital ulcers due to other conditions may be coinfected with *H. ducreyi*.

Treatment

- Antibiotics (various)

Treatment of chancroid should be started promptly, without waiting for test results. One of the following is recommended:

- A single-dose of azithromycin 1 g po or ceftriaxone 250 mg IM
- Erythromycin 500 mg po qid for 7 days
- Ciprofloxacin 500 mg po bid for 3 days

Patients treated for other causes of genital ulcers should be given antibiotics that also treat chancroid if chancroid is suspected and laboratory testing is impractical. Treatment of patients with HIV coinfection, particularly with single-dose regimens, may be ineffective. In these patients, ulcers may require up to 2 wk to heal, and lymphadenopathy may resolve more slowly.

Buboes can safely be aspirated for diagnosis or incised for symptomatic relief if patients are also given effective antibiotics.

Sex partners should be examined, and patients should have a serologic test for syphilis and HIV in 3 mo.

CHLAMYDIAL, MYCOPLASMAL, AND UREAPLASMAL MUCOSAL INFECTIONS

Sexually transmitted urethritis, cervicitis, proctitis, and pharyngitis not due to gonorrhea are caused predominantly by chlamydiae and infrequently by *mycoplasmas* or *Ureaplasma* sp. Chlamydiae may also cause salpingitis, epididymitis, perihepatitis, neonatal conjunctivitis, and infant pneumonia. Untreated chlamydial salpingitis can become chronic, causing minimal symptoms but having serious consequences. Diagnosis is by culture, immunoassay for antigens, or nucleic acid–based tests (NAT). Treatment is with single-dose azithromycin or a week of ofloxacin, levofloxacin, erythromycin, or a tetracycline.

Several organisms can cause nongonococcal sexually transmitted cervicitis in women and urethritis, proctitis, and pharyngitis in both sexes. These organisms include

- *Chlamydia trachomatis* (responsible for about 50% of such cases of urethritis and most cases of mucopurulent cervicitis)
- *Mycoplasma genitalium*
- *Ureaplasma urealyticum*
- *Trichomonas vaginalis* (trichomoniasis)

Chlamydiae may also cause lymphogranuloma venereum. The imprecise term "nonspecific urethritis" can be used, but only if tests for chlamydiae and gonococci are negative and no other pathogen is identified.

Symptoms and Signs

Men develop symptomatic urethritis after a 7- to 28-day incubation period, usually beginning with mild dysuria, discomfort in the urethra, and a clear to mucopurulent discharge. Discharge may be slight, and symptoms may be mild but are frequently more marked early in the morning; then, the urethral meatus is often red and blocked with dried secretions, which may also stain underclothes. Occasionally, onset is more acute and severe, with severe dysuria, frequency, and a copious, purulent discharge that simulates gonococcal urethritis. Infection may progress to epididymitis. After rectal or orogenital contact with an infected person, proctitis or pharyngitis may develop.

Women are usually asymptomatic, although vaginal discharge, dysuria, increased urinary frequency and urgency, pelvic pain, dyspareunia, and symptoms of urethritis may occur. Cervicitis with yellow, mucopurulent exudate and cervical ectopy (expansion of the red endocervical epithelium onto the vaginal surfaces of the cervix) are characteristic. PID (salpingitis and pelvic peritonitis) may cause lower abdominal discomfort (typically bilateral) and marked tenderness when the abdomen, adnexa, and cervix are palpated. Long-term consequences of PID include ectopic pregnancy and infertility. Fitz-Hugh-Curtis syndrome (perihepatitis) may cause right upper quadrant pain, fever, and vomiting.

Chlamydiae may be transferred to the eye, causing acute conjunctivitis.

Reactive arthritis caused by immunologic reactions to genital and intestinal infections is an infrequent complication of chlamydial infections in adults. Reactive arthritis sometimes causes skin and eye lesions and noninfectious recurrent urethritis.

Infants born to women with chlamydial cervicitis may develop chlamydial pneumonia or ophthalmia neonatorum (neonatal conjunctivitis).

Diagnosis

- NAT of cervical, urethral, pharyngeal, or rectal exudate or urine

Chlamydial, mycoplasmal, or ureaplasmal infection is suspected in patients with symptoms of urethritis, salpingitis, cervicitis, or unexplained proctitis, but similar symptoms can also result from gonococcal infection.

If clinical evidence for urethritis is uncertain, the Center for Disease Control and Prevention's 2015 STDs Treatment Guidelines state that urethritis can be documented by any of the following:

- Mucoid, mucopurulent, or purulent discharge observed during examination
- ≥ 10 WBCs per high-power field in spun first-void urine
- A positive leukocyte esterase test on first-void urine
- ≥ 2 WBCs per oil immersion field in Gram-stained urethral secretions

Samples of cervical or vaginal specimens or male urethral or rectal exudates are obtained to check for chlamydiae. Urine samples can be used as an alternative to cervical or urethral specimens. Throat and rectal swabs are needed to test for infection at those sites.

Commercially available NAT for chlamydial DNA may be done on nonamplified samples or samples amplified using one of several nucleic acid amplification techniques. Tests are usually done on swab samples, but NAATs are highly sensitive and specific and can also be done on urine, eliminating the need for doing an uncomfortable swab of the urethra or cervix. In general, samples from the throat and rectum should be tested only in laboratories that have verified the use of these tests for those anatomic sites. Amplification techniques should be routinely used for screening and diagnosis in patients at high risk (eg, unprotected sex with new or multiple partners, history of prior sexually transmitted disease, exchanging sex for drugs or money).

Because other STDs (particularly gonococcal infection) often coexist, patients who have symptomatic urethritis should also be tested for gonorrhea. Testing for other STDs, including serologic testing for syphilis and HIV, should also be considered.

Detection of mycoplasmas and *Ureaplasma* sp is currently impractical in routine practice; some commercial NAAT assays are being developed for mycoplasma but may not be widely available.

In the US, confirmed cases of chlamydial infection, gonorrhea, and syphilis must be reported to the public health system.

Screening: Urine testing using NAAT is especially useful for screening asymptomatic people at high risk of STDs because genital examination is not necessary. Screening recommendations vary by sex, age, sexual practices, and setting.

Nonpregnant women (including women who have sex with women) are screened annually if they

- Are sexually active and ≤ 24 yr
- Have a history of a prior STD
- Engage in high-risk sexual behavior (eg, have a new sex partner or multiple sex partners, engage in sex work, use condoms inconsistently)
- Have a partner who engages in high-risk behavior

Pregnant women are screened during their initial prenatal visit; those ≤ 24 yr or with risk factors are screened again during the 3rd trimester.

Heterosexually active men are not routinely screened except for those in situations with a high prevalence of chlamydial infection, including those with multiple sex partners, patients at adolescent or STD clinics, and men entering correctional facilities.

Men who have sex with men are screened if they have been sexually active within the previous year (for insertive intercourse, urine screen; for receptive intercourse, rectal swab; and for oral intercourse, pharyngeal swab).

(See also the US Preventive Services Task Force's summary of recommendations regarding screening for chlamydial infection at www.uspreventiveservicestaskforce.org.)

Treatment

- Oral antibiotics (preferably azithromycin)
- Empiric treatment for gonorrhea if it has not been excluded
- Treatment of sex partners

Uncomplicated documented or suspected chlamydial, ureaplasmal, or mycoplasmal infections are treated with one of the following:

- A single dose of azithromycin 1 g po
- Doxycycline 100 mg po bid for 7 days
- Erythromycin as the base 500 mg po or as ethylsuccinate 800 mg qid for 7 days
- Ofloxacin 300 mg po bid for 7 days
- Levofloxacin 500 mg po once/day for 7 days

Azithromycin (given as a single dose) is preferred to drugs that require multiple doses over 7 days.

For pregnant women, azithromycin 1 g po once should be used.

These regimens do not reliably treat gonorrhea, which coexists in many patients with chlamydial infections. Therefore, treatment should include a single dose of ceftriaxone 250 mg IM if gonorrhea has not been excluded.

Patients who relapse (about 10%) are usually coinfected with microbes that do not respond to antichlamydial therapy, or they were reinfected since treatment. They should be retested for chlamydial infection and gonorrhea and, if possible, for trichomoniasis. They should be treated with azithromycin unless they were treated with it before. If azithromycin has been ineffective, moxifloxacin should be tried. In areas where trichomoniasis is prevalent, empiric treatment with metronidazole is recommended unless PCR indicates patients are negative for trichomoniasis.

Current sex partners should be treated. Patients should abstain from sexual intercourse until they and their partners have been treated for ≥ 1 wk.

If chlamydial genital infections are untreated, symptoms and signs subside within 4 wk in about two thirds of patients. However, in women, asymptomatic cervical infection may persist, resulting in chronic endometritis, salpingitis, or pelvic peritonitis and their sequelae—pelvic pain, infertility, and increased risk of ectopic pregnancy. Because chlamydial infections can have serious long-term consequences for women, even when symptoms are mild or absent, detecting the infection in women and treating them and their sex partners is crucial.

KEY POINTS

- Sexually acquired chlamydial, mycoplasmal, and ureaplasmal infections may affect the urethra, cervix, adnexa, throat, or rectum.
- Diagnose using NAATs.
- Also test for coinfection with other STDs, including gonorrhea, syphilis, and HIV infection.
- Screen high-risk, asymptomatic patients for chlamydial infection.
- Use an antibiotic regimen that also treats gonorrhea if it has not been excluded.

GENITAL WARTS

(Anogenital Warts; Condylomata Acuminata; Venereal Warts)

Genital warts are lesions of the skin or mucous membranes of the genitals caused by certain types of human papillomavirus (HPV). Some types of HPV cause flat warts in the cervical canal or anus; infection with certain HPV types can lead to cancer. Diagnosis of external warts is based on their clinical appearance. Multiple treatments exist, but few are highly effective unless applied repeatedly over weeks to months. Genital warts may resolve without treatment in immunocompetent patients but may persist and spread widely in patients with decreased cell-mediated immunity (eg, due to pregnancy or HIV infection).

In the US, an estimated 1.4 million people have genital warts at any given time, and about 360,000 new cases of genital warts occur each year. In the US, there are about 14 million new cases of sexually transmitted HPV infection each year. By age 50, about 80% of sexually active women have been infected with genital HPV at least once.

Most HPV infections clear spontaneously within 1 to 2 yr, but some persist.

Etiology

There are > 100 known types of HPV. Some cause common skin warts. Some infect primarily the skin and mucosa of the anogenital region.

Important manifestations of anogenital HPV include

- Genital warts (condyloma acuminatum)
- Intraepithelial neoplasia and carcinoma of the cervix, anus, or penis
- Bladder and oral cancers
- Bowenoid papulosis

Condylomata acuminata are benign anogenital warts most often caused by HPV types 6 and 11. Low- and high-grade intraepithelial neoplasia and carcinoma may be caused by HPV. Virtually all cervical cancer is caused by HPV; about 70% is caused by types 16 and 18, and many of the rest result from types 31, 33, 35, and 39. HPV types that affect mainly the anogenital area can be transmitted to the oropharynx by orogenital contact; type 16 appears responsible for many cases of oropharyngeal cancer. HPV types 16 and 18 can also cause cancer in other areas, including the vulva, vagina, and penis.

HPV is transmitted from lesions during skin-to-skin contact. The types that affect the anogenital region are usually transmitted sexually by penetrative vaginal or anal intercourse, but digital, oral, and nonpenetrative genital contact may be involved.

Genital warts are more common among immunocompromised patients. Growth rates vary, but pregnancy, immunosuppression, or maceration of the skin may accelerate the growth and spread of warts.

Symptoms and Signs

Warts appear after an incubation period of 1 to 6 mo.

Visible anogenital warts are usually soft, moist, minute pink or gray polyps (raised lesions) that

- Enlarge
- May become pedunculated
- Have rough surfaces
- May occur in clusters

The warts are usually asymptomatic, but some patients have itching, burning, or discomfort.

In men, warts occur most commonly under the foreskin, on the coronal sulcus, within the urethral meatus, and on the penile shaft (see Plate 78). They may occur around the anus and in the rectum, especially in homosexual men.

In women, warts occur most commonly on the vulva, vaginal wall, cervix, and perineum (see Plate 77); the urethra and anal region may be affected.

HPV types 16 and 18 usually cause flat endocervical or anal warts that are difficult to see and diagnose clinically.

Diagnosis

- Clinical evaluation, sometimes including colposcopy, anoscopy, or both

Genital warts are usually diagnosed clinically. Their appearance usually differentiates them from condyloma lata of secondary syphilis (which are flat-topped) and from carcinomas. However, serologic tests for syphilis should be done initially and after 3 mo. Biopsies of atypical, bleeding, ulcerated, or persistent warts may be necessary to exclude carcinoma.

Endocervical and anal warts can be visualized only by colposcopy and anoscopy. Applying a 3 to 5% solution of acetic acid for a few minutes before colposcopy causes warts to whiten and enhances visualization and detection of small warts.

NAATs for HPV DNA confirm the diagnosis and allow typing of HPV, but their role in HPV management is not yet clear.

Treatment

- Mechanical removal (eg, by cryotherapy, electrocauterization, laser, or surgical excision)
- Topical treatment (eg, with antimitotics, caustics, or interferon inducers)

No treatment of anogenital warts is completely satisfactory, and relapses are frequent and require retreatment. In immunocompetent people, genital warts may resolve without treatment. In immunocompromised patients, warts may be less responsive to treatment.

Because no treatment is clearly more efficacious than others, treatment of anogenital warts should be guided by other considerations, mainly wart size, number, and anatomic site; patient preference; cost of treatment; convenience; adverse effects; and the practitioner's experience (see the Centers for Disease Control and Prevention's 2015 STDs Treatment Guidelines: Anogenital Warts at www.cdc.gov).

Genital warts may be removed by cryotherapy, electrocauterization, laser, or surgical excision; a local or general anesthetic is used depending on the size and number to be removed. Removal with a resectoscope may be the most effective treatment; a general anesthetic is used.

Topical antimitotics (eg, podophyllotoxin, podophyllin, 5-fluorouracil), caustics (eg, trichloroacetic acid), interferon inducers (eg, imiquimod), and sinecatechins (a newer botanical product with an unknown mechanism) are widely used but usually require multiple applications over weeks to months and are frequently ineffective. Before topical treatments are applied, surrounding tissue should be protected with petroleum jelly. Patients should be warned that after treatment, the area may be painful.

Interferon alfa (eg, interferon alfa-2b, interferon alfa-n3), intralesionally or IM, has cleared intractable lesions on the skin and genitals, but optimal administration and long-term effects are unclear. Also, in some patients with bowenoid papulosis of the genitals (caused by type 16 HPV), lesions initially disappeared after treatment with interferon alfa but reappeared as invasive cancers.

For intraurethral lesions, thiotepa (an alkylating drug), instilled in the urethra, is effective. In men, 5-fluorouracil applied bid to tid is highly effective for urethral lesions, but rarely, it causes swelling, leading to urethral obstruction.

Endocervical lesions should not be treated until Papanicolaou (Pap) test results rule out other cervical abnormalities (eg, dysplasia, cancer) that may dictate additional treatment.

By removing the moist underside of the prepuce, circumcision may prevent recurrences in uncircumcised men.

Sex partners of women with endocervical warts and of patients with bowenoid papulosis should be counseled and screened regularly for HPV-related lesions. A similar approach can be used for HPV in the rectum.

Current sex partners of people with genital warts should be examined and, if infected, treated.

Prevention

A **9-valent vaccine** and a **quadrivalent vaccine** that protect against the 2 types of HPV (types 6 and 11) that cause > 90% of visible genital warts are available. These vaccines also protect against the 2 types of HPV (types 16 and 18) that cause most cervical cancers. The 9-valent vaccine also protects against other types of HPV (types 31, 33, 45, 52, and 58) that cause about 15% of cervical cancers.

A **bivalent vaccine** that protects against only types 16 and 18 is also available.

The HPV vaccine (9-valent, quadrivalent, or bivalent—see Table 291–3 on p. 2467) is recommended for girls and women aged 9 to 26 yr for prevention of initial infection. Three doses are given, preferably at age 11 to 12 yr. The vaccine should be administered before onset of sexual activity, but girls and women who are sexually active should still be vaccinated.

Only the 9-valent or quadrivalent vaccine is recommended for males. Three doses of the vaccine are recommended for boys at age 11 to 12; boys aged 13 to 21 who have not completed the 3-dose series should also be given the vaccine. The vaccine is also recommended for men up to age 26 who have sex with men or whose immune system is compromised; it may be given to men aged 22 to 26 if they have not completed the 3-dose series.

Because of the location of these warts, condoms may not fully protect against infection.

KEY POINTS

- Genital warts are caused by a few types of human papillomavirus (HPV).
- HPV types 16 and 18 cause about 70% of cervical cancers and can cause cancer in other areas, including the vulva, vagina, penis, and oropharynx.
- Diagnose warts by inspection; HPV testing is available, but its role in HPV management is unclear.
- Remove warts mechanically or using various topical treatments.
- HPV vaccination is recommended for children and young adults of both sexes.

GONORRHEA

Gonorrhea is caused by the bacteria *Neisseria gonorrhoeae*. It typically infects epithelia of the urethra, cervix, rectum, pharynx, or conjunctivae, causing irritation or pain and purulent discharge. Dissemination to skin and joints, which is uncommon, causes sores on the skin, fever, and migratory polyarthritis or pauciarticular septic arthritis. Diagnosis is by microscopy, culture, or nucleic acid amplification tests (NAATs). Several oral or injectable antibiotics can be used, but drug resistance is an increasing problem.

N. gonorrhoeae is a gram-negative diplococcus that occurs only in humans and is almost always transmitted by sexual contact. Urethral and cervical infections are most common, but infection in the pharynx or rectum can occur after oral or anal intercourse, and conjunctivitis may follow contamination of the eye.

After an episode of vaginal intercourse, likelihood of transmission from women to men is about 20%, but from men to women, it may be higher. Neonates can acquire conjunctival infection during passage through the birth canal (see p. 2629), and children may acquire gonorrhea as a result of sexual abuse.

In 10 to 20% of women, cervical infection ascends via the endometrium to the fallopian tubes (salpingitis) and pelvic peritoneum, causing pelvic inflammatory disease (PID). Chlamydiae or intestinal bacteria may also cause PID. Gonorrheal cervicitis is commonly accompanied by dysuria or inflammation of Skene ducts and Bartholin glands. In a small fraction of men, ascending urethritis progresses to epididymitis.

Disseminated gonococcal infection (DGI) due to hematogenous spread occurs in < 1% of cases, predominantly in women. DGI typically affects the skin, tendon sheaths, and joints. Pericarditis, endocarditis, meningitis, and perihepatitis occur rarely.

Coinfection with *Chlamydia trachomatis* occurs in 15 to 25% of infected heterosexual men and 35 to 50% of women.

Symptoms and Signs

About 10 to 20% of infected women and very few infected men are asymptomatic. About 25% of men have minimal symptoms.

Male urethritis has an incubation period from 2 to 14 days. Onset is usually marked by mild discomfort in the urethra, followed by more severe penile tenderness and pain, dysuria, and a purulent discharge. Urinary frequency and urgency may develop as the infection spreads to the posterior urethra. Examination detects a purulent, yellow-green urethral discharge, and the meatus may be inflamed.

Epididymitis usually causes unilateral scrotal pain, tenderness, and swelling. Rarely, men develop abscesses of Tyson and Littre glands, periurethral abscesses, or infection of Cowper glands, the prostate, or the seminal vesicles.

Cervicitis usually has an incubation period of > 10 days. Symptoms range from mild to severe and include dysuria and vaginal discharge. During pelvic examination, clinicians may note a mucopurulent or purulent cervical discharge, and the cervical os may be red and bleed easily when touched with the speculum. Urethritis may occur concurrently; pus may be expressed from the urethra when the symphysis pubis is pressed or from Skene ducts or Bartholin glands. Rarely, infections in sexually abused prepubertal girls cause dysuria, purulent vaginal discharge, and vulvar irritation, erythema, and edema.

PID occurs in 10 to 20% of infected women. PID may include salpingitis, pelvic peritonitis, and pelvic abscesses and may cause lower abdominal discomfort (typically bilateral), dyspareunia, and marked tenderness on palpation of the abdomen, adnexa, or cervix.

Fitz-Hugh-Curtis syndrome is gonococcal (or chlamydial) perihepatitis that occurs predominantly in women and causes right upper quadrant abdominal pain, fever, nausea, and vomiting, often mimicking biliary or hepatic disease.

Rectal gonorrhea is usually asymptomatic. It occurs predominantly in men practicing receptive anal intercourse and can occur in women who participate in anal sex. Symptoms include rectal itching, a cloudy rectal discharge, bleeding, and constipation—all of varying severity. Examination with a proctoscope may detect erythema or mucopurulent exudate on the rectal wall.

Gonococcal pharyngitis is usually asymptomatic but may cause sore throat. *N. gonorrhoeae* must be distinguished from *N. meningitidis* and other closely related organisms that are often present in the throat without causing symptoms or harm.

DGI, also called the arthritis-dermatitis syndrome, reflects bacteremia and typically manifests with fever, migratory pain or joint swelling (polyarthritis), and pustular skin lesions. In some patients, pain develops and tendons (eg, at the wrist or ankle) redden or swell. Skin lesions (see Plate 73) occur typically on the arms or legs, have a red base, and are small, slightly painful, and often pustular. Genital gonorrhea, the usual source of disseminated infection, may be asymptomatic. DGI can mimic other disorders that cause fever, skin lesions, and polyarthritis (eg, the prodrome of hepatitis B infection or meningococcemia); some of these other disorders also cause genital symptoms (eg, reactive arthritis).

Gonococcal septic arthritis is a more localized form of DGI that results in a painful arthritis with effusion, usually of 1 or 2 large joints such as the knees, ankles, wrists, or elbows. Some patients present with or have a history of skin lesions of DGI. Onset is often acute, usually with fever, severe joint pain, and limitation of movement. Infected joints are swollen, and the overlying skin may be warm and red.

Diagnosis

- Gram staining and culture
- Nucleic acid–based testing

Gonorrhea is diagnosed when gonococci are detected via microscopic examination using Gram stain, culture, or a nucleic acid–based test of genital fluids, blood, or joint fluids (obtained by needle aspiration).

Gram stain is sensitive and specific for gonorrhea in men with urethral discharge; gram-negative intracellular diplococci typically are seen. Gram stain is much less accurate for infections of the cervix, pharynx, and rectum and is not recommended for diagnosis at these sites.

Culture is sensitive and specific, but because gonococci are fragile and fastidious, samples taken using a swab need to be rapidly plated on an appropriate medium (eg, modified Thayer-Martin) and transported to the laboratory in a CO_2-containing environment. Blood and joint fluid samples should be sent to the laboratory with notification that gonococcal infection is suspected. Because NAATs have replaced culture in most laboratories, finding a laboratory that can provide culture and sensitivity testing may be difficult and require consultation with a public health or infectious disease specialist.

NAATs may be done on genital, rectal, or oral swabs. Most tests simultaneously detect gonorrhea and chlamydial infection and then differentiate between them in a subsequent specific test. NAATs further increase the sensitivity adequately to enable testing of urine samples in both sexes.

In the US, confirmed cases of gonorrhea, chlamydial infection, and syphilis must be reported to the public health system. Serologic tests for syphilis and HIV and NAAT to screen for chlamydial infection should also be done.

Men with urethritis: Men with obvious discharge may be treated presumptively if likelihood of follow-up is questionable or if clinic-based diagnostic tools are not available.

Samples for Gram staining can be obtained by touching a swab or slide to the end of the penis to collect discharge. Gram stain does not identify chlamydiae, so urine or swab samples for NAAT are obtained.

Women with genital symptoms or signs: A cervical swab should be sent for culture or NAAT. If a pelvic examination is not possible, NAAT of a urine sample or self-collected vaginal swab can detect gonococcal (and chlamydial) infections rapidly and reliably.

Pharyngeal or rectal exposures (either sex): Swabs of the affected area are sent for culture or NAAT.

Arthritis, DGI, or both: An affected joint should be aspirated, and fluid should be sent for culture and routine analysis (arthrocentesis). Patients with skin lesions, systemic symptoms, or both should have blood, urethral, cervical, and rectal cultures or NAAT. In about 30 to 40% of patients with DGI, blood cultures are positive during the first week of illness. With gonococcal arthritis, blood cultures are less often positive, but cultures of joint fluids are usually positive. Joint fluid is usually cloudy to purulent because of large numbers of WBCs (typically > 20,000/μL).

Screening: Asymptomatic patients considered at high risk of STD can be screened by NAAT of urine samples, thus not requiring invasive procedures to collect samples from genital sites.

Nonpregnant women (including women who have sex with women) are screened annually if they

- Are sexually active and ≤ 24 yr
- Have a history of a prior STD
- Engage in high-risk sexual behavior (eg, have a new sex partner or multiple sex partners, engage in sex work, use condoms inconsistently)
- Have a partner who engages in high-risk behavior

Pregnant women are screened during their initial prenatal visit and again during the 3rd trimester if they are ≤ 24 yr or have risk factors.

Heterosexually active men are not routinely screened unless they are considered at high risk (eg, those with multiple sex partners, patients at adolescent or STD clinics, men entering correctional facilities).

Men who have sex with men are screened if they have been sexually active within the previous year (for insertive intercourse, urine screen; for receptive intercourse, rectal swab; and for oral intercourse, pharyngeal swab).

(See also the US Preventive Services Task Force's summary of recommendations regarding screening for gonorrhea at www.uspreventiveservicestaskforce.org.)

Treatment

- For uncomplicated infection, a single dose of ceftriaxone plus azithromycin
- For DGI with arthritis, a longer course of parenteral antibiotics
- Concomitant treatment for chlamydial infection
- Treatment of sex partners

Uncomplicated gonococcal infection of the urethra, cervix, rectum, and pharynx is treated with the following:

- Preferred: A single dose of ceftriaxone 250 mg IM plus azithromycin 1 g po once (an alternative to azithromycin is doxycycline 100 mg po bid for 7 days)
- Second choice: A single dose of cefixime 400 mg po plus azithromycin 1 g po once

Patients who are allergic to cephalosporins, are treated with one of the following:

- Gemifloxacin 320 mg po plus azithromycin 2 g po
- Gentamicin 240 mg IM plus azithromycin 2 g po

Monotherapy and previous oral regimens of fluoroquinolones (eg, ciprofloxacin, levofloxacin, ofloxacin) or cefixime are no longer recommended because of increasing drug resistance. Test of cure is recommended only for patients treated with an alternative regimen for pharyngeal infections.

DGI with gonococcal arthritis is initially treated with IM or IV antibiotics (eg, ceftriaxone 1 g IM or IV q 24 h, ceftizoxime 1 g IV q 8 h, cefotaxime 1 g IV q 8 h) continued for 24 to 48 h once symptoms lessen, followed by 4 to 7 days of oral therapy. Antichlamydial therapy is also routinely given.

Gonococcal arthritis does not usually require joint drainage. Initially, the joint is immobilized in a functional position. Passive range-of-motion exercises should be started as soon as patients can tolerate them. Once pain subsides, more active exercises, with stretching and muscle strengthening, should begin. Over 95% of patients treated for gonococcal arthritis recover complete joint function. Because sterile joint fluid accumulations (effusions) may persist for prolonged periods, an anti-inflammatory drug may be beneficial.

Posttreatment cultures are unnecessary if symptomatic response is adequate. However, for patients with symptoms for > 7 days, specimens should be obtained, cultured, and tested for antimicrobial sensitivity.

Patients should abstain from sexual activity until treatment is completed to avoid infecting sex partners.

PEARLS & PITFALLS

- To limit development of drug resistance, experts no longer recommend monotherapy for gonococcal infection.

Sex partners: All sex partners who have had sexual contact with the patient within 60 days should be tested for gonorrhea and other STDs and treated if results are positive. Sex partners with contact within 2 wk should be treated presumptively for gonorrhea (epidemiologic treatment).

Expedited partner therapy (EPT) involves giving patients a prescription or drugs to deliver to their partner. EPT may enhance partner adherence and reduce treatment failure due to reinfection. It may be most appropriate for partners of women with gonorrhea or chlamydial infection. However, a health care visit is preferable to ascertain histories of drug allergies and to screen for other STDs.

KEY POINTS

- Gonorrhea typically causes uncomplicated infection of the urethra, cervix, rectum, pharynx, and/or conjunctivae.
- Sometimes gonorrhea spreads to the adnexa, causing salpingitis, or disseminates to skin and/or joints, causing skin sores or septic arthritis.
- Diagnose using NAAT, but culture and sensitivity testing should be done when needed to detect antimicrobial resistance.
- Screen asymptomatic, high-risk patients using NAAT.
- Treat uncomplicated infection with a single dose of ceftriaxone 250 mg IM plus azithromycin 1 g po once.

GRANULOMA INGUINALE

(Donovanosis)

Granuloma inguinale is a rare, progressive infection of genital and perineal skin caused by *Klebsiella* (formerly *Calymmatobacterium*) *granulomatis*. The disease is characterized by slowly progressive skin lesions that are beefy red, raised, painless, and often ulcerated; regional lymphadenopathy is uncommon. Diagnosis is by clinical criteria and microscopy. Treatment is with antibiotics, usually tetracyclines, macrolides, or trimethoprim/sulfamethoxazole.

Infections with *K. granulomatis* are extremely rare but have been previously reported in areas such as Papua New Guinea, Australia, southern Africa, the Caribbean, and parts of Brazil and India.

Symptoms and Signs

Sites of infection are

- Penis, scrotum, groin, and thighs in men (see Plate 80)
- Vulva, vagina, and perineum in women (see Plate 79)
- Anus and buttocks in patients who engage in anal-receptive intercourse
- Face in both sexes

After an incubation period of about 1 to 12 wk, a painless, red skin nodule slowly enlarges, becoming a raised, beefy red, moist, smooth, foul-smelling lesion. The lesion slowly enlarges, often ulcerates, and may spread to other skin areas. Lesions heal slowly, with scarring. Secondary infections with other bacteria are common and can cause extensive tissue destruction. Lymphadenopathy is uncommon.

Occasionally, granuloma inguinale spreads through the bloodstream to the bones, joints, or liver; without treatment, anemia, wasting, and uncommonly death may occur.

Diagnosis

- Microscopic examination showing Donovan bodies in fluid from a lesion

Granuloma inguinale is suspected in patients from endemic areas with characteristic lesions.

Diagnosis is confirmed microscopically by the presence of Donovan bodies (numerous bacilli in the cytoplasm of macrophages shown by Giemsa or Wright stain) in smears of fluid from scrapings from the edge of lesions. These smears contain many plasma cells.

Biopsy specimens are taken if the diagnosis is unclear or if adequate tissue fluid cannot be obtained because lesions are dry, sclerotic, or necrotic. The bacteria do not grow on ordinary culture media.

Treatment

- Antibiotics (various)

Many oral antibiotics kill the bacteria, but tetracyclines, macrolides, and trimethoprim/sulfamethoxazole (TMP/SMX) are most effective, followed by ceftriaxone, aminoglycosides, fluoroquinolones, and chloramphenicol.

Recommended oral regimens include

- Doxycycline 100 mg bid for 3 wk
- TMP/SMX 160/800 mg bid for 3 wk
- Erythromycin 500 mg qid for 3 wk
- Azithromycin 1 g/wk for 3 wk

IV or IM antibiotics (eg, ceftriaxone) are an alternative.

Response to treatment should begin within 7 days, but healing of extensive disease may be slow and lesions may recur, requiring longer treatment. HIV-infected patients may also require prolonged or intensive treatment. After apparently successful treatment, follow-up should continue for 6 mo.

Current sex partners should be examined and, if infected, treated.

LYMPHOGRANULOMA VENEREUM

Lymphogranuloma venereum (LGV) is a disease caused by 3 unique strains of *Chlamydia trachomatis* and characterized by a small, often asymptomatic skin lesion, followed by regional lymphadenopathy in the groin or pelvis. Alternatively, if acquired by anal sex, it may manifest as severe proctitis. Without treatment, LGV may cause obstruction of lymph flow and chronic swelling of genital tissues. Diagnosis is by clinical signs, but laboratory confirmation with serologic or immunofluorescent testing is usually possible. Treatment is 21 days of a tetracycline or erythromycin.

LGV is caused by serotypes L1, L2, and L3 of the bacteria *Chlamydia trachomatis*. These serotypes differ from the chlamydial serotypes that cause trachoma, inclusion conjunctivitis, urethritis, and cervicitis because they can invade and reproduce in regional lymph nodes.

LGV occurs sporadically in the US but is endemic in parts of Africa, India, Southeast Asia, South America, and the Caribbean. It is diagnosed much more often in men than women.

Symptoms and Signs

The **1st stage** begins after an incubation period of about 3 days with a small skin lesion at the site of entry. It may cause the overlying skin to break down (ulcerate) but heals so quickly that it may pass unnoticed.

The **2nd stage** usually begins in men after about 2 to 4 wk, with the inguinal lymph nodes on one or both sides enlarging and forming large, tender, sometimes fluctuant masses (buboes). The buboes stick to deeper tissues and cause the overlying skin to become inflamed, sometimes with fever and malaise. In women, backache or pelvic pain is common; the initial lesions may be on the cervix or upper vagina, resulting in enlargement and inflammation of deeper perirectal and pelvic lymph nodes. Multiple draining sinus tracts may develop and discharge pus or blood.

In the **3rd stage,** lesions heal with scarring, but sinus tracts can persist or recur. Persistent inflammation due to untreated infection obstructs the lymphatic vessels, causing swelling and skin sores.

People who engage in receptive anal sex may have severe proctitis or proctocolitis with bloody purulent rectal discharge during the 1st stage. In the chronic stages, colitis simulating Crohn disease may cause tenesmus and strictures in the rectum or pain due to inflamed pelvic lymph nodes. Proctoscopy may detect diffuse inflammation, polyps, and masses or mucopurulent exudate—findings that resemble inflammatory bowel disease.

Diagnosis

- Antibody detection
- Sometimes nucleic acid amplification testing (NAAT)

LGV is suspected in patients who have genital ulcers, swollen inguinal lymph nodes, or proctitis and who live in, have visited, or have sexual contact with people from areas where infection is common. LGV is also suspected in patients with buboes, which may be mistaken for abscesses caused by other bacteria.

Diagnosis has usually been made by detecting antibodies to chlamydial endotoxin (complement fixation titers > 1:64 or microimmunofluorescence titers > 1:256) or by genotyping using a PCR-based NAAT. Antibody levels are usually elevated at presentation or shortly thereafter and remain elevated. Direct tests for chlamydial antigens with immunoassays (eg, enzyme-linked immunosorbent assay [ELISA]) or with immunofluorescence using monoclonal antibodies to stain pus or NAATs may be available through reference laboratories (eg, Centers for Disease Control and Prevention in the US).

All sex partners should be evaluated.

After apparently successful treatment, patients should be followed for 6 mo.

Treatment

- Oral tetracyclines or erythromycin
- Possibly drainage of buboes for symptomatic relief

Doxycycline 100 mg po bid, erythromycin 500 mg po qid, or tetracycline 500 mg po qid, each for 21 days, are effective for early disease. Azithromycin 1 g po once/wk for 1 to 3 wk is probably effective, but neither it nor clarithromycin has been adequately evaluated.

Swelling of damaged tissues in later stages may not resolve despite elimination of the bacteria. Buboes may be drained by needle or surgically if necessary for symptomatic relief, but most patients respond quickly to antibiotics. Buboes and sinus tracts may require surgery, but rectal strictures can usually be dilated.

Current sex partners, if infected, are treated.

SEXUALLY TRANSMITTED ENTERIC INFECTIONS

Various pathogens—bacterial (*Shigella*, *Campylobacter*, or *Salmonella*), viral (hepatitis A, B, and C viruses), and parasitic (*Giardia* sp or amebae)—are transmitted via sexual practices, especially those that can involve fecal-oral contamination. In order of decreasing risk, these practices are

- Oral-rectal
- Anal-genital
- Oral-genital
- Genital-genital intercourse

Although some of the above bacterial and parasitic pathogens may cause proctitis, they usually cause infection higher in the intestinal tract; symptoms include diarrhea, fever, bloating, nausea, and abdominal pain. Multiple infections are frequent, especially in people who have many sex partners and who engage in sexual practices that lead to direct or indirect oral-rectal contact.

Most of these pathogens can cause infections without symptoms; asymptomatic infection is the rule with *Entamoeba dispar* (formerly, nonpathogenic *Entamoeba histolytica*), which commonly occurs in homosexual men.

For diagnosis and treatment of these infections, see elsewhere in The Manual.

SYPHILIS

Syphilis is caused by the spirochete *Treponema pallidum* and is characterized by 3 sequential clinical, symptomatic stages separated by periods of asymptomatic latent infection. Common manifestations include genital ulcers, skin lesions, meningitis, aortic disease, and neurologic syndromes. Diagnosis is by serologic tests and adjunctive tests selected based on the disease stage. Penicillin is the drug of choice.

Syphilis is caused by *T. pallidum*, a spirochete that cannot survive for long outside the human body. *T. pallidum* enters through the mucous membranes or skin, reaches the regional lymph nodes within hours, and rapidly spreads throughout the body.

Syphilis occurs in primary, secondary, and tertiary stages (see Table 202–2), with long latent periods between them. Infected people are contagious during the first 2 stages.

Infection is usually transmitted by sexual contact (including genital, orogenital, and anogenital) but may be transmitted nonsexually by skin contact or transplacentally— see p. 2625). Risk of transmission is about 30% from a single sexual encounter with a person who has primary syphilis and 60 to 80% from an infected mother to a fetus. Infection does not lead to immunity against reinfection.

Symptoms and Signs

Syphilis may manifest at any stage and may affect multiple or single organs, mimicking many other disorders. Syphilis may be accelerated by coexisting HIV infection; in these cases, eye involvement, meningitis, and other neurologic complications are more common and more severe.

Primary syphilis: After an incubation period of 3 to 4 wk (range 1 to 13 wk), a primary lesion (chancre—see Plate 85) develops at the site of inoculation. The initial red papule quickly forms a chancre, usually a painless ulcer with a firm base; when rubbed, it produces clear fluid containing numerous spirochetes. Nearby lymph nodes may be enlarged, firm, and nontender.

Chancres can occur anywhere but are most common on the following:

- Penis, anus, and rectum in men
- Vulva, cervix, rectum, and perineum in women
- Lips or mouth in either sex

About half of infected women and one third of infected men are unaware of the chancre because it causes few symptoms. Chancres in the rectum or mouth, usually occurring in men, are often unnoticed.

The chancre usually heals in 3 to 12 weeks. Then, people appear to be completely healthy.

Secondary syphilis: The spirochete spreads in the bloodstream, producing widespread mucocutaneous lesions (see Plate 86), lymph node swelling, and, less commonly, symptoms in other organs. Symptoms typically begin 6 to 12 wk after the chancre appears; about 25% of patients still have a chancre. Fever, loss of appetite, nausea, and fatigue are common. Headache (due to meningitis), hearing loss (due to otitis), balance problems (due to labyrinthitis), visual disturbances (due to retinitis or uveitis), and bone pain (due to periostitis) can also occur.

Over 80% of patients have mucocutaneous lesions; a wide variety of rashes and lesions occur, and any body surface can be affected. Without treatment, lesions may disappear in a few days to weeks, persist for months, or return after healing, but all eventually heal, usually without scarring.

Syphilitic dermatitis is usually symmetric and more marked on the palms and soles. The individual lesions are round, often scale, and may coalesce to produce larger lesions, but they generally do not itch or hurt. After lesions resolve, the affected areas may be lighter or darker than normal. If the scalp is involved, alopecia areata often occurs.

Condyloma lata are hypertrophic, flattened, dull pink or gray papules at mucocutaneous junctions and in moist areas of the skin (eg, in the perianal area, under the breasts); lesions are extremely infectious. Lesions of the mouth, throat, larynx, penis, vulva, or rectum are usually circular, raised, and often gray to white with a red border.

Secondary syphilis can affect many other organs:

- About half of patients have lymphadenopathy, usually generalized, with nontender, firm, discrete nodes, and often hepatosplenomegaly.
- About 10% of patients have lesions in other organs, such as the eyes (uveitis), bones (periostitis), joints, meninges, kidneys (glomerulitis), liver (hepatitis), or spleen.
- About 10 to 30% of patients have mild meningitis, but < 1% have meningeal symptoms, which can include headache, neck stiffness, cranial nerve lesions, deafness, and eye inflammation (eg, optic neuritis, retinitis).

However, acute or subacute meningitis is more common among patients with HIV infection and may manifest as meningeal symptoms or strokes due to intracranial vasculitis.

Latent period: Latent syphilis can be early (< 1 yr after infection) or late (≥ 1 yr after infection).

Table 202–2. CLASSIFICATION OF SYPHILIS

STAGE	DESCRIPTION	SYMPTOMS AND SIGNS
Acquired		
Primary	Contagious	Chancre (a small, usually painless skin sore), regional lymphadenopathy
Secondary	Contagious Occurs weeks to months after the primary stage	Rashes (which may be confused with those due to several other disorders), sores on mucous membranes, hair loss, fever, many other symptoms
Latent	Asymptomatic; not contagious May persist indefinitely or be followed by late-stage disease	**Early latent syphilis** (infection < 1 yr duration), sometimes with recurrence of infectious lesions **Late latent syphilis** (infection ≥ 1 yr duration), rarely with recurrences; positive serologic tests
Late or tertiary	Symptomatic; not contagious	Clinically classified as benign tertiary syphilis, cardiovascular syphilis, or neurosyphilis (eg, asymptomatic, meningovascular, or parenchymatous neurosyphilis; tabes dorsalis)
Congenital*		
Early	Symptomatic Occurring up to age 2 yr	Overt disease
Late	Symptomatic Occurring later in life	Hutchinson teeth, eye or bone abnormalities

*Can also exist in a permanently latent (asymptomatic) state.

Symptoms and signs are absent, but antibodies, detected by serologic tests for syphilis (STS) persist. Because symptoms of primary and secondary syphilis are often minimal or ignored, patients frequently are first diagnosed during the latent stage when routine blood tests for syphilis are done.

Syphilis may remain latent permanently, but relapses with contagious skin or mucosal lesions may occur during the early latent period.

Patients are often given antibiotics for other disorders, which may cure latent syphilis and may account for the rarity of late-stage disease in developed countries.

Late or tertiary syphilis: About one third of untreated people develop late syphilis, although not until years to decades after the initial infection. Lesions may be clinically classified as benign tertiary syphilis, cardiovascular syphilis, or neurosyphilis.

Benign tertiary gummatous syphilis usually develops within 3 to 10 yr of infection and may involve the skin, bones, and internal organs. Gummas are soft, destructive, inflammatory masses that are typically localized but may diffusely infiltrate an organ or tissue; they grow and heal slowly and leave scars.

Benign tertiary syphilis of bone results in either inflammation or destructive lesions that cause a deep, boring pain, characteristically worse at night.

Cardiovascular syphilis usually manifests 10 to 25 yr after the initial infection as aneurysmal dilation of the ascending aorta, insufficiency of the aortic valve, or narrowing of the coronary arteries. Pulsations of the dilated aorta may cause symptoms by compressing or eroding adjacent structures in the chest. Symptoms include brassy cough, and obstruction of breathing due to pressure on the trachea, hoarseness due to vocal cord paralysis resulting from compression of the left laryngeal nerve, and painful erosion of the sternum and ribs or spine.

Neurosyphilis has several forms:

- Asymptomatic neurosyphilis
- Meningovascular neurosyphilis
- Parenchymatous neurosyphilis
- Tabes dorsalis

Asymptomatic neurosyphilis causes mild meningitis in about 15% of patients originally diagnosed as having latent syphilis, in 25 to 40% of those with secondary syphilis, in 12% of those with cardiovascular syphilis, and in 5% of those with benign tertiary syphilis. Without treatment, it evolves to symptomatic neurosyphilis in 5%. If CSF examination does not detect evidence of meningitis 2 yr after the initial infection, neurosyphilis is unlikely to develop.

Meningovascular neurosyphilis results from inflammation of large- to medium-sized arteries of the brain or spinal cord; symptoms typically occur 5 to 10 yr after infection and range from none to strokes. Initial symptoms may include headache, neck stiffness, dizziness, behavioral abnormalities, poor concentration, memory loss, lassitude, insomnia, and blurred vision. Spinal cord involvement may cause weakness and wasting of shoulder-girdle and arm muscles, slowly progressive leg weakness with urinary or fecal incontinence or both, and, rarely, sudden paralysis of the legs due to thrombosis of spinal arteries.

Parenchymatous neurosyphilis (general paresis, or dementia paralytica) results when chronic meningoencephalitis causes destruction of cortical parenchyma. It usually develops 15 to 20 yr after initial infection and typically does not affect patients before their 40s or 50s. Behavior progressively deteriorates, sometimes mimicking a mental disorder or dementia. Irritability, difficulty concentrating, deterioration of memory, defective judgment, headaches, insomnia, fatigue, and lethargy are common; seizures, aphasia, and transient hemiparesis are possible. Hygiene and grooming deteriorate. Patients may become emotionally unstable and depressed and have delusions of grandeur with lack of insight; wasting may occur. Tremors of the mouth, tongue, outstretched hands, and whole body may occur; other signs include pupillary abnormalities, dysarthria, hyperreflexia, and, in some patients, extensor plantar responses. Handwriting is usually shaky and illegible.

Tabes dorsalis (locomotor ataxia) involves slow, progressive degeneration of the posterior columns and nerve roots. It typically develops 20 to 30 yr after initial infection; mechanism is unknown. Usually, the earliest, most characteristic symptom is an intense, stabbing (lightning) pain in the back and legs that recurs irregularly. Gait ataxia, hyperesthesia, and paresthesia may produce a sensation of walking on foam rubber. Loss of bladder sensation leads to urine retention, incontinence, and recurrent infections. Erectile dysfunction is common.

Most patients with tabes dorsalis are thin and have characteristic sad facies and Argyll Robertson pupils (pupils that accommodate for near vision but do not respond to light). Optic atrophy may occur. Examination of the legs detects hypotonia, hyporeflexia, impaired vibratory and joint position sense, ataxia in the heel-shin test, absence of deep pain sensation, and Romberg sign. Tabes dorsalis tends to be intractable even with treatment. Visceral crises (episodic pain) are a variant of tabes dorsalis; paroxysms of pain occur in various organs, most commonly in the stomach (causing vomiting) but also in the rectum, bladder, and larynx.

Other lesions: Syphilitic ocular and otic manifestations can occur at any stage of the disease.

Ocular syndromes can affect virtually any part of the eye; they include interstitial keratitis, uveitis (anterior, intermediate, and posterior), chorioretinitis, retinitis, retinal vasculitis, and cranial nerve and optic neuropathies. Cases of ocular syphilis have occurred among HIV-infected men who have sex with men. Several cases resulted in significant morbidity, including blindness. Patients with ocular syphilis are at risk of neurosyphilis.

Otosyphilis may affect the cochlea (causing hearing loss and tinnitus) or vestibular system (causing vertigo and nystagmus).

Trophic lesions, secondary to hypoesthesia of the skin or periarticular tissues, may develop in the later stages. Trophic ulcers may develop on the soles of the feet and penetrate as deeply as the underlying bone.

Neurogenic arthropathy (Charcot joints), a painless joint degeneration with bony swelling and abnormal range of movement, is a classic manifestation of neuropathy.

Diagnosis

- Serologic reaginic tests (rapid plasma reagin [RPR] or Venereal Disease Research Laboratory [VDRL]) for screening blood and diagnosing CNS infections
- Serologic treponemal tests (eg, fluorescent treponemal antibody absorption or microhemagglutination assay for antibodies to *T. pallidum*)

(See also the US Preventive Services Task Force's summary of recommendations regarding screening for syphilis infection at www.uspreventiveservicestaskforce.org.)

Syphilis should be suspected in patients with typical mucocutaneous lesions or unexplained neurologic disorders, particularly in areas where the infection is prevalent. In such areas, it should also be considered in patients with a broad range of unexplained findings. Because clinical manifestations are so diverse and advanced stages are now relatively rare in most developed countries, syphilis may escape recognition. Patients with HIV and syphilis may have atypical or accelerated disease.

Diagnostic test selection depends on which stage of syphilis is suspected. Neurologic infection is best detected by and followed with quantitative reaginic tests of CSF. Cases must be reported to public health agencies.

Diagnostic tests for syphilis: Tests include serologic tests for syphilis (STS), which consist of

- Screening (a reaginic, or nontreponemal) tests
- Confirmatory (treponemal) tests
- Darkfield microscopy

T. pallidum cannot be grown in vitro. Traditionally, reaginic tests have been done first, and positive results are confirmed by a treponemal test. Some laboratories now reverse this sequence; they do newer, inexpensive treponemal tests first and confirm positive results using a nontreponemal test.

Nontreponemal (reaginic) tests use lipid antigens (cardiolipin from bovine hearts) to detect reagin (human antibodies that bind to lipids). The Venereal Disease Research Laboratory (VDRL) and rapid plasma reagin (RPR) tests are sensitive, simple, and inexpensive reaginic tests that are used for screening but are not completely specific for syphilis. Results may be presented qualitatively (eg, reactive, weakly reactive, borderline, or nonreactive) and quantitatively as titers (eg, positive at 1:16 dilution).

Many disorders other than treponemal infections (eg, SLE, antiphospholipid antibody syndromes) can produce a positive (biologically false-positive) reagin test result. CSF reaginic tests are reasonably sensitive for early disease but less so for late neurosyphilis. CSF reagin tests can be used to diagnose neurosyphilis or to monitor response to treatment by measuring antibody titers.

Treponemal tests detect antitreponemal antibodies qualitatively and are very specific for syphilis. They include the following:

- Fluorescent treponemal antibody absorption (FTA-ABS) test
- Microhemagglutination assay for antibodies to *T. pallidum* (MHA-TP)
- *T. pallidum* hemagglutination assay (TPHA)
- *T. pallidum* enzyme immunoassay (TP-EIA)
- Chemoluminescence immunoassays (CLIA)

If they do not confirm treponemal infection after a positive reaginic test, the reaginic result is deemed biologically false-positive. Treponemal tests of CSF are controversial, but some authorities believe the FTA-ABS test is sensitive.

Neither reaginic nor treponemal tests become positive until 3 to 6 wk after the initial infection. Thus, a negative result is common in early primary syphilis and does not exclude syphilis until after 6 wk. Reaginic titers decline after effective treatment, becoming negative by 1 yr in primary and by 2 yr in secondary syphilis. Treponemal tests usually remain positive for many decades, despite effective treatment and thus cannot be used to assess effectiveness.

Choice of tests and interpretation of test results depends on various factors, including previous syphilis, possible exposure to syphilis, and results of testing.

If patients have had syphilis, a reaginic test is done. A 4-fold increase in titer suggests new infection or failed treatment.

If patients have not had syphilis, treponemal and reaginic tests are done. Test results determine the next steps:

- Positive results on both tests: These results suggest new infection.
- Positive results on the treponemal test, but negative results on the reaginic test: A second treponemal test is done to confirm the positive test. If reaginic test results are repeatedly negative, treatment is not indicated.
- Positive results on treponemal test, negative results on the reaginic test, but history suggests recent exposure: A reaginic test is repeated 2 to 4 wk after exposure to make sure any new infection is detected.

Darkfield microscopy directs light obliquely through a slide of exudate from a chancre or lymph node aspirate to directly visualize spirochetes. Although the skills and equipment required are not usually available, darkfield microscopy is the most sensitive and specific test for early primary syphilis. The spirochetes appear against a dark background as bright, motile, narrow coils that are about 0.25 µm wide and 5 to 20 µm long. They must be distinguished morphologically from nonpathogenic spirochetes, which may be part of the normal flora, especially of the mouth. Therefore, darkfield examination of intraoral specimens for syphilis is not done.

Primary syphilis: Primary syphilis is usually suspected based on relatively painless genital (but occasionally extragenital) ulcers. Syphilitic ulcers should be differentiated from other sexually transmitted genital lesions (see Table 202–1). Coinfections with 2 ulcer-causing pathogens (eg, herpes simplex virus plus *T. pallidum*) are not rare.

Darkfield microscopy of exudate from a chancre or lymph node aspirate may be diagnostic. If results are negative or the test is unavailable, a reaginic STS is done. If results are negative or the test cannot be done immediately but a skin lesion has been present for < 3 wk (before the STS becomes positive) and an alternate diagnosis seems unlikely, treatment may be instituted, and the STS repeated in 2 to 4 wk.

Patients with syphilis should be tested for other STDs, including HIV infection, at diagnosis and 6 mo later.

Secondary syphilis: Because syphilis can mimic many diseases, it should be considered when any cutaneous eruption or mucosal lesion is undiagnosed, particularly if patients have any of the following:

- Generalized lymphadenopathy
- Lesions on the palms or soles
- Condyloma lata
- Risk factors (eg, HIV, multiple sex partners)

Clinically, secondary syphilis may be mistaken for a drug eruption, rubella, infectious mononucleosis, erythema multiforme, pityriasis rubra pilaris, fungal infection, or, particularly, pityriasis rosea. Condyloma lata may be mistaken for warts, hemorrhoids, or pemphigus vegetans; scalp lesions may be mistaken for ringworm or idiopathic alopecia areata.

Secondary syphilis is excluded by a negative reaginic STS, which is virtually always reactive during this stage, often with a high titer. A compatible syndrome with a positive STS (reaginic or treponemal) warrants treatment. Uncommonly, this combination represents latent syphilis coexisting with another skin disease. Patients with secondary syphilis should be tested for other STDs and for asymptomatic neurosyphilis.

Latent syphilis: Asymptomatic, latent syphilis is diagnosed when reaginic and treponemal STSs are positive in the absence of symptoms or signs of active syphilis. Such patients should have a thorough examination, particularly genital, skin, neurologic, and cardiovascular examinations, to exclude secondary and tertiary syphilis.

Criteria for early latent syphilis include during the prior year, a documented conversion from negative to positive treponemal test, a newly positive nontreponemal test, or a sustained (> 2-wk) 4-fold or greater increase in reaginic test titers plus any of the following:

- Unequivocal symptoms of primary or secondary syphilis
- A sex partner with documented primary, secondary, or early latent syphilis
- No possible exposure except during the previous 12 mo

Patients who have latent syphilis but do not fulfill the above criteria have late latent syphilis.

Treatment and serologic follow-up for up to several years may be needed to ensure the success of therapy because reaginic STS titers decrease slowly.

Latent acquired syphilis must be differentiated from latent congenital syphilis, latent yaws, and other treponemal infections.

Late or tertiary syphilis: Patients with symptoms or signs of tertiary syphilis (particularly unexplained neurologic abnormalities) require STS. If the test is reactive, the following should be done:

- Lumbar puncture for CSF examination (including reaginic STS)
- Imaging of the brain and aorta
- Screening of any other organ systems clinically suspected to be involved

At this stage of syphilis, a reaginic STS is nearly always positive, except in a few cases of tabes dorsalis.

In **benign tertiary syphilis,** differentiation from other inflammatory mass lesions or ulcers may be difficult without biopsy.

Cardiovascular syphilis is suggested by symptoms and signs of aneurysmal compression of adjacent structures, particularly stridor or hoarseness.

Syphilitic aortic aneurysm is suggested by aortic insufficiency without aortic stenosis and, on chest x-ray, by widening of the aortic root and linear calcification on the walls of the ascending aorta. Diagnosis of aneurysm is confirmed with aortic imaging (transesophageal echocardiography, CT, or MRI).

In **neurosyphilis,** most symptoms and signs, except for Argyll Robertson pupil, are nonspecific, so that diagnosis relies heavily on a high index of clinical suspicion. Asymptomatic neurosyphilis is diagnosed based on abnormal CSF (typically, lymphocytic pleocytosis and elevated protein) and a reactive CSF reaginic test. In parenchymatous neurosyphilis, the CSF reaginic and serum treponemal tests are reactive, and CSF typically has lymphocytic pleocytosis and elevated protein. If present, HIV may confound the diagnosis because it causes mild pleocytosis and various other neurologic symptoms.

If **ocular syphilis** is diagnosed, CSF testing for neurosyphilis should be done.

In **tabes dorsalis,** serum reaginic tests may be negative if patients have been previously treated, but serum treponemal tests are usually positive. CSF usually has lymphocytic pleocytosis and elevated protein, and sometimes reaginic or treponemal test results are positive; however, in many treated patients, CSF is normal.

Treatment

- Benzathine penicillin G for most infections
- Aqueous penicillin for ocular syphilis or neurosyphilis
- Treatment of sex partners

The treatment of choice in all stages of syphilis and during pregnancy is the sustained-release penicillin benzathine penicillin (Bicillin L-A). The combination of benzathine and procaine penicillin (Bicillin C-R) should not be used.

All sex partners within the past 3 mo (if primary syphilis is diagnosed) and within 1 yr (if secondary syphilis is diagnosed) should be evaluated and, if infected, treated.

PEARLS & PITFALLS

- Use only pure benzathine penicillin (Bicillin L-A) for syphilis; do not use the similarly named combination of benzathine and procaine penicillin (Bicillin C-R).

Primary, secondary, and latent syphilis: Benzathine penicillin G 2.4 million units IM given once produces blood levels that are sufficiently high for 2 wk to cure primary, secondary, and early (< 1 yr) latent syphilis. Doses of 1.2 million units are usually given in each buttock to reduce local reactions.

Additional injections of 2.4 million units should be given 7 and 14 days later for late (> 1 yr) latent syphilis or latent syphilis of unknown duration because treponemes occasionally persist in the CSF after single-dose regimens. Treatment is the same regardless of HIV status.

For nonpregnant patients with a significant penicillin allergy (anaphylactic, bronchospastic, or urticarial), the first alternative is doxycycline 100 mg po bid for 14 days (28 days for late latent syphilis or latent syphilis of unknown duration). Azithromycin 2 g po in a single dose is effective for primary, secondary, or early latent syphilis caused by susceptible strains. However, a single mutation that increases resistance is increasingly common in many parts of the world, including the US, and results in unacceptably high failure rates.

Azithromycin should not be used to treat pregnant women or late latent syphilis. Pregnant patients with a penicillin allergy should be hospitalized and desensitized to penicillin.

Ceftriaxone 1 g IM or IV once/day for 10 to 14 days has been effective in some patients with early syphilis and may be effective at later stages, but optimal dose and duration of therapy are unknown.

Late or tertiary syphilis: Benign or cardiovascular tertiary syphilis can be treated in the same way as late latent syphilis.

For **ocular syphilis or neurosyphilis,** aqueous penicillin 3 to 4 million units IV q 4 h (best penetrates the CNS but may be impractical) or procaine penicillin G 2.4 million units IM once/day plus 500 mg probenecid po qid is recommended; both drugs are given for 10 to 14 days, followed by benzathine penicillin 2.4 million units IM once/wk for up to 3 wk to provide total duration of therapy comparable to that for late latent syphilis. For patients who have penicillin allergies, ceftriaxone 2 g IM or IV once/day for 14 days can be effective, but cross-sensitivity with cephalosporins may be a concern. The alternative is penicillin desensitization because azithromycin and doxycycline have not been adequately evaluated in patients with neurosyphilis.

Treatment of **asymptomatic neurosyphilis** appears to prevent the development of new neurologic deficits. Patients with neurosyphilis may be given oral or IM antipsychotics to help control paresis.

Patients with **tabes dorsalis** and lightning pains should be given analgesics as needed; carbamazepine 200 mg po tid or qid sometimes helps.

Jarisch-Herxheimer reaction (JHR): Most patients with primary or secondary syphilis, especially those with secondary syphilis, have a JHR within 6 to 12 h of initial treatment. It typically manifests as malaise, fever, headache, sweating, rigors, anxiety, or a temporary exacerbation of the syphilitic lesions. The mechanism is not understood, and JHR may be misdiagnosed as an allergic reaction.

JHR usually subsides within 24 h and poses no danger. However, patients with general paresis or a high CSF cell count may have a more serious reaction, including seizures or strokes, and should be warned and observed accordingly.

Unanticipated JHR may occur if patients with undiagnosed syphilis are given antitreponemal antibiotics for other infections.

Posttreatment surveillance: After treatment, patients should have

- Examinations and reaginic tests at 3, 6, and 12 mo and annually thereafter until the test is nonreactive or until a durable 4-fold reduction in titer is achieved
- For neurosyphilis, syphilis testing every 6 mo until syphilis cell count is normal

The importance of repeated tests to confirm cure should be explained to patients before treatment. Examinations and reaginic tests should be done at 3, 6, and 12 mo after treatment and annually thereafter until the test is nonreactive. Failure of titers to decline by 4-fold at 6 mo suggests treatment failure. After successful treatment, primary lesions heal rapidly, and plasma reaginic titers fall and usually become qualitatively negative within 9 to 12 mo.

In about 15% of patients with primary or secondary syphilis treated as recommended, the reaginic titer does not decrease by 4-fold—the criterion used to define response at 1 yr after treatment. These patients should be followed clinically and serologically; they should also be evaluated for HIV infection. If follow-up cannot be ensured, CSF should be checked for neurosyphilis (because unrecognized neurosyphilis may be the cause of treatment failure), or patients should be retreated with benzathine penicillin 2.4 million units IM once/wk for 3 wk.

Treponemal tests may remain positive for decades or permanently and should not be measured to monitor progress. Serologic or clinical relapse, usually affecting the nervous system, may occur after 6 to 9 mo, but the cause may be reinfection rather than relapse.

Patients with neurosyphilis require CSF testing at 6-mo intervals until the CSF cell count is normal. In HIV-infected patients, persisting CSF pleocytosis may represent effects of HIV rather than persisting neurosyphilis. Normal CSF cell count, negative CSF and serum reaginic test results, and negative neurologic examination findings for 2 yr indicates probable cure. If any of the following is present, retreatment with a more intensive regimen of antibiotics is indicated:

- CSF cell count that remains abnormal for > 2 yr
- A serum reaginic test that remains reactive for > 2 yr
- An increasing serum reaginic test titer
- Clinical relapse

KEY POINTS

- Syphilis has 3 sequential clinical, symptomatic stages separated by periods of asymptomatic latent infection.
- A characteristic skin lesion (chancre) typically appears at the site of primary infection.
- Subsequently, almost any organ can be affected, but skin, mucous membranes, eyes, bone, aorta, meninges, and the brain are commonly affected.
- Diagnose using a nontreponemal (reaginic) test (eg, RPR, VDRL), and confirm positive results using a treponemal antibody test.
- Treat with penicillin whenever possible.
- Report cases of syphilis to public health agencies.

TRICHOMONIASIS

Trichomoniasis is infection of the vagina or male genital tract with *Trichomonas vaginalis*. It can be asymptomatic or cause urethritis, vaginitis, or occasionally cystitis, epididymitis, or prostatitis. Diagnosis is by direct microscopic examination, dipstick tests, or nucleic acid amplification tests (NAATs) of vaginal secretions or by urine or urethral culture. Patients and sex partners are treated with metronidazole or tinidazole.

T. vaginalis is a flagellated, sexually transmitted protozoan that more often infects women (about 20% of women of reproductive age) than men. Infection may be asymptomatic in either sex, but asymptomatic is the rule for men. In men, the organism may persist for long periods in the GU tract without causing symptoms and may be transmitted unwittingly to sex partners. Trichomoniasis may account for up to 5% of nongonococcal, nonchlamydial urethritis in men in some areas.

Coinfection with gonorrhea and other STDs is common.

Symptoms and Signs

In women, symptoms range from none to copious, yellow-green, frothy vaginal discharge with soreness of the vulva and perineum, dyspareunia, and dysuria. Asymptomatic infection may become symptomatic at any time as the vulva and perineum become inflamed and edema develops in the labia. The vaginal walls and surface of the cervix may have punctate, red "strawberry" spots. Urethritis and possibly cystitis may also occur.

Men are usually asymptomatic; however, sometimes urethritis results in a discharge that may be transient, frothy, or purulent or that causes dysuria and frequency, usually early in the morning. Often, urethritis is mild and causes only minimal urethral irritation and occasional moisture at the urethral meatus, under the foreskin, or both. Epididymitis and prostatitis are rare complications.

Diagnosis

- Microscopic examination of vaginal secretions, dipstick tests, or NAATs
- Culture of urine or urethral swabs from men

Trichomoniasis is suspected in women with vaginitis, in men with urethritis, and in their sex partners. Suspicion is high if symptoms persist after patients have been evaluated and treated for other infections such as gonorrhea and chlamydial, mycoplasmal, and ureaplasmal infections.

In women, diagnosis is based on clinical criteria and point of care (POC) testing. One of the following POC tests may be done:

- Direct microscopic examination of vaginal secretions
- Immunochromographic flow dipstick tests
- NAAT

Microscopic examination is the simplest method and enables clinicians to test for trichomoniasis and bacterial vaginosis at the same time. Tests for both infections should be done because they cause similar symptoms and/or may coexist. Vaginal secretions are obtained from the posterior fornix. The pH is measured. Secretions are then placed on 2 slides; they are diluted with 10% K hydroxide on one slide (KOH wet mount) and with 0.9% NaCl on the other (saline wet mount). For the whiff test, the KOH wet mount is checked for a fishy odor, which results from amines produced in trichomonas vaginitis or bacterial vaginosis. The saline wet mount is examined microscopically as soon as possible to detect trichomonads, which can become immotile and more difficult to recognize within minutes after slide preparation. (Trichomonads are pear-shaped with flagella, often motile, and average 7 to 10 μm—about the size of WBCs—but occasionally reach 25 μm.) If trichomoniasis is present, numerous neutrophils are also present. Trichomoniasis is also commonly diagnosed by seeing the organism when a Papanicolaou (Pap) test is done.

Alternatively, **immunochromographic flow dipstick tests** or **NAAT,** which are available from some laboratories, may be done. In women, these tests are more sensitive than microscopic examination or culture. Also, NAAT can be configured to simultaneously detect other organisms or other STDs such as chlamydial infection or gonorrhea.

Culture of urine or urethral swabs is the only validated test for detecting *T. vaginalis* in men. In men, microscopy of urine is insensitive, and NAAT and dipstick tests have not been rigorously validated; however, epidemiologic studies suggest that for NAAT, urethral swabs are better than urine.

As with diagnosis of any STD, patients with trichomoniasis should be tested to exclude other common STDs such as gonorrhea and chlamydial infection.

Treatment

- Oral metronidazole or tinidazole
- Treatment of sex partners

Metronidazole or tinidazole 2 g po in a single dose cures up to 95% of women if sex partners are treated simultaneously. Effectiveness of single-dose regimens in men is not as clear, so treatment is typically with metronidazole or tinidazole 500 mg po bid for 5 to 7 days.

If infection persists in women and reinfection by sex partners has been excluded, women are retreated first with metronidazole or tinidazole 2 g po once or metronidazole 500 mg bid for 7 days. If the initial retreatment regimen fails, metronidazole or tinidazole 2 g once/day for 5 days may be effective.

Metronidazole may cause leukopenia, disulfiram-like reactions to alcohol, or candidal superinfections. It is relatively contraindicated during early pregnancy, although it may not be dangerous to the fetus after the 1st trimester. Tinidazole has not been established as safe during pregnancy and so is not used.

Sex partners should be seen and treated for trichomoniasis with tinidazole 2 g in a single dose or metronidazole 500 mg bid for 5 days and should be screened for other STDs. If poor adherence to follow-up by sex partners is likely, treatment can be initiated in sex partners of patients with documented trichomoniasis without confirming the diagnosis in the partner.

KEY POINTS

- Trichomoniasis can be asymptomatic, particularly in men, or cause vaginitis or sometimes urethritis.
- In women, diagnose by microscopic examination of vaginal secretions, dipstick tests, or NAAT.
- In symptomatic men, diagnose by culture of urine, urethral swab, or possibly NAAT.
- Treat patients and their sex partners with oral metronidazole or tinidazole.

203 Spirochetes

BEJEL, PINTA, AND YAWS

Bejel, pinta, and yaws (endemic treponematoses) are chronic, tropical, nonvenereal spirochetal infections spread by body contact. Symptoms of bejel are mucous membrane and cutaneous lesions, followed by bone and skin gummas. Yaws causes periostitis and dermal lesions. Pinta lesions are confined to the dermis. Diagnosis is clinical and epidemiologic. Treatment is with penicillin.

The family Spirochaetales is distinguished by the helical shape of the bacteria. They are too thin to be visualized using routine microscopy but can be viewed using darkfield microscopy. There are 3 genera: *Treponema*, *Leptospira*, and *Borrelia*.

For bejel, pinta, and yaws, the causative agents are

- Bejel: *Treponema pallidum* subsp *endemicum*
- Yaws: *T. pallidum* subsp *pertenue*
- Pinta: *T. carateum*

These *Treponema* species are morphologically and serologically indistinguishable from the agent of syphilis, *T. pallidum* subsp *pallidum*. As in syphilis, the typical course is an initial mucocutaneous lesion followed by diffuse secondary lesions, a latent period, and late destructive disease.

Transmission is by close skin contact—sexual or not—primarily between children living in conditions of poor hygiene. Bejel (endemic syphilis) occurs mainly in arid countries of the eastern Mediterranean, southwest Asia, and North Africa. Transmission results from mouth-to-mouth contact or sharing eating and drinking utensils. Yaws (frambesia) is the most prevalent of the endemic treponematoses and occurs in humid equatorial countries where transmission is favored by scanty clothing and skin trauma. Pinta, which is more limited in geographical distribution, occurs among the natives of Mexico, Central America, and South America and is not very contagious. Transmission probably requires contact with broken skin.

Unlike *T. pallidum*, other human treponemal subspecies are not transmitted via blood or transplacentally.

Symptoms and Signs

Bejel begins in childhood as a mucous patch (usually on the buccal mucosa), which may go unnoticed, or as stomatitis at the angles of the lips. These painless lesions may resolve spontaneously but are usually followed by papulosquamous and erosive papular lesions of the trunk and extremities that are similar to yaws. Periostitis of the leg bones is common. Later, gummatous lesions of the nose and soft palate develop.

Yaws, after an incubation period of several weeks, begins at the site of inoculation as a red papule that enlarges, erodes, and ulcerates (primary yaws). The surface resembles a strawberry, and the exudate is rich in spirochetes. Local lymph nodes may be enlarged and tender. The lesion heals but is followed after months to a year by successive generalized eruptions that resemble the primary lesion (secondary yaws). These lesions often develop in moist areas of the axillae, skinfolds, and mucosal surfaces; they heal slowly and may recur. Keratotic lesions may develop on the palms and soles, causing painful ulcerations (crab yaws). Five to 10 yr later, destructive lesions (tertiary yaws) may develop; they include the following:

- Periostitis (particularly of the tibia)
- Proliferative exostoses of the nasal portion of the maxillary bone (goundou)
- Juxta-articular nodules
- Gummatous skin lesions
- Ultimately, mutilating facial ulcers, particularly around the nose (gangosa)

Pinta lesions are confined to the dermis. They begin at the inoculation site as a small papule that enlarges and becomes hyperkeratotic; they develop mainly on the extremities, face, and neck. After 3 to 9 mo, further thickened and flat lesions (pintids) appear all over the body and over bony prominences. Still later, some lesions become slate blue or depigmented, resembling vitiligo. Pinta lesions typically persist if not treated.

Diagnosis

- Clinical evaluation

Diagnosis of endemic treponematoses is based on the typical appearance of lesions in people from endemic areas.

Serologic tests for syphilis (the Venereal Disease Research Laboratory [VDRL] and fluorescent treponemal antibody absorption tests) are positive; thus, differentiation from venereal syphilis is clinical. Early lesions are often darkfield-positive for spirochetes and are indistinguishable from *T. pallidum* subsp *pallidum*.

Treatment

- Penicillin

Active disease is treated with 1 dose of penicillin benzathine 1.2 million units IM. Children < 45 kg should receive 600,000 units IM. A single dose of azithromycin 30 mg/kg po (maximum 2 g) or doxycycline 100 mg po bid for 14 days is an alternative for penicillin-allergic adults.

Public health control includes active case finding and treatment of family and close contacts with penicillin benzathine or doxycycline to prevent infection from developing.

KEY POINTS

- The *Treponema* species that cause bejel, pinta, and yaws are morphologically and serologically indistinguishable from the agent of syphilis, *T. pallidum* subsp *pallidum*.
- Disease is spread by close body contact, typically between children living in conditions of poor hygiene.
- As in syphilis, the typical course is an initial mucocutaneous lesion, followed by diffuse secondary lesions, a latent period, and late destructive disease.
- Serologic tests for syphilis (including fluorescent treponemal antibody tests) are positive; thus, differentiation from venereal syphilis is clinical.
- Give 1 dose of penicillin benzathine IM or, for penicillin-allergic adults, 2 wk of doxycycline 100 mg po bid.
- Treat close contacts with antibiotics.

LEPTOSPIROSIS

Leptospirosis is an infection caused by one of several pathogenic serotypes of the spirochete *Leptospira*. Symptoms are biphasic. Both phases involve acute febrile episodes; the 2nd phase sometimes includes hepatic, renal, and meningeal involvement. Diagnosis is by darkfield microscopy, culture, and serologic testing. Treatment is with doxycycline or penicillin.

The family Spirochaetales is distinguished by the helical shape of the bacteria. They are too thin to be visualized using routine microscopy but can be viewed using darkfield microscopy. There are 3 genera: *Treponema*, *Leptospira*, and *Borrelia*.

Leptospirosis, a zoonosis occurring in many domestic and wild animals, may cause inapparent illness or serious, even fatal disease. Human infections are rare in the US.

Leptospira are maintained in nature through chronic renal infection of carrier animals—commonly rats, dogs, cattle, horses, sheep, goat, and pigs. These animals can shed leptospires in their urine for years. Dogs and rats are probably common sources of human infection.

Human infections are acquired by direct contact with infected urine or tissue or indirectly by contact with contaminated water or soil. Abraded skin and exposed mucous membranes (conjunctival, nasal, oral) are the usual entry portals. Leptospirosis can be an occupational disease (eg, of farmers or sewer and abattoir workers), but in the US, most patients are exposed incidentally during recreational activities (eg, swimming in contaminated freshwater). Outbreaks have been reported outside the US after heavy rainfall or flooding.

Cases of leptospirosis must be reported to the CDC. The 40 to 100 known annual US cases occur mainly in late summer and early fall. Because distinctive clinical features are lacking, probably many more cases are not diagnosed and reported.

Symptoms and Signs

The incubation period ranges from 2 to 20 (usually 7 to 13) days.

Leptospirosis is characteristically biphasic.

The **septicemic phase** starts abruptly, with headache, severe muscular aches, chills, fever, cough, pharyngitis, chest pain, and, in some patients, hemoptysis. Conjunctival suffusion usually appears on the 3rd or 4th day. Splenomegaly and hepatomegaly are uncommon. This phase lasts 4 to 9 days, with recurrent chills and fever that often spikes to > 39° C. Defervescence follows.

The **2nd, or immune, phase** occurs between the 6th and 12th day of illness, correlating with appearance of antibodies in serum. Fever and earlier symptoms recur, and meningitis may develop. Iridocyclitis, optic neuritis, and peripheral neuropathy occur infrequently.

If acquired during pregnancy, leptospirosis, even during the convalescent period, may cause abortion.

Weil syndrome (icteric leptospirosis) is a severe form with jaundice and usually azotemia, anemia, diminished consciousness, and continued fever. Onset is similar to that of less severe forms. However, hemorrhagic manifestations, which are due to capillary injury and include epistaxis, petechiae, purpura, and ecchymoses, then develop and rarely progress to subarachnoid, adrenal, or GI hemorrhage. Thrombocytopenia may occur. Signs of hepatocellular and renal dysfunction appear from the 3rd to 6th day. Renal abnormalities include proteinuria, pyuria, hematuria, and azotemia. Hepatocellular damage is minimal, and healing is complete.

Mortality is nil in anicteric patients. With jaundice, the mortality rate is 5 to 10%; it is higher in patients > 60 yr.

Diagnosis

- Blood cultures
- Serologic testing
- Sometimes PCR

Similar symptoms can result from viral meningoencephalitis, hemolytic fever with renal syndrome due to hantaviruses, other spirochetal infections, influenza, and hepatitis. The history of biphasic illness may help differentiate leptospirosis.

Leptospirosis should be considered in any patient with FUO if they might have been exposed to leptospires.

Patients with suspected leptospirosis should have blood cultures, acute and convalescent (3- to 4-wk) antibody titers, CBC, serum chemistries, and liver function tests.

Meningeal findings mandate lumbar puncture; the CSF cell count is between 10 and 1000/μL (usually < 500/μL), with predominantly mononuclear cells. CSF glucose is normal; protein is < 100 mg/dL. CSF bilirubin levels are higher than serum bilirubin levels.

The peripheral blood WBC count is normal or slightly elevated in most patients but may reach 50,000/μL in severely ill patients with jaundice. The presence of > 70% neutrophils helps differentiate leptospirosis from viral illnesses. Serum bilirubin is elevated out of proportion to elevations in serum aminotransferases. In jaundiced patients, bilirubin levels are usually < 20 mg/dL (< 342 μmol/L) but may reach 40 mg/dL (684 μmol/L) in severe infection.

Leptospirosis is confirmed if leptospires are isolated from clinical specimens or seen in fluids or tissues. Blood and CSF cultures are likely to be positive during the 1st wk of illness, when leptospires may be present and before antibody titers are detectable; urine cultures are likely to be positive during wk 1 to 3 of illness. The laboratory should be notified that leptospirosis is suspected because special media and prolonged incubation are required.

Leptospirosis is also confirmed by either of the following:

- *Leptospira* agglutination antibody titer increases by ≥ 4-fold (microscopic agglutination test on paired samples obtained ≥ 2 wk apart).
- When only a single specimen is available, titer is ≥ 1:800 in patients with typical symptoms and signs (or ≥ 1:400 or even ≥ 1:100 in regions where the prevalence of leptospirosis is low).

Molecular assays, such as PCR, can also confirm the diagnosis rapidly during the early phase of the illness. An IgM enzyme-linked immunosorbent assay (ELISA) detects infections within 3 to 5 days, but positive results should be confirmed by definitive testing (cultures, microscopic agglutination test, PCR).

Treatment

- Penicillin
- Doxycycline

Antibiotic therapy is most effective when begun early in the infection.

In **severe illness**, one of the following is recommended:

- Penicillin G 5 to 6 million units IV q 6 h
- Ampicillin 500 to 1000 mg IV q 6 h

In **less severe cases**, one of the following may be given for 5 to 7 days:

- Doxycycline 100 mg po q 12 h
- Ampicillin 500 to 750 mg po q 6 h
- Amoxicillin 500 mg po q 6 h

In severe cases, supportive care, including fluid and electrolyte therapy, is also important.

Patient isolation is not required, but urine must be handled and disposed of carefully.

Doxycycline 200 mg po given once/wk during a period of known geographic exposure prevents disease.

KEY POINTS

- Leptospirosis is a zoonosis that occurs in many domestic and wild animals (particularly dogs and rats); human infections are rare and are acquired by contact with infected urine or tissue or contaminated water or soil.
- There are 2 phases of illness: septicemic and immune.
- The septicemic phase starts abruptly with headache, severe muscular aches, fever to > 39° C, chills, cough, sore throat, and sometimes hemoptysis; this phase lasts 4 to 9 days.
- The immune phase occurs between the 6th and 12th day of illness when antibodies appear in serum; fever and other symptoms recur, and some patients develop meningitis.
- Weil syndrome is a severe form with jaundice and usually azotemia, anemia, diminished consciousness, and sometimes hemorrhagic manifestations.
- Diagnose using blood cultures, CSF (in patients with meningeal findings), urine cultures, serologic tests, and PCR.
- Treat severe illness with parenteral penicillin G or ampicillin and less severe cases with oral doxycycline, ampicillin, or amoxicillin.

LYME DISEASE

Lyme disease is a tick-transmitted infection caused by the spirochete *Borrelia burgdorferi*. Early symptoms include an erythema migrans rash, which may be followed weeks to months later by neurologic, cardiac, or joint abnormalities. Diagnosis is primarily clinical in early-stage disease, but serologic testing can help diagnose cardiac, neurologic, and rheumatologic complications that occur later in the disease. Treatment is with antibiotics such as doxycycline or ceftriaxone.

The family Spirochaetales is distinguished by the helical shape of the bacteria. They are too thin to be visualized using routine microscopy but can be viewed using darkfield microscopy. There are 3 genera: *Treponema*, *Leptospira*, and *Borrelia*.

Epidemiology

Lyme disease was recognized in 1976 because of close clustering of cases in Lyme, Connecticut and is now the most commonly reported tick-borne illness in the US. It has been reported in 49 states, but > 90% of cases occur from Maine to Virginia and in Wisconsin, Minnesota, and Michigan. On the West Coast, most cases occur in northern California and Oregon. Lyme disease also occurs in Europe, across the former Soviet Union, and in China and Japan. Onset is usually in the summer and early fall. Most patients are children and young adults living in heavily wooded areas.

Lyme disease is transmitted primarily by 4 *Ixodes* sp worldwide:

- *Ixodes scapularis* (the deer tick) in the northeastern and north central US
- *I. pacificus* in the western US
- *I. ricinus* in Europe
- *I. persulcatus* in Asia

In the US, the white-footed mouse is the primary animal reservoir for *Borrelia burgdorferi* and the preferred host for nymphal and larval forms of the deer tick (see Fig. 188–1 on p. 1552). Deer are hosts for adult ticks but do not carry *Borrelia*. Other mammals (eg, dogs) can be incidental hosts and can develop Lyme disease. In Europe, sheep are hosts for the adult tick.

Pathophysiology

B. burgdorferi enters the skin at the site of the tick bite. After 3 to 32 days, the organisms migrate locally in the skin around the bite, spread via the lymphatics to cause regional adenopathy or disseminate in blood to organs or other skin sites. Initially, an inflammatory reaction (erythema migrans) occurs before significant antibody response to infection (serologic conversion).

Symptoms and Signs

Lyme disease has 3 stages:

- Early localized
- Early disseminated
- Late

The early and late stages are usually separated by an asymptomatic interval.

Early localized: Erythema migrans (EM—see Plate 74), the hallmark and best clinical indicator of Lyme disease, is the first sign of the disease. It occurs in at least 75% of patients, beginning as a red macule or papule at the site of the tick bite, usually on the proximal portion of an extremity or the trunk (especially the thigh, buttock, or axilla), between 3 and 32 days after a tick bite. Because tick nymphs are so small, most patients do not realize that they have been bitten.

The area expands, often with clearing between the center and periphery resembling a bull's eye, to a diameter ≤ 50 cm. Darkening erythema may develop in the center, which may be hot to the touch and indurated. Without therapy, EM typically fades within 3 to 4 wk.

Evanescent lesions may appear as EM resolves. Mucosal lesions do not occur. Apparent recurrences of EM lesions after treatment are caused by reinfection, rather than relapse, because the genotype identified in the new lesion differs from that of the original infecting organism.

Early disseminated: Symptoms of early-disseminated disease begin days or weeks after the appearance of the primary lesion, when the bacteria spread through the body. Soon after onset, nearly half of untreated patients develop multiple, usually smaller annular secondary skin lesions without indurated centers. Cultures of biopsy samples of these secondary lesions have been positive, indicating dissemination of infection.

Patients also develop a musculoskeletal, flu-like syndrome, consisting of malaise, fatigue, chills, fever, headache, stiff neck, myalgias, and arthralgias that may last for weeks. Because symptoms are often nonspecific, the diagnosis is frequently missed if EM is absent; a high index of suspicion is required. Frank arthritis is rare at this stage. Less common are backache, nausea and vomiting, sore throat, lymphadenopathy, and splenomegaly.

Symptoms are characteristically intermittent and changing, but malaise and fatigue may linger for weeks. Some patients develop symptoms of fibromyalgia. Resolved skin lesions may reappear faintly, sometimes before recurrent attacks of arthritis, in late-stage disease.

Neurologic abnormalities develop in about 15% of patients within weeks to months of EM (generally before arthritis occurs), commonly last for months, and usually resolve completely. Most common are lymphocytic meningitis (CSF pleocytosis of about 100 cells/μL) or meningoencephalitis, cranial neuritis (especially Bell palsy, which may be bilateral), and sensory or motor radiculoneuropathies, alone or in combination.

Myocardial abnormalities occur in about 8% of patients within weeks of EM. They include fluctuating degrees of atrioventricular block (1st-degree, Wenckebach, or 3rd-degree) and, rarely, myopericarditis with chest pain, reduced ejection fractions, and cardiomegaly.

Late: In untreated Lyme disease, the late stage begins months to years after initial infection. Arthritis develops in about 60% of patients within several months, occasionally up to 2 yr, of disease onset (as defined by EM). Intermittent swelling and pain in a few large joints, especially the knees, typically recur for several years. Affected knees commonly are much more swollen than painful; they are often hot, but rarely red. Baker cysts may form and rupture. Malaise, fatigue, and low-grade fever may precede or accompany arthritis attacks. In about 10% of patients, knee involvement is chronic (unremittent for ≥ 6 mo).

Other late findings (occurring years after onset) include an antibiotic-sensitive skin lesion (acrodermatitis chronica atrophicans) and chronic CNS abnormalities, either polyneuropathy or a subtle encephalopathy with mood, memory, and sleep disorders.

Diagnosis

- Clinical evaluation, supported by acute and convalescent serologic testing

EM is usually diagnosed clinically because it develops before serologic tests become positive.[1]

Cultures of blood and relevant body fluids (eg, CSF, joint fluid) may be obtained, primarily to diagnose other pathogens.

Acute (IgM) and convalescent (IgG) antibody titers 2 wk apart may be helpful; positive enzyme-linked immunosorbent assay (C6 ELISA) titers should be confirmed by Western blot. However, seroconversion may be late (eg, > 4 wk) or occasionally absent (eg, if patients received prior antibiotic therapy), and positive IgG titers alone represent previous exposure. If only IgM bands are detected on Western blot, especially long after exposure, the results are often false positive. PCR testing of CSF or synovial fluid is often positive when those sites are involved.

Consequently, diagnosis of Lyme disease depends on both test results and the presence of typical findings. A classic EM rash strongly suggests Lyme disease, particularly when supported by other elements (eg, recent tick bite, exposure to endemic area, typical systemic symptoms).

In areas where Lyme disease is endemic, many patients report arthralgias, fatigue, difficulty concentrating, or other nonspecific symptoms. Few patients who have these symptoms but have had no history of EM or other symptoms of early-localized or early-disseminated Lyme disease actually have Lyme disease. In such patients, elevated IgG titers (with normal IgM titers) indicate past exposure, not current or persistent infection, and may, if misinterpreted, lead to long and unnecessary courses of antibiotic therapy. There is no evidence linking *B. burgdorferi* infection to this fibromyalgia-like or chronic fatigue–like syndrome, often termed chronic Lyme disease.

Differential diagnosis: In the absence of rash, diagnosis is more difficult.

Early-disseminated disease may mimic juvenile idiopathic arthritis in children and reactive arthritis and atypical rheumatoid arthritis in adults. Findings that are often present in rheumatoid arthritis but not Lyme disease include morning stiffness, subcutaneous nodules, iridocyclitis, mucosal lesions, rheumatoid factor, and antinuclear antibodies. Late-stage Lyme disease lacks axial involvement, which distinguishes it from spondyloarthropathies with peripheral joint involvement.

In the US, human granulocytic anaplasmosis (a rickettsial infection) and babesiosis are also transmitted by *I. scapularis* and have a common geographic distribution in the northeastern and upper Midwest. Patients ill with any one of the diseases transmitted by *I. scapularis* may be concurrently infected with the other diseases it transmits; however, clinical coinfection with anaplasmosis is rare. A clinician should suspect that patients with Lyme disease also have

- Babesiosis if they have hemolytic anemia and thrombocytopenia
- Human granulocytic anaplasmosis if they have elevated aminotransferase levels, leukopenia, inclusion bodies in neutrophils, and/or thrombocytopenia

Acute rheumatic fever is considered in the occasional patient with migratory polyarthralgias and either an increased PR interval or chorea (as a manifestation of meningoencephalitis). However, patients with Lyme disease rarely have heart murmurs or evidence of a preceding streptococcal infection.

Human monocytotropic ehrlichiosis, which is caused by *Ehrlichia chaffeensis* and transmitted by the Lone Star tick, *Amblyomma americanum*, occurs mainly in the southeastern and south-central US and is unlikely to be confused with Lyme disease.

In southern and mid-Atlantic states, bites from the *A. americanum* tick may result in an EM-like rash accompanied by nonspecific self-limited systemic symptoms and signs. No specific infectious agent has yet been identified as the cause of this disorder (called southern tick-associated rash illness).

Lyme disease may cause Bell palsy and, in summer, can manifest with a musculoskeletal aseptic meningitis syndrome that mimics other causes of lymphocytic meningitis or that mimics peripheral neuropathies.

1. Sanchez E, Vannier E, Wormser GP, et al: Diagnosis, treatment, and prevention of Lyme disease, human granulocytic anaplasmosis, and babesiosis: a review. *JAMA* 315(16):1767–1777, 2016. doi:10:1001/jama.2016.2284.

Treatment

- Multiple alternatives that vary with stage of disease but typically include amoxicillin, doxycycline, and ceftriaxone

Most features of Lyme disease respond to antibiotics, but treatment of early disease is most successful. In late-stage disease, antibiotics eradicate the bacteria, relieving the arthritis in most people. However, a few genetically predisposed people have persistent arthritis even after the infection has been eliminated because of continued inflammation. Table 203–1 shows adult treatment regimens for various presentations of Lyme disease. Treatment in children is similar except that doxycycline is avoided in children < 8 yr and doses are adjusted based on weight (see Table 184–3 on p. 1497).

For symptomatic relief, NSAIDs may be used. Complete heart block may require a temporary pacemaker. Tense knee joints due to effusions require aspiration. Some genetically predisposed patients with arthritis of the knee that persists despite antibiotic therapy may respond to arthroscopic synovectomy.

Prevention

Precautions against tick bite should be taken by people in endemic areas. Deer tick nymphs, which attack humans, are small and difficult to see. Once attached to the skin, they gorge on blood for days. Transmission of *B. burgdorferi* does not usually occur until the infected tick has been in place for > 36 h. Thus, searching for ticks after potential exposure and removing them promptly can help prevent infection.

Routine use of antibiotic prophylaxis to prevent Lyme disease after a recognized tick bite is not recommended. Patients with a known tick bite can easily be instructed to monitor the bite site and seek care if rash or other symptoms occur; the diagnostic dilemma of Lyme is most prominent when there is no history of tick bite. A single dose of doxycycline 200 mg po has been shown to reduce the likelihood of Lyme disease after a deer tick bite. According to the 2006 Infectious Diseases Society of America (IDSA) guidelines, antibiotic prophylaxis should be offered only when all the following circumstances exist:[1]

- The attached tick can be reliably identified as an adult or nymphal *I. scapularis* tick.
- The tick is estimated to have been attached ≥ 36 h (based on degree of engorgement of the tick with blood or time of exposure).
- Prophylaxis can be started within 72 h of tick removal.
- Patients live in or have visited an area where ≥ 20% of these ticks are infected with *B. burgdorferi* (generally only in parts of New England, parts of the mid-Atlantic states, and parts of Minnesota and Wisconsin).
- Doxycycline is not contraindicated; it is contraindicated in pregnant or lactating women, children < 8 yr, and people who have had an allergic reaction to a tetracycline antibiotic.

1. Wormser GP, Dattwyler RJ, Shapiro ED, et al: The clinical assessment, treatment, and prevention of Lyme disease, human granulocytic anaplasmosis, and babesiosis: Clinical practice guidelines by the Infectious Diseases Society of America. *Clin Infect Dis* 43(9):1089–1134, 2006.

KEY POINTS

- In the US, > 90% of Lyme disease cases occur from Maine to Virginia and in Wisconsin, Minnesota, and Michigan; *Ixodes scapularis* (the deer tick) is the primary vector in these areas.
- In the US, the white-footed mouse is the primary animal reservoir for *Borrelia burgdorferi* and the preferred host for nymphal and larval forms of the deer tick; deer are hosts for adult ticks but do not carry *Borrelia*.
- Lyme disease has 3 stages: early localized, early disseminated, and late.
- Erythema migrans is the first and best clinical indicator; it occurs in ≥ 75% of patients.
- In endemic areas, few patients who have arthralgias, fatigue, difficulty concentrating, or other nonspecific symptoms but who have had no history of EM or other symptoms of early-localized or early-disseminated Lyme disease actually have Lyme disease.
- Diagnose clinically if typical rash is present; otherwise, do acute and convalescent serologic testing (ELISA confirmed by Western blot).
- Treat with oral or parenteral antibiotics depending on disease manifestations.

RAT-BITE FEVER

Rat-bite fever is caused by either *Streptobacillus moniliformis* or *Spirillum minus*. Symptoms of the streptobacillary form include fever, rash, and arthralgias. The spirillary form causes relapsing fever, rash, and regional lymphadenitis. Diagnosis is clinical and confirmed by culture and sometimes rising antibody titers. Treatment is with penicillin or doxycycline.

Rat-bite fever is transmitted to humans in up to 10% of rat bites. However, there may be no history of rat bite. Rat-bite fever is most commonly caused by rat bites but can be caused

Table 203–1. GUIDELINES FOR ANTIBIOTIC TREATMENT OF LYME DISEASE IN ADULTS*

DRUG	DOSAGE
Early Lyme disease[†]	
Amoxicillin	500 mg po tid for 14–21 days
Doxycycline	100 mg po bid for 14–21 days
Cefuroxime axetil	500 mg po bid for 14–21 days
Neurologic manifestations	
Bell palsy (no other neurologic abnormalities):	
Doxycycline	As for early disease
Meningitis (with or without radiculoneuropathy or encephalitis)[‡]:	
Ceftriaxone	2 g IV once/day for 14–28 days
Cefotaxime	2 g IV q 8 h for 14–28 days
Penicillin G	3–4 million units IV q 4 h for 14–28 days
Doxycycline	100–200 mg po bid for 14–28 days
Cardiac manifestations	
Ceftriaxone	2 g IV once/day for 14–21 days
Penicillin G	3–4 million units IV q 4 h for 14–21 days
Doxycycline	100 mg po bid for 14–21 days[§]
Amoxicillin	500 mg po tid for 14–21 days[§]
Arthritis (no neurologic involvement)[‖]	
Amoxicillin	500 mg po tid for 28 days
Doxycycline	100 mg po bid for 28 days
Cefuroxime axetil	500 mg po bid for 28 days
Ceftriaxone	2 g IV once/day for 28 days
Penicillin G	3–4 million units IV q 4 h for 28 days
Acrodermatitis chronica atrophicans	
Amoxicillin	500 mg po tid for 21 days
Doxycycline	100 mg po bid for 21 days

*Pregnant women may receive amoxicillin 500 mg tid for 21 days. No treatment is necessary for pregnant women who are seropositive but asymptomatic.

†Without neurologic, cardiac, or joint involvement. For early Lyme disease limited to a single erythema migrans lesion, 10 days is sufficient.

‡Optimal duration of therapy has not been established. There are no controlled trials of therapy > 4 wk for any neurologic manifestation of Lyme disease.

§For mild carditis with 1st-degree heart block, PR interval ≤ 30 sec, and normal ventricular function.

‖Treatment begins with an oral regimen, which is repeated if response is inadequate. If there was no response or symptoms worsen, parenteral ceftriaxone is given.

Adapted from Wormser GP, Dattwyler RJ, Shapiro ED, et al: The clinical assessment, treatment, and prevention of Lyme disease, human granulocytic anaplasmosis, and babesiosis: clinical practice guidelines by the Infectious Diseases Society of America. *Clinical Infectious Diseases* 43:1089–1134, 2006.

by the bite of any rodent or of a carnivore that preys on rodents. Both the streptobacillary and spirillary forms affect mainly urban dwellers living in crowded conditions and biomedical laboratory personnel. In the US and Europe, rat-bite fever is usually due to *Streptobacillus moniliformis*; in Asia, it is usually due to the spirochete *Spirillum minus*.

Streptobacillary rat-bite fever: Streptobacillary rat-bite fever is caused by the pleomorphic gram-negative bacillus *S. moniliformis*, an organism present in the oropharynx of healthy rats. Epidemics have been associated with ingestion of unpasteurized milk contaminated by *S. moniliformis* (Haverhill fever), but infection is usually a consequence of a bite by a wild rat or mouse. Other rodents and weasels have also been implicated.

The primary wound usually heals promptly, but after an incubation period of 1 to 22 (usually < 10) days, a viral-like syndrome develops abruptly, causing chills, fever, vomiting, headache, and back and joint pains. Most patients develop a morbilliform, petechial, or vesicular rash on the hands and feet about 3 days later. Polyarthralgia or arthritis, usually affecting the large joints asymmetrically, develops in many patients within 1 wk and, if untreated, may persist for several days or months. Fever may return, occurring irregularly over a period of weeks to months.

Bacterial endocarditis and abscesses in the brain or other tissues are rare but serious. Some patients have infected pericardial effusion and infected amniotic fluid.

Haverhill fever (erythema arthriticum epidemicum) resembles percutaneously acquired rat-bite fever, but with more prominent pharyngitis and vomiting.

Diagnosis of streptobacillary rat-bite fever is confirmed by culturing the organism from blood or joint fluid. Measurable agglutinins develop during the 2nd or 3rd wk and are diagnostically important if the titer increases. PCR or enzyme-linked immunosorbent assay (ELISA) tests may be helpful. The WBC count ranges between 6,000 and 30,000/μL. Nontreponemal syphilis serologic tests (Venereal Disease Research Laboratory [VDRL] or rapid plasma reagin [RPR] tests) may be falsely positive. The streptobacillary form usually can be differentiated clinically from the spirillary form.

Treatment of streptobacillary rat-bite fever involves one of the following given for 7 to 10 days:

- Amoxicillin 1 g po q 8 h
- Procaine penicillin G 600,000 units IM q 12 h
- Penicillin V 500 mg po qid

Erythromycin 500 mg po qid may be used for patients allergic to penicillin. Doxycycline 100 mg q 12 h for 14 days is an alternative.

Patients with *S. moniliformis* endocarditis require high-dose penicillin G plus either streptomycin or gentamicin.

Untreated, rat bite fever has a case fatality rate of about 10%.

Spirillary rat-bite fever (sodoku): *S. minus* infection is acquired through a rat bite or occasionally a mouse bite. Ingestion of the organism does not cause disease. The wound usually heals promptly, but inflammation recurs at the site after 4 to 28 (usually > 10) days, accompanied by a relapsing fever and regional lymphadenitis. A roseolar-urticarial rash sometimes develops but is less prominent than the streptobacillary rash. Systemic symptoms commonly accompany fever, but arthritis is rare. In untreated patients, 2- to 4-day cycles of fever usually recur for 4 to 8 wk, but febrile episodes rarely recur for > 1 yr.

Diagnosis of spirillary rat-bite fever is by

- Direct visualization or culture of *Spirillum* from blood smears or tissue from lesions or lymph nodes
- Giemsa stain or darkfield examination of blood from inoculated mice

Direct visualization is required because *S. minus* cannot be cultured on synthetic media. The WBC count ranges between 5,000 and 30,000/μL.

The VDRL results are false-positive in half the patients. The disease may easily be confused with malaria or *Borrelia recurrentis* infection; both are characterized by relapsing fever.

Treatment of spirillary rat-bite fever is the same as for the streptobacillary form.

RELAPSING FEVER

(Tick, Recurrent, or Famine Fever)

Relapsing fever is a recurring febrile disease caused by several species of the spirochete *Borrelia* and transmitted by lice or ticks. Symptoms are recurrent febrile episodes with headache, myalgia, and vomiting lasting 3 to 5 days, separated by intervals of apparent recovery. Diagnosis is clinical, confirmed by staining of peripheral blood smears. Treatment is with a tetracycline or erythromycin.

The family Spirochaetales is distinguished by the helical shape of the bacteria. They are too thin to be visualized using routine microscopy but can be viewed using darkfield microscopy. There are 3 genera: *Treponema*, *Leptospira*, and *Borrelia*.

The insect vector may be soft ticks of the genus *Ornithodoros* or the human body louse, depending on geographic location.

Louse-borne relapsing fevers are rare in the US; they are endemic only in northeast Africa (Ethiopia, Sudan, Eritrea, Somalia) and were recently diagnosed in Europe in refugees from these African countries. Louse-borne relapsing fever tends to occur in epidemics, particularly in regions affected by war, and in refugee camps. The louse is infected by feeding on a febrile patient; humans are the only reservoir. If the louse is crushed on a new host, *Borrelia* are released and can enter abraded skin or bites. Intact lice do not transmit disease.

Tick-borne relapsing fevers are endemic in the Americas, Africa, Asia, and Europe. In the US, the disease is generally confined to the western states, where occurrence is highest between May and September. Ticks acquire the spirochetes from rodent reservoirs. Humans are infected when spirochetes in the tick's saliva or excreta enter the skin rapidly as the tick bites. Infection is more likely to be acquired by people sleeping in rodent-infested cabins in the mountains.

Congenital infection with *Borrelia* has also been reported.

The case fatality rate is generally < 5% with treatment but may be considerably higher in very young, pregnant, old, malnourished, or debilitated people or during epidemics of louse-borne fever.

Symptoms and Signs

Because the tick feeds transiently and painlessly at night and does not remain attached for a long time, most patients do not report a history of tick bite but may report an overnight exposure to caves or rustic dwellings.

When present, louse infestation is usually obvious.

The incubation period ranges from 3 to 11 days (median, 6 days).

The clinical manifestations of tick-borne and louse-borne relapsing fever are very similar. Symptoms correspond to the level of bacteremia and, after several days, resolve when *Borrelia* are cleared from the blood. Bacteremia and symptoms then return after a 1-wk afebrile period. Symptoms are less severe with each subsequent return. A single relapse characterizes louse-borne relapsing fever, and up to 10 relapses may occur in tick-borne relapsing fever.

Sudden chills mark the onset, followed by high fever, tachycardia, severe headache, nausea, vomiting, muscle and joint pain, and often delirium. An eschar may be present at the site of the tick bite. An erythematous macular or purpuric rash may appear early over the trunk and extremities. Conjunctival, subcutaneous, or submucous hemorrhages may be present. Fever remains high for 3 to 5 days, then clears abruptly, indicating a turning point in the disease. The duration of illness ranges from 1 to 54 days (median, 18 days). Later in the several weeks' course of the disease, jaundice, hepatomegaly, splenomegaly, myocarditis, and heart failure may occur, especially in louse-borne disease.

Other symptoms may include ophthalmitis, iridocyclitis, exacerbation of asthma, and erythema multiforme. Neurologic complications (eg, meningitis, meningoencephalitis, radiculomyelitis) may occur; they are more common in tick-borne relapsing fever. Spontaneous abortion can occur.

Patients are usually asymptomatic for several days to ≥ 1 wk between the initial episode and the first relapse. Relapses, related to the cyclic development of the parasites, occur with a sudden return of fever and often arthralgia and all the former symptoms and signs. Jaundice is more common during relapse. The illness clears as before, but 2 to 10 similar episodes may follow at intervals of 1 to 2 wk. The episodes become progressively less severe, and patients eventually recover as they develop immunity.

Diagnosis

- Darkfield microscopy

The diagnosis of relapsing fever is suggested by recurrent fever and confirmed by visualization of spirochetes in the blood during a febrile episode. The spirochetes may be seen on darkfield examination or Wright- or Giemsa-stained thick and thin blood smears. (Acridine orange stain for examining blood or tissue is more sensitive than Wright or Giemsa stain.) Serologic tests are unreliable. Mild polymorphonuclear leukocytosis may occur. Serologic tests for syphilis and Lyme disease may be falsely positive.

Differential diagnosis includes Lyme arthritis, malaria, dengue, yellow fever, leptospirosis, typhus, influenza, and enteric fevers.

Treatment

- Tetracycline, doxycycline, or erythromycin

In relapsing fever transmitted by ticks, tetracycline or erythromycin 500 mg po q 6 h is given for 5 to 10 days. For louse-transmitted relapsing fever, a single 500-mg oral dose of either drug is effective. Doxycycline 100 mg po q 12 h for 5 to 10 days is also effective. Children < 8 yr are given erythromycin estolate 10 mg/kg po tid.

When vomiting or severe disease precludes oral administration or when the CNS is affected, parenteral ceftriaxone 2 g/day for 10 to 14 days or doxycycline 1 to 2 mg/kg IV q 12 to 24 h may be given to adults or children > 8 yr. Children < 8 yr are given penicillin G 25,000 units/kg IV q 6 h.

Therapy should be started early during fever. A Jarisch-Herxheimer reaction may occur within 2 h of starting therapy. Severity of the Jarisch-Herxheimer reaction may be lessened by giving acetaminophen 650 mg po 2 h before and 2 h after the first dose of doxycycline or erythromycin.

Dehydration and electrolyte imbalance should be corrected with parenteral fluids. Acetaminophen with oxycodone or hydrocodone may be used for severe headache. Nausea and vomiting should be treated with prochlorperazine 5 to 10 mg po or IM once/day to qid. If heart failure occurs, specific therapy is indicated.

KEY POINTS

- Relapsing fever is caused by several *Borrelia* species and is transmitted by lice or ticks.
- Patients have sudden chills, high fever, severe headache, nausea, vomiting, muscle and joint pain, and often delirium and/or a rash on the trunk and extremities; jaundice, hepatomegaly, splenomegaly, myocarditis, and heart failure may occur, especially in louse-borne disease.
- Untreated patients have 2 to 10 relapses at 1- to 2-wk intervals; relapses manifest with a sudden return of fever and often arthralgia and all the former symptoms and signs, although they may be less severe.
- Diagnose using darkfield microscopy or Wright- or Giemsa-stained thick and thin blood smears; serologic tests are unreliable.
- Treat with tetracycline, doxycycline, or erythromycin.

204 Trematodes (Flukes)

Flukes are parasitic flatworms that infect the blood vessels, GI tract, lungs, or liver. They are often categorized according to the organ system they invade:

- *Clonorchis sinensis*, *Fasciola hepatica*, and *Opisthorchis* sp: Liver
- *Fasciolopsis buski*, *Heterophyes heterophyes*, and related organisms: Lumen of the GI tract
- *Paragonimus westermani* and related species: Lungs and other organs such as the CNS
- *Schistosoma* sp: Vasculature of the GI or GU system

CLONORCHIASIS

(Chinese or Oriental Liver Fluke Infection)

Clonorchiasis is infection with the liver fluke *Clonorchis sinensis*. Infection is acquired by eating undercooked freshwater fish. Symptoms include fever, chills, epigastric pain, tender hepatomegaly, diarrhea, and mild jaundice. Diagnosis is by identifying eggs in the feces or duodenal contents. Treatment is with praziquantel or albendazole.

Flukes are parasitic flatworms that infect various parts of the body (eg, blood vessels, GI tract, lungs, liver) depending on the species.

Clonorchis is endemic in the Far East, especially in Korea, Japan, Taiwan, and southern China, and infection occurs elsewhere among immigrants and people eating fish imported from endemic areas.

Pathophysiology

Adult forms of *C. sinensis* live in the bile ducts. Eggs are passed in the stool and ingested by snails. Cercariae (free-swimming larvae) released from infected snails subsequently infect a variety of freshwater fish. Humans become infected by eating raw, undercooked, dried, salted, or pickled fish containing encysted metacercariae (resting or maturing stage). Metacercariae are released in the duodenum, enter the common bile duct through the ampulla of Vater, and migrate to smaller intrahepatic ducts (or occasionally the gallbladder and pancreatic ducts), where they mature into adults in about 1 mo. The adults may live ≥ 20 yr and grow to about 10 to 25 mm by 3 to 5 mm.

Symptoms and Signs

Light infections are usually asymptomatic. In the acute phase, heavier infections can cause fever, chills, epigastric pain, tender hepatomegaly, mild jaundice, and eosinophilia. Later, diarrhea may occur. Chronic cholangitis in heavy infections may progress to atrophy of liver parenchyma, portal fibrosis, and cirrhosis. Jaundice may occur if a mass of flukes obstructs the biliary tree. Other complications include suppurative cholangitis, cholelithiasis, pancreatitis, and, late in the course, cholangiocarcinoma.

Diagnosis

- Microscopic examination of stool

Diagnosis of clonorchiasis is by finding eggs in the feces or duodenal contents. The eggs are difficult to distinguish from those of *Opisthorchis*. Occasionally, the diagnosis is made by identifying adult flukes in surgical specimens or by doing percutaneous transhepatic cholangiography.

Other tests are nondiagnostic but may be abnormal; alkaline phosphatase, bilirubin, and eosinophil counts may be elevated.

A plain abdominal x-ray occasionally shows intrahepatic calcification. Hepatic ultrasonography, CT, MRI, ERCP, or cholangiography may show ductal irregularities and evidence of scarring.

Treatment

- Praziquantel or albendazole

Treatment of clonorchiasis is with praziquantel 25 mg/kg po tid for 2 days or albendazole 10 mg/kg po once/day for 7 days.

Biliary obstruction may require surgery.

Prevention involves thoroughly cooking freshwater fish from endemic waters and not eating it raw, pickled, or wine-soaked.

FASCIOLIASIS

Fascioliasis is infection with the liver fluke *Fasciola hepatica*, which is acquired by eating contaminated watercress or other water plants.

Flukes are parasitic flatworms that infect various parts of the body (eg, blood vessels, GI tract, lungs, liver) depending on the species.

F. hepatica is the sheep and cattle liver fluke. Incidental human fascioliasis, acquired by eating watercress contaminated by sheep or cattle dung, occurs in Europe, Africa, China, and South America but is rare in the US.

In acute infection, immature flukes migrate through the intestinal wall, the peritoneal cavity, the liver capsule, and the parenchyma of the liver before entering the biliary ducts where they mature to adulthood in about 3 to 4 mo.

Symptoms and Signs

Acute infection causes abdominal pain, hepatomegaly, nausea, vomiting, intermittent fever, urticaria, eosinophilia, malaise, and weight loss due to liver damage.

Chronic infection may be asymptomatic or lead to intermittent abdominal pain, cholelithiasis, cholangitis, obstructive jaundice, or pancreatitis.

Heavy infection can cause sclerosing cholangitis and biliary cirrhosis. Ectopic lesions may occur in the intestinal wall, lungs, or other organs. Pharyngeal fascioliasis has been reported after consumption of infected raw liver in the Middle East.

Diagnosis

- Antibody assays
- Microscopic examination of stool or duodenal or biliary material for eggs

CT frequently shows hypodense lesions in the liver during the acute stage of infection. Ultrasonography, CT, MRI, ERCP, or cholangiography can detect biliary tract abnormalities in chronic disease.

Antibody detection assays are useful in

- The early stages of infection before eggs are produced
- Chronic infection when egg production is sporadic or low

Loss of detectable antibodies occurs 6 to 12 mo after cure.

In chronic infections, eggs may be recovered from the stool or from duodenal or biliary materials. The eggs are indistinguishable from those of *Fasciolopsis buski.* In endemic areas, eggs can also be seen in stool after ingestion of infected animal livers. Thus, patients should be asked to follow a liver-free diet for several days before their stool is examined.

Treatment

- Triclabendazole or nitazoxanide

Treatment of fascioliasis is with triclabendazole (10 mg/kg po once after meals or, for severe infections, twice 12 to 24 h apart); it is available from the Centers for Disease Control and Prevention (CDC) as an investigational drug. An alternative is nitazoxanide 500 mg bid po for 7 days.

Treatment failures are common with praziquantel.

FASCIOLOPSIASIS

Fasciolopsiasis is infection with the intestinal fluke *Fasciolopsis buski*, which is acquired by eating aquatic plants.

Flukes are parasitic flatworms that infect various parts of the body (blood vessels, GI tract, lungs, liver) depending on the species.

F. buski is present in the intestine of pigs in many parts of Asia and the Indian subcontinent.

Human infection is acquired by eating aquatic plants (eg, water chestnuts) that bear infectious metacercariae (encysted stage). Adult worms attach to and ulcerate the mucosa of the proximal small bowel. They grow to about 20 to 75 mm by 8 to 20 mm. Adults have a life span of about 1 yr.

Most infections are light and asymptomatic, but heavy infections may cause diarrhea, abdominal pain, fever, and signs of malabsorption or intestinal obstruction.

Diagnosis of fasciolopsiasis is made by finding eggs or, less commonly, adult worms in the feces. The eggs are indistinguishable from those of *Fasciola hepatica.*

Treatment of fasciolopsiasis is with praziquantel 25 mg/kg po once (WHO) or tid for 1 day (CDC).

HETEROPHYIASIS AND RELATED TREMATODE INFECTIONS

Heterophyiasis is infection with the intestinal fluke *Heterophyes heterophyes*, which is acquired by eating infected raw or undercooked fish from freshwater or brackish water.

Flukes are parasitic flatworms that infect various parts of the body (eg, blood vessels, GI tract, lungs, liver) depending on the species.

Heterophyes heterophyes is endemic in the Far East, Middle East, and Egypt.

Infection is acquired by eating infected raw or undercooked fish from freshwater or brackish water containing metacercariae (encysted stage). After ingestion, metacercariae excyst and attach to the mucosa of the small intestine. There, they develop into adults, growing to about 1.0 to 1.7 mm by 0.3 to 0.4 mm.

Infection with *Metagonimus yokogawai*, a related trematode, has been reported after eating raw or undercooked freshwater or brackish fish in the Far East, Siberia, Manchuria, the Balkan states, Israel, and Spain. Intestinal infection with *Nanophyetus salmincola* has been reported after ingestion of raw or undercooked salmon.

Adult flukes can cause abdominal pain and diarrhea.

Diagnosis of heterophyiasis is by finding eggs in the feces. The eggs of *H. heterophyes* are indistinguishable from those of *M. yokogawai* and similar to those of *Clonorchis* and *Opisthorchis*.

Treatment of heterophyiasis is with praziquantel 25 mg/kg po tid for 1 day for *H. heterophyes* and *M. yokogawai* and 20 mg/kg po tid for 1 day for *N. salmincola*.

OPISTHORCHIASIS

Opisthorchiasis is infection with *Opisthorchis viverrini* (Southeast Asian liver fluke) or *O. felineus* (cat liver fluke), which are acquired by eating infected raw or undercooked fish.

Flukes are parasitic flatworms that infect various parts of the body (eg, blood vessels, GI tract, lungs, liver) depending on the species.

Opisthorchiasis due to *O. viverrini* occurs mainly in northeast Thailand, Laos, and Cambodia; *O. felineus* occurs mainly in Europe and Asia, including the former Soviet Union. The life cycle of *Opisthorchis* requires both snails and fish. Human disease resembles clonorchiasis and is acquired by eating raw or undercooked freshwater fish that contains infectious metacercariae (encysted stage). After ingestion, metacercariae excyst and ascend through the ampulla of Vater into the biliary ducts, where they attach to the mucosa and mature. Adult flukes grow to 5 to 10 mm by 1 to 2 mm (*O. viverrini*) or 7 to 12 mm by 2 to 3 mm (*O. felineus*).

Most infections are subclinical. Symptoms of opisthorchiasis include vague GI discomfort, diarrhea, and constipation. In chronic infection, symptoms may be more severe; hepatomegaly and undernutrition may be present. Rare complications include cholecystitis, cholangitis, and cholangiocarcinoma.

Diagnosis of opisthorchiasis is by finding eggs in the feces. Ultrasonography, CT, MRI, cholangiography, or ERCP may show biliary tract abnormalities.

The **treatment** of choice for opisthorchiasis is

- Praziquantel 25 mg/kg po tid for 2 days

Infection can be prevented by cooking freshwater fish.

PARAGONIMIASIS

(Endemic Hemoptysis; Oriental Lung Fluke Infection)

Paragonimiasis is infection with the lung fluke *Paragonimus westermani* and related species. Humans are infected by eating raw, pickled, or poorly cooked freshwater crustaceans. Symptoms include chronic cough, chest pain, dyspnea, and hemoptysis. Allergic skin reactions and CNS abnormalities due to ectopic flukes, including seizures, aphasia, paresis, and visual disturbances, can also occur. Diagnosis is by identifying eggs in sputum, stool, or pleural or peritoneal fluid. Serologic tests are also available. Praziquantel is the treatment of choice.

Flukes are parasitic flatworms that infect various parts of the body (eg, blood vessels, GI tract, lungs, liver) depending on the species.

Although > 30 species of *Paragonimus* exist and 10 have been reported to infect humans, *P. westermani* is the most frequent cause of disease. The most important endemic areas are in the Far East, principally Korea, Japan, Taiwan, the highlands of China, and the Philippines. Endemic foci with other *Paragonimus* spp exist in West Africa and in parts of South and Central America. *P. kellicotti* has caused human infection in North America.

Pathophysiology

Eggs passed in sputum or feces develop for 2 to 3 wk in freshwater before miracidia (first larval stage) hatch. The miracidia invade snails; there, they develop, multiply, and eventually emerge as cercariae (free-swimming larvae). Cercariae penetrate freshwater crabs or crayfish and encyst to form metacercariae. Humans become infected by eating raw, pickled, or poorly cooked crustaceans. Metacercariae excyst in the human GI tract, penetrate the intestinal wall, and move into the peritoneal cavity, then through the diaphragm into the pleural cavity; they enter lung tissue, become encapsulated, and develop into hermaphroditic adult worms, which produce eggs. Adult worms grow to about 7.5 to 12 mm by 4 to 6 mm. From the lungs, eggs exit the body in the sputum that is coughed up and spit out or swallowed and passed in stool.

Worms may also reach the brain, liver, lymph nodes, skin, and spinal cord and develop there. However, in these organs, the life cycle cannot be completed because the eggs have no way to exit the body. Adult flukes may persist for 20 to 25 yr.

Other hosts include pigs, dogs, and a variety of feline species.

Symptoms and Signs

During invasion and migration of the flukes, diarrhea, abdominal pain, fever, cough, urticaria, hepatosplenomegaly, pulmonary abnormalities, and eosinophilia may develop.

During the chronic phase, the lungs are damaged most, but other organs may be involved. Manifestations of pulmonary infection develop slowly and include chronic cough, chest pain, hemoptysis, and dyspnea; the clinical picture resembles and is often confused with TB. Cerebral infections manifest as space-occupying lesions, often within a year after the onset of pulmonary disease. Seizures, aphasia, paresis, and visual disturbances occur. Migratory allergic skin lesions similar to those of cutaneous larva migrans are common in infections with *P. skrjabini* but also occur with other species.

Diagnosis

- Microscopic examination of sputum and stool
- Serologic tests to detect antibodies

Diagnosis of paragonimiasis is by identifying the characteristic large operculated eggs in sputum or stool. Occasionally, eggs may be found in pleural or peritoneal fluid. Eggs may be difficult to find because they are released intermittently and in small numbers. Concentration techniques increase sensitivity.

Serologic tests to detect antibodies are useful in light infections and in the diagnosis of extrapulmonary paragonimiasis.

X-rays provide ancillary information but are not diagnostic; chest x-rays and CT may show a diffuse infiltrate, nodules, annular ring shadow lesions, cavitations, linear opacities, lung abscesses, pleural effusion, and pneumothorax.

Treatment

- Praziquantel

Praziquantel 25 mg/kg po tid for 2 days is the drug of choice for paragonimiasis.

Triclabendazole is an acceptable treatment in areas where it is available; dosage is 10 mg/kg po once postprandially or, for severe infections, 2 doses of 10 mg/kg given postprandially 12 h apart.

Praziquantel is used to treat extrapulmonary infections, but multiple courses may be required.

For cerebral infections, a short course of corticosteroids may be given with praziquantel to reduce the inflammatory response induced by dying flukes.

Surgery may be needed to excise skin lesions or, rarely, brain cysts.

The best prevention is to avoid eating raw or undercooked freshwater crabs and crayfish from endemic waters.

SCHISTOSOMIASIS

(Bilharziasis)

Schistosomiasis is infection with blood flukes of the genus *Schistosoma*, which are acquired transcutaneously by swimming or wading in contaminated freshwater. The organisms infect the vasculature of the GI or GU system. Acute symptoms are dermatitis, followed several weeks later by fever, chills, nausea, abdominal pain, diarrhea, malaise, and myalgia. Chronic symptoms vary with species but include bloody diarrhea (eg, with *S. mansoni* and *S. japonicum*) or hematuria (eg, with *S. haematobium*). Diagnosis is by identifying eggs in stool, urine, or biopsy specimens. Serologic tests may be sensitive and specific but do not provide information about the worm burden or clinical status. Treatment is with praziquantel.

Flukes are parasitic flatworms that infect various parts of the body (eg, blood vessels, GI tract, lungs, liver) depending on the species.

Etiology

Schistosomiasis is by far the most important trematode infection. *Schistosoma* is the only trematode that invades through the skin; all other trematodes infect only via ingestion. About 200 million people are infected worldwide.

Five species of schistosomes infect humans; all have similar life cycles involving freshwater snails. *S. haematobium* causes urinary tract disease; the other *Schistosoma* sp cause intestinal disease.

Geographic distribution differs by species:

- *S. haematobium:* Widely distributed over the African continent with smaller foci in the Middle East, Turkey, and India
- *S. mansoni:* Widespread in Africa, foci in Middle East, and the only species in the Western Hemisphere in parts of South America and some Caribbean islands
- *S. japonicum:* Asia, mainly in China, the Philippines, Thailand, and Indonesia.
- *S. mekongi:* Southeast Asia
- *S. intercalatum:* Central and West Africa

Humans are the main reservoir of infection. Dogs, cats, rodents, pigs, horses, and goats are reservoirs for *S. japonicum*, and dogs are reservoirs for *S. mekongi*. The disease may be imported in travelers and immigrants from endemic areas, but transmission does not occur within the US and Canada.

Pathophysiology

Adult worms live and copulate within venules of the mesentery (typically *S. japonicum* and *S. mansoni*) or bladder (typically *S. haematobium*—see Fig. 204–1). Some eggs penetrate the intestinal or bladder mucosa and are passed in stool or urine; other eggs remain within the host organ or are transported through the portal system to the liver and occasionally to other sites (eg, lungs, CNS, spinal cord). Excreted eggs hatch in freshwater, releasing miracidia (first larval stage), which enter snails. After multiplication, thousands of free-swimming cercariae are released.

Cercariae penetrate human skin within a few minutes after exposure and transform into schistosomula, which travel through the bloodstream to the liver, where they mature into adults. The adults then migrate to their ultimate home in the intestinal veins or the venous plexus of the GU tract.

Eggs appear in stool or urine 1 to 3 mo after cercarial penetration.

Estimates of the adult worm life span range from 3 to 7 yr. The females range in size from 7 to 20 mm; males are slightly smaller.

Symptoms and Signs

Acute schistosome dermatitis: Most infections are asymptomatic. A pruritic papular rash (cercarial dermatitis) can develop where cercariae penetrate the skin in previously sensitized people.

Acute Katayama fever: Katayama fever may occur with onset of egg laying, typically 2 to 4 wk after heavy exposure. Symptoms include fever, chills, cough, nausea, abdominal pain, malaise, myalgia, urticarial rashes, and marked eosinophilia, resembling serum sickness. Manifestations are more common and usually more severe in visitors than in residents of endemic areas and typically last for several weeks.

Chronic schistosomiasis: Chronic schistosomiasis results primarily from host responses to eggs retained in tissues. Early on, intestinal mucosal ulcerations caused by *S. mansoni* or *S. japonicum* may bleed and result in bloody diarrhea. As lesions progress, focal fibrosis, strictures, fistulas, and papillomatous growths may develop in the intestine.

Granulomatous reactions to eggs of *S. mansoni* and *S. japonicum* in the liver usually do not compromise liver function, but they may cause fibrosis and cirrhosis, which can lead to portal hypertension and subsequent hematemesis due to esophageal varices.

Eggs in the lungs may produce granulomas and focal obliterative arteritis, which may ultimately result in pulmonary hypertension and cor pulmonale.

With *S. haematobium*, ulcerations in the bladder wall may cause dysuria, hematuria, and urinary frequency. Over time, chronic cystitis develops. Strictures may lead to hydroureter and hydronephrosis. Papillomatous masses in the bladder are common, and squamous cell carcinoma may develop. Blood loss from both GI and GU tracts frequently results in anemia.

Secondary bacterial infection of the GU tract is common, and persistent *Salmonella* septicemia may occur with *S. mansoni*. Several species, notably *S. haematobium*, can cause genital disease in both men and women, resulting in numerous symptoms

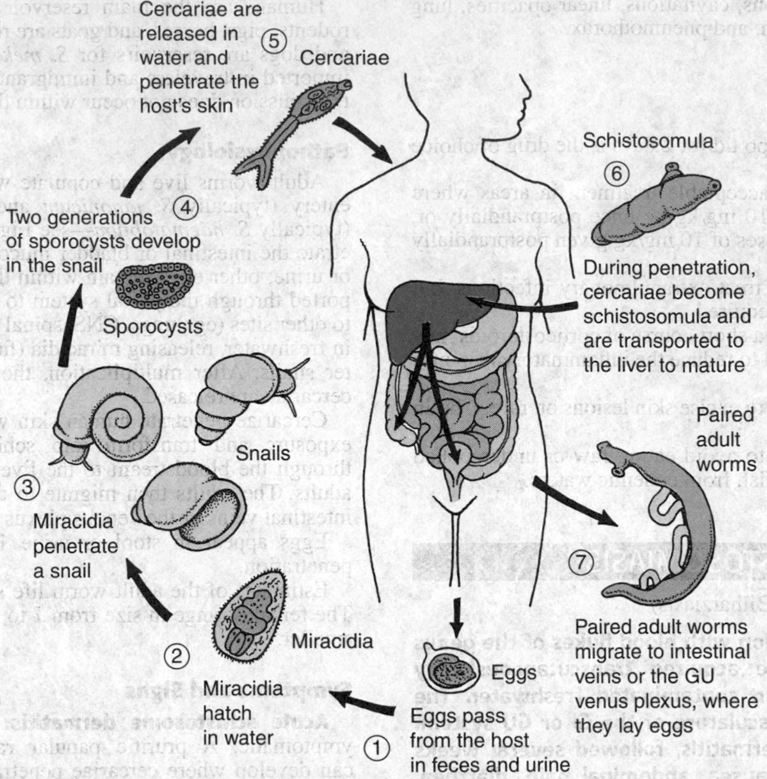
Cercariae are released in water and penetrate the host's skin
5
Cercariae
Schistosomula
6
Two generations of sporocysts develop in the snail
4
Sporocysts
During penetration, cercariae become schistosomula and are transported to the liver to mature
Paired adult worms
Snails
3
Miracidia penetrate a snail
7
Paired adult worms migrate to intestinal veins or the GU venus plexus, where they lay eggs
Miracidia
2
Eggs
Miracidia hatch in water
Eggs pass from the host in feces and urine
1

Fig. 204–1. Simplified *Schistosoma* life cycle.

including infertility. Neurologic complications can occur even in light *Schistosoma* infections. Eggs or adult worms lodged in the spinal cord can cause transverse myelitis, and those in the brain can produce focal lesions and seizures.

Diagnosis

- Microscopic examination of stool or urine (*S. haematobium*) for eggs
- Serologic tests

Stool or urine (*S. haematobium*, occasionally *S. japonicum*) is examined for eggs. Repeated examinations using concentration techniques may be necessary. Geography is a primary determinant of species, so a history of exposure should be communicated to the laboratory. If the clinical picture suggests schistosomiasis but no eggs are found after repeated examination of urine or feces, intestinal or bladder mucosa can be biopsied to check for eggs.

Depending on the antigens used, serologic tests may be sensitive and specific for infection, but they do not provide information about worm burden, clinical status, or prognosis.

Treatment

- Praziquantel

Single-day oral treatment with praziquantel (20 mg/kg bid for *S. haematobium*, *S. mansoni*, and *S. intercalatum*; 20 mg/kg tid for *S. japonicum* and *S. mekongi*) is recommended. Praziquantel is effective against adult schistosomes, but not developing schistosomula, which are present early in infection. Thus, for travelers, treatment is delayed for 6 to 8 wk after the last exposure. Adverse effects of praziquantel are generally mild and include abdominal pain, diarrhea, headache, and dizziness. Therapeutic failures have been reported, but it is difficult to determine whether they are due to reinfection or drug-resistant strains. If eggs are present at the time of diagnosis, follow-up examination 1 to 2 mo after treatment is suggested to help confirm cure. Treatment is repeated if eggs are still present.

Treatment of Katayama fever is uncertain. Praziquantel is not particularly effective early in infection; corticosteroids can ameliorate severe symptoms.

Patients should be examined for living eggs 3 and 6 mo after treatment. Retreatment is indicated if egg excretion has not decreased markedly.

Prevention

Scrupulously avoiding contact with contaminated freshwater prevents infection.

Freshwater used for bathing should be boiled for at least 1 min and then cooled before bathing. However, water that has been held in a storage tank for at least 1 to 2 days should be safe without boiling.

People who are accidentally exposed to possibly contaminated water (eg, by falling into a river) should vigorously dry off with a towel to attempt to remove any parasites before they penetrate the skin.

The sanitary disposal of urine and feces reduces the likelihood of infection.

Adult residents of endemic areas are more resistant to reinfection than children, suggesting the possibility of acquired immunity.

Vaccine development is under way.

KEY POINTS

- *Schistosoma* is the only trematode that invades through the skin; about 200 million people are infected worldwide.
- Cercariae mature in the liver, and adults migrate to their ultimate home in the intestinal veins or the venous plexus of the GU tract.
- Organisms in the liver cause a granulomatous reaction that can lead to fibrosis and cirrhosis.
- Organisms in the intestine can cause bloody diarrhea, and organisms in the bladder can cause hematuria and chronic cystitis.
- Treat with praziquantel.
- To prevent infection, avoid contact with fresh water in endemic areas.

Dermatitis Caused by Avian and Animal Schistosomes

(Cercarial Dermatitis; Clam Digger's Itch; Swimmer's Itch)

Cercarial dermatitis, a skin condition, occurs when *Schistosoma* sp that cannot develop in humans penetrate the skin during contact with contaminated freshwater or brackish water.

Cercariae of *Schistosoma* sp that infect birds and mammals other than humans can penetrate the skin. Although the organisms do not develop in humans, humans may become sensitized and develop pruritic maculopapular, then vesicular skin lesions at the site of penetration. Skin lesions may be accompanied by a systemic febrile response that runs for 5 to 7 days and resolves spontaneously.

Cercarial dermatitis occurs worldwide. In North America, ocean-related schistosome dermatitis (clam digger's itch) occurs on all Atlantic, Gulf, Pacific, and Hawaiian coasts. It is common in muddy flats off Cape Cod. Freshwater schistosome dermatitis (swimmer's itch) is common in the Great Lakes region.

Diagnosis of cercarial dermatitis is based on clinical findings. Most cases do not require medical attention.

Treatment of cercarial dermatitis is symptomatic with cool compresses, baking soda, or antipruritic lotions. Topical corticosteroids can also be used.

205 Viruses

Viruses are the smallest parasites, typically ranging from 0.02 to 0.3 μm, although several very large viruses up to 1 μm long (megavirus, pandoravirus) have recently been discovered. Viruses depend completely on cells (bacterial, plant, or animal) to reproduce. Viruses have an outer cover of protein and sometimes lipid, an RNA or DNA core, and sometimes enzymes needed for the first steps of viral replication.

Viruses are classified principally according to the nature and structure of their genome and their method of replication, not according to the diseases they cause. Thus, there are DNA viruses and RNA viruses; each type may have single or double strands of genetic material. Single-strand RNA viruses are further divided into those with (+) sense and (-) sense RNA. DNA viruses typically replicate in the host cell nucleus, and RNA viruses typically replicate in the cytoplasm. However, certain single-strand, (+) sense RNA viruses termed retroviruses use a very different method of replication.

Retroviruses use reverse transcription to create a double-stranded DNA copy (a provirus) of their RNA genome, which is inserted into the genome of their host cell. Reverse transcription is accomplished using the enzyme reverse transcriptase, which the virus carries with it inside its shell. Examples of retroviruses are the human immunodeficiency viruses and the human T-cell leukemia viruses. Once the provirus is integrated into the host cell DNA, it is transcribed using typical cellular mechanisms to produce viral proteins and genetic material. If the infected cell belongs to the germline, the integrated provirus can become established as an endogenous retrovirus that is transmitted to offspring. The sequencing of the human genome revealed that at least 1% of the human genome consists of endogenous retroviral sequences, representing past encounters with retroviruses during the course of human evolution. A few endogenous human retroviruses have remained transcriptionally active and produce functional proteins (eg, the syncytins that contribute to the structure of the human placenta). Some experts speculate that some disorders of uncertain etiology, such as multiple sclerosis, certain autoimmune disorders, and various cancers, may be caused by endogenous retroviruses.

Because RNA transcription does not involve the same error-checking mechanisms as DNA transcription, RNA viruses, particularly retroviruses, are particularly prone to mutation.

For infection to occur, the virus first attaches to the host cell at one or one of several receptor molecules on the cell surface. The viral DNA or RNA then enters the host cell and separates from the outer cover (uncoating) and replicates inside the host cell in a process that requires specific enzymes. The newly synthesized viral components then assemble into a complete virus particle. The host cell typically dies, releasing new viruses that infect other host cells. Each step of viral replication involves different enzymes and substrates and offers an opportunity to interfere with the process of infection.

The consequences of viral infection vary considerably. Many infections cause acute illness after a brief incubation period, but some are asymptomatic or cause minor symptoms that may not be recognized except in retrospect. Many viral infections are cleared by the body's defenses, but some remain in a latent state, and some cause chronic disease. In latent infection, viral RNA or DNA remains in host cells but does not replicate or cause disease for a long time, sometimes for many years. Latent viral infections may be transmissible during the asymptomatic period, facilitating person-to-person spread. Sometimes a trigger (particularly immunosuppression) causes reactivation. Common viruses that remain latent include herpesviruses, HIV, and papovaviruses. Chronic viral infections are characterized by continuous, prolonged viral shedding; examples are congenital infection with rubella virus or with cytomegalovirus and persistent hepatitis B or C. HIV can cause both latent and chronic infections.

Some disorders are caused by viral reactivation in the CNS after a very long latency period. These diseases include progressive multifocal leukoencephalopathy (due to the JC virus, a polyomavirus), subacute sclerosing panencephalitis (due to measles virus), and progressive rubella panencephalitis (due to rubella virus). Variant Creutzfeldt-Jakob disease and bovine spongiform encephalopathy were formerly termed slow viral diseases because they have lengthy incubations (years), but they are now known to be caused by prions; prions are proteinaceous disease-causing agents that are not bacterial, fungal, or viral and that contain no genetic material (see p. 1997).

Several hundred different viruses infect humans. Viruses that infect primarily humans often spread via respiratory and enteric excretions. Some are transmitted sexually and through transfer of blood (eg, via transfusion, mucosal contact, or puncture by a contaminated needle) or through transplantation of tissue. Many viruses are transmitted via rodent or arthropod vectors, and bats have recently been identified as hosts for almost all mammalian viruses, including some responsible for certain serious human infections (eg, severe acute respiratory syndrome [SARS]). Viruses exist worldwide, but their spread is limited by inborn resistance, prior immunizing infections or vaccines, sanitary and other public health control measures, and prophylactic antiviral drugs.

Zoonotic viruses (see p. 1480) pursue their biologic cycles chiefly in animals; humans are secondary or accidental hosts. These viruses are limited to areas and environments able to support their nonhuman natural cycles of infection (vertebrates, arthropods, or both).

Viruses and cancer: Some viruses are oncogenic and predispose to certain cancers:

- Papillomavirus: Cervical, penile, vaginal, anal, oropharyngeal, and esophageal carcinomas
- Human T-lymphotropic virus 1: Certain types of human leukemia and lymphoma
- Epstein-Barr virus: Nasopharyngeal carcinoma, Burkitt lymphoma, Hodgkin lymphoma, and lymphomas in immunosuppressed organ transplant recipients
- Hepatitis B and C viruses: Hepatocellular carcinoma
- Human herpesvirus 8: Kaposi sarcoma, primary effusion lymphomas, and multicentric Castleman disease (a lymphoproliferative disorder)

Diagnosis

Some viral disorders can be diagnosed clinically (eg, by well-known viral syndromes such as measles, rubella, roseola infantum, erythema infectiosum, and chickenpox) or epidemiologically (eg, during epidemic outbreaks such as influenza, norovirus infection, and mumps). Definitive laboratory diagnosis is necessary mainly when specific treatment may be helpful or when the agent may be a public health threat (eg, HIV). Typical hospital laboratories can test for some viruses, but for less common disorders (eg, rabies, Eastern equine encephalitis, human parvovirus B19), specimens must be sent to state health laboratories or the Centers for Disease Control and Prevention.

Serologic examination during acute and convalescent stages is sensitive and specific, but slow; more rapid diagnosis can sometimes be made using culture, PCR, or viral antigen tests. Histopathology with electron (not light) microscopy can sometimes help. For specific diagnostic procedures, see p. 1443.

Viral genomes are small; the genome of RNA viruses ranges from 3.5 kilobases (some retroviruses) to 27 kilobases (some reoviruses), and the genome of DNA viruses ranges from 5 kilobases (some parvoviruses) to 280 kilobases (some poxviruses). This manageable size together with the current advances in nucleotide sequencing technology means that partial and whole virus genome sequencing will become an essential component in epidemiologic investigations of disease outbreaks.

Treatment

Antiviral drugs: Progress in the use of antiviral drugs is occurring rapidly. Antiviral chemotherapy can be directed at various phases of viral replication: It can interfere with viral particle attachment to host cell membranes or uncoating of viral nucleic acids, inhibit a cellular receptor or factor required for viral replication, or block specific virus-coded enzymes and proteins that are produced in the host cells and that are essential for viral replication but not for normal host cell metabolism.

Antiviral drugs are most often used therapeutically or prophylactically against herpesviruses (including cytomegalovirus—see p. 1616), respiratory viruses (see p. 1683), and HIV (see p. 1627). However, some drugs are effective against many different kinds of viruses. Some drugs active against HIV are used for other viral infections such as hepatitis B.

Interferons: Interferons are compounds released from infected host cells in response to viral or other foreign antigens. There are many different interferons, which have numerous effects such as blocking translation and transcription of viral RNA and stopping viral replication without disturbing normal host cell function. Interferons are sometimes given attached to polyethylene glycol (pegylated formulations), allowing slow, sustained release of the interferon.

Viral disorders sometimes treated with interferon therapy include

- Chronic hepatitis B and C
- Condyloma acuminata
- Kaposi sarcoma

Adverse effects of interferons include fever, chills, weakness, and myalgia, typically starting 7 to 12 h after the first injection and lasting up to 12 h. Depression, hepatitis, and, when high doses are used, bone marrow suppression are also possible.

Prevention

Vaccines: Vaccines (see p. 1448) work by stimulating immunity. Viral vaccines in general use include hepatitis A, hepatitis B, human papillomavirus, influenza, Japanese encephalitis, measles, mumps, poliomyelitis, rabies, rotavirus, rubella, tick-borne encephalitis, varicella, and yellow fever. Adenovirus and smallpox vaccines are available but used only in high-risk groups (eg, military recruits).

Viral diseases can be eradicated by good vaccines. Smallpox was eradicated in 1978, and the cattle plague rinderpest (caused by a virus closely related to human measles virus) was eradicated in 2011. Poliomyelitis has been eradicated from all but a few countries where logistics and religious sentiment continue to impede vaccination. Measles has been eradicated from some parts of the world, notably the Americas, but because measles is highly contagious and vaccination coverage is incomplete even in regions where it is considered eradicated, final eradication is not imminent. The prospects for eradication of other more intractable virus infections (such as HIV) are presently uncertain.

Immune globulins: Immune globulins (see p. 1460) are available for passive immune prophylaxis in limited situations. They can be used preexposure (eg, for hepatitis A), postexposure (eg, for rabies or hepatitis), and for treating disease (eg, eczema vaccinatum).

Protective measures: Many viral infections can be prevented by commonsense protective measures (which vary depending on the transmission mode of a given agent). Important measures include hand washing, appropriate food preparation and water treatment, avoidance of contact with sick people, and safe-sex practices. For infections with an insect vector (eg, mosquitoes, ticks), avoiding the vector is important.

TYPES OF VIRAL DISORDERS

Categorizing viral infections by the organ system most commonly affected (eg, lungs, GI tract, skin, liver, CNS, mucous membranes) can be clinically useful, although certain viral disorders (eg, mumps) are hard to categorize. Many specific viruses and the disorders they cause are also discussed elsewhere in THE MANUAL.

Respiratory infections: The most common viral infections are probably URIs. Respiratory infections are more likely to cause severe symptoms in infants, the elderly, and patients with a lung or heart disorder.

Respiratory viruses include the epidemic influenza viruses (A and B), H5N1 and H7N9 avian influenza A viruses, parainfluenza viruses 1 through 4, adenoviruses, respiratory syncytial virus A and B, human metapneumovirus, and rhinoviruses (see Table 205–1 and Respiratory Viruses on p. 1683). In 2012, a novel coronavirus, Middle East respiratory syndrome coronavirus (MERS-CoV—see MERS on p. 1690), appeared in Kuwait; it can cause severe acute respiratory illness and is sometimes fatal. Respiratory viruses are typically spread from person to person by contact with infected respiratory droplets.

GI infections: Gastroenteritis is usually caused by viruses (see p. 124) and transmitted from person to person by the oral-fecal route. Age group primarily affected depends on the virus:

- Rotavirus: Children
- Norovirus: Older children and adults
- Astrovirus: Usually infants and young children
- Adenovirus 40 and 41: Infants
- Coronavirus-like agents: Infants

Table 205–1. SOME RESPIRATORY VIRUSES

PRINCIPAL SYNDROMES	PREVALENCE AND DISTRIBUTION	SPECIFIC THERAPY	SPECIFIC PREVENTION*
Epidemic influenza viruses A, B, and C and avian influenza viruses			
Influenza AFRD Acute bronchitis and pneumonia Croup	A and B: Epidemic, occasionally pandemic C: Endemic Global	A and B: Oseltamivir or zanamivir	A and B: Vaccine, oseltamivir or zanamivir
	Avian H5N1 and avian H7N9: Poultry associated	Oseltamivir	Avoiding contact with birds
Parainfluenza viruses 1–4			
AFRD (children) Acute bronchitis and pneumonia Croup	1: Local epidemics 1, 2, and 3: Widespread in children	None	Vaccines under investigation
Adenoviruses			
AFRD (children) Acute respiratory disease (adults) Acute pharyngoconjunctival fever Epidemic keratoconjunctivitis Viral pneumonia Acute follicular conjunctivitis Diarrhea Hemorrhagic cystitis	Global Mostly children	None	Vaccine containing types 4 and 7 for epidemics in military populations
Respiratory syncytial virus and human metapneumovirus			
Lower respiratory illness (infants) Mild upper respiratory illness (adults)	Widespread in children	Ribavirin sometimes used in immunocompromised patients	Palivizumab IM† monthly (for certain infants at high risk of RSV infection)
Rhinoviruses			
Common cold Acute coryza with or without fever	Universal, especially during cold months	None	None

*Nonspecific precautions (eg, avoidance of infected patients and insect and animal vectors, routine hygiene measures) are also recommended.
†Unlike RSV-IVIG, palivizumab does not interfere with immunizations (eg, MMR, chickenpox).
AFRD = acute febrile respiratory disease; IVIG = IV immune globulin; MMR = measles, mumps, and rubella; RSV = respiratory syncytial virus.

Local epidemics may occur in children, particularly during colder months.

The main symptoms are vomiting and diarrhea.

No specific treatment is recommended, but supportive care, particularly rehydration, is important.

A rotavirus vaccine that is effective against most pathogenic strains is part of the recommended infant vaccination schedule (see Table 291–2 on p. 2462). Hand washing and good sanitation measures can help prevent spread.

Exanthematous infections: Some viruses cause only skin lesions (as in molluscum contagiosum and warts—see p. 1082); others also cause systemic manifestations or lesions elsewhere in the body (see Table 205–2). Transmission is typically from person to person; alphaviruses have a mosquito vector.

Table 205–2. SOME EXANTHEMATOUS VIRUSES

PRINCIPAL SYNDROMES	PREVALENCE AND DISTRIBUTION	SPECIFIC THERAPY	SPECIFIC PREVENTION*
Rubeola virus			
Measles Encephalomyelitis CNS involvement (rare)	Global Incidence decreasing because of vaccine	None	Vaccines
Rubella virus			
German measles Birth defects due to infection during pregnancy	Universal	None	Vaccines
Human parvovirus B19			
Erythema infectiosum (fifth disease) Rash, malaise, arthritis Hydrops fetalis (infection during pregnancy) Anemia (in immunocompromised hosts or patients with hemoglobinopathies)	Sporadic outbreaks	IVIG (for severe anemia)	None
Human herpesvirus type 6			
Roseola infantum (exanthem subitum)	Widespread Affects young children	None	None
Varicella-zoster virus			
Chickenpox	Before vaccine, almost universal in children, occasionally in adults	Acyclovir, famciclovir, valacyclovir	Immune globulins, vaccine
Zoster	Common in adults, resulting from reactivation of latent virus	Acyclovir, famciclovir, valacyclovir	Vaccine
Variola			
Smallpox	Natural disease eradicated	Cidofovir† Smallpox vaccine up to 4 days after exposure	Vaccine Cidofovir†
Alphaviruses (some)			
Chikungunya disease (acute febrile illness followed by more chronic polyarthritis)	Transmitted by *Aedes* mosquitoes Africa, Southeast Asia, India, Europe	None	None
Mayaro disease (a dengue-like disease)	Mosquito-borne South America, Trinidad	None	None
Molluscum contagiosum virus			
Molluscum contagiosum papules	Genital (adults) Exposed skin (children) More severe (AIDS patients)	Cryotherapy, curettage	None

*Nonspecific precautions (eg, avoidance of infected patients and insect and animal vectors, routine hygiene measures) are also recommended.
†Based on animal studies.
IVIG = IV immune globulin.

Table 205–3. VIRAL HEPATITIS

PRINCIPAL SYNDROMES	PREVALENCE AND DISTRIBUTION	SPECIFIC THERAPY	SPECIFIC PREVENTION*
Hepatitis A (acute)	Widespread, often epidemic	None	γ-Globulin, vaccine
Hepatitis B (acute and chronic)	Widespread	Interferon, other antivirals, including nucleoside analogs (eg, entecavir) and nucleotide analogs (eg, tenofovir disoproxil fumarate)	Screening for hepatitis B surface antigen Vaccine, γ- or hyperimmune globulin
Hepatitis C (acute and chronic)	Widespread	Interferon, ribavirin	Screening for hepatitis C
Hepatitis D (delta)	Endemic pockets in several countries Parenteral drug users at relatively high risk Can infect only in the presence of hepatitis B	Interferon	None
Hepatitis E	Outbreaks Developing world Severe during pregnancy	None	Vaccine (not available in US)

*Nonspecific precautions (eg, avoidance of body fluids of infected patients, aseptic precautions, routine hygiene measures) are also recommended.

Hepatic infections: At least 5 specific viruses (hepatitis A, B, C, D, and E viruses) can cause hepatitis; each causes a specific type of hepatitis (see Table 205–3 and see p. 222). Hepatitis D virus can infect only when h410epatitis B is present. Transmission is from person to person by contact with infected blood or body secretions or by the fecal-oral route for hepatitis A and E.

Other viruses can affect the liver as part of their disease process. Common examples are cytomegalovirus, Epstein-Barr virus, and yellow fever virus. Less common examples are echovirus, coxsackievirus, and herpes simplex, rubeola, rubella, and varicella viruses.

Neurologic infections: Most cases of encephalitis are caused by viruses (see Table 205–4 and p. 1850). Many of these viruses are transmitted to humans by blood-eating arthropods, mainly mosquitoes and ticks (see p. 1480); these viruses are called arboviruses (arthropod-borne viruses). For such infections, prevention includes avoiding mosquito and tick bites.

Hemorrhagic fevers: Certain viruses cause fever and a bleeding tendency (see Table 205–5 and p. 1480). Transmission may involve mosquitoes, ticks, or contact with infected animals (eg, rodents, monkeys, bats) and people. Prevention involves avoiding the means of transmission.

Cutaneous or mucosal infections: Some viruses cause skin or mucosal lesions that recur and may become chronic (see Table 205–6). Mucocutaneous infections are the most common type of herpes simplex virus infection (see p. 1621). Human papillomavirus causes warts (see p. 1082); some subtypes cause anogenital and oropharyngeal cancer (see pp. 1702 and 2251). Transmission is by person-to-person contact.

Multisystem diseases: Enteroviruses, which include coxsackieviruses and echoviruses (see p. 1538), can cause various multisystem syndromes, as can cytomegaloviruses (see Table 205–7 and p. 1620). Transmission is by the fecal-oral route.

Nonspecific febrile illness: Some viruses cause nonspecific symptoms, including fever, malaise, headaches, and myalgia (see Table 183–1 on p. 1482 and Table 205–8). Transmission is usually by an insect or arthropod vector.

Rift Valley fever rarely progresses to ocular disorders, meningoencephalitis, or a hemorrhagic form (which has a 50% mortality rate).

Table 205–4. SOME NEUROLOGIC VIRUSES

PRINCIPAL SYNDROMES	PREVALENCE AND DISTRIBUTION	SPECIFIC THERAPY	SPECIFIC PREVENTION*
Polioviruses			
Poliomyelitis (acute flaccid paralysis) Aseptic meningitis	Global Incidence now low because of vaccine	None	Vaccines: Live (oral), killed (injected)
Alphaviruses (some), mosquito-borne			
Western equine encephalitis	North and South America	None	None
Eastern equine encephalitis	North and South America	None	Vaccine available to protect equines only
Venezuelan equine encephalitis	Gulf states to South America	None	Vaccine available for equines Investigational vaccine used in laboratory workers at risk
Flaviviruses (some), mosquito-borne			
Japanese encephalitis	Southeast Asia, Japan, Korea, China, India, Philippines, eastern former Soviet Union	None	Vaccine
Murray Valley encephalitis	Australia, New Guinea	None	None
St. Louis encephalitis	North and South America	None	None
West Nile virus encephalitis	Africa, Middle East, southern France, former Soviet Union, India, Indonesia, US	None	Screening blood and blood products for the virus
Flaviviruses (some), tick-borne			
Powassan encephalitis	Canada, northeastern US	None	None
Tick-borne encephalitis	Eastern and Central Europe, Balkans, former Soviet Union Outbreaks that coincide with periods of tick activity	None	Vaccine available in Europe and Russia
Bunyaviruses (some), mosquito-borne			
California encephalitis and related types (eg, La Crosse encephalitis)	Probably worldwide Common in Midwestern and eastern US Symptomatic infection primarily in children	None	None
Arenaviruses (some)			
Lymphocytic choriomeningitis	US, Europe, possibly elsewhere Chief reservoir: House mouse Primarily in adults during autumn and winter	None	None
Rabies virus			
Rabies	Worldwide	None	Vaccine Postexposure rabies immune globulin

*Nonspecific precautions (eg, avoidance of contaminated food and water and insect and animal vectors, routine hygiene measures) are also recommended.

Table 205–5. SOME VIRUSES THAT CAUSE HEMORRHAGIC FEVER

PRINCIPAL SYNDROMES	DISTRIBUTION	SPECIFIC THERAPY	SPECIFIC PREVENTION*
Flaviviruses (some)			
Omsk hemorrhagic fever	Former Soviet Union (Siberia)	None	None
Kyasanur Forest disease	India	None	None
Yellow fever	Africa, Central and South America	None	Vaccine for travelers to endemic areas and for populations experiencing an outbreak
Dengue fever	Tropics and subtropics, worldwide	None	None
Bunyaviruses (some)			
Hemorrhagic fever with renal syndrome due to Hantaan, Puumala, Dobrava (Belgrade), or Seoul virus	Northern Asia, Europe, southwestern US	Ribavirin	None
Filoviruses			
Lake Victoria marburgvirus disease	Africa	None	None
Sudan ebolavirus disease	Africa, Sumatra	None	None
Bundibugyo ebolavirus disease	Uganda	None	None
Zaire ebolavirus disease	Zaire	None	None
Reston ebolavirus disease	Philippines	None	None
Arenaviruses (some)			
Lassa fever Bolivian hemorrhagic fever (due to Machupo virus) Argentinian hemorrhagic fever (due to Junin virus) Venezuelan hemorrhagic fever (due to Guanarito virus) Brazilian hemorrhagic fever (due to Sabia virus)	South America, Africa (only Lassa fever)	Ribavirin Convalescent plasma for all except Lassa fever	Vaccine for Argentinian hemorrhagic fever under investigation
Lujo virus disease	Zambia	None	None
Nairovirus			
Crimean-Congo hemorrhagic fever	Former Soviet Union, western Pakistan, Africa, Asia, Middle East, Eastern Europe	Ribavirin Possibly convalescent plasma	Vaccine available in Eastern Europe

*Nonspecific precautions (eg, avoidance of the means of transmission, routine hygiene measures) are also recommended

Table 205–6. SOME VIRUSES THAT CAUSE RECURRENT OR CHRONIC SKIN OR MUCOSAL LESIONS

PRINCIPAL SYNDROMES	PREVALENCE	SPECIFIC THERAPY	SPECIFIC PREVENTION*
Herpes simplex virus			
Herpes labialis Herpetic gingivostomatitis Dermatitis Keratoconjunctivitis Encephalitis Vulvovaginitis Neonatal disseminated disease	Labial: Recurrent, almost universal Gingivostomatitis: Frequent in infants and children	Acyclovir, famciclovir, valacyclovir, penciclovir	Neonatal infection: Treatment of maternal infection; suppressive therapy beginning at 36 wk of gestation if patients have a history of recurrent HSV; cesarean delivery if lesions or prodromal symptoms are present at time of delivery
Human papillomavirus			
Warts (verrucae) Genital warts Cervical, anogenital, and oropharyngeal cancer	Universal Common, often recurrent	Cryotherapy, interferon (possibly for genital), podophyllin (genital), imiquimod	Vaccine for the 4 subtypes of HPV most commonly associated with cancers and genital warts Condoms

*Nonspecific precautions (eg, routine hygiene measures, safe-sex practices) are also recommended.

Table 205–7. SOME VIRUSES THAT CAUSE MULTISYSTEM DISEASE

PRINCIPAL SYNDROMES	DISTRIBUTION AND PREVALENCE	SPECIFIC THERAPY	SPECIFIC PREVENTION*
Coxsackieviruses			
Herpangina Epidemic pleurodynia Aseptic meningitis Meningoencephalitis Neonatal sepsis Myocarditis Pericarditis AFRD (children) Paralysis Fever and exanthem	Varies with types Most people infected Increased during warm months in temperate climates and year round in the tropics and in children Person-to-person spread usually via the fecal-oral route	None	None
Echoviruses† and high-numbered enteroviruses			
Aseptic meningitis Fever and exanthem Meningoencephalitis Neonatal sepsis Paralysis Myocarditis Pericarditis	As for coxsackieviruses	None	None
Cytomegalovirus			
Congenital defects (cytomegalic inclusion disease) Hepatitis (cytomegalovirus mononucleosis) In immunocompromised patients (including those with AIDS): Retinitis, GI disorders, CNS disorders, pneumonia	Widespread Congenital Common among immunocompromised patients	Ganciclovir, foscarnet, cidofovir, sometimes immune globulin (eg, in organ transplant recipients with pneumonia)	Ganciclovir, foscarnet

*Nonspecific precautions (eg, adequate sanitation, hand washing) are also recommended.

†Echovirus types 10, 21, 22, and 28 have been reclassified; these numbers are no longer used. More recently described enteroviruses have been designated as types 68 to 72.

AFRD = acute febrile respiratory disease.

Table 205–8. SOME VIRUSES THAT CAUSE NONSPECIFIC ACUTE FEBRILE ILLNESS

PRINCIPAL SYNDROMES	DISTRIBUTION	SPECIFIC THERAPY*	SPECIFIC PREVENTION†
Colorado tick fever virus (coltivirus)			
Colorado tick fever, with leukopenia and thrombocytopenia	Western US, Canada	None	None
Phleboviruses (some)			
Phlebotomus (sandfly) fever	Mediterranean basin, Balkans, Middle East, Pakistan, India, China, eastern Africa, Panama, Brazil	None	None
Rift Valley fever	Eastern Africa, Egypt	None	Vaccine for livestock Human vaccine under investigation
Severe fever with thrombocytopenia syndrome	China, Korea, Japan	None	None

*Treatment is usually supportive.

†Nonspecific precautions (eg, avoidance of the means of transmission, routine hygiene measures, screening of bone marrow used for transplantation) are also recommended.

SECTION 16

Psychiatric Disorders

206 Approach to the Patient with Mental Symptoms

Patients with mental complaints or concerns or disordered behavior present in a variety of clinical settings, including primary care and emergency treatment centers. Complaints or concerns may be new or a continuation of a history of mental problems. Complaints may be related to coping with a physical condition or be the direct effects of a physical condition. The method of assessment depends on whether the complaints constitute an emergency or are reported in a scheduled visit. In an emergency, a physician may have to focus on more immediate history, symptoms, and behavior to be able to make a management decision. In a scheduled visit, a more thorough assessment is appropriate.

ROUTINE PSYCHIATRIC ASSESSMENT

Assessment includes a general medical and psychiatric history and a mental status examination. (See also the American Psychiatric Association's Psychiatric Evaluation of Adults Quick Reference Guide at http://psychiatryonline.org.)

History

The physician must determine whether the patient can provide a history, ie, whether the patient readily and coherently responds to initial questions. If not, information is sought from family, caregivers, or other collateral sources (eg, police). Even when a patient is communicative, close family members, friends, or caseworkers may provide information that the patient has omitted. Receiving information that is not solicited by the physician does not violate patient confidentiality. Previous psychiatric assessments, treatments, and degree of adherence to past treatments are reviewed, and records from such care are obtained as soon as possible.

Conducting an interview hastily and indifferently with closed-ended queries (following a rigid system review) often prevents patients from revealing relevant information. Tracing the history of the presenting illness with open-ended questions, so that patients can tell their story in their own words, takes a similar amount of time and enables patients to describe associated social circumstances and reveal emotional reactions.

The interview should first explore what prompted the need (or desire) for psychiatric assessment (eg, unwanted or unpleasant thoughts, undesirable behavior), including how much the presenting symptoms affect the patient or interfere with the patient's social, employment, and interpersonal functioning. The interviewer then attempts to gain a broader perspective on the patient's personality by reviewing significant life events—current and past—and the patient's responses to them (see Table 206–1). Psychiatric, medical, social, and developmental history is also reviewed. A review of systems to check for other symptoms not described in the psychiatric history is important. Focusing only on the presenting symptoms may result in missing either psychiatric or medical comorbidities.

The personality profile that emerges may suggest traits that are adaptive (eg, resilience, conscientiousness) or maladaptive (eg, self-centeredness, dependency, poor tolerance of frustration) and may show the coping mechanisms used. The interview may reveal obsessions (unwanted and distressing thoughts or impulses), compulsions (urges to do irrational or apparently useless acts), and delusions (fixed false beliefs) and may

Table 206–1. AREAS TO COVER IN THE INITIAL PSYCHIATRIC ASSESSMENT

AREA	SOME ELEMENTS
Psychiatric history	Known diagnoses Previous treatments, including drugs and hospitalizations
Medical history	Known disorders and chronic conditions New-onset physical symptoms Current drugs and treatments
Social history	Education level and educational history (eg, grades, difficulties making it through school) Marital history, including quality and stability of marriage or marriages or significant relationships Employment history, including stability and effectiveness at work Legal history, including arrests and incarcerations Living arrangements (eg, alone, with family, in group home or shelter, on street) Pattern of social life (eg, quality and frequency of interaction with friends and family)
Family health history	Known diagnoses, including mental disorders
Response to the usual vicissitudes of life	Divorce, job loss, death of friends and family, illness, other failures, setbacks, and losses Behavior while driving
Developmental history	Family composition and atmosphere during childhood Behavior during schooling Handling of different family and social roles Sexual adaptation and experiences
Daily conduct	Use or abuse of alcohol, drugs, and tobacco
Potential for harm to self or others	Suicidal thoughts, plans, and intent Prior suicide attempts and means used Intent to harm others

determine whether distress is expressed in physical symptoms (eg, headache, abdominal pain), mental symptoms (eg, phobic behavior, depression), or social behavior (eg, withdrawal, rebelliousness). The patient should also be asked about attitudes regarding psychiatric treatments, including drugs and psychotherapy, so that this information can be incorporated into the treatment plan.

The interviewer should establish whether a physical condition or its treatment is causing or worsening a mental condition. In addition to having direct effects (eg, symptoms, including mental ones), many physical conditions cause enormous stress and require coping mechanisms to withstand the pressures related to the condition. Many patients with severe physical conditions experience some kind of adjustment disorder, and those with underlying mental disorders may become unstable.

Observation during an interview may provide evidence of mental or physical disorders. Body language may reveal evidence of attitudes and feelings denied by the patient. For example, does the patient fidget or pace back and forth despite denying anxiety? Does the patient seem sad despite denying feelings of depression? General appearance may provide clues as well. For example, is the patient clean and well-kept? Is a tremor or facial droop present?

Mental Status Examination

A mental status examination uses observation and questions to evaluate several domains of mental function, including speech, emotional expression, thinking and perception, and cognitive functions. Brief standardized screening questionnaires are available for assessing certain components of the mental status examination, including those specifically designed to assess orientation and memory. Such standardized assessments can help identify the most important symptoms and provide a baseline for measuring response to treatment. However, screening questionnaires cannot take the place of a broader, more detailed mental status examination (see Sidebar 220–1 on p. 1836).

General appearance should be assessed for unspoken clues to underlying conditions. Patients' appearance can help determine whether they are unable to care for themselves (eg, they appear undernourished, disheveled, or dressed inappropriately for the weather or have significant body odor), are unable or unwilling to comply with social norms (eg, they are garbed in socially inappropriate clothing), or have engaged in substance abuse or attempted self-harm (eg, they have an odor of alcohol, scars suggesting IV drug abuse or self-inflicted injury).

Speech can be assessed by noting spontaneity, syntax, rate, and volume. A patient with depression may speak slowly and softly, whereas a patient with mania may speak rapidly and loudly. Abnormalities such as dysarthrias and aphasias may indicate a physical cause of mental status changes, such as head injury, stroke, brain tumor, or multiple sclerosis.

Emotional expression can be assessed by asking patients to describe their feelings. The patient's tone of voice, posture, hand gestures, and facial expressions are all considered. Mood (emotions patients report) and affect (emotional state interviewer notes) should be assessed. Discrepancies between mood and affect should be noted.

Thinking and perception can be assessed by noticing not only what is communicated but also how it is communicated. Abnormal content may take the form of delusions (false, fixed beliefs), ideas of reference (notions that everyday occurrences have special meaning or significance personally intended for or directed to the patient), or obsessions (persistent ideas, feelings, impulses, preoccupations). The physician can assess whether ideas seem to be linked and goal-directed and whether transitions from one thought to the next are logical. Psychotic or manic patients may have disorganized thoughts or an abrupt flight of ideas.

Cognitive functions include the patient's level of alertness; attentiveness or concentration; orientation to person, place, and time; memory; abstract reasoning; insight; and judgment. Abnormalities of cognition most often occur with delirium or dementia or with substance abuse or withdrawal but can also occur with depression.

MEDICAL ASSESSMENT OF THE PATIENT WITH MENTAL SYMPTOMS

Medical assessment of patients with mental symptoms seeks to identify 3 things:

- Physical disorders *mimicking* mental disorders
- Physical disorders *accompanying* mental disorders
- Physical disorders *caused by* mental disorders or their treatment

Numerous physical disorders cause symptoms mimicking specific mental disorders (see Table 206–2). Other physical disorders may not mimic specific mental syndromes but instead change mood and energy.

Table 206–2. SELECTED MENTAL SYMPTOMS DUE TO PHYSICAL DISORDERS

MENTAL SYMPTOM	PHYSICAL DISORDER*
Confusion, delirium, disorientation	Cerebral arteritis, including that caused by SLE
	CNS infection (eg, encephalitis, meningitis, toxoplasmosis)
	Complex partial seizures
	Dehydration
	Drug overdose, including prescription drug overdose
	Electrolyte abnormalities
	Fever
	Hypoglycemia
	Hypothermia
	Hypothyroidism
	Hypoxia
	Liver failure
	Mass lesion (eg, tumor, hematoma)
	Renal failure
	Sepsis
	Thyroid disorders
	Vascular infarct
	Vitamin deficiency
Cognitive impairment, behavioral instability	Alzheimer and other dementias
	HIV/AIDS
	Lyme disease
	Mass lesion
	Multiple sclerosis
	Neurosyphilis
	Parkinson disease
	Subdural hematoma
	SLE
	Thyroid disorders
	Vascular infarct
	Vitamin deficiency

Table 206–2. SELECTED MENTAL SYMPTOMS DUE TO PHYSICAL DISORDERS (*Continued*)

MENTAL SYMPTOM	PHYSICAL DISORDER*
Delusions	Multiple sclerosis Polysubstance abuse Seizure disorders
Depression	Brain tumor Cancer treatments, including interferon Cushing syndrome Dementia Diabetes mellitus Hypothyroidism Multiple sclerosis Sarcoidosis Sleep apnea
Euphoria, mania	Brain tumor Multiple sclerosis Polysubstance abuse
Hallucinations	Encephalitis Mass lesion Migraine Polysubstance abuse Seizure disorders
Insomnia	Circadian rhythm disorders Dyspnea or hypoxia Gastroesophageal reflux disease (GERD) Hyperthyroidism Periodic leg movement disorder or restless legs syndrome Pain syndromes
Irritability	Analgesic withdrawal Multiple sclerosis Vitamin B_{12} deficiency
Memory impairment	Alcohol abuse Hypothyroidism Multiple sclerosis Vitamin deficiency
Mood symptoms	HIV/AIDS Hypothyroidism Multiple sclerosis Stroke Substance abuse
Personality change	Mass lesion Multiple sclerosis Seizure disorders SLE
Psychosis (eg, hallucinations)	Brain tumor Dementia Electrolyte abnormalities Migraine Multiple sclerosis Polysubstance abuse Sarcoidosis Sensory loss SLE Syphilis

*In addition, numerous drugs and toxins may cause mental symptoms.

Many drugs cause mental symptoms; the most common classes of drug causes are

- CNS-active drugs (eg, anticonvulsants, antidepressants, antipsychotics, sedative/hypnotics, stimulants)
- Anticholinergics (eg, antihistamines)
- Corticosteroids

Numerous other therapeutic drugs and drug classes have also been implicated; they include some classes that may not ordinarily be considered (eg, antibiotics, antihypertensives). Drugs of abuse, particularly alcohol, amphetamines, cocaine, hallucinogens, and phencyclidine (PCP), particularly in overdose, are also frequent causes of mental symptoms. Withdrawal from alcohol, barbiturates, or benzodiazepines may cause mental symptoms (eg, anxiety) in addition to symptoms of physical withdrawal.

Patients with a mental disorder may develop a physical disorder (eg, meningitis, diabetic ketoacidosis) that causes new or worsened mental symptoms. Thus, a clinician should not assume that all mental symptoms in patients with a known mental disorder are due to that disorder. The clinician may need to be proactive in addressing possible physical causes for mental symptoms, especially in patients unable to describe their physical health because they have psychosis or dementia.

Patients presenting for psychiatric care occasionally have undiagnosed physical disorders that are not the cause of their mental symptoms but nonetheless require evaluation and treatment. Such disorders may be unrelated (eg, hypertension, angina) or caused by the mental disorder (eg, undernutrition due to inanition resulting from chronic psychosis) or its treatment (eg, hypothyroidism due to lithium, hyperlipidemia secondary to atypical antipsychotics).

Evaluation

Medical assessment by history, physical examination, and often brain imaging and laboratory testing is required for patients with

- New-onset mental symptoms (ie, no prior history of similar symptoms)
- Qualitatively different or unexpected symptoms (ie, in a patient with a known or stable mental disorder)
- Mental symptoms that begin at an unexpected age

The goal is to diagnose underlying and concomitant physical disorders rather than to make a specific psychiatric diagnosis.

History: History of present illness should note the nature of symptoms and their onset, particularly whether onset was sudden or gradual and whether symptoms followed any possible precipitants (eg, trauma, starting or stopping of a drug or abused substance). The clinician should ask whether patients have had previous episodes of similar symptoms, whether a mental disorder has been diagnosed and treated, and, if so, whether patients have stopped taking their drugs.

Review of systems seeks symptoms that suggest possible causes:

- Vomiting, diarrhea, or both: Dehydration, electrolyte disturbance
- Palpitations: Hyperthyroidism, drug effects including withdrawal
- Polyuria and polydipsia: Diabetes mellitus
- Tremors: Parkinson disease, withdrawal syndromes
- Difficulty walking or speaking: Multiple sclerosis, Parkinson disease, stroke
- Headache: CNS infection, complex migraine, hemorrhage, mass lesion

- Fever, cough, dysuria, vomiting, or diarrhea: Systemic infection
- Weight loss: Infection, cancer, inflammatory bowel disease, hyperthyroidism
- Paresthesias and weakness: Vitamin deficiency, stroke, demyelinating disease
- Relapsing and remitting neurologic symptoms: Multiple sclerosis, vasculitis

Past medical history should identify known chronic physical disorders that can cause mental symptoms (eg, thyroid, liver, or kidney disease; diabetes; HIV infection). All prescription and OTC drugs should be reviewed, and patients should be queried about any alcohol or illicit substance use (amount and duration). Family history of physical disorders, particularly of thyroid disease and multiple sclerosis, is assessed. Risk factors for infection (eg, unprotected sex, needle sharing, recent hospitalization, residence in a group facility) are noted.

Physical examination: Vital signs are reviewed, particularly for fever, tachypnea, hypertension, and tachycardia. Mental status is assessed (see Sidebar 220–1 on p. 1836), particularly for signs of confusion or inattention. A full physical examination is done, although the focus is on signs of infection (eg, meningismus, lung congestion, flank tenderness), the neurologic examination (including gait testing and weakness), and funduscopy to detect signs of increased intracranial pressure (eg, papilledema, loss of venous pulsations). Signs of liver disease (eg, jaundice, ascites, spider angiomas) should be noted. The skin is carefully inspected for self-inflicted wounds or other evidence of external trauma (eg, bruising).

Interpretation of findings: The findings from the history and physical examination help interpret possible causes and guide testing and treatment.

Confusion and inattention (reduced clarity of awareness of the environment—see p. 1871), especially if of sudden onset, fluctuating, or both, indicate the presence of a physical disorder. However, the converse is not true (ie, a clear sensorium does not confirm that the cause is a mental disorder). Other findings that suggest a physical cause include

- Abnormal vital signs (eg, fever, tachycardia, tachypnea)
- Meningeal signs
- Abnormalities noted during the neurologic examination, including aphasia
- Disturbance of gait, balance, or both
- Incontinence

Some findings help suggest a specific cause, especially when symptoms and signs are new or have changed from a long-standing baseline. Dilated pupils (particularly if accompanied by flushed, hot, dry skin) suggest anticholinergic drug effects. Constricted pupils suggest opioid drug effects or pontine hemorrhage. Rotary or vertical nystagmus suggests PCP intoxication, and horizontal nystagmus often accompanies diphenylhydantoin toxicity. Garbled speech or inability to produce speech suggests a brain lesion (eg, stroke). A preceding history of relapsing-remitting neurologic symptoms, particularly when a variety of nerves appear to be involved, suggests multiple sclerosis or vasculitis. Stocking-glove paresthesias may indicate thiamin or vitamin B_{12} deficiency. In patients with hallucinations, the type of hallucination is not particularly diagnostic except that command hallucinations or voices commenting on the patient's behavior probably represent a mental disorder.

Symptoms that began shortly after significant trauma or after beginning a new drug may be due to those events. Drug or alcohol abuse may or may not be the cause of mental symptoms; about 40 to 50% of patients with a mental disorder also have substance abuse (dual diagnosis).

Testing: Patients typically should have

- Pulse oximetry
- Fingerstick glucose testing
- Measurement of therapeutic drug levels
- Urine drug screen
- Blood alcohol level
- CBC
- Urinalysis

If patients with a known mental disorder have an exacerbation of their typical symptoms and they have no medical complaints, a normal sensorium, and a normal physical examination (including vital signs, pulse oximetry, and fingerstick glucose testing), they do not typically require further laboratory testing. Most other patients should have

- HIV testing

Many clinicians also measure

- Serum electrolytes (including Ca and Mg), BUN, and creatinine
- ESR or C-reactive protein

Electrolyte and renal function tests may be diagnostic and help inform subsequent drug management (eg, for drugs that require adjustment in patients with renal insufficiency).

Other tests are commonly done based on specific findings:

- Head CT: Patients with new-onset mental symptoms or with delirium, headache, history of recent trauma, or focal neurologic findings (eg, weakness of an extremity)
- Lumbar puncture: Patients with meningeal signs or with normal head CT findings plus fever, headache, or delirium
- Thyroid function tests: Patients taking lithium, those with symptoms or signs of thyroid disease, and those > 40 yr with new-onset mental symptoms (particularly females or patients with a family history of thyroid disease)
- Chest x-ray: Patients with low oxygen saturation, fever, productive cough, or hemoptysis
- Blood cultures: Seriously ill patients with fever
- Liver function tests: Patients with symptoms or signs of liver disease, with a history of alcohol or drug abuse, or with no obtainable history

Less often, findings may suggest testing for SLE, syphilis, demyelinating disorders, Lyme disease, or vitamin B_{12} or thiamin deficiency, especially in patients presenting with signs of dementia.

BEHAVIORAL EMERGENCIES

Patients who are experiencing severe changes in mood, thoughts, or behavior or severe, potentially life-threatening drug adverse effects need urgent assessment and treatment. Nonspecialists are often the first care providers for outpatients and inpatients on medical units, but whenever possible, such cases should also be evaluated by a psychiatrist.

When a patient's mood, thoughts, or behavior is highly unusual or disorganized, assessment must first determine whether the patient is a

- Threat to self
- Threat to others

The threat to self can include inability to care for self (leading to self-neglect) or suicidal behavior (see p. 1806). Self-neglect is a particular concern for patients with psychotic disorders, dementia, or substance abuse because their ability to obtain food, clothing, and appropriate protection from the elements is impaired.

Patients posing a threat to others include those who are actively violent (ie, actively assaulting staff members, throwing and breaking things), those who appear belligerent and hostile (ie, potentially violent), and those who do not appear threatening to the examiner and staff members but express intent to harm another person (eg, spouse, neighbor, public figure). It is also important to identify caregivers who cannot safely and adequately care for their dependents.

Causes: Aggressive, violent patients are often psychotic and have diagnoses such as polysubstance abuse, schizophrenia, delusional disorder, or acute mania. Other causes include physical disorders that cause acute delirium (see Table 206–2), a chronic organic brain disorder (eg, dementia) and intoxication with alcohol or other substances, particularly methamphetamine, cocaine, and sometimes PCP and club drugs (eg, MDMA [3,4-methylenedioxymethamphetamine]). A prior history of violence or aggression is a strong predictor of future episodes.

General Principles

Management typically occurs simultaneously with evaluation, particularly evaluation for a possible physical disorder (see p. 1736); it is a mistake to assume that the cause of abnormal behavior is a mental disorder or intoxication, even in patients who have a known psychiatric diagnosis or an odor of alcohol. Because patients are often unable or unwilling to provide a clear history, other collateral sources of information (eg, family members, friends, caseworkers, medical records) must be identified and consulted immediately. The clinician must be aware that patient violence may be directed at the treatment team and other patients.

Actively violent patients must first be restrained by

- Physical means
- Drugs (chemical restraint)
- Both

Such interventions are done to prevent harm to patients and others and to allow evaluation of the cause of the behavior (eg, by taking vital signs and doing blood tests). Once the patient is restrained, close monitoring, sometimes involving constant observation by a trained sitter, is required. Medically stable patients may be placed in a safe seclusion room. Although clinicians must be aware of legal issues regarding involuntary treatment (see Sidebar 206–1), such issues must not delay potentially lifesaving interventions.

Potentially violent patients require measures to defuse the situation. Measures that may help reduce agitation and aggressiveness include

- Moving patients to a calm, quiet environment (eg, a seclusion room, when available)
- Removing objects that could be used to inflict harm to self or others
- Expressing sympathetic concern for patients and their complaints
- Responding in a confident yet supportive manner
- Inquiring what can be done to resolve the cause of the anger

Speaking directly—mentioning that patients seem angry or upset, asking them if they intend to hurt someone—acknowledges their feelings and may elicit information; it does not make them more likely to act out.

Counterproductive measures include

- Challenging the validity of patients' fears and complaints
- Issuing threats (eg, to call police, to commit them)
- Speaking in a condescending manner
- Attempting to deceive patients (eg, hiding drugs in food, promising them they will not be restrained)

Staff and public safety: When hostile, aggressive patients are interviewed, staff safety must be considered. Most hospitals have a policy to search for weapons (manually, with metal detectors, or both) on patients presenting with disordered behavior. When possible, patients should be assessed in an area with safety features such as security cameras, metal detectors, and interview rooms that are visible to staff members.

Patients who are hostile but not yet violent typically do not assault staff members randomly; rather, they assault staff members who anger or appear threatening to them. Doors to rooms should be left open. Staff members may also avoid appearing threatening by sitting on the same level as patients. Staff members may avoid angering patients by not responding to their hostility in kind, with loud, angry remarks or arguing. If patients nonetheless become increasingly agitated and violence appears impending, staff members should simply leave the room and summon sufficient additional staff to provide a show of force, which sometimes deters patients. Typically, at least 4 or 5 people should be present (some preferably young and male). However, the team should not bring restraints into the room

Sidebar 206–1. Regulatory Issues in Use of Physical Restraints in Aggressive, Violent Patients

Use of physical restraints should be considered a last resort, when other steps have not sufficiently controlled aggressive, potentially violent behavior. When restraints are needed for such a situation, they are legal in all states as long as their use is properly ordered and documented in the patient's medical record. Restraints have the advantage of being immediately removable, whereas drugs may alter symptoms enough or in a way that delays assessment.

The Joint Commission on Accreditation of Healthcare Organizations guidelines for use of restraints in the psychiatric setting state that restraints must be applied under the direction of a licensed independent practitioner (LIP). The LIP must assess the patient within the first hour of restraint placement. The order for continued restraint of adults may be written for up to 4 h at a time. The patient must be evaluated by an LIP or registered nurse during the 4-h interval and before further continuation of the restraint order. At 8 h, the LIP must reevaluate the patient in person before continuing the restraint order. Children aged 9–17 yr must be assessed every 2 h, and those < 9 yr, every hour.

Hospital accreditation standards require that patients in restraints be continuously observed by a trained sitter. Immediately after restraints have been applied, the patient must be monitored for signs of injury; circulation, range of motion, nutrition and hydration, vital signs, hygiene, and elimination are also monitored. Physical and mental comfort and readiness for discontinuation of restraints as appropriate are also assessed. These assessments should be done every 15 min.

Seclusion and restraints should be used simultaneously only under special circumstances and with continuous monitoring.

unless they are definitely to be applied; seeing restraints may further agitate patients.

Verbal threats must be taken seriously. In most states, when a patient expresses the intention to harm a particular person, the evaluating physician is required to warn the intended victim and to notify a specified law enforcement agency. Specific requirements vary by state. Typically, state regulations also require reporting of suspected abuse of children, the elderly, and spouses.

Physical Restraints

Use of physical restraints is controversial and should be considered only when other methods have failed and a patient continues to pose a significant risk of harm to self or others. Restraints may be needed to hold the patient long enough to administer drugs, do a complete assessment, or both. Because restraints are applied without the patient's consent, certain legal and ethical issues should be considered (see Sidebar 206–1).

Restraints are used to

- Prevent clear, imminent harm to the patient or others
- Prevent the patient's medical treatment from being significantly disrupted (eg, by pulling out tubes or IVs) when consent to the treatment has been provided
- Prevent damage to physical surroundings, staff members, or other patients
- Prevent a patient who requires involuntary treatment from leaving (when a locked room is unavailable)

Restraints should not be used for

- Punishment
- Convenience of staff members (eg, to prevent wandering)

Caution is required in overtly suicidal patients, who could use the restraint as a suicide device.

Procedure: Restraints should be applied only by staff members adequately trained in correct techniques and in protecting patient rights and safety.

First, adequate staff are assembled in the room, and patients are informed that restraints must be applied. Patients are encouraged to cooperate to avoid a struggle. However, once the clinician has determined that restraints are necessary, there is no negotiation, and patients are told that restraints will be applied whether or not they agree. Some actually understand and appreciate having external limits on their behavior. In preparation for applying restraints, one person is assigned to each extremity and another to the patient's head. Then, each person simultaneously grasps their assigned extremity and places the patient supine on the bed; one physically fit person can typically control a single extremity of even large, violent patients (provided all extremities are grasped at the same time). However, an additional person is needed to apply the restraints. Rarely, upright patients who are extremely combative may first need to be sandwiched between 2 mattresses.

Leather restraints are preferred. One restraint is applied to each ankle and wrist and attached to the bed frame, not the rail. Restraints are not applied around the chest, neck, or head, and gags (eg, to prevent spitting and swearing) are forbidden. Patients who remain combative in restraints (eg, attempting to upset the stretcher, bite, or spit) require chemical restraint.

Complications: Agitated or violent people brought to the hospital by police are almost always in restraints (eg, handcuffs). Occasionally, young, healthy people have died in police restraints before or shortly after hospital arrival. The cause is often unclear but probably involves some combination of overexertion with subsequent metabolic derangement and hyperthermia, drug use, aspiration of stomach contents into the respiratory system, embolism in people left in restraints for a long time, and occasionally serious underlying medical disorders. Death is more likely if people are restrained in the hobble position, with one or both wrists shackled to the ankles behind their back; this type of restraint may cause asphyxia and should be avoided. Because of these complications, violent patients presenting in police custody should be evaluated promptly and thoroughly and not dismissed as mere sociobehavioral problems.

Chemical Restraints

Drug therapy, if used, should target control of specific symptoms.

Drugs: Patients can usually be rapidly calmed or tranquilized using

- Benzodiazepines
- Antipsychotics (typically a conventional antipsychotic, but a 2nd-generation drug may be used)

These drugs are better titrated and act more rapidly and reliably when administered IV (see Table 206–3), but IM administration may be necessary when IV access cannot be achieved in struggling patients. Both classes of drug are effective sedatives for agitated, violent patients. Benzodiazepines are probably preferred for stimulant drug overdoses and for alcohol and benzodiazepine drug withdrawal syndromes, and antipsychotics are preferred for clear exacerbations of known mental disorders. Sometimes a combination of both drugs is more effective; when large doses of one drug have not had the full desired effect, using another drug class instead of continuing to increase the dose of the first drug may limit adverse effects.

Table 206–3. DRUG THERAPY FOR AGITATED OR VIOLENT PATIENTS

DRUG	DOSAGE	COMMENTS
Lorazepam	0.5–2 mg q 1 h IM (deltoid) or IV prn	IV is preferred because absorption from IM injection may be erratic. Respiratory depression is possible.
Haloperidol	1–10 mg po, IM (deltoid), or IV q 1 h prn (1–2.5 mg for mild agitation and for frail or older patients; 2.5–5 mg for moderate agitation; 5–10 mg for severe agitation)	The drug is usually required only if psychosis is clear. The drug can make some substance intoxications (eg, with PCP) worse and may cause dystonia. A liquid concentrate may be used for rapid absorption if the patient can take the drug po. Respiratory depression does not occur.
Ziprasidone	10–20 mg IM (may repeat 10-mg dose q 2 h or 20-mg dose q 4 h; maximum, 40 mg/day)	ECG monitoring may be needed. Concomitant use with carbamazepine and ketoconazole should be avoided.

Table 206–4. TREATMENT OF ACUTE ADVERSE EFFECTS OF ANTIPSYCHOTICS

SYMPTOMS	TREATMENT	COMMENTS
Acute dystonic reactions (eg, oculogyric crisis, torticollis)	Benztropine 2 mg IV or IM (may be repeated once in 20 min) Diphenhydramine 50 mg IV or IM q 20 min for 2 doses	Benztropine 2 mg po may prevent dystonia when given with an antipsychotic.
Laryngeal dystonia	Lorazepam 4 mg IV over 10 min, then 1–2 mg IV slowly	Intubation may be needed.
Akinesia, severe parkinsonian tremors, bradykinesia	Benztropine 1–2 mg po bid Diphenhydramine 25–50 mg po tid	In patients with akinesia, the antipsychotic may have to be stopped, and one with a lower potency used.
Akathisia (with other extrapyramidal symptoms)	Amantadine 100–150 mg po bid Benztropine 1–2 mg po bid Biperiden 1–4 mg po bid Procyclidine 2.5–10 mg po bid Propranolol 10–30 mg po tid Trihexyphenidyl 2–7 mg po bid or 1–5 mg po tid (or for the sustained-release form, 2–7 mg bid)	The causative drug should be stopped, or a lower dose used.
Akathisia associated with extreme anxiety	Lorazepam 1 mg tid po Clonazepam 0.5 mg bid po	—

Adverse effects of benzodiazepines: Parenteral benzodiazepines, particularly in the doses sometimes needed for extremely violent patients, may cause respiratory depression. Airway management with intubation and assisted ventilation may be required. The benzodiazepine antagonist, flumazenil, may be used, but caution is required because if sedation is significantly reversed, the original behavioral problem may reappear.

Benzodiazepines sometimes lead to further disinhibition of behavior.

Adverse effects of antipsychotic drugs: Antipsychotics, particularly dopamine-receptor antagonists, at therapeutic as well as toxic doses, can have acute extrapyramidal adverse effects (see Table 206–4), including acute dystonia and akathisia (an unpleasant sensation of motor restlessness). These adverse effects may be dose dependent and may resolve once the drug is stopped. Several antipsychotics, including thioridazine, haloperidol, olanzapine, risperidone, and ziprasidone, can cause long QT interval syndrome and ultimately increase the risk of fatal arrhythmias. Neuroleptic malignant syndrome is also a possibility (see p. 3018). For other adverse effects, see Table 213–1 on p. 1792.

Legal Considerations

Patients with severe changes in mood, thoughts, or behavior are usually hospitalized when their condition is likely to deteriorate without psychiatric intervention and when appropriate alternatives are not available.

Consent and involuntary treatment: If patients refuse hospitalization, the physician must decide whether to hold them against their will. Doing so may be necessary to ensure the immediate safety of the patient or of others or to allow completion of an assessment and implementation of treatment. Criteria and procedures for involuntary hospitalization vary by jurisdiction. Usually, temporary restraint requires a physician or psychologist and one additional clinician, family member, or close contact to certify that the patient has a mental disorder, is a danger to self or to others, and refuses voluntary treatment. Physicians should obtain consent to drug treatment of minor children from parents or guardians.

Danger to self includes but is not limited to

- Suicidal ideation or attempts
- Failure to attend to basic needs, including nutrition, shelter, and needed drugs

In most jurisdictions, knowledge of intent to commit suicide requires a healthcare practitioner to act immediately to prevent the suicide, for example, by notifying the police or another responsible agency.

Danger to others includes

- Expressing homicidal intent
- Placing others in peril
- Failing to provide for the needs or safety of dependents because of the mental disorder

207 Anxiety and Stressor-Related Disorders

Everyone periodically experiences fear and anxiety. Fear is an emotional, physical, and behavioral response to an immediately recognizable external threat (eg, an intruder, a car spinning on ice). Anxiety is a distressing, unpleasant emotional state of nervousness and uneasiness; its causes are less clear. Anxiety is less tied to the exact timing of a threat; it can be anticipatory before a threat, persist after a threat has passed, or occur without an identifiable threat. Anxiety is often accompanied by physical changes and behaviors similar to those caused by fear.

Some degree of anxiety is adaptive; it can help people prepare, practice, and rehearse so that their functioning is improved and can help them be appropriately cautious in potentially dangerous situations. However, beyond a certain level, anxiety causes dysfunction and undue distress. At this point, it is maladaptive and considered a disorder.

Anxiety occurs in a wide range of physical and mental disorders, but it is the predominant symptom of several. Anxiety disorders are more common than any other class of psychiatric disorder. However, they often are not recognized and consequently not treated. Left untreated, chronic maladaptive anxiety can contribute to or interfere with treatment of some general medical disorders.

Mental distress that occurs immediately or shortly after experiencing or witnessing an overwhelming traumatic event is no longer classified as an anxiety disorder. Such disorders are now classified as trauma- and stressor-related disorders (see Acute Stress Disorder on p. 1746 and Posttraumatic Stress Disorder on p. 1747).

Etiology

The causes of anxiety disorders are not fully known, but both psychiatric and general medical factors are involved. Many people develop anxiety disorders without any identifiable antecedent triggers. Anxiety can be a response to environmental stressors, such as the ending of a significant relationship or exposure to a life-threatening disaster.

Some general medical disorders can directly cause anxiety; they include the following:

- Hyperthyroidism
- Pheochromocytoma
- Hyperadrenocorticism
- Heart failure
- Arrhythmias
- Asthma
- COPD

Other causes include use of drugs; effects of corticosteroids, cocaine, amphetamines, and even caffeine can mimic anxiety disorders. Withdrawal from alcohol, sedatives, and some illicit drugs can also cause anxiety.

Symptoms and Signs

Anxiety can arise suddenly, as in panic, or gradually over many minutes, hours, or even days. Anxiety may last from a few seconds to years; longer duration is more characteristic of anxiety disorders. Anxiety ranges from barely noticeable qualms to complete panic. The ability to tolerate a given level of anxiety varies from person to person.

Anxiety disorders can be so distressing and disruptive that depression may result. Alternatively, an anxiety disorder and a depressive disorder may coexist, or depression may develop first, with symptoms and signs of an anxiety disorder occurring later.

Diagnosis

- Exclusion of other causes
- Assessment of severity

Deciding when anxiety is so dominant or severe that it constitutes a disorder depends on several variables, and physicians differ at what point they make the diagnosis. Physicians must first use history, physical examination, and appropriate laboratory tests to determine whether anxiety is due to a general medical disorder or drug. They must also determine whether anxiety is better accounted for by another mental disorder.

An anxiety disorder is present and merits treatment if the following apply:

- Other causes are not identified.
- Anxiety is very distressing.
- Anxiety interferes with functioning.
- Anxiety does not stop spontaneously within a few days.

Diagnosis of a specific anxiety disorder is based on its characteristic symptoms and signs. Clinicians usually use specific criteria of the *Diagnostic and Statistical Manual of Mental Disorders*, Fifth Edition (DSM-5), which describes the specific symptoms and requires exclusion of other causes of symptoms.

A family history of anxiety disorders helps in making the diagnosis because some patients appear to inherit a predisposition to the same anxiety disorders that their relatives have, as well as a general susceptibility to other anxiety disorders. However, some patients appear to acquire the same disorders as their relatives through learned behavior.

Treatment

Treatments vary for the different anxiety disorders, but typically involve a combination of psychotherapy specific for the disorder and drug treatment. The most common drug classes used are the benzodiazepines and SSRIs.

GENERALIZED ANXIETY DISORDER

Generalized anxiety disorder (GAD) is characterized by excessive anxiety and worry that is present more days than not for ≥ 6 mo about a number of activities or events. The cause is unknown, although it commonly coexists in people who have alcohol abuse, major depression, or panic disorder. Diagnosis is based on history and physical examination. Treatment is psychotherapy, drug therapy, or both.

GAD is common, affecting about 3% of the population within a 1-yr period. Women are twice as likely to be affected as men. The disorder often begins in childhood or adolescence but may begin at any age.

Symptoms and Signs

The focus of the worry is not restricted as it is in other psychiatric disorders (eg, to having a panic attack, being embarrassed in public, or being contaminated); the patient has multiple worries, which often shift over time. Common worries include work and family responsibilities, money, health, safety, car repairs, and chores.

The course is usually fluctuating and chronic, and worsens during stress. Most patients with GAD have one or more other comorbid psychiatric disorders, including major depression, specific phobia, social phobia, and panic disorder.

Diagnosis

- Clinical criteria

Diagnosis is clinical based on criteria in the *Diagnostic and Statistical Manual of Mental Disorders*, Fifth Edition (DSM-5). Patients have excessive anxiety and worries about a number of activities or events. Patients have difficulty controlling

Table 207–1. BENZODIAZEPINES

DRUG	STARTING ORAL DOSE	MAINTENANCE ORAL DOSE*	ONSET/DURATION
Alprazolam†	0.25 mg bid Extended-release: 0.5 mg once/day	1 mg tid Extended-release: 3 mg once/day	Intermediate/intermediate
Chlordiazepoxide‡	5 mg tid	25 mg tid	Intermediate/long
Clonazepam†	0.25 mg once/day	1 mg tid	Intermediate/long
Clorazepate‡	7.5 mg bid	7.5 mg tid or 15 mg bid Single-dose (sustained release): 22.5 mg once/day after stabilized on 7.5 mg tid	Rapid/long
Diazepam‡	2 mg tid	5 mg tid	Rapid/long
Lorazepam	0.5 mg tid	1 mg tid	Intermediate/short
Oxazepam	10 mg tid	15 mg qid	Slow/short

*Maintenance dose can vary and depends on individual response.
†An oral disintegrating tablet or wafer is available. Onset does not differ from other formulations. Although these tablets disintegrate in the mouth, they are absorbed in the stomach and intestine, as are standard tablets.
‡Generally, these drugs are not recommended in the elderly because of a long half-life.

the worries, which occur more days than not for ≥ 6 mo. The worries must also be associated with ≥ 3 of the following:

- Restlessness or a keyed-up or on-edge feeling
- Easily fatigability
- Difficulty concentrating
- Irritability
- Muscle tension
- Disturbed sleep

Also, the anxiety and worry cannot be accounted for by substance use or another medical disorder (eg, hyperthyroidism).

Treatment

- Antidepressants and often benzodiazepines

Certain antidepressants, including SSRIs (eg, escitalopram, starting dose of 10 mg po once/day) and serotonin-norepinephrine reuptake inhibitors (eg, venlafaxine extended-release, starting dose 37.5 mg po once/day) are effective but typically only after being taken for at least a few weeks. Benzodiazepines (anxiolytics—see Table 207–1) in small to moderate doses are also often and more rapidly effective, although sustained use may lead to physical dependence. One strategy involves starting with concomitant use of a benzodiazepine and an antidepressant. Once the antidepressant becomes effective, the benzodiazepine is tapered.

Buspirone is also effective; the starting dose is 5 mg po bid or tid. However, buspirone can take at least 2 wk before it begins to help.

Psychotherapy, usually cognitive-behavioral therapy, can be both supportive and problem-focused. Relaxation and biofeedback may be of some help, although few studies have documented their efficacy.

PANIC ATTACKS AND PANIC DISORDER

A panic attack is the sudden onset of a discrete, brief period of intense discomfort, anxiety, or fear accompanied by somatic and/or cognitive symptoms. Panic disorder is occurrence of repeated panic attacks typically accompanied by fears about future attacks or changes in behavior to avoid situations that might predispose to attacks. Diagnosis is clinical. Isolated panic attacks may not require treatment. Panic disorder is treated with drug therapy, psychotherapy (eg, exposure therapy, cognitive-behavioral therapy), or both.

Panic attacks are common, affecting as many as 11% of the population in a single year. Most people recover without treatment; a few develop panic disorder.

Panic disorder is uncommon, affecting 2 to 3% of the population in a 12-mo period. Panic disorder usually begins in late adolescence or early adulthood and affects women about 2 times more often than men.

Symptoms and Signs

A panic attack involves the sudden onset of intense fear or discomfort accompanied by at least 4 of the 13 symptoms listed in Table 207–2. Symptoms usually peak within 10 min and dissipate within minutes thereafter, leaving little for a physician to observe. Although uncomfortable—at times extremely so—panic attacks are not medically dangerous.

Panic attacks may occur in any anxiety disorder, usually in situations tied to the core features of the disorder (eg, a person with a phobia of snakes may panic at seeing a snake). Such panic attacks are termed expected. Unexpected panic attacks are those that occur spontaneously, without any apparent trigger.

Most people with panic disorder anticipate and worry about another attack (anticipatory anxiety) and avoid places or situations where they have previously panicked. People with panic disorder often worry that they have a dangerous heart, lung, or brain disorder and repeatedly visit their family physician or an emergency department seeking help. Unfortunately, in these settings, attention is often focused on general medical symptoms, and the correct diagnosis sometimes is not made.

Many people with panic disorder also have symptoms of major depression.

Table 207–2. SYMPTOMS OF A PANIC ATTACK

Cognitive
Fear of dying
Fear of going crazy or of losing control
Feelings of unreality, strangeness (derealization), or detachment from the self (depersonalization)
Somatic
Chest pain or discomfort
Dizziness, unsteady feelings, or faintness
Feeling of choking
Flushes or chills
Nausea or abdominal distress
Numbness or tingling sensations
Palpitations or accelerated heart rate
Sensations of shortness of breath or smothering
Sweating
Trembling or shaking

Diagnosis

- Clinical criteria

Panic disorder is diagnosed after physical disorders that can mimic anxiety are eliminated and when symptoms meet diagnostic criteria stipulated in the *Diagnostic and Statistical Manual of Mental Disorders*, Fifth Edition (DSM-5). Patients must have recurrent panic attacks (frequency is not specified) in which ≥ 1 attack has been followed by one or both of the following for ≥ 1 mo:

- Persistent worry about having additional panic attacks or worry about their consequences (eg, losing control, going crazy)
- Maladaptive behavioral response to the panic attacks (eg, avoiding common activities such as exercise or social situations to try to prevent further attacks)

Treatment

- Often antidepressants, benzodiazepines, or both
- Often nondrug measures (eg, exposure therapy, cognitive-behavioral therapy)

Some people recover without treatment, particularly if they continue to confront situations in which attacks have occurred. For others, especially without treatment, panic disorder follows a chronic waxing and waning course.

Patients should be told that treatment usually helps control symptoms. If avoidance behaviors have not developed, reassurance, education about anxiety, and encouragement to continue to return to and remain in places where panic attacks have occurred may be all that is needed. However, with a long-standing disorder that involves frequent attacks and avoidance behaviors, treatment is likely to require drug therapy combined with more intensive psychotherapy.

Drugs: Many drugs can prevent or greatly reduce anticipatory anxiety, phobic avoidance, and the number and intensity of panic attacks:

- **Antidepressants:** The different classes—SSRIs, serotonin-norepinephrine reuptake inhibitors (SNRIs), serotonin modulators, tricyclics (TCAs), and monoamine oxidase inhibitors (MAOIs)—are similarly effective. However, SSRIs and SNRIs offer a potential advantage of fewer adverse effects in comparison with other antidepressants.
- **Benzodiazepines:** These anxiolytics (see Table 207–1) work more rapidly than antidepressants but are more likely to cause physical dependence and such adverse effects as somnolence, ataxia, and memory problems. For some patients, long-term use of benzodiazepines is the only effective treatment.
- **Antidepressants plus benzodiazepines:** These drugs are sometimes used in combination initially; the benzodiazepine is slowly tapered after the antidepressant becomes effective (although some patients respond only to the combination treatment).

Panic attacks often recur when drugs are stopped.

Psychotherapy: Different forms of psychotherapy are effective.

Exposure therapy, in which patients confront their fears, helps diminish the fear and complications caused by fearful avoidance. For example, patients who fear that they will faint during a panic attack are asked to spin in a chair or to hyperventilate until they feel dizzy or faint, thereby learning that they will not faint during an attack.

Cognitive-behavioral therapy involves teaching patients to recognize and control their distorted thinking and false beliefs and to modify their behavior so that it is more adaptive. For example, if patients describe acceleration of their heart rate or shortness of breath in certain situations or places and fear that they are having a heart attack, they are taught the following:

- Not to avoid those situations
- To understand that their worries are unfounded
- To respond instead with slow, controlled breathing or other methods that promote relaxation

SPECIFIC PHOBIC DISORDERS

Specific phobic disorders consist of persistent, unreasonable, intense fears (phobias) of specific situations, circumstances, or objects. The fears provoke anxiety and avoidance. The causes of phobias are unknown. Phobic disorders are diagnosed based on history. Treatment is mainly with exposure therapy.

A specific phobia is fear of and anxiety about a particular situation or object (see Table 207–3). The situation or object is usually avoided when possible, but if exposure occurs, anxiety quickly develops. The anxiety may intensify to the level of a panic attack (see p. 1743). People with specific phobias typically recognize that their fear is unreasonable and excessive.

Specific phobias are the most common anxiety disorders. Some of the most common are fear of animals (zoophobia), heights (acrophobia), and thunderstorms (astraphobia or brontophobia). Specific phobias affect about 13% of women and 4% of men during any 12-mo period. Some cause little inconvenience—as when city dwellers fear snakes (ophidiophobia), unless they are asked to hike in an area where snakes are found. However, other phobias interfere severely with functioning—as when people who must work on an upper floor of a skyscraper fear closed, confined places (claustrophobia), such as elevators. Fear of blood (hemophobia), injections (trypanophobia), needles or other sharp objects (belonephobia), or injury (traumatophobia) occurs to some degree in at least 5% of the population. People with a phobia of blood, needles, or injury, unlike those with other phobias or anxiety disorders, can actually faint because an excessive vasovagal reflex causes bradycardia and orthostatic hypotension.

Symptoms and Signs

Symptoms depend on the type of phobic disorder.

Table 207–3. SOME COMMON PHOBIAS*

PHOBIA	DEFINITION
Acrophobia	Fear of heights
Amathophobia	Fear of dust
Astraphobia	Fear of thunder and lightning
Aviophobia	Fear of flying
Belonephobia	Fear of needles, pins, or other sharp objects
Brontophobia	Fear of thunder
Claustrophobia	Fear of confined spaces
Eurotophobia	Fear of female genitals
Gephyrophobia	Fear of crossing bridges
Hydrophobia	Fear of water
Odontiatophobia	Fear of dentists
Phartophobia	Fear of passing gas in a public place
Phasmophobia	Fear of ghosts
Phobophobia	Fear of having fears or developing a phobia
Triskaidekaphobia	Fear of all things associated with the number 13
Trypanophobia	Fear of injections
Zoophobia	Fear of animals (usually spiders, snakes, or mice)

*There are over 500 named phobias, listed at the Phobia List web site (www.phobialist.com/). Most are extremely rare.

Diagnosis

Diagnosis is clinical based on criteria in the *Diagnostic and Statistical Manual of Mental Disorders*, Fifth Edition (DSM-5).

Patients have marked, persistent (≥ 6 mo) fear of or anxiety about a specific situation or object, plus all of the following:

- The situation or object nearly always triggers immediate fear or anxiety.
- Patients actively avoid the situation or object.
- The fear or anxiety is out of proportion to the actual danger (taking into account sociocultural norms).
- The fear, anxiety, and/or avoidance cause significant distress or significantly impair social or occupational functioning.

Also, the fear and anxiety cannot be more correctly characterized as a different mental disorder (eg, agoraphobia, social anxiety, a stress disorder).

Treatment

- Exposure therapy
- Sometimes limited use of a benzodiazepine or β-blocker

The prognosis for untreated specific phobias varies because certain uncommon situations or objects (eg, snakes, caves) are easy to avoid, whereas other situations or objects (eg, bridges, thunderstorms) are common and difficult to avoid.

Exposure therapy: Because many phobic disorders involve avoidance, exposure therapy, a specific psychotherapy, is the treatment of choice. With structure and support from a clinician who prescribes exposure homework, patients seek out, confront, and remain in contact with what they fear and avoid until their anxiety is gradually relieved through a process called habituation. Because most patients know their fears are excessive and may be embarrassed by their fears, they are usually willing to participate in this therapy—ie, to avoid avoiding.

Typically, clinicians begin with a moderate exposure (eg, patients are asked to closely approach the feared object). If patients describe acceleration of their heart rate or shortness of breath when they encounter the feared situation or object, they may be taught to respond with slow, controlled breathing or other methods that promote relaxation. Or, they may be asked to note when their heart rate accelerated and shortness of breath began and when the response returned toward normal. When patients feel comfortable at one level of exposure, the exposure level is increased (eg, to touching the feared object). Clinicians continue to increase the exposure level until patients can tolerate normal interaction with the situation or object (eg, ride in an elevator, cross a bridge). Exposure can increase as rapidly as patients tolerate it; sometimes only a few sessions are needed.

Exposure therapy helps > 90% of patients who carry it out faithfully and is almost always the only treatment needed for specific phobias.

Drugs: Short-term therapy with a benzodiazepine (eg, lorazepam 0.5 to 1.0 mg po) or a β-blocker (propranolol is generally preferred—10 to 40 mg po), ideally about 1 to 2 h before the exposure, is occasionally useful when exposure to an object or situation cannot be avoided (eg, when a person who has a phobia of flying must fly on short notice) or when exposure therapy is either unwanted or has not been successful.

SOCIAL PHOBIA

(Social Anxiety Disorder)

Social phobia is fear of and anxiety about being exposed to certain social or performance situations. These situations are avoided or endured with substantial anxiety.

Social phobia affects about 9% of women and 7% of men during any 12-mo period, but the lifetime prevalence may be at least 13%. Men are more likely than women to have the most severe form of social anxiety, avoidant personality disorder (see p. 1777).

Fear and anxiety in people with social phobia often centers on being embarrassed or humiliated if they fail to meet expectations. Often, the concern is that their anxiety will be apparent through sweating, blushing, vomiting, or trembling (sometimes as a quavering voice) or that the ability to keep a train of thought or find words to express themselves will be lost. Usually, the same activity done alone causes no anxiety.

Situations in which social phobia is common include public speaking, acting in a theatrical performance, and playing a musical instrument. Other potential situations include eating with others, meeting new people, having a conversation, signing a document before witnesses, or using public bathrooms. A more generalized type of social phobia causes anxiety in a broad array of social situations.

Most people recognize that their fears are unreasonable and excessive.

Diagnosis

- Clinical criteria

Diagnosis is clinical based on criteria in the *Diagnostic and Statistical Manual of Mental Disorders*, Fifth Edition (DSM-5).

To meet the DSM-5 criteria for diagnosis, patients must have a marked, persistent (≥ 6 mo) fear of or anxiety about one or more social situations in which they may be scrutinized by others. Fear must involve a negative evaluation by others (eg, that patients will be humiliated, embarrassed, or rejected or will offend others). In addition, all of the following should be present:

- The same social situations nearly always trigger fear or anxiety.
- Patients actively avoid the situation.
- The fear or anxiety is out of proportion to the actual threat (taking into account sociocultural norms).
- The fear, anxiety, and/or avoidance cause significant distress or significantly impair social or occupational functioning.

Also, the fear and anxiety cannot be more correctly characterized as a different mental disorder (eg, agoraphobia, panic disorder, body dysmorphic disorder).

Treatment

- Cognitive-behavioral therapy
- Sometimes an SSRI

Social phobia is almost always chronic, and treatment is needed.

Cognitive-behavioral therapy is effective for social phobia. Cognitive-behavioral therapy involves teaching patients to recognize and control their distorted thinking and false beliefs as well as instructing them on exposure therapy (controlled exposure to the anxiety-provoking situation—see p. 1745).

SSRIs and benzodiazepines are effective for social phobia, but SSRIs are probably preferable in most cases because unlike benzodiazepines, they are unlikely to interfere with cognitive-behavioral therapy.

β-Blockers may be used to reduce the increased heart rate, trembling, and sweating experienced by patients who are distressed by performing in public, but these drugs do not reduce anxiety.

AGORAPHOBIA

Agoraphobia is fear of and anticipatory anxiety about being trapped in situations or places without a way to escape easily and without help if intense anxiety develops.

The situations are avoided, or they may be endured but with substantial anxiety. About 30 to 50% of people with agoraphobia also have panic disorder (see p. 1743).

Agoraphobia without panic disorder affects about 2% of women and 1% of men during any 12-mo period. Peak age at onset is the early 20s; first appearance after age 40 is unusual.

Common examples of situations or places that create fear and anxiety include standing in line at a bank or at a supermarket checkout, sitting in the middle of a long row in a theater or classroom, and using public transportation, such as a bus or an airplane. Some people develop agoraphobia after a panic attack in a typical agoraphobic situation. Others simply feel uncomfortable in such a situation and may never or only later have panic attacks there. Agoraphobia often interferes with function and, if severe enough, can cause people to become housebound.

Diagnosis

- Clinical criteria

Diagnosis is clinical based on criteria in the *Diagnostic and Statistical Manual of Mental Disorders*, Fifth Edition (DSM-5).

To meet the DSM-5 criteria for diagnosis, patients must have marked, persistent (≥ 6 mo) fear of or anxiety about ≥ 2 of the following situations:

- Using public transportation
- Being in open spaces (eg, parking lot, marketplace)
- Being in an enclosed place (eg, shop, theater)
- Standing in line or being in a crowd
- Being alone outside the home

Fear must involve thoughts that escape from the situation might be difficult or that patients would receive no help if they became incapacitated by fear or a panic attack. In addition, all of the following should be present:

- The same situations nearly always trigger fear or anxiety.
- Patients actively avoid the situation and/or require the presence of a companion.
- The fear or anxiety is out of proportion to the actual threat (taking into account sociocultural norms).
- The fear, anxiety, and/or avoidance cause significant distress or significantly impair social or occupational functioning.

Also, the fear and anxiety cannot be more correctly characterized as a different mental disorder (eg, social anxiety disorder, body dysmorphic disorder).

Treatment

- Cognitive-behavioral therapy
- Sometimes an SSRI

If untreated, agoraphobia usually waxes and wanes in severity. Agoraphobia may disappear without formal treatment, possibly because some affected people conduct their own form of exposure therapy. But if agoraphobia interferes with functioning, treatment is needed.

Cognitive-behavioral therapy is effective for agoraphobia. Cognitive-behavioral therapy involves teaching patients to recognize and control their distorted thinking and false beliefs as well as instructing them on exposure therapy (see p. 1745).

Many patients with agoraphobia benefit from drug therapy with an SSRI.

OVERVIEW OF TRAUMA AND STRESSOR-RELATED DISORDERS

Trauma- and stressor-related disorders involve exposure to a traumatic or stressful event. Specific disorders include acute stress disorder (ASD) and posttraumatic stress disorder (PTSD). ASD and PTSD are similar except that ASD typically begins immediately after the trauma and lasts from 3 days to 1 mo, whereas PTSD lasts for > 1 mo, either as a continuation of ASD or as a separate occurrence up to 6 mo after the trauma.

Previously, trauma- and stressor-related disorders were considered anxiety disorders (see p. 1741). However, they are now considered distinct because many patients do not have anxiety but instead have symptoms of anhedonia or dysphoria, anger, aggression, or dissociation.

ACUTE STRESS DISORDER

Acute stress disorder (ASD) is a brief period of intrusive recollections occurring within 4 wk of witnessing or experiencing an overwhelming traumatic event.

In ASD, people have been through a traumatic event, experiencing it directly (eg, as a serious injury or the threat of death) or indirectly (eg, witnessing events happening to others, learning of events that occurred to close family members or friends). People have recurring recollections of the trauma, avoid stimuli that remind them of the trauma, and have increased arousal. Symptoms begin within 4 wk of the traumatic event and last a minimum of 3 days but, unlike PTSD, last no more than 1 mo. People with this disorder may experience dissociative symptoms.

Diagnosis

- Clinical criteria

Diagnosis is based on criteria recommended by the *Diagnostic and Statistical Manual of Mental Disorders*, Fifth Edition (DSM-5); these criteria include intrusion symptoms, negative mood, and dissociative, avoidance, and arousal symptoms.

To meet the criteria for diagnosis, patients must have been exposed directly or indirectly to a traumatic event, and ≥ 9 of the following must be present for a period of 3 days up to 1 mo:

- Recurrent, involuntary, and intrusive distressing memories of the event
- Recurrent distressing dreams of the event
- Dissociative reactions (eg, flashbacks) in which patients feel as if the traumatic event is recurring
- Intense psychologic or physiologic distress when reminded of the event (eg, by its anniversary, by sounds similar to those heard during the event)
- Persistent inability to experience positive emotions (eg, happiness, satisfaction, loving feelings)
- An altered sense of reality (eg, feeling in a daze, time slowing, altered perceptions)
- Inability to remember an important part of the traumatic event
- Efforts to avoid distressing memories, thoughts, or feelings associated with the event
- Efforts to avoid external reminders (people, places, conversations, activities, objects, situations) associated with the event
- Sleep disturbance
- Irritability or angry outbursts
- Hypervigilance
- Difficulty concentrating
- Exaggerated startle response

In addition, manifestations must cause significant distress or significantly impair social or occupational functioning and not be attributable to the physiologic effects of a substance or another medical disorder.

Treatment

- Nondrug measures

Many people recover once they are removed from the traumatic situation, shown understanding and empathy, and given an opportunity to describe the event and their reaction to it.

To prevent or minimize this disorder, some experts recommend systematic debriefing to assist people who were involved in or witnessed a traumatic event as they process what has happened and reflect on its effect. In one approach to debriefing, the event is referred to as the critical incident, and the debriefing is referred to as critical incident stress debriefing (CISD). Other experts have expressed concern and some studies show that CISD may not be as helpful as supportive, empathic interviewing, may be quite distressful for some patients, and may even impede natural recovery.

Drugs to assist sleep may help, but other drugs are generally not indicated.

POSTTRAUMATIC STRESS DISORDER

Posttraumatic stress disorder (PTSD) is recurring, intrusive recollections of an overwhelming traumatic event; recollections last > 1 mo and begin within 6 mo of the event. The pathophysiology of the disorder is incompletely understood. Symptoms also include avoidance of stimuli associated with the traumatic event, nightmares, and flashbacks. Diagnosis is based on history. Treatment consists of exposure therapy and drug therapy.

When terrible things happen, many people are lastingly affected; in some, the effects are so persistent and severe that they are debilitating and constitute a disorder. Generally, events likely to evoke PTSD are those that invoke feelings of fear, helplessness, or horror. These events may be experienced directly (eg, as a serious injury or the threat of death) or indirectly (eg, witnessing others being seriously injured, killed, or threatened with death; learning of events that occurred to close family members or friends). Combat, sexual assault, and natural or man-made disasters are common causes of PTSD.

Lifetime prevalence approaches 9%, with a 12-mo prevalence of about 4%.

Symptoms and Signs

Most commonly, patients have frequent, unwanted memories replaying the triggering event. Nightmares of the event are common. Much rarer are transient waking dissociative states in which events are relived as if happening (flashback), sometimes causing patients to react as if in the original situation (eg, loud noises such as fireworks might trigger a flashback of being in combat, which in turn might cause patients to seek shelter or prostrate themselves on the ground for protection).

Patients avoid stimuli associated with the trauma and often feel emotionally numb and disinterested in daily activities.

Sometimes symptoms represent a continuation of acute stress disorder (see p. 1746), or they may occur separately, beginning up to 6 mo after the trauma. Sometimes full expression of symptoms is delayed, occurring many months or even years after the traumatic event.

Depression, other anxiety disorders, and substance abuse are common among patients with chronic PTSD.

In addition to trauma-specific anxiety, patients may experience guilt because of their actions during the event or because they survived when others did not.

Diagnosis

- Clinical criteria

Diagnosis is clinical based on criteria in the *Diagnostic and Statistical Manual of Mental Disorders*, Fifth Edition (DSM-5).

To meet the criteria for diagnosis, patients must have been exposed directly or indirectly to a traumatic event and have symptoms from each of the following categories for a period ≥ 1 mo.

Intrusion symptoms (≥ 1 of the following):

- Having recurrent, involuntary, intrusive, disturbing memories
- Having recurrent disturbing dreams (eg, nightmares) of the event
- Acting or feeling as if the event were happening again, ranging from having flashbacks to completely losing awareness of the present surroundings
- Feeling intense psychologic or physiologic distress when reminded of the event (eg, by its anniversary, by sounds similar to those heard during the event)

Avoidance symptoms (≥ 1 of the following):

- Avoiding thoughts, feelings, or memories associated with the event
- Avoiding activities, places, conversations, or people that trigger memories of the event

Negative effects on cognition and mood (≥ 2 of the following):

- Memory loss for significant parts of the event (dissociative amnesia)
- Persistent and exaggerated negative beliefs or expectations about oneself, others, or the world
- Persistent distorted thoughts about the cause or consequences of the trauma that lead to blaming self or others
- Persistent negative emotional state (eg, fear, horror, anger, guilt, shame)
- Markedly diminished interest or participation in significant activities
- A feeling of detachment or estrangement from others
- Persistent inability to experience positive emotions (eg, happiness, satisfaction, loving feelings)

Altered arousal and reactivity (≥ 2 of the following):

- Difficulty sleeping
- Irritability or angry outbursts
- Reckless or self-destructive behavior
- Problems with concentration
- Increased startle response
- Hypervigilance

In addition, manifestations must cause significant distress or significantly impair social or occupational functioning and not be attributable to the physiologic effects of a substance or another medical disorder.

Treatment

- Exposure therapy or other psychotherapy, including supportive psychotherapy
- SSRI or other drug therapy

If untreated, chronic PTSD often diminishes in severity without disappearing, but some people remain severely impaired.

The primary form of psychotherapy used, exposure therapy (see p. 1745), involves exposure to situations that the person avoids because they may trigger recollections of the trauma. Repeated exposure in fantasy to the traumatic experience itself usually lessens distress after some initial increase in discomfort.

Eye movement desensitization and reprocessing (EMDR) is a form of exposure therapy. For this therapy, patients are asked to follow the therapist's moving finger while they imagine being exposed to the trauma.

Stopping certain ritual behaviors, such as excessive washing to feel clean after a sexual assault, also helps.

Drug therapy, particularly with SSRIs (see p. 1762), is effective. Prazosin appears helpful in reducing nightmares. Mood stabilizers and atypical antipsychotics are sometimes prescribed, but support for their use is scant.

Because the anxiety is often intense, supportive psychotherapy plays an important role. Therapists must be openly empathic and sympathetic, recognizing and acknowledging patients' mental pain and the reality of the traumatic events. Therapists must also encourage patients to face the memories through desensitizing exposure and learning techniques to control anxiety. For survivor guilt, psychotherapy aimed at helping patients understand and modify their self-critical and punitive attitudes may be helpful.

208 Dissociative Disorders

Everyone occasionally experiences a failure in the normal automatic integration of memories, perceptions, identity, and consciousness. For example, people may drive somewhere and then realize that they do not remember many aspects of the drive because they are preoccupied with personal concerns, a program on the radio, or conversation with a passenger. Typically, such a failure, referred to as nonpathologic dissociation, does not disrupt everyday activities.

In contrast, people with a dissociative disorder may totally forget a series of normal behaviors occupying minutes or hours and may sense a missing period of time in their experience. In dissociative disorders, the normal integration of consciousness, memory, perceptions, identity, emotion, body representation, motor control, and behavior is disrupted, and continuity of self is lost.

People may experience the following:

- Unbidden intrusions into awareness with loss of continuity of experience, including feelings of detachment from self (depersonalization) and/or the surroundings (derealization) and fragmentation of identity
- Memory loss for important personal information (dissociative amnesia)

Dissociative disorders frequently develop after overwhelming stress. Such stress may be generated by traumatic events or by intolerable inner conflict. Dissociative disorders are related to trauma- and stressor-related disorders; acute stress disorder and posttraumatic stress disorder can cause dissociative symptoms (eg, amnesia, flashbacks, numbing, depersonalization/derealization).

DEPERSONALIZATION/DEREALIZATION DISORDER

Depersonalization/derealization disorder is a type of dissociative disorder that consists of persistent or recurrent feelings of being detached (dissociated) from one's body or mental processes, usually with a feeling of being an outside observer of one's life (depersonalization), or of being detached from one's surroundings (derealization). The disorder is often triggered by severe stress. Diagnosis is based on symptoms after other possible causes are ruled out. Treatment consists of psychotherapy plus drug therapy for any comorbid depression and/or anxiety.

About 50% of the general population have had at least one transient experience of depersonalization or derealization in their lifetime. However, only about 2% of people ever meet the criteria for having depersonalization/derealization disorder.

Depersonalization or derealization can also occur as a symptom in many other mental disorders as well as in physical disorders such as seizure disorders (ictal or postictal). When depersonalization or derealization occurs independently of other mental or physical disorders, is persistent or recurrent, and impairs functioning, depersonalization/derealization disorder is present.

Depersonalization/derealization disorder occurs equally in men and women. Mean age at onset is 16 yr. The disorder may begin during early or middle childhood; only 5% of cases start after age 25, and the disorder rarely begins after age 40.

Etiology

People with depersonalization/derealization disorder often have experienced severe stress, particularly emotional abuse or neglect, during childhood. Other stressors include being physically abused, witnessing domestic violence, having a severely impaired or mentally ill parent, and having a family member or close friend die unexpectedly.

Episodes can be triggered by interpersonal, financial, or occupational stress; depression; anxiety; or use of illicit drugs, particularly marijuana, ketamine, or hallucinogens.

Symptoms and Signs

Symptoms of depersonalization/derealization disorder are usually episodic and wax and wane in intensity. Episodes may last for only hours or days or for weeks, months, or sometimes years. But in some patients, symptoms are constantly present at an unchanging intensity for years or decades.

Depersonalization symptoms include

- Feeling detached from one's body, mind, feelings, and/or sensations

Patients feel like an outside observer of their life. Many patients also say they feel unreal or like a robot or automaton (having no control over what they do or say). They may feel emotionally and physically numb and have flattened affect; some describe themselves as the "walking dead." Some patients cannot recognize or describe their emotions (alexithymia). They feel disconnected from their memories and are unable to remember them clearly.

Derealization symptoms include

- Feeling detached from the surroundings (eg, people, objects, everything), which seem unreal

Patients may feel as if they are in a dream or a fog or as if a glass wall or veil separates them from their surroundings. The world seems lifeless, colorless, or artificial. Subjective distortion of the world is common. For example, objects may appear blurry or unusually clear; they may seem flat or smaller or larger than they are. Sounds may seem louder or softer than they are; time may seem to be going too slow or too fast.

Symptoms are almost always distressing and, when severe, profoundly intolerable. Anxiety and depression are common. Some patients fear that they have irreversible brain damage or that they are going crazy. Others obsess about whether they really exist or repeatedly check to determine whether their perceptions are real. However, patients always retain the knowledge that their unreal experiences are not real but rather are just the way that they feel (ie, they have intact reality testing). This awareness differentiates depersonalization disorder from a psychotic disorder, in which such insight is always lacking.

Diagnosis

- Clinical criteria

Diagnosis of depersonalization/derealization disorder is clinical, based on criteria in the *Diagnostic and Statistical Manual of Mental Disorders*, Fifth Edition (DSM-5):

- Patients have persistent or recurrent episodes of depersonalization, derealization, or both.
- Patients know that their unreal experiences are not real (ie, they have an intact sense of reality).
- Symptoms cause significant distress or significantly impair social or occupational functioning.

Also, the symptoms cannot be better accounted for by another disorder (eg, seizures, ongoing substance abuse, panic disorder, major depressive disorder, another dissociative disorder).

MRI and EEG are done to rule out physical causes, particularly if symptoms or progression is atypical (eg, if symptoms began after age 40 yr). Urine toxicology tests may also be indicated.

Psychologic tests and special structured interviews and questionnaires are helpful.

Prognosis

Patients often improve without intervention. Complete recovery is possible for many patients, especially if symptoms result from treatable or transient stresses or have not been protracted. In others, depersonalization and derealization become more chronic and refractory.

Even persistent or recurrent depersonalization or derealization symptoms may cause only minimal impairment if patients can distract themselves from their subjective sense of self by keeping their mind busy and focusing on other thoughts or activities. Some patients become disabled by the chronic sense of estrangement, by the accompanying anxiety or depression, or both.

Treatment

- Psychotherapy

Treatment of depersonalization/derealization disorder must address all stresses associated with onset of the disorder as well as earlier stresses (eg, childhood abuse or neglect), which may have predisposed patients to late onset of depersonalization and/or derealization.

Various psychotherapies (eg, psychodynamic psychotherapy, cognitive-behavioral therapy) are successful for some patients:

- **Cognitive techniques** can help block obsessive thinking about the unreal state of being.
- **Behavioral techniques** can help patients engage in tasks that distract them from the depersonalization and derealization.
- **Grounding techniques** use the 5 senses (eg, by playing loud music or placing a piece of ice in the hand) to help patients feel more connected to themselves and the world and feel more real in the moment.
- **Psychodynamic therapy** helps patients deal with negative feelings, underlying conflicts, or experiences that make certain affects intolerable to the self and thus dissociated.
- **Moment-to-moment tracking and labeling of affect and dissociation** in therapy sessions works well for some patients.

Various drugs have been used, but none have clearly demonstrable efficacy. However, some patients are apparently helped by SSRIs, lamotrigine, opioid antagonists, anxiolytics, and stimulants. However, these drugs may work largely by targeting other mental disorders (eg, anxiety, depression) that are often associated with or precipitated by depersonalization and derealization.

DISSOCIATIVE AMNESIA

Dissociative amnesia is a type of dissociative disorder that involves inability to recall important personal information that would not typically be lost with ordinary forgetting. It is usually caused by trauma or stress. Diagnosis is based on history after ruling out other causes of amnesia. Treatment is psychotherapy, sometimes combined with hypnosis or drug-facilitated interviews.

The information lost would normally be part of conscious awareness and would be described as autobiographic memory.

Although the forgotten information may be inaccessible to consciousness, it sometimes continues to influence behavior (eg, a woman who was raped in an elevator refuses to ride in elevators even though she cannot recall the rape).

Dissociative amnesia is probably underdetected. Prevalence is not well-established; in one small US community study, the 12-mo prevalence was 1.8% (1% in men; 2.6% in women).

The amnesia appears to be caused by traumatic or stressful experiences endured or witnessed (eg, physical or sexual abuse, rape, combat, genocide, natural disasters, death of a loved one, financial troubles) or by tremendous internal conflict (eg, turmoil over guilt-ridden impulses, apparently unresolvable interpersonal difficulties, criminal behaviors).

Symptoms and Signs

The main symptom of dissociative amnesia is memory loss that is inconsistent with normal forgetfulness. The amnesia may be

- Localized
- Selective
- Generalized

Rarely, dissociative amnesia is accompanied by purposeful travel or bewildered wandering, called fugue (from the Latin word *fugere* "to flee").

Localized amnesia involves being unable to recall a specific event or events or a specific period of time; these gaps in memory are usually related to trauma or stress. For example, patients may forget the months or years of being abused as a child or the days spent in intense combat. The amnesia may not manifest for hours, days, or longer after the traumatic period. Usually, the forgotten time period, which can range from minutes to decades, is clearly demarcated. Typically, patients experience one or more episodes of memory loss.

Selective amnesia involves forgetting only some of the events during a certain period of time or only part of a traumatic event. Patients may have localized and selective amnesia.

In **generalized amnesia**, patients forget their identify and life history—eg, who they are, where they went, to whom they spoke, and what they did, said, thought, experienced, and felt. Some patients can no longer access well-learned skills and lose formerly known information about the world. Generalized dissociative amnesia is rare; it is more common among combat veterans, people who have been sexually assaulted, and people experiencing extreme stress or conflict. Onset is usually sudden.

In **systematized amnesia,** patients forget information in a specific category, such as all information about a particular person or about their family.

In **continuous amnesia,** patients forget each new event as it occurs.

Most patients are partly or completely unaware that they have gaps in their memory. They become aware only when personal identity is lost or when circumstances make them aware—eg, when others tell them or ask them about events they cannot remember.

Patients seen shortly after they become amnestic may appear confused. Some are very distressed; others are indifferent. If those who are unaware of their amnesia present for psychiatric help, they may do so for other reasons.

Patients have difficulty forming and maintaining relationships.

Some patients report flashbacks, as occur in posttraumatic stress disorder (PTSD); flashbacks may alternate with amnesia for the contents of the flashbacks. Some patients develop PTSD later, especially when they become aware of the traumatic or stressful events that triggered their amnesia.

Depressive and functional neurologic symptoms are common, as are suicidal and other self-destructive behaviors. Risk of suicidal behaviors may be increased when amnesia resolves suddenly and patients are overwhelmed by the traumatic memories.

Dissociative fugue: Dissociative fugue is an uncommon phenomenon that sometimes occurs in dissociative amnesia.

Dissociative fugue often manifests as sudden, unexpected, purposeful travel away from home or as bewildered wandering. Patients, having lost their customary identity, leave their family and job. A fugue may last from hours to months, occasionally longer. If the fugue is brief, they may appear simply to have missed some work or come home late. If the fugue lasts several days or longer, they may travel far from home, assume a new name and identity, and begin a new job, unaware of any change in their life.

Many fugues appear to represent disguised wish fulfillment or the only permissible way to escape from severe distress or embarrassment, especially for people with a rigid conscience. For example, a financially distressed executive leaves a hectic life and lives as a farmhand in the country.

During the fugue, patients may appear and act normal or only mildly confused. However, when the fugue ends, patients report suddenly finding themselves in the new situation with no memory of how they came to be there or what they have been doing. They often feel shame, discomfort, grief, and/or depression. Some are frightened, especially if they cannot remember what happened during the fugue. These manifestations may bring them to the attention of medical or legal authorities. Most people eventually recall their past identity and life, although recalling may be a lengthy process; a very few remember nothing or almost nothing about their past indefinitely.

Often, a fugue state is not diagnosed until patients abruptly return to their pre-fugue identity and are distressed to find themselves in unfamiliar circumstances. The diagnosis is usually made retrospectively, based on documentation of the circumstances before travel, the travel itself, and the establishment of an alternate life.

Diagnosis

- Clinical criteria

Diagnosis of dissociative amnesia is clinical, based on criteria in the *Diagnostic and Statistical Manual of Mental Disorders*, Fifth Edition (DSM-5):

- Patients cannot recall important personal information (usually trauma- or stress-related) that would not typically be lost with ordinary forgetting.
- Symptoms cause significant distress or significantly impair social or occupational functioning.

Also, the symptoms cannot be better accounted for by the effects of a drug or another disorder (eg, partial complex seizures, traumatic brain injury, posttraumatic stress disorder, another dissociative disorder).

Diagnosis requires a medical and psychiatric examination to rule out other possible causes. Initial evaluation should include

- MRI to rule out structural causes
- EEG to rule out a seizure disorder
- Blood and urine tests to rule out toxic causes, such as illicit drug use

Psychologic testing can help better characterize the nature of the dissociative experiences.

Prognosis

Sometimes memories return quickly, as can happen when patients are taken out of the traumatic or stressful situation (eg, combat). In other cases, amnesia, particularly in patients with dissociative fugue, persists for a long time. The capacity for dissociation may decrease with age.

Most patients recover their missing memories, and amnesia resolves. However, some are never able to reconstruct their missing past. The prognosis is determined mainly by the patient's life circumstances, particularly stresses and conflicts associated with the amnesia, and by the patient's overall mental adjustment.

Treatment

- To recover memory, a supportive environment and sometimes hypnosis or a drug-induced hypnotic state
- Psychotherapy to deal with issues associated with recovered memories

If memory of only a very short time period is lost, supportive treatment of dissociative amnesia is usually adequate, especially if patients have no apparent need to recover the memory of some painful event.

Treatment for more severe memory loss begins with creation of a safe and supportive environment. This measure alone frequently leads to gradual recovery of missing memories. When it does not or when the need to recover memories is urgent, questioning patients while they are under hypnosis or, rarely, in a drug-induced (barbiturate or benzodiazepine) semihypnotic state can be successful. These strategies must be done gently because the traumatic circumstances that stimulated memory loss are likely to be recalled and to be very upsetting. The questioner also must carefully phrase questions so as not to suggest the existence of an event and risk creating a false memory.

The accuracy of memories recovered with such strategies can be determined only by external corroboration. However, regardless of the degree of historical accuracy, filling in the gap as much as possible is often therapeutically useful in restoring continuity to the patient's identity and sense of self and in creating a cohesive narrative.

Once the amnesia is lifted, treatment helps with the following:

- Giving meaning to the underlying trauma or conflict
- Resolving problems associated with the amnestic episode
- Enabling patients to move on with their life

If patients have experienced dissociative fugue, psychotherapy, sometimes combined with hypnosis or drug-facilitated interviews, may be used to try to restore memory; these efforts are often unsuccessful. Regardless, a psychiatrist can help patients explore how they handle the types of situations, conflicts, and emotions that precipitated the fugue and thus develop better responses to those events and help prevent fugue from recurring.

DISSOCIATIVE IDENTITY DISORDER

Dissociative identity disorder, formerly called multiple personality disorder, is a type of dissociative disorder characterized by ≥ 2 personality states (also called alters, self-states, or identities) that alternate. The disorder includes inability to recall everyday events, important personal information, and/or traumatic or stressful events, all of which would not typically be lost with ordinary forgetting. The cause is almost invariably overwhelming childhood trauma. Diagnosis is based on history, sometimes with hypnosis or drug-facilitated interviews. Treatment is long-term psychotherapy, sometimes with drug therapy for comorbid depression and/or anxiety.

How overt the different identities are varies. They tend to be more overt when people are under extreme stress. What is known by one identity may or may not be known by another; ie, one identity may have amnesia for events experienced by other identities. Some identities appear to know and interact with others in an elaborate inner world, and some identities interact more than others.

In one small US community study, the 12-mo prevalence of dissociative identity disorder was 1.5%, with men and women affected almost equally. The disorder may begin at any age, from early childhood to late life.

Dissociative identity disorder has a possession and nonpossession form.

In the **possession form**, the identities usually manifest as though they were an outside agent, typically a supernatural being or spirit (but sometimes another person), who has taken control of the person, causing the person to speak and act in a very different way. In such cases, the different identities are very overt (readily noticed by others). In many cultures, similar possession states are a normal part of cultural or spiritual practice and are not considered dissociative identity disorder. The possession form that occurs in dissociative identity disorder differs in that the alternate identity is unwanted and occurs involuntarily, it causes substantial distress and impairment, and it manifests in times and places that violate cultural and/or religious norms.

Nonpossession forms tend to be less overt. People may feel a sudden alteration in their sense of self, perhaps feeling as though they were observers of their own speech, emotions, and actions, rather than the agent. Many also have recurrent dissociative amnesia.

Etiology

Dissociative identity disorder usually occurs in people who experienced overwhelming stress during childhood.

Children are not born with a sense of a unified identity; it develops from many sources and experiences. In overwhelmed children, many parts of what should have blended together remain separate. Chronic and severe abuse (physical, sexual, or emotional) and neglect during childhood are frequently reported by and documented in patients with dissociative identity disorder (in the US, Canada, and Europe, about 90% of patients). Some patients have not been abused but have experienced an important early loss (such as death of a parent), serious medical illness, or other overwhelmingly stressful events.

In contrast to most children who achieve cohesive, complex appreciation of themselves and others, severely mistreated children may go through phases in which different perceptions, memories, and emotions of their life experiences are kept segregated. Over time, such children may develop an increasing ability to escape the mistreatment by "going away" or retreating into their own mind. Each developmental phase or traumatic experience may be used to generate a different identity.

On standardized tests, people with this disorder have high scores for susceptibility to hypnosis and dissociation (ability to uncouple one's memories, perceptions, or identity from conscious awareness).

Symptoms and Signs

Several symptoms are characteristic of dissociative identity disorder.

Multiple identities: In the **possession form,** the multiple identities are readily apparent to family members and associates. Patients speak and act in an obviously different manner, as though another person or being has taken over. The new identity may be that of another person (often someone who has died, perhaps in a dramatic fashion) or that of a supernatural spirit (often a demon or god), who may demand punishment for past actions.

In the **nonpossession form,** the different identities are often not as apparent to observers. Instead, patients experience feelings of depersonalization; ie, they feel unreal, removed from self, and detached from their physical and mental processes. Patients say that they feel like an observer of their life, as if they were watching themselves in a movie over which they have no control (loss of personal agency). They may think that their body feels different (eg, like that of a small child or someone of the opposite sex) and does not belong to them. They may have sudden thoughts, impulses, and emotions that do not seem to belong to them and that may manifest as multiple confusing thought streams or as voices. Some manifestations may be noticed by observers. For example, patients' attitudes, opinions, and preferences (eg, regarding food, clothing, or interests) may suddenly change, then change back.

Amnesia: Patients typically have dissociative amnesia. It typically manifests as

- Gaps in memory of past personal events (eg, periods of time during childhood or adolescence, death of a relative)
- Lapses in dependable memory (eg, what happened today, well-learned skills such as how to use a computer)
- Discovery of evidence of things that they have done but have no memory of doing

Periods of time may be lost. Patients may discover objects in their shopping bag or samples of handwriting that they cannot account for or recognize. They may also find themselves in different places from where they last remember being and have no idea why or how they got there. Unlike patients with posttraumatic stress disorder, patients with dissociative identity disorder forget everyday events as well as stressful or traumatic ones.

Patients vary in their awareness of the amnesia. Some try to hide it. The amnesia may be noticed by others when patients cannot remember things they have said and done or important personal information, such as their own name.

Other symptoms: In addition to hearing voices, patients with dissociative identity disorder may have visual, tactile, olfactory, and gustatory hallucinations. Thus, patients may be misdiagnosed with a psychotic disorder. However, these hallucinatory symptoms differ from the typical hallucinations of psychotic disorders such as schizophrenia. Patients with dissociative identity disorder experience these symptoms as coming from an alternate identity (eg, as if someone else was wanting to cry with their eyes).

Depression, anxiety, substance abuse, self-injury, self-mutilation, nonepileptic seizures, and suicidal behavior are common, as is sexual dysfunction.

The switching of identities and the amnestic barriers between them frequently result in chaotic lives. Generally, patients try to minimize their symptoms and the effect they have on others.

Diagnosis

- Clinical criteria
- Detailed interviews, sometimes with hypnosis or facilitated by drugs

Diagnosis of dissociative identity disorder is clinical, based on criteria in the *Diagnostic and Statistical Manual of Mental Disorders*, Fifth Edition (DSM-5):

- Patients have ≥ 2 personality states or identities (disruption of identity), with substantial discontinuity in their sense of self and sense of agency.
- Patients have gaps in their memory for everyday events, important personal information, and traumatic events—information that would not typically be lost with ordinary forgetting.
- Symptoms cause significant distress or significantly impair social or occupational functioning.

Also, the symptoms cannot be better accounted for by another disorder (eg, complex partial seizures, bipolar disorder, posttraumatic stress disorder, another dissociative disorder), by the effects of alcohol intoxication, by broadly accepted cultural or religious practices, or, in children, by fantasy play (eg, an imaginary friend).

The diagnosis requires knowledge of and specific questions about dissociative phenomena. Prolonged interviews, hypnosis, or drug-facilitated (barbiturate or benzodiazepine) interviews are sometimes used, and patients may be asked to keep a journal between visits. All of these measures encourage a shift of identities during the evaluation. The clinician may over time attempt to map out the different identities and their interrelationships. Specially designed structured interviews and questionnaires can be very helpful, especially for clinicians who have less experience with this disorder.

The clinician may also attempt to directly contact other identities by asking to speak to the part of the mind involved in behaviors that patients cannot remember or that seem to be done by someone else.

Malingering (intentional feigning of physical or psychologic symptoms motivated by an external incentive) should be considered if gain could be a motive (eg, to escape accountability for actions or responsibilities). However, malingerers tend to overreport well-known symptoms of the disorder (eg, dissociative amnesia) and underreport others. They also tend to create stereotypical alternate identities. In contrast to patients who have the disorder, malingerers usually seem to enjoy the idea of having the disorder; in contrast, patients with dissociative identity disorder often try to hide it. When clinicians suspect that the disorder is faked, cross-checking information from multiple sources may detect inconsistencies that preclude the diagnosis.

Prognosis

Impairment in dissociative identity disorder varies widely. It may be minimal in highly functioning patients; in these patients, relationships (eg, with their children, spouse, or friends) may be impaired more than occupational functioning. With treatment, relational, social, and occupational functioning may improve, but some patients respond very slowly to treatment and may need long-term supportive treatment.

Symptoms wax and wane spontaneously, but dissociative identity disorder does not resolve spontaneously. Patients can be divided into groups based on their symptoms:

- Symptoms are mainly dissociative and posttraumatic. These patients generally function well and recover completely with treatment.
- Dissociative symptoms are combined with prominent symptoms of other disorders, such as personality disorders, mood disorders, eating disorders, and substance abuse disorders. These patients improve more slowly, and treatment may be less successful or longer and more crisis-ridden.
- Patients not only have severe symptoms due to coexisting mental disorders but may also remain deeply emotionally attached to their abusers. These patients can be challenging to treat, often requiring longer treatments that typically aim to help control symptoms more than to achieve integration.

Treatment

- Supportive care, including drug treatment as needed for associated symptoms
- Psychotherapy focused on long-term integration of identity states when possible

Integration of the identity states is the most desirable outcome of treatment of dissociative identity disorder. Drugs are widely used to help manage symptoms of depression, anxiety, impulsivity, and substance abuse but do not relieve dissociation per se; treatment to achieve integration centers on psychotherapy. For patients who cannot or will not strive for integration, treatment aims to facilitate cooperation and collaboration among the identities and to reduce symptoms.

The first priority of psychotherapy is to stabilize patients and ensure safety, before evaluating traumatic experiences and exploring problematic identities and reasons for dissociations. Some patients benefit from hospitalization, during which continuous support and monitoring are provided as painful memories are addressed.

Hypnosis may help with accessing the identities, facilitating communication among them, and stabilizing and interpreting them. Modified exposure techniques can be used to gradually desensitize patients to traumatic memories, which are sometimes tolerated only in small fragments.

As the reasons for dissociations are addressed and worked through, therapy can move toward reconnecting, integrating, and rehabilitating the patient's alternate selves, relationships, and social functioning. Some integration occurs spontaneously during treatment. Integration can be encouraged by negotiating with and arranging the unification of the identities or can be facilitated using hypnotic suggestion and guided imagery.

Patients who have been traumatized, particularly during childhood, may expect further abuse during therapy and develop complex transference reactions to their therapist. Discussing these understandable feelings is an important component of effective psychotherapy.

209 Eating Disorders

Eating disorders involve a persistent disturbance of eating or of behavior related to eating that

- Alters consumption or absorption of food
- Significantly impairs physical health and/or psychosocial functioning

Specific eating disorders include

- Anorexia nervosa
- Avoidant/restrictive food intake disorder
- Binge eating disorder
- Bulimia nervosa
- Pica
- Rumination disorder

See the American Psychiatric Association's Practice Guidelines: Treatment of Patients With Eating Disorders, 3rd Edition (http://psychiatryonline.org), its corresponding Guideline Watch (August 2012), and guidelines from the National Institute for Clinical Excellence (NICE–www.nice.org.uk).

Avoidant/restrictive food intake disorder: In this disorder, patients avoid eating food or restrict their food intake to such an extent that they have ≥ 1 of the following:

- Significant weight loss or, in children, failure to grow as expected
- Significant nutritional deficiency
- Dependence on enteral feeding (ie, via a feeding tube) or oral nutritional supplements
- Markedly disturbed psychosocial functioning

Criteria for the disorder include that the food restriction is not caused by unavailability of food, a cultural practice (eg, religious fasting), physical illness, medical treatment (eg, radiation therapy, chemotherapy), or another eating disorder—particularly anorexia nervosa or bulimia nervosa—and that there is no evidence of a disturbed perception of body weight or shape. However, patients who have a physical disorder that causes decreased food intake but who maintain the decreased intake for much longer than typically expected and to a degree requiring specific intervention may be considered to have avoidant/restrictive food intake disorder.

Avoidant/restrictive food intake disorder typically begins during childhood and may initially resemble the picky eating that is common during childhood—when children refuse to eat certain foods or foods of a certain color, consistency, or odor. However, such food fussiness, unlike avoidant/restrictive food intake disorder, usually involves only a few food items, and the child's appetite, overall food intake, and growth and development are normal. In avoidant/restrictive food intake disorder, nutritional deficiencies can be life threatening, and social functioning (eg, participating in family meals) can be markedly impaired.

When patients first present, clinicians must exclude physical illness as well as other mental disorders that impair appetite and/or intake, including other eating disorders, depression, schizophrenia, and factitious disorder imposed on another.

Behavioral therapy is commonly used to help patients normalize their eating.

Pica: Pica is persistent eating of nonnutritive, nonfood material for ≥ 1 mo when it is not developmentally appropriate (eg, in children < 2 yr, who frequently mouth and ingest a variety of objects) nor part of a cultural tradition (eg, of folk medicine, religious rites, or common practice, such as ingestion of clay (kaolin) in the Georgia Piedmont). Patients tend to eat nontoxic materials (eg, paper, clay, dirt, hair, chalk, string, wool), and usually ingestion does not cause significant medical harm. However, some patients develop complications such as GI obstruction by impacted material, lead poisoning from eating paint chips, and parasitic infestation from eating dirt.

Pica itself rarely impairs social functioning, but it often occurs in people with other mental disorders that do impair functioning (eg, autism, intellectual disability, schizophrenia). Pica is also common during pregnancy. Swallowing objects in an attempt to cause self-harm or to falsify illness (see p. 1804) is not considered pica.

Rumination disorder: In rumination disorder, patients repeatedly regurgitate food after eating, but they have no nausea or involuntary retching. The food may be spit out or reswallowed; some patients rechew the food before reswallowing. The behavior must occur over a period of ≥ 1 mo and must not be caused by a GI disorder that can lead to regurgitation (eg, gastroesophageal reflux, Zenker diverticulum) or by another eating disorder such as anorexia nervosa. Regurgitation occurs several times a week, typically daily.

The regurgitation is volitional (although patients may report not being able to restrain themselves) and often can be directly observed by the clinician. Some patients are aware that the behavior is socially undesirable and attempt to disguise it by putting a hand over their mouth or limiting their food intake. Patients who spit out the regurgitated material or who significantly limit their intake may lose weight or develop nutritional deficiencies.

ANOREXIA NERVOSA

Anorexia nervosa is characterized by a relentless pursuit of thinness, a morbid fear of obesity, a distorted body image, and restriction of intake relative to requirements, leading to a significantly low body weight. Diagnosis is clinical. Most treatment is with some form of psychologic therapy. Olanzapine may help with weight gain.

Anorexia nervosa occurs predominantly in girls and young women. Onset is usually during adolescence and rarely after age 40.

The etiology is unknown. Other than being female, few risk factors have been identified. In Western society, obesity is considered unattractive and unhealthy, and the desire to be thin is pervasive, even among children. More than 50% of prepubertal girls diet or take other measures to control their weight. Excessive concern about weight or a history of dieting appears to indicate increased risk, and some genetic predisposition probably exists. Studies of identical twins have shown a concordance of < 50%; concordance is lower in fraternal twins. Family and social factors probably play a role. Many patients belong to middle or upper socioeconomic classes, are meticulous and compulsive, have average intelligence, and have very high standards for achievement and success.

Two types of anorexia nervosa are recognized:

- Restricting type: Patients restrict food intake but do not regularly engage in binge eating or purging behavior; some patients exercise excessively.
- Binge-eating/purging type: Patients regularly binge eat and then induce vomiting and/or misuse laxatives, diuretics, or enemas.

Binges are defined as consumption of a much larger amount of food than most people would eat in a similar time period under similar circumstances with loss of control (ie, perceived inability to resist or stop eating).

Pathophysiology

Endocrine abnormalities are common; they include low levels of gonadal hormones, mildly reduced levels of thyroxine (T_4) and triiodothyronine (T_3), and increased cortisol secretion. Menses usually cease, but cessation of menses is no longer a criterion for diagnosis. Bone mass declines. In severely undernourished patients, virtually every major organ system may be affected. Susceptibility to infections is typically not increased.

Dehydration and metabolic alkalosis may occur, and serum K and/or Na may be low; all are aggravated by induced vomiting and laxative or diuretic use.

Cardiac muscle mass, chamber size, and output decrease; mitral valve prolapse is commonly detected. Some patients have prolonged QT intervals (even when corrected for heart rate), which, with the risks imposed by electrolyte disturbances, may predispose to tachyarrhythmias. Sudden death, most likely due to ventricular tachyarrhythmias, may occur.

Symptoms and Signs

Anorexia nervosa may be mild and transient or severe and long-standing.

Most patients are lean but are concerned that they are overweight or that specific body areas (eg, thighs, buttocks) are too fat. They persist in efforts to lose weight despite reassurances and warnings from friends and family members that they are thin or even significantly underweight, and they view any weight gain as an unacceptable failure of self-control. Preoccupation and anxiety about weight increase even as emaciation develops.

Anorexia is a misnomer because appetite often remains until patients become significantly cachectic. Patients are preoccupied with food:

- They study diets and calories.
- They hoard, conceal, and waste food.
- They collect recipes.
- They prepare elaborate meals for other people.

Patients often exaggerate their food intake and conceal behavior, such as induced vomiting. Binge-eating/purging occurs in 30 to 50% of patients. The others simply restrict their food intake.

Many patients with anorexia nervosa also exercise excessively to control weight. Even patients who appear cachectic tend to remain very active (including pursuing vigorous exercise programs).

Reports of bloating, abdominal distress, and constipation are common. Patients usually lose interest in sex. Depression occurs frequently.

Common physical findings include bradycardia, low BP, hypothermia, lanugo hair or slight hirsutism, and edema. Body fat is greatly reduced. Patients who vomit frequently may have eroded dental enamel, painless salivary gland enlargement, and/or an inflamed esophagus.

Diagnosis

- Clinical criteria

Not recognizing the seriousness of the low body weight and restrictive eating are prominent features of anorexia nervosa, and patients resist evaluation and treatment. They are usually brought to the physician's attention by family members or by intercurrent illness.

Clinical criteria for diagnosis include the following:

- Restriction of food intake resulting in a significantly low body weight
- Fear of obesity (stated specifically by the patient or manifested as behavior that interferes with weight gain)
- Body image disturbance (misperception of body weight and/or appearance) or denial of illness

In adults, low body weight is defined using the BMI. BMI of < 17 kg/m^2 is considered significantly low; BMI 17 to < 18.5 kg/m^2 may be significantly low depending on the patient's starting point. For children and adolescents, the BMI percentile for age is used; the 5th percentile is usually given as the cutoff. However, children above the 5th percentile who have not maintained their projected growth trajectory may also be considered to meet the criteria; BMI percentile for age tables and standard growth charts are available from the CDC (see CDC Growth Charts at www.cdc.gov).

Patients may otherwise appear well. The key to diagnosis is eliciting from them an intense fear of fatness that is not diminished by weight loss.

Differential diagnosis: Another mental disorder, such as schizophrenia or primary depression, may cause weight loss and reluctance to eat, but these disorders are not associated with anorexia nervosa.

Rarely, an unrecognized severe physical disorder may cause substantial weight loss. Disorders to consider include malabsorption syndromes (eg, due to inflammatory bowel disease or celiac disease), new-onset type 1 diabetes, adrenal insufficiency, and cancer. Amphetamine abuse may cause similar symptoms.

Prognosis

Mortality rates are high, approaching 10% per decade among affected people who come to clinical attention; unrecognized mild disease probably rarely leads to death. With treatment, half of patients regain most or all of lost weight, and any endocrine and other complications are reversed. About one fourth have intermediate outcomes and may relapse. The remaining one fourth have a poor outcome, including relapses and persistent physical and mental complications. Children and adolescents treated for anorexia nervosa have better outcomes than adults.

Treatment

- Nutrition supplementation
- Psychologic therapy (eg, cognitive-behavioral treatment)
- For adolescents, family therapy

Treatment may require life-saving short-term intervention to restore body weight. When weight loss has been severe or rapid or when weight has fallen below about 75% of recommended weight, prompt restoration of weight becomes critical, and hospitalization should be considered. If any doubt exists, patients should be hospitalized. Outpatient treatments may include varying degrees of support and supervision and commonly involve a team of practitioners.

Nutritional supplementation, which begins by providing about 30 to 40 kcal/kg/day, can produce weight gains of up to 1.5 kg/wk during inpatient care and 0.5 kg/wk during outpatient care. Oral feedings using solid foods are best, but very resistant, undernourished patients occasionally require nasogastric feedings. Elemental Ca 1200 to 1500 mg/day and vitamin D 600 to 800 IU/day are commonly prescribed for bone loss.

Once nutritional, fluid, and electrolyte status has been stabilized, long-term treatment begins. Outpatient psychologic therapy is the cornerstone of treatment. Treatments should emphasize behavioral outcomes such as normalized eating and weight. Treatment should continue for a full year after weight is restored. Results are best in adolescents who have had the disorder < 6 mo. Family therapy, particularly using the Maudsley model, is useful for adolescents. This model has 3 phases:

- Family members are taught how to refeed the adolescent (eg, through a supervised family meal) and thus restore the adolescent's weight (in contrast to earlier approaches, this model does not assign blame to the family or the adolescent).
- Control over eating is gradually returned to the adolescent.
- After the adolescent is able to maintain the restored weight, therapy focuses on engendering a healthy adolescent identity.

Treatment is complicated by patients' abhorrence of weight gain and denial of illness. The physician should attempt to provide a calm, concerned, stable relationship while encouraging a reasonable caloric intake.

Although psychologic therapy is primary, drugs are sometimes helpful. Second-generation antipsychotics (eg, olanzapine up to 10 mg po once/day) may help produce weight gain and relieve anxiety.

KEY POINTS

- Patients with anorexia nervosa have an intense fear of gaining weight or becoming fat that persists despite all evidence to the contrary.
- In the restricting type, patients restrict food intake and sometimes exercise excessively but do not regularly engage in binge eating or purging.
- In the binge-eating/purging type, patients regularly binge eat and then induce vomiting and/or misuse laxatives, diuretics, or enemas in an attempt to purge themselves of food.
- In adults, BMI is very low, and in adolescents BMI percentile is low or decreasing significantly.
- Nutritional deficiency disorders are common, and death can occur.
- Treat with nutritional supplementation, cognitive-behavioral therapy, and, for adolescents, family therapy; 2nd-generation antipsychotics (eg, olanzapine) may be helpful.

BINGE EATING DISORDER

Binge eating disorder is characterized by recurrent episodes of consuming large amounts of food with a feeling of loss of control. It is not followed by inappropriate compensatory behavior, such as self-induced vomiting or laxative abuse. Diagnosis is clinical. Treatment is with cognitive-behavioral therapy or sometimes interpersonal psychotherapy.

Binge eating disorder affects about 3.5% of women and 2% of men in the general population. Unlike bulimia nervosa, binge eating disorder occurs most commonly among overweight and obese people because it contributes to excessive caloric intake; it may be present in ≥ 30% of patients in some weight reduction programs. Compared with people with anorexia nervosa or bulimia nervosa, those with binge eating disorder are older and more likely to be male.

People with binge eating disorder are distressed by it. Clinical depression and preoccupation with body shape, weight, or both are more common in obese people with binge eating disorder than in obese people who are not binge eaters.

Diagnosis

- Clinical criteria

Clinical criteria for diagnosis require binge eating once/wk for at least 3 mo and a sense of lack of control over eating, plus the presence of ≥ 3 of the following:

- Eating much more rapidly than normal
- Eating until feeling uncomfortably full
- Eating large amounts of food when not feeling physically hungry
- Eating alone because of embarrassment
- Feeling disgusted, depressed, or guilty after overeating

Binge eating disorder is differentiated from bulimia nervosa (which also involves binge eating) by the absence of compensatory behaviors (eg, self-induced vomiting, use of laxatives or diuretics, excessive exercise, fasting).

Treatment

- Cognitive-behavioral therapy (CBT)
- Sometimes interpersonal psychotherapy (IPT)
- Consideration of drug therapy with SSRIs or weight-loss drugs

CBT is the most researched and best supported treatment. Both CBT and IPT result in remission rates of ≥ 60%; improvement is usually well-maintained over the long-term. These treatments do not produce significant weight loss in obese patients.

Conventional behavioral weight loss treatment has short-term effectiveness in reducing binge eating, but patients tend to relapse. Antidepressant drugs also have short-term effectiveness in eliminating binge eating, but long-term effectiveness is unknown. Appetite-suppressing drugs (eg, topiramate) or weight-loss drugs (eg, orlistat) may be additionally helpful.

BULIMIA NERVOSA

Bulimia nervosa is characterized by recurrent episodes of binge eating followed by some form of inappropriate compensatory behavior such as purging (self-induced vomiting, laxative or diuretic abuse), fasting, or driven exercise; episodes must occur at least 1 time/wk for 3 mo. Diagnosis is based on history and examination. Treatment is with psychologic therapy and antidepressants.

Bulimia nervosa affects about 1.6% of adolescent and young women and 0.5% of men of comparable age. Those affected are persistently and overly concerned about body shape and weight. Unlike patients with anorexia nervosa, those with bulimia nervosa are usually of normal or above-normal weight.

Pathophysiology

Serious fluid and electrolyte disturbances, especially hypokalemia, occur occasionally. Extremely rarely, the stomach ruptures or the esophagus is torn during a binge or purge episode, leading to life-threatening complications.

Because substantial weight loss does not occur, the serious nutritional deficiencies that occur with anorexia nervosa are not present. Cardiomyopathy may result from long-term abuse of syrup of ipecac if used to induce vomiting.

Symptoms and Signs

Patients typically describe binge-purge behavior. Binges involve rapid consumption of an amount of food definitely larger than most people would eat in a similar period of time under similar circumstances (eg, the amount considered excessive for a normal meal vs a holiday meal may differ) accompanied by feelings of loss of control.

Patients tend to consume sweet, high-fat foods (eg, ice cream, cake). The amount of food consumed in a binge varies, sometimes involving thousands of calories. Binges tend to be episodic, are often triggered by psychosocial stress, may occur as often as several times a day, and are usually carried out in secret.

Binge eating is followed by compensatory behaviors: self-induced vomiting, use of laxatives or diuretics, excessive exercise, and/or fasting.

Patients are typically of normal weight; a minority are overweight or obese. However, patients are excessively concerned about their body weight and/or shape; they are often dissatisfied with their bodies and think that they need to lose weight.

Most symptoms and physical complications result from purging. Self-induced vomiting may lead to erosion of dental enamel of the front teeth, painless parotid (salivary) gland enlargement, and an inflamed esophagus. Physical signs include

- Swollen parotid glands
- Scars on the knuckles (from induced vomiting)
- Dental erosion

Patients with bulimia nervosa tend to be more aware of and remorseful or guilty about their behaviors than those with anorexia nervosa and are more likely to acknowledge their concerns when questioned by a sympathetic clinician. They are also less socially isolated and more prone to impulsive behavior, drug and alcohol abuse, and overt depression. Anxiety (eg, concerning weight and/or social situations) and anxiety disorders may be more common among these patients.

Diagnosis

- Clinical criteria

Clinical criteria for diagnosis include the following:

- Recurrent episodes of binge eating (the uncontrolled consumption of unusually large amounts of food) that are accompanied by feelings of loss of control over eating and that occur at least once/wk for 3 mo
- Recurrent inappropriate compensatory behavior to influence body weight (at least once/wk for 3 mo)
- Self-evaluation unduly influenced by body shape and weight concerns

Treatment

- Cognitive-behavioral therapy (CBT)
- Interpersonal psychotherapy (IPT)
- SSRIs

CBT is the treatment of choice. Therapy usually involves 16 to 20 individual sessions over 4 to 5 mo, although it can also be done as group therapy. Treatment aims to increase motivation for change, replace dysfunctional dieting with a regular and flexible pattern of eating, decrease undue concern with body shape and weight, and prevent relapse. CBT eliminates binge eating and purging in about 30 to 50% of patients. Many others show improvement; some drop out of treatment or do not respond. Improvement is usually well-maintained over the long-term.

In IPT, the emphasis is on helping patients identify and alter current interpersonal problems that may be maintaining the eating disorder. The treatment is both nondirective and noninterpretive and does not focus directly on eating disorder symptoms. IPT can be considered an alternative when CBT is unavailable.

SSRIs used alone reduce the frequency of binge eating and vomiting, although long-term outcomes are unknown. SSRIs are also effective in treating comorbid anxiety and depression. Fluoxetine 60 mg po once/day is recommended (this dose is higher than that typically used for depression).

KEY POINTS

- Bulimia nervosa involves recurrent episodes of binge eating followed by inappropriate compensatory behavior such as self-induced vomiting, laxative or diuretic abuse, fasting, or excessive exercise.
- Unlike patients with anorexia nervosa, patients rarely lose much weight or develop nutritional deficiencies.
- Recurrent self-induced vomiting may erode dental enamel and/or cause esophagitis.
- Cognitive-behavioral therapy is used, sometimes along with an SSRI.

210 Mood Disorders

(For mood disorders in children, see p. 2716.)

Mood disorders are emotional disturbances consisting of prolonged periods of excessive sadness, excessive joyousness, or both. Mood disorders are categorized as

- Depressive
- Bipolar

Anxiety and related disorders also affect mood (see p. 1741).

Sadness and joy (elation) are part of everyday life. Sadness is a universal response to defeat, disappointment, and other discouraging situations. Joy is a universal response to success, achievement, and other encouraging situations. Grief, a form of sadness, is considered a normal emotional response to a loss. Bereavement refers specifically to the emotional response to death of a loved one.

A mood disorder is diagnosed when sadness or elation is overly intense and persistent, is accompanied by a requisite number of other mood disorder symptoms, and significantly impairs the person's capacity to function. In such cases, intense sadness is termed depression, and intense elation is termed mania. Depressive disorders are characterized by depression; bipolar disorders are characterized by varying combinations of depression and mania.

Lifetime risk of suicide for people with a depressive disorder is 2 to 15%, depending on severity of the disorder. Risk is further increased in the following cases:

- At the start of treatment, when psychomotor activity is returning to normal but mood is still dark
- During mixed bipolar states
- At personally significant anniversaries
- By severe anxiety
- By alcohol and substance use

Other complications of mood disorders include

- Disability ranging from mild to complete inability to function, maintain social interaction, and participate in routine activities
- Impaired food intake
- Severe anxiety
- Alcoholism
- Other drug dependencies

DEPRESSIVE DISORDERS

Depressive disorders are characterized by sadness severe enough or persistent enough to interfere with function and often by decreased interest or pleasure in activities. Exact cause is unknown but probably involves heredity, changes in neurotransmitter levels, altered neuroendocrine function, and psychosocial factors. Diagnosis is based on history. Treatment usually consists of drugs, psychotherapy, or both and sometimes electroconvulsive therapy.

The term depression is often used to refer to any of several depressive disorders. Some are classified in the *Diagnostic and Statistical Manual of Mental Disorders*, Fifth Edition (DSM-5) by specific symptoms:

- Major depressive disorder (often called major depression)
- Persistent depressive disorder (dysthymia)
- Other specified or unspecified depressive disorder

Others are classified by etiology:

- Premenstrual dysphoric disorder
- Depressive disorder due to another medical condition
- Substance/medication-induced depressive disorder

Depressive disorders occur at any age but typically develop during the mid-teens, 20s, or 30s. In primary care settings, as many as 30% of patients report depressive symptoms, but < 10% have major depression.

Demoralization and grief: The term depression is often used to describe the low or discouraged mood that results from disappointments (eg, financial calamity, natural disaster, serious illness) or losses (eg, death of a loved one). However, better terms for such moods are demoralization and grief.

The negative feelings of demoralization and grief, unlike those of depression, occur in waves that tend to be tied to thoughts or reminders of the inciting event, resolve when circumstances or events improve, may be interspersed with periods of positive emotion and humor, and are not accompanied by pervasive feelings of worthlessness and self-loathing. The low mood usually lasts days rather than weeks or months, and suicidal thoughts and prolonged loss of function are much less likely.

However, events and stressors that cause demoralization and grief can also precipitate a major depressive episode, particularly in vulnerable people (eg, those with a past history or family history of major depression).

Etiology

Exact cause of depressive disorders is unknown, but genetic and environmental factors contribute.

Heredity accounts for about half of the etiology (less so in late-onset depression). Thus, depression is more common among 1st-degree relatives of depressed patients, and concordance between identical twins is high. Also, genetic factors probably influence the development of depressive responses to adverse events.

Other theories focus on changes in neurotransmitter levels, including abnormal regulation of cholinergic, catecholaminergic (noradrenergic or dopaminergic), and serotonergic (5-hydroxytryptamine) neurotransmission. Neuroendocrine dysregulation may be a factor, with particular emphasis on 3 axes: hypothalamic-pituitary-adrenal, hypothalamic-pituitary-thyroid, and growth hormone.

Psychosocial factors also seem to be involved. Major life stresses, especially separations and losses, commonly precede episodes of major depression; however, such events do not usually cause lasting, severe depression except in people predisposed to a mood disorder.

People who have had an episode of major depression are at higher risk of subsequent episodes. People who are less resilient and/or who have anxious tendencies may be more likely to develop a depressive disorder. Such people often do not develop the social skills to adjust to life pressures. Depression may also develop in people with other mental disorders.

Women are at higher risk, but no theory explains why. Possible factors include the following:

- Greater exposure to or heightened response to daily stresses
- Higher levels of monoamine oxidase (the enzyme that degrades neurotransmitters considered important for mood)
- Higher rates of thyroid dysfunction
- Endocrine changes that occur with menstruation and at menopause

In **peripartum-onset depression,** symptoms develop during pregnancy or within 4 wk after delivery (postpartum depression); endocrine changes have been implicated, but the specific cause is unknown.

In **seasonal affective disorder,** symptoms develop in a seasonal pattern, typically during autumn or winter; the disorder tends to occur in climates with long or severe winters.

Depressive symptoms or disorders may accompany various physical disorders, including thyroid disorders, adrenal gland disorders, benign and malignant brain tumors, stroke, AIDS, Parkinson disease, and multiple sclerosis (see Table 210–1).

Certain drugs, such as corticosteroids, some beta-blockers, interferon, and reserpine, can also result in depressive disorders. Abuse of some recreational drugs (eg, alcohol, amphetamines) can lead to or accompany depression. Toxic effects or withdrawal of drugs may cause transient depressive symptoms.

Symptoms and Signs

Depression causes cognitive, psychomotor, and other types of dysfunction (eg, poor concentration, fatigue, loss of sexual desire, loss of interest or pleasure in nearly all activities that were previously enjoyed, sleep disturbances), as well as a depressed mood. People with a depressive disorder frequently have thoughts of suicide and may attempt suicide. Other mental symptoms or disorders (eg, anxiety and panic attacks) commonly coexist, sometimes complicating diagnosis and treatment.

Patients with all forms of depression are more likely to abuse alcohol or other recreational drugs in an attempt to self-treat sleep disturbances or anxiety symptoms; however, depression is a less common cause of alcoholism and drug abuse than was once thought. Patients are also more likely to become heavy smokers and to neglect their health, increasing the risk of development or progression of other disorders (eg, COPD).

Depression may reduce protective immune responses. Depression increases risk of cardiovascular disorders, MIs, and stroke, perhaps because in depression, cytokines and factors that increase blood clotting are elevated and heart rate variability is decreased—all potential risk factors for cardiovascular disorders.

Major depression (unipolar disorder): Patients may appear miserable, with tearful eyes, furrowed brows, down-turned corners of the mouth, slumped posture, poor eye contact, lack of facial expression, little body movement, and speech changes (eg, soft voice, lack of prosody, use of monosyllabic words). Appearance may be confused with Parkinson disease. In some patients, depressed mood is so deep that tears dry up; they report that they are unable to experience usual emotions and feel that the world has become colorless and lifeless.

Nutrition may be severely impaired, requiring immediate intervention.

Some depressed patients neglect personal hygiene or even their children, other loved ones, or pets.

For diagnosis, ≥ 5 of the following must have been present nearly every day during the same 2-wk period, and one of them must be depressed mood or loss of interest or pleasure:

- Depressed mood most of the day
- Markedly diminished interest or pleasure in all or almost all activities for most of the day
- Significant (> 5%) weight gain or loss or decreased or increased appetite
- Insomnia (often sleep-maintenance insomnia) or hypersomnia
- Psychomotor agitation or retardation observed by others (not self-reported)
- Fatigue or loss of energy
- Feelings of worthlessness or excessive or inappropriate guilt
- Diminished ability to think or concentrate or indecisiveness
- Recurrent thoughts of death or suicide, a suicide attempt, or a specific plan for committing suicide

Persistent depressive disorder: Depressive symptoms that persist for ≥ 2 yr without remission are classified as persistent depressive disorder (PDD), a category that consolidates disorders formerly termed chronic major depressive disorder and dysthymic disorder.

Symptoms typically begin insidiously during adolescence and may persist for many years or decades. The number of symptoms often fluctuates above and below the threshold for major depressive episode.

Affected patients may be habitually gloomy, pessimistic, humorless, passive, lethargic, introverted, hypercritical of self and others, and complaining. Patients with PDD are also more likely to have underlying anxiety, substance use, or personality (ie, borderline personality) disorders.

For diagnosis, patients must have had a depressed mood for most of the day for more days than not for ≥ 2 yr plus ≥ 2 of the following:

- Poor appetite or overeating
- Insomnia or hypersomnia
- Low energy or fatigue
- Low self-esteem
- Poor concentration or difficulty making decisions
- Feelings of hopelessness

Table 210–1. SOME CAUSES OF SYMPTOMS OF DEPRESSION AND MANIA

TYPE OF DISORDER	DEPRESSION	MANIA
Connective tissue	SLE	Rheumatic fever SLE
Endocrine	Addison disease Cushing syndrome Diabetes mellitus Hyperparathyroidism Hyperthyroidism Hypothyroidism Hypopituitarism Hypogonadism	Hyperthyroidism
Infectious	AIDS General paresis (parenchymatous neurosyphilis) Influenza Infectious mononucleosis TB Viral hepatitis Viral pneumonia	AIDS General paresis Influenza St. Louis encephalitis
Neoplastic	Cancer of the head of the pancreas Disseminated carcinomatosis	—
Neurologic	Cerebral tumors Complex partial seizures (temporal lobe) Head trauma Multiple sclerosis Parkinson disease Sleep apnea Stroke (left frontal)	Complex partial seizures (temporal lobe) Diencephalic tumors Head trauma Huntington disease Multiple sclerosis Stroke
Nutritional	Pellagra Pernicious anemia	—
Other*	Coronary artery disease Fibromyalgia Renal failure or hepatic failure	—
Pharmacologic	Amphetamine withdrawal Amphotericin B Anticholinesterase insecticides Barbiturates Beta-blockers (some, eg, propranolol) Cimetidine Corticosteroids Cycloserine Estrogen therapy Indomethacin Interferon Mercury Methyldopa Metoclopramide Oral contraceptives Phenothiazines Reserpine Thallium Vinblastine Vincristine	Amphetamines Certain antidepressants Bromocriptine Cocaine Corticosteroids Levodopa Methylphenidate Sympathomimetic drugs
Mental	Alcoholism and other substance use disorders Antisocial personality disorder Anxiety disorders Borderline personality disorder Dementing disorders in the early phase Schizophrenic disorders	—

*Depression commonly occurs in these disorders, but no causal relationship has been established.

Premenstrual dysphoric disorder: Premenstrual dysphoric disorder involves mood and anxiety symptoms that are clearly related to the menstrual cycle, with onset during the premenstrual phase and a symptom-free interval after menstruation. Symptoms must be present during most menstrual cycles during the past year.

Manifestations are similar to those of premenstrual syndrome (see p. 2292) but are more severe, causing clinically significant distress and/or marked impairment of social or occupational functioning. The disorder may begin any time after menarche; it may worsen as menopause approaches but ceases after menopause. Prevalence is estimated at 2 to 6% of menstruating women in a given 12-mo interval.

For diagnosis, patients must have ≥ 5 symptoms during the week before menstruation. Symptoms must begin to remit within a few days after onset of menses and become minimal or absent in the week after menstruation. Symptoms must include ≥ 1 of the following:

- Marked mood swings (eg, suddenly feeling sad or tearful)
- Marked irritability or anger or increased interpersonal conflicts
- Marked depressed mood, feelings of hopelessness, or self-deprecating thoughts
- Marked anxiety, tension, or an on-edge feeling

In addition, ≥ 1 of the following must be present:

- Decreased interest in usual activities
- Difficulty concentrating
- Low energy or fatigue
- Marked change in appetite, overeating, or specific food cravings
- Hypersomnia or insomnia
- Feeling overwhelmed or out of control
- Physical symptoms such as breast tenderness or swelling, joint or muscle pain, a feeling of being bloated, and weight gain

Other depressive disorder: Clusters of symptoms with characteristics of a depressive disorder that do not meet the full criteria for other depressive disorders but that cause clinically significant distress or impairment of functioning are classified as other depressive (specified or unspecified) disorder.

Included are recurrent periods of dysphoria with ≥ 4 other depressive symptoms that last < 2 wk in people who have never met criteria for another mood disorder (eg, recurrent brief depression) and depressive periods that last longer but that include insufficient symptoms for diagnosis of another depressive disorder.

Specifiers: Major depression and PPD may include one or more specifiers that describe additional manifestations during a depressive episode:

- **Anxious distress:** Patients feel tense and unusually restless; they have difficulty concentrating because they worry or fear that something awful may happen, or they feel that they may lose control of themselves.
- **Mixed features:** Patients also have ≥ 3 manic or hypomanic symptoms (eg, elevated mood, grandiosity, greater talkativeness than usual, flight of ideas, decreased sleep).
- **Melancholic:** Patients have lost pleasure in nearly all activities or do not respond to usually pleasurable stimuli. They may be despondent and despairing, feel excessive or inappropriate guilt, or have early morning awakenings, marked psychomotor retardation or agitation, and significant anorexia or weight loss.
- **Atypical:** Patients' mood temporarily brightens in response to positive events (eg, a visit from children). They also have ≥ 2 of the following: overreaction to perceived criticism or rejection, feelings of leaden paralysis (a heavy or weighted-down feeling, usually in the extremities), weight gain or increased appetite, and hypersomnia.
- **Psychotic:** Patients have delusions and/or hallucinations. Delusions often involve having committed unpardonable sins or crimes, harboring incurable or shameful disorders, or being persecuted. Hallucinations may be auditory (eg, hearing accusatory or condemning voices) or visual. If only voices are described, careful consideration should be given to whether the voices represent true hallucinations.
- **Catatonic:** Patients have severe psychomotor retardation, engage in excessive purposeless activity, and/or withdraw; some patients grimace and mimic speech (echolalia) or movement (echopraxia).
- **Peripartum onset:** Onset is during pregnancy or in the 4 wk after delivery. Psychotic features may be present; infanticide is often associated with psychotic episodes involving command hallucinations to kill the infant or delusions that the infant is possessed.
- **Seasonal pattern:** Episodes occur at a particular time of year, most often fall or winter.

Diagnosis

- Clinical criteria (DSM-5)
- CBC, electrolytes, and TSH, vitamin B_{12}, and folate levels to rule out physical disorders that can cause depression

Diagnosis of depressive disorders is based on identification of the symptoms and signs and the clinical criteria described above. To help differentiate depressive disorders from ordinary mood variations, there must be significant distress or impairment in social, occupational, or other important areas of functioning.

Several brief questionnaires are available for screening. They help elicit some depressive symptoms but cannot be used alone for diagnosis. Specific close-ended questions help determine whether patients have the symptoms required by DSM-5 criteria for diagnosis of major depression.

Severity is determined by the degree of pain and disability (physical, social, occupational) and by duration of symptoms. A physician should gently but directly ask patients about any thoughts and plans to harm themselves or others, any previous threats of and/or attempts at suicide, and other risk factors. Psychosis and catatonia indicate severe depression. Melancholic features indicate severe or moderate depression. Coexisting physical conditions, substance abuse disorders, and anxiety disorders may add to severity.

Differential diagnosis: Depressive disorders must be distinguished from demoralization and grief. Other mental disorders (eg, anxiety disorders) can mimic or obscure the diagnosis of depression. Sometimes more than one disorder is present. Major depression (unipolar disorder) must be distinguished from bipolar disorder.

In elderly patients, depression can manifest as dementia of depression (formerly called pseudodementia), which causes many of the symptoms and signs of dementia such as psychomotor retardation and decreased concentration. However, early dementia may cause depression. In general, when the diagnosis is uncertain, treatment of a depressive disorder should be tried.

Differentiating chronic depressive disorders, such as dysthymia, from substance abuse disorders may be difficult, particularly because they can coexist and may contribute to each other.

Physical disorders must also be excluded as a cause of depressive symptoms. Hypothyroidism often causes symptoms of depression and is common, particularly among the elderly. Parkinson disease, in particular, may manifest with symptoms that mimic depression (eg, loss of energy, lack of expression, paucity of movement). A thorough neurologic examination is needed to exclude this disorder.

Testing: No laboratory findings are pathognomonic for depressive disorders. Tests for limbic-diencephalic dysfunction are rarely indicated or helpful. However, laboratory testing is necessary to exclude physical conditions that can cause depression. Tests include CBC, TSH levels, and routine electrolyte, vitamin B_{12}, and folate levels. Testing for illicit drug use is sometimes appropriate.

Treatment

- Support
- Psychotherapy
- Drugs

Symptoms may remit spontaneously, particularly when they are mild or of short duration. Mild depression may be treated with general support and psychotherapy. Moderate to severe depression is treated with drugs, psychotherapy, or both and sometimes electroconvulsive therapy. Some patients require a combination of drugs. Improvement may not be apparent until after 1 to 4 wk of drug treatment.

Depression, especially in patients who have had > 1 episode, is likely to recur; therefore, severe cases often warrant long-term maintenance drug therapy.

Most people with depression are treated as outpatients. Patients with significant suicidal ideation, particularly when family support is lacking, require hospitalization, as do those with psychotic symptoms or physical debilitation.

In patients with **substance abuse disorders,** depressive symptoms often resolve within a few months of stopping substance use. Antidepressant treatment is much less likely to be effective while substance abuse continues.

If a **physical disorder** or **drug toxicity** could be the cause, treatment is directed first at the underlying disorder. However, if the diagnosis is in doubt or if symptoms are disabling or include suicidal ideation or hopelessness, a therapeutic trial with an antidepressant or a mood-stabilizing drug may help.

Initial support: Until definite improvement begins, a physician may need to see patients weekly or biweekly to provide support and education and to monitor progress. Telephone calls may supplement office visits.

Patients and loved ones may be worried or embarrassed about the idea of having a mental disorder. The physician can help by explaining that depression is a serious medical disorder caused by biologic disturbances and requires specific treatment and that the prognosis with treatment is good. Patients and loved ones should be reassured that depression does not reflect a character flaw (eg, laziness, weakness). Telling patients that the path to recovery often fluctuates helps them put feelings of hopelessness in perspective and improves adherence.

Encouraging patients to gradually increase simple activities (eg, taking walks, exercising regularly) and social interactions must be balanced with acknowledging their desire to avoid activities. The physician can suggest that patients avoid self-blame and explain that dark thoughts are part of the disorder and will go away.

Psychotherapy: Numerous controlled trials have shown that psychotherapy, particularly cognitive-behavioral therapy and interpersonal therapy, is effective in patients with major depressive disorder, both to treat acute symptoms and to decrease the likelihood of relapse. Patients with mild depression tend to have better outcomes than those with more severe depression, but the magnitude of improvement is greater in those with more severe depression.

Drug therapy (see also p. 1762): Several drug classes and drugs can be used to treat depression:

- Selective serotonin reuptake inhibitors (SSRIs)
- Serotonin modulators (5-HT_2 blockers)
- Serotonin-norepinephrine reuptake inhibitors
- Norepinephrine-dopamine reuptake inhibitor
- Heterocyclic antidepressants
- Monoamine oxidase inhibitors (MAOIs)
- Melatonergic antidepressant

Choice of drug may be guided by past response to a specific antidepressant. Otherwise, SSRIs are often the initial drugs of choice. Although the different SSRIs are equally effective for typical cases, certain properties of the drugs make them more or less appropriate for certain patients.

Electroconvulsive therapy (ECT): The following are often treated with ECT if drugs are ineffective:

- Severe suicidal depression
- Depression with agitation or psychomotor retardation
- Delusional depression
- Depression during pregnancy

Patients who have stopped eating may need ECT to prevent death. ECT is particularly effective for psychotic depression.

Response to 6 to 10 ECT treatments is usually dramatic and may be lifesaving. Relapse after ECT is common, and drug therapy is often maintained after ECT is stopped.

Phototherapy: Phototherapy is best known for its effects on seasonal depression but appears to be equally effective for nonseasonal depression.

Treatment can be provided at home with 2,500 to 10,000 lux at a distance of 30 to 60 cm for 30 to 60 min/day (longer with a less intense light source).

In patients who go to sleep late at night and rise late in the morning, phototherapy is most effective in the morning, sometimes supplemented with 5 to 10 min of exposure between 3 PM and 7 PM. For patients who go to sleep and rise early, phototherapy is most effective between 3 PM and 7 PM.

Other therapies: Psychostimulants (eg, dextroamphetamine, methylphenidate) are sometimes used, often with antidepressants; however, they have not been studied in controlled clinical trials.

Medicinal herbs are used by some patients. St. John's wort may be effective for mild depression, although data are contradictory. St. John's wort may interact with other antidepressants and other drugs. Some placebo-controlled studies of omega-3 supplementation, used as augmentation or as monotherapy, have suggested that eicosapentaenoic acid 1 to 2 g once/day has useful antidepressant effects.

Vagus nerve stimulation involves intermittently stimulating the vagus nerve via an implanted pulse generator. It may be useful for depression refractory to other treatments but usually takes 3 to 6 mo to be effective.

The use of **repetitive transcranial magnetic stimulation (rTMS)** for the acute treatment of major depressive disorder has substantial support from controlled trials. Low-frequency rTMS may be applied to the right dorsolateral prefrontal cortex (DLPC), and high-frequency rTMS can be applied to the left DLPC. The most common adverse effects are headaches and scalp discomfort; both occur more often when high-frequency rather than low-frequency rTMS is used.

Deep brain stimulation targeting the subgenual cingulate or the anterior ventral internal capsule/ventral striatum has had promising results in uncontrolled case series.[1] Controlled trials are under way.

1. Bergfeld IO, Mantione M, Hoogendoorn MLC, et al: Deep brain stimulation of the ventral anterior limb of the internal capsule for treatment-resistant depression: A randomized clinical trial. *JAMA Psychiatry* 1:73(5): 456–64, 2016. doi: 10.1001/jamapsychiatry.2016.0152.

KEY POINTS

- Depression is a common disorder that involves depressed mood and/or near-complete loss of interest or pleasure in activities that were previously enjoyed; somatic (eg, weight change, sleep disturbance) and cognitive manifestations (eg, difficulty concentrating) are common.
- Depression may markedly impair the ability to function at work and to interact socially; risk of suicide is significant.
- Sometimes depressive symptoms are caused by physical disorders (eg, thyroid or adrenal gland disorders, benign or malignant brain tumors, stroke, AIDS, Parkinson disease, multiple sclerosis) or use of certain drugs (eg, corticosteroids, some beta-blockers, interferon, some recreational drugs).
- Diagnosis is based on clinical criteria; physical disorders must be ruled out by clinical evaluation and selected testing (eg, CBC; electrolyte, TSH, B_{12}, and folate levels).
- Treatment involves psychotherapy and usually drugs; SSRIs are usually tried first, and if they are ineffective, other drugs that affect serotonin and/or norepinephrine may be tried.

DRUG TREATMENT OF DEPRESSION

Several drug classes and drugs can be used to treat depression:

- Selective serotonin reuptake inhibitors (SSRIs)
- Serotonin modulators (5-HT_2 blockers)
- Serotonin-norepinephrine reuptake inhibitors
- Norepinephrine-dopamine reuptake inhibitor
- Heterocyclic antidepressants
- Monoamine oxidase inhibitors (MAOIs)
- Melatonergic antidepressant

Choice of drug may be guided by past response to a specific antidepressant. Otherwise, SSRIs are often the initial drugs of choice. Although the different SSRIs are equally effective for typical cases, certain properties of the drugs make them more or less appropriate for certain patients.

Selective Serotonin Reuptake Inhibitors (SSRIs)

These drugs prevent reuptake of serotonin (5-hydroxytryptamine [5-HT]). SSRIs include citalopram, escitalopram, fluoxetine, fluvoxamine, paroxetine, sertraline, and vilazodone. Although these drugs have the same mechanism of action, differences in their clinical properties make selection important. SSRIs have a wide therapeutic margin; they are relatively easy to administer, with little need for dose adjustment (except for fluvoxamine).

By preventing reuptake of 5-HT presynaptically, SSRIs result in more 5-HT to stimulate postsynaptic 5-HT receptors. SSRIs are selective to the 5-HT system but not specific for the different 5-HT receptors. They stimulate 5-HT_1 receptors, with antidepressant and anxiolytic effects, but they also stimulate 5-HT_2 receptors, commonly causing anxiety, insomnia, and sexual dysfunction, and 5-HT_3 receptors, commonly causing nausea and headache. Thus, SSRIs can paradoxically relieve and cause anxiety.

A few patients may seem more agitated, depressed, and anxious within a week of starting SSRIs or increasing the dose. Patients and their loved ones should be warned of this possibility and instructed to call the physician if symptoms worsen with treatment. This situation should be closely monitored because some patients, especially younger children and adolescents, become increasingly suicidal if agitation, increased depression, and anxiety are not detected and rapidly treated. Several analyses of the FDA database of industry-sponsored trials led to a black box warning that antidepressants in general are associated with an increased risk of emergence of suicidal ideas and suicide attempts in patients aged ≤ 24 yr. Subsequent analyses of FDA and other data have cast doubt on this conclusion.[1]

Sexual dysfunction (especially difficulty achieving orgasm but also decreased libido and erectile dysfunction) occurs in one-third or more of patients. Some SSRIs cause weight gain. Others, especially fluoxetine, may cause anorexia in the first few months. SSRIs have few anticholinergic, adrenolytic, and cardiac conduction effects. Sedation is minimal or nonexistent, but in the early weeks of treatment, some patients tend to be sleepy during the day. Loose stools or diarrhea occurs in some patients.

Drug interactions are relatively uncommon; however, fluoxetine, paroxetine, and fluvoxamine can inhibit cytochrome P-450 (CYP450) isoenzymes, which can lead to serious drug interactions. For example, these drugs can inhibit the metabolism of certain beta-blockers, including propranolol and metoprolol, potentially resulting in hypotension and bradycardia.

Discontinuation symptoms (eg, irritability, anxiety, nausea) can occur if the drug is stopped abruptly; such effects are less likely with fluoxetine.

1. Gibbons RD, Brown CH, Hur K, et al: Suicidal thoughts and behavior with antidepressant treatment: Reanalysis of the randomized placebo-controlled studies of fluoxetine and venlafaxine. *Arch Gen Psychiatry* 69(6):580–587, 2012. Clarification and additional information. *Arch Gen Psychiatry* 70(8):881, 2013.

Serotonin Modulators (5-HT_2 Blockers)

These drugs block primarily the 5-HT_2 receptor and inhibit reuptake of 5-HT and norepinephrine. Serotonin modulators include

- Trazodone
- Mirtazapine

Serotonin modulators have antidepressant and anxiolytic effects but do not cause sexual dysfunction.

Trazodone does not inhibit 5-HT reuptake presynaptically. It has caused priapism (in 1/1000) and, as an alpha-1 noradrenergic blocker, may cause orthostatic (postural) hypotension. It is very sedating, so its use in antidepressant doses (> 200 mg/day) is limited. It is most often given in 50- to 100-mg doses at bedtime to depressed patients with insomnia.

Mirtazapine inhibits 5-HT reuptake and blocks alpha-2 adrenergic autoreceptors, as well as 5-HT_2 and 5-HT_3 receptors. The result is increased serotonergic function and increased noradrenergic function without sexual dysfunction or nausea. It has no cardiac adverse effects, has minimal interaction with drug-metabolizing liver enzymes, and is generally well-tolerated, although it does cause sedation and weight gain, mediated by H_1 (histamine) blockade.

Serotonin-Norepinephrine Reuptake Inhibitors

These drugs (eg, desvenlafaxine, duloxetine, levomilnacipran, venlafaxine, vortioxetine) have a dual 5-HT and norepinephrine mechanism of action, as do tricyclic antidepressants.

However, their toxicity approximates that of SSRIs. Nausea is the most common problem during the first 2 wk; modest dose-dependent increases in BP occur with high doses. Discontinuation symptoms (eg, irritability, anxiety, nausea) often occur if the drug is stopped suddenly.

Duloxetine resembles venlafaxine in effectiveness and adverse effects.

Norepinephrine-Dopamine Reuptake Inhibitor

By mechanisms not clearly understood, these drugs favorably influence catecholaminergic, dopaminergic, and noradrenergic function. They do not affect the 5-HT system.

Bupropion is currently the only drug in this class. It can help depressed patients with concurrent attention-deficit/hyperactivity disorder or cocaine dependence and those trying to stop smoking. Bupropion causes hypertension in a very few patients but has no other effects on the cardiovascular system. Bupropion can cause seizures in 0.4% of patients taking doses > 150 mg tid (or > 200 mg sustained-release [SR] bid or > 450 mg extended-release [XR] once/day); risk is increased in patients with bulimia. Bupropion does not have sexual adverse effects and interacts little with coadministered drugs, although it does inhibit the CYP2D6 hepatic enzyme. Agitation, which is common, is considerably attenuated by using the SR or XR form.

Heterocyclic Antidepressants

This group of drugs, once the mainstay of treatment, includes tricyclic (tertiary amines amitriptyline and imipramine and their secondary amine metabolites nortriptyline and desipramine), modified tricyclic, and tetracyclic antidepressants.

Acutely, heterocyclic antidepressants increase the availability of primarily norepinephrine and, to some extent, 5-HT by blocking reuptake in the synaptic cleft. Long-term use downregulates alpha-1 adrenergic receptors on the postsynaptic membrane—a possible final common pathway of their antidepressant activity.

Although effective, these drugs are now rarely used because overdose causes toxicity and they have more adverse effects than other antidepressants. The more common adverse effects of heterocyclics are due to their muscarinic-blocking, histamine-blocking, and alpha-1 adrenolytic actions. Many heterocyclics have strong anticholinergic properties and are thus unsuitable for the elderly and for patients with benign prostatic hypertrophy, glaucoma, or chronic constipation. All heterocyclics, particularly maprotiline and clomipramine, lower the threshold for seizures.

Monoamine Oxidase Inhibitors (MAOIs)

These drugs inhibit the oxidative deamination of the 3 classes of biogenic amines (norepinephrine, dopamine, 5-HT) and other phenylethylamines.

Their primary value is for treating refractory or atypical depression when SSRIs, tricyclic antidepressants, and sometimes even electroconvulsive therapy are ineffective.

MAOIs marketed as antidepressants in the US (eg, phenelzine, tranylcypromine, isocarboxazid) are irreversible and nonselective (inhibiting MAO-A and MAO-B). Another MAOI (selegiline), which inhibits only MAO-B at lower doses, is available as a patch.

Hypertensive crises can occur if MAOIs that inhibit MAO-A and MAO-B are ingested concurrently with a sympathomimetic drug or food containing tyramine or dopamine. This effect is called the cheese reaction because mature cheese has a high tyramine content. MAOIs are used infrequently because of concern about this reaction. The lower dosage of the selegiline patch is considered safe to use without specific dietary restrictions, unless the dosage must be higher than starting levels (a 6-mg patch). More selective and reversible MAOIs (eg, moclobemide, befloxatone), which inhibit MAO-A, are relatively free of these interactions but are not available in the US.

To prevent hypertension and febrile crises, patients taking MAOIs should avoid sympathomimetic drugs (eg, pseudoephedrine), dextromethorphan, reserpine, and meperidine as well as malted beers, Chianti wines, sherry, liqueurs, and overripe or aged foods that contain tyramine or dopamine (eg, fava or broad beans, yeast extracts, canned figs, raisins, yogurt, cheese, sour cream, soy sauce, pickled herring, caviar, liver, banana peel, extensively tenderized meats). Patients can carry 25-mg tablets of chlorpromazine and, as soon as signs of such a hypertensive reaction occur, take 1 or 2 tablets as they head to the nearest emergency department.

Common adverse effects include erectile dysfunction (least common with tranylcypromine), anxiety, nausea, dizziness, insomnia, pedal edema, and weight gain.

MAOIs should not be used with other classes of antidepressants, and at least 2 wk (5 wk with fluoxetine, which has a long half-life) should elapse between use of the 2 classes of drugs. MAOIs used with antidepressants that affect the 5-HT system (eg, SSRIs) may cause neuroleptic malignant syndrome (malignant hyperthermia, muscle breakdown, renal failure, seizures, and eventual death).

Patients who are taking MAOIs and who also need antiasthmatic or antiallergic drugs, a local anesthetic, or a general anesthetic should be treated by a psychiatrist plus an internist, a dentist, or an anesthesiologist with expertise in neuropsychopharmacology.

Melatonergic Antidepressant

Agomelatine is a melatonergic (MT1/MT2) agonist and a 5-HT_{2C} receptor antagonist. It is used for major depressive episodes.

Agomelatine has fewer adverse effects than most antidepressants and does not cause daytime sedation, insomnia, weight gain, or sexual dysfunction. It is not addictive and does not cause withdrawal symptoms. It may cause headache, nausea and diarrhea. It may also increase liver enzyme levels, and these levels should be measured before therapy is started and every 6 wk thereafter. It is contraindicated in patients with hepatic dysfunction.

Agomelatine is taken at bedtime at a dose of 25 mg.

Drug Choice and Administration

Choice of drug may be guided by past response to a specific antidepressant. Otherwise, SSRIs are often the initial drugs of choice. Although the different SSRIs are equally effective for typical cases, certain properties of the drugs make them more or less appropriate for certain patients (see Table 210–2).

If one SSRI is ineffective, another SSRI can be substituted, or an antidepressant from a different class may be used instead. Tranylcypromine 20 to 30 mg po bid is often effective for depression refractory to sequential trials of other antidepressants; it should be given by a physician experienced in using MAOIs. Psychologic support of patients and loved ones is particularly important in refractory cases.

Insomnia, a common adverse effect of SSRIs, is treated by reducing the dose or adding a low dose of trazodone or another sedating antidepressant. Initial nausea and loose stools usually resolve, but throbbing headaches do not always go away, necessitating a change in drug class. An SSRI should be stopped if it causes agitation. When decreased libido, impotence, or anorgasmia occur during SSRI therapy, dose reduction or a

Table 210–2. ANTIDEPRESSANTS

DRUG	STARTING DOSE*	THERAPEUTIC DOSAGE RANGE	PRECAUTIONS
SSRIs			Cause discontinuation symptoms if stopped abruptly (less likely with fluoxetine)
Citalopram	20 mg once/day	20–40 mg	Lower potential for drug interactions because it has less effect on CYP450 isoenzymes Risk of QT-interval prolongation that limits doses to ≤ 40 mg/day
Escitalopram	10 mg once/day	10–20 mg	Lower potential for drug interactions because it has less effect on CYP450 isoenzymes
Fluoxetine	10 mg once/day	20–60 mg	Has very long half-life Less likely to cause discontinuation symptoms The only antidepressant proven effective in children
Fluvoxamine	50 mg once/day	100–200 mg	Can cause clinically significant elevation of theophylline, warfarin, and clozapine blood levels Has potential for interactions between its active metabolites and HCAs, carbamazepine, antipsychotics, or type IC antiarrhythmics Has CYP450 profile similar to fluoxetine
Paroxetine	20 mg once/day 25 mg CR once/day	20–50 mg 25–62.5 mg CR	Has potential for interactions between its active metabolites and HCAs, carbamazepine, antipsychotics, or type IC antiarrhythmics Has CYP450 profile similar to fluoxetine Of SSRIs, may cause the most weight gain
Sertraline	50 mg once/day	50–200 mg	Of SSRIs, has highest incidence of loose stools
Vilazodone	10 mg po once/day for 7 days, then increase to 20 mg daily for 7 days	10–40 mg (titrate by 5–10 mg q 7 days)	May increase risk of bleeding if the drug is taken with aspirin, other NSAIDs, or other drugs that affect coagulation Should not be stopped abruptly; reduce dose gradually
Serotonin modulators (5-HT$_2$ blockers)			
Mirtazapine	15 mg once/day	15–45 mg	Causes weight gain and sedation Has fewer sexual adverse effects than SSRIs and serotonin-norepinephrine reuptake inhibitors
Trazodone	50 mg tid	150–300 mg	May cause priapism May cause orthostatic hypotension
Serotonin-norepinephrine reuptake inhibitors			Cause discontinuation symptoms if stopped abruptly
Desvenlafaxine	50 mg once/day	50–100 mg	May increase BP or HR (control BP before initiating the drug and monitor BP and HR while patients are taking the drug)
Duloxetine	20 mg bid	60–120 mg	Modest dose-dependent increase in systolic and diastolic BP May cause mild urinary hesitancy in males Less potential for drug-drug interactions because it has less effect on CYP450 isoenzymes
Levomilnacipran	20 mg once/day for 2 days, then 40 mg once/day	40–120 mg (increase dose in increments of 40 mg/day at intervals of ≥ 2 days; not to exceed 120 mg/day)	May increase BP or HR (control BP before initiating the drug and monitor BP and HR while patients are taking the drug) May increase risk of bleeding (caution required if the drug is taken with aspirin, other NSAIDs, or anticoagulants) Can affect urinary hesitation or retention (caution required in patients with obstructive urinary disorders; stop the drug if symptoms develop)
Venlafaxine	25 mg tid 37.5 mg XR once/day	75–375 mg 72–225 mg XR	Modest dose-dependent increase in diastolic BP Dual norepinephrine and 5-HT reuptake effect at about 150 mg Rarely, increase in systolic BP (not dose-dependent) If stopped, should be tapered slowly Less potential for drug-drug interactions because it has less effect on CYP450 isoenzymes
Vortioxetine	5–10 mg once/day	10–20 mg	Should caution patients about increased risk of bleeding when the drug is taken with aspirin, other NSAIDs, or other drugs that affect coagulation or bleeding

Table 210–2. ANTIDEPRESSANTS (*Continued*)

DRUG	STARTING DOSE*	THERAPEUTIC DOSAGE RANGE	PRECAUTIONS
Norepinephrine-dopamine reuptake inhibitor			
Bupropion	100 mg bid 150 mg SR once/day 150 mg XL once/day	200–450 mg	Contraindicated in patients who have bulimia or who are seizure-prone May interact with HCAs, increasing the risk of seizures May cause dose-dependent recent memory loss
Heterocyclics			Contraindicated in patients with coronary artery disease, certain arrhythmias, angle-closure glaucoma, benign prostatic hypertrophy, or esophageal hiatus hernia Can cause orthostatic hypotension leading to falls and fractures, potentiate the effect of alcohol, and raise the blood level of antipsychotics With significant overdose, potentially lethal
Amitriptyline	50 mg once/day	150–300 mg	Causes weight gain
Amoxapine	50 mg bid	150–400 mg	Can have extrapyramidal adverse effects
Clomipramine	25 mg once/day	100–250 mg	Lowers seizure threshold at doses of > 250 mg/day
Desipramine	25 mg once/day	150–300 mg	—
Doxepin	25 mg once/day	150–300 mg	Causes weight gain
Imipramine	25 mg once/day	150–300 mg	May cause excessive sweating and nightmares
Maprotiline	75 mg once/day	150–225 mg	Increased risk of seizures with rapid dose escalation at high doses
Nortriptyline	25 mg once/day	50–150 mg	Effective within the therapeutic window
Protriptyline	5 mg tid	15–60 mg	Has long half-life (74 h)
Trimipramine	50 mg once/day	150–300 mg	Causes weight gain
MAOIs			Serotonergic syndrome possible when taken with an SSRI Hypertensive crisis possible when taken with other antidepressants, sympathomimetic or other selective drugs, or certain foods and beverages With significant overdose, potentially lethal
Isocarboxazid	10 mg bid	30–60 mg	Causes orthostatic hypotension
Phenelzine	15 mg tid	45–90 mg	Causes orthostatic hypotension
Selegiline, transdermal	6 mg once/day	12 mg	Can cause application site reactions and insomnia
Tranylcypromine	10 mg bid	30–60 mg	Causes orthostatic hypotension Has amphetamine-type stimulant effects and modest abuse potential
Melatonergic antidepressant			
Agomelatine ($5\text{-}HT_{2C}$ receptor antagonist)	25 mg once/day at bedtime	25–50 mg	Should be stopped immediately if symptoms or signs of potential liver injury develop or if serum transaminases increase to > 3 times the upper limit of normal

*All drugs are given orally except for transdermal selegiline.

CR = continuous release; CYP450 = cytochrome P-450 system; HCAs = heterocyclic antidepressants; HR = heart rate; 5-HT = 5-hydroxytryptamine (serotonin); MAOIs = monoamine oxidase inhibitors; SR = sustained release; XL = extended release; XR = extended release.

change to a serotonin modulator or a norepinephrine-dopamine reuptake inhibitor may help.

SSRIs, which tend to stimulate many depressed patients, should be given in the morning. Giving the entire heterocyclic antidepressant dose at bedtime usually makes sedatives unnecessary, minimizes adverse effects during the day, and improves adherence. MAOIs are usually given in the morning and early afternoon to avoid excessive stimulation.

Therapeutic response with most classes of antidepressants usually occurs in about 2 to 3 wk (sometimes as early as 4 days or as late as 8 wk). For a first episode of mild or moderate depression, the antidepressant should be given for 6 mo, then tapered gradually over 2 mo. If the episode is severe or is a recurrence or if there is suicidal risk, the dose that produces full remission should be continued during maintenance.

For psychotic depression, the combination of an antidepressant and an antipsychotic is more effective than either used alone. Patients who have recovered from psychotic depression are at higher risk of relapse than those who had nonpsychotic depression, so prophylactic treatment is particularly important.

Continued therapy with an antidepressant for 6 to 12 mo (up to 2 yr in patients > 50) is usually needed to prevent relapse.

Most antidepressants, especially SSRIs, should be tapered off (by decreasing the dose by about 25%/wk) rather than stopped abruptly; stopping SSRIs abruptly may result in discontinuation syndrome (nausea, chills, muscles aches, dizziness, anxiety, irritability, insomnia, fatigue). The likelihood and severity of withdrawal varies inversely with the half-life of the SSRI.

BIPOLAR DISORDERS

Bipolar disorders are characterized by episodes of mania and depression, which may alternate, although many patients have a predominance of one or the other. Exact cause is unknown, but heredity, changes in the level of brain neurotransmitters, and psychosocial factors may be involved. Diagnosis is based on history. Treatment consists of mood-stabilizing drugs, sometimes with psychotherapy.

Bipolar disorders usually begin in the teens, 20s, or 30s. Lifetime prevalence is about 4%. Rates of bipolar I disorder are about equal for men and women.

Bipolar disorders are classified as

- **Bipolar I disorder:** Defined by the presence of at least one full-fledged (ie, disrupting normal social and occupational function) manic episode and usually depressive episodes
- **Bipolar II disorder:** Defined by the presence of major depressive episodes with at least one hypomanic episode but no full-fledged manic episodes
- **Unspecified bipolar disorder:** Disorders with clear bipolar features that do not meet the specific criteria for other bipolar disorders

In **cyclothymic disorder**, patients have prolonged (> 2-yr) periods that include both hypomanic and depressive episodes; however, these episodes do not meet the specific criteria for a bipolar disorder.

Etiology

Exact cause of bipolar disorder is unknown. Heredity plays a significant role. There is also evidence of dysregulation of serotonin and norepinephrine. Psychosocial factors may be involved. Stressful life events are often associated with initial development of symptoms and later exacerbations, although cause and effect have not been established.

Certain drugs can trigger exacerbations in some patients with bipolar disorder; these drugs include

- Sympathomimetics (eg, cocaine, amphetamines)
- Alcohol
- Certain antidepressants (eg, tricyclics, MAOIs)

Symptoms and Signs

Bipolar disorder begins with an acute phase of symptoms, followed by a repeating course of remission and relapse. Remissions are often complete, but many patients have residual symptoms, and for some, the ability to function at work is severely impaired. Relapses are discrete episodes of more intense symptoms that are manic, depressive, hypomanic, or a mixture of depressive and manic features.

Episodes last anywhere from a few weeks to 3 to 6 mo.

Cycles—time from onset of one episode to that of the next—vary in length among patients. Some patients have infrequent episodes, perhaps only a few over a lifetime, whereas others have rapid-cycling forms (usually defined as ≥ 4 episodes/yr). Only a minority alternate back and forth between mania and depression with each cycle; in most, one or the other predominates to some extent.

Patients may attempt or commit suicide. Lifetime incidence of suicide in patients with bipolar disorder is estimated to be at least 15 times that of the general population.

Mania: A manic episode is defined as ≥ 1 wk of a persistently elevated, expansive, or irritable mood and persistently increased goal-directed activity or energy plus ≥ 3 additional symptoms:

- Inflated self-esteem or grandiosity
- Decreased need for sleep
- Greater talkativeness than usual
- Flight of ideas or racing of thoughts
- Distractibility
- Increased goal-directed activity
- Excessive involvement in activities with high potential for painful consequences (eg, buying sprees, foolish business investments)

Manic patients may be inexhaustibly, excessively, and impulsively involved in various pleasurable, high-risk activities (eg, gambling, dangerous sports, promiscuous sexual activity) without insight into possible harm. Symptoms are so severe that they cannot function in their primary role (occupation, school, housekeeping). Unwise investments, spending sprees, and other personal choices may have irreparable consequences.

Patients in a manic episode may be exuberant and flamboyantly or colorfully dressed and often have an authoritative manner with a rapid, unstoppable flow of speech. Patients may make clang associations (new thoughts that are triggered by word sounds rather than meaning). Easily distracted, patients may constantly shift from one theme or endeavor to another. However, they tend to believe they are in their best mental state.

Lack of insight and an increased capacity for activity often lead to intrusive behavior and can be a dangerous combination. Interpersonal friction results and may cause patients to feel that they are being unjustly treated or persecuted. As a result, patients may become a danger to themselves or to other people. Accelerated mental activity is experienced as racing thoughts by patients and is observed as flights of ideas by the physician.

Manic psychosis is a more extreme manifestation, with psychotic symptoms that may be difficult to distinguish from schizophrenia. Patients may have extreme grandiose or persecutory delusions (eg, of being Jesus or being pursued by the FBI), occasionally with hallucinations. Activity level increases markedly; patients may race about and scream, swear, or sing. Mood lability increases, often with increasing irritability. Full-blown delirium (delirious mania) may appear, with complete loss of coherent thinking and behavior.

Hypomania: A hypomanic episode is a less extreme variant of mania involving a distinct episode that lasts ≥ 4 days with behavior that is distinctly different from the patient's usual non-depressed self and that includes ≥ 3 of the additional symptoms listed above under mania.

During the hypomanic period, mood brightens, the need for sleep decreases, and psychomotor activity accelerates. For some patients, hypomanic periods are adaptive because they produce high energy, creativity, confidence, and supernormal social functioning. Many do not wish to leave the pleasurable, euphoric state. Some function quite well, and in most, functioning is not markedly impaired. However, in some patients, hypomania manifests as distractibility, irritability, and labile mood, which the patient and others find less attractive.

Depression: A depressive episode has features typical of major depression; the episode must include ≥ 5 of the following during the same 2-wk period, and one of them must be depressed mood or loss of interest or pleasure:

- Depressed mood most of the day
- Markedly diminished interest or pleasure in all or almost all activities for most of the day
- Significant (> 5%) weight gain or loss or decreased or increased appetite
- Insomnia (often sleep-maintenance insomnia) or hypersomnia
- Psychomotor agitation or retardation observed by others (not self-reported)
- Fatigue or loss of energy
- Feelings of worthlessness or excessive or inappropriate guilt
- Diminished ability to think or concentrate or indecisiveness
- Recurrent thoughts of death or suicide, a suicide attempt, or specific plan for suicide

Psychotic features are more common in bipolar depression than in unipolar depression.

Mixed features: An episode of mania or hypomania is designated as having mixed features if ≥ 3 depressive symptoms are present for most days of the episode. This condition is often difficult to diagnose and may shade into a continuously cycling state; the prognosis is worse than that in a pure manic or hypomanic state.

Risk of suicide during mixed episodes is particularly high.

Diagnosis

- Clinical criteria (*Diagnostic and Statistical Manual of Mental Disorders*, Fifth Edition)
- Thyroxine (T_4) and TSH levels to exclude hyperthyroidism
- Exclusion of stimulant drug abuse clinically or by urine testing

Diagnosis of bipolar disorder is based on identification of symptoms of mania or hypomania as described above, plus a history of remission and relapse. Symptoms must be severe enough to markedly impair social or occupational functioning or to require hospitalization to prevent harm to self or others.

Some patients who present with depressive symptoms may have previously experienced hypomania or mania but do not report it unless they are specifically questioned. Skillful questioning may reveal morbid signs (eg, excesses in spending, impulsive sexual escapades, stimulant drug abuse), although such information is more likely to be provided by relatives. A structured inventory such as the Mood Disorder Questionnaire may be useful. All patients must be asked gently but directly about suicidal ideation, plans, or activity.

Similar acute manic or hypomanic symptoms may result from stimulant abuse or physical disorders such as hyperthyroidism or pheochromocytoma. Patients with hyperthyroidism typically have other physical symptoms and signs, but thyroid function testing (T_4 and TSH levels) is a reasonable screen for new patients. Patients with pheochromocytoma are markedly hypertensive; if they are not, testing is not indicated. Other disorders less commonly cause symptoms of mania, but depressive symptoms may occur in a number of disorders (see Table 210–1).

A review of substance use (especially of amphetamines and cocaine) and urine drug screening can help identify drug causes. However, because drug use may simply have triggered an episode in a patient with bipolar disorder, seeking evidence of symptoms (manic or depressive) not related to drug use is important.

Some patients with schizoaffective disorder have manic symptoms, but such patients rarely return to normal between episodes, and they, unlike most patients with mania, do not show interest in connecting with other people.

Patients with bipolar disorder may also have anxiety disorders (eg, social phobia, panic attacks, obsessive-compulsive disorders), possibly confusing the diagnosis.

Treatment

- Mood stabilizers (eg, lithium, certain anticonvulsants), a 2nd-generation antipsychotic, or both
- Support and psychotherapy

Treatment of bipolar disorder usually has 3 phases:

- Acute: To stabilize and control the initial, sometimes severe manifestations
- Continuation: To attain full remission
- Maintenance or prevention: To keep patients in remission

Although most patients with hypomania can be treated as outpatients, severe mania or depression often requires inpatient management.

Drug treatment of bipolar disorder (see also p. 1768): Drugs for bipolar disorder include

- Mood stabilizers: Lithium and certain anticonvulsants, especially valproate, carbamazepine, and lamotrigine
- 2nd-generation antipsychotics: Aripiprazole, lurasidone, olanzapine, quetiapine, risperidone, and ziprasidone

These drugs are used alone or in combination for all phases of treatment, although at different dosages.

Choice of drug treatment for bipolar disorder can be difficult because all drugs have significant adverse effects, drug interactions are common, and no drug is universally effective. Selection should be based on what has previously been effective and well-tolerated in a given patient. If there is no prior experience (or it is unknown), choice is based on the patient's medical history (vis-à-vis the adverse effects of the specific mood stabilizer) and the severity of symptoms.

Specific antidepressants (eg, SSRIs) are sometimes added for severe depression, but their effectiveness is controversial; they are not recommended as sole therapy for depressive episodes.

Other treatments: **Electroconvulsive therapy** (ECT) is sometimes used for depression refractory to treatment and is also effective for mania.

Phototherapy can be useful in treating seasonal bipolar I or bipolar II disorder (with autumn-winter depression and spring-summer hypomania). It is probably most useful as augmentative therapy.

Education and psychotherapy: Enlisting the support of loved ones is crucial to preventing major episodes.

Group therapy is often recommended for patients and their partner; there, they learn about bipolar disorder, its social sequelae, and the central role of mood stabilizers in treatment.

Individual psychotherapy may help patients better cope with problems of daily living and adjust to a new way of identifying themselves.

Patients, particularly those with bipolar II disorder, may not adhere to mood-stabilizer regimens because they believe that these drugs make them less alert and creative. The physician can explain that decreased creativity is relatively uncommon because mood stabilizers usually provide opportunity for a more even performance in interpersonal, scholastic, professional, and artistic pursuits.

Patients should be counseled to avoid stimulant drugs and alcohol, to minimize sleep deprivation, and to recognize early signs of relapse. If patients tend to be financially extravagant, finances should be turned over to a trusted family member. Patients with a tendency to sexual excesses should be given information about conjugal consequences (eg, divorce) and infectious risks of promiscuity, particularly AIDS.

Support groups (eg, the Depression and Bipolar Support Alliance [DBSA]) can help patients by providing a forum to share their common experiences and feelings.

KEY POINTS

- Bipolar disorder is a cyclic condition that involves episodes of mania with or without depression (bipolar 1) or hypomania plus depression (bipolar 2).
- Bipolar disorder markedly impairs the ability to function at work and to interact socially, and risk of suicide is significant; however, mild manic states (hypomania) are sometimes adaptive because they can produce high energy, creativity, confidence, and supernormal social functioning.
- Length and frequency of cycles vary among patients; some patients have only a few over a lifetime, whereas others have ≥ 4 episodes/yr (rapid-cycling forms).
- Only a few patients alternate back and forth between mania and depression during each cycle; in most cycles, one or the other predominates.
- Diagnosis is based on clinical criteria, but stimulant abuse and physical disorders such as hyperthyroidism or pheochromocytoma must be ruled out by examination and testing.
- Treatment depends on the manifestations and their severity but typically involves mood stabilizers (eg, lithium, valproate, carbamazepine, lamotrigine) and/or 2nd-generation antipsychotics (eg, aripiprazole, lurasidone, olanzapine, quetiapine, risperidone, ziprasidone).

DRUG TREATMENT OF BIPOLAR DISORDER

Drug Selection and Use

Choice of drug can be difficult because all drugs have significant adverse effects, drug interactions are common, and no drug is universally effective. Selection should be based on what has previously been effective and well-tolerated in a given patient. If there is no prior experience (or it is unknown), choice is based on the patient's medical history (vis-à-vis the adverse effects of the specific mood stabilizer) and the severity of symptoms.

For **severe manic psychosis,** in which immediate patient safety and management is compromised, urgent behavioral control usually requires a sedating 2nd-generation antipsychotic, sometimes supplemented initially with a benzodiazepine such as lorazepam or clonazepam 2 to 4 mg IM or po tid.

For **less severe acute episodes** in patients without contraindications (eg, renal disorders), lithium is a good first choice for both mania and depressive episodes. Because its onset is slow (4 to 10 days), patients with significant symptoms may also be given an anticonvulsant or a 2nd-generation antipsychotic.

For **patients with depression,** lamotrigine may be a good choice of anticonvulsant.

For **bipolar depression,** the best evidence suggests using quetiapine or lurasidone alone or the combination of fluoxetine and olanzapine.

Once remission is achieved, preventive treatment with mood stabilizers is indicated for all bipolar I patients. If episodes recur during maintenance treatment, clinicians should determine whether adherence is poor and, if so, whether nonadherence preceded or followed recurrence. Reasons for nonadherence should be explored to determine whether a change in mood stabilizer type or dosing would render treatment more acceptable.

Lithium

As many as two thirds of patients with uncomplicated bipolar disorder respond to lithium, which attenuates bipolar mood swings but has no effect on normal mood.

Whether lithium or another mood stabilizer is being used, breakthroughs are more likely in patients who have mixed states, rapid-cycling forms of bipolar disorder, comorbid anxiety, substance abuse, or a neurologic disorder.

Lithium carbonate is started at 300 mg po bid or tid and titrated, based on steady-state blood levels and tolerance, to a range of 0.8 to 1.2 mEq/L. Levels should be drawn after 5 days at a stable dose and 12 h after the last dose. Target drug levels for maintenance are lower, about 0.6 to 0.7 mEq/L. Higher maintenance levels are more protective against manic (but not depressive) episodes but have more adverse effects. Adolescents, whose glomerular function is excellent, need higher doses; elderly patients need lower doses.

Lithium can cause sedation and cognitive impairment directly or indirectly (by causing hypothyroidism) and often exacerbates acne and psoriasis. The most common acute, mild adverse effects are fine tremor, fasciculation, nausea, diarrhea, polyuria, polydipsia, and weight gain (partly attributed to drinking high-calorie beverages). These effects are usually transient and often respond to decreasing the dose slightly, dividing the dose (eg, tid), or using slow-release forms. Once dosage is established, the entire dose should be given after the evening meal. This dosing may improve adherence. A beta-blocker (eg, atenolol 25 to 50 mg po once/day) can control severe tremor; however, some beta-blockers (eg, propranolol) may worsen depression.

Acute lithium toxicity is manifested initially by gross tremor, increased deep tendon reflexes, persistent headache, vomiting, and confusion and may progress to stupor, seizures, and arrhythmias. Toxicity is more likely to occur in the following:

- Elderly patients
- Patients with decreased creatinine clearance
- Those with sodium loss (eg, due to fever, vomiting, diarrhea, or use of diuretics)

Thiazide diuretics, ACE inhibitors, and NSAIDs other than aspirin may contribute to hyperlithemia. Lithium blood levels should be measured every 6 mo and whenever the dose is changed.

Long-term adverse effects of lithium include

- Hypothyroidism, particularly when there is a family history of hypothyroidism
- Renal damage involving the distal tubule (mainly in patients with a history of renal parenchymal disease)

Therefore, TSH levels should be monitored when lithium is started and annually thereafter if there is a family history of thyroid dysfunction or every other year for all other patients. Levels should also be measured whenever symptoms suggest thyroid dysfunction (including when mania recurs) because hypothyroidism may blunt the effect of mood stabilizers. BUN and creatinine should be measured at baseline, 2 or 3 times during the first 6 mo, and then once or twice a year.

Anticonvulsants

Anticonvulsants that act as mood stabilizers, especially valproate and carbamazepine, are often used for acute mania and for mixed states (mania and depression). Lamotrigine is effective for mood-cycling and for depression. The precise mechanism of action for anticonvulsants in bipolar disorder is unknown but may involve gamma-aminobutyric acid mechanisms and ultimately G-protein signaling systems. Their main advantages over lithium include a wider therapeutic margin and lack of renal toxicity.

For **valproate**, a loading dose of 20 to 30 mg/kg is given, then 250 to 500 mg po tid (extended-release formulation can be used); target blood levels are between 50 and 125 μg/mL. This approach does not result in more adverse effects than does gradual titration. Adverse effects include nausea, headache, sedation, dizziness, and weight gain; rare serious effects include hepatotoxicity and pancreatitis.

Carbamazepine should not be loaded; it should be started at 200 mg po bid and be increased gradually in 200-mg/day increments to target levels between 4 and 12 μg/mL (maximum, 800 mg bid). Adverse effects include nausea, dizziness, sedation, and unsteadiness. Very severe effects include aplastic anemia and agranulocytosis.

Lamotrigine is started at 25 mg po once/day for 2 wk, then 50 mg once/day for 2 wk, then 100 mg/day for 1 wk, and then can be increased by 50 mg each week as needed up to 200 mg once/day. Dosage is lower for patients taking valproate and higher for patients taking carbamazepine. Lamotrigine can cause rash and, rarely, the life-threatening Stevens-Johnson syndrome, particularly if the dosage is increased more rapidly than recommended. While taking lamotrigine, patients should be encouraged to report any new rash, hives, fever, swollen glands, sores in the mouth and on the eyes, and swelling of the lips or tongue.

Antipsychotics

Acute manic psychosis is being increasingly managed with 2nd-generation antipsychotics, such as

- Risperidone (usually 2 to 3 mg po bid)
- Olanzapine (usually 5 to 10 mg po bid)
- Quetiapine (200 to 400 mg po bid)
- Ziprasidone (40 to 80 mg po bid)
- Aripiprazole (10 to 30 mg po once/day)

In addition, evidence suggests that these drugs may enhance the effects of mood stabilizers after the acute phase.

Although any of these drugs may have extrapyramidal adverse effects and cause akathisia, risk is lower with more sedating drugs such as quetiapine and olanzapine. Less immediate adverse effects include substantial weight gain and development of the metabolic syndrome (including weight gain, excess abdominal fat, insulin resistance, and dyslipidemia); risk may be lower with the least sedating 2nd-generation antipsychotics, ziprasidone and aripiprazole.

For extremely hyperactive psychotic patients with poor food and fluid intake, an antipsychotic given IM plus supportive care in addition to lithium or an anticonvulsant may be appropriate.

Precautions During Pregnancy

Lithium use during pregnancy has been associated with an increased risk of cardiovascular malformations (particularly Ebstein anomaly). However, the absolute risk of this particular malformation is quite low. Taking lithium during pregnancy appears to increase the relative risk of any congenital anomaly by about 2-fold, a risk similar to the 2- to 3-fold increased risk of congenital anomalies associated with use of carbamazepine or lamotrigine and is substantially lower than the risk associated with use of valproate.

With **valproate**, risk of neural tube defects and other congenital malformations appears to be 2 to 7 times higher than that with other commonly used anticonvulsants. Valproate increases the risk of neural tube defects, congenital heart defects, genitourinary anomalies, musculoskeletal abnormalities, and cleft lip or palate. Also, cognitive outcomes (eg, IQ scores) in children of women who took valproate during pregnancy are worse than those with other anticonvulsants; risk appears to be dose-related. Valproate also appears to increase risk of attention-deficit/hyperactivity disorder and autism spectrum disorders.[1]

Extensive study of the use of 1st-generation antipsychotics and tricyclic antidepressants during early pregnancy has not revealed causes for concern. The same appears to be true of SSRIs, except for paroxetine. Data about the risks of 2nd-generation antipsychotics to the fetus are sparse as yet, even though these drugs are being more widely used for all phases of bipolar disorder.

Use of drugs (particularly lithium and SSRIs) before parturition may have carry-over effects on neonates.

Treatment decisions are complicated by the fact that with unplanned pregnancy, teratogenic effects may already have taken place by the time practitioners become aware of the issue. Consultation with a perinatal psychiatrist should be considered. In all cases, discussing the risks and benefits of treatment with patients is important.

1. Tomson T, Battino D, Perucca E: Valproic acid after five decades of use in epilepsy: Time to reconsider the indications of a time-honoured drug. *Lancet Neurol* 15(2): 210–218, 2016. Epub ahead of print (2015 Dec 3). doi: 10.1016/S1474-4422(15)00314-2.

CYCLOTHYMIC DISORDER

Cyclothymic disorder is characterized by hypomanic and mini-depressive periods that last a few days, follow an irregular course, and are less severe than those in bipolar disorder; these symptom periods must occur for more than half the days during a period of ≥ 2 yr. Diagnosis is clinical and based on history. Management consists primarily of education, although some patients with functional impairment require drug therapy.

Cyclothymic disorder is commonly a precursor of bipolar II disorder. However, it can also occur as extreme moodiness without becoming a major mood disorder.

In **chronic hypomania,** a form rarely seen clinically, elated periods predominate, with habitual reduction of sleep to < 6 h. People with this form are constantly overcheerful, self-assured, overenergetic, full of plans, improvident, overinvolved, and meddlesome; they rush off with restless impulses and may act in an overfamiliar manner with people.

For some people, cyclothymic and chronic hypomanic dispositions contribute to success in business, leadership, achievement, and artistic creativity; however, they more often have serious detrimental interpersonal and social consequences. Consequences often include instability with an uneven work and schooling history, impulsive and frequent changes of residence, repeated romantic or marital breakups, and an episodic abuse of alcohol and drugs.

Diagnosis of cyclothymic disorder is clinical and based on history.

Treatment

- Supportive care
- Sometimes a mood stabilizer

Patients should be taught how to live with the extremes of their temperamental inclinations; however, living with cyclothymic disorder is not easy because interpersonal relationships are often stormy. Jobs with flexible hours are advised. Patients with artistic inclinations should be encouraged to pursue careers in the arts because the excesses and fragility of cyclothymia may be better tolerated there.

The decision to use a mood stabilizer (eg, lithium; certain anticonvulsants, especially valproate, carbamazepine, and lamotrigine) depends on the balance between functional impairment and the social benefits or creative spurts that patients may experience. Divalproex 500 to 1000 mg po once/day is often better tolerated than equivalent doses of lithium.

Antidepressants should be avoided unless depressive symptoms are severe and prolonged because switching and rapid cycling are risks.

Support groups can help patients by providing a forum to share their common experiences and feelings.

211 Obsessive-Compulsive and Related Disorders

OBSESSIVE-COMPULSIVE DISORDER

Obsessive-compulsive disorder (OCD) is characterized by recurrent, persistent, unwanted, and intrusive thoughts, urges, or images (obsessions) and/or by repetitive behaviors or mental acts that patients feel driven to do (compulsions) to try to lessen or prevent the anxiety that obsessions cause. Diagnosis is based on history. Treatment consists of psychotherapy (specifically, exposure and response prevention), drug therapy (specifically, SSRIs or clomipramine), or, especially in severe cases, both.

OCD is slightly more common among women than men and affects about 1 to 2% of the population. Up to 30% of people with OCD also have a past or current tic disorder (see p. 2776).

Symptoms and Signs

Obsessions are unwanted, intrusive thoughts, urges, or images, the presence of which usually cause marked distress or anxiety. The dominant theme of the obsessive thoughts may be harm, risk to self or others, danger, contamination, doubt, loss, or aggression. For example, patients may obsess about becoming contaminated with dirt or germs unless they wash their hands for ≥ 2 h a day. The obsessions are not pleasurable. Thus, patients try to ignore and/or suppress the thoughts, urges, or images. Or they try to neutralize them by performing a compulsion.

Compulsions (often called rituals) are excessive, repetitive, purposeful behaviors that affected people feel they must do to prevent or reduce the anxiety caused by their obsessive thoughts or to neutralize their obsessions. Examples are

- Washing (eg, handwashing, showering)
- Checking (eg, that the stove is turned off, that doors are locked)
- Counting (eg, repeating a behavior a certain number of times)
- Ordering (eg, arranging tableware or workspace items in a specific pattern)

Most rituals, such as hand washing or checking locks, are observable, but some mental rituals, such as silent repetitive counting or statements muttered under the breath, are not. Typically, the compulsive rituals must be done in a precise way according to rigid rules. The rituals may or may not be connected realistically to the feared event. When connected realistically (eg, showering to avoid being dirty, checking the stove to prevent fire), the compulsions are clearly excessive—eg, showering for hours each day or always checking the stove 30 times before leaving the house. In all cases, the obsessions and/or compulsions must be time-consuming (> 1 h/day, often much more) or cause patients significant distress or impairment in functioning; at their extreme, obsessions and compulsions may be incapacitating.

The degree of insight varies. Most people with OCD recognize to some degree that the beliefs underlying their obsessions are not realistic (eg, that they really will not get cancer if they touch an ashtray). However, occasionally, insight is completely lacking (ie, patients are convinced that the beliefs underlying their obsessions are true and that their compulsions are reasonable).

Because people with this disorder fear embarrassment or stigmatization, they often conceal their obsessions and rituals. Relationships often deteriorate, and performance in school or at work may decline. Depression is a common secondary feature.

Diagnosis

- Clinical criteria

Diagnosis is clinical, based on the presence of obsessions, compulsions, or both. The obsessions or compulsions must be time-consuming or cause clinically significant distress or impairment of functioning.

Treatment

- Exposure and ritual prevention therapy
- SSRI or clomipramine

Exposure and ritual prevention therapy is often effective; its essential element is gradually exposing patients to situations or people that trigger the anxiety-provoking obsessions and rituals while requiring them not to perform their rituals. This approach allows the anxiety triggered by exposure to diminish through habituation. Improvement often continues for years, especially in patients who master the approach and use it even after formal treatment has ended. However, some patients have incomplete responses (as some also do to drugs).

Certain antidepressants, including SSRIs (see p. 1762) and clomipramine (a tricyclic antidepressant with potent serotonergic effects), are often very effective. Patients often require higher doses than are typically needed for depression and most anxiety disorders. Many experts believe that combining exposure and ritual prevention with drug therapy is best, especially for severe cases.

KEY POINTS

- Obsessions are intrusive, unwanted thoughts, images, or urges that usually cause marked distress or anxiety.
- Compulsions are excessive, repetitive rituals that people feel they must do to reduce the anxiety caused by their obsessive thoughts or to neutralize their obsessions.
- Obsessions and/or compulsions must be time-consuming (> 1 h/day, often much more) or cause patients significant distress or impairment in functioning.
- Treat by gradually exposing patients to situations that trigger the anxiety-provoking obsessions and rituals while requiring them not to perform their rituals.
- Giving an SSRI or clomipramine may also help.

BODY DYSMORPHIC DISORDER

Body dysmorphic disorder is characterized by preoccupation with ≥ 1 perceived defects in physical appearance that are not apparent or appear only slight to other people. The preoccupation with appearance must cause clinically significant distress or impairment in social, occupational, academic, or other aspects of functioning. And at some point, patients must repetitively and excessively perform ≥ 1 behaviors (eg, mirror checking, comparing their appearance with that of other people) in response to the preoccupation with appearance. Diagnosis is based on history. Treatment consists of drug therapy (specifically, SSRIs or clomipramine), psychotherapy (specifically, cognitive-behavioral therapy), or both.

Body dysmorphic disorder usually begins during adolescence and may be somewhat more common among women. At any given point in time, about 2% of people have the disorder.

Symptoms and Signs

Symptoms may develop gradually or abruptly. Although intensity may vary, the disorder is thought usually to be chronic unless patients are appropriately treated. Concerns commonly involve the face or head but may involve any body part or any number of parts and may change from one part to another over time. For example, patients may be concerned about thinning hair, acne, wrinkles, scars, vascular markings, color of their complexion, or excessive facial or body hair. Or they may focus on the shape or size of the nose, eyes, ears, mouth, breasts, buttocks, legs, or other body part. Men (and rarely women) may have a form of the disorder called muscle dysmorphia, which involves preoccupation with the idea that their body is not sufficiently lean and muscular. Patients may describe the disliked body parts as looking ugly, unattractive, deformed, hideous, or monstrous.

Patients usually spend many hours a day worrying about their perceived defects and often mistakenly believe that people take special note of or mock them because of these defects. Most check themselves often in mirrors, others avoid mirrors, and still others alternate between the 2 behaviors.

Other common compulsive behaviors include excessive grooming, skin picking (to remove or fix perceived skin defects), reassurance seeking (about the perceived defects), and clothes changing. Most try to camouflage their perceived defects—eg, by growing a beard to hide perceived scars or by wearing a hat to cover slightly thinning hair. Many undergo dermatologic, dental, surgical, or other cosmetic treatment to correct their perceived defects, but such treatment is usually unsuccessful and may intensify their preoccupation. Men with muscle dysmorphia may use androgen supplements, which can be dangerous.

Because people with body dysmorphic disorder feel self-conscious about their appearance, they may avoid going out in public. For most, social, occupational, academic, and other aspects of functioning are impaired—often substantially—because of their concerns about appearance. Some leave their homes only at night; others, not at all. Social isolation, depression, repeated hospitalization, and suicidal behavior are common.

The degree of insight varies, but it is usually poor or absent. That is, patients genuinely believe that the disliked body part probably (poor insight) or definitely (absent insight) looks abnormal, ugly, or unattractive.

Diagnosis

- Clinical criteria

Because many patients are too embarrassed and ashamed to reveal their symptoms, the disorder may go undiagnosed for years. It is distinguished from normal concerns about appearance because the preoccupations are time-consuming and cause significant distress, impairment in functioning, or both.

Diagnosis is based on history. If the only concern is body shape and weight, an eating disorder may be the more accurate diagnosis (see p. 1753); if the only concern is the appearance of sex characteristics, a diagnosis of gender dysphoria may be considered (see p. 1797).

Criteria include the following:

- Preoccupation with one or more perceived defects in appearance that are not observable or appear slight to others
- Performance of repetitive behaviors (eg, mirror checking, excessive grooming) in response to the appearance concerns
- The preoccupation causes significant distress or impairs social, occupational or other areas of functioning

Treatment

- SSRIs and clomipramine
- Cognitive-behavioral therapy

Certain antidepressants, including SSRIs (see p. 1762) and clomipramine (a tricyclic antidepressant with potent serotonergic effects), are often very effective. Patients often require higher doses than are typically needed for depression and most anxiety disorders.

Cognitive-behavioral therapy that is tailored to the specific symptoms of body dysmorphic disorder is currently the psychotherapy of choice. Cognitive approaches and exposure and ritual prevention are essential elements of therapy. Clinicians have patients face situations they fear or avoid while refraining from performing their rituals. Because most patients have poor or absent insight, motivational interviewing is often needed to increase their willingness to participate and stay in treatment.

Many experts believe that combining exposure and ritual prevention with drug therapy is best for severe cases.

KEY POINTS

- Patients are preoccupied with ≥ 1 perceived defects in their physical appearance that are not apparent or appear only slight to other people.
- In response to the appearance concerns, patients perform repetitive behaviors (eg, mirror checking, excessive grooming) and/or take measures to camouflage or remove the perceived defect.
- Patients typically have poor or absent insight and genuinely believe that the disliked body area looks abnormal or unattractive.
- Treat using cognitive-behavioral therapy involving cognitive approaches and ritual prevention, as well as drug therapy with an SSRI or clomipramine.

HOARDING DISORDER

Hoarding disorder is characterized by persistent difficulty discarding or parting with possessions, regardless of their actual value. This difficulty results in the accumulation of possessions that congest and clutter living areas to the point that the intended use of the areas is substantially compromised.

Hoarding disorder often begins at a mild level during adolescence and gradually worsens with age, causing clinically significant impairment by the mid-30s. At any given point in time, an estimated 2 to 6% of people have this disorder.

Symptoms and Signs

The disorder is typically chronic, with little or no waxing and waning of symptoms or spontaneous remission. Patients have a strong need to save items, and they experience significant distress when parting with the items or contemplating parting with them. Patients accumulate a large number of items for which they have inadequate space; the items congest and clutter the living space so much that large areas become unusable, except for storing hoarded items. For example, stacks of hoarded newspapers may fill the sink and cover the countertops and stove in the kitchen, preventing these areas from being used to prepare meals.

Animal hoarding is a form of hoarding disorder in which patients accumulate a large number of animals and do not provide adequate nutrition, sanitation, and veterinary care despite deterioration of the animals (eg, weight loss, illness) and/or environment (eg, extreme overcrowding, highly unsanitary conditions).

Degree of insight varies. Some patients recognize that the hoarding-related beliefs and behaviors are problematic, others do not.

Diagnosis

- Clinical criteria

Hoarding is distinguished from transient accumulation and clutter (eg, as when property is inherited) by its persistence and other features; in addition, patients resist giving away or selling hoarded items. Collectors (eg, of books, figurines), like hoarders, can acquire and keep a large number of items, but in contrast to hoarding, collections are organized and systematic and do not significantly impair functioning or the safety of the home environment.

Diagnostic criteria include the following;

- Patients have persistent difficulty discarding or parting with possessions, regardless of their actual value.
- The difficulty discarding is due to the perceived need to save the items and to the distress associated with discarding them.
- The accumulated possessions congest and clutter active living areas (ie, not basements or storage areas) and substantially compromise the intended use of these areas.
- The hoarding causes significant distress or impairs social, occupational, or other areas of functioning.

Treatment

- SSRIs
- Cognitive-behavioral therapy

SSRIs may be helpful, although data on their efficacy are limited. Cognitive-behavioral therapy that is tailored to treat the specific hoarding symptoms may also be helpful.

TRICHOTILLOMANIA

(Hair-Pulling Disorder)

Trichotillomania is characterized by recurrent pulling out of one's hair resulting in hair loss.

Patients with trichotillomania repeatedly pull or pluck out their hair for noncosmetic reasons. Most commonly, they pull hair from their scalp, eyebrows, and/or eyelids, but any body hair may be pulled out. Sites of hair pulling may change over time.

For some patients, this activity is somewhat automatic (ie, without full awareness); others are more conscious of the activity. Hair pulling is not triggered by obsessions or concerns about appearance but may be preceded by a feeling of tension or anxiety that is relieved by the hair pulling, which is often then followed by a feeling of gratification.

Hair pulling typically begins just before or after puberty. At any given point in time, about 1 to 2% of people have the disorder. About 90% of them are female.

Symptoms and Signs

Hair pulling is usually chronic, with waxing and waning of symptoms.

Patterns of hair loss vary from patient to patient. Some have areas of complete alopecia or missing eyelashes and/or eyebrows; others merely have thinned hair.

A range of behaviors (rituals) may accompany hair pulling. Patients may search fastidiously for a particular kind of hair to pull; they may try to ensure that hair is pulled out in a particular way. They may roll the hair between their fingers, pull the strands between their teeth, or bite the hair once it is pulled. Many patients swallow their hair.

Patients may feel embarrassed by or ashamed of their appearance. Many try to camouflage the hair loss by covering the bald areas (eg, wearing wigs or scarfs). Some patients pull out hair from widely scattered areas to disguise the loss. They may avoid situations in which other people may see the hair loss; typically, they do not pull hair out in front of others, except for family members.

Some patients pull hair from others or from pets or pull strands from fibrous materials (eg, clothing, blankets). Most patients also have other body-focused repetitive behaviors, such as skin picking or nail biting.

Diagnosis

- Clinical criteria

Diagnostic criteria typically include the following:

- Removing hair
- Making repeated attempts to stop the hair pulling
- Experiencing significant distress or impairment from the activity

The distress can include feelings of embarrassment or shame (eg, at loss of control of one's behavior, at the cosmetic consequences of the hair loss).

Treatment

- SSRIs or clomipramine
- Cognitive-behavioral therapy

SSRIs or clomipramine (a tricyclic antidepressant with potent serotonergic effects) may be useful for coexisting depression or anxiety disorders. For hair pulling, clomipramine appears to be more effective than desipramine (a tricyclic antidepressant that inhibits reuptake of norepinephrine). However, SSRIs have been disappointing. Some evidence suggests that *N*-acetylcysteine (a partial glutamatergic agonist) is effective. There is also limited evidence that low-dose dopamine blockers are effective, but risk:benefit ratio must be carefully assessed.

Cognitive-behavioral therapy that is tailored to treat the specific symptoms of hair-pulling disorder is currently the psychotherapy of choice. For example, habit reversal, a predominantly behavioral therapy, can be used; it includes awareness training (eg, self-monitoring, identification of triggers for the behavior), stimulus control (modifying situations—eg, avoiding triggers—to reduce the likelihood of initiating pulling), and competing response training (substituting other behaviors for hair pulling).

EXCORIATION DISORDER

(Skin-Picking)

Excoriation disorder is characterized by recurrent picking of one's skin resulting in skin lesions.

Patients with excoriation disorder repeatedly pick at or scratch their skin for noncosmetic reasons (ie, not to remove a lesion that they perceive as unattractive or possibly cancerous). Some patients pick at healthy skin; others pick at minor lesions such as calluses, pimples, or scabs.

Some patients pick at their skin somewhat automatically (ie, without full awareness); others are more conscious of the activity. The picking is not triggered by obsessions or concerns about appearance but may be preceded by a feeling of tension or anxiety that is relieved by the picking, which often is also accompanied by a feeling of gratification.

Skin picking often begins during adolescence, although it may begin at various ages. At any given point in time, about 1 to 2% of people have the disorder. About 75% of them are female.

Symptoms and Signs

Skin picking is usually chronic, with waxing and waning of symptoms. Sites of skin picking may change over time. Patterns of skin picking vary from patient to patient. Some have multiple areas of scarring; others focus on only a few lesions. Many patients try to camouflage the skin lesions with clothing or makeup.

Skin picking may be accompanied by a range of behaviors or rituals. Patients may search fastidiously for a particular kind of scab to pull; they may try to ensure that the scab is pulled off in a particular way (using either fingers or an implement) and may bite or swallow the scab once it has been pulled off.

Patients may feel embarrassed by or ashamed of the appearance of the skin-picking sites. Patients may avoid situations in which others may see the skin lesions and typically do not pick in front of others, except for family members. Some patients may pick the skin of other people. Many also have other body-focused repetitive behaviors, such as hair pulling or nail biting.

Diagnosis

- Clinical criteria

To meet diagnostic criteria, patients must typically

- Cause visible skin lesions (although some patients try to camouflage lesions with clothing or makeup)
- Make repeated attempts to stop the picking
- Experience significant distress or impairment from the activity

The distress can include feelings of embarrassment or shame (eg, at loss of control of one's behavior, at the cosmetic consequences of the skin lesions).

Treatment

- SSRIs
- Cognitive-behavioral therapy

SSRIs may be useful for coexisting depression or anxiety disorders, and some evidence suggests that these drugs can also reduce skin picking to some degree.

Cognitive-behavioral therapy that is tailored to treat the specific symptoms of skin-picking disorder is currently the psychotherapy of choice. For example, habit reversal, a predominantly behavioral therapy, can be used; it includes awareness training (eg, self-monitoring, identification of triggers for the behavior), stimulus control (modifying situations—eg, avoiding triggers—to reduce the likelihood of initiating picking), and competing response training (substituting other behaviors for skin picking).

BODY-FOCUSED REPETITIVE BEHAVIOR DISORDER

Body-focused repetitive behavior disorder is characterized by body-focused repetitive behaviors (eg, nail biting, lip biting, cheek chewing) and attempts to stop the behaviors.

Body-focused repetitive behavior disorder is an example of another specified obsessive-compulsive and related disorder. Patients with this disorder repeatedly engage in body-focused activities (eg, nail biting, lip biting, cheek chewing).

Some patients engage in these activities somewhat automatically (ie, without full awareness); others are more conscious of the activity. The behaviors are not triggered by obsessions or concerns about appearance but may be preceded by a feeling of tension or anxiety that is relieved by the behavior, which is often also accompanied by a feeling of gratification.

Severe nail biting or nail picking (onychotillomania) can cause significant nail deformities (eg, washboard deformity, or habit-tic nails) and subungual hemorrhages.

Diagnosis

To meet diagnostic criteria, patients must typically

- Have body-focused repetitive behaviors other than hair pulling or skin picking
- Make repeated attempts to reduce or stop the behaviors
- Experience significant distress or impairment from the behaviors

Treatment

Treatment includes drugs (eg, SSRIs) and cognitive-behavioral therapy. It is similar to that for trichotillomania (hair-pulling disorder—see p. 1772) and excoriation disorder.

OLFACTORY REFERENCE SYNDROME

Olfactory reference syndrome is an example of another specified obsessive-compulsive and related disorder (see p. 1770). Patients with this disorder are preoccupied with a distressing or impairing belief that they emit a foul or offensive body odor, which is not perceived by others. The preoccupation is usually accompanied by repetitive behaviors (eg, smelling themselves, excessive showering).

212 Personality Disorders

Personality disorders in general are pervasive, enduring patterns of perceiving, reacting, and relating that cause significant distress or functional impairment. Personality disorders vary significantly in their manifestations, but all are believed to be caused by a combination of genetic and environmental factors. Many gradually become less severe with age, but certain traits may persist to some degree after the acute symptoms that prompted the diagnosis of a disorder abate. Diagnosis is clinical. Treatment is with psychosocial therapies and sometimes drug therapy.

Personality traits represent patterns of thinking, perceiving, reacting, and relating that are relatively stable over time.

Personality disorders exist when these traits become so pronounced, rigid, and maladaptive that they impair work and/or interpersonal functioning. These social maladaptations can cause significant distress in people with personality disorders and in those around them. For people with personality disorders (unlike many others who seek counseling), the distress caused by the consequences of their socially maladaptive behaviors is usually the reason they seek treatment, rather than any discomfort with their own thoughts and feelings. Thus, clinicians must initially help patients see that their personality traits are the root of the problem.

Personality disorders usually start to become evident during late adolescence or early adulthood, and their traits and symptoms vary considerably in how long they persist; many resolve with time.

The *Diagnostic and Statistical Manual of Mental Disorders*, Fifth Edition (DSM-5) lists 10 distinct types of personality disorders. Some types (eg, antisocial, borderline) tend to lessen or resolve as people age; others (eg, obsessive-compulsive, schizotypal) are less likely to do so.

About 10% of the general population and up to half of psychiatric patients in hospital units and clinics have a personality disorder. Overall, there are no clear distinctions in terms of sex, socioeconomic class, and race. However, in antisocial personality disorder, men outnumber women 6:1. In borderline personality disorder, women outnumber men 3:1 (but only in clinical settings, not in the general population).

For most personality disorders, levels of heritability are about 50%, which is similar to or higher than that of many other major psychiatric disorders. This degree of heritability argues against the common assumption that personality disorders are character flaws primarily shaped by an adverse environment.

The direct healthcare costs and indirect costs of lost productivity associated with personality disorders, particularly borderline and obsessive-compulsive personality disorder, are significantly greater than similar costs associated with major depressive disorder or generalized anxiety disorder.

Types of Personality Disorders

DSM-5 groups the 10 types of personality disorders into 3 clusters (A, B, and C), based on similar characteristics. However, the clinical usefulness of these clusters has not been established.

Cluster A is characterized by appearing odd or eccentric. It includes the following personality disorders with their distinguishing features:

- Paranoid: Mistrust and suspicion
- Schizoid: Disinterest in others
- Schizotypal: Eccentric ideas and behavior

Cluster B is characterized by appearing dramatic, emotional, or erratic. It includes the following personality disorders with their distinguishing features:

- Antisocial: Social irresponsibility, disregard for others, deceitfulness, and manipulation of others for personal gain
- Borderline: Intolerance of being alone and emotional dysregulation
- Histrionic: Attention seeking
- Narcissistic: Underlying dysregulated, fragile self-esteem and overt grandiosity

Cluster C is characterized by appearing anxious or fearful. It includes the following personality disorders with their distinguishing features:

- Avoidant: Avoidance of interpersonal contact due to rejection sensitivity
- Dependent: Submissiveness and a need to be taken care of
- Obsessive-compulsive: Perfectionism, rigidity, and obstinacy

Symptoms and Signs

According to DSM-5, personality disorders are primarily problems with

- Self-identity
- Interpersonal relationships

Self-identity problems may manifest as an unstable self-image (eg, people fluctuate between seeing themselves as kind or cruel) or as inconsistencies in values, goals, and appearance (eg, people are deeply religious while in church but profane and disrespectful elsewhere).

Interpersonal issues typically manifest as failing to develop or sustain close relationships and/or being insensitive to others (eg, unable to empathize).

People with personality disorders often seem inconsistent, confusing, and frustrating to people around them (including clinicians). These people may have difficulty knowing the boundaries between themselves and others. Their self-esteem may be inappropriately high or low. They may have inconsistent, detached, overemotional, abusive, or irresponsible styles of parenting, which can lead to physical and mental problems in their spouse or children.

People with personality disorders may not recognize that they have problems.

Diagnosis

- Clinical criteria (DSM-5)

Once clinicians suspect a personality disorder, they evaluate cognitive, affective, interpersonal, and behavioral tendencies using specific diagnostic criteria. More sophisticated and empirically rigorous diagnostic tools are available for more specialized and academic clinicians.

Diagnosis of a personality disorder requires the following:

- A persistent, inflexible, pervasive pattern of maladaptive traits involving ≥ 2 of the following: cognition (ways or

perceiving and interpreting self, others, and events), affectivity, interpersonal functioning, and impulse control
- Significant distress or impaired functioning resulting from the maladaptive pattern
- Stability and early onset (during adolescence or early adulthood) of the pattern

Also, other possible causes of the symptoms (eg, other mental health disorders, substance use, head trauma) must be excluded.

For a personality disorder to be diagnosed in patients < 18 yr, the pattern must have been present for ≥ 1 yr, except for antisocial personality disorders, which cannot be diagnosed in patients < 18 yr.

Because many patients with a personality disorder lack insight into their condition, clinicians may need to obtain history from clinicians who have treated these patients previously, other practitioners, family members, friends, or others who have contact with them.

Treatment

- Psychotherapy

The gold standard of treatment for personality disorders is psychotherapy. Both individual and group psychotherapy are effective for many of these disorders if the patient is seeking treatment and is motivated to change.

Typically, personality disorders are not very responsive to drugs, although some drugs can effectively target specific symptoms (eg, depression, anxiety).

Disorders that often coexist with personality disorders (eg, mood, anxiety, substance abuse, somatic symptom, and eating disorders) can make treatment challenging, lengthening time to remission, increasing risk of relapse, and decreasing response to otherwise effective treatment. For treatment recommendations for each disorder, see Table 212–1.

General principles of treatment: In general, treatment of personality disorders aims to

- Reduce subjective distress
- Enable patients to understand that their problems are internal to themselves
- Decrease significantly maladaptive and socially undesirable behaviors
- Modify problematic personality traits

Reducing subjective distress (eg, anxiety, depression) is the first goal. These symptoms often respond to increased psychosocial support, which often includes moving the patient out of highly stressful situations or relationships. Drug therapy may also help relieve stress. Reduced stress makes treating the underlying personality disorder easier.

An effort to enable patients to see that their problems are internal should be made early. Patients need to understand

Table 212–1. TREATMENT OF PERSONALITY DISORDERS

DIAGNOSIS	PSYCHOTHERAPY	DRUGS
Paranoid	Supportive psychotherapy Cognitive-behavioral therapy	Antidepressants Atypical antipsychotics
Schizoid	Supportive psychotherapy Social skills training	—
Schizotypal	Supportive psychotherapy Social skills training Cognitive-behavioral therapy for anxiety management	Antipsychotics
Antisocial*	Cognitive-behavioral therapy Contingency management	Antidepressants (SSRIs) Mood stabilizers (lithium, valproate)
Borderline	General psychiatric management and other structured clinical management approaches Supportive psychotherapy Dialectical behavioral therapy Mentalization-based treatment Transference-focused psychotherapy Schema-focused therapy Systems training for emotional predictability and problem solving	Mood stabilizers (lamotrigine, topiramate) for mood symptoms, impulsivity, and anxiety Atypical antipsychotics for transient psychotic symptoms and anger problems Antidepressants (not harmful but limited efficacy) Avoidance of benzodiazepines and stimulants
Histrionic	Psychodynamic psychotherapy	—
Narcissistic	Psychodynamic psychotherapy Mentalization-based treatment Transference-focused psychotherapy	—
Avoidant	Psychodynamic psychotherapy Supportive psychotherapy Cognitive-behavioral therapy	Antidepressants (MAOIs, SSRIs) Anxiolytics
Dependent	Psychodynamic psychotherapy Cognitive-behavioral therapy	Antidepressants (MAOIs, SSRIs)
Obsessive-compulsive	Psychodynamic psychotherapy Cognitive-behavioral therapy	Antidepressants (SSRIs)

*There is controversy about whether antisocial personality disorder is treatable.

that their problems with work or relationships are caused by their problematic ways of relating to the world (eg, to tasks, to authority, or in intimate relationships). Achieving such understanding requires a substantial amount of time, patience, and commitment on the part of a clinician. Clinicians also need a basic understanding of the patient's areas of emotional sensitivity and usual ways of coping. Family members and friends can help identify problems of which patients and clinicians would otherwise be unaware.

Maladaptive and undesirable behaviors (eg, recklessness, social isolation, lack of assertiveness, temper outbursts) should be dealt with quickly to minimize ongoing damage to jobs and relationships. Behavioral change is most important for patients with the following personality disorders:

- Borderline
- Antisocial
- Avoidant

Behavior can typically be improved within months by group therapy and behavior modification; limits on behavior must often be established and enforced. Sometimes patients are treated in a day hospital or residential setting. Self-help groups or family therapy can also help change socially undesirable behaviors. Because family members and friends can act in ways that either reinforce or diminish the patient's problematic behavior or thoughts, their involvement is helpful; with coaching, they can be allies in treatment.

Modifying problematic personality traits (eg, dependency, distrust, arrogance, manipulativeness) takes a long time—typically > 1 yr. The cornerstone for effecting such change is

- Individual psychotherapy

During therapy, clinicians try to identify interpersonal problems as they occur in the patient's life. Clinicians then help patients understand how these problems are related to their personality traits and provide skills training to develop new, better ways of interacting. Typically, clinicians must repeatedly point out the undesirable behaviors and their consequences before patients become aware of them to help patients change their maladaptive behaviors and mistaken beliefs. Although clinicians should act with sensitivity, they should be aware that kindness and sensible advice by themselves do not change personality disorders.

KEY POINTS

- Personality disorders involve rigid, maladaptive personality traits that are marked enough to cause significant distress or to impair work and/or interpersonal functioning.
- Treatments become effective only after patients see that their problems are within themselves, not just externally caused.
- Psychosocial therapies are the main treatment.
- Drugs help control specific symptoms only in selected cases—eg, to control significant anxiety, angry outbursts, and depression.
- Personality disorders are often resistant to change, but many gradually become less severe over time.

ANTISOCIAL PERSONALITY DISORDER

Antisocial personality disorder (ASPD) is characterized by a pervasive pattern of disregard for consequences and for the rights of others. Diagnosis is by clinical criteria. Treatment may include cognitive-behavioral therapy, antipsychotic drugs, and antidepressants.

People with antisocial personality disorder commit unlawful, deceitful, exploitative, reckless acts for personal profit or pleasure and without remorse; they may do the following:

- Justify or rationalize their behavior (eg, thinking losers deserve to lose, looking out for number one)
- Blame the victim for being foolish or helpless
- Be indifferent to the exploitative and harmful effects of their actions on others

Reported prevalence varies but is probably about 1 to 3.6% of the general population. It is more common among men than among women (6:1), and there is a strong heritable component. Prevalence decreases with age, suggesting that patients can learn over time to change their maladaptive behavior and try to build a life.

Comorbidities are common. Most patients also have a substance use disorder (and about half of those with a substance use disorder meet criteria for antisocial personality disorder). Patients with antisocial personality disorder often also have an impulse control disorder, attention-deficit/hyperactivity disorder, or borderline personality disorder.

Etiology

Both genetic and environmental factors (eg, abuse during childhood) contribute to the development of antisocial personality disorder. A possible mechanism is impulsive aggression, related to abnormal serotonin transporter functioning. Disregard for the pain of others during early childhood has been linked to antisocial behavior during late adolescence.

Antisocial personality disorder is more common among 1st-degree relatives of patients with the disorder than among the general population. Risk of developing this disorder is increased in both adopted and biologic children of parents with the disorder.

If conduct disorder accompanied by attention-deficit/hyperactivity disorder develops before age 10 yr, risk of developing antisocial personality disorder during adulthood is increased. Risk of conduct disorder evolving into antisocial personality disorder may be increased when parents abuse or neglect the child or are inconsistent in discipline or in parenting style (eg, switching from warm and supportive to cold and critical).

Symptoms and Signs

Patients with antisocial personality disorder may express their disregard for others and for the law by destroying property, harassing others, or stealing. They may deceive, exploit, con, or manipulate people to get what they want (eg, money, power, sex). They may use an alias.

These patients are impulsive, not planning ahead and not considering the consequences for or the safety of self or others. As a result, they may suddenly change jobs, homes, or relationships. They may speed when driving and drive while intoxicated, sometimes leading to accidents. They may consume excessive amounts of alcohol or take illegal drugs that may have harmful effects.

Patients with antisocial personality disorder are socially and financially irresponsible. They may change jobs with no plan for getting another. They may not seek employment when opportunities are available. They may not pay their bills, default on loans, or not pay child support.

These patients are often easily provoked and physically aggressive; they may start fights or abuse their spouse or partner. In sexual relationships, they may be irresponsible and exploit their partner and be unable to remain monogamous.

Remorse for actions is lacking. Patients with antisocial personality disorder may rationalize their actions by blaming those they hurt (eg, they deserved it) or the way life is (eg, unfair).

They are determined not to be pushed around and to do what they think is best for themselves at any cost.

These patients lack empathy for others and may be contemptuous of or indifferent to the feelings, rights, and suffering of others.

Patients with antisocial personality disorder tend to have a high opinion of themselves and may be very opinionated, self-assured, or arrogant. They may be charming, voluble, and verbally facile in their efforts to get what they want.

Diagnosis

- Clinical criteria (*Diagnostic and Statistical Manual of Mental Disorders*, Fifth Edition [DSM-5])

For a diagnosis of antisocial personality disorder, patients must have persistent disregard for the rights of others, as shown by ≥ 3 of the following:

- Disregarding the law, indicated by repeatedly committing acts that are grounds for arrest
- Being deceitful, indicated by lying repeatedly, using aliases, or conning others for personal gain or pleasure
- Acting impulsively or not planning ahead
- Being easily provoked or aggressive, indicated by constantly getting into physical fights or assaulting others
- Recklessly disregarding their safety or the safety of others
- Consistently acting irresponsibly, indicated by quitting a job with no plans for another one or not paying bills
- Not feeling remorse, indicated by indifference to or rationalization of hurting or mistreating others

Also, patients must have evidence that a conduct disorder has been present since age 15 yr. Antisocial personality disorder is diagnosed only in people ≥ 18 yr.

Differential diagnosis: Antisocial personality disorder should be distinguished from the following:

- **Substance use disorder:** Determining whether impulsivity and irresponsibility result from substance use disorder or from antisocial personality disorder can be difficult but is possible based on a review of the patient's history, including early history, to check for periods of sobriety. Sometimes antisocial personality disorder can be diagnosed more easily after a coexisting substance use disorder is treated, but antisocial personality disorders can be diagnosed even when substance use disorder is present.
- **Conduct disorder:** Conduct disorder has a similar pervasive pattern of violating social norms and laws, but conduct disorder must be present before age 15.
- **Narcissistic personality disorder:** Patients are similarly exploitative and lacking in empathy, but they tend not to be aggressive and deceitful as occurs in antisocial personality disorder.
- **Borderline personality disorder:** Patients are similarly manipulative but do so to be nurtured rather than to get what they want (eg, money, power) as occurs in antisocial personality disorder.

Treatment

- In some cases, cognitive-behavioral therapy and mood stabilizers and antidepressants

There is no evidence that any particular treatment leads to long-term improvement. Thus, treatment aims to reach some other short-term goal, such as avoiding legal consequences, rather than changing the patient. Contingency management (ie, giving or withholding what patients want depending on their behavior) is indicated.

Aggressive patients with prominent impulsivity and labile affect may benefit from treatment with cognitive-behavioral therapy or drugs (eg, lithium, valproate, SSRIs). Antipsychotics can help, but there is less evidence for its use.

AVOIDANT PERSONALITY DISORDER

Avoidant personality disorder (AVPD) is characterized by the avoidance of social situations or interactions that involve risk of rejection, criticism, or humiliation. Diagnosis is by clinical criteria. Treatment is with psychotherapy, anxiolytics, and antidepressants.

People with avoidant personality disorder have intense feelings of inadequacy and cope maladaptively by avoiding any situations in which they may be evaluated negatively.

Between 1 to 5.2% of the general population are estimated to have avoidant personality disorders; it is more common among women than among men.

Comorbidities are common. Patients often also have major depressive disorder, dysthymia, obsessive-compulsive disorder, or an anxiety disorder (eg, panic disorder, particularly social phobia [social anxiety disorder]). They may also have another personality disorder (eg, dependent, borderline). Patients with social phobia and avoidant personality disorder have more severe symptoms and disability than those with either disorder alone.

Etiology

Research suggests that experiences of rejection and marginalization during childhood and innate traits of social anxiousness and avoidance may contribute to avoidant personality disorder. Avoidance in social situations has been detected as early as about age 2 yr.

Symptoms and Signs

Patients with avoidant personality disorder avoid social interaction, including those at work, because they fear that they will be criticized or rejected or that people will disapprove of them, as in the following situations:

- They may refuse a promotion because they fear co-workers will criticize them.
- They may avoid meetings.
- They avoid making new friends unless they are sure they will be liked.

These patients assume people will be critical and disapproving until rigorous tests proving the contrary are passed. Thus, before joining a group and forming a close relationship, patients with this disorder require repeated assurances of support and uncritical acceptance.

Patients with avoidant personality disorder long for social interaction but fear placing their well-being in the hands of others. Because these patients limit their interactions with people, they tend to be relatively isolated and do not have a social network that could help them when they need it.

These patients are very sensitive to anything slightly critical, disapproving, or mocking because they constantly think about being criticized or rejected by others. They are vigilant for any sign of a negative response to them. Their tense, anxious appearance may elicit mockery or teasing, thus seeming to confirm their self-doubts.

Low self-esteem and a sense of inadequacy inhibit these patients in social situations, especially new ones. Interactions with new people are inhibited because patients think of themselves as socially inept, unappealing, and inferior to others. They tend to be quiet and timid and try to disappear because they tend to think that if they say anything, others will say it is wrong. They are reluctant to talk about themselves lest they be mocked or humiliated. They worry they will blush or cry when they are criticized.

Patients with avoidant personality disorder are very reluctant to take personal risks or participate in new activities for similar reasons. In such cases, they tend to exaggerate the dangers and use minimal symptoms or other problems to explain their avoidance. They may prefer a limited lifestyle because of their need for security and certainty.

Diagnosis

- Clinical criteria (*Diagnostic and Statistical Manual of Mental Disorders*, Fifth Edition [DSM-5])

For a diagnosis of avoidant personality disorder, patients must have a persistent pattern of avoiding social contact, feeling inadequate, and being hypersensitive to criticism and rejection, as shown by ≥ 4 of the following:

- Avoidance of job-related activities that involve interpersonal contact because they fear that they will be criticized or rejected or that people will disapprove of them
- Unwillingness to get involved with people unless they are sure of being liked
- Reserve in close relationships because they fear ridicule or humiliation
- Preoccupation with being criticized or rejected in social situations
- Inhibition in new social situations because they feel inadequate
- A view of self as socially incompetent, unappealing, or inferior to others
- Reluctance to take personal risks or participate in any new activity because they may be embarrassed

Also, symptoms must have begun by early adulthood.

Differential diagnosis: Avoidant personality disorder must be distinguished from the following 2 disorders:

- **Social phobia:** Differences between social phobia and avoidant personality disorder are subtle. Avoidant personality disorder involves more pervasive anxiety and avoidance than social phobia, which is often specific to situations that may result in public embarrassment (eg, public speaking, performing on stage). However, social phobia may involve a broader avoidance pattern and thus may be hard to distinguish. The 2 disorders often occur together.
- **Schizoid personality disorder:** Both disorders are characterized by social isolation. However, patients with schizoid personality disorder become isolated because they are disinterested in others, whereas those with avoidant personality disorder become isolated because they are hypersensitive to possible rejection or criticism by others.

Other personality disorders may be similar in some ways to avoidant personality disorder but can be distinguished by characteristic features (eg, by a need to be cared for in dependent personality disorder vs avoidance of rejection and criticism in avoidant personality disorder).

Treatment

- Cognitive-behavioral therapy focused on social skills
- Supportive psychotherapy
- Psychodynamic psychotherapy
- Anxiolytics and antidepressants

General treatment of avoidant personality disorder is similar to that for all personality disorders.

Patients with avoidant personality disorder often avoid treatment.

Effective therapies for patients with both social phobia and avoidant personality disorder include

- Cognitive-behavioral therapy that focuses on acquisition of social skills, done in groups
- Other group therapies if the group consists of people with the same difficulties

Patients with avoidant personality disorder benefit from

- Individual therapies that are supportive and sensitive to the patient's hypersensitivities toward others

Psychodynamic psychotherapy, which focuses on underlying conflicts, may be helpful.

Effective drug therapy includes monoamine oxidase inhibitors (MAOIs), SSRIs, and anxiolytics, which help reduce anxiety enough to enable patients to expose themselves to new social situations.

BORDERLINE PERSONALITY DISORDER

Borderline personality disorder (BPD) is characterized by a pervasive pattern of instability and hypersensitivity in interpersonal relationships, instability in self-image, extreme mood fluctuations, and impulsivity. Diagnosis is by clinical criteria. Treatment is with psychotherapy and drugs.

Patients with borderline personality disorder have an intolerance of being alone; they make frantic efforts to avoid abandonment and generate crises, such as making suicidal gestures in a way that invites rescue and caregiving by others.

Reported prevalence of borderline personality disorder varies but is probably between 1.7 to 3% in the general population, but up to 15 to 20% in patients being treated for mental health disorders. In clinical settings, 75% of patients with this disorder are female, but in the general population, the ratio of men to women is 1:1.

Comorbidities are complex. Patients often have a number of other disorders, particularly depression, anxiety disorders (eg, panic disorder), and posttraumatic stress disorder, as well as eating disorders and substance use disorders.

Etiology

Stresses during early childhood may contribute to the development of borderline personality disorder. A childhood history of physical and sexual abuse, neglect, separation from caregivers, and/or loss of a parent is common among patients with borderline personality disorder.

Certain people may have a genetic tendency to have pathologic responses to environment life stresses, and borderline personality disorder clearly appears to have a heritable component. First-degree relatives of patients with borderline personality disorder are 5 times more likely to have the disorder than the general population. Disturbances in regulatory functions of the brain and neuropeptide systems may also contribute but are not present in all patients with borderline personality disorder.

Symptoms and Signs

When patients with borderline personality disorder feel that they are being abandoned or neglected, they feel intense fear or anger. For example, they may become panicky or furious when someone important to them is a few minutes late or cancels an engagement.

They think that this abandonment means that they are bad. They fear abandonment partly because they do not want to be alone.

These patients tend to change their view of others abruptly and dramatically. They may idealize a potential caregiver or lover early in the relationship, demand to spend a lot of time together, and share everything. Suddenly, they may feel that the person does not care enough, and they become disillusioned; then they may belittle or become angry with the person. This shift from idealization to devaluation reflects black-and-white thinking (splitting, polarization of good and bad).

Patients with borderline personality disorder can empathize with and care for a person but only if they feel that another person will be there for them whenever needed.

Patients with this disorder have difficulty controlling their anger and often become inappropriate and intensely angry. They may express their anger with biting sarcasm, bitterness, or angry tirades, often directed at their caregiver or lover for neglect or abandonment. After the outburst, they often feel ashamed and guilty, reinforcing their feeling of being bad.

Patients with borderline personality disorder may also abruptly and dramatically change their self-image, shown by suddenly changing their goals, values, opinions, careers, or friends. They may be needy one minute and righteously angry about being mistreated the next. Although they usually see themselves as bad, they sometimes feel that they do not exist at all—eg, when they do not have someone who cares for them. They often feel empty inside.

The changes in mood (eg, intense dysphoria, irritability, anxiety) usually last only a few hours and rarely last more than a few days; they may reflect the extreme sensitivity to interpersonal stresses in patients with borderline personality disorder.

Patients with borderline personality disorder often sabotage themselves when they are about to reach a goal. For example, they may drop out of school just before graduation, or they may ruin a promising relationship.

Impulsivity leading to self-harm is common. These patients may gamble, engage in unsafe sex, binge eat, drive recklessly, abuse substances, or overspend. Suicidal behaviors, gestures, and threats and self-mutilation (eg, cutting, burning) are very common. Although many of these self-destructive acts are not intended to end life, risk of suicide in these patients is 40 times that of the general population; About 8 to 10% of these patients die by suicide. These self-destructive acts are usually triggered by rejection by, possible abandonment by, or disappointment in a caregiver or lover. Patients may self-mutilate to compensate for their being bad or to reaffirm their ability to feel during a dissociative episode.

Dissociative episodes, paranoid thoughts, and sometimes psychotic-like symptoms (eg, hallucinations, ideas of reference) may be triggered by extreme stress, usually fear of abandonment, whether real or imagined. These symptoms are temporary and usually not severe enough to be considered a separate disorder.

Symptoms lessen in most patients; relapse rate is very low. However, functional status does not usually improve as dramatically.

Diagnosis

- Clinical criteria (*Diagnostic and Statistical Manual of Mental Disorders*, Fifth Edition [DSM-5])

For a diagnosis of borderline personality disorder, patients must have persistent pattern of unstable relationships, self-image, and emotions (ie, emotional dysregulation) and pronounced impulsivity, as shown by ≥ 5 of the following:

- Desperate efforts to avoid abandonment (actual or imagined)
- Unstable, intense relationships that alternate between idealizing and devaluing the other person
- An unstable self-image or sense of self
- Impulsivity in ≥ 2 areas that could harm themselves (eg, unsafe sex, binge eating, reckless driving)
- Repeated suicidal behavior, gestures, or threats or self-mutilation
- Rapid changes in mood, lasting usually only a few hours and rarely more than a few days
- Persistent feelings of emptiness
- Inappropriately intense anger or problems controlling anger
- Temporary paranoid thoughts or severe dissociative symptoms triggered by stress

Also, symptoms must have begun by early adulthood but can occur during adolescence.

Differential diagnosis: Borderline personality disorder is most commonly misdiagnosed as bipolar disorder because of the wide fluctuations in mood, behavior, and sleep. However, in borderline personality disorder, mood and behavior change rapidly in response to stressors, especially interpersonal ones, whereas in bipolar disorder, moods are more sustained and less reactive.

Other personality disorders share similar manifestations. Patients with histrionic personality disorder or narcissistic personality disorder can be attention-seeking and manipulative, but those with borderline personality disorder also see themselves as bad and feel empty. Some patients meet criteria for more than one personality disorder.

Borderline personality disorder can be distinguished from mood and anxiety disorders based on the negative self-image, insecure attachments, and sensitivity to rejection that are prominent features of borderline personality disorder and are usually absent in patients with a mood or anxiety disorder.

Differential diagnosis for borderline personality disorder also includes substance abuse disorders and posttraumatic stress disorder; many disorders in the differential diagnosis of borderline personality disorder coexist with it.

Treatment

- Psychotherapy
- Drugs

General treatment of borderline personality disorder is the same as that for all personality disorders.

Identifying and treating coexisting disorders is important for effective treatment of borderline personality disorder.

Psychotherapy: The main treatment for borderline personality disorder is psychotherapy.

Many psychotherapeutic interventions are effective in reducing suicidal behaviors, ameliorating depression, and improving function in patients with this disorder.

Cognitive-behavioral therapy focuses on emotional dysregulation and lack of social skills. It includes the following:

- Dialectical behavioral therapy (a combination of individual and group sessions with therapists acting as behavior coaches and available on call around the clock)
- Systems training for emotional predictability and problem solving (STEPPS)

Other interventions focus on disturbances in the ways patients emotionally experience themselves and others. These interventions include the following:

- Mentalization-based treatment
- Transference-focused psychotherapy
- Schema-focused therapy

Mentalization refers to people's ability to reflect on and understand their own state of mind and the state of mind of others. Mentalization is thought to be learned through a secure attachment to the caregiver. Mentalization-based treatment helps patients do the following:

- Effectively regulate their emotions (eg, calm down when upset)
- Understand how they contribute to their problems and difficulties with others
- Reflect on and understand the minds of others

It thus helps them relate to others with empathy and compassion.

Transference-focused psychotherapy centers on the interaction between patient and therapist. The therapist asks questions and helps patients think about their reactions so that they can examine their exaggerated, distorted, and unrealistic images of self during the session. The current moment (eg, how patients are relating to their therapist) is emphasized rather than the past. For example, when a timid, quiet patient suddenly becomes hostile and argumentative, the therapist may ask whether the patient noticed a shift in feelings and then ask the patient to think about how the patient was experiencing the therapist and self when things changed. The purpose is

- To enable patients to develop a more stable and realistic sense of self and others
- To relate to others in a healthier way through transference to the therapist

Schema-focused therapy is an integrative therapy that combines cognitive-behavioral therapy, attachment theory, psychodynamic concepts, and emotion-focused therapies. It focuses on lifelong maladaptive patterns of thinking, feeling, behaving and coping (called schemas), affective change techniques, and the therapeutic relationship, with limited reparenting. The purpose is help patients change their schemas. Therapy has 3 stages:

- Assessment: Identifying the schemas
- Awareness: Recognizing the schemas when they are operating in daily life
- Behavioral change: Replacing negative thoughts, feelings, and behaviors with healthier ones

Some of these interventions are specialized and require specialized training and supervision. However, some interventions do not; one such intervention, which is designed for the general practitioner, is

- General (or good) psychiatric management

This intervention uses individual therapy once a week and sometimes drugs.

Supportive psychotherapy is also useful. The goal is to establish an emotional, encouraging, supportive relationship with the patient and thus help the patient develop healthy defense mechanisms, especially in interpersonal relationships.

Drugs: Drugs work best when used sparingly and systematically for specific symptoms.

SSRIs are usually well-tolerated; chance of a lethal overdose is minimal. However, SSRIs are only marginally effective for depression and anxiety in patients with borderline personality disorder.

The following drugs are effective in ameliorating symptoms of borderline personality disorder:

- Mood stabilizers such as lamotrigine: For depression, anxiety, mood lability, and impulsivity
- Antipsychotics: For anxiety, anger, and cognitive symptoms, including transient stress-related cognitive distortions (eg, paranoid thoughts, black-and-white thinking, severe cognitive disorganization)

Benzodiazepines and stimulants also may help relieve symptoms but are not recommended because dependency and drug diversion are risks.

DEPENDENT PERSONALITY DISORDER

Dependent personality disorder (DPD) is characterized by a pervasive, excessive need to be taken care of, leading to submissiveness and clinging behaviors. Diagnosis is by clinical criteria. Treatment is with psychotherapy and possibly antidepressants.

In patients with dependent personality disorder, the need to be taken care of results in loss of their autonomy and interests. Because they are intensely anxious about taking care of themselves, they become excessively dependent and submissive.

About 0.7% of the general population are estimated to have dependent personality disorder; it is more common among women.

Comorbidities are common. Patients often also have a depressive disorder (major depressive disorder or dysthymia), an anxiety disorder, an alcohol use disorder, or another personality disorder (eg, borderline, histrionic).

Etiology

Information about the causes of dependent personality disorder is limited. Cultural factors, negative early experiences, and biologic vulnerabilities associated with anxiety are thought to contribute to the development of dependent personality disorder. Familial traits such as submissiveness, insecurity, and self-effacing behavior may also contribute.

Symptoms and Signs

Patients with dependent personality disorder do not think they can take care of themselves. They use submissiveness to try to get other people to take care of them.

Patients with this disorder typically require much reassurance and advice when making ordinary decisions. They often let others, often one person, take responsibility for many aspects of their life. For example, they may depend on their spouse to tell them what to wear, what kind of job to look for, and with whom to associate.

These patients consider themselves inferior and tend to belittle their abilities; they take any criticism or disapproval as proof of their incompetence, further undermining their confidence.

It is difficult for them to express disagreement with others because they fear losing support or approval. They may agree to something they know is wrong rather than risk losing the help of others. Even when anger is appropriate, they do not get angry at friends and co-workers for fear of losing their support.

Because these patients are sure that they cannot do anything on their own, they have difficulty starting a new task and working independently, and they avoid tasks that require taking responsibility. They present themselves as incompetent and needing constant help and reassurance. When reassured that a competent person is supervising and approving of them, these patients tend to function adequately. However, they do not want to appear too competent lest they be abandoned. As a result, their career may be harmed. They perpetuate their dependency because they tend not to learn skills of independent living.

These patients go to great lengths to obtain care and support (eg, doing unpleasant tasks, submitting to unreasonable demands, tolerating physical, sexual, or emotional abuse). Being alone makes them feel extremely uncomfortable or afraid because they fear they cannot take care of themselves.

Patients with this disorder tend to interact socially with only the few people they depend on. When a close relationship ends, patients with this disorder immediately try to find a replacement. Because of their desperate need to be taken care of, they are not discriminating in choosing a replacement.

These patients fear abandonment by those they depend on, even when there is no reason to.

Diagnosis

- Clinical criteria (*Diagnostic and Statistical Manual of Mental Disorders*, Fifth Edition [DSM-5])

For a diagnosis of dependent personality disorder, patients must have a persistent, excessive need to be taken of, resulting in submissiveness and clinging, as shown by ≥ 5 of the following:

- Difficulty making daily decisions without an inordinate amount of advice and reassurance from other people
- A need to have others be responsible for most important aspects of their life
- Difficulty expressing disagreement with others because they fear loss of support or approval
- Difficulty starting projects on their own because they are not confident in their judgment and/or abilities (not because they lack motivation or energy)
- Willingness to go to great lengths (eg, do unpleasant tasks) to obtain support from others
- Feelings of discomfort or helplessness when they are alone because they fear they cannot take of themselves
- An urgent need to establish a new relationship with someone who will provide care and support when a close relationship ends
- Unrealistic preoccupation with fears of being left to take care of themselves

Also, symptoms must have begun by early adulthood.

Differential diagnosis: Several other personality disorders are characterized by hypersensitivity to rejection. However, they can be distinguished from dependent personality disorder based on characteristic features, as follows:

- **Borderline personality disorder:** Patients with this disorder are too frightened to submit to the same degree of control as patients with dependent personality disorder. Patients with borderline personality disorder, unlike those with dependent personality disorder, vacillate between submissiveness and rageful hostility.
- **Avoidant personality disorder:** Patients with this disorder are also be too frightened to submit to the same degree of control as patients with dependent personality disorder. Patients with avoidant personality disorder withdraw until they are sure they will be accepted without criticism; in contrast, those with dependent personality disorder seek out and try to maintain relationships with others.
- **Histrionic personality disorder:** Patients with this disorder seek attention rather than reassurance (as do those with dependent personality disorder), but they are more disinhibited. They are more flamboyant and actively seek attention; those with dependent personality disorder are self-effacing and shy.

Dependent personality disorder should be distinguished from the dependency that is present in other psychiatric disorders (eg, mood disorders, panic disorder, agoraphobia).

Treatment

- Cognitive-behavioral therapy
- Psychodynamic psychotherapy
- Possibly antidepressants

General treatment of dependent personality disorder is similar to that for all personality disorders.

Psychodynamic psychotherapy and cognitive-behavioral therapy that focus on examining fears of independence and difficulties with assertiveness can help patients with dependent personality disorder. Clinicians should be careful not to promote dependency in the therapy relationship.

Evidence about drug therapy for dependent personality disorder is sparse. MAOIs, which are effective in avoidant personality disorder, may be effective, as may SSRIs.

Benzodiazepines are not used because patients with dependent personality disorder have an increased risk of drug dependency.

HISTRIONIC PERSONALITY DISORDER

Histrionic personality disorder (HPD) is characterized by a pervasive pattern of excessive emotionality and attention seeking. Diagnosis is by clinical criteria. Treatment is with psychodynamic psychotherapy.

Patients with histrionic personality disorder use their physical appearance, acting in inappropriately seductive or provocative ways, to gain the attention of others. They lack a sense of self-direction and are highly suggestible, often acting submissively to retain the attention of others.

About 1.5 to 3% of the general population are estimated to have histrionic personality disorder; it is more common among women than among men.

Comorbidities are common, particularly other personality disorders (antisocial, borderline, narcissistic), suggesting that these disorders share a biologic vulnerability or casting doubt on whether histrionic personality disorder is a separate disorder. Some patients also have somatic symptom disorder, which may be the reason they present for evaluation. Major depressive disorder, dysthymia, and conversion disorder may also coexist.

Symptoms and Signs

Patients with histrionic personality disorder continually demand to be the center of attention and often become depressed when they are not. They are often lively, dramatic, enthusiastic, and flirtatious and sometimes charm new acquaintances.

These patients often dress and act in inappropriately seductive and provocative ways, not just with potential romantic interests, but in many contexts (eg, work, school). They want to impress others with their appearance and so are often preoccupied with how they look.

Expression of emotion may be shallow (turned off and on too quickly) and exaggerated. They speak dramatically, expressing strong opinions, but with few facts or details to support their opinions.

Patients with histrionic personality disorder are easily influenced by others and by current trends. They tend to be too trusting, especially of authority figures who, they think, may be able to solve all their problems. They often think relationships are closer than they appear. They crave novelty and tend to bore easily. Thus, they may change jobs and friends frequently. Delayed gratification is very frustrating to them, so their actions are often motivated by obtaining immediate satisfaction.

Achieving emotional or sexual intimacy may be difficult. Patients may, often without being aware of it, play a role (eg, victim). They may try to control their partner using seductiveness or emotional manipulations while becoming very dependent on the partner.

Diagnosis

- Clinical criteria (*Diagnostic and Statistical Manual of Mental Disorders*, Fifth Edition [DSM-5])

For a diagnosis of histrionic personality disorder, patients must have a persistent pattern of excessive emotionality and attention seeking, as shown by ≥ 5 of the following:

- Discomfort when they are not the center of attention
- Interaction with others that is inappropriately sexually seductive or provocative
- Rapidly shifting and shallow expression of emotions
- Consistent use of physical appearance to call attention to themselves
- Speech that is extremely impressionistic and vague
- Self-dramatization, theatricality, and extravagant expression of emotion
- Suggestibility (easily influenced by others or situations)
- Interpretation of relationships as more intimate than in reality

Also, symptoms must have begun by early adulthood.

Differential diagnosis: Histrionic personality disorders can be distinguished from other personality disorders based on characteristic features:

- **Narcissistic:** Patients with narcissistic personality disorder also seek attention, but they, unlike those with histrionic personality disorder, want to feel admired or elevated by it; patients with histrionic personality disorder are not so picky about the kind of attention they get and do not mind being thought cute or silly.
- **Borderline:** Patients with borderline personality disorder consider themselves bad and experience emotions intensely and deeply; those with histrionic personality disorder do not see themselves as bad, even though their dependence on the reaction of others may stem from poor self-esteem.
- **Dependent:** Patients with dependent personality disorder, like those with histrionic personality disorder, try to be near others but are more anxious, inhibited, and submissive (because they are worried about rejection); patients with histrionic personality disorder are less inhibited and more flamboyant.

Differential diagnosis for histrionic personality disorder also includes somatic symptom disorder and illness anxiety disorder.

Treatment

- Psychodynamic psychotherapy

General treatment of histrionic personality disorder is the same as that for all personality disorders.

Little is known about the efficacy of cognitive-behavioral therapy and drug therapy for histrionic personality disorder.

Psychodynamic psychotherapy, which focuses on underlying conflicts, may be tried. The therapist may start by encouraging patients to substitute speech for behavior, and thus, patients can understand themselves and communicate with others in a less dramatic way. Then, the therapist can help patients realize how their histrionic behaviors are a maladaptive way to attract the attention of others and to manage their self-esteem.

NARCISSISTIC PERSONALITY DISORDER

Narcissistic personality disorder (NPD) is characterized by a pervasive pattern of grandiosity, need for adulation, and lack of empathy. Diagnosis is by clinical criteria. Treatment is with psychodynamic psychotherapy.

Because patients with narcissistic personality disorder have difficulty regulating self-esteem, they need praise and affiliations with special people or institutions; they also tend to devalue other people so that they can maintain a sense of superiority.

About 0.5% of the general population are estimated to have narcissistic personality disorders; it is more common among men than among women.

Comorbidities are common. Patients often also have a depressive disorder (eg, major depressive disorder, dysthymia), anorexia nervosa, a substance use disorder (especially cocaine), or another personality disorder (histrionic, borderline, paranoid).

Etiology

Little research about biologic factors that contribute to narcissistic personality disorder has been done, although there appears to be a significant heritable component. Some theories posit that caregivers may not have treated the child appropriately—for example, by being overly critical or by excessively praising, admiring, or indulging the child.

Some patients with this disorder have special gifts or talents and become used to associating their self-image and sense of self with the admiration and esteem of others.

Symptoms and Signs

Patients with narcissistic personality disorder overestimate their abilities and exaggerate their achievements. They think they are superior, unique, or special. Their overestimation of their own worth and achievements often implies an underestimation of the worth and achievements of others.

These patients are preoccupied with fantasies of great achievements—of being admired for their overwhelming intelligence or beauty, of having prestige and influence, or of experiencing a great love. They feel they should associate only with others as special and talented as themselves, not ordinary people. This association with extraordinary people is used to support and enhance their self-esteem.

Because patients with narcissistic disorder need to be admired, their self-esteem depends on the positive regard of others and is thus usually very fragile. People with this disorder are often watching to see what others think of them and evaluating how well they are doing. They are sensitive to and bothered by the criticism of others and by failure, which makes them feel humiliated and defeated. They may respond with rage or contempt, or they may viciously counterattack. Or they may withdraw or outwardly accept the situation in an effort to protect their sense of self-importance (grandiosity). They may avoid situations in which they can fail.

Diagnosis

- Clinical criteria (*Diagnostic and Statistical Manual of Mental Disorders*, Fifth Edition [DSM-5])

For a diagnosis of narcissistic personality disorder, patients must have a persistent pattern of grandiosity, need for admiration, and lack of empathy, as shown by ≥ 5 of the following:

- An exaggerated, unfounded sense of their own importance and talents (grandiosity)

- Preoccupation with fantasies of unlimited achievements, influence, power, intelligence, beauty, or perfect love
- Belief that they are special and unique and should associate only with people of the highest caliber
- A need to be unconditionally admired
- A sense of entitlement
- Exploitation of others to achieve their own goals
- A lack of empathy
- Envy of others and a belief that others envy them
- Arrogance and haughtiness

Also, symptoms must have begun by early adulthood.

Differential diagnosis: Narcissistic personality disorders can be distinguished from the following disorders:

- **Bipolar disorder:** Patients with narcissistic personality disorder often present with depression and, because of their grandiosity, may be misdiagnosed as bipolar. Such patients may have depression, but their persistent need to elevate themselves above others distinguishes them from those with bipolar disorder. Also, in narcissistic personality disorder, changes in mood are triggered by insults to self-esteem.
- **Antisocial personality disorder:** Exploitation of others to promote themselves is characteristic of both personality disorders. However, the motives are different. Patients with antisocial personality disorder exploit others for material gain; those with narcissistic personality disorder exploit others to maintain their self-esteem.
- **Histrionic personality disorder:** Seeking the attention of others is characteristic of both personality disorders. But patients with narcissistic personality disorder, unlike those with histrionic personality disorder, disdain doing anything cute and silly to get attention; they wish to be admired.

Treatment

- Psychodynamic psychotherapy

General treatment of narcissistic personality disorder is the same as that for all personality disorders.

Psychodynamic psychotherapy, which focuses on underlying conflicts, can be effective. Some approaches developed for borderline personality disorder may be effectively adapted for use in patients with narcissistic personality disorder. They include

- Mentalization-based treatment
- Transference-focused psychotherapy

These approaches focus on disturbances in the ways patients emotionally experience themselves and others.

Cognitive-behavioral therapy may appeal to patients with narcissistic personality disorder because they may find the opportunity to increase mastery appealing; their need for praise may enable a therapist to shape their behavior. Some patients with narcissistic personality disorder find manualized cognitive-behavioral approaches too simplistic or generic for their special needs.

OBSESSIVE-COMPULSIVE PERSONALITY DISORDER

Obsessive-compulsive personality disorder (OCPD) is characterized by a pervasive preoccupation with orderliness, perfectionism, and control (with no room for flexibility) that ultimately slows or interferes with completing a task. Diagnosis is by clinical criteria. Treatment is with psychodynamic psychotherapy, cognitive-behavioral therapy, and SSRIs.

Because patients with obsessive-compulsive personality disorder need to be in control, they tend to be solitary in their endeavors and to mistrust the help of others.

About 2.1% of the general population are estimated to have obsessive-compulsive personality disorder; it is more common among men.

Familial traits of compulsivity, restricted range of emotion, and perfectionism are thought to contribute to this disorder.

Comorbidities may be present. Patients often also have a depressive disorder (major depressive disorder or dysthymia) or an alcohol use disorder.

Symptoms and Signs

Symptoms of obsessive-compulsive personality disorder may lessen over a year, but their persistence during the long term has not been studied.

In patients with obsessive-compulsive personality disorder, preoccupation with order, perfectionism, and control of themselves and situations interferes with flexibility, effectiveness, and openness. Rigid and stubborn in their activities, these patients insist that everything be done in specific ways.

To maintain a sense of control, patients focus on rules, minute details, procedures, schedules, and lists. As a result, the main point of a project or activity is lost. These patients repeatedly check for mistakes and pay extraordinary attention to detail. They do not make good use of their time, often leaving the most important tasks until the end. Their preoccupation with the details and making sure everything is perfect can endlessly delay completion. They are unaware of how their behavior affects their co-workers. When focused on one task, these patients may neglect all other aspects of their life.

Because these patients want everything done in a specific way, they have difficulty delegating tasks and working with others. When working with others, they may make detailed lists about how a task should be done and become upset if a co-worker suggests an alternative way. They may reject help even when they are behind schedule.

Patients with obsessive-compulsive personality disorder are excessively dedicated to work and productivity; their dedication is not motivated by financial necessity. As a result, leisure activities and relationships are neglected. They may think they have no time to relax or go out with friends; they may postpone a vacation so long that it does not happen, or they may feel they must take work with them so that they do not waste time. Time spent with friends, when it occurs, tends to be in a formally organized activity (eg, a sport). Hobbies and recreational activities are considered important tasks requiring organization and hard work to master; the goal is perfection.

These patients plan ahead in great detail and do not wish to consider changes. Their relentless rigidity may frustrate co-workers and friends.

Expression of affection is also tightly controlled. These patients may relate to others in a formal, stiff, or serious way. Often, they speak only after they think of the perfect thing to say. They may focus on logic and intellect and be intolerant of emotional or expressive behavior.

These patients may be overzealous, picky, and rigid about issues of morality, ethics, and values. They apply rigid moral principles to themselves and to others and are harshly self-critical. They are rigidly deferential to authorities and insist on exact compliance to rules, with no exceptions for extenuating circumstances.

Diagnosis

- Clinical criteria (*Diagnostic and Statistical Manual of Mental Disorders*, Fifth Edition [DSM-5])

For a diagnosis of obsessive-compulsive personality disorder, patients must have a persistent pattern of preoccupation with order, perfectionism, and control of self, others, and situations, as shown by ≥ 4 of the following:

- Preoccupation with details, rules, schedules, organization, and lists
- A striving to do something perfectly that interferes with completion of the task
- Excessive devotion to work and productivity (not due to financial necessity), resulting in neglect of leisure activities and friends
- Excessive conscientiousness, fastidiousness, and inflexibility regarding ethical and moral issues and values
- Unwillingness to throw out worn-out or worthless objects, even those with no sentimental value
- Reluctance to delegate or work with other people unless those people agree to do things exactly as the patients want
- A miserly approach to spending for themselves and others because they see money as something to be saved for future disasters
- Rigidity and stubbornness

Also, symptoms must have begun by early adulthood.

Differential diagnosis: Obsessive-compulsive personality disorder should be distinguished from the following disorders:

- **Obsessive-compulsive disorder (OCD—see also p. 1770):** Patients with OCD have true obsessions (repetitive, unwanted, intrusive thoughts that cause marked anxiety) and compulsions (ritualistic behaviors that they feel they must do to control their obsessions). Patients with OCD are often distressed by their lack of control over compulsive drives; in patients with obsessive-compulsive personality disorder, the need for control is driven by their preoccupation with order so their behavior, values, and feelings are acceptable and consistent with their sense of self.
- **Avoidant personality disorder:** Both avoidant and obsessive-compulsive personality disorders are characterized by social isolation; however, in patients with obsessive-compulsive personality disorder, isolation results from giving priority to work and productivity rather than relationships, and these patients mistrust others only because of their potential to intrude on the patients' perfectionism.
- **Schizoid personality disorder:** Both schizoid and obsessive-compulsive personality disorders are characterized by a seeming formality in interpersonal relationships and by detachment. However, the motives are different: a basic incapability for intimacy in patients with schizoid personality disorder vs discomfort with emotions and dedication to work in patients with obsessive-compulsive personality disorder.

Treatment

- Psychodynamic psychotherapy
- Cognitive-behavioral therapy
- SSRIs

General treatment of obsessive-compulsive personality disorder is similar to that for all personality disorders.

Information about treatment for obsessive-compulsive personality disorder is sparse. Also, treatment is complicated by the patient's rigidity, obstinacy, and need for control, which can be frustrating for therapists.

Psychodynamic therapy and cognitive-behavioral therapy can help patients with obsessive-compulsive personality disorder. Sometimes during therapy, the patient's interesting, detailed, intellectualized conversation may seem psychologically oriented, but it is void of affect and does not lead to change.

SSRIs may be useful.

PARANOID PERSONALITY DISORDER

Paranoid personality disorder (PPD) is characterized by a pervasive pattern of unwarranted distrust and suspicion of others that involves interpreting their motives as malicious. Diagnosis is by clinical criteria. Treatment is with cognitive-behavioral therapy.

Patients with paranoid personality disorder distrust others and assume that others intend to harm or deceive them, even when they have no or insufficient justification for these feelings.

From 0.4 to 5.1% of the general population and 9.7% of the clinical population are estimated to have paranoid personality disorder. There is some evidence of increased prevalence in families. Some evidence suggests a link between this disorder and emotional and/or physical abuse and victimization during childhood.

Comorbidities are common. Paranoid personality disorder is rarely the sole diagnosis. Common comorbidities include thought disorders (eg, schizophrenia), anxiety disorders (eg, social phobia [social anxiety disorder]), posttraumatic stress disorder, alcohol use disorders, or another personality disorder (eg, borderline).

Symptoms and Signs

Patients with paranoid personality disorder suspect that others are planning to exploit, deceive, or harm them. They feel that they may be attacked at any time and without reason. Even though there is little or no evidence, they persist in maintaining their suspicions and thoughts.

Often, these patients think that others have greatly and irreversibly injured them. They are hypervigilant for potential insults, slights, threats, and disloyalty and look for hidden meanings in remarks and actions. They closely scrutinize others for evidence to support their suspicions. For example, they may misinterpret an offer of help as implication that they are unable to do the task on their own. If they think that they have been insulted or injured in any way, they do not forgive the person who injured them. They tend to counterattack or to become angry in response to these perceived injuries. Because they distrust others, they feel a need to be autonomous and in control.

These patients are hesitant to confide in or develop close relationships with others because they worry that the information may be used against them. They doubt the loyalty of friends and the faithfulness of their spouse or partner. They can be extremely jealous and may constantly question the activities and motives of their spouse or partner in an effort to justify their jealousy.

Thus, patients with paranoid personality disorder can be difficult to get along with. When others respond negatively to them, they take these responses as confirmation of their original suspicions.

Diagnosis

- Clinical criteria (*Diagnostic and Statistical Manual of Mental Disorders*, Fifth Edition [DSM-5])

For a diagnosis of paranoid personality disorder, patients must have a persistent distrust and suspiciousness of others, as shown by ≥ 4 of the following:

- Unjustified suspicion that other people are exploiting, injuring, or deceiving them
- Preoccupation with unjustified doubts about the reliability of their friends and co-workers
- Reluctance to confide in others lest the information be used against them
- Misinterpretation of benign remarks or events as having hidden belittling, hostile, or threatening meaning
- Holding of grudges for insults, injuries, or slights
- Readiness to think that their character or reputation has been attacked and quickness to react angrily or to counterattack
- Recurrent, unjustified suspicions that their spouse or partner is unfaithful

Also, symptoms must have begun by early adulthood.

Differential diagnosis: Clinicians can usually distinguish paranoid personality disorder from other personality disorders by the pervasiveness of its paranoia regarding others (eg, as opposed to the more transient paranoia of borderline personality) and by the core feature of each disorder:

- Schizoid: Disinterest (as opposed to the mistrust in paranoid)
- Schizotypal: Eccentric ideas, speech, and behavior
- Borderline: Dependency
- Narcissistic: Grandiosity
- Antisocial: Exploitation
- Avoidant: Fear of rejection

Paranoid personality disorder can be distinguished from delusional disorder (persecutory type), schizophrenia, and a mood disorder with psychotic features because in these disorders, episodes of psychotic symptoms (eg, delusions, hallucinations) are prominent.

Treatment

- Cognitive-behavioral therapy

General treatment of paranoid personality disorder is the same as that for all personality disorders.

No treatments have been proved effective for paranoic personality disorder.

The overall high level of suspicion and mistrust in patients make establishing rapport difficult. Expressing recognition of any validity in patients' suspicions may facilitate an alliance between patient and clinician. This alliance may then enable patients to participate in cognitive-behavioral therapy or be willing to take any drugs (eg, antidepressants, atypical antipsychotics) prescribed to treat specific symptoms. Atypical antipsychotics may help decrease anxiety.

SCHIZOID PERSONALITY DISORDER

Schizoid personality disorder (ScPD) is characterized by a pervasive pattern of detachment from and general disinterest in social relationships and a limited range of emotions in their interpersonal relationships. Diagnosis is by clinical criteria. Treatment is with cognitive-behavioral therapy.

In schizoid personality disorder, the ability to relate to others meaningfully is limited.

About 1 to 3% of the general population are estimated to have schizoid personality disorder. This disorder may be more common among people with a family history of schizophrenia or schizotypal personality disorder.

Comorbidities are common. Up to half of patients have had at least one episode of major depression. They often also have other personality disorders, most commonly schizotypal, paranoid, borderline, or avoidant.

Etiology

Having caregivers who were emotionally cold, neglecting, and detached during childhood may contribute to the development of schizoid personality disorder by fueling the child's feeling that interpersonal relationships are not satisfying.

Symptoms and Signs

Patients with schizoid personality disorder seem to have no desire for close relationships with other people, including relatives. They have no close friends or confidants, except sometimes a 1st-degree relative. They rarely date and often do not marry. They prefer being by themselves, choosing activities and hobbies that do not require interaction with others (eg, computer games). Sexual activity with others is of little, if any, interest to them. They also seem to experience less enjoyment from sensory and bodily experiences (eg, walking on the beach).

These patients do not seem bothered by what others think of them—whether good or bad. Because they do not notice normal clues of social interaction, they may seem socially inept, aloof, or self-absorbed. They rarely react (eg, by smiling or nodding) or show emotion in social situations. They have difficulty expressing anger, even when they are provoked. They do not react appropriately to important life events and may seem passive in response to changes in circumstances. As a result, they may seem to have no direction to their life.

Rarely, when these patients feel comfortable exposing themselves, they admit that they feel pain, especially in social interactions.

Symptoms of schizoid personality disorder tend to remain stable over time, more so than those of other personality disorders.

Diagnosis

- Clinical criteria (*Diagnostic and Statistical Manual of Mental Disorders*, Fifth Edition [DSM-5])

For a diagnosis of schizoid personality disorder, patients must have a persistent detachment from and general disinterest in social relationships and limited expression of emotions in interpersonal interactions, as shown by ≥ 4 of the following:

- No desire for or enjoyment of close relationships, including those with family members
- Strong preference for solitary activities
- Little, if any, interest in sexual activity with another person
- Enjoyment of few, if any, activities
- Lack of close friends or confidants, except possibly 1st-degree relatives
- Apparent indifference to the praise or criticism of others
- Emotional coldness, detachment, or flattened affect

Also, symptoms must have begun by early adulthood.

Differential diagnosis: Clinicians should distinguish schizoid personality disorder from the following:

- **Schizophrenia and related disorders (see p. 1787):** Patients with schizoid personality disorder do not have cognitive or perceptual disturbances (eg, paranoia, hallucinations).
- **Autism spectrum disorders (see p. 2698):** Social impairment and stereotyped behaviors or interests are less prominent in patients with schizoid personality disorder.

- **Schizotypal personality disorder:** This disorder is characterized by distorted perceptions and thinking; these features are absent in schizoid personality disorder.
- **Avoidant personality disorder:** Social isolation in schizoid personality disorder is due to pervasive detachment from and general disinterest in social relationships whereas in avoidant personality disorder, it is due to fear of being embarrassed or rejected.

Treatment

- Social skills training

General treatment of schizoid personality disorder is the same as that for all personality disorders.

No controlled studies have been published about psychotherapies or drug therapy for schizoid personality disorder.

Generally, efforts to share interest in nonpersonal topics (eg, possessions, collections, hobbies) that appeal to people who prefer solitary pursuits can help establish a relationship with a patient and perhaps facilitate a therapeutic interaction.

Cognitive-behavioral approaches that focus on acquiring social skills may also help patients change.

Because patients with schizoid personality disorder lack interest in other people, they may not be motivated to change.

SCHIZOTYPAL PERSONALITY DISORDER

Schizotypal personality disorder is characterized by a pervasive pattern of intense discomfort with and reduced capacity for close relationships, by distorted cognition and perceptions, and by eccentric behavior. Diagnosis is by clinical criteria. Treatment is with antipsychotic drugs, antidepressants and cognitive-behavioral therapy.

In schizotypal personality disorder, cognitive experiences reflect a more florid departure from reality (eg, ideas of reference, paranoid ideas, bodily illusions, magical thinking) and a greater disorganization of thought and speech than occurs in other personality disorders.

Reported prevalence varies but is probably about 1 to 2% of the general population.

Comorbidities are common. Over half of patients with schizotypal personality disorder have had ≥ 1 episode of major depressive disorder, and 30 to 50% of them have major depressive disorder when schizotypal personality disorder is diagnosed. These patients often also have a substance abuse disorder.

Etiology

Etiology of schizotypal personality disorder is thought to be primarily biologic because it shares many of the brain-based abnormalities characteristic of schizophrenia. It is more common among 1st-degree relatives of people with schizophrenia or another psychotic disorder.

Symptoms and Signs

Patients with schizotypal personality disorder do not have close friends or confidants, except for 1st-degree relatives, They are very uncomfortable relating to people. They interact with people if they have to but prefer not to because they feel like they are different and do not belong. However, they may say their lack of relationships makes them unhappy. They are very anxious in social situations, especially unfamiliar ones. Spending more time in a situation does not ease their anxiety.

These patients often incorrectly interpret ordinary occurrences as having special meaning for them (ideas of reference). They may be superstitious or think they have special paranormal powers that enable them to sense events before they happen or to read other people's minds. They may think that they have magical control over others, thinking that they cause other people to do ordinary things (eg, feeding the dog), or that performing magical rituals can prevent harm (eg, washing their hands 3 times can prevent illness).

Speech may be odd. It may be excessively abstract or concrete or contain odd phrases or use phrases or words in odd ways. They often dress oddly or in an unkempt way (eg, wearing ill-fitting or dirty clothes) and have odd mannerisms. They may ignore ordinary social conventions (eg, not make eye contact), and because they do not understand usual social cues, they may interact with others inappropriately or stiffly.

Patients with schizotypal personality disorder are often suspicious and may think others are out to get them.

Diagnosis

- Clinical criteria (*Diagnostic and Statistical Manual of Mental Disorders*, Fifth Edition [DSM-5])

For a diagnosis of schizotypal personality disorder, patients must have intense discomfort with and decreased capacity for close relationships, as shown by ≥ 5 of the following:

- Ideas of reference (notions that everyday occurrences have special meaning or significance personally intended for or directed to themselves) but not *delusions* of reference (which are similar but held with greater conviction)
- Odd beliefs or magical thinking (eg, believing in clairvoyance, telepathy, or a sixth sense; being preoccupied with paranormal phenomena)
- Unusual perceptional experiences (eg, hearing a voice whispering their name)
- Odd thought and speech (eg, that is vague, metaphorical, excessively elaborate, or stereotyped)
- Suspicions or paranoid thoughts
- Incongruous or limited affect
- Odd, eccentric, or peculiar behavior and/or appearance
- Lack of close friends or confidants, except for 1st-degree relatives
- Excessive social anxiety that does not lessen with familiarity and is related mainly to paranoid fears

Also, symptoms must have begun by early adulthood.

Differential diagnosis: The primary diagnostic challenge is to differentiate schizotypal personality disorder from major thought disorders (eg, schizophrenia, bipolar or depressive disorder with psychotic features), which typically have more severe, bizarre, and persistent manifestations and are accompanied by delusions and hallucinations.

Schizotypal personality disorder can be distinguished from paranoid and schizoid personality disorder because patients with these personality disorders do not have odd, disorganized thought and behavior.

Treatment

- Antipsychotic drugs and antidepressants
- Cognitive-behavioral therapy

General treatment of schizotypal personality disorder is the same as that for all personality disorders.

The primary treatment for schizotypal personality disorder is drugs. Antipsychotics lessen anxiety and psychotic-like symptoms; antidepressants may also help lessen anxiety in patients with schizotypal personality disorder.

Cognitive-behavioral therapy that focuses on acquiring social skills and managing anxiety can help. Such therapy can also increase patients' awareness of how their own behavior may be perceived.

Supportive psychotherapy is also useful. The goal is to establish an emotional, encouraging, supportive relationship with the patient and thus help the patient develop healthy defense mechanisms, especially in interpersonal relationships.

213 Schizophrenia and Related Disorders

Schizophrenia and related disorders—brief psychotic disorder, delusional disorder, schizoaffective disorder, schizophreniform disorder, and schizotypal personality disorder—are characterized by psychotic symptoms and often by negative symptoms and/or cognitive dysfunction.

Psychotic symptoms include delusions, hallucinations, disorganized thinking and speech, and bizarre and inappropriate motor behavior (including catatonia).

Negative symptoms refer to a decrease in or lack of normal emotions and behaviors, such as having a flattened affect and lack of motivation.

Cognitive dysfunction in these disorders affects mainly sustained attention and working memory.

BRIEF PSYCHOTIC DISORDER

Brief psychotic disorder consists of delusions, hallucinations, or other psychotic symptoms for at least 1 day but < 1 mo, with eventual return to normal premorbid functioning. It is typically caused by severe stress in susceptible people.

Brief psychotic disorder is uncommon. Preexisting personality disorders (eg, paranoid, histrionic, narcissistic, schizotypal, borderline) predispose to its development. A major stressor, such as loss of a loved one, may precipitate the disorder.

The disorder causes at least one psychotic symptom:

- Delusions
- Hallucinations
- Disorganized speech
- Grossly disorganized or catatonic behavior

Brief psychotic disorder is not diagnosed if a psychotic mood disorder, a schizoaffective disorder, schizophrenia, a physical disorder, or an adverse drug effect (prescribed or illicit) better accounts for the symptoms.

Differentiating between brief psychotic disorder and schizophrenia in a patient without any prior psychotic symptoms is based on duration of symptoms; if the duration exceeds 1 mo, the patient no longer meets required diagnostic criteria for brief psychotic disorder.

Treatment of brief psychotic disorder is similar to treatment of an acute exacerbation of schizophrenia; supervision and short-term treatment with antipsychotics may be required.

Relapse is common, but patients typically function well between episodes and have few or no symptoms.

DELUSIONAL DISORDER

Delusional disorder is characterized by delusions (false beliefs) that persist for at least 1 mo, without other symptoms of schizophrenia.

Delusional disorder is distinguished from schizophrenia by the presence of delusions without other symptoms of schizophrenia. The delusions may be

- Nonbizarre: They involve situations that could occur, such as being followed, poisoned, infected, loved at a distance, or deceived by one's spouse or lover.
- Bizarre: They involve implausible situations such as believing that someone removed their internal organs without leaving a scar.

In contrast to schizophrenia, delusional disorder is relatively uncommon. Onset generally occurs in middle or late adult life. Psychosocial functioning is not as impaired as it is in schizophrenia, and impairments usually arise directly from the delusional belief.

When delusional disorder occurs in elderly patients, it is sometimes called paraphrenia. It may coexist with mild dementia. The physician must be careful to distinguish delusions from elder abuse being reported by a mildly demented elderly patient.

Symptoms and Signs

Delusional disorder may arise from a preexisting paranoid personality disorder. In such people, a pervasive distrust and suspiciousness of others and their motives begin in early adulthood and extend throughout life.

Early symptoms may include the feeling of being exploited, preoccupation with the loyalty or trustworthiness of friends, a tendency to read threatening meanings into benign remarks or events, persistent bearing of grudges, and a readiness to respond to perceived slights.

Several subtypes of delusional disorder are recognized:

- **Erotomanic:** Patients believe that another person is in love with them. Efforts to contact the object of the delusion through telephone calls, letters, surveillance, or stalking are common. People with this subtype may have conflicts with the law related to this behavior.
- **Grandiose:** Patients believe they have a great talent or have made an important discovery.
- **Jealous:** Patients believe that their spouse or lover is unfaithful. This belief is based on incorrect inferences supported by dubious evidence. They may resort to physical assault.
- **Persecutory:** Patients believe that they are being plotted against, spied on, maligned, or harassed. They may repeatedly attempt to obtain justice through appeals to courts and other government agencies and may resort to violence in retaliation for the imagined persecution.
- **Somatic:** The delusion relates to a bodily function; eg, patients believe they have a physical deformity, odor, or parasite.

Patients' behavior is not obviously bizarre or odd, and apart from the possible consequences of their delusions (eg, social isolation or stigmatization, marital or work difficulties), patients' functioning is not markedly impaired.

Diagnosis

- Clinical evaluation

Diagnosis depends largely on making a clinical assessment, obtaining a thorough history, and ruling out other specific conditions associated with delusions (eg, substance abuse, Alzheimer disease, obsessive-compulsive disorder, delirium, other schizophrenia spectrum disorders).

Assessment of dangerousness, especially the extent to which patients are willing to act on their delusion, is very important.

Prognosis

Delusional disorder does not usually lead to severe impairment or change in personality, but delusional concerns may gradually progress. Most patients can remain employed.

Treatment

- Establishment of an effective physician–patient relationship
- Management of complications
- Sometimes antipsychotics

Treatment aims to establish an effective physician–patient relationship and to manage complications. Substantial lack of insight is a challenge to treatment.

If patients are assessed to be dangerous, hospitalization may be required.

Insufficient data are available to support the use of any particular drug, although antipsychotics sometimes suppress symptoms.

A long-term treatment goal of shifting the patient's major area of concern away from the delusional locus to a more constructive and gratifying area is difficult but reasonable.

PSYCHOTIC DISORDER DUE TO ANOTHER MEDICAL CONDITION

Psychotic disorder due to another medical condition is hallucinations or delusions that are caused by another medical disorder.

Psychosis refers to symptoms such as delusions, hallucinations, disorganized thinking and speech, and bizarre and inappropriate motor behavior (including catatonia) that indicate loss of contact with reality.

This diagnosis applies when psychosis is due to the physiologic effects of a medical condition. Examples are psychotic behavior or olfactory hallucinations that are sometimes associated with temporal lobe epilepsy and the contralateral neglect syndrome that is sometimes caused by parietal lobe lesions.

Other medical disorders that may cause psychosis include CNS tumors and infections, stroke, migraine, and various endocrine disorders.

The diagnosis is not used if patients have a psychologically mediated response to medical illness (eg, ICU psychosis), psychosis due to the effects of drugs or drug withdrawal, or delirium caused by a medical condition.

It is essential to establish a temporal relationship between the medical and psychotic condition (ie, they begin and end at the same time).

Treating the medical condition often reduces the severity of psychotic symptoms, but some patients also need specific treatment of the psychotic symptoms.

OTHER SCHIZOPHRENIA SPECTRUM AND PSYCHOTIC DISORDERS

Some significant episodes of psychotic symptoms do not fulfill criteria for other diagnoses in the schizophrenia spectrum.

Psychosis refers to symptoms such as delusions, hallucinations, disorganized thinking and speech, and bizarre and inappropriate motor behavior (including catatonia) that indicate loss of contact with reality.

Other psychotic disorders are categorized as

- Other specified schizophrenia spectrum and other psychotic disorders
- Unspecified schizophrenia spectrum and other psychotic disorders

These categories refer to symptoms that are typical of a schizophrenia spectrum or other psychotic disorder (eg, delusions, hallucinations, disorganized thinking and speech, catatonic behavior), that cause substantial social and occupational distress and impairment, but that do not meet the full criteria for any specific disorder. These categories sometimes apply early in a schizophrenia spectrum disorder before it has fully manifested.

The category psychotic disorder not otherwise specified is no longer used.

A disorder is classified as specified if the clinician chooses to specify how the characteristics of the symptoms do not meet the criteria for a specific disorder. For example, a patient may have persistent auditory hallucinations with no other symptoms, thus not meeting criteria for schizophrenia, which requires 2 psychotic manifestations.

The unspecified category is used when the information needed to make a diagnosis is insufficient (eg, in an emergency department).

Antipsychotic drugs and psychiatric referral may be used as needed.

SCHIZOAFFECTIVE DISORDER

Schizoaffective disorder is characterized by significant mood symptoms, psychosis, and other symptoms of schizophrenia. It is differentiated from schizophrenia by occurrence of ≥ 1 episodes of depressive or manic symptoms.

Psychosis refers to symptoms such as delusions, hallucinations, disorganized thinking and speech, and bizarre and inappropriate motor behavior (including catatonia) that indicate loss of contact with reality.

Schizoaffective disorder is considered when a psychotic patient also demonstrates mood symptoms. The diagnosis requires that significant mood symptoms (depressive or manic) be present for a majority of the total duration of illness, concurrent with ≥ 2 symptoms of schizophrenia (delusions, hallucinations, disorganized speech, grossly disorganized or catatonic behavior, negative symptoms).

Differentiating schizoaffective disorder from schizophrenia and mood disorders may require longitudinal assessment of symptoms and symptom progression.

The prognosis is somewhat better than that for schizophrenia but worse than that for mood disorders.

Treatment

- Often a combination of drugs, psychotherapy, and community support

Because schizoaffective disorder often leads to long-term disability, comprehensive treatment (including drugs, psychotherapy, and community support) is often required.

For treatment of the manic type, antipsychotics combined with lithium, carbamazepine, or valproate may be more effective than antipsychotics alone.

For treatment of the depressive type, a 2nd-generation antipsychotic is given first. Then, once positive psychotic symptoms are stabilized, an antidepressant should be introduced; SSRIs are preferred because of their safety profile.

SCHIZOPHRENIA

Schizophrenia is characterized by psychosis (loss of contact with reality), hallucinations (false perceptions), delusions (false beliefs), disorganized speech and behavior, flattened affect (restricted range of emotions), cognitive deficits (impaired reasoning and problem solving), and occupational and social dysfunction. The cause is unknown, but evidence for a genetic component is strong. Symptoms usually begin in adolescence or early adulthood. One or more episodes of symptoms must last ≥ 6 mo before the diagnosis is made. Treatment consists of drug therapy, psychotherapy, and rehabilitation.

Psychosis refers to symptoms such as delusions, hallucinations, disorganized thinking and speech, and bizarre and inappropriate motor behavior (including catatonia) that indicate loss of contact with reality.

Worldwide, the prevalence of schizophrenia is about 1%. The rate is comparable among men and women and relatively constant cross-culturally. The rate is higher among lower socioeconomic classes in urban areas, perhaps because its disabling effects lead to unemployment and poverty. Similarly, a higher prevalence among single people may reflect the effect of illness or illness precursors on social functioning.

The average age at onset is early to mid-20s in women and somewhat earlier in men; about 40% of males have their first episode before age 20. Onset is rare in childhood, but early-adolescent onset or late-life onset (when it is sometimes called paraphrenia) may occur.

Etiology

Although its specific cause is unknown, schizophrenia has a biologic basis, as evidenced by

- Alterations in brain structure (eg, enlarged cerebral ventricles, thinning of the cortex, decreased size of the anterior hippocampus and other brain regions)
- Changes in neurotransmitters, especially altered activity of dopamine and glutamate

Some experts suggest that schizophrenia occurs in people with neurodevelopmental vulnerabilities and that the onset, remission, and recurrence of symptoms are the result of interactions between these enduring vulnerabilities and environmental stressors.

Neurodevelopmental vulnerability: Vulnerability may result from

- Genetic predisposition
- Intrauterine, birth, or postnatal complications
- Viral CNS infections

Maternal exposure to famine and influenza during the 2nd trimester of pregnancy, birth weight < 2500 g, Rh incompatibility during a 2nd pregnancy, and hypoxia increase risk.

Although most people with schizophrenia do not have a family history, genetic factors have been implicated. People who have a 1st-degree relative with schizophrenia have about a 10% risk of developing the disorder, compared with a 1% risk among the general population. Monozygotic twins have a concordance of about 50%.

Sensitive neurologic and neuropsychiatric tests suggest that aberrant smooth-pursuit eye tracking, impaired cognition and attention, and deficient sensory gating occur more commonly among patients with schizophrenia than among the general population. These markers (endophenotypes) also occur among 1st-degree relatives of people with schizophrenia and may represent the inherited component of vulnerability.

Environmental stressors: Stressors can trigger the emergence or recurrence of symptoms in vulnerable people. Stressors may be primarily biochemical (eg, substance abuse, especially marijuana) or social (eg, becoming unemployed or impoverished, leaving home for college, breaking off a romantic relationship, joining the Armed Forces); however, these stressors are not causative. There is no evidence that schizophrenia is caused by poor parenting.

Protective factors that may mitigate the effect of stress on symptom formation or exacerbation include good social support, coping skills, and antipsychotics.

Symptoms and Signs

Schizophrenia is a chronic illness that may progress through several phases, although duration and patterns of phases can vary. Patients with schizophrenia tend to develop psychotic symptoms an average of 12 to 24 mo before presenting for medical care.

Symptoms of schizophrenia typically impair the ability to function and often markedly interfere with work, social relationships, and self-care. Unemployment, isolation, deteriorated relationships, and diminished quality of life are common outcomes.

Phases of schizophrenia: In the **premorbid phase**, patients may show no symptoms or may have impaired social competence, mild cognitive disorganization or perceptual distortion, a diminished capacity to experience pleasure (anhedonia), and other general coping deficiencies. Such traits may be mild and recognized only in retrospect or may be more noticeable, with impairment of social, academic, and vocational functioning.

In the **prodromal phase**, subclinical symptoms may emerge; they include withdrawal or isolation, irritability, suspiciousness, unusual thoughts, perceptual distortions, and disorganization.[1] Onset of overt schizophrenia (delusions and hallucinations) may be sudden (over days or weeks) or slow and insidious (over years).

In the **middle phase**, symptomatic periods may be episodic (with identifiable exacerbations and remissions) or continuous; functional deficits tend to worsen.

In the **late illness phase**, the illness pattern may be established, and disability may stabilize or even diminish.

Symptom categories in schizophrenia: Generally, symptoms are categorized as

- Positive: An excess or distortion of normal functions
- Negative: Diminution or loss of normal functions and affect
- Disorganized: Thought disorders and bizarre behavior
- Cognitive: Deficits in information processing and problem solving

Patients may have symptoms from one or all categories.

Positive symptoms can be further categorized as

- Delusions
- Hallucinations

Delusions are erroneous beliefs that are maintained despite clear contradictory evidence. There are several types of delusions:

- Persecutory delusions: Patients believe they are being tormented, followed, tricked, or spied on.
- Delusions of reference: Patients believe that passages from books, newspapers, song lyrics, or other environmental cues are directed at them.
- Delusions of thought withdrawal or thought insertion: Patients believe that others can read their mind, that their thoughts are being transmitted to others, or that thoughts and impulses are being imposed on them by outside forces.

Delusions in schizophrenia tend to be bizarre—ie, clearly implausible and not derived from ordinary life experiences (eg, believing that someone removed their internal organs without leaving a scar).

Hallucinations are sensory perceptions that are not perceived by anyone else. They may be auditory, visual, olfactory, gustatory, or tactile, but auditory hallucinations are by far the most common. Patients may hear voices commenting on their behavior, conversing with one another, or making critical and abusive comments. Delusions and hallucinations may be extremely vexing to patients.

Negative (deficit) symptoms include

- Blunted affect: The patient's face appears immobile, with poor eye contact and lack of expressiveness.
- Poverty of speech: The patient speaks little and gives terse replies to questions, creating the impression of inner emptiness.
- Anhedonia: There is a lack of interest in activities and increased purposeless activity.
- Asociality: There is a lack of interest in relationships.

Negative symptoms often lead to poor motivation and a diminished sense of purpose and goals.

Disorganized symptoms, which can be considered a type of positive symptom, involve

- Thought disorders
- Bizarre behaviors

Thinking is disorganized, with rambling, non–goal-directed speech that shifts from one topic to another. Speech can range from mildly disorganized to incoherent and incomprehensible. Bizarre behavior may include childlike silliness, agitation, and inappropriate appearance, hygiene, or conduct. Catatonia is an extreme example of bizarre behavior, which can include maintaining a rigid posture and resisting efforts to be moved or engaging in purposeless and unstimulated motor activity.

Cognitive deficits include impairment in the following:

- Attention
- Processing speed
- Working memory
- Abstract thinking
- Problem solving
- Understanding of social interactions

The patient's thinking may be inflexible, and the ability to problem solve, understand the viewpoints of other people, and learn from experience may be diminished. Severity of cognitive impairment is a major determinant of overall disability.

Subtypes of schizophrenia: Some experts classify schizophrenia into deficit and nondeficit subtypes based on the presence and severity of negative symptoms, such as blunted affect, lack of motivation, and diminished sense of purpose.

Patients with the **deficit subtype** have prominent negative symptoms unaccounted for by other factors (eg, depression, anxiety, an understimulating environment, drug adverse effects).

Those with the **nondeficit subtype** may have delusions, hallucinations, and thought disorders but are relatively free of negative symptoms.

The previously recognized subtypes of schizophrenia (paranoid, disorganized, catatonic, residual, undifferentiated) have not proved valid or reliable and are no longer used.

Suicide: About 5 to 6% of patients with schizophrenia commit suicide, and about 20% attempt it; many more have significant suicidal ideation. Suicide is the major cause of premature death among people with schizophrenia and explains, in part, why on average the disorder reduces life span by 10 yr.

Risk may be especially high for young men with schizophrenia and a substance use disorder. Risk is also increased in patients who have depressive symptoms or feelings of hopelessness, who are unemployed, or who have just had a psychotic episode or been discharged from the hospital.

Patients who have late onset and good premorbid functioning—the very patients with the best prognosis for recovery—are also at the greatest risk of suicide. Because these patients retain the capacity for grief and anguish, they may be more prone to act in despair based on a realistic recognition of the effect of their disorder.

Violence: Schizophrenia is a relatively modest risk factor for violent behavior. Threats of violence and minor aggressive outbursts are far more common than seriously dangerous behavior.

Patients more likely to engage in significant violence include those with substance abuse, persecutory delusions, or command hallucinations and those who do not take their prescribed drugs. A very few severely depressed, isolated, paranoid patients attack or murder someone whom they perceive as the single source of their difficulties (eg, an authority, a celebrity, their spouse).

1. Tsuang MT, Van Os J, Tandon R, et al: Attenuated psychosis syndrome in DSM-5. *Schizophr Res* 150(1): 31–35, 2013.

Diagnosis

- Clinical criteria (*Diagnostic and Statistical Manual of Mental Disorders*, Fifth Edition [DSM-5])
- Combination of history, symptoms, and signs

If the first episode of schizophrenia that meets criteria for the disorder is recognized early and treated, outcome is better.

No definitive test for schizophrenia exists. Diagnosis is based on a comprehensive assessment of history, symptoms, and signs. Information from collateral sources, such as family members, friends, teachers, and co-workers, is often important.

According to the DSM-5, the diagnosis requires both of the following:

- ≥ 2 characteristic symptoms (delusions, hallucinations, disorganized speech, disorganized behavior, negative symptoms) for a significant portion of a 6-mo period (symptoms must include at least one of the first 3)
- Prodromal or attenuated signs of illness with social, occupational, or self-care impairments evident for a 6-mo period that includes 1 mo of active symptoms

Differential diagnosis: Psychosis due to other medical disorders or to substance abuse must be ruled out by history and examination that includes laboratory tests and neuroimaging (see p. 1736). Although some patients with schizophrenia have structural brain abnormalities present on imaging, these abnormalities are insufficiently specific to have diagnostic value.

Other mental disorders with similar symptoms include several that are related to schizophrenia:

- Brief psychotic disorder
- Delusional disorder
- Schizoaffective disorder
- Schizophreniform disorder
- Schizotypal personality disorder.

In addition, mood disorders can cause psychosis in some people.

Certain personality disorders (especially schizotypal) cause symptoms similar to those of schizophrenia, although they are usually milder and do not involve psychosis.

Prognosis

The earlier treatment is started, the better the outcome.

During the first 5 yr after onset of symptoms, functioning may deteriorate and social and work skills may decline, with progressive neglect of self-care. Negative symptoms may increase in severity, and cognitive functioning may decline. Thereafter, the level of disability tends to plateau. Some evidence suggests that severity of illness may lessen in later life, particularly among women. Spontaneous movement disorders may develop in patients who have severe negative symptoms and cognitive dysfunction, even when antipsychotics are not used.

Schizophrenia can occur with other mental disorders. When associated with significant obsessive-compulsive symptoms, prognosis is particularly poor; with symptoms of borderline personality disorder, prognosis is better. About 80% of people with schizophrenia experience one or more episodes of major depression at some time in their life.

For the first year after diagnosis, prognosis is closely related to adherence to prescribed psychoactive drugs.

Overall, one-third of patients achieve significant and lasting improvement; one-third improve somewhat but have intermittent relapses and residual disability; and one-third are severely and permanently incapacitated. Only about 15% of all patients fully return to their pre-illness level of functioning.

Factors associated with a good prognosis include

- Good premorbid functioning (eg, good student, strong work history)
- Late and/or sudden onset of illness
- Family history of mood disorders other than schizophrenia
- Minimal cognitive impairment
- Few negative symptoms
- Shorter duration of untreated psychosis

Factors associated with a poor prognosis include

- Young age at onset
- Poor premorbid functioning
- Family history of schizophrenia
- Many negative symptoms
- Longer duration of untreated psychosis

Men have poorer outcomes than women; women respond better to treatment with antipsychotics.

Substance abuse is a significant problem in up to 50% of patients with schizophrenia. Anecdotal evidence suggests that use of marijuana and other hallucinogens is highly disruptive for patients with schizophrenia and should be strongly discouraged. Comorbid substance abuse is a significant predictor of poor outcome and may lead to drug nonadherence, repeated relapse, frequent rehospitalization, declining function, and loss of social support, including homelessness.

Treatment

- Antipsychotic drugs
- Rehabilitation, including community support services
- Psychotherapy

The time between onset of psychotic symptoms and first treatment correlates with the rapidity of initial treatment response and quality of treatment response. When treated early, patients tend to respond more quickly and fully. Without ongoing use of antipsychotics after an initial episode, 70 to 80% of patients have a subsequent episode within 12 mo. Continuous use of antipsychotics can reduce the 1-yr relapse rate to about 30%. Drug treatment is continued for 1 to 2 yr after a first episode. If patients have been ill longer, it is given for many years.

General goals for schizophrenia treatment are to

- Reduce the severity of psychotic symptoms
- Prevent recurrences of symptomatic episodes and associated deterioration of functioning
- Help patients function at the highest level possible

Antipsychotics, rehabilitation with community support services, and psychotherapy are the major components of treatment. Because schizophrenia is a long-term and recurrent illness, teaching patients illness self-management skills is a significant overall goal. Providing information about the disorder (psychoeducation) to parents can reduce the relapse rate.

Drugs are divided into conventional antipsychotics and 2nd-generation antipsychotics (SGAs) based on their specific neurotransmitter receptor affinity and activity. SGAs may offer some advantages both in terms of modestly greater efficacy (although recent evidence casts doubt on SGAs' advantage as a class) and reduced likelihood of an involuntary movement disorder and related adverse effects. However, risk of metabolic syndrome (excess abdominal fat, insulin resistance, dyslipidemia, and hypertension) is greater with SGAs than with conventional antipsychotics. Several antipsychotics in both classes can cause long QT syndrome and ultimately increase the risk of fatal arrhythmias; these drugs include thioridazine, haloperidol, olanzapine, risperidone, and ziprasidone.

Conventional antipsychotics: Conventional antipsychotics (see Table 213–1) act primarily by blocking the dopamine-2 receptor (dopamine-2 blockers).

Conventional antipsychotics can be classified as high, intermediate, or low potency. High-potency antipsychotics have a higher affinity for dopamine receptors and less for alpha-adrenergic and muscarinic receptors. Low-potency antipsychotics, which are rarely used, have less affinity for dopamine receptors and relatively more affinity for alpha-adrenergic, muscarinic, and histaminic receptors.

Different drugs are available in tablet, liquid, and short- and long-acting IM preparations. A specific drug is selected primarily based on the following:

- Adverse effect profile
- Required route of administration
- The patient's previous response to the drug

Table 213–1. CONVENTIONAL ANTIPSYCHOTICS

DRUG	DAILY DOSE (RANGE)*	USUAL ADULT DOSE	COMMENTS
Chlorpromazine†,‡	30–800 mg	400 mg po at bedtime	Prototypic low-potency drug Also available as a rectal suppository
Thioridazine‡	150–800 mg	400 mg po at bedtime	Only drug with an absolute maximum (800 mg/day) because it causes pigmentary retinopathy at higher doses and has a significant anticholinergic effect Warning about QTc prolongation added to label
Trifluoperazine†,‡	2–40 mg	10 mg po at bedtime	—
Fluphenazine†,‡	0.5–40 mg	7.5 mg po at bedtime	Also available as fluphenazine decanoate and fluphenazine enanthate, which are IM depot forms (dose equivalents are not available)
Perphenazine†,‡	12–64 mg	16 mg po at bedtime	—
Loxapine	20–250 mg	60 mg po at bedtime	Has affinity for dopamine-2 and 5-hydroxytryptamine (serotonin)-2 receptors
Molindone	15–225 mg	60 mg po at bedtime	Possibly associated with weight reduction
Thiothixene†,‡	8–60 mg	10 mg po at bedtime	Has high incidence of akathisia
Haloperidol†,‡	1–15 mg	8 mg po at bedtime	Prototypic high-potency drug Haloperidol decanoate available as an IM depot Akathisia common
Pimozide	1–10 mg	3 mg po at bedtime	Approved only for Tourette syndrome

*Current recommended dosing for conventional antipsychotics is to initiate at low range of displayed values and titrate upwards gradually to a single dose; dosing at bedtime is recommended. There is no evidence that rapid dose escalation is more effective.
†These drugs are available in an IM form for acute treatment.
‡These drugs are available as an oral concentrate.
QTc = QT interval corrected for heart rate.

Some antipsychotics are available as long-acting depot preparations (see Table 213–2). These preparations are useful for eliminating drug nonadherence. They may also help patients who, because of disorganization, indifference, or denial of illness, cannot reliably take daily oral drugs.

Conventional antipsychotics have several adverse effects, such as sedation, cognitive blunting, dystonia and muscle stiffness, tremors, elevated prolactin levels, weight gain, and lowered seizure threshold in patients with seizures or at risk of seizures (for treatment of adverse effects, see Table 206–4 on p. 1741). Akathisia (motor restlessness) is particularly unpleasant and may lead to nonadherence; it can be treated with propranolol.

These drugs may also cause tardive dyskinesia, an involuntary movement disorder most often characterized by puckering of the lips and tongue, writhing of the arms or legs, or both. For patients taking conventional antipsychotics, the incidence of tardive dyskinesia is about 5% each year of drug exposure. In about 2%, tardive dyskinesia is severely disfiguring. In some patients, tardive dyskinesia persists indefinitely, even after the drug is stopped. Because of this risk, patients receiving long-term maintenance therapy should be evaluated at least every 6 mo. Rating instruments, such as the Abnormal Involuntary Movement Scale, may be used (see Table 213–3). Patients who have schizophrenia and who continue to require an antipsychotic drug may be treated with clozapine or quetiapine, which are SGAs.

Neuroleptic malignant syndrome, a rare but potentially fatal adverse effect, is characterized by rigidity, fever, autonomic instability, and elevated CK.

About 30% of patients with schizophrenia do not respond to conventional antipsychotics. They may respond to clozapine, an SGA.

Second-generation antipsychotics: About 95% of all antipsychotics prescribed are SGAs.

SGAs block dopamine receptors more selectively than conventional antipsychotics, decreasing the likelihood of extrapyramidal (motor) adverse effects. Although greater binding to serotonergic receptors was initially thought to contribute to the

Table 213–2. DEPOT ANTIPSYCHOTIC DRUGS

DRUG*	DOSAGE	PEAK LEVEL†
Aripiprazole, long-acting, injectable	300–400 mg q mo	5–7 days
Fluphenazine decanoate	12.5–50 mg q 2–4 wk	1 day
Fluphenazine enanthate	12.5–50 mg q 1–2 wk	2 days
Haloperidol decanoate	25–150 mg q 28 days (3–5 wk range is acceptable)	7 days
Olanzapine pamoate‡	210–300 mg q 2 wk or 300–405 mg q 4 wk	7 days
Risperidone microspheres§	12.5–50 mg q 2 wk	35 days

*Drugs are given IM with Z-track technique.
†Time until peak level after a single dose is listed.
‡Olanzapine pamoate may cause rare, but significant sedation so patients must be observed for 3 h after the injection.
§Because of a 3-wk lag time between first injection and achievement of adequate blood levels, patients should continue taking oral antipsychotics for 3 wk after the first injection. Assessment of tolerability with oral risperidone is recommended before initiating therapy.

Table 213–3. ABNORMAL INVOLUNTARY MOVEMENT SCALE

Before or after completing the scoring, clinicians should do the following:

1. Observe patient's gait on the way into the room.
2. Have patient remove gum or dentures if ill-fitting.
3. Determine whether patient is aware of any movements.
4. Have patient sit on a firm, armless chair with hands on knees, legs slightly apart, and feet flat on the floor. Now and throughout the examination, look at the entire body for movements.
5. Have patient sit with hands unsupported, dangling over the knees.
6. Ask patient to open mouth twice. Look for tongue movements.
7. Ask patient to stick out the tongue twice.
8. Ask patient to tap thumb against each finger for 15 sec with each hand. Observe face and legs.
9. Have patient stand with arms extended forward.

Rate each of the following items on a 0 to 4 scale for the greatest severity observed:

0 = none
1 = minimal, may be extreme normal
2 = mild
3 = moderate
4 = severe

Movements that occur only on activation are given 1 point less than those that occur spontaneously.

CATEGORY	ITEM	RANGE OF POSSIBLE SCORES
Facial and oral movements	Muscles of facial expression	0 1 2 3 4
	Lips and perioral area	0 1 2 3 4
	Jaw	0 1 2 3 4
	Tongue	0 1 2 3 4
Extremity movements	Arms	0 1 2 3 4
	Legs	0 1 2 3 4
Trunk movements	Neck, shoulders, and hips	0 1 2 3 4
Global judgment	Severity of abnormal movements	0 1 2 3 4
	Incapacitation due to abnormal movements	0 1 2 3 4
	Patient's awareness of abnormal movements (0 = unaware; 4 = severe distress)	0 1 2 3 4

Adapted from Guy W: *ECDEU [Early Clinical Drug Evaluation Unit] Assessment Manual for Psychopharmacology*. Rockville (MD), National Institute of Health, Psychopharmacology Research Branch, 1976. Copyright 1976 by US Department of Health, Education and Welfare.

efficacy of SGAs, studies suggest this binding is unrelated to efficacy or adverse effect profile.

SGAs also do the following:

- Tend to alleviate positive symptoms
- May lessen negative symptoms to a greater extent than do conventional antipsychotics (although such differences have been questioned)
- May cause less cognitive blunting
- Are less likely to have extrapyramidal adverse effects
- Have a lower risk of causing tardive dyskinesia
- Increase prolactin slightly or not at all (except risperidone, which increases prolactin as much as do conventional antipsychotics)

SGAs may appear to lessen negative symptoms because they are less likely to have parkinsonian adverse effects than conventional antipsychotics.

Clozapine, the first SGA, is the only SGA shown to be effective in up to 50% of patients resistant to conventional antipsychotics. Clozapine reduces negative symptoms, has few or no motor adverse effects, and has minimal risk of causing tardive dyskinesia, but it has other adverse effects, including sedation, hypotension, tachycardia, weight gain, type 2 diabetes, and increased salivation. It also may cause seizures in a dose-dependent fashion. The most serious adverse effect is agranulocytosis, which can occur in about 1% of patients. Consequently, frequent monitoring of WBCs (done weekly for the first 6 mo and every 2 wk thereafter, then once/mo after a year) is required, and clozapine is generally reserved for patients who have responded inadequately to other drugs.

Newer SGAs (see Table 213–4) provide some of the benefits of clozapine without the risk of agranulocytosis and are generally preferable to conventional antipsychotics for treatment of an acute episode and for prevention of recurrence. However, in a large, long-term, controlled clinical trial, symptom relief using any of 4 SGAs (olanzapine, risperidone, quetiapine, ziprasidone) was no greater than that with perphenazine, a conventional antipsychotic with anticholinergic effects. In a follow-up study, patients who left the study prematurely were randomized to one of the 3 other study SGAs or to clozapine; this study demonstrated a clear advantage of clozapine over the other SGAs. Hence, clozapine seems to be the only effective treatment for patients who have failed treatment with a conventional antipsychotic or an SGA. However, clozapine remains underused, probably because of lower tolerability and need for continuous blood monitoring.

Table 213–4. SECOND-GENERATION ANTIPSYCHOTICS*

DRUG	DOSE RANGE	USUAL ADULT DOSE	COMMENTS†
Aripiprazole	10–30 mg po	15 mg po	Dopamine-2 partial agonist Low risk of metabolic syndrome
Asenapine	5–10 mg sublingually bid	10 mg sublingually bid	Given sublingually with no food to be consumed for 10 min afterward (tablet should not be swallowed)
Brexpiprazole	2–4 mg po	2–4 mg po	Dopamine-2 partial agonist Low risk of metabolic syndrome Helps with major depression Dose titrated with • 1 mg given on days 1–4 • 2 mg given on days 5–7 • 4 mg given on day 8 (maximum dose: 4 mg)
Cariprazine	1.5–6 mg po	3–6 mg po	Low risk of metabolic syndrome Most common adverse effects: Somnolence, upset stomach Dose titrated with • 1.5 mg given on day 1 • 3 mg given on day 2
Clozapine	150–450 mg po bid	400 mg po at bedtime	First SGA Only one with demonstrated efficacy in patients unresponsive to other antipsychotics Frequent WBC counts required because agranulocytosis is a risk Increased risk of seizures and metabolic syndrome
Iloperidone	1–12 mg po bid	12 mg po once/day	Because of possible orthostatic hypotension, titrated over 4 days when initiated
Lurasidone	40–160 mg po once/day	80 mg po once/day	Given once/day with food Lower doses used in patients with liver impairment
Olanzapine	10–20 mg po at bedtime	15 mg po at bedtime	Most common adverse effects: Somnolence, metabolic syndrome, and dizziness
Paliperidone	3–12 mg po at bedtime	6 mg po at bedtime	Metabolite of risperidone Similar to risperidone
Quetiapine	150–375 mg po bid Extended-release: 400–800 mg po at bedtime	200 mg po bid	Low potency allowing a wide dosing range May cause metabolic syndrome No anticholinergic effect Dose titration required because of blocking of alpha-2 receptors Bid dosing required for immediate-release formulation; extended release given once at bedtime
Risperidone	4–10 mg po at bedtime	4 mg po at bedtime	May cause extrapyramidal symptoms at doses > 6 mg, dose-dependent prolactin elevation, or metabolic syndrome
Ziprasidone	40–80 mg po bid	80 mg po bid	Inhibition of serotonin and norepinephrine reuptake, possibly with antidepressant effects Shortest half-life of new drugs Requires bid dosing with food IM form available for acute treatment Low risk of metabolic syndrome

*Monitoring for metabolic syndrome and type 2 diabetes is recommended for this class of antipsychotics.
†All SGAs have been associated with increased mortality in elderly patients with dementia.
SGA = second-generation antipsychotic.

Newer SGAs are very similar to each other in efficacy but differ in adverse effects, so drug choice is based on individual response and on other drug characteristics. For example, olanzapine, which has a relatively high rate of sedation, may be prescribed for patients with prominent agitation or insomnia; less sedating drugs might be preferred for patients with lethargy. A 4- to 8-wk trial is usually required to assess efficacy. After acute symptoms have stabilized, maintenance treatment is initiated; for it, the lowest dose that prevents symptom recurrence is used. Aripiprazole, olanzapine, and risperidone are available in a long-acting injectable formulation.

Weight gain, hyperlipidemia, and elevated risk of type 2 diabetes are the major adverse effects of SGAs. Thus, before treatment with SGAs is begun, all patients should be screened for risk factors, including personal or family history of diabetes, weight, waist circumference, BP, and fasting plasma glucose and lipid profile. Those found to have or be at significant risk of metabolic syndrome may be better treated with ziprasidone or aripiprazole than the other SGAs. Patient and family education regarding symptoms and signs of diabetes, including polyuria, polydipsia, weight loss, and diabetic ketoacidosis (nausea, vomiting, dehydration, rapid respiration, clouding of sensorium), should be provided. In addition, nutritional and physical activity counseling should be provided to all patients when they start taking an SGA. All patients taking an SGA require periodic monitoring of weight, body mass index, and fasting plasma glucose and referral for specialty evaluation if they develop hyperlipidemia or type 2 diabetes.

Rehabilitation and community support services: Psychosocial skill training and vocational rehabilitation programs help many patients work, shop, and care for themselves; manage a household; get along with others; and work with mental health-care practitioners.

Supported employment, in which patients are placed in a competitive work setting and provided with an on-site job coach to promote adaptation to work, may be particularly valuable. In time, the job coach acts only as a backup for problem solving or for communication with employers.

Support services enable many patients with schizophrenia to reside in the community. Although most can live independently, some require supervised apartments where a staff member is present to ensure drug adherence. Programs provide a graded level of supervision in different residential settings, ranging from 24-h support to periodic home visits. These programs help promote patient autonomy while providing sufficient care to minimize the likelihood of relapse and need for inpatient hospitalization. Assertive community treatment programs provide services in the patient's home or other residence and are based on high staff-to-patient ratios; treatment teams directly provide all or nearly all required treatment services.

Hospitalization or crisis care in a hospital alternative may be required during severe relapses, and involuntary hospitalization may be necessary if patients pose a danger to themselves or others. Despite the best rehabilitation and community support services, a small percentage of patients, particularly those with severe cognitive deficits and those poorly responsive to drug therapy, require long-term institutional or other supportive care.

Cognitive remediation therapy helps some patients. This therapy is designed to improve neurocognitive function (eg, attention, working memory, executive functioning) and to help patients learn or relearn how to do tasks. This therapy may enable patients to function better.

Psychotherapy: The goal of psychotherapy is to develop a collaborative relationship between the patients, family members, and physician so that patients can learn to understand and manage their illness, take drugs as prescribed, and handle stress more effectively.

Although individual psychotherapy plus drug therapy is a common approach, few empirical guidelines are available. Psychotherapy that begins by addressing the patient's basic social service needs, provides support and education regarding the nature of the illness, promotes adaptive activities, and is based on empathy and a sound dynamic understanding of schizophrenia is likely to be most effective. Many patients need empathic psychologic support to adapt to what is often a lifelong illness that can substantially limit functioning.

In addition to individual psychotherapy, there has been significant development of cognitive behavioral therapy for schizophrenia. For example, this therapy, done in an individual or a group setting, can focus on ways to diminish delusional thoughts.

For patients who live with their families, psychoeducational family interventions can reduce the rate of relapse. Support and advocacy groups, such as the National Alliance on Mental Illness, are often helpful to families.

KEY POINTS

- Schizophrenia is characterized by psychosis, hallucinations, delusions, disorganized speech and behavior, flattened affect, cognitive deficits, and occupational and social dysfunction.
- Suicide is the most common cause of premature death.
- Threats of violence and minor aggressive outbursts are far more common than seriously dangerous behavior.
- Treat with antipsychotic drugs early, basing selection primarily on adverse effect profile, required route of administration, and the patient's previous response to the drug.
- Psychotherapy helps patients understand and manage their illness, take drugs as prescribed, and handle stress more effectively.
- With treatment, one-third of patients achieve significant and lasting improvement; one-third improve somewhat but have intermittent relapses and residual disability; and one-third are severely and permanently incapacitated.

SCHIZOPHRENIFORM DISORDER

Schizophreniform disorder is characterized by symptoms identical to those of schizophrenia but that last ≥ 1 mo but < 6 mo.

Psychosis refers to symptoms such as delusions, hallucinations, disorganized thinking and speech, and bizarre and inappropriate motor behavior (including catatonia) that indicate loss of contact with reality.

At presentation, schizophrenia is likely to be suspected. Psychosis secondary to substance abuse or to a physical disorder must also be ruled out. Differentiating between schizophreniform disorder and schizophrenia in a patient without any prior psychotic symptoms is based on duration of symptoms. If duration of symptoms or disability exceeds 6 mo, the patient no longer meets required diagnostic criteria for schizophreniform disorder, and the diagnosis is likely to be schizophrenia, although the acute psychosis may also evolve into a psychotic mood disorder, such as bipolar disorder or schizoaffective disorder. Longitudinal observation is often required to establish the diagnosis and appropriate treatment.

Treatment with antipsychotics and supportive psychosocial care is indicated. After symptoms resolve, drug treatment is continued for 12 mo and then gradually tapered while closely monitoring for the return of psychotic symptoms.

SHARED PSYCHOSIS

Shared psychosis occurs when people acquire a delusion from someone with whom they have a close personal relationship.

Psychosis refers to symptoms such as delusions, hallucinations, disorganized thinking and speech, and bizarre and inappropriate motor behavior (including catatonia) that indicate loss of contact with reality.

Shared psychosis (previously termed folie à deux) is now considered a subset of delusional disorder. It usually occurs in a person or group of people (usually a family) who are related to a person with a significant delusional disorder or schizophrenia. The prevalence of shared psychosis is not known, but the disorder appears to be rare. The patient with the primary disorder is usually the socially dominant member in the relationship and imposes the delusion on or convinces the patient with the secondary disorder of the unusual beliefs.

Identifying who in the relationship has the primary psychosis is important because the person with the secondary disorder typically does not maintain the delusional beliefs when separated from the person with the primary disorder.

Counseling and therapy can usually help people who have a shared psychosis. Usually, the person with the psychotic symptoms needs drug treatment.

SUBSTANCE-/MEDICATION-INDUCED PSYCHOTIC DISORDER

Substance-/medication-induced psychotic disorder is characterized by hallucinations and/or delusions due to the direct effects of a substance or withdrawal from a substance in the absence of delirium.

Episodes of substance-induced psychosis are common in emergency departments and crisis centers. There are many precipitating substances, including alcohol, amphetamines, cannabis, cocaine, hallucinogens, opioids, phencyclidine (PCP), and sedative/hypnotics. To be considered substance-induced psychosis, the hallucinations and delusions should be in excess of those that typically accompany simple substance intoxication or withdrawal, although the patient may also be intoxicated or withdrawing.

Symptoms are often brief, resolving shortly after the causative drug is cleared, but psychosis triggered by amphetamines, cocaine, or PCP may persist for many weeks. Because some young people with prodromal or early-stage schizophrenia use substances that can induce psychosis, it is important to obtain a thorough history, particularly to seek evidence of prior mental symptoms before concluding that acute psychosis is due to substance use.

Treatment

- A calm environment
- Often a benzodiazepine or antipsychotic

In most substance-induced psychoses, stopping the substance and giving an anxiolytic or antipsychotic drug is effective.

For psychosis due to dopamine-stimulating drugs such as amphetamine, an antipsychotic drug is most effective.

For psychosis due to drugs such as LSD, quiet observation may be all that is needed.

For substances with actions that do not involve dopamine, observation may be all that is needed, or an anxiolytic may help.

214 Sexuality, Gender Dysphoria, and Paraphilias

(For sexual dysfunction in men, see p. 2134; for sexual dysfunction in women, see p. 2302.)

Accepted norms of sexual behavior and attitudes vary greatly within and among different cultures. Healthcare practitioners should never be judgmental of sexual behaviors, even under societal pressure. Generally, what is normal and abnormal cannot be defined medically. However, when sexual behavior or difficulties cause significant distress for a patient or the patient's partner or cause harm, treatment is warranted.

Societal attitudes about sexuality and gender: Societal attitudes about sexuality and gender change with time, as has occurred with the following:

- **Masturbation:** Once widely regarded as a perversion and a cause of mental disorders, masturbation is now recognized as a normal sexual activity throughout life. It is considered abnormal only when it inhibits partner-oriented behavior, is done in public, or is sufficiently compulsive to cause distress. About 97% of males and 80% of females masturbate. Although masturbation is harmless, guilt created by the disapproval and punitive attitudes of other people may cause considerable distress and impair sexual performance. Masturbation often continues at some level even in a sexually healthy relationship.
- **Homosexuality:** Homosexuality has not been considered a disorder by the American Psychiatric Association for > 4 decades. About 4 to 5% of the population identify themselves as exclusively homosexual for their entire lives. Like heterosexuality, homosexuality results from complex biologic and environmental factors leading to an ability to become sexually aroused by people of the same sex. Like heterosexuality, homosexuality is not a matter of choice.
- **Promiscuity:** Frequent sexual activity with many partners, often involving anonymous or one-time-only encounters, may indicate a diminished capacity for intimacy. However, promiscuity is not in itself evidence of a psychosexual disorder. Casual sex is common in Western cultures, although the fear of AIDS, herpes simplex infections, and other sexually transmitted diseases has resulted in a decrease.
- **Extramarital sex:** Most cultures discourage extramarital sexual activity but accept premarital or nonmarital sexual activity as normal. In the US, most people engage in sexual activity before marriage or without marriage as part of the trend toward more sexual freedom in developed countries. Extramarital sex occurs frequently among married people despite social taboos. This behavior has the potential to pass diseases to unsuspecting spouses and sex partners.
- **Gender identity:** Gender identity is the subjective sense of knowing to which gender one belongs. There is growing cultural recognition that some people do not fit—nor necessarily wish to fit—into the traditional male-female dichotomy.

Influence of parents on sexuality: Accepted norms of sexual behavior and attitudes are influenced greatly by parents.

A forbidding, puritanical rejection of physical affection, including touching, by a parent engenders guilt and shame in children and inhibits their capacity for enjoying sex and developing healthy intimate relationships as adults.

Relations with parents may be damaged by

- Excessive emotional distance
- Punitive behaviors
- Overt seductiveness and sexual exploitation

Children exposed to verbal and physical hostility, rejection, and cruelty are likely to develop problems with sexual and emotional intimacy. For example, love and sexual arousal may become dissociated, so that although emotional bonds can be formed with people from the same social class or intellectual circle, sexual relationships can be formed only with those for whom there is no emotional intimacy, typically those who are perceived to be of a lower class or in some way depreciated (eg, prostitutes, anonymous partners).

Role of the healthcare practitioner: Well-informed health care practitioners can offer sensitive, disciplined advice on sexuality and should not miss opportunities for helpful intervention. Behaviors that place patients at risk of sexually transmitted diseases must be addressed. Practitioners have an opportunity to recognize and address psychosexual issues, including sexual dysfunction (see pp. 2134 and 2302), gender dysphoria, and paraphilias.

GENDER DYSPHORIA AND TRANSSEXUALISM

Gender dysphoria is characterized by a strong, persistent cross-gender identification; people believe they are victims of a biologic accident and are cruelly imprisoned in a body incompatible with their subjective gender identity. Those with the most extreme form of gender dysphoria may be referred to as transsexuals.

Sex, gender, and identity: Sex and gender are not the same thing.

- **Sex** refers to a person's biologic status: male, female, or intersex.
- **Sexual identity** refers to the sex to which a person is sexually attracted.
- **Gender identity** is the subjective sense of knowing to which gender one belongs; ie, whether people regard themselves as male, female, transgender, or another identifying term (eg, genderqueer).
- **Gender role** is the objective, public expression of gender identity and includes everything that people say and do to indicate to themselves and to others the degree to which they are the gender that they identify with.

Gender role behaviors fall on a continuum of traditional masculinity or femininity, with a growing cultural recognition that some people do not fit—nor necessarily wish to fit—into the traditional male-female dichotomy.

Western cultures are more tolerant of gender-nonconforming (tomboyish) behaviors in young girls (generally not considered a gender disorder) than effeminate or "sissy" behaviors in boys. Many boys role-play as girls or mothers, including trying on their sister's or mother's clothes. Usually, this behavior is part of normal development. Gender nonconformity in children is not considered a disorder and rarely persists into adulthood or leads to gender dysphoria, although nonconforming boys may be more likely to become homosexual or bisexual.

Gender dysphoria: For most people, there is congruity between their biologic (birth) sex, gender identity, and gender role. However, those with gender dysphoria experience some degree of incongruity between their birth sex and their gender identity.

Gender incongruity itself is not considered a disorder. However, when the perceived mismatch between birth sex and felt gender identity causes significant distress or disability, a diagnosis of gender dysphoria may be appropriate. The distress is typically a combination of anxiety, depression, and irritability. People with severe gender dysphoria, often referred to as transsexuals, may experience severe, disturbing, and long-standing symptoms and have a strong wish to change their body medically and/or surgically to make their body more closely align with their gender identity. However, labeling this condition "gender dysphoria" can add to the distress; patients should be reassured that the term is not intended to be judgmental. Transsexualism appears to occur in about 1 of 11,900 male and 1 of 30,000 female births.

Some scholars argue that this diagnosis is primarily a medical condition, akin to disorders of sex development, and not a mental disorder at all. Conversely, some members of the transgender community consider even extreme forms of gender nonconformity to be simply a normal variant in human gender identity and expression.

Etiology

Although biologic factors (eg, genetic complement, prenatal hormonal milieu) largely determine gender identity, the formation of a secure, unconflicted gender identity and gender role is also influenced by social factors (eg, the character of the parents' emotional bond, the relationship that each parent has with the child). Some studies show a higher concordance rate for gender dysphoria in monozygotic twins than in dizygotic twins, suggesting that there is a heritable component.

Rarely, transsexualism is associated with genital ambiguity (intersex conditions [disorders of sex development]) or a genetic abnormality (eg, Turner syndrome, Klinefelter syndrome).

When sex labeling and rearing are confusing (eg, in cases of ambiguous genitals or genetic syndromes altering genital appearance, such as androgen insensitivity syndromes), children may become uncertain about their gender identity or role, although the level of importance of environmental factors remains controversial. However, when sex labeling and rearing are unambiguous, even the presence of ambiguous genitals may not affect a child's gender identity development.

Symptoms and Signs

Gender dysphoria symptoms in children: Childhood gender dysphoria often manifests by age 2 to 3 yr. Children commonly do the following:

- Prefer cross-dressing
- Insist that they are of the other sex
- Wish that they would wake up as the other sex
- Prefer participating in the stereotypical games and activities of the other sex
- Have negative feelings toward their genitals

For example, a young girl may insist she will grow a penis and become a boy; she may stand to urinate. A boy may fantasize about being female and avoid rough-and-tumble play and competitive games. He may sit to urinate and wish to be rid of his penis and testes. For boys, distress at the physical changes of puberty is often followed by a request during adolescence for feminizing somatic treatments. Most children with gender dysphoria are not evaluated until they are age 6 to 9, at a point when gender dysphoria is already chronic.

Gender dysphoria symptoms in adults: Although most transsexuals have gender dysphoria symptoms or experience a sense of being different in early childhood, some do not present until adulthood. Male-to-female transsexuals may first be cross-dressers and only later in life come to accept their cross-gender identity.

Marriage and military service are common among transsexuals who seek to run from their cross-gender (transgender) feelings. Once they accept their cross-gender feelings, many transsexuals adopt a convincing public cross-gender role.

Some birth-sex male transsexuals are satisfied with mastering a more feminine appearance and obtaining female identification cards (eg, driver's license) to help them work and live in society as women. Others experience problems, which may include anxiety, depression, and suicidal behavior. These problems may be related to societal and family stressors associated with lack of acceptance of gender-nonconforming behaviors.

Diagnosis

- Specific *Diagnostic and Statistical Manual of Mental Disorders*, Fifth Edition (DSM-5) criteria

Diagnosis in all age groups: Gender dysphoria is expressed differently in different age groups. But for diagnosis in all age groups, DSM-5 criteria require the presence of both of the following:

- Marked incongruity between birth sex and felt gender identity (cross-gender identification) that has been present for ≥ 6 mo
- Clinically significant distress or functional impairment resulting from this incongruity

Diagnosis in children: In addition to the characteristics required for all age groups, children must have ≥ 6 of the following:

- A strong desire to be or insistence that they are the other gender (or some other gender)
- A strong preference for dressing in clothing typical of the opposite gender and, in girls, resistance to wearing typically feminine clothing
- A strong preference for cross-gender roles when playing
- A strong preference for toys, games, and activities typical of the other gender
- A strong preference for playmates of the other gender
- A strong rejection of toys, games, and activities typical of the gender that matches their birth sex
- A strong dislike of their anatomy
- A strong desire for the primary and/or secondary sex characteristics that match their felt gender identity

Cross-gender identification must not be merely a desire for perceived cultural advantages of being the other sex. For example, a boy who says he wants to be a girl so that he will receive the same special treatment his younger sister receives is not likely to have gender dysphoria.

Diagnosis in adolescents and adults: In addition to the characteristics required for all age groups, adolescents and adults must have ≥ 1 of the following:

- A strong desire to be rid of (or for young adolescents, prevent the development of) their primary and/or secondary sex characteristics
- A strong desire for the primary and/or secondary sex characteristics that match their felt gender
- A strong desire to be the other gender (or some other gender)
- A strong desire to be treated like another gender
- A strong belief that they have the typical feelings and reactions of another gender

Diagnosis in adults focuses on determining whether there is significant distress or obvious impairment in social, occupational, or other important areas of functioning. Gender nonconformity alone is insufficient for diagnosis.

Treatment

- Psychotherapy
- For certain motivated patients, cross-sex hormone therapy and sometimes sex reassignment surgery

Gender-nonconforming behavior, such as cross-dressing, may not require treatment if it occurs without concurrent psychologic distress or functional impairment.

When treatment is required, it is aimed at helping patients adapt to rather than trying to dissuade them from their identity. Attempts at altering gender identity in adults have not proved effective and are now considered unethical.

Most transsexuals who request treatment are birth-sex males who claim a female gender identity and regard their genitals and masculine features with repugnance. However, as treatments have improved, female-to-male transsexualism is increasingly seen in medical and psychiatric practice, although the incidence in Western cultures is about one third of that for male-to-female transsexualism.

Transsexuals' primary objective in seeking medical help is not to obtain psychologic treatment but to obtain hormones and genital surgery that will make their physical appearance approximate their felt gender identity. The combination of psychotherapy, hormonal reassignment, living at least a year in the felt gender, and sex reassignment surgery may be curative when the disorder is appropriately diagnosed and clinicians follow the internationally accepted standards of care for the treatment of gender identity disorders, available from the World Professional Association for Transgender Health (WPATH).

Although patients with gender dysphoria are no longer required to have psychotherapy before consideration of cross-sex hormonal and surgical procedures, mental healthcare practitioners can do the following to help patients make decisions:

- Assess and treat comorbid disorders (eg, depression, substance use disorders)
- Help patients deal with the negative effects of stigma (eg, disapproval, discrimination)
- Help patients find a gender expression that is comfortable
- If applicable, facilitate gender role changes and coming out

Male-to-female transsexualism: Feminizing hormones in moderate doses (eg, estradiol transdermal patches 0.1 to 0.15 mg/day) plus electrolysis, voice therapy, and other feminizing treatments may make the adjustment to a female gender role more stable. Feminizing hormones have significant beneficial effects on the symptoms of gender dysphoria, often before there are any visible changes in secondary sexual characteristics (eg, breast growth, decreased facial and body hair growth, redistribution of fat to the hips). Feminizing hormones, even without psychologic support or surgery, are all some patients need to make them feel sufficiently comfortable as a female.

Sex reassignment surgery is requested by many male-to-female transsexuals. Surgery involves removal of the penis and testes and creation of an artificial vagina. A part of the glans penis is retained as a clitoris, which is usually sexually sensitive and retains the capacity for orgasm in most cases.

The decision to pursue sex reassignment surgery often raises important social problems for patients. Many of these patients are married and have children. A parent or spouse who changes sex and gender role will likely have substantial adjustment issues in intimate relationships and may lose loved ones in the process. In follow-up studies, genital surgery has helped some transsexuals live happier and more productive lives and so is justified in highly motivated, appropriately assessed and treated transsexuals who have completed at least 1 yr of living full-time in the opposite gender role.

Participation in gender support groups, available in most large cities, is usually helpful.

Female-to-male transsexualism: Female-to-male patients often ask for mastectomy early because it is difficult to live in the male gender role with a large amount of breast tissue; breast binding often makes breathing difficult.

Then, hysterectomy and oophorectomy may be done after a course of androgenic hormones (eg, testosterone ester preparations 300 to 400 mg IM q 3 wk or equivalent doses of androgen transdermal patches or gels). Testosterone preparations permanently deepen the voice, induce a more masculine muscle and fat distribution, induce clitoromegaly, and promote growth of facial and body hair.

Patients may opt for one of the following:

- An artificial phallus (neophallus) to be fashioned from skin transplanted from the inner forearm, leg, or abdomen (phalloplasty)
- A micropenis to be fashioned from fat tissue removed from the mons pubis and placed around the testosterone-hypertrophied clitoris (metoidioplasty)

Surgery may help certain patients achieve greater adaptation and life satisfaction. Similar to male-to-female transsexuals, female-to-male transsexuals should live in the male gender role for at least 1 yr before irreversible genital surgery.

Anatomic results of neophallus surgical procedures are often less satisfactory in terms of function and appearance than neovaginal procedures for male-to-female transsexuals, possibly resulting in relatively fewer requests for genital sex reassignment surgery from female-to-male transsexuals.

Complications are common, especially in procedures that involve extending the urethra into the neophallus.

OVERVIEW OF PARAPHILIC DISORDERS

(Paraphilias)

Paraphilic disorders are recurrent, intense, sexually arousing fantasies, urges, or behaviors that are distressing or disabling and that involve inanimate objects, children or nonconsenting adults, or suffering or humiliation of oneself or the partner with the potential to cause harm.

Paraphilias involve sexual arousal to atypical objects, situations, and/or targets (eg, children, corpses, animals). However, some sexual activities that seem unusual to another person or a healthcare practitioner do not constitute a paraphilic disorder simply because they are unusual. People may have paraphilic interests but not meet the criteria for a paraphilic disorder.

The unconventional sexual arousal patterns in paraphilias are considered pathologic disorders only when both of the following apply:

- They are intense and persistent.
- They cause significant distress or impairment in social, occupational, or other important areas of functioning, or they harm or have the potential to harm others (eg, children, nonconsenting adults)

People with a paraphilic disorder may have an impaired or a nonexistent capacity for affectionate, reciprocal emotional and sexual intimacy with a consenting partner. Other aspects of personal and emotional adjustment may be impaired as well.

The pattern of disturbed erotic arousal is usually fairly well developed before puberty. At least 3 processes are involved:

- Anxiety or early emotional trauma interferes with normal psychosexual development.
- The standard pattern of arousal is replaced by another pattern, sometimes through early exposure to highly charged sexual experiences that reinforce the person's experience of sexual pleasure.
- The pattern of sexual arousal often acquires symbolic and conditioning elements (eg, a fetish symbolizes the object of arousal but may have been chosen because the fetish was accidentally associated with sexual curiosity, desire, and excitement).

Whether all paraphilic development results from these psychodynamic processes is controversial, and some evidence of altered brain functioning and functional anatomy is present in some paraphilias (eg, pedophilia).

In most cultures, paraphilias are far more common among males. Biologic reasons for the unequal distribution may exist but are poorly defined.

Dozens of paraphilias have been described, but most are uncommon or rare. The most common are

- Pedophilia
- Voyeurism
- Transvestic fetishism
- Exhibitionism

Others include sexual masochism disorder and sexual sadism disorder.

Some paraphilias (such as pedophilia) are illegal and may result in being imprisoned and being labeled and registered as a sex offender for life. Some of these offenders also have significant personality disorders (eg, antisocial, narcissistic), which make treatment difficult.

Often, more than one paraphilic disorder is present.

FETISHISTIC DISORDER

(Fetishism)

Fetishism is use of an inanimate object (the fetish) as the preferred method of producing sexual excitement. However, in common parlance, the word is often used to describe particular sexual interests, such as sexual role-playing, preference for certain physical characteristics, and preferred sexual activities or objects. Fetishistic disorder refers to recurrent, intense sexual arousal from use of an inanimate object or from a very specific focus on a nongenital body part (or parts) that causes significant distress or functional impairment.

Fetishism is a form of paraphilia, but most people who have fetishism do not meet the clinical criteria for a paraphilic disorder, which require that the person's behavior, fantasies, or intense urges result in clinically significant distress or functional impairment. The condition must also have been present for ≥ 6 mo.

There are many fetishes; common fetishes include aprons, shoes, leather or latex items, and women's underclothing. The fetish may replace typical sexual activity with a partner or may be integrated into sexual activity with a willing partner. Minor fetishistic behavior as an adjunct to consensual sexual behavior is not considered a disorder because distress, disability, and significant dysfunction are absent. More intense, obligatory, and highly compulsive fetishistic arousal patterns and behaviors may cause problems in a relationship or become all-consuming and destructive in a person's life.

Fetishes may include clothing of the opposite sex (eg, women's undergarments), but if sexual arousal occurs mainly from *wearing* that clothing (ie, cross-dressing) rather than using it in some other way, the paraphilia is considered transvestism).

Treatment of fetishism may include psychotherapy, drugs, or both. SSRIs have been used with limited success in some patients who request treatment.

TRANSVESTIC DISORDER

(Transvestism)

Transvestism involves recurrent and intense sexual arousal from cross-dressing, which may manifest as fantasies, urges, or behaviors. Transvestic disorder is transvestism that causes significant distress or significant functional impairment.

Transvestism is a type of paraphilia, but most cross-dressers do not meet the clinical criteria for a paraphilic disorder; these criteria require that the person's fantasies, intense urges, or behaviors cause distress, impair functioning, or harm others. The condition must also have been present for ≥ 6 mo.

Cross-dresser is a more common and acceptable term than transvestite. Cross-dressing and transvestic disorder are extremely rare in birth-sex females.

Heterosexual males who dress in women's clothing typically begin such behavior during late childhood. This behavior is associated, at least initially, with intense sexual arousal. Sexual arousal that is produced by the clothing itself is considered a form of fetishism and may occur with or independent of cross-dressing.

Personality profiles of cross-dressing men are generally similar to age- and race-matched norms.

When their partner is cooperative, cross-dressing men may engage in sexual activity in partial or full feminine attire. When their partner is not cooperative, they may feel anxiety, depression, guilt, and shame because of their desire to cross-dress. In response to these feelings, these men often purge their wardrobe of female clothing.

Treatment

- Social and support groups
- Sometimes psychotherapy

Most cross-dressers do not present for treatment. Those who do are usually brought in by an unhappy spouse, referred by courts, or self-referred out of concern about experiencing negative social and employment consequences. Some cross-dressers present for treatment of comorbid gender dysphoria, substance abuse, or depression.

Social and support groups for men who cross-dress are often very helpful.

No drugs are reliably effective.

Psychotherapy, when indicated, is aimed at self-acceptance and modulating risky behaviors.

Later in life, sometimes in their 50s or 60s, cross-dressing men may present for medical care because of gender dysphoria symptoms and may then meet diagnostic criteria for gender dysphoria.

EXHIBITIONISTIC DISORDER

(Exhibitionism)

Exhibitionism is characterized by achievement of sexual excitement through genital exposure, usually to an unsuspecting stranger. It may also refer to a strong desire to be observed by other people during sexual activity. Exhibitionistic disorder involves acting on these urges with a nonconsenting person or experiencing significant distress or functional impairment because of such urges and impulses.

Exhibitionism is a form of paraphilia, but most people who have exhibitionism do not meet the clinical criteria for a paraphilic disorder, which require that a person's behavior, fantasies, or intense urges result in clinically significant distress or impaired functioning or cause harm to others (which in exhibitionism includes acting on the urges with a nonconsenting person). The condition must also have been present for ≥ 6 mo.

Estimated prevalence in men is 2 to 4%; it is lower in women. Few females are diagnosed with exhibitionistic disorder; society sanctions some exhibitionistic behaviors in females (through media and entertainment venues).

Exhibitionists (usually male) may masturbate while exposing or fantasizing about exposing themselves to others. They may be aware of their need to surprise, shock, or impress the unwilling observer. The victim is almost always a female adult or a child of either sex. Actual sexual contact is rarely sought, and physical harm to the unsuspecting witness is unusual.

Onset is usually during adolescence; occasionally, the first act occurs during preadolescence or middle age.

About 30% of apprehended male sex offenders are exhibitionists. They have the highest recidivism rate of all sex offenders; about 20 to 50% are re-arrested.

Most exhibitionists are married, but the marriage is often troubled by poor social and sexual adjustment, including frequent sexual dysfunction.

Exhibitionists may also have a personality disorder or conduct disorder.

For some people, exhibitionism is expressed as a strong desire to have other people watch their sexual acts. What appeals to such people is not the act of surprising an audience but rather of being seen by a consenting audience. People with this form of exhibitionism may make pornographic films or become adult entertainers. They are rarely troubled by this desire and thus may not have a psychiatric disorder.

Treatment

- Psychotherapy, support groups, and SSRIs
- Sometimes antiandrogen drugs

When laws are broken and sex offender status is conferred, treatment usually begins with psychotherapy, support groups, and SSRIs.

If these drugs are ineffective and if the disorder is severe, drugs that reduce testosterone levels and thus reduce libido should be considered. These drugs are referred to as antiandrogens, although the most commonly used drugs do not actually block the effects of testosterone. These drugs include gonadotropin-releasing hormone (GnRH) agonists (eg, leuprolide) and depot medroxyprogesterone acetate; both decrease pituitary production of luteinizing hormone (LH) and follicle-stimulating hormone (FSH). Full informed consent and appropriate monitoring of liver function and serum testosterone levels are required.

Recidivism rates are high. Effectiveness of treatment is monitored based on self-report, penile plethysmography, and arrest records.

VOYEURISTIC DISORDER

(Voyeurism)

Voyeurism is achievement of sexual arousal by observing people who are naked, disrobing, or engaging in sexual activity. When observation is of unsuspecting people, this sexual behavior often leads to problems with the law and relationships. Voyeuristic disorder involves acting on voyeuristic urges or fantasies with a nonconsenting person or experiencing significant distress or functional impairment because of such urges and impulses.

Voyeurism is form of paraphilia, but most people who have voyeuristic interests do not meet the clinical criteria for a paraphilic disorder, which require that the person's behavior, fantasies, or intense urges result in clinically significant distress or impaired functioning or cause harm to others (which in voyeurism includes acting on the urges with a nonconsenting person). The condition must also have been present for ≥ 6 mo.

Desire to watch others in sexual situations is common and not in itself abnormal. Voyeurism usually begins during adolescence or early adulthood. Adolescent voyeurism is generally viewed more leniently; few teenagers are arrested. When voyeurism is pathologic, voyeurs spend considerable time seeking out viewing opportunities, often to the exclusion of fulfilling important responsibilities in their life. Orgasm is usually achieved by masturbating during or after the voyeuristic activity. Voyeurs do not seek sexual contact with the people being observed.

In many cultures, voyeurs have ample legal opportunities to watch sexual activity. However, voyeuristic behaviors are the most common of sexual behaviors that may result in a brush with the law.

Up to 12% of males and 4% of females may meet clinical criteria for voyeuristic disorder; most do not seek medical evaluation and treatment.

Treatment

- Psychotherapy, support groups, and SSRIs
- Sometimes antiandrogen drugs

When laws are broken and sex offender status is conferred, treatment usually begins with therapy, support groups, and SSRIs.

If these drugs are ineffective and if the disorder is severe, drugs that reduce testosterone levels and thus reduce libido should be considered. These drugs are referred to as antiandrogens, although the most commonly used drugs do not actually block the effects of testosterone. Drugs include gonadotropin-releasing hormone (GnRH) agonists (eg, leuprolide) and depot medroxyprogesterone acetate; both decrease pituitary production of luteinizing hormone (LH) and follicle-stimulating hormone (FSH) and thus reduce testosterone production. Full informed consent and appropriate monitoring of liver function and serum testosterone levels are required.

SEXUAL MASOCHISM DISORDER

Sexual masochism is intentional participation in an activity that involves being humiliated, beaten, bound, or otherwise abused to experience sexual excitement. Sexual masochism disorder is sexual masochism that causes significant distress or significantly impairs functioning.

Sexual masochism is form of paraphilia, but most people who have masochistic interests do not meet clinical criteria for a paraphilic disorder, which require that the person's behavior, fantasies, or intense urges result in clinically significant distress or impairment. The condition must also have been present for ≥ 6 mo.

Sadomasochistic fantasies and sexual behavior between consenting adults is very common. Masochistic activity tends to be ritualized and long-standing. For most participants, the humiliation and beating are simply acted out; participants know that it is a game and carefully avoid actual humiliation or injury. However, some masochists increase the severity of their activity with time, potentially leading to serious injury or death.

Masochistic activities may be the preferred or exclusive mode of producing sexual excitement. People may act out their masochistic fantasies on themselves—for example, by

- Binding themselves
- Piercing their skin
- Applying electrical shocks
- Burning themselves

Or they may seek out a partner who may be a sexual sadist. Activities with a partner include being

- Bound
- Blindfolded
- Spanked
- Flagellated (whipped)
- Humiliated by being urinated or defecated on
- Forced to cross-dress
- Part of a simulated rape

As with all paraphilias, diagnosis of a disorder is warranted only if there is clinically significant distress or functional impairment.

Treatment of this disorder is often ineffective.

Autoerotic asphyxiation (asphyxiophilia): Asphyxiophilia is considered a subtype of sexual masochism disorder.

In this disorder, people restrict their breathing (partial asphyxiation) at or near the time of orgasm to enhance the experience. Typically, people use articles of clothing (eg, scarves, underwear) as a ligature to choke themselves. The ligature is often suspended from an object in the room (eg, doorknob, bedpost).

Loss of consciousness can occur rapidly because obstruction of venous return from the brain impairs cerebral perfusion even before hypoxia and hypercarbia become significant. People who asphyxiate themselves in such a way that the ligature does not release if they lose consciousness can have permanent brain damage or die.

SEXUAL SADISM DISORDER

Sexual sadism is infliction of physical or psychologic suffering (eg, humiliation, terror) on another person to stimulate sexual excitement and orgasm. Sexual sadism disorder is sexual sadism that causes significant distress or significant functional impairment or is acted on with a nonconsenting person.

People with sexual sadism disorder have either acted on the intense urges or have debilitating or distressing fantasies with sexually sadistic themes. The condition must also have been present for ≥ 6 mo.

Sexual sadism is form of paraphilia but mild sadistic sexual behavior is a common sexual practice between consenting adults, is usually limited in scope, is not harmful, and does not meet the clinical criteria for a paraphilic disorder, which require that a person's behavior, fantasies, or intense urges result in clinically significant distress or functional impairment or cause harm to others. However, in some people, the behaviors escalate to the point of harm. When sadism becomes pathologic is a matter of degree.

Most sexual sadists have persistent fantasies in which sexual excitement results from suffering inflicted on the partner, consenting or not. When practiced with nonconsenting partners, sexual sadism constitutes criminal activity and is likely to continue until the sadist is apprehended. However, sexual sadism is not synonymous with rape, a complex amalgam of sex and power over the victim. Sexual sadism is diagnosed in < 10% of rapists but is present in 37 to 75% of people who have committed sexually motivated homicides.

Sexual sadism is particularly dangerous when associated with antisocial personality disorder. This combination of disorders is particularly recalcitrant to any form of psychiatric treatment.

PEDOPHILIC DISORDER

(Pedophilia)

Pedophilic disorder is characterized by recurrent, intense sexually arousing fantasies, urges, or behaviors involving prepubescent or young adolescents (usually ≤ 13 yr); it is diagnosed only when people are ≥ 16 yr and ≥ 5 yr older than the child who is the target of the fantasies or behaviors.

Pedophilia is form of paraphilia that causes harm to others and is thus considered a a paraphilic disorder.

Sexual offenses against children constitute a significant proportion of reported criminal sexual acts. For older adolescents (ie, 17 to 18 yr old), ongoing sexual interest or involvement with a 12- or 13-yr-old may not meet the clinical criteria for a disorder. However, legal criteria may be different from psychiatric criteria. For example, sexual activity between a 19-yr-old and a 16-yr-old may be a crime and not a pedophilic disorder, depending on the jurisdiction. Diagnostic age guidelines apply to Western cultures and not to the many cultures where sexual activity, marriage, and childbearing are accepted at much younger ages than in the West.

Most pedophiles are male. Attraction may be to young boys, girls, or both. But pedophiles prefer opposite-sex to same-sex children 2:1. In most cases, the adult is known to the child and may be a family member, stepparent, or a person with authority (eg, a teacher). Looking or touching seems more prevalent than genital contact. Pedophiles may be attracted only to children (exclusive) or also adults (nonexclusive); some are attracted only to children who are related to them (incest).

Predatory pedophiles, many of whom have antisocial personality disorder, may use force and threaten to physically harm the child or the child's pets if the abuse is disclosed.

The course of pedophilia is chronic, and perpetrators often have or develop substance abuse or dependence and depression. Pervasive family dysfunction, a personal history of sexual abuse, and marital conflict are common. Other comorbid disorders include attention deficit disorder, depression, anxiety disorders, and posttraumatic stress disorder.

Diagnosis

- Clinical evaluation

Extensive use of child pornography is a reliable marker of sexual attraction to children and may be the only indicator of the disorder. However, use of child pornography by itself does not meet criteria for pedophilic disorder, although it is typically illegal.

If a patient denies sexual attraction to children but circumstances suggest otherwise, certain diagnostic tools can help confirm such attraction. Tools include penile plethysmography (men), vaginal photoplethysmography (women), and viewing time of standardized erotic materials; however, possession of such material, even for diagnostic purposes, may be illegal in certain jurisdictions.

Clinical criteria for diagnosis (based on *Diagnostic and Statistical Manual of Mental Disorders*, Fifth Edition [DSM-5]) are

- Recurrent, intense sexually arousing fantasies, urges, or behaviors involving a prepubescent child or children (usually ≤ 13 yr) have been present for ≥ 6 mo.
- The person has acted on the urges or is greatly distressed or impaired by the urges and fantasies.
- The person is ≥ 16 yr and ≥ 5 yr older than the child who is the target of the fantasies or behaviors (but excluding an older adolescent who is in an ongoing relationship with a 12- or 13-yr-old).

Identifying a patient as a potential pedophile sometimes poses an ethical crisis for healthcare practitioners. However, health care practitioners have a responsibility to protect the community of children. Practitioners should know the reporting requirements in their state. If practitioners have reasonable suspicion of child sexual or physical abuse, the law requires that it be reported to authorities. Reporting requirements vary by state (see Child Welfare Information Gateway at www.childwelfare.gov).

Treatment

- Psychotherapy
- Treatment of comorbid disorders
- Drug treatment (eg, antiandrogens, SSRIs)

Long-term individual or group psychotherapy is usually necessary and may be especially helpful when it is part of multimodal treatment that includes social skills training, treatment of comorbid physical and mental disorders, and drug treatment.

Treatment is less effective when court ordered, although many adjudicated sex offenders have benefited from treatments, such as group psychotherapy plus antiandrogens.

Some pedophiles who are committed to treatment and monitoring can refrain from pedophilic activity and can be reintegrated into society. These results are more likely when no other psychiatric disorders, particularly personality disorders, are present.

Drugs: In the US, the treatment of choice is

- IM medroxyprogesterone acetate

By blocking pituitary production of luteinizing hormone (LH) and follicle-stimulating hormone (FSH), medroxyprogesterone reduces testosterone production and thus reduces libido. Typical doses are medroxyprogesterone 200 mg IM 2 to 3 times/wk for 2 wk, followed by 200 mg 1 to 2 times/wk for 4 wk, then 200 mg q 2 to 4 wk.

The gonadotropin-releasing hormone (GnRH) agonist, leuprolide, which reduces pituitary production of LH and FSH and thus reduces testosterone production, is also an option and requires less frequent IM injections (at 1- to 6 mo- intervals). Cyproterone, which blocks testosterone receptors, is used in Europe. Serum testosterone should be monitored and maintained in the normal female range (< 62 ng/dL) in male patients. Treatment is usually long-term because deviant fantasies usually recur weeks to months after treatment is stopped. Liver function tests should be done, and BP, bone mineral density, and CBC should be monitored as required.

The usefulness of antiandrogens in female pedophiles is less well established.

In addition to antiandrogens, SSRIs (eg, high-dose fluoxetine 60 to 80 mg once/day or fluvoxamine 200 to 300 mg po once/day) may be useful.

Drugs are most effective when used as part of a multimodal treatment program.

215 Somatic Symptom and Related Disorders

Somatization is the expression of mental phenomena as physical (somatic) symptoms. Disorders characterized by somatization extend in a continuum from those in which symptoms develop unconsciously and nonvolitionally to those in which symptoms develop consciously and volitionally. This continuum includes

- Somatic symptom and related disorders
- Factitious disorders
- Malingering (the latter is not a psychiatric disorder)

In all of the disorders, patients focus prominently on somatic concerns. Thus, somatization typically leads patients to seek medical evaluation and treatment rather than psychiatric care.

Somatic symptom disorder and related disorders are characterized by persistent physical symptoms that are associated with excessive or maladaptive thoughts, feelings, and behaviors in response to these symptoms and associated health concerns. These disorders are distressing and often impair social, occupational, academic, or other aspects of functioning. They include

- Conversion disorder
- Factitious disorders
- Illness anxiety disorder
- Psychological factors affecting other medical conditions
- Somatic symptom disorder

Somatic symptom disorder and illness anxiety disorder are the most common.

Factitious disorders involve the falsification of physical or psychologic symptoms and/or signs in the absence of obvious external incentives (eg, obtaining time off from work, disability payments, or drugs of abuse; avoiding military service or criminal prosecution). The term Munchausen syndrome is no longer used for factitious disorders.

Malingering is intentional feigning of physical or psychologic symptoms motivated by an external incentive, which distinguishes malingering from factitious disorders.

CONVERSION DISORDER

Conversion disorder consists of neurologic symptoms or deficits that develop unconsciously and nonvolitionally and usually involve motor or sensory function. The manifestations are incompatible with known pathophysiologic mechanisms or anatomic pathways. Onset, exacerbation, or maintenance of conversion symptoms is commonly attributed to mental factors, such as stress. Diagnosis is based on history after excluding physical disorders as the cause. Treatment begins by establishing a consistent, supportive physician–patient relationship; psychotherapy can help, as may hypnosis.

Conversion disorder is a form of somatization—the expression of mental phenomena as physical (somatic) symptoms.

Conversion disorder tends to develop during late childhood to early adulthood but may occur at any age. It is more common among women.

Symptoms and Signs

Symptoms of conversion disorder often develop abruptly, and onset can often be linked to a stressful event. Typically, symptoms involve apparent deficits in voluntary motor or sensory function but sometimes include shaking movements and impaired consciousness (suggesting seizures) and abnormal limb posturing (suggesting another neurologic or general physical disorder). For example, patients may present with impaired coordination or balance, weakness, paralysis of an arm or a leg, loss of sensation in a body part, seizures, unresponsiveness, blindness, double vision, deafness, aphonia, difficulty swallowing, sensation of a lump in the throat, or urinary retention.

Patients may have a single episode or sporadic repeated ones; symptoms may become chronic. Typically, episodes are brief.

Diagnosis

- Clinical evaluation

The diagnosis of conversion disorder is considered only after a comprehensive medical examination and tests to rule out neurologic or general medical disorders that can fully account for the symptoms and their effects. An important characteristic is that the symptoms and signs are not consistent with neurologic disease. For example, they may not follow anatomic distributions (eg, sensory deficits that involve parts of multiple nerve roots), or findings may vary at different examinations or when assessed in different ways, as in the following:

- A patient may have marked weakness of plantar flexion when tested in bed but can walk normally on tiptoes.
- In a supine patient, the examiner's hand under the heel of a "paralyzed" leg detects downward pressure when the patient lifts the unaffected leg against resistance (Hoover sign).
- Tremor changes or disappears when the patient is distracted (eg, by having the patient copy a rhythmic movement with the unaffected hand).
- Resistance to eye opening is detected during an apparent seizure.
- A visual field deficit is tubular (tunnel vision).

Also, to meet criteria for being a disorder, the symptoms must be severe enough to cause significant distress or impair social, occupational, or other important areas of functioning.

Treatment

- Sometimes hypnosis or cognitive-behavioral therapy

A consistently trustful and supportive physician-patient relationship is essential. Collaborative treatment that involves a psychiatrist and a physician from another field (eg, neurologist, internist) seems most helpful. After the physician has excluded a general medical disorder and reassured patients that the symptoms do not indicate a serious underlying disorder, patients may begin to feel better, and symptoms may fade.

The following treatments may help:

- Hypnosis may help by enabling patients to control the effects of stress and their mental state on their bodily functions.
- Narcoanalysis is a rarely used procedure similar to hypnosis except that patients are given a sedative to induce a state of semisleep.
- Psychotherapy, including cognitive-behavioral therapy, is effective for some people.

Any coexisting psychiatric disorders (eg, depression) should be treated.

FACTITIOUS DISORDER IMPOSED ON SELF

Factitious disorder is falsification of physical or psychologic symptoms without an obvious external incentive; the motivation for this behavior is to assume the sick role. Symptoms can be acute, dramatic, and convincing. Patients often wander from one physician or hospital to another for treatment. The cause is unknown, although stress and a severe personality disorder, most often borderline personality disorder, are often implicated. Diagnosis is clinical. There are no clearly effective treatments.

Factitious disorder imposed on self was previously called Munchausen syndrome, particularly when manifestations were dramatic and severe. Factitious disorder imposed on another person may also occur.

These patients initially and sometimes chronically become the responsibility of medical or surgical clinics. Nevertheless, the disorder is a mental problem, is more complex than simple dishonest simulation of symptoms, and is associated with severe emotional difficulties.

Patients may have prominent borderline personality features and are usually intelligent and resourceful. They know how to simulate disease and are sophisticated regarding medical practices. They differ from malingerers because, although their deceits and simulations are conscious and volitional, there are no obvious external incentives (eg, economic gain) for their behavior. It is unclear what they gain beyond medical attention for their suffering, and their motivations and quest for attention are largely unconscious and obscure.

Patients may have an early history of emotional and physical abuse. Patients may also have experienced a severe illness during childhood or had a seriously ill relative. Patients appear to have problems with their identity as well as unstable relationships. Feigning illness may be a way to increase or protect self-esteem by blaming failures on their illness, by being associated with prestigious physicians and medical centers, and/or by appearing unique, heroic, or medically knowledgeable and sophisticated.

Symptoms and Signs

Patients with factitious disorder imposed on self may complain of or simulate physical symptoms that suggest certain disorders (eg, abdominal pain suggesting an acute surgical abdomen, hematemesis). Patients often know many associated symptoms and features of the disorder that they are feigning (eg, that pain from an MI may radiate to the left arm or jaw or be accompanied by diaphoresis).

Sometimes they simulate or induce physical findings (eg, pricking a finger to contaminate a urine specimen with blood, injecting bacteria under their skin to produce fever or abscess; in such cases, *Escherichia coli* is often the infecting organism). Their abdominal wall may be crisscrossed by scars from exploratory laparotomies, or a digit or a limb may have been amputated.

Diagnosis

- Clinical evaluation

Diagnosis of factitious disorder imposed on self is based on history and examination, along with any tests necessary to exclude physical disorders and demonstration of exaggeration, fabrication, simulation, and/or induction of physical symptoms. The behavior must occur in the absence of obvious external incentives (eg, time off work, financial compensation for injury).

Treatment

- No clearly effective treatments

Treatment of factitious disorder imposed on self is usually challenging, and there are no clearly effective treatments. Patients may obtain initial relief by having their treatment demands met, but their symptoms typically escalate, ultimately surpassing what physicians are willing or able to do. Confrontation or refusal to meet treatment demands often results in angry reactions, and patients usually move from one physician or hospital to another (called peregrination).

Recognizing the disorder and requesting psychiatric or psychologic consultation early is important, so that risky invasive testing, surgical procedures, and excessive or unwarranted use of drugs can be avoided.

A nonaggressive, nonpunitive, nonconfrontational approach should be used to present the diagnosis of factitious disorder to patients. To avoid suggesting guilt or reproach, a physician can present the diagnosis as a cry for help. Alternatively, some experts recommend providing mental health treatment without requiring patients to admit their role in causing their illness. In either case, conveying to the patient that the physician and patient can cooperatively resolve the problem is helpful.

Factitious Disorder Imposed on Another

Factitious disorder imposed on another is falsification of manifestations of an illness in another person, typically done by caregivers to someone in their care.

Previously, this disorder was known as factitious disorder by proxy or Munchausen syndrome by proxy. In factitious disorder imposed on another, people, usually caregivers such as a parent, intentionally produce or falsify physical or psychologic symptoms or signs in a person in their care (usually a child), rather than in themselves (as in factitious disorder imposed on self).

The caregiver falsifies history and may injure the child with drugs or other agents or add blood or bacterial contaminants to urine specimens to simulate disease. The caregiver seeks medical care for the child and appears to be deeply concerned and protective. The child typically has a history of frequent hospitalizations, usually for a variety of nonspecific symptoms, but no firm diagnosis. Victimized children may be seriously ill and sometimes die.

As with factious disorder imposed on self, the caregiver's behavior must occur in the absence of obvious external incentives (eg, to cover up signs of child abuse).

ILLNESS ANXIETY DISORDER

Illness anxiety disorder is preoccupation with and fear of having or acquiring a serious disorder. Diagnosis is confirmed when fears and symptoms (if any) persist for ≥ 6 mo despite reassurance after a thorough medical evaluation. Treatment includes establishing a consistent, supportive physician-patient relationship; cognitive-behavioral therapy and serotonin reuptake inhibitors may help.

Illness anxiety disorder (previously called hypochondriasis, a term that has been abandoned because of its pejorative connotation) most commonly begins during early adulthood and appears to occur equally among men and women.

The patient's fears may derive from misinterpreting nonpathologic physical symptoms or normal bodily functions (eg, borborygmi, abdominal bloating and crampy discomfort, awareness of heartbeat, sweating).

Symptoms and Signs

Patients with illness anxiety disorder are so preoccupied with the idea that they are or might become ill that their illness anxiety impairs social and occupational functioning or causes significant distress. Patients may or may not have physical symptoms, but if they do, their concern is more about the possible implications of the symptoms than the symptoms themselves.

Some patients examine themselves repeatedly (eg, looking at their throat in a mirror, checking their skin for lesions). They are easily alarmed by new somatic sensations. Some patients visit physicians frequently (care-seeking type); others rarely seek medical care (care-avoidant type).

The course is often chronic—fluctuating in some, steady in others. Some patients recover.

Diagnosis

- Clinical evaluation

The diagnosis of illness anxiety disorder is based on criteria from the *Diagnostic and Statistical Manual of Mental Disorders*, Fifth Edition (DSM-5), including the following:

- The patient is preoccupied with having or acquiring a serious illness.
- The patient has no or minimal somatic symptoms.
- The patient is highly anxious about health and easily alarmed about personal health issues.
- The patient repeatedly checks health status or maladaptively avoids doctor appointments and hospitals.
- The patient has been preoccupied with illness for ≥ 6 mo, although the specific illness feared may change during that time period.
- Symptoms are not better accounted for by depression or another mental disorder.

Patients who have significant somatic symptoms and are primarily concerned about the symptoms themselves are diagnosed with somatic symptom disorder.

Treatment

- Sometimes serotonin reuptake inhibitors or cognitive-behavioral therapy

Patients can benefit from having a trustful relationship with a caring, reassuring physician. If symptoms are not adequately relieved, patients may benefit from a psychiatric referral while they continue under the care of the primary physician.

Treatment with serotonin reuptake inhibitors may be helpful, as may cognitive-behavioral therapy.

PSYCHOLOGICAL FACTORS AFFECTING OTHER MEDICAL CONDITIONS

Psychological factors affecting other medical conditions is diagnosed when psychologic or behavioral factors adversely affect the course or outcome of an existing medical condition.

Patients have one or more clinically significant psychologic or behavior factors that adversely affect an existing medical disorder (eg, diabetes mellitus, heart disease) or symptom (eg, pain). These factors may increase the risk of suffering, death, or disability; aggravate an underlying medical condition; or result in hospitalization or emergency department visit. Abnormal psychologic or behavioral responses to a medical condition that do not affect medical outcome are considered an adjustment disorder.

Psychologic or behavior factors that can adversely affect a medical disorder include

- Denial of the significance or severity of symptoms
- Poor adherence to prescribed testing and treatment

Patients may present as treatment failures or with aggravation of medical conditions associated with stress (eg, Takotsubo cardiomyopathy).

Patient education and psychotherapeutic intervention can help.

SOMATIC SYMPTOM DISORDER

Somatic symptom disorder is characterized by multiple persistent physical complaints that are associated with excessive and maladaptive thoughts, feelings, and behaviors related to those symptoms. The symptoms are not intentionally produced or feigned and may or may not accompany known medical illness. Diagnosis is based on history from the patient and occasionally from family members. Treatment focuses on establishing a consistent, supportive physician–patient relationship that avoids exposing the patient to unnecessary diagnostic testing and therapies.

Some previously distinct somatic disorders—somatization disorder, undifferentiated somatoform disorder, hypochondriasis, and somatoform pain disorder—are now considered somatic symptom disorders. All have common features, including somatization—the expression of mental phenomena as physical (somatic) symptoms.

The symptoms may or may not be associated with another medical problem; symptoms no longer have to be medically unexplained but are characterized by the patient having disproportionately excessive thoughts, feelings, and concerns about them. Sometimes the symptoms are normal body sensations or discomfort that do not signify a serious disorder.

Patients are commonly unaware of their underlying mental problem and believe that they have physical ailments, so they typically continue to pressure physicians for additional or repeated tests and treatments even after results of a thorough evaluation have been negative.

Symptoms and Signs

Recurring physical complaints usually begin before age 30; most patients have multiple somatic symptoms, but some have only one severe symptom, typically pain. Severity may fluctuate, but symptoms persist and rarely remit for any extended period. The symptoms themselves or excessive worry about them is distressing or disrupts daily life. Some patients become overtly depressed.

When somatic symptom disorder accompanies another medical disorder, patients overrespond to the implications of the medical disorder; for example, patients who have had complete physical recovery from an uncomplicated MI may continue to behave as invalids or constantly worry about having another MI.

Whether or not symptoms are related to another medical disorder, patients worry excessively about the symptoms and their possible catastrophic consequences and are very difficult to reassure. Attempts at reassurance are often interpreted as the physician not taking their symptoms seriously.

Health concerns often assume a central and sometimes all-consuming role in a patient's life. Patients are very anxious about their health and frequently seem unusually sensitive to adverse drug effects.

Any body part may be affected, and specific symptoms and their frequency vary among cultures. Whatever the manifestations, the essence of somatic symptom disorder is the patient's excessive or maladaptive thoughts, feelings, or behaviors in response to the symptoms.

Patients may become dependent on others, demanding help and emotional support and becoming angry when they feel their needs are not met. They may also threaten or attempt suicide. Often dissatisfied with their medical care, they typically go from one physician to another or seek treatment from several physicians concurrently.

The intensity and persistence of symptoms may reflect a strong desire to be cared for. Symptoms may help patients avoid responsibilities but may also prevent pleasure and act as punishment, suggesting underlying feelings of unworthiness and guilt.

Diagnosis

- Usually clinical criteria

Symptoms must be distressing or disruptive of daily life for > 6 mo and be associated with at least one of the following:

- Disproportionate and persistent thoughts about the seriousness of the symptoms
- Persistently high anxiety about health or the symptoms
- Excessive time and energy spent on the symptoms or health concerns

At first presentation, physicians take an extensive history (sometimes conferring with family members) and do a thorough examination and often testing to determine whether a medical disorder is the cause. Because patients with somatic symptom disorder may develop concurrent physical disorders, appropriate examinations and tests should also be done when symptoms change significantly or when objective signs develop. However, once a medical disorder has clearly been excluded or a mild disorder has been identified and treated, physicians should avoid repeating tests; patients are rarely reassured by negative test results and may interpret continued testing as confirmation that the physician is uncertain the diagnosis is benign.

Illness anxiety disorder has similar manifestations except that physical symptoms are absent or minimal. Somatic symptom disorder is distinguished from generalized anxiety disorder, conversion disorder, and major depression by the predominance, multiplicity, and persistence of physical symptoms and the accompanying excessive thoughts, feelings, and behaviors.

Treatment

- Cognitive-behavioral therapy

Patients, even those who have a satisfactory relationship with a primary physician, are commonly referred to a psychiatrist. Pharmacologic treatment of concurrent mental disorders (eg, depression) may help; however, the primary intervention is psychotherapy, particularly cognitive-behavioral therapy.

Patients also benefit from having a supportive relationship with a primary care physician, who coordinates all of their health care, offers symptomatic relief, sees them regularly, and protects them from unnecessary tests and procedures.

216 Suicidal Behavior and Self-Injury

SUICIDAL BEHAVIOR

Suicidal behavior includes completed suicide and attempted suicide. Thoughts and plans about suicide are referred to as suicide ideation.

Completed suicide is a suicidal act that results in death. Attempted suicide is a nonfatal, self-directed, potentially injurious act intended to result in death. A suicide attempt may or may not result in injury. Nonsuicidal self-injury (NSSI) is a self-inflicted act that causes pain or superficial damage but is not intended to cause death. (See also the American Psychiatric Association's Practice Guideline for the Assessment and Treatment of Patients With Suicidal Behaviors at http://psychiatryonline.org.)

Epidemiology

Statistics on suicidal behavior are based mainly on death certificates and inquest reports and underestimate the true incidence. To provide more reliable information, the CDC established the National Violent Death Reporting System (NVDRS); it is a state-based system that collects facts about each violent incident from various sources to provide a clearer understanding of the causes of violent deaths (homicides and suicides). The NVDRS is currently in place in 40 states.

In the US, suicide is the 10th leading cause of death, with a death rate of 13.8/100,000 and almost 41,000 completed suicides in 2015. In the US, 121 people die by suicide per day. As a cause of death, it ranks as follows:

- 2nd among people aged 15 to 34 yr
- 3rd among those aged 10 to 14
- 4th among those aged 35 to ≥ 44

The age group with the highest suicide rate is now people aged 45 to 64 yr, resulting from a recent significant increase. Why this rate has increased is unknown; however, the following may have contributed:

- Years ago, as teenagers, this group had a higher rate of depression than older groups, and researchers predicted the suicide rate would rise as they aged.
- This rate includes the increased number of suicides in the military and veterans (20% of suicides are in that group).
- This rate may reflect increased abuse of prescription and nonprescription drugs and a response to the poor economy.

The second highest rate of suicide is in people > 85 yr.

In recent years, youth suicide rates decreased after more than a decade of steady increase, only to start climbing again.

In all age groups, male deaths by suicide outnumber female deaths 3.5 to 1. The reasons are unclear, but possible explanations include

- Men are less likely to seek help when they are distressed.
- Men have a higher prevalence of alcohol and drug abuse, which leads to suicidal tendencies.
- Men are more aggressive and use more lethal means when attempting suicide.
- The number of suicides in men includes suicides in the military and veterans who have a higher proportion of men to women.

In 2015, >1.1 million people reported making a suicide attempt. About 25 attempts are made for every death that occurs by suicide. Many make repeated attempts. Only 5 to 10% of people who make an attempt eventually die by suicide; however in the elderly, 1 in every 4 suicide attempts ends in death. Women attempt suicide 2 to 3 times more often than men; among girls aged 15 to 19 yr, there may be 100 attempts to every 1 attempt among boys of the same age.

A suicide note is left by about 1 in 6 people who complete suicide. The content may indicate the reasons for the suicide (including a mental disorder).

Copycat suicide or suicide contagion accounts for about 10% of the suicides. Group suicides are extremely rare, as are murder/suicides. Rarely, people commit an act (eg, brandish a weapon) that forces law enforcement agents to kill them—called suicide by police.

Etiology

Suicidal behaviors usually result from the interaction of several factors. The primary remediable risk factor in suicide is

- Depression

The amount of time spent in an episode of depression is the strongest predictor of suicide. Also, suicide appears to be more common when severe anxiety is part of major depression or bipolar depression. Risk of suicidal thoughts and attempts may increase after antidepressant drugs are started (see pp. 1809 and 2718).

Other risk factors for suicide (see Table 216–1) include the following:

- Most other serious mental disorders
- Use of alcohol, drugs of abuse, and prescription pain drugs

Table 216–1. RISK FACTORS AND WARNING SIGNS FOR SUICIDE

TYPE	SPECIFIC FACTORS
Demographic data	Male Age 45–64
Social situation	Personally significant anniversaries Unemployment or financial difficulties, particularly if causing a drastic fall in economic status Recent separation, divorce, or widowhood Recent arrest or trouble with the law Social isolation with real or imagined unsympathetic attitude of relatives or friends
History of suicidality	Previous suicide attempt Making detailed suicide plans, taking steps to implement the plan (obtaining gun, pills), and taking precautions against being discovered Family history of suicide or a mental disorder
Clinical features	Depressive illness, especially at onset Marked motor agitation, restlessness, and anxiety with severe insomnia Marked feelings of guilt, inadequacy, and hopelessness; perception of being a burden to others (burdensomeness); self-denigration; nihilistic delusion Delusion or near-delusional conviction of a physical disorder (eg, cancer, a heart disorder, sexually transmitted disease) or other delusions (eg, delusions of poverty) Command hallucinations Impulsive, hostile personality A chronic, painful, or disabling physical disorder, especially in formerly healthy patients
Drug use	Alcohol or drug abuse (including abuse of prescription drugs), especially if recent use has increased Use of drugs that may contribute to suicidal behavior (eg, abruptly stopping paroxetine and certain other antidepressants can result in increased depression and anxiety, which in turn increases risk of suicidal behavior)

- Previous suicide attempts
- Serious physical disorders, especially in the elderly
- Personality disorders
- Unemployment and economic downturns
- Traumatic childhood experiences
- Family history of suicide and/or mental disorders

Death by suicide is more common among people with a mental disorder than among age- and sex-matched controls.

Some people with schizophrenia die by suicide, sometimes because of depression, to which these people are prone. The suicide method may be bizarre and violent. Attempted suicide among these people is more common than previously thought.

Alcohol and drugs of abuse may increase disinhibition and impulsivity as well as worsen mood—a potentially lethal combination. About 30% of people who attempt suicide have consumed alcohol before the attempt, and about half of them were intoxicated at the time. Alcoholics are at increased risk of suicide even when they are sober.

Serious physical disorders, especially those that are chronic and painful, contribute to about 20% of suicides in the elderly.

People with personality disorders are prone to suicide—especially emotionally immature people with a borderline or an antisocial personality disorder because they tolerate frustration poorly and react to stress impetuously, with violence and aggression.

Certain social factors (eg, sex partner problems, bullying, recent arrest, trouble with the law) appear to be associated with suicide. Often after such events, suicide is the last resort for these already distressed people.

Traumatic childhood experiences, particularly the stresses of sexual or physical abuse or parental deprivation, are associated with suicide attempts and perhaps completed suicide.

Suicide runs in families, so a family history of suicide, suicide attempts, or mental disorders is associated with an increased risk of suicide in susceptible people.

Methods

Choice of method for suicide is determined by many things, including cultural factors and availability as well as the seriousness of intent. Some methods (eg, jumping from heights) make survival virtually impossible, whereas others (eg, drug ingestion) may allow rescue. However, using a method that proves not to be fatal does not necessarily imply that the intent was less serious.

A bizarre method suggests an underlying psychosis.

Drug ingestion is the most common method used in suicide attempts. Violent methods, such as shooting and hanging, are uncommon among attempted suicides.

Some methods, such as driving over cliffs, can endanger others.

For completed suicides, men most commonly use firearms (56%), followed by hanging, poisoning, jumping from a height, and cutting. Women most often use poisoning (37%), followed by firearms, hanging, jumping from a height, and drowning.

Management

A healthcare practitioner who foresees the likelihood of suicide in a patient is, in most jurisdictions, required to inform an empowered agency to intervene. Failure to do so can result in criminal and civil actions. Such patients should not be left alone until they are in a secure environment. They should be transported to a secure environment (often a psychiatric facility) by trained professionals (eg, ambulance, police).

Any suicidal act, regardless of whether it is a gesture or an attempt, must be taken seriously. Every person with a serious self-injury should be evaluated and treated for the physical injury. If an overdose of a potentially lethal drug is confirmed, immediate steps are taken to prevent absorption and expedite excretion, administer any available antidote, and provide supportive treatment (see p. 3053).

Initial assessment can be done by any healthcare practitioner trained in the assessment and management of suicidal behavior. However, all patients require psychiatric assessment as soon as possible. A decision must be made as to whether patients need to be admitted and whether involuntary commitment or restraint is necessary. Patients with a psychotic disorder and some with severe depression and an unresolved crisis should be admitted to a psychiatric unit. Patients with manifestations of potentially confounding medical disorders (eg, delirium, seizures, fever) may need to be admitted to a medical unit with appropriate suicide precautions.

After a suicide attempt, the patient may deny any problems because the severe depression that led to the suicidal act may be followed by a short-lived mood elevation. Nonetheless, the risk of later, completed suicide is high unless the patient's disorder is treated.

Psychiatric assessment identifies some of the problems that contributed to the attempt and helps the physician plan appropriate treatment. It consists of the following:

- Establishing rapport
- Understanding the suicide attempt, its background, the events preceding it, and the circumstances in which it occurred
- Inquiring about symptoms of mental disorders that are associated with suicide
- Fully assessing the patient's mental state, with particular emphasis on identifying depression, anxiety, agitation, panic attacks, severe insomnia, other mental disorders, and alcohol or drug abuse (many of these problems require specific treatment in addition to crisis intervention)
- Thoroughly understanding personal and family relationships, which are often pertinent to the suicide attempt
- Interviewing close family members and friends
- Inquiring about the presence of a firearm in the house (except in Florida, where such inquiry is forbidden by law)
- Helping patients identify triggers to suicide planning and develop plans to deal with suidical thoughts when they occur

Prevention

Prevention requires identifying at-risk people and initiating appropriate interventions (see Table 216–1).

Although some attempted or completed suicides are a surprise and shock, even to close relatives and associates, clear warnings may have been given to family members, friends, or healthcare practitioners. Warnings are often explicit, as when patients actually discuss plans or suddenly write or change a will. However, warnings can be more subtle, as when patients make comments about having nothing to live for or being better off if dead.

On average, primary care physicians encounter ≥ 6 potentially suicidal people in their practice each year. About 77% of people who die by suicide were seen by a physician within 1 yr before killing themselves, and about 32% had been under the care of a mental health care practitioner during the preceding year. Because severe and painful physical disorders, substance abuse, and mental disorders (particularly depression) are often a factor in suicide, recognizing these possible factors and initiating appropriate treatment are important contributions a physician can make to suicide prevention.

Each depressed patient should be questioned about thoughts of suicide. The fear that such inquiry may implant the idea of self-destruction is baseless. Inquiry helps the physician obtain a clearer picture of the depth of the depression, encourages constructive discussion, and conveys the physician's awareness of the patient's deep despair and hopelessness.

Even people threatening imminent suicide (eg, those who call and declare that they are going to take a lethal dose of a drug or who threaten to jump from a high height) may have some desire to live. The physician or another person to whom they appeal for help must support the desire to live.

Emergency psychiatric aid for suicidal people includes the following:

- Establishing a relationship and open communication with them
- Inquiring about current and past psychiatric care and drugs currently being taken
- Helping sort out the problem that has caused the crisis
- Offering constructive help with the problem

- Beginning treatment of the underlying mental disorder
- Referring them to an appropriate place for follow-up care as soon as possible
- Discharging low-risk patients in the company of a loved one or a dedicated and understanding friend
- Providing these patients with the telephone number for Lifeline: 1-800-273-TALK (8255)

Treatment of depression and risk of suicide: The combination of antidepressants and some proven short-term psychotherapy is the ideal treatment for depression.

People with depression have a significant risk of suicide and should be carefully monitored for suicidal behaviors and ideation. Risk of suicide may be increased early in the treatment of depression, when psychomotor retardation and indecisiveness have been ameliorated but the depressed mood is only partially lifted. When antidepressants are started or when doses are increased, a few patients experience agitation, anxiety, and increasing depression, which may increase suicidality.

Recent public health warnings about the possible association between use of antidepressants (particularly paroxetine) and suicidal thoughts and attempts in children, adolescents, and young adults have led to a significant reduction (> 30%) in antidepressant prescriptions to these populations. However, youth suicide rates increased by 14% during the same period. Thus, by discouraging drug treatment of depression, these warnings may have temporarily resulted in more, not fewer, deaths by suicide. Together, these findings suggest that the best approach is to encourage treatment, but with appropriate precautions such as

- Dispensing antidepressants in sublethal amounts
- More frequent visits early in treatment
- Giving a clear warning to patients and to family members and significant others to be alert for worsening symptoms or suicidal ideation
- Instructing patients, family members, and significant others to immediately call the prescribing clinician or seek care elsewhere if symptoms worsen or suicidal ideation occurs

Effect of Suicide

Any suicidal act has a marked emotional effect on all involved. The physician, family members, and friends may feel guilt, shame, and remorse at not having prevented a suicide, as well as anger toward the deceased or others. The physician can provide valuable assistance to the deceased's family members and friends in dealing with their feelings of guilt and sorrow.

Physician Aid in Dying

Physician aid in dying (formerly, assisted suicide) refers to the assistance given by physicians to people who wish to end their life. It is controversial and is legal in only 5 states (Oregon, Washington, Montana, Vermont, California) and Canada; it is possible only when rules for its use are well worked out. Nonetheless, patients with painful, debilitating, and untreatable conditions may initiate a discussion about it with a physician.

Physician aid in dying may pose difficult ethical issues for physicians.

NONSUICIDAL SELF-INJURY

Nonsuicidal self-injury (NSSI) is a self-inflicted act that causes pain or superficial damage but is not intended to cause death.

Although the methods used sometimes overlap with those of suicide attempts (eg, cutting the wrists with a razor blade), NSSI is distinct from suicide because patients do not intend the acts to be lethal. Patients may specifically state a lack of intent, or the lack may be inferred by their repeated use of clearly nonlethal methods. Despite the lack of immediate lethality, long-term risk of suicide attempts and of suicide is increased, and thus, NSSI should not be dismissed lightly.

The most common examples of NSSI include

- Cutting or stabbing the skin with a sharp object (eg, knife, razor blade, needle)
- Burning the skin (typically with a cigarette)

Patients often injure themselves repeatedly in a single session, creating multiple lesions in the same location, typically in a visible and/or accessible area (eg, forearms, front of thighs). The behavior is often repeated, resulting in extensive patterns of scarring. Patients are often preoccupied with thoughts about the injurious acts.

NSSI tends to start in the early teens, and prevalence is more evenly distributed between the sexes than that of suicidal behavior. The natural history is unclear, but the behavior appears to decrease after young adulthood.

The motivations for NSSI are unclear, but self-injury may be a way to reduce tension or negative feelings, a way to resolve interpersonal difficulties, self-punishment for perceived faults, or a plea for help. Some patients view the self-injury as a positive activity and thus tend not to seek or accept counseling.

NSSI is often accompanied by other disorders, particularly borderline personality disorder, antisocial personality disorder, eating disorders, and substance abuse.

Diagnosis

- Exclusion of suicidal behavior
- Assessment of self-injury

Diagnosis of NSSI must exclude suicidal behavior.

Assessment of NSSI, as for suicidal behavior, is essential before treatment begins.

Facilitating discussion of the self-injury with the patient is essential to adequate assessment and helps physicians plan treatment. Physicians can facilitate such discussions by doing the following:

- Validating the patient's experience by communicating that they have heard the patient and take the patient's experiences seriously
- Understanding the patient's emotions (eg, confirming that the patient's emotions and actions are understandable in light of the patient's circumstances)

Assessment should include the following:

- Determining what type of injury and how many types of injury the patient has inflicted
- Determining how often NSSI occurs and how long it has been occurring
- Determining the function of NSSI for the patient
- Checking for coexisting psychiatric disorders
- Estimating the risk of a suicide attempt
- Determining how willing the patient is to participate in treatment

Treatment

- Sometimes certain forms of psychotherapy
- Treatment of coexisting disorders

The following psychotherapies may be useful for treating NSSI:

- Dialectical behavioral therapy (DBT)
- Emotion regulation group therapy (ERGT)

DBT involves individual and group therapy for 1 yr. ERGT is done in a 14-wk group setting.

No drugs have been approved for the treatment of NSSI. However, naltrexone and certain atypical antipsychotics have been effective in some patients.

Coexisting psychiatric disorders (eg, depression, eating disorders, substance abuse, borderline personalty disorder, antisocial personality disorder) should be treated appropriately. Patients should be referred to an appropriate healthcare practitioner as needed.

Follow-up appointments should be scheduled.

217 Substance-Related Disorders

Substance-related disorders involve drugs that directly activate the brain's reward system. The activation of the reward system typically causes feelings of pleasure; the specific pleasurable feelings evoked vary widely depending on the drug. These drugs are divided into 10 different classes that have different, although not completely distinct, pharmacologic mechanisms. The classes of drugs include

- Alcohol
- Caffeine
- Cannabis
- Hallucinogens (eg, LSD, phencyclidine, psilocybin)
- Inhalants (volatile hydrocarbons [eg, paint thinner, certain glues])
- Opioids (eg, fentanyl, heroin, morphine, oxycodone)
- Sedatives, hypnotics, and anxiolytics (eg, lorazepam, secobarbital)
- Stimulants (eg, amphetamines, cocaine)
- Tobacco
- Other (eg, anabolic steroids)

This classification is not based on whether a drug is legal (eg, alcohol, caffeine), illegal (eg, hallucinogens), or available by prescription (eg, morphine, lorazepam). Specific details regarding these drugs and their effects are discussed elsewhere in THE MANUAL.

The term narcotic is a legal and colloquial term. Originally, it referred to drugs that caused narcosis (insensibility or stupor), particularly opioid drugs (eg, opium, opium derivatives). However, the term is currently used so inconsistently (eg, the US government classifies the stimulant drug cocaine as a narcotic) that the term has little scientific or medical meaning.

Classification of substance-related disorders: Substance-related disorders are typically divided into

- Substance-induced disorders
- Substance use disorders

Substance-induced disorders involve the direct effects of a drug, typically including

- Intoxication
- Withdrawal
- Substance-induced mental disorders

Substance use disorders involve a pathologic pattern of behaviors in which patients continue to use a substance despite experiencing significant problems related to its use. There may also be physiologic manifestations, including changes in brain circuitry. The common terms "addiction," "abuse," and "dependence" are too loosely and variably defined to be very useful in systematic diagnosis; "substance use disorder" is more comprehensive and has fewer negative connotations.

Drugs in the 10 classes vary in how likely they are to cause a substance use disorder. The likelihood is termed **addiction liability** and depends upon a combination of factors including

- Route of administration
- Rate at which the drug crosses the blood-brain barrier and stimulates the reward pathway
- Time to onset of effect
- Ability to induce tolerance and/or withdrawal symptoms

Scheduled drugs: In the US, the Comprehensive Drug Abuse Prevention and Control Act of 1970 and subsequent modifications require the pharmaceutical industry to maintain physical security of and strict record keeping for certain classes of drugs (controlled substances—see Table 217–1). Controlled substances are divided into 5 schedules (or classes) on the basis of their potential for abuse, accepted medical use, and accepted safety under medical supervision. The schedule classification determines how a substance must be controlled.

- Schedule I: These substances have a high addiction liability, no accredited medical use, and a lack of accepted safety. They can be used only under government-approved research conditions.
- Schedule II to IV: Going from schedule II to IV, these drugs have progressively less addiction liability. They have an accredited medical use. Prescriptions for these drugs must bear the physician's federal Drug Enforcement Administration (DEA) license number.
- Schedule V: These substances have the least addiction liability. Some Schedule V drugs do not require a prescription.

State schedules may vary from federal schedules.

SUBSTANCE-INDUCED DISORDERS

Substance-induced disorders are a type of substance-related disorder that involve the direct effects of a drug; they include

- Intoxication
- Withdrawal
- Substance-induced mental disorders

Substance-related disorders that involve pathologic patterns of behavior related to drug use (eg, patients continue to use a substance despite experiencing significant problems related to use of that substance) are considered substance use disorders. The common terms "addiction," "abuse," and "dependence" are too loosely and variably defined to be useful in systematic diagnosis.

The specific manifestations and treatment of intoxication and withdrawal vary by the substance or substance class and are discussed elsewhere in THE MANUAL.

Table 217–1. SOME EXAMPLES OF CONTROLLED SUBSTANCES*

SCHEDULE	EXAMPLES
I†	Cathinone (khat) and methcathinone, GHB, heroin (and some other opioids), LSD, MDMA, psilocybin, synthetic cannabinoids
II	Amphetamines, barbiturates (short-acting), cocaine, hydrocodone (including hydrocodone combination products), hydromorphone, methadone, methylphenidate, morphine and other strong opioid agonists, oxycodone, phencyclidine
III	Anabolic steroids, barbiturates (intermediate-acting), buprenorphine, dihydrocodeine, dronabinol, ketamine, paregoric
IV	Barbiturates (long-acting), benzodiazepines, chloral hydrate, modafinil, meprobamate, pentazocine, propoxyphene, zolpidem
V	Cough suppressants containing small amounts of codeine, pregabalin

*The Drug Enforcement Administration maintains a complete alphabetical listing of controlled substances.
†Cannot be prescribed.
GHB = gamma hydroxybutyrate; LSD = lysergic acid diethylamide; MDMA = methylenedioxymethamphetamine.

Intoxication: Intoxication refers to development of a reversible substance-specific syndrome of mental and behavioral changes that may involve altered perception, euphoria, cognitive impairment, impaired judgment, impaired physical and social functioning, mood lability, belligerence, or a combination. Taken to the extreme, intoxication can lead to overdose, significant morbidity, and risk of death.

Withdrawal: Withdrawal refers to substance-specific physiologic effects, symptoms, and behavioral changes that are caused by stopping or reducing the intake of a substance. To be classified as a substance-withdrawal disorder, the syndrome must cause the patient significant distress and/or impair functioning (eg, social, occupational). Most patients with withdrawal recognize that re-administering the substance will reduce their symptoms.

Although some patients with a withdrawal syndrome have a substance use disorder, some drugs, particularly opioids, sedative/hypnotics, and stimulants, can result in withdrawal symptoms even when taken as prescribed for legitimate medical reasons and for relatively brief periods (< 1 wk for opioids). Withdrawal symptoms that develop following appropriate medical use are not considered criteria for diagnosis of a substance use disorder.

Substance-induced mental disorders: Substance-induced mental disorders are mental changes produced by substance use or withdrawal that resemble independent mental disorders (eg, depression, psychosis, anxiety, or neurocognitive disorders).

To be considered substance-induced, the substance involved must be known to be capable of causing the disorder. Substances can be members of the 10 classes of drug that typically cause substance-related disorders or many others (eg, anticholinergics and corticosteroids may cause temporary psychotic syndromes). In addition, the mental disorder should

- Appear within 1 mo of substance intoxication or withdrawal
- Cause significant distress or impaired functioning
- Not have manifested *before* use of the substance
- Not occur solely during acute delirium caused by the substance
- Not persist for a substantial period of time*

*Certain neurocognitive disorders caused by alcohol, inhalants, or sedative-hypnotics and perceptual disorders caused by hallucinogens may be long-lasting.

SUBSTANCE USE DISORDERS

Substance use disorders are a type of substance-related disorder that involve a pathologic pattern of behaviors in which patients continue to use a substance despite experiencing significant problems related to its use. There may also be physiologic manifestations, including changes in brain circuitry.

The substances involved are typically members of the 10 classes of drug that typically cause substance-related disorders. These substances all directly activate the brain reward system and produce feelings of pleasure. The activation may be so intense that patients intensely crave the substance and neglect normal activities to obtain and use it.

The common terms "addiction," "abuse," and "dependence" have often been used with regard to substance use, but these terms are too loosely and variably defined to be very useful in systematic diagnosis. Substance use disorder is more comprehensive and has fewer negative connotations.

Recreational and illicit substance use: Use of illegal drugs, although problematic because it is illegal, does not always involve a substance use disorder. Conversely, legal substances, such as alcohol and prescription drugs (and cannabis in an increasing number of US states), may be involved in a substance use disorder. Problems caused by use of prescription and illegal drugs cut across all socioeconomic groups.

Recreational drug use, although typically not sanctioned by society, is not a new phenomenon, and has existed in some form or another for centuries. People have used drugs for a variety of reasons:

- To alter or enhance mood
- As part of religious ceremonies
- To obtain spiritual enlightenment
- To enhance performance

Some users apparently are unharmed; they tend to use drugs episodically in relatively small doses, precluding clinical toxicity and development of tolerance and physical dependence. Many recreational drugs (eg, crude opium, alcohol, marijuana, caffeine, hallucinogenic mushrooms, coca leaf) are "natural" (ie, close to plant origin); they contain a mixture of relatively low concentrations of psychoactive compounds and are not isolated psychoactive compounds.

Etiology

People usually progress from experimentation to occasional use and then to heavy use and sometimes a substance use disorder. This progression is complex and only partially understood. The process depends on interaction between the drug, user, and setting.

Drug: Drugs in the 10 classes vary in how likely they are to cause a substance use disorder. The likelihood is termed addiction liability. Addiction liability depends upon a combination of factors including

- Route of administration
- Rate at which the drug crosses the blood-brain barrier and stimulates the reward pathway
- Time to onset of effect
- Ability to induce tolerance and/or withdrawal symptoms

In addition, substances that are legally and/or readily available (eg, alcohol, tobacco) are more likely to be used initially and thus risk progression to problematic use. Further, as perception of the risk in using a particular substance diminishes, there may be subsequent experimentation and/or recreational use of the drug, increasing exposures to substances of abuse. Fluctuations in perception of risk are influenced by multiple factors, including findings regarding medical and psychiatric sequelae of use and social outcomes.

During treatment of medical illness or following surgical or dental procedures, patients are routinely prescribed opioids. A substantial portion of these drugs go unused, representing a significant source for children, adolescents, and adults who wish to use them for nonmedical purposes. In response, there has been increased emphasis on the need to prescribe opioid drugs in lower amounts more appropriate to the likely duration of pain, promotion of safe storage of leftover drugs, and expansion of prescription take-back programs.

User: Predisposing factors in users include the following:

- Physical characteristics
- Personal characteristics
- Circumstances and disorders

Physical characteristics likely include genetic factors. However, although researchers have long tried to identify specific factors, they have found few biochemical or metabolic differences between people who do and do not develop substance use disorder.

Personal characteristics are not clearly a strong factor, although people with low levels of self-control (impulsivity) or high levels of risk-taking and novelty-seeking may have an increased risk of developing substance use disorder. However, the concept of the addictive personality that has variously been described by some behavioral scientists has little scientific evidence to back it.

A number of circumstances and coexisting disorders appear to increase risk. For example, people who are sad, emotionally distressed, or socially alienated may find these feelings are temporarily relieved by a drug; this can lead to increased use and sometimes a substance use disorder. Patients with other, unrelated psychiatric disorders are at increased risk of developing a substance use disorder. Patients with chronic pain (eg, back pain, pain due to sickle cell disease, neuropathic pain, fibromyalgia) often require opioid drugs for relief; many subsequently develop a substance use disorder. However, in many of these patients, nonopioid drugs and other treatments do not adequately relieve pain and suffering.

Setting: Cultural and social factors are very important in initiating and maintaining (or relapsing to) substance use. Observing family members (eg, parents, older siblings) and peers using substances increases risk that people will begin using substances. Peers are a particularly powerful influence among adolescents (see p. 2821). People who are trying to stop using a substance find it much more difficult if they are around others who also use that substance.

Physicians may inadvertently contribute to harmful use of psychoactive drugs by overzealously prescribing them to relieve stress. Many social factors, including mass media, contribute to patients' expectation that drugs should be used to relieve all distress.

Diagnosis

- Specific criteria

Diagnosis of substance use disorder is based on identifying a pathologic pattern of behaviors in which patients continue to use a substance despite experiencing significant problems related to its use. There are 11 criteria divided into four categories.

Impaired control over use

- The person takes the substance in larger amounts or for a longer time than originally planned
- The person desires to stop or cut down use of the substance
- The person spends substantial time obtaining, using, or recovering from the effects of the substance
- The person has an intense desire (craving) to use the substance

Social impairment

- The person fails to fulfill major role obligations at work, school, or home
- The person continues to use the substance even though it causes (or worsens) social or interpersonal problems
- The person gives up or reduces important social, occupational, or recreational activity because of substance use

Risky use

- The person uses the substance in physically hazardous situations (eg, when driving or in dangerous social circumstances)
- The person continues to use the substance despite knowing it is worsening a medical or psychologic problem

Pharmacologic symptoms*

- Tolerance: The person needs to progressively increase the drug dose to produce intoxication or the desired effect, or the effect of a given dose decreases over time
- Withdrawal: Untoward physical effects occur when the drug is stopped or when it is counteracted by a specific antagonist

*Note that some drugs, particularly opioids, sedative/hypnotics, and stimulants, can result in tolerance and/or withdrawal symptoms even when taken as prescribed for legitimate medical reasons and for relatively brief periods (< 1 wk for opioids). Withdrawal symptoms that develop following such appropriate medical use do not count as criteria for diagnosis of a substance use disorder.

People who have ≥ 2 of these criteria within a 12-month period are considered to have a substance use disorder. The severity of the substance use disorder is determined by the number of symptoms:

- Mild: 2 to 3 criteria
- Moderate: 4 to 5 criteria
- Severe: ≥ 6 criteria

Treatment

- Varies depending on substance and circumstances

Treating substance use disorder is challenging and includes one or more of the following: acute detoxification, prevention and management of withdrawal, cessation (or rarely, reduction) of use, maintenance of abstinence. Different treatment phases may be managed with drugs and/or counseling and support. Specific measures and issues are discussed under the specific substance elsewhere in The Manual.

With increasing evidence and greater understanding of the biologic processes underlying compulsive drug taking, substance use disorders have become much more firmly established as medical illnesses. As such, these illnesses are amenable to various forms of treatment, including support groups (Alcoholics Anonymous and other Twelve Step programs); psychotherapy (eg, motivational enhancement therapy, cognitive-behavioral therapy, relapse prevention); and medications, ranging from agonist therapy (eg, nicotine replacement therapy for tobacco use disorder, methadone and buprenorphine for opioid use disorder) to novel approaches currently under investigation. Focus on accurate identification of patients with substance use disorders and referral for specialty treatment will help greatly in reducing individual consequences as well as societal impact.

KEY POINTS

- Substance use disorder involves a pathologic pattern of behaviors in which patients continue to use a substance despite experiencing significant problems related to its use.
- Manifestations are categorized into impaired control over use, social impairment, risky use, and pharmacologic symptoms.
- The terms "addiction," "abuse," and "dependence" are vague and value-laden; it is preferable to speak of substance use disorder and focus on the specific manifestations and their severity.
- The consequences and treatment of substance use disorder vary greatly depending on the substance.

SECTION 17

Neurologic Disorders

218 Approach to the Neurologic Patient

Patients with neurologic symptoms are approached in a stepwise manner termed the neurologic method, which consists of the following:

- Identifying the anatomic location of the lesion or lesions causing symptoms
- Identifying the pathophysiology involved
- Generating a differential diagnosis
- Selecting specific, appropriate tests

Identifying the anatomy and pathophysiology of the lesion through careful history taking and an accurate neurologic examination markedly narrows the differential diagnosis and thus the number of tests needed. This approach should not be replaced by reflex ordering of CT, MRI, and other laboratory testing; doing so leads to error and unnecessary cost.

To identify the anatomic location, the examiner considers questions such as

- Is the lesion in one or multiple locations?
- Is the lesion confined to the nervous system, or is it part of a systemic disorder?
- What part of the nervous system is affected?

Specific parts of the nervous system to be considered include the cerebral cortex, subcortical white matter, basal ganglia, thalamus, cerebellum, brain stem, spinal cord, brachial or lumbosacral plexus, peripheral nerves, neuromuscular junction, and muscle.

Once the location of the lesion is identified, categories of pathophysiologic causes are considered. They include

- Vascular
- Infectious
- Neoplastic
- Degenerative
- Traumatic
- Toxic-metabolic
- Immune-mediated

When appropriately applied, the neurologic method provides an orderly approach to even the most complex case, and clinicians are far less likely to be fooled by neurologic mimicry—eg, when symptoms of an acute stroke are actually due to a brain tumor or when rapidly ascending paralysis suggesting Guillain-Barré syndrome is actually due to spinal cord compression.

History

The history is the most important part of the neurologic evaluation. Patients should be put at ease and allowed to tell their story in their own words. Usually, a clinician can quickly determine whether a reliable history is forthcoming or whether a family member should be interviewed instead.

History of present illness should include the following:

- Specific questions clarify the quality, intensity, distribution, duration, and frequency of each symptom.
- What aggravates and attenuates the symptom and whether past treatment was effective should be determined.
- Asking the patient to describe the order in which symptoms occur can help identify the cause.
- Specific disabilities should be described quantitatively (eg, walks at most 25 ft before stopping to rest), and their effect on the patient's daily routine noted.

Past medical history and a **complete review of systems** are essential because neurologic complications are common in other disorders, especially alcoholism, diabetes, cancer, vascular disorders, and HIV infection.

Family history is important because migraine and many metabolic, muscle, nerve, and neurodegenerative disorders are inherited.

Social, occupational, and travel history provide information about unusual infections and exposure to toxins and parasites.

Sometimes neurologic symptoms and signs are functional or hysterical, reflecting a psychiatric disorder. Typically, such symptoms and signs do not conform to the rules of anatomy and physiology, and the patient is often depressed or unusually frightened. However, functional and physical disorders sometimes coexist, and distinguishing them can be challenging.

Physical Examination and Testing

A physical examination to evaluate all body systems is done, but the focus is on the nervous system (neurologic examination). The neurologic examination, discussed in Ch. 220, includes the following:

- Mental status
- Cranial nerves
- Motor system
- Muscle strength
- Gait, stance, and coordination
- Sensation
- Reflexes
- Autonomic nervous system

In many situations, a cerebrovascular examination also is done.

Diagnostic tests may be needed to confirm a diagnosis or exclude other possible disorders.

219 Symptoms of Neurologic Disorders

MEMORY LOSS

Memory loss is a common complaint in the primary care setting. It is particularly common among the elderly but also may be reported by younger people. Sometimes family members rather than the patient report the memory loss (typically in an elderly person, often one with dementia).

Clinicians and patients are often concerned that the memory loss indicates impending dementia. Such concern is based on the common knowledge that the first sign of dementia typically is memory loss. However, most memory loss does not represent the onset of dementia.

The most common and earliest complaints of memory loss usually involve

- Difficulty remembering names and the location of car keys or other commonly used items

As memory loss becomes more severe, people may not remember to pay bills or keep appointments. People with severe memory loss may have dangerous lapses, such as forgetting to turn off a stove, to lock the house when leaving, or to keep track of an infant or child they are supposed to watch. Other symptoms (eg, depression, confusion, personality change, difficulty with activities of daily living) may be present depending on the cause of memory loss.

Etiology

The **most common causes** of memory loss (see Table 219–1) are

- Age-associated memory impairment (most common)
- Mild cognitive impairment
- Dementia
- Depression

Age-associated memory impairment refers to the worsening of memory that occurs with aging. In people with this condition, it takes longer to form new memories (eg, a new neighbor's name, a new computer password) and to learn new complex information and tasks (eg, work procedures, computer programs). Age-associated memory impairment leads to occasional forgetfulness (eg, misplacing car keys) or embarrassment. However, cognition is not impaired. Given sufficient time to think and answer questions, patients with this condition can usually do so, indicating intact memory and cognitive functions.

Patients with **mild cognitive impairment** have actual memory loss, rather than the sometimes slow memory retrieval from relatively preserved memory storage in age-matched controls. Mild cognitive impairment tends to affect short-term (also called episodic) memory first. Patients have trouble

Table 219–1. CHARACTERISTICS OF COMMON CAUSES OF MEMORY LOSS

CAUSE	SUGGESTIVE FINDINGS	DIAGNOSTIC APPROACH
Age-associated memory impairment	Occasional forgetfulness (eg, of names or location of car keys) but no other impairment of memory Normal cognitive function	Clinical evaluation
Mild cognitive impairment	Memory impaired Daily function not affected Other aspects of cognition intact	Clinical evaluation Sometimes neuropsychiatric testing
Dementia	Memory impaired Daily function affected (eg, finding their way around the neighborhood, or doing usual tasks at work) Impairment of at least 1 other aspect of cognition: • Impaired reasoning and handling of complex tasks (executive function) and poor judgment (eg, being unable to manage bank account, making poor financial decisions) • Aphasia (language dysfunction), causing difficulty finding words and/or naming objects • Visuospatial dysfunction (eg, inability to recognize faces or common objects) • Personality and behavioral changes (eg, suspicion, anxiety, agitation)	Clinical evaluation Sometimes neuropsychiatric testing
Depression	Memory loss often correlated with severity of mood disturbance Sometimes sleep disturbance, loss of appetite, psychomotor slowing Often present in patients with dementia, mild cognitive impairment, or age-associated memory impairment	Clinical evaluation
Drug use (eg, of anticholinergic drugs, antidepressants, opioids, psychoactive drugs, or sedatives)	Use of causative drug Often recent initiation of drug therapy, an increase in drug dose, or slowing of drug clearance (eg, caused by decrease in renal or liver function)	Typically a trial of stopping or changing the suspected causative drug

remembering recent conversations, the location of commonly used items, and appointments. However, memory for remote events is typically intact, as is attention (also called working memory—patients can repeat lists of items and do simple calculations). The definition of mild cognitive impairment is evolving; mild cognitive impairment is now sometimes defined as impairment in memory and/or other cognitive functions that is not severe enough to affect daily function. Up to 50% of patients with mild cognitive impairment develop dementia within 3 yr.

Patients with **dementia** have memory loss plus evidence of cognitive and behavioral dysfunction (see p. 1874). For example, they may have difficulty with finding words and/or naming objects (aphasia), doing previously learned motor activities (apraxia), or planning and organizing everyday tasks, such as meals, shopping, and bill paying (impaired executive function). Their personality may change; for example, they may become uncharacteristically irritable, anxious, agitated, and/or inflexible.

Depression is common among patients with dementia. However, depression itself can cause memory loss that simulates dementia (pseudodementia). Such patients usually have other features of depression.

Delirium is an acute confusional state, which may be caused by a severe infection, a drug (adverse effect), or drug withdrawal (see p. 1871). Patients with delirium have impaired memory, but the main reason they present is usually severe global changes in mental status and cognitive dysfunction, not memory loss.

Evaluation

The highest priority is

- To identify delirium, which requires rapid treatment

The evaluation then focuses on distinguishing the few cases of mild cognitive impairment and early dementia from the greater number with age-associated memory impairment or simply normal forgetfulness.

Full evaluation for dementia usually requires more time than the 20 to 30 min that is commonly allotted for an office visit.

History: History should, when possible, be taken from the patient and family members separately. Cognitively impaired patients may not be able to provide a detailed, accurate history, and family members may not feel free to give a candid history with the patient listening.

History of present illness should include a description of the specific types of memory loss (eg, forgetting words or names, getting lost) and their onset, severity, and progression. The clinician should determine how much symptoms affect day-to-day function at work and at home. Important associated findings involve changes in language use, eating, sleeping, and mood.

Review of systems should identify neurologic symptoms that may suggest a specific type of dementia, such as the following:

- Parkinsonian symptoms in Lewy body dementia
- Focal deficits in vascular dementia
- Inability to look upward and falling in progressive supranuclear palsy
- Choreiform movements in Huntington disease
- Gait disturbance in normal-pressure hydrocephalus
- Balance problems and difficulty with fine motor movements in vitamin B_{12} deficiency

Past medical history should include known disorders and complete prescription and OTC drug use history.

Family and social histories should include the patient's baseline levels of intelligence, education, employment, and social functioning. Previous and current substance abuse is noted. Family history of dementia or early mild cognitive impairment is queried.

Physical examination: In addition to a general examination, a complete neurologic examination (see p. 1835) is done, with detailed mental status testing.

Mental status testing assesses the following by asking the patient to do certain tasks:

- Orientation (give their name, the date, and their location)
- Attention and concentration (eg, repeat a list of words, do simple calculations, spell "world" backwards)
- Short-term memory (eg, repeat a list of 3 or 4 items after 5, 10, and 30 min)
- Language (eg, name common objects)
- Praxis and executive function (eg, follow a multiple-stage command)
- Constructional praxis (eg, copy a design or draw a clock face)

Various scales can be used to test these components. The most common way to test these components (see also Sidebar 220–1 on p. 1836) is with the Mini-Mental Status Examination, which requires about 7 min to administer.

Red flags: The following findings are of particular concern:

- Impaired daily function
- Loss of attention or altered level of consciousness
- Symptoms of depression (eg, loss of appetite, psychomotor slowing, suicidal ideation)

Interpretation of findings: Presence of actual memory loss and impairment of daily function and other cognitive functions help differentiate age-related memory changes, mild cognitive impairment, and dementia.

Mood disturbance is present in patients with depression but is also common in patients with dementia or mild cognitive impairment. Thus, differentiating depression from dementia can be difficult until memory loss becomes more severe or unless other neurologic deficits (eg, aphasia, agnosia, apraxia) are evident.

Inattention helps differentiate delirium from early dementia. In most patients with delirium, memory loss is not the presenting symptom. Nonetheless, delirium must be excluded before a diagnosis of dementia is made.

One particularly helpful clue is how the patient came to medical attention. If the patient initiates the medical evaluation because of worries about becoming forgetful, age-associated memory impairment is the likely cause. If a family member initiates a medical evaluation for a patient who is less worried about memory loss than the family, dementia is much more likely than when the patient initiates the evaluation.

Testing: Diagnosis is primarily clinical. However, any brief mental status examination is affected by the patient's intelligence and educational level and has limited accuracy. For example, patients with high educational levels can score falsely high, and those with low levels can score falsely low.

If the diagnosis is unclear, more accurate, formal neuropsychologic testing can be done; results have higher diagnostic accuracy.

If a drug is the suspected cause, the drug can be stopped or another drug substituted as a diagnostic trial.

Treating apparently depressed patients may facilitate differentiation between depression and mild cognitive impairment.

If patients have neurologic abnormalities (eg, weakness, altered gait, involuntary movements), MRI or CT is required.

For most patients, serum vitamin B_{12} measurement and thyroid functions tests are needed to exclude vitamin B_{12} deficiency and thyroid disorders, which are reversible causes of impaired memory.

If patients have delirium or dementia, further testing should be done to determine the cause.

Treatment

Patients with age-associated memory impairment should be reassured. Some generally healthful measures are often recommended to help maintain function and possibly decrease the risk of dementia.

Patients with depression are treated with drugs and/or psychotherapy.

Patients with memory loss and signs of depression should be treated with nonanticholinergic antidepressants, preferably SSRIs. Memory loss tends to resolve as depression does.

Delirium is treated by correcting the underlying condition.

Rarely, dementia is reversible with a specific treatment (eg, supplementary vitamin B_{12}, thyroid hormone replacement, shunting for normal-pressure hydrocephalus).

Other patients with memory loss are treated supportively.

General measures: The following can be recommended for patients who are worried about memory loss:

- Regular exercise
- Consumption of a healthy diet with lots of fruits and vegetables
- Sufficient sleep
- Not smoking
- Use of alcohol only in moderation
- Participation in social and intellectually stimulating activities
- Regular physical examinations
- Stress management
- Prevention of head injury

These measures, with control of BP, cholesterol levels, and plasma glucose levels, also tend to reduce risk of cardiovascular disorders. Some evidence suggests that these measures may reduce risk of dementia, but this effect has not been proved.

Some experts recommend learning new things (eg, a new language, a new musical instrument), doing mental exercises (eg, memorizing lists; doing word puzzles; playing chess, bridge, or other games that use strategy), reading, working on the computer, or doing crafts (eg, knitting, quilting). These activities may help maintain or improve cognitive function, possibly because they strengthen neuronal connections and promote new connections.

Patient safety: Occupational and physical therapists can evaluate the home of impaired patients for safety with the goal of preventing falls and other accidents. Protective measures (eg, hiding knives, unplugging the stove, removing the car, confiscating car keys) may be required. Some states require physicians to notify the Department of Motor Vehicles of patients with dementia. If patients wander, signal monitoring systems can be installed, or patients can be registered in the Safe Return program. Information is available from the Alzheimer's Association (Safe Return program).

Ultimately, assistance (eg, housekeepers, home health aides) or a change of environment (eg, living facility without stairs, assisted-living facility, skilled nursing facility) may be indicated.

Environmental measures: Environmental measures can help patients with dementia.

Patients with dementia usually function best in familiar surroundings, with frequent reinforcement of orientation (including large calendars and clocks), a bright, cheerful environment, and a regular routine. The room should contain sensory stimuli (eg, radio, television, night-light).

In institutions, staff members can wear large name tags and repeatedly introduce themselves. Changes in surroundings, routines, or people should be explained to patients precisely and simply, omitting nonessential procedures.

Frequent visits by staff members and familiar people encourage patients to remain social. Activities can help; they should be enjoyable and provide some stimulation but not involve too many choices or challenges. Exercises to improve balance and maintain cardiovascular tone can also help reduce restlessness, improve sleep, and manage behavior. Occupational therapy and music therapy help maintain fine motor control and provide nonverbal stimulation. Group therapy (eg, reminiscence therapy, socialization activities) may help maintain conversational and interpersonal skills.

Drugs: Eliminating or limiting drugs with CNS activity often improves function. Sedating and anticholinergic drugs, which tend to worsen dementia, should be avoided.

The cholinesterase inhibitors donepezil, rivastigmine, and galantamine are somewhat effective in improving cognitive function in patients with Alzheimer disease or Lewy body dementia (see Table 219–2) and may be useful in other forms of dementia. Memantine, an NMDA (*N*-methyl-D-aspartate) antagonist, can be used in moderate to severe dementia.

Donepezil may provide temporary improvement in memory for patients with mild cognitive impairment, but the benefit appears to be modest. No other drug is recommended to enhance cognition or memory in patients with mild cognitive impairment.

Geriatric Essentials

Mild cognitive impairment is common with aging. Prevalence is between 14 and 18% after age 70.

Dementia is one of the most common causes of institutionalization, morbidity, and mortality among the elderly.

Table 219–2. DRUGS USED TO TREAT ALZHEIMER DISEASE AND SOMETIMES OTHER FORMS OF DEMENTIA

DRUG NAME	STARTING DOSE	MAXIMUM DOSE	COMMENTS
Donepezil	5 mg once/day	23 mg once/day	Generally well-tolerated but can cause nausea or diarrhea
Galantamine	4 mg bid Extended-release: 8 mg once/day in the AM	12 mg bid Extended-release: 24 mg once/day in the AM	Possibly more beneficial for behavioral symptoms than other drugs Modulates nicotinic receptors and appears to stimulate release of acetylcholine and enhances its effect
Memantine	5 mg bid	10 mg bid	Appears to slow disease progression
Rivastigmine	Liquid or capsule: 1.5 mg bid Patch: 4.6 mg/24 h	Liquid or capsule: 6 mg bid Patch: 13.3 mg/24 h	Available in liquid solution and a patch

Aging itself accounts for most of the risk of dementia. Prevalence of dementia is

- About 1% at age 60 to 64
- 30 to 50% at age > 85
- 60 to 80% among elderly nursing home residents

KEY POINTS

- Memory loss and dementia are common and are common sources of worry in the elderly.
- Age-associated memory impairment is common, causing slowing, but not deterioration, of memory and cognition.
- Diagnosis is primarily by clinical criteria, particularly mood, attention, presence of true memory loss, and effect on daily function.
- A complete drug history is critical because sedating and anticholinergic drugs can cause memory loss that can be reversed by stopping the drug.
- Self-reported memory loss is usually not due to dementia.
- Delirium must be ruled out before diagnosing dementia.

MUSCLE CRAMPS

A muscle cramp (charley horse) is a sudden, brief, involuntary, painful contraction of a muscle or group of muscles. Cramps commonly occur in healthy people (usually middle-aged and elderly people), sometimes during rest, but particularly during or after exercise or at night (including during sleep). Leg cramps at night usually occur in the calf and cause plantar flexion of the foot and toes.

Other disorders can simulate cramps:

- **Dystonias** can cause muscle spasm, but symptoms are usually more sustained and recurrent and involve muscles other than those affected by typical leg cramps (eg, neck, hand, face, muscles throughout the body).
- **Tetany** can cause muscle spasm, but spasm is usually more sustained (often with repetitive brief muscle twitches); it is usually bilateral and diffuse, but isolated carpopedal spasm may occur.
- **Muscle ischemia** during exertion in patients with peripheral arterial disease (claudication) may cause calf pain, but this pain is due to inadequate blood flow to muscles, and the muscles do not contract as with a cramp.
- **Illusory cramps** are the sensation of cramps in the absence of muscle contraction or ischemia.

Causes

The most common types of leg cramps are

- Benign idiopathic leg cramps (leg cramps in the absence of a causative disorder, typically at night)
- Exercise-associated muscle cramping (cramps during or immediately after exercise)

Although almost everyone has muscle cramps at some time, certain factors increase the risk and severity of cramps. They include the following:

- Tight calf muscles (eg, due to lack of stretching, inactivity, or sometimes chronic lower leg edema)
- Dehydration
- Electrolyte abnormalities (eg, low body levels of potassium or magnesium)
- Neurologic or metabolic disorders
- Drugs (see Table 219–3)

Evaluation

Evaluation focuses on recognition of what is treatable. In many cases, a disorder contributing to cramps has already been diagnosed or causes other symptoms that are more troublesome than cramps.

Cramps must be differentiated from claudication and dystonias; clinical evaluation is usually adequate.

History: History of present illness should elicit a description of cramps, including their duration, frequency, location, apparent triggers, and any associated symptoms. Symptoms that may be related to neurologic or muscle disorders can include muscle stiffness, weakness, pain, and loss of sensation. Factors that can contribute to dehydration or electrolyte or body fluid imbalances (eg, vomiting, diarrhea, excessive exercise and sweating, recent dialysis, diuretic use, pregnancy) are recorded.

Review of systems should seek symptoms of possible causes, including the following:

- Amenorrhea or menstrual irregularity: Pregnancy-related leg cramps
- Cold intolerance with weight gain and skin changes: Hypothyroidism
- Weakness: Neurologic disorders
- Pain or loss of sensation: Peripheral neuropathies or radiculopathies

Past medical history should include any disorders that can cause cramps. A complete drug history, including use of alcohol, is taken.

Physical examination: General examination should include the skin, looking for stigmata of alcoholism, nonpitting edema or loss of eyebrow hair (suggesting hypothyroidism), and changes in skin moisture or turgor. A neurologic examination, including deep tendon reflexes, is done.

Pulses should be palpated, and BP measured in all extremities. A weak pulse or low ankle:brachial BP ratio in an affected limb may indicate ischemia.

Red flags: The following findings are of particular concern:

- Upper extremity or truncal involvement
- Hyperreflexia
- Muscle weakness
- Fasciculations
- Alcoholism
- Hypovolemia
- Pain or loss of sensation in a peripheral nerve, plexus, or root distribution

Interpretation of findings: Focal cramps suggest benign idiopathic leg cramps, exercise-associated muscle cramping, musculoskeletal abnormalities, peripheral nervous system causes, or an early degenerative disorder that can be asymmetric, such as a motor neuron disorder. Focal hyporeflexia suggests a peripheral neuropathy, plexopathy, or radiculopathy.

In patients with diffuse cramps (particularly those who are tremulous), hyperreflexia suggests a systemic cause (eg, ionized hypocalcemia; sometimes alcoholism, a motor neuron disorder, or a drug, although effects on deep tendon reflexes can vary by drug). Generalized hyporeflexia can suggest hypothyroidism and sometimes alcoholism or be a normal finding, particularly in the elderly.

A normal examination and compatible history suggests benign idiopathic leg cramps or exercise-associated muscle cramping.

Testing: Testing is done as indicated by abnormal clinical findings. No tests are routinely done.

Table 219–3. SOME DRUGS AND DISORDERS ASSOCIATED WITH MUSCLE CRAMPS

CAUSE	SUGGESTIVE FINDINGS	DIAGNOSIS CONFIRMED BY
Drugs		
Contributory drugs: ARBs, cisplatin, clofibrate, diuretics, donepezil, drugs with β-adrenergic agonist effects (including bronchodilators and some beta-blockers), lovastatin, oral contraceptives, pyrazinamide, raloxifene, stimulants (eg, amphetamines, caffeine, cocaine, ephedrine, nicotine, pseudoephedrine), teriparatide, tolcapone, vincristine **Withdrawal syndromes:** Alcohol, barbiturates, benzodiazepines, sedative-hypnotics	In patients taking a causative drug	Clinical evaluation, including sometimes trial of withdrawal of suspected drug
Disorders		
Extracellular fluid volume depletion and/or electrolyte abnormalities (eg, ionized hypocalcemia, low body potassium or magnesium)	Sometimes excessive sweating, vomiting, diarrhea, use of a diuretic, signs of dehydration Sometimes occurring during or after hemodialysis or during late pregnancy (probably related to low body magnesium)	Sometimes serum potassium, magnesium, and/or ionized calcium
Metabolic disorders (eg, alcoholism, hypothyroidism)	Alcoholism: History of overuse; sometimes ascites, gynecomastia, spider angiomas, testicular atrophy Hypothyroidism: Cold intolerance, constipation, fatigue, sluggish reflexes	Alcoholism: Clinical evaluation Hypothyroidism: Thyroid function testing
Peripheral neuropathies Plexopathies Radiculopathies Motor neuron disease Myopathies	Weakness, sensory loss, pain, and/or hyporeflexia in a peripheral nerve, plexus, or nerve root distribution Fasciculations In motor neuron disease, weakness that begins in one hand or foot	Clinical evaluation Sometimes EMG, nerve conduction studies, and/or spinal cord MRI
Musculoskeletal abnormalities	Tight calf muscles, a history of prolonged sitting In patients with structural disorders (eg, flat feet, genu recurvatum)	Clinical evaluation
Exercise-associated muscle cramping	Cramping of involved muscles during exercise or in the few hours after exercise	Clinical evaluation
Benign idiopathic leg cramps	Unprovoked and unexplained cramps, typically in calf muscles and at night Usually tight calf muscles	Clinical evaluation

ARBs = angiotensin II receptor blockers; EMG = electromyography.

Blood glucose, renal function tests, and electrolyte levels, including calcium and magnesium, should be measured if patients have diffuse cramps of unknown cause, particularly if hyperreflexia is present.

Ionized calcium and ABGs (to confirm respiratory alkalosis) are measured if patients have tetany.

Electromyography is done if cramped muscles are weak.

MRI of the brain and often spinal cord is done if muscle weakness is diffuse.

Treatment

- Stretching

Underlying conditions are treated when identified.

If a cramp occurs, stretching the affected muscles often relieves the cramp. For example, to relieve a calf cramp, patients can use their hand to pull the toes and foot upward (dorsiflexion).

Prevention

Measures to prevent cramps include the following:

- Not exercising immediately after eating
- Gently stretching the muscles before exercising or going to bed
- Drinking plenty of fluids (particularly beverages that contain potassium) after exercise
- Not consuming stimulants (eg, caffeine, nicotine, ephedrine, pseudoephedrine)
- Not smoking

The runner's stretch is most useful. A person stands with one leg forward and bent at the knee and the other leg behind and the knee straight—a lunge position. The hands can be placed on the wall for balance. Both heels remain on the floor. The knee of the front leg is bent further until a stretch is felt along the back of the other leg. The greater the distance between the two feet and the more the front knee is bent, the greater the stretch.

The stretch is held for 30 sec and repeated 5 times. The set of stretches is repeated on the other side.

Most of the drugs often prescribed to prevent cramps (eg, calcium supplements, quinine, magnesium, benzodiazepines) are not recommended. Most have no demonstrated efficacy. Quinine has been effective in some trials but is usually not recommended because of occasional serious side effects (eg, arrhythmias, thrombocytopenia, thrombotic thrombocytopenic purpura [TTP] and hemolytic-uremic syndrome [HUS], severe allergic reactions). Mexiletine sometimes helps, but whether using it is worth the risk of adverse effects is unclear. These effects include nausea, vomiting, heartburn, dizziness, and tremor.

KEY POINTS

- Leg cramps are common.
- The most common causes are benign idiopathic leg cramps and exercise-associated muscle cramping.
- Cramps must be differentiated from claudication and dystonias; clinical evaluation is usually adequate.
- Stretching can help relieve and prevent cramps.
- Drug therapy is usually not recommended.

NUMBNESS

"Numbness" can be used by patients to describe various symptoms, including loss of sensation, abnormal sensations, and weakness or paralysis. However, numbness is actually loss of sensation, either partial (hypesthesia) or complete (anesthesia). Numbness may involve the 3 major sensory modalities—light touch, pain and temperature sensation, and position and vibration sensation—to the same or different degrees.

Numbness is often accompanied by abnormal sensations of tingling (pins-and-needles) unrelated to a sensory stimulus (paresthesias). Other manifestations (eg, pain, extremity weakness, nonsensory cranial nerve dysfunction) may also be present depending on the cause.

Adverse effects of chronic numbness include

- Difficulty walking and driving
- Increased risk of falls

In addition, infections, diabetic foot ulcers, and injuries may not be recognized, leading to delayed treatment.

Pathophysiology

Anatomy: Sensory processing areas within the brain connect with cranial nerves or spinal cord sensory pathways. Sensory fibers exiting the spinal cord join just outside the cord to form dorsal nerve roots (except for C1—see Fig. 240–1 on p. 2027). These 30 dorsal sensory roots join with corresponding motor ventral roots to form spinal nerves. Branches of the cervical and lumbosacral spinal nerves join more distally to form plexuses and then branch into nerve trunks. The intercostal nerves do not form plexuses; these nerves correspond to their segment of origin in the spinal cord. The term peripheral nerve refers to the part of the nerve distal to the nerve root and plexus.

Nerve roots from the most distal spinal cord segments descend within the spinal column below the end of the spinal cord, forming the cauda equina. The cauda equina supplies sensation to the legs, pubic, perineal, and sacral areas (saddle area).

The spinal cord is divided into functional segments (levels) that correspond approximately to the attachments of the pairs of spinal nerve roots. The area of skin supplied mostly by a particular spinal nerve is the dermatome corresponding to that spinal segment (see Fig. 220–1 on p. 1839).

Mechanisms: Numbness can occur from dysfunction anywhere along the pathway from the sensory receptors up to and including the cerebral cortex. Common mechanisms include the following:

- Ischemia (eg, brain infarction, spinal cord infarction, vasculitis)
- Demyelinating disorders (eg, multiple sclerosis, Guillain-Barré syndrome)
- Mechanical nerve compression (eg, by tumors or a herniated disk [nucleus pulposus], in carpal tunnel syndrome)
- Infections (eg, HIV, leprosy)
- Toxins or drugs (eg, heavy metals, certain chemotherapy drugs)
- Metabolic disorders (eg, diabetes, chronic kidney disease, thiamin deficiency, vitamin B_{12} deficiency)
- Immune-mediated disorders (eg, postinfectious inflammation, such as transverse myelitis)
- Degenerative disorders (eg, hereditary neuropathies)

Etiology

There are many causes of numbness. Although there is some overlap, dividing the causes based on the pattern of numbness can be helpful (see Table 219–4).

Evaluation

Because so many disorders can cause numbness, a sequential evaluation is done.

- First, the distribution of numbness is used to localize the part of the nervous system that is involved.
- Then, other clinical features—particularly rate of onset, associated neurologic symptoms and signs, and symmetry—further narrow the differential diagnosis and thus guide further questions and tests to diagnose specific causative disorders.

Although in practice certain elements of the history are typically asked selectively (eg, patients with a typical stroke syndrome are not usually asked at length about risk factors for polyneuropathy and vice versa), many of the potentially relevant components of the history are presented here for informational purposes.

History: History of present illness should include using an open-ended question to ask patients to describe numbness. Symptom onset, duration, and time course should be ascertained. Most important are

- The location of numbness
- Associated neurologic symptoms (eg, paresis, dysesthesias, sphincter dysfunction such as incontinence or retention, dysphasia, visual loss, diplopia, dysphagia, cognitive decline)

Possible precipitating causes (eg, compression of an extremity, trauma, recent intoxication or sleeping in an awkward position, symptoms of infection) are sought.

Review of systems should identify symptoms of causative disorders. Some examples are

- Back and/or neck pain: Osteoarthritis- or RA-associated herniated disk or spinal cord compression
- Fever and/or rash: Infectious neuropathy, infectious radiculopathy, brain infection, or rheumatic disorders
- Headache: Brain tumor, stroke, or encephalopathy
- Joint pain: Rheumatic disorders
- Undernutrition: Vitamin B_{12} deficiency
- Excessive intake of high-mercury seafood: Polyneuropathy

Table 219–4. SOME CAUSES OF NUMBNESS

CAUSE	SUGGESTIVE FINDINGS	DIAGNOSTIC APPROACH
Unilateral numbness of both limbs*		
Cortical dysfunction (eg, stroke, tumor, multiple sclerosis, degenerative brain disorders)	Facial and body sensations lost on the same side, plus loss of cortical sensation (eg, agraphesthesia, astereognosis, extinction) Usually nonsensory neurologic deficits (eg, weakness, hyperreflexia, ataxia)	MRI or CT
Upper brain stem or thalamus dysfunction (eg, stroke, tumor, abscess)	Facial and body sensations lost on the same side Often cranial nerve deficits (eg, oculomotor nerve palsy on the side opposite the numbness in some upper brain stem strokes)	MRI (preferred for brain stem dysfunction) or CT
Lower brain stem dysfunction (eg, stroke, tumor, degenerative brain disorders)	Facial and body sensations lost on opposite sides (crossed face-body distribution) Often cranial nerve deficits	MRI
Bilateral numbness of the limbs or trunk		
Transverse myelopathy† (eg, spinal cord compression, transverse myelitis)	Loss of sensory, motor, and reflex function below a specific spinal segment Autonomic dysfunction (eg, bowel, bladder, and erectile dysfunction; anhidrosis)	MRI
Dorsal column spinal cord dysfunction (eg, multiple sclerosis, vitamin B_{12} deficiency, tabes dorsalis)	Disproportionate loss of vibration and position sensation In vitamin B_{12} deficiency, bilateral and symmetric findings (usually due to spinal cord dysfunction, although peripheral neuropathy may contribute)	MRI Vitamin B_{12} level, CSF cell count and protein, CSF and blood tests for syphilis
Compression of the cauda equina—also called cauda equina syndrome† (eg, due to a herniated disk or spinal or vertebral metastases)	Numbness affecting primarily the perineum (saddle area) Often urinary retention, fecal incontinence, and/or loss of sphincter reflexes (eg, anal wink, bulbocavernosus)	MRI
Polyneuropathies such as • Axonal polyneuropathies (eg, those associated with drugs, diabetes, chronic kidney disease, metabolic disorders) • Demyelinating polyneuropathies (eg, Guillain-Barré syndrome, chronic inflammatory demyelinating polyneuropathy, toxic or drug-related demyelinating polyneuropathy)	Bilateral, roughly symmetric, mostly distal (stocking-glove distribution) paresthesias and sensory deficits Sometimes weakness and hyporeflexia (eg, in demyelinating polyneuropathies)	Electrodiagnostic testing Laboratory testing based on suspected disorder
Multiple mononeuropathy—also called mononeuritis multiplex (eg, associated with connective tissue disorders, infection, or metabolic disorders such as diabetes)	Numbness with or without pain Usually motor and reflex deficits in the distribution of multiple peripheral nerves, sometimes affecting specific nerves sequentially (but may be clinically indistinguishable from stocking-glove distribution)	Usually electrodiagnostic testing and laboratory testing based on suspected disorder
Numbness of part of a single limb		
Radiculopathy‡ (eg, a herniated disk, bone compression due to OA or RA, carcinomatous meningitis, infectious radiculopathy)	Pain (sometimes like an electric shock), sensory and often motor and/or reflex deficits in a nerve root distribution (see Table 236–5 on p. 1989) Pain possibly worsened by moving the spine or a Valsalva maneuver	MRI or CT Sometimes electrodiagnostic testing

Table 219–4. SOME CAUSES OF NUMBNESS (*Continued*)

CAUSE	SUGGESTIVE FINDINGS	DIAGNOSTIC APPROACH
Plexopathy (eg, brachial or lumbar plexopathy, brachial neuritis, thoracic outlet compression syndrome)	Sensory deficits, pain, and motor deficits in part of a limb (sometimes most of a limb) in a distribution larger than that caused by radiculopathy or single mononeuropathy	Electrodiagnostic testing MRI unless the cause is trauma or suspected brachial neuritis
Single mononeuropathy (eg, carpal, cubital, radial, and tarsal tunnel syndromes; ulnar, radial, and peroneal nerve palsies)	Numbness (with or without pain) and motor and reflex deficits in the distribution of a single peripheral nerve	Clinical evaluation Sometimes electrodiagnostic testing

*Only a single entire limb may be affected; the trunk may be affected.
†Conus medullaris syndrome is a transverse myelopathy at about the L1 level. Findings are similar to those of cauda equina syndrome.
‡Findings may be bilateral.
OA = osteoarthritis.

Past medical history should identify known conditions that can cause numbness, particularly the following:

- Diabetes or chronic kidney disease: Polyneuropathy
- Infections such as HIV, syphilis, or Lyme disease: Infectious peripheral neuropathy or brain infection
- Coronary artery disease, atrial fibrillation, atherosclerosis, or smoking: Stroke
- Osteoarthritis or RA: Radiculopathy

Family history should include information about any familial neurologic disorders. Drug and social history should include use of all drugs and substances and occupational exposures to toxins.

Physical examination: A complete neurologic examination is done, emphasizing the location and neurologic territories of deficits in reflex, motor, and sensory function. In general, reflex testing is the most objective examination, and sensory testing is the most subjective; often, the area of sensory loss cannot be precisely defined.

Red flags: The following findings are of particular concern:

- Sudden onset (eg, within minutes or hours) of numbness
- Sudden or rapid onset (eg, within hours or days) of weakness
- Dyspnea
- Signs of cauda equina or conus medullaris syndrome (eg, saddle anesthesia, incontinence, loss of anal wink reflex)
- Neurologic deficits below a spinal segment
- Loss of sensation on both the face and body (on the same side or opposite sides)

Interpretation of findings: The **anatomic pattern of symptoms** suggests the location of the lesion but is often not specific. In general,

- Numbness of part of one limb: Peripheral nervous system lesion
- Unilateral numbness of both limbs (with or without the trunk): Brain lesion
- Bilateral numbness below a specific dermatomal level: Transverse myelopathy (a spinal cord lesion)
- Bilateral numbness not corresponding to a specific dermatomal level: Polyneuropathy, multiple mononeuropathy, or a patchy spinal cord or brain disorder

More specific localizing patterns include the following:

- Stocking-glove distribution: When motor signs are minimal or absent, usually an axonal polyneuropathy; when accompanied by weakness and spasticity (eg, hyperreflexia, increased tone, extensor plantar response), sometimes cervical spondylosis or a demyelinating polyneuropathy or demyelinating lesion of the spinal cord
- Single dermatomal distribution: Nerve root lesion (radiculopathy)
- Single extremity with more than one nerve or nerve root affected: Plexus lesion (plexopathy)
- Multiple related or unrelated peripheral nerves: Multiple mononeuropathy
- Loss of sensation affecting position and vibration disproportionately: Dysfunction of the dorsal columns or a demyelinating peripheral neuropathy
- Saddle area distribution: Conus medullaris syndrome or compression of the cauda equina (cauda equina syndrome)
- Crossed face-body distribution (ie, face and body affected on different sides): Lower brain stem lesion
- Ipsilateral face and body distribution: Upper brain stem, thalamic, or cortical lesion

Findings that indicate involvement of multiple anatomic areas (eg, both brain and spinal cord lesions) suggest more than one lesion (eg, multiple sclerosis, metastatic tumors, multifocal degenerative brain or spinal cord disorders) or more than one causative disorder.

The **rate of symptom onset** helps suggest likely pathophysiology:

- Nearly instantaneous (usually seconds, occasionally minutes): Ischemic or traumatic
- Hours to days: Infectious or toxic-metabolic
- Days to weeks: Infectious, toxic-metabolic, or immune-mediated
- Weeks to months: Neoplastic or degenerative

Degree of symmetry also provides clues. Highly symmetric involvement suggests a systemic cause (eg, a metabolic, toxic, drug-related, infectious, or postinfectious cause; vitamin deficiency). Clearly asymmetric involvement suggests a structural cause (eg, tumor, trauma, stroke, peripheral plexus or nerve compression, a focal or multifocal degenerative disorder).

After location of the lesion, rate of onset, and degree of symmetry have been determined, the list of potential specific diagnoses is much smaller, so that focusing on clinical features that differentiate among them is practical (see Table 219–4). For example, if initial evaluation suggests an axonal polyneuropathy, subsequent evaluation focuses on features of each of the many possible drugs, toxins, and disorders that can cause these polyneuropathies.

Testing: Testing is required unless the diagnosis is clinically obvious and conservative treatment is elected (eg, in some cases of carpal tunnel syndrome, for a herniated disk or traumatic neuropraxia). Test selection is based on anatomic location of the suspected cause:

- Peripheral nerves or nerve roots: Nerve conduction studies and electromyography (electrodiagnostic testing)
- Brain or spinal cord: MRI

Electrodiagnostic tests can help differentiate between neuropathies and plexopathies (lesions distal to the nerve root) and more proximal lesions (eg, radiculopathies) and between types of polyneuropathies (eg, axonal and demyelinating, hereditary and acquired).

If clinical findings suggest a structural lesion of the brain or spinal cord or a radiculopathy, MRI is usually indicated. CT is usually a second choice but may be particularly helpful if MRI is not available soon enough (eg, in emergencies).

After the lesion is localized, subsequent testing can focus on specific disorders (eg, metabolic, infectious, toxic, autoimmune, or other systemic disorders). For example, if findings indicate a polyneuropathy, subsequent tests typically include CBC, electrolytes, renal function tests, rapid plasma reagin test, and measurement of fasting plasma glucose, hemoglobin A_{1C}, vitamin B_{12}, folate, and thyroid-stimulating hormone. Some clinicians include serum protein electrophoresis.

Treatment

Treatment is directed at the disorder causing numbness.

Patients with insensitive feet, particularly if circulation is impaired, should take precautions to prevent and recognize injury. Socks and well-fitting shoes are needed when walking, and shoes must be inspected for hidden foreign material before wear. The feet should be inspected frequently for ulcers and signs of infection. Patients with insensitive hands or fingers must be alert when handling potentially hot or sharp objects.

Patients with diffuse sensory loss or loss of position sense should be referred to a physical therapist for gait training. Precautions to prevent falls should be taken.

Driving skill should be monitored.

KEY POINTS

- Use an open-ended question to ask patients to describe their numbness.
- The anatomic pattern and time course of symptoms helps narrow the list of possible diagnoses.
- If part of a limb is numb, suspect a peripheral nerve, plexus, or nerve root lesion.
- If both limbs are numb on one side, with or without numbness of the trunk on the same side, suspect a brain lesion.
- If patients have bilateral numbness below a specific spinal cord segment, particularly with motor and reflex deficits, suspect a transverse myelopathy.
- If patients have bilateral numbness not corresponding to a spinal cord segment, suspect a polyneuropathy, multiple mononeuropathy, or a patchy spinal cord or brain lesion.
- If numbness occurs in a stocking-glove distribution, suspect an axonal polyneuropathy.
- If numbness occurs nearly instantaneously in the absence of trauma, suspect an acute ischemic event.
- Consider doing electrodiagnostic studies for suspected peripheral nervous system causes and MRI for CNS causes.

WEAKNESS

Weakness is one of the most common reasons patients present to primary care clinicians. Weakness is loss of muscle strength, although many patients also use the term when they feel generally fatigued or have functional limitations (eg, due to pain or limited joint motion) even though muscle strength is normal.

Weakness may affect a few or many muscles and develop suddenly or gradually. Other symptoms may be present depending on the cause. Weakness of specific muscle groups can cause disorders of eye movement, dysarthria, dysphagia, or respiratory weakness.

Pathophysiology

Voluntary movement is initiated in the cerebral motor cortex, at the posterior aspect of the frontal lobe. The neurons involved (upper motor or corticospinal tract neurons) synapse with neurons in the spinal cord (lower motor neurons). Lower motor neurons transmit impulses to the neuromuscular junction to initiate muscle contraction.

Common mechanisms of weakness thus include dysfunction of

- Upper motor neurons (corticospinal and corticobulbar tract lesions)
- Lower motor neurons (eg, due to peripheral polyneuropathies or anterior horn cell lesions)
- Neuromuscular junction
- Muscle (eg, due to myopathies)

The location of certain lesions correlates with physical findings:

- Upper motor neuron dysfunction disinhibits lower motor neurons, resulting in increased muscle tone (spasticity) and increased muscle stretch reflexes (hyperreflexia). An extensor plantar (Babinski) reflex is specific for corticospinal tract dysfunction. However, upper motor neuron dysfunction can decrease tone and reflexes if motor paralysis is sudden and severe (eg, in spinal cord transection, in which tone first decreases, then increases gradually over days to weeks) or if the lesion damages the motor cortex of the precentral gyrus and not nearby motor association areas.
- Lower motor neuron dysfunction disrupts reflex arcs, causing hyporeflexia and decreased muscle tone (flaccidity), and may cause fasciculations; with time, muscles atrophy.
- Peripheral polyneuropathies tend to be most noticeable in the longest nerves (ie, weakness is more prominent in the distal limb than the proximal and in legs more than arms) and produce signs of lower motor neuron dysfunction (eg, decreased reflexes and muscle tone).
- The most common disorder of the neuromuscular junction—myasthenia gravis—typically causes fluctuating weakness that worsens with activity and lessens with rest.
- Diffuse muscle dysfunction (eg, in myopathies) tends to be most noticeable in the largest muscle groups (proximal muscles).

Etiology

The many causes of muscle weakness are categorized by location of the lesion (see Table 219–5). Usually, lesions in a given location manifest with similar clinical findings. However, some disorders have characteristics of lesions in more than one location. For example, patients with amyotrophic lateral sclerosis (ALS) may have findings of both upper and lower motor neuron dysfunction. Disorders of the spinal cord may affect

Table 219–5. SOME CAUSES OF MUSCLE WEAKNESS

CAUSE	SUGGESTIVE FINDINGS	DIAGNOSTIC APPROACH*
Brain upper motor neuron lesions		
Brain tumors Multiple sclerosis Stroke	Increased muscle tone, hyperreflexia, extensor plantar (Babinski) reflex Possibly more stiffness and loss of fine motor control (finger dexterity) than weakness (hand grip)	Brain imaging with CT or MRI
Myelopathies (involving upper or lower motor neuron dysfunction or both)		
Spinal cord compression (eg, due to spondylosis, epidural tumor, hematoma, or abscess) Cauda equina syndrome Spinal cord ischemia or infarction Autoimmune disorders (eg, multiple sclerosis, neuromyelitis optica, vasculitis) Infections (eg, HTLV-1, HIV, syphilis, human herpes simplex 6, EBV, varicella-zoster) Spinocerebellar atrophies Subacute combined degeneration Transverse myelitis Copper deficiency	Dysfunction of upper motor neurons, lower motor neurons, or both Commonly erectile dysfunction, incontinence of bowel and bladder, absence of sphincter reflexes (eg, anal wink, bulbocavernosus) Progressive limb weakness and fatigability, clumsiness, spasticity (legs first, then arms with gradual spinal cord compression) Classically dermatomal sensory level	**Tests to help identify the cause:** Possibly including vitamin B_{12} level, HIV test, ANA, RPR, NMO-IgG autoantibody (anti–aquaporin-4 antibody), HTLV-1 or VDRL, genetic testing, serum copper and ceruloplasmin, Spinal cord MRI, CT myelography, or both CSF analysis (eg, protein, VDRL, IgG index, oligoclonal banding, viral titers, PCR) Somatosensory evoked potentials
Motor neuron disorders (upper, lower, or both)		
Amyotrophic lateral sclerosis Inherited motor neuron diseases (eg, spinal muscular or spinocerebellar atrophies, including Kennedy disease) Myelopathies Postpoliomyelitis syndrome Progressive bulbar palsy Viral polio-like disorders	Progressive weakness and fatigability, clumsiness, spasticity (upper motor neuron) Hyporeflexia or flaccidity (lower motor neuron) Muscle atrophy (lower motor neuron) Fasciculations (lower motor neuron) Gynecomastia, diabetes, and testicular atrophy (Kennedy disease)	Electromyography and brain and spinal cord MRI, CT myelography, or both **Other tests:** Possibly including 24-h urine heavy metal screen to exclude lead neuropathy, anti-GM1 antibody titers (for multifocal motor neuropathy), and genetic testing (eg, for Kennedy disease)
Polyneuropathies (mostly, peripheral polyneuropathies)[†]		
Alcohol-related neuropathy Critical illness polyneuropathy Demyelinating neuropathies (eg, CIDP, Guillain-Barré syndrome) Diabetic neuropathy Drug-induced neuropathies (eg, by vincristine, cisplatin, or statins) Hereditary neuropathies Infectious neuropathies (eg, diphtheria, hepatitis C, HIV/AIDS, Lyme disease, syphilis) Multifocal motor neuropathy Sarcoidosis Toxic neuropathies (eg, heavy metals) Vitamin deficiency (eg, thiamin, vitamin B_6 or B_{12})	Hyporeflexia, sometimes fasciculations If chronic, muscle atrophy In peripheral polyneuropathy, disproportionate weakness of most distal muscles and often sensory deficits in the same (stocking-glove) distribution (common exceptions include CIDP, which affects proximal and distal nerves and muscles equally)	**Tests to confirm the presence of neuropathy:** Electrodiagnostic tests **Tests to help identify the cause:** Possibly including plasma glucose, 2-h oral glucose tolerance test, hemoglobin A_{1c} (HbA_{1c}), RPR, HIV test, folate, vitamin B_{12}, serum protein immunofixation electrophoresis, chest CT and serum ACE level (for sarcoidosis), 24-h urine heavy metals screen, anti-MAG antibodies (present in some demyelinating neuropathies), anti-GM1 antibody titers (for multifocal motor neuropathy), and genetic testing
Neuromuscular junction disorders		
Botulism Eaton-Lambert syndrome Myasthenia gravis Organophosphate poisoning Tick paralysis	Weakness that fluctuates in intensity (eg, in myasthenia gravis or Eaton-Lambert syndrome) Often, prominent bulbar findings (eg, in myasthenia gravis, botulism, or organophosphate poisoning) Sometimes hyporeflexia (eg, in Eaton-Lambert syndrome, tick paralysis, or organophosphate poisoning)	**Tests to confirm mechanism:** Electrodiagnostic testing **Other testing as needed to help determine specific disorder** (eg, acetylcholine receptor antibody, edrophonium testing for suspected myasthenia gravis)

Table continues on the following page.

Table 219–5. SOME CAUSES OF MUSCLE WEAKNESS (*Continued*)

CAUSE	SUGGESTIVE FINDINGS	DIAGNOSTIC APPROACH*
Myopathies		
Alcoholic myopathy Channelopathies Corticosteroid myopathy Cushing syndrome Hereditary muscle disorders (eg, muscular dystrophies) Hypocalcemia Hypokalemia Hypomagnesemia Hypophosphatemia Hypothyroid myopathy Metabolic myopathies Polymyositis or dermatomyositis Rhabdomyolysis Statin-induced myopathy Thyrotoxic myopathy Viral myositis	Disproportionate weakness of proximal muscles (equally) If chronic, muscle wasting With some types, muscle tenderness	**Tests to confirm mechanism:** Electrodiagnostic testing, muscle enzymes (eg, CK, aldolase), and sometimes MRI to confirm muscle atrophy, hypertrophy, or pseudohypertrophy **Tests to help identify the cause:** Possibly including muscle biopsy with special stains and genetic testing for certain hereditary disorders
Generalized muscle wasting due to illness and disuse		
Burns Cancer Prolonged bed rest Sepsis Starvation	Diffuse muscle atrophy, normal sensation and reflexes, no fasciculations Clinically apparent risk factors	Clinical evaluation

*Testing may vary; additional testing may be indicated depending on which disorders are clinically suspected.
†Multiple mononeuropathy (mononeuritis multiplex), if sufficiently widespread, may cause deficits clinically similar to those of diffuse polyneuropathies.
ANA = antinuclear antibodies; anti-GM1 = anti-ganglioside monosialic acid; anti-MAG = antimyelin-associated glycoprotein; CIDP = chronic inflammatory demyelinating polyneuropathy; EBV = Epstein-Barr virus; HTLV = human T-lymphotropic virus; NMO-IgG = neuromyelitis optica antibody; RPR = rapid plasma reagin; VDRL = Venereal Disease Research Laboratory.

tracts from upper motor neurons, lower motor neurons (anterior horn cells), or both.

Common causes of **focal weakness** include

- Stroke (the most common cause of unilateral weakness)
- Neuropathies, including those that are caused by trauma or entrapment (eg, carpal tunnel syndrome) and that are immune-mediated (eg, Bell palsy)
- Spinal root entrapment (eg, herniated intervertebral disk)
- Spinal cord compression (eg, cervical spondylosis, epidural cancer metastasis, trauma)
- Multiple sclerosis

Temporary focal weakness may occur as part of postictal (Todd) paralysis, which usually resolves over several hours, or result from hypoglycemia; with treatment, hypoglycemia and the resulting weakness resolve.

The most common causes of **generalized weakness** are

- Deconditioning due to inactivity (disuse atrophy) resulting from illness or frailty, especially in the elderly
- Generalized muscle wasting due to prolonged immobilization in an ICU (ICU myopathy)
- Critical illness polyneuropathy (ICU neuropathy)
- Common myopathies (eg, alcoholic myopathy, hypokalemia, corticosteroid myopathy)
- Use of paralytic drugs in a critical care patient

Fatigue: Many patients report weakness when their problem is fatigue (see p. 3214). Fatigue can prevent maximal effort and muscle performance during strength testing.

Common causes of fatigue include acute severe illness of almost any cause, cancers, chronic infections (eg, HIV, hepatitis, endocarditis, mononucleosis), endocrine disorders, renal failure, hepatic failure, heart failure, and anemia.

Patients with fibromyalgia, depression, or chronic fatigue syndrome may report weakness or fatigue but have no defined objective abnormalities.

Evaluation

Evaluation should try to distinguish true muscular weakness from fatigue, then check for findings that help establish the mechanism (eg, whether weakness is caused by dysfunction of the brain, spinal cord, plexuses, peripheral nerves, neuromuscular junction, or muscles) and, when possible, the cause.

History: History of present illness should begin with open-ended questions, asking patients to describe in detail what they are experiencing as weakness. Then, specific questions can be asked, particularly about the ability to do specific tasks, including brushing teeth or hair, speaking, swallowing, rising from a chair, climbing stairs, and walking.

Clinicians should also ask about the onset (sudden or gradual) and progression (eg, constant, worsening, intermittent) of symptoms. Close questioning is needed to differentiate sudden onset from sudden recognition; patients may suddenly recognize symptoms only after slowly progressive weakness crosses a threshold that prevents them from doing some normally routine task (eg, walking, tying shoes).

Important associated symptoms include sensory changes, double vision, memory loss, difficulty using language, seizures, and headaches. Factors that worsen weakness, such as heat (suggesting multiple sclerosis) or repetitive use of a muscle (suggesting myasthenia gravis), are noted.

Review of systems should seek symptoms suggesting possible causes, including the following:

- Rash: Dermatomyositis, Lyme disease, or syphilis
- Fevers: Chronic infection
- Muscle pain: Myositis
- Neck pain: Cervical myelopathy
- Vomiting or diarrhea: Botulism
- Shortness of breath: Heart failure, a pulmonary disorder, or anemia
- Anorexia and weight loss: Cancer or other chronic illness
- Change in color of urine: Porphyria or a liver or kidney disorder
- Heat or cold intolerance: Thyroid dysfunction
- Depressed mood, poor concentration, anxiety, and loss of interest in usual activities: Mood disorder

Past medical history should identify known disorders that can cause weakness or fatigue, including thyroid, liver, kidney, or adrenal disorders; cancer or risk factors for cancer (paraneoplastic syndromes—eg, Eaton-Lambert syndrome) such as heavy smoking; osteoarthritis (cervical myelopathy); and infections.

Clinicians should assess risk factors for possible causes, including those for infection (eg, unprotected sexual intercourse, blood transfusions, exposure to TB) and stroke (eg, hypertension, atrial fibrillation, atherosclerosis).

Complete drug history should be reviewed.

Family history should include known hereditary disorders (eg, hereditary muscle disorders, channelopathies, metabolic myopathies, hereditary neuropathies) and presence of similar symptoms in family members (suggesting a possible unrecognized hereditary disorder). Hereditary motor neuropathies often go unrecognized in families because of variable, incomplete phenotypic expression. Hammer toes, high arches in the feet, and poor performance in sports may indicate an undiagnosed hereditary motor neuropathy.

Social history should note the following:

- Use of alcohol: Suggesting alcoholic myopathy
- Illicit drug use: Suggesting increased risk of HIV/AIDS, bacterial infections, TB, or stroke due to cocaine use
- Occupational or other exposure to toxins (eg, organophosphate insecticides, heavy metals, industrial solvents)
- Recent travel: Suggesting Lyme disease, tick paralysis, diphtheria, or a parasitic infection
- Social stressors: Suggesting depression

Physical examination: A complete neurologic and muscle examination is done to identify localizing or diagnostic findings. Key findings usually involve

- Cranial nerves
- Motor function
- Reflexes

Cranial nerve examination (see also p. 1835) includes inspection of the face for gross asymmetry and ptosis; mild facial asymmetry can be normal. Extraocular movements and facial muscles, including masseters (for strength), are tested. Palatal weakness is suggested by a nasal voice quality; testing the gag reflex and looking at the palate directly are less helpful. Tongue weakness is suggested by inability to clearly articulate certain consonants (eg, saying "ta-ta-ta") and slurring of speech (lingual dysarthria). Mild asymmetry during tongue protrusion may be normal. Sternocleidomastoid and trapezius strength is tested by having the patient rotate the head and shrug the shoulders against resistance. The patient is asked to blink repeatedly to see whether blinking fatigues.

Motor examination (see also p. 1837) includes inspection, assessment of tone, and strength testing. The body is inspected for kyphoscoliosis (sometimes suggesting chronic weakness of paraspinal muscles) and for surgical and traumatic scars. Dystonic posturing (eg, torticollis) may interfere with movement, mimicking weakness. Muscles are inspected for fasciculations and atrophy; both may begin focally or asymmetrically in ALS. Fasciculations may be most visible in the tongue in patients with advanced ALS. Diffuse atrophy may be most evident in the hands, face, and shoulder girdle.

Muscle tone is assessed using passive motion. Tapping a muscle (eg, hypothenar) may induce fasciculations in neuropathies or a myotonic contraction in myotonic dystrophy.

Strength testing (see also p. 1838) should include muscles that are proximal, distal, extensor, and flexor. Some tests of large, proximal muscles include standing from a sitting position; squatting and rising; and flexing, extending, and turning the head against resistance. Motor strength is often rated on a 0 to 5 scale:

0: No visible muscle contraction
1: Visible muscle contraction with no limb movement
2: Limb movement but not against gravity
3: Movement against gravity but not resistance
4: Weakness against resistance
5: Full strength

Although these numbers seem objective, rating strength between 3 and 5 (the typical levels during early weakness, when diagnosis usually occurs) is rather subjective; if symptoms are unilateral, comparison with the unaffected side improves discrimination. Describing specifically what the patient can or cannot do is often more useful than simply assigning a number for level of weakness, particularly for assessing changes in weakness over time. A cognitive deficit may cause motor impersistence (inability to focus attention on completing a motor task), motor perseveration, apraxia, or incomplete effort. Malingering and other functional weakness is often characterized by give-way weakness, in which normal strength of effort suddenly gives way.

Coordination testing (see also p. 1838) includes finger-to-nose and heel-to-shin maneuvers and toe-heel tandem gait to check for cerebellar dysfunction, which can accompany cerebellar stroke, vermian atrophy (eg, due to alcohol abuse), some hereditary spinocerebellar ataxias, multiple sclerosis, and the Miller Fisher variant of Guillain-Barré syndrome.

Gait is observed for the following:

- Ignition failure (temporary freezing in place when starting to walk, followed by festination): Parkinson disease
- Apraxia, as when feet stick to the floor: Normal-pressure hydrocephalus or other frontal lobe disorders
- Festination: Parkinson disease
- Limb asymmetry, as when patients drag a leg, have reduced arm swing, or both: Hemispheric stroke
- Ataxia: Midline cerebellar disease
- Instability during turns: Parkinsonism

Walking on the toes and heels is tested; distal muscle weakness makes these maneuvers difficult. Walking on the heels is particularly difficult when corticospinal tract lesions are the cause of weakness. Spastic gait is notable for scissoring (legs flexed slightly at the hips and knees, giving the appearance of crouching, with the knees and thighs hitting or crossing in a scissors-like movement) and walking on the toes. A steppage gait and foot drop may occur with peroneal nerve palsy.

Sensation is tested (see also p. 1838); sensory deficits can help localize some lesions causing weakness (eg, sensory level localizes the lesion to a spinal cord segment) or suggest certain specific causes of weakness (eg, distal sensory loss helps confirm clinical suspicion of Guillain-Barré syndrome).

A bandlike tingling and pressure is a spinal cord sign that occurs with both intrinsic and extrinsic lesions.

Reflexes are tested (see also p. 1839). If deep tendon reflexes appear absent, they may be elicited by augmentation with Jendrassik maneuver (eg, trying to pull the hands apart while they are clasped together). Hyporeflexia may be normal, particularly with aging, but findings should be symmetric and augmentation should elicit reflexes that are otherwise absent. The plantar reflex (extensor, flexor) is tested. The following responses suggest certain disorders or locations of lesions:

- The classic Babinski reflex (the great toe extends and the other toes fan apart) is highly specific for a corticospinal tract lesion.
- A normal jaw jerk and hyperreflexic arms and legs suggest a cervical lesion affecting the corticospinal tract, usually cervical stenosis.
- Anal tone, anal wink reflex, or both are reduced or absent in spinal cord injury but are preserved in ascending paralysis due to Guillain-Barré syndrome.
- Abdominal reflexes are absent below the level of spinal cord injury.
- A cremasteric reflex can test the integrity of the upper lumbar cord and roots in males.

Evaluation also includes

- Testing for back tenderness to percussion (present with vertebral inflammation, some vertebral tumors, and epidural abscess)
- Straight leg raising (painful with sciatica)
- Checking for scapular winging (suggesting weakness of the shoulder girdle muscles)

General examination: If patients have no objective motor weakness, the general examination is particularly important; in such patients, nonneuromuscular disorders should be sought.

Signs of respiratory distress (eg, tachypnea, weak inspiration) are noted. The skin is examined for jaundice, pallor, rash, and striae. Other important findings during inspection include the moon facies of Cushing syndrome and the parotid enlargement, smooth hairless skin, ascites, and vascular spiders of chronic alcohol use.

The neck, axillae, and inguinal area should be palpated for adenopathy; any thyromegaly is noted.

Heart and lungs are auscultated for crackles, wheezes, prolonged expiration, murmurs, and gallops.

The abdomen is palpated for masses, including, if spinal cord dysfunction is possible, a grossly enlarged bladder.

A rectal examination is done to check for heme-positive stool. Joint range of motion is assessed.

If tick paralysis is suspected, the skin, particularly the scalp, should be thoroughly inspected for ticks.

Red flags: The following findings are of particular concern:

- Weakness that becomes severe over a few days or less
- Dyspnea
- Inability to raise the head against gravity
- Bulbar symptoms (eg, difficulty chewing, talking, and swallowing)
- Loss of ambulation

Interpretation of findings: The history helps differentiate weakness from fatigue, defines the time course of the illness, and gives clues to the anatomic pattern of weakness. Weakness and fatigue tend to cause different symptoms:

- **Weakness:** Patients typically complain that they cannot do specific tasks. They may also report limb heaviness or stiffness. Weakness usually has a particular pattern in time, anatomy, or both.
- **Fatigue:** Fatigue reported as weakness tends to have no temporal pattern (eg, "tired all of the time") or anatomic pattern (eg, "weak everywhere"); complaints center more on being tired than on being unable to do specific tasks.

The **temporal pattern** of symptoms is useful.

- Weakness that becomes severe within minutes or less is usually caused by severe trauma or stroke; in stroke, weakness is usually unilateral and can be mild or severe. Sudden weakness, numbness, and severe pain localized to a limb are more likely caused by local arterial occlusion and limb ischemia, which can be differentiated by vascular assessment (eg, pulse, color, temperature, capillary refill, differences in Doppler-measured limb BPs). Spinal cord compression can also cause paralysis that evolves over minutes (but usually over hours or days) and is readily distinguished by incontinence and clinical findings of a discrete cord sensory and motor level.
- Weakness that progresses steadily over hours to days may be caused by acute or subacute disorders (eg, spinal cord compression, transverse myelitis, spinal cord ischemia or hemorrhage, Guillain-Barré syndrome, sometimes muscle wasting caused by a critical illness, rhabdomyolysis, botulism, organophosphate poisoning).
- Weakness that progresses over weeks to months may be caused by subacute or chronic disorders (eg, cervical myelopathy, most inherited and acquired polyneuropathies, myasthenia gravis, motor neuron disorders, acquired myopathies, most tumors).
- Weakness that fluctuates from day to day may be caused by multiple sclerosis and sometimes metabolic myopathies.
- Weakness that fluctuates over the course of a day may be caused by myasthenia gravis, Eaton-Lambert syndrome, or periodic paralysis.

The **anatomic pattern** of weakness is characterized by specific motor tasks that are difficult to do. Anatomic patterns suggest certain diagnoses:

- Proximal muscle weakness impairs reaching upward (eg, combing hair, lifting objects over the head), ascending stairs, or getting up from a sitting position; this pattern is typical of myopathies.
- Distal muscle weakness impairs tasks such as stepping over a curb, holding a cup, writing, buttoning, or using a key; this pattern is typical of polyneuropathies and myotonic dystrophy. Many disorders (eg, chronic inflammatory demyelinating polyneuropathy, Guillain-Barré syndrome, myasthenia gravis, radiculopathies, Eaton-Lambert syndrome) cause proximal and distal weakness, but one pattern may be more prominent at first.
- Bulbar weakness can cause facial weakness, dysarthria, and dysphagia, with or without impairment of ocular movements; these manifestations are typical of certain neuromuscular disorders, such as myasthenia gravis, Eaton-Lambert syndrome, or botulism, but also certain motor neuron disorders, such as ALS or progressive supranuclear bulbar palsy.

Physical examination further helps localize the lesion. First, general patterns are discerned:

- Weakness primarily of proximal muscles suggests myopathy.
- Weakness accompanied by hyperreflexia and increased muscle tone suggests upper motor neuron (corticospinal or other

motor tract) dysfunction, particularly if an extensor plantar (Babinski) reflex is present.

- Disproportionate impairment of fine finger dexterity (eg, fine pincer movements, playing the piano) with relatively preserved grip strength indicates selective disruption of the corticospinal (pyramidal) tract.
- Complete paralysis accompanied by absent reflexes and severely depressed muscle tone (flaccidity) occurs in sudden, severe spinal cord injury (spinal shock).
- Weakness accompanied by hyporeflexia, decreased muscle tone (with or without fasciculations), and chronic muscle atrophy suggests lower motor neuron dysfunction.
- Weakness that is most noticeable in muscles innervated by the longest nerves (ie, distal more than proximal, legs more than arms), particularly with loss of distal sensation, suggests lower motor neuron dysfunction due to peripheral polyneuropathy.
- Absence of neurologic abnormalities (ie, normal reflexes, no muscle wasting or fasciculations, normal strength or poor effort during strength testing) or poor effort in patients with tiredness or with weakness that has no temporal or anatomic pattern suggests fatigue rather than true muscular weakness. However, if weakness is intermittent and is absent at the time of examination, abnormalities may be missed.

Additional findings can help localize the lesion more precisely. For example, weakness accompanied by upper motor signs plus other signs such as aphasia, mental status abnormalities, or other cortical dysfunction suggests a brain lesion. Unilateral upper motor neuron signs (spasticity, hyperreflexia, extensor plantar response) and weakness involving an arm and a leg on the same side of the body suggest a contralateral hemispheric lesion, most often a stroke. Upper or lower motor neuron signs (or both) plus loss of sensation below a segmental spinal cord level and loss of bowel or bladder control (or both) suggest a spinal cord lesion. Weakness with lower motor neuron signs may result from a disorder affecting one or more peripheral nerves; such a disorder has very specific patterns of weakness (eg, wristdrop in radial nerve injury). When the brachial or lumbosacral plexus is damaged, motor, sensory, and reflex deficits are often patchy and do not follow any one peripheral nerve pattern.

Determination of a specific causative disorder: Sometimes combinations of findings suggest a cause (see Table 219–6).

If **no symptoms or signs of true weakness** (eg, characteristic anatomic and temporal pattern, objective signs) are present and patients complain only of overall weakness, fatigue, or lack of energy, clinicians should consider nonneurologic disorders. However, among elderly patients who feel too weak to walk, determining the contribution of muscle weakness may be difficult because gait dysfunction is often multifactorial (see p. 1834).

Patients with many disorders may be functionally limited but lack true loss of muscle strength. For example, cardiopulmonary dysfunction or anemia can cause fatigue due to dyspnea or exercise intolerance. Joint dysfunction (eg, due to arthritis) or muscle pain (eg, due to polymyalgia rheumatica or fibromyalgia) may make doing physical tasks difficult. These and other physical disorders that cause complaints of weakness (eg, influenza, infectious mononucleosis, renal failure) typically are already diagnosed or are suggested by findings during the history, physical examination, or both.

In general, if history and physical examination do not detect abnormalities suggesting physical disorders, these disorders are unlikely; disorders that cause constant, generalized fatigue with no physiologic temporal or anatomic pattern (eg, depression, chronic fatigue syndrome) should be considered.

Testing: Testing may be unnecessary in patients with fatigue rather than weakness. Although many tests can be done if patients have true muscular weakness, such testing is often only adjunctive.

If **no true weakness** is present, other clinical findings (eg, dyspnea, pallor, jaundice, heart murmur), if present, are used to guide testing.

If patients have no abnormal clinical findings, test results are unlikely to be abnormal. In such cases, testing practices vary widely. If done, initial tests usually include some combination of CBC, electrolytes (including calcium and magnesium), glucose, kidney and liver function tests, thyroid-stimulating hormone (TSH), ESR, and hepatitis C serologic testing.

If **sudden or severe general weakness or any respiratory symptoms** are present, forced vital capacity and maximal

Table 219–6. FINDINGS RELATED TO WEAKNESS SUGGESTING A SPECIFIC DISORDER

FINDINGS	DISORDERS TO CONSIDER
Rapidly progressive generalized weakness; prominent ophthalmoplegia, dysarthria, and dysphagia, particularly if preceded by gastroenteritis	Botulism
Symptoms and signs suggesting dissemination of lesions in time and space, history of relapses and remissions, monocular visual loss due to optic neuritis, diplopia due to internuclear ophthalmoplegia	Multiple sclerosis
Acute or chronic weakness, dysarthria, dysphagia, hyporeflexia, excessive cholinergic symptoms and signs (eg, salivation, lacrimation, urination, pupillary constriction, abdominal cramping, diarrhea, bradycardia)	Organophosphate poisoning
Unilateral weakness, upper motor neuron signs	Single brain lesion, such as acute stroke (ischemic or hemorrhagic), tumor, or abscess
Chronic progressive quadriparesis, upper motor neuron signs, preserved cranial nerves, normal jaw jerk	Cervical myelopathy due to spondylosis
Prominent extraocular muscle palsy (possibly only diplopia during extreme gaze)	Myasthenia gravis, botulism, Miller Fisher variant of Guillain-Barré syndrome
Fatigability detected by sequential testing (eg, eye blinking)	Myasthenia gravis
Asymmetric limb weakness, dysarthria, dysphagia, prominent tongue fasciculations	Amyotrophic lateral sclerosis

inspiratory force must be tested to assess risk of acute ventilatory failure. Patients with vital capacity < 15 mL/kg or inspiratory force < 20 cm H_2O are at increased risk.

If **true weakness** is present (and usually after risk of acute ventilatory failure is assessed), initial testing typically focuses on determining the mechanism of weakness. Unless the cause is obvious, routine laboratory tests (CBC, electrolytes [including calcium and magnesium], glucose, kidney and liver function tests, TSH, ESR, hepatitis C serologic testing) are usually done.

If **brain upper motor neuron dysfunction** is suspected as the cause of weakness, the key test is MRI. CT is used when MRI testing is not possible (eg, in patients with a cardiac pacemaker).

If **myelopathy** is suspected, MRI can detect lesions in the spinal cord. It also detects other causes of paralysis that may mimic myelopathy, including lesions of the cauda equina, spinal roots, and brachial and lumbosacral plexuses. CT myelography may be used when MRI testing is not available. Other tests are done (see Table 219–5). CSF analysis may be unnecessary for some disorders diagnosed during imaging (eg, epidural tumor) and is contraindicated if CSF block (eg, due to epidural spinal cord compression) is suspected.

If **polyneuropathies, myopathies, or neuromuscular junction disorders** are suspected, the key tests that help differentiate these mechanisms of weakness are electrodiagnostic studies (electromyography and nerve conduction studies).

After nerve injury, changes in nerve conduction and muscle denervation can take up to a few weeks to develop, so electrodiagnostic studies may not help when the disorder is acute. However, these studies can help differentiate among certain acute disorders, such as acute demyelinating neuropathy (eg, Guillain-Barré syndrome), acute botulism, and other acute neuromuscular junction disorders.

If **myopathy** is suspected (suggested by muscle weakness, muscle cramping, and pain), muscle enzymes (eg, CK, aldolase, LDH) may be measured. Elevated levels are consistent with myopathy but can also be high in neuropathies (reflecting muscle atrophy) and very high in ischemic rhabdomyolysis. Also, levels may not be high in all myopathies. Regular crack cocaine use can also cause chronically moderately elevated CK levels (mean value, 400 IU/L).

Clinicians can use MRI to identify muscle inflammation, as occurs in inflammatory myopathies. Muscle biopsy may be necessary ultimately to diagnose myopathy or myositis. MRI or electromyography can help find a suitable site for muscle biopsy. However, needlestick artifact can mimic muscle pathology and must be avoided; thus, biopsy should never be done in the same muscle tested by electromyography.

Genetic testing can help confirm certain hereditary myopathies.

If **motor neuron disorders** (eg, ALS) are suspected, tests include electromyography and nerve conduction studies to confirm the diagnosis and exclude treatable disorders that mimic motor neuron disorders (eg, chronic inflammatory demyelinating polyneuropathy, multifocal motor neuropathy with conduction block). Brain MRI may show degeneration of the corticospinal tracts when ALS is advanced. Spinal cord MRI (or CT myelography) is done routinely to rule out spinal cord compression or other myelopathies (see Table 219–5).

Testing for specific disorders may be needed:

- If findings suggest myasthenia gravis, edrophonium test and serologic testing (eg, acetylcholine receptor antibody levels, sometimes anti–muscle-specific tyrosine kinase antibodies)
- If findings suggest vasculitis, autoantibody testing
- If family history suggests a hereditary disorder, genetic testing
- If findings suggest polyneuropathy, other tests (see Table 219–5)
- If myopathy is unexplained by drugs, metabolic, or endocrine disorders, possibly muscle biopsy

Treatment

Causes are treated. For patients with life-threatening, acute weakness, ventilatory support may be needed.

Physical and occupational therapy can help people adapt to permanent weakness and minimize loss of function.

Geriatrics Essentials

Some decrease in deep tendon reflexes is normal with aging, but asymmetry or absence of these reflexes with augmentation is abnormal.

Because the elderly are more likely to have preexisting sarcopenia, bed rest can cause debilitating muscle wasting rapidly, sometimes after only several days.

The elderly take more drugs and are more susceptible to drug-induced myopathies, neuropathies, and fatigue; thus, drugs are a common cause of weakness in the elderly.

Feeling too weak to walk often has multiple causes. Factors may include the following:

- Muscle weakness (eg, caused by stroke, use of certain drugs, myelopathy due to cervical spondylosis, or muscle atrophy)
- Hydrocephalus
- Parkinsonism
- Painful arthritis
- Age-related loss of neural networks mediating postural stability (vestibular system, proprioceptive pathways), coordination (cerebellum, basal ganglia), vision, and praxis (frontal lobe)

Evaluation should focus on reversible factors.

Physical therapy and rehabilitation are generally helpful no matter what the etiology of the weakness is.

KEY POINTS

- Distinguish loss of muscle strength from a feeling of fatigue.
- If fatigue has no anatomic or temporal pattern of weakness in patients with a normal physical examination, suspect chronic fatigue syndrome, an as yet undiscovered systemic illness (eg, severe anemia, hypothyroidism, Addison disease), a psychologic problem (eg, depression), or an adverse drug effect.
- If patients have true muscle weakness, first focus on determining whether weakness is caused by dysfunction of the brain, spinal cord, plexuses, peripheral nerves, neuromuscular junction, or muscles.
- If patients have hyperreflexia and increased muscle tone (spasticity), particularly if Babinski reflex is present, suspect an upper motor neuron (eg, corticospinal tract) lesion in the brain or spinal cord; MRI is usually required.
- If patients have hyporeflexia, decreased muscle tone, muscle atrophy, and muscle fasciculations, suspect a lower motor neuron lesion.
- If patients have hyporeflexia and predominantly distal muscle weakness, particularly with distal sensory deficits or paresthesias, suspect polyneuropathy.
- If patients have difficulty climbing stairs, combing hair, and standing up with predominantly proximal muscle weakness and intact sensation, suspect myopathy.
- Physical therapy is usually helpful in improving strength no matter the cause.

220 Neurologic Examination

The neurologic examination begins with careful observation of the patient entering the examination area and continues during history taking. The patient should be assisted as little as possible, so that difficulties in function can become apparent. The patient's speed, symmetry, and coordination while moving to the examining table are noted, as are posture and gait. The patient's demeanor, dress, and responses provide information about mood and social adaptation. Abnormal or unusual speech, use of language, or praxis; neglect of space; unusual posturing; and other disorders of movement may be apparent before formal testing.

As information is obtained, a skilled examiner may include certain components of the examination and exclude others based on a preliminary hypothesis about the anatomy and pathophysiology of the problem. If the examiner is less skilled, complete neurologic screening is done.

The neurologic examination includes the following:

- Mental status
- Cranial nerves
- Motor system
- Muscle strength
- Gait, stance, and coordination
- Sensation
- Reflexes
- Autonomic nervous system

Although a detailed neurologic examination can take considerable time, the fundamentals can be completed in about 4 min and can detect deficits in any of the major components. Abnormal findings trigger a more detailed examination of that component.

HOW TO ASSESS MENTAL STATUS

The patient's attention span is assessed first; an inattentive patient cannot cooperate fully and hinders testing. Any hint of cognitive decline requires examination of mental status (see Sidebar 220–1), which involves testing multiple aspects of cognitive function, such as the following:

- Orientation to time, place, and person
- Attention and concentration
- Memory
- Verbal and mathematical abilities
- Judgment
- Reasoning

Loss of orientation to person (ie, not knowing one's own name) occurs only when obtundation, delirium, or dementia is severe; when it occurs as an isolated symptom, it suggests malingering.

Insight into illness and fund of knowledge in relation to educational level are assessed, as are affect and mood. Vocabulary usually correlates with educational level.

The patient is asked to do the following:

- Follow a complex command that involves 3 body parts and discriminates between right and left (eg, "Put your right thumb in your left ear, and stick out your tongue")
- Name simple objects and parts of those objects (eg, glasses and lens, belt and belt buckle)
- Name body parts and read, write, and repeat simple phrases (if deficits are noted, other tests of aphasia are needed)

Spatial perception can be assessed by asking the patient to imitate simple and complex finger constructions and to draw a clock, cube, house, or interlocking pentagons; the effort expended is often as informative as the final product. This test may identify impersistence, perseveration, micrographia, and hemispatial neglect.

Praxis (cognitive ability to do complex motor movements) can be assessed by asking the patient to use a toothbrush or comb, light a match, or snap the fingers.

HOW TO ASSESS THE CRANIAL NERVES

1st cranial nerve: Smell, a function of the 1st (olfactory) cranial nerve, is usually evaluated only after head trauma or when lesions of the anterior fossa (eg, meningioma) are suspected or patients report abnormal smell or taste.

The patient is asked to identify odors (eg, soap, coffee, cloves) presented to each nostril while the other nostril is occluded. Alcohol, ammonia, and other irritants, which test the nociceptive receptors of the 5th (trigeminal) cranial nerve, are used only when malingering is suspected.

2nd cranial nerve: For the 2nd (optic) cranial nerve, visual acuity is tested using a Snellen chart for distance vision or a handheld chart for near vision; each eye is assessed individually, with the other eye covered.

Color perception is tested using standard pseudoisochromatic Ishihara or Hardy-Rand-Ritter plates that have numbers or figures embedded in a field of specifically colored dots.

Visual fields are tested by directed confrontation in all 4 visual quadrants. Direct and consensual pupillary responses are tested. Funduscopic examination is also done.

3rd, 4th, and 6th cranial nerves: For the 3rd (ocolomotor), 4th (trochlear), and 6th (abducens) cranial nerves, eyes are observed for symmetry of movement, globe position, asymmetry or droop of the eyelids (ptosis), and twitches or flutters of globes or lids. Extraocular movements controlled by these nerves are tested by asking the patient to follow a moving target (eg, examiner's finger, penlight) to all 4 quadrants (including across the midline) and toward the tip of the nose; this test can detect nystagmus and palsies of ocular muscles. Brief fine amplitude nystagmus at end-lateral gaze is normal.

Anisocoria or differences in pupillary size should be noted in a dimly lit room. The pupillary light response is tested for symmetry and briskness.

5th cranial nerve: For the 5th (trigeminal) nerve, the 3 sensory divisions (ophthalmic, maxillary, mandibular) are evaluated by using a pinprick to test facial sensation and by brushing a wisp of cotton against the lower or lateral cornea to evaluate the corneal reflex. If facial sensation is lost, the angle of the jaw should be examined; sparing of this area (innervated by spinal root C2) suggests a trigeminal deficit. A weak blink due to facial weakness (eg, 7th cranial nerve paralysis) should be distinguished from depressed or absent corneal sensation, which is common in contact lens wearers. A patient with facial weakness feels the cotton wisp normally on both sides, even though blink is decreased.

Trigeminal motor function is tested by palpating the masseter muscles while the patient clenches the teeth and by asking the patient to open the mouth against resistance. If a pterygoid muscle is weak, the jaw deviates to that side when the mouth is opened.

Sidebar 220–1. Examination of Mental Status

The mental status examination is an assessment of current mental capacity through evaluation of general appearance, behavior, any unusual or bizarre beliefs and perceptions (eg, delusions, hallucinations), mood, and all aspects of cognition (eg, attention, orientation, memory).

Examination of mental status is done in anyone with an altered mental status or evolving impairment of cognition whether acute or chronic. Many screening tools are available; the following are particularly useful:

- Montreal Cognitive Assessment (MOCA) for general screening because it covers a broad array of cognitive functions
- Mini-Mental State Examination when evaluating patients for Alzheimer disease because it focuses on testing memory

Baseline results are recorded, and the examination is repeated yearly and whenever a change in mental status is suspected.

Patients should be told that recording of mental status is routine and that they should not be embarrassed by its being done.

The examination is done in a quiet room, and the examiner should make sure that patients can hear the questions clearly. Patients who do not speak English as their primary language should be questioned in the language they speak fluently.

Mental status examination evaluates different areas of cognitive function. The examiner must first establish that patients are attentive—eg, by assessing their level of attention while the history is taken or by asking them to immediately repeat 3 words. Testing an inattentive patient further is not useful.

The parameters of cognitive function to be tested and examples of how to test them include the following:

Orientation	Test the 3 parameters of orientation: • Person (What is your name?) • Time (What is today's date?) • Place (What is the name of this place?)
Short-term memory	Ask the patient to recall 3 objects after about 2 to 5 min.
Long-term memory	Ask the patient a question about the past, such as "What color suit did you wear at your wedding?" or "What was the make of your first car?"
Math	Use any simple mathematical test. Serial 7s are common: The patient is asked to start with 100 and to subtract 7, then 7 from 93, etc. Alternatively, ask how many nickels are in $1.35.
Word finding	Ask the patient to name as many objects in a single category, such as articles of clothing or animals, as possible in 1 min.
Attention and concentration	Ask the patient to spell a 5-letter word forward and backward. "World" is commonly used.
Naming objects	Present an object, such as a pen, book, or ruler, and ask the patient to name the object and a part of it.
Following commands	Start with a 1-step command, such as "Touch your nose with your right hand." Then test a 3-step command, such as "Take this piece of paper in your right hand. Fold it in half. Put the paper on the floor."
Writing	Ask the patient to write a sentence. The sentence should contain a subject and an object and should make sense. Spelling errors should be ignored.
Spatial orientation	Ask the patient to draw a house or a clock and mark the clock with a specific time. Or ask the patient to draw 2 intersecting pentagons.
Abstract reasoning	Ask the patient to identify a unifying theme between 3 or 4 objects (eg, all are fruit, all are vehicles of transportation, all are musical instruments). Ask the patient to interpret a moderately challenging proverb, such as "People who live in glass houses should not throw stones."
Judgment	Ask the patient about a hypothetical situation requiring good judgment, such as "What would you do if you found a stamped letter on the sidewalk?" Placing it in the mailbox is the correct answer; opening the letter suggests a personality disorder.

7th cranial nerve: The 7th (facial) cranial nerve is evaluated by checking for hemifacial weakness. Asymmetry of facial movements is often more obvious during spontaneous conversation, especially when the patient smiles or, if obtunded, grimaces at a noxious stimulus; on the weakened side, the nasolabial fold is depressed and the palpebral fissure is widened. If the patient has only lower facial weakness (ie, furrowing of the forehead and eye closure are preserved), etiology of 7th nerve weakness is central rather than peripheral.

Taste in the anterior two thirds of the tongue can be tested with sweet, sour, salty, and bitter solutions applied with a cotton swab first on one side of the tongue, then on the other.

Hyperacusis, indicating weakness of the stapedius muscle, may be detected with a vibrating tuning fork held next to the ear.

8th cranial nerve: Because the 8th (vestibulocochlear, acoustic, auditory) cranial nerve carries auditory and vestibular input, evaluation involves

- Hearing tests
- Vestibular function tests

Hearing is first tested in each ear by whispering something while occluding the opposite ear. Any suspected loss should prompt formal audiologic testing to confirm findings and help differentiate conductive hearing loss from sensorineural hearing loss (see p. 813). The Weber and Rinne tests may be done at the bedside to attempt to differentiate the two, but they are difficult to do effectively except in specialized settings.

Vestibular function can be evaluated by testing for nystagmus (see Sidebar 91–1 on p. 785). The presence and characteristics (eg, direction, duration, triggers) of nystagmus help identify vestibular disorders and sometimes differentiate central from peripheral vertigo. Vestibular nystagmus has 2 components:

- A slow component caused by vestibular input
- A quick, corrective component that causes movement in the opposite direction (called beating)

The direction of the nystagmus is defined by the direction of the quick component because it is easier to see. Nystagmus may be rotary, vertical, or horizontal and may occur spontaneously, with gaze, or with head motion.

When trying to differentiate central from peripheral causes of vertigo, the following guidelines are reliable and should be considered at the onset:

- There are no central causes of unilateral hearing loss because peripheral sensory input from the 2 ears is combined virtually instantaneously as the peripheral nerves enter the pons.
- There are no peripheral causes of CNS signs. If a CNS sign (eg cerebellar ataxia) appears at the same time as the vertigo, the localization is virtually certain to be central.

Evaluation of vertigo using nystagmus testing is particularly useful in the following situations:

- When patients are having vertigo during the examination
- When patients have acute vestibular syndrome
- When patients have episodic, positional vertigo

If patients have acute vertigo during the examination, nystagmus is usually apparent during inspection. However, visual fixation can suppress nystagmus. In such cases, the patient is asked to wear +30 diopter or Frenzel lenses to prevent visual fixation so that nystagmus, if present, can be observed. Clues that help differentiate central from peripheral vertigo in these patients include the following:

- If nystagmus is absent with visual fixation but present with Frenzel lenses, it is probably peripheral.
- If nystagmus changes direction (eg, from one side to the other when, for example, the direction of gaze changes), it is probably central. However, absence of this finding does not exclude central causes.

If nystagmus is peripheral, the eyes beat away from the dysfunctional side.

When evaluating patients with acute vestibular syndrome (rapid onset of severe vertigo, nausea and vomiting, spontaneous nystagmus, and postural instability), the most important maneuver to help differentiate central vertigo from peripheral vertigo is the head thrust maneuver. With the patient sitting, the examiner holds the patient's head and asks the patient to focus on an object, such as the examiner's nose. The examiner then suddenly and rapidly turns the patient's head about 20° to the right or left. Normally, the eyes stay focused on the object (via the vestibular ocular reflex). Other findings are interpreted as follows:

- If the eyes temporarily move away from the object and then a frontal corrective saccade returns the eyes to the object, nystagmus is probably peripheral (eg, vestibular neuronitis). The vestibular apparatus on one side is dysfunctional. The faster the head is turned, the more obvious is the corrective saccade.
- If the eyes stay focused on the object and there is no need for a corrective saccade, nystagmus is probably central (eg, cerebellar stroke).

When vertigo is episodic and provoked by positional change, the Dix-Hallpike (or Barany) maneuver is done to test for obstruction of the posterior semicircular canal with displaced otoconial crystals (ie, for benign paroxysmal positional vertigo [BPPV]). In this maneuver, the patient sits upright on the examining table. The patient is rapidly lowered backward to a supine position with the head extended 45° below the horizontal plane (over the edge of the examining table) and rotated 45° to one side (eg, to the right side). Direction and duration of nystagmus and development of vertigo are noted. The patient is returned to an upright position, and the maneuver is repeated with rotation to the other side. Nystagmus secondary to BPPV has the following nearly pathognomonic characteristics:

- A latency period of 5 to 10 sec
- Usually, vertical (upward-beating) nystagmus when the eyes are turned away from the affected ear and rotary nystagmus when the eyes are turned toward the affected ear
- Nystagmus that fatigues when the Dix-Hallpike maneuver is repeated

In contrast, positional vertigo and nystagmus related to CNS dysfunction have no latency period and do not fatigue.

The Epley canalith repositioning maneuver (see Fig. 95–2 on p. 821). can be done for both sides to help confirm the diagnosis of BPPV. If the patient has BPPV, there is a high probability (up to 90%) that the symptoms will disappear after the Epley maneuver, and results of a repeat Dix-Hallpike maneuver will then be negative.

9th and 10th cranial nerves: The 9th (glossopharyngeal) and 10th (vagus) cranial nerves are usually evaluated together. Whether the palate elevates symmetrically when the patient says "ah" is noted. If one side is paretic, the uvula is lifted away from the paretic side. A tongue blade can be used to touch one side of the posterior pharynx, then the other, and symmetry of the gag reflex is observed; bilateral absence of the gag reflex is common among healthy people and may not be significant.

In an unresponsive, intubated patient, suctioning the endotracheal tube normally triggers coughing.

If hoarseness is noted, the vocal cords are inspected. Isolated hoarseness (with normal gag and palatal elevation) should prompt a search for lesions (eg, mediastinal lymphoma, aortic aneurysm) compressing the recurrent laryngeal nerve.

11th cranial nerve: The 11th (spinal accessory) cranial nerve is evaluated by testing the muscles it supplies:

- For the sternocleidomastoid, the patient is asked to turn the head against resistance supplied by the examiner's hand while the examiner palpates the active muscle (opposite the turned head).
- For the upper trapezius, the patient is asked to elevate the shoulders against resistance supplied by the examiner.

12th cranial nerve: The 12th (hypoglossal) cranial nerve is evaluated by asking the patient to extend the tongue and inspecting it for atrophy, fasciculations, and weakness (deviation is toward the side of a lesion).

HOW TO ASSESS THE MOTOR SYSTEM

The limbs and shoulder girdle should be fully exposed, then inspected for the following:

- Atrophy
- Hypertrophy
- Asymmetric development
- Fasciculations
- Myotonia
- Tremor
- Other involuntary movements, including chorea (brief, jerky movements), athetosis (continuous, writhing movements), and myoclonus (shocklike contractions of a muscle)

Passive flexion and extension of the limbs in a relaxed patient provide information about muscle tone.

Atrophy is indicated by decreased muscle bulk, but bilateral atrophy or atrophy in large or concealed muscles, unless advanced, may not be obvious. In the elderly, loss of some muscle mass is common.

Hypertrophy occurs when one muscle must work harder to compensate for weakness in another; pseudohypertrophy occurs when muscle tissue is replaced by excessive connective tissue or nonfunctional material (eg, amyloid).

Fasciculations (brief, fine, irregular twitches of the muscle visible under the skin) are relatively common. Although they can occur in normal muscle, particularly in calf muscles of the elderly, fasciculations frequently indicate lesions of the lower motor neuron (eg, nerve degeneration or injury and regeneration).

Myotonia (slowed relaxation of muscle after a sustained contraction or direct percussion of the muscle) indicates myotonic dystrophy and may be demonstrated by inability to quickly open a clenched hand.

Increased resistance followed by relaxation (clasp-knife phenomenon) and spasticity indicates upper motor neuron lesions.

Lead-pipe rigidity (uniform rigidity throughout the range of motion), often with cogwheeling, suggests a basal ganglia disorder.

HOW TO ASSESS MUSCLE STRENGTH

Patients who report weakness may mean fatigue, clumsiness, or true muscle weakness. Thus, the examiner must define the precise character of symptoms, including exact location, time of occurrence, precipitating and ameliorating factors, and associated symptoms and signs.

Limbs are inspected for weakness (when extended, a weak limb drifts downward), tremor, and other involuntary movements. The strength of specific muscle groups is tested against resistance, and one side of the body is compared with the other. However, pain may preclude a full effort during strength testing.

With hysterical or factitious weakness, resistance to movement may be initially normal, followed by a sudden giving way, or patients may not use supporting muscles appropriately. For example, patients with true deltoid weakness use accessory muscles that tilt their trunk and neck away from the weak deltoid because they want to prevent the examiner from overcoming their weakness. In contrast, in patients with factitious deltoid weakness (eg, due to malingering), the shoulder and head tilt toward the weak deltoid as the muscle is overcome, indicating their lack of effort.

Subtle weakness may be indicated by decreased arm swing while walking, pronator drift in an outstretched arm, decreased spontaneous use of a limb, an externally rotated leg, slowing of rapid alternating movements, or impairment of fine dexterity (eg, ability to fasten a button, open a safety pin, or remove a match from its box).

Strength should be graded. The following scale, originally developed by The Medical Research Council of the United Kingdom, is now used universally:

0: No visible muscle contraction
1: Visible muscle contraction with no or trace movement
2: Limb movement, but not against gravity
3: Movement against gravity but not resistance
4: Movement against at least some resistance supplied by the examiner
5: Full strength

The difficulty with this and similar scales is the large range in strength possible between grades 4 and 5.

Distal strength can be semiquantitatively measured with a handgrip ergometer or with an inflated BP cuff squeezed by the patient.

Functional testing often provides a better picture of the relationship between strength and disability. As the patient does various maneuvers, deficiencies are noted and quantified as much as possible (eg, number of squats done or steps climbed). Rising from a squatting position or stepping onto a chair tests proximal leg strength; walking on the heels and on tiptoe tests distal strength. Pushing with the arms to get out of a chair indicates quadriceps weakness. Swinging the body to move the arms indicates shoulder girdle weakness. Rising from the supine position by turning prone, kneeling, and using the hands to climb up the thighs and slowly push erect (Gowers sign) suggests pelvic girdle weakness.

HOW TO ASSESS GAIT, STANCE, AND COORDINATION

Normal gait, stance, and coordination require integrity of the motor, vestibular, cerebellar, and proprioceptive pathways (see also p. 1928). A lesion in any of the pathways causes characteristic deficits:

- Patients with cerebellar ataxia require a wide gait for stability.
- Footdrop causes a steppage gait (lifting the leg higher than normal to avoid catching the foot on surface irregularities).
- Pelvic muscle weakness causes waddling.
- Spastic leg causes scissoring and circumduction.
- Patients with impaired proprioception must constantly observe placement of their feet to avoid tripping or falling.

Coordination can be tested with finger-to-nose or knee-to-shin maneuvers, which help detect ataxic movements.

HOW TO ASSESS SENSATION

For the **ability to sense a sharp object,** the best screening test uses a safety pin or other sharp object to lightly prick the face, torso, and 4 limbs; the patient is asked whether the pinprick feels the same on both sides and whether the sensation is dull or sharp. The sharp object is discarded after use to avoid potential transmission of bloodborne disorders (eg, HIV infection, hepatitis).

Cortical sensory function is evaluated by asking the patient to identify a familiar object (eg, coin, key) placed in the palm of the hand (stereognosis) and numbers written on the palm (graphesthesia) and to distinguish between 1 and 2 simultaneous, closely placed pinpricks on the fingertips (2-point discrimination).

Another indicator of impaired cortical sensory function is extinction, which is inability to identify a stimulus on one side—one that can be identified when one side of the body is tested at a time—when both sides of the body are tested simultaneously. For example, when extinction is present, patients report feeling sensation on only one side when simultaneously touched on both sides even though they can feel sensation on both sides when one side is tested at a time.

Temperature sense is usually tested with a cold tuning fork.

Joint position sense is tested by moving the terminal phalanges of the patient's fingers, then the toes, up or down a few degrees. If the patient cannot identify these tiny movements with eyes closed, larger up-and-down movements are tried before testing the next most proximal joints (eg, testing the ankles if toe movement is not perceived).

Pseudoathetosis refers to involuntary writhing, snakelike movements of a limb that result from severe loss of position sense; motor pathways, including those of the basal ganglia, are preserved. The brain cannot sense where the limb is in space so the limb moves on its own, and the patient must use vision to control the limb's movements. Typically, when the eyes are closed, the patient cannot locate the limb in space.

Inability to stand with feet together and eyes closed (Romberg test) indicates impaired position sense in the lower extremities. When cerebellar disease is present, the patient tries to stand with the feet apart but as close together as possible without falling and only then closes the eyes. Rarely, a positive result is due to severe bilateral loss of vestibular function (eg, aminoglycoside toxicity).

To test **vibration sense,** the examiner places a finger under the patient's distal interphalangeal joint and presses a lightly tapped 128-cycle tuning fork on top of the joint. The patient should note the end of vibration about the same time as the examiner, who feels it through the patient's joint.

Light touch is tested with a cotton wisp.

If sensation is impaired, the anatomic pattern suggests location of the lesion (see Figs. 220–1, 220–2, and 220–3):

- Stocking-glove distribution: Distal peripheral nerves
- Single dermatomal or nerve branch distribution: Isolated nerves (mononeuritis multiplex) or nerve roots (radiculopathy)
- Patchy sensory, motor, and reflex deficits in a limb: Brachial or pelvic plexus
- Sensation reduced below a certain dermatomal level: Spinal cord
- Saddle area sensory loss: Cauda equina
- Crossed face-body pattern: Brain stem
- Hemisensory loss: Brain
- Midline hemisensory loss: Thalamus or functional (psychiatric)

Location of the lesion is confirmed by determining whether motor weakness and reflex changes follow a similar pattern.

HOW TO ASSESS REFLEXES

Deep tendon reflexes: Deep tendon (muscle stretch) reflex testing evaluates afferent nerves, synaptic connections within the spinal cord, motor nerves, and descending motor pathways. Lower motor neuron lesions (eg, affecting the anterior horn cell, spinal root, or peripheral nerve) depress reflexes; upper motor neuron lesions (ie, non–basal ganglia disorders anywhere above the anterior horn cell) increase reflexes.

Reflexes tested include the following:

- Biceps (innervated by C5 and C6)
- Radial brachialis (by C6)
- Triceps (by C7)
- Distal finger flexors (by C8)
- Quadriceps knee jerk (by L4)
- Ankle jerk (by S1)
- Jaw jerk (by the 5th cranial nerve)

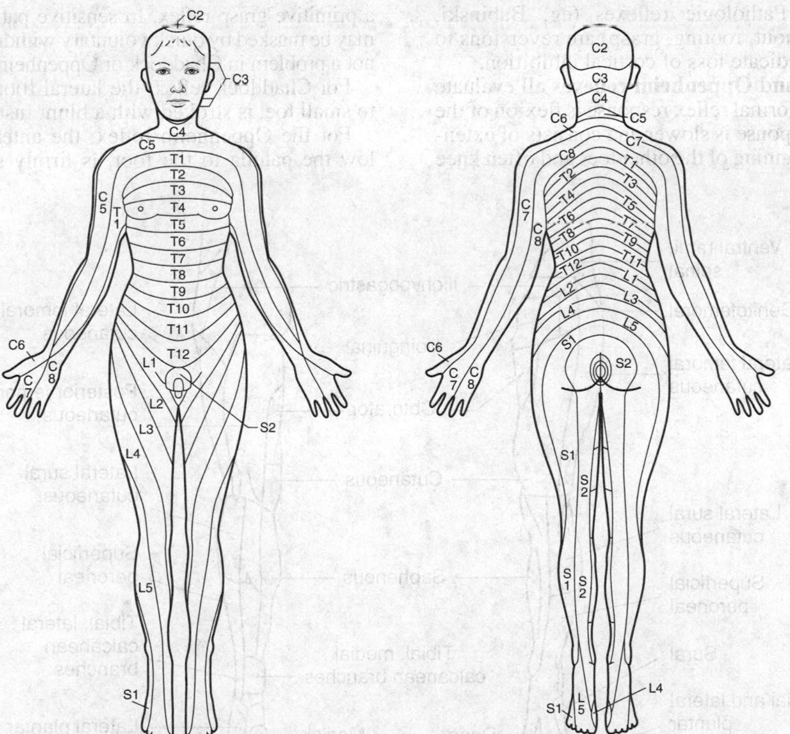

Fig. 220–1. Sensory dermatomes. In the anterior chest, T2 and C4 dermatomes usually adjoin one another (over or excluding C5 and T1, which cover mostly the arms). (Redrawn from Keegan JJ, Garrett FD, *Anatomical Record* 102:409–437, 1948; used with permission of The Wistar Institute, Philadelphia, Pennsylvania.)

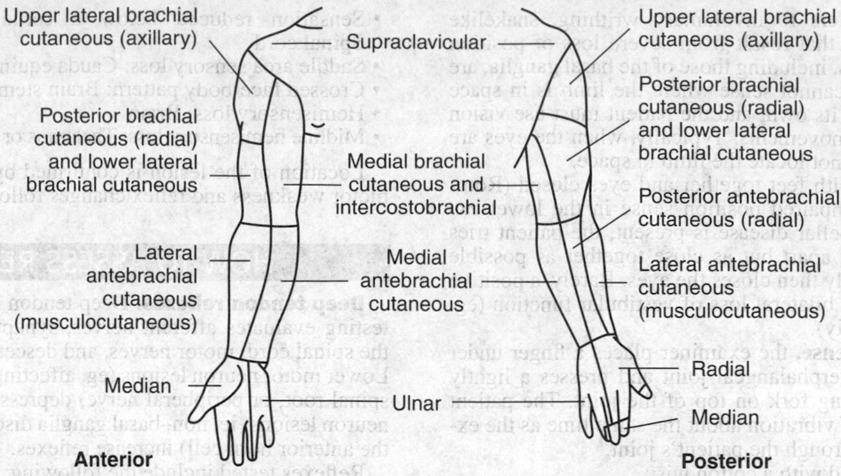

Fig. 220–2. Cutaneous nerve distribution: upper limb. (Redrawn from *Anatomy,* ed. 5, edited by R O' Rahilly. Philadelphia, WB Saunders Company, 1986; used with permission.)

Any asymmetric increase or depression is noted. Jendrassik maneuver can be used to augment hypoactive reflexes: The patient locks the hands together and pulls vigorously apart as a tendon in the lower extremity is tapped. Alternatively, the patient can push the knees together against each other, while the upper limb tendon is tested.

Pathologic reflexes: Pathologic reflexes (eg, Babinski, Chaddock, Oppenheim, snout, rooting, grasp) are reversions to primitive responses and indicate loss of cortical inhibition.

Babinski, Chaddock, and Oppenheim reflexes all evaluate the plantar response. The normal reflex response is flexion of the great toe. An abnormal response is slower and consists of extension of the great toe with fanning of the other toes and often knee and hip flexion. This reaction is of spinal reflex origin and indicates spinal disinhibition due to an upper motor neuron lesion.

For Babinski reflex, the lateral sole of the foot is firmly stroked from the heel to the ball of the foot with a tongue blade or end of a reflex hammer. The stimulus must be noxious but not injurious; stroking should not veer too medially, or it may inadvertently induce a primitive grasp reflex. In sensitive patients, the reflex response may be masked by quick voluntary withdrawal of the foot, which is not a problem in Chaddock or Oppenheim reflex testing.

For Chaddock reflex, the lateral foot, from lateral malleolus to small toe, is stroked with a blunt instrument.

For the Oppenheim reflex, the anterior tibia, from just below the patella to the foot, is firmly stroked with a knuckle.

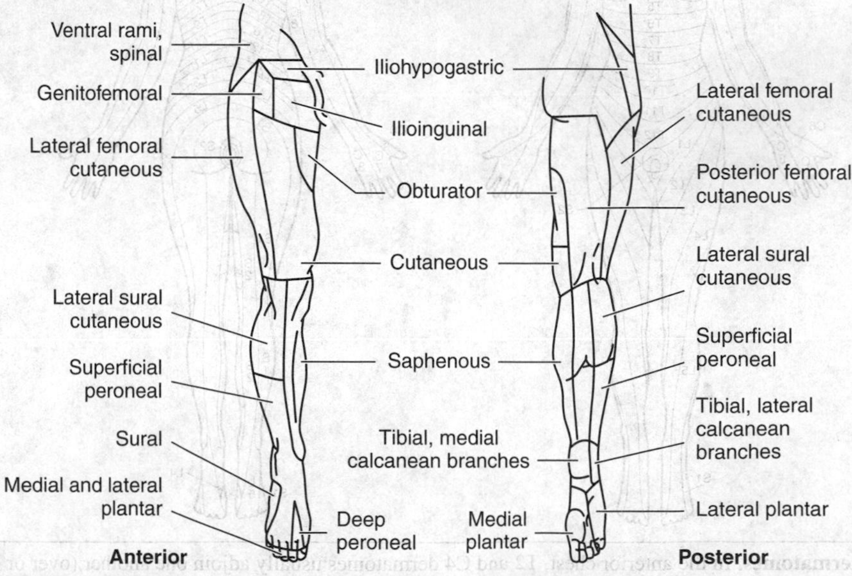

Fig. 220–3. Cutaneous nerve distribution: lower limb. (Redrawn from *Anatomy,* ed. 5, edited by R O' Rahilly. Philadelphia, WB Saunders Company, 1986; used with permission.)

The Oppenheim test may be used with the Babinski test or the Chaddock test to make withdrawal less likely.

The **snout reflex** is present if tapping a tongue blade across the lips causes pursing of the lips.

The **rooting reflex** is present if stroking the lateral upper lip causes movement of the mouth toward the stimulus.

The **grasp reflex** is present if gently stroking the palm of the patient's hand causes the fingers to flex and grasp the examiner's finger.

The **palmomental reflex** is present if stroking the palm of the hand causes contraction of the ipsilateral mentalis muscle of the lower lip.

Hoffmann sign is present if flicking down on the nail on the 3rd or 4th finger elicits involuntary flexion of the distal phalanx of the thumb and index finger.

Tromner sign is similar to the Hoffman sign, but the finger is flicked upward.

For the **glabellar sign**, the forehead is tapped to induce blinking; normally, each of the first 5 taps induces a single blink, then the reflex fatigues. Blinking persists in patients with diffuse cerebral dysfunction.

Other reflexes: Testing for **clonus** (rhythmic, rapid alternation of muscle contraction and relaxation caused by sudden, passive tendon stretching) is done by rapid dorsiflexion of the foot at the ankle. Sustained clonus indicates an upper motor neuron disorder.

The **superficial abdominal reflex** is elicited by lightly stroking the 4 quadrants of the abdomen near the umbilicus with a wooden cotton applicator stick or similar tool. The normal response is contraction of the abdominal muscles causing the umbilicus to move toward the area being stroked. Stroking the skin toward the umbilicus is recommended to rule out the possibility that movement was caused by the skin being dragged by the stroking. Depression of this reflex may be due to a central lesion, obesity, or lax skeletal muscles (eg, after pregnancy); its absence may indicate spinal cord injury.

Sphincteric reflexes may be tested during the rectal examination. To test sphincteric tone (S2 to S4 nerve root levels), the examiner inserts a gloved finger into the rectum and asks the patient to squeeze it. Alternatively, the perianal region is touched lightly with a cotton wisp; the normal response is contraction of the external anal sphincter (anal wink reflex). Rectal tone typically becomes lax in patients with acute spinal cord injury or cauda equine syndrome.

For the **bulbospongiosus reflex**, which tests S2 to S4 levels, the dorsum of the penis is tapped; normal response is contraction of the bulbospongiosus muscle.

For the **cremasteric reflex**, which tests the L2 level, the medial thigh 7.6 cm (3 in) below the inguinal crease is stroked upward; normal response is elevation of the ipsilateral testis.

HOW TO ASSESS THE AUTONOMIC NERVOUS SYSTEM

Assessment of the autonomic nervous system involves checking for the following:

- Postural hypotension
- Heart rate changes in response to the Valsalva maneuver
- Decreased or absent sweating
- Evidence of Horner syndrome (unilateral ptosis, pupillary constriction, facial anhidrosis)

Disturbances of bowel, bladder, sexual, and hypothalamic function should be noted.

CEREBROVASCULAR EXAMINATION

In a patient presenting with acute stroke, radial pulse and BP in the 2 arms are compared to check for painless aortic dissection, which can occlude a carotid artery and cause stroke. The skin, sclerae, fundi, oral mucosae, and nail beds are inspected for hemorrhages and evidence of cholesterol or septic emboli.

Auscultation over the heart can detect new or evolving murmurs and arrhythmias. Bruits over the cranium may indicate an arteriovenous malformation or fistula or, occasionally, redirected blood flow across the circle of Willis after carotid occlusion. Auscultation over the carotid arteries can detect bruits near the bifurcation; vigorous palpation should be avoided. By running the bell of the stethoscope down the neck toward the heart, the examiner may identify a change in character that can distinguish a bruit from a systolic heart murmur. Decreased vigor of the carotid upstroke or a bruit that continues into diastole suggests severe stenosis.

Peripheral pulses are palpated to check for peripheral vascular disease. The temporal arteries are palpated; enlargement or tenderness may suggest temporal arteritis.

221 Neurologic Tests and Procedures

COMPUTED TOMOGRAPHY IN NEUROLOGIC DISORDERS

CT provides rapid, noninvasive imaging of the brain and skull. CT is superior to magnetic resonance imaging (MRI) in visualizing fine bone detail in (but not the contents of) the posterior fossa, base of the skull, and spinal canal.

Noncontrast CT is used to rapidly detect acute hemorrhage and various gross structural changes without concern about contrast allergy or renal failure.

A radiopaque contrast agent helps detect brain tumors and abscesses. With an intrathecal agent, CT can outline abnormalities encroaching on the brain stem, spinal cord, or spinal nerve roots (eg, meningeal carcinoma, herniated disk) and may detect a syrinx in the spinal cord.

CT angiography using a contrast agent can show the cerebral blood vessels, obviating the need for MRI or angiography.

Adverse effects of contrast agents include allergic reactions and contrast nephropathy (see p. 3222).

ELECTROENCEPHALOGRAPHY

Electrodes are distributed over the brain to detect electrical changes associated with

- Seizure disorders
- Sleep disorders
- Metabolic or structural encephalopathies

Twenty electrodes are distributed symmetrically over the scalp.

The normal awake electroencephalography (EEG) shows 8- to 12-Hz, 50-μV sinusoidal alpha waves that wax and wane over the occipital and parietal lobes and > 12-Hz, 10- to 20-μV beta waves frontally, interspersed with 4- to 7-Hz, 20- to 100-uV theta waves.

The EEG is examined for asymmetries between the 2 hemispheres (suggesting a structural disorder), for excessive slowing (appearance of 1- to 4-Hz, 50- to 350-μV delta waves, as occurs in depressed consciousness, encephalopathy, and dementia), and for abnormal wave patterns.

Abnormal wave patterns may be nonspecific (eg, epileptiform sharp waves) or diagnostic (eg, 3-Hz spike and wave discharges for absence seizures, 1-Hz periodic sharp waves for Creutzfeldt-Jakob disease).

The EEG is particularly useful for appraising episodic altered consciousness of uncertain etiology.

If a seizure disorder is suspected and the routine EEG is normal, maneuvers that electrically activate the cortex (eg, hyperventilation, photic stimulation, sleep, sleep deprivation) can sometimes elicit evidence of a seizure disorder. Nasopharyngeal leads can sometimes detect a temporal lobe seizure focus when the EEG is otherwise uninformative. Continuous ambulatory monitoring of the EEG (with or without video monitoring) over 24 h can often determine whether fleeting memory lapses, subjective auras, or unusual episodic motor behavior is due to seizure activity.

If clinicians need to determine whether an episode is a seizure or a psychiatric disorder, a video camera may be used to monitor the patient while EEG is done in the hospital. This technique (called video EEG) is also used before surgery to see what type of seizure results from an abnormality in a particular epileptogenic focus.

ELECTROMYOGRAPHY AND NERVE CONDUCTION STUDIES

When determining whether weakness is due to a nerve, muscle, or neuromuscular junction disorder is clinically difficult, these studies can identify the affected nerves and muscles.

Electromyography: In electromyography (EMG), a needle is inserted in a muscle, and electrical activity is recorded while the muscle is contracting and resting. Normally, resting muscle is electrically silent; with minimal contraction, action potentials of single motor units appear. As contraction increases, the number of potentials increases, forming an interference pattern.

Denervated muscle fibers are recognized by increased activity with needle insertion and abnormal spontaneous activity (fibrillations and fasciculations); fewer motor units are recruited during contraction, producing a reduced interference pattern. Surviving axons branch to innervate adjacent muscle fibers, enlarging the motor unit and producing giant action potentials.

In muscle disorders, individual fibers are affected without regard to their motor units; thus, amplitude of their potentials is diminished, but the interference pattern remains full.

Nerve conduction studies: In nerve conduction studies, a peripheral nerve is stimulated with electrical shocks at several points along its course to a muscle, and the time to initiation of contraction is recorded. The time an impulse takes to traverse a measured length of nerve determines conduction velocity. The time required to traverse the segment nearest the muscle is called distal latency. Similar measurements can be made for sensory nerves. Nerve conduction studies test large, myelinated nerves, not thinly myelinated or unmyelinated nerves.

In neuropathy, conduction is often slowed, and the response pattern may show a dispersion of potentials due to unequal involvement of myelinated and unmyelinated axons. However, when neuropathies affect only small umyelinated or thinly myelinated fibers (or when weakness is due to a muscle disorder), results are typically normal.

A nerve can be repeatedly stimulated to evaluate the neuromuscular junction for fatigability (eg, a progressive decremental response occurs in myasthenia gravis).

LUMBAR PUNCTURE

(Spinal Tap)

Lumbar puncture is used to do the following:

- Evaluate intracranial pressure and CSF composition (see Table 221–1)
- Therapeutically reduce intracranial pressure (eg, idiopathic intracranial hypertension)
- Administer intrathecal drugs or a radiopaque contrast agent for myelography

Relative contraindications include

- Infection at the puncture site
- Bleeding diathesis
- Increased intracranial pressure due to an intracranial mass lesion, obstructed CSF outflow (eg, due to aqueductal stenosis or Chiari I malformation), or spinal cord CSF blockage (eg, due to tumor cord compression)

If papilledema or focal neurologic deficits are present, CT or MRI should be done before lumbar puncture to rule out presence of a mass that could precipitate transtentorial or cerebellar herniation (see Fig. 221–1).

Lumbar puncture procedure: For the procedure, the patient is typically in the left lateral decubitus position. A cooperative patient is asked to hug the knees and curl up as tightly as possible. Assistants may have to hold patients who cannot maintain this position, or the spine may be flexed better by having patients, particularly obese patients, sit on the side of the bed and lean over a bedside tray table.

An area 20 cm in diameter is washed with iodine, then wiped with alcohol to remove the iodine and prevent its introduction into the subarachnoid space. A lumbar puncture needle with stylet is inserted into the L3-to-L4 or L4-to-L5 interspace (the L4 spinous process is typically on a line between the posterior-superior iliac crests); the needle is aimed rostrally toward the patient's umbilicus and always kept parallel to the floor. Entrance into the subarachnoid space is often accompanied by a discernible pop; the stylet is withdrawn to allow CSF to flow out.

Opening pressure is measured with a manometer; 4 tubes are each filled with about 2 to 10 mL of CSF for testing. The puncture site is then covered with a sterile adhesive strip.

A post–lumbar puncture headache occurs in about 10% of patients.

CSF color: Normal CSF is clear and colorless; ≥ 300 cells/μL produces cloudiness or turbidity.

Bloody fluid may indicate a traumatic puncture (pushing the needle in too far, into the venous plexus along the anterior spinal canal) or subarachnoid hemorrhage. A traumatic puncture is distinguished by

- Gradual clearing of the CSF between the 1st and 4th tubes (confirmed by decreasing RBC count)
- Absence of xanthochromia (yellowish CSF due to lysed RBCs) in a centrifuged sample
- Fresh, uncrenated RBCs

With intrinsic subarachnoid hemorrhage, the CSF remains uniformly bloody throughout collection; xanthochromia is

Table 221–1. CEREBROSPINAL FLUID ABNORMALITIES IN VARIOUS DISORDERS

CONDITION	PRESSURE*	WBCs/μL*	PREDOMINANT CELL TYPE	GLUCOSE	PROTEIN*
Normal	100–200 mm H_2O	0–3	L	50–100 mg/dL (2.78–5.55 mmol/L)	20–45 mg/dL
Acute bacterial meningitis	↑	100–10,000	PMN	↓	> 100 mg/dL†
Subacute meningitis (eg, due to TB, *Cryptococcus* infection, sarcoidosis, leukemia, or carcinoma)	N or ↑	100–700	L	↓	↑
Acute syphilitic meningitis	N or ↑	25–2000	L	N	↑
Paretic neurosyphilis	N or ↑	15–2000	L	N	↑
Lyme disease of CNS	N or ↑	0–500	L	N	N or ↑
Brain abscess or tumor	N or ↑	0–1000	L	N	↑
Viral infections	N or ↑	100–2000	L	N	N or ↑
Idiopathic intracranial hypertension	↑	N	L	N	N or ↓
Cerebral hemorrhage	↑	Bloody	RBC	N	↑
Cerebral thrombosis	N or ↑	0–100	L	N	N or ↑
Spinal cord tumor	N	0–50	L	N	N or ↑
Multiple sclerosis	N	0–50	L	N	N or ↑
Guillain-Barré syndrome	N	0–100	L	N	> 100 mg/dL
Lead encephalopathy	↑	0–500	L	N	↑

*Figures given for pressure, cell count, and protein are approximations; exceptions are common. Similarly, PMNs may predominate in disorders usually characterized by lymphocyte response, especially early in the course of viral infections or tuberculous meningitis. Alterations in glucose are less variable and more reliable.

†Up to 14% of patients may have a CSF protein level < 100 mg/dL in the initial lumbar puncture sample.

L = lymphocyte; N = normal; PMN = polymorphonuclear leukocyte; ↑= increased; ↓ = decreased.

often present if several hours have passed after ictus; and RBCs are usually older and crenated. Faintly yellow fluid may also be due to senile chromogens, severe jaundice, or increased protein (> 100 mg/dL).

CSF cell count and glucose and protein levels: Cell count and differential and glucose and protein levels aid in the diagnosis of many neurologic disorders (see Table 221–1).

Normally, CSF:blood glucose ratio is about 0.6, and except in severe hypoglycemia, CSF glucose is typically > 50 mg/dL (> 2.78 mmol/L).

Increased CSF protein (> 50 mg/dL) is a sensitive but nonspecific index of disease; protein increases to > 500 mg/dL in purulent meningitis, advanced TB meningitis, complete block by spinal cord tumor, or a bloody puncture. Special examinations

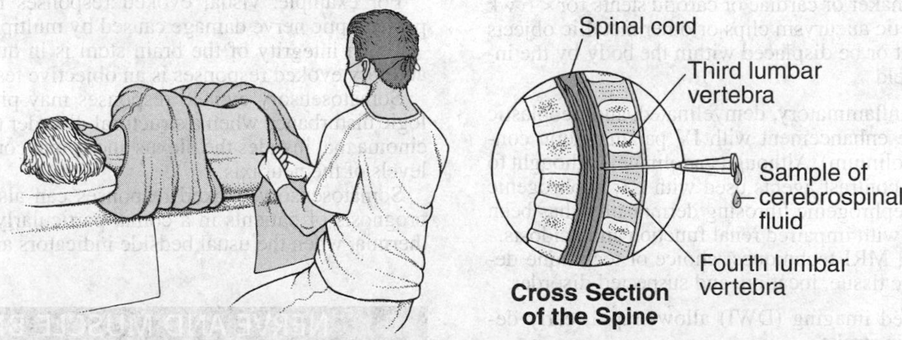

Fig. 221–1. Lumbar puncture. For the procedure, the patient is typically in the left lateral decubitus position. A lumbar puncture needle with stylet is inserted into the L3-to-L4 or L4-to-L5 interspace (the L4 spinous process is typically on a line between the posterior-superior iliac crests); the needle is aimed rostrally toward the patient's umbilicus and always kept parallel to the floor. Entrance into the subarachnoid space is often accompanied by a discernible pop; the stylet is withdrawn to allow CSF to flow out.

for globulin (normally < 15%), oligoclonal banding, and myelin basic protein aid in diagnosis of a demyelinating disorder.

CSF staining, testing, and culture: If infection is suspected, the centrifuged CSF sediment is stained for bacteria (Gram stain), for TB (acid-fast stain or immunofluorescence), and for *Cryptococcus* sp (India ink). Larger amounts of fluid (10 mL) improve the chances of detecting the pathogen, particularly acid-fast bacilli and certain fungi, in stains and cultures. In early meningococcal meningitis or severe leukopenia, CSF protein may be too low for bacterial adherence to the glass slide during Gram staining, producing a false-negative result. Mixing a drop of aseptic serum with CSF sediment prevents this problem. When hemorrhagic meningoencephalitis is suspected, a wet mount is used to search for amebas. Latex particle agglutination and coagglutination tests may allow rapid bacterial identification, especially when stains and cultures are negative (eg, in partially treated meningitis). CSF should be cultured aerobically and anaerobically and for acid-fast bacilli and fungi.

Except for enteroviruses, viruses are seldom isolated from the CSF. Viral antibody panels are available.

Venereal Disease Research Laboratories (VDRL) testing and cryptococcal antigen testing are often routinely done. PCR tests for herpes simplex virus and other CNS pathogens are increasingly available.

MAGNETIC RESONANCE IMAGING IN NEUROLOGIC DISORDERS

Magnetic resonance imaging (MRI) provides better resolution of neural structures than CT. This difference is most significant clinically for visualizing the following:

- Cranial nerves
- Brain stem lesions
- Abnormalities of the posterior fossa
- Spinal cord

CT images of these regions are often marred by bony streak artifacts. MRI is especially valuable for identifying spinal abnormalities (eg, tumor, abscess) compressing the spinal cord and requiring emergency intervention. Also, MRI is better for detecting demyelinating plaques, early infarction, subclinical brain edema, cerebral contusions, incipient transtentorial herniation, abnormalities of the craniocervical junction, and syringomyelia.

MRI is **contraindicated** if patients

- Have had a pacemaker or cardiac or carotid stents for < 6 wk
- Have ferromagnetic aneurysm clips or other metallic objects that may overheat or be displaced within the body by the intense magnetic field

Visualization of inflammatory, demyelinated, and neoplastic lesions may require enhancement with IV paramagnetic contrast agents (eg, gadolinium). Although gadolinium is thought to be much safer than contrast agents used with CT, nephrogenic systemic fibrosis (nephrogenic fibrosing dermopathy) has been reported in patients with impaired renal function and acidosis.

There are several MRI techniques; choice of technique depends on the specific tissue, location, and suspected disorder:

- Diffusion-weighted imaging (DWI) allows rapid, early detection of ischemic stroke.
- Perfusion-weighted imaging (PWI) can detect areas of hypoperfusion in early ischemic stroke but cannot yet reliably distinguish areas with benign oligemia from those with injurious hypoperfusion that results in infarction.
- Diffusion tensor imaging (DTI) is an extension of DWI that can show white matter tracts in 3 dimensions (tractography) and can be used to monitor the integrity of CNS tracts affected by aging and disease.
- Double inversion recovery (DIR), used in research centers, can detect demyelination of gray matter better than other MRI techniques; gray matter demyelination is now considered common in multiple sclerosis.
- Functional MRI (fMRI) shows which brain regions are activated (shown by increased flow of oxygenated blood) by a specific cognitive or motor task, but its clinical use is still being defined.

Magnetic resonance angiography (MRA) uses MRI with or without a contrast agent to show cerebral vessels and major arteries and their branches in the head and neck. Although MRA has not replaced cerebral angiography, it is used when cerebral angiography cannot be done (eg, because the patient refuses or has increased risk). As a check for stroke, MRA tends to exaggerate severity of arterial narrowing and thus does not usually miss occlusive disease of large arteries.

Magnetic resonance venography (MRV) uses MRI to show the major veins and dural sinuses of the cranium. MRV obviates the need for cerebral angiography in diagnosing cerebral venous thrombosis and is useful for monitoring thrombus resolution and guiding the duration of anticoagulation.

Magnetic resonance spectroscopy can measure metabolites in the brain regionally to distinguish tumors from abscess or stroke.

MEASUREMENT OF EVOKED RESPONSES

Visual, auditory, or tactile stimuli are used to activate corresponding areas of the cerebral cortex, resulting in focal cortical electrical activity. Ordinarily, these small potentials are lost in EEG background noise, but computer processing cancels out the noise to reveal a waveform. Latency, duration, and amplitude of the evoked responses indicate whether the tested sensory pathway is intact.

Evoked responses are particularly useful for the following:

- Detecting clinically inapparent deficits in a demyelinating disorder
- Appraising sensory systems in infants
- Substantiating deficits suspected to be histrionic
- Following the subclinical course of disease

For example, visual evoked responses may detect unsuspected optic nerve damage caused by multiple sclerosis.

When integrity of the brain stem is in question, brain stem auditory evoked responses is an objective test.

Somatosensory evoked responses may pinpoint the physiologic disturbance when a structural disorder (eg, metastatic carcinoma that invades the plexus and spinal cord) affects multiple levels of the neuraxis.

Somatosensory evoked responses can also help predict the prognosis of patients in a coma, particularly those with hypothermia, when the usual bedside indicators are unclear.

NERVE AND MUSCLE BIOPSY

Nerve and muscle biopsy are usually done simultaneously. Nerve biopsy can help differentiate axonal from demyelinating polyneuropathies when other tests are inconclusive. A nerve supplying the affected area should be chosen. If polyneuropathy may be caused by vasculitis, the sample should include skin to increase the chances of finding a characteristic vascular abnormality. If the biopsy shows that nerve endings are lost, skin punch biopsy can help confirm small-fiber polyneuropathy.

Muscle biopsy can help confirm myopathies.

OTHER NEUROLOGIC IMAGING STUDIES

Cerebral catheter angiography: X-rays taken after a radiopaque agent is injected via an intra-arterial catheter show individual cerebral arteries and venous structures of the brain. With digital data processing (digital subtraction angiography), small amounts of agent can produce high-resolution images.

Cerebral angiography supplements CT and MRI in delineating the site and vascularity of intracranial lesions; it has been the gold standard for diagnosing stenotic or occluded arteries, congenitally absent vessels, aneurysms, and arteriovenous malformations. Vessels as small as 0.1 mm can be visualized. However, its use has decreased dramatically with the advent of MRA and CT angiography. It is still routinely used when cerebral vasculitis is suspected and when angiographic interventions (eg, angioplasty, stent placement, intra-arterial thrombolysis, aneurysm obliteration) may be necessary.

Duplex Doppler ultrasonography: This noninvasive procedure can assess dissection, stenosis, occlusion, and ulceration of the carotid bifurcation. It is safe and rapid, but it does not provide the detail of angiography. It is preferable to periorbital Doppler ultrasonography and oculoplethysmography for evaluating patients with carotid artery transient ischemic attacks and is useful for following an abnormality over time.

Transcranial Doppler ultrasonography helps evaluate residual blood flow after brain death, vasospasm of the middle cerebral artery after subarachnoid hemorrhage, and vertebrobasilar stroke.

Echoencephalography: Ultrasonography can be used at the bedside (usually in the neonatal ICU) to detect hemorrhage and hydrocephalus in children < 2 yr.

CT has replaced echoencephalography in older children and adults.

Myelography: X-rays are taken after a radiopaque agent is injected into the subarachnoid space via lumbar puncture. MRI has replaced myelography for evaluation of intraspinal abnormalities, but CT myelography is still done when MRI is unavailable.

Contraindications are the same as those for lumbar puncture.

Myelography may exacerbate the effects of spinal cord compression, especially if too much fluid is removed too rapidly. Rarely, myelography results in inflammation of the arachnoid membranes around the spinal nerves (arachnoiditis), which may cause chronic pain and paresthesias in the lower back and extremities.

222 Autonomic Nervous System

The autonomic nervous system (ANS) regulates physiologic processes. Regulation occurs without conscious control, ie, autonomously. The 2 major divisions are the

- Sympathetic system
- Parasympathetic system

Disorders of the ANS cause autonomic insufficiency or failure and can affect any system of the body.

Anatomy

The ANS receives input from parts of the CNS that process and integrate stimuli from the body and external environment. These parts include the hypothalamus, nucleus of the solitary tract, reticular formation, amygdala, hippocampus, and olfactory cortex.

The sympathetic and parasympathetic systems each consist of 2 sets of nerve bodies:

- Preganglionic: This set is located in the CNS, with connections to another set in ganglia outside the CNS.
- Postganglionic: This set has efferent fibers that go from the ganglia to effector organs (see Fig. 222–1).

Sympathetic: The preganglionic cell bodies of the sympathetic system are located in the intermediolateral horn of the spinal cord between T1 and L2 or L3.

The sympathetic ganglia are adjacent to the spine and consist of the vertebral (sympathetic chain) and prevertebral ganglia, including the superior cervical, celiac, superior mesenteric, inferior mesenteric, and aorticorenal ganglia.

Long fibers run from these ganglia to effector organs, including the following:

- Smooth muscle of blood vessels, viscera, lungs, scalp (piloerector muscles), and pupils
- Heart
- Glands (sweat, salivary, and digestive)

Parasympathetic: The preganglionic cell bodies of the parasympathetic system are located in the brain stem and sacral portion of the spinal cord. Preganglionic fibers exit the brain stem with the 3rd, 7th, 9th, and 10th (vagus) cranial nerves and exit the spinal cord at S2 and S3; the vagus nerve contains about 75% of all parasympathetic fibers.

Parasympathetic ganglia (eg, ciliary, sphenopalatine, otic, pelvic, and vagal ganglia) are located within the effector organs, and postganglionic fibers are only 1 or 2 mm long. Thus, the parasympathetic system can produce specific, localized responses in effector organs, such as the following:

- Blood vessels of the head, neck, and thoracoabdominal viscera
- Lacrimal and salivary glands
- Smooth muscle of glands and viscera (eg, liver, spleen, colon, kidneys, bladder, genitals)
- Muscles of the pupil

Physiology

The autonomic nervous system controls BP, heart rate, body temperature, weight, digestion, metabolism, fluid and electrolyte balance, sweating, urination, defecation, sexual response, and other processes. Many organs are controlled primarily by either the sympathetic or parasympathetic system, although they may receive input from both; occasionally, functions are reciprocal (eg, sympathetic input increases heart rate; parasympathetic decreases it).

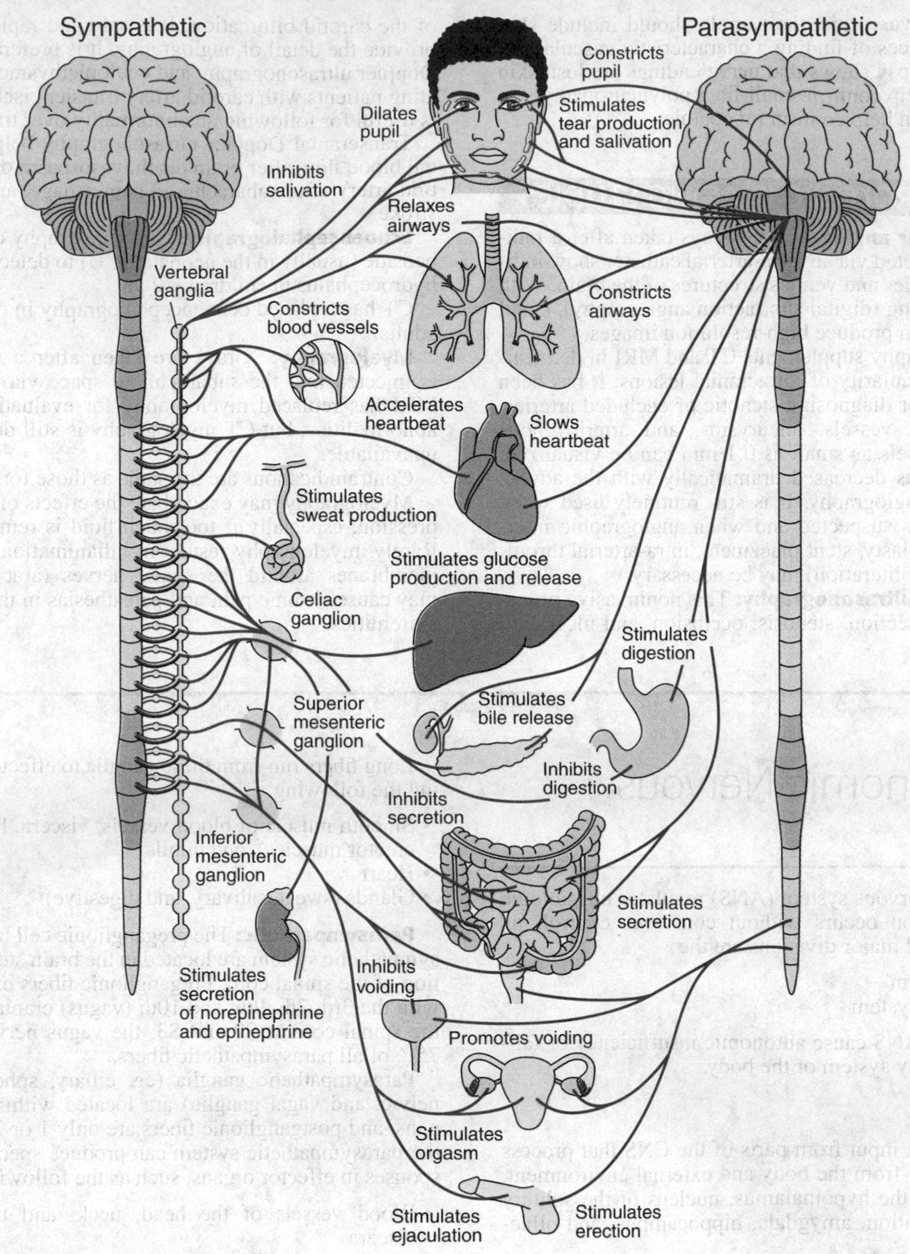

Fig. 222–1. The autonomic nervous system.

The **sympathetic nervous system** is catabolic; it activates fight-or-flight responses.

The **parasympathetic nervous system** is anabolic; it conserves and restores (see Table 222–1).

Two major neurotransmitters in the ANS are

- **Acetylcholine:** Fibers that secrete acetylcholine (cholinergic fibers) include all preganglionic fibers, all postganglionic parasympathetic fibers, and some postganglionic sympathetic fibers (those that innervate piloerectors, sweat glands, and blood vessels).
- **Norepinephrine:** Fibers that secrete norepinephrine (adrenergic fibers) include most postganglionic sympathetic fibers. Sweat glands on the palms and soles also respond to adrenergic stimulation to some degree.

There are different subtypes of adrenergic receptors and cholinergic receptors, which vary by location.

Table 222–1. DIVISIONS OF THE AUTONOMIC NERVOUS SYSTEM

DIVISION	EFFECTS
Sympathetic	Increases the following: • Heart rate and contractility • Bronchodilation • Hepatic glycogenolysis and glucose release • BMR • Muscular strength Causes sweaty palms Decreases less immediately life-preserving functions (eg, digestion) Controls ejaculation
Parasympathetic	Stimulates GI secretions and motility (including evacuation) Slows heart rate Reduces BP Controls erection

Etiology of Autonomic Insufficiency

Disorders causing autonomic insufficiency or failure can originate in the peripheral or central nervous system and may be primary or secondary to other disorders.

The **most common causes** of autonomic insufficiency are

- Peripheral neuropathies
- Aging
- Parkinson disease

Other causes include

- Autoimmune autonomic neuropathy
- Multiple system atrophy
- Pure autonomic failure
- Spinal cord disorders
- Drugs
- Disorders of the neuromuscular junction (eg, botulism, Lambert-Eaton syndrome)

Evaluation of Autonomic Insufficiency

History: Symptoms suggesting autonomic insufficiency include

- Orthostatic intolerance (development of symptoms such as light-headedness that is relieved by sitting down) due to orthostatic hypotension or postural orthostatic tachycardia syndrome
- Heat intolerance
- Loss of bladder and bowel control
- Erectile dysfunction (an early symptom)

Other possible symptoms include dry eyes and dry mouth, but they are less specific.

Physical examination: Important parts of the examination include the following:

- **Postural BP and heart rate:** In a normally hydrated patient, a sustained (eg, > 1 min) decrease of ≥ 20 mm Hg in systolic BP or a decrease of ≥ 10 mm Hg in diastolic BP with standing indicates orthostatic hypotension. Heart rate change with respiration and standing should be noted; absence of physiologic sinus arrhythmia and failure of heart rate to increase with standing indicate autonomic insufficiency. In contrast, patients with postural tachycardia syndrome, a benign disorder, typically have postural tachycardia without hypotension.
- **Eye examination:** Miosis and mild ptosis (Horner syndrome) suggest a sympathetic lesion. A dilated, unreactive pupil (Adie pupil) suggests a parasympathetic lesion.
- **GU and rectal reflexes:** Abnormal GU and rectal reflexes may indicate ANS deficits. Testing includes the cremasteric reflex (normally, stroking the upper inner thigh results in retraction of the testes), anal wink reflex (normally, stroking perianal skin results in contraction of the anal sphincter), and bulbocavernosus reflex (normally, squeezing the glans penis or clitoris results in contraction of the anal sphincter). In practice, the GU and rectal reflexes are rarely tested because laboratory testing is much more reliable.

Laboratory testing: If patients have symptoms and signs suggesting autonomic insufficiency, sudomotor, cardiovagal, and adrenergic testing is usually done to help determine severity and distribution of the insufficiency.

Sudomotor testing includes the following:

- **Quantitative sudomotor axon-reflex test:** This test evaluates integrity of postganglionic fibers. The fibers are activated by iontophoresis using acetylcholine. Standard sites on the leg and wrist are tested, and the volume of sweat is then measured. The test can detect decreased or absent sweat production.
- **Thermoregulatory sweat test:** This test evaluates both preganglionic and postganglionic pathways. After a dye is applied to the skin, patients enter a closed compartment that is heated to cause maximal sweating. Sweating causes the dye to change color, so that areas of anhidrosis and hypohidrosis are apparent and can be calculated as a percentage of BSA.

Cardiovagal testing evaluates heart rate response (via ECG rhythm strip) to deep breathing and to the Valsalva maneuver. If the ANS is intact, heart rate varies with these maneuvers; normal responses to deep breathing and the Valsalva ratio vary by age.

Adrenergic testing evaluates response of beat-to-beat BP to the following:

- **Head-up tilt:** Blood is shifted to dependent parts, causing reflex responses in BP and heart rate. This test helps differentiate autonomic neuropathies from postural orthostatic tachycardia syndrome.
- **Valsalva maneuver:** This maneuver increases intrathoracic pressure and reduces venous return, causing changes in BP and heart rate that reflect vagal and adrenergic baroreflex function.

With the head-up tilt test and Valsalva maneuvers, the pattern of responses is an index of adrenergic function.

Plasma norepinephrine levels can be measured with patients supine and then after they stand for > 5 min. Normally, levels increase after standing. If patients have autonomic insufficiency, levels may not increase with standing and may be low in the supine position, particularly in postganglionic disorders (eg, autonomic neuropathy, pure autonomic failure).

AUTONOMIC NEUROPATHIES

Autonomic neuropathies are peripheral nerve disorders with disproportionate involvement of autonomic fibers.

The best known autonomic neuropathies are those accompanying peripheral neuropathy due to diabetes, amyloidosis, or autoimmune disorders.

Autoimmune autonomic neuropathy is an idiopathic disorder that often develops after a viral infection; onset may be subacute.

Autonomic insufficiency is usually a late manifestation in alcoholic neuropathy.

Other causes can include toxins, drugs, and paraneoplastic syndromes.

Symptoms and Signs

Common symptoms of autonomic neuropathies include orthostatic hypotension, neurogenic bladder, erectile dysfunction, gastroparesis, and intractable constipation. When somatic fibers are involved, sensory loss in a stocking-and-glove distribution and distal weakness may occur (see also p. 1978).

Diagnosis

- Clinical evaluation

Diagnosis of autonomic neuropathy is based on demonstration of autonomic failure and of a specific cause of neuropathy (eg, diabetes, amyloidosis).

Autoimmune autonomic neuropathy may be suspected after a viral infection. Ganglionic anti–acetylcholine receptor antibody A_3 is present in about half of patients with autoimmune autonomic neuropathy and is occasionally present in patients with other autonomic neuropathies.

Treatment

- Treatment of underlying disorders

Underlying disorders are treated.

Autoimmune autonomic neuropathy may respond to immunotherapy; plasma exchange or IV gamma-globulin can be used for more severe cases.

HORNER SYNDROME

Horner syndrome is ptosis, miosis, and anhidrosis due to dysfunction of cervical sympathetic output.

Etiology

Horner syndrome results when the cervical sympathetic pathway running from the hypothalamus to the eye is disrupted. The causative lesion may be primary (including congenital) or secondary to another disorder.

Lesions are usually divided into the following:

- Central (eg, brain stem ischemia, syringomyelia, brain tumor)
- Peripheral (eg, Pancoast tumor, cervical adenopathy, neck and skull injuries, aortic or carotid dissection, thoracic aortic aneurysm)

Peripheral lesions may be preganglionic or postganglionic in origin.

Symptoms and Signs

Symptoms include ptosis, miosis, anhidrosis, and hyperemia of the affected side.

In the congenital form, the iris does not become pigmented and remains blue-gray.

Diagnosis

- Cocaine eye drop test
- MRI or CT to diagnose cause

Instilling eyedrops can help confirm and characterize Horner syndrome. First, cocaine (4 to 5%) or apraclonidine (0.5%) drops are put in both eyes:

- Cocaine: Cocaine blocks the synaptic reuptake of norepinephrine and causes the pupil of the unaffected eye to dilate. If a postganglionic lesion (peripheral Horner syndrome) is present, the pupil of the affected eye does not dilate because the postganglionic nerve terminals have degenerated; the result is increased anisocoria. If the lesion is below the superior cervical ganglion (preganglionic or central Horner syndrome) and the postganglionic fibers are intact, the pupil of the affected eye also dilates, and anisocoria decreases.
- Apraclonidine: Apraclonidine is a weak alpha-adrenergic agonist that minimally dilates the pupil of a normal eye. If a postganglionic lesion is present (peripheral Horner syndrome), the pupil of the affected eye dilates much more than that of the unaffected eye because the iris dilator muscle of the affected eye has lost its sympathetic innervation and has developed adrenergic supersensitivity. As a result, anisocoria decreases. (However, results may be falsely normal if the causative lesion is acute.) If the lesion is preganglionic (or a central Horner syndrome), the pupil of the affected eye does not dilate because the iris dilator muscle does not develop adrenergic supersensitivity; as a result, anisocoria increases.

If results suggest Horner syndrome, hydroxyamphetamine (1%) can be put in both eyes 48 h later to help locate the lesion. Hydroxyamphetamine works by causing norepinephrine to be released from the presynaptic terminals. It has no effect if postganglionic lesions are present because these lesions cause postganglionic terminals to degenerate. Thus, when hydroxyamphetamine is applied, the following occur:

- Postganglionic lesion: The pupil of the affected eye does not dilate, but the pupil of the unaffected eye dilates, resulting in increased anisocoria.
- Central or preganglionic lesion: The pupil of the affected eye dilates normally or more than it normally does, and the pupil of the unaffected eye dilates normally, resulting in decreased or unchanged anisocoria. (However, postganglionic lesions sometimes produce the same results.)

Hydroxyamphetamine testing is done less frequently than testing with apraclonidine, partly because hydroxyamphetamine tends to be available less often. For results to be valid, hydroxyamphetamine testing must be delayed until at least 24 h after apraclonidine instillation.

Patients with Horner syndrome require MRI or CT of the brain, spinal cord, chest, or neck, depending on clinical suspicion.

Treatment

- Treatment of the cause

The cause, if identified, is treated; there is no treatment for primary Horner syndrome.

KEY POINTS

- Horner syndrome causes ptosis, miosis, and anhidrosis.
- It results from a central or peripheral lesion (preganglionic or postganglionic) that disrupts the cervical sympathetic pathway, which runs from the hypothalamus to the eye.
- Instill cocaine, apraclonidine, and/or hydroxyamphetamine in both eyes to confirm the diagnosis of Horner syndrome and help locate the lesion (preganglionic or postganglionic).
- Treat the cause, if identified; there is no treatment for primary Horner syndrome.

MULTIPLE SYSTEM ATROPHY

Multiple system atrophy (MSA) is a relentlessly progressive neurodegenerative disorder causing pyramidal, cerebellar, and autonomic dysfunction. It includes 3 disorders previously thought to be distinct: olivopontocerebellar atrophy, striatonigral degeneration, and Shy-Drager syndrome. Symptoms include hypotension, urinary retention, constipation, ataxia, rigidity, and postural instability. Diagnosis is clinical. Treatment is symptomatic, with volume expansion, compression garments, and vasoconstrictor drugs.

MSA affects about twice as many men as women. Mean age at onset is about 53 yr; after symptoms appear, patients live about 9 to 10 yr.

Etiology

Etiology of MSA is unknown, but neuronal degeneration occurs in several areas of the brain; the area and amount damaged determine initial symptoms. A characteristic finding is cytoplasmic inclusion bodies containing alpha-synuclein within oligodendroglial cells.

MSA is a synucleinopathy (due to synuclein deposition); synuclein can also accumulate in patients with Parkinson disease, pure autonomic failure, or Lewy body dementia. Synuclein is a neuronal and glial cell protein that can aggregate into insoluble fibrils and form Lewy bodies.

Symptoms and Signs

Initial symptoms of MSA vary but include a combination of

- Parkinsonism unresponsive to levodopa
- Cerebellar abnormalities
- Symptoms due to autonomic insufficiency

Parkinsonian symptoms: Parkinsonian symptoms predominate in striatonigral degeneration. They include rigidity, bradykinesia, postural instability, and jerky postural tremor. High-pitched, quavering dysarthria is common.

In contrast to Parkinson disease, MSA usually does not usually cause resting tremor and dyskinesia, and symptoms respond poorly and transiently to levodopa.

Cerebellar abnormalities: Cerebellar abnormalities predominate in olivopontocerebellar atrophy. They include ataxia, dysmetria, dysdiadochokinesia (difficulty performing rapidly alternating movements), poor coordination, and abnormal eye movements.

Autonomic symptoms: Typically, autonomic insufficiency causes orthostatic hypotension (symptomatic fall in BP when a person stands, often with syncope), urinary retention or incontinence, constipation, and erectile dysfunction.

Other autonomic symptoms, which may occur early or late, include decreased sweating, difficulty breathing and swallowing, fecal incontinence, and decreased tearing and salivation.

REM sleep behavior disorder (eg, speech or skeletal muscle movement during REM sleep) and respiratory stridor are common. Patients are often unaware of REM sleep behavior disorder.

Patients may have nocturnal polyuria; contributing factors may include a circadian decrease in arginine vasopressin and treatments used to increase blood volume.

Diagnosis

- Clinical evaluation (parkinsonism or cerebellar symptoms that respond poorly to levodopa plus autonomic insufficiency)
- MRI

Diagnosis of MSA is suspected clinically, based on the combination of autonomic insufficiency and parkinsonism or cerebellar symptoms. Similar symptoms may result from Parkinson disease, Lewy body dementia, pure autonomic failure, autonomic neuropathies, progressive supranuclear palsy, multiple cerebral infarcts, or drug-induced parkinsonism.

No diagnostic test is definitive, but some (eg, MRI, nuclear imaging with ^{123}I-metaiodobenzylguanidine [MIBG], autonomic tests) help confirm clinical suspicion of MSA—for example, if

- MRI shows characteristic changes in the midbrain, pons, or cerebellum.
- MIBG scans show intact innervation of the heart.
- Autonomic tests indicate generalized autonomic failure.

Treatment

- Supportive care

There is no specific treatment for MSA, but symptoms are managed as follows:

- **Orthostatic hypotension:** Treatment includes intravascular volume expansion with salt and water supplementation and sometimes fludrocortisone 0.1 to 0.4 mg po once/day. Use of compression garments for the lower body (eg, abdominal binder, compression stockings) and alpha-adrenoreceptor stimulation with midodrine 10 mg po tid may help. However, midodrine also increases peripheral vascular resistance and supine BP, which may be problematic. Raising the head of the bed about 10 cm reduces nocturnal polyuria and supine hypertension and may reduce morning orthostatic hypotension. Alternatively, droxidopa may be used; its action is similar to that of midodrine, but duration of action is longer.
- **Parkinsonism:** Levodopa/carbidopa 25/100 mg po at bedtime may be tried to relieve rigidity and other parkinsonian symptoms, but this combination is usually ineffective or provides modest benefit.
- **Urinary incontinence:** If the cause is detrusor hyperreflexia, oxybutynin chloride 5 mg po tid or tolterodine 2 mg po bid may be used. Tamsulosin 0.4 to 0.8 mg once/day may be effective for urinary urgency. Alternatively, the beta-3 adrenergic agonist mirabegron 25 to 50 mg once/day can be used; unlike tamsulosin, mirabegron does not worsen orthostatic hypotension.
- **Urinary retention:** Many patients must self-catheterize their bladder.
- **Constipation:** A high-fiber diet and stool softeners can be used; for refractory cases, enemas may be necessary.
- **Erectile dysfunction:** Drugs such as sildenafil 50 mg po prn or tadalafil 2.5 to 5 mg once/day and various physical means can be used.

KEY POINTS

- MSA can include parkinsonian symptoms, cerebellar abnormalities, and autonomic insufficiency in various degrees of severity.
- Diagnose this disorder based on clinical, autonomic, and MRI findings, but consider Parkinson disease, Lewy body dementia, pure autonomic failure, autonomic neuropathies, progressive supranuclear palsy, multiple cerebral infarcts, and drug-induced parkinsonism, which can all cause similar symptoms.
- Use treatments specific for the symptoms present.

PURE AUTONOMIC FAILURE

Pure autonomic failure results from neuronal loss in autonomic ganglia, causing orthostatic hypotension and other autonomic symptoms.

Pure autonomic failure, previously called idiopathic orthostatic hypotension or Bradbury-Eggleston syndrome, denotes generalized autonomic failure without CNS involvement. This disorder differs from multiple system atrophy because it lacks central or preganglionic involvement. Pure autonomic failure affects more women, tends to begin during a person's 40s or 50s, and does not result in death.

Pure autonomic failure is a synucleinopathy (due to synuclein deposition); synuclein can also accumulate in patients with Parkinson disease, multiple system atrophy, or Lewy body dementia. (Synuclein is a neuronal and glial cell protein that can aggregate into insoluble fibrils and form Lewy bodies.) Some patients with pure autonomic failure eventually develop multiple system atrophy or Lewy body dementia.

Symptoms and Signs

The main symptom is

- Orthostatic hypotension

There may be other autonomic symptoms, such as decreased sweating, heat intolerance, urinary retention, bladder spasms (possibly causing incontinence), erectile dysfunction, fecal incontinence or constipation, and pupillary abnormalities.

Diagnosis

- Clinical evaluation

Diagnosis of pure autonomic failure is by exclusion. The norepinephrine level is usually < 100 pg/mL supine and does not increase with standing. Postural orthostatic tachycardia syndrome can be differentiated because with standing, it does not usually cause hypotension, the norepinephrine level increases, and heart rate increases by > 30 beats/min or to 120 beats/min within 10 min.

Treatment

- Symptomatic treatment

Treatment of pure autonomic failure is symptomatic:

- **Orthostatic hypotension:** Volume expansion, vasopressors, and support hose
- **Constipation:** High-fiber diet and stool softeners
- **Bladder spasms:** Bladder antispasmodics
- **Urinary retention:** Possibly self-catheterization of the bladder
- **Sweating abnormalities:** Avoidance of hot conditions

KEY POINTS

- Pure autonomic failure, like Parkinson disease, multiple system atrophy, and Lewy body dementia, is a synucleinopathy.
- The main symptom is orthostatic hypotension.
- Diagnose by excluding other disorders that cause similar symptoms.
- Use treatments specific for the symptoms present.

223 Brain Infections

Brain infections may manifest as follows:

- Diffuse infection, resulting in encephalitis, sometimes affecting specific areas on the brain
- Inflammation of the brain secondary to meningeal infections or parameningeal infections
- Focal infection (eg, due to a brain abscess or to fungal or parasitic brain infections)

Encephalitis is most commonly due to viruses, such as herpes simplex, herpes zoster, cytomegalovirus, or West Nile virus. HIV infection and prion diseases can also affect the brain diffusely.

Slow virus infections, such as progressive multifocal leukoencephalopathy (caused by the JC virus) or subacute sclerosing panencephalitis (caused by the measles virus) also affect the brain; they are characterized by a long incubation and a prolonged course.

Certain noninfectious disorders can mimic encephalitis. An example is anti-NMDA (*N*-methyl-D-aspartate) receptor encephalitis, which involves an autoimmune attack on neuronal membrane proteins.

Multifocal brain involvement may also be a manifestation of acute diffuse disseminated encephalomyelitis (a postinfectious syndrome).

BRAIN ABSCESS

A brain abscess is an intracerebral collection of pus. Symptoms may include headache, lethargy, fever, and focal neurologic deficits. Diagnosis is by contrast-enhanced MRI or CT. Treatment is with antibiotics and usually CT-guided stereotactic aspiration or surgical drainage.

An abscess forms when an area of cerebral inflammation becomes necrotic and encapsulated by glial cells and fibroblasts. Edema around the abscess may increase intracranial pressure.

Etiology

A brain abscess can result from

- Direct extension of cranial infections (eg, osteomyelitis, mastoiditis, sinusitis, subdural empyema)
- Penetrating head wounds (including neurosurgical procedures)
- Hematogenous spread (eg, in bacterial endocarditis, congenital heart disease with right-to-left shunt, or IV drug abuse)
- Unknown causes

The bacteria involved are usually anaerobic and sometimes mixed, often including anaerobes, such as *Bacteroides* and anaerobic and microaerophilic streptococci. Staphylococci are common after cranial trauma, neurosurgery, or endocarditis. Enterobacteriaceae may be isolated in chronic ear infections.

Fungi (eg, *Aspergillus*) and protozoa (eg, *Toxoplasma gondii*, particularly in HIV-infected patients) can cause abscesses.

Symptoms and Signs

Symptoms result from increased intracranial pressure and mass effect. Classically, headache, nausea, vomiting, lethargy, seizures, personality changes, papilledema, and focal neurologic deficits develop over days to weeks; however, in some patients, these manifestations are subtle or absent until late in the clinical course.

Fever, chills, and leukocytosis may develop before the infection is encapsulated, but they may be absent at presentation or subside over time.

Diagnosis

- Contrast-enhanced MRI or, if unavailable, contrast-enhanced CT

When symptoms suggest an abscess, contrast-enhanced MRI or, if unavailable, contrast-enhanced CT is done. A fully developed abscess appears as an edematous mass with ring enhancement, which may be difficult to distinguish from a tumor or occasionally infarction; CT-guided aspiration, culture, surgical excision, or a combination may be necessary.

Culturing pus aspirated from the abscess can make targeted antibiotic therapy of the abscess possible. However, antibiotics should not be withheld until culture results are available.

Lumbar puncture is not done because it may precipitate transtentorial herniation and because CSF findings are nonspecific (see Table 221–1 on p. 1843).

Treatment

- Antibiotics (initially cefotaxime or ceftriaxone, plus metronidazole for *Bacteroides* sp or vancomycin for *Staphylococcus aureus* based on suspicion, then as guided by culture and susceptibility testing)
- Usually CT-guided stereotactic aspiration or surgical drainage
- Sometimes corticosteroids, anticonvulsants, or both

All patients receive antibiotics for a minimum of 4 to 8 wk. Initial empiric antibiotics include cefotaxime 2 g IV q 4 h or ceftriaxone 2 g IV q 12 h; both are effective against streptococci, Enterobacteriaceae, and most anaerobes, but not against *Bacteroides fragilis*. If clinicians suspect *Bacteroides* sp, metronidazole 15 mg/kg (loading dose) followed by 7.5 mg/kg IV q 6 h is also required. If *S. aureus* is suspected, vancomycin 1 g q 12 h is used (with cefotaxime or ceftriaxone) until sensitivity to nafcillin (2 g q 4 h) is determined. Response to antibiotics is best monitored by serial MRI or CT.

Drainage (CT-guided stereotactic or open) provides optimal therapy and is necessary for most abscesses that are solitary and surgically accessible, particularly those > 2 cm in diameter. If abscesses are < 2 cm in diameter, antibiotics alone may be tried, but abscesses must then be monitored with serial MRI or CT; if abscesses enlarge after being treated with antibiotics, surgical drainage is indicated.

Patients with increased intracranial pressure may benefit from a short course of high-dose corticosteroids (dexamethasone 10 mg IV once, then 4 mg IV q 6 h for 3 or 4 days).

Anticonvulsants are sometimes recommended to prevent seizures.

KEY POINTS

- Brain abscess can result from direct extension (eg, of mastoiditis, osteomyelitis, sinusitis, or subdural empyema), penetrating wounds (including neurosurgery), or hematogenous spread.
- Headache, nausea, vomiting, lethargy, seizures, personality changes, papilledema, and focal neurologic deficits develop over days to weeks; fever may be absent at presentation.
- Do contrast-enhanced MRI or, if unavailable, contrast-enhanced CT.
- Treat all brain abscesses with antibiotics (usually initially with ceftriaxone or cefotaxime plus metronidazole if clinicians suspect *Bacteroides* sp or with vancomycin if they suspect *S. aureus*), typically followed by CT-guided stereotactic aspiration or surgical drainage.
- If abscesses are < 2 cm in diameter, they may be treated with antibiotics alone but must then be monitored periodically with MRI or CT; if abscesses enlarge after being treated with antibiotics, surgical drainage is indicated.

ENCEPHALITIS

Encephalitis is inflammation of the parenchyma of the brain, resulting from direct viral invasion. Acute disseminated encephalomyelitis is brain and spinal cord inflammation caused by a hypersensitivity reaction to a virus or another foreign protein. Both disorders are usually triggered by viruses. Symptoms include fever, headache, and altered mental status, often accompanied by seizures or focal neurologic deficits. Diagnosis requires CSF analysis and neuroimaging. Treatment is supportive and, for certain causes, includes antiviral drugs.

Etiology

Encephalitis is usually a primary manifestation or a secondary (postinfectious) immunologic complication of viral infection.

Primary viral infection: Viruses causing primary encephalitis directly invade the brain. These infections may be

- Epidemic (eg, due to arbovirus, echovirus, coxsackievirus, or poliovirus [in some underdeveloped countries])
- Sporadic (eg, due to cytomegalovirus or to herpes simplex, varicella-zoster, lymphocytic choriomeningitis, rabies, or mumps virus)

Mosquito-borne arboviral encephalitides infect people during the spring, summer, and early fall when the weather is warm (see Table 223–1). Incidence in the US varies from 150 to > 4000 cases yearly, mostly in children. Most cases occur during epidemics.

In the US, the most common sporadic encephalitis is caused by herpes simplex virus (HSV); hundreds to several thousand cases occur yearly. Most are due to HSV-1, but HSV-2 may be more common among immunocompromised patients. HSV encephalitis occurs at any time of the year, tends to affect patients < 20 or > 40 yr, and is often fatal if untreated.

Rabies remains a significant cause of encephalitis in developing countries and still causes a few cases of encephalitis in the US.

Primary encephalitis can occur as a late consequence of a viral infection. The best known types are

- HIV-associated encephalopathy and dementia (see p. 1884)
- Subacute sclerosing panencephalitis (which occurs years after a measles infection and is thought to represent reactivation of the original infection; it is now rare in Western countries—see p. 2766)
- Progressive multifocal leukoencephalopathy (PML), which is caused by reactivation of JC virus (see p. 1856)

Table 223–1. SOME ARBOVIRAL ENCEPHALITIDES IN THE US

VIRUS	DISTRIBUTION	MORTALITY RATE	COMMENTS
Chikungunya virus	Florida, Puerto Rico, the US Virgin Islands Common in Africa, India, Guam, Southeast Asia, New Guinea, China, Mexico, Central America Reunion Islands, limited areas of Europe	—	Should be considered in US travelers who develop encephalitis after visiting endemic areas Can lead to severe encephalitis and even death, especially in infants and people > 65
La Crosse virus (California virus)	Primarily in the north central US but geographically widespread	Probably < 1%	Is probably underrecognized Accounts for most cases of arbovirus encephalitis in children
St. Louis encephalitis virus	Mostly in the central and eastern US	—	Until 1975, occurred every 10 yr; is now rare
West Nile virus	Throughout the US	About 9% of patients with CNS involvement	As of 2009, spread from the East Coast, where it first appeared in 1999, to all of the western states
Eastern equine encephalitis virus	Eastern US	About 50–70%	Occurs as small epidemics every 10–20 yr, mainly among young children and people > 55
Western equine encephalitis virus	—	—	For unknown reasons, has largely disappeared from the US since 1988
Zika virus	Florida South America, Central America, Caribbean Islands, Pacific Islands, Cape Verde (a nation of islands off the northwest coast of Africa), Southeast Asia	—	May cause a dengue-like illness and has been implicated in causing Guillain-Barré syndrome, severe brain damage, and microcephaly in infants of infected mothers

Immunologic reaction: Encephalitis can occur as a secondary immunologic complication of certain viral infections or vaccinations. Inflammatory demyelination of the brain and spinal cord can occur 1 to 3 wk later (as acute disseminated encephalomyelitis); the immune system attacks one or more CNS antigens that resemble proteins of the infectious agent. The most common causes of this complication used to be measles, rubella, chickenpox, and mumps (all now uncommon because childhood vaccination is widespread); smallpox vaccine; and live-virus vaccines (eg, the older rabies vaccines prepared from sheep or goat brain). In the US, most cases now result from influenza A or B virus, enteroviruses, Epstein-Barr virus, hepatitis A or B virus, or HIV.

Encephalopathies caused by autoantibodies to neuronal membrane proteins (eg, *N*-methyl-D-aspartate [NMDA] receptors) may mimic viral encephalitis.

Pathophysiology

In acute encephalitis, inflammation and edema occur in infected areas throughout the cerebral hemispheres, brain stem, cerebellum, and, occasionally, spinal cord. Petechial hemorrhages may be present in severe infections. Direct viral invasion of the brain usually damages neurons, sometimes producing microscopically visible inclusion bodies. Severe infection, particularly untreated HSV encephalitis, can cause brain hemorrhagic necrosis.

Acute disseminated encephalomyelitis is characterized by multifocal areas of perivenous demyelination and absence of virus in the brain.

Symptoms and Signs

Symptoms include fever, headache, and altered mental status, often accompanied by seizures and focal neurologic deficits. A GI or respiratory prodrome may precede these symptoms. Meningeal signs are typically mild and less prominent than other manifestations.

Status epilepticus, particularly convulsive status epilepticus, or coma suggests severe brain inflammation and a poor prognosis.

Olfactory seizures, manifested as an aura of foul smells (rotten eggs, burnt meat), indicate temporal lobe involvement and suggest HSV encephalitis.

Diagnosis

- MRI
- CSF testing

Encephalitis is suspected in patients with unexplained alterations in mental status. Clinical presentation and differential diagnoses may suggest certain diagnostic tests, but MRI and CSF analysis (including PCR for HSV and other viruses) are usually done, typically with other tests (eg, serologic tests) to identify the causative virus. Despite extensive testing, the cause of many cases of encephalitis remains unknown.

MRI: Contrast-enhanced MRI is sensitive for early HSV encephalitis, showing edema in the orbitofrontal and temporal areas, which HSV typically infects. MRI shows demyelination in progressive multifocal leukoencephalopathy and may show basal ganglia and thalamic abnormalities in West Nile and eastern equine encephalitis. MRI can also exclude lesions that mimic viral encephalitis (eg, brain abscess, sagittal sinus thrombosis).

CT is much less sensitive than MRI for HSV encephalitis but can help because it is rapidly available and can exclude disorders that make lumbar puncture risky (eg, mass lesions, hydrocephalus, cerebral edema).

CSF testing: If encephalitis is present, CSF is characterized by lymphocytic pleocytosis, normal glucose, mildly elevated protein, and an absence of pathogens after Gram staining and culture (similar to CSF in aseptic meningitis). Pleocytosis may be polymorphonuclear in severe infections. CSF abnormalities may not develop until 8 to 24 h after onset of symptoms. Hemorrhagic necrosis can introduce RBCs into CSF and elevate protein. CSF glucose levels may be low when the cause is varicella-zoster virus or lymphocytic choriomeningitis virus.

PCR testing of CSF is the diagnostic test of choice for HSV-1, HSV-2, varicella-zoster virus, cytomegalovirus, enteroviruses, and JC virus. PCR for HSV in CSF is particularly sensitive and specific. However, results may not be available rapidly, and despite advances in technology, false-negative and false-positive results may still occur because of a variety of conditions; not all are technical failures (eg, the blood in a mildly traumatic CSF tap may inhibit the PCR amplification step). False-negative results can occur early in HSV-1 encephalitis; in such cases, testing should be repeated in 48 to 72 h.

CSF viral cultures grow enteroviruses but not most other viruses. For this reason, CSF viral cultures are rarely used in diagnosis.

CSF viral IgM titers are often useful for diagnosing acute infection, especially West Nile encephalitis, for which they are more reliable than PCR. CSF IgG and IgM titers may be more sensitive than PCR for varicella-zoster virus encephalitis. Paired acute and convalescent serologic tests of CSF and blood must be drawn several weeks apart; they can detect an increase in viral titers specific for certain viral infections.

Brain biopsy: Brain biopsy may be indicated for patients who

- Are worsening
- Are responding poorly to treatment with acyclovir or another antimicrobial
- Have a lesion that is still undiagnosed

However, brain biopsy has a low yield unless it targets an abnormality seen on MRI or CT.

Prognosis

Recovery from viral encephalitis may take a very long time. Mortality rate varies with cause, but severity of epidemics due to the same virus varies during different years. Permanent neurologic deficits are common among patients who survive severe infection.

Treatment

- Supportive care
- Acyclovir for HSV or varicella-zoster virus encephalitis

Supportive therapy for encephalitis includes treatment of fever, dehydration, electrolyte disorders, and seizures. Euvolemia should be maintained.

Until HSV encephalitis and varicella-zoster virus encephalitis are excluded, acyclovir 10 mg/kg IV q 8 h should be started promptly and continued usually for 14 days or until infection with these viruses is excluded. Acyclovir is relatively nontoxic but can cause liver function abnormalities, bone marrow suppression, and transient renal failure. Giving acyclovir IV slowly over 1 h with adequate hydration helps prevent nephrotoxicity.

Because a bacterial CNS infection is often difficult to exclude when patients who appear seriously ill present, empiric antibiotics are often given until bacterial meningitis is excluded.

If encephalitis is due to an immunologic reaction, treatment may include corticosteroids (prednisone or methylprednisolone) and plasma exchange or IV immune globulin.

KEY POINTS

- Viruses that cause epidemic or sporadic infections can invade and infect brain parenchyma (causing encephalitis) and/or trigger postinfectious inflammatory demyelination (acute disseminated encephalomyelitis).
- Encephalitis causes fever, headache, and altered mental status, often accompanied by seizures and focal neurologic deficits.
- Do contrast-enhanced MRI and CSF testing.
- Until HSV encephalitis and varicella-zoster virus encephalitis are excluded, promptly treat with acyclovir and continue usually for 14 days or until infection with these viruses is excluded.

RABIES

Rabies is a viral encephalitis transmitted by the saliva of infected bats and certain other infected mammals. Symptoms include depression and fever, followed by agitation, excessive salivation, and hydrophobia. Diagnosis is by serologic tests or biopsy. Vaccination is indicated for people at high risk of exposure. Postexposure prophylaxis (PEP) involves wound care and passive and active immunoprophylaxis and, if promptly and meticulously executed, almost always prevents human rabies. Otherwise, the disorder is almost universally fatal. Treatment is supportive.

Rabies causes > 55,000 human deaths worldwide annually, mostly in Latin America, Africa, and Asia, where canine rabies is endemic. In the US, vaccination of domestic animals has reduced rabies cases in people to < 3/yr, mostly transmitted by infected bats. Infected raccoons, skunks, and foxes can also transmit rabies.

Rabid animals transmit the infection through their saliva, usually by biting. Rarely, the virus can enter through a skin abrasion or across mucous membranes of the eyes, nose, or mouth. The virus travels from the site of entry via peripheral nerves to the spinal cord (or to the brain stem when the face is bitten), then to the brain. It then spreads from the CNS via peripheral nerves to other parts of the body. Involvement of the salivary glands and oral mucosa is responsible for transmissibility.

Symptoms and Signs

Pain or paresthesias may develop at the site of the bite. Rapidity of progression depends on the viral inoculum and proximity of the wound to the brain. The incubation period averages 1 to 2 mo but may be > 1 yr.

Initial symptoms are nonspecific: fever, headache, and malaise. Within days, encephalitis (furious rabies; in 80%) or paralysis (dumb rabies; in 20%) develops. Encephalitis causes restlessness, confusion, agitation, bizarre behavior, hallucinations, and insomnia. Salivation is excessive, and attempts to drink cause painful spasms of the laryngeal and pharyngeal muscles (hydrophobia). In the paralytic form, ascending paralysis and quadriplegia develop without delirium and hydrophobia.

Diagnosis

- Skin biopsy
- Sometimes PCR testing of fluid or tissue samples

Rabies is suspected in patients with encephalitis or ascending paralysis and a history of an animal bite or exposure to bats; bat bites may be superficial and overlooked.

Direct fluorescence antibody testing of a biopsy specimen of skin from the nape of the neck is the diagnostic test of choice. Diagnosis can also be made by PCR of CSF, saliva, or tissue. Specimens tested for rabies antibodies include serum and CSF.

CT, MRI, and EEG are normal or show nonspecific changes.

Treatment

- Supportive care

Treatment once rabies has developed is only supportive and includes heavy sedation (eg, with ketamine and midazolam) and comfort measures. Death usually occurs 3 to 10 days after symptoms begin. Few patients have survived; many received immunoprophylaxis before onset of symptoms. There is evidence that giving rabies vaccine and immune globulin *after* clinical rabies develops may cause more rapid deterioration.

Experimental therapies with ribavirin, amantadine, interferon-alfa, and other drugs are sometimes tried in desperation.

Prevention

Rabid animals can often be recognized by their strange behavior; they may be agitated and vicious, weak, or paralyzed and may show no fear of people. Nocturnal animals (eg, bats, skunks, raccoons) may be out during the day. Bats may make unusual noises and have difficulty flying. An animal suspected of having rabies should not be approached. Local health authorities should be contacted to remove the animal.

Because bats are an important reservoir for rabies virus in the US and because bat bites may be hard to detect, contact with a bat is an absolute indication for PEP.

Recommendations for preexposure and PEP are available.[1]

Preexposure rabies prophylaxis: Human diploid cell rabies vaccine (HDCV) is safe and recommended for preexposure prophylaxis for people at risk, including veterinarians, animal handlers, spelunkers, workers who handle the virus, and travelers to endemic areas.

A total of three 1-mL doses are given IM, one each on days 0, 7, and between day 21 and 28. Vaccination provides lifetime protection to some degree. However, protection decreases with time; if exposure is likely to continue, serologic testing every 6 mo (for continuous exposure) or every 2 yr (for frequent exposure) is recommended, and a booster dose of vaccine is given if the antibody titer is below a certain level.

Postexposure rabies prophylaxis: Exposure is considered to be a bite that breaks the skin or any contact between mucous membrane or broken skin and animal saliva. If exposure occurs, prompt, meticulously executed prophylaxis almost always prevents human rabies. The wound is cleansed immediately and thoroughly with soap and water or benzalkonium chloride. Deep puncture wounds are flushed with soapy water using moderate pressure. Wounds are usually left open.

PEP with rabies vaccine and rabies immune globulin (RIG) is given depending on the biting animal and circumstances (see Table 223–2). PEP is begun, and the animal's brain is tested for virus. Local or state health departments or the CDC usually conduct testing and can advise on other treatment issues.

PEARLS & PITFALLS

- Consider raccoons, skunks, or foxes that have bitten a person rabid.
- Because bat bites can be tiny and hard to detect, give the rabies vaccine and RIG to anyone who has had contact with a bat.

For PEP, RIG 20 IU/kg is infiltrated around the wound for passive immunization; if injection volume is too much for distal areas (eg, fingers, nose), some RIG may be given IM.[2] This treatment is accompanied by HDCV for active immunization. HDCV is given in a series of four 1-mL IM injections (deltoid area is preferred), beginning on the day of exposure (day 0), in a limb other than the one used for RIG. Subsequent injections occur on days 3, 7, and 14; immunosuppressed patients receive a 5th dose on day 28. Rarely, a serious systemic or neuroparalytic reaction occurs; then, completion of vaccination is weighed against the patient's risk of developing rabies. Rabies antibody titer is measured to help assess risk of stopping vaccination.

PEP for a person previously vaccinated against rabies includes 1-mL IM injections of HDCV on days 0 and 3 but no RIG.

1. ACIP: Human Rabies Prevention—United States, 2008 Recommendations of the Advisory Committee on Immunization Practices. *Morbidity and Mortality Weekly Report* 57(RR03):1–26,28, 2008,
2. ACIP: (Advisory Committee on Immunization Practices) recommendations: Use of a reduced (4-dose) vaccine schedule for PEP to prevent human rabies. *Morbidity and Mortality Weekly Report* 59(RR02):1–9, 2010.

KEY POINTS

- Worldwide, rabies still causes tens of thousands of deaths yearly, mostly in Latin America, Africa, and Asia, where canine rabies is endemic.
- In the US, rabies kills only a few people yearly; it is usually transmitted by bats, but possibly by racoons, skunks, or foxes.
- Pain and/or paresthesias at the bite site are followed by encephalitis (causing restlessness and agitation) or by ascending paralysis.
- Biopsy neck skin or do PCR of saliva, CSF, or tissue if patients have unexplained encephalitis or ascending paralysis.
- Treat patients supportively.
- Before exposure, give the rabies vaccine to people at risk (eg, veterinarians, animal handlers, spelunkers, workers who handle the virus, travelers to endemic areas).
- After exposure, thoroughly clean and debride wounds, then give the rabies vaccine and RIG.
- Raccoons, skunks, or foxes that have bitten a person should be regarded as rabid; because bat bites can be minute and hard to detect, contact with a bat is an absolute indication for RIG.

Table 223–2. RABIES POSTEXPOSURE PROPHYLAXIS

ANIMAL TYPE	EVALUATION AND DISPOSITION OF ANIMAL	POSTEXPOSURE PROPHYLAXIS*
Skunks, raccoons, bats,† foxes, and most other carnivores	Regarded as rabid unless proved negative by laboratory tests‡	Consider immediate vaccination and RIG.
Dogs, cats, and ferrets	Healthy and available for 10 days of observation	Do not begin immunoprophylaxis unless animal develops symptoms of rabies.§
	Unknown (escaped)	Consult public health officials.¶
	Rabid or suspected rabid	Vaccinate immediately. Consider RIG.
Livestock, small rodents (eg, squirrels, hamsters, guinea pigs, gerbils, chipmunks, rats, mice), lagomorphs (rabbits, hares), large rodents (eg, woodchucks, beavers), and other mammals	Considered individually	Consult public health officials. Immunoprophylaxis is almost never required for bites of squirrels, hamsters, guinea pigs, gerbils, chipmunks, rats, mice, other small rodents, or lagomorphs.

*Clean all bites immediately with soap and water.

†Because detecting bat bites is difficult, vaccination is indicated if a bite is reasonably likely, as when a person awakens with a bat in the room or a young child is found with a bat.

‡The animal should be euthanized and tested as soon as possible. Holding for observation is not recommended. Vaccine is stopped if rabies immunofluorescence tests of the animal are negative. Offspring from matings between wild animals and domestic dogs or cats are considered wild animals, and euthanasia and rabies testing is considered the safest approach. An exception may be animals described as wolf-dogs, which may be dogs; in such cases, consulting public health officials before euthanizing and testing the animal is recommended.

§If the animal remains healthy during the 10-day observation period, it was not infective at the time of the bite. However, treatment with RIG and human diploid cell rabies vaccine (HDCV) is begun at the first sign of rabies in a dog, cat, or ferret that has bitten someone. A symptomatic animal should be immediately euthanized and tested.

¶If expert consultation is not available locally and rabies is possible, immediate vaccination should be considered.

Adapted from Human Rabies Prevention—United States, 2008 Recommendations of the Advisory Committee on Immunization Practices. *Morbidity and Mortality Weekly Report* 57(RR03):1–26,28, 2008.

HELMINTHIC BRAIN INFECTIONS

Parasitic helminthic worms infect the CNS of millions of people in developing countries. Infected people who visit or immigrate to nonendemic areas, including the US, may present there. Worms may cause meningitis, encephalitis, cerebral masses, hydrocephalus, stroke, and myelopathy.

Neurocysticercosis: Among about 20 helminths that can cause neurologic disorders, the pork tapeworm Taenia solium causes by far the most cases in the Western Hemisphere. The resulting disorder is neurocysticercosis. After a person eats food contaminated with the worm's eggs, larvae migrate to tissues, including the brain, spinal cord, and CSF pathways, and form cysts. Cyst diameter rarely exceeds 1 cm in neural parenchyma but may exceed 5 cm in CSF spaces.

Brain parenchymal cysts cause few symptoms until death of the worms triggers local inflammation, gliosis, and edema, causing seizures (most commonly), cognitive or focal neurologic deficits, or personality changes. Larger cysts in CSF pathways may cause obstructive hydrocephalus. Cysts may rupture into CSF, inducing acute or subacute eosinophilic meningitis. Mortality rate for symptomatic neurocysticercosis is up to 50%.

Neurocysticercosis is suspected in patients who live in or have come from developing countries and who have eosinophilic meningitis or unexplained seizures, cognitive or focal deficits, or personality changes. It is suggested by multiple calcified cystic lesions seen on CT or MRI; a contrast agent may enhance the lesions. Diagnosis requires serum and CSF serologic tests and occasionally cyst biopsy.

Albendazole (7.5 mg/kg po q 12 h for 8 to 30 days; maximum daily dose, 800 mg) is the antihelminthic drug of choice. Alternatively, praziquantel 20 to 33 mg/kg po tid may be given for 30 days. Dexamethasone 8 mg once/day IV or po for the first 2 to 4 days may lessen the acute inflammatory response as the worms die. Antihelminthic therapy can cause serious morbidity in patients with a large number of cysts and may not help patients with a single cyst. Treatment must be carefully individualized.

Short- or long-term anticonvulsant treatment may be required. Surgical excision of cysts and ventricular shunts may also be required.

Other helminthic infections: In schistosomiasis, necrotizing eosinophilic granulomas develop in the brain, causing seizures, increased intracranial pressure, and diffuse and focal neurologic deficits.

Large, solitary echinococcal cysts can cause focal deficits and, occasionally, seizures.

Coenurosis, caused by tapeworm larvae, usually produces grapelike cysts that may obstruct CSF outflow in the 4th ventricle. Symptoms require several years to develop and, if the brain is involved, include increased intracranial pressure, seizures, loss of consciousness, and focal neurologic deficits.

Gnathostomiasis, a rare infection by larvae of the nematode *Gnathostoma* sp, results in necrotic tracts surrounded by inflammation along the nerve roots, spinal cord, and brain or in subarachnoid hemorrhage, causing low-grade fever, stiff neck, photophobia, headache, migratory neurologic deficits (occasionally affecting the 6th or 7th cranial nerve), and paralysis.

PROGRESSIVE MULTIFOCAL LEUKOENCEPHALOPATHY

Progressive multifocal leukoencephalopathy (PML) is caused by reactivation of the JC virus. The disease usually occurs in patients with impaired cell-mediated immunity, particularly patients with HIV infection. PML results in subacute and progressive CNS demyelination, multifocal neurologic deficits, and death, usually within a year. Diagnosis is with MRI plus CSF PCR. In AIDS patients, highly active antiretroviral therapy may slow down the progression, and patients taking immunosuppressants may improve when those drugs are withdrawn. Treatment is otherwise supportive.

Etiology

PML is caused by reactivation of the JC virus, a ubiquitous human papovavirus that is typically acquired during childhood and remains latent in the kidneys and possibly other sites (eg, mononuclear cells, CNS). The reactivated virus has a tropism for oligodendrocytes. Most patients who develop PML have depressed cell-mediated immunity due to AIDS (the most common risk factor), reticuloendothelial system disorders (eg, leukemia, lymphoma), or other conditions (eg, Wiskott-Aldrich syndrome, organ transplantation).

The risk in AIDS increases with increasing HIV viral load; prevalence of PML has decreased because of widespread use of more effective antiretrovirals. Increasingly, PML is occurring as a complication of immunomodulatory therapy (eg, monoclonal antibodies, such as natalizumab and rituximab). Measuring serum antibodies to JC virus (JC virus index) may help assess the risk of PML in patients taking natalizumab.

Symptoms and Signs

Clumsiness may be the first symptom. Hemiparesis is the most common finding. Aphasia, dysarthria, and hemianopia are also common. Multifocal cortical damage produces cognitive impairment in two thirds of patients. Sensory, cerebellar, and brain stem deficits may be present.

Headaches and convulsive seizures are rare and occur most often in patients with AIDS.

Gradual, relentless progression culminates in death, usually 1 to 9 mo after symptoms begin.

Diagnosis

- MRI
- CSF testing for JC viral DNA

PML is suspected in patients with unexplained progressive brain dysfunction, particularly in those with depressed cell-mediated immunity.

Provisional diagnosis of PML is made by contrast-enhanced MRI, which shows single or multiple white matter lesions on T2-weighted images. A contrast agent enhances, usually faintly and peripherally, 5 to 15% of lesions. CT may show low-density, nonenhancing lesions but is significantly less sensitive than MRI.

CSF is analyzed for JC viral DNA using PCR; a positive result with compatible neuroimaging findings is nearly pathognomonic. Routine CSF analysis is usually normal.

Serologic tests are not helpful. Stereotaxic biopsy can provide a definitive diagnosis but is rarely warranted.

Treatment

- Supportive care

Treatment of PML is mainly supportive.

Experimental use of drugs such as cidofovir and other antivirals has failed to provide benefit. Antiretroviral therapy (ART) in AIDS patients has improved outcome in PML, increasing the 1-yr survival rate from 10 to 50%. However, patients treated with aggressive antiretroviral therapy may develop immune reconstitution inflammatory syndrome (IRIS). In IRIS, the recovering immune system produces an intense inflammatory response against the JC virus, thus worsening symptoms. Imaging done after IRIS develops shows greater contrast enhancement of the lesions and may show significant cerebral edema. Corticosteroids may be helpful. Depending on the severity of IRIS and of AIDS, clinicians may decide to withdraw ART.

Withdrawal of immunosuppressants may result in clinical improvement. However, patients who stop taking these drugs are also at risk of developing IRIS.

If PML develops in patients taking natalizumab, another immunomodulatory drug, or an immunosuppressant, the drug should be stopped, and plasma exchange should be done to remove residual circulating drug.

KEY POINTS

- Reactivation of the ubiquitous JC virus, usually due to impaired cell-mediated immunity, leads to PML.
- PML commonly causes clumsiness, hemiparesis, aphasia, dysarthria, hemianopia, and cognitive impairment.
- Do MRI and test CSF for JC virus DNA in patients who have impaired cell-mediated immunity and unexplained progressive brain dysfunction.
- Treat patients supportively, and manage underlying disorders as indicated (eg, by stopping natalizumab, another immunomodulatory drug, or an immunosuppressant or by initiating antiretroviral therapy, watching closely for development of IRIS).

INTRACRANIAL EPIDURAL ABSCESS AND SUBDURAL EMPYEMA

Epidural abscess is a collection of pus between the dura mater and skull. Subdural empyema is a collection of pus between the dura mater and the underlying arachnoid mater. Symptoms of epidural abscess include fever, headache, vomiting, and sometimes lethargy, focal neurologic deficits, seizures, and/or coma. Symptoms of subdural empyema include fever, vomiting, impaired consciousness, and rapid development of neurologic signs suggesting widespread involvement of one cerebral hemisphere. Diagnosis is by contrast-enhanced MRI or, if MRI is not available, contrast-enhanced CT. Treatment is with surgical drainage and antibiotics.

Etiology

Cranial epidural abscess and subdural empyema are usually complications of sinusitis (especially frontal, ethmoidal, or sphenoidal), but they can follow ear infections, cranial trauma or surgery, or, rarely, bacteremia. Pathogens are similar to those that cause brain abscess (eg, *Staphylococcus aureus*, *Bacteroides fragilis*).

In children < 5 yr, the usual cause is bacterial meningitis; because childhood meningitis is now uncommon, childhood subdural empyema is uncommon.

Complications: Epidural abscess may extend into the subdural space to cause subdural empyema. Both epidural abscess and subdural empyema may progress to meningitis, cortical venous thrombosis, or brain abscess. Subdural empyema can rapidly spread to involve an entire cerebral hemisphere.

Symptoms and Signs

Fever, headache, lethargy, focal neurologic deficits (often indicating subdural empyema when rapidly developing deficits suggest widespread involvement of one cerebral hemisphere), and seizures usually evolve over several days.

Patients with intracranial epidural abscess may also develop a subperiosteal abscess and osteomyelitis of the frontal bone (Pott puffy tumor), and patients with subdural empyema develop meningeal signs. In epidural abscess and subdural empyema, vomiting and papilledema are common.

Without treatment, coma and death occur rapidly.

Diagnosis

- Contrast-enhanced MRI

Diagnosis of epidural abscess or subdural empyema is by contrast-enhanced MRI or, if MRI is not available, by contrast-enhanced CT. Blood and surgical specimens are cultured aerobically and anaerobically.

Lumbar puncture provides little useful information and may precipitate transtentorial herniation. If intracranial epidural abscess or subdural empyema is suspected (eg, based on symptom duration of several days, focal deficits, or risk factors) in patients with meningeal signs, lumbar puncture is contraindicated until neuroimaging excludes a mass lesion. In infants, a subdural tap may be diagnostic and may relieve pressure.

Treatment

- Surgical drainage
- Antibiotics

Emergency surgical drainage of the epidural abscess or subdural empyema and any underlying fluid in the sinuses should be done.

Pending culture results, antibiotic coverage is the same as antibiotics used to treat brain abscess (eg, cefotaxime, ceftriaxone, metronidazole, vancomycin on p. 1922) except in young children, who may require other antibiotics for any accompanying meningitis (see Tables 231–4 and 231–6 on pp. 1921 and 1923).

Anticonvulsants and measures to reduce intracranial pressure may be needed.

KEY POINTS

- Epidural abscess and subdural empyema may progress to meningitis, cortical venous thrombosis, or brain abscess; subdural empyema can rapidly spread to involve an entire cerebral hemisphere.
- Fever, headache, lethargy, focal neurologic deficits, and seizures usually evolve over several days; vomiting and papilledema are common.
- Without treatment, coma and death occur rapidly.
- Use contrast-enhanced MRI or, if MRI is not available, contrast-enhanced CT to diagnose epidural abscess or subdural empyema.
- Lumbar puncture provides little useful information and may precipitate transtentorial herniation.
- Drain the epidural abscess or subdural empyema and any underlying fluid in the sinuses as soon as possible, and treat with antibiotics (eg, cefotaxime, ceftriaxone, metronidazole, vancomycin).

224 Coma and Impaired Consciousness

Coma is unresponsiveness from which the patient cannot be aroused. Impaired consciousness refers to similar, less severe disturbances of consciousness; these disturbances are not considered coma. The mechanism for coma or impaired consciousness involves dysfunction of both cerebral hemispheres or of the reticular activating system (RAS—also known as the ascending arousal system). Causes may be structural or nonstructural (eg, toxic or metabolic disturbances). Damage may be focal or diffuse. Diagnosis is clinical; identification of cause requires laboratory tests and neuroimaging. Treatment is immediate stabilization and specific management of the cause. For long-term coma, adjunctive treatment includes passive range-of-motion exercises, enteral feedings, and measures to prevent pressure ulcers.

Decreased or impaired consciousness or alertness refers to decreased responsiveness to external stimuli. Severe impairment includes

- **Coma:** The patient cannot be aroused, and the eyes do not open in response to any stimulation.
- **Stupor:** The patient can be awakened only by vigorous physical stimulation.

Less severely impaired levels of consciousness are often labeled as lethargy or, if more severe, obtundation. However, differentiation between less severely impaired levels is often imprecise; the label is less important than a precise clinical description (eg, "the best level of response is partial limb withdrawal to nail bed pressure"). Delirium differs because cognitive disturbances (in attention, cognition, and level of consciousness) fluctuate more; also, delirium is usually reversible.

Pathophysiology

Maintaining alertness requires intact function of the cerebral hemispheres and preservation of arousal mechanisms in the RAS (also known as the ascending arousal system)—an extensive network of nuclei and interconnecting fibers in the upper pons, midbrain, and posterior diencephalon. Therefore, the mechanism of impaired consciousness must involve both cerebral hemispheres or dysfunction of the RAS.

To impair consciousness, cerebral dysfunction must be bilateral; unilateral cerebral hemisphere disorders are not sufficient, although they may cause severe neurologic deficits. However, rarely, a unilateral massive hemispheric focal lesion (eg, left middle cerebral artery stroke) impairs consciousness if the contralateral hemisphere is already compromised or if it results in compression of the contralateral hemisphere (eg, by causing edema).

Usually, RAS dysfunction results from a condition that has diffuse effects, such as toxic or metabolic disturbances (eg, hypoglycemia, hypoxia, uremia, drug overdose). RAS dysfunction can also be caused by focal ischemia (eg, certain upper brain stem infarcts), hemorrhage, or direct, mechanical disruption.

Any condition that increases intracranial pressure (ICP) may decrease cerebral perfusion pressure, resulting in secondary brain ischemia. Secondary brain ischemia may affect the RAS or both cerebral hemispheres, impairing consciousness.

When brain damage is extensive, brain herniation (see Fig. 224–1 and Table 224–1) contributes to neurologic deterioration because it does the following:

- Directly compresses brain tissue
- Increases ICP
- May lead to hydrocephalus
- Results in neuronal and vascular cell dysfunction

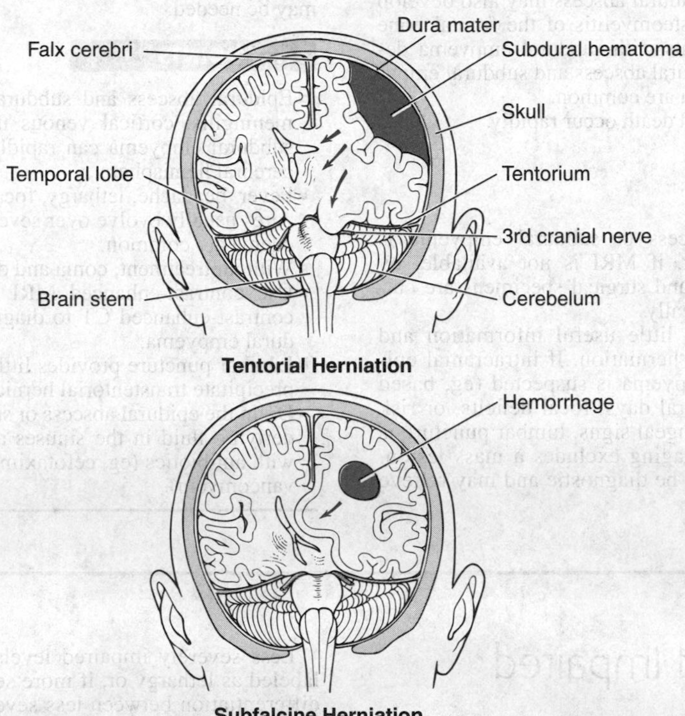

Fig. 224–1. Brain herniation. Because the skull is rigid after infancy, intracranial masses or swelling may increase ICP, sometimes causing protrusion (herniation) of brain tissue through one of the rigid intracranial barriers (tentorial notch, falx cerebri, foramen magnum). When ICP is increased sufficiently, regardless of the cause, Cushing reflex and other autonomic abnormalities can occur. Cushing reflex includes systolic hypertension with increased pulse pressure, irregular respirations, and bradycardia. Brain herniation is life-threatening.

Transtentorial herniation: The medial temporal lobe is squeezed by a unilateral mass across and under the tentlike tentorium that supports the temporal lobe. The herniating lobe compresses the following structures:

- **Ipsilateral 3rd cranial nerve (often first) and posterior cerebral artery**
- **As herniation progresses, the ipsilateral cerebral peduncle**
- **In about 5% of patients, the contralateral 3rd cranial nerve and cerebral peduncle**
- **Eventually, the upper brain stem and the area in or around the thalamus**

Subfalcine herniation: The cingulate gyrus is pushed under the falx cerebri by an expanding mass high in a cerebral hemisphere. In this process, one or both anterior cerebral arteries become trapped, causing infarction of the paramedian cortex. As the infarcted area expands, patients are at risk of transtentorial herniation, central herniation, or both.

Central herniation: Both temporal lobes herniate through the tentorial notch because of bilateral mass effects or diffuse brain edema. Ultimately, brain death occurs.

Upward transtentorial herniation: This type can occur when an infratentorial mass (eg, tumor, cerebellar hemorrhage) compresses the brain stem, kinking it and causing patchy brain stem ischemia. The posterior 3rd ventricle becomes compressed. Upward herniation also distorts the mesencephalon vasculature, compresses the veins of Galen and Rosenthal, and causes superior cerebellar infarction due to occlusion of the superior cerebellar arteries.

Tonsillar herniation: Usually, the cause is an expanding infratentorial mass (eg, cerebellar hemorrhage). The cerebellar tonsils, forced through the foramen magnum, compress the brain stem and obstruct CSF flow.

Table 224–1. EFFECTS OF BRAIN HERNIATION

TYPE OF HERNIATION	MECHANISM*	FINDINGS
Transtentorial	Compression of ipsilateral 3rd cranial nerve	Unilateral dilated, fixed pupil Oculomotor paresis
	Compression of the posterior cerebral artery	Contralateral homonymous hemianopia Absence of blinking in response to visual threat from the hemianopic side in obtunded patients
	Compression of the contralateral 3rd cranial nerve and cerebral peduncle (indented by the tentorium to form Kernohan notch)	Contralateral dilated pupil and oculomotor paresis Ipsilateral hemiparesis
	Compression of the ipsilateral cerebral peduncle	Contralateral hemiparesis
	Eventually, compression of the upper brain stem and the area in and around the thalamus	Impaired consciousness Abnormal breathing patterns Fixed, unequal pupils
	Further compromise of the brain stem	Loss of oculocephalic reflex Loss of oculovestibular reflex Loss of corneal reflexes Decerebrate posturing
Subfalcine (cingulate)	Trapping of one or both anterior cerebral arteries, causing infarction of the paramedian cortex	Leg paralysis
	Expansion of infarcted area	Edema Increased ICP Increased risk of transtentorial herniation, central herniation, or both
Central	Bilateral, more or less symmetric damage to the midbrain	Pupils fixed in midposition Decerebrate posturing Many of the same symptoms as transtentorial herniation
	Further compromise of the brain stem	Loss of all brain stem reflexes Disappearance of decerebrate posturing Cessation of respirations Brain death
Upward transtentorial	Compression of the posterior 3rd ventricle	Hydrocephalus, which increases ICP
	Distortion of the mesencephalon vasculature Compression of the veins of Galen and Rosenthal Superior cerebellar infarction due to occlusion of the superior cerebellar arteries	Early: Nausea, vomiting, occipital headache, ataxia Later: Somnolence, breathing abnormalities, patchy and progressive loss of brain stem reflexes
	Posterior fossa mass (eg, cerebellar hemorrhage)	Ataxia, dysarthria
	Progression	Increasing somnolence Respiratory irregularities Patchy but progressive loss of brain stem reflexes
Tonsillar	Compression of the brain stem Obstruction of CSF flow	Acute hydrocephalus (with impaired consciousness, headache, vomiting, and meningismus) Dysconjugate eye movements Later, abrupt respiratory and cardiac arrest

*Not all mechanisms occur in every patient.

In addition to the direct effects of increased ICP on neuronal and vascular cells, cellular pathways of apoptosis and autophagy (which are forms of programmed cell death or destruction) can become activated.

Impaired consciousness may progress to coma and ultimately to brain death.

Etiology

Coma or impaired consciousness may result from structural disorders, which typically cause focal damage, or nonstructural disorders, which most often cause diffuse damage (see Table 224–2).

Psychiatric disorders (eg, psychogenic unresponsiveness) can mimic impaired consciousness, are volitional, and can be distinguished from true impaired consciousness by neurologic examination.

Symptoms and Signs

Consciousness is decreased to varying degrees. Repeated stimuli arouse patients only briefly or not at all.

Table 224–2. COMMON CAUSES OF COMA OR IMPAIRED CONSCIOUSNESS

CAUSE	EXAMPLES
Focal	
Structural disorders	Brain abscess Brain tumor Head trauma (eg, concussion, cerebral lacerations or contusions, epidural or subdural hematoma) Hydrocephalus (acute) Intraparenchymal hemorrhage Subarachnoid hemorrhage Upper brain stem infarct or hemorrhage
Nonstructural disorders	Seizures (eg, nonconvulsive status epilepticus) or a postictal state caused by an epileptogenic focus
Diffuse	
Metabolic and endocrine disorders	Diabetic ketoacidosis Hepatic encephalopathy Hypercalcemia Hypercapnia Hyperglycemia Hypernatremia Hypoglycemia Hyponatremia Hypothyroidism Hypoxia Uremia Wernicke encephalopathy
Infections	Encephalitis Meningitis Sepsis
Other disorders	Diffuse axonal injury Hypertensive encephalopathy Hyperthermia or hypothermia
Drugs	Alcohol CNS stimulants Sedatives Other CNS depressants
Toxins	Carbon monoxide

Depending on the cause, other symptoms develop (see Table 224–3):

- **Eye abnormalities:** Pupils may be dilated, pinpoint, or unequal. One or both pupils may be fixed in midposition. Eye movement may be dysconjugate or absent (oculomotor paresis) or involve unusual patterns (eg, ocular bobbing, ocular dipping, opsoclonus). Homonymous hemianopia may be present. Other abnormalities include absence of blinking in response to visual threat (almost touching the eye), as well as loss of the oculocephalic reflex (the eyes do not move in response to head rotation), the oculovestibular reflex (the eyes do not move in response to caloric stimulation), and corneal reflexes.
- **Autonomic dysfunction:** Patients may have abnormal breathing patterns (Cheyne-Stokes or Biot respirations), sometimes with hypertension and bradycardia (Cushing reflex). Abrupt respiratory and cardiac arrest may occur.
- **Motor dysfunction:** Abnormalities include flaccidity, hemiparesis, asterixis, multifocal myoclonus, decorticate posturing (elbow flexion and shoulder adduction with leg extension), and decerebrate posturing (limb extension and internal shoulder rotation).
- **Other symptoms:** If the brain stem is compromised, nausea, vomiting, meningismus, occipital headache, ataxia, and increasing somnolence can occur.

Diagnosis

- History
- General physical examination
- Neurologic examination, including eye examination
- Laboratory tests (eg, pulse oximetry, bedside glucose measurement, blood and urine tests)
- Immediate neuroimaging
- Sometimes measurement of ICP
- If diagnosis is unclear, lumbar puncture or EEG

Impaired consciousness is diagnosed if repeated stimuli arouse patients only briefly or not at all. If stimulation triggers primitive reflex movements (eg, decerebrate or decorticate posturing), impaired consciousness may be deepening into coma.

Diagnosis and initial stabilization (airway, breathing, and circulation) should occur simultaneously. Temperature is measured to check for hypothermia or hyperthermia; if either is present, treatment is started immediately. Glucose levels must be measured at bedside to identify low levels, which should also be corrected immediately. If trauma is involved, the neck is immobilized until clinical history, physical examination, or imaging tests exclude an unstable injury and damage to the cervical spine.

History: Medical identification bracelets or the contents of a wallet or purse may provide clues (eg, hospital identification card, drugs). Relatives, paramedics, police officers, and any witnesses should be questioned about the circumstances and environment in which the patient was found; containers that may have held food, alcohol, drugs, or poisons should be examined and saved for identification (eg, drug identification aided by a poison center) and possible chemical analysis.

Relatives should be asked about the following:

- The onset and time course of the problem (eg, whether seizure, headache, vomiting, head trauma, or drug ingestion was observed; how quickly symptoms appeared; whether the course has been progressive or waxing and waning)
- Baseline mental status
- Recent infections and possible exposure to infections
- Recent travel
- Ingestions of unusual meals
- Psychiatric problems and symptoms
- Drug history
- Alcohol and other substance use
- Previous illnesses
- The last time the patient was normal
- Any hunches they may have about what might be the cause (eg, possible occult overdose, possible occult head trauma due to recent intoxication)

Medical records should be reviewed if available.

General physical examination: Physical examination should be focused and efficient and should include thorough examination of the head and face, skin, and extremities. Signs of head trauma include periorbital ecchymosis (raccoon eyes), ecchymosis behind the ear (Battle sign), hemotympanum, instability of the maxilla, and CSF rhinorrhea and otorrhea. Scalp contusions and small bullet holes can be missed unless the head is carefully inspected.

If unstable injury and cervical spine damage have been excluded, passive neck flexion is done; stiffness suggests subarachnoid hemorrhage or meningitis.

Table 224–3. FINDINGS BY LOCATION*

LOCATION	ABNORMAL FINDINGS
Bilateral hemispheric damage or dysfunction*	Symmetric tone and response (flexor or extensor) to pain Myoclonus (possible) Periodic cycling of breathing
Supratentorial mass compressing the brain stem	Ipsilateral 3rd cranial nerve palsy with unilateral dilated, fixed pupil and oculomotor paresis Sometimes contralateral homonymous hemianopia and absent blinking response to visual threat Contralateral hemiparesis
Brain stem lesion	Early abnormal pupillary and oculomotor signs Abnormal oculocephalic reflex Abnormal oculovestibular reflex Asymmetrical motor responses Decorticate rigidity (usually due to an upper brain stem lesion) or decerebrate rigidity (usually due to a bilateral midbrain or pontine lesion) Hyperventilation (due to a midbrain or upper pontine lesion)
Midbrain lesion	Pupils locked in midposition with loss of light reflexes (due to a structural or metabolic disorder that causes loss of both sympathetic and parasympathetic pupillary tone)
Toxic-metabolic dysfunction*	Spontaneous, conjugate roving eye movements in mild coma Fixed eye position in deeper coma Abnormal oculovestibular reflex Multifocal myoclonus Asterixis (may be considered a type of negative myoclonus) Decorticate and decerebrate rigidity or flaccidity

*Not all of the findings occur in all cases. Brain stem reflexes and pupillary light responses may be intact in patients with bilateral hemispheric damage or dysfunction or toxic-metabolic dysfunction; however, hypothermia, sedative overdose, or use of an anesthetic can cause partial loss of brain stem reflexes.

Findings may suggest a cause:

- Hypothermia: Environmental exposure, near-drowning, sedative overdose, Wernicke encephalopathy, or, in the elderly, sepsis
- Hyperthermia: Heatstroke
- Fever, petechial or purpuric rash, hypotension, or severe extremity infections (eg, gangrene of one or more toes): Sepsis or CNS infection
- Needle marks: Drug overdose (eg, of opioids or insulin)
- A bitten tongue: Seizure
- Breath odor: Alcohol, other drug intoxication, or diabetic ketoacidosis

Neurologic examination: The neurologic examination determines whether the brain stem is intact and where the lesion is located within the CNS. The examination focuses on the following:

- Level of consciousness
- Eyes
- Motor function
- Deep tendon reflexes

Level of consciousness is evaluated by attempting to wake patients first with verbal commands, then with nonnoxious stimuli, and finally with noxious stimuli (eg, pressure to the supraorbital ridge, nail bed, or sternum).

The Glasgow Coma Scale (see Table 224–4) was developed to assess patients with head trauma. For head trauma, the score assigned by the scale is valuable prognostically. For coma or impaired consciousness of any cause, the scale is used because it is a relatively reliable, objective measure of the severity of unresponsiveness and can be used serially for monitoring. The scale assigns points based on responses to stimuli.

Eye opening, facial grimacing, and purposeful withdrawal of limbs from a noxious stimulus indicate that consciousness is not greatly impaired. Asymmetric motor responses to pain or deep tendon reflexes may indicate a focal hemispheric lesion.

As impaired consciousness deepens into coma, noxious stimuli may trigger stereotypic reflex posturing.

- **Decorticate posturing** can occur in structural or metabolic disorders and indicates hemispheric damage with preservation of motor centers in the upper portion of the brain stem (eg, rubrospinal tract).
- **Decerebrate posturing** indicates that the upper brain stem motor centers, which facilitate flexion, have been structurally damaged and that only the lower brain stem centers (eg, vestibulospinal tract, reticulospinal tract), which facilitate extension, are responding to sensory stimuli.

Decerebrate posturing may also occur, although less often, in diffuse disorders such as anoxic encephalopathy.

Flaccidity without movement indicates that the lower brain stem is not affecting movement, regardless of whether the spinal cord is damaged. It is the worst possible motor response.

Asterixis and multifocal myoclonus suggest metabolic disorders such as uremia, hepatic encephalopathy, hypoxic encephalopathy, and drug toxicity.

Psychogenic unresponsiveness can be differentiated because although voluntary motor response is typically absent, muscle tone and deep tendon reflexes remain normal, and all brain stem reflexes are preserved. Vital signs are usually not affected.

Eye examination: The following are evaluated:

- Pupillary responses
- Extraocular movements
- Fundi
- Other neuro-ophthalmic reflexes

Table 224–4. GLASGOW COMA SCALE*

AREA ASSESSED	RESPONSE	POINTS
Eye opening	Open spontaneously; open with blinking at baseline	4
	Open to verbal command, speech, or shout	3
	Open in response to pain applied to the limbs or sternum	2
	None	1
Verbal	Oriented	5
	Confused conversation but able to answer questions	4
	Inappropriate responses; words discernible	3
	Incomprehensible speech	2
	None	1
Motor	Obeys commands for movement	6
	Responds to pain with purposeful movement	5
	Withdraws from pain stimuli	4
	Responds to pain with abnormal flexion (decorticate posturing)	3
	Responds to pain with abnormal extension (decerebrate posturing)	2
	None	1

*Combined scores < 8 are typically regarded as coma.
Adapted from Teasdale G, Jennett B: Assessment of coma and impaired consciousness. A practical scale. *Lancet* 2:81–84, 1974.

Pupillary responses and **extraocular movements** provide information about brain stem function (see Table 224–5). One or both pupils usually become fixed early in coma due to structural lesions, but pupillary responses are often preserved until very late when coma is due to diffuse metabolic disorders (called toxic-metabolic encephalopathy), although responses may be sluggish. If one pupil is dilated, other causes of anisocoria should be considered; they include past ocular trauma, certain headaches, and use of a scopolamine patch.

The **fundi** should be examined. Papilledema may indicate increased ICP but may take many hours to appear. Increased ICP can cause earlier changes in the fundi, such as disk hypermia, dilated capillaries, blurring of the medial disk margins, and sometimes hemorrhages. Subhyaloid hemorrhage may indicate subarachnoid hemorrhage.

The **oculocephalic reflex** is tested by the doll's-eye maneuver in unresponsive patients: The eyes are observed while the head is passively rotated from side to side or flexed and extended. *This maneuver should not be attempted if cervical spine instability is suspected.*

- If the reflex is present, the maneuver causes the eyes to move in the opposite direction of head rotation, flexion, or extension, indicating that the oculovestibular pathways in the brain stem are intact. Thus, in a supine patient, the eyes continue to look straight up when the head is turned side to side.
- If the reflex is absent, the eyes do not move and thus point in whatever direction the head is turned, indicating the oculovestibular pathways are disrupted. The reflex is also absent in most patients with psychogenic unresponsiveness because visual fixation is conscious.

If the patient is unconscious and the oculocephalic reflex is absent or the neck is immobilized, oculovestibular (cold caloric) testing is done. After integrity of the tympanic membrane is confirmed, the patient's head is elevated 30°, and with a syringe connected to a flexible catheter, the examiner irrigates the external auditory canal with 50 mL of ice water over a 30-sec period.

- If both eyes deviate toward the irrigated ear, the brain stem is functioning normally, suggesting mildly impaired consciousness.
- If nystagmus away from the irrigated ear also occurs, the patient is conscious and psychogenic unresponsiveness is likely. In conscious patients, 1 mL of ice water is often enough to induce ocular deviation and nystagmus. Thus, if psychogenic unresponsiveness is suspected, a small amount of water should be used (or caloric testing should not be done) because cold caloric testing can induce severe vertigo, nausea, and vomiting in conscious patients.
- If the eyes do not move or movement is dysconjugate after irrigation, the integrity of the brain stem is uncertain and the coma is deeper. Prognosis may be less favorable.

PEARLS & PITFALLS

- If muscle tone, deep tendon reflexes, and the response to the doll's-eye maneuver are normal, suspect psychogenic unresponsiveness.

Certain patterns of eye abnormalities and other findings may suggest brain herniation (see Fig. 224–1 and Table 224–1).

Respiratory patterns: The spontaneous respiratory rate and pattern should be documented unless emergency airway intervention is required. It may suggest a cause.

- Periodic cycling of breathing (Cheyne-Stokes or Biot respiration) may indicate dysfunction of both hemispheres or of the diencephalon.
- Hyperventilation (central neurogenic hyperventilation) with respiratory rates of > 40 breaths/min may indicate midbrain or upper pontine dysfunction.
- An inspiratory gasp with respiratory pauses of about 3 sec after full inspiration (apneustic breathing) typically indicates pontine or medullary lesions; this type of breathing often progresses to respiratory arrest.

Testing: Initially, pulse oximetry, fingerstick plasma glucose measurements, and cardiac monitoring are done.

Blood tests should include a comprehensive metabolic panel (including at least serum electrolytes, BUN, creatinine, and calcium levels), CBC with differential and platelets, liver function tests, and ammonia level.

ABGs are measured, and if carbon monoxide toxicity is suspected, carboxyhemoglobin level is measured.

Blood and urine should be obtained for culture and routine toxicology screening; serum ethanol level is also measured. Other toxicology screening panels and additional toxicology tests (eg, serum drug levels) are done based on clinical suspicion.

ECG (12-lead) should be done.

Table 224–5. INTERPRETATION OF PUPILLARY RESPONSE AND EYE MOVEMENTS

AREA ASSESSED	FINDING	INTERPRETATION
Pupils	Sluggish light reactivity retained until all other brain stem reflexes are lost	Diffuse cellular cerebral dysfunction (toxic-metabolic encephalopathy)
	Unilateral pupillary dilation, pupil unreactive to light	3rd cranial nerve compression (eg, in transtentorial herniation), usually due to an ipsilateral lesion (see p. 899)
	Pupils fixed in midposition	Midbrain dysfunction due to structural damage (eg, infarction, hemorrhage) Central herniation Severe metabolic depression by drugs or toxins (all other brain stem reflexes are also absent)
	Constricted pupils (1 mm wide)	Massive pontine hemorrhage Toxicity due to opioids or certain insecticides (eg, organophosphates, carbamates)
Eye movements	Early abnormal pupillary and oculomotor signs	Primary brain stem lesion
	Spontaneous, conjugate roving eye movements but intact brain stem reflexes	Early toxic-metabolic encephalopathy
	Gaze preference to one side	Brain stem lesion on the opposite side Cerebral hemisphere lesion on the same side
	Absent eye movements	Further testing required (eg, oculocephalic and oculovestibular reflexes) Possibly toxicity due to phenobarbital or phenytoin, Wernicke encephalopathy, botulism, or brain death

If the cause is not immediately apparent, noncontrast head CT should be done as soon as possible to check for masses, hemorrhage, edema, evidence of bone trauma, and hydrocephalus. Initially, noncontrast CT rather than contrast CT is preferred to rule out brain hemorrhage. MRI can be done instead if immediately available, but it is not as quick as newer-generation CT scanners and may not be as sensitive for traumatic bone injuries (eg, skull fractures). Contrast CT can then be done if noncontrast CT is not diagnostic. MRI or contrast CT may detect isodense subdural hematomas, multiple metastases, sagittal sinus thrombosis, herpes encephalitis, or other causes missed by noncontrast CT. A chest x-ray should also be taken.

If coma is unexplained after MRI or CT and other tests, lumbar puncture (spinal tap) is done to check opening pressure and to exclude infection, subarachnoid hemorrhage, and other abnormalities. However, MRI or CT images should also be reviewed for intracranial masses, obstructive hydrocephalus, and other abnormalities that could obstruct CSF flow or the ventricular system and thus significantly increase ICP. Such abnormalities contraindicate lumbar puncture. Suddenly lowering CSF pressure, as can occur during lumbar puncture, in patients with increased ICP could trigger brain herniation; however, this outcome is rare.

CSF analysis includes cell and differential counts, protein, glucose, Gram staining, cultures, and sometimes, based on clinical suspicion, specific tests (eg, cryptococcal antigen test, cytology, measurement of tumor markers, Venereal Disease Research Laboratory [VDRL] tests, PCR for herpes simplex, visual or spectrophotometric determination of xanthochromia).

If increased ICP is suspected, pressure is measured. Hyperventilation, managed by an ICU specialist, should be considered. Hyperventilation causes hypocapnia, which in turn decreases cerebral blood flow globally through vasoconstriction. Reduction in Pco_2 from 40 mm Hg to 30 mm Hg can reduce ICP by about 30%. Pco_2 should be maintained at 25 mm Hg to 30 mm Hg, but aggressive hyperventilation to < 25 mm Hg should be avoided because this approach may reduce cerebral blood flow excessively and result in cerebral ischemia.

If pressure is increased, it is monitored continuously (see p. 528).

If diagnosis remains uncertain, EEG may be done. In most comatose patients, EEG shows slowing and reductions in wave amplitude that are nonspecific but often occur in toxic-metabolic encephalopathy. However, EEG monitoring (eg, in the ICU) is increasingly identifying nonconvulsive status epilepticus. In such cases, the EEG may show spikes, sharp waves, or spike and slow complexes.

Prognosis

Prognosis depends on the cause, duration, and depth of the impairment of consciousness. For example, absent brain stem reflexes indicates a poor prognosis after cardiac arrest, but not always after a sedative overdose. In general, if unresponsiveness lasts < 6 h, prognosis is more favorable.

After coma, the following prognostic signs are considered favorable:

- Early return of speech (even if incomprehensible)
- Spontaneous eye movements that can track objects
- Normal resting muscle tone
- Ability to follow commands

If the cause is a reversible condition (eg, sedative overdose, some metabolic disorders such as uremia), patients may lose all brain stem reflexes and all motor response and yet recover fully. After trauma, a Glasgow Coma Scale score of 3 to 5 may indicate fatal brain damage, especially if pupils are fixed or oculovestibular reflexes are absent.

After cardiac arrest, clinicians must exclude major confounders of coma, including sedatives, neuromuscular blockade, hypothermia, metabolic derangements, and severe liver or kidney failure. If brain stem reflexes are absent at day 1 or lost later, testing for brain death is indicated. Prognosis is poor if patients have any of the following:

- Myoclonic status epilepticus (bilaterally synchronous twitching of axial structures, often with eye opening and upward deviation of the eyes) that occurs within 24 to 48 h after cardiac arrest
- No pupillary light reflexes 24 to 72 h after cardiac arrest
- No corneal reflexes 72 h after cardiac arrest
- Extensor posturing or no response elicited by painful stimuli 72 h after cardiac arrest
- No N20 on somatosensory evoked potentials (SSEP) or a serum neuron-specific enolase level of > 33 μg/L

If patients were treated with hypothermia, 72 h should be added to the times above because hypothermia slows recovery. If any of the above criteria is met, outcome is usually (but not always) poor; thus, whether to withdraw life support may be a difficult decision.

Patients may also have nonneurologic complications, depending on the cause of impaired consciousness. For example, a drug or disorder causing metabolic coma may also cause hypotension, arrhythmias, MI, or pulmonary edema. Prolonged immobilization may also result in complications (eg, pulmonary embolism, pressure ulcers, UTI).

Treatment

- Immediate stabilization (airway, breathing, circulation, or ABCs)
- Supportive measures, including, when necessary, control of ICP
- Admission to an ICU
- Treatment of underlying disorder

Airway, breathing, and circulation must be ensured immediately. Hypotension must be corrected. Patients are admitted to the ICU so that respiratory and neurologic status can be monitored.

Because some patients in coma are undernourished and susceptible to Wernicke encephalopathy, thiamin 100 mg IV or IM should be given routinely. If plasma glucose is low, patients should be given 50 mL of 50% dextrose IV.

If opioid overdose is suspected, naloxone 2 mg IV is given.

If trauma is involved, the neck is immobilized until damage to the cervical spine is ruled out.

If a recent (within about 1 h) drug overdose is possible, gastric lavage can be done through a large-bore orogastric tube (eg, ≥ 32 Fr) after endotracheal intubation. Activated charcoal can then be given via the orogastric tube.

Coexisting disorders and abnormalities are treated as indicated. For example, metabolic abnormalities are corrected. Core body temperature may need to be corrected (eg, cooling for severe hyperthermia, warming for hypothermia).

Endotracheal intubation: Patients with any of the following require endotracheal intubation to prevent aspiration and ensure adequate ventilation:

- Infrequent, shallow, or stertorous respirations
- Low O_2 saturation (determined by pulse oximetry or ABG measurements)
- Impaired airway reflexes
- Severe unresponsiveness (including most patients with a Glasgow Coma Scale score ≤ 8)

If increased ICP is suspected, intubation should be done via rapid-sequence oral intubation (using a paralytic drug) rather than via nasotracheal intubation; nasotracheal intubation in a patient who is breathing spontaneously causes more coughing and gagging, thus increasing ICP, which is already increased because of intracranial abnormalities.

To minimize the increase in ICP that may occur when the airway is manipulated, some clinicians recommend giving lidocaine 1.5 mg/kg IV 1 to 2 min before giving the paralytic. Patients are sedated before the paralytic is given. Etomidate is a good choice in hypotensive or trauma patients because it has minimal effects on BP; IV dose is 0.3 mg/kg for adults (or 20 mg for an average-sized adult) and 0.2 to 0.3 mg/kg for children. Alternatively, if hypotension is absent and unlikely and if propofol is readily available, propofol 0.2 to 1.5 mg/kg may be used. Succinylcholine 1.5 mg/kg IV is typically used as a paralytic. However, use of paralytics is minimized and, whenever possible, avoided because they can mask neurologic findings and changes.

Pulse oximetry and ABGs (if possible, end-tidal CO_2) should be used to assess adequacy of oxygenation and ventilation.

ICP control: If ICP is increased, intracranial and cerebral perfusion pressure should be monitored (see p. 528), and pressures should be controlled. The goal is to maintain ICP at ≤ 20 mm Hg and cerebral perfusion pressure at 50 to 70 mm Hg. Cerebral venous drainage can be enhanced (thus lowering ICP) by elevating the head of the bed to 30° and by keeping the patient's head in a midline position.

Control of increased ICP involves several strategies:

- **Sedation:** Sedatives may be necessary to control agitation, excessive muscular activity (eg, due to delirium), or pain, which can increase ICP. Propofol is often used in adults (contraindicated in children) because onset and duration of action are quick; dose is 0.3 mg/kg/h by continuous IV infusion, titrated gradually up to 3 mg/kg/h as needed. An initial bolus is not used. The most common adverse effect is hypotension. Prolonged use at high doses can cause pancreatitis. Benzodiazepines (eg, midazolam, lorazepam) can also be used. Because sedatives can mask neurologic findings and changes, their use should be minimized and, whenever possible, avoided. Antipsychotics should be avoided if possible because they can delay recovery. Sedatives are not used to treat agitation and delirium due to hypoxia; O_2 is used instead.
- **Hyperventilation:** Hyperventilation causes hypocapnia, which causes vasoconstriction, thus decreasing cerebral blood flow globally. Reduction in Pco_2 from 40 to 30 mm Hg can reduce ICP about 30%. Hyperventilation that reduces Pco_2 to 28 to 33 mm Hg decreases ICP for only about 30 min and is used by some clinicians as a temporary measure until other treatments take effect. Aggressive hyperventilation to < 25 mm Hg should be avoided because it may reduce cerebral blood flow excessively and result in cerebral ischemia. Other measures to control increased ICP may be used.
- **Hydration:** Isotonic fluids are used. Providing free water through IV fluids (eg, 5% dextrose, 0.45% saline) can aggravate cerebral edema and should be avoided. Fluids may be restricted to some degree, but patients should be kept euvolemic. If patients have no signs of dehydration or fluid overload, IV fluids with normal saline can be started at 50 to 75 mL/h. The rate can be increased or decreased based on serum Na, osmolality, urine output, and signs of fluid retention (eg, edema).
- **Diuretics:** Serum osmolality should be kept at 295 to 320 mOsm/kg. Osmotic diuretics (eg, mannitol) may be given IV to lower ICP and maintain serum osmolality. These drugs do not cross the blood-brain barrier. They pull water

from brain tissue across an osmotic gradient into plasma, eventually leading to equilibrium. Effectiveness of these drugs decreases after a few hours. Thus, they should be reserved for patients whose condition is deteriorating or used preoperatively for patients with hematomas. Mannitol 20% solution is given 0.5 to 1 g/kg IV (2.5 to 5 mL/kg) over 15 to 30 min, then given as often as needed (usually q 6 to 8 h) in a dose ranging from 0.25 to 0.5 g/kg (1.25 to 2.5 mL/kg). Mannitol must be used cautiously in patients with severe coronary artery disease, heart failure, renal insufficiency, or pulmonary vascular congestion because mannitol rapidly expands intravascular volume. Because osmotic diuretics increase renal excretion of water relative to sodium, prolonged use of mannitol may result in water depletion and hypernatremia. Furosemide 1 mg/kg IV can decrease total body water, particularly when transient hypervolemia associated with mannitol is to be avoided. Fluid and electrolyte balance should be monitored closely while osmotic diuretics are used. A 3% saline solution is another potential osmotic agent to control ICP.

- **BP control:** Systemic antihypertensives are needed only when hypertension is severe (> 180/95 mm Hg). How much BP is reduced depends on the clinical context. Systemic BP needs to be high enough to maintain cerebral perfusion pressure even when ICP increases. Hypertension can be managed by titrating a nicardipine drip (5 mg/h, increased by 2.5 mg q 5 min to a maximum of 15 mg/h) or by boluses of labetalol (10 mg IV over 1 to 2 min, repeated q 10 min to a maximum of 150 mg).
- **Corticosteroids:** These drugs are usually helpful for patients with a brain tumor or brain abscess, but they are ineffective for patients with head trauma, cerebral hemorrhage, ischemic stroke, or hypoxic brain damage after cardiac arrest. Corticosteroids increase plasma glucose; this increase may worsen the effects of cerebral ischemia and complicate management of diabetes mellitus. After an initial dose of dexamethasone 20 to 100 mg, 4 mg once/day appears to be effective while minimizing adverse effects. Dexamethasone can be given IV or po.

If ICP continues to increase despite other measures to control it, the following may be used:

- **Pentobarbital coma:** Pentobarbital can reduce cerebral blood flow and metabolic demands. However, its use is controversial because the effect on clinical outcome is not consistently beneficial, and treatment with pentobarbital can lead to complications (eg, hypotension). In some patients with refractory intracranial hypertension that does not respond to standard hypercapnia and hyperosmolar therapy, pentobarbital can improve functional outcome. Coma is induced by giving pentobarbital 10 mg/kg IV over 30 min, followed by 5 mg/kg/h for 3 h, then 1 mg/kg/h. The dose may be adjusted to suppress bursts of EEG activity, which is continuously monitored. Hypotension is common and is managed by giving fluids and, if necessary, vasopressors. Other possible adverse effects include arrhythmias, myocardial depression, and impaired uptake or release of glutamate.
- **Decompressive craniotomy:** Craniotomy with duraplasty can be done to provide room for brain swelling. This procedure can prevent deaths, but overall functional outcome may not improve much. It may be most useful for large cerebral infarcts with impending herniation, particularly in patients < 50 yr.

Long-term care: Patients require meticulous long-term care. Stimulants, sedatives, and opioids should be avoided.

Enteral feeding is started with precautions to prevent aspiration (eg, elevation of the head of the bed); a percutaneous endoscopic jejunostomy tube is placed if necessary.

Early, vigilant attention to skin care, including checking for breakdown especially at pressure points, is required to prevent pressure ulcers. Topical ointments to prevent desiccation of the eyes are beneficial.

Passive range-of-motion exercises done by physical therapists and taping or dynamic flexion splitting of the extremities may prevent contractures. Measures are also taken to prevent UTIs and deep venous thrombosis.

Geriatric Essentials

Elderly patients may be more susceptible to coma, altered consciousness, and delirium because of many factors, including the following:

- Less cognitive reserve due to age-related brain effects and/or preexisting brain disorders
- Higher risk of drug interactions affecting the brain due to polypharmacy
- Higher risk of drug accumulation and drug effects on the brain due to age-related decreased function of organs responsible for drug metabolism
- Higher risk of incorrect drug dosing due to polypharmacy with complex dosing regimens

Relatively minor problems, such as dehydration and UTIs, can alter consciousness in the elderly.

In elderly patients, mental status and communications skills are more likely to be compromised, making lethargy and obtundation harder to recognize.

Age-related decreases in cognitive reserve and neuroplasticity can impair recovery from brain injury.

KEY POINTS

- Coma and impaired consciousness require dysfunction of both cerebral hemispheres or dysfunction of the reticular activating system.
- Manifestations include abnormalities of the eyes (eg, abnormal conjugate gaze, pupillary responses, and/or oculocephalic or oculovestibular reflexes), vital signs (eg, abnormal respirations), and motor function (eg, flaccidity, hemiparesis, asterixis, multifocal myoclonus, decorticate or decerebrate posturing).
- Taking a complete history of prior events is critical; ask witnesses and relatives about the time course for the change in mental status and about possible causes (eg, recent travel, ingestion of unusual meals, exposure to possible infections, drug or alcohol use, possible trauma).
- Do a general physical examination, including thorough examination of the head and face, skin, and extremities and a complete neurologic examination (focusing on level of consciousness, the eyes, motor function, and deep tendon reflexes), followed by appropriate blood and urine tests, toxicology screening, and fingerstick plasma glucose measurements.
- Do noncontrast CT as soon as the patient has been stabilized.
- Ensure adequate airway, breathing, and circulation.
- Give IV or IM thiamin and IV glucose if plasma glucose is low and IV naloxone if opioid overdose is suspected.
- Control ICP using various strategies, which may include sedatives (as needed) to control agitation, temporary hyperventilation, fluids and diuretics to maintain euvolemia, and antihypertensives to control BP.

VEGETATIVE STATE AND MINIMALLY CONSCIOUS STATE

A vegetative state is absence of responsiveness and awareness due to overwhelming dysfunction of the cerebral hemispheres, with sufficient sparing of the diencephalon and brain stem to preserve autonomic and motor reflexes and sleep-wake cycles. Patients may have complex reflexes, including eye movements, yawning, and involuntary movements to noxious stimuli, but show no awareness of self or environment. A minimally conscious state, unlike a vegetative state, is characterized by some evidence of awareness of self and/or the environment, and patients tend to improve. Diagnosis is clinical. Treatment is mainly supportive. Prognosis for patients with persistent deficits is typically bleak.

The vegetative state is a chronic condition that preserves the ability to maintain BP, respiration, and cardiac function, but not cognitive function. Hypothalamic and medullary brain stem functions remain intact to support cardiorespiratory and autonomic functions and are sufficient for survival if medical and nursing care is adequate. The cortex is severely damaged (eliminating cognitive function), but the reticular activating system (RAS) remains functional (making wakefulness possible). Midbrain or pontine reflexes may or may not be present. Patients have no awareness of self and interact with the environment only via reflexes. Seizure activity may be present but not be clinically evident.

Traditionally, a vegetative state that lasts > 1 mo is considered to be a persistent vegetative state. However, a diagnosis of persistent vegetative state does not imply permanent disability because in very rare cases (eg, after traumatic brain injury), patients can improve, reaching a minimally conscious state or a higher level of consciousness.

The **most common causes** are

- Traumatic brain injury
- Diffuse cerebral hypoxia

However, any disorder that results in brain damage can cause a vegetative state. Typically, a vegetative state occurs because the function of the brain stem and diencephalon resumes after coma, but cortical function does not.

In the minimally conscious state, unlike the vegetative state, there is evidence that patients are aware of themselves and/or their environment. Patients also tend to improve (ie, gradually become more conscious), but improvement is limited. This state may be the first indication of brain damage or may follow a vegetative state as people recover some function. Patients can transition between the vegetative state and minimally conscious state, sometimes for years after the original brain damage.

Symptoms and Signs

Vegetative state: Patients show no evidence of awareness of self or environment and cannot interact with other people. Purposeful responses to external stimuli are absent, as are language comprehension and expression.

Signs of an intact reticular formation (eg, eye opening) and an intact brain stem (eg, reactive pupils, oculocephalic reflex) are present. Sleep-wake cycles occur but do not necessarily reflect a specific circadian rhythm and are not associated with the environment. More complex brain stem reflexes, including yawning, chewing, swallowing, and, uncommonly, guttural vocalizations, are also present. Arousal and startle reflexes may be preserved; eg, loud sounds or blinking with bright lights may elicit eye opening. Eyes may water and produce tears. Patients may appear to smile or frown. Spontaneous roving eye movements—usually slow, of constant velocity, and without saccadic jerks—may be misinterpreted as volitional tracking and can be misinterpreted by family members as evidence of awareness.

Patients cannot react to visual threat and cannot follow commands. The limbs may move, but the only purposeful motor responses that occur are primitive (eg, grasping an object that contacts the hand). Pain usually elicits a motor response (typically decorticate or decerebrate posturing), but no purposeful avoidance. Patients have fecal and urinary incontinence. Cranial nerve and spinal reflexes are typically preserved.

Rarely, brain activity, detected by functional MRI or EEG, indicates a response to questions and commands even though there is no behavioral response. The extent of patients' actual awareness is not yet known. In most patients who have such brain activity, the vegetative state resulted from traumatic brain injury, not hypoxic encephalopathy.

Minimally conscious state: Fragments of meaningful interaction with the environment are preserved. Patients may establish eye contact, purposefully grasp at objects, respond to commands in a stereotypic manner, or answer with the same word.

Diagnosis

- Clinical criteria after sufficient observation
- Neuroimaging

A vegetative state is suggested by characteristic findings (eg, no purposeful activity or comprehension) plus signs of an intact reticular formation. Diagnosis is based on clinical criteria. However, neuroimaging is indicated to rule out treatable disorders.

The vegetative state must be distinguished from the minimally conscious state. Both states can be permanent or temporary, and the physical examination may not reliably distinguish one from the other. Sufficient observation is needed. If observation is too brief, evidence of awareness may be overlooked. Some patients with severe Parkinson disease are misdiagnosed as being in a vegetative state.

CT or MRI can differentiate an ischemic infarct, an intracerebral hemorrhage, and a mass lesion involving the cortex or the brain stem. MR angiography can be used to visualize the cerebral vasculature after exclusion of a cerebral hemorrhage. Diffusion-weighted MRI is becoming the preferred imaging modality for following ongoing ischemic changes in the brain.

PET and SPECT can be used to assess cerebral function (rather than brain anatomy). If the diagnosis of persistent vegetative state is in doubt, PET or SPECT should be done.

EEG is useful in assessing cortical dysfunction and identifying occult seizure activity.

Prognosis

Vegetative state: Prognosis varies somewhat by cause and duration of the vegetative state. Prognosis may be better if the cause is a reversible metabolic condition (eg, toxic encephalopathy) than if the cause is neuronal death due to extensive hypoxia and ischemia or another condition. Also, younger patients may recover more motor function than older patients but not more cognition, behavior, or speech.

Recovery from a vegetative state is unlikely after 1 mo if brain damage is nontraumatic and after 12 mo if brain damage is traumatic. Even if some recovery occurs after these intervals, most patients are severely disabled. Rarely, improvement occurs late; after 5 yr, about 3% of patients recover the ability to communicate and comprehend, but even fewer can live independently; no patients regain normal function.

If a vegetative state persists, most patients die within 6 mo of the original brain damage. The cause is usually pulmonary infection, UTI, or multiple organ failure, or death may be sudden and of unknown cause. For most of the rest, life expectancy is about 2 to 5 yr; only about 25% of patients live > 5 yr. A few patients live for decades.

Minimally conscious state: Most patients tend to recover consciousness but to a limited extent depending on how long the minimally conscious state has lasted. The longer it has lasted, the less chance of patients recovering higher cortical function. Prognosis may be better if the cause is traumatic brain injury.

Rarely, patients regain clear but limited awareness after years of coma, called awakenings by the news media.

Treatment

- Supportive care

Supportive care is the mainstay of treatment for patients in a vegetative state or minimally conscious state; it should include the following:

- Preventing systemic complications due to immobilization (eg, pneumonia, UTI, thromboembolic disease)
- Providing good nutrition
- Preventing pressure ulcers
- Providing physical therapy to prevent limb contractures

Vegetative state has no specific treatment. Decisions about life-sustaining care should involve social services, the hospital ethics committee, and family members. Maintaining patients, especially those without advanced directives to guide decisions about terminating treatment, in a prolonged vegetative state raises ethical and other (eg, resource utilization) questions.

Most patients in a minimally conscious state do not respond to specific treatments. However, rarely, treatment with zolpidem can cause dramatic and repeated improvement in neurologic responsiveness for as long as the drug is continued.

KEY POINTS

- Vegetative state is typically characterized by absence of responsiveness and awareness due to overwhelming dysfunction of the cerebral hemispheres, intact brain stem function, and sometimes the simulation of awareness despite its absence.
- Minimally conscious state differs from vegetative state in that patients have some interaction with the environment and tend to improve over time.
- Diagnosis requires exclusion of other disorders and often prolonged observation, particularly to differentiate vegetative state, minimally conscious state, and Parkinson disease.
- Prognosis tends to be poor, particularly for patients in a vegetative state.
- Treatment is mainly supportive.

LOCKED-IN SYNDROME

Locked-in syndrome is a state of wakefulness and awareness with quadriplegia and paralysis of the lower cranial nerves, resulting in inability to show facial expression, move, speak, or communicate, except by coded eye movements.

Locked-in syndrome typically results from a pontine hemorrhage or infarct that causes quadriplegia and disrupts and damages the lower cranial nerves and the centers that control horizontal gaze. Other disorders that result in severe widespread motor paralysis (eg, Guillain-Barré syndrome) and cancers that involve the posterior fossa and the pons are less common causes.

Patients have intact cognitive function and are awake, with eye opening and normal sleep-wake cycles. They can hear and see. However, they cannot move their lower face, chew, swallow, speak, breathe, move their limbs, or move their eyes laterally. Vertical eye movement is possible; patients can open and close their eyes or blink a specific number of times to answer questions.

Diagnosis

- Clinical evaluation

Diagnosis is primarily clinical. Because patients lack the motor responses (eg, withdrawal from painful stimuli) usually used to measure responsiveness, they may be mistakenly thought to be unconscious. Thus, all patients who cannot move should have their comprehension tested by requesting eye blinking or vertical eye movements.

As in vegetative state, neuroimaging is indicated to rule out treatable disorders. Brain imaging with CT or MRI is done and helps identify the pontine abnormality. PET, SPECT, or functional MRI may be done to further assess cerebral function if the diagnosis is in doubt.

In patients with locked-in syndrome, EEG shows normal sleep-wake patterns.

Prognosis

Prognosis depends on the cause and the subsequent level of support provided. For example, locked-in syndrome due to transient ischemia or a small stroke in the vertebrobasilar artery distribution may resolve completely. When the cause (eg, Guillain-Barré syndrome) is partly reversible, recovery can occur over months but is seldom complete.

Favorable prognostic features include

- Early recovery of lateral eye movements
- Early recovery of evoked potentials in response to magnetic stimulation of the motor cortex

Irreversible or progressive disorders (eg, cancers that involve the posterior fossa and the pons) are usually fatal.

Treatment

- Supportive care

Supportive care is the mainstay of treatment for patients with locked-in syndrome and should include the following:

- Preventing systemic complications due to immobilization (eg, pneumonia, UTI, thromboembolic disease)
- Providing good nutrition
- Preventing pressure ulcers
- Providing physical therapy to prevent limb contractures

There is no specific treatment.

Speech therapists may help establish a communication code using eye blinks or movements.

Because cognitive function is intact and communication is possible, patients should make their own health care decisions.

Some patients with locked-in syndrome communicate with each other via the Internet using a computer terminal controlled by eye movements and other means.

BRAIN DEATH

Brain death is loss of function of the entire cerebrum and brain stem, resulting in coma, no spontaneous respiration, and loss of all brain stem reflexes. Spinal reflexes, including deep tendon, plantar flexion, and withdrawal reflexes, may remain. Recovery does not occur.

The concept of brain death developed because ventilators and drugs can perpetuate cardiopulmonary and other body functions despite complete cessation of all cerebral activity. The concept that brain death (ie, total cessation of integrated brain function, especially that of the brain stem) constitutes a person's death has been accepted legally and culturally in most of the world.

Diagnosis

- Serial determination of clinical criteria
- Apnea testing
- Sometimes EEG, brain vascular imaging, or both

For a physician to declare brain death, a known structural or metabolic cause of brain damage must be present, and use of potentially anesthetizing or paralyzing drugs, especially self-administered, must be ruled out.

Hypothermia < 35° C must be increased slowly to > 36° C, and if status epilepticus is suspected, EEG should be done. Sequential testing over 6 to 24 h is typically done (see Table 224–6).

Examination includes

- Assessment of pupil reactivity
- Assessment of oculovestibular, oculocephalic, and corneal reflexes
- Apnea testing

Sometimes EEG or tests of brain perfusion are used to confirm absence of brain activity or brain blood flow and thus provide additional evidence to family members, but these tests are not usually required. They are indicated when apnea testing is not hemodynamically tolerated and when only one neurologic examination is desirable (eg, to expedite organ procurement for transplantation).

Table 224–6. GUIDELINES FOR DETERMINING BRAIN DEATH (IN PATIENTS > 1 YR)

All 9 items must be confirmed to declare brain death:

1. Reasonable efforts were made to notify the patient's next of kin or another person close to the patient.
2. Cause of coma is known and sufficient to account for irreversible loss of all brain function.
3. CNS depressant drugs, hypothermia (< 35° C), and hypotension (MAP < 55 mm Hg) have been excluded. No neuromuscular blockers contribute to the neurologic findings.
4. Any observed movements can be attributed entirely to spinal cord function.
5. The cough reflex, pharyngeal reflexes, or both are tested and shown to be absent.
6. Corneal and pupillary light responses are absent.
7. No caloric responses follow ice water siphoned against the tympanic membrane.
8. An apnea test of a minimum of 8 min shows no respiratory movements with a documented increase in $Paco_2$ of > 20 mm Hg from pretest baseline.

PROCEDURE: Apnea testing is done by disconnecting the ventilator from the endotracheal tube. O_2 (6 L/min) can be supplied by diffusion from a cannula placed through the endotracheal tube. Despite the ventilatory stimulus of the passively rising $Paco_2$, no spontaneous respirations are seen over an 8- to 12-min period.

NOTE: The apnea test should be done with extreme caution to minimize risks of hypoxia and hypotension, particularly in potential organ donors. If arterial BP falls significantly during the test, the test should be stopped, and an arterial blood sample drawn to determine whether $Paco_2$ has risen either to > 55 mm Hg or has increased by > 20 mm Hg. This finding validates the clinical diagnosis of brain death.

9. At least one of the following 4 criteria has been established:
   a. Items 2–8 have been confirmed by 2 examinations separated by at least 6 h.
   b. Items 2–8 have been confirmed AND
      - An EEG shows electrocortical silence.
      - A 2nd examination at least 2 h after the 1st confirms items 2–8.
   c. Items 2–8 have been confirmed AND
      - Conventional angiography, transcranial Doppler ultrasonography, or technetium-99m hexamethylpropyleneamine oxime brain scanning shows no intracranial blood flow.
      - A 2nd examination at least 2 h after the first confirms items 2–8.
   d. If any of items 2–8 cannot be determined because the injury or condition prohibits evaluation (eg, extensive facial injury precludes caloric testing), the following criteria apply:
      - Items that are assessable are confirmed.
      - Conventional angiography, transcranial Doppler ultrasonography, or technetium-99m hexamethylpropyleneamine oxime brain scanning shows no intracranial blood flow.
      - A 2nd examination 6 h after the first confirms all assessable items.

MAP = mean arterial pressure.
Adapted from the American Academy of Neurology Guidelines (1995).

Prognosis

The diagnosis of brain death is equivalent to the person's death. No one who meets the criteria for brain death recovers.

After brain death is confirmed, all supporting cardiac and respiratory treatments are ended. Cessation of ventilatory support results in terminal arrhythmias. Spinal motor reflexes may occur during terminal apnea; they include arching of the back, neck turning, stiffening of the legs, and upper extremity flexion (the so-called Lazarus sign). Family members who wish to be present when the ventilator is shut off need to be warned of such reflex movements.

225 Craniocervical Junction Abnormalities

Craniocervical junction abnormalities are congenital or acquired abnormalities of the occipital bone, foramen magnum, or first two cervical vertebrae that decrease the space for the lower brain stem and cervical cord. These abnormalities can result in neck pain; syringomyelia; cerebellar, lower cranial nerve, and spinal cord deficits; and vertebrobasilar ischemia. Diagnosis is by MRI or CT. Treatment often involves reduction, followed by stabilization via surgery or an external device.

Neural tissue is flexible and susceptible to compression. Craniocervical junction abnormalities can cause or contribute to cervical spinal cord or brain stem compression; some abnormalities and their clinical consequences include the following:

- Fusion of the atlas (C1) and occipital bone: Spinal cord compression if the anteroposterior diameter of the foramen magnum behind the odontoid process is < 19 mm
- Basilar invagination (upward bulging of the occipital condyles): A short neck and compression that can affect the cerebellum, brain stem, lower cranial nerves, and spinal cord
- Atlantoaxial subluxation or dislocation (displacement of the atlas anteriorly in relation to the axis): Acute or chronic spinal cord compression
- Klippel-Feil malformation (fusion of cervical vertebrae): Deformity and limited motion of the neck but usually no neurologic consequences
- Platybasia (flattening of the skull base so that the angle formed by the intersection of the clival and anterior fossa planes is > 135°), seen on lateral skull imaging: Usually, no symptoms or cerebellar or spinal cord deficits

Etiology

Craniocervical junction abnormalities can be congenital or acquired.

Congenital: Congenital abnormalities may be specific structural abnormalities or general or systemic disorders that affect skeletal growth and development. Many patients have multiple abnormalities.

Structural abnormalities include the following:

- Os odontoideum (anomalous bone that replaces all or part of the odontoid process)
- Atlas assimilation (congenital fusion of the atlas and occipital bone)
- Congenital Klippel-Feil malformation (eg, with Turner or Noonan syndrome), often associated with atlanto-occipital anomalies
- Atlas hypoplasia
- Chiari malformations (descent of the cerebellar tonsils or vermis into the cervical spinal canal, sometimes associated with platybasia)

General or systemic disorders that affect skeletal growth and development and involve the craniocervical junction include the following:

- Achondroplasia (impaired epiphyseal bone growth, resulting in shortened, malformed bones) sometimes causes the foramen magnum to narrow or fuse with the atlas and thus may compress the spinal cord or brain stem.
- Down syndrome, Morquio syndrome (mucopolysaccharidosis IV), or osteogenesis imperfecta can cause atlantoaxial subluxation or dislocation.

Acquired: Acquired causes include injuries and disorders.

- Injuries may involve bone, ligaments, or both and are usually caused by vehicle or bicycle accidents, falls, and particularly diving; some injuries are immediately fatal.
- RA (the most common disease cause) and Paget disease of the cervical spine can cause atlantoaxial dislocation or subluxation, basilar invagination, or platybasia.
- Metastatic tumors that affect bone can cause atlantoaxial dislocation or subluxation.
- Slowly growing craniocervical junction tumors (eg, meningioma, chordoma) can impinge on the brain stem or spinal cord.

Symptoms and Signs

Symptoms and signs can occur after a minor neck injury or spontaneously and may vary in progression. Presentation varies by degree of compression and by structures affected. The most common manifestations are

- Neck pain, often with headache
- Symptoms and signs of spinal cord compression

Neck pain often spreads to the arms and may be accompanied by headache (commonly, occipital headache radiating to the skull vertex); it is attributed to compression of the C2 root and the greater occipital nerve and to local musculoskeletal dysfunction. Neck pain and headache usually worsen with head movement and can be precipitated by coughing or bending forward. If patients with Chiari malformation have hydrocephalus, being upright may aggravate the hydrocephalus and result in headaches.

Spinal cord compression involves the upper cervical cord. Deficits include spastic paresis in the arms, legs, or both, caused by compression of motor tracts. Joint position and vibration senses (posterior column function) are commonly impaired. Tingling down the back, often into the legs, with neck flexion (Lhermitte sign) may occur. Uncommonly, pain and temperature senses (spinothalamic tract function) are impaired in a stocking-glove pattern.

Neck appearance, range of motion, or both can be affected by some abnormalities (eg, platybasia, basilar invagination, Klippel-Feil malformation). The neck may be short, webbed (with a skinfold running approximately from the sternocleidomastoid to the shoulder), or in an abnormal position (eg, torticollis in Klippel-Feil malformation). Range of motion may be limited.

Brain compression (eg, due to platybasia, basilar invagination, or craniocervical tumors) may cause brain stem, cranial nerve, and cerebellar deficits. Brain stem and cranial nerve deficits include sleep apnea, internuclear ophthalmoplegia (ipsilateral weakness of eye adduction plus contralateral horizontal nystagmus in the abducting eye with lateral gaze), downbeat nystagmus (fast component downward), hoarseness, dysarthria, and dysphagia. Cerebellar deficits usually impair coordination.

Vertebrobasilar ischemia can be triggered by changing head position. Symptoms may include intermittent syncope, drop attacks, vertigo, confusion or altered consciousness, weakness, and visual disturbance.

Syringomyelia (cavity in the central part of the spinal cord) is common in patients with Chiari malformation. It may cause segmental flaccid weakness and atrophy, which first appear or are most severe in the distal upper extremities; pain and temperature senses may be lost in a capelike distribution over the neck and proximal upper extremities, but light touch is preserved.

Diagnosis

- MRI or CT of the brain and upper spinal cord

A craniocervical abnormality is suspected when patients have pain in the neck or occiput plus neurologic deficits referable to the lower brain stem, upper cervical spinal cord, or cerebellum. Lower cervical spine disorders can usually be distinguished clinically (based on level of spinal cord dysfunction) and by neuroimaging.

Neuroimaging: If a craniocervical abnormality is suspected, MRI or CT of the upper spinal cord and brain, particularly the posterior fossa and craniocervical junction, is done. Acute or suddenly progressive deficits are an emergency, requiring immediate imaging. Sagittal MRI best identifies associated neural lesions (eg, hindbrain, cerebellar, spinal cord, and vascular abnormalities; syringomyelia) and soft-tissue lesions. CT shows bone structures more accurately than MRI and may be done more easily in an emergency.

If MRI and CT are unavailable, plain x-rays—lateral view of the skull showing the cervical spine, anteroposterior view, and oblique views of the cervical spine—are taken.

If MRI is unavailable or inconclusive and CT is inconclusive, CT myelography (CT after intrathecal injection of a radiopaque dye) is done. If MRI or CT suggests vascular abnormalities, magnetic resonance angiography or vertebral angiography is done.

Treatment

- Reduction and immobilization
- Sometimes surgical decompression, fixation, or both

If neural structures are compressed, treatment consists of reduction (traction or changes in head position to realign the craniocervical junction and thus relieve neural compression). After reduction, the head and neck are immobilized. *Acute or suddenly progressive spinal cord compression requires emergency reduction.*

For most patients, reduction involves skeletal traction with a crown halo ring and weight of up to about 4 kg. Reduction with traction may take 5 to 6 days. If reduction is achieved, the neck is immobilized in a halo vest for 8 to 12 wk; then x-rays must be taken to confirm stability.

If reduction does not relieve neural compression, surgical decompression, using a ventral or a dorsal approach, is necessary. If instability persists after decompression, posterior fixation (stabilization) is required. For some abnormalities (eg, due to RA), external immobilization alone is rarely successful; if it is unsuccessful, posterior fixation or anterior decompression and stabilization are required.

Several different methods of instrumentation (eg, plates or rods with screws) can be used for temporary stabilization until bones fuse and stability is permanent. In general, all unstable areas must be fused.

Bone disease: Radiation therapy and a hard cervical collar often help patients with metastatic bone tumors. Calcitonin, mithramycin, and bisphosphonates may help patients with Paget disease.

KEY POINTS

- Craniocervical junction abnormalities are congenital or acquired abnormalities of the occipital bone, foramen magnum, or first two cervical vertebrae that decrease the space for the lower brain stem and cervical cord.
- Suspect a craniocervical junction abnormality if patients have pain in the neck or occiput plus neurologic deficits referable to the lower brain stem, upper cervical spinal cord, or cerebellum.
- Diagnose craniocervical abnormalities using MRI or CT of the brain and upper spinal cord.
- Reduce and immobilize compressed neural structures.
- Treat most patients with traction immobilization or surgery.

226 Delirium and Dementia

Delirium (sometimes called acute confusional state) and dementia are the most common causes of cognitive impairment, although affective disorders (eg, depression) can also disrupt cognition. Delirium and dementia are separate disorders but are sometimes difficult to distinguish. In both, cognition is disordered; however, the following helps distinguish them:

- **Delirium** affects mainly attention.
- **Dementia** affects mainly memory.

Other specific characteristics also help distinguish the 2 disorders (see Table 226–1):

- **Delirium** is typically caused by acute illness or drug toxicity (sometimes life threatening) and is often reversible.
- **Dementia** is typically caused by anatomic changes in the brain, has slower onset, and is generally irreversible.

Delirium often develops in patients with dementia. Mistaking delirium for dementia in an elderly patient—a common clinical error—must be avoided, particularly when delirium is superimposed on chronic dementia. No laboratory test can definitively establish the cause of cognitive impairment; a thorough history

Table 226–1. DIFFERENCES BETWEEN DELIRIUM AND DEMENTIA*

FEATURE	DELIRIUM	DEMENTIA
Onset	Sudden, with a definite beginning point	Slow and gradual, with an uncertain beginning point
Duration	Days to weeks, although it may be longer	Usually permanent
Cause	Almost always another condition (eg, infection, dehydration, use or withdrawal of certain drugs)	Usually a chronic brain disorder (eg, Alzheimer disease, Lewy body dementia, vascular dementia)
Course	Usually reversible	Slowly progressive
Effect at night	Almost always worse	Often worse
Attention	Greatly impaired	Unimpaired until dementia has become severe
Level of consciousness	Variably impaired	Unimpaired until dementia has become severe
Orientation to time and place	Varies	Impaired
Use of language	Slow, often incoherent, and inappropriate	Sometimes difficulty finding the right word
Memory	Varies	Lost, especially for recent events
Need for medical attention	Immediate	Required but less urgently

*Differences are generally true and helpful diagnostically, but exceptions are not rare. For example, traumatic brain injury occurs suddenly but may result in severe, permanent dementia; hypothyroidism may produce the slowly progressive picture of dementia but be completely reversible with treatment.

and physical examination as well as knowledge of baseline function are essential.

DELIRIUM

Delirium is an acute, transient, usually reversible, fluctuating disturbance in attention, cognition, and consciousness level. Causes include almost any disorder or drug. Diagnosis is clinical, with laboratory and usually imaging tests to identify the cause. Treatment is correction of the cause and supportive measures.

Delirium may occur at any age but is more common among the elderly. At least 10% of elderly patients who are admitted to the hospital have delirium; 15 to 50% experience delirium at some time during hospitalization. Delirium is also common after surgery and among nursing home residents and ICU patients. When delirium occurs in younger people, it is usually due to drug use or a life-threatening systemic disorder.

Delirium is sometimes called acute confusional state or toxic or metabolic encephalopathy.

Delirium and dementia are separate disorders but are sometimes difficult to distinguish. In both, cognition is disordered; however, the following helps distinguish them:

- **Delirium** affects mainly attention, is typically caused by acute illness or drug toxicity (sometimes life-threatening), and is often reversible.
- **Dementia** affects mainly memory, is typically caused by anatomic changes in the brain, has slower onset, and is generally irreversible.

Other specific characteristics also help distinguish the 2 disorders (see Table 226–1).

Etiology

The **most common causes** of delirium are the following:

- Drugs, particularly anticholinergics, psychoactive drugs, and opioids
- Dehydration
- Infection

Many other conditions can cause delirium (see Table 226–2). In about 10 to 20% of patients, no cause is identified.

Predisposing factors include brain disorders (eg, dementia, stroke, Parkinson disease), advanced age, sensory impairment (eg, impaired vision or hearing), alcohol intoxication, and multiple coexisting disorders.

Precipitating factors include use of drugs (particularly ≥ 3 new drugs), infection, dehydration, shock, hypoxia, anemia, immobility, undernutrition, use of bladder catheters (whether urinary retention is present or not), hospitalization, pain, sleep deprivation, and emotional stress. Unrecognized liver or kidney failure may cause drug toxicity and delirium by impairing the metabolism and reducing the clearance of a previously well-tolerated drug.

Recent exposure to anesthesia also increases risk, especially if exposure is prolonged and if anticholinergics are given during surgery. After surgery, pain and the use of opioid analgesics can also contribute to delirium. Decreased sensory stimuli at night may trigger delirium in at-risk patients.

For elderly patients in an ICU, risk of delirium (ICU psychosis) is particularly high. Nonconvulsive status epilepticus is being increasingly recognized as a cause of altered mental status in ICU patients.

Pathophysiology

Mechanisms are not fully understood but may involve

- Reversible impairment of cerebral oxidative metabolism
- Multiple neurotransmitter abnormalities
- Generation of cytokines

Table 226–2. CAUSES OF DELIRIUM

CATEGORY	EXAMPLES
Neurologic causes	
Cerebrovascular disorders	Hemorrhagic stroke, ischemic stroke, transient ischemia attack
Migraine	Confusional migraine (migraine that alters consciousness)
Inflammation or infection	Acute demyelinating encephalomyelitis, brain abscess, CNS vasculitis, encephalitis, meningitis, meningoencephalitis
Seizure disorders	Nonconvulsive status epilepticus, postictal state
Trauma	Subdural hematoma, traumatic brain injury
Tumor	Meningeal carcinomatosis, primary or metastatic brain tumor
Nonneurologic causes	
Drugs	Anticholinergics, antiemetics, antihistamines (eg, diphenhydramine), antihypertensives, some antimicrobials, antipsychotics, antispasmodics, benzodiazepines, cardiovascular drugs (often beta-blockers), cimetidine, corticosteroids, digoxin, dopamine agonists, hypnotics, muscle relaxants, NSAIDs, opioids, recreational drugs, sedatives, tricyclic antidepressants
Endocrine disorders	Adrenal or pituitary insufficiency, Cushing syndrome, hyperparathyroidism, hyperthyroidism, hypothyroidism
Hematologic disorders	Hyperviscosity syndrome, leukemic blast cell crisis, polycythemia, thrombocytosis
Infections	Fever, pneumonia, sepsis, systemic infections, UTIs
Injuries	Burns, electrical injuries, fat embolism, heatstroke, hypothermia
Metabolic disorders	Acid-base disturbances, fluid and electrolyte abnormalities (eg, dehydration, hypercalcemia, hypernatremia, hypocalcemia, hyponatremia, hypomagnesemia), hepatic or uremic encephalopathy, hyperosmolality, hyperglycemia, hyperthermia, hypoglycemia, hypoxia, Wernicke encephalopathy
Vascular or circulatory disorders	Anemia, cardiac arrhythmias, heart failure, hypoperfusion states, shock
Vitamin deficiency	Thiamin deficiency, vitamin B_{12} deficiency
Withdrawal syndromes	Alcohol, barbiturates, benzodiazepines, opioids
Other causes	Change of environment, fecal impaction, hypertensive encephalopathy, liver failure, long stays in an ICU, mental disorders, postoperative states, sensory deprivation, sleep deprivation, toxins that affect the CNS, urinary retention

Stress of any kind upregulates sympathetic tone and downregulates parasympathetic tone, impairing cholinergic function and thus contributing to delirium. The elderly are particularly vulnerable to reduced cholinergic transmission, increasing their risk of delirium.

Regardless of the cause, the cerebral hemispheres or arousal mechanisms of the thalamus and brain stem reticular activating system become impaired.

Symptoms and Signs

Delirium is characterized primarily by

- Difficulty focusing, maintaining, or shifting attention (inattention)

Consciousness level fluctuates; patients are disoriented to time and sometimes place or person. They may have hallucinations, delusions, and paranoia. Confusion regarding day-to-day events and daily routines is common, as are changes in personality and affect. Thinking becomes disorganized, and speech is often disordered, with prominent slurring, rapidity, neologisms, aphasic errors, or chaotic patterns.

Symptoms of delirium fluctuate over minutes to hours; they may lessen during the day and worsen at night.

Other symptoms may include inappropriate behavior, fearfulness, and paranoia. Patients may become irritable, agitated, hyperactive, and hyperalert, or they may become quiet, withdrawn, and lethargic. Very elderly people with delirium tend to become quiet and withdrawn—changes that may be mistaken for depression. Some patients alternate between the two.

Usually, patterns of sleeping and eating are grossly distorted.

Because of the many cognitive disturbances, insight is poor, and judgment is impaired.

Other symptoms and signs depend on the cause.

Diagnosis

- Mental status examination
- Standard diagnostic criteria to confirm delirium
- Thorough history
- Directed physical examination and selective testing to determine cause

Delirium, particularly in elderly patients, is often overlooked by clinicians. Clinicians should consider delirium in any elderly patient who presents with impairment in memory or attention.

PEARLS & PITFALLS

- Consider delirium as well as dementia in elderly patients with impaired memory.

Mental status examination: Patients with any sign of cognitive impairment require a formal mental status examination (see Sidebar 220–1 on p. 1836).

Attention is assessed first. Simple tests include immediate repetition of the names of 3 objects, digit span (ability to repeat 7 digits forward and 5 backward), and naming the days of the week forward and backward. Inattention (patient does not register directions or other information) must be distinguished from poor short-term memory (patient registers information but rapidly forgets it). Further cognitive testing is futile for patients who cannot register information.

After initial assessment, standard diagnostic criteria, such as the *Diagnostic and Statistical Manual of Mental Disorders, 5th Edition* (DSM-5) or Confusion Assessment Method (CAM), may be used.

The following features are required for diagnosis of delirium using DSM-5 criteria:

- Disturbance in attention (eg, difficulty focusing or following what is said) and awareness (ie, reduced orientation to the environment)
- The disturbance develops over a short period of time (over hours to days) and tends to fluctuate during the day.
- Acute change in cognition (eg, deficits of memory, language, perception, thinking)

In addition, there must be evidence from the history, physical examination, and/or laboratory testing suggesting that the disturbance is caused by a medical disorder, a substance (including drugs or toxins), or substance withdrawal.

CAM uses the following criteria:

- An altered level of consciousness (eg, hyperalert, lethargic, stuporous, comatose) or disorganized thinking (eg, rambling, irrelevant conversation, illogical flow of ideas)

History: History is obtained by interviewing family members, caregivers, and friends. It can determine whether the change in mental status is recent and is distinct from any baseline dementia (see Table 226–1). The history helps distinguish a mental disorder from delirium. Mental disorders, unlike delirium, almost never cause inattention or fluctuating consciousness, and onset of mental disorders is nearly always subacute.

Sundowning (behavioral deterioration during evening hours), which is common among institutionalized patients with dementia, may be difficult to differentiate; newly symptomatic deterioration should be presumed to be delirium until proved otherwise.

History should also include use of alcohol and all illicit, OTC, and prescription drugs, focusing particularly on drugs with anticholinergic and/or other CNS effects and on new additions, discontinuations, or changes in dose, including overdosing. Nutritional supplements (eg, herbal products) should also be included.

Physical examination: Examination, particularly in patients who are not fully cooperative, should focus on the following:

- Vital signs
- Hydration status
- Potential foci for infection
- Skin and head and neck
- Neurologic examination

Findings can suggest a cause, as with the following:

- Fever, meningismus, or Kernig and Brudzinski signs suggest CNS infection.
- Tremor and myoclonus suggest uremia, liver failure, drug intoxication, or certain electrolyte disorders (eg, hypocalcemia, hypomagnesemia).
- Ophthalmoplegia and ataxia suggest Wernicke-Korsakoff syndrome.
- Focal neurologic abnormalities (eg, cranial nerve palsies, motor or sensory deficits) or papilledema suggests a structural CNS disorder.
- Scalp or facial lacerations, bruising, swelling, and other signs of head trauma suggest traumatic brain injury.

Testing: Testing usually includes

- CT or MRI
- Tests for suspected infections (eg, CBC, blood cultures, chest x-ray, urinalysis)
- Evaluation for hypoxia (pulse oximetry or arterial blood gases)
- Measurement of electrolytes, BUN, creatinine, plasma glucose, and blood levels of any drugs suspected to be having toxic effects
- A urine drug screen

If the diagnosis is unclear, further testing may include liver function tests; measurement of serum calcium and albumin, thyroid-stimulating hormone (TSH), vitamin B_{12}, ESR, and antinuclear antibody (ANA); and a test for syphilis (eg, rapid plasma reagin [RPR] or Venereal Disease Research Laboratory [VDRL] test).

If the diagnosis is still unclear, testing may include CSF analysis (particularly to rule out meningitis, encephalitis, or subarachnoid hemorrhage), measurement of serum ammonia, and testing to check for heavy metals.

If nonconvulsive seizure activity, including status epilepticus, is suspected (suggested by subtle motor twitches, automatisms, and a fluctuating pattern of bewilderment and drowsiness), EEG monitoring should be done.

Prognosis

Morbidity and mortality rates are high in patients who have delirium and are admitted to the hospital or who develop delirium during hospitalization; 35 to 40% of hospitalized patients with delirium die within 1 yr. These rates may be high partly because such patients tend to be older and to have other serious disorders.

Delirium due to certain conditions (eg, hypoglycemia, drug or alcohol intoxication, infection, iatrogenic factors, drug toxicity, electrolyte imbalance) typically resolves rapidly with treatment. However, recovery may be slow (days to even weeks or months), especially in the elderly, resulting in longer hospital stays, increased risk and severity of complications, increased costs, and long-term disability. Some patients never fully recover from delirium. For up to 2 yr after delirium occurs, risk of cognitive and functional decline, institutionalization, and death is increased.

Treatment

- Correction of the cause and removal of aggravating factors
- Supportive care
- Management of agitation

Correcting the cause (eg, treating infection, giving fluids and electrolytes for dehydration) and removing aggravating factors (eg, stopping drugs) may result in resolution of delirium. Nutritional deficiencies (eg, of thiamin or vitamin B_{12}) should be corrected, and good nutrition and hydration should be provided.

General measures: The environment should be stable, quiet, and well-lit and include visual cues to orient the patient (eg, calendar, clocks, family photographs). Frequent reorientation and reassurance by hospital staff or family members may also help. Sensory deficits should be minimized (eg, by replacing hearing-aid batteries, by encouraging patients who need eyeglasses or hearing aids to use them).

Approach to treatment should be interdisciplinary (with a physician, physical and occupational therapists, nurses, and social workers); it should involve strategies to enhance mobility and range of motion, treat pain and discomfort, prevent skin breakdown, ameliorate incontinence, and minimize risk of aspiration.

Agitation may threaten the well-being of the patient, a caregiver, or a staff member. Simplifying drug regimens and avoiding use of IV lines, bladder catheters, and physical restraints (particularly in the long-term care setting) as much as possible can help prevent exacerbation of agitation and reduce risk of injury. However, in certain circumstances, physical restraints may be needed to prevent patients from harming themselves or others. Restraints should be applied by a staff member trained in their use; they should be released at least every 2 h to prevent injury and discontinued as soon as possible. Use of hospital-employed assistants (sitters) as constant observers may help avoid the need for restraints.

Explaining the nature of delirium to family members can help them cope. They should be told that delirium is usually reversible but that cognitive deficits often take weeks or months to abate after resolution of the acute illness.

Drugs: Drugs, typically low-dose haloperidol (0.5 to 1.0 mg po, IV, or IM once, then repeated q 1 to 2 h as needed), may lessen agitation or psychotic symptoms; occasionally, much higher doses are necessary. However, drugs do not correct the underlying problem and may prolong or exacerbate delirium. Second-generation (atypical) antipsychotics (eg, risperidone 0.5 to 3 mg po q 12 h, olanzapine 2.5 to 15 mg po once/day, quetiapine 25 to 200 mg po q 12 h) may be preferred because they have fewer extrapyramidal adverse effects; however, long-term use in patients with dementia may increase risk of stroke and death. These drugs are not typically given IV or IM.

Benzodiazepines (eg, lorazepam 0.5 to 1.0 mg po or IV once, then repeated q 1 to 2 h as needed) are the drugs of choice for delirium caused by withdrawal from alcohol or benzodiazepines. Their onset of action is more rapid (5 min after parenteral administration) than antipsychotics. Benzodiazepines should be avoided if delirium results from other conditions because these drugs worsen confusion and sedation.

Prevention

Because delirium greatly worsens prognosis for hospitalized patients, prevention should be emphasized. Hospital staff members should be trained to take measures to maintain orientation, mobility, and cognition and to ensure sleep, good nutrition and hydration, and sufficient pain relief, particularly in elderly patients. Family members can be encouraged to help with these strategies.

The number and doses of drugs should be reduced if possible.

KEY POINTS

- Delirium, which is very common among hospitalized elderly patients, is often caused by drugs, dehydration, and infections (eg, UTI) but can have many other causes.
- Consider delirium in elderly patients, particularly those presenting with impaired memory or attention.
- History taken from family members, caregivers, and friends and mental status examination are key to recognizing delirium.
- Thoroughly assess patients with delirium for possible neurologic and systemic causes and triggers.
- Do a thorough drug review, and stop any potentially contributory drugs.
- About 35 to 40% of hospitalized patients with delirium die within 1 yr.
- Treat the cause of delirium, and provide supportive care, including sedation when necessary.

DEMENTIA

Dementia is chronic, global, usually irreversible deterioration of cognition. Diagnosis is clinical; laboratory and imaging tests are usually used to identify treatable causes. Treatment is supportive. Cholinesterase inhibitors can sometimes temporarily improve cognitive function.

Dementia may occur at any age but affects primarily the elderly. It accounts for more than half of nursing home admissions.

Dementias can be classified in several ways:

- Alzheimer or non-Alzheimer type
- Cortical or subcortical
- Irreversible or potentially reversible
- Common or rare

Dementia should not be confused with delirium although cognition is disordered in both. The following helps distinguish them:

- **Dementia** affects mainly memory, is typically caused by anatomic changes in the brain, has slower onset, and is generally irreversible.
- **Delirium** affects mainly attention, is typically caused by acute illness or drug toxicity (sometimes life threatening), and is often reversible.

Other specific characteristics also help distinguish the 2 disorders (see Table 226–1).

Etiology

Dementias may result from primary diseases of the brain or other conditions (see Table 226–3).

The most common types of dementia are

- Alzheimer disease (see p. 1878)
- Vascular dementia (see p. 1887)
- Lewy body dementia (see p. 1885)
- Frontotemporal dementias (see p. 1883)
- HIV-associated dementia (see p. 1884)

Dementia also occurs in patients with Parkinson disease, Huntington disease, progressive supranuclear palsy, Creutzfeldt-Jakob disease, Gerstmann-Sträussler-Scheinker syndrome, other prion disorders, and neurosyphilis. Patients can have > 1 type (mixed dementia).

Some structural brain disorders (eg, normal-pressure hydrocephalus, subdural hematoma), metabolic disorders (eg, hypothyroidism, vitamin B_{12} deficiency), and toxins (eg, lead) cause a slow deterioration of cognition that may resolve with treatment. This impairment is sometimes called reversible dementia, but some experts restrict the term dementia to irreversible cognitive deterioration.

Depression may mimic dementia (and was formerly called pseudodementia); the 2 disorders often coexist. However, depression may be the first manifestation of dementia.

Age-associated memory impairment refers to changes in cognition that occur with aging; these changes are not dementia.

Table 226–3. CLASSIFICATION OF SOME DEMENTIAS

CLASSIFICATION	EXAMPLES
Beta-amyloid deposits and neurofibrillary tangles	Alzheimer disease
Tau abnormalities	Chronic traumatic encephalopathy Corticobasal ganglionic degeneration Frontotemporal dementia (including Pick disease) Progressive supranuclear palsy
Alpha-synuclein abnormalities	Lewy body dementia Parkinson disease dementia
Huntingtin gene mutation	Huntington disease
Cerebrovascular disease	Binswanger disease Lacunar disease Multi-infarct dementia Strategic single-infarct dementia
Ingestion of drugs or toxins	Alcohol-associated dementia Dementia due to exposure to heavy metals
Infections	**Fungal:** Dementia due to cryptococcosis **Spirochetal:** Dementia due to syphilis or Lyme disease **Viral:** HIV-associated dementia, postencephalitis syndromes
Prion disorders	Alzheimer disease Amyotrophic lateral sclerosis Creutzfeldt-Jakob disease Frontotemporal dementia Huntington disease Parkinson disease Variant Creutzfeldt-Jakob disease
Structural brain disorders	Brain tumors Chronic subdural hematomas Normal-pressure hydrocephalus
Other potentially reversible disorders	Depression Hypothyroidism Vitamin B_{12} deficiency

The elderly have a relative deficiency in recall, particularly in speed of recall, compared with recall during their youth. However, this change does not affect daily functioning.

Mild cognitive impairment causes greater memory loss than age-associated memory impairment; memory and sometimes other cognitive functions are worse in patients with this disorder than in age-matched controls, but daily functioning is typically not affected. In contrast, dementia impairs daily functioning. Up to 50% of patients with mild cognitive impairment develop dementia within 3 yr.

Any **disorder** may exacerbate cognitive deficits in patients with dementia. Delirium often occurs in patients with dementia.

Drugs, particularly benzodiazepines and anticholinergics (eg, some tricyclic antidepressants, antihistamines, antipsychotics, benztropine), may temporarily cause or worsen symptoms of dementia, as may alcohol, even in moderate amounts. New or progressive kidney or liver failure may reduce drug clearance and cause drug toxicity after years of taking a stable drug dose (eg, of propranolol).

Prion mechanisms (see p. 1997) appear to be involved in most or all neurodegenerative disorders that first manifest in the elderly. A normal cellular protein sporadically (or via an inherited mutation) becomes misfolded into a pathogenic form or prion. The prion then acts as a template, causing other proteins to misfold similarly. This process occurs over years and in many parts of the CNS. Many of these prions become insoluble and, like amyloid, cannot be readily cleared by the cell. Evidence implies prion or similar mechanisms in Alzheimer disease (strongly), as well as in Parkinson disease, Huntington disease, frontotemporal dementia (FTD), and amyotrophic lateral sclerosis. These prions are not as infectious as those in Creutzfeld-Jacob disease, but they can be transmitted.

Symptoms and Signs

Dementia impairs cognition globally. Onset is gradual, although family members may suddenly notice deficits (eg, when function becomes impaired). Often, loss of short-term memory is the first sign. At first, early symptoms may be indistinguishable from those of age-associated memory impairment or mild cognitive impairment.

Although symptoms of dementia exist in a continuum, they can be divided into

- Early
- Intermediate
- Late

Personality changes and behavioral disturbances may develop early or late. Motor and other focal neurologic deficits occur at different stages, depending on the type of dementia; they occur early in vascular dementia and late in Alzheimer disease. Incidence of seizures is somewhat increased during all stages.

Psychosis—hallucinations, delusions, or paranoia—occurs in about 10% of patients with dementia, although a higher percentage may experience these symptoms temporarily.

Early dementia symptoms: Recent memory is impaired; learning and retaining new information become difficult. Language problems (especially with word finding), mood swings, and personality changes develop. Patients may have progressive difficulty with independent activities of daily living (eg, balancing their checkbook, finding their way around, remembering where they put things). Abstract thinking, insight, or judgment may be impaired. Patients may respond to loss of independence and memory with irritability, hostility, and agitation.

Functional ability may be further limited by the following:

- Agnosia: Impaired ability to identify objects despite intact sensory function
- Apraxia: Impaired ability to do previously learned motor activities despite intact motor function
- Aphasia: Impaired ability to comprehend or use language

Although early dementia may not compromise sociability, family members may report strange behavior accompanied by emotional lability.

Intermediate dementia symptoms: Patients become unable to learn and recall new information. Memory of remote events is reduced but not totally lost. Patients may require help with basic activities of daily living (eg, bathing, eating, dressing, toileting).

Personality changes may progress. Patients may become irritable, anxious, self-centered, inflexible, or angry more easily, or they may become more passive, with a flat affect, depression, indecisiveness, lack of spontaneity, or general withdrawal from social situations.

Behavior disorders may develop: Patients may wander or become suddenly and inappropriately agitated, hostile, uncooperative, or physically aggressive.

By this stage, patients have lost all sense of time and place because they cannot effectively use normal environmental and social cues. Patients often get lost; they may be unable to find their own bedroom or bathroom. They remain ambulatory but are at risk of falls or accidents secondary to confusion.

Altered sensation or perception may culminate in psychosis with hallucinations and paranoid and persecutory delusions.

Sleep patterns are often disorganized.

Late (severe) dementia symptoms: Patients cannot walk, feed themselves, or do any other activities of daily living; they may become incontinent. Recent and remote memory is completely lost. Patients may be unable to swallow. They are at risk of undernutrition, pneumonia (especially due to aspiration), and pressure ulcers. Because they depend completely on others for care, placement in a long-term care facility often becomes necessary. Eventually, patients become mute.

Because such patients cannot relate any symptoms to a physician and because elderly patients often have no febrile or leukocytic response to infection, a physician must rely on experience and acumen whenever a patient appears ill.

End-stage dementia results in coma and death, usually due to infection.

Diagnosis

- Differentiation of delirium from dementia by history and neurologic examination (including mental status)
- Identification of treatable causes clinically and by laboratory testing and neuroimaging
- Sometimes formal neuropsychologic testing

Recommendations about diagnosis of dementia are available from the American Academy of Neurology.

Distinguishing type or cause of dementia can be difficult; definitive diagnosis often requires postmortem pathologic examination of brain tissue. Thus, clinical diagnosis focuses on distinguishing dementia from delirium and other disorders and identifying the cerebral areas affected and potentially reversible causes.

Dementia must be distinguished from the following:

- **Delirium:** Distinguishing between dementia and delirium is crucial (because delirium is usually reversible with prompt treatment) but can be difficult. Attention is assessed first. If a patient is inattentive, the diagnosis is likely to be delirium, although advanced dementia also severely impairs attention. Other features that suggest delirium rather than dementia (eg, duration of cognitive impairment—see Table 226–1) are determined by the history, physical examination, and tests for specific causes.
- **Age-associated memory impairment:** Memory impairment does not affect daily functioning. If affected people are given enough time to learn new information, their intellectual performance is good.
- **Mild cognitive impairment:** Memory and/or other cognitive functions are impaired, but impairment is not severe enough to interfere with daily activities.
- **Cognitive symptoms related to depression:** This cognitive disturbance resolves with treatment of depression. Depressed older patients may experience cognitive decline, but unlike patients with dementia, they tend to exaggerate their memory loss and rarely forget important current events or personal matters. Neurologic examinations are normal except for signs of psychomotor slowing. When tested, patients with depression make little effort to respond, but those with dementia often try hard but respond incorrectly. When depression and dementia coexist, treating depression does not fully restore cognition.

Clinical criteria: The most recent National Institute on Aging–Alzheimer's Association diagnostic guidelines specify that a general diagnosis of dementia requires all of the following:

- Cognitive or behavioral (neuropsychiatric) symptoms interfere with the ability to function at work or do usual daily activities.
- These symptoms represent a decline from previous levels of functioning.
- These symptoms are not explained by delirium or a major psychiatric disorder.

The cognitive or behavioral impairment should be diagnosed based on a combination of history from the patient and from someone who knows the patient plus assessment of cognitive function (a bedside mental status examination *or*, if bedside testing is inconclusive, formal neuropsychologic testing). In addition, the impairment should involve ≥ 2 of the following domains:

- Impaired ability to acquire and remember new information (eg, asking repetitive questions, frequently misplacing objects or forgetting appointments)
- Impaired reasoning and handling of complex tasks and poor judgment (eg, being unable to manage bank account, making poor financial decisions)
- Language dysfunction (eg, difficulty thinking of common words, errors speaking and/or writing)
- Visuospatial dysfunction (eg, inability to recognize faces or common objects)
- Changes in personality, behavior, or comportment.

If cognitive impairment is confirmed, history and physical examination should then focus on signs of treatable disorders that cause cognitive impairment (eg, vitamin B_{12} deficiency, neurosyphilis, hypothyroidism, depression—see Table 226–2).

Assessment of cognitive function: The **Mini-Mental Status Examination** (see Sidebar 220–1 on p. 1836) is often used as a bedside screening test. When delirium is absent, the presence of multiple deficits, particularly in patients with an average or a higher level of education, suggests dementia. The best screening test for memory is a short-term memory test (eg, registering 3 objects and recalling them after 5 min); patients with dementia fail this test. Another test of mental status assesses the ability to name objects within categories (eg, lists of animals, plants, or pieces of furniture). Patients with dementia struggle to name a few; those without dementia easily name many.

Neuropsychologic testing should be done when history and bedside mental status testing are not conclusive. It evaluates mood as well as multiple cognitive domains. It takes 1 to 3 h to complete and is done or supervised by a neuropsychologist. Such testing helps primarily in differentiating the following:

- Age-associated memory impairment, mild cognitive impairment, and dementia, particularly when cognition is only slightly impaired or when the patient or family members are anxious for reassurance
- Dementia and focal syndromes of cognitive impairment (eg, amnesia, aphasia, apraxia, visuospatial difficulties, impairment of executive function) when the distinction is not clinically evident

Testing may also help characterize specific deficits due to dementia, and it may detect depression or a personality disorder that is contributing to poor cognitive performance.

Laboratory testing: Tests should include TSH and vitamin B_{12} levels. Routine CBC and liver function tests are sometimes recommended, but yield is very low.

If clinical findings suggest a specific disorder, other tests (eg, for HIV or syphilis) are indicated. Lumbar puncture is rarely needed but should be considered if a chronic infection or neurosyphilis is suspected. Other tests may be used to exclude causes of delirium.

Biomarkers for Alzheimer disease can be useful in research settings but are not yet routine in clinical practice. For example, in CSF, the tau level increases and beta-amyloid decreases as Alzheimer disease progresses. Also, routine genetic testing for the apolipoprotein E4 allele (apo ε4) is not recommended. (For people with 2 ε4 alleles, the risk of developing Alzheimer disease by age 75 is 10 to 30 times that for people without the allele.)

Neuroimaging: CT or MRI should be done in the initial evaluation of dementia or after any sudden change in cognition or mental status. Neuroimaging can identify potentially reversible structural disorders (eg, normal-pressure hydrocephalus, brain tumors, subdural hematoma) and certain metabolic disorders (eg, Hallervorden-Spatz disease, Wilson disease).

Occasionally, EEG is useful (eg, to evaluate episodic lapses in attention or bizarre behavior).

Functional MRI or single-photon emission CT can provide information about cerebral perfusion patterns and help with differential diagnosis (eg, in differentiating Alzheimer disease from FTD and Lewy body dementia).

Amyloid radioactive tracers that bind specifically to beta-amyloid plaques (eg, Pittsburgh compound B [PiB], florbetapir, flutemetamol, florbetaben) have been used with PET to image amyloid plaques in patients with mild cognitive impairment or dementia. This testing should be used when the cause of cognitive impairment (eg, mild cognitive impairment or dementia) is uncertain after a comprehensive evaluation and when Alzheimer disease is a diagnostic consideration. Determining amyloid status via PET is expected to increase the certainty of diagnosis and management.

Prognosis

Dementia is usually progressive. However, progression rate varies widely and depends on the cause. Dementia shortens life expectancy, but survival estimates vary.

Treatment

- Measures to ensure safety
- Provision of appropriate stimulation, activities, and cues for orientation
- Elimination of drugs with sedating or anticholinergic effects
- Possibly cholinesterase inhibitors and memantine
- Assistance for caregivers
- Arrangements for end-of-life care

Recommendations about treatment of dementia are available from the American Academy of Neurology. Measures to ensure patient safety and to provide an appropriate environment are essential to treatment, as is caregiver assistance. Several drugs are available.

Patient safety: Occupational and physical therapists can evaluate the home for safety; the goals are to prevent accidents (particularly falls), to manage behavior disorders, and to plan for change as dementia progresses.

How well patients function in various settings (ie, kitchen, automobile) should be evaluated using simulations. If patients have deficits and remain in the same environment, protective measures (eg, hiding knives, unplugging the stove, removing the car, confiscating car keys) may be required. Some states require physicians to notify the Department of Motor Vehicles of patients with dementia because at some point, such patients can no longer drive safely.

If patients wander, signal monitoring systems can be installed, or patients can be registered in the Safe Return program. Information is available from the Alzheimer's Association.

Ultimately, assistance (eg, housekeepers, home health aides) or a change of environment (living facilities without stairs, assisted-living facility, skilled nursing facility) may be indicated.

Environmental measures: Patients with mild to moderate dementia usually function best in familiar surroundings.

Whether at home or in an institution, the environment should be designed to help preserve feelings of self-control and personal dignity by providing the following:

- Frequent reinforcement of orientation
- A bright, cheerful, familiar environment
- Minimal new stimulation
- Regular, low-stress activities

Orientation can be reinforced by placing large calendars and clocks in the room and establishing a routine for daily activities; medical staff members can wear large name tags and repeatedly introduce themselves. Changes in surroundings, routines, or people should be explained to patients precisely and simply, omitting nonessential procedures. Patients require time to adjust and become familiar with the changes. Telling patients about what is going to happen (eg, about a bath or feeding) may avert resistance or violent reactions. Frequent visits by staff members and familiar people encourage patients to remain social.

The **room** should be reasonably bright and contain sensory stimuli (eg, radio, television, night-light) to help patients remain oriented and focus their attention. Quiet, dark, private rooms should be avoided.

Activities can help patients function better; those related to interests before dementia began are good choices. Activities should be enjoyable, provide some stimulation, but not involve too many choices or challenges.

Exercise to reduce restlessness, improve balance, and maintain cardiovascular tone should be done daily. Exercise can also help improve sleep and manage behavior disorders.

Occupational therapy and **music therapy** help maintain fine motor control and provides nonverbal stimulation.

Group therapy (eg, reminiscence therapy, socialization activities) may help maintain conversational and interpersonal skills.

Drugs: Eliminating or limiting drugs with CNS activity often improves function. Sedating and anticholinergic drugs, which tend to worsen dementia, should be avoided.

The **cholinesterase inhibitors** donepezil, rivastigmine, and galantamine are somewhat effective in improving cognitive function in patients with Alzheimer disease or Lewy body dementia and may be useful in other forms of dementia. These drugs inhibit acetylcholinesterase, increasing the acetylcholine level in the brain.

Memantine, an NMDA (*N*-methyl-D-aspartate) antagonist, may help slow the loss of cognitive function in patients with moderate to severe dementia and may be synergistic when used with a cholinesterase inhibitor.

Drugs to control behavior disorders (eg, antipsychotics) have been used. Patients with dementia and signs of depression should be treated with nonanticholinergic antidepressants, preferably SSRIs.

Caregiver assistance: Immediate family members are largely responsible for care of a patient with dementia (see p. 2899). Nurses and social workers can teach them and other caregivers how to best meet the patient's needs (eg, how to deal with daily care and handle financial issues); teaching should be ongoing. Other resources (eg, support groups, educational materials, Internet web sites) are available.

Caregivers may experience substantial stress. Stress may be caused by worry about protecting the patient and by frustration, exhaustion, anger, and resentment from having to do so much to care for someone. Health care practitioners should watch for early symptoms of caregiver stress and burnout and, when needed, suggest support services (eg, social worker, nutritionist, nurse, home health aide).

If a patient with dementia has an unusual injury, the possibility of elder abuse should be investigated.

End-of-life issues: Because insight and judgment deteriorate in patients with dementia, appointment of a family member, guardian, or lawyer to oversee finances may be necessary. Early in dementia, before the patient is incapacitated, the patient's wishes about care should be clarified, and financial and legal arrangements (eg, durable power of attorney, durable power of attorney for health care) should be made. When these documents are signed, the patient's capacity should be evaluated, and evaluation results recorded (see p. 3210). Decisions about artificial feeding and treatment of acute disorders are best made before the need develops.

In advanced dementia, palliative measures may be more appropriate than highly aggressive interventions or hospital care.

KEY POINTS

- Dementia, unlike age-associated memory loss and mild cognitive impairment, causes cognitive impairments that interfere with daily functioning.
- Be aware that family members may report sudden onset of symptoms only because they suddenly recognized gradually developing symptoms.
- Consider reversible causes of cognitive decline, such as structural brain disorders (eg, normal-pressure hydrocephalus, subdural hematoma), metabolic disorders (eg, hypothyroidism, vitamin B_{12} deficiency), drugs, depression, and toxins (eg, lead).
- Do bedside mental status testing and, if necessary, formal neuropsychologic testing to confirm that cognitive function is impaired in ≥ 2 domains.
- Recommend or help arrange measures to maximize patient safety, to provide a familiar and comfortable environment for the patient, and to provide support for caregivers.
- Consider adjunctive drug therapy, and recommend making end-of-life arrangements.

ALZHEIMER DISEASE

Alzheimer disease causes progressive cognitive deterioration and is characterized by beta-amyloid deposits and neurofibrillary tangles in the cerebral cortex and subcortical gray matter.

Alzheimer disease, a neurocognitive disorder, is the most common cause of dementia; it accounts for 60 to 80% of dementias in the elderly. In the US, an estimated 13% of people ≥ 65 and 45% of people ≥ 85 have Alzheimer disease. The disease is twice as common among women as among men, partly because women have a longer life expectancy. Prevalence in industrialized countries is expected to increase as the proportion of the elderly increases.

Etiology

Most cases are sporadic, with late onset (≥ 65 yr) and unclear etiology. Risk of developing the disease is best predicted by age. However, about 5 to 15% of cases are familial; half of these cases have an early (presenile) onset (< 65 yr) and are typically related to specific genetic mutations.

At least 5 distinct genetic loci, located on chromosomes 1, 12, 14, 19, and 21, influence initiation and progression of Alzheimer disease.

Mutations in genes for the amyloid precursor protein, presenilin I, and presenilin II may lead to autosomal dominant forms of Alzheimer disease, typically with presenile onset. In affected patients, the processing of amyloid precursor protein is altered, leading to deposition and fibrillar aggregation of beta-amyloid; beta-amyloid is the main component of senile plaques, which consist of degenerated axonal or dendritic processes, astrocytes, and glial cells around an amyloid core. Beta-amyloid may also alter kinase and phosphatase activities in ways that eventually lead to hyperphosphorylation of tau and formation of neurofibrillary tangles.

Other genetic determinants include the apolipoprotein (apo) E alleles (ε). Apo E proteins influence beta-amyloid deposition, cytoskeletal integrity, and efficiency of neuronal repair. Risk of Alzheimer disease is substantially increased in people with 2 ε4 alleles and may be decreased in those who have the ε2 allele. For people with 2 ε4 alleles, risk of developing Alzheimer disease by age 75 is about 10 to 30 times that for people without the allele.

Variants in *SORL1* may also be involved; they are more common among people with late-onset Alzheimer disease.

These variants may cause the gene to malfunction, possibly resulting in increased production of beta-amyloid.

The relationship of other factors (eg, low hormone levels, metal exposure) and Alzheimer disease is under study, but no definite causal links have been established.

Pathophysiology

The 2 pathologic hallmarks of Alzheimer disease are

- Extracellular beta-amyloid deposits (in senile plaques)
- Intracellular neurofibrillary tangles (paired helical filaments)

The beta-amyloid deposition and neurofibrillary tangles lead to loss of synapses and neurons, which results in gross atrophy of the affected areas of the brain, typically starting at the mesial temporal lobe.

The mechanism by which beta-amyloid peptide and neurofibrillary tangles cause such damage is incompletely understood. There are several theories.

The **amyloid hypothesis** posits that progressive accumulation of beta-amyloid in the brain triggers a complex cascade of events ending in neuronal cell death, loss of neuronal synapses, and progressive neurotransmitter deficits; all of these effects contribute to the clinical symptoms of dementia.

Prion mechanisms have been identified in Alzheimer disease. In prion diseases, a normal cell-surface brain protein called prion protein becomes misfolded into a pathogenic form termed a prion. The prion then causes other prion proteins to misfold similarly, resulting in a marked increase in the abnormal proteins, which leads to brain damage. In Alzheimer disease, it is thought that the beta-amyloid in cerebral amyloid deposits and tau in neurofibrillary tangles have prion-like, self-replicating properties.

Symptoms and Signs

Patients have symptoms and signs of dementia.

The **most common first manifestation** is

- Loss of short-term memory (eg, asking repetitive questions, frequently misplacing objects or forgetting appointments)

Other cognitive deficits tend to involve multiple functions, including the following:

- Impaired reasoning, difficulty handling complex tasks, and poor judgment (eg, being unable to manage bank account, making poor financial decisions)
- Language dysfunction (eg, difficulty thinking of common words, errors speaking and/or writing)
- Visuospatial dysfunction (eg, inability to recognize faces or common objects)

The disease progresses gradually but may plateau for periods of time.

Behavior disorders (eg, wandering, agitation, yelling, persecutory ideation) are common.

Diagnosis

- Similar to that of other dementias
- Formal mental status examination
- History and physical examination
- Laboratory testing
- Neuroimaging

Generally, diagnosis of Alzheimer disease is similar to that of other dementias (see p. 1876).

Evaluation includes a thorough history and standard neurologic examination. Clinical criteria are 85% accurate in establishing the diagnosis and differentiating Alzheimer disease from other forms of dementia, such as vascular dementia and Lewy body dementia.

Traditional diagnostic criteria for Alzheimer disease include all of the following:

- Dementia established clinically and documented by a formal mental status examination
- Deficits in ≥ 2 areas of cognition
- Gradual onset (ie, over months to years, rather than days or weeks) and progressive worsening of memory and other cognitive functions
- No disturbance of consciousness
- Onset after age 40, most often after age 65
- No systemic or brain disorders (eg, tumor, stroke) that could account for the progressive deficits in memory and cognition

However, deviations from these criteria do not exclude a diagnosis of Alzheimer disease, particularly because patients may have mixed dementia.

The most recent National Institute on Aging–Alzheimer's Association diagnostic guidelines also include biomarkers for the pathophysiologic process of Alzheimer disease:

- A low level of beta-amyloid in CSF
- Beta-amyloid deposits in the brain detected by PET imaging using radioactive tracer that binds specifically to beta-amyloid plaques (eg, Pittsburgh compound B [PiB], florbetapir)

Other biomarkers indicate downstream neuronal degeneration of injury:

- Elevated levels of tau protein in CSF
- Decreased cerebral metabolism in the temporoparietal cortex measured using PET with fluorine-18 (^{18}F) labeled deoxyglucose (fluorodeoxyglucose, or FDG)
- Local atrophy in the medial, basal, and lateral temporal lobes and the medial parietal cortex, detected by MRI

These findings increase the probability that dementia is due to Alzheimer disease. However, the guidelines do not advocate routine use of these biomarkers for diagnosis because standardization and availability are limited at this time. Also, they do not recommend routine testing for the apo ε4 allele.

Differential diagnosis: Distinguishing Alzheimer disease from other dementias is difficult. Assessment tools (eg, Hachinski Ischemic Score—see Table 226-4) can help distinguish vascular dementia from Alzheimer disease. Fluctuations in cognition, parkinsonian symptoms, well-formed visual hallucinations, and relative preservation of short-term memory suggest Lewy body dementia rather than Alzheimer disease (see Table 226–5).

Patients with Alzheimer disease are often better-groomed and neater than patients with other dementias.

Prognosis

Although progression rate varies, cognitive decline is inevitable. Average survival from time of diagnosis is 7 yr, although this figure is debated. Average survival from the time patients can no longer walk is about 6 mo.

Treatment

- Generally similar to that of other dementias
- Possibly cholinesterase inhibitors and memantine

Safety and supportive measures are the same as that of all dementias. For example, the environment should be bright, cheerful, and familiar, and it should be designed to reinforce orientation (eg, placement of large clocks and calendars in the room).

Table 226–4. MODIFIED HACHINSKI ISCHEMIC SCORE

FEATURE	POINTS*
Abrupt onset of symptoms	2
Stepwise deterioration (eg, decline-stability-decline)	1
Fluctuating course	2
Nocturnal confusion	1
Personality relatively preserved	1
Depression	1
Somatic complaints (eg, body aches, chest pain)	1
Emotional lability	1
History or presence of hypertension	1
History of stroke	2
Evidence of coexisting atherosclerosis (eg, PAD, MI)	1
Focal neurologic symptoms (eg, hemiparesis, homonymous hemianopia, aphasia)	2
Focal neurologic signs (eg, unilateral weakness, sensory loss, asymmetric reflexes, Babinski sign)	2

*Total score is determined:

- < 4 suggests primary dementia (eg, Alzheimer disease).
- 4–7 is indeterminate.
- > 7 suggests vascular dementia.

PAD = peripheral arterial disease.

Measures to ensure patient safety (eg, signal monitoring systems for patients who wander) should be implemented.

Drugs to treat Alzheimer disease: Cholinesterase inhibitors modestly improve cognitive function and memory in some patients. Four are available; generally, donepezil, rivastigmine, and galantamine are equally effective, but tacrine is rarely used because of its hepatotoxicity. Donepezil is a first-line drug because it has once/day dosing and is well-tolerated. The recommended dose is 5 mg once/day for 4 to 6 wk, then increased to 10 mg once/day. Donepezil 23 mg once/day dose may be more effective than the traditional 10 mg/day dose for moderate to severe Alzheimer disease. Treatment should be continued if functional improvement is apparent after several months, but otherwise it should be stopped. The most common adverse effects are GI (eg, nausea, diarrhea). Rarely, dizziness and cardiac arrhythmias occur. Adverse effects can be minimized by increasing the dose gradually (see Table 226–6).

Memantine, an *N*-methyl-D-aspartate receptor antagonist, appears to improve cognition and functional capacity of patients with moderate to severe Alzheimer disease. The dose is 5 mg po once/day, which is increased to 10 mg po bid over about 4 wk. For patients with renal insufficiency, the dose should be reduced or the drug should be avoided. Memantine can be used with a cholinesterase inhibitor.

Efficacy of high-dose vitamin E (1000 IU po once/day or bid), selegiline, NSAIDs, *Ginkgo biloba* extracts, and statins is unclear. Estrogen therapy does not appear useful in prevention or treatment and may be harmful.

Prevention

Preliminary, observational evidence suggests that risk of Alzheimer disease may be decreased by the following:

- Continuing to do challenging mental activities (eg, learning new skills, doing crossword puzzles) well into old age
- Exercising
- Controlling hypertension
- Lowering cholesterol levels
- Consuming a diet rich in omega-3 fatty acids and low in saturated fats
- Drinking alcohol in modest amounts

However, there is no convincing evidence that people who do not drink alcohol should start drinking to prevent Alzheimer disease.

Table 226–5. DIFFERENCES BETWEEN ALZHEIMER DISEASE AND LEWY BODY DEMENTIA

FEATURE	ALZHEIMER DISEASE	LEWY BODY DEMENTIA
Pathology	Senile plaques, neurofibrillary tangles, and beta-amyloid deposits in the cerebral cortex and subcortical gray matter	Lewy bodies in neurons of the cortex
Epidemiology	Affects twice as many women	Affects twice as many men
Inheritance	Familial in 5–15% cases	Rarely familial
Day-to-day fluctuation	Some	Prominent
Short-term memory	Lost early in the disease	Less affected Deficits in alertness and attention more than in memory acquisition
Parkinsonian symptoms	Very rare, occurring late in the disease Normal gait	Prominent, obvious early in the disease Axial rigidity and unstable gait
Autonomic dysfunction	Rare	Common
Hallucinations	Occur in about 20% of patients, usually when disease is moderately advanced	Occur in about 80%, usually when disease is early Most commonly, visual
Adverse effects with antipsychotics	Common Possible worsening of symptoms of dementia	Common Acute worsening of extrapyramidal symptoms, which may be severe or life-threatening

Table 226–6. DRUGS FOR ALZHEIMER DISEASE

DRUG NAME	STARTING DOSE	MAXIMUM DOSE	COMMENTS
Donepezil	5 mg once/day	23 mg once/day (for moderate to severe Alzheimer disease)	Generally well-tolerated but can cause nausea or diarrhea
Galantamine	4 mg bid Extended-release: 8 mg once/day in the AM	12 mg bid Extended-release: 24 mg once/day in the AM	Possibly more beneficial for behavioral symptoms than other drugs Modulates nicotinic receptors and appears to stimulate release of acetylcholine and enhances its effect
Memantine	5 mg bid	10 mg bid	Used in patients with moderate to severe Alzheimer disease
Rivastigmine	Liquid or capsule: 1.5 mg bid Patch: 4.6 mg/24 h	Liquid or capsule: 6 mg bid Patch: 13.3 mg/24 h	Available in liquid solution and a patch

KEY POINTS

- Although genetic factors can be involved, most cases of Alzheimer disease are sporadic, with risk predicted best by patient age.
- Differentiating Alzheimer disease from other causes of dementia (eg, vascular dementia, Lewy body dementia) can be difficult but is often best done using clinical criteria, which are 85% accurate in establishing the diagnosis.
- Treat Alzheimer disease similarly to other dementias.

BEHAVIORAL AND PSYCHOLOGIC SYMPTOMS OF DEMENTIA

Disruptive actions are common among patients with dementia and are the primary reason for up to 50% of nursing home admissions. Disruptive actions include wandering, restlessness, yelling, throwing, hitting, refusing treatment, incessantly questioning, disrupting work of staff members, insomnia, and crying. Behavioral and psychologic symptoms of dementia have not been well characterized, and their treatment is poorly understood.

Deciding what actions constitute a behavioral symptom is highly subjective. Tolerability (what actions caregivers can tolerate) depends partly on the patient's living arrangements, particularly safety. For example, wandering may be tolerable if a patient lives in a safe environment (with locks and alarms on all doors and gates); however, if the patient lives in a nursing home or hospital, wandering may be intolerable because it disturbs other patients or interferes with the operation of the institution.

Many behaviors (eg, wandering, repeatedly questioning, being uncooperative) are better tolerated during the day. Whether sundowning (exacerbation of disruptive behaviors at sundown or early evening) represents decreased tolerance by caregivers or true diurnal variation is unknown. In nursing homes, 12 to 14% of patients with dementia act disruptively more often during the evening than during the day.

Etiology

Behavioral and psychologic symptoms may result from functional changes related to dementia:

- Reduced inhibition of inappropriate behaviors (eg, patients may undress in public places)
- Misinterpretation of visual and auditory cues (eg, they may resist treatment, which they perceive as an assault)
- Impaired short-term memory (eg, they repeatedly ask for things already received)
- Reduced ability or inability to express needs (eg, they wander because they are lonely, frightened, or looking for something or someone)

Patients with dementia often adapt poorly to the regimentation of institutional living. Mealtimes, bedtimes, and toileting times are not individualized. For many elderly patients with dementia, behavioral and psychologic symptoms develop or worsen after they are moved to a more restrictive, unfamiliar environment.

Physical problems (eg, pain, shortness of breath, urinary retention, constipation, physical abuse) can exacerbate behavioral and psychologic symptoms partly because patients may be unable to adequately communicate what the problem is. Physical problems can lead to delirium, and delirium superimposed on chronic dementia may worsen the behavioral symptom.

Evaluation

- Characterization of behaviors (eg, by Cohen-Mansfield Agitation Inventory)
- Recording of specific behaviors
- Evaluation for coexisting depression and psychosis

The best approach is to characterize and classify the behavior, rather than to label all such behaviors agitation, a term with too many meanings to be useful. The Cohen-Mansfield Agitation Inventory is commonly used; it classifies behaviors as follows:

- **Physically aggressive:** For example, hitting, pushing, kicking, biting, scratching, or grabbing people or things
- **Physically nonaggressive:** For example, handling things inappropriately, hiding things, dressing or undressing inappropriately, pacing, repeating mannerisms or sentences, acting restless, or trying to go elsewhere
- **Verbally aggressive:** For example, cursing, making strange noises, screaming, or having temper outbursts
- **Verbally nonaggressive:** For example, complaining, whining, constantly requesting attention, not liking anything, interrupting with relevant or irrelevant remarks, or being negative or bossy

The following information should be recorded:

- Specific behaviors
- Precipitating events (eg, feeding, toileting, drug administration, visits)
- Time the behavior started and resolved should be recorded

This information helps identify changes in pattern or intensity of a behavior and makes planning a management strategy easier.

If behavior changes, a physical examination should be done to exclude physical disorders and physical abuse, but environmental changes (eg, a different caregiver) should also be noted because they, rather than a patient-related factor, may be the reason.

Depression, common among patients with dementia, may affect behavior and must be identified. It may first manifest as an abrupt change in cognition, decreased appetite, deterioration in mood, a change in sleep pattern (often hypersomnolence), withdrawal, decreased activity level, crying spells, talk of death and dying, sudden development of irritability or psychosis, or other sudden changes in behavior. Often, depression is suspected first by family members.

Psychotic behavior must also be identified because management differs. Presence of delusions or hallucinations indicates psychosis. Delusions and hallucinations must be distinguished from disorientation, fearfulness, and misunderstanding, which are common among patients with dementia:

- Delusions without paranoia may be confused with disorientation, but delusions are usually fixed (eg, a nursing home is repeatedly called a prison), and disorientation varies (eg, a nursing home is called a prison, a restaurant, and a home).
- Hallucinations occur without external sensory stimuli; hallucinations should be distinguished from illusions, which involve misinterpreting external sensory stimuli (eg, cellular phones, pagers).

Treatment

- Environmental measures and caregiver support
- Drugs only when necessary

Management of behavioral and psychologic symptoms of dementia is controversial and has been inadequately studied. Supportive measures are preferred; however, drugs are commonly used.

Environmental measures: The environment should be safe and flexible enough to accommodate behaviors that are not dangerous. Signs to help patients find their way and doors equipped with locks or alarms can help ensure the safety of patients who wander. Flexible sleeping hours and organization of beds can help patients with sleeping problems.

Measures used to treat dementia generally also help minimize behavioral symptoms:

- Providing cues about time and place
- Explaining care before giving it
- Encouraging physical activity

If an institution cannot provide an appropriate environment for a particular patient, transferring the patient to one that can may be preferable to drug treatment.

Caregiver support: Providing caregiver support is crucial. Learning how dementia leads to behavioral and psychologic symptoms and how to respond to disruptive behavior can help family members and other caregivers provide care for and cope with the patient better.

Learning how to manage stress, which may be considerable, is essential. Stressed caregivers should be referred to support services (eg, social workers, caregiver support groups, home health aides) and should be told how to obtain respite care if such care is available.

Family members who are caregivers should be monitored for depression, which occurs in nearly half of them. Depression in caregivers should be treated promptly.

Use of drugs: Drugs that improve cognition (eg, cholinesterase inhibitors) may also help manage behavioral and psychologic symptoms in patients with dementia. However, drugs directed primarily at behavior (eg, antipsychotics) are used only when other approaches are ineffective and when drugs are essential for safety. The need for continued treatment should be reassessed at least every month. Drugs should be selected to target the most intolerable behaviors.

Antidepressants, preferably SSRIs, should be prescribed only for patients with signs of depression.

Antipsychotics: Antipsychotics are often used even though their efficacy has been shown only in psychotic patients. Other patients are unlikely to benefit and are likely to experience adverse effects, particularly extrapyramidal symptoms. Tardive dyskinesia or tardive dystonia may develop; these conditions often do not resolve when the dose is reduced or the drug is stopped.

Choice of antipsychotic depends on relative toxicity. Of conventional antipsychotics, haloperidol is relatively nonsedating and has less potent anticholinergic effects but is most likely to cause extrapyramidal symptoms; thioridazine and thiothixene are less likely to cause extrapyramidal symptoms but are more sedating and have more anticholinergic effects than haloperidol.

Second-generation (atypical) antipsychotics (eg, aripiprazole, olanzapine, quetiapine, risperidone) are minimally anticholinergic and cause fewer extrapyramidal symptoms than conventional antipsychotics; however, these drugs, used for an extended period, may be associated with an increased risk of hyperglycemia and all-cause mortality. Also, they may increase risk of stroke in elderly patients who have dementia-related psychosis.

If antipsychotics are used, they should be given in a low dose (eg, olanzapine 2.5 to 15 mg po once/day; risperidone 0.5 to 3 mg po q 12 h; haloperidol 0.5 to 1.0 mg po, IV, or IM bid or as needed) and for a short time.

Other drugs: Anticonvulsants, particularly valproate, may be useful in controlling impulsive behavioral outbursts.

Sedatives (eg, a short-acting benzodiazepine such as lorazepam 0.5 mg po q 12 h as needed) are sometimes used in the short term to alleviate event-related anxiety, but such treatment is not recommended for the long term.

KEY POINTS

- What constitutes disruptive behavior is subjective and variable, yet behavioral disturbances are the reason for up to 50% of nursing home admissions.
- Behavior often deteriorates when patients are moved from their familiar home environment.
- Behavioral disturbances may be triggered by a physical problem that the patient cannot communicate.
- Categorize behavioral disturbances using the Cohen-Mansfield Agitation Inventory.
- Recognize signs of depression, such as abrupt changes in cognition, decreased appetite, deterioration in mood, a change in sleep pattern (often hypersomnolence), withdrawal, decreased activity level, crying spells, talk of death and dying, and sudden development of irritability or psychosis.
- Treat using environmental measures, avoiding drugs when possible.

CHRONIC TRAUMATIC ENCEPHALOPATHY

(Dementia Pugilistica)

Chronic traumatic encephalopathy (CTE) is a progressive degenerative brain disorder that may occur after repetitive head trauma or blast injuries.

Dementia pugilistica, identified in boxers in the 1920s, and CTE, a more recent term, are thought to be the same disorder. CTE has been widely studied. It occurs in some retired professional football players and other athletes who have had repetitive head trauma and in some soldiers with brain damage secondary to closed head injuries due to blast trauma.

Why only certain people who have repetitive head trauma develop CTE and what the risks of developing it are after various amounts of head trauma (eg, how many, how much force) are currently unknown. About 3% of athletes who have had multiple (even apparently minor) concussions develop CTE.

Pathologically, CTE is characterized by the deposition of hyperphosphorylated tau protein as neurofibrillary tangles, most prominently in the perivascular spaces, cortical sulcal depths, and subpial and periventricular areas.

Symptoms and Signs

Initial symptoms of CTE typically include ≥ 1 of the following:

- Mood disturbance: Depression, irritability, and/or hopelessness
- Behavioral abnormalities: Impulsivity, explosivity, and/or aggression
- Cognitive impairment: Memory impairment, executive dysfunction, and/or dementia
- Motor abnormalities: Parkinsonism, ataxia, and/or dysarthria

There are two distinct clinical courses:

- Mood disturbances and behavioral abnormalities develop during young adulthood (eg, during the patient's 30s), and cognitive impairment develops later.
- Cognitive impairment develops later in life (eg, during the patient's 60s), and mood disturbances and behavioral abnormalities may develop after cognitive impairment.

Diagnosis

- Clinical criteria

Criteria for clinical diagnosis of CTE include the following:

- A history of head trauma
- Symptoms and signs consistent with CTE
- Absence of a more likely explanation of clinical findings

These criteria are also used in research.

Results of routine neuroimaging such as CT or MRI are usually normal. Currently, there are no objective, validated in vivo biomarkers of CTE.

A definitive diagnosis of CTE is based on neuropathologic examination during autopsy.

Treatment

- Supportive measures

There is no specific treatment. Supportive measures, as for other dementias, may help. For example, the environment should be bright, cheerful, and familiar, and it should be designed to reinforce orientation (eg, placement of large clocks and calendars in the room). Measures to ensure patient safety (eg, signal monitoring systems for patients who wander) should be implemented.

Prevention

Preventive measures are the most important intervention. Because CTE typically results from repeated head injury, people who have had a concussion are advised to rest and to gradually return to sports activity. Those who have had several concussions should be advised of the risks of continued play.

FRONTOTEMPORAL DEMENTIA

Frontotemporal dementia (FTD) refers to sporadic and hereditary disorders that affect the frontal and temporal lobes, including Pick disease.

Dementia is chronic, global, usually irreversible deterioration of cognition. FTD accounts for up to 10% of dementias. Age at onset is typically younger (age 55 to 65) than in Alzheimer disease. FTDs affect men and women about equally.

Pick disease is a term used to describe pathologic changes in FTD, including severe atrophy, neuronal loss, gliosis, and presence of abnormal neurons (Pick cells) containing inclusions (Pick bodies).

About half of FTDs are inherited; most mutations involve chromosome 17q21-22 and result in abnormalities of the microtubule-binding tau protein; thus, FTDs are considered tauopathies. Some experts classify supranuclear palsy and corticobasal degeneration with FTDs because they share similar pathology and gene mutations affecting the tau protein. Symptoms, gene mutations, and pathologic changes may not correspond to each other. For example, the same mutation causes FTD symptoms in one family member but symptoms of corticobasal degeneration in another.

Dementia should not be confused with delirium although cognition is disordered in both. The following helps distinguish them:

- **Dementia** affects mainly memory, is typically caused by anatomic changes in the brain, has slower onset, and is generally irreversible.
- **Delirium** affects mainly attention, is typically caused by acute illness or drug toxicity (sometimes life threatening), and is often reversible.

Other specific characteristics also help distinguish the dementia and delirium (see Table 226–1).

Symptoms and Signs

Generally, FTD affects personality, behavior, and usually language function (syntax and fluency) more and memory less than does Alzheimer disease. Abstract thinking and attention (maintaining and shifting) are impaired; responses are disorganized. Orientation is preserved, but retrieval of information may be impaired. Motor skills are generally preserved. Patients have difficulty sequencing tasks, although visuospatial and constructional tasks are affected less.

Frontal release signs (grasp, root, suck, snout, and palmomental reflexes and glabellar sign—see p. 1889) appear late in the disease but also occur in other dementias.

Some patients develop motor neuron disease with generalized muscle atrophy, weakness, fasciculations, bulbar symptoms (eg, dysphagia, dysphonia, difficulty chewing), and increased risk of aspiration pneumonia and early death.

Behavioral (frontal) variant FTD: Social behavior and personality change because the orbitobasal frontal lobe is affected. Patients become impulsive and lose their social inhibitions (eg, they may shoplift); they neglect personal hygiene.Some have Klüver-Bucy syndrome, which involves emotional blunting, hypersexual activity, hyperorality (eg, bulimia, sucking and smacking of lips), and visual agnosias. Impersistence (impaired concentration), inertia, and mental rigidity appear.

Behavior becomes repetitive and stereotyped (eg, patients may walk to the same location every day). Patients may pick up and manipulate random objects for no reason (called utilization behavior). Verbal output is reduced; echolalia, perseveration (inappropriate repetition of a response), and eventually mutism occur.

Primary progressive aphasia: Language function deteriorates because of asymmetric (worse on left) anterolateral temporal lobe atrophy; the hippocampus and memory are relatively spared. Most patients present with difficulty finding words. Attention (eg, digit span) may be severely impaired. Many patients have aphasia, with decreased fluency and difficulty comprehending language; hesitancy in speech production and dysarthria are also common. In some patients, aphasia is the only symptom for ≥ 10 yr; in others, global deficits develop within a few years.

Semantic dementia is a type of primary progressive aphasia. When the left side of the brain is affected most, the ability to comprehend words is progressively lost. Speech is fluent but lacks meaning; a generic or related term may be used instead of the specific name of an object. When the right side is affected most, patients have progressive anomia (inability to name objects) and prosopagnosia (inability to recognize familiar faces). They cannot remember topographic relationships. Some patients with semantic dementia also have Alzheimer disease.

Diagnosis

- Generally similar to diagnosis of other dementias
- Additional clinical evaluation to differentiate from some other dementias

A general diagnosis of dementia requires all of the following:

- Cognitive or behavioral (neuropsychiatric) symptoms interfere with the ability to function at work or do usual daily activities.
- These symptoms represent a decline from previous levels of functioning.
- These symptoms are not explained by delirium or a major psychiatric disorder.

Diagnosis of FTD is suggested by typical clinical findings (eg, social disinhibition or impaired language function with relative sparing of memory).

As for other dementias, cognitive deficits are evaluated. Evaluation involves taking a history from the patient and from someone who knows the patient plus doing a bedside mental status examination *or*, if bedside testing is inconclusive, formal neuropsychologic testing (see p. 1877).

CT and MRI are done to determine location and extent of brain atrophy and to exclude other possible causes (eg, brain tumors, abscesses, stroke). FTDs are characterized by severely atrophic, sometimes paper-thin gyri in the temporal and frontal lobes. However, MRI or CT may not show these changes until late in FTD. Thus, FTDs and Alzheimer disease can usually be differentiated more easily by clinical criteria. For example, primary progressive aphasia differs from Alzheimer disease in that memory and visuospatial function are preserved and syntax and fluency are impaired.

PET with fluorine-18 (^{18}F)–labeled deoxyglucose (fluorodeoxyglucose, or FDG may help differentiate Alzheimer disease from FTD by showing the location of hypometabolic areas. In Alzheimer disease, these areas are located in the posterior temporoparietal association cortex and posterior cingulate cortex; in FTD, they are located in the anterior regions—in the frontal lobes, anterior temporal cortex, and anterior cingulate cortex.

Prognosis

FTDs usually progress gradually, but progression rate varies; if symptoms are limited to speech and language, progression to general dementia may be slower.

Treatment

- Supportive measures

There is no specific treatment. Treatment is generally supportive. For example, the environment should be bright, cheerful, and familiar, and it should be designed to reinforce orientation (eg, placement of large clocks and calendars in the room). Measures to ensure patient safety (eg, signal monitoring systems for patients who wander) should be implemented.

Symptoms are treated as needed.

HIV-ASSOCIATED DEMENTIA

HIV-associated dementia is chronic cognitive deterioration due to brain infection by HIV.

Dementia is chronic, global, usually irreversible deterioration of cognition. HIV-associated dementia (AIDS dementia complex) may occur in the late stages of HIV infection (see p. 1627). Unlike almost all other forms of dementia, it tends to occur in younger people.

Dementia should not be confused with delirium (see p. 1871) although cognition is disordered in both. The following helps distinguish them:

- **Dementia** affects mainly memory, is typically caused by anatomic changes in the brain, has slower onset, and is generally irreversible.
- **Delirium** affects mainly attention, is typically caused by acute illness or drug toxicity (sometimes life-threatening), and is often reversible.

Other specific characteristics also help distinguish the 2 disorders (see Table 226–1).

Purely HIV-associated dementia is caused by neuronal damage by the HIV virus. However, in patients with HIV infection, dementia may result from other disorders, some of which may be treatable. These disorders include other infections, such as secondary infection with JC virus causing progressive multifocal leukoencephalopathy and CNS lymphoma. Other opportunistic infections (eg, cryptococcal meningitis, other fungal meningitis, some bacterial infections, TB meningitis, viral infections, toxoplasmosis) may also contribute.

In purely HIV-associated dementia, subcortical pathologic changes result when infected macrophages or microglial cells infiltrate into the deep gray matter (ie, basal ganglia, thalamus) and white matter.

Prevalence of dementia in late-stage HIV infection ranges from 7 to 27%, but 30 to 40% may have milder forms. Incidence is inversely proportional to CD4 count.

Symptoms and Signs

Symptoms and signs may be similar to those of other dementias. Early manifestations include

- Slowed thinking and expression
- Difficulty concentrating
- Apathy

Insight is preserved, and manifestations of depression are few. Motor movements are slowed; ataxia and weakness may be evident.

Abnormal neurologic signs may include

- Paraparesis
- Lower-extremity spasticity
- Ataxia
- Extensor-plantar responses

Mania or psychosis is sometimes present.

Diagnosis

- Clinical evaluation
- Measurement of CD4 count and HIV viral load
- Prompt evaluation, including MRI and usually lumbar puncture, when deterioration is acute

HIV-associated dementia should be suspected in patients who have

- Symptoms of dementia
- Known HIV infection or symptoms or risk factors suggesting HIV infection

If patients known to have HIV infection have symptoms suggesting dementia, a general diagnosis of dementia is confirmed based on the usual criteria, including the following:

- Cognitive or behavioral (neuropsychiatric) symptoms interfere with the ability to function at work or do usual daily activities.
- These symptoms represent a decline from previous levels of functioning.
- These symptoms are not explained by delirium or a major psychiatric disorder.

Evaluation of cognitive function involves taking a history from the patient and from someone who knows the patient plus doing a bedside mental status examination *or*, if bedside testing is inconclusive, formal neuropsychologic testing (see p. 1877).

If patients with symptoms of dementia are *not* known to have HIV infection but have risk factors for HIV infection, they are tested for HIV.

In patients with HIV infection or suspected HIV-associated dementia, CD4 count and HIV viral load are measured. In patients with suspected or confirmed HIV and dementia, these values help determine how likely HIV-associated dementia (and CNS lymphoma and other HIV-associated CNS infections) is to be contributing to dementia. In patients who have HIV infection but not dementia, these values help determine how likely HIV-associated dementia is to develop.

If patients have dementia and HIV infection, other processes can cause or contribute to worsening dementia symptoms. Thus, the cause of cognitive decline, particularly sudden, severe decline—whether due to HIV or another infection—must be identified as soon as possible.

MRI, with and without contrast, should be done to identify other causes of dementia, and if MRI does not identify any contraindication to lumbar puncture, lumbar puncture should also be done.

Late-stage findings of HIV-associated dementia may include diffuse nonenhancing white matter hyperintensities, cerebral atrophy, and ventricular enlargement.

Prognosis

Patients with HIV infection and untreated dementia have a worse prognosis (average life expectancy of 6 mo) than those without dementia.

Treatment

- Antiretroviral therapy

The primary treatment of HIV-associated dementia is antiretroviral therapy, which increases CD4 counts and improves cognitive function.

Supportive measures are similar to those for other dementias. For example, the environment should be bright, cheerful, and familiar, and it should be designed to reinforce orientation (eg, placement of large clocks and calendars in the room). Measures to ensure patient safety (eg, signal monitoring systems for patients who wander) should be implemented.

Symptoms are treated as necessary.

LEWY BODY DEMENTIA AND PARKINSON DISEASE DEMENTIA

Lewy body dementia is chronic cognitive deterioration characterized by cellular inclusions called Lewy bodies in the cytoplasm of cortical neurons. Parkinson disease dementia is cognitive deterioration characterized by Lewy bodies in the substantia nigra; it develops late in Parkinson disease.

Dementia is chronic, global, usually irreversible deterioration of cognition. Lewy body dementia is the 3rd most common dementia. Age of onset is typically > 60.

Lewy bodies are spherical, eosinophilic, neuronal cytoplasmic inclusions composed of aggregates of α-synuclein, a synaptic protein. They occur in the cortex of some patients with primary Lewy body dementia. Neurotransmitter levels and neuronal pathways between the striatum and the neocortex are abnormal.

Lewy bodies also occur in the substantia nigra of patients with Parkinson disease, and dementia (Parkinson disease dementia) may develop late in the disease. About 40% of patients with Parkinson disease develop Parkinson disease dementia, usually after age 70 and about 10 to 15 yr after Parkinson disease has been diagnosed.

Because Lewy bodies occur in Lewy body dementia and in Parkinson disease dementia, some experts think that the 2 disorders may be part of a more generalized synucleinopathy affecting the central and peripheral nervous systems. Lewy bodies sometimes occur in patients with Alzheimer disease, and patients with Lewy body dementia may have neuritic plaques and neurofibrillary tangles. Lewy body dementia, Parkinson disease, and Alzheimer disease overlap considerably. Further research is needed to clarify the relationships among them.

Both Lewy body dementia and Parkinson disease dementia have a progressive course with a poor prognosis.

Dementia should not be confused with delirium although cognition is disordered in both. The following usually helps distinguish dementia from delirium:

- **Dementia** affects mainly memory, is typically caused by anatomic changes in the brain, has slower onset, and is generally irreversible.
- **Delirium** affects mainly attention, is typically caused by acute illness or drug toxicity (sometimes life threatening), and is often reversible.

Other specific characteristics also help distinguish the dementia and delirium (see Table 226–1).

Symptoms and Signs

Lewy body dementia: Initial cognitive deterioration in Lewy body dementia resembles that of other dementias (see p. 1875); it involves deterioration in memory, attention, and executive function and behavioral problems.

Extrapyramidal symptoms (typically including rigidity, bradykinesia, and gait instability) occur (see also Movement and Cerebellar Disorders on p. 1928). However, in Lewy body dementia (unlike in Parkinson disease), cognitive and extrapyramidal symptoms usually begin within 1 yr of each other. Also, the extrapyramidal symptoms differ from those of Parkinson disease. In Lewy body dementia, tremor does not occur early, rigidity of axial muscles with gait instability occurs early, and deficits tend to be symmetric. Repeated falls are common.

Fluctuating cognitive function is a relatively specific feature of Lewy body dementia. Periods of being alert, coherent, and oriented may alternate with periods of being confused and unresponsive to questions, usually over a period of days to weeks but sometimes during the same interview.

Memory is impaired, but the impairment appears to result more from deficits in alertness and attention than in memory acquisition; thus, short-term recall is affected less than digit span memory (ability to repeat 7 digits forward and 5 backward).

Patients may stare into space for long periods. Excessive daytime drowsiness is common.

Visuospatial and visuoconstructional abilities (tested by block design, clock drawing, or figure copying) are affected more than other cognitive deficits.

Visual hallucinations are common and often threatening, unlike the benign hallucinations of Parkinson disease. Auditory, olfactory, and tactile hallucinations are less common. Delusions occur in 50 to 65% of patients and are often complex and bizarre, compared with the simple persecutory ideation common in Alzheimer disease.

Autonomic dysfunction is common, and unexplained syncope may result. Autonomic dysfunction may occur simultaneously with or occur after onset of cognitive deficits. Extreme sensitivity to antipsychotics is typical.

Many patients have FTD (REM) sleep behavior disorder, a parasomnia characterized by vivid dreams without the usual physiologic paralysis of skeletal muscles during REM sleep. As a result, dreams may be acted out, sometimes injuring the bed partner.

Parkinson disease dementia: In Parkinson disease dementia (unlike in Lewy body dementia), cognitive impairment that leads to dementia typically begins 10 to 15 yr after motor symptoms have appeared.

Parkinson disease dementia may affect multiple cognitive domains including attention, memory, and visuospatial, constructional, and executive functions. Executive dysfunction typically occurs earlier and is more common in Parkinson disease dementia than in Alzheimer disease.

Psychiatric symptoms (eg, hallucinations, delusions) appear to be less frequent and/or less severe than in Lewy body dementia.

In Parkinson disease dementia, postural instability and gait abnormalities are more common, motor decline is more rapid, and falls are more frequent than in Parkinson disease without dementia.

Diagnosis

- Clinical criteria
- Neuroimaging to rule out other disorders

Diagnosis is clinical, but sensitivity and specificity are poor. A general diagnosis of dementia requires all of the following:

- Cognitive or behavioral (neuropsychiatric) symptoms interfere with the ability to function at work or do usual daily activities.
- These symptoms represent a decline from previous levels of functioning.
- These symptoms are not explained by delirium or a major psychiatric disorder.

Evaluation of cognitive function involves taking a history from the patient and from someone who knows the patient plus doing a bedside mental status examination *or*, if bedside testing is inconclusive, formal neuropsychologic testing (see p. 1877).

Diagnosis of Lewy body dementia is considered probable if 2 of the following 3 features are present and is considered possible if only one is present:

- Fluctuations in cognition
- Visual hallucinations
- Parkinsonism

Supportive evidence consists of repeated falls, syncope, REM sleep disorder, and sensitivity to antipsychotics.

Overlap of symptoms in Lewy body dementia and Parkinson disease dementia may complicate diagnosis. When motor deficits (eg, tremor, bradykinesia, rigidity) precede and are more severe than cognitive impairment, Parkinson disease dementia is usually diagnosed. When early cognitive impairment (particularly executive dysfunction) and behavioral disturbances predominate, Lewy body dementia is usually diagnosed.

Because patients with Lewy body dementia often have impaired alertness, which is more characteristic of delirium than dementia, evaluation for delirium should be done, particularly for common causes such as

- Drugs, particularly anticholinergics, psychoactive drugs, and opioids
- Dehydration
- Infection

CT and MRI show no characteristic changes but are helpful initially in ruling out other causes of dementia. PET with fluorine-18 (^{18}F)–labeled deoxyglucose (fluorodeoxyglucose, or FDG) and single-photon emission CT (SPECT) with ^{123}I-FP-CIT (*N*-3-fluoropropyl-2β-carbomethoxy-3β-[4-iodophenyl]-tropane), a fluoroalkyl analog of cocaine, may help identify Lewy body dementia but are not routinely done.

Definitive diagnosis requires autopsy samples of brain tissue.

Treatment

- Supportive care

Treatment is generally supportive. For example, the environment and should be bright, cheerful, and familiar, and it should be designed to reinforce orientation (eg, placement of large clocks and calendars in the room). Measures to ensure patient safety (eg, signal monitoring systems for patients who wander) should be implemented.

Troublesome symptoms can be treated.

Drugs: Cholinesterase inhibitors may improve cognitive function and may be helpful.

Rivastigmine, a cholinesterase inhibitor, can be used to treat Lewy body dementia and Parkinson disease dementia. A starting dose of 1.5 mg po bid may be titrated upward as needed to 6 mg bid to try to improve cognition. Other cholinesterase inhibitors may also be used.

In about half of patients, extrapyramidal symptoms respond to antiparkinsonian drugs, but psychiatric symptoms may worsen. If such drugs are needed, levodopa is preferred.

In Lewy body dementia, traditional antipsychotics, even at very low doses, tend to acutely worsen extrapyramidal symptoms and are best avoided.

KEY POINTS

- Because Lewy bodies occur in Lewy body dementia and in Parkinson disease, some experts hypothesize that the 2 disorders are part of the same synucleinopathy affecting the central and peripheral nervous systems.
- Suspect Lewy body dementia if dementia develops nearly simultaneously with parkinsonian features and when dementia is accompanied by fluctuations in cognition, loss of attention, psychiatric symptoms (eg, visual hallucinations; complex, bizarre delusions), and autonomic dysfunction.
- Suspect Parkinson disease dementia if dementia begins years after parkinsonian features, particularly if executive dysfunction occurs early.
- Consider use of rivastigmine and sometimes other cholinesterase inhibitors to try to improve cognition.

NORMAL-PRESSURE HYDROCEPHALUS

Normal-pressure hydrocephalus is characterized by gait disturbance, urinary incontinence, dementia, enlarged brain ventricles, and normal or slightly elevated CSF pressure.

Normal-pressure hydrocephalus is thought to result from a defect in CSF resorption in arachnoid granulations. This disorder accounts for up to 6% of dementias; dementia is chronic, global, usually irreversible deterioration of cognition.

Dementia should not be confused with delirium although cognition is disordered in both. The following helps distinguish them:

- **Dementia** affects mainly memory, is typically caused by anatomic changes in the brain, has slower onset, and is generally irreversible.
- **Delirium** affects mainly attention, is typically caused by acute illness or drug toxicity (sometimes life-threatening), and is often reversible.

Other specific characteristics also help distinguish dementia and delirium (see Table 226–1).

Symptoms and Signs

The **gait disturbance** in normal-pressure hydrocephalus is usually nonspecific unsteadiness and impaired balance, although a magnetic gait (the feet appear to stick to the floor) is considered the characteristic gait disturbance.

Dementia may not occur until late in the disorder. The most common early symptoms of dementia are disturbances of executive function and attention; memory tends to become impaired later.

Urinary incontinence is common.

Diagnosis

- Clinical evaluation
- Neuroimaging
- Sometimes removal of CSF

The classic symptoms (gait disturbance, urinary incontinence, and dementia), even combined, are nonspecific for normal-pressure hydrocephalus, particularly in the elderly. For example, some forms of vascular dementia can cause dementia, gait disturbance, and, less commonly, urinary incontinence.

A general diagnosis of dementia requires all of the following:

- Cognitive or behavioral (neuropsychiatric) symptoms interfere with the ability to function at work or do usual daily activities.
- These symptoms represent a decline from previous levels of functioning.
- These symptoms are not explained by delirium or a major psychiatric disorder.

Evaluation of cognitive function involves taking a history from the patient and from someone who knows the patient plus doing a bedside mental status examination *or*, if bedside testing is inconclusive, formal neuropsychologic testing (see p. 1877).

Brain imaging may show ventricular enlargement disproportionate to cortical atrophy; this finding is nonspecific but may support the diagnosis of normal-pressure hydrocephalus.

Lumbar puncture with removal of 30 to 50 mL of CSF can be done as a diagnostic trial. Improvement in gait, continence, and cognition after removal helps confirm the diagnosis, but improvement may not be evident until several hours after removal. Additional CSF may leak out after lumbar puncture, sometimes contributing to neurologic improvement.

Treatment

- Sometimes ventriculoperitoneal shunting

Ventriculoperitoneal shunting is useful for patients with acceptable surgical risks. Improvements after lumbar puncture to remove CSF, done during diagnosis, may predict the response to shunting. In several case series (but in no randomized trials), patients improved substantially, typically in gait, continence, and daily functioning, after shunting; improvement in cognition was less common.

VASCULAR DEMENTIA

Vascular dementia is acute or chronic cognitive deterioration due to diffuse or focal cerebral infarction that is most often related to cerebrovascular disease.

Dementia is chronic, global, usually irreversible deterioration of cognition. Vascular dementia is the 2nd most common cause of dementia among the elderly. It is more common among men and usually begins after age 70. It occurs more often in people who have vascular risk factors (eg, hypertension, diabetes mellitus, hyperlipidemia, smoking) and in those who have had several strokes. Many people have both vascular dementia and Alzheimer disease.

Dementia should not be confused with delirium (see p. 1871), although cognition is disordered in both. The following helps distinguish them:

- **Dementia** affects mainly memory, is typically caused by anatomic changes in the brain, has slower onset, and is generally irreversible.
- **Delirium** affects mainly attention, is typically caused by acute illness or drug toxicity (sometimes life threatening), and is often reversible.

Other specific characteristics also help distinguish the 2 disorders (see Table 226–1).

Etiology

Vascular dementia typically occurs when multiple small cerebral infarcts (or sometimes hemorrhages) cause enough neuronal or axonal loss to impair brain function.

Vascular dementias include the following:

- **Multiple lacunar infarction:** Small blood vessels are affected. Multiple lacunar infarcts occur deep within hemispheric white and gray matter.
- **Multi-infarct dementia:** Medium-sized blood vessels are affected.
- **Strategic single-infarct dementia:** A single infarct occurs in a crucial area of the brain (eg, angular gyrus, thalamus).
- **Binswanger dementia (subcortical arteriosclerotic encephalopathy):** This uncommon variant of small-vessel dementia is associated with severe, poorly controlled hypertension and systemic vascular disease. It causes diffuse and irregular loss of axons and myelin with widespread gliosis, tissue death due to an infarction, or loss of blood supply to the white matter of the brain.

Symptoms and Signs

Symptoms and signs of vascular dementia are similar to those of other dementias (eg, memory loss, impaired executive function, difficulty initiating actions or tasks, slowed thinking, personality and mood changes, language deficits). However, compared with Alzheimer disease, vascular dementia tends to cause memory loss later and to affect executive function earlier. Also, symptoms can vary depending on where the infarcts occur.

Unlike other dementias, multiple-infarct dementia tends to progress in discrete steps; each episode is accompanied by intellectual decline, sometimes followed by modest recovery. Subcortical vascular dementia caused by small-vessel ischemic damage (which includes multiple lacunar infarction and Binswanger dementia) tends to cause small, incremental deficits; thus, the decline appears to be gradual.

As the disease progresses, focal neurologic deficits often develop:

- Exaggeration of deep tendon reflexes
- Extensor plantar response
- Gait abnormalities
- Weakness of an extremity
- Hemiplegias
- Pseudobulbar palsy with pathologic laughing and crying
- Other signs of extrapyramidal dysfunction
- Aphasias

Cognitive loss may be focal. For example, short-term memory may be less affected than in other dementias. Because loss may be focal, patients may retain more aspects of mental function. Thus, they may be more aware of their deficits, and depression may be more common than in other dementias.

Diagnosis

- Generally similar to diagnosis of other dementias
- Neuroimaging

Diagnosis of vascular dementia is similar to that of other dementias (see p. 1876). A general diagnosis of dementia requires all of the following:

- Cognitive or behavioral (neuropsychiatric) symptoms interfere with the ability to function at work or do usual daily activities.
- These symptoms represent a decline from previous levels of functioning.
- These symptoms are not explained by delirium or a major psychiatric disorder.

Evaluation of cognitive function involves taking a history from the patient and from someone who knows the patient plus doing a bedside mental status examination *or*, if bedside testing is inconclusive, formal neuropsychologic testing (see p. 1877).

Differentiation of vascular dementia from other dementia is based on clinical judgment. Factors that suggest vascular dementia (or Alzheimer disease with cerebrovascular disease) include the following:

- Evidence of brain infarcts
- High Hachinski Ischemic Score
- Clinical features characteristic of vascular dementia (eg, prominent executive dysfunction, mild or absent memory loss)

Confirmation of vascular dementia requires a history of stroke or evidence of a vascular cause for dementia detected by neuroimaging. If focal neurologic signs or evidence of cerebrovascular disease is present, a thorough evaluation for stroke should be done.

CT and MRI may show bilateral multiple infarcts in the dominant hemisphere and limbic structures, multiple lacunar strokes, or periventricular white-matter lesions extending into the deep white matter. In Binswanger dementia, imaging shows leukoencephalopathy in the cerebrum semiovale adjacent to the cortex, often with multiple lacunae affecting structures deep in the gray matter (eg, basal ganglia, thalamic nuclei).

The Hachinski Ischemic Score is sometimes used to help differentiate vascular dementia from Alzheimer disease (see Table 226–4).

Prognosis

The 5-yr mortality rate is 61%, which is higher than that for most forms of dementia, presumably because other atherosclerotic disorders coexist.

Treatment

- Safety and supportive measures
- Management of vascular risk factors, including smoking cessation

Safety and supportive measures are similar to those of other dementias. For example, the environment should be bright, cheerful, and familiar, and it should be designed to reinforce orientation (eg, placement of large clocks and calendars in the room). Measures to ensure patient safety (eg, signal monitoring systems for patients who wander) should be implemented.

Troublesome symptoms can be treated.

Managing vascular risk factors (eg, hypertension, diabetes, hyperlipidemia) may slow the progression of vascular dementia and help prevent future strokes, which could cause more cognitive impairment. Management includes the following:

- BP control
- Cholesterol-lowering therapy
- Regulation of plasma glucose (90 to 150 mg/dL)
- Smoking cessation

Drugs, such as cholinesterase inhibitors and memantine, may be helpful in some dementias. Cholinesterase inhibitors may improve cognitive function. Memantine, an NMDA (*N*-methyl-D-aspartate) antagonist, may help slow the loss of cognitive function in patients with moderate to severe dementia and may be synergistic when used with a cholinesterase inhibitor.

However, efficacy of cholinesterase inhibitors and memantine is uncertain in vascular dementia. Nonetheless, a trial of these drugs is reasonable because elderly patients with vascular dementia may also have Alzheimer disease.

Adjunctive drugs for depression, psychosis, and sleep disorders are useful.

KEY POINTS

- Vascular dementia can occur as a series of discrete episodes (which may seem like a gradual decline) or in a single episode.
- Focal neurologic signs may help differentiate vascular dementia from other dementias.
- Confirm that dementia is vascular based on a history of stroke or neuroimaging findings that suggest a vascular cause.
- Control vascular risk factors, and if Alzheimer disease could also be present, treat with cholinesterase inhibitors and memantine.

227 Demyelinating Disorders

Myelin sheaths cover many nerve fibers in the central and peripheral nervous system; they accelerate axonal transmission of neural impulses. Disorders that affect myelin interrupt nerve transmission; symptoms may reflect deficits in any part of the nervous system.

Myelin formed by oligodendroglia in the CNS differs chemically and immunologically from that formed by Schwann cells peripherally. Thus, some myelin disorders (eg, Guillain-Barré syndrome, chronic inflammatory demyelinating polyneuropathy, some other peripheral nerve polyneuropathies) tend to affect primarily the peripheral nerves, and others affect primarily the CNS (see Table 227–1). The most commonly affected areas in the CNS are the brain, spinal cord, and optic nerves.

Demyelination is often secondary to an infectious, ischemic, metabolic, or hereditary disorder or to a toxin (eg, alcohol, ethambutol). In primary demyelinating disorders, cause is unknown, but an autoimmune mechanism is suspected because the disorder sometimes follows a viral infection or viral vaccination.

Demyelination tends to be segmental or patchy, affecting multiple areas simultaneously or sequentially. Remyelination often occurs, with repair, regeneration, and complete recovery

Table 227–1. DISORDERS THAT CAN CAUSE CNS DEMYELINATION

CATEGORY	DISORDERS
Hereditary disorders	Phenylketonuria and other aminoacidurias Tay-Sachs disease, Niemann-Pick disease, and Gaucher disease Hurler syndrome Krabbe disease and other leukodystrophies* Adrenoleukodystrophies* Adrenomyeloneuropathy* Leber hereditary optic atrophy and related mitochondrial disorders
Hypoxia and ischemia	Carbon monoxide toxicity and other syndromes of delayed hypoxic cerebral demyelination Progressive subcortical ischemic demyelination
Nutritional deficiencies	Osmotic demyelination syndrome† (formerly called central pontine myelinolysis) Demyelination of the corpus callosum (Marchiafava-Bignami disease) Vitamin B_{12} deficiency
Direct viral invasion of CNS	Progressive multifocal leukoencephalopathy Subacute sclerosing panencephalitis Tropical spastic paraparesis/HTLV-1–associated myelopathy
Primary demyelinating disorders	Recurrent, progressive disorders (multiple sclerosis and its variants) Monophasic disorders such as optic neuritis, acute transverse myelitis, acute disseminated encephalomyelitis, and acute hemorrhagic leukoencephalitis Neuromyelitis optica
Toxins	Alcohol Ethambutol

*Some subtypes may also cause peripheral demyelination.
†Osmotic demyelination syndrome may also be caused by sodium fluxes.
HTLV-1 = human T-lymphotropic virus 1.

of neural function. However, extensive myelin loss is usually followed by axonal degeneration and often cell body degeneration; both may be irreversible.

Demyelination should be considered in any patient with unexplained neurologic deficits. Primary demyelinating disorders are suggested by the following:

- Diffuse or multifocal deficits
- Sudden or subacute onset, particularly in young adults
- Onset within weeks of an infection or vaccination
- Deficits that wax and wane
- Symptoms suggesting a specific demyelinating disorder (eg, unexplained optic neuritis or internuclear ophthalmoplegia suggesting multiple sclerosis)

Specific tests and treatment depend on the specific disorder.

MULTIPLE SCLEROSIS

Multiple sclerosis (MS) is characterized by disseminated patches of demyelination in the brain and spinal cord. Common symptoms include visual and oculomotor abnormalities, paresthesias, weakness, spasticity, urinary dysfunction, and mild cognitive symptoms. Typically, neurologic deficits are multiple, with remissions and exacerbations gradually producing disability. Diagnosis requires clinical or MRI evidence of ≥ 2 characteristic neurologic lesions that are separated in both time and space (location in the CNS). Treatment includes corticosteroids for acute exacerbations, immunomodulatory drugs to prevent exacerbations, and supportive measures.

MS is believed to involve an immunologic mechanism. One postulated cause is infection by a latent virus (possibly a human herpesvirus such as Epstein-Barr virus), which, when activated, triggers a secondary autoimmune response. An increased incidence among certain families and presence of human leukocyte antigen (HLA) allotypes (HLA-DR2) suggests genetic susceptibility. MS is more common among people who spend their first 15 yr of life in temperate climates (1/2000) than in those who spend them in the tropics (1/10,000). One explanation is that lower levels of vitamin D are associated with an increased risk of MS, and vitamin D levels correlate with the degree of sun exposure, which is lower in temperate climates. Cigarette smoking also appears to increase risk.

Age at onset ranges from 15 to 60 yr, typically 20 to 40 yr; women are affected somewhat more often.

Neuromyelitis optica (Devic disease), previously considered a variant of MS, is now recognized as a separate disorder.

Pathophysiology

Localized areas of demyelination (plaques) occur, with destruction of oligodendroglia, perivascular inflammation, and chemical changes in lipid and protein constituents of myelin in and around the plaques. Axonal damage is possible, but cell bodies tend to be relatively preserved.

Fibrous gliosis develops in plaques that are disseminated throughout the CNS, primarily in white matter, particularly in the lateral and posterior columns (especially in the cervical regions), optic nerves, and periventricular areas. Tracts in the midbrain, pons, and cerebellum are also affected. Gray matter in the cerebrum and spinal cord can be affected but to a much lesser degree.

Symptoms and Signs

MS is characterized by varied CNS deficits, with remissions and recurring exacerbations. Exacerbations average about 1 every 2 yr, but frequency varies greatly.

Although MS may progress and regress unpredictably, there are typical patterns of progression:

- **Relapsing-remitting pattern:** Exacerbations alternate with remissions, when partial or full recovery occurs or symptoms are stable. Remissions may last months or years. Exacerbations can occur spontaneously or can be triggered by an infection such as influenza.
- **Primary progressive pattern:** The disease progresses gradually with no remissions, although there may be temporary plateaus during which the disease does not progress. Unlike in the relapsing-remitting pattern, there are no clear exacerbations.
- **Secondary progressive pattern:** This pattern begins with relapses alternating with remissions (relapsing-remitting pattern), followed by gradual progression of the disease.
- **Progressive relapsing pattern:** The disease progresses gradually, but progression is interrupted by sudden, clear relapses. This pattern is rare.

The most common initial symptoms are the following:

- Paresthesias in one or more extremities, in the trunk, or on one side of the face
- Weakness or clumsiness of a leg or hand
- Visual disturbances (eg, partial loss of vision and pain in one eye due to retrobulbar optic neuritis, diplopia due to internuclear ophthalmoplegia, scotomas)

Other common early symptoms include slight stiffness or unusual fatigability of a limb, minor gait disturbances, difficulty with bladder control, vertigo, and mild affective disturbances; all usually indicate scattered CNS involvement and may be subtle. Fatigue is common. Excess heat (eg, warm weather, a hot bath, fever) may temporarily exacerbate symptoms and signs (Uhthoff phenomenon).

Mild cognitive symptoms are common. Apathy, poor judgment, or inattention may occur. Affective disturbances, including emotional lability, euphoria, or, most commonly, depression, are common. Depression may be reactive or partly due to cerebral lesions of MS. A few patients have seizures.

Cranial nerves: Unilateral or asymmetric optic neuritis and bilateral internuclear ophthalmoplegia are typical. Optic neuritis causes loss of vision (ranging from scotomas to blindness), eye pain during eye movement, and sometimes abnormal visual fields, a swollen optic disk, or a partial or complete afferent pupillary defect.

Internuclear ophthalmoplegia (INO) results if there is a lesion in the medial longitudinal fasciculus connecting the 3rd, 4th, and 6th nerve nuclei. During horizontal gaze, adduction of one eye is decreased, with nystagmus of the other (abducting) eye; convergence is intact. In MS, INO is typically bilateral; unilateral INO is often caused by ischemic stroke.

Rapid, small-amplitude eye oscillations in straight-ahead (primary) gaze (pendular nystagmus) are uncommon but characteristic of MS. Vertigo is common. Intermittent unilateral facial numbness or pain (resembling trigeminal neuralgia), palsy, or spasm may occur. Mild dysarthria may occur, caused by bulbar weakness, cerebellar damage, or disturbance of cortical control. Other cranial nerve deficits are unusual but may occur secondary to brain stem injury.

Motor: Weakness is common. It usually reflects corticospinal tract damage in the spinal cord, affects the lower extremities preferentially, and is bilateral and spastic.

Deep tendon reflexes (eg, knee and ankle jerks) are usually increased, and an extensor plantar response (Babinski sign) and clonus are often present. Spastic paraparesis produces a stiff, imbalanced gait; in advanced cases, it may confine patients to a wheelchair. Painful flexor spasms in response to sensory stimuli (eg, bedclothes) may occur late. Cerebral or cervical spinal cord lesions may result in hemiparesis, which sometimes is the presenting symptom.

Reduced mobility increases the risk of osteoporosis.

Cerebellar: In advanced MS, cerebellar ataxia plus spasticity may be severely disabling; other cerebellar manifestations include slurred speech, scanning speech (slow enunciation with a tendency to hesitate at the beginning of a word or syllable), and Charcot triad (intention tremor, scanning speech, and nystagmus).

Sensory: Paresthesias and partial loss of any type of sensation are common and often localized (eg, to one or both hands or legs).

Various painful sensory disturbances (eg, burning or electric shocklike pains) can occur spontaneously or in response to touch, especially if the spinal cord is affected. An example is Lhermitte sign, an electric shocklike pain that radiates down the spine or into the legs when the neck is flexed.

Objective sensory changes tend to be transient and difficult to demonstrate early in the disease.

Spinal cord: Involvement commonly causes bladder dysfunction (eg, urinary urgency or hesitancy, partial retention of urine, mild urinary incontinence). Constipation, erectile dysfunction in men, and genital anesthesia in women may occur. Frank urinary and fecal incontinence may occur in advanced MS.

Progressive myelopathy, a variant of MS, causes spinal cord motor weakness but no other deficits.

Diagnosis

- Clinical criteria
- Brain and spinal MRI
- Sometimes CSF IgG levels and evoked potentials

MS is suspected in patients with optic neuritis, INO, or other symptoms that suggest MS, particularly if deficits are multifocal or intermittent. If MS is suspected, brain MRI and spinal MRI are done.

MRI is the most sensitive imaging test for MS and can exclude other treatable disorders that may mimic MS, such as nondemyelinating lesions at the junction of the spinal cord and medulla (eg, subarachnoid cyst, foramen magnum tumors). Gadolinium-contrast enhancement can distinguish actively inflamed from older plaques. The sensitivity of MRI is increased by giving twice the dose of contrast agent (which is standard practice) and delaying scanning (double-dose delayed scanning). Also, higher-field MRI magnets (3 to 7 Tesla) can distinguish perivenular MS plaques from nonspecific white-matter lesions.

MS must be distinguished from the following:

- Clinically isolated syndromes (consisting of only a single clinical manifestation typical of MS)
- Radiologically isolated syndrome (MRI findings typical of MS that are incidentally noted in patients with no clinical manifestations)

MS can be distinguished because diagnosis of MS requires evidence of CNS lesions that are separated in both time and space (location in the CNS). For example, any of the following can indicate separation in time:

- A history of exacerbations and remissions
- MRI that shows simultaneous enhancing and nonenhancing lesions, even if patients are asymptomatic
- A new lesion on a subsequent MRI in patients with a previous lesion

Either of the following can indicate separation in space:

- Enhancing MRI lesions in ≥ 2 areas typically affected by MS (eg, the periventricular, juxtacortical, or infratentorial areas or spinal cord)
- Clinical evidence of a lesion at another time, such as a previous or subsequent deficit typical of MS

Additional testing: If MRI plus clinical findings are not diagnostic, additional testing may be necessary to objectively demonstrate separate neurologic abnormalities. Such testing may include evoked potentials and, occasionally, CSF examination or blood tests.

Evoked potentials (delays in electrical responses to sensory stimulation) are often more sensitive for MS than symptoms or signs. Visual evoked responses are sensitive and particularly helpful in patients with no confirmed cranial lesions (eg, those with lesions only in the spinal cord). Somatosensory evoked potentials and brain stem auditory evoked potentials are sometimes also measured.

CSF examination is being done less frequently (because the diagnosis can usually be based on MRI) but can be helpful if MRI plus clinical findings are inconclusive or if infection (eg, CNS Lyme disease) must be ruled out. CSF tests include opening pressure, cell count and differential, protein, glucose, IgG, oligoclonal bands, and usually myelin basic protein and albumin. IgG is usually increased as a percentage of CSF components, such as protein (normally < 11%) or CSF albumin (normally < 27%). IgG levels correlate with disease severity. Oligoclonal IgG bands can usually be detected by electrophoresis of CSF. Myelin basic protein may be elevated during active demyelination. CSF lymphocyte count and protein content may be slightly increased.

Blood tests may be necessary. Sometimes systemic disorders (eg, SLE) and infections (eg, Lyme disease) can mimic MS and should be excluded with specific blood tests. Blood tests to measure an IgG antibody specific for neuromyelitis optica (aquaporin-4 antibody [also known as NMO-IgG]) may be done to differentiate that disorder from MS.

Prognosis

The course is highly varied and unpredictable. In most patients, especially when MS begins with optic neuritis, remissions can last months to > 10 yr.

Most patients who have a clinically isolated syndrome eventually develop MS, with a second lesion becoming evident or MRI detecting a lesion, usually 2 to 4 yr after the initial symptoms begin. Treatment with disease-modifying drugs can delay this progression. If patients have a radiologically isolated syndrome, progression to MS is a risk, but further study of this risk is needed.

If the initial brain or spinal MRI shows more extensive disease, patients may be at risk of earlier disability, as may patients who have motor, bowel, and/or bladder symptoms when they present. Some patients, such as men with onset in middle age and with frequent exacerbations, can become rapidly incapacitated. Cigarette smoking may accelerate disease progression.

Life span is shortened only in very severe cases.

Treatment

- Corticosteroids for acute exacerbations
- Immunomodulators to prevent exacerbations
- Baclofen or tizanidine for spasticity
- Gabapentin or tricyclic antidepressants for pain
- Supportive care

Goals for treatment of MS include the following:

- Shortening acute exacerbations
- Decreasing frequency of exacerbations
- Relieving symptoms
- Maintaining the patient's ability to walk (which is particularly important)

Disease-modifying drugs: Acute exacerbations that cause objective deficits sufficient to impair function (eg, loss of vision, strength, or coordination) are treated with brief courses of corticosteroids (eg, prednisone 60 to 100 mg po once/day tapered over 2 to 3 wk, methylprednisolone 500 to 1000 mg IV once/day for 3 to 5 days). Some evidence indicates that IV corticosteroids shorten acute exacerbations, slow progression, and improve MRI measures of disease.

Immunomodulatory therapy, such as interferons (IFNs) or glatiramer, decreases the frequency of acute exacerbations and delays eventual disability. Typical regimens include the following:

- Interferon beta-1b 8 million IU sc every other day
- Interferon beta-1a 6 million IU (30 mcg) IM weekly
- Interferon beta-1a 44 mcg sc 3 times weekly

Common adverse effects of IFNs include flu-like symptoms and depression (which tend to decrease over time), development of neutralizing antibodies after months of therapy, and cytopenias.

Glatiramer acetate 20 mg sc once/day or 40 mg sc 3 times/wk (given ≥ 48 h apart) may be used. The oral immunomodulatory drugs fingolimod 0.5 mg po once/day, teriflunomide 14 mg po once/day, and dimethyl fumarate 240 mg po bid, have recently become available for the treatment of relapsing forms of MS.

There is no consensus regarding choice of disease-modifying immunomodulatory therapy; many experts recommend patient education and shared decision making. Treatment with disease-modifying drugs is indicated for a clinically isolated syndrome (eg, optic neuritis) as well as for definite MS.

The immunosuppressant mitoxantrone, 12 mg/m^2 IV q 3 mo for 24 mo, may be helpful, particularly for progressive MS that is refractory to other treatments.

Natalizumab, an anti–alpha-4 integrin antibody, inhibits passage of leukocytes across the blood-brain barrier; given as a monthly infusion, it reduces number of exacerbations and new brain lesions but may increase the risk of progressive multifocal leukoencephalopathy.

Recently, alemtuzumab, an anti-CD52 humanized monoclonal antibody given IV, has been shown to be effective in the treatment of MS. However, because it increases risk of autoimmune disorders, serious infusion reactions, and certain cancers, alemtuzumab is usually used only when treatment with ≥ 2 other drugs has been ineffective.

If immunomodulatory drugs are ineffective, monthly IV immune globulin may help.

Immunosuppressants other than mitoxantrone (eg, methotrexate, azathioprine, mycophenolate, cyclophosphamide, cladribine) have been used for more severe, progressive MS but are controversial.

Plasma exchange and hematopoietic stem cell transplantation may be somewhat useful for severe, intractable disease.

Symptom control: Other treatments can be used to control specific symptoms:

- **Spasticity** is treated with escalating doses of baclofen 10 to 20 mg po tid to qid or tizanidine 4 to 8 mg po tid. Gait training and range-of-motion exercises can help weak, spastic limbs.
- **Painful paresthesias** are usually treated with gabapentin 100 to 800 mg po tid or pregabalin 25 to 150 mg po bid; alternatives include tricyclic antidepressants (eg, amitriptyline 25 to 75 mg po at bedtime, desipramine 25 to 100 mg po at bedtime if amitriptyline has intolerable anticholinergic effects), carbamazepine 200 mg po tid, as well as other anticonvulsants, and opioids.
- **Depression** is treated with counseling and antidepressants.
- **Bladder dysfunction** is treated based on its underlying mechanism.
- **Fatigue** can be treated with amantadine 100 mg po tid, modafinil 100 to 300 mg po once/day, armodafinil 150 to 250 mg po once/day, or extended-release amphetamine 10 to 30 mg once/day.

Supportive care: Encouragement and reassurance help.

Regular exercise (eg, stationary biking, treadmill, swimming, stretching, balance exercises), with or without physical therapy, is recommended, even for patients with advanced MS, because exercise conditions the heart and muscles, reduces spasticity, prevents contractures and falls, and has psychologic benefits.

Vitamin D supplements (800 to 1000 units daily) may decrease the risk of disease progression. Serum vitamin D levels should be monitored to make sure that dosing is adequate. Vitamin D also reduces the risk of osteoporosis, particularly in patients at increased risk because mobility is decreased or they take corticosteroids.

Patients should maintain as normal and active a life as possible but should avoid overwork, fatigue, and exposure to excess heat. Cigarette smoking should be stopped.

Vaccination does not appear to increase risk of exacerbations.

Debilitated patients require measures to prevent pressure ulcers and UTIs; intermittent urinary self-catheterization may be necessary.

KEY POINTS

- MS involves demyelination of the CNS; MS may progress unpredictably but has several typical patterns of progression.
- The most common symptoms are paresthesias, weakness or clumsiness, and visual symptoms, but a wide variety of symptoms are possible.
- MS is confirmed if MRI and clinical findings establish characteristic lesions that are separate in time and space; however, progression to MS is likely if patients have even a single characteristic clinical deficit or possibly a single radiologic lesion.
- Treat patients with corticosteroids (for severe exacerbations) and immunomodulatory drugs (to delay or prevent exacerbations).
- Treat patients supportively, using drugs to treat symptoms (eg, spasticity, painful paresthesias, depression, bladder dysfunction, fatigue) when warranted.

NEUROMYELITIS OPTICA

(Devic Disease)

Neuromyelitis optica (NMO) is a demyelinating disorder that affects only the eyes and spinal cord.

NMO causes acute optic neuritis (see p. 248), sometimes bilateral, plus demyelination of the cervical or thoracic spinal cord. It was previously considered to be a variant of MS but is now recognized as a different disorder.

Symptoms include visual loss, muscle spasms, paraparesis or quadriparesis, and incontinence.

Diagnosis

- Brain and spinal cord MRI
- Visual evoked potentials

Diagnosis of NMO usually includes brain and spinal cord MRI and visual evoked potentials.

NMO is distinguished from MS because it affects several contiguous spinal segments of the spinal cord, whereas MS typically affects a single segment. Also unlike in MS, cerebral white matter lesions are uncommon in NMO.

Blood tests to measure an IgG antibody specific for NMO (aquaporin-4 antibody [also known as NMO-IgG]) may be done to differentiate it from MS.

Treatment

- Corticosteroids and immunomodulatory or immunosuppressive treatments

There is no cure. However, treatment can prevent, slow, or decrease the severity of exacerbations.

Methylprednisolone and azathioprine are often used together. Plasma exchange may help people who do not respond to corticosteroids.

Rituximab, an anti–B-cell antibody, reduces IgG production and appears to stabilize the disease.

Treatment of symptoms is similar to that for MS. Baclofen or tizanidine may relieve muscle spasms.

228 Function and Dysfunction of the Cerebral Lobes

The cerebrum is divided by a longitudinal fissure into 2 hemispheres, each containing 5 discrete lobes:

- Frontal
- Parietal
- Temporal
- Occipital
- Insula

The frontal, temporal, parietal, and occipital lobes cover the brain's surface; the insula is hidden under the Sylvian fissure (see Fig. 228–1). Although specific functions are attributed to each lobe, most activities require coordination of multiple areas in both hemispheres. For example, although the occipital lobe is essential to visual processing, parts of the parietal, temporal, and frontal lobes on both sides also process complex visual stimuli.

Function is extensively lateralized. Visual, tactile, and motor activities of the left side of the body are directed predominantly by the right hemisphere and vice versa. Certain complex functions involve both hemispheres but are directed predominantly by one (cerebral dominance). For example, the left hemisphere is typically dominant for language, and the right is dominant for spatial attention.

The cerebral cortex contains

- The primary sensory area
- The primary motor area
- Multiple association areas, including heteromodal association areas

The **primary sensory areas** receive somesthetic, auditory, visual, olfactory, and gustatory stimuli from specialized sensory organs and peripheral receptors. Sensory stimuli are further processed in association areas that relate to one or more senses.

The **primary motor cortex** generates volitional body movements; motor association areas help plan and execute complex motor activity.

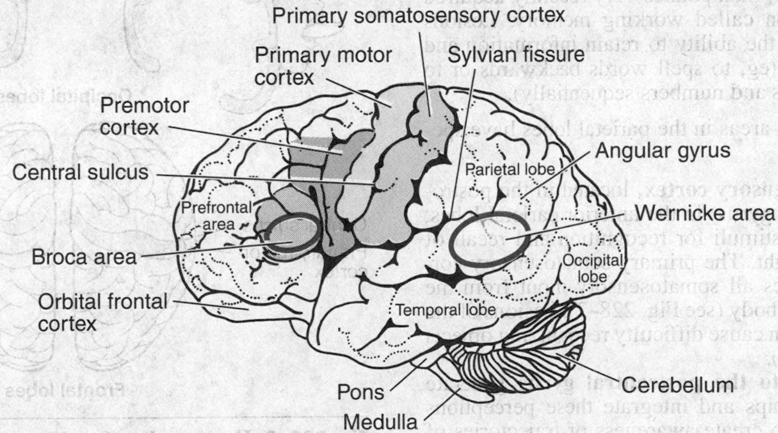

Fig. 228–1. Areas of the brain.

Heteromodal association areas are not restricted to any single motor or sensory function but receive convergent information from multiple sensory and motor areas of the brain. Heteromodal association areas in the frontal, temporal, and parietal lobes integrate sensory data, motor feedback, and other information with instinctual and acquired memories. This integration facilitates learning and creates thought, expression, and behavior.

Frontal lobes: The frontal lobes are anterior to the central sulcus. They are essential for planning and executing learned and purposeful behaviors; they are also the site of many inhibitory functions. There are several functionally distinct areas in the frontal lobes:

- The **primary motor cortex** is the most posterior part of the precentral gyrus. The primary motor cortex on one side controls all moving parts on the contralateral side of the body (shown on a spatial map called a homunculus—see Fig. 228–2); 90% of motor fibers from each hemisphere cross the midline in the brain stem. Thus, damage to the motor cortex of one hemisphere causes weakness or paralysis mainly on the contralateral side of the body.
- The **medial frontal cortex** (sometimes called the medial prefrontal area) is important in arousal and motivation. If lesions in this area are large and extend to the most anterior part of the cortex (frontal pole), patients sometimes become abulic (apathetic, inattentive, and markedly slow to respond).
- The **orbital frontal cortex** (sometimes called the orbital prefrontal area—see Fig. 228–1) helps modulate social behaviors. Patients with orbital frontal lesions can become emotionally labile, indifferent to the implications of their actions, or both. They may be alternately euphoric, facetious, vulgar, and indifferent to social nuances. Bilateral acute trauma to this area may make patients boisterously talkative, restless, and socially intrusive. The disinhibition and abnormal behaviors that can occur with aging and in many types of dementia probably result from degeneration of the frontal lobe, particularly the orbital frontal cortex.
- The **left posteroinferior frontal cortex** (sometimes called the Broca area or posteroinferior prefrontal area—see Fig. 228–1) controls expressive language function. Lesions in this area cause expressive aphasia (impaired expression of words).
- The **dorsolateral frontal cortex** (sometimes called the dorsolateral prefrontal area) manipulates very recently acquired information—a function called working memory. Lesions in this area can impair the ability to retain information and process it in real time (eg, to spell words backwards or to alternate between letters and numbers sequentially).

Parietal lobes: Several areas in the parietal lobes have specific functions.

- The **primary somatosensory cortex,** located in the postrolandic area (postcentral gyrus) in the anterior parietal lobes, integrates somesthetic stimuli for recognition and recall of form, texture, and weight. The primary somatosensory cortex on one side receives all somatosensory input from the contralateral side of the body (see Fig. 228–2). Lesions of the anterior parietal lobe can cause difficulty recognizing objects by touch (astereognosis).
- **Areas posterolateral to the postcentral gyrus** generate visual-spatial relationships and integrate these perceptions with other sensations to create awareness of trajectories of moving objects. These areas also mediate proprioception (awareness of the position of body parts in space).
- **Parts of the midparietal lobe of the dominant hemisphere** are involved in abilities such as calculation, writing, left-right orientation, and finger recognition. Lesions in the angular gyrus can cause deficits in writing, calculating, left-right disorientation, and finger-naming (Gerstmann syndrome).
- The **nondominant parietal lobe** integrates the contralateral side of the body with its environment, enabling people to be aware of this environmental space, and is important for abilities such as drawing. Acute injury to the nondominant parietal lobe may cause neglect of the contralateral side (usually the left), resulting in decreased awareness of that part of the body, its environment, and any associated injury to that side (anosognosia). For example, patients with large right parietal lesions may deny the existence of left-sided paralysis. Patients with smaller lesions may lose the ability to do learned motor tasks (eg, dressing, other well-learned activities)—a spatial-manual deficit called apraxia.

Temporal lobes: The temporal lobes are integral to auditory perception, receptive components of language, visual memory, declarative (factual) memory, and emotion. Patients with right temporal lobe lesions commonly lose the ability to interpret nonverbal auditory stimuli (eg, music). Left temporal lobe lesions interfere greatly with the recognition, memory, and formation of language.

Patients with epileptogenic foci in the medial limbic-emotional parts of the temporal lobe commonly have complex partial seizures, characterized by uncontrollable feelings and autonomic, cognitive, or emotional dysfunction. Occasionally, such patients have personality changes, characterized by humorlessness, philosophic religiosity, and obsessiveness. Patients may have olfactory hallucinations and hypergraphia (an overwhelming urge to write).

Occipital lobes: The occipital lobes contain

- The primary visual cortex
- Visual association areas

Lesions in the primary visual cortex lead to a form of central blindness called Anton syndrome; patients become unable to

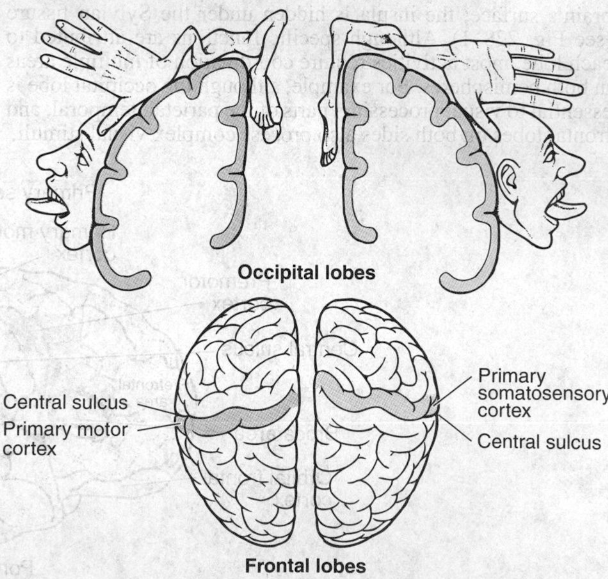

Fig. 228–2. Homunculus. Specific parts of the cortex control specific motor and sensory functions on the contralateral side of the body. The amount of cortical space given to a body part varies; eg, the area of the cortex that controls the hand is larger than the area that controls the shoulder. The map of these parts is called the homunculus ("little person").

recognize objects by sight and are generally unaware of their deficits, often confabulating descriptions of what they see.

Seizures involving the occipital lobe can cause visual hallucinations, often consisting of lines or meshes of color superimposed on the contralateral visual field.

Insula: The insula integrates sensory and autonomic information from the viscera. It plays a role in certain language functions, as evidenced by aphasia in patients with some insular lesions. The insula processes aspects of pain and temperature sensation and possibly taste.

Pathophysiology

Cerebral dysfunction may be focal or global. Focal and global processes may also affect subcortical systems, altering arousal (eg, causing stupor or coma) or integration of thought (eg, causing delirium).

Focal dysfunction usually results from structural abnormalities (eg, tumors, stroke, trauma, malformations, gliosis, demyelination). Manifestations depend on the lesion's location, size, and development rate. Lesions that are < 2 cm in diameter or that develop very slowly may be asymptomatic. Larger lesions, rapidly developing lesions (over weeks or months rather than years), and lesions that simultaneously affect both hemispheres are more likely to become symptomatic. Focal lesions in white matter can interrupt the connectivity between brain areas and cause the disconnection syndrome (inability to do a task that requires coordinated activity of ≥ 2 brain regions, despite retention of basic functions of each region).

Global dysfunction is caused by toxic-metabolic disorders or sometimes by diffuse inflammation, vasculopathy, major trauma, or disseminated cancer; these disorders affect multiple dimensions of cerebral function.

Recovery: Recovery from brain injury depends in part on the following characteristics of the brain:

- Plasticity of the remaining cerebrum
- Redundancy

Plasticity (ability of an area of the brain to alter its function) of the cerebrum varies from person to person and is affected by age and general health. Plasticity is most prominent in the developing brain. For example, if the dominant hemisphere language areas are severely damaged before age 8 yr, the opposite hemisphere can often assume near-normal language function. Although capacity for recovery from brain injury is considerable after the first decade of life, severe damage more often results in permanent deficits. Gross reorganization of brain function after injury in adults is uncommon, although plasticity remains operative in certain specific areas of the brain throughout life.

Redundancy refers to the ability of more than one area of the brain to perform the same function.

Cerebral dysfunction syndromes: Specific syndromes include

- Agnosia
- Amnesia (including transient global amnesia)
- Aphasia
- Apraxia

Psychiatric conditions (eg, depression, psychosis, anxiety disorders) sometimes include similar elements. Dysarthria, a neuromotor disorder, may cause symptoms similar to those of aphasia.

Diagnosis

- Clinical evaluation
- Often neuropsychologic testing

In general, diagnosis of cerebral dysfunction is clinical, often assisted by neuropsychologic testing.

Diagnosis of the cause usually requires laboratory tests (blood and sometimes CSF analysis) and brain imaging, either structural (CT, MRI) or functional (PET, single-photon emission CT).

AGNOSIA

Agnosia is inability to identify an object using one or more of the senses. Diagnosis is clinical, often including neuropsychologic testing, with brain imaging (eg, CT, MRI) to identify the cause. Prognosis depends on the nature and extent of damage and patient age. There is no specific treatment, but speech and occupational therapy may help patients compensate.

Agnosias are uncommon. They result from damage to (eg, by infarct, tumor, abscess, or trauma) or degeneration of areas of the brain that integrate perception, memory, and identification (eg, Alzheimer disease, Parkinson disease dementia).

Types

Discrete brain lesions can cause different forms of agnosia, which may involve any sense. Typically, only one sense is affected. Examples are hearing (auditory agnosia—the inability to identify objects through sound such as a ringing telephone), taste (gustatory agnosia), smell (olfactory agnosia), touch (tactile agnosia), and sight (visual agnosia).

Other forms of agnosia involve very specific and complex processes within one sense.

Prosopagnosia is inability to identify well-known faces, including those of close friends, or to otherwise distinguish individual objects among a class of objects, despite the ability to identify generic facial features and objects.

Anosognosia often accompanies damage to the right, nondominant parietal lobe (which is usually due to an acute stroke or traumatic brain injury). Patients with multiple impairments can be unaware of one impairment but fully aware of others. Patients with anosognosia may deny their motor deficit, insisting that nothing is wrong even when one side of their body is completely paralyzed. When shown the paralyzed body part, patients may deny that it is theirs.

In an often related phenomenon, patients ignore the paralyzed or desensitized body parts (hemi-inattention) or the space around them (hemineglect). Hemineglect most often involves the left side of the body.

Lesions in the parietal lobe can also cause somatosensory agnosia. Patients with somatosensory agnosia have difficulty identifying a familiar object (eg, key, safety pin) that is placed in the hand on the side of the body opposite the damage. However, when they look at the object, they immediately recognize and can identify it.

Occipitotemporal lesions may cause

- An inability to recognize familiar places (environmental agnosia)
- Visual disturbances (visual agnosia)
- Color blindness (achromatopsia)

Right-sided temporal lesions may cause

- An inability to interpret sounds (auditory agnosia)
- Impairment of music perception (amusia)

Diagnosis

- Bedside and neuropsychologic testing
- Brain imaging

At bedside, patients are asked to identify common objects through sight, touch, or another sense. If hemineglect is suspected, patients are asked to identify the paralyzed parts of their body or objects in their hemivisual fields.

Physical examination is done to detect primary deficits in individual senses or in the ability to communicate that may interfere with testing for agnosias. For example, if light touch is defective, patients may not sense an object even when cortical function is intact. Also, aphasias may interfere with patient's expression. Neuropsychologic testing may help identify more subtle agnosias.

Brain imaging (eg, CT or MRI with or without angiographic protocols) is required to characterize a central lesion (eg, infarct, hemorrhage, mass) and to check for atrophy suggesting a degenerative disorder.

Prognosis

Recovery from agnosia may be influenced by the

- Type, size, and location of lesions
- Degree of impairment
- Patient age
- Effectiveness of therapy

Most recovery occurs within the first 3 mo but may continue to a variable degree up to a year.

Treatment

- Treatment of the cause
- Speech or occupational therapy

When possible, the cause of agnosia is treated (eg, surgery and/or antibiotics for cerebral abscess, surgery and/or radiation for brain tumor).

Rehabilitation with speech or occupational therapists can help patients learn to compensate for their deficits.

KEY POINTS

- Agnosias are uncommon but may affect any sense.
- Diagnose agnosias by asking patients to identify objects or, for subtle agnosias, by doing neuropsychologic tests.
- Do brain imaging to characterize the causative lesion.
- Recommend rehabilitation with speech or occupational therapy to help patients compensate for deficits.

AMNESIAS

Amnesia is partial or total inability to recall past experiences. It may result from traumatic brain injury, degeneration, metabolic disorders, seizures, or psychologic disturbances. Diagnosis is clinical but often includes neuropsychologic testing and brain imaging (eg, CT, MRI). Treatment is directed at the cause.

Processing of memories involves the following:

- Registration (taking in new information)
- Encoding (forming associations, time stamps, and other processes necessary for retrieval)
- Retrieval

Deficits in any of these steps can cause amnesia. Amnesia, by definition, results from impairment of memory functions, not impairment of other functions (eg, attention, motivation, reasoning, language), which may cause similar symptoms.

Amnesia can be classified as follows:

- **Retrograde:** Amnesia for events *before* the causative event
- **Anterograde:** Inability to store new memories *after* the causative event
- **Sense-specific:** Amnesia for events processed by one sense—eg, an agnosia

Amnesia may be

- Transient (as occurs after brain trauma)
- Fixed (as occurs after a serious event such as encephalitis, global ischemia, or cardiac arrest)
- Progressive (as occurs with degenerative dementias, such as Alzheimer disease)

Memory deficits more commonly involve facts (declarative memory) and, less commonly, skills (procedural memory).

Etiology

Amnesia can result from diffuse cerebral impairment, bilateral lesions, or multifocal injuries that impair memory-storage areas in the cerebral hemispheres.

Predominant pathways for declarative memory are located along the medial parahippocampal region and hippocampus as well as in the inferomedial temporal lobes, orbital surface of the frontal lobes (basal forebrain), and diencephalon (which contains the thalamus and hypothalamus). Of these structures, the following are critical:

- Hippocampal gyri
- Hypothalamus
- Nuclei of the basal forebrain
- Dorsomedial thalamic nuclei

The amygdaloid nucleus contributes emotional amplifications to memory. The thalamic intralaminar nuclei and brain stem reticular formation stimulate the imprinting of memories. Bilateral damage to the mediodorsal nuclei of the thalamus severely impairs recent memory and the ability to form new memories.

Amnesia may be caused by

- Thiamin deficiency (by causing Wernicke encephalopathy or Korsakoff psychosis) in patients with chronic alcohol abuse or severe undernutrition
- Traumatic brain injury
- Seizures
- Global brain anoxia or ischemia
- Encephalitis
- Embolic occlusion at the top of the basilar artery (top of the basilar artery embolism)
- Degenerative dementias such as Alzheimer disease
- Various drug intoxications (eg, chronic solvent sniffing, amphotericin B or lithium toxicity)
- Hypothalamic tumors
- Psychologic trauma or stress

Posttraumatic amnesias for the periods immediately before and after concussion or moderate or severe head trauma seem to result from medial temporal lobe injury. Moderate or severe trauma may affect larger areas of memory storage and recall, as can many diffuse cerebral disorders that cause dementia.

Psychologic disturbances of memory (as occurs in dissociative amnesia—see p. 1750) result from extreme psychologic trauma or stress.

Benign senescent forgetfulness (age-associated memory impairment) refers to the memory loss that occurs with normal aging. People with benign senescent forgetfulness gradually develop noticeable problems with memory, often first for names, then for events, and occasionally for spatial relationships.

Benign senescent forgetfulness has no proven relationship to dementia, although some similarities are hard to overlook.

Amnestic mild cognitive impairment (amnestic MCI) may be present in people who have a subjective memory problem, who do worse on objective memory tests, but who otherwise have intact cognition and daily function. People with amnestic MCI are more likely to develop Alzheimer disease than age-matched people without memory problems.

Diagnosis

- Bedside testing

Simple bedside tests (eg, 3-item recall, location of objects previously hidden in the room) and formal tests (eg, word list learning tests such as the California Verbal Learning Test and the Buschke Selective Reminding Test) can help identify verbal memory loss. Assessment of nonverbal memory is more difficult but may include recall of visual designs or a series of tones.

Clinical findings usually suggest causes and any necessary tests.

Treatment

- Treatment directed at the cause

Any underlying disorder or psychologic cause must be treated. However, some patients with acute amnesia improve spontaneously. Certain disorders that cause amnesia (eg, Alzheimer disease, Korsakoff psychosis, herpes encephalitis) can be treated; however, treatment of the underlying disorder may or may not lessen the amnesia.

Cholinergic drugs (eg, donepezil) may improve memory slightly and temporarily in patients with Alzheimer disease; these drugs are often also tried when another dementia is the cause. Otherwise, no specific measures can hasten recovery or improve the outcome.

KEY POINTS

- Amnesias have various causes, including traumatic brain injury, degenerative dementias, metabolic disorders, seizures, and psychologic trauma or stress.
- Diagnose amnesia clinically using bedside tests (eg, 3-item recall) or formal tests (eg, word list learning tests).
- Treat the cause of amnesia.

TRANSIENT GLOBAL AMNESIA

Transient global amnesia is anterograde and usually retrograde amnesia that begins suddenly and lasts up to 24 h. Diagnosis is primarily clinical but includes laboratory tests and CT, MRI, or both to evaluate central circulation. The amnesia typically remits spontaneously but may recur. There is no specific treatment, but underlying abnormalities are corrected.

Most (75%) cases of transient global amnesia occur in people aged 50 to 70; this disorder rarely occurs in patients < 40.

Etiology

The etiology of transient global amnesia is not clear. Suggested mechanisms include those related to migraine, hypoxia and/or ischemia, venous flow abnormalities, or seizures, as well as psychologic factors.

Recent data suggest that vulnerability of CA1 neurons to metabolic stress is pivotal; the resulting damage triggers a cascade of changes that lead to impaired hippocampal function.

A distinct benign form of transient global amnesia can follow excessive alcohol ingestion, moderately large sedative doses of barbiturates, use of several illicit drugs, or sometimes relatively small doses of benzodiazepines (especially midazolam and triazolam).

Events that can trigger transient global amnesia include

- Sudden immersion in cold or hot water
- Physical exertion
- Emotional or psychologic stress
- Pain
- Medical procedures
- Sexual intercourse
- A Valsalva maneuver

Symptoms and Signs

Patients often present after a triggering event.

The classic presentation in transient global amnesia is

- Abrupt onset of severe anterograde amnesia

But a less severe retrograde amnesia may be the presenting symptom. Episodes usually last for 1 to 8 h but may last from 30 min to 24 h (rarely). Patients are often disoriented to time and place but usually not to personal identity. Many patients are anxious or agitated and may repeatedly ask questions about transpiring events. Language function, attention, visual-spatial skills, and social skills are retained. Impairments gradually resolve as the episode subsides.

The **benign transient amnesia after substance ingestion** is distinct because it

- Is selectively retrograde (ie, for events during and preceding intoxication)
- Relates specifically to drug-accompanied events
- Does not cause confusion (once acute intoxication resolves)
- Recurs only if similar amounts of the same drug are ingested

Diagnosis

- Primarily clinical evaluation
- Brain imaging

Diagnosis of transient global amnesia is primarily clinical. Neurologic examination typically does not detect any abnormalities other than disturbed memory. Brain ischemia must be ruled out (see p. 2038).

Laboratory tests should include CBC, coagulation tests, and evaluation for hypercoagulable states.

Brain CT, brain MRI, or both are usually done. High-resolution diffusion-weighted MRI should be done to rule out brain ischemia if it is suspected; MRI may show focal hyperintense lesions correlating with restricted diffusion in the lateral hippocampus. During the first 24 h after symptom onset, MRI detects hippocampal lesions in only 12% of patients. Detection increases to 81% if MRI is done 3 days later and uses thinner 3-mm sections and higher b-values. Why lesions are more visible 3 days later is unknown.

EEG usually shows nonspecific abnormalities and is unnecessary unless a seizure is suspected or episodes recur.

Prognosis

Prognosis is good. Symptoms typically last < 24 h. As the disorder resolves, the amnesia lessens, but memory for events during the episode may be lost.

Usually, episodes do not recur, unless the cause is seizures or migraines. Overall lifetime recurrence rate is about 5 to 25%.

Risk of stroke is not increased.

Treatment

- Treatment of the cause if possible

No specific treatment is indicated for transient global amnesia. However, any underlying condition should be treated.

KEY POINTS

- Transient global amnesia usually affects patients aged 50 to 70.
- Do high-resolution diffusion-weighted brain MRI to exclude brain ischemia as a cause.
- Although memories that were lost may not be recovered, memory function tends to resolve within 24 h, and episodes usually do not recur.

APHASIA

Aphasia is language dysfunction that may involve impaired comprehension or expression of words or nonverbal equivalents of words. It results from dysfunction of the language centers in the cerebral cortex and basal ganglia or of the white matter pathways that connect them. Diagnosis is clinical, often including neuropsychologic testing, with brain imaging (CT, MRI) to identify cause. Prognosis depends on the cause and extent of damage and on patient age. There is no specific treatment, but speech therapy may promote recovery.

In right-handed people and about two-thirds of left-handed people, language function resides in the left hemisphere. In the other third of left-handed people, much of language function resides in the right hemisphere. Cortical areas responsible for language function include

- Posterosuperior temporal lobe (which contains the Wernicke area)
- Adjacent inferior parietal lobe
- Posteroinferior part of the frontal lobe just anterior to the motor cortex (Broca area)
- Subcortical connection between those regions

Damage to any part of this roughly triangular area (eg, by infarct, tumor, trauma, or degeneration) interferes with some aspect of language function.

Prosody (quality of rhythm and emphasis that adds meaning to speech) is usually influenced by both hemispheres but is sometimes affected by dysfunction of the nondominant hemisphere alone.

Aphasia is distinct from developmental disorders of language and from dysfunction of the motor pathways and muscles that produce speech (dysarthria).

Etiology

Aphasia usually results from disorders that do not cause progressive damage (eg, stroke, head trauma, encephalitis); in such cases, aphasia does not worsen. It sometimes results from a progressive disorder (eg, enlarging brain tumor, dementia); in such cases, aphasia progressively worsens.

Types

Aphasia is broadly divided into receptive and expressive aphasia.

- **Receptive (sensory, fluent, or Wernicke) aphasia:** Patients cannot comprehend words or recognize auditory, visual, or tactile symbols. It is caused by a disorder of the posterosuperior temporal gyrus of the language-dominant hemisphere (Wernicke area). Often, alexia (loss of the ability to read words) is also present.
- **Expressive (motor, nonfluent, or Broca) aphasia:** The ability to produce words is impaired, but comprehension and ability to conceptualize are relatively preserved. It is due to a disorder that affects the dominant left frontal or frontoparietal area, including the Broca area. It often causes agraphia (loss of the ability to write) and impairs oral reading.

There are other types of aphasia (see Table 228–1), which may overlap considerably. No aphasia classification system is ideal. Describing the types of deficits is often the most precise way to describe a particular aphasia.

Symptoms and Signs

Wernicke aphasia: Patients speak normal words fluently, often including meaningless phonemes, but do not know their meaning or relationships. The result is a jumble of words or "word salad." Patients are typically unaware that their speech is incomprehensible to others.

A right visual field cut commonly accompanies Wernicke aphasia because the visual pathway is near the affected area.

Broca aphasia: Patients can comprehend and conceptualize relatively well, but their ability to form words is impaired. Usually, the impairment affects speech production and writing (agraphia, dysgraphia), greatly frustrating patients' attempts to communicate. However, spoken and written communication makes sense to the patient.

Broca aphasia may include anomia (inability to name objects) and impaired prosody.

Diagnosis

- Exclusion of other communication problems
- Bedside and neuropsychologic testing
- Brain imaging

Verbal interaction can typically identify gross aphasias. However, the clinician should try to differentiate aphasias from communication problems that stem from severe dysarthria or from impaired hearing, vision (eg, when assessing reading), or motor writing ability.

Initially, Wernicke aphasia may be mistaken for delirium. However, Wernicke aphasia is a pure language disturbance without other features of delirium (eg, fluctuating level of consciousness, hallucinations, inattention).

Bedside testing to identify specific deficits should include assessment of the following:

- **Spontaneous speech:** Speech is assessed for fluency, number of words spoken, ability to initiate speech, presence of spontaneous errors, word-finding pauses, hesitations, and prosody.
- **Naming:** Patients are asked to name objects. Those who have difficulty naming often use circumlocutions (eg, "what you use to tell time" for "clock").
- **Repetition:** Patients are asked to repeat grammatically complex phrases (eg, "no ifs, ands, or buts").

Table 228–1. TYPES OF APHASIA

TYPE	LOCATION OF CAUSATIVE LESION*	COMMON CAUSES	SPEECH PATTERN
Anomic	Lesion (usually small) anywhere in the left-hemisphere language areas	Various disorders	Anomia in oral language (leading to empty, circumlocutory, paraphasic speech) and in written language, fluent speech, good auditory and reading comprehension, normal repetition
Broca (nonfluent, expressive, motor)	Large lesion in the left frontal or frontoparietal area, including the Broca area	Infarction Hemorrhage Trauma Tumor	Anomia in oral and written language, nonfluent speech (with slow, effortful production, short phrase length, impaired prosody, and reduced use of prepositions and conjunctions), good comprehension, impaired repetition, impaired writing (agraphia)
Wernicke (fluent, receptive, sensory)	Large lesion in the left temporoparietal area, including the Wernicke area	Infarction Tumor	Anomia in oral and written language, fluent speech (with paraphasias, a variety of grammatical forms, but often conveying little meaning), poor auditory and written comprehension, impaired repetition, errors in reading (alexia), agraphia
Conduction	Subcortical lesion in the left hemisphere, often under the superior temporal gyrus or under the inferior parietal lobe	Infarction Hemorrhage Tumor	Anomia (with prominent paraphasias), otherwise fluent speech, good comprehension, impaired repetition (with frequent paraphasias), good reading comprehension Writing unaffected
Global	Large lesion in the left frontotemporoparietal area, including the Broca and Wernicke areas	Infarction Hemorrhage Trauma Tumor	Severe anomia in oral and written language, nonfluent speech (often with sparse output), poor comprehension, impaired repetition, alexia, agraphia
Transcortical motor	Lesion in the left frontal area, excluding the Broca and Wernicke areas	Infarction Encephalitis Hemorrhage Trauma Tumor	Similar to Broca aphasia except with normal repetition Articulation often unaffected
Transcortical sensory	Lesion in the temporoparietal area, excluding the Broca and Wernicke areas	Infarction Encephalitis Hemorrhage Trauma Tumor	Similar to Wernicke aphasia, except with normal repetition

*Causative lesion is in the language-dominant (usually left) hemisphere.

- **Comprehension:** Patients are asked to point to objects named by the clinician, carry out one-step and multistep commands, and answer simple and complex yes-or-no questions.
- **Reading and writing:** Patients are asked to write spontaneously and to read aloud. Reading comprehension, spelling, and writing in response to dictation are assessed.

Formal cognitive testing by a neuropsychologist or speech and language therapist may detect finer levels of dysfunction and assist in planning treatment and assessing potential for recovery. Various formal tests for diagnosing aphasia (eg, Boston Diagnostic Aphasia Examination, Western Aphasia Battery, Boston Naming Test, Token Test, Action Naming Test) are available.

Brain imaging (eg, CT, MRI; with or without angiographic protocols) is required to characterize the lesion (eg, infarct, hemorrhage, mass). Further tests are done to determine the etiology of the lesion (eg, stroke evaluation) as indicated.

Prognosis

Recovery is influenced by the following:

- Cause
- Size and location of lesions
- Extent of language impairment
- Response to therapy
- To a lesser degree, the age, education, and general health of the patient

Children < 8 yr often regain language function after severe damage to either hemisphere. After that age, most recovery occurs within the first 3 mo, but improvement continues to a variable degree up to a year.

Treatment

- Treatment of cause
- Speech therapy
- Augmentative communication devices

Treatment of certain lesions can be very effective (eg, corticosteroids if a mass lesion causes vasogenic edema). The effectiveness of treating aphasia itself is unclear, but most clinicians think that treatment by qualified speech therapists helps and that patients treated soon after onset improve the most.

Patients who cannot recover basic language skills and caregivers of such patients are sometimes able to convey messages with augmentative communication devices (eg, a book or communication board that contains pictures or symbols of a patient's daily needs, computer-based devices).

KEY POINTS

- Language function resides in the left hemisphere in right-handed people and in two thirds of left-handed people.
- Describe a particular aphasia by describing the types of deficits because types of aphasia overlap and no classification system is ideal.
- Evaluate the patient's ability to name, repeat, comprehend, read, and write at the bedside, do brain imaging, and consider neuropsychologic testing.
- Treat the cause when possible, and recommend speech therapy.

APRAXIA

Apraxia is inability to execute purposeful, previously learned motor tasks, despite physical ability and willingness, as a result of brain damage. Diagnosis is clinical, often including neuropsychologic testing, with brain imaging (eg, CT, MRI) to identify cause. Prognosis depends on the cause and extent of damage and patient age. There is no specific treatment, but physical and occupational therapy may modestly improve functioning and patient safety.

Apraxia results from brain damage (eg, by infarct, tumor, or trauma) or degeneration, usually in the parietal lobes or their connections, which retain memories of learned movement patterns. Less commonly, apraxia results from damage to other areas of the brain, such as the premotor cortex (the part of the frontal lobe anterior to the motor cortex), other parts of the frontal lobe, or the corpus callosum, or from diffuse damage related to degenerative dementias.

Symptoms and Signs

Patients cannot conceptualize or do learned complex motor tasks despite having intact motor, sensory, and coordination systems and being able to do the individual component movements. For example, patients with constructional apraxia may be unable to copy a simple geometric shape despite being able to see and recognize the stimulus, hold and use a pen, and understand the task. Typically, patients do not recognize their deficits.

Diagnosis

- Bedside and neuropsychologic testing
- Brain imaging

Bedside tests include asking patients to do or imitate common learned tasks (eg, saluting, stopping or starting to walk, combing hair, striking and blowing out a match, opening a lock with a key, using a screwdriver or scissors, taking a deep breath and holding it). Strength and range of motion must be assessed to exclude motor weakness and musculoskeletal abnormalities as the cause of symptoms.

Neuropsychologic testing or assessment by a physical or occupational therapist may help identify more subtle apraxias.

Caregivers should be asked about the patient's ability to do activities of daily living, especially those that involve household tools (eg, correct and safe use of eating utensils, toothbrush, kitchen utensils to prepare a meal, hammer, and scissors) and writing.

Brain imaging (eg, CT, MRI; with or without angiographic protocols) is required to diagnose and characterize central lesions (eg, infarct, hemorrhage, mass, focal atrophy).

Prognosis

In general, patients become dependent, requiring help with activities of daily living and at least some degree of supervision. Patients with stroke may have a stable course and even improve somewhat.

Treatment

- Physical and occupational therapy

There is no specific medical treatment. Drugs that slow the symptomatic progression of dementia do not appear beneficial.

Physical and occupational therapy may modestly improve functioning but is more often useful for making the environment safer and for providing devices that help patients circumvent the primary deficit.

KEY POINTS

- Affected patients cannot conceptualize or do learned complex motors tasks despite being able to do the individual component movements.
- Ask patients to do common tasks at the bedside, recommend neuropsychologic testing, and do brain imaging.
- Consider recommending supportive physical and occupational therapy.

229 Headache

APPROACH TO THE PATIENT WITH HEADACHE

Headache is pain in any part of the head, including the scalp, face (including the orbitotemporal area), and interior of the head. Headache is one of the most common reasons patients seek medical attention.

Pathophysiology

Headache is due to activation of pain-sensitive structures in or around the brain, skull, face, sinuses, or teeth.

Etiology

Headache may occur as a primary disorder or be secondary to another disorder.

Primary headache disorders include the following:

- Migraine
- Cluster headache (including chronic paroxysmal hemicrania, hemicrania continua, and short-lasting unilateral

neuralgiform headache with conjunctival injection and tearing—sometimes collectively called trigeminal autonomic cephalalgias)
- Tension-type headache

Secondary headache has numerous causes (see Table 229–1). Overall, the **most common causes of headache** are

- Tension-type headache
- Migraine

Some causes of headache are common; others are important to recognize because they are dangerous, require specific treatment, or both (see Table 229–2).

Evaluation

Evaluation of headache focuses on

- Determining whether a secondary headache is present
- Checking for symptoms that suggest a serious cause

If no cause or serious symptoms are identified, evaluation focuses on diagnosing primary headache disorders.

History: History of present illness includes questions about headache location, duration, severity, onset (eg, sudden, gradual), and quality (eg, throbbing, constant, intermittent, pressure-like). Exacerbating and remitting factors (eg, head position, time of day, sleep, light, sounds, physical activity, odors, chewing) are noted. If the patient has had previous or recurrent headaches, the previous diagnosis (if any) needs to be identified, and whether the current headache is similar or different needs to be determined. For recurrent headaches, age at onset, frequency of episodes, temporal pattern (including any relationship to phase of menstrual cycle), and response to treatments (including OTC treatments) are noted.

Review of systems should seek symptoms suggesting a cause, including

- Vomiting: Migraine or increased intracranial pressure
- Fever: Infection (eg, encephalitis, meningitis, sinusitis)
- Red eye and/or visual symptoms (halos, blurring): Acute angle-closure glaucoma
- Visual field deficits, diplopia, or blurring vision: Ocular migraine, brain mass lesion, or idiopathic intracranial hypertension
- Lacrimation and facial flushing: Cluster headache
- Rhinorrhea: Sinusitis
- Pulsatile tinnitus: Idiopathic intracranial hypertension
- Preceding aura: Migraine
- Focal neurologic deficit: Encephalitis, meningitis, intracerebral hemorrhage, subdural hematoma, tumor, or other mass lesion
- Seizures: Encephalitis, tumor, or other mass lesion
- Syncope at headache onset: Subarachnoid hemorrhage
- Myalgias and/or vision changes (in people > 55 yr): Giant cell arteritis

Past medical history should identify risk factors for headache, including exposure to drugs, substances (particularly caffeine), and toxins (see Table 229–1); recent lumbar puncture (LP); immunosuppressive disorders or IV drug use (risk of infection); hypertension (risk of brain hemorrhage); cancer (risk of brain metastases); and dementia, trauma, coagulopathy, or use of anticoagulants or ethanol (risk of subdural hematoma).

Family and social history should include any family history of headaches, particularly because migraine headache may be undiagnosed in family members.

To streamline data collection, clinicians can ask patients to fill out a headache questionnaire that covers most of the relevant medical history pertinent to diagnosis of headache. Patients may complete the questionnaire before their visit and bring the results with them.

Physical examination: Vital signs, including temperature, are measured. General appearance (eg, whether restless or calm in a dark room) is noted. A general examination, with a focus on the head and neck, and a full neurologic examination are done.

The scalp is examined for areas of swelling and tenderness. The ipsilateral temporal artery is palpated, and both temporomandibular joints are palpated for tenderness and crepitance while the patient opens and closes the jaw.

The eyes and periorbital area are inspected for lacrimation, flushing, and conjunctival injection. Pupillary size and light responses, extraocular movements, and visual fields are assessed. The fundi are checked for spontaneous venous pulsations and papilledema. If patients have vision-related symptoms or eye abnormalities, visual acuity is measured. If the conjunctiva is red, the anterior chamber and cornea are examined with a slit lamp if possible, and intraocular pressure is measured.

The nares are inspected for purulence. The oropharynx is inspected for swellings, and the teeth are percussed for tenderness.

Neck is flexed to detect discomfort, stiffness, or both, indicating meningismus. The cervical spine is palpated for tenderness.

Table 229–1. DISORDERS CAUSING SECONDARY HEADACHE

CAUSE	EXAMPLES
Extracranial disorders	Carotid or vertebral artery dissection (which also causes neck pain)
	Dental disorders (eg, infection, temporomandibular joint dysfunction)
	Glaucoma
	Sinusitis
Intracranial disorders	Brain tumors and other masses
	Chiari type I malformation
	CSF leak with low-pressure headache
	Hemorrhage (intracerebral, subdural, subarachnoid)
	Idiopathic intracranial hypertension
	Infections (eg, abscess, encephalitis, meningitis, subdural empyema)
	Meningitis, noninfectious (eg, carcinomatous, chemical)
	Obstructive hydrocephalus
	Vascular disorders (eg, vascular malformations, vasculitis, venous sinus thrombosis)
Systemic disorders	Acute severe hypertension
	Bacteremia
	Fever
	Giant cell arteritis
	Hypercapnia
	Hypoxia (including altitude sickness)
	Viral infections
	Viremia
Drugs and toxins	Analgesic overuse
	Caffeine withdrawal
	Carbon monoxide
	Hormones (eg, estrogen)
	Nitrates
	Proton pump inhibitors

Table 229–2. SOME CHARACTERISTICS OF HEADACHE DISORDERS BY CAUSE

CAUSE	SUGGESTIVE FINDINGS	DIAGNOSTIC APPROACH
Primary headache disorders*		
Cluster headache	Unilateral orbitotemporal attacks, often at the same time of day Deep, severe, lasting 30–180 min Often with lacrimation, facial flushing, or Horner syndrome; restlessness	Clinical evaluation
Migraine headache	Frequently unilateral and pulsating, lasting 4–72 h Occasionally with aura Usually nausea, photophobia, sonophobia, or osmophobia Worse with activity, preference to lie in the dark, resolution with sleep	Clinical evaluation
Tension-type headache	Frequent or continuous, mild, bilateral, and viselike occipital or frontal pain that spreads to entire head Worse at end of day	Clinical evaluation
Secondary headache		
Acute angle-closure glaucoma	Unilateral frontal or orbital Halos around lights, decreased visual acuity, conjunctival injection, vomiting	Tonometry
Altitude sickness	Light-headedness, anorexia, nausea, vomiting, fatigue, irritability, difficulty sleeping In patients who have recently gone to a high altitude (including flying ≥ 6 h in an airplane)	Clinical evaluation
Encephalitis	Fever, altered mental status, seizures, focal neurologic deficits	MRI, CSF analysis
Giant cell arteritis	Age > 55 Unilateral throbbing pain, pain when combing hair, visual disturbances, jaw claudication, fever, weight loss, sweats, temporal artery tenderness, proximal myalgias	ESR, temporal artery biopsy, usually neuroimaging
Idiopathic intracranial hypertension	Migraine-like headache, diplopia, pulsatile tinnitus, loss of peripheral vision, papilledema	Neuroimaging (preferably MRI with magnetic resonance venography), followed by measurement of CSF opening pressure and cell count culture and analysis
Intracerebral hemorrhage	Sudden onset Vomiting, focal neurologic deficits, altered mental status	Neuroimaging
Medication overuse headache	Headache with variable location and intensity Present > 15 days/mo Often present on awakening Typically develops after overuse of analgesics taken for an episodic headache disorder	Clinical evaluation
Meningitis	Fever, meningismus, altered mental status	CSF analysis, often preceded by CT
Post-lumbar puncture and other low-pressure headaches	Intense headaches, often with meningismus and/or vomiting Worsened by sitting or standing and alleviated only by lying completely flat	Clinical evaluation
Sinusitis	Positional facial or tooth pain, fever, purulent rhinorrhea	Clinical evaluation, sometimes CT
Subarachnoid hemorrhage	Peak intensity a few seconds after headache onset (thunderclap headache) Vomiting, syncope, obtundation, meningismus	Neuroimaging, followed by CSF analysis if it is not contraindicated and imaging is not diagnostic
Subdural hematoma (chronic)	Sleepiness, altered mental status, hemiparesis, loss of spontaneous venous pulsations, papilledema Presence of risk factors (eg, older age, coagulopathy, dementia, anticoagulant use, ethanol abuse)	Neuroimaging
Tumor or mass	Eventually altered mental status, seizures, vomiting, diplopia when looking laterally, loss of spontaneous venous pulsations or papilledema, focal neurologic deficits	Neuroimaging

* Primary headaches are usually recurrent.

Red flags: The following findings are of particular concern:

- Neurologic symptoms or signs (eg, altered mental status, weakness, diplopia, papilledema, focal neurologic deficits)
- Immunosuppression or cancer
- Meningismus
- Onset of headache after age 50
- Thunderclap headache (severe headache that peaks within a few seconds)
- Symptoms of giant cell arteritis (eg, visual disturbances, jaw claudication, fever, weight loss, temporal artery tenderness, proximal myalgias)
- Systemic symptoms (eg, fever, weight loss)
- Progressively worsening headache
- Red eye and halos around lights

Interpretation of findings: If similar headaches recur in patients who appear well and have a normal examination, the cause is rarely ominous. Headaches that have recurred since childhood or young adulthood suggest a primary headache disorder. If headache type or pattern clearly changes in patients with a known primary headache disorder, secondary headache should be considered.

Most single symptoms of primary headache disorders other than aura are nonspecific. A combination of symptoms and signs is more characteristic (see Table 229–2).

Red flag findings suggest a cause (see Table 229–3).

Testing: Most patients can be diagnosed without testing. However, some serious disorders may require urgent or immediate testing. Some patients require tests as soon as possible.

CT (or MRI) should be done as soon as possible in patients with any of the following findings:

- Thunderclap headache
- Altered mental status
- Meningismus
- Papilledema
- Signs of sepsis (eg, rash, shock)
- Acute focal neurologic deficit
- Severe hypertension (eg, systolic > 220 mm Hg or diastolic > 120 mm Hg on consecutive readings)

In addition, if meningitis, subarachnoid hemorrhage, or encephalitis is being considered, LP and CSF analysis should be done, if not contraindicated by imaging results. Patients with a thunderclap headache require CSF analysis even if CT and examination findings are normal as long as LP is not contraindicated by imaging results.

Tonometry should be done if findings suggest acute narrow-angle glaucoma (eg, visual halos, nausea, corneal edema, shallow anterior chamber).

Other testing should be done within hours or days, depending on the acuity and seriousness of findings and suspected causes.

Neuroimaging, usually MRI, should be done if patients have any of the following:

- Focal neurologic deficit of subacute or uncertain onset
- Age > 50 yr
- Weight loss
- Cancer
- HIV infection or AIDS
- Change in an established headache pattern
- Diplopia

ESR should be done if patients have visual symptoms, jaw or tongue claudication, temporal artery signs, or other findings suggesting giant cell arteritis.

CT of the paranasal sinuses is done to rule out complicated sinusitis if patients have a moderately severe systemic illness (eg, high fever, dehydration, prostration, tachycardia) and findings suggesting sinusitis (eg, frontal, positional headache; epistaxis; purulent rhinorrhea).

LP and CSF analysis are done if headache is progressive and findings suggest idiopathic intracranial hypertension (eg, transient obscuration of vision, diplopia, pulsatile intracranial tinnitus) or chronic meningitis (eg, persistent low-grade fever, cranial neuropathies, cognitive impairment, lethargy, vomiting).

Treatment

Treatment of headache is directed at the cause.

Geriatrics Essentials

New-onset headache after age 50 should be considered a secondary disorder until proven otherwise.

Table 229–3. MATCHING RED FLAG FINDINGS WITH A CAUSE FOR HEADACHE

SUGGESTIVE FINDINGS	CAUSES
Neurologic symptoms or signs (eg, altered mental status, confusion, neurogenic weakness, diplopia, papilledema, focal neurologic deficits)	Encephalitis, subdural hematoma, subarachnoid or intracerebral hemorrhage, tumor, other intracranial mass, increased intracranial pressure
Immunosuppression or cancer	CNS infection, metastases
Meningismus	Meningitis, subarachnoid hemorrhage, subdural empyema
Onset of headache after age 50	Increased risk of a serious cause (eg, tumor, giant cell arteritis)
Thunderclap headache (severe headache that peaks within a few seconds)	Subarachnoid hemorrhage
Combination of fever, weight loss, visual disturbances, jaw claudication, temporal artery tenderness, and proximal myalgias	Giant cell arteritis
Systemic symptoms (eg, fever, weight loss)	Sepsis, hyperthyroidism, cancer
Progressively worsening headache	Secondary headache
Red eye and halos around lights	Acute angle-closure glaucoma

KEY POINTS

- Recurrent headaches that began at a young age in patients with a normal examination are usually benign.
- Neuroimaging is recommended as soon as possible for patients with altered mental status, seizures, papilledema, focal neurologic deficits, or thunderclap headache.
- CSF analysis is required for patients with meningismus and usually, after neuroimaging, for immunosuppressed patients.
- Patients with thunderclap headache require CSF analysis even if CT and examination findings are normal.

CLUSTER HEADACHE

Cluster headaches cause excruciating, unilateral periorbital or temporal pain, with ipsilateral autonomic symptoms (ptosis, lacrimation, rhinorrhea, nasal congestion). Diagnosis is clinical. Acute treatment is with parenteral triptans, dihydroergotamine, or oxygen. Prevention is with verapamil, lithium, topiramate, divalproex, or a combination.

Cluster headache affects primarily men, typically beginning at age 20 to 40; prevalence in the US is 0.4%. Usually, cluster headache is episodic; for 1 to 3 mo, patients experience ≥ 1 attack/day, followed by remission for months to years. Some patients have cluster headaches without remission.

Pathophysiology is unknown, but the periodicity suggests hypothalamic dysfunction.

Alcohol intake triggers cluster headache during the attack period but not during remission.

Symptoms and Signs

Symptoms of cluster headache are distinctive. Attacks often occur at the same time each day, often awakening patients from sleep. When attacks occur, pain is always unilateral and occurs on the same side of the head in an orbitotemporal distribution. It is excruciating, peaking within minutes; it usually subsides spontaneously within 30 min to 1 h. Patients are agitated, restlessly pacing the floor, unlike migraine patients who prefer to lie quietly in a darkened room. The restlessness can be so severe that it leads to bizarre behavior (eg, banging the head on a wall).

Autonomic features, including nasal congestion, rhinorrhea, lacrimation, facial flushing, and Horner syndrome, are prominent and occur on the same side as the headache.

Diagnosis

- Clinical evaluation

Diagnosis of cluster headache is based on the distinctive symptom pattern and exclusion of intracranial abnormalities.

Other unilateral primary headache syndromes with autonomic symptoms, which are sometimes grouped together with cluster headache as trigeminal autonomic cephalgias, should be excluded:

- SUNCT (short-lasting unilateral neuralgiform headache with conjunctival injection and tearing): Attacks are very brief (5 to 250 sec) and occur at high frequency (up to 200 attacks/day).
- Chronic paroxysmal hemicrania: Attacks are more frequent (> 5/day) and much briefer (usually just minutes) than in cluster headache.
- Hemicrania continua: Moderately severe continuous unilateral head pain occurs with superimposed brief episodes of more intense pain.

Chronic paroxysmal hemicrania and hemicrania continua, unlike SUNCT and cluster headache (and migraine), respond dramatically to indomethacin, but not to other NSAIDs.

Treatment

- For aborting attacks, parenteral triptans, dihydroergotamine, or 100% oxygen
- For long-term prophylaxis, verapamil, lithium, topiramate, divalproex, or a combination

Acute attacks of cluster headache can be aborted with either a parenteral triptan or dihydroergotamine and/or 100% oxygen given by nonrebreathing face mask.

All patients require preventive drugs because cluster headache is frequent, severe, and incapacitating. Prednisone (eg, 60 mg po once/day) or a greater occipital nerve block (with a local anesthetic and a corticosteroid) can provide prompt temporary prevention while preventive drugs with slower onset of action (eg, verapamil, lithium, topiramate, divalproex) are initiated.

KEY POINTS

- Typically, cluster headache causes excruciating unilateral periorbital or temporal pain, with ipsilateral ptosis, lacrimation, rhinorrhea, and/or nasal congestion, in men aged 20 to 40 yr.
- Usually, patients experience ≥ 1 attack/day for 1 to 3 mo, followed by remission for months to years.
- Diagnose cluster headache based on clinical findings.
- To abort attacks, give a parenteral triptan or dihydroergotamine (see Table 229–4) and/or 100% oxygen by a nonrebreathing face mask.
- To prevent attacks, use prednisone or a greater occipital nerve block for short-term relief and verapamil, lithium, topiramate, and/or divalproex for long-term relief.

IDIOPATHIC INTRACRANIAL HYPERTENSION

(Benign Intracranial Hypertension; Pseudotumor Cerebri)

Idiopathic intracranial hypertension causes increased intracranial pressure without a mass lesion or hydrocephalus, probably by obstructing venous drainage; CSF composition is normal.

Idiopathic intracranial hypertension typically occurs in women of childbearing age. Incidence is 1/100,000 in normal-weight women but 20/100,000 in obese women. Intracranial pressure is elevated (> 250 mm H_2O); the cause is unknown but probably involves obstruction of cerebral venous outflow, possibly because venous sinuses are smaller than normal.

In children, this disorder sometimes develops after corticosteroids are stopped or after children have taken large amounts of tetracycline.

Symptoms and Signs

Almost all patients have a daily or near daily generalized headache of fluctuating intensity, at times with nausea. They may also have transient obscuration of vision, diplopia (due to 6th cranial nerve dysfunction), and pulsatile intracranial tinnitus. Vision loss begins peripherally and may not be noticed by patients until late in the course. Permanent vision loss is the most serious consequence. Once vision is lost, it usually does not return, even if ICP is reduced.

Table 229–4. DRUGS FOR MIGRAINE AND CLUSTER HEADACHES*

DRUG	DOSAGE	COMMENTS
Prevention		
Amitriptyline	10–100 mg po at bedtime	Used only for migraines Has anticholinergic effects; causes weight gain Helpful for patients with insomnia Small doses often effective
Beta-blockers	Atenolol 25–100 mg po once/day Metoprolol 50–200 mg po once/day Nadolol 20–160 mg po once/day Propranolol 20–160 mg po bid Timolol 5–20 mg po once/day	Used only for migraines Only beta-blockers without intrinsic sympathomimetic activity used Avoided in patients with bradycardia, hypotension, diabetes, or asthma
Divalproex	Regular-release: 250–500 mg po bid Extended-release: 500–1000 mg po once/day	Can cause alopecia, GI upset, hepatic dysfunction, thrombocytopenia, tremor, and weight gain
Lithium	300 mg po bid to qid	Used only for cluster headaches May cause weakness, thirst, tremor, and polyuria Periodic checking of drug levels required
OnabotulinumtoxinA	—	First-line treatment for chronic migraine
Topiramate	50–200 mg po usually once/day	Can cause weight loss and CNS adverse effects (eg, confusion, depression)
Verapamil[†]	240 mg once/day to tid	Most useful for patients with cluster headache Can cause hypotension and constipation
Treatment		
Dihydroergotamine	0.5–1 mg sc or IV 4 mg/mL nasal spray	Can cause nausea Contraindicated in patients with hypertension or coronary artery disease Cannot be used concurrently with triptans Pulmonary-inhaled formulation under development
Triptans[‡]	Almotriptan 12.5 mg po Eletriptan 20–40 mg po Frovatriptan 2.5 mg po Naratriptan 2.5 mg po Rizatriptan 10 mg po Sumatriptan 50–100 mg po, 5–20 mg nasal spray, 6 mg sc, or one 6.5-mg transdermal patch, followed, if needed, by a 2nd patch after 2 h (not to exceed 2 patches in 24 h) Zolmitriptan 2.5–5 mg po or 5 mg nasal spray	Can cause flushing, paresthesias, and sense of pressure in chest or throat Can repeat doses up to 3 times/day if headache recurs Contraindicated in patients with coronary artery disease, uncontrolled hypertension, hemiplegic migraine, or intracranial vascular disease Injections or nasal spray used for cluster headache
Valproate	500–1000 mg IV	Usually for patients who cannot tolerate triptans or vasoconstrictors With long-term use, can cause alopecia, GI upset, hepatic dysfunction, thrombocytopenia, tremor, and weight gain

*Drugs can be used for either type of headache unless specified otherwise.
[†]The regular-release formulation is usually used.
[‡]Triptans are given once, then repeated as needed.

Bilateral papilledema is common; a few patients have unilateral or no papilledema. In some asymptomatic patients, papilledema is discovered during routine ophthalmoscopic examination. Neurologic examination may detect partial 6th cranial nerve palsy but is otherwise unremarkable.

PEARLS & PITFALLS

- If clinical findings suggest idiopathic intracranial hypertension, check visual fields and optic fundi, even when patients have no visual symptoms.

Diagnosis

- MRI with magnetic resonance venography
- Lumbar puncture

If clinical findings suggest idiopathic intracranial hypertension, clinicians should check visual fields and optic fundi, even in patients with no visual symptoms.

Diagnosis is suspected clinically and established by brain imaging (preferably MRI with magnetic resonance venography) that has normal results (except for venous transverse), followed, if not contraindicated, by lumbar puncture with CSF testing that indicates elevated opening pressure and normal CSF composition.

Use of certain drugs and certain disorders can produce a clinical picture resembling idiopathic intracranial hypertension and should be excluded (see Table 229–5).

Treatment

- Acetazolamide
- Weight loss
- Drugs used for migraine, especially topiramate

Idiopathic intracranial hypertension occasionally resolves without treatment.

Treatment of idiopathic intracranial hypertension is aimed at the following:

- Reducing pressure
- Preserving vision
- Relieving symptoms

The carbonic anhydrase inhibitor acetazolamide (250 mg po qid) is used as a diuretic.

Obese patients are encouraged to lose weight, which may help reduce intracranial pressure.

Serial lumbar punctures are controversial but are sometimes used, particularly if, while waiting for definitive treatment, vision is threatened.

Any potential causes (disorders or drugs) are corrected or eliminated if possible.

Drugs used for migraine (particularly topiramate, which also inhibits carbonic anhydrase) may relieve headache. NSAIDs can be used as needed.

If vision deteriorates despite treatment, one of the following may be indicated:

- Optic nerve sheath fenestration
- Shunting (lumboperitoneal or ventriculoperitoneal)
- Endovascular venous stenting

Bariatric surgery with sustained weight loss may cure the disorder in obese patients who were otherwise unable to lose weight.

Table 229–5. CONDITIONS ASSOCIATED WITH PAPILLEDEMA AND RESEMBLING IDIOPATHIC INTRACRANIAL HYPERTENSION

CONDITION	EXAMPLES
Obstruction of cerebral venous drainage	Cerebral venous sinus thrombosis Jugular vein thrombosis
Disorders	Addison disease COPD Hypoparathyroidism Iron deficiency anemia if severe Obesity (usually in young women) Polycystic ovary syndrome Renal failure Right ventricular heart failure with pulmonary hypertension Sleep apnea
Drugs	Anabolic steroids Corticosteroid withdrawal after prolonged use Growth hormone in patients with a deficiency Nalidixic acid Nitrofurantoin Tetracycline and its derivatives Vitamin A toxicity

Frequent ophthalmologic assessment (including quantitative visual fields) is required to monitor response to treatment; testing visual acuity is not sensitive enough to warn of impending vision loss.

KEY POINTS

- Consider idiopathic intracranial hypertension if patients, particularly overweight women, have a daily generalized headache with or without visual symptoms; check visual fields and optic fundi.
- Diagnose based on results of brain imaging (preferably MRI with venography) and, if not contraindicated, lumbar puncture.
- Advise weight loss if needed and treat with acetazolamide.
- Do frequent ophthalmologic assessments (including quantitative visual fields) to monitor response to treatment.

MIGRAINE

Migraine is an episodic primary headache disorder. Symptoms typically last 4 to 72 h and may be severe. Pain is often unilateral, throbbing, worse with exertion, and accompanied by symptoms such as nausea and sensitivity to light, sound, or odors. Auras occur in about 25% of patients, usually just before but sometimes after the headache. Diagnosis is clinical. Treatment is with triptans, dihydroergotamine, antiemetics, and analgesics. Preventive regimens include lifestyle modifications (eg, of sleeping habits or diet) and drugs (eg, beta-blockers, amitriptyline, topiramate, divalproex).

Epidemiology

Migraine is the most common cause of recurrent moderate to severe headache; 1-yr prevalence is 18% for women and 6% for men in the US. Migraine most commonly begins during puberty or young adulthood, waxing and waning in frequency and severity over the ensuing years; it often diminishes after age 50. Studies show familial aggregation of migraine.

Evidence based on evaluation of veterans of the Iraq and Afghanistan conflicts suggests that migraine may frequently develop after mild traumatic brain injury.

Pathophysiology

Migraine is thought to be a neurovascular pain syndrome with altered central neuronal processing (activation of brain stem nuclei, cortical hyperexcitability, and spreading cortical depression) and involvement of the trigeminovascular system (triggering neuropeptide release, which causes painful inflammation in cranial vessels and the dura mater).

Many potential migraine triggers have been identified; they include the following:

- Drinking red wine
- Skipping meals
- Excessive afferent stimuli (eg, flashing lights, strong odors)
- Weather changes
- Sleep deprivation
- Stress
- Hormonal factors, particularly menstruation
- Certain foods

Head trauma, neck pain, or temporomandibular joint dysfunction sometimes triggers or exacerbates migraine.

Fluctuating estrogen levels are a potent migraine trigger. Many women have onset of migraine at menarche, severe attacks during menstruation (menstrual migraine), and worsening during menopause. For most women, migraines remit during pregnancy (but sometimes they worsen during the 1st or 2nd trimester); they worsen after childbirth, when estrogen levels decrease rapidly.

Oral contraceptives and other hormone therapy occasionally trigger or worsen migraine and have been associated with stroke in women who have migraine with aura.

Familial hemiplegic migraine, a rare subtype of migraine, is associated with genetic defects on chromosomes 1, 2, and 19. The role of genes in the more common forms of migraine is under study.

Symptoms and Signs

Often, a **prodrome** (a sensation that a migraine is beginning) heralds attacks. The prodrome may include mood changes, loss of appetite, nausea, or a combination.

An **aura** precedes attacks in about 25% of patients. Auras are temporary neurologic disturbances that can affect sensation, balance, muscle coordination, speech, or vision; they last minutes to an hour. The aura may persist after headache onset. Most commonly, auras involve visual symptoms (fortification spectra—eg, binocular flashes, arcs of scintillating lights, bright zigzags, scotomata). Paresthesias and numbness (typically starting in one hand and marching to the ipsilateral arm and face), speech disturbances, and transient brain stem dysfunction (causing, for example, ataxia, confusion, or even obtundation) are less common than visual auras. Some patients have an aura with little or no headache.

Headache varies from moderate to severe, and attacks last from 4 h to several days, typically resolving with sleep. The pain is often unilateral but may be bilateral, most often in a frontotemporal distribution, and is typically described as pulsating or throbbing.

Migraine is more than a headache. Associated symptoms such as nausea (and occasionally vomiting), photophobia, sonophobia, and osmophobia are prominent. Patients report difficulty concentrating during attacks. Routine physical activity usually aggravates migraine headache; this effect, plus the photophobia and sonophobia, encourages most patients to lie in a dark, quiet room during attacks. Severe attacks can be incapacitating, disrupting family and work life.

Attacks vary significantly in frequency and severity. Many patients have several types of headache, including milder attacks without nausea or photophobia; they may resemble tension-type headache but are a forme fruste of migraine.

Chronic migraines: Patients with episodic migraine can develop chronic migraine. These patients have headaches ≥ 15 days/mo. This headache disorder used to be called combination or mixed headache because it had features of migraine and tension-type headache. These headaches often develop in patients who overuse drugs for acute treatment of headaches.

Other symptoms: Other, rare forms of migraine can cause other symptoms:

- **Basilar artery migraine** causes combinations of vertigo, ataxia, visual field loss, sensory disturbances, focal weakness, and altered level of consciousness.
- **Hemiplegic migraine,** which may be sporadic or familial, causes unilateral weakness.

Diagnosis

- Clinical evaluation

Diagnosis of migraine is based on characteristic symptoms and a normal physical examination, which includes a thorough neurologic examination.

Red flag findings that suggest an alternate diagnosis (even in patients known to have migraine) include the following:

- Pain that reaches peak intensity within a few seconds or less (thunderclap headache)
- Onset after age 50
- Headaches that increase in intensity or frequency for weeks or longer
- History of cancer (brain metastases) or an immunosuppressive disorder (eg, HIV infection, AIDS)
- Fever, meningismus, altered mental status, or a combination
- Persistent focal neurologic deficits
- Papilledema
- A clear change in an established headache pattern

Patients with characteristic symptoms and no red flag findings do not require testing. Patients with red flag findings often require brain imaging and sometimes lumbar puncture.

Common diagnostic errors include the following:

- Not realizing that migraine often causes bilateral pain and is not always described as throbbing
- Misdiagnosing migraine as sinus headache or eyestrain because of autonomic and visual symptoms of migraine
- Assuming that any headache in patients known to have migraine represents another migraine attack (a thunderclap headache or a change in the previous headache pattern may indicate a new, potentially serious disorder)
- Mistaking migraine with aura for a transient ischemic attack, especially when the aura occurs without headache, in older people
- Diagnosing a thunderclap headache as migraine because a triptan relieves it (a triptan can also relieve a headache due to subarachnoid hemorrhage)

Several unusual disorders can mimic migraine with aura:

- Dissection of the carotid or vertebral artery
- Cerebral vasculitis
- Moyamoya disease
- CADASIL (cerebral autosomal dominant arteriopathy with subcortical infarcts and leukoencephalopathy)
- MELAS (mitochondrial encephalopathy, lactic acidosis, and strokelike episodes) syndrome

Prognosis

For some patients, migraine is an infrequent, tolerable inconvenience. For others, it is a devastating disorder resulting in frequent periods of incapacity, loss of productivity, and severely impaired quality of life.

Treatment

- Elimination of triggers
- For stress, behavioral interventions
- For mild headaches, acetaminophen or NSAIDs
- For severe attacks, triptans or dihydroergotamine plus a dopamine antagonist antiemetic

A thorough explanation of the disorder helps patients understand that although migraine cannot be cured, it can be controlled, enabling them to better participate in treatment.

Patients are urged to keep a written headache diary to document the number and timing of attacks, possible triggers, and response to treatment. Identified triggers are eliminated when possible. Patients should be encouraged to avoid triggers, and clinicians recommend behavioral interventions (biofeedback, stress management, psychotherapy) to manage migraine when stress is a major trigger or when analgesics are being overused.

Treatment of acute migraine headache is based on frequency, duration, and severity of attacks. It may include analgesics, antiemetics, triptans, and/or dihydroergotamine.[1]

Mild to moderate attacks: NSAIDs or acetaminophen is used. Analgesics containing opioids, caffeine, or butalbital are helpful for infrequent, mild attacks but are prone to being overused, sometimes leading to a type of daily headache syndrome called medication overuse headache.

An antiemetic alone may be used to relieve mild or moderate attacks.

Severe attacks: If mild attacks evolve into incapacitating migraine or if attacks are severe from the onset, triptans are used. Triptans are selective serotonin 1B,1D receptor agonists. They are not analgesic per se but specifically block the release of vasoactive neuropeptides that trigger migraine pain. Triptans are most effective when taken at the onset of attacks. They are available in oral, intranasal, and sc forms (see Table 229–4); sc forms are more effective but have more adverse effects. Overuse of triptans can also lead to medication overuse headache. When nausea is prominent, combining a triptan with an antiemetic at the onset of attacks is effective.

IV fluids (eg, 1 to 2 L of 0.9% normal saline solution) can help relieve headache and increase a sense of well-being, especially in patients who are dehydrated from vomiting.

IV dihydroergotamine with a dopamine antagonist antiemetic (eg, metoclopramide 10 mg IV, prochlorperazine 5 to 10 mg IV) helps abort very severe, persistent attacks. Dihydroergotamine is also available in an sc form and as a nasal spray. A pulmonary-delivery formulation is being developed.

Triptans and dihydroergotamine can cause coronary artery constriction and are thus contraindicated in patients with coronary artery disease or uncontrolled hypertension; these drugs must be used with caution in elderly patients and in patients with vascular risk factors.

A good response to dihydroergotamine or a triptan should not be interpreted as diagnostic for migraine because these drugs may relieve headache due to subarachnoid hemorrhage and other structural abnormalities.

Prochlorperazine suppositories (25 mg) or tablets (10 mg) are an option for patients who cannot tolerate triptans and other vasoconstrictors.

Opioids should be used as a last resort (rescue drug) for severe headache when other measures are ineffective.

Chronic migraines: The same drugs used to prevent episodic migraine are used to treat chronic migraine. Also, supporting evidence is strong for onabotulinumtoxinA and, to a lesser extent, topiramate.

1. Marmura MJ, Silberstein SD, Schwedt TJ: The acute treatment of migraine in adults: The American Headache Society evidence assessment of migraine pharmacotherapies. *Headache* 55(1):3–20, 2015.

Prevention

Daily preventive therapy is warranted when frequent migraines interfere with activity despite acute treatment. Some experts consider onabotulinumtoxinA the drug of choice.

For patients who use analgesics frequently (eg, > 2 days/wk), particularly those with medication overuse headache, preventive drugs (see Table 229–4) should be combined with a program for stopping overused analgesics. Choice of drug can be guided by coexisting disorders, as for the following:

- A small bedtime dose of amitriptyline for patients with insomnia
- A beta-blocker for patients with anxiety or coronary artery disease
- Topiramate, which can induce weight loss, for obese patients or for patients who wish to avoid weight gain
- Divalproex for patients with mania

KEY POINTS

- Migraine is a common primary headache disorder with multiple potential triggers.
- Symptoms can include throbbing unilateral or bilateral pain, nausea, sensitivity to sensory stimuli (eg, light, sounds, smells), nonspecific prodromal symptoms, and temporary neurologic symptoms that precede headache (auras).
- Diagnose migraine based on clinical findings; if patients have red flag findings, tests are often needed.
- Involve patients in their care, including avoiding triggers and using biofeedback, stress management, and psychotherapy as appropriate.
- Treat most headaches with analgesics, IV dihydroergotamine, or triptans.
- If attacks are frequent and interfere with activities, use preventive therapy (eg, onabotulinumtoxinA, amitriptyline, a beta-blocker, topiramate, divalproex).

POST–LUMBAR PUNCTURE AND OTHER LOW-PRESSURE HEADACHES

Low-pressure headaches result from reduction in CSF volume and pressure due to lumbar puncture (LP) or spontaneous or traumatic CSF leaks.

Removal of CSF by LP reduces CSF volume and pressure, as do spontaneous or traumatic CSF leaks.

Headache after LP is common, usually occurring hours to a day or two afterward, and can be severe. Younger patients with a small body mass are at greatest risk. Using small, noncutting needles reduces risk. The amount of CSF removed and duration of recumbency after LP do not affect incidence.

Spontaneous CSF leaks may result when a nerve root arachnoid diverticulum or cyst along the spinal canal ruptures. Coughing or sneezing may cause the rupture. CSF may leak after certain head or facial injuries (eg, basilar skull fractures).

Headache results when head elevation while sitting or standing stretches the pain-sensitive basal meninges. Headaches are intense, postural, and often accompanied by neck pain, meningismus, and vomiting. Headache is alleviated only by lying completely flat.

Diagnosis

- Clinical evaluation

Post-LP headache is clinically obvious, and testing is rarely needed; other low-pressure headaches may require brain imaging. MRI with gadolinium often shows diffuse enhancement of the pachymeninges and, in severe cases, downward sagging of the brain.

CSF pressure is typically low or unobtainable if patients have been upright for any length of time.

Treatment

- Hydration and caffeine
- Usually an epidural blood patch

The first line of treatment for post-LP headache is

- Recumbency
- Hydration
- An elastic abdominal binder
- Caffeine
- Analgesics as needed

However, if post-LP headache persists after a day of such treatment, an epidural blood patch (injection of a few mL of the patient's clotted venous blood into the lumbar epidural space) is usually effective. A blood patch may also be effective for spontaneous or traumatic CSF leaks, which rarely require surgical closure.

SHORT-LASTING UNILATERAL NEURALGIFORM HEADACHE WITH CONJUNCTIVAL INJECTION AND TEARING

Short-lasting unilateral neuralgiform headache with conjunctival injection and tearing (SUNCT) is a rare headache disorder characterized by extremely frequent attacks of unilateral head pain and autonomic activation.

SUNCT, like cluster headache, is a primary headache disorder characterized by unilateral pain in the trigeminal nerve distribution and by autonomic manifestations. As such, SUNCT and cluster headaches are sometimes grouped together as trigeminal autonomic cephalgias.

In SUNCT, pain paroxysms are typically periorbital, are extremely frequent (up to 200/day), and last from 5 to 250 sec. Conjunctival injection is often the most prominent autonomic feature; tearing may also be obvious.

Diagnosis

- Clinical evaluation

Diagnosis of SUNCT is clinical.

SUNCT should be distinguished from trigeminal neuralgia, which causes similar symptoms; SUNCT differs in that

- It has no refractory period.
- Pain occurs predominantly in the ophthalmic division of the trigeminal nerve.
- Attacks are not triggered by cutaneous stimuli.
- Indomethacin does not relieve symptoms, as it does in some other headache disorders.

Treatment

- For acute attacks, IV lidocaine
- For prevention, anticonvulsants and/or occipital nerve stimulation or blockade

Treatment of SUNCT can include IV lidocaine for acute attacks and, for prevention, anticonvulsants (eg, lamotrigine, topiramate, gabapentin) and occipital nerve stimulation or blockade.

TENSION-TYPE HEADACHE

(Tension Headache)

Tension-type headache causes mild generalized pain without the incapacity, nausea, or photophobia associated with migraine.

Tension-type headaches may be episodic or chronic:

- **Episodic tension-type headaches** occur < 15 days/mo. Episodic tension-type headache is very common; most patients obtain relief with OTC analgesics and do not seek medical attention.
- **Chronic tension-type headaches** occur ≥ 15 days/mo.

Symptoms and Signs

The pain is usually mild to moderate and often described as viselike. These headaches originate in the occipital or frontal region bilaterally and spread over the entire head.

Unlike migraine headaches, tension-type headaches are not accompanied by nausea and vomiting and are not made worse by physical activity, light, sounds, or smells. Potential triggers for chronic tension-type headache include sleep disturbances, stress, temporomandibular joint dysfunction, neck pain, and eyestrain.

Episodic headaches may last 30 min to several days. They typically start several hours after waking and worsen as the day progresses. They rarely awaken patients from sleep.

Chronic headaches may vary in intensity throughout the day but are almost always present.

Diagnosis

- Clinical evaluation

Diagnosis of tension-type headache is based on characteristic symptoms and a normal physical examination, which includes a neurologic examination. Potential triggers for chronic tension-type headache should be identified and treated.

Tension-type headache should be distinguished from a forme fruste of migraine, which many patients with migraine have; these headaches have only some features of migraine and resemble tension-type headache, but they are mild and respond to migraine-specific drugs.

If severe headaches are thought to be tension-type headaches, the diagnosis should be reconsidered because severe tension-type headaches are rare.

PEARLS & PITFALLS

- Reconsider the diagnosis of tension-type headache if headache is severe.

Treatment

- Analgesics
- Sometimes behavioral and psychologic interventions

Some drugs used to prevent migraine (see Table 229–4), particularly amitriptyline, can help prevent chronic tension-type headache.

For most mild to moderate tension-type headaches, OTC analgesics (eg, aspirin, acetaminophen) can provide relief. Massaging the affected area may help.

Behavioral and psychologic interventions (eg, relaxation and stress management techniques) are often used and are effective, especially when combined with drug treatment.

230 Intracranial and Spinal Tumors

Intracranial tumors may involve the brain or other structures (eg, cranial nerves, meninges). The tumors usually develop during early or middle adulthood but may develop at any age; they are becoming more common among the elderly. Brain tumors are found in about 2% of routine autopsies.

Some tumors are benign, but because the cranial vault allows no room for expansion, even benign tumors can cause serious neurologic dysfunction or death.

Classification

There are 2 types of brain tumors:

- Primary tumors: Originate in the brain either in the brain parenchyma (eg, gliomas, medulloblastomas, ependymomas) or in extraneural structures (eg, meningiomas, acoustic neuromas, other schwannomas)
- Secondary brain tumors (brain metastases): Originate in tissues outside the brain and spread to the brain

Brain metastases are about 10 times more common than primary tumors.

PEARLS & PITFALLS

- Brain metastases are about 10 times more common than primary brain tumors.

Type of tumor varies somewhat by site (see Table 230–1) and patient age (see Table 230–2).

Pathophysiology

Neurologic dysfunction may result from the following:

- Invasion and destruction of brain tissue by the tumor
- Direct compression of adjacent tissue by the tumor
- Increased intracranial pressure (because the tumor occupies space within the skull)
- Bleeding within or outside the tumor
- Cerebral edema
- Obstruction of dural venous sinuses (especially by bone or extradural metastatic tumors)
- Obstruction of CSF drainage (occurring early with 3rd-ventricle or posterior fossa tumors)
- Obstruction of CSF absorption (eg, when leukemia or carcinoma involves the meninges)
- Obstruction of arterial flow
- Rarely, paraneoplastic syndromes (see p. 1175)

A malignant tumor can develop new internal blood vessels, which can bleed or become occluded, resulting in necrosis and neurologic dysfunction that mimics stroke.

Benign tumors grow slowly. They may become quite large before causing symptoms, partly because often there is no cerebral edema. Malignant primary tumors grow rapidly but rarely spread beyond the CNS. Death results from local tumor growth and thus can result from benign as well as malignant tumors. Therefore, distinguishing between benign and malignant is prognostically less important for brain tumors than for other tumors.

Symptoms and Signs

Symptoms caused by primary tumors and metastatic tumors are the same. Many symptoms result from increased intracranial pressure:

- Headache
- Deterioration in mental status
- Focal brain dysfunction

Headache is the most common symptom. Headache may be most intense when patients awake from deep non-REM sleep (usually several hours after falling asleep) because hypoventilation, which increases cerebral blood flow and thus intracranial pressure, is usually maximal during non-REM sleep. Headache is also progressive and may be worsened by recumbency or the Valsalva maneuver. When intracranial pressure is very high, the headache may be accompanied by vomiting, sometimes with little nausea preceding it. Papilledema develops in about 25% of patients with a brain tumor but may be absent even when intracranial pressure is increased. In infants and very young children, increased intracranial pressure may enlarge the head. If intracranial pressure increases sufficiently, brain herniation occurs (see Fig. 224–1 on p. 1858).

Deterioration in mental status is the 2nd most common symptom. Manifestations include drowsiness, lethargy, personality changes, disordered conduct, and impaired cognition, particularly with malignant brain tumors. Generalized seizures may occur, more often with primary than metastatic brain tumors. Impaired consciousness (see p. 1857) can result from herniation, brain stem dysfunction, or diffuse bilateral cortical dysfunction. Airway reflexes may be impaired.

Focal brain dysfunction causes some symptoms. Focal neurologic deficits, endocrine dysfunction, or focal seizures (sometimes with secondary generalization) may develop depending on the tumor's location (see Table 230–1). Focal deficits often suggest the tumor's location. However, sometimes focal deficits do not correspond to the tumor's location. Such deficits, called false localizing signs, include the following:

- Unilateral or bilateral lateral rectus palsy (with paresis of eye abduction) due to increased intracranial pressure compressing the 6th cranial nerve
- Ipsilateral hemiplegia due to compression of the contralateral cerebral peduncle against the tentorium (Kernohan notch)
- Ipsilateral visual field defect due to ischemia in the contralateral occipital lobe

Some tumors cause meningeal inflammation, resulting in subacute or chronic meningitis (see p. 1917).

Diagnosis

- T1-weighted MRI with gadolinium or CT with contrast

Early-stage brain tumors are often misdiagnosed. A brain tumor should be considered in patients with any of the following:

- Progressive focal or global deficits of brain function
- New seizures
- Persistent, unexplained, recent-onset headaches, particularly if worsened by sleep
- Evidence of increased intracranial pressure (eg, papilledema, unexplained vomiting)
- Pituitary or hypothalamic endocrinopathy

Table 230–1. COMMON LOCALIZING MANIFESTATIONS OF BRAIN TUMORS

TUMOR SITE	FINDINGS	COMMON PRIMARY TUMOR TYPES*
Anterior corpus callosum	Cognitive impairment	Astrocytoma Oligodendroglioma
Basal ganglia	Hemiparesis (contralateral), movement disorders	Astrocytoma
Brain stem	Unilateral or bilateral motor or sensory loss, cranial nerve deficits (eg, gaze palsies, hearing loss, vertigo, palatal paresis, facial weakness), ataxia, intention tremor, nystagmus	Astrocytoma (most often juvenile pilocytic astrocytoma)
Cerebellopontine angle	Tinnitus and hearing loss (both ipsilateral), vertigo, loss of vestibular response to caloric stimulation If tumor is large, ataxia, loss of facial sensation and facial weakness (both ipsilateral), possibly other cranial nerve or brain stem deficits	Acoustic neuroma Meningioma Schwannoma
Cerebellum	Ataxia, nystagmus, tremor, hydrocephalus with suddenly increased intracranial pressure	Astrocytoma Ependymoma Medulloblastoma
2nd cranial (optic) nerve	Loss of vision	Astrocytoma (most often juvenile pilocytic astrocytoma)
5th cranial (trigeminal) nerve	Loss of facial sensation, jaw weakness	Meningioma
Frontal lobe	Generalized or focal (contralateral) seizures, gait disorders, urinary urgency or incontinence, impaired attention and cognition and apathy (particularly if tumor is bilateral), hemiparesis Expressive aphasia if tumor is in dominant hemisphere Anosmia if tumor is at base of lobe	Astrocytoma Oligodendroglioma
Hypothalamus	Eating and drinking disorders (eg, polydipsia), precocious puberty (especially in boys), hypothermia	Astrocytoma
Occipital lobe	Generalized seizures with visual aura, visual hallucinations, hemianopia or quadrantanopia (contralateral)	Astrocytoma Oligodendroglioma
Parietal lobe	Deficits in position sensation and in 2-point discrimination (contralateral), anosognosia (no recognition of bodily defects), denial of illness, hemianopia (contralateral), generalized or focal seizures, inability to perceive (extinguishing of) a contralateral stimulus when stimuli are applied to both sides of the body (called double simultaneous stimulation) Receptive aphasia if tumor is in dominant hemisphere	Astrocytoma Oligodendroglioma
Pineal region	Paresis of upward gaze, ptosis, loss of pupillary light and accommodation reflexes, sometimes hydrocephalus with suddenly increased intracranial pressure	Germ cell tumor Pineocytoma (rare)
Pituitary or suprasellar region	Endocrinopathies, monocular visual loss, headache without increased intracranial pressure, bitemporal hemianopia	Craniopharyngioma Pituitary adenoma Pituitary carcinoma (rare)
Temporal lobe	Complex partial seizures, generalized seizures with or without aura, hemianopia (contralateral), mixed expressive and receptive aphasia or anomia	Astrocytoma Oligodendroglioma
Thalamus	Sensory impairment (contralateral)	Astrocytoma

*Similar manifestations may result from brain parenchymal metastases or from tumors around the dura (eg, metastatic tumors; meningeal tumors such as meningiomas, sarcomas, or gliomas) or skull lesions (eg, granulomas, hemangiomas, osteitis deformans, osteomas, xanthomas) that compress the underlying brain.

Similar findings can result from other intracranial masses (eg, abscess, aneurysm, arteriovenous malformation, intracerebral hemorrhage, subdural hematoma, granuloma, parasitic cysts such as neurocysticercosis) or ischemic stroke.

A complete neurologic examination, neuroimaging, and chest x-rays (for a source of metastases) should be done. T1-weighted MRI with gadolinium is the study of choice. CT with contrast agent is an alternative. MRI usually detects low-grade astrocytomas and oligodendrogliomas earlier than CT and shows brain structures near bone (eg, the posterior fossa) more clearly. If whole-brain imaging does not show sufficient detail in the target area (eg, sella turcica, cerebellopontine angle, optic nerve), closely spaced images or other special views of the area are obtained. If neuroimaging is normal but increased intracranial

Table 230–2. COMMON TUMORS

AGE GROUP	PRIMARY	METASTASES
Children	Cerebellar astrocytomas and medulloblastomas Ependymomas Gliomas of the brain stem or optic nerve Germinomas Congenital tumors*	Neuroblastoma (usually epidural) Leukemia (meningeal)
Adults	Meningiomas Schwannomas Primary lymphomas Gliomas of the cerebral hemispheres, particularly glioblastoma multiforme, anaplastic astrocytoma, low-grade astrocytoma, and oligodendroglioma	Bronchogenic carcinoma Adenocarcinoma of the breast Malignant melanoma Any cancer that has spread to the lungs

*Congenital tumors include craniopharyngiomas, chordomas, germinomas, teratomas, dermoid cysts, angiomas, and hemangioblastomas.

pressure is suspected, idiopathic intracranial hypertension (see p. 1904) should be considered and lumbar puncture done.

Radiographic clues to the type of tumor, mainly location (see Table 230–1) and pattern of enhancement on MRI, may be inconclusive; brain biopsy, sometimes excisional biopsy, may be required. Specialized tests (eg, molecular and genetic tumor markers in blood and CSF) can help in some cases; eg, in patients with AIDS, Epstein-Barr virus titers in CSF typically increase as CNS lymphoma develops.

Treatment

- Airway protection
- Dexamethasone for increased intracranial pressure
- Mannitol for herniation
- Definitive therapy with excision, radiation therapy, chemotherapy, or a combination

Patients in a coma or with impaired airway reflexes require endotracheal intubation (see p. 554). Brain herniation due to tumors is treated with mannitol 25 to 100 g infused IV, a corticosteroid (eg, dexamethasone 16 mg IV, followed by 4 mg po or IV q 6 h), and endotracheal intubation. Mass lesions should be surgically decompressed as soon as possible.

Increased intracranial pressure due to tumors but without herniation is treated with corticosteroids (eg, dexamethasone as for herniation above or prednisone 30 to 40 mg po bid).

Treatment of the brain tumor depends on pathology and location (for acoustic neuroma, see p. 819). Surgical excision should be used for diagnosis (excisional biopsy) and symptom relief. It may cure benign tumors. For tumors infiltrating the brain parenchyma, treatment is multimodal. Radiation therapy is required, and chemotherapy appears to benefit some patients.

Treatment of metastatic tumors includes radiation therapy and sometimes stereotactic radiosurgery. For patients with a single metastasis, surgical excision of the tumor before radiation therapy improves outcome.

End-of-life issues: If brain tumors are expected to soon be fatal, end-of-life issues should be considered (see p. 3175).

Cranial Radiation Therapy and Neurotoxicity

Radiation therapy may be directed diffusely to the whole head for diffuse or multicentric tumors or locally for well-demarcated tumors. Localized brain radiation therapy may be conformal, targeting the tumor with the aim of sparing normal brain tissue, or stereotactic, involving brachytherapy, a gamma knife, or a linear accelerator. In brachytherapy, radioactive stable iodine ($^{125}I_3$) or iridium-192 ($^{192}Ir_4$) is implanted in or near the tumor. Gliomas are treated with conformal radiation therapy; a gamma knife or linear accelerator is useful for metastases. Giving radiation daily tends to maximize efficacy and minimize neurotoxicity damage to normal CNS tissue (see p. 3093).

Degree of neurotoxicity depends on

- Cumulative radiation dose
- Individual dose size
- Duration of therapy
- Volume of tissue irradiated
- Individual susceptibility

Because susceptibility varies, prediction of radiation neurotoxicity is imprecise. Symptoms can develop in the first few days (acute) or months of treatment (early-delayed) or several months to years after treatment (late-delayed). Rarely, radiation causes gliomas, meningiomas, or peripheral nerve sheath tumors years after therapy.

Acute radiation neurotoxicity: Typically, acute neurotoxicity involves headache, nausea, vomiting, somnolence, and sometimes worsening focal neurologic signs in children and adults. It is particularly likely if intracranial pressure is high. Using corticosteroids to lower intracranial pressure can prevent or treat acute toxicity. Acute toxicity lessens with subsequent treatments.

Early-delayed neurotoxicity: In children or adults, early-delayed neurotoxicity can cause encephalopathy, which must be distinguished by MRI or CT from worsening or recurrent brain tumor. It occurs in children who have received prophylactic whole-brain radiation therapy for leukemia; they develop somnolence, which lessens spontaneously over several days to weeks, possibly more rapidly if corticosteroids are used.

After radiation therapy to the neck or upper thorax, early-delayed neurotoxicity can result in a myelopathy, characterized by Lhermitte sign (an electric shock-like sensation radiating down the back and into the legs when the neck is flexed). The myelopathy resolves spontaneously.

Late-delayed neurotoxicity: After diffuse brain radiation therapy, many children and adults develop late-delayed neurotoxicity if they survive long enough. The most common cause in children is diffuse therapy given to prevent leukemia or to treat medulloblastoma. After diffuse therapy, the main symptom is progressive dementia; adults also develop an unsteady gait. MRI or CT shows cerebral atrophy.

After localized therapy, neurotoxicity more often involves focal neurologic deficits. MRI or CT shows a mass that may be enhanced by contrast agent and that may be difficult to distinguish from recurrence of the primary tumor. Excisional biopsy of the mass is diagnostic and often ameliorates symptoms.

Late-delayed myelopathy can develop after radiation therapy for extraspinal tumors (eg, due to Hodgkin lymphoma). It is characterized by progressive paresis and sensory loss, often as a Brown-Séquard syndrome (ipsilateral paresis and proprioceptive sensory loss, with contralateral loss of pain and temperature sensation). Most patients eventually become paraplegic.

GLIOMAS

Gliomas are primary tumors that originate in brain parenchyma. Symptoms and diagnosis are similar to those of other brain tumors. Treatment involves surgical excision, radiation therapy, and, for some tumors, chemotherapy. Excision rarely cures.

Gliomas include astrocytomas, oligodendrogliomas, medulloblastomas, and ependymomas. Many gliomas infiltrate brain tissue diffusely and irregularly.

Astrocytomas are the most common gliomas. They are classified, in ascending order of malignancy, as

- Grade 1 or 2: Low-grade astrocytomas
- Grade 3: Anaplastic astrocytomas
- Grade 4: Glioblastomas, including glioblastoma multiforme, the most malignant

Low-grade or anaplastic astrocytomas tend to develop in younger patients and can evolve into glioblastomas (secondary glioblastomas). Glioblastomas contain chromosomally heterogeneous cells. They can develop de novo (primary glioblastomas), usually in middle-aged or elderly people. Primary and secondary glioblastomas have distinct genetic characteristics, which can change as the tumors evolve. Some astrocytomas contain oligodendroglioma cells; patients with these tumors (called oligoastrocytomas) have a better prognosis than those with pure astrocytomas.

Oligodendrogliomas are among the most benign gliomas. They affect mainly the cerebral cortex, particularly the frontal lobes. Some oligodendrogliomas are characterized by deletion of the p arm of chromosome 1 (1p deletion), deletion of the q arm of chromosome 19 (19q deletion), or both. These deletions predict longer survival and better response to radiation therapy and chemotherapy. Anaplastic oligodendrogliomas are a more malignant form of oligodendrogliomas and are managed accordingly.

Medulloblastomas and **ependymomas** usually develop near the 4th ventricle. Medulloblastomas develop mainly in children and young adults. Ependymomas, which are uncommon, develop mainly in children. Both types of tumors predispose to obstructive hydrocephalus.

Symptoms and signs vary by location (see Table 230–1). Diagnosis is the same as that of other brain tumors.

Treatment

- Surgical excision
- Radiation therapy
- Chemotherapy for some types

Anaplastic astrocytomas and glioblastomas: Treatment involves surgery, radiation therapy, and chemotherapy to reduce tumor mass. Excising as much tumor as possible is safe, prolongs survival, and improves neurologic function.

After surgery, patients receive a full tumor dose of radiation therapy (60 Gy over 6 wk); ideally, conformal radiation therapy, which targets the tumor and spares normal brain tissue, is used.

For glioblastomas, chemotherapy with temozolomide is now routinely given with radiation therapy. The dose is 75/mg/m^2/day (including weekend days when radiation is skipped) for 42 days, then 150 mg/m^2 po once/day for 5 days/mo during the next month, followed by 200 mg/m^2 po once/day for 5 days/mo in subsequent months for a total of 6 to 12 mo. During treatment with temozolomide, trimethoprim/sulfamethoxazole 800 mg/160 mg is given 3 times/wk to prevent *Pneumocystis jirovecii* pneumonia.

Patients receiving chemotherapy require a CBC at varying intervals.

Implantation of chemotherapy wafers during surgical resection may be appropriate for some patients.

Investigational therapies (eg, stereotactic radiosurgery, new chemotherapeutic drugs, gene or immune therapy, radiation therapy plus temozolomide) should also be considered.

After conventional multimodal treatment, the survival rate for patients with glioblastomas is about 50% at 1 yr, 25% at 2 yr, and 10 to 15% at 5 yr. Prognosis is better in the following cases:

- Patients are < 45 yr.
- Histology is anaplastic astrocytoma (rather than glioblastoma multiforme).
- Initial excision improves neurologic function and leaves minimal or no residual tumor.

With standard treatment, the median survival time is about 30 mo for patients with anaplastic astrocytoma and about 15 mo for patients with glioblastomas.

Low-grade astrocytomas: These tumors are excised if possible, followed by radiation therapy. When radiation therapy should begin is controversial. Early treatment may maximize efficacy but may cause brain damage earlier.

With treatment, 5-yr survival rate is about 40 to 50%.

Oligodendrogliomas: Treatment involves excision and radiation therapy, similar to low-grade astrocytomas. Chemotherapy is sometimes also used.

With treatment, 5-yr survival rate is about 50 to 60%.

Medulloblastomas: Treatment involves whole-brain radiation therapy using about 35 Gy, a posterior fossa boost using 15 Gy, and spinal cord radiation therapy using about 35 Gy. Chemotherapy may be given as adjunctive therapy and for recurrences. Several drugs are effective for certain patients; these drugs include nitrosoureas, procarbazine, vincristine alone or in combination, intrathecal methotrexate, combination chemotherapy (eg, mechlorethamine, vincristine [Oncovin], procarbazine, plus prednisone [MOPP]), cisplatin, and carboplatin. However, no regimen is consistently effective.

With treatment, survival rates are at least 50% at 5 yr and about 40% at 10 yr.

Ependymomas: Usually, surgery to excise the tumor and open CSF pathways is done, followed by radiation therapy. For histologically benign ependymomas, radiation therapy is directed at the tumor; for more malignant tumors with residual tumor after surgery, whole-brain radiation therapy is used. For tumors with evidence of dissemination, radiation therapy is directed at the whole brain and spinal cord.

How much of the tumor can be excised may predict survival best. With treatment, overall 5-yr survival rate is about 50%; however, for patients with no residual tumor, the 5-yr survival rate is > 70%.

KEY POINTS

- Gliomas are primary tumors that originate in brain parenchyma; they include astrocytomas, oligodendrogliomas, medulloblastomas, and ependymomas.
- Gliomas vary in location, degree of malignancy, treatment, and prognosis.

MENINGIOMAS

Meningiomas are benign tumors of the meninges that can compress adjacent brain tissue. Symptoms depend on the tumor's location. Diagnosis is by MRI with contrast agent. Treatment may include excision, stereotactic radiosurgery, and sometimes radiation therapy.

Meningiomas, particularly those < 2 cm in diameter, are among the most common intracranial tumors. Meningiomas are the only brain tumor more common among women. These tumors tend to occur between ages 40 and 60 but can occur during childhood. These benign tumors can develop wherever there is dura, most commonly over the convexities near the venous sinuses, along the base of the skull, and in the posterior fossa and rarely within ventricles. Multiple meningiomas may develop. Meningiomas compress but do not invade brain parenchyma. They can invade and distort adjacent bone. There are many histologic types; all follow a similar clinical course, and some become malignant.

Symptoms and Signs

Symptoms depend on which part of the brain is compressed and thus on the tumor's location (see Table 230–3). Midline tumors in the elderly can cause dementia with few other focal neurologic findings.

Diagnosis

- MRI

Diagnosis is similar to that of other brain tumors, usually by MRI with a paramagnetic contrast agent. Bone abnormalities

Table 230–3. SYMPTOMS OF MENINGIOMAS BY SITE

SITE	FINDINGS
Base of skull	Visual loss Oculomotor palsies Exophthalmos
Cerebral convexities	Focal seizures Cognitive deficits Ultimately, signs of increased intracranial pressure
Clivus and apical petrous bone	Gait disturbance Limb ataxia Deficits referable to the 5th, 7th, and 8th cranial nerves
Foramen magnum	Ipsilateral suboccipital pain Paresis that begins in the ipsilateral arm and progresses to the ipsilateral leg, then to the contralateral leg and arm Sometimes Lhermitte sign Cranial nerve deficits (eg, dysphagia, dysarthria, nystagmus, diplopia, facial hypoesthesia)
Olfactory groove	Anosmia Sometimes papilledema and visual loss
Parasagittal or falx	Spastic paresis or sensory loss, usually beginning in the contralateral leg, but occasionally bilateral Cognitive deficits
Posterior fossa tentorial tumors that extend superiorly or inferiorly	Hydrocephalus
Sphenoid wing:	
Medial (growing into the cavernous sinus)	Oculomotor palsies Facial numbness
Middle (growing anteriorly into the orbit)	Visual loss Exophthalmos
Lateral (as a globular mass or a meningioma en plaque*)	Seizures Headaches
Tuberculum sellae	Visual loss Bone changes sometimes visible with imaging

*Meningioma en plaque involves spread into the dura, with dural thickening and invasion of adjacent bone; the tumor sometimes grows into the temporal bone.

(eg, brain atrophy, hyperostosis around the cerebral convexities, changes in the tuberculum sellae) may be seen incidentally on CT or plain x-rays.

Treatment

- For symptomatic or enlarging meningiomas, surgical excision or radiation therapy

For asymptomatic small meningiomas, particularly in older adults, monitoring with serial neuroimaging is sufficient.

Symptomatic or enlarging meningiomas should be excised if possible. If they are large, encroach on blood vessels (usually surrounding veins), or are close to critical brain areas (eg, brain stem), surgery may cause more damage than the tumor and is thus deferred.

Stereotactic radiosurgery is used for surgically inaccessible meningiomas and electively for other meningiomas. It is also used when tumor tissue remains after surgical excision or when patients are elderly.

If stereotactic radiosurgery is impossible or if a meningioma recurs, radiation therapy may be useful.

KEY POINTS

- Meningiomas are tumors of the meninges that are usually but not always benign.
- They typically occur between ages 40 and 60 and are more common among women.
- Symptoms vary greatly depending on the location of the tumor.
- Excise symptomatic or enlarging tumors; use stereotactic radiosurgery if tumor remains after excision or cannot be excised completely.

PINEAL REGION TUMORS

Most pineal region tumors are germ cell tumors.

Common primary pineal region tumors include germ cell tumors: germinomas (most common), choriocarcinomas, yolk-sac tumors, and teratomas. Less common primary pineal tumors include pineocytomas and the rare malignant pineoblastomas.

Pineal region tumors tend to occur during childhood but can occur at any age.

These tumors may increase intracranial pressure by compressing the aqueduct of Sylvius. They may also cause paresis of upward gaze, ptosis, and loss of pupillary light and accommodation reflexes by compressing the pretectum rostral to the superior colliculi (Parinaud syndrome). These tumors may cause precocious puberty, especially in boys, probably because the hypothalamus is compressed.

CSF β-human chorionic gonadotropin or α-fetoprotein may be elevated, depending on the tumor type. Elevated levels suggest the diagnosis; levels may be measured to monitor response to treatment.

Prognosis and treatment depend on tumor histology. Radiation therapy, chemotherapy, radiosurgery, and surgery are used alone or in combination. Germinomas are very sensitive to radiation therapy and are often cured.

PITUITARY TUMORS

Most pituitary tumors are adenomas. Symptoms include headache and endocrinopathies; endocrinopathies result when the tumor produces hormones or destroys hormone-producing tissue. Diagnosis is by MRI. Treatment includes correction of any endocrinopathy and surgery, radiation therapy, and dopaminergic agonists.

Most tumors of the pituitary and suprasellar region are pituitary adenomas. Rarely, pituitary tumors are carcinomas. Meningiomas, craniopharyngiomas, metastases, and dermoid cysts may also develop in the region of the sella turcica.

Adenomas may be secretory or nonsecretory. Secretory adenomas produce pituitary hormones; many secretory adenomas are < 10 mm in size (microadenomas). Secretory adenomas can be classified by histologic staining characteristics (eg, acidophilic, basophilic, chromophobe [nonstaining]). The hormone produced often correlates with these characteristics; eg, acidophilic adenomas overproduce growth hormone, and basophilic adenomas overproduce ACTH. The hormone most commonly overproduced is prolactin.

Any tumor that grows out of the pituitary can compress optic nerve tracts, including the chiasm. Tumors may also compress or destroy pituitary or hypothalamic tissue, impairing hormone production or secretion.

Symptoms and Signs

Headache may result from an enlarging pituitary adenoma, even when intracranial pressure is not increased. Visual manifestations such as bitemporal hemianopia, unilateral optic atrophy, and contralateral hemianopia may develop if a tumor compresses optic nerve tracts (see Fig. 114–1 on p. 946).

Many patients present with an endocrinopathy due to hormone deficiency or excess:

- Diabetes insipidus if less vasopressin is released because the hypothalamus is compressed
- Amenorrhea and galactorrhea in women and, less commonly, erectile dysfunction and gynecomastia in men if prolactin is overproduced
- Gigantism before puberty or acromegaly after puberty if growth hormone is overproduced
- Cushing syndrome if ACTH is overproduced

Rarely, hemorrhage into a pituitary tumor causes pituitary apoplexy, with sudden headache, ophthalmoplegia, and visual loss.

Diagnosis

- MRI with 1-mm slices

Pituitary tumors are suspected in patients with unexplained headaches, characteristic visual abnormalities, or endocrinopathies. Neuroimaging with 1-mm thick slices is done. MRI is usually much more sensitive than CT, particularly for microadenomas.

Treatment

- Surgical excision when possible
- For endocrinopathies, drug treatment

Endocrinopathies are treated.

Pituitary tumors that produce ACTH, growth hormone, or thyroid-stimulating hormone are surgically excised, usually using a transsphenoidal approach. Sometimes, particularly for surgically inaccessible or multifocal tumors, radiation therapy is required.

Adenomas that produce prolactin are treated with dopaminergic agonists (eg, bromocriptine, pergolide, cabergoline), which lower blood levels and often shrink the tumor. Surgery and radiation therapy are usually unnecessary.

KEY POINTS

- Most pituitary tumors are adenomas, which may be secretory or nonsecretory.
- Secretory adenomas may cause diabetes insipidus, galactorrhea, Cushing syndrome, or gigantism or acromegaly.
- Any pituitary tumor may compress optic nerve tracts, causing bitemporal hemianopia, unilateral optic atrophy, or contralateral hemianopia.
- Excise tumors and treat endocrinopathies; adenomas that produce prolactin may require only treatment with dopaminergic agonists.

PRIMARY BRAIN LYMPHOMAS

Primary brain lymphomas originate in neural tissue and are usually B-cell tumors. Diagnosis requires neuroimaging and sometimes CSF analysis (including Epstein-Barr titers) or brain biopsy. Treatment includes corticosteroids, chemotherapy, and radiation therapy.

Incidence of primary brain lymphomas is increasing, particularly among immunocompromised patients and the elderly. Lymphomas tend to infiltrate the brain diffusely, often as multicentric masses adjacent to the ventricles, but may occur as solitary brain masses. Lymphomas may also occur in the meninges, uvea, or vitreous humor. Most are B-cell tumors, often immunoblastic. The Epstein-Barr virus may contribute to development of lymphomas in immunocompromised patients. Most patients do not develop subsequent systemic lymphoma.

Diagnosis

- MRI
- Sometimes CSF analysis or biopsy

MRI can suggest the diagnosis. MRI may be unable to distinguish cerebral toxoplasmosis (which is common among patients with AIDS) from lymphoma.

If there are meningeal signs, CSF is examined; it may contain lymphoma cells. In immunocompromised patients, Epstein-Barr virus DNA may be detected in CSF. If CSF does not contain lymphoma cells or Epstein-Barr virus DNA, guided-needle or open biopsy is required. Because lymphoma is initially highly sensitive to corticosteroids, giving these drugs just before biopsy may cause the lesion to disappear, resulting in a false-negative biopsy.

Treatment

- Corticosteroids
- Chemotherapy
- Radiation therapy

Most primary brain lymphomas are difficult to cure because they infiltrate the brain diffusely. Usually, corticosteroids result in rapid improvement initially. Many chemotherapy regimens, particularly those containing methotrexate (delivered as high-dose IV infusions), are effective; with methotrexate, median survival may approach 4 yr. Methotrexate can also be delivered intrathecally, usually via an sc intraventricular device (Ommaya reservoir). The drug is sometimes infused into the carotid artery after general anesthesia is induced and 25% mannitol is given IV to open the blood-brain barrier.

Chemotherapy regimens may be followed by radiation therapy, usually after 12 to 16 wk but sometimes delayed until the tumor recurs. The delay helps reduce radiation toxicity.

SPINAL CORD TUMORS

Spinal cord tumors may develop within the spinal cord parenchyma, directly destroying tissue, or outside the cord parenchyma, often compressing the cord or nerve roots. Symptoms include progressive back pain and neurologic deficits referable to the spinal cord or spinal nerve roots. Diagnosis is by MRI. Treatment may include corticosteroids, surgical excision, and radiation therapy.

Spinal cord tumors may be intramedullary (within the cord parenchyma) or extramedullary (outside the parenchyma).

Intramedullary tumors: The most common are gliomas (eg, ependymomas, low-grade astrocytomas). Intramedullary tumors infiltrate and destroy cord parenchyma; they may extend over multiple spinal cord segments or result in a syrinx (see p. 2033).

Extramedullary tumors: These tumors may be intradural or extradural. Most intradural tumors are benign, usually meningiomas and neurofibromas, which are the most common primary spinal tumors. Most extradural tumors are metastatic, usually from carcinomas of the lungs, breasts, prostate, kidneys, or thyroid or from lymphoma (eg, Hodgkin lymphoma, lymphosarcoma, reticulum cell sarcoma).

Intradural and extradural tumors cause neurologic damage by compressing the spinal cord or nerve roots. Most extradural tumors invade and destroy bone before compressing the cord.

Symptoms and Signs

Pain is an early symptom, especially for extradural tumors. It is progressive, unrelated to activity, and worsened by recumbency. Pain may occur in the back, radiate along the sensory distribution of a particular dermatome (radicular pain), or both. Usually, neurologic deficits referable to the spinal cord eventually develop. Common examples are spastic weakness, incontinence, and dysfunction of some or all of the sensory tracts at a particular segment of the spinal cord and below. Deficits are usually bilateral.

Many patients with extramedullary tumors present with pain, but some present with sensory deficits of the distal lower extremities, segmental neurologic deficits, symptoms of spinal cord compression, or a combination. Symptoms of spinal cord compression can worsen rapidly and result in paraplegia and loss of bowel and bladder control. Symptoms of nerve root compression are also common; they include pain and paresthesias followed by sensory loss, muscular weakness, and, if compression is chronic, muscle wasting, which occurs along the distribution of the affected roots.

Diagnosis

- MRI

Patients with segmental neurologic deficits or suspected spinal cord compression require emergency diagnosis and treatment.

The following suggest spinal tumors:

- Progressive, unexplained, or nocturnal back or radicular pain
- Segmental neurologic deficits
- Unexplained neurologic deficits referable to the spinal cord or nerve roots
- Unexplained back pain in patients with primary tumors of the lungs, breasts, prostate, kidneys, or thyroid or with lymphoma

Diagnosis is by MRI of the affected area of the spinal cord. CT with myelography is an alternative but is less accurate.

If MRI does not show a spinal cord tumor, clinicians consider other spinal masses (eg, abscesses, arteriovenous malformations—see p. 2029) and paravertebral tumors. Spinal x-rays, taken for other reasons, may show bone destruction, widening of the vertebral pedicles, or distortion of paraspinal tissues, especially if the tumor is metastatic.

Treatment

- Corticosteroids
- Excision, radiation therapy, or both

For patients with neurologic deficits, corticosteroids (eg, dexamethasone 100 mg IV, then 10 mg po qid) are begun immediately to reduce spinal cord edema and preserve function. Tumors compressing the spinal cord are treated as soon as possible.

Some well-localized primary spinal cord tumors can be excised surgically. Deficits resolve in about half of these patients. If tumors cannot be surgically excised, radiation therapy is used, with or without surgical decompression. Compressive metastatic extradural tumors are usually surgically excised from the vertebral body, then treated with radiation therapy. Noncompressive metastatic extradural tumors may be treated with radiation therapy alone but may require excision if radiation therapy is ineffective.

KEY POINTS

- Spinal cord tumors may be intramedullary (within the cord parenchyma) or extramedullary (outside the parenchyma).
- Extramedullary tumors may be intradural or extradural.
- Most intradural tumors are benign meningiomas and neurofibromas, which are the most common primary spinal tumors; most extradural tumors are metastatic.
- Give corticosteroids to patients with neurologic deficits.
- Surgically excise spinal cord tumors and/or use radiation therapy.

231 Meningitis

Meningitis is inflammation of the meninges and subarachnoid space. It may result from infections, other disorders, or reactions to drugs. Severity and acuity vary. Findings typically include headache, fever, and nuchal rigidity, Diagnosis is by CSF analysis. Treatment includes antimicrobial drugs as indicated plus adjunctive measures.

Meningitis may be classified as acute, subacute, chronic, or recurrent. It may also be classified by its cause: bacteria, viruses, fungi, protozoa, or, occasionally, noninfectious conditions. But the most clinically useful categories of meningitis are

- Acute bacterial meningitis
- Viral meningitis
- Noninfectious meningitis
- Recurrent meningitis
- Subacute and chronic meningitis

Acute bacterial meningitis is particularly serious and rapidly progressive. Viral and noninfectious meningitides are usually self-limited. Subacute and chronic meningitides usually follow a more indolent course than other meningitides, but determining the cause can be difficult.

Aseptic meningitis, an older term, is sometimes used synonymously with viral meningitis; however, it usually refers to acute meningitis caused by anything other than the bacteria that typically cause acute bacterial meningitis. Thus, aseptic meningitis can be caused by viruses, noninfectious conditions (eg, drugs, disorders), or, occasionally, other organisms (eg, *Borrelia burgdorferi* in Lyme disease, *Treponema pallidum* in syphilis).

Symptoms and Signs

Symptoms and signs of the different types of meningitis may vary, particularly in severity and acuity. However, all types tend to cause the following (except in infants):

- Headache
- Fever
- Nuchal rigidity (meningismus)

Patients may appear lethargic or obtunded.

Nuchal rigidity, a key indicator of meningeal irritation, is resistance to passive or volitional neck flexion. Nuchal rigidity may take time to develop. Clinical tests for it, from least to most sensitive, are

- Kernig sign (resistance to passive knee extension)
- Brudzinski sign (full or partial flexion of the hips and knees when the neck is flexed)
- Difficulty touching the chin to the chest with the mouth closed
- Difficulty touching the forehead or chin to the knee

Nuchal rigidity can be distinguished from neck stiffness due to cervical spine osteoarthritis or influenza with severe myalgia. In these disorders, neck movement in all directions is usually affected. In contrast, nuchal rigidity due to meningeal irritation affects mostly neck flexion; thus, the neck can usually be rotated but cannot be flexed.

Diagnosis

- CSF analysis

Diagnosis is mainly by CSF analysis. Because meningitis can be serious and lumbar puncture is a safe procedure, lumbar puncture should usually be done if there is any suspicion of meningitis. CSF findings tend to differ by the type of meningitis but can overlap.

If patients have signs suggesting increased intracranial pressure (ICP) or a mass effect (eg, focal neurologic deficits, papilledema, deterioration in consciousness, seizures, especially if patients have HIV infection or are immunocompromised), neuroimaging—typically, contrast-enhanced CT or MRI—is done before lumbar puncture. In such patients, lumbar puncture may cause brain herniation.

Also, if a bleeding disorder is suspected, lumbar puncture is not done until the bleeding disorder is excluded or controlled.

When lumbar puncture is deferred, blood cultures should be obtained, followed immediately by empiric treatment with antibiotics. After ICP has been lowered and if no mass is detected, lumbar puncture can be done.

If the skin over the needle insertion site is infected or if a subcutaneous or parameningeal lumbar infection is suspected, the needle is inserted at a different site.

Treatment

- Antimicrobial therapy as indicated
- Adjunctive treatments

Infectious meningitis is treated with antimicrobial therapy as indicated clinically.

Adjunctive treatments for meningitis can include

- Supportive measures
- Treatment of complications or of associated disorders
- Removal of causative drugs
- For bacterial meningitis, corticosteroids

ACUTE BACTERIAL MENINGITIS

Acute bacterial meningitis is rapidly progressive bacterial infection of the meninges and subarachnoid space. Findings typically include headache, fever, and nuchal rigidity. Diagnosis is by CSF analysis. Treatment is with antibiotics and corticosteroids given as soon as possible.

Pathophysiology

Most commonly, bacteria reach the subarachnoid space and meninges via hematogenous spread. Bacteria may also reach the meninges from nearby infected structures or through a congenital or acquired defect in the skull or spine.

Because WBCs, immunoglobulins, and complement are normally sparse or absent from CSF, bacteria initially multiply without causing inflammation. Later, bacteria release endotoxins, teichoic acid, and other substances that trigger an inflammatory response with mediators such as WBCs and TNF. Typically in CSF, levels of protein increase, and because bacteria consume glucose and because less glucose is transported into the CSF, glucose levels decrease.

Inflammation in the subarachnoid space is accompanied by cortical encephalitis and ventriculitis. Complications are common and may include

- Hydrocephalus (in some patients)
- Arterial or venous infarcts due to inflammation and thrombosis of arteries and veins in superficial and sometimes deep areas of brain
- Abducens palsy due to inflammation of the 6th cranial nerve
- Deafness due to inflammation of the 8th cranial nerve or structures in the middle ear
- Subdural empyema
- Increased intracranial pressure (ICP) due to cerebral edema
- Brain herniation (the most common cause of death during the acute stages)
- Systemic complications (which are sometimes fatal), such as septic shock, disseminated intravascular coagulation (DIC), or hyponatremia due to syndrome of inappropriate antidiuretic hormone secretion (SIADH)

Etiology

Likely causes of bacterial meningitis depend on

- Patient age
- Route of entry
- Immune status of the patient

Age (see Table 231–1): In **children and young adults,** the most common causes of bacterial meningitis are

- *Neisseria meningitidis*
- *Streptococcus pneumoniae*

N. meningitidis meningitis occasionally causes death within hours. Sepsis caused by *N. meningitidis* sometimes results in bilateral adrenal hemorrhagic infarction (Waterhouse-Friderichsen syndrome).

Haemophilus influenzae type B, previously the most common cause of meningitis in children < 6 yr and overall, is now a rare cause in the US and Western Europe, where the *H. influenzae* vaccine is widely used. However, in areas where it is not widely used, *H. influenzae* is a common cause, particularly in children aged 2 mo to 6 yr.

In **middle-aged adults** and in **the elderly**, the most common cause of bacterial meningitis is

- *S. pneumoniae*

Less commonly, *N. meningitidis* causes meningitis in middle-aged and older adults. As host defenses decline with age, patients may develop meningitis due to *L. monocytogenes* or gram-negative bacteria.

In people of all ages, *Staphylococcus aureus* occasionally causes meningitis.

Route (see Table 231–2): Routes of entry include the following:

- By hematogenous spread (the most common route)
- From infected structures in or around the head (eg, sinuses, middle ear, mastoid process), sometimes associated with a CSF leak
- Through a penetrating wound
- After a neurosurgical procedure (eg, if a ventricular shunt becomes infected)
- Through congenital or acquired defects in the skull or spine

Having any of the above conditions increases the risk of acquiring meningitis.

Immune status: Overall, the most common causes of bacterial meningitis in immunocompromised patients are

- *S. pneumoniae*
- *L. monocytogenes*
- *Pseudomonas aeruginosa*
- *Mycobacterium tuberculosis*
- *N. meningitidis*
- Gram-negative bacteria

Table 231–1. CAUSES OF BACTERIAL MENINGITIS BY PATIENT AGE

AGE GROUP	BACTERIA
Children and young adults	*Neisseria meningitidis* *Streptococcus pneumoniae* *Staphylococcus aureus** *Haemophilus influenzae* (rare in developed countries but still seen in countries where the *H. influenzae* type B vaccine is not widely used)
Middle-aged adults	*S. pneumoniae* *S. aureus** *N. meningitidis* (less common in this age group)
The elderly	*S. pneumoniae* *S. aureus** *Listeria monocytogenes* Gram-negative bacteria

**S. aureus* occasionally causes severe meningitis in patients of all ages. It is the most common cause of meningitis that develops after a penetrating head wound.

Table 231–2. CAUSES OF BACTERIAL MENINGITIS BY ROUTE

ROUTE	BACTERIA
Infection in or around the head (eg, sinusitis, otitis, mastoiditis), sometimes with a CSF leak	*Streptococcus pneumoniae* *Haemophilus influenzae* Anaerobic and microaerophilic streptococci *Bacteroides* sp *Staphylococcus aureus*
Penetrating head wound	*S. aureus*
Damaged skin (eg, skin infections, abscesses, pressure ulcers, large burns)	*S. aureus*
An infected shunt	*S. epidermidis*
A neurosurgical procedure	Gram-negative bacteria (eg, *Klebsiella pneumoniae, Acinetobacter calcoaceticus, Escherichia coli*)

But the most likely bacteria depend on the type of immune deficiency:

- Defects in cell-mediated immunity (eg, in AIDS, Hodgkin lymphoma, or drug-induced immunosuppression): *L. monocytogenes* or mycobacteria
- Defects in humoral immunity or splenectomy: *S. pneumoniae* or, less frequently, *N. meningitidis* (both can cause fulminant meningitis)
- Neutropenia: *P. aeruginosa* or gram-negative enteric bacteria

In very young infants (particularly premature infants) and the elderly, T-cell immunity may be weak; thus, these age groups are at risk of meningitis due to *L. monocytogenes*.

Symptoms and Signs

In most cases, bacterial meningitis begins with 3 to 5 days of insidiously progressive nonspecific symptoms including malaise, fever, irritability, and vomiting. However, meningitis may be more rapid in onset and can be fulminant, making bacterial meningitis one of the few disorders in which a previously healthy young person may go to sleep with mild symptoms and never awaken.

Typical meningeal symptoms and signs include

- Fever
- Tachycardia
- Headache
- Photophobia
- Changes in mental status (eg, lethargy, obtundation)
- Nuchal rigidity (although not all patients report it)
- Sometimes, when *Staphylococcus aureus* is the cause, back pain

Seizures occur early in up to 40% of children with acute bacterial meningitis and may occur in adults. Up to 12% of patients present in coma. Severe meningitis may cause papilledema, but papilledema may be absent early, even when ICP is increased.

Accompanying systemic infection by the organism may cause

- Rashes, petechiae, or purpura (which suggest meningococcemia)
- Pulmonary consolidation (often in meningitis due to *S. pneumoniae*)
- Heart murmurs (which suggest endocarditis—eg, often caused by *S. aureus* or *S. pneumoniae*)

Atypical presentations in adults: Fever and nuchal rigidity may be absent or mild in immunocompromised or elderly patients and in alcoholics. Often, in the elderly, the only sign is confusion in those who were previously alert or altered responsiveness in those who have dementia. In such patients, starting appropriate antibiotics before head CT or MRI may be prudent.

If bacterial meningitis develops after a neurosurgical procedure, symptoms often take days to develop.

Diagnosis

■ CSF analysis

As soon as acute bacterial meningitis is suspected, blood cultures and lumbar puncture for CSF analysis (unless contraindicated) are done.

- If bacterial meningitis is suspected and the patient is very ill, antibiotics and corticosteroids are given immediately, even before lumbar puncture.
- If bacterial meningitis is suspected and lumbar puncture will be delayed pending CT or MRI, antibiotics and corticosteroids should be started after blood cultures but before neuroimaging is done; the need for confirmation should not delay treatment.

Clinicians should suspect bacterial meningitis in patients with typical symptoms and signs, usually fever, changes in mental status, and nuchal rigidity. However, clinicians must be aware that symptoms and signs are different in neonates and infants and may be absent or initially mild in the elderly, alcoholics, and immunocompromised patients. Diagnosis can be challenging in the following patients:

- Those who have had a neurosurgical procedure because such procedures can also cause changes in mental status and neck stiffness
- The elderly and alcoholics because changes in mental status may be due to metabolic encephalopathy (which may have multiple causes) or to falls and subdural hematomas

Focal seizures or focal neurologic deficits may indicate a focal lesion such as a brain abscess.

Because untreated bacterial meningitis is lethal, tests should be done if there is even a small chance of meningitis. Testing is particularly helpful in infants, the elderly, alcoholics, immunocompromised patients, and patients who had neurosurgical procedure because symptoms may be atypical.

PEARLS & PITFALLS

- Do a lumbar puncture even if findings are not specific for meningitis, particularly in infants, the elderly, alcoholics, immunocompromised patients, and patients who have had neurosurgery.

If findings suggest acute bacterial meningitis, routine tests include

- CSF analysis
- CBC and differential
- Metabolic panel
- Blood cultures plus PCR (if available)

Lumbar puncture: Unless contraindicated, lumbar puncture is done immediately to obtain CSF for analysis, the mainstay of diagnosis.

Contraindications to immediate lumbar puncture are signs suggesting markedly increased ICP or an intracranial mass effect (eg, due to edema, hemorrhage, or tumor); typically, these signs include

- Focal neurologic deficits
- Papilledema
- Deterioration in consciousness
- Seizures (within 1 wk of presentation)
- Immunocompromise
- History of CNS disease (eg, mass lesion, stroke, focal infection)

In such cases, lumbar puncture may cause brain herniation and thus is deferred until neuroimaging (typically CT or MRI) is done to check for increased ICP or a mass effect. When lumbar puncture is deferred, treatment is best begun immediately (after blood sampling for culture and before neuroimaging). After ICP, if increased, has been lowered or if no mass effect is detected, lumbar puncture can be done.

CSF should be sent for analysis: cell count, protein, glucose, Gram staining, culture, PCR (if available), and other tests as indicated clinically. Simultaneously, a blood sample should be drawn and sent to have the CSF:blood glucose ratio determined. CSF cell count should be determined as soon as possible because WBCs may adhere to the walls of the collecting tube, resulting in a falsely low cell count; in extremely purulent CSF, WBCs may lyse.

Typical CSF findings (see Table 231–3) in bacterial meningitis include

- Increased pressure
- Fluid that is often turbid
- A high WBC count (consisting predominantly of PMNs)
- Elevated protein
- A low CSF:blood glucose ratio

A CSF:blood glucose level of < 50% suggests possible meningitis. A CSF glucose level of ≤ 18 mg/dL or a CSF:blood glucose ratio of < 0.23 strongly suggests bacterial meningitis. However, changes in CSF glucose may lag 30 to 120 min behind changes in blood glucose. In acute bacterial meningitis, an elevated protein level (usually 100 to 500 mg/dL) indicates blood-brain barrier injury.

CSF cell count and protein and glucose levels in patients with acute bacterial meningitis are not always typical. Atypical CSF findings may include

- Normal in early stages except for the presence of bacteria
- Predominance of lymphocytes in about 14% of patients, particularly in neonates with gram-negative meningitis, patients with meningitis due to *L. monocytogenes*, and some patients with partially treated bacterial meningitis
- Normal glucose in about 9% of patients
- Normal WBC counts in severely immunosuppressed patients

Identification of the causative bacteria involves Gram staining, culture, and, when available, PCR. Gram staining provides information rapidly, but the information is limited. For bacteria to be reliably detected with Gram stain, about 10^5 bacteria/mm^3 must be present. Results may be falsely negative if CSF is handled carelessly, if bacteria are not adequately resuspended after CSF has been allowed to

Table 231–3. CSF FINDINGS IN MENINGITIS

CONDITION	PREDOMINANT CELL TYPE*	PROTEIN*	GLUCOSE*	SPECIFIC TESTS
Normal CSF	**All lymphocytes (0–5 cells/μL)**	**< 40 mg/dL**	**> 50% of blood glucose**	**None**
Bacterial meningitis	Leukocytes (usually PMNs), often greatly increased	Elevated	< 50% of blood glucose (may be extremely low)	Gram staining (yield is high if 10^5 colony-forming units of bacteria/ mL are present) Bacterial culture PCR if available
Viral meningitis	Lymphocytes (may be mixed; PMNs and lymphocytes during the first 24–48 h)	Elevated	Usually normal	PCR (to check for enteroviruses or herpes simplex, herpes zoster, or West Nile virus) IgM (to check for West Nile virus or other arboviruses)
†Tuberculous meningitis	PMNs and lymphocytes (usually pleocytosis)	Elevated	< 50% of blood glucose (may be extremely low)	Acid-fast staining PCR Mycobacterial culture (ideally using a CSF sample of ≥ 30 mL) Interferon-γ tests of serum and (if available) CSF
Fungal meningitis	Usually lymphocytes	Elevated	< 50% of blood glucose (may be extremely low)	Cryptococcal antigen test Serologic tests for *Coccidioides immitis* or *Histoplasma* sp antigen, especially if patients have recently spent time in an endemic area Fungal culture (ideally using a CSF sample of ≥ 30 mL) India ink (for *Cryptococcus* sp)

*Changes in cell count, glucose, and protein may be minimal in severely immunocompromised patients.

†In tuberculous meningitis, CSF acid-fast staining can be insensitive, sensitivity of PCR is only about 50%, and culture requires up to 8 wk. Positive CSF interferon-γ tests indicate tuberculous meningitis, but serum interferon-γ tests may only indicate prior infection. Thus, confirming a diagnosis of tuberculous meningitis is difficult, and if it is strongly suspected, even if not confirmed, it is treated presumptively.

‡A small number of cells vmay be present normally in neonates or after a seizure.

PCR = polymerase chain reaction; PMNs = polymorphonuclear neutrophils.

settle, or if errors in decolorization or reading of the slide occur.

Diagnosis of the specific bacteria and determination of antibiotic sensitivity requires bacterial culture. If clinicians suspect an anaerobic infection or other unusual bacteria, they should tell the laboratory before samples are plated for cultures. Prior antibiotic therapy can reduce the yield from Gram staining and culture. PCR, if available, may be a useful adjunctive test, especially in patients who have already received antibiotics.

Until the cause of meningitis is confirmed, other tests using samples of CSF or blood may be done to check for other causes of meningitis, such as viruses (particularly herpes simplex), fungi, and cancer cells.

Other tests: Samples from other sites suspected of being infected (eg, urinary or respiratory tract) are also cultured.

Prognosis

For children < 19 yr, the mortality rate may be as low as 3% but is often higher; survivors may be deaf and neuropsychologically impaired. The mortality rate is about 17% for adults < 60 yr but up to 37% in those > 60. Community-acquired meningitis due to *S. aureus* has a mortality rate of 43%.

In general, mortality rate correlates with depth of obtundation or coma. Factors associated with a poor prognosis include

- Age > 60 yr
- Coexisting debilitating disorders
- A low Glasgow coma score at admission (see Tables 224–4 on p. 1862 and 349–1 on p. 2929)
- Focal neurologic deficits
- A low CSF cell count
- Increased CSF pressure (particularly)

Table 231–4. INITIAL ANTIBIOTICS FOR ACUTE BACTERIAL MENINGITIS

PATIENT GROUP	SUSPECTED BACTERIA	PROVISIONAL ANTIBIOTICS
Age		
< 3 mo	*Streptococcus agalactiae* *Escherichia coli* or other gram-negative bacteria *Listeria monocytogenes* *Staphylococcus aureus**	Ampicillin *plus* Ceftriaxone or cefotaxime
3 mo–18 yr	*Neisseria meningitidis* *S. pneumoniae* *S. aureus** *Haemophilus influenzae*‡	Cefotaxime or ceftriaxone *plus* Vancomycin
18–50 yr	*S. pneumoniae* *N. meningitidis* *S. aureus**	Ceftriaxone or cefotaxime *plus* Vancomycin
> 50 yr	*S. pneumoniae* *L. monocytogenes* *S. aureus* Gram-negative bacteria *N. meningitidis* (unusual in this age group)	Ceftriaxone or cefotaxime *plus* Ampicillin *plus* Vancomycin
Route		
Sinusitis, otitis, CSF leaks	*S. pneumoniae*† *H. influenzae* Gram-negative bacteria including *Pseudomonas aeruginosa* Anaerobic or microaerophilic streptococci *Bacteroides fragilis* *S. aureus**	Vancomycin *plus* Ceftazidime or meropenem *plus* Metronidazole
Penetrating head wounds, neurosurgical procedures, shunt infections	*S. aureus* *S. epidermidis* Gram-negative bacteria including *P. aeruginosa* *S. pneumoniae*	Vancomycin *plus* Ceftazidime
Immune status		
AIDS, other conditions that impair cell-mediated immunity	*S. pneumoniae* *L. monocytogenes* Gram-negative bacteria including *P. aeruginosa* *S. aureus**	Ampicillin *plus* Ceftazidime *plus* Vancomycin

**S. aureus* is an uncommon cause of meningitis except when the route is a penetrating head wound or a neurosurgical procedure. However, it can cause meningitis in all patient groups. Thus, vancomycin or other antistaphylococcal antibiotics should be given if clinicians think that these bacteria are a possible, even if unlikely, cause.

†*S. pneumoniae* is the most common causative bacteria in patients with a CSF leak or acute otitis. Such patients may be treated with vancomycin and ceftriaxone or cefotaxime. However, when meningitis is accompanied by subdural empyema or develops after a neurosurgical procedure, other bacteria, including *P. aeruginosa*, are more likely to be present; in such cases, initial treatment should include vancomycin plus ceftazidime plus metronidazole.

‡*H. influenzae*should be considered in children < 5 yr with no record of *H. influenzae* type b conjugate vaccination.

Seizures and a low CSF:serum glucose ratio may also indicate a poor prognosis.

Treatment

- Antibiotics
- Corticosteroids to decrease cerebral inflammation and edema

Antibiotics are the mainstay of therapy. In addition to antibiotics, treatment includes measures to decrease brain and cranial nerve inflammation and increased ICP.

Most patients are admitted to an ICU.

Antibiotics: Antibiotics must be bactericidal for the causative bacteria and must be able to penetrate the blood-brain barrier.

If patients appear ill and findings suggest meningitis, antibiotics (see Table 231–4) and corticosteroids are started as soon as blood cultures are drawn and even before lumbar puncture. Also, if lumbar puncture is delayed pending neuroimaging results, antibiotic and corticosteroid treatment begins before neuroimaging.

PEARLS & PITFALLS

- If patients appear ill and acute meningitis is suspected, treat them with antibiotics and corticosteroids as soon as blood for cultures is drawn.

Appropriate empiric antibiotics depend on the patient's age and immune status and route of infection (see Table 231–5). In general, clinicians should use antibiotics that are effective against *S. pneumoniae*, *N. meningitidis*, and *S. aureus*. Sometimes (eg, in neonates and some immunosuppressed patients), herpes simplex encephalitis cannot be excluded; thus, acyclovir is added. Antibiotic therapy may need to be modified based on results of culture and sensitivity testing.

Commonly used antibiotics (see Table 231–6) include

- 3rd-generation cephalosporins for *S. pneumoniae* and *N. meningitidis*
- Ampicillin for *L. monocytogenes*
- Vancomycin for penicillin-resistant strains of *S. pneumoniae* and for *S. aureus*

Table 231–5. SPECIFIC ANTIBIOTICS FOR ACUTE BACTERIAL MENINGITIS

BACTERIA	AGE GROUP	ANTIBIOTICS*	COMMENTS
Gram-positive bacteria (unidentified)	Children and adults	Vancomycin *plus* Ceftriaxone (cefotaxime) and ampicillin†	—
Gram-negative bacilli (unidentified)	Children and adults	Cefotaxime (or ceftriaxone, meropenem, or ceftazidime) *plus* Gentamicin, tobramycin, or amikacin‡ if systemic infection is suspected	—
Haemophilus influenzae type b	Children and adults	Ceftriaxone (cefotaxime)	—
Neisseria meningitidis	Children and adults	Ceftriaxone (cefotaxime)	Penicillin G is used for susceptible strains after sensitivities are known.
Streptococcus pneumoniae	Children and adults	Vancomycin and ceftriaxone (cefotaxime)	Penicillin G may be used for susceptible strains after sensitivities are known.
Staphylococcus aureus and *S. epidermidis*	Children and adults	Vancomycin with or without rifampin	Vancomycin is used for methicillin-resistant strains, or nafcillin or oxacillin may be used after sensitivities are known. Rifampin is added if no improvement occurs with vancomycin or nafcillin.
Listeria sp	Children and adults	Ampicillin (penicillin G) *or* Trimethoprim/sulfamethoxazole‡	Penicillin G is used for susceptible strains after sensitivities are known. Trimethoprim/sulfamethoxazole is used in patients who are allergic to penicillin.
Enteric gram-negative bacteria (eg, *Escherichia coli*, *Klebsiella* sp, *Proteus* sp)	Children and adults	Ceftriaxone (cefotaxime) *plus* Gentamicin, tobramycin, or amikacin‡ if systemic infection is suspected	—
Pseudomonas sp	Children and adults	Meropenem (ceftazidime or cefepime), usually alone but sometimes with an aminoglycoside *or* Aztreonam	—

*Alternative antibiotics are in parentheses.

†If gram-positive bacteria are pleomorphic, ampicillin is included to cover *Listeria* sp.

‡Amikacin is used in areas where gentamicin resistance is common. Because aminoglycosides have poor CSF penetration, they are infrequently used for treatment of meningitis. When required, they may have to be given intrathecally or via an Ommaya reservoir, especially in patients with *Pseudomonas* meningitis. When aminoglycosides are used, renal function should be monitored.

Table 231–6. COMMON IV ANTIBIOTIC DOSAGES FOR ACUTE BACTERIAL MENINGITIS*

ANTIBIOTIC	DOSAGE	
	CHILDREN > 1 MO	ADULTS
Ceftriaxone	50 mg/kg q 12 h	2 g q 12 h
Cefotaxime	50 mg/kg q 6 h	2 g q 4–6 h
Ceftazidime	50 mg/kg q 8 h	2 g q 8 h
Cefepime	2 g q 12 h	2 g q 8–12 h
Ampicillin	75 mg/kg q 6 h	2–3 g q 4 h
Penicillin G	4 million units q 4 h	4 million units q 4 h
Nafcillin and oxacillin	50 mg/kg q 6 h	2 g q 4 h
Vancomycin†	15 mg/kg q 6 h	10–15 mg/kg q 8 h
Meropenem	40 mg/kg q 8 h	2 g q 8 h
Gentamicin and tobramycin†	2.5 mg/kg q 8 h	2 mg/kg q 8 h
Amikacin†	10 mg/kg q 8 h	7.5 mg/kg q 12 h
Rifampin	6.7 mg/kg q 8 h	600 mg q 24 h

*For neonatal dosages, see Table 314–1 on p. 2620.
†Renal function should be monitored.

Corticosteroids: Dexamethasone is used to decrease cerebral and cranial nerve inflammation and edema; it should be given when therapy is started. Adults are given 10 mg IV; children are given 0.15 mg/kg IV. Dexamethasone is given immediately before or with the initial dose of antibiotics and q 6 h for 4 days. Use of dexamethasone is best established for patients with pneumococcal meningitis.

Other measures: The effectiveness of other measures is less well-proved.

Patients presenting with papilledema or signs of impending brain herniation are treated for increased ICP:

- Elevation of the head of the bed to 30°
- Hyperventilation to a PCO_2 of 27 to 30 mm Hg to cause intracranial vasoconstriction
- Osmotic diuresis with IV mannitol

Usually, adults are given mannitol 1 g/kg IV bolus over 30 min, repeated prn q 3 to 4 h or 0.25 g/kg q 2 to 3 h, and children are given 0.5 to 2.0 g/kg over 30 min, repeated prn.

Additional measures can include

- IV fluids
- Anticonvulsants
- Treatment of concomitant infections
- Treatment of specific complications (eg, corticosteroids for Waterhouse-Friderichsen syndrome, surgical drainage for subdural empyema)

Prevention

Use of vaccines for *H. influenzae* type B and, to a lesser extent, for *N. meningitidis* and *S. pneumoniae* has reduced the incidence of bacterial meningitis.

Physical measures: Keeping patients in respiratory isolation (using droplet precautions) for the first 24 h of therapy can help prevent meningitis from spreading. Gloves, masks, and gowns are used.

Vaccination: Vaccination can prevent certain types of bacterial meningitis.

A **conjugated pneumococcal vaccine** effective against 13 serotypes, including > 80% of organisms that cause meningitis, is recommended for all children (see Table 291–2 on p. 2462).

Routine vaccination against *H. influenzae* type b is highly effective and begins at age 2 mo.

A **quadrivalent meningococcal vaccine** is given to

- Children who are 2 to 10 yr if they have an immunodeficiency or functional asplenia
- All children at age 11 to 12 yr
- Older children, college students living in dormitories, and military recruits who have not had the vaccine previously
- Travelers to or residents of endemic areas
- Laboratory personnel who routinely handle meningococcal specimens

During a meningitis epidemic, the population at risk (eg, college students, a small town) must be identified, and its size must be determined before proceeding to mass vaccination. The effort is expensive and requires public education and support, but it saves lives and reduces morbidity.

The meningococcal vaccine does not protect against serotype B meningococcal meningitis; this information should be kept in mind when a vaccinated patient presents with symptoms of meningitis.

Chemoprophylaxis: Anyone who has prolonged face-to-face contact with a patient who has meningitis (eg, household or day care contacts, medical personnel and other people who are exposed to the patient's oral secretions) should be given postexposure chemoprophylaxis.

For **meningococcal meningitis,** chemoprophylaxis consists of one of the following:

- Rifampin 600 mg (for children > 1 mo, 10 mg/kg; for children < 1 mo, 5 mg/kg) po q 12 h for 4 doses
- Ceftriaxone 250 mg (for children < 15 yr, 125 mg) IM for 1 dose
- For adults, a fluoroquinolone (ciprofloxacin or levofloxacin 500 mg or ofloxacin 400 mg) po for 1 dose

For **meningitis due to *H. influenzae* type b**, chemoprophylaxis is rifampin 20 mg/kg po once/day (maximum: 600 mg/day) for 4 days. There is no consensus on whether children < 2 yr require prophylaxis for exposure at day care.

Chemoprophylaxis is not usually needed for contacts of patients with other types of bacterial meningitis.

KEY POINTS

- Common causes include *N. meningitidis* and *S. pneumoniae* in children and adults and *Listeria* sp in infants and the elderly; *S. aureus* occasionally causes meningitis in people of all ages.
- Typical features may be absent or subtle in infants, alcoholics, the elderly, immunocompromised patients, and patients who develop meningitis after a neurosurgical procedure.
- If patients have focal neurologic deficits, obtundation, seizures, or papilledema (suggesting increased ICP or an intracranial mass effect), defer lumbar puncture pending results of neuroimaging.
- Treat acute bacterial meningitis as soon as possible, even before the diagnosis is confirmed.
- Common empirically chosen antibiotic regimens often include 3rd-generation cephalosporins (for *S. pneumoniae* and *N. meningitidis*), ampicillin (for *L. monocytogenes*), and vancomycin (for penicillin-resistant strains of *S. pneumoniae* and for *S. aureus*).
- Routine vaccination for *S. pneumoniae* and *N. meningitidis* and chemoprophylaxis against *N. meningitidis* help prevent meningitis.

VIRAL MENINGITIS

Viral meningitis tends to be less severe than acute bacterial meningitis. Findings include headache, fever, and nuchal rigidity. Diagnosis is by CSF analysis. Treatment is with supportive measures, acyclovir for suspected herpes simplex, and antiretroviral drugs for suspected HIV infection.

Viral meningitis is sometimes used synonymously with aseptic meningitis. However, aseptic meningitis usually refers to acute meningitis caused by anything other than the bacteria that typically cause acute bacterial meningitis. Thus, aseptic meningitis can be caused by viruses, noninfectious conditions (eg, drugs, disorders), fungi, or, occasionally, other organisms (eg, in Lyme disease, in syphilis).

Causes

Viral meningitis usually results from hematogenous spread, but meningitis due to herpes simplex virus type 2 (HSV-2) can also result from reactivation of latent infection.

The most common cause of viral meningitis is

- Enteroviruses

For many viruses that cause meningitis (unlike the bacteria that cause acute bacterial meningitis), incidence is seasonal (see Table 231–7).

Symptoms and Signs

Viral meningitis, like acute bacterial meningitis, usually begins with symptoms that suggest viral infection (eg, fever, myalgias, GI or respiratory symptoms), followed by symptoms and signs of meningitis (headache, fever, nuchal rigidity). Manifestations tend to resemble those of bacterial meningitis but are usually less severe (eg, nuchal rigidity may be less pronounced). However, findings are sometimes severe enough to suggest acute bacterial meningitis.

Diagnosis

- CSF analysis (cell count, protein, glucose)
- PCR of CSF and sometimes IgM
- Sometimes PCR and/or culture of blood, a throat swab, nasopharyngeal secretions, or stool

Diagnosis of viral meningitis is based on analysis of CSF obtained by lumbar puncture (preceded by neuroimaging if increased intracranial pressure or a mass is suspected). Typically, protein is slightly increased but less than that in acute bacterial meningitis (eg, < 150 mg/dL); however, the protein level can be very high in West Nile virus meningitis. Glucose is usually normal or only slightly lower than normal. Other findings include pleocytosis with a lymphocytic predominance. Nonetheless, no

Table 231–7. COMMON CAUSES OF VIRAL MENINGITIS

VIRUS	MECHANISM OF TRANSMISSION	SEASONAL INCIDENCE
Enteroviruses (eg, coxsackieviruses, echoviruses	Fecal-oral spread (eg, via contaminated food, in swimming pools)	Summer to early autumn Sometimes sporadic cases throughout year
*Herpes simplex, usually virus type 2	Close contact with a person actively shedding the virus	None
Varicella-zoster virus	Inhalation of respiratory droplets from or by contact with an infected person	None
Western equine virus† Venezuelan equine virus†	Mosquito	Summer to early autumn
West Nile virus St. Louis virus	Mosquito	Summer to early autumn
California encephalitis virus La Crosse virus	Mosquito	Summer to early autumn
Colorado tick fever virus (unusual)	Ticks	Late spring to early summer
Lymphocytic choriomeningitis virus	Airborne‡	Autumn to winter
HIV-1 HIV-2	Contact with body fluids of an infected person	None§

*Herpes simplex type 2 meningitis may occur as an isolated instance or may recur.
†Western equine and Venezuelan equine viruses have been associated with meningitis, but no cases have been reported in the US in recent years.
‡Lymphocytic choriomeningitis virus is associated with exposure to infected wild mice (the natural host for this virus) and is most common during autumn or winter when mice tend to move indoors. Infection may also occur year-round when the cause is exposure to infected pet hamsters.
§Meningitis due to HIV usually begins early in the course of systemic infection—when seroconversion occurs.

combination of findings in CSF cells, protein, and glucose can rule out bacterial meningitis.

CSF viral culture is insensitive and not routinely done. PCR can be used to detect some viruses in CSF (enteroviruses and herpes simplex, herpes zoster, West Nile viruses). Measurement of IgM in CSF is more sensitive than PCR in diagnosing suspected West Nile virus or other arboviruses.

Viral serologic tests, PCR, or culture of samples taken from other areas (eg, blood, a throat swab, nasopharyngeal secretions, stool) may help identify the causative virus.

PEARLS & PITFALLS

- If patients appear seriously ill, treat them for acute bacterial meningitis until it is ruled out, even if the cause is suspected to be viral.

Treatment

- Supportive measures
- Acyclovir (for suspected herpes simplex or herpes zoster) and antiretroviral drugs (for HIV infection)

If patients appear seriously ill and if acute bacterial seems possible (even if viral meningitis is suspected), appropriate antibiotics and corticosteroids are started immediately (without waiting for test results) and continued until bacterial meningitis is ruled out (ie, CSF is shown to be sterile).

Viral meningitis usually resolves spontaneously over weeks or, occasionally (eg, in West Nile virus meningitis or lymphocytic choriomeningitis), months. Treatment is mainly supportive.

Acyclovir is efficacious in treating herpes simplex meningitis and can be used to treat herpes zoster meningitis. If either of these viruses is suspected or if herpes simplex encephalitis is at all suspected, most clinicians begin empiric treatment with acyclovir and, if PCR is negative for these viruses, then stop the drug.

Pleconaril is only modestly efficacious for meningitis due to enteroviruses and is not available for routine clinical use.

Patients with HIV meningitis are treated with antiretroviral drugs.

KEY POINTS

- Viral meningitis begins with symptoms typical of a viral illness, followed by headache, fever, and nuchal rigidity, but is rarely as severe as acute bacterial meningitis.
- Enteroviruses are the most common cause, usually during summer or early autumn.
- CSF findings (usually lymphocytic pleocytosis, near normal glucose, and slightly increased protein) cannot exclude acute bacterial meningitis.
- Treat patients for acute bacterial meningitis until that diagnosis is ruled out.
- Treatment is mainly supportive; patients with herpes simplex or herpes zoster meningitis may be treated with acyclovir.

NONINFECTIOUS MENINGITIS

Meningitis is occasionally caused by noninfectious conditions (eg, noninfectious disorders, drugs, vaccines). Many cases of noninfectious meningitis are subacute or chronic (see Table 231–8).

Noninfectious meningitis causes symptoms (eg, headache, fever, nuchal rigidity) that are similar to those caused by other kinds of meningitis. Severity and acuity can vary, but noninfectious meningitis tends to be less severe than acute bacterial meningitis.

Table 231–8. SOME NONINFECTIOUS CAUSES OF MENINGITIS

TYPE	EXAMPLES
Disorders	Metastatic cancer Sarcoidosis Behçet syndrome SLE Sjögren syndrome RA Rupture of an intracranial cysticercal or epidermoid cyst
Drugs with anti-inflammatory or immune-modulating effects	Azathioprine Cyclosporine Cytosine arabinoside IVIG Muromonab-CD3 (OKT3) NSAIDs (most commonly, ibuprofen)
Other drugs	Certain antibiotics (eg, ciprofloxacin, isoniazid, penicillin, trimethoprim/sulfamethoxazole) Carbamazepine Phenazopyridine Ranitidine
Substances injected into the subarachnoid space	Anesthetics Antibiotics Chemotherapy drugs Radiopaque dyes
Vaccines	Pertussis Rabies Smallpox

Diagnosis of noninfectious meningitis is based on analysis of CSF obtained by lumbar puncture (preceded by neuroimaging if increased ICP or an intracranial mass effect is suspected). CSF findings may include

- Lymphocytic or neutrophilic pleocytosis
- Elevated protein
- Usually normal glucose

Causative disorders are treated, and causative drugs are stopped. Otherwise, treatment is supportive.

If patients appear seriously ill, appropriate antibiotics and corticosteroids are started immediately (without waiting for tests results) and continued until acute bacterial meningitis is ruled out (ie, CSF is shown to be sterile).

RECURRENT MENINGITIS

Recurrent meningitis is usually caused by bacteria, viruses, or noninfectious conditions.

Recurrent viral meningitis: Recurrent viral meningitis is most often due to

- Herpes simplex virus type 2 (HSV-2; called Mollaret meningitis)

Typically when HSV-2 is the cause, patients have ≥ 3 episodes of fever, nuchal rigidity, and CSF lymphocytic pleocytosis; each episode lasts from 2 to 5 days, then resolves spontaneously. Patients can also have other neurologic deficits (eg, altered sensorium, seizures, cranial nerve palsies).

The cause is treated if possible. Mollaret meningitis is treated with acyclovir. Most patients recover fully.

Recurrent acute bacterial meningitis: Acute bacterial meningitis may recur if it is acquired via a congenital or acquired defect at the skull base or in the spine and that defect is not corrected. If the cause is an injury, meningitis may not develop until many years later.

If patients have recurrent bacterial meningitis, clinicians should thoroughly check for such defects. High-resolution CT can usually show defects in the skull. Clinicians should check the patient's lower back for a dimple or tuft of hair, which may indicate a defect in the spine (eg, spina bifida).

Rarely, recurrent bacterial meningitis (usually due to *Streptococcus pneumoniae* or *Neisseria meningitidis*) results from a deficiency in the complement system. Treatment is the same as that used in patients without complement deficits. Vaccination against *S. pneumoniae* and *N. meningitidis* (repeated every 3 yr) may reduce likelihood of infection.

Other recurrent meningitides: Acute meningitis secondary to NSAIDs or other drugs may recur when the causative drug is used again.

SUBACUTE AND CHRONIC MENINGITIS

Subacute meningitis develops over days to a few weeks. Chronic meningitis lasts ≥ 4 wk. Possible causes include fungi, *Mycobacterium tuberculosis*, rickettsiae, spirochetes, *Toxoplasma gondii*, HIV, enteroviruses, and disorders such as autoimmune rheumatic disorders (eg, SLE, RA) and cancer. Symptoms and signs are similar to those of other meningitides but more indolent. Cranial nerve palsies and infarction (due to vasculitis) may occur. Diagnosis requires analysis of a large volume of CSF (typically obtained via repeated lumbar punctures) and sometimes biopsy or ventricular or cisternal puncture. Treatment is directed at the cause.

Chronic meningitis may last > 25 yr. Rarely, chronic meningitis has a protracted benign course, then resolves spontaneously.

Subacute and chronic meningitis may result from a wide variety of organisms and conditions (see Table 231–9).

Tuberculous meningitis: *M. tuberculosis* are aerobic bacteria that replicate in host cells; thus, control of these bacteria depends largely on T cell-mediated immunity (see p. 1650). These bacteria may infect the CNS during primary or reactivated infection. In developed countries, meningitis usually results from reactivated infection.

Meningeal symptoms usually develop over days to a few weeks but may develop much more rapidly or gradually. Characteristically, *M. tuberculosis* causes a basilar meningitis that results in 3 complications:

- Hydrocephalus due to obstruction of the foramina of Luschka and Magendi or the aqueduct of Sylvius
- Vasculitis, sometimes causing arterial or venous occlusion and stroke
- Cranial nerve deficits, particularly of cranial nerves II, VII, and VIII

Diagnosis of tuberculous meningitis may be difficult. There may be no evidence of systemic tuberculosis. Inflammation of the basilar meninges, shown by contrast-enhanced CT or MRI, suggests the diagnosis.

Characteristically, CSF findings include

- Mixed pleocytosis with lymphocytic predominance
- Low glucose
- Elevated protein (see Table 231–3)

Occasionally, the first CSF abnormality is extremely low glucose.

Detecting the causative organism is often difficult because

- CSF acid-fast staining is ≤ 30% sensitive.
- CSF mycobacterial cultures are only about 70% sensitive and require up to 6 wk.
- CSF PCR is about 50 to 70% sensitive.

An automated rapid nucleic acid amplification test called Xpert MTB/RIF has been recommended by the WHO for the diagnosis of tuberculous meningitis. This test detects *M. tuberculosis* DNA and resistance to rifampicin in CSF specimens.

Because tuberculous meningitis has a rapid and destructive course and because diagnostic tests are limited, this infection should be treated based on clinical suspicion. Currently, the WHO recommends treatment with isoniazid, rifampin, pyrazinamide, and ethambutol for 2 mo followed by isoniazid and rifampin for 6 to 7 mo (see p. 1654). Corticosteroids

Table 231–9. MAJOR INFECTIOUS CAUSES OF SUBACUTE OR CHRONIC MENINGITIS

ORGANISMS	CIRCUMSTANCES
Bacteria	
Mycobacteria: (*Mycobacterium tuberculosis*, rarely other mycobacteria)	—
Spirochetes: Lyme disease, syphilis, rarely leptospirosis	For Lyme disease, East Coast, upper Midwest, California, Oregon
Brucella sp	Associated with livestock Unusual in the US or other developed countries
Ehrlichia sp	—
Leptospira sp	Associated with exposure to urine of rats, mice, and other animals Unusual in Western countries
Fungi	
Cryptococcus neoformans	—
C. gattii	Predominantly northern Pacific coast Appears to have a widespread distribution
Coccidioides immitis	Southwestern US
Histoplasma capsulatum	Central and Eastern US
Blastomyces sp	Predominantly Central and Eastern US
Sporothrix sp (unusual)	No geographic distribution, but infection associated with rose thorns or brush
Parasites	
Toxoplasma gondii	—
Viruses	
Retroviruses: HIV, HTLV-1	In patients with known HIV or risk factors
Enteroviruses	In patients with a congenital immunodeficiency syndrome

(prednisone or dexamethasone) may be added if patients present with stupor, coma, or neurologic deficits.

Meningitis due to spirochetes: Lyme disease (see p. 1715) is a chronic spirochetal infection caused by *Borrelia burgdorferi* in the US and by *B. afzelii* and *B. garinii* in Europe. The disease is spread by *Ixodes* ticks, usually the deer tick in the US. In the US, 12 states account for 95% of cases. The states include mid-Atlantic and northeastern coastal states, Wisconsin, California, Oregon, and Washington. Up to 8% of children and some adults who contract Lyme disease develop meningitis. The meningitis may be acute or chronic; usually, it begins more slowly than acute viral meningitis.

Clues to the diagnosis include

- Time spent in wooded areas and travel to an endemic area (including in Europe)
- History of erythema migrans or other symptoms of Lyme disease
- Unilateral or bilateral facial palsy (common in Lyme disease but rare in most viral meningitides)
- Papilledema (well-described in children with Lyme disease but rare in viral meningitis)

CSF findings typically include

- Lymphocytic pleocytosis
- Moderately elevated protein
- Normal glucose

Diagnosis of Lyme disease is based on serologic tests with enzyme-linked immunosorbent assay (ELISA), followed by Western blot analysis to confirm. In some laboratories, false-positive rates may be unacceptably high.

Treatment of Lyme meningitis is with cefotaxime or ceftriaxone given over 14 days. Doses for cefotaxime are 150 to 200 mg/kg/day IV in 3 to 4 divided doses (eg, 50 mg tid to qid) for children and 2 g IV q 8 h for adults. Doses for ceftriaxone are 50 to 75 mg/kg/day IV (2 g maximum) once/day for children and 2 g IV once/day for adults. Clinicians should remember that concomitant anaplasmosis or babesiosis is possible in patients with severe disease.

Syphilitic meningitis is less common; it is usually a feature of meningovascular syphilis. The meningitis may be acute or chronic. It may be accompanied by complications such as cerebrovascular arteritis (possibly causing thrombosis with ischemia or infarction), retinitis, cranial nerve deficits (especially of the 7th cranial nerve), or myelitis.

CSF findings may include pleocytosis (usually lymphocytic), elevated protein, and low glucose. These abnormalities may be more pronounced in patients with AIDS.

Diagnosis of syphilitic meningitis is based on serum and CSF serologic tests, followed by fluorescent treponemal antibody absorption (FTA-ABS) testing to confirm. MR angiography and cerebral angiography may accurately differentiate between parenchymal disease and arteritis.

Patients with syphilitic meningitis are treated with aqueous penicillin 12 to 24 million units IV/day given in divided doses q 4 h (eg, 2 to 4 million units q 4 h) for 10 to 14 days.

Cryptococcal meningitis: Cryptococcal meningitis is the most common cause of chronic meningitis in the Western hemisphere and the most common opportunistic infection in patients with AIDS (see on p. 1572). Common causes of cryptococcal meningitis in the US are

- *Cryptococcus neoformans* var. *neoformans* (serotype D strains)
- *C. neoformans* var. *grubii* (serotype A strains)

C. neoformans var. *grubii* causes 90% of cases. *C. neoformans* can be in soil, trees, and pigeon or other bird excreta. Meningitis due to *C. neoformans* usually develops in immunocompromised patients but occasionally develops in patients without apparent underlying disease.

Another cryptococcal species, *C. gattii*, has caused meningitis in the Pacific region and Washington state; it may cause meningitis in people with a normal immune status.

Cryptococci cause a basilar meningitis with hydrocephalus and cranial nerve deficits; vasculitis is less common. Meningeal symptoms usually begin insidiously, at times with protracted relapses and remissions.

CSF findings typically include

- Lymphocytic pleocytosis
- Elevated protein
- Low glucose

However, cellular response may be minimal or absent in patients with advanced AIDS or another severe immunocompromised state.

Diagnosis of cryptococcal meningitis is based on cryptococcal antigen tests and fungal culture; diagnostic yield with these tests is 80 to 90%. India ink preparation, which has a sensitivity of 50%, may also be used.

Patients who have *C. neoformans* meningitis but do not have AIDS are traditionally treated with the synergistic combination of 5-fluorocytosine and amphotericin B. Patients with cryptococcal meningitis and AIDS are treated with amphotericin B plus flucytosine (if tolerated) followed by fluconazole.

Fungal meningitis that develops after epidural methylprednisolone injection: Occasionally, outbreaks of fungal meningitis have occurred in patients given spinal epidural injections of methylprednisolone. In each case, the drug had been prepared by a compounding pharmacy, and there were significant violations of sterile technique during drug preparation.

The first outbreak in the United States (in 2002) resulted in 5 cases of meningitis. The most recent outbreak (in 2012) resulted in 414 cases of meningitis, stroke, myelitis, or other fungal infection-related complications and in 31 deaths. Outbreaks have also occurred in Sri Lanka (7 cases) and Minnesota (1 case). Most cases were caused by *Exophiala dermatitidis* in 2002 and by *Exserohilum rostratum* in 2012; a few cases were caused by *Aspergillus* or *Cladosporium* sp.

The meningitis tends to develop insidiously, often with infection at the base of the brain; blood vessels may be affected, resulting in vasculitis and stroke. Headache is the most common presenting symptoms, followed by altered cognition, nausea or vomiting, or fever. Symptoms may be delayed by as much as 6 mo after the epidural injection. Signs of meningeal irritation are absent in about one-third of patients.

Typical CSF findings include

- Neutrophilic pleocytosis
- Elevated protein
- Frequently low glucose

The most sensitive test for *Exserohilum* meningitis is a PCR test, available through the Centers for Disease Control and Prevention; in a few cases, the diagnosis can be based on culture.

Aspergillus meningitis may be suspected if galactomannan levels in CSF are elevated; diagnosis is based on culture.

Meningitis due to *Exophiala* or *Exserohilum* sp is rare, and definitive treatment is not known. However, voriconazole 6 mg/kg/day IV is recommended initially. Drug dosage should be adjusted based on blood levels of the drug. Liver enzyme and Na levels should be measured periodically during the 2 to 3 wk after initiation of treatment. Prognosis is guarded, and appropriate treatment does not guarantee survival.

Other fungal meningitides: *Coccidioides*, *Histoplasma*, *Blastomyces*, *Sporothrix*, and *Candida* sp may all cause chronic meningitis similar to that caused by *C. neoformans*. *Coccidioides* sp are confined to the American Southwest (predominantly southern Utah, New Mexico, Arizona, and California). *Histoplasma* and *Blastomyces* sp occur predominantly in the central and eastern US. Thus, if patients with subacute meningeal symptoms reside in or travel to this region, clinicians should suspect the appropriate fungal causes.

CSF findings typically include

- Lymphocytic pleocytosis
- Elevated protein
- Low glucose

Candida sp may also cause polymorphonuclear pleocytosis.

Coccidioidal meningitis tends to resist treatment and may require lifelong treatment with fluconazole. Voriconazole and amphotericin B have also been used. Treatment of the other fungal meningitides is usually with amphotericin B.

Other causes of chronic meningitis: Rarely, other infectious organisms and some noninfectious disorders (see Table 231–8) cause chronic meningitis. Noninfectious causes include

- Cancer
- Autoimmune rheumatic disorders including SLE, RA, and Sjögren syndrome
- Intracranial arteritis
- Neurosarcoidosis
- Behçet syndrome
- Chronic idiopathic meningitis:

Chronic idiopathic meningitis: Occasionally, chronic, usually lymphocytic meningitis persists for months or even years, but no organisms are identified; and death does not result. In some patients, the meningitis eventually remits spontaneously. Generally, empiric trials of antifungal drugs or corticosteroids have not been helpful.

Chronic meningitis in patients with HIV infection: Meningitis is common among HIV-infected patients. Most CSF abnormalities result from HIV, which invades the CNS early in the course of the infection. Onset of meningitis and meningeal symptoms often coincides with seroconversion. Meningitis may then remit or follow a steady or fluctuating course.

However, many other organisms can cause chronic meningitis in patients with HIV infection. They include *C. neoformans* (the most common), *M. tuberculosis*, *Treponema pallidum*, *B. burgdorferi*, *Toxoplasma gondii*, *Coccidioides immitis*, and other fungi. CNS lymphoma can also cause findings similar to those of meningitis in these patients.

Regardless of the cause, parenchymal lesions may develop.

Diagnosis

- CSF analysis

Clinical findings are often nonspecific. However, a careful search for a systemic infection or disorder may suggest a cause for meningitis. Also, sometimes risk factors (eg, immunocompromise, HIV infection or risk factors for it, recent time spent in endemic areas) and occasionally specific neurologic deficits (eg, particular cranial nerve deficits) suggest specific causes, such as *C. neoformans* meningitis in HIV-infected patients or *C. immitis* infections in patients living in the southwestern US.

Typically, CSF findings include lymphocytic pleocytosis. In many of the infections that cause chronic meningitis, CSF contains only a few of the organisms, making identification of the cause difficult. Thus, diagnosis based on CSF findings may require multiple large samples over time, particularly for cultures. CSF analysis commonly includes

- Aerobic and anaerobic bacterial culture
- Mycobacterial and fungal culture
- Cryptococcal antigen testing
- Antigen or serologic testing
- Special stains (eg, acid-fast staining, India ink)
- Cytology

If CSF findings do not provide a diagnosis and meningitis is causing morbidity or is progressive, more invasive testing (eg, cisternal or ventricular puncture, biopsy) is indicated. Occasionally, organisms are recovered from ventricular or cisternal CSF when lumbar CSF is negative.

MRI or CT may be done to identify focal areas of inflammation for biopsy; blind meningeal biopsy has a very low yield.

Treatment

- Treatment of the cause

Treatment is directed at the cause (for mycobacterial, spirochetal, and fungal meningitides, see above; for other causes, see elsewhere in THE MANUAL).

KEY POINTS

- Consider risk factors (eg, time spent in endemic areas, HIV infection or risk factors for it, immunocompromise, autoimmune rheumatic disorders) to help identify likely causes.
- Carefully checking for a systemic infection or disorder may provide the diagnosis.
- Many samples may be needed for CSF analysis because CSF may contain few of the causative organisms; sometimes diagnosis requires cisternal or ventricular puncture and/or biopsy.

232 Movement and Cerebellar Disorders

Voluntary movement requires complex interaction of the corticospinal (pyramidal) tracts, basal ganglia, and cerebellum (the center for motor coordination) to ensure smooth, purposeful movement without extraneous muscular contractions.

The **pyramidal tracts** pass through the medullary pyramids to connect the cerebral cortex to lower motor centers of the brain stem and spinal cord.

The **basal ganglia** (caudate nucleus, putamen, globus pallidus, subthalamic nucleus, and substantia nigra) form the extrapyramidal system. They are located deep in the forebrain and direct their output mainly rostrally through the thalamus to the cerebral cortex (see Fig. 232–1).

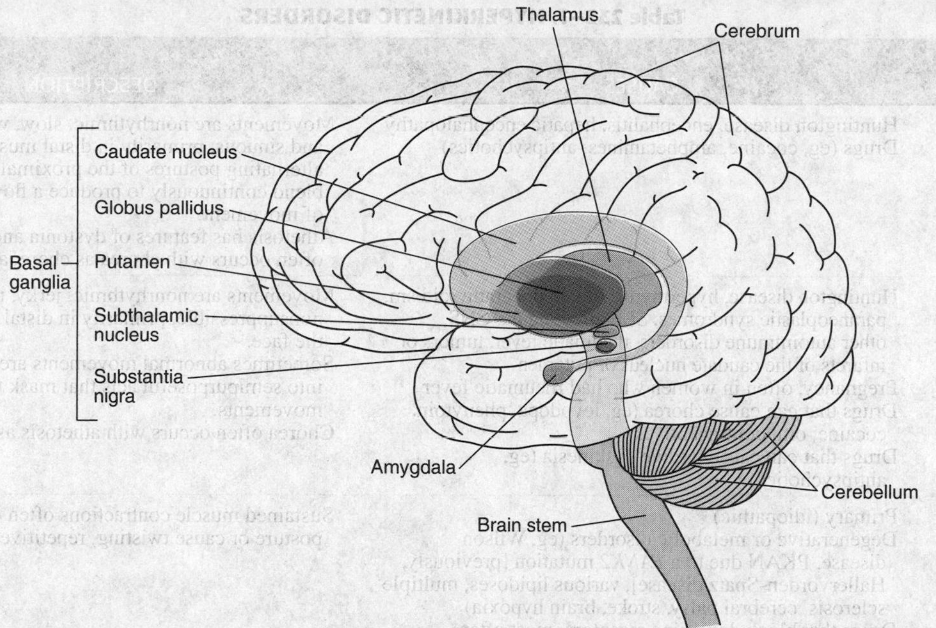

Fig. 232–1. Basal ganglia.

Most neural lesions that cause movement disorders occur in the extrapyramidal system; thus, movement disorders are sometimes called extrapyramidal disorders.

Classification

Movement disorders are commonly classified as those with

- Decreased or slow movement (hypokinetic disorders)
- Increased movement (hyperkinetic disorders)

The **classic and most common hypokinetic disorder** is

- Parkinson disease (PD)

Hyperkinetic disorders refer to

- Tremor
- Myoclonus
- Dystonia
- Chorea (including hemiballismus [rapid chorea] and athetosis [slow chorea])
- Tics

However, this classification does not account for overlap between categories (eg, tremors that occur in PD).

Hyperkinetic disorders: Hyperkinetic disorders (see Fig. 232–2 and Table 232–1) can be

- Rhythmic
- Nonrhythmic

Rhythmic disorders are primarily tremors—regular alternating or oscillatory movements, which can occur mainly at rest, while maintaining a position, and/or during attempted movement. However, in some cases, a tremor, though rhythmic, is irregular, as occurs when tremor is associated with dystonic disorders.

Nonrhythmic hyperkinetic disorders can be

- Slow (eg, athetosis)
- Sustained (eg, dystonias)
- Rapid (eg, myoclonus, chorea, tics, hemiballismus)

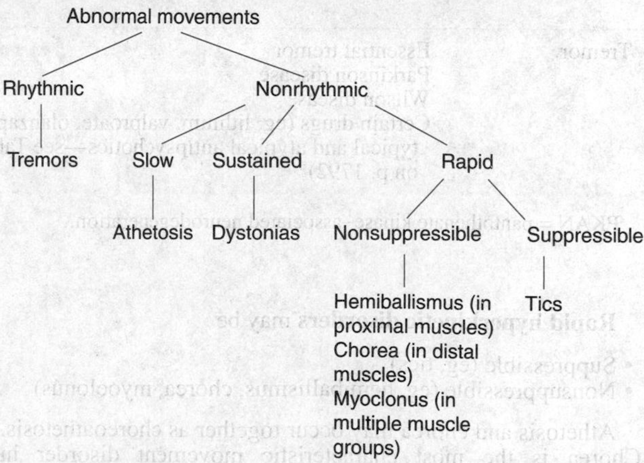

Fig. 232–2. Classification of common hyperkinetic disorders.

Table 232–1. HYPERKINETIC DISORDERS

ABNORMAL MOVEMENT	CAUSES	DESCRIPTION
Athetosis	Huntington disease, encephalitis, hepatic encephalopathy Drugs (eg, cocaine, amphetamines, antipsychotics)	Movements are nonrhythmic, slow, writhing, and sinuous, primarily in distal muscles; alternating postures of the proximal limbs often blend continuously to produce a flowing stream of movement. Athetosis has features of dystonia and chorea and often occurs with chorea as choreoathetosis.
Chorea	Huntington disease, hyperthyroidism, hypoparathyroidism, paraneoplastic syndromes, SLE affecting the CNS, other autoimmune disorders, rheumatic fever, tumors or infarcts of the caudate nucleus or putamen Pregnancy, often in women who had rheumatic fever Drugs that can cause chorea (eg, levodopa, phenytoin, cocaine, oral contraceptives) Drugs that can cause tardive dyskinesia (eg, antipsychotics)	Movements are nonrhythmic, jerky, rapid, and nonsuppressible, primarily in distal muscles or the face. Sometimes abnormal movements are incorporated into semipurposeful acts that mask the involuntary movements. Chorea often occurs with athetosis as choreoathetosis.
Dystonias	Primary (idiopathic) Degenerative or metabolic disorders (eg, Wilson disease, PKAN due to a *PANK2* mutation [previously, Hallervorden-Spatz disease], various lipidoses, multiple sclerosis, cerebral palsy, stroke, brain hypoxia) Drugs that block dopamine receptors, most often antipsychotics (eg, phenothiazines, thioxanthenes, butyrophenones) or antiemetics	Sustained muscle contractions often distort body posture or cause twisting, repetitive movements.
Hemiballismus	Lesions (most often due to stroke) in the contralateral subthalamic nucleus or in connecting afferent or efferent pathways	Movements are nonrhythmic, rapid, nonsuppressible, violent, and flinging.
Myoclonus	Various causes	Very rapid and jerky, nonsuppressible, shocklike twitches occur; they may be focal, segmental, or generalized.
Tics	**Primary:** Tourette syndrome (see p. 2776) **Secondary:** Huntington disease, neuroacanthocytosis, PKAN, infections, stroke, drugs (eg, methylphenidate, cocaine, amphetamines, dopamine antagonists [which can cause tardive dyskinesias])	Movements are nonrhythmic, stereotypical, rapid, and repetitive; characteristically, patients have an urge to do them and feel brief relief after doing them. Tics can be suppressed only for brief periods and with conscious effort. Tics may be motor or phonatory; they may be simple (eg, eye blinking, growling, clearing the throat) or complex (eg, shoulder shrugging, arm swinging, shouting words or sentences, including obscenities).
Tremor	Essential tremor Parkinson disease Wilson disease Certain drugs (eg, lithium, valproate, olanzapine, other typical and atypical antipsychotics—see Table 213–1 on p. 1792)	Movements are regular, mostly rhythmic, and oscillatory.

PKAN = pantothenate kinase–associated neurodegeneration.

Rapid hyperkinetic disorders may be

- Suppressible (eg, tics)
- Nonsuppressible (eg, hemiballismus, chorea, myoclonus)

Athetosis and chorea may occur together as choreoathetosis. Chorea is the most characteristic movement disorder in Huntington disease.

Multiple motor and phonatory tics are the defining feature of Tourette syndrome (see p. 2776).

CHOREA, ATHETOSIS, AND HEMIBALLISMUS

Chorea is a nonrhythmic, jerky, rapid, nonsuppressible involuntary movement, mostly of the distal muscles and face; movements may be incorporated into semipurposeful acts that mask the involuntary movements. Athetosis (slow chorea) is nonrhythmic, slow, writhing,

sinuous movements predominantly in distal muscles, often alternating with postures of the proximal limbs. Hemiballismus is unilateral rapid, nonrhythmic, non-suppressible, wildly flinging movement of the proximal arm and/or leg; rarely, such movement occurs bilaterally (ballismus). Hemiballismus may be considered a severe form of chorea.

Chorea and athetosis are defined by clinical manifestations; many experts believe that when they occur together (as choreoathetosis), athetosis is a dystonia superimposed on chorea. Chorea and athetosis result from impaired inhibition of thalamocortical neurons by the basal ganglia. Excess dopaminergic activity may be the mechanism.

Clinicians should seek and treat the cause of chorea whenever possible.

Huntington disease is the most common degenerative disorder causing chorea. In Huntington disease, drugs that suppress dopaminergic activity, such as antipsychotics (eg, risperidone, olanzapine), and dopamine-depleting drugs (eg, reserpine, tetrabenazine) can be used to treat chorea. Antipsychotics may also help by lessening the neuropsychiatric symptoms commonly associated with Huntington disease (eg, impulsivity, anxiety, psychotic behavior). However, improvement may be limited and transient. These drugs may be judiciously used to treat choreas without a definable cause.

Other causes of chorea include

- Hyperthyroidism
- Hypoparathyroidism
- Hyperglycemia
- Use of oral contraceptives
- Pregnancy
- SLE that affects the CNS
- Drugs (eg, levodopa in patients with PD, phenytoin, cocaine)
- Tardive dyskinesia (due to use of typical and most atypical antipsychotics)
- Autoimmune disorders
- Paraneoplastic syndromes

Sydenham chorea can occur in rheumatic fever and may be the first symptom of it. A tumor or an infarct in the striatum (caudate or putamen) can cause acute unilateral chorea (hemichorea). Sydenham chorea and chorea due to infarcts of the caudate nucleus often lessen over time without treatment.

Chorea due to hyperthyroidism or another metabolic cause (eg, hyperglycemia) usually lessens when thyroid function or blood glucose level is normalized.

Chorea in patients > 60 should be thoroughly evaluated to identify the cause (eg, toxic, metabolic, autoimmune, paraneoplastic).

Chorea gravidarum occurs during pregnancy, often in patients who have had rheumatic fever. Chorea usually begins during the 1st trimester and resolves spontaneously at or after delivery. If treatment before delivery is necessary because chorea is severe, barbiturates are indicated because they have fewer fetal risks than other drugs used to manage chorea. Rarely, a similar disorder occurs in women taking oral contraceptives.

Hemiballismus is caused by a lesion, usually an infarct, in or around the contralateral subthalamic nucleus. Although disabling, hemiballismus is usually self-limited, lasting 6 to 8 wk. If severe, it can be treated with an antipsychotic for 1 to 2 mo.

DYSTONIAS

Dystonias are sustained involuntary muscle contractions of antagonistic muscle groups in the same body part, leading to abnormal posturing or jerky, twisting, intermittent spasms that can resemble tremors, athetosis, or choreoathetosis. Dystonias can be primary or secondary and can be generalized, focal, or segmental. Diagnosis is clinical. Botulinum toxin injections are used to treat focal or segmental dystonias. Treatment of severe generalized dystonia may require a combination of oral anticholinergic drugs, muscle relaxants, and benzodiazepines. Severe segmental or generalized dystonia that is refractory to treatment may require surgery.

Dystonia may be

- Primary (idiopathic)
- Secondary to CNS disorders or drugs

CNS disorders that can cause dystonias include

- Wilson disease
- Pantothenate kinase-associated neurodegeneration [PKAN] associated with *PANK2* mutations [previously, Hallervorden-Spatz disease]
- Various lipidoses
- Multiple sclerosis
- Cerebral palsy
- Stroke
- Brain hypoxia

Drugs that most commonly cause dystonias include

- Antipsychotics (eg, phenothiazines, thioxanthenes, butyrophenones)
- Antiemetics (eg, metoclopramide, prochlorperazine)

Disordered movement that appears to be athetosis or choreoathetosis may be caused by dystonia.

Classification

Dystonias are classified based on

- Etiology
- Clinical features

Etiology is categorized as

- **Inherited:** Has a proven genetic origin (previously known as primary) and includes disorders with autosomal dominant, autosomal recessive, or X-linked inheritance
- **Idiopathic:** Can be familial or sporadic
- **Acquired:** Associated with neuroanatomic abnormalities due to other disorders

Clinical features include the following:

- **Onset:** Can occur at any age, from infancy to late adulthood
- **Body distribution:** May be focal (limited to one body part), segmental (involving ≥ 2 more contiguous body parts, such as the upper and lower face or face and neck), multifocal (involving ≥ 2 noncontiguous body parts, such as the neck and leg), generalized (involving the trunk plus 2 different body parts), or hemicorporal (involving half the body; also called hemidystonia)
- **Temporal pattern:** May be static, progressive, paroxysmal, or persistent and may have diurnal variability or be triggered by certain tasks (task-specific dystonia)

- **Isolated** (no evidence of another movement disorder) or **combined** (accompanied by other involuntary movements [other than tremor], but predominantly dystonia)

PEARLS & PITFALLS

- Consider antipsychotic and antiemetic drugs as causes of sudden, unexplained dystonia.

Primary generalized dystonia (DYT1 dystonia): This rare dystonia is progressive and characterized by sustained, often bizarre postures. It is often inherited as an autosomal dominant disorder with partial penetrance due to mutations in the *DYT1* gene; in some family members, the gene is minimally expressed. Asymptomatic siblings of patients (carriers) may have a forme fruste of the disorder.

Symptoms of primary generalized dystonia usually begin in childhood with inversion and plantar flexion of the foot while walking. At first, the dystonia may affect only the trunk or leg but often progresses to affect the whole body, usually moving cephalad. Patients with the most severe form may become twisted into grotesque, nearly fixed postures and ultimately be confined to a wheelchair. Symptoms that begin during adulthood usually affect only the face or arms.

Mental function is usually preserved.

Dopa-responsive dystonia: This rare dystonia is hereditary. Symptoms of dopa-responsive dystonia usually begin during childhood. Typically, one leg is affected first. As a result, children tend to walk on tiptoes. Symptoms worsen at night. Walking becomes progressively more difficult, and arms and legs are affected. However, some children have only mild symptoms, such as muscle cramps after exercise. Sometimes symptoms appear later in life and resemble those of PD. Movements may be slow, balance may be difficult to maintain, and a tremor may occur in the hands during rest.

Symptoms lessen dramatically when low doses of levodopa are used. If levodopa relieves the symptoms, the diagnosis is confirmed.

Focal dystonias: These dystonias affect a single body part. They typically start during adulthood, after ages 20 to 30.

Initially, the posturing may be intermittent or task-specific (and thus is sometimes described as spasms). The movements tend to be more prominent during action and less so at rest, but these differences lessen over time, often resulting in distortion of the affected body part and severe disability. However, pain is uncommon except in focal primary dystonia of the neck (cervical dystonia) and in the dystonias that occur when response to levodopa starts to wear off in PD (most often affecting the lower limb, eg, causing inversion of the foot).

Occupational dystonia consists of task-specific focal dystonic spasms triggered by performing skilled acts (eg, writer's cramp, musician´s dystonia, the yips in golfers).

Spasmodic dysphonia consists of a strained, hoarse, or creaky voice due to focal dystonia of the laryngeal muscles.

Cervical dystonia manifests with involuntary tonic contractions or intermittent spasms of neck muscles.

Segmental dystonias: These dystonias affect ≥ 2 contiguous body parts.

Meige syndrome (blepharospasm plus oromandibular dystonia) consists of involuntary blinking, jaw grinding, and grimacing, usually beginning during late adulthood. It must be distinguished from the buccal-lingual-facial chorea of tardive dyskinesia and tardive dystonia (a variant of tardive dyskinesia).

Diagnosis

- Clinical evaluation

Diagnosis of dystonia is clinical.

Treatment

- For generalized dystonia, anticholinergic drugs, muscle relaxants, or both
- For focal or segmental dystonia, botulinum toxin injections to paralyze muscles
- Sometimes a neurosurgical procedure

For **generalized dystonia,** an anticholinergic drug (trihexyphenidyl 2 to 10 mg po tid, benztropine 3 to 15 mg po once/day) is most commonly used; the dose is slowly titrated to target. A muscle relaxant (usually baclofen), a benzodiazepine (eg, clonazepam), or both may provide adjunctive benefit.

Generalized dystonia that is severe or does not respond to drugs may be treated with deep brain stimulation of the globus pallidus interna (GPi), a stereotactic neurosurgical procedure. In some cases, stereotactic unilateral ablative surgery of the GPi is indicated.

For **focal or segmental dystonias or for generalized dystonia that affects mainly one body part,** the treatment of choice is

- Purified botulinum toxin type A or B injected into the affected muscles, done with or without electromyographic guidance and by an experienced practitioner

Botulinum toxin weakens excessive muscular contractions through chemodenervation, but it does not alter the abnormal brain circuitry that causes dystonia. Toxin injection is most effective for blepharospasm and torticollis but can be very effective for most other forms of focal dystonia. Dosage varies greatly. Treatments must be repeated every 3 to 4 mo because the toxin's duration of activity is limited. However, in a few cases, when the toxin is repeatedly injected, this treatment becomes less effective because neutralizing antibodies against the toxin protein develop; not all antibodies that develop neutralize the toxin.

KEY POINTS

- Dystonias cause abnormal postures and/or twisting, jerky movements.
- Focal dystonias are common and usually begin during adulthood.
- Generalized dystonia is usually secondary to a disorder or drug and rarely a primary disorder.
- Diagnosis is clinical.
- Treat generalized dystonias with anticholinergic drugs and/or muscle relaxants; treat focal or segmental dystonias and generalized dystonias that affect mainly one body part with botulinum toxin injections.

CERVICAL DYSTONIA

(Spasmodic Torticollis)

Cervical dystonia is characterized by involuntary tonic contractions or intermittent spasms of neck muscles. The cause is usually unknown. Diagnosis is clinical. Treatment can include physical therapy, drugs, and selective denervation of neck muscles with surgery or locally injected botulinum toxin.

In cervical dystonia, contraction of the neck muscles causes the neck to turn from its usual position. It is the most common dystonia.

Spasmodic (adult-onset) torticollis is the most common form of cervical dystonia. It is usually idiopathic. A few patients have a family history, and in some of them (eg, those with dystonia-6 [DYT6], dystonia-7 [DYT7], or dystonia-25 [DYT25; associated with the *GNAL* gene]), a genetic cause has been identified. Some of these patients have other dystonias (eg, of the eyelids, face, jaw, or hand).

Cervical dystonia can be

- Congenital
- Secondary to other conditions such as lesions of the brain stem or basal ganglia or use of dopamine-blocking drugs (eg, haloperidol)

Rarely, dystonia has a psychogenic cause. In this type of dystonia, pathophysiology is not well understood; however, changes in brain function have been detected by functional neuroimaging. In many cases, an emotional stressor or an abnormal core of beliefs is identified as a trigger. In such cases, a multidisciplinary team, including a neurologist, psychiatrist, and psychologist, is necessary.

Symptoms and Signs

Cervical dystonia symptoms may begin at any age but usually begin between ages 20 and 60, with a peak between ages 30 and 50.

Symptoms usually begin gradually; rarely, they begin acutely and progress rapidly. Sometimes symptoms begin with a tremor that rotates the neck (in a no-no gesture).

The cardinal symptom is

- Painful tonic contractions or intermittent spasms of the sternocleidomastoid, trapezius, and other neck muscles, usually unilaterally, that result in an abnormal head position

Unilateral sternocleidomastoid muscle contraction causes the head to rotate to the opposite side. Rotation may involve any plane but almost always has a horizontal component. Besides rotational tilting (torticollis), the head can tilt laterally (laterocollis), forward (anterocollis), or backward (retrocollis, common when dopamine-blocking drugs are the cause).

Patients may discover sensory or tactile tricks that lessen the dystonic posturing or tremor (eg, touching the face on the side contralateral to the deviation). During sleep, muscle spasms disappear.

Spasmodic torticollis ranges from mild to severe. Usually, it progresses slowly for 1 to 5 yr, then plateaus. About 10 to 20% of patients recover spontaneously within 5 yr of onset (usually in milder cases with onset at a younger age). However, it may persist for life and can result in restricted movement and postural deformity.

Diagnosis

- Clinical evaluation

The diagnosis of cervical dystonia is based on characteristic symptoms and signs and exclusion of alternative diagnoses, including the following:

- **Tardive dyskinesia** can cause torticollis but can usually be distinguished by a history of chronic antipsychotic use and involuntary movements in muscles outside of the neck.
- **Basal ganglia disorders** and occasionally **CNS infections** can cause movement disorders but usually also involve other muscles; CNS infections are usually acute and cause other symptoms.
- **Neck infections or tumors** are usually differentiated by features of the primary process.
- **Antipsychotics and other drugs** can cause acute torticollis, but the symptoms usually develop in hours and resolve within days after the drug is stopped.

Treatment

- Physical measures
- Sometimes botulinum toxin or oral drugs

Spasms can sometimes be temporarily inhibited by physical therapy and massage, including sensory biofeedback techniques (eg, slight tactile pressure to the jaw on the same side as head rotation) and any light touch.

Drugs: Injections of botulinum toxin type A or B into the dystonic muscles can reduce painful spasms for 1 to 4 mo in about 70% of patients, restoring a more neutral position of the head. However, in a few cases, when the toxin is repeatedly injected, it becomes less effective because neutralizing antibodies against the toxin develop.

Oral drugs can usually relieve pain, but they suppress dystonic movements in only about 25 to 33% of patients. These drugs include

- Anticholinergic drugs, such as trihexyphenidyl 10 to 25 mg po once/day or bid (but adverse effects may limit their use)
- Benzodiazepines (particularly clonazepam 0.5 mg po bid)
- Baclofen
- Carbamazepine

All drugs should be started in low doses (eg, trihexyphenidyl 2 mg po tid). Doses should be increased until symptoms are controlled or intolerable adverse effects (particularly likely in the elderly) develop.

Surgery: Surgery is controversial. The most successful surgical approach selectively severs nerves to affected neck muscles, permanently weakening or paralyzing them. Results are favorable when the procedure is done at centers with extensive experience.

KEY POINTS

- Spasmodic torticollis is a common adult-onset cervical dystonia and is usually idiopathic.
- Diagnosis is clinical and involves exclusion of tardive dyskinesia, basal ganglia disorders, CNS infections, neck infections and tumors, and drugs.
- Treatment is most often physical measures, botulinum toxin injection, and/or oral drugs.

FRAGILE X–ASSOCIATED TREMOR/ATAXIA SYNDROME

Fragile X–associated tremor/ataxia syndrome (FXTAS) is a genetic disorder affecting mostly men and causing tremor, ataxia, and dementia. Tremor is a common early symptom that is followed by ataxia, parkinsonism, and eventually dementia. Diagnosis is confirmed by genetic testing. Tremor can often be relieved with primidone, propranolol, and/or antiparkinsonian drugs.

FXTAS affects about 1/3000 men > 50. It results from a premutation (50 to 200 CGG repeats) in the Fragile X mental retardation (*FMR1*) gene on the X chromosome. Fragile X syndrome, the most common form of intellectual disability in males, develops when the mutation is full (> 200 repeats).

People with the premutation are considered carriers. Daughters (but not sons) of men with the premutation inherit the premutation. These daughters' children (grandchildren of the men with the FXTAS premutation) have a 50% chance of inheriting the premutation, which can expand into a full mutation when passed from mother to child (and thus cause Fragile X syndrome).

FXTAS develops in about 30% of men with the premutation and in < 5% of women with the premutation.

Risk of developing FXTAS increases with age.

Symptoms and Signs

FXTAS symptoms become noticeable in late adulthood. The more CGG repeats, the more severe the symptoms and the earlier the onset.

Tremor, often misdiagnosed as essential tremor, is a common early symptom. Patients develop ataxia (which progressively worsens), then parkinsonism, and eventually dementia.

PEARLS & PITFALLS

- Consider FXTAS in patients diagnosed with essential tremor if they develop ataxia or signs of parkinsonism.

Dementia begins with loss of short-term memory, slowed thought, and difficulty problem solving. Depression, anxiety, impatience, hostility, and mood lability may develop.

Peripheral neuropathy is often present, causing loss of sensation and reflexes in the feet. Dysautonomia (eg, orthostatic hypotension) may occur. In later stages, bladder and bowel control may be lost.

Life expectancy after motor symptoms develop ranges from about 5 to 25 yr.

In women with the premutation, symptoms are usually less severe, possibly because the presence of another X chromosome is protective. These women have an increased risk of early menopause, infertility, and ovarian dysfunction.

Diagnosis

- Genetic testing

If FXTAS is suspected, patients should be asked whether any of their grandchildren have intellectual disability and whether their daughters have had early menopause or infertility. Also, grandparents of patients that have Fragile X syndrome should be asked whether they have symptoms suggesting FXTAS; if so, genetic counseling is recommended for their children and/or grandchildren, except for the patient known to have Fragile X syndrome.

MRI is done; it may identify the characteristic increased signal in the middle cerebellar peduncles.

Diagnosis of FXTAS is confirmed by genetic testing.

Treatment

- Primidone, propranolol, and/or antiparkinsonian drugs

The tremor in FXTAS can often be relieved with primidone, propranolol, and/or antiparkinsonian drugs.

KEY POINTS

- FXTAS affects about 1/3000 men > 50; Fragile X syndrome, the most common cause of intellectual disability in males, develops from a related gene mutation.
- Ask patients whether any of their grandchildren have intellectual disability and whether their daughters have had early menopause or infertility, and ask grandparents of patients with Fragile X syndrome whether they have symptoms suggesting FXTAS.
- Do genetic testing to confirm the diagnosis.
- Treat tremor with primidone, propranolol, and/or antiparkinsonian drugs.

HUNTINGTON DISEASE

(Chronic Progressive Chorea; Hereditary Chorea; Huntington Chorea)

Huntington disease is an autosomal dominant disorder characterized by chorea, neuropsychiatric symptoms, and progressive cognitive deterioration, usually beginning during middle age. Diagnosis is by genetic testing. First-degree relatives should be offered genetic counseling before genetic tests are done. Treatment is supportive.

Huntington disease affects both sexes equally.

Pathophysiology

The caudate nucleus atrophies, the inhibitory medium spiny neurons in the corpus striatum degenerate, and levels of the neurotransmitters γ-aminobutyric acid (GABA) and substance P decrease.

Huntington disease results from a mutation in the *huntingtin* (*HTT*) gene (on chromosome 4), causing abnormal repetition of the DNA sequence CAG, which codes for the amino acid glutamine. The resulting gene product, a large protein called huntingtin, has an expanded stretch of polyglutamine residues, which accumulate within neurons and lead to disease via unknown mechanisms. The more CAG repeats, the earlier the onset of disease and the more severe its expression (phenotype). The number of repeats can increase with successive generations and, over time, lead to increasingly severe phenotypes within a family (called anticipation).

Symptoms and Signs

Symptoms and signs of Huntington disease develop insidiously, starting at about age 35 to 40, depending on phenotype severity.

Dementia or psychiatric disturbances (eg, depression, apathy, irritability, anhedonia, antisocial behavior, full-blown bipolar or schizophreniform disorder) develop before or simultaneously with the movement disorder.

Abnormal movements appear; they include chorea, myoclonic jerks, and pseudo-tics (one cause of tourettism). Tourettism refers to Tourette-like symptoms that result from a neurologic disorder or use of a drug.

Typical features include a bizarre, puppet-like gait, facial grimacing, inability to intentionally move the eyes quickly without blinking or head thrusting (oculomotor apraxia), and inability to sustain a motor act (motor impersistence), such as tongue protrusion or grasping.

Huntington disease progresses, making walking impossible and swallowing difficult; it results in severe dementia. Most patients eventually require institutionalization. Death usually occurs 13 to 15 yr after symptoms begin.

Diagnosis

- Clinical evaluation, confirmed by genetic testing
- Neuroimaging

Diagnosis of Huntington disease is based on typical symptoms and signs plus a positive family history and is confirmed by genetic testing that measures the number of CAG repeats (for interpretation of results, see Table 232–2).

Table 232–2. GENETIC TESTING FOR HUNTINGTON DISEASE

NUMBER OF CAG REPEATS	INTERPRETATION
≤ 26	Normal
27–35	Normal but unstable (increased risk that children will have Huntington disease)
36–39	Abnormal with variable penetrance; unstable (in some studies, most patients had symptoms and signs)
≥ 40	Abnormal with complete penetrance

Neuroimaging helps identify caudate atrophy and often some frontal-predominant cortical atrophy.

Treatment

- Supportive measures
- Genetic counseling for relatives

Because Huntington disease is progressive, end-of-life care should be discussed early.

Treatment of Huntington disease is supportive.

Antipsychotics may partially suppress chorea and agitation. Antipsychotics include

- Chlorpromazine 25 to 300 mg po tid
- Haloperidol 5 to 45 mg po bid
- Risperidone 0.5 to 3 mg po bid
- Olanzapine 5 to 10 mg po once/day
- Clozapine 12.5 to 100 mg po once/day or bid

In patients taking clozapine, WBC counts must be done frequently because agranulocytosis is a risk. The antipsychotic dose is increased until intolerable adverse effects (eg, lethargy, parkinsonism) develop or symptoms are controlled.

Alternatively, **tetrabenazine** may be used. The dose is started at 12.5 mg po once/day and increased to 12.5 mg bid in the 2nd wk, 12.5 mg tid in the 3rd wk, and 12.5 mg po qid in the 4th wk. Doses of > 12.5 mg po qid (total dose of 50 mg po/day) are given in tid doses; the total dose is increased 12.5 mg/day weekly. The maximum dose is 33.3 mg po tid (total dose of 100 mg/day). Doses are increased sequentially as needed to control symptoms or until intolerable adverse effects occur. Adverse effects can include excessive sedation, akathisia, parkinsonism, and depression. Depression is treated with antidepressants.

Therapies currently under study aim to reduce glutamatergic neurotransmission via the *N*-methyl-D-aspartate receptor and to bolster mitochondrial energy production. Treatments that aim to increase GABAergic function in the brain have been ineffective.

People who have 1st-degree relatives with Huntington disease, particularly women of childbearing age and men considering having children, should be offered genetic counseling and genetic testing. Genetic counseling should be offered before genetic testing because the ramifications of Huntington disease are so profound.

KEY POINTS

- Huntington disease, an autosomal dominant disorder that affects either sex, usually causes dementia and chorea during middle age.
- If symptoms and family history suggest the diagnosis, provide genetic counseling before genetic testing, and consider neuroimaging.
- Treat symptoms and discuss end-of-life care as soon as possible.
- Offer counselling and genetic testing to 1st-degree relatives, particularly potential parents.

MYOCLONUS

Myoclonus is a brief, shocklike contraction of a muscle or group of muscles. Diagnosis is clinical and sometimes confirmed by electromyographic testing. Treatment includes correction of reversible causes and, when necessary, oral drugs to relieve symptoms.

Myoclonus may be

- Focal
- Segmental (contiguous areas)
- Multifocal (noncontiguous areas)
- Generalized

It may be physiologic or pathologic.

Physiologic myoclonus may occur when a person is falling asleep and during early sleep phases (called hypnic myoclonus). Hypnic myoclonus can be focal, multifocal, segmental, or generalized and may resemble a startle reaction. Another type of physiologic myoclonus is hiccuping (diaphragmatic myoclonus).

Pathologic myoclonus can result from various disorders and drugs (see Table 232–3). The most common causes are

- Hypoxia
- Drug toxicity
- Metabolic disturbances

Other causes include degenerative disorders affecting the basal ganglia and some dementias.

Classification of myoclonus: Myoclonus may be classified based on the site of origin as follows:

- **Cortical:** This type of myoclonus is associated with cerebral cortex damage or epilepsy. Photic visual stimuli or touching may trigger myoclonic jerks, which may cause abnormalities on an EEG (eg, focal or generalized spike-and-wave or polyspike-and-wave epileptiform discharges, giant somatosensory evoked potentials). The myoclonic jerks may be less evident at rest but aggravated during motor action.
- **Subcortical:** This type of myoclonus is associated with disorders that affect the basal ganglia. It is similar to cortical myoclonus. However, there are no EEG abnormalities or giant somatosensory evoked potentials, and photic visual stimuli are not a trigger.
- **Reticular:** This type of myoclonus is thought to originate in the brain stem. It is similar to hyperexplexia (hypertonia and an exaggerated startle reaction). But in reticular myoclonus, unlike in hyperexplexia, myoclonus frequently occurs spontaneously and is more likely to be triggered by touching the distal limbs rather than the head, face and/or upper chest. Reticular myoclonus can also be triggered by movement. Myoclonic jerks usually affect the whole body, with muscles on both sides of the body affected simultaneously.
- **Peripheral:** This type of myoclonus results from damage to peripheral nerves, nerve roots, or plexuses. It is characterized by rhythmic or semirhythmic jerks. Hemifacial spasm is an example of peripheral myoclonus.

Table 232–3. CAUSES OF MYOCLONUS

CAUSE	EXAMPLES
Degeneration of the basal ganglia	Lewy body dementia Huntington disease Parkinson disease Progressive supranuclear palsy
Dementias	Alzheimer disease Creutzfeldt-Jakob disease Progressive myoclonic encephalopathies (eg, mitochondrial disorders, certain types of epilepsy, such as sialidosis, neuronal ceroid lipofuscinosis, and Unverricht-Lundborg disease)
Metabolic disturbances	Hypercapnia Hyperglycemia, nonketotic Hypocalcemia Hypoglycemia Hypomagnesemia Hyponatremia Liver failure Uremia
Physical and hypoxic encephalopathies	Electric shock Heatstroke Hypoxia Traumatic brain injury
Toxic encephalopathies	DDT Heavy metals (including bismuth) Methyl bromide
Viral encephalopathies	Encephalitis lethargica Herpes simplex encephalitis Postinfectious encephalitis Subacute sclerosing panencephalitis
Drugs	Antihistamines* Carbamazepine* Cephalosporins* Levodopa† Lithium* MAO inhibitors* Opioids (usually dose related) Penicillin* Phenytoin* Tricyclic antidepressants* SSRIs* Valproate*

*At toxic or high doses.
†With long-term treatment; dose-related.
DDT = dichlorodiphenyltrichloroethane; MAO = monoamine oxidase.

Classifying myoclonus based on site of origin is thought to be the most helpful when choosing the most effective treatment.

Symptoms and Signs

Myoclonus can vary in amplitude, frequency, and distribution.

Muscle jerks may occur spontaneously or be induced by a stimulus (eg, sudden noise, movement, light, visual threat).

Myoclonus that occurs when patients are suddenly startled (startle myoclonus) may be an early symptom of Creutzfeldt-Jacob disease.

Myoclonus due to severe closed head trauma or hypoxic-ischemic brain damage may worsen with purposeful movements (action myoclonus) or may occur spontaneously when movement is limited because of injury.

Myoclonus due to metabolic disturbances may be multifocal, asymmetric, and stimulus-induced; it usually involves facial or proximal limb muscles. If the disturbance persists, generalized myoclonic jerks and, ultimately, seizures may occur.

Diagnosis

- Clinical evaluation

Diagnosis of myoclonus is clinical. Testing is done based on clinically suspected causes.

Treatment

- Correcting the metabolic disturbance or other cause if possible
- Stopping or reducing the dose of the causative drug
- Drug therapy to relieve symptoms

Treatment of myoclonus begins with correction of underlying metabolic disturbances or other causes if correctable. If a drug is the cause, the drug is stopped, or the dose is reduced.

For symptom relief, clonazepam 0.5 to 2 mg po tid is often effective. Valproate 250 to 500 mg po bid or levetiracetam 250 to 500 mg po once/day to bid may be effective; rarely, other anticonvulsants help. Doses of clonazepam or valproate may need to be lower in the elderly.

Site of origin for myoclonus can help guide treatment. For example, valproate, levetiracetam, and piracetam tend to be effective in cortical myoclonus but ineffective in other types of myoclonus. Clonazepam may be effective in all types of myoclonus. In some cases, a combination of drugs is necessary.

Many types of myoclonus respond to the serotonin precursor 5-hydroxytryptophan (initially, 25 mg po qid, increased to 150 to 250 mg po qid), which must be used with the oral decarboxylase inhibitor carbidopa (50 mg every morning and 25 mg at noon or 50 mg every evening and 25 mg at bedtime).

KEY POINTS

- Myoclonus is a brief, shocklike muscle contraction that can vary in severity and distribution.
- Myoclonus can be physiologic (eg, hiccuping, sleep-related muscle contractions) or secondary to various brain disorders, systemic disorders, or drugs.
- If a metabolic disturbance is the cause, correct it, and when necessary, give drugs (eg, clonazepam, valproate, levetiracetam) to relieve symptoms.

PARKINSON DISEASE

Parkinson disease (PD) is a slowly progressive, degenerative disorder characterized by resting tremor, stiffness (rigidity), slow and decreased movement (bradykinesia), and gait and/or postural instability. Diagnosis is clinical. Treatment aims to restore dopaminergic function in the brain with levodopa plus carbidopa and/or other drugs (eg, dopamine agonists, MAO type B [MAO-B] inhibitors, amantadine). For refractory, disabling symptoms in patients without dementia, stereotactic deep brain stimulation or lesional surgery and levodopa and an apomorphine pump may help.

Parkinson disease affects about

- 0.4% of people > 40 yr
- 1% of people ≥ 65 yr
- 10% of people ≥ 80 yr

The mean age at onset is about 57 yr.

PD is usually idiopathic.

Rarely, PD begins during childhood or adolescence (juvenile parkinsonism). Onset between ages 21 and 40 yr is sometimes called young or early-onset PD. Genetic causes are more likely in juvenile and early-onset PD; these forms may differ from later-onset PD because they progress more slowly and are very sensitive to dopaminergic treatments and because most disability results from nonmotor symptoms such as depression, anxiety, and pain.

Secondary parkinsonism is brain dysfunction that is characterized by basal ganglia dopaminergic blockade and that is similar to PD, but it is caused by something other than PD (eg, drugs, cerebrovascular disease, trauma, postencephalitic changes).

Atypical parkinsonism refers to a group of neurodegenerative disorders that have some features similar to those of PD but have some different clinical features, a worse prognosis, a modest or no response to levodopa, and a different pathology (eg, neurodegenerative disorders such as multiple system atrophy, progressive supranuclear palsy, dementia with Lewy bodies, corticobasal degeneration).

Pathophysiology

Synuclein is a neuronal and glial cell protein that can aggregate into insoluble fibrils and form Lewy bodies.

The **pathologic hallmark of PD** is

- Synuclein-filled Lewy bodies in the nigrostriatal system

However, synuclein can accumulate in many other parts of the nervous system, including the dorsal motor nucleus of the vagus nerve, basal nucleus of Meynert, hypothalamus, neocortex, olfactory bulb, sympathetic ganglia, and myenteric plexus of the GI tract. Lewy bodies appear in a temporal sequence, and many experts believe that PD is a relatively late development in a systemic synucleinopathy. Other synucleinopathies (synuclein deposition disorders) include dementia with Lewy bodies and multiple system atrophy. PD may share features of other synucleinopathies, such as autonomic dysfunction and dementia.

Rarely, PD occurs without Lewy bodies (eg, in a form due to a mutation in the *PARK 2* gene).

In PD, pigmented neurons of the substantia nigra, locus ceruleus, and other brain stem dopaminergic cell groups degenerate. Loss of substantia nigra neurons results in depletion of dopamine in the dorsal aspect of the putamen (part of the basal ganglia—see Fig. 232–1) and causes many of the motor manifestations of PD.

Etiology

A genetic predisposition is likely, at least in some cases of PD. About 10% of patients have a family history of PD. Several abnormal genes have been identified. Inheritance is autosomal dominant for some genes and autosomal recessive for others.

In genetic forms, age at onset tends to be younger, but the course is typically more benign than that of later-onset, presumably nongenetic PD.

Symptoms and Signs

In most patients, symptoms of PD begin insidiously.

A **resting tremor** of one hand is often the first symptom. The tremor is characterized as follows:

- Slow and coarse
- Maximal at rest, lessening during movement, and absent during sleep
- Amplitude increased by emotional tension or fatigue
- Often involving the wrist and fingers, sometimes involving the thumb moving against the index finger (pill rolling), as when people roll a pill in their hand or handle a small object

Usually, the hands or feet are affected first, most often asymmetrically. The jaw and tongue may also be affected, but not the voice. Tremor may become less prominent as the disease progresses.

Rigidity develops independently of tremor in many patients. When a clinician moves a rigid joint, semirhythmic jerks due to variations in the intensity of the rigidity occur, producing a ratchet-like effect (cogwheel rigidity).

Slow movements (bradykinesia) are typical. Movement also becomes decreased in amplitude (hypokinesia) and difficult to initiate (akinesia).

Rigidity and hypokinesia may contribute to muscle aches and sensations of fatigue. The face becomes masklike (hypomimic), with an open mouth and reduced blinking. Excessive drooling (sialorrhea) may contribute to disability. Speech becomes hypophonic, with characteristic monotonous, sometimes stuttering dysarthria.

Hypokinesia and impaired control of distal muscles cause micrographia (writing in very small letters) and make activities of daily living increasingly difficult. Without warning, voluntary movement, including walking, may suddenly halt (called freezing of gait).

Postural instability may develop, resulting in falls, which occur later in PD. Patients have difficulty starting to walk, turning, and stopping. They shuffle, taking short steps, holding their arms flexed to the waist, and swinging their arms little or not at all with each stride. Steps may inadvertently quicken, while stride length progressively shortens; this gait abnormality, called festination, is often a precursor to freezing of gait. A tendency to fall forward (propulsion) or backward (retropulsion) when the center of gravity is displaced results from loss of postural reflexes. Posture becomes stooped.

Dementia (see p. 1885) develops in about one-third of patients, usually late in PD. Early predictors of its development are visuospatial impairment (eg, getting lost while driving) and decreased verbal fluency.

Sleep disorders are common. Insomnia may result from nocturia or from the inability to turn in bed. Rapid eye movement (REM) sleep behavior disorder may develop; in this disorder, violent bursts of physical activity occur during REM sleep because the paralysis that normally occurs during REM sleep is absent. Sleep deprivation may exacerbate depression and cognitive impairment, as well as contribute to excessive daytime sleepiness. Recently, studies have shown that REM sleep behavior disorder is a marker of synucleinopathies and indicates higher risk of developing Lewy body dementia or PD dementia.

Neurologic symptoms unrelated to parkinsonism commonly develop because synucleinopathy occurs in other areas of the central, peripheral, and autonomic nervous systems. The following are examples:

- Almost universal sympathetic denervation of the heart, contributing to orthostatic hypotension
- Esophageal dysmotility, contributing to dysphagia and increased risk of aspiration
- Lower bowel dysmotility, contributing to constipation
- Urinary hesitancy and/or urgency, potentially leading to incontinence (common)
- Anosmia (common)

In some patients, some of these symptoms occur before the motor symptoms of PD and frequently worsen over time.

Seborrheic dermatitis is also common.

Diagnosis

- Mainly clinical evaluation, based on motor symptoms

Diagnosis of PD is clinical. PD is suspected in patients with characteristic unilateral resting tremor, decreased movement, or rigidity. During finger-to-nose coordination testing, the tremor disappears (or attenuates) in the limb being tested.

During the neurologic examination, patients cannot perform rapidly alternating or rapid successive movements well. Sensation and strength are usually normal. Reflexes are normal but may be difficult to elicit because of marked tremor or rigidity.

Slowed and decreased movement due to PD must be differentiated from decreased movement and spasticity due to lesions of the corticospinal tracts. Unlike PD, corticospinal tract lesions cause

- Paresis (weakness or paralysis), preferentially in distal antigravity muscles
- Hyperreflexia
- Extensor plantar responses (Babinski sign)
- Spasticity that increases muscle tone in proportion to the rate and degree of stretch placed on a muscle until resistance suddenly melts away (clasp-knife phenomenon)

The diagnosis of PD is supported by the presence of other signs such as infrequent blinking, lack of facial expression, impaired postural reflexes, and gait abnormalities.

In the elderly, other possible causes of decreased spontaneous movements or a short-stepped gait, such as severe depression, hypothyroidism, or use of antipsychotics or certain antiemetics, must be excluded before PD is diagnosed.

To help distinguish PD from secondary or atypical parkinsonism, clinicians often test responsiveness to levodopa. A large, sustained response strongly supports PD. A modest or no response to levodopa at doses of at least 1200 mg/day suggests another form of parkinsonism. Causes of secondary or atypical parkinsonism can be identified by

- A thorough history, including occupational, drug, and family history
- Evaluation for neurologic deficits characteristic of disorders other than PD
- Neuroimaging when patients have atypical features (eg, early falls, early cognitive impairment, ideomotor apraxia [inability to imitate hand gestures], hyperreflexia)

Treatment

- Carbidopa/levodopa (mainstay of treatment)
- Amantadine, MAO type B (MAO-B) inhibitors, or, in few patients, anticholinergic drugs
- Dopamine agonists
- Catechol *O*-methyltransferase (COMT) inhibitors, always used with levodopa, particularly when response to levodopa is wearing off
- Surgery if drugs do not sufficiently control symptoms or have intolerable adverse effects
- Exercise and adaptive measures

Many oral drugs are commonly used to relieve symptoms of PD (see Table 232–4).

Levodopa is the most effective treatment. However, when PD is advanced, sometimes soon after diagnosis, response to levodopa can wear off, causing fluctuations in motor symptoms and dyskinesias (see below). To reduce the time levodopa is taken and thus minimize these effects, clinicians can consider treating younger patients who have mild disability with the following:

- MAO-B inhibitors (selegiline, rasagiline)
- Dopamine agonists (eg, pramipexole, ropinirole, rotigotine)
- Amantadine (which is also the best option when trying to decrease peak-dose dyskinesias)

However, if these drugs do not sufficiently control symptoms, clinicians should promptly initiate levodopa because it can usually greatly improve quality of life. Evidence now suggests that levodopa becomes ineffective because of disease progression rather than cumulative exposure to levodopa, as was previously believed, so early use of levodopa probably does not hasten the drug's ineffectiveness.

Doses are often reduced in the elderly. Drugs that cause or worsen symptoms, particularly antipsychotics, are avoided.

Levodopa: Levodopa, the metabolic precursor of dopamine, crosses the blood-brain barrier into the basal ganglia, where it is decarboxylated to form dopamine. Coadministration of the peripheral decarboxylase inhibitor carbidopa prevents levodopa from being decarboxylated into dopamine outside the brain (peripherally), thus lowering the levodopa dosage required to produce therapeutic levels in the brain and minimizing adverse effects due to dopamine in the peripheral circulation.

Levodopa is most effective at relieving bradykinesia and rigidity, although it often substantially reduces tremor.

Common short-term adverse effects of levodopa are

- Nausea
- Vomiting
- Light-headedness

Common long-term adverse effects include

- Mental and psychiatric abnormalities (eg, delirium with confusion, paranoia, visual hallucinations, punding [complex, repetitive, stereotyped behaviors])
- Motor dysfunction (eg, dyskinesias, motor fluctuations)

Hallucinations and paranoia occur most often in the elderly and in patients who have cognitive impairment or dementia.

The dose that causes dyskinesias tends to decrease as the disease progresses. Over time, the dose that is needed for therapeutic benefit and the one that causes dyskinesia converge.

Dosage of carbidopa/levodopa is increased every 4 to 7 days as tolerated until maximum benefit is reached or adverse effects develop. The risk of adverse effects may be minimized by starting at a low dose, such as half of a 25/100 mg of carbidopa/levodopa tablet tid or qid (12.5/50 mg tid or qid), and increasing slowly to about one, two, or three 25/100-mg tablets qid. Preferably, levodopa should not be given with food because protein can reduce absorption of levodopa.

If peripheral adverse effects of levodopa (eg, nausea, vomiting, postural light-headedness) predominate, increasing the amount of carbidopa may help. Carbidopa doses up to 150 mg are safe and do not decrease the efficacy of levodopa. Most patients with PD require 400 to 1200 mg/day of levodopa in divided doses every 2 to 5 h, but some patients with malabsorption require up to 3000 mg/day.

A dissolvable immediate-release oral form of carbidopa/levodopa can be taken without water; this form is useful for patients who have difficulty swallowing. Doses are the same as for nondissolvable immediate-release carbidopa/levodopa.

A controlled-release preparation of carbidopa/levodopa is available; however, it is usually used only to treat nighttime

Table 232–4. SOME COMMONLY USED ORAL ANTIPARKINSONIAN DRUGS

DRUG	STARTING DOSE	AVERAGE DAILY DOSE AND MAXIMUM DOSE WHEN APPLICABLE	MAJOR ADVERSE EFFECTS
Dopamine precursors			
Carbidopa/levodopa 10/100, 25/100, or 25/250 mg (immediate-release or dissolvable)	1/2–1 tablet of 25/100 mg tid or qid	1–3 tablets of 25/100 mg qid	**Central:** Drowsiness, confusion, orthostatic hypotension, psychotic disturbances, nightmares, dyskinesia **Peripheral:** Nausea, anorexia, flushing abdominal cramping, palpitations **With sudden discontinuation:** Neuroleptic malignant syndrome
Carbidopa/levodopa 25/100 or 50/200 mg (controlled-release; recommended only for nighttime [not daytime] symptoms)	1 tablet of 25/100 mg at bedtime	2 tablets of 50/200 mg at bedtime	
Antiviral drug			
Amantadine	100 mg once/day	100–200 mg bid	Confusion, urinary retention, leg edema, elevated intraocular pressure, livedo reticularis **Rarely, with discontinuation or a decrease in dose:** Neuroleptic malignant syndrome
Dopamine agonists			
Pramipexole	0.125 mg tid	0.5–1 mg tid Maximum dose: 4.5 mg/day Extended-release formulation: Can be dosed once or twice/day	Nausea, vomiting, somnolence, orthostatic hypotension, dyskinesia, confusion, hallucinations, delirium, psychosis, gambling, obsessive-compulsive behavior **With sudden discontinuation:** Withdrawal syndrome or neuroleptic malignant syndrome
Ropinirole	0.25 mg tid	3–4 mg tid Maximum dose: 24 mg/day Extended-release formulation: Can be dosed once/day	
Anticholinergic drugs*			
Benztropine	0.5 mg at night	1 mg bid–2 mg tid	Dry mouth, urinary retention, constipation, blurred vision **Particularly in the elderly:** Confusion, delirium, impaired thermoregulation due to decreased sweating
Trihexyphenidyl	1 mg tid	2–5 mg tid	
Monoamine oxidase type B (MAO-B) inhibitors			
Rasagiline	0.5 mg once/day	1–2 mg once/day	Nausea, insomnia, somnolence, edema
Selegiline†	5 mg once/day	5 mg bid	Possible potentiation of nausea, insomnia, confusion, and dyskinesias when given with levodopa
Catechol *O*-methyltransferase (COMT) inhibitors			
Entacapone‡	200 mg with each dose of levodopa	200 mg with each dose of levodopa Maximum dose: 200 mg 8 times/day	**Due to increased bioavailability of levodopa**: Dyskinesias, nausea, confusion, hallucinations **Unrelated to levodopa**: Back pain, diarrhea, changes in color of urine With tolcapone, risk of liver toxicity (rare)
Tolcapone	100 mg tid	100–200 mg tid	

*Anticholinergic drugs should preferably not be used in the elderly. Because these drugs have adverse effects and because recent findings suggest that these drugs may increase tau pathology and neurodegeneration, their use should be limited.

†Selegiline is also available in a formulation designed for buccal absorption.

‡Entacapone is also available in a triple combination tablet (carbidopa, levodopa, and entacapone).

symptoms because when taken with food, it can be absorbed erratically and it is present longer in the stomach than immediate-release forms.

Occasionally, levodopa must be used to maintain motor function despite levodopa-induced hallucinations or delirium.

Psychosis has been treated with oral quetiapine or clozapine; these drugs, unlike other antipsychotics (eg, risperidone, olanzapine, all typical psychotics), do not aggravate parkinsonian symptoms. Quetiapine can be started at 25 mg at night and increased in 25-mg increments every 1 to 3 days up to 400 mg at night or 200 bid. Although clozapine is most effective, its use is limited because agranulocytosis is a risk (estimated to occur in 1% of patients). When clozapine is used, the dose is 12.5 to 50 mg once/day to 12.5 to 25 mg bid. CBC is done weekly for 6 mo and every 2 wk for another 6 mo and then every 4 wk thereafter. However, the frequency may vary depending on the WBC count. Recent evidence suggests that pimavanserin is efficacious for psychotic symptoms and does not aggravate parkinsonian symptoms; also, drug monitoring does not appear necessary. Pending further confirmation of efficacy and safety, pimavanserin may become the drug of choice for psychosis in PD.

After 2 to 5 yr of treatment, most patients experience fluctuations in their response to levodopa, and symptom control may fluctuate unpredictably between effective and ineffective (on-off fluctuations), as response to levodopa starts to wear off. Symptoms may occur before the next scheduled dose (called off effects). The dyskinesias and off effects result from a combination of the pharmacokinetic properties of levodopa, particularly its short half-life (because it is an oral drug), and disease progression.

Dyskinesias result mainly from disease progression and are not directly related to cumulative exposure to levodopa, as previously believed. Disease progression is associated with pulsatile administration of oral levodopa, which sensitizes and changes glutamatergic receptors, especially NMDA (*N*-methyl-D-aspartate) receptors. Eventually, the period of improvement after each dose shortens, and drug-induced dyskinesias result in swings from akinesia to dyskinesias. Traditionally, such swings are managed by keeping the levodopa dose as low as possible and using dosing intervals as short as every 1 to 2 h, which are highly impractical. Alternative methods to decrease the off (akinetic) times include adjunctive use of dopamine agonists, as well as COMT and/or MAO inhibitors; amantadine can reliably manage dyskinesias.

A formulation of levodopa/carbidopa intestinal gel (available in Europe) can be given using a pump connected to a feeding tube inserted in the proximal small bowel. This formulation is being studied as treatment for patients who have severe motor fluctuations or dyskinesias that cannot be relieved by drugs and who are not candidates for deep brain stimulation. This formulation appears to greatly reduce the off times and increase quality of life.

Amantadine: Amantadine is most often used to do the following:

- Ameliorate dyskinesias secondary to levodopa
- Lessen tremors

Amantadine is useful as monotherapy for early, mild parkinsonism and later can be used to augment levodopa's effects. It may augment dopaminergic activity, anticholinergic effects, or both. Amantadine is also an NMDA-receptor antagonist and thus may help slow the progression of PD and dyskinesias. If used as monotherapy, amantadine often loses its effectiveness after several months.

Dopamine agonists: These drugs directly activate dopamine receptors in the basal ganglia. They include

- Pramipexole (0.75 to 4.5 mg/day po)
- Ropinirole (3 to 6 mg/day po up to 24 mg/day)
- Rotigotine (given transdermally)
- Apomorphine (given by injection)

Bromocriptine may still be used in some countries, but in North America, its use is largely limited to treatment of pituitary adenomas because it increases the risk of cardiac valve fibrosis and pleural fibrosis.

Pergolide, an older ergot-derived dopamine agonist, was taken off the market because it increased the risk of cardiac valve fibrosis.

Oral dopamine agonists can be used as monotherapy but, as such, are rarely effective for more than a few years. Using these drugs early in treatment, with small doses of levodopa, may be useful in patients at high risk of dyskinesias and on-off effects (eg, in patients < 60 yr). However, dopamine agonists may be useful at all stages of the disease, including as adjunctive therapy in later stages. Adverse effects may limit the use of oral dopamine agonists. In 1 to 2% of patients, these drugs may cause compulsive gambling, excessive shopping, hypersexuality, or overeating, requiring dose reduction or withdrawal of the causative drug and possibly avoidance of the drug class.

Rotigotine, given transdermally once/day, provides more continuous dopaminergic stimulation than drugs given via other routes. It was recently reintroduced in the US after technical problems with the patch technology were resolved. Dose starts at 2 mg once/day and is usually increased to 6 mg once/day. Outside the US, higher doses may be recommended.

Apomorphine is an injectable dopamine agonist used as rescue therapy when off effects are frequent and severe. Onset of action is rapid (5 to 10 min), but duration is short (60 to 90 min). Apomorphine 2 to 6 mg sc can be given up to 5 times/day as needed. A 2-mg test dose is given first to check for orthostatic hypotension. BP is checked in the supine and standing positions before treatment and 20, 40, and 60 min afterward. Other adverse effects are similar to those of other dopamine agonists. Nausea can be prevented by starting trimethobenzamide 300 mg po tid 3 days before apomorphine and continuing it for the first 2 mo of treatment.

Apomorphine given by subcutaneous pump is available in some countries; it can be used instead of a levodopa pump in patients who have advanced PD and who are not candidates for functional surgery.

Selective MAO-B inhibitors: These drugs include selegiline and rasagiline.

Selegiline inhibits one of the 2 major enzymes that break down dopamine in the brain, thereby prolonging the action of each dose of levodopa. In some patients with mild off effects, selegiline helps prolong levodopa's effectiveness. Used initially as monotherapy, selegiline controls mild symptoms; as a result, use of levodopa can be delayed by about 1 yr. A dose of 5 mg po bid does not cause hypertensive crisis, which, because of the drug's amphetamine-like metabolites, is sometimes triggered when patients taking a nonselective MAO inhibitor consume tyramine in foods (eg, some cheeses). Although virtually free of adverse effects, selegiline can potentiate levodopa-induced dyskinesias, mental and psychiatric adverse effects, and nausea, requiring reduction in the levodopa dose. Selegiline is also available in a formulation designed for buccal absorption (zydis-selegiline).

Rasagiline inhibits the same enzymes as selegiline. It is effective and well-tolerated in early and late disease; uses of rasagiline 1 to 2 mg po once/day are similar to those of selegiline. Unlike selegiline, it does not have amphetamine-like metabolites, so theoretically, risk of a hypertensive crisis when patients consume tyramine is lower with rasagiline.

Anticholinergic drugs: Anticholinergic drugs can be used as monotherapy in early disease and later to supplement levodopa. They are most effective for tremor. Doses are increased very slowly. Adverse effects may include cognitive impairment and dry mouth, which are particularly troublesome for the elderly and may be the principal problem with use of these drugs. Thus, anticholinergic drugs are usually used only in young patients with tremor-predominant PD or with some dystonic components. Rarely, they are used as adjunctive treatment in elderly patients without cognitive impairment or psychiatric disorders.

Recent studies using a mouse model indicate that use of anticholinergic drugs should be limited because these drugs appear to increase tau pathology and neurodegeneration; degree of increase correlates with the drug's central anticholinergic activity.[1]

Commonly used anticholinergic drugs include benztropine and trihexyphenidyl.

Antihistamines with anticholinergic effects (eg, diphenhydramine 25 to 50 mg po bid to qid, orphenadrine 50 mg po once/day to qid) are occasionally useful for treating tremor.

Anticholinergic tricyclic antidepressants (eg, amitriptyline 10 to 150 mg po at bedtime), if used for depression, may be useful as an adjunct to levodopa.

Catechol *O*-methyltransferase (COMT) inhibitors: These drugs (eg, entacapone, tolcapone) inhibit the breakdown of levodopa and dopamine and therefore appear to be useful adjuncts to levodopa. They are used commonly in patients who have been taking levodopa for a long time when response to levodopa is progressively wearing off at the end of dosing intervals (known as wearing-off effects).

Entacapone can be used in combination with levodopa and carbidopa. For each dose of levodopa taken, 200 mg of entacapone is given, to a maximum of 200 mg 8 times/day.

Tolcapone is a more potent COMT inhibitor because it can cross the blood-brain barrier; however, it is less commonly used because rarely, liver toxicity has been reported. It is an appropriate option if entacapone does not sufficiently control off effects. The dose for tolcapone is increased gradually from 100 up to 200 mg tid. Liver enzymes must be monitored periodically. Tolcapone should be stopped if ALT or AST levels increase to twice the upper limit of the normal range or higher or if symptoms and signs suggest that the liver is damaged.

Surgery: If drugs are ineffective and/or have intolerable adverse effects, surgery, including deep brain stimulation and lesional surgery, may be considered.

For patients with levodopa-induced dyskinesias or significant motor fluctuations, deep brain stimulation of the subthalamic nucleus or globus pallidus interna is often recommended to modulate overactivity in the basal ganglia and to thus decrease parkinsonian symptoms in patients with PD. For patients with tremor only, stimulation of the ventralis intermediate nucleus of the thalamus is sometimes recommended; however, because most patients also have other symptoms, stimulation of the subthalamic nucleus, which relieves tremor as well as other symptoms, is usually preferred.

Lesional surgery aims to stop overactivity directed to the thalamus from the globus pallidus interna or to control tremor in patients with tremor-predominant PD if thalamotomy is planned. However, lesional surgery is not reversible and cannot be modulated over time; bilateral lesional surgery is not recommended because it can have severe adverse effects such as dysphagia and dysarthria. Lesional surgery involving the subthalamic nucleus is contraindicated because it causes severe ballismus.

Patients with cognitive impairment, dementia, or a psychiatric disorder are not suitable candidates for surgery because neurosurgery can exacerbate cognitive impairment and psychiatric disorders, and the risk of additional mental impairment outweighs the benefits of any improvement in motor function.

Focused ultrasound therapy: Focused ultrasound therapy is used to is used to destroy a small amount of tissue that is interfering with motor function. Tremor control is its main goal. Focused ultrasound therapy remains experimental but may be available in the future.

Physical measures: Maximizing activity is a goal. Patients should increase daily activities to the greatest extent possible. If they cannot, physical or occupational therapy, which may involve a regular exercise program, may help condition them physically. Therapists may teach patients adaptive strategies and help them make appropriate adaptations in the home (eg, installing grab bars to reduce the risk of falls).

To prevent or relieve constipation (which may result from the disease, antiparkinsonian drugs, and/or inactivity), patients should consume a high-fiber diet, exercise when possible, and drink adequate amounts of fluids. Dietary supplements (eg, psyllium) and stimulant laxatives (eg, bisacodyl 10 to 20 mg po once/day) can help.

Caregiver and end-of-life issues: Because PD is progressive, patients eventually need help with normal daily activities. Caregivers should be directed to resources that can help them learn about the physical and psychologic effects of PD and about ways to help the patient function as well as possible. Because such care is tiring and stressful, caregivers should be encouraged to contact support groups for social and psychologic support.

Eventually, most patients with PD become severely disabled and immobile. They may be unable to eat, even with assistance. Because swallowing becomes increasingly difficult, death due to aspiration pneumonia is a risk. For some patients, a nursing home may be the best place for care.

Before people with PD are incapacitated, they should establish advance directives, indicating what kind of medical care they want at the end of life.

1. Yoshiyama Y, Kojima A, Itoh K, Uchiyama T, Arai K: Anticholinergics boost the pathological process of neurodegeneration with increased inflammation in a tauopathy mouse model. *Neurobiol Dis* 45(1):329–336, 2012. doi: 10.1016/j.nbd.2011.08.017.

KEY POINTS

- PD is a synucleinopathy and thus can overlap with other synucleinopathies (eg, dementia with Lewy bodies, multiple system atrophy).
- Suspect PD based on characteristic features: resting tremor, muscle rigidity, slow and decreased movement, and postural and gait instability.
- Distinguish PD from disorders that cause similar symptoms based mainly on the history and physical examination results, but also test responsiveness to levodopa; sometimes neuroimaging is useful.
- Typically, use levodopa/carbidopa (the mainstay of treatment), but other drugs (amantadine, dopamine agonists, MAO-B inhibitors, COMT inhibitors) may be used before and/or with levodopa/carbidopa.
- Consider surgical procedures, such as deep brain stimulation, if patients have symptoms refractory to optimal drug therapy and do not have cognitive impairment or a psychiatric disorder.

SECONDARY AND ATYPICAL PARKINSONISM

Secondary parkinsonism refers to a group of disorders that have features similar to those of Parkinson disease (PD) but have a different etiology. Atypical parkinsonism refers to a group of neurodegenerative disorders other than PD that have some features of PD but have some different clinical features and a different pathology. Diagnosis is by clinical evaluation and response to levodopa. Treatment is directed at the cause when possible.

Parkinsonism results from drugs, disorders other than PD, or exogenous toxins.

In **secondary parkinsonism,** the mechanism is blockade of or interference with dopamine's action in the basal ganglia. The most common cause of secondary parkinsonism is

- Use of drugs that decrease dopaminergic activity

These drugs include antipsychotics (eg, phenothiazine, thioxanthene, butyrophenone), antiemetics (eg, metoclopramide, prochlorperazine), and drugs (see Table 232–5) that deplete dopamine (eg, tetrabenazine, reserpine).

Atypical parkinsonism encompasses neurodegenerative disorders such as progressive supranuclear palsy, diffuse Lewy body dementia, corticobasal degeneration, and multiple system atrophy.

Symptoms and Signs

Parkinsonism causes the same symptoms as PD (eg, resting tremor, rigidity, bradykinesia, postural instability).

Diagnosis

- Clinical evaluation, response to levodopa therapy, and, for differential diagnosis, sometimes neuroimaging

To differentiate PD from secondary or atypical parkinsonism, clinicians note whether levodopa results in dramatic improvement, suggesting PD.

Causes of parkinsonism can be identified by the following:

- A thorough history, including occupational, drug, and family history
- Evaluation for neurologic deficits characteristic of neurodegenerative disorders other than PD
- Neuroimaging when indicated

Deficits that suggest neurodegenerative disorders other than PD include gaze palsies, signs of corticospinal tract dysfunction (eg, hyperreflexia), myoclonus, autonomic dysfunction (if early or severe), cerebellar ataxia, prominent dystonia, ideomotor apraxia (inability to mimic hand motions), early dementia, early falls, and confinement to a wheelchair.

Treatment

- Treatment of the cause

The cause of secondary parkinsonism is corrected or treated if possible, sometimes resulting in clinical improvement or disappearance of symptoms.

Drugs used to treat PD are often ineffective or have only transient benefit. But amantadine or an anticholinergic drug (eg, benztropine) may ameliorate parkinsonism secondary to use of antipsychotic drugs. However, because these drugs may increase tau pathology and neurodegeneration, their use should be limited.[1]

Physical measures to maintain mobility and independence are useful (as for PD). Maximizing activity is a goal. Patients should increase daily activities to the greatest extent possible. If they cannot, physical or occupational therapy, which may involve a regular exercise program, may help condition them physically. Therapists may teach patients adaptive strategies, help them make appropriate adaptations in the home (eg, installing grab bars to reduce the risk of falls), and recommend adaptive devices that may be useful.

Good nutrition is essential.

1. Yoshiyama Y, Kojima A, Itoh K, Uchiyama T, Arai K: Anticholinergics boost the pathological process of neurodegeneration with increased inflammation in a tauopathy mouse model. *Neurobiol Dis* 45(1):329–336, 2012. doi: 10.1016/j.nbd.2011.08.017.

KEY POINTS

- Parkinsonism can be caused by drugs, toxins, neurodegenerative disorders, and other disorders that affect the brain (eg, stroke, tumor, infection, trauma, hypoparathyroidism).
- Suspect parkinsonism based on the clinical evaluation and differentiate it from PD based on lack of response to levodopa; neuroimaging may be needed.
- Check for deficits that suggest a neurodegenerative disorder other than PD.
- Correct or treat the cause if possible, and recommend physical measures to maintain mobility.

PROGRESSIVE SUPRANUCLEAR PALSY

(Steele-Richardson-Olszewski Syndrome)

Progressive supranuclear palsy is a rare, degenerative CNS disorder that progressively impairs voluntary eye movements and causes bradykinesia, muscular rigidity with progressive axial dystonia, pseudobulbar palsy, and dementia. Diagnosis is clinical. Treatment focuses on relieving symptoms.

The cause of progressive supranuclear palsy is unknown.

Neurons in the basal ganglia and brain stem degenerate; neurofibrillary tangles containing an abnormally phosphorylated tau protein are also present. Multiple lacunar strokes in the basal ganglia and deep white matter can resemble progressive supranuclear palsy; however, cerebrovascular disease is nondegenerative and progresses more gradually.

Symptoms and Signs

Symptoms of progressive supranuclear palsy usually begin in late middle age.

The first symptom may be

- Difficulty looking up or down without moving the neck or difficulty climbing up and down stairs

Voluntary eye movements, particularly vertical, are difficult, but reflexive eye movements are unaffected.

Movements are slowed, muscles become rigid, and axial dystonia develops. Patients tend to fall backward.

Dysphagia and dysarthria with emotional lability (pseudobulbar palsy) are common. Resting tremor may develop.

Dementia eventually occurs.

Many patients become incapacitated within about 5 yr and die within about 10 yr.

Table 232–5. SOME CAUSES OF SECONDARY AND ATYPICAL PARKINSONISM

CAUSE	COMMENTS
Neurodegenerative disorders	
Amyotrophic lateral sclerosis–parkinsonism-dementia complex of Guam	Responds poorly to antiparkinsonian drugs
Corticobasal degeneration	Begins asymmetrically, usually after age 60 Causes cortical and basal ganglia signs, often with apraxia, dystonia, myoclonus, and alien limb syndrome (movement of a limb that seems independent of the patient's conscious control) Causes immobility after about 5 yr and death after about 10 yr Responds poorly to antiparkinsonian drugs
Dementia (eg, Alzheimer disease, chromosome 17–linked frontotemporal dementias, diffuse Lewy body dementia)	Parkinsonism often preceded by dementia most typically with • Prominent memory loss (Alzheimer disease) • Language impairment (frontotemporal dementias) • Visuospatial impairment (diffuse Lewy body dementia)
Multiple system atrophy	May include prominent autonomic dysfunction May include prominent cerebellar dysfunction May include severe parkinsonian features, usually with poor response to levodopa Often causes early falls and balance problems Responds poorly to antiparkinsonian drugs
Progressive supranuclear palsy	First manifests with gait and balance problems In its classic form, causes progressive ophthalmoparesis, starting with impairment of downward gaze Responds poorly to antiparkinsonian drugs
Spinocerebellar ataxias (usually type 2 or 3)	Usually first manifests with imbalance and poor coordination Responds poorly to antiparkinsonian drugs
Other disorders	
Cerebrovascular disease	Manifests with rigidity and bradykinesia or akinesia (akinetic-rigid syndrome) that predominantly involves the lower extremities, with prominent gait disturbance and symmetric symptoms Rarely responds to antiparkinsonian drugs
Brain tumors near the basal ganglia	Manifests with hemiparkinsonism (ie, restricted to one side of the body)
Repeated traumatic brain injury	Often causes dementia (as in dementia pugilistica)
Hydrocephalus	Usually characterized by normal CSF pressure (normal-pressure hydrocephalus) and caused by various mechanisms Rarely caused by obstructed CSF flow with increased CSF pressure (obstructive hydrocephalus)
Hypoparathyroidism	Causes calcification of the basal ganglia May cause chorea and athetosis
Viral encephalitis (eg, West Nile encephalitis), infectious or postinfectious autoimmune	Can cause parkinsonism transiently during the acute phase or, rarely, permanently (eg, postencephalitic parkinsonism after the epidemic of encephalitis lethargica in 1915–1926) In postencephalitic parkinsonism, forced, sustained deviation of the head and eyes (oculogyric crises); other dystonias; autonomic instability; depression; and personality changes
Drugs	
Antipsychotics	Can cause reversible* parkinsonism
Meperidine analog (*N*-MPTP)[†]	Can cause sudden, irreversible parkinsonism Occurs in IV drug users
Metoclopramide Reserpine Lithium, long-term use	Can cause reversible* parkinsonism May be dose-dependent or related to susceptibility (risk factors include older age and female sex) With lithium, sometimes results in cerebellar dysfunction

Table continues on the following page.

Table 232–5. SOME CAUSES OF SECONDARY AND ATYPICAL PARKINSONISM (*Continued*)

CAUSE	COMMENTS
Toxins	
Carbon monoxide	Can cause irreversible parkinsonism
Methanol	As contaminated moonshine, can cause hemorrhagic necrosis of the basal ganglia
Manganese	Can cause parkinsonism with dystonia and cognitive changes when toxicity is chronic Usually related to occupation (eg, welding) but can result from abuse of methcathinone (in bath salts made from ephedrine)

*When drugs are withdrawn, symptoms usually resolve within a few weeks, although they may persist for months.
†*N*-MPTP results from unsuccessful attempts to produce meperidine for illicit use.
N-MPTP = *N*-methyl-4-phenyl-1,2,3,6-tetrahydropyridine.

Diagnosis

- Clinical evaluation

Diagnosis of progressive supranuclear palsy is clinical.

MRI is usually done to exclude other disorders. In advanced cases, MRI shows a characteristic decrease in midbrain size that is best seen on midsagittal views and that causes the midbrain to be shaped like a hummingbird or emperor penguin. On axial views, the midbrain may resemble a morning glory.[1]

1. Adachi M, Kawanami T, Ohshima H, et al: Morning glory sign: a particular MR finding in progressive supranuclear palsy. *Magn Reson Med Sci* 3(3):125–132, 2004.

Treatment

- Supportive care

Treatment of progressive supranuclear palsy focuses on relieving symptoms but is unsatisfactory. Occasionally, levodopa and/or amantadine partially relieve rigidity. Physical and occupational therapy may help improve mobility and function and reduce the risk of falls.

Because progressive supranuclear palsy is fatal, patients should be encouraged to prepare advance directives soon after the disorder is diagnosed. These directives should indicate what kind of medical care people want at the end of life.

TREMOR

Tremors are involuntary, rhythmic, oscillatory movements of reciprocal, antagonistic muscle groups, typically involving the hands, head, face, vocal cords, trunk, or legs. Diagnosis is clinical. Treatment depends on the cause and type of tremor and may involve avoidance of triggers (physiologic), propranolol or primidone (essential), physical therapy (cerebellar), levodopa (parkinsonian), and possibly deep brain stimulation or thalamotomy (disabling and drug-refractory).

Tremor may be

- Normal (physiologic)
- Pathologic

Physiologic tremor, usually barely perceptible, becomes noticeable in many people during physical or mental stress.

Tremors vary in

- Pattern of occurrence (eg, intermittent, constant)
- Severity
- Acuity (eg, gradual, abrupt)

The severity of tremor may not be related to the seriousness of the underlying disorder. For example, essential tremor is generally thought of as benign and should not shorten life, but symptoms can be disabling, and cerebellar degeneration has detected in some neuropathologic studies.

Pathophysiology

Various lesions in the brain stem, extrapyramidal system, or cerebellum can cause tremors. Neural dysfunction or lesions that cause tremor may result from injury, ischemia, metabolic abnormalities, or a neurodegenerative disorder. Sometimes tremor is a familial condition (eg, essential tremor).

Classification: Tremor is classified primarily based on when it occurs:

- **Resting tremors** are visible at rest and occur when a body part is completely supported against gravity. Resting tremors are minimal or absent during activity. They occur at a frequency of 3 to 6 cycles/sec (Hz).
- **Action tremors** are maximal when a body part is moved voluntarily. Action tremors may or may not change in severity as a target is reached; they can occur at very different frequencies, but the frequency is always < 13 Hz. Action tremors include kinetic, intention, and postural tremors.
- **Kinetic tremors** appear in the last part of a movement toward a target; amplitude is low.
- **Intention tremors** occur during voluntary movement toward a target, but amplitude is high and frequency is low during the complete movement, while the tremor worsens as the target is reached (as seen in finger-to-nose testing); they occur at a frequency of 3 to 10 Hz.
- **Postural tremors** are maximal when a limb is maintained in a fixed position against gravity (eg, holding the arms stretched out); they occur at a frequency of 5 to 8 Hz. Sometimes they are modified by specific positions or tasks, which may indicate their origin; for example, dystonia may trigger a tremor (dystonic tremor).

Complex tremors can have components of more than one type of tremor.

Tremor can also be classified based on whether it is

- Physiologic (within the range of normal)
- A primary disorder (essential tremor, Parkinson disease)
- Secondary to a disorder (eg, stroke)

Tremor is usually described based on frequency of oscillations (rapid or slow) and amplitude of movement (fine or coarse).

Etiology

Physiologic tremor: Physiologic tremor occurs in otherwise healthy people. It is an action or postural tremor that tends to affect both hands about equally; amplitude is usually fine. It is often noticeable only when certain stressors are present. These stressors include

- Anxiety
- Fatigue
- Exercise
- Sleep deprivation
- Withdrawal of alcohol or certain other CNS depressant drugs (eg, benzodiazepines, opioids)
- Certain disorders (eg, hyperthyroidism), when symptomatic
- Consumption of caffeine or recreational drugs such as cocaine, amphetamines, or phencyclidine
- Use of certain therapeutic drugs, such as theophylline, beta-adrenergic agonists, corticosteroids, and valproate

Pathologic (nonphysiologic) tremor: There are many causes (see Table 232–6), but the most common are

- For action or postural tremors: Essential tremor
- For resting tremors: Parkinson disease
- For intention tremors: Cerebellar dysfunction (eg, due to a stroke, trauma, or multiple sclerosis)

Drugs (see Table 232–7) can cause or aggravate different types of tremor. Low doses of some sedatives (eg, alcohol) may relieve some tremors (eg, essential and physiologic tremor); higher doses may cause or exacerbate tremor.

Evaluation

Because the diagnosis of tremor is largely clinical, a meticulous history and physical examination are essential.

History: History of present illness should cover

- Acuity of onset (eg, gradual, abrupt)
- Age at onset
- Body parts affected
- Provoking factors (eg, movement, rest, standing)
- Alleviating or exacerbating factors (eg, alcohol, caffeine, stress, anxiety)

If onset is abrupt, patients should be asked about potential triggering events (eg, recent trauma or illness, use of a new drug).

Review of systems should seek symptoms of causative disorders, including

- Multiple episodic neurologic problems: Multiple sclerosis
- Recent sudden onset of motor weakness, language difficulties, or dysarthria: Stroke
- Confusion and fever: Meningitis, encephalitis, brain abscess, or brain tumor
- Muscle rigidity, gait and postural problems, and slowness of movement: Parkinson disease or other forms of parkinsonism
- Weight loss, increased appetite, palpitations, diarrhea, and heat intolerance: Hyperthyroidism
- Sensory deficits: Peripheral neuropathy
- Agitation and hallucinations: Alcohol withdrawal or drug toxicity

Past medical history should cover conditions associated with tremor (see Table 232–6). Family history should include questions about tremor in 1st-degree relatives. The drug profile should be reviewed for causative drugs (see Table 232–7), and patients should be asked specifically about caffeine intake and alcohol and recreational drug use (particularly recent discontinuation).

Physical examination: A complete and extensive neurologic examination is mandatory and should include evaluation of mental status, cranial nerves, motor and sensory function, gait, muscle stretch reflexes, and cerebellar function (with

Table 232–6. SOME CAUSES OF TREMOR

CAUSE	SUGGESTIVE FINDINGS	DIAGNOSTIC APPROACH
Action tremor		
Alcohol or drug withdrawal (eg, of benzodiazepines or opioids)	Agitation and fine tremor starting 24–72 h after the last use of alcohol or the drug (eg, a benzodiazepine) Sometimes hypertension, tachycardia, or fever, especially in hospitalized patients	Clinical evaluation
Drug-induced	History of drug use	Amelioration of tremor after stopping the drug
Endocrinologic, metabolic, and toxic abnormalities: • Anoxic encephalopathy • Heavy metal poisoning • Hepatic encephalopathy • Hyperparathyroidism • Hyperthyroidism • Hypoglycemia • Pheochromocytoma • Uremic encephalopathy	Tremor plus altered level of consciousness (suggesting encephalopathy) and an obvious underlying disorder (eg, renal or hepatic failure) Exophthalmos, hyperreflexia, tachycardia, heat intolerance (suggesting hyperthyroidism) Extreme, refractory hypertension (suggesting pheochromocytoma)	TSH level 24-h urine collection to check for metanephrines and to measure ammonia level, BUN, glucose level, and calcium and PTH levels Heavy metal testing

Table continues on the following page.

Table 232–6. SOME CAUSES OF TREMOR (*Continued*)

CAUSE	SUGGESTIVE FINDINGS	DIAGNOSTIC APPROACH
Essential tremor	Progressively persistent coarse or fine, slow (4–8 Hz) tremor, usually symmetric and affecting both upper extremities and sometimes the head and voice, particularly in patients with a family history of tremor	Clinical evaluation
Physiologic tremor	Fine, rapid (8–13 Hz) tremor that occurs in otherwise healthy people and may be enhanced by certain drugs or conditions (see above) Usually suppression of tremor with low doses of alcohol and other sedatives	Clinical evaluation
Resting tremor		
Drug-induced parkinsonism	History of drug use	Amelioration of tremor after stopping the drug
Parkinson disease	Low-frequency (3–5 Hz) alternating tremor, often of the thumb against the index finger (pill rolling) but sometimes also affecting the chin or a leg Usually accompanied by other symptoms, such as micrographia, bradykinesia (slow movement), cogwheel rigidity, and shuffling gait Often no family history of Parkinson tremor and no reduction in tremor after alcohol consumption	Specific clinical criteria Good response to empiric trial of dopaminergic drugs
Intention tremor		
Cerebellar lesions: • Abscess • Friedreich ataxia • Hemorrhage • Multiple sclerosis • Spinocerebellar degeneration • Stroke • TBI • Tumor	Low-frequency (< 4 Hz) tremor that usually occurs unilaterally with ataxia, dysmetria, dysdiadochokinesia (inability to perform rapid alternating movements), and dysarthria In some patients, family history of the disorder (eg, Friedreich ataxia)	MRI of the brain
Drug-induced	History of drug use	Amelioration of tremor after stopping the drug
Complex tremors		
Holmes tremor (midbrain, red nucleus, rubral, or thalamic tremor)	Irregular, low-frequency (< 4.5 Hz) tremor predominantly in the proximal limbs Combination of rest, postural, and intention tremors caused by midbrain lesions (eg, due to stroke or multiple sclerosis) near the red nucleus Sometimes signs of ataxia and weakness	MRI of the brain
Neuropathic tremor: • Chronic relapsing polyneuropathy • Guillain-Barré syndrome • Diabetes • IgM neuropathy	Variable tremor type and frequency, usually postural and intention tremor in the affected extremities Other signs of peripheral neuropathy	Electromyography
Psychogenic tremor	Abrupt onset and/or spontaneous remission of complex mixed-type tremor with changing characteristics Increased by attention and lessened by distraction of patient	Clinical evaluation
Wilson disease	Variable tremor type (usually in the proximal arm) in children or young adults, often with signs of hepatic failure, rigidity, clumsy gait, dysarthria, inappropriate grinning, drooling, and neuropsychiatric signs	24-h urine collection to measure copper level; serum ceruloplasmin Slit-lamp examination to check for Kayser-Fleischer rings around the iris (caused by copper deposition)

PTH = parathyroid hormone; TBI = traumatic brain injury; TSH = thyroid-stimulating hormone.

Table 232–7. SOME DRUG CAUSES OF TREMOR BY TYPE

DRUG	POSTURAL TREMOR	RESTING TREMOR (DRUG-INDUCED PARKINSONISM)	INTENTION TREMOR
Amiodarone*	√		
Amitriptyline*	√		
Amphotericin B		√	
Beta-agonists (inhaled)*	√		√
Caffeine*	√		
Calcitonin	√		
Cimetidine	√		
Cocaine*	√		
Cyclosporine*	√		√
Cytarabine	√		√
Epinephrine			√
Ethanol*	√	√	√
Haloperidol*	√	√	
Ifosfamide	√		√
Interferon-alfa	√		
Lithium*	√	√	√
MDMA (Ecstasy)	√		
Medroxyprogesterone	√	√	
Metoclopramide*		√	
Mexiletine	√		
Nicotine*	√		
Procainamide	√		
Reserpine	√	√	
SSRIs*	√	√	
Tacrolimus	√		√
Tamoxifen	√		
Theophylline*	√		
Thioridazine*	√	√	
Thyroxine*	√		
Valproate*	√	√	
Vidarabine			√

*More common cause of tremor.
MDMA = methylenedioxymethamphetamine.
Data from Morgan JC, Sethi KD: Drug-induced tremors. *The Lancet Neurology* 4:866–876, 2005.

observation of finger-to-nose, shin-to-heel, and rapid alternating hand movements. The examiner should test muscles for rigidity by moving the limbs through their range of motion.

Vital signs should be reviewed for tachycardia, hypertension, or fever. General examination should note any cachexia, psychomotor agitation, and absence of facial expressions (which may indicate bradykinesia). The thyroid should be palpated for nodules and enlargement, and any signs of exophthalmus or eyelid lag should be noted.

Focused examination should note distribution and frequency of the tremor while

- The affected body parts are at rest and fully supported (eg, in the patient's lap).
- The patient assumes certain postures (eg, holding the arms outstretched).
- The patient is walking or doing tasks with the affected body part.

The examiner should note whether the tremor changes during mental distraction tasks (eg, serial subtraction of 7 from 100). The quality of the voice should be observed while the patient sustains a long note.

Red flags: The following findings are of particular concern:

- Abrupt onset
- Onset in people < 50 and with no family history of benign tremor
- Other neurologic deficits (eg, change in mental status, motor weakness, cranial nerve palsy, ataxic gait, dysarthria)
- Tachycardia and agitation

Interpretation of findings: Clinical findings help suggest a cause (see Table 232–6).

Tremor type and onset are useful clues:

- **Resting tremors** usually indicate Parkinson disease, particularly when they are unilateral or when tremor is isolated to the chin, voice, or leg.
- **Intention tremors** suggest a cerebellar disorder but may result from multiple sclerosis or Wilson disease.
- **Postural tremor** suggests physiologic or essential tremor if onset is gradual; it suggests a toxic or metabolic disorder if onset is sudden.

Severe essential tremor is often confused with Parkinson disease but can usually be distinguished by specific characteristics (see Table 232–8). Occasionally, the 2 syndromes overlap (mixed essential tremor–Parkinson disease).

The following findings may help suggest causes:

- Sudden onset is most typical of psychogenic tremor.
- Stepwise progression suggests an ischemic vascular disorder or multiple sclerosis
- Development of tremor after use of a new drug suggests that the drug is the cause.
- Onset of tremor with agitation, tachycardia, and hypertension within 24 to 72 h of hospitalization may suggest withdrawal from alcohol, a sedative, or an illicit substance.

Gait is observed. Gait abnormalities may suggest multiple sclerosis, stroke, Parkinson disease, or a cerebellar disorder. Gait is characteristically narrow-based and shuffling in Parkinson disease and wide-based and ataxic in cerebellar disorders. The gait may have histrionic or inconsistent qualities in patients with psychogenic tremor. In patients with essential tremor, gait is often normal, but tandem gait (placing heel to toe) may be abnormal.

Complex tremor that decreases with mental distraction or whose frequency entrains to a volitional tapping rhythm by an unaffected body part (maintaining 2 different volitional movement frequencies simultaneously in 2 different body parts is difficult) suggests a psychogenic tremor.

Testing: In most patients, history and physical examination are sufficient to identify the likely etiology. However, MRI or CT of the brain should be done if

- Tremor onset is acute.
- Progression is rapid.
- Neurologic signs suggest stroke, a demyelinating disorder, or a structural lesion.

When the cause of tremor is unclear (based on history and physical examination findings), the following are done:

- Thyroid-stimulating hormone (TSH) and thyroxine (T_4) are measured to check for hyperthyroidism.
- Calcium and parathyroid hormone are measured to check for hyperparathyroidism.
- Glucose testing is done to rule out hypoglycemia.

In patients with toxic encephalopathy, the underlying condition is usually readily apparent, but measurement of BUN and ammonia levels can help confirm the diagnosis. Measurement of free metanephrines in plasma is indicated in patients with unexplained refractory hypertension; serum ceruloplasmin and urinary copper levels should be measured if patients are < 40 and have tremor with an unclear cause (with or without parkinsonism) and no family history of benign tremor.

Although electromyography (EMG) can differentiate true tremor from other movement disorders (eg, myoclonus, clonus, epilepsia partialis continua), it is rarely required. However, EMG may help establish peripheral neuropathy as a potential cause of tremor if a neuropathy is clinically suspected.

Treatment

Physiologic tremors: No treatment is necessary unless symptoms are bothersome. Avoiding triggers (such as caffeine, fatigue, sleep deprivation, drugs, and, when possible, stress and anxiety) can help prevent or reduce symptoms.

Physiologic tremor enhanced by alcohol withdrawal or hyperthyroidism responds to treatment of the underlying condition.

Oral benzodiazepines (eg, diazepam 2 to 10 mg, lorazepam 1 to 2 mg, oxazepam 10 to 30 mg) given tid or qid may be useful for people with tremor and chronic anxiety, but continuous use should be avoided. Propranolol 20 to 80 mg po qid (and other beta-blockers) is often effective for tremor enhanced by drugs or acute anxiety (eg, stage fright).

Table 232–8. SOME CHARACTERISTICS DIFFERENTIATING PARKINSON DISEASE FROM ESSENTIAL TREMOR

CHARACTERISTIC	PARKINSON DISEASE	ESSENTIAL TREMOR
Tremor type	Resting tremor	Postural and intention tremors
Age	Older age (> 60)	All age groups
Family history	Usually negative	Positive in > 60% of patients
Alcohol	Not beneficial	Often beneficial
Tremor onset	Unilateral	Bilateral
Muscle tone	Cogwheel rigidity	Normal
Facial expression	Decreased	Normal
Gait	Decreased arm swing	Normal or mild imbalance
Tremor latency	Longer (8–9 sec)	Shorter (1–2 sec)

Essential tremors: Propranolol 20 to 80 mg po qid (or other beta-blockers) is often effective, as is primidone 50 to 250 mg po tid. For some patients, a small amount of alcohol is effective; however, alcohol is not routinely recommended for treatment because abuse is a risk.

Second-line drugs are topiramate 25 to 100 mg po bid and gabapentin 300 mg po bid or tid. Benzodiazepines may be added if other drugs do not control the tremor.

Cerebellar tremors: No effective drug is available; physical therapy (eg, weighting the affected limbs, teaching patients to brace the proximal limb during activity) sometimes helps.

Parkinsonian tremors: Parkinson disease is treated.

Levodopa is usually the treatment of choice for most parkinsonian tremors.

Anticholinergic drugs may be considered in certain cases, but their adverse effects (decreased mental concentration, dry mouth, dry eyes, urinary retention and the possibility that they enhance tau pathology) may outweigh their benefits, particularly in the elderly.

Other drugs include dopamine agonists (eg, pramipexole, ropinirole), MAO type B inhibitors (selegiline, rasagiline), COMT inhibitors (entacapone, tolcapone—used only in combination with levodopa), and amantadine.

Disabling tremor: For severe, disabling, drug-refractory essential tremor, surgical management with unilateral stereotactic thalamotomy or chronic unilateral or bilateral thalamic deep brain stimulation may be considered.

Dystonic tremor may respond better to functional neurosurgery targeting the internal portion of the globus pallidus.

In Parkinson disease, tremor substantially lessens after thalamic, internal globus pallidus, or subthalamic nucleus deep brain stimulation.

Although these techniques are widely available, they should be used only after reasonable drug therapy has failed and only in patients who do not have substantial cognitive or psychiatric impairment.

Geriatrics Essentials: Tremor

Many elderly patients attribute development of tremor to normal aging and may not seek medical attention. Although essential tremor is more prevalent among the elderly, a thorough history and physical examination are required to rule out other causes and to determine whether the symptoms are severe enough to justify drug or surgical treatment.

Comparatively low doses of drugs may exacerbate tremor in the elderly, and adjusting doses of chronically used drugs (eg, amiodarone, metoclopramide, SSRIs, thyroxine) to the lowest effective dose should be considered. Similarly, elderly patients are more vulnerable to adverse effects of drugs used to treat tremor; thus, these drugs should be used cautiously in the elderly, usually at lower dosages than are otherwise considered optimal. If possible, anticholinergic drugs should not be used in the elderly.

Tremor can significantly affect functional ability in the elderly, particularly if they have other physical or cognitive impairments. Physical and occupational therapy can provide simple coping strategies, and assistive devices may help maintain quality of life.

KEY POINTS

- Tremor can be classified as resting or action (which includes intention, kinetic, and postural tremors).
- The most common causes of tremor include physiologic tremor, essential tremor, and Parkinson disease.
- History and physical examination can typically identify the etiology of tremor.
- Consider Parkinson disease if patients have a resting tremor, consider essential or physiologic tremor if they have a postural or an action tremor, and consider cerebellar tremor if they have an intention tremor.
- If tremor begins abruptly or occurs in patients who are < 50 and do not have a family history of benign tremor, evaluate them promptly and thoroughly.
- Treat according to the cause and type of tremor: avoidance of triggers (physiologic), propranolol or primidone (essential), physical therapy (cerebellar), usually levodopa (parkinsonian), and possibly deep brain stimulation (disabling and drug-refractory).

CEREBELLAR DISORDERS

Cerebellar disorders have numerous causes, including congenital malformations, hereditary ataxias, and acquired conditions. Symptoms vary with the cause but typically include ataxia (impaired muscle coordination). Diagnosis is clinical and often by imaging and sometimes genetic testing. Treatment is usually supportive unless the cause is acquired and reversible.

The cerebellum has 3 parts:

- **Archicerebellum (vestibulocerebellum):** It includes the flocculonodular lobe, which is located in the medial zone. The archicerebellum helps maintain equilibrium and coordinate eye, head, and neck movements; it is closely interconnected with the vestibular nuclei.
- **Midline vermis (paleocerebellum):** It helps coordinate trunk and leg movements. Vermis lesions result in abnormalities of stance and gait.
- **Lateral hemispheres (neocerebellum):** They control quick and finely coordinated limb movements, predominantly of the arms.

There is growing consensus that in addition to coordination, the cerebellum controls some aspects of memory, learning, and cognition.

Ataxia is the archetypal sign of cerebellar dysfunction, but many other motor abnormalities may occur (see Table 232–9).

Etiology

Congenital malformations: Such malformations are almost always sporadic, often occurring as part of complex malformation syndromes (eg, Dandy-Walker malformation) that affect other parts of the CNS.

Malformations manifest early in life and are nonprogressive. Manifestations vary markedly depending on the structures involved; ataxia is usually present.

Hereditary ataxias: Hereditary ataxias may be autosomal recessive or autosomal dominant. Autosomal recessive ataxias include Friedreich ataxia (the most prevalent), ataxia-telangiectasia, abetalipoproteinemia, ataxia with isolated vitamin E deficiency, and cerebrotendinous xanthomatosis.

Friedreich ataxia results from a gene mutation causing abnormal repetition of the DNA sequence GAA in the gene that codes for the mitochondrial protein frataxin. Inheritance is autosomal recessive. Decreased frataxin levels lead to mitochondrial iron overload and impaired mitochondrial function.

In Friedreich ataxia, gait unsteadiness begins between ages 5 and 15; it is followed by upper-extremity ataxia, dysarthria, and paresis, particularly of the lower extremities. Mental function

Table 232–9. SIGNS OF CEREBELLAR DISORDERS

DEFICIT	MANIFESTATION
Ataxia	Reeling, wide-based gait
Decomposition of movement	Inability to correctly sequence fine, coordinated acts
Dysarthria	Inability to articulate words correctly, with slurring and inappropriate phrasing
Dysdiadochokinesia	Inability to perform rapid alternating movements
Dysmetria	Inability to control range of movement
Hypotonia	Decreased muscle tone
Nystagmus	Involuntary, rapid oscillation of the eyeballs in a horizontal, vertical, or rotary direction, with the fast component maximal toward the side of the cerebellar lesion
Scanning speech	Slow enunciation with a tendency to hesitate at the beginning of a word or syllable
Tremor	Rhythmic, alternating, oscillatory movement of a limb as it approaches a target (intention tremor) or of proximal musculature when fixed posture or weight bearing is attempted (postural tremor)

often declines. Tremor, if present, is slight. Reflexes and vibration and position senses are lost. Talipes equinovarus (clubfoot), scoliosis, and progressive cardiomyopathy are common. By their late 20s, patients may be confined to a wheelchair. Death, often due to arrhythmia or heart failure, usually occurs by middle age.

Spinocerebellar ataxias (SCAs) are the main autosomal dominant ataxias. Classification of these ataxias has been revised many times recently as knowledge about genetics increases. Currently, at least 43 different gene loci are recognized; about 10 involve expanded DNA sequence repeats. Some involve a repetition of the DNA sequence CAG that codes for the amino acid glutamine, similar to that in Huntington disease.

Manifestations of SCAs vary. Some of the most common SCAs affect multiple areas in the central and peripheral nervous systems; neuropathy, pyramidal signs, and restless leg syndrome, as well as ataxia, are common. Some SCAs usually cause only cerebellar ataxia.

SCA type 3, formerly known as Machado-Joseph disease, may be the most common dominantly inherited SCA worldwide. Symptoms include ataxia, parkinsonism, and possibly dystonia, facial twitching, ophthalmoplegia, and peculiar bulging eyes.

Acquired conditions: Acquired ataxias may result from nonhereditary neurodegenerative disorders (eg, multiple system atrophy), systemic disorders, multiple sclerosis, cerebellar strokes, repeated traumatic brain injury, or toxin exposure, or they may be idiopathic. Systemic disorders include alcoholism (alcoholic cerebellar degeneration), celiac disease, heatstroke, hypothyroidism, and vitamin E deficiency. Toxins include carbon monoxide, heavy metals, lithium, phenytoin, and certain solvents. Toxic levels of certain drugs (eg, anticonvulsants) can cause cerebellar dysfunction and ataxia.

In children, primary brain tumors (medulloblastoma, cystic astrocytoma) may be the cause; the midline cerebellum is the most common site of such tumors. Rarely, in children, reversible diffuse cerebellar dysfunction follows viral infections.

Diagnosis

- Clinical evaluation
- Typically MRI
- Sometimes genetic testing

Diagnosis of cerebellar disorders is clinical and includes a thorough family history and search for acquired systemic disorders.

Neuroimaging, typically MRI, is done. Genetic testing is done if family history is suggestive.

Treatment

- Treatment of the cause if possible
- Usually only supportive

Some systemic disorders (eg, hypothyroidism, celiac disease) and toxin exposure can be treated; occasionally, surgery for structural lesions (tumor, hydrocephalus) is beneficial. However, treatment is usually only supportive.

233 Neuro-ophthalmologic and Cranial Nerve Disorders

Dysfunction of certain cranial nerves may affect the eye, pupil, optic nerve, or extraocular muscles and their nerves; thus, they can be considered cranial nerve disorders, neuro-ophthalmologic disorders, or both. Neuro-ophthalmologic disorders may also involve dysfunction of the central pathways that control and integrate ocular movement and vision. Cranial nerve disorders can also involve dysfunction of smell, vision, chewing, facial sensation or expression, taste, hearing, balance, swallowing, phonation, head turning and shoulder elevation, or tongue movements (see Table 233–1). One or more cranial nerves may be affected.

Causes and symptoms of neuro-ophthalmologic and cranial nerve disorders overlap. Both types of disorders can result from tumors, inflammation, trauma, systemic disorders, and degenerative or other processes, causing such symptoms as vision loss, diplopia, ptosis, pupillary abnormalities, periocular pain, facial pain, or headache.

Table 233–1. CRANIAL NERVES

NERVE	FUNCTION	POSSIBLE FINDINGS	POSSIBLE CAUSES*
Olfactory (1st)	Provides sensory input for smell	Anosmia	Head trauma Nasal disorders (eg, allergic rhinitis) Neurodegenerative disorders (eg, Alzheimer disease, Parkinson disease) Paranasal sinusitis Tumors of the cranial fossa, nasal cavity, and paranasal sinuses
Optic (2nd)	Provides sensory input for vision	Amaurosis fugax (transient monocular blindness), unilateral loss of superior or inferior visual field	Embolism of the ophthalmic artery Ipsilateral internal carotid disease Embolism of retinal arteries
		Anterior ischemic optic neuropathy	Crowded optic disk morphology (called disk at risk) Complications after cataract extraction Connective tissue disease that causes arteritis (eg, temporal arteritis, antiphospholipid antibody syndrome) Diabetes Hypotension or hypovolemia if severe Ipsilateral internal carotid artery obstruction Phosphodiesterase type 5 (PDE5) inhibitors (eg, sildenafil, tadalafil, vardenafil) Retinal artery embolism
		Optic neuritis (papillitis and retrobulbar)	Acute demyelinating disease (eg, multiple sclerosis, neuromyelitis optica) Bacterial infections (eg, TB, syphilis, Lyme disease) Postinfectious or disseminated encephalomyelitis Uveitis Viral infections (eg, HIV, herpes simplex, hepatitis B, cytomegalovirus)
		Toxic-nutritional optic neuropathy (toxic amblyopia)	Drugs (chloramphenicol, ethambutol, isoniazid, streptomycin, sulfonamides, digitalis, chlorpropamide, ergot, disulfiram) Methanol ingestion Nutritional deprivation if severe Organic mercury Vitamin B_{12} deficiency
		Bitemporal hemianopia	Craniopharyngioma Meningioma of tuberculum sellae Saccular aneurysm in the cavernous sinus Suprasellar extension of pituitary adenoma
Oculomotor (3rd)	Raises eyelids Moves eyes up, down, and medially Adjusts amount of light entering eyes Focuses lenses	Palsies	Aneurysm of posterior communicating artery Ischemia of the 3rd cranial nerve (often due to small-vessel disease as occurs in diabetes) or its fascicle in the midbrain Transtentorial herniation due to intracranial mass (eg, subdural hematoma, tumor, abscess)
Trochlear (4th)	Moves eye in and down via the superior oblique muscle	Palsies	Often idiopathic Head trauma Infarction often due to small-vessel disease (eg, in diabetes) Tentorial meningioma Pinealoma

Table continues on the following page.

Table 233–1. CRANIAL NERVES (*Continued*)

NERVE	FUNCTION	POSSIBLE FINDINGS	POSSIBLE CAUSES*
		Myokymia of the superior oblique muscle (typically with brief episodic ocular movements that cause subjective visual shimmering, ocular trembling, and/or tilted vision)	Entrapment of the trochlear nerve by a vascular loop (similar to the pathophysiology of trigeminal neuralgia)
Trigeminal (5th)			
• Ophthalmic division	Provides sensory input from the eye surface, tear glands, scalp, forehead, and upper eyelids	Neuralgia	Vascular loop compressing the nerve root Multiple sclerosis (occasionally) Lesions of cavernous sinus or superior orbital fissure
• Maxillary and mandibular divisions	Provides sensory input from the teeth, gums, lip, lining of palate, and skin of the face	Neuralgia	Lesions of cavernous sinus or superior orbital fissure Multiple sclerosis (occasionally) Vascular loop compressing the nerve root
	Moves masticatory muscles (chewing, grinding the teeth)	Neuropathy	Carcinomatous or lymphomatous meningitis Connective tissue disorders Meningiomas, schwannomas, or metastatic tumors at the skull base
Abducens (6th)	Moves the eye outward (abduction) via the lateral rectus muscle	Palsies	Often idiopathic Head trauma Increased intracranial pressure Infarction (may be mononeuritis multiplex) Infections or tumors affecting the meninges Multiple sclerosis Nasopharyngeal carcinoma Pontine or cerebellar tumors Pontine infarction Wernicke encephalopathy
Facial (7th)	Moves muscles of facial expression Proximal branches: Innervate tear glands and salivary glands and provide sensory input for taste on the anterior two-thirds of the tongue	Palsies	Vestibular schwannoma Basilar skull fracture Bell palsy Guillain-Barré syndrome Infarcts and tumors of the pons Lyme disease Melkersson-Rosenthal syndrome Ramsay Hunt syndrome Sarcoidosis Tumors that invade the temporal bone Uveoparotid fever (Heerfordt syndrome)
		Hemifacial spasm	Artery loop compressing the nerve root
Vestibulocochlear (8th)	Provides sensory input for equilibrium and hearing	Tinnitus, vertigo, sense of fullness in the ear, and hearing loss	Meniere disease Barotrauma
		Benign paroxysmal positional vertigo	Otolithic aggregation in the posterior or horizontal semicircular canal, related to aging and/or trauma Infection (occasionally)
		Vestibular neuronitis	Viral infection
		Hearing loss or disturbance	Acoustic neuromas Aging Barotrauma Cerebellopontine angle tumors Congenital rubella infection Exposure to loud noises Hereditary disorders Meningitis Viral infection (possibly)

Table 233–1. CRANIAL NERVES (*Continued*)

NERVE	FUNCTION	POSSIBLE FINDINGS	POSSIBLE CAUSES*
Glossopharyngeal (9th)	Provides sensory input from the pharynx, tonsils, posterior tongue, and carotid arteries	Glossopharyngeal neuralgia	Ectatic artery or tumor (less common) compressing the nerve
	Moves muscles of swallowing and salivary glands Helps regulate BP	Glossopharyngeal neuropathy	Tumor or aneurysm in the posterior fossa or jugular foramen
Vagus (10th)	Moves vocal cords and muscles for swallowing Transmits impulses to the heart and smooth muscles of visceral organs	Hoarseness, dysphonia, and dysphagia Vasovagal syncope	Entrapment of recurrent laryngeal nerve by mediastinal tumor Herpes zoster Infectious or carcinomatous meningitis Medullary tumors or ischemia (eg, lateral medullary syndrome)
Accessory (11th)	Turns the head Shrugs the shoulders	Partial or complete paralysis of the sternocleidomastoid and trapezius	Iatrogenic (eg, due to lymph node biopsy in posterior triangle of the neck) Idiopathic Trauma Tumors at the skull base or near the meninges
Hypoglossal (12th)	Moves the tongue	Atrophy and fasciculation of tongue	Intramedullary lesions (eg, motor neuron disease, tumors) Lesions of the basal meninges or occipital bones (eg, platybasia, Paget disease of skull base) Surgical trauma (eg, due to endarterectomy) Motor neuron disease (eg, amyotrophic lateral sclerosis)

*Disorders that cause diffuse motor paralysis (eg, myasthenia gravis, botulism, variant Guillain-Barré syndrome, poliomyelitis with bulbar involvement) often affect cranial nerves. Amyotrophic lateral sclerosis may cause prominent tongue fasciculations.

Diagnosis

Evaluation includes the following:

- Detailed questioning about symptoms
- Examination of the visual system
- Tests to detect nystagmus (see Sidebar 91–1 on p. 785)
- Examination of the cranial nerves

Visual system examination includes ophthalmoscopy and testing of visual acuity, visual fields (see Table 107–1 on p. 895), pupils (see Table 233–2), and eye movements (ocular motility—see Table 233–3). As part of this testing, the 2nd, 3rd, 4th, and 6th cranial nerves are examined (see also p. 1835). Neuroimaging with CT or MRI is also usually required.

The following parts of the visual examination are of particular interest in diagnosing neuro-ophthalmologic and cranial nerve disorders.

Pupils are inspected for size, equality, and regularity. Normally, the pupils constrict promptly (within 1 sec) and equally during accommodation and during exposure to direct light and to light directed at the other pupil (consensual light reflex). Testing pupillary response to consensual light via a swinging flashlight test can determine whether a defect is present. Normally, the degree of pupillary constriction does not change as the flashlight is swung from eye to eye.

- If a **relative afferent defect** (deafferented pupil, afferent pupillary defect, or Marcus Gunn pupil) is present, the pupil paradoxically dilates when the flashlight swings to the side of the defect. A deafferented pupil constricts in response to consensual but not to direct light.
- If an **efferent defect** is present, the pupil responds sluggishly or does not respond to both direct and consensual light.

Eye movements are checked by having the patient hold the head steady while tracking the examiner's finger as it moves to the far right, left, upward, downward, diagonally to either side, and inward toward the patient's nose (to assess accommodation). However, such examination may miss mild paresis of ocular movement sufficient to cause diplopia.

Diplopia may indicate a defect in bilateral coordination of eye movements (eg, in neural pathways) or in the 3rd (oculomotor), 4th (trochlear), or 6th (abducens) cranial nerve. If diplopia persists when one eye is closed (monocular diplopia), the cause is probably a nonneurologic eye disorder. If diplopia disappears when either eye is closed (binocular diplopia), the cause is probably a disorder of ocular motility. The 2 images are furthest apart when the patient looks in the direction served by the paretic eye muscle (eg, to the left when the left lateral rectus muscle is paretic). The eye that, when closed, eliminates the more peripheral image is paretic. Placing a red glass over one eye can help identify the paretic eye. When the red glass covers the paretic eye, the more peripheral image is red.

Treatment

Treatment of neuro-ophthalmologic and cranial disorders depends on the cause.

Table 233–2. COMMON PUPILLARY ABNORMALITIES

FINDING	EXPLANATION
Asymmetry of 1–2 mm between pupils, preserved light responses, and no symptoms	Normal variant (physiologic anisocoria)
Asymmetry, impaired light responses, and preserved response to accommodation (light-near dissociation or Argyll Robertson pupil)	Neurosyphilis (possibly)
Bilateral constriction	Opioids Miotic eye drops for glaucoma (most common; causing unilateral constriction if single eye is dosed) Pontine hemorrhage Organophosphate or cholinergic toxins
Bilateral dilation with preserved light reflexes	Hyperadrenergic states (eg, withdrawal syndromes, drugs such as sympathomimetics or cocaine, thyrotoxicosis)
Bilateral dilation with impaired direct light response	Mydriatic eye drops such as sympathomimetics (eg, phenylephrine) and cycloplegics (eg, cyclopentolate, tropicamide, homatropine, atropine) Brain herniation Hypoxic or ischemic encephalopathy
Unilateral dilation with afferent pupillary defect	Lesions of the eye, retina, or 2nd cranial (optic) nerve
Unilateral dilation with efferent pupillary defect	Third cranial (oculomotor) nerve palsies, often due to compression (eg, due to aneurysm of the posterior communicating artery or to transtentorial herniation) Iris trauma (also irregular pupil) Mydriatic eye drops*
Unilateral dilation with minimal or slow direct and consensual light reflexes and pupil constriction in response to accommodation	Tonic (Adie) pupil†

*Transtentorial herniation and use of mydriatic eye drops can often be distinguished by instilling a drop of pilocarpine ocular solution into the dilated pupil; no constriction in response suggests mydriatic eye drops.

†Tonic pupil is permanent but nonprogressive abnormal dilation of the pupil due to damage of the ciliary ganglion. It typically occurs in women aged 20 to 40. Onset is usually sudden. The only findings are slight blurring of vision, impaired dark adaptation, and sometimes absent deep tendon reflexes.

CONJUGATE GAZE PALSIES

A conjugate gaze palsy is inability to move both eyes in a single horizontal (most commonly) or vertical direction.

Gaze palsies most commonly affect horizontal gaze; some affect upward gaze, and fewer affect downward gaze.

Horizontal gaze palsies: Conjugate horizontal gaze is controlled by neural input from the cerebral hemispheres, cerebellum, vestibular nuclei, and neck. Neural input from these sites converges at the horizontal gaze center (paramedian pontine reticular formation) and is integrated into a final command to the adjacent 6th cranial nerve nucleus, which controls the lateral rectus on the same side, and, via the medial longitudinal fasciculus (MLF), to the contralateral 3rd cranial nerve nucleus and the medial rectus it controls. Inhibitory signals to opposing eye muscles occur simultaneously.

The most common and devastating impairment of horizontal gaze results from pontine lesions that affect the horizontal gaze

Table 233–3. COMMON DISTURBANCES OF OCULAR MOTILITY

CLINICAL FINDING	SYNDROME	COMMON CAUSES
Pareses		
Paresis of horizontal gaze in one direction	Conjugate horizontal gaze palsy	Lesion in the ipsilateral pontine horizontal gaze center or in the contralateral frontal cortex
Paresis of horizontal gaze in both directions	Complete (bilateral) horizontal gaze palsy	Wernicke encephalopathy Large bilateral pontine lesion affecting both horizontal gaze centers
Bilateral paresis of all horizontal eye movements except for abduction of the eye contralateral to the lesion; convergence unaffected	One-and-a-half syndrome	Lesion in the medial longitudinal fasciculus and ipsilateral pontine horizontal gaze center

Table 233–3. COMMON DISTURBANCES OF OCULAR MOTILITY (*Continued*)

CLINICAL FINDING	SYNDROME	COMMON CAUSES
Unilateral or bilateral paresis of eye adduction in horizontal lateral gaze but not in convergence	Internuclear ophthalmoplegia	Lesion in the medial longitudinal fasciculus
Bilateral paresis of upward eye movement with dilated pupils, loss of the pupillary light response despite preservation of pupillary accommodation and constriction with convergence, downward gaze preference, and downbeating nystagmus	Parinaud syndrome (a type of conjugate vertical gaze palsy)	Pineal tumor Dorsal midbrain infarct
Bilateral paresis of downward eye movements	Conjugate downward gaze palsy	Progressive supranuclear palsy
Unilateral eye deviation (resting position is down and out); unilateral paresis of eye adduction, elevation, and depression; ptosis; and often a dilated pupil	3rd cranial nerve palsy	Aneurysms Oculomotor nerve or midbrain ischemia Trauma Transtentorial herniation
Unilateral paresis of downward and inward (nasal) eye movement, which may be subtle, causing symptoms (difficulty looking down and inward) Head tilt sign (patient tilts the head to the side opposite the affected eye)	4th cranial nerve palsy	Idiopathic Head trauma Ischemia Congenital
Unilateral paresis of eye abduction	6th cranial nerve palsy	Idiopathic Infarct Vasculitis Increased intracranial pressure Wernicke encephalopathy Multiple sclerosis
Skew deviation (vertical misalignment of the eyes)	Partial and unequal involvement of 3rd cranial nerve nuclei, vertical gaze center, or median longitudinal fasciculus	Brain stem lesion anywhere from midbrain to medulla
Weakness or restriction of all extraocular muscles	External ophthalmoplegia	Dysfunction of eye muscles or of neuromuscular junction Usually caused by the following: • Myasthenia gravis • Graves disease • Botulism • Mitochondrial myopathies (eg, Kearn-Sayre syndrome) • Oculopharyngeal dystrophy • Myotonic dystrophy • Orbital pseudotumor
Involuntary or abnormal movements		
Rhythmic involuntary movements, usually bilateral	Nystagmus	See Sidebar 91–1 on p. 895
Fast downward jerk and slow upward return to midposition	Ocular bobbing	Extensive pontine destruction or dysfunction
Gaze overshoot followed by several oscillations	Ocular dysmetria	Cerebellar pathway disorders
Burst of rapid horizontal oscillations about a point of fixation	Ocular flutter	Many causes: • Postanoxic encephalopathy • Occult neuroblastoma • Paraneoplastic effects • Ataxia-telangiectasia • Viral encephalitis • Toxic effects of drugs
Rapid, conjugate, multidirectional, chaotic movements, often with widespread myoclonus	Opsoclonus	Many causes (same as for ocular flutter, above)

center and the 6th cranial nerve nucleus. Strokes are a common cause, resulting in loss of horizontal gaze ipsilateral to the lesion. In palsies due to stroke, the eyes may not move in response to any stimulus (eg, voluntary or vestibular). Milder palsies may cause only nystagmus or inability to maintain fixation.

Another common cause is a lesion in the contralateral cerebral hemisphere rostral to the frontal gyrus. These lesions are typically caused by a stroke. The resulting palsy usually abates with time. Horizontal conjugate gaze mediated by brain stem reflexes (eg, in response to cold-water caloric stimulation) is preserved.

Vertical gaze palsies: Upward and downward gaze depends on input from fiber pathways that ascend from the vestibular system through the MLF on both sides to the 3rd and 4th cranial nerve nuclei, the interstitial nucleus of Cajal, and the rostral interstitial nucleus of the MLF. A separate system descends, presumably from the cerebral hemispheres, through the midbrain pretectum to the 3rd and 4th cranial nerve nuclei. The rostral interstitial nucleus of the MLF integrates the neural input into a final command for vertical gaze.

Vertical gaze becomes more limited with aging.

Vertical gaze palsies commonly result from midbrain lesions, usually infarcts and tumors. In upward vertical gaze palsies, the pupils may be dilated, and vertical nystagmus occurs during upward gaze.

Parinaud syndrome (dorsal midbrain syndrome), a conjugate upward vertical gaze palsy, may result from a pineal tumor or, less commonly, a tumor or infarct of the midbrain pretectum. This syndrome is characterized by impaired upward gaze, lid retraction (Collier sign), downward gaze preference (setting-sun sign), convergence-retraction nystagmus, and dilated pupils (about 6 mm) that respond poorly to light but better to accommodation (light-near dissociation).

Downward gaze palsies: Impaired downward gaze with preservation of upward gaze usually indicates progressive supranuclear palsy; other causes are rare.

INTERNUCLEAR OPHTHALMOPLEGIA

Internuclear ophthalmoplegia is characterized by paresis of eye adduction in horizontal gaze but not in convergence. It can be unilateral or bilateral.

During horizontal gaze, the **medial longitudinal fasciculus** (MLF) on each side of the brain stem enables abduction of one eye to be coordinated with adduction of the other. The MLF connects the following structures:

- 6th cranial nerve nucleus (which controls the lateral rectus, responsible for abduction)
- Adjacent horizontal gaze center (paramedian pontine reticular formation)
- Contralateral 3rd cranial nerve nucleus (which controls the medial rectus, responsible for adduction)

The MLF also connects the vestibular nuclei with the 3rd and 4th cranial nerve nuclei.

Internuclear ophthalmoplegia results from a lesion in the MLF. In young people, the disorder is commonly caused by multiple sclerosis and may be bilateral. In the elderly, internuclear ophthalmoplegia is typically caused by stroke and is unilateral. Rarely, the cause is Arnold-Chiari malformation, neurosyphilis, Lyme disease, tumor, head trauma, nutritional disorders (eg, Wernicke encephalopathy, pernicious anemia), or drug intoxication (eg, with tricyclic antidepressants or opioids).

If a lesion in the MLF blocks signals from the horizontal gaze center to the 3rd cranial nerve, the eye on the affected side cannot adduct (or adducts weakly) past the midline. The affected eye adducts normally in convergence because convergence does not require signals from the horizontal gaze center. This finding distinguishes internuclear ophthalmoplegia from 3rd cranial nerve palsy, which impairs adduction in convergence (this palsy also differs because it causes limited vertical eye movement, ptosis, and pupillary abnormalities).

During horizontal gaze to the side opposite the affected eye, images are horizontally displaced, causing diplopia; nystagmus often occurs in the abducting eye. Sometimes vertical bilateral nystagmus occurs during attempted upward gaze.

Treatment is directed at the underlying disorder.

One-and-a-half syndrome: This uncommon syndrome occurs if a lesion affects the horizontal gaze center and the MLF on the same side. The eye affected by the lesion cannot move horizontally to either side, but the eye on the side opposite the lesion can abduct; convergence is unaffected.

Causes of one-and-a-half syndrome include multiple sclerosis, infarction, hemorrhage, and tumor.

With treatment (eg, radiation therapy for a tumor, treatment of multiple sclerosis), improvement may occur but is often limited after infarction.

THIRD CRANIAL NERVE DISORDERS

Third cranial nerve disorders can impair ocular motility, pupillary function, or both. Symptoms and signs include diplopia, ptosis, and paresis of eye adduction and of upward and downward gaze. If the pupil is affected, it is dilated, and light reflexes are impaired. If the pupil is affected or patients are increasingly unresponsive, neuroimaging is done as soon as possible.

Etiology

Third cranial (oculomotor) nerve disorders that cause palsies and affect the pupil commonly result from

- Aneurysms (especially of the posterior communicating artery)
- Transtentorial brain herniation
- Less commonly, meningitis affecting the brain stem (eg, TB meningitis)

The most common cause of palsies that spare the pupil, particularly partial palsies, is

- Ischemia of the 3rd cranial nerve (usually due to diabetes or hypertension) or of the midbrain

Occasionally, a posterior communicating artery aneurysm causes oculomotor palsy and spares the pupil.

Symptoms and Signs

Diplopia and ptosis (drooping of the upper eyelid) occur. The affected eye may deviate slightly out and down in straight-ahead gaze; adduction is slow and may not proceed past the midline. Upward gaze is impaired. When downward gaze is attempted, the superior oblique muscle causes the eye to adduct slightly and rotate.

The pupil may be normal or dilated; its response to direct and to consensual light may be sluggish or absent (efferent defect). Mydriasis (pupil dilation) may be an early sign.

Diagnosis

- Clinical evaluation
- CT or MRI

Differential diagnosis includes

- Midbrain lesions that disrupt the oculomotor fascicle (Claude syndrome, Benedict syndrome)
- Leptomeningeal tumor or infection
- Cavernous sinus disease (giant carotid aneurysm, fistula, or thrombosis)
- Intraorbital structural lesions (eg, orbital mucormycosis) that restrict ocular motility
- Ocular myopathies (eg, due to hyperthyroidism or mitochondrial disorders)
- Disorders of the neuromuscular junction (eg, due to myasthenia gravis or botulism)

Differentiation may be clinical. Exophthalmos or enophthalmos, a history of severe orbital trauma, or an obviously inflamed orbit suggests an intraorbital structural disorder. Graves orbitopathy (ophthalmopathy) should be considered in patients with bilateral ocular paresis, paresis of upward gaze or abduction, exophthalmos, lid retraction, lid lag during downward gaze (Graefe sign), and a normal pupil.

CT or MRI is required. If a patient has a dilated pupil and a sudden, severe headache (suggesting ruptured aneurysm) or is increasingly unresponsive (suggesting herniation), CT is done immediately. If ruptured aneurysm is suspected and CT (or MRI) does not show blood or is not available rapidly, other tests, such as lumbar puncture, magnetic resonance angiography, CT angiography, or cerebral angiography, are indicated. Cavernous sinus disease and orbital mucormycosis require immediate MRI imaging for timely treatment.

Treatment

Treatment depends on the cause.

FOURTH CRANIAL NERVE PALSY

Fourth cranial nerve palsy impairs the superior oblique muscle, causing paresis of vertical gaze, mainly in adduction.

Fourth cranial (trochlear) nerve palsy is often idiopathic. Few causes have been identified. Causes include closed head injury (common), which may cause unilateral or bilateral palsies, and infarction due to small-vessel disease (eg, in diabetes). Rarely, this palsy results from aneurysms, tumors (eg, tentorial meningioma, pinealoma), or multiple sclerosis.

Because the superior oblique muscle is paretic, the eyes do not adduct normally. Patients see double images, one above and slightly to the side of the other; thus, going down stairs, which requires looking down and inward, is difficult. However, tilting the head to the side opposite the palsied muscle can compensate and eliminate the double images.

Examination may detect subtle impaired ocular motility, causing symptoms but not signs.

Oculomotor exercises or prism glasses may help restore concordant vision. Surgery may eventually be needed.

SIXTH CRANIAL NERVE PALSY

(Abducens Nerve Palsy)

Sixth cranial nerve palsy affects the lateral rectus muscle, impairing eye abduction. The eye may be slightly adducted when the patient looks straight ahead. The palsy may be secondary to nerve infarction, Wernicke encephalopathy, trauma, infection, or increased intracranial pressure, or it may be idiopathic. Determining the cause requires MRI and often lumbar puncture and evaluation for vasculitis.

Etiology

Sixth cranial (abducens) nerve palsy typically results from small-vessel disease, particularly in diabetics as part of a disorder called mononeuritis multiplex (multiple mononeuropathy). It may result from ischemia, hypertension (sometimes), or compression of the nerve by lesions in the cavernous sinus (eg, nasopharyngeal tumors), orbit, or base of the skull. The palsy may also result from increased intracranial pressure, head trauma, or both. Other causes include meningitis, meningeal carcinomatosis, Wernicke encephalopathy, aneurysm, vasculitis, multiple sclerosis, pontine stroke, and, rarely, low CSF pressure headache (eg, after lumbar puncture). Children with respiratory infection may have recurrent palsy. However, the cause of an isolated 6th cranial nerve palsy is often not identified.

Symptoms and Signs

Symptoms of 6th cranial nerve palsy include binocular horizontal diplopia when looking to the side of the paretic eye. Because the tonic action of the medial rectus muscle is unopposed, the eye is slightly adducted when the patient looks straight ahead. The eye abducts sluggishly, and even when abduction is maximal, the lateral sclera is exposed. With complete paralysis, the eye cannot abduct past midline.

Palsy resulting from nerve compression by a hemorrhage (eg, due to head trauma or intracranial bleeding), a tumor, or an aneurysm in the cavernous sinus causes severe head pain, chemosis (conjunctival edema), anesthesia in the distribution of the 1st division of the 5th cranial nerve, optic nerve compression with vision loss, and paralysis of the 3rd, 4th, and 6th cranial nerves. Both sides are typically affected, although unevenly.

Diagnosis

- MRI
- If vasculitis is suspected, ESR, antinuclear antibodies, and rheumatoid factor

A 6th nerve palsy is usually obvious, but the cause is not. If retinal venous pulsations are seen during ophthalmoscopy, increased intracranial pressure is unlikely.

CT is often done because it is often immediately available. However, MRI is the test of choice; MRI provides greater resolution of the orbits, cavernous sinus, posterior fossa, and cranial nerves. If imaging results are normal but meningitis or increased intracranial pressure is suspected, lumbar puncture is done.

If vasculitis is suspected clinically, evaluation begins with measurement of ESR, antinuclear antibodies, and rheumatoid factor.

In children, if increased intracranial pressure is excluded, respiratory infection is considered.

Treatment

In many patients, 6th cranial nerve palsies resolve once the underlying disorder is treated. Idiopathic palsy and ischemic palsy usually abate within 2 mo.

TRIGEMINAL NEURALGIA

(Tic Douloureux)

Trigeminal neuralgia is severe paroxysmal, lancinating facial pain due to a disorder of the 5th cranial nerve. Diagnosis is clinical. Treatment is usually with carbamazepine or gabapentin; sometimes surgery is required.

Trigeminal neuralgia affects mainly adults, especially the elderly.

Etiology

Trigeminal neuralgia is usually caused by

- An intracranial artery (eg, anterior inferior cerebellar artery, ectatic basilar artery)
- Less often, a venous loop that compresses the 5th cranial (trigeminal) nerve at its root entry zone into the brain stem

Other **less common causes** include compression by a tumor and occasionally a multiple sclerosis plaque at the root entry zone, but these causes are usually distinguished by accompanying sensory and other deficits.

Other disorders that cause similar symptoms (eg, multiple sclerosis) are sometimes considered to be trigeminal neuralgia and sometimes not. Recognizing the cause is what is important.

The mechanism is unclear. One theory suggests that nerve compression causes local demyelination, which may result in ectopic impulse generation and/or disinhibition of central pain pathways involving the spinal trigeminal nucleus.

Symptoms and Signs

Pain occurs along the distribution of one or more sensory divisions of the trigeminal nerve, most often the maxillary. The pain is paroxysmal, lasting seconds up to 2 min, but attacks may recur rapidly. It is lancinating, excruciating, and sometimes incapacitating. Pain is often precipitated by stimulating a facial trigger point (eg, by chewing, brushing the teeth, or smiling). Sleeping on that side of the face is often intolerable.

Diagnosis

- Clinical evaluation

Symptoms are almost pathognomonic. Thus, some other disorders that cause facial pain can be differentiated clinically:

- Chronic paroxysmal hemicrania (Sjaastad syndrome) is differentiated by longer (5 to 8 min) attacks of pain and its dramatic response to indomethacin.
- Postherpetic pain is differentiated by its constant duration (without paroxysms), typical antecedent rash, scarring, and predilection for the ophthalmic division.
- Migraine, which may cause atypical facial pain, is differentiated by pain that is more prolonged and often throbbing.

Neurologic examination is normal in trigeminal neuralgia. Thus, neurologic deficits (usually loss of facial sensation) suggest that the trigeminal neuralgia–like pain is caused by another disorder (eg, tumor, stroke, multiple sclerosis plaque, vascular malformation, other lesions that compress the trigeminal nerve or disrupt its brain stem pathways).

Treatment

- Usually anticonvulsants

Carbamazepine 200 mg po tid or qid is usually effective for long periods; it is begun at 100 mg po bid, increasing the dose by 100 to 200 mg/day until pain is controlled (maximum daily dose 1200 mg). If carbamazepine is ineffective or has adverse effects, one of the following may be tried:

- Oxcarbazepine 150 to 300 mg po bid
- Gabapentin 300 to 600 mg po tid (300 mg po once on day 1, 300 mg po bid on day 2, 300 mg po tid on day 3, then increasing dose as needed to 1200 mg po tid)
- Phenytoin 100 to 200 mg po bid (beginning with 100 mg po bid, then increasing as needed)
- Baclofen 10 to 30 mg po tid (beginning with 5 to 10 mg po tid, then increasing as needed by about 5 mg/day)
- Amitriptyline 25 to 150 mg po taken at bedtime (beginning with 25 mg, then increasing by 25-mg increments each week as needed)

Peripheral nerve block provides temporary relief.

If pain is severe despite these measures, neuroablative treatments are considered; however, efficacy may be temporary, and improvement may be followed by recurrent pain that is more severe than the preceding episodes. In a posterior fossa craniectomy, a small pad can be placed to separate the pulsating vascular loop from the trigeminal root (called microvascular decompression, or the Jannetta procedure). In radiosurgery, a gamma knife can be used to cut the proximal trigeminal nerve. Electrolytic or chemical lesions or balloon compression of the trigeminal (gasserian) ganglion can be made via a percutaneous stereotactically positioned needle. Occasionally, the trigeminal nerve fibers between the gasserian ganglion and brain stem are cut. Sometimes, as a last resort to relieve intractable pain, the trigeminal nerve is destroyed.

HEMIFACIAL SPASM

Hemifacial spasm refers to unilateral painless, synchronous contractions of facial muscles due to dysfunction of the 7th cranial (facial) nerve and/or its motor nucleus.

Hemifacial spasm usually results from nerve compression by a pulsating blood vessel, similar to that in trigeminal neuralgia.

Unilateral, involuntary, painless contractions of facial muscles usually begin in the eyelid, then spread to the cheek and mouth. Contractions may be intermittent at first but may become almost continuous.

The pulsating blood vessel is often visible on MRI, but diagnosis of hemifacial spasm is ultimately clinical. Focal seizures, blepharospasm, and tics cause similar symptoms and should be considered.

The most effective treatment for hemifacial spasm is

- Injection of botulinum toxin (botulinum toxin type A or botulinum toxin type B)

Treatments for trigeminal neuralgia (eg, anticonvulsants, baclofen, amitriptyline, surgery) can also be used.

FACIAL NERVE PALSY

(Bell Palsy)

Facial nerve (7th cranial nerve) palsy is often idiopathic (formerly called Bell palsy). Idiopathic facial nerve palsy is sudden, unilateral peripheral facial nerve palsy. Symptoms of facial nerve palsy are hemifacial paresis of the upper and lower face. Tests (eg, chest x-ray, serum ACE level) are done to diagnose treatable causes. Treatment may include lubrication of the eye, intermittent use of an eye patch, and, for idiopathic facial nerve palsy, corticosteroids.

Etiology

Historically, Bell palsy was thought to be idiopathic facial nerve (peripheral 7th cranial nerve) palsy. However, facial nerve palsy is now considered a clinical syndrome with its own differential diagnosis, and the term "Bell palsy" is not always considered synonymous with idiopathic facial nerve palsy. About half the cases of facial nerve palsy are idiopathic.

The mechanism for idiopathic facial nerve palsy is presumably swelling of the facial nerve due to an immune or viral disorder. Recent evidence suggests that herpes simplex virus infection is the most common cause and that herpes zoster may be the second most common viral cause. Other viral causes include coxsackievirus, cytomegalovirus, adenovirus, and the Epstein-Barr, mumps, rubella, and influenza B viruses. The swollen nerve is maximally compressed as it passes through the labyrinthine portion of the facial canal, resulting in ischemia and paresis.

Various other disorders (eg, Lyme disease, sarcoidosis) can cause facial nerve palsy.

Pathophysiology

The facial muscles are innervated peripherally (infranuclear innervation) by the ipsilateral 7th cranial nerve and centrally (supranuclear innervation) by the contralateral cerebral cortex. Central innervation tends to be bilateral for the upper face (eg, forehead muscles) and unilateral for the lower face. As a result, both central and peripheral lesions tend to paralyze the lower face (see Plate 87). However, peripheral lesions (facial nerve palsy) tend to affect the upper face more than central lesions (eg, stroke) do.

Symptoms and Signs

Pain behind the ear often precedes facial paresis in idiopathic facial nerve palsy. Paresis, often with complete paralysis, develops within hours and is usually maximal within 48 to 72 h. Patients may report a numb or heavy feeling in the face. The affected side becomes flat and expressionless; the ability to wrinkle the forehead, blink, and grimace is limited or absent. In severe cases, the palpebral fissure widens and the eye does not close, often irritating the conjunctiva and drying the cornea.

Sensory examination is normal, but the external auditory canal and a small patch behind the ear (over the mastoid) may be painful to the touch. If the nerve lesion is proximal to the geniculate ganglion, salivation, taste, and lacrimation may be impaired, and hyperacusis may be present.

Diagnosis

- Clinical evaluation
- Chest x-ray or CT and serum ACE levels to check for sarcoidosis
- MRI if onset was gradual or other neurologic deficits are present
- Other testing if indicated by clinical findings

Facial nerve palsy is diagnosed based on clinical evaluation. There are no specific diagnostic tests. Facial nerve palsy can be distinguished from a central facial nerve lesion (eg, due to hemispheric stroke or tumor), which causes weakness primarily of the lower face, sparing the forehead muscle and allowing patients to wrinkle their forehead; also, patients with central lesions can usually furrow their brow and close their eyes tightly.

Other disorders that cause peripheral facial nerve palsies include the following:

- Geniculate herpes (Ramsay Hunt syndrome, which is due to herpes zoster)
- Middle ear or mastoid infections
- Sarcoidosis
- Lyme disease
- Petrous bone fractures
- Carcinomatous or leukemic nerve invasion
- Chronic meningitis
- Cerebellopontine angle or glomus jugulare tumors
- Diabetes

The other disorders that cause peripheral facial nerve palsy typically develop more slowly than idiopathic facial nerve palsy and may have other distinguishing symptoms or signs. Thus, if patients have any other neurologic symptoms or signs or if symptoms developed gradually, MRI should be done.

In idiopathic facial nerve palsy, MRI may show contrast enhancement of the facial nerve at or near the geniculate ganglion or along the entire course of the nerve. However, its enhancement may reflect other causes, such as meningeal tumor. If the paralysis progresses over weeks to months, the likelihood of a tumor (eg, most commonly schwannoma) compressing the facial nerve increases. MRI can also help exclude other structural disorders causing facial nerve palsy. CT, usually negative in Bell palsy, is done if a fracture is suspected or if MRI is not immediately available and stroke is possible.

In addition, acute and convalescent serologic tests for Lyme disease are done if patients have been in a geographic area where ticks and Lyme disease are endemic.

For all patients, a chest x-ray is taken or CT is done and serum ACE is measured to check for sarcoidosis. Serum glucose is measured. Viral titers are not helpful.

Prognosis

In idiopathic facial nerve palsy, the extent of nerve damage determines outcome. If some function remains, full recovery typically occurs within several months. Nerve conduction studies and electromyography are done to help predict outcome. The likelihood of complete recovery after total paralysis is 90% if nerve branches in the face retain normal excitability to supramaximal electrical stimulation and is only about 20% if electrical excitability is absent.

Regrowth of nerve fibers may be misdirected, innervating lower facial muscles with periocular fibers and vice versa. The result is contraction of unexpected muscles during voluntary facial movements (synkinesia) or crocodile tears during salivation. Chronic disuse of the facial muscles may lead to contractures.

Treatment

- Protection for the cornea
- Corticosteroids for idiopathic facial nerve palsy

Corneal drying must be prevented by frequent use of natural tears, isotonic saline, or methylcellulose drops and by intermittent use of tape or a patch to help close the eye, particularly during sleep. Tarsorrhaphy is occasionally required.

In idiopathic facial nerve palsy, corticosteroids, if begun within 48 h after onset, result in faster and more complete recovery.[1] Prednisone 60 to 80 mg po once/day is given for 1 wk, then decreased gradually over the 2nd wk. Antiviral drugs effective against herpes simplex virus (eg, valacyclovir 1 g po tid for 7 to 10 days, famciclovir 500 mg po tid for 5 to 10 days, acyclovir 400 mg po 5 times/day for 10 days) have been prescribed, but recent data suggest that antiviral drugs provide no benefit.

1. Gronseth GS, Paduga R: Evidence-based guideline update: Steroids and antivirals for Bell palsy: Report of the Guideline Development Subcommittee of the American Academy of Neurology. *Neurology* 79:2209–2213, 2012.

KEY POINTS

- In facial nerve palsy, patients cannot move the upper and lower part of their face on one side; in contrast, central facial nerve lesions (eg, due to stroke) affect primarily the lower face.
- Cause of idiopathic facial nerve palsy is unclear, but evidence is increasingly implicating herpes viruses.
- Diagnosis is clinical, but if onset is not clearly acute, MRI should be done.
- If given early, corticosteroids are helpful for idiopathic facial nerve palsy; antivirals probably provide no benefit.

GLOSSOPHARYNGEAL NEURALGIA

Glossopharyngeal neuralgia is characterized by recurrent attacks of severe pain in the 9th and 10th cranial nerve distribution (posterior pharynx, tonsils, back of the tongue, middle ear, under the angle of the jaw). Diagnosis is clinical. Treatment is usually with carbamazepine or gabapentin.

Glossopharyngeal neuralgia sometimes results from nerve compression by an aberrant, pulsating artery similar to that in trigeminal neuralgia and hemifacial spasm. The nerve may be compressed in the neck by an elongated styloid process (Eagle syndrome). Rarely, the cause is a tumor in the cerebellopontine angle or the neck, a peritonsillar abscess, a carotid aneurysm, or a demyelinating disorder. Often, no cause is identified.

Glossopharyngeal neuralgia is rare, more commonly affecting men, usually after age 40.

Symptoms and Signs

As in trigeminal neuralgia, paroxysmal attacks of unilateral brief, excruciating pain occur spontaneously or are precipitated when areas innervated by the glossopharyngeal nerve are stimulated (eg, by chewing, swallowing, coughing, talking, yawning, or sneezing). The pain, lasting seconds to a few minutes, usually begins in the tonsillar region or at the base of the tongue and may radiate to the ipsilateral ear. Occasionally, increased vagus nerve activity causes sinus arrest with syncope; episodes may occur daily or once every few weeks.

Diagnosis

- Clinical evaluation, often including response to anesthetics
- MRI

Diagnosis of glossopharyngeal neuralgia is clinical.

Glossopharyngeal neuralgia is distinguished from trigeminal neuralgia by the location of the pain. Also, in glossopharyngeal neuralgia, swallowing or touching the tonsils with an applicator tends to precipitate pain, and applying lidocaine to the throat temporarily eliminates spontaneous or evoked pain.

MRI is done to exclude tonsillar, pharyngeal, and cerebellopontine angle tumors and metastatic lesions in the anterior cervical triangle. Local nerve blocks done by an ENT physician can help distinguish between carotidynia, superior laryngeal neuralgia, and pain caused by tumors.

Treatment

- Usually anticonvulsants

Treatment of glossopharyngeal neuralgia is the same as that for trigeminal neuralgia. If oral drugs are ineffective, local anesthetics can provide relief. For example, topical cocaine applied to the pharynx may provide temporary relief, and surgery to decompress the nerve from a pulsating artery may be necessary. If pain is restricted to the pharynx, surgery can be restricted to the extracranial part of the nerve. If pain is widespread, surgery must involve the intracranial part of the nerve.

234 Neurotransmission

A neuron generates and propagates an action potential along its axon, then transmits this signal across a synapse by releasing neurotransmitters, which trigger a reaction in another neuron or an effector cell (eg, muscle cells, most exocrine and endocrine cells). The signal may stimulate or inhibit the receiving cell, depending on the neurotransmitter and receptor involved.

In the CNS, interconnections are complex. An impulse from one neuron to another may pass from axon to cell body, axon to dendrite (a neuron's receiving branches), cell body to cell body, or dendrite to dendrite. A neuron can simultaneously receive many impulses—excitatory and inhibitory—from other neurons and integrate simultaneous impulses into various patterns of firing.

Propagation: Action potential propagation along an axon is electrical, caused by the exchanges of Na^+ and K^+ ions across the axonal membrane. A particular neuron generates the same action potential after each stimulus, conducting it at a fixed velocity along the axon. Velocity depends on axonal diameter and degree of myelination and ranges from 1 to 4 m/sec in small unmyelinated fibers to 75 m/sec in large myelinated ones. Propagation speed is higher in myelinated fibers because the myelin cover has regular gaps (nodes of Ranvier) where the axon is exposed. The electrical impulse jumps from one node to the next, skipping the myelinated section of the axon. Thus, disorders that alter the myelin cover (eg, multiple sclerosis) interfere with impulse propagation, causing various neurologic symptoms.

Transmission: Impulse transmission is chemical, caused by release of specific neurotransmitters from the nerve ending (terminal). Neurotransmitters diffuse across the synaptic cleft and bind briefly to specific receptors on the adjoining neuron or effector cell. Depending on the receptor, the response may be excitatory or inhibitory.

One type of synapse, the electrical synapse, does not involve neurotransmitters; ion channels directly connect the cytoplasm of the presynaptic and postsynaptic neurons. This type of transmission is the fastest.

The nerve cell body produces enzymes that synthesize most neurotransmitters, which are stored in vesicles at the nerve terminal (see Fig. 234–1). The amount in one vesicle (usually several thousand molecules) is a quantum. A membrane action potential arriving at the terminal opens axonal Ca channels; Ca inflow releases neurotransmitter molecules from many vesicles by fusing the vesicle membranes to the nerve terminal

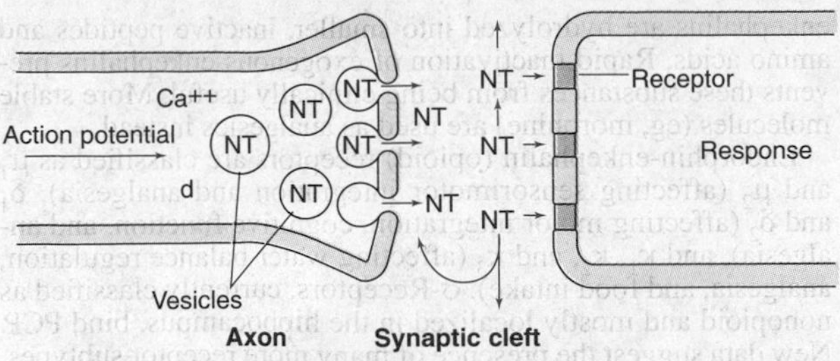

Fig. 234–1. Neurotransmission. Action potentials open the axonal Ca channels (not shown). Ca^{++} activates release of neurotransmitters (NT) from vesicles where they are stored. NT molecules fill the synaptic cleft. Some bind to postsynaptic receptors, initiating a response. The others are pumped back into the axon and stored or diffuse into the surrounding tissues.

membrane. Membrane fusion generates an opening through which the molecules are expelled into the synaptic cleft via exocytosis.

The amount of neurotransmitters (NT) in the terminal is typically independent of nerve activity and kept relatively constant by modifying uptake of neurotransmitter precursors or the activity of enzymes involved in neurotransmitter synthesis or destruction. Stimulation of presynaptic receptors can decrease presynaptic neurotransmitter synthesis, and blockade can increase it.

The neurotransmitter-receptor interaction must be terminated quickly to allow rapid, repeated activation of receptors. One of the following can happen to NT that have interacted with receptors:

- They can be quickly pumped back into the presynaptic nerve terminals by active, ATP-dependent processes (reuptake).
- They can be destroyed by enzymes near the receptors.
- They can diffuse into the surrounding area and be removed.

NT taken up by the nerve terminals are repackaged in vesicles for reuse.

Receptors: Neurotransmitter receptors are protein complexes that span the cell membrane. Their nature determines whether a given neurotransmitter is excitatory or inhibitory. Receptors that are continuously stimulated by NT or drugs become desensitized (downregulated); those that are not stimulated by their neurotransmitter or are chronically blocked by drugs become supersensitive (upregulated). Downregulation or upregulation of receptors strongly influences the development of tolerance and physical dependence. These concepts are particularly important in organ or tissue transplantation, in which denervation deprives receptors of their neurotransmitter. Withdrawal symptoms can be explained at least in part by a rebound phenomenon due to altered receptor affinity or density.

Most NT interact primarily with postsynaptic receptors, but some receptors are located on presynaptic neurons, providing fine control of neurotransmitter release.

One family of receptors, termed ionotropic receptors (eg, *N*-methyl-D-glutamate, kinate-quisqualate, nicotinic acetylcholine, glycine, and γ-aminobutyric acid [GABA] receptors), consist of ion channels that open when bound to the neurotransmitter and effect a very rapid response. In the other family, termed metabotropic receptors (eg, serotonin, α- and β-adrenergic, and dopaminergic receptors), neurotransmitters interact with G proteins and activate another molecule (2nd messenger such as cAMP) that catalyzes a chain of events through protein phosphorylation Ca mobilization, or both; cellular changes mediated by 2nd messengers are slower and permit finer tuning of the rapid ionotropic neurotransmitter response. Far more neurotransmitters activate specific receptors than 2nd messengers.

Major Neurotransmitters and Receptors

At least 100 substances can act as neurotransmitters; about 18 are of major importance. Several occur in slightly different forms.

Glutamate and aspartate: These amino acids are the major excitatory neurotransmitters in the CNS. They occur in the cortex, cerebellum, and spinal cord. In neurons, synthesis of nitric oxide (NO) increases in response to glutamate. Excess glutamate can be toxic, increasing intracellular Ca, free radicals, and proteinase activity. These neurotransmitters may contribute to tolerance to opioid therapy and mediate hyperalgesia.

Glutamate receptors are classified as NMDA (*N*-methyl-D-aspartate) receptors and non-NMDA receptors. Phencyclidine (PCP, also known as angel dust) and memantine (used to treat Alzheimer disease) bind to NMDA receptors.

GABA: GABA is the major inhibitory neurotransmitter in the brain. It is an amino acid derived from glutamate, which is decarboxylated by glutamate decarboxylase. After interaction with its receptors, GABA is actively pumped back into nerve terminals and metabolized. Glycine, which resembles GABA in its action, occurs principally in interneurons (Renshaw cells) of the spinal cord and in circuits that relax antagonist muscles.

GABA receptors are classified as $GABA_A$ (activating chloride channels) and $GABA_B$ (potentiating cAMP formation). $GABA_A$ receptors are the site of action for several neuroactive drugs, including benzodiazepines, barbiturates, picrotoxin, and muscimol. $GABA_B$ receptors are activated by baclofen, used to treat muscle spasms (eg, in multiple sclerosis).

Serotonin: Serotonin (5-hydroxytryptamine, or 5-HT) is generated by the raphe nucleus and midline neurons of the pons and upper brain stem. Tryptophan is hydroxylated by tryptophan hydroxylase to 5-hydroxytryptophan, then decarboxylated to serotonin. Serotonin levels are controlled by the uptake of tryptophan and intraneuronal monoamine oxidase (MAO), which breaks down serotonin. Ultimately, serotonin is excreted in the urine as 5-hydroxyindoacetic acid or 5-HIAA.

Serotoninergic (5-HT) receptors (with at least 15 subtypes) are classified as 5-HT_1 (with 4 subtypes), 5-HT_2, and 5-HT_3. Selective serotonin receptor agonists (eg, sumatriptan) can abort migraines.

Acetylcholine: Acetylcholine is the major neurotransmitter of the bulbospinal motor neurons, autonomic preganglionic fibers, postganglionic cholinergic (parasympathetic) fibers, and many neurons in the CNS (eg, basal ganglia, motor cortex). It is synthesized from choline and acetyl coenzyme A by choline acetyltransferase, and its action is rapidly terminated via local hydrolysis to choline and acetate by acetylcholinesterase. Acetylcholine levels are regulated by choline acetyltransferase and by choline uptake. Levels of this neurotransmitter are decreased in patients with Alzheimer disease.

Cholinergic receptors are classified as nicotinic N_1 (in the adrenal medulla and autonomic ganglia) or N_2 (in skeletal muscle) or muscarinic M_1 through M_5 (widely distributed in the CNS). M_1 occurs in the autonomic nervous system, striatum, cortex, and hippocampus; M_2 occurs in the autonomic nervous system, heart, intestinal smooth muscle, hindbrain, and cerebellum.

Dopamine: Dopamine interacts with receptors on some peripheral nerve fibers and many central neurons (eg, in the substantia nigra, midbrain, ventral tegmental area, and hypothalamus). The amino acid tyrosine is taken up by dopaminergic neurons and converted by tyrosine hydroxylase to 3,4-dihydroxyphenylalanine (dopa), which is decarboxylated by aromatic-L-amino-acid decarboxylase to dopamine. After release and interaction with receptors, dopamine is actively pumped back (reuptake) into the nerve terminal. Tyrosine hydroxylase and MAO (which breaks down dopamine) regulate dopamine levels in nerve terminals.

Dopaminergic receptors are classified as D_1 through D_5. D_3 and D_4 receptors play a role in thought control (limiting the negative symptoms of schizophrenia); D_2 receptor activation controls the extrapyramidal system. However, receptor affinity does not predict functional response (intrinsic activity). For example, ropinirole, which has high affinity for the D_3 receptor, has intrinsic activity via activation of D_2 receptors.

Norepinephrine: Norepinephrine is the neurotransmitter of most postganglionic sympathetic fibers and many central neurons (eg, in the locus caeruleus and hypothalamus). The precursor tyrosine is converted to dopamine, which is hydroxylated by dopamine β-hydroxylase to norepinephrine. After release and interaction with receptors, some norepinephrine is degraded by catechol *O*-methyltransferase (COMT), and the remainder is actively taken back into the nerve terminal, where it is degraded by MAO. Tyrosine hydroxylase, dopamine β-hydroxylase, and MAO regulate intraneuronal norepinephrine levels.

Adrenergic receptors are classified as α_1 (postsynaptic in the sympathetic system), α_2 (presynaptic in the sympathetic system and postsynaptic in the brain), β_1 (in the heart), or β_2 (in other sympathetically innervated structures).

Endorphins and enkephalins: Endorphins and enkephalins are opioids. Endorphins are large polypeptides that activate many central neurons (eg, in the hypothalamus, amygdala, thalamus, and locus caeruleus). The cell body contains a large polypeptide called pro-opiomelanocortin, the precursor of α-, β-, and γ-endorphins. This polypeptide is transported down the axon and cleaved into fragments; one is β-endorphin, contained in neurons that project to the periaqueductal gray matter, limbic structures, and major catecholamine-containing neurons in the brain. After release and interaction with receptors, β-endorphin is hydrolyzed by peptidases.

Met-enkephalin and leu-enkephalin are small polypeptides present in many central neurons (eg, in the globus pallidus, thalamus, caudate, and central gray matter). Their precursor, proenkephalin, is formed in the cell body, then split by specific peptidases into the active peptides. These substances are also localized in the spinal cord, where they modulate pain signals. The NTs of pain signals in the posterior horn of the spinal cord are glutamate and substance P. Enkephalins decrease the amount of neurotransmitter released and hyperpolarize (make more negative) the postsynaptic membrane, reducing the generation of action potentials and pain perception at the level of the postcentral gyrus. After release and interaction with peptidergic receptors, enkephalins are hydrolyzed into smaller, inactive peptides and amino acids. Rapid inactivation of exogenous enkephalins prevents these substances from being clinically useful. More stable molecules (eg, morphine) are used as analgesics instead.

Endorphin-enkephalin (opioid) receptors are classified as μ_1 and μ_2 (affecting sensorimotor integration and analgesia), δ_1 and δ_2 (affecting motor integration, cognitive function, and analgesia), and κ_1, κ_2, and κ_3 (affecting water balance regulation, analgesia, and food intake). σ-Receptors, currently classified as nonopioid and mostly localized in the hippocampus, bind PCP. New data suggest the presence of many more receptor subtypes, with pharmacologic implications. Components of the molecular precursor to the receptor protein can be rearranged during receptor synthesis to produce several receptor variants (eg, 27 splice variants of the μ opioid receptor). Also, 2 receptors can combine (dimerize) to form a new receptor.

Other neurotransmitters: Dynorphins are a group of 7 peptides with similar amino acid sequences. They, like enkephalins, are opioids.

Substance P, a peptide, occurs in central neurons (in the habenula, substantia nigra, basal ganglia, medulla, and hypothalamus) and is highly concentrated in the dorsal root ganglia. Its release is triggered by intense afferent painful stimuli. It modulates the neural response to pain and mood; it modulates nausea and vomiting through the activation of NK1A receptors that are localized in the brain stem.

Nitric oxide (NO) is a labile gas that mediates many neuronal processes. It is generated from arginine by NO synthase. Neurotransmitters that increase intracellular Ca^{++} (eg, substance P, glutamate, acetylcholine) stimulate NO synthesis in neurons that express NO synthetase. NO may be an intracellular messenger; it may diffuse out of a cell into a 2nd neuron and produce physiologic responses (eg, long-term potentiation [strengthening of certain presynaptic and postsynaptic responses—a form of learning]) or enhance glutamate (NMDA-receptor–mediated) neurotoxicity (eg, in Parkinson disease, stroke, or Alzheimer disease).

Substances with less firmly established roles in neurotransmission include histamine, vasopressin, vasoactive intestinal peptide, carnosine, bradykinin, cholecystokinin, bombesin, somatostatin, corticotropin-releasing factor, neurotensin, and possibly adenosine.

Disorders Associated With Defects in Neurotransmission

Disorders or substances that alter the production, release, reception, breakdown, or reuptake of neurotransmitters or that change the number and affinity of receptors can cause neurologic or psychiatric symptoms and cause disease (see Table 234–1). Drugs that modify neurotransmission can alleviate many of these disorders (eg, Parkinson disease, depression).

Table 234–1. EXAMPLES OF DISORDERS ASSOCIATED WITH DEFECTS IN NEUROTRANSMISSION

DISORDER	PATHOPHYSIOLOGY	TREATMENT
Neurotransmitter imbalance		
Alzheimer disease	Extracellular β-amyloid deposits, intracellular neurofibrillary tangles, and senile plaques, particularly in the limbic system (eg, hippocampus), in the association area of the cortex, and in neurons that synthesize and use acetylcholine (eg, in the basal nucleus of Meynert and its wide projections to the cortex)	Cholinesterase inhibitors (donepezil, rivastigmine, galantamine) delay synaptic degradation of acetylcholine and thus modestly improve cognitive function and memory. Memantine, an NMDA-receptor antagonist, may slow progression of the disease and increase autonomy.

Table 234–1. EXAMPLES OF DISORDERS ASSOCIATED WITH DEFECTS IN NEUROTRANSMISSION (*Continued*)

DISORDER	PATHOPHYSIOLOGY	TREATMENT
Anxiety	May reflect reduced activity of GABA, perhaps due to imbalance of endogenous inhibitors, stimulators of the GABA receptor, or both May also involve imbalances in norepinephrine and 5-HT responses	Benzodiazepines increase the probability of opening Cl^- channels modulated by GABA through $GABA_A$ receptor activation. SSRIs are the drugs of choice for long-term treatment because tolerance to benzodiazepines can develop.
Autism	Possible hyperserotonemia, which occurs in 30–50% of autistic people, with no evidence of central 5-HT abnormalities	SSRIs and risperidone may be helpful.
Brain injury	Injury (eg, trauma, hypoxia, prolonged seizures) stimulating excessive release of excitatory neurotransmitters (eg, glutamate) and accumulation of intracellular Ca^{++}, which contribute to neuronal death	In experimental models of ischemia and injury, Ca channel blockers, glycine, and older NMDA-receptor antagonists (eg, dextromethorphan, ketamine) may reduce the extent of neuronal loss, but these drugs are not effective in people. Memantine, a newer NMDA-receptor antagonist, is under study.
Depression	Complex abnormalities in cholinergic, catechol-aminergic (noradrenergic, dopaminergic) and serotonergic (5-HT) transmission Possible involvement of other hormones and neuropeptides (eg, substance P, dopamine, acetylcholine, GABA)	Antidepressants downregulate receptors indirectly or directly by inhibiting reuptake of 5-HT (as with SSRIs) and norepinephrine or dopamine or by blocking MAO. Blockade of $5\text{-HT}_{2A/2C}$ (a type of 5-HT receptor abundant in the prefrontal area) may increase the efficacy of SSRIs (eg, trazodone).
Seizure disorders	Seizures consisting of sudden synchronous high-frequency firing by localized groups of neurons in certain brain areas, perhaps caused by increased activity of glutamate or reduced activity of GABA	Phenytoin, lamotrigine, carbamazepine, valproate, topiramate, and some other anticonvulsants (eg, zonisamide, oxcarbazepine) stabilize voltage-dependent Na channels. Ethosuximide and gabapentin decrease certain Ca currents. Phenytoin also reduces excessive neurotransmitter release. Lamotrigine may decrease levels of glutamate and aspartate. Phenobarbital and benzodiazepines enhance GABA activation by affecting the $GABA_A$ receptor–Cl channel complex. Tiagabine blocks GABA glial uptake. Valproate increases levels of GABA. Topiramate increases GABA activity.
Huntington disease (chorea)	Major neuronal damage in the cortex and striatum due to polyglutamine expansion (encoded by CAG repeat), produced by an abnormal gene on chromosome 4 (the abnormal gene overproduces the protein huntingtin, which may combine with molecules that induce excessive stimulation of cells by excitatory amino acid neurotransmitters such as glutamate)	No specific treatment exists, but drugs that block NMDA receptors may block the toxic effects of excess glutamate. GABA-mimetic drugs are ineffective.
Mania	Increased norepinephrine and dopamine activity, reduced 5-HT levels, and abnormal glutamate neurotransmission	Lithium is the traditional first choice. It reduces norepinephrine release and increases 5-HT synthesis. Valproate and lamotrigine are beneficial, possibly by normalizing glutamate transmission. Topiramate blocks voltage-dependent Na channels, augments GABA activity at some subtypes of the $GABA_A$ receptor, antagonizes the AMPA/kainate subtype of the glutamate receptor, and inhibits the carbonic anhydrase enzyme, particularly isozymes II and IV. Gabapentin is thought to bind to the $\alpha2\delta$ subunit (1 and 2) of the voltage-dependent Ca channel in the CNS. Carbamazepine and oxcarbazepine stabilize voltage dependent Na+ channels.
Neuroleptic malignant syndrome	Blockage of dopamine (D_2) receptors by drugs (eg, antipsychotic drugs, methylphenidate) or abrupt withdrawal of a dopaminergic agonist, resulting in muscle rigidity, fever, change in mental status, and autonomic instability	Treatment with a D_2 agonist (eg, bromocriptine) reverses the disordered neurotransmission. Other drugs are also used as needed (eg, dantrolene, a direct muscular blocker, is used to block the muscle spasms).

Table continues on the following page.

Table 234–1. EXAMPLES OF DISORDERS ASSOCIATED WITH DEFECTS IN NEUROTRANSMISSION (*Continued*)

DISORDER	PATHOPHYSIOLOGY	TREATMENT
Pain	Tissue injury, which causes release of substance P and glutamate in the posterior horn of the spinal cord and release of other macromolecules that mediate pain signals, such as calcitonin gene-related protein, neurokinin A, and bradykinin, which are localized primarily in the lamina II and IV of the spinal cord Further modulation of these signals by endorphins (in the spinal cord) and by 5-HT and norepinephrine (in the descending pathways that originate in the brain)	NSAIDs inhibit prostaglandin synthesis selectively (with COX-2 inhibitors—eg, celecoxib, parecoxib) or nonselectively (with COX-1 and -2 inhibitors—eg, ibuprofen, naproxen) and reduce pain impulse formation. Opioid analgesics (eg, morphine) activate endorphin-enkephalin (μ, δ, and κ) receptors, reducing pain impulse transmission.
Parkinsonism	Inhibition of the dopaminergic system due to blockage of dopaminergic receptors by antipsychotic drugs	Anticholinergic drugs reduce cholinergic activity and restore balance between cholinergic and dopaminergic systems.
Parkinson disease	Loss of dopaminergic neurons of the pars compacta in the substantia nigra and other areas, with reduced levels of dopamine and metenkephalin, altering the dopamine/acetylcholine balance and resulting in striatal acetylcholine overactivity	L-Dopa reaches the synaptic cleft, is taken up by the axon, and is decarboxylated to dopamine, which is secreted into the cleft to activate dendritic dopamine receptors. Amantadine increases the presynaptic release of dopamine; dopamine agonists stimulate dopamine receptors, although bromocriptine, pramipexole, and ropinirole bind only to D_2, D_3, and D_4 dopamine receptor subtypes. Anticholinergic drugs reduce activity of the cholinergic system, restoring the balance of dopamine and acetylcholine. MAO-B inhibitors prevent reuptake of dopamine, increasing its levels. Selegiline, an MAO-B inhibitor, blocks dopamine breakdown and thus prolongs the response to levodopa and allows the dosage of carbidopa/levodopa to be reduced. Catechol *O*-methyltransferase (COMT) inhibitors also inhibit dopamine breakdown.
Schizophrenia	Increased presynaptic release, synthesis of dopamine, sensitivity or density of postsynaptic dopamine receptors, or a combination	Antipsychotic drugs block dopamine receptors and reduce dopaminergic overactivity to normal. Haloperidol preferentially blocks D_2 and D_3 receptors (high affinity) and D_4 receptors (low affinity) in mesocortical areas. Clozapine has a high affinity for binding D_4 and 5-HT_2 receptors, suggesting 5-HT system involvement in the pathogenesis of schizophrenia and its response to treatment. Clozapine has a significant risk of leukopenia. Olanzapine and risperidone, similar to haloperidol, also have high affinity for 5-HT_2 and D_2 receptors.
Tardive dyskinesia	Hypersensitive dopamine receptors due to chronic blockade by antipsychotic drugs	Reducing doses of antipsychotics may reduce hypersensitivity of dopamine receptors; however, in some cases, changes can be irreversible.
Normal neurotransmitters but nonfunctional receptors		
Myasthenia gravis	Reflects inactivation of acetylcholine receptors and postsynaptic histochemical changes at the neuromuscular junction due to autoimmune reactions	Anticholinesterase drugs inhibit acetylcholinesterase, increase acetylcholine levels at the junction, and stimulate remaining receptors, increasing muscle activity.
Decreased neuronal uptake of neurotransmitters		
Amyotrophic lateral sclerosis	Destruction of upper and lower motor neurons, possibly caused in part by glutamate neurotoxicity	Riluzole, which inhibits glutamate transmission, modestly extends survival.
Normal neurotransmitters but ion channel defects		
Episodic ataxias	Defective voltage-gated K channels, causing distal rippling and incoordination (myokymia)	Treatment with acetazolamide is effective in some types of episodic ataxia.
Hyperkalemic periodic paralysis	Decreased Na channel inactivation	Severe attacks may be terminated by Ca gluconate, glucose, and insulin.
Hypokalemic periodic paralysis	Defective voltage-gated Ca channels	Acute attacks can be terminated by K salts. Acetazolamide is effective for prevention.

Table 234–1. EXAMPLES OF DISORDERS ASSOCIATED WITH DEFECTS IN NEUROTRANSMISSION (*Continued*)

DISORDER	PATHOPHYSIOLOGY	TREATMENT
Lambert-Eaton syndrome*	Antibodies that decrease presynaptic release of acetylcholine	Corticosteroids, 3,4-diaminopyridine (DAP), guanidine, IVIG, and plasmapheresis can be helpful.
Paramyotonia congenita	Defective voltage-gated Na channels, causing cold-induced myotonia and episodic weakness	Mexiletine (a Na channel blocker) and acetazolamide (a carbonic anhydrase inhibitor) may be helpful.
Rasmussen encephalitis	Postviral production of antibodies to glutamate receptors, affecting glutamate-gated channels Most distinctive form of epilepsia partialis continua	Corticosteroids and antiviral drugs are usually ineffective. Functional hemispherectomy can control seizures if spontaneous remission does not occur.
Startle disease (hyperexplexia, stiff baby syndrome)	Mutation in the gene for the α1 subunit of the glycine-gated channel Characterized by stiffness, nocturnal myoclonus, and an exaggerated startle reflex, with hyperreflexia and falling	Clonazepam or certain other anticonvulsants (eg, phenytoin, phenobarbital, diazepam, valproate) may result in improvement.
Poisoning		
Botulism	Inhibition of acetylcholine release from motor neurons by toxin from *Clostridium botulinum*	No specific drug therapy exists. Tiny amounts of the toxin are used to treat certain dystonias, spasticity, neuropathic pain, and migraines or cosmetically to reduce skin wrinkles.
Mushroom poisoning	*Amanita muscaria:* Contains ibotenic acid (which has effects similar to those of glutamate) and a metabolite similar to muscimol (which has effects similar to those of GABA) *Inocybe* and *Clitocybe* spp: Stimulation of muscarinic receptors by muscarine and related compounds	Treatment is supportive because no drugs reverse the effects on neurotransmission. Atropine helps reverse muscarinic manifestations.
Organophosphates	Irreversible inhibition of acetylcholinesterase and marked increase in acetylcholine levels in synaptic cleft	Pralidoxime removes toxin from acetylcholinesterase and helps reverse nicotinic as well as muscarinic manifestations. Atropine helps rapidly reverse muscarinic effects.
Snake venom from *Bungarus multicinctus* (Taiwanese banded krait)	Blocks acetylcholine receptors at neuromuscular junction by α-*Bungarus* toxin	Antivenom appears to be effective and is available.

*Eaton-Lambert syndrome is an antibody-mediated paraneoplastic syndrome that typically occurs in small cell lung cancer. It can be present before the tumor manifests.

CRF = corticotropin (ACTH)-releasing factor; GABA = γ-aminobutyric acid; 5-HT = serotonin; IVIG = IV immune globulin; MAO = monoamine oxidase; MAO-B = MAO type B; NMDA = *N*-methyl-D-aspartate; PIP_2 = phosphatidylinositol 4,5-bisphosphate.

235 Pain

Pain is the most common reason patients seek medical care. Pain has sensory and emotional components and is often classified as acute or chronic. Acute pain is frequently associated with anxiety and hyperactivity of the sympathetic nervous system (eg, tachycardia, increased respiratory rate and BP, diaphoresis, dilated pupils). Chronic pain does not involve sympathetic hyperactivity but may be associated with vegetative signs (eg, fatigue, loss of libido, loss of appetite) and depressed mood. People vary considerably in their tolerance for pain.

Pathophysiology

Acute pain, which usually occurs in response to tissue injury, results from activation of peripheral pain receptors and their specific A delta and C sensory nerve fibers (nociceptors).

Chronic pain (see p. 1973) related to ongoing tissue injury is presumably caused by persistent activation of these fibers. However, the severity of tissue injury does not always predict the severity of chronic or acute pain. Chronic pain may also result from ongoing damage to or dysfunction of the peripheral or central nervous system (which causes neuropathic pain—see p. 1975).

Nociceptive pain may be somatic or visceral. Somatic pain receptors are located in skin, subcutaneous tissues, fascia, other connective tissues, periosteum, endosteum, and joint capsules. Stimulation of these receptors usually produces sharp or dull localized pain, but burning is not uncommon if the skin or subcutaneous tissues are involved. Visceral pain receptors are located in most viscera and the surrounding connective tissue. Visceral pain due to obstruction of a hollow organ is poorly localized, deep, and cramping and may be referred to remote cutaneous sites. Visceral pain due to injury of organ capsules or other deep connective tissues may be more localized and sharp.

Psychologic factors modulate pain intensity to a highly variable degree. Thoughts and emotions have an important role in the perception of pain. Many patients who have chronic pain also have psychologic distress, especially depression and anxiety. Because certain syndromes characterized as psychiatric disorders (eg, some somatic symptom disorders—see p. 1805) are defined by self-reported pain, patients with poorly explained pain are often mischaracterized as having a psychiatric disorder and are thus deprived of appropriate care.

Pain impairs multiple cognitive domains including attention, memory, concentration, and content of thought, possibly by demanding cognitive resources.

Many pain syndromes are multifactorial. For example, chronic low back pain and most cancer pain syndromes have a prominent nociceptive component but may also involve neuropathic pain (due to nerve damage).

Pain transmission and modulation: Pain fibers enter the spinal cord at the dorsal root ganglia and synapse in the dorsal horn. From there, fibers cross to the other side and travel up the lateral columns to the thalamus and then to the cerebral cortex.

Repetitive stimulation (eg, from a prolonged painful condition) can sensitize neurons in the dorsal horn of the spinal cord so that a lesser peripheral stimulus causes pain (wind-up phenomenon). Peripheral nerves and nerves at other levels of the CNS may also be sensitized, producing long-term synaptic changes in cortical receptive fields (remodeling) that maintain exaggerated pain perception.

Substances released when tissue is injured, including those involved in the inflammatory cascade, can sensitize peripheral nociceptors. These substances include vasoactive peptides (eg, calcitonin gene-related protein, substance P, neurokinin A) and other mediators (eg, prostaglandin E_2, serotonin, bradykinin, epinephrine).

The pain signal is modulated at multiple points in both segmental and descending pathways by many neurochemical mediators, including endorphins (eg, enkephalin) and monoamines (eg, serotonin, norepinephrine). These mediators interact in poorly understood ways to increase, sustain, shorten, or reduce the perception of and response to pain. They mediate the potential benefit of CNS-active drugs (eg, opioids, antidepressants, anticonvulsants, membrane stabilizers) that interact with specific receptors and neurochemicals in the treatment of chronic pain.

Psychologic factors are important modulators. They not only affect how patients speak about pain (eg, in a stoic, irritable, or complaining way) and how they behave in response to it (eg, whether they grimace), but they also generate neural output that modulates neurotransmission along pain pathways. Psychologic reaction to protracted pain interacts with other CNS factors to induce long-term changes in pain perception.

Geriatrics Essentials

In the elderly, the most common causes of pain are musculoskeletal disorders. However, pain is often chronic and multifactorial, and the causes may not be clear.

NSAIDs: Risk of ulcers and GI bleeding due to NSAIDs for people > 65 is 3 to 4 times higher than that for middle-aged people. Risk depends on drug dose and duration of therapy. Elderly patients at high risk of GI adverse effects may benefit from concomitant use of cytoprotective drugs (usually, a proton pump inhibitor; occasionally, the prostaglandin misoprostol).

The newly recognized risk of cardiovascular toxicity, which presumably occurs with nonselective COX-1 and COX-2 inhibitors (coxibs) and with selective coxibs, is particularly relevant to the elderly, who are more likely to have cardiovascular risk factors (eg, a history of MI or cerebrovascular or peripheral vascular disease).

Both nonselective and selective NSAIDs can impair renal function and cause Na and water retention; they should be used cautiously in the elderly, particularly in those who have a renal or hepatic disorder, heart failure, or hypovolemia. Rarely, NSAIDs cause cognitive impairment and personality changes in the elderly. Indomethacin causes more confusion in the elderly than other NSAIDs and should be avoided.

Given the overall greater risk of serious toxicity in the elderly, low doses of NSAIDs should be used if possible, and using short-term therapy or interrupted therapy to confirm effectiveness should be considered. NSAIDs are most likely to relieve pain generated by inflammation. Naproxen may be preferred because it appears to have a lower risk of cardiovascular adverse effects than other commonly prescribed NSAIDs.

Opioids: In the elderly, opioids have a longer half-life and possibly a greater analgesic effect than in younger patients. In elderly patients with chronic pain, short-term use of opioids appears to reduce pain and improve physical functioning but to impair mental function. Opioid-related constipation and urinary retention tend to be more problematic in the elderly. Risk of fracture during the first 2 wk of treatment is higher with opioids than with NSAIDs in the elderly.

Compared with other opioids, transdermal buprenorphine, an opioid agonist/antagonist, has a more favorable risk:benefit profile in elderly patients with renal insufficiency.

EVALUATION OF PAIN

Clinicians should evaluate the cause, severity, and nature of the pain and its effect on activities, mood, cognition, and sleep. Evaluation of the cause of acute pain (eg, back pain, chest pain—see elsewhere in THE MANUAL) differs from that of chronic pain (see p. 1973).

The history should include the following information about the pain:

- Quality (eg, burning, cramping, aching, deep, superficial, boring, shooting)
- Severity
- Location
- Radiation pattern
- Duration
- Timing (including pattern and degree of fluctuation and frequency of remissions)
- Exacerbating and relieving factors

The patient's level of function should be assessed, focusing on activities of daily living (eg, dressing, bathing), employment, avocations, and personal relationships (including sexual).

The patient's perception of pain can represent more than the disorder's intrinsic physiologic processes. What pain means to the patient should be determined, with emphasis on psychologic issues, depression, and anxiety. Reporting pain is more socially acceptable than reporting anxiety or depression, and appropriate therapy often depends on sorting out these divergent perceptions. Pain and suffering should also be distinguished, especially in cancer patients (see p. 1194); suffering may be due as much to loss of function and fear of impending death as to pain. Whether secondary gain (external, incidental benefits of a disorder—eg, time off, disability payments) contributes to pain or pain-related disability should be considered. The patient should be asked whether litigation is ongoing or financial compensation for injury will be sought. A personal or family history of chronic pain can often illuminate the current problem. Whether family members perpetuate chronic pain (eg, by constantly asking about the patient's health) should be considered.

Patients and sometimes family members and caregivers should be asked about the use, efficacy, and adverse effects of prescription and OTC drugs and other treatments and about alcohol and recreational or illicit drug use.

Pain severity: Pain severity should be assessed before and after potentially painful interventions. In verbal patients, self-report is the gold standard, and external signs of pain or distress (eg, crying, wincing, rocking) are secondary. For patients who have difficulty communicating and for young children, nonverbal indicators (behavioral and sometimes physiologic) may need to be the primary source of information.

Formal measures (see Fig. 235–1) include verbal category scales (eg, mild, moderate, severe), numeric scales, and the Visual Analog Scale (VAS). For the numeric scale, patients are asked to rate their pain from 0 to 10 (0 = no pain; 10 = "the worst pain ever"). For the VAS, patients make a hash mark representing their degree of pain on an unmarked 10-cm line with the left side labeled "no pain" and the right side labeled "unbearable pain." The pain score is distance in mm from the left end of the line. Children and patients with limited literacy or known developmental problems may select from images of faces ranging from smiling to contorted with pain or from fruits of varying sizes to convey their perception of pain severity. When measuring pain, the examiner should specify a time period (eg, "on average during the past week").

Demented and aphasic patients: Assessing pain in patients with disorders affecting cognition, speech, or language (eg, dementia, aphasia) can be difficult. Pain is suggested by facial grimacing, frowning, or repetitive eye blinking. Sometimes caregivers can describe behaviors that suggest pain (eg, sudden social withdrawal, irritability, grimacing). Pain should be considered in patients who have difficulty communicating

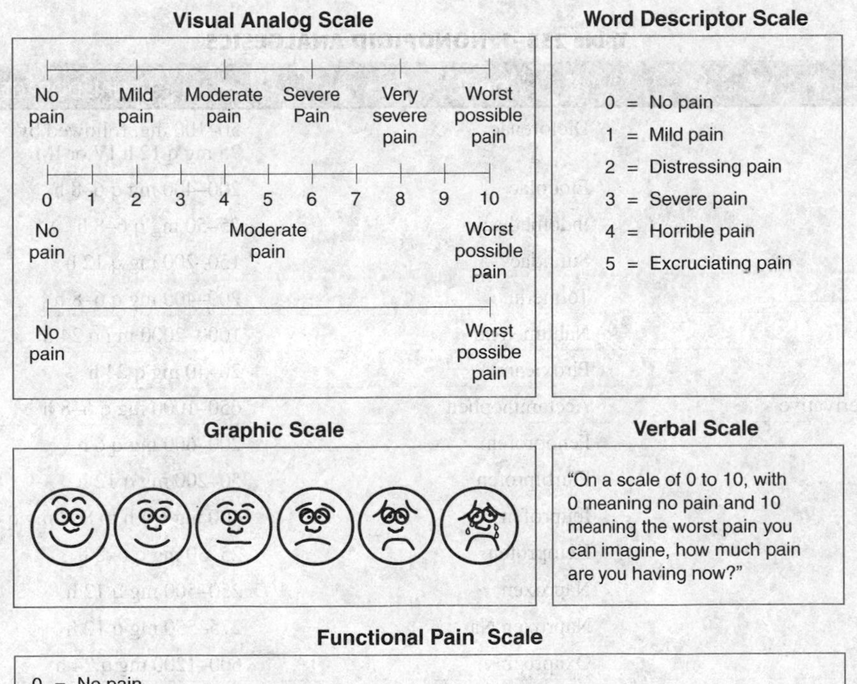

Fig. 235–1. Some pain scales for quantifying pain as it is occurring. For the Functional Pain Scale, examiners should clearly explain to the patient that functional limitations are relevant to the evaluation only if they are due to the pain being evaluated; treatment aims to relieve pain as much as possible, at least to a tolerable level (0–2). Adapted from the American Geriatrics Society (AGS) Panel on Chronic Pain in Older Persons: The management of chronic pain in older persons. *Journal of the American Geriatrics Society* 46:635–651, 1998; used with permission; from Gloth FM III, Scheve AA, Stober CV, et al: The functional pain scale (FPS): Reliability, validity, and responsiveness in a senior population. *Journal of the American Medical Directors Association* 2(3):110–114, 2001; and from Gloth FM III: Assessment. In *Handbook of Pain Relief in Older Adults: An Evidence-Based Approach*, edited by FM Gloth III. Totowa (NJ), Humana Press, 2003, p. 17; used with permission; copyright © FM Gloth, III, 2000.

and who inexplicably change their behavior. Many patients who have difficulty communicating can communicate meaningfully when an appropriate pain scale is used. For example, the Function Pain Scale has been validated and can be used in nursing home patients who have Mini-Mental State Examination scores of ≥ 17.

Patients receiving neuromuscular blockade: No validated instruments are available to assess pain when neuromuscular blockade is used to facilitate mechanical ventilation. If the patient is given a sedative, the dose can be adjusted until there is no evidence of consciousness. In such cases, specific analgesics are not needed. If, however, the patient is sedated but continues to have evidence of consciousness (eg, blinking, some eye movement response to command), pain treatment should be considered based on the degree of pain usually caused by the condition (eg, burns, trauma). If a potentially painful procedure (eg, turning a bedbound patient) is required, pretreatment with the selected analgesic or anesthetic should be given.

TREATMENT OF PAIN

Nonopioid and opioid analgesics are the main drugs used to treat pain. Antidepressants, anticonvulsants, and other CNS-active drugs may also be used for chronic or neuropathic pain and are first-line therapy for some conditions. Neuraxial infusion, nerve stimulation, injection therapies, and neural blockade can help selected patients. Cognitive-behavioral interventions (eg, changes in relationships in the home; systematic use of relaxation techniques, hypnosis, or biofeedback; graduated exercise) may reduce pain and pain-related disability and help patients cope.

Nonopioid Analgesics

Acetaminophen and NSAIDs are often effective for mild to moderate pain (see Table 235–1). Of these, only ketorolac and diclofenac can be given parenterally. Nonopioids do not cause physical dependence or tolerance.

Table 235–1. NONOPIOID ANALGESICS

CLASS	DRUG	USUAL DOSAGE RANGE*
Indoles	Diclofenac	50–100 mg, followed by 50 mg q 8 h 75 mg q 12 h IV or IM
	Etodolac	200–400 mg q 6–8 h
	Indomethacin	25–50 mg q 6–8 h
	Sulindac	150–200 mg q 12 h
	Tolmetin	200–400 mg q 6–8 h
Naphthylalkanone	Nabumetone	1000–2000 mg q 24 h
Oxicam	Piroxicam	20–40 mg q 24 h
Para-aminophenol derivative	Acetaminophen	650–1000 mg q 6–8 h
Propionic acids	Fenoprofen	200–600 mg q 6 h
	Flurbiprofen	50–200 mg q 12 h
	Ibuprofen	400 mg q 4 h to 800 mg q 6 h
	Ketoprofen	25–50 mg q 6–8 h
	Naproxen	250–500 mg q 12 h
	Naproxen Na	275–550 mg q 12 h
	Oxaprozin	600–1200 mg q 24 h
Salicylates	Aspirin	650–1000 mg q 4–6 h
	Choline Mg trisalicylate	870 mg q 12 h
	Diflunisal	250–500 mg q 8–12 h
	Salsalate	750–2000 mg q 12 h
Fenamates	Meclofenamate	50–100 mg q 6–8 h
	Mefenamic acid	250 mg q 6 h
Pyrazole	Phenylbutazone	100 mg q 6–8 h up to 7 days
Pyrrolo-pyrrolo derivative	Ketorolac	15–30 mg IV or IM q 6 h or 20, followed by 10 mg q 4–6 h for maximum 5 days
Selective COX-2 inhibitor	Celecoxib	100–200 mg q 12 h

*Route is oral, except for ketorolac and diclofenac, which can be given parenterally.

Acetaminophen has no anti-inflammatory or antiplatelet effects and does not cause gastric irritation.

NSAIDs include nonselective COX (COX-1 and COX-2) inhibitors and selective coxibs; all are effective analgesics. Aspirin is the least expensive but has prolonged antiplatelet effects. Coxibs have lowest risk of ulcer formation and GI upset. However, when a coxib is used with low-dose aspirin, it may have no GI benefit over other NSAIDs.

Studies suggest that inhibition of COX-2, which occurs with both nonselective COX inhibitors and coxibs, has a prothrombotic effect that can increase risk of MI, stroke, and claudication. This effect appears to be drug-related, as well as dose- and duration-related. Although there is some evidence that the risk is very low with some of the nonselective COX inhibitors (eg, ibuprofen, naproxen) and coxibs (celecoxib) and although data are still limited, it is prudent to consider the potential for prothrombotic effects as a risk of all NSAID therapy, suggesting that all NSAIDs should be used cautiously in patients with clinically significant atherosclerosis or multiple cardiovascular risk factors.

If an NSAID is likely to be used only short-term, significant adverse effects are unlikely, regardless of the drug used. Some clinicians use a coxib first whenever therapy is likely to be long-term (eg, months) because the risk of GI adverse effects is lower; others limit coxib use to patients predisposed to GI adverse effects (eg, the elderly, patients taking corticosteroids, those with a history of peptic ulcer disease or GI upset due to other NSAIDs) and those who are not doing well with nonselective NSAIDs or who have a history of intolerance to them.

All NSAIDs should be used cautiously in patients with renal insufficiency; coxibs are not renal-sparing.

If initial recommended doses provide inadequate analgesia, a higher dose is given, up to the conventional safe maximum dose. If analgesia remains inadequate, the drug should be stopped. If pain is not severe, another NSAID may be tried because response varies from drug to drug. It is prudent during long-term NSAID therapy to monitor for occult blood in stool and changes in CBC, electrolytes, and hepatic and renal function.

Topical NSAIDs may be applied directly to the painful region for disorders such as osteoarthritis and minor sprains, strains, and contusions. A 1.5% solution of diclofenac has been shown to effectively treat pain and limited joint function caused by osteoarthritis of the knees; dose is 40 drops (1.2 mL) applied qid to each affected knee. Other topical diclofenac formulations that may be useful for local pain relief include a patch (applied bid over the affected area) or a 1% gel (2 g qid for the upper extremities or 4 g qid for the lower extremities).

Opioid Analgesics

"Opioid" is a generic term for natural or synthetic substances that bind to specific opioid receptors in the CNS, producing an agonist action. Opioids are also called narcotics—a term originally used to refer to any psychoactive substance that induces sleep. Opioids have both analgesic and sleep-inducing effects, but the 2 effects are distinct from each other.

Some opioids used for analgesia have both agonist and antagonist actions. Potential for abuse among those with a known history of abuse or addiction may be lower with agonist-antagonists than with pure agonists, but agonist-antagonist drugs have a ceiling effect for analgesia and induce a withdrawal syndrome in patients already physically dependent on opioids.

In general, acute pain is best treated with short-acting pure agonist drugs, and chronic pain, when treated with opioids, should be treated with long-acting opioids (see Tables 235–2 and 235–3). Because of the higher doses in many long-acting formulations, these drugs have a higher risk of serious adverse effects (eg, death due to respiratory depression) in opioid-naive patients.

Table 235–2. OPIOID ANALGESICS

DRUG	ADULT DOSE*	PEDIATRIC DOSE†	COMMENTS
Opioid agonists in combination products‡ for moderate pain			
Codeine	Oral: 30–60 mg q 4 h	0.5–1 mg/kg	—
Hydrocodone	Oral: 5–10 mg q 4–6 h	0.135 mg/kg	Similar to codeine
Opioid agonists for moderate-to-severe pain			
Fentanyl	Transdermal: 12 or 25 mcg/h q 3 days Transmucosal: 100–200 mcg q 2–4 h Intranasal: 100–200 mcg q 2–4 h	Transmucosal: 5–15 mcg/kg	May trigger less histamine release and thus may cause less hypotension than other opioids Transdermal 12 mcg/h patch useful for opioid-naive patients; other doses used only for patients who have been stabilized on opioids Supplemental analgesia required at first because peak analgesia does not occur until 18–24 h after application Short-acting transmucosal forms used for breakthrough pain in adults and for conscious sedation in children
Hydromorphone	Oral: 2–4 mg q 4–6 h Parenteral: 0.5–1 mg q 4–6 h Extended-release: 8–32 mg q 24 h	—	Short half-life
	Rectal: 3 mg q 6–8 h	—	Rectal form used at bedtime
Levorphanol	Oral: 2 mg q 6–8 h Parenteral: 2 mg q 6–8 h	—	Long half-life

Table continues on the following page.

Table 235–2. OPIOID ANALGESICS (*Continued*)

DRUG	ADULT DOSE*	PEDIATRIC DOSE†	COMMENTS
Meperidine	Oral: 50–300 mg q 4 h Parenteral: 50–150 mg q 4 h	1.1–1.75 mg/kg	Not preferred because its active metabolite (normeperidine) causes dysphoria and CNS excitation (eg, myoclonus, tremulousness, seizures) and accumulates for days after dosing is begun, particularly in patients with renal failure
Methadone	Oral: 2.5–10 mg q 6–8 h Parenteral: 2.5–5 mg q 6–8 h	—	Used for treatment of heroin withdrawal, long-term maintenance treatment of opioid addiction, and analgesia for chronic pain Establishment of a safe, effective dose for analgesia complicated by its long half-life (usually much longer than duration of analgesia) Requires close monitoring for several days or more after amount or frequency of dose is increased because serious toxicity can occur as the plasma level rises to steady state
Morphine	Oral immediate-release: 10–30 mg q 4 h Oral controlled-release: 15 mg q 12 h Oral sustained-release: 30 mg q 24 h Parenteral: 5–10 mg q 4 h	0.05–0.2 mg/kg q 4 h	Standard of comparison Triggers histamine release more often than other opioids, causing itching
Oxycodone‡	Oral: 5–10 mg q 4 h Oral controlled-release: 10–20 mg q 12 h	—	Also in combination products containing acetaminophen or aspirin
Oxymorphone	Oral: 5 mg q 4 h Oral controlled-release: 5–10 mg q 12 h IM or sc: 1–1.5 mg q 4 h IV: 0.5 mg q 4 h Rectal: 5 mg q 4–6 h	—	May trigger less histamine release than other opioids
Opioid agonist-antagonists§			
Buprenorphine	IV or IM: 0.3 mg q 6 h Sublingual: 2 mg q 12 h Transdermal patch: 5–20 mcg/h applied once/wk (in European Union, doses may exceed 20 mcg/h)	Use only in patients > 13 yr (same as adult dose)	Psychotomimetic effects (eg, delirium) less prominent than those of other agonist-antagonists, but other effects similar Respiratory depression that may not be fully reversible with naloxone Sublingual buprenorphine used occasionally for chronic pain; may be used for agonist therapy of opioid addiction
Butorphanol	IV: 1 (0.5–2) mg q 3–4 h IM: 2 (1–4) mg q 3–4 h Nasal: 1 mg (1 spray), repeated in 1 h prn	Not recommended	2-dose nasal sequence, repeated q 3–4 h if needed
Nalbuphine	Parenteral: 10 mg q 3–6 h	Not recommended	Psychotomimetic effects less prominent than those of pentazocine but more prominent than those of morphine
Pentazocine	Oral: 50–100 mg q 3–4 h Parenteral: 30 mg q 3–4 h (not to exceed 360 mg/day)	Not recommended	Usefulness limited by ceiling effect for analgesia at higher doses, by potential for opioid withdrawal in patients physically dependent on opioid agonists, and by risk of psychotomimetic effects, especially for nontolerant, nonphysically dependent patients with acute pain Available in tablets combined with naloxone, aspirin, or acetaminophen Can cause confusion and anxiety, especially in the elderly

*Starting doses are for opioid-naive patients. Patients with opioid tolerance or severe pain may require higher doses.
†Not all drugs are appropriate for analgesia in children.
‡These opioid agonists may be combined into a single pill with acetaminophen, aspirin, or ibuprofen.
§Opioid agonist-antagonists are not usually used for chronic pain and are rarely drugs of choice for the elderly.

Opioid analgesics are useful in managing acute and chronic pain. They are sometimes underused in patients with severe acute pain or with pain and a terminal disorder such as cancer, resulting in needless pain and suffering. Reasons for undertreatment include

- Underestimation of the effective dose
- Overestimation of the risk of adverse effects

Generally, opioids should not be withheld when treating acute, severe pain; however, simultaneous treatment of the condition causing the pain usually limits the duration of severe pain and the need for opioids to a few days or less. Also, opioids should generally not be withheld when treating cancer pain; in such cases, adverse effects can be prevented or managed, and addiction is less of a concern.

In patients with chronic noncancer pain, nonopioid therapy should be tried first (see Treatment on p. 1975). Opioids should be used when the benefit of pain reduction outweighs the risk of adverse effects and of drug misuse. If nonopioid therapy has been unsuccessful, opioid therapy should be considered. In such cases, obtaining informed consent may help clarify the goals, expectations, and risks of treatment and facilitate education and counseling about misuse. Patients receiving chronic (> 3 mo) opioid therapy should be regularly assessed for pain control, adverse effects, and signs of misuse. If patients have persistent severe pain despite increasing opioid doses, do not adhere to the terms of treatment, or have deteriorating physical or mental function, opioid therapy should be tapered and stopped.

Physical dependence (development of withdrawal symptoms when a drug is stopped) should be assumed to exist in all patients treated with opioids for more than a few days. Thus, opioids should be used as briefly as possible, and in dependent patients, the dose should be tapered to control withdrawal symptoms when opioids are no longer necessary. Patients with pain due to an acute, transient disorder (eg, fracture, burn, surgical procedure) should be switched to a nonopioid drug as soon as possible. Dependence is distinct from addiction, which, although it does not have a universally accepted definition, typically involves compulsive use and overwhelming involvement with the drug including craving, loss of control over use, and use despite harm.

Table 235–3. EQUIANALGESIC DOSES OF OPIOID ANALGESICS*

DRUG	IM (mg)	ORAL (mg)
Butorphanol	2	—
Codeine	130	200
Hydromorphone	1.5	7.5
Levorphanol	2	4
Meperidine	75	300
Methadone	10	20
Morphine	10	30
Nalbuphine	10	—
Oxycodone	15†	20
Oxymorphone	1	15
Pentazocine	60	180

*Equivalences are based on single-dose studies influenced by clinical experience. Cross-tolerance between drugs is incomplete, so when one drug is substituted for another, the equianalgesic dose should be reduced by 50%; methadone should be reduced by 75–90%.

†Parental oxycodone is available in Europe but not in the US.

Route of administration: Almost any route can be used. The oral or transdermal route is preferred for long-term use; both are effective and provide stable blood levels. Modified-release oral and transdermal forms allow less frequent dosing, which is particularly important for providing overnight relief.

The IV route provides the most rapid onset and thus the easiest titration, but duration of analgesia is short. Large, rapid fluctuations in blood levels (bolus effect) can lead to toxicity at peak levels early in the dosing interval or later to breakthrough pain at trough levels. Continuous IV infusion, sometimes with patient-controlled supplemental doses, eliminates this effect but requires an expensive pump; this approach is used most often for postoperative pain.

The IM route provides analgesia longer than IV but is painful, and absorption can be erratic; it is not recommended. Long-term continuous sc infusion can be used, particularly for cancer pain.

Transmucosal (sublingual) formulations of fentanyl are now available. Lozenges are used for sedation in children and as treatment of breakthrough pain in patients with cancer.

Intraspinal opioids (eg, morphine 5 to 10 mg epidurally or 0.5 to 1 mg intrathecally for acute pain) can provide relief, which is prolonged when a hydrophilic drug such as morphine is used; they are typically used postoperatively. Implanted infusion devices can provide long-term neuraxial infusion. These devices can also be used with other drugs (eg, local anesthetics, clonidine, ziconotide).

Dosing and titration: Initial dose is modified according to the patient's response; it is increased incrementally until analgesia is satisfactory or adverse effects limit treatment. Sedation and respiratory rate are monitored when opioids are given parenterally to relatively opioid-naive patients. For opioid-naive patients in particular, opioid therapy should start with a short-acting drug because many longer-acting opioids are more potent.

Because of methadone's variable pharmacokinetics, this drug should be started at a low dose, and the dose should not be increased more often than once/wk.

The elderly are more sensitive to opioids and are predisposed to adverse effects; opioid-naive elderly patients typically require lower doses than younger patients. Neonates, especially when premature, are also sensitive to opioids because they lack adequate metabolic pathways to eliminate them.

For moderate, transient pain, an opioid may be given prn. For severe or ongoing pain, doses should be given regularly, without waiting for severe pain to recur; supplemental doses are given as needed when treating cancer pain. The doses for patients with chronic noncancer pain are typically decided case by case.

For patient-controlled analgesia, a bolus dose (in a postoperative setting, typically morphine 1 mg q 6 min) is provided when patients push a button; a baseline infusion (eg, morphine 0.5 to 1 mg/h) may or may not be given. The physician controls the amount and interval of the bolus. Patients with prior opioid exposure or with chronic pain require a higher bolus and baseline infusion dose; the infusion dose is further adjusted based on response.

Patients with dementia cannot use patient-controlled analgesia, nor can young children; however, adolescents often can.

During long-term treatment, the effective opioid dose can remain constant for prolonged periods. Some patients need intermittent dose escalation, typically in the setting of physical changes that suggest an increase in the pain (eg, progressive neoplasm). Fear of tolerance should not inhibit appropriate early, aggressive use of an opioid. If a previously adequate dose becomes inadequate, that dose must usually be increased by 30 to 100% to control pain.

Nonopioid analgesics (eg, acetaminophen, NSAIDs) are often given concomitantly. Products containing both drugs are convenient, but the nonopioid may limit upward titration of the opioid dose.

Adverse effects: In opioid-naive patients, adverse effects common at the start of therapy include

- Sedation and mental clouding
- Nausea and vomiting
- Itching
- Respiratory depression (rare with appropriate doses)

Because steady-state plasma levels are not approached until 4 to 5 half-lives have passed, drugs with a long half-life (particularly levorphanol and methadone) have a risk of delayed toxicity as plasma levels rise. Modified-release opioids typically require several days to approach steady-state levels.

In the elderly, opioids tend to have more adverse effects (commonly, constipation and sedation or mental clouding). Falls are a particular risk in the elderly. Opioids may cause urinary retention in men with benign prostatic hyperplasia.

Although tolerance to opioid-induced sedation, mental clouding, and nausea usually develops within days, tolerance to opioid-induced constipation and urinary retention usually occurs much more slowly. Any adverse effect may be persistent in some patients; constipation is particularly likely to persist.

Opioids should be used cautiously in patients with certain disorders:

- Hepatic disorders because drug metabolism is delayed, particularly with modified-release preparations
- COPD because respiratory depression is a risk
- Some neurologic disorders, such as dementia and encephalopathy, because delirium is a risk
- Severe renal insufficiency because metabolites may accumulate and cause problems; accumulation least likely with fentanyl and methadone

Constipation is common among patients who take opioids for more than a few days. For prevention in predisposed patients (eg, the elderly), dietary fiber and fluids should be increased, and a stimulant laxative (eg, senna—see p. 72) should be given. Persisting constipation can be managed with Mg citrate 90 mL po q 2 to 3 days, lactulose 15 mL po bid, or propylethylene glycol powder (dose is adjusted as needed). Some patients require regular enemas. If patients receiving palliative care have constipation refractory to fluids, fiber, and laxatives, methylnaltrexone 8 to 12 mg sc every other day may help by antagonizing opioid receptors only in the bowel.

Patients should not drive and should take precautions to prevent falls and other accidents for a period of time after initiation of opioids and after an increase in dose. Patients and family members should be instructed to contact the physician if patients experience sedation. If sedation impairs quality of life, certain stimulant drugs may be given intermittently (eg, before a family gathering or other event that requires alertness) or, to some patients, regularly. Drugs that can be effective are methylphenidate (initially, 5 to 10 mg po bid), dextroamphetamine (initially, 2.5 to 10 mg po bid), or modafinil (initially, 100 to 200 mg po once/day). These drugs are typically given in the morning and as needed later. The maximum dose of methylphenidate seldom exceeds 60 mg/day. For some patients, caffeine-containing beverages provide enough stimulation. Stimulants may also potentiate analgesia.

Nausea can be treated with hydroxyzine 25 to 50 mg po q 6 h, metoclopramide 10 to 20 mg po q 6 h, or an antiemetic phenothiazine (eg, prochlorperazine 10 mg po or 25 mg rectally q 6 h).

Itching is caused by histamine release and may be relieved by an antihistamine (eg, diphenhydramine, 25 to 50 mg po or IV).

Respiratory depression is rare with conventional doses and with long-term use. If it occurs acutely, ventilatory assistance may be needed until the opioid's effect can be reversed by an opioid antagonist. Long-term use of opioids may lead to sleep-related breathing disorders including obstructive sleep apnea and, less commonly, central sleep apnea, irregular respiration, and periods of sustained hypoventilation.

For urinary retention, double voiding or using the Credé method during voiding may help; some patients benefit from adding an α-adrenergic blocker such as tamsulosin 0.4 mg po once/day (starting dose).

Opioids can cause neuroendocrine effects, typically reversible hypogonadism. Symptoms may include fatigue, loss of libido, infertility due to low levels of sex hormones, and, in women, amenorrhea.

Some drugs have unique risks. For example, rapid-acting fentanyl preparations (eg, lozenge, effervescent oral tablet, intranasal spray) have a high risk of dose-related adverse effects in opioid-naive patients with chronic noncancer pain such as migraine; these drugs should not be started until patients require a 24-h morphine dose with analgesic potency equal to 60 mg of oral morphine. Methadone should not be used in patients at risk of QT-interval prolongation.

Opioid misuse, diversion, and abuse: Opioids are now the leading cause of accidental death and fatal drug overdose in the US. Risk of fatal drug overdose increases significantly when opioid analgesics are used with benzodiazepines. Also, rates of misuse, diversion, and abuse (aberrant drug-taking behaviors—see p. 3246) are increasing.

Opioid misuse may be intentional or unintentional. It includes any use that contradicts medical advice or deviates from what is prescribed.

Diversion involves selling or giving a prescribed drug to others.

Abuse refers to recreational or nontherapeutic use (eg, euphoria, other psychotropic effects).

Addiction, typically marked by impaired control and craving, refers to compulsive use despite harm and negative consequences.

When considering prescribing opioid therapy, particularly chronic therapy, clinicians should evaluate patients for risk factors for abuse and diversion and counsel them against intentional and inadvertent misuse. Risk factors include

- Patient history of alcohol or drug abuse
- Family history of alcohol or drug abuse
- Major psychiatric disorder (current or past)

If risk factors are present, treatment may still be appropriate; however, clinicians should use more stringent measures to prevent abuse and addiction. Measures include prescription of only small amounts (requiring frequent visits for refills), urine drug screening to monitor treatment adherence (ie, to confirm that patients are taking the drugs and not diverting them), no refills for "lost" prescriptions, and use of tamper-resistant opioid formulations that have been developed to deter abuse by chewing or by crushing and injecting oral preparations. Clinicians may need to refer problematic patients to a pain specialist or an addiction medicine specialist experienced in pain management.

To avoid misuse of their drug by others, patients should keep opioids in a safe place and dispose of any unused drugs by returning them to the pharmacy. All patients should be counseled regarding the risks of combining opioids with alcohol and anxiolytics and self-adjustment of dosing.

Opioid antagonists: Opioid antagonists are opioid-like substances that bind to opioid receptors but produce little or no agonist activity. They are used mainly to reverse symptoms of opioid overdose, particularly respiratory depression.

Naloxone acts in < 1 min when given IV and slightly less rapidly when given IM. It can also be given sublingually or endotracheally. Duration of action is about 60 to 120 min. However, opioid-induced respiratory depression usually lasts longer than the duration of antagonism; thus, *repeated doses of naloxone and close monitoring are necessary*. The dose for acute opioid overdosage is 0.4 mg IV q 2 to 3 min prn. For patients receiving long-term opioid therapy, naloxone should be used only to reverse respiratory depression and must be given more cautiously to avoid precipitating withdrawal or recurrent pain. A reasonable regimen is 1 mL of a dilute solution (0.4 mg in 10 mL saline) IV q 1 to 2 min, titrated to adequate respirations (not alertness).

Nalmefene is similar to naloxone, but its duration of action is about 4 to 8 h. Nalmefene is occasionally used to ensure prolonged opioid reversal.

Naltrexone, an orally bioavailable opioid antagonist, is given as adjunctive therapy in opioid and alcohol addiction. It is long-acting and generally well-tolerated.

Adjuvant Analgesic Drugs

Many drugs are used as adjuvant analgesics, including anticonvulsants (eg, gabapentin, pregabalin), antidepressants (eg, tricyclics, duloxetine, venlafaxine, bupropion), and many others (see Table 235–4). These drugs have many uses, most notably to relieve pain with a neuropathic component.

Gabapentin is the most widely used drug for such purposes. For effective analgesia, the dose should usually be > 600 mg tid, and many patients need a higher dose.

Pregabalin is similar to gabapentin but has more stable pharmacokinetics; some patients who do not respond well to gabapentin do respond to pregabalin and vice versa.

Duloxetine is a mixed mechanism (serotonin and norepinephrine) reuptake inhibitor, which appears to be effective for diabetic neuropathic pain, fibromyalgia, chronic low back pain, and chemotherapy-induced neuropathy.

Topical drugs are also widely used. Capsaicin cream, topical NSAIDs, other compounded creams (eg, local anesthetics), and a lidocaine 5% patch have little risk of adverse effects; they should be considered for many types of pain.

Neural Blockade

Interrupting nerve transmission in peripheral or central pain pathways via drugs or physical methods provides short-term and sometimes long-term relief. Neuroablation (pathway destruction) is used rarely; it is typically reserved for patients with an advanced disorder and a short life expectancy.

Local anesthetic drugs (eg, lidocaine) can be given IV, intrathecally, intrapleurally, transdermally, sc, or epidurally. Epidural analgesia using local anesthetics or opioids is particularly useful for some types of postoperative pain. Long-term epidural drug administration is occasionally used for patients with localized pain and a short life expectancy. Generally, for long-term neuraxial infusion, an intrathecal route via an implanted pump is preferred.

Neuroablation involves interrupting a nociceptive pathway surgically or using radiofrequency energy to produce a lesion. The procedure is used mainly for cancer pain. Somatic pain is more responsive than visceral pain. Neuroablation of the ascending spinothalamic tract (cordotomy) is usually used; it provides relief for several years, although numbness and dysesthesias develop. Neuroablation of the dorsal roots (rhizotomy) is used when a specific dermatome can be identified.

Neuromodulation

Stimulation of neural tissues may decrease pain, presumably by activating endogenous pain modulatory pathways. The most commonly used noninvasive method is transcutaneous electrical nerve stimulation (TENS), which applies a small current to the skin. Evidence supports treatment of certain types of neuropathic pain (eg, chronic leg pain after spine surgery) using an electrode placed epidurally to stimulate the spinal cord. Also, electrodes may be implanted along peripheral nerves and ganglia in patients with certain headache syndromes or chronic neuralgia. Stimulation of brain structures (deep brain stimulation, motor cortex stimulation) has also been used, but evidence of benefit is slight.

CHRONIC PAIN

Chronic pain is pain that persists or recurs for > 3 mo, persists > 1 mo after resolution of an acute tissue injury, or accompanies a nonhealing lesion. Causes include chronic disorders (eg, cancer, arthritis, diabetes), injuries (eg, herniated disk, torn ligament), and many primary pain disorders (eg, neuropathic pain, fibromyalgia, chronic headache). Various drugs and psychologic treatments are used.

Unresolved, long-lasting disorders (eg, cancer, RA, herniated disk) that produce ongoing nociceptive stimuli may account completely for chronic pain. Alternatively, injury, even mild injury, may lead to long-lasting changes (sensitization) in the nervous system—from peripheral receptors to the cerebral cortex—that may produce persistent pain in the absence of ongoing nociceptive stimuli. With sensitization, discomfort that is due to a nearly resolved disorder and might otherwise be perceived as mild or trivial is instead perceived as significant pain. Psychologic factors may also amplify persistent pain. Thus, chronic pain commonly appears out of proportion to identifiable physical processes. In some cases (eg, chronic back pain after injury), the original precipitant of pain is obvious; in others (eg, chronic headache, atypical facial pain, chronic abdominal pain), the precipitant is remote or occult.

In most patients, physical processes are undeniably involved in sustaining chronic pain and are sometimes (eg, in cancer pain) the main factor. However, even in these patients, psychologic factors usually also play a role. Patients who have to continually prove that they are sick to obtain medical care, insurance coverage, or work relief may unconsciously reinforce their pain perceptions, particularly when litigation is involved. This response differs from malingering, which is conscious exaggeration of symptoms for secondary gain (eg, time off, disability payments). Various factors in the patient's environment (eg, family members, friends) may reinforce behaviors that perpetuate chronic pain.

Chronic pain can lead to or exacerbate psychologic problems (eg, depression). Distinguishing psychologic cause from effect is often difficult.

Symptoms and Signs

Chronic pain often leads to vegetative signs (eg, lassitude, sleep disturbance, decreased appetite, loss of taste for food, weight loss, diminished libido, constipation), which develop

Table 235–4. DRUGS FOR NEUROPATHIC PAIN

CLASS/DRUG	DOSE*	COMMENTS
Anticonvulsants†		
Carbamazepine	200–400 mg bid	Monitor WBCs when starting treatment First-line treatment for trigeminal neuralgia
Gabapentin	300 mg bid–1200 mg tid	Preferred drug in this class; starting dose usually 300 mg once/day
Phenytoin	300 mg once/day	Limited data; 2nd-line drug
Pregabalin	75–300 mg bid	Mechanism similar to gabapentin but more stable pharmacokinetics
Valproate	250–500 mg bid	Limited data, but strong support for treatment of headache
Antidepressants		
Amitriptyline	10–25 mg at bedtime	May increase dose to 75–150 mg over 1–2 wk, particularly if significant depression is present; may not need high doses Not recommended for the elderly or patients with a heart disorder because it has strong anticholinergic effects
Desipramine	10–25 mg at bedtime	Better tolerated than amitriptyline May increase dose to 150 mg or sometimes higher
Duloxetine	30 mg bid	Better tolerated than tricyclic antidepressants
Central α_2-adrenergic agonists		
Clonidine	0.1 mg once/day	Also can be used transdermally or intrathecally
Tizanidine	2–20 mg bid	Less likely to cause hypotension than clonidine
Corticosteroids		
Dexamethasone	0.5–4 mg qid	Used only for pain with an inflammatory component
Prednisone	5–60 mg once/day	Used only for pain with an inflammatory component
NMDA-receptor antagonists		
Memantine	10–30 mg once/day	Limited evidence of efficacy
Dextromethorphan	30–120 mg qid	Usually considered 2nd-line
Oral Na channel blockers		
Mexiletine	150 mg once/day to 300 mg q 8 h	Used only for neuropathic pain For patients with a significant heart disorder, cardiac evaluation considered before the drug is started
Topical		
Capsaicin 0.025–0.075%	tid	Some evidence of efficacy in neuropathic pain and arthritis
EMLA®	tid, under occlusive dressing if possible	Usually considered for a trial if a lidocaine patch is ineffective; expensive
Lidocaine 5%	Daily	Available as patch
Other		
Baclofen	20–60 mg bid	May act via $GABA_B$ receptor Helpful in trigeminal neuralgia; used in other types of neuropathic pain
Pamidronate	60–90 mg/mo	Evidence of efficacy in complex regional pain syndrome

*Route is oral unless otherwise indicated.

†Newer anticonvulsants have fewer adverse effects.

EMLA = eutectic mixture of local anesthetics; GABA = γ-aminobutyric acid; NMDA = *N*-methyl-D-aspartate.

gradually. Constant, unremitting pain may lead to depression and anxiety and interfere with almost all activities. Patients may become inactive, withdraw socially, and become preoccupied with physical health. Psychologic and social impairment may be severe, causing virtual lack of function.

Some patients, particularly those without a clear-cut ongoing cause, have a history of failed medical and surgical treatments, multiple (and duplicative) diagnostic tests, use of many drugs (sometimes involving abuse or addiction), and inappropriate use of health care.

Diagnosis

- Evaluation for physical cause initially and if symptoms change

A physical cause should always be sought—even if a prominent psychologic contribution to the pain is likely. Physical processes associated with the pain should be evaluated appropriately and characterized. However, once a full evaluation is done, repeating tests in the absence of new findings is not useful. The best approach is often to stop testing and focus on relieving pain and restoring function.

The effect of pain on the patient's life should be evaluated; evaluation by an occupational therapist may be necessary. Formal psychiatric evaluation should be considered if a coexisting psychiatric disorder (eg, major depression) is suspected as cause or effect.

Treatment

- Often multimodal therapy (eg, analgesics, physical methods, psychologic treatments)

Specific causes should be treated. Early, aggressive treatment of acute pain is always preferable and may limit or prevent sensitization and remodeling and hence prevent progression to chronic pain.

Drugs or physical methods may be used. Psychologic and behavioral treatments are usually helpful. Many patients who have marked functional impairment or who do not respond to a reasonable attempt at management by their physician benefit from the multidisciplinary approach available at a pain clinic.

Many patients prefer to have their pain treated at home, even though an institution may offer more advanced modalities of pain management. Also, pain control may be compromised by certain practices in institutions; for example, they restrict visiting hours, use of televisions and radios (which provide useful distraction), and use of heating pads (for fear of thermal injury).

Drugs: Analgesics include NSAIDs, opioids, and adjuvant analgesics (eg, antidepressants, anticonvulsants—see p. 1973 and Table 235–4). One or more drugs may be appropriate. Adjuvant analgesics are most commonly used for neuropathic pain. For persistent, moderate-to-severe pain that impairs function, opioids should be considered after determining the following:

- What conventional treatment practice is
- Whether other treatments are reasonable
- Whether the patient has an unusually high risk of adverse effects from an opioid
- Whether the patient is at risk of misuse, diversion, or abuse (aberrant drug-taking behaviors)

When prescribing opioids for chronic pain, physicians should take several steps:

- Provide education and counseling about misuse: Topics should include the risks of combining opioids with alcohol and anxiolytics, self-adjustment of dosing, and the need for safe, secure storage of drugs. Patients should also be taught how to correctly dispose of unused drugs; they should be instructed not to share opioids and to contact their physician if they experience sedation.
- Evaluate patients for risk of misuse, diversion, and abuse: Risk factors include prior or current alcohol or drug abuse, a family history of alcohol or drug abuse, and a prior or current major psychiatric disorder. Presence of risk factors does not always contraindicate opioid use. However, if patients have risk factors, they should be referred to a pain management specialist, or the physician should take special precautions to deter misuse, diversion, and abuse; these measures can include prescribing only small amounts (requiring frequent visits for refills), not refilling prescriptions allegedly lost, and using urine drug screening to confirm that the prescribed opioid is being taken and not diverted to others.
- Obtain informed consent, when possible, to help clarify the goals, expectations, and risks of treatment, as well as the possible use of nonopioid treatment alternatives.
- Regularly reassess the extent of pain reduction, functional improvement, and adverse effects, and look for signs suggesting misuse, diversion, or abuse

As pain lessens, patients usually need help reducing use of opioids. If depression coexists with pain, antidepressants should be used.

Depending on the condition, trigger point injection, joint or spinal injections, nerve blocks, or neuraxial infusion may be appropriate.

Physical methods: Many patients benefit from physical therapy or occupational therapy. Spray-and-stretch techniques can relieve myofascial trigger points. Some patients require an orthosis. Spinal cord stimulation may be appropriate.

Psychologic treatments: Behavioral treatments can improve patient function, even without reducing pain. Patients should keep a diary of daily activities to pinpoint areas amenable to change. The physician should make specific recommendations for gradually increasing physical activity and social engagement. Activities should be prescribed in gradually increasing units of time; pain should not, if at all possible, be allowed to abort the commitment to greater function. When activities are increased in this way, reports of pain often decrease.

Various cognitive techniques of pain control (eg, relaxation training, distraction techniques, hypnosis, biofeedback) may be useful. Patients may be taught to use distraction by guided imagery (organized fantasy evoking calm and comfort—eg, imagining resting on a beach or lying in a hammock). Other cognitive-behavioral techniques (eg, self-hypnosis) may require training by specialists.

Behavior of family members or fellow workers that reinforces pain behavior (eg, constant inquiries about the patient's health or insistence that the patient do no chores) should be discouraged. The physician should avoid reinforcing pain behavior, discourage maladaptive behaviors, applaud progress, and provide pain treatment while emphasizing return of function.

KEY POINTS

- Nociceptive stimuli, sensitization of the nervous system, and psychologic factors can contribute to chronic pain.
- Distinguishing between the psychologic causes and effects of chronic pain may be difficult.
- Seek a physical cause even if psychologic factors are prominent, and always evaluate the effect of pain on the patient's life.
- Treat poorly controlled pain with multimodal therapy (eg, appropriate physical, psychologic, behavioral, and interventional treatments; drugs).

NEUROPATHIC PAIN

Neuropathic pain results from damage to or dysfunction of the peripheral or central nervous system, rather than stimulation of pain receptors. Diagnosis is suggested by pain out of proportion to tissue injury, dysesthesia (eg, burning, tingling), and signs of nerve injury detected

during neurologic examination. Although neuropathic pain responds to opioids, treatment is often with adjuvant drugs (eg, antidepressants, anticonvulsants, baclofen, topical drugs).

Pain can develop after injury to any level of the nervous system, peripheral or central; the sympathetic nervous system may be involved (causing sympathetically maintained pain). Specific syndromes include postherpetic neuralgia (see p. 1625), root avulsions, painful traumatic mononeuropathy, painful polyneuropathy (particularly due to diabetes—see p. 1260), central pain syndromes (potentially caused by virtually any lesion at any level of the nervous system), postsurgical pain syndromes (eg, postmastectomy syndrome, postthoracotomy syndrome, phantom limb pain), and complex regional pain syndrome (reflex sympathetic dystrophy and causalgia).

Etiology

Peripheral nerve injury or dysfunction can result in neuropathic pain. Examples are mononeuropathies (eg, carpal tunnel syndrome, radiculopathy), plexopathies (typically caused by nerve compression, as by a neuroma, tumor, or herniated disk), and polyneuropathies (typically caused by various metabolic neuropathies—see Table 236–1 on p. 1979). Mechanisms presumably vary and may involve an increased number of Na channels on regenerating nerves.

Central neuropathic pain syndromes appear to involve reorganization of central somatosensory processing; the main categories are deafferentation pain and sympathetically maintained pain. Both are complex and, although presumably related, differ substantially.

Deafferentation pain is due to partial or complete interruption of peripheral or central afferent neural activity. Examples are postherpetic neuralgia, central pain (pain after CNS injury), and phantom limb pain (pain felt in the region of an amputated body part—see p. 3258). Mechanisms are unknown but may involve sensitization of central neurons, with lower activation thresholds and expansion of receptive fields.

Sympathetically maintained pain depends on efferent sympathetic activity. Complex regional pain syndrome (CRPS) sometimes involves sympathetically maintained pain. Other types of neuropathic pain may have a sympathetically maintained component. Mechanisms probably involve abnormal sympathetic-somatic nerve connections (ephapses), local inflammatory changes, and changes in the spinal cord.

Symptoms and Signs

Dysesthesias (spontaneous or evoked burning pain, often with a superimposed lancinating component) are typical, but pain may also be deep and aching. Other sensations—eg, hyperesthesia, hyperalgesia, allodynia (pain due to a nonnoxious stimulus), and hyperpathia (particularly unpleasant, exaggerated pain response)—may also occur. Symptoms are long-lasting, typically persisting after resolution of the primary cause (if one was present) because the CNS has been sensitized and remodeled.

Diagnosis

- Clinical evaluation

Neuropathic pain is suggested by its typical symptoms when nerve injury is known or suspected. The cause (eg, amputation, diabetes) may be readily apparent. If not, the diagnosis often can be assumed based on the description. Pain that is ameliorated by sympathetic nerve block is sympathetically maintained pain.

Treatment

- Multimodal therapy (eg, psychologic treatments, physical methods, antidepressants or anticonvulsants, sometimes surgery)

Without concern for diagnosis, rehabilitation, and psychosocial issues, treatment has a limited chance of success. For peripheral nerve lesions, mobilization is needed to prevent trophic changes, disuse atrophy, and joint ankylosis. Surgery may be needed to alleviate compression. Psychologic factors must be constantly considered from the start of treatment. Anxiety and depression must be treated appropriately. When dysfunction is entrenched, patients may benefit from the comprehensive approach provided by a pain clinic.

Several classes of drugs are moderately effective (see Table 235–4), but complete or near-complete relief is unlikely. Antidepressants and anticonvulsants are most commonly used. Evidence of efficacy is strong for several antidepressants and anticonvulsants.

Opioid analgesics can provide some relief but are generally less effective than for acute nociceptive pain; adverse effects may prevent adequate analgesia. Topical drugs and a lidocaine-containing patch may be effective for peripheral syndromes.

Other potentially effective treatments include

- Spinal cord stimulation by an electrode placed epidurally for certain types of neuropathic pain (eg, chronic leg pain after spine surgery)
- Electrodes implanted along peripheral nerves and ganglia for certain chronic neuralgias
- Sympathetic blockade, which is usually ineffective, except for some patients with CRPS

KEY POINTS

- Neuropathic pain can result from efferent activity or from interruption of afferent activity.
- Consider neuropathic pain if patients have dysesthesia or if pain is out of proportion to tissue injury and nerve injury is suspected.
- Treat patients using multiple modalities (eg, psychologic treatments, physical methods, antidepressants or anticonvulsants, analgesics, surgery), and recommend rehabilitation as appropriate.

COMPLEX REGIONAL PAIN SYNDROME

(Reflex Sympathetic Dystrophy and Causalgia)

Complex regional pain syndrome (CRPS) is chronic neuropathic pain that follows soft-tissue or bone injury (type I) or nerve injury (type II) and lasts longer and is more severe than expected for the original tissue damage. Other manifestations include autonomic changes (eg, sweating, vasomotor abnormalities), motor changes (eg, weakness, dystonia), and trophic changes (eg, skin or bone atrophy, hair loss, joint contractures). Diagnosis is clinical. Treatment includes drugs, physical therapy, and sympathetic blockade.

CRPS type I was previously known as reflex sympathetic dystrophy, and type II was known as causalgia. Both types occur most often in young adults and are 2 or 3 times more common among women.

Etiology

CRPS type I typically follows an injury (usually of a hand or foot), most commonly after crush injuries, especially in a lower limb. It may follow amputation, acute MI, stroke, or cancer (eg, lung, breast, ovary, CNS); no precipitant is apparent in about 10% of patients. CRPS type II is similar to type I but involves overt damage to a peripheral nerve.

Pathophysiology

Pathophysiology is unclear, but peripheral nociceptor and central sensitization and release of neuropeptides (substance P, calcitonin gene-related peptide) help maintain pain and inflammation. The sympathetic nervous system is more involved in CRPS than in other neuropathic pain syndromes: Central sympathetic activity is increased, and peripheral nociceptors are sensitized to norepinephrine (a sympathetic neurotransmitter); these changes may lead to sweating abnormalities and poor blood flow due to vasoconstriction. Nonetheless, only some patients respond to sympathetic manipulation (ie, central or peripheral sympathetic blockade).

Symptoms and Signs

Symptoms vary greatly and do not follow a pattern; they include sensory, focal autonomic (vasomotor or sudomotor), and motor abnormalities.

Pain—burning or aching—is common. It does not follow the distribution of a single peripheral nerve; it may worsen with changes in environment or emotional stress. Allodynia and hyperalgesia may occur. Pain often causes patients to limit use of an extremity.

Cutaneous vasomotor changes (eg, red, mottled, or ashen color; increased or decreased temperature) and sudomotor abnormalities (dry or hyperhidrotic skin) may be present. Edema may be considerable and locally confined. Other symptoms include trophic abnormalities (eg, shiny, atrophic skin; cracking or excess growth of nails; bone atrophy; hair loss) and motor abnormalities (weakness, tremors, spasm, dystonia with fingers fixed in flexion or equinovarus position of foot). Range of motion is often limited, sometimes leading to joint contractures. Symptoms may interfere with fitting a prosthesis after amputation.

Psychologic distress (eg, depression, anxiety, anger) is common, fostered by the poorly understood cause, lack of effective therapy, and prolonged course.

Diagnosis

- Clinical evaluation

The following clinical criteria must be present to establish the diagnosis of CRPS:

- Occurrence of pain (usually burning)
- Allodynia or hyperalgesia
- Focal autonomic dysregulation (vasomotor or sudomotor abnormalities)
- No evidence of another disorder that could explain the symptoms

If another disorder is present, CRPS should be considered possible or probable.

Other symptoms and findings may support the diagnosis: edema, trophic abnormalities, or a change in temperature of the affected area. Thermography may be used to document the temperature change if clinical evaluation is equivocal and if this finding would help establish the diagnosis. Bone changes (eg, demineralization on x-ray, increased uptake on a triple-phase radionuclide bone scan) may be detected and are usually evaluated only if the diagnosis is equivocal. However, imaging tests may also be abnormal after trauma in patients without CRPS.

Sympathetic nerve block (cervical stellate ganglion or lumbar) can be used for diagnosis and treatment. However, false-positive and false-negative results are common because not all CRPS pain is sympathetically maintained and nerve block may also affect nonsympathetic fibers. In another test of sympathetic involvement, a patient is given IV infusions of saline (placebo) or phentolamine 1 mg/kg over 10 min while pain scores are recorded; a decrease in pain after phentolamine but not placebo indicates sympathetically maintained pain.

Prognosis

Prognosis varies and is difficult to predict. CRPS may remit or remain stable for years; in a few patients, it progresses, spreading to other areas of the body.

Treatment

- Multimodal therapy (eg, drugs, physical therapy, sympathetic blockade, psychologic treatments, neuromodulation, mirror therapy)

Treatment is complex and often unsatisfactory, particularly if begun late. It includes drugs, physical therapy, sympathetic blockade, psychologic treatments, and neuromodulation. Few controlled trials have been done.

Many of the drugs used for neuropathic pain, including tricyclic antidepressants, anticonvulsants, and corticosteroids (see Table 235–4), may be tried; none is known to be superior. Long-term treatment with opioid analgesics may be useful for selected patients.

In some patients with sympathetically maintained pain, regional sympathetic blockade relieves pain, making physical therapy possible. Oral analgesics (NSAIDs, opioids, and various adjuvant analgesics) may also relieve pain sufficiently to allow rehabilitation.

For neuromodulation, implanted spinal cord stimulators are being increasingly used. Transcutaneous electrical nerve stimulation (TENS), applied at multiple locations with different stimulation parameters, should be given a long trial. Implanted stimulation systems targeting peripheral nerves (eg, occipital nerve stimulation for some headache syndromes) may be beneficial. Other methods of neuromodulation include brisk rubbing of the affected part (counterirritation) and acupuncture. No one form of neuromodulation is known to be more effective than another, and a poor response to one form does not mean a poor response to another.

Neuraxial infusion with opioids, anesthetics, and clonidine may help, and intrathecal baclofen has reduced dystonia in a few patients.

Physical therapy is essential. Goals include strengthening, increased range of motion, and vocational rehabilitation.

Mirror therapy has been reported to benefit patients with CRPS type 1 due to phantom limb pain or stroke. Patients straddle a large mirror between their legs. The mirror reflects the image of the unaffected limb and hides the affected (painful or missing) limb, giving patients the impression that they have 2 normal limbs. Patients are instructed to move their painful or missing limb while viewing the reflected image of their normal limb attempting the same movement. Most patients who do this exercise for 30 min/day for 4 wk report a substantial reduction in pain.

KEY POINTS

- CRPS may follow injury (to soft tissue, bone, or nerve), amputation, acute MI, stroke, or cancer or have no apparent precipitant.
- Diagnose CRPS if patients have neuropathic pain, allodynia or hyperalgesia, and focal autonomic dysregulation when no other cause is identified.
- Prognosis is unpredictable, and treatment is often unsatisfactory.
- Treat as early as possible using multiple modalities (eg, drugs used for neuropathic pain, physical therapy, sympathetic blockade, psychologic treatments, neuromodulation, mirror therapy).

236 Peripheral Nervous System and Motor Unit Disorders

The peripheral nervous system refers to parts of the nervous system outside the brain and spinal cord. It includes the cranial nerves and spinal nerves from their origin to their end. The anterior horn cells, although technically part of the CNS, are sometimes discussed with the peripheral nervous system because they are part of the motor unit.

Motor neuron dysfunction results in muscle weakness or paralysis. Sensory neuron dysfunction results in abnormal or lost sensation. Some disorders are progressive and fatal.

Anatomy

A motor unit consists of

- An anterior horn cell
- Its motor axon
- The muscle fibers it innervates
- The connection between them (neuromuscular junction)

The anterior horn cells are located in the gray matter of the spinal cord and thus are technically part of the CNS. In contrast to the motor system, the cell bodies of the afferent sensory fibers lie outside the spinal cord, in dorsal root ganglia.

Nerve fibers outside the spinal cord join to form anterior (ventral) motor roots and posterior (dorsal) sensory root nerve roots. The ventral and dorsal roots combine to form a spinal nerve. Thirty of the 31 pairs of spinal nerves have dorsal and ventral roots; C1 has no sensory root (see Fig. 240–1 on p. 2027).

The spinal nerves exit the vertebral column via an intervertebral foramen. Because the spinal cord is shorter than the vertebral column, the more caudal the spinal nerve, the further the foramen is from the corresponding cord segment. Thus, in the lumbosacral region, nerve roots from lower cord segments descend within the spinal column in a near-vertical sheaf, forming the cauda equina. Just beyond the intervertebral foramen, spinal nerves branch into several parts.

Branches of the cervical and lumbosacral spinal nerves anastomose peripherally into plexuses, then branch into nerve trunks that terminate up to 1 m away in peripheral structures (see Fig. 236–1 on p. 1995). The intercostal nerves are segmental.

The term peripheral nerve refers to the part of a spinal nerve distal to the root and plexus. Peripheral nerves are bundles of nerve fibers. They range in diameter from 0.3 to 22 μm. Schwann cells form a thin cytoplasmic tube around each fiber and further wrap larger fibers in a multilayered insulating membrane (myelin sheath).

Physiology

The myelin sheath enhances impulse conduction. The largest and most heavily myelinated fibers conduct quickly; they convey motor, touch, and proprioceptive impulses. The less myelinated and unmyelinated fibers conduct more slowly; they convey pain, temperature, and autonomic impulses.

Because nerves are metabolically active tissues, they require nutrients, supplied by blood vessels called the vasa nervorum.

Etiology

Peripheral nerve disorders can result from damage to or dysfunction of the one of the following:

- Cell body
- Myelin sheath
- Axons
- Neuromuscular junction

Disorders can be genetic or acquired (due to toxic, metabolic, traumatic, infectious, or inflammatory conditions—see Table 236–1).

Peripheral neuropathies may affect

- One nerve (mononeuropathy)
- Several discrete nerves (multiple mononeuropathy, or mononeuritis multiplex)
- Multiple nerves diffusely (polyneuropathy)
- A plexus (plexopathy)
- A nerve root (radiculopathy)

More than one site can be affected; eg, in the most common variant of Guillain-Barré syndrome, multiple segments of cranial nerves, usually the 2 facial nerves, may be affected.

Pathophysiology

Because sensory and motor cell bodies are in different locations, a nerve cell body disorder typically affects either the sensory or motor component but rarely both.

Damage: Damage to the myelin sheath (demyelination) slows nerve conduction. Demyelination affects mainly heavily myelinated fibers, causing large-fiber sensory dysfunction (buzzing and tingling sensations), motor weakness, and diminished reflexes. The hallmark of acquired demyelinating polyneuropathy is severe motor weakness with minimal atrophy.

Because the vasa nervorum do not reach the center of a nerve, centrally located fascicles are most vulnerable to vascular disorders (eg, vasculitis, ischemia). These disorders result in small-fiber sensory dysfunction (sharp pain and burning sensations), motor weakness proportional to atrophy, and less severe reflex abnormalities than in other nerve disorders. The distal two-thirds of a limb is affected most. Initially, deficits tend to be asymmetric because the vasculitic or ischemic process is

Table 236–1. SOME CAUSES OF PERIPHERAL NERVOUS SYSTEM DISORDERS

SITE	TYPE	EXAMPLES
Motor neuron*	Hereditary	Spinal muscular atrophy types I–IV
	Acquired, acute	Polio, infections due to coxsackievirus and other enteroviruses (rare), West Nile virus infection
	Acquired, chronic	Amyotrophic lateral sclerosis, paraneoplastic syndrome, postpolio syndrome, progressive bulbar palsy
Nerve root	Hereditary	Neurofibroma
	Acquired	Herniated disk, infections, metastatic cancer, spinal foraminal stenosis, trauma
Plexus	Acquired	Acute brachial neuritis, diabetes mellitus, hematoma, local tumors (eg, schwannoma), metastatic cancer, neurofibromatosis (rare), traction during birth, severe trauma
Peripheral nerve	Entrapment	Carpal tunnel syndrome, cubital tunnel syndrome, radial nerve palsy, peroneal nerve palsy, tarsal tunnel syndrome
	Hereditary	Hereditary adult-onset neuropathies, hereditary sensory and motor neuropathies, hereditary sensory and autonomic neuropathies
	Infectious	Hepatitis C, herpes zoster, HIV infection, Lyme disease, syphilis In developing nations: Diphtheria, leprosy, parasite infections
	Inflammatory	Chronic inflammatory demyelinating polyradiculoneuropathy, Guillain-Barré syndrome and variants
	Ischemic	Femoral nerve infarction (diabetic amyotrophy), vasculitis causing multiple mononeuropathy (mononeuritis multiplex)
	Toxic-metabolic	Amyloidosis, diabetes mellitus, dysproteinemic neuropathy, chronic excessive alcohol consumption with undernutrition (particularly deficiency of B vitamins), ICU neuropathy, leukodystrophies (rare), renal insufficiency, toxins (eg, arsenic, lead, mercury, thallium, chemotherapy drugs, pyridoxine toxicity)
Neuromuscular junction	—	Botulism in infants, congenital myasthenia (very rare), Eaton-Lambert syndrome, myasthenia gravis, toxic or drug induced neuromuscular junction dysfunction (eg, due to exposure to insecticides or nerve gas, abnormally high Mg levels, or use of neuromuscular blockers)
Muscle fiber	Dystrophies	Distal muscular dystrophy (late distal hereditary myopathy; rare), Duchenne muscular dystrophy and related dystrophies, fascioscapulohumeral muscular dystrophy, limb-girdle muscular dystrophy, oculopharyngeal dystrophy (rare)
	Channelopathies (myotonic)	Familial periodic paralysis, myotonia congenita (Thomsen disease), myotonic dystrophy (Steinert disease)
	Congenital	Central core disease, centronuclear myopathy, nemaline myopathy (very rare)
	Endocrine	Acromegaly, Cushing syndrome, diabetes mellitus, hypothyroidism, thyrotoxic myopathy
	Inflammatory	Infection (viral more than bacterial), polymyositis and dermatomyositis
	Metabolic	Acid maltase deficiency, alcoholism, carnitine deficiency, glycogen storage and lipid storage diseases (rare), hypokalemia

*Lower motor neuron disorders (eg, spinal muscular atrophies) technically involve the CNS because the cell body of the motor neuron (anterior horn cell) is located in the spinal cord.

Adapted from Tandan R, Bradley WA: Amyotrophic lateral sclerosis. Part I: Clinical features, pathology and ethical issues in management. *Annals of Neurology* 18:271–280, 1985; used with permission of Little, Brown and Company.

random. However, multiple infarcts may later coalesce, causing symmetric deficits (multiple mononeuropathy).

Toxic-metabolic or genetic disorders usually begin symmetrically. Immune-mediated processes may be symmetric or, early in rapidly evolving processes, asymmetric.

Damage to the axon transport system for cellular constituents, especially microtubules and microfilaments, causes significant axon dysfunction. First affected are the smaller fibers (because they have greater metabolic requirements) at the most distal part of the nerve. Then, axonal degeneration slowly ascends, producing the characteristic distal-to-proximal pattern of symptoms (stocking-glove sensory loss, followed by weakness).

Recovery: Damage to the myelin sheath (eg, by injury or Guillain-Barré syndrome) can often be repaired by surviving Schwann cells in about 6 to 12 wk.

After axonal damage, the fiber regrows within the Schwann cell tube at about 1 mm/day once the pathologic process ends. However, regrowth may be misdirected, causing aberrant innervation (eg, of fibers in the wrong muscle, of a touch receptor at the wrong site, or of a temperature instead of a touch receptor).

Regeneration is impossible when the cell body dies and is unlikely when the axon is completely lost.

Evaluation

- Deficits defined by history and examination
- Attention to clinical clues to peripheral nervous system disorders
- Usually nerve conduction studies and electromyography
- Sometimes nerve or skin punch biopsy
- Genetic testing (for hereditary neuropathies)

Clinical evaluation: History should focus on type of symptom, onset, progression, and location, as well as information about potential causes (eg, family history, toxic exposures, past medical disorders).

Physical and neurologic examination should further define the type of deficit (eg, motor deficit, type of sensory deficit, combination). Sensation (using pinprick and temperature for small fibers; using vibration and proprioception tests for large fibers), motor strength, and deep tendon reflexes are evaluated. Cranial nerve as well as central and peripheral nerve function is evaluated. Whether motor weakness is proportional to the degree of atrophy is noted, as are type and distribution of reflex abnormalities. Autonomic function is evaluated.

Physicians should suspect a peripheral nervous system disorder based on the pattern and type of neurologic deficits, especially if deficits are localized to particular nerve roots, spinal nerves, plexuses, specific peripheral nerves, or a combination. These disorders are also suspected in patients with mixed sensory and motor deficits, with multiple foci, or with a focus that is incompatible with a single anatomic site in the CNS.

Physicians should also suspect peripheral nervous system disorders in patients with generalized or diffuse weakness but no sensory deficits; in these cases, peripheral nervous system disorders may be overlooked because they are not the most likely cause of such symptoms. Clues that a peripheral nervous system disorder may be the cause of generalized weakness include the following:

- Patterns of generalized weakness that suggest a specific cause (eg, predominant ptosis and diplopia, which suggest early myasthenia gravis)
- Symptoms and signs other than weakness that suggest a specific disorder or group of disorders (eg, cholinergic effects, which suggest organophosphate poisoning)
- Deficits in a stocking-glove distribution, which suggest diffuse axonal disorders or polyneuropathy
- Fasciculations
- Hypotonia
- Muscle wasting without hyperreflexia
- Weakness that is progressive, chronic, and unexplained

Clues that the cause may not be a peripheral nervous system disorder include

- Hyperreflexia
- Hypertonia

These deficits suggest an upper motor neuron disorder as the cause of weakness. Hyporeflexia is consistent with peripheral nervous system deficits but is nonspecific. For example, cervical spinal cord compression can mimic Guillain-Barré syndrome, particularly in patients with preexisting neuropathy.

Although many exceptions are possible, certain clinical clues may also suggest possible causes of peripheral nervous system deficits (see Table 236–2).

Clinical assessment narrows diagnostic possibilities and guides further testing.

Testing: Usually, nerve conduction studies and electromyography (EMG—collectively called electrodiagnostic testing)

Table 236–2. CLINICAL CLUES TO CAUSES OF PERIPHERAL NERVOUS SYSTEM* DISORDERS

FINDING	CAUSE TO CONSIDER
Symmetric, diffuse deficits	Diffuse disorders (eg, toxic-metabolic, hereditary, infectious, or inflammatory disorders; most immune-mediated disorders)
Unilateral deficits	Focal disorders (eg, mononeuropathies, plexopathies)
Deficits localized to one or more peripheral nervous system structures (eg, nerve root, spinal nerve, nerve plexus, single peripheral nerve, ≥ 2 discrete nerves in separate areas [multiple mononeuropathy])	Lesion in a peripheral nervous system structure
Stocking-glove distribution of deficits	Diffuse peripheral polyneuropathies, possibly axonal
Disproportionate weakness of proximal muscles (eg, difficulty climbing stairs or combing hair) with no sensory deficits	Diffuse muscle dysfunction, as occurs in diffuse myopathies Possibly disorders of the neuromuscular junction if eye movements are affected
Chronic, progressive weakness affecting mostly distal muscles with no sensory deficits	Motor neuron disease
Buzzing and tingling with motor weakness and decreased reflexes	Demyelination
Profound proximal and distal motor weakness with minimal atrophy	Acquired demyelinating polyneuropathy
Deficient pain and temperature sensation; painful, often burning sensations	Vascular disorders (eg, vasculitis, ischemia, hypercoagulable states)
Weakness proportional to atrophy; disproportionately mild reflex abnormalities, usually more distal than proximal	

*Lower motor neuron disorders (eg, spinal muscular atrophies) technically involve the CNS because the cell body of the motor neuron (anterior horn cell) is located in the spinal cord.

are done. These tests help identify level of involvement (nerve, plexus, root) and distinguish demyelinating disorders (very slow conduction) from axonal disorders. Other testing, such as imaging, depends on whether a CNS lesion must be ruled out (eg, MRI if all limbs are affected, to rule out cervical spinal cord compression).

Nerve biopsy is occasionally done to help differentiate demyelinating from vasculitic large-fiber neuropathies. If vasculitis is a consideration, the biopsy specimen should include skin and muscle to increase the likelihood of a definitive diagnosis. If a small-fiber neuropathy is suspected, skin punch biopsy can be done; loss of nerve endings supports that diagnosis.

PEARLS & PITFALLS

- If clinical findings and electrodiagnostic test results are inconclusive, do a biopsy (nerve biopsy for suspected large-fiber neuropathy or skin punch biopsy for suspected small-fiber neuropathy).
- If all limbs are affected, consider MRI to rule out cervical spinal cord compression.

Genetic testing is indicated if a hereditary neuropathy is suspected.

Patients with weakness but no sensory deficits are evaluated for weakness. Electrodiagnostic testing helps differentiate peripheral nervous system disorders from other causes of weakness and helps differentiate among peripheral nervous system disorders (eg, root, plexus, peripheral nerve, neuromuscular junction, muscle fiber). It also helps differentiate between axonal and demyelinating peripheral neuropathies.

Treatment

- Treatment of underlying disorder
- Supportive care, often by a multidisciplinary team

Treatment is directed at the underlying disorder when possible. Otherwise, treatment is supportive. A multidisciplinary team approach helps patients cope with progressive neurologic disability:

- Physical therapists may help patients maintain muscle function.
- Occupational therapists can recommend adaptive braces and walking devices to help with activities of daily living.
- Speech and language therapists may provide alternative communication devices.
- If pharyngeal weakness develops, a speech therapist or a multidisciplinary team that specializes in swallowing problems can help assess risk of aspiration and recommend measures for prevention (eg, precautions for oral feeding and/or need for tube feedings).
- A gastroenterologist may recommend percutaneous endoscopic gastrostomy.
- If respiratory weakness develops, forced vital capacity is measured, and pulmonary or intensive care specialists help assess whether intensive care, noninvasive respiratory support (eg, bilevel positive airway pressure), and tracheostomy with full ventilatory support are needed.

Early in fatal disorders, health care practitioners must talk frankly with patients, family members, and caregivers to determine the level of intervention acceptable. Patients are encouraged to put their decisions in writing (advance directives) before they become incapacitated. These decisions should be reviewed and confirmed at various stages of the disorder.

KEY POINTS

- Peripheral nervous system disorders are often suspected based on clinical findings (eg, stocking-glove distribution, hyporeflexia, distal muscle weakness and wasting, localization to a peripheral nerve distribution).
- If patients have profound motor weakness with minimal atrophy and areflexia, consider acquired demyelinating polyneuropathy.
- If patients have abnormal pain and temperature sensation and atrophy in proportion to weakness (sometimes with disproportionate preservation of reflexes), consider a vasculitic or ischemic neuropathy.
- If patients have chronic progressive muscle weakness, fasciculations, muscle atrophy, and no sensory deficits, consider MND.
- Nerve conduction studies and EMG help identify level of involvement (root, plexus, peripheral nerve, neuromuscular junction, muscle fiber) and help distinguish demyelinating from axonal disorders.

DISORDERS OF NEUROMUSCULAR TRANSMISSION

Disorders of neuromuscular transmission affect the neuromuscular junction. They may involve

- Postsynaptic receptors (eg, in myasthenia gravis)
- Presynaptic release of acetylcholine (eg, in botulism)
- Breakdown of acetylcholine within the synapse (eg, due to drugs or neurotoxic chemicals)

Common features of these disorders include fluctuating fatigue and muscle weakness with no sensory deficits.

Some disorders that affect other areas of the body primarily (eg, stiff-person syndrome, Isaacs syndrome) have neuromuscular manifestations.

Eaton-Lambert syndrome: Eaton-Lambert syndrome is due to impaired acetylcholine release from presynaptic nerve terminals (see p. 1175).

Botulism: Also due to impaired release of acetylcholine from presynaptic nerve terminals, botulism develops when toxin produced by *Clostridium botulinum* spores irreversibly binds to a specific receptor (synaptotagmin II) on the presynaptic terminal cholinergic nerve endings (see also p. 1464). The result is severe weakness, sometimes with respiratory compromise and difficulty swallowing. Other systemic symptoms may include mydriasis, dry mouth, constipation, urinary retention, and tachycardia due to unopposed sympathetic nervous system activity (anticholinergic syndrome). These systemic findings are absent in myasthenia gravis.

In botulism, electromyography detects a mild decremental response to low-frequency (2- to 3-Hz) repetitive nerve stimulation but a pronounced incremental response after 10 sec of exercise or with rapid (50-Hz) repetitive nerve stimulation.

Drugs or toxic chemicals: Cholinergic drugs, organophosphate insecticides, and most nerve gases (eg, sarin) block neuromuscular transmission by excessive acetylcholine action that depolarizes postsynaptic receptors. Miosis, bronchorrhea, abdominal cramps, diarrhea, and myasthenic-like weakness (cholinergic syndrome) result.

Aminoglycoside and polypeptide antibiotics decrease presynaptic acetylcholine release and sensitivity of the postsynaptic membrane to acetylcholine. At high serum levels, these antibiotics may increase neuromuscular block in patients with latent myasthenia gravis. Long-term penicillamine treatment may cause a reversible syndrome that clinically and electromyographically resembles myasthenia gravis. Excessive magnesium po or IV (with blood levels approaching 8 to 9 mg/dL) can also induce severe weakness resembling a myasthenic syndrome.

Treatment consists of eliminating the drug or toxic chemical and providing necessary respiratory support and intensive nursing care. Atropine 0.4 to 0.6 mg po tid decreases bronchial secretions in patients with cholinergic excess. Higher doses (eg, 2 to 4 mg IV q 5 min) may be necessary for organophosphate insecticide or nerve gas poisoning.

ISAACS SYNDROME

(Neuromyotonia)

Isaacs syndrome causes neuromuscular manifestations, including myokymia.

Isaacs syndrome is a peripheral nerve hyperexcitability syndrome, generally thought to be a voltage-gated potassium channelopathy; it sometimes occurs as a paraneoplastic syndrome. It may also accompany other disorders (eg, myasthenia gravis, thymoma, Hashimoto thyroiditis, vitamin B_{12} deficiency, celiac disease, connective tissue disorders) or can be inherited.

Cause of Isaacs syndrome is unknown. Abnormalities are thought to originate in a peripheral nerve because they are abolished by curare but usually persist after general anesthesia.

The limbs are most affected. The sine qua non is myokymia—continuous muscle twitching described as bag-of-worms movements. Other symptoms include fasciculations, carpopedal spasms, intermittent cramps, increased sweating, and pseudomyotonia (impaired relaxation after a strong muscle contraction but without the typical waxing-and-waning electromyography [EMG] abnormality of true myotonia).

Diagnosis

- Clinical evaluation
- Results of nerve conduction and EMG studies

The diagnosis of Isaacs syndrome is based on the above clinical findings, and results of nerve conduction and EMG studies, which show characteristic abnormalities; these abnormalities include after-discharges on nerve conductions studies and, on needle EMG studies, fasciculation potentials, myokymic discharges, neuromyotonic discharges, fibrillation potentials, and cramp discharges, most prominent in distal limb muscles.

Laboratory testing should include tests for the striational, voltage-gated calcium channel, gliadin, glutamic acid decarboxylase (GAD), muscle AChR, and voltage-gated potassium channel antibodies.

Treatment

- Drugs to relieve symptoms
- Plasma exchange or IV immune globulin (IVIG)

Drugs that may relieve symptoms of Isaac syndrome include carbamazepine, phenytoin, gabapentin, mexiletine (experience is limited), valproate, lamotrigine, and clonazepam.

Plasma exchange and, to a lesser degree, IVIG are usually beneficial and are often used with prednisone and azathioprine.

STIFF-PERSON SYNDROME

(Stiff-Man Syndrome)

Stiff-person syndrome is a CNS disorder that causes progressive muscle stiffness and spasms.

Stiff-person syndrome (formerly called stiff-man syndrome) affects the CNS but has neuromuscular manifestations.

Most patients with stiff-person syndrome have antibodies against GAD, the enzyme involved in the production of the inhibitory neurotransmitter GABA (gamma-aminobutyric acid). However, stiff-person syndrome may be

- Autoimmune
- Paraneoplastic
- Idiopathic

The **autoimmune type** often occurs with type 1 diabetes, as well as other autoimmune disorders including thyroiditis, vitiligo, and pernicious anemia. Autoantibodies against several proteins involved in GABA synapses are present in the autoimmune type, affecting primarily inhibitory neurons that originate in the anterior horn of the spinal cord.

In the **paraneoplastic type**, antiamphiphysin antibodies are often present; anti-GAD and anti-Ri antibodies may be present. This type is commonly associated with breast cancer but may also occur in patients with lung, renal, thyroid, or colon cancer or lymphoma.

Clinical manifestations are similar in all types. Muscle stiffness, rigidity, and spasms progress insidiously in the trunk and abdomen and, to a lesser degree, in the legs and arms. Patients are otherwise normal, and examination detects only muscle hypertrophy and stiffness. Electromyography (EMG) shows only the electrical activity of normal contraction.

Diagnosis of stiff person syndrome is based on recognizing the symptoms and is supported by antibody testing, response to diazepam, and results of EMG studies, which show continuous motor unit activity in agonist and antagonist muscles.

Treatment

- Diazepam or baclofen
- Possibly IV immune globulin (IVIG)

Only symptomatic therapy is available. Diazepam is the drug of choice; it most consistently relieves muscle stiffness. If diazepam is ineffective, baclofen, given orally or intrathecally, can be considered.

Corticosteroids are reportedly effective but have many long-term adverse effects.

Results of plasma exchange are inconsistent, but IVIG appears to result in improvement lasting up to a year.

GUILLAIN-BARRÉ SYNDROME

(Acute Idiopathic Polyneuritis; Acute Inflammatory Demyelinating Polyradiculoneuropathy)

Guillain-Barré syndrome is an acute, usually rapidly progressive but self-limited inflammatory polyneuropathy characterized by muscular weakness and mild distal sensory loss. Cause is thought to be autoimmune. Diagnosis is clinical. Treatment includes IV immune globulin (IVIG), plasma exchange, and, for severe cases, mechanical ventilation.

Guillain-Barré syndrome is the most common acquired inflammatory neuropathy. There are several variants.

Although the cause is not fully understood, it is thought to be autoimmune. In some variants, demyelination predominates; other variants affect the axon.

In about two-thirds of patients, Guillain-Barré syndrome begins 5 days to 3 wk after a banal infectious disorder, surgery, or vaccination. Infection is the trigger in > 50% of patients; common pathogens include *Campylobacter jejuni*, enteric viruses, herpesviruses (including cytomegalovirus and Epstein-Barr virus), and *Mycoplasma* spp. A cluster of cases followed the swine flu vaccination program in 1976, but the association was later shown to be spurious, due to ascertainment bias.

Symptoms and Signs

Flaccid weakness predominates in most patients; it is always more prominent than sensory abnormalities and may be most prominent proximally. Relatively symmetric weakness with paresthesias usually begins in the legs and progresses to the arms, but it occasionally begins in the arms or head. In 90% of patients, weakness is usually maximal at 3 to 4 wk. Deep tendon reflexes are lost. Sphincters are usually spared. Weakness remains the same for a variable period of time, typically for about a week, then resolves.

Facial and oropharyngeal muscles are weak in > 50% of patients with severe disease. Dehydration and undernutrition may result. Respiratory paralysis severe enough to require endotracheal intubation and mechanical ventilation occurs in 5 to 10%.

A few patients (possibly with a variant form) have significant, life-threatening autonomic dysfunction causing BP fluctuations, inappropriate ADH secretion, cardiac arrhythmias, GI stasis, urinary retention, and pupillary changes.

An unusual variant (Fisher variant, or Miller-Fisher syndrome) may cause only ophthalmoparesis, ataxia, and areflexia.

Diagnosis

- Clinical evaluation
- Electrodiagnostic testing
- CSF analysis

Diagnosis of Guillain-Barré syndrome is primarily clinical.

Differential diagnosis: Similar acute weakness can result from myasthenia gravis, botulism, poliomyelitis (mainly outside the US), tick paralysis, West Nile virus infection, and metabolic neuropathies, but these disorders can usually be distinguished as follows:

- **Myasthenia gravis** is intermittent and worsened by exertion.
- **Botulism** may cause fixed dilated pupils (in 50%) and prominent cranial nerve dysfunction with normal sensation.
- **Poliomyelitis** usually occurs in epidemics.
- **Tick paralysis** causes ascending paralysis but spares sensation.
- **West Nile virus** causes headache, fever, and asymmetric flaccid paralysis but spares sensation.
- **Metabolic neuropathies** occur with a chronic metabolic disorder.

Testing: Tests for infectious disorders and immune dysfunction, including tests for hepatitis and HIV and serum protein electrophoresis, are done.

If Guillain-Barré syndrome is suspected, patients should be admitted to a hospital for electrodiagnostic testing (nerve conduction studies and electromyography), CSF analysis, and monitoring by measuring forced vital capacity every 6 to 8 h. Initial electrodiagnostic testing detects slow nerve conduction velocities and evidence of segmental demyelination in two-thirds of patients; however, normal results do not exclude the diagnosis and should not delay treatment.

CSF analysis may detect albuminocytologic dissociation (increased protein but normal WBC count), but it may not appear for up to 1 wk and does not develop in 10% of patients.

Rarely, cervical spinal cord compression—particularly when polyneuropathy coexists (causing or contributing to hyporeflexia) and bulbar involvement is not prominent—may mimic Guillain-Barré syndrome; in such cases, MRI should be done.

Prognosis

Guillain-Barré syndrome is fatal in < 2%. Most patients improve considerably over a period of months, but about 30% of adults and even more children have some residual weakness at 3 yr. Patients with residual defects may require retraining, orthopedic appliances, or surgery.

After initial improvement, 3 to 10% of patients develop chronic inflammatory demyelinating polyneuropathy (CIDP).

Treatment

- Intensive supportive care
- IVIG or plasma exchange

Guillain-Barré syndrome is a medical emergency, requiring constant monitoring and support of vital functions, typically in an ICU. Forced vital capacity should be measured frequently so that respiration can be assisted if necessary; if vital capacity is < 15 mL/kg, endotracheal intubation is indicated. Inability to lift the head off the pillow by flexing the neck is another danger sign; it frequently develops simultaneously with phrenic nerve (diaphragm) weakness.

If oral fluid intake is difficult, IV fluids are given as needed to maintain a urine volume of at least 1 to 1.5 L/day. Extremities should be protected from trauma and from the pressure of bed rest.

Heat therapy helps relieve pain, making early physical therapy possible. Immobilization, which may cause ankylosis and contractures, should be avoided. Passive full-range joint movement should be started immediately, and active exercises should be initiated when acute symptoms subside. Heparin 5000 units sc bid helps prevent deep venous thrombosis in bed-bound patients.

Given early, IVIG 400 mg/kg IV once/day for 5 consecutive days is the treatment of choice; it has some benefit up to 1 mo from disease onset.

Plasma exchange helps when done early; it is used if IVIG is ineffective. Plasma exchange is relatively safe, shortens the disease course and hospital stay, and reduces mortality risk and incidence of permanent paralysis. Plasma exchange removes any previously administered IVIG, negating its benefits, and so should never be done during or soon after use of IVIG. Waiting at least 2 to 3 days after stopping IVIG is recommended.

PEARLS & PITFALLS

- Do not give corticosteroids in Guillain-Barré syndrome because they may worsen outcome.

Corticosteroids do not improve and may worsen the outcome.

KEY POINTS

- Guillain-Barré syndrome typically begins with an ascending, relatively symmetric flaccid weakness.
- Initially, distinguish other disorders that cause similar symptoms (eg, myasthenia gravis, botulism, tick paralysis, West Nile virus infection, metabolic neuropathies; outside the US, poliomyelitis) based on history and examination results.
- Do electrodiagnostic testing and CSF analysis, even though diagnosis is primarily clinical.
- About 70% of patients recover completely, but 3 to 10% develop CIDP.
- Intensive supportive care is key to recovery.
- Try IVIG first, then if it is ineffective, plasma exchange.

CHRONIC INFLAMMATORY DEMYELINATING POLYNEUROPATHY

(Chronic Acquired Demyelinating Polyneuropathy; Chronic Relapsing Polyneuropathy)

Chronic inflammatory demyelinating polyneuropathy (CIDP) is an immune-mediated polyneuropathy characterized by symmetric weakness of proximal and distal muscles and by progression continuing > 2 mo.

Symptoms of CIDP resemble those of Guillain-Barré syndrome. However, progression for > 2 mo differentiates CIDP from Guillain-Barré syndrome, which is monophasic and self-limited. CIDP develops in 3 to 10% of patients with Guillain-Barré syndrome.

Symptoms and Signs

CIDP typically starts insidiously and may slowly worsen or follow a pattern of relapses and recovery; between relapses, recovery may be partial or complete. Flaccid weakness, usually in the limbs, predominates in most patients; it is typically more prominent than sensory abnormalities (eg, paresthesias of hands and feet). Deep tendon reflexes are lost.

In most patients, autonomic function is affected less than it is in Guillain-Barré syndrome, Also, weakness may be asymmetric and progress more slowly than in Guillain-Barré syndrome.

Diagnosis

- CSF analysis and electrodiagnostic tests

Testing includes CSF analysis and electrodiagnostic tests. Results are similar to those in Guillain-Barré syndrome, including albuminocytologic dissociation (increased protein but normal WBC count) and demyelination, detected by electrodiagnostic testing.

Nerve biopsy, which can also detect demyelination, is seldom needed.

Treatment

- IV immune globulin (IVIG)
- Plasma exchange
- Corticosteroids

Often, deciding which therapy to offer first is difficult.

IVIG is better tolerated than corticosteroids and has fewer adverse effects, but IVIG may be associated with earlier deterioration after treatment is stopped. Subcutaneous IG may be as effective as IVIG.

Plasma exchange is the most invasive of the 3 options and thus offered last.

Immunosuppressants (eg, azathioprine) may be helpful and can reduce corticosteroid dependence.

Treatment may be needed for a long time.

KEY POINTS

- Although symptoms of CIDP resemble those of Guillain-Barré syndrome, the two can be differentiated based on how long symptoms have continued to progress (ie, > 2 mo for CIDP).
- Symptoms start insidiously and may slowly worsen or follow a pattern of relapses and recovery.
- CNS analysis and electrodiagnostic test results are similar to those of Guillain-Barré syndrome.
- Treat with IVIG and corticosteroids, but in severe cases, consider plasma exchange; immunosuppressants may help and can reduce dependence on corticosteroids.

HEREDITARY NEUROPATHIES

Hereditary neuropathies include a variety of congenital degenerative peripheral neuropathies.

Hereditary neuropathies are classified as

- Motor and sensory
- Sensory and autonomic
- Motor

Hereditary neuropathies may be primary or secondary to other hereditary disorders, including Refsum disease, porphyria, and Fabry disease.

Motor and sensory neuropathies: There are 3 main types (I, II, and III); all begin in childhood. Some less common types begin at birth and result in greater disability.

Types I and II (varieties of Charcot-Marie-Tooth disease, also called peroneal muscular atrophy) are the most common; they are usually autosomal dominant disorders but can be X-linked. Type I results from a duplication (extra copy) of the peripheral myelin protein-22 gene (*PMP22*), located on the short arm of chromosome 17.

Types I and II are characterized by weakness and atrophy, primarily in peroneal and distal leg muscles. Patients often have a family history of neuropathy. Natural history varies: Some patients are asymptomatic and have only slowed conduction velocities (detected on nerve conduction studies); others are more severely affected.

Patients with type I may present in middle childhood with footdrop and slowly progressive distal muscle atrophy, causing stork leg deformity. Intrinsic muscle wasting in the hands begins later. Vibration, pain, and temperature sensation decreases in a stocking-glove pattern. Deep tendon reflexes are absent. High pedal arches or hammertoes may be the only signs in family members who are carriers. Nerve conduction velocities are slow, and distal latencies are prolonged. Segmental demyelination and remyelination occur. Enlarged peripheral nerves may be palpated. The disease progresses slowly and does not affect life span. In one subtype, males have severe symptoms, and females have mild symptoms or may be unaffected.

Type II evolves more slowly; weakness usually develops later in life. Patients have relatively normal nerve conduction velocities but low amplitude sensory nerve action potentials and compound muscle action potentials. Biopsies detect axonal (wallerian) degeneration.

Type III (hypertrophic interstitial neuropathy, Dejerine-Sottas disease), a rare autosomal recessive disorder, begins in childhood with progressive weakness and sensory loss and absent deep tendon reflexes. Although initially it resembles Charcot-Marie-Tooth disease, the motor weakness progresses more quickly. Demyelination and remyelination occur, producing enlarged peripheral nerves and onion bulbs, detected by nerve biopsy.

Sensory and autonomic neuropathies: Hereditary sensory and autonomic neuropathies are rare. Five types have been described.

Loss of distal pain and temperature sensation is more prominent than loss of vibratory and position sense. The main complication is foot mutilation due to pain insensitivity, resulting in a high risk of infections and osteomyelitis.

Diagnosis

- Clinical evaluation
- Electrodiagnostic testing

The characteristic distribution of motor weakness, foot deformities, and family history suggests the diagnosis, which should be confirmed by electrodiagnostic testing.

Genetic analysis is available.

Treatment

- Supportive care

Bracing helps correct footdrop; orthopedic surgery to stabilize the foot may help.

Physical therapy (to strengthen muscles) and occupational therapy may help; vocational counseling may help prepare young patients to maintain vocational skills despite disease progression.

KEY POINTS

- Hereditary neuropathies may affect motor and sensory nerves, sensory nerves, sensory and autonomic nerves, or only motor nerves.
- There are 3 main types, which vary in severity and rate of progression; all begin in childhood.
- Use braces to correct footdrop and recommend physical and occupational therapy to help patients maintain function; sometimes orthopedic surgery is needed.

HEREDITARY MOTOR NEUROPATHY WITH LIABILITY TO PRESSURE PALSIES

(Tomaculous Neuropathy)

In hereditary motor neuropathy with liability to pressure palsies (HNPP), nerves become increasingly sensitive to pressure and stretch.

In HNPP, nerves lose their myelin sheath and do not conduct nerve impulses normally. Inheritance is usually autosomal dominant. In 80%, the cause is loss of one copy of peripheral myelin protein-22 gene (*PMP22*), located on the short arm of chromosome 17. Two copies of the gene are needed for normal function.

Incidence of HNPP is estimated to be 2 to 5/100,000.

Symptoms and Signs

Usually, symptoms start during adolescence or young adulthood, but they may start at any age.

Peroneal nerve palsy with footdrop, ulnar nerve palsy, and carpal tunnel syndrome commonly develop. The pressure palsies can be mild or severe and last from minutes to months. Numbness and weakness occur in affected areas.

After an episode, about half of affected people completely recover, and symptoms are mild in most of the rest.

Diagnosis

- Electrodiagnostic testing
- Genetic testing

HNPP should be suspected in patients with any of the following:

- Recurrent compression mononeuropathies
- Multiple mononeuropathy of unknown origin
- Symptoms suggesting recurrent demyelinating polyneuropathy
- A family history of carpal tunnel syndrome

Electrodiagnostic testing and genetic testing aid in diagnosis; rarely, biopsy is required.

Treatment

- Supportive care

Treatment of HNPP involves avoiding or modifying activities that cause symptoms. Wrist splints and elbow pads can reduce pressure, prevent reinjury, and allow the nerve to repair the myelin over time.

Surgery is rarely indicated.

AMYOTROPHIC LATERAL SCLEROSIS AND OTHER MOTOR NEURON DISEASES

(Lou Gehrig Disease; Charcot Syndrome)

Amyotrophic lateral sclerosis (ALS) and other motor neuron diseases (MNDs) are characterized by steady, relentless, progressive degeneration of corticospinal tracts, anterior horn cells, bulbar motor nuclei, or a combination. Symptoms vary in severity and may include muscle weakness and atrophy, fasciculations, emotional lability, and respiratory muscle weakness. Diagnosis involves nerve conduction studies, electromyography (EMG), and exclusion of other disorders via MRI and laboratory tests. Treatment is supportive.

ALS is the most common MND. MNDs may involve the CNS as well as the peripheral nervous system. Usually, etiology is unknown. Nomenclature and symptoms vary according to the part of the motor system most affected.

Myopathies have similar features but are disorders of the muscle membrane, contractile apparatus, or organelles.

MNDs can be classified as upper and lower; some disorders (eg, ALS) have features of both. MNDs are more common among men, most often appearing during their 50s.

Symptoms and Signs

Upper MNDs (eg, primary lateral sclerosis) affect neurons of the motor cortex, which extend to the brain stem (corticobulbar tracts) or spinal cord (corticospinal tracts). Generally, symptoms consist of stiffness, clumsiness, and awkward movements, usually affecting first the mouth, throat, or both, then spreading to the limbs.

Lower MNDs affect the anterior horn cells or cranial nerve motor nuclei or their efferent axons to the skeletal muscles. In bulbar palsies, only the cranial nerve motor nuclei in the brain stem (bulbar nuclei) are affected. Patients usually present with facial weakness, dysphagia, and dysarthria. When anterior horn cells of spinal (not cranial) nerves are affected, as in spinal muscular atrophies, symptoms usually include muscle weakness and atrophy, fasciculations (visible muscle twitches), and muscle cramps, initially in a hand, a foot, or the tongue. Poliomyelitis, an enteroviral infection that attacks anterior horn cells, and postpolio syndrome are also lower MNDs.

Physical findings help differentiate upper from lower MNDs (see Table 236–3) and weakness due to lower MNDs from that due to myopathy (see Table 236–4).

ALS: Most patients with ALS present with random, asymmetric symptoms, consisting of cramps, weakness, and muscle atrophy of the hands (most commonly) or feet. Weakness progresses to the forearms, shoulders, and lower limbs. Fasciculations, spasticity, hyperactive deep tendon reflexes, extensor plantar reflexes, clumsiness, stiffness of movement, weight

Table 236–3. DISTINGUISHING UPPER FROM LOWER MOTOR NEURON LESIONS

FEATURE	UPPER LESION	LOWER LESION
Reflexes	Hyperactive	Diminished or absent
Atrophy	Absent*	Present
Fasciculations	Absent	Present
Tone	Increased	Decreased or absent

*May appear with prolonged disuse of limbs.

loss, fatigue, and difficulty controlling facial expression and tongue movements soon follow.

Other symptoms include hoarseness, dysphagia, and slurred speech; because swallowing is difficult, salivation appears to increase, and patients tend to choke on liquids.

Late in the disorder, a pseudobulbar affect occurs, with inappropriate, involuntary, and uncontrollable excesses of laughter or crying. Sensory systems, consciousness, cognition, voluntary eye movements, sexual function, and urinary and anal sphincters are usually spared.

Death is usually caused by failure of the respiratory muscles; 50% of patients die within 3 yr of onset, 20% live 5 yr, and 10% live 10 yr. Survival for > 30 yr is rare. In progressive bulbar palsy with ALS (bulbar-variant ALS), deterioration and death occur more rapidly.

Progressive bulbar palsy: The muscles innervated by cranial nerves and corticobulbar tracts are predominantly affected, causing progressive difficulty with chewing, swallowing, and talking; nasal voice; reduced gag reflex; fasciculations and weak movement of the facial muscles and tongue; and weak palatal movement. Aspiration is a risk. A pseudobulbar affect with emotional lability may occur if the corticobulbar tract is affected.

Commonly, the disorder spreads, affecting extrabulbar segments; then it is called bulbar-variant ALS.

Patients with dysphagia have a very poor prognosis; respiratory complications due to aspiration frequently result in death within 1 to 3 yr.

Progressive muscular atrophy: In many cases, especially those with childhood onset, inheritance is autosomal recessive. Other cases are sporadic. The disorder can develop at any age.

Anterior horn cell involvement occurs alone or is more prominent than corticospinal involvement, and progression tends to be more benign than that of other MNDs.

Fasciculations may be the earliest manifestation. Muscle wasting and marked weakness begin in the hands and progress to the arms, shoulders, and legs, eventually becoming generalized. Patients may survive ≥ 25 yr.

PEARLS & PITFALLS

- Suspect ALS or another MND in patients who have features of upper and/or lower neuron weakness (eg, extensor plantar responses plus atrophy and fasciculations).

Primary lateral sclerosis and progressive pseudobulbar palsy: Muscle stiffness and signs of distal motor weakness gradually increase, affecting the limbs in primary lateral sclerosis and the lower cranial nerves in progressive pseudobulbar palsy. Fasciculations and muscle atrophy may follow many years later. These disorders usually take several years to result in total disability.

Diagnosis

- Electrodiagnostic tests
- MRI of the brain and, if no cranial nerve involvement, cervical spine
- Laboratory tests to check for other, treatable causes

Diagnosis is suggested by progressive, generalized motor weakness without significant sensory abnormalities.

Differential diagnosis: Other disorders that cause pure muscle weakness should be ruled out:

- Disorders of neuromuscular transmission
- Various myopathies (including noninflammatory and drug-induced)
- Spinal muscular atrophies (mostly in children)
- Polymyositis
- Dermatomyositis
- Thyroid and adrenal disorders
- Electrolyte abnormalities (eg, hypokalemia, hypercalcemia, hypophosphatemia)
- Various infections (eg, syphilis, Lyme disease, hepatitis C)
- Autoimmune-mediated motor neuropathies

When cranial nerves are affected, a treatable cause is less likely. Upper and lower motor neuron signs plus weakness in facial muscles strongly suggest ALS.

PEARLS & PITFALLS

- If cranial nerves are affected and findings are compatible with ALS, a treatable alternative cause is less likely.

Testing: Electrodiagnostic tests should be done to check for evidence of disorders of neuromuscular transmission or demyelination. Such evidence is not present in MNDs; nerve conduction velocities are usually normal until late in the disease. Needle EMG is the most useful test, showing fibrillations, positive waves, fasciculations, and sometimes giant motor units, even in unaffected limbs.

Brain MRI is required. When there is no clinical or EMG evidence of cranial nerve motor weakness, MRI of the cervical spine is indicated to exclude structural lesions.

Laboratory tests are done to check for treatable causes. Tests include CBC, electrolytes, creatine kinase, and thyroid function tests.

Table 236–4. DISTINGUISHING THE CAUSE OF MUSCLE WEAKNESS: LOWER MOTOR NEURON DYSFUNCTION VS MYOPATHY*

FEATURE	LOWER MOTOR NEURON DYSFUNCTION	MYOPATHY*
Distribution of weakness	Distal > proximal	Proximal > distal
Fasciculations	May be present	Absent
Reflexes	Diminished	Often preserved

*Nerve function intact.
> = more affected than.

Serum and urine protein electrophoresis with immunofixation is done to check for a paraprotein that is rarely associated with MNDs. Discovering an underlying paraproteinemia may indicate that the MND is paraneoplastic, and treatment of the paraproteinemia may ameliorate the MND.

Antimyelin-associated glycoprotein (MAG) antibodies are associated with a demyelinating motor neuropathy, which may mimic ALS.

A 24-h urine collection is done to check for heavy metals in patients who may have been exposed to them.

Lumbar puncture may be done to exclude other clinically suspected disorders; if WBCs or the protein level is elevated, an alternative diagnosis is likely.

Serum Venereal Disease Research Laboratories (VDRL) tests, ESR, and measurement of certain antibodies (rheumatoid factor, Lyme titer, HIV, hepatitis C virus, antinuclear [ANA], anti-Hu [to check for anti-Hu paraneoplastic syndrome]) are indicated only if suggested by risk factors or history.

Genetic testing (eg, for superoxide dismutase gene mutation or genetic abnormalities that cause spinal muscular atrophies) and enzyme measurements (eg, hexosaminidase A) should not be done unless patients are interested in genetic counseling; disorders detected by these tests have no known specific treatments.

Treatment

- Supportive care
- Riluzole for bulbar variant ALS

There is no specific treatment for MNDs. However, an antiglutamate drug, riluzole 50 mg po bid, prolongs life by 2 to 3 mo in patients with bulbar variant ALS.

A multidisciplinary team approach helps patients cope with progressive neurologic disability.

The following drugs may help reduce symptoms:

- For spasticity, baclofen
- For cramps, quinine or phenytoin
- To decrease saliva production, a strong anticholinergic drug (eg, glycopyrrolate, amitriptyline, benztropine, trihexyphenidyl, transdermal hyoscine, atropine)
- For pseudobulbar affect, amitriptyline, fluvoxamine, or a combination of dextromethorphan and quinidine

In patients with progressive bulbar palsy, surgery to improve swallowing has had limited success.

KEY POINTS

- Consider an MND in patients who have diffuse upper and/or lower motor weakness without sensory abnormalities.
- Suspect ALS in patients with upper and lower motor neuron signs plus weakness in facial muscles.
- Do MRI of the brain and electrodiagnostic and laboratory testing to exclude other disorders.
- The mainstay of treatment is supportive measures (eg, multidisciplinary support to help cope with disability; drug treatment for symptoms such as spasticity, cramps, and pseudobulbar affect).

MYASTHENIA GRAVIS

Myasthenia gravis involves episodic muscle weakness and easy fatigability caused by autoantibody- and cell-mediated destruction of acetylcholine receptors. It is more common among young women but may occur in men or women at any age. Symptoms worsen with muscle activity and lessen with rest. Diagnosis is by measurement of serum acetylcholine receptor antibody levels, EMG, and sometimes IV edrophonium challenge, which briefly lessens the weakness. Treatment includes anticholinesterase drugs, immunosuppressants, corticosteroids, plasma exchange, IVIG, and possibly thymectomy.

Myasthenia gravis develops most commonly in women aged 20 to 40.

Myasthenia gravis results from an autoimmune attack on postsynaptic acetylcholine receptors, which disrupts neuromuscular transmission. The trigger for autoantibody production is unknown, but the disorder is associated with abnormalities of the thymus, autoimmune hyperthyroidism, and other autoimmune disorders (eg, RA, SLE, pernicious anemia).

The role of the thymus in myasthenia is unclear, but 65% of patients have thymic hyperplasia, and 10% have a thymoma. About half of the thymomas are malignant.

Precipitating factors for myasthenia gravis include

- Infection
- Surgery
- Certain drugs (eg, aminoglycosides, quinine, magnesium sulfate, procainamide, calcium channel blockers)

Abnormal antibodies: Only about 10 to 20% of patients with generalized myasthenia have no antibodies to acetylcholine receptors (AChRs) in serum; up to 50% of these AChR antibody–negative patients have antibodies to muscle-specific receptor tyrosine kinase (MuSK), a surface membrane enzyme that helps AChR molecules aggregate during development of the neuromuscular junction. However, anti-MuSK antibodies do not occur in most patients with AChR antibodies or with isolated ocular myasthenia.

The clinical significance of anti-MuSK antibodies is still under study, but patients with these antibodies are much less likely to have thymic hyperplasia or a thymoma, may be less responsive to anticholinesterase drugs, and may require more aggressive early immunotherapy than patients who have AChR antibodies.

Uncommon forms: Ocular myasthenia gravis involves only extraocular muscles. It represents about 15% of cases.

Congenital myasthenia is a rare autosomal recessive disorder that begins in childhood. It is not immune-mediated and results from presynaptic or postsynaptic abnormalities, including the following:

- Reduced acetylcholine resynthesis due to choline acetyltransferase deficiency
- End-plate acetylcholinesterase deficiency
- Structural abnormalities in the postsynaptic receptor

Ophthalmoplegia is common.

Neonatal myasthenia affects 12% of infants born to women with myasthenia gravis. It is due to IgG antibodies that passively cross the placenta. It causes generalized muscle weakness, which resolves in days to weeks as antibody titers decline. Thus, treatment is usually supportive.

Symptoms and Signs

The most common symptoms are ptosis, diplopia, and muscle weakness after use of the affected muscle. Weakness resolves when the affected muscles are rested but recurs when they are used again.

Ocular muscles are affected initially in 40% of patients and eventually in 85% and are the only muscles affected in 15%. If generalized myasthenia is going to develop after ocular symptoms, it usually does so within the first 3 yr.

Hand grip may alternate between weak and normal (milkmaid's grip). Neck muscles may become weak. Proximal limb weakness is common. Some patients present with bulbar symptoms (eg, altered voice, nasal regurgitation, choking, dysphagia). Sensation and deep tendon reflexes are normal. Manifestations fluctuate in intensity over minutes to hours to days.

Myasthenic crisis, a severe generalized quadriparesis or life-threatening respiratory muscle weakness, occurs in about 15 to 20% of patients at least once in their life. It is often due to a supervening infection that reactivates the immune system. Once respiratory insufficiency begins, respiratory failure may occur rapidly.

Cholinergic crisis is muscular weakness that can result when the dose of anticholinesterase drugs (eg, neostigmine, pyridostigmine) is too high. A mild crisis may be difficult to differentiate from worsening myasthenia. Severe cholinergic crisis can usually be differentiated because it, unlike myasthenia gravis, results in increased lacrimation and salivation, tachycardia, and diarrhea.

Diagnosis

- Bedside tests
- AChR antibody levels, electromyography (EMG), or both

The diagnosis of myasthenia gravis is suggested by symptoms and signs and confirmed by tests.

Bedside testing: The traditional anticholinesterase test, done at bedside and using the short-acting (< 5 min) drug edrophonium, is positive in most patients who have myasthenia with overt weakness. However, this test should only be done in patients with obvious ptosis or ophthalmoparesis; these deficits must be present to be able to clearly see improvement to normal strength and thus provide unequivocal objective evidence of a positive test result. For the test, patients are asked to exercise the affected muscle until fatigue occurs (eg, to hold the eyes open until ptosis occurs); then, edrophonium 2 mg IV is given. If no adverse reaction (eg, bradycardia, atrioventricular block) occurs within 30 sec, another 8 mg is given. Rapid (< 2 min) recovery of muscle function is a positive result. However, this test is not ideal for the following reasons:

- A positive result is not definitive for myasthenia gravis because such improvement may occur in other neuromuscular disorders.
- Results may be equivocal, particularly if the test is done in patients without obvious ptosis or ophthalmoparesis.
- During the test, weakness due to cholinergic crisis may worsen; thus, resuscitation equipment and atropine (as an antidote) must be available during the test.

Because weakness due to myasthenia lessens in cooler temperature, patients with ptosis can be tested using the ice pack test. For this test, an icepack is applied to a patient's closed eyes for 2 min, then removed. A positive result is full or partial resolution of ptosis. The ice pack test usually does not work if patients have ophthalmoparesis.

Patients with opthalmoparesis can be tested using the rest test. For this test, patients are asked to lie quietly in a dark room for 5 min with their eyes closed. If ophthalmoparesis resolves after this rest, the result is positive.

PEARLS & PITFALLS

- Try the ice pack or rest test before the anticholinesterase test.
- Do the anticholinesterase test only if patients have obvious ptosis or ophthalmoparesis (to get unequivocal results).

Antibody testing and EMG: Even if a bedside test is unequivocally positive, one or both of the following are required to confirm the diagnosis:

- Serum AChR antibody levels
- EMG

AChR antibodies are present in 80 to 90% of patients with generalized myasthenia but in only 50% with the ocular form. Antibody levels do not correlate with disease severity. Up to 50% of patients without AChR antibodies test positive for anti-MuSK antibodies.

EMG using repetitive stimuli (2 to 3/sec) shows a > 10% decrease in amplitude of the compound muscle action potential response in 60% of patients. Single-fiber EMG can detect abnormal neuromuscular transmission in > 95%.

Further testing: Once myasthenia is diagnosed, CT or MRI of the thorax should be done to check for thymic hyperplasia and a thymoma.

Other tests should be done to screen for autoimmune disorders frequently associated with myasthenia gravis (eg, pernicious anemia, autoimmune hyperthyroidism, RA, SLE).

Patients in myasthenic crisis should be evaluated for an infectious trigger. Bedside pulmonary function tests (eg, forced vital capacity) help detect impending respiratory failure.

Treatment

- Anticholinesterase drugs to relieve symptoms
- Corticosteroids, immunomodulating treatments (eg, IV immune globulin [IVIG], plasma exchange), immunosuppressant drugs, and thymectomy to lessen the autoimmune reaction
- Supportive care

In patients with congenital myasthenia, anticholinesterase drugs and immunomodulating treatments are not beneficial and should be avoided. Patients with respiratory failure require intubation and mechanical ventilation.

Symptomatic treatment: Anticholinesterase drugs are the mainstay of symptomatic treatment but do not alter the underlying disease process. Moreover, they rarely relieve all symptoms, and myasthenia may become refractory to these drugs.

Pyridostigmine is begun at 60 mg po q 3 to 4 h and titrated up to a maximum of 120 mg/dose based on symptoms. When parenteral therapy is necessary (eg, because of dysphagia), neostigmine (1 mg = 60 mg of pyridostigmine) may be substituted. Anticholinesterase drugs can cause abdominal cramps and diarrhea, which are treated with oral atropine 0.4 to 0.6 mg (given with pyridostigmine or neostigmine) or propantheline 15 mg tid to qid.

Patients who have been responding well to treatment and then deteriorate require respiratory support because they may have cholinergic crisis, and anticholinesterase drugs must be stopped for several days.

Immunomodulating treatment: Immunosuppressants interrupt the autoimmune reaction and slow the disease course, but they do not relieve symptoms rapidly. After being given IVIG 400 mg/kg once/day for 5 days, 70% of patients improve in 1 to 2 wk. Effects may last 1 to 2 mo. Plasma exchange (eg, 5 exchanges of 3 to 5 L plasma over 7 to 14 days) can have similar effects.

Corticosteroids are necessary as maintenance therapy for many patients but have little immediate effect in myasthenic crisis. Over half of patients worsen acutely after starting high-dose corticosteroids. Initially, prednisone 10 mg po once/day is given; dose is increased by 10 mg weekly up to 60 mg, which is given for about 2 mo, then tapered slowly. Improvement may take several months; then, the dose should be reduced to the minimum necessary to control symptoms.

Azathioprine 2.5 to 3.5 mg/kg po once/day may be as effective as corticosteroids, although significant benefit may not occur for many months. Cyclosporine 2 to 2.5 mg/kg po bid may allow the corticosteroid dose to be reduced. These drugs require the usual precautions.

Other drugs that may be beneficial include methotrexate, cyclophosphamide, and mycophenolate mofetil. For patients with refractory disease, monoclonal antibodies (eg, rituximab, eculizumab) may be beneficial but are costly.

Thymectomy may be indicated for patients with generalized myasthenia if they are < 80 yr; it should be done in all patients with a thymoma. Subsequently, in 80%, remission occurs or the maintenance drug dose can be lowered.

Plasma exchange or IVIG is useful for myasthenic crisis and, for patients unresponsive to drugs, before thymectomy.

KEY POINTS

- Consider myasthenia gravis in patients with ptosis, diplopia, and muscle weakness after use of the affected muscle.
- To confirm the diagnosis, measure serum levels of AChR antibody (usually present in myasthenia gravis), do EMG, or both.
- After the diagnosis is confirmed, test for thymic hyperplasia, thymomas, hyperthyroidism, and autoimmune disorders, which commonly accompany myasthenia gravis.
- For most patients, use anticholinesterase drugs to relieve symptoms and immunomodulating treatment to slow disease progression and help relieve symptoms; do not use these treatments in patients with congenital myasthenia.
- If patients suddenly deteriorate after responding well to treatment, provide respiratory support and stop anticholinesterase drugs for several days.

NERVE ROOT DISORDERS

(Radiculopathies)

Nerve root disorders result in segmental radicular deficits (eg, pain or paresthesias in a dermatomal distribution, weakness of muscles innervated by the root). Diagnosis may require neuroimaging, electrodiagnostic testing, and systemic testing for underlying disorders. Treatment depends on the cause but includes symptomatic relief with NSAIDs, other analgesics, and corticosteroids.

Nerve root disorders are precipitated by acute or chronic pressure on a nerve root in or adjacent to the spinal column (see Fig. 240–1 on p. 2027).

Etiology

The most common cause is

- A herniated intervertebral disk

Bone changes due to RA or osteoarthritis, especially in the cervical and lumbar areas, may also compress isolated nerve roots.

Less commonly, carcinomatous meningitis causes patchy multiple root dysfunction. Rarely, spinal mass lesions (eg, epidural abscesses and tumors, spinal meningiomas, neurofibromas) may manifest with radicular symptoms instead of the usual symptoms of spinal cord dysfunction.

Diabetes can cause a painful thoracic or extremity radiculopathy by causing ischemia of the nerve root.

Infectious disorders, such as those due to mycobacteria (eg, TB), fungi (eg, histoplasmosis), or spirochetes (eg, Lyme disease, syphilis), sometimes affect nerve roots. Herpes zoster infection usually causes a painful radiculopathy with dermatomal sensory loss and characteristic rash, but it may cause a motor radiculopathy with segmental weakness and reflex loss. Cytomegalovirus-induced polyradiculitis is a complication of AIDS.

Symptoms and Signs

Radiculopathies tend to cause characteristic radicular syndromes of pain and segmental neurologic deficits based on the cord level of the affected root (see Table 236–5). Muscles innervated by the affected motor root become weak and atrophy; they also may be flaccid with fasciculations. Sensory root involvement causes sensory impairment in a dermatomal distribution. Corresponding segmental deep tendon reflexes may be diminished or absent. Electric shock-like pains may radiate along the affected nerve root's distribution.

Pain may be exacerbated by movements that transmit pressure to the nerve root through the subarachnoid space (eg, moving the spine, coughing, sneezing, doing the Valsalva maneuver).

Lesions of the cauda equina, which affect multiple lumbar and sacral roots, cause radicular symptoms in both legs and may impair sphincter and sexual function.

Findings indicating spinal cord compression include the following:

- A sensory level (an abrupt change in sensation below a horizontal line across the spine)
- Flaccid paraparesis or quadriparesis
- Reflex abnormalities below the site of compression
- Early-onset hyporeflexia followed later by hyperreflexia
- Sphincter dysfunction

Table 236–5. SYMPTOMS OF COMMON RADICULOPATHIES BY CORD LEVEL

LEVEL	SYMPTOMS
C6	Pain in the trapezius ridge and tip of the shoulder, often radiating to the thumb, with paresthesias and sensory impairment in the same areas Weakness of biceps Decreased biceps brachii and brachioradialis reflexes
C7	Pain in the shoulder blade and axilla, radiating to the middle finger Weakness of triceps Decreased triceps brachii reflex
T (any)	Bandlike dysesthesias around the thorax
L5	Pain in the buttock, posterior lateral thigh, calf, and foot Footdrop with weakness of the anterior tibial, posterior tibial, and peroneal muscles Sensory loss over the shin and dorsal foot
S1	Pain along the posterior aspect of the leg and buttock Weakness of the medial gastrocnemius muscle with impaired ankle plantar flexion Loss of ankle jerk Sensory loss over the lateral calf and foot

Diagnosis

- Neuroimaging
- Sometimes electrodiagnostic tests

Radicular symptoms require MRI or CT of the affected area. Myelography is needed only if MRI is contraindicated (eg, because of an implanted pacemaker or presence of other metal) and CT is inconclusive. The area imaged depends on symptoms and signs; if the level is unclear, electrodiagnostic tests should be done to localize the affected root, but they cannot identify the cause.

If imaging does not detect an anatomic abnormality, CSF analysis is done to check for infectious or inflammatory causes, and fasting plasma glucose is measured to check for diabetes.

Treatment

- Treatment of the cause and of pain

Specific causes are treated.

Acute pain requires appropriate analgesics (eg, acetaminophen, NSAIDs, sometimes opioids). NSAIDs are particularly useful for disorders that involve inflammation. Muscle relaxants, sedatives, and topical treatments rarely provide additional benefit. If symptoms are not relieved with nonopioid analgesics, corticosteroids can be given systemically or as an epidural injection; however, analgesia tends to be modest and temporary. Methylprednisolone may be given, tapered over 6 days, starting with 24 mg po daily and decreased by 4 mg a day.

Management of chronic pain can be difficult; acetaminophen and NSAIDs are often only partly effective, and chronic use of NSAIDs has substantial risks. Opioids have a high risk of addiction. Tricyclic antidepressants and anticonvulsants may be effective, as may physical therapy and consultation with a mental health practitioner. For a few patients, alternative medical treatments (eg, transdermal electrical nerve stimulation, spinal manipulation, acupuncture, medicinal herbs) may be tried if all other treatments are ineffective.

KEY POINTS

- Suspect a nerve root disorder in patients who have segmental deficits such as sensory abnormalities in a dermatomal distribution (eg, pain, paresthesias) and/or motor abnormalities (eg, weakness, atrophy, fasciculations, hyporeflexia) at a nerve root level.
- If patients have a sensory level, bilateral flaccid weakness, and/or sphincter dysfunction, suspect spinal cord compression.
- If clinical findings suggest radiculopathy, do MRI or CT.
- Use analgesics and sometimes corticosteroids for acute pain, and consider other drugs and other treatments, as well as analgesics, for chronic pain.

HERNIATED NUCLEUS PULPOSUS

(Herniated, Ruptured, or Prolapsed Intervertebral Disk)

Herniated nucleus pulposus is prolapse of an intervertebral disk through a tear in the surrounding annulus fibrosus. The tear causes pain; when the disk impinges on an adjacent nerve root, a segmental radiculopathy with paresthesias and weakness in the distribution of the affected root results. Diagnosis is usually by MRI or CT. Treatment of mild cases is with analgesics as needed. Bed rest is rarely indicated. Patients with progressive or severe neurologic deficits, intractable pain, or sphincter dysfunction may require immediate or elective surgery (eg, diskectomy, laminectomy).

Spinal vertebrae are separated by cartilaginous disks consisting of an outer annulus fibrosus and an inner nucleus pulposus. When degenerative changes (with or without trauma) result in protrusion or rupture of the nucleus through the annulus fibrosus in the lumbosacral or cervical area, the nucleus is displaced posterolaterally or posteriorly into the extradural space.

Radiculopathy occurs when the herniated nucleus compresses or irritates the nerve root. Posterior protrusion may compress the cord or cauda equina, especially in a congenitally narrow spinal canal (spinal stenosis). In the lumbar area, > 80% of disk ruptures affect L5 or S1 nerve roots; in the cervical area, C6 and C7 are most commonly affected.

Herniated disks are common.

Symptoms and Signs

Herniated disks often cause no symptoms, or they may cause symptoms and signs in the distribution of affected nerve roots. Pain usually develops suddenly, and back pain is typically relieved by bed rest. In contrast, nerve root pain caused by an epidural tumor or abscess begins more insidiously, and back pain is worsened by bed rest.

In patients with lumbosacral herniation, straight-leg raises stretch the lower lumbar roots and exacerbate back or leg pain (bilateral if disk herniation is central); straightening the knee while sitting also causes pain.

Cervical herniation causes pain during neck flexion or tilting. Cervical cord compression, if chronic, manifests with spastic paresis of the lower limbs and, if acute, causes quadriparesis.

Cauda equina compression often results in urine retention or incontinence due to loss of sphincter function.

Diagnosis

- MRI or CT

MRI or CT can identify the cause and precise level of the lesion. Rarely (ie, when MRI is contraindicated and CT is inconclusive), CT myelography is necessary. Electrodiagnostic testing may help identify the involved root.

Because an asymptomatic herniated disk is common, the clinician must carefully correlate symptoms with MRI abnormalities before invasive procedures are considered.

Treatment

- Conservative treatment initially
- Invasive procedures if neurologic deficits are progressive or severe
- Immediate surgical evaluation if the spinal cord is compressed

Because a herniated disk desiccates and shrinks over time, symptoms tend to abate regardless of treatment. Up to 85% of patients with back pain—regardless of cause—recover without surgery within 6 wk.

Conservative treatment: Treatment of a herniated disk should be conservative, unless neurologic deficits are progressive or severe. Heavy or vigorous physical activity is restricted, but ambulation and light activity (eg, lifting objects < 2.5 to 5 kg [≈ 5 to 10 lb] using correct techniques) are permitted as tolerated; prolonged bed rest (including traction) is contraindicated.

Acetaminophen, NSAIDs, or other analgesics should be used as needed to relieve pain. If symptoms are not relieved with nonopioid analgesics, corticosteroids can be given systemically or as an epidural injection; however, analgesia tends to be modest and temporary. Methylprednisolone may be given, tapered over 6 days, starting with 24 mg po daily and decreased by 4 mg a day.

Physical therapy and home exercises can improve posture and strengthen back muscles and thus reduce spinal movements that further irritate or compress the nerve root.

Invasive procedures: Invasive procedures should be considered if

- Lumbar radiculopathies result in persistent or worsening neurologic deficits, particularly objective deficits (eg, weakness, reflex deficits).
- Patients have severe, intractable nerve root pain or sensory deficits.

Microscopic diskectomy and laminectomy with surgical removal of herniated material are usually the procedures of choice. Percutaneous approaches to remove bulging disk material are still being evaluated.

Dissolving herniated disk material with local injections of the enzyme chymopapain is not recommended.

Lesions acutely compressing the spinal cord or cauda equina (eg, causing urine retention or incontinence) require immediate surgical evaluation (see p. 2031).

If cervical radiculopathies result in signs of spinal cord compression, surgical decompression is needed immediately; otherwise, it is done electively when nonsurgical treatments are ineffective.

KEY POINTS

- Herniated disks are common and usually affect nerve roots at C6, C7, L5, or S1.
- If symptoms develop suddenly and back pain is relieved with rest, suspect a herniated disk rather than an epidural tumor or abscess.
- Recommend analgesics, light activity as tolerated, and exercises to improve posture and strength; however, if pain or deficits are severe or worsening, consider invasive procedures.

PERIPHERAL NEUROPATHY

Peripheral neuropathy is dysfunction of one or more peripheral nerves (the part of a nerve distal to the root and plexus). It includes numerous syndromes characterized by varying degrees of sensory disturbances, pain, muscle weakness and atrophy, diminished deep tendon reflexes, and vasomotor symptoms, alone or in any combination. Initial classification is based on history and physical examination. Electromyography and nerve conduction studies (electrodiagnostic testing) help localize the lesion and determine whether the pathophysiology is primarily axonal (often metabolic) or demyelinating (often autoimmune). Treatment is aimed mainly at the cause.

Peripheral neuropathy may affect

- A single nerve (mononeuropathy)
- ≥ 2 discrete nerves in separate areas (multiple mononeuropathy)
- Many nerves simultaneously suggesting a diffuse process (polyneuropathy)

MONONEUROPATHIES

Single mononeuropathies are characterized by sensory disturbances and weakness in the distribution of the affected nerve. Diagnosis is clinical but may require confirmation with electrodiagnostic tests. Treatment is directed at the cause, sometimes with splinting, NSAIDs, corticosteroid injections, and, for severe cases of nerve entrapment, surgery.

Trauma is the most common cause of acute mononeuropathy and may occur as follows:

- Violent muscular activity or forcible overextension of a joint may cause focal neuropathy, as may repeated small traumas (eg, tight gripping of small tools, excessive vibration from air hammers).
- Prolonged, uninterrupted pressure at bony prominences can cause pressure neuropathy, usually affecting superficial nerves (ulnar, radial, peroneal), particularly in thin people; such pressure may occur during sound sleep, intoxication, bicycle riding, or anesthesia.
- Compression of nerves in narrow passageways causes entrapment neuropathy (eg, in carpal tunnel syndrome).
- Nerve compression by a tumor, hyperostosis, a cast, crutches, or prolonged cramped postures (eg, during gardening) may cause compression paralysis.

Hemorrhage that compresses a nerve, exposure to cold or radiation, or direct tumor invasion may also cause neuropathy.

Compression of a nerve may be transient (eg, caused by an activity) or fixed (eg, caused by a mass or anatomic abnormality).

Symptoms and Signs

Single mononeuropathies are characterized by pain, weakness, and paresthesias in the distribution of the affected nerve or nerves. Pure motor nerve involvement begins with painless weakness; pure sensory nerve involvement begins with sensory disturbances and no weakness.

Carpal tunnel syndrome: Carpal tunnel syndrome (see also p. 288) may be unilateral or bilateral. It results from compression of the median nerve in the volar aspect of the wrist between the transverse superficial carpal ligament and the flexor tendons of the forearm muscles.

The compression causes paresthesias in the radial-palmar aspect of the hand and pain in the wrist and palm. Pain may be referred to the forearm and shoulder. Pain may be more severe at night. A sensory deficit in the palmar aspect of the first 3 fingers may follow, and the muscles that control thumb abduction and opposition may become weak and atrophied.

Sensory symptoms due to carpal tunnel syndrome are similar to those due to C6 root dysfunction secondary to cervical radiculopathy.

Peroneal nerve palsy: Peroneal nerve palsy is usually caused by compression of the nerve against the lateral aspect of the fibular neck. It is most common among emaciated bedbound patients and thin people who habitually cross their legs.

Peroneal nerve palsy causes footdrop (weakened dorsiflexion and eversion of the foot) and, occasionally, a sensory deficit in the anterolateral aspect of the lower leg and the dorsum of the foot or in the web space between the 1st and 2nd metatarsals.

L5 radiculopathy can cause similar deficits but, unlike peroneal nerve palsy, tends to weaken hip abduction by the gluteus medius.

Radial nerve palsy: Radial nerve palsy (Saturday night palsy) is caused by compression of the nerve against the humerus, as when the arm is draped over the back of a chair for a long time (eg, during intoxication or deep sleep).

Typical symptoms of radial nerve palsy include wristdrop (weakness of the wrist and finger extensors) and sensory loss in the dorsal aspect of the first dorsal interosseous muscle.

C7 radiculopathy can cause similar motor deficits.

Ulnar nerve palsy: Ulnar nerve palsy at the elbow is often caused by trauma to the nerve in the ulnar groove of the elbow by repeated leaning on the elbow or by asymmetric bone growth after a childhood fracture (tardy ulnar palsy). The ulnar nerve can also be compressed at the cubital tunnel (sometimes causing cubital tunnel syndrome).

Compression at the level of the elbow can cause paresthesias and a sensory deficit in the 5th digit and medial half of the 4th digit; the thumb adductor, 5th digit abductor, and interosseus muscles are weak and may be atrophied. Severe chronic ulnar palsy causes a clawhand deformity.

Sensory symptoms due to ulnar nerve palsy are similar to those due to C8 root dysfunction secondary to cervical radiculopathy; however, radiculopathy normally affects the more proximal aspects of the C8 dermatome.

Diagnosis

- Clinical evaluation
- Electrodiagnostic testing if clinical diagnosis is inconclusive

Symptoms and examination findings may be nearly pathognomonic.

Electrodiagnostic tests are usually done to clarify the diagnosis, particularly when clinical findings are inconclusive—for example,

- To distinguish sensory symptoms due to ulnar nerve palsy from C8 root dysfunction due to cervical radiculopathy
- To distinguish sensory symptoms due to carpal tunnel syndrome from C6 root dysfunction due to cervical radiculopathy

Electrodiagnostic tests also help localize the lesion, assess severity, and estimate prognosis.

Treatment

- Various treatments depending on the cause

Underlying disorders are treated.

Treatment of compression neuropathy depends on cause:

- **Fixed compression** (eg, by tumor) often must be relieved surgically.
- For **transient compression,** rest, heat, limited courses of NSAIDs in doses that reduce inflammation (eg, ibuprofen 800 mg tid), and avoidance or modification of the causative activity usually relieve symptoms.
- For **carpal tunnel syndrome,** conservative therapy includes splinting the wrist, oral or injected corticosteroids, and ultrasound. For refractory cases, surgical release is usually effective.

Braces or splints are often used pending resolution to prevent contractures.

Surgery should be considered when progression occurs despite conservative treatment.

KEY POINTS

- If findings indicate that a single nerve is affected, trauma is the most likely cause.
- Do electrodiagnostic tests if necessary to distinguish mononeuropathies from radiculopathies and other disorders that cause similar symptoms.
- For transient nerve compression, advising patients to avoid the causative activity may be all that is needed.

MULTIPLE MONONEUROPATHY

(Mononeuritis Multiplex)

Multiple mononeuropathies are characterized by sensory disturbances and weakness in the distribution of the affected nerve or nerves.

Multiple mononeuropathy is usually secondary to

- Connective tissue disorders (eg, polyarteritis nodosa, SLE, other types of vasculitis, Sjögren syndrome, RA)
- Sarcoidosis
- Metabolic disorders (eg, diabetes, amyloidosis)
- Infectious disorders (eg, Lyme disease, HIV infection, leprosy)

However, diabetes usually causes sensorimotor distal polyneuropathy.

Multiple mononeuropathies are characterized by pain, weakness, and paresthesias in the distribution of the affected nerve or nerves. Pure motor nerve involvement begins with painless weakness; pure sensory nerve involvement begins with sensory disturbances and no weakness. Multiple mononeuropathy is often asymmetric at first; nerves may be involved all at once or progressively. Extensive involvement of many nerves may simulate polyneuropathy.

Symptoms and examination findings may be nearly pathognomonic. When they are not, electrodiagnostic testing is done to establish the diagnosis, localize the lesion, assess severity, and estimate prognosis.

Underlying disorders are treated.

POLYNEUROPATHY

A polyneuropathy is a diffuse peripheral nerve disorder that is not confined to the distribution of a single nerve or a single limb and typically is relatively symmetrical bilaterally. Electrodiagnostic tests should always be done to classify the nerve structures involved, distribution, and severity of the disorder and thus help identify the cause. Treatment is directed toward correcting the cause.

Some polyneuropathies (eg, due to lead toxicity, dapsone use, tick bite, porphyria, or Guillain-Barré syndrome) affect primarily motor fibers; others (eg, due to dorsal root ganglionitis of cancer, leprosy, AIDS, diabetes mellitus, or chronic pyridoxine intoxication) affect primarily sensory fibers. Some disorders (eg, Guillain-Barré syndrome, Lyme disease, diabetes, diphtheria) can also affect cranial nerves. Certain drugs and toxins can affect sensory or motor fibers or both (see Table 236–6).

Symptoms and Signs

Symptoms of polyneuropathy may appear suddenly or develop slowly and become chronic depending on the cause. Because pathophysiology and symptoms are related, polyneuropathies are often classified by area of dysfunction:

- Myelin
- Vasa nervorum
- Axon

Polyneuropathies may be acquired or inherited.

Myelin dysfunction: Myelin dysfunction (demyelinating) polyneuropathies most often result from a parainfectious immune response triggered by encapsulated bacteria (eg, *Campylobacter* sp), viruses (eg, enteric or influenza viruses, HIV), or

Table 236–6. TOXIC CAUSES OF POLYNEUROPATHIES

TYPE OF NEUROPATHY	CAUSES
Axonal motor	Gangliosides, tetanus, tick paralysis With prolonged exposure, lead, mercury
Axonal sensorimotor	Acrylamide, alcohol (ethanol), allyl chloride, arsenic, cadmium, carbon disulfide, chlorphenoxy compounds, ciguatoxin, colchicine, cyanide, dapsone, disulfiram, DMAPN, ethylene oxide, lithium, methyl bromide, nitrofurantoin, organophosphates, PCBs, PNU, podophyllin, saxitoxin, Spanish toxic oil, taxol, tetrodotoxin, thallium, trichloroethylene, TOCP, vinca alkaloids
Axonal sensory	Almitrine, bortezomib, chloramphenicol, dioxin, doxorubicin, ethambutol, ethionamide, etoposide, gemcitabine, glutethimide, hydralazine, ifosfamide, interferon alfa, isoniazid, lead, metronidazole, misonidazole, nitrous oxide, nucleosides (didanosine [ddI], stavudine [d4T], zalcitabine [ddC]), phenytoin, platinum analogs, propafenone, pyridoxine, statins, thalidomide
Demyelinating	Buckthorn, chloroquine, diphtheria, hexachlorophene, muzolimine, perhexiline, procainamide, tacrolimus tellurium, zimeldine
Mixed	Amiodarone, ethylene glycol, gold, hexacarbons, *n*-hexane, sodium cyanate, suramin

DMAPN = dimethylaminopropionitrile; PCBs = polychlorinated biphenyls; PNU = *N*-3 pyridylmethyl-*N′*-p-nitrophenyl urea; TOCP = triorthocresyl phosphate.

vaccines (eg, influenza vaccine). Presumably, antigens in these agents cross-react with antigens in the peripheral nervous system, causing an immune response (cellular, humoral, or both) that culminates in varying degrees of myelin dysfunction.

In acute cases (eg, in Guillain-Barré syndrome—see p. 1982), rapidly progressive weakness and respiratory failure may develop. In chronic inflammatory demyelinating polyneuropathy, symptoms may recur or progress over months and years (see p. 1984).

Myelin dysfunction usually results in large-fiber sensory disturbances (paresthesias), significant muscle weakness greater than expected for degree of atrophy, and greatly diminished reflexes. Trunk musculature and cranial nerves may be involved. Demyelination typically occurs along the entire length of a nerve, causing proximal and distal symptoms. There may be side-to-side asymmetries, and the upper body may be affected before the lower body, or vice versa. Muscle bulk and tone are relatively preserved.

Vasa nervorum compromise: Chronic arteriosclerotic ischemia, vasculitis, infections, and hypercoagulable states can compromise the vascular supply to nerves, causing nerve infarction.

Usually, small-fiber sensory and motor dysfunction occurs first. Patients typically have painful, often burning sensory disturbances. Pain and temperature sensation are deficient.

Vasa nervorum involvement (eg, caused by vasculitis or infections) can begin as multiple mononeuropathies, which, when many nerves are affected bilaterally, can look like polyneuropathy. Abnormalities tend to be asymmetric early in the disorder and rarely affect the proximal one third of the limb or trunk muscles. Cranial nerve involvement is rare, except in diabetes, which commonly affects the 3rd cranial (oculomotor) nerve. Later, if nerve lesions coalesce, symptoms and signs may appear symmetric.

Dysautonomia and skin changes (eg, atrophic, shiny skin) sometimes occur.

Muscle weakness tends to be proportional to atrophy, and reflexes are rarely lost completely.

Axonopathy: Axonopathies tend to be distal; they may be symmetric or asymmetric.

Symmetric axonopathies result most often from toxic-metabolic disorders. Common causes include the following:

- Diabetes mellitus
- Chronic renal insufficiency
- Adverse effects of chemotherapy drugs (eg, vinca alkaloids)

Axonopathy may result from nutritional deficiencies (most commonly, of thiamin or vitamin B_6, B_{12}, or E) or from excess intake of vitamin B_6 or alcohol. Less common metabolic causes include hypothyroidism, porphyria, sarcoidosis, and amyloidosis. Other causes include certain infections (eg, Lyme disease), drugs (eg, nitrous oxide), and exposure to certain chemicals (eg, Agent Orange, *n*-hexane) or heavy metals (eg, lead, arsenic, mercury).

In a paraneoplastic syndrome associated with small-cell lung cancer, loss of dorsal root ganglia and their sensory axons results in subacute sensory neuropathy.

Primary axon dysfunction may begin with symptoms of large- or small-fiber dysfunction or both. Usually, the resulting neuropathy has a distal symmetric, stocking-glove distribution; it evenly affects the lower extremities before the upper extremities and progresses symmetrically from distal to proximal areas.

Asymmetric axonopathy can result from parainfectious or vascular disorders.

Diagnosis

- Electrodiagnostic tests
- Laboratory tests, determined by suspected type of neuropathy

Polyneuropathy is suspected in patients with diffuse or multifocal sensory deficits, weakness without hyperreflexia, or both. However, if findings are relatively diffuse but began asymmetrically, the cause may be multiple mononeuropathy.

PEARLS & PITFALLS

- If findings are consistent with polyneuropathy, try to determine whether symptoms began asymmetrically (possibly suggesting multiple mononeuropathy).

Clinical findings, particularly tempo of onset, help clinicians diagnose and identify the cause of polyneuropathy, as in the following:

- Asymmetric neuropathies suggest a disorder affecting the myelin sheath or vasa nervorum.
- Symmetric, distal neuropathies suggest toxic or metabolic causes.

- Slowly progressive, chronic neuropathies tend to be inherited or due to long-term toxic exposure or metabolic disorders.
- Acute neuropathies suggest an autoimmune cause, vasculitis, a toxin, an infection, or a postinfectious cause or possibly a drug or cancer.
- Rash, skin ulcers, and Raynaud syndrome in patients with an asymmetric axonal neuropathy suggest a hypercoagulable state or parainfectious or autoimmune vasculitis.
- Weight loss, fever, lymphadenopathy, and mass lesions suggest a tumor or paraneoplastic syndrome.

Axonopathies should be considered in all patients with polyneuropathy.

Electrodiagnostic tests: Regardless of clinical findings, electromyography (EMG) and nerve conduction studies are necessary to classify the type of neuropathy. At a minimum, EMG of both lower extremities should be done to assess for asymmetry and full extent of axon loss.

Because EMG and nerve conduction studies assess primarily large myelinated fibers in distal limb segments, EMG may be normal in patients with proximal myelin dysfunction (eg, early in Guillain-Barré syndrome) and in patients with primarily small-fiber dysfunction. In such cases, quantitative sensory or autonomic testing or skin punch biopsy may be done depending on the presenting symptoms.

Laboratory tests: Baseline laboratory tests for all patients include CBC, electrolytes, renal function tests, rapid plasma reagin test, a 2-h glucose tolerance test, and measurement of fasting plasma glucose, HbA_{1C}, vitamin B_{12}, folate, and thyroid-stimulating hormone. Some clinicians include serum protein electrophoresis. The need for other tests is determined by polyneuropathy subtype. When EMG and clinical differentiation are inconclusive, tests for all subtypes may be necessary.

For **acute myelin dysfunction neuropathies,** the approach is the same as that for Guillain-Barré syndrome; forced vital capacity is measured to check for incipient respiratory failure. In acute or chronic myelin dysfunction, tests for infectious disorders and immune dysfunction, including tests for hepatitis and HIV and serum protein electrophoresis, are done. A lumbar puncture should also be done; myelin dysfunction due to an autoimmune response often causes albuminocytologic dissociation: increased CSF protein (> 45 mg%) but normal WBC count (≤ 5/μL).

For **vasa nervorum compromise or asymmetric axonal polyneuropathies,** tests for hypercoagulable states and parainfectious or autoimmune vasculitis, particularly if suggested by clinical findings, should be done; the minimum is

- ESR
- Serum protein electrophoresis
- Measurement of rheumatoid factor, antinuclear antibodies, and serum CK

CK may be elevated when rapid onset of disease results in muscle injury.

Other tests depend on the suspected cause:

- Coagulation studies (eg, protein C, protein S, antithrombin III, anticardiolipin antibody, and homocysteine levels) should be done only if personal or family history suggests a hypercoagulable state.
- Tests for sarcoidosis, hepatitis C, or granulomatosis with polyangiitis (formerly known as Wegener granulomatosis) should be done only if symptoms and signs suggest one of these disorders.
- If no cause is identified, nerve and muscle biopsy should be done.

An affected sural nerve is usually biopsied. A muscle adjacent to the biopsied sural nerve or a quadriceps, biceps brachii, or deltoid muscle may be biopsied. The muscle should be one with moderate weakness that has not been tested by needle EMG (to avoid misinterpretation of needle artifacts). An abnormality is more often detected when the contralateral muscle has EMG abnormalities, particularly when the neuropathy is somewhat symmetric. Nerve biopsies are useful in symmetric and asymmetric polyneuropathies but are particularly useful in asymmetric axonopathies.

If initial tests do not identify the cause of distal symmetric axonopathies, a 24-h urine collection is tested for heavy metals, and urine protein electrophoresis is done. If chronic heavy metal poisoning is suspected, testing of hairs from the pubis or axillary region may help.

Whether tests for other causes are needed depends on history and physical examination findings.

Treatment

- Treatment directed at the cause
- Supportive care

Treatment of polyneuropathy focuses on correcting the causes when possible; a causative drug or toxin can be eliminated, or a dietary deficiency corrected. Although these actions may halt progression and lessen symptoms, recovery is slow and may be incomplete.

If the cause cannot be corrected, treatment focuses on minimizing disability and pain. Physical and occupational therapists can recommend useful assistive devices. Tricyclic antidepressants such as amitriptyline or anticonvulsants such as gabapentin are useful for relief of neuropathic pain (eg, diabetic burning feet).

For **myelin dysfunction polyneuropathies,** immune system–modifying treatments are usually used:

- Plasma exchange or IV immune globulin (IVIG) for acute myelin dysfunction
- Plasma exchange or IVIG, corticosteroids, and/or antimetabolite drugs for chronic myelin dysfunction

KEY POINTS

- Suspect polyneuropathy if patients have diffuse sensory deficits, weakness without hyperreflexia, or both.
- Consider a hereditary cause, long-term toxic exposure, or a metabolic disorder if patients have a slowly progressive chronic polyneuropathy.
- Consider toxic or metabolic causes if patients have a symmetric distal neuropathy.
- Consider disorders that affect the myelin sheath or vasa nervorum if patients have an asymmetric polyneuropathy.
- Consider a demyelinating disorder if patients have polyneuropathy with profound motor weakness, minimal atrophy, and hyporeflexia.
- Consider vasa nervorum compromise if patients have polyneuropathy, pain and temperature sensation abnormalities, atrophy in proportion to weakness, and sometimes disproportionate preservation of reflexes.
- Consider axonopathies in all patients with polyneuropathy.

BRACHIAL PLEXUS AND LUMBOSACRAL PLEXUS DISORDERS

Disorders of the brachial or lumbosacral plexus cause a painful mixed sensorimotor disorder of the corresponding limb.

Because several nerve roots intertwine within the plexus (see Fig. 236–1), the symptom pattern does not fit the distribution of individual roots or nerves. Disorders of the rostral brachial plexus affect the shoulders, those of the caudal brachial plexus affect the hands, and those of the lumbosacral plexus affect the legs.

Plexus disorders (plexopathies) are usually due to physical compression or injury:

- In infants, traction during birth
- In adults, usually trauma (typically, for the brachial plexus, a fall that forces the head away from the shoulder) or invasion by metastatic cancer (typically, breast or lung cancer for the brachial plexus and intestinal or GU tumors for the lumbosacral plexus)

In patients receiving anticoagulants, a hematoma may compress the lumbosacral plexus. Neurofibromatosis occasionally involves a plexus. Other causes include postradiation fibrosis (eg, after radiation therapy for breast cancer) and diabetes.

Acute brachial neuritis (neuralgic amyotrophy, Parsonage-Turner syndrome) occurs primarily in men and typically in young adults, although it can occur at any age. Cause is unknown, but viral or immunologic inflammatory processes are suspected.

Symptoms and Signs

Manifestations of plexus disorders include extremity pain and motor or sensory deficits that do not correspond to an isolated nerve root or peripheral nerve distribution.

For **acute brachial neuritis,** symptoms include severe supraclavicular pain, weakness, and diminished reflexes, with minor sensory abnormalities in the distribution of the brachial plexus.

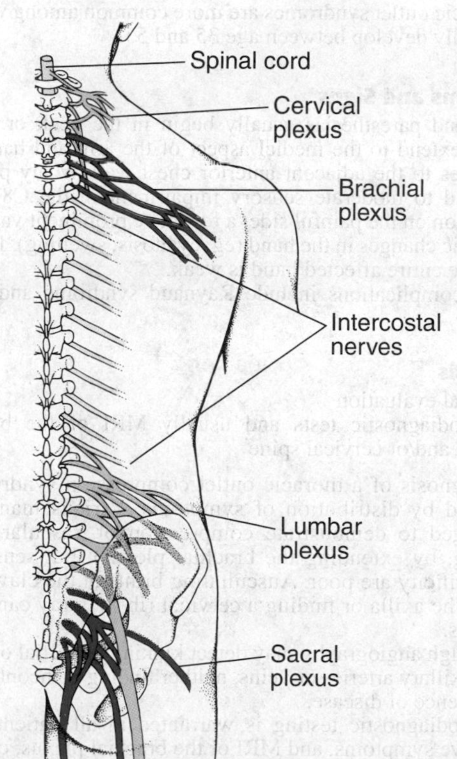

Fig. 236–1. Plexuses.

Usually, weakness develops and reflexes decrease as pain resolves. Severe weakness develops within 3 to 10 days, then typically regresses over the next few months. The most commonly affected muscles are the serratus anterior (causing winging of the scapula), other muscles innervated by the upper trunk, and muscles innervated by the anterior interosseous nerve (in the forearm—patients may not be able to make an *o* with the thumb and index finger).

Diagnosis

- Electromyography (EMG) and nerve conduction studies
- Usually MRI or CT of the appropriate plexus

Diagnosis of a plexus disorder is suggested by clinical findings. EMG and nerve conduction studies should be done to clarify the anatomic distribution (including possible nerve root involvement).

MRI or CT of the appropriate plexus and adjacent spine is done to detect abnormalities such as tumors and hematomas. MRI or CT is indicated for all nontraumatic plexopathies except typical cases of brachial neuritis.

Treatment

- Treatment directed at the cause

Corticosteroids, although commonly prescribed, have no proven benefit.

Surgery may be indicated for injuries, hematomas, and benign or metastatic tumors. Metastases should also be treated with radiation therapy, chemotherapy, or both.

Glycemic control can benefit patients with diabetic plexopathy.

KEY POINTS

- Plexopathies are usually caused by compression or injury.
- Suspect acute brachial neuritis if patients have severe supraclavicular pain, followed by weakness and hyporeflexia that develop within days and resolve over months.
- Suspect a plexopathy if pain or peripheral neurologic deficits do not correspond to a nerve root or peripheral nerve distribution.
- In most cases, do EMG and MRI or CT.
- Treat the cause.

SPINAL MUSCULAR ATROPHIES

Spinal muscular atrophies (SMAs) include several types of hereditary disorders characterized by skeletal muscle wasting due to progressive degeneration of anterior horn cells in the spinal cord and of motor nuclei in the brain stem. Manifestations may begin in infancy or childhood. They vary by the specific type and may include hypotonia; hyporeflexia; difficulty sucking, swallowing, and breathing; unmet developmental milestones; and, in more severe types, very early death. Diagnosis is by genetic testing. Treatment is supportive.

SMAs usually result from autosomal recessive mutations of a single gene locus on the short arm of chromosome 5, causing a homozygous deletion. They may involve the CNS and thus are not purely peripheral nervous system disorders.

There are 4 main types.

Type I spinal muscular atrophy (Werdnig-Hoffmann disease) is present in utero and becomes symptomatic by about age

6 mo. Affected infants have hypotonia (often notable at birth), hyporeflexia, tongue fasciculations, and pronounced difficulty sucking, swallowing, and eventually breathing. Death, usually due to respiratory failure, occurs within the first year in 95% and by age 4 yr in all.

In **type II (intermediate) spinal muscular atrophy,** symptoms usually manifest between 3 and 15 mo of age; < 25% of affected children learn to sit, and none walk or crawl. Children have flaccid muscle weakness and fasciculations, which may be hard to see in young children. Deep tendon reflexes are absent. Dysphagia may be present. Most children are confined to a wheelchair by age 2 to 3 yr. The disorder is often fatal in early life, frequently resulting from respiratory complications. However, progression can stop spontaneously, leaving children with permanent, nonprogressive weakness and a high risk of severe scoliosis and its complications.

Type III spinal muscular atrophy (Wohlfart-Kugelberg-Welander disease) usually manifests between age 15 mo and 19 yr. Findings are similar to those of type I, but progression is slower and life expectancy is longer; some patients have a normal life span. Some familial cases are secondary to specific enzyme defects (eg, hexosaminidase deficiency). Symmetric weakness and wasting progress from proximal to distal areas and are most evident in the legs, beginning in the quadriceps and hip flexors. Later, arms are affected. Life expectancy depends on whether respiratory complications develop.

Type IV spinal muscular atrophy can be recessive, dominant, or X-linked, with adult onset (age 30 to 60 yr) and slow progression of primarily proximal muscle weakness and wasting. Differentiating this disorder from ALS that involves predominantly lower motor neurons may be difficult.

Diagnosis

- Electrodiagnostic testing
- Genetic testing

A diagnosis of spinal muscular atrophy should be suspected in patients with unexplained muscle wasting and flaccid weakness, particularly in infants and children.

Electromyography (EMG) and nerve conduction studies should be done; muscles innervated by cranial nerves should be included. Conduction is normal, but affected muscles, which are often clinically unaffected, are denervated.

Definitive diagnosis is by genetic testing, which detects the causative mutation in about 95% of patients.

Muscle biopsy is done occasionally. Serum enzymes (eg, CK, aldolase) may be slightly increased.

Amniocentesis, done if family history is positive, is often diagnostic.

Treatment

- Supportive care

There is no specific treatment; treatment is mainly supportive. Physical therapy, braces, and special appliances can benefit patients with static or slowly progressive disease by preventing scoliosis and contractures. Adaptive devices available through physical and occupational therapists may improve children's independence and self-care by enabling them to feed themselves, write, or use a computer.

KEY POINTS

- If infants and children have unexplained muscle wasting and flaccid weakness, evaluate them for SMAs.
- EMG shows muscle denervation.
- Use genetic testing to confirm the presence and type of spinal muscular atrophy.
- Refer patients to physical and occupational therapists, who may help patients learn to function more independently.

THORACIC OUTLET COMPRESSION SYNDROMES

Thoracic outlet compression syndromes (TOS) are a group of poorly defined disorders characterized by pain and paresthesias in a hand, the neck, a shoulder, or an arm. They appear to involve compression of the brachial plexus (and perhaps the subclavian vessels) as these structures traverse the thoracic outlet. Diagnostic techniques have not been established. Treatment includes physical therapy, analgesics, and, in severe cases, surgery.

Pathogenesis is often unknown but sometimes involves compression of the lower trunk of the brachial plexus (and perhaps the subclavian vessels) as these structures traverse the thoracic outlet below the scalene muscles and over the 1st rib, before they enter the axilla, but this involvement is unclear. Compression may be caused by

- A cervical rib
- An abnormal 1st thoracic rib
- Abnormal insertion or position of the scalene muscles
- A malunited clavicle fracture

Thoracic outlet syndromes are more common among women and usually develop between age 35 and 55.

Symptoms and Signs

Pain and paresthesias usually begin in the neck or shoulder and extend to the medial aspect of the arm and hand and sometimes to the adjacent anterior chest wall. Many patients have mild to moderate sensory impairment in the C8 to T1 distribution on the painful side; a few have prominent vascular-autonomic changes in the hand (eg, cyanosis, swelling). In even fewer, the entire affected hand is weak.

Rare complications include Raynaud syndrome and distal gangrene.

Diagnosis

- Clinical evaluation
- Electrodiagnostic tests and usually MRI of the brachial plexus and/or cervical spine

A diagnosis of a thoracic outlet compression syndrome is suggested by distribution of symptoms. Various maneuvers are alleged to demonstrate compression of vascular structures (eg, by extending the brachial plexus), but sensitivity and specificity are poor. Auscultating bruits at the clavicle or apex of the axilla or finding a cervical rib by x-ray can aid in diagnosis.

Although angiography may detect kinking or partial obstruction of axillary arteries or veins, neither finding is incontrovertible evidence of disease.

Electrodiagnostic testing is warranted in all patients with suggestive symptoms, and MRI of the brachial plexus, cervical spine, or both is usually also necessary.

Treatment

- Physical therapy and analgesics
- In severe cases, surgery

Most patients without objective neurologic deficits respond to physical therapy, NSAIDs, and low-dose tricyclic antidepressants.

If cervical ribs or subclavian artery compression is identified, an experienced specialist should decide whether surgery is necessary. With few exceptions, surgery should be reserved for patients who have significant or progressive neurovascular deficits and do not respond to conservative treatment.

KEY POINTS

- Consider these syndromes if patients have unexplained pain and paresthesias that begin in the neck or shoulder and extend down the medial arm.
- Do electrodiagnostic tests and usually MRI of the brachial plexus and/or cervical spine.
- Treat most patients with analgesics and physical therapy.
- Consider surgery if patients have a cervical rib or subclavian artery compression and neurovascular deficits that progress despite conservative treatments.

237 Prion Diseases

(Transmissible Spongiform Encephalopathies)

Prion diseases are progressive, fatal, and untreatable degenerative brain disorders.

Prominent types include

- Creutzfeldt-Jakob disease (CJD), the prototypic example (usually sporadic)
- Variant CJD (vCJD; acquired by eating prion-contaminated meat)
- Variably protease-sensitive prionopathy (VPSPr; sporadic)
- Gerstmann Sträussler-Scheinker disease (GSS; inherited)
- Fatal insomnia (FI; includes a sporadic and an inherited form)
- Kuru (acquired by ritual cannibalism)

A recently identified type is prion disease associated with diarrhea and autonomic neuropathy, which is inherited.

Prion diseases result from misfolding of a normal cell-surface brain protein called cellular prion protein (PrP^C), whose exact function is unknown. Misfolded prion proteins are called prions or scrapie PrP (PrP^{Sc}—from the name of the prototypic prion disease of sheep).

Prions (PrP^{Sc}) are pathogenic and often infectious. They produce prion disease by

- Self-replicating: PrP^{Sc} induces conformational transformation of PrP^C, creating duplicate PrP^{Sc}, which, in a chain reaction, induces further transformation of PrP^C into PrP^{Sc}. This transformation process spreads PrP^{Sc} to various regions of the brain.
- Causing neuronal cell death
- Being transmissible

Normal PrP^C is water soluble and protease sensitive, but a large percentage of PrP^{Sc} is water insoluble and markedly resistant to protease degradation (similar to beta-amyloid in Alzheimer disease, which PrP^{Sc} resembles), resulting in slow but inexorable cellular accumulation and neuronal cell death. Accompanying pathologic changes include gliosis and characteristic histologic vacuolar (spongiform) changes, resulting in dementia and other neurologic deficits. Symptoms and signs develop months to years after the initial exposure to PrP^{Sc}.

Prion diseases should be considered in all patients with dementia, especially if it progresses rapidly.

Transmission of prion diseases: Prion diseases originate

- Sporadically (apparently starting spontaneously, without a known cause)
- Via genetic inheritance (familial)
- Via infectious transmission

Sporadic prion diseases are the most common, with a worldwide annual incidence of about 1/1 million people. How PrP^{Sc} first forms is unknown.

Familial prion diseases are caused by defects in the *PrP* gene, which is contained in the short arm of chromosome 20. The genetic mutations causing prion diseases are autosomal dominant; ie, they cause disease when they are inherited from only one parent. Also, penetrance is variable; ie, depending on the type of mutation, a variable percentage of carriers of the mutation have clinical signs of the disease during their lifetime. Some gene defects cause familial CJD, some cause GSS, and others cause diseases with mixed features of CJD and GSS. To date, researchers have identified only one mutation that causes fatal familial insomnia (FFI), the familial form of fatal insomnia. The *PrP* gene mutations alter the amino acid sequence of PrP^C, causing it to misfold and become PrP^{Sc}. Small abnormalities in specific codons (nucleotide sequences that are the building blocks of genes), which on their own do not cause disease, may determine the predominant symptoms and rate of disease progression in familial and other prion diseases.[1]

Infectiously transmitted prion diseases are rare. They can be transmitted

- From person to person: Iatrogenically, via organ and tissue transplants, use of contaminated surgical instruments, or, rarely, blood transfusion (as in vCJD); or via cannibalism (as in kuru)
- From animal to person: Via ingestion of contaminated beef (as in vCJD)

Prion diseases are not known to be contagious through casual person-to-person contact.

Prion diseases occur in many mammals (eg, mink, elk, deer, domestic sheep and cattle) and can be transmitted between species via the food chain. However, transmission from animals to humans has been observed only in vCJD, after people consumed beef from cattle with bovine spongiform encephalopathy (BSE, or mad cow disease).

In several western US states, Canada, and now South Korea and Norway,[2] there is concern that chronic wasting disease (CWD), the prion disease of elk and deer, may be transmissible to people who hunt, butcher, or eat the affected animals. Although transmission of CWD from animals to humans is unlikely, recent data indicate that the barriers between species may be weakened when CWD has been transmitted from animal to animal several times (as may happen in the wild).[3]

1. Gambetti P, Kong Q, Zou W, et al: Sporadic and familial CJD: Classification and characterisation. *Br Med Bull* 66(1):213–239, 2003. doi: https://doi.org/10.1093/bmb/66.1.213.
2. Benestad SL, Mitchell G, Simmons M, et al: First case of chronic wasting disease in Europe in a Norwegian free-ranging reindeer. *Vet Res* 47(1):88, 2016. doi: 10.1186/s13567-016-0375-4.
3. Barria MA, Telling GC, Gambetti P, et al: Generation of a new form of human PrP^{Sc} in vitro by interspecies transmission from cervid prions. *J Biol Chem* 4;286(9): 7490–7495, 2011. doi: 10.1074/jbc.M110.198465.

Treatment of Prion Diseases

- Supportive care

There is no treatment for prion diseases. Treatment is supportive.

Patients should be encouraged to prepare advance directives (eg, preferred end-of-life care) soon after the disorder is diagnosed.

Genetic counseling may be recommended for family members of patients with a familial prion disease.

Prevention of Prion Diseases

Prions resist standard disinfection techniques and may be a risk to other patients and to surgeons, pathologists, or technicians who handle contaminated tissues or instruments.

Transmission can be prevented by taking precautions when handling infected tissues and by using appropriate techniques to clean contaminated instruments. Using one of the following procedures is recommended:

- Steam autoclaving at 132° C for 1 h
- Immersion in sodium hydroxide 1 N (normal) or 10% sodium hypochlorite solution for 1 h

CREUTZFELDT-JAKOB DISEASE

(Subacute Spongiform Encephalopathy)

Creutzfeldt-Jakob disease (CJD) is the most common human prion disease. It occurs worldwide and has several forms and subtypes. CJD symptoms include dementia, myoclonus, and other CNS deficits; death usually occurs between 4 mo and 2 yr after infection, depending on the CJD form and subtype. Treatment is supportive.

CJD has three forms:[1]

- Sporadic (sCJD)
- Familial
- Acquired

sCJD is the most common type, accounting for about 85% of cases. sCJD typically affects people > 40 yr (median, about 60 yr).

Familial CJD occurs in about 5 to 15% of cases. Inheritance is autosomal dominant; age at onset is usually earlier than that in sCJD, and disease duration is longer.

Acquired CJD probably accounts for < 1% of cases. It has occurred after the ingestion of beef contaminated by prions (in variant CJD [vCJD]). Iatrogenic CJD (iCJD) has been acquired via use of cadaveric corneal or dural transplants, stereotactic intracerebral electrodes, or growth hormone prepared from human pituitary glands.[2] About half of iCJD cases involve changes similar to those of Alzheimer disease, suggesting that in iCJD, a disorder that resembles Alzheimer disease (in addition to CJD) can be acquired iatrogenically.[3]

Variant CJD (vCJD): vCJD is a rare acquired form of CJD. Most cases have occurred in the United Kingdom (UK), which had 178 cases as of November 2016, compared with 53 cases in all other European and non-European countries. vCJD occurs after ingestion of beef from cattle with bovine spongiform encephalopathy (BSE), also called mad cow disease.

In vCJD, symptoms develop at a younger average age (< 30 yr) than in sCJD. In recent cases, the incubation period (time between ingestion of contaminated beef and development of symptoms) has been 12 to > 20 yr.

In the early 1980s, because of relaxed regulations for processing animal by-products, contaminated tissue, probably from sheep infected with scrapie or cattle infected with BSE, introduced the scrapie prion protein (PrP^{Sc}) into cattle feed. Hundreds of thousands of cattle developed BSE. Despite widespread exposure, relatively few people who ate meat from affected cattle developed vCJD.

Because the incubation period in BSE is long, a connection between BSE and contaminated feed was not recognized in the UK until BSE had become an epidemic. The BSE epidemic came under control after a massive slaughter of cattle and after changes in the rendering procedures, which drastically reduced contamination of meat by nervous system tissue. In the UK, the annual number of new cases of vCJD, which peaked in 2000, has steadily declined, with only 2 cases after 2011.

Four cases of vCJD have been linked to blood transfusion; they occurred in people who received transfusions between 1996 and 1999. In the UK, about 1/2000 people may carry vCJD (based on examination of a large number of appendix tissue samples) but have no symptoms; these people may transmit the disease if they donate blood or have a surgical procedure. Whether there is a latent pool of people who have received contaminated blood transfusions and who are thus at risk of later development of vCJD is unclear. However, new blood donor referral criteria related to vCJD may further reduce the risk of vCJD transmission by blood transfusion, which is already very low outside of France and the UK.

Although no case of vCJD originating in North America has been reported, BSE has been reported in a few North American cattle (4 in the US and 19 in Canada).

1. Gambetti P, Kong Q, Zou W, et al: Sporadic and familial CJD: Classification and characterisation. *Br Med Bull* 66(1):213–239, 2003. doi: https://doi.org/10.1093/bmb/66.1.213.
2. Ritchie DL, Barria MA, Peden, AH, et al: UK Iatrogenic CJD: investigating human prion transmission across genotypic barriers using human tissue-based and molecular approaches. *Acta Neuropathol* 2016. [Epub ahead of print]
3. Jaunmuktane Z, Mead S, Ellis M, et al: Evidence for human transmission of amyloid-β pathology and cerebral amyloid angiopathy. *Nature* 525:247–250, 2015. doi:10.1038/nature15369.

Symptoms and Signs

About 70% of patients with CJD present with memory loss and confusion, which eventually develop in all patients; 15 to 20% present with incoordination and ataxia, which often develop early in the disease. Myoclonus provoked by noise or other sensory stimuli (startle myoclonus) often develops in the middle to late stages of disease. People with vCJD present with psychiatric symptoms (eg, anxiety, depression), rather than memory loss. Later symptoms are similar in both forms.

Although dementia, ataxia, and myoclonus are most characteristic, other neurologic abnormalities (eg, hallucinations, seizures, neuropathy, various movement disorders) can occur.

Ocular disturbances (eg, visual field defects, diplopia, dimness or blurring of vision, visual agnosia) are common in sCJD.

Diagnosis

- Diffusion-weighted MRI
- CSF markers
- Exclusion of other disorders

CJD should be considered in elderly patients with rapidly progressive dementia, especially if accompanied by myoclonus or ataxia. However, other disorders can mimic CJD and must be considered; they include

- CNS vasculitis
- Rapidly progressive Alzheimer disease
- Hashimoto encephalopathy (an autoimmune encephalopathy that is characterized by high thyroid antibody levels and that responds to corticosteroids)
- Intravascular lymphoma (a rare lymphoma)
- Encephalitis that affects the limbic system, brain stem, and cerebellum
- Lewy body dementia
- Intoxication with lithium or bismuth

CJD is suspected in symptomatic younger patients when they have been exposed to prion-contaminated beef in the UK or other at-risk countries or who have a family history of CJD (familial CJD). Rarely, sCJD develops in young patients, but in such patients, other diseases must be excluded.

Diagnosis of CJD may be difficult.

The best noninvasive diagnostic test for CJD is

- Diffusion-weighted MRI

It can detect evolving patchy areas of hyperintensity (bright areas) in the cortical ribbon, which strongly suggest CJD.

Proteins 14-3-3, brain-specific enolase, and tau are commonly increased in CSF but are not specific for CJD. A relatively new CSF test, called real-time quaking-induced conversion (RT-QuIC), amplifies and detects minimal amounts of prion activity in CSF; this test appears to be more accurate than previous CSF tests.[1] A similar test can reliably detect evidence of vCJD by identifying prions in urine.

EEG is done. Results are positive in about 70% of patients with CJD; EEG shows characteristic periodic sharp waves, but this pattern typically occurs late in the disease and may be transient.

Brain biopsy is usually unnecessary.

1. Foutz A, Appleby BS, Hamlin C, et al: Diagnostic and prognostic value of human prion detection in cerebrospinal fluid. *Ann Neurol* 81(1):79–92, 2017. doi: 10.1002/ana.24833.

Prognosis

Death typically occurs after 6 to 12 mo, commonly due to pneumonia. Life expectancy in vCJD is longer (averaging 1.5 yr).

Treatment

- Supportive care

There is no treatment for CJD. Treatment is supportive.

Prevention

Because there is no effective treatment, prevention of transmissible CJD is essential.

Workers handling fluids and tissues from patients suspected of having CJD must wear gloves and avoid mucous membrane exposure. Contaminated skin can be disinfected by applying 4% sodium hydroxide for 5 to 10 min, followed by extensive washing with water.

Steam autoclaving at 132° C for 1 h or immersion in sodium hydroxide 1 N (normal) or 10% sodium hypochlorite solution for 1 h is recommended for materials that come in contact with tissues of patients with suspected or confirmed CJD. Standard methods of sterilization (eg, exposure to formalin) are ineffective.

The US Department of Agriculture (USDA) currently carries out BSE surveillance for 2000 to 5000 cattle/mo. In 2004, a positive BSE case in the US caused testing to be expanded to an average of 1000 cattle/day, but testing was later reduced to 40,000/yr (0.1% of the cattle that are slaughtered).

KEY POINTS

- CJD is the most common human prion disease; the sporadic form accounts for about 85% of cases.
- Acquired CJD, which probably accounts for < 1% of CJD cases, can result from ingesting beef contaminated by prions (in variant CJD [vCJD]) or can be acquired iatrogenically.
- Most cases of vCJD have occurred in the United Kingdom (178 cases as of November 2016, with only 2 since 2011); 53 cases have occurred in all other European and non-European countries.
- About 70% of patients with CJD present with memory loss and confusion, which eventually develop in all patients; 15 to 20% present with incoordination and ataxia.
- Consider CJD in elderly patients with rapidly progressive dementia, especially if they also have myoclonus or ataxia, and suspect it in symptomatic younger patients who have been exposed to prion-contaminated beef or who have a family history of CJD.
- Do diffusion-weighted MRI to check for evolving patchy areas of hyperintensity in the cortical ribbon, which strongly suggest CJD; also consider doing an RT-QuIC test on CSF.
- Death typically occurs after 6 to 12 mo, but life expectancy in vCJD is longer, averaging 1.5 yr.
- Steam autoclaving or immersing contaminated materials in sodium hydroxide or sodium hypochlorite is recommended to prevent spread.

FATAL INSOMNIA

(Fatal Familial Insomnia; Sporadic Fatal Insomnia)

Fatal insomnia, which includes fatal familial insomnia and sporadic fatal insomnia, are rare hereditary or sporadic prion disorders causing difficulty sleeping, motor dysfunction, and death.

Fatal familial insomnia (FFI) results from an autosomal dominant mutation in the *PrP* gene. Average age at onset is 40 yr (ranging from the late 20s to the early 70s). Life expectancy is 7 to 73 mo. Early symptoms of FFI include increasing difficulty falling asleep and maintaining sleep, as well as cognitive decline, ataxia, and psychiatric symptoms. Sympathetic hyperactivity (eg, hypertension, tachycardia, hyperthermia, sweating) may occur later.

Sporadic fatal insomnia (sFI) lacks a *PrP* gene mutation. Average age at onset is slightly older and life expectancy is slightly longer than in FFI. Early symptoms include cognitive decline and ataxia. Sleep abnormalities are not commonly reported but can usually be observed during a sleep study.

Fatal insomnia should be considered as a rare possibility when patients have rapidly progressive cognitive impairment accompanied by behavioral or mood changes, ataxia, and sleep disturbances. Suspicion of FFI or sFI should prompt a sleep study by polysomnography. Genetic testing can confirm the diagnosis of the familial form. MRI and measurement of 14-3-3 protein and tau in CSF are not useful, but polysomnography and PET (which shows thalamic hypometabolism) can confirm the diagnosis.

There is only supportive treatment for fatal insomnia.

GERSTMANN-STRÄUSSLER-SCHEINKER DISEASE

Gerstmann-Sträussler-Scheinker (GSS) disease is an autosomal dominant prion brain disease that typically begins during middle age.

GSS occurs worldwide and is about 100-fold less common than CJD. It develops at an earlier age (40 vs 60 yr), and average life expectancy is longer (5 yr vs 6 mo).

Patients have cerebellar dysfunction with unsteady gait, dysarthria, and nystagmus. Gaze palsies, deafness, dementia, parkinsonism, hyporeflexia, and extensor plantar responses are also common. Myoclonus is much less common than in CJD.

GSS should be considered in patients with characteristic symptoms and signs and a family history, particularly if they are ≤ 45 yr. Genetic testing can confirm the diagnosis.

There is only supportive treatment for GSS.

KURU

Kuru is a rare prion brain disease endemic to Papua, New Guinea, and thought to be spread by ritual cannibalism.

Although ritual cannibalism ended in the 1950s, 11 new cases of kuru have been reported between 1996 and 2004, suggesting an incubation period that may exceed 50 yr.

Symptoms of kuru begin with tremors (resembling shivering) and ataxia. Movement disorders such as choreoathetosis, fasciculations, and myoclonus develop later, followed by dementia.

CSF testing does not appear to be useful. Few other test results have been reported. No diagnostic abnormalities have been identified in the *PrP* gene of people with kuru. However, a *PrP* gene variation that protects against prion disease has been identified in people in the Papua population who have not contracted kuru.[1] Autopsy can show typical PrP^{Sc}-containing plaques, with the greatest density in the cerebellum.

Death usually occurs within 2 yr after symptoms begin; cause of death is usually pneumonia or infection due to pressure sores.

There is only supportive treatment for kuru.

1. Asante EA, Smidak M, Grimshaw A, et al: A naturally occurring variant of the human prion protein completely prevents prion disease. *Nature* 522(7557):478–481, 2015. doi: 10.1038/nature14510.

PRION DISEASE ASSOCIATED WITH DIARRHEA AND AUTONOMIC NEUROPATHY

Prion disease associated with diarrhea and autonomic neuropathy describes a novel inherited prion disease that manifests with peripheral rather than CNS symptoms.

This disease was identified in 2013 in an extended British family.

This disease differs from other prion diseases because

- Prion amyloid is not limited to the CNS but is distributed in peripheral nerves and internal organs; thus, peripheral symptoms predominate initially, and CNS symptoms occur late.
- It is associated with a novel mutation in the prion gene (Y163X mutation) that results in truncation of the mutated prion protein; thus, the mutated protein lacks the anchor that typically tethers the prion protein to cell membranes, presumably favoring the prion protein's floating in body fluids and migrating to other tissues.

This new prion disease shows that a novel mutation can radically change where the abnormal proteins deposit and which symptoms they cause, and it suggests that the diagnosis of prion disease should be considered in patients with unexplained chronic diarrhea and neuropathy or with an unexplained syndrome similar to familial amyloid polyneuropathy (which causes autonomic and peripheral neuropathy).

Symptoms begin in early adulthood; they include chronic watery diarrhea, autonomic failure (eg, urinary retention, urinary incontinence, orthostatic hypotension), and a primarily sensory peripheral polyneuropathy. Cognitive decline and seizures occur when patients are in their 40s or 50s.

The disease progresses over decades; patients may live up to 30 yr after symptoms develop.

There is only symptomatic treatment for this disorder.

VARIABLY PROTEASE-SENSITIVE PRIONOPATHY

Variably protease-sensitive prionopathy (VPSPr) is a rare sporadic prion disease (identified in 2008).

VPSPr occurs in 2 to 3/100 million people.

VPSPr resembles Gerstmann-Sträussler-Scheinker disease (GSS) in terms of the characteristics of the abnormal prion protein (PrP^{Sc}). However, unlike in GSS, no mutations in the prion protein gene have been identified.

Clinical manifestations differ from those of CJD, and the PrP^{Sc} is less resistant to digestion by proteases; some variants are more sensitive to proteases than others, hence the name: variably protease-sensitive.

Patients present with psychiatric symptoms, speech deficits (aphasia and/or dysarthria), and cognitive impairment. Ataxia and parkinsonism can develop. Average age at onset is 70 yr, and duration of survival is 24 mo. About 40% of patients have a family history of dementia.

Diagnosis of VPSPr is difficult. MRI, EEG, and tests for 14-3-3 protein and tau are usually not helpful, and no mutations have been observed in the coding region of the PrP gene.

There is only supportive treatment for VPSPr.

238 Seizure Disorders

A seizure is an abnormal, unregulated electrical discharge that occurs within the brain's cortical gray matter and transiently interrupts normal brain function. A seizure typically causes altered awareness, abnormal sensations, focal involuntary movements, or convulsions (widespread violent involuntary contraction of voluntary muscles). Diagnosis may be clinical and involves results of neuroimaging, laboratory testing, and EEG for new-onset seizures or anticonvulsant levels for previously diagnosed seizure disorders. Treatment includes elimination of the cause if possible, anticonvulsants, and surgery (if anticonvulsants are ineffective).

About 2% of adults have a seizure at some time during their life. Two thirds of these people never have another one.

Definitions: Terminology can be confusing.

Epilepsy (also called epileptic seizure disorder) is a chronic brain disorder characterized by recurrent (≥ 2) seizures that are unprovoked (ie, not related to reversible stressors) and that occur > 24 h apart. A single seizure is not considered an epileptic seizure. Epilepsy is often idiopathic, but various brain disorders, such as malformations, strokes, and tumors, can cause symptomatic epilepsy.

Symptomatic epilepsy is epilepsy due to a known cause (eg, brain tumor, stroke). The seizures it causes are called symptomatic epileptic seizures. Such seizures are most common among neonates (see p. 2774) and the elderly.

Cryptogenic epilepsy is epilepsy assumed to be due to a specific cause, but whose specific cause is currently unknown.

Nonepileptic seizures are provoked by a temporary disorder or stressor (eg, metabolic disorders, CNS infections, cardiovascular disorders, drug toxicity or withdrawal, psychogenic disorders). In children, fever can provoke a seizure (febrile seizures—see p. 2772).

Psychogenic nonepileptic seizures (pseudoseizures) are symptoms that simulate seizures in patients with psychiatric disorders but that do not involve an abnormal electrical discharge in the brain.

Table 238–1. CAUSES OF SEIZURES

CONDITION	EXAMPLES
Autoimmune disorders	Cerebral vasculitis, anti-NMDA receptor encephalitis, multiple sclerosis (rarely)
Cerebral edema	Eclampsia, hypertensive encephalopathy
Cerebral ischemia or hypoxia	Cardiac arrhythmias, carbon monoxide toxicity, nonfatal drowning, near suffocation, stroke, vasculitis
Head trauma*	Birth injury, blunt or penetrating injuries
CNS infections	AIDS, brain abscess, falciparum malaria, meningitis, neurocysticercosis, neurosyphilis, rabies, tetanus, toxoplasmosis, viral encephalitis
Congenital or developmental abnormalities	Cortical malformations, genetic disorders (eg, fifth day fits†, lipid storage diseases such as Tay-Sachs disease), neuronal migration disorders (eg, heterotopias), phenylketonuria
Drugs and toxins‡	Cause seizures: Camphor, ciprofloxacin, cocaine and other CNS stimulants, cyclosporine, imipenem, lead, pentylenetetrazol, picrotoxin, strychnine, tacrolimus Lower seizure threshold: Aminophylline, antidepressants (particularly tricyclics), sedating antihistamines, antimalarial drugs, some antipsychotics (eg, clozapine), buspirone, fluoroquinolones, theophylline When blood levels of phenytoin are very high, a paradoxical increase in seizure frequency
Expanding intracranial lesions	Hemorrhage, hydrocephalus, tumors
Hyperpyrexia	Drug toxicity (eg, with amphetamines or cocaine), fever, heatstroke
Metabolic disturbances	Commonly, hypocalcemia (eg, secondary to hypoparathyroidism), hypoglycemia, hyponatremia Less commonly, aminoacidurias, hepatic or uremic encephalopathy, hyperglycemia, hypomagnesemia, hypernatremia In neonates, vitamin B_6 (pyridoxine) deficiency
Neurocutaneous disorders	Neurofibromatosis, tuberous sclerosis
Pressure-related	Decompression illness, hyperbaric oxygen treatments
Withdrawal syndromes	Alcohol, anesthetics, barbiturates, benzodiazepines

*Posttraumatic seizures occur in 25 to 75% of patients who have brain contusion, skull fracture, intracranial hemorrhage, prolonged coma, or focal neurologic deficits.

†Fifth day fits (benign neonatal seizures) are tonic-clonic seizures occurring between 4 and 6 days of age in otherwise healthy infants; one form is inherited.

‡When given in toxic doses, various drugs can cause seizures.

NMDA = *N*-methyl-D-aspartate.

Etiology

Common causes of seizures (see Table 238–1) vary by age of onset:

- Before age 2: Fever, birth or developmental defects, birth injuries, and metabolic disorders
- Ages 2 to 14: Idiopathic seizure disorders
- Adults: Cerebral trauma, alcohol withdrawal, tumors, strokes, and an unknown cause (in 50%)
- The elderly: Tumors and strokes

In **reflex epilepsy**, a rare disorder, seizures are triggered predictably by an external stimulus, such as repetitive sounds, flashing lights, video games, music, or even touching certain parts of the body.

In cryptogenic epilepsy and often in refractory epilepsy, a rare but increasingly identified cause is anti-NMDA (*N*-methyl-D-aspartate) receptor encephalitis, especially in young women. This disorder also causes psychiatric symptoms, a movement disorder, and CSF pleocytosis. Ovarian teratoma occurs in about 60% of women with anti-NMDA receptor encephalitis. Removal of the teratoma (if present) and immunotherapy control the seizures much better than anticonvulsants.

Classification

Seizures are classified as generalized or partial.

Generalized: In generalized seizures, the aberrant electrical discharge diffusely involves the entire cortex of both hemispheres from the onset, and consciousness is usually lost. Generalized seizures result most often from metabolic disorders and sometimes from genetic disorders. Generalized seizures include the following:

- Infantile spasms
- Absence seizures
- Tonic-clonic seizures
- Tonic seizures
- Atonic seizures
- Myoclonic seizures (eg, in juvenile myoclonic epilepsy)

Partial seizures: In partial seizures, the excess neuronal discharge occurs in one cerebral cortex, and most often results from structural abnormalities. Partial seizures may be

- Simple (no impairment of consciousness)
- Complex (reduced but not complete loss of consciousness)

Partial seizures may evolve into a generalized seizure (called secondary generalization), which causes loss of consciousness. Secondary generalization occurs when a partial seizure spreads and activates the entire cerebrum bilaterally. Activation may occur so rapidly that the initial partial seizure is not clinically apparent or is very brief.

A revised terminology for partial seizures has been proposed.[1] In this system, partial seizures are called focal seizures, and the following terms are used for subtypes:

- For simple partial seizures: Focal seizures without impairment of consciousness or awareness
- For complex partial seizures: Focal seizures with impairment of consciousness or awareness
- For secondarily generalized partial seizures: Focal seizures evolving to a bilateral or convulsive seizure

This terminology is not yet in common use.

1. Berg AT, Berkovic SF, Brodie MJ, et al: Revised terminology and concepts for organization of seizures and epilepsies: Report of the ILAE [International League Against Epilepsy] Commission on Classification and Terminology, 2005–2009. *Epilepsia* 51:676–685, 2010.

Symptoms and Signs

An **aura** may precede seizures. Auras are simple partial seizures that begin focally. Auras may consist of motor activity or sensory, autonomic, or psychic sensations (eg, paresthesias, a rising epigastric sensation, abnormal smells, a sensation of fear, a déjà vu or jamais vu sensation). In jamais vu, a familiar place or experience feels very unfamiliar—the opposite of déjà vu.

Most seizures end spontaneously in 1 to 2 min.

A **postictal state** often follows generalized seizures; it is characterized by deep sleep, headache, confusion, and muscle soreness; this state lasts from minutes to hours. Sometimes the postictal state includes Todd paralysis (a transient neurologic deficit, usually weakness, of the limb contralateral to the seizure focus).

Most patients appear neurologically normal between seizures, although high doses of the drugs used to treat seizure disorders, particularly anticonvulsants, can reduce alertness. Any progressive mental deterioration is usually related to the neurologic disorder that caused the seizures rather than to the seizures themselves.

Occasionally, seizures are unremitting, as in status epilepticus.

Partial seizures: There are several types of partial seizures.

Simple partial seizures cause motor, sensory, or psychomotor symptoms without loss of consciousness. Specific symptoms reflect the affected area of the brain (see Table 238–2). In jacksonian seizures, focal motor symptoms begin in one

Table 238–2. MANIFESTATIONS OF PARTIAL SEIZURES BY SITE

FOCAL MANIFESTATION	SITE OF DYSFUNCTION
Bilateral tonic posture	Frontal lobe (supplementary motor cortex)
Simple movements (eg, limb twitching, jacksonian march)	Contralateral frontal lobe
Head and eye deviation with posturing	Supplementary motor cortex
Abnormal taste sensation (dysgeusia)	Insula
Visceral or autonomic abnormalities (eg, epigastric aura, salivation)	Insular-orbital-frontal cortex
Olfactory hallucinations	Anteromedial temporal lobe
Chewing movements, salivation, speech arrest	Amygdala, opercular region
Complex behavioral automatisms	Temporal lobe
Unusual behavior suggesting a psychiatric cause or sleep disorder	Frontal lobe
Visual hallucinations (formed images)	Posterior temporal lobe or amygdala-hippocampus
Localized sensory disturbances (eg, tingling or numbness of a limb or half the body)	Parietal lobe (sensory cortex)
Visual hallucinations (unformed images)	Occipital lobe

hand, then march up the arm (jacksonian march). Other focal seizures affect the face first, then spread to an arm and sometimes a leg. Some partial motor seizures begin with an arm raising and the head turning toward the raised arm (called fencing posture).

Epilepsia partialis continua, a rare disorder, causes focal motor seizures that usually involve the arm, hand, or one side of the face; seizures recur every few seconds or minutes for days to years at a time. The cause is usually

- In adults: A structural lesion (eg, stroke)
- In children: A focal cerebral cortical inflammatory process (eg, Rasmussen encephalitis), possibly caused by a chronic viral infection or by autoimmune processes

PEARLS & PITFALLS

- Consider partial seizures in patients with transient, unexplained, recurrent abnormalities that appear psychiatric (eg, hallucinations, complex behavioral automatisms, speech arrest, reduced responsiveness while staring).

Complex partial seizures are often preceded by an aura. During the seizure, patients may stare. Consciousness is impaired, but patients have some awareness of the environment (eg, they purposefully withdraw from noxious stimuli). The following may also occur:

- Oral automatisms (involuntary chewing or lip smacking)
- Limb automatisms (eg, automatic purposeless movements of the hands)
- Utterance of unintelligible sounds without understanding what they say
- Resistance to assistance
- Tonic or dystonic posturing of the extremity contralateral to the seizure focus
- Head and eye deviation, usually in a direction contralateral to the seizure focus
- Bicycling or pedaling movements of the legs if the seizure emanates from the medial frontal or orbitofrontal head regions

Motor symptoms subside after 1 to 2 min, but confusion and disorientation may continue for another 1 or 2 min. Postictal amnesia is common. Patients may lash out if restrained during the seizure or while recovering consciousness if the seizure generalizes. However, unprovoked aggressive behavior is unusual.

Left temporal lobe seizures may cause verbal memory abnormalities; right temporal lobe seizures may cause visual spatial memory abnormalities.

Generalized seizures: Consciousness is usually lost, and motor function is abnormal from the onset.

Infantile spasms are characterized by sudden flexion and adduction of the arms and forward flexion of the trunk (see also p. 2773). Seizures last a few seconds and recur many times a day. They occur only in the first 5 yr of life, then are replaced by other types of seizures. Developmental defects are usually present.

Typical absence seizures (formerly called petit mal seizures) consist of 10- to 30-sec loss of consciousness with eyelid fluttering; axial muscle tone may or may not be lost. Patients do not fall or convulse; they abruptly stop activity, then just as abruptly resume it, with no postictal symptoms or knowledge that a seizure has occurred. Absence seizures are genetic and occur predominantly in children. Without treatment, such seizures are likely to occur many times a day. Seizures often occur when patients are sitting quietly, can be precipitated by hyperventilation, and rarely occur during exercise. Neurologic and cognitive examination results are usually normal.

Atypical absence seizures usually occur as part of the Lennox-Gastaut syndrome, a severe form of epilepsy that begins before age 4 yr. They differ from typical absence seizures as follows:

- They last longer.
- Jerking or automatic movements are more pronounced.
- Loss of awareness is less complete.

Many patients have a history of damage to the nervous system, developmental delay, abnormal neurologic examination results, and other types of seizures. Atypical absence seizures usually continue into adulthood.

Atonic seizures occur most often in children, usually as part of Lennox-Gastaut syndrome. Atonic seizures are characterized by brief, complete loss of muscle tone and consciousness. Children fall or pitch to the ground, risking trauma, particularly head injury.

Tonic seizures occur most often during sleep, usually in children. The cause is usually the Lennox-Gastaut syndrome. Tonic (sustained) contraction of axial muscles may begin abruptly or gradually, then spread to the proximal muscles of the limbs. Tonic seizures usually last 10 to 15 sec. In longer tonic seizures, a few, rapid clonic jerks may occur as the tonic phase ends.

Tonic-clonic seizures may be

- Primarily generalized
- Secondarily generalized

Primarily generalized seizures typically begin with an outcry; they continue with loss of consciousness and falling, followed by tonic contraction, then clonic (rapidly alternating contraction and relaxation) motion of muscles of the extremities, trunk, and head. Urinary and fecal incontinence, tongue biting, and frothing at the mouth sometimes occur. Seizures usually last 1 to 2 min. There is no aura.

Secondarily generalized tonic-clonic seizures begin with a simple partial or complex partial seizure, then progress to resemble other generalized seizures.

Myoclonic seizures are brief, lightning-like jerks of a limb, several limbs, or the trunk. They may be repetitive, leading to a tonic-clonic seizure. The jerks may be bilateral or unilateral. Unlike other seizures with bilateral motor movements, consciousness is not lost unless the myoclonic seizure progresses into a generalized tonic-clonic seizure.

Juvenile myoclonic epilepsy is an epilepsy syndrome characterized by myoclonic, tonic-clonic, and absence seizures. It typically appears during adolescence. Seizures begin with a few bilateral, synchronous myoclonic jerks, followed in 90% of cases by generalized tonic-clonic seizures. They often occur when patients awaken in the morning, especially after sleep deprivation or alcohol use. Absence seizures may occur in one third of patients.

Febrile seizures occur, by definition, with fever and in the absence of intracranial infection; they are considered a type of provoked seizure (see also p. 2772). They affect about 4% of children aged 3 mo to 5 yr. Benign febrile seizures are brief, solitary, and generalized tonic-clonic in appearance. Complicated febrile seizures are focal, last > 15 min, or recur ≥ 2 times in < 24 h. Overall, 2% of patients with febrile seizures develop a subsequent seizure disorder. However, incidence of seizure disorders and risk of recurrent febrile seizures are much greater among children with any of the following:

- Complicated febrile seizures
- Preexisting neurologic abnormalities
- Onset before age 1 yr
- A family history of seizure disorders

Status epilepticus: Status epilepticus has 2 forms: convulsive and nonconvulsive.

Generalized convulsive status epilepticus involves at least one of the following:

- Tonic-clonic seizure activity lasting > 5 to 10 min
- ≥ 2 seizures between which patients do not fully regain consciousness

The previous definition of > 30-min duration was revised to encourage more prompt identification and treatment. Untreated generalized seizures lasting > 60 min may result in permanent brain damage; longer-lasting seizures may be fatal. Heart rate and temperature increase. Generalized convulsive status epilepticus has many causes, including head trauma and rapid withdrawal of anticonvulsants.

Nonconvulsive status epilepticus includes complex partial status epilepticus and absence status epilepticus. They often manifest as prolonged episodes of mental status changes. EEG may be required for diagnosis.

Diagnosis

- Clinical evaluation
- For new-onset seizures, neuroimaging, laboratory testing, and usually EEG
- For known seizure disorders, usually anticonvulsant levels
- For new-onset or known seizure disorders, other testing as clinically indicated

Evaluation must determine whether the event was a seizure vs another cause of obtundation (eg, a pseudoseizure, syncope), then identify possible causes or precipitants. Patients with new-onset seizures are evaluated in an emergency department; they can sometimes be discharged after thorough evaluation. Those with a known seizure disorder may be evaluated in a physician's office.

History: Patients should be asked about unusual sensations, suggesting an aura and thus a seizure, and about typical seizure manifestations. Patients typically do not remember generalized seizures, so a description of the seizure itself must be obtained from witnesses.

Manifestations of other conditions, such as sudden global brain ischemia (eg, due to ventricular arrhythmia), can resemble those of a seizure, including loss of consciousness and some myoclonic jerks.

PEARLS & PITFALLS

- In patients who suddenly lose consciousness, consider global brain ischemia (eg, due to ventricular arrhythmia), even if observers report myoclonic jerks.

History should include information about the first and any subsequent seizures (eg, duration, frequency, sequential evolution, longest and shortest interval between seizures, aura, postictal state, precipitating factors). All patients should be asked about risk factors for seizures:

- Prior head trauma or CNS infection
- Known neurologic disorders
- Drug use or withdrawal, particularly of recreational drugs
- Alcohol withdrawal
- Nonadherence to anticonvulsants
- Family history of seizures or neurologic disorders

Patients should also be asked about rare triggers (eg, repetitive sounds, flashing lights, video games, touching certain parts of the body) and about sleep deprivation, which can lower the seizure threshold.

Physical examination: In patients who have lost consciousness, a bitten tongue, incontinence (eg, urine or feces in clothing), or prolonged confusion after loss of consciousness suggest seizure.

In pseudoseizures, generalized muscular activity and lack of response to verbal stimuli may at first glance suggest generalized tonic-clonic seizures. However, pseudoseizures can usually be distinguished from true seizures by clinical characteristics:

- Pseudoseizures often last longer (several minutes or more).
- Postictal confusion tends to be absent.
- Typical tonic phase activity, followed by clonic phase, usually does not occur.
- The progression of muscular activity does not correspond to true seizure patterns (eg, jerks moving from one side to the other and back [nonphysiologic progression], exaggerated pelvic thrusting).
- Intensity may wax and wane.
- Vital signs, including temperature, usually remain normal.
- Patients often actively resist passive eye opening.

Physical examination rarely indicates the cause when seizures are idiopathic but may provide clues when seizures are symptomatic (see Table 238–3).

Testing: Testing is done routinely, but normal results do not necessarily exclude a seizure disorder. Thus, the diagnosis may ultimately be clinical. Testing depends on results of the history and neurologic examination.

If patients have a known seizure disorder and examination results are normal or unchanged, little testing is required except

Table 238–3. CLINICAL CLUES TO THE CAUSES OF SYMPTOMATIC SEIZURES

FINDING	POSSIBLE CAUSE
Fever and stiff neck	Meningitis Subarachnoid hemorrhage Meningoencephalitis
Papilledema	Increased intracranial pressure
Loss of spontaneous venous pulsations (noted during funduscopy)	Increased intracranial pressure (specificity is 80–90%*)
Focal neurologic defects (eg, asymmetry of reflexes or muscle strength)	Structural abnormality (eg, tumor, stroke) Postictal paralysis
Generalized neuromuscular irritability (eg, tremulousness, hyperreflexia)	Drug toxicity (eg, sympathomimetics) Withdrawal syndromes (eg, of alcohol or sedatives) Certain metabolic disorders (eg, hypocalcemia, hypomagnesemia)
Skin lesions (eg, axillary freckling or café-au-lait spots, hypomelanotic skin macules, shagreen patches)	Neurocutaneous disorders (eg, neurofibromatosis, tuberous sclerosis)

*Spontaneous venous pulsations are absent in all patients with increased intracranial pressure; these pulsations are also absent in 10–20% of people with normal intracranial pressure, but sometimes only temporarily.

for blood anticonvulsant levels. Additional testing is indicated if patients have symptoms or signs of a treatable disorder such as trauma, infection, or a metabolic disorder.

If seizures are new-onset or if examination results are abnormal for the first time, neuroimaging is required. Patients with new-onset seizures or atypical manifestations also require laboratory testing, including blood tests (serum electrolytes, BUN, creatinine, glucose, Ca, Mg, and P levels), and liver function tests. Other tests may be done based on disorders that are suspected clinically:

- Meningitis or CNS infection with normal neuroimaging results: Lumbar puncture is required.
- Unreported use of recreational drugs that can cause or contribute to seizures: Drug screens may be done, although this practice is controversial because positive results do not indicate causality and test results can be inaccurate.
- Cryptogenic epilepsy: Testing for the anti-NMDA receptor antibody should be considered, especially in young women (as many as 26% may test positive); a positive result suggests anti-NMDA receptor encephalitis.

Neuroimaging (typically head CT, but sometimes MRI) is usually done immediately to exclude a mass or hemorrhage. Some experts say that CT can be deferred and possibly avoided in children with typical febrile seizures whose neurologic status rapidly returns to normal.

Follow-up MRI is recommended when CT is negative. It provides better resolution of brain tumors and abscesses and can detect cortical dysplasias, cerebral venous thrombosis, and herpes encephalitis. An epilepsy-protocol MRI of the head uses high-resolution coronal T1 and T2 sequences, which can detect hippocampal atrophy or sclerosis. MRI can detect some common causes of seizures, such as malformations of cortical development in young children and mesial temporal sclerosis, traumatic gliosis, and small tumors in adults.

EEG is critical in the diagnosis of epileptic seizures, particularly of complex partial or absence status epilepticus, when EEG may be the most definitive indication of a seizure. EEG may detect epileptiform abnormalities (spikes, sharp waves, spike and slow-wave complexes, polyspike and slow-wave complexes). Epileptiform abnormalities may be bilateral, symmetric, and synchronous in patients with primarily generalized seizures and may be localized in patients with partial seizures. EEG findings may include the following:

- Epileptiform abnormalities in temporal lobe foci between seizures (interictal) in complex partial seizures originating in the temporal lobe
- Interictal bilateral symmetric bursts of 4- to 7-Hz epileptiform activity in primarily generalized tonic-clonic seizures
- Focal epileptiform discharges in secondarily generalized seizures
- Spikes and slow-wave discharges occurring bilaterally at a rate of 3/sec and usually a normal interictal EEG in typical absence seizures
- Slow spike and wave discharges usually at a rate of < 2.5/sec, typically with interictal disorganization of background activity and diffuse slow waves, in atypical absence seizures
- Bilateral polyspike and wave abnormality at a rate of 4- to 6-Hz in juvenile myoclonic epilepsy

However, normal EEG cannot exclude the diagnosis of epileptic seizures, which must be made clinically. EEG is less likely to detect abnormalities if seizures are infrequent. The initial EEG may detect an epileptiform abnormality in only 30 to 55% of patients with a known epileptic seizure disorder. Serial EEG may detect epileptiform abnormalities in up to 80 to 90% of such patients. In general, serial EEG with extended recording times and with tests done after sleep deprivation greatly increases the chance of detecting epileptiform abnormalities in patients with epileptic seizures.

Inpatient combined video-EEG monitoring, usually for 2 to 7 days, records EEG activity and clinical behavior simultaneously. It is the most sensitive EEG testing available and is thus useful in differentiating epileptic from nonepileptic seizures.

If surgical resection of areas of epileptic foci is being considered, advanced imaging tests to identify such areas are available in epilepsy centers. Functional MRI can identify functioning cortex and guide surgical resection. If EEG and MRI do not clearly identify the epileptic focus, magnetoencephalography with EEG (called magnetic source imaging) may localize the lesion, avoiding the need for invasive intraoperative mapping procedures. Single-photon emission CT (SPECT) during the peri-ictal period may detect increased perfusion in the seizure focus and help localize the area to be surgically removed. Because injection of contrast is required at the time of seizure, patients must be admitted for continuous EEG-video monitoring when SPECT is done during the peri-ictal period.

Neuropsychologic testing may help identify functional deficits before and after surgery and help predict social and psychologic prognosis and capacity for rehabilitation.

Prognosis

With treatment, seizures are eliminated in one third of patients with epileptic seizures, and frequency of seizures is reduced by > 50% in another third. About 60% of patients whose seizures are well-controlled by drugs can eventually stop the drugs and remain seizure-free.

Epileptic seizures are considered resolved when patients have been seizure-free for 10 yr and have not taken anticonvulsants for the last 5 yr of that time period.

Sudden unexplained death in epilepsy (SUDEP) is a rare complication of unknown cause.

Treatment

- Elimination of the cause if possible
- Avoidance of or precautions during situations when loss of consciousness could be life-threatening
- Drugs to control seizures
- Surgery if ≥ 2 drugs in therapeutic doses do not control seizures

Optimal treatment of seizures is to eliminate the causes whenever possible.

If the cause cannot be corrected or identified, anticonvulsants are often required, particularly after a 2nd seizure; usefulness of anticonvulsants after a single seizure is controversial, and risks and benefits should be discussed with the patient. Because the risk of a subsequent seizure is low, drugs may be withheld until a 2nd seizure occurs, particularly in children. In children, certain anticonvulsants cause important behavior and learning problems.

During a generalized tonic-clonic seizure, injury should be prevented by loosening clothing around the neck and placing a pillow under the head. Attempting to protect the tongue is futile and likely to damage the patient's teeth or the rescuer's fingers. Patients should be rolled onto their left side to prevent aspiration. These measures should be taught to the patient's family members and coworkers.

Because partial seizures can become generalized, patients are at risk of losing consciousness and thus should be advised to take certain precautions. Until seizures are controlled, patients should refrain from activities in which loss of consciousness could be life-threatening (eg, driving, swimming, climbing, operating power tools, bathing in a bathtub). After seizures are completely controlled (typically for > 6 mo), many such activities can be resumed if appropriate safeguards (eg, lifeguards) are used, and patients should be encouraged to lead a normal life, including exercise and social activities.

In a few states, physicians must report patients with seizures to the Department of Motor Vehicles. However, most states allow automobile driving after patients have been seizure-free for 6 mo to 1 yr.

Patients should be advised to avoid cocaine and some other illicit drugs (eg, phencyclidine, amphetamines), which can trigger seizures, and to avoid alcohol. Some drugs (eg, haloperidol, phenothiazines) may lower seizure threshold and should be avoided if possible.

Family members must be taught a commonsense approach toward the patient. Overprotection should be replaced with sympathetic support that lessens negative feelings (eg, of inferiority or self-consciousness); invalidism should be prevented.

Institutional care is rarely advisable and should be reserved for severely cognitively impaired patients and for patients with seizures so frequent and violent despite drug treatment that they cannot be cared for elsewhere.

Acute seizures and status epilepticus: Most seizures remit spontaneously in several minutes or less and do not require emergency drug treatment. However, status epilepticus and most seizures lasting > 5 min require drugs to terminate the seizures, with monitoring of respiratory status. Endotracheal intubation is necessary if there is any indication of airway compromise.

The sooner anticonvulsant therapy is started, the better and the more easily seizures are controlled.

IV access should be quickly obtained, and patients are given lorazepam 0.05 to 0.1 mg/kg IV (typically a 4-mg IV dose for adults) at a rate of 2 mg/min. Larger doses are sometimes required. After lorazepam is given, a second, longer-acting anticonvulsant is indicated.

There is no consensus or evidence-based guideline indicating which longer-acting anticonvulsant is preferred. Many experts choose one of the following:

- Fosphenytoin 15 to 20 PE (phenytoin equivalents)/kg IV, given at a rate of 100 to 150 PE/min
- Phenytoin 15 to 20 mg/kg IV, given at a rate of 50 mg/min

If seizures persist after these doses are used, an additional 5 to 10 PE/kg of fosphenytoin or 5 to 10 mg/kg of phenytoin can be given.

Alternative anticonvulsants include the following:

- Valproate 20 to 40 mg/kg IV (loading dose) over 30 min followed by 4 to 8 mg/kg po tid
- Levetiracetam 1500 to 3000 mg IV over 25 min, then 1500 mg po bid

If IV access cannot be obtained, options include IM fosphenytoin and sublingual or rectal benzodiazepines.

Seizures that persist after use of lorazepam and phenytoin (or another 2nd anticonvulsant) define refractory status epilepticus.

Recommendations for a 3rd anticonvulsant vary and include phenobarbital, propofol, midazolam, levetiracetam, and valproate. Dose of phenobarbital is 15 to 20 mg/kg IV at 100 mg/min (3 mg/kg/min in children); continued seizures require another 5- to 10-mg/kg dose. A loading dose of valproate 20 to 40 mg/kg IV is an alternative.

At this point, if status epilepticus has not abated, intubation and general anesthesia are necessary. The optimal anesthetic to use is controversial, but many physicians use propofol 1 to 2 mg/kg at 100 mg/min or pentobarbital 5 to 8 mg/kg (loading dose) followed by infusion of 2 to 4 mg/kg/h until EEG manifestations of seizure activity have been suppressed. Inhalational anesthetics are rarely used.

After initial treatment, the cause of status epilepticus must be identified and treated.

Posttraumatic seizures: Drugs are given to prevent seizures if head injury causes significant structural injury (eg, large contusions or hematomas, brain laceration, depressed skull fracture) or a Glasgow Coma Scale (GCS) score of < 10. These drugs reduce risk of seizures during the first week after injury but do not prevent permanent posttraumatic epilepsy months or years later. They should be stopped after 1 wk unless seizures occur.

If seizures begin > 1 wk after head injury, long-term treatment with drugs is required.

Long-term drug therapy: Anticonvulsants may be required indefinitely, but many types of seizures (eg, most febrile seizures, seizures due to alcohol withdrawal, seizures that do not recur) do not require treatment with anticonvulsants.

No single drug controls all types of seizures, and different patients require different drugs. Some patients require multiple drugs. The drugs preferred vary according to type of seizure (see Table 238–4). For more detailed drug-specific information, see Anticonvulsant Choice for Long-Term Treatment on p. 2007.

Surgery: About 10 to 20% of patients have intractable seizures refractory to medical treatment and are potential surgical candidates. If seizures originate from a focal, resectable area in the brain, resection of the epileptic focus usually improves seizure control markedly. If the focus is in the anteromesial temporal lobe, resection eliminates seizures in about 60% of patients. After surgical resection, some patients remain seizure-free without taking anticonvulsants, but many still require the drugs, but in reduced doses and possibly as monotherapy.

Because surgery requires extensive testing and monitoring, these patients are best treated in specialized epilepsy centers.

Vagus nerve stimulation: Intermittent electrical stimulation of the left vagus nerve with an implanted pacemaker-like device (vagus nerve stimulator) is used as an adjunct to drug therapy in patients who have intractable seizures and are not candidates for epilepsy surgery. This procedure reduces the number of partial seizures by ≥ 50% in about 40%. After the device is programmed, patients can activate it with a magnet to abort an imminent seizure.

Adverse effects of vagus nerve stimulation include deepening of the voice during stimulation, cough, and hoarseness. Complications are minimal.

Duration of effectiveness is unclear.

KEY POINTS

- Common causes of seizures include birth defects or injuries, developmental defects, and metabolic disorders in children < 2 yr; idiopathic seizure disorders in children 2 to 14 yr; head trauma, alcohol withdrawal, tumors, and strokes in adults; and tumors and strokes in the elderly.
- Loss of consciousness is likely to be caused by seizures if patients have bitten their tongue, are incontinent (eg, urine or feces in clothing), or are confused for a long time after loss of consciousness.
- Evaluate patients with seizures for signs of possible causes (eg, fever, stiff neck, focal neurologic deficits, neuromuscular irritability and hyperreflexia, papilledema), and test accordingly.
- Evaluate all patients who have new or unexplained seizures with neuroimaging, EEG, and blood tests.

- Talk to patients about how to avoid or minimize seizure triggers and how to reduce risk of seizure complications (eg, by not driving and not swimming alone).
- Anticonvulsants may be required indefinitely, but many types of seizures (eg, most febrile seizures, seizures due to alcohol withdrawal, seizures that do not recur) do not require anticonvulsant treatment.
- Consider surgery if therapeutic doses of ≥ 2 anticonvulsants do not control seizures.

DRUG TREATMENT OF SEIZURES

No single drug controls all types of seizures, and different patients require different drugs. Some patients require multiple drugs. (See also the practice guideline for the treatment of refractory epilepsy from the American Academy of Neurology and the American Epilepsy Society.)

Principles of Long-Term Treatment

There are some general principles for using anticonvulsants:

- A single drug, usually the 1st or 2nd one tried, controls epileptic seizures in about 60% of patients.
- If seizures are difficult to control from the outset (in 30 to 40% of patients), ≥ 2 drugs may eventually be required.
- If seizures are intractable (refractory to an adequate trial of ≥ 2 drugs), patients should be referred to an epilepsy center to determine whether they are candidates for surgery.

Some drugs (eg, phenytoin, valproate), given IV or orally, reach the targeted therapeutic range very rapidly. Others (eg, lamotrigine, topiramate) must be started at a relatively low dose and gradually increased over several weeks to the standard therapeutic dose, based on the patient's lean body mass. Dose should be tailored to the patient's tolerance of the drug. Some patients have symptoms of drug toxicity when blood drug levels are low; others tolerate high levels without symptoms. If seizures continue, the daily dose is increased by small increments.

The appropriate dose of any drug is the lowest dose that stops all seizures and has the fewest adverse effects, regardless of blood drug level. Blood drug levels are only guidelines. Once drug response is known, following the clinical course is more useful than measuring blood levels.

If toxicity develops before seizures are controlled, the dose is reduced to the pretoxicity dose. Then, another drug is added at a low dose, which is gradually increased until seizures are controlled. Patients should be closely monitored because the 2 drugs can interact, interfering with either drug's rate of metabolic degradation. The initial drug is then slowly tapered and eventually withdrawn completely.

Use of multiple drugs should be avoided if possible because incidence of adverse effects, poor adherence, and drug interactions increases significantly. Adding a 2nd drug helps about 10% of patients, but incidence of adverse effects more than doubles. The blood level of anticonvulsants is altered by many other drugs, and vice versa. Physicians should be aware of all potential drug-drug interactions before prescribing a new drug.

Once seizures are controlled, the drug should be continued without interruption until patients have been seizure-free for at least 2 yr. At that time, stopping the drug may be considered. Most of these drugs can be tapered by 10% every 2 wk. Relapse is more likely in patients who have had any of the following:

- A seizure disorder since childhood
- Need for > 1 drug to be seizure-free
- Previous seizures while taking an anticonvulsant
- Partial or myoclonic seizures
- Underlying static encephalopathy
- Abnormal EEG results within the last year
- Structural lesions (seen on imaging studies)

Of patients who relapse, about 60% do so within 1 yr, and 80% within 2 yr. Patients who have a relapse when they are not taking anticonvulsants should be treated indefinitely.

Anticonvulsant Choice for Long-Term Treatment

The drugs preferred vary according to type of seizure (see Table 238–4). For more detailed drug-specific information, see p. 2009. Traditionally, drugs have been separated into older and newer groups based on when they became available. However, some so-called newer drugs have been available for many years now.

Broad-spectrum anticonvulsants (which are effective for partial seizures and various types of generalized seizures) include lamotrigine, levetiracetam, topiramate, valproate, and zonisamide.

For **partial seizures** and **generalized tonic-clonic seizures,** the newer anticonvulsants (eg, clobazam, clonazepam, ezogabine, felbamate, lacosamide, lamotrigine, levetiracetam, oxcarbazepine, pregabalin, tiagabine, topiramate, zonisamide) are no more effective than the established drugs. However, the newer drugs tend to have fewer adverse effects and to be better tolerated.

Infantile spasms, atonic seizures, and **myoclonic seizures** are difficult to treat. Valproate or vigabatrin is preferred, followed by clonazepam. For infantile spasms, corticosteroids for 8 to 10 wk are often effective. The optimal regimen is controversial. ACTH 20 to 60 units IM once/day may be used. A ketogenic diet (a very high fat diet that induces ketosis) may help but is difficult to maintain.

For **juvenile myoclonic epilepsy,** life-long treatment is usually recommended. Carbamazepine, oxcarbazepine, or gabapentin can exacerbate the seizures.

For **febrile seizures,** drugs are not recommended unless children have a subsequent seizure in the absence of febrile illness. Previously, many physicians gave phenobarbital or other anticonvulsants to children with complicated febrile seizures to prevent nonfebrile seizures from developing, but this treatment does not appear effective, and long-term use of phenobarbital reduces learning capacity.

For **seizures due to alcohol withdrawal,** drugs are not recommended. Instead, treating the withdrawal syndrome tends to prevent seizures. Treatment usually includes a benzodiazepine.

Adverse effects: The different adverse effects of anticonvulsants may influence the choice of anticonvulsant for an individual patient. For example, anticonvulsants that cause weight gain (eg, valproate) may not be the best option for an overweight patient, and topiramate or zonisamide may not be suitable for patients with history of kidney stones.

Some adverse effects of anticonvulsants can be minimized by increasing the dose gradually.

Overall, the newer anticonvulsants have advantages, such as better tolerability, less sedation, and fewer drug interactions.

All anticonvulsants may cause an allergic scarlatiniform or morbilliform rash.

Some types of seizures may be worsened by anticonvulsants. For example, pregabalin and lamotrigine may worsen myoclonic seizures; carbamazepine may worsen absence, myoclonic, and atonic seizures.

Other adverse effects vary by drug (see pp. 2009–2012).

Anticonvulsant use during pregnancy: Anticonvulsants are associated with an increased risk of teratogenicity.

Table 238–4. CHOICE OF DRUGS FOR SEIZURES

TYPE	DRUGS	USE
Primarily generalized tonic-clonic seizures	Divalproex Valproate	First-line monotherapy
	Lamotrigine Levetiracetam Topiramate	2nd-line monotherapy or adjunctive therapy
	Perampanel Zonisamide	Adjunctive therapy
	Phenobarbital	Although effective, often considered 2nd-line monotherapy because it is sedating and can cause behavioral and learning problems in children
Partial seizures with or without secondary generalization	Carbamazepine Lamotrigine Levetiracetam Oxcarbazepine Fosphenytoin Phenytoin Topiramate	First-line monotherapy
	Divalproex Eslicarbazepine Gabapentin Lacosamide Perampanel Pregabalin Valproate Zonisamide	2nd-line monotherapy or adjunctive therapy
	Clobazam Ezogabine Felbamate Tiagabine Vigabatrin	3rd-line monotherapy or adjunctive therapy
	Phenobarbital	Although effective, often considered less desirable because it is sedating and can cause behavioral problems in children
Typical absence seizures	Divalproex Ethosuximide Lamotrigine Valproate	First-line monotherapy
	Clobazam Levetiracetam Topiramate Zonisamide	Also effective
Atypical absence seizures Absence seizures associated with other seizure types	Divalproex Felbamate Lamotrigine Topiramate Valproate	First-line monotherapy
	Clonazepam	Also effective, but often development of tolerance
	Acetazolamide	Reserved for refractory cases
Infantile spasms Atonic seizures Myoclonic seizures	Divalproex Valproate Vigabatrin	First-line monotherapy; risk of irreversible visual field defects
	Clonazepam	2nd-line
Tonic and/or atonic seizures in Lennox-Gastaut syndrome	Divalproex Lamotrigine Topiramate Valproate	First-line monotherapy
	Clobazam Felbamate Zonisamide	Sometimes alternative or adjunctive therapy for atonic seizures

Table 238–4. CHOICE OF DRUGS FOR SEIZURES (*Continued*)

TYPE	DRUGS	USE
Juvenile myoclonic epilepsy	Divalproex Valproate	First-line monotherapy
	Lamotrigine Levetiracetam Topiramate Zonisamide	2nd-line monotherapy or adjunctive therapy
Unclassifiable seizures	Divalproex Valproate	First-line monotherapy
	Lamotrigine	2nd-line monotherapy
	Levetiracetam Topiramate Zonisamide	3rd-line monotherapy or adjunctive therapy

Fetal antiepileptic drug syndrome (cleft lip, cleft palate, cardiac defects, microcephaly, growth retardation, developmental delay, abnormal facies, limb or digit hypoplasia) occurs in 4% of children of women who take anticonvulsants during pregnancy.

Yet, because uncontrolled generalized seizures during pregnancy can lead to fetal injury and death, continued treatment with drugs is generally advisable (see p. 2399). Women should be informed of the risks of anticonvulsants to the fetus, and the risk should be put in perspective: Alcohol is more toxic to the developing fetus than any anticonvulsant. Taking folate supplements before conception helps reduce risk of neural tube defects and should be recommended to all women who are of childbearing age and who take anticonvulsants.

Many anticonvulsants decrease folate and B_{12} serum levels; oral vitamin supplements can prevent this effect.

Risk of teratogenicity is less with monotherapy and varies by anticonvulsant; none is completely safe during pregnancy (see p. 2399). Risk with carbamazepine, phenytoin, and valproate is relatively high; there is evidence that they have caused congenital malformations in humans (see Table 283–1 on p. 2360). Risk of neural tube defects is somewhat greater with valproate than other commonly used anticonvulsants. Risk with some of the newer drugs (eg, lamotrigine) seems to be less.

Specific Anticonvulsants

Dosing for adults is based on a weight of 70 kg if not specified.

Acetazolamide: This drug is indicated for refractory absence seizures.

Dosage is

- Adults: 4 to 15 mg/kg po bid (not to exceed 1g/day)
- Children: 4 to 15 mg/kg po bid (not to exceed 1g/day)

Therapeutic and toxic levels are

- Therapeutic: 8 to 14 µg/mL (34 to 59 µmol/L)
- Toxic: > 25 µg/mL (> 106 µmol/L)

Adverse effects include renal calculi, dehydration, and metabolic acidosis.

Carbamazepine: This drug is indicated for partial, generalized, and mixed seizures but not absence, myoclonic, or atonic seizures.

Dosage is

- Adults: 200 to 600 mg po bid (starting dose is the same for regular and extended-release tablets)
- Children < 6 yr: 5 to 10 mg/kg po bid (tablets) or 2.5 to 5 mg/kg po qid (suspension)
- Children 6 to 12 yr: 100 mg po bid (tablets) or 2.5 mL (50 mg) po qid (suspension)
- Children > 12 yr: 200 mg po bid (tablets) or 5 mL (100 mg) po qid (suspension)

Therapeutic and toxic levels are

- Therapeutic: 4 to 12 µg/mL (17 to 51 µmol/L)
- Toxic: > 14 µg/mL (> 59 µmol/L)

Adverse effects include diplopia, dizziness, nystagmus, GI upset, dysarthria, lethargy, a low WBC count (3000 to 4000/µL), and severe rash (in 5%). Idiosyncratic adverse effects include granulocytopenia, thrombocytopenia, liver toxicity, and aplastic anemia.

If people have the HLA-B*1502 allele, particularly Asians, risk of severe rash (Stevens-Johnson syndrome or toxic-epidermal necrolysis) is higher than the usual rate of 5%. Thus, before prescribing carbamazepine, clinicians should test for HLAs, at least in Asians.

CBC should be monitored routinely for the first year of therapy. Decreases in WBC count and dose-dependent neutropenia (neutrophil count < 1000/µL) are common. Sometimes, if no other drug can be readily substituted, decreasing the dose can manage these effects. However, if the WBC count decreases rapidly, carbamazepine should be stopped.

Clobazam: This drug is indicated for absence seizures; it is indicated as adjunctive therapy for tonic or atonic seizures in Lennox-Gastaut syndrome and for refractory partial seizures with or without secondary generalization.

Dosage is

- Adults: 5 mg to 20 mg po bid
- Children: 5 to 10 mg po bid (up to 20 mg po bid in children > 30 kg)

Therapeutic levels are not clearly defined.

Adverse effects include somnolence, sedation, constipation, ataxia, suicidal thoughts, drug dependency, irritability, and dysphagia.

Clonazepam: This drug is indicated for atypical absence seizures in Lennox-Gastaut syndrome, atonic and myoclonic seizures, infantile spasms, and possibly absence seizures refractory to ethosuximide.

Dosage is

- Adults: Initially, 0.5 mg po tid, up to 5 to 7 mg po tid for maintenance (maximum: 20 mg/day)
- Children: Initially, 0.01 mg/kg po bid to tid (maximum: 0.05 mg/kg/day), increased by 0.25 to 0.5 mg every 3 days until seizures are controlled or adverse effects occur (usual maintenance dose: 0.03 to 0.06 mg/kg po tid)

Therapeutic and toxic levels are

- Therapeutic: 25 to 30 ng/mL
- Toxic: > 80 ng/mL

Adverse effects include drowsiness, ataxia, behavioral abnormalities, and partial or complete tolerance to beneficial effects (usually in 1 to 6 mo); serious reactions rare.

Divalproex: This drug is a compound composed of sodium valproate and valproic acid and has the same indications as valproate; ie, it is indicated for absence seizures (typical and atypical), partial seizures, tonic-clonic seizures, myoclonic seizures, juvenile myoclonic epilepsy, infantile spasms, and neonatal or febrile seizures. It is also indicated for tonic or atonic seizures in Lennox-Gastaut syndrome.

Dosage is

- Adults: 5 mg/kg po tid, increased slowly—eg, by 1.67 to 3.33 mg/kg po tid at weekly intervals, especially if other drugs are being taken (maximum: 20 mg/kg tid)
- Children: Initially, 5 mg/kg po bid or tid, increased by 5 to 10 mg/kg/day at weekly intervals (usual maintenance dose: 10 to 20 mg/kg po tid)

Children may be given delayed (slow)-release tablets for once/day dosing. The total daily dose is 8 to 20% higher than that for the regular tablets. Delayed-release divalproex may have fewer adverse effects, possibly improving adherence.

Therapeutic and toxic levels are

- Therapeutic levels: 50 to 100 μg/mL (347 to 693 μmol/L) before the AM dose
- Toxic levels: > 150 μg/mL (> 1041 μmol/L)

Adverse effects include nausea and vomiting, GI intolerance, weight gain, reversible alopecia (in 5%), transient drowsiness, transient neutropenia, and tremor. Hyperammonemic encephalopathy may occur idiosyncratically. Rarely, fatal hepatic necrosis occurs, particularly in young neurologically impaired children treated with multiple anticonvulsants. Risk of neural tube defects is somewhat greater with valproate than other commonly used anticonvulsants.

Because hepatic side effects are possible, patients taking divalproex should have liver function tests every 3 mo for 1 yr; if serum transaminases or ammonia levels increase significantly (> 2 times the upper limit of normal), the drug should be stopped. An increase in ammonia up to 1.5 times the upper limit of normal can be tolerated safely.

Ethosuximide: This drug is indicated for absence seizures.

Dosage is

- Adults: 250 mg po bid, increased in 250-mg increments every 4 to 7 days (usual maximum: 1500 mg/day)
- Children 3 to 6 yr: 250 mg po once/day (usual maximum: 20 to 40 mg/kg/day)
- Children > 6 yr: Initially, 250 mg po bid, increased by 250 mg/day as needed every 4 to 7 days (usual maximum: 1500 mg/day)

Therapeutic and toxic levels are

- Therapeutic: 40 to 100 μg/mL (283 to 708 μmol/L)
- Toxic: > 100 μg/mL (> 708 μmol/L)

Toxic levels have not been well-established.

Adverse effects include nausea, lethargy, dizziness, and headache. Idiosyncratic adverse effects include leukocytopenia or pancytopenia, dermatitis, and SLE.

Eslicarbazepine: This drug is indicated for treatment of partial seizures as monotherapy or adjunctive therapy.

Dosage is

- Initially, 400 mg po once/day, increased by 400 mg to 600 mg/day at weekly intervals to a recommended maintenance dose of 800 to 1600 mg once/day

Eslicarbazepine is not indicated for use in patients < 18 yr.

Adverse effects include dizziness, diplopia, somnolence, hyponatremia, suicidal ideation, and dermatologic reactions, including Stevens-Johnson syndrome.

Ezogabine: This drug is indicated for partial seizures as 3rd-line monotherapy or adjunctive therapy.

Dosage is

- Adults: 200 to 400 mg po tid

Ezogabine is not indicated for use in patients < 18 yr.

No significant relationship between blood levels and pharmacologic effect has been observed.

Adverse effects include urinary retention, neuropsychiatric symptoms (eg, confusion, psychosis, hallucinations, suicidal thoughts), retinal abnormalities, QT prolongation, dizziness, and somnolence.

Felbamate: This drug is indicated for refractory partial seizures and atypical absence seizures in Lennox-Gastaut syndrome.

Dosage is

- Adults: Initially, 400 mg po tid (maximum: 3600 mg/day)
- Children: Initially, 15 mg/kg/day po (maximum: 45 mg/kg/day)

Therapeutic and toxic levels are

- Therapeutic: 30 to 60 μg/mL (125 to 250 μmol/L)
- Toxic: Not applicable

Adverse effects include headache, fatigue, liver failure, and, rarely, aplastic anemia. Written informed consent is required from the patient.

Fosphenytoin: This drug is indicated for status epilepticus. It also has the same indications as IV phenytoin. They include tonic-clonic seizures, complex partial seizures, prevention of seizures secondary to head trauma, and convulsive status epilepticus.

Dosage is

- Adults: 10 to 20 phenytoin equivalents (PE)/kg IV or IM once (maximum infusion rate: 150 PE/min)
- Children: Same as that for adults

Heart rate and BP must be monitored if the maximum infusion rate is used, but not at slower rates.

Therapeutic and toxic levels are

- Therapeutic: 10 to 20 μg/mL (40 to 80 μmol/L)
- Toxic: > 25 μg/mL (> 99 μmol/L)

Adverse effects include ataxia, dizziness, somnolence, headache, pruritus, and paresthesias.

Gabapentin: This drug is indicated as adjunctive therapy for partial seizures in patients aged 3 to 12 yr and as adjunctive therapy for partial seizures with or without secondarily generalized tonic-clonic seizures in patients aged ≥ 12 yr.

Dosage is

- Adults: 300 mg po tid (usual maximum: 1200 mg tid)
- Children 3 to 12 yr: 12.5 to 20 mg/kg po bid (usual maximum: 50 mg/kg bid)
- Children ≥ 12 yr: 300 mg po tid (usual maximum: 1200 mg tid)

Therapeutic and toxic levels have not been determined.

Adverse effects include drowsiness, dizziness, weight gain, and headache and, in patients aged 3 to 12 yr, somnolence, aggressive behavior, mood lability, and hyperactivity.

Lacosamide: This drug is indicated as 2nd-line monotherapy or adjunctive therapy for partial seizures in patients ≥ 17 yr.

Dosage is

- Adults: 100 to 200 mg po bid

Lacosamide is not indicated for use in children < 17 yr.

Therapeutic and toxic levels are

- Therapeutic: 5 to 10 ug/mL
- Toxic: Not well-established

Adverse effects include dizziness, diplopia, and suicidal thoughts.

Lamotrigine: This drug is indicated as adjunctive therapy for partial seizures in patients ≥ 2 yr, generalized seizures in Lennox-Gastaut syndrome, and primarily generalized tonic-clonic seizures. In patients ≥ 16 yr, lamotrigine is used as substitution monotherapy for partial or secondarily generalized seizures after a concomitantly used enzyme-inducing anticonvulsant (eg, carbamazepine, phenytoin, phenobarbital) or valproate is stopped.

The metabolism of the lamotrigine is increased by enzyme-inducing anticonvulsants and decreased by enzyme-inhibiting anticonvulsants (eg, valproate). Valproate inhibits a broad-spectrum of hepatic enzymes. Lamotrigine may have a special synergistic effect when used with valproate.

Dosage in adults is

- With enzyme-inducing anticonvulsants and without valproate: 50 mg po once/day for 2 wk, followed by 50 mg po bid for 2 wk, then increased by 100 mg/day every 1 to 2 wk to the usual maintenance dose (150 to 250 mg po bid)
- With valproate and with or without enzyme-inducing anticonvulsants: 25 mg po once every other day for 2 wk, followed by 25 mg po once/day for 2 wk, then increased by 25 to 50 mg/day every 1 to 2 wk to the usual maintenance dose (100 mg po once/day to 200 mg po bid)

Dosage in patients < 16 yr is

- With enzyme-inducing anticonvulsants and without valproate: Initially, 1 mg/kg po bid for 2 wk, followed by 2.5 mg/kg po bid for 2 wk, then 5 mg/kg po bid (usual maximum: 15 mg/kg or 250 mg/day)
- With enzyme-inducing anticonvulsants and valproate: Initially, 0.1 mg/kg po bid for 2 wk, followed by 0.2 mg/kg po bid for 2 wk, then 0.5 mg/kg po bid (usual maximum: 5 mg/kg or 250 mg/day)
- With valproate and without enzyme-inducing anticonvulsants: Initially, 0.1 to 0.2 mg/kg po bid for 2 wk, followed by 0.1 to 0.25 mg/kg po bid for 2 wk, then 0.25 to 0.5 mg/kg po bid (usual maximum: 2 mg/kg or 150 mg/day)

No significant relationship between blood levels and pharmacologic effect has been observed.

Common adverse effects include headache, dizziness, drowsiness, insomnia, fatigue, nausea, vomiting, diplopia, ataxia, tremor, menstrual abnormalities, and rash (in 2 to 3%), which sometimes progresses to Stevens-Johnson syndrome (in 1/50 to 100 children and 1/1000 adults). Risk of rash can be reduced by increasing the dosage more slowly, especially if lamotrigine is added to valproate. Lamotrigine may exacerbate myoclonic seizures in adults.

Levetiracetam: This drug is indicated as adjunctive therapy for the following: partial seizures in patients ≥ 4 yr, primarily generalized tonic-clonic seizures in patients > 6 yr, myoclonic seizures in patients > 12 yr, and juvenile myoclonic epilepsy.

Dosage is

- Adults: 500 mg po bid (maximum: 2000 mg bid)
- Children: 250 mg po bid (maximum: 1500 mg bid)

No significant relationship between blood levels and pharmacologic effect has been observed.

Adverse effects include fatigue, weakness, ataxia, and mood and behavioral changes.

Oxcarbazepine: This drug is indicated for partial seizures in patients aged 4 to 16 yr as adjunctive therapy and for partial seizures in adults.

Dosage is

- Adults: 300 mg po bid, increased by 300 mg bid at weekly intervals as needed to 1200 mg po bid
- Children: Initially, 4 to 15 mg/kg po bid, then increased over 2 wk to 15 mg/kg po bid (the usual maintenance dose)

The **therapeutic level** is

- 15 to 25 µg/mL

Adverse effects include fatigue, nausea, abdominal pain, headache, dizziness, somnolence, leukopenia, diplopia, and hyponatremia (in 2.5%).

Perampanel: This drug is indicated as adjunctive therapy for partial seizures and primarily generalized tonic-clonic seizures in people who have epilepsy and are ≥ 12 yr.

Dosage is

- Initially, 2 mg po once/day, increased by 2 mg/day at weekly intervals, based on clinical response and tolerability, until reaching the recommended maintenance dose of 8 to 12 mg once/day for partial seizures and 8 mg once/day for primarily generalized seizures

Perampanel is not indicated for use in children < 12 yr.

Adverse effects include aggressiveness, mood and behavioral changes, suicidal ideation, dizziness, and gait disturbances.

Phenobarbital: This drug is indicated for generalized tonic-clonic seizures, partial seizures, status epilepticus, and neonatal seizures.

Dosage is usually once/day, but divided doses may be used. For all indications except status epilepticus, dose is

- Adults: 1.5 to 4 mg/kg po at bedtime
- Neonates: 3 to 4 mg/kg po once/day, then increased (based on clinical response and blood levels)
- Infants: 5 to 8 mg/kg po once/day
- Children 1 to 5 yr: 3 to 5 mg/kg po once/day
- Children 6 to 12 yr: 4 to 6 mg/kg po once/day

Dosage for status epilepticus is

- Adults: 15 to 20 mg/kg IV (maximum infusion rate: 60 mg/min or 2 mg/kg/min)
- Children: 10 to 20 mg/kg IV (maximum infusion rate: 100 mg/min or 2 mg/kg/min)

Therapeutic and toxic levels are

- Therapeutic: 10 to 40 µg/mL (43 to 129 µmol/L)
- Toxic: > 40 µg/mL (> 151 µmol/L)

Adverse effects include drowsiness, nystagmus, ataxia, and learning difficulties and, in children, paradoxical hyperactivity. Idiosyncratic adverse effects include anemia and rash.

Phenytoin: This drug is indicated for secondarily generalized tonic-clonic seizures, complex partial seizures, and convulsive status epilepticus. It is also used to prevent seizures secondary to head trauma.

Dosage for all indications except status epilepticus is

- Adults: 4 to 7 mg/kg po at bedtime
- Neonates: Initially, 2.5 mg/kg po bid (usual maintenance: 2.5 to 4 mg/kg po bid)

Dosage for status epilepticus is

- Adults: 15 to 20 mg/kg IV
- Children 6 mo to 3 yr: 8 to10 mg/kg IV
- Children 4 to 6 yr: 7.5 to 9 mg/kg IV
- Children 7 to 9 yr: 7 to 8 mg/kg IV
- Children 10 to 16 yr: 6 to 7 mg/kg IV

The maximum infusion rate is 1 to 3 mg/kg/min for children (up to 16 yr) and 50 mg/min for adults.

Therapeutic and toxic levels are

- Therapeutic: 10 to 20 μg/mL (40 to 80 μmol/L)
- Toxic: > 25 μg/mL (> 99 μmol/L)

Adverse effects include megaloblastic anemia, gingival hyperplasia, hirsutism, adenopathy, and loss of bone density. Folic acid supplements (0.5 mg/day) can markedly lessen gingival hyperplasia. At high blood levels, phenytoin can cause nystagmus, ataxia, dysarthria, lethargy, irritability, nausea, vomiting, and confusion. Idiosyncratic adverse effects include rash, exfoliative dermatitis, and, rarely, exacerbation of seizures.

Pregabalin: This drug is indicated as adjunctive therapy for partial seizures.

Dosage is

- Adults: Initially, 50 mg po tid or 75 mg po bid, increased as needed and tolerated to 200 mg po tid or 300 mg po bid (maximum: 600 mg/day)

Pregabalin is not indicated for use in children < 18 yr.

No significant relationship between blood levels and pharmacologic effect has been observed.

Adverse effects include dizziness, somnolence, ataxia, blurred vision, diplopia, tremor, and weight gain. Pregabalin may exacerbate myoclonic seizures.

Tiagabine: This drug is indicated as adjunctive therapy for partial seizures in patients ≥ 12 yr.

Dosage is

- Adults: 4 mg once/day po, increased by 4 to 8 mg/day at weekly intervals to 28 mg po bid or 14 mg po qid (maximum: 56 mg/day)
- Children ≥ 12 yr: 4 mg po once/day, increased by 4 mg/day as needed at weekly intervals to 16 mg po bid or 8 mg po qid (maximum: 32 mg/day)

No significant relationship between blood levels and pharmacologic effect has been observed.

Adverse effects include dizziness, light-headedness, confusion, slowed thinking, fatigue, tremor, sedation, nausea, and abdominal pain.

Topiramate: This drug is indicated for partial seizures in patients ≥ 2 yr, for atypical absence seizures, and as 2nd-line monotherapy or adjunctive therapy for primarily generalized tonic-clonic seizures.

Dosage is

- Adults: 50 mg po once/day, increased by 25 to 50 mg/day every 1 to 2 wk (usual maximum: 200 mg bid)
- Children 2 to 16 yr: 0.5 to 1.5 mg/kg po bid (maximum: 25 mg/day)

Therapeutic level is

- 5 to 20 mg/mL (probably)

Adverse effects include decreased concentration, paresthesias, fatigue, speech dysfunction, confusion, anorexia, weight loss, reduced sweating, metabolic acidosis, nephrolithiasis (in 1 to 5%), and psychosis (in 1%).

Valproate: This drug is indicated for absence seizures (typical and atypical), partial seizures, tonic-clonic seizures, myoclonic seizures, juvenile myoclonic epilepsy, infantile spasms, and neonatal or febrile seizures. It is also indicated for tonic or atonic seizures in Lennox-Gastaut syndrome. Valproate inhibits a broad-spectrum of hepatic enzymes.

Dosage is

- Adults: 5 mg/kg po tid, increased slowly—eg, by 1.67 to 3.33 mg/kg tid at weekly intervals, especially if other drugs are being taken (maximum: 20 mg/kg tid)
- Children: Initially, 5 mg/kg po bid or tid, increased by 5 to 10 mg/kg/day at weekly intervals (usual maintenance: 10 to 20 mg/kg tid)

Therapeutic and toxic levels are

- Therapeutic levels: 50 to 100 μg/mL (347 to 693 μmol/L) before the AM dose
- Toxic levels: > 150 μg/mL (> 1041 μmol/L)

Adverse effects include nausea and vomiting, GI intolerance, weight gain, reversible alopecia (in 5%), transient drowsiness, transient neutropenia, and tremor. Hyperammonemic encephalopathy may occur idiosyncratically. Rarely, fatal hepatic necrosis occurs, particularly in young neurologically impaired children treated with multiple anticonvulsants. Risk of neural tube defects is somewhat greater with valproate than other commonly used anticonvulsants.

Because hepatic adverse effects are possible, patients taking valproate should have liver function tests every 3 mo for 1 yr; if serum transaminases or ammonia levels increase significantly (> 2 times the upper limit of normal), the drug should be stopped. An increase in ammonia up to 1.5 times the upper limit of normal can be tolerated safely.

Vigabatrin: This drug is indicated as adjunctive therapy for partial seizures; it is also indicated for infantile spasms.

Dosage is

- Adults: Initially, 0.5 to 1.0 g/day po, increased by 0.5 to 1.0 g every 1 to 2 wk to usual maintenance dose of 2 to 4 g/day
- Children: Titrated up to 100 mg/kg/day po in 1 wk, then usual maintenance dose of 100 to150 mg/kg/day

No significant relationship between blood levels and pharmacologic effect has been observed.

Adverse effects include drowsiness, dizziness, headache, fatigue, and irreversible visual field defects (requires regular visual field evaluations).

Zonisamide: This drug is indicated as adjunctive therapy for partial seizures in patients ≥ 16 yr; it is also indicated as alternative or adjunctive therapy for tonic or atonic seizures in Lennox-Gastaut syndrome.

Dosage is

- Adults: 100 mg po once/day, increased up to 100 mg/day every 2 wk (maximum: 300 mg bid)

Zonisamide is not commonly used in children < 16 yr.

Therapeutic and toxic levels are

- Therapeutic levels: 15 to 40 μg/mL (at > 30 μg/mL, CNS adverse effects are possibly increased)
- Toxic levels: > 40 μg/mL

Adverse effects include sedation, fatigue, dizziness, ataxia, confusion, cognitive impairment (eg, impaired word finding), weight loss, anorexia, and nausea. Less commonly, zonisamide causes depression, psychosis, urinary calculi, and oligohidrosis.

239 Sleep and Wakefulness Disorders

Almost half of all people in the US report sleep-related problems. Disordered sleep can cause emotional disturbance, memory difficulty, poor motor skills, decreased work efficiency, and increased risk of traffic accidents. It can even contribute to cardiovascular disorders and mortality.

APPROACH TO THE PATIENT WITH A SLEEP OR WAKEFULNESS DISORDER

The most commonly reported sleep-related symptoms are insomnia and excessive daytime sleepiness (EDS).

- **Insomnia** is difficulty falling or staying asleep, early awakening, or a sensation of unrefreshing sleep.
- **EDS** is the tendency to fall asleep during normal waking hours.

EDS is not a disorder but a symptom of various sleep-related disorders. Insomnia can be a disorder, even if it exists in the context of other disorders, or can be a symptom of other disorders. Parasomnias are abnormal sleep-related events (eg, night terrors, sleepwalking—see p. 2024).

Pathophysiology

There are 2 states of sleep, each marked by characteristic physiologic changes:

- **Nonrapid eye movement (NREM):** NREM sleep constitutes about 75 to 80% of total sleep time in adults. It consists of 3 stages (N1 to N3) in increasing depth of sleep. Slow, rolling eye movements, which characterize quiet wakefulness and early stage N1 sleep, disappear in deeper sleep stages. Muscle activity also decreases. Stage N3 is referred to as deep sleep because arousal threshold is high; people may perceive this stage as high-quality sleep.
- **Rapid eye movement (REM):** REM sleep follows each cycle of NREM sleep. It is characterized by low-voltage fast activity on the EEG and postural muscle atonia. Respiration rate and depth fluctuate dramatically. Most dreams occur during REM sleep.

Progression through the 3 stages, typically followed by a brief interval of REM sleep, occurs cyclically 5 to 6 times a night (see Fig. 239–1). Brief periods of wakefulness (stage W) occur periodically.

Individual sleep requirements vary widely, ranging from 6 to 10 h/24 h. Infants sleep a large part of the day; with aging, total sleep time and deep sleep tend to decrease, and sleep becomes more interrupted. In the elderly, stage N3 may disappear. These changes may account for increasing EDS and fatigue with aging, but their clinical significance is unclear.

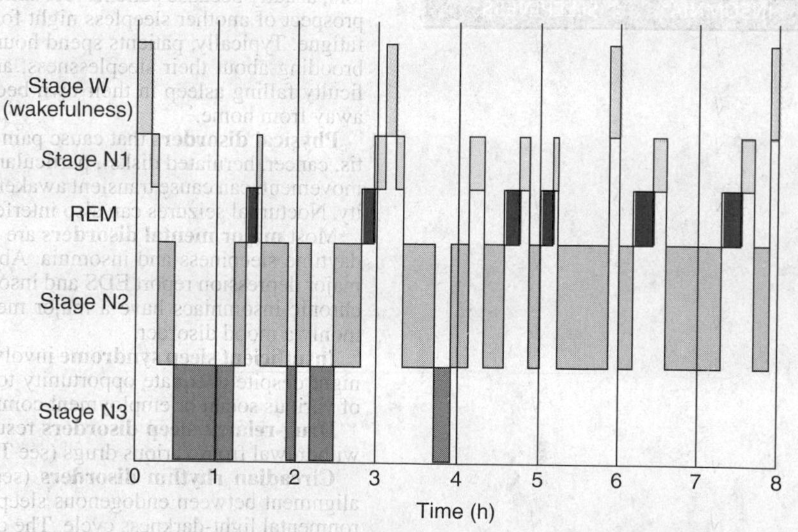

Fig. 239–1. Typical sleep pattern in young adults. Rapid eye movement (REM) sleep occurs cyclically throughout the night every 90–120 min. Brief periods of wakefulness (stage W) occur periodically. Sleep time is spent as follows:

- Stage N1: 2–5%
- Stage N2: 45–55%
- Stage N3: 13–23%
- REM: 20–25%

Etiology

Some disorders can cause either insomnia or EDS (sometimes both), and some cause one or the other (see Table 239–1).

Insomnia (see p. 2022) is most often caused by

- An insomnia disorder (eg, adjustment sleep disorder, psychophysiologic insomnia)
- Inadequate sleep hygiene
- Psychiatric disorders, particularly mood, anxiety, and substance use disorders
- Miscellaneous medical disorders such as cardiopulmonary disorders, musculoskeletal conditions, and chronic pain

Excessive daytime sleepiness (see p. 2022) is most often caused by

- Insufficient sleep syndrome
- Obstructive sleep apnea (OSA)
- Miscellaneous medical, neurologic, and psychiatric disorders
- Circadian rhythm disorders such as jet lag and shift work sleep disorders

Inadequate sleep hygiene refers to behaviors that are not conducive to sleep (see Table 239–5 on p. 2017). They include

- Consumption of caffeine or sympathomimetic or other stimulant drugs (typically near bedtime, but even in the afternoon for people who are particularly sensitive)
- Exercise or excitement (eg, a thrilling TV show) late in the evening
- An irregular sleep-wake schedule

Table 239–1. SOME CAUSES OF INSOMNIA AND EXCESSIVE DAYTIME SLEEPINESS

DISORDER	INSOMNIA	EXCESSIVE DAYTIME SLEEPINESS
Inadequate sleep hygiene	√	√
Adjustment insomnia	√	
Psychophysiologic insomnia	√	
Physical or mental sleep disorders	√	√
Insufficient sleep syndrome		√
Drug-dependent and drug-induced sleep disorders	√	√
Obstructive sleep apnea		√
Central sleep apnea syndrome	√	
Circadian rhythm sleep disorders	√	√
Narcolepsy		√
Periodic limb movement disorder	√	√
Restless legs syndrome	√	

√ = commonly present (but insomnia and/or excessive daytime sleepiness can occur in any of these disorders).

Table 239–2. SOME DRUGS THAT INTERFERE WITH SLEEP

CAUSE	EXAMPLE
Drug use	Alcohol Anticonvulsants (eg, phenytoin) Antimetabolite chemotherapy Certain antidepressants of the SSRI, SNRI, MAOI, and TCA classes CNS stimulants (eg, amphetamines, caffeine) Oral contraceptives Propranolol Steroids (anabolic steroids, corticosteroids) Thyroid hormone preparations
Drug withdrawal	Alcohol Certain antidepressants of the SSRI, SNRI, MAOI, and TCA classes CNS depressants (eg, barbiturates, opioids, sedatives) Illicit drugs (eg, cocaine, heroin, marijuana, phencyclidine)

MAOI = monoamine oxidase inhibitor; SNRI = serotonin-norepinephrine reuptake inhibitor; TCA = tricyclic antidepressant.

Patients who compensate for lost sleep by sleeping late or by napping further fragment their nocturnal sleep.

Adjustment insomnia results from acute emotional stressors (eg, job loss, hospitalization) that disrupt sleep.

Psychophysiologic insomnia is insomnia (regardless of cause) that persists well beyond resolution of precipitating factors, usually because patients feel anticipatory anxiety about the prospect of another sleepless night followed by another day of fatigue. Typically, patients spend hours in bed focusing on and brooding about their sleeplessness, and they have greater difficulty falling asleep in their own bedroom than falling asleep away from home.

Physical disorders that cause pain or discomfort (eg, arthritis, cancer, herniated disks), particularly those that worsen with movement, can cause transient awakenings and poor sleep quality. Nocturnal seizures can also interfere with sleep.

Most **major mental disorders** are associated with excessive daytime sleepiness and insomnia. About 80% of patients with major depression report EDS and insomnia; conversely, 40% of chronic insomniacs have a major mental disorder, most commonly a mood disorder.

Insufficient sleep syndrome involves not sleeping enough at night despite adequate opportunity to do so, typically because of various social or employment commitments.

Drug-related sleep disorders result from chronic use of or withdrawal from various drugs (see Table 239–2).

Circadian rhythm disorders (see p. 2021) result in misalignment between endogenous sleep-wake rhythms and environmental light-darkness cycle. The cause may be external (eg, jet lag disorder, shift work disorder) or internal (eg, delayed or advanced sleep phase disorder).

Central sleep apnea (see p. 514) consists of repeated episodes of breathing cessation or shallow breathing during sleep, lasting at least 10 sec and caused by diminished respiratory effort. The disorder typically manifests as insomnia or as disturbed and unrefreshing sleep.

Obstructive sleep apnea (OSA—see p. 514) consists of episodes of partial or complete closure of the upper airway during sleep, leading to cessation of breathing for ≥ 10 sec. Most patients snore, and sometimes patients awaken, gasping. These episodes disrupt sleep and result in a feeling of unrefreshing sleep and EDS.

Narcolepsy (see p. 2023) is characterized by chronic EDS, often with cataplexy, sleep paralysis, and hypnagogic or hypnopompic hallucinations:

- **Cataplexy** is momentary muscular weakness or paralysis without loss of consciousness that is evoked by sudden emotional reactions (eg, mirth, anger, fear, joy, surprise). Weakness may be confined to the limbs (eg, patients may drop the rod when a fish strikes their line) or may cause a limp fall during hearty laughter (as in "weak with laughter") or sudden anger.
- **Sleep paralysis** is the momentary inability to move when just falling asleep or immediately after awakening.
- **Hypnagogic and hypnopompic phenomena** are vivid auditory or visual illusions or hallucinations that occur when just falling asleep (hypnagogic) or, less often, immediately after awakening (hypnopompic).

Periodic limb movement disorder (PLMD—see p. 2025) is characterized by repetitive (usually every 20 to 40 sec) twitching or kicking of the lower extremities during sleep. Patients usually complain of interrupted nocturnal sleep or EDS. They are typically unaware of the movements and brief arousals that follow, and they have no abnormal sensations in the extremities.

Restless legs syndrome (RLS—see p. 2025) is characterized by an irresistible urge to move the legs and, less frequently, the arms, usually accompanied by paresthesias (eg, creeping or crawling sensations) in the limbs when reclining. To relieve symptoms, patients move the affected extremity by stretching, kicking, or walking. As a result, they have difficulty falling asleep, repeated nocturnal awakenings, or both.

Evaluation

History: History of present illness should include duration and age at onset of symptoms and any events (eg, a life or work change, new drug, new medical disorder) that coincided with onset. Symptoms during sleeping and waking hours should be noted.

The quality and quantity of sleep are identified by determining

- Bedtime
- Latency of sleep (time from bedtime to falling asleep)
- Number and time of awakenings
- Final morning awakening and arising times
- Frequency and duration of naps

Having patients keep a sleep log for several weeks is more accurate than questioning them. Bedtime events (eg, food or alcohol consumption, physical or mental activity) should be evaluated. Intake of and withdrawal from drugs, alcohol, caffeine, and nicotine as well as level and timing of physical activity should also be included.

If EDS is the problem, severity should be quantified based on the propensity for falling asleep in different situations (eg, resting comfortably vs when driving a car). The Epworth Sleepiness Scale (ESS—see Table 239–3) may be used; a cumulative score ≥ 10 represents abnormal daytime sleepiness.

Review of systems should check for symptoms of specific sleep disorders, including

- Snoring, interrupted breathing patterns, and other nocturnal respiratory disturbances (sleep apnea syndromes)
- Depression, anxiety, mania, and hypomania (mental sleep disorders)

Table 239–3. EPWORTH SLEEPINESS SCALE

Situation
Sitting and reading
Watching TV
Sitting inactive in a public place
Riding as a car passenger for 1 h continuously
Lying down to rest in the afternoon
Sitting and talking to someone
Sitting quietly after lunch (no alcohol)
Sitting in a car stopped for a few minutes in traffic

For each situation, probability of dozing is self-rated as none (0), slight (1), moderate (2), or high (3). A score of ≥ 10 suggests abnormal daytime sleepiness.

- Restlessness in the legs, an irresistible desire to move them, and jerking leg movements (RLS)
- Cataplexy, sleep paralysis, and hypnagogic phenomena (narcolepsy)

Bed partners or other family members can best identify some of these symptoms.

Past medical history should check for known disorders that can interfere with sleep, including COPD, asthma, heart failure, hyperthyroidism, gastroesophageal reflux, neurologic disorders (particularly movement and degenerative disorders), and painful disorders (eg, RA). Risk factors for OSA include obesity, heart disorders, hypertension, stroke, smoking, snoring, and nasal trauma. Drug history should include questions about use of any drugs associated with sleep disturbance (see Table 239–2).

Physical examination: The physical examination is useful mainly for identifying signs associated with OSA:

- Obesity with fat distributed around the neck or midriff
- Large neck circumference (≥ 43.2 cm in males, ≥ 40.6 cm in females)
- Mandibular hypoplasia and retrognathia
- Nasal obstruction
- Enlarged tonsils, tongue, uvula, or soft palate (Mallampati score 3 or 4—see Fig. 239–2)
- Decreased pharyngeal patency
- Increased obstruction of uvula and soft palate by the tongue
- Redundant pharyngeal mucosa

The chest should be examined for expiratory wheezes and kyphoscoliosis. Signs of right ventricular failure should be noted. A thorough neurologic examination should be done.

Red flags: The following findings are of particular concern:

- Falling asleep while driving or other potentially dangerous situations
- Repeated sleep attacks (falling asleep without warning)
- Breathing interruptions or awakening with gasping reported by bed partner
- Unstable cardiac or pulmonary status
- Recent stroke
- Status cataplecticus (continuous cataplexy attacks)
- History of violent behaviors or injury to self or others during asleep
- Frequent sleepwalking or other out-of-bed behavior

Interpretation of findings: Inadequate sleep hygiene and situational stressors are usually apparent in the history. EDS that disappears when sleep time is increased (eg, on weekends or vacations) suggests inadequate sleep syndrome. EDS that is accompanied by cataplexy, hypnagogic/hypnopompic hallucinations, or sleep paralysis suggests narcolepsy.

Difficulty falling asleep (sleep-onset insomnia) should be distinguished from difficulty maintaining sleep and early awakening (sleep maintenance insomnia).

Sleep-onset insomnia suggests delayed sleep phase syndrome, chronic psychophysiologic insomnia, RLS, or childhood phobias.

Sleep maintenance insomnia suggests major depression, central or OSA, PLMD, or aging.

Falling asleep early and awakening early suggest advanced sleep phase syndrome.

Clinicians should suspect OSA in patients with significant snoring, frequent awakenings, and other risk factors. The STOP-BANG score can help predict risk of obstructive sleep apnea (see Table 239–4).

Testing: Tests are usually done when specific symptoms or signs suggest OSA, nocturnal seizures, narcolepsy, PLMD, or other disorders whose diagnosis relies on identification of characteristic polysomnographic findings. Tests are also done when the clinical diagnosis is in doubt or when response to initial presumptive treatment is inadequate. If symptoms or signs strongly suggest certain causes (eg, RLS, poor sleep habits, transient stress, shift work disorder), testing is not required.

Polysomnography is particularly useful when OSA, narcolepsy, nocturnal seizures, PLMD, or parasomnias are suspected. It also helps clinicians evaluate violent and potentially injurious sleep-related behaviors. It monitors brain activity (via EEG), eye movements, heart rate, respirations, O_2 saturation, and muscle tone and activity during sleep. Video recording may be used to identify abnormal movements during sleep. Polysomnography is typically done in a sleep laboratory; equipment for home use has been devised but is intended to help diagnose only OSA, not any other sleep disorders.

The **multiple sleep latency test** assesses speed of sleep onset in 5 daytime nap opportunities 2 h apart during the patient's typical daytime. Patients lie in a darkened room and are asked to sleep. Onset and stage of sleep (including REM) are monitored by polysomnography to determine the degree of sleepiness. This test's main use is in the diagnosis of narcolepsy.

For the **maintenance of wakefulness test,** patients are asked to stay awake in a quiet room during 4 wakefulness opportunities 2 h apart while they sit in a bed or a recliner. This test is probably a more accurate measure of ability to remain awake in everyday situations.

Patients with EDS may require laboratory tests of renal, liver, and thyroid function.

Table 239–4. STOP-BANG RISK SCORE FOR OBSTRUCTIVE SLEEP APNEA

ITEM EVALUATED	FINDING
*S*noring	Loud snoring (louder than talking or loud enough to be heard through a closed door)
*T*ired	Often fatigue or sleepiness during the daytime
*O*bserved	Observed to stop breathing during sleep
B*P*	High BP or current treatment for hypertension
*B*MI	> 35 kg/m^2
*A*ge	> 50 yr
*N*eck circumference	> 40 cm (> 15 3/4 in)
*G*ender	Male

≥ 3 findings = high risk of OSA.
< 3 findings = low risk of OSA.
BMI = body mass index; OSA = obstructive sleep apnea.

Treatment

Specific conditions are treated. Good sleep hygiene (see Table 239–5) is important whatever the cause and is often the only treatment patients with mild problems need.

Hypnotics: General guidelines for use of hypnotics (see Table 239–6) aim at minimizing abuse, misuse, and addiction.

For commonly used hypnotics, see Table 239–7. All hypnotics (except ramelteon, low-dose doxepin, and suvorexant) act at the benzodiazepine recognition site on the γ-aminobutyric (GABA) receptor and augment the inhibitory effects of GABA.

Hypnotics differ primarily in elimination half-life and onset of action. Drugs with a short half-life are used for sleep-onset insomnia. Drugs with a longer half-life are useful for both sleep-onset and sleep maintenance insomnia, or, in the case of low-dose doxepin, only for sleep maintenance insomnia. Some hypnotics (eg, older benzodiazepines) have greater potential for daytime carryover effects, especially after prolonged use and/or in the elderly. New drugs with a very short duration of action (low-dose sublingual zolpidem) can be taken in the middle of the night, during a nocturnal awakening, as long as patients stay in bed for at least 4 h after use.

Patients who experience daytime sedation, incoordination, or other daytime effects should avoid activities requiring alertness (eg, driving), and the dose should be reduced, the drug stopped, or, if needed, another drug used. Other adverse effects include amnesia, hallucinations, incoordination, and falls.

Recently approved hypnotics include suvorexant and tasimelteon.

Suvorexant is a new treatment for insomnia that acts by blocking brain orexin receptors, thereby blocking orexin-induced wakefulness signals and enabling sleep initiation. Recommended dose is 10 mg, taken no more than once/night and taken within 30 min of going to bed, with at least 7 h before the planned time of awakening. The dose can be increased but should not to exceed 20 mg once/day. The most common adverse effect is somnolence.

Tasimelteon, a melatonin receptor agonist, can increase nighttime sleep duration and decrease daytime sleep duration in totally blind patients who have non–24-h sleep-wake syndrome. The dose is 20 mg once/day before bedtime, at the same time every night. The most common adverse effects are headaches and abnormal dreams or nightmares. Tasmelteon does not appear to have abuse potential.

Hypnotics should be used cautiously in patients with pulmonary insufficiency. In the elderly, any hypnotic, even in small doses, can cause restlessness, excitement, or exacerbation of delirium and dementia. Rarely, hypnotics can cause complex sleep-related behaviors, such as sleepwalking and even sleep driving; use of higher-than-recommended doses and concurrent consumption of alcoholic beverages may increase risk of such behaviors. Rarely, severe allergic reactions occur.

Prolonged use is typically discouraged because tolerance can develop (see p. 3238) and because abrupt discontinuation

Table 239–5. SLEEP HYGIENE

MEASURE	IMPLEMENTATION
Regular sleep/wake schedule	Bedtime and particularly wake-up time should be the same each day, including weekends. Patients should not spend excessive time in bed.
Appropriate use of the bed	Limiting time in bed improves sleep continuity. If unable to fall sleep within 20 min, patients should get out of bed and return when sleepy. The bed should not be used for activities other than sleep or sex (eg, not for reading, eating, watching television, or paying bills).
Avoidance of daytime naps, except by shift workers, the elderly, and patients with narcolepsy	Daytime naps may aggravate sleeplessness in patients with insomnia. However, naps decrease the need for stimulants in patients with narcolepsy and improve performance in shift workers. Naps should be taken at the same time each day and limited to 30 min.
Regular routine before bedtime	A pattern of activities—brushing teeth, washing, setting the alarm clock—can set the mood for sleep. Bright lights should be avoided before bedtime and during nocturnal awakenings.
Sleep-conducive environment	The bedroom should be dark, quiet, and reasonably cool; it should be used only for sleep and sexual activity. Heavy curtains or a sleep mask can eliminate light, and earplugs, fans, or white-noise devices can help eliminate disturbing noise.
Pillows	Pillows between the knees or under the waist can increase comfort. For patients with back problems, helpful positions include lying supine with a large pillow under the knees and sleeping on one side with a pillow between the knees.
Regular exercise	Exercise promotes sleep and reduces stress, but if done in the late evening, it can stimulate the nervous system and interfere with falling asleep.
Relaxation	Stress and worry interfere with sleep. Reading or taking a warm bath before bedtime can aid relaxation. Techniques such as visual imagery, progressive muscle relaxation, and breathing exercises can be used. Patients should not watch the clock.
Avoidance of stimulants and diuretics	Drinking alcoholic or caffeinated beverages, smoking, eating caffeinated foods (eg, chocolate), and taking appetite suppressants or prescription diuretics—especially near bedtime—should be avoided.
Bright light exposure while awake	Light exposure during the day can help rectify circadian rhythms, but if light exposure is too close to bedtime, it can interfere with sleep.

can cause rebound insomnia or even anxiety, tremor, and seizures. These effects are more common with benzodiazepines (particularly triazolam) and less common with nonbenzodiazepines. Difficulties can be minimized by using the lowest effective dose for brief periods and by tapering the dose before stopping the drug (see also p. 3239). Nevertheless, many patients with chronic insomnia require long-term treatment with hypnotics; such treatment should not be withheld because chronic sleeplessness by itself can disrupt emotional and physical well-being.

Other sedatives: Many drugs not specifically indicated for insomnia are used to induce and maintain sleep.

Alcohol is used by many patients to help with sleep, but alcohol is a poor choice because after prolonged use and at higher doses, it produces unrefreshing, disturbed sleep with frequent nocturnal awakenings, often increasing daytime sleepiness. Alcohol can further impair respiration during sleep in patients with OSA and other pulmonary disorders such as COPD.

OTC antihistamines (eg, doxylamine, diphenhydramine) can induce sleep. However, efficacy is unpredictable, and these drugs have adverse effects such as daytime sedation, confusion, urinary retention, and other systemic anticholinergic effects, which are particularly worrisome in the elderly.

Antidepressants taken in low doses at bedtime (eg, doxepin 25 to 50 mg, paroxetine 5 to 20 mg, trazodone 50 mg, trimipramine 75 to 200 mg) may improve sleep. However, antidepressants should be used in these low doses mainly when standard hypnotics are not tolerated (rare) or in higher (antidepressant) doses when depression is present. Ultra low dose doxepin (3 or 6 mg) is indicated for sleep maintenance insomnia.

Melatonin is a hormone that is secreted by the pineal gland (and that occurs naturally in some foods). Darkness stimulates secretion, and light inhibits it. By binding with melatonin receptors in the suprachiasmatic nucleus, melatonin mediates circadian rhythms, especially during physiologic sleep onset. Oral

Table 239–6. GUIDELINES FOR THE USE OF HYPNOTICS

Define a clear indication and treatment goal.
Prescribe the lowest effective dose.
Except for specific hypnotics and patients, limit duration of use to a few weeks.
Individualize the dose for each patient.
Use lower doses in patients also taking a CNS depressant, in the elderly, and in patients with hepatic or renal disorders.
Avoid* if patients have sleep apnea or respiratory disorders or a history of sedative abuse, if they are drinking alcohol, or if they are pregnant.
For patients who need longer-term treatment, consider intermittent therapy.
Avoid abruptly stopping the drug if possible (ie, taper it).
Re-evaluate drug treatment regularly; assess efficacy and adverse events.

*Ramelteon is an exception; it can be given to patients with mild to moderate OSA or COPD or a history of sedative abuse. Low-dose doxepin also has no abuse liability.

Table 239–7. ORAL HYPNOTICS IN COMMON USE

DRUG	HALF LIFE* (h)	DOSE†	COMMENTS
Benzodiazepine receptor agonists: Benzodiazepines			
Triazolam	1.5–5.5	0.25–0.5 mg	May cause anterograde amnesia; high likelihood of tolerance and rebound after repeated use
Temazepam	9.5–12.4	7.5–15 mg	Longest latency for sleep induction
Estazolam	10–24	0.5–2 mg	Effective for sleep induction and maintenance
Quazepam	39–100	7.5–15 mg	High lipophilicity, which may mitigate residual sedation in first 7–10 days of continuous use
Flurazepam	47–100	15–30 mg	High risk of next-day residual sedation; not recommended for the elderly
Benzodiazepine receptor agonists: Nonbenzodiazepines			
Zaleplon	1	5–20 mg	Ultrashort-acting; can be given for sleep-onset insomnia or after nocturnal awakening (if patients can spend at least 4 h in bed after taking the drug) When given at normal bedtime, least likely to have residual effects
Zolpidem, tablets	2.5	Men: 5–10 mg Women: 5 mg	Effective for sleep-onset insomnia only
Zolpidem oral spray‡	2.7	Men: 5 mg, 10 mg Women: 5 mg	Used for sleep-onset insomnia
Zolpidem, extended-release	2.8	Men: 6.25–12.5 mg Women: 6.25 mg	Effective for sleep-onset insomnia and sleep maintenance insomnia; no tolerance with up to 6 mo of use 3 to 7 nights/wk
Zolpidem, sublingual‡	2.9	At bedtime: Men: 5 mg, 10 mg Women: 5 mg Middle of the night: Men: 3.5 mg Women: 1.75 mg	More rapid onset of action than zolpidem tablets Higher doses used for sleep-onset insomnia Lower doses used for early awakening (should not be taken unless patients can spend at least 4 h in bed after taking the drug)
Eszopiclone	6	1–3 mg	Effective for sleep-onset insomnia and sleep maintenance insomnia; no tolerance with up to 6 mo nightly use
Melatonin receptor agonists			
Ramelteon	1–5	8 mg	Useful only for sleep-onset insomnia; one of a few hypnotics that are not associated with abuse liability Can be safely given to patients with mild to moderate OSA or COPD No difficulties with long-term use
Tricyclic antidepressants			
Doxepin, ultra low dose	15.3	3 mg, 6 mg	Indicated for sleep maintenance insomnia; no abuse liability

*Includes parent and active metabolites. Arranged in order from shortest to longest half-life.
†Dose given at bedtime.
‡Newer forms of zolpidem.

melatonin (typically 0.5 to 5 mg at bedtime) may be effective for sleep problems due to delayed sleep phase syndrome. When used to treat this disorder, it must be taken at the appropriate time (a few hours before the evening increase in endogenous melatonin secretion—in early evening for most people, typically 3 to 5 h before the intended bedtime) and at a low dose of 0.5 to 1 mg; taken at the wrong time, it can aggravate sleep problems.

For other forms of insomnia, melatonin's efficacy is largely unproved, and its safety is in question because it appears to stimulate coronary artery changes in animals. Nevertheless, worrisome adverse effects have not been reported after widespread use. Available preparations of melatonin are unregulated, so content and purity cannot be ensured, and the effects of long-term use are unknown. Its use should be supervised by a physician.

KEY POINTS

- Poor sleep hygiene and situational disruptors (eg, shift work, emotional stressors) cause many cases of insomnia.
- Consider medical disorders (eg, sleep apnea syndromes, pain disorders) and psychiatric disorders (eg, mood disorders) as possible causes.
- Usually, consider sleep studies (eg, polysomnography) when sleep apnea syndromes, periodic limb movements, or other sleep disorders are suspected, when the clinical diagnosis is in doubt, or when response to initial presumptive treatment is inadequate.
- Use hypnotics and sedatives with caution in the elderly.
- Good sleep hygiene may be the only treatment needed by patients with mild insomnia problems.

SNORING

Snoring is a raspy noise produced in the nasopharynx during sleep. It is quite common, occurring in about 57% of men and 40% of women; prevalence increases with age. However, because a bed partner's perception of and response to snoring is highly subjective and because snoring varies from night to night, prevalence estimates vary widely.

The sound ranges from barely audible to an extremely bothersome noise that may be loud enough to hear in another room. Snoring is distressing usually to others (typically a bed partner or roommate trying to sleep) rather than the snorer; uncommonly, snorers wake up to the sound of their own snoring.

Snoring can have significant social consequences. It can cause strife between bed partners or roommates; rarely, snorers have been assaulted and even murdered because of their snoring.

Other symptoms such as frequent awakening, gasping or choking during sleep, excessive daytime sleepiness (EDS), and morning headache may also be present, depending on the severity, cause, and consequences of the snoring.

Pathophysiology

Snoring results from airflow-induced flutter of soft tissues of the nasopharynx, particularly the soft palate. As in any fluttering physical structure (eg, a flag), flutter in the nasopharynx develops depending on interacting factors, including the mass, stiffness, and attachments of the fluttering element and the velocity and direction of airflow. The fact that people do not snore while awake suggests that sleep-induced muscular relaxation is at least part of the etiology because muscle tone is the only component of flutter that can change during sleep; tissue mass and attachments do not change. Furthermore, if pharyngeal dilators cannot keep the airway open in response to the negative intraluminal pressure induced by inspiration, the upper airway narrows, increasing local airflow velocity (for a given inspiratory volume). The increased flow velocity promotes flutter directly and decreases intraluminal pressure, further enhancing airway closure and thus promoting flutter and snoring.

Snoring is more likely to occur in airways that are already compromised by structural factors, including

- Micrognathia or retrognathia
- Nasal septal deviation
- Rhinitis that causes tissue swelling
- Obesity

Etiology

Primary snoring: Primary snoring is snoring that is not accompanied by awakening or excessive arousals, limitation of airflow, oxygen desaturation, or arrhythmias during sleep and that occurs in people who do not have EDS. Arousals are brief transitions to lighter sleep or awakenings that last < 15 sec and are usually not noticed.

Sleep-disordered breathing: Snoring is sometimes a manifestation of sleep-disordered breathing, which covers a spectrum ranging from upper airway resistance syndrome to obstructive sleep apnea (OSA—see p. 514). Each has similar upper airway obstructive pathophysiology but differs in degree and clinical consequences of the airway obstruction. The clinical consequences involve mainly disturbances of sleep and/or airflow.

Patients with **OSA** have ≥ 5 episodes of apnea or hypopnea per hour during sleep (apnea/hypopnea index [AHI]) plus ≥ 1 of the following:

- Daytime sleepiness, unintentional sleep episodes, unrefreshing sleep, fatigue, or insomnia
- Awakening with breath holding, gasping, or choking
- Reports by a bed partner of loud snoring, breathing interruptions, or both during the patient's sleep

OSA can be categorized by severity: mild (5 to 15 episodes/hr), moderate (16 to 30 episodes/hr), or severe (> 30 episodes/hr).

Upper airway resistance syndrome causes EDS or other manifestations but does not meet full criteria for OSA.

Complications: Although snoring itself has no known adverse physiologic effects, OSA may have consequences (eg, hypertension, stroke, heart disorders, diabetes).

Risk factors: Risk factors for snoring include

- Older age
- Obesity
- Use of alcohol or other sedatives
- Chronic nasal congestion or blockage
- A small or posteriorly displaced jaw
- Male sex
- Postmenopausal status
- Black race
- Pregnancy
- Abnormal structures that can block airflow (eg, large tonsils, a deviated nasal septum, nasal polyps)

There may also be familial risk.

Evaluation

The primary goal is to identify snorers who are at high risk of having OSA. Many snorers do not have OSA, but most patients with OSA snore (the precise proportion is not known).

Because several important manifestations of OSA are noticed mainly by others, bed partners or roommates should also be interviewed when possible.

History: History of present illness should cover severity of snoring, including its frequency, duration, and loudness. Also, the degree that snoring affects the bed partner should be noted. A snoring severity scale may be used.

Review of systems should seek symptoms suggesting OSA, such as the presence of sleep disturbance as indicated by

- Number of awakenings
- Witnessed apneic or gasping/choking episodes
- Presence of unrefreshing sleep or morning headaches
- EDS

The ESS (see Table 239–3) can be used to quantify daytime sleepiness. The STOP-BANG score (see Table 239–4) is a useful tool to predict risk of OSA for patients who snore.

Past medical history should note presence of disorders that may be associated with OSA, particularly hypertension, coronary ischemia, heart failure, stroke, gastroesophageal reflux disease (GERD), atrial fibrillation, depression, obesity (especially morbid obesity), and diabetes. Patients are asked how much alcohol they consume and when it is consumed in relation to bedtime. Drug history may identify sedating or muscle-relaxing drugs.

Physical examination: Examination should begin by measuring height and weight, with calculation of body mass index (BMI).

The rest of the examination is of limited use and focuses on inspecting the nose and mouth for evidence of obstruction. Signs include

- Nasal polyps and engorged turbinates
- A high, arched palate
- Enlargement of the tongue, tonsils, or uvula
- A small or posteriorly displaced mandible

A Mallampati score of 3 or 4 (only the base or none of the uvula is visible during oral inspection—see Fig. 239–2) suggests increased risk of OSA.

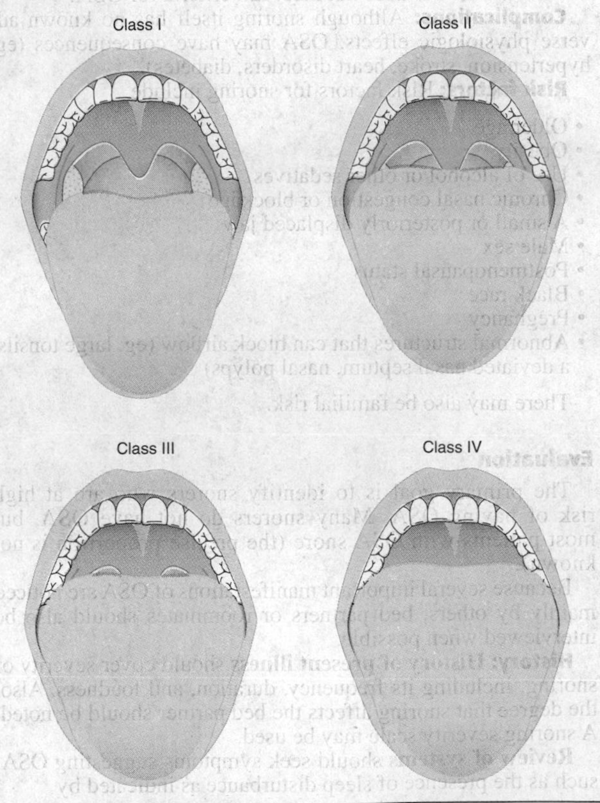

Fig. 239–2. Mallampati scoring. Modified Mallampati scoring is as follows:

- Class 1: Tonsils, uvula, and soft palate are fully visible.
- Class 2: Hard and soft palate, upper portion of tonsils, and uvula are visible.
- Class 3: Soft and hard palate and base of the uvula are visible.
- Class 4: Only the hard palate is visible.

Red flags: The following findings are of particular concern:

- Witnessed apnea or choking during sleep
- Morning headaches
- Epworth sleepiness score ≥ 10
- BMI ≥ 35
- Very loud, constant snoring

Interpretation of findings: The clinical evaluation is not completely reliable for diagnosis of OSA but can be suggestive. Red flag findings clearly correlate with OSA. However, all of these findings occur along a continuum, and there is no widespread agreement on cut-off points and relative weighting. Nonetheless, the more red flag findings a patient has and the more severe they are, the greater the likelihood of OSA.

Testing: Testing is done when a diagnosis of OSA is suspected; it consists of polysomnography (PSG—see p. 2016). However, because snoring is so common, PSG should be done only when clinical suspicion for OSA is significant. A reasonable approach is to test patients who have red flag findings (particularly witnessed apnea) as well as those who have several red flag elements that do not quite meet the listed scores.

People with no symptoms or signs of sleep disturbance other than snoring do not need to be tested but should be clinically monitored for development of such manifestations.

Treatment

Treatment of snoring associated with other conditions, such as chronic nasal obstruction and OSA (see p. 516), are discussed elsewhere in The Manual.

Overall, treatment includes general measures to manage risk factors plus physical methods to open the airways and/or stiffen the involved structures.

General measures: Several general measures can be used for primary snoring. Their efficacy has not been well-evaluated, primarily because perception of snoring is highly subjective; However, particular patients may benefit. Measures include

- Avoiding alcohol and sedating drugs for several hours before bedtime
- Sleeping with the head elevated (best accomplished by using bed- or body-positioning devices such as wedges)
- Losing weight
- Using earplugs
- Implementing alternate sleeping arrangements (eg, separate rooms)
- Treating any nasal congestion (eg, with decongestant and/or corticosteroid sprays or with elastic strips that hold the nares open)

Oral appliances: Oral appliances are worn only during sleep; they include mandibular advancement devices and tongue-retaining devices. These appliances must be fitted by specially trained dentists. They are helpful for patients with mild to moderate OSA and are generally regarded as highly effective for simple snoring, although studies into this area are scant.

Adverse effects include temporomandibular joint (TMJ) discomfort, dental misalignment, and excessive salivation, but most patients tolerate the devices well.

Mandibular advancement devices are most commonly used. These devices push the mandible and tongue forward relative to the maxilla and thus reduce airway collapse during sleep. These devices may be fixed or adjustable; with adjustable devices, how far the mandible is advanced can be adjusted incrementally after the initial fitting to optimize results. Adjustable devices are more effective than fixed devices.

Tongue-retaining devices (TRD) use suction to maintain the tongue in an anterior position. TRDs are more uncomfortable and probably less effective than mandibular advancement devices.

Continuous positive airway pressure (CPAP): CPAP devices maintain a constant positive pressure in the upper airway via a small mask applied to the nose or nose and mouth (see p. 516). By eliminating the need for negative pressure during inspiration, CPAP prevents the narrowing or collapse of the airways at that time. It thus provides very effective relief of OSA and is effective for primary snoring. However, its use in primary snoring is limited because third-party reimbursement for this use is lacking and because patients are not sufficiently motivated. Although patients are often willing to use a CPAP device nightly to avoid the significant symptoms and long-term consequences of OSA, they are less willing to use the device to manage primary snoring, whose consequences are primarily social.

Surgery: Because reduced nasal patency promotes snoring, surgically correcting specific causes of airway compromise (eg, nasal polyps, hypertrophied tonsils, deviated septum) would seem to be a reasonable way to decrease snoring. However, studies have not yet substantiated this theory.

Various pharyngeal surgical procedures that alter the structure of the palate and sometimes the uvula have been developed for OSA. Some are also useful for nonapneic snoring.

Uvulopalatopharyngoplasty can be highly effective for snoring, although effects may not last beyond a few years. It is an inpatient procedure requiring general anesthesia; thus, its usefulness for snoring alone is limited.

Therefore, a number of outpatient procedures that can be done using a local anesthetic have been developed:

- **Laser-assisted uvuloplasty** is less invasive than uvulopalatopharyngoplasty. Although some patients report benefit, its usefulness in treating snoring has not been proved.
- For **injection snoreplasty**, a sclerotherapeutic agent is injected into the submucosa of the soft palate to stiffen it and the uvula. Its usefulness for snoring alone requires further study.
- For **radiofrequency ablation**, a probe is used to introduce thermal energy into the soft palate. Studies have shown its usefulness for snoring, but further study is needed.
- **Palatal implants**, made of polyethylene, can be placed into the soft palate to stiffen it. Three small implants are used. Their usefulness for snoring alone has not been proved.

KEY POINTS

- Only some snorers have OSA, but most patients who have OSA snore.
- Clinical risk factors such as nocturnal apneic or choking episodes, daytime sleepiness, and a high BMI help identify patients at risk of OSA and thus in need of testing with PSG.
- Recommend general measures to reduce snoring (eg, avoiding alcohol and sedating drugs, sleeping with the head elevated, losing weight).
- Consider specific measures such as mandibular advancement devices, uvulopalatopharyngoplasty, palate-altering procedures, and CPAP to treat snoring due to OSA.

CIRCADIAN RHYTHM SLEEP DISORDERS

Circadian rhythm sleep disorders are caused by desynchronization between internal sleep-wake rhythms and the light-darkness cycle. Patients typically have insomnia, excessive daytime sleepiness, or both, which typically resolve as the body clock realigns itself. Diagnosis is clinical. Treatment depends on the cause.

In circadian rhythm disorders, endogenous sleep-wake rhythms (body clock) and the external light-darkness cycle become misaligned (desynchronized). The cause may be internal (eg, delayed or advanced sleep phase syndrome) or external (eg, jet lag, shift work).

If the cause is external, other circadian body rhythms, including temperature and hormone secretion, can become out of sync with the light-darkness cycle (external desynchronization) and with one another (internal desynchronization); in addition to insomnia and excessive sleepiness, these alterations may cause nausea, malaise, irritability, and depression. Risk of cardiovascular and metabolic disorders may also be increased.

Repetitive circadian shifts (eg, due to frequent long-distance travel or rotating shift work) are particularly difficult to adapt to, especially when the shifts change in a counterclockwise direction. Counterclockwise shifts are those that shift awakening and sleeping times earlier (eg, when flying eastward, when rotating shifts from days to nights to evenings). Symptoms resolve over several days or, in some patients (eg, the elderly), over a few weeks or months, as rhythms readjust. Because light is a strong synchronizer of circadian rhythms, exposure to bright light (sunlight or artificial light of 5,000 to 10,000 lux intensity) after the desired awakening time and the use of sunglasses to decrease light exposure before the desired bedtime speed readjustment. Melatonin before bedtime may help (see p. 2017).

Patients with circadian rhythm disorders often misuse alcohol, hypnotics, and stimulants.

Circadian rhythm disorders include the following:

- Circadian rhythm sleep disorder, jet lag type (jet lag disorder)
- Circadian rhythm sleep disorder, shift work type (shift work disorder)
- Circadian rhythm sleep disorder, altered sleep phase types

Circadian rhythm sleep disorder, jet lag type (jet lag disorder): This syndrome is caused by rapid travel across > 2 time zones. Eastward travel (advancing the sleep cycle) causes more severe symptoms than westward travel (delaying sleep).

If possible, travelers should gradually shift their sleep-wake schedule before travel to approximate that of their destination, and after arriving in the new locale, they should maximize exposure to daylight during the day (particularly in the morning) and exposure to darkness before bedtime. Short-acting hypnotics and/or wake-promoting drugs (eg, modafinil) may be used for brief periods after arrival.

Circadian rhythm sleep disorder, shift work type (shift work disorder): Severity of symptoms is proportional to the

- Frequency of shift changes
- Magnitude of each change
- Number of consecutive nights worked
- Length of shifts
- Frequency of counterclockwise (sleep advancing) changes

Fixed-shift work (ie, full-time night or evening) is preferable; rotating shifts should go clockwise (ie, day to evening to night). However, even fixed-shift workers have difficulties because daytime noise and light interfere with sleep quality, and workers often shorten sleep times to participate in social or family events.

Shift workers should maximize their exposure to bright light (sunlight or, for night workers, specially constructed bright artificial lightboxes) at times when they should be awake and ensure that the bedroom is as dark and quiet as possible during sleep. Wearing sunglasses during the morning commute home in anticipation of sleep is also useful. Sleep masks and white-noise devices are helpful. Melatonin before bedtime can also help. When symptoms persist and interfere with functioning, judicious use of hypnotics with a short half-life and wake-promoting drugs is appropriate.

Circadian rhythm sleep disorder, altered sleep phase types: In these syndromes, patients have normal sleep quality and duration with a 24-h circadian rhythm cycle, but the cycle is out of sync with desired or necessary wake times. Less commonly, the cycle is not 24 h, and patients awaken and sleep earlier or later each day. If able to follow their natural cycle, patients have no symptoms.

- **Delayed sleep phase syndrome:** Patients consistently go to sleep and awaken late (eg, 3 AM and 10 AM). This pattern is more common during adolescence. If required to awaken earlier for work or school, excessive daytime sleepiness results; patients often present because school performance is poor or they miss morning classes. They can be distinguished from people who stay up late by choice because they cannot fall asleep earlier even if they try. Mild phase delay (< 3 h) is treated by progressive earlier arising plus morning bright light therapy, perhaps with melatonin 4 to 5 h before the desired bedtime. An alternative method is to progressively delay bedtime and awakening time by 1 to 3 h/day until the correct sleep and wake times are reached.
- **Advanced sleep phase syndrome:** This syndrome (early to bed and early to rise) is more common among the elderly and responds to treatment with bright light in the evening and light-preventing goggles in the morning.
- **Non–24-h sleep-wake syndrome:** Much less common, this syndrome is characterized by a free-running sleep-wake rhythm. The sleep-wake cycle commonly remains constant in length but is > 24 h, resulting in a delay of sleep and wake times by 1 to 2 h each day. This disorder is more common among blind people. Tasimelteon, a melatonin receptor agonist, can increase nighttime sleep duration and decrease daytime sleep duration in totally blind patients who have this disorder. The dose is 20 mg once/day before bedtime, at the same time every night.

INSOMNIA AND EXCESSIVE DAYTIME SLEEPINESS

Many sleep disorders manifest with insomnia and usually excessive daytime sleepiness (EDS).

- **Insomnia** is difficulty falling or staying asleep, early awakening, or a sensation of unrefreshing sleep.
- **EDS** is the tendency to fall asleep during normal waking hours.

Sleep disorders may be caused by factors inside the body (intrinsic) or outside the body (extrinsic).

Inadequate sleep hygiene: Sleep is impaired by certain behaviors. They include

- Consumption of caffeine or sympathomimetic or other stimulant drugs (typically near bedtime, but even in the afternoon for people who are particularly sensitive)
- Exercise or excitement (eg, a thrilling TV show) late in the evening
- An irregular sleep-wake schedule

Patients who compensate for lost sleep by sleeping late or by napping further fragment nocturnal sleep.

Insomniacs should adhere to a regular awakening time and avoid naps regardless of the amount of nocturnal sleep.

Adequate sleep hygiene can improve sleep (see Table 239–5).

Adjustment insomnia: Acute emotional stressors (eg, job loss, hospitalization) can cause insomnia. Symptoms typically remit shortly after the stressors abate; insomnia is usually transient and brief. Nevertheless, if daytime sleepiness and fatigue develop, especially if they interfere with daytime functioning, short-term treatment with hypnotics is warranted. Persistent anxiety may require specific treatment.

Psychophysiologic insomnia: Insomnia, regardless of cause, may persist well beyond resolution of precipitating factors, usually because patients feel anticipatory anxiety about the prospect of another sleepless night followed by another day of fatigue. Typically, patients spend hours in bed focusing on and brooding about their sleeplessness, and they have greater difficulty falling asleep in their own bedroom than falling asleep away from home.

Optimal treatment combines

- Cognitive-behavioral strategies
- Hypnotics

Although **cognitive-behavioral strategies** are more difficult to implement and take longer, effects are longer lasting, up to 2 yr after treatment is ended. These strategies include

- Sleep hygiene (particularly restriction of time in bed—see Table 239–5)
- Education
- Relaxation training
- Stimulus control
- Cognitive therapy

Hypnotics are suitable for patients who need rapid relief and whose insomnia has had daytime effects, such as EDS and fatigue. These drugs must not be used indefinitely in most cases.

Physical sleep disorders: Physical disorders may interfere with sleep and cause insomnia and EDS. Disorders that cause pain or discomfort (eg, arthritis, cancer, herniated disks), particularly those that worsen with movement, cause transient awakenings and poor sleep quality. Nocturnal seizures can also interfere with sleep.

Treatment is directed at the underlying disorder and symptom relief (eg, with bedtime analgesics).

Mental sleep disorders: Most major mental disorders can cause insomnia and EDS. About 80% of patients with major depression report these symptoms. Conversely, 40% of chronic insomniacs have a major mental disorder, most commonly a mood disorder.

Patients with depression may have initial sleeplessness or sleep maintenance insomnia. Sometimes in the depressed phase of bipolar disorder and in seasonal affective disorder, sleep is uninterrupted, but patients complain of unrelenting daytime fatigue.

If depression is accompanied by sleeplessness, antidepressants that provide more sedation (eg, citalopram, paroxetine, mirtazapine) may help patients sleep. These drugs are used at regular, not low, doses to ensure correction of the depression. However, clinicians should note that these drugs are not predictably sedating and may have activating properties. In addition, the sedation provided may outlast its usefulness, causing EDS, and these drugs may have other adverse effects, such as weight gain. Alternatively, any antidepressant may be used with a hypnotic.

If depression is accompanied by EDS, antidepressants with activating qualities (eg, bupropion, venlafaxine, certain SSRIs such as fluoxetine and sertraline) may be chosen.

Insufficient sleep syndrome (sleep deprivation): Patients with this syndrome do not sleep enough at night, despite adequate opportunity to do so, to stay alert when awake. The cause is usually various social or employment commitments. This syndrome is probably the most common cause of EDS, which disappears when sleep time is increased (eg, on weekends or vacations). After long periods of sleep deprivation, weeks or months of extended sleep are needed to restore daytime alertness.

Drug-related sleep disorders: Insomnia and EDS can result from chronic use of CNS stimulants (eg, amphetamines, caffeine), hypnotics (eg, benzodiazepines), other sedatives, antimetabolite chemotherapy, anticonvulsants (eg, phenytoin), oral contraceptives, methyldopa, propranolol, alcohol, and thyroid hormone preparations (see Table 239–2). Commonly prescribed hypnotics can cause irritability and apathy and reduce mental alertness. Many psychoactive drugs can induce abnormal movements during sleep.

Insomnia can develop during withdrawal of CNS depressants (eg, barbiturates, opioids, sedatives), tricyclic antidepressants, monoamine oxidase inhibitors, or illicit drugs (eg, cocaine, heroin, marijuana, phencyclidine). Abrupt withdrawal of hypnotics or sedatives can cause nervousness, tremors, and seizures.

NARCOLEPSY

Narcolepsy is characterized by chronic excessive daytime sleepiness, often with sudden loss of muscle tone (cataplexy). Other symptoms include sleep paralysis and hypnagogic and hypnopompic hallucinations. Diagnosis is by polysomnography and multiple sleep latency testing. Treatment is with modafinil, various stimulants, or Na oxybate for excessive daytime sleepiness and with certain antidepressants for associated symptoms.

The cause is unknown. In Europe, Japan, and the US, incidence is 0.2 to 1.6/1000. Narcolepsy is equally common in both sexes.

Narcolepsy is strongly associated with specific HLA haplotypes, and children of patients with narcolepsy have a 40-fold increased risk, suggesting a genetic cause. However, concordance in twins is low (25%), suggesting a prominent role for environmental factors, which often trigger the disorder. The neuropeptide hypocretin-1 is deficient in CSF of narcoleptic animals and most human patients, suggesting that the cause may be HLA-associated autoimmune destruction of hypocretin-containing neurons in the lateral hypothalamus.

Narcolepsy features dysregulation of the timing and control of REM sleep. Therefore, REM sleep intrudes into wakefulness and into the transition from wakefulness to sleep. Many symptoms of narcolepsy result from postural muscle paralysis and vivid dreaming, which characterize REM.

There are 2 types:

- Type 1: Narcolepsy due to hypocretin deficiency and accompanied by cataplexy (momentary muscular weakness or paralysis evoked by sudden emotional reactions)
- Type 2: Narcolepsy with normal hypocretin levels and without cataplexy

Symptoms and Signs

The main symptoms are

- Excessive daytime sleepiness
- Cataplexy
- Hypnagogic and hypnopompic hallucinations
- Sleep paralysis

About 10% of patients have all 4 of these symptoms. Nocturnal sleep is often also disturbed, and some patients develop hypersomnia (prolonged sleep times).

Symptoms usually begin in adolescents or young adults without prior illness, although onset can be precipitated by an illness, a stressor, or a period of sleep deprivation. Once established, narcolepsy persists throughout life; life span is unaffected.

Excessive daytime sleepiness (EDS): EDS can occur anytime. Sleep episodes vary from few to many per day, and each may last minutes or hours. Patients can resist the desire to sleep only temporarily but can be roused as readily as from normal sleep. Sleep tends to occur during monotonous conditions (eg, reading, watching television, attending meetings) but may also occur during complex tasks (eg, driving, speaking, writing, eating).

Patients may also experience sleep attacks—episodes of sleep that strike without warning. Patients may feel refreshed when they awaken yet fall asleep again in a few minutes.

Nighttime sleep may be unsatisfying and interrupted by vivid, frightening dreams.

Consequences include low productivity, breaches in interpersonal relationships, poor concentration, low motivation, depression, a dramatic reduction in quality of life, and potential for physical injury (particularly due to motor vehicle collisions).

Cataplexy: Momentary muscular weakness or paralysis occurs without loss of consciousness; it is evoked by sudden emotional reactions, such as mirth, anger, fear, joy, or, often, surprise.

Weakness may be confined to the limbs (eg, patients may drop the rod when a fish strikes their line) or may cause a limp fall during hearty laughter (as in "weak with laughter") or sudden anger. Cataplexy can also affect other muscles: The jaw may droop, facial muscles may flicker, eyes may close, the head may nod, and speech may be slurred. These attacks resemble the loss of muscle tone that occurs during REM sleep.

Cataplexy occurs in about three fourths of patients.

Sleep paralysis: Patients are momentarily unable to move as they are just falling asleep or immediately after they awaken. These occasional episodes may be very frightening. They resemble the motor inhibition that accompanies REM sleep.

Sleep paralysis occurs in about one fourth of patients but also in some healthy children and, less commonly, in healthy adults.

Hypnagogic or hypnopompic hallucinations: Particularly vivid auditory or visual illusions or hallucinations may occur when just falling asleep (hypnagogic) or, less often, immediately after awakening (hypnopompic). They are difficult to distinguish from intense reverie and are somewhat similar to vivid dreams, which are normal in REM sleep.

Hypnagogic hallucinations occur in about one-third of patients, are common among healthy young children, and occasionally occur in healthy adults.

Diagnosis

- Polysomnography (PSG)
- Multiple sleep latency testing (MSLT)

A delay of 10 yr from onset to diagnosis is common.

A history of cataplexy strongly suggests narcolepsy in patients with EDS.

In patients with EDS, nocturnal PSG, followed by MSLT, can confirm a diagnosis of narcolepsy when the findings include the following:

- Sleep-onset REM episodes during at least 2 of 5 daytime nap opportunities or one during daytime nap opportunities plus one during the preceding nocturnal polysomnogram
- Average sleep latency (time to fall asleep) of ≤ 8 min
- No other diagnostic abnormalities on nocturnal PSG

Narcolepsy type 1 is diagnosed if patients also have cataplexy; type 2 is diagnosed if patients do not have cataplexy.

The maintenance of wakefulness test does not help with diagnosis but does help monitor treatment efficacy.

Other disorders that can cause chronic EDS are usually suggested by the history and physical examination; brain imaging and blood and urine tests can confirm the diagnosis. These disorders include space-occupying lesions affecting the hypothalamus or upper brain stem, increased intracranial pressure, and certain forms of encephalitis. Hypothyroidism, hyperglycemia, hypoglycemia, anemia, uremia, hypercapnia, hypercalcemia, hepatic failure, and seizure disorders can also cause EDS with or without hypersomnia. Acute, relatively brief EDS and hypersomnia commonly accompany acute systemic disorders such as influenza.

The **Kleine-Levin syndrome,** a very rare disorder in adolescent boys, causes episodic hypersomnia and hyperphagia. Etiology is unclear but may be an autoimmune response to an infection.

Treatment

- Modafinil
- Methylphenidate and its derivatives, amphetamine derivatives, or Na oxybate
- Certain REM-suppressant antidepressants

Some patients who have occasional episodes of sleep paralysis or hypnagogic and hypnopompic hallucinations, infrequent and partial cataplexy, and mild EDS need no treatment. For others, stimulant drugs and anticataplectic drugs are used. Patients should also get enough sleep at night and take brief naps (< 30 min) at the same time every day (typically afternoon).

Modafinil, a long-acting wake-promoting drug, can help patients with mild to moderate EDS. The mechanism of action is unclear. Typically, modafinil 100 to 200 mg po is given in the morning. Dose is increased to 400 mg as needed. Doses > 400 mg have not been shown to be more effective. If effects do not last into the evening, a small 2nd dose (eg, 100 mg) at noon or 1 PM may be used, although this dose sometimes interferes with nocturnal sleep. Alternatively, a short-acting form of methylphenidate can be added in the afternoon on a regular or as-needed basis.

Adverse effects of modafinil include nausea and headache, which are mitigated by lower initial doses and slower titration. Modafinil can lower the effectiveness of oral contraceptives and has abuse potential, although it is low. Rarely, serious rashes and Stevens-Johnson syndrome have developed in patients taking modafinil. If serious reactions develop, the drug should be stopped permanently.

Armodafinil, the *R*-enantiomer of modafinil, has similar benefits and adverse effects; dosage is 150 or 250 mg po once in the morning.

Methylphenidate or **amphetamine derivatives** are usually used instead of or with modafinil if patients do not respond to modafinil. Methylphenidate 5 mg po bid to 20 mg po tid is especially useful for immediate management because modafinil's onset is delayed. Methamphetamine 5 to 20 mg po bid or dextroamphetamine 5 mg po bid to 20 mg po tid may be used; all are available in long-acting preparations and therefore can be dosed once/day in many patients. They can also be used on an as-needed basis for patients already taking modafinil because their onset is rapid and duration is relatively short. Adverse effects include agitation, hypertension, tachycardia, and mood changes (eg, manic reactions); abuse potential is high.

Pemoline, although less addictive than amphetamines, is not recommended because it may be hepatotoxic and liver enzymes must be monitored every 2 wk.

Na oxybate can also be used to treat EDS and cataplexy. A dose of 2.25 g po is taken at bedtime while in bed, followed by the same dose 2.5 to 4 h later. The maximum dose is 9 g/night. Adverse effects include headache, nausea, dizziness, nasopharyngitis, somnolence, vomiting, urinary incontinence, and sometimes sleepwalking. Na oxybate is a schedule III drug and has potential for abuse and dependence. It is contraindicated in patients with succinic semialdehyde dehydrogenase deficiency and should not be used in patients with untreated respiratory disorders.

Tricyclic antidepressants (particularly clomipramine, imipramine, and protriptyline) and **SSRIs** (eg, venlafaxine, fluoxetine) are useful in treating cataplexy, sleep paralysis, and hypnagogic and hypnopompic hallucinations. Clomipramine 25 to 150 mg po once/day in the morning seems to be the most potent anticataplectic but should be taken only during the day to reduce nocturnal arousal.

KEY POINTS

- Narcolepsy may be caused by autoimmune destruction of hypocretin-containing neurons in the lateral hypothalamus in genetically at-risk patients.
- The main symptoms are EDS, cataplexy, hypnagogic and hypnopompic hallucinations, and sleep paralysis.
- Confirm the diagnosis by PSG and MSLT.
- EDS usually responds to modafinil (sometimes used with methylphenidate, an amphetamine derivative) or to Na oxybate.
- Tricyclic antidepressants and SSRIs may be useful for cataplexy, sleep paralysis, and hypnagogic and hypnopompic hallucinations.

IDIOPATHIC HYPERSOMNIA

Idiopathic hypersomnia is excessive daytime sleepiness with or without a long sleep time; it is differentiated from narcolepsy by lack of cataplexy, hypnagogic hallucinations, and sleep paralysis.

Idiopathic hypersomnia is not well characterized. Cause is presumed to be CNS dysfunction.

Excessive daytime sleepiness is the main symptom; sleep time may or may not be prolonged.

Diagnosis

- History or sleep logs
- Sleep tests

In idiopathic hypersomnia with a long sleep time, the history or sleep logs indicate > 10 h of nocturnal sleep; in idiopathic hypersomnia without a long sleep time, it is > 6 h but < 10 h. In both cases, polysomnography shows no evidence of other sleep abnormalities. Multiple sleep latency testing shows short sleep latencies (< 8 min) with fewer than 2 REM periods.

Treatment

- Similar to that of narcolepsy

Treatment is similar to that of narcolepsy, except that anticataplectic drugs are unnecessary.

PARASOMNIAS

Parasomnias are undesirable behaviors that occur during entry into sleep, during sleep, or during arousal from sleep. Diagnosis is clinical. Treatment may include drugs and psychotherapy.

For many of these disorders, history and physical examination can confirm the diagnosis.

Somnambulism: Sitting, walking, or other complex behavior occurs during sleep, usually with the eyes open but without evidence of recognition. Somnambulism is most common during late childhood and adolescence and occurs after and during arousal from NREM stage N3 sleep. Prior sleep deprivation and poor sleep hygiene increase the likelihood of these episodes, and risk is higher for 1st-degree relatives of patients with the disorder. Episodes may be triggered by factors that cause arousals during sleep (eg, caffeine, other stimulant drugs and substances, behaviors that disrupt sleep) or that enhance N3 sleep (eg, prior sleep deprivation, excessive exercise).

Patients may mumble repetitiously, and some injure themselves on obstacles or stairs. Patients do not remember dreaming after awakening or the following morning and usually do not remember the episode.

Treatment is directed at eliminating the triggers for these episodes. It also involves protecting patients from injury—eg, by using electronic alarms to awaken patients when they leave the bed, using a low bed, and removing sharp objects from the bedside and obstacles from the bedroom. Occasionally, patients are advised to sleep on mattresses on the floor.

Benzodiazepines, particularly clonazepam 0.5 to 2 mg po, at bedtime typically help if behavioral measures are not completely effective.

Sleep (night) terrors: During the night, patients suddenly scream, flail, and appear to be frightened and intensely activated. Episodes can lead to sleepwalking. Patients are difficult to awaken. Sleep terrors are more common among children and occur after arousal from N3 sleep; thus, they do not represent nightmares. In adults, sleep terrors can be associated with mental difficulties or alcoholism.

For children, parental reassurance is often the mainstay of treatment. If daily activities are affected (eg, if school work deteriorates), intermediate- or long-acting oral benzodiazepines (eg, clonazepam 1 to 2 mg, diazepam 2 to 5 mg) at bedtime may help. Adults may benefit from psychotherapy or drug treatment.

Nightmares: Children are more likely to have nightmares than adults. Nightmares occur during REM sleep, more commonly when fever, excessive fatigue, or mental distress is present or after alcohol has been ingested.

Treatment is directed at any underlying mental distress.

REM sleep behavior disorder: Verbalization (sometimes profane) and often violent movements (eg, waving the arms, punching, kicking) occur during REM sleep. These behaviors may represent acting out dreams by patients who, for unknown reasons, do not have the atonia normally present during REM sleep. Patients are aware of having vivid dreams when they awaken after the behaviors.

This disorder is more common among the elderly, particularly those with CNS degenerative disorders (eg, Parkinson or Alzheimer disease, vascular dementia, olivopontocerebellar degeneration, multiple system atrophy, progressive supranuclear palsy). Similar behavior can occur in patients who have narcolepsy or who take norepinephrine reuptake inhibitors (eg, atomoxetine, reboxetine, venlafaxine). Cause is usually unknown. Some patients develop Parkinson disease years after REM sleep behavior disorder is diagnosed.

Diagnosis may be suspected based on symptoms reported by patients or the bed partner. Polysomnography can usually confirm the diagnosis. It may detect excessive motor activity during REM; audiovisual monitoring may document abnormal body movements and vocalizations. A neurologic examination is done to rule out neurodegenerative disorders. If an abnormality is detected, CT or MRI may be done.

Treatment is with clonazepam 0.5 to 2 mg po at bedtime. Most patients need to take the drug indefinitely to prevent recurrences; potential for tolerance or abuse is low. Bed partners should be warned about the possibility of harm and may wish to sleep in another bed until symptoms resolve. Sharp objects should be removed from the bedside.

Sleep-related leg cramps: Muscles of the calf or foot muscles often cramp during sleep in otherwise healthy middle-aged and elderly patients.

Diagnosis is based on the history and lack of physical signs or disability.

Prevention includes stretching the affected muscles for several minutes before sleep. Stretching as soon as cramps occur relieves symptoms promptly and is preferable to drug treatment. Numerous drugs (eg, quinine, Ca and Mg supplements, diphenhydramine, benzodiazepines, mexiletine) have been used; none is likely to be effective, and adverse effects may be significant (particularly with quinine and mexiletine). Avoiding caffeine and other sympathetic stimulants may help.

PERIODIC LIMB MOVEMENT DISORDER AND RESTLESS LEGS SYNDROME

Periodic limb movement disorder (PLMD) and restless legs syndrome (RLS) are characterized by abnormal motions of and sometimes sensations in the lower or upper extremities, which may interfere with sleep.

PLMD and RLS are more common during middle and older age; > 80% of patients with RLS also have PLMD.

The mechanism is unclear but may involve abnormalities in dopamine neurotransmission in the CNS. The disorders can occur

- In isolation
- During drug withdrawal
- With use of stimulants, certain antidepressants, or dopamine antagonists
- During pregnancy
- In patients with chronic renal or hepatic failure, iron deficiency, anemia, diabetes mellitus, a neurologic disorder (eg, multiple sclerosis, Parkinson disease), or other disorders

In primary RLS, heredity may be involved; more than one third of patients with primary RLS have a family history of it. Risk factors may include a sedentary lifestyle, smoking, and obesity.

Periodic leg movement disorder is common among people with narcolepsy and REM behavior disorder.

Symptoms and Signs

PLMD is characterized by repetitive (usually every 20 to 40 sec) twitching or kicking of the lower or upper extremities during sleep. Patients usually complain of interrupted nocturnal sleep or excessive daytime sleepiness. They are typically unaware of the movements and brief arousals that follow and have no abnormal sensations in the extremities.

RLS is a sensorimotor disorder characterized by an irresistible urge to move the legs, arms, or, less commonly, other body parts, usually accompanied by paresthesias (eg, creeping or crawling sensations) and sometimes pain in the upper or lower extremities; symptoms are more prominent when patients are inactive or recline and peak in severity around bedtime. To relieve symptoms, patients move the affected extremity by stretching, kicking, or walking. As a result, they have difficulty falling asleep, repeated nocturnal awakenings, or both.

Diagnosis

- For RLS, history alone
- For PLMD, history of disturbed sleep or excessive daytime sleepiness and polysomnography

Diagnosis may be suggested by the patient's or bed partner's history. For example, patients with PLMD typically have insomnia, excessive daytime sleepiness, and/or excessive twitching just before sleep onset or during sleep.

Polysomnography is necessary to confirm the diagnosis of PLMD, which is usually apparent as repetitive bursts of electromyographic activity. Polysomnography may be also done after RLS is diagnosed to determine whether patients also have PLMD, but polysomnography is not necessary for diagnosis of RLS itself.

Patients with either disorder should be evaluated medically for disorders that can contribute (eg, with blood tests for anemia and iron deficiency and with hepatic and renal function tests).

Treatment

- For RLS: Pramipexole, ropinirole, a rotigotine patch, or gabapentin enacarbil, plus iron supplements if ferritin is < 50 ng/mL
- For PLMD: Usually the same treatments as for RLS

For RLS, numerous drugs (eg, dopaminergic drugs, benzodiazepines, anticonvulsants, vitamins and minerals) are used.

Dopaminergic drugs, although often effective, may have adverse effects such as augmentation (RLS symptoms that worsen before the next drug dose is given and that affect other body parts such as the arms), rebound (symptoms that worsen after the drug is stopped or after the effects of the drug dissipate), nausea, orthostatic hypotension, and insomnia. Three dopamine agonists, pramipexole, ropinirole, and rotigotine (used as a patch), are effective and have few serious adverse effects other than augmentation:

- Pramipexole 0.125 mg po is given 2 h before onset of moderate to severe symptoms and is increased, as needed, by 0.125 mg po q 2 nights until symptoms are relieved (maximum dose 0.5 mg).
- Ropinirole 0.25 mg po is given 1 to 3 h before onset of symptoms and is increased, as needed, by 0.25 mg nightly (maximum dose 4 mg).
- The rotigotine patch (1 mg/24 h) is initially applied any time during the day; dosage is increased as needed by 1 mg/24 h at weekly intervals, up to 3 mg/24 h.

Levodopa/carbidopa may be used, but other drugs, which are less likely to cause augmentation and rebound symptoms, are usually preferred.

Gabapentin may help relieve RLS symptoms and is used when RLS is accompanied by pain. Dosing begins with 300 mg at bedtime and can be increased by 300 mg weekly (maximum dose 900 mg po tid). However, this drug is not approved for the treatment of RLS.

Gabapentin enacarbil, a prodrug of gabapentin, may help relieve RLS symptoms and is approved for this indication. The recommended dose is 600 mg once/day taken with food at about 5 PM. Its most common adverse effects include somnolence and dizziness.

Pregabalin, a nondopaminergic $\alpha 2\delta$ ligand, may help relieve RLS symptoms; augmentation is less likely to occur than with pramipexole. Pregabalin may also be useful for RLS accompanied by pain. For RLS, a dose of 300 mg once/day has been used. Dizziness and somnolence are the most common adverse effects. However, use of this drug to treat RLS has not been extensively studied.

Benzodiazepines may improve sleep continuity but do not reduce limb movements; they should be used cautiously to avoid tolerance and daytime sleepiness.

Opioids may also work for patients with RLS and pain but are used as a last resort because of tolerance, adverse effects, and abuse potential.

Ferritin levels should be obtained, and if levels are low (< 50 μg/L), supplementation with ferrous sulfate 325 mg plus 100 to 200 mg of vitamin C at bedtime is warranted. Patients should exercise good sleep hygiene.

For PLMD, there are no specific treatments, but the treatments for RLS are usually used and often help. However, treatments require further study.

KEY POINTS

- PLMD is repetitive twitching or kicking of the lower or upper extremities during sleep, often interrupting nocturnal sleep and causing excessive daytime sleepiness.
- RLS is characterized by an irresistible urge to move the legs, arms, or, less commonly, other body parts, usually accompanied by paresthesias, often causing difficulty falling asleep and/or repeated nocturnal awakenings.
- Diagnose RLS clinically, but if PLMD is suspected, consider polysomnography.
- PMLD has no specific treatments, but those used for RLS often help.
- For RLS, try dopaminergic drugs or gabapentin enacarbil, which are often effective.

240 Spinal Cord Disorders

Spinal cord disorders can cause permanent severe neurologic disability. For some patients, such disability can be avoided or minimized if evaluation and treatment are rapid.

Spinal cord disorders usually result from conditions extrinsic to the cord, such as the following:

- Compression due to spinal stenosis
- Herniated disk
- Tumor
- Abscess
- Hematoma

Less commonly, disorders are intrinsic to the cord. Intrinsic disorders include spinal cord infarction, hemorrhage, transverse myelitis, HIV infection, poliovirus infection, West Nile virus infection, syphilis (which can cause tabes dorsalis), trauma, vitamin B_{12} deficiency (which causes subacute combined degeneration), decompression sickness, lightning injury (which can cause keraunoparalysis), radiation therapy (which can cause myelopathy), syrinx, and spinal cord tumor. Arteriovenous malformations may be extrinsic or intrinsic. Copper deficiency

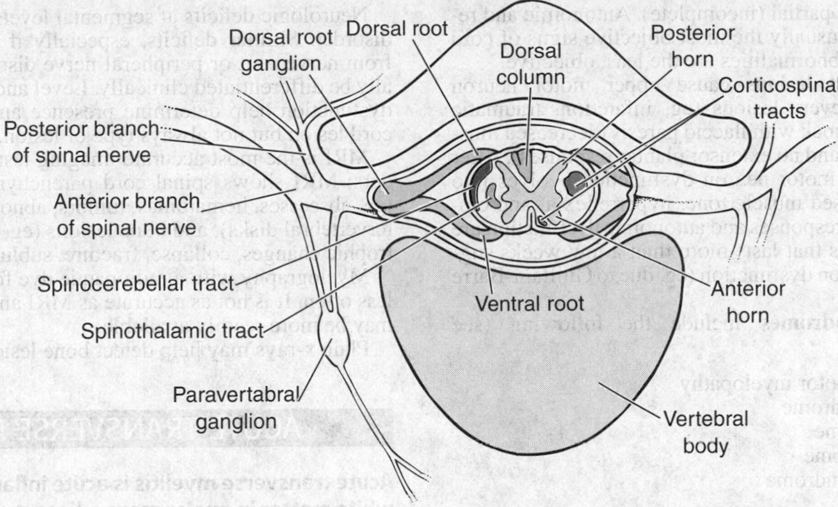

Fig. 240–1. Spinal nerve.

may result in myelopathy similar to that caused by vitamin B_{12} deficiency.

Spinal nerve roots outside of the spinal cord may also be damaged (see p. 1989).

Anatomy

The spinal cord extends caudally from the medulla at the foramen magnum and terminates at the upper lumbar vertebrae, usually between L1 and L2, where it forms the conus medullaris. In the lumbosacral region, nerve roots from lower cord segments descend within the spinal column in a nearly vertical sheaf, forming the cauda equina.

The white matter at the cord's periphery contains ascending and descending tracts of myelinated sensory and motor nerve fibers. The central H-shaped gray matter is composed of cell bodies and nonmyelinated fibers (see Fig. 240–1). The anterior (ventral) horns of the "H" contain lower motor neurons, which receive impulses from the motor cortex via the descending corticospinal tracts and, at the local level, from internuncial neurons and afferent fibers from muscle spindles. The axons of the lower motor neurons are the efferent fibers of the spinal nerves. The posterior (dorsal) horns contain sensory fibers that originate in cell bodies in the dorsal root ganglia. The gray matter also contains many internuncial neurons that carry motor, sensory, or reflex impulses from dorsal to ventral nerve roots, from one side of the cord to the other, or from one level of the cord to another.

The spinothalamic tract transmits pain and temperature sensation contralaterally in the spinal cord; most other tracts transmit information ipsilaterally. The cord is divided into functional segments (levels) corresponding approximately to the attachments of the 31 pairs of spinal nerve roots.

Symptoms and Signs

Neurologic dysfunction due to spinal cord disorders occurs at the involved spinal cord segment (see Table 240–1) and at all segments below it. The exception is the central cord syndrome (see Table 240–2), which may spare segments below.

Spinal cord disorders cause various patterns of deficits depending on which nerve tracts within the cord or which spinal roots outside the cord are damaged. Disorders affecting spinal nerves, but not directly affecting the cord, cause sensory or motor abnormalities or both only in the areas supplied by the affected spinal nerves.

Spinal cord dysfunction causes

- Paresis
- Loss of sensation
- Reflex changes
- Autonomic dysfunction (eg, bowel, bladder, and erectile dysfunction; loss of sweating)

Table 240–1. EFFECTS OF SPINAL CORD DYSFUNCTION BY SEGMENTAL LEVEL

LOCATION OF LESION*	POSSIBLE EFFECTS
At or above C5	Respiratory paralysis Quadriplegia
Between C5 and C6	Paralysis of legs, wrists, and hands Weakness of shoulder abduction and elbow flexion Loss of biceps jerk reflex Loss of brachioradialis deep tendon reflex
Between C6 and C7	Paralysis of legs, wrists, and hands, but shoulder movement and elbow flexion usually possible
Between C7 and C8	Loss of triceps jerk reflex Paralysis of legs and hands
At C8 to T1	Horner syndrome (constricted pupil, ptosis, facial anhidrosis) Paralysis of legs
Between T1 and conus medullaris	Paralysis of legs

*Abbreviations refer to vertebrae; the cord is shorter than the spine, so that moving down the spine, cord segments and vertebral levels are increasingly out of alignment.

At all levels of cord injury, deep tendon reflexes are altered (initially decreased and later becoming brisk) below the level of the lesion, bowel and bladder control is lost, and sensation is lost below the level of injury.

Dysfunction may be partial (incomplete). Autonomic and reflex abnormalities are usually the most objective signs of cord dysfunction; sensory abnormalities are the least objective.

Corticospinal tract lesions cause upper motor neuron dysfunction. Acute, severe lesions (eg, infarction, traumatic lesions) cause spinal shock with flaccid paresis (decreased muscle tone, hyporeflexia, and no extensor plantar responses). After days or weeks, upper motor neuron dysfunction evolves into spastic paresis (increased muscle tone, hyperreflexia, and clonus). Extensor plantar responses and autonomic dysfunction are present. Flaccid paresis that lasts more than a few weeks suggests lower motor neuron dysfunction (eg, due to Guillain-Barré syndrome).

Specific cord syndromes include the following (see Table 240–2):

- Transverse sensorimotor myelopathy
- Brown-Séquard syndrome
- Central cord syndrome
- Anterior cord syndrome
- Conus medullaris syndrome

Cauda equina syndrome, which involves damage to nerve roots at the caudal end of the cord, is not a spinal cord syndrome. However, it mimics conus medullaris syndrome, causing distal leg paresis and sensory loss in and around the perineum and anus (saddle anesthesia), as well as bladder, bowel, and pudendal dysfunction (eg, urinary retention, urinary frequency, urinary or fecal incontinence, erectile dysfunction, loss of rectal tone, abnormal bulbocavernosus and anal wink reflexes). In cauda equina syndrome (unlike in spinal cord injury), muscle tone and deep tendon reflexes are decreased in the legs.

Diagnosis

- MRI

Neurologic deficits at segmental levels suggest a spinal cord disorder. Similar deficits, especially if unilateral, may result from nerve root or peripheral nerve disorders, which can usually be differentiated clinically. Level and pattern of spinal cord dysfunction help determine presence and location of a spinal cord lesion but not always type of lesion.

MRI is the most accurate imaging test for spinal cord disorders; MRI shows spinal cord parenchyma, soft-tissue lesions (eg, abscesses, hematomas, tumors, abnormalities involving intervertebral disks), and bone lesions (eg, erosion, severe hypertrophic changes, collapse, fracture, subluxation, tumors).

Myelography with a radiopaque dye followed by CT is used less often. It is not as accurate as MRI and is more invasive but may be more readily available.

Plain x-rays may help detect bone lesions.

ACUTE TRANSVERSE MYELITIS

Acute transverse myelitis is acute inflammation of gray and white matter in one or more adjacent spinal cord segments, usually thoracic. Causes include multiple sclerosis, neuromyelitis optica, infections, autoimmune or postinfectious inflammation, vasculitis, and certain drugs. Symptoms include bilateral motor, sensory, and sphincter deficits below the level of the lesion. Diagnosis is usually by MRI, CSF analysis, and blood tests. IV corticosteroids and plasma exchange may be helpful early. Otherwise, treatment is with supportive measures and correction of any causes.

Acute transverse myelitis is most commonly due to multiple sclerosis but can occur with vasculitis, mycoplasmal infections, Lyme disease, syphilis, TB, or viral meningoencephalitis or in

Table 240–2. SPINAL CORD SYNDROMES

SYNDROME	CAUSE	SYMPTOMS AND SIGNS
Anterior cord syndrome	Lesions disproportionately affecting the anterior spinal cord, commonly due to infarction (eg, caused by occlusion of the anterior spinal artery)	Malfunction of all tracts except the posterior columns, thus sparing position and vibratory sensation
Brown-Séquard syndrome (rare)	Unilateral spinal cord lesions, typically due to penetrating trauma	Ipsilateral paresis Ipsilateral loss of touch, position, and vibratory sensation Contralateral loss of pain and temperature sensation*
Central cord syndrome affecting the cervical spinal cord	Lesions affecting the center of the cervical spinal cord, mainly central gray matter (including spinothalamic tracts, which cross), commonly due to trauma, syrinx, or tumors in the central spinal cord	Paresis tending to be more severe in the upper extremities than in the lower extremities and sacral regions Tendency to lose pain and temperature sensation in a capelike distribution over the upper neck, shoulders, and upper trunk, with light touch, position, and vibratory sensation relatively preserved (dissociated sensory loss)
Conus medullaris syndrome	Lesions around L1	Distal leg paresis Perianal and perineal loss of sensation (saddle anesthesia) Erectile dysfunction Urinary retention, frequency, or incontinence Fecal incontinence Hypotonic anal sphincter Abnormal bulbocavernosus and anal wink reflexes
Transverse myelopathy	Lesions affecting all or most tracts of the spinal cord at ≥ 1 segmental levels	Deficits in all functions mediated by the spinal cord (because all tracts are affected to some degree)

*Occasionally, only part of one side of the spinal cord malfunctions (partial Brown-Séquard syndrome).

patients taking amphetamines, IV heroin, or antiparasitic or antifungal drugs. Transverse myelitis occurs with optic neuritis in neuromyelitis optica (Devic disease), once considered a variant of multiple sclerosis but now considered a distinct disorder.

The mechanism of transverse myelitis is often unknown, but some cases follow viral infection or vaccination, suggesting an autoimmune reaction. Inflammation tends to involve the spinal cord diffusely at one or more levels, affecting all spinal cord functions.

Symptoms and Signs

Pain in the neck, back, or head may occur. A bandlike tightness around the chest or abdomen, weakness, tingling, numbness of the feet and legs, and difficulty voiding develop over hours to a few days. Deficits may progress over several more days to a complete transverse sensorimotor myelopathy, causing paraplegia, loss of sensation below the lesion, urinary retention, and fecal incontinence. Occasionally, position and vibration sensation are spared, at least initially.

The syndrome occasionally recurs in patients with multiple sclerosis, SLE, or antiphospholipid syndrome.

Diagnosis

- MRI and CSF analysis
- Other tests to identify treatable causes

Diagnosis of acute transverse myelitis is suggested by transverse sensorimotor myelopathy with segmental deficits. Guillain-Barré syndrome can be distinguished because it does not localize to a specific spinal segment.

Diagnosis requires MRI and CSF analysis. MRI typically shows cord swelling if transverse myelitis is present and can help exclude other treatable causes of spinal cord dysfunction (eg, spinal cord compression). CSF usually contains monocytes, protein content is slightly increased, and IgG index is elevated (normal, ≤ 0.85).

A test for a marker for neuromyelitis optica IgG (NMO-IgG)—an autoantibody that targets the astrocyte water channel protein aquaporin-4—is highly specific and helps distinguish neuromyelitis optica from multiple sclerosis.

Tests for treatable causes should include chest x-ray; PPD; serologic tests for mycoplasma, Lyme disease, and HIV; vitamin B_{12}, folate, zinc, and copper levels; ESR; antinuclear antibodies; and CSF and blood Venereal Disease Research Laboratory (VDRL) tests. History may suggest a drug as a cause.

Brain MRI is done; multiple sclerosis develops in 50% of patients who have multiple periventricular T2 bright lesions and in 5% who do not have them.

Prognosis

Generally, the more rapid the progression is, the worse the prognosis. Pain suggests more intense inflammation. About one third of patients recover, one-third retain some weakness and urinary urgency, and one third are bedbound and incontinent.

Multiple sclerosis eventually develops in about 10 to 20% of the patients in whom the cause is initially unknown.

Treatment

- Treatment of the cause
- Sometimes corticosteroids

Treatment of acute transverse myelitis is directed at the cause or associated disorder but is otherwise supportive.

In idiopathic cases, high-dose corticosteroids are often given and sometimes followed by plasma exchange because the cause may be autoimmune. Efficacy of such a regimen is uncertain.

KEY POINTS

- Autoimmune and demyelinating disorders, infections, and drugs can inflame tissues in spinal cord segments, causing transverse myelitis, which may progress to complete transverse sensorimotor myelopathy.
- Do MRI of the spinal cord, CSF analysis, testing for neuromyelitis optica IgG, and other tests for treatable causes (eg, infections, nutritional deficiencies).
- Treat the cause if identified, and, if no cause is evident, consider corticosteroids and plasma exchange.

SPINAL CORD ARTERIOVENOUS MALFORMATIONS

Arteriovenous malformations (AVMs) in or around the spinal cord can cause cord compression, ischemia, parenchymal hemorrhage, subarachnoid hemorrhage, or a combination. Symptoms may include gradually progressive, ascending, or waxing and waning segmental neurologic deficits; radicular pain; and sudden back pain with sudden segmental neurologic deficits. Diagnosis is by MRI. Treatment is with surgery or stereotactic radiosurgery and may include angiographic embolization.

AVMs are the most common spinal vascular malformations. Most are thoracolumbar, posterior, and outside the cord (extramedullary). The rest are cervical or upper thoracic and often inside the cord (intramedullary). AVMs may be small and localized or may affect up to half the cord. They may compress or even replace normal spinal cord parenchyma, or they may rupture, causing focal or generalized hemorrhage.

Symptoms and Signs

A cutaneous angioma sometimes overlies a spinal AVM. AVMs commonly compress

- Nerve roots, causing pain that radiates down the distribution of a nerve root (radicular pain)
- The spinal cord, causing segmental neurologic deficits that gradually progress or that wax and wane

Combined lower and upper motor neuron deficits are common. AVMs may rupture into the spinal cord parenchyma, causing sudden, severe back pain and sudden segmental neurologic deficits. Rarely, high cervical AVMs rupture into the subarachnoid space, causing subarachnoid hemorrhage with sudden and severe headache, nuchal rigidity, and impaired consciousness.

Diagnosis

- Imaging

Spinal cord AVMs may be detected incidentally during imaging. AVMs are suspected clinically in patients with unexplained segmental neurologic deficits or subarachnoid hemorrhage, particularly those who have sudden, severe back pain or cutaneous midline angiomas.

Diagnosis of AVMs is by MRI (usually done first), then magnetic resonance angiography, and then selective arteriography. Occasionally, myelography plus CT is used.

Treatment

- Surgery if spinal cord function is threatened

Surgery is indicated if spinal cord function is threatened, but expertise in specialized microtechniques is required. Stereotactic radiosurgery is helpful if the AVM is small and located in a surgically inaccessible location. Angiographic embolization occludes feeder arteries and often precedes surgical removal or stereotactic radiosurgery.

CERVICAL SPONDYLOSIS AND SPONDYLOTIC CERVICAL MYELOPATHY

Cervical spondylosis is osteoarthritis of the cervical spine causing stenosis of the canal and sometimes cervical myelopathy due to encroachment of bony osteoarthritic growths (osteophytes) on the lower cervical spinal cord, sometimes with involvement of lower cervical nerve roots (radiculomyelopathy). Diagnosis is by MRI or CT. Treatment may involve NSAIDs and a soft cervical collar or cervical laminectomy.

Cervical spondylosis due to osteoarthritis is common. Occasionally, particularly when the spinal canal is congenitally narrow (< 10 mm), osteoarthritis leads to stenosis of the canal and bony impingement on the cord, causing compression and myelopathy (functional disturbance of the spinal cord). Hypertrophy of the ligamentum flavum can aggravate this effect. Osteophytes in the neural foramina, most commonly between C5 and C6 or C6 and C7, can cause radiculopathy (a nerve root disorder). Manifestations vary according to the neural structures involved but commonly include pain.

Symptoms and Signs

Cord compression commonly causes gradual spastic paresis, paresthesias, or both in the hands and feet and may cause hyperreflexia. Neurologic deficits may be asymmetric, nonsegmental, and aggravated by cough or Valsalva maneuvers. After trauma, people with cervical spondylosis may develop a central cord syndrome (see Table 240–2).

Eventually, muscle atrophy and flaccid paresis may develop in the upper extremities at the level of the lesion, with spasticity below the level of the lesion.

Nerve root compression commonly causes early radicular pain; later, there may be weakness, hyporeflexia, and muscle atrophy.

Diagnosis

- MRI or CT

Cervical spondylosis is suspected when characteristic neurologic deficits occur in patients who are elderly, have osteoarthritis, or have radicular pain at the C5 or C6 levels.

Diagnosis of cervical spondylosis is by MRI or CT.

Treatment

- For cord involvement or refractory radiculopathy, cervical laminectomy
- For radiculopathy only, NSAIDs and a soft cervical collar

For patients with cord involvement, cervical laminectomy is usually needed; a posterior approach can relieve the compression but leaves anterior compressive osteophytes and may result in spinal instability and kyphosis. Thus, an anterior approach with spinal fusion is generally preferred.

Patients with only radiculopathy may try nonsurgical treatment with NSAIDs and a soft cervical collar; if this approach is ineffective, surgical decompression may be required.

HEREDITARY SPASTIC PARAPARESIS

Hereditary spastic paraparesis is a group of rare hereditary disorders characterized by progressive, spinal, nonsegmental, spastic leg paresis, sometimes with intellectual disability, seizures, and other extraspinal deficits. Diagnosis is clinical and sometimes by genetic testing. Treatment is symptomatic, including drugs to relieve spasticity.

The genetic basis of hereditary spastic paraparesis varies and, for many forms, is unknown. In all forms, the descending corticospinal tracts and, to a lesser extent, the dorsal columns and spinocerebellar tracts degenerate, sometimes with loss of anterior horn cells.

Onset can be at any age, from the first year of life to old age, depending on the specific genetic form.

Symptoms and Signs

Symptoms and signs of hereditary spastic paraparesis include spastic leg paresis, with progressive gait difficulty, hyperreflexia, clonus, and extensor plantar responses. Sensation and sphincter function are usually spared. The arms may also be affected. Deficits are not localized to a spinal cord segment.

In some forms, patients also have extraspinal neurologic deficits (eg, spinocerebellar and ocular symptoms, extrapyramidal symptoms, optic atrophy, retinal degeneration, intellectual disability, dementia, polyneuropathy).

Diagnosis

- Clinical evaluation

Hereditary spastic paraparesis is suggested by a family history and any signs of spastic paraparesis.

Diagnosis of hereditary spastic paraparesis is by exclusion of other causes and sometimes by genetic testing.

Treatment

- Symptomatic, including drugs to relieve spasticity

Treatment for all forms of hereditary spastic paraparesis is symptomatic. Baclofen 10 mg po bid, increased as needed up to 40 mg po bid, is given for spasticity. Alternatives include diazepam, clonazepam, dantrolene, botulinum toxin (botulinum toxin type A or botulinum toxin type B), and tizanidine.

Physical therapy and exercise can help maintain mobility and muscle strength, improve range of motion and endurance, reduce fatigue, and prevent spasms. Some patients benefit from using splints, a cane, or crutches.

SPINAL CORD INFARCTION

(Ischemic Myelopathy)

Spinal cord infarction usually results from ischemia originating in an extravertebral artery. Symptoms include sudden and severe back pain, followed immediately by rapidly progressive bilateral flaccid limb weakness and loss of sensation, particularly for pain and temperature. Diagnosis is by MRI. Treatment is generally supportive.

The primary vascular supply for the posterior third of the spinal cord is the posterior spinal arteries; for the anterior two thirds, it is the anterior spinal artery. The anterior spinal artery has only a few feeder arteries in the upper cervical region and one large feeder (the artery of Adamkiewicz) in the lower thoracic region. The feeder arteries originate in the aorta.

Because collateral circulation for the anterior spinal artery is sparse in places, certain cord segments (eg, those around the 2nd to 4th thoracic segments) are especially vulnerable to ischemia. Injury to an extravertebral feeder artery or the aorta (eg, due to atherosclerosis, dissection, or clamping during surgery) causes infarction more commonly than do intrinsic disorders of spinal arteries. Thrombosis is an uncommon cause, and polyarteritis nodosa is a rare cause.

Symptoms and Signs

Sudden pain in the back with tightness radiating circumferentially is followed within minutes by segmental bilateral flaccid weakness and sensory loss. Pain and temperature sensation are disproportionately impaired. The anterior spinal artery is typically affected, resulting in the anterior cord syndrome (see Table 240–2). Position and vibration sensation, conducted by the posterior columns, and often light touch are relatively spared. If the infarct is small and affects primarily tissue farthest away from an occluded artery (toward the center of the cord), a central cord syndrome is also possible. Neurologic deficits may partially resolve after the first few days.

Diagnosis

- MRI

Infarction is suspected when severe back pain and characteristic deficits develop suddenly.

Diagnosis of spinal cord infarction is by MRI. Acute transverse myelitis, spinal cord compression, and demyelinating disorders may cause similar findings but are usually more gradual and are excluded by MRI and by CSF analysis.

Treatment

- Supportive care

Occasionally, the cause of infarction (eg, aortic dissection, polyarteritis nodosa) can be treated, but often the only possible treatment is supportive.

SPINAL CORD COMPRESSION

Various lesions can compress the spinal cord, causing segmental sensory, motor, reflex, and sphincter deficits. Diagnosis is by MRI. Treatment is directed at relieving compression.

Compression is caused far more commonly by lesions outside the spinal cord (extramedullary) than by lesions within it (intramedullary).

Compression may be

- Acute
- Subacute
- Chronic

Acute compression develops within minutes to hours. It is often due to trauma (eg, vertebral crush fracture with displacement of fracture fragments, acute disk herniation, metastatic tumor, severe bone or ligamentous injury causing hematoma, vertebral subluxation or dislocation). It is occasionally due to abscess and rarely due to spontaneous epidural hematoma. Acute compression may follow subacute and chronic compression, especially if the cause is abscess or tumor.

Subacute compression develops over days to weeks. It is usually caused by a metastatic extramedullary tumor, a subdural or an epidural abscess or hematoma, or a cervical or, rarely, thoracic herniated disk.

Chronic compression develops over months to years. It is commonly caused by bony protrusions into the cervical, thoracic, or lumbar spinal canal (eg, due to osteophytes or spondylosis, especially when the spinal canal is narrow, as occurs in spinal stenosis). Compression can be aggravated by a herniated disk and hypertrophy of the ligamentum flavum. Less common causes include arteriovenous malformations and slow-growing extramedullary tumors.

Atlantoaxial subluxation and other craniocervical junction abnormalities may cause acute, subacute, or chronic spinal cord compression.

Lesions that compress the spinal cord may also compress nerve roots or, rarely, occlude the spinal cord's blood supply, causing spinal cord infarction.

Symptoms and Signs

Acute or advanced spinal cord compression causes segmental deficits, paraparesis or quadriparesis, hyporeflexia (when acute) followed by hyperreflexia, extensor plantar responses, loss of sphincter tone (with bowel and bladder dysfunction), and sensory deficits. Subacute or chronic compression may begin with local back pain, often radiating down the distribution of a nerve root (radicular pain), and sometimes hyperreflexia and loss of sensation. Sensory loss may begin in the sacral segments. Complete loss of function may follow suddenly and unpredictably, possibly resulting from secondary spinal cord infarction.

Spinal percussion tenderness is prominent if the cause is metastatic carcinoma, abscess, or hematoma.

Intramedullary lesions tend to cause poorly localized burning pain rather than radicular pain and to spare sensation in sacral dermatomes. These lesions usually result in spastic paresis.

Diagnosis

- MRI or CT myelography

Spinal cord compression is suggested by spinal or radicular pain with reflex, motor, or sensory deficits, particularly at a segmental level.

PEARLS & PITFALLS

- Image the spinal cord immediately if patients have sudden spinal or radicular pain with reflex, motor, or sensory deficits, particularly at a segmental level.

MRI is done immediately if available. If MRI is unavailable, CT myelography is done; a small amount of iohexol (a nonionic, low osmolar radiopaque dye) is introduced via a lumbar puncture and allowed to run cranially to check for complete CSF block. If a block is detected, a radiopaque dye is introduced via a cervical puncture to determine the rostral extension of the block. If traumatic bone abnormalities (eg, fracture, dislocation, subluxation) that require immediate spinal immobilization are suspected, plain spinal x-rays can be done. However, CT detects bone abnormalities better.

Treatment

- Relief of compression

Treatment of spinal cord compression is directed at relieving pressure on the cord. Incomplete or very recent complete loss of function may be reversible, but complete loss of function rarely is; thus, *for acute compression, diagnosis and treatment must occur immediately.*

If compression is due to a tumor, IV dexamethasone 100 mg is given immediately, followed by 25 mg q 6 h and immediate surgery or radiation therapy.

Surgery is indicated in the following cases:

- Neurologic deficits worsen despite nonsurgical treatment.
- A biopsy is needed.
- The spine is unstable.
- Tumors recur after radiation therapy.
- An abscess or a compressive subdural or epidural hematoma is suspected.

KEY POINTS

- Spinal cord compression is usually secondary to an extrinsic mass.
- Manifestations may include back and radicular pain (early) and segmental sensory and/or motor deficits, altered reflexes, extensor plantar responses, and loss of sphincter tone (with bowel and bladder dysfunction).
- Do MRI or CT myelography immediately.
- To relieve pressure on the cord, do surgery or give corticosteroids as soon as possible.

SPINAL EPIDURAL ABSCESS

A spinal epidural abscess is an accumulation of pus in the epidural space that can mechanically compress the spinal cord. Diagnosis is by MRI or, if unavailable, myelography followed by CT. Treatment involves antibiotics and sometimes drainage of the abscess.

Spinal epidural abscesses usually occur in the thoracic or lumbar regions. An underlying infection is often present; it may be remote (eg, endocarditis, furuncle, dental abscess) or contiguous (eg, vertebral osteomyelitis, pressure ulcer, retroperitoneal abscess). In about one-third of cases, the cause cannot be determined. The most common causative organism is *Staphylococcus aureus*, followed by *Escherichia coli* and mixed anaerobes. Occasionally, the cause is a tuberculous abscess of the thoracic spine (Pott disease). Rarely, a similar abscess occurs in the subdural space.

Symptoms and Signs

Symptoms of spinal epidural abscess begin with local or radicular back pain and percussion tenderness, which become severe; pain may be worsened by recumbency. Fever is common. Spinal cord compression may develop; compression of lumbar spinal roots may cause cauda equina syndrome, with neurologic deficits resembling those of conus medullaris syndrome (eg, leg paresis, saddle anesthesia, bladder and bowel dysfunction—see Table 240–2). Deficits progress over hours to days.

Diagnosis

- MRI

Because rapid treatment is necessary to prevent or minimize neurologic deficits, clinicians should consider spinal epidural abscess if patients have significant atraumatic back pain, particularly when there is focal percussion tenderness over the spine, or if they have a fever or have had a recent infection or dental procedure. Characteristic neurologic deficits are more specific but may occur later, so delaying imaging until these neurologic deficits are present can make a poor outcome more likely.

Diagnosis of spinal epidural abscess is by MRI; myelography followed by CT may be used if MRI is not available. Samples from blood and infected areas are cultured.

Lumbar puncture is contraindicated because it may trigger cord herniation if the abscess completely obstructs CSF flow. Plain x-rays are not routinely indicated but show osteomyelitis in about one third of patients. ESR is elevated, but this finding is nonspecific.

Treatment

- Antibiotics
- If abscess causes neurologic compromise, immediate drainage

Antibiotics with or without parenteral needle aspiration may be sufficient; however, abscesses causing neurologic compromise (eg, paresis, bowel or bladder dysfunction) are surgically drained immediately. Pus is gram-stained and cultured. Pending culture results, antibiotics to cover staphylococcus and anaerobes are given as for brain abscess. If the abscess developed after a neurosurgical procedure, an aminoglycoside is added to cover gram-negative bacteria.

SPINAL SUBDURAL OR EPIDURAL HEMATOMA

A spinal subdural or epidural hematoma is an accumulation of blood in the subdural or epidural space that can mechanically compress the spinal cord. Diagnosis is by MRI or, if not immediately available, by CT myelography. Treatment is with immediate surgical drainage.

Spinal subdural or epidural hematoma (usually thoracic or lumbar) is rare but may result from back trauma, anticoagulant or thrombolytic therapy, or, in patients with bleeding diatheses, lumbar puncture.

Symptoms and Signs

Symptoms of a spinal subdural or epidural hematoma begin with local or radicular back pain and percussion tenderness; they are often severe. Spinal cord compression may develop; compression of lumbar spinal roots may cause cauda equina syndrome and lower extremity paresis. Deficits progress over minutes to hours.

Diagnosis

- MRI

Hematoma is suspected in patients with acute, nontraumatic spinal cord compression or sudden, unexplained lower extremity paresis, particularly if a possible cause (eg, trauma, bleeding diathesis) is present.

Diagnosis is by MRI or, if MRI is not immediately available, by CT myelography.

Treatment

- Drainage

Treatment of a spinal subdural or epidural hematoma is immediate surgical drainage.

Patients taking coumarin anticoagulants are given phytonadione (vitamin K_1) 2.5 to 10 mg sc and fresh frozen plasma as needed to normalize INR. Patients with thrombocytopenia are given platelets.

SYRINX OF THE SPINAL CORD OR BRAIN STEM

A syrinx is a fluid-filled cavity within the spinal cord (syringomyelia) or brain stem (syringobulbia). Predisposing factors include craniocervical junction abnormalities, previous spinal cord trauma, and spinal cord tumors. Symptoms include flaccid weakness of the hands and arms and deficits in pain and temperature sensation in a capelike distribution over the back and neck; light touch and position and vibration sensation are not affected. Diagnosis is by MRI. Treatment includes correction of the cause and surgical procedures to drain the syrinx or otherwise open CSF flow.

Syrinxes usually result from lesions that partially obstruct CSF flow. At least half of syrinxes occur in patients with congenital abnormalities of the craniocervical junction (eg, herniation of cerebellar tissue into the spinal canal, called Chiari malformation), brain (eg, encephalocele), or spinal cord (eg, myelomeningocele). For unknown reasons, these congenital abnormalities often expand during the teen or young adult years. A syrinx can also develop in patients who have a spinal cord tumor, scarring due to previous spinal trauma, or no known predisposing factors. About 30% of people with a spinal cord tumor eventually develop a syrinx.

Syringomyelia is a paramedian, usually irregular, longitudinal cavity. It commonly begins in the cervical area but may extend downward along the entire length of the spinal cord.

Syringobulbia, which is rare, usually occurs as a slitlike gap within the lower brain stem and may disrupt or compress the lower cranial nerve nuclei or ascending sensory or descending motor pathways.

Symptoms and Signs

Symptoms of a syrinx usually begin insidiously between adolescence and age 45.

Syringomyelia develops in the center of the spinal cord, causing a central cord syndrome (see Table 240–2). Pain and temperature sensory deficits occur early but may not be recognized for years. The first abnormality recognized may be a painless burn or cut. Syringomyelia typically causes weakness, atrophy, and often fasciculations and hyporeflexia of the hands and arms; a deficit in pain and temperature sensation in a capelike distribution over the shoulders, arms, and back is characteristic. Light touch and position and vibration sensation are not affected. Later, spastic leg weakness develops. Deficits may be asymmetric.

Syringobulbia may cause vertigo, nystagmus, unilateral or bilateral loss of facial sensation, lingual atrophy and weakness, dysarthria, dysphagia, hoarseness, and sometimes peripheral sensory or motor deficits due to medullary compression.

Diagnosis

- MRI of spinal cord and brain with gadolinium

A syrinx is suggested by an unexplained central cord syndrome or other characteristic neurologic deficits, particularly pain and temperature sensory deficits in a capelike distribution.

MRI of the entire spinal cord and brain is done. Gadolinium enhancement is useful for detecting any associated tumor.

Treatment

- Sometimes surgical decompression

Underlying problems (eg, craniocervical junction abnormalities, postoperative scarring, spinal tumors) are corrected when possible. Surgical decompression of the foramen magnum and upper cervical cord is the only useful treatment, but surgery usually cannot reverse severe neurologic deterioration.

TROPICAL SPASTIC PARAPARESIS/ HTLV-1–ASSOCIATED MYELOPATHY

Tropical spastic paraparesis/HTLV-1–associated myelopathy (TSP/HAM) is a slowly progressive viral immune-mediated disorder of the spinal cord caused by the human T-lymphotropic virus 1 (HTLV-1). It causes spastic weakness of both legs. Diagnosis is by serologic and PCR tests of serum and CSF. Treatment includes supportive care and possibly immunosuppressive therapies.

The HTLV-1 retrovirus is transmitted via sexual contact, IV drug use, or exposure to infected blood or from mother to child via breastfeeding. It is most common among prostitutes, IV drug users, hemodialysis patients, and people from endemic areas such as equatorial regions, southern Japan, and parts of South America.

TSP/HAM affects < 2% of HTLV-1 carriers. It is more common among women; this finding is consistent with the higher prevalence of HTLV-1 infection in women. HTLV-2 may cause a similar disorder.

The virus resides in T cells in blood and CSF. CD4+ memory T cells, CD8+ cytotoxic T cells, and macrophages infiltrate the perivascular areas and parenchyma of the spinal cord; astrocytosis occurs. For several years after onset of neurologic symptoms, inflammation of spinal gray and white matter progresses, causing preferential degeneration of the lateral and posterior columns. Myelin and axons in the anterior columns are also lost.

Symptoms and Signs

Spastic weakness develops gradually in both legs, with extensor plantar responses and bilateral symmetric loss of position and vibratory sensation in the feet. Achilles tendon reflexes are often absent. Urinary incontinence and urgency are common.

Symptoms usually progress over several years.

Diagnosis

- Serologic and PCR tests of serum and CSF

TSP/HAM is suggested by typical neurologic deficits that are otherwise unexplained, particularly in patients with risk factors.

Serum and CSF serologic tests, PCR tests, and spinal cord MRI are indicated. If CSF-to-serum ratio of HTLV-1 antibodies is > 1 or if PCR detects HTLV-1 antigen in CSF, the diagnosis is very likely. Protein and Ig levels in CSF may also be elevated, often with oligoclonal bands; lymphocytic pleocytosis occurs in up to 50% of patients. Spinal cord lesions often appear hyperintense on T2-weighted MRI.

Treatment

- Immunomodulatory or immunosuppressive therapies

No treatment has proved effective, but interferon alfa, IV immune globulin, and oral methylprednisolone may have some benefit.

Treatment of spasticity is symptomatic (eg, with baclofen or tizanidine).

241 Stroke

Strokes are a heterogeneous group of disorders involving sudden, focal interruption of cerebral blood flow that causes neurologic deficit. Strokes can be

- Ischemic (80%), typically resulting from thrombosis or embolism
- Hemorrhagic (20%), resulting from vascular rupture (eg, subarachnoid hemorrhage, intracerebral hemorrhage)

Transient stroke symptoms (typically lasting < 1 h) without evidence of acute cerebral infarction (based on diffusion-weighted MRI) are termed a transient ischemic attack (TIA).

In the US, stroke is the 4th most common cause of death and the most common cause of neurologic disability in adults.

Strokes involve the arteries of the brain (see Fig. 241–1), either the anterior circulation (branches of the internal carotid artery) or the posterior circulation (branches of the vertebral and basilar arteries).

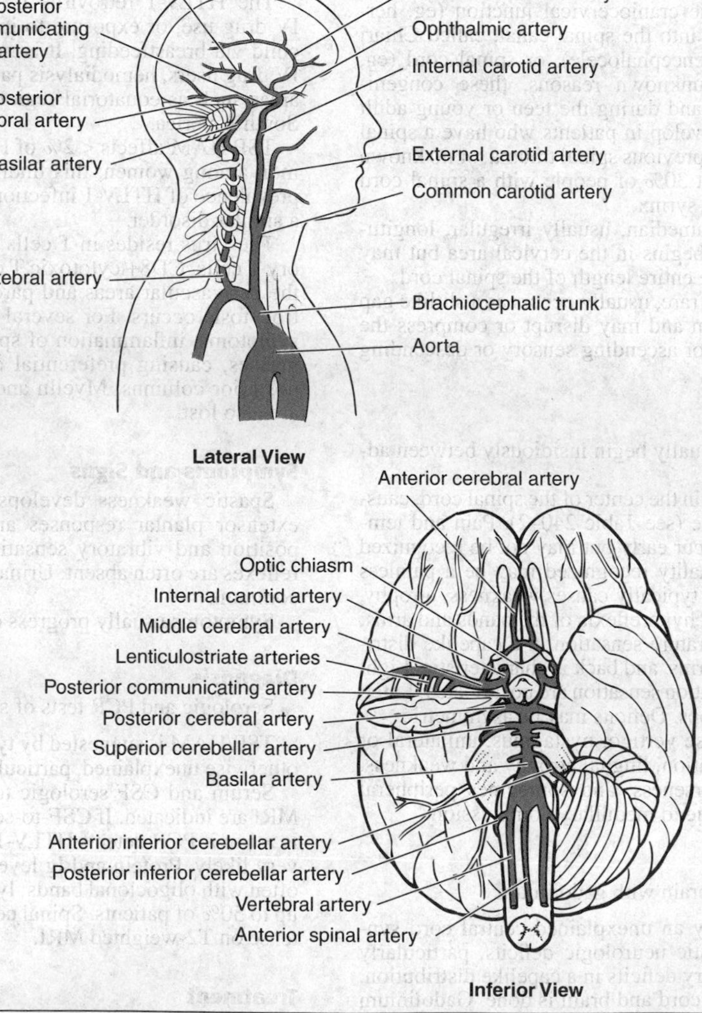

Fig. 241–1. Arteries of the brain. The anterior cerebral artery supplies the medial portions of the frontal and parietal lobes and corpus callosum. The middle cerebral artery supplies large portions of the frontal, parietal, and temporal lobe surfaces. Branches of the anterior and middle cerebral arteries (lenticulostriate arteries) supply the basal ganglia and anterior limb of the internal capsule. The vertebral and basilar arteries supply the brain stem, cerebellum, posterior cerebral cortex, and medial temporal lobe. The posterior cerebral arteries bifurcate from the basilar artery to supply the medial temporal (including the hippocampus) and occipital lobes, thalamus, and mammillary and geniculate bodies. Anterior circulation and posterior circulation communicate in the circle of Willis.

Risk factors: The following are the modifiable factors that contribute the most to increased risk of stroke:

- Hypertension
- Cigarette smoking
- Dyslipidemia
- Diabetes
- Insulin resistance[1]
- Abdominal obesity
- Alcoholism
- Lack of physical activity
- High-risk diet (eg, high in saturated fats, trans fats, and calories)
- Psychosocial stress (eg, depression)
- Heart disorders (particularly disorders that predispose to emboli, such as acute MI, infective endocarditis, and atrial fibrillation)
- Hypercoagulability (thrombotic stroke only)
- Intracranial aneurysms (subarachnoid hemorrhage only)
- Use of certain drugs (eg, cocaine, amphetamines)
- Vasculitis

Unmodifiable risk factors include the following:

- Prior stroke
- Older age
- Family history of stroke
- Male sex

1. Kernan WN, Viscoli CM, Furie KL, et al: Pioglitazone after ischemic stroke or transient ischemic attack. *N Engl J Med* 374(14):1321–1331, 2016. doi: 10.1056/NEJMoa1506930.

Symptoms and Signs

Initial symptoms of stroke occur suddenly. Generally, they include numbness, weakness, or paralysis of the contralateral limbs and the face; aphasia; confusion; visual disturbances in one or both eyes (eg, transient monocular blindness); dizziness or loss of balance and coordination; and headache.

Neurologic deficits reflect the area of brain involved (see Table 241–1). Anterior circulation stroke typically causes unilateral symptoms. Posterior circulation stroke can cause unilateral or bilateral deficits and is more likely to affect consciousness, especially when the basilar artery is involved.

Systemic or autonomic disturbances (eg, hypertension, fever) occasionally occur.

Other manifestations, rather than neurologic deficits, often suggest the type of stroke. For example,

- Sudden, severe headache suggests subarachnoid hemorrhage.
- Impaired consciousness or coma, often accompanied by headache, nausea, and vomiting, suggests increased intracranial pressure, which can occur 48 to 72 h after large ischemic strokes and earlier in many hemorrhagic strokes; fatal brain herniation may result.

Complications: Stroke complications can include sleep problems, confusion, depression, incontinence, atelectasis, pneumonia, and swallowing dysfunction, which can lead to aspiration, dehydration, or undernutrition. Immobility can lead to thromboembolic disease, deconditioning, sarcopenia, UTIs, pressure ulcers, and contractures.

Daily functioning (including the ability to walk, see, feel, remember, think, and speak) may be decreased.

Evaluation

Evaluation aims to establish the following:

- Whether stroke has occurred
- Whether stroke is ischemic or hemorrhagic
- Whether emergency treatment is required
- What the best strategies for preventing subsequent strokes are
- Whether and how to pursue rehabilitation

Table 241–1. SELECTED STROKE SYNDROMES

SYMPTOMS AND SIGNS	SYNDROME
Contralateral hemiparesis (maximal in the leg), urinary incontinence, apathy, confusion, poor judgment, mutism, grasp reflex, gait apraxia	Anterior cerebral artery (uncommon)
Contralateral hemiparesis (worse in the arm and face than in the leg), dysarthria, hemianesthesia, contralateral homonymous hemianopia, aphasia (if the dominant hemisphere is affected) or apraxia and sensory neglect (if the nondominant hemisphere is affected)	Middle cerebral artery (common)
Contralateral homonymous hemianopia, unilateral cortical blindness, memory loss, unilateral 3rd cranial nerve palsy, hemiballismus	Posterior cerebral artery
Monocular loss of vision (amaurosis)	Ophthalmic artery (a branch of the internal carotid artery)
Unilateral or bilateral cranial nerve deficits (eg, nystagmus, vertigo, dysphagia, dysarthria, diplopia, blindness), truncal or limb ataxia, spastic paresis, crossed sensory and motor deficits*, impaired consciousness, coma, death (if basilar artery occlusion is complete), tachycardia, labile BP	Vertebrobasilar system
Absence of cortical deficits plus one of the following: • Pure motor hemiparesis • Pure sensory hemianesthesia • Ataxic hemiparesis • Dysarthria–clumsy hand syndrome	Lacunar infarcts

*Ipsilateral facial sensory loss or motor weakness with contralateral body hemianesthesia or hemiparesis indicates a lesion at the pons or medulla.

Stroke is suspected in patients with any of the following:

- Sudden neurologic deficits compatible with brain damage in an arterial territory
- A particularly sudden, severe headache
- Sudden, unexplained coma
- Sudden impairment of consciousness

Glucose is measured at bedside to rule out hypoglycemia.

If stroke is still suspected, immediate neuroimaging is required to differentiate hemorrhagic from ischemic stroke and to detect signs of increased intracranial pressure. CT is sensitive for intracranial blood but may be normal or show only subtle changes during the first hours of symptoms after anterior circulation ischemic stroke. CT also misses some small posterior circulation strokes. MRI is sensitive for intracranial blood and may detect signs of ischemic stroke missed by CT, but CT can usually be done more rapidly. If CT does not confirm clinically suspected stroke, diffusion-weighted MRI can usually detect ischemic stroke.

If consciousness is impaired and lateralizing signs are absent or equivocal, further tests to check for other causes are done.

After the stroke is identified as ischemic or hemorrhagic, tests are done to determine the cause. Patients are also evaluated for coexisting acute general disorders (eg, infection, dehydration, hypoxia, hyperglycemia, hypertension). Patients are asked about depression, which commonly occurs after stroke. A dysphagia team evaluates swallowing; sometimes a barium swallow study is necessary.

Treatment

- Stabilization
- Reperfusion for some ischemic strokes
- Supportive measures and treatment of complications
- Strategies to prevent future strokes

Stabilization may need to precede complete evaluation. Comatose or obtunded patients (eg, Glasgow Coma Score ≤ 8) may require airway support. If increased intracranial pressure is suspected, intracranial pressure monitoring and measures to reduce cerebral edema may be necessary.

Specific acute treatments vary by type of stroke. They may include reperfusion (eg, recombinant tissue plasminogen activator, thrombolysis, mechanical thrombectomy) for some ischemic strokes.

Providing supportive care, correcting coexisting abnormalities (eg, fever, hypoxia, dehydration, hyperglycemia, sometimes hypertension), and preventing and treating complications are vital during the acute phase and convalescence (see Table 241–2); these measures clearly improve clinical outcomes.[1] During convalescence, measures to prevent aspiration, deep venous thrombosis, UTIs, pressure ulcers, and undernutrition may be necessary. Passive exercises, particularly of paralyzed limbs, and breathing exercises are started early to prevent contractures, atelectasis, and pneumonia.

After a stroke, most patients require rehabilitation (occupational and physical therapy) to maximize functional recovery. Some need additional therapies (eg, speech therapy, feeding restrictions). For rehabilitation, an interdisciplinary approach is best.

Depression after stroke may require antidepressants; many patients benefit from counseling.

Modifying risk factors through lifestyle changes (eg, stopping cigarette smoking) and drug therapy (eg, for hypertension) can help delay or prevent subsequent strokes. Other stroke prevention strategies are chosen based on the patient's risk factors. For ischemic stroke prevention, strategies may include procedures (eg, carotid endarterectomy, stent placement), antiplatelet therapy, and anticoagulation.

Table 241–2. STRATEGIES TO PREVENT AND TREAT STROKE COMPLICATIONS

Applying intermittent external compression devices when anticoagulants are contraindicated and providing frequent active and passive leg exercises
Turning bedridden patients frequently, with special attention to pressure sites
Passively moving limbs at risk of contractures and placing them in the appropriate resting positions, using splints if necessary
Ensuring adequate fluid intake and nutrition, including evaluating patients for swallowing difficulties and providing nutritional support as necessary
Giving small doses of enoxaparin 40 mg sc q 24 h or heparin 5000 U sc q 12 h, when not contraindicated, to prevent deep venous thrombosis and pulmonary embolism
Encouraging early ambulation (as soon as vital signs are normal), with close monitoring
Maximizing lung function (eg, smoking cessation, deep breathing exercises, respiratory therapy, measures to prevent aspiration in patients with dysphagia)
Looking for and treating infections early, especially pneumonia, UTIs, and skin infections
Managing urinary bladder problems in bedbound patients, preferably without using an indwelling catheter
Promoting risk factor modification (eg, smoking cessation, weight loss, healthful diet)
Prescribing early rehabilitation (eg, active and passive exercises, range-of-motion exercises)
Compassionately discussing residual function, prognosis for recovery, and strategies to compensate for lost function with the patient
Encouraging maximum independence through rehabilitation
Encouraging the patient and family members to contact stroke support groups for social and psychologic support

1. Jauch EC, Saver JL, Adams HP Jr, et al: Guidelines for the early management of patients with acute ischemic stroke: A guideline for healthcare professionals from the American Heart Association/American Stroke Association. *Stroke* 44(3):870–947, 2013. doi: 10.1161/STR.0b013e318284056a.

ISCHEMIC STROKE

Ischemic stroke is sudden neurologic deficits that result from focal cerebral ischemia associated with permanent brain infarction (eg, positive results on diffusion-weighted MRI). Common causes are (from most to least common) atherothrombotic occlusion of large arteries; cerebral embolism (embolic infarction); nonthrombotic occlusion of small, deep cerebral arteries (lacunar infarction); and

proximal arterial stenosis with hypotension that decreases cerebral blood flow in arterial watershed zones (hemodynamic stroke). Diagnosis is clinical, but CT or MRI is done to exclude hemorrhage and confirm the presence and extent of stroke. Thrombolytic therapy may be useful acutely in certain patients. Depending on the cause of stroke, carotid endarterectomy or stenting, antiplatelet drugs, or warfarin may help reduce risk of subsequent strokes.

Etiology

The following are the modifiable risk factors that contribute the most to increased risk of ischemic stroke:

- Hypertension
- Cigarette smoking
- Dyslipidemia
- Diabetes
- Insulin resistance[1]
- Abdominal obesity
- Alcoholism
- Lack of physical activity
- High-risk diet (eg, high in saturated fats, trans fats, and calories)
- Psychosocial stress (eg, depression)
- Heart disorders (particularly disorders that predispose to emboli, such as acute MI, infective endocarditis, and atrial fibrillation)
- Use of certain drugs (eg, cocaine, amphetamines)
- Hypercoagulability
- Vasculitis

Unmodifiable risk factors include the following:

- Prior stroke
- Older age
- Family history of stroke
- Male sex

Ischemia usually results from thrombi or emboli. Even infarcts classified as lacunar based on clinical criteria (morphology, size, and location) often involve small thrombi or emboli.

Thrombosis: Atherothrombotic occlusion of large arteries (thrombus superimposed on an atherosclerotic artery) is the most common cause of ischemic stroke.

Atheromas, particularly if ulcerated, predispose to thrombi. Atheromas can occur in any major cerebral artery and are common at areas of turbulent flow, particularly at the carotid bifurcation. Partial or complete thrombotic occlusion occurs most often at the main trunk of the middle cerebral artery and its branches but is also common in the large arteries at the base of the brain, in deep perforating arteries, and in small cortical branches. The basilar artery and the segment of the internal carotid artery between the cavernous sinus and supraclinoid process are often occluded.

Less common causes of thrombosis include vascular inflammation secondary to disorders such as acute or chronic meningitis, vasculitic disorders, and syphilis; dissection of intracranial arteries or the aorta; hypercoagulability disorders (eg, antiphospholipid syndrome, hyperhomocysteinemia); hyperviscosity disorders (eg, polycythemia, thrombocytosis, hemoglobinopathies, plasma cell disorders); and rare disorders (eg, fibromuscular dysplasia, moyamoya disease, Binswanger disease). Older oral contraceptive formulations increase risk of thrombosis. In children, sickle cell disease is a common cause of ischemic stroke.

Embolism: Emboli may lodge anywhere in the cerebral arterial tree.

Emboli may originate as cardiac thrombi, especially in the following conditions:

- Atrial fibrillation
- Rheumatic heart disease (usually mitral stenosis)
- Post-MI
- Vegetations on heart valves in bacterial or marantic endocarditis
- Prosthetic heart valves
- Mechanical circulatory assist devices (eg, left ventricular assist device, or LVAD)[2]

Other sources include clots that form after open-heart surgery and atheromas in neck arteries or in the aortic arch. Rarely, emboli consist of fat (from fractured long bones), air (in decompression sickness), or venous clots that pass from the right to the left side of the heart through a patent foramen ovale with shunt (paradoxical emboli). Emboli may dislodge spontaneously or after invasive cardiovascular procedures (eg, catheterization). Rarely, thrombosis of the subclavian artery results in embolic stroke in the vertebral artery or its branches.

Lacunar infarcts: Ischemic stroke can also result from lacunar infarcts. These small (≤ 1.5 cm) infarcts result from nonatherothrombotic obstruction of small, perforating arteries that supply deep cortical structures; the usual cause is lipohyalinosis (degeneration of the media of small arteries and replacement by lipids and collagen). Whether emboli cause lacunar infarcts is controversial.

Lacunar infarcts tend to occur in elderly patients with diabetes or poorly controlled hypertension.

Other causes: Any factor that impairs systemic perfusion (eg, carbon monoxide toxicity, severe anemia or hypoxia, polycythemia, hypotension) increases risk of all types of ischemic strokes. A stroke may occur along the borders between territories of arteries (watershed areas); in such areas, blood supply is normally low, particularly if patients have hypotension and/or if major cerebral arteries are stenotic.

Less commonly, ischemic stroke results from vasospasm (eg, during migraine, after subarachnoid hemorrhage, after use of sympathomimetic drugs such as cocaine or amphetamines) or venous sinus thrombosis (eg, during intracranial infection, postoperatively, peripartum, secondary to a hypercoagulability disorder).

1. Kernan WN, Viscoli CM, Furie KL, et al: Pioglitazone after ischemic stroke or transient ischemic attack. *N Engl J Med* 374(14):1321–1331, 2016. doi: 10.1056/NEJMoa1506930.
2. Morgan JA, Brewer RJ, Nemeh HW, et al: Stroke while on long-term left ventricular assist device support: incidence, outcome, and predictors. *ASAIO* J 60(3):284–289, 2014. doi: 10.1097/MAT.0000000000000074.

Pathophysiology

Inadequate blood flow in a single brain artery can often be compensated for by an efficient collateral system, particularly between the carotid and vertebral arteries via anastomoses at the circle of Willis and, to a lesser extent, between major arteries supplying the cerebral hemispheres. However, normal variations in the circle of Willis and in the caliber of various collateral vessels, atherosclerosis, and other acquired arterial lesions can interfere with collateral flow, increasing the chance that blockage of one artery will cause brain ischemia.

Some neurons die when perfusion is < 5% of normal for > 5 min; however, the extent of damage depends on the severity of ischemia. If it is mild, damage proceeds slowly; thus, even if perfusion is 40% of normal, 3 to 6 h may elapse before brain tissue is completely lost. However, if severe ischemia persists > 15 to 30 min, all of the affected tissue dies (infarction). Damage occurs more rapidly during hyperthermia and more slowly during hypothermia. If tissues are ischemic but not yet irreversibly damaged, promptly restoring blood flow may reduce or reverse injury. For example, intervention may be able to salvage the moderately ischemic areas (penumbras) that often surround areas of severe ischemia (these areas exist because of collateral flow).

Mechanisms of ischemic injury include

- Edema
- Microvascular thrombosis
- Programmed cell death (apoptosis)
- Infarction with cell necrosis

Inflammatory mediators (eg, IL-1B, tumor necrosis factor-alpha) contribute to edema and microvascular thrombosis. Edema, if severe or extensive, can increase intracranial pressure.

Many factors may contribute to necrotic cell death; they include loss of ATP stores, loss of ionic homeostasis (including intracellular calcium accumulation), lipid peroxidative damage to cell membranes by free radicals (an iron-mediated process), excitatory neurotoxins (eg, glutamate), and intracellular acidosis due to accumulation of lactate.

Symptoms and Signs

Symptoms and signs of ischemic stroke depend on the part of brain affected. Patterns of neurologic deficits often suggest the affected artery (see Table 241–1), but correlation is often inexact.

Deficits may become maximal within several minutes of onset, typically in embolic stroke. Less often, deficits evolve slowly, usually over 24 to 48 h (called evolving stroke or stroke in evolution), typically in atherothrombotic stroke. In most evolving strokes, unilateral neurologic dysfunction (often beginning in one arm, then spreading ipsilaterally) extends without causing headache, pain, or fever. Progression is usually stepwise, interrupted by periods of stability. A stroke is considered submaximal when after it is complete, there is residual function in the affected area, suggesting viable tissue at risk of damage.

Embolic strokes often occur during the day; headache may precede neurologic deficits. Thrombi tend to occur during the night and thus are first noticed on awakening.

Lacunar infarcts may produce one of the classic lacunar syndromes (eg, pure motor hemiparesis, pure sensory hemianesthesia, ataxic hemiparesis, dysarthria–clumsy hand syndrome); signs of cortical dysfunction (eg, aphasia) are absent. Multiple lacunar infarcts may result in multi-infarct dementia.

A seizure may occur at stroke onset, more often with embolic than thrombotic stroke. Seizures may also occur months to years later; late seizures result from scarring or hemosiderin deposition at the site of ischemia.

Deterioration during the first 48 to 72 h after onset of symptoms, particularly progressively impaired consciousness, results more often from cerebral edema than from extension of the infarct. Unless the infarct is large or extensive, function commonly improves within the first few days; further improvement occurs gradually for up to 1 yr.

Diagnosis

- Primarily clinical evaluation
- Neuroimaging and bedside glucose testing
- Evaluation to identify the cause

Diagnosis of ischemic stroke is suggested by sudden neurologic deficits referable to a specific arterial territory. Ischemic stroke must be distinguished from other causes of similar focal deficits (sometimes called stroke mimics), such as

- Hypoglycemia
- Postictal [Todd] paralysis (a transient neurologic deficit, usually weakness, of the limb contralateral to the seizure focus)
- Hemorrhagic stroke
- Rarely, migraine

Headache, coma or stupor, and vomiting are more likely with hemorrhagic stroke.

Differentiating clinically between the types of stroke is imprecise; however, some clues based on symptom progression, time of onset, and type of deficit can help.

Although diagnosis is clinical, neuroimaging and bedside glucose testing are mandatory. CT is done first to exclude intracerebral hemorrhage, subdural or epidural hematoma, and a rapidly growing, bleeding, or suddenly symptomatic tumor. CT evidence of even a large anterior circulation ischemic stroke may be subtle during the first few hours; changes may include effacement of sulci or the insular cortical ribbon, loss of the gray-white junction between cortex and white matter, and a dense middle cerebral artery sign. Within 6 to 12 h of ischemia, medium-sized to large infarcts start to become visible as hypodensities; small infarcts (eg, lacunar infarcts) may be visible only with MRI. Diffusion-weighted MRI (highly sensitive for early ischemia) can be done immediately after initial CT neuroimaging.

Distinction between lacunar, embolic, and thrombotic stroke based on history, examination, and neuroimaging is not always reliable, so tests to identify common or treatable causes and risk factors for all of these types of strokes are routinely done. Patients should be evaluated for the following categories of causes and risk factors:

- Cardiac (eg, atrial fibrillation, potential structural sources of emboli)
- Vascular (eg, critical arterial stenosis)
- Blood (eg, hypercoagulability)

For **cardiac causes**, testing typically includes ECG, telemetry or Holter monitoring, serum troponin, and transthoracic or transesophageal echocardiography.

For **vascular causes**, testing may include magnetic resonance angiography (MRA), CT angiography (CTA), carotid and transcranial duplex ultrasonography, and conventional angiography. The choice and sequence of testing is individualized, based on clinical findings. MRA, CTA, and carotid ultrasonography all show the anterior circulation; however, MRA and CTA provide better images of the posterior circulation than carotid ultrasonography. MRA is generally preferred to CTA if patients can remain still during MRA (to avoid motion artifact).

For **blood-related causes** (eg, thrombotic disorders), blood tests are done to assess their contribution and that of other causes. Routine testing typically includes CBC, platelet count, PT/PTT, fasting blood glucose, and lipid profile.

Depending on which causes are clinically suspected, additional tests may include measurement of homocysteine, testing for thrombotic disorders (antiphospholipid antibodies, protein S, protein C, antithrombin III, factor V Leiden), testing for rheumatic disorders (eg, antinuclear antibodies, rheumatoid factor, ESR), syphilis serologic testing, Hb electrophoresis, and a urine drug screen for cocaine and amphetamines.

A cause cannot be identified for some strokes (cryptogenic strokes).

Prognosis

Stroke severity and progression are often assessed using standardized measures such as the National Institutes of Health (NIH) Stroke Scale (see Table 241–3); the score on this scale correlates with extent of functional impairment and prognosis. During the first days, progression and outcome can be difficult to predict. Older age, impaired consciousness, aphasia, and brain stem signs suggest a poor prognosis. Early improvement and younger age suggest a favorable prognosis.

About 50% of patients with moderate or severe hemiplegia and most with milder deficits have a clear sensorium and eventually can take care of their basic needs and walk adequately. Complete neurologic recovery occurs in about 10%. Use of the affected limb is usually limited, and most deficits that remain after 12 mo are permanent. Patients who have had a stroke are at high risk of subsequent strokes and each tends to worsen neurologic function. About 25% of patients who recover from a first stroke have another stroke within 5 yr.

After an ischemic stroke, about 20% of patients die in the hospital; mortality rate increases with age.

Treatment

- General stroke treatments
- Acute antihypertensive therapy only in certain circumstances
- Antiplatelet therapy
- For acute treatment, sometimes reperfusion with recombinant tissue plasminogen activator (IV or thrombolysis-in-situ), and/or mechanical thrombectomy
- Sometimes anticoagulation
- Long-term control of risk factors
- Sometimes carotid endarterectomy or stenting

Acute stroke treatment: Guidelines for early management of stroke are available from the American Heart Association and American Stroke Association. Patients with acute ischemic strokes are usually hospitalized. Supportive measures may be needed during initial evaluation and stabilization.

Table 241–3. THE NATIONAL INSTITUTES OF HEALTH STROKE SCALE*

CRITERION	FINDING	SCORE	CRITERION	FINDING	SCORE
Level of consciousness (LOC)	Alert	0	Motor leg function (score for both left and right sides)	No drift	0
	Drowsy	1		Drift	1
	Stuporous	2		No resistance to gravity	2
	Comatose	3		No effort against gravity	3
LOC questions†	Answers both correctly	0		No movement	4
	Answers one correctly	1	Limb ataxia	Absent	0
	Answers both incorrectly	2		Present in 1 limb	1
LOC commands‡	Obeys both correctly	0		Present in 2 limbs	2
	Obeys one correctly	1		Untestable	—
	Obeys both incorrectly	2	Sensory	Normal	0
Gaze	Normal	0		Mild to moderate loss	1
	Partial gaze palsy	1		Severe loss	2
	Forced deviation	2	Best language function	No aphasia	0
Visual field	No visual loss	0		Mild to moderate aphasia	1
	Partial hemianopia	1		Severe aphasia	2
	Complete hemianopia	2		Mute	3
	Bilateral hemianopia	3	Dysarthria	Normal articulation	0
Facial palsy	None	0		Mild to moderate dysarthria	1
	Minor	1		Severe dysarthria (unintelligible or worse)	2
	Partial	2		Untestable	—
	Complete	3	Neglect	No neglect	0
Motor arm function (score for both left and right sides)	No drift	0		Partial neglect	1
	Drift	1		Complete neglect	2
	No resistance to gravity	2			
	No effort against gravity	3			
	No movement	4			

*Total score is the sum of the scores for individual items.
†Patients are asked their age and the current month.
‡Patients are asked to open and close the eyes and to make a fist.

Perfusion of an ischemic brain area may require a high BP because autoregulation is lost; thus, BP should not be decreased except in the following cases:

- BP is > 220 mm Hg systolic or > 120 mm Hg diastolic on 2 successive readings > 15 min apart.
- There are signs of other end-organ damage (eg, aortic dissection, acute MI, pulmonary edema, hypertensive encephalopathy, retinal hemorrhages, acute renal failure).
- Use of recombinant tPA and/or mechanical thrombectomy is likely.

To lower BP, clinicians can give nicardipine 2.5 mg/h IV initially; dose is increased by 2.5 mg/h q 5 min to a maximum of 15 mg/h as needed to decrease systolic BP by 10 to 15%. Alternatively, IV labetalol 20 mg IV can be given over 2 min; if response is inadequate, 40 to 80 mg can be given every 10 min up to a total dose of 300 mg.

Patients with presumed thrombi or emboli may be treated with one or a combination of the following:

- tPA, thrombolysis-in-situ, and/or mechanical thrombectomy[1]
- Antiplatelet drugs
- Anticoagulants

Most patients are not candidates for thrombolytic therapy; they should be given an antiplatelet drug (usually aspirin 325 mg po) when they are admitted to the hospital. Contraindications to antiplatelet drugs include aspirin-induced or NSAID-induced asthma or urticaria, other hypersensitivity to aspirin or to tartrazine, acute GI bleeding, G6PD deficiency, and use of warfarin.

Recombinant tPA can be used for patients with acute ischemic stroke up to 3 h after symptom onset if they have no contraindications to tPA (see Table 241–4). Some experts recommend using tPA up to 4.5 h after symptom onset; however, between 3 h and 4.5 h after symptom onset, additional exclusion criteria apply (see Table 241–4). Although tPA can cause fatal or other symptomatic brain hemorrhage, patients treated with tPA strictly according to protocols still have a higher likelihood of functional neurologic recovery. Only physicians experienced in stroke management should use tPA to treat patients with acute stroke; inexperienced physicians are more likely to violate protocols, resulting in more brain hemorrhages and deaths. When tPA is given incorrectly (eg, when given despite the presence of exclusion criteria), risk of hemorrhage due to tPA is high mainly for patients who have had stroke; risk of brain hemorrhage is very low (about 0.5%; 95% confidence interval of 0 to 2.0%)[2] for patients who have had a stroke mimic. If experienced physicians are not available on site, consultation with an expert at a stroke center (including video evaluation of the patient [telemedicine]), if possible, may enable these physicians to use tPA. Because most poor outcomes result from failure to strictly adhere to the protocol, a checklist of inclusion and exclusion criteria should be used.

tPA must be given within 4.5 h of symptom onset—a difficult requirement. Because the precise time of symptom onset may not be known, clinicians must start timing from the moment the patient was last observed to be well.

Before treatment with tPA, the following are required:

- Brain hemorrhage must be excluded by CT.
- Systolic BP must be < 185 mm Hg.
- Diastolic BP must be < 110 mm Hg.

Antihypertensive drugs (IV nicardipine, IV labetalol) may be given as above.

Dose of tPA is 0.9 mg/kg IV (maximum dose 90 mg); 10% is given by rapid IV injection, and the remainder by constant infusion over 60 min. Vital signs are closely monitored for 24 h after treatment, and BP is maintained below 185 mm Hg systolic and 110 mm Hg diastolic. Any bleeding complications are

Table 241–4. EXCLUSION CRITERIA FOR USE OF TISSUE PLASMINOGEN ACTIVATOR IN STROKE

Exclusion criteria < 3 h after symptom onset
Intracranial hemorrhage on CT scan
Multilobar infarct (hypodensity in more than one third of the territory supplied by the middle cerebral artery) on CT scan
Presentation suggesting subarachnoid hemorrhage even if CT is negative
History of intracranial hemorrhage
Intracranial aneurysm, arteriovenous malformation, or tumor
History of stroke or head trauma within the past 3 mo
Systolic BP >185 mm Hg or diastolic BP > 110 mm Hg after antihypertensive treatment
Arterial puncture at noncompressible site or lumbar puncture in the past 7 days
Active internal bleeding
Suspected bleeding disorder
Platelet count < 100,000/μL
Use of heparin within 48 h and elevated PTT
Current use of oral anticoagulants, INR > 1.7, or PT > 15
Serum glucose < 50 mg/dL (< 2.8 mmol/L)
Current use of a direct thrombin inhibitor or direct factor Xa inhibitor with evidence of anticoagulant effect, detected by tests such as PTT, INR, and appropriate factor Xa activity assays
Plasma glucose < 50 or > 400 mg/dL (< 2.78 or > 22.2 mmol/L)
Bacterial endocarditis or suspected pericarditis
Relative exclusion criteria*
Rapidly decreasing symptoms
Major surgery or serious trauma in the past 14 days
GI or urinary tract hemorrhage in the past 21 days
Seizure at onset with postictal residual neurologic deficits
Pregnancy
Acute MI in the past 3 mo
Additional exclusion criteria 3–4.5 h after symptom onset
Age > 80 yr
Use of oral anticoagulants regardless of INR
Baseline NIH stroke score > 25
A history of both stroke and diabetes mellitus

*Jauch EC, Saver JL, Adams HP Jr, et al: Guidelines for the early management of patients with acute ischemic stroke: A guideline for healthcare professionals from the American Heart Association/American Stroke Association. Stroke 44 (3):870–947, 2013. doi: 10.1161/STR.0b013e318284056a.

NIH = National Institutes of Health.

aggressively managed. Anticoagulants and antiplatelet drugs are not used within 24 h of treatment with tPA.

Thrombolysis-in-situ (angiographically directed intra-arterial thrombolysis) of a thrombus or embolus can sometimes be used for major strokes if symptoms began < 6 h ago, particularly for strokes that are due to large occlusions in the middle cerebral artery and cannot be treated with IV recombinant tPA. Clots in the basilar artery may be intra-arterially lysed up to 12 h after stroke onset, sometimes even later depending on the clinical circumstances. This treatment, although standard of care in some large stroke centers, is often unavailable in other hospitals.

Mechanical thrombectomy (angiographically directed intra-arterial removal of a thrombus or embolus by a stent retriever device) is often used to treat patients who have had a severe stroke and have an NIH stroke score ≥ 6 when IV and/or intra-arterial thrombolysis has been ineffective; it must be done within 6 h of symptom onset.[1] Mechanical thrombectomy may be part of standard of care in large stroke centers. It should not be used outside of a stroke center and should not be used instead of IV recombinant tPA within 4.5 h of onset of symptoms in eligible patients with acute ischemic stroke. Devices used to remove thrombi are being improved, and recent models reestablish perfusion in 90 to 100% of patients. It is unclear whether clinical outcomes are better after successful mechanical reperfusion than after treatment with IV tPA; evidence suggests that the earlier reperfusion is achieved, the better the outcome regardless how it is achieved.

In some stroke centers, IV tPA, thrombolysis in situ, and/or mechanical thrombectomy are sometimes done based on imaging criteria (tissue-based criteria) rather than on time after symptom onset (time-based criteria). Tissue-based criteria can be used when time of symptom onset cannot be established (eg, if a patient awakens with stroke symptoms after sleeping several hours or if a patient has aphasia and cannot provide a time frame). To determine eligibility, clinicians use imaging to identify potentially salvageable brain tissue (also called penumbral tissue). The volume of infarcted tissue identified by diffusion-weighted MRI is compared with the volume of at-risk underperfused tissue identified by perfusion-weighted MRI or CT. A sizeable mismatch between the volumes identified by diffusion-weighted and perfusion-weighted imaging suggests that substantial penumbral tissue may still be rescued, and thus thrombolysis and/or thrombectomy is indicated. However, time-based criteria are still used in clinical practice; studies to determine whether outcomes are better using tissue- or time-based criteria are ongoing.

Anticoagulation with heparin or low molecular weight heparin is used for stroke caused by cerebral venous thrombosis and is sometimes used for emboli due to atrial fibrillation and for stroke due to presumed progressive thrombosis if it continues to evolve despite use of antiplatelet drugs and cannot be treated any other way (eg, with tPA or invasive methods). In one large series, outcomes after treatment of basilar artery thrombosis with IV heparin plus IV tPA were as good as or better than those after treatment with endovascular therapies. Warfarin is begun simultaneously with heparin. Before anticoagulation, hemorrhage must be excluded by CT. Constant weight-based heparin infusion (see Fig. 61–2 on p. 496) is used to increase PTT to 1.5 to 2 times baseline values until warfarin has increased the INR to 2 to 3 (3 in hypercoagulable disorders). Because warfarin predisposes to bleeding and is continued after hospital discharge, its use should be restricted to patients who are likely to comply with dosage and monitoring requirements and who are not prone to falls.

Long-term stroke treatment: Supportive care is continued during convalescence. Controlling hyperglycemia and fever can limit brain damage after stroke, leading to better functional outcomes.

Long-term management also focuses on prevention of recurrent stroke (secondary prevention). Modifiable risk factors (eg, hypertension, diabetes, smoking, alcoholism, dyslipidemia, obesity) are treated. Reducing systolic BP may be more effective when the target BP is < 120 mm Hg rather than the typical level (< 140 mm Hg).

Extracranial carotid endarterectomy or stenting is indicated for patients with recent nondisabling, submaximal stroke attributed to an ipsilateral carotid obstruction of 70 to 99% of the arterial lumen or to an ulcerated plaque if life expectancy is at least 5 yr. In other symptomatic patients (eg, patients with TIAs), endarterectomy or stenting with antiplatelet therapy is indicated for carotid obstruction of ≥ 60% with or without ulceration if life expectancy is at least 5 yr. These procedures should be done by surgeons and interventionists who have a successful record with the procedure (ie, morbidity and mortality rate of < 3%) in the hospital where it will be done. If carotid stenosis is asymptomatic, endarterectomy or stenting is beneficial only when done by very experienced surgeons or interventionists, and that benefit is likely to be small. For many patients, carotid stenting with an emboli-protection device (a type of filter) is preferred to endarterectomy, particularly if patients are < 70 yr and have a high surgical risk. Carotid endarterectomy and stenting are equally effective for stroke prevention. In the periprocedural period, MI is more likely after endarterectomy, and recurrent stroke is more likely after stenting.

Extracranial vertebral angioplasty and/or stenting can be used in certain patients with recurrent symptoms of vertebrobasilar ischemia despite optimal medical treatment and a vertebral artery obstruction of 50 to 99%.

Intracranial major artery angioplasty and/or stenting is considered investigational for patients with recurrent stroke or TIA symptoms despite optimal medical treatment and a 50 to 99% obstruction of a major intracranial artery.

Endovascular closure of a patent foramen ovale does not appear to be more effective for preventing strokes than medical management, but studies are ongoing.

Oral antiplatelet drugs are used to prevent subsequent noncardioembolic (atherothrombotic, lacunar, cryptogenic) strokes (secondary prevention). The following may be used:

- Aspirin 81 or 325 mg once/day
- Clopidogrel 75 mg once/day
- The combination product aspirin 25 mg/extended-release dipyridamole 200 mg bid

In patients taking warfarin, antiplatelet drugs additively increase risk of bleeding and are thus usually avoided; however, aspirin is occasionally used simultaneously with warfarin in certain high-risk patients. Clopidogrel is indicated for patients who are allergic to aspirin. If ischemic stroke recurs or if a coronary artery stent becomes blocked while patients are taking clopidogrel, clinicians should suspect impaired metabolism of clopidogrel (ineffective conversion of clopidogrel to its active form because CYP2C19 activity is reduced); a test to determine CYP2C19 status (eg, genetic testing for CYP450 polymorphisms) is recommended. If impaired metabolism is confirmed, aspirin or the combination product aspirin/extended-release dipyridamole is a reasonable alternative.

If patients have had a TIA or minor stroke, clopidogrel plus aspirin given within 24 h of symptom onset appears more effective than aspirin alone for reducing risk of stroke in the first 90 days and does not increase risk of hemorrhage. However, prolonged (eg, > 6 mo) use of clopidogrel plus aspirin is avoided because it has no advantage over aspirin alone in long-term secondary stroke prevention and results in more bleeding complications. Clopidogrel plus aspirin before and for ≥ 30 days after stenting is indicated, usually for ≤ 6 mo; if patients cannot tolerate clopidogrel, ticlopidine 250 mg bid can be substituted.

Oral anticoagulants are indicated for secondary prevention of cardioembolic strokes (as well as primary prevention). Adjusted-dose warfarin (a vitamin K antagonist) with a target INR of 2 to 3 is used for certain patients with nonvalvular or valvular atrial fibrillation. A target INR of 2.5 to 3.5 is used if patients have a mechanical prosthetic cardiac valve. Efficacious alternatives to warfarin for patients with nonvalvular atrial fibrillation include the following new anticoagulants:

- Dabigatran (a direct thrombin inhibitor) 150 mg bid in patients without severe renal failure (creatinine clearance < 15 mL/min) and/or liver failure (elevated INR)
- Apixaban (a direct factor Xa inhibitor) 5 mg bid in patients ≥ 80 yr, in patients with serum creatinine ≥ 1.5 mg/dL and creatinine clearance ≥ 25 mL/min, or as an alternative to aspirin in patients who cannot take warfarin
- Rivaroxaban (a direct factor Xa inhibitor) 20 mg once/day for patients without severe renal failure (creatinine clearance < 15 mL/min)

The main advantage of these new anticoagulants is ease of use (eg, no need to check anticoagulation level with a blood test after the initial dose or to use a parenteral anticoagulant such as unfractionated heparin given by continuous infusion when transitioning from parenteral to oral anticoagulants). Their main disadvantage is lack of an antidote to reverse anticoagulation in case a hemorrhagic complication occurs; the exception is dabigatran, for which idarucizumab is an antidote.[3] Efficacy and safety of combining any of these new anticoagulants with an antiplatelet drug have not been established.

Statins are used to prevent recurrent strokes; lipid levels must be decreased by substantial amounts. Atorvastatin 80 mg once/day is recommended for patients with evidence of atherosclerotic stroke and LDL (low-density lipoprotein) cholesterol ≥ 100 mg/dL. A reasonable LDL cholesterol target is a 50% reduction or a level of < 70 mg/dL. Other statins (eg, simvastatin, pravastatin) may be also used.

1. Powers WJ, Derdeyn CP, Biller J, et al: 2015 American Heart Association/American Stroke Association focused update of the 2013 Guidelines for the Early Management of Patients With Acute Ischemic Stroke regarding endovascular treatment: A guideline for healthcare professionals From the American Heart Association/American Stroke Association. *Stroke* 46(10):3020–3035, 2015. doi: 10.1161/STR.0000000000000074.
2. Tsivgoulis G, Zand R, Katsanos AH, et al: Safety of intravenous thrombolysis in stroke mimics: prospective 5-year study and comprehensive meta-analysis. *Stroke* 46(5):1281–1287, 2015. doi: 10.1161/STROKEAHA.115.009012.
3. Pollack CV Jr, Reilly PA, Eikelboom, J, et al: Idarucizumab for dabigatran reversal. *N Engl J Med* 373:511–520, 2015. doi: 10.1056/NEJMoa1502000.

KEY POINTS

- Differentiate ischemic stroke from hypoglycemia, postictal paralysis, hemorrhagic stroke, and migraine.
- Although clinical differentiation is imprecise, some clues to help differentiate between common types of stroke include symptom progression (maximal deficits within minutes of onset with embolic vs sometimes stepwise or slow onset with thrombotic), time of onset (day with embolic vs night with thrombotic), and type of deficits (eg, specific syndromes and absence of cortical signs with lacunar infarcts).
- Test patients for cardiac causes (including atrial fibrillation) and arterial stenosis, and do blood tests (eg, for thrombotic, rheumatic, and other disorders as indicated).
- In general, do not aggressively reduce BP soon after acute ischemic stroke.
- To determine eligibility for tPA, use a checklist and, when available consult an expert, either in person or via telemedicine.
- To prevent future ischemic strokes, control modifiable risk factors and treat, when appropriate, with antiplatelet therapy, statin therapy, and/or endarterectomy or stenting.

TRANSIENT ISCHEMIC ATTACK

A transient ischemic attack (TIA) is focal brain ischemia that causes sudden, transient neurologic deficits and is not accompanied by permanent brain infarction (eg, negative results on diffusion-weighted MRI). Diagnosis is clinical. Carotid endarterectomy or stenting, antiplatelet drugs, and anticoagulants decrease risk of stroke after certain types of TIA.

TIA is similar to ischemic stroke except that symptoms usually last < 1 h; most TIAs last < 5 min. Infarction is very unlikely if deficits resolve within 1 h. As shown by diffusion-weighted MRI and other studies, deficits that resolve spontaneously within 1 to 24 h are often accompanied by infarction and are thus no longer considered TIAs.

TIAs are most common among the middle-aged and elderly. TIAs markedly increase risk of stroke, beginning in the first 24 h.

Etiology

Risk factors for TIA are the same as those for ischemic stroke. Modifiable risk factors include the following:

- Alcoholism
- Hypertension
- Cigarette smoking
- Dyslipidemia
- Diabetes
- Insulin resistance[1]
- Obesity
- Lack of physical activity
- High-risk diet (eg, high in saturated fats, trans fats, and calories)
- Psychosocial stress (eg, depression)
- Heart disorders (particularly disorders that predispose to emboli, such as acute MI, infective endocarditis, and atrial fibrillation)
- Use of certain drugs (eg, cocaine, amphetamines)
- Hypercoagulability
- Vasculitis

Unmodifiable risk factors include the following:

- Prior stroke
- Older age
- Family history of stroke
- Male sex

Most TIAs are caused by emboli, usually from carotid or vertebral arteries, although most of the causes of ischemic stroke can also result in TIAs.

Uncommonly, TIAs result from impaired perfusion due to severe hypoxemia, reduced oxygen-carrying capacity of blood (eg, profound anemia, carbon monoxide poisoning), or increased blood viscosity (eg, severe polycythemia), particularly in brain arteries with preexisting stenosis. Systemic hypotension does not usually cause cerebral ischemia unless it is severe or arterial stenosis preexists because autoregulation maintains brain blood flow at near-normal levels over a wide range of systemic BPs.

In **subclavian steal syndrome,** a subclavian artery stenosed proximal to the origin of the vertebral artery "steals" blood from the vertebral artery (in which blood flow reverses) to supply the arm during exertion, causing signs of vertebrobasilar ischemia.

Occasionally, TIAs occur in children with a severe cardiovascular disorder that produces emboli or a very high Hct.

1. Kernan WN, Viscoli CM, Furie KL, et al: Pioglitazone after Ischemic stroke or transient ischemic attack. *N Engl J Med* 374(14):1321–1ß331, 2016. doi: 10.1056/NEJMoa1506930.

Symptoms and Signs

Neurologic deficits are similar to those of strokes (see Table 241–1 on p. 2035). Transient monocular blindness (amaurosis fugax), which usually lasts < 5 min, may occur when the ophthalmic artery is affected.

Symptoms of TIAs begin suddenly, usually last 2 to 30 min, then resolve completely. Patients may have several TIAs daily or only 2 or 3 over several years. Symptoms are usually similar in successive carotid attacks but vary somewhat in successive vertebrobasilar attacks.

Diagnosis

- Resolution of stroke-like symptoms within 1 h
- Neuroimaging
- Evaluation to identify the cause

TIAs are diagnosed retrospectively when sudden neurologic deficits referable to ischemia in an arterial territory resolve within 1 h.

Isolated peripheral facial nerve palsy, loss of consciousness, or impaired consciousness does not suggest TIA. TIAs must be distinguished from other causes of similar symptoms, such as

- Hypoglycemia
- Migraine aura
- Postictal [Todd] paralysis (a transient neurologic deficit, usually weakness, of the limb contralateral to the seizure focus)

Because an infarct, a small hemorrhage, and even a mass lesion cannot be excluded clinically, neuroimaging is required. Usually, CT is the study most likely to be immediately available. However, CT may not identify infarcts for > 24 h. MRI usually detects evolving infarction within hours. Diffusion-weighted MRI is the most accurate imaging test to rule out an infarct in patients with presumed TIA but is not always available.

The cause of a TIA is sought as for causes of ischemic strokes; evaluation includes tests for carotid stenosis, cardiac sources of emboli, atrial fibrillation, and hematologic abnormalities and screening for stroke risk factors. Because risk of subsequent ischemic stroke is high and immediate, evaluation proceeds rapidly, usually on an inpatient basis. It is not clear which patients, if any, can be safely discharged from the emergency department. Risk of stroke after TIA or minor stroke is highest within the first 24 to 48 h, so if either is suspected, patients are typically admitted to the hospital for telemetry and evaluation.

Treatment

- Prevention of strokes

Treatment of TIAs is aimed at preventing strokes; antiplatelet drugs and statins are used. Carotid endarterectomy or arterial angioplasty plus stenting can be useful for some patients, particularly those who have no neurologic deficits but who are at high risk of stroke. Anticoagulation is indicated if cardiac sources of emboli are present.

Modifying stroke risk factors, when possible, may prevent stroke.

KEY POINTS

- A focal neurologic deficit that resolves within 1 h is almost always a TIA.
- Test as for ischemic stroke.
- Use the same treatments used for secondary prevention of ischemic stroke (eg, antiplatelet drugs, statins, sometimes carotid endarterectomy or arterial angioplasty plus stenting).

INTRACEREBRAL HEMORRHAGE

Intracerebral hemorrhage is focal bleeding from a blood vessel in the brain parenchyma. The cause is usually hypertension. Typical symptoms include focal neurologic deficits, often with abrupt onset of headache, nausea, and impairment of consciousness. Diagnosis is by CT or MRI. Treatment includes BP control, supportive measures, and, for some patients, surgical evacuation.

Most intracerebral hemorrhages occur in the basal ganglia, cerebral lobes, cerebellum, or pons. Intracerebral hemorrhage may also occur in other parts of the brain stem or in the midbrain.

Etiology

Intracerebral hemorrhage usually results from rupture of an arteriosclerotic small artery that has been weakened, primarily by chronic arterial hypertension. Such hemorrhages are usually large, single, and catastrophic. Other modifiable risk factors that contribute to arteriosclerotic hypertensive intracerebral hemorrhages include cigarette smoking, obesity, and a high-risk diet (eg, high in saturated fats, trans fats, and calories). Use of cocaine or, occasionally, other sympathomimetic drugs can cause transient severe hypertension leading to hemorrhage.

Less often, intracerebral hemorrhage results from congenital aneurysm, arteriovenous or other vascular malformation (see Sidebar 241–1), trauma, mycotic aneurysm, brain infarct (hemorrhagic infarction), primary or metastatic brain tumor, excessive anticoagulation, blood dyscrasia, intracranial arterial dissection, moyamoya disease, or a bleeding or vasculitic disorder.

Lobar intracerebral hemorrhages (hematomas in the cerebral lobes, outside the basal ganglia) usually result from angiopathy due to amyloid deposition in cerebral arteries (cerebral amyloid angiopathy), which affects primarily the elderly. Lobar hemorrhages may be multiple and recurrent.

Sidebar 241–1. Vascular Lesions in the Brain

Common brain vascular lesions include arteriovenous malformations and aneurysms.

Arteriovenous malformations (AVMs): AVMs are tangled, dilated blood vessels in which arteries flow directly into veins. AVMs occur most often at the junction of cerebral arteries, usually within the parenchyma of the frontal-parietal region, frontal lobe, lateral cerebellum, or overlying occipital lobe. AVMs also can occur within the dura. AVMs can bleed or directly compress brain tissue; seizures or ischemia may result.

Neuroimaging may detect them incidentally; contrast or noncontrast CT can usually detect AVMs > 1 cm, but the diagnosis is confirmed with MRI. Occasionally, a cranial bruit suggests an AVM. Conventional angiography is required for definitive diagnosis and determination of whether the lesion is operable.

Superficial AVMs > 3 cm in diameter are usually obliterated by a combination of microsurgery, radiosurgery, and endovascular surgery. AVMs that are deep or < 3 cm in diameter are treated with stereotactic radiosurgery, endovascular therapy (eg, preresection embolization or thrombosis via an intra-arterial catheter), or coagulation with focused proton beams.

Aneurysms: Aneurysms are focal dilations in arteries. They occur in about 5% of people.

Common contributing factors may include arteriosclerosis, hypertension, and hereditary connective tissue disorders (eg, Ehlers-Danlos syndrome, pseudoxanthoma elasticum, autosomal dominant polycystic kidney syndrome). Occasionally, septic emboli cause mycotic aneurysms.

Brain aneurysms are most often < 2.5 cm in diameter and saccular (noncircumferential); sometimes they have one or more small, thin-walled, outpouchings (berry aneurysm).

Most aneurysms occur along the middle or anterior cerebral arteries or the communicating branches of the circle of Willis, particularly at arterial bifurcations. Mycotic aneurysms usually develop distal to the first bifurcation of the arterial branches of the circle of Willis.

Many aneurysms are asymptomatic, but a few cause symptoms by compressing adjacent structures. Ocular palsies, diplopia, squint, or orbital pain may indicate pressure on the 3rd, 4th, 5th, or 6th cranial nerves. Visual loss and a bitemporal field defect may indicate pressure on the optic chiasm.

Aneurysms may bleed into the subarachnoid space, causing subarachnoid hemorrhage. Before rupture, aneurysms occasionally cause sentinel (warning) headaches due to painful expansion of the aneurysm or to blood leaking into the subarachnoid space. Actual rupture causes a sudden severe headache called a thunderclap headache.

Neuroimaging may detect aneurysms incidentally.

Diagnosis of aneurysms requires angiography, CT angiography, or magnetic resonance angiography.

If < 7 mm, asymptomatic aneurysms in the anterior circulation rarely rupture and do not warrant the risks of immediate treatment. They can be monitored with serial imaging. If aneurysms are larger, are in the posterior circulation, or cause symptoms due to bleeding or due to compression of neural structures, endovascular therapy, if feasible, can be tried.

Pathophysiology

Blood from an intracerebral hemorrhage accumulates as a mass that can dissect through and compress adjacent brain tissues, causing neuronal dysfunction. Large hematomas increase intracranial pressure. Pressure from supratentorial hematomas and the accompanying edema may cause transtentorial brain herniation (see Fig. 224–1 on p. 1858), compressing the brain stem and often causing secondary hemorrhages in the midbrain and pons.

If the hemorrhage ruptures into the ventricular system (intraventricular hemorrhage), blood may cause acute hydrocephalus. Cerebellar hematomas can expand to block the 4th ventricle, also causing acute hydrocephalus, or they can dissect into the brain stem. Cerebellar hematomas that are > 3 cm in diameter may cause midline shift or herniation.

Herniation, midbrain or pontine hemorrhage, intraventricular hemorrhage, acute hydrocephalus, or dissection into the brain stem can impair consciousness and cause coma and death.

Symptoms and Signs

Symptoms of intracerebral hemorrhage typically begin with sudden headache, often during activity. However, headache may be mild or absent in the elderly. Loss of consciousness is common, often within seconds or a few minutes. Nausea, vomiting, delirium, and focal or generalized seizures are also common.

Neurologic deficits are usually sudden and progressive. Large hemorrhages, when located in the hemispheres, cause hemiparesis; when located in the posterior fossa, they cause cerebellar or brain stem deficits (eg, conjugate eye deviation or ophthalmoplegia, stertorous breathing, pinpoint pupils, coma).

Large hemorrhages are fatal within a few days in about half of patients. In survivors, consciousness returns and neurologic deficits gradually diminish to various degrees as the extravasated blood is resorbed. Some patients have surprisingly few neurologic deficits because hemorrhage is less destructive to brain tissue than infarction.

Small hemorrhages may cause focal deficits without impairment of consciousness and with minimal or no headache and nausea. Small hemorrhages may mimic ischemic stroke.

Diagnosis

- Neuroimaging

Diagnosis of intracerebral hemorrhage is suggested by sudden onset of headache, focal neurologic deficits, and impaired consciousness, particularly in patients with risk factors.

Intracerebral hemorrhage must be distinguished from

- Ischemic stroke
- Subarachnoid hemorrhage
- Other causes of acute neurologic deficits (eg, seizure, hypoglycemia)

Blood glucose level should be measured at the bedside immediately.

Immediate CT or MRI is necessary. Neuroimaging is usually diagnostic. If neuroimaging shows no hemorrhage but subarachnoid hemorrhage is suspected clinically, lumbar puncture is necessary. CT angiography, done within hours of bleeding onset, may show areas where contrast extravasates into the clot (spot sign); this finding indicates that bleeding is continuing and suggests that the hematoma will expand and the outcome will be poor.

Treatment

- Supportive measures
- Sometimes surgical evacuation (eg, for many cerebellar hematomas > 3 cm)

Treatment includes supportive measures and control of modifiable risk factors.

Anticoagulants and antiplatelet drugs are contraindicated. If patients have used anticoagulants, the effects are reversed when possible by giving fresh frozen plasma, prothrombin complex concentrate, vitamin K, or platelet transfusions as indicated. Hemodialysis can remove about 60% of dabigatran.

As recommended by the American Heart Association and American Stroke Association 2015 guidelines, hypertension can be safely lowered to systolic BP 140 mm Hg if systolic BP is between 150 mm Hg and 220 mm Hg and if acute antihypertensive treatment is not contraindicated.[1] If systolic BP is > 220 mm Hg, hypertension can be treated aggressively with a continuous IV infusion; in such cases, systolic BP must be monitored frequently. Nicardipine 2.5 mg/h IV is given initially; dose is increased by 2.5 mg/h q 5 min to a maximum of 15 mg/h as needed to decrease systolic BP by 10 to 15%.

Cerebellar hemisphere hematomas that are > 3 cm in diameter may cause midline shift or herniation, so surgical evacuation is often lifesaving. Early evacuation of large lobar cerebral hematomas may also be lifesaving, but rebleeding occurs frequently, sometimes increasing neurologic deficits. Early evacuation of deep cerebral hematomas is seldom indicated because surgical mortality is high and neurologic deficits are usually severe. Anticonvulsants are not typically used prophylactically; they are used only if patients have had a seizure.

1. Hemphill JC, Greenberg SM, Anderson CS, et al: Guidelines for the management of spontaneous intracerebral hemorrhage: A guideline for healthcare professionals from the American Heart Association/American Stroke Association. *Stroke* 46:2032–2060, 2015. https://doi.org/10.1161/STR.0000000000000069.

KEY POINTS

- With intracerebral hemorrhage, sudden, severe symptoms (eg, sudden headache, loss of consciousness, vomiting) are common, but headache may be absent (particularly in the elderly), and small hemorrhages may mimic ischemic stroke.
- Do CT or MRI and a bedside glucose test immediately.
- Essential supportive care may include reversing anticoagulation and decreasing BP if systolic BP is > 150 mm Hg; if systolic BP is > 220 mm Hg, consider aggressively reducing BP by continuously infusing nicardipine IV.
- Consider surgical evacuation for large lobar cerebral hematomas and hematomas > 3 cm in a cerebellar hemisphere.

SUBARACHNOID HEMORRHAGE

Subarachnoid hemorrhage is sudden bleeding into the subarachnoid space. The most common cause of spontaneous bleeding is a ruptured aneurysm. Symptoms include sudden, severe headache, usually with loss or impairment of consciousness. Secondary vasospasm (causing focal brain ischemia), meningismus, and hydrocephalus (causing persistent headache and obtundation) are common. Diagnosis is by CT or MRI; if neuroimaging is normal, diagnosis is by CSF analysis. Treatment is with supportive measures and neurosurgery or endovascular measures, preferably in a comprehensive stroke center.

Etiology

Subarachnoid hemorrhage is bleeding between the arachnoid and pia mater. In general, head trauma is the most common cause, but traumatic subarachnoid hemorrhage is usually considered a separate disorder. Spontaneous (primary) subarachnoid hemorrhage usually results from ruptured aneurysms. A congenital intracranial saccular or berry aneurysm is the cause in about 85% of patients. Bleeding may stop spontaneously. Aneurysmal hemorrhage may occur at any age but is most common from age 40 to 65.

Less common causes are mycotic aneurysms, arteriovenous malformations, and bleeding disorders.

Pathophysiology

Blood in the subarachnoid space causes a chemical meningitis that commonly increases intracranial pressure for days or a few weeks. Secondary vasospasm may cause focal brain ischemia; about 25% of patients develop signs of a TIA or ischemic stroke. Brain edema is maximal and risk of vasospasm and subsequent infarction (called angry brain) is highest between 72 h and 10 days. Secondary acute hydrocephalus is also common. A 2nd rupture (rebleeding) sometimes occurs, most often within about 7 days.

Symptoms and Signs

Headache is usually severe, peaking within seconds. Loss of consciousness may follow, usually immediately but sometimes not for several hours. Severe neurologic deficits may develop and become irreversible within minutes or a few hours. Sensorium may be impaired, and patients may become restless. Seizures are possible. Usually, the neck is not stiff initially unless the cerebellar tonsils herniate. However, within 24 h, chemical meningitis causes moderate to marked meningismus, vomiting, and sometimes bilateral extensor plantar responses. Heart or respiratory rate is often abnormal.

Fever, continued headaches, and confusion are common during the first 5 to 10 days. Secondary hydrocephalus may cause headache, obtundation, and motor deficits that persist for weeks. Rebleeding may cause recurrent or new symptoms.

Diagnosis

- Usually noncontrast CT and, if negative, lumbar puncture

Diagnosis of subarachnoid hemorrhage is suggested by characteristic symptoms. Testing should proceed as rapidly as possible, before damage becomes irreversible.

Noncontrast CT is done within 6 h of symptom onset. MRI is comparably sensitive but less likely to be immediately available. False-negative results occur if volume of blood is small or if the patient is so anemic that blood is isodense with brain tissue.

If subarachnoid hemorrhage is suspected clinically but not identified by neuroimaging or if neuroimaging is not immediately available, lumbar puncture is done. Lumbar puncture is contraindicated if increased intracranial pressure is suspected because the sudden decrease in CSF pressure may lessen the tamponade of a clot on the ruptured aneurysm, causing further bleeding.

PEARLS & PITFALLS

- Suspect subarachnoid hemorrhage if headache reaches peak, severe intensity within seconds of onset or causes loss of consciousness.
- Do lumbar puncture if subarachnoid hemorrhage is suspected clinically but CT shows no hemorrhage or is not available; however, lumbar puncture is contraindicated if increased intracranial pressure is suspected.

CSF findings suggesting subarachnoid hemorrhage include

- Numerous RBCs
- Xanthochromia
- Increased pressure

RBCs in CSF may also be caused by traumatic lumbar puncture. Traumatic lumbar puncture is suspected if the RBC count decreases in tubes of CSF drawn sequentially during the same lumbar puncture. About 6 h or more after a subarachnoid hemorrhage, RBCs become crenated and lyse, resulting in a xanthochromic CSF supernatant and visible crenated RBCs (noted during microscopic CSF examination); these findings usually indicate that subarachnoid hemorrhage preceded the lumbar puncture. If there is still doubt, hemorrhage should be assumed, or the lumbar puncture should be repeated in 8 to 12 h.

In patients with subarachnoid hemorrhage, conventional cerebral angiography is done as soon as possible after the initial bleeding episode; alternatives include magnetic resonance angiography and CT angiography. All 4 arteries (2 carotid and 2 vertebral arteries) should be injected because up to 20% of patients (mostly women) have multiple aneurysms.

On ECG, subarachnoid hemorrhage may cause ST-segment elevation or depression. It can cause syncope, mimicking MI. Other possible ECG abnormalities include prolongation of the QRS or QT intervals and peaking or deep, symmetric inversion of T waves.

Prognosis

About 35% of patients die after the first aneurysmal subarachnoid hemorrhage; another 15% die within a few weeks because of a subsequent rupture. After 6 mo, a 2nd rupture occurs at a rate of about 3%/yr. In general, prognosis is grave with an aneurysm, better with an arteriovenous malformation, and best when 4-vessel angiography does not detect a lesion, presumably because the bleeding source is small and has sealed itself. Among survivors, neurologic damage is common, even when treatment is optimal.

Treatment

- Treatment in a comprehensive stroke center
- Nicardipine if mean arterial pressure is > 130 mm Hg
- Nimodipine to prevent vasospasm
- Occlusion of causative aneurysms

Patients with subarachnoid hemorrhage should be treated in a comprehensive stroke center whenever possible.

Hypertension should be treated only if mean arterial pressure is > 130 mm Hg; euvolemia is maintained, and IV nicardipine is titrated as for intracerebral hemorrhage (see p. 2043).

Bed rest is mandatory. Restlessness and headache are treated symptomatically. Stool softeners are given to prevent constipation, which can lead to straining.

Anticoagulants and antiplatelet drugs are contraindicated.

Vasospasm is prevented by giving nimodipine 60 mg po q 4 h for 21 days to prevent vasospasm, but BP needs to be maintained in the desirable range (usually considered to be a mean arterial pressure of 70 to 130 mm Hg and a systolic pressure of 120 to 185 mm Hg).

If clinical signs of acute hydrocephalus occur, ventricular drainage should be considered.

Aneurysms are occluded to reduce risk of rebleeding. Detachable endovascular coils can be inserted during angiography to occlude the aneurysm. Alternatively, if the aneurysm is accessible, surgery to clip the aneurysm or bypass its blood flow can be done, especially for patients with an evacuable hematoma or acute hydrocephalus. If patients are arousable, most vascular neurosurgeons operate within the first 24 h to minimize risk of rebleeding and risks due to angry brain. If > 24 h have elapsed, some neurosurgeons delay surgery until 10 days have passed; this approach decreases risks due to angry brain but increases risk of rebleeding and overall mortality.

KEY POINTS

- Possible complications after subarachnoid hemorrhage include chemical meningitis, vasospasm, hydrocephalus, rebleeding, and brain edema.
- Suspect subarachnoid hemorrhage if headache is severe at onset and reaches peak intensity within seconds or causes loss of consciousness.
- If subarachnoid hemorrhage is confirmed, scan both carotid and both vertebral arteries using conventional cerebral angiography, magnetic resonance angiography or CT angiography because many patients have multiple aneurysms.
- If possible, send patients to a comprehensive stroke center for treatment.

SECTION 18

Genitourinary Disorders

242 Approach to the Genitourinary Patient

EVALUATION OF THE RENAL PATIENT

In patients with renal disorders, symptoms and signs may be nonspecific, absent until the disorder is severe, or both. Findings can be local (eg, reflecting kidney inflammation or mass), result from the systemic effects of kidney dysfunction, or affect urination (eg, changes in urine itself or in urine production).

History

History plays a limited role because symptoms are nonspecific.

Hematuria is relatively specific for a GU disorder, but patients who report red urine may instead have one of the following:

- Myoglobinuria
- Hemoglobinuria
- Porphyrinuria
- Porphobilinuria
- Food-induced urine coloring (some foods, eg, beets, rhubarb, sometimes food coloring, may make urine appear red)
- Drug-induced urine coloring (some drugs, most commonly phenazopyridine, but sometimes cascara, diphenylhydantoin, rifampin, methyldopa, phenacetin, phenindione, phenolphthalein, phenothiazines, and senna may make urine appear dark yellow to orange or red)

High concentrations of urinary protein cause frothy or sudsy urine. Urinary frequency (voiding more often) should be distinguished from polyuria (voiding a larger amount than normal) in patients who report excessive urination. Nocturia may be a feature of either but is often the result of excess fluid intake too close to bedtime, prostate enlargement, or chronic kidney disease. Family history is useful for identifying inheritance patterns and risk of polycystic kidney disease or other hereditary nephropathies (eg, hereditary nephritis, thin basement membrane disease, nail-patella syndrome, cystinuria, hyperoxaluria).

Physical Examination

Patients with moderate or severe chronic kidney disease sometimes appear pale, wasted, or ill. Deep (Kussmaul) respiration suggests hyperventilation in response to metabolic acidosis with acidemia.

Chest examination: Pericardial and pleuritic friction rubs may be signs of uremia.

Abdominal examination: Visual fullness of the upper abdomen is an unusual, nonspecific finding of polycystic kidney disease. It may also indicate a kidney or abdominal mass or hydronephrosis. A soft, lateralizing bruit is occasionally audible in the epigastrium or the flank in renal artery stenosis; presence of a diastolic component increases the probability of renovascular hypertension.

Pain elicited by mild striking of the back, flanks, and angle formed by the 12th rib and lumbar spine with a fist (costovertebral tenderness) may indicate pyelonephritis or urinary tract obstruction (eg, due to calculi). Normal kidneys are not usually palpable. However, in some women, the lower pole of the right kidney can occasionally be felt with palpation during deep inspiration, and large kidneys or masses can sometimes be felt without special maneuvers. In neonates, the kidneys can be felt with the thumbs when the thumbs are placed anterior and the fingers posterior to the costovertebral angle.

Transillumination can distinguish solid from cystic renal masses in some children < 1 yr if the kidney and mass are manipulated against the abdominal wall.

Skin examination: Chronic kidney disease can cause any of the following:

- Xerosis due to sebaceous and eccrine sweat gland atrophy
- Pallor due to anemia
- Hyperpigmentation due to melanin deposition
- Sallow or yellow-brown skin due to urochrome deposition
- Petechiae or ecchymoses due to platelet dysfunction
- Excoriation due to itching caused by hyperphosphatemia or uremia

Uremic frost, the deposition of white-to-tan urea crystals on the skin after sweat evaporation, is rare.

Neurologic examination: Patients with acute renal failure may be drowsy, confused, or inattentive; speech may be slurred. Asterixis can be detected in handwriting or by observation of outstretched hands maximally extended at the wrists; after several seconds in this position, a hand flap in the flexor direction is asterixis. Asterixis suggests one of the following:

- Chronic kidney disease
- Chronic liver failure
- CO_2 narcosis
- Toxic encephalopathy

Testing

Urinalysis and measurement of serum creatinine are the initial steps in evaluation of renal disorders. Other urine, blood, and imaging tests (eg, ultrasonography, CT, MRI) are done in specific circumstances. Ideally, after the urethral meatus is cleaned, the urine specimen is collected midstream (clean-catch specimen) during the first void of the morning; the urine should be examined immediately because delays can lead to changes in test results. Bladder catheterization or suprapubic aspiration can be used for collection when urine cannot be obtained by spontaneous voiding or when vaginal material contaminates the urine specimen. However, the trauma of catheterization may falsely increase the number of RBCs in the specimen, so catheterization is usually avoided if the outcome of interest is microscopic hematuria. A specimen from a catheter collection bag is not acceptable for microscopic or bacteriologic tests.

Urinalysis: A complete urinalysis includes the following:

- Inspection for color, appearance, and odor
- Measurement of pH, specific gravity, protein, glucose, RBCs, nitrites, and WBC esterase by dipstick reagents
- Microscopic analysis for casts, crystals, and cells (urine sediment)

Bilirubin and urobilinogen, although standard parts of many dipstick tests, no longer play significant roles in evaluation of renal or hepatic disorders.

Color is the most obvious of urine attributes, and observation of color is an integral part of urinalysis (see Table 242–1). Urine color may suggest possible causes and help direct additional testing.

Table 242–1. CAUSES OF URINE COLOR CHANGES

COLOR	CAUSE
Red, orange, or brown	Bilirubin Drugs (eg, cascara, diphenylhydantoin, levodopa, methyldopa, phenacetin, phenazopyridine, phenindione, phenolphthalein, phenothiazines, rifampin, senna) Foods (eg, beets) Free myoglobin Porphyrins RBCs
Cloudy white	Infection (pyuria) Lymph (chyluria) due to filariasis or to obstructed retroperitoneal lymphatics Precipitated phosphate crystals
Green	Drugs (eg, amitriptyline, methylene blue, propofol) *Pseudomonas* infection
Purple (rare)	Gram-negative bacteria in urinary catheters*
Dark brown or black	Melanoma†

*Rarely, urine in collection bags of catheterized, bedbound patients turns purple (purple urine bag syndrome) when urinary gram-negative bacteria metabolize a tryptophan metabolite (indican) in alkaline urine into indigo; this reaction is clinically insignificant.

†Caused by oxidation of excessive homogentisic acid or melanogen when urine is exposed to air for several hours.

Odor, often unintentionally noted during visual inspection, conveys useful information only in rare cases of inherited disorders of amino acid metabolism when urine has a distinctive smell (eg, maple syrup in maple syrup urine disease, sweaty feet in isovaleric acidemia, tomcat urine in multiple carboxylase deficiency [see Table 315–9 on p. 2652]).

pH is normally 5.0 to 6.0 (range 4.5 to 8.0). Measuring with a glass pH electrode is recommended when precise values are necessary for decision making, as when diagnosing renal tubular acidosis; in these cases, a layer of mineral oil should be added to the urine specimen to prevent escape of CO_2. Delay in processing a specimen may elevate pH because ammonia is released as bacteria break down urea. Infection with urease-producing pathogens can spuriously increase pH.

Specific gravity provides a rough measure of urine concentration (osmolality). Normal range is 1.001 to 1.035; values may be low in the elderly or in patients with impaired renal function, who are less able to concentrate urine. It is measured by hydrometer or refractometer or estimated with a dipstick. Accuracy of the dipstick test is controversial, but the test may be sufficient for patients who have calculi and are advised to self-monitor urine concentration to maintain dilute urine. Specific gravity by dipstick may be spuriously elevated when urine pH is < 6 or low when pH is > 7. Hydrometer and refractometer measurements may be elevated by high levels of large molecules (eg, radiopaque contrast agent, albumin, glucose, carbenicillin) in the urine.

Protein, detected by standard dipstick tests, reflects mainly urinary albumin concentration, classified as negative (< 10 mg/dL), trace (15 to 30 mg/dL), or 1+ (30 to 100 mg/dL) through 4+ (> 500 mg/dL). Microalbuminuria, an important marker for renal complications in patients with diabetes, is not detected by standard dipsticks, but special microalbumin dipsticks are available. Light-chain proteins (eg, due to multiple myeloma) also are not detected. Significance of proteinuria depends on total protein excretion rather than protein concentration estimated by dipstick; thus, when proteinuria is detected with dipstick testing, quantitative measures of urinary protein should be done. False-negative results can be caused by dilute urine. False-positive results can be caused by any of the following:

- High pH (> 9)
- Presence of cells
- Radiopaque contrast agents
- Concentrated urine

Glucose usually appears in the urine when serum glucose increases to > 180 mg/dL (> 10.1 mmol/L) and renal function is normal. Threshold for detection by urine dipstick is 50 mg/dL (2.8 mmol/L). Any amount is abnormal. Falsely low or negative results can result from any of the following:

- Ascorbic acid
- Ketones
- Aspirin
- Levodopa
- Tetracycline
- Very high urine pH
- Dilute urine

Hematuria is detected when RBCs lyse on a dipstick test strip, releasing Hb and causing a color change. Range is from negative (0) to 4+. Trace blood (corresponding to 3 to 5 RBCs/high-power field [HPF]) is normal under some circumstances (eg, exercise) in some people. Because the test strip reagent reacts with Hb, free Hb (eg, due to intravascular hemolysis) or myoglobin (eg, due to rhabdomyolysis) causes a positive result. Hemoglobinuria and myoglobinuria can be distinguished from hematuria by the absence of RBCs on microscopic examination and by the pattern of color change on the test strip. RBCs create a dotted or speckled pattern; free Hb and myoglobin create a uniform color change. Povidone iodine causes false-positive results (uniform coloring); ascorbic acid causes false-negative results.

Nitrites are produced when bacteria reduce urinary nitrates derived from amino acid metabolism. Nitrites are not normally present and signify bacteriuria. The test is either positive or negative. False-negative results may occur with any of the following:

- Infection with certain pathogens that cannot convert nitrate to nitrite (eg, *Enterococcus faecalis*, *Neisseria gonorrhoeae*, *Mycobacterium tuberculosis*, *Pseudomonas* sp)
- Urine that has not stayed long enough (< 4 h) in the bladder
- Low urinary excretion of nitrate
- Enzymes (of certain bacteria) that reduce nitrates to nitrogen
- High urine urobilinogen level
- Presence of ascorbic acid
- Urine pH < 6.0

Nitrites are used mainly with WBC esterase testing to monitor patients with recurrent urine infections, particularly children with vesicoureteral reflux, and sometimes to confirm the diagnosis of uncomplicated UTI in women of childbearing age.

WBC esterase is released by lysed neutrophils. Its presence in urine reflects acute inflammation, most commonly due to bacterial infection but sometimes due to interstitial nephritis, nephrolithiasis, or renal TB. Threshold for detection is about 5 WBCs/HPF, and test results range from negative to 4+. The test is not very sensitive for detection of infection. Contamination of a urine specimen with vaginal flora is the most common cause of false-positive results. False-negative results may result from any of the following:

- Very dilute urine
- Glycosuria
- Urobilinogen
- Use of phenazopyridine, nitrofurantoin, rifampin, or large amounts of vitamin C

WBC esterase is used mainly with nitrite testing to monitor patients with recurrent urine infections and sometimes to diagnose uncomplicated UTI in women of childbearing age. If both tests are negative, the likelihood of a positive urine culture is small.

Microscopic analysis: Detection of solid elements (cells, casts, crystals) requires microscopic analysis, ideally done immediately after voiding, and dipstick testing. The specimen is prepared by centrifuging 10 to 15 mL of urine at 1500 to 2500 rpm for 5 min. The supernatant is fully decanted; a small amount of urine remains with the residue at the bottom of the centrifuge tube. The residue can be mixed back into solution by gently agitating the tube or tapping the bottom. A single drop is pipetted onto a slide and covered with a coverslip. For routine microscopic analysis, staining is optional. The specimen is examined under reduced light with the low-power objective and under full-intensity light with the high-power objective; the latter is typically used for semiquantitative estimates (eg, 10 to 15 WBCs/HPF). Polarized light is used to identify some crystals and lipids in the urine. Phase-contrast microscopy enhances identification of cells and casts.

Epithelial cells (renal tubular, transitional, squamous cells) frequently are found in urine; most common are squamous cells lining the end of the urethra and contaminants from the vagina. Only renal tubular cells are diagnostically important; however, except when found in casts, they are difficult to distinguish from transitional cells. A few renal tubular cell casts appear in normal urine, but a large number suggests tubular injury (eg, acute tubular necrosis, tubulointerstitial nephritis, nephrotoxins, nephrotic syndrome).

RBCs < 3/HPF may be normal (< 5/HPF is sometimes normal, eg, after exercise), and any isolated hematuria should be interpreted in clinical context. On microscopic analysis, glomerular RBCs are smaller and dysmorphic, with spicules, folding, and blebs; nonglomerular RBCs retain their normal shape and size.

WBCs < 5/HPF may be normal; special staining can distinguish eosinophils from neutrophils. Pyuria is defined as > 5 WBCs/HPF in a sample of centrifuged urine.

Lipiduria is most characteristic of the nephrotic syndrome; renal tubular cells absorb filtered lipids, which appear microscopically as oval fat bodies, and cholesterol, which produces a Maltese cross pattern under polarized light. Lipids and cholesterol can also be free floating or incorporated into casts.

Crystals in urine are common and usually clinically insignificant (see Table 242–2). Crystal formation depends on all of the following:

- Urine concentration of crystal constituents
- pH
- Absence of crystallization inhibitors

Drugs are an underrecognized cause of crystals (see Table 242–3).

Casts are made up of glycoprotein of unknown function (Tamm-Horsfall protein) secreted from the thick ascending loop of Henle. They are cylindrical and have regular margins. Their presence indicates renal origin, which may be helpful diagnostically. Types of casts differ in constituents and appearance (see Table 242–4).

Other urine tests: Other tests are useful in specific instances.

Total protein excretion can be measured in a 24-h collection or can be estimated by the protein/creatinine ratio, which, in a random urine sample, correlates well with values in g/1.73 m² BSA from a 24-h collection (eg, 400 mg/dL protein and 100 mg/dL creatinine in a random sample equal 4 g/1.73 m² in a 24-h collection). The protein/creatinine ratio is less accurate when creatinine excretion is significantly increased (eg, in muscular athletes) or decreased (eg, in cachexia).

Microalbuminuria is albumin excretion persistently between 30 and 300 mg/day (20 to 200 μg/min); lesser amounts are considered within the range of normal, and amounts > 300 mg/day (> 200 μg/min) are considered overt proteinuria. Use of the urine albumin/urine creatinine ratio is a reliable and more convenient screening test because it avoids timed urine specimens and correlates well with 24-h values. A value > 30 mg/g (> 0.03 mg/mg) suggests microalbuminuria. The reliability of the test is best when a midmorning specimen is used, vigorous exercise is avoided before the test, because vigorous exercise can cause transient dipstick positivity for protein, and unusual creatinine production (in cachectic or very muscular

Table 242–2. COMMON TYPES OF URINARY CRYSTALS

TYPE	APPEARANCE	COMMENTS
Calcium oxalate	Occur in several shapes but are most easily recognized when they form small, octahedral, envelope-like shapes	When present in large numbers, strongly suggest ethylene glycol poisoning or, rarely, short bowel syndrome, hereditary oxalosis and oxaluria, or high doses of vitamin C Important in evaluation as potential constituents of calculi
Cystine	Perfect hexagons, sometimes alone as flat plates or as overlapping crystals of varying sizes	Diagnostic of cystinuria, a rare hereditary cause of calculi
Magnesium ammonium phosphate	May resemble coffin lids or quartz crystals	Often occur in normal alkaline urine or in urine of patients with struvite calculi
Uric acid	May be diamond- or needle-shaped or rhomboid, although uric acid may be amorphous	Often present in acidic, cool, highly concentrated urine May indicate mild dehydration in neonates or tumor lysis syndrome in patients with cancer or renal failure

Table 242–3. DRUGS THAT CAUSE CRYSTAL FORMATION

DRUG	CRYSTAL DESCRIPTION
Acyclovir	Birefringent, needle-shaped May be free or engulfed in leukocytes
Ampicillin	Needle-shaped Best seen under polarized light
Indinavir	Starburst-shaped or individual needle-shaped crystals Best seen under polarized light
Sulfa	Needle-shaped or fan-shaped; may cluster Best seen under polarized light

patients) is not present. Microalbuminuria can occur in all of the following:

- Diabetes mellitus
- Hypertension
- Renal allograft dysfunction
- Preeclampsia
- UTI
- Chronic kidney disease

Microalbuminuria is an early stage of diabetic kidney disease in both type 1 and 2 diabetes; the progression of renal disease is more predictable in type 1 than 2 disease. Microalbuminuria is a risk factor for cardiovascular disorders and early cardiovascular mortality independent of diabetes or hypertension.

Sulfosalicylic acid (SSA) test strips can be used to detect protein other than albumin (eg, immunoglobulins in multiple myeloma) when dipstick urine tests are negative; urine supernatant mixed with SSA becomes turbid if protein is present. The test is semiquantitative with a scale of 0 (no turbidity) to 4+ (flocculent precipitates). Readings are falsely elevated by radiopaque contrast agents.

Ketones spill into urine with ketonemia, but use of test strips to measure urinary ketones is no longer widely recommended because they measure only acetoacetic acid and acetone, not beta-hydroxybutyric acid. Thus, a false-negative result is possible even without an exogenous cause (eg, vitamin C, phenazopyridine, *N*-acetylcysteine); direct measurement of serum ketones is more accurate. Ketonuria is caused by endocrine and metabolic disorders and does not reflect renal dysfunction.

Osmolality, the total number of solute particles per unit mass (mOsm/kg [mmol/kg]), can be measured directly by osmometer. Normally, osmolality is 50 to 1200 mOsm/kg. Measurement is most useful for evaluating hypernatremia, hyponatremia,

Table 242–4. URINARY CASTS

TYPE	DESCRIPTION	SIGNIFICANCE
Plain casts		
Hyaline	Glycoprotein matrix consisting mainly of Tamm-Horsfall protein secreted by tubules	Nonspecific Can be present in normal urine or in patients with low urine flow (eg, due to dehydration, after diuretic therapy), physiologic stress, an acute renal disorder plus other abnormalities, or a chronic renal disorder (as broad casts formed in dilated tubules)
Waxy	Glycoprotein matrix with degraded protein Formed in atrophic tubules Highly refractile with waxy appearance	Present in advanced chronic kidney disease
Casts with inclusions		
RBC	Glycoprotein matrix with RBCs Often appears red-orange	Virtually pathognomonic of glomerulonephritis Occurs extremely rarely in patients with cortical necrosis or acute tubular injury or in runners with hematuria
Epithelial cell	Protein matrix variably filled with tubular cells	Occurs in acute tubular injury, glomerulonephritis, or nephrotic syndrome
WBC	Protein matrix variably filled with WBCs	Suggests pyelonephritis but can indicate other causes of tubulointerstitial inflammation May occur in proliferative glomerulonephritis
Granular	Glycoprotein matrix with protein or cellular debris	Occasionally occurs after exercise or dehydration when renal function is normal More often indicates acute tubular necrosis
Pigment	Tubular cell or granular casts with pigment stain	Usually occurs in acute kidney injury due to hemolysis or rhabdomyolysis or in acute tubular necrosis
Fatty	Fat droplets or oval fat bodies (cholesterol produces a Maltese cross pattern in polarized light)	May occur in various types of tubulointerstitial disorders In large numbers, strongly suggests nephrotic syndrome
Mixed	Hyaline cast with various cells (eg, RBCs, WBCs, tubular cells)	Usually occurs in proliferative glomerulonephritis
Pseudocasts		
—	Clumped urates, WBCs, bacteria, hair, glass fragments, cloth fiber, or artifacts	Important not to confuse with true casts, which are cylindrical and shaped like renal tubules

syndrome of inappropriate antidiuretic hormone secretion (SIADH), and diabetes insipidus.

Electrolyte measurements help diagnose specific disorders. Sodium (Na) level can help distinguish whether volume depletion (urine Na < 10 mEq/L) or acute tubular necrosis (urine Na > 40 mEq/L) is the cause of acute renal insufficiency or failure. The fractional excretion of Na (FE_{Na}) is the percentage of filtered Na that is excreted. It is calculated as the ratio of excreted to filtered Na, which can be simplified to the following:

$$FE_{Na} = \frac{(U_{Na})(P_{Cr})}{(P_{Na})(U_{Cr})} \times 100\%$$

where U_{Na} is urine Na, P_{Na} is plasma Na, P_{Cr} is plasma creatinine, and UCr is urine creatinine.

This ratio is a more reliable measure than U_{Na} alone because U_{Na} levels between 10 and 40 mEq/L are nonspecific. FE_{Na} < 1% suggests prerenal causes, such as volume depletion; however, acute glomerulonephritis or certain types of acute tubular necrosis (eg, rhabdomyolysis, radiocontrast-induced renal failure) and acute partial obstruction can result in FE_{Na} < 1%. A value > 1% suggests acute tubular necrosis or acute interstitial nephritis.

Other useful measurements include the following:

- Fractional excretion of HCO_3 in evaluation of renal tubular acidosis
- Cl levels and urine anion gap for diagnosis of metabolic alkalosis and metabolic acidosis
- K levels in determining the cause of hypokalemia or hyperkalemia
- Levels of calcium, magnesium, uric acid, oxalate, citrate, and cystine in evaluation of calculi

Eosinophils, cells that stain bright red or pink-white with Wright or Hansel staining, most commonly indicate one of the following:

- Acute interstitial nephritis
- Rapidly progressive glomerulonephritis
- Acute prostatitis
- Renal atheroembolism

Cytology is used for the following:

- To screen for cancer in high-risk populations (eg, petrochemical workers)
- To evaluate painless hematuria in the absence of glomerular disease (suggested by the absence of dysmorphic RBCs, proteinuria, and renal failure)
- To check for recurrence after bladder tumor resection

Sensitivity is about 90% for carcinoma in situ; however, sensitivity is considerably lower for low-grade transitional cell carcinomas. Inflammatory or reactive hyperplastic lesions or cytotoxic drugs for carcinoma may produce false-positive results. Accuracy for detecting bladder tumors may be increased by vigorous bladder lavage with a small volume of 0.9% saline solution (50 mL pushed in and then aspirated by syringe through a catheter). Cells collected in the saline are concentrated and examined.

Gram stain and cultures with susceptibility testing are indicated when GU tract infections are suspected; a positive result must be interpreted in the clinical context (see p. 2175).

Amino acids are normally filtered and reabsorbed by the proximal tubules. They may appear in urine when a hereditary or acquired tubular transport defect (eg, Fanconi syndrome, cystinuria) is present. Measuring type and amount of amino acids may help in the diagnosis of certain types of calculi, renal tubular acidosis, and inherited disorders of metabolism.

Blood tests: Blood tests are useful in evaluation of renal disorders.

Serum creatinine values > 1.3 mg/dL (> 114 μmol/L) in men and > 1 mg/dL (> 90 μmol/L) in women are usually abnormal. Serum creatinine depends on creatinine generation as well as renal creatinine excretion. Because creatinine turnover increases with higher muscle mass, muscular people have higher serum creatinine levels and elderly and undernourished people have lower levels.

Serum creatinine may also be increased in the following conditions:

- Use of ACE inhibitors and angiotensin II receptor blockers
- Consumption of large amounts of meat
- Use of some drugs (cimetidine, trimethoprim, cefoxitin, flucytosine)

ACE inhibitors and angiotensin II receptor blockers reversibly decrease GFR and increase serum creatinine because they vasodilate efferent more than afferent glomerular arterioles, mainly in people who are dehydrated or are receiving diuretics. In general, serum creatinine alone is not a good indicator of kidney function. The Cockcroft and Gault formula and the Modification of Diet in Renal Disease formula estimate GFR based on serum creatinine and other parameters and more reliably evaluate kidney function.

BUN/creatinine ratio is used to distinguish prerenal from renal or postrenal (obstructive) azotemia; a value > 15 is considered abnormal and may occur in prerenal and postrenal azotemia. However, BUN is affected by protein intake and by several nonrenal processes (eg, trauma, infection, GI bleeding, corticosteroid use) and, although suggestive, is generally inconclusive as evidence of renal dysfunction.

Cystatin C, a serine proteinase inhibitor that is produced by all nucleated cells and filtered by the kidneys, can also be used to evaluate kidney function. Its plasma concentration is independent of sex, age, and body weight. Testing is not always available, and values are not standardized across laboratories.

Serum electrolytes (eg, Na, K, HCO_3) may become abnormal and the anion gap (Na – [Cl + HCO_3]) may increase in acute kidney injury and chronic kidney disease. Serum electrolytes should be monitored periodically.

CBC may detect anemia in chronic kidney disease or, rarely, polycythemia in renal cell carcinoma or polycystic kidney disease. Anemia is often multifactorial (mainly due to erythropoietin deficiency and sometimes worsened or caused by blood loss in dialysis circuits or the GI tract); it may be microcytic or normocytic, and may be hypochromic or normochromic.

Renin, a proteolytic enzyme, is stored in the juxtaglomerular cells of the kidneys. Renin secretion is stimulated by reduced blood volume and renal blood flow and is inhibited by Na and water retention. Plasma renin is assayed by measuring renin activity as the amount of angiotensin I generated per hour. Specimens should be drawn from well-hydrated, Na- and potassium-replete patients. Plasma renin, aldosterone, cortisol, and ACTH should be measured in evaluation of all of the following:

- Adrenal insufficiency
- Hyperaldosteronism
- Refractory hypertension

The plasma aldosterone/renin ratio calculated from measurements obtained with the patient in an upright posture is the best screening test for hyperaldosteronism, provided that plasma renin activity is > 0.5 ng/mL/h and aldosterone is > 12 to 15 ng/dL.

Evaluating Kidney Function

Kidney function is evaluated using values calculated from formulas based on results of blood and urine tests.

GFR: Glomerular filtration rate (GFR), the volume of blood filtered through the kidney per minute, is the best overall measure of kidney function; it is expressed in mL/min. Because normal GFR increases with increasing body size, a correction factor using body surface area (BSA) typically is applied. This correction is necessary to compare a patient's GFR to normal and to define different stages of chronic kidney disease. Given the mean normal BSA of 1.73 m^2, the correction factor is 1.73/patient BSA; adjusted GFR results are then expressed as mL/min/1.73 m^2.

Normal GFR in young, healthy adults is about 120 to 130 mL/min/1.73 m^2 and declines with age to about 75 mL/min/1.73 m^2 at age 70. Chronic kidney disease is defined by a GFR < 60 mL/min/1.73 m^2 for > 3 mo. The standard for GFR measurement is inulin clearance. Inulin is neither absorbed nor secreted by the renal tubule and therefore it is the ideal marker for evaluation of kidney function. However, its measurement is cumbersome and, therefore, is mostly used in research settings.

Creatinine clearance: Creatinine is produced at a constant rate by muscle metabolism and is freely filtered by the glomeruli and also is secreted by the renal tubules. Because creatinine is secreted, creatinine clearance (CrCl) overestimates GFR by about 10 to 20% in people with normal kidney function and by up to 50% in patients with advanced renal failure; thus, use of CrCl to estimate GFR in chronic kidney disease is discouraged.

Using a timed (usually 24-h) urine collection, CrCl can be calculated as

$$\text{CrCl} = \text{UCr} \times \frac{\text{UVol}}{\text{PCr}}$$

where UCr is urine creatinine in mg/mL, UVol is urine volume in mL/min of collection (1440 min for a full 24-h collection), and PCr is plasma creatinine in mg/mL.

Estimating creatinine clearance: Because serum creatinine by itself is inadequate for evaluation of kidney function, several formulas have been devised to estimate CrCl using serum creatinine and other factors.

The **Cockcroft and Gault** formula can be used to estimate CrCl. It uses age, lean body weight, and serum creatinine level. It is based on the premise that daily creatinine production is 28 mg/kg/day with a decrease of 0.2 mg/yr of age.

$$\text{CrCl}_{(\text{est})} = \frac{(140 - \text{age [yr]})\ (\text{lean body wt [kg]})}{(72)\ (\text{serum creatinine [mg/dL]})}\ (\times\ 0.85 \text{ if female})$$

The **Modification of Diet in Renal Disease (MDRD)** study formula (current 4-factor formula) can also be used, although it requires a calculator or computer:

$$\text{CrCl}_{(\text{est})} = 186 \times (\text{serum creatinine})^{-1.154} \times (\text{age})^{-0.203} \times 0.742\ (\text{if female}) \times 1.210\ (\text{if black})$$

The **Chronic Kidney Disease Epidemiology Collaboration (CKD-EPI) formula** provides a lower sensitivity but a higher specificity for detecting a GFR less than 60 mL/min per 1.73 m^2, and may be more useful in evaluating patients with normal or near-normal kidney function. Like the Cockcroft and Gault and MDRD equations, it is also based on the serum creatinine level.

$$\text{eGFR} = 141 \times \min\left(\frac{S_{Cr}}{k}, 1\right)^{\alpha} \times \max\left(\frac{S_{Cr}}{k}, 1\right)^{-1.209} \times 0.993^{\text{age}} \times 1.018\ [\text{if female}] \times 1.159\ [\text{if black}]$$

where S_{Cr} is serum creatinine in mg/dL, kappa (κ) is 0.7 for females and 0.9 for males, α is −0.329 for females and −0.411 for males, min indicates the minimum of S_{Cr}/κ or 1, and max indicates the maximum of S_{Cr}/κ or 1.

A calculator is available from the National Kidney Foundation (www.kidney.org).

EVALUATION OF THE UROLOGIC PATIENT

Urologic patients may have symptoms referable to the kidneys as well as to other parts of the GU tract.

History

Pain originating in the kidneys or ureters is usually vaguely localized to the flanks or lower back and may radiate into the ipsilateral iliac fossa, upper thigh, testis, or labium. Typically, pain caused by calculi is colicky and may be prostrating; it is more constant if caused by infection. Acute urinary retention distal to the bladder causes agonizing suprapubic pain; chronic urinary retention causes less pain and may be asymptomatic. Dysuria is a symptom of bladder or urethral irritation. Prostatic pain manifests as vague discomfort or fullness in the perineal, rectal, or suprapubic regions.

Symptoms of bladder obstruction in men include urinary hesitancy, straining, decrease in force and caliber of the urinary stream, and terminal dribbling. Incontinence has various forms. Enuresis after age 3 to 4 yr may be a symptom of urethral stenosis in girls, posterior urethral valves in boys, psychologic distress, or, if onset is new, infection.

Pneumaturia (air passed with urine) suggests a vesicovaginal, vesicoenteric, or ureteroenteric fistula; the last 2 may be caused by diverticulitis, Crohn disease, abscess, or colon cancer. Pneumaturia could also be due to emphysematous pyelonephritis.

Physical Examination

Physical examination focuses on the costovertebral angle, abdomen, rectum, groin, and genitals. In women with urinary symptoms, pelvic examination is usually done.

Costovertebral angle: Pain elicited by blunt striking of the back, flanks, and angle formed by the 12th rib and lumbar spine with a fist (costovertebral tenderness) may indicate pyelonephritis, calculi, or urinary tract obstruction.

Abdomen: Visual fullness of the upper abdomen is an extremely rare and nonspecific finding of hydronephrosis or a kidney or abdominal mass. Dullness to percussion in the lower abdomen suggests bladder distention; normally, even a full bladder cannot be percussed above the symphysis pubis. Bladder palpation can be used to confirm distention and urinary retention.

Rectum: During digital rectal examination, prostatitis may be detected as a boggy, tender prostate. Focal nodules and less discrete hard areas must be distinguished from prostate cancer. The prostate may be symmetrically enlarged, rubbery, and nontender with benign prostatic hyperplasia.

Groin and genitals: Inguinal and genital examination should be done with patients standing. Inguinal hernia or adenopathy may explain scrotal or groin pain. Gross asymmetry, swelling, erythema, or discoloration of the testes may indicate infection, torsion, tumor, or other mass. Horizontal testicular lie (bell-clapper deformity) indicates increased risk of testicular torsion. Elevation of one testis (normally the left is lower) may be a sign of testicular torsion. The penis is examined with and without retracting the foreskin. Inspection of the penis can detect

- Hypospadias or epispadias in young boys
- Peyronie disease in men
- Priapism, ulcers, and discharge in either group

Palpation may reveal an inguinal hernia. Cremasteric reflex may be absent with testicular torsion. Location of masses in relation to the testis and the degree and location of tenderness may help differentiate among testicular masses (eg, spermatoceles, epididymitis, hydroceles, tumors). If swelling is present, the area should be transilluminated to help determine whether the swelling is cystic or solid. Fibrous plaques on the penile shaft are signs of Peyronie disease.

Testing

Urinalysis is critical for evaluating urologic disorders. Imaging tests (eg, ultrasonography, CT, MRI) are frequently required. For semen testing, see p. 2269.

Bladder tumor antigen testing for transitional cell cancer of the urinary tract is more sensitive than urinary cytology in detecting low-grade cancer; it is not sensitive enough to replace endoscopic examination. Urine cytology is the best test to detect high-grade cancer.

Prostate-specific antigen (PSA) is a glycoprotein with unknown function produced by prostatic epithelial cells. Levels can be elevated in prostate cancer and in some common noncancerous disorders (eg, benign prostatic hyperplasia, infection, trauma). PSA is measured to detect recurrence of cancer after treatment; its widespread use for cancer screening is controversial.

243 Symptoms of Genitourinary Disorders

DYSURIA

Dysuria is painful or uncomfortable urination, typically a sharp, burning sensation. Some disorders cause a painful ache over the bladder or perineum. Dysuria is an extremely common symptom in women, but it can occur in men and can occur at any age.

Pathophysiology

Dysuria results from irritation of the bladder trigone or urethra. Inflammation or stricture of the urethra causes difficulty in starting urination and burning on urination. Irritation of the trigone causes bladder contraction, leading to frequent and painful urination. Dysuria most frequently results from an infection in the lower urinary tract, but it could also be caused by an upper UTI. Impaired renal concentrating ability is the main reason for frequent urination in upper UTIs.

Etiology

Dysuria is typically caused by urethral or bladder inflammation, although perineal lesions in women (eg, from vulvovaginitis or herpes simplex virus infection) can be painful when exposed to urine. Most cases are caused by infection, but sometimes noninfectious inflammatory disorders are responsible (see Table 243–1).

Overall, the **most common causes** of dysuria are

- Cystitis
- Urethritis due to a sexually transmitted disease (STD)

Evaluation

History: History of present illness should cover duration of symptoms and whether they have occurred in the past. Important accompanying symptoms include fever, flank pain, urethral or vaginal discharge, and symptoms of bladder irritation (frequency, urgency) or obstruction (hesitancy, dribbling). Patients should be asked whether the urine is bloody, cloudy, or malodorous and the nature of any discharge (eg, thin and watery or thick and purulent). Clinicians should also ask whether patients have recently engaged in unprotected intercourse, have applied potential irritants to the perineum, have had recent urinary instrumentation (eg, cystoscopy, catheterization, surgery), or might be pregnant.

Review of systems should seek symptoms of a possible cause, including back or joint pain and eye irritation (connective tissue disorder) and GI symptoms, such as diarrhea (reactive arthritis).

Past medical history should note prior urinary infections (including those during childhood) and any known abnormality of the urinary tract, including a history of kidney stones. As with any potentially infectious illness, a history of an immunocompromised state (including HIV/AIDS) or recent hospitalization is important.

Physical examination: Examination begins with review of vital signs, particularly to note the presence of fever.

Skin, mucosa, and joints are examined for lesions suggesting reactive arthritis (eg, conjunctivitis, oral ulcers, vesicular or crusting lesions of palms, soles, and around nails, joint tenderness). The flank is percussed for tenderness over the kidneys. The abdomen is palpated for tenderness over the bladder.

Women should have a pelvic examination to detect perineal inflammation or lesions and vaginal or cervical discharge (see on p. 2315). Swabs for STD testing and wet mount should be obtained at this time rather than doing a 2nd examination.

Men should undergo external inspection to detect penile lesions and discharge; the area under the foreskin should be examined. Testes and epididymis are palpated to detect tenderness or swelling. Rectal examination is done to palpate the prostate for size, consistency, and tenderness.

Red flags: The following findings are of particular concern:

- Fever
- Flank pain or tenderness
- Recent instrumentation
- Immunocompromised patient
- Recurrent episodes (including frequent childhood infections)
- Known urinary tract abnormality
- Male sex

Table 243–1. SOME CAUSES OF DYSURIA

CAUSE	SUGGESTIVE FINDINGS	DIAGNOSTIC APPROACH
Infectious disorders*		
Cervicitis	Often cervical discharge History of unprotected intercourse	STD testing
Cystitis	Typically urinary frequency and urgency Sometimes bloody or malodorous urine Bladder tenderness	Clinical evaluation with or without urinalysis unless red flags† are present
Epididymo-orchitis	Tender, swollen epididymis	Clinical evaluation
Prostatitis	Enlarged, tender prostate Often history of obstructive symptoms	Clinical evaluation
Urethritis	Usually visible discharge History of unprotected intercourse	STD testing
Vulvovaginitis	Vaginal discharge Erythema of labia and introitus	Clinical evaluation, urinalysis, and culture to rule out UTI Consideration of catheterization to minimize contamination of specimen
Inflammatory disorders		
Contact irritant or allergen (eg, spermicide, lubricant, latex condom), foreign bodies in the bladder, parasites, calculi, chemotherapy (cyclophosphamide), and radiation	External inflammation Clinical history Family history	Clinical evaluation Urinalysis Imaging of the urinary tract and pelvis
Interstitial cystitis	Chronic symptoms No other, more common causes found	Cystoscopy
Spondyloarthropathies (eg, reactive arthritis, Behçet syndrome)	Preceding GI or joint symptoms or both Sometimes skin and mucosal lesions	Clinical evaluation STD testing
Other disorders		
Atrophic vaginitis	Postmenopausal (including estrogen deficiencies due to drugs, surgery, or radiation) Often dyspareunia Atrophy or erythema of vaginal folds Vaginal discharge	Clinical evaluation
Tumors (usually bladder, prostate, or urethral cancer)	Long-standing symptoms Usually hematuria without pyuria or infection	Cystoscopy, urine cytology Possible prostate biopsy or bladder biopsy

*Common pathogens include nonsexually transmitted bacteria (mostly *Escherichia coli*, *Staphylococcus saphrophyticus*, *Enterococcus* sp, *Klebsiella* sp, and *Proteus* sp) and sexually transmitted pathogens (eg, *Neisseria gonorrhoeae*, *Chlamydia trachomatis*, *Ureaplasma urealyticum*, *Trichomonas vaginalis*, herpes simplex virus).

†Red flags are fever, flank pain or tenderness, recent instrumentation of the GU tract, immunocompromised patient, recurrent episodes, known urologic abnormalities, and male sex.

STD = sexually transmitted disease.

Interpretation of findings: Some findings are highly suggestive (see Table 243–1). In young, healthy women with dysuria and significant symptoms of bladder irritation, cystitis is the most likely cause. Visible urethral or cervical discharge suggests an STD. Thick purulent material is usually gonococcal; thin or watery discharge is nongonococcal. Vaginitis and the ulcerative lesions of herpes simplex virus infection are typically apparent on inspection. In men, a very tender prostate suggests prostatitis, and a tender, swollen epididymis suggests epididymitis. Other findings also are helpful but may not be diagnostic; eg, women with findings of vulvovaginitis may also have a UTI or another cause of dysuria. Diagnosis of UTI based on symptoms is less accurate in the elderly.

Findings suggestive of infection are more concerning in patients with red flag findings. Fever, flank pain, or both suggest an accompanying pyelonephritis. History of frequent UTIs should raise concern for an underlying anatomic abnormality or compromised immune status. Infections following hospitalization or instrumentation may indicate an atypical or resistant pathogen.

Testing: No single approach is uniformly accepted. Many clinicians presumptively give antibiotics for cystitis without any testing (sometimes not even urinalysis) in young, otherwise healthy women presenting with classic dysuria, frequency, and urgency and without red flag findings. Others evaluate everyone with a clean-catch midstream urine sample for urinalysis and culture. Some clinicians defer culture unless dipstick testing detects WBCs. In women of childbearing age, a pregnancy test is done (UTI during pregnancy is of concern because it may increase the risk of preterm labor or premature rupture of the membranes). Vaginal discharge warrants a wet mount. Many clinicians routinely obtain samples of cervical (women) or urethral (men) exudate for STD testing (gonococcus and chlamydia culture or PCR) because many infected patients do not have a typical presentation.

A finding of > 10^5 bacteria colony-forming units (CFU)/mL suggests infection. In symptomatic patients, sometimes counts as low as 10^2 or 10^3 CFUs indicate UTI. WBCs detected with urinalysis in patients with sterile cultures are nonspecific and may occur with an STD, vulvovaginitis, prostatitis, TB, tumor, interstitial nephritis, or other causes. RBCs detected with urinalysis in patients with no WBCs and sterile cultures may be due to cancer, calculus, foreign body, glomerular abnormalities, or recent instrumentation of the urinary tract.

Cystoscopy and imaging of the urinary tract may be indicated to check for obstruction, anatomic abnormalities, cancer, or other problems in patients who have no response to antibiotics, recurrent symptoms, or hematuria without infection. Rectovesicular fistula should be considered in men with recurrent lower urinary tract infections or those with polymicrobial infections. Pregnant patients, males, older patients, and patients with prolonged or recurrent dysuria need closer attention and a more thorough investigation.

Treatment

Treatment is directed at the cause. Many clinicians do not treat dysuria in women without red flag findings if no cause is apparent based on examination and the results of a urinalysis. If treatment is decided upon, a 3-day course of trimethoprim/sulfamethoxazole or trimethoprim alone is recommended. Because they can cause tendinopathy, fluoroquinolones should not be used for uncomplicated UTIs whenever possible. Some clinicians give presumptive treatment for an STD in men with similarly unremarkable findings; other clinicians await STD test results, particularly in reliable patients.

Acute, intolerable dysuria due to cystitis can be relieved somewhat by phenazopyridine 100 to 200 mg po tid for the first 24 to 48 h. This drug turns urine red-orange and may stain undergarments; patients should be cautioned not to confuse this effect with progression of infection or hematuria. Complicated UTI requires 10 to 14 days of treatment with an antibiotic that is effective against gram-negative organisms, particularly *Escherichia coli*.

KEY POINTS

- Dysuria is not always caused by a bladder infection.
- STDs should be considered.

HEMATOSPERMIA

Hematospermia is blood in semen. It is often frightening to patients but is usually benign. Men sometimes mistake hematuria or blood from a sexual partner for hematospermia.

Pathophysiology

Semen is composed of sperm from the distal epididymis and fluids from the seminal vesicles, prostate, and Cowper and bulbourethral glands. Thus, a lesion anywhere along this pathway could introduce blood into the semen.

Etiology

Most cases of hematospermia are

- Idiopathic and benign

Such cases resolve spontaneously within a few days to a few months.

The most common known cause is

- Prostate biopsy

Less common causes include other instrumentation, benign prostatic hyperplasia, infections (eg, prostatitis, urethritis, epididymitis), and prostate cancer (in men > 35 to 40 yr). Occasionally, tumors of the seminal vesicles and testes are associated with hematospermia. Hemangiomas of the prostatic urethra or spermatic duct may cause massive hematospermia.

Schistosoma haematobium, a parasitic fluke that causes significant disease in Africa, parts of the Middle East, and southeast Asia, can invade the urinary tract, causing hematuria and not infrequently hematospermia. Schistosomiasis is a consideration only in men who have spent time in areas where the disorder is endemic. TB is also an uncommon cause of hematospermia.

Evaluation

History: History of present illness should note the duration of symptoms. Patients who do not volunteer information should be asked specifically about a recent prostate biopsy. Important associated symptoms include hematuria, difficulty starting or stopping urine flow, nocturia, burning with urination, and penile discharge. Association with sexual activity should also be noted.

Review of systems should seek symptoms of causative disorders, including easy bruising, frequent nosebleeds, and excessive gum bleeding with tooth brushing or dental procedures (hematologic disorders), and fevers, chills, night sweats, bone pain, or weight loss (prostate infection or cancer).

Past medical history should specifically ask about known disorders of the prostate, history of or exposure to TB or HIV, risk factors for STDs (eg, unprotected intercourse, multiple sex partners), known bleeding disorders, and known disorders that predispose to bleeding (eg, cirrhosis). Drug history should note use of anticoagulants or antiplatelet drugs. Patients should be asked about any family history of prostate cancer and travel to regions where schistosomiasis is endemic.

Physical examination: The external genitals should be inspected and palpated for signs of inflammation (erythema, mass, tenderness), particularly along the course of the epididymis. A digital rectal examination is done to examine the prostate for enlargement, tenderness, or a lump.

Red flags: The following findings are of particular concern:

- Symptoms lasting > 1 mo in the absence of a recent prostate biopsy
- Palpable lesion along the epididymis or in the prostate
- Travel to a region where schistosomiasis is prevalent
- Systemic symptoms (eg, fevers, weight loss, night sweats)

Interpretation of findings: Patients whose symptoms followed prostate biopsy can be reassured that the hematospermia is harmless and will go away.

Healthy, young patients with a brief duration of hematospermia, an otherwise normal history and examination, and no travel history likely have an idiopathic disorder.

Patients with abnormal findings on prostate examination may have prostate cancer, benign prostatic hyperplasia, or prostatitis. Urethral discharge suggests an STD.

Epididymal tenderness suggests an STD or rarely TB (more likely in patients with risk factors of exposure or who are immunocompromised).

Characteristic findings of a bleeding disorder or use of drugs that increase risk of bleeding suggests a precipitating cause but does not rule out an underlying disorder.

Testing: In most cases, especially in men < 35 to 40 yr, hematospermia is almost always benign. If no significant abnormality is found on physical examination (including digital rectal examination), urinalysis, urine culture, and STD testing are done, but no further workup is necessary.

Patients who may have a more serious underlying disorder and should have testing include those who have

- A longer duration of symptoms (> 1 mo)
- Hematuria
- Obstructive urinary symptoms
- Abnormal examination findings
- Fevers, weight loss, or night sweats

These findings are of particular concern in men > 40 yr. Testing includes urinalysis, urine culture, prostate-specific antigen (PSA) testing, and transrectal ultrasonography (TRUS). Occasionally, MRI and cystoscopy are needed. Semen inspection and analysis are rarely done, but it can be useful when travel history suggests possible exposure to *S. haematobium*.

Treatment

Treatment is directed at the cause if known. For almost all men, reassurance that hematospermia is not a sign of cancer and does not affect sexual function is the only intervention necessary. If prostatitis is suspected, it can be treated with trimethoprim/sulfamethoxazole or other antibiotic for 4 to 6 wk. Because they can cause tendinopathy, fluoroquinolones should not be used for uncomplicated urinary tract infections whenever possible.

KEY POINTS

- Most cases are idiopathic or follow prostate biopsy.
- Testing is required mainly for patients with prolonged symptoms or abnormal examination findings.
- Schistosomiasis should be considered in patients who have traveled to endemic areas.

ISOLATED HEMATURIA

Hematuria is RBCs in urine, specifically > 3 RBCs per high-power field on urine sediment examination. Urine may be red, bloody, or cola-colored (gross hematuria with oxidation of blood retained in the bladder) or not visibly discolored (microscopic hematuria). Isolated hematuria is urinary RBCs without other urine abnormalities (eg, proteinuria, casts).

Red urine is not always due to RBCs. Red or reddish brown discoloration may result from the following:

- Hb or myoglobin in urine
- Porphyria (most types)
- Foods (eg, beets, rhubarb, sometimes food coloring)
- Drugs (most commonly phenazopyridine, but sometimes cascara, diphenylhydantoin, methyldopa, phenacetin, phenindione, phenolphthalein, phenothiazine, and senna)

Pathophysiology

RBCs may enter urine from anywhere along the urinary tract—from the kidneys, collecting system and ureters, prostate, bladder, and urethra.

Etiology

Most cases involve transient microscopic hematuria that is self-limited and idiopathic. Transient microscopic hematuria is particularly common in children, present in up to 5% of their urine samples. There are numerous specific causes (see Table 243–2).

The **most common specific causes** differ somewhat by age, but overall the most common are

- UTI
- Prostatitis
- Urinary calculi (in adults)

Vigorous exercise may cause transient hematuria. Cancer and prostate disease are a concern mainly in patients > 50, although younger patients with risk factors may develop cancer.

Glomerular disorders can be a cause at all ages. Glomerular disorders may represent a primary renal disorder (acquired or hereditary) or be secondary to many causes, including infections (eg, group A beta-hemolytic streptococcal infection), connective tissue disorders and vasculitis (eg, SLE at all ages, immunoglobulin A–associated vasculitis [Henoch-Schönlein purpura] in children), and blood disorders (eg, mixed cryoglobulinemia, serum sickness). Worldwide, IgA nephropathy is the most common form of glomerulonephritis.

Schistosoma haematobium, a parasitic fluke that causes significant disease in Africa (and, to a lesser extent, in India and parts of the Middle East), can invade the urinary tract, causing hematuria. Schistosomiasis is considered only if people have spent time in endemic areas. *Mycobacterium tuberculosis* may also infect the lower or upper urinary tract and cause hematuria, occasionally causing urethral strictures.

Evaluation

History: History of present illness includes duration of hematuria and any previous episodes. Urinary obstructive symptoms (eg, incomplete emptying, nocturia, difficulty starting or stopping) and irritative symptoms (eg, irritation, urgency, frequency, dysuria) should be noted. Patients should be asked about the presence of pain and its location and severity and whether they have vigorously exercised.

Review of systems should seek symptoms of possible causes, including joint pain and rashes (connective tissue disorder). Presence of fever, night sweats, or weight loss should also be noted.

Past medical history should include questions about any recent infections, particularly a sore throat that may indicate a group A beta-hemolytic streptococcal infection. Conditions known to cause urinary tract bleeding (particularly kidney calculi, sickle cell disease or trait, and glomerular disorders) should be sought. Also, conditions that predispose to a glomerular disorder, such as a connective tissue disorder (particularly SLE and RA), endocarditis, shunt infections, and abdominal abscesses, should be identified. Risk factors for GU cancer should be identified, including smoking (the most significant), drugs (eg, cyclophosphamide, phenacetin), and exposure to industrial chemicals (eg, nitrates, nitrilotriacetate, nitrites, trichloroethylene).

Family history should identify relatives with known polycystic kidney disease, a glomerular disorder, or GU cancer. Patients should be asked about travel to areas where schistosomiasis is endemic, and TB risk factors should be assessed. Drug history should note use of anticoagulants, antiplatelet drugs (although controlled anticoagulation itself does not cause hematuria), and heavy analgesic use.

Physical examination: Vital signs should be reviewed for fever and hypertension.

The heart should be auscultated for murmurs (suggesting endocarditis).

The abdomen should be palpated for masses; flanks should be percussed for tenderness over the kidneys. In men, a digital rectal examination should be done to check for prostate enlargement, nodules, and tenderness.

Table 243–2. SOME COMMON SPECIFIC CAUSES OF HEMATURIA

CAUSE	SUGGESTIVE FINDINGS	DIAGNOSTIC APPROACH*
Infection	Urinary irritative symptoms, with or without fever	Urinalysis and culture
Calculi	Sudden-onset, usually colicky, severe flank or abdominal pain, sometimes with vomiting	Abdominal CT without contrast or ultrasonography of the abdomen
Glomerular disease (numerous forms)	In many patients, hypertension, edema, or both Possibly red or dark (cola-colored) urine Sometimes preceding infection, family history of renal disorders, or connective tissue disorder Usually proteinuria	Urinalysis Urine sediment examination for RBC cast and dysmorphic RBCs Serologic tests Renal biopsy
Genitourinary cancer (bladder, kidney, prostate, ureter)	Mainly in patients > 50 or with risk factors (smoking, family history, chemical or drug [eg, phenacetin, cyclophosphamide] exposures) Sometimes voiding symptoms with bladder cancer Often systemic symptoms with renal cell carcinoma	In all patients without another obvious cause, cystoscopy and possible bladder biopsy; if prostate cancer suspected PSA and possibly prostate biopsy
Prostatic hyperplasia	Mainly in patients > 50 Often, urinary obstructive symptoms Palpably enlarged prostate	PSA Measurement of postvoid residual urine volume Ultrasonography of pelvis
Prostatitis	Mainly in patients > 50 Often, urinary irritative and obstructive symptoms Painful, tender prostate with acute infection	Clinical evaluation Sometimes transrectal ultrasonography or cystoscopy
Polycystic kidney disease	Chronic flank or abdominal pain Hypertension Large kidneys	Ultrasonography or noncontrast CT/MRI of the abdomen
Renal papillary infarction or necrosis	Often in people with sickle cell disease or trait (eg, blacks, mainly children and young adults, often with known disease) Sometimes heavy analgesic use (analgesic nephropathy)	Sometimes sickle cell preparation and Hb electrophoresis
Endometriosis	Hematuria coinciding with menses	Clinical evaluation
Trauma (blunt or penetrating)	Usually, presentation as injury rather than as hematuria	CT of the abdomen and pelvis
Loin pain–hematuria syndrome	Flank pain Hematuria	Urinalysis and CT
Nutcracker syndrome	Hematuria Left testicular pain Varicocele	CT angiography

*All patients require urinalysis and evaluation of renal function; older patients require imaging of kidneys and pelvis.
PSA = prostate-specific antigen.

The face and extremities should be inspected for edema (suggesting a glomerular disorder), and the skin should be inspected for rashes (suggesting vasculitis, SLE, or immunoglobulin A–associated vasculitis).

Red flags: The following findings are of particular concern:

- Gross hematuria and concurrent proteinuria
- Persistent microscopic hematuria, especially in older patients
- Age > 50
- Hypertension and edema
- Systemic symptoms (eg, fever, night sweats, weight loss)

Interpretation of findings: Clinical manifestations of the various causes overlap significantly, so urine and often blood tests are required. Depending on results, imaging tests may then be needed. However, some clinical findings provide helpful clues (see Table 243–2).

- Blood clots in urine essentially rule out a glomerular disorder. Glomerular disorders are often accompanied by edema, hypertension, or both; symptoms may be preceded by an infection (particularly a group A beta-hemolytic streptococcal infection in children).
- Calculi usually manifest with excruciating, colicky pain. Less severe, more continuous pain is more likely to result from infection, cancer, polycystic kidney disease, glomerulonephritis, and loin pain–hematuria syndrome.
- Urinary irritative symptoms suggest bladder or prostate infection but may accompany certain cancers (mainly bladder and prostate).

- Urinary obstructive symptoms usually suggest prostate disease.
- An abdominal mass suggests polycystic kidney disease or renal cell carcinoma.
- A family history of nephritis, sickle cell disease or trait, or polycystic kidney disease suggests that as a cause.
- Travel to Africa, the Middle East, or India suggests the possibility of schistosomiasis.
- Systemic symptoms (eg, fever, night sweats, weight loss) may indicate cancer or subacute infection (eg, TB) or an autoimmune (connective tissue) disorder.

On the other hand, some common findings (eg, prostate enlargement, excessive anticoagulation), although potential causes of hematuria, should not be assumed to be the cause without further evaluation.

Testing: Before testing proceeds, true hematuria should be distinguished from red urine by urinalysis. In women with vaginal bleeding, the specimen should be obtained by straight catheterization to avoid contamination by a nonurinary source of blood. Red urine without RBCs suggests myoglobinuria or hemoglobinuria, porphyria, or ingestion of certain drugs or foods. Generally, the presence of hematuria should be confirmed by testing a 2nd specimen.

Presence of casts, protein, or dysmorphic RBCs (unusually shaped, with spicules, folding, and blebs) indicates a glomerular disorder. WBCs or bacteria suggest an infectious etiology. However, because urinalysis shows predominantly RBCs in some patients with cystitis, urine culture is usually done. A positive culture result warrants treatment with antibiotics. If hematuria resolves after treatment and no other symptoms are present, no further evaluation is required for patients < 50, especially women.

If patients < 50 (including children) have only microscopic hematuria and no urine findings suggesting a glomerular disorder, no clinical manifestations suggesting a cause, and no risk factors for cancer, they can be observed, with urinalysis repeated every 6 to 12 mo. If hematuria is persistent, ultrasonography or CT with contrast is suggested.

Patients < 50 with gross hematuria or unexplained systemic symptoms require ultrasonography or CT of the abdomen and pelvis.

If urine or clinical findings suggest a glomerular disorder, renal function is evaluated by measuring BUN, serum creatinine, and electrolytes; doing a urinalysis; and periodically determining the urine protein/creatinine ratio. Further evaluation of a glomerular disorder may require serologic tests, kidney biopsy, or both.

All patients ≥ 50 require cystoscopy, as do patients who are < 50 but have risk factors, such as a family history of cancer, or systemic symptoms. Men ≥ 50 require testing for PSA; those with elevated levels require further evaluation for prostate cancer.

Treatment

Treatment is directed at the cause.

KEY POINTS

- Red urine should be differentiated from true hematuria (RBCs in urine).
- Urinalysis and urine sediment examination help differentiate glomerular from nonglomerular causes.
- Risk of serious disease increases with aging and with duration and degree of hematuria.
- Cystoscopy and imaging tests are usually needed for patients > 50 or for younger patients with systemic symptoms or risk factors for cancer.

POLYURIA

Polyuria is urine output of > 3 L/day; it must be distinguished from urinary frequency, which is the need to urinate many times during the day or night but in normal or less-than-normal volumes. Either problem can include nocturia.

Pathophysiology

Water homeostasis is controlled by a complex balance of water intake (itself a matter of complex regulation), renal perfusion, glomerular filtration and tubular reabsorption of solutes, and reabsorption of water from the renal collecting ducts.

When water intake increases, blood volume increases and blood osmolality decreases, decreasing release of ADH (also referred to as argininevasopressin) from the hypothalamic-pituitary system. Because ADH promotes water reabsorption in the renal collecting ducts, decreased levels of ADH increase urine volume, allowing blood osmolality to return to normal.

Additionally, high amounts of solutes within the renal tubules cause a passive osmotic diuresis (solute diuresis) and thus an increase in urine volume. The classic example of this process is the glucose-induced osmotic diuresis in uncontrolled diabetes mellitus, when high urinary glucose levels (> 250 mg/dL) exceed tubular reabsorption capacity, leading to high glucose levels in the renal tubules; water follows passively, resulting in glucosuria and increased urine volume.

Therefore, polyuria results from any process that involves

- Sustained increase in water intake (polydipsia)
- Decreased ADH secretion (central diabetes insipidus)
- Decreased peripheral ADH sensitivity (nephrogenic diabetes insipidus)
- Solute diuresis

Etiology

The most common cause of polyuria in adults is

- Taking diuretics

The most common cause of polyuria (see Table 243–3) in adults and children is

- Uncontrolled diabetes mellitus

In the absence of diabetes mellitus, the most common causes are

- Primary polydipsia
- Central diabetes insipidus
- Nephrogenic diabetes insipidus

Evaluation

History: History of present illness should include the amounts of fluid consumed and voided to distinguish between polyuria and urinary frequency. If polyuria is present, patients should be asked about the age at onset, rate of onset (eg, abrupt vs gradual), and any recent clinical factors that may cause polyuria (eg, IV fluids, tube feedings, resolution of urinary obstruction, stroke, head trauma, surgery). Patients should be asked about their degree of thirst.

Review of systems should seek symptoms suggesting possible causes, including dry eyes and dry mouth (Sjögren syndrome) and weight loss and night sweats (cancer).

Past medical history should be reviewed for conditions associated with polyuria, including diabetes mellitus, psychiatric disorders, sickle cell disease, sarcoidosis, amyloidosis, and hyperparathyroidism. A family history of polyuria and excessive

Table 243–3. SOME CAUSES OF POLYURIA

CAUSE	SUGGESTIVE FINDINGS	DIAGNOSTIC APPROACH*
Water diuresis†		
Central diabetes insipidus (partial or complete) • Inherited • Acquired (due to injury, tumors, or other lesions)	Abrupt or chronic onset of thirst and polyuria Sometimes follows trauma, pituitary surgery, or hypoxic or ischemic cerebrovascular insult or occurs during the first few weeks of life	Laboratory tests Water deprivation test with ADH challenge ADH measurement when diagnosis remains unclear
Nephrogenic diabetes insipidus • Amyloidosis • Drugs (lithium, cidofovir, foscarnet) • Hypercalcemia (due to cancer, hyperparathyroidism, or granulomatous disease) • Inherited disorders • Sickle cell disease • Sjögren syndrome	Gradual onset of thirst and polyuria in a patient with a history of lithium use for bipolar disorder or with hypercalcemia related to hyperparathyroidism, or in a child with family members who drink excess amounts of water with an underlying paraneoplastic disorder, or during the first few years of life	Laboratory tests Water deprivation test with ADH challenge
Polydipsia • Primary (hypothalamic lesions in the hypothalamic thirst center) • Psychogenic	Anxious, middle-aged woman History of psychiatric illnesses Infiltrating lesions of the hypothalamus (usually sarcoidosis)	Laboratory tests Water deprivation test with ADH challenge
Excessive hypotonic IV fluid administration	Hospitalized patient receiving IV fluids Possibly edema	Resolution after fluids stopped or rate of administration decreased
Diuretic use	Recent initiation of diuretic for volume overload (eg, due to heart failure or peripheral edema) Patients who are likely to surreptitiously use diuretics for weight loss (eg, those with eating disorders or concerns about weight, athletes, adolescents)	Clinical evaluation
Adipsic diabetes insipidus	Polyuria without excessive thirst Sometimes lesions in the hypothalamic region, such as a germinoma or craniopharyngioma, or recent anterior communicating artery repair	Sometimes hyperosmolality (eg, 300 to 340 mOsm/kg) and hypernatremia without excessive thirst
Gestational diabetes insipidus (resulting from increased ADH metabolism)	Polydipsia (with excessive thirst) and polyuria that develop for the first time during the 3rd trimester	Inappropriately normal plasma Na (normally decreases by about 5 mEq/L in late pregnancy) with urine osmolality lower than plasma osmolality Resolution 2–3 wk postpartum
Solute diuresis†		
Uncontrolled diabetes mellitus	Thirst and polyuria in a young child or in an obese adult with family history of type 2 diabetes	Finger-stick glucose measurement
Isotonic or hypertonic saline infusions	Hospitalized patient receiving IV fluids	Laboratory tests (eg, 24 h urine collection showing total osmole excretion [osmolality × urine volume]) Stopping or slowing rate of administration (to confirm that polyuria resolves)
High-protein tube feedings	Any patient receiving tube feedings	Switching to tube feedings with lower protein content (to confirm that polyuria resolves)
Relief of urinary tract obstruction	Polyuria after bladder catheterization in a patient with bladder outlet obstruction	Clinical evaluation

*Most patients should have measurement of urine and plasma osmolarity and serum sodium.
†Urine osmolality is typically < 300 mOsm/kg in water diuresis and > 300 mOsm/kg in solute diuresis.
ADH = antidiuretic hormone.

water drinking should be noted. Drug history should note use of any drugs associated with nephrogenic diabetes insipidus (see Table 243–3) and agents that increase urine output (eg, diuretics, alcohol, caffeinated beverages).

Physical examination: The general examination should note signs of obesity (as a risk factor for type 2 diabetes mellitus) or undernutrition or cachexia that might reflect an underlying cancer or an eating disorder plus surreptitious diuretic use.

The head and neck examination should note dry eyes or dry mouth (Sjögren syndrome). Skin examination should note the presence of any hyperpigmented or hypopigmented lesions, ulcers, or subcutaneous nodules that may suggest sarcoidosis. Comprehensive neurologic examination should note any focal deficits that suggest an underlying neurologic insult and assess mental status for indications of a thought disorder. Volume status should be assessed. Extremities should be examined for edema.

Red flags: The following findings are of particular concern:

- Abrupt onset or onset during the first few years of life
- Night sweats, cough, and weight loss, especially when there is an extensive smoking history
- Psychiatric disorder

Interpretation of findings: History can often distinguish polyuria from frequency, but rarely a 24-h urine collection may be needed.

Clinical evaluation may suggest a cause (see Table 243–3), but testing is usually necessary. Diabetes insipidus is suggested by a history of cancer or chronic granulomatous disease (due to hypercalcemia), use of certain drugs (lithium, cidofovir, foscarnet, ifosfamide), and less common conditions (eg, sickle cell disease, renal amyloidosis, sarcoidosis, Sjögren syndrome) that have manifestations that are often more prominent than and precede the polyuria.

Abrupt onset of polyuria at a precise time suggests central diabetes insipidus, as does preference for extremely cold or iced water. Onset during the first few years of life is typically related to inherited central or nephrogenic diabetes insipidus or uncontrolled type 1 diabetes mellitus. Polyuria caused by solute diuresis is suggested by a history of diabetes mellitus. Psychogenic polydipsia is more common in patients with a history of a psychiatric disorder (primarily bipolar disorder, or schizophrenia) rather than as an initial manifestation.

Testing: Once excess urine output has been verified by history or measurements, serum or fingerstick glucose determination should be done to rule out uncontrolled diabetes.

If hyperglycemia is not present, then testing is required:

- Serum and urine chemistries (electrolytes, calcium)
- Serum and urine osmolality and sometimes plasma ADH level

These tests look for hypercalcemia, hypokalemia (due to surreptitious diuretic use), and hypernatremia or hyponatremia:

- Hypernatremia (sodium > 142 mEq/L) suggests excess free water loss due to central or nephrogenic diabetes insipidus.
- Hyponatremia (sodium < 137 mEq/L) suggests excess free water intake secondary to polydipsia.
- Urine osmolality is typically < 300 mOsm/kg with water diuresis and > 300 mOsm/kg with solute diuresis.

If the diagnosis remains unclear, then measurement of serum and urine sodium and osmolality in response to a **water deprivation test** and exogenous ADH administration should be done. Because serious dehydration may result from this testing, the test should be done only while patients are under constant supervision; hospitalization is usually required. Additionally, patients in whom psychogenic polydipsia is suspected must be observed to prevent surreptitious drinking.

Various protocols can be used in water deprivation tests. Each protocol has some limitations. Typically, the test is started in the morning by weighing the patient, obtaining venous blood to determine serum electrolyte concentrations and osmolality, and measuring urine osmolality. Voided urine is collected hourly, and its osmolality is measured. Dehydration is continued until orthostatic hypotension and postural tachycardia appear, ≥ 5% of the initial body weight has been lost, or the urinary concentration does not increase > 30 mOsm/kg in sequentially voided specimens. Serum electrolytes and osmolality are again determined, and 5 units of aqueous vasopressin are injected sc. Urine for osmolality measurement is collected one final time 60 min postinjection, and the test is terminated.

A normal response produces maximum urine osmolality after dehydration (> 700 mOsm/kg), and osmolality does not increase more than an additional 5% after injection of vasopressin.

In **central diabetes insipidus,** patients are typically unable to concentrate urine to greater than the plasma osmolality but are able to increase their urine osmolality after vasopressin administration. The increase in urine osmolality is 50 to 100% in central diabetes insipidus vs 15 to 45% with partial central diabetes insipidus.

In **nephrogenic diabetes insipidus,** patients are unable to concentrate urine to greater than the plasma osmolality and show no additional response to vasopressin administration. Occasionally in partial nephrogenic diabetes insipidus, the increase in urine osmolality can be up to 45%, but overall these numbers are much lower than those that occur in partial central diabetes insipidus (usually < 300 mOsm/kg).

In **psychogenic polydipsia,** urine osmolality is < 100 mOsm/kg. Decreasing water intake gradually will lead to decreasing urine output, increasing plasma and urine osmolality and serum sodium concentration.

Measurement of circulating ADH is the most direct method of diagnosing central diabetes insipidus. Levels at the end of the water deprivation test (before the vasopressin injection) are low in central diabetes insipidus and appropriately elevated in nephrogenic diabetes insipidus. However, ADH levels are not routinely available. In addition, water deprivation is so accurate that direct measurement of ADH is rarely necessary. If measured, ADH levels should be checked at the beginning of the water deprivation test, when the patient is well hydrated; ADH levels should increase as intravascular volume decreases.

Treatment

Treatment varies by cause.

KEY POINTS

- Use of diuretics and uncontrolled diabetes mellitus are common causes of polyuria.
- In the absence of diabetes mellitus and diuretic use, the most common causes of chronic polyuria are primary polydipsia, central diabetes insipidus, and nephrogenic diabetes insipidus.
- Hypernatremia can indicate central or nephrogenic diabetes insipidus.
- Hyponatremia is more characteristic of polydipsia.
- Abrupt onset of polyuria suggests central diabetes insipidus.
- A water deprivation test can help with diagnosis but should only be done with the patient under close supervision.

PRIAPISM

Priapism is painful, persistent, abnormal erection unaccompanied by sexual desire or excitation. It is most common in boys 5 to 10 yr and in men age 20 to 50 yr.

Pathophysiology

The penis is composed of 3 corporeal bodies: 2 corpora cavernosa and 1 corpus spongiosum. Erection is the result of smooth muscle relaxation and increased arterial flow into the corpora cavernosa, causing engorgement and rigidity.

Ischemic priapism: Most cases of priapism involve failure of detumescence and are most commonly due to failure of venous outflow (ie, low flow), also known as ischemic priapism. Severe pain from ischemia occurs after 4 h. If prolonged > 4 h, priapism can lead to corporeal fibrosis and subsequent erectile dysfunction or even penile necrosis and gangrene.

Stuttering priapism is a recurrent form of ischemic priapism with repeated episodes and intervening periods of detumescence.

Nonischemic priapism: Less commonly, priapism is due to unregulated arterial inflow (ie, high flow), usually as a result of formation of an arterial fistula after trauma. Nonischemic priapism is not painful and does not lead to necrosis. Subsequent erectile dysfunction is common.

Etiology

In adults, the most common cause (see Table 243–4) is

- Drug therapy for erectile dysfunction

In children, the most common causes are

- Hematologic disorders (eg, sickle cell disease, less commonly leukemia)

In many cases, priapism may be idiopathic and recurrent.

Evaluation

Priapism requires urgent treatment to prevent chronic complications (primarily erectile dysfunction). Evaluation and treatment should be done simultaneously.

History: History of present illness should cover the duration of erection, presence of partial or complete rigidity, presence or absence of pain, and any recent or past genital trauma. The drug history should be reviewed for offending drugs, and patients should be directly asked about the use of recreational drugs and drugs used to treat erectile dysfunction.

Review of systems should seek symptoms suggesting a cause, including dysuria (UTIs), urinary hesitancy or frequency (prostate cancer), fever and night sweats (leukemia), and lower-extremity weakness (spinal cord pathology).

Past medical history should identify known conditions associated with priapism (see Table 243–4), particularly hematologic disorders. Patients should be asked about a family history of hemoglobinopathies (sickle cell disease or thalassemia).

Physical examination: A focused genital examination should be done to evaluate extent of rigidity and tenderness and determine whether the glans and corpus spongiosum are also affected. Penile or perineal trauma and signs of infection, inflammation, or gangrenous change should be noted.

The general examination should note any psychomotor agitation, and the head and neck examination should look for pupillary dilation associated with stimulant use. The abdomen and suprapubic area should be palpated to detect any masses or splenomegaly, and a digital rectal examination should be done to detect prostatic enlargement or other pathology. Neurologic examination is useful to detect any signs of lower-extremity weakness or saddle paresthesias that might indicate spinal pathology.

Red flags: The following findings are of particular concern:

- Pain
- Priapism in a child
- Recent trauma
- Fever and night sweats

Interpretation of findings: In most cases, the clinical history reveals a history of drug treatment for erectile dysfunction, illicit drug use, or a history of sickle cell disease or trait; in these cases, no testing is indicated.

In patients with ischemic priapism, physical examination typically reveals complete rigidity with pain and tenderness of the corpus cavernosa and sparing of the glans and corpus spongiosum. By contrast, nonischemic priapism is painless and nontender, and the penis may be partially or completely rigid.

Testing: If the cause is not obvious, screening is done for hemoglobinopathies, leukemia, lymphoma, UTI, and other causes:

- CBC
- Urinalysis and culture
- Hb electrophoresis in blacks and men of Mediterranean descent

Many clinicians also do drug screening, intracavernosal ABG testing, and duplex ultrasonography. Penile duplex ultrasonography will show little or absent cavernosal blood flow in men with ischemic priapism and normal to high cavernosal blood flow in men with nonischemic priapism. Ultrasonography may also reveal anatomic abnormalities, such as cavernous arterial fistula or pseudoaneurysm, which usually indicate nonischemic priapism. Occasionally, MRI with contrast is useful to demonstrate arteriovenous fistulas or aneurysms.

Treatment

Treatment is often difficult and sometimes unsuccessful, even when the etiology is known. Whenever possible, patients should be referred to an emergency department; patients should preferably be seen and treated urgently by a urologist. Other disorders should be treated. For example, priapism often resolves when sickle cell crisis is treated. Measures used to treat priapism itself depend on the type.

Ischemic priapism: Treatment should begin immediately, typically with aspiration of blood from the base of one of the corpora cavernosa using a nonheparinized syringe, often with saline irrigation and intracavernous injection of the alpha-receptor agonist phenylephrine. For phenylephrine injections, 1 mL of 1% phenylephrine (10 mg/mL) is added to 19 mL of 0.9% saline to make 500 mcg/mL; 100 to 500 mcg (0.2 to 1 mL) is injected every 5 to 10 min until relief occurs or a total dose of 1000 mcg is given. Before aspiration or injection, anesthesia is provided with a dorsal nerve block or local infiltration.

If these measures are unsuccessful or if priapism has lasted > 48 h (and is thus unlikely to resolve with these measures), a surgical shunt can be created between the corpus cavernosum and glans penis or corpus spongiosum and another vein.

Stuttering priapism: Stuttering priapism, when acute, is treated in the same way as other forms of ischemic priapism. There is a report of several cases caused by sickle cell disease that responded to a single oral dose of sildenafil. Treatments

Table 243–4. SOME CAUSES OF PRIAPISM

CAUSE	SUGGESTIVE FINDINGS	DIAGNOSTIC APPROACH
Drugs for erectile dysfunction: • Alprostadil (injected, intraurethral) • Papaverine (injected) • Phentolamine (injected) • Phosphodiesterase type 5 (PDE-5) inhibitors (avanafil, sildenafil, tadalafil, vardenafil)	Painful ischemic priapism in men with history of treatment for erectile dysfunction	Clinical evaluation
Recreational drugs: • Amphetamines • Cocaine	Painful ischemic priapism and psychomotor agitation and anxiety	Clinical evaluation Sometimes toxicology screen
Other drugs: • Beta-blockers (prazosin, tamsulosin, terazosin) • Anticoagulants (warfarin) • Antihypertensives (nifedipine) • Antipsychotics* • Corticosteroids • Hypoglycemics (tolbutamide) • Lithium • Methaqualone • Trazodone	Painful ischemic priapism in men undergoing treatment for another medical disorder	Clinical evaluation
Hematologic disorders: • Leukemia • Lymphoma • Sickle cell disease (rarely, sickle cell trait) • Thalassemia	Young males, often of African or Mediterranean descent	CBC Hb electrophoresis
Locally advanced prostate cancer Any metastatic disease	Men > 50 with history of increasing symptoms of bladder outlet obstruction	PSA testing CT
Spinal cord stenosis or compression Continuous epidural infusions	Concomitant lower-extremity weakness	CT or MRI of the spine
Trauma (resulting in unregulated arterial inflow or arterial fistula formation)	Nonischemic, nonpainful priapism in men with recent trauma	Penile duplex ultrasonography Angiography MRI
Rare causes: • Cerebrospinal disorder (eg, syphilis, tumor) • Genital infection and inflammation (eg, prostatitis, urethritis, cystitis), especially if complicated by a bladder calculus • Pelvic hematoma or tumor • Pelvic vein thrombosis • Total parenteral nutrition • Carbon monoxide poisoning	Various	Various

*All atypical antipsychotics may cause priapism.

that may help prevent recurrences of stuttering priapism include antiandrogen therapy with gonadotropin-releasing hormone agonists, estrogen, bicalutamide, flutamide, phosphodiesterase type-5 inhibitors, and ketoconazole. The goal of antiandrogen therapy is to decrease the plasma testosterone level to < 10% of normal. Digoxin, terbutaline, gabapentin, and hydroxyurea have also been tried with some success.

Nonischemic priapism: Conservative therapy (eg, ice packs and analgesics) is usually successful; if not, selective embolization or surgery is indicated.

Refractory priapism: If other treatments are ineffective, a penile prosthesis can be placed.

KEY POINTS

- Priapism requires urgent evaluation and treatment.
- Drugs (prescription and recreational) and sickle cell disease are the most common causes.
- Acute treatment is with alpha-agonists, needle decompression, or both.

PROTEINURIA

Proteinuria is protein, usually albumin, in urine. High concentrations of protein cause frothy or sudsy urine. In many renal disorders, proteinuria occurs with other urinary abnormalities (eg, hematuria). Isolated proteinuria is urinary protein without other symptoms or urinary abnormalities.

Pathophysiology

Although the glomerular basement membrane is a very effective barrier against larger molecules (eg, most plasma proteins, primarily albumin), a small amount of protein passes through the capillary basement membranes into the glomerular filtrate. Some of this filtered protein is degraded and reabsorbed by the proximal tubules, but some is excreted in the urine. The upper limit of normal urinary protein excretion is considered to be 150 mg/day, which can be measured in a 24-h urine collection or estimated by random urine protein/creatinine ratio (values > 0.3 are abnormal); for albumin it is about 30 mg/day. Albumin excretion between 30 and 300 mg/day (20 to 200 μg/min) is considered microalbuminuria, and higher levels are considered macroalbuminuria. Mechanisms of proteinuria may be categorized as

- Glomerular
- Tubular
- Overflow
- Functional

Glomerular proteinuria results from glomerular disorders, which typically involve increased glomerular permeability; this permeability allows increased amounts of plasma proteins (sometimes very large amounts) to pass into the filtrate.

Tubular proteinuria results from renal tubulointerstitial disorders that impair reabsorption of protein by the proximal tubule, causing proteinuria (mostly from smaller proteins such as immunoglobulin light chains rather than albumin). Causative disorders are often accompanied by other defects of tubular function (eg, HCO_3 wasting, glucosuria, aminoaciduria) and sometimes by glomerular pathology (which also contributes to the proteinuria).

Overflow proteinuria occurs when excessive amounts of small plasma proteins (eg, immunoglobulin light chains produced in multiple myeloma) exceed the reabsorptive capacity of the proximal tubules.

Functional proteinuria occurs when increased renal blood flow (eg, due to exercise, fever, high-output heart failure) delivers increased amounts of protein to the nephron, resulting in increased protein in the urine (usually < 1 g/day). Functional proteinuria reverses when renal blood flow returns to normal.

Orthostatic proteinuria is a benign condition (most common among children and adolescents) in which proteinuria occurs mainly when the patient is upright. Thus, urine typically contains more protein during waking hours (when people are more often upright) than during sleep. It has a very good prognosis and requires no special intervention.

Consequences: Proteinuria caused by renal disorders usually is persistent (ie, present on serial testing) and, when in the nephrotic range, can cause significant protein wasting. Presence of protein in the urine is toxic to the kidneys and causes renal damage.

Etiology

Causes can be categorized by mechanism. The most common causes of proteinuria are glomerular disorders, typically manifesting as nephrotic syndrome (see Table 243–5).

The most common causes of proteinuria (and nephrotic syndrome) in adults are

- Focal segmental glomerulosclerosis
- Membranous nephropathy
- Diabetic nephropathy

Table 243–5. CAUSES OF PROTEINURIA

MECHANISM	EXAMPLES
Glomerular	Primary glomerular disorders (eg, membranous nephropathy, minimal change disease, focal segmental glomerulosclerosis) Secondary glomerular disorders (eg, diabetic nephropathy, preeclampsia, postinfectious glomerulonephritis, lupus nephritis, amyloidosis)
Tubular	Fanconi syndrome Acute tubular necrosis Tubulointerstitial nephritis Polycystic kidney disease
Overflow	Acute monocytic leukemia with lysozymuria Monoclonal gammopathy Multiple myeloma Myelodysplastic syndromes
Functional	Fever Heart failure Intense exercise or activity
Unknown	Orthostatic

The most common causes in children are

- Minimal change disease (in young children)
- Focal segmental glomerulosclerosis (in older children)

Evaluation

History and physical examination: History of present illness may reveal symptoms of fluid overload or hypoalbuminemia, such as eye puffiness upon awakening and leg or abdominal swelling. Proteinuria itself may cause heavy foaming of the urine. However, patients with proteinuria and no obvious fluid overload may not report any symptoms.

Review of systems seeks symptoms suggesting cause, including red or brown urine (glomerulonephritis) or bone pain (myeloma). Patients are asked about existing conditions that can cause proteinuria, including recent serious illness (particularly with fever), intense physical activity, known renal disorders, diabetes, pregnancy, sickle cell disease, SLE, and cancer (particularly myeloma and related disorders).

Physical examination is of limited use, but vital signs should be reviewed for increased BP, suggesting glomerulonephritis. The examination should seek signs of peripheral edema and ascites, reflective of fluid overload or low serum albumin.

Testing: Urine dipstick primarily detects albumin. Precipitation techniques, such as heating and sulfosalicylic acid test strips, detect all proteins. Thus, isolated proteinuria detected incidentally is usually albuminuria. Dipstick testing is relatively insensitive for detection of microalbuminuria, so a positive urine dipstick test usually suggests overt proteinuria. Dipstick testing is also unlikely to detect excretion of smaller proteins characteristic of tubular and overflow proteinuria.

Patients with a positive dipstick test (for protein or any other component) should have routine microscopic urinalysis. Abnormalities on urinalysis (eg, casts and dysmorphic RBCs suggesting glomerulonephritis; glucose, ketones, or both suggesting diabetes) or disorders suggested by history and physical examination (eg, peripheral edema suggesting a glomerular disorder) require further workup.

If urinalysis is otherwise normal, further testing can be deferred pending repeat urine protein assessment. If proteinuria is no longer present, particularly in patients who have had recent intense exercise, fever, or heart failure exacerbation, functional proteinuria is likely. Persistent proteinuria is a sign of a glomerular disorder and requires further testing and referral to a nephrologist. Further testing includes CBC; measurement of serum electrolytes, BUN, creatinine, and glucose; determination of GFR (see p. 2055); quantification of urinary protein (by 24-h measurement or random urine protein/creatinine ratio); and evaluation of kidney size (by ultrasonography or CT). In most patients with glomerulopathy, proteinuria is in the nephrotic range (> 3.5 g/day or urine protein/creatinine ratio > 2.7).

Other testing is usually done to determine the cause of a glomerular disorder, including lipid profile, complement levels, cryoglobulins, hepatitis B and C serology, antinuclear antibody testing, urine and serum protein electrophoresis, HIV testing, and rapid plasma reagin testing for syphilis. If these noninvasive tests are not diagnostic (as is often the case), renal biopsy is necessary. Unexplained proteinuria and renal failure, especially in older patients, could be due to myelodysplastic disorders (eg, multiple myeloma) or amyloidosis.

Among patients < 30 yr, orthostatic proteinuria should be considered. Diagnosis requires 2 urine collections, one done from 7 AM to 11 PM (day sample) and the other from 11 PM to 7 AM (night sample). The diagnosis is confirmed if the urinary protein exceeds normal values in the day sample (or if urine protein/creatinine ratio is > 0.3) and does not in the night sample.

Treatment

Treatment is directed at the cause.

PAINLESS SCROTAL MASS

A painless scrotal mass is often noticed by the patient but may be an incidental finding on routine physical examination.

Scrotal pain and painful scrotal masses or swelling can be caused by testicular torsion, appendiceal torsion, epididymitis, epididymo-orchitis, scrotal abscess, trauma, strangulated inguinal hernias, orchitis, and Fournier gangrene.

Etiology

There are several causes (see Table 243–6) of a painless scrotal mass but the most common include the following:

- Hydrocele
- Nonincarcerated inguinal hernia
- Varicocele (present in up to 20% of adult men)

Less common causes include spermatocele, hematocele, fluid overload, and occasionally testicular cancer. Testicular cancer is the most concerning cause of a painless scrotal mass. Although it is rare compared with the other listed causes, it is the most common solid cancer in men < 40 yr; because it responds well to treatment, prompt recognition is important.

Evaluation

History: History of present illness should address duration of symptoms, the effect of upright position and increase in intra-abdominal pressure, and presence and characteristics of associated symptoms such as pain.

Review of systems should seek symptoms suggesting possible causes, including abdominal pain, anorexia, or vomiting (inguinal hernia with intermittent strangulation); dyspnea and leg swelling (right heart failure); abdominal distention (ascites); and decreased libido, feminization, and infertility (testicular atrophy with bilateral varicoceles).

Past medical history should identify existing disorders that can cause masses (eg, right heart failure, ascites causing bilateral lymphedema); known scrotal disorders (eg, testicular tumor or epididymitis causing hydrocele); past history of pelvic surgery or radiation, and inguinal hernia.

Physical examination: Physical examination includes evaluation for systemic disorders that can cause edema (eg, heart failure, ascites) and detailed inguinal and genital examination.

Inguinal and genital examination should be done with patients standing and recumbent. The inguinal area is inspected and palpated, particularly for reducible masses. The testes, epididymides, and spermatic cords should be palpated for swelling, masses, and tenderness. Careful palpation can usually localize a discrete mass to one of these structures. Nonreducible masses should be transilluminated to help determine whether they are cystic or solid.

Red flags: The following findings are of particular concern:

- Nonreducible mass that obscures normal spermatic cord structures
- Mass that is part of or attached to the testis and does not transilluminate

Interpretation of findings: A nonreducible mass that obscures normal spermatic cord structures suggests an incarcerated inguinal hernia. If a mass is part of or attached to the testis and does not transilluminate, testicular cancer is possible.

Other clinical characteristics can provide important clues (see Table 243–6). For example, a mass that transilluminates is probably cystic (eg, hydrocele, spermatocele). A mass that disappears or becomes smaller when recumbent suggests varicocele, inguinal hernia, or communicating hydrocele. The presence of a hydrocele makes assessment for other scrotal masses by examination difficult. Rarely, a varicocele persists when the patient is recumbent or is present on the right side; either finding suggests inferior vena caval obstruction.

Testing: Clinical evaluation may be diagnostic (eg, in varicocele, lymphedema, inguinal hernia); otherwise, testing is typically done. Ultrasonography is done when

- The diagnosis is uncertain
- Usually when hydrocele is present (to diagnose causative scrotal lesions)
- The mass does not transilluminate

If ultrasonography confirms a solid testicular mass, further testing is done for testicular cancer (see p. 2103), including the following:

- Beta-human chorionic gonadotropin level (hCG)
- Alpha-fetoprotein level
- LDH level
- CT of the abdomen

Treatment

Treatment is directed at the cause. Not all masses require treatment. If inguinal hernia is suspected, reduction can be attempted (see p. 90).

KEY POINTS

- A nonreducible mass that obscures normal spermatic cord structures suggests an incarcerated inguinal hernia.
- A solid mass, one that does not transilluminate, or both mandates evaluation for testicular cancer.
- The cause of a hydrocele must be determined.

Table 243–6. SOME CAUSES OF A PAINLESS SCROTAL MASS

CAUSE	SUGGESTIVE FINDINGS	DIAGNOSTIC APPROACH
Hydrocele (communicating) usually in patients with inguinal hernias	Cystic swelling Increase in size when upright or when intra-abdominal pressure increases Usually congenital Transilluminates	Clinical evaluation Ultrasonography if diagnosis is uncertain
Hydrocele (noncommunicating)	Cystic swelling Does not change in size with changes in position of intra-abdominal pressure Often a simultaneous scrotal abnormality (eg, tumor, epididymitis) Transilluminates	Clinical evaluation Usually ultrasonography
Spermatocele	Cystic mass at the upper pole of the testis, adjacent to epididymis Transilluminates	Clinical evaluation Ultrasonography if diagnosis is uncertain
Inguinal hernia	Increases in size when upright or when intra-abdominal pressure increases May disappear when recumbent or be reducible or compressible Possibly bowel sounds Absence of normal spermatic cord structures above the mass Possibly palpable in the inguinal canal	Clinical evaluation
Varicocele	Palpable when standing (enhanced with Valsalva), feeling like a bag of worms Usually on left side Possibly pain and fullness when standing Possibly testicular atrophy	Clinical evaluation
Hematocele	Tender swelling Risk factors (eg, trauma, surgery, bleeding disorder or use of anticoagulants)	Usually ultrasonography
Fluid overload	Diffuse, bilateral enlargement of scrotal sac Often pitting Often causative disorder evident (eg, heart failure, ascites) Transilluminates	Clinical evaluation Ultrasonography if diagnosis is uncertain
Lymphedema (eg, from filariasis, congenital, idiopathic, after pelvic radiation or cancer [eg, prostate, bladder, testicular])	Diffuse scrotal swelling Often nonpitting	Clinical evaluation Imaging (CT/Ultrasonography) if diagnosis is uncertain
Testicular cancer	Mass attached to or part of testis Is solid or does not transilluminate Possibly dull, aching pain or acute pain due to hemorrhage	Ultrasonography of scrotum Alpha-fetoprotein Beta-human chorionic gonadotropin LDH CT of the abdomen

SCROTAL PAIN

Scrotal pain can occur in males of any age, from neonates to the elderly.

Etiology

The most common causes of scrotal pain include

- Testicular torsion
- Torsion of the testicular appendage
- Epididymitis

There are a number of less common causes (see Table 243–7). Age, onset of symptoms, and other findings can help determine the cause.

Evaluation

Expeditious evaluation, diagnosis, and treatment are required because untreated testicular torsion may cause loss of a testis.

History: History of present illness should determine location (unilateral or bilateral), onset (acute or subacute), and duration of pain. Important associated symptoms include fever, dysuria, penile discharge, and presence of scrotal mass. Patients should be asked about preceding events, including injury, straining or lifting, and sexual contact.

Review of systems should seek symptoms of causative disorders, including purpuric rash, abdominal pain, and arthralgias (immunoglobulin A–associated vasculitis [Henoch-Schönlein purpura]); intermittent scrotal masses, groin swelling,

Table 243–7. SOME CAUSES OF SCROTAL PAIN

CAUSE	SUGGESTIVE FINDINGS	DIAGNOSTIC APPROACH
Testicular torsion	Sudden onset of severe, unilateral, constant pain Cremasteric reflex absent Asymmetric, transversely oriented, high-riding testis on affected side Typically occurring in neonates and postpubertal boys but can occur in adults	Color Doppler ultrasonography
Appendiceal torsion (a vesicular nonpedunculated structure attached to the cephalic pole of the testis)	Subacute onset of pain over several days Pain in the upper pole of testis Cremasteric reflex present Possibly reactive hydrocele, blue dot sign (blue or black spot under the skin on superior aspect of testis or epididymis) Typically occurs in boys aged 7–14 yr	Color Doppler ultrasonography
Epididymitis or epididymo-orchitis, usually infectious, with gram-negative organisms in prepubertal boys and older men or, in sexually active men, STD Can be noninfectious, resulting from urine reflux into ejaculatory ducts	Acute or subacute onset of pain in the epididymis and sometimes also the testis Possibly urinary frequency, dysuria, recent lifting or straining Cremasteric reflex present Often scrotal induration, swelling, erythema Sometimes penile discharge Typically occurring in postpubertal boys and men	Urinalysis and culture Nucleic acid amplification tests for *Neisseria gonorrhoeae* and *Chlamydia trachomatis*
Postvasectomy, acute and chronic (postvasectomy pain syndrome)	History of vasectomy Pain during intercourse, ejaculation, or both Pain during physical exertion Tender or full epididymis	Clinical evaluation
Trauma	Clear history of trauma to the genitals Often swelling, possible intratesticular hematoma or hematocele	Color Doppler ultrasonography
Inguinal hernia (strangulated)	Long history of painless swelling (often known diagnosis of hernia) with acute or subacute pain Scrotal mass, usually large, compressible, possibly with audible bowel sounds Not reducible	Clinical evaluation
Immunoglobulin A–associated vasculitis (Henoch-Schönlein purpura)	Palpable purpura (typically of lower extremities and buttocks), arthralgia, arthritis, abdominal pain, renal disease Typically occurring in boys aged 3–15 yr	Clinical evaluation Sometimes biopsy of skin lesions
Polyarteritis nodosa	Fever, weight loss, abdominal pain, hypertension, edema Skin lesions including palpable purpura and subcutaneous nodules Can be acute or chronic May cause testicular ischemia and infarction Most common in men aged 40–50 yr	Angiography Sometimes biopsy of affected organ
Referred pain (abdominal aortic aneurysm, urolithiasis, lower lumbar or sacral nerve root impingement, retrocecal appendicitis, retroperitoneal tumor, postherniorrhaphy pain)	Normal scrotal examination Sometimes abdominal tenderness depending on cause	Directed by examination findings and suspected cause
Orchitis (usually viral—eg, mumps; rubella; coxsackievirus, echovirus, or parvovirus infection)	Scrotal and abdominal pain, nausea, fever Unilateral or bilateral swelling, erythema of scrotum	Acute and convalescent viral titers
Fournier gangrene (necrotizing fasciitis of the perineum)	Severe pain, fever, toxic appearance, erythema, blistering or necrotic lesions Sometimes palpable subcutaneous gas Sometimes history of recent abdominal surgery More common in older men with diabetes, peripheral vascular disease, or both	Clinical evaluation

or both (inguinal hernia); fever and parotid gland swelling (mumps orchitis); and flank pain or hematuria (renal calculus).

Past medical history should identify known disorders that may cause referred pain, including hernias, abdominal aortic aneurysm, renal calculi, and risk factors for serious disorders, including diabetes and peripheral vascular disease (Fournier gangrene).

Physical examination: Physical examination begins with a review of vital signs and assessment of the severity of pain. Examination focuses on the abdomen, inguinal region, and genitals.

The abdomen is examined for tenderness and masses (including bladder distention). Flanks are percussed for costovertebral angle tenderness.

Inguinal and genital examination should be done with the patient standing. Inguinal area is inspected and palpated for adenopathy, swelling, or erythema. Examination of the penis should note ulcerations, urethral discharge, and piercings and tattoos (sources of bacterial infections). Scrotal examination should note asymmetry, swelling, erythema or discoloration, and positioning of the testes (horizontal vs vertical, high vs low). Cremasteric reflex should be tested bilaterally. The testes, epididymides, and spermatic cords should be palpated for swelling and tenderness. If swelling is present, the area should be transilluminated to help determine whether the swelling is cystic or solid.

Red flags: The following findings are of particular concern:

- Sudden onset of pain; exquisite tenderness; and a high-riding, horizontally displaced testis (testicular torsion)
- Inguinal or scrotal nonreducible mass with severe pain, vomiting, and constipation (incarcerated hernia)
- Scrotal or perineal erythema, necrotic or blistered skin lesions, and toxic appearance (Fournier gangrene)
- Sudden onset of pain, hypotension, weak pulse, pallor, dizziness, and confusion (ruptured abdominal aortic aneurysm)

Interpretation of findings: The focus is to distinguish causes that require immediate treatment from others. Clinical findings provide important clues (see Table 243–7).

Aortic catastrophes and Fournier gangrene occur primarily in patients > 50 yr; the other conditions that require immediate treatment can occur at any age. However, testicular torsion is most common in neonates and postpubertal boys, torsion of the testicular appendage occurs most commonly in prepubertal boys (7 to 14 yr), and epididymitis is most common in adolescents and adults.

Severe, sudden onset of pain suggests testicular torsion or renal calculus. Pain from epididymitis, incarcerated hernia, or appendicitis is of more gradual onset. Patients with torsion of the testicular appendage present with moderate pain that develops over a few days; pain is localized to the upper pole. Bilateral pain suggests infection (eg, orchitis, particularly if accompanied by fever and viral symptoms) or a referred cause. Flank pain that radiates to the scrotum suggests renal calculus or, in men > 55 yr, abdominal aortic aneurysm.

Normal findings on scrotal and perineal examination suggest referred pain. Attention must then be directed to extrascrotal disorders, particularly appendicitis, renal calculi, and, in men > 55, abdominal aortic aneurysm.

Abnormal scrotal and perineal examination findings often suggest a cause. Sometimes, early in epididymitis, tenderness and induration may be localized to the epididymis; early in torsion, the testis may be clearly high-riding, with a horizontal lie and the epididymis not particularly tender. However, frequently the testis and epididymis are both swollen and tender, there is scrotal edema, and it is not possible to differentiate epididymitis from torsion by palpation. However, the cremasteric reflex is absent in torsion, as are findings of a STD (eg, purulent urethral discharge); the presence of both of these findings makes epididymitis quite likely.

Sometimes, a scrotal mass caused by a hernia may be palpable in the inguinal canal; in other cases, hernia can be difficult to distinguish from testicular swelling.

Painful erythema of the scrotum with no tenderness of the testes or epididymides should raise suspicion of infection, either cellulitis or early Fournier gangrene.

A vasculitic rash, abdominal pain, and arthralgias are consistent with a systemic vasculitis syndrome such as immunoglobulin A–associated vasculitis or polyarteritis nodosa.

Testing: Testing is typically done.

- Urinalysis and culture (all patients)
- STD testing (all patients with positive urinalysis, discharge, or dysuria)
- Color Doppler ultrasonography to rule out torsion (no clear-cut alternate cause)
- Other testing as suggested by findings (see Table 243–7)

Urinalysis and culture are always required. Findings of UTI (eg, pyuria, bacteriuria) suggest epididymitis. Patients with findings that suggest UTI and patients with urethral discharge or dysuria should be tested for STDs as well as other bacterial causes of UTI.

Timely diagnosis of testicular torsion is critical. If findings are highly suggestive of torsion, immediate surgical exploration is done in preference to testing. If findings are equivocal and there is no clear alternate cause of acute scrotal pain, color Doppler ultrasonography is done. If Doppler ultrasonography is not available, radionuclide scanning may be used but is less sensitive and specific.

Treatment

Treatment is directed at the cause and can range from emergency surgery (testicular torsion) to bed rest (torsion of the testicular appendage). If testicular torsion is present, prompt surgery (< 12 h after presentation) is generally required. Delayed surgery may lead to testicular infarction, long-term testicular damage, or the loss of a testis. Surgical detorsion of the testis relieves the pain immediately, and simultaneous bilateral orchiopexy prevents recurrence of torsion.

Analgesics, such as morphine or other opioids, are indicated for the relief of acute pain. Antibiotics are indicated for cases of bacterial epididymitis or orchitis.

Geriatrics Essentials

Testicular torsion is uncommon in older men, and when present, the manifestations are usually atypical and therefore diagnosis is delayed. Epididymitis, orchitis, and trauma are more common in older men. Occasionally, inguinal hernia, colon perforation, or renal colic may cause scrotal pain in elderly men.

KEY POINTS

- Always consider testicular torsion in patients with acute scrotal pain, particularly in children and adolescents; quick, accurate diagnosis is essential.
- Other common causes of scrotal pain are torsion of the testicular appendage and epididymitis.
- Color Doppler ultrasonography is usually done when the diagnosis is unclear.
- Normal findings on scrotal and perineal examination suggest referred pain.

URINARY FREQUENCY

Urinary frequency is the need to urinate many times during the day, at night (nocturia), or both but in normal or less-than-normal volumes. Frequency may be accompanied by a sensation of an urgent need to void (urinary urgency). Urinary frequency is distinguished from polyuria, which is urine output of > 3 L/day.

Pathophysiology

Urinary frequency usually results from disorders of the lower GU tract. Inflammation of the bladder, urethra, or both causes a sensation of the need to urinate. However, this sensation is not relieved by emptying the bladder, so once the bladder is emptied, patients continue trying to void but pass only small volumes of urine.

Etiology

There are many causes of urinary frequency (see Table 243–8), but the most common include

- UTIs
- Urinary incontinence
- Benign prostatic hyperplasia
- Urinary tract calculi

Evaluation

History: History of present illness should first ask about the amounts of fluid consumed and voided to distinguish between urinary frequency and polyuria. If urinary frequency is present, patients are asked about acuity of onset, presence or absence of

Table 243–8. SOME CAUSES OF URINARY FREQUENCY

CAUSE	SUGGESTIVE FINDINGS	DIAGNOSTIC APPROACH
Benign prostatic hyperplasia or prostate cancer	Progressive onset of urinary hesitancy, incontinence, poor urine stream, a sensation of incomplete voiding	Rectal examination Ultrasonography Cystometry
Cystocele	Urinary incontinence Sensation of vaginal fullness Pain or urinary leakage during sexual intercourse	Pelvic examination Voiding cystourethrography
Drugs and substances • Caffeine • Alcohol • Diuretics	Urinary frequency in an otherwise healthy patient	Empiric elimination of offending substance (to confirm that frequency resolves)
Pregnancy	3rd trimester of pregnancy	Clinical evaluation
Prostatitis	Urgency, dysuria, nocturia, purulent urethral discharge with fever, chills, low back pain, myalgia, arthralgia, and perineal fullness Prostate tender to palpation	Rectal examination Culture of secretions after prostatic massage
Radiation cystitis	History of radiation therapy of the lower abdomen, prostate, or perineum for treatment of cancer	Clinical evaluation Cystoscopy and biopsy
Reactive arthritis	Asymmetric arthritis of knees, ankles, and metatarsophalangeal joints Unilateral or bilateral conjunctivitis Small, painless ulcers on the mouth, tongue, glans penis, palms, and soles 1–2 wk after sexual contact	STD testing
Spinal cord injury or lesion	Lower-extremity weakness, decreased anal sphincter tone, absent anal wink reflex Loss of sensation at a segmental level Injury usually clinically obvious	MRI of the spine
Urethral stricture	Hesitancy, tenesmus, reduced caliber and force of the urine stream	Urethrography
Urinary incontinence	Unintentional passage of urine, particularly when bending, coughing, or sneezing	Cystometry
Urinary tract calculi	Colicky flank or groin pain	Urinalysis for hematuria Ultrasonography or CT of the kidneys, ureters, and bladder
UTIs	Dysuria and foul-smelling urine, sometimes fever, confusion, and flank pain, particularly in women and girls Dysuria and frequency in young sexually active men (which suggests an STD)	Urinalysis and culture STD testing
Bladder detrusor overactivity	Nocturia, urge incontinence, weak urinary stream, and sometimes urinary retention	Cystometry

STD = sexually transmitted disease.

irritative symptoms (eg, irritation, urgency, dysuria), obstructive symptoms (eg, hesitancy, poor flow, sensation of incomplete voiding, nocturia), and recent sexual contacts.

Review of systems should cover symptoms suggestive of a cause, including fever, flank or groin pain, and hematuria (infection); missed menses, breast swelling, and morning sickness (pregnancy); and arthritis and conjunctivitis (reactive arthritis).

Past medical history should ask about known causes, including prostate disease and previous pelvic radiation therapy or surgeries. Drugs and diet are reviewed for the use of agents that increase urine output (eg, diuretics, alcohol, caffeinated beverages).

Physical examination: Examination focuses on the GU system.

Any urethral discharge or any lesions consistent with STDs are noted. Rectal examination in men should note the size and consistency of the prostate and rectal tone; pelvic examination in women should note the presence of any cystocele. Patients should be instructed to cough while the urethra is observed for signs of urinary leakage.

The costovertebral angle should be palpated for tenderness, and the abdominal examination should note the presence of any masses or suprapubic tenderness.

Neurologic examination should test for lower-extremity weakness and loss of sensation.

Red flags: The following findings are of particular concern:

- Lower-extremity weakness or signs of spinal cord damage (eg, loss of sensation at a segmental level, loss of anal sphincter tone and anal wink reflex)
- Fever and back pain

Interpretation of findings: Dysuria suggests frequency is due to UTI or calculi. Prior pelvic surgery suggests incontinence. Weak urine stream, nocturia, or both suggests BPH. Urinary frequency in an otherwise healthy young patient may be due to excessive intake of alcohol or caffeinated beverages. Gross hematuria suggests UTI and calculi in younger patients and genitourinary cancer in older patients.

Testing: All patients require urinalysis and culture, which are easily done and can detect infection and hematuria.

Cytoscopy, cystometry, and urethrography can be done to diagnose cystitis, bladder outlet obstruction, and cystocele. PSA level determination, ultrasonography, and prostate biopsy may be required, especially in older men, to differentiate BPH from prostate cancer.

Treatment

Treatment varies by cause.

Geriatrics Essentials

Urinary frequency in elderly men is often caused by bladder neck obstruction secondary to prostate enlargement or cancer. These patients usually require postvoid residual urine volume determination. UTI or use of diuretics may be a cause in both sexes.

KEY POINTS

- UTI is the most common cause in children and women.
- Prostate disease is a common cause in men > 50 yr.
- Excessive intake of caffeine can cause urinary frequency in healthy people.

244 Genitourinary Tests and Procedures

BLADDER CATHETERIZATION

Bladder catheterization is used to do the following:

- Obtain urine for examination
- Measure residual urine volume
- Relieve urinary retention or incontinence
- Deliver radiopaque contrast agents or drugs directly to the bladder
- Irrigate the bladder

Catheterization may be urethral or suprapubic.

Catheters: Catheters vary by caliber, tip configuration, number of ports, balloon size, type of material, and length.

Caliber is standardized in French (F) units—also known as Charrière (Ch) units. Each unit is 0.33 mm, so a 14-F catheter is 4.6 mm in diameter. Sizes range from 12 to 24 F for adults and 8 to 12 F for children. Smaller catheters are usually sufficient for uncomplicated urinary drainage and useful for urethral strictures and bladder neck obstruction; bigger catheters are indicated for bladder irrigation and some cases of hemorrhage (eg, postoperatively or in hemorrhagic cystitis) and pyuria because clots could obstruct smaller caliber catheters.

Tips are straight in most catheters (eg, Robinson, whistle-tip) and are used for intermittent urethral catheterization (ie, catheter is removed immediately after bladder drainage). Foley catheters have a straight tip and an inflatable balloon for self-retention. Other self-retaining catheters may have an expanded tip shaped like a mushroom (de Pezzer catheter) or a 4-winged perforated mushroom (Malecot catheter); they are used in suprapubic catheterization or nephrostomy. Elbowed (coudé) catheters, which may have balloons for self-retention, have a bent tip to ease catheterization through strictures or obstructions (eg, prostatic obstruction).

Ports are present in all catheters used for continuous urinary drainage. Many catheters have ports for balloon inflation, irrigation, or both (eg, 3-way Foley).

Balloons on self-retaining catheters have different volumes, from 2.5 to 5 mL in balloons intended for use in children and from 10 to 30 mL in balloons used in adults. Larger balloons and catheters are generally used to manage bleeding; traction on the catheter pulls the balloon against the base of the bladder and puts pressure on vessels, decreasing bleeding but potentially causing ischemia.

Stylets are flexible metal guides inserted through the catheter to give stiffness and to facilitate insertion through strictures or obstructions and should only be used by physicians experienced with the technique.

Catheter material chosen depends on the intended use. Plastic, latex, or polyvinyl chloride catheters are for intermittent use. Latex with silicone, hydrogel, or silver alloy–coated polymer (to diminish bacterial colonization) catheters are for continuous use. Silicone catheters are used in patients with latex allergy.

Urethral catheterization: A urethral catheter can be inserted by any health care practitioner and sometimes by patients themselves. No prior patient preparation is necessary; thus, the bladder is catheterized through the urethra unless the urethral route is contraindicated.

Relative contraindications are the following:

- Urethral strictures
- Current UTI
- Urethral reconstruction or bladder surgery
- Urethral trauma

After the urethral meatus is carefully cleaned with an antibacterial solution, using strict sterile technique, the catheter is lubricated with sterile gel and gently advanced through the urethra into the bladder. Lidocaine gel may be injected through the male urethra before the catheter is passed to help relieve discomfort.

Complications of bladder catheterization include all of the following:

- Urethral or bladder trauma with bleeding or microscopic hematuria (common)
- UTI (common)
- Creation of false passages
- Scarring and strictures
- Bladder perforation (rare)

Catheter-associated UTIs tend to increase morbidity, mortality, healthcare costs, and hospital length of stay. Recommendations for how to minimize the rates of these UTIs include the following:

- Restricting the use of urethral catheterization to indications that are clearly medically necessary (eg, not solely to minimize the number of bedside visits by healthcare providers made to empty urinals)
- Removing catheters as soon possible
- Using strictly aseptic technique during catheter insertion
- Maintaining sterility and closure of the drainage system

Suprapubic catheterization: Suprapubic catheterization via percutaneous cystostomy is done by a urologist or another experienced physician. No prior patient preparation is necessary. General indications include need for long-term bladder drainage and inability to pass a catheter through the urethra or contraindication to catheter use when bladder catheterization is necessary.

Contraindications include the following:

- Inability to define bladder location clinically or ultrasonographically
- An empty bladder
- Suspected pelvic or lower abdominal adhesions (eg, after pelvic or lower abdominal surgery or radiation therapy)

After the abdomen above the pubic area is numbed with a local anesthetic, a spinal needle is inserted into the bladder; ultrasound guidance is used if available. A catheter is then placed through a special trocar or over a guide wire threaded through the spinal needle. Prior lower abdominal surgery and previous radiation therapy contraindicate blind insertion. Complications include UTI, intestinal injury, and bleeding.

BIOPSY OF THE KIDNEYS, BLADDER, AND PROSTATE

Biopsy requires a trained specialist (nephrologist, urologist, or interventional radiologist).

Renal biopsy: Indications for diagnostic biopsy include unexplained nephritic or nephrotic syndrome or acute kidney injury. Biopsy is occasionally done to assess response to treatment. Relative contraindications include bleeding diathesis and uncontrolled hypertension. Mild preoperative sedation with a benzodiazepine may be needed. Complications are rare but may include renal bleeding, requiring transfusion or radiologic or surgical intervention.

Bladder biopsy: Bladder biopsy is indicated to diagnose certain disorders (eg, bladder cancer, sometimes interstitial cystitis or schistosomiasis) and occasionally to assess response to treatment. Contraindications include bleeding diathesis and acute tuberculous cystitis. Preoperative antibiotics are necessary only if active UTI is present. The biopsy instrument is inserted into the bladder through a cystoscope; rigid or flexible instruments can be used. The biopsy site is cauterized to prevent bleeding. A drainage catheter is left in place to facilitate healing and drainage of clots. Complications include excessive bleeding, UTI, and bladder perforation.

Prostate biopsy: Prostate biopsy is usually done to diagnose prostate cancer. Contraindications include bleeding diathesis, acute prostatitis, and UTIs. Patient preparation includes stopping aspirin, antiplatelet drugs, and anticoagulants one week before biopsy; preoperative antibiotics (usually a fluoroquinolone); and an enema to clear the rectum. With the patient in a lateral position, the prostate is located by palpation or, preferably, transrectal ultrasonography. Overlying structures (perineum or rectum) are anesthetized, a spring-loaded biopsy needle is inserted into the prostate, and usually 12 tissue cores are obtained. Complications include the following:

- Urosepsis
- Hemorrhage
- Urinary retention
- Hematuria
- Hematospermia (often for 3 to 6 mo after biopsy)

CYSTOSCOPY

Cystoscopy is insertion of a rigid or flexible fiberoptic instrument into the bladder.

Indications include the following:

- Helping diagnose urologic disorders (eg, bladder tumors, calculi)
- Treating urethral strictures
- Accessing the bladder for ureteral x-rays or placement of JJ stents (stents with coiled ends placed in the renal pelvis and bladder)

The main contraindication is active UTI.

Cystoscopy is usually done in an outpatient setting with use of local anesthesia (urethral application of 2% lidocaine gel) or, when necessary, conscious sedation or general anesthesia. Complications include UTI, bleeding, and bladder and/or urethral trauma.

GENITOURINARY IMAGING TESTS

Imaging tests are often used to evaluate patients with renal and urologic disorders.

Plain X-Rays Without Contrast

Abdominal x-rays without radiopaque contrast agents may be done to check for positioning of ureteral stents or to monitor position and growth of kidney stones. However, for initial diagnosis of urolithiasis, plain x-rays are less sensitive than CT and lack anatomic detail, so they are not the study of choice.

X-Rays With Use of Contrast

Images taken after administration of water-soluble contrast agents highlight the kidneys and urinary collecting system. Nonionic iso-osmolal agents (eg, iohexol, iopamidol) are now widely used; they have fewer adverse effects than older hyperosmolal agents but still pose a risk of acute renal injury (contrast nephropathy—see p. 3222).

In urography, an x-ray is taken after IV, percutaneous antegrade or retrograde, or cystoscopic retrograde administration of a radiopaque contrast agent. Primary contraindications for all patients are iodine allergy and risk factors for contrast nephropathy.

IVU (IV urography or pyelography): IVU has been largely superseded by rapid multidimensional CT and MRI with or without a contrast agent. When IVU is done, abdominal compression may improve visualization of the renal pelvis and proximal ureters (with application) and distal ureters (after release). Additional x-rays at 12 and 24 h after contrast administration may be indicated for detection of postrenal obstruction or hydronephrosis.

Percutaneous antegrade urography: For percutaneous antegrade urography, a radiopaque contrast agent is introduced through an existing nephrostomy tube or, less commonly, through percutaneous puncture of the renal pelvis guided by fluoroscopy. Occasionally, a ureterostomy or an ileal conduit can be used. Antegrade urography is used in the following circumstances:

- When retrograde urography is unsuccessful (eg, because of tumor obstruction at the bladder level)
- When large kidney calculi requiring percutaneous surgery must be evaluated
- When transitional cell carcinoma of the upper collecting system is suspected
- When patients cannot tolerate general anesthesia or the degree of sedation required for retrograde urography

Complications relate to puncture and placement of the catheter in the GU tract and include bleeding, infection, injury to the lungs or colon, hematuria, pain, and prolonged urinary extravasation.

Retrograde urography: Retrograde urography uses cystoscopy and ureteral catheterization to introduce a radiopaque contrast agent directly into the ureters and renal collecting system. Sedation or general anesthesia is required. This technique can be used when CT and MRI with IV contrast agents are contraindicated (eg, in chronic kidney disease) or unavailable or when results are equivocal (eg, in renal insufficiency).

It is also useful for detailed examination of the pelvicaliceal collecting system and ureters to check for injury, stricture, or fistula. Overdistention and backflow from a kidney into the venous system may distort calyces and obscure details. Risk of infection is higher than that with other types of urography. Acute ureteral edema and secondary stricture formation are rare complications.

Cystourethrography: For cystourethrography, the radiopaque contrast agent is introduced directly into the urethra and bladder. This technique provides more details than other imaging studies for evaluation of the following:

- Vesicoureteral reflux
- Urinary incontinence
- Recurrent UTIs
- Urethral strictures
- Suspected urethral or bladder trauma

Voiding cystourethrography is done during urination and is primarily used to image the posterior urethra (eg, for strictures or valves). No patient preparation is necessary. Adverse effects include UTIs and urosepsis.

Angiography: Conventional catheter angiography has been largely replaced by noninvasive vascular imaging (eg, magnetic resonance angiography, CT angiography, ultrasonography, radionuclide scanning). Remaining indications include renal vein renin imaging, and, among patients with renal artery stenosis, angioplasty and stent placement. Arteriography is also rarely used for evaluation and treatment of renal hemorrhage and before kidney-sparing surgery. Digital subtraction angiography is no longer used when rapid-sequence multidimensional CT or helical (spiral) CT is available.

Ultrasonography

Ultrasonography can provide useful images of many GU structures without exposing patients to ionizing radiation. Images are interpreted as they are acquired, so the technician can focus on concerning areas and obtain additional information if necessary. Its main disadvantages are the need for a skilled operator and the time required. A full bladder helps provide better images of certain structures but no other preparation is needed.

Structures that can be imaged and common indications include the following:

- Kidneys: For hydronephrosis, stones, and tumors
- Bladder: For bladder volumes (eg, postvoid volume, assessed immediately after voiding; in suspected urinary retention due to bladder outlet obstruction), diverticula, and stones
- Scrotum: For hydroceles, spermatoceles, testicular tumors, varicoceles, and (with Doppler blood flow measurement) for testicular torsion
- Prostate: To measure prostate volume (eg, to help assess benign prostatic hyperplasia or interpret prostate-specific antigen results) and to guide needle biopsy
- Penis: To help evaluate Peyronie disease; with Doppler, to assess blood flow (when evaluating erectile dysfunction)
- Urethra: To measure length and caliber of urethral strictures

Computed Tomography

CT provides a broad view of the urinary tract and surrounding structures. Conventional or helical scanners are used for most purposes with or without IV contrast agents. Use of contrast agents with either technique resembles IVU but provides additional detail. Previously, in trauma patients, there was concern that use of contrast would make it difficult to distinguish abdominal hemorrhage from urinary tract disruption, but with modern imaging techniques and protocols, this distinction can be made. Helical CT without a contrast agent is the study of choice for imaging of calculi; dual-energy scanners may provide additional information that can help determine stone composition.

The main disadvantage of CT is that it exposes patients to a relatively large dose of ionizing radiation. CT angiography is a less invasive alternative to conventional angiography (see p. 3223).

Magnetic Resonance Imaging

Compared with CT, MRI is safer for patients at risk of contrast nephropathy, does not expose patients to ionizing radiation, and provides superior soft-tissue detail (but images bones and calculi poorly). MRI is contraindicated in patients with ferromagnetic metal (ie, containing iron) implants and magnetically activated or electronically controlled devices (eg, cardiac pacemakers).

Also, due to the risk of nephrogenic systemic fibrosis, MRI with gadolinium contrast is contraindicated in patients with GFR < 30 mL/min. The most common urologic application of MRI is evaluation of renal cysts and small renal masses. Endorectal MRI provides excellent anatomic detail of the prostate and may be useful in diagnosing and managing prostate cancer in the future, but these uses are currently investigational. MRI is also helpful in imaging blood vessels (eg, for renal artery stenosis and renal vein thrombosis), and its use is increasing as MRI becomes more widely available.

Radionuclide Scanning

Cortical tracers that bind to proximal tubular cells (eg, technetium-99m dimercaptosuccinic acid [^{99m}Tc DMSA]) are used to image the renal parenchyma. Excretory tracers that are rapidly filtered and excreted into urine (eg, iodine-125 iothalmate, ^{99m}Tc diethylenetriamine pentaacetic acid [DTPA], ^{99m}Tc mercaptoacetyltriglycine-3 [MAG3]) are used to assess GFR and overall renal perfusion. Radionuclide scanning can be used to evaluate renal function when use of IV contrast is undesirable. Radionuclide scanning also provides more information than does IVU or cross-sectional imaging about the following:

- Segmental renal emboli
- Renal parenchymal scarring due to vesicoureteral reflux
- Functional significance of renal artery stenosis
- Kidney function in living donors before transplantation

^{99m}Tc pertechnetate can be used to image blood flow to the testes and to distinguish torsion from epididymitis in patients with acute testicular pain, although Doppler ultrasonography is used more commonly because it is quicker. No patient preparation is necessary for radionuclide scanning, but patients should be asked about known allergies to the tracer.

URETHRAL DILATION

Urethral dilation is used to treat the following:

- Urethral strictures
- Meatal stenosis

Contraindications include untreated infection and bleeding diathesis. Dilation can be done using various techniques, such as by inflating a balloon or by inserting progressively larger instruments called sounds. Usually, lidocaine gel, a local anesthetic, is first introduced into the penis. Typically, after dilation a urethral catheter is left in place temporarily to facilitate healing. Sometimes patients are asked to insert an instrument into their own urethra periodically at home.

245 Acute Kidney Injury

(Acute Renal Failure)

Acute kidney injury (AKI) is a rapid decrease in renal function over days to weeks, causing an accumulation of nitrogenous products in the blood (azotemia). It often results from inadequate renal perfusion due to severe trauma, illness, or surgery but is sometimes caused by a rapidly progressive, intrinsic renal disease. Symptoms include anorexia, nausea, and vomiting. Seizures and coma may occur if the condition is untreated. Fluid, electrolyte, and acid-base disorders develop quickly. Diagnosis is based on laboratory tests of renal function, including serum creatinine. Urinary indices, urinary sediment examination, and often imaging and other tests are needed to determine the cause. Treatment is directed at the cause but also includes fluid and electrolyte management and sometimes dialysis.

In all cases of AKI, creatinine and urea build up in the blood over several days, and fluid and electrolyte disorders develop. The most serious of these disorders are hyperkalemia and fluid overload (possibly causing pulmonary edema). Phosphate retention leads to hyperphosphatemia. Hypocalcemia is thought to occur because the impaired kidney no longer produces calcitriol and because hyperphosphatemia causes calcium phosphate precipitation in the tissues. Acidosis develops because hydrogen ions cannot be excreted. With significant uremia, coagulation may be impaired, and pericarditis may develop. Urine output varies with the type and cause of AKI.

Etiology

Causes of AKI (see Table 245–1) can be classified as

- Prerenal
- Renal
- Postrenal

Prerenal azotemia is due to inadequate renal perfusion. The main causes are

- ECF volume depletion
- Cardiovascular disease

Prerenal conditions cause about 50 to 80% of AKI but do not cause permanent kidney damage (and hence are potentially reversible) unless hypoperfusion is severe enough to cause tubular ischemia. Hypoperfusion of an otherwise functioning kidney leads to enhanced reabsorption of sodium and water, resulting in oliguria with high urine osmolality and low urine sodium.

Renal causes of AKI involve intrinsic kidney disease or damage. Renal causes are responsible for about 10 to 40% of cases. Disorders may involve the glomeruli, tubules, or interstitium. Overall, the most common causes are

- Prolonged renal ischemia
- Nephrotoxins (including IV use of iodinated radiopaque contrast agents).

Glomerular disease reduces glomerular filtration rate (GFR) and increases glomerular capillary permeability to proteins; it may be inflammatory (glomerulonephritis) or the result of vascular damage due to ischemia or vasculitis.

Tubules also may be damaged by ischemia and may become obstructed by cellular debris, protein or crystal deposition, and cellular or interstitial edema. Tubular damage impairs reabsorption of sodium, so urinary sodium tends to be elevated, which is helpful diagnostically.

Table 245–1. MAJOR CAUSES OF ACUTE KIDNEY INJURY

CAUSE	EXAMPLES
Prerenal	
ECF volume depletion	Excessive diuresis, hemorrhage, GI losses, loss of intravascular fluid into the extravascular space (due to ascites, peritonitis, pancreatitis, or burns), loss of skin and mucus membranes, renal salt- and water-wasting states
Low cardiac output	Cardiomyopathy, MI, cardiac tamponade, pulmonary embolism, pulmonary hypertension, positive-pressure mechanical ventilation
Low systemic vascular resistance	Septic shock, liver failure, antihypertensive drugs
Increased renal vascular resistance	NSAIDs, cyclosporine, tacrolimus, hypercalcemia, anaphylaxis, some anesthetics, renal artery obstruction, renal vein thrombosis, sepsis, hepatorenal syndrome
Decreased efferent arteriolar tone (leading to decreased GFR from reduced glomerular transcapillary pressure, especially in patients with bilateral renal artery stenosis)	ACE inhibitors or angiotensin II receptor blockers
Renal	
Acute tubular injury	Ischemia (prolonged or severe prerenal state): Surgery, hemorrhage, arterial or venous obstruction, NSAIDs, cyclosporine, tacrolimus, amphotericin B Toxins: Aminoglycosides, amphotericin B, foscarnet, ethylene glycol, hemoglobin (as in hemoglobinuria), myoglobin (as in myoglobinuria), ifosfamide, heavy metals, methotrexate, radiopaque contrast agents, streptozotocin
Acute glomerulonephritis	ANCA-associated: Crescentic glomerulonephritis, microscopic polyangiitis, granulomatosis with polyangiitis Anti-GBM glomerulonephritis: Goodpasture syndrome Immune-complex: Lupus glomerulonephritis, postinfectious glomerulonephritis, cryoglobulinemic glomerulonephritis
Acute tubulointerstitial nephritis	Drug reaction (eg, beta-lactams, NSAIDs, sulfonamides, ciprofloxacin, thiazide diuretics, furosemide, cimetidine, phenytoin, allopurinol), pyelonephritis, papillary necrosis
Acute vascular nephropathy	Vasculitis, malignant hypertension, thrombotic microangiopathies, systemic sclerosis, atheroembolism
Infiltrative diseases	Lymphoma, sarcoidosis, leukemia
Postrenal	
Tubular precipitation	Uric acid (tumor lysis), sulfonamides, triamterene, acyclovir, indinavir, methotrexate, calcium oxalate (ethylene glycol ingestion), myeloma protein, myoglobin
Ureteral obstruction	Intrinsic: Calculi, clots, sloughed renal tissue, fungus ball, edema, cancer, congenital defects Extrinsic: Cancer, retroperitoneal fibrosis, ureteral trauma during surgery or high impact injury
Bladder obstruction	Mechanical: Benign prostatic hyperplasia, prostate cancer, bladder cancer, urethral strictures, phimosis, paraphimosis, urethral valves, obstructed indwelling urinary catheter Neurogenic: Anticholinergic drugs, upper or lower motor neuron lesion

ANCA = antineutrophil cytoplasmic antibody; GBM = glomerular basement membrane.

Interstitial inflammation (nephritis) usually involves an immunologic or allergic phenomenon. These mechanisms of tubular damage are complex and interdependent, rendering the previously popular term acute tubular necrosis an inadequate description.

Postrenal azotemia (obstructive nephropathy) is due to various types of obstruction in the voiding and collecting parts of the urinary system and is responsible for about 5 to 10% of cases. Obstruction can also occur within the tubules when crystalline or proteinaceous material precipitates and is often grouped with postrenal failure because the mechanism is obstructive.

Obstructed ultrafiltrate, in tubules or more distally, increases pressure in the urinary space of the glomerulus, reducing GFR. Obstruction also affects renal blood flow, initially increasing the flow and pressure in the glomerular capillary by reducing afferent arteriolar resistance. However, within 3 to 4 h, the renal blood flow is reduced, and by 24 h, it has fallen to < 50% of normal because of increased resistance of renal vasculature. Renovascular resistance may take up to a week to return to normal after relief of a 24-h obstruction.

To produce significant azotemia, obstruction at the level of the ureter requires involvement of both ureters unless the patient has only a single functioning kidney.

Bladder outlet obstruction is probably the most common cause of sudden, and often total, cessation of urinary output in men.

Symptoms and Signs

Initially, weight gain and peripheral edema may be the only findings. Often, predominant symptoms are those of the underlying illness or those caused by the surgical complication that precipitated renal deterioration.

Symptoms of uremia may develop later as nitrogenous products accumulate. Such symptoms include

- Anorexia
- Nausea
- Vomiting
- Weakness
- Myoclonic jerks
- Seizures
- Confusion
- Coma

Asterixis and hyperreflexia may be present on examination. Chest pain (typically worse with inspiration or when recumbent), a pericardial friction rub, and findings of pericardial tamponade may occur if uremic pericarditis is present. Fluid accumulation in the lungs may cause dyspnea and crackles on auscultation.

Other findings depend on the cause. Urine may be cola-colored in glomerulonephritis or myoglobinuria. A palpable bladder may be present with outlet obstruction. The costovertebral angle may be tender if the kidney is acutely enlarged.

Changes in urine output: Prerenal causes typically manifest with oliguria, not anuria. Anuria usually occurs only in obstructive uropathy or, less commonly, in bilateral renal artery occlusion, acute cortical necrosis, or rapidly progressive glomerulonephritis.

A relatively preserved urine output of 1 to 2.4 L/day is initially present in most renal causes.

In acute tubular injury, output may have 3 phases:

- The **prodromal phase,** with usually normal urine output, varies in duration depending on causative factors (eg, the amount of toxin ingested, the duration and severity of hypotension).
- The **oliguric phase,** with output typically between 50 and 400 mL/day, lasts an average of 10 to 14 days but varies from 1 day to 8 wk. However, many patients are never oliguric. Nonoliguric patients have lower mortality and morbidity and less need for dialysis.
- In the **postoliguric phase,** urine output gradually returns to normal, but serum creatinine and urea levels may not fall for several more days. Tubular dysfunction may persist for a few days or weeks and is manifested by sodium wasting, polyuria (possibly massive) unresponsive to vasopressin, or hyperchloremic metabolic acidosis.

Diagnosis

- Serum creatinine
- Urinary sediment
- Urinary diagnostic indices
- Postvoid residual bladder volume if postrenal cause suspected

AKI is suspected when urine output falls or serum BUN and creatinine rise. Evaluation should determine the presence and type of AKI and seek a cause. Blood tests generally include CBC, BUN, creatinine, and electrolytes (including calcium and phosphate). Urine tests include sodium and creatinine concentration and microscopic analysis of sediment. Early detection and treatment increase the chances of reversing renal failure and in some cases preventing it.

A progressive daily rise in serum creatinine is diagnostic of AKI. Serum creatinine can increase by as much as 2 mg/dL/day (180 μmol/L/day), depending on the amount of creatinine produced (which varies with lean body mass) and total body water. A rise of > 2 mg/dL/day suggests overproduction due to rhabdomyolysis.

Urea nitrogen may increase by 10 to 20 mg/dL/day (3.6 to 7.1 mmol urea/L/day), but BUN may be misleading because it is frequently elevated in response to increased protein catabolism resulting from surgery, trauma, corticosteroids, burns, transfusion reactions, parenteral nutrition, or GI or internal bleeding.

When creatinine is rising, 24-h urine collection for creatinine clearance and the various formulas used to calculate creatinine clearance from serum creatinine are inaccurate and should not be used in estimating GFR, because the rise in serum creatinine concentration is a delayed function of GFR decline.

Other laboratory findings are progressive acidosis, hyperkalemia, hyponatremia, and anemia. Acidosis is ordinarily moderate, with a plasma bicarbonate content of 15 to 20 mmol/L. Serum potassium concentration increases slowly, but when catabolism is markedly accelerated, it may rise by 1 to 2 mmol/L/day. Hyponatremia usually is moderate (serum sodium, 125 to 135 mmol/L) and correlates with a surplus of water. Normochromic-normocytic anemia with an Hct of 25 to 30% is typical.

Hyperphosphatemia and hypocalcemia are common in AKI and may be profound in patients with rhabdomyolysis or tumor lysis syndrome. Profound hypocalcemia in rhabdomyolysis apparently results from the combined effects of calcium deposition in necrotic muscle, reduced calcitriol production, resistance of bone to parathyroid hormone (PTH), and hyperphosphatemia. During recovery from AKI following rhabdomyolysis-induced acute tubular necrosis, hypercalcemia may supervene as renal calcitriol production increases, the bone becomes responsive to PTH, and calcium deposits are mobilized from damaged tissue. Hypercalcemia during recovery from AKI is otherwise uncommon.

Determination of cause: Immediately reversible prerenal or postrenal causes must be excluded first. ECF volume depletion and obstruction are considered in all patients. The drug history must be accurately reviewed and all potentially renal toxic drugs stopped. Urinary diagnostic indices (see Table 245 2) are helpful in distinguishing prerenal azotemia from acute tubular injury, which are the most common causes of AKI in hospitalized patients.

Table 245–2. URINARY DIAGNOSTIC INDICES IN PRERENAL AZOTEMIA AND ACUTE TUBULAR INJURY

INDEX	PRERENAL	TUBULAR INJURY
U/P osmolality	> 1.5	1–1.5
Urine Na (mmol/L)	< 10	> 40
Fractional excretion of Na (FE_{Na})*	< 1%	> 1%
Renal failure index†	< 1	> 2
BUN/creatinine ratio	> 20	< 10

*U/P Na ÷ U/P creatinine.

†Urine Na ÷ U/P creatinine ratio.

AGN = acute glomerulonephritis; Na = sodium; U/P = urine-to-plasma ratio.

Adapted from Miller TR, Anderson RJ, Linas SL, et al: Urinary diagnostic indices in acute renal failure. *Annals of Internal Medicine* 89(1):47–50, 1978; used with permission of the American College of Physicians and the author.

Prerenal causes are often apparent clinically. If so, correction of an underlying hemodynamic abnormality should be attempted. For example, in hypovolemia, volume infusion can be tried, in heart failure, diuretics and afterload reducing drugs can be tried, and in liver failure, octreotide can be tried. Abatement of AKI confirms a prerenal cause.

Postrenal causes should be sought in most cases of AKI. Immediately after the patient voids, bedside ultrasonography of the bladder is done (or, alternatively, a urinary catheter is placed) to determine the residual urine in the bladder. A postvoid residual urine volume > 200 mL suggests bladder outlet obstruction, although detrusor muscle weakness and neurogenic bladder may also cause residual volume of this amount. The catheter may be kept in for the first day to monitor hourly output but is removed once oliguria is confirmed (if bladder outlet obstruction is not present) to decrease risk of infection.

Renal ultrasonography is then done to diagnose more proximal obstruction. However, sensitivity for obstruction is only 80 to 85% when ultrasonography is used because the collecting system is not always dilated, especially when the condition is acute, an intrarenal pelvis is present, the ureter is encased (eg, in retroperitoneal fibrosis or neoplasm), or the patient has concomitant hypovolemia. If obstruction is strongly suspected, noncontrast CT can establish the site of obstruction and guide therapy.

The **urinary sediment** may provide etiologic clues. A normal urine sediment occurs in prerenal azotemia and sometimes in obstructive uropathy. With renal tubular injury, the sediment characteristically contains tubular cells, tubular cell casts, and many granular casts (often with brown pigmentation). Urinary eosinophils suggest allergic tubulointerstitial nephritis, but the diagnostic accuracy of this finding is limited. RBC casts indicate glomerulonephritis or vasculitis but rarely may occur in acute tubular necrosis.

Renal causes are sometimes suggested by clinical findings. Patients with glomerulonephritis often have edema, marked proteinuria (nephrotic syndrome), or signs of arteritis in the skin and retina, often without a history of intrinsic renal disease. Hemoptysis suggests granulomatosis with polyangiitis or Goodpasture syndrome. Certain rashes (eg, erythema nodosum, cutaneous vasculitis, discoid lupus) suggest cryoglobulinemia, SLE, or immunoglobulin A-associated vasculitis. Tubulointerstitial nephritis, drug allergy, and possibly microscopic polyangiitis are suggested by a history of drug ingestion and a maculopapular or purpuric rash.

To further differentiate renal causes, antistreptolysin-O and complement titers, antinuclear antibodies, and antineutrophil cytoplasmic antibodies are determined. Renal biopsy may be done if the diagnosis remains elusive (see Table 245–3).

Imaging: In addition to renal ultrasonography, other imaging tests are occasionally of use. In evaluating for ureteral obstruction, noncontrast CT is preferred over antegrade and retrograde urography. In addition to its ability to delineate soft-tissue structures and calcium-containing calculi, CT can detect nonradiopaque calculi.

Contrast agents should be avoided if possible. However, renal arteriography or venography may sometimes be indicated if vascular causes are suggested clinically. Magnetic resonance angiography was increasingly being used for diagnosing renal artery stenosis as well as thrombosis of both arteries and veins because MRI used gadolinium, which was thought to be safer than the iodinated contrast agents used in angiography and contrast-enhanced CT. However, recent evidence suggests that gadolinium may be involved in the pathogenesis of nephrogenic systemic fibrosis, a serious complication that occurs in patients with AKI as well as chronic kidney disease. Thus, gadolinium should be avoided if possible in patients with reduced renal function.

Kidney size, as determined with imaging tests, is helpful to know, because a normal or enlarged kidney favors reversibility, whereas a small kidney suggests chronic renal insufficiency.

Prognosis

Although many causes are reversible if diagnosed and treated early, the overall survival rate remains about 50% because many patients with AKI have significant underlying disorders (eg, sepsis, respiratory failure). Death is usually the result of these disorders rather than AKI itself. Most survivors have adequate kidney function. About 10% require dialysis or transplantation—half right away and the others as renal function slowly deteriorates.

Treatment

- Immediate treatment of pulmonary edema and hyperkalemia
- Dialysis as needed to control hyperkalemia, pulmonary edema, metabolic acidosis, and uremic symptoms
- Adjustment of drug regimen
- Usually restriction of water, sodium, phosphate, and potassium intake, but provision of adequate protein
- Possibly phosphate binders and sodium polystyrene sulfonate

Table 245–3. CAUSES OF ACUTE KIDNEY INJURY BASED ON LABORATORY FINDINGS

BLOOD TEST	FINDING	POSSIBLE DIAGNOSIS
Antiglomerular basement membrane antibodies	Positive	Goodpasture syndrome
Antineutrophil cytoplasmic antibodies	Positive	Small-vessel vasculitis (granulomatosis with polyangiitis or microscopic angiitis)
Antinuclear antibodies or antibodies to double-stranded DNA	Positive	SLE
Antistreptolysin-O or antibodies to streptokinase or hyaluronidase	Positive	Poststreptococcal glomerulonephritis
CK or myoglobin level	Markedly elevated	Rhabdomyolysis
Complement titers	Low	Postinfectious glomerulonephritis, SLE, subacute bacterial endocarditis, cholesterol embolization
Protein electrophoresis (serum)	Monoclonal spike	Multiple myeloma
Uric acid level	Elevated	Cancer or tumor lysis syndrome (leading to uric acid crystals) Prerenal acute kidney injury

Emergency treatment: Life-threatening complications are addressed, preferably in a critical care unit. Pulmonary edema is treated with oxygen, IV vasodilators (eg, nitroglycerin), diuretics (often ineffective in AKI), or dialysis.

Hyperkalemia is treated as needed with IV infusion of 10 mL of 10% calcium gluconate, 50 g of dextrose, and 5 to 10 units of insulin. These drugs do not reduce total body potassium, so further (but slower acting) treatment is needed (eg, sodium polystyrene sulfonate, dialysis).

Although correction of an anion gap metabolic acidosis with sodium bicarbonate is controversial, correction of the nonanion gap portion of severe metabolic acidosis (pH < 7.20) is less controversial. The nonanion gap portion may be treated with IV sodium bicarbonate in the form of a slow infusion (≤ 150 mEq sodium bicarbonate in 1 L of 5% D/W at a rate of 50 to 100 mL/h). Using the delta delta gradient calculation, a normal-anion gap metabolic acidosis plus a high anion-gap metabolic acidosis yields a negative delta delta gradient; sodium bicarbonate is given to raise the serum bicarbonate until the delta delta gradient reaches zero. Because variations in body buffer systems and the rate of acid production are hard to predict, calculating the amount of bicarbonate needed to achieve a full correction is usually not recommended. Instead, bicarbonate is given via continuous infusion and the anion gap is monitored serially.

Hemodialysis or **hemofiltration** is initiated when

- Severe electrolyte abnormalities cannot otherwise be controlled (eg, potassium > 6 mmol/L)
- Pulmonary edema persists despite drug treatment
- Metabolic acidosis is unresponsive to treatment
- Uremic symptoms occur (eg, vomiting thought to be due to uremia, asterixis, encephalopathy, pericarditis, seizures)

BUN and creatinine levels are probably not the best guides for initiating dialysis in AKI. In asymptomatic patients who are not seriously ill, particularly those in whom return of renal function is considered likely, dialysis can be deferred until symptoms occur, thus avoiding placement of a central venous catheter with its attendant complications.

General measures: Nephrotoxic drugs are stopped, and all drugs excreted by the kidneys (eg, digoxin, some antibiotics) are adjusted; serum levels are useful.

Daily water intake is restricted to a volume equal to the previous day's urine output plus measured extrarenal losses (eg, vomitus) plus 500 to 1000 mL/day for insensible loss. Water intake can be further restricted for hyponatremia or increased for hypernatremia. Although weight gain indicates excess fluid, water intake is not decreased if serum sodium remains normal; instead, dietary sodium is restricted.

Sodium and potassium intake is minimized except in patients with prior deficiencies or GI losses. An adequate diet should be provided, including daily protein intake of about 0.8 g/kg. If oral or enteral nutrition is impossible, parenteral nutrition is used; however, in AKI, risks of fluid overload, hyperosmolality, and infection are increased by IV nutrition. Calcium salts (calcium carbonate, calcium acetate) or synthetic non–calcium-containing phosphate binders before meals help maintain serum phosphate at < 5 mg/dL (< 1.78 mmol/L).

If needed to help maintain serum potassium at < 6 mmol/L in the absence of dialysis (eg, if other therapies, such as diuretics, fail to lower potassium), a cation-exchange resin, sodium polystyrene sulfonate, is given 15 to 60 g po or rectally 1 to 4 times/day as a suspension in water or in a syrup (eg, 70% sorbitol).

An indwelling bladder catheter is rarely needed and should be used only when necessary because of an increased risk of UTI and urosepsis.

In many patients, a brisk and even dramatic diuresis after relief of obstruction is a physiologic response to the expansion of ECF during obstruction and does not compromise volume status. However, polyuria accompanied by the excretion of large amounts of sodium, potassium, magnesium, and other solutes may cause hypokalemia, hyponatremia, hypernatremia (if free water is not provided), hypomagnesemia, or marked contraction of ECF volume with peripheral vascular collapse. In this postoliguric phase, close attention to fluid and electrolyte balance is mandatory. Overzealous administration of salt and water after relief of obstruction can prolong diuresis. When postoliguric diuresis occurs, replacement of urine output with 0.45% saline at about 75% of urine output prevents volume depletion and the tendency for excessive free water loss while allowing the body to eliminate excessive volume if this is the cause of the polyuria.

Prevention

AKI can often be prevented by maintaining normal fluid balance, blood volume, and BP in patients with trauma, burns, or severe hemorrhage and in those undergoing major surgery. Infusion of isotonic saline and blood may be helpful.

Use of contrast agents should be minimized, particularly in at-risk groups (eg, the elderly and patients with preexisting renal insufficiency, volume depletion, diabetes, or heart failure). If contrast agents are necessary, risk can be lowered by minimizing volume of the IV contrast agent, using nonionic and low osmolal or iso-osmolal contrast agents, avoiding NSAIDs, and pretreating with normal saline at 1 mL/kg/h IV for 12 h before the test. Infusion of isotonic sodium bicarbonate before and after contrast administration has also been used successfully instead of normal saline. *N*-acetylcysteine 600 mg po bid the day before and the day of IV contrast administration has been used to prevent contrast nephropathy, but reports of its efficacy are conflicting.

Before cytolytic therapy is initiated in patients with certain neoplastic diseases (eg, lymphoma, leukemia), treatment with rasburicase or allopurinol should be considered along with increasing urine flow by increasing oral or IV fluids to reduce urate crystalluria. Making the urine more alkaline (by giving oral or IV sodium bicarbonate or acetazolamide) has been recommended by some but is controversial because it may also induce urinary calcium phosphate precipitation and crystalluria, which may worsen AKI.

The renal vasculature is very sensitive to endothelin, a potent vasoconstrictor that reduces renal blood flow and GFR. Endothelin is implicated in progressive renal damage, and endothelin receptor antagonists have successfully slowed or even halted experimental renal disease. Antiendothelin antibodies and endothelin-receptor antagonists are being studied to protect the kidney against ischemic AKI.

KEY POINTS

- Causes of AKI can be prerenal (eg, kidney hypoperfusion), renal (eg, direct effects on the kidney), or postrenal (eg, urinary tract obstruction distal to the kidneys).
- With AKI, consider ECF volume depletion and nephrotoxins, obtain urinary diagnostic indices and measure bladder residual volume to identify obstruction.
- Avoid using IV contrast in imaging studies.
- Initiate hemodialysis or hemofiltration as needed for pulmonary edema, hyperkalemia, metabolic acidosis, or uremic symptoms unresponsive to other treatments.
- Minimize risk of AKI in patients at risk by maintaining normal fluid balance, avoiding nephrotoxins (including contrast agents) when possible, and taking precautions such as giving fluids or drugs when contrast or cytolytic therapy is necessary.

246 Benign Prostate Disease

BENIGN PROSTATIC HYPERPLASIA

(Benign Prostatic Hypertrophy)

Benign prostatic hyperplasia (BPH) is nonmalignant adenomatous overgrowth of the periurethral prostate gland. Symptoms are those of bladder outlet obstruction—weak stream, hesitancy, urinary frequency, urgency, nocturia, incomplete emptying, terminal dribbling, overflow or urge incontinence, and complete urinary retention. Diagnosis is based primarily on digital rectal examination and symptoms; cystoscopy, transrectal ultrasonography, urodynamics, or other imaging studies may also be needed. Treatment options include 5 alpha-reductase inhibitors, alpha-blockers, tadalafil, and surgery.

Using the criteria of a prostate volume > 30 mL and a moderate or high American Urological Association Symptom Score (see Table 246–1), the prevalence of BPH in men aged 55 to 74 without prostate cancer is 19%. But if voiding criteria of a maximal urinary flow rate < 10 mL/sec and a postvoid residual urine volume > 50 mL are included, the prevalence is only 4%. Based on autopsy studies, the prevalence of BPH increases from 8% in men aged 31 to 40 yr to 40 to 50% in men aged 51 to 60 yr and to > 80% in men > 80 yr.

The etiology is unknown but probably involves hormonal changes associated with aging.

Pathophysiology

Multiple fibroadenomatous nodules develop in the periurethral region of the prostate, probably originating within the periurethral glands rather than in the true fibromuscular prostate (surgical capsule), which is displaced peripherally by progressive growth of the nodules.

As the lumen of the prostatic urethra narrows and lengthens, urine outflow is progressively obstructed. Increased pressure associated with micturition and bladder distention can progress to hypertrophy of the bladder detrusor, trabeculation, cellule formation, and diverticula. Incomplete bladder emptying causes stasis and predisposes to calculus formation and infection. Prolonged urinary tract obstruction, even if incomplete, can cause hydronephrosis and compromise renal function.

Symptoms and Signs

Lower urinary tract symptoms: Symptoms of BPH include progressive lower urinary tract symptoms (LUTS):

- Urinary frequency
- Urgency
- Nocturia
- Hesitancy
- Intermittency

Frequency, urgency, and nocturia are due to incomplete emptying and rapid refilling of the bladder. Decreased size and force of the urinary stream cause hesitancy and intermittency.

Pain and dysuria are usually not present. Sensations of incomplete emptying, terminal dribbling, overflow incontinence, or complete urinary retention may ensue. Straining to void can cause congestion of superficial veins of the prostatic

Table 246–1. AMERICAN UROLOGICAL ASSOCIATION SYMPTOM SCORE FOR BENIGN PROSTATIC HYPERPLASIA

	SCORE					
OVER ABOUT THE PAST MONTH	Never	< 20% of the Time	< 50% of the Time	About 50% of the Time	> 50% of the Time	Almost Always
How often have you had a sensation of not emptying your bladder completely after you finish urinating?	0	1	2	3	4	5
How often have you had to urinate again < 2 h after you finished urinating?	0	1	2	3	4	5
How often have you stopped and started again several times when urinating?	0	1	2	3	4	5
How often have you found it difficult to postpone urination?	0	1	2	3	4	5
How often has your urinary stream been weak?	0	1	2	3	4	5
How often have you had to push or strain to begin urination?	0	1	2	3	4	5
How many times did you most typically get up to urinate between going to bed at night and waking in the morning?	none = 0	once = 1	twice = 2	3 times = 3	4 times = 4	≥ 5 times = 5
American Urological Association symptom score = total ______.						

Adapted from Barry MJ, Fowler FJ, O'Leary MP, et al: The American Urological Association symptom index for benign prostatic hyperplasia. *Journal of Urology* 148:1549, 1992.

urethra and trigone, which may rupture and cause hematuria. Straining also may acutely cause vasovagal syncope and, over the long term, may cause dilation of hemorrhoidal veins or inguinal hernias.

Urinary retention: Some patients present with sudden, complete urinary retention, with marked abdominal discomfort and bladder distention. Retention may be precipitated by any of the following:

- Prolonged attempts to postpone voiding
- Immobilization
- Exposure to cold
- Use of anesthetics, anticholinergics, sympathomimetics, opioids, or alcohol

Symptom scores: Symptoms can be quantitated by scores, such as the 7-question American Urological Association Symptom Score (see Table 246–1). This score also allows doctors to monitor symptom progression:

- Mild symptoms: Scores 1 to 7
- Moderate symptoms: Scores 8 to 19
- Severe symptoms: Scores 20 to 35

Digital rectal examination: On digital rectal examination, the prostate usually is enlarged and nontender, has a rubbery consistency, and in many cases has lost the median furrow. However, prostate size as detected with digital rectal examination may be misleading; an apparently small prostate may cause obstruction. If distended, the urinary bladder may be palpable or percussible during abdominal examination.

Diagnosis

- Digital rectal examination
- Urinalysis and urine culture
- Prostate-specific antigen level
- Sometimes uroflowmetry and bladder ultrasonography

The lower urinary tract symptoms of BPH can also be caused by other disorders, including infection and prostate cancer. Furthermore, BPH and prostate cancer may coexist. Although palpable prostate tenderness suggests infection, digital rectal examination findings in BPH and cancer often overlap. Although cancer may cause a stony, hard, nodular, irregularly enlarged prostate, most patients with cancer, BPH, or both have a benign-feeling, enlarged prostate. Thus, testing should be considered for patients with symptoms or palpable prostatic abnormalities.

Typically, urinalysis and urine culture are done, and serum prostate-specific antigen (PSA) levels are measured. Men with moderate or severe symptoms of obstruction may also have uroflowmetry (an objective test of urine volume and flow rate) with measurement of postvoid residual volume by bladder ultrasonography. Flow rate < 15 mL/sec suggests obstruction, and postvoid residual volume > 100 mL suggests retention.

PSA levels: Interpreting PSA levels can be complex. The PSA level is moderately elevated in 30 to 50% of patients with BPH, depending on prostate size and degree of obstruction, and is elevated in 25 to 92% of patients with prostate cancer, depending on the tumor volume.

In patients without cancer, serum PSA levels > 1.5 ng/mL usually indicate a prostate volume ≥ 30 mL. If the PSA is elevated (level is > 4 ng/mL), further discussion/shared decision making regarding other tests or biopsy is recommended.

For men < 50 or those at high risk of prostate cancer, a lower cutoff (PSA > 2.5 ng/mL) may be used. Other measures, including rate of PSA increase, free-to-bound PSA ratio, and other markers, may be useful (a full discussion of prostate cancer screening and diagnosis is elsewhere).

Other testing: Transrectal biopsy is usually done with ultrasound guidance. Transrectal ultrasonography can also measure prostate volume.

Clinical judgment must be used to evaluate the need for further testing. Contrast imaging studies (eg, CT, IVU) are rarely necessary unless the patient has had a UTI with fever or obstructive symptoms have been severe and prolonged. Upper urinary tract abnormalities that usually result from bladder outlet obstruction include upward displacement of the terminal portions of the ureters (fish hooking), ureteral dilation, and hydronephrosis. If an upper tract imaging study is warranted due to pain or elevated serum creatinine level, ultrasonography may be preferred because it avoids radiation and IV contrast exposure.

Treatment

- Avoidance of anticholinergics, sympathomimetics, and opioids
- Use of alpha-adrenergic blockers (eg, terazosin, doxazosin, tamsulosin, alfuzosin), 5 alpha-reductase inhibitors (finasteride, dutasteride), or, if there is concomitant erectile dysfunction, the phosphodiesterase type 5 inhibitor tadalafil
- Transurethral resection of the prostate or a less invasive procedure

Urinary retention: Urinary retention requires immediate decompression. Passage of a standard urinary catheter is first attempted; if a standard catheter cannot be passed, a catheter with a coudé tip may be effective. If this catheter cannot be passed, flexible cystoscopy or insertion of filiforms and followers (guides and dilators that progressively open the urinary passage) may be necessary (this procedure should usually be done by a urologist). Suprapubic percutaneous decompression of the bladder may be used if transurethral approaches are unsuccessful.

Drug therapy: For partial obstruction with troublesome symptoms, all anticholinergics, sympathomimetics, and opioids should be stopped, and any infection should be treated with antibiotics.

For patients with mild to moderate obstructive symptoms, alpha-adrenergic blockers (eg, terazosin, doxazosin, tamsulosin, alfuzosin) may decrease voiding problems. The 5 alpha-reductase inhibitors (finasteride, dutasteride) may reduce prostate size, decreasing voiding problems over months, especially in patients with larger (> 30 mL) glands. A combination of both classes of drugs is superior to monotherapy. For men with concomitant erectile dysfunction, daily tadalafil may help relieve both conditions. Many OTC complementary and alternative agents are promoted for treatment of BPH, but none, including the thoroughly studied saw palmetto, has been shown to be more efficacious than placebo.

Surgery: Surgery is done when patients do not respond to drug therapy or develop complications such as recurrent UTI, urinary calculi, severe bladder dysfunction, or upper tract dilation. Transurethral resection of the prostate (TURP) is the standard. Erectile function and continence are usually retained, although about 5 to 10% of patients experience some postsurgical problems, most commonly retrograde ejaculation. The incidence of erectile dysfunction after TURP is between 1 and 35%, and the incidence of incontinence is about 1 to 3%. About 10% of men undergoing TURP need the procedure repeated within 10 yr because the prostate continues to grow. Various laser ablation techniques are being used as alternatives to TURP. Larger prostates (usually > 75 g) require open surgery via a suprapubic or retropubic approach. All surgical methods require postoperative catheter drainage for 1 to 7 days.

Other procedures: Less invasive procedures include microwave thermotherapy, electrovaporization, high-intensity focused ultrasonography, transurethral needle ablation, radiofrequency vaporization, pressurized heated water injection therapy, urethral lift, and intraurethral stents. The circumstances under which these procedures should be used have not been firmly established, but those done in the physician's office (microwave thermotherapy and radiofrequency procedures) are being more commonly used and do not require use of general or regional anesthesia. Their long-term ability to alter the natural history of BPH is under study.

KEY POINTS

- BPH is extremely common with aging but only sometimes causes symptoms.
- Acute urinary retention can develop with exposure to cold, prolonged attempts to postpone voiding, immobilization, or use of anesthetics, anticholinergics, sympathomimetics, opioids, or alcohol.
- Evaluate patients with a digital rectal examination and usually urinalysis, urine culture, and PSA.
- In men with BPH, avoid use of anticholinergics, sympathomimetics, and opioids.
- Consider relieving troublesome obstructive symptoms with alpha-adrenergic blockers (eg, terazosin, doxazosin, tamsulosin, alfuzosin), 5 alpha-reductase inhibitors (finasteride, dutasteride), or, if there is concomitant erectile dysfunction, tadalafil.
- Consider TURP or ablation if BPH causes complications (eg, recurrent calculi, bladder dysfunction, upper tract dilation) or if bothersome symptoms are drug resistant.

PROSTATITIS

Prostatitis refers to a disparate group of disorders that manifests with a combination of predominantly irritative or obstructive urinary symptoms and perineal pain. Some cases result from bacterial infection of the prostate gland and others, which are more common, from a poorly understood combination of noninfectious inflammatory factors, spasm of the muscles of the urogenital diaphragm, or both. Diagnosis is clinical, along with microscopic examination and culture of urine samples obtained before and after prostate massage. Treatment is with an antibiotic if the cause is bacterial. Nonbacterial causes are treated with warm sitz baths, muscle relaxants, and anti-inflammatory drugs or anxiolytics.

Etiology

Prostatitis can be bacterial or, more commonly, nonbacterial. However, differentiating bacterial and nonbacterial causes can be difficult, particularly in chronic prostatitis.

Bacterial prostatitis can be acute or chronic and is usually caused by typical urinary pathogens (eg, *Klebsiella*, *Proteus*, *Escherichia coli*) and possibly by *Chlamydia*. How these pathogens enter and infect the prostate is unknown. Chronic infections may be caused by sequestered bacteria that antibiotics have not eradicated.

Nonbacterial prostatitis can be inflammatory or noninflammatory. The mechanism is unknown but may involve incomplete relaxation of the urinary sphincter and dyssynergic voiding. The resultant elevated urinary pressure may cause urine reflux into the prostate (triggering an inflammatory response) or increased pelvic autonomic activity leading to chronic pain without inflammation.

Classification

Prostatitis is classified into 4 categories (see Table 246–2). These categories are differentiated by clinical findings and by the presence or absence of signs of infection and inflammation in 2 urine samples. The first sample is a midstream collection. Then digital prostate massage is done, and patients void immediately; the first 10 mL of urine constitutes the 2nd sample. Infection is defined by bacterial growth in urine culture;

Table 246–2. NIH CONSENSUS CLASSIFICATION SYSTEM FOR PROSTATITIS

NUMBER	CATEGORY	CHARACTERISTICS	URINE FINDING	PREMASSAGE	POSTMASSAGE
I	Acute bacterial prostatitis	Acute symptoms of urinary infection	WBC	+/−	+
			Bacteria	+/−	+
II	Chronic bacterial prostatitis	Recurrent urinary infection with same organism	WBC	+/−	+
			Bacteria	+/−	+
III	Chronic prostatitis/chronic pelvic pain syndrome	Primarily symptoms of pain, voiding, and sexual dysfunction			
IIIa	Inflammatory		WBC	−	+
			Bacteria	−	−
IIIb	Noninflammatory*		WBC	−	−
			Bacteria	−	−
IV	Asymptomatic inflammatory prostatitis	Discovered incidentally during urologic evaluation (eg, prostate biopsy, seminal fluid analysis) for other conditions	WBC	−	+
			Bacteria	−	−

*Previously called prostatodynia.
+/− = possibly present; + = present; − = absent.
Data from Krieger JN, Nyberg L, Nickel JC: NIH consensus definition and classification of prostatitis. *JAMA* 282:236–237, 1999.

inflammation is defined by the presence of WBCs in urine. The use of the term prostatodynia for prostatitis without inflammation is discouraged.

Symptoms and Signs

Symptoms vary by category but typically involve some degree of urinary irritation or obstruction and pain. Irritation is manifested by frequency and urgency, obstruction, a sensation of incomplete bladder emptying, a need to void again shortly after voiding, or nocturia. Pain is typically in the perineum but may be perceived at the tip of the penis, lower back, or testes. Some patients report painful ejaculation.

Acute bacterial prostatitis often causes such systemic symptoms as fever, chills, malaise, and myalgias. The prostate is exquisitely tender and focally or diffusely swollen, boggy, indurated, or a combination. A generalized sepsis syndrome may result, characterized by tachycardia, tachypnea, and sometimes hypotension.

Chronic bacterial prostatitis manifests with recurrent episodes of infection with or without complete resolution between bouts. Symptoms and signs tend to be milder than in acute prostatitis.

Chronic prostatitis/chronic pelvic pain syndrome typically has pain as the predominant symptom, often including pain with ejaculation. The discomfort can be significant and often markedly interferes with quality of life. Symptoms of urinary irritation or obstruction also may be present. On examination, the prostate may be tender but usually is not boggy or swollen. Clinically, inflammatory and noninflammatory types of chronic prostatitis/chronic pelvic pain syndrome are similar.

Asymptomatic inflammatory prostatitis causes no symptoms and is discovered incidentally during evaluation for other prostate diseases when WBCs are present in the urine.

Diagnosis

- Urinalysis
- Prostate massage except possibly in acute bacterial prostatitis

Diagnosis of type I, II, or III prostatitis is suspected clinically. Similar symptoms can result fromurethritis, perirectal abscess, or UTI. Examination is helpful diagnostically only in acute bacterial prostatitis.

Febrile patients with typical symptoms and signs of acute bacterial prostatitis usually have WBCs and bacteria in a midstream urine sample. Prostate massage to obtain a postmassage urine sample is thought to be unnecessary and possibly dangerous in these patients (although danger remains unproved) because bacteremia can be induced. For the same reason, rectal examination should be done gently. Blood cultures should be obtained in patients who have fever and severe weakness, confusion, disorientation, hypotension, or cool extremities. For afebrile patients, urine samples before and after massage are adequate for diagnosis.

For patients with acute or chronic bacterial prostatitis who do not respond favorably to antibiotics, transrectal ultrasonography and sometimes cystoscopy may be necessary to rule out prostatic abscess or destruction and inflammation of the seminal vesicles.

For patients with types II, III, and IV (nonacute prostatitis) disease, additional tests that can be considered are cystoscopy and urine cytology (if hematuria is also present) and urodynamic measurements (if there is suspicion of neurologic abnormalities or detrusor-sphincter dyssynergia).

Treatment

- Treatment varies significantly with etiology

Acute bacterial prostatitis: Nontoxic patients can be treated at home with antibiotics, bed rest, analgesics, stool softeners, and hydration. Therapy with a fluoroquinolone (eg, ciprofloxacin 500 mg po bid or ofloxacin 300 mg po bid) is usually effective and can be given until culture and sensitivity results are known. If the clinical response is satisfactory, treatment is continued for about 30 days to prevent chronic bacterial prostatitis.

If sepsis is suspected, the patient is hospitalized and given broad-spectrum antibiotics IV (eg, ampicillin plus gentamicin). Antibiotics are started after the appropriate cultures are taken and continued until the bacterial sensitivity is known. If the clinical response is adequate, IV therapy is continued until the patient is afebrile for 24 to 48 h, followed by oral therapy usually for 4 wk.

Adjunctive therapies include NSAIDs and potentially alpha-blockers (if bladder emptying is poor) and supportive measures such as sitz baths. Rarely, prostate abscess develops, requiring surgical drainage.

Chronic bacterial prostatitis: Chronic bacterial prostatitis is treated with oral antibiotics such as fluoroquinolones for at least 6 wk. Therapy is guided by culture results; empiric antibiotic treatment for patients with equivocal or negative culture results has a low success rate. Other treatments include anti-inflammatory drugs, muscle relaxants (eg, cyclobenzaprine to possibly relieve spasm of the pelvic muscles), alpha-adrenergic blockers, and other symptomatic measures, such as sitz baths.

Chronic prostatitis/chronic pelvic pain syndrome: Treatment is difficult and often unrewarding. In addition to considering any and all of the above treatments, anxiolytics (eg, SSRIs, benzodiazepines), sacral nerve stimulation, biofeedback, prostatic massage, and minimally invasive prostatic procedures (such as microwave thermotherapy) have been attempted with varying results.

Asymptomatic inflammatory prostatitis: Asymptomatic prostatitis requires no treatment.

KEY POINTS

- Prostatitis can be an acute or chronic bacterial infection or a more poorly understood group of disorders typically characterized by irritative and obstructive urinary symptoms, urogenital diaphragm muscle spasm, and perineal pain.
- Treat patients who have chronic bacterial prostatitis and nontoxic patients who have acute bacterial prostatitis with a fluoroquinolone and symptomatic measures.
- Hospitalize patients who have acute bacterial prostatitis and systemic symptoms that suggest sepsis and give broad-spectrum antibiotics such as ampicillin plus gentamicin.
- For men with chronic prostatitis or chronic pelvic pain syndrome, consider anxiolytics (eg, SSRIs, benzodiazepines), sacral nerve stimulation, biofeedback, prostatic massage, and minimally invasive prostatic procedures (eg, microwave thermotherapy).

PROSTATE ABSCESS

Prostate abscesses are focal purulent collections that develop as complications of acute bacterial prostatitis.

The usual infecting organisms are aerobic gram-negative bacilli or, less frequently, *Staphylococcus aureus*.

Symptoms

Common symptoms include

- Urinary frequency
- Dysuria
- Urinary retention

Perineal pain, evidence of acute epididymitis, hematuria, and a purulent urethral discharge are less common. Fever is sometimes present.

Rectal examination may disclose prostate tenderness and fluctuance, but prostate enlargement is often the only abnormality, and sometimes the gland feels normal.

Diagnosis

- Prostate ultrasonography and possibly cystoscopy

Abscess is suspected in patients with persistent perineal pain and continued or recurrent UTIs despite antimicrobial therapy. Such patients should undergo prostate ultrasonography and possibly cystoscopy.

Many abscesses, however, are discovered unexpectedly during prostate surgery or endoscopy; bulging of a lateral lobe into the prostatic urethra or rupture during instrumentation reveals the abscess. Although pyuria and bacteriuria are common, urine may be normal. Blood cultures are positive in some patients.

Treatment

- Antibiotics
- Drainage

Treatment involves appropriate antibiotics plus drainage by transurethral evacuation or transperineal aspiration and drainage. Pending culture results, empiric antibiotic therapy is begun with a fluoroquinolone (eg, ciprofloxacin).

247 Chronic Kidney Disease

(Chronic Renal Failure)

Chronic kidney disease (CKD) is long-standing, progressive deterioration of renal function. Symptoms develop slowly and in advanced stages include anorexia, nausea, vomiting, stomatitis, dysgeusia, nocturia, lassitude, fatigue, pruritus, decreased mental acuity, muscle twitches and cramps, water retention, undernutrition, peripheral neuropathies, and seizures. Diagnosis is based on laboratory testing of renal function, sometimes followed by renal biopsy. Treatment is primarily directed at the underlying condition but includes fluid and electrolyte management, blood pressure control, treatment of anemia, various types of dialysis, and kidney transplantation.

Prevalence of CKD (stages 1 through 5) in the US adult general population is estimated at 14.8% (NHANES 2011–2014 database).

Etiology

CKD may result from any cause of renal dysfunction of sufficient magnitude (see Table 247–1).

The **most common causes** in the US in order of prevalence are

- Diabetic nephropathy
- Hypertensive nephrosclerosis
- Various primary and secondary glomerulopathies

Metabolic syndrome, in which hypertension and type 2 diabetes are present, is a large and growing cause of renal damage.

Pathophysiology

CKD is initially described as diminished renal reserve or renal insufficiency, which may progress to renal failure (end-stage renal disease). Initially, as renal tissue loses function, there are few noticeable abnormalities because the remaining tissue increases its performance (renal functional adaptation).

Decreased renal function interferes with the kidneys' ability to maintain fluid and electrolyte homeostasis. The ability to concentrate urine declines early and is followed by decreases in ability to excrete excess phosphate, acid, and potassium. When renal failure is advanced (GFR ≤ 15 mL/min/1.73 m^2), the ability to effectively dilute or concentrate urine is lost; thus, urine osmolality is usually fixed at about 300 to 320 mOsm/kg,

Table 247–1. MAJOR CAUSES OF CHRONIC KIDNEY DISEASE

CAUSE	EXAMPLES
Chronic tubulointerstitial nephropathies	See Table 258–3 on p. 2169
Glomerulopathies (primary)	Focal segmental glomerulosclerosis Idiopathic crescentic glomerulonephritis IgA nephropathy Membranoproliferative glomerulonephritis Membranous nephropathy
Glomerulopathies associated with systemic disease	Amyloidosis Diabetes mellitus Anti-GBM antibody disease (also known as Goodpasture syndrome) Granulomatosis with polyangiitis Hemolytic-uremic syndrome Mixed cryoglobulinemia Postinfectious glomerulonephritis SLE
Hereditary nephropathies	Autosomal dominant interstitial kidney disease (medullary cystic kidney disease) Hereditary nephritis (Alport syndrome) Nail-patella syndrome Polycystic kidney disease
Hypertension	Hypertensive nephrosclerosis
Obstructive uropathy	Benign prostatic hyperplasia Posterior urethral valves Retroperitoneal fibrosis Ureteral obstruction (congenital, calculi, cancer) Vesicoureteral reflux
Renal macrovascular disease (vasculopathy of renal arteries and veins)	Renal artery stenosis caused by atherosclerosis or fibromuscular dysplasia

close to that of plasma (275 to 295 mOsm/kg), and urinary volume does not respond readily to variations in water intake.

Creatinine and urea: Plasma concentrations of creatinine and urea (which are highly dependent on glomerular filtration) begin a hyperbolic rise as GFR diminishes. These changes are minimal early on. When the GFR falls below 15 mL/min/1.73 m^2 (normal > 90 mL/min/1.73 m^2), creatinine and urea levels are high and are usually associated with systemic manifestations (uremia). Urea and creatinine are not major contributors to the uremic symptoms; they are markers for many other substances (some not yet well defined) that cause the symptoms.

Sodium and water: Despite a diminishing GFR, sodium and water balance is well maintained by increased fractional excretion of sodium in urine and a normal response to thirst. Thus, the plasma sodium concentration is typically normal, and hypervolemia is infrequent unless dietary intake of sodium or water is very restricted or excessive. Heart failure can occur due to sodium and water overload, particularly in patients with decreased cardiac reserve.

Potassium: For substances whose secretion is controlled mainly through distal nephron secretion (eg, potassium), renal adaptation usually maintains plasma levels at normal until renal failure is advanced or dietary potassium intake is excessive. Potassium-sparing diuretics, ACE inhibitors, beta-blockers, NSAIDs, cyclosporine, tacrolimus, trimethoprim/sulfamethoxazole, pentamidine, or angiotensin II receptor blockers may raise plasma potassium levels in patients with less advanced renal failure.

Calcium and phosphate: Abnormalities of calcium, phosphate, parathyroid hormone (PTH), and vitamin D metabolism can occur, as can renal osteodystrophy. Decreased renal production of calcitriol contributes to hypocalcemia. Decreased renal excretion of phosphate results in hyperphosphatemia. Secondary hyperparathyroidism is common and can develop in renal failure before abnormalities in calcium or phosphate concentrations occur. For this reason, monitoring PTH in patients with moderate CKD, even before hyperphosphatemia occurs, has been recommended.

Renal osteodystrophy (abnormal bone mineralization resulting from hyperparathyroidism, calcitriol deficiency, elevated serum phosphate, or low or normal serum calcium) usually takes the form of increased bone turnover due to hyperparathyroid bone disease (osteitis fibrosa) but can also involve decreased bone turnover due to adynamic bone disease (with increased parathyroid suppression) or osteomalacia. Calcitriol deficiency may cause osteopenia or osteomalacia.

pH and bicarbonate: Moderate acidosis (plasma bicarbonate content 15 to 20 mmol/L) is characteristic. Acidosis causes muscle wasting due to protein catabolism, bone loss due to bone buffering of acid, and accelerated progression of kidney disease.

Anemia: Anemia is characteristic of moderate to advanced CKD (≥ stage 3). The anemia of CKD is normochromic-normocytic, with an Hct of 20 to 30% (35 to 40% in patients with polycystic kidney disease). It is usually caused by deficient erythropoietin production due to a reduction of functional renal mass (see p. 1094). Other causes include deficiencies of iron, folate, and vitamin B_{12}.

Symptoms and Signs

Patients with mildly diminished renal reserve are asymptomatic. Even patients with mild to moderate renal insufficiency may have no symptoms despite elevated BUN and creatinine. Nocturia is often noted, principally due to failure to concentrate the urine. Lassitude, fatigue, anorexia, and decreased mental acuity often are the earliest manifestations of uremia.

With more severe renal disease (eg, estimated glomerular filtration rate [eGFR] < 15 mL/min/1.73 m^2), neuromuscular symptoms may be present, including coarse muscular twitches, peripheral sensory and motor neuropathies, muscle cramps, hyperreflexia, restless legs syndrome, and seizures (usually the result of hypertensive or metabolic encephalopathy).

Anorexia, nausea, vomiting, weight loss, stomatitis, and an unpleasant taste in the mouth are almost uniformly present. The skin may be yellow-brown. Occasionally, urea from sweat crystallizes on the skin (uremic frost). Pruritus may be especially uncomfortable. Undernutrition leading to generalized tissue wasting is a prominent feature of chronic uremia.

In advanced CKD, pericarditis and GI ulceration and bleeding may occur. Hypertension is present in > 80% of patients with advanced CKD and is usually related to hypervolemia. Heart failure caused by hypertension or coronary artery disease and renal retention of sodium and water may lead to dependent edema and/or dyspnea.

Diagnosis

- Electrolytes, BUN, creatinine, phosphate, calcium, CBC
- Urinalysis (including urinary sediment examination)
- Quantitative urine protein (24-h urine protein collection or spot urine protein to creatinine ratio)
- Ultrasonography
- Sometimes renal biopsy

CKD is usually first suspected when serum creatinine rises. The initial step is to determine whether the renal failure is acute, chronic, or acute superimposed on chronic (ie, an acute disease that further compromises renal function in a patient with CKD—see Table 247–2). The cause of renal failure is also determined. Sometimes determining the duration of renal failure helps determine the cause; sometimes it is easier to determine the cause than the duration, and determining the cause helps determine the duration.

Testing includes urinalysis with examination of the urinary sediment, electrolytes, urea nitrogen, creatinine, phosphate, calcium, and CBC. Sometimes specific serologic tests are needed to determine the cause. Distinguishing acute kidney injury from CKD is most helped by a history of an elevated creatinine level or abnormal urinalysis. Urinalysis findings depend on the nature of the underlying disorder, but broad (> 3 WBC diameters wide) or especially waxy (highly refractile) casts often are prominent in advanced renal failure of any cause.

An ultrasound examination of the kidneys is usually helpful in evaluating for obstructive uropathy and in distinguishing acute kidney injury from CKD based on kidney size. Except in certain conditions (see Table 247–1), patients with CKD have small shrunken kidneys (usually < 10 cm in length) with thinned, hyperechoic cortex. Obtaining a precise diagnosis becomes increasingly difficult as renal function reaches values close to those of end-stage renal disease. The definitive diagnostic tool is renal biopsy, but it is not recommended when ultrasonography indicates small, fibrotic kidneys; high procedural risk outweighs low diagnostic yield.

Classification: Staging CKD is a way of quantifying its severity. CKD has been classified into 5 stages.

- Stage 1: Normal GFR (≥ 90 mL/min/1.73 m^2) plus either persistent albuminuria or known structural or hereditary renal disease
- Stage 2: GFR 60 to 89 mL/min/1.73 m^2
- Stage 3a: 45 to 59 mL/min/1.73 m^2
- Stage 3b: 30 to 44 mL/min/1.73 m^2
- Stage 4: GFR 15 to 29 mL/min/1.73 m^2
- Stage 5: GFR < 15 mL/min/1.73 m^2

Table 247–2. DISTINGUISHING ACUTE KIDNEY INJURY FROM CHRONIC KIDNEY DISEASE

FINDING	COMMENT
Decreased kidney function (estimated glomerular filtration rate [eGFR] < 60 mL/min/1.73 m^2) for ≥ 3 mo	Most reliable evidence of CKD
Renal sonogram showing small kidneys	Usually CKD
Renal sonogram showing normal or enlarged kidneys	May be AKI or some forms of CKD (diabetic nephropathy, acute hypertensive nephrosclerosis, polycystic kidney disease, myeloma, rapidly progressive glomerulonephritis, infiltrative diseases [eg, lymphoma, leukemia, amyloidosis], obstruction)
Oliguria, daily increases in serum creatinine and BUN	Probably AKI or AKI superimposed on CKD
No anemia	Probably AKI or CKD due to polycystic kidney disease
Severe anemia, hyperphosphatemia, and hypocalcemia	Possibly CKD but may be AKI
Subperiosteal erosions on radiography	Probably CKD
Chronic symptoms or signs (eg, fatigue, nausea, pruritus, nocturia, hypertension)	Usually CKD

AKI = acute kidney injury; CKD = chronic kidney disease.

GFR (in mL/min/1.73 m^2) in CKD can be estimated by the MDRD equation: $186.3 \times (\text{serum creatinine})^{-1.154} \times (\text{age})^{-0.203}$. The result is multiplied by 0.742 if the patient is female and by 1.21 if the patient is African American. For female African Americans, the result is multiplied by 0.742 × 1.21 (0.898). This calculation is not very accurate for patients who are older and sedentary, very obese, or very thin. Alternatively, GFR can be estimated using the Cockcroft-Gault equation (see p. 2055) to approximate creatinine clearance; this equation tends to overestimate GFR by 10 to 40%.

The Chronic Kidney Disease Epidemiology Collaboration (CKD-EPI) formula is more accurate than the MDRD and Cockcroft and Gault formulas, particularly for patients with a GFR near normal values. The CKD-EPI equation (see p. 2055) yields fewer falsely positive results indicating CKD and predicts outcome better than the other formulas.

Prognosis

Progression of CKD is predicted in most cases by the degree of proteinuria. Patients with nephrotic-range proteinuria (> 3 g/24 h or urine protein/creatinine ratio > 3) usually have a poorer prognosis and progress to renal failure more rapidly. Progression may occur even if the underlying disorder is not active. In patients with urine protein < 1.5 g/24 h, progression usually occurs more slowly if at all. Hypertension, acidosis, and hyperparathyroidism are associated with more rapid progression as well.

Treatment

- Control of underlying disorders
- Possible restriction of dietary protein, phosphate, and potassium
- Vitamin D supplements
- Treatment of anemia
- Treatment of contributing comorbidities (eg, heart failure, diabetes mellitus, nephrolithiasis, prostatic hypertrophy)
- Doses of all drugs adjusted as needed
- Dialysis for severely decreased GFR if symptoms and signs not adequately managed by medical interventions
- Maintaining sodium bicarbonate level at 23 mmol/L

Underlying disorders and contributory factors must be controlled. In particular, controlling hyperglycemia in patients with diabetic nephropathy and controlling hypertension in all patients substantially slows deterioration of GFR.

For **hypertension**, recent guidelines suggest a target BP of < 140/90 mm Hg, but some authors continue to recommend about 110 to 130/ < 80 mm Hg. ACE inhibitors and angiotensin II receptor blockers decrease the rate of decline in GFR in patients with most causes of CKD, particularly those with proteinuria. Increasing evidence suggests that, compared with either drug alone, combined use of ACE inhibitors and angiotensin II receptor blockers increases incidence of complications and does not slow decline in renal function, even though combined use does reduce proteinuria more.

Activity need not be restricted, although fatigue and lassitude usually limit a patient's capacity for exercise. Pruritus may respond to dietary phosphate restriction and phosphate binders if serum phosphate is elevated.

Nutrition: Severe protein restriction in renal disease is controversial. However, moderate restriction (0.8 g/kg/day) among patients with eGFR < 60 mL/min/1.73 m^2 without nephrotic syndrome is safe and easy for most patients to tolerate. Some experts recommend 0.6 g/kg/day for patients with diabetes and for patients without diabetes if GFR is < 25 mL/min/1.73 m^2. Many uremic symptoms markedly lessen when protein catabolism and urea generation are reduced. Also, rate of progression of CKD may slow down. Sufficient carbohydrate and fat are given to meet energy requirements and prevent ketosis. Patients for whom < 0.8 g/kg/day has been prescribed should be closely followed by a dietician.

Because dietary restrictions may reduce necessary vitamin intake, patients should take a multivitamin containing water-soluble vitamins. Administration of vitamin A and E is unnecessary. Vitamin D in the form of 1,25-dihydroxy vitamin D (calcitriol) or its analogs should be given as indicated by PTH concentrations. Dose is determined by stage of CKD, PTH concentration, and phosphate concentrations (see Table 247–3). Target levels for calcium are 8.4 to 9.5 mg/dL (2.10 to 2.37 mmol/L); for the calcium-phosphate product, < 55 mg^2/dL^2.

A typical starting dose is calcitriol (or a calcitriol analog) 0.25 mcg po once/day or 1 to 4 mcg 2 times/wk. PTH levels are not corrected to normal because doing so risks precipitating adynamic bone disease.

Table 247–3. TARGET LEVELS FOR PTH AND PHOSPHATE IN CHRONIC KIDNEY DISEASE

CHRONIC KIDNEY DISEASE STAGE	PTH (pg/mL)	PHOSPHATE (mg/dL [mmol/L])
3	35–70	2.7–4.6 (0.87–1.49)
4	70–110	2.7–4.6 (0.87–1.49)
5	150–300	3.5–5.5 (1.13–1.78)

PTH = parathyroid hormone.

Dyslipidemia should be addressed (see p. 1303). Dietary modification may be helpful for hypertriglyceridemia. In patients with hypercholesterolemia, a statin is effective. Fibric acid derivatives (clofibrate, gemfibrozil) may increase risk of rhabdomyolysis in patients with CKD, especially if taken with statin drugs, whereas ezetimibe (which reduces cholesterol absorption) appears relatively safe. Correction of hypercholesterolemia is intended to reduce risk of cardiovascular disease, which is increased in patients with CKD.

Fluid and electrolytes: Water intake is restricted only when serum sodium concentration is < 135 mmol/L or there is heart failure or severe edema.

Sodium restriction of < 2 g/day is recommended for CKD patients with eGFR < 60 mL/m/1.73 m^2 who have hypertension, volume overload, or proteinuria.

Potassium restriction is individualized based on serum level, eGFR, dietary customs, and use of drugs that increase potassium levels (eg, ACE, ARBs, or potassium-sparing diuretics). Typically, potassium restriction is not needed with eGFR > 30 mL/min/1.73 m.^{2} Treatment of mild to moderate hyperkalemia (5.1 to 6 mmol/L) entails dietary restriction (including avoiding salt substitutes), correction of metabolic acidosis, and use of potassium-lowering diuretics and gastrointestinal cation exchangers. Severe hyperkalemia (> 6 mmol/L) warrants urgent treatment.

Phosphate restriction of 0.8 to 1 g/day of dietary intake is typically sufficient to normalize serum phosphate level in patients with eGFR < 60 mL/min/1.73 m^2. Additional intestinal phosphate binders (calcium-containing or non-calcium-containing) may be necessary for adequate control of hyperphosphatemia, which has been associated with increased cardiovascular risk. Noncalcium-containing binders are preferred in patients with hypercalcemia, suspected adynamic bone disease, or evidence of vascular calcification on imaging. If calcium-containing binders are prescribed, then the total dietary and medication sources of calcium should not exceed 2000 mg/day in patients with eGFR < 60 mL/min/1.73 m^2.

Metabolic acidosis should be treated to bring serum bicarbonate to normal (> 23 mmol/L) to help reverse or slow muscle wasting, bone loss, and progression of CKD. Acidosis can be corrected with oral alkali sources such as sodium bicarbonate or an alkaline-ash diet (primarily fruits and vegetables). Sodium bicarbonate 1 to 2 g po bid is given and amount is increased gradually until bicarbonate concentration is about 23 mmol/L or until evidence of sodium overloading prevents further therapy. If the alkaline-ash diet is used, serum potassium is monitored because fruits and vegetables contain potassium.

Anemia and coagulation disorders: Anemia is a common complication of moderate to advanced CKD (≥ stage 3), and, when severe, is treated with erythropoiesis-stimulating agents (ESA), such as recombinant human erythropoietin (eg, epoetin alfa). Due to risk of cardiovascular complications, including stroke, thrombosis, and death, the lowest dose of these agents needed to keep the Hb between 10 and 11 g/dL is used. Because of increased iron utilization with stimulated erythropoiesis, iron stores must be replaced, often requiring parenteral iron. Iron concentrations, iron-binding capacity, and ferritin concentrations should be followed closely. Target transferrin saturation (TSAT), calculated by dividing serum iron by total iron binding capacity and multiplying by 100%, should be > 20%. Target ferritin in patients not on dialysis is >100 ng/mL. Transfusion should not be done unless anemia is severe (Hb < 8 g/dL) or causes symptoms.

The bleeding tendency in CKD rarely needs treatment. Cryoprecipitate, RBC transfusions, desmopressin 0.3 to 0.4 mcg/kg (20 mcg maximum) in 20 mL of isotonic saline IV over 20 to 30 min, or conjugated estrogens 2.5 to 5 mg po once/day help when needed. The effects of these treatments last 12 to 48 h, except for conjugated estrogens, which may last for several days.

Heart failure: Symptomatic heart failure is treated with sodium restriction and diuretics. Loop diuretics such as furosemide usually are effective even when renal function is markedly reduced, although large doses may be needed. If left ventricular function is depressed, ACE inhibitors (or ARBs) and beta-blockers (carvedilol or metoprolol) should be used. Aldosterone receptor antagonists are recommended in patients with advanced stages of heart failure. Digoxin may be added, but the dosage must be reduced based on degree of renal function.

Moderate or severe hypertension should be treated to avoid its deleterious effects on cardiac and renal function. Patients who do not respond to sodium restriction (1.5 g/day), should receive diuretics. Loop diuretics (eg, furosemide 80 to 240 mg po bid) may be combined with thiazide diuretics (eg, chlorthalidone 12.5 to 100 mg po once/day, hydrochlorothiazide 25 to 100 mg po in one to two divided doses/day, metolazone 2.5 to 20 mg po once/day) if hypertension or edema is not controlled. Even in renal failure, the combination of a thiazide diuretic with a loop diuretic is quite potent and must be used with caution to avoid overdiuresis.

Occasionally, dialysis may be required to control heart failure. If reduction of the ECF volume does not control BP, conventional antihypertensives are added. Azotemia may increase with such treatment and may be necessary for adequate control of heart failure and/or hypertension.

Drugs: Renal excretion of drugs is often impaired in patients with renal failure. Common drugs that require revised dosing include penicillins, cephalosporins, aminoglycosides, fluoroquinolones, vancomycin, and digoxin. Hemodialysis reduces the serum concentrations of some drugs, which should be supplemented after hemodialysis. It is strongly recommended that physicians consult a reference on drug dosing in renal failure before prescribing drugs to these very vulnerable patients. Some appropriate references include

- CKD and Drug Dosing: Information for Providers (at www.niddk.nih.gov)
- Drug Dosing Adjustments in Patients with CKD (at www.aafp.org)
- Drug dosing consideration in patients with acute and CKD—A clinical update from Kidney Disease: Improving Global Outcomes (KDIGO—www.kdigo.org)

Most experts recommend avoiding NSAIDs in patients with CKD because they may worsen renal function, exacerbate hypertension, and precipitate electrolyte disturbances.

Certain drugs should be avoided entirely in patients with CKD with eGFR < 60 mL/min/1.73m^2. They include nitrofurantoin and phenazopyridine. The MRI contrast agent gadolinium has been associated with the development of nephrogenic systemic fibrosis in some patients; because risk is particularly high if patients have estimated GFR < 30 mL/min/1.73m^2, gadolinium should be avoided whenever possible in these patients.

Dialysis: Dialysis is usually initiated at the onset of either of the following:

- Uremic symptoms (eg, anorexia, nausea, vomiting, weight loss, pericarditis, pleuritis)
- Difficulty controlling fluid overload, hyperkalemia, or acidosis with drugs and lifestyle interventions

These problems typically occur when the estimated GFR reaches ≤ 10 mL/min in a patient without diabetes or ≤ 15 mL/min in a patient with diabetes; patients whose estimated GFR values are near these values should be closely monitored so that these signs and symptoms are recognized early. Dialysis is best anticipated so that preparations can be made and urgent insertion of a hemodialysis catheter can be avoided. Such preparations usually begin when the patient is in early to mid stage 4 CKD; preparation allows time for patient education, selection of the type of dialysis, and timely creation of an arteriovenous fistula or placement of a peritoneal dialysis catheter. (For dialysis preparation, see p. 2145.)

PEARLS & PITFALLS

- Begin preparation for dialysis, kidney transplantation, or palliative care during early to mid stage 4 CKD to allow adequate time for patient education and selection of treatment modality, along with any associated preparatory procedures.

Transplantation: If a living kidney donor is available, better long-term outcomes occur when a patient receives the transplanted kidney early, even before beginning dialysis. Patients who are transplant candidates but have no living donor should be placed on the waiting list of their regional transplant center early, because wait times may exceed several years in many regions of the US.

KEY POINTS

- Common causes of CKD in the US are diabetic nephropathy (the most common), hypertensive nephrosclerosis, glomerulopathies, and metabolic syndrome.
- Effects of CKD can include hypocalcemia, hyperphosphatemia, metabolic acidosis, anemia, secondary hyperparathyroidism, and renal osteodystrophy.
- Distinguish CKD from acute kidney injury based on history, clinical findings, routine laboratory tests, and ultrasonography.
- Control underlying disorders (eg, diabetes) and BP levels (usually with an ACE inhibitor or angiotensin II receptor blocker).
- Give supplemental vitamin D and/or sodium bicarbonate and restrict potassium and phosphate as needed.
- Treat heart failure, anemia, and other complications.
- Educate patients with advanced CKD on treatment options (dialysis, kidney transplantation, or palliative care) early, to allow adequate time for planning.
- Initiate dialysis for patients with severely decreased eGFR when signs and symptoms are inadequately controlled with drugs and lifestyle interventions.

248 Cystic Kidney Disease

Cystic kidney disease may be congenital or acquired. Congenital disorders may be inherited as autosomal dominant disorders or autosomal recessive disorders or have other causes (eg, sporadic mutations, chromosomal abnormalities, teratogens). Some are part of a malformation syndrome (see Table 248–1).

ACQUIRED RENAL CYSTS

Acquired renal cysts are simple cysts that must be distinguished from more serious causes of cystic disease.

Acquired cysts are usually simple, ie, they are round and sharply demarcated with smooth walls. They may be solitary or multiple.

Solitary renal cysts: Isolated cysts are most often detected incidentally on imaging studies; they are distinguished from other cystic renal disorders and renal masses, such as renal cell carcinoma, which is typically irregular or multiloculated with complex features such as irregular walls, septae, and areas of unclear demarcation or calcification. Their cause is unknown. They are generally clinically insignificant but rarely can cause hematuria or become infected.

Multiple renal cysts: Multiple cysts are most common in patients with chronic kidney disease, especially patients undergoing dialysis for many years. Cause is unknown, but the cysts may be due to compensatory hyperplasia of residually functioning nephrons. More than 50 to 80% of patients receiving dialysis for > 10 yr develop acquired cystic disease (with multiple acquired cysts). Usual criterion for diagnosis is ≥ 4 cysts in each kidney detected with ultrasonography or CT. This disorder can usually be differentiated from autosomal dominant polycystic kidney disease by the absence of family history and by small or normal-sized kidneys.

Acquired cysts are usually asymptomatic, but occasional patients develop hematuria, renal or perirenal hemorrhage, infection, or flank pain. Acquired cysts are significant mainly because patients have a higher incidence of renal cell carcinoma; whether the cysts become malignant is unknown. For this reason, some physicians periodically screen patients with acquired cysts for renal carcinoma using ultrasonography or CT. Cysts that cause persistent bleeding or infection may require percutaneous drainage or, rarely, partial or complete nephrectomy.

AUTOSOMAL DOMINANT POLYCYSTIC KIDNEY DISEASE

Polycystic kidney disease (PKD) is a hereditary disorder of renal cyst formation causing gradual enlargement of both kidneys, sometimes with progression to renal failure. Almost all forms are caused by a familial genetic mutation. Symptoms and signs include flank and abdominal pain, hematuria, and hypertension. Diagnosis is by CT or ultrasonography. Treatment is symptomatic before renal failure and with dialysis or transplantation afterward.

Table 248–1. MAJOR GROUPS OF CYSTIC NEPHROPATHIES

DISORDER	CLINICAL FEATURES
Autosomal dominant	
Autosomal dominant polycystic kidney disease	Flank and abdominal pain Hematuria Hypertension Large kidneys with multiple bilateral cysts Extrarenal cysts (liver, pancreas, intestine) Cerebral aneurysms Diverticulosis Abdominal wall hernias ESRD during adulthood if at all
Branchio-oto-renal syndrome (Melnick-Fraser syndrome)	Branchial fistulas and cysts Preauricular pits or tags Hearing loss
Familial renal hamartomas	Primary hyperparathyroidism Ossifying fibromas of the jaw
Autosomal dominant tubulointerstitial kidney disease (ADTKD)	Small to normal-sized kidneys Polydipsia and polyuria Absent-to-mild proteinuria Bland urinary sediment No severe hypertension during early stages Nocturia or enuresis in children ESRD during adulthood Sometimes gout
Oral-facial-digital syndrome	Partial clefts in lip, tongue, and alveolar ridges Hypoplasia of nasal cartilage Microcysts in kidneys
Tuberous sclerosis	Benign tumors of the brain, kidneys, and skin Angiomyolipomas of the kidneys
Von Hippel–Lindau disease	Hemangioblastoma proliferation in the retina, brain, spinal cord, and adrenal glands Renal cell carcinoma Pheochromocytoma
Autosomal recessive	
Alström syndrome	Obesity Type 2 diabetes mellitus Retinitis pigmentosa
Autosomal recessive polycystic kidney disease	Large kidneys with multiple bilateral cysts Hepatic fibrosis Hypertension ESRD during childhood
Bardet-Biedl syndrome	Male hypogonadism Intellectual disability Retinopathy Obesity Polydactyly
Ellis–van Creveld syndrome	Short-limb dwarfism Polydactyly Heart defects frequently
Ivemark syndrome	Spleen agenesis Cyanotic heart disease Gut malrotation
Jeune syndrome (asphyxiating thoracic dystrophy)	Dwarfism involving the chest, arms, and legs
Joubert syndrome	Intellectual disability Hypotonia Irregular breathing Eye movement abnormalities

Table continues on the following page.

Table 248–1. MAJOR GROUPS OF CYSTIC NEPHROPATHIES (*Continued*)

DISORDER	CLINICAL FEATURES
Meckel-Gruber syndrome	Occipital encephalocele Polydactyly Craniofacial dysplasia
Nephronophthisis	Small to normal-sized kidneys Polydipsia and polyuria Mild proteinuria with benign urinary sediment ESRD possibly during childhood
Zellweger syndrome (cerebrohepatorenal syndrome)	Brain and liver defects Developmental delay High serum iron and copper levels Hypotonia
Other congenital*	
Cysts of nontubular origin (includes glomerular, subcapsular, and pyelocalyceal cysts)	Various clinical characteristics
Malformation syndromes	Various clinical characteristics
Medullary sponge kidney	Tubular dilations and cysts of collecting ducts Associated renal tubular acidosis type 1 and renal calculi Does not progress to ESRD
Multicystic dysplastic kidney	Unilateral nonreniform mass of cysts and connective tissue, with typically absent functioning renal tissue
Renal cystic dysplasia	Associated with urinary structural obstruction or metanephric malformation Degree of dysplasia asymmetric between kidneys
Trisomy 18	Profound developmental delay Malformations of the head, face, hands, and feet
Acquired	
Acquired cystic disease	Multiple cysts Associated with long-term dialysis, usually after > 10 yr High risk of renal cell carcinoma
Cysts associated with tumors	For example, with renal cell carcinoma or nephroblastoma
Solitary simple cysts	Low risk of chronic kidney disease and hypertension Associated with aging

*Caused by, eg, sporadic mutations, chromosomal abnormalities, teratogens, or unknown mechanisms.
ESRD = end-stage renal disease.

Etiology

Inheritance of PKD is

- Autosomal dominant
- Recessive
- Sporadic (rare)

Autosomal dominant polycystic kidney disease (ADPKD) has an incidence of 1/1000 and accounts for about 5% of patients with end-stage renal disease requiring renal replacement therapy. Clinical manifestations are rare before adulthood, but penetrance is essentially complete; all patients ≥ 80 yr have some signs. In contrast, autosomal recessive PKD is rare; incidence is 1/10,000. It frequently causes renal failure during childhood (see p. 2537).

In 86 to 96% of cases, ADPKD is caused by mutations in the *PKD1* gene on chromosome 16, which codes for the protein polycystin 1; most other cases are caused by mutations in the *PKD2* gene on chromosome 4, which codes for polycystin 2. A few familial cases are unrelated to either locus.

Pathophysiology

Polycystin 1 may regulate tubular epithelial cell adhesion and differentiation; polycystin 2 may function as an ion channel, with mutations causing fluid secretion into cysts. Mutations in these proteins may alter the function of renal cilia, which enable tubular cells to sense flow rates. A leading hypothesis proposes that tubular cell proliferation and differentiation are linked to flow rate and that ciliary dysfunction may thus lead to cystic transformation.

Early in the disorder, tubules dilate and slowly fill with glomerular filtrate. Eventually, the tubules separate from the functioning nephron and fill with secreted rather than filtered fluid, forming cysts. Hemorrhage into cysts may occur, causing hematuria. Patients are also at higher risk of acute pyelonephritis, cyst infections, and urinary calculi (in 20%). Vascular sclerosis and interstitial fibrosis eventually develop via unknown mechanisms and typically affect < 10% of tubules; nonetheless, renal failure develops in about 35 to 45% of patients by age 60.

Extrarenal manifestations are common:

- Hepatic cysts are present in most patients; these typically do not affect liver function.
- Patients also have a higher incidence of pancreatic and intestinal cysts, colonic diverticula, and inguinal and abdominal wall hernias.
- Valvular heart disorders (most often mitral valve prolapse and aortic regurgitation) can be detected by cardiac ultrasonography in 25 to 30% of patients; other valvular disorders may be due to collagen abnormalities.
- Aortic regurgitation results from aortic root dilation due to arterial wall changes (including aortic aneurysm).
- Coronary artery aneurysms occur.
- Cerebral aneurysms are present in about 4% of young adults and up to 10% of elderly patients. Aneurysms rupture in 65 to 75% of patients, usually before age 50; risk factors include family history of aneurysm or rupture, larger aneurysms, and poorly controlled hypertension.

Symptoms and Signs

ADPKD usually causes no symptoms initially; one half of patients remain asymptomatic, never develop renal insufficiency or failure, and are never diagnosed. Most patients who develop symptoms do so by the end of their 20s.

Symptoms include low-grade flank, abdominal, and lower back pain due to cystic enlargement and symptoms of infection. Acute pain, when it occurs, is usually due to hemorrhage into cysts or passage of a calculus. Fever is common with acute pyelonephritis, and rupture of cysts into the retroperitoneal space may cause a fever that can last for weeks. Hepatic cysts may cause right upper quadrant pain if they enlarge or become infected.

Valvular disorders rarely cause symptoms but occasionally cause heart failure and require valvular replacement.

Symptoms and signs of unruptured cerebral aneurysm can be absent or may include headache, nausea and vomiting, and cranial nerve deficits; these manifestations warrant immediate intervention (see Sidebar 241–1 on p. 2044).

Signs are nonspecific and include hematuria and hypertension (each in about 40 to 50%) and, in 20% of patients, proteinuria in the subnephrotic range (< 3.5g/24 h in adults). Anemia is less common than in other types of chronic kidney disease, presumably because erythropoietin production is preserved. In advanced disease, the kidneys may become grossly enlarged and palpable, causing fullness in the upper abdomen and flank.

Diagnosis

- Ultrasonography
- Sometimes CT or MRI or genetic testing

The diagnosis of polycystic kidney disease is suspected in patients with the following:

- A positive family history
- Typical symptoms or signs
- Cysts detected incidentally on imaging studies

Patients should be counseled before undergoing diagnostic testing, particularly if they are asymptomatic. For example, many authorities recommend against testing asymptomatic young patients because no disease-modifying treatment is effective at this age and diagnosis has potential negative effects on ability to obtain life insurance on favorable terms and on mood.

Diagnosis is usually by imaging, showing extensive and bilateral cystic changes throughout the kidneys, which are typically enlarged and have a moth-eaten appearance due to cysts that displace functional tissue. These changes develop with age and are less often present or obvious in younger patients.

Ultrasonography is usually done first. If ultrasonography results are inconclusive, CT or MRI, which are both more sensitive (particularly when done using contrast), is done. MRI is especially useful for measuring cyst and kidney volume. These measurements predict risk of progression to chronic kidney disease and end-stage renal disease, often before changes in routine laboratory studies. For example, cyst size and kidney size predict 8 yr risk of chronic kidney disease more accurately than age, degree of proteinuria, or serum BUN, or creatinine. Urinalysis, renal function tests, and CBC are done, but results are not specific.

Urinalysis detects mild proteinuria and microscopic or macroscopic hematuria. Gross hematuria may be due to a dislodged calculus or to hemorrhage from a ruptured cyst. Pyuria is common even without bacterial infection; thus diagnosis of infection should be based on culture results and clinical findings (eg, dysuria, fever, flank pain) as well as urinalysis. Initially, BUN and creatinine are normal or only mildly elevated, but they slowly increase, especially when hypertension is present. Rarely, CBC detects polycythemia.

Patients with symptoms of cerebral aneurysm require high-resolution CT or magnetic resonance angiography. However, most experts do not recommend routine screening for cerebral aneurysm in asymptomatic patients. A reasonable approach is to screen patients with ADPKD who have a family history of hemorrhagic stroke or cerebral aneurysm.

Genetic testing for PKD mutations is currently reserved for any of the following:

- Patients with suspected PKD and no known family history
- Patients with inconclusive results on imaging
- Younger patients (eg, age < 30, in whom imaging results are often inconclusive) in whom the diagnosis must be made (eg, a potential kidney donor)

Genetic counseling is recommended for 1st-degree relatives of patients with ADPKD.

Prognosis

By age 75, 50 to 75% of patients with ADPKD require renal replacement therapy (dialysis or transplantation). On average, glomerular filtration rate (GFR) declines by about 5 mL/min/year after the fourth decade of life. Predictors of more rapid progression to renal failure include the following:

- Earlier age at diagnosis
- Male sex
- Sickle cell trait
- PKD1 genotype
- Larger or rapidly increasing kidney size
- Gross hematuria
- Hypertension
- Being black
- Increasing proteinuria

ADPKD does not increase risk of renal cancer, but if patients with ADPKD develop renal cancer, it is more likely to be bilateral. Renal cancer rarely causes death. Patients usually die of heart disease (sometimes valvular), disseminated infection, or ruptured cerebral aneurysm.

Treatment

- Control of complications (eg, hypertension, infection, renal failure)
- Supportive measures

Strict BP control is essential. Typically an ACE inhibitor or angiotensin receptor blocker is used. In addition to controlling BP, these drugs help block angiotensin and aldosterone, growth factors that contribute to renal scarring and loss of renal function. UTIs should be treated promptly. Percutaneous aspiration of cysts may help relieve severe pain due to hemorrhage or compression but has no effect on long-term outcome. Nephrectomy is an option to relieve severe symptoms due to massive kidney enlargement (eg, pain, hematuria) or recurrent UTIs.

Hemodialysis, peritoneal dialysis, or kidney transplantation is required in patients who develop chronic renal failure. ADPKD does not recur in grafts. With dialysis, patients with ADPKD maintain higher Hb levels than any other group of patients with renal failure.

Mammalian target of rapamycin (mTOR) inhibitors may slow the increase in kidney volume but not the decline in renal function; thus, they are not typically used in routine practice.

Tolvaptan, a vasopressin receptor 2 antagonist, is a drug that may benefit patients with ADPKD, but its use is not yet recommended. Tolvaptan appears to slow increase in renal volume and decline in renal function, but it can cause adverse effects via free water diuresis (eg, thirst, polydipsia, polyuria) that can make adherence difficult. Also, tolvaptan has been reported to cause severe liver failure, and data on long-term outcomes are not yet sufficient to confirm a favorable benefit/harm balance.

In children with autosomal dominant PKD, early use of pravastatin may slow the progression of structural kidney disease.[1]

1. Cadnapaphornchai MA, George DM, McFann K, et al: Effect of pravastatin on total kidney volume, left ventricular mass index, and microalbuminuria in pediatric autosomal dominant polycystic kidney disease. *Clin J Am Soc Nephrol* 9(5):889-896, 2014.

KEY POINTS

- ADPKD occurs in about 1/1000 people.
- About half of patients have no manifestations, but in others symptoms of back or abdominal pain, hematuria and/or hypertension develop gradually, usually beginning before age 30; 35 to 45% develop renal failure by age 60.
- Extrarenal manifestations are common and include cerebral and coronary artery aneurysms, cardiac valve disease, and cysts in the liver, pancreas, and intestines.
- Diagnose PKD based on imaging studies and clinical findings, reserving genetic testing for patients with no family history, with inconclusive results on imaging, or who are young and in whom the diagnosis will affect management.
- Do not routinely screen asymptomatic patients for ADPKD or asymptomatic patients who have ADPKD for cerebral aneurysms.
- Arrange genetic counseling for 1st-degree relatives of patients with ADPKD.
- Give ACE inhibitors or angiotensin receptor blockers for hypertension and to help prevent renal scarring and dysfunction; treat other complications as they arise, and consider use of tolvaptan.

CONGENITAL RENAL CYSTIC DYSPLASIA

Congenital renal cystic dysplasia is a broad category of congenital malformations involving metanephric malformation or congenital obstructive uropathies.

Congenital renal cystic dysplasia affects one or both kidneys. Renal cystic dysplasia may be an isolated congenital anomaly, or it may be part of a malformation syndrome (ie, associated with other clinical features—see Table 248–1). Associated urologic abnormalities may include ureteropelvic and ureterovesicular junction obstruction, neurogenic bladder, ureterocele, posterior urethral valves, and prune-belly syndrome (a triad of abdominal wall muscle defects, urinary tract abnormalities [eg, dilated ureters, enlarged bladder and urethra], and bilateral cryptorchidism).

Symptoms and signs vary by how much renal parenchyma is preserved and whether involvement is unilateral or bilateral. Some degree of renal insufficiency or renal failure may develop. Congenital renal cystic dysplasia is commonly discovered by ultrasonography prenatally or during early childhood.

Prognosis is highly unpredictable due to an inability to quantify residual functional parenchyma. Treatment is surgical correction of any associated GU abnormalities and, if renal insufficiency or renal failure is present, renal replacement therapy.

MEDULLARY SPONGE KIDNEY

Medullary sponge kidney is formation of diffuse, bilateral medullary cysts caused by abnormalities in pericalyceal terminal collecting ducts.

The cause of medullary sponge kidney is unknown, but genetic transmission occurs in < 5% of cases.

Most patients are asymptomatic, and the disorder usually remains undiagnosed. It predisposes to calculus formation (often with increased urinary calcium excretion) and UTI, so the most common presenting symptoms are the following:

- Renal colic
- Hematuria
- Dysuria

Medullary sponge kidney is benign, and long-term prognosis is excellent. Obstruction by renal calculi may transiently reduce GFR and increase serum creatinine.

Diagnosis

- CT or IVU

The diagnosis is suspected in patients with recurrent calculi or UTIs or on the basis of incidental radiographic findings such as medullary nephrocalcinosis and dilated contrast-filled collecting ducts. Urinalysis typically shows evidence of incomplete distal renal tubular acidosis (overt metabolic acidosis is rare) and decreased urine-concentrating ability in patients without symptomatic polyuria.

Diagnosis is generally confirmed by CT, but IVU can be used. Ultrasonography is not helpful because cysts are small and located deep in the medulla.

Treatment

- Control of complications (eg, UTI, renal calculi)

Treatment is indicated only for UTIs and for recurrent calculus formation. Thiazide diuretics (eg, hydrochlorothiazide 25 mg po once/day) and high fluid intake may inhibit calculus formation by reducing urinary calcium excretion and preventing urinary stasis. These effects may reduce incidence of obstructive complications in patients with recurrent calculi.

NEPHRONOPHTHISIS AND AUTOSOMAL DOMINANT TUBULOINTERSTITIAL KIDNEY DISEASE

Nephronophthisis and autosomal dominant tubulointerstitial kidney disease (ADTKD) are inherited disorders that cause cysts restricted to the renal medulla or corticomedullary border and, eventually, end-stage renal disease.

Nephronophthisis and ADTKD are grouped together because they share many features. Pathologically, they can cause cysts restricted to the renal medulla or corticomedullary border, as well as a triad of tubular atrophy, tubular basement membrane disintegration, and interstitial fibrosis. Cysts may or may not be present and are a result of tubular dilation. They probably share similar mechanisms, although these are not well characterized. Features of both disorders include the following:

- A vasopressin (ADH)-resistant urine-concentrating defect that leads to polyuria and polydipsia
- Sodium wasting severe enough to require supplementation
- Anemia
- A tendency toward mild proteinuria and a benign urinary sediment
- Eventually, end-stage renal disease (ESRD)

Key differences between nephronophthisis and medullary cystic kidney disease include inheritance patterns and age at onset of chronic kidney disease.

Nephronophthisis

Inheritance is autosomal recessive. Nephronophthisis accounts for up to 15% of chronic kidney disease with renal failure in children and young adults (< 20 yr). There are 3 types:

- Infantile, median age at onset 1 yr
- Juvenile, median age at onset 13 yr
- Adolescent, median age at onset 19 yr

Eleven gene mutations have been identified in patients with nephronophthisis. Mutations of the *NPHP1* gene are the most common, identified in about 30 to 60% of patients. About 10% of patients with nephronophthisis also have other manifestations, including retinitis pigmentosa, hepatic fibrosis, intellectual disability, and other neurologic abnormalities.

ESRD often develops during childhood and causes growth restriction and bone disease. However, in many patients, these problems develop slowly over years and are so well compensated for that they are not recognized as abnormal until significant uremic symptoms appear. Hypertension sometimes develops.

Diagnosis

- Imaging, genetic testing, or both

The diagnosis should be suspected in children with the following, particularly if the urinary sediment is benign:

- Polydipsia and polyuria
- Progressively decreasing renal function, particularly without hypertension
- Associated extrarenal findings
- Anemia out of proportion to the degree of renal failure

Proteinuria is usually absent. Diagnosis is confirmed by imaging, but cysts often occur only late in disease. Ultrasonography, CT, or MRI may show smooth renal outlines with normal-sized or small kidneys, loss of corticomedullary differentiation, and multiple cysts at the corticomedullary junction. Hydronephrosis is typically absent. Genetic testing is available.

Treatment

- Supportive care

In early disease, treatment involves management of hypertension, electrolyte and acid-base disorders, and anemia. Children with growth restriction may respond to nutritional supplements and growth hormone therapy. Ultimately, all patients develop renal failure and require dialysis or transplantation.

Autosomal Dominant Tubulointerstitial Kidney Disease

ADTKD (previously known as medullary cystic kidney disease) is a group of uncommon genetic disorders. A consensus

Table 248–2. AUTOSOMAL DOMINANT TUBULOINTERSTITIAL KIDNEY DISEASE: GENE-BASED CLASSIFICATION

CAUSAL GENE	PREVIOUS TERMINOLOGY	CHARACTERISTICS
Uromodulin (*UMOD*)	Uromodulin kidney disease (UKD) Uromodulin-associated kidney disease (UAKD) Familial juvenile hyperuricemic nephropathy (FJHN) Medullary cystic kidney disease type 2 (CKD2)	Rarely presents in childhood Early gout with hyperuricemia
Mucin-1 (*MUC1*)	Mucin-1 kidney disease (MKD) Medullary cystic kidney disease type 1 (MCKD1)	No childhood presentation
Renin (*REN*)	Familial juvenile hyperuricemic nephropathy type 2 (FJHN2)	Frequent childhood presentation Mild hypotension Risk for acute kidney injury Risk for anemia, hyperuricemia, and hyperkalemia
Hepatocyte nuclear factor-1 beta (*HNF1B*)	Maturity-onset diabetes mellitus of the Young type 5 (MODY5) Renal cyst and diabetes syndrome (RCAD)	Frequent childhood presentation Prenatal ultrasound findings Genital abnormalities Pancreatic atrophy Hypomagnesemia, hypokalemia Liver enzyme test abnormalities

report[1] from Kidney Disease Improving Global Outcomes (KDIGO) has proposed classifying these disorders based on the causative gene, of which 4 are currently known (see Table 248–2).

Histopathologic changes common to these disorders include

- Interstitial fibrosis
- Tubular atrophy
- Thickening of tubular basement membranes
- Possible cyst formation as a result of tubular dilation
- Absence of complement and immunoglobulin staining on immunofluorescence

ADTKD affects people in their 30s through 70s. About 15% of patients have no family history, suggesting a sporadic new mutation. Hypertension is common but usually only modest and typically does not precede the onset of kidney dysfunction. Hyperuricemia and gout is common and can precede the onset of significant renal insufficiency. ESRD typically develops at age 30 to 50. ADTKD should be suspected in patients with the following, particularly if the urinary sediment is benign:

- Polydipsia and polyuria
- Gout at a young age
- Family history of gout and chronic kidney disease

Proteinuria is absent to mild. Results of imaging studies have many similarities to that of nephronophthisis; however, renal medullary cysts are only sometimes visible. Genetic testing can confirm the diagnosis. Kidney biopsy may be necessary in at least one affected family member.

Treatment is generally similar to that of nephronophthisis. Allopurinol can help control gout.

1. Eckardt K-U, Alper SL, Antignac C, et al: Autosomal dominant tubulointerstitial kidney disease: diagnosis, classification, and management—A KDIGO consensus report. *Kidney Int* 88:676–683, 2015.

KEY POINTS

- Nephronophthisis and ADTKD cause inability to concentrate urine (with polydipsia and polyuria), sodium wasting, anemia, and ESRD.
- Nephronophthisis is autosomal recessive and causes ESRD during childhood, whereas ADTKD is autosomal dominant and causes ESRD at age 30 to 50.
- Obtain renal imaging and, when available, genetic testing.
- Treat associated disorders and treat kidney disease supportively.

249 Genitourinary Cancer

GU cancers (bladder, penile, prostate, kidney and renal pelvic, testicular, ureteral, and urethral) account for about 40% of cancers in men (primarily as prostate cancer) and 5.6% in women.

BLADDER CANCER

Bladder cancer is usually transitional cell (urothelial) carcinoma. Patients usually present with hematuria (most commonly) or irritative voiding symptoms such as frequency and/or urgency; later, urinary obstruction can cause pain. Diagnosis is by cystoscopy and biopsy. Treatment is with fulguration, transurethral resection, intravesical instillations, radical surgery, chemotherapy, or a combination.

In the US, > 79,000 new cases of bladder cancer and about 16,000 deaths occur each year. Bladder cancer is the 4th most common cancer among men and is less common among women; male:female incidence is about 3:1. Bladder cancer is more common among whites than blacks, and incidence increases with age.

Risk factors include the following:

- Smoking (the most common risk factor, causing ≥ 50% of new cases)
- Excess phenacetin use (analgesic abuse)
- Long-term cyclophosphamide use
- Chronic irritation (eg, in schistosomiasis, by chronic catheterization, or by bladder calculi)
- Exposure to hydrocarbons, tryptophan metabolites, or industrial chemicals, notably aromatic amines (aniline dyes, such as naphthylamine used in the dye industry) and chemicals used in the rubber, electric, cable, paint, and textile industries

Types of bladder cancer include

- Transitional cell carcinomas (urothelial carcinoma), which account for > 90% of bladder cancers. Most are papillary carcinomas, which tend to be superficial and well-differentiated and to grow outward; sessile tumors are more insidious, tending to invade early and metastasize.
- Squamous cell carcinomas, which are less common and usually occur in patients with parasitic bladder infestation or chronic mucosal irritation.
- Adenocarcinomas, which may occur as primary tumors or rarely reflect metastasis from intestinal carcinoma. Metastasis should be ruled out.

In > 40% of patients, tumors recur at the same or another site in the bladder, particularly if tumors are large or poorly differentiated or if several tumors are present. Bladder cancer tends to metastasize to the lymph nodes, lungs, liver, and bone. Expression of mutations in tumor gene *p53* may be associated with progression and resistance to chemotherapy.

In the bladder, carcinoma in situ is high grade but noninvasive and usually multifocal; it tends to recur.

Symptoms and Signs

Most patients present with unexplained hematuria (gross or microscopic). Some patients present with anemia, and hematuria is detected during evaluation. Irritative voiding symptoms (dysuria, burning, frequency) and pyuria are also common at presentation. Pelvic pain occurs with advanced cancer, when a pelvic mass may be palpable.

Diagnosis

- Cystoscopy with biopsy
- Urine cytology

Bladder cancer is suspected clinically. Urine cytology, which may detect malignant cells, may be done. Cystoscopy (see p. 2073) and biopsy of abnormal areas are usually also done initially because these tests are needed even if urine cytology is negative. Urinary antigen tests are available but are not routinely recommended for use in diagnosis. They are used sometimes if cancer is suspected but cytology results are negative.

For low-stage (stage T1 or more superficial) tumors, which comprise 70 to 80% of bladder cancers, cystoscopy with biopsy is sufficient for staging. However, if biopsy shows the tumor is more invasive than a superficial flat tumor, then additional biopsy, including of muscle tissue, is done. If a tumor is found to invade muscle (≥ stage T2), abdominal and pelvic CT and chest x-ray are done to determine tumor extent and evaluate for metastases. Patients with invasive tumors undergo bimanual examination (rectal examination in men, rectovaginal examination in women) while under anesthesia for cystoscopy and biopsy. The standard TNM (tumor, node, metastasis) staging system is used (Tables 249–1 and 249–2).

Prognosis

Superficial bladder cancer (stage Ta or T1) rarely causes death. Carcinoma in situ (stage Tis) may be more aggressive. For patients with invasion of the bladder musculature, the 5-yr survival rate is about 50%, but adjuvant chemotherapy may improve these results. Generally, prognosis for patients with progressive or recurrent invasive bladder cancer is poor. Prognosis for patients with squamous cell carcinoma or adenocarcinoma of the bladder is also poor because these cancers are usually highly infiltrative and often detected at an advanced stage.

Treatment

- Transurethral resection and intravesical chemotherapy (for superficial cancers)
- Cystectomy (for invasive cancers)

Superficial cancers: Superficial cancers can be completely removed by transurethral resection or fulguration. Repeated bladder instillations of chemotherapeutic drugs, such as mitomycin C, may reduce risk of recurrence. For carcinoma in situ and other high-grade, superficial, transitional cell carcinomas, immunotherapeutic treatments, such as BCG instillation after transurethral resection is generally more effective than chemotherapy instillations. Instillation can be done at intervals from weekly to monthly over 1 to 3 yr.

Invasive cancers: Tumors that penetrate the muscle (ie, ≥ stage T2) usually require radical cystectomy (removal of bladder and adjacent structures) with concomitant urinary diversion; partial cystectomy is possible for < 5% of patients. Cystectomy is being done with increasing frequency after initial chemotherapy in patients with locally advanced disease. Extended lymph node dissection at the time of surgery can increase survival rates. Urinary diversion traditionally involves routing urine through an ileal conduit to an abdominal stoma and collecting it in an external drainage bag. Alternatives such as orthotopic neobladder or continent cutaneous diversion are becoming common and are appropriate for many, patients. For both procedures, an internal reservoir is constructed from the intestine. For the orthotopic neobladder, the reservoir is connected to the urethra. Patients empty the reservoir by relaxing the pelvic floor muscles and increasing abdominal pressure, so that urine passes through the urethra almost naturally. Most patients maintain urinary control during the day, but some incontinence may occur at night. For continent cutaneous urinary diversion, the reservoir is connected to a continent abdominal stoma. Patients empty the reservoir by self-catheterization at regular intervals throughout the day.

Bladder preservation protocols that combine chemotherapy and radiation therapy may be appropriate for some older patients or those who refuse more aggressive surgery. These protocols may provide 5-yr survival rates of 36 to 74%.

Patients should be monitored every 3 to 6 mo for progression or recurrence.

Metastatic and recurrent cancers: Metastases require chemotherapy, which is frequently effective but rarely curative unless metastases are confined to lymph nodes. Combination chemotherapy may prolong life in patients with metastatic disease. For patients who are cisplatin-ineligible or have progressed after receiving cisplatin-based regimens, newer immunotherapies using PD-1 and PD-L1 inhibitors have been approved.

Treatment of recurrent cancer depends on clinical stage and site of recurrence and previous treatment. Recurrence after transurethral resection of superficial tumors is usually treated with a 2nd resection or fulguration.

Table 249–1. AJCC/TNM* STAGING OF BLADDER CANCER

STAGE	TUMOR	REGIONAL LYMPH NODE METASTASIS	DISTANT METASTASIS
0a	Ta	N0	M0
0is	Tis	N0	M0
I	T1	N0	M0
II	T2a	N0	M0
	T2b	N0	M0
III	T3a	N0	M0
	T3b	N0	M0
	T4a	N0	M0
IV	T4b	N0	M0
	Any T	N1–N3	M0
	Any T	Any N	M1

*For AJCC/TMN definitions, see Table 249–2.

AJCC = American Joint Commission on Cancer; T = primary tumor; N = regional lymph node metastasis; M = distant metastasis.

Data from Edge SB, Byrd DR, Compton CC, et al: *AJCC Cancer Staging Manual*, 7th ed. New York, Springer, 2010.

Table 249–2. TMN DEFINITIONS FOR BLADDER CANCER

FEATURE	DEFINITION
Primary tumor	
Ta	Noninvasive papillary
Tis	Flat tumors (carcinoma in situ)
T1	Invades subepithelial connective tissue
T2	Invades muscle
T2a	Invades superficial muscle (inner half)
T2b	Invades deep muscle (outer half)
T3	Invades perivesical tissue
T3a	Invades perivesical tissue microscopically
T3b	Invades perivesical tissue macroscopically (extravesical mass)
T4	Invades adjacent organs
T4a	Invades prostate, uterus, or vagina
T4b	Invades pelvic or abdominal wall
Regional lymph node metastasis	
NX	Not assessable
N0	No lymph node metastases
N1	Single node in true pelvis
N2	≥ 2 nodes in true pelvis
N3	≥ 1 common iliac node
Distant metastasis	
M0	No distant metastases
M1	Distant metastases

TMN = tumor, node, metastasis.
Data from Edge SB, Byrd DR, Compton CC, et al: *AJCC Cancer Staging Manual*, 7th ed. New York, Springer, 2010.

KEY POINTS

- Risk of bladder cancer increases with smoking, phenacetin or cyclophosphamide use, chronic irritation, or exposure to certain chemicals.
- Transitional (urothelial) cell carcinoma is > 90% of bladder cancers.
- Suspect bladder cancer in patients with unexplained hematuria or other urinary symptoms (particularly middle-aged or older men).
- Diagnose bladder cancer via cystoscopic biopsy and, if there is muscle invasion, do imaging studies for staging.
- Remove superficial cancers by transurethral resection or fulguration, followed by repeated bladder instillations of drugs.
- If cancer penetrates the muscle, treat with radical cystectomy with urinary diversion.

PENILE CANCER

Most penile cancers are squamous cell carcinomas; they usually occur in uncircumcised men, particularly those with poor local hygiene. Diagnosis is by biopsy. Treatment includes excision.

Human papillomavirus, particularly types 16 and 18, plays a role in etiology. Premalignant lesions include erythroplasia of Queyrat, Bowen disease, and bowenoid papulosis. Erythroplasia of Queyrat (affecting the glans or inner prepuce) and Bowen disease (affecting the shaft) progress to invasive squamous cell carcinoma in 5 to 10% of patients; bowenoid papulosis does not appear to do so. The 3 lesions have different clinical manifestations and biologic effects but are virtually the same histologically; they may be more appropriately called intraepithelial neoplasia or carcinoma in situ.

Symptoms and Signs

Most squamous cell carcinomas originate on the glans, in the coronal sulcus, or under the foreskin. They usually begin as a small erythematous lesion and may be confined to the skin for a long time. These carcinomas may be fungating and exophytic or ulcerative and infiltrative. The latter type metastasizes more commonly, usually to the superficial and deep inguinofemoral and pelvic nodes. Metastases to distant sites (eg, lungs, liver, bone, brain) are rare until late in the disease.

Most patients present with a sore that has not healed, subtle induration of the skin, or sometimes a pus-filled or warty growth. The sore may be shallow or deep with rolled edges. Many patients do not notice the cancer or do not report it promptly. Pain is uncommon. Inguinal nodes may be enlarged due to inflammation and secondary infection.

Diagnosis

If cancer is suspected, biopsy is required; if possible, tissue under the lesion should be sampled. CT or MRI helps in staging localized cancer, checking for invasion of the corpora, and evaluating lymph nodes.

Treatment

- Excision
- For small lesions, sometimes topical treatment

Untreated penile cancer progresses, typically causing death within 2 yr. Treated early, penile cancer can usually be cured.

Topical treatment with 5-fluourouracil or imiquod and laser ablation are effective for small, superficial lesions. Circumcision is preferred for lesions of the foreskin. Wide excision is preferred for recurrent lesions or in patients who cannot reliably follow-up. Mohs surgery can be done instead of wide excision where available.

Invasive and high-grade lesions require more radical resection. Partial penectomy is appropriate if the tumor can be completely excised with adequate margins, leaving a penile stump that permits urination and sexual function. Total penectomy is required for large infiltrative lesions. If tumors are high-grade or invade the corpora cavernosa, bilateral ilioinguinal lymphadenectomy is required. The role of radiation therapy has not been established. For advanced, invasive cancer, palliation may include surgery and radiation therapy, but cure is unlikely. Chemotherapy for advanced cancer has had limited success.

KEY POINTS

- Penile cancer is usually squamous or another skin cancer.
- Consider penile cancer with any nonhealing sore, induration, or purulent or warty penile growth, particularly in uncircumcised men.
- Diagnose penile cancer by biopsy and treat it by excision.

PROSTATE CANCER

Prostate cancer is usually adenocarcinoma. Symptoms are usually absent until tumor growth causes hematuria and/or obstruction with pain. Diagnosis is suggested by digital rectal examination or prostate-specific antigen measurement and confirmed by biopsy. Screening is controversial and should involve shared decision making. Prognosis for most patients with prostate cancer, especially when it is localized or regional (usually before symptoms develop), is very good; more men die with prostate cancer than of it. Treatment is with prostatectomy, radiation therapy, palliative measures (eg, hormonal therapy, radiation therapy, chemotherapy), or, for many elderly and even carefully selected younger patients, active surveillance.

Adenocarcinoma of the prostate is the most common nondermatologic cancer in men > 50 in the US. In the US, about 161,360 new cases and about 26,730 deaths (2017 estimates) occur each year. Incidence increases with each decade of life; autopsy studies show prostate cancer in 15 to 60% of men age 60 to 90 yr, with incidence increasing with age. The lifetime risk of being diagnosed with prostate cancer is 1 in 6. Median age at diagnosis is 72, and > 75% of prostate cancers are diagnosed in men > 65. Risk is highest for black men.

Sarcoma of the prostate is rare, occurring primarily in children. Undifferentiated prostate cancer, squamous cell carcinoma, and ductal transitional carcinoma also occur infrequently. Prostatic intraepithelial neoplasia is considered a possible premalignant histologic change.

Hormonal influences contribute to the course of adenocarcinoma but almost certainly not to other types of prostate cancer.

Symptoms and Signs

Prostate cancer usually progresses slowly and rarely causes symptoms until advanced. In advanced disease, hematuria and symptoms of bladder outlet obstruction (eg, straining, hesitancy, weak or intermittent urine stream, a sense of incomplete emptying, terminal dribbling) may appear. Bone pain, pathologic fractures, or spinal cord compression may result from osteoblastic metastases to bone (commonly pelvis, ribs, vertebral bodies).

Diagnosis

- Screening by digital rectal examination and prostate-specific antigen
- Assessment of abnormalities by transrectal needle biopsy
- Grading by histology
- Staging by CT and bone scanning

Sometimes stony-hard induration or nodules are palpable during digital rectal examination (DRE), but the examination is often normal; induration and nodularity suggest cancer but must be differentiated from granulomatous prostatitis, prostate calculi, and other prostate disorders. Extension of induration to the seminal vesicles and lateral fixation of the gland suggest locally advanced prostate cancer. Prostate cancers detected by DRE tend to be large, and > 50% extend through the capsule.

Diagnosis of prostate cancer requires histologic confirmation, most commonly by transrectal ultrasound (TRUS)–guided needle biopsy, which can be done in an office with use of local anesthesia. Hypoechoic areas are more likely to represent cancer. Occasionally, prostate cancer is diagnosed incidentally in tissue removed during surgery for benign prostatic hyperplasia (BPH).

Screening: Most cancers today are found by screening with serum prostate-specific antigen (PSA) levels (and sometimes DRE). Screening is commonly done annually in men > 50 yr but is sometimes begun earlier for men at high risk (eg, those with a family history of prostate cancer and black men). Screening is not usually recommended for men with a life expectancy < 10 to 15 yr. Abnormal findings are further investigated with biopsy.

It is still not certain whether screening decreases morbidity or mortality or whether any gains resulting from screening outweigh the decreases in quality of life resulting from treatment of asymptomatic cancers. Screening is recommended by some professional organizations and discouraged by others. Most patients with newly diagnosed prostate cancers have a normal DRE, and serum PSA measurement is not ideal as a screening test. Although PSA is elevated in 25 to 92% of patients with prostate cancer (depending on tumor volume), it also is moderately elevated in 30 to 50% of patients with BPH (depending on prostate size and degree of obstruction), in some smokers, and for several weeks after prostatitis. A level of ≥ 4 ng/mL has traditionally been considered an indication for biopsy in men > 50 yr (in younger patients, levels > 2.5 ng/mL probably warrant biopsy because BPH, the most common cause of PSA elevation, is rare in younger men). Although very high levels are significant (suggesting extracapsular extension of the tumor or metastases) and likelihood of cancer increases with increasing PSA levels, there is no cut-off below which there is no risk.

In asymptomatic patients, positive predictive value for cancer is 67% for PSA > 10 ng/mL and 25% for PSA 4 to 10 ng/mL; recent evidence indicates a 15% prevalence of cancer in men ≥ 55 yr with PSA < 4 ng/mL and a 10% incidence with PSA between 0.6 and 1.0 ng/mL. However, cancer present in men with lower levels tends to be smaller (often < 1 mL) and of lower grade, although high-grade cancer (Gleason score 7 to 10) can be present at any level of PSA; perhaps 15% of cancers manifesting with PSA < 4 ng/mL are high grade. Although it appears that a cut-off of 4 ng/mL will miss some potentially serious cancers, the cost and morbidity resulting from the increased number of biopsies necessary to find them is unclear.

The decision whether to biopsy may be helped by other PSA-related factors, even in the absence of a family history of prostate cancer. For example, the rate of change in PSA (PSA velocity) should be < 0.75 ng/mL/yr (lower in younger patients). Biopsy is indicated for PSA velocities > 0.75 ng/mL/yr.

Assays that determine the free-to-total PSA ratio and complex PSA are more tumor-specific than standard total PSA measurements and may reduce the frequency of biopsies in patients without cancer. Prostate cancer is associated with less free PSA; no standard cut-off has been established, but generally, levels < 10 to 20% warrant biopsy. Other isoforms of PSA and new markers for prostate cancer are being studied. None of these other uses of PSA answers all of the concerns about possibly triggering too many biopsies. Many new tests (eg, urinary prostate cancer antigen 3 [PCA-3], Prostate Health Index, 4Kscore, Select MDX, Confirm MDX) are under evaluation as aids to screening decisions.

Clinicians should discuss the risks and benefits of PSA testing with patients. Some patients prefer to eradicate cancer at all costs no matter how low the potential for progression and possible metastasis and may prefer annual PSA testing. Others may value quality of life highly and can accept some uncertainty; they may prefer less frequent (or no) PSA testing.

Grading and staging: Grading, based on the resemblance of tumor architecture to normal glandular structure, helps define the aggressiveness of the tumor. Grading takes into account histologic heterogeneity in the tumor. The Gleason score is commonly used. The most prevalent pattern and the next most prevalent pattern are each assigned a grade of 1 to 5, and the two grades are added to produce a total score. Most experts consider a score ≤ 6 to be well differentiated, 7 moderately differentiated, and 8 to 10 poorly differentiated.

The lower the score, the less aggressive and invasive is the tumor and the better is the prognosis. For localized tumors, the Gleason score helps predict the likelihood of capsular penetration, seminal vesicle invasion, and spread to lymph nodes.

Elimination of Gleason patterns 1 and 2 as well as patient confusion surrounding a score of 6 on a 2–10 point scale representing the lowest grade of disease has led to the use of a new grading terminology accepted by the WHO in 2016:

- Grade group 1 = Gleason 3+3
- Grade group 2 = Gleason 3+4
- Grade group 3 = Gleason 4+3
- Grade group 4 = Gleason 8
- Grade group 5 = Gleason 9 and 10

Gleason score, clinical stage, and PSA level together (using tables or nomograms) predict pathologic stage and prognosis better than any of them alone.

Prostate cancer is staged to define extent of the tumor (Tables 249–3 and 249–4). Transrectal ultrasonography (TRUS) may provide information for staging, particularly about capsular penetration and seminal vesicle invasion. Patients with clinical stage T1c to T2a tumors, low Gleason score (≤ 7), and PSA < 10 ng/mL usually get no additional staging tests before proceeding to treatment. Radionuclide bone scans are rarely helpful for finding bone metastases (they are frequently abnormal because of the trauma of arthritic changes) until the PSA is > 20 ng/mL or unless the Gleason score is high (ie, ≥ 8 or [4 +3]). CT (or MRI) of the abdomen and pelvis is commonly done to assess pelvic and retroperitoneal lymph nodes if the Gleason score is 8 to 10 and the PSA is > 10 ng/mL, or if the PSA is > 20 ng/mL with any Gleason score. Suspect lymph nodes can be further evaluated by using needle biopsy. An MRI with endorectal coil may also help define the local extent of the tumor in patients with locally advanced prostate cancer (stage T3). The role of In-111 capromab pendetide scanning for staging is evolving but is certainly not needed for early, localized disease. Elevated serum acid phosphatase—especially the enzymatic assay—correlates well with the presence of metastases, particularly in lymph nodes. However, this enzyme may also be elevated in BPH (and is slightly elevated after vigorous prostatic massage), multiple myeloma, Gaucher disease, and hemolytic anemia. It is rarely used today to guide treatment or to follow patients after treatment, especially because its value when done as a radioimmune assay (the way it is usually done) has not been established. Reverse transcriptase–PCR assays for circulating prostate cancer cells are being studied as staging and prognostic tools.

Risk of cancer spread is considered low if

- Stage is ≤ T2a
- Gleason score is ≤ 6
- PSA level is ≤ 10 ng/mL

T2b tumor, Gleason score 7, or PSA > 10 ng/mL are considered intermediate risk by most experts. T2c tumor, Gleason score ≥ 8, or PSA > 20 ng/mL (or 2 intermediate risk factors) are generally high risk.

Risk of cancer spread can be estimated by tumor stage, Gleason score, and PSA level:

- Low risk: Stage ≤ T2a, Gleason score ≤ 6, and PSA level ≤ 10 ng/mL
- Intermediate risk: Stage T2b, Gleason score = 7, or PSA level ≥ 10 and ≤ 20 ng/mL
- High risk: Stage ≥ T2c, Gleason score ≥ 8, or PSA ≥ 20 ng/mL

Both acid phosphatase and PSA levels decrease after treatment and increase with recurrence, but PSA is the most sensitive marker for monitoring cancer progression and response to treatment and has virtually replaced acid phosphatase for this purpose.

Table 249–3. AJCC/TMN* STAGING OF PROSTATE CANCER

STAGE	TUMOR	REGIONAL LYMPH NODE METASTASIS	DISTANT METASTASIS	PROSTATE-SPECIFIC ANTIGEN LEVEL	GLEASON SCORE
I	T1a–T1c	N0	M0	< 10 ng/mL	≤ 6
	T2a	N0	M0	< 10 ng/mL	≤ 6
	T1–T2a	N0	M0	Unknown	Unknown
IIA	T1a–T1c	N0	M0	< 20 ng/mL	7
	T1a–T1c	N0	M0	≥10 ng/mL but < 20 ng/mL	≤ 6
	T2a	N0	M0	≥ 10 ng/ml but < 20 ng/mL	≤ 6
	T2a	N0	M0	< 20 ng/mL	7
	T2b	N0	M0	< 20 ng/mL	≤ 7
	T2b	N0	M0	Unknown	Unknown
IIB	T2c	N0	M0	Any	Any
	T1–T2	N0	M0	≥ 20 ng/mL	Any
	T1–T2	N0	M0	Any PSA	≥ 8
III	T3a–T3b	N0	M0	Any PSA	Any Gleason
IV	T4	N0	M0	Any PSA	Any Gleason
	Any T	N1	M0	Any PSA	Any Gleason
	Any T	Any N	M1	Any PSA	Any Gleason

*For AJCC/TMN definitions, see Table 249–4.

AJCC = American Joint Commission on Cancer; PSA = prostate-specific antigen; TNM = tumor, node, metastasis.

Adapted from Edge SB, Byrd DR, Compton CC, et al: *AJCC Cancer Staging Manual*, 7th ed. New York, Springer, 2010.

Table 249–4. TNM DEFINITIONS FOR PROSTATE CANCER

FEATURE	DEFINITION
Primary tumor	
T1	Clinically inapparent by palpation or imaging
T1a	Incidentally found in ≤ 5% of resected tissue
T1b	Incidentally found in > 5% of resected tissue
T1c	Identified by needle biopsy done for elevated PSA level
T2	Is palpable or reliably visible by imaging Limited to prostate
T2a	Involves ≤ 50% of one lobe
T2b	Involves > 50% of one lobe and spares the other lobe
T2c	Involves both lobes
T3	Extends through the prostatic capsule
T3a	Extends through the prostatic capsule unilaterally or bilaterally
T3b	Invades seminal vesicles
T4	Is fixed or invades adjacent structures other than seminal vesicles
Regional lymph node metastasis	
NX	Not assessed
N0	None
N1	Present
Distant metastasis	
M0	None
M1	Present

AJCC = American Joint Commission on Cancer; PSA = prostate-specific antigen; TMN = tumor, node, metastasis.

Data from Edge SB, Byrd DR, Compton CC, et al: *AJCC Cancer Staging Manual*, 7th ed. New York, Springer, 2010.

Prognosis

Prognosis for most patients with prostate cancer, especially when it is localized or regional, is very good. Life expectancy for elderly men with prostate cancer may differ little from age-matched men without prostate cancer, depending on their age and comorbidities. For many patients, long-term local control, or even cure, is possible. Potential for cure, even when cancer is clinically localized, depends on the tumor's grade and stage. Without early treatment, patients with high-grade, poorly differentiated cancer have a poor prognosis. Undifferentiated prostate cancer, squamous cell carcinoma, and ductal transitional carcinoma respond poorly to conventional therapies. Metastatic cancer has no cure. Median life expectancy with metastatic disease is 1 to 3 yr, although some patients live for many years.

Treatment

- For localized cancer within the prostate, surgery or radiation therapy
- For cancer outside of the prostate, palliation with hormonal therapy, radiation therapy, or chemotherapy
- For some men who have low-risk cancers, active surveillance without treatment

Treatment is guided by PSA level, grade and stage of tumor, patient age, coexisting disorders, and life expectancy. The goal of therapy can be

- Active surveillance
- Local (aimed at cure)
- Systemic (aimed at decreasing or limiting tumor extent)

Most patients, regardless of age, prefer definitive therapy if cancer is potentially curable. However, therapy is palliative rather than definitive if cancer has spread outside the prostate because cure is unlikely. Watchful waiting can be used for men unlikely to benefit from definitive therapy (eg, because of older age or comorbidity); these patients are treated with palliative measures if symptoms develop.

Active surveillance: Active surveillance is appropriate for many asymptomatic patients > 70 with low-risk, or possibly even intermediate-risk, localized prostate cancer or if life-limiting disorders coexist; in these patients, risk of death due to other causes is greater than that due to prostate cancer. This approach requires periodic DRE, PSA measurement, and monitoring of symptoms. In healthy younger men with low-risk cancer, active surveillance also requires periodic repeat biopsies. The optimal interval between biopsies has not been established, but most experts agree that it should be ≥ 1 yr, possibly less frequently if biopsies have been repeatedly negative. If the cancer progresses, treatment is required. About 30% of patients undergoing active surveillance eventually require therapy. In elderly men, active surveillance results in the same overall survival rate as prostatectomy; however, patients who had surgery have a significantly lower risk of distant metastases and disease-specific mortality.

Local therapies: Local therapy is aimed at curing prostate cancer and may thus also be called definitive therapy. Radical prostatectomy, some forms of radiation therapy, and cryotherapy are options. Careful counseling concerning the risks and benefits of these treatments and considerations of patient-specific characteristics (age, health, tumor characteristics) are critical in decision making.

Radical **prostatectomy** (removal of prostate with seminal vesicles and regional lymph nodes) is probably best for patients < 70 with a tumor confined to the prostate. Prostatectomy is appropriate for some elderly men, based on life expectancy, coexisting disorders, and ability to tolerate surgery and anesthesia. Prostatectomy is done through an incision in the lower abdomen. More recently, a robot-assisted laparoscopic approach has been developed that minimizes blood loss and hospital stay but has not been shown to alter morbidity or mortality. Complications include urinary incontinence (in about 5 to 10%), bladder neck contracture or urethral stricture (in about 7 to 20%), erectile dysfunction (in about 30 to 100%—heavily dependent on age and current function), and rectal injury (in 1 to 2%). Nerve-sparing radical prostatectomy reduces the likelihood of erectile dysfunction but cannot always be done, depending on tumor stage and location.

Cryotherapy (destruction of prostate cancer cells by freezing with cryoprobes, followed by thawing) is less well established; long-term outcomes are unknown. Adverse effects include bladder outlet obstruction, urinary incontinence, erectile dysfunction, and rectal pain or injury. Cryotherapy is not commonly the therapy of choice in the US but may be used if radiation therapy is unsuccessful.

Standard external beam **radiation therapy** usually delivers 70 Gy in 7 wk, but this technique has been supplanted by conformal 3-dimensional radiation therapy and by intensity modulated radiation therapy (IMRT), which safely deliver doses approaching 80 Gy to the prostate; data indicate that the rate of local control is higher, especially for high-risk patients. Some decrease in erectile function occurs in at least 40%. Other adverse effects include radiation proctitis, cystitis, diarrhea, fatigue, and possibly urethral strictures, particularly in patients with a prior history of transurethral resection of the prostate. Results with radiation therapy and prostatectomy were shown to be comparable, up to 10 yr after treatment in the ProtecT trial. Newer forms of radiation therapy such as proton therapy are more costly, and the benefits in men with prostate cancer are not clearly established. External beam radiation therapy also has a role if cancer is left after radical prostatectomy or if the PSA level begins to rise after surgery and no metastasis can be found.

Brachytherapy involves the implantation of radioactive seeds into the prostate through the perineum. These seeds emit a burst of radiation over a finite period (usually 3 to 6 mo) and are then inert. Research protocols are examining whether high-quality implants used as monotherapy or implants plus external beam radiation therapy are superior for intermediate-risk patients. Brachytherapy also decreases erectile function, although onset may be delayed and patients may be more responsive to phosphodiesterase type 5 inhibitors than patients whose neurovascular bundles are resected or injured during surgery. Urinary frequency, urgency, and, less often, retention are common but usually subside over time. Other adverse effects include increased bowel movements; rectal urgency, bleeding, or ulceration; and prostatorectal fistulas.

If cancer localized to the prostate is high risk, various therapies may need to be combined (eg, for high-risk prostate cancer treated with external beam radiation, addition of hormonal therapy).

Systemic therapies: If cancer has spread beyond the prostate gland, cure is unlikely; systemic treatment aimed at decreasing or limiting tumor extent is usually given.

Patients with a locally advanced tumor or metastases may benefit from androgen deprivation by castration, either surgically with bilateral orchiectomy or medically with luteinizing hormone-releasing hormone (LHRH) agonists, such as leuprolide, goserelin, triptorelin, histrelin, and buserelin, with or without radiation therapy. LHRH antagonists (eg, degarelix) can also lower the testosterone level, usually more rapidly than LHRH agonists. LHRH agonists and LHRH antagonists usually reduce serum testosterone almost as much as bilateral orchiectomy.

Hormone-sensitive metastatic prostate cancer has been shown to have increased survival if abiraterone and prednisone are added to standard therapy.

All androgen deprivation treatments cause loss of libido and erectile dysfunction and may cause hot flushes. LHRH agonists may cause PSA levels to increase temporarily. Some patients benefit from adding antiandrogens (eg, flutamide, bicalutamide, nilutamide, cyproterone acetate [not available in US]) for total androgen blockade. Combined androgen blockade usually refers to LHRH agonists plus antiandrogens, but its benefits appear minimally better than those of an LHRH agonist (or degarelix or orchiectomy) alone. Another approach is intermittent androgen blockade, which purports to delay emergence of androgen-independent prostate cancer and helps to limit some adverse effects of androgen deprivation. Total androgen ablation is given until PSA levels are reduced (usually to undetectable levels), then stopped. Treatment is started again when PSA levels rise above a certain threshold, although the ideal threshold is not yet defined. The optimal schedules for treatment and time off treatment have not been determined and vary widely among practitioners. Androgen deprivation may impair quality of life significantly (eg, self-image, attitude toward the cancer and its treatment, energy levels) and cause osteoporosis, anemia, and loss of muscle mass with long-term treatment. Exogenous estrogens are rarely used because they have a risk of cardiovascular and thromboembolic complications.

Hormonal therapy is effective in metastatic prostate cancer for a limited amount of time. Cancer that progresses (indicated by an increasing PSA level) despite a testosterone level consistent with castration (< 50 ng/dL) is classified as **castrate-resistant prostate cancer.** Treatments that prolong survival in castrate-resistant prostate cancer (many identified since 2010) include docetaxel (a taxane chemotherapy drug), sipuleucel-T (a vaccine designed to induce immunity against prostate cancer cells), abiraterone (which blocks androgen synthesis in the tumor as well as in the testes and adrenal glands), enzalutamide (which blocks binding of androgens to their receptors), and cabazitaxel (a taxane chemotherapy drug that may have activity in tumors that have become resistant to docetaxel). Some data suggest that sipuleucel-T should be used at the earliest sign of castrate-resistant prostate cancer. In general, treatments for castrate-resistant prostate cancer are being tried earlier during the course of prostate cancer. However, choice of treatment may involve many factors, and few data may be available to help predict results; thus patient education and shared decision making are recommended.

To help treat and prevent complications due to **bone metastases** (eg, pathologic fractures, pain, spinal cord compression), an osteoclast inhibitor (eg, denosumab, zoledronic acid) can be used. Traditional external beam radiation therapy has been used to treat individual bone metastases. Radium-233, which emits alpha radiation, was recently found to prolong survival as well as prevent complications due to bone metastases in men with castrate-resistant prostate cancer.

KEY POINTS

- Prostate cancer develops very commonly with aging but is not always clinically important.
- Symptoms develop only after the cancer has enlarged enough to be more difficult to cure.
- Complications due to bone metastases are common and consequential.
- Diagnose prostate cancer by TRUS-guided needle biopsy.
- Discuss advantages and disadvantages of screening in men > age 50 with life expectancy > 10 or 15 yr.
- For localized prostate cancer, consider local, curative treatment (eg, prostatectomy, radiation therapy) and active surveillance.
- For cancer that has spread beyond the prostate, consider systemic treatments (eg, various hormonal therapies, sipuleucel-T, taxane chemotherapy).
- For bone metastases, consider radium-233 and osteoclast inhibitors.

RENAL CELL CARCINOMA

(Adenocarcinoma of the Kidneys)

Renal cell carcinoma (RCC) is the most common renal cancer. Symptoms can include hematuria, flank pain, a palpable mass, and FUO. However, symptoms are often absent, so the diagnosis is usually suspected based on incidental findings. Diagnosis is confirmed by CT or MRI and occasionally by biopsy. Treatment is with surgery for early disease and targeted therapy, an experimental protocol, or palliative therapy for advanced disease.

RCC, an adenocarcinoma, accounts for 90 to 95% of primary malignant renal tumors. Less common primary renal tumors include transitional cell carcinoma, Wilms tumor (most often in children—see p. 2783), and sarcoma.

In the US, about 65,000 cases of RCC and pelvic tumors and 13,000 deaths occur each year. RCC occurs slightly more often in men (male:female incidence is about 3:2). People affected are usually between 50 and 70 yr. Risk factors include the following:

- Smoking, which doubles the risk (in 20 to 30% of patients)
- Obesity
- Excess use of phenacetin
- Acquired cystic kidney disease in dialysis patients
- Exposure to certain radiopaque dyes, asbestos, cadmium, and leather tanning and petroleum products
- Some familial syndromes, particularly von Hippel–Lindau disease

RCC can trigger thrombus formation in the renal vein, which occasionally propagates into the vena cava. Tumor invasion of the vein wall is uncommon. RCC metastasizes most often to the lymph nodes, lungs, adrenal glands, liver, brain, and bone.

Symptoms and Signs

Symptoms usually do not appear until late, when the tumor may already be large and metastatic. Gross or microscopic hematuria is the most common manifestation, followed by flank pain, FUO, and a palpable mass. Sometimes hypertension results from segmental ischemia or pedicle compression. Paraneoplastic syndromes occur in 20% of patients. Polycythemia can result from increased erythropoietin activity. However, anemia may also occur. Hypercalcemia is common and may require treatment (see p. 1285). Thrombocytosis, cachexia, or secondary amyloidosis may develop.

Diagnosis

- CT with contrast or MRI

Most often, a renal mass is detected incidentally during abdominal imaging (eg, CT, ultrasonography) done for other reasons. Otherwise, diagnosis is suggested by clinical findings and confirmed by abdominal CT before and after injection of a radiocontrast agent or by MRI. A renal mass that is enhanced by radiocontrast strongly suggests RCC. CT and MRI also provide information about local extension and nodal and venous involvement. MRI provides further information about extension into the renal vein and vena cava and has replaced inferior vena cavography. Ultrasonography and IVU may show a mass but provide less information about the characteristics of the mass and extent of disease than do CT or MRI. Often, nonmalignant and malignant masses can be distinguished radiographically, but sometimes surgery is needed for confirmation. Needle biopsy does not have sufficient sensitivity when findings are equivocal; it is recommended only when there is an infiltrative pattern instead of a discrete mass, when the renal mass may be a metastasis from another known cancer, or sometimes to confirm a diagnosis before chemotherapy for metastases.

Three-dimensional CT, CT angiography, or magnetic resonance angiography is used before surgery, particularly before nephron-sparing surgery, to define the nature of RCC, to more accurately determine the number of renal arteries present, and to delineate the vascular pattern. These imaging techniques have replaced aortography and selective renal artery angiography.

A chest x-ray and liver function tests are essential. If chest x-ray is abnormal, chest CT is done. If alkaline phosphatase is elevated, bone scanning is needed. Serum electrolytes, BUN, creatinine, and Ca are measured. BUN and creatinine are unaffected unless both kidneys are diseased.

Staging: Information from the evaluation makes preliminary staging possible. The TNM (tumor, node, metastasis) system has been recently refined to be precise (Tables 249–5 and 249–6). At diagnosis, RCC is localized in 45%, locally invasive in about 33%, and spread to distant organs in 25%.

Prognosis

Five-year survival rates range from about 81% for the American Joint Commission on Cancer (AJCC) stage grouping I (T1 N0 M0) to 8% for stage grouping IV (T4 or M1). Prognosis is poor for patients with metastatic or recurrent RCC because treatments are usually ineffective for cure, although they may be useful for palliation.

Treatment

- For early RCC, surgical treatment
- For advanced RCC, palliative therapies or experimental protocols

Curative treatments: Radical nephrectomy (removal of kidney, adrenal gland, perirenal fat, and Gerota fascia) is standard treatment for localized RCC and provides a reasonable chance for cure. Results with open or laparoscopic procedures are comparable; recovery is easier with laparoscopic procedures. Nephron-sparing surgery (partial nephrectomy) is possible and appropriate for many patients, even in patients with a normal contralateral kidney if the tumor is < 4 to 7 cm. Nonsurgical destruction of renal tumors via freezing (cryosurgery) or thermal energy (radiofrequency ablation) are not currently recommended as primary treatment. They are being done in highly selected patients, but long-term data about efficacy and indications are not yet available.

Table 249–5. AJCC/TNM* STAGING OF RENAL CELL CARCINOMA

STAGE	TUMOR	REGIONAL LYMPH NODE METASTASIS	DISTANT METASTASIS
I	T1	N0	M0
II	T2	N0	M0
III	T1 or T2	N1	M0
	T3	N0 or N1	M0
IV	T4	Any N	M0
	Any T	Any N	M1

*For AJCC/TMN definitions, see Table 249–6.

AJCC = American Joint Commission on Cancer; TNM = tumor, node, metastasis.

Adapted from Edge SB, Byrd DR, Compton CC, et al: *AJCC Cancer Staging Manual,* 7th ed. New York, Springer, 2010.

Table 249–6. TMN DEFINITIONS FOR RENAL CELL CARCINOMA

FEATURE	DEFINITION
Primary tumor	
T1	≤ 7 cm in greatest dimension Limited to kidney
T1a	≤ 4 cm in greatest dimension
T1b	> 4 cm but ≤ 7 cm in greatest dimension
T2	≥ 7 cm in greatest dimension Limited to kidney
T2a	> 7 cm but ≤ 10 cm in greatest dimension
T2b	> 10 cm in greatest dimension
T3	Extends into major veins or invades perinephric tissues but not beyond Gerota fascia or into the adrenal gland
T3a	Extends into renal veins or its segmental branches or invades perirenal and/or renal sinus fat, but not beyond Gerota fascia
T3b	Grossly extends into the vena cava below the diaphragm
T3c	Grossly extends into vena cava above the diaphragm or invades the wall of the vena cava
T4	Invades beyond Gerota fascia, including contiguous extension into the ipsilateral adrenal gland (non-contiguous extension into an adrenal gland is considered a metastasis)
Regional lymph node metastasis	
NX	Not assessable
N0	None
N1	Present
Distant metastasis	
M0	None
M1	Present

AJCC = American Joint Commission on Cancer; TMN = tumor, node, metastasis.

Data from Edge SB, Byrd DR, Compton CC, et al: *AJCC Cancer Staging Manual,* 7th ed. New York, Springer, 2010.

For tumors involving the renal vein and vena cava, surgery may be curative if no nodal or distant metastases exist.

If both kidneys are affected, partial nephrectomy of one or both kidneys is preferable to bilateral radical nephrectomy if technically feasible.

Radiation therapy is no longer combined with nephrectomy.

Palliative treatments: Palliation can include nephrectomy, tumor embolization, and possibly external beam radiation therapy. Resection of metastases offers palliation and, if metastases are limited in number, prolongs life in some patients, particularly those with a long interval between initial treatment (nephrectomy) and development of metastases. Although metastatic RCC is traditionally characterized as radioresistant, radiation therapy can be palliative when RCC is metastatic in bone.

For some patients, drug therapy reduces tumor size and prolongs life. About 10 to 20% of patients respond to interferon alfa-2b or IL-2, although the response is long-lasting in < 5%. Many targeted therapies have shown efficacy for advanced tumors: sunitinib, sorafenib, bevacizumab, pazopanib, cabozantinib, axitinib, and lenvatinib (tyrosine kinase inhibitors) and temsirolimus and everolimus, which inhibit the mammalian target of rapamycin (mTOR).

For metastatic RCC that has progressed on targeted therapy, nivolumab (a monoclonal antibody against PD-1) has been shown to improve overall survival by 5.4 mo (25.0 vs. 19.6 mo) compared to everolimus in patients who had been treated with one or more tyrosine kinase inhibitors.

Other treatments are experimental. They include stem cell transplantation, other interleukins, antiangiogenesis therapy (eg, thalidomide), and vaccine therapy. Traditional chemotherapeutic drugs, alone or combined, and progestins are ineffective. Cytoreductive nephrectomy before systemic therapy, or as a delayed surgical procedure to remove the primary tumor after response in the metastases, is commonly done in patients healthy enough to undergo it.

Increased knowledge of genetic subtypes of RCC is leading to evolving management recommendations that are more specific.

KEY POINTS

- RCC, an adenocarcinoma, accounts for 90 to 95% of primary malignant renal tumors.
- Symptoms (most often gross or microscopic hematuria) usually do not develop until the tumor is large or metastatic, so incidental discovery is common.
- Diagnose RCC by MRI or contrast-enhanced CT and do a chest x-ray and liver function tests.
- Treat most localized RCC by radical nephrectomy.
- Treat advanced RCC with palliative surgery, radiation therapy, targeted drug therapies, and/or interferon alfa-2b or IL-2.

RENAL METASTASES

Nonrenal cancers may metastasize to the kidneys. The most common cancers that metastasize to the kidney are melanomas and solid tumors, particularly lung, breast, stomach, gynecologic, intestinal, and pancreatic. Leukemia and lymphoma may invade the kidneys, which then appear enlarged, often asymmetrically.

Despite extensive interstitial involvement, symptoms are rare, and renal function may not change from baseline. Proteinuria is absent or insignificant, and blood urea and creatinine levels rarely increase unless a complication (eg, uric acid nephropathy, hypercalcemia, bacterial infection) occurs.

Renal metastases are usually discovered during evaluation of the primary tumor or incidentally during abdominal imaging. If there is no known primary tumor, diagnosis proceeds as for RCC (see p. 2100).

Treatment is systemic therapy for the primary tumor and, rarely, surgery; however, partial nephrectomy may be necessary to guide choice of systemic therapy in cases where core needle biopsy is unable to provide sufficient tissue.

RENAL PELVIC AND URETERAL CANCERS

Cancers of the renal pelvis and ureters are usually transitional cell carcinomas (TCCs) and occasionally squamous cell

carcinomas. Symptoms include hematuria and sometimes pain. Diagnosis is by CT, cytology, and sometimes biopsy. Treatment is surgery.

TCC of the renal pelvis accounts for about 7 to 15% of all kidney tumors. TCC of the ureters accounts for about 4% of upper tract tumors. Risk factors are the same as those for bladder cancer (smoking, excess phenacetin use, long-term cyclophosphamide use, chronic irritation, exposure to certain chemicals). Also, inhabitants of the Balkans with endemic familial nephropathy are inexplicably predisposed to develop upper tract TCC.

Symptoms and Signs

Most patients present with hematuria; dysuria and frequency may occur if the bladder also is involved. Colicky pain may accompany obstruction (see p. 2137). Uncommonly, hydronephrosis results from a renal pelvic tumor.

Diagnosis

- Ultrasonography or CT with contrast
- Cytology or histology

In patients with unexplained urinary tract symptoms, typically ultrasonography or CT with contrast is done. If the diagnosis cannot be excluded, cytologic or histologic analysis is done for confirmation. Ureteroscopy is done when biopsy of the upper tract is needed or when urine cytology is positive but no source of the malignant cells is obvious. Abdominal and pelvic CT and chest x-ray are done to determine tumor extent and to check for metastases.

Prognosis

Prognosis depends on depth of penetration into or through the uroepithelial wall, which is difficult to determine. Likelihood of cure is > 90% for patients with a superficial, localized tumor but is 10 to 15% for those with a deeply invasive tumor. If tumors penetrate the wall or distant metastases occur, cure is unlikely.

Treatment

- Excision or ablation
- Posttreatment surveillance with cystoscopy

Usual treatment is radical nephroureterectomy, including excision of a cuff of bladder. Partial ureterectomy is indicated in some carefully selected patients (eg, patients with a distal ureteral tumor, decreased renal function, or a solitary kidney). Laser fulguration for accurately staged and adequately visualized renal pelvic or low-grade ureteral tumors is sometimes possible. Occasionally, a drug, such as mitomycin C or BCG, is instilled. However, efficacy of laser therapy and chemotherapy has not been established. Checkpoint inhibitors of the PD-1/PD-L1 may prove to be a useful adjuvant treatment in cisplatin-ineligible patients with upper tract urethral cancer.

Periodic cystoscopy is indicated because renal pelvic and ureteral cancers tend to recur in the bladder, and such recurrence, if detected at an early stage, may be treated by fulguration, transurethral resection, or intravesical instillations. Management of metastases is the same as that for metastatic bladder cancer.

KEY POINTS

- Risk of renal pelvis and ureteral cancers increases with smoking, phenacetin or cyclophosphamide use, chronic irritation, or exposure to certain chemicals.
- Do ultrasonography or CT with contrast if urinary tract symptoms are unexplained.
- Confirm the diagnosis histologically.
- Excise or ablate tumors, usually using radical nephroureterectomy, and monitor patients with periodic cystoscopy.

TESTICULAR CANCER

Testicular cancer begins as a scrotal mass, which is usually not painful. Diagnosis is by ultrasonography. Treatment is with orchiectomy and sometimes lymph node dissection, radiation therapy, chemotherapy, or a combination, depending on histology and stage.

Testicular cancer is the most common solid cancer in males aged 15 to 35, with about 8000 cases annually, but only about 400 deaths. Incidence is 2.5 to 20 times higher in patients with cryptorchidism. This excess risk is decreased or eliminated if orchiopexy is done before age 10 yr. Cancer can also develop in the contralateral normally descended testis. The cause of testicular cancer is unknown.

Most testicular cancers originate in primordial germ cells. Germ cell tumors are categorized as seminomas (40%) or nonseminomas (tumors containing any nonseminomous elements). Nonseminomas include teratomas, embryonal carcinomas, endodermal sinus tumors (yolk sac tumors), and choriocarcinomas. Histologic combinations are common; eg, teratocarcinoma contains teratoma plus embryonal carcinoma. Functional interstitial cell carcinomas of the testis are rare.

Even patients with apparently localized tumors may have occult nodal or visceral metastases. For example, almost 30% of patients with nonseminomas will relapse with nodal or visceral metastases if they undergo no treatment after orchiectomy. Risk of metastases is highest for choriocarcinoma and lowest for teratoma.

Tumors originating in the epididymis, testicular appendages, and spermatic cord are usually benign fibromas, fibroadenomas, adenomatoid tumors, and lipomas. Sarcomas, most commonly rhabdomyosarcoma, occur occasionally, primarily in children.

Symptoms and Signs

Most patients present with a scrotal mass, which is painless or sometimes associated with dull, aching pain. In a few patients, hemorrhage into the tumor may cause acute local pain and tenderness. Many patients discover the mass themselves after minor scrotal trauma.

Diagnosis

- Ultrasonography for scrotal masses
- Exploration if testicular mass is present
- Staging by abdominal, pelvic, and chest CT as well as tissue examination

Many patients discover the mass themselves during self-examination. Monthly self-examination should be encouraged among young men.

The origin and nature of scrotal masses must be determined accurately because most testicular masses are malignant, but most extratesticular masses are not; distinguishing between the two during physical examination may be difficult. Scrotal ultrasonography can confirm testicular origin. If a testicular mass is confirmed, serum markers α-fetoprotein and β-human chorionic gonadotropin should be measured and a chest x-ray taken. Then, inguinal exploration is indicated; the spermatic cord is exposed and clamped before the abnormal testis is manipulated.

If cancer is confirmed, abdominal, pelvic, and chest CT is needed for clinical staging using the standard TNM (tumor,

Table 249–7. AJCC/TNM* STAGING OF TESTICULAR CANCER

STAGE	TUMOR	REGIONAL LYMPH NODE METASTASIS	DISTANT METASTASIS	SERUM TUMOR MARKERS
0	pTis	N0	M0	S0
I	pT1–pT4	N0	M0	SX
IA	pT1	N0	M0	S0
IB	pT2	N0	M0	S0
	pT3	N0	M0	S0
	pT4	N0	M0	S0
IS	Any pT/pTX	N0	M0	S1–S3
II	Any pT/pTX	N1–N3	M0	SX
IIA	Any pT/pTX	N1	M0	S0
	Any pT/pTX	N1	M0	S1
IIB	Any pT/pTX	N2	M0	S0
	Any pT/pTX	N2	M0	S1
IIC	Any pT/pTX	N3	M0	S0
	Any pT/pTX	N3	M0	S1
III	Any pT/pTX	Any N	M1	SX
IIIA	Any pTp/TX	Any N	M1a	S0–S1
IIIB	Any pT/pTX	N1–N3	M0	S2
	Any pT/pTX	Any N	M1a	S2
IIIC	Any pT/pTX	N1–N3	M0	S3
	Any pT/pTX	Any N	M1a	S3
	Any pT/pTX	Any N	M1b	Any S

*For AJCC/TNM staging definitions, see Table 249–8.

Adapted from Edge SB, Byrd DR, Compton CC, et al: *AJCC Cancer Staging Manual*, 7th ed. New York, Springer, 2010.

node, metastasis) system (Tables 249–7 and 249–8). Tissue obtained during treatment (usually radical inguinal orchiectomy) helps provide important histopathologic information, particularly about the proportion of histologic types and presence of intratumoral vascular or lymphatic invasion. Such information can predict the risk of occult lymph node and visceral metastases. Patients with nonseminomas have about a 30% risk of recurrence despite normal x-rays and serum markers and having what appears to be localized disease. Seminomas recur in about 15% of such patients.

Prognosis

Prognosis depends on histology and extent of the tumor. The 5-yr survival rate is > 95% for patients with a seminoma or nonseminoma localized to the testis or with a nonseminoma and low-volume metastases in the retroperitoneum. The 5-yr survival rate for patients with extensive retroperitoneal metastases or with pulmonary or other visceral metastases ranges from 48% (for some nonseminomas) to > 80%, depending on site, volume, and histology of the metastases, but even patients with advanced disease at presentation may be cured.

Treatment

- Radical inguinal orchiectomy
- Radiation therapy for seminomas
- Usually retroperitoneal lymph node dissection for nonseminomas

Radical inguinal orchiectomy is the cornerstone of treatment and helps provide important diagnostic information; it also helps formulate the subsequent treatment plan. A cosmetic testicular prosthesis may be placed during orchiectomy. Silicone prostheses are not widely available because of the problems with silicone breast implants. However, saline implants have been developed. For men who wish to retain reproductive capacity, sperm banking is potentially available in anticipation of radiation therapy or chemotherapy.

Radiation therapy: Standard treatment for seminoma after unilateral orchiectomy is radiation therapy, usually 20 to 40 Gy (higher dose is used for patients with a nodal mass) to the para-aortic regions up to the diaphragm. The ipsilateral ilioinguinal region is no longer routinely treated. Occasionally, the mediastinum and left supraclavicular regions are also irradiated, depending on clinical stage. However, in stage I disease, single-dose carboplatin has largely replaced radiation therapy due to concerns of long-term cardiovascular toxicity with radiation. There is no role for radiation therapy in nonseminoma.

Lymph node dissection: For nonseminomas, many experts consider standard treatment to be retroperitoneal lymph node dissection. For clinical stage 1 tumors in patients who have no prognostic factors that predict relapse, an alternative is active surveillance (frequent serum marker measurements, chest x-rays, CT). Intermediate-sized retroperitoneal nodal masses may require retroperitoneal lymph node dissection and chemotherapy (eg, bleomycin, etoposide, cisplatin), but the optimal sequence is undecided.

Table 249–8. TMN AND SERUM MARKER DEFINITIONS FOR TESTICULAR CANCER

FEATURE	DEFINITION
Tumor	
pTX	Not assessable
pT0	No evidence of primary tumor (eg, scar in testis)
pTis	Intratubular germ cell tumors (carcinoma in situ)
pT1	Limited to testis and epididymis without vascular or lymphatic invasion May invade tunica albuginea but not tunica vaginalis
pT2	Limited to testis and epididymis with vascular or lymphatic invasion, or extends through tunica albuginea and involves tunica vaginalis
pT3	Invades spermatic cord with or without vascular or lymphatic invasion
pT4	Invades scrotum with or without vascular or lymphatic invasion
Regional lymph node metastasis	
NX	Not assessable
N0	None
N1	≥ 1 node, all ≤ 2 cm in greatest dimension
N2	≥ 1 node > 2 cm but ≤ 5 cm in greatest dimension, with or without other nodes ≤ 5 cm in greatest dimension
N3	≥ 1 node > 5 cm in greatest dimension
Distant metastasis	
M0	None
M1	Present
M1a	Nonregional nodal or lung metastasis
M1b	Distant metastasis other than nonregional lymph nodes or lung
Serum markers	
SX	Markers not available or not measured
S0	Levels within normal limits
S1	LDH < 1.5 × the upper limit of normal for the LDH assay *and* hCG < 5000 mIu/mL *and* AFP < 1000 ng/mL
S2	LDH = 1.5–10 × upper limit of normal for the LDH assay *or* hCG 5000–50,000 mIu/mL *or* AFP 1000–10,000 ng/mL
S3	LDH > 10 × upper limit of normal for the LDH assay *or* hCG > 50,000 mIu/mL *or* AFP >10,000 ng/mL

AFP = alpha fetoprotein; AJCC = American Joint Commission on Cancer; hCG = human chorionic gonadotropin; p = pathologic staging; pT = primary tumor; N = regional lymph nodes (assessed clinically); M = distant metastases; S = serum tumor markers.

Data from Edge SB, Byrd DR, Compton CC, et al: *AJCC Cancer Staging Manual*, 7th ed. New York, Springer, 2010.

Lymph node dissection is done laparoscopically at some centers. The most common adverse effect of lymph node dissection overall is failure to ejaculate. However, a nerve-sparing dissection is often possible, particularly for early-stage tumors, which usually preserves ejaculation.

Chemotherapy: Nodal masses > 5 cm, lymph node metastases above the diaphragm, or visceral metastases require initial platinum-based combination chemotherapy followed by surgery for residual masses. Such treatment commonly controls the tumor long term. Fertility is often impaired, but no risk to the fetus has been proved if pregnancy does occur.

Surveillance: Surveillance is appropriate for some patients, although many clinicians do not offer this option because it requires rigorous follow-up protocols and excellent patient adherence to be safe. It is more commonly offered to patients at low risk of relapse. High-risk patients usually get retroperitoneal lymph node dissections or, in some centers, 2 courses of chemotherapy after orchiectomy instead of surgery.

Recurrences: Nonseminoma recurrences are usually treated with chemotherapy, although delayed retroperitoneal lymph node dissection may be appropriate for some patients with nodal relapse and no evidence of visceral metastases. Surveillance is not used as often for seminomas because the morbidity of 2 wk of radiation therapy is so low and the results in preventing late relapse so high that there is less reason to try to avoid treatment.

KEY POINTS

- Testicular cancer is the most common solid cancer in males aged 15 to 35 but is often curable, particularly seminoma.
- Assess scrotal masses by ultrasonography and if they are testicular, do a chest x-ray and measure α-fetoprotein and β-human chorionic gonadotropin.
- Do radical inguinal orchiectomy, usually with radiation therapy (for seminomas) and retroperitoneal lymph node dissection (for nonseminomas).

URETHRAL CANCER

Urethral cancer is rare and occurs in both sexes; it may be squamous or transitional cell carcinoma or, occasionally, adenocarcinoma.

Most patients are age ≥ 50. Certain strains of human papillomavirus have been implicated in certain cases. Urethral tumors invade adjacent structures early and thus tend to be advanced when diagnosed. External groin or pelvic (obturator) lymph nodes are usually the first sites of metastasis.

Symptoms and Signs

Most women present with hematuria and obstructive voiding symptoms or urinary retention. Most have a history of urinary frequency or urethral syndrome (hypersensitivity of the pelvic floor muscles). Most men present with symptoms of urethral stricture; only a few present with hematuria or a bloody discharge. Sometimes if the tumor is advanced, a mass is felt.

Diagnosis

Diagnosis is suggested clinically and confirmed by cystourethroscopy. Biopsy may be required to differentiate urethral carcinoma, prolapse, and caruncle. CT or MRI is used for staging.

Prognosis

Prognosis depends on the precise location in the urethra and extent of the cancer, particularly depth of invasion. The 5-yr survival rates are > 60% for patients with distal tumors and 10 to 20% for patients with proximal tumors. Recurrence rate is > 50%.

Treatment

- Usually excision or ablation

For superficial or minimally invasive distal tumors in the anterior urethra, treatment is with surgical excision, radiation therapy (interstitial or a combination of interstitial and external beam), fulguration, or laser ablation. Larger and more deeply invasive anterior tumors and proximal tumors in the posterior urethra require multimodal therapy with radical surgery and urinary diversion, usually in combination with radiation therapy. Surgery includes bilateral pelvic and sometimes inguinal lymph node dissection, often with removal of part of the symphysis pubis and inferior pubic rami. The value of chemotherapy, which is sometimes used, has not been established.

250 Glomerular Disorders

The hallmark of glomerular disorders is proteinuria, which is often in the nephrotic range (≥ 3 g/day).

Glomerular disorders are classified based on urine changes as those that manifest predominantly with

- Nephrotic range proteinuria, and nephrotic urine sediment (fatty casts, oval fat bodies, but few cells or cellular casts)
- Hematuria, usually in combination with proteinuria (which may be nephrotic range); the RBCs are usually dysmorphic and often there are RBC or mixed cellular casts (nephritic urine sediment)

Nephrotic syndrome is nephrotic urine sediment plus edema and hypoalbuminemia (typically with hypercholesterolemia and hypertriglyceridemia).

Nephritic syndrome is nephritic urine sediment with or without hypertension, elevated serum creatinine, and oliguria.

Several glomerular disorders typically manifest with features of both nephritic and nephrotic syndromes. These disorders include, but are not limited to, fibrillary and immunotactoid glomerulopathies, membranoproliferative glomerulonephritis (GN), and lupus nephritis.

The pathophysiology of nephritic and nephrotic disorders differs substantially, but their clinical overlap is considerable—eg, several disorders may manifest with the same clinical picture—and the presence of hematuria or proteinuria does not itself predict response to treatment or prognosis.

Disorders tend to manifest at different ages (see Table 250–1) although there is much overlap. The disorders may be

- Primary (idiopathic)
- Secondary (see Tables 250–2 and 250–4 on p. 2114)

Table 250–1. GLOMERULAR DISORDERS BY AGE AND MANIFESTATIONS

AGE (YR)	NEPHRITIC SYNDROME	NEPHROTIC SYNDROME	MIXED NEPHRITIC AND NEPHROTIC SYNDROME
< 15	Mild PIGN IgA nephropathy Thin basement membrane disease Hereditary nephritis IgA–associated vasculitis Lupus nephritis	Congenital nephrotic syndromes Minimal change disease Focal segmental glomerulosclerosis Lupus nephritis (membranous subtype)	Lupus nephritis Membranoproliferative GN
15–40	IgA nephropathy Thin basement membrane disease Lupus nephritis Hereditary nephritis RPGN PIGN	Focal segmental glomerulosclerosis Lupus nephritis (membranous subtype) Minimal change disease Membranous nephropathy Diabetic nephropathy Preeclampsia Late PIGN IgA nephropathy	Membranoproliferative GN Fibrillary and immunotactoid GN* IgA nephropathy Lupus nephritis RPGN
> 40	IgA nephropathy RPGN Vasculitides PIGN	Focal segmental glomerulosclerosis Membranous nephropathy Diabetic nephropathy Minimal change disease IgA nephropathy Amyloidosis (primary) Light chain deposition disease Benign hypertensive arteriolar nephrosclerosis (protein excretion is usually < 1 g/day) Late PIGN	IgA nephropathy Fibrillary and immunotactoid GN* RPGN

*More commonly manifests as nephrotic syndrome.
GN = glomerulonephritis; PIGN = postinfectious glomerulonephritis; RPGN = rapidly progressive glomerulonephritis.
Adapted from Rose BD: *Pathophysiology of Renal Disease*, ed. 2. New York, McGraw-Hill, 1987, p. 167.

Table 250–2. CAUSES OF GLOMERULONEPHRITIS

TYPE	EXAMPLES
Primary	
Idiopathic	Fibrillary and immunotactoid GN Idiopathic crescentic GN IgA nephropathy Membranoproliferative GN
Secondary	
Bacterial*	Group A beta-streptococcal infection *Mycoplasma* infection *Neisseria meningitidis* infection *Salmonella typhi* infection Staphylococcal infections (especially bacterial endocarditis) *Streptococcus pneumoniae* infection Visceral abscesses (due to *Escherichia coli* or *Pseudomonas*, *Proteus*, *Klebsiella*, or *Clostridium* sp) Sepsis
Parasitic*	Loiasis Malaria (due to *Plasmodium falciparum* or *P. malariae*) Schistosomiasis (due to *Schistosoma mansoni*)
Viral*	Coxsackievirus infection Cytomegalovirus infection Epstein-Barr virus infection Hepatitis B Hepatitis C Herpes zoster Measles Mumps Varicella
Other infectious and postinfectious causes	Fungal infections (due to *Candida albicans* or *Coccidioides immitis*) Rickettsial infection
Connective tissue disorders	Eosinophilic granulomatosis with polyangiitis Granulomatosis with polyangiitis IgA–associated vasculitis Microscopic polyangiitis Polyarteritis nodosa SLE
Drug-induced disorders	SLE (rarely due to hydralazine or procainamide) Hemolytic-uremic syndrome (due to quinine, cisplatin, gemcitabine, or mitomycin C)
Hematologic dyscrasias	Mixed IgG-IgM cryoglobulinemia Serum sickness Thrombotic thrombocytopenic purpura–hemolytic-uremic syndrome
Glomerular basement membrane diseases	Goodpasture syndrome
Hereditary disorders	Hereditary nephritis Thin basement membrane disease

*Infectious and postinfectious causes.
GN = glomerulonephritis.

Diagnosis

- Serum creatinine level and urinalysis

A glomerular disorder is usually suspected when screening or diagnostic testing reveals an elevated serum creatinine level and abnormal urinalysis (hematuria with or without casts, proteinuria, or both). Approach to the patient involves distinguishing predominant-nephritic from predominant-nephrotic features and identifying likely causes by patient age, accompanying illness (see Tables 250–1 and 250–4 on p. 2114), and other elements of the history (eg, time course, systemic manifestations, family history).

Renal biopsy is indicated when diagnosis is unclear from history or when histology influences choice of treatment and outcomes (eg, lupus nephritis).

OVERVIEW OF NEPHRITIC SYNDROME

Nephritic syndrome is defined by hematuria, variable degrees of proteinuria, usually dysmorphic RBCs, and often RBC casts on microscopic examination of urinary sediment. Often ≥ 1 of the following elements are present: edema, hypertension, elevated serum creatinine, and oliguria. It has both primary and secondary causes. Diagnosis is based on history, physical examination, and sometimes renal biopsy. Treatment and prognosis vary by cause.

Nephritic syndrome is a manifestation of glomerular inflammation (glomerulonephritis [GN]) and occurs at any age. Causes differ by age (see Table 250–1), and mechanisms differ by cause. The syndrome can be

- Acute (serum creatinine rises over many weeks or less)
- Chronic (renal insufficiency may progress over years)

Nephritic syndrome can also be

- Primary (idiopathic)
- Secondary

Acute glomerulonephritis: Postinfectious GN is the prototype of acute GN, but the condition may be caused by other glomerulopathies and by systemic disorders such as connective tissue disorders and hematologic dyscrasias (see Table 250–2).

Rapidly progressive GN is another acute GN.

Chronic GN: Chronic GN has features similar to those of acute GN but develops slowly and may cause mild to moderate proteinuria. Examples include

- IgA nephropathy
- Hereditary nephritis
- Thin basement membrane disease

HEREDITARY NEPHRITIS

(Alport Syndrome)

Hereditary nephritis is a genetically heterogeneous disorder characterized by nephritic syndrome (ie, hematuria, proteinuria, hypertension, eventual renal insufficiency) often with sensorineural deafness and, less commonly, ophthalmologic symptoms. Cause is a gene mutation affecting type IV collagen. Diagnosis is by history, including family history, urinalysis, and biopsy (renal or skin). Treatment is the same as that of chronic kidney disease, sometimes including kidney transplantation.

Hereditary nephritis is a nephritic syndrome caused by a mutation in the COL4A5 gene that encodes the alpha-5 chain of type IV collagen and results in altered type IV collagen strands. The mechanism by which collagen alteration causes a glomerular disorder is unknown, but impaired structure and function are presumed; in most families, thickening and thinning of the glomerular and tubular basement membranes occur, with multilamination of the lamina densa in a focal or local distribution (basket-weave pattern). Glomerular scarring and interstitial fibrosis eventually result.

The disorder is most commonly inherited in X-linked fashion, although autosomal recessive and, rarely, autosomal dominant varieties exist. Cases with X-linked inheritance may be clinically categorized as

- Juvenile form: Renal insufficiency develops between 20 and 30 yr
- Adult form: Renal insufficiency develops in people > 30 yr

Symptoms and Signs

Classic X-linked disease in males and autosomal recessive disease are clinically similar. Patients develop renal symptoms and signs similar to those of acute nephritic syndrome (eg, microscopic hematuria, hypertension, eventually gross hematuria with proteinuria) and progress to renal insufficiency between ages 20 and 30 (juvenile forms).

Sensorineural hearing loss frequently is present, affecting higher frequencies; it may not be noticed during early childhood.

Ophthalmologic abnormalities—cataracts (most common), anterior lenticonus (a regular conical protrusion on the anterior aspect of the lens due to thinning of the lens capsule), spherophakia (spherical lens deformation that can predispose to lens subluxation), nystagmus, retinitis pigmentosa, blindness—also occur but less frequently than hearing loss.

X-linked disease occurs in heterozygous women, who, because they have one normal X chromosome, usually have less severe, more slowly progressing symptoms than men.

Some men with X-linked disease develop renal insufficiency after age 30 with hearing loss that occurs late or is mild, and autosomal dominant disease typically does not cause renal failure until age ≥ 45 yr (adult forms).

In patients with X-linked Alport syndrome, sensorineural hearing loss usually manifests in childhood, whereas renal disease often does not manifest until adulthood.

Other nonrenal manifestations rarely include polyneuropathy and thrombocytopenia.

Diagnosis

- Urinalysis
- Renal biopsy

Diagnosis is suggested in patients who have microscopic hematuria on urinalysis or recurrent episodes of gross hematuria, particularly if an abnormality of hearing or vision or a family history of chronic kidney disease is present.

Urinalysis and usually renal biopsy are done. In addition to dysmorphic RBCs, the urine may contain protein, WBCs, and casts of various types. Nephrotic syndrome occurs rarely. No distinguishing histologic changes are seen on light microscopy. The diagnosis can be confirmed by any of the following:

- Renal biopsy with immunostaining for the subtypes of type IV collagen
- Characteristic disorganization of the lamina densa with variable thickening and thinning of the glomerular capillary basement membrane seen using electron microscopy
- Skin biopsy with immunostaining for the type IV collagen subtypes in a patient with a positive family history

A combination of immunostaining and electron microscopy is often needed to distinguish hereditary nephritis from some forms of thin basement membrane disease. Although not yet widely available, molecular techniques for evaluating DNA gene mutations or mRNA may become the diagnostic techniques of choice.

Treatment

- Same as that for other causes of chronic kidney disease
- Kidney transplantation

Treatment is indicated only when uremia occurs; its management is the same as that for other causes of chronic kidney disease. Anecdotal reports suggest that ACE inhibitors or angiotensin II receptor blockers may slow progression of renal disease. Transplantation has been successful, but antiglomerular basement membrane antibody disease may occur, usually only in males, in the transplanted kidney. Genetic counseling is indicated.

KEY POINTS

- Consider hereditary nephritis if patients have hematuria plus a hearing and/or vision abnormality or a family history of chronic kidney disease.
- Confirm the diagnosis by biopsy of the kidney or sometimes skin and immunostaining for type IV collagen subtypes.
- Treat chronic kidney disease and consider transplantation.

IMMUNOGLOBULIN A NEPHROPATHY

(IgA Nephropathy; Berger Disease)

IgA nephropathy is deposition of IgA immune complexes in glomeruli, manifesting as slowly progressive hematuria, proteinuria, and, often, renal insufficiency. Diagnosis is based on urinalysis and renal biopsy. Prognosis is generally good. Treatment options include ACE inhibitors, angiotensin II receptor blockers, corticosteroids, immunosuppressants, and omega-3 polyunsaturated fatty acids.

IgA nephropathy is a nephritic syndrome, a form of chronic GN characterized by the deposition of IgA immune complexes in glomeruli. It is the most common form of GN worldwide. It occurs at all ages, with a peak onset in the teens and 20s; affects men 2 to 6 times more frequently than women; and is more common in whites and Asians than in blacks. Prevalence estimates for IgA kidney deposits are 5% in the US, 10 to 20% in southern Europe and Australia, and 30 to 40% in Asia. However, some people with IgA deposits do not develop clinical disease.

Cause is unknown, but evidence suggests that there may be several mechanisms, including

- Increased IgA1 production
- Defective IgA1 glycosylation causing increased binding to mesangial cells
- Decreased IgA1 clearance
- A defective mucosal immune system
- Overproduction of cytokines stimulating mesangial cell proliferation

Familial clustering has also been observed, suggesting genetic factors at least in some cases.

Renal function is initially normal, but symptomatic renal disease may develop. A few patients present with acute kidney injury or chronic kidney disease, severe hypertension, or nephrotic syndrome.

Symptoms and Signs

The most common manifestations are persistent or recurrent macroscopic hematuria or asymptomatic microscopic hematuria with mild proteinuria. Flank pain and low-grade fever may accompany acute episodes. Other symptoms are usually not prominent.

Gross hematuria usually begins 1 or 2 days after a febrile mucosal (upper respiratory, sinus, enteral) illness, thus mimicking acute postinfectious GN, except the onset of hematuria is earlier (coinciding with or immediately after the febrile illness).

Rapidly progressive GN is the initial manifestation in < 10% of patients.

Diagnosis

- Urinalysis
- Sometimes renal biopsy

Diagnosis is suggested by any of the following:

- Gross hematuria, particularly within 2 days of a febrile mucosal illness or with flank pain
- Incidentally noted findings on urinalysis
- Occasionally, rapidly progressive GN

When manifestations are moderate or severe, diagnosis is confirmed by biopsy.

Urinalysis demonstrates microscopic hematuria, usually with dysmorphic RBCs and occasionally RBC casts. Mild proteinuria (< 1 g/day) is typical and may occur without hematuria; nephrotic syndrome develops in ≤ 20%. Serum creatinine level is usually normal.

Renal biopsy shows granular deposition of IgA and complement (C3) on immunofluorescent staining in an expanded mesangium with foci of segmental proliferative or necrotizing lesions. Importantly, mesangial IgA deposits are nonspecific and also occur in many other disorders, including immunoglobulin A–associated vasculitis, cirrhosis, inflammatory bowel disease, psoriasis, HIV infection, lung cancer, and several connective tissue disorders.

Glomerular IgA deposition is a primary feature of immunoglobulin A-associated vasculitis, and it may be indistinguishable from IgA nephropathy based on biopsy specimens, leading to speculation that immunoglobulin A–associated vasculitis may be a systemic form of IgA nephropathy. However, immunoglobulin A–associated vasculitis is clinically distinct from IgA nephropathy, usually manifesting as hematuria, purpuric rash, arthralgias, and abdominal pain.

Other serum immunologic tests are usually unnecessary. Complement concentrations are usually normal. Plasma IgA concentration may be elevated, and circulating IgA-fibronectin complexes are present; however, these findings are not helpful diagnostically.

Prognosis

IgA nephropathy usually progresses slowly; renal insufficiency and hypertension develop within 10 yr in 15 to 20% of patients. Progression to end-stage renal disease occurs in 25% of patients after 20 yr. When IgA nephropathy is diagnosed in childhood, prognosis is usually good. However, persistent hematuria invariably leads to hypertension, proteinuria, and renal insufficiency. Risk factors for progressive deterioration in renal function include the following:

- Proteinuria > 1 g/day
- Elevated serum creatinine level
- Uncontrolled hypertension
- Persistent microscopic hematuria
- Extensive fibrotic changes in the glomerulus or interstitium
- Crescents on biopsy

Treatment

- Often ACE inhibitors or angiotensin II receptor blockers for hypertension, serum creatinine > 1.2 mg/dL, or macroalbuminuria (urinary protein > 300 mg/day) and with a target urinary protein of < 500 mg/day
- Corticosteroids for progressive disease, including increasing proteinuria especially into the nephrotic range, or increasing serum creatinine level
- Corticosteroids and cyclophosphamide for proliferative injury or rapidly progressive GN
- Transplantation rather than dialysis if possible

Normotensive patients with intact renal function (serum creatinine < 1.2 mg/dL) and only mild proteinuria (< 0.5 g/day) usually are not treated. Patients with renal insufficiency or more severe proteinuria and hematuria are usually offered treatment, which ideally should be started before significant renal insufficiency develops.

Angiotensin inhibition in IgA nephropathy: ACE inhibitors or angiotensin II receptor blockers are used on the premise that they reduce BP, proteinuria, and glomerular fibrosis. Patients with the DD genotype for the ACE gene may be at greater risk of disease progression but may also be more likely to respond to ACE inhibitors or angiotensin II receptor blockers. For patients with hypertension, ACE inhibitors or angiotensin II receptor blockers are the antihypertensives of choice even for relatively mild chronic kidney disease.

Corticosteroids and immunosuppressants in IgA nephropathy: Corticosteroids have been used for many years, but benefit is not well documented. One protocol uses methylprednisolone 1 g IV once/day for 3 days at the beginning of months 1, 3, and 5 plus prednisone 0.5 mg/kg po every other day for 6 mo. Another regimen uses prednisone beginning 1 mg/kg po once/day with dose gradually tapered over 6 mo.

Because of the risk of adverse effects, corticosteroids should probably be reserved for patients with any of the following:

- Worsening or persistent proteinuria (> 1 g/day), especially if in the nephrotic range despite maximal ACE inhibitor or angiotensin II receptor blocker therapy
- Increasing serum creatinine level

Combinations of IV corticosteroids and cyclophosphamide plus oral prednisone are used for severe disease, such as proliferative or crescentic (rapidly progressive) nephropathy. Evidence for mycophenolate mofetil is conflicting; it should not be used as first-line treatment. None of these drugs, however, prevents recurrence in transplant patients. Immunosuppressive therapy should also be avoided in patients with advanced fibrotic kidney disease, which is not reversible.

Other treatments: Omega-3 polyunsaturated fatty acids (eg, 4 to 12 g/day), available in fish oil supplements, have been used to treat IgA nephropathy, but data on efficacy are contradictory. Mechanism of effect may include alterations in inflammatory cytokines.

Other interventions have been tried to lower IgA overproduction and to inhibit mesangial proliferation. Elimination of gluten, dairy products, eggs, and meat from the diet; tonsillectomy; and immune globulin 1 g/kg IV 2 days/mo for 3 mo followed by immune globulin 0.35 mL/kg of 16.5% solution IM q 2 wk for 6 mo all theoretically reduce IgA production. Heparin, dipyridamole, and statins are just a few examples of in vitro mesangial cell inhibitors. Data supporting any of these interventions are limited or absent, and none can be recommended for routine treatment.

Kidney transplantation is better than dialysis because of excellent long-term disease-free survival. The condition recurs in ≤ 15% of graft recipients.

KEY POINTS

- IgA nephropathy is the most common cause of GN worldwide and is common among young adults, whites, and Asians.
- Consider the diagnosis in patients with unexplained signs of GN, particularly when it occurs within 2 days of a febrile mucosal illness or with flank pain.
- Treat patients who have creatinine > 1.2 mg/dL or proteinuria > 300 mg/day with ACE inhibitors or angiotensin II blockers.
- Reserve corticosteroids for patients with worsening renal function or proteinuria (> 1 g/day) despite maximal ACE inhibitor or angiotensin II blocker treatment.
- Treat patients who have proliferative injury or rapidly progressive GN with corticosteroids and cyclophosphamide.

POSTINFECTIOUS GLOMERULONEPHRITIS

(Poststreptococcal Glomerulonephritis; Nonstreptococcal Postinfectious Glomerulonephritis)

Postinfectious glomerulonephritis occurs after infection, usually with a nephritogenic strain of group A beta-hemolytic streptococcus. Diagnosis is suggested by history and urinalysis and confirmed by finding a low complement level and sometimes by antibody testing. Prognosis is excellent. Treatment is supportive.

Etiology

Postinfectious glomerulonephritis, a nephritic syndrome, is the most common cause of a glomerular disorder in children between 5 and 15 yr; it is rare in children < 2 yr and uncommon in adults > 40 yr.

Most cases are caused by nephritogenic strains of group A beta-hemolytic streptococci, most notably type 12 (which causes pharyngitis) and type 49 (which causes impetigo); an estimated 5 to 10% of patients with streptococcal pharyngitis and about 25% of those with impetigo develop PIGN. A latency period of 6 to 21 days between infection and GN onset is typical, but latency may extend up to 6 wk.

Less common pathogens are nonstreptococcal bacteria, viruses, parasites, rickettsiae, and fungi (see Table 250–2). Bacterial endocarditis and ventriculoatrial shunt infections are additional important conditions in which PIGN develops; ventriculoperitoneal shunts are more resistant to infection.

The mechanism is unknown, but microbial antigens are thought to bind to the glomerular basement membrane and activate primarily the alternate complement pathway both directly and via interaction with circulating antibodies, causing glomerular damage, which may be focal or diffuse. Alternatively, circulating immune complexes could precipitate on the glomerular basement membrane.

Symptoms and Signs

Symptoms and signs range from asymptomatic hematuria (in about 50%) and mild proteinuria to full-blown nephritis with microscopic or gross hematuria (cola-colored, brown, smoky, or frankly bloody urine), proteinuria (sometimes nephrotic-range), oliguria, edema, hypertension, and renal insufficiency. Fever is unusual and suggests persistent infection.

Renal failure that causes fluid overload with heart failure and severe hypertension requiring dialysis affects 1 to 2% of patients and may manifest as a pulmonary-renal syndrome with hematuria and hemoptysis.

Uncommonly, nephrotic syndrome may persist after resolution of severe disease.

Clinical manifestations of nonstreptococcal PIGN may mimic other disorders (eg, polyarteritis nodosa, renal emboli, antimicrobial drug–induced acute interstitial nephritis).

Diagnosis

- Clinical evidence of recent infection
- Urinalysis typically showing dysmorphic RBCs, RBC casts, proteinuria, WBCs, and renal tubular cells
- Often hypocomplementemia

Streptococcal PIGN is suggested by history of pharyngitis or impetigo plus either typical symptoms of PIGN or incidental findings on urinalysis. Demonstration of hypocomplementemia is essentially confirmatory.

Tests done to confirm the diagnosis depend on clinical findings. Antistreptolysin O, antihyaluronidase, and antideoxyribonuclease (anti-DNAase) antibodies are commonly measured. Serum creatinine and complement levels (C3 and total hemolytic complement activity) are also usually measured; however, in patients with typical clinical findings, some tests can be omitted. Sometimes other tests are done. Biopsy confirms the diagnosis but is rarely necessary.

Antistreptolysin O level, the most common laboratory evidence of recent streptococcal infection, increases and remains elevated for several months in about 75% of patients with pharyngitis and in about 50% of patients with impetigo, but it is not specific. The streptozyme test, which additionally measures antihyaluronidase, antideoxyribonuclease, and other titers detects 95% of recent streptococcal pharyngitis and 80% of skin infections.

Urinalysis typically shows proteinuria (0.5 to 2 g/m^2/day); dysmorphic RBCs; WBCs; renal tubular cells; and possibly RBC, WBC, and granular casts. Random (spot) urinary protein/creatinine ratio is usually between 0.2 and 2 (normal, < 0.2) but may occasionally be in the nephrotic range (≥ 3).

Serum creatinine may rise rapidly but usually peaks below a level requiring dialysis.

C3 and total hemolytic complement activity (CH50) levels fall during active disease and return to normal within 6 to 8 wk in 80% of PIGN cases; C1q, C2, and C4 levels are only minimally decreased or remain normal. Cryoglobulinemia may appear and persist for several months, whereas circulating immune complexes are detectable for only a few weeks.

Biopsy specimens show enlarged and hypercellular glomeruli, initially with neutrophilic infiltration and later with mononuclear infiltration. Epithelial cell hyperplasia is a common early, transient feature. Microthrombosis may occur; if damage is severe, hemodynamic changes due to cellular proliferation and edema of the glomerulus cause oliguria, occasionally accompanied by epithelial crescents (formed within Bowman space from epithelial cell hyperplasia). Endothelial and mesangial cells multiply, and the mesangial regions often are greatly expanded by edema and contain neutrophils, dead cells, cellular debris, and subepithelial deposits of electron-dense material.

Immunofluorescence microscopy usually shows immune complex deposition with IgG and complement in a granular pattern. On electron microscopy, these deposits are semilunar or hump-shaped and are located in the subepithelial area. The presence of these deposits and of small subendothelial and mesangial deposits initiates a complement-mediated inflammatory reaction that leads to glomerular damage. The major antigen is probably Zymogen cysteine proteinase exotoxin B (Zymogen/SPE B).

Prognosis

Normal renal function is retained or regained by 85 to 95% of patients. GFR usually returns to normal over 1 to 3 mo, but proteinuria may persist for 6 to 12 mo and microscopic hematuria for several years. Transient changes in urinary sediment may recur with minor URIs. Renal cellular proliferation disappears within weeks, but residual sclerosis is common. In 10% of adults and 1% of children, PIGN evolves into rapidly progressive GN.

Treatment

- Supportive care

Treatment is supportive and may include restriction of dietary protein, sodium, and fluid and, in more severe cases, treatment of edema and hypertension. Dialysis is occasionally necessary. Antimicrobial therapy is preventive only when given within 36 h of infection and before GN becomes established.

KEY POINTS

- Consider PIGN in young patients who have had pharyngitis or impetigo plus signs of GN.
- Biopsy confirms the diagnosis but is rarely necessary; demonstration of hypocomplementemia is essentially confirmatory.
- Supportive treatment usually leads to recovery of kidney function.

RAPIDLY PROGRESSIVE GLOMERULONEPHRITIS

(Crescentic Glomerulonephritis)

Rapidly progressive glomerulonephritis (RPGN) is acute nephritic syndrome accompanied by microscopic glomerular crescent formation with progression to renal failure within weeks to months. Diagnosis is based on history, urinalysis, serologic tests, and renal biopsy. Treatment is with corticosteroids, with or without cyclophosphamide, and sometimes plasma exchange.

RPGN, a type of nephritic syndrome, is accompanied by extensive glomerular crescent formation (which can be seen in a biopsy specimen) that, if untreated, progresses to end-stage renal disease over weeks to months. It is relatively uncommon, affecting 10 to 15% of patients with glomerulonephritis (GN), and occurs predominantly in patients 20 to 50 yr. Types and causes are classified by findings using immunofluorescence microscopy and serologic tests (eg anti-GBM antibody, anti-neutrophil cytoplasmic antibody [ANCA]—see Table 250–3).

Antiglomerular basement membrane antibody disease: Antiglomerular basement membrane (GBM) antibody disease (type 1 RPGN) is autoimmune GN and accounts for up to 10% of RPGN cases. It may arise when respiratory exposures (eg, cigarette smoke, viral URI) or some other stimulus exposes alveolar capillary collagen, triggering formation of anticollagen antibodies. The anticollagen antibodies cross-react with GBM, fixing complement and triggering a cell-mediated inflammatory response in the kidneys and usually the lungs.

Table 250–3. CLASSIFICATION OF RAPIDLY PROGRESSIVE GLOMERULONEPHRITIS BASED ON IMMUNOFLUORESCENCE MICROSCOPY

TYPE	PERCENTAGE OF RPGN CASES	CAUSES
Type 1: Anti-GBM antibody–mediated	≤ 10%	Anti-GBM GN (without lung hemorrhage*) Goodpasture syndrome (with lung hemorrhage)
Type 2: Immune complex	≤ 40%	Postinfectious causes: • Antistreptococcal antibodies (eg, poststreptococcal GN) • Infective endocarditis • Vascular prosthetic nephritis • Viral hepatitis B infection • Visceral abscess or sepsis Connective tissue disorders: • Anti-DNA autoantibodies (eg, lupus nephritis) • IgA immune complexes (eg, immunoglobulin A–associated vasculitis GN) • Mixed IgG-IgM cryoglobulins (eg, cryoglobulinemic GN) Other glomerulopathies: • IgA nephropathy • Membranoproliferative GN • Idiopathic crescentic GN (rare)
Type 3: Pauci-immune	≤ 50%	Eosinophilic granulomatosis with polyangiitis Pulmonary necrotizing granulomas (eg, granulomatosis with polyangiitis) Renal-limited disease (eg, idiopathic crescentic GN) Microscopic polyangiitis
Type 4: Double-antibody positive	Rare	Same as for as types 1 and 3

*When the lung is also affected, anti-GBM glomerulonephritis is called Goodpasture syndrome.
GBM = glomerular basement membrane; GN = glomerulonephritis; RPGN = rapidly progressive glomerulonephritis.

The term Goodpasture syndrome refers to a combination of GN and alveolar hemorrhage in the presence of anti-GBM antibodies. GN without alveolar hemorrhage in the presence of anti-GBM antibodies is called anti-GBM glomerulonephritis. Immunofluorescent staining of renal biopsy tissue demonstrates linear IgG deposits.

Immune complex RPGN: Immune complex RPGN (type 2 RPGN) complicates numerous infectious and connective tissue disorders and also occurs with other primary glomerulopathies. Immunofluorescent staining demonstrates nonspecific granular immune deposits. The condition accounts for up to 40% of RPGN cases. Pathogenesis is usually unknown.

Pauci-immune RPGN: Pauci-immune RPGN (type 3 RPGN) is distinguished by the absence of immune complex or complement deposition on immunofluorescent staining. It constitutes up to 50% of all RPGN cases. Almost all patients have elevated antineutrophil cytoplasmic antibodies (ANCAs, usually anti-proteinase 3-ANCA or myeloperoxidase-ANCA) and systemic vasculitis.

Double-antibody disease: Double-antibody disease (type 4 RPGN) has features of types 1 and 3, with the presence of anti-GBM and ANCA antibodies. It is rare.

Idiopathic RPGN: Idiopathic cases are rare. They include patients with either of the following:

- Immune complexes (similar to type 2) but no obvious cause such as infection, connective tissue disorder, or glomerular disorder
- Pauci-immune features (similar to type 3) but absence of ANCA antibodies

Symptoms and Signs

Manifestations are usually insidious, with weakness, fatigue, fever, nausea, vomiting, anorexia, arthralgia, and abdominal pain. Some patients present similarly to those with PIGN, with abrupt-onset hematuria. About 50% of patients have edema and a history of an acute influenza-like illness within 4 wk of onset of renal failure, usually followed by severe oliguria. Nephrotic syndrome is present in 10 to 30%. Hypertension is uncommon and rarely severe. Patients with anti-GBM antibody disease may have pulmonary hemorrhage, which can manifest with hemoptysis or be detectable only by finding diffuse alveolar infiltrates on chest x-ray (pulmonary-renal syndrome or diffuse alveolar hemorrhage syndrome).

Diagnosis

- Progressive renal failure over weeks to months
- Nephritic urinary sediment
- Serologic testing
- Serum complement levels
- Renal biopsy

Diagnosis is suggested by acute kidney injury in patients with hematuria and dysmorphic RBCs or RBC casts. Testing includes serum creatinine, urinalysis, CBC, serologic tests, and renal biopsy. Diagnosis is usually by serologic tests and renal biopsy.

Serum creatinine is almost always elevated.

Urinalysis shows hematuria is always present, and RBC casts are usually present. Telescopic sediment (ie, sediment with multiple elements, including WBCs, dysmorphic RBCs, and WBC, RBC, granular, waxy, and broad casts) is common.

On **CBC,** anemia is usually present, and leukocytosis is common.

Serologic testing should include anti-GBM antibodies (anti-GBM antibody disease); antistreptolysin O antibodies, anti-DNA antibodies, or cryoglobulins (immune complex RPGN); and ANCA titers (pauci-immune RPGN).

Complement measurement may be useful in suspected immune complex RPGN because hypocomplementemia is common.

Early **renal biopsy** is essential. The feature common to all types of RPGN is focal proliferation of glomerular epithelial cells, sometimes interspersed with numerous neutrophils, that forms a crescentic cellular mass (crescents) and that fills Bowman space in > 50% of glomeruli. The glomerular tuft usually appears hypocellular and collapses. Necrosis within the tuft or involving the crescent may occur and may be the most prominent abnormality. In such patients, histologic evidence of vasculitis should be sought.

Immunofluorescence microscopy findings differ for each type:

- In anti-GBM antibody disease (type 1), linear or ribbon-like deposition of IgG along the GBM is most prominent and is often accompanied by linear and sometimes granular deposition of C3.
- In immune complex RPGN (type 2), immunofluorescence reveals diffuse, irregular mesangial IgG and C3 deposits.
- In pauci-immune RPGN (type 3), immune staining and deposits are not detected. However, fibrin occurs within the crescents, regardless of the fluorescence pattern.
- In double antibody RPGN (type 4), linear staining of the GBM is present (similar to type 1).
- In idiopathic RPGN some patients have immune complexes (similar to those of type 2) and others have absence of immune staining and deposits (similar to type 3).

Prognosis

Spontaneous remission is rare, and 80 to 90% of untreated patients progress to end-stage renal disease within 6 mo. Prognosis improves with early treatment.

Favorable prognostic factors include RPGN caused by the following:

- Anti-GBM disease if treated early, especially when treated before oliguria occurs and when creatinine level is < 7 mg/dL
- PIGN
- SLE
- Granulomatosis with polyangiitis
- Microscopic polyangiitis

Unfavorable prognostic factors include the following:

- Age > 60 yr
- Oliguric renal failure
- Higher serum creatinine level
- Circumferential crescents in > 75% of glomeruli
- Among patients with pauci-immune RPGN, no response to treatment

About 30% of patients with pauci-immune RPGN do not respond to treatment; among nonresponders, about 40% require dialysis, and 33% die within 4 yr. In contrast, among patients who respond to treatment, < 20% of patients require dialysis, and about 3% die.

Patients with double-antibody disease appear to have a renal prognosis somewhat better than patients with only anti-GBM antibody disease and worse than patients with pauci-immune RPGN.

Patients who recover normal renal function after RPGN demonstrate residual histologic changes principally in glomeruli, consisting chiefly of hypercellularity, with little or no sclerosis within the glomerular tuft or the epithelial cells and minimal fibrosis of the interstitium.

Death is usually due to infectious or cardiac causes, providing that a uremic death is prevented by dialysis.

Treatment

- Corticosteroids
- Cyclophosphamide
- Plasma exchange

Treatment varies by disease type, although no regimens have been rigorously studied. Therapy should be instituted early, ideally when serum creatinine is < 5 mg/dL and before the biopsy shows crescentic involvement of all glomeruli or organizing crescents as well as fibrotic interstitium and atrophic tubules. Treatment becomes less effective as these features become more prominent and may be harmful in some patients (eg, the elderly, patients with infection).

Treatment varies by disease type, although no regimens have been rigorously studied.

Corticosteroids and cyclophosphamide are usually given. For immune complex and pauci-immune RPGN, corticosteroids (methylprednisolone 1 g IV once/day over 30 min for 3 to 5 days followed by prednisone 1 mg/kg po once/day) may reduce serum creatinine levels or delay dialysis for > 3 yr in 50% of patients.

Cyclophosphamide 1.5 to 2 mg/kg po once/day is usually given and may particularly benefit ANCA-positive patients; monthly pulse regimens may cause fewer adverse effects (eg, leukopenia, infection) than oral therapy because of reduced cumulative dosing, but their role is not defined. Prednisone and cyclophosphamide are typically started concurrent with plasma exchange for anti-GBM antibody disease and continued to minimize new antibody formation. Patients with idiopathic disease are usually treated with corticosteroids and cyclophosphamide, but data regarding efficacy are scarce.

Plasma exchange (daily 3- to 4-L exchanges for 14 days) is recommended for anti-GBM antibody disease. Plasma exchange should also be considered for immune complex and pauci-immune ANCA-associated RPGN with pulmonary hemorrhage or severe renal dysfunction on presentation (serum creatinine > 5.7 mg/dL or dialysis dependency). Plasma exchange is believed to be effective because it rapidly removes free antibody, intact immune complexes, and mediators of inflammation (eg, fibrinogen, complement).

Lymphocytapheresis, a technique to remove peripheral lymphocytes from circulation, may benefit pauci-immune RPGN but requires further investigation.

Kidney transplantation is effective for all types, but disease may recur in the graft; risk diminishes with time. In anti-GBM antibody disease, the anti-GBM titers should be undetectable for at least 12 mo before transplantation. For patients with pauci-immune RPGN, disease activity should be quiescent for at least 6 mo before transplantation; ANCA titers do not need to be suppressed.

KEY POINTS

- Consider RPGN if patients have acute kidney injury with hematuria and dysmorphic RBCs or RBC casts, particularly with subacute constitutional or nonspecific symptoms (eg, fatigue, fever, anorexia, arthralgia, abdominal pain).
- Do serologic tests and early renal biopsy.
- Initiate treatment early, with corticosteroids, cyclophosphamide, and often plasma exchange.
- Consider kidney transplantation after disease activity is controlled.

THIN BASEMENT MEMBRANE DISEASE

(Benign Familial Hematuria)

Thin basement membrane disease is diffuse thinning of the glomerular basement membrane from a width of 300 to 400 nm in normal subjects to 150 to 225 nm.

Thin basement membrane disease is a type of nephritic syndrome. It is hereditary and usually transmitted in autosomal dominant fashion. Not all genetic mutations have been characterized, but in some families with thin basement membrane disease there is a mutation in the type IV collagen α4 gene. Prevalence is estimated to be 5 to 9%.

Symptoms and Signs

Most patients are asymptomatic and are incidentally noted to have microscopic hematuria on routine urinalysis, although mild proteinuria and gross hematuria are occasionally present. Renal function is typically normal, but a few patients develop progressive renal failure for unknown reasons. Recurrent flank pain, similar to that in IgA nephropathy, is a rare manifestation.

Diagnosis

- Clinical evaluation
- Sometimes renal biopsy

Diagnosis is based on family history and findings of hematuria without other symptoms or pathology, particularly if asymptomatic family members also have hematuria. Renal biopsy is unnecessary but is often done as part of a hematuria evaluation. Early on, thin basement membrane disease may be difficult to differentiate from hereditary nephritis because of histologic similarities.

Treatment

- For frequent gross hematuria, flank pain, or proteinuria, ACE inhibitors or angiotensin II receptor blockers

Long-term prognosis is excellent, and no treatment is necessary in most cases. Patients with frequent gross hematuria, flank pain, or proteinuria (eg, urine protein/creatinine ratio of > 0.2) may benefit from ACE inhibitors or angiotensin receptor II blockers, which may lower intraglomerular pressure.

OVERVIEW OF NEPHROTIC SYNDROME

Nephrotic syndrome is urinary excretion of > 3 g of protein/day due to a glomerular disorder plus edema and hypoalbuminemia. It is more common among children and has both primary and secondary causes. Diagnosis is by determination of urine protein/creatinine ratio in a random urine sample or measurement of urinary protein in a 24-h urine collection; cause is diagnosed based on history, physical examination, serologic testing, and renal biopsy. Prognosis and treatment vary by cause.

Etiology

Nephrotic syndrome occurs at any age but is more prevalent in children (primarily minimal change disease), mostly between ages 1½ and 4 yr. Congenital nephrotic syndromes appear during the first year of life. At younger ages (< 8 yr), boys are affected more often than girls, but both are affected equally at older ages. Causes differ by age (see Table 250–1) and may be primary or secondary (see Table 250–4).

The **most common primary causes** are the following:

- Minimal change disease
- Focal segmental glomerulosclerosis
- Membranous nephropathy

Secondary causes account for < 10% of childhood cases but > 50% of adult cases, most commonly the following:

- Diabetic nephropathy
- Preeclampsia

Amyloidosis, an underrecognized cause, is responsible for 4% of cases.

HIV-associated nephropathy is a type of focal segmental glomerulosclerosis that occurs in patients with AIDS.

Pathophysiology

Proteinuria occurs because of changes to capillary endothelial cells, the glomerular basement membrane (GBM), or podocytes, which normally filter serum protein selectively by size and charge.

The mechanism of damage to these structures is unknown in primary and secondary glomerular diseases, but evidence suggests that T cells may up-regulate a circulating permeability factor or down-regulate an inhibitor of permeability factor in response to unidentified immunogens and cytokines. Other possible factors include hereditary defects in proteins that are integral to the slit diaphragms of the glomeruli, activation of complement leading to damage of the glomerular epithelial cells and loss of the negatively charged groups attached to proteins of the GBM and glomerular epithelial cells.

Complications of nephrotic syndrome: The disorder results in urinary loss of macromolecular proteins, primarily albumin but also opsonins, immunoglobulins, erythropoietin, transferrin, hormone-binding proteins (including thyroid-binding globulin and vitamin D-binding protein), and antithrombin III. Deficiency of these and other proteins contribute to a number of complications (see Table 250–5); other physiologic factors also play a role.

Table 250–4. CAUSES OF NEPHROTIC SYNDROME

CAUSES	EXAMPLES
Primary causes	
Idiopathic	Fibrillary and immunotactoid GN Focal segmental glomerulosclerosis IgA nephropathy* Membranoproliferative GN Membranous nephropathy Minimal change disease Rapidly progressive GN*
Secondary causes	
Metabolic	Amyloidosis Diabetes mellitus
Immunologic	Cryoglobulinemia Erythema multiforme Immunoglobulin A–associated vasculitis* Microscopic polyangiitis Serum sickness Sjögren syndrome SLE*
Idiopathic	Castleman disease Sarcoidosis
Neoplastic	Carcinoma (eg, bronchus, breast, colon, stomach, kidney) Leukemia Lymphomas Melanoma Multiple myeloma
Drug-related	Gold Heroin Interferon alfa Lithium NSAIDs Mercury Pamidronate Penicillamine Probenecid
Bacterial†	Infective endocarditis Leprosy Syphilis
Protozoan†	Filariasis Helminthic infections Loiasis Malaria Schistosomiasis (due to *Schistosoma haematobium*) Toxoplasmosis
Viral†	Epstein-Barr virus infection Hepatitis B and C Herpes zoster HIV infection
Allergic	Antitoxins Insect stings Poison ivy or oak Snake venoms
Genetic syndromes	Congenital nephrotic syndromes • Diffuse mesangial sclerosis • Finnish type, ie, nephrin defect • Corticosteroid-resistant nephrotic syndrome (podocin defect) • Denys-Drash syndrome • Familial FSGS • Nail-patella syndrome Fabry disease Familial FSGS Hereditary nephritis* Sickle cell disease
Physiologic	Adaptation to reduced nephrons Morbid obesity Oligomeganephronia
Miscellaneous	Chronic allograft nephropathy Malignant hypertension Preeclampsia

*More commonly manifests as nephritic syndrome.
†Infectious and postinfectious causes.
FSGS = focal segmental glomerulonephritis;
GN = glomerulonephritis.

Table 250–5. COMPLICATIONS OF NEPHROTIC SYNDROME

COMPLICATION	CONTRIBUTING FACTORS
Edema (including ascites and pleural effusions)	Generalized capillary leak, due to hypoalbuminemia with decreased oncotic pressure Possibly renal sodium retention
Infection (especially cellulitis and, in 2 to 6%, spontaneous bacterial peritonitis)	Unknown Possibly loss of opsonins and immunoglobulins
Anemia	Loss of erythropoietin and transferrin
Changes in thyroid function test results (among patients previously hypothyroid, increased dose requirement for thyroid replacement hormone)	Loss of thyroid-binding globulin
Hypercoagulability and thromboembolism (especially renal vein thrombosis and pulmonary embolism, which occur in up to 5% of children and 40% of adults)	Loss of antithrombin III Increased hepatic synthesis of clotting factors Platelet abnormalities Hyperviscosity caused by hypovolemia
Protein undernutrition in children (sometimes with brittle hair and nails, alopecia, and stunted growth)	Loss of proteins Decreased hepatic production Sometimes decreased oral intake secondary to mesenteric edema
Dyslipidemia	Increased hepatic lipoprotein synthesis
Coronary artery disease in adults	Dyslipidemia with atherosclerosis Hypertension Hypercoagulability
Hypertension in adults	Renal sodium retention
Bone disorder	Corticosteroid use
Chronic kidney disease	Unknown Possibly hypovolemia, interstitial edema, and use of NSAIDs
Proximal tubular dysfunction (acquired Fanconi syndrome), with glucosuria, aminoaciduria, potassium depletion, phosphaturia, renal tubular acidosis, bicarbonaturia, hypercitraturia, and uricosuria	Toxic effects on proximal tubular cells secondary to large amounts of protein that they reabsorb

Symptoms and Signs

Primary symptoms include anorexia, malaise, and frothy urine (caused by high concentrations of protein).

Fluid retention may cause

- Dyspnea (pleural effusion or laryngeal edema)
- Arthralgia (hydrarthrosis)
- Abdominal pain (ascites or, in children, mesenteric edema)

Corresponding signs may develop, including peripheral edema and ascites. Edema may obscure signs of muscle wasting and cause parallel white lines in fingernail beds (Muehrcke lines).

Other symptoms and signs are attributable to the many complications of nephrotic syndrome (see Table 250–5).

Diagnosis

- Urine random (spot) protein/creatinine ratio ≥ 3 or proteinuria ≥ 3 g/24 h
- Serologic testing and renal biopsy unless the cause is clinically obvious

Diagnosis is suspected in patients with edema and proteinuria on urinalysis and confirmed by random (spot) urine protein and creatinine levels or 24-h measurement of urinary protein. The cause may be suggested by clinical findings (eg, SLE, preeclampsia, cancer); when the cause is unclear, additional (eg, serologic) testing and renal biopsy are indicated.

Urine testing: A finding of significant **proteinuria** (3 g protein in a 24-h urine collection) is diagnostic (normal excretion is < 150 mg/day). Alternatively, the protein/creatinine ratio in a random urine specimen usually reliably estimates grams of protein/1.73 m^2 BSA in a 24-h collection (eg, values of 40 mg/dL protein and 10 mg/dL creatinine in a random urine sample are equivalent to the finding of 4 g/1.73 m^2 in a 24-h specimen).

Calculations based on random specimens may be less reliable when creatinine excretion is high (eg, during athletic training) or low (eg, in cachexia). However, calculations based on random specimens are usually preferred to 24-h collection because random collection is more convenient and less prone to error (eg, due to lack of adherence); more convenient testing facilitates monitoring changes that occur during treatment.

Besides proteinuria, **urinalysis** may demonstrate casts (hyaline, granular, fatty, waxy, or epithelial cell). Lipiduria, the presence of free lipid or lipid within tubular cells (oval fat bodies), within casts (fatty casts), or as free globules, suggests a glomerular disorder causing nephrotic syndrome. Urinary cholesterol can be detected with plain microscopy and demonstrates a Maltese cross pattern under crossed polarized light; Sudan staining must be used to show triglycerides.

Adjunctive testing in nephrotic syndrome: Adjunctive testing helps characterize severity and complications.

- BUN and creatinine concentrations vary by degree of renal impairment.
- Serum albumin often is < 2.5 g/dL.
- Total cholesterol and triglyceride levels are typically increased.

It is not routinely necessary to measure levels of alpha- and gamma-globulins, immunoglobulins, hormone-binding proteins, ceruloplasmin, transferrin, and complement components, but these levels may also be low.

Testing for secondary causes of nephrotic syndrome: The role of testing for secondary causes of nephrotic syndrome (see Table 250–4) is controversial because yield may be low. Tests are best done as indicated by clinical context. Tests may include the following:

- Serum glucose or glycosylated Hb (HbA_{1c})
- Antinuclear antibodies
- Hepatitis B and C serologic tests
- Serum or urine protein electrophoresis
- Cryoglobulins
- Rheumatoid factor
- Serologic test for syphilis (eg, rapid plasma reagin)
- HIV antibody test
- Complement levels (CH50, C3, C4)

Test results may alter management and preclude the need for biopsy. For example, demonstration of cryoglobulins suggests mixed cryoglobulinemia (eg, from chronic inflammatory disorders such as SLE, Sjögren syndrome, or hepatitis C virus infection), and demonstration of a monoclonal protein on serum or urine protein electrophoresis suggests a monoclonal gammopathy (eg, multiple myeloma), especially in patients > 50 yr who have anemia.

Renal biopsy is indicated in adults to diagnose the disorder causing idiopathic nephrotic syndrome. Idiopathic nephrotic syndrome in children is most likely minimal change disease and is usually presumed without biopsy unless the patient fails to improve during a trial of corticosteroids. Specific biopsy findings are discussed under the individual disorders.

Prognosis

Prognosis varies by cause. Complete remissions may occur spontaneously or with treatment. The prognosis generally is favorable in corticosteroid-responsive disorders.

In all cases, prognosis may be worse in the presence of the following:

- Infection
- Hypertension
- Significant azotemia
- Hematuria
- Thromboses in cerebral, pulmonary, peripheral, or renal veins

The recurrence rate is high in kidney transplantation patients with focal segmental glomerulosclerosis, IgA nephropathy, and membranoproliferative glomerulonephritis (especially type 2).

Treatment

- Treatment of causative disorder
- Angiotensin inhibition
- Na restriction
- Statins
- Diuretics for excessive fluid overload
- Rarely, nephrectomy

Treatment of disorder causing nephrotic syndrome: Treatment of underlying disorders may include prompt treatment of infections (eg, staphylococcal endocarditis, malaria, syphilis, schistosomiasis), allergic desensitization (eg, for poison oak or ivy and insect antigen exposures), and stopping drugs (eg, gold, penicillamine, NSAIDs); these measures may cure nephrotic syndrome in specific instances.

Proteinuria treatment: Angiotensin inhibition (using ACE inhibitors or angiotensin II receptor blockers) is indicated to reduce systemic and intraglomerular pressure and proteinuria. These drugs may cause or exacerbate hyperkalemia in patients with moderate to severe renal insufficiency.

Protein restriction is no longer recommended because of lack of demonstrated effect on progression.

Edema treatment: Sodium restriction (< 2 g sodium, or about 100 mmol/day) is recommended for patients with symptomatic edema.

Loop diuretics are usually required to control edema but may worsen preexisting renal insufficiency and hypovolemia, hyperviscosity, and hypercoagulability and thus should be used only if sodium restriction is ineffective or there is evidence of intravascular fluid overload. In severe cases, of nephrotic syndrome, IV albumin infusion followed by a loop diuretic may also be given to control edema.

Dyslipidemia treatment: Statins are indicated for dyslipidemia.

Limitation of saturated fat and cholesterol intake is recommended to help control dyslipidemia.

Hypercoagulability treatment: Anticoagulants are indicated for treatment of thromboembolism, but few data exist to support their use as primary prevention.

Management of infection risk: All patients should receive pneumococcal vaccination if not otherwise contraindicated.

Nephrectomy for nephrotic syndrome: Rarely, bilateral nephrectomy is necessary in severe nephrotic syndrome because of persistent hypoalbuminemia. The same result can sometimes be achieved by embolizing the renal arteries with coils, thus avoiding surgery in high-risk patients. Dialysis is used as necessary.

KEY POINTS

- Nephrotic syndrome is most common in young children, usually idiopathic, and most often minimal change disease.
- In adults, nephrotic syndrome is usually secondary, most often to diabetes or preeclampsia.
- Consider nephrotic syndrome in patients, particularly young children, with unexplained edema or ascites.
- Confirm nephrotic syndrome by finding spot protein/creatinine ratio ≥ 3 or urinary protein ≥ 3 g/24 h.
- Do tests for secondary causes and renal biopsy selectively, based on clinical findings.
- Assume minimal change disease if a child with idiopathic nephrotic syndrome improves after treatment with corticosteroids.
- Treat the causative disorder and with angiotensin inhibition, Na restriction, and often diuretics and/or statins.

CONGENITAL NEPHROTIC SYNDROMES

Congenital and infantile nephrotic syndromes are those that manifest during the first year of life. They include diffuse mesangial sclerosis and Finnish-type nephrotic syndrome.

Nephrotic syndrome is more prevalent among children than adults.

Congenital and infantile nephrotic syndromes are generally rare inherited defects in glomerular filtration. Symptoms are centered around proteinuria, edema, and hypoproteinemia. These diseases are best diagnosed by their gene mutations, because their presentations and histopathologies are not sufficiently specific. Early, aggressive treatment may include ACE inhibitors, angiotensin receptor II blockers, and NSAIDs (eg, indomethacin) for proteinuria; diuretics, IV albumin, and fluid restriction for edema; and antibiotics, anticoagulation, and hypernutrition. Nephrectomy, followed by dialysis or kidney transplantation, may be necessary to stop the proteinuria.

Diffuse mesangial sclerosis: This nephrotic syndrome is rare. Inheritance is variable. It is caused by a mutation in the *PLCE1* gene, which codes for phospholipase C epsilon. Progression to end-stage renal failure occurs by age 2 or 3 yr.

Patients with severe proteinuria may require bilateral nephrectomy because of severe hypoalbuminemia; dialysis should be initiated early to ameliorate nutritional deficits and mitigate failure to thrive. The disorder usually recurs in a renal graft.

Finnish-type nephrotic syndrome: This syndrome is an autosomal recessive disorder that affects 1/8200 Finnish neonates and is caused by a mutation in the *NPHS1* gene, which codes for a podocytic slit-diaphragm protein (nephrin).

Finnish-type nephrotic syndrome is rapidly progressive and usually necessitates dialysis within 1 yr. Most patients die within 1 yr, but a few have been supported nutritionally until renal failure occurs and then managed with dialysis or transplantation. However, the disorder may recur in a renal graft.

Other congenital nephrotic syndromes: Several other rare congenital nephrotic syndromes are now genetically characterized. These disorders include

- Corticosteroid-resistant nephrotic syndrome (defective *NPHS2* gene coding for podocin),
- Familial focal segmental glomerulosclerosis (defective *ACTN 4* gene coding for alpha-actin 4),
- Denys-Drash syndrome, which is characterized by diffuse mesangial sclerosis, male pseudohermaphroditism, and Wilms tumor (defective *WT1* gene)

DIABETIC NEPHROPATHY

Diabetic nephropathy is glomerular sclerosis and fibrosis caused by the metabolic and hemodynamic changes of diabetes mellitus (see p. 1253). It manifests as slowly progressive albuminuria with worsening hypertension and renal insufficiency. Diagnosis is based on history, physical examination, urinalysis, and urine albumin/creatinine ratio. Treatment is strict glucose control, angiotensin inhibition (using ACE inhibitors or angiotensin II receptor blockers), and control of BP and lipids.

(See also Diabetic Nephropathy on p. 1260)

Diabetic nephropathy (DN) is the most common cause of nephrotic syndrome in adults. Diabetic nephropathy is also the most common cause of end-stage renal disease in the US, accounting for up to 80% of cases. The prevalence of renal failure is probably about 40% among patients with type 1 diabetes mellitus. The prevalence of renal failure among patients with type 2 diabetes mellitus is usually stated as 20 to 30%, but this figure is probably low. Renal failure is particularly common in certain ethnic groups, such as blacks, Mexican-Americans, Polynesians, and Pima Indians. Other risk factors include the following:

- Duration and degree of hyperglycemia
- Hypertension
- Dyslipidemia
- Cigarette smoking
- Certain polymorphisms affecting the renin-angiotensin-aldosterone axis
- Family history of diabetic nephropathy
- Genetic variables (decreased number of glomeruli)

Because type 2 diabetes is often present for several years before being recognized, nephropathy often develops < 10 yr after diabetes is diagnosed.

Renal failure usually takes ≥ 10 yr after the onset of nephropathy to develop.

Pathophysiology

Pathogenesis begins with small vessel disease. Pathophysiology is complex, involving glycosylation of proteins, hormonally influenced cytokine release (eg, transforming growth factor-beta), deposition of mesangial matrix, and alteration of glomerular hemodynamics. Hyperfiltration, an early functional abnormality, is only a relative predictor for the development of renal failure.

Hyperglycemia causes glycosylation of glomerular proteins, which may be responsible for mesangial cell proliferation and matrix expansion and vascular endothelial damage. The glomerular basement membrane classically becomes thickened.

Lesions of diffuse or nodular intercapillary glomerulosclerosis are distinctive; areas of nodular glomerulosclerosis may be referred to as Kimmelstiel-Wilson lesions. There is marked hyalinosis of afferent and efferent arterioles as well as arteriosclerosis; interstitial fibrosis and tubular atrophy may be present. Only mesangial matrix expansion appears to correlate with progression to end-stage renal disease.

DN begins as glomerular hyperfiltration (increased GFR); GFR normalizes with early renal injury and mild hypertension, which worsens over time. Microalbuminuria, urinary excretion of albumin in a range of 30 to 300 mg albumin/day, then occurs. Urinary albumin in these concentrations is called microalbuminuria because detection of proteinuria by dipstick on routine urinalysis usually requires > 300 mg albumin/day. Microalbuminuria progresses to macroalbuminuria (proteinuria > 300 mg/day at a variable course, usually over years. Nephrotic syndrome (proteinuria ≥ 3 g/day) precedes end-stage renal disease, on average, by about 3 to 5 yr, but this timing is also highly variable.

Other urinary tract abnormalities commonly occurring with DN that may accelerate the decline of renal function include papillary necrosis, type IV renal tubular acidosis, and UTIs. In DN, the kidneys are usually of normal size or larger (> 10 to 12 cm in length).

Symptoms and Signs

DN is asymptomatic in early stages. Sustained microalbuminuria is the earliest warning sign. Hypertension and some measure of dependent edema eventually develop in most untreated patients.

In later stages, patients may develop symptoms and signs of uremia (eg, nausea, vomiting, anorexia) earlier (ie, with higher GFR) than do patients without DN, possibly because the combination of end-organ damage due to diabetes (eg, neuropathy) and renal failure worsens symptoms.

Diagnosis

- Yearly screening of all patients with diabetes with random urine albumin/creatinine ratio
- Urinalysis for signs of other renal disorders (eg, hematuria, RBC casts)

The diagnosis is suspected in patients with diabetes who have proteinuria, particularly if they have diabetic retinopathy (indicating small vessel disease) or risk factors for DN. Other renal disorders should be considered if there are any of the following:

- Heavy proteinuria with only a brief history of diabetes
- Absence of diabetic retinopathy
- Rapid onset of heavy proteinuria
- Gross hematuria
- RBC casts
- Rapid decline in GFR
- Small kidney size

Urinary protein: Patients are tested for proteinuria by routine urinalysis; if proteinuria is present, testing for microalbuminuria is unnecessary because the patient already has macroalbuminuria suggestive of diabetic renal disease. In patients without proteinuria on urinalysis, an albumin/creatinine ratio should be calculated from a mid-morning urine specimen. A ratio ≥ 0.03 mg/mg (≥ 30 mg/g) indicates microalbuminuria if it is present on at least 2 of 3 specimens within 3 to 6 mo and if it cannot be explained by infection or exercise.

Some experts recommend that microalbuminuria be measured from a 24-h urine collection, but this approach is less convenient, and many patients have difficulty accurately collecting a specimen. The random urine albumin/creatinine ratio overestimates 24-h collection of microalbuminuria in up to 30% of patients > 65 due to reduced creatinine production from reduced muscle mass. Inaccurate results can also occur in very muscular patients or if vigorous exercise precedes urine collection.

For most patients with diabetes who have proteinuria, the diagnosis is clinical. Renal biopsy can confirm the diagnosis but is rarely necessary.

Screening: Patients with type 1 diabetes without known renal disease should be screened for proteinuria and, if proteinuria is absent on routine urinalysis, for microalbuminuria, beginning 5 yr after diagnosis and at least annually thereafter.

Patients with type 2 diabetes should be screened at the time of diagnosis and annually thereafter.

Prognosis

Prognosis is good for patients who are meticulously treated and monitored. Such care is often difficult in practice, however, and most patients slowly lose renal function; even prehypertension (BP 120 to 139/80 to 89 mm Hg) or stage 1 hypertension (BP 140 to 159/90 to 99 mm Hg) may accelerate injury. Systemic atherosclerotic disease (stroke, MI, peripheral arterial disease) predicts an increase in mortality.

Treatment

- Maintenance of glycosylated Hb (HbA_{1c}) ≤ 7.0
- Aggressive BP control, beginning with angiotensin inhibition

Blood glucose control: Primary treatment is strict glucose control to maintain HbA_{1c} ≤ 7.0; maintenance of euglycemia reduces microalbuminuria but may not retard disease progression once DN is well established.

Blood pressure control: Glucose control must also be accompanied by strict control of BP to < 130/80 mm Hg, although some experts now recommend BP < 140/90 mm Hg. Some suggest BP should be 110 to 120/65 to 80 mm Hg, particularly in patients with protein excretion of > 1 g/day; however, others claim that BP values < 120/85 mm Hg are associated with increased cardiovascular mortality and heart failure.

Angiotensin inhibition is first-line therapy. Thus, ACE inhibitors or angiotensin II receptor blockers are the antihypertensives of choice; they reduce BP and proteinuria and slow the progression of DN. ACE inhibitors are usually less expensive, but angiotensin II receptor blockers can be used instead if ACE inhibitors cause persistent cough. Treatment should be started when microalbuminuria is detected regardless of whether hypertension is present; some experts recommend drugs be used even before signs of renal disease appear.

Diuretics are required by most patients in addition to angiotensin inhibition to reach target BP levels. Dose should be decreased if symptoms of orthostatic hypotension develop or serum creatinine increases by more than 30%.

Nondihydropyridine calcium channel blockers (diltiazem and verapamil) are also antiproteinuric and renoprotective and can be used if proteinuria does not meaningfully decrease when target BP is reached or as alternatives for patients with hyperkalemia or other contraindications to ACE inhibitors or angiotensin II receptor blockers.

In contrast, dihydropyridine calcium channel blockers (eg, nifedipine, felodipine, amlodipine) do not reduce proteinuria, although they are useful adjuncts for BP control and may be cardioprotective in combination with ACE inhibitors. ACE inhibitors and nondihydropyridine calcium channel blockers have greater antiproteinuric and renoprotective effects when used together, and their antiproteinuric effect is enhanced by sodium restriction. Nondihydropyridine calcium channel blockers should be used with caution in patients taking beta-blockers because of the potential to worsen bradycardia.

Dyslipidemia: Dyslipidemia should also be treated.

Statins should be used as first-line therapy for dyslipidemia treatment in patients with DN because they reduce cardiovascular mortality and urinary protein.

Other treatments: Dietary protein restriction yields mixed results. The American Diabetes Association recommends that people with diabetes and overt nephropathy be restricted to 0.8 to 1.2 g protein/kg/day. Significant protein restriction is not recommended.

Vitamin D supplementation, typically with cholecalciferol (vitamin D_3).

Sodium bicarbonate, given to maintain a serum bicarbonate concentration > 22 mEq/L, may slow disease progression in patients with chronic kidney disease and metabolic acidosis.

Treatments for edema can include the following:

- Dietary sodium restriction (eg, < 2 g/day)
- Fluid restriction
- Loop diuretics, as needed, with careful titration to avoid hypovolemia

Kidney transplantation: Kidney transplantation with or without simultaneous or subsequent pancreas transplantation is an option for patients with end-stage renal disease. The 5-yr survival rate for patients with type 2 diabetes receiving a kidney transplant is almost 60%, compared with 2% for dialysis-dependent patients who do not undergo transplantation (though this statistic probably represents significant selection bias). Kidney allograft survival rate is > 85% at 2 yr.

KEY POINTS

- Diabetic nephropathy is very common, asymptomatic until late, and should be considered in all patients with diabetes.
- Periodically screen all patients with diabetes with urinalysis and, if proteinuria is absent, albumin/creatinine ratio calculated from a mid-morning urine specimen.
- Treat BP aggressively, usually beginning with angiotensin inhibition.
- Control glucose to maintain HbA_{1c} at ≤ 7.0.

FOCAL SEGMENTAL GLOMERULOSCLEROSIS

Focal segmental glomerulosclerosis is scattered (segmental) mesangial sclerosis that begins in some but not all (focal) glomeruli and eventually involves all glomeruli. It is most often idiopathic but may be secondary to use of heroin or other drugs, HIV infection, obesity, sickle cell disease, atheroembolic disease, or nephron loss (eg, in reflux nephropathy, subtotal nephrectomy, or renal dysgenesis). It manifests mainly in adolescents but also in young and middle-aged adults. Patients have insidious onset of proteinuria, mild hematuria, hypertension, and azotemia. Diagnosis is confirmed by renal biopsy. Treatment is with angiotensin inhibition and, for idiopathic disease, corticosteroids and sometimes cytotoxic drugs.

Focal segmental glomerulosclerosis (FSGS) is now the most common cause of idiopathic (or primary) nephrotic syndrome among adults in the US. It is especially common in black men. Though usually idiopathic, FSGS can occur in association with other factors (secondary FSGS), including drugs (eg, heroin, lithium, interferon alfa, pamidronate, cyclosporine, or NSAIDs [causing analgesic nephropathy]), atheroembolic disease affecting the kidneys, obesity, HIV infection (see p. 2120), and disorders causing nephron loss (eg, reflux nephropathy, subtotal nephrectomy, renal dysgenesis [eg oligomeganephronia: renal hypoplasia with a decreased number of nephrons]). Familial cases exist.

In FSGS, because charge as well as size ultrafiltration barriers are defective, proteinuria is typically nonselective, affecting high molecular-weight proteins (eg, Igs) as well as albumin. Kidneys tend to be small.

Symptoms and Signs

FSGS patients commonly present with heavy proteinuria, hypertension, renal dysfunction, edema, or a combination. Sometimes the only sign is asymptomatic proteinuria that is not in nephrotic range. Microscopic hematuria is occasionally present.

Diagnosis

- Renal biopsy, when possible, with immunostaining and electron microscopy

FSGS is suspected in patients with nephrotic syndrome, proteinuria, or renal dysfunction with no obvious cause, particularly patients who have disorders or use drugs associated with FSGS.

Urinalysis is done and BUN, serum creatinine, and 24-h urinary protein excretion are measured.

Diagnosis is confirmed by renal biopsy, which shows focal and segmental hyalinization of the glomeruli, often with immunostaining showing IgM and complement (C3) deposits in a nodular and coarse granular pattern. Electron microscopy reveals diffuse effacement of podocyte foot processes in idiopathic cases but may show patchy effacement in secondary cases. Global sclerosis may be visible, along with secondary atrophic glomeruli. Biopsy may be falsely negative if areas of focal abnormalities are not sampled.

Prognosis

Prognosis is poor. Spontaneous remissions occur in < 10% of patients. Renal failure occurs in > 50% of patients within 10 yr; in 20%, end-stage renal disease occurs within 2 yr despite treatment and is more likely if patients have significant tubulointerstitial fibrosis. The disorder is more rapidly progressive in adults than in children.

The presence of segmental sclerosis consistently at the glomerular pole where the tubule originates (tip lesion) may portend a more favorable response to corticosteroid therapy. Another variant, in which the capillary walls are wrinkled or collapsed (collapsing FSGS, which is typical in association with IV drug abuse or HIV infection), suggests more severe disease and rapid progression to renal failure. Pregnancy may exacerbate FSGS.

FSGS may recur after kidney transplantation; proteinuria sometimes returns within hours of transplantation. Of patients whose transplant was for end-stage renal disease caused by FSGS, about 8 to 30% lose their graft due to recurrent FSGS; risk is highest in young children, patients who are not black, patients who develop renal failure < 3 yr after disease onset, patients with mesangial proliferation, and patients with repeat transplants when the diagnosis before the first transplant was primary FSGS. Familial forms of FSGS rarely recur after transplantation.

Heroin addicts with nephrotic syndrome due to FSGS can experience complete remission if they cease taking heroin early in the disease.

Treatment

- Angiotensin inhibition
- Corticosteroids and sometimes cytotoxic drugs for idiopathic FSGS
- Kidney transplantation for patients with end-stage renal disease

Treatment often is not effective. Patients with FSGS should be treated with angiotensin inhibition (with an ACE inhibitor or an angiotensin II receptor blocker) unless contraindicated by angioedema or hyperkalemia. Patients with nephrotic syndrome should be treated with a statin.

In idiopathic FSGS, a trial of immunosuppressive therapy is indicated if proteinuria reaches the nephrotic range or if renal function worsens, especially if kidney biopsy reveals a tip lesion. In contrast, patients with secondary FSGS, collapsing FSGS, or advanced tubulointerstitial fibrosis on renal biopsy are generally not treated with immunosuppression because they tend to not respond; instead, the primary disorder is treated.

Immunosuppressive therapy: Corticosteroids (eg, prednisone 1 mg/kg po once/day or 2 mg/kg every other day) are recommended for at least 2 mo, although some experts recommend use for up to 9 mo. Response rates of 30 to 50% have been reported with prolonged therapy and vary by the histologic classification of FSGS. After a 2-wk remission of proteinuria, the corticosteroid is slowly tapered over ≥ 2 mo. Secondary and familial cases, collapsing FSGS, and advanced tubulointerstitial fibrosis are more likely to be corticosteroid-resistant.

If only slight improvement or relapse occurs with corticosteroid therapy, remission may be induced with cyclosporine 1.5 to 2 mg/kg po bid for 6 mo or, alternatively, mycophenolate mofetil 750 to 1000 mg po bid for 6 mo in patients > 1.25 m^2 BSA or 600 mg/m^2 BSA bid up to 1000 mg bid.

In patients with contraindications to high-dose corticosteroids (eg, diabetes, osteoporosis), cyclosporine can be given along with a lower dose of corticosteroids (eg, prednisone 0.15 mg/kg po once/day).

An alternative is plasma exchange with tacrolimus immunosuppression.

KEY POINTS

- Suspect FSGS if patients have nephrotic syndrome, proteinuria, or renal dysfunction with no obvious cause, particularly patients who have disorders or use drugs associated with FSGS.
- When possible, confirm FSGS by renal biopsy with immunostaining and electron microscopy.
- Consider treatment with corticosteroids and possibly cyclosporine or mycophenolate mofetil if FSGS is idiopathic and proteinuria reaches the nephrotic range or renal function worsens.

HIV-ASSOCIATED NEPHROPATHY

HIV-associated nephropathy is characterized by clinical findings similar to those of focal segmental glomerulosclerosis and often biopsy features of collapsing glomerulopathy (a variant of focal segmental glomerulosclerosis).

HIV-associated nephropathy (HIVAN), a type of nephrotic syndrome seems to be more common among black patients with HIV who are injection drug users or have been poorly compliant with antiretroviral therapy. Infection of renal cells with HIV may contribute.

Most clinical findings are similar to those of focal segmental glomerulosclerosis, but hypertension is less common and the kidneys remain enlarged.

Most patients experience rapid progression to end-stage renal disease within 1 to 4 mo.

Diagnosis

- Renal biopsy

HIVAN is suspected in patients with nephrotic syndrome or nephropathy who have AIDS or symptoms of AIDS. HIVAN should be distinguished from the many other disorders that occur with higher frequency in HIV-infected patients and cause renal disease, such as thrombotic microangiopathy (hemolytic-uremic syndrome and thrombotic thrombocytopenic purpura), immune complex–mediated glomerulonephritis, and drug-induced interstitial nephritis (due to indinavir and ritonavir) and rhabdomyolysis (due to statins).

Ultrasonography, if done, shows that the kidneys are enlarged and highly echogenic.

Renal biopsy typically is done. Light microscopy shows capillary collapse of varying severity (collapsing glomerulopathy) and differing degrees of increased mesangial matrix. Tubular cells show marked degenerative changes and tubular atrophy or microcytic dilation. Interstitial immune cell infiltrate, fibrosis, and edema are common. Tubular reticular inclusions, similar to those in SLE, are found within endothelial cells but are now rare with more effective HIV therapy.

Normotension and persistently enlarged kidneys help to differentiate HIVAN from focal segmental glomerulosclerosis.

Treatment

- Highly active antiretroviral therapy (HAART) and ACE inhibitors

Control of the HIV infection may help minimize renal damage; in fact, HIVAN is rare in patients taking HAART with well-controlled HIV infection. ACE inhibitors are probably of some benefit. The role of corticosteroids is not well defined. Dialysis is usually required. At some centers, outcomes after transplantation have been excellent.

MEMBRANOUS NEPHROPATHY

(Membranous Glomerulonephritis)

Membranous nephropathy is deposition of immune complexes on the glomerular basement membrane (GBM) with GBM thickening. Cause is usually unknown, although secondary causes include drugs, infections, autoimmune disorders, and cancer. Manifestations include insidious onset of edema and heavy proteinuria with benign urinary sediment, normal renal function, and normal or elevated BP. Diagnosis is by renal biopsy. Spontaneous remission is common. Treatment of patients at high risk of progression is usually with corticosteroids and cyclophosphamide or chlorambucil.

The M-type phospholipase A2 receptor (PLA2R) in the glomerular podocyte has been identified as the major target antigen in deposited immune-complexes.

Membranous nephropathy (MN) mostly affects adults, in whom it is a common cause of nephrotic syndrome.

Etiology

MN is usually idiopathic, but it may be secondary to any of the following:

- Drugs (eg, gold, penicillamine, NSAIDs)
- Infections (eg, hepatitis B or C virus infection, syphilis, HIV infection)
- Autoimmune disorders (eg, SLE)
- Thyroiditis
- Cancer
- Parasitic diseases (eg, malaria, schistosomiasis, leishmaniasis)

Depending on the patient's age, 4 to 20% have an underlying cancer, including solid cancers of the lung, colon, stomach, breast, or kidney; Hodgkin or non-Hodgkin lymphoma; chronic lymphocytic leukemia; and melanoma.

MN is rare in children and, when it occurs, is usually due to hepatitis B virus infection or SLE.

Renal vein thrombosis is more frequent in MN and is usually asymptomatic, but may manifest with flank pain, hematuria, and hypertension. It may progress to pulmonary embolism.

Symptoms and Signs

Patients typically present with edema and nephrotic-range proteinuria and occasionally with microscopic hematuria and hypertension. Symptoms and signs of a disorder causing MN (eg, a cancer) may be present initially.

Diagnosis

- Renal biopsy
- Evaluation for secondary causes

Diagnosis is suggested by development of nephrotic syndrome, particularly in patients who have potential causes of MN. The diagnosis is confirmed by biopsy.

Proteinuria is in the nephrotic range in 80%. Laboratory testing is done as indicated for nephrotic syndrome. The GFR, if measured, is normal or decreased.

Immune complexes are seen as dense deposits on electron microscopy (see Fig. 250–1). Subepithelial dense deposits occur with early disease, with spikes of lamina densa between the deposits. Later, deposits appear within the GBM, and marked thickening occurs. A diffuse, granular pattern of IgG deposition occurs along the GBM without cellular proliferation, exudation, or necrosis.

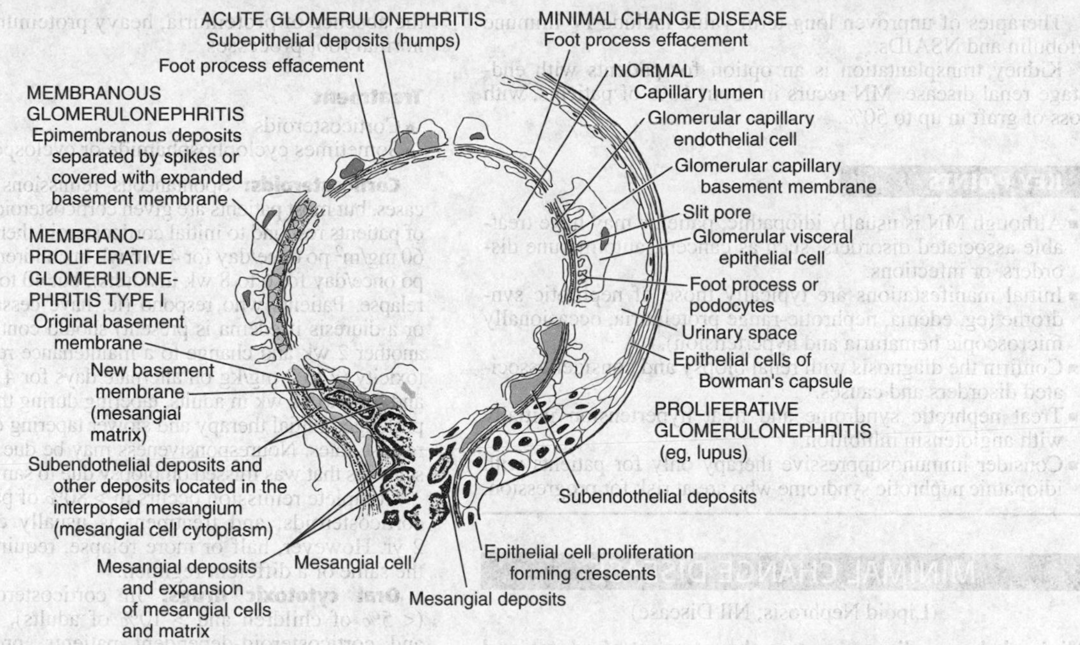

Fig. 250–1. Electron microscopic features in immunologic glomerular disorders.

Diagnosis of cause: Evaluation of patients diagnosed with MN usually includes the following:

- A search for occult cancer, particularly in a patient who has lost weight, has unexplained anemia or heme-positive stools, or is elderly
- Consideration of drug-induced MN
- Hepatitis B and C serologic testing
- Antinuclear antibody testing

The search for occult cancer is usually limited to age-appropriate screening (eg, colonoscopy for patients age > 50 or with other symptoms or risk factors, mammography for women age > 40, prostate-specific antigen measurement for men age > 50 [age > 40 for blacks], chest x-ray and possibly chest CT for patients at risk of lung cancer).

Prognosis

About 25% of patients undergo spontaneous remission, 25% develop persistent, non-nephrotic–range proteinuria, 25% develop persistent nephrotic syndrome, and 25% progress to end-stage renal disease. Women, children, and young adults with non-nephrotic–range proteinuria and patients with persistently normal renal function 3 yr after diagnosis tend to have little disease progression. More than 50% of patients with nephrotic-range proteinuria who are asymptomatic or who have edema that can be controlled with diuretics will have a partial or complete remission within 3 to 4 yr.

Risk of progression to renal failure is highest among patients with

- Persistent proteinuria ≥ 8 g/day, particularly men age > 50 yr
- An elevated serum creatinine level at presentation or diagnosis
- Biopsy evidence of substantial interstitial inflammation

Treatment

- Treatment of secondary causes and of nephrotic syndrome as indicated
- Immunosuppressive therapy for patients at high risk of progression
- Kidney transplantation for patients with end-stage renal disease

Primary treatment is that of the causes. Among patients with idiopathic MN, asymptomatic patients with non-nephrotic–range proteinuria do not require treatment; renal function should be monitored periodically (eg, twice yearly when apparently stable).

Patients with nephrotic-range proteinuria who are asymptomatic or who have edema that can be controlled with diuretics should be treated for nephrotic syndrome.

Patients with hypertension should be given an ACE inhibitor or angiotensin II receptor blocker; these drugs may also benefit patients without hypertension by reducing proteinuria.

Immunosuppressive therapy: Immunosuppressants should be considered only for patients with symptomatic idiopathic nephrotic syndrome and for those most at risk of progressive disease. However, there is no strong evidence that adults with nephrotic syndrome benefit long-term from immunosuppressive therapy. Older and chronically ill patients are at greater risk of infectious complications due to immunosuppressants.

No consensus protocol exists, but historically, a common regimen included corticosteroids, followed by chlorambucil. However, this regimen is not often used currently. Most experts favor use of combinations of cyclophosphamide and corticosteroids because of their better safety profile.

For patients who are intolerant of cytotoxic drugs or who do not respond to them, cyclosporine 4 to 6 mg/kg po once/day for 4 mo or rituximab 375 mg/m^2 IV once/wk for 4 wk may be beneficial.

Therapies of unproven long-term value include IV immune globulin and NSAIDs.

Kidney transplantation is an option for patients with end-stage renal disease. MN recurs in about 10% of patients, with loss of graft in up to 50%.

KEY POINTS

- Although MN is usually idiopathic, patients may have treatable associated disorders, such as cancers, autoimmune disorders, or infections.
- Initial manifestations are typically those of nephrotic syndrome (eg, edema, nephrotic-range proteinuria, occasionally microscopic hematuria and hypertension).
- Confirm the diagnosis with renal biopsy and consider associated disorders and causes.
- Treat nephrotic syndrome and treat hypertension initially with angiotensin inhibition.
- Consider immunosuppressive therapy only for patients with idiopathic nephrotic syndrome who are at risk for progression.

MINIMAL CHANGE DISEASE

(Lipoid Nephrosis; Nil Disease)

Minimal change disease causes abrupt onset of edema and heavy proteinuria, mostly in children. Renal function is typically normal. Diagnosis is based on clinical findings or renal biopsy. Prognosis is excellent. Treatment is with corticosteroids or, in patients who do not respond, cyclophosphamide or cyclosporine.

Minimal change disease (MCD) is the most common cause of nephrotic syndrome in children 4 to 8 yr (80 to 90% of childhood nephrotic syndrome), but it also occurs in adults (10 to 20% of adult nephrotic syndrome). The cause is almost always unknown, although rare cases may occur secondary to drug use (especially NSAIDs) and hematologic cancers (especially Hodgkin lymphoma).

Symptoms and Signs

MCD causes nephrotic syndrome, usually without hypertension or azotemia; microscopic hematuria occurs in about 20% of patients, mainly adults. Azotemia can occur in secondary cases and in patients > 60 yr. Albumin is lost in the urine of patients with MCD more so than larger serum proteins probably because MCD causes changes in the charge barrier that affect albumin selectively.

Diagnosis

- In adults with idiopathic nephrotic syndrome, renal biopsy

In children, the following:

- Sudden onset of unexplained nephrotic-range proteinuria that is mainly albumin
- Normal renal function
- Non-nephritic urine sediment
- Renal biopsy in atypical cases

Renal biopsy is required in atypical cases and in adults. Electron microscopy demonstrates edema with diffuse swelling (effacement) of foot processes of the epithelial podocytes (see Fig. 250–1). Complement and Ig deposits are absent on immunofluorescence. Although effacement is not observed in the absence of proteinuria, heavy proteinuria may occur with normal foot processes.

Treatment

- Corticosteroids
- Sometimes cyclophosphamide or cyclosporine

Corticosteroids: Spontaneous remissions occur in 40% of cases, but most patients are given corticosteroids. About 80 to 90% of patients respond to initial corticosteroid therapy (eg, prednisone 60 mg/m^2 po once/day for 4 to 6 wk in children and 1 to 1.5 mg/kg po once/day for 6 to 8 wk in adults), but 40 to 73% of responders relapse. Patients who respond (ie, have cessation of proteinuria or a diuresis if edema is present) should continue prednisone for another 2 wk and change to a maintenance regimen to minimize toxicity (2 to 3 mg/kg on alternate days for 4 to 6 wk in children and for 8 to 12 wk in adults, tapering during the next 4 mo). More prolonged initial therapy and slower tapering of prednisone lower relapse rates. Nonresponsiveness may be due to underlying focal sclerosis that was missed on biopsy due to sampling error.

Complete remission occurs in > 80% of patients treated with corticosteroids, and treatment is usually continued for 1 to 2 yr. However, half or more relapse, requiring treatment with the same or a different regimen.

Oral cytotoxic drugs: In corticosteroid nonresponders (< 5% of children and > 10% of adults), frequent relapsers, and corticosteroid-dependent patients, prolonged remission may be achieved with an oral cytotoxic drug (usually cyclophosphamide 2 to 3 mg/kg once/day for 12 wk or chlorambucil 0.15 mg/kg once/day for 8 wk). However, these drugs may suppress gonadal function (most serious in prepubertal adolescents), cause hemorrhagic cystitis, have mutagenic potential, and suppress bone marrow and lymphocyte function. Dosage should be monitored with frequent CBCs, and hemorrhagic cystitis should be sought by urinalysis. Adults, particularly if older or hypertensive, are more prone to adverse effects from these cytotoxic drugs. Another alternative is cyclosporine 3 mg/kg po bid, adjusted to obtain a whole-blood trough concentration of 50 to 150 μg/L (40 to 125 nmol/L).

Patients responsive to cyclosporine frequently relapse when the drug is stopped.

Other treatment: Most patients who are unresponsive to these interventions respond to alternative therapies, including ACE inhibitors, thioguanine, levamisole, azathioprine, and mycophenolate mofetil; < 5% progress to renal failure.

KEY POINTS

- MCD accounts for most cases of nephrotic syndrome in children and is usually idiopathic.
- Suspect MCD in children who have sudden onset of nephrotic range proteinuria with normal renal function and a non-nephritic urine sediment.
- Confirm the diagnosis by renal biopsy in adults and atypical childhood cases.
- Treatment with corticosteroids is usually sufficient.

FIBRILLARY AND IMMUNOTACTOID GLOMERULOPATHIES

Fibrillary and immunotactoid glomerulopathies are rare conditions defined pathologically by organized deposition of nonamyloid microfibrillar or microtubular structures within the renal mesangium and basement membrane.

Fibrillary and immunotactoid glomerulopathies are thought by some experts to be related disorders. They are found in about 0.6% of renal biopsy specimens, occur equally in men and women, and have been described in patients ≥ 10 yr. Average age at diagnosis is about 45. Mechanism is unknown, although deposition of immunoglobulin, particularly IgG kappa and lambda light chains and complement (C3), suggests immune system dysfunction. Patients may have accompanying cancer, paraproteinemia, cryoglobulinemia, plasma cell dyscrasia, hepatitis C infection, or SLE, or they may have a primary renal disease without evidence of systemic disease.

All patients have proteinuria, > 60% in the nephrotic range. Microscopic hematuria is present in about 60%; hypertension, in about 70%. Slightly > 50% have renal insufficiency at presentation.

Diagnosis

- Renal biopsy

Diagnosis is suggested by laboratory data and confirmed by renal biopsy. If nephrotic syndrome is present, testing is done as for other cases of nephrotic syndrome.

Urinalysis usually shows features of nephritic syndrome and nephrotic syndrome.

Serum C3 and C4 are usually measured and are occasionally decreased.

Light microscopy of a biopsy specimen shows mesangial expansion by amorphous eosinophilic deposits and mild mesangial hypercellularity. Various other changes may be present on light microscopy (eg, crescent formation, membranoproliferative patterns). Congo red staining is negative for amyloid. Immunostaining reveals IgG and C3 and sometimes kappa and lambda light chains in the area of the deposits.

Electron microscopy shows glomerular deposits consisting of extracellular, elongated, nonbranching microfibrils or microtubules. In fibrillary glomerulonephritis, the diameter of the microfibrils and microtubules varies from 20 to 30 nm. In immunotactoid glomerulonephritis, the diameter of the microfibrils and microtubules varies from 30 to 50 nm. In contrast, in amyloidosis, fibrils are 8 to 12 nm.

Some experts distinguish immunotactoid from fibrillary glomerulopathy by the presence of microtubular (as opposed to smaller microfibrillar) structures in the deposits; others distinguish them by the presence of a related systemic illness. For example, a lymphoproliferative disorder, monoclonal gammopathy, cryoglobulinemia, or SLE may suggest immunotactoid glomerulonephritis.

Prognosis

The conditions are usually slowly progressive with renal insufficiency, progressing to end-stage renal disease in 50% of patients within 2 to 4 yr. A more rapid decline is predicted by the presence of hypertension, nephrotic-range proteinuria, and renal insufficiency at presentation.

Treatment

- Evidence is lacking, but consider ACE inhibitors or angiotensin II receptor blockers, immunosuppressants, and/or corticosteroids

Evidence to support specific treatments is lacking although ACE inhibitors and angiotensin II receptor blockers may be used to reduce proteinuria. Immunosuppressants have been used based on anecdotal evidence but are not a mainstay of therapy; success may be greater with corticosteroids when serum complement is decreased. The disorder may recur after transplantation.

MEMBRANOPROLIFERATIVE GLOMERULONEPHRITIS

(Lobular Glomerulonephritis; Mesangiocapillary Glomerulonephritis)

Membranoproliferative glomerulonephritis is a heterogeneous group of disorders that share mixed nephritic and nephrotic features and microscopic findings. They mostly affect children. Cause is immune complex deposition that is idiopathic or secondary to a systemic disorder. Diagnosis is by renal biopsy. Prognosis is generally poor. Treatment, when indicated, is with corticosteroids and antiplatelet drugs.

Membranoproliferative glomerulonephritis is a group of immune-mediated disorders characterized histologically by glomerular basement membrane (GBM) thickening and proliferative changes on light microscopy. There are 3 types, each of which may have primary (idiopathic) or secondary causes. Primary forms affect children and young adults between ages 8 and 30 and account for 10% of cases of nephrotic syndrome in children; secondary forms tend to affect adults > 30. Men and women are affected equally. Reported familial cases of some types suggest genetic factors play a role in at least some cases. Many factors contribute to hypocomplementemia.

Membranoproliferative glomerulonephritis type I: Type I (mesangial proliferation with immune deposits) accounts for 80 to 85% of cases. The idiopathic form is rare. Type I most commonly occurs secondary to one of the following:

- Systemic immune complex disorder (eg, SLE, mixed cryoglobulinemia, Sjögren syndrome)
- Chronic infection (eg, bacterial endocarditis, HIV infection, hepatitis B or C infection, visceral abscess, ventriculoatrial shunt infection)
- Cancer (eg, chronic lymphocytic leukemia, lymphomas, melanoma)
- Other disorders (eg, partial lipodystrophy, C2 or C3 deficiencies, sarcoidosis, thrombotic microangiopathies)

Membranoproliferative glomerulonephritis type II: Type II (similar to type I with less mesangial proliferation and with GBM dense deposits) accounts for 15 to 20%. It is probably an autoimmune disorder in which an IgG autoantibody (C3 nephritic factor) binds C3 convertase, rendering C3 resistant to inactivation; immunofluorescent staining identifies C3 around dense deposits and in mesangium.

Membranoproliferative glomerulonephritis type III: Type III is thought to be a disorder similar to type I and accounts for few cases. Cause is unknown but may be related to immune complex (IgG, C3) deposition. An IgG autoantibody against the terminal component of complement is found in 70% of patients. Subepithelial deposits can occur focally and appear to disrupt the GBM.

Symptoms and Signs

Symptoms and signs are those of nephrotic syndrome in 60 to 80% of cases. Symptoms and signs of nephritic syndrome (acute glomerulonephritis) are presenting features in 15 to 20% of cases of type I and III disease and in a higher percentage of type II disease. At diagnosis, 30% of patients have hypertension and 20% have renal insufficiency; hypertension often develops even before GFR declines.

Patients with type II disease have a greater incidence of ocular abnormalities (basal laminar drusen, diffuse retinal pigment alterations, diskiform macular detachment, choroidal neovascularization), which ultimately impair vision.

Diagnosis

- Renal biopsy
- Serum complement profile
- Serologic tests

Diagnosis is confirmed by renal biopsy. The location of immune complex deposits can help differentiate between types; typically subendothelial and mesangial in type I, intramembranous in type II, and subepithelial in type III. Other tests are also done.

Serum complement profiles are more frequently abnormal in membranoproliferative glomerulonephritis than in other glomerular disorders and provide supportive evidence of the diagnosis (see Table 250–6). C3 levels are often low. In type I disease, the classic complement pathway is activated and C3 and C4 are decreased. C3 may be decreased more often than C4 at diagnosis and decreases further during follow-up, but eventually normalizes. In type II disease, the alternate complement pathway is activated and C3 is more frequently and severely reduced than in type I while C4 levels are normal. In type III disease, C3 is reduced but C4 is normal. C3 nephritic factor is detectable in 80% of patients with type II and in some patients with type I disease. Terminal complement nephritic factor is detectable in 20% of patients with type I, rarely in patients with type II, and 70% of patients with type III disease.

Serologic tests (eg, for SLE, hepatitis B and C virus, and cryoglobulinemia) are warranted to check for secondary causes of type I disease.

CBC, often obtained in the course of diagnostic evaluation, demonstrates normochromic-normocytic anemia, often out of proportion to the stage of renal insufficiency (possibly because of hemolysis), and thrombocytopenia from platelet consumption.

Prognosis

Prognosis is good if a condition causing secondary membranoproliferative glomerulonephritis is successfully treated. Idiopathic type I membranoproliferative glomerulonephritis often progresses slowly; type II progresses more rapidly. In general, the long-term prognosis is poor. End-stage renal disease occurs in 50% of patients at 10 yr and in 90% at 20 yr. Spontaneous remission occurs in < 5% with type II. Type I membranoproliferative glomerulonephritis recurs in 30% of kidney transplantation patients; type II recurs in 90% but, despite this high recurrence rate, leads to graft loss only infrequently. Outcome tends to be worse if proteinuria is in the nephrotic range.

Treatment

- Corticosteroids for children with nephrotic-range proteinuria
- Dipyridamole and aspirin for adults
- Kidney transplantation for patients with end-stage renal disease

Underlying disorders are treated when possible. Specific therapy is probably not indicated for patients with non-nephrotic-range proteinuria, which usually suggests slow progression.

Among **children** with nephrotic-range proteinuria, treatment with corticosteroids (eg, prednisone 2.5 mg/kg po once/day on alternate days [maximum 80 mg/day]) for 1 yr, followed by tapering to a maintenance dose of 20 mg on alternate days for 3 to 10 yr, may stabilize renal function. However, corticosteroid treatment may retard growth and cause hypertension.

Among **adults,** dipyridamole 225 mg po once/day with aspirin 975 mg po once/day for 1 yr may stabilize renal function at 3 to 5 yr, but at 10 yr there is no difference from placebo. Studies of antiplatelet therapy yield inconsistent results.

Alternate therapies are sometimes substituted for the usual treatments (eg, corticosteroids could exacerbate underlying hepatitis C). Alternative therapies include pegylated interferon alfa-2a or pegylated interferon alfa-2b (with addition of ribavirin if creatinine clearance is > 50 mL/min) for hepatitis C virus–associated disease and plasma exchange with corticosteroids for concomitant severe cryoglobulinemia or rapidly progressive glomerulonephritis. ACE inhibitors may decrease proteinuria and help control hypertension.

KEY POINTS

- Membranoproliferative glomerulonephritis is a group of immune-mediated disorders with some common histologic features.
- Patients most often present with nephrotic syndrome, but they may present with nephritic syndrome.
- Confirm the diagnosis with renal biopsy and obtain serum complement profile and serologic tests.
- Treat children who have nephrotic range proteinuria with corticosteroids.

Table 250–6. SERUM COMPLEMENT PROFILES IN MEMBRANOPROLIFERATIVE GLOMERULONEPHRITIS

TYPE	COMPLEMENT PROFILE	COMMENTS
Type I	Classic complement pathway activated C3: Decreased C4: Decreased	C3 may be decreased more often than C4 at diagnosis, decreases further during follow-up, and eventually normalizes. C3 nephritic factor can be detected in some patients. Terminal complement nephritic factor can be detected in 20% of patients.
Type II	Alternate complement pathway activated C3: Frequently and severely reduced C4: Normal	C3 nephritic factor can be detected in 80% of patients. Terminal complement nephritic factor can rarely be detected.
Type III	C3: Reduced C4: Normal	Terminal complement nephritic factor can be detected in 70% of patients.

LUPUS NEPHRITIS

Lupus nephritis is glomerulonephritis caused by SLE. Clinical findings include hematuria, nephrotic-range proteinuria, and, in advanced stages, azotemia. Diagnosis is based on renal biopsy. Treatment is of the underlying disorder and usually involves corticosteroids and cytotoxic or other immunosuppressant drugs.

Lupus nephritis is diagnosed in about 50% of patients with SLE (see p. 262) and typically develops within 1 yr of diagnosis. However, the total incidence is probably > 90%, because renal biopsy in patients with suspected SLE without clinical evidence of renal disease shows changes of glomerulonephritis (GN).

Pathophysiology

Pathophysiology involves immune complex deposition with development of glomerulonephritis. The immune complexes consist of

- Nuclear antigens (especially DNA)
- High-affinity complement-fixing IgG antinuclear antibodies
- Antibodies to DNA

Subendothelial, intramembranous, subepithelial, or mesangial deposits are characteristic. Wherever immune complexes are deposited, immunofluorescence staining is positive for complement and for IgG, IgA, and IgM in varying proportions. Epithelial cells may proliferate, forming crescents.

Classification of lupus nephritis is based on histologic findings (see Table 250–7).

Antiphospholipid syndrome nephropathy (APLS): This syndrome may occur with or without lupus nephritis in up to one-third of patients with SLE. The syndrome occurs in the absence of any other autoimmune process in 30 to 50% of affected patients. In antiphospholipid antibody syndrome, circulating lupus anticoagulant causes microthrombi, endothelial damage, and cortical ischemic atrophy. Antiphospholipid syndrome nephropathy increases a patient's risk of hypertension and renal insufficiency or failure compared with lupus nephritis alone.

Symptoms and Signs

The most prominent symptoms and signs are those of SLE; patients who present with renal disease may have edema, foaming urine, hypertension, or a combination.

Diagnosis

- Urinalysis and serum creatinine (all patients with SLE)
- Renal biopsy

Diagnosis is suspected in all patients with SLE, particularly in patients who have proteinuria, microscopic hematuria, RBC casts, or hypertension. Diagnosis is also suspected in patients with unexplained hypertension, elevated serum creatinine levels, or abnormalities on urinalysis who have clinical features suggesting SLE.

Urinalysis is done and serum creatinine is measured.

Table 250–7. CLASSIFICATION OF LUPUS NEPHRITIS

CLASS	DESCRIPTION	HISTOLOGIC FINDINGS*	CLINICAL FINDINGS	RENAL PROGNOSIS
I	Minimal mesangial	Normal (although immune complexes are sometimes visible using immunofluorescence or electron microscopy)	None	Excellent
II	Mesangial proliferative	Immune complexes in the mesangium only and mesangial hypercellularity	Possibly microscopic hematuria, proteinuria, or both	Excellent
III	Focal proliferative	Endocapillary and extracapillary cellular proliferation and inflammation in < 50% of glomeruli, usually in a segmental distribution	Usually hematuria and proteinuria Possibly hypertension, nephrotic syndrome, and elevated serum creatinine	Variable
IV	Diffuse proliferative[†]	Endocapillary and extracapillary cellular proliferation and inflammation in > 50% of glomeruli	Usually hematuria and proteinuria Frequently hypertension, nephrotic syndrome, and elevated serum creatinine	Variable
V	Membranous	Thickening of the glomerular basement membrane with subepithelial and intramembranous immune complex deposition	Usually nephrotic syndrome Sometimes microscopic hematuria or hypertension Serum creatinine usually normal or slightly elevated	Poorly defined
VI	Sclerosing	Sclerosis of > 90% of glomerular capillaries	Bland urinary sediment and end-stage renal disease or slowly increasing serum creatinine	Poor

*Using light microscopy.
[†]Most common form.

If either is abnormal, **renal biopsy** is usually done to confirm the diagnosis and classify the disorder histologically. Histologic classification helps determine prognosis and direct treatment.

Some of the histologic subtypes are similar to other glomerulopathies; eg, membranous lupus nephritis is histologically similar to idiopathic membranous nephropathy and diffuse proliferative lupus nephritis is histologically similar to type I membranoproliferative glomerulonephritis. Overlap between these categories is substantial, and patients may progress from one class to another.

Renal function and SLE activity should be monitored regularly. A rising serum creatinine level reflects deteriorating renal function, while a falling serum complement level or a rising anti-DNA antibody titer suggests increased disease activity.

Prognosis

Class of nephritis influences renal prognosis (see Table 250–7), as do other renal histologic features. Renal biopsies are scored with a chronicity index and with a semiquantitative activity score.

Black patients with lupus nephritis are also at higher risk of progression to end-stage renal disease.

Patients with lupus nephritis are at high risk of cancers, primarily B-cell lymphomas. Risk of atherosclerotic complications (eg, coronary artery disease, ischemic stroke) is also high, because of frequent vasculitis, hypertension, dyslipidemia, and use of corticosteroids.

Treatment

- Angiotensin inhibition for hypertension or proteinuria
- Cyclophosphamide and prednisone for active, potentially reversible nephritis
- Kidney transplantation for patients with end-stage renal disease

Angiotensin inhibition with an ACE inhibitor or angiotensin II receptor blocker is indicated for patients with even mild hypertension (eg, BP > 130/80 mm Hg) or proteinuria. Also, dyslipidemia and risk factors for atherosclerosis should be treated aggressively.

Immunosuppression: Treatment is toxic and thus is reserved for nephritis that has the following characteristics:

- Is active
- Has the potential for a poor prognosis
- Is potentially reversible

Activity is estimated by the activity score as well as clinical criteria (eg, urine sediment, increasing urine protein, increasing serum creatinine). Many experts believe that a mild to moderate chronicity score, because it suggests reversibility, should provoke more aggressive therapy than a more severe chronicity score. Nephritis with the potential for deterioration and for reversibility is usually class III or IV; it is unclear whether class V nephritis warrants aggressive treatment.

The **activity score** describes the degree of inflammation. The score is based on cellular proliferation, fibrinoid necrosis, cellular crescents, hyaline thrombi, wire loop lesions, glomerular leukocyte infiltration, and interstitial mononuclear cell infiltration. The activity score is less well correlated with disease progression, and is used, rather, to help identify active nephritis.

The **chronicity index** describes the degree of scarring. It is based on presence of glomerular sclerosis, fibrous crescents, tubular atrophy, and interstitial fibrosis. The chronicity index predicts progression of lupus nephritis to renal failure. A mild to moderate chronicity score suggests at least partially reversible disease, whereas more severe chronicity scores may indicate irreversible disease.

Many experts believe that a mild to moderate chronicity score, because it suggests reversibility, should provoke more aggressive therapy than a more severe chronicity score. Nephritis with the potential for deterioration and for reversibility is usually class III or IV; it is unclear whether class V nephritis warrants aggressive treatment.

Treatment for proliferative lupus nephritis usually combines cytotoxic drugs, corticosteroids, and sometimes other immunosuppressants.

One **induction** regimen consists of cyclophosphamide, which is usually given in IV boluses (monthly for up to 6 mo) beginning with 0.75 g/m^2 in a saline solution over 30 to 60 min and, assuming a WBC count > 3000/μL, increasing to a maximum of 1 g/m^2. Oral or IV fluid administration to create rapid urine flow minimizes the bladder toxicity of cyclophosphamide, as does mesna (see Table 33–2 on p. 265).

Another induction regimen uses mycophenolate mofetil with a target dose of 3 g/day. Prednisone is also begun at 60 to 80 mg po once/day and tapered according to response to 20 to 25 mg every other day over 6 to 12 mo. The amount of prednisone is determined by the extrarenal manifestations and number of relapses. Relapses are usually treated with increasing doses of prednisone. Both induction regimens are equally efficacious, although systemic toxicity may be less with mycophenolate mofetil than with cyclophosphamide.

Many experts are replacing the more toxic cyclophosphamide **maintenance** regimens (after induction with 6 or 7 monthly IV cyclophosphamide doses) with protocols using mycophenolate mofetil 500 mg to 1 g po bid or, as a second choice, azathioprine 2 mg/kg po once/day (maximum 150 to 200 mg/day). Chlorambucil, cyclosporine, and tacrolimus have also been used, but relative efficacies are not clear. Low-dose prednisone 0.05 to 0.2 mg/kg po once/day is continued and titrated based on disease activity. Duration of maintenance therapy is at least 1 yr.

Other treatments: Anticoagulation is of theoretical benefit for patients with antiphospholipid syndrome nephropathy, but the value of such treatment has not been established.

Kidney transplantation is an option for patients with end-stage renal disease due to lupus nephritis. Recurrent disease in the graft is uncommon (< 5%), but risk may be increased in blacks, females, and younger patients.

KEY POINTS

- Nephritis, although clinically evident in only 50%, occurs in probably > 90% of patients with SLE.
- Do urinalysis and measure serum creatinine in all patients with lupus and do renal biopsy if an unexplained abnormality is found in either.
- Initiate angiotensin inhibition for even mild hypertension and treat atherosclerotic risk factors aggressively.
- Treat active, potentially reversible nephritis with corticosteroids plus cyclophosphamide and/or mycophenolate mofetil.

251 Male Reproductive Endocrinology and Related Disorders

Male sexual development and hormonal function depend on a complex feedback circuit involving the hypothalamus-pituitary-testes modulated by the central nervous system. Male sexual dysfunction (see p. 2134) can be secondary to hypogonadism, neurovascular disorders, drugs, or other disorders.

Physiology

The hypothalamus produces gonadotropin-releasing hormone (GnRH), which is released in a pulsatile fashion every 60 to 120 min. Its target organ, the anterior pituitary gland, responds to each pulse of GnRH by producing a corresponding pulse of luteinizing hormone (LH) and, to a lesser degree, follicle-stimulating hormone (FSH). If the GnRH pulses do not occur with the proper amplitude, frequency, and diurnal variation, hypogonadism may result. (idiopathic hypogonadotropic hypogonadism). Continuous (as opposed to pulsatile) stimulation by GnRH agonists (eg, as a treatment for advanced prostate cancer) actually suppresses pituitary release of LH and FSH and thus testosterone production.

The Leydig cells of the testes respond to LH by producing between 5 and 10 mg of testosterone daily. Testosterone levels are highest in early morning and lowest during the evening hours; however, in older men, this diurnal pattern may be blunted.

Testosterone is synthesized from cholesterol through several intermediate compounds, including dehydroepiandrosterone (DHEA) and androstenedione. Circulating testosterone is mostly protein-bound, about 40% avidly bound to sex hormone–binding globulin (SHBG) and 58% loosely bound to albumin. Thus, only about 2% of circulating testosterone is bioavailable as free testosterone.

In target tissues, about 4 to 8% of testosterone is converted to a more potent metabolite, dihydrotestosterone (DHT), by the enzyme 5α-reductase. DHT has important trophic effects in the prostate and mediates androgenic alopecia. In adults, spermatogenesis requires adequate intratesticular testosterone, but the role of DHT in spermatogenesis is unclear.

Testosterone and DHT have metabolic and other effects, including

- Stimulating protein anabolism (increasing muscle mass and bone density)
- Stimulating renal erythropoietin production (increasing red blood cell mass)
- Stimulating bone marrow stem cells (modulating the immune system)
- Causing cutaneous effects (ie, sebum production, hair growth)
- Causing neural effects (ie, affecting cognition, increasing libido and possibly aggression)

Testosterone undergoes conversion to estradiol as well as to DHT; estradiol mediates most of testosterone's action on organs such as bones and the brain.

Testosterone, DHT, and estradiol provide negative feedback on the hypothalamic-pituitary axis. In males, estradiol is the main inhibitor of LH production, whereas both estradiol and inhibin B, a peptide produced by Sertoli cells of the testes, inhibit production of FSH. In the presence of testosterone, FSH stimulates the Sertoli cells and induces spermatogenesis. In spermatogenesis, each germinal cell (spermatogonium), located adjacent to the Sertoli cells, undergoes differentiation into 16 primary spermatocytes, each of which generates 4 spermatids. Each spermatid matures into a spermatozoon. Spermatogenesis takes 72 to 74 days and yields about 100 million new spermatozoa each day. Upon maturation, spermatozoa are released into the rete testis, where they migrate to the epididymis and eventually to the vas deferens. Migration requires an additional 14 days. During ejaculation, spermatozoa are mixed with secretions from the seminal vesicles, prostate, and bulbourethral glands.

Sexual Differentiation, Adrenarche, and Puberty

In the embryo, the presence of a Y chromosome triggers development and growth of the testes, which begin secreting testosterone and a müllerian duct inhibitor by about 7 wk of gestation. Testosterone virilizes the wolffian duct (which develops into the epididymis, vas deferens, and seminal vesicles). DHT promotes development of the external genitals. Testosterone levels peak in the 2nd trimester and fall to almost zero by birth. Testosterone production rises briefly during the first 6 mo of life, after which testosterone levels remain low until puberty.

LH and FSH are elevated at birth but fall to low levels within a few months, remaining low or undetectable throughout the prepubertal years. Through an unknown mechanism, blood levels of the adrenal androgens DHEA and DHEA sulfate begin to increase several years before puberty. Their conversion to testosterone in small amounts initiates pubic and axillary hair growth (adrenarche). Adrenarche can occur as early as 9 or 10 yr of age.

The mechanisms that initiate puberty are unclear, although early in puberty the hypothalamus becomes less sensitive to the inhibitory effects of sex hormones. This desensitization increases secretion of LH and FSH, corresponding to pulsatile GnRH secretion, and stimulating testosterone and sperm production. In boys, the increased testosterone levels cause pubertal changes, the first of which is growth of the testes and scrotum. Later, penile length, muscle mass, and bone density increase; the voice deepens; and pubic and axillary hair becomes denser and thicker (see Fig. 251–1).

Effects of Aging

Both hypothalamic secretion of GnRH and the response of Leydig cells to FSH and LH diminish with aging. In the elderly, Leydig cells decrease in number as well. Beginning at about age 30, a man's serum total testosterone levels decline by 1 to 2%/yr. Men aged 70 to 80 tend to have serum testosterone levels that are about one half to two thirds of those of men in their 20s. In addition, SHBG levels increase with aging, causing an even greater decline in serum free and bioavailable testosterone. FSH and LH levels tend to be normal or high-normal. These age-related changes are referred to as the andropause, although there are no abrupt changes in hormone levels (and corresponding symptoms) as occur in the menopause. The decline in testosterone may contribute to a combination of symptoms that has been termed **androgen deficiency of the aging male** (ADAM), which includes

- Age-related muscle loss
- Increased fat deposition
- Osteopenia
- Loss of libido and erectile function
- Cognitive decline

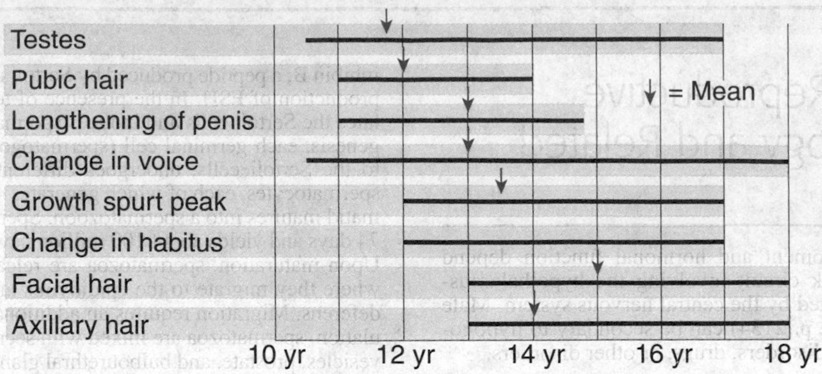

Fig. 251-1. Puberty—when male sexual characteristics develop. Bars indicate normal ranges. No mean is available for change in habitus.

If men have these symptoms plus low serum testosterone, they are diagnosed with hypogonadism and are eligible for treatment with supplemental testosterone.

Testosterone supplementation in men with low-normal levels of testosterone is controversial. Some experts recommend a trial of testosterone supplementation in older men with symptoms or signs of hypogonadism and whose serum testosterone levels are slightly below the lower limit of normal. No data favor any of the testosterone preparations specifically for use in ADAM, although daily transcutaneous applications appear to be the most physiologic and best tolerated.

MALE HYPOGONADISM

Hypogonadism is defined as testosterone deficiency with associated symptoms or signs, deficiency of spermatozoa production, or both. It may result from a disorder of the testes (primary hypogonadism) or of the hypothalamic-pituitary axis (secondary hypogonadism). Both may be congenital or acquired as the result of aging, disease, drugs, or other factors. Additionally, a number of congenital enzyme deficiencies cause varying degrees of target organ androgen resistance. Diagnosis is confirmed by hormone levels. Treatment varies with etiology but typically includes GnRH, gonadotropin, or testosterone replacement.

Etiology

Primary hypogonadism involves failure of the testes to respond to FSH and LH. When primary hypogonadism affects testosterone production, testosterone is insufficient to inhibit production of FSH and LH; hence, FSH and LH levels are elevated. The most common cause of primary hypogonadism is Klinefelter syndrome. It involves seminiferous tubule dysgenesis and a 47,XXY karyotype (see p. 2493).

Secondary hypogonadism is failure of the hypothalamus to produce GnRH or of the pituitary gland to produce enough FSH and LH. In secondary hypogonadism, testosterone levels are low and levels of FSH and LH are low or inappropriately normal. Any acute systemic illness can cause temporary secondary hypogonadism. Some syndromes of hypogonadism have both primary and secondary causes (mixed hypogonadism). Table 251–1 lists some common causes of hypogonadism by category.

Some syndromes of hypogonadism (eg, cryptorchidism, some systemic disorders) affect spermatozoon production more than testosterone levels.

Symptoms and Signs

Age at onset of testosterone deficiency dictates the clinical presentation: congenital, childhood-onset, or adult-onset hypogonadism.

Congenital hypogonadism may be of 1st-, 2nd-, or 3rd-trimester onset. Congenital hypogonadism of 1st-trimester onset results in inadequate male sexual differentiation. Complete absence of testosterone's effects results in normal-appearing female external genitals. Partial testosterone deficiency results in abnormalities ranging from ambiguous external genitals to hypospadias. Second- or 3rd-trimester onset of testosterone deficiency results in microphallus and undescended testes.

Childhood-onset testosterone deficiency (see p. 2571) has few consequences and usually is unrecognized until puberty is delayed. Untreated hypogonadism impairs development of secondary sexual characteristics. As adults, affected patients have poor muscle development, a high-pitched voice, a small scrotum, decreased phallic and testicular growth, sparse pubic and axillary hair, and an absence of body hair. They may develop gynecomastia and eunuchoidal body proportions (span > height by 5 cm and pubic to floor length > crown to pubic length by > 5 cm) because of delayed fusion of the epiphyses and continued long bone growth.

Adult-onset testosterone deficiency has varied manifestations depending on the degree and duration of the deficiency. Decreased libido; erectile dysfunction; decline in cognitive skills, such as visual-spatial interpretation; sleep disturbances; vasomotor instability (in acute, severe male hypogonadism); and mood changes, such as depression and anger, are common. Decreased lean body mass, increased visceral fat, testicular atrophy, osteopenia, gynecomastia, and sparse body hair typically take months to years to develop. Testosterone deficiency may increase the risk of coronary artery disease.

Diagnosis

- Testing, beginning with FSH, LH, and testosterone levels

Congenital and childhood-onset hypogonadism are often suspected because of developmental abnormalities or delayed puberty. Adult-onset hypogonadism should be suspected on the basis of symptoms or signs but is easily missed because these clinical markers are insensitive and nonspecific. Klinefelter

Table 251–1. CAUSES* OF HYPOGONADISM

TYPE	CONGENITAL CAUSES	ACQUIRED CAUSES
Primary (testicular)	Klinefelter syndrome Anorchia (bilateral) Cryptorchidism Myotonic dystrophy Enzymatic defects in testosterone synthesis Leydig cell aplasia Noonan syndrome	Chemotherapy or radiation therapy Testicular infection (eg, mumps, echovirus, flavivirus) High doses of antiandrogen drugs (eg, cimetidine, spironolactone, ketoconazole, flutamide, cyproterone)
Secondary (hypothalamic-pituitary)	Idiopathic hypogonadotropic hypogonadism Kallmann syndrome Prader-Willi syndrome Dandy-Walker malformation Isolated LH deficiency	Any acute systemic illness Hypopituitarism (tumor, infarction, infiltrative disease, infection, trauma, irradiation) Hyperprolactinemia Iron overload (hemochromatosis) Certain drugs (eg, estrogens, psychoactive drugs, metoclopramide, opioids, leuprolide, goserelin, triptorelin, newer androgen biosynthesis inhibitors for prostate cancer) Cushing syndrome Cirrhosis Morbid obesity Idiopathic
Mixed	—	Aging Alcoholism Systemic disease (eg, uremia, liver failure, AIDS, sickle cell disease) Drugs (ethanol, corticosteroids)

*In approximate order of frequency.

syndrome should be considered in adolscent males in whom puberty is delayed, young men with hypogonadism, and all adult men with very small testes. Hypogonadism requires confirmatory testing (see Fig. 251–2).

Diagnosis of primary and secondary hypogonadism: Increases in FSH and LH are more sensitive for primary hypogonadism than are decreases in testosterone levels. Levels of FSH and LH also help determine whether hypogonadism is primary or secondary. High gonadotropin levels, even with low-normal testosterone levels, indicate primary hypogonadism, whereas gonadotropin levels that are low or lower than expected for the level of testosterone indicate secondary hypogonadism. Alternatively, in boys of short stature with delayed puberty, low testosterone plus low gonadotropin levels might result from constitutional delay of puberty. Elevation of serum FSH with normal levels of serum testosterone and LH often occurs when spermatogenesis is impaired but testosterone production is normal. The cause of hypogonadism is often evident clinically. Primary hypogonadism requires no further testing, although some clinicians do a karyotype to definitively diagnose Klinefelter syndrome.

Total (and, when possible, free) serum testosterone, serum FSH, and serum LH levels are measured simultaneously. The normal range for total testosterone is 300 to 1000 ng/dL (10.5 to 35 nmol/L). The testosterone level should be drawn in the morning (before 10:00 AM) to confirm hypogonadism. Because of the increase in SHBG with aging, total testosterone level is a less sensitive indicator of hypogonadism after age 50. Although serum free testosterone more accurately reflects functional testosterone levels, its measurement requires equilibrium dialysis, which is technically difficult and not widely available.

Some commercially available kits, including the analog free testosterone assay, attempt to measure serum free testosterone levels, but the results are often inaccurate, particularly in conditions (such as type 2 diabetes, obesity, and hypothyroidism) that alter SHBG levels. Free testosterone levels can be calculated based on SHBG, albumin, and testosterone values; there are calculators available online at http://www.issam.ch.

Because of the pulsatile secretion of FSH and LH, these hormones are sometimes measured as a pooled sample of 3 venipunctures taken at 20-min intervals, but these pooled samples seldom add clinically important information compared with a single blood sample. Serum FSH and LH levels are usually ≤ 5 mIU/mL before puberty and between 5 and 15 mIU/mL in adulthood.

Semen analysis should be done in all men who are seeking fertility treatment. In adolescents or adults, a semen sample collected by masturbation after 2 days of abstinence from ejaculation provides an excellent index of seminiferous tubular function. A normal semen sample (WHO standards) has a volume of > 1.5. mL with > 20 million sperm/mL, of which 50% are of normal morphology and are motile (see also p. 2269).

Evaluation of secondary hypogonadism: Because any systemic illness can temporarily decrease levels of testosterone, FSH, and LH, secondary hypogonadism should be confirmed by measuring these levels again at least 4 wk after resolution of the systemic illness. To confirm secondary hypogonadism in adolescents, the GnRH stimulation test may be considered. If levels of FSH and LH increase in response to IV GnRH, puberty is simply delayed. If levels do not increase, true hypogonadism is likely.

To help determine the cause of confirmed secondary hypogonadism, testing should include serum prolactin level (to screen for pituitary adenoma—see p. 1915) and transferrin saturation (to screen for hemochromatosis—see p. 1138). Sella imaging with MRI or CT is done to exclude a pituitary macroadenoma or other mass in men with any of the following:

- Age < 60 yr with no other identified cause for hypogonadism
- Very low total testosterone levels (< 200 ng/dL)
- Elevated prolactin levels
- Symptoms consistent with a pituitary tumor (eg, headache, visual symptoms)

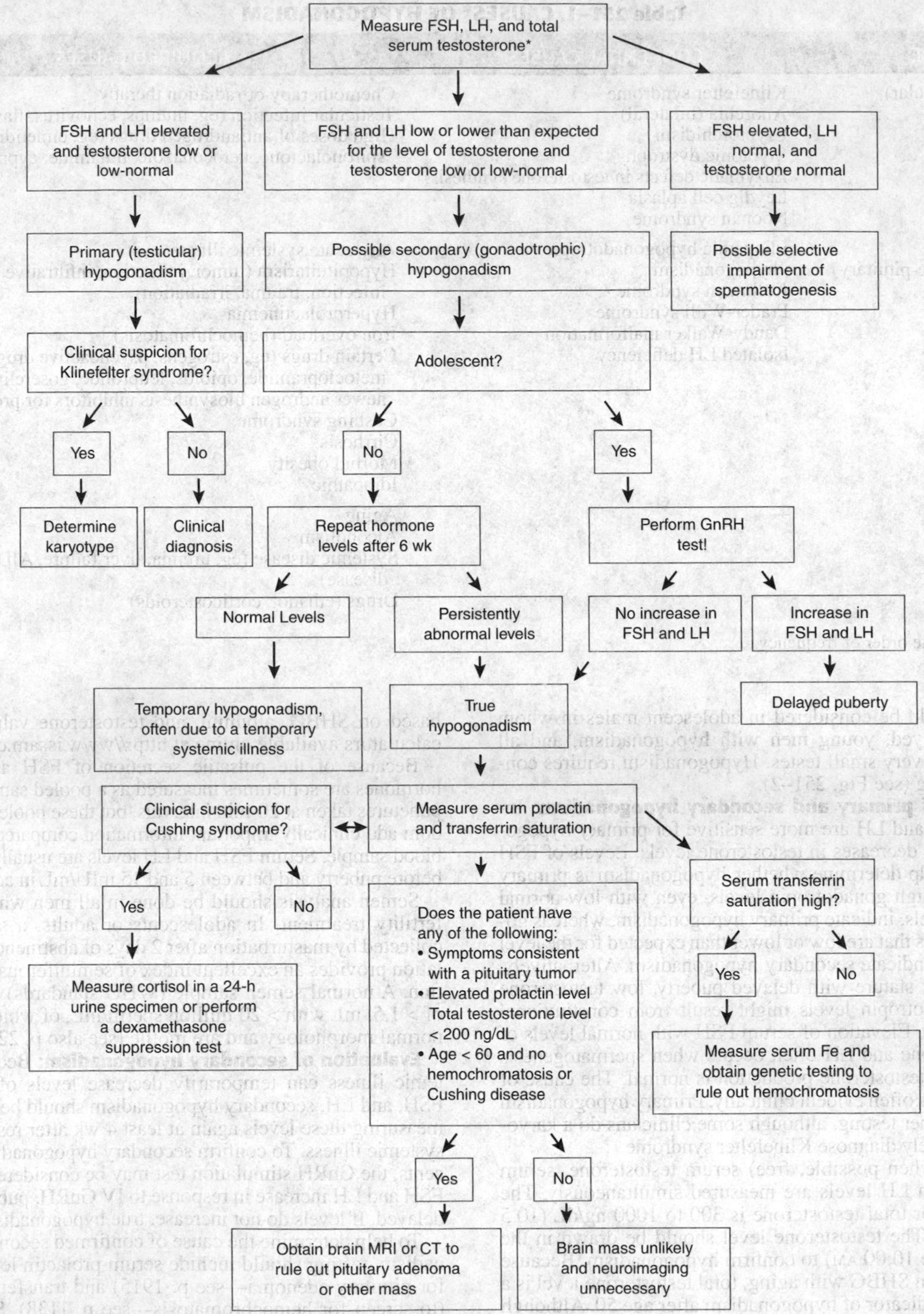

*Total testosterone has lower sensitivity for hypogonadism in men aged > 50 yr. If the test for free and weekly bound testosterone is available, levels are measured. If not, levels are calculated.
*Recommended by some physicians.

Fig. 251–2. Laboratory evaluation of male hypogonadism. Fe = iron; FSH = follicle-stimulating hormone; GnRH = gonadotropin-releasing hormone; LH = luteinizing hormone.

Also, if there are symptoms or signs of Cushing syndrome, 24-h urine collection for free cortisol or a dexamethasone suppression test is done (see p. 1240). If no abnormalities are identified, the diagnosis is acquired idiopathic secondary hypogonadism.

Treatment

- Testosterone therapy
- Gonadotropin replacement therapy for restoration of fertility due to secondary hypogonadism

Treatment is directed toward providing adequate androgen replacement conveniently and safely. Although patients with primary hypogonadism will not become fertile with any endocrine therapy, patients with secondary hypogonadism often become fertile with gonadotropin therapy. Testosterone formulations discussed here are those available in the US. Other formulations may be available in other countries.

Testosterone replacement therapy (TRT): Because exogenous testosterone impairs spermatogenesis, TRT should be avoided, when possible, in secondary hypogonadism or when subsequent fertility is a concern (unless there is irreversible primary testicular failure). Treatment of secondary hypogonadism in boys with gonadotropin replacement therapy (see below) usually stimulates androgen production as well as spermatogenesis.

TRT can be used for males who

- Have no signs of puberty
- Are near age 15
- Have had secondary hypogonadism excluded

They may be given long-acting testosterone enanthate 50 mg IM once/mo for 4 to 8 mo. These low doses cause some virilization without restricting adult height. Older adolescents with testosterone deficiency receive long-acting testosterone enanthate or testosterone cypionate at a dose that is increased gradually over 18 to 24 mo from 50 to 100 to 200 mg IM q 1 to 2 wk. Transcutaneous gel may also be used, although it is more expensive, could possibly be transferred to others during intimate contact, and is more difficult to accurately dose. It is reasonable to convert older adolescents to testosterone gel preparations at adult dosages when their IM dosage has reached the equivalent of 100 to 200 mg q 2 wk.

Adults with established testosterone deficiency may benefit from replacement therapy. Treatment slows the course of osteopenia, muscle loss, vasomotor instability, loss of libido, depression, and occasionally erectile dysfunction. The effects of testosterone on coronary artery disease are not well understood. TRT may improve coronary artery blood flow and may decrease the risk of coronary artery disease; however, concerns that TRT increases risk of cardiovascular events have been raised. Options for replacement therapy include

- Testosterone gel 1% or 1.62% (5 to 10 g of gel daily to deliver 5 to 10 mg of testosterone daily)
- Transdermal axillary solution (60 mg once/day)
- A buccal mucosal lozenge (30 mg bid)
- Transdermal testosterone patch (4 mg once/day)
- A new nasal formulation (one spray of 5.5 mg in each nostril tid)
- Subcutaneous testosterone implants (75 mg/pellet) given as 4 to 6 units placed q 3 to 6 mo
- IM testosterone enanthate or cypionate (100 mg q 7 days or 200 mg q 10 to 14 days)

Testosterone gel maintains physiologic blood levels more consistently than other treatments, but IM or patch systems are sometimes preferred because of their lower cost. Oral formulations are unpredictably absorbed.

Potential adverse effects of testosterone and its analogs include

- Erythrocytosis (particularly in men ≥ 50 yr receiving IM testosterone)
- Venous thromboembolism unrelated to erythrocytosis
- Acne
- Gynecomastia
- Low sperm count

Very rarely prostatic enlargement or edema occurs. Prostatic obstructive symptoms are rare. Currently, replacing testosterone enough to achieve physiologic levels is not thought to cause new prostate cancer or accelerate growth or spread of localized prostate cancer, and TRT is thought to have a minimal effect on serum prostate-specific antigen (PSA) levels in men with benign prostatic hyperplasia and in men with treated prostate cancer. However, product inserts do state that TRT is contraindicated in men with prostate cancer, and men who have or are at high risk of prostate cancer should be counseled and carefully followed with digital rectal examinations and PSA measurements while taking TRT. A prostate biopsy may be needed if PSA elevation persists after TRT is stopped. Hypogonadal men suspected of having prostate cancer should seek consultation with an expert. Oral formulations carry risks of hepatocellular dysfunction and hepatic adenoma.

Men taking supplemental testosterone should be monitored periodically. Hct, PSA, and testosterone levels should be measured quarterly during the first year of TRT and semiannually thereafter. Digital rectal examination should be offered at the same times. If Hct is ≥ 54%, the testosterone dose should be reduced. Significant increases in PSA level should prompt consideration of prostate biopsy in men who would otherwise be candidates for prostate cancer diagnosis and treatment.

Treatment of infertility due to hypogonadism: Infertility, which has many possible causes other than hypogonadism, is discussed in full on p. 2269. Infertility due to primary hypogonadism does not respond to hormonal therapy. Men with primary hypogonadism occasionally have a few intratesticular sperm that can be harvested with various microsurgical techniques and used to fertilize an egg by assisted reproductive technique (eg, intracytoplasmic injection).

Infertility due to secondary hypogonadism usually responds to gonadotropin replacement therapy. Other symptoms of secondary hypogonadism respond well to testosterone replacement therapy alone. If secondary hypogonadism results from pituitary disease, gonadotropin replacement therapy usually is successful. Therapy begins with replacement of LH and FSH. LH replacement is initiated using human chorionic gonadotropin (hCG) at doses of 1500 IU sc 3 times/wk. FSH replacement, which is expensive, uses human menotropic gonadotropin or human recombinant FSH, at doses of 150 IU 3 times/wk. Doses may be adjusted based on the results of periodic testing with semen analysis and levels of serum FSH, LH, and testosterone. Once an adequate sperm count is achieved, FSH can be stopped and hCG monotherapy continued.

Most men who have secondary hypogonadism due to a hypothalamic defect (eg, idiopathic hypogonadotropic hypogonadism, Kallmann syndrome) become fertile with treatment despite sperm counts that are low (eg, < 5 million/mL). When LH and FSH treatment is ineffective, pulsatile GnRH replacement therapy (q 2 h sc by a programmable minipump), although less readily available, might be more effective. Most (80 to 90%) of men respond successfully to these regimens.

KEY POINTS

- Levels of FSH and LH help differentiate between primary hypogonadism (high levels) and secondary hypogonadism (low or inappropriately normal levels).
- Age-related symptoms of male hypogonadism include inadequate sexual differentiation (congenital), delayed puberty (childhood onset), and various nonspecific symptoms such as decreased libido, erectile dysfunction, cognitive decline, decrease in percentage of lean body mass, sleep disturbances, and mood changes (adult onset).
- Free testosterone levels, which can be calculated and sometimes measured, better reflect gonadal sufficiency than do total testosterone levels.
- Diagnosis can be approached systematically, using an algorithm.
- TRT can relieve symptoms of hypogonadism but does not restore fertility.
- Gonadotropin replacement therapy can usually restore fertility in men with secondary hypogonadism.

GYNECOMASTIA

Gynecomastia is hypertrophy of breast glandular tissue in males. It must be differentiated from pseudogynecomastia, which is increased breast fat, but no enlargement of breast glandular tissue.

Pathophysiology

During infancy and puberty, enlargement of the male breast is normal (physiologic gynecomastia). Enlargement is usually transient, bilateral, smooth, firm, and symmetrically distributed under the areola; breasts may be tender. Physiologic gynecomastia that develops during puberty usually resolves within about 6 mo to 2 yr. Similar changes may occur during old age and may be unilateral or bilateral. Most of the enlargement is due to proliferation of stroma, not of breast ducts. The mechanism is usually a decrease in androgen effect or an increase in estrogen effect (eg, decrease in androgen production, increase in estrogen production, androgen blockade, displacement of estrogen from sex-hormone binding globulin, androgen receptor defects).

PEARLS & PITFALLS

- During infancy and puberty, bilateral, symmetric, smooth, firm, and tender enlargement of breast tissue under the areola is normal.

If evaluation reveals no cause for gynecomastia, it is considered idiopathic. The cause may not be found because gynecomastia is physiologic or because there is no longer any evidence of the inciting event.

Etiology

In infants and boys, the most common cause is

- Physiologic gynecomastia

In men, the most common causes are (see Table 251–2)

- Persistent pubertal gynecomastia
- Idiopathic gynecomastia
- Drugs (particularly spironolactone, anabolic steroids, and antiandrogens—see Table 251–3)

Table 251–2. SOME CAUSES OF GYNECOMASTIA

CAUSE	SUGGESTIVE FINDINGS	DIAGNOSTIC APPROACH
Chronic kidney disease	History of chronic kidney disease	Serum electrolytes, BUN, and creatinine Urinalysis Possibly urine culture and urinary levels of Na, K, and creatinine
Cirrhosis	Often history of liver disease, alcohol use, or both Ascites, spider angiomas, dilated abdominal veins	Routine laboratory testing Sometimes liver biopsy
Drugs (see Table 251–3)	History of use	Trial of stopping the drug
Feminizing adrenocortical tumor	Palpable mass, testicular atrophy	Imaging (MRI or CT)
Hyperthyroidism	Tremor, heat intolerance, diarrhea, tachycardia, weight loss, goiter, exophthalmos	Thyroid function tests
Hypogonadism	Prepubertal onset: Underdeveloped secondary sexual characteristics Postpubertal onset: Decreased libido, erectile dysfunction, mood changes, decreased muscle and increased fat mass, osteopenia, testicular atrophy, mild cognitive changes	Serum FSH, LH, and testosterone levels (see p. 2128)
Paraneoplastic ectopic production of human chorionic gonadotropin (hCG)	Possibly signs of primary tumor or symptoms and signs of hypogonadism	Evaluation for suspected primary tumor
Testicular tumors	Testicular mass Possibly symptoms and signs of hypogonadism	Ultrasonography
Feeding after undernutrition	Muscle and fat wasting, hair loss, skin changes, frequent infections, fatigue, signs of vitamin deficiencies (eg, osteopenia)	Clinical evaluation Selective laboratory testing
Idiopathic gynecomastia	No abnormal findings other than gynecomastia, no symptoms, no apparent cause	Repeat clinical evaluation in 6 mo Possibly serum testosterone level

FSH = follicle-stimulating hormone; LH = luteinizing hormone.

Table 251–3. COMMON DRUG CAUSES OF GYNECOMASTIA*

CATEGORY	DRUGS
Drugs that inhibit androgen synthesis or activity	Cyproterone (an antiandrogen) Dutasteride and finasteride (5α-reductase inhibitors) Goserelin, histrelin, leuprolide, and triptorelin (LH-RH agonists) Flutamide, bicalutamide, enzalutamide, and nilutamide (antiandrogens used to treat prostate cancer)
Antimicrobials	Efavirenz Ethionamide Isoniazid Ketoconazole Metronidazole
Antineoplastic drugs	Alkylating drugs Imatinib Methotrexate Vinca alkaloids
Cardiovascular drugs	ACE inhibitors (eg, captopril, enalapril) Amiodarone Ca channel blockers (eg, nifedipine, diltiazem) Methyldopa Reserpine Spironolactone
CNS-acting drugs	Diazepam Haloperidol Methadone Phenothiazines Tricyclic antidepressants
Antiulcer drugs†	Cimetidine Ranitidine Omeprazole
Hormones	Androgens Anabolic steroids Estrogens Human growth hormone
Recreational drugs	Amphetamines Ethanol Heroin Marijuana
OTC herbal drugs	Lavender oil Tea tree oils
Other drugs	Auranofin Diethylpropion Domperidone Metoclopramide Phenytoin Penicillamine Sulindac Theophylline

*Not all drugs that have been associated with gynecomastia have been shown to cause gynecomastia through challenge-rechallenge testing.

†Drugs are listed in order of frequency of association.

Breast cancer, which is uncommon in males, may cause unilateral breast abnormalities but is rarely confused with gynecomastia.

Evaluation

History: History of present illness should help clarify the duration of breast enlargement, whether secondary sexual characteristics are fully developed, the relationship between onset of gynecomastia and puberty, and the presence of any genital symptoms (eg, decreased libido, erectile dysfunction) and breast symptoms (eg, pain, nipple discharge).

Review of systems should seek symptoms that suggest possible causes, such as

- Weight loss and fatigue (cirrhosis, undernutrition, chronic kidney disease, hyperthyroidism)
- Skin discoloration (chronic kidney disease, cirrhosis)
- Hair loss and frequent infections (undernutrition)
- Fragility fractures (undernutrition, hypogonadism)
- Mood and cognitive changes (hypogonadism)
- Tremor, heat intolerance, and diarrhea (hyperthyroidism)

Past medical history should address disorders that can cause gynecomastia and include a history of all prescribed and OTC drugs.

Physical examination: Complete examination is done, including assessment of vital signs, skin, and general appearance. The neck is examined for goiter. The abdomen is examined for ascites, venous distention, and suspected adrenal masses. Development of secondary sexual characteristics (eg, the penis, pubic hair, and axillary hair) is assessed. The testes are examined for masses or atrophy.

The breasts are examined while patients are recumbent with their hands behind the head. Examiners bring their thumb and forefinger together from opposite sides of the nipple until they meet. Any nipple discharge is noted. Lumps are assessed and characterized in terms of location, consistency, fixation to underlying tissues, and skin changes. The axilla is examined for lymph node involvement in men who have breast lumps.

Red flags: The following findings are of particular concern:

- Localized or eccentric breast swelling, particularly with nipple discharge, fixation to the skin, or hard consistency
- Symptoms or signs of hypogonadism (eg, delayed puberty, testicular atrophy, decreased libido, erectile dysfunction, decreased proportion of lean body mass, loss of visual-spatial abilities)
- Symptoms or signs of hyperthyroidism (eg, tremor, tachycardia, sweating, heat intolerance, weight loss)
- Testicular mass
- Recent onset of painful, tender gynecomastia in an adult

Interpretation of findings: With pseudogynecomastia, the examiner feels no resistance between the thumb and forefinger until they meet at the nipple. In contrast, with gynecomastia, a rim of tissue > 0.5 cm in diameter surrounds the nipple symmetrically and is similar in consistency to the nipple itself. Breast cancer is suggested by swelling with any of the following characteristics:

- Eccentric unilateral location
- Firm or hard consistency
- Fixation to skin or fascia
- Nipple discharge
- Skin dimpling
- Nipple retraction
- Axillary lymph node involvement

Table 251–4. INTERPRETATION OF SOME FINDINGS IN GYNECOMASTIA

FINDING	POSSIBLE CAUSES
Tachycardia, tremor, goiter, exophthalmos	Hyperthyroidism
Weight loss	Chronic kidney disease Cirrhosis Hyperthyroidism Refeeding after undernutrition
Fragile skin	Chronic kidney disease Undernutrition
Ascites, vascular spiders	Cirrhosis
Underdeveloped secondary sexual characteristics	Hypogonadism (prepubertal onset)
Skin discoloration	Chronic kidney disease Cirrhosis
Testicular atrophy	Cirrhosis Hypogonadism (postpubertal onset)
Testicular mass	Testicular (Leydig cell) tumor

Gynecomastia in an adult that is of recent onset and causes pain is more often caused by a hormonal abnormality (eg, tumor, hypogonadism) or drugs. Other examination findings may also be helpful (see Table 251–4).

Testing: If breast cancer is suspected, mammography should be done. If another disorder is suspected, appropriate testing should be done (see Table 251–2). Extensive testing is often unnecessary, especially for patients in whom the gynecomastia is chronic and detected only during physical examination. Because hypogonadism is somewhat common with aging, some authorities recommend measuring the serum testosterone level in older men, particularly if other findings suggest hypogonadism. However, in adults with recent onset of painful gynecomastia without a drug or evident pathologic cause, measurement of serum levels of LH, FSH, testosterone, estradiol, and hCG are recommended. Patients with physiologic or idiopathic gynecomastia are evaluated again in 6 mo.

Treatment

In most cases, no specific treatment is needed because gynecomastia usually remits spontaneously or disappears after any causative drug (except perhaps anabolic steroids) is stopped or underlying disorder is treated. Some clinicians try tamoxifen 10 mg po bid if pain and tenderness are very troublesome in men or adolescents, but this treatment is not always effective. Tamoxifen may also help prevent gynecomastia in men being treated with high-dose antiandrogen (eg, bicalutamide) therapy for prostate cancer; breast radiation therapy is an alternative. Resolution of gynecomastia is unlikely after 12 mo. Thus, after 12 mo, if cosmetic appearance is unacceptable, surgical removal of excess breast tissue (eg, suction lipectomy alone or with cosmetic surgery) may be used.

KEY POINTS

- Gynecomastia must be differentiated from increased fat tissue in the breast.
- Gynecomastia is often physiologic or idiopathic.
- A wide variety of drugs can cause gynecomastia.
- Patients should be evaluated for clinically suspected genital or systemic disorders.

252 Male Sexual Dysfunction

There are 4 main components of male sexual function:

- Libido
- Erection
- Ejaculation
- Orgasm

Sexual dysfunction is a problem with one of these components that interferes with interest in or ability to engage in sexual intercourse. Many drugs and numerous physical and psychologic disorders affect sexual function.

Libido

Libido is the conscious component of sexual function. Decreased libido manifests as a lack of sexual interest or a decrease in the frequency and intensity of sexual thoughts, either spontaneous or in response to erotic stimuli. Libido is sensitive to testosterone levels as well as to general nutrition, health, and drugs.

Conditions particularly likely to decrease libido include hypogonadism, chronic kidney disease, and depression; up to 25% of men with diabetes may meet the definition of hypogonadism.

Drugs that potentially decrease libido include weak androgen receptor antagonists (eg, spironolactone, cimetidine), luteinizing hormone-releasing hormone (LHRH) agonists (eg, leuprolide, goserelin, buserelin) and antagonists (eg, degarelix) used to treat prostate cancer, antiandrogens used to treat prostate cancer (eg, flutamide, bicalutamide), 5α-reductase inhibitors (eg, finasteride, dutasteride) used to treat benign prostatic hyperplasia, some antihypertensives, and virtually all drugs that are active in the CNS (eg, SSRIs, tricyclic antidepressants, antipsychotics). Loss of libido due to SSRIs or tricyclic antidepressants sometimes is reversible with the addition of bupropion or trazodone.

Erection

Erection is a neurovascular response to certain psychologic and/or tactile stimuli. Higher cortical input and a sacral parasympathetic reflex arc mediate the erectile response. Neural output travels through the cavernous nerves, which traverse the posterolateral aspect of the prostate. Terminating in the penile vasculature, these nonadrenergic, noncholinergic nerves liberate nitric oxide, a gas. Nitric oxide diffuses into penile arterial smooth muscle cells, causing increased production of cyclic GMP, which relaxes the arteries and allows more blood to flow through them and into the corpora cavernosa. As the corpora fill with blood, intracavernous pressure increases, which compresses surrounding venules, causing veno-occlusion and decreased venous outflow. The increased inflow of blood and decreased outflow further increase intracavernous pressure, contributing to erection. Many factors affect the ability to have an erection (see below).

Ejaculation and Orgasm

Ejaculation is controlled by the sympathetic nervous system. Neural stimulation of the α-adrenergic receptors in the male adnexa (eg, penis, testes, perineum, prostate, seminal vesicles) causes contractions of the epididymis, vas deferens, seminal vesicles, and prostate that transport semen to the posterior urethra. Then, rhythmic contractions of the pelvic floor muscles result in pulsatile ejaculation of the accumulated seminal fluid. At the same time, the neck of the bladder closes, preventing retrograde ejaculation of semen into the bladder. SSRIs and alpha blockers may delay or inhibit ejaculation by receptor inhibition at these sites.

Orgasm is the pleasurable sensation that occurs in the brain generally simultaneously with ejaculation. Anorgasmia may be a physical phenomenon due to decreased penile sensation (eg, from neuropathy) or a neuropsychologic phenomenon due to psychiatric disorders or psychoactive drugs.

Ejaculatory dysfunction: Ejaculatory dysfunction is reduced or absent semen volume. It may result from retrograde ejaculation, which may occur in men with diabetes or as a complication of bladder neck surgery or transurethral resection of the prostate. It also may result from sympathetic interruption, either due to surgery (eg, retroperitoneal lymph node dissection) or to drugs (eg, guanethidine, phentolamine, phenoxybenzamine, thioridazine). Radical prostatectomy (removal of the prostate gland plus the seminal vesicles and regional lymph nodes) eliminates any ejaculation because removing the seminal vesicles and prostate eliminates semen production.

Premature ejaculation: Premature ejaculation is defined as ejaculation occurring sooner than desired by the man or his partner and causing distress to the couple. It is usually caused by sexual inexperience, anxiety, and other psychologic factors instead of disease. It can be treated successfully with sex therapy, tricyclic antidepressants, and SSRIs.

ERECTILE DYSFUNCTION

(Impotence)

Erectile dysfunction is the inability to attain or sustain an erection satisfactory for sexual intercourse. Most erectile dysfunction is related to vascular, neurologic, psychologic, and hormonal disorders; drug use can also be a cause. Evaluation typically includes screening for underlying disorders and measuring testosterone levels. Treatment options include oral phosphodiesterase inhibitors, intraurethral or intracavernosal prostaglandins, vacuum erection devices, and surgical implants.

Erectile dysfunction (ED; formerly called impotence) affects up to 20 million men in the US. The prevalence of partial or complete ED is > 50% in men aged 40 to 70, and prevalence increases with aging. Most affected men can be successfully treated.

Etiology

There are 2 types of ED:

- Primary ED, the man has never been able to attain or sustain an erection
- Secondary ED, acquired later in life by a man who previously was able to attain erections

Primary ED is rare and is almost always due to psychologic factors or clinically obvious anatomic abnormalities.

Secondary ED is more common, and > 90% of cases have an organic etiology. Many men with secondary ED develop reactive psychologic difficulties that compound the problem.

Psychologic factors, whether primary or reactive, must be considered in every case of ED. Psychologic causes of primary ED include guilt, fear of intimacy, depression, or anxiety. In secondary ED, causes may relate to performance anxiety, stress, or depression. Psychogenic ED may be situational, involving a particular place, time, or partner.

The **major organic causes of ED** are

- Vascular disorders
- Neurologic disorders

These disorders often stem from atherosclerosis or diabetes.

The most common **vascular cause** is atherosclerosis of cavernous arteries of the penis, often caused by smoking and diabetes. Atherosclerosis and aging decrease the capacity for dilation of arterial blood vessels and smooth muscle relaxation, limiting the amount of blood that can enter the penis (see p. 2134). Veno-occlusive dysfunction permits venous leakage, which results in inability to maintain erection.

Priapism, usually associated with trazodone use, cocaine abuse, and sickle cell disease, may cause penile fibrosis and lead to ED by causing fibrosis of penile veins that interferes with drainage.

Neurologic causes include stroke, partial complex seizures, multiple sclerosis, peripheral and autonomic neuropathies, and spinal cord injuries. Diabetic neuropathy and surgical injury are particularly common causes.

Complications of pelvic surgery (eg, radical prostatectomy [even with nerve-sparing techniques], radical cystectomy, transurethral resection of the prostate, rectal cancer surgery) are other common causes. Other causes include hormonal disorders, drugs, pelvic radiation, and structural disorders of the penis (eg, Peyronie disease). Prolonged perineal pressure (as occurs during bicycle riding) or pelvic or perineal trauma can cause ED.

Any endocrinopathy or aging associated with testosterone deficiency (hypogonadism) may decrease libido and cause ED. However, erectile function only rarely improves with normalization of serum testosterone levels because most affected men also have neurovascular causes of ED.

Numerous drug causes are possible (see Table 252–1). Alcohol can cause temporary ED.

Diagnosis

- Clinical evaluation
- Screening for depression
- Testosterone level

Evaluation should include history of drug (including prescription drugs and herbal products) and alcohol use, pelvic surgery and trauma, smoking, diabetes, hypertension, and atherosclerosis and symptoms of vascular, hormonal, neurologic, and psychologic disorders. Satisfaction with sexual relationships should be explored, including evaluation of partner interaction and partner sexual dysfunction (eg, atrophic vaginitis, dyspareunia, depression).

It is vital to screen for depression, which may not always be apparent. The Beck Depression Scale or, in older men, the Yesavage Geriatric Depression Scale is easy to administer and may be useful.

Examination is focused on the genitals and extragenital signs of hormonal, neurologic, and vascular disorders. Genitals are

Table 252–1. COMMONLY USED DRUGS THAT CAN CAUSE ERECTILE DYSFUNCTION

CLASS	DRUGS
Antihypertensives	β-Blockers, clonidine, loop diuretics (probably), spironolactone, thiazide diuretics
CNS drugs	Alcohol, anxiolytics, cocaine, monoamine oxidase inhibitors, opioids, SSRIs, tricyclic antidepressants
Others	Amphetamines, 5α-reductase inhibitors, antiandrogens, cancer chemotherapy drugs, anticholinergics, cimetidine, estrogens, luteinizing hormone-releasing hormone agonists and antagonists

examined for anomalies, signs of hypogonadism, and fibrous bands or plaques (Peyronie disease). Poor rectal tone, decreased perineal sensation, or abnormal bulbocavernosus reflexes may indicate neurologic dysfunction. Diminished peripheral pulses suggest vascular dysfunction.

A psychologic cause should be suspected in young healthy men with abrupt onset of ED, particularly if onset is associated with a specific emotional event or if the dysfunction occurs only in certain settings. A history of ED with spontaneous improvement also suggests psychologic origin (psychogenic ED). Men with psychogenic ED usually have normal nocturnal erections and erections upon awakening, whereas men with organic ED often do not.

Testing

Laboratory assessment should include measurement of morning testosterone level; if the level is low or low-normal, prolactin and luteinizing hormone (LH) should be measured. Evaluation for occult diabetes, dyslipidemias, hyperprolactinemia, thyroid disease, and Cushing syndrome should be done based on clinical suspicion.

Currently, duplex ultrasonography after intracavernous injection of a vasoactive drug such as prostaglandin E_1 is most often used to evaluate penile vasculature. Normal values include a peak systolic flow velocity > 20 cm/sec and a resistive index > 0.8. Resistive index is the difference between peak systolic velocity and end-diastolic velocity divided by peak systolic velocity. Rarely, in selected patients for whom penile revascularization surgery is being considered after pelvic trauma, dynamic infusion cavernosography and cavernosometry may be done.

Treatment

- Treatment of underlying causes
- Drugs, usually oral phosphodiesterase inhibitors
- Vacuum erection device or intracavernosal or intraurethral prostaglandin E_1 (2nd-line treatment)
- If other treatments fail, surgical implantation of penile prosthesis

Underlying organic disorders (eg, diabetes, hypogonadism, Peyronie disease) require appropriate treatment. Drugs that are temporally related to onset of ED should be stopped or switched. Depression may require treatment. For all patients, reassurance and education (including of the patient's partner whenever possible) are important.

For further therapy, an oral phosphodiesterase inhibitor is tried first. If necessary, another noninvasive method, such as a vacuum erection device or intracavernosal or intraurethral prostaglandin E_1 is tried next. Invasive treatments are used only when noninvasive methods fail. All drugs and devices should be tried ≥ 5 times before being considered ineffective.

Drugs for ED: First-line treatment of ED is usually an oral phosphodiesterase inhibitor. Other drugs used include intracavernosal or intraurethral prostaglandin E_1. However, because almost all patients prefer oral drug therapy, oral drugs are used unless they are contraindicated or not tolerated.

Oral phosphodiesterase inhibitors selectively inhibit cyclic guanosine monophosphate (cGMP)–specific phosphodiesterase type 5 (PDE5), the predominant phosphodiesterase isoform in the penis. These drugs include sildenafil, vardenafil, avanafil, and tadalafil (see Table 252–2). By preventing the hydrolysis

Table 252–2. ORAL PHOSPHODIESTERASE TYPE 5 INHIBITORS FOR ERECTILE DYSFUNCTION

DRUG	DOSE*	ONSET OF ACTION	COMMENTS
Avanafil	50, 100, or 200 mg	30 min	Can be taken 15 min before intercourse
Sildenafil	Initial: 50 mg Maintenance: 25–100 mg (most men respond best to 100 mg)	60 min	Duration: ≈ 4 h
Tadalafil	10–20 mg	60 min	Duration of action: 24–48 h
Tadalafil, low-dose	2.5–5 mg	60 min	For daily use, taken at about the same time each day, without regard to timing of sexual activity For daily use in patients who also need treatment of benign prostatic hyperplasia
Vardenafil	10–20 mg	60 min	Duration of action: ≈ 4 h
Vardenafil, orally disintegrating form	10 mg	30 min	Can be taken 30 min before intercourse

*PDE5 inhibitors should be taken on an empty stomach at least 1 h before sexual intercourse except as noted. Maximum frequency is once/day unless otherwise noted.

PDE5 = phosphodiesterase type 5.

of cGMP, these drugs promote the cGMP-dependent smooth muscle relaxation that is essential for normal erection. Although vardenafil and tadalafil are more selective for the penile vasculature than sildenafil, clinical responses and adverse effects of these drugs are similar. In comparative clinical trials, these drugs show comparable efficacy (60 to 75%).

All PDE5 inhibitors cause direct coronary vasodilation and potentiate the hypotensive effects of other nitrates, including those used to treat coronary artery disease as well as recreational amyl nitrate ("poppers"). Thus, the concomitant use of nitrates and PED5 inhibitors can be dangerous and should be avoided. Patients who only occasionally use nitrates (eg, for rare bouts of angina) should discuss the risks, selection, and proper timing of possible PDE5 inhibitor use with a cardiologist.

Adverse effects of PDE5 inhibitors include flushing, visual abnormalities, hearing loss, dyspepsia and headache. Sildenafil and vardenafil may cause abnormal color perception (blue haze). Tadalafil use has been linked with myalgias. Rarely, nonarteritic ischemic optic neuropathy (NAION) has been associated with PDE5 inhibitor use, but a causal relationship has not been established. All PDE5 inhibitors should be administered cautiously and at lower initial dosages to patients receiving α-blockers (eg, prazosin, terazosin, doxazosin, tamsulosin) because of the risk of hypotension. Patients taking an α-blocker should wait at least 4 h before using a PDE5 inhibitor. Rarely, PDE5 inhibitors cause priapism.

Alprostadil (prostaglandin E_1), self-administered via intraurethral insertion or intracavernosal injection, can produce erections with a mean duration of 30 to 60 min. Intracavernous alprostadil may be compounded with papaverine and phentolamine for increased efficacy when necessary. Excessive dosing may cause priapism in ≤ 1% of patients and genital or pelvic pain in about 10%. Office teaching and monitoring by the physician helps achieve optimal and safe use, including minimizing the risk of prolonged erection. Intraurethral therapy is less effective at producing satisfactory erection (up to 60% of men) than intracavernosal injection (up to 90%). Combination therapy with a PDE5 inhibitor and intraurethral alprostadil may be useful for some patients who fail to respond to oral PDE5 inhibitors alone.

Mechanical devices for ED: Men who can develop but not sustain an erection may use a constriction ring to help maintain erection; an elastic ring is placed around the base of the erect penis, preventing early loss of erection. Men who cannot achieve erection can first use a vacuum erection device that draws blood into the penis via suction, after which an elastic ring is placed at the base of the penis to maintain the erection. Bruising of the penis, coldness of the tip of the penis, and lack of spontaneity are some drawbacks to this modality. These devices can also be combined with drug therapy if needed.

Surgery for ED: If drugs and vacuum devices fail, surgical implantation of a penile prosthesis can be considered. Prostheses include semirigid silicone rods and saline-filled multicomponent inflatable devices. Both models carry the risks of general anesthesia, infection, and prosthesis erosion or malfunction. With experienced surgeons, the long-term rate of infection or malfunction is well below 5% and the rate of patient and partner satisfaction is > 95%.

KEY POINTS

- Vascular, neurologic, psychologic, and hormonal disorders and sometimes drug use can compromise achievement of satisfactory erections.
- Evaluate all men with ED for hormonal, neurologic, and vascular disorders and depression.
- Measure testosterone levels and consider other testing based on clinical findings.
- Treat underlying disorders and use an oral PDE5 inhibitor if necessary.
- If those measures are ineffective, consider intracavernosal or intraurethral prostaglandin E_1 or use of a vacuum device; surgical implantation of a penile prosthesis is the final line of treatment.

253 Obstructive Uropathy

(Urinary Tract Obstruction)

Obstructive uropathy is structural or functional hindrance of normal urine flow, sometimes leading to renal dysfunction (obstructive nephropathy). Symptoms, less likely in chronic obstruction, may include pain radiating to the T11 to T12 dermatomes and abnormal voiding (eg, difficulty voiding, anuria, nocturia, and/or polyuria). Diagnosis is based on results of bladder catheterization, cystourethroscopy, and imaging (eg, ultrasonography, CT, pyelography), depending on the level of obstruction. Treatment, depending on cause, may require prompt drainage, instrumentation, surgery (eg, endoscopy, lithotripsy), hormonal therapy, or a combination of these modalities.

The prevalence of obstructive uropathy, depending on the cause, ranges from five in 10,000 to five in 1,000. The condition has a bimodal distribution. In childhood, it is due mainly to congenital anomalies of the urinary tract. Incidence then declines until after age 60, when incidence rises, particularly in men because of the increased incidence of benign prostatic hyperplasia (BPH) and prostate cancer. Overall, obstructive uropathy is responsible for about 4% of end-stage renal disease. Hydronephrosis is found at postmortem examination in 2 to 4% of patients.

Etiology

Many conditions can cause obstructive uropathy, which may be acute or chronic, partial or complete, and unilateral or bilateral (see Table 253–1).

The **most common causes** differ by age:

- Children: Anatomic abnormalities (including posterior urethral valves or stricture and stenosis at the ureterovesical or ureteropelvic junction)
- Young adults: Calculi
- Older adults: BPH or prostate cancer, retroperitoneal or pelvic tumors (including metastatic cancer), and calculi

Obstruction may occur at any level, from the renal tubules (casts, crystals) to the external urethral meatus. Proximal to the obstruction, effects may include increased intraluminal

Table 253–1. CAUSES OF OBSTRUCTIVE UROPATHY

LOCATION	EXAMPLES
Anatomic abnormalities	
Bladder	Contracture of the vesical neck
Ureters	Polyp Stricture
Urethra	Abnormal anterior or posterior valve Diverticulum Injury (eg, due to pelvic fracture or straddle injury) Meatal stenosis Paraphimosis Phimosis Stricture
Compression due to extrinsic masses or processes	
Female reproductive system	Abscess Gartner duct cyst Pregnancy Tubo-ovarian abscess Tumor (cervical, ovarian) Uterine prolapse
GI tract	Appendiceal abscess Crohn disease (via inflammation or abscess) Cyst Diverticular abscess Tumor
GU tract	Benign prostatic hyperplasia Fibrosed chronic prostatitis Periurethral abscess Prostate cancer
Blood vessels	Aberrant blood vessels Aneurysm Puerperal ovarian vein thrombophlebitis Retrocaval ureter
Retroperitoneum	Fibrosis (idiopathic, surgical, drug-induced) Hematoma Lymphocele Lymphoma Metastatic tumor (eg, breast, prostate, testicular) Pelvic lipomatosis Sarcoidosis TB
Functional abnormalities	
Bladder	Bladder neck dysfunction Drug-induced bladder dysfunction (eg, by anticholinergic drugs) Nervous system dysfunction causing neurogenic bladder
Ureters	Ureteropelvic or ureterovesical junction dysfunction
Mechanical obstruction of the lumen of the urinary tract	
Renal pelvis or ureters	Blood clot Fungus ball Sloughed renal papillae Urolithiasis Urothelial carcinoma
Renal tubule	Uric acid crystals

pressure, urinary stasis, UTI, or calculus formation (which may also exacerbate or cause obstruction). Obstruction is much more common in males (usually due to BPH), but acquired and congenital urethral strictures and meatal stenosis occur in both males and females. In females, urethral obstruction may occur secondary to a primary or metastatic tumor or as a result of stricture formation after radiation therapy, surgery, or urologic instrumentation (usually repeated dilation).

Pathophysiology

Pathologic findings consist of dilation of the collecting ducts and distal tubules and chronic tubular atrophy with little glomerular damage. Dilation takes 3 days from the onset of obstructive uropathy to develop; before then, the collecting system is relatively noncompliant and less likely to dilate. Obstructive uropathy without dilation can also occur when fibrosis or a retroperitoneal tumor encases the collecting systems, when obstructive uropathy is mild and renal function is not impaired, and in the presence of an intrarenal pelvis.

Obstructive nephropathy: Obstructive nephropathy is renal dysfunction (renal insufficiency, renal failure, or tubulointerstitial damage) resulting from urinary tract obstruction. The mechanism involves, among many factors, increased intratubular pressure, local ischemia, and, often, UTI. If obstruction is bilateral, nephropathy may result in renal insufficiency. Renal insufficiency may rarely occur when obstruction is unilateral because autonomic-mediated vascular or ureteral spasm may affect the functioning kidney.

The time and rate at which irreversible damage to the kidney (or kidneys) develops after obstruction depends on so many factors that it is hard to predict. To prevent irreversible damage, obstruction of the urinary tract should be diagnosed and treated as promptly as possible.

Symptoms and Signs

Symptoms and signs vary with the site, degree, and rapidity of onset of obstructive uropathy.

Pain is common when obstruction acutely distends the bladder, collecting system (ie, the ureter, renal pelvis, and renal calyces), or renal capsule. Upper ureteral or renal pelvic lesions cause flank pain or tenderness, whereas lower ureteral obstruction causes pain that may radiate to the ipsilateral testis or labium. The distribution of kidney and ureteral pain is usually along T11 to T12. Acute complete ureteral obstruction (eg, an obstructing ureteral calculus) may cause severe pain accompanied by nausea and vomiting. A large fluid load (eg, from drinking alcoholic or caffeinated beverages, or osmotic diuresis due to an IV contrast agent) causes dilation and pain if urine production increases to a level greater than the flow rate through the area of obstruction.

Pain is typically minimal or absent with partial or slowly developing obstructive uropathy (eg, congenital ureteropelvic junction obstruction, pelvic tumor). Hydronephrosis may occasionally cause a palpable flank mass, particularly in massive hydronephrosis of infancy and childhood.

Urine volume does not diminish in unilateral obstruction unless it occurs in the only functioning kidney (solitary kidney). Absolute anuria occurs with complete obstruction at the level of the bladder or urethra. Partial obstruction at that level may cause difficulty voiding or abnormalities of the urine stream. In partial obstruction, urine output is often normal and is rarely increased. Increased urine output with polyuria and nocturia occur if the ensuing nephropathy causes impaired renal concentrating capacity and sodium reabsorption. Long-standing nephropathy may also result in hypertension.

Infection complicating obstruction may cause dysuria, pyuria, urinary urgency and frequency, referred kidney and ureteral pain, costovertebral angle tenderness, fever, and, occasionally, septicemia.

Diagnosis

- Urinalysis and serum electrolytes, BUN, and creatinine
- Bladder catheterization or bedside ultrasonographic estimation of bladder volume after voiding, sometimes followed by cystourethroscopy and voiding cystourethrography for suspected urethral obstruction
- Imaging for suspected ureteral or more proximal obstruction or for hydronephrosis without apparent obstruction

Obstructive uropathy should be considered in patients with any of the following:

- Diminished or absent urine output
- Unexplained renal insufficiency
- Pain that suggests distention in the urinary tract
- A pattern of oliguria or anuria alternating with polyuria

The history may suggest symptoms of BPH, prior cancer (eg, prostate, kidney, ureteral, bladder, gynecologic, colorectal), or urolithiasis. Because early relief of obstruction usually achieves the best outcome, diagnosis should be as rapid as possible.

Urinalysis and serum chemistries (serum electrolytes, BUN, creatinine) should be done. Other tests are done depending on symptoms and suspected level of obstruction. Infection with urinary obstruction requires immediate evaluation and treatment.

In an asymptomatic patient with long-standing obstructive uropathy, urinalysis may be normal or reveal only a few casts, WBCs, or RBCs. In a patient with acute renal failure who has a normal urinalysis, bilateral obstructive nephropathy should be considered.

If serum chemistries indicate renal insufficiency, obstruction is probably bilateral and severe or complete. Other findings in bilateral obstruction with nephropathy may include hyperkalemia. Hyperkalemia may result from type 1 renal tubular acidosis due to decreased hydrogen ion and potassium secretion by distal segments of the nephron.

Evaluation of suspected urethral obstruction: If urine output is diminished or if there is a distended bladder or suprapubic pain, bladder catheterization should be done. If catheterization results in a normal flow of urine or if the catheter is difficult to pass, a urethral obstruction (eg, prostatic enlargement, urethral valve, or urethral stricture) is suspected. In the absence of palpable bladder distention and inability to void, obstruction can be confirmed by bedside ultrasonography to determine bladder volume after voiding; volume of > 50 mL (slightly higher among older adults) suggests obstruction. Patients with such findings should have cystourethroscopy and children should usually have voiding cystourethrography (see p. 2073).

Voiding cystourethrography (VCUG) shows nearly all bladder neck and urethral obstructions as well as vesicoureteral reflux, adequately displaying the anatomy and the volume of urine left in the bladder after voiding (postvoiding residual volume). It is most commonly done in children to diagnose anatomic or congenital abnormalities. However, it may be done in adults if a urethral stricture is suspected.

If symptoms of urethral obstruction are absent or if cystourethroscopy and VCUG show no obstruction, the site of obstruction is presumed to be at the ureters or proximal to them.

Evaluation of ureteral or more proximal obstruction: Patients undergo imaging tests to detect the presence and site of obstruction. The choice and sequencing of tests depend on the clinical scenario.

Abdominal ultrasonography is the initial imaging test of choice in most patients without urethral abnormalities because it avoids potential allergic and toxic complications of contrast agents and allows assessment of associated renal parenchymal atrophy. Ultrasonography is aimed at detection of hydronephrosis. However, the false-positive rate is 25% if only minimal criteria (visualization of the collecting systems) are considered in the diagnosis. Also, absence of hydronephrosis (and false-negative results) can occur if obstruction is early (in the first few days) or mild or if retroperitoneal fibrosis or tumor encases the collecting system, preventing dilation of the ureter.

CT is sensitive for diagnosing obstructive nephropathy and is used when obstruction cannot be shown by ultrasonography or by intravenous urography. Unenhanced helical CT is the modality of choice for obstruction due to ureteral calculi. CT urography done with and without contrast is particularly useful in the evaluation of hematuria. Thinning of the renal parenchyma suggests more chronic obstruction.

Duplex Doppler ultrasonography can usually show unilateral obstructive uropathy in the first few days of acute obstruction before the collecting system dilates by detecting an increased resistive index (a reflection of increased renal vascular resistance) in the affected kidney. This modality is less useful in obesity and in bilateral obstruction, which cannot be distinguished from intrinsic renal disease.

Excretory urography (contrast urography, intravenous pyelography [IVP], intravenous urography [IVU]) has been largely superseded by CT and MRI (with or without contrast). However, when CT cannot identify the level of obstructive uropathy and when acute obstructive uropathy is thought to be caused by calculi, sloughed papillae, or a blood clot, IVU or retrograde pyelography may be indicated.

Antegrade or retrograde pyelography is preferred to studies that involve vascular administration of contrast agents in patients with azotemia. Retrograde studies are done through a cystoscope, whereas antegrade studies require placement of a catheter into the renal pelvis percutaneously. Patients with intermittent obstruction should be studied when they are having symptoms; otherwise, the obstruction may be missed.

Radionuclide scans also require some renal function but can detect obstruction without the use of contrast agents. When a kidney is assessed as nonfunctioning, a radionuclide scan can determine perfusion and identify functional renal parenchyma. Because this test cannot detect specific areas of obstruction, it is mainly used in conjunction with diuresis renography to evaluate hydronephrosis without apparent obstruction.

MRI can be used when avoiding ionizing radiation is important (eg, in young children or pregnant women). However, it is inferior in accuracy to ultrasonography or CT, particularly in detection of calculi.

Evaluation of hydronephrosis without apparent obstruction: Testing may be necessary to determine whether back or flank pain is caused by obstruction in patients who have hydronephrosis but no obvious obstruction revealed by other imaging tests. Testing may also be done to detect otherwise unrecognized obstruction in patients with incidentally recognized hydronephrosis.

In **diuretic renography,** a loop diuretic (eg, furosemide 0.5 mg/kg IV) is given before a radionuclide renal scan. The patient must have sufficient renal function to respond to the diuretic. If obstruction is present, the rate of washout of the radionuclide (or contrast agent) from the time the tracer appears in the renal pelvis is reduced to a half-life of > 20 min (normal is < 15 min). On rare occasions, if the renogram is negative or equivocal but the patient is symptomatic, a perfusion pressure flow study is done via percutaneous insertion of a catheter into the dilated renal pelvis, followed by fluid perfusion into the pelvis at 10 mL/min.

The patient is in a prone position. If obstructive uropathy is present, in spite of the marked increase in urine flow, the rate of washout of the radionuclide during renal scanning is delayed, and there will be further dilation of the collecting system and elevation of the renal pelvic pressure to > 22 mm Hg during perfusion.

A renogram or perfusion study that causes pain similar to the patient's initial complaint is interpreted as positive. If the perfusion study is negative, the pain probably has a nonrenal cause. False-positive and false-negative results are common for both tests.

Prognosis

Most obstruction can be corrected, but a delay in therapy can lead to irreversible renal damage. How long it takes for nephropathy to develop and how reversible nephropathy is vary depending on the underlying pathology, the presence or absence of UTI, and the degree and duration of the obstruction. In general, acute renal failure due to a ureteral calculus is reversible, with adequate return of renal function. With chronic progressive obstructive uropathy, renal dysfunction may be partially or completely irreversible. Prognosis is worse if UTI remains untreated.

Treatment

- Relief of obstruction

Treatment consists of eliminating the obstruction by surgery, instrumentation (eg, endoscopy, lithotripsy), or drug therapy (eg, hormonal therapy for prostate cancer). Prompt drainage of hydronephrosis is indicated if renal function is compromised, UTI persists, or pain is uncontrollable or persistent. Immediate drainage is indicated if obstruction is accompanied by infection. Lower obstructive uropathy may require catheter or more proximal drainage. Indwelling ureteral catheters can be placed for acute or long-term drainage in selected patients.

Temporary drainage using a percutaneous nephrostomy technique may be needed in severe obstructive uropathy, UTI, or calculi.

Intensive treatment for UTI and renal failure is imperative.

In the case of hydronephrosis without evident obstruction, surgery should be considered if the patient has pain and a positive diuretic renogram. However, no therapy is necessary in an asymptomatic patient with a negative diuretic renogram or with a positive diuretic renogram but normal renal function.

KEY POINTS

- Common causes in children include congenital anomalies, in young adults, calculi, and in older men benign prostatic hypertrophy.
- Consequences can include renal insufficiency and infection.
- Pain is common when organs are acutely distended in the upper GU tract (commonly felt in the flank) or the bladder (commonly felt in the testes, suprapubic area, or labia).
- Suspect obstructive uropathy when patients have unexplained renal insufficiency, decreased urine output, pain that suggests obstruction, or oliguria or anuria alternating with polyuria.
- For suspected lower tract obstruction, catheterize the bladder, then consider cystourethroscopy and, in selected cases, VCUG.
- For suspected upper tract obstruction, do imaging studies (eg, abdominal ultrasonography, CT, duplex Doppler ultrasonography, intravenous pyelography, MRI).
- Relieve obstruction promptly, particularly if patients also have UTI.

254 Penile and Scrotal Disorders

For priapism, see p. 2064. For a painless scrotal mass, see p. 2067. For penile cancer, see p. 2096. For testicular cancer, see p. 2103. For congenital anomalies of the penis and male urethra, see p. 2536. For cryptorchidism, see p. 2535. For testicular and scrotal anomalies, see p. 2538.

BALANITIS, POSTHITIS, AND BALANOPOSTHITIS

Balanitis is inflammation of the glans penis, posthitis is inflammation of the prepuce, and balanoposthitis is inflammation of both.

Inflammation of the head of the penis has both infectious and noninfectious causes (see Table 254–1). Often, no cause can be found.

Balanitis usually leads to posthitis except in circumcised patients.

Balanoposthitis is predisposed to by

- Diabetes mellitus
- Phimosis (tight, nonretractable prepuce)

Phimosis interferes with adequate hygiene. Subpreputial secretions may become infected with anaerobic bacteria, resulting in inflammation.

Chronic balanoposthitis increases the risk of

- Balanitis xerotica obliterans
- Phimosis
- Paraphimosis
- Cancer

Symptoms and Signs

Pain, irritation, and a subpreputial discharge often occur 2 or 3 days after sexual intercourse. Phimosis, superficial ulcerations, and inguinal adenopathy may follow.

Diagnosis

- Clinical evaluation and selective testing

History should include investigation of latex condom use. The skin should be examined for lesions that suggest a dermatosis capable of genital involvement. Patients should be tested for both infectious and noninfectious causes, especially candidiasis. Blood should be tested for glucose.

Treatment

- Hygiene and treatment of specific causes
- Sometimes subpreputial irrigation
- Sometimes circumcision

Table 254–1. CAUSES OF PENILE INFLAMMATION

CATEGORY	EXAMPLES
Infectious	Candidiasis Chancroid Chlamydial urethritis Gonococcal urethritis Herpes simplex virus infection Molluscum contagiosum Scabies Syphilis, primary or secondary Trichomoniasis
Noninfectious	Balanitis xerotica obliterans Contact dermatitis Fixed drug eruptions Lichen planus Lichen simplex chronicus Psoriasis Reactive arthritis* Seborrheic dermatitis

*Reactive arthritis can cause shallow, painless ulcers of the glans (balanitis circinata).

Hygiene measures should be instituted and specific causes treated. Subpreputial irrigation to remove secretions and detritus may be necessary. If phimosis persists after inflammation has resolved, circumcision should be considered.

CUTANEOUS PENILE LESIONS

Common skin disorders and infections can cause cutaneous penile lesions (see Table 254–2).

Balanitis xerotica obliterans: This lesion, another name for lichen sclerosus et atrophicus in men, is an indurated, blanched area near the tip of the glans surrounding and often constricting the meatus. It results from chronic inflammation and may lead to phimosis, paraphimosis, or urethral stricture. Topical drugs, including corticosteroids, tacrolimus, antibiotics, and anti-inflammatory drugs, may be used, but their efficacy is limited. Surgery is required in severe cases.

Table 254–2. CAUSES OF CUTANEOUS PENILE LESIONS

CATEGORY	CAUSE
Common skin disorders	Allergic or irritant contact dermatitis Balanitis xerotica obliterans Carcinoma in situ: Erythroplasia of Queyrat, Bowen disease Fixed drug eruptions Papulosquamous or systemic disorders Psoriasis Squamous cell carcinoma
Sexually transmitted diseases*	Chancroid Genital herpes Genital warts (condylomata acuminata) Granuloma inguinale Syphilis
Rare infectious causes	Fungal infections Herpes zoster Lymphogranuloma venereum TB

*See also p. 1699.

Carcinoma in situ: Carcinoma in situ can include

- Erythroplasia of Queyrat
- Bowen disease of the penis
- Paget disease of the nipple
- Bowenoid papulosis

Erythroplasia of Queyrat and Bowen disease of the penis are well-circumscribed areas of reddish, velvety pigmentation in the genital area, usually on the glans or at the corona, primarily in uncircumcised men.

Paget disease of the nipple (not to be confused with Paget disease of bone) is a rare intraepithelial adenocarcinoma that can occur in extramammary locations, including the penis.

Bowenoid papulosis involves smaller, often multiple papules on the shaft of the penis.

These conditions are considered intraepithelial neoplasia or carcinoma in situ and should be biopsied.

Treatment consists of 5% fluorouracil cream, local excision, or laser therapy. Close follow-up is indicated.

Penile lichen planus: This lesion occurs as small papules or macules, sometimes annular, on the glans or shaft and may be mistaken for pemphigoid or erythema multiforme. Pruritus is common.

Penogingival syndrome in men (and vulvovaginal gingival syndrome in women) is a more severe form of erosive lichen planus. It occurs on both oral and genital mucosa. Ulcers may develop and cause pain.

Lichen planus usually resolves spontaneously. If asymptomatic, it may not require treatment. Topical corticosteroids may help relieve symptoms.

Pearly penile papules: These papules are small, harmless angiofibromas that appear on the corona of the penis as dome-shaped or hairlike projections and tend to be skin-colored. They may also appear on the distal shaft. They are common, occurring in up to 10% of men. They are not associated with human papillomavirus, although they may be mistaken for genital warts. Treatment is not required.

Contact dermatitis of the penis: Contact dermatitis of the penis has become more common with the widespread use of latex condoms. Dermatitis appears as red, pruritic lesions, sometimes with weeping or fissures. Treatment is with topical corticosteroids and use of nonlatex condoms (but not natural condoms, which do not provide adequate protection against HIV). Mild OTC corticosteroids can be tried first, with use of middle or high potency prescription preparations as needed.

EPIDIDYMITIS

Epididymitis is inflammation of the epididymis, occasionally accompanied by inflammation of the testis (epididymo-orchitis). Scrotal pain and swelling usually occur unilaterally. Diagnosis is based on physical examination. Treatment is with antibiotics, analgesics, and scrotal support.

Etiology

Bacterial epididymitis: Most epididymitis (and epididymo-orchitis) is caused by bacteria. When inflammation involves the vas deferens, vasitis ensues. When all spermatic cord structures also are involved, the diagnosis is funiculitis. Rarely, epididymal abscess, scrotal extra-epididymal abscess, pyocele (accumulation of pus within a hydrocele), or testicular infarction occurs.

In men < 35 yr, most cases are due to a sexually transmitted pathogen, especially *Neisseria gonorrhoeae* or *Chlamydia trachomatis*. Infection may begin as urethritis.

In men > 35 yr, most cases are due to gram-negative coliform bacilli and typically occur in patients with urologic abnormalities, indwelling catheters, or recent urologic procedures.

Tuberculous epididymitis and syphilitic gummas are rare in the US except in immunocompromised (eg, HIV-infected) patients.

Nonbacterial epididymitis: Viral causes (eg, cytomegalovirus infection) and mycotic causes (eg, actinomycosis, blastomycosis) of epididymitis are rare in the US except in immunocompromised (eg, HIV-infected) patients. Epididymitis and epididymo-orchitis of noninfectious etiology may be due to chemical irritation secondary to a retrograde flow of urine into the epididymis, which may occur with Valsalva maneuver (eg, with heavy lifting) or after local trauma.

Symptoms and Signs

Scrotal pain occurs in both bacterial and nonbacterial epididymitis. Pain can be severe and is sometimes referred to the abdomen. In bacterial epididymitis, patients may also have fever, nausea, or urinary symptoms. Urethral discharge may be present if the cause is urethritis.

Physical examination reveals swelling, induration, marked tenderness, and sometimes erythema of a portion of or all of the affected epididymis and, sometimes, the adjacent testis. Sepsis is suggested by fever, tachycardia, hypotension, and a toxic appearance.

Diagnosis

- Clinical evaluation
- Sometimes urethral swab and urine culture

Diagnosis of epididymitis is confirmed by finding swelling and tenderness of the epididymis. However, unless findings are clearly isolated to the epididymis, testicular torsion must also be considered, particularly in patients < 30 yr; immediate color Doppler ultrasonography is indicated. A GU consultation is indicated if the cause is unclear or the disorder is recurrent.

PEARLS & PITFALLS

- In males with acute scrotal pain, exclude testicular torsion unless findings are clearly limited to the epididymis.

Urethritis suggests that the cause of epididymitis is a sexually transmitted pathogen, and a urethral swab is sent for gonococcus and chlamydia culture or PCR. Otherwise, the infecting organism usually can be identified by urine culture. Urinalysis and culture are normal in nonbacterial causes.

Treatment

- Antibiotics
- Supportive measures

Epididymitis treatment consists of bed rest, scrotal elevation (eg, with a jockstrap when upright) to decrease repetitive, minor bumps, scrotal ice packs, anti-inflammatory analgesics, and a broad-spectrum antibiotic such as ciprofloxacin 500 mg po bid or levofloxacin 500 mg po once/day for 21 to 30 days. Alternatively, doxycycline 100 mg po bid or trimethoprim/sulfamethoxazole double-strength (160/800 mg) po bid may be used.

If sepsis is suspected, an aminoglycoside such as tobramycin 1 mg/kg IV q 8 h or a 3rd-generation cephalosporin such as ceftriaxone 1 to 2 g IV once/day may be useful until the infecting organism and its sensitivities are known.

Abscess and pyocele usually require surgical drainage.

Recurrent bacterial epididymitis secondary to incurable chronic urethritis or prostatitis occasionally can be prevented by vasectomy. An epididymectomy, occasionally done for chronic epididymitis, may not relieve symptoms.

Patients who must continuously wear an indwelling urethral catheter are prone to develop recurrent epididymitis and epididymo-orchitis. In such cases, placement of a suprapubic cystostomy or institution of a self-catheterization regimen may be useful.

Treatment of nonbacterial epididymitis includes the above general measures, but antimicrobial therapy is not warranted. Nerve block of the spermatic cord with local anesthesia can relieve symptoms in severe, persistent cases.

KEY POINTS

- The most common causes of epididymitis are bacteria: *Neisseria gonorrhoeae* and *Chlamydia trachomatis* in younger men and adolescents, and gram-negative coliform bacilli in older men.
- Tenderness affects the epididymis and often the testis.
- Diagnose epididymitis clinically and exclude testicular torsion by clinical findings or, if necessary, by color Doppler ultrasonography.
- For most cases, give antibiotics (eg, for outpatient treatment, a fluoroquinolone, doxycycline, or trimethoprim/sulfamethoxazole) and treat pain.

ORCHITIS

Orchitis is infection of the testes, typically with mumps virus. Symptoms are testicular pain and swelling. Diagnosis is clinical. Treatment is symptomatic. Antibiotics are given if bacterial infection is identified.

Isolated orchitis (ie, infection localized to the testes) is nearly always viral in origin, and most cases are due to mumps. Rare causes include congenital syphilis, TB, leprosy, echovirus infection, lymphocytic choriomeningitis, coxsackievirus infection, infectious mononucleosis, varicella, and infection with group B arborviruses. Most bacterial orchitis is the result of severe bacterial epididymitis extending to the testis (epididymo-orchitis).

Orchitis develops in 20 to 25% of males with mumps; 80% of cases occur in patients < 10 yr. Two-thirds of cases are unilateral and one-third bilateral. Sixty percent of patients with mumps orchitis develop testicular atrophy in at least one testis. Atrophy is unrelated to fertility or to the severity of the orchitis. The incidence of tumor does not appear to be increased, but unilateral disease diminishes fertility in one-fourth of men after unilateral mumps orchitis and in two-thirds of men who have had bilateral disease.

Symptoms and Signs

Unilateral mumps orchitis develops acutely between 4 and 7 days after parotid swelling in mumps. In 30% of cases, the disease spreads to the other testis in 1 to 9 days. Pain may be of any degree of severity. In addition to pain and swelling of the testes, systemic symptoms may develop, such as malaise, fever, nausea, headache, and myalgias. Testicular examination reveals tenderness, enlargement, and induration of the testis and edema and erythema of the scrotal skin.

Other infectious agents cause similar symptoms with speed of onset and intensity related to their pathogenicity.

Diagnosis

- Clinical evaluation and selective testing
- Color Doppler ultrasonography to rule out other causes of acute scrotum

History and physical examination usually indicate the diagnosis of orchitis. Urgent differentiation of orchitis from testicular torsion and other causes of acute scrotal swelling and pain is accomplished with color Doppler ultrasonography.

Mumps can be confirmed by serum immunofluorescence antibody testing. Other infectious agents may be identified by urine culture or serology.

Treatment

- Analgesic measures
- Antibiotics if bacterial infection

Supportive care with analgesics and hot or cold packs is sufficient if bacterial infection has been ruled out. Bacterial infections (usually causing epididymo-orchitis) are treated with appropriate antibiotics.

Urologic follow-up is recommended.

PEYRONIE DISEASE

Peyronie disease is fibrosis of the cavernous sheaths leading to contracture of the investing fascia of the corpora, resulting in a deviated and sometimes painful erection.

Peyronie disease occurs in adults. The cause is unknown but appears to be similar to that of Dupuytren contracture and may be related to past trauma, possibly during intercourse. The contracture usually results in deviation of the erect penis to the involved side, occasionally causes painful erections, and may prevent penetration. Fibrosis may extend into the corpus cavernosum, compromising tumescence distally.

Diagnosis is made clinically. Ultrasound or other examination of the erect penis may be used to document the fibrosis.

Resolution may occur spontaneously over many months. Mild Peyronie disease that does not cause sexual dysfunction does not need treatment.

Treatment

- Oral vitamin E and K para-aminobenzoate
- Surgical replacement of fibrosis with patch graft
- Local injections of verapamil, high-potency corticosteroids, or collagenase clostridium histolyticum
- Ultrasound or radiation therapy or a prosthesis

Treatment results are unpredictable. Oral vitamin E and K para-aminobenzoate have had varied success. Surgical removal of the fibrosis and replacement with a patch graft may be successful or may result in further scarring and exaggeration of the defect. A series of local injections of verapamil or high-potency corticosteroids into the plaque may be effective, but oral corticosteroids are not. For a penile curvature of > 30° accompanied by a palpable plaque, one or more injections of collagenase clostridium histolyticum into the plaque followed by manual penile remodeling may be used.

Ultrasound treatments can stimulate blood flow, which may prevent further scarring. Radiation therapy may decrease pain; however, radiation often worsens tissue damage. To assist penetration, a penile prosthesis may be implanted but may require a patch procedure to straighten the penis.

PHIMOSIS AND PARAPHIMOSIS

Phimosis is inability to retract the foreskin. Paraphimosis is entrapment of the foreskin in the retracted position; it is a medical emergency.

Phimosis: Phimosis is normal in children and typically resolves by age 5. Treatment is not required in the absence of complications such as balanitis, UTIs, urinary outlet obstruction, unresponsive dermatologic disease, or suspicion of carcinoma.

Betamethasone cream 0.05% bid to tid applied to the tip of the foreskin and the area touching the glans for 3 mo is often effective. Stretching the foreskin gently with 2 fingers or over an erect penis for 2 to 3 wk with care not to cause paraphimosis is also successful. If conservative measures are ineffective, circumcision is the preferred surgical option.

In adults, phimosis may result from balanoposthitis or prolonged irritation. Risk of UTI, penile cancer, HIV, and sexually transmitted diseases is increased. The usual treatment is circumcision.

Paraphimosis: Paraphimosis can occur when the foreskin is left retracted (behind the glans penis). Retraction may occur during catheterization or physical examination. If the retracted foreskin is somewhat tight, it functions as a tourniquet, causing the glans to swell, both blocking the foreskin from returning to its normal position and worsening the constriction.

PEARLS & PITFALLS

- Always remember to reduce the foreskin after urethral catheterization.

Paraphimosis should be regarded as an emergency, because constriction leads quickly to vascular compromise and necrosis of the glans penis. Firm circumferential compression of the glans with the hand may relieve edema sufficiently to allow the foreskin to be restored to its normal position. If this technique is ineffective, a dorsal slit done using a local anesthetic relieves the condition temporarily. Circumcision is then done when edema has resolved.

TESTICULAR TORSION

Testicular torsion is an emergency condition due to rotation of the testis and consequent strangulation of its blood supply. Symptoms are acute scrotal pain and swelling, nausea, and vomiting. Diagnosis is based on physical examination and confirmed by color Doppler ultrasonography. Treatment is immediate manual detorsion followed by surgical intervention.

Anomalous development of the tunica vaginalis and spermatic cord can lead to incomplete fixation of the testis to the tunica vaginalis (bell-clapper deformity—see Fig. 254–1). This anomaly predisposes the testis to twisting on its cord

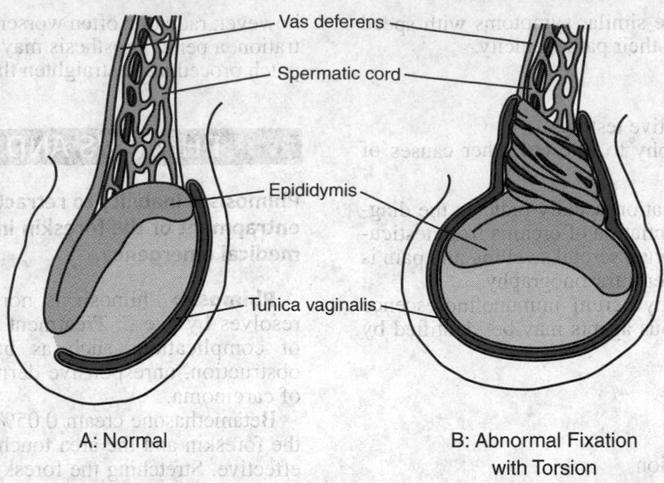

Fig. 254–1. Abnormal testicular fixation leading to torsion. Typically, the anterior two-thirds of each testis is covered by the tunica vaginalis, where fluids can accumulate. The tunica vaginalis attaches to the posterolateral surface of the testes and limits their movement within the scrotum. If the fixation is too high (anterior and cephalad), the testes can move more freely and torsion is more likely. A: Fixation is normal. B: Fixation is too high, allowing the testis to rotate transversely and resulting in torsion.

spontaneously or after trauma. The predisposing anomaly is present in about 12% of males. Torsion is most common between the ages of 12 and 18, with a secondary peak in infancy. It is uncommon in men > age 30. It is more common in the left testis.

Symptoms and Signs

Immediate symptoms are rapid onset of severe local pain, nausea, and vomiting, followed by scrotal edema and induration. Fever and urinary frequency may be present. The testis is tender and may be elevated and horizontal. The contralateral testis may also be horizontal because the anatomic defect is usually bilateral. The cremasteric reflex is usually absent on the affected side. Sometimes, torsion can spontaneously resolve and then recur, which may appear to suggest a less acute onset. Usually, however, the onset and resolution of pain is very rapid with each episode.

Diagnosis

- Clinical evaluation
- Often color Doppler ultrasonography

Torsion must be rapidly identified. Similar symptoms result mainly from epididymitis. With epididymitis, pain and swelling are usually less acute and initially localized to the epididymis. However, in both conditions, generalized swelling and tenderness often develop, making it difficult to distinguish torsion from epididymitis. A clinical diagnosis usually is sufficient to proceed to treatment.

An equivocal diagnosis may be resolved by immediate imaging if available. Color Doppler ultrasonography of the scrotum is preferred. Radioisotope scrotal scanning is also diagnostic but takes longer and is less useful.

Treatment

- Manual detorsion
- Surgery: Urgently if detorsion is unsuccessful, otherwise electively

Immediate manual detorsion without imaging can be attempted during the initial examination; its success is variable. Because testes usually rotate inward, for detorsion the testis is rotated in an outward direction (eg, for the left testis, detorsion is clockwise when viewed from the front—underneath the testis). More than one rotation may be needed to resolve the torsion; pain relief guides the procedure.

If detorsion fails, immediate surgery is indicated, because exploration within a few hours offers the only hope of testicular salvage. Testicular salvage drops rapidly from 80 to 100% at 6 to 8 h to near zero at 12 h. Fixation of the contralateral testis is also done to prevent torsion on that side. When manual detorsion is successful, bilateral testicular fixation is done electively.

KEY POINTS

- Testicular torsion typically causes rapid onset of severe scrotal pain, nausea, and vomiting, followed by scrotal edema and induration.
- Neither urinary frequency or fever rule out testicular torsion, but the cremasteric reflex is usually absent.
- Treat patients with suggestive clinical findings; reserve imaging studies for cases with equivocal findings.
- Rotate the affected testicle outward and, if not successful, arrange for immediate surgery.

URETHRAL STRICTURE

Urethral stricture is scarring that obstructs the anterior urethral lumen.

Urethral stricture can be

- Congenital
- Acquired

Anything that damages the urethral epithelium or corpus spongiosum can cause acquired stricture.

Common causes include

- Trauma
- Sexually transmitted diseases such as gonorrhea
- Unknown causes (idiopathic strictures)

Trauma, the most common cause, may result from a straddle injury or, occasionally, an iatrogenic injury (eg, after traumatic endoscopy or catheterization).

Less common causes include

- Lichen sclerosis
- Urethritis (usually chronic or untreated)

Symptoms and Signs

Symptoms may not develop until the urethral lumen has been decreased considerably. Strictures may cause a double urine stream, obstructive voiding symptoms (eg, weak urinary stream, hesitancy, incomplete emptying), or recurrent UTIs (including prostatitis).

A urethral diverticulum may develop, sometimes accompanied by abscess formation and, rarely, a fistula with extravasation of urine into the scrotum and perineum.

Diagnosis

- Retrograde urethrography or cystoscopy

Urethral stricture is usually suspected when urethral catheterization is difficult. It should also be considered in males with gradual onset of obstructive symptoms or recurrent UTIs, particularly if they have risk factors or are young.

Diagnosis of urethral stricture is usually confirmed by retrograde urethrography or cystoscopy.

Treatment

- Dilation or internal urethrotomy
- Self-catheterization
- Open urethroplasty

Treatment is determined by the type of urethral obstruction. Often, dilation or endoscopy (internal urethrotomy) is done. However, with certain types of strictures (eg, complicated strictures, such as very long or recurrent strictures or strictures that persist despite initial treatments), dilation and endoscopy should be avoided; daily self-catheterization may be indicated.

Open urethroplasty may be indicated if the stricture is localized and causes recurrent problems.

255 Renal Replacement Therapy

Renal replacement therapy (RRT) replaces nonendocrine kidney function in patients with renal failure and is occasionally used for some forms of poisoning. Techniques include intermittent hemodialysis, continuous hemofiltration and hemodialysis, and peritoneal dialysis. All modalities exchange solute and remove fluid from the blood, using dialysis and filtration across permeable membranes.

RRT does not correct the endocrine abnormalities (decreased erythropoietin and 1,25-dihydroxyvitamin D3 production) of renal failure. During dialysis, serum solute (eg, sodium, chloride, potassium, bicarbonate, calcium, magnesium, phosphate, urea, creatinine, uric acid) diffuses passively between fluid compartments down a concentration gradient (diffusive transport). During filtration, serum water passes between compartments down a hydrostatic pressure gradient, dragging solute with it (convective transport). The two processes are often used in combination (hemodiafiltration). Hemoperfusion is a rarely used technique that removes toxins by flowing blood over a bed of adsorbent material (usually a resin compound or charcoal).

Dialysis and filtration can be done intermittently or continuously. Continuous therapy is used almost exclusively for acute kidney injury. Continuous therapy is sometimes better tolerated than intermittent therapy in unstable patients because solute and water are removed more slowly. All forms of RRT except peritoneal dialysis require vascular access; continuous techniques require a direct arteriovenous or venovenous circuit.

The choice of technique depends on multiple factors, including the primary need (eg, solute or water removal or both), underlying indication (eg, acute or chronic kidney failure, poisoning), vascular access, hemodynamic stability, availability, local expertise, and patient preference and capability (eg, for home dialysis). Table 255–1 lists indications and contraindications for the common forms of RRT.

Care of patients requiring long-term RRT ideally involves a nephrologist, a psychiatrist, a social worker, a renal dietitian, dialysis nurses, a vascular surgeon (or other surgeon skilled in peritoneal dialysis catheter placement), and the transplant surgical team. Patient assessment should begin when end-stage renal failure is anticipated but before RRT is needed, so that care can be coordinated and patients can be educated about their options, evaluated for resources and needs, and have vascular access created.

Psychosocial evaluation is important because RRT makes patients socially and emotionally vulnerable. It interrupts routine work, school, and leisure activities; creates anger, frustration, tension, and guilt surrounding dependency; and alters body image because of reduced physical energy, loss of or change in sexual function, changed appearance due to access surgery, dialysis catheter placement, needle marks, bone disease, or other physical deterioration. Some patients react to these feelings by nonadherence or by being uncooperative with the treatment team.

Personality traits that improve prognosis for successful long-term adjustment include adaptability, independence, self-control, tolerance for frustration, and optimism. Emotional stability, family encouragement, consistent treatment team support, and patient and family participation in decision making are also important. Programs that encourage patient independence and maximal resumption of former life interests are more successful in decreasing psychosocial problems.

HEMODIALYSIS

(Intermittent Hemodialysis)

In hemodialysis, a patient's blood is pumped into a dialyzer containing 2 fluid compartments configured as bundles of hollow fiber capillary tubes or as parallel, sandwiched sheets of

Table 255–1. INDICATIONS AND CONTRAINDICATIONS TO COMMON RENAL REPLACEMENT THERAPIES

RENAL REPLACEMENT THERAPY	INDICATIONS	CONTRAINDICATIONS
Hemodialysis	Renal insufficiency or failure (acute or chronic) with any of the following that cannot otherwise be controlled: • Fluid overload (including refractory heart failure) • Hyperkalemia • Hypercalcemia • Metabolic acidosis • Pericarditis • Uremic symptoms • GFR* < 10 mL/min/1.73 m^2 BSA (chronic kidney disease, no diabetes) • GFR* < 15 mL/min/1.73 m^2 BSA (chronic kidney disease, diabetes) • Some poisonings	Uncooperative or hemodynamically unstable patient
Peritoneal dialysis	Same indications as for hemodialysis (except for poisonings) in patients who • Have inadequate vascular access *or* • Prefer self-therapy	**Absolute:** • Loss of peritoneal function • Adhesions that limit dialysate flow • Recent abdominal wounds • Abdominal fistulas • Abdominal wall defects that prevent effective dialysis or increase infection risk (eg, irreparable inguinal or diaphragmatic hernia, bladder extrophy) • Patient's condition not amenable to dialysis **Relative:** • Abdominal wall infection • Frequent episodes of diverticulitis • Inability to tolerate large volumes of peritoneal dialysate • Inflammatory bowel disease • Ischemic colitis • Morbid obesity • Peritoneal leaks • Severe undernutrition
Hemoperfusion	Poisoning or toxicity (eg, due to barbiturates, many antidepressants, ethchlorvynol, meprobamate, paraquat, glutethimide, metals such as lithium and barium, or toxic doses of aminoglycosides or cardiovascular drugs)	Uncooperative or hemodynamically unstable patient

*For calculation of GFR, see p. 2055.
BSA = body surface area.
GFR = glomerular filtration rate.

semipermeable membranes. In either configuration, blood in the first compartment is pumped along one side of a semipermeable membrane while a crystalloid solution (dialysate) is pumped along the other side, in a separate compartment, in the opposite direction.

Concentration gradients of solute between blood and dialysate lead to desired changes in the patient's serum solutes, such as a reduction in urea nitrogen and creatinine; an increase in bicarbonate; and equilibration of sodium, chloride, potassium, and magnesium. The dialysate compartment is under negative pressure relative to the blood compartment and has a higher osmolality to prevent filtration of dialysate into the bloodstream and to remove the excess fluid from the patient. The dialyzed blood is then returned to the patient.

The patient is usually systemically anticoagulated during hemodialysis to prevent blood from clotting in the dialysis machine. However, hemodialysis treatment may also be done with regional anticoagulation of the dialysis circuit (using heparin or trisodium citrate) or with saline flush, in which 50 to 100 mL of saline every 15 to 30 min clears the dialysis circuit of any blood clots.

The immediate objectives of hemodialysis are to correct electrolyte and fluid imbalances and remove toxins. Longer term objectives in patients with renal failure are to

- Optimize the patient's functional status, comfort, and BP
- Prevent complications of uremia
- Prolong survival

The optimal "dose" of hemodialysis is uncertain, but most patients do well with 3 to 5 h of hemodialysis 3 times/wk. One way to assess the adequacy of each session is by measuring BUN before and after each session. A ≥ 65% decrease of BUN from predialysis level ([predialysis BUN − postdialysis BUN]/predialysis BUN × 100% is ≥ 65%) indicates an adequate session. Specialists may use other, more calculation-intensive formulas, such as KT/V ≥ 1.2 (where K is the urea clearance of the dialyzer in mL/min, T is dialysis time in minutes, and V is volume of distribution of urea [which is about equal to total body water] in mL). Hemodialysis dose can be increased by increasing time on dialysis, blood flow, membrane surface area, and membrane porosity. Nightly hemodialysis sessions (6 to 8 h, 5 to 6 days/wk) and short (1.5 to 2.5 h) daily sessions, when available, are used selectively for patients who have any of the following:

- Excessive fluid gain between dialysis sessions
- Frequent hypotension during dialysis
- Poorly controlled BP
- Hyperphosphatemia that is otherwise difficult to control

These daily sessions are most economically feasible if patients can do hemodialysis at home.

Vascular access:

- Surgically created arteriovenous fistula (preferred)
- Central vein catheter

Hemodialysis is usually done through a surgically created arteriovenous fistula.

A **central vein catheter** can be used for dialysis if an arteriovenous fistula has not yet been created or is not ready for use or if creation of an arteriovenous fistula is impossible. The primary disadvantages of central vein catheters are a relatively narrow caliber that does not allow for blood flow high enough to achieve optimal clearance and a high risk of catheter site infection and thrombosis. Central venous catheterization for hemodialysis is best done by using the right internal jugular vein. Most internal jugular vein catheters remain useful for 2 to 6 wk if strict aseptic skin care is practiced and if the catheter is used only for hemodialysis. Catheters with a subcutaneous tunnel and fabric cuff have a longer life span (29 to 91% functional at 1 yr) and may be useful for patients in whom creation of an arteriovenous fistula is impossible.

Surgically created arteriovenous fistulas are better than central venous catheters because they are more durable and less likely to become infected. But they are also prone to complications (thrombosis, infection, aneurysm or pseudoaneurysm). A newly created fistula may take 2 to 3 mo to mature and become usable. However, additional time may be needed for fistula revision, so in patients with chronic kidney disease, the fistula is best created at least 6 mo before the anticipated need for dialysis. The surgical procedure anastomoses the radial, brachial, or femoral artery to an adjacent vein in an end-of-the-vein to the side-of-the-artery fashion. When the adjacent vein is not suitable for access creation, a piece of prosthetic graft is used. For patients who have poor veins, an autogenous saphenous vein graft is also an option.

Vascular access complications: Complications of vascular access include

- Infection
- Stenosis
- Thrombosis (often in a stenotic passage)
- Aneurysm or pseudoaneurysm

These complications significantly limit the quality of hemodialysis that can be delivered, increase long-term morbidity and mortality, and are common enough that patients and practitioners should be vigilant for suggestive changes. These changes include pain, edema, erythema, breaks in the skin overlying the access, absence of bruit and pulse in the access, hematoma around the access, and prolonged bleeding from the dialysis cannula puncture site. Infection is treated with antibiotics, surgery, or both.

The fistula may be monitored for signs of impending failure by serial Doppler dilution blood flow measurements, thermal or urea dilution techniques, or by measurement of the static venous chamber pressures. One of these tests is usually recommended at least monthly. Treatment of stenosis, thrombosis, pseudoaneurysm, or aneurysm may involve angioplasty, stenting, or surgery.

Dialysis complications: Complications are listed in Table 255–2.

The **most common complication of dialysis** is

- Hypotension

Hypotension has multiple causes, including too-rapid water removal, osmotic fluid shifts across cell membranes, acetate in the dialysate, heat-related vasodilation, allergic reactions, sepsis, and underlying conditions (eg, autonomic neuropathy, cardiomyopathy with poor ejection fraction, myocardial ischemia, arrhythmias).

Other frequent complications include

- Restless leg syndrome
- Cramps
- Pruritus
- Nausea and vomiting
- Headache
- Chest and back pain

In most cases, these complications occur for unknown reasons, but some may be part of a first-use syndrome (when the patient's blood is exposed to cuprophane or cellulose membranes in the dialyzer) or dialysis dysequilibrium syndrome, a syndrome thought to be caused by too rapid removal of urea and other osmolytes from the serum, causing osmotic movement of fluid into the brain. More severe cases of dialysis dysequilibrium manifest as disorientation, restlessness, blurred vision, confusion, seizures, and even death.

Dialysis-related amyloidosis affects patients who have been on hemodialysis for years and manifests as carpal tunnel syndrome, bone cysts, arthritis, and cervical spondyloarthropathy. Dialysis-related amyloidosis is believed to be less common with the high-flux dialyzers in wide use today because beta-2 microglobulin (the protein causing the amyloidosis) is removed more effectively with these dialyzers.

Prognosis: Overall adjusted annual mortality in hemodialysis-dependent patients tends to be about 20%. The 5-yr survival rate is lower for patients with diabetes than for patients with glomerulonephritis. Death is generally mostly attributable to cardiovascular disease, followed by infection and withdrawal from hemodialysis. Blacks have usually had a higher survival rate in all age groups. Nonhemodialysis contributors to mortality include comorbidities (eg, hyperparathyroidism, diabetes, undernutrition, other chronic disorders), older age, and late referral for dialysis.

CONTINUOUS HEMOFILTRATION AND HEMODIALYSIS

Continuous hemofiltration and hemodialysis procedures filter and dialyze blood without interruption. The principal advantage is the ability to remove large volumes of fluid while avoiding the hypotensive episodes caused by intermittent hemodialysis and its intermittent removal of large volumes of fluid. These procedures are therefore indicated for managing patients with acute kidney injury who are hemodynamically unstable, who must receive large volumes of fluid (eg, patients with multiple organ system failure or shock who require hyperalimentation or vasopressor drips), or both.

Table 255–2. COMPLICATIONS OF RENAL REPLACEMENT THERAPY

TYPE	HEMODIALYSIS	PERITONEAL DIALYSIS
Cardiovascular	Air embolism Angina Arrhythmia Cardiac arrest (rare) Cardiac tamponade Hypotension*	Arrhythmia Hypotension* Pulmonary edema
Infectious	Bacteremia Colonization of temporary central venous catheters Exit-site infection of both tunneled and temporary central venous catheters Endocarditis Meningitis Osteomyelitis Sepsis Vascular access cellulitis or abscess	Catheter exit site infection* Peritonitis*
Mechanical	Obstruction of the arteriovenous fistula due to thrombosis or infection Stenosis or thrombosis of the subclavian vein or superior vena cava due to recurrent use of subclavian and internal jugular vein catheters	Catheter obstruction by clots, fibrin, omentum, or fibrous encasement Dialysate leakage around the catheter Dissection of fluid into the abdominal wall Hematoma in the pericatheter tract Perforation of a viscus by the catheter
Metabolic	Hypoglycemia in diabetics who use insulin Hypokalemia Hyponatremia or hypernatremia Iron loss	Hypoalbuminemia Hyperglycemia Hyperlipidemia Obesity
Pulmonary	Dyspnea due to anaphylactic reaction to hemodialysis membrane Hypoxia when acetate buffered dialysate is used	Atelectasis Pleural effusion Pneumonia
Miscellaneous	Amyloid deposits Catheter-related hemorrhage Fever due to bacteremia, pyrogens, or overheated dialysate Hemorrhage (GI, intracranial, retroperitoneal, intraocular) Insomnia Muscle cramps* Pruritus Restlessness Seizures	Abdominal and inguinal hernias Catheter-related intra-abdominal bleeding Hypothermia Peritoneal sclerosis Seizures

*Most common complications overall.

In continuous hemofiltration, water and solutes up to 20,000 daltons in molecular weight filter from the blood by convection through a permeable membrane; the filtrate is discarded, and the patient must receive infusions of physiologically balanced water and electrolytes. A dialysis circuit can be added to the filter to improve solute clearance. Procedures may be

- Arteriovenous
- Venovenous

In **arteriovenous procedures,** the femoral artery is cannulated, and arterial pressure pushes blood through the filter into the femoral vein. Filtration rates are typically low, especially in hypotensive patients.

In **continuous venovenous procedures,** a pump is required to push blood from one large vein (femoral, subclavian, or internal jugular) through the dialysis circuit and back into the venous circulation. Using a double-lumen catheter, blood is drawn from and returned to the same vein.

The arteriovenous route has the advantage of a simple system without the requirement of a pump but may give unreliable blood flows in hypotensive patients. Advantages of the venovenous route include better control of BP and filtration rate with smoother removal of fluid. Also, the venovenous route requires cannulation of only one vessel. Neither procedure is proven more effective than the other.

Both procedures require anticoagulation, most commonly regional rather than systemic. With regional citrate anticoagulation, blood leaving the patient is infused with citrate, which binds calcium to prevent coagulation; calcium is then reinfused as the blood returns from the machine to the patient. This method avoids the complications of systemic heparinization. However, not all patients can receive citrate.[1]

1. Acute Kidney Injury Work Group. KDIGO clinical practice guideline for acute kidney injury. *Kidney Int Suppl* 2(1):89–115, 2012.

PERITONEAL DIALYSIS

Peritoneal dialysis uses the peritoneum as a natural permeable membrane through which water and solutes can equilibrate. Compared to hemodialysis, peritoneal dialysis is

- Less physiologically stressful
- Does not require vascular access
- Can be done at home
- Allows patients much greater flexibility

However, peritoneal dialysis requires much more patient involvement than in-center hemodialysis. Maintaining sterile technique is important. Of the total estimated resting splanchnic blood flow of 1200 mL/min, only about 70 mL/min comes into contact with the peritoneum, so solute equilibration occurs much more slowly than in hemodialysis. But because solute and water clearance is a function of contact time and peritoneal dialysis is done nearly continuously, efficacy in terms of solute removal is equivalent to that obtained with hemodialysis.

In general, dialysate is instilled through a catheter into the peritoneal space, is left to dwell, and then drained. In the double-bag technique, the patient drains the fluid instilled in the abdomen in one bag and then infuses fluid from the other bag into the peritoneal cavity.

Peritoneal dialysis can be done manually or using an automated device.

Manual methods include the following:

- Continuous ambulatory peritoneal dialysis (CAPD) does not require a machine to do the exchanges. A typical adult infuses 2 to 3 L (children, 30 to 40 mL/kg) of dialysate 4 to 5 times/day. Dialysate is allowed to remain for 4 h during the day and 8 to 12 h at night. The solution is manually drained. Flushing the infusion set before filling reduces peritonitis rates.
- Intermittent peritoneal dialysis (IPD) is simple, achieves higher solute clearance than automated IPD, and is useful chiefly in the treatment of acute kidney injury (AKI). In adults, 2 to 3 L (in children, 30 to 40 mL/kg) of dialysate, warmed to 37° C, is infused over 10 to 15 min, allowed to dwell in the peritoneal cavity for 30 to 40 min, and drained in about 10 to 15 min. Multiple exchanges may be needed over 12 to 48 h.

Automated peritoneal dialysis (APD) is becoming the most popular form of peritoneal dialysis. It uses an automated device to do multiple nighttime exchanges, sometimes with a daytime dwell. There are 3 types:

- Continuous cyclic peritoneal dialysis (CCPD) uses a long (12 to 15 h) daytime dwell and 3 to 6 nighttime exchanges done with an automated cycler.
- Nocturnal intermittent peritoneal dialysis (NIPD) involves nighttime exchanges and leaves the patient's peritoneal cavity without dialysate during the day.
- Tidal peritoneal dialysis (TPD) involves leaving some dialysate fluid (often more than half) in the peritoneum from one exchange to the next, resulting in greater patient comfort and avoiding the problems (eg, frequent repositioning) resulting from inability to completely drain dialysate. TPD may be done with or without a daytime dwell.

Some patients require both CAPD and CCPD to achieve adequate clearances.

Access: Peritoneal dialysis requires intraperitoneal access, usually via a soft silicone rubber or porous polyurethane catheter. The catheter may be implanted in the operating room under direct visualization or at the bedside by blind insertion of a trocar or under visualization through a peritoneoscope. Most catheters incorporate a polyester fabric cuff that allows tissue ingrowth from the skin or preperitoneal fascia, ideally resulting in a watertight, bacteria-impervious seal and preventing introduction of organisms along the catheter tract. Allowing 10 to 14 days between catheter implantation and use improves healing and reduces the frequency of early pericatheter leakage of dialysate. Double-cuff catheters are better than single-cuff catheters. Also, a caudally directed exit site (the opening of the tunnel through which the catheter enters the peritoneal cavity) lowers the incidence of exit site infections (eg, by collecting less water while showering).

Once access is established, the patient undergoes a peritoneal equilibration test, in which dialysate drained after a 4-h dwell time is analyzed and compared with serum to determine solute clearance rates. This procedure helps determine the patient's peritoneal transport characteristics, the dose of dialysis required, and the most appropriate technique. In general, adequacy is defined as a weekly $KT/V \geq 1.7$ (where K is the urea clearance in mL/min, T is dialysis time in minutes, and V is volume of distribution of urea [which is about equal to total body water] in mL).

Complications of Peritoneal Dialysis

The most important and common complications of peritoneal dialysis (see Table 255–2) are

- Peritonitis
- Catheter tunnel exit-site infection

Peritonitis: Peritonitis symptoms and signs include abdominal pain, cloudy peritoneal fluid, fever, nausea, and tenderness to palpation.

Diagnosis of peritonitis is made by clinical criteria and testing. A sample of peritoneal fluid is obtained for Gram stain, culture, and WBC count with differential. Gram stain is often unrevealing, but cultures are positive in > 90%. About 90% also have > 100 WBCs/μL, usually neutrophils (lymphocytes with fungal peritonitis). Negative cultures and WBC counts < 100/μL do not exclude peritonitis, so treatment is indicated if peritonitis is suspected based on clinical or laboratory criteria and should begin immediately, before culture results are available. Peritoneal fluid studies may be falsely negative due to prior antibiotic use, infection limited to the catheter exit site or tunnel, or sampling of too little fluid.

PEARLS & PITFALLS

- If peritonitis is suspected based on clinical criteria, start treatment immediately regardless of laboratory findings.

Empiric treatment should be adapted to microbial resistance patterns of a given facility, but typical recommendations are for initial treatment with drugs active against gram-positive organisms, eg, either vancomycin or a 1st-generation cephalosporin, plus drugs active against gram-negative organisms, such as a 3rd-generation cephalosporin (eg, ceftazidime) or an aminoglycoside (eg, gentamicin). Doses are adjusted for renal failure. Drugs are adjusted based on the result of peritoneal dialysis fluid culture. Antibiotic therapy is usually given IV or intraperitoneally (IP) for peritonitis and orally for exit-site infections. Patients with peritonitis are admitted to the hospital if IV treatment is necessary or if hemodynamic instability or other significant complications arise.

Most cases of peritonitis respond to prompt antibiotic therapy. If peritonitis does not respond to antibiotics within 5 days or is caused by recurrence of the same organism or by fungi, the dialysis catheter is removed.

Catheter tunnel exit-site infection: Catheter tunnel exit-site infection manifests as tenderness over the tunnel or at the exit site along with crusting, erythema, or drainage. Diagnosis is clinical. Treatment of infection without drainage is topical antiseptics (eg, povidone iodine, chlorhexidine); if ineffective, vancomycin is usually used empirically, with culture results guiding subsequent therapy.

Prognosis

Overall, 5-yr survival rate in peritoneal dialysis patients is slightly better than that of hemodialysis patients (about 41% in peritoneal dialysis compared to 35% in hemodialysis).

MEDICAL ASPECTS OF LONG-TERM RENAL REPLACEMENT THERAPY

All patients undergoing long-term RRT develop accompanying metabolic and other disorders. These disorders require appropriate attention and adjunctive treatment. Approach varies by patient but typically includes nutritional modifications and management of multiple metabolic abnormalities (see also p. 2086).

Diet: Diet should be carefully controlled. Generally, hemodialysis patients tend to be anorexic and should be encouraged to eat a daily diet of 35 kcal/kg ideal body weight (in children, 40 to 70 kcal/kg/day depending on age and activity). Daily sodium intake should be limited to 2 g (88 mEq), potassium to 2.3 g (60 mEq), and phosphate to 800 to 1000 mg. Fluid intake is limited to 1000 to 1500 mL/day and monitored by measuring weight gain between dialysis treatments. Patients undergoing peritoneal dialysis need a protein intake of 1.25 to 1.5 g/kg/day (compared with 1.0 to 1.2 g/kg/day in hemodialysis patients) to replace peritoneal losses (8.4 +/- 2.2 g/day). Survival is best among patients (both hemodialysis and peritoneal dialysis) who maintain a serum albumin > 3.5 g/dL; serum albumin is the best predictor of survival in these patients.

Anemia of renal failure: The anemia that occurs in renal failure should be treated with recombinant human erythropoietin and iron supplementation (see p. 2087). Because the absorption of oral iron is limited, many patients require IV iron during hemodialysis. (Sodium ferric gluconate and iron sucrose are preferred to iron dextran, which has a higher incidence of anaphylaxis.) Iron stores are assessed using serum iron, total iron-binding capacity, and serum ferritin. Typically, iron stores are assessed before the start of erythropoietin therapy and thereafter every other month. Iron deficiency is the most common reason for erythropoietin resistance. However, some dialysis patients who have received multiple blood transfusions have iron overload and should not be given iron supplements.

Coronary artery disease: Risk factors for coronary artery disease must be managed aggressively because many patients who require RRT have hypertension, dyslipidemia, or diabetes; smoke cigarettes; and ultimately die of cardiovascular disease. Continuous peritoneal dialysis is more effective than hemodialysis in removing fluid. As a result, hypertensive patients require fewer antihypertensive drugs. Hypertension can also be controlled in about 80% of hemodialysis patients by filtration alone. Antihypertensive drugs are required in the remaining 20%. Treatment of dyslipidemia, diabetes management, and smoking cessation are very important.

Hyperphosphatemia: Hyperphosphatemia, a consequence of phosphate retention due to low GFR, increases risk of soft-tissue calcification, especially in coronary arteries and heart valves, when Ca × PO_4 > 50 to 55. It also stimulates development of secondary hyperparathyroidism. Initial treatment is calcium-based antacids (eg, calcium carbonate 1.25 g po tid, calcium acetate 667 to 2001 mg po tid with meals), which function as phosphate binders and reduce phosphate levels. Constipation and abdominal bloating are complications of chronic use. Patients should be monitored for hypercalcemia.

Sevelamer carbonate 800 to 3200 mg or lanthanum carbonate 250 to 1000 mg or sucroferric oxyhydroxide 500 to 1000 mg with each meal is an option for patients who develop hypercalcemia while taking calcium-containing phosphate binders. Some patients (eg, those hospitalized with AKI and very high serum phosphate concentrations) require addition of aluminum-based phosphate binders, but these drugs should be used short-term only (eg, 1 to 2 wk as needed) to prevent aluminum toxicity.

Hypocalcemia and secondary hyperparathyroidism: These complications often coexist as a result of impaired renal production of vitamin D. Treatment of hypocalcemia is with calcitriol either orally (0.25 to 1.0 μg po once/day) or IV (1 to 3 μg in adults and 0.01 to 0.05 μg/kg in children per dialysis treatment). Treatment can increase serum phosphate level and should be withheld until the level is normalized to avoid soft-tissue calcification. Doses are titrated to suppress parathyroid hormone (PTH) levels, usually to 150 to 300 pg/mL (PTH reflects bone turnover better than serum calcium). Oversuppression decreases bone turnover and leads to adynamic bone disease, which carries a high risk of fracture. The vitamin D analogs doxercalciferol and paricalcitol have less effect on calcium and phosphate absorption from the gut but suppress PTH equally well. Early hints that these drugs may reduce mortality compared with calcitriol require confirmation.

Cinacalcet, a calcimimetic drug, increases sensitivity of parathyroid calcium-sensing receptors to calcium and may also be indicated for hyperparathyroidism, but its role in routine practice has yet to be defined. Its ability to decrease PTH levels by as much as 75% may decrease the need for parathyroidectomy in these patients.

Aluminum toxicity: Toxicity is a risk in hemodialysis patients who are exposed to aluminum-contaminated dialysate (now uncommon) and aluminum-based phosphate binders. Manifestations are osteomalacia, microcytic anemia (iron-resistant), and probably dialysis dementia (a constellation of memory loss, dyspraxia, hallucinations, facial grimaces, myoclonus, seizures, and a characteristic EEG).

Aluminum toxicity should be considered in patients receiving RRT who develop osteomalacia, iron-resistant microcytic anemia, or neurologic manifestations such as memory loss, dyspraxia, hallucinations, facial grimaces, myoclonus, or seizures. Diagnosis is by measurement of plasma aluminum before and 2 days after IV infusion of deferoxamine 5 mg/kg. Deferoxamine chelates aluminum, releasing it from tissues and increasing the blood level among patients with aluminum toxicity. A rise in aluminum level of ≥ 50 μg/L suggests toxicity. Aluminum-related osteomalacia can also be diagnosed by needle biopsy of bone (requires special stains for aluminum).

Treatment is avoidance of aluminum-based binders plus IV or intraperitoneal deferoxamine.

PEARLS & PITFALLS

- Consider aluminum toxicity in RRT patients with osteomalacia, iron-resistant microcytic anemia, or neurologic symptoms.

Bone disease: Renal osteodystrophy is abnormal bone mineralization. It has multiple causes, including vitamin D deficiency, elevated serum phosphate, secondary hyperparathyroidism, chronic metabolic acidosis, and aluminum toxicity. Treatment is that of the cause.

Vitamin deficiencies: Vitamin deficiencies result from dialysis-related loss of water-soluble vitamins (eg, B, C, folate) and can be replenished with daily multivitamin supplements.

Calciphylaxis: Calciphylaxis is a rare disorder of systemic arterial calcification causing ischemia and necrosis in localized areas of the fat and skin of the trunk, buttocks, and lower extremities. Cause is unknown, though hyperparathyroidism, vitamin D supplementation, and elevated calcium (Ca) and phosphate (PO_4) levels are thought to contribute. It manifests as painful, violaceous, purpuric plaques and nodules that ulcerate, form eschars, and become infected. It is often fatal. Treatment is usually supportive. Several cases have been reported in which sodium thiosulfate given IV at the end of dialysis 3 times/wk along with aggressive efforts to reduce the serum Ca × PO_4 product has resulted in considerable improvement.

Constipation: Constipation is a minor but troubling aspect of long-term RRT and, because of resulting bowel distention, may interfere with catheter drainage in peritoneal dialysis. Many patients require osmotic (eg, sorbitol) or bulk (eg, psyllium) laxatives. Laxatives containing magnesium or phosphate should be avoided.

256 Renal Transport Abnormalities

(See also Congenital Renal Transport Abnormalities on p. 2540.)

Many substances are secreted or reabsorbed in the renal tubule system, including electrolytes, protons, bicarbonate molecules, glucose, uric acid, amino acids, and free water. Dysfunction of these processes can result in clinical syndromes.

Syndromes are inherited, acquired, or both. Some syndromes almost always manifest in childhood, including

- Bartter syndrome (see p. 2540)
- Gitelman syndrome (see p. 2540)
- Cystinuria (see p. 2541)
- Hartnup disease (see p. 2542)
- Hypophosphatemic rickets (see p. 2543)

Other syndromes affecting renal tubules may manifest in either adults or children, including

- Fanconi syndrome
- Liddle syndrome
- Nephrogenic diabetes insipidus
- Pseudohypoaldosteronism type I
- Renal glucosuria
- Renal tubular acidosis

FANCONI SYNDROME

Fanconi syndrome consists of multiple defects in renal proximal tubular reabsorption, causing glucosuria, phosphaturia, generalized aminoaciduria, and bicarbonate wasting. It may be hereditary or acquired. Symptoms in children are failure to thrive, growth retardation, and rickets. Symptoms in adults are osteomalacia and muscle weakness. Diagnosis is by showing glucosuria, phosphaturia, and aminoaciduria. Treatment is sometimes bicarbonate and potassium replacement, removal of offending nephrotoxins, and measures directed at renal failure.

Etiology

Fanconi syndrome can be

- Hereditary
- Acquired

Hereditary Fanconi syndrome: This disorder usually accompanies another genetic disorder, particularly cystinosis. Cystinosis is an inherited (autosomal recessive) metabolic disorder in which cystine accumulates within cells and tissues (and is not excreted to excess in the urine as occurs in cystinuria). Besides renal tubular dysfunction, other complications of cystinosis include eye disorders, hepatomegaly, hypothyroidism, and other manifestations.

Fanconi syndrome may also accompany Wilson disease, hereditary fructose intolerance, galactosemia, oculocerebrorenal syndrome (Lowe syndrome), mitochondrial cytopathies, and tyrosinemia. Inheritance patterns vary with the associated disorder.

Acquired Fanconi syndrome: This disorder may be caused by various drugs, including certain cancer chemotherapy drugs (eg, ifosfamide, streptozocin), antiretrovirals (eg, didanosine, cidofovir), and outdated tetracycline. All of these drugs are nephrotoxic. Acquired Fanconi syndrome also may occur after renal transplantation and in patients with multiple myeloma, amyloidosis, intoxication with heavy metals or other chemicals, or vitamin D deficiency.

Pathophysiology

Various defects of proximal tubular transport function occur, including impaired resorption of glucose, phosphate, amino acids, bicarbonate, uric acid, water, potassium, and sodium. The aminoaciduria is generalized, and, unlike that in cystinuria, increased cystine excretion is a minor component. The basic pathophysiologic abnormality is unknown but may involve a mitochondrial disturbance. Low levels of serum phosphate cause rickets, which is worsened by decreased proximal tubular conversion of vitamin D to its active form.

Symptoms and Signs

In hereditary Fanconi syndrome, the chief clinical features—proximal tubular acidosis, hypophosphatemic rickets, hypokalemia, polyuria, and polydipsia—usually appear in infancy.

When Fanconi syndrome occurs because of cystinosis, failure to thrive and growth retardation are common. The retinas show patchy depigmentation. Interstitial nephritis develops, leading to progressive renal failure that may be fatal before adolescence.

In acquired Fanconi syndrome, adults present with the laboratory abnormalities of renal tubular acidosis (RTA) type 2—see Table 256–1 on p. 2155, hypophosphatemia, and hypokalemia. They may present with symptoms of bone disease (osteomalacia) and muscle weakness.

Diagnosis

- Urine testing for glucose, phosphates, and amino acids

Diagnosis is made by showing the abnormalities of renal function, particularly glucosuria (in the presence of normal serum glucose), phosphaturia, and aminoaciduria. In cystinosis, slit-lamp examination may show cystine crystals in the cornea.

Treatment

- Sometimes sodium bicarbonate or potassium bicarbonate or sodium citrate or potassium citrate
- Sometimes potassium supplementation

Other than removing the offending nephrotoxin, there is no specific treatment.

Acidosis may be lessened by giving tablets or solutions of sodium bicarbonate or potassium bicarbonate or sodium citrate or potassium citrate, eg, Shohl's solution (sodium citrate and citric acid; 1 mL is equivalent to 1 mmol of bicarbonate) given 1 mEq/kg bid to tid or 5 to 15 mL after meals and at bedtime.

Potassium depletion may require replacement therapy with a potassium-containing salt.

Hypophosphatemic rickets can be treated.

Kidney transplantation has been successful in treating renal failure. However, when cystinosis is the underlying disease, progressive damage may continue in other organs and eventually result in death.

KEY POINTS

- Multiple defects impair proximal tubular reabsorption of glucose, phosphate, amino acids, bicarbonate, uric acid, water, potassium, and sodium.
- Fanconi syndrome is usually caused by a drug or accompanies another genetic disorder.
- In hereditary Fanconi syndrome, proximal tubular acidosis, hypophosphatemic rickets, hypokalemia, polyuria, and polydipsia usually appear in infancy.
- Test urine for glucosuria (particularly in the presence of normal serum glucose), phosphaturia, and aminoaciduria.
- Treat by giving combinations as needed of potassium or sodium with either bicarbonate or citrate, or sometimes with just a supplemental potassium salt.

LIDDLE SYNDROME

Liddle syndrome is a rare hereditary disorder involving increased activity of the epithelial sodium channel (ENaC) which causes the kidneys to excrete potassium but retain too much sodium and water, leading to hypertension. Symptoms are of hypertension, fluid retention, and metabolic alkalosis. Diagnosis is through measurement of urinary electrolytes. Potassium-sparing diuretics provide the best treatment.

Liddle syndrome is a rare autosomal dominant disorder of renal epithelial transport that clinically resembles primary aldosteronism, with hypertension and hypokalemic metabolic alkalosis and with low plasma renin and aldosterone levels. The syndrome results from an inherently increased activity of the epithelial sodium channels, located on the luminal membrane in the collecting tubule, which accelerates sodium resorption and potassium secretion (underactivity of epithelial sodium channels causes sodium excretion and potassium retention—see p. 2153).

Patients with Liddle syndrome present at age < 35 yr. Hypertension and symptoms and signs of hypokalemia and metabolic alkalosis occur.

Diagnosis

- Urine sodium level
- Plasma renin and aldosterone levels

Diagnosis is suggested by the presence of hypertension in a young patient, particularly one with a positive family history. Low urine sodium (< 20 mEq), low plasma renin and aldosterone levels, and response to empiric treatment usually are considered sufficient to confirm the diagnosis. Definitive diagnosis can be achieved through genetic testing.

Treatment

- Triamterene or amiloride

Triamterene 100 to 200 mg po bid and amiloride 5 to 20 mg po once/day are both effective because they close sodium channels. Spironolactone is ineffective.

NEPHROGENIC DIABETES INSIPIDUS

Nephrogenic diabetes insipidus (NDI) is an inability to concentrate urine due to impaired renal tubule response to vasopressin (ADH), which leads to excretion of large amounts of dilute urine. It can be inherited or occur secondary to conditions that impair renal concentrating ability. Symptoms and signs include polyuria and those related to dehydration and hypernatremia. Diagnosis is based on measurement of urine osmolality changes after water deprivation and administration of exogenous vasopressin. Treatment consists of adequate free water intake, thiazide diuretics, NSAIDs, and a low-salt, low-protein diet.

NDI is characterized by inability to concentrate urine in response to vasopressin. Central diabetes insipidus is characterized by lack of vasopressin. Either type of diabetes insipidus may be complete or partial.

Etiology

NDI can be

- Inherited
- Acquired

Inherited NDI: The most common inherited NDI is an X-linked trait with variable penetrance in heterozygous females that affects the arginine vasopressin (AVP) receptor 2 gene. Heterozygous females may have no symptoms or a variable degree of polyuria and polydipsia, or they may be as severely affected as males.

In rare cases, NDI is caused by an autosomal recessive or autosomal dominant mutation that affects the aquaporin-2 gene and can affect both males and females.

Acquired NDI: Acquired NDI can occur when disorders (many of which are tubulointerstitial diseases) or drugs disrupt the medulla or distal nephrons and impair urine concentrating ability, making the kidneys appear insensitive to vasopressin. These disorders include the following:

- Autosomal dominant polycystic kidney disease
- Nephronophthisis and medullary cystic kidney disease complex
- Sickle cell nephropathy

- Release of obstructing periureteral fibrosis
- Medullary sponge kidney
- Pyelonephritis
- Hypercalcemia
- Amyloidosis
- Sjögren syndrome
- Bardet-Biedl syndrome
- Certain cancers (eg, myeloma, sarcoma)
- Many drugs, especially lithium, but also others (eg, demeclocycline, amphotericin B, dexamethasone, dopamine, ifosfamide, ofloxacin, orlistat)
- Possibly chronic hypokalemic nephropathy

Acquired NDI can also be idiopathic. A mild form of acquired NDI can occur in any patient who is elderly or sick or who has acute or chronic renal insufficiency.

In addition, certain clinical syndromes can resemble NDI:

- The placenta can secrete vasopressinase during the 2nd half of pregnancy (a syndrome called gestational diabetes insipidus).
- After pituitary surgery, some patients secrete an ineffective ADH precursor rather than vasopressin.

Symptoms and Signs

Generation of large amounts of dilute urine (3 to 20 L/day) is the hallmark. Patients typically have a good thirst response, and serum sodium remains near normal. However, patients who do not have good access to water or who cannot communicate thirst (eg, infants, elderly patients with dementia) typically develop hypernatremia due to extreme dehydration. Hypernatremia may cause neurologic symptoms, such as neuromuscular excitability, confusion, seizures, or coma.

Diagnosis

- 24-h urine volume and osmolality
- Serum electrolytes
- Water deprivation test

NDI is suspected in any patient with polyuria. In infants, polyuria may be noticed by the caregivers; if not, the first manifestation may be dehydration.

Initial testing includes 24-h urine collection (without fluid restriction) for volume and osmolality, and serum electrolytes.

Patients with NDI excrete > 50 mL/kg of urine/day (polyuria). If urine osmolality is < 300 mOsm/kg (water diuresis), central diabetes insipidus or NDI is likely. With NDI, urine osmolality is typically < 200 mOsm/kg despite clinical signs of hypovolemia (normally, urine osmolality is high in patients with hypovolemia). If osmolality is > 300 mOsm/kg, solute diuresis is likely. Glucosuria and other causes of solute diuresis must be excluded.

Serum sodium is mildly elevated (142 to 145 mEq/L) in patients with adequate free water intake but can be dramatically elevated in patients who do not have adequate access to free water.

Water deprivation test: The diagnosis is confirmed by a water deprivation test, which assesses the maximum urine concentrating ability and response to exogenous vasopressin.

During the test, urine volume and osmolality are measured hourly and serum osmolality is measured every 2 h. After 3 to 6 h of water deprivation, the maximal osmolality of urine in patients with NDI is abnormally low (< 300 mOsm/kg). NDI can be distinguished from central diabetes insipidus (lack of vasopressin) by administering exogenous vasopressin (aqueous vasopressin 5 units sc or desmopressin 10 mcg intranasally) and measuring urine osmolality. In patients with central diabetes insipidus, urine osmolality increases 50 to 100% over the 2 h after administration of exogenous vasopressin (15 to 45% in partial central diabetes insipidus). Patients with NDI usually have only a minimal rise in urine osmolality (< 50 mOsm/kg; up to 45% in partial NDI).

Prognosis

Infants with inherited NDI may develop brain damage with permanent intellectual disability if treatment is not started early. Even with treatment, physical growth is often delayed in affected children presumably because of frequent dehydration. All complications of NDI except for ureteral dilation are preventable with adequate water intake.

Treatment

- Adequate free water intake
- Restriction of dietary salt and protein
- Correction of the cause
- Sometimes a thiazide diuretic, an NSAID, or amiloride

Treatment consists of ensuring adequate free water intake; providing a low-salt, low-protein diet; and correcting the cause or stopping any likely nephrotoxin. Serious sequelae are rare if patients can drink at will.

If symptoms persist despite these measures, drugs can be given to lower urine output. Thiazide diuretics (eg, hydrochlorothiazide 25 mg po once/day or bid) can paradoxically reduce urine output by diminishing water delivery to vasopressin-sensitive sites in the collecting tubules. NSAIDs (eg, indomethacin) or amiloride can also help.

KEY POINTS

- Patients with NDI are unable to concentrate urine due to impaired renal tubule response to vasopressin.
- They typically pass large volumes of dilute urine, are appropriately thirsty and have near-normal serum sodium levels.
- Minimize preventable neurologic sequelae by considering inherited NDI in infants with polyuria or affected family members.
- Measure 24-h urine volume and osmolality and serum electrolytes.
- Confirm the diagnosis with a water deprivation test.
- Ensure adequate free water intake, restrict dietary salt and protein, and use a thiazide diuretic or amiloride as needed.

PSEUDOHYPOALDOSTERONISM TYPE I

Pseudohypoaldosteronism type I is a group of rare hereditary disorders that cause the kidneys to retain too much potassium but excrete too much sodium and water, leading to hypotension. Symptoms may result from hypotension, hypovolemia, hyponatremia, and hyperkalemia. Treatment is with a high sodium diet and sometimes fludrocortisone.

There are 3 types of pseudohypoaldosteronism:

- Autosomal recessive pseudohypoaldosteronism type I
- Autosomal dominant pseudohypoaldosteronism type I
- Pseudohypoaldosteronism type II

Inheritance is autosomal recessive or autosomal dominant.

Pseudohypoaldosteronism type I resembles other forms of hypoaldosteronism except that aldosterone levels are high.

The very rare pseudohypoaldosteronism type II is not discussed here.

Autosomal recessive pseudohypoaldosteronism type I: The autosomal recessive form tends to be severe and permanent. Infants are resistant to the effects of aldosterone due to mutations causing decreased activity of the epithelial sodium channels (ENaC) located on the luminal membrane of the collecting tubule (overactivity of ENaC causes potassium excretion and sodium retention—see p. 2152). The sodium channel in tissues other than the kidneys may be affected, leading to a miliary rash and/or complications similar to those of cystic fibrosis.

Autosomal dominant pseudohypoaldosteronism type 1: Children are resistant to mineralocorticoids due to mutations of the mineralocorticoid receptor. The autosomal dominant form is usually less severe, affecting mainly the mineralocorticoid receptor in the kidney, and may resolve somewhat as children age.

Diagnosis

- Plasma renin and aldosterone levels

The diagnosis is suspected based on clinical findings of hypovolemia, high serum potassium, low serum sodium, high renin and aldosterone levels, particularly in infants with a positive family history. The diagnosis is confirmed by genetic testing.

Treatment

- High-sodium diet and sometimes fludrocortisone

A high-sodium diet helps maintain volume and BP and increases excretion of potassium. If diet is ineffective, fludrocortisone 0.5 to 1.0 mg po bid or 1 to 2 mg po once/day can be given.

RENAL GLUCOSURIA

(Renal Glycosuria)

Renal glucosuria is glucose in the urine without hyperglycemia; it results from either an acquired or an inherited, isolated defect in glucose transport or occurs with other renal tubule disorders.

Renal glucosuria is the excretion of glucose in the urine in the presence of normal plasma glucose levels.

Renal glucosuria can be inherited. This form usually involves a reduction in the glucose transport maximum (the maximum rate at which glucose can be resorbed) and subsequent escape of glucose in the urine. The inherited disorder is usually transmitted as an incompletely recessive trait (heterozygotes have modest glucosuria).

Renal glucosuria may occur without any other abnormalities of renal function or as part of a generalized defect in proximal tubule function (Fanconi syndrome). It also may occur with various systemic disorders, including cystinosis, Wilson disease, hereditary tyrosinemia, and oculocerebrorenal syndrome (Lowe syndrome).

Symptoms

Renal glucosuria is asymptomatic and without serious sequelae. However, if there is an associated generalized defect in proximal tubular function, symptoms and signs may include hypophosphatemic rickets, volume depletion, short stature, muscle hypotonia, and ocular changes of cataracts or glaucoma (oculocerebrorenal syndrome) or Kayser-Fleischer rings (Wilson disease). With such findings, transport defects other than glucosuria should be sought.

Diagnosis

- Urinalysis
- 24-h urine collection

The disorder is typically initially noted on routine urinalysis. Diagnosis is based on finding glucose in a 24-h urine collection (when the diet contains 50% carbohydrate) in the absence of hyperglycemia (serum glucose < 140 mg/dL). To confirm that the excreted sugar is glucose and to exclude pentosuria, fructosuria, sucrosuria, maltosuria, galactosuria, and lactosuria, the glucose oxidase method should be used for all laboratory measurements. Some experts require a normal result on an oral glucose tolerance test for the diagnosis.

Treatment

- No treatment needed

Isolated renal glucosuria is benign; no treatment is necessary.

RENAL TUBULAR ACIDOSIS

Renal tubular acidosis (RTA) is acidosis and electrolyte disturbances due to impaired renal hydrogen ion excretion (type 1), impaired bicarbonate resorption (type 2), or abnormal aldosterone production or response (type 4). (Type 3 is extremely rare and is not discussed.) Patients may be asymptomatic, display symptoms and signs of electrolyte derangements, or progress to chronic kidney disease. Diagnosis is based on characteristic changes in urine pH and electrolytes in response to provocative testing. Treatment corrects pH and electrolyte imbalances using alkaline agents, electrolytes, and, rarely, drugs.

RTA defines a class of disorders in which excretion of hydrogen ions or reabsorption of filtered bicarbonate is impaired, leading to a chronic metabolic acidosis with a normal anion gap. Hyperchloremia is usually present, and secondary derangements may involve other electrolytes, such as potassium (frequently) and calcium (rarely—see Table 256–1).

Chronic RTA is often associated with structural damage to renal tubules and may progress to chronic kidney disease.

Type 1 (distal) RTA: Type 1 is impairment in hydrogen ion secretion in the distal tubule, resulting in a persistently high urine pH (> 5.5) and systemic acidosis. Plasma bicarbonate is frequently < 15 mEq/L, and hypokalemia, hypercalciuria, and decreased citrate excretion are often present. Hypercalciuria is the primary abnormality in some familial cases, with calcium-induced tubulointerstitial damage causing distal RTA. Nephrocalcinosis and nephrolithiasis are possible complications of hypercalciuria and hypocitraturia if urine is relatively alkaline.

This syndrome is rare. Sporadic cases occur most often in adults and may be primary (nearly always in women) or secondary. Familial cases usually first manifest in childhood and are most often autosomal dominant. Secondary type 1 RTA may result from drugs, kidney transplantation, or various disorders:

- Autoimmune disease with hypergammaglobulinemia, particularly Sjögren syndrome or RA
- Kidney transplantation
- Nephrocalcinosis
- Medullary sponge kidney
- Chronic obstructive uropathy
- Drugs (mainly amphotericin B, ifosfamide, and lithium)
- Cirrhosis
- Sickle cell anemia

Table 256–1. SOME FEATURES OF DIFFERENT TYPES OF RENAL TUBULAR ACIDOSIS*

FEATURE	TYPE 1	TYPE 2	TYPE 4
Incidence	Rare	Very rare	Common
Mechanism	Impaired hydrogen ion excretion	Impaired bicarbonate resorption	Decrease in aldosterone secretion or activity
Plasma bicarbonate (mEq/L)	Frequently < 15, occasionally < 10	Usually 12–20	Usually > 17
Plasma potassium	Usually low but tends to normalize with alkalinization	Usually low and decreased further by alkalinization	High
Urine pH	> 5.5	> 7 if plasma bicarbonate is normal < 5.5 if plasma bicarbonate is depleted (eg, < 15 mEq/L)	< 5.5

*Type 3 is very rare.

Potassium level may be high in patients with chronic obstructive uropathy or sickle cell anemia.

Type 2 (proximal) RTA: Type 2 is impairment in bicarbonate resorption in the proximal tubules, producing a urine pH > 7 if plasma bicarbonate concentration is normal, and a urine pH < 5.5 if plasma bicarbonate concentration is already depleted as a result of ongoing losses.

This syndrome may occur as part of a generalized dysfunction of proximal tubules and patients can have increased urinary excretion of glucose, uric acid, phosphate, amino acids, citrate, calcium, potassium, and protein. Osteomalacia or osteopenia (including rickets in children) may develop. Mechanisms may include hypercalciuria, hyperphosphaturia, alterations in vitamin D metabolism, and secondary hyperparathyroidism.

Type 2 RTA is very rare and most often occurs in patients who have one of the following:

- Fanconi syndrome
- Light chain nephropathy due to multiple myeloma
- Various drug exposures (usually acetazolamide, sulfonamides, ifosfamide, outdated tetracycline, or streptozocin)

It sometimes has other etiologies, including vitamin D deficiency, chronic hypocalcemia with secondary hyperparathyroidism, kidney transplantation, heavy metal exposure, and other inherited diseases (eg, fructose intolerance, Wilson disease, oculocerebrorenal syndrome [Lowe syndrome], cystinosis).

Type 4 (generalized) RTA: Type 4 results from aldosterone deficiency or unresponsiveness of the distal tubule to aldosterone. Because aldosterone triggers sodium resorption in exchange for potassium and hydrogen, there is reduced potassium excretion, causing hyperkalemia and reduced acid excretion. Hyperkalemia may decrease ammonia excretion, contributing to metabolic acidosis. Urine pH is usually appropriate for serum pH (usually < 5.5 when there is serum acidosis). Plasma bicarbonate is usually > 17 mEq/L. This disorder is the most common type of RTA. It typically occurs sporadically secondary to impairment in the renin-aldosterone-renal tubule axis (hyporeninemic hypoaldosteronism), which occurs in patients with the following:

- Diabetic nephropathy
- Chronic interstitial nephritis

Other factors that can contribute to type 4 RTA include the following:

- ACE inhibitor use
- Aldosterone synthase type I or II deficiency
- Angiotensin II receptor blocker use
- Chronic kidney disease, usually due to diabetic nephropathy or chronic interstitial nephritis
- Congenital adrenal hyperplasia, particularly 21-hydroxylase deficiency
- Critical illness
- Cyclosporine use
- Heparin use (including low molecular weight heparins)
- HIV nephropathy (due, possibly in part, to infection with *Mycobacterium avium* complex or cytomegalovirus)
- Interstitial renal damage (eg, due to SLE, obstructive uropathy, or sickle cell disease)
- Potassium-sparing diuretics (eg, amiloride, eplerenone, spironolactone, triamterene)
- NSAID use
- Obstructive uropathy
- Other drugs (eg, pentamidine, trimethoprim)
- Primary adrenal insufficiency
- Pseudohypoaldosteronism (type I or II)
- Volume expansion (eg, in acute glomerulonephritis or chronic kidney disease)

Symptoms and Signs

RTA is usually asymptomatic. Severe electrolyte disturbances are rare but can be life threatening.

Nephrolithiasis and nephrocalcinosis are possible, particularly with type 1 RTA.

Signs of ECF volume depletion may develop from urinary water loss accompanying electrolyte excretion in type 2 RTA.

People with type 1 or type 2 RTA may show symptoms and signs of hypokalemia, including muscle weakness, hyporeflexia, and paralysis. Bony involvement (eg, bone pain and osteomalacia in adults and rickets in children) may occur in type 2 and sometimes in type 1 RTA.

Type 4 RTA is usually asymptomatic with only mild acidosis, but cardiac arrhythmias or paralysis may develop if hyperkalemia is severe.

Diagnosis

- Suspected in patients with metabolic acidosis with normal anion gap or with unexplained hyperkalemia
- Serum and urine pH, electrolyte levels, and osmolalities
- Often, testing after stimulation (eg, with ammonium chloride, bicarbonate, or a loop diuretic)

RTA is suspected in any patient with unexplained metabolic acidosis (low plasma bicarbonate and low blood pH) with normal anion gap. Type 4 RTA should be suspected in patients who have persistent hyperkalemia with no obvious cause, such as potassium supplements, potassium-sparing diuretics, or chronic kidney disease. ABG sampling is done to help confirm RTA and to exclude respiratory alkalosis as a cause of compensatory metabolic acidosis. Serum electrolytes, BUN, creatinine, and urine pH are measured in all patients. Further tests and sometimes provocative tests are done, depending on which type of RTA is suspected:

- **Type 1 RTA** is confirmed by a urine pH that remains > 5.5 during systemic acidosis. The acidosis may occur spontaneously or be induced by an acid load test (administration of ammonium chloride 100 mg/kg po). Normal kidneys reduce urine pH to < 5.2 within 6 h of acidosis.
- **Type 2 RTA** is diagnosed by measurement of the urine pH and fractional bicarbonate excretion during a bicarbonate infusion (sodium bicarbonate 0.5 to 1.0 mEq/kg/h IV). In type 2, urine pH rises above 7.5, and the fractional excretion of bicarbonate is > 15%. Because IV bicarbonate can contribute to hypokalemia, potassium supplements should be given in adequate amounts before infusion.
- **Type 4 RTA** is confirmed by a history of a condition that could be associated with type 4 RTA, chronically elevated potassium, and normal or mildly decreased bicarbonate. In most cases plasma renin activity is low, aldosterone concentration is low, and cortisol is normal.

Treatment

- Varies by type
- Often alkali therapy
- Treatment of concomitant abnormalities related to potassium, calcium, and phosphate metabolism

Treatment consists of correction of pH and electrolyte balance with alkali therapy. Failure to treat RTA in children slows growth.

Alkaline agents such as sodium bicarbonate, potassium bicarbonate, or sodium citrate help achieve a relatively normal plasma bicarbonate concentration (22 to 24 mEq/L). Potassium citrate can be substituted when persistent hypokalemia is present or, because sodium increases calcium excretion, when calcium calculi are present.

Vitamin D (eg, ergocalciferol 800 IU po once/day) and oral calcium supplements (elemental calcium 500 mg po tid, eg, as calcium carbonate, 1250 mg po tid) may also be needed to help reduce skeletal deformities resulting from osteomalacia or rickets.

Type 1 RTA: Adults are given sodium bicarbonate or sodium citrate 0.25 to 0.5 mEq/kg po q 6 h. In children, the total daily dose may need to be as much as 2 mEq/kg q 8 h; this dose can be adjusted as the child grows. Potassium supplementation is usually not required when the dehydration and secondary aldosteronism are corrected with bicarbonate therapy.

Type 2 RTA: Plasma bicarbonate cannot be restored to the normal range, but bicarbonate replacement should exceed the acid load of the diet (eg, sodium bicarbonate 1 mEq/kg po q 6 h in adults or 2 to 4 mEq/kg q 6 h in children) to maintain serum bicarbonate at about 22 to 24 mEq/L because lower levels risk growth disturbance. However, excess bicarbonate replacement increases potassium bicarbonate losses in the urine. Thus, citrate salts can be substituted for sodium bicarbonate and may be better tolerated.

Potassium supplements or potassium citrate may be required in patients who become hypokalemic when given sodium bicarbonate but is not recommended in patients with normal or high serum potassium levels. In difficult cases, treatment with low-dose hydrochlorothiazide 25 mg po bid may stimulate proximal tubule transport functions. In cases of generalized proximal tubule disorder, hypophosphatemia and bone disorders are treated with phosphate and vitamin D supplementation to normalize the plasma phosphate concentration.

Type 4 RTA: Hyperkalemia is treated with volume expansion, dietary potassium restriction, and potassium-wasting diuretics (eg, furosemide 20 to 40 mg po once/day or bid titrated to effect). Alkalinization is often unnecessary. A few patients need mineralocorticoid replacement therapy (fludrocortisone 0.1 to 0.2 mg po once/day, often higher in hyporeninemic hypoaldosteronism); mineralocorticoid replacement should be used with caution because it may exacerbate underlying hypertension, heart failure, or edema.

KEY POINTS

- RTA is a class of disorders in which excretion of hydrogen ions or reabsorption of filtered bicarbonate is impaired, leading to a chronic metabolic acidosis with a normal anion gap.
- RTA is usually due to abnormal aldosterone production or response (type 4), or less often, due to impaired hydrogen ion excretion (type 1) or impaired bicarbonate resorption (type 2).
- Consider RTA if patients have metabolic acidosis with a normal anion gap or unexplained hyperkalemia.
- Check ABG and serum electrolytes, BUN, and creatinine, and urine pH.
- Do other testing to confirm type of RTA (eg, acid load test for type 1, bicarbonate infusion for type 2).
- Treat using alkali therapy and measures to correct low serum potassium in type 2 and sometimes type 1 RTA, and using potassium restriction or potassium-wasting diuretics in type 4 RTA; give other electrolytes as needed.

257 Renovascular Disorders

BENIGN HYPERTENSIVE ARTERIOLAR NEPHROSCLEROSIS

Benign hypertensive arteriolar nephrosclerosis is progressive renal impairment caused by chronic, poorly controlled hypertension. Symptoms and signs of chronic kidney disease may develop (eg, anorexia, nausea, vomiting, pruritus, somnolence or confusion), as may signs of end-organ damage secondary to hypertension. Diagnosis is primarily clinical, supported by ultrasonography and routine laboratory test findings. Treatment is strict BP control and support of renal function.

Benign hypertensive arteriolar nephrosclerosis results when chronic hypertension damages small blood vessels, glomeruli, renal tubules, and interstitial tissues. As a result, progressive chronic kidney disease develops.

Benign nephrosclerosis progresses to end-stage renal disease in only a small percentage of patients. However, because chronic hypertension and benign nephrosclerosis are common, benign nephrosclerosis is one of the most common diagnoses in patients with end-stage renal disease. It is termed benign to distinguish it from malignant arteriolar nephrosclerosis, which is a synonym for hypertensive emergency.

Risk factors include

- Older age
- Poorly controlled moderate to severe hypertension
- Other renal disorders (eg, diabetic nephropathy)

Blacks are at increased risk; it is unclear if the risk is increased because poorly treated hypertension is more common among blacks or because blacks are more genetically susceptible to hypertension-induced renal damage.

Symptoms and Signs

Symptoms and signs of chronic kidney disease, such as anorexia, nausea, vomiting, pruritus, somnolence or confusion, weight loss, and an unpleasant taste in the mouth, may develop. Signs of hypertension-related end-organ damage may occur in the vasculature of the eyes and in the skin, CNS, and periphery.

Diagnosis

- History of hypertension
- Blood tests indicating renal failure
- Signs of hypertensive end-organ damage
- No other cause of chronic kidney disease

The diagnosis may be suspected when routine blood tests indicate deteriorating renal function (eg, elevated creatinine and BUN, hyperphosphatemia) in a hypertensive patient. Diagnosis is usually inferred because of the history and evidence of hypertension-related end-organ damage (eg, retinal changes, left ventricular hypertrophy) on physical examination. Hypertension should be present before onset of proteinuria and renal failure, and there should be no other clinically suspected cause of renal failure.

Urine testing should not suggest other causes of renal failure (eg, glomerulonephritis, hypertensive emergency). On urinalysis, there should be few cells or casts in the sediment, and protein excretion is usually < 1 g/day (it is occasionally higher and in the nephrotic range).

Ultrasonography should be done to exclude other causes of renal failure. It may show that kidney size is reduced. Renal biopsy is done only if the diagnosis remains unclear.

Prognosis

Prognosis usually depends on adequacy of BP control and degree of renal failure. Usually, renal impairment progresses slowly; after 5 to 10 yr, only 1 to 2% of patients develop clinically significant renal dysfunction.

Treatment

- BP control

Treatment involves strict BP control. The BP goal is < 140/90 mm Hg, according to JNC 8 guidelines.[1] Most experts suggest using an angiotensin II receptor blocker or an ACE inhibitor for patients who have proteinuria. Calcium channel blockers and thiazide diuretics can be used as first-line drugs; most patients require combination therapy for BP control. Weight loss, exercise, and salt and water restriction also help control BP. Chronic kidney disease should be managed.

1. James PA, Oparil S, Carter BL, et al. 2014 Evidence-based guideline for the management of high blood pressure in adults: Report from the panel members appointed to the Eighth Joint National Committee (JNC 8). *JAMA* 311(5):507–520, 2014.

KEY POINTS

- Chronic hypertension can cause benign hypertensive arteriolar nephrosclerosis, resulting in chronic kidney disease and, infrequently, end-stage renal disease.
- Suspect the diagnosis if chronic hypertension precedes onset of renal insufficiency.
- Do ultrasonography to check for other causes of renal failure.
- Treat most patients with an ACE inhibitor or angiotensin II receptor blocker and possibly other drugs.

RENAL ARTERY STENOSIS AND OCCLUSION

Renal artery stenosis is a decrease in blood flow through one or both of the main renal arteries or their branches. Renal artery occlusion is a complete blockage of blood flow through one or both of the main renal arteries or its branches. Stenosis and occlusion are usually due to thromboemboli, atherosclerosis, or fibromuscular dysplasia. Symptoms of acute occlusion include steady, aching flank pain, abdominal pain, fever, nausea, vomiting, and hematuria. Acute kidney injury may develop. Chronic, progressive stenosis causes refractory hypertension and may lead to chronic kidney disease. Diagnosis is by imaging tests (eg, CT angiography, magnetic resonance angiography). Treatment of acute occlusion is with anticoagulation and sometimes fibrinolytics and surgical or catheter-based embolectomy, or a combination. Treatment of chronic, progressive stenosis includes angioplasty with stenting or surgical bypass.

Renal hypoperfusion results in renovascular hypertension, renal failure, and, if complete occlusion occurs, renal infarction and necrosis.

Etiology

Occlusion may be acute or chronic. Acute occlusion is usually unilateral. Chronic occlusion may be unilateral or bilateral.

Acute renal artery occlusion: The most common cause is thromboembolism. Emboli may originate in the heart (due to atrial fibrillation, after MI, or from vegetations due to bacterial endocarditis) or the aorta (as atheroemboli); less often, fat or tumor emboli are the cause. Thrombosis may occur in a renal artery spontaneously or after trauma, surgery, angiography, or angioplasty. Other causes of acute occlusion include aortic dissection and rupture of a renal artery aneurysm.

Rapid, total occlusion of large renal arteries for 30 to 60 min results in infarction. The infarct is typically wedge-shaped, radiating outward from the affected vessel.

Chronic progressive renal artery stenosis: About 90% of cases are due to atherosclerosis, which is usually bilateral. Almost 10% of cases are due to fibromuscular dysplasia (FMD), which is commonly unilateral. Less than 1% of cases result from Takayasu arteritis, Kawasaki disease, neurofibromatosis type 1, aortic wall hematoma, or aortic dissection.

Atherosclerosis develops primarily in patients > 50 (more often men) and usually affects the aortic orifice or proximal segment of the renal artery. Chronic progressive stenosis tends to become clinically evident after about 10 yr of atherosclerosis, causing renal atrophy and chronic kidney disease.

FMD is pathologic thickening of the arterial wall, most often of the distal main renal artery or the intrarenal branches. The thickening tends to be irregular and can involve any layer (but most often the media). This disorder develops primarily in younger adults, particularly in women aged 20 to 50. It is more common among 1st-degree relatives of patients with FMD and among people with the ACE1 gene.

Symptoms and Signs

Manifestations depend on rapidity of onset, extent, whether unilateral or bilateral, and duration of renal hypoperfusion. Stenosis of one renal artery is often asymptomatic for a considerable time.

Acute complete occlusion of one or both renal arteries causes steady and aching flank pain, abdominal pain, fever, nausea, and vomiting. Gross hematuria, oliguria, or anuria may occur; hypertension is rare. After 24 h, symptoms and signs of acute kidney injury may develop. If the cause was thromboembolic, features of thromboembolism at other sites (eg, blue toes, livedo reticularis, retinal lesions on funduscopic examination) also may be present.

Chronic progressive stenosis causes hypertension, which may begin at an atypical age (eg, < 30 yr or after age 50 yr) and which may be refractory to control despite use of multiple antihypertensives. Physical examination may detect an abdominal bruit or signs of atherosclerosis. Symptoms and signs of chronic kidney disease develop slowly.

Diagnosis

- Clinical suspicion
- Imaging

Diagnosis is suspected in patients with renal failure and who have

- Symptoms of acute renal artery occlusion
- Symptoms or signs of thromboembolism
- Hypertension that begins before age 30 or is refractory to treatment with > 3 antihypertensive drugs

Blood and urine tests are done to confirm renal failure. Diagnosis is confirmed by imaging tests (see Table 257–1). Which tests are done depends on the patient's renal function and other characteristics and on test availability.

Some tests (CT angiography, arteriography, digital subtraction angiography) require an IV ionic radiocontrast agent, which may be nephrotoxic; this risk is lower with the nonionic hypo-osmolar or iso-osmolar contrast agents that are now in widespread use (see p. 3222). Magnetic resonance angiography (MRA) requires the use of gadolinium contrast; in patients with severe chronic kidney disease, gadolinium contrast carries the risk of nephrogenic systemic fibrosis, a condition that closely resembles systemic sclerosis and that has no satisfactory method of treatment.

When results of other tests are inconclusive or negative but clinical suspicion is strong, arteriography is necessary for definitive diagnosis. Arteriography may also be needed before invasive interventions.

When a thromboembolic disorder is suspected, ECG (to detect atrial fibrillation) and hypercoagulability studies may be needed to identify treatable embolic sources. Transesophageal echocardiography is done to detect atheromatous lesions in the ascending and thoracic aorta and cardiac sources of thrombi or valvular vegetations.

Blood and urine tests are nondiagnostic but are done to confirm renal failure, indicated by elevated creatinine and BUN and by hyperkalemia. Leukocytosis, gross or microscopic hematuria, and proteinuria may also be present.

Treatment

- Restoration of vascular patency in acute occlusions and, if patients have refractory hypertension or potential for renal failure, in chronic stenosis

Treatment depends on the cause.

Acute renal artery occlusion: A renal thromboembolic disorder may be treated with a combination of anticoagulation, fibrinolytics, and surgical or catheter-based embolectomy. Treatment within 3 h of symptom onset is likely to improve renal function. However, complete recovery is unusual, and early and late mortality rates are high because of extrarenal embolization or underlying atherosclerotic heart disease.

Patients presenting within 3 h may benefit from fibrinolytic (thrombolytic) therapy (eg, streptokinase, alteplase) given IV or by local intra-arterial infusion. However, such rapid diagnosis and treatment are rare.

All patients with a thromboembolic disorder require anticoagulation with IV heparin, unless contraindicated. Long-term anticoagulation with oral warfarin can be initiated simultaneously with heparin if no invasive intervention is planned. Anticoagulation should be continued for at least 6 to 12 mo—indefinitely for patients with a recurrent thromboembolic disorder or a hypercoagulability disorder.

Surgery to restore vascular patency has a higher mortality rate than fibrinolytic therapy and has no advantage in recovery of renal function. However, surgery, particularly if done within the first few hours, is preferred for patients with traumatic renal artery thrombosis. If patients with nontraumatic, severe renal failure do not recover function after 4 to 6 wk of drug therapy, surgical revascularization (embolectomy) can be considered, but it helps only a few.

If the cause is thromboemboli, the source should be identified and treated appropriately.

Chronic progressive renal artery stenosis: Treatment is indicated for patients who meet one or more of the following 5 criteria:

- Hypertension refractory to medical treatment with ≥ 3 drugs
- Deterioration of renal function despite optimal medical therapy
- A short duration of BP elevation prior to the diagnosis of renovascular disease
- Recurrent flash pulmonary edema
- Unexplained rapid progression of renal insufficiency

Treatment is with percutaneous transluminal angioplasty (PTA) plus stent placement or with surgical bypass of the stenotic segment. Surgery is usually more effective than PTA for atherosclerotic occlusion; it cures or attenuates hypertension in 60 to 70% of patients. However, surgery is considered only if patients have complex anatomic lesions or if PTA is unsuccessful, particularly with repeated in-stent restenosis. PTA is preferred for FMD; risk is minimal, success rate is high, and restenosis rate is low.

Renovascular hypertension: Treatments are typically ineffective unless vascular patency (see p. 736) is restored. However, the 2014 CORAL study showed that renal-artery stenting plus medical therapy had no significant benefit over medical therapy alone for preventing adverse cardiovascular or renal events.[1] ACE inhibitors, angiotensin II receptor blockers, or renin inhibitors can be used in unilateral and, if GFR is monitored closely, in bilateral renal artery stenosis. These drugs can reduce GFR and increase serum BUN and creatinine levels. If GFR de-

Table 257–1. IMAGING TESTS FOR DIAGNOSIS OF RENAL ARTERY STENOSIS OR OCCLUSION

TEST	ADVANTAGES	DISADVANTAGES
CT angiography	Noninvasive Fast Generally available	Requires IV iodinated contrast, which may be nephrotoxic
MR angiography	Highly accurate Noninvasive Safe in patients with GFR > 60 mL/min and possibly GFR 30—60 mL/min	Requires gadolinium contrast, which increases risk of nephrogenic systemic fibrosis
Doppler ultrasonography	Noninvasive, highly accurate Provides information about renal function	Operator-dependent, time-consuming, and not always available; limited accuracy in obese patients
Radionuclide renography	Noninvasive Images renal blood flow	More accurate in unilateral than in bilateral stenosis; more accurate when captopril is used; at least 10% false-positive and false-negative rates, even when captopril is used Usually not used as the initial test
Arteriography	Diagnostic gold standard Provides anatomic detail for surgical and invasive radiologic procedures	Invasive Risk of atheroembolism (due to arterial catheterization) and contrast-induced nephropathy
Digital subtraction angiography	Noninvasive Uses less iodinated contrast than arteriography	Requires iodinated contrast, but in smaller amounts than arteriography
Carbon dioxide angiography	No need for contrast agent	Relatively unavailable

creases enough to increase serum creatinine, calcium channel blockers (eg, amlodipine, felodipine) or vasodilators (eg, hydralazine, minoxidil) should be added or substituted.

1. Cooper CJ, Murphy TP, Cutlip DE, et al: Stenting and medical therapy for atherosclerotic renal-artery stenosis. *N Engl J Med* 370(1):13–22, 2014.

KEY POINTS

- Renal artery stenosis or occlusion may be acute (usually due to thromboembolism) or chronic (usually due to atherosclerosis or FMD).
- Suspect acute occlusion if patients have steady, aching flank or abdominal pain, and sometimes fever, nausea and vomiting, and/or gross hematuria.
- Suspect chronic occlusion in patients who develop unexplained severe or early-onset hypertension.
- Confirm the diagnosis with vascular imaging.
- Restore vascular patency for patients who have acute occlusion and for selected patients (eg, with severe complications or refractory disease) who have chronic occlusion.
- Hypertension may be difficult to control until vascular patency is restored, but begin treatment with ACE inhibitors, angiotensin II receptor blockers, or renin inhibitors; closely monitor GFR; and substitute calcium channel blockers or vasodilators if GFR decreases.

RENAL ATHEROEMBOLISM

Renal atheroembolism is occlusion of renal arterioles by atherosclerotic emboli, causing progressive chronic kidney disease. It results from rupture of atheromatous plaques. Symptoms are those of renal failure; symptoms and signs of widespread arterial embolic disease may be present. Diagnosis is by renal biopsy. Long-term prognosis is usually poor. Treatment aims to prevent further embolization.

Atheromatous plaque rupture usually results from manipulation of the aorta or other large arteries during vascular surgery, angioplasty, or arteriography. Spontaneous plaque rupture, which occurs most often in patients who have diffuse erosive atherosclerosis or who are being treated with anticoagulants or fibrinolytics, is rare.

Atheroemboli tend to cause incomplete occlusion with secondary ischemic atrophy rather than renal infarction. A foreign body immune reaction often follows embolization, leading to continued deterioration in renal function for 3 to 8 wk. Acute renal impairment may also result from massive or recurrent episodes of embolization.

Symptoms and Signs

Symptoms are usually those of acute or chronic renal dysfunction with uremia (see p. 2077). Renal atheroembolism rarely causes hypertension. Abdominal pain, nausea, and vomiting can result from concomitant compromised arterial microcirculation of abdominal organs (eg, pancreas, GI tract). Sudden blindness and formation of bright yellow retinal plaques (Hollenhorst plaques) can result from emboli in retinal arterioles.

Signs of widespread peripheral embolism (eg, livedo reticularis, painful muscle nodules, overt gangrene, which is often referred to as the trash syndrome) are sometimes present.

Diagnosis

- Clinical suspicion
- Imaging (usually renal ultrasonography)
- Sometimes, renal biopsy
- Location of source of emboli

Diagnosis is suggested by worsening renal function in a patient with recent manipulation of the aorta, particularly if there are signs of atheroemboli. Differential diagnosis includes contrast-induced and drug-induced nephropathy. An imaging study (usually ultrasonography) should be done.

If suspicion of atheroembolism remains high, percutaneous renal biopsy is done; it has a sensitivity of about 75%. Diagnosis is important because there may be treatable causes of emboli in the absence of vascular obstruction. Cholesterol crystals in the emboli dissolve during tissue fixation, leaving pathognomonic biconcave, needle-shaped clefts in the occluded vessel. Sometimes skin, muscle, or GI biopsy can provide the same information and indirectly help establish the diagnosis.

Blood and urine tests can confirm the diagnosis of acute kidney injury or chronic kidney disease but do not establish cause. Urinalysis typically shows microscopic hematuria and minimal proteinuria; however, proteinuria is occasionally in the nephrotic range (> 3 g/day). Eosinophilia, eosinophiluria, and transient hypocomplementemia may be present.

If renal or systemic emboli recur and their source is unclear, transesophageal echocardiography is done to detect atheromatous lesions in the ascending and thoracic aorta and cardiac sources of emboli; dual helical CT may help characterize the ascending aorta and aortic arch.

Prognosis

Patients with renal atheroemboli have a poor overall prognosis.

Treatment

- Treatment of embolic source when possible
- Supportive measures
- Modification of risk factors

Sometimes the source of emboli can be treated (eg, anticoagulation for patients with emboli from a cardiac source and atrial fibrillation and for patients in whom a clot becomes a source of new emboli). However, no direct treatment of existing renal emboli is effective. Corticosteroids, antiplatelet drugs, vasodilators, and plasma exchange are not helpful. There is no demonstrated benefit of anticoagulation, and, according to most experts, its use may actually enhance atheroembolism.

Treatment of renal dysfunction includes control of hypertension and management of electrolytes and fluid status; sometimes dialysis is required. Modifying risk factors for atherosclerosis may slow its progression and induce regression. Strategies include management of hypertension, hyperlipidemia, and diabetes; smoking cessation; and encouragement of regular aerobic exercise and good nutrition (see p. 653).

KEY POINTS

- Renal atheroembolism usually results from manipulation of the aorta during vascular surgery, angioplasty, or arteriography, and not from spontaneous atherosclerotic embolization.
- Suspect the diagnosis if renal function deteriorates after the aorta or another large artery is manipulated.
- Confirm the diagnosis based on clinical findings and occasionally with percutaneous renal biopsy.
- Treat supportively, correcting modifiable risk factors and, when possible treating the embolic source. However, the overall prognosis remains poor.

RENAL CORTICAL NECROSIS

Renal cortical necrosis is destruction of cortical tissue resulting from renal arteriolar injury and leading to chronic kidney disease. This rare disorder typically occurs in neonates and in pregnant or postpartum women when sepsis or pregnancy complications occur. Symptoms and signs include gross hematuria, flank pain, decreased urine output, fever, and symptoms of uremia. Symptoms of the underlying disorder may predominate. Diagnosis is by MRI, CT, isotopic renal scanning, or renal biopsy. Mortality rate at 1 yr is > 20%. Treatment is directed at the underlying disorder and at preserving renal function.

In renal cortical necrosis, which may be patchy or diffuse, bilateral renal arteriolar injury results in destruction of cortical tissues and acute kidney injury. Renal cortical tissues eventually calcify. The juxtamedullary cortex, medulla, and the area just under the capsule are spared.

Etiology

Injury usually results from reduced renal artery perfusion secondary to vascular spasm, microvascular injury, or intravascular coagulation.

About 10% of cases occur in infants and children. Pregnancy complications increase risk of this disorder in neonates and in women, as does sepsis. Other causes (eg, disseminated intravascular coagulation [DIC]) are less common (see Table 257–2).

Table 257–2. CAUSES OF RENAL CORTICAL NECROSIS

PATIENT GROUP	CAUSES
Neonates	Abruptio placentae (causes about 50% of cases) Congenital heart disease (severe) Dehydration Fetomaternal transfusion Hemolytic anemia (severe) Perinatal asphyxia Renal vein thrombosis Sepsis
Children	Dehydration Hemolytic-uremic syndrome Sepsis Shock
Pregnant and postpartum women	Pregnancy complications (cause > 50% of cases): Abruptio placentae, amniotic fluid embolism, intrauterine fetal death, placenta previa, preeclampsia, puerperal sepsis, uterine hemorrhage Sepsis (causes about 30%)
Others	Burns Disseminated intravascular coagulation Drugs (eg, NSAIDs) Hyperacute renal allograft rejection Incompatible blood transfusion Nephrotoxic contrast agents Pancreatitis Poisoning (eg, phosphorus, arsenic) Sepsis Snakebite Trauma

Symptoms and Signs

Gross hematuria, flank pain, and sometimes decreased urine output or abrupt anuria occur. Fever is common, and chronic kidney disease with hypertension develops. However, these symptoms are often overshadowed by symptoms of the underlying disorder.

Diagnosis

- Imaging, usually with CT angiography

Diagnosis is suspected when typical symptoms occur in patients with a potential cause.

Imaging tests can sometimes confirm the diagnosis. CT angiography is usually preferred despite the risks of using an iodinated contrast agent. Because of the risk of nephrogenic systemic fibrosis, use of MRA with gadolinium contrast is not recommended in these patients, who usually have severe renal dysfunction.

An alternative is isotopic renal scanning using diethylenetriamine penta-acetic acid. It shows enlarged, nonobstructed kidneys, with little or no renal blood flow. Renal biopsy is done only if the diagnosis is unclear and no contraindications exist. It provides definitive diagnosis and prognostic information.

Urinalysis, CBC, liver function tests, and serum electrolytes and renal function tests are done routinely. These tests often confirm renal dysfunction (eg, indicated by elevated creatinine and BUN and by hyperkalemia) and may suggest a cause. Severe electrolyte abnormalities may be present depending on the cause (eg, hyperkalemia, hyperphosphatemia, hypocalcemia). CBC often detects leukocytosis (even when sepsis is not the cause) and may detect anemia and thrombocytopenia if hemolysis, DIC, or sepsis is the cause. Transaminases may be increased in relative hypovolemic states (eg, septic shock, postpartum hemorrhage). If DIC is suspected, coagulation studies are done. They may detect low fibrinogen levels, increased fibrin-degradation products, and increasing PT/INR and PTT. Urinalysis typically detects proteinuria and hematuria.

Prognosis

Prognosis of renal cortical necrosis was poor in the past, with mortality > 50% in the first year. More recently, with aggressive supportive therapy, 1-yr mortality can be about 20%, and up to 20% of survivors may recover some renal function.

Treatment

Treatment is directed at the underlying disorder and at preserving renal function (eg, with early dialysis).

KEY POINTS

- Renal cortical necrosis is rare, typically occurring in neonates and in pregnant or postpartum women with sepsis or pregnancy complications.
- Suspect the diagnosis in patients at risk who develop typical symptoms (eg, gross hematuria, flank pain, decreased urine output, fever, hypertension).
- Confirm the diagnosis with renal vascular imaging, usually CT angiography.
- Treat the underlying disorder.

RENAL VEIN THROMBOSIS

Renal vein thrombosis is thrombotic occlusion of one or both main renal veins, resulting in acute kidney injury or chronic kidney disease. Common causes include nephrotic syndrome, primary hypercoagulability disorders, malignant renal tumors, extrinsic compression, trauma, and rarely inflammatory bowel disease. Symptoms of renal failure and sometimes nausea, vomiting, flank pain, gross hematuria, decreased urine output, or systemic manifestations of venous thromboembolism may occur. Diagnosis is by CT, MRA, or renal venography. With treatment, prognosis is generally good. Treatment is anticoagulation, support of renal function, and treatment of the underlying disorder. Some patients benefit from thrombectomy or nephrectomy.

Etiology

Renal vein thrombosis usually results from local and systemic hypercoagulability due to nephrotic syndrome associated with membranous nephropathy (most often), minimal change disease, or membranoproliferative glomerulonephritis. The risk of thrombosis due to nephrotic syndrome appears to be proportional to the severity of the hypoalbuminemia. Overly aggressive diuresis or prolonged high-dose corticosteroid treatment may contribute to thrombosis of the renal vein in patients with these conditions.

Other causes include

- Allograft rejection
- Amyloidosis
- Diabetic nephropathy
- Estrogen therapy
- Pregnancy
- Primary hypercoagulability disorders (eg, antithrombin III deficiency, protein C or S deficiency, factor V Leiden mutation, prothrombin G20210A mutation)
- Renal vasculitis
- Sickle cell nephropathy
- SLE

Less common causes are related to reduced renal vein blood flow and include malignant renal tumors that extend into the renal veins (typically renal cell carcinoma), extrinsic compression of the renal vein or inferior vena cava (eg, by vascular abnormalities, tumor, retroperitoneal disease, ligation of the inferior vena cava, aortic aneurysm), oral contraceptive use, trauma, dehydration, and, rarely, thrombophlebitis migrans and cocaine abuse.

Symptoms and Signs

Usually, onset of renal dysfunction is insidious. However, onset may be acute, causing renal infarction with nausea, vomiting, flank pain, gross hematuria, and decreased urine output.

When the cause is a hypercoagulability disorder, signs of venous thromboembolic disorders (eg, deep venous thrombosis, pulmonary embolism) may occur. When the cause is a renal cancer, its signs (eg, hematuria, weight loss) predominate.

Diagnosis

- Vascular imaging

Renal vein thrombosis should be considered in patients with renal infarction or any unexplained deterioration in renal function, particularly in patients with the nephrotic syndrome or other risk factors.

The traditional diagnostic test of choice and the standard is venography of the inferior vena cava; this test is diagnostic, but it may mobilize clots. Because of the risks of conventional venography, magnetic resonance venography and Doppler ultrasonography are being used increasingly. Magnetic resonance venography can be done if GFR > 30 mL/min. Doppler ultrasonography sometimes detects renal vein thrombosis but has high false-negative and false-positive rates. Notching of the ureter due to dilated collateral veins is a characteristic finding in some chronic cases.

CT angiography provides good detail with high sensitivity and specificity and is fast but requires administration of a radiocontrast agent, which may be nephrotoxic. Serum electrolytes and urinalysis are done and confirm deterioration of renal function.

Microscopic hematuria is often present. Proteinuria may be in the nephrotic range.

If no cause is apparent, testing for hypercoagulability disorders should be initiated (see p. 1206). Renal biopsy is nonspecific but may detect a coexisting renal disorder.

Prognosis

Death is rare and usually related to complications such as pulmonary embolism and those due to nephrotic syndrome or a malignant tumor.

Treatment

- Treatment of underlying disorder
- Anticoagulation
- Sometimes percutaneous catheter-directed thrombectomy or thrombolysis

The underlying disorder should be treated.

Treatment options for renal vein thrombosis include anticoagulation with heparin, thrombolysis, and catheter-directed or surgical thrombectomy. Long-term anticoagulation with low molecular weight heparin or oral warfarin should be started immediately if no invasive intervention is planned. Anticoagulation minimizes risk of new thrombi, promotes recanalization of vessels with existing clots, and improves renal function. Anticoagulation should be continued for at least 6 to 12 mo and, if a hypercoagulability disorder (eg, persistent nephrotic syndrome) is present, indefinitely.

Use of a percutaneous catheter for thrombectomy or thrombolysis is currently recommended. Surgical thrombectomy is rarely used but should be considered in patients with acute bilateral renal vein thrombosis and acute kidney injury who cannot be treated with percutaneous catheter thrombectomy and/or thrombolysis.

Nephrectomy is done only if infarction is total (in certain cases) or if the underlying disorder warrants it.

KEY POINTS

- The most common cause of renal vein thrombosis is nephrotic syndrome associated with membranous nephropathy.
- Consider renal vein thrombosis in patients with renal infarction or any unexplained deterioration in renal function, particularly those who have the nephrotic syndrome or other risk factors.
- Confirm the diagnosis with vascular imaging, usually magnetic resonance venography (if GFR > 30 mL/min) or Doppler ultrasonography.
- Treat the underlying disorder and initiate anticoagulation, thrombolysis, or thrombectomy.

258 Tubulointerstitial Diseases

Tubulointerstitial diseases are clinically heterogeneous disorders that share similar features of tubular and interstitial injury. In severe and prolonged cases, the entire kidney may become involved, with glomerular dysfunction and even renal failure. The primary categories of tubulointerstitial disease are

- Acute tubular necrosis
- Acute or chronic tubulointerstitial nephritis

Contrast nephropathy is acute tubular necrosis caused by an iodinated radiocontrast agent.

Analgesic nephropathy, reflux nephropathy, and myeloma kidney are types of chronic tubulointerstitial nephritis.

Tubulointerstitial disorders can also result from metabolic disturbances and exposure to toxins.

Pathophysiology

The kidneys are exposed to unusually high concentrations of toxins. The kidneys have the highest blood supply of all tissues (about 1.25 L/min or 25% of cardiac output), and unbound solutes leave the circulation via glomerular filtration at ≥ 100 mL/min; as a result, toxic agents are delivered at a rate 50 times that of other tissues and in much higher concentrations. When urine is concentrated, the luminal surfaces of tubular cells may be exposed to molecule concentrations 300 to 1000 times greater than those of plasma. The fine brush border of proximal tubular cells exposes an enormous surface area. A countercurrent flow mechanism increases ionic concentration of the interstitial fluid of the medulla (and thereby increases urine concentration) up to 4 times the plasma concentration.

In addition, factors can affect cellular vulnerability after exposure to toxins:

- Tubular transport mechanisms separate drugs from their binding proteins, which normally protect cells from toxicity.
- Transcellular transport exposes the interior of the cell and its organelles to newly encountered chemicals.
- Binding sites of some agents (eg, sulfhydryl groups) may facilitate entry but retard exit (eg, heavy metals).
- Chemical reactions (eg, alkalinization, acidification) may alter transport in either direction.
- Blockade of transport receptors may alter tissue exposure (eg, diuresis from blockade of adenosine A1 such as with aminophylline) receptors may decrease exposure).
- The kidneys have the highest oxygen and glucose consumption per gram of tissue and are therefore vulnerable to toxins affecting cell energy metabolism.

ACUTE TUBULAR NECROSIS

Acute tubular necrosis (ATN) is kidney injury characterized by acute tubular cell injury and dysfunction. Common causes are hypotension or sepsis that causes renal hypoperfusion and nephrotoxic drugs. The condition is asymptomatic unless it causes renal failure. The

diagnosis is suspected when azotemia develops after a hypotensive event, severe sepsis, or drug exposure and is distinguished from prerenal azotemia by laboratory testing and response to volume expansion. Treatment is supportive.

Etiology

Common causes of ATN include the following:

- Renal hypoperfusion, most often caused by hypotension or sepsis (ischemic ATN; most common, especially in patients in an ICU)
- Nephrotoxins
- Major surgery (often due to multiple factors)

Other causes of ATN include

- Third-degree burns covering > 15% of BSA
- The heme pigments myoglobin and hemoglobin (caused by either rhabdomyolysis or massive hemolysis)
- Other endogenous toxins, resulting from disorders such as tumor lysis or multiple myeloma
- Poisons, such as ethylene glycol
- Herbal and folk remedies, such as ingestion of fish gallbladder in Southeast Asia

Common nephrotoxins include the following:

- Aminoglycosides
- Amphotericin B
- Cisplatin and other chemotherapy drugs
- Radiocontrast (particularly ionic high osmolar agents given IV in volumes > 100 mL—see p. 2164)
- NSAIDs (especially when concurrent with poor renal perfusion or other nephrotoxic agents)
- Colistimethate
- Calcineurin inhibitors (eg, cyclosporine, tacrolimus, used systemically)

Massive volume loss, particularly in patients with septic or hemorrhagic shock, pancreatitis, or major surgery, increases the risk of ischemic ATN; patients with serious comorbidities are at highest risk.

Major surgery and advanced hepatobiliary disease increase the risk of aminoglycoside toxicity. Certain drug combinations (eg, aminoglycosides with amphotericin B) may be especially nephrotoxic. NSAIDs may cause several types of intrinsic kidney disease, including ATN.

Toxic exposures cause patchy, segmental, tubular luminal occlusion with casts and cellular debris or segmental tubular necrosis.

ATN is more likely to develop in patients with the following:

- Preexisting chronic kidney disease
- Diabetes mellitus
- Preexisting hypovolemia or poor renal perfusion
- Older age

Symptoms and Signs

ATN is usually asymptomatic but may cause symptoms or signs of acute kidney injury, typically oliguria initially if ATN is severe. However, urine output may not be reduced if ATN is less severe (eg, typical in aminoglycoside-induced ATN).

Diagnosis

- Differentiation from prerenal azotemia, based mainly on laboratory findings and, in the case of blood or fluid loss, response to volume expansion

ATN is suspected when serum creatinine rises ≥ 0.5 mg/dL/day above baseline after an apparent trigger (eg, hypotensive event, exposure to a nephrotoxin); the rise in creatinine may occur 1 to 2 days after certain exposures (eg, IV radiocontrast) but be more delayed after exposure to other nephrotoxins (eg, aminoglycosides).

ATN must be differentiated from prerenal azotemia because treatment differs. In prerenal azotemia, renal perfusion is decreased enough to elevate serum BUN out of proportion to creatinine, but not enough to cause ischemic damage to tubular cells. Prerenal azotemia can be caused by direct intravascular fluid loss (eg, due to hemorrhage, GI tract losses, urinary losses) or by a relative decrease in effective circulating volume *without* loss of total body fluid (eg, in heart failure, portal hypertension with ascites). If fluid loss is the cause, volume expansion using IV normal saline solution increases urine output and normalizes serum creatinine level. If ATN is the cause, IV saline typically causes no increase in urine output and no rapid change in serum creatinine. Untreated prerenal azotemia may progress to ischemic ATN.

Laboratory findings also help distinguish ATN from prerenal azotemia (see Table 258–1).

Prognosis

In otherwise healthy patients, short-term prognosis is good when the underlying insult is corrected; serum creatinine

Table 258–1. LABORATORY FINDINGS DISTINGUISHING ACUTE TUBULAR NECROSIS FROM PRERENAL AZOTEMIA

TEST*	ACUTE TUBULAR NECROSIS	PRERENAL AZOTEMIA
Rate of creatinine rise	0.3–0.5 mg/dL/day	Variable and fluctuates
BUN/creatinine ratio	10–15:1	> 20:1
Urine osmolality (mOsm/kg)	< 450 (usually < 350)	> 500
Urine specific gravity	≤ 1.010	> 1.020
Urine sodium (mEq/L)	> 40	< 20
Urine/plasma creatinine ratio	< 20	> 40
Fractional excretion of sodium (%)	> 2	< 1
Urinary sediment	Muddy brown granular casts, epithelial cell casts, free epithelial cells, or a combination	Normal or with hyaline casts

*Criteria may not apply in patients with chronic kidney disease or recent diuretic use.

typically returns to normal or near-normal within 1 to 3 wk. In sick patients, even when acute kidney injury is mild, morbidity and mortality are increased. Prognosis is better in patients who do not require ICU care (32% mortality) than in those who do (72% mortality). Predictors of mortality include mainly

- Decreased urine volume (eg, anuria, oliguria)
- Severity of the underlying disorder
- Severity of coexisting disorders

Patients who survive ATN have an increased risk of chronic kidney disease.

Cause of death is usually infection or the underlying disorder.

Treatment

- Supportive care

Treatment is supportive and includes stopping nephrotoxins whenever possible, maintaining euvolemia, providing nutritional support, and treating infections (preferably with drugs that are not nephrotoxic). Diuretics may be used to maintain urine output in oliguric ATN but are of unproven benefit and do not alter the course of kidney injury; there is no evidence to support use of mannitol or dopamine. General management of acute kidney injury is discussed elsewhere.

PEARLS & PITFALLS

- Diuretics may help maintain urinary output in patients with ATN but do not alter the course of kidney injury.

Prevention

Prevention includes the following:

- Maintaining euvolemia and renal perfusion in critically ill patients
- Avoiding nephrotoxic drugs when possible
- Closely monitoring renal function when nephrotoxic drugs must be used
- Taking measures to prevent contrast nephropathy
- Among patients with diabetes, controlling blood glucose levels

There is no evidence that loop diuretics, mannitol, or dopamine helps prevent or alter the course of established ATN.

KEY POINTS

- ATN can develop after various disorders or triggers decrease renal perfusion or expose the kidneys to toxins.
- Other than oliguria in severe cases, symptoms do not develop unless and until renal failure develops.
- Differentiate ATN from prerenal azotemia by the response to volume expansion and by urine and blood chemistry tests and calculations derived from them.
- Correct the cause of ATN as soon as possible to achieve a good short-term prognosis.
- Stop nephrotoxins, maintain euvolemia, and treat infection and undernutrition.

ANALGESIC NEPHROPATHY

Analgesic nephropathy (AN) is chronic tubulointerstitial nephritis caused by cumulative lifetime use of large amounts (eg, ≥ 2 kg) of certain analgesics. Patients present with kidney injury and usually non-nephrotic proteinuria and bland urinary sediment or sterile pyuria. Hypertension, anemia, and impaired urinary concentration occur as renal insufficiency develops. Papillary necrosis occurs late. Diagnosis is based on a history of analgesic use and results of noncontrast CT. Treatment is stopping the causative analgesic.

AN, a type of chronic interstitial nephritis, was originally described in conjunction with overuse of combination analgesics containing phenacetin (typically with aspirin, acetaminophen, codeine, or caffeine). However, despite removal of phenacetin from the market, AN continued to occur. Studies to identify the causal agent are equivocal, but acetaminophen, aspirin, and other NSAIDs have been implicated. Mechanism is unclear. Whether COX-2 inhibitors cause AN is not known, but these drugs probably can cause acute tubulointerstitial nephritis and nephrotic syndrome due to minimal change disease or membranous nephropathy.

AN predominates in women (peak incidence, 50 to 55 yr) and, in the US, is responsible for 3 to 5% of cases of end-stage renal disease (13 to 20% in Australia and South Africa).

Symptoms and Signs

Patients present with kidney injury and usually non-nephrotic proteinuria with a bland urinary sediment or sterile pyuria. Hypertension, anemia, and impaired urinary concentration are common once renal insufficiency develops.

Flank pain and hematuria and passage of a renal papilla (causing upper urinary tract obstruction) are signs of papillary necrosis that occur late in the course of disease.

Chronic complaints of musculoskeletal pain, headache, malaise, and dyspepsia may be related to long-term analgesic use rather than AN.

Diagnosis

- History of chronic analgesic use
- CT

Analgesic nephropathy diagnosis is based on history of chronic analgesic use and noncontrast CT. CT signs of AN are the following:

- Decreased renal size
- Bumpy contours, defined as at least 3 indentations in the normally convex outline of the kidney
- Papillary calcifications

The combination of these findings has a sensitivity of 85% and a specificity of 93% for early diagnosis, but these specificity and sensitivity numbers are based on studies done when use of phenacetin-containing analgesics was widespread.

Treatment

- Stopping analgesic use

Renal function stabilizes when analgesics are stopped unless kidney injury is advanced, in which case it may progress to chronic kidney disease. Patients with AN are at greater risk of transitional cell carcinomas of the urinary tract.

CONTRAST NEPHROPATHY

Contrast nephropathy is worsening of renal function after IV administration of radiocontrast and is usually temporary. Diagnosis is based on a progressive rise in serum creatinine 24 to 48 h after contrast is given. Treatment

is supportive. Volume loading with isotonic saline before and after contrast administration may help in prevention.

Contrast nephropathy is acute tubular necrosis (ATN) caused by an iodinated radiocontrast agent, all of which are nephrotoxic. However, risk is lower with newer contrast agents, which are nonionic and have a lower osmolality than older agents, whose osmolality is about 1400 to 1800 mOsm/kg. For example, 2nd-generation, low-osmolal agents (eg, iohexol, iopamidol, ioxaglate) have an osmolality of about 500 to 850 mOsm/kg, which is still higher than blood osmolality. Iodixanol, the first of the even newer iso-osmolal agents, has an osmolality of 290 mOsm/kg, about equal to that of blood.

The precise mechanism of radiocontrast toxicity is unknown but is suspected to be some combination of renal vasoconstriction and direct cytotoxic effects, perhaps through formation of reactive O_2 species, causing ATN.

Most patients have no symptoms. Renal function usually later returns to normal.

Risk factors for contrast nephropathy: Risk factors for nephrotoxicity are the following:

- Older age
- Preexisting chronic kidney disease
- Diabetes mellitus
- Heart failure
- Multiple myeloma
- High doses (eg, > 100 mL) of a hyperosmolar contrast agent (eg, during percutaneous coronary interventions)
- Factors that reduce renal perfusion, such as volume depletion or the concurrent use of NSAIDs, diuretics, or ACE inhibitors
- Concurrent use of nephrotoxic drugs (eg, aminoglycosides)
- Liver failure

Diagnosis

- Serum creatinine measurement

Diagnosis is based on a progressive rise in serum creatinine 24 to 48 h after a contrast study.

After femoral artery catheterization, contrast nephropathy may be difficult to distinguish from renal atheroembolism. Factors that can suggest renal atheroemboli include the following:

- Delay in onset of increased creatinine > 48 h after the procedure
- Presence of other atheroembolic findings (eg, livedo reticularis of the lower extremities or bluish discoloration of the toes)
- Persistently poor renal function that may deteriorate in a stepwise fashion
- Transient eosinophilia or eosinophiluria and low C3 complement levels (measured if atheroemboli are seriously considered)

Treatment

- Supportive care

Treatment is supportive.

Prevention

Preventing contrast nephropathy involves avoiding contrast when possible (eg, not using CT to diagnose appendicitis) and, when contrast is necessary for patients with risk factors, using a nonionic agent with the lowest osmolality at a low dose.

When contrast is given, mild volume expansion with isotonic saline (ie, 154 mEq/L) is ideal; 1 mL/kg/h is given beginning 6 to 12 h before contrast is given and continued for 6 to 12 h after the procedure. A sodium bicarbonate ($NaHCO_3$) solution may also be infused but has no proven advantage over normal saline. Volume expansion may be most helpful in patients with mild preexisting renal disease and exposure to a low dose of contrast. Volume expansion should be avoided in heart failure. Nephrotoxic drugs are avoided before and after the procedure.

Acetylcysteine, an antioxidant, is sometimes given for patients at high risk but has no proven benefit. Protocols vary, but acetylcysteine, 600 mg po bid the day before and the day of the procedure, may be given, combined with saline infusion.

Periprocedural continuous venovenous hemofiltration has no proven benefit compared with other less invasive strategies in preventing acute kidney injury in patients who have chronic kidney disease and who require high doses of contrast and also is not practical. Therefore, this procedure is not recommended. Patients undergoing regular hemodialysis for end-stage renal disease who require contrast do not typically need supplementary, prophylactic hemodialysis after the procedure unless they have significant residual renal function (eg, produce > 100 mL/day of urine).

KEY POINTS

- Although most patients recover from use of iodinated radiocontrast without clinical consequences, all such radiocontrast is nephrotoxic.
- Suspect contrast nephropathy if serum creatinine increases 24 to 48 h after a contrast study.
- Decrease the risk of contrast nephropathy, particularly in patients at risk, by minimizing the use and volume of contrast and expanding volume when possible.

HEAVY METAL NEPHROPATHY

Exposure to heavy metals and other toxins can result in tubulointerstitial disorders.

Heavy metals (eg, lead, cadmium, copper) and other toxins can cause a form of chronic interstitial nephritis.

Lead nephropathy: Chronic tubulointerstitial nephritis results as lead accumulates in proximal tubular cells.

Short-term lead exposure causes proximal tubular dysfunction, including decreased urate secretion and hyperuricemia (urate is the substrate for saturnine gout), aminoaciduria, and renal glucosuria.

Chronic lead exposure (ie, for 5 to ≥ 30 yr) causes progressive tubular atrophy and interstitial fibrosis, with renal insufficiency, hypertension, and gout. However, chronic low-level exposure may cause renal insufficiency and hypertension independent of tubulointerstitial disease. The following groups are at highest risk:

- Children exposed to lead paint dust or chips
- Welders
- Battery workers
- Drinkers of high-proof distilled (moonshine) alcohol

Exposed children may develop nephropathy during adulthood. Common findings include a bland urinary sediment and hyperuricemia disproportionate to the degree of renal insufficiency:

- Serum urate > 9 mg/dL with serum creatinine < 1.5 mg/dL
- Serum urate > 10 mg/dL with serum creatinine 1.5 to 2 mg/dL
- Serum urate > 12 mg/dL with serum creatinine > 2 mg/dL

Diagnosis is usually made by measuring whole blood lead levels. Alternatively, x-ray fluorescence may be used to detect increased bone lead concentrations, which reflect high cumulative lead exposure.

Treatment with chelation therapy can stabilize renal function, but recovery may be incomplete.

Cadmium nephropathy: Cadmium exposure due to contaminated water, food, or tobacco and, mainly, due to workplace exposures can cause nephropathy. It can also cause a glomerulopathy that is usually asymptomatic.

Early manifestations of cadmium nephropathy are those of tubular dysfunction, including low molecular weight tubular proteinuria (eg, beta2-microglobulin), aminoaciduria, and renal glucosuria. Symptoms and signs, when they occur, are attributable to chronic kidney disease. Renal disease follows a dose-response curve.

Diagnosis of cadmium nephropathy is likely with the following:

- History of occupational exposure to cadmium
- Increased levels of urinary beta2-microglobulin (missed by urinary dipstick protein testing but detected using radioimmunoassay)
- Increased urinary cadmium levels (> 7 μg/g creatinine)

Treatment is elimination of cadmium exposure; note that chelation with EDTA may aggravate renal toxicity in acute cadmium poisoning but has been used successfully in cases of chronic cadmium exposure. Tubular proteinuria usually is irreversible.

Other heavy metal nephropathies: Other heavy metals that are nephrotoxic include

- Copper
- Gold
- Uranium
- Arsenic
- Iron
- Mercury
- Bismuth
- Chromium

All of these metals cause tubular damage and dysfunction (eg, tubular proteinuria, aminoaciduria) as well as tubular necrosis, but glomerulopathies may predominate with some compounds (mercury, gold).

Treatment involves removal of the patient from further exposure and either or both of the following:

- Chelating agents (copper, arsenic, bismuth)
- Dialysis (chromium, arsenic, bismuth), often used when chelation fails or simultaneously with chelation for severe arsenic poisoning

METABOLIC NEPHROPATHIES

Tubulointerstitial disorders can result from several metabolic disturbances.

Several metabolic disturbances can cause tubulointerstitial nephritis.

Acute urate nephropathy: This disorder is not a true form of acute tubulointerstitial nephritis but rather an intraluminal obstructive uropathy caused by uric acid crystal deposition within the lumen of renal tubules; acute oliguric or anuric kidney injury results.

The **most common cause** of acute urate nephropathy is

- Tumor lysis syndrome after treatment of lymphoma, leukemia, or other myeloproliferative disorders

Other causes of acute urate nephropathy include seizures, treatment of solid tumors, rare primary disorders of urate overproduction (hypoxanthine-guanine phosphoribosyltransferase deficiency), and disorders of urate overexcretion due to decreased proximal tubule reabsorption (Fanconi-like syndromes).

Disorders of urate overproduction and overexcretion are rare.

Typically, no symptoms are present.

Diagnosis is suspected when acute kidney injury occurs in patients with marked hyperuricemia (> 15 mg/dL). Urinalysis results may be normal or may show urate crystals.

Prognosis for complete recovery of renal function is excellent if treatment is initiated rapidly.

In patients with normal cardiac and renal function, treatment is usually with allopurinol plus aggressive IV hydration with normal saline. Supportive measures are indicated. Hemodialysis may be recommended to remove excess circulating urate in severe cases where diuresis cannot be induced with a loop diuretic and IV saline. Alkalinization with a sodium bicarbonate infusion is no longer recommended because even though it increases solubility of urate, it risks tubular precipitation of calcium phosphate salts.

Prevention of acute urate nephropathy is indicated for patients at high risk (eg, those at risk of tumor lysis syndrome). Prevention is by use of allopurinol 300 mg po bid to tid plus saline loading to maintain a urine output > 2.5 L/day before chemotherapy or radiation therapy. Urate oxidase (rasburicase), which catalyzes urate to a much more soluble compound, is also preventive and is being more commonly used in patients with severe hyperuricemia. However, patients given rasburicase must be carefully monitored because the drug must be given IV and can cause anaphylaxis, hemolysis, and other adverse effects.

Chronic urate nephropathy: This condition is chronic tubulointerstitial nephritis caused by deposition of sodium urate crystals in the medullary interstitium in patients with chronic hyperuricemia. Sequelae are chronic inflammation and fibrosis, with ensuing chronic renal insufficiency and renal failure. Chronic urate nephropathy was once common in patients with tophaceous gout but is now rare because gout is more often effectively treated.

Suggestive but nonspecific findings include a bland urine sediment and hyperuricemia disproportionate to the degree of renal insufficiency:

- Urate > 9 mg/dL with serum creatinine < 1.5 mg/dL
- Urate > 10 mg/dL with serum creatinine 1.5 to 2 mg/dL
- Urate > 12 mg/dL with serum creatinine > 2 mg/dL

Many causes of tubulointerstitial diseases may have these findings, lead nephropathy being the most common.

Treatment of chronic urate nephropathy is that of hyperuricosuria.

Hyperoxaluria: Hyperoxaluria is a common cause of nephrolithiasis but an uncommon cause of acute and chronic tubulointerstitial nephritis. Causes and prevention of hyperoxaluria are discussed elsewhere.

Hypercalcemia: Hypercalcemia causes nephropathy by 2 mechanisms.

Severe (> 12 mg/dL) temporary hypercalcemia may cause reversible renal insufficiency by renal vasoconstriction and natriuresis-induced volume depletion.

Long-standing hypercalcemia and hypercalciuria lead to chronic tubulointerstitial nephritis with calcification and necrosis of tubular cells, interstitial fibrosis, and calcification (nephrocalcinosis). Common associated findings include

- Nephrolithiasis
- Renal tubular acidosis
- Nephrogenic diabetes insipidus

Diagnosis is based on presence of hypercalcemia and unexplained renal insufficiency; nephrocalcinosis can be detected by ultrasonography or noncontrast CT.

Treatment is management of hypercalcemia.

Chronic hypokalemia: Chronic hypokalemia of a moderate to severe degree may cause nephropathy with impaired urinary concentration and vacuolation of proximal tubular cells and occasionally of distal tubular cells. Diagnosis is suggested by history of prolonged severe hypokalemia. Renal biopsy is not usually required in the diagnostic evaluation of these patients; however, chronic interstitial inflammatory changes, fibrosis, and renal cysts have been found in renal biopsies of patients with hypokalemia of ≥ 1 mo.

Treatment consists of correction of the underlying disorder and oral potassium supplements. Although the hypokalemia as well as the number and size of the cysts are reversible, the chronic tubulointerstitial nephropathy and renal insufficiency may be irreversible.

MYELOMA-RELATED KIDNEY DISEASE

(Myeloma Cast Nephropathy; Myeloma Kidney)

Patients with multiple myeloma overproduce monoclonal Ig light chains (Bence Jones proteins); these light chains are filtered by glomeruli, are nephrotoxic, and, in their various forms (free, tubular casts, amyloid), can damage virtually all areas of the kidney parenchyma. Diagnosis is by urine tests (sulfosalicylic acid test or protein electrophoresis) or renal biopsy. Treatment focuses on the multiple myeloma and ensuring adequate urine flow. Myeloma-related kidney disease is rarely caused by Ig heavy chains.

Tubulointerstitial disease and glomerular damage are the most common types of renal damage. The mechanisms by which light chains damage nephrons directly are unknown. Hypercalcemia contributes to renal insufficiency by decreasing renal blood flow.

Tubulointerstitial disease: Types of tubulointerstitial renal disorders in multiple myeloma include

- Myeloma kidney (myeloma cast nephropathy)
- Acquired Fanconi syndrome (proximal tubular disease)
- Interstitial light chain deposition, causing acute tubular necrosis (ATN)

Light chains saturate the reabsorptive capacity of the proximal tubule, reach the distal nephron, and combine with filtered proteins and Tamm-Horsfall mucoprotein (secreted by cells of the thick ascending limb of Henle) to form obstructive casts. The term myeloma kidney or myeloma cast nephropathy generally refers to renal insufficiency caused by the tubulointerstitial damage that results. Factors that predispose to cast formation include the following:

- Low urine flow
- Radiocontrast agents
- Hyperuricemia
- NSAIDs
- Elevation of luminal sodium chloride concentration (eg, due to a loop diuretic)
- Increased intratubular calcium due to the hypercalcemia that often occurs secondary to bone lysis in multiple myeloma

Other types of tubulointerstitial lesions that occur with Bence Jones proteinuria include proximal tubular transport dysfunction, causing Fanconi syndrome, and light chain interstitial deposition with inflammatory infiltrates and active tubular damage, which can cause ATN.

Glomerulopathies: Types of glomerular renal disorders in multiple myeloma include

- Primary (AL) amyloidosis
- Light chain deposition disease (LCDD)
- Heavy chain deposition, rarely

AL amyloidosis results in glomerular deposition of AL amyloid in the mesangial, subepithelial, or subendothelial areas or a combination. Amyloid deposition is with randomly oriented, nonbranching fibrils composed of the variable regions of lambda light chains. LCDD, which also can occur with lymphoma and macroglobulinemia, is glomerular deposition of nonpolymerized light chains (ie, without fibrils), generally the constant regions of kappa chains.

Rarely, a nonproliferative, noninflammatory glomerulopathy that causes nephrotic-range proteinuria can develop in advanced myeloma-related renal disease. A proliferative glomerulonephritis occasionally develops as an early form of LCDD with progression to membranoproliferative glomerulonephritis and nodular glomerulopathy reminiscent of diabetic nephropathy; nephrotic-range proteinuria is common.

Symptoms and Signs

Symptoms and signs are predominantly those of the myeloma (eg, skeletal pain, pathologic fractures, diffuse osteoporosis, bacterial infections, hypercalcemia, normochromic-normocytic anemia out of proportion to the degree of renal failure).

Diagnosis

- Urine sulfosalicylic acid test or urine protein electrophoresis (myeloma kidney)
- Biopsy (glomerulopathy)

Diagnosis of myeloma-related kidney disease is suggested by the following combination of findings:

- Renal insufficiency
- Bland urine sediment
- Negative or trace positive dipstick for protein (unless urine albumin is elevated in a patient with an accompanying nephrotic syndrome)
- Elevated total urinary protein

The diagnosis should be suspected even in patients without a history of or findings suggesting multiple myeloma, particularly if total urinary protein is elevated out of proportion to urinary albumin). Total urinary protein is measured over 24 h (and is often elevated enough to suggest nephrotic syndrome) or as a spot measurement (eg, using the urine sulfosalicylic acid test); urinary albumin is measured by dipstick.

Diagnosis of light chain tubulointerstitial disease (myeloma kidney) is confirmed by a markedly positive urine sulfosalicylic acid test suggesting significant nonalbumin proteins, by urine protein electrophoresis (UPEP), or both.

Diagnosis of glomerulopathy is confirmed by renal biopsy. Renal biopsy may demonstrate light chain deposition in 30 to 50% of patients with myeloma despite the absence of detectable serum or urine paraproteins by immunoelectrophoresis.

Prognosis

Kidney disease is a major predictor of overall prognosis in multiple myeloma. Prognosis is good for patients with tubulointerstitial and glomerular LCDD who receive treatment. Prognosis is worse for patients with AL amyloidosis, in whom amyloid deposition continues and progresses to renal failure in most cases. In either form without treatment, virtually all renal lesions progress to renal failure.

Treatment

- Management of multiple myeloma
- Prevention of volume depletion and maintenance of a high urine flow rate

Management of multiple myeloma and prevention of volume depletion (eg, using normal saline for volume expansion) to maintain a high urine flow rate are the primary treatments. In addition, factors that worsen renal function (eg, hypercalcemia, hyperuricemia, use of nephrotoxic drugs) should be avoided or treated.

Several measures are often recommended but are of unproved efficacy. Plasma exchange may be tried to remove light chains. Alkalinization of the urine to help change the net charge of the light chain and reduce charge interaction with Tamm-Horsfall mucoprotein may make the light chains more soluble. Colchicine may be given to decrease secretion of Tamm-Horsfall mucoprotein into the lumen and to decrease the interaction with light chains, thus decreasing toxicity. Loop diuretics may be avoided to prevent volume depletion and high distal sodium concentrations that can worsen myeloma-related kidney disease.

KEY POINTS

- Patients with multiple myeloma can sustain tubulointerstitial or glomerular damage by various mechanisms.
- Suspect myeloma-related kidney disease if patients have unexplained renal insufficiency, bland urinary sediment, and/or increased non-albumin urinary proteins.
- Treat myeloma and maintain euvolemia.

TUBULOINTERSTITIAL NEPHRITIS

Tubulointerstitial nephritis is primary injury to renal tubules and interstitium resulting in decreased renal function. The acute form is most often due to allergic drug reactions or to infections. The chronic form occurs with a diverse array of causes, including genetic or metabolic disorders, obstructive uropathy, and chronic exposure to environmental toxins or to certain drugs and herbs. Diagnosis is suggested by history and urinalysis and often confirmed by biopsy. Treatment and prognosis vary by the etiology and potential reversibility of the disorder at the time of diagnosis.

Etiology

Tubulointerstitial nephritis can be primary, but a similar process can result from glomerular damage or renovascular disorders.

Primary tubulointerstitial nephritis may be

- Acute (see Table 258–2)
- Chronic (see Table 258–3)

Acute tubulointerstitial nephritis: Acute tubulointerstitial nephritis (ATIN) involves an inflammatory infiltrate and edema affecting the renal interstitium that often develops over days to

Table 258–2. CAUSES OF ACUTE TUBULOINTERSTITIAL NEPHRITIS

CAUSE	EXAMPLES
Drugs*	
Antibiotics	Beta-lactam antibiotics (the most common cause) Ciprofloxacin Ethambutol Indinavir Isoniazid Macrolides Minocycline Rifampin Tetracycline Trimethoprim/sulfamethoxazole Vancomycin
Anticonvulsants	Carbamazepine Phenobarbital Phenytoin Valproate
Diuretics	Bumetanide Furosemide Thiazides Triamterene
NSAIDs	Diclofenac Fenoprofen Ibuprofen Indomethacin Naproxen
Other	Allopurinol Aristolochic acid[†] Captopril Cimetidine Interferon alfa Lansoprazole Mesalamine Omeprazole Ranitidine
Metabolic disorders	
Hyperoxalaturia	Ethylene glycol poisoning
Hyperuricosuria	Tumor lysis syndrome
Renal parenchymal infection	
Bacterial	*Brucella* sp *Corynebacterium diphtheriae* *Legionella* sp *Leptospira* sp *Mycobacterium* sp *Mycoplasma* sp *Rickettsia* sp *Salmonella* sp Staphylococci Streptococci *Treponema pallidum* *Yersinia* sp
Fungal	*Candida* sp
Parasitic	*Toxoplasma gondii*

Table 258–2. CAUSES OF ACUTE TUBULOINTERSTITIAL NEPHRITIS (*Continued*)

CAUSE	EXAMPLES
Viral	Cytomegalovirus Epstein-Barr virus Hantavirus Hepatitis C virus HIV Mumps Polyomavirus
Other conditions	
Idiopathic without and with uveitis	—
Immunologic	Cryoglobulinemia Granulomatosis with polyangiitis Idiopathic hypocomplementemic interstitial nephritis IgA nephropathy IgG4-related tubulointerstitial nephritis Renal transplant rejection Sarcoidosis Sjögren syndrome SLE (rare)
Neoplastic	Lymphoma Myeloma

*Most common causative drugs are listed; > 120 drugs are implicated.

†Contained in some medicinal herbs used in traditional Chinese medicine.

months. Over 95% of cases result from infection or an allergic drug reaction.

ATIN causes acute kidney injury; severe cases, delayed therapy, or continuance of an offending drug can lead to permanent injury and chronic kidney disease.

Renal-ocular syndrome, ATIN plus uveitis, also occurs and is idiopathic.

Chronic tubulointerstitial nephritis: Chronic tubulointerstitial nephritis (CTIN) arises when chronic tubular insults cause gradual interstitial infiltration and fibrosis, tubular atrophy and dysfunction, and a gradual deterioration of renal function, usually over years. Concurrent glomerular involvement (glomerulosclerosis) is much more common in CTIN than in ATIN.

Causes of CTIN are myriad; they include immunologically mediated disorders, infections, reflux or obstructive nephropathy, drugs, and other disorders. CTIN due to toxins, metabolic derangements, hypertension, and inherited disorders results in symmetric and bilateral disease; when CITN is due to other causes, renal scarring may be unequal and involve only one kidney. Some well-characterized forms of CTIN include and

- Analgesic nephropathy
- Metabolic nephropathies
- Heavy metal nephropathy
- Reflux nephropathy
- Myeloma kidney

Hereditary cystic kidney diseases are discussed elsewhere.

Table 258–3. CAUSES OF CHRONIC TUBULOINTERSTITIAL NEPHRITIS

CAUSE	EXAMPLES
Balkan nephropathy	—
Cystic diseases	Acquired cystic disease Medullary cystic disease Medullary sponge kidney Nephronophthisis Polycystic kidney disease*
Drugs	Analgesics* Antineoplastics (cisplatin and nitrosourea) Chinese herbs (due to aristolochic acid†) Immunosuppressants (cyclosporine* and tacrolimus) Lithium*
Granulomatous	Granulomatosis with polyangiitis Inflammatory bowel disease Sarcoidosis TB
Hematologic	Aplastic anemia Leukemia Lymphoma Multiple myeloma* Sickle cell anemia
Hereditary nephropathy associated with hyperuricemia and gout	—
Idiopathic	—
Immunologic	Amyloidosis Cryoglobulinemia Goodpasture syndrome IgA nephropathy Renal transplant rejection Sarcoidosis Sjögren syndrome SLE
Infection	Renal parenchymal: • Pyelonephritis • Hantavirus—Puumula type infection (nephropathia epidemica) Systemic
Mechanical	Obstructive uropathy Reflux nephropathy*
Metabolic	Chronic hypokalemia Cystinosis Fabry disease Hypercalcemia, hypercalciuria Hyperoxaluria Hyperuricemia*, hyperuricosuria
Radiation nephritis	—
Toxins	Aristolochic acid† Heavy metals (eg, arsenic, bismuth, cadmium, chromium, copper, gold, iron, lead, mercury, uranium)
Vascular	Atheroembolism Hypertension Renal vein thrombosis

*Common causes.

†Contained in some medicinal herbs used in traditional Chinese medicine.

Symptoms and Signs

Acute tubulointerstitial nephritis: Symptoms and signs of ATIN may be nonspecific and are often absent unless symptoms and signs of renal failure develop. Many patients develop polyuria and nocturia (due to a defect in urinary concentration and sodium reabsorption).

ATIN symptom onset may be as long as several weeks after initial toxic exposure or as soon as 3 to 5 days after a 2nd exposure; extremes in latency range from 1 day with rifampin to 18 mo with an NSAID. Fever and urticarial rash are characteristic early manifestations of drug-induced ATIN, but the classically described triad of fever, rash, and eosinophilia is present in < 10% of patients with drug-induced ATIN. Abdominal pain, weight loss, and bilateral renal enlargement (caused by interstitial edema) may also occur in ATIN and with fever may mistakenly suggest renal cancer or polycystic kidney disease. Peripheral edema and hypertension are uncommon unless renal failure occurs.

Chronic tubulointerstitial nephritis: Symptoms and signs are generally absent in CTIN unless renal failure develops. Edema usually is not present, and BP is normal or only mildly elevated in the early stages. Polyuria and nocturia may develop.

Diagnosis

- Risk factors
- In ATIN, active urinary sediment with sterile pyuria
- Sometimes renal biopsy
- Usually imaging to exclude other causes

Few clinical and routine laboratory findings are specific for tubulointerstitial nephritis. Thus, suspicion should be high when the following are present:

- Typical symptoms or signs
- Risk factors, particularly a temporal relationship between onset and use of a potentially causative drug
- Characteristic urinalysis findings, particularly sterile pyuria
- Modest proteinuria, usually < 1 g/day (except with use of NSAIDs, which may cause nephrotic-range proteinuria, 3.5 g/day)
- Evidence of tubular dysfunction (eg, renal tubular acidosis, Fanconi syndrome)
- Concentrating defect out of proportion to the degree of renal failure

Eosinophiluria cannot be relied upon to make or exclude the diagnosis, but the absence of eosinophils makes the diagnosis less likely (high negative predictive value). Other tests (eg, imaging) are usually necessary to differentiate ATIN or CTIN from other disorders. A presumptive clinical diagnosis of ATIN is often made based on the specific findings mentioned above, but renal biopsy is necessary to establish a definitive diagnosis.

Acute tubulointerstitial nephritis: Urinalysis that shows signs of active kidney inflammation (active urinary sediment), including RBCs, WBCs, and WBC casts, and absence of bacteria on culture (sterile pyuria) is typical; marked hematuria and dysmorphic RBCs are uncommon. Eosinophiluria has traditionally been thought to suggest ATIN; however, the presence or absence of urinary eosinophils is not particularly useful diagnostically. Proteinuria is usually minimal but may reach nephrotic range with combined ATIN-glomerular disease induced by NSAIDs, ampicillin, rifampin, interferon alfa, or ranitidine.

Blood test findings of tubular dysfunction include hypokalemia (caused by a defect in potassium reabsorption) and a nonanion gap metabolic acidosis (caused by a defect in proximal tubular bicarbonate reabsorption or in distal tubular acid excretion).

Ultrasonography, radionuclide scanning, or both may be needed to differentiate ATIN from other causes of acute kidney injury, such as ATN. In ATIN, ultrasonography may show kidneys that are greatly enlarged and echogenic because of interstitial inflammatory cells and edema. Radionuclide scans may show kidneys avidly taking up radioactive gallium-67 or radionuclide-labeled WBCs. Positive scans strongly suggest ATIN (and indicate that ATN is less likely), but a negative scan does not exclude ATIN.

Renal biopsy is usually reserved for patients with the following:

- An uncertain diagnosis
- Progressive renal injury
- No improvement after potential causative drugs are stopped
- Findings suggesting early disease
- Drug-induced ATIN for which corticosteroid therapy is under consideration

In ATIN, glomeruli are usually normal. The earliest finding is interstitial edema, typically followed by interstitial infiltration with lymphocytes, plasma cells, eosinophils, and a few polymorphonuclear leukocytes. In severe cases, inflammatory cells can be seen invading the space between the cells lining the tubular basement membrane (tubulitis); in other specimens, granulomatous reactions resulting from exposure to beta-lactam antibiotics, sulfonamides, mycobacteria, or fungi may be seen. The presence of noncaseating granulomas suggests sarcoidosis. Immunofluorescence or electron microscopy seldom reveals any pathognomonic changes.

Chronic tubulointerstitial nephritis: Findings of CTIN are generally similar to those of ATIN, although urinary RBCs and WBCs are uncommon. Because CTIN is insidious in onset and interstitial fibrosis is common, imaging tests may show small kidneys with evidence of scarring and asymmetry.

In CTIN, renal biopsy is not often done for diagnostic purposes but has helped characterize the nature and progression of tubulointerstitial disease. Glomeruli vary from normal to completely destroyed. Tubules may be absent or atrophied. Tubular lumina vary in diameter but may show marked dilation, with homogeneous casts. The interstitium contains varying degrees of inflammatory cells and fibrosis. Nonscarred areas appear almost normal. Grossly, the kidneys are small and atrophic.

Prognosis

Acute tubulointerstitial nephritis: In drug-induced ATIN, renal function usually recovers within 6 to 8 wk when the causative drug is stopped, although some residual scarring is common. Recovery may be incomplete, with persistent azotemia above baseline. Prognosis is usually worse if ATIN is caused by NSAIDs than by other drugs. When other factors cause ATIN, histologic changes usually are reversible if the cause is recognized and removed; however, some severe cases progress to fibrosis and chronic kidney disease. Regardless of cause, irreversible injury is suggested by the following:

- Diffuse rather than patchy interstitial infiltrate
- Significant interstitial fibrosis
- Delayed response to prednisone
- Acute kidney injury lasting > 3 wk

Chronic tubulointerstitial nephritis: In CTIN, prognosis depends on the cause and on the ability to recognize and stop the process before irreversible fibrosis occurs. Many genetic (eg, cystic kidney disease), metabolic (eg, cystinosis), and toxic (eg, heavy metal) causes may not be modifiable, in which case CTIN usually evolves to end-stage renal disease.

Treatment

- Treatment of cause (eg, stopping the causative drug)
- Corticosteroids for immune-mediated and sometimes drug-induced ATIN

Treatment of both ATIN and CTIN is management of the cause.

For immunologically induced ATIN and sometimes drug-induced ATIN, corticosteroids (eg, prednisone 1 mg/kg po once/day with gradual tapering of the dose over 4 to 6 wk) may accelerate recovery.

For drug-induced ATIN, corticosteroids are most effective when given within 2 wk of stopping the causative drugs. NSAID-induced ATIN is less responsive to corticosteroids than other drug-induced ATIN. ATIN should be proven by biopsy before corticosteroids are started.

Treatment of CTIN often requires supportive measures such as controlling BP and treating anemia associated with kidney disease. In patients with CTIN and progressive renal injury, ACE inhibitors or angiotensin II receptor blockers may slow disease progression but should not be used together because of an additive risk of hyperkalemia and accelerating disease progression.

PEARLS & PITFALLS

- In patients with chronic tubulointerstitial nephritis, ACE inhibitors and angiotensin II receptor blockers should not be used together because of the additive risk of hyperkalemia and acceleration of disease progression.

KEY POINTS

- Causes of CTIN are myriad and much more diverse than ATIN (usually caused by an allergic reaction to a drug or by an infection).
- Symptoms are often absent or nonspecific, particularly in CTIN.
- Suspect the diagnosis based on risk factors and urinary sediment, exclude other causes using imaging, and sometimes confirm the diagnosis by biopsy.
- Stop causative drugs, treat any other causes, and provide supportive treatment.
- Treat biopsy-proven immune-mediated and sometimes drug-induced ATIN with corticosteroids (within 2 wk of stopping any causative drugs).

VESICOURETERAL REFLUX AND REFLUX NEPHROPATHY

Reflux nephropathy is renal scarring presumably induced by vesicoureteral reflux of infected urine into the renal parenchyma. The diagnosis is suspected in children with UTI or a family history of reflux nephropathy, or if a prenatal ultrasound shows hydronephrosis. Diagnosis is by voiding cystourethrography or radionuclide cystography. Children with moderate or severe reflux are treated with prophylactic antibiotics or surgical correction.

(See also Vesicoureteral Reflux on p. 2539.)

Reflux nephropathy is a type of chronic tubulointerstitial nephritis (see p. 2181). Traditionally, the mechanism of renal scarring has been thought to be chronic pyelonephritis. However, reflux is probably the single most important factor, and factors unrelated to reflux or pyelonephritis (eg, congenital factors) can contribute.

Vesicoureteral reflux (VUR) affects about 1% of neonates and 30 to 45% of young children with a febrile UTI; it is common among children with renal scars and, for unknown reasons, is less common among black children than white children. Familial predisposition is common. Children with gross reflux (up to the renal pelvis plus ureteral dilation) are at highest risk of scarring and subsequent chronic kidney disease.

Reflux requires incompetent ureterovesical valves or mechanical obstruction in the lower urinary tract. Young children with shorter intravesical portions of the ureter are most susceptible; normal growth usually results in spontaneous cessation of intrarenal and vesicoureteral reflux by age 5. New scars in children > 5 yr are unusual but may occur after acute pyelonephritis.

Symptoms and Signs

Few symptoms and signs other than occasional UTI are present in young children, and the diagnosis is often overlooked until adolescence, when patients present with some combination of the following:

- Polyuria
- Nocturia
- Hypertension
- Symptoms and signs of renal insufficiency

Diagnosis

- Initial screening with ultrasonography
- Voiding cystourethrography or radionuclide cystography

Reflux nephropathy may be suspected prenatally or postnatally. Initial screening is done with ultrasonography, which is highly sensitive.

Diagnosis and staging of reflux nephropathy (prenatal or postnatal presentation) are ultimately made with voiding cystourethrography (VCUG), which can demonstrate the degree of ureteral dilation. Radionuclide cystography (RNC) can also be used; it provides less anatomic detail than VCUG but involves less radiation exposure. Renal scarring is diagnosed with technetium-99m–labeled dimercaptosuccinic acid (DMSA) radionuclide scanning.

Prenatal diagnosis: The diagnosis is suspected prenatally if ultrasonography, done because of a family history or for unrelated reasons, shows hydronephrosis; 10 to 40% of such patients are diagnosed postnatally with VUR.

Postnatal diagnosis: VUR is suspected postnatally in patients with any of the following:

- UTI at age ≤ 3 yr
- Febrile UTI at age ≤ 5 yr
- Recurrent UTIs in children
- UTI in males

- Strong family history, such as a sibling with VUR (controversial)
- Adults (or children > 5 yr) with recurrent UTI in whom renal ultrasonography reveals scarring or a urinary tract anatomic abnormality

Laboratory abnormalities may include proteinuria, Na wasting, hyperkalemia, metabolic acidosis, renal insufficiency, or a combination.

Testing for these patients is with RNC or VCUG. Because these tests involve catheterization (and risk of UTI) as well as radiation exposure, thresholds for obtaining them can be controversial. Some experts recommend VCUG or RNC only if family history is strong or if postnatal renal ultrasonography is markedly or persistently abnormal; however, it is not clear whether renal ultrasonography is sufficiently sensitive to detect VUR. DMSA scanning may be done for infants or children with UTIs as listed above.

In older children in whom reflux is no longer active, VCUG may not show reflux, although DMSA scanning shows scarring; cystoscopy can demonstrate evidence of previous reflux at ureteral orifices. Thus, DMSA scanning and cystoscopy may be done if prior reflux is suspected but not confirmed.

Renal biopsy at this late stage shows CTIN and focal glomerulosclerosis, which may cause mild (1 to 1.5 g/day) to nephrotic-range (3.5 g/day) proteinuria.

Treatment

- Usually prophylactic antibiotics
- Surgical treatment if VUR is moderate or severe

Treatment of reflux nephropathy is based on the unproven assumption that decreasing reflux and UTIs prevents renal scarring. Children with very mild VUR require no treatment, but they should be closely observed for symptoms of UTI.

Children with moderate reflux are usually given antibiotics. However, drug therapy predisposes to new episodes of acute pyelonephritis, and it is not clear whether prophylactic antibiotics are more effective than close observation.

Patients with severe reflux are at higher risk of renal insufficiency and are usually given antibiotic prophylaxis or undergo surgical interventions, including ureteral reimplantation or endoscopic injection of materials behind the ureter to prevent reflux (bladder contraction during voiding compresses the ureter between the bladder and the material). Incidence of new renal scars is similar in patients treated with surgery and with drugs.

Reflux spontaneously resolves in about 80% of young children within 5 yr.

KEY POINTS

- Consider reflux nephropathy in children < 5 yr with UTIs or a family history, particularly among boys or if patients have fever or recurrent UTIs.
- If reflux nephropathy is suspected, do ultrasonography; if abnormal, consider VCUG or, to minimize radiation exposure, RNC.
- Consider prophylactic antibiotics and, if reflux is severe, surgical treatment.
- Consensus is lacking for certain recommendations, such as when and how to image patients for diagnosis and when to prescribe prophylactic antibiotics.
- Reflux spontaneously resolves in about 80% of young children within 5 yr.

259 Urinary Calculi

(Nephrolithiasis; Stones; Urolithiasis)

Urinary calculi are solid particles in the urinary system. They may cause pain, nausea, vomiting, hematuria, and, possibly, chills and fever due to secondary infection. Diagnosis is based on urinalysis and radiologic imaging, usually noncontrast helical CT. Treatment is with analgesics, antibiotics for infection, medical expulsive therapy, and, sometimes, shock wave lithotripsy or endoscopic procedures.

About 1/1000 adults in the US is hospitalized annually because of urinary calculi, which are also found in about 1% of all autopsies. Up to 12% of men and 5% of women will develop a urinary calculus by age 70. Calculi vary from microscopic crystalline foci to calculi several centimeters in diameter. A large calculus, called a staghorn calculus, can fill an entire renal calyceal system.

Etiology

About 85% of calculi in the US are composed of calcium, mainly calcium oxalate (see Table 259–1); 10% are uric acid; 2% are cystine; most of the remainder are magnesium ammonium phosphate (struvite).

General risk factors include disorders that increase urinary salt concentration, either by increased excretion of calcium or uric acid salts, or by decreased excretion of urinary citrate.

For **calcium calculi,** risk factors vary by population. The main risk factor in the US is hypercalciuria, a hereditary condition present in 50% of men and 75% of women with calcium calculi; thus, patients with a family history of calculi are at increased risk of recurrent calculi. These patients have normal serum calcium, but urinary calcium is elevated > 250 mg/day (> 6.2 mmol/day) in men and > 200 mg/day (> 5.0 mmol/day) in women.

Hypocitruria (urinary citrate < 350 mg/day [1820 μmol/day]), present in about 40 to 50% of calcium calculi-formers, promotes calcium calculi formation because citrate normally binds urinary calcium and inhibits the crystallization of calcium salts.

About 5 to 8% of calculi are caused by renal tubular acidosis. About 1 to 2% of patients with calcium calculi have primary hyperparathyroidism. Rare causes of hypercalciuria are sarcoidosis, vitamin D intoxication, hyperthyroidism, multiple myeloma, metastatic cancer, and hyperoxaluria.

Hyperoxaluria (urinary oxalate > 40 mg/day [> 440 μmol/day]) can be primary or caused by excess ingestion of oxalate-containing foods (eg, rhubarb, spinach, cocoa, nuts, pepper, tea) or by excess oxalate absorption due to various enteric diseases

Table 259–1. COMPOSITION OF URINARY CALCULI

COMPOSITION	PERCENTAGE OF ALL CALCULI	COMMON CAUSES
Calcium oxalate	70	Hypercalciuria Hyperparathyroidism Hypocitruria Renal tubular acidosis
Calcium phosphate	15	Hypercalciuria Hyperparathyroidism Hypocitruria Renal tubular acidosis
Cystine	2	Cystinuria
Magnesium ammonium phosphate (struvite)	3	UTI caused by urea-splitting bacteria
Uric acid	10	Urine pH < 5.5 Occasionally hyperuricosuria

(eg, bacterial overgrowth syndromes, chronic pancreatic or biliary disease) or ileojejunal (eg, bariatric) surgery.

Other risk factors include taking high doses of vitamin C (ie, > 2000 mg/day), a calcium-restricted diet (possibly because dietary calcium binds dietary oxalate), and mild hyperuricosuria. Mild hyperuricosuria, defined as urinary uric acid > 800 mg/day (> 5 mmol/day) in men or > 750 mg/day (> 4 mmol/day) in women, is almost always caused by excess intake of purine (in proteins, usually from meat, fish, and poultry); it may cause calcium oxalate calculus formation (hyperuricosuric calcium oxalate nephrolithiasis).

Uric acid calculi most commonly develop as a result of increased urine acidity (urine pH < 5.5), or rarely with severe hyperuricosuria (urinary uric acid > 1500 mg/day [> 9 mmol/day]), which crystallizes undissociated uric acid. Uric acid crystals may comprise the entire calculus or, more commonly, provide a nidus on which calcium or mixed calcium and uric acid calculi can form.

Cystine calculi occur only in the presence of cystinuria.

Magnesium ammonium phosphate calculi (struvite, infection calculi) indicate the presence of a UTI caused by urea-splitting bacteria (eg, *Proteus* sp, *Klebsiella* sp). The calculi must be treated as infected foreign bodies and removed in their entirety. Unlike other types of calculi, magnesium ammonium phosphate calculi occur 3 times more frequently in women.

Rare causes of urinary calculi include indinavir, melamine, triamterene, and xanthine.

Pathophysiology

Urinary calculi may remain within the renal parenchyma or renal collecting system or be passed into the ureter and bladder. During passage, calculi may irritate the ureter and may become lodged, obstructing urine flow and causing hydroureter and sometimes hydronephrosis. Common areas of lodgment include the following:

- Ureteropelvic junction
- Distal ureter (at the level of the iliac vessels)
- Ureterovesical junction

Larger calculi are more likely to become lodged. Typically, a calculus must have a diameter > 5 mm to become lodged. Calculi ≤ 5 mm are likely to pass spontaneously.

Even partial obstruction causes decreased glomerular filtration, which may persist briefly after the calculus has passed. With hydronephrosis and elevated glomerular pressure, renal blood flow declines, further worsening renal function. Generally, however, in the absence of infection, permanent renal dysfunction occurs only after about 28 days of complete obstruction.

Secondary infection can occur with long-standing obstruction, but most patients with calcium-containing calculi do not have infected urine.

Symptoms and Signs

Large calculi remaining in the renal parenchyma or renal collecting system are often asymptomatic unless they cause obstruction and/or infection. Severe pain, often accompanied by nausea and vomiting, usually occurs when calculi pass into the ureter and cause acute obstruction. Sometimes gross hematuria also occurs.

Pain (renal colic) is of variable intensity but is typically excruciating and intermittent, often occurs cyclically, and lasts 20 to 60 min. Nausea and vomiting are common. Pain in the flank or kidney area that radiates across the abdomen suggests upper ureteral or renal pelvic obstruction. Pain that radiates along the course of the ureter into the genital region suggests lower ureteral obstruction. Suprapubic pain along with urinary urgency and frequency suggests a distal ureteral, ureterovesical, or bladder calculus (see p. 2138).

On examination, patients may be in obvious extreme discomfort, often ashen and diaphoretic. Patients with renal colic may be unable to lie still and may pace, writhe, or constantly shift position. The abdomen may be somewhat tender on the affected side as palpation increases pressure in the already-distended kidney (costovertebral angle tenderness), but peritoneal signs (guarding, rebound, rigidity) are lacking.

For some patients, the first symptom is hematuria or either gravel or a calculus in the urine. Other patients may have symptoms of a UTI, such as fever, dysuria, or cloudy or foul-smelling urine.

Diagnosis

- Clinical differential diagnosis
- Urinalysis
- Imaging
- Determination of calculus composition

The symptoms and signs may suggest other diagnoses, such as

- **Peritonitis** (eg, due to appendicitis, ectopic pregnancy, or pelvic inflammatory disease): Pain is usually constant, and patients lie still because movement worsens pain; patients often also have rebound tenderness or rigidity.
- **Cholecystitis:** May cause colicky pain, usually in the epigastrium or right upper quadrant, often with Murphy sign.
- **Bowel obstruction:** May cause colicky abdominal pain and vomiting, but the pain is usually bilateral and not located primarily in the flank or along the ureter.
- **Pancreatitis:** May cause upper abdominal pain and vomiting, but the pain is usually constant, may be bilateral, and is usually not along the flank or ureter.

With most of these disorders, urinary symptoms are uncommon and other symptoms may suggest which organ system is actually involved (eg, vaginal discharge or bleeding in pelvic disorders among females). Dissecting aortic aneurysm must be considered, particularly in the elderly, because, if a renal artery is affected, it can cause hematuria, pain that radiates along a ureteral distribution, or both. Other considerations in the general evaluation of acute abdominal pain are discussed on p. 83.

PEARLS & PITFALLS

- Giving fluid (oral or IV) does not speed the passage of urinary calculi.

Patients suspected of having a calculus causing colic require urinalysis and usually an imaging study. If a calculus is confirmed, evaluation of the underlying disorder, including calculus composition testing, is required.

Urinalysis: Macroscopic or microscopic hematuria is common, but urine may be normal despite multiple calculi. Pyuria with or without bacteria may be present. Pyuria suggests infection, particularly if combined with suggestive clinical findings, such as foul-smelling urine or a fever. A calculus and various crystalline substances may be present in the sediment. If so, further testing is usually necessary because the composition of the calculus and crystals cannot be determined conclusively by microscopy. The only exception is when typical hexagonal crystals of cystine are found in a concentrated, acidified specimen, confirming cystinuria.

Imaging tests: Noncontrast helical CT is the initial imaging study. This study can detect the location of a calculus as well as the degree of obstruction. Moreover, helical CT may also reveal another cause of the pain (eg, aortic aneurysm). For patients who have recurrent calculi, cumulative radiation exposure from multiple CT scans is a concern. However, the routine use of low-dose renal CT can meaningfully reduce cumulative radiation dose with little loss of sensitivity.[1] For patients with typical symptoms, ultrasonography or plain abdominal x-rays can usually confirm presence of a calculus with minimal or no radiation exposure. MRI may not identify calculi.

Although most urinary calculi are demonstrable on plain x-ray, neither their presence nor their absence obviates the need for more definitive imaging, so this study can be avoided except in some patients with suspected recurrent calculi. Both renal ultrasonography and excretory urography (previously called intravenous urography) can identify calculi and hydronephrosis. However, ultrasonography is less sensitive for small or ureteral calculi in patients without hydronephrosis, and excretory urography is time consuming and exposes the patient to the risk of IV contrast agents. These studies are generally used when helical CT is unavailable.

Identifying the cause: The calculus is obtained by straining the urine (or, if necessary, during operative removal) and sent to the laboratory for stone analysis. Some calculi are brought in by patients. Urine specimens that show microscopic crystals are sent for crystallography.

In patients with a single calcium calculus and no additional risk factors for calculi, evaluation to exclude hyperparathyroidism is sufficient. Evaluation entails urinalysis and determination of plasma calcium concentration on 2 separate occasions. Predisposing factors, such as recurrent calculi, a diet high in animal protein, or use of vitamin C or D supplements, should be sought.

Patients with a strong family history of calculi, conditions that might predispose to calculi formation (eg, sarcoidosis, bone metastases, multiple myeloma), or conditions that would make it difficult to treat calculi (eg, solitary kidney, urinary tract anomalies) require evaluation for all possible causative disorders and risk factors. This evaluation should include serum electrolytes, uric acid, and calcium on 2 separate occasions. Follow-up determination of parathyroid hormone levels is done if necessary. Urine tests should include routine urinalysis and 2 separate 24-h urine collections to determine urine volume, pH, and excretion of calcium, uric acid, citrate, oxalate, sodium, and creatinine.[2]

Treatment

- Analgesia
- Facilitate calculus passage, eg, with alpha-receptor blockers such as tamsulosin (described as medical expulsive therapy)
- For persistent or infection-causing calculi, complete removal using primarily endoscopic techniques

Analgesia: Renal colic may be relieved with opioids, such as morphine and, for a rapid onset, fentanyl. Ketorolac 30 mg IV is rapidly effective and nonsedating. Vomiting usually resolves as pain decreases, but persistent vomiting can be treated with an antiemetic (eg, ondansetron 10 mg IV).

Medical expulsive therapy: Although increasing fluids (either oral or IV) has traditionally been recommended, increased fluid administration has not been proven to speed the passage of calculi. Patients with calculi < 1 cm in diameter who have no infection or obstruction, whose pain is controlled with analgesics, and who can tolerate liquids can be treated at home with analgesics and alpha-receptor blockers (eg, tamsulosin 0.4 mg po once/day) to facilitate calculus passage. Calculi that have not passed within 6 to 8 wk typically require removal. In patients with infection and obstruction, initial treatment is relief of obstruction with a ureteral stent and treatment of the infection followed by removal of calculi as soon as possible.

Calculus removal: The technique used for removal depends on the location and size of the calculus. Techniques include shock wave lithotripsy and, to ensure complete removal or for larger calculi, endoscopic techniques. Endoscopic techniques may involve rigid or flexible ureteroscopes (endoscopes) and may involve direct-vision removal (basketing), fragmentation with some sort of lithotripsy device (eg, pneumatic, ultrasonic, laser), or both.

For **symptomatic calculi** < 1 cm in diameter in the renal collecting system or proximal ureter, shock wave lithotripsy is a reasonable first option for therapy.

For **larger calculi** or if shock wave lithotripsy is unsuccessful, ureteroscopy (done in a retrograde fashion) with holmium laser lithotripsy is usually used. Sometimes removal is possible using an endoscope inserted anterograde through the kidney. For renal stones > 2 cm, percutaneous nephrolithotomy, with insertion of a nephroscope directly into the kidney, is the treatment of choice.

For **midureteral calculi**, ureteroscopy with holmium laser lithotripsy is usually the treatment of choice. Shock wave lithotripsy is an alternative.

For **distal ureteral calculi**, endoscopic techniques (ureteroscopy), such as direct removal and use of intracorporeal lithotripsy (eg, pneumatic, electrohydraulic, laser), are considered by many to be the procedures of choice. Shock wave lithotripsy can also be used.

Calculus dissolution: Uric acid calculi in the upper or lower urinary tract occasionally may be dissolved by prolonged alkalinization of the urine with potassium citrate 20 mEq po bid to tid, but chemical dissolution of calcium calculi is not possible and of cystine calculi is difficult.

Prevention

In a patient who has passed a first calcium calculus, the likelihood of forming a 2nd calculus is about 15% at 1 yr, 40% at 5 yr, and 80% at 10 yr. Drinking large amounts of fluids—8 to 10 ten-ounce (300-milliliter) glasses a day—is recommended for prevention of all stones. Recovery and analysis of the calculus, measurement of calculus-forming substances in the urine, and the clinical history are needed to plan other prophylactic measures.

In < 3% of patients, no metabolic abnormality is found. These patients seemingly cannot tolerate normal amounts of calculus-forming salts in their urine without crystallization. Thiazide diuretics, potassium citrate, and increased fluid intake may reduce their calculus production rate.

For **hypercalciuria,** patients may receive thiazide diuretics (eg, chlorthalidone 25 mg po once/day or indapamide 1.25 mg po once/day) to lower urine calcium excretion and thus prevent urinary supersaturation with calcium oxalate. Patients are encouraged to increase their fluid intake to ≥ 3 L/day. A diet that is low in sodium and high in potassium is recommended. Even with a high potassium intake, supplementation with potassium citrate is recommended to prevent hypokalemia. Restriction of dietary animal protein is also recommended.

For patients with **hypocitruria,** potassium citrate (20 mEq po bid) enhances citrate excretion. A normal calcium intake (eg, 1000 mg or about 2 to 3 dairy servings per day) is recommended, and calcium restriction is avoided. Oral orthophosphate has not been thoroughly studied.

Hyperoxaluria prevention varies. Patients with small-bowel disease can be treated with a combination of high fluid intake, calcium loading (usually in the form of calcium citrate 400 mg po bid with meals), cholestyramine, and a low-oxalate, low-fat diet. Hyperoxaluria may respond to pyridoxine 100 to 200 mg po once/day, possibly by increasing transaminase activity, because this activity is responsible for the conversion of glyoxylate, the immediate oxalate precursor, to glycine.

In **hyperuricosuria,** intake of animal protein should be reduced. If the diet cannot be changed, allopurinol 300 mg each morning lowers uric acid production. For uric acid calculi, the urine pH must be increased to between 6 and 6.5 by giving an oral alkalinizing drug that contains potassium (eg, potassium citrate 20 mEq bid) along with increased fluid intake.

Infection with **urea-splitting bacteria** requires culture-specific antibiotics and complete removal of all calculi. If eradication of infection is impossible, long-term suppressive therapy (eg, with nitrofurantoin) may be necessary. In addition, acetohydroxamic acid can be used to reduce the recurrence of struvite calculi.

To prevent recurrent **cystine calculi,** urinary cystine levels must be reduced to < 250 mg cystine/L of urine. Any combination of increasing urine volume along with reducing cystine excretion (eg, with alpha-mercaptopropionylglycine or penicillamine) should reduce the urinary cystine concentration.

1. Zilberman DE, Tsivian M, Lipkin ME, et al. Low dose computerized tomography for detection of urolithiasis—its effectiveness in the setting of the urology clinic. *J Urol* 185(3):910–914, 2011.
2. Pearle MS, Goldfarb DS, Assimos DG, et al. Medical management of kidney stones—AUA guideline. *J Urology* 192(2):316–324, 2014.

KEY POINTS

- 85% of urinary calculi are calcium, mainly calcium oxalate (see Table 259–1); 10% are uric acid; 2% are cystine; and most of the remainder are magnesium ammonium phosphate (struvite).
- Larger calculi are more likely to obstruct; however, obstruction can occur even with small ureteral calculi (ie, 2 to 5 mm).
- Symptoms include hematuria, symptoms of infection, and renal colic.
- Test usually with urinalysis, imaging, and if the calculus can later be retrieved, determination of calculus composition.
- Give analgesics and drugs to facilitate calculus passage (eg, alpha-receptor blockers) acutely and remove calculi that cause infection or persist endoscopically.
- Decrease the risk of subsequent calculus formation by treating with measures such as thiazide diuretics, potassium citrate, increases in fluid intake, and decreases in dietary animal protein, depending on calculus composition.

260 Urinary Tract Infections

(See also Urinary Tract Infection in Children on p. 2742.)

Urinary tract infections (UTIs) can be divided into upper tract infections, which involve the kidneys (pyelonephritis), and lower tract infections, which involve the bladder (cystitis), urethra (urethritis), and prostate (prostatitis). However, in practice, and particularly in children, differentiating between the sites may be difficult or impossible. Moreover, infection often spreads from one area to the other. Although urethritis and prostatitis are infections that involve the urinary tract, the term UTI usually refers to pyelonephritis and cystitis.

Most cystitis and pyelonephritis are caused by bacteria. The most common nonbacterial pathogens are fungi (usually candidal species), and, less commonly, mycobacteria, viruses, and parasites. Nonbacterial pathogens usually affect patients who are immunocompromised; have diabetes, obstruction, or structural urinary tract abnormalities; or have had recent urinary tract instrumentation.

Other than adenoviruses (implicated in hemorrhagic cystitis), viruses have no major contribution to UTI in immunocompetent patients.

The predominant parasitic causes of UTIs are filariasis, trichomoniasis, leishmaniasis, malaria, and schistosomiasis. Of the parasitic diseases, only trichomoniasis is common in the US, usually as a sexually transmitted disease (STD).

Urethritis is usually caused by an STD. Prostatitis is usually caused by a bacterium and is sometimes caused by an STD.

BACTERIAL URINARY TRACT INFECTIONS

Bacterial UTIs can involve the urethra, prostate, bladder, or kidneys. Symptoms may be absent or include urinary frequency, urgency, dysuria, lower abdominal pain, and flank pain. Systemic symptoms and even sepsis may occur with kidney infection. Diagnosis is based on analysis and culture of urine. Treatment is with antibiotics and removal of any urinary tract catheters and obstructions.

Among adults aged 20 to 50 yr, UTIs are about 50-fold more common in women. In women in this age group, most UTIs are cystitis or pyelonephritis. In men of the same age, most UTIs are urethritis or prostatitis. The incidence of UTI increases in patients > 50 yr, but the female:male ratio decreases because of the increasing frequency of prostate enlargement and instrumentation in men.

Pathophysiology

The urinary tract, from the kidneys to the urethral meatus, is normally sterile and resistant to bacterial colonization despite frequent contamination of the distal urethra with colonic bacteria. The major defense against UTI is complete emptying of the bladder during urination. Other mechanisms that maintain the tract's sterility include urine acidity, vesicoureteral valve, and various immunologic and mucosal barriers.

About 95% of UTIs occur when bacteria ascend the urethra to the bladder and, in the case of pyelonephritis, ascend the ureter to the kidney. The remainder of UTIs are hematogenous. Systemic infection can result from UTI, particularly in the elderly. About 6.5% of cases of hospital-acquired bacteremia are attributable to UTI.

Uncomplicated UTI is usually considered to be cystitis or pyelonephritis that occurs in premenopausal adult women with no structural or functional abnormality of the urinary tract and who are not pregnant and have no significant comorbidity that could lead to more serious outcomes. Also, some experts consider UTIs to be uncomplicated even if they affect postmenopausal women or patients with well-controlled diabetes. In men, most UTIs occur in children or elderly patients, are due to anatomic abnormalities or instrumentation, and are considered complicated.

The rare UTIs that occur in men aged 15 to 50 yr are usually in men who have unprotected anal intercourse or in those who have an uncircumcised penis, and they are generally considered uncomplicated. UTIs in men this age who do not have unprotected anal intercourse or an uncircumcised penis are very rare and, although also considered uncomplicated, warrant evaluation for urologic abnormalities.

Complicated UTI can involve either sex at any age. It is usually considered to be pyelonephritis or cystitis that does not fulfill criteria to be considered uncomplicated. A UTI is considered complicated if the patient is a child, is pregnant, or has any of the following:

- A structural or functional urinary tract abnormality and obstruction of urine flow
- A comorbidity that increases risk of acquiring infection or resistance to treatment, such as poorly controlled diabetes, chronic kidney disease, or immunocompromise.
- Recent instrumentation or surgery of the urinary tract

Risk factors: Risk factors for development of UTI in women include the following:

- Sexual intercourse
- Diaphragm and spermicide use
- Antibiotic use
- New sex partner within the past year
- History of UTIs in 1st-degree female relatives
- History of recurrent UTIs
- First UTI at early age

Even use of condoms that are spermicide-coated increases risk of UTI in women. The increased risk of UTI in women using antibiotics or spermicides probably occurs because of alterations in vaginal flora that allow overgrowth of *Escherichia coli*. In elderly women, soiling of the perineum due to fecal incontinence increases risk.

Anatomic, structural, and functional abnormalities are risk factors for UTI. A common consequence of anatomic abnormality is vesicoureteral reflux (VUR), which is present in 30 to 45% of young children with symptomatic UTI. VUR is usually caused by a congenital defect that results in incompetence of the ureterovesical valve. VUR can also be acquired in patients with a flaccid bladder due to spinal cord injury or after urinary tract surgery. Other anatomic abnormalities predisposing to UTI include urethral valves (a congenital obstructive abnormality), delayed bladder neck maturation, bladder diverticulum, and urethral duplications.

Structural and functional urinary tract abnormalities that predispose to UTI usually involve obstruction of urine flow and poor bladder emptying. Urine flow can be compromised by calculi and tumors. Bladder emptying can be impaired by neurogenic dysfunction (see p. 2185), pregnancy, uterine prolapse, cystocele, and prostatic enlargement. UTI caused by congenital factors manifests most commonly during childhood. Most other risk factors are more common in the elderly.

Other risk factors for UTI include instrumentation (eg, bladder catheterization, stent placement, cystoscopy) and recent surgery.

Etiology

The bacteria that most often cause cystitis and pyelonephritis are the following:

- Enteric, usually gram-negative aerobic bacteria (most often)
- Gram-positive bacteria (less often)

In normal GU tracts, strains of *Escherichia coli* with specific attachment factors for transitional epithelium of the bladder and ureters account for 75 to 95% of cases. The remaining gram-negative urinary pathogens are usually other enterobacteria, typically *Klebsiella* or *Proteus mirabilis*, and occasionally *Pseudomonas aeruginosa*. Among gram-positive bacteria, *Staphylococcus saprophyticus* is isolated in 5 to 10% of bacterial UTIs. Less common gram-positive bacterial isolates are *Enterococcus faecalis* (group D streptococci) and *Streptococcus agalactiae* (group B streptococci), which may be contaminants, particularly if they were isolated from patients with uncomplicated cystitis.

In hospitalized patients, *E. coli* accounts for about 50% of cases. The gram-negative species *Klebsiella*, *Proteus*, *Enterobacter*, *Pseudomonas*, and *Serratia* account for about 40%, and the gram-positive bacterial cocci, *E. faecalis*, *S. saprophyticus*, and *Staphylococcus aureus* account for the remainder.

Classification

Urethritis: Infection of the urethra with bacteria (or with protozoa, viruses, or fungi) occurs when organisms that gain access to it acutely or chronically colonize the numerous periurethral glands in the bulbous and pendulous portions of the male urethra and in the entire female urethra. The sexually transmitted pathogens *Chlamydia trachomatis* (see p. 1701), *Neisseria gonorrhoeae* (see p. 1704), *Trichomonas vaginalis* (see p. 1712), and herpes simplex virus are common causes in both sexes.

Cystitis: Cystitis is infection of the bladder. It is common in women, in whom cases of uncomplicated cystitis are usually preceded by sexual intercourse (honeymoon cystitis). In men, bacterial infection of the bladder is usually complicated and usually results from ascending infection from the urethra or prostate or is secondary to urethral instrumentation. The most common cause of recurrent cystitis in men is chronic bacterial prostatitis.

Acute urethral syndrome: Acute urethral syndrome, which occurs in women, is a syndrome involving dysuria, frequency, and pyuria (dysuria-pyuria syndrome), which thus resembles cystitis. However, in acute urethral syndrome (unlike in cystitis), routine urine cultures are either negative or show colony counts that are lower than the traditional criteria for diagnosis of bacterial cystitis. Urethritis is a possible cause because causative organisms include *Chlamydia trachomatis* and *Ureaplasma urealyticum*, which are not detected on routine urine culture.

Noninfectious causes have been proposed, but supporting evidence is not conclusive, and most noninfectious causes usually cause little or no pyuria. Possible noninfectious causes include anatomic abnormalities (eg, urethral stenosis), physiologic abnormalities (eg, pelvic floor muscle dysfunction), hormonal imbalances (eg, atrophic urethritis), localized trauma, GI system symptoms, and inflammation.

Asymptomatic bacteriuria: Asymptomatic bacteriuria is absence of UTI signs or symptoms in a patient whose urine culture satisfies criteria for UTI. Pyuria may or may not be present. Because it is asymptomatic, such bacteriuria is found mainly when high-risk patients are screened or when urine culture is done for other reasons.

Screening patients for asymptomatic bacteriuria is indicated for those at risk of complications if the bacteriuria is untreated. Such patients include

- Pregnant women at 12 to 16 wks' gestation or at the first prenatal visit, if later (because of the risk of symptomatic UTI, including pyelonephritis, during pregnancy; and adverse pregnancy outcomes, including low-birth-weight neonate and premature delivery) (See the US Preventive Services Task Force Reaffirmation Recommendation Statement.)
- Patients who have had a kidney transplant within the previous 6 mo
- Young children with gross VUR
- Before certain invasive GU procedures that can cause mucosal bleeding (eg, transurethral resection of the prostate)

Certain patients (eg, postmenopausal women; patients with controlled diabetes; patients with ongoing use of urinary tract foreign objects such as stents, nephrostomy tubes, and indwelling catheters) often have persistent asymptomatic bacteriuria and sometimes pyuria. However, such patients should not be screened because they are at low risk of complicated UTI due to the bacteriuria and thus do not require treatment. Also, in patients with indwelling catheters, treatment often fails to clear the bacteriuria and only leads to development of highly antibiotic-resistant organisms.

Acute pyelonephritis: Pyelonephritis is bacterial infection of the kidney parenchyma. The term should not be used to describe tubulointerstitial nephropathy unless infection is documented. In women, about 20% of community-acquired bacteremias are due to pyelonephritis. Pyelonephritis is uncommon in men with a normal urinary tract.

In 95% of cases of pyelonephritis, the cause is ascension of bacteria through the urinary tract. Although obstruction (eg, strictures, calculi, tumors, neurogenic bladder, VUR) predisposes to pyelonephritis, most women with pyelonephritis have no demonstrable functional or anatomic defects. In men, pyelonephritis is always due to some functional or anatomic defect. Cystitis alone or anatomic defects may cause reflux. The risk of bacterial ascension is greatly enhanced when ureteral peristalsis is inhibited (eg, during pregnancy, by obstruction, by endotoxins of gram-negative bacteria). Pyelonephritis is common in young girls and in pregnant women after bladder catheterization.

Pyelonephritis not caused by bacterial ascension is caused by hematogenous spread, which is particularly characteristic of virulent organisms such as *S. aureus*, *P. aeruginosa*, *Salmonella* species, and *Candida* species.

The affected kidney is usually enlarged because of inflammatory PMNs and edema. Infection is focal and patchy, beginning in the pelvis and medulla and extending into the cortex as an enlarging wedge. Cells mediating chronic inflammation appear within a few days, and medullary and subcortical abscesses may develop. Normal parenchymal tissue between foci of infection is common.

Papillary necrosis may be evident in acute pyelonephritis associated with diabetes, obstruction, sickle cell disease, pyelonephritis in renal transplants, pyelonephritis due to candidiasis, or analgesic nephropathy.

Although acute pyelonephritis is frequently associated with renal scarring in children, similar scarring in adults is not detectable in the absence of reflux or obstruction.

Symptoms and Signs

Elderly patients and patients with a neurogenic bladder or an indwelling catheter may present with sepsis and delirium but without symptoms referable to the urinary tract.

When symptoms are present, they may not correlate with the location of the infection within the urinary tract because there is considerable overlap; however, some generalizations are useful.

In **urethritis,** the main symptoms are dysuria and, primarily in men, urethral discharge. Discharge can be purulent, whitish, or mucoid. Characteristics of the discharge, such as the amount of purulence, do not reliably differentiate gonococcal from nongonococcal urethritis.

Cystitis onset is usually sudden, typically with frequency, urgency, and burning or painful voiding of small volumes of urine. Nocturia, with suprapubic pain and often low back pain, is common. The urine is often turbid, and microscopic (or rarely gross) hematuria can occur. A low-grade fever may develop. Pneumaturia (passage of air in the urine) can occur when infection results from a vesicoenteric or vesicovaginal fistula or from emphysematous cystitis.

In **acute pyelonephritis,** symptoms may be the same as those of cystitis. One-third of patients have frequency and dysuria. However, with pyelonephritis, symptoms typically include chills, fever, flank pain, colicky abdominal pain, nausea, and vomiting. If abdominal rigidity is absent or slight, a tender, enlarged kidney is sometimes palpable. Costovertebral angle percussion tenderness is generally present on the infected side. In urinary tract infection in children, symptoms often are meager and less characteristic.

Diagnosis

- Urinalysis
- Sometimes urine culture

Diagnosis by culture is not always necessary. If done, diagnosis by culture requires demonstration of significant bacteriuria in properly collected urine.

Urine collection: If an STD is suspected, a urethral swab for STD testing is obtained prior to voiding. Urine collection is then by clean-catch or catheterization.

To obtain a **clean-catch, midstream specimen,** the urethral opening is washed with a mild, nonfoaming disinfectant and air dried. Contact of the urinary stream with the mucosa should be minimized by spreading the labia in women and by pulling back the foreskin in uncircumcised men. The first 5 mL of urine is not captured; the next 5 to 10 mL is collected in a sterile container.

A **specimen obtained by catheterization** is preferable in older women (who typically have difficulty obtaining a clean-catch specimen) and in women with vaginal bleeding or discharge. Many clinicians also use catheterization to obtain a specimen if evaluation includes a pelvic examination. Diagnosis in patients with indwelling catheters is discussed elsewhere (see p. 2181).

Testing, particularly culturing, should be done within 2 h of specimen collection; if not, the sample should be refrigerated.

Urine testing: Microscopic examination of urine is useful but not definitive. Pyuria is defined as ≥ 8 WBCs/μL of uncentrifuged urine, which corresponds to 2 to 5 WBCs/high-power field in spun sediment. Most truly infected patients have > 10 WBCs/μL. The presence of bacteria in the absence of pyuria, especially when several strains are found, is usually due to contamination during sampling. Microscopic hematuria occurs in up to 50% of patients, but gross hematuria is uncommon. WBC casts, which may require special stains to differentiate from renal tubular casts, indicate only an inflammatory reaction; they can be present in pyelonephritis, glomerulonephritis, and noninfective tubulointerstitial nephritis.

Pyuria in the absence of bacteriuria and of UTI is possible, for example, if patients have nephrolithiasis, a uroepithelial tumor, appendicitis, or inflammatory bowel disease or if the sample is contaminated by vaginal WBCs. Women who have dysuria and pyuria but without significant bacteriuria have the urethral syndrome or dysuria-pyuria syndrome.

Dipstick tests also are commonly used. A positive nitrite test on a freshly voided specimen (bacterial replication in the container renders results unreliable if the specimen is not tested rapidly) is highly specific for UTI, but the test is not very sensitive. The leukocyte esterase test is very specific for the presence of > 10 WBCs/μL and is fairly sensitive. In adult women with uncomplicated UTI with typical symptoms, most clinicians consider positive microscopic and dipstick tests sufficient; in these cases, given the likely pathogens, cultures are unlikely to change treatment but add significant expense.

Cultures are recommended in patients whose characteristics and symptoms suggest complicated UTI or an indication for treatment of bacteriuria. Common examples include the following:

- Pregnant women
- Postmenopausal women
- Men
- Prepubertal children
- Patients with urinary tract abnormalities or recent instrumentation
- Patients with immunosuppression or significant comorbidities
- Patients whose symptoms suggest pyelonephritis or sepsis
- Patients with recurrent UTIs (≥ 3/yr)

Samples containing large numbers of epithelial cells are contaminated and unlikely to be helpful. An uncontaminated specimen must be obtained for culture. Culture of a morning specimen is most likely to detect UTI. Samples left at room temperature for > 2 h can give falsely high colony counts due to continuing bacterial proliferation. Criteria for culture positivity include isolation of a single bacterial species from a midstream, clean catch, or catheterized urine specimen.

For **asymptomatic bacteriuria,** criteria for culture positivity based on the guidelines of the Infectious Diseases Society of America (see Guidelines for the Diagnosis and Treatment of Asymptomatic Bacteriuria in Adults at www.idsociety.org) are

- Two consecutive clean-catch, voided specimens (for men, one specimen) from which the same bacterial strain is isolated in colony counts of $> 10^5$/mL
- Among women or men, in a catheter-obtained specimen, a single bacterial species is isolated in colony counts of $> 10^2$/mL

For **symptomatic patients,** culture criteria are

- Uncomplicated cystitis in women: $> 10^3$/mL
- Uncomplicated cystitis in women: $> 10^2$/mL *(This quantification may be considered to improve sensitivity to E. coli.)*
- Acute, uncomplicated pyelonephritis in women: $> 10^4$/mL
- Complicated UTI: $> 10^5$/mL in women; or $> 10^4$/mL in men or from a catheter-derived specimen in women
- Acute urethral syndrome: $> 10^2$/mL of a single bacterial species

Any positive culture result, regardless of colony count, in a sample obtained via suprapubic bladder puncture should be considered a true positive.

In midstream urine, *E. coli* in mixed flora may be a true pathogen.[1]

Occasionally, UTI is present despite lower colony counts, possibly because of prior antibiotic therapy, very dilute urine (specific gravity < 1.003), or obstruction to the flow of grossly infected urine. Repeating the culture improves the diagnostic accuracy of a positive result, ie, may differentiate between a contaminant and a true positive result.

Infection localization: Clinical differentiation between upper and lower UTI is impossible in many patients, and testing is not usually advisable. When the patient has high fever, costovertebral angle tenderness, and gross pyuria with casts, pyelonephritis is highly likely. The best noninvasive technique for differentiating bladder from kidney infection appears to be the response to a short course of antibiotic therapy. If the urine has not cleared after 3 days of treatment, pyelonephritis should be sought.

Symptoms similar to those of cystitis and urethritis can occur in patients with vaginitis, which may cause dysuria due to the passage of urine across inflamed labia. Vaginitis can often be distinguished by the presence of vaginal discharge, vaginal odor, and dyspareunia.

Other testing: Seriously ill patients require evaluation for sepsis, typically with CBC, electrolytes, lactate, BUN, creatinine, and blood cultures. Patients with abdominal pain or tenderness are evaluated for other causes of an acute abdomen.

Patients who have dysuria/pyuria but no bacteriuria should have testing for an STD, typically using nucleic acid-based testing of swabs from the urethra and cervix (see p. 1701).

Most adults do not require assessment for structural abnormalities unless the following occur:

- The patient has ≥ 2 episodes of pyelonephritis.
- Infections are complicated.
- Nephrolithiasis is suspected.
- There is painless gross hematuria or new renal insufficiency.
- Fever persists for ≥ 72 h.

Urinary tract imaging choices include ultrasonography, CT, and IVU. Occasionally, voiding cystourethrography, retrograde urethrography, or cystoscopy is warranted. Urologic investigation is not routinely needed in women with symptomatic cystitis or asymptomatic recurrent cystitis, because findings do not influence therapy. Children with UTI often require imaging.

1. Hooton TM, Roberts PL, Cox ME, Stapleton AE. Voided midstream urine culture and acute cystitis in premenopausal women. *N Engl J Med* 369(20):1883–1891, 2013.

Treatment

- Antibiotics
- Occasionally surgery (eg, to drain abscesses, correct underlying structural abnormalities, or relieve obstruction)

All forms of symptomatic bacterial UTI require antibiotics. For patients with troublesome dysuria, phenazopyridine may help control symptoms until the antibiotics do (usually within 48 h).

Choice of antibiotic should be based on the patient's allergy and adherence history, local resistance patterns (if known), antibiotic availability and cost, and patient and provider tolerance for risk of treatment failure. Propensity for inducing antibiotic resistance should also be considered. When urine culture is done, choice of antibiotic should be modified when culture and sensitivity results are available to the most narrow-spectrum drug effective against the identified pathogen.

Surgical correction is usually required for obstructive uropathy, anatomic abnormalities, and neuropathic urinary tract lesions such as compression of the spinal cord. Catheter drainage of an obstructed urinary tract aids in prompt control of UTI. Occasionally, a renal cortical abscess or perinephric abscess requires surgical drainage. Instrumentation of the lower urinary tract in the presence of infected urine should be deferred if possible. Sterilization of the urine before instrumentation and antibiotic therapy for 3 to 7 days after instrumentation can prevent life-threatening urosepsis.

Urethritis: Sexually active patients with symptoms are usually treated presumptively for STDs pending test results. A typical regimen is ceftriaxone 250 mg IM plus either azithromycin 1 g po once or doxycycline 100 mg po bid for 7 days. All sex partners within 60 days should be evaluated. Men diagnosed with urethritis should be tested for HIV and syphilis in accordance with the Centers for Disease Control and Prevention's 2015 Sexually Transmitted Diseases Treatment Guidelines.

Cystitis: First-line treatment of uncomplicated cystitis is nitrofurantoin 100 mg po bid for 5 days (it is contraindicated if creatinine clearance is < 60 mL/min), trimethoprim/sulfamethoxazole (TMP/SMX) 160/800 mg po bid for 3 days, or fosfomycin 3 g po once. Less desirable choices include a fluoroquinolone or a beta-lactam antibiotic. If cystitis recurs within a week or two, a broader spectrum antibiotic (eg, a fluoroquinolone) can be used and the urine should be cultured.

Complicated cystitis should be treated with empiric broad-spectrum antibiotics chosen based on local pathogens and resistance patterns and adjusted based on culture results. Urinary tract abnormalities must also be managed.

Acute urethral syndrome: Treatment depends on clinical findings and urine culture results:

- Women with dysuria, pyuria, and colony growth of > 10^2/mL of a single bacterial species on urine culture can be treated as for uncomplicated cystitis.
- Women who have dysuria and pyuria with no bacteriuria should be evaluated for an STD (including for *N. gonorrhoeae* and *C. trachomatis*).
- Women who have dysuria but neither pyuria nor bacteriuria do not have the true urethral syndrome. They should be evaluated for noninfectious causes of dysuria. Evaluation may include therapeutic trials, for example, of behavioral treatments (eg, biofeedback and pelvic musculature relaxation), surgery (for urethral stenosis), and drugs (eg, hormone replacement for suspected atrophic urethritis, anesthetics, antispasmodics).

Asymptomatic bacteriuria: Typically, asymptomatic bacteriuria in patients with diabetes, elderly patients, or patients with chronically indwelling bladder catheters should not be treated. However, patients at risk of complications from asymptomatic bacteriuria (see p. 2177) should have any treatable causes addressed and be given antibiotics as for cystitis. In pregnant women, only a few antibiotics can be safely used. Oral beta-lactams, sulfonamides, and nitrofurantoin are considered safe in early pregnancy, but trimethoprim should be avoided during the 1st trimester, and sulfamethoxazole should be avoided during the 3rd trimester, particularly near parturition. Patients with untreatable obstructive problems (eg, calculi, reflux) may require long-term suppressive therapy.

Acute pyelonephritis: Antibiotics are required. Outpatient treatment with oral antibiotics is possible if all of the following criteria are satisfied:

- Patients are expected to be adherent
- Patients are immunocompetent
- Patients have no nausea or vomiting or evidence of volume depletion or septicemia
- Patients have no factors suggesting complicated UTI

Ciprofloxacin 500 mg po bid for 7 days and levofloxacin 750 mg po once/day for 5 days are 1st-line antibiotics if < 10% of the uropathogens in the community are resistant. A 2nd option is usually TMP/SMX 160/800 mg po bid for 14 days. However, local sensitivity patterns should be considered because in some parts of the US, > 20% of *E. coli* are resistant to sulfa.

Patients not eligible for outpatient treatment should be hospitalized and given parenteral therapy selected on the basis of local sensitivity patterns. First-line antibiotics are usually renally excreted fluoroquinolones, such as ciprofloxacin and levofloxacin. Other choices, such as ampicillin plus gentamicin, broad-spectrum cephalosporins (eg, ceftriaxone, cefotaxime, cefepime), aztreonam, beta-lactam/beta-lactam inhibitor combinations (ampicillin/sulbactam, ticarcillin/clavulanate, piperacillin/tazobactam), and imipenem/cilastatin, are usually reserved for patients with more complicated pyelonephritis (eg, with obstruction, calculi, resistant bacteria, or a hospital-acquired infection) or recent urinary tract instrumentation.

Parenteral therapy is continued until defervescence and other signs of clinical improvement occur. In > 80% of patients, improvement occurs within 72 h. Oral therapy can then begin, and the patient can be discharged for the remainder of a 7- to 14-day treatment course. Complicated cases require longer courses of IV antibiotics with total duration of 2 to 3 wk and urologic correction of anatomic defects.

Outpatient management can be considered in pregnant women with pyelonephritis, but only if symptoms are mild, close follow-up is available, and (preferably) pregnancy is < 24 wk gestation. Outpatient treatment is with cephalosporins (eg, ceftriaxone 1 to 2 g IV or IM, then cephalexin 500 mg po qid for 10 days). Otherwise, 1st-line IV antibiotics include cephalosporins, aztreonam, or ampicillin plus gentamicin. If pyelonephritis is severe, possibilities include piperacillin/tazobactam or meropenem. Fluoroquinolones and TMP/SMX should be avoided. Because recurrence is common, some authorities recommend prophylaxis after the acute infection resolves with nitrofurantoin 100 mg po or cephalexin 250 mg po every night during the remainder of the pregnancy and for 4 to 6 wk after pregnancy.

Prevention

In women who experience ≥ 3 UTIs/yr, behavioral measures are recommended, including increasing fluid intake, avoiding spermicides and diaphragm use, not delaying urination, wiping front to back after defecation, avoiding douching, and urinating immediately after sexual intercourse. Although some evidence shows that cranberry products prevent UTI in women, others do not; the optimal dose is unknown; and they can have high amounts of oxalates (possibly increasing risk of oxalate stones). Thus, most experts do not recommend use of cranberry products for prevention of symptomatic UTI in women. (For further details, see the 2012 Cochrane review article by Jepson et al., Cranberries for preventing UTIs at www.ncbi.nlm.nih.gov.)

If these techniques are unsuccessful, antibiotic prophylaxis should be considered. Common options are continuous and postcoital prophylaxis.

Continuous prophylaxis commonly begins with a 6 mo trial. If UTI recurs after 6 mo of prophylactic therapy, prophylaxis may be reinstituted for 2 or 3 yr. Choice of antibiotic depends on susceptibility patterns of prior infections. Common options are TMP/SMX 40/200 mg po once/day or 3 times/wk, nitrofurantoin 50 or 100 mg po once/day, cephalexin 125 to 250 mg po once/day, and fosfomycin 3 g po q 10 days. Fluoroquinolones are effective but are not usually recommended because resistance is increasing. Also, fluoroquinolones are contraindicated in pregnant women and children. Nitrofurantoin is contraindicated if creatinine clearance is < 60 mL/min. Long-term use can rarely cause damage to the lungs, liver, and nervous system.

Postcoital prophylaxis in women may be more effective if UTIs are temporally related to sexual intercourse. Usually, a single dose of one of the drugs used for continuous prophylaxis (other than fosfomycin) is effective.

Contraception is recommended for women using a fluoroquinolone because these drugs can potentially injure a fetus. Although concern exists that antibiotics may decrease the effectiveness of oral contraceptives, pharmacokinetic studies have not shown a significant or consistent effect. Nonetheless, some experts still recommend that women who use oral contraceptives use barrier contraceptives while they are taking antibiotics.

In **pregnant women,** effective prophylaxis of UTI is similar to that in nonpregnant women, including use of postcoital prophylaxis. Appropriate patients include those with acute pyelonephritis during a pregnancy, patients with > 1 episode (despite treatment) of UTI or bacteriuria during pregnancy, and patients who required prophylaxis for recurrent UTI before pregnancy.

In **postmenopausal women,** antibiotic prophylaxis is similar to that described previously. Additionally, topical estrogen therapy markedly reduces the incidence of recurrent UTI in women with atrophic vaginitis or atrophic urethritis.

KEY POINTS

- The most common causes of bacterial UTI and UTI overall are *E. coli* and other gram-negative enteric bacteria.
- Do not test for or treat asymptomatic bacteriuria except in pregnant women, immunocompromised patients, or before an invasive urologic procedure.
- In general, culture urine in suspected complicated UTI but not in uncomplicated cystitis.
- Test patients for structural abnormalities if infections recur or are complicated, nephrolithiasis is suspected, there is painless hematuria or new renal insufficiency, or fever persists for ≥ 72 h.
- If available, consider local resistance patterns when choosing antibiotic therapy for UTI.
- For women with ≥ 3 UTIs/yr despite behavioral prophylactic measures, consider continuous or postcoital antibiotic prophylaxis.

CATHETER-ASSOCIATED URINARY TRACT INFECTIONS

A catheter-associated UTI (CAUTI) is a UTI in which the positive culture was taken when an indwelling urinary catheter had been in place for > 2 calendar days. Patients with indwelling bladder catheters are predisposed to bacteriuria and UTIs. Symptoms may be vague or may suggest sepsis. Diagnosis depends on the presence of symptoms. Testing includes urinalysis and culture after the catheter has been removed and a new one inserted. The most effective preventive measures are avoiding unnecessary catheterization and removing catheters as soon as possible.

Bacteria can enter the bladder during the insertion of the catheter, through the catheter lumen, or from around the outside of the catheter. A biofilm develops around the outside of the catheter and on the uroepithelium. Bacteria enter this biofilm, which protects them from the mechanical flow of urine, host defenses, and antibiotics, making bacterial elimination difficult. Even with thoroughly aseptic catheter insertion and care, the chance of developing significant bacteriuria is 3 to 10% every day the catheter is indwelling. Of patients who develop bacteriuria, 10 to 25% develop symptoms of UTI. Fewer develop sepsis.

Risk factors for UTI include duration of catheterization, female sex, diabetes mellitus, opening a closed system, and suboptimal aseptic techniques. Indwelling bladder catheters can also predispose to fungal UTI.

UTI can also develop in women during the days after a catheter has been removed.

Symptoms and Signs

Patients with CAUTI cannot have some of the symptoms typical of UTIs (dysuria, frequency), but they may complain of feeling the need to urinate or of suprapubic discomfort. However, such symptoms of lower tract UTI may also be caused by obstruction of the catheter or development of bladder calculi. Symptoms of acute or chronic pyelonephritis may also develop without the typical urinary tract symptoms. Patients may have nonspecific symptoms such as malaise, fever, flank pain, anorexia, altered mental status, and signs of sepsis.

Diagnosis

- Urinalysis and urine culture for patients with symptoms or at high risk of sepsis

Testing is done only in patients who might require treatment, including those who have symptoms and those at high risk of developing sepsis, such as

- Patients with granulocytopenia
- Organ transplant patients taking immunosuppressants
- Pregnant women
- Patients undergoing urologic surgery

Diagnostic testing includes urinalysis and urine culture. If bacteremia is suspected, blood cultures are done. Urine cultures should be done, preferably after replacing the catheter (to avoid culturing colonizing bacteria), then by a direct needle stick of the catheter, all done with aseptic technique, so that contamination of the specimen is minimized.

In women who have had a catheter removed, urine culture within 48 h is recommended regardless of whether symptoms occur.

Treatment

- Antibiotics

Asymptomatic, low-risk patients are not treated. Symptomatic and high-risk patients are treated using antibiotics and supportive measures. The catheter should be replaced when treatment begins. Choice of empiric antibiotic is as for acute pyelonephritis. Sometimes vancomycin is added to the regimen. Subsequently, antibiotics with the narrowest spectrum of activity, based on culture and sensitivity testing, should be used. Optimal duration is not well established but 7 to 14 days is reasonable in patients who had a satisfactory clinical response, including resolution of systemic manifestations.

Asymptomatic women and men with recent catheter removal who have UTI diagnosed by urine culture should be treated based on the culture results. Optimal duration of treatment is not known.

Prevention

The most effective preventive measures are avoiding catheterization and removing catheters as soon as possible. Optimizing aseptic technique and maintaining a closed drainage system also reduce risk. How often and even whether to routinely change indwelling catheters is unknown. Intermittent catheterization carries less risk than use of an indwelling catheter and should be used instead whenever feasible. Antibiotic prophylaxis and antibiotic-coated catheters are no longer recommended for patients who require long-term indwelling catheters.

KEY POINTS

- Long-term use of indwelling bladder catheters increases risk of bacteriuria, although bacteriuria is usually asymptomatic.
- Symptomatic UTI may manifest with systemic symptoms (eg, fever, altered mental status, decreased BP) and few or no symptoms typical of UTIs.
- Do urinalysis and urine culture if patients have symptoms or are at high risk of sepsis (eg, because of immunocompromise).
- Treat similarly to other complicated UTIs.
- Whenever possible, avoid use of catheters or remove them at the first opportunity.

CHRONIC PYELONEPHRITIS

(Chronic Infective Tubulointerstitial Nephritis)

Chronic pyelonephritis is continuing pyogenic infection of the kidney that occurs almost exclusively in patients with major anatomic abnormalities. Symptoms may be absent or may include fever, malaise, and flank pain. Diagnosis is with urinalysis, culture, and imaging tests. Treatment is with antibiotics and correction of any structural disorders.

Reflux of infected urine into the renal pelvis is the usual mechanism. Causes include obstructive uropathy, struvite calculi, and, most commonly, vesicoureteral reflux (VUR).

Pathologically there is atrophy and calyceal deformity with overlying parenchymal scarring. Chronic pyelonephritis may progress to chronic kidney disease. Patients with chronic pyelonephritis may have residual foci of infection that may predispose to bacteremia or, among kidney transplant patients, seed the urinary tract and transplanted kidney.

Xanthogranulomatous pyelonephritis (XPN) is an unusual variant that appears to represent an abnormal inflammatory response to infection. Giant cells, lipid-laden macrophages, and cholesterol clefts account for the yellow color of the infected tissue. The kidney is enlarged, and perirenal fibrosis and adhesions to adjacent retroperitoneal structures are common. The disorder is almost always unilateral and most often occurs in middle-aged women with a history of recurrent UTIs. Long-term urinary tract obstruction (usually by a calculus) and infection increase risk. The most common pathogens are *Proteus mirabilis* and *Escherichia coli*.

Symptoms and Signs

Symptoms and signs are often vague and inconsistent. Some patients have fever, flank or abdominal pain, malaise, or anorexia. In XPN, a unilateral mass can usually be palpated.

Diagnosis

- Urinalysis and urine culture
- Imaging

Chronic pyelonephritis is suspected in patients with a history of recurrent UTIs and acute pyelonephritis. However, most patients, except for children with VUR, do not have such a history. Sometimes the diagnosis is suspected because typical findings are incidentally noted on an imaging study. Symptoms, because they are vague and nonspecific, may not suggest the diagnosis.

Urinalysis and urine culture and usually imaging tests are done. Urinary sediment is usually scant, but renal epithelial cells, granular casts, and occasionally WBC casts are present. Proteinuria is almost always present and can be in the nephrotic range if VUR causes extensive renal damage. When both kidneys are involved, defects in concentrating ability and hyperchloremic acidosis may appear before significant azotemia occurs. Urine culture may be sterile or positive, usually for gram-negative organisms.

Initial imaging is usually with ultrasonography, helical CT, or IVU. The hallmark of chronic pyelonephritis (usually with reflux or obstruction) on imaging is classically a large, deep, segmental, coarse cortical scar usually extending to one or more of the renal calyces. The upper pole is the most common site. Renal cortex is lost, and the renal parenchyma thins. Uninvolved renal tissue may hypertrophy locally with segmental enlargement. Ureteral dilation may be present, reflecting the changes induced by chronic severe reflux. Similar changes can occur with urinary tract TB.

In **XPN,** urine cultures almost always grow *P. mirabilis* or *E. coli.* CT imaging is done to detect calculi or other obstruction. Imaging shows an avascular mass with a variable degree of extension around the kidney. Sometimes, to differentiate cancer (eg, renal cell carcinoma), biopsy may be required, or tissue removed during nephrectomy can be examined.

Prognosis

The course of chronic pyelonephritis is extremely variable, but the disease typically progresses very slowly. Most patients have adequate renal function for ≥ 20 yr after onset. Frequent exacerbations of acute pyelonephritis, although controlled, usually further deteriorate renal structure and function. Continued obstruction predisposes to or perpetuates pyelonephritis and increases intrapelvic pressure, which damages the kidney directly.

Treatment

If obstruction cannot be eliminated and recurrent UTIs are common, long-term therapy with antibiotics (eg, TMP/SMX, trimethoprim, a fluoroquinolone, nitrofurantoin) is useful and may be required indefinitely. Complications of uremia or hypertension must be treated appropriately.

For XPN, an initial course of antibiotics should be given to control local infection, followed by en bloc nephrectomy with removal of all involved tissue.

Patients undergoing renal transplantation who have chronic pyelonephritis may require nephrectomy before the transplant.

KEY POINTS

- Chronic pyelonephritis usually affects patients predisposed to urinary reflux into the renal pelvis (eg, by VUR, obstructive uropathy, or struvite calculi).
- Suspect chronic pyelonephritis if patients have recurrent acute pyelonephritis, but the diagnosis is often first suspected based on incidental findings on imaging.
- Obtain an imaging study (ultrasonography, helical CT, or IVU).
- If obstruction cannot be relieved, consider long-term antibiotic prophylaxis.

FUNGAL URINARY TRACT INFECTIONS

Fungal infections of the urinary tract primarily affect the bladder and kidneys.

Species of *Candida*, the most common cause, are normal commensals in humans. *Candida* colonization differs from infection in that infection produces tissue reaction. All invasive fungi (eg, *Cryptococcus neoformans*, *Aspergillus* sp, *Mucoraceae* sp, *Histoplasma capsulatum*, *Blastomyces* sp, *Coccidioides immitis*) may infect the kidneys as part of systemic or disseminated mycotic infection. Their presence alone indicates infection.

Lower UTI with *Candida* usually occurs in patients with urinary catheters, typically after antibiotic therapy, although candidal and bacterial infections frequently occur simultaneously. *C. albicans* prostatitis occurs infrequently in patients with diabetes, usually after instrumentation.

Renal candidiasis is usually spread hematogenously and commonly originates from the GI tract. Ascending infection is possible and occurs mainly in patients with nephrostomy tubes, other permanent indwelling devices, and stents. At high risk are patients with diabetes and those who are immunocompromised because of tumor, AIDS, chemotherapy, or immunosuppressants. A major source of candidemia in such high-risk hospitalized patients is an indwelling intravascular catheter. Renal transplantation increases the risk because of the combination of indwelling catheters, stents, antibiotics, anastomotic leaks, obstruction, and immunosuppressive therapy.

Complications of candidal infection can include emphysematous cystitis or pyelonephritis and fungus balls in the renal pelvis, ureter, or bladder. Bezoars may form in the bladder. Lower or upper urinary tract obstruction may occur. Papillary necrosis and intrarenal and perinephric abscesses may form. Although renal function often declines, severe renal failure is rare without postrenal obstruction.

Symptoms and Signs

Most patients with candiduria are asymptomatic. Whether *Candida* can cause urethral symptoms (mild urethral itching, dysuria, watery discharge) in men is uncertain. Rarely, dysuria in women is caused by candidal urethritis, but it may result from the urine coming into contact with periurethral tissue that is inflamed due to candidal vaginitis.

Among **lower UTIs,** cystitis due to *Candida* may result in frequency, urgency, dysuria, and suprapubic pain. Hematuria is common. In patients with poorly controlled diabetes, pneumaturia due to emphysematous cystitis has occurred. Fungus balls or bezoars may cause symptoms of urethral obstruction.

Most patients with **renal candidiasis** that is hematogenously spread lack symptoms referable to the kidneys but may have antibiotic-resistant fever, candiduria, and unexplained deteriorating renal function. Fungus ball elements in the ureter and renal pelvis frequently cause hematuria and urinary obstruction. Occasionally, papillary necrosis or intrarenal or perinephric abscesses cause pain, fever, hypertension, and hematuria. Patients may have manifestations of candidiasis in other sites (eg, CNS, skin, eyes, liver, spleen).

Diagnosis

- Urine culture
- Evidence of tissue reaction (in cystitis) or pyelonephritis

Candida UTI is considered in patients with predisposing factors and symptoms suggesting UTI and in all patients with candidemia. *Candida* should be suspected in men with symptoms of urethritis only when all other causes of urethritis have been excluded.

Diagnosis of *Candida* UTI is by culture, usually from urine. The level at which candiduria reflects true *Candida* UTI and not merely colonization or contamination is unknown. Differentiating *Candida* colonization from infection requires evidence of tissue reaction.

Cystitis is usually diagnosed in high-risk patients with candiduria by the presence of bladder inflammation or irritation, as evidenced by pyuria. Cystoscopy and ultrasonography of the kidneys and bladder may help detect bezoars and obstruction.

Renal candidiasis is considered in patients with fever, candiduria, or passage of fungus balls. Severe renal failure suggests postrenal obstruction. Imaging of the urinary tract may help reveal the degree of involvement. Blood cultures for *Candida* are often negative.

Unexplained candiduria should prompt evaluation of the urinary tract for structural abnormalities.

Treatment

- Only for symptomatic or high-risk patients
- Fluconazole or, for resistant organisms, amphotericin B; sometimes flucytosine is added

Fungal colonization of catheters does not require treatment. Asymptomatic candiduria rarely requires therapy. Candiduria should be treated in the following:

- Symptomatic patients
- Neutropenic patients
- Patients with renal allografts
- Patients who are undergoing urologic manipulation

Urinary stents and Foley catheters should be removed (if possible). For symptomatic cystitis, treatment is with fluconazole 200 mg po once/day. For pyelonephritis, fluconazole 200 to 400 mg po once/day is preferred. Therapy in both cases should be for 2 wk. For fungi resistant to fluconazole, amphotericin B is recommended at dose of 0.3 to 0.6 mg/kg IV once/day for 2 wk for cystitis and 0.5 to 0.7 mg/kg IV once/day for 2 wk for pyelonephritis.

For resistant pyelonephritis, flucytosine 25 mg/kg po qid is added to the regimen if patients have adequate renal function; if not, the dose should be modified based on creatinine clearance (see p. 1564).

Flucytosine may help eradicate candiduria due to non-*albicans* species of *Candida*; however, resistance may emerge rapidly when this compound is used alone. Bladder irrigation with amphotericin B may transiently clear candiduria but is no longer indicated for cystitis or pyelonephritis. Even with apparently successful local or systemic antifungal therapy for candiduria, relapse is frequent, and this likelihood is increased by continued use of a urinary catheter. Clinical experience with using voriconazole to treat UTIs is scant.

KEY POINTS

- Fungal UTI affects mainly patients who have urinary tract obstruction or instrumentation, immunocompromise (including diabetes), or both.
- Suspect fungal UTI in patients at risk or with candidemia who have clinical or laboratory findings consistent with UTI.
- Use antifungal drug therapy only if patients will undergo urologic manipulation or have symptoms, neutropenia, or renal allografts.

261 Voiding Disorders

(See also Urinary Incontinence in Children on p. 2613.)

Voiding disorders affect urine storage or release because both are controlled by the same neural and urinary tract mechanisms. The result is incontinence or retention.

For normal urinary function, the autonomic and voluntary nervous systems must be intact, and muscles of the urinary tract must be functional. Normally, bladder filling stimulates stretch receptors in the bladder wall to send impulses via spinal nerves S2 to S4 to the spinal cord, then to the sensory cortex, where the need to void is perceived. A threshold volume, which differs from person to person, triggers awareness of the need to void. However, the external urinary sphincter at the bladder outlet is under voluntary control and usually remains contracted until a person decides to urinate.

The micturition inhibitory center in the frontal lobe also helps control urination. When the decision is made, voluntary signals in the motor cortex initiate urination. These impulses are transmitted to the pontine micturition center, which coordinates simultaneous signals to contract detrusor smooth muscle throughout the bladder (via parasympathetic cholinergic nerve fibers) and to relax the internal sphincter (via alpha sympathetic nerve fibers) and striated muscle of the external sphincter and pelvic floor (see Fig. 261–1). In addition to normal urinary function, continence and normal voiding require normal cognitive function (including motivation), mobility, access to a toilet, and manual dexterity.

Damage to or dysfunction of any of the components involved in voiding can cause urinary incontinence or retention.

INTERSTITIAL CYSTITIS

Interstitial cystitis is noninfectious bladder inflammation that causes pain (suprapubic, pelvic, and abdominal), urinary frequency, and urgency with incontinence. Diagnosis is by history and exclusion of other disorders clinically and by cystoscopy and biopsy. With treatment, most patients improve, but cure is rare. Treatment varies but includes dietary changes, bladder training, pentosan, analgesics, and intravesical therapies.

Incidence of interstitial cystitis is unknown, but the disorder appears to be more common than once thought and may underlie other clinical syndromes (eg, chronic pelvic pain). Whites are more susceptible, and 90% of cases occur in women.

Cause is unknown, but pathophysiology may involve loss of protective urothelial mucin, with penetration of urinary potassium and other substances into the bladder wall, activation of sensory nerves, and smooth muscle damage. Mast cells may mediate the process, but their role is unclear.

Symptoms and Signs

Interstitial cystitis is initially asymptomatic, but symptoms appear and worsen over years as the bladder wall is damaged. Suprapubic and pelvic pressure or pain occurs, usually with urinary frequency (up to 60 times/day) or urgency. These symptoms worsen as the bladder fills and diminish when patients void; in some people, symptoms worsen during ovulation, menstruation, seasonal allergies, physical or emotional stress, or sexual intercourse. Foods with high potassium content (eg, citrus fruits, chocolate, caffeinated drinks, tomatoes) may cause exacerbations. Tobacco, alcohol, and spicy foods may worsen symptoms. If the bladder wall becomes scarred, bladder compliance and capacity decrease, causing or worsening urinary urgency and frequency.

Diagnosis

- Clinical evaluation
- Cystoscopy with possible biopsy

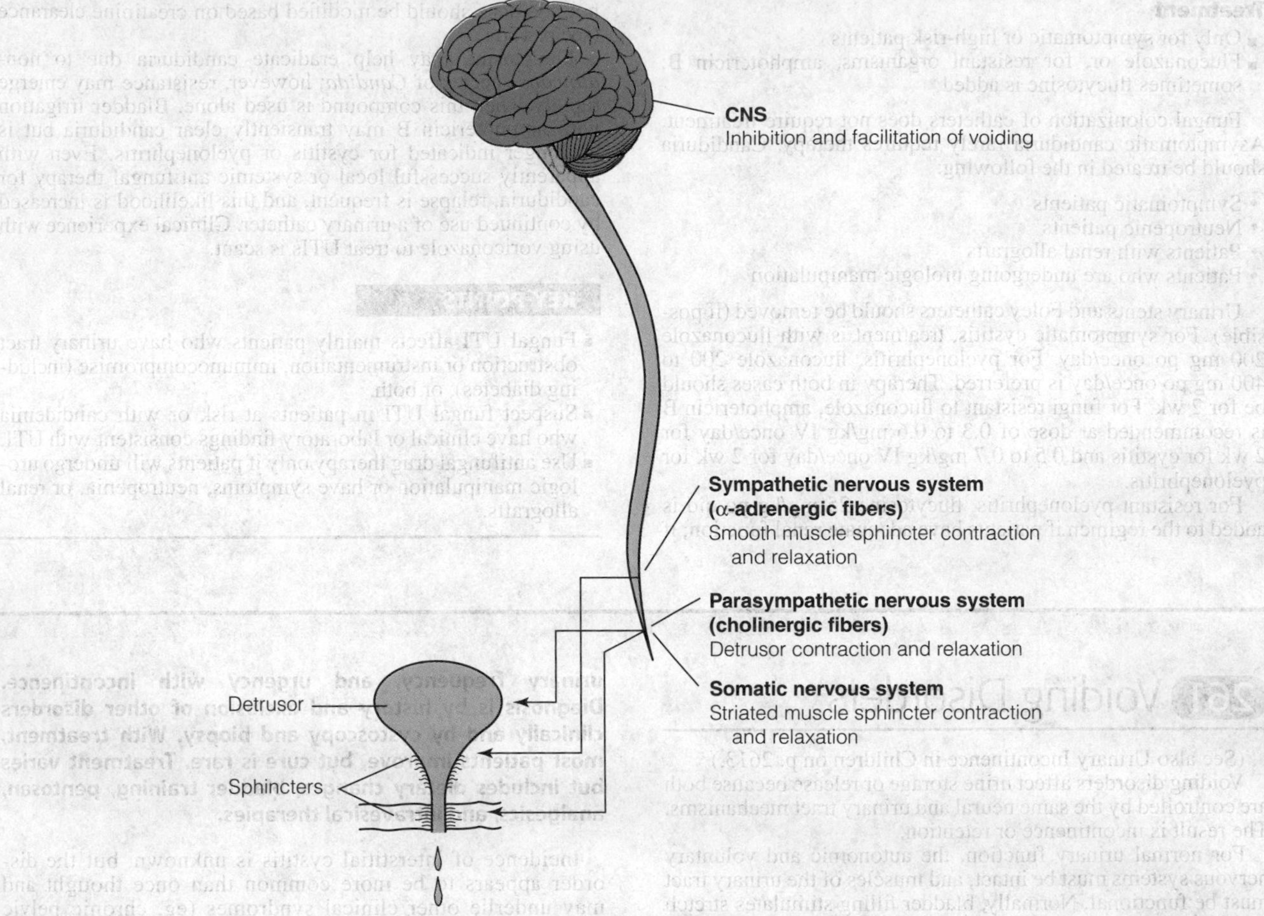

Fig. 261–1. Normal micturition occurs when bladder contraction is coordinated with urethral sphincter relaxation. The CNS inhibits voiding until the appropriate time and coordinates and facilitates input from the lower urinary tract to start and complete voiding. The sympathetic system contracts the smooth muscle sphincter. The parasympathetic nervous system contracts the bladder detrusor muscle through cholinergic fibers. The somatic nervous system contracts the striated muscle sphincter through cholinergic fibers from the pudendal nerve. (Adapted from DuBeau CE, Resnick NM with the Massachusetts Department of Health EDUCATE project collaborators: *Urinary Incontinence in the Older Adult: An Annotated Speaker/Teacher Kit*, 1993; used with permission of the authors.)

Diagnosis is suggested by symptoms after testing has excluded more common disorders that cause similar symptoms (eg, UTIs, pelvic inflammatory disease, chronic prostatitis or prostatodynia, diverticulitis). Cystoscopy is necessary and sometimes reveals benign bladder (Hunner) ulcers; biopsy is required to exclude bladder cancer. Assessment of symptoms with a standardized symptom scale or during intravesical potassium chloride infusion (potassium sensitivity testing) may improve diagnostic accuracy but is not yet routine practice.

Treatment

- Lifestyle modification
- Bladder training
- Drugs (eg, pentosan polysulfate sodium, tricyclic antidepressants, NSAIDs, dimethyl sulfoxide instillation)
- Surgery as a last resort

Lifestyle modification: Up to 90% of patients improve with treatment, but cure is rare. Treatment should involve avoidance of tobacco, alcohol, foods with high potassium content, and spicy foods.

Choice of treatment: In addition to lifestyle modification, bladder training, drugs, intravesical therapies, and surgery are used as needed. Stress reduction and biofeedback (to strengthen pelvic floor muscles, eg, with Kegel exercises) may help. No treatment has been proved effective, but a combination of ≥ 2 nonsurgical treatments is recommended before surgery is considered.

Drug therapies: The most commonly used drug is pentosan polysulfate sodium, a heparin-like molecule similar to urothelial glycosaminoglycan; doses of 100 mg po tid may help restore the bladder's protective surface lining. Improvement may not be noticed for 2 to 4 mo. Intravesical instillation of 15 mL of a solution containing 100 mg of pentosan or 40,000 units of heparin plus 80 mg of lidocaine and 3 mL of sodium bicarbonate may benefit patients unresponsive to oral drugs. Tricyclic antidepressants (eg, imipramine 25 to 50 mg po once/day) and NSAIDs in standard doses may relieve pain. Antihistamines (eg, hydroxyzine 10 to 50 mg once before bedtime) may help by directly inhibiting mast cells or by blocking allergic triggers.

Dimethyl sulfoxide instilled into the bladder through a catheter and retained for 15 min may deplete substance P and trigger mast cell granulation; 50 mL q 1 to 2 wk for 6 to 8 wk, repeated as needed, relieves symptoms in up to one half of patients. Intravesical instillation of BCG and hyaluronic acid are under study.

Surgical and other procedures: Bladder hydrodistention, cystoscopic resection of a Hunner ulcer, and sacral nerve root (S3) stimulation help some patients.

Surgery (eg, partial cystectomy, bladder augmentation, neobladder, and urinary diversion) is a last resort for patients with intolerable pain refractory to all other treatments. Outcome is unpredictable; in some patients, symptoms persist.

KEY POINTS

- Interstitial cystitis is noninfectious bladder inflammation that tends to cause chronic pelvic pain and urinary frequency.
- Diagnosis requires exclusion of other causes for symptoms (eg, UTIs, pelvic inflammatory disease, chronic prostatitis or prostatodynia, diverticulitis), cystoscopy, and biopsy.
- Cure is rare, but up to 90% of patients improve with treatment.
- Treatments can include diet modification, bladder training, and drugs (eg, pentosan polysulfate sodium, tricyclic antidepressants, NSAIDs, dimethyl sulfoxide instillation).
- Surgery is a last resort for patients with intolerable pain refractory to all other treatments.

NEUROGENIC BLADDER

Neurogenic bladder is bladder dysfunction (flaccid or spastic) caused by neurologic damage. Symptoms can include overflow incontinence, frequency, urgency, urge incontinence, and retention. Risk of serious complications (eg, recurrent infection, vesicoureteral reflux, autonomic dysreflexia) is high. Diagnosis involves imaging and cystoscopy or urodynamic testing. Treatment involves catheterization or measures to trigger urination.

Any condition that impairs bladder and bladder outlet afferent and efferent signaling can cause neurogenic bladder. Causes may involve the CNS (eg, stroke, spinal injury, meningomyelocele, amyotrophic lateral sclerosis), peripheral nerves (eg, diabetic, alcoholic, or vitamin B_{12} deficiency neuropathies; herniated disks; damage due to pelvic surgery), or both (eg, Parkinson disease, multiple sclerosis, syphilis). Bladder outlet obstruction (eg, due to benign prostatic hyperplasia, prostate cancer, fecal impaction, or urethral strictures) often coexists and may exacerbate symptoms.

In **flaccid (hypotonic) neurogenic bladder**, volume is large, pressure is low, and contractions are absent. It may result from peripheral nerve damage or spinal cord damage at the S2 to S4 level. After acute cord damage, initial flaccidity may be followed by long-term flaccidity or spasticity, or bladder function may improve after days, weeks, or months.

In **spastic bladder,** volume is typically normal or small, and involuntary contractions occur. It usually results from brain damage or spinal cord damage above T12. Precise symptoms vary by site and severity of the lesion. Bladder contraction and external urinary sphincter relaxation are typically uncoordinated (detrusor-sphincter dyssynergia).

Mixed patterns (flaccid and spastic bladder) may be caused by many disorders, including syphilis, diabetes mellitus, brain or spinal cord tumors, stroke, ruptured intervertebral disk, and demyelinating or degenerative disorders (eg, multiple sclerosis, amyotrophic lateral sclerosis).

Symptoms and Signs

Overflow incontinence is the primary symptom in patients with a flaccid bladder. Patients retain urine and have constant overflow dribbling. Men typically also have erectile dysfunction.

Patients with spastic bladder may have frequency, nocturia, and spastic paralysis with sensory deficits; most have intermittent bladder contractions causing urine leakage and, unless they lack sensation, urgency. In patients with detrusor-sphincter dyssynergia, sphincter spasm during voiding may prevent complete bladder emptying.

Common complications include recurrent UTIs and urinary calculi. Hydronephrosis with vesicoureteral reflux may occur because the large urine volume puts pressure on the vesicoureteral junction, causing dysfunction with reflux and, in severe cases, nephropathy. Patients with high thoracic or cervical spinal cord lesions are at risk of autonomic dysreflexia (a life-threatening syndrome of malignant hypertension, bradycardia or tachycardia, headache, piloerection, and sweating due to unregulated sympathetic hyperactivity). This disorder may be triggered by acute bladder distention (due to urinary retention) or bowel distention (due to constipation or fecal impaction).

Diagnosis

- Postvoid residual volume
- Renal ultrasonography
- Serum creatinine
- Usually cystography, cystoscopy, and cystometrography with urodynamic testing

Diagnosis is suspected clinically. Usually, postvoid residual volume is measured, renal ultrasonography is done to detect hydronephrosis, and serum creatinine is measured to assess renal function.

Further studies are often not done in patients who are not able to self-catheterize or ask to go to the bathroom (eg, severely debilitated elderly or post-stroke patients).

In patients with hydronephrosis or nephropathy who are not severely debilitated, cystography, cystoscopy, and cystometrography with urodynamic testing are usually recommended and may guide further therapy.

- **Cystography** is used to evaluate bladder capacity and detect ureteral reflux.
- **Cystoscopy** is used to evaluate duration and severity of retention (by detecting bladder trabeculations) and to check for bladder outlet obstruction.
- **Cystometrography** can determine whether bladder volume and pressure are high or low; if done during the recovery phase of flaccid bladder after spinal cord injury, it can help evaluate detrusor functional capacity and predict rehabilitation prospects (see p. 2190).

Urodynamic testing of voiding flow rates with sphincter electromyography can show whether bladder contraction and sphincter relaxation are coordinated.

Treatment

- Catheterization
- Increased fluid intake
- Drugs
- Surgery if conservative measures fail

Prognosis is good if the disorder is diagnosed and treated before kidneys are damaged.

Specific treatment involves catheterization or measures to trigger urination. General treatment includes renal function monitoring, control of UTIs, high fluid intake to decrease risk of UTIs and urinary calculi (although this measure may exacerbate incontinence), early ambulation, frequent changes of position, and dietary calcium restriction to inhibit calculus formation.

Catheterization: For flaccid bladder, especially if the cause is an acute spinal cord injury, immediate continuous or intermittent catheterization is needed. Intermittent self-catheterization is preferable to indwelling urethral catheterization, which has a high risk of recurrent UTIs and, in men, a high risk of urethritis, periurethritis, prostatic abscesses, and urethral fistulas. Suprapubic catheterization may be used if patients cannot self-catheterize.

Drug and other therapies: For spastic bladder, treatment depends on the patient's ability to retain urine. Patients who can retain normal volumes can use techniques to trigger voiding (eg, applying suprapubic pressure, scratching the thighs); anticholinergics may be effective. For patients who cannot retain normal volumes, treatment is the same as that of urge incontinence (see p. 2190), including drugs (see Table 261–3 on p. 2191) and sacral nerve stimulation.

Surgery: Surgery is a last resort. It is usually indicated if patients have had or are at risk of severe acute or chronic sequelae or if social circumstances, spasticity, or quadriplegia prevents use of continuous or intermittent bladder drainage. Sphincterotomy (for men) converts the bladder into an open draining conduit. Sacral (S3 and S4) rhizotomy converts a spastic into a flaccid bladder. Urinary diversion may involve an ileal conduit or ureterostomy.

An artificial, mechanically controlled urinary sphincter, surgically inserted, is an option for patients who have adequate bladder capacity, good bladder emptying, and upper extremity motor skills and who can comply with instructions for use of the device; if patients do not comply, life-threatening situations (eg, renal failure, urosepsis) can result.

KEY POINTS

- Damage to the neural pathways that control voiding can render the bladder too flaccid or spastic.
- Flaccid bladder tends to cause overflow incompetence.
- Spastic bladder tends to cause frequency, urge incontinence and, particularly with detrusor-sphincter dyssynergia, retention.
- Measure postvoid residual volume, do renal ultrasonography and serum creatinine measurement, and in many patients, do cystography, cystoscopy, and cystometrography with urodynamic testing.
- Treatment for flaccid bladder includes increased fluid intake and intermittent self-catheterization.
- Treatment for spastic bladder may include measures to trigger urination and/or measures used to treat urge incontinence (including drugs).

URINARY INCONTINENCE IN ADULTS

Urinary incontinence is involuntary loss of urine; some experts consider it present only when a patient thinks it is a problem. The disorder is greatly underrecognized and underreported. Many patients do not report the problem to their physician, and many physicians do not ask about incontinence specifically. Incontinence can occur at any age but is more common among the elderly and among women, affecting about 30% of elderly women and 15% of elderly men.

Incontinence greatly reduces quality of life by causing embarrassment, stigmatization, isolation, and depression. Many elderly patients are institutionalized because incontinence is a burden to caregivers. In bedbound patients, urine irritates and macerates skin, contributing to sacral pressure ulcer formation. Elderly people with urgency are at increased risk of falls and fractures.

Types: Incontinence may manifest as near-constant dribbling or as intermittent voiding with or without awareness of the need to void. Some patients have extreme urgency (irrepressible need to void) with little or no warning and may be unable to inhibit voiding until reaching a bathroom. Incontinence may occur or worsen with maneuvers that increase intra-abdominal pressure. Postvoid dribbling is extremely common and probably a normal variant in men. Identifying the clinical pattern is sometimes useful, but causes often overlap and much of treatment is the same.

Urge incontinence is uncontrolled urine leakage (of moderate to large volume) that occurs immediately after an urgent, irrepressible need to void. Nocturia and nocturnal incontinence are common. Urge incontinence is the most common type of incontinence in the elderly but may affect younger people. It is often precipitated by use of a diuretic and is exacerbated by inability to quickly reach a bathroom. In women, atrophic vaginitis, common with aging, contributes to thinning and irritation of the urethra and urgency.

Stress incontinence is urine leakage due to abrupt increases in intra-abdominal pressure (eg, with coughing, sneezing, laughing, bending, or lifting). Leakage volume is usually low to moderate. It is the 2nd most common type of incontinence in women, largely because of complications of childbirth and development of atrophic urethritis. Men can develop stress incontinence after procedures such as radical prostatectomy. Stress incontinence is typically more severe in obese people because of pressure from abdominal contents on the top of the bladder.

Overflow incontinence is dribbling of urine from an overly full bladder. Volume is usually small, but leaks may be constant, resulting in large total losses. Overflow incontinence is the 2nd most common type of incontinence in men.

Functional incontinence is urine loss due to cognitive or physical impairments (eg, due to dementia or stroke) or environmental barriers that interfere with control of voiding. For example, the patient may not recognize the need to void, may not know where the toilet is, or may not be able to walk to a remotely located toilet. Neural pathways and urinary tract mechanisms that maintain continence may be normal.

Mixed incontinence is any combination of the above types. The most common combinations are urge with stress incontinence and urge or stress with functional incontinence.

Etiology

The disorder tends to differ among age groups. With aging, bladder capacity decreases, ability to inhibit urination declines, involuntary bladder contractions (detrusor overactivity) occur more often, and bladder contractility is impaired. Thus, voiding becomes more difficult to postpone and tends to be incomplete. Postvoid residual volume increases, probably to ≤ 100 mL (normal < 50 mL). Endopelvic fascia weakens.

In postmenopausal women, decreased estrogen levels lead to atrophic urethritis and atrophic vaginitis and to decreasing urethral resistance, length, and maximum closure pressure.

In men, prostate size increases, partially obstructing the urethra and leading to incomplete bladder emptying and strain on the detrusor muscle. These changes occur in many normal, continent elderly people and may facilitate incontinence but do not cause it.

In younger patients, incontinence often begins suddenly, may cause little leakage, and usually resolves quickly with little or no treatment. Often, incontinence has one cause in younger patients but has several in the elderly.

Conceptually, categorization into reversible (transient) or established causes may be useful. However, causes and mechanisms often overlap and occur in combination.

Transient incontinence: There are several causes of transient incontinence (see Table 261–1). A useful mnemonic for many transient causes is DIAPPERS (with an extra P): *D*elirium, *I*nfection (commonly, symptomatic UTIs), *A*trophic urethritis and vaginitis, *P*harmaceuticals (eg, those with alpha-adrenergic, cholinergic, or anticholinergic properties; diuretics; sedatives), *P*sychiatric disorders (especially depression), *E*xcess urine output (polyuria), *R*estricted mobility, and *S*tool impaction.

Established incontinence: Established incontinence is caused by a persistent problem affecting nerves or muscles. Mechanisms usually used to describe these problems are bladder outlet incompetence or obstruction, detrusor overactivity or underactivity, detrusor-sphincter dyssynergia, or a combination (see Table 261–2). However, these mechanisms are also involved in some transient causes.

Outlet incompetence is a common cause of stress incontinence. In women, it is usually due to weakness of the pelvic floor or of the endopelvic fascia. Such weakness commonly results from multiple vaginal deliveries, pelvic surgery (including hysterectomy), age-related changes (including atrophic urethritis), or a combination. As a result, the vesicourethral junction descends, the bladder neck and urethra become hypermobile, and pressure in the urethra falls below that of the bladder. In men, a common cause is damage to the sphincter or to the bladder neck and posterior urethra after radical prostatectomy.

Outlet obstruction is a common cause of incontinence in men, although most men with obstruction are not incontinent. Obstruction in men commonly results from benign prostatic hyperplasia, prostate cancer, or urethral stricture. In both sexes, fecal impaction can cause obstruction. In women, outlet obstruction can result from previous surgery for incontinence or from a prolapsed cystocele that causes the urethra to kink during straining to void.

Obstruction leads to a chronically overdistended bladder, which loses its ability to contract; then the bladder does not empty completely, resulting in overflow. Obstruction also may lead to detrusor overactivity and urge incontinence. If the detrusor muscle loses its ability to contract, overflow incontinence may follow. Some causes of outlet obstruction (eg, large bladder diverticula, cystoceles, bladder infections, calculi, and tumors) are reversible.

Detrusor overactivity is a common cause of urge incontinence in elderly and younger patients. The detrusor muscle contracts intermittently for no apparent reason, usually when the bladder is partially or nearly full. Detrusor overactivity may be idiopathic or may result from dysfunction of the frontal micturition inhibitory center (commonly due to age-related changes, dementia, or stroke) or outlet obstruction. Detrusor overactivity (hyperactivity) with impaired contractility is a variant of urge incontinence characterized by urgency, frequency, a weak flow rate, urinary retention, bladder trabeculation, and a postvoid residual volume of > 50 mL. This variant may mimic prostatism in men or stress incontinence in women.

Detrusor underactivity causes urinary retention and overflow incontinence in about 5% of patients with incontinence. It may be caused by injury to the spinal cord or to nerve roots supplying the bladder (eg, by disk compression, tumor, or surgery), by peripheral or autonomic neuropathies, or by other neurologic disorders (see Table 261–2). Anticholinergics and opioids greatly decrease detrusor contractility; these drugs are common transient causes. The detrusor may become underactive in men with chronic outlet obstruction as the detrusor is replaced by fibrosis and connective tissue, preventing the bladder from emptying even when the obstruction is removed. In women, detrusor underactivity is usually idiopathic. Less severe detrusor weakness is common among elderly women. Such weakness does not cause incontinence but can complicate treatment if other causes of incontinence coexist.

Detrusor-sphincter dyssynergia (loss of coordination between bladder contraction and external urinary sphincter relaxation) may cause outlet obstruction, with resultant overflow incontinence. Dyssynergia is often due to a spinal cord lesion that interrupts pathways to the pontine micturition center, which coordinates sphincter relaxation and bladder contraction. Rather than relaxing when the bladder contracts, the sphincter contracts, obstructing the bladder outlet. Dyssynergia causes severe trabeculation, diverticula, a "Christmas tree" deformation of the bladder, hydronephrosis, and renal failure.

Functional impairment (eg, cognitive impairment, reduced mobility, reduced manual dexterity, coexisting disorders, lack of motivation), particularly in the elderly, may contribute to established incontinence but rarely causes it.

Evaluation

Most patients, embarrassed to mention incontinence, do not volunteer information about it, although they may mention related symptoms (eg, frequency, nocturia, hesitancy). All adults should therefore be screened with a question such as "Do you ever leak urine?"

Clinicians should not assume that incontinence is irreversible just because it is long-standing. Also, urinary retention must be excluded before treatment for detrusor overactivity is started.

PEARLS & PITFALLS

- Most patients are embarrassed to mention incontinence, so ask all adults about incontinence.

History: History focuses on duration and patterns of voiding, bowel function, drug use, and obstetric and pelvic surgical history. A voiding diary can provide clues to causes. Over 48 to 72 h, the patient or caregiver records volume and time of each void and each incontinent episode in relation to associated activities (especially eating, drinking, and drug use) and during sleep. The amount of urine leakage can be estimated as drops, small, medium, or soaking; or by pad tests (measuring the weight of urine absorbed by feminine pads or incontinence pads during a 24-h period).

If the volume of most nightly voids is much smaller than functional bladder capacity (defined as the largest single voided volume recorded in the diary), the cause is a sleep-related problem (patients void because they are awake anyway) or a bladder abnormality (patients without bladder dysfunction or a sleep-related problem awaken to void only when the bladder is full).

Of men with obstructive symptoms (hesitancy, weak urinary stream, intermittency, feeling of incomplete bladder emptying), about one third have detrusor overactivity without obstruction.

Urgency or an abrupt gush of urine without warning or without preceding increase in intra-abdominal pressure (often called reflex or unconscious incontinence) typically indicates detrusor

Table 261–1. CAUSES OF TRANSIENT INCONTINENCE

CAUSE	COMMENTS
GI disorders	
Fecal impaction	Mechanism may involve mechanical disturbance of the bladder or urethra. Patients usually present with urge or overflow incontinence, typically with fecal incontinence.
GU disorders	
Atrophic urethritis Atrophic vaginitis	Thinning of urethral and vaginal epithelium and submucosa may cause local irritation and decrease urethral resistance, length, and maximum closure pressure with loss of the mucosal seal. These disorders are usually characterized by urgency and occasionally by scalding dysuria.
Urinary calculi Foreign bodies	Bladder irritation precipitates spasm.
UTIs	Only symptomatic UTIs cause incontinence. Dysuria and urgency can prevent patients from reaching the toilet before voiding.
Neuropsychiatric disorders	
Delirium Depression Psychosis	Awareness of the need or ability to void is impaired.
Restricted mobility	
Weakness Injury Use of physical restraints	Access to toilet is impaired.
Systemic disorders	
Excess urine output due to various disorders (eg, diabetes insipidus, diabetes mellitus)	Frequency, urgency, and nocturia can result.
Drugs	
Alcohol	Alcohol has a diuretic effect and can cause sedation, delirium, or immobility, which can result in functional incontinence.
Caffeine (eg, in coffee, tea, cola and some other soft drinks, cocoa, chocolate, and energy drinks)	Urine production and output are increased, causing polyuria, frequency, urgency, and nocturia.
Alpha-adrenergic antagonists (eg, alfuzosin, doxazosin, prazosin, tamsulosin, terazosin)	Bladder neck muscle in women or prostate smooth muscle in men is lax, sometimes causing stress incontinence.
Anticholinergics (eg, antihistamines, antipsychotics, benztropine, tricyclic antidepressants)	Bladder contractility can be impaired, sometimes causing urinary retention and overflow incontinence. These drugs also can cause delirium, constipation, and fecal impaction.
Calcium channel blockers (eg, diltiazem, nifedipine, verapamil)	Detrusor contractility is decreased, sometimes causing urinary retention and overflow incontinence, nocturia due to peripheral edema, constipation, and fecal impaction.
Diuretics (eg, bumetanide, furosemide, [not thiazides])	Urine production and output are increased, causing polyuria, frequency, urgency, and nocturia.
Hormone therapy (systemic estrogen/progestin therapy)	Collagen in the paraurethral connective tissues is degraded, causing ineffective urethral closure.
Misoprostol	Misoprostol relaxes the urethra and thus may cause stress incontinence.
Opioids	Opioids cause urinary retention, constipation, fecal impaction, sedation, and delirium.
Psychoactive drugs (eg, antipsychotics, benzodiazepines, sedative-hypnotics, tricyclic antidepressants)	Awareness of the need to void is blunted, and dexterity and mobility are decreased. These drugs can precipitate delirium.

Table 261–2. CAUSES OF ESTABLISHED INCONTINENCE

URODYNAMIC DIAGNOSIS	SOME NEUROLOGIC CAUSES	SOME NONNEUROLOGIC CAUSES
Bladder outlet incompetence	Lower motor neuron lesion (rare) In men, radical prostatectomy*	Intrinsic sphincter deficiency Urethral hypermobility In women, multiple vaginal deliveries, pelvic surgery (eg, hysterectomy), age-related changes (eg, atrophic urethritis) In men, prostate surgery
Bladder outlet obstruction	Spinal cord lesion causing detrusor-sphincter dyssynergia (rare)	Anterior urethral stricture Urethral diverticula (rarely) or large bladder diverticula (very rarely) Bladder calculi Bladder neck suspension surgery In women, cystocele (if large) In men, benign prostatic hyperplasia or prostate cancer
Detrusor overactivity	Alzheimer disease Spinal cord injury/dysfunction Multiple sclerosis Stroke	Bladder carcinoma Cystitis Idiopathic Outlet obstruction or incompetence
Detrusor underactivity	Autonomic neuropathy (eg, due to diabetes, alcoholism, or vitamin B_{12} deficiency) Disk compression Plexopathy Spinal neural tube defect (less often, may cause overactivity) Surgical damage (eg, anteroposterior resection) Tumor	Chronic bladder outlet obstruction Idiopathic (common among women)
Detrusor-sphincter dyssynergia	Spinal cord lesion Brain lesion affecting pathways to the pontine micturition center	Voiding dysfunction of childhood (poor relaxation of the sphincter with bladder contraction can result from the fear of bed wetting or soiling of clothes)

*Other prostate surgical procedures rarely cause established incontinence.

overactivity. The term overactive bladder is sometimes used to describe urinary urgency (with or without incontinence) that is often accompanied by urinary frequency and nocturia.

Physical examination: Neurologic, pelvic, and rectal examinations are the focus.

Neurologic examination involves assessing mental status, gait, and lower extremity function and checking for signs of peripheral or autonomic neuropathy, including orthostatic hypotension. Neck and upper extremities should be checked for signs of cervical spondylosis or stenosis. The spinal column should be checked for evidence of prior surgeries and for deformities, dimples, or hair tufts suggesting neural tube defects.

Innervation of the external urethral sphincter, which shares the same sacral roots as the anal sphincter, can be tested by assessing:

- Perineal sensation
- Volitional anal sphincter contraction (S2 to S4)
- The anal wink reflex (S4 to S5), which is anal sphincter contraction triggered by lightly stroking perianal skin
- The bulbocavernosus reflex (S2 to S4), which is anal sphincter contraction triggered by pressure on the glans penis or clitoris

However, the absence of these reflexes is not necessarily pathologic.

Pelvic examination in women can identify atrophic vaginitis and urethritis, urethral hypermobility, and pelvic floor weakness with or without pelvic organ prolapse. Pale, thin vaginal mucosae with loss of rugae indicate atrophic vaginitis. Urethral hypermobility can be seen during coughing when the posterior vaginal wall is stabilized with a speculum. A cystocele, an enterocele, a rectocele, or uterine prolapse suggests pelvic floor weakness (see p. 2294). When the opposite wall is stabilized with a speculum, bulging of the anterior wall indicates a cystocele, and bulging of the posterior wall indicates a rectocele or enterocele. Pelvic floor weakness does not suggest a cause, unless a large, prolapsed cystocele is present.

Rectal examination can identify fecal impaction, rectal masses, and, in men, prostate nodules or masses. Prostate size should be noted but correlates poorly with outlet obstruction. Suprapubic palpation and percussion to detect bladder distention are usually of little value except in extreme acute cases of urinary retention.

Urinary stress testing can be done on the examination table if stress incontinence is suspected; this method has a sensitivity and specificity of > 90%. The bladder must be full; a patient sits upright or close to upright with the legs spread, relaxes the perineal area, and coughs vigorously once:

- Immediate leakage that starts and stops with the cough confirms stress incontinence.
- Delayed or persistent leakage suggests detrusor overactivity triggered by the cough.

If cough triggers incontinence, the maneuver can be repeated while the examiner places 1 or 2 fingers inside the vagina to elevate the urethra (Marshall-Bonney test); incontinence that is corrected by this maneuver may respond to surgery.

- Results can be false-positive if patients have an abrupt urge to void during the test.
- Results can be false-negative if patients do not relax, the bladder is not full, the cough is not strong, or a large cystocele is present (in women). In women with large cystoceles, the test should be repeated with the patient supine and the cystocele reduced, if possible.

Testing:

- Urinalysis, urine culture
- Serum BUN, creatinine
- Postvoid residual volume
- Sometimes urodynamic testing

Urinalysis, urine culture, and measurement of BUN and serum creatinine are required. Other tests may include serum glucose and calcium (with albumin for estimation of protein-free calcium levels) if the voiding diary suggests polyuria, electrolytes if patients are confused, and vitamin B_{12} levels if clinical findings suggest a neuropathy.

Postvoid residual volume should be determined by catheterization or ultrasonography (preferred). Postvoid residual volume plus voided volume estimates total bladder capacity and helps assess bladder proprioception. A volume < 50 mL is normal; < 100 mL is usually acceptable in patients > 65 but abnormal in younger patients; and > 100 mL may suggest detrusor underactivity or outlet obstruction.

Urodynamic testing is indicated when clinical evaluation combined with the appropriate tests is not diagnostic or when abnormalities must be precisely characterized before surgery.

Cystometry may help diagnose urge incontinence, but sensitivity and specificity are unknown. Sterile water is introduced into the bladder in 50-mL increments using a 50-mL syringe and a 12- to 14-F urethral catheter until the patient experiences urgency or bladder contractions, detected by changes in fluid level in the syringe. If < 300 mL causes urgency or contractions, detrusor overactivity and urge incontinence are likely.

Peak urinary flow rate testing with a flow meter is used to confirm or exclude outlet obstruction in men. Results depend on initial bladder volume, but a peak flow rate of < 12 mL/sec with a urinary volume of ≥ 200 mL and prolonged voiding suggest outlet obstruction or detrusor underactivity. A rate of ≥ 12 mL/sec excludes obstruction and may suggest detrusor overactivity. During testing, patients are instructed to place their hand on their abdomen to check for straining during urination, especially if stress incontinence is suspected and surgery is contemplated. Straining suggests detrusor weakness that may predispose patients to postoperative retention.

In cystometrography, pressure-volume curves and bladder sensation are recorded while the bladder is filled with sterile water; provocative testing (with bethanechol or ice water) is used to stimulate bladder contractions.

Electromyography of perineal muscle is used to assess sphincter innervation and function. Urethral, abdominal, and rectal pressures may be measured.

Pressure-flow video studies, usually done with voiding cystourethrography, can correlate bladder contraction, bladder neck competency, and detrusor-sphincter synergy, but equipment is not widely available.

Treatment

- Bladder training
- Kegel exercises
- Drugs

Specific causes are treated, and drugs that can cause or worsen incontinence are stopped or the dosing schedule is altered (eg, a diuretic dose is timed so that a bathroom is near when the drug takes effect). Other treatment is based on type of incontinence. Regardless of type and cause, some general measures are usually helpful.

General measures: Patients are instructed to limit fluid intake at certain times (eg, before going out, 3 to 4 h before bedtime), to avoid fluids that irritate the bladder (eg, caffeine-containing fluids), and to drink 48 to 64 oz (1500 to 2000 mL) of fluid a day (because concentrated urine irritates the bladder).

Some patients, especially those with restricted mobility or cognitive impairment, benefit from a portable commode. Others use absorbent pads or specialized padded undergarments. These products can greatly improve the quality of life of patients and their caregivers. However, they should not be substituted for measures that can control or eliminate incontinence, and they must be changed often to avoid skin irritation and development of UTIs.

Bladder training: Patients may benefit from bladder training (to change voiding habits) and changes in fluid intake. Bladder training usually involves timed voiding (every 2 to 3 h) while awake. Over time, this interval can be increased to every 3 to 4 h while awake. Prompted voiding is used for cognitively impaired patients; they are asked about every 2 h whether they need to void or whether they are wet or dry. A voiding diary helps establish how often and when voiding is indicated and whether patients can sense a full bladder.

Kegel exercises: Pelvic muscle exercises (eg, Kegel exercises) are often effective, especially for stress incontinence. Patients must contract the pelvic muscles (pubococcygeus and paravaginal) rather than the thigh, abdominal, or buttock muscles. The muscles are contracted for 10 sec, then relaxed for 10 sec 10 to 15 times tid. Re-instruction is often necessary, and biofeedback is often useful. In women < 75 yr, cure rate is 10 to 25%, and improvement occurs in an additional 40 to 50%, especially if patients are motivated; do the exercises as instructed; and receive written instructions, follow-up visits for encouragement, or both.

Pelvic floor electrical stimulation is an automated version of Kegel exercises; it uses electrical current to inhibit detrusor overactivity and contract pelvic muscles. Advantages are improved compliance and contraction of the correct pelvic muscles, but benefits over behavioral changes alone are unclear.

Drugs: Drugs are often useful (see Table 261–3). Such drugs include anticholinergics and antimuscarinics, which relax the detrusor, and alpha-agonists, which increase sphincter tone. Drugs with strong anticholinergic effects should be used judiciously in the elderly. Alpha-antagonists and 5-alpha-reductase inhibitors may be used to treat outlet obstruction in men with urge or overflow incontinence.

Urge incontinence: Treatment aims to reduce detrusor overactivity; it begins with bladder training, Kegel exercises, and relaxation techniques. Biofeedback can be used with these treatments. Drugs may also be needed, as may intermittent self-catheterization (eg, when postvoid residual volume is large). Infrequently, sacral nerve stimulation, intravesical therapies, and surgery are used.

Bladder training helps patients tolerate and ultimately inhibit detrusor contractions. Regular voiding intervals are gradually lengthened (eg, 30 min every 3 days that urinary control is maintained) to improve tolerance of detrusor contractions. **Relaxation techniques** can improve emotional and physical responses to the urge to void. Relaxing, standing in place or sitting down (rather than rushing to the toilet), and tightening pelvic floor muscles can help patients suppress the urge to void.

Table 261–3. DRUGS USED TO TREAT INCONTINENCE

DRUG	MECHANISMS	DOSE	COMMENTS
Bladder outlet incompetence in stress incontinence			
Duloxetine	Centrally acting serotonin and norepinephrine reuptake inhibition	20–40 mg po bid to 80 mg po once/day	Duloxetine increases urinary sphincter striated muscle tone. It appears to be effective, but experience with it is limited.
Imipramine	Tricyclic antidepressant, anticholinergic, and alpha-agonist effects	25 mg po at night; may be increased in increments of 25 mg to a maximum dose of 150 mg	Imipramine is useful for nocturia and mixed incontinence caused by detrusor overactivity and bladder outlet incompetence.
Pseudoephedrine	Alpha-agonist effects	30–60 mg po q 6 h	Pseudoephedrine stimulates urethral smooth muscle contraction. Adverse effects include insomnia, anxiety, and, in men, urinary retention. This drug is not recommended for people with heart disorders, hypertension, glaucoma, diabetes, hyperthyroidism, or benign prostatic hyperplasia.
Bladder outlet obstruction in men with urge or overflow incontinence			
Alfuzosin	Alpha-adrenergic blockade	10 mg po once/day	In men, alpha-adrenergic blockers relieve symptoms of outlet obstruction, may reduce postvoid residual volume and outlet resistance, and may increase urinary flow rate. Effect occurs within days to weeks. Adverse effects include hypotension, fatigue, asthenia, and dizziness.
Doxazosin		1–8 mg po once/day	
Prazosin		0.5–2 mg po bid	
Silodosin		4–8 mg po once/day	
Tamsulosin		0.4–0.8 mg po once/day	
Terazosin		1–10 mg po once/day	
Dutasteride	5-Alpha-reductase inhibition	0.5 mg po once/day	Dutasteride and finasteride reduce prostate size and obstructive symptoms and make transurethral resection of prostate glands > 50 g less likely to be needed. Adverse effects are minimal and consist of sexual dysfunction (eg, decreased libido, erectile dysfunction).
Finasteride		5 mg po once/day	
Tadalafil	Not established	5 mg po once/day	Tadalafil is also used to treat erectile dysfunction. If possible, it should not be used in patients taking nitrates or alpha-adrenergic blockers.
Detrusor overactivity in urge or stress incontinence*			
Darifenacin	Anticholinergic effects, selective M_3 muscarinic antagonism	Extended-release: 7.5 mg po once/day	Adverse effects are similar to those of oxybutynin but, because of bladder selectivity, may be less severe.
Dicyclomine	Smooth muscle relaxation, anticholinergic effects	10–20 mg po tid to qid	Dicyclomine has not been well-studied.
Fesoterodine	Anticholinergic effects, selective M_3 muscarinic antagonism	4–8 mg po once/day	This prodrug has the same active metabolite as tolterodine. The dose should not exceed 4 mg once/day in patients with renal impairment. Adverse effects are similar to those of oxybutynin.
Flavoxate	Smooth muscle relaxation	100–200 mg po tid to qid	Flavoxate is usually ineffective. Adverse effects include nausea, vomiting, dry mouth, and blurred vision. Adverse effects are tolerable with doses of up to 1200 mg/day.

Table continues on the following page.

Table 261–3. DRUGS USED TO TREAT INCONTINENCE (*Continued*)

DRUG	MECHANISMS	DOSE	COMMENTS
Hyoscyamine	Anticholinergic effects	Tablet or liquid: 0.125–0.25 mg po qid Extended-release tablet: 0.375 mg po bid	Hyoscyamine has not been well-studied.
Imipramine	Tricyclic antidepressant, anticholinergic, and alpha-agonist effects	25 mg po at night; may be increased in increments of 25 mg to a maximum dose of 150 mg	Imipramine is useful for nocturia and mixed incontinence caused by detrusor overactivity and bladder outlet incompetence.
Mirabegron	Beta-3 adrenergic agonist	25–50 mg po once/day	Mirabegron is used to treat overactive bladder (urgency with or without urge incontinence and usually with urinary frequency). It may increase BP.
OnabotulinumtoxinA (botulinum toxin product)	Blockage of neuromuscular transmission by binding to receptor sites on nerve terminals and inhibiting the release of acetylcholine	100 units (for overactive bladder) or 200 units (for urinary incontinence due to neurogenic detrusor overactivity [neurogenic urge incontinence]) injected into the detrusor as often as q 12 wk as needed	OnabotulinumtoxinA is injected cystoscopically. It is used to treat adults with overactive bladder or neurogenic urge incontinence if they have an inadequate response to or cannot tolerate anticholinergic drugs.
Oxybutynin	Smooth muscle relaxation; anticholinergic, nonselective muscarinic, and local anesthetic effects	Immediate-release: 2.5–5 mg po tid to qid Extended-release: 5–30 mg po once/day Transdermal patch: 3.9 mg twice/wk Transdermal gel (10%): 100 mg in a 1-g sachet applied once/day Transdermal gel 3%: 3 pumps applied once/day	Oxybutynin is the most effective drug used to treat detrusor overactivity responsible for urge or stress incontinence. Efficacy may increase over time. Adverse effects include anticholinergic effects (eg, dry mouth, constipation), which may interfere with adherence and worsen incontinence. Adverse effects are less severe with extended-release and transdermal forms.
Propantheline	Anticholinergic effects	7.5–15 mg po 4–6 times/day	Propantheline has largely been replaced by newer drugs that have fewer adverse effects. This drug must be taken on an empty stomach.
Solifenacin	Anticholinergic effects, selective M_1 and M_3 muscarinic antagonism	Extended-release: 5–10 mg po once/day	Adverse effects are similar to those of oxybutynin but, because of bladder selectivity, may be less severe.
Tolterodine	Anticholinergic effects, selective M_3 muscarinic antagonism	Immediate-release: 1–2 mg po bid Extended-release: 2–4 mg po once/day	Efficacy and adverse effects are similar to those of oxybutynin, but long-term experience is limited. Because M_3 receptors are targeted, adverse effects are less severe than those of oxybutynin. Dose reduction is needed in patients with severe renal impairment.
Trospium	Anticholinergic effects	Immediate-release: 20 mg po bid (20 mg once/day in renal insufficiency)	Adverse effects are similar to those of oxybutynin. Dose reduction is needed in patients with severe renal impairment.
Detrusor underactivity in overflow incontinence			
Bethanechol	Cholinergic effects	10–50 mg po q 6 h	Bethanechol is usually ineffective. Adverse effects include flushing, tachycardia, abdominal cramps, and malaise.

*Drugs with anticholinergic effects should be used judiciously in the elderly.

Drugs (see Table 261–3) should supplement, not replace, behavioral changes. The most commonly used are oxybutynin and tolterodine; both are anticholinergic and antimuscarinic and are available in extended-release forms that can be taken po once/day. Oxybutynin is available as a skin patch that is changed twice/wk as well as topical gels that are applied to the skin daily.

Newer drugs with anticholinergic and antimuscarinic properties include solifenacin and darifenacin, which are taken po once/day, and trospium, which is taken once/day or bid. Drugs may be required to suppress urgency symptoms due to detrusor overactivity (hyperactivity) with impaired contractility. Drugs with a rapid onset of action (eg, immediate-release oxybutynin) can be used prophylactically if incontinence occurs at predictable times. Combinations of drugs may increase both efficacy and adverse effects, possibly limiting this approach in the elderly. OnabotulinumtoxinA is administered via cystoscopic injection into the detrusor muscle and is useful in treating urge incontinence refractory to other treatments in patients with neurologic causes (eg, multiple sclerosis, spinal cord dysfunction).

Sacral nerve stimulation is indicated for patients with severe urge incontinence refractory to other treatments. It is thought to work by centrally inhibiting bladder sensory afferents. The procedure begins with percutaneous nerve stimulation of the S3 nerve roots for at least 3 days; if patients respond, a neurostimulator is permanently implanted under the buttock skin. Posterior tibial nerve stimulation (PTNS) is a similar technique of electrical neuromodulation for the treatment of voiding dysfunction that was developed as a less invasive alternative to traditional sacral nerve stimulation. A needle is inserted above the medial malleolus near the posterior tibial nerve followed by the application of low voltage stimulation in 30-min sessions given weekly for 10 to 12 wk. The durability of PTNS is uncertain.

Rarely, **intravesical instillation of capsaicin or resiniferatoxin** (a capsaicin analog) is used when urge incontinence results from spinal cord injuries and other CNS disorders. This experimental treatment desensitizes C-fiber bladder afferents responsible for reflex bladder emptying.

Surgery is a last resort, usually used only for younger patients with severe urge incontinence refractory to other treatments. Augmentation cystoplasty, in which a section of intestine is sewn into the bladder to increase bladder capacity, is most common. Intermittent self-catheterization may be required if augmentation cystoplasty results in weak bladder contractions or poor coordination of abdominal pressure (Valsalva maneuver) with sphincter relaxation. Detrusor myomectomy may be done to decrease undesired bladder contractions. As a last resort, a urinary diversion can be created to divert the urine away from the bladder. Choice of procedure is based on presence of other disorders, physical limitations, and patient preference.

Stress incontinence: Treatment includes bladder training and Kegel exercises. Drugs, surgery, other procedures, or, in women, occlusive devices are also usually needed. Treatment is generally directed at outlet incompetence but includes treatments for urge incontinence if detrusor overactivity is present. Avoiding physical stresses that provoke incontinence can help. Losing weight may help lessen incontinence in obese patients.

Drugs (see Table 261–3) include pseudoephedrine, which may be useful in women with outlet incompetence; imipramine, which may be used for mixed stress and urge incontinence or for either separately; and duloxetine. If stress incontinence is due to atrophic urethritis, topical estrogen (0.3 mg conjugated or 0.5 mg estradiol once/day for 3 wk, then twice/wk after) is often effective.

Surgery and other procedures provide the best chance of cure when noninvasive treatments are ineffective. Bladder neck suspension is used to correct urethral hypermobility. Suburethral slings, injection of periurethral bulking agents, or surgical insertion of an artificial sphincter is used to treat sphincter deficiency. Choice depends on the patient's ability to tolerate surgery and need for other surgeries (eg, hysterectomy, cystocele repair) and on local experience.

Occlusive devices may be used in elderly women with or without bladder or uterine prolapse if surgical risks are high or if prior surgery for stress incontinence was ineffective. Various mesh slings can be used. Pessaries may be effective; they elevate the bladder neck, elevate the vesicourethral junction, and increase urethral resistance by pressing the urethra against the pubic symphysis. Newer, possibly more acceptable alternatives include silicone suction caps over the urethral meatus, intraurethral occlusive devices inserted with an applicator, and intravaginal bladder neck support prostheses. Removable intraurethral plugs are under study.

Exercise regimens using vaginal cones—in which progressively heavier cones are inserted into the vagina and retained for 15 min bid by contracting pelvic floor muscles—are also under study.

Overflow incontinence: Treatment depends on whether the cause is outlet obstruction, detrusor underactivity, or both.

Outlet obstruction due to benign prostatic hyperplasia or cancer is treated with drugs or surgery; that due to urethral stricture is treated with dilation or stenting. Cystoceles in women are treated with surgery or can be reduced using a pessary; unilateral suture removal or urethral adhesiolysis may be effective if cystoceles resulted from surgery. If urethral hypermobility coexists, bladder neck suspension should be done.

Detrusor underactivity requires bladder decompression (reduction of residual volume) by intermittent self-catheterization or, rarely, temporary use of an indwelling catheter (see Bladder Catheterization on p. 2072). Several weeks of decompression may be required to restore bladder function. If bladder function is not fully restored, maneuvers to augment voiding are used. Examples include

- Double voiding
- Valsalva maneuver
- Application of suprapubic pressure [Credé method] during voiding

A completely acontractile detrusor requires intermittent self-catheterization or use of an indwelling catheter. Using antibiotics or methenamine mandelate to prevent UTIs in patients who require intermittent self-catheterization is controversial but probably indicated if patients have frequent symptomatic UTIs or a valvular or orthopedic prosthesis. Such prophylaxis is not helpful with indwelling catheters.

Additional treatments that may induce bladder contraction and promote emptying include electrical stimulation and the cholinergic agonist bethanechol. However, bethanechol is usually ineffective and has adverse effects (see Table 261–3).

Refractory incontinence: Absorbent pads, special undergarments, and intermittent self-catheterization may be needed. Indwelling urethral catheters are an option for patients who cannot walk to the toilet or who have urinary retention and cannot self-catheterize; these catheters are not recommended for urge incontinence because they may exacerbate detrusor contractions. If a catheter is necessary (eg, to allow healing of a pressure ulcer in patients with refractory detrusor overactivity), a narrow catheter with a small balloon should be used because it will minimize irritability; irritability can force urine out, even around a catheter.

For men who can comply with treatment, condom catheters may be preferable because they reduce risk of UTIs; however, these catheters may cause skin breakdown and reduce motivation to become dry. New external collection devices may be effective in women. If involuntary bladder contractions persist, oxybutynin or tolterodine can be used. If mobility is restricted, measures to prevent skin irritation and breakdown due to urine are essential (see p. 1069).

KEY POINTS

- Because patients often do not volunteer that they are incontinent, ask about it specifically.
- Incontinence is not a normal consequence of aging and should always be investigated.
- The 4 types of urinary incontinence are urge, stress, overflow, and functional.
- Even some longstanding causes of incontinence are reversible.
- Do at least a urinalysis, urine culture, serum BUN and creatinine, and measurement of postvoid residual volume on all incontinent patients.
- Consider bladder training and Kegel exercises.
- Direct drug therapy toward correcting the mechanism of bladder dysfunction.

URINARY RETENTION

Urinary retention is incomplete emptying of the bladder or cessation of urination; it may be

- Acute
- Chronic

Causes include impaired bladder contractility, bladder outlet obstruction, detrusor-sphincter dyssynergia (lack of coordination between bladder contraction and sphincter relaxation), or a combination.

Retention is most common among men, in whom prostate abnormalities or urethral strictures cause outlet obstruction. In either sex, retention may be due to drugs (particularly those with anticholinergic effects, including many OTC drugs), severe fecal impaction (which increases pressure on the bladder trigone), or neurogenic bladder in patients with diabetes, multiple sclerosis, Parkinson disease, or prior pelvic surgery resulting in bladder denervation.

Urinary retention can be asymptomatic or cause urinary frequency, a sense of incomplete emptying, and urge or overflow incontinence. It may cause abdominal distention and pain. When retention develops slowly, pain may be absent. Long-standing retention predisposes to UTI and can increase bladder pressure, causing obstructive uropathy.

Diagnosis

- Measurement of postvoid residual volume

Diagnosis is obvious in patients who cannot void. In those who can void, incomplete bladder emptying is diagnosed by postvoid catheterization or ultrasonography showing an elevated residual urine volume. A volume < 50 mL is normal; < 100 mL is usually acceptable in patients > 65 but abnormal in younger patients. Other tests (eg, urinalysis, blood tests, ultrasonography, urodynamic testing, cystoscopy, cystography) are done based on clinical findings.

Treatment

- Urethral catheterization and treatment of cause

Relief of acute urinary retention requires urethral catheterization. Subsequent treatment depends on cause. In men with benign prostatic hypertrophy, drugs (usually alpha-adrenergic blockers or 5-alpha-reductase inhibitors) or surgery may help decrease bladder outlet resistance.

No treatment is effective for impaired bladder contractility; however, reducing outlet resistance with alpha-adrenergic blockers may increase bladder emptying.

Intermittent self-catheterization or indwelling catheterization is often required. An indwelling suprapubic tube or urinary diversion is a last resort.

KEY POINTS

- Mechanisms include impaired bladder contractility, bladder outlet obstruction, and detrusor-sphincter dyssynergia.
- Incomplete retention is diagnosed by a postvoid residual volume > 50 mL (> 100 mL in patients > 65).
- Prescribe urethral catheterization and treat the cause of retention.

SECTION 19

Gynecology and Obstetrics

262 Approach to the Gynecologic Patient

Most women, particularly those seeking general preventive care, require a complete history and physical examination as well as a gynecologic evaluation.

Gynecologic evaluation may be necessary to assess a specific problem such as pelvic pain, vaginal bleeding, or vaginal discharge. Women also need routine gynecologic evaluations, which may be provided by a gynecologist, an internist, or a family practitioner; evaluations are recommended every year for all women who are sexually active or > 18 yr. Obstetric evaluation focuses on issues related to pregnancy.

Many women expect their gynecologist to provide general as well as gynecologic health care. General medical care may include counseling on general health and routine screening for the following:

- Hypertension
- Dyslipidemia
- Diabetes
- Depression
- Tobacco use
- Alcohol use
- Drug use

For more information, see Well-Woman Task Force: Components of the Well-Woman Visit (http://journals.lww.com).

History

Gynecologic history consists of a description of the problem prompting the visit (chief complaint, history of present illness); menstrual, obstetric, and sexual history; and history of gynecologic symptoms, disorders, and treatments.

Current symptoms are explored using open-ended questions followed by specific questions about the following:

- Pelvic pain (location, duration, character, quality, triggering and relieving factors)
- Abnormal vaginal bleeding (quantity, duration, relation to the menstrual cycle)
- Vaginal discharge (color, odor, consistency), irritation, or both

Patients of reproductive age are asked about symptoms of pregnancy (eg, morning sickness, breast tenderness, delayed menses).

Menstrual history includes the following:

- Age at menarche
- Number of days of menses
- Length and regularity of the interval between cycles
- Start date of the last menstrual period (LMP)
- Dates of the preceding period (previous menstrual period, or PMP)
- Color and volume of flow
- Any symptoms that occur with menses (eg, cramping, loose stools)

Usually, menstrual fluid is medium or dark red, and flow lasts for 5 (± 2) days, with 21 to 35 days between menses; average blood loss is 30 mL (range, 13 to 80 mL), with the most bleeding on the 2nd day. A saturated pad or tampon absorbs 5 to 15 mL. Cramping is common on the day before and on the first day of menses. Vaginal bleeding that is painless, scant, and dark, is abnormally brief or prolonged, or occurs at irregular intervals suggests absence of ovulation (anovulation).

Obstetric history includes dates and outcomes of all pregnancies and previous ectopic or molar pregnancies.

Sexual history should be obtained in a professional and nonjudgmental way and includes the following:

- Frequency of sexual activity
- Number and sex of partners
- Use of contraception
- Participation in unsafe sex
- Effects of sexual activity (eg, pleasure, orgasm, dyspareunia)

Past gynecologic history includes questions about previous gynecologic symptoms (eg, pain), signs (eg, vaginal bleeding, discharge), and known diagnoses, as well the results of any testing.

Screening for domestic violence should be routine. Methods include self-administered questionnaires and a directed interview by a staff member or physician. In patients who do not admit to experiencing abuse, findings that suggest past abuse include the following:

- Inconsistent explanations for injuries
- Delay in seeking treatment for injuries
- Unusual somatic complaints
- Psychiatric symptoms
- Frequent emergency department visits
- Head and neck injuries
- Prior delivery of a low-birth-weight infant

Physical Examination

The examiner should explain the examination, which includes a breast examination and abdominal and pelvic examinations, to the patient.

For the **pelvic examination**, the patient lies supine on an examination table with her legs in stirrups and is usually draped. A chaperone is usually required, particularly when the examiner is male, and may also provide assistance.

The pelvic examination includes the following:

- External examination
- Speculum examination
- Bimanual examination
- Rectal examination (sometimes)

A pelvic examination is indicated for

- Symptomatic patients (eg, those with pelvic pain)
- Asymptomatic patients with specific indications (eg, need for cervical cancer screening)

Some experts recommend that patients < 21 yr have pelvic examinations only when medically indicated and that patients ≥ 21 yr have pelvic examinations annually. However, no evidence supports or refutes pelvic examinations for asymptomatic, low-risk patients. Thus, for such patients, the decision about how often these examinations should be done should be made after the health care practitioner and patient discuss the issues.

External examination: The pubic area and hair are inspected for lesions, folliculitis, and lice. The perineum is inspected for redness, swelling, excoriations, abnormal pigmentation, and lesions (eg, ulcers, pustules, nodules, warts, tumors). Structural abnormalities due to congenital malformations or female genital mutilation are noted. A vaginal opening that is < 3 cm may indicate infibulation, a severe form of genital mutilation.

Next, the introitus is palpated between the thumb and index finger for cysts or abscesses in Bartholin glands. While spreading the labia and asking the patient to bear down, the examiner checks the vaginal opening for signs of pelvic relaxation: an anterior bulge (suggesting cystocele), a posterior bulge (suggesting rectocele), and displacement of the cervix toward the introitus (suggesting prolapsed uterus).

Speculum examination: Before the speculum examination, the patient is asked to relax her legs and hips and breathe deeply.

The speculum is sometimes kept warm with a heating pad and may be moistened or lubricated before insertion, particularly when the vagina is dry. If a Papanicolaou (Pap) test or cervical culture is planned, the speculum is rinsed with warm water; lubricants have traditionally been avoided, but current-generation water-based lubricants can be used to increase patient comfort.

A gloved finger is inserted into the vagina to determine the position of the cervix. Then, the speculum is inserted with the blades nearly in the vertical plane (at about 1 and 7 o'clock) while widening the vagina by pressing 2 fingers on the posterior vaginal wall (perineal body). The speculum is fully inserted toward the cervix, then rotated so that the handle is down, and gently opened; it is pulled back as needed to visualize the cervix.

When the cervix is seen, the blades are positioned so that the posterior blade is deeper than the cervix (in the posterior fornix) and the anterior blade is allowed to rise gently and rest anterior to the cervix (in the anterior fornix). The examiner should take care to open the anterior blade slowly and gently and not to pinch the labia or perineum as the speculum is opened.

Normally, the cervix is pink and shiny, and there is no discharge.

A specimen for the Pap test is taken from the endocervix and external cervix with a brush and plastic spatula or with a cervical sampler that can simultaneously collect cells from the cervical canal and the transition zone; the specimen is rinsed in a liquid, producing a cell suspension to be analyzed for cancerous cells and human papillomavirus. Specimens for detection of sexually transmitted diseases (STDs) are taken from the endocervix. The speculum is withdrawn, taking care not to pinch the labia with the speculum blades.

Bimanual examination: Before the bimanual examination, the patient is asked to relax her legs and hips and breathe deeply.

The index and middle fingers of the dominant hand are inserted into the vagina to just below the cervix. The other hand is placed just above the pubic symphysis and gently presses down to determine the size, position, and consistency of the uterus and, if possible, the ovaries.

Normally, the uterus is about 6 cm by 4 cm and tilts anteriorly (anteversion), but it may tilt posteriorly (retroversion) to various degrees. The uterus may also be bent at an angle anteriorly (anteflexion) or posteriorly (retroflexion). The uterus is movable and smooth; irregularity suggests uterine fibroids (leiomyomas).

Normally, the ovaries are about 2 cm by 3 cm in young women and are not palpable in postmenopausal women. With ovarian palpation, mild nausea and tenderness are normal.

Significant pain when the cervix is gently moved from side to side (cervical motion tenderness) suggests pelvic inflammation.

Rectal examination: After bimanual palpation, the examiner palpates the rectovaginal septum by inserting the index finger in the vagina and the middle finger in the rectum.

Children: The examination should be adjusted according to children's psychosexual development and is usually limited to inspection of the external genitals. Young children can be examined on their mother's lap. Older children can be examined in the knee-chest position or on their side with one knee drawn up to their chest. Vaginal discharge can be collected, examined, and cultured.

Sometimes a small catheter attached to a syringe of saline is used to obtain washings from the vagina. If cervical examination is required, a fiberoptic vaginoscope, cystoscope, or flexible hysteroscope with saline lavage should be used.

In children, pelvic masses may be palpable in the abdomen.

Adolescents: For adolescents who are not sexually active, the examination is similar to that of children.

Some experts recommend that patients < 21 yr have pelvic examinations only when medically indicated (eg, if a patient has a persistent, symptomatic vaginal discharge).

All sexually active girls and those who are no longer active but have a history of a sexually transmitted disease may be offered a pelvic examination. However, clinicians can often check for STDs using a urine sample or a vaginal swab and thus avoid doing a speculum examination.

Sexually active girls should also be screened annually for chlamydial infection and gonorrhea.

Pubertal status is assessed.

During the visit, information about contraception should be offered as appropriate, and recommendations for the human papillomavirus (HPV) vaccine should be discussed. Clinicians should allow time for girls to speak privately about personal concerns (eg, contraception, safe sex, menstrual problems)

Testing

Testing is guided by the symptoms present.

Pregnancy testing: Most women who are of reproductive age and have gynecologic symptoms are tested for pregnancy.

Urine assays of the beta-subunit of human chorionic gonadotropin (beta-hCG) are specific and highly sensitive; they become positive within about 1 wk of conception. Serum assays are specific and even more sensitive.

Screening tests for cervical cancer: Tests used for cervical cancer screening include

- Papanicolaou (Pap) test
- Human papillomavirus (HPV) test

Specimens of cervical cells taken for the Pap test are examined for signs of cervical cancer; the same specimen may be tested for HPV. Screening tests are done routinely for most of a woman's life (see also Cervical Cancer Screening Guidelines for Average-Risk Women at www.cdc.gov).

For most women, frequency of screening depends mainly on the woman's age and results of previous tests:

- From age 21 to 30: Usually every 3 yr for the Pap test (HPV testing is not generally recommended)
- Age 30 to 65: Every 3 yr if only a Pap test is done or every 5 yr if a Pap test and an HPV test are done (more frequently in women at high risk of cervical cancer)
- After age 65: No more testing if test results have been normal in the preceding 10 yr

Pap tests should be resumed if a woman has a new sex partner; it should be continued if she has several sex partners.

For women with certain indications (eg, women with HIV infection), more frequent screening may be required, and screening may be started at a younger age.

Microscopic examination of vaginal secretions: This examination helps identify vaginal infections (eg, trichomoniasis, bacterial vaginosis, yeast infection).

Microbiologic testing: Culture or molecular methods (eg, PCR) are used to analyze specimens for specific STD organisms (eg, *Neisseria gonorrhoeae*, *Chlamydia trachomatis*) if patients have symptoms or risk factors; in some practices, such analysis is always done. Specimens may be obtained from urogenital sites including the endocervix (obtained during the Pap test) and urine. (See also the US Preventive Services Task Force practice guidelines screening for gonorrhea and screening for chlamydial infection at www.uspreventiveservicetaskforce.org.)

Cervical mucus inspection: Bedside inspection of a cervical mucus specimen by a trained examiner can provide information about the menstrual cycle and hormone states; this information may help in assessment of infertility and time of ovulation.

The specimen is placed on a slide, allowed to dry, and assessed for degree of microscopic crystallization (ferning), which reflects levels of circulating estrogens. Just before ovulation, cervical mucus is clear and copious with abundant ferning because estrogen levels are high. Just after ovulation, cervical mucus is thick and ferns little.

Imaging tests: Imaging of suspected masses and other lesions usually involves ultrasonography, which may be done in the office; both transvaginal and transabdominal probes are used.

MRI is highly specific but expensive.

CT is usually less desirable because it is somewhat less accurate, involves significant radiation exposure, and often requires a radiopaque agent.

Laparoscopy: This surgical procedure can detect structural abnormalities too small to be detected by imaging, as well as abnormalities on the surfaces of internal organs (eg, endometriosis, inflammation, scarring). It is also used to sample tissue.

Culdocentesis: Culdocentesis, now rarely used, is needle puncture of the posterior vaginal fornix to obtain fluid from the cul-de-sac (which is posterior to the uterus) for culture and for tests to detect blood from a ruptured ectopic pregnancy or ovarian cyst.

Endometrial aspiration: This procedure is done if women > 35 have unexplained vaginal bleeding. A thin, flexible, plastic suction curette is inserted through the cervix to the level of the uterine fundus; dilation is often not required. Suction is applied to the device, which is turned 360° and moved up and down a few times to sample different parts of the endometrial cavity. Sometimes the uterus must be stabilized with a cervical tenaculum.

Other tests: Pituitary and hypothalamic hormones and ovarian hormones may be measured when infertility is evaluated or when abnormalities are suspected.

Other tests may be done for specific clinical indications. They include the following:

- Colposcopy: Examination of the vagina and cervix with a magnifying lens (eg, to identify areas that require biopsy)
- Endocervical curettage: Insertion of a curet to obtain tissue from deep inside the cervical canal (eg, used with colposcopy-directed biopsy to diagnose cervical cancer)
- Dilation and curettage (D & C): Spreading of the vaginal walls with a speculum and insertion of a curet to remove tissue from the endometrium or the uterine contents by scraping or scooping (eg, to treat incomplete abortions)
- Hysterosalpingography: Fluoroscopic imaging of the uterus and fallopian tubes after injection of a radiopaque agent into the uterus (eg, to remove pelvic and intrauterine lesions, which may interfere with fertilization or implantation or cause dysmenorrhea)
- Hysteroscopy: Insertion of a thin viewing tube (hysteroscope) through the vagina and cervix into the uterus (used to view the interior of the uterus and identify abnormalities and/or to do some surgical procedures using instruments threaded through the laparoscope)
- Loop electrical excision procedure (LEEP): Use of a thin wire loop that conducts an electrical current to remove tissue (eg, for biopsy or as treatment)
- Sonohysterography (saline infusion sonography): Injection of isotonic fluid through the cervix into the uterus during ultrasonography (eg, to detect and evaluate small endometrial polyps, other uterine abnormalities, and tubal lesions)

263 Symptoms of Gynecologic Disorders

PELVIC MASS

A pelvic mass may be detected during routine gynecologic examination.

Etiology

Pelvic masses may originate from gynecologic organs (cervix, uterus, uterine adnexa) or from other pelvic organs (intestine, bladder, ureters, skeletal muscle, bone).

Type of mass tends to vary by age group.

In **infants**, in utero maternal hormones may stimulate development of adnexal cysts during the first few months of life. This effect is rare.

At **puberty,** menstrual fluid may accumulate and form a vaginal mass (hematocolpos) because outflow is obstructed. The cause is usually an imperforate hymen; other causes include congenital malformations of the uterus, cervix, or vagina.

In **women of reproductive age,** the most common cause of symmetric uterine enlargement is pregnancy, which may be unsuspected. Another common cause is fibroids, which may extend outward. Common adnexal masses include graafian follicles (usually 5 to 8 cm) that develop normally but do not release an egg (called functional ovarian cysts). These cysts often resolve spontaneously within a few months. Adnexal masses may also result from ectopic pregnancy, ovarian cancer, fallopian tube cancer, benign tumors (eg, benign cystic teratomas), or hydrosalpinges. Endometriosis can cause single or multiple masses anywhere in the pelvis, usually on the ovaries.

In **postmenopausal women,** masses are more likely to be cancerous. Many benign ovarian masses (eg, endometriomas, myomas) depend on ovarian hormone secretion and thus become less common after menopause.

Evaluation

History: General medical and complete gynecologic histories are obtained. Findings may suggest a cause:

- Vaginal bleeding and pelvic pain: Ectopic pregnancy or, rarely, gestational trophoblastic disease
- Dysmenorrhea: Endometriosis or uterine fibroids

- In young girls, precocious puberty: A masculinizing or feminizing ovarian tumor
- In women, virilization: A masculinizing ovarian tumor
- Menometrorrhagia or postmenopausal bleeding: A feminizing ovarian tumor

Examination: During the general examination, the examiner should look for signs of nongynecologic (eg, GI, endocrine) disorders and for ascites. A complete gynecologic examination is done.

Distinguishing uterine from adnexal masses may be difficult. Endometriomas are usually adnexal masses. Advanced endometriosis can manifest as nonmobile cul-de-sac masses. Adnexal cancers, benign tumors (eg, benign cystic teratomas), and adnexal masses due to ectopic pregnancy are often mobile. Hydrosalpinges are usually fluctuant, tender, nonmobile, and sometimes bilateral.

In young girls, pelvic organ masses may be palpable in the abdomen because the pelvis is too small to contain a large mass.

Testing: If the presence or origin (gynecologic vs nongynecologic) of a mass cannot be determined clinically, an imaging test can usually do so. Usually, pelvic ultrasonography is done first. If it does not clearly delineate size, location, and consistency of the mass, another imaging test (eg, CT, MRI) may. Ovarian masses with radiographic characteristics of cancer (eg, a solid component, surface excrescences, irregular shape) require needle aspiration or biopsy. Tumor markers may help in the diagnosis of specific tumors.

Women of reproductive age are tested for pregnancy; if the test is positive, ultrasonography or other imaging is not always necessary unless ectopic pregnancy is suspected. In women of reproductive age, simple, thin-walled cystic adnexal masses that are 5 to 8 cm (usually graafian follicular cysts) do not require further investigation unless they persist for > 3 menstrual cycles or are accompanied by moderate to severe pain.

KEY POINTS

- Type of pelvic mass tends to vary by age group.
- In women of reproductive age, the most common cause of symmetric uterine enlargement is pregnancy; other common causes of pelvic masses are fibroids and functional ovarian cysts.
- In postmenopausal women, masses are more likely to be cancerous.
- In women of reproductive age, do a pregnancy test.
- If clinical evaluation is inconclusive, do an imaging test; usually, pelvic ultrasonography is done first.

PELVIC PAIN

Pelvic pain is discomfort in the lower torso; it is a common complaint in women. It is considered separately from perineal pain, which occurs in the external genitals and nearby perineal skin.

Etiology

Pelvic pain may originate in reproductive organs (cervix, uterus, uterine adnexa) or other organs. Sometimes the cause is unknown.

Gynecologic disorders: Some gynecologic disorders (see Table 263–1) cause cyclic pain (ie, pain recurring during the same phase of the menstrual cycle). In others, pain is a discrete event unrelated to menstrual cycles. Whether onset of pain is sudden or gradual helps discriminate between the two.

Overall, the most common gynecologic causes of pelvic pain include

- Dysmenorrhea
- Ovulation (mittelschmerz)
- Endometriosis

Uterine fibroids can cause pelvic pain if they are degenerating or if their located in the uterus results in excessive bleeding or cramping. Most uterine fibroids do not cause pain.

Nongynecologic disorders: Nongynecologic disorders that can cause pelvic pain may be

- GI (eg, tumors, constipation, high perirectal abscess)
- Urinary (eg, cystitis, interstitial cystitis, calculi)
- Musculoskeletal (eg, diastasis of the pubic symphysis due to previous vaginal deliveries, abdominal muscle strains)
- Psychogenic (eg, somatization; effects of previous physical, psychologic, or sexual abuse)

The most common is difficult to specify.

Evaluation

Evaluation of pelvic pain must be expeditious because some causes of pelvic pain (eg, ectopic pregnancy, adnexal torsion) require immediate treatment.

Pregnancy should be excluded in women of childbearing age regardless of stated history.

History: History of present illness should include gynecologic history (gravity, parity, menstrual history, history of sexually transmitted disease) and onset, duration, location, and character of pain. Quality, acuity, severity, and location of pain and its relationship to the menstrual cycle are noted and can suggest the most likely causes. Important associated symptoms include vaginal bleeding or discharge and symptoms of hemodynamic instability (eg, dizziness, light-headedness, syncope or near-syncope).

Review of systems should seek symptoms suggesting possible causes, including the following:

- Morning sickness, breast swelling or tenderness, or missed menses: Pregnancy
- Fever and chills: Infection
- Abdominal pain, nausea, vomiting, or change in stool habits: GI disorders
- Urinary frequency, urgency, or dysuria: Urinary disorders

Past medical history should note history of infertility, ectopic pregnancy, pelvic inflammatory disease, urolithiasis, diverticulitis, and any GI or GU cancers. Any previous abdominal or pelvic surgery should be noted.

Physical examination: The physical examination begins with review of vital signs for signs of instability (eg, fever, hypotension) and focuses on abdominal and pelvic examinations.

The abdomen is palpated for tenderness, masses, and peritoneal signs. Rectal examination is done to check for tenderness, masses, and occult blood. Location of pain and any associated findings may provide clues to the cause (see Table 263–2).

Pelvic examination includes inspection of external genitals, speculum examination, and bimanual examination. The cervix is inspected for discharge, uterine prolapse, and cervical stenosis or lesions. Bimanual examination should assess cervical motion tenderness, adnexal masses or tenderness, and uterine enlargement or tenderness.

Table 263–1. SOME GYNECOLOGIC CAUSES OF PELVIC PAIN

CAUSE	SUGGESTIVE FINDINGS	DIAGNOSTIC APPROACH*
Related to menstrual cycle		
Dysmenorrhea	Sharp or crampy pain a few days before or at onset of menses, often with headache, nausea, constipation, diarrhea, or urinary frequency Symptoms usually peaking in 24 h but sometimes persisting for 2–3 days after onset of menses	Clinical evaluation
Endometriosis	Sharp or crampy pain before and during early menses, often with dysmenorrhea, dyspareunia, or painful defecation May eventually cause pain unrelated to the menstrual cycle In advanced stages, sometimes uterine retroversion, tenderness, decreased mobility Sometimes a fixed pelvic mass (possibly an endometrioma) or tender nodules noted during bimanual vaginal and rectovaginal examination	Clinical evaluation Laparoscopy
Mittelschmerz	Sudden onset of severe, sharp pain, most intense at onset and abating over 1–2 days Often accompanied by light spotty vaginal bleeding Occurring midcycle (during ovulation), caused by mild, brief peritoneal irritation due to a ruptured follicular cyst	Clinical evaluation Diagnosis of exclusion
Unrelated to menstrual cycle		
Pelvic inflammatory disease	Gradual onset of pelvic pain, mucopurulent cervical discharge Sometimes fever, dysuria, dyspareunia Typically, marked cervical motion tenderness and adnexal tenderness Rarely, an adnexal mass (eg, abscess)	Clinical evaluation Cervical culture Sometimes pelvic ultrasonography (if abscess is suspected)
Ruptured ovarian cyst	Sudden onset of pain, most severe at onset and often rapidly decreasing over a few hours Sometimes with slight vaginal bleeding, nausea, vomiting, and peritoneal signs	Clinical evaluation Sometimes pelvic ultrasonography
Ruptured ectopic pregnancy	Sudden onset of localized, constant (not crampy) pain, often with vaginal bleeding and sometimes syncope or hemorrhagic shock Closed cervical os Sometimes acute abdominal distention or tender adnexal mass	Quantitative beta-hCG measurement Pelvic ultrasonography Sometimes laparoscopy or laparotomy
Acute degeneration of uterine fibroid	Sudden onset of pain, vaginal bleeding Most common during the first 12 wk of pregnancy or after delivery or termination of a pregnancy	Pelvic ultrasonography
Adnexal torsion	Sudden onset of severe, unilateral pain, occasionally colicky (because of intermittent torsion) Often with nausea, vomiting, peritoneal signs, and cervical motion tenderness Presence of risk factors (eg, pregnancy, induction of ovulation, ovarian enlargement to > 4 cm)	Pelvic ultrasonography with color Doppler flow studies Sometimes laparoscopy or laparotomy
Uterine cancer or ovarian cancer	Gradual onset of pain, vaginal discharge (which precedes bleeding), abnormal vaginal bleeding (eg, postmenopausal bleeding, premenopausal recurrent metrorrhagia) Rarely, a palpable pelvic mass	Pelvic ultrasonography Biopsy Sometimes additional tests such as hysteroscopy or saline-infusion sonohysterography to help identify abnormalities in the endometrium
Adhesions	Gradual onset of pelvic pain (often becoming chronic) or dyspareunia in patients who have had abdominal surgery or sometimes pelvic infections No vaginal bleeding or discharge Sometimes nausea and vomiting (suggesting intestinal obstruction)	Clinical evaluation Diagnosis of exclusion Sometimes abdominal obstruction series (flat and upright abdominal x-rays)
Spontaneous abortion	Vaginal bleeding associated with crampy lower abdominal pain or back pain during early pregnancy and accompanied by other symptoms of early pregnancy, such as breast tenderness, nausea, and delayed menses	Clinical evaluation Pregnancy test Pelvic ultrasonography to assess viability of pregnancy

*Pelvic examination, urinalysis, and a urine or serum pregnancy test should be done. Most patients with acute or significant recurrent symptoms require pelvic ultrasonography.

Beta-hCG = beta subunit of human chorionic gonadotropin.

Red flags: The following findings are of particular concern:

- Syncope or hemorrhagic shock (eg, tachycardia, hypotension)
- Peritoneal signs (rebound, rigidity, guarding)
- Postmenopausal vaginal bleeding
- Fever or chills
- Sudden severe pain with nausea, vomiting, diaphoresis, or agitation

Interpretation of findings: Acuity and severity of pelvic pain and its relationship to menstrual cycles can suggest the most likely causes (see Table 263–1). Quality and location of pain and associated findings also provide clues (see Table 263–2). However, findings can be nonspecific. For example, endometriosis can result in a wide variety of findings.

Testing: All patients with pelvic pain should have

- Urinalysis
- Urine pregnancy test

If a patient is pregnant, ectopic pregnancy is assumed until excluded by ultrasonography or, if ultrasonography is unclear, by other tests (see p. 2324). If a suspected pregnancy may be < 5 wk, a serum pregnancy test should be done; a urine pregnancy test may not be sensitive enough to rule out pregnancy that early in gestation.

Other testing depends on which disorders are clinically suspected. If a patient cannot be adequately examined (eg, because of pain or inability to cooperate) or if a mass is suspected, pelvic ultrasonography is done. If the cause of severe or persistent pain remains unidentified, laparoscopy is done.

Pelvic ultrasonography using a vaginal probe can be a useful adjunct to pelvic examination; it can better define a mass or help diagnose a pregnancy after 5 wk gestation (ie, 1 wk after a missed menstrual period). For example, free pelvic fluid and a positive pregnancy test plus no evidence of an intrauterine pregnancy help confirm ectopic pregnancy.

Treatment

The underlying disorder is treated when possible.

Pelvic pain is initially treated with oral NSAIDs. Patients who do not respond well to one NSAID may respond to another. If NSAIDs are ineffective, other analgesics or hypnosis may be tried.

Musculoskeletal pain may also require rest, heat, physical therapy, or, for fibromyalgia, injection of tender points with 0.5% bupivacaine or 1% lidocaine.

If patients have intractable pain, hysterectomy can be done, but it may be ineffective.

Geriatrics Essentials

Pelvic pain symptoms in elderly women may be vague. Careful review of systems with attention to bowel and bladder function is essential.

Table 263–2. SOME CLUES TO DIAGNOSIS OF PELVIC PAIN

FINDING	POSSIBLE DIAGNOSIS
Syncope or hemorrhagic shock	Ruptured ectopic pregnancy Possibly a ruptured ovarian cyst
Vaginal discharge, fever, bilateral pain and tenderness	Pelvic inflammatory disease
Severe, intermittent colicky pain (sometimes with nausea), which may develop and reach peak intensity within seconds or minutes	Adnexal torsion Renal colic Ectopic pregnancy
Nausea followed by anorexia, fever, and right-sided pain	Appendicitis
Constipation, diarrhea, relief or worsening of pain during defecation	GI disorder
Left lower quadrant pain in women > 40	Diverticulitis
Generalized abdominal tenderness or peritoneal signs	Peritonitis (eg, due to appendicitis, diverticulitis, another GI disorder, pelvic inflammatory disease, adnexal torsion, or rupture of an ovarian cyst or ectopic pregnancy)
Tenderness in the anterior vaginal wall	Lower urinary tract disorder (eg, interstitial cystitis), causing bladder or urethral pain
Uterine fixation detected by bimanual examination	Adhesions Endometriosis Late-stage cancer
Tender adnexal mass or tenderness with cervical motion	Ectopic pregnancy Pelvic inflammatory disease Ovarian cyst or tumor Adnexal torsion
Tenderness of the pubic bone in parous women, particularly if pain occurs during ambulation	Diastasis of the pubic symphysis
Acute, painful defecation plus localized, tender, fluctuant mass felt during internal or external rectal examination; with or without fever	Perirectal abscess
Gross or microscopic rectal blood	GI disorder
Chronic painful defecation plus localized, firm woody mass felt during internal or external rectal examination; without fever	Severe endometriosis Late-stage cervical cancer

In elderly women, common causes of pelvic pain may be different because some disorders that cause pelvic pain become more common as women age, particularly after menopause. These disorders include

- Cystitis
- Constipation
- Pelvic relaxation syndromes
- Many cancers of the reproductive tract, including cancers of the endometrium, fallopian tubes, ovaries, and vagina

A sexual history should be obtained; clinicians often do not realize that many women remain sexually active throughout their life. Whether a woman's partner is living should be determined before inquiring about sexual activity. In elderly women, vaginal irritation, itching, urinary symptoms, or bleeding may occur secondary to sexual intercourse. Such problems often resolve after a few days of pelvic rest.

Acute loss of appetite, weight loss, dyspepsia, or a sudden change in bowel habits may be signs of ovarian or uterine cancer and requires thorough clinical evaluation.

KEY POINTS

- Pelvic pain is common and may have a gynecologic or nongynecologic cause.
- Pregnancy should be ruled out in women of childbearing age.
- Quality, acuity, severity, and location of pain and its relationship to the menstrual cycle can suggest the most likely causes.
- Dysmenorrhea is a common cause of pelvic pain but is a diagnosis of exclusion.

VAGINAL BLEEDING

Abnormal vaginal bleeding includes

- Menses that are excessive (menorrhagia or hypermenorrhea) or too frequent (polymenorrhea)
- Bleeding that is unrelated to menses, occurring irregularly between menses (metrorrhagia)
- Bleeding that is excessive during menses and occurs irregularly between menses (menometrorrhagia)
- Postmenopausal bleeding (ie, > 6 mo after the last normal menses)

Vaginal bleeding may also occur during early pregnancy (see p. 2326) or late pregnancy (see p. 2332).

Vaginal bleeding can originate anywhere in the genital tract, including the vulva, vagina, cervix, and uterus. When vaginal bleeding originates in the uterus, it is called abnormal uterine bleeding (AUB—see p. 2285).

Pathophysiology

Most abnormal vaginal bleeding involves

- Hormonal abnormalities in the hypothalamic-pituitary-ovarian axis (most common)
- Structural, inflammatory, or other gynecologic disorders (eg, tumors)
- Bleeding disorders (uncommon)

With hormonal causes, ovulation does not occur or occurs infrequently. During an anovulatory cycle, the corpus luteum does not form, and thus the normal cyclical secretion of progesterone does not occur. Without progesterone, estrogen causes the endometrium to continue to proliferate, eventually outgrowing its blood supply. The endometrium then sloughs and bleeds incompletely, irregularly, and sometimes profusely or for a long time.

Etiology

Causes in adults (see Table 263–3) and children (see Table 263–4) vary.

During the reproductive years, common causes of vaginal bleeding in women who are not known to be pregnant include

- AUB, particularly anovulatory bleeding
- Complications of an early, undiagnosed pregnancy
- Submucous myoma
- Midcycle bleeding associated with ovulation
- Breakthrough bleeding while women are taking oral contraceptives

Anovulatory uterine bleeding is the most common cause of abnormal vaginal bleeding during the reproductive years.

Table 263–3. SOME CAUSES OF ABNORMAL VAGINAL BLEEDING IN ADULT WOMEN

CATEGORY	CONDITIONS
Early pregnancy* and related complications	Spontaneous abortion (patients may present immediately during the abortion or later because of bleeding due to retained products of conception) Ectopic pregnancy
Late pregnancy* and related complications	Abruptio placentae Gestational trophoblastic disease Placental polyps Placenta previa
Structural gynecologic disorders	Adenomyosis Vaginal cancer, cervical cancer, or endometrial cancer Endometrial hyperplasia Endometriosis Fibroids (submucosal or prolapsed) Polyps of the cervix or endometrium
Other gynecologic disorders	Atrophic vaginitis Cervicitis Foreign body in the vagina Injury of the cervix, vagina, or vulva Vaginitis
Ovulatory disorders	Anovulatory bleeding Functional ovarian cysts (may be a sign of anovulation) Polycystic ovary syndrome
Endocrine disorders	Hyperprolactinemia Thyroid disorders (eg, hypothyroidism)
Bleeding disorders	Coagulation disorders (eg, due to drugs, liver disorders, or hereditary disorders) Platelet disorders
Contraception and hormone therapy	Depot medroxyprogesterone injections Hormone replacement therapy Intrauterine devices Levonorgestrel implants Oral contraceptives, particularly when doses are missed or when long-cycle regimens or progestin only is used

*At presentation, patients may not suspect pregnancy of any stage (including recent spontaneous abortion).

Table 263–4. COMMON CAUSES OF VAGINAL BLEEDING IN CHILDREN

AGE GROUP	CAUSES
Infants	In utero endometrial stimulation by transplacental estrogens (causes minimal bleeding during the first 2 wk of life)
Older children	Precocious puberty with premature menses Prolapse of the urethral meatus Trauma (including sexual abuse) Tumors (eg, sarcoma botryoides, cervical adenocarcinoma secondary to DES exposure) Vaginal foreign body Warts, cervical or vaginal

DES = diethylstilbestrol.

Causes of AUB in nonpregnant women of reproductive age may be classified as structural or nonstructural as in the PALM-COEIN classification system (see Fig. 263–1).[1,2] PALM-COEIN is a mnemonic for the structural causes (PALM) and the nonstructural (COEIN) causes.

Vaginitis, foreign bodies, trauma, and sexual abuse are common causes of vaginal bleeding before menarche.

1. Practice bulletin no. 128: Diagnosis of abnormal uterine bleeding in reproductive-aged women. *Obstet Gynecol* 120(1):197–206, 2012. doi: 10.1097/AOG.0b013e318262e320.
2. Practice bulletin no. 136: Management of abnormal uterine bleeding associated with ovulatory dysfunction. *Obstet Gynecol* 122(1):176–185, 2013. doi: 10.1097/01.AOG.0000431815.52679.bb.

Evaluation

Unrecognized pregnancy must be suspected and diagnosed in women of childbearing age because some causes of bleeding during pregnancy (eg, ectopic pregnancy) are life-threatening.

History: History of present illness should include quantity (eg, by number of pads used per day or hour) and duration of bleeding, as well as the relationship of bleeding to menses and intercourse. Clinicians should ask about the following:

- Menstrual history, including date of last normal menstrual period, age at menarche and menopause (when appropriate), cycle length and regularity, and quantity and duration of typical menstrual bleeding
- Previous episodes of abnormal bleeding, including frequency, duration, quantity, and pattern (cyclicity) of bleeding
- Sexual history, including possible history of rape or sexual assault

Review of systems should seek symptoms of possible causes, including the following:

- Missed menses, breast swelling, and nausea: Pregnancy-related bleeding
- Abdominal pain, light-headedness, and syncope: Ectopic pregnancy or ruptured ovarian cyst
- Chronic pain and weight loss: Cancer
- Easy bruising and excessive bleeding due to toothbrushing, minor lacerations, or venipuncture: A bleeding disorder

Past medical history should identify disorders known to cause bleeding, including a recent spontaneous or therapeutic abortion and structural disorders (eg, uterine fibroids, ovarian cysts). Clinicians should identify risk factors for endometrial cancer, including obesity, diabetes, hypertension, prolonged unopposed estrogen use (ie, without progesterone), and polycystic ovary syndrome. Drug history should include specific questions about hormone use.

If sexual abuse of a child is suspected, a structured forensic interview based on the National Institute of Child Health and Human Development (NICHD) Protocol can be used. It helps the child report information about the experienced event and improves the quality of information obtained.

Physical examination: Vital signs are reviewed for signs of hypovolemia (eg, tachycardia, tachypnea, hypotension).

During the general examination, clinicians should look for signs of anemia (eg, conjunctival pallor) and evidence of possible causes of bleeding, including the following:

- Warm and moist or dry skin, eye abnormalities, tremor, abnormal reflexes, or goiter: A thyroid disorder
- Hepatomegaly, jaundice, asterixis (flapping tremor of the wrist), or splenomegaly: A liver disorder
- Nipple discharge: Hyperprolactinemia
- Low body mass index and loss of subcutaneous fat: Possibly anovulation

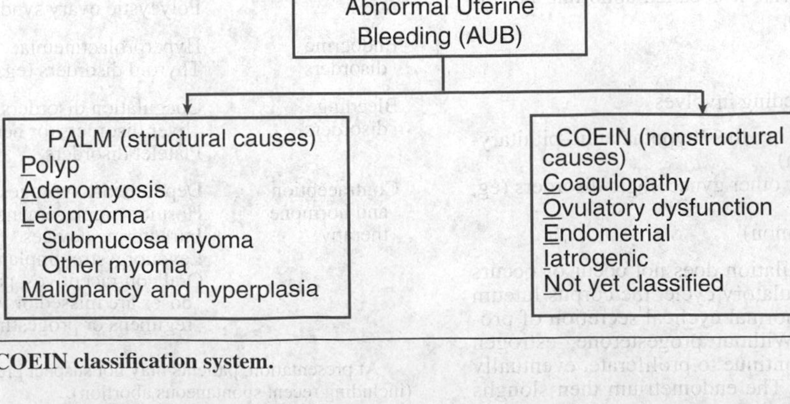

Abnormal Uterine Bleeding (AUB)

PALM (structural causes)
Polyp
Adenomyosis
Leiomyoma
Submucosa myoma
Other myoma
Malignancy and hyperplasia

COEIN (nonstructural causes)
Coagulopathy
Ovulatory dysfunction
Endometrial
Iatrogenic
Not yet classified

Fig. 263–1. PALM-COEIN classification system.

- High body mass index and excess subcutaneous fat: Androgen or estrogen excess or polycystic ovary syndrome
- Hirsutism, acne, obesity, and enlarged ovaries: Polycystic ovary syndrome
- Easy bruising, petechiae, purpura, or mucosal (eg, gingival) bleeding: A bleeding disorder
- In children, breast development and presence of pubic and axillary hair: Puberty
- In children, difficulty walking or sitting; bruises or tears around the genitals, anus, or mouth; and/or vaginal discharge or pruritus: Sexual abuse

The abdomen is examined for distention, tenderness, and masses (particularly an enlarged uterus). If the uterus is enlarged, auscultation for fetal heart sounds is done.

A complete gynecologic examination is done unless abdominal examination suggests a late-stage pregnancy; then, digital pelvic examination is contraindicated until placental position is determined. In all other cases, speculum examination helps identify lesions of the urethra, vagina, and cervix. Bimanual examination is done to evaluate uterine size and ovarian enlargement. If no blood is present in the vagina, rectal examination is done to determine whether bleeding is GI in origin.

Red flags: The following findings are of particular concern:

- Hemorrhagic shock (tachycardia, hypotension)
- Premenarchal and postmenopausal vaginal bleeding
- Vaginal bleeding in pregnant patients
- Excessive bleeding
- In children, difficulty walking or sitting; bruises or tears around the genitals, anus, or mouth; and/or vaginal discharge or pruritus

Interpretation of findings: Significant hypovolemia or hemorrhagic shock is unlikely except with ruptured ectopic pregnancy or, rarely, ovarian cyst (particularly when a tender pelvic mass is present).

In **children,** breast development and pubic or axillary hair suggest precocious puberty and premature menses. In those without such findings, the possibility of sexual abuse should be investigated unless an explanatory lesion or foreign body is obvious.

In **women of reproductive age,** examination may detect a causative gynecologic lesion or other findings suggesting a cause. If younger patients taking hormone therapy have no apparent abnormalities during examination and bleeding is spotty, bleeding is probably related to the hormone therapy. If the problem is excessive menstrual bleeding only, a uterine disorder or bleeding diathesis should be considered. Inherited bleeding disorders may initially manifest as heavy menstrual bleeding beginning at menarche or during adolescence.

In **postmenopausal women,** gynecologic cancer should be suspected.

If abnormal bleeding does not result from any of the usual causes, it may be related to changes in the hormonal control of the menstrual cycle.

Testing: All women of reproductive age require

- A urine pregnancy test

During early pregnancy (before 5 wk), a urine pregnancy test may not be sensitive enough. Urine contaminated with blood may lead to false results. A qualitative serum beta subunit of human chorionic gonadotropin (beta-hCG) test should be done if the urine test is negative and pregnancy is suspected. Vaginal bleeding during pregnancy requires a specific approach (see pp. 2326 and 2332).

Blood tests include CBC if bleeding is unusually heavy (eg, > 1 pad or tampon/h) or has lasted at least several days or if findings suggest anemia or hypovolemia. If anemia is identified and is not obviously due to iron deficiency (eg, based on microcytic, hypochromic RBC indices), iron studies are done.

Thyroid-stimulating hormone and prolactin levels are usually measured, even when galactorrhea is absent.

If a bleeding disorder is suspected, von Willebrand factor, platelet count, PT, and PTT are determined.

If polycystic ovary syndrome is suspected, testosterone and dehydroepiandrosterone sulfate (DHEAS) levels are measured.

Imaging includes transvaginal ultrasonography if women have any of the following:

- Age > 35
- Risk factors for endometrial cancer
- Bleeding that continues despite use of empiric hormone therapy

Focal thickening of the endometrium that is detected during screening ultrasonography may require hysteroscopy or saline-infusion sonohysterography to identify small intrauterine masses (eg, endometrial polyps, submucous myomas).

Other testing includes endometrial sampling if examination and ultrasonography are inconclusive in women with any of the following:

- Age > 35
- Risk factors for cancer
- Endometrial thickening > 4 mm

Sampling can be done by aspiration or, if the cervical canal requires dilation, by D & C. In postmenopausal women, hysteroscopy with D & C is recommended so that the entire uterine cavity can be assessed.

Treatment

Hemorrhagic shock is treated. Women with iron deficiency anemia may require supplemental oral iron.

Definitive treatment of vaginal bleeding is directed at the cause. Typically, hormones, usually oral contraceptives, are first-line treatment for anovulatory AUB.

Geriatrics Essentials

Postmenopausal bleeding (bleeding > 6 mo after menopause) is abnormal in most women and requires further evaluation to exclude cancer unless it clearly results from withdrawal of exogenous hormones.

In women not taking exogenous hormones, the most common cause of postmenopausal bleeding is endometrial and vaginal atrophy.

In some older women, physical examination of the vagina can be difficult because lack of estrogen leads to increased friability of the vaginal mucosa, vaginal stenosis, and sometimes adhesions in the vagina. For these patients, a pediatric speculum may be more comfortable.

KEY POINTS

- Pregnancy must be excluded in women of reproductive age even when history does not suggest it.
- Anovulatory uterine bleeding is the most common cause of abnormal vaginal bleeding during the reproductive years.
- Vaginitis, foreign bodies, trauma, and sexual abuse are common causes of vaginal bleeding before menarche.
- Postmenopausal vaginal bleeding needs further evaluation to exclude cancer as the cause.

VAGINAL ITCHING AND DISCHARGE

Vaginal itching (pruritus), discharge, or both result from infectious or noninfectious inflammation of the vaginal mucosa (vaginitis—see p. 2311), often with inflammation of the vulva (vulvovaginitis). Symptoms may also include irritation, burning, erythema, and sometimes dysuria and dyspareunia. Symptoms of vaginitis are one of the most common gynecologic complaints.

Pathophysiology

Some vaginal discharge is normal, particularly when estrogenlevels are high. Estrogen levels are high in the following situations:

- A few days before ovulation
- During the first 2 wk of life (because maternal estrogens are transferred before birth)
- During the few months before menarche and during pregnancy (when estrogen production increases)
- With use of drugs that contain estrogen or that increase estrogen production (eg, some fertility drugs)

However, irritation, burning, and pruritus are never normal.

Normally in women of reproductive age, *Lactobacillus* sp is the predominant constituent of normal vaginal flora. Colonization by these bacteria keeps vaginal pH in the normal range (3.8 to 4.2), thereby preventing overgrowth of pathogenic bacteria. Also, high estrogen levels maintain vaginal thickness, bolstering local defenses.

Factors that predispose to overgrowth of bacterial vaginal pathogens include

- Use of antibiotics (which may decrease lactobacilli)
- Alkaline vaginal pH due to menstrual blood, semen, or a decrease in lactobacilli
- Poor hygiene
- Frequent douching
- Pregnancy
- Diabetes mellitus
- An intravaginal foreign body (eg, a forgotten tampon or vaginal pessary)

Etiology

The most common causes vary by patient age (see Table 263–5).

Children: Vaginitis usually involves infection with GI tract flora (nonspecific vulvovaginitis). A common contributing factor in girls aged 2 to 6 yr is poor perineal hygiene (eg, wiping from back to front after bowel movements, not washing their hands after bowel movements).

Table 263–5. SOME CAUSES OF VAGINAL PRURITUS AND DISCHARGE

CAUSE	SUGGESTIVE FINDINGS	DIAGNOSTIC APPROACH*
Children		
Poor perineal hygiene	Pruritus, vulvovaginal erythema, vaginal odor, sometimes dysuria, no discharge	Diagnosis of exclusion
Chemical irritation (eg, soaps, bubble baths)	Vulvovaginal erythema and soreness, often recurrent and accompanied by pruritus and dysuria	Clinical evaluation
Foreign bodies (often toilet paper)	Vaginal discharge, usually with a foul odor and vaginal spotting	Clinical evaluation (may require a topical anesthetic or procedural sedation)
Infections (eg, candidal, pinworm, streptococcal, staphylococcal)	Pruritus and vaginal discharge with vulvar erythema and swelling, often with dysuria Worsening of pruritus at night (suggesting pinworm infection) Significant erythema and vulvar edema with discharge (suggesting streptococcal or staphylococcal infection)	Microscopic examination of vaginal secretions for yeast and hyphae and culture to confirm Examination of vulva and anus for pinworms
Sexual abuse	Vulvovaginal soreness, bloody or malodorous vaginal discharge Often, vague and nonspecific medical complaints (eg, fatigue, abdominal pain) or behavior changes (eg, temper tantrums)	Clinical evaluation Cultures or PCR for sexually transmitted diseases Measures to ensure the child's safety and a report to state authorities if abuse is suspected
Women of reproductive age		
Bacterial vaginosis	Malodorous (fishy), thin, gray vaginal discharge with pruritus and irritation Erythema and edema uncommon	Criteria for diagnosis (3 of 4): • Gray discharge • Vaginal secretion pH > 4.5 • Fishy odor to discharge • Clue cells seen during microscopic examination
Candidal infection	Vulvar and vaginal irritation, edema, pruritus Discharge that resembles cottage cheese and adheres to the vaginal wall Sometimes worsening of symptoms after intercourse and before menses Sometimes recent antibiotic use or history of diabetes	Clinical evaluation plus • Vaginal pH < 4.5 • Yeast or hyphae identified on a wet mount or KOH preparation Sometimes culture

Table 263–5. SOME CAUSES OF VAGINAL PRURITUS AND DISCHARGE (*Continued*)

CAUSE	SUGGESTIVE FINDINGS	DIAGNOSTIC APPROACH*
Trichomonal infection	Yellow-green, frothy vaginal discharge, often with a fishy odor Often soreness, erythema, and edema of the vulva and vagina Sometimes dysuria and dyspareunia Sometimes punctate, red "strawberry" spots on the vaginal walls or cervix Mild cervical motion tenderness often detected during bimanual examination	Motile, pear-shaped flagellated organisms seen during microscopic examination Rapid diagnostic assay for *Trichomonas*, if available
Foreign bodies (often a forgotten tampon)	Extremely malodorous, often profuse vaginal discharge, often with vaginal erythema, dysuria, and sometimes dyspareunia Object visible during examination	Clinical evaluation
Pelvic inflammatory disease	Abdominal or pelvic pain Fever Cervical motion and/or adnexal tenderness	Cultures or PCR for sexually transmitted diseases
Postmenopausal women		
Atrophic (inflammatory) vaginitis	Dyspareunia, scant discharge, thin and dry vaginal tissue	Clinical evaluation plus • Vaginal pH > 6 • No fishy odor to discharge • Increased number of neutrophils, parabasal cells, and cocci and decreased number of bacilli seen during microscopic examination
Vaginal cancer, cervical cancer, or endometrial cancer	Gradual onset of pain, a watery or bloody vaginal discharge (which precedes bleeding), abnormal vaginal bleeding (eg, postmenopausal bleeding, premenopausal recurrent metrorrhagia) Often no other symptoms until the cancer is advanced Sometimes weight loss Rarely, a palpable pelvic mass	Pelvic ultrasonography Biopsy
Chemical vulvitis due to irritation from urine or feces	Diffuse redness Risk factors (eg, incontinence, restriction to bed rest)	Clinical evaluation
All ages		
Hypersensitivity reactions	Vulvovaginal erythema, edema, pruritus (often intense), vaginal discharge History of recent use of hygiene sprays or perfume, bath water additives, topical treatment for candidal infections, fabric softeners, bleaches, or laundry soaps	Clinical evaluation Trial of avoidance
Inflammatory (eg, pelvic radiation, oophorectomy, chemotherapy)†	Purulent vaginal discharge, dyspareunia, dysuria, irritation Sometimes pruritus, erythema, burning pain, mild bleeding Thin, dry vaginal tissue	Diagnosis of exclusion based on history and risk factors Vaginal pH > 6 Negative whiff test Granulocytes and parabasal cells seen during microscopic examination
Enteric fistulas (complication of delivery, pelvic tumors, pelvic surgery, or inflammatory bowel disease)	Malodorous vaginal discharge with passage of feces from vagina	Direct visualization or palpation of the fistula in the lower part of the vagina CT with contrast Endoscopy
Skin disorders (eg, psoriasis, lichen sclerosus, tinea versicolor)	Characteristic genital and extragenital skin findings	Clinical evaluation Biopsy

*If discharge is present, microscopic examination of a saline wet mount and KOH preparation and cultures or PCR for sexually transmitted organisms are done (unless a noninfectious cause such as allergy or a foreign body is obvious).

†Such inflammatory conditions are an uncommon cause of vaginitis.

KOH = Potassium hydroxide.

Chemicals in bubble baths or soaps may cause inflammation and pruritus of the vulva, which often recur. Foreign bodies may cause nonspecific vaginitis, often with a scant bloody discharge.

Women of reproductive age: Vaginitis is usually infectious. The most common types are

- Bacterial vaginosis
- Candidal vaginitis
- Trichomonal vaginitis (usually sexually transmitted)

Sometimes another infection (eg, gonorrhea, chlamydial infection) causes a discharge. These infections often also cause pelvic inflammatory disease (see p. 2315).

Genital herpes sometimes causes vaginal itching but typically manifests with pain and ulceration (see p. 1623).

Vaginitis may also result from foreign bodies (eg, a forgotten tampon). Inflammatory noninfectious vaginitis is uncommon.

Postmenopausal women: In postmenopausal women (see also p. 2211), atrophic vaginitis is a common cause.

Other causes of discharge include vaginal cancer, cervical cancer, and endometrial cancer and, in women who are incontinent or bedbound, chemical vulvitis.

Women of all ages: At any age, conditions that predispose to vaginal or vulvar infection include

- Fistulas between the intestine and genital tract (which allow intestinal flora to seed the genital tract)
- Pelvic radiation or tumors (which break down tissue and thus compromise normal host defenses)

Fistulas are usually obstetric in origin (due to vaginal birth trauma or a complication of episiotomy infection) but are sometimes due to inflammatory bowel disease or pelvic tumors or occur as a complication of pelvic surgery (eg, hysterectomy, anal surgery).

Noninfectious vulvitis accounts for up to 30% of vulvovaginitis cases. It may result from hypersensitivity or irritant reactions to various agents, including hygiene sprays or perfumes, menstrual pads, laundry soaps, bleaches, fabric softeners, and sometimes spermicides, vaginal creams or lubricants, latex condoms, vaginal contraceptive rings, and diaphragms.

Evaluation

History: History of present illness includes nature of symptoms (eg, pruritus, burning, pain, discharge), duration, and intensity. If vaginal discharge is present, patients should be asked about the color and odor of the discharge and any exacerbating and remitting factors (particularly those related to menses and intercourse). They should also be asked about use of hygiene sprays or perfumes, spermicides, vaginal creams or lubricants, latex condoms, vaginal contraceptive rings, and diaphragms.

Review of systems should seek symptoms suggesting possible causes, including the following:

- Fever or chills and abdominal or suprapubic pain: Pelvic inflammatory disease (PID) or cystitis
- Polyuria and polydipsia: New-onset diabetes

Past medical history should note risk factors for candidal infection (eg, recent antibiotic use, diabetes, HIV infection, other immunosuppressive disorders), fistulas (eg, Crohn disease, GU or GI cancer, pelvic or rectal surgery, lacerations during delivery), and sexually transmitted diseases (eg, unprotected intercourse, multiple partners).

If sexual abuse of a child is suspected, a structured forensic interview based on the NICHD Protocol can be used. It helps the child report information about the experienced event and improves the quality of information obtained.

Physical examination: Physical examination focuses on the pelvic examination.

The external genitals are examined for erythema, excoriations, and swelling. A water-lubricated speculum is used to check the vaginal walls for erythema, discharge, and fistulas. The cervix is inspected for inflammation (eg, trichomoniasis) and discharge. Vaginal pH is measured, and samples of secretions are obtained for testing. A bimanual examination is done to identify cervical motion tenderness and adnexal or uterine tenderness (indicating PID).

Red flags: The following findings are of particular concern:

- Trichomonal vaginitis in children (suggesting sexual abuse)
- Fecal discharge (suggesting a fistula, even if not seen)
- Fever or pelvic pain
- Bloody discharge in postmenopausal women

Interpretation of findings: Often, the history and physical examination help suggest a diagnosis (see Table 263–5), although there can be much overlap.

In **children,** a vaginal discharge suggests a foreign body in the vagina. If no foreign body is present and children have trichomonal vaginitis, sexual abuse is likely. If they have unexplained vaginal discharge, cervicitis, which may be due to a sexually transmitted disease, should be considered. Nonspecific vulvovaginitis is a diagnosis of exclusion.

In **women of reproductive age,** discharge due to vaginitis must be distinguished from normal discharge:

- Normal vaginal discharge is commonly milky white or mucoid, odorless, and nonirritating; it can result in vaginal wetness that dampens underwear.
- Bacterial vaginosis produces a thin, gray discharge with a fishy odor.
- A trichomonal infection produces a frothy, yellow-green vaginal discharge and causes vulvovaginal soreness.
- Candidal vaginitis produces a white discharge that resembles cottage cheese, often increasing the week before menses; symptoms worsen after sexual intercourse.

Contact irritant or allergic reactions cause significant irritation and inflammation with comparatively minimal discharge.

Discharge due to cervicitis (eg, due to PID) can resemble that of vaginitis. Abdominal pain, cervical motion tenderness, or cervical inflammation suggests PID.

In **women of all ages,** vaginal pruritus and discharge may result from skin disorders (eg, psoriasis, lichen sclerosus, tinea versicolor), which can usually be differentiated by history and skin findings.

Discharge that is watery, bloody, or both may result from vulvar, vaginal, or cervical cancer; cancers can be differentiated from vaginitis by examination and biopsy.

In atrophic vaginitis, discharge is scant and may be watery and thin or thick and yellowish. Dyspareunia is common, and vaginal tissue appears thin and dry.

Testing: All patients require the following in-office testing:

- pH
- Wet mount
- Potassium hydroxide (KOH) preparation

Testing for gonorrhea and chlamydial infections is typically done unless a noninfectious cause (eg, allergy, foreign body) is obvious.

Vaginal secretions are tested using pH paper with 0.2 intervals from pH 4.0 to 6.0. Then, a cotton swab is used to place secretions on 2 slides; secretions are diluted with 0.9% sodium chloride on one slide (saline wet mount) and with 10% KOH on the other (KOH preparation).

The KOH preparation is sniffed (whiff test) for a fishy odor, which results from amines produced in trichomonal vaginitis and bacterial vaginosis. The slide is examined using a microscope; KOH dissolves most cellular material except yeast hyphae, making identification easier.

The saline wet mount is examined using a microscope as soon as possible to detect motile trichomonads, which can become immotile and more difficult to recognize within minutes after slide preparation.

If clinical criteria and in-office test results are inconclusive, the discharge may be cultured for fungi and trichomonads.

Treatment

Any specific cause is treated.

The vulva should be kept as clean as possible. Soaps and unnecessary topical preparations (eg, feminine hygiene sprays) should be avoided. If a soap is needed, a hypoallergenic soap should be used. Intermittent use of ice packs or warm sitz baths (with or without baking soda) may reduce soreness and pruritus. If chronic vulvar inflammation is due to being bedbound or incontinent, better vulvar hygiene may help.

If symptoms are moderate or severe or do not respond to other measures, drugs may be needed. For pruritus, topical corticosteroids (eg, 1% hydrocortisone bid prn) can be applied to the vulva but not into the vagina. Oral antihistamines lessen pruritus and cause drowsiness, helping patients sleep.

Prepubertal girls should be taught good perineal hygiene (eg, wiping front to back after bowel movements and voiding, washing their hands, avoiding fingering the perineum).

Geriatrics Essentials

In postmenopausal women, a marked decrease in estrogen causes vaginal thinning (atrophic vaginitis), increasing vulnerability to infection and inflammation. Other common causes of decreased estrogen in older women include oophorectomy, pelvic radiation, and certain chemotherapy drugs.

In atrophic vaginitis, inflammation often results in an abnormal discharge, which is scant and may be watery and thin or thick and yellowish. Dyspareunia is common, and vaginal tissue appears thin and dry.

Poor hygiene (eg, in patients who are incontinent or bedbound) can lead to chronic vulvar inflammation due to chemical irritation by urine or feces.

Bacterial vaginosis, candidal vaginitis, and trichomonal vaginitis are uncommon among postmenopausal women but may occur in those with risk factors.

After menopause, risk of cancer increases, and a bloody or watery discharge is more likely to be due to cancer; thus, any vaginal discharge in postmenopausal women should be promptly evaluated.

KEY POINTS

- Vaginal complaints are often nonspecific.
- Causes of vaginal pruritus and itching vary depending on the patient's age.
- Most patients require measurement of vaginal pH and microscopic examination of secretions; if needed, culture for sexually transmitted organisms is done.
- In postmenopausal women, any vaginal discharge should be promptly evaluated.

264 Benign Gynecologic Lesions

ADNEXAL TORSION

Adnexal torsion is twisting of the ovary and sometimes the fallopian tube, interrupting the arterial supply and causing ischemia.

Adnexal torsion is uncommon, occurring most often during reproductive years. It usually indicates an ovarian abnormality.

Risk factors for adnexal torsion include the following:

- Pregnancy
- Induction of ovulation
- Ovarian enlargement to > 4 cm (particularly by benign tumors)

Benign tumors are more likely to cause torsion than malignant ones. Torsion of normal adnexa, which is rare, is more common among children than adults.

Typically, one ovary is involved, but sometimes the fallopian tube is also involved. Adnexal torsion can cause peritonitis.

Symptoms and Signs

Torsion causes sudden, severe pelvic pain and sometimes nausea and vomiting. For days or occasionally weeks before the sudden pain, women may have intermittent, colicky pain, presumably resulting from intermittent torsion that spontaneously resolves. Cervical motion tenderness, a unilateral tender adnexal mass, and peritoneal signs are usually present.

Diagnosis

- Color Doppler transvaginal ultrasonography

Adnexal torsion is suspected based on typical symptoms (ie, intermittent, severe pelvic pain) and unexplained peritoneal signs plus severe cervical motion tenderness or an adnexal mass. The pain may be unilateral.

Diagnosis of adnexal torsion is usually confirmed by color Doppler transvaginal ultrasonography.

Treatment

- Surgery to salvage the ovary

If adnexal torsion is suspected or confirmed by ultrasonography, laparoscopy or laparotomy is done immediately to attempt to salvage the ovary and fallopian tube by untwisting them. Salpingo-oophorectomy is required for nonviable or necrotic tissue. If an ovarian cyst or mass is present and the ovary can be salvaged, cystectomy is done. Otherwise, oophorectomy is required.

KEY POINTS

- Adnexal torsion, which is uncommon, is more likely to result from benign tumors than from malignant ones.
- Torsion causes sudden, severe pelvic pain and sometimes nausea and vomiting; it may be preceded by days or occasionally weeks of intermittent, colicky pain, presumably resulting from intermittent torsion.
- Suspect adnexal torsion based on symptoms, and confirm by Doppler transvaginal ultrasonography.
- Immediately attempt to salvage the ovary and fallopian tube by untwisting them via laparoscopy or laparotomy; if nonviable or necrotic tissue or an ovarian cyst or mass is present, surgery (salpingo-oophorectomy, cystectomy) is required.

BARTHOLIN GLAND CYSTS

Bartholin gland cysts are mucus-filled and occur on either side of the vaginal opening (see Plate 88). They are the most common large vulvar cysts. Symptoms of large cysts include vulvar irritation, dyspareunia, pain during walking, and vulvar asymmetry. Bartholin gland cysts may form abscesses, which are painful and usually red. Diagnosis is by physical examination. Large cysts and abscesses require drainage and sometimes excision; abscesses require antibiotics.

Bartholin glands are round, very small, nonpalpable, and located deep in the posterolateral vaginal orifice. Obstruction of the Bartholin duct causes the gland to enlarge with mucus, resulting in a cyst. Cause of obstruction is usually unknown. Rarely, the cysts result from a sexually transmitted disease (eg, gonorrhea).

These cysts develop in about 2% of women, usually those in their 20s. With aging, cysts are less likely to develop.

A cyst may become infected, forming an abscess. Methicillin-resistant *Staphylococcus aureus* (MRSA) is becoming more common in such infections (and in other vulvar infections).

Vulvar cancers rarely originate in Bartholin glands.

Symptoms and Signs

Most Bartholin gland cysts are asymptomatic, but large cysts can be irritating, interfering with sexual intercourse and walking. Most cysts are nontender, unilateral, and palpable near the vaginal orifice. Cysts distend the affected labia majora, causing vulvar asymmetry.

Abscesses cause severe vulvar pain and sometimes fever; they are tender and typically erythematous. A vaginal discharge may be present. Sexually transmitted diseases may coexist.

Diagnosis

- Clinical evaluation

Diagnosis of Bartholin gland cysts is usually by physical examination. A sample of discharge, if present, may be tested for sexually transmitted diseases. Abscess fluid should be cultured.

In women > 40, biopsy must be done to exclude vulvar cancer.

Treatment

- Surgery for symptomatic cysts and for all cysts in women > 40

In women < 40, asymptomatic cysts do not require treatment. Mild symptoms may resolve when sitz baths are used. Otherwise, symptomatic cysts may require surgery. Abscesses also require surgery. Because cysts often recur after simple drainage, surgery aims to produce a permanent opening from the duct to the exterior. Usually, one of the following is done:

- **Catheter insertion:** A small balloon-tipped catheter may be inserted, inflated, and left in the cyst for 4 to 6 wk; this procedure stimulates fibrosis and produces a permanent opening.
- **Marsupialization:** The everted edges of the cyst are sutured to the exterior.

Recurrent cysts may require excision.

In women > 40, newly developed cysts must be surgically explored and biopsied (to exclude vulvar cancer) or removed. Cysts that have been present for years and have not changed in appearance do not require biopsy or surgical removal unless symptoms are present.

Abscesses are also treated with oral antibiotic regimens that cover MRSA (eg, trimethoprim 160 mg/sulfamethoxazole 800 mg bid or amoxicillin/clavulanate 875 mg po bid for 1 wk) plus clindamycin (300 mg po qid for 1 wk).

KEY POINTS

- For most Bartholin gland cysts, the cause of ductal obstruction is unknown; rarely, cysts result from a sexually transmitted disease.
- Cysts may become infected, often with MRSA, and form an abscess.
- In women > 40, biopsy newly developed cysts to exclude vulvar cancer or remove them.
- If cysts cause symptoms, treat surgically (eg, with catheter insertion, marsupialization, and/or excision).

BENIGN OVARIAN MASSES

Benign ovarian masses include functional cysts and tumors; most are asymptomatic.

Functional cysts: There are 2 types of functional cysts:

- **Follicular cysts:** These cysts develop from graafian follicles.
- **Corpus luteum cysts:** These cysts develop from the corpus luteum. They may hemorrhage into the cyst cavity, distending the ovarian capsule or rupturing into the peritoneum.

Most functional cysts are < 1.5 cm in diameter; few exceed 5 cm. Functional cysts usually resolve spontaneously over days to weeks. Functional cysts are uncommon after menopause.

Polycystic ovary syndrome is usually defined as a clinical syndrome, not by the presence of ovarian cysts. But ovaries typically contain many 2- to 6-mm follicular cysts and sometimes contain larger cysts that contain atretic cells.

Benign tumors: Benign ovarian tumors usually grow slowly and rarely become malignant. They include the following:

- **Benign cystic teratomas:** These tumors are also called dermoid cysts because although derived from all 3 germ cell layers, they consist mainly of ectodermal tissue.
- **Fibromas:** These slow-growing tumors are usually < 7 cm in diameter.
- **Cystadenomas:** These tumors are most commonly serous or mucinous.

Symptoms and Signs

Most functional cysts and benign tumors are asymptomatic. Sometimes they cause menstrual abnormalities. Hemorrhagic corpus luteum cysts may cause pain or signs of peritonitis, particularly when they rupture. Occasionally, severe abdominal pain results from adnexal torsion of a cyst or mass, usually > 4 cm.

Ascites and rarely pleural effusion may accompany fibromas.

Diagnosis

- Transvaginal ultrasonography
- Sometimes tests for tumor markers

Masses are usually detected incidentally but may be suggested by symptoms and signs. A pregnancy test is done to exclude ectopic pregnancy. Transvaginal ultrasonography can usually confirm the diagnosis. If results are indeterminate, MRI or CT may help.

Masses with radiographic characteristics of cancer (eg, cystic and solid components, surface excrescences, multilocular appearance, irregular shape) require excision.

Tests for tumor markers are done if a mass requires excision or if ovarian cancer is being considered. One commercially available product tests for 5 tumor markers (beta-2 microglobulin, cancer antigen [CA] 125 II, apolipoprotein A-1, prealbumin, transferrin) and may help determine the need for surgery. Tumor markers are best used for monitoring response to treatment rather than for screening, for which they lack adequate sensitivity, specificity, and predictive values. For example, tumor marker values may be falsely elevated in women who have endometriosis, uterine fibroids, peritonitis, cholecystitis, pancreatitis, inflammatory bowel disease, or various cancers.

In women of reproductive age, simple, thin-walled cystic adnexal masses 5 to 8 cm (usually follicular) without characteristics of cancer do not require further evaluation unless they persist for > 3 menstrual cycles.

Treatment

- Removal of selected cysts
- Sometimes oophorectomy

Many functional cysts < 5 cm resolve without treatment; serial ultrasonography is done to document resolution. Fibromas and cystadenomas require treatment.

Masses with radiographic characteristics of cancer are excised.

If technically feasible, cyst removal from the ovary (ovarian cystectomy) via laparoscopy or laparotomy may be necessary for the following:

- Most cysts that are ≥ 10 cm and that persist for > 3 menstrual cycles
- Cystic teratomas < 10 cm
- Hemorrhagic corpus luteum cysts with peritonitis
- Fibromas and other solid tumors

Oophorectomy is done for the following:

- Fibromas that cannot be removed by cystectomy
- Cystadenomas
- Cystic teratomas > 10 cm
- Cysts that cannot be surgically removed separately from the ovary
- Most cysts that are detected in postmenopausal women and that are > 5 cm

KEY POINTS

- Functional cysts tend to be small (usually < 1.5 cm in diameter), to occur in premenopausal woman, and to resolve spontaneously.
- Functional cysts and benign tumors are usually asymptomatic.
- Exclude ectopic pregnancy by doing a pregnancy test.
- Excise masses that have radiographic characteristics of cancer (eg, cystic and solid components, surface excrescences, multilocular appearance, irregular shape).
- Excise certain cysts and benign tumors, including cysts that do not spontaneously resolve.

CERVICAL MYOMAS

Cervical myomas are smooth, benign tumors of the cervix.

Cervical myomas are uncommon. Uterine myomas (fibroids—see p. 2309) usually coexist. Large cervical myomas may partially obstruct the urinary tract or may prolapse into the vagina. Prolapsed myomas sometimes ulcerate, become infected, bleed, or a combination.

Symptoms and Signs

Most cervical myomas eventually cause symptoms. The most common symptom is bleeding, which may be irregular or heavy, sometimes causing anemia. Dyspareunia may occur. Infection may cause pain, bleeding, or discharge.

Rarely, prolapse causes a feeling of pressure or a mass in the pelvis.

Urinary outflow obstruction causes hesitancy, dribbling, or urinary retention; UTIs may develop.

Diagnosis

- Physical examination

Diagnosis of cervical myomas is by physical examination. Cervical myomas, particularly if prolapsed, may be visible with use of a speculum. Some are palpable during bimanual examination.

Transvaginal ultrasonography is done only for the following:

- To confirm an uncertain diagnosis
- To exclude urinary outflow obstruction
- To identify additional myomas

Hb or Hct is measured to exclude anemia. Cervical cytology is done to exclude cervical cancer.

Treatment

- Removal of symptomatic myomas

Treatment of cervical myomas is similar to that of fibroids. Small, asymptomatic myomas are not treated. Most symptomatic cervical myomas are removed by myomectomy (particularly if childbearing capacity is important) or, if myomectomy is technically difficult, by hysterectomy. Prolapsed myomas should be removed transvaginally if possible.

KEY POINTS

- Cervical myomas are benign.
- Most cervical myomas eventually cause symptoms, mainly bleeding; large myomas may partially block the urinary tract or prolapse into the vagina.
- Diagnose cervical myomas by physical examination and sometimes transvaginal ultrasonography.
- Surgically remove symptomatic cervical myomas, usually by myomectomy but, if myomectomy is not possible, by hysterectomy.

CERVICAL POLYPS

Cervical polyps are common benign growths of the cervix and endocervix.

Cervical polyps occur in about 2 to 5% of women. They usually originate in the endocervical canal. Endocervical polyps may be caused by chronic inflammation. They rarely become malignant.

Symptoms and Signs

Most cervical polyps are asymptomatic. Endocervical polyps may bleed between menses or after intercourse or become infected, causing purulent vaginal discharge (leukorrhea).

Endocervical polyps are usually reddish pink, glistening, and < 1 cm in all dimensions; they may be friable.

Diagnosis

- Speculum examination

Diagnosis of cervical polyps is by speculum examination.

Treatment

- Excision

Polyps that cause bleeding or discharge should be removed. Excision can be done in the office by grasping the base with forceps and twisting off the polyp (polypectomy). Polypectomy does not require anesthetics. Bleeding after excision is rare and can be controlled with chemical cautery. Cervical cytology should be done.

If bleeding or discharge persists after treatment, endometrial biopsy is done to exclude cancer.

KEY POINTS

- Cervical polyps rarely become malignant.
- Most are asymptomatic, but some cause bleeding or become infected, causing purulent vaginal discharge.
- Diagnose by speculum examination.
- If polyps cause symptoms, remove them; if bleeding or discharge persists after removal, biopsy is required to exclude cancer.

CERVICAL STENOSIS

Cervical stenosis is stricture of the internal cervical os.

Cervical stenosis may be congenital or acquired.

The **most common acquired causes of cervical stenosis** are

- Menopause
- Cervical surgery (eg, conization, cautery)
- Endometrial ablation procedures to treat uterine abnormalities that cause menorrhagia
- Cervical or uterine cancer
- Radiation therapy

Cervical stenosis may be complete or partial.

It may result in the following:

- Hematometra (accumulation of blood in the uterus)
- In premenopausal women, retrograde flow of menstrual blood into the pelvis, possibly causing endometriosis
- Pyometra (accumulation of pus in the uterus), particularly in women with cervical or uterine cancer

Symptoms and Signs

Common symptoms in premenopausal women include amenorrhea, dysmenorrhea, abnormal bleeding, and infertility. Postmenopausal women may be asymptomatic for long periods.

Hematometra or pyometra may cause uterine distention or sometimes a palpable mass.

Diagnosis

- Clinical evaluation

Cervical stenosis may be suspected based on symptoms and signs (particularly development of amenorrhea or dysmenorrhea after cervical surgery) or on inability to obtain endocervical cells or an endometrial sample for diagnostic tests (eg, for a Papanicolaou [Pap] test).

Diagnosis of complete stenosis is established if a 1- to 2-mm diameter probe cannot be passed into the uterine cavity.

If cervical stenosis causes symptoms or uterine abnormalities (eg, hematometra, pyometra), cervical cytology and endometrial biopsy or D & C should be done to exclude cancer. For postmenopausal women with no history of abnormal Pap tests and for women without symptoms or uterine abnormalities, no further evaluation is needed.

Treatment

- Dilation and stenting if symptomatic

Treatment of cervical stenosis is indicated only if symptoms or uterine abnormalities are present and typically involves cervical dilation and placement of cervical stent.

KEY POINTS

- Cervical stenosis may be congenital or acquired (eg, caused by menopause, cervical surgery, endometrial ablation, cervical or uterine cancer, or radiation therapy).
- Cervical stenosis can cause amenorrhea, dysmenorrhea, abnormal bleeding, and infertility in premenopausal women; postmenopausal women may be asymptomatic for long periods of time.
- Suspect cervical stenosis based on symptoms and signs or on inability to obtain endocervical or endometrial samples for tests; inability to pass a 1- to 2-mm diameter probe into the uterine cavity confirms complete stenosis.
- If symptoms or uterine abnormalities (eg, hematometra, pyometra) are present, exclude cancer by cervical cytology and endometrial biopsy or D & C, then dilate the cervix and place a stent.

SKENE DUCT CYST

Skene duct cysts develop adjacent to the distal urethra, sometimes causing perineal discharge, dyspareunia, urinary obstruction, or abscess formation.

Skene glands (periurethral or paraurethral glands) are located adjacent to the distal urethra. Cysts form if the duct is obstructed, usually because the gland is infected. They occur mainly in adults. Cysts may form abscesses or cause urethral obstruction and recurrent UTIs.

Most Skene duct cysts are < 1 cm and asymptomatic. Some are larger and cause dyspareunia. The first symptoms may be those of urinary outflow obstruction (eg, hesitancy, dribbling, retention) or of UTIs. Abscesses are painful, swollen, tender, and erythematous but usually do not cause fever.

Diagnosis

- Clinical evaluation

Diagnosis of Skene duct cysts is usually clinical. Most symptomatic cysts and abscesses are palpable adjacent to the distal urethra; however, a diverticulum of the distal urethra may be clinically indistinguishable, requiring ultrasonography or cystoscopy for differentiation.

Treatment

- Surgical excision if the cyst causes symptoms

Symptomatic cysts are excised. Abscesses are treated initially with oral broad-spectrum antibiotics (eg, cephalexin 500 mg q 6 h for 7 to 10 days) and are excised or marsupialized.

KEY POINTS

- Skene duct cysts form if the duct is obstructed, usually because the gland is infected.
- Cysts may form abscesses, obstruct the urethra, and/or cause recurrent UTIs.
- Most are small and asymptomatic; large cysts may cause dyspareunia.
- Diagnose Skene duct cysts by physical examination and, if needed, by ultrasonography or cystoscopy.
- Excise symptomatic cysts, and treat abscesses with broad-spectrum antibiotics and excision or marsupialization.

UTERINE ADENOMYOSIS

Uterine adenomyosis is the presence of endometrial glands and stroma in the uterine musculature; it tends to cause a diffusely enlarged uterus.

In adenomyosis, the ectopic endometrial tissue tends to induce diffuse uterine enlargement (globular uterine enlargement). The uterus may double or triple in size but typically does not exceed the size of a uterus at 12 wk gestation.

True prevalence is unknown, partly because making the diagnosis is difficult. However, adenomyosis is most often detected incidentally in women who are being evaluated for endometriosis, fibroids, or pelvic pain. Higher parity increases risk.

Symptoms and Signs

Common symptoms of uterine adenomyosis are heavy menstrual bleeding, dysmenorrhea, and anemia. Chronic pelvic pain may also be present.

Symptoms may resolve after menopause.

Diagnosis

- Usually ultrasonography or MRI

Uterine adenomyosis is suggested by symptoms and diffuse uterine enlargement in patients without endometriosis or fibroids. Transvaginal ultrasonography and MRI are commonly used for diagnosis, although definitive diagnosis requires histology after hysterectomy.

Needle biopsy is done only occasionally (eg, when endometrial cancer needs to be excluded); its accuracy can be limited, primarily by sampling error.

Treatment

- Hysterectomy

The most effective treatment for uterine adenomyosis is hysterectomy.

Hormonal treatments similar to those used to treat endometriosis may be tried. Treatment with oral contraceptives can be tried but is usually unsuccessful. A levonorgestrel-releasing IUD may help control dysmenorrhea and bleeding.

KEY POINTS

- In uterine adenomyosis, the uterus may double or triple in size.
- It commonly causes heavy menstrual bleeding, dysmenorrhea, and anemia and may cause chronic pelvic pain; symptoms may resolve after menopause.
- Diagnose by transvaginal ultrasonography and/or MRI; however, definitive diagnosis requires histology after hysterectomy.
- The most effective treatment is hysterectomy, but hormonal treatments (eg, oral contraceptives) can be tried.

VULVAR ENDOMETRIOMAS

Vulvar endometriomas are rare, painful cysts that result from extrauterine implantation of functioning endometrial tissue (endometriosis) in the vulva.

Rarely, endometriosis occurs in the vulva (or the vagina), sometimes producing cysts (endometriomas), often at the site of previous surgery or a wound (eg, episiotomy, laceration during childbirth).

Endometriomas usually develop in the midline. They may be painful, particularly during intercourse. During menstruation, pain increases and endometriomas may enlarge. Endometriomas are tender and may appear blue. They can rupture, causing severe pain.

Diagnosis of vulvar endometriomas is by physical examination and biopsy.

Treatment of vulvar endometriomas involves excision.

VULVAR INCLUSION AND EPIDERMAL CYSTS

Vulvar inclusion cysts contain epithelial tissue; vulvar epidermal cysts develop from sebaceous glands. Both cysts eventually enlarge with cellular debris and sometimes become infected.

Inclusion cysts are the most common vulvar cysts; they may also occur in the vagina. They may result from trauma (eg, laceration, episiotomy repair) that entraps viable epithelial tissue below the surface, or they may develop spontaneously.

Epidermal cysts result from obstruction of sebaceous gland ducts.

Uninfected cysts are usually asymptomatic but occasionally cause irritation; they are white or yellow and usually < 1 cm. Infected cysts may be red and tender and cause dyspareunia.

Diagnosis of vulvar cysts is clinical.

Treatment of vulvar cysts, indicated only for symptomatic cysts, is excision. A local anesthetic can be used for a single lesion. For multiple lesions, regional or general anesthesia may be preferred.

265 Breast Disorders

Breast symptoms (eg, masses, nipple discharge, pain) are common, accounting for > 15 million physician visits/yr. Although > 90% of symptoms have benign causes, breast cancer is always a concern. Because breast cancer is common and may mimic benign disorders, the approach to all breast symptoms and findings is to conclusively exclude or confirm cancer.

Evaluation

History: History includes the following:

- Duration of symptoms
- Relation of symptoms to menses and pregnancy
- Presence and type of pain, discharge, and skin changes
- Use of drugs, including hormone therapy
- Personal and family history of breast cancer
- Date and results of last mammogram

Breast examination: Principles of examination are similar for physician and patient.

Breasts are inspected for asymmetry in shape, nipple inversion, bulging, and dimpling (see Fig. 265–1A and B for usual positions). Although size differential is common, each breast should have a regular contour. An underlying cancer is sometimes detected by having the patient press both hands against the hips or the palms together in front of the forehead (see Fig. 265–1C and D). In these positions, the pectoral muscles are contracted, and a subtle dimpling of the skin may appear if a growing tumor has entrapped a Cooper ligament.

The nipples are squeezed to check for a discharge and determine its source (eg, whether it is multiductal).

The axillary and supraclavicular lymph nodes are most easily examined with the patient seated or standing (see Fig. 265–1E). Supporting the patient's arm during the axillary examination allows the arm to be fully relaxed so that nodes deep within the axilla can be palpated.

The breast is palpated with the patient seated and again with the patient supine, the ipsilateral arm above the head, and a pillow under the ipsilateral shoulder (see Fig. 265–1F). The latter position is also used for breast self-examination; the patient examines the breast with her contralateral hand. Having the patient roll to one side, so that the breast on the examined side falls medially, may help differentiate breast and chest wall tenderness because the chest wall can be palpated separately from breast tissue.

The breast should be palpated with the palmar surfaces of the 2nd, 3rd, and 4th fingers, moving systematically in a small circular pattern from the nipple to the outer edges (see Fig. 265–1G). Precise location and size (measured with a caliper) of any abnormality should be noted on a drawing of the breast, which becomes part of the patient's record. A written description of the consistency of the abnormality and degree to which it can be distinguished from surrounding breast tissue should also be included. Detection of abnormalities during physical examination may mean that a biopsy is needed, even if imaging shows no abnormalities.

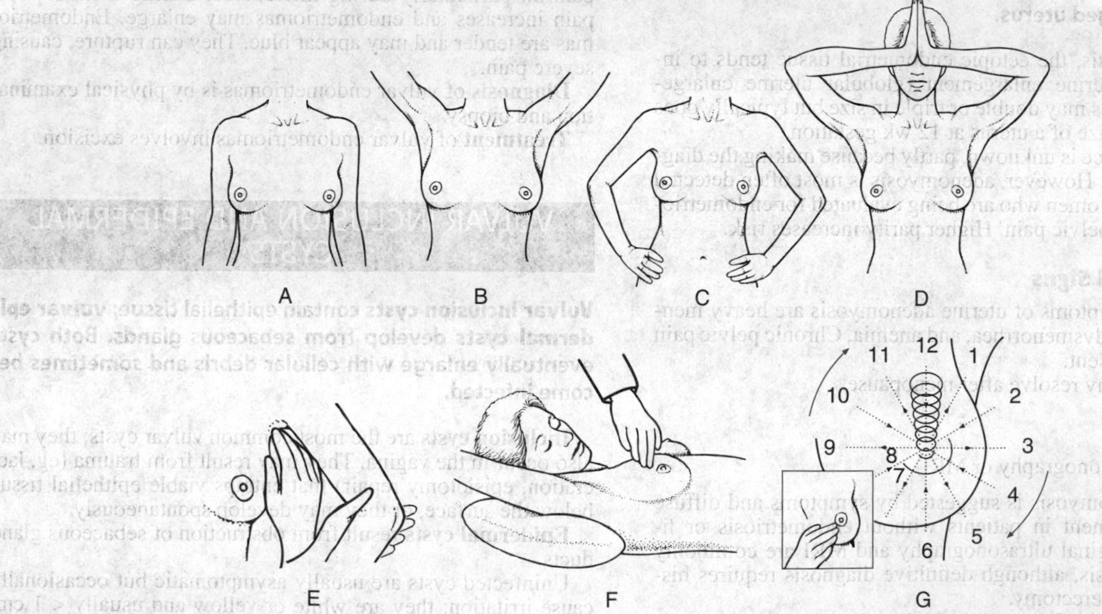

Fig. 265–1. Breast examination. Positions include the patient seated or standing (A) with arms at sides; (B) with arms raised over the head, elevating the pectoral fascia and breasts; (C) with hands pressed firmly against hips; or (D) with palms pressed together in front of the forehead, contracting the pectoral muscles. (E) Palpation of axilla; arm supported as shown, relaxing the pectoral muscles. (F) Patient supine with pillow under the shoulder and with the arm raised above the head on the side being examined. (G) Palpation of breast in a circular pattern from the nipple outward.

Testing: Imaging tests are used for

- Screening: Testing of asymptomatic women to detect early cancer
- Diagnosis: Evaluation of breast abnormalities (eg, masses, nipple discharge)

All women should be screened for breast cancer. All professional societies and groups agree on this concept, although they differ on the recommended age at which to start screening and the precise frequency of screening.

Screening mammography recommendations for average-risk women vary but generally, screening starts at age 40 or 50 and is repeated every year or two until age 75 or until life expectancy is < 10 yr (see p. 2219 and Table 265–1). Mammography is more effective in older women because with aging, fibroglandular tissue in breasts tends to be replaced with fatty tissue, which can be more easily distinguished from abnormal tissue. Mammography is less sensitive in women with dense breast tissue; some states mandate informing patients that they have dense breast tissue when it is detected by screening mammography.

In mammography, low-dose x-rays of both breasts are taken in 1 (oblique) or 2 views (oblique and craniocaudal). Only about 10 to 15% of abnormalities detected result from cancer. Accuracy of mammography depends partly on the techniques used and experience of the mammographer; false-negative results may exceed 15%. Some centers use computer analysis of digital mammography images to help in diagnosis. Such systems are not recommended for stand-alone diagnosis, but they appear to improve sensitivity for detecting small cancers by radiologists.

Breast tomosynthesis (3-dimensional mammography) done with digital mammography increases the rate of cancer detection slightly and decreases the rate of recall imaging; this test is helpful for women with dense breast tissue. However, the test exposes women to almost twice as much radiation as traditional mammography.

Diagnostic mammography is used to do the following:

- Evaluate masses, pain, and nipple discharge
- Determine size and location of a lesion and provide images of surrounding tissues and lymph nodes
- Guide biopsy
- After surgery, image the breast and the excised mass to help determine whether excision was complete

Diagnostic mammography requires more views than screening mammography. Views include magnified views and spot compression views, which provide better visualization of suspect areas.

Ultrasonography can be used to do the following:

- Diagnose breast abnormalities
- Identify abnormal axillary nodes that may require core biopsy
- Stage breast cancer
- Evaluate abnormalities detected by MRI or mammography (eg, determine whether they are solid or cystic)

MRI can be used to do the following:

- Diagnose breast abnormalities
- Before surgery, accurately determine tumor size, chest wall involvement, and number of tumors
- Identify abnormal axillary lymph nodes (to help stage breast cancer)

For women at high risk of breast cancer (eg, with a *BRCA* gene mutation or a calculated lifetime risk of breast cancer of ≥ 15 to 20%), screening should include MRI in addition to clinical breast examination and mammography. MRI is not considered appropriate for screening women with average or slightly increased risk.

BREAST CANCER

Breast cancer most often involves glandular breast cells in the ducts or lobules. Most patients present with an asymptomatic mass discovered during examination or screening mammography. Diagnosis is confirmed by biopsy. Treatment usually includes surgical excision, often with radiation therapy, with or without adjuvant chemotherapy, hormonal therapy, or both.

About 252,710 new cases of invasive breast cancer and about 40,610 deaths from it are expected in 2017. In addition, about 63,410 new cases of in situ breast cancer are expected in 2017. Breast cancer is the 2nd leading cause of cancer death in women (after lung cancer).

Male breast cancer accounts for about 1% of total cases; about 2470 new cases of invasive breast cancer and 460 deaths from it are expected in 2017. In men, manifestations, diagnosis, and management are the same, although men tend to present later.

Table 265–1. RECOMMENDATIONS FOR BREAST CANCER SCREENING MAMMOGRAPHY IN WOMEN WITH AVERAGE RISK

RECOMMENDATIONS	USPSTF	ACS	ACP	AAFP	ACOG	ACR	NCCN
Initiation age (yr)	50	45	50*	50*	40	40	40
Frequency (yr)	2	Yearly until age 54, then every 2 yr	1–2	2	1	1	1
Cessation age (yr)	75	When life expectancy is < 10 yr	75	75	75[†]	75[†]	75[†]

*Women aged 40–50: Counseling about risks and benefits of mammography is recommended, and testing may be done based on risk and patient preference.

[†]Women age ≥ 75: Screening may be done if life expectancy is good or the patient requests it.

AAFP = American Academy of Family Physicians; ACOG = American College of Obstetricians and Gynecologists; ACP = American College of Physicians; ACR = American College of Radiology; ACS = American Cancer Society; NCCN = National Comprehensive Cancer Network; USPSTF = US Preventive Services Task Force.

Risk Factors

For women in the US, cumulative risk of developing breast cancer is 12% (1 in 8) by age 95, and risk of dying of it is about 4%. Much of the risk is incurred after age 60 (see Table 265–2). These statistics can be misleading because most people die before age 95, and cumulative risk of developing the cancer in any 20-yr period is considerably lower.

Factors that may affect breast cancer risk include the following:

- **Age:** The strongest risk factor for breast cancer is age. Most breast cancers occur in women > 50.
- **Family history:** Having a 1st-degree relative (mother, sister, daughter) with breast cancer doubles or triples the risk of developing the cancer, but breast cancer in more distant relatives increases the risk only slightly. When ≥ 2 first-degree relatives have breast cancer, risk may be 5 to 6 times higher.
- **Breast cancer gene mutation:** About 5% of women with breast cancer carry a mutation in one of the 2 known breast cancer genes, *BRCA1* or *BRCA2*. If relatives of such a woman also carry the mutation, they have a 50 to 85% lifetime risk of developing breast cancer. Women with *BRCA1* mutations also have a 20 to 40% lifetime risk of developing ovarian cancer; risk among women with *BRCA2* mutations is increased less. Women without a family history of breast cancer in at least two 1st-degree relatives are unlikely to carry this mutation and thus do not require screening for *BRCA1* and *BRCA2* mutations. Men who carry a *BRCA2* mutation also have an increased risk of developing breast cancer. The mutations are more common among Ashkenazi Jews. Women with *BRCA1* or *BRCA2* mutations may require closer surveillance or preventive measures, such as taking tamoxifen or raloxifene or undergoing double mastectomy.
- **Personal history:** Having had in situ or invasive breast cancer increases risk. Risk of developing cancer in the contralateral breast after mastectomy is about 0.5 to 1%/yr of follow-up.
- **Gynecologic history:** Early menarche, late menopause, or late first pregnancy increases risk. Women who have a first pregnancy after age 30 are at higher risk than those who are nulliparous.
- **Breast changes:** History of a lesion that required a biopsy increases risk slightly. Women with multiple breast masses but no histologic confirmation of a high-risk pattern should not be considered at high risk. Benign lesions that may slightly increase risk of developing invasive breast cancer include complex fibroadenoma, moderate or florid hyperplasia (with or without atypia), sclerosing adenosis, and papilloma. Risk is about 4 or 5 times higher than average in patients with atypical ductal or lobular hyperplasia and about 10 times higher if they also have a family history of invasive breast cancer in a 1st-degree relative. Increased breast density seen on screening mammography is associated with an increased risk of breast cancer.
- **Lobular carcinoma in situ (LCIS):** Having LCIS increases the risk of developing invasive carcinoma in either breast by about 25 times; invasive carcinoma develops in about 1 to 2% of patients with LCIS annually.
- **Use of oral contraceptives:** Oral contraceptive use increases risk very slightly (by about 5 more cases per 100,000 women). Risk increases primarily during the years of contraceptive use and tapers off during the 10 yr after stopping. Risk is highest in women who began to use contraceptives before age 20 (although absolute risk is still very low).
- **Hormone therapy:** Postmenopausal hormone (estrogen plus a progestin) therapy appears to increase risk modestly after only 3 yr of use.[1] After 5 yr of use, the increased risk is about 7 or 8 more cases per 10,000 women for each year of use (about a 24% increase in relative risk). Use of estrogen alone does not appear to increase risk of breast cancer (as reported in the Women's Health Initiative). Selective estrogen-receptor modulators (eg, raloxifene) reduce the risk of developing breast cancer.
- **Radiation therapy:** Exposure to radiation therapy before age 30 increases risk. Mantle-field radiation therapy for Hodgkin lymphoma about quadruples risk of breast cancer over the next 20 to 30 yr.
- **Diet:** Diet may contribute to development or growth of breast cancers, but conclusive evidence about the effect of a particular diet (eg, one high in fats) is lacking. Obese postmenopausal women are at increased risk, but there is no evidence that dietary modification reduces risk. For obese women who are menstruating later than normal, risk may be decreased.
- **Lifestyle factors:** Smoking and alcohol may contribute to a higher risk of breast cancer. Women are counseled to stop smoking and to reduce alcohol consumption.

The Breast Cancer Risk Assessment Tool (BCRAT) or (Gail model), can be used to calculate a women's 5-yr and lifetime risk of developing breast cancer (see Breast Cancer Risk Assessment Tool).

1. Writing Group for the Women's Health Initiative Investigators: Risks and benefits of estrogen plus progestin in healthy postmenopausal women: Principal results from the Women's Health Initiative randomized controlled trial. *JAMA* 288(3):321–333, 2002.

Pathology

Most breast cancers are epithelial tumors that develop from cells lining ducts or lobules; less common are nonepithelial cancers of the supporting stroma (eg, angiosarcoma, primary

Table 265–2. RISK OF BEING DIAGNOSED WITH INVASIVE BREAST CANCER

AGE (YR)	10-YR RISK (%)	20-YR RISK (%)	30-YR RISK (%)	LIFETIME RISK (%)	LIFETIME RISK OF DYING OF INVASIVE BREAST CANCER (%)
30	0.4	1.9	4.1	12.5	2.8
40	1.4	3.7	6.8	12.2	2.8
50	2.3	5.5	8.8	11.1	2.6
60	3.5	6.9	8.9	9.4	2.4
70	3.9	6.2	—	6.7	2.0

Data from 2010–12. Based on the seer.cancer.gov web site. Accessed on February 22, 2016.

stromal sarcomas, phyllodes tumor). Cancers are divided into carcinoma in situ and invasive cancer.

Carcinoma in situ is proliferation of cancer cells within ducts or lobules and without invasion of stromal tissue. There are 2 types:

- **Ductal carcinoma in situ (DCIS):** About 85% of carcinoma in situ are this type. DCIS is usually detected only by mammography. It may involve a small or wide area of the breast; if a wide area is involved, microscopic invasive foci may develop over time.
- **Lobular carcinoma in situ (LCIS):** LCIS is often multifocal and bilateral. There are 2 types: classic and pleomorphic. Classic LCIS is not malignant but increases risk of developing invasive carcinoma in either breast. This nonpalpable lesion is usually detected via biopsy; it is rarely visualized with mammography. Pleomorphic LCIS behaves more like DCIS; it should be excised to negative margins.

Invasive carcinoma is primarily adenocarcinoma. About 80% is the infiltrating ductal type; most of the remaining cases are infiltrating lobular. Rare types include medullary, mucinous, metaplastic, and tubular carcinomas. Mucinous carcinoma tends to develop in older women and to be slow growing. Women with these types of breast cancer have a much better prognosis than women with other types of invasive breast cancer.

Inflammatory breast cancer is a fast-growing, often fatal cancer. Cancer cells block the lymphatic vessels in breast skin; as a result, the breast appears inflamed, and the skin appears thickened, resembling orange peel (peau d'orange). Usually, inflammatory breast cancer spreads to the lymph nodes in the armpit. The lymph nodes feel like hard lumps. However, often no mass is felt in the breast itself because this cancer is dispersed throughout the breast.

Paget disease of the nipple (see also p. 1017—not to be confused with the metabolic bone disease also called Paget disease) is a form of DCIS that extends into the skin over the nipple and areola, manifesting with a skin lesion (eg, an eczematous or a psoriaform lesion). Characteristic malignant cells called Paget cells are present in the epidermis. Women with Paget disease of the nipple often have underlying invasive or in situ cancer.

Pathophysiology

Breast cancer invades locally and spreads through the regional lymph nodes, bloodstream, or both. Metastatic breast cancer may affect almost any organ in the body—most commonly, lungs, liver, bone, brain, and skin.

Most skin metastases occur near the site of breast surgery; scalp metastases are also common. Metastatic breast cancer frequently appears years or decades after initial diagnosis and treatment.

Hormone receptors: Estrogen and progesterone receptors, present in some breast cancers, are nuclear hormone receptors that promote DNA replication and cell division when the appropriate hormones bind to them. Thus, drugs that block these receptors may be useful in treating tumors with the receptors. About two thirds of postmenopausal patients have an estrogen-receptor positive (ER+) tumor. Incidence of ER+ tumors is lower among premenopausal patients.

Another cellular receptor is human epidermal growth factor receptor 2 (HER2; also called HER2/neu or ErbB2); its presence correlates with a poorer prognosis at any given stage of cancer.

Symptoms and Signs

Many breast cancers are discovered as a mass by the patient or during routine physical examination or mammography. Less commonly, the presenting symptom is breast pain or enlargement or a nondescript thickening in the breast.

Paget disease of the nipple manifests as skin changes, including erythema, crusting, scaling, and discharge; these changes usually appear so benign that the patient ignores them, delaying diagnosis for a year or more. About 50% of patients with Paget disease of the nipple have a palpable mass at presentation.

A few patients with breast cancer present with signs of metastatic disease (eg, pathologic fracture, pulmonary dysfunction).

A common finding during physical examination is asymmetry or a dominant mass—a mass distinctly different from the surrounding breast tissue. Diffuse fibrotic changes in a quadrant of the breast, usually the upper outer quadrant, are more characteristic of benign disorders; a slightly firmer thickening in one breast but not the other may be a sign of cancer.

More advanced breast cancers are characterized by fixation of the mass to the chest wall or to overlying skin, by satellite nodules or ulcers in the skin, or by exaggeration of the usual skin markings resulting from skin edema caused by invasion of dermal lymphatic vessels (so-called peau d'orange). Matted or fixed axillary lymph nodes suggest tumor spread, as does supraclavicular or infraclavicular lymphadenopathy.

Inflammatory breast cancer is characterized by peau d'orange, erythema, and enlargement of the breast, often without a mass, and has a particularly aggressive course.

Screening

All women should be screened for breast cancer.[1] All professional societies and groups agree on this concept, although they differ on the recommended age at which to start screening and the precise frequency of screening.

Screening modalities include

- Mammography (including digital and 3-dimensional)
- Clinical breast examination (CBE) by health care practitioners
- MRI (for high-risk patients)
- Monthly breast self-examination (BSE)

Mammography: In mammography, low-dose x-rays of both breasts are taken in 1 (oblique) or 2 views (oblique and craniocaudal).

Mammography is more accurate in older women, partly because with aging, fibroglandular tissue in breasts tends to be replaced with fatty tissue, which can be more easily distinguished from abnormal tissue. Mammography is less sensitive in women with dense breast tissue, and some states mandate informing patients that they have dense breast tissue when it is detected by screening mammography.

Screening mammography guidelines for women with average risk of breast cancer vary, but generally, screening starts at age 40 or 50 and is repeated every year or two until age 75 or life expectancy is < 10 yr (see Table 265–1). Clinicians should make sure that patients understand what their individual risk of breast cancer is and ask patients their preference for testing.

The Breast Cancer Risk Assessment Tool (BCRAT), or Gail Model, can be used to calculate a woman's 5-yr and lifetime risk of developing breast cancer (see Breast Cancer Risk Assessment Tool at www.cancer.gov/bcrisktool). A woman is considered at average risk if her lifetime risk of breast cancer is < 15%.

Concerns about when and how often to do screening mammography include

- Accuracy
- Risks and costs

Only about 10 to 15% of abnormalities detected on screening mammography result from cancer—an 85 to 90% false-positive rate. False-negative results may exceed 15%. Many of the false-positives are caused by benign lesions (eg, cysts, fibroadenomas), but there are new concerns about detecting lesions that meet histologic definitions of cancer but do not develop into invasive cancer during a patient's lifetime.

Accuracy depends partly on the techniques used and experience of the mammographer. Some centers use computer analysis of digitized mammography images (full-field digital mammography) to help in diagnosis. Such systems may be slightly more sensitive for invasive cancers in women < 50 when results are interpreted by radiologists, but probably not when interpreted primarily via computer detection.

Although mammography uses low doses of radiation, radiation exposure has cumulative effects on cancer risk. When radiologic screening is started at a young age, risk of cancer is increased.

Costs include not only the cost of imaging itself but the costs and risks of diagnostic tests needed to evaluate false-positive imaging results.

Breast examination: The value of routine clinical or BSE remains controversial. Some societies such as the American Cancer Society and the US Preventive Services Task Force recommend against either modality for routine screening in average-risk women. Other societies including the American College of Obstetricians and Gynecologists advocate clinical and BSE as important components of screening for breast cancer.

CBE is usually part of routine annual care for women > 40.[1] In the US, CBE augments rather than replaces screening mammography. However, in some countries where mammography is considered too expensive, CBE is the sole screen; reports on its effectiveness in this role vary.

BSE alone has not been shown to reduce mortality rate, but evidence of its usefulness is mixed, and it is widely practiced. Because a negative BSE may tempt some women to forego mammography or CBE, the need for these procedures should be reinforced when BSE is taught. Patients should be instructed to do BSE on the same day each month. For menstruating women, 2 or 3 days after menses ends is recommended because breasts are less likely to be tender and swollen.

MRI: MRI is thought to be better than CBE or mammography for screening women with a high (eg, > 15%) risk of breast cancer, such as those with a *BRCA* gene mutation. For these women, screening should include MRI as well as mammography and CBE. MRI has higher sensitivity but may be less specific. Because specificity is lower, MRI is not considered appropriate for screening women with average or slightly increased risk.

1. The American College of Obstetricians and Gynecologists: Practice bulletin no. 122: Breast cancer screening. *Obstet Gynecol* 118(2), part 1:372–382, 2011.

Diagnosis

- Screening by mammography, breast examination, ultrasonography, and/or MRI
- Biopsy, including analysis for estrogen and progesterone receptors and for HER2 protein

Testing is required to differentiate benign lesions from cancer. Because early detection and treatment of breast cancer improves prognosis, this differentiation must be conclusive before evaluation is terminated.

If advanced cancer is suspected based on physical examination, biopsy should be done first; otherwise, the approach is as for breast mass (see p. 2226). All lesions that could be cancer should be biopsied. A prebiopsy bilateral mammogram may help delineate other areas that should be biopsied and provides a baseline for future reference. However, mammogram results should not alter the decision to do a biopsy if that decision is based on physical findings.

PEARLS & PITFALLS

- Mammogram results should not alter the decision to do a biopsy if that decision is based on physical findings.

Biopsy: Percutaneous core biopsy is preferred to surgical biopsy. Core biopsy can be done guided by imaging or palpation (freehand). Routinely, stereotactic biopsy (needle biopsy guided by mammography done in 2 planes and analyzed by computer to produce a 3-dimensional image) or ultrasound-guided biopsy is being used to improve accuracy. Clips are placed at the biopsy site to identify it.

If core biopsy is not possible (eg, the lesion is too posterior), surgical biopsy can be done; a guidewire is inserted, using imaging for guidance, to help identify the biopsy site.

Any skin taken with the biopsy specimen should be examined because it may show cancer cells in dermal lymphatic vessels.

The excised specimen should be x-rayed, and the x-ray should be compared with the prebiopsy mammogram to determine whether all of the lesion has been removed. Mammography is repeated when the breast is no longer tender, usually 6 to 12 wk after biopsy, to confirm removal of the lesion.

Evaluation after cancer diagnosis: After cancer is diagnosed, evaluation is usually done in consultation with an oncologist, who helps determine which of the many possible tests are needed for a specific patient.

Part of a positive biopsy specimen should be analyzed for estrogen and progesterone receptors and for HER2 protein.

Cells from blood or saliva should be tested for *BRCA1* and *BRCA2* genes when

- Family history includes multiple cases of early-onset breast cancer.
- Ovarian cancer develops in patients with a family history of breast or ovarian cancer.
- Breast and ovarian cancers occur in the same patient.
- Patients have an Ashkenazi Jewish heritage.
- Family history includes a single case of male breast cancer.
- Breast cancer develops at age < 45.
- The cancer does not have estrogen or progesterone receptors or overexpression of HER2 protein (triple negative breast cancer).

Chest x-ray, CBC, liver function tests, and serum calcium levels should be done to check for metastatic disease.

An oncologist should be consulted to determine whether to measure serum carcinoembryonic antigen (CEA), cancer antigen (CA) 15-3, or CA 27-29 and whether bone scanning should be done.

For **bone scanning,** common indications include the following:

- Bone pain
- Elevated serum alkaline phosphatase
- Stage III or IV cancer

Abdominal CT is done if patients have any of the following:

- Abnormal liver function results
- Abnormal abdominal or pelvic examination
- Stage III or IV cancer

Table 265–3. STAGING OF BREAST CANCER

STAGE	TUMOR	REGIONAL LYMPH NODE/DISTANT METASTASIS
0	Tis	N0/M0
IA	T1*	N0/M0
IB	T0	N1mi/M0
	T1*	N1mi/M0
IIA	T0	N1†/M0
	T1*	N1†/M0
	T2	N0/M0
IIB	T2	N1/M0
	T3	N0/M0
IIIA	T0	N2/M0
	TI*	N2/M0
	T2	N2/M0
	T3	N1/M0
	T3	N2/M0
IIIB	T4	N0/M0
	T4	N1/M0
	T4	N2/M0
IIIC	Any T	N3/M0
IV	Any T	Any N/M1

*T1 includes T1mi.

†Here, N1 excludes N1mi.

Tis = carcinoma in situ or Paget disease of the nipple with no tumor (Paget disease with a tumor is classified by tumor size); T1 = tumor ≤ 2 cm; T1mi = tumor ≤ 0.1 cm; T2 = tumor > 2 but < 5 cm; T3 = tumor > 5 cm; T4 = any size with extension to chest wall or skin and with ulceration or skin nodules or inflammatory cancer. Larger tumors are more likely to be node-positive, but they also confer a worse prognosis independent of nodal status.

NX = Nearby nodes not assessable (for example, because removed previously); N0 = no spread to nearby nodes; N1 = spread to 1–3 movable, low or midaxillary nodes; N1mi = N1 nodes with micrometastases (> 0.2 mm and/or 200 cells, but none > 2 mm); N2 = any of the following:

- Spread to low or midaxillary nodes that are fixed or matted
- Spread to internal mammary nodes but not axillary nodes as detected by clinical examination or imaging

N3 = any of the following:

- Spread to internal mammary nodes plus axillary nodes as detected by clinical examination or imaging
- Spread to infraclavicular nodes
- Spread to supraclavicular nodes

M0 = no metastases; M1 = metastases present.

Adapted from the American Joint Committee on Cancer, *AJCC Cancer Staging Manual, Seventh Edition (2010)*. Springer New York, Inc.

Chest CT is done if patients have either of the following:

- Pulmonary symptoms such as shortness of breath
- Stage III or IV cancer

MRI is often used by surgeons for preoperative planning; it can accurately determine tumor size, chest wall involvement, and number of tumors.

Grading and staging: Grading is based on histologic examination of the tissue taken during biopsy.

Staging follows the TNM (tumor, node, metastasis) classification (see Table 265–3). Because clinical examination and imaging have poor sensitivity for nodal involvement, staging is refined during surgery, when regional lymph nodes can be evaluated. However, if patients have palpably abnormal axillary nodes, preoperative ultrasonography-guided fine needle aspiration or core biopsy may be done:

- If results are positive, axillary lymph node dissection is typically done during the definitive surgical procedure.
- If results are negative, a sentinel lymph node biopsy, a less aggressive procedure, may be done instead.

Prognosis

Long-term prognosis depends on tumor stage. Nodal status (including number and location of nodes) correlates with disease-free and overall survival better than any other prognostic factor.

The 5-yr survival rate (from the National Cancer Institute's Surveillance, Epidemiology, and End Results [SEER] Program) depends on cancer stage:

- Localized (confined to primary site): 98.6%
- Regional (confined to regional lymph nodes): 84.9%
- Distant (metastasized): 25.9%

Poor prognosis is associated with the following other factors:

- **Young age:** Prognosis appears worse for patients diagnosed with breast cancer during their 20s and 30s than for patients diagnosed during middle age.
- **Larger primary tumor:** Larger tumors are more likely to be node-positive, but they also confer a worse prognosis independent of nodal status.
- **High-grade tumor:** Patients with poorly differentiated tumors have a worse prognosis.
- **Absence of estrogen and progesterone receptors:** Patients with ER+ tumors have a somewhat better prognosis and are more likely to benefit from hormone therapy. Patients with progesterone receptors on a tumor may also have a better prognosis. Patients with both estrogen and progesterone receptors on a tumor may have a better prognosis than those who have only one of these receptors, but this benefit is not clear.
- **Presence of HER2 protein:** When the *HER2* gene (*HER2/neu* [*erb-b2*]) is amplified, HER2 is overexpressed, increasing cell growth and reproduction and often resulting in more aggressive tumor cells. Overexpression of HER2 is an independent risk factor for a poor prognosis; it may also be associated with high histologic grade, ER− tumors, greater proliferation, and larger tumor size, which are all poor prognostic factors.
- **Presence of** *BRCA* genes: For any given stage, patients with the *BRCA1* gene appear to have a worse prognosis than those with sporadic tumors, perhaps because they have a higher proportion of high-grade, hormone receptor–negative cancers. Patients with the *BRCA2* gene probably have the same

prognosis as those without the genes if the tumors have similar characteristics. With either gene, risk of a 2nd cancer in remaining breast tissue is increased (to perhaps as high as 40%).

Treatment

- Surgery
- Usually radiation therapy
- Systemic therapy: Hormone therapy, chemotherapy, or both

For most types of breast cancer, treatment involves surgery, radiation therapy, and systemic therapy. Choice of treatment depends on tumor and patient characteristics (see Table 265–4). Recommendations for surgery are evolving.

Surgery: Surgery consists of mastectomy or breast-conserving surgery plus radiation therapy.

Mastectomy is removal of the entire breast and includes the following types:

- **Skin-sparing mastectomy**: Spares the pectoral muscles and enough skin to cover the wound, making breast reconstruction much easier, and spares axillary lymph nodes
- **Nipple-sparing mastectomy:** Same as skin-sparing mastectomy plus spares the nipple and areola
- **Simple mastectomy:** Spares the pectoral muscles and axillary lymph nodes
- **Modified radical mastectomy**: Spares the pectoral muscles and removes some axillary lymph nodes
- **Radical mastectomy**: Removes axillary lymph nodes and the pectoral muscles

Radical mastectomy is rarely done unless the cancer has invaded the pectoral muscles.

Table 265–4. TREATMENT BY TYPE OF BREAST CANCER

TYPE	POSSIBLE TREATMENTS
DCIS	Mastectomy Breast-conserving surgery in some patients (with lesions confined to one quadrant) with or without* radiation therapy Hormone therapy for some patients
LCIS, classic	Surgical excision to exclude cancer If negative, observation with regular examinations and mammograms Tamoxifen or, for some postmenopausal women, raloxifene or aromatase inhibitors to reduce risk of invasive cancer Bilateral prophylactic mastectomy (rarely)
LCIS, pleomorphic	Surgical excision to negative margins Chemoprevention with tamoxifen or raloxifene for some patients
Stages I and II (early-stage) cancer	Preoperative chemotherapy if tumor is > 5 cm or fixed to the chest wall Breast-conserving surgery, followed by radiation therapy Mastectomy with or without breast reconstruction Systemic therapy (eg, postoperative chemotherapy, hormonal therapy, trastuzumab, a combination) based on results of tumor tests (eg, analysis for hormone receptors and HER2 protein)
Stage III (locally advanced) cancer, including inflammatory breast cancer	Preoperative systemic therapy, usually chemotherapy Breast-conserving surgery or mastectomy if tumor is resectable after preoperative therapy Mastectomy for inflammatory breast cancer Usually, postoperative radiation therapy Postoperative chemotherapy, hormonal therapy, or both
Stage IV (metastatic) cancer	If cancer is symptomatic and multifocal, hormone therapy, ovarian ablation therapy, or chemotherapy If HER2 is overexpressed, trastuzumab For brain metastases, local skin recurrences, or isolated, symptomatic bone metastases, radiation therapy For bone metastases, IV bisphosphonates to reduce bone loss and bone pain
Paget disease of the nipple	Usually, based on underlying breast cancer if any Occasionally, local excision only
Locally recurrent breast cancer	Mastectomy or surgical resection (if mastectomy has already been done), sometimes preceded by chemotherapy or hormone therapy Radiation therapy for some patients Chemotherapy or hormone therapy
Phyllodes tumors if malignant	Wide excision Sometimes radiation therapy Mastectomy if the mass is large or histology suggests cancer

*Wide excision or breast-conserving surgery may be used alone, especially if the lesion is < 2.5 cm and histologic characteristics are favorable, or with radiation therapy if size and histologic characteristics are less favorable.

DCIS = ductal carcinoma in situ; LCIS = lobular carcinoma in situ.

Breast-conserving surgery includes the following:

- Lumpectomy
- Wide excision
- Quadrantectomy (see Fig. 265–2)

For patients with invasive cancer, survival rates do not differ significantly whether mastectomy or breast-conserving surgery plus radiation therapy is used.

Thus, patient preference can guide choice of treatment within limits. The main advantage of breast-conserving surgery plus radiation therapy is less extensive surgery and opportunity to keep the breast. In 15% of patients thus treated, cosmetic results are excellent. However, the need for total removal of the tumor with a tumor-free margin overrides cosmetic considerations.

With both types of surgery, axillary lymph nodes are typically evaluated. Methods include

- Axillary lymph node dissection (ALND)
- Sentinel lymph node biopsy (SLNB)

ALND is a fairly extensive procedure that involves removal of as many axillary nodes as possible; adverse effects, particularly lymphedema, are common. Most clinicians now first do SLNB unless biopsy of clinically suspect nodes detected cancer. Routine use of ALND is not justified because the main value of lymph node removal is diagnostic, not therapeutic, and SLNB has ≥ 95% sensitivity for axillary node involvement.

For SLNB, blue dye and/or radioactive colloid is injected around the breast, and a gamma probe (and when dye is used, direct inspection) is used to locate the nodes the substance drains into. Because these nodes are the first to receive the tracers, they are considered the most likely to receive any metastatic cells and are thus called sentinel nodes. If any of the sentinel nodes contain cancer cells, ALND may be necessary, based on numerous factors such as tumor stage, hormone receptor status, number of involved nodes, extranodal extension, and patient characteristics. Some surgeons do frozen section analysis during SLNB and get prior agreement for ALND in case nodes are positive; others await standard pathology results and do ALND as a 2nd procedure if needed.

Some physicians use preoperative chemotherapy to shrink the tumor before removing it and applying radiation therapy; thus, some patients who might otherwise have required mastectomy can have breast-conserving surgery. Early data suggest that this approach does not affect survival.

Radiation therapy after mastectomy significantly reduces incidence of local recurrence on the chest wall and in regional lymph nodes and may improve overall survival in patients with primary tumors > 5 cm or with involvement of ≥ 4 axillary nodes. Adverse effects of radiation therapy (eg, fatigue, skin changes) are usually transient and mild. Late adverse effects (eg, lymphedema, brachial plexopathy, radiation pneumonitis, rib damage, secondary cancers, cardiac toxicity) are less common.

Impaired lymphatic drainage of the ipsilateral arm often occurs after axillary node removal (ALND or SLNB) or radiation therapy, sometimes resulting in substantial swelling due to lymphedema. Magnitude of the effect is roughly proportional to the number of nodes removed; thus, SLNB causes less lymphedema than ALND. The lifetime risk of lymphedema after ALND is about 25%. However, even with SLNB, there is a 6% lifetime risk of lymphedema. To reduce risk of lymphedema, practitioners usually avoid giving IV infusions on the affected side. Wearing compression garments and preventing infection in the affected limbs (eg, by wearing gloves during yard work) are important. Avoiding ipsilateral BP measurement and venipuncture is sometimes also recommended, even though supporting evidence is minimal.

If lymphedema develops, a specially trained therapist must treat it. Special massage techniques used once or twice daily may help drain fluid from congested areas toward functioning lymph basins; low-stretch bandaging is applied immediately

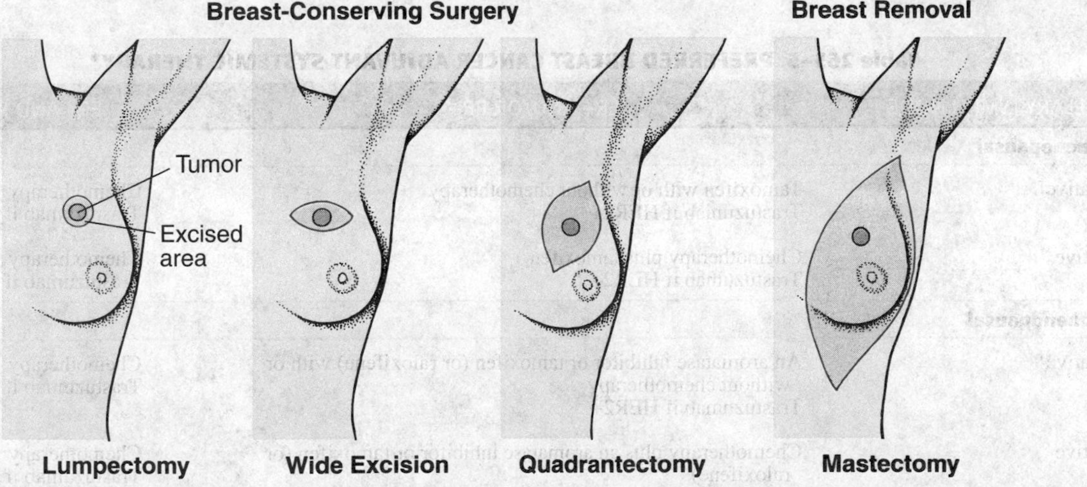

Fig. 265–2. Surgery for breast cancer Surgery for breast cancer consists of 2 main options:

- Breast-conserving surgery, which includes lumpectomy (removal of a small amount of surrounding normal tissue), wide excision (partial mastectomy; removal of a somewhat larger amount of the surrounding normal tissue), and quadrantectomy (removal of 1/4 of the breast)
- Mastectomy (removal of all breast tissue)

after manual drainage, and patients should exercise daily as prescribed. After the lymphedema lessens, typically in 1 to 4 wk, patients continue daily exercise, overnight bandaging of the affected limb indefinitely.

Reconstructive procedures include the following:

- Prosthetic reconstruction: Placement of a silicone or saline implant, sometimes after a tissue expander is used
- Autologous reconstruction: Muscle flap transfer (using the latissimus dorsi, gluteus maximus, or the lower rectus abdominis) or muscle-free flap transfer

Breast reconstruction can be done during the initial mastectomy or later as a separate procedure. Timing of surgery depends on patient preference as well as the need for adjuvant therapy such as radiation therapy. Advantages of breast reconstruction include improved mental health in patients who have a mastectomy. Disadvantages include surgical complications and possible long-term adverse effects of implants.

Adjuvant systemic therapy: (See also NCCN Clinical Practice Guideline: Breast Cancer at www.nccn.org.)

Patients with LCIS are often treated with daily oral tamoxifen. For postmenopausal women, raloxifene or an aromatase inhibitor is an alternative.

For patients with invasive cancer, chemotherapy or hormone therapy is usually begun soon after surgery and continued for months or years; these therapies delay or prevent recurrence in almost all patients and prolong survival in some. However, some experts believe that these therapies are not necessary for many small (< 0.5 to 1 cm) tumors with no lymph node involvement (particularly in postmenopausal patients) because the prognosis is already excellent. If tumors are > 5 cm, adjuvant systemic therapy may be started before surgery.

Relative reduction in risk of recurrence and death with chemotherapy or hormone therapy is the same regardless of the clinical-pathologic stage of the cancer. Thus, absolute benefit is greater for patients with a greater risk of recurrence or death (ie, a 20% relative risk reduction reduces a 10% recurrence rate to 8% but a 50% rate to 40%). Adjuvant chemotherapy reduces annual odds of death (relative risk) on average by 25 to 35% for premenopausal patients; for postmenopausal patients, the reduction is about half of that (9 to 19%), and the absolute benefit in 10-yr survival is much smaller.

Postmenopausal patients with ER– tumors benefit the most from adjuvant chemotherapy (see Table 265–5). Predictive genomic testing of the primary breast cancer is being used increasingly to stratify risk in patients and to determine whether combination chemotherapy or hormone therapy alone is indicated. Common prognostic tests include

- The 21-gene recurrence score assay (based on Oncotype Dx™)
- The Amsterdam 70-gene profile (MammaPrint®)
- The 50-gene risk of recurrence score (PAM50 assay)

Combination chemotherapy regimens are more effective than a single drug. Dose-dense regimens given for 4 to 6 mo are preferred; in dose-dense regimens, the time between doses is shorter than that in standard-dose regimens. There are many regimens: a commonly used one is ACT (doxorubicin plus cyclophosphamide followed by paclitaxel). Acute adverse effects depend on the regimen but usually include nausea, vomiting, mucositis, fatigue, alopecia, myelosuppression, cardiotoxicity, and thrombocytopenia. Growth factors that stimulate bone marrow (eg, filgrastim, pegfilgrastim) are commonly used to reduce risk of fever and infection due to chemotherapy. Long-term adverse effects are infrequent with most regimens; death due to infection or bleeding is rare (< 0.2%).

High-dose chemotherapy plus bone marrow or stem cell transplantation offers no therapeutic advantage over standard therapy and should not be used.

If tumors overexpress HER2 (HER2+), adding the humanized monoclonal antibody trastuzumab to chemotherapy provides substantial benefit. Trastuzumab is usually continued for a year, although the optimal duration of therapy is unknown. A serious potential adverse effect is a decreased cardiac ejection fraction.

Table 265–5. PREFERRED BREAST CANCER ADJUVANT SYSTEMIC THERAPY*

AXILLARY LYMPH NODE	ER+ AND/OR PR+	ER– AND PR–
Premenopausal		
Negative†	Tamoxifen with or without chemotherapy Trastuzumab if HER2+	Chemotherapy Trastuzumab if HER2+
Positive	Chemotherapy plus tamoxifen Trastuzumab if HER2+	Chemotherapy Trastuzumab if HER2+
Postmenopausal		
Negative†	An aromatase inhibitor or tamoxifen (or raloxifene) with or without chemotherapy Trastuzumab if HER2+	Chemotherapy Trastuzumab if HER2+
Positive	Chemotherapy plus an aromatase inhibitor or tamoxifen (or raloxifene) Trastuzumab if HER2+	Chemotherapy Trastuzumab if HER2+

*For all protocols involving chemotherapy, enrollment in a clinical trial is often considered.
†Treatment of node-negative tumors also depends on tumor size and grade.
ER = estrogen receptor; HER2 = human epidermal growth factor receptor 2; PR = progesterone receptor.

With hormone therapy (eg, tamoxifen, raloxifene, aromatase inhibitors), benefit depends on estrogen and progesterone receptor expression; benefit is

- Greatest when tumors have expressed estrogen and progesterone receptors
- Nearly as great when they have only estrogen receptors
- Minimal when they have only progesterone receptors
- Absent when they have neither receptor

In patients with ER+ tumors, particularly low-risk tumors, hormone therapy may be used instead of chemotherapy.

- **Tamoxifen:** This drug competitively binds with estrogen receptors. Adjuvant tamoxifen for 5 yr reduces annual odds of death by about 25% in premenopausal and postmenopausal women regardless of axillary lymph node involvement; treatment for 2 yr is not as effective. If tumors have estrogen receptors, treatment for 10 yr appears to prolong survival and reduce recurrence risk compared with 5 yr of treatment. Tamoxifen can induce or exacerbate menopausal symptoms but reduces incidence of contralateral breast cancer and lowers serum cholesterol. Tamoxifen increases bone density in postmenopausal women and may reduce risk of fractures and ischemic heart disease. However, it significantly increases risk of developing endometrial cancer; reported incidence is 1% in postmenopausal women after 5 yr of use. Thus, if such women have spotting or bleeding, they must be evaluated for endometrial cancer. Nonetheless, the improved survival for women with breast cancer far outweighs increased risk of death due to endometrial cancer. Risk of thromboembolism is also increased.
- **Aromatase inhibitors:** These drugs (anastrozole, exemestane, letrozole) block peripheral production of estrogen in postmenopausal women. More effective than tamoxifen, these drugs are becoming the preferred treatment for early-stage hormone receptor–positive cancer in postmenopausal patients. Letrozole may be used in postmenopausal women who have completed tamoxifen treatment. Optimal duration of aromatase inhibitor therapy is uncertain. A recent trial showed that extending treatment to 10 yr resulted in a lower rate of breast cancer recurrence and higher rate of disease-free survival. There was no change in overall survival (and a higher rate of fractures and osteoporosis) in patients treated for an extended time.

Raloxifene, although indicated for prevention, is not indicated for treatment.

Metastatic disease: Any indication of metastases should prompt immediate evaluation. Treatment of metastases increases median survival by 6 mo or longer. These treatments (eg, chemotherapy), although relatively toxic, may palliate symptoms and improve quality of life. Thus, the decision to be treated may be highly personal.

Choice of therapy depends on the following:

- Hormone-receptor status of the tumor
- Length of the disease-free interval (from remission to manifestation of metastases)
- Number of metastatic sites and organs affected
- Patient's menopausal status

Systemic hormone therapy or chemotherapy is usually used to treat symptomatic metastatic disease. Initially, patients with multiple metastatic sites outside the CNS should be given systemic therapy. If metastases are asymptomatic, there is no proof that treatment substantially increases survival, and it may reduce quality of life.

Hormone therapy is preferred over chemotherapy for patients with any of the following:

- ER+ tumors
- A disease-free interval of > 2 yr
- Disease that is not immediately life threatening

In premenopausal women, tamoxifen is often used first. Reasonable alternatives include ovarian ablation by surgery, radiation therapy, and use of a luteinizing-releasing hormone agonist (eg, buserelin, goserelin, leuprolide). Some experts combine ovarian ablation with tamoxifen or an aromatase inhibitor. In postmenopausal women, aromatase inhibitors are being increasingly used as primary hormone therapy. If the cancer initially responds to hormone therapy but progresses months or years later, additional forms of hormone therapy (eg, progestins, the antiestrogen fulvestrant) may be used sequentially until no further response occurs.

The most effective **chemotherapy drugs** are capecitabine, doxorubicin (including its liposomal formulation), gemcitabine, the taxanes paclitaxel and docetaxel, and vinorelbine. Response rate to a combination of drugs is higher than that to a single drug, but survival is not improved and toxicity is increased. Thus, some oncologists use single drugs sequentially.

For tumors that overexpress HER2, **trastuzumab** is effective in treating and controlling visceral metastatic sites. It is used alone or with hormone therapy or chemotherapy.

Lapatinib is being used increasingly. Its role is evolving.

Radiation therapy alone may be used to treat isolated, symptomatic bone lesions or local skin recurrences not amenable to surgical resection. Radiation therapy is the most effective treatment for brain metastases, occasionally providing long-term control.

Palliative mastectomy is sometimes an option for patients with stable metastatic breast cancer.

IV bisphosphonates (eg, pamidronate, zoledronate) decrease bone pain and bone loss and prevent or delay skeletal complications due to bone metastases. About 10% of patients with bone metastases eventually develop hypercalcemia, which can also be treated with IV bisphosphonates.

End-of-life issues: For patients with metastatic breast cancer, quality of life may deteriorate, and the chances that further treatment will prolong life may be small. Palliation may eventually become more important than prolongation of life (see p. 3177).

Cancer pain can be adequately controlled with appropriate drugs, including opioid analgesics. Other symptoms (eg, constipation, difficulty breathing, nausea) should also be treated.

Psychologic and spiritual counseling should be offered.

Patients with metastatic breast cancer should be encouraged to update their will and to prepare advance directives, indicating the type of care they desire in case they are no longer able to make such decisions.

Prevention

Chemoprevention with tamoxifen or raloxifene may be indicated for women with the following:

- Age > 35 and previous LCIS or atypical ductal or lobular hyperplasia
- Presence of *BRCA1* or *BRCA2* mutations
- Age 35 to 59 yr and a 5-yr risk of developing breast cancer > 1.66%, based on the multivariable Gail model, which includes the women's current age, age at menarche, age at first live childbirth, number of 1st-degree relatives with breast cancer, and results of prior breast biopsies

A computer program to calculate breast cancer risk by the Gail model is available from the National Cancer Institute (NCI) at 1-800-4CANCER and on the NCI web site (www.cancer.gov). Recommendations of the U.S. Preventive Services Task Force (USPSTF) for chemoprevention of breast cancer are available at the USPSTF web site (www.uspreventiveservicestaskforce.org).

Patients should be informed of risks before beginning chemoprevention. Risks of tamoxifen include uterine cancer, thromboembolic complications, cataracts, and possibly stroke. Risks are higher for older women. Raloxifene appears to be about as effective as tamoxifen in postmenopausal women and to have a lower risk of uterine cancer, thromboembolic complications, and cataracts. Raloxifene, like tamoxifen, may also increase bone density. Raloxifene should be considered as an alternative to tamoxifen for chemoprevention in postmenopausal women.

KEY POINTS

- Breast cancer is the 2nd leading cause of cancer death in women; cumulative risk of developing breast cancer by age 95 is 12%.
- Factors that greatly increase risk include breast cancer in close relatives (particularly if a *BRCA* gene mutation is present), atypical ductal or lobular hyperplasia, LCIS, and significant exposure to chest radiation therapy before age 30.
- Screen women by doing CBE, mammography (beginning at age 50 and often at age 40), and, for women at high risk, MRI.
- Factors suggesting a poorer prognosis include younger age, absence of estrogen and progesterone receptors, and presence of HER2 protein or *BRCA* genes.
- For most women, treatment requires surgical removal, lymph node sampling, systemic therapy (hormone therapy or chemotherapy), and radiation therapy.
- Treat with hormone therapy (eg, tamoxifen, an aromatase inhibitor) if tumors have hormone receptors.
- Consider treating metastatic disease to relieve symptoms (eg, with chemotherapy, hormone therapy, or, for bone metastases, radiation therapy or bisphosphonates), even though survival is unlikely to be prolonged.
- Consider chemoprevention with tamoxifen or raloxifene for women at high risk.

BREAST MASSES

(Breast Lumps)

The term breast mass is preferred over lump for a palpably discrete area of any size. A breast mass may be discovered by patients incidentally or during breast self-examination or by the clinician during routine physical examination.

Masses may be painless or painful and are sometimes accompanied by nipple discharge or skin changes.

Etiology

Although breast cancer is the most feared cause, most (about 90%) breast masses are nonmalignant. The most common causes include

- Fibrocystic changes
- Fibroadenomas

Fibrocystic changes (previously, fibrocystic disease) is a catchall term that refers to mastalgia, breast cysts, and nondescript masses (usually in the upper outer part of the breast); these findings may occur in isolation or together. Breasts have a nodular and dense texture and are frequently tender when palpated. Fibrocystic changes cause the most commonly reported breast symptoms and have many causes. Fibrocystic changes are not associated with increased risk of cancer.

Repeated stimulation by estrogen and progesterone may contribute to fibrocystic changes, which are more common among women who had early menarche, who had their first live birth at age > 30, or who are nulliparous.

Fibroadenomas are typically smooth, rounded, mobile, painless masses; they may be mistaken for cancer. They usually develop in women during their reproductive years and may decrease in size over time. Juvenile fibroadenoma, a variant, occurs in adolescents, and unlike fibroadenomas in older women, these fibroadenomas continue to grow over time. Simple fibroadenoma does not appear to increase risk of breast cancer; complex fibroadenoma may increase risk slightly.

Breast infections (mastitis) cause pain, erythema, and swelling; an abscess can produce a discrete mass. Infections are extremely rare except during the puerperium (postpartum) or after penetrating trauma. They may occur after breast surgery. Puerperal mastitis, usually due to *Staphylococcus aureus*, can cause massive inflammation and severe breast pain, sometimes with an abscess. If infection occurs under other circumstances, an underlying cancer should be sought promptly.

Galactocele is a round, easily movable milk-filled cyst that usually occurs up to 6 to 10 mo after lactation stops. Such cysts rarely become infected.

Cancers of various types can manifest as a mass. About 5% of patients have pain.

Evaluation

History: History of present illness should include how long the mass has been present and whether it comes and goes or is painful. Previous occurrence of a mass and the outcome of its evaluation should be queried.

Review of systems should determine whether nipple discharge is present and, if present, whether it is spontaneous or only in response to breast manipulation and whether it is clear, milky, or bloody. Symptoms of advanced cancer (eg, weight loss, malaise, bone pain) should be sought.

Past medical history should include risk factors for breast cancer, including previous diagnosis of breast cancer, history of radiation therapy to the chest area before age 30 (eg, for Hodgkin lymphoma). Family history should note breast cancer in a 1st-degree relative (mother, sister, daughter) and, if family history is positive, whether the relative carried one of the 2 known breast cancer genes, *BRCA1* or *BRCA2*.

Physical examination: Examination focuses on the breast and adjacent tissue. The breast is inspected for skin changes over the area of the mass and for nipple discharge. Skin changes include erythema, rash, exaggeration of normal skin markings, and trace edema sometimes termed peau d'orange (orange peel).

The mass is palpated for size, tenderness, consistency (ie, hard or soft, smooth or irregular), and mobility (whether it feels freely mobile or fixed to the skin or chest wall). The axillary, supraclavicular, and infraclavicular areas are palpated for masses and adenopathy.

Red flags: Certain findings are of particular concern:

- Mass fixed to the skin or chest wall
- Stony hard, irregular mass
- Skin dimpling
- Matted or fixed axillary lymph nodes

- Bloody or spontaneous nipple discharge
- Thickened, erythematous skin

Interpretation of findings: Painful, tender, rubbery masses in women who have a history of similar findings and who are of reproductive age suggest fibrocystic changes.

Red flag findings suggest cancer. However, the characteristics of benign and malignant lesions, including presence or absence of risk factors, overlap considerably. For this reason and because failure to recognize cancer has serious consequences, most patients require testing to more conclusively exclude breast cancer.

Testing: Initially, physicians try to differentiate solid from cystic masses because cysts are rarely cancerous. Typically, ultrasonography is done. Lesions that appear cystic are sometimes aspirated (eg, when they cause symptoms), and solid masses are evaluated with mammography followed by imaging-guided biopsy. Some physicians evaluate all masses with needle aspiration; if no fluid is obtained or if aspiration does not eliminate the mass, mammography followed by imaging-guided biopsy is done.

Fluid aspirated from a cyst is sent for cytology only under the following circumstances:

- It is turbid or grossly bloody.
- Minimal fluid is obtained.
- A mass remains after aspiration.

Patients are reexamined in 4 to 8 wk. If the cyst is no longer palpable, it is considered benign. If the cyst has recurred, it is reaspirated, and any fluid is sent for cytology regardless of appearance. A 3rd recurrence or persistence of the mass after initial aspiration (even if cytology was negative) requires biopsy.

Treatment

Treatment is directed at the cause.

A fibroadenoma is usually removed if it grows or causes symptoms. Fibroadenomas can usually be excised using a local anesthetic, but they frequently recur. Patients who have fibroadenomas that are not excised should be checked periodically for changes. After patients have had several fibroadenomas established as benign, they may decide against having subsequent ones excised. Because juvenile fibroadenomas tend to grow, they should be removed.

Acetaminophen, NSAIDs, and athletic bras (to reduce trauma) can be used to relieve symptoms of fibrocystic changes. Vitamin E and evening primrose oil may be somewhat effective.

KEY POINTS

- Most breast masses are not cancer.
- Clinical features of benign and malignant disease overlap so much that testing should usually be done.

MASTALGIA

(Breast Pain)

Mastalgia is common and can be localized or diffuse and unilateral or bilateral.

Etiology

Localized breast pain is usually caused by a focal disorder that causes a mass, such as a breast cyst, or an infection (eg, mastitis, abscess). Most breast cancers do not cause pain.

Diffuse bilateral pain may be caused by fibrocystic changes or, uncommonly, diffuse bilateral mastitis. However, diffuse bilateral pain is very common in women without breast abnormalities. The most common causes are

- Hormonal changes that cause breast tissue proliferation (eg, during the luteal phase or early pregnancy, in women taking estrogens or progestins)
- Large, pendulous breasts that stretch Cooper ligaments

Evaluation

History: History of present illness should address the temporal pattern of pain and its nature (focal or diffuse, unilateral or bilateral). The relation between chronic or recurrent pain and menstrual cycle phase should be ascertained.

Review of systems should seek other symptoms suggesting pregnancy (eg, abdominal enlargement, amenorrhea, morning nausea) or fibrocystic changes (eg, presence of many masses).

Past medical history should cover disorders that could cause diffuse pain (eg, fibrocystic changes) and use of estrogens and progestins.

Physical examination: Examination focuses on the breast and adjacent tissue, looking for abnormalities such as skin changes including erythema, rash, exaggeration of normal skin markings, and trace edema sometimes termed peau d'orange (orange peel), and signs of infection, such as redness, warmth, and tenderness.

Red flags: The following are of particular concern:

- Signs of infection

Interpretation of findings: Absence of abnormal findings suggests that pain is due to hormonal changes or large, pendulous breasts. Abnormal findings may suggest other specific problems.

Testing: Pregnancy testing should be done if pain is unexplained and has lasted less than several months, particularly if other symptoms or signs are consistent with pregnancy.

Other testing is indicated infrequently—only if physical findings suggest another problem that requires testing.

Treatment

For menstrual-related mastalgia, acetaminophen or an NSAID is usually effective. If pain is severe, a brief course of danazol or tamoxifen may be given. These drugs inhibit estrogen and progesterone. If estrogen or a progestin is being taken, stopping may be necessary.

For pregnancy-related breast pain, wearing a firm, supportive brassiere, taking acetaminophen, or both, can help.

Recent evidence suggests that evening primrose oil, vitamin E, or both used together may reduce the severity of mastalgia.

KEY POINTS

- Diffuse, bilateral breast pain is usually caused by hormonal changes or large, pendulous breasts and causes no abnormal physical findings.

NIPPLE DISCHARGE

Nipple discharge is a common complaint in women who are not pregnant or breastfeeding, especially during the reproductive years. Nipple discharge is not necessarily abnormal, even among postmenopausal women, although it is always abnormal in men.

Nipple discharge can be serous (yellow), mucinous (clear and watery), milky, sanguineous (bloody), purulent, multicolored and sticky, or serosanguineous (pink). It may occur spontaneously or only in response to breast manipulation.

Pathophysiology

Nipple discharge may be breast milk or an exudate produced by a number of conditions.

Breast milk production in nonpregnant and nonlactating women (galactorrhea) typically involves an elevated prolactin level, which stimulates glandular tissue of the breast. However, only some patients with elevated prolactin levels develop galactorrhea (see p. 1320).

Etiology

Most frequently, nipple discharge has a benign cause (see Table 265–6). Cancer (usually intraductal carcinoma or invasive ductal carcinoma) causes < 10% of cases. The rest result from benign ductal disorders (eg, intraductal papilloma, mammary duct ectasia, fibrocystic changes), endocrine disorders, or breast abscesses or infections. Of these causes, intraductal papilloma is probably the most common; it is also the most common cause of a bloody nipple discharge without a breast mass.

Endocrine causes involve elevation of prolactin levels, which has numerous causes.

Evaluation

History: History of present illness should include the following:

- Whether the current discharge is unilateral or bilateral
- What its color is
- How long it has lasted
- Whether it is spontaneous or occurs only with nipple stimulation
- Whether a mass or breast pain is present

Review of systems should seek symptoms suggesting possible causes, including the following:

- Fever: Mastitis or breast abscess
- Cold intolerance, constipation, or weight gain: Hypothyroidism
- Amenorrhea, infertility, headache, or visual disturbances: Pituitary tumor
- Ascites or jaundice: Liver disorders

Past medical history should include possible causes of hyperprolactinemia, including chronic renal failure, pregnancy, liver disorders, and thyroid disorders, as well as history of infertility, hypertension, depression, breastfeeding, menstrual patterns, and cancer. Clinicians should ask specifically about drugs that can cause prolactin release such as oral contraceptives, antihypertensive drugs (eg, methyldopa, reserpine, verapamil), H_2-antagonists (eg, cimetidine, ranitidine), opioids, and dopamine D_2 antagonists (eg, many psychoactive drugs, including phenothiazines and tricyclic antidepressants).

Physical examination: Physical examination focuses on the breasts. The breasts are inspected for symmetry, dimpling of the skin, erythema, swelling, color changes in the nipple and skin, and crusting, ulceration, or retraction of the nipple. The breasts are palpated for masses and evidence of lymphadenopathy in the axillary or supraclavicular region. If there is no spontaneous discharge, the area around the nipples is systematically palpated to try to stimulate a discharge and to identify any particular location associated with the discharge.

Table 265–6. SOME CAUSES OF NIPPLE DISCHARGE

CAUSE	SUGGESTIVE FINDINGS	DIAGNOSTIC APPROACH
Benign breast disorders		
Intraductal papilloma (most common cause)	Unilateral bloody (or guaiac-positive) or serosanguinous discharge	Evaluation as for breast mass
Mammary duct ectasia	Unilateral or often bilateral bloody (or guaiac-positive), serosanguinous, or multicolored (purulent, gray, or milky) discharge	Evaluation as for breast mass
Fibrocystic changes	A mass, often rubbery and tender, usually in premenopausal women Possibly a serous, green, or white discharge Possibly a history of other masses	Evaluation as for breast mass
Abscess or infection	Acute onset with pain, tenderness, or erythema With abscess, a tender mass and possibly purulent discharge	Clinical evaluation If discharge does not resolve with treatment, evaluation as for breast mass
Breast cancer		
Most often, intraductal carcinoma or invasive ductal carcinoma	May have a palpable mass, skin changes, or lymphadenopathy Sometimes bloody or guaiac-positive discharge	If suspected, evaluation as for breast mass
Hyperprolactinemia		
Many causes (see Table 170–3 on p. 1321)	Often bilateral, milky not bloody discharge with multiple ducts involved and no masses Possibly menstrual irregularities or amenorrhea If a pituitary lesion is the cause, possibly signs of CNS mass (visual field changes, headache) or other endocrinopathy	Prolactin level, TSH, review of drug use If prolactin or TSH is elevated, MRI of head

TSH = thyroid-stimulating hormone.

A bright light and magnifying lens can help assess whether the nipple discharge is uniductal or multiductal.

Red flags: Certain findings are of particular concern:

- Spontaneous discharge
- Age ≥ 40
- Unilateral discharge
- Bloody or guaiac-positive discharge
- Palpable mass
- Male sex

Interpretation of findings: Important differentiating points are

- Whether a mass is present
- Whether the discharge involves one or both breasts
- Whether the discharge is bloody (including guaiac-positive)

If a mass is present, cancer must be considered. Because cancer rarely involves both breasts or multiple ducts at presentation, a bilateral, guaiac-negative discharge suggests an endocrine cause. However, if the discharge is guaiac-positive, even if bilateral, cancer must be considered.

Presence of a breast mass, a bloody (or guaiac-positive) discharge, a spontaneous unilateral discharge, or history of an abnormality on a mammogram or an ultrasound scan requires follow-up with a surgeon who is experienced with breast disorders.

For other suggestive findings, see Table 265–6.

Testing: If endocrine causes are suspected, the following are measured:

- Prolactin level
- Thyroid-stimulating hormone (TSH) level

If discharge is guaiac-positive, the following is done:

- Cytology

If there is a palpable mass, evaluation as for breast mass is done, usually beginning with

- Ultrasonography

Lesions that appear cystic are sometimes aspirated, and solid masses or any that remain after aspiration are evaluated with mammography followed by imaging-guided biopsy.

If there is no mass but cancer is otherwise suspected or if other tests are indeterminate, the following is done:

- Mammography

Abnormal results are evaluated by biopsy-guided imaging. If mammography and ultrasonography do not identify a source and the discharge is spontaneous and comes from a single duct or breast, ductography (contrast-enhanced imaging of the milk duct) can be done.

Treatment

Treatment is based on the cause.

If the cause is benign and the discharge is persistent and annoying, the terminal duct can be excised on an outpatient basis.

KEY POINTS

- Nipple discharge is most often benign.
- Bilateral, multiductal, guaiac-negative discharge is usually benign and has an endocrine etiology.
- Spontaneous, unilateral discharge requires diagnostic testing; this type of discharge may be cancer, particularly if it is bloody (or guaiac-positive).
- Presence of a breast mass, a bloody (or guaiac-positive) discharge, or history of an abnormality on a mammogram or an ultrasound scan requires follow-up with a surgeon who is experienced with breast disorders.

PHYLLODES TUMOR

(Cystosarcoma Phyllodes)

Phyllodes tumor is a nonepithelial breast tumor that may be benign or malignant.

Tumors are frequently large (4 to 5 cm) at diagnosis. About half are malignant, accounting for < 1% of breast cancers. Between 20% and 35% of these tumors recur locally, and distant metastases occur in 10 to 20% of patients.

Usual treatment is wide excision, but a mastectomy may be more appropriate if the mass is large or histology suggests cancer. Radiation therapy may be recommended in some cases.

Prognosis is good unless metastases (usually pulmonary) are present.

266 Domestic Violence and Rape

MEDICAL EXAMINATION OF THE RAPE VICTIM

Although legal and medical definitions vary, rape is typically defined as oral, anal, or vaginal penetration that involves threats or force against an unwilling person. Such penetration, whether wanted or not, is considered statutory rape if victims are younger than the age of consent. Sexual assault is rape or any other sexual contact that results from coercion, including seduction of a child through offers of affection or bribes; it also includes being touched, grabbed, kissed, or shown genitals. Rape and sexual assault, including childhood sexual assault, are common; the lifetime prevalence estimates for both ranges from 2 to 30% but tends to be about 15 to 20%. However, actual prevalence may be higher because rape and sexual assault tend to be underreported.

Typically, rape is an expression of aggression, anger, or need for power; psychologically, it is more violent than sexual. Nongenital or genital injury occurs in about 50% of rapes of females.

Females are raped and sexually assaulted more often than males. Male rape is often committed by another man, often in prison. Males who are raped are more likely than females to be physically injured, to be unwilling to report the crime, and to have multiple assailants.

Symptoms and Signs

Rape may result in the following:

- Extragenital injury
- Genital injury
- Psychologic symptoms
- Sexually transmitted diseases (STDs—eg, hepatitis, syphilis, gonorrhea, chlamydial infection, trichomoniasis, HIV infection [rarely])
- Pregnancy (uncommonly)

Most physical injuries are relatively minor, but some lacerations of the upper vagina are severe. Additional injuries may result from being struck, pushed, stabbed, or shot.

Psychologic symptoms of rape are potentially the most prominent. In the short term, most patients experience fear, nightmares, sleep problems, anger, embarrassment, shame, guilt, or a combination. Immediately after an assault, patient behavior can range from talkativeness, tenseness, crying, and trembling to shock and disbelief with dispassion, quiescence, and smiling. The latter responses rarely indicate lack of concern; rather, they reflect avoidance reactions, physical exhaustion, or coping mechanisms that require control of emotion. Anger may be displaced onto hospital staff members.

Friends, family members, and officials often react judgmentally, derisively, or in another negative way. Such reactions can impede recovery after an assault.

Eventually, most patients recover; however, long-range effects of rape may include posttraumatic stress disorder (PTSD—see p. 1747), particularly among women. PTSD is an anxiety disorder; symptoms include re-experiencing (eg, flashbacks, intrusive upsetting thoughts or images), avoidance (eg, of trauma-related situations, thoughts, and feelings), and hyperarousal (eg, sleep difficulties, irritability, concentration problems). Symptoms last for > 1 mo and significantly impair social and occupational functioning.

Evaluation

Goals of rape evaluation are

- Medical assessment and treatment of injuries and assessment, treatment, and prevention of pregnancy and STDs
- Collection of forensic evidence
- Psychologic evaluation
- Psychologic support

If patients seek advice before medical evaluation, they are told not to throw out or change clothing, wash, shower, douche, brush their teeth, or use mouthwash; doing so may destroy evidence.

Whenever possible, all people who are raped are referred to a local rape center, often a hospital emergency department; such centers are staffed by specially trained practitioners (eg, sexual assault nurse examiners). Benefits of a rape evaluation are explained, but patients are free to consent to or decline the evaluation. The police are notified if patients consent. Most patients are greatly traumatized, and their care requires sensitivity, empathy, and compassion. Females may feel more comfortable with a female physician; a female staff member should accompany all males evaluating a female. Patients are provided privacy and quiet whenever possible.

A form (sometimes part of a rape kit) is used to record legal evidence and medical findings (for typical elements in the form, see Table 266–1); it should be adapted to local requirements. Because the medical record may be used in court, results should be written legibly and in nontechnical language that can be understood by a jury.

History and examination: Before beginning, the examiner asks the patient's permission. Because recounting the events often frightens or embarrasses the patient, the examiner must be reassuring, empathetic, and nonjudgmental and should not rush the patient. Privacy should be ensured. The examiner elicits specific details, including

- Type of injuries sustained (particularly to the mouth, breasts, vagina, and rectum)
- Any bleeding from or abrasions on the patient or assailant (to help assess the risk of transmission of HIV and hepatitis)
- Description of the attack (eg, which orifices were penetrated, whether ejaculation occurred or a condom was used)
- Assailant's use of aggression, threats, weapons, and violent behavior
- Description of the assailant

Many rape forms include most or all of these questions (see Table 266–1). The patient should be told why questions are being asked (eg, information about contraceptive use helps determine risk of pregnancy after rape; information about previous coitus helps determine validity of sperm testing).

The examination should be explained step by step as it proceeds. Results should be reviewed with the patient. When feasible, photographs of possible injuries are taken. The mouth, breasts, genitals, and rectum are examined closely. Common sites of injury include the labia minora and posterior vagina. Examination using a Wood's lamp may detect semen or foreign debris on the skin. Colposcopy is particularly sensitive for subtle genital injuries. Some colposcopes have cameras attached, making it possible to detect and photograph injuries simultaneously. Whether use of toluidine blue to highlight areas of injury is accepted as evidence varies by jurisdiction.

Testing and evidence collection: Routine testing includes a pregnancy test and serologic tests for syphilis, hepatitis B, and HIV; if done within a few hours of rape, these tests provide information about pregnancy or infections present before the rape but not those that develop after the rape. Vaginal discharge is examined to check for trichomonal vaginitis and bacterial vaginosis; samples from every penetrated orifice (vaginal, oral, or rectal) are obtained for gonorrheal and chlamydial testing. If the patient has amnesia for events around the time of rape, drug screening for flunitrazepam (the date rape drug) and gamma hydroxybutyrate should be considered. Testing for drugs of abuse and alcohol is controversial because evidence of intoxication may be used to discredit the patient.

Follow-up tests for the following are done:

- At 6 wk: Gonorrhea, chlamydial infection, human papillomavirus infection (initially using a cervical sample from a Papanicolaou test), syphilis, and hepatitis
- At 90 days: HIV infection
- At 6 mo: Syphilis, hepatitis, and HIV infection

However, testing for STDs is controversial because evidence of preexisting STDs may be used to discredit the patient in court.

If the vagina was penetrated and the pregnancy test was negative at the first visit, the test is repeated within the next 2 wk. Patients with lacerations of the upper vagina, especially children, may require laparoscopy to determine depth of the injury.

Table 266–1. TYPICAL EXAMINATION FOR ALLEGED RAPE

CATEGORY	SPECIFICS
General information	Demographic data about the patient Name, address, and phone number of the guardian if the patient is under age Name of police officer, badge number, and department Date, time, and location of examination
History	Circumstances of attack, including • Date, time, and location (familiar to patient?) • Information about assailants (number, name if known, description) • Use of threats, restraints, or weapon • Type of sexual contact (vaginal, oral, rectal; use of condom?) • Types of extragenital injuries sustained • Occurrence of bleeding (patient or assailant) • Occurrence and location of ejaculation by the assailant Activities of the patient after the attack, such as • Douching or bathing • Use of a tampon or sanitary napkin • Urination or defecation • Changing of clothing • Eating or drinking • Use of toothpaste, mouthwash, enemas, or drugs Last menstrual period Date of previous coitus and time, if recent Contraceptive history (eg, oral contraceptives, intrauterine device)
Physical examination	General (extragenital) trauma to any area Genital trauma to the perineum, hymen, vulva, vagina, cervix, or anus Foreign material on the body (eg, stains, hair, dirt, twigs) Examination with Wood's lamp or colposcopy when available
Data collection	Condition of clothing (eg, damaged, stained, foreign material adhering) Small samples of clothing, including an unstained sample, given to the police or laboratory Hair samples, including loose hairs adhering to the patient or clothing, semen-encrusted pubic hair, and clipped scalp and pubic hairs of the patient (at least 10 of each for comparison) Semen taken from the cervix, vagina, rectum, mouth, and thighs Blood taken from the patient Dried samples of the assailant's blood taken from the patient's body and clothing Urine Saliva Smears of buccal mucosa Fingernail clippings and scrapings Other specimens, as indicated by the history or physical examination
Laboratory testing	Acid phosphatase to detect presence of sperm* Saline suspension from the vagina† (for sperm motility) Semen analysis for sperm morphology and presence of A, B, or H blood group substances‡ Baseline serologic test for syphilis in the patient§ Baseline testing for STDs in the patient§ Blood typing (using blood from the patient and dried samples of the assailant's blood) Urine testing, including drug screen‖ and pregnancy tests Other tests, as indicated by the history or physical examination
Treatment, referral, physician's clinical comments	Specify
Witness to examination	Signature
Disposition of evidence	Name of the person who delivered the evidence and the person who received it Date and time of delivery and receipt

*This test is particularly useful if the assailant had a vasectomy, is oligospermic, or used a condom, which may cause sperm to be absent. If the test cannot be done immediately, a specimen should be placed in a freezer.

†This test should be done by the examining physician if it can be done in time to detect motile sperm.

‡In 80% of cases, blood group substances are found in semen.

§This test is not recommended by all authorities because evidence of preexisting STDs may be used to discredit the patient in court.

‖Many authorities recommend not including comments or tests regarding the presence of alcohol or drugs in the patient because evidence of intoxication may be used to discredit the patient in court.

Evidence that can provide proof of rape is collected; it typically includes clothing; smears of the buccal, vaginal, and rectal mucosa; combed samples of scalp and pubic hair as well as control samples (pulled from the patient); fingernail clippings and scrapings; blood and saliva samples; and, if available, semen (see Table 266–1). Many types of evidence collection kits are available commercially, and some states recommend specific kits. Evidence is often absent or inconclusive after showering, changing clothes, or activities that involve sites of penetration, such as douching. Evidence becomes weaker or disappears as time passes, particularly after > 36 h; however, depending on the jurisdiction, evidence may be collected up to 7 days after rape.

A chain of custody, in which evidence is in the possession of an identified person at all times, must be maintained. Thus, specimens are placed in individual packages, labeled, dated, sealed, and held until delivery to another person (typically, law enforcement or laboratory personnel), who signs a receipt. In some jurisdictions, samples for DNA testing to identify the assailant are collected.

Treatment

- Psychologic support or intervention
- Prophylaxis for STDs and possibly hepatitis B or HIV infection
- Possibly emergency contraception

After the evaluation, the patient is provided with facilities to wash, change clothing, use mouthwash, and urinate or defecate if needed. A local rape crisis team can provide referrals for medical, psychologic, and legal support services.

Most injuries are minor and are treated conservatively. Vaginal lacerations may require surgical repair.

Psychologic support: Sometimes examiners can use common sense measures (eg, reassurance, general support, nonjudgmental attitude) to relieve strong emotions of guilt or anxiety. Possible psychologic and social effects are explained, and the patient is introduced to a specialist trained in rape crisis intervention. Because the full psychologic effects cannot always be ascertained at the first examination, follow-up visits are scheduled at 2-wk intervals. Severe psychologic effects (eg, persistent flashbacks, significant sleep disruption, fear leading to significant avoidance) or psychologic effects still present at follow-up visits warrant psychiatric or psychologic referral.

Family members and friends can provide vital support, but they may need help from rape crisis specialists in handling their own negative reactions.

PTSD can be effectively treated psychosocially and pharmacologically (see p. 1747).

Prevention of infections: Routine empiric prophylaxis for STDs consists of ceftriaxone 125 mg IM in a single dose (for gonorrhea), metronidazole 2 g po in a single dose (for trichomoniasis and bacterial vaginosis), and either doxycycline 100 mg po bid for 7 days or azithromycin 1 g po once (for chlamydial infection). Alternatively, azithromycin 2 g po (which covers gonorrhea and chlamydial infection) can be given with metronidazole 2 g po, both as a single dose.

Empiric prophylactic treatment of hepatitis B and HIV after rape is controversial. For hepatitis B, the CDC recommends hepatitis B vaccination unless the patient has been previously vaccinated and has documented immunity. The vaccine is repeated 1 and 6 mo after the first dose. Hepatitis B immune globulin (HBIG) is not given. For HIV, most authorities recommend offering prophylaxis; however, the patient should be told that on average, the risk after rape from an unknown assailant is only about 0.2%. Risk may be higher with any of the following:

- Anal penetration
- Bleeding (assailant or victim)
- Male-male rape
- Rape by multiple assailants (eg, male victims in prisons)
- Rape in areas with a high prevalence of HIV infection

Treatment is best begun < 4 h after penetration and should not be given after > 72 h. Usually, a fixed-dose combination of zidovudine (ZDV) 300 mg and lamivudine (3TC) 150 mg is given bid for 4 wk if exposure appears low risk. If risk is higher, a protease inhibitor is added (see p. 1641).

Prevention of pregnancy: Although pregnancy caused by rape is rare (except in the few days before ovulation), emergency contraception (see p. 2245) should be offered to all women with a negative pregnancy test. Usually, oral contraceptives are used; if used > 72 h after rape, they are much less likely to be effective. An antiemetic may help if nausea develops. An intrauterine device may be effective if used up to 10 days after rape. If pregnancy results from rape, the patient's attitude toward the pregnancy and abortion should be determined, and if appropriate, the option of elective termination should be discussed.

DOMESTIC VIOLENCE

- Domestic violence includes physical, sexual, and psychologic abuse between intimate partners.
- The victim is usually a woman.
- Physical injuries, psychologic problems, social isolation, loss of a job, financial difficulties, and even death can result.
- Keeping safe—for example, having a plan of escape—is the most important consideration.

Domestic violence includes physical, sexual, and psychologic abuse between people who live together, including intimate partners, parents and children, children and grandparents, and siblings. It occurs among people of all cultures, races, occupations, income levels, and ages. In the United States, as many as 30% of marriages are considered physically aggressive.

Women are more commonly victims of domestic violence than are men. About 95% of people who seek medical attention as a result of domestic violence are women, and perhaps 400,000 to 500,000 of women's visits to the emergency department each year are for injuries related to domestic violence. Women are more likely to be severely assaulted or killed by a male partner than by anyone else. Each year in the United States, about 2 million women are severely beaten by their partner.

Physical abuse is the most obvious form of domestic violence. It may include hitting, slapping, kicking, punching, breaking bones, pulling hair, pushing, and twisting arms. The victim may be deprived of food or sleep. Weapons, such as a gun or knife, may be used to threaten or cause injury.

Sexual assault is also common: 33 to 50% of women who are physically assaulted by their partner are also sexually assaulted by their partner. Sexual assault involves the use of threats or force to coerce sexual contact and includes unwanted touching, grabbing, or kissing.

Psychologic abuse may be even more common than physical abuse and may precede it. Psychologic abuse involves any nonphysical behavior that undermines or belittles the victim or that enables the perpetrator to control the victim. Psychologic abuse can include abusive language, social isolation, and financial control. Usually, the perpetrator uses language to demean, degrade, humiliate, intimidate, or threaten the victim in private or in public. The perpetrator may make the victim think she is crazy or make her feel guilty or responsible, blaming her for the abusive relationship. The perpetrator may also humiliate the victim in terms of her sexual performance, physical appearance, or both.

The perpetrator may try to partly or completely isolate the victim by controlling the victim's access to friends, relatives, and other people. Control may include forbidding direct, written, telephone, or e-mail contact with others. The perpetrator may use jealousy to justify his actions.

Often, the perpetrator withholds money to control the victim. The victim may depend on the perpetrator for most or all of her money. The perpetrator may maintain control by preventing the victim from getting a job, by keeping information about their finances from her, and by taking money from her.

After an incident of abuse, the perpetrator may beg for forgiveness and promise to change and stop the abusive behavior. However, typically, the abuse continues and often escalates.

Effects

A victim of domestic violence may be physically injured. Physical injuries can include bruises, black eyes, cuts, scratches, broken bones, lost teeth, and burns. Injuries may prevent the victim from going to work regularly, causing her to lose her job. Injuries, as well as the abusive situation, may embarrass the victim, causing her to isolate herself from family and friends. The victim may also have to move often—a financial burden—to escape the perpetrator. Sometimes the perpetrator kills the victim.

As a result of domestic violence, many victims have psychologic problems. Such problems include PTSD, substance abuse, anxiety, and depression. About 60% of battered women are depressed. Women who are more severely battered are more likely to develop psychologic problems. Even when physical abuse decreases, psychologic abuse often continues, reminding the woman that she can be physically abused at any time. Abused women may feel that psychologic abuse is more damaging than physical abuse. Psychologic abuse increases the risk of depression and substance abuse.

Sidebar 266–1. Children Who Witness Domestic Violence

Each year, at least 3.3 million children are estimated to witness physical or verbal abuse in their homes. These children may develop problems such as excessive anxiety or crying, fearfulness, difficulty sleeping, depression, social withdrawal, and difficulty in school. Also, children may blame themselves for the situation. Older children may run away from home. Boys who see their father abuse their mother may be more likely to become abusive adults. Girls who see their father abuse their mother may be more likely to tolerate abuse as adults. The perpetrator may also physically hurt the children. In homes where domestic violence is present, children are much more likely to be physically mistreated.

Management

In cases of domestic violence, the most important consideration is safety. During a violent incident, the victim should try to move away from areas in which she can be trapped or in which the perpetrator can obtain weapons, such as the kitchen. If she can, the victim should promptly call 911 or the police and leave the house. The victim should have any injuries treated and documented with photographs. She should teach her children not to get in the middle of a fight and when and how to call for help.

Developing a safety plan is important. It should include where to go for help, how to get away, and how to access money. The victim should also make and hide copies of official documents (such as children's birth certificates, social security cards, insurance cards, and bank account numbers). She should keep an overnight bag packed in case she needs to leave quickly.

Sometimes the only solution is to leave the abusive relationship permanently, because domestic violence tends to continue, especially among very aggressive men. Also, even when physical abuse decreases, psychologic abuse may persist. The decision to leave is not simple. After the perpetrator knows the victim has decided to leave, the victim's risk of serious harm and death may be greatest. At this time, the victim should take additional steps (such as obtaining a restraining or protection order) to protect herself and her children. Help is available through shelters for battered women, support groups, the courts, and a national hotline (1-800-799-SAFE or, for TTY, 1-800-787-3224).

267 Endometriosis

In endometriosis, functioning endometrial tissue is implanted in the pelvis outside the uterine cavity. Symptoms depend on location of the implants and may include dysmenorrhea, dyspareunia, infertility, dysuria, and pain during defecation. Severity of symptoms is not related to disease stage. Diagnosis is by direct visualization and sometimes biopsy, usually via laparoscopy. Treatments include anti-inflammatory drugs, drugs to suppress ovarian function and endometrial tissue growth, surgical ablation and excision of endometriotic implants, and, if disease is severe and no childbearing is planned, hysterectomy alone or hysterectomy plus bilateral salpingo-oophorectomy.

Endometriosis is usually confined to the peritoneal or serosal surfaces of pelvic organs, commonly the ovaries, broad ligaments, posterior cul-de-sac, and uterosacral ligaments. Less common sites include the fallopian tubes, serosal surfaces of the small and large intestines, ureters, bladder, vagina, cervix, surgical scars, and, more rarely, the lung, pleura, and pericardium.

Bleeding from peritoneal implants is thought to initiate sterile inflammation, followed by fibrin deposition, adhesion formation, and, eventually, scarring, which distorts peritoneal surfaces of organs, leading to pain and distorted pelvic anatomy.

Reported prevalence varies but is probably about

- 6 to 10% in all women
- 25 to 50% in infertile women
- 75 to 80% in women with chronic pelvic pain

Average age at diagnosis is 27, but endometriosis also occurs among adolescents.

Etiology and Pathophysiology

The most widely accepted hypothesis for the pathophysiology of endometriosis is that endometrial cells are transported from the uterine cavity during menstruation and subsequently become implanted at ectopic sites. Retrograde flow of menstrual tissue through the fallopian tubes is common and could transport endometrial cells intra-abdominally; the lymphatic or circulatory system could transport endometrial cells to distant sites (eg, the pleural cavity).

Another hypothesis is coelomic metaplasia: Coelomic epithelium is transformed into endometrium-like glands.

Microscopically, endometriotic implants consist of glands and stroma identical to intrauterine endometrium. These tissues contain estrogen and progesterone receptors and thus usually grow, differentiate, and bleed in response to changes in hormone levels during the menstrual cycle; also, these tissues can produce estrogen and prostaglandins. Implants may become self-sustaining or regress, as may occur during pregnancy (probably because progesterone levels are high). Ultimately, the implants cause inflammation and increase the number of activated macrophages and the production of proinflammatory cytokines.

The increased incidence in 1st-degree relatives of women with endometriosis suggests that heredity is a factor.

In patients with severe endometriosis and distorted pelvic anatomy, the infertility rate is high, possibly because the distorted anatomy and inflammation interfere with mechanisms of ovum pickup, oocyte fertilization, and tubal transport.

Some patients with minimal endometriosis and normal pelvic anatomy are also infertile; reasons for impaired fertility are unclear but may include the following:

- Increased incidence of luteinized unruptured ovarian follicle syndrome (trapped oocyte)
- Increased peritoneal prostaglandin production or peritoneal macrophage activity that may affect sperm and oocyte function
- Nonreceptive endometrium (because of luteal phase dysfunction or other abnormalities)

Potential risk factors for endometriosis are

- Family history of 1st-degree relatives with endometriosis
- Delayed childbearing or nulliparity
- Early menarche
- Late menopause
- Shortened menstrual cycles (< 27 days) with menses that are heavy and prolonged (> 8 days)
- Müllerian duct defects
- Exposure to diethylstilbestrol in utero

Potential protective factors seem to be

- Multiple births
- Prolonged lactation
- Late menarche
- Use of low-dose oral contraceptives (continuous or cyclic)
- Regular exercise (especially if begun before age 15, if done for > 4 h/wk, or both)

Symptoms and Signs

Cyclic midline pelvic pain, specifically pain preceding or during menses (dysmenorrhea) and during sexual intercourse (dyspareunia), is typical and can be progressive and chronic (lasting > 6 mo). Adnexal masses and infertility are also typical. Interstitial cystitis with suprapubic or pelvic pain, urinary frequency, and urge incontinence is common. Intermenstrual bleeding is possible.

Some women with extensive endometriosis are asymptomatic; some with minimal disease have incapacitating pain. Dysmenorrhea is an important diagnostic clue, particularly if it begins after several years of relatively pain-free menses. Symptoms often lessen or resolve during pregnancy.

Symptoms can vary depending on location of implants.

- Large intestine: Pain during defecation, abdominal bloating, diarrhea or constipation, or rectal bleeding during menses
- Bladder: Dysuria, hematuria, suprapubic or pelvic pain (particularly during urination), urinary frequency, urge incontinence, or a combination
- Ovaries: Formation of an endometrioma (a 2- to 10-cm cystic mass localized to an ovary), which occasionally ruptures or leaks, causing acute abdominal pain and peritoneal signs
- Adnexal structures: Formation of adnexal adhesions, resulting in a pelvic mass or pain
- Extrapelvic structures: Vague abdominal pain (sometimes)

Pelvic examination may be normal, or findings may include a retroverted and fixed uterus, enlarged or tender ovaries, fixed ovarian masses, thickened rectovaginal septum, induration of the cul-de-sac, nodules on the uterosacral ligament, and/or adnexal masses. Rarely, lesions can be seen on the vulva or cervix or in the vagina, umbilicus, or surgical scars.

Diagnosis

- Direct visualization, usually during pelvic laparoscopy
- Sometimes biopsy

Diagnosis of endometriosis is suspected based on typical symptoms but must be confirmed by direct visualization and sometimes biopsy, usually via pelvic laparoscopy but sometimes via laparotomy, vaginal examination, sigmoidoscopy, or cystoscopy. Biopsy is not required, but results may help with the diagnosis. Macroscopic appearance (eg, clear, red, brown, black) and size of implants vary during the menstrual cycle. However, typically, areas of endometriosis on the pelvic peritoneum are punctate red, blue, or purplish brown spots that are > 5 mm, often called powder burn lesions. Microscopically, endometrial glands and stroma are usually present. Stromal elements in the absence of glandular elements indicate a rare variant of endometriosis called stromal endometriosis.

Imaging tests (eg, ultrasonography) are not specific or adequate for diagnosis. However, they sometimes show the extent of endometriosis and thus can be used to monitor the disorder once it is diagnosed. The serum cancer antigen 125 level may be elevated, but obtaining this level is usually neither helpful nor specific in diagnosis or management. Testing for other infertility disorders may be indicated.

Staging the disorder helps physicians formulate a treatment plan and evaluate response to therapy. According to the

Table 267–1. STAGES OF ENDOMETRIOSIS

STAGE	CLASSIFICATION	DESCRIPTION
I	Minimal	A few superficial implants
II	Mild	More and slightly deeper implants
III	Moderate	Many deep implants, small endometriomas on one or both ovaries, and some filmy adhesions
IV	Severe	Many deep implants, large endometriomas on one or both ovaries, and many dense adhesions, sometimes with the rectum adhering to the back of the uterus

American Society for Reproductive Medicine, endometriosis may be classified as stage I (minimal), II (mild), III (moderate), or IV (severe), based on

- Number, location, and depth of implants
- Presence of endometriomas and filmy or dense adhesions (see Table 267–1)

The endometriosis fertility index (EFI) has been developed to stage endometriosis-associated infertility; this system can help predict pregnancy rates after various treatments. Factors used to score the EFI include

- The woman's age
- The number of years she has been infertile
- History or absence of prior pregnancies
- The least-function score for both fallopian tubes, fimbria, and ovaries
- The American Society for Reproductive Medicine endometriosis (lesion and total) scores

Treatment

- NSAIDs for discomfort
- Drugs to suppress ovarian function
- Conservative surgical resection or ablation of endometriotic tissue, with or without drugs
- Total abdominal hysterectomy with or without bilateral salpingo-oophorectomy if disease is severe and the patient has completed childbearing

Symptomatic medical treatment begins with analgesics (usually NSAIDs) and hormonal contraceptives. More definitive treatment must be individualized based on the patient's age, symptoms, and desire to preserve fertility and on the extent of the disorder.

Conservative surgical treatment of endometriosis is excision or ablation of endometriotic implants and removal of pelvic adhesions during laparoscopy.

Drugs and conservative surgery are used mainly to control symptoms. In most patients, endometriosis recurs within 6 mo to 1 yr after drugs are stopped unless ovarian function is permanently and completely ablated. Endometriosis may also recur after conservative surgery.

Total abdominal hysterectomy with or without bilateral salpingo-oophorectomy is considered definitive treatment of endometriosis. It helps prevent complications and modify the course of disease as well as relieving symptoms; however, it can recur.

Drug therapy: Drugs that suppress ovarian function inhibit the growth and activity of endometriotic implants. These drugs include the following (see Table 267–2):

- Continuous combination oral contraceptives: Commonly used
- Progestins: Used only in women who cannot take combination oral contraceptives
- Gonadotropin-releasing hormone (GnRH) agonists: Used only if women cannot take combination oral contraceptives or if treatment with combination oral contraceptives is ineffective
- Danazol: Used only if women cannot take combination oral contraceptives or if treatment with combination oral contraceptives is ineffective

GnRH agonists temporarily suppress estrogen production by the ovaries; however, treatment is limited to ≤ 6 mo because long-term use may result in bone loss. If treatment lasts > 4 to 6 mo, a progestin or a bisphosphonate may be used concurrently (as add-back therapy) to minimize bone loss. If endometriosis recurs, women may need to be treated again.

Danazol, a synthetic androgen and an antigonadotropin, inhibits ovulation. However, its androgenic adverse effects limit its use.

Cyclic or continuous **combination oral contraceptives** given after danazol or GnRH agonists may slow disease progression and are warranted for women who wish to delay childbearing.

Drug treatment does not change fertility rates in women with minimal or mild endometriosis.

Surgery: Most women with moderate to severe endometriosis are treated most effectively by ablating or excising as many implants as possible while restoring pelvic anatomy and preserving fertility as much as possible. Superficial endometriotic implants can be ablated. Deep, extensive implants should be excised.

Specific indications for laparoscopic surgery and hysterectomy include

- Moderate to severe pelvic pain that does not respond to drugs
- Presence of endometriomas
- Significant pelvic adhesions
- Fallopian tube obstruction
- A desire to maintain fertility
- Pain during intercourse

Lesions are usually removed via a laparoscope; peritoneal or ovarian lesions can sometimes be electrocauterized, excised, or, uncommonly, vaporized with a laser. Endometriomas should be removed because removal prevents recurrence more effectively than drainage. After this treatment, fertility rates are inversely proportional to the severity of endometriosis. If resection is incomplete, GnRH agonists are sometimes given during the perioperative period, but whether these drugs increase fertility rates is unclear. Laparoscopic resection of the uterosacral ligaments with electrocautery or a laser may reduce midline pelvic pain.

Rectovaginal endometriosis, the most severe form of the disease, can be treated with the usual treatments for endometriosis; however, colonoscopic resection or surgery may be required to prevent obstruction of the colon.

Hysterectomy with or without ovarian conservation should usually be reserved for patients who have moderate to severe

Table 267–2. DRUGS USED TO TREAT ENDOMETRIOSIS

DRUG	DOSAGE	ADVERSE EFFECTS
Combination estrogen/progestin oral contraceptive		
Ethinyl estradiol 20 mcg plus a progestin Ethinyl estradiol 10 mcg plus a progestin	Continuous, prolonged use (1 tablet once/day for 3–4 cycles, then stopped for 4 days) or cyclic use (as directed for contraception, usually not taken for several days to 1 wk each mo)	Abdominal swelling, breast tenderness, increased appetite, edema, nausea, breakthrough bleeding, deep venous thrombosis, MI, stroke, peripheral vascular disease, mood changes
Progestins		
Levonorgestrel-releasing intrauterine device (IUD)	About 20 mcg/day, decreasing progressively over 5 yr to 10 mcg (delivered by IUD)	Irregular uterine bleeding, sometimes amenorrhea (developing over time)
Medroxyprogesterone acetate	20–30 mg po once/day for 6 mo, followed by 100 mg IM q 2 wk for 2 mo, then 200 mg IM monthly for 4 mo	Breakthrough bleeding, emotional lability, depression, atrophic vaginitis, weight gain
Norethindrone acetate	2.5–5 mg po at bedtime	Irregular uterine bleeding, emotional lability, depression, weight gain
Androgen		
Danazol	100–400 mg po bid for 3–6 mo	Weight gain, acne, lowering of voice, hirsutism, hot flushes, atrophic vaginitis, edema, muscle cramps, breakthrough bleeding, decreased breast size, emotional lability, liver dysfunction, carpal tunnel syndrome, adverse effects on lipid levels
GnRH agonists*		
Leuprolide†	1 mg sc once/day	Hot flushes, atrophic vaginitis, bone demineralization, emotional lability, joint stiffness, headaches, weakness, myalgias, reduced libido
Leuprolide depot	3.75 mg IM q 28 days *or* 11.25 mg IM q 3 mo	Same as for sc
Nafarelin	200–400 mcg intranasally bid	Hot flushes, atrophic vaginitis, bone demineralization, emotional lability, headaches, acne, decreased libido, joint stiffness, vaginal dryness

*Treatment is limited to ≤ 6 mo.

†Leuprolide is often given with a progestin such as norethindrone acetate (2.5–5 mg po once/day) to prevent bone loss and reduce hot flushes during treatment.

GnRH = gonadotropin-releasing hormone.

pelvic pain, who have completed childbearing, and who prefer a definitive procedure. Hysterectomy is done to remove adhesions or implants that adhere to the uterus or cul-de-sac. If women < 50 require hysterectomy with bilateral salpingo-oophorectomy, supplemental estrogen should be considered (eg, to prevent menopausal symptoms). However, concomitant continuous progestin therapy (eg, medroxyprogesterone acetate 2.5 mg po once/day) is often recommended because if estrogen is given alone, residual tissue may grow, resulting in recurrence. If symptoms persist after salpingo-oophorectomy in women > 50, continuous progestin therapy alone (norethindrone acetate 2.5 to 5 mg, medroxyprogesterone acetate 5 mg po once/day, micronized progesterone 100 to 200 mg po at bedtime) can be tried.

KEY POINTS

- Endometriosis is a common cause of cyclic and chronic pelvic pain, dysmenorrhea, dyspareunia, and infertility.
- The stage of endometriosis does not correlate with severity of symptoms.
- Confirm the diagnosis usually by laparoscopy; a biopsy is not mandatory but may aid in the diagnosis.
- Treat pain (eg, with NSAIDs) and, depending on patient fertility goals, usually use drugs that suppress ovarian function to inhibit the growth and activity of endometriotic implants.
- For moderate to severe endometriosis, consider ablating or excising as many implants as possible while restoring normal pelvic anatomy.

268 Family Planning

A couple's decision to begin, prevent, or interrupt a pregnancy may be influenced by many factors including maternal medical disorders, risks involved in the pregnancy, and socioeconomic factors.

One or both members of a couple can use contraception to prevent pregnancy temporarily or sterilization to prevent pregnancy permanently. If contraception fails, abortion (termination of pregnancy) may be considered.

OVERVIEW OF CONTRACEPTION

Among contraceptive users in the US, the most commonly used methods are oral contraceptives (OCs—28%), female sterilization (27.1%), male condoms (16.1%), male sterilization (9.9%), intrauterine devices (IUDs—5.5%), withdrawal (coitus interruptus—5.2%), progestin injections (3.2%), vaginal contraceptive rings (2.4%), subdermal progestin implants (< 1%), contraceptive transdermal patches (< 1%), fertility awareness methods (periodic abstinence—< 1%), and female barrier methods (< 1%—see Table 268–1).

In the first year of use, pregnancy rates with typical use are

- < 1% with methods unrelated to coitus and not requiring user involvement (IUDs, subdermal progestin implants, sterilization)
- About 6 to 9% with hormonal contraceptive methods unrelated to coitus and requiring user involvement (oral contraceptives, progestin injection, transdermal patch, vaginal ring)
- > 10% with coitus-related methods (eg, condoms, diaphragms, fertility awareness methods, spermicides, withdrawal)

Pregnancy rates tend to be higher during the first year of use and decrease in subsequent years as users become more

Table 268–1. COMPARISON OF COMMON CONTRACEPTIVE METHODS

TYPE	PREGNANCY RATE IN FIRST YEAR OF USE: WITH PERFECT USE	PREGNANCY RATE IN FIRST YEAR OF USE: WITH TYPICAL USE	PREGNANCY RATE WITH CONTINUED USE	REQUIREMENTS FOR USE	SELECTED DISADVANTAGES
Hormonal					
Oral contraceptives (OCs)*	0.3%	9%	67%	Pill taken daily Progestin-only pills: Taken at the same time of day	Fluid retention, irregular bleeding, breast tenderness, nausea and vomiting, headache, multiple drug interactions **Combination OCs:** Increased risk of venous thromboembolism **Progestin-only OCs:** Similar to those of contraceptive implants
Progestin injection	0.2%	6 %	56%	Injection q 3 mo	Amenorrhea, irregular bleeding, weight gain
Subdermal progestin implant	0.05%	0.05%	84%	Implant q 3 yr	Amenorrhea, irregular bleeding
Transdermal patch	0.3%	9%	67%	Weekly application and removal	Similar to OCs Local irritation
Vaginal ring	0.3%	9%	67%	Monthly application (inserted vaginally) and removal	Similar to OCs
Barrier					
Cervical cap with spermicide	—	8% (higher among parous women)	N/A	Must be used with each coital act 3 sizes (size chosen based on the woman's pregnancy history) Should be left in the vagina for ≥ 6 h after intercourse	Possibly vaginal irritation or ulceration if left in place for > 48 h

Table continues on the following page.

Table 268–1. COMPARISON OF COMMON CONTRACEPTIVE METHODS (*Continued*)

TYPE	PREGNANCY RATE IN FIRST YEAR OF USE: WITH PERFECT USE	PREGNANCY RATE IN FIRST YEAR OF USE: WITH TYPICAL USE	PREGNANCY RATE WITH CONTINUED USE	REQUIREMENTS FOR USE	SELECTED DISADVANTAGES
Condom, male[†]	2%	18%	43%	Must be used with each coital act	Requires cooperative partner Allergic reactions
Condom, female[†]	5%	21%	41%	Must be used with each coital act	Allergic reactions
Contraceptive sponge (containing sustained-release spermicide)	9% for nulliparous women 20% for parous women	12% for nulliparous women 24% for parous women	36%	Must be used with each coital act May be inserted 24 h before intercourse Must remain in place for ≥ 6 h after intercourse	Allergic reactions, vaginal dryness or irritation
Diaphragm with spermicide	6%	12%	57%	Must be used with each coital act Must be inserted ≤ 6 h before intercourse May be left in place 6–24 h after intercourse	Occasionally vaginal irritation Increased incidence of UTIs
Other					
Intrauterine devices (IUDs)	**Levonorgestrel-releasing IUDs:** 0.3–0.5% (LNg14 [3-yr IUD]) or 0.2% (LNg20 [5-yr IUD]) **Copper-bearing T380A IUDs:** 0.6%	**Levonorgestrel-releasing IUDs:** Same as perfect use **Copper-bearing T380A IUDs:** 8%	78–80%	**Levonorgestrel-releasing IUDs:** Insertion q 3 yr or 5 yr (depending on type) **Copper-bearing T380A IUDs:** Insertion q 10 yr	Spontaneous expulsion, uterine perforation (rare) **Levonorgestrel-releasing IUDs:** Irregular bleeding, amenorrhea **Copper-bearing T380A IUDs:** Increased menstrual blood loss, pelvic pain
Fertility awareness–based methods (periodic abstinence)	0.45% or higher, depending on method	24%	47%	Training, effort, and multiple steps required for the more effective methods	No likely systemic or significant local adverse effects
Withdrawal method	4%	22%	46%	Must be used with each coital act	Requires cooperative partner
Sterilization, female	0.5%	Same as perfect use	100%	Requires a procedure (typically done in an operating room but sometimes in an office)	Considered permanent Backup contraceptive method required while waiting for confirmation of sterility after office procedures (3 mo)
Sterilization, male	0.15%	Same as perfect use	100%	Requires a procedure (done in an office) and a local anesthetic	Considered permanent Backup contraceptive method required while waiting for confirmation of sterility (3 mo)

*Oral contraceptives (OCs) have health benefits other than contraception.
†Condoms protect both partners against sexually transmitted diseases.
N/A = not applicable.

familiar with the contraceptive method they have chosen. Also, as women age, fertility declines. For fertile couples trying to conceive, the pregnancy rate is about 85% after 1 yr if no contraceptive method is used.

Despite the higher pregnancy rate associated with condom use, experts recommend that condoms always be worn during intercourse because they protect against sexually transmitted diseases (STDs). Most importantly, they help protect against HIV. For most effective contraception, other birth control methods should be used with condoms.

If contraception fails, emergency contraception may help prevent an unintended pregnancy. Emergency contraception should not be used as a regular form of contraception.

ORAL CONTRACEPTIVES

Oral contraceptives (OCs) mimic ovarian hormones. Once ingested, they inhibit the release of gonadotropin-releasing hormone (GnRH) by the hypothalamus, thus inhibiting the release of the pituitary hormones that stimulate ovulation. OCs also affect the lining of the uterus and cause the cervical mucus to thicken, making it impervious to sperm. If used consistently and correctly, OCs are an effective form of contraception.

OCs may be a combination of the hormone estrogen and a progestin or a progestin alone.

For most **combination OCs**, an active pill (estrogen plus progestin) is taken daily for 21 to 24 days. Then, an inactive (placebo) pill is taken daily for 4 to 7 days to allow for withdrawal bleeding. In some products, the placebo pill contains iron and folate (folic acid); in others, this pill is not truly inactive but contains 10 mcg of ethinyl estradiol.

Most combination OCs contain 10 to 35 mcg of ethinyl estradiol. This dose is considered low. Low-dose OCs are usually preferred to high-dose OCs (50 mcg of estrogen) because low-dose OCs appear equally effective and have fewer adverse effects, except for a higher incidence of irregular vaginal bleeding during the first few months of use. One new product uses estradiol valerate instead of ethinyl estradiol. The doses of estrogen and progestin are the same throughout the month in some combination OCs (monophasic pills); they change throughout the month in others (multiphasic pills).

All combination OCs have similar efficacy; the pregnancy rate after 1 yr is 0.3% with perfect use and about 9% with typical (ie, inconsistent) use.

To be effective, **progestin-only OCs** must be taken at the same time of day, every day. No inactive pills are included. Progestin-only OCs provide effective contraception primarily by thickening the cervical mucus and preventing sperm from passing through the cervical canal and endometrial cavity to fertilize the egg. In some cycles, these OCs also suppress ovulation, but this effect is not the primary mechanism of action. Common side effects include irregular bleeding. Progestin-only OCs are commonly prescribed when women wish to take OCs but estrogen is contraindicated. Pregnancy rates with perfect and typical use of progestin-only OCs are similar to those with combination OCs.

OCs may be started at any time in a woman's life up until menopause. However, combination OCs must be used with caution in some women (for more information, see the US Medical Eligibility Criteria for Contraceptive Use at www.cdc.gov/mmwr). Use of combination OCs is contraindicated by the following:

- < 21 days postpartum or < 42 days postpartum if risk of venous thromboembolism is high
- Smoking > 15 cigarettes/day in women > 35
- Current or past breast cancer
- Severe decompensated cirrhosis, hepatocellular adenoma, or liver cancer
- Venous thromboembolism (deep venous thrombosis or pulmonary embolism), thrombogenic mutation, or SLE with unknown or positive antiphospholipid antibody status
- Migraine with aura or migraine of any type in women > 35
- Hypertension
- Ischemic heart disease
- Peripartum cardiomyopathy
- Diabetes for > 20 yr or with vascular disease (eg, neuropathy, nephropathy, retinopathy)
- History of malabsorptive bariatric surgery
- Valvular heart disorders with complications
- Solid-organ transplantation with complications
- Current or medically treated gallbladder disease or a history of contraceptive-related cholestasis
- Hypertriglyceridemia
- Acute viral hepatitis

Adverse effects: Although OCs may have some adverse effects, the overall risk of these events is small.

OCs may cause breakthrough bleeding (which may resolve with time or when the estrogen dose is increased) or amenorrhea; amenorrhea, if not acceptable, may resolve when the progestin dose is decreased. In some women, ovulation remains inhibited for a few months after they stop taking OCs. OCs do not adversely affect the outcome of pregnancy when conception occurs during or after their use.

Estrogens increase aldosterone production and cause Na retention, which can cause dose-related, reversible increases in BP and in weight (up to about 2 kg). Weight gain may be accompanied by bloating, edema, and breast tenderness. Most progestins used in OCs are related to 19-nortestosterone and are androgenic. Norgestimate, etonogestrel, and desogestrel are less androgenic than levonorgestrel, norethindrone, norethindrone acetate, and ethynodiol diacetate. Androgenic effects may include acne, nervousness, and an anabolic effect resulting in weight gain. If a woman gains > 4.5 kg/yr, a less androgenic OC should be used. Newer 4th-generation antiandrogenic progestins include dienogest and drospirenone (related to spironolactone, a diuretic).

The incidence of deep venous thrombosis and thromboembolism (eg, pulmonary embolism) increases as the estrogen dose is increased. With OCs that contain 10 to 35 mcg of estrogen, risk is 2 to 4 times the risk at baseline. However, this increased risk is still much lower than the risk associated with pregnancy. A wide variety of progestins in combination OCs may also affect this risk. OCs that contain levonorgestrel appear to lower this risk, and OCs that contain drospirenone or desogestrel may increase it. Risk is probably increased because production of clotting factors in the liver and platelet adhesion are increased. If deep vein thrombosis or pulmonary embolism is suspected in a woman taking OCs, OCs should be stopped immediately until results of diagnostic tests can confirm or exclude the diagnosis. Also, OCs should be stopped as soon as possible before any major surgery that requires immobilization for a long time. Women with a family history of idiopathic venous thromboembolism should not use OCs that contain estrogen.

Current use of OCs does not increase the risk of breast cancer, nor does former use in women aged 35 to 65. Also, risk is not increased in high-risk groups (eg, women with certain benign breast disorders or a family history of breast cancer).

Risk of cervical cancer is slightly increased in women who have used OCs for > 5 yr, but this risk decreases to baseline 10 yr after stopping OCs. Whether this risk is related to a hormonal effect or to behaviors (ie, not using barrier contraception) is unclear.

Although increased stroke risk has been attributed to OCs, low-dose combination OCs do not appear to increase risk of stroke in healthy, normotensive, nonsmoking women. Nonetheless, if focal neurologic symptoms, aphasia, or other symptoms that may herald stroke develop, OCs should be stopped.

CNS effects of OCs include nausea, vomiting, headache, depression, and sleep disturbances.

Although progestins may cause reversible, dose-related insulin resistance, use of OCs with a low progestin dose rarely results in hyperglycemia. Serum high-density lipoprotein (HDL) cholesterol levels may decrease when OCs with a high progestin dose are used but usually only increase when OCs with low progestin and estrogen doses are used. The estrogen in OCs increases triglyceride levels and can exacerbate preexisting hypertriglyceridemia. Most alterations in serum levels of other metabolites are not clinically significant. Thyroxine-binding globulin capacity may increase in OC users; however, free thyroxine levels, thyroid-stimulating hormone levels, and thyroid function are not affected.

Levels of pyridoxine, folate, B complex vitamins, ascorbic acid, Ca, manganese, and zinc decrease in OC users; vitamin A levels increase. None of these effects is clinically significant, and vitamin supplementation is not advised as an adjunct to OC use.

Recent evidence indicates that low-dose OCs do not increase the risk of developing gallstones. However, women who previously developed cholestasis when they were using OCs should not take OCs again. Women who have had cholestasis of pregnancy (idiopathic recurrent jaundice of pregnancy) may become jaundiced if they take OCs, and OCs should be used cautiously in these women.

Rarely, benign hepatic adenomas, which can spontaneously rupture, develop. Incidence increases as duration of use and OC dose increase; adenomas usually regress spontaneously after OCs are stopped.

Melasma occurs in some women; it is accentuated by sunlight and disappears slowly after OCs are stopped. Because treatment is difficult (see p. 1063), OCs are stopped when melasma first appears. OCs do not increase risk of melanoma.

Benefits: OCs have some very important health benefits. High- and low-dose combination OCs decrease the risk of endometrial and ovarian cancers by about 50% for at least 20 yr after OCs are stopped. They also decrease the risk of benign ovarian tumors, abnormal vaginal bleeding, dysmenorrhea, osteoporosis, premenstrual dysphoric disorder, iron deficiency anemia, benign breast disorders, and functional ovarian cysts. Ectopic pregnancy and salpingitis, which can impair fertility, occur less frequently in OC users.

Drug interactions: Although OCs can slow the metabolism of certain drugs (eg, meperidine), these effects are not clinically important.

Some drugs can induce liver enzymes (eg, cytochrome P-450 enzymes) that accelerate transformation of OCs to less biologically active metabolites. Women who take these drugs should not be given OCs concurrently unless other contraceptive methods are unavailable or unacceptable. These drugs include certain anticonvulsants (most commonly phenytoin, carbamazepine, barbiturates, primidone, topiramate, and oxcarbazepine), ritonavir-boosted protease inhibitors, rifampin, and rifabutin. Lamotrigine should not be used with OCs because OCs can decrease lamotrigine levels and affect seizure control.

Initiation: Before OCs are started, clinicians should take a thorough medical, social, and family history to check for potential contraindications to use. BP is measured, and a urine pregnancy test is done. OCs should not be prescribed unless BP is normal and results of the urine pregnancy test are negative. A physical examination, although often done when OCs are started, is not required. However, a physical examination is recommended within 1 yr of OC initiation. A follow-up visit in 3 mo may be useful for discussing potential adverse effects and for rechecking BP. OCs can be prescribed for 13 mo at a time.

OCs may be started on the same day as the contraceptive office visit (often called the quick-start method). The day of the week and time in the menstrual cycle are not important to when OCs are started. However, if OCs are started > 5 days after the first day of menses, women should use a backup contraceptive method (eg, condoms) for the first 7 days of OC use.

Progestin-only OCs must be taken every day, at the same time every day. If > 27 h elapse between doses of a progestin-only OC, women should use a backup contraceptive method for 7 days in addition to taking the OC daily. For combination OC, timing is not as stringent. However, if combined OC users miss taking a pill, they are advised to take 2 pills the next day. If they forget to take a pill for 2 days, they should resume taking the OC each day and should use a backup contraceptive method for 7 days.

After a 1st-trimester spontaneous or induced abortion, combination OCs may be started immediately. For deliveries at 12 to 28 wk gestation, combination OCs may be started within 1 wk. After a delivery at > 28 wk, combination OCs should not be started until > 21 days after delivery because risk of thromboembolism is additionally increased during the postpartum period. If women are exclusively breastfeeding (feeding on demand including night feedings and not supplementing with other foods) or if their risk of venous thromboembolism is increased (eg, because of a recent cesarean delivery), use of combination OCs should be delayed 42 days. In 98% of women who are exclusively breastfeeding and in whom menses does not resume, pregnancy does not occur for 6 mo postpartum even when no contraception is used. However, these women are often advised to start using contraception within 3 mo after delivery.

Progestin-only OCs may be used immediately postpartum.

If women have a history of a liver disorder, tests to confirm normal liver function should be done before OCs are prescribed. Women at risk of diabetes (eg, those who have a family history, who have had gestational diabetes, who have had high-birth-weight infants, or who have physical signs of insulin resistance such as acanthosis nigricans—see Plate 27) require plasma glucose screening and a complete serum lipid profile annually. Use of low-dose OCs is not contraindicated by abnormal glucose or lipid test results, except for triglycerides > 250 mg/dL. Most women with diabetes mellitus may take combination OCs; exceptions are those who have vascular complications (eg, neuropathy, retinopathy, nephropathy) and those who have had diabetes for > 20 yr.

KEY POINTS

- All combination OCs (estrogen plus a progestin) are equally effective; formulations with a low estrogen dose are preferred because they have fewer adverse effects.
- Progestin-only OCs may cause irregular bleeding and must be taken at the same time every day.
- Women may take OCs continuously until menopause if they have no contraindications.
- Combination OCs increase the risk of thrombotic disorders, but this risk is less than that associated with pregnancy.
- OCs do not increase the overall risk of breast cancer.
- Before OCs are prescribed, a thorough patient history is required; a physical examination is not required but ideally should be done within 1 yr after OCs are started.

TRANSDERMAL AND VAGINAL RING HORMONAL CONTRACEPTIVES

A quick-start protocol, similar to that used for OCs, can be used for transdermal (patch) and vaginal ring contraceptives. If either contraceptive method is started at any time other than the first 5 days of menses, a backup contraceptive method should be used concurrently for 7 days.

Transdermal contraceptives: A 20-cm^2 transdermal patch delivers 150 mcg of the progestin norelgestromin (the active metabolite of norgestimate) and 20 mcg of ethinyl estradiol daily into the systemic circulation for 7 days. After 1 wk, the patch is removed, and a new patch is applied to a different area of the skin. After 3 patches are used, no patch is used for the 4th wk to allow for withdrawal bleeding.

Hormone blood levels of estrogen and progestin are much more constant with the patch than with OCs. Overall, contraceptive efficacy, incidence of bleeding, and adverse effects with the patch are similar to those with OCs, but patient adherence may be better with the patch because it is applied weekly rather than taken daily. The patch may be less effective in obese women who weigh > 90 kg.

Women should be advised to use a backup contraceptive method concurrently for 7 days if > 2 days have elapsed since a new patch was to be applied.

Vaginal ring contraceptives: In the US, only one type of vaginal ring is currently available. This vaginal ring is flexible, soft, and transparent; it comes in only one size and is 58 mm in diameter and 4 mm thick. Each ring releases 15 mcg of ethinyl estradiol (estrogen) and 120 mcg of etonogestrel (progestin) daily. These hormones are absorbed through the vaginal epithelium. When a vaginal ring is used, hormone blood levels are relatively constant.

Women insert and remove the ring themselves; no fitting by a physician is required. The ring is typically left in place for 3 wk, then removed for 1 wk to allow for withdrawal bleeding. However, each ring contains enough hormone to effectively inhibit ovulation for up to 5 wk. Thus, the ring may be used continuously and replaced with a new ring every 5 wk. With continuous use, breakthrough bleeding is more common, and the possibility of this adverse effect should be explained to women who are considering continuous use.

Contraceptive efficacy and adverse effects with vaginal rings are similar to those of OCs, but adherence may be better with rings because they are inserted monthly rather than taken daily.

Women may wish to remove the vaginal ring at times other than the week for withdrawal bleeding. However, if the ring is removed for > 3 h, women should be advised to use a backup contraceptive method concurrently for 7 days.

PROGESTIN CONTRACEPTIVE INJECTIONS

Depot medroxyprogesterone acetate (DMPA) is a long-acting injectable formulation of medroxyprogesterone acetate in a crystalline suspension. Pregnancy rates in the first year are 0.2% with perfect use and about 6% with typical use (ie, delays between injections).

DMPA may be given as an IM (150 mg) or sc injection (104 mg) q 3 mo. The injection site is not to be massaged because doing so may increase the rate of absorption. Effective contraceptive hormonal serum levels are usually attained as early as 24 h after injection and are maintained for at least 14 wk although levels may remain effective for up to 16 wk. If the interval between injections is > 16 wk, a pregnancy test should be done to rule out pregnancy before the next injection is given. DMPA may be started immediately (a quick-start protocol) if DMPA is given within the first 5 to 7 days of the menstrual cycle. If it is not started during this time frame, a backup contraceptive method should be used concurrently for 7 days. DMPA may also be given immediately after a spontaneous or induced abortion or immediately postpartum regardless of breastfeeding status.

The most common adverse effect of DMPA is irregular vaginal bleeding. In the 3 mo after the first DMPA injection, about 30% of women have amenorrhea. Another 30% have spotting or irregular bleeding (usually light) > 11 days/mo. Despite these bleeding abnormalities, anemia does not usually result. With continued use, bleeding tends to decrease. After 2 yr, about 70% of DMPA users have amenorrhea. Because DMPA has a long duration of action, ovulation may be delayed for up to 18 mo after the last injection. After ovulation occurs, fertility is usually rapidly restored.

Women typically gain 1.5 to 4 kg during the first year of DMPA use and continue to gain weight thereafter. Because changes in appetite rather than metabolism are thought to be responsible, women who want to take DMPA are usually advised to limit caloric intake and increase energy expenditure.

Headache is a common reason for stopping DMPA, but severity tends to decrease over time. Most women using DMPA do not have headaches, and preexisting tension headaches and migraines usually do not worsen.

Mild, reversible deterioration of glucose tolerance and lipid profile may occur. Although bone mineral density may decrease when estrogen levels are low, there is no evidence of increased fracture risk, and bone scanning is not recommended for women who use DMPA. Adolescent and young women who use DMPA, like those who do not, should consume 1500 mg of Ca and 400 units of vitamin D daily; supplements should be taken if necessary.

Unlike combination OCs, DMPA does not increase the risk of hypertension. Progestins are not believed to increase the risk of thromboembolism; however, some evidence suggests that use of DMPA may double the risk of thromboembolism. However, this association is not well-established, and DMPA is currently considered safe for women with contraindications to estrogen use.

DMPA does not appear to increase the risk of breast, ovarian, or invasive cervical cancer. DMPA reduces the risk of endometrial cancer, pelvic inflammatory disease, and iron deficiency anemia. Some evidence suggests DMPA may reduce the incidence of painful crisis in women with sickle cell disease.

DMPA may be an appropriate contraceptive option for women with a seizure disorder.

Other contraceptive injections are available elsewhere in the world.

SUBDERMAL CONTRACEPTIVE IMPLANTS

Only one progestin implant is available in the US; it is a 4-cm, match-sized single-rod implant that can be inserted through a trocar subdermally at the groove between the bicep and tricep. No skin incision is required. The implant releases etonogestrel (a progestin) at an average rate of 50 mcg/day at 12 mo. The implant provides effective contraception for up to 3 yr. Before inserting or removing this implant, health care practitioners must complete 3 h of manufacturer-sponsored training. The implant currently available is bioequivalent to the previously used implant but is designed to be radiopaque to make it easier to locate at the time of removal. Also, the insertion applicator is easier to use, so that the implant is less likely to be inserted too deeply.

A subdermal implant may be inserted at any time during the menstrual cycle. However, if unprotected intercourse has occurred within the past month, another contraceptive method should be used concurrently until pregnancy can be reliably excluded by a negative pregnancy test or by the subsequent occurrence of menses. If the implant is inserted during the first 5 days of menstrual cycle, no backup contraceptive method is needed. If it is not inserted during this time frame, a backup contraceptive method should be used concurrently for at least 3 days. The implant may be inserted immediately after spontaneous or induced abortion or immediately postpartum regardless of breastfeeding status.

The most common adverse effects are similar to those of other progestins (irregular vaginal bleeding, amenorrhea, headache). Removing the implant, which should be done no later than 3 yr after insertion, requires a skin incision. After implant removal, ovarian activity normalizes immediately.

Other contraceptive implants are available elsewhere in the world.

BARRIER CONTRACEPTIVES

Barrier contraceptives include vaginal spermicides (foams, creams, suppositories), condoms, diaphragms, cervical caps, and contraceptive sponges.

Spermicides: Vaginal foams, creams, and suppositories contain agents that provide a chemical barrier to sperm by damaging sperm cell membranes and thus preventing fertilization. Most spermicides contain nonoxynol-9 and are available without a prescription. These products are similar in efficacy; the pregnancy rate is 19% with perfect use and 28% with typical (ie, inconsistent) use.

Spermicides should be placed in the vagina at least 10 to 30 min before sexual intercourse and reapplied before each coital act. Because their efficacy is limited, spermicides are often used with other barrier methods. Spermicides do not reliably protect against STDs. Also, spermicidal agents may cause vaginal irritation that increases the risk of HIV transmission. For this reason, condoms are no longer lubricated with nonoxynol-9.

Condoms: Condom use reliably reduces the risk of STDs, including HIV infection. Condoms may be made of latex, polyurethane, silicone rubber, and lamb intestine. Lamb-intestine condoms are impenetrable to sperm but not to many of the viruses that can cause serious infections (eg, HIV). Thus, latex and polyurethane condoms are preferred. Condoms also protect against human papilloma virus (HPV), thus reducing the risk of precancerous cervical lesions.

The male condom is the only reversible male contraceptive method other than withdrawal, which has higher contraceptive failure rates.

The male condom is applied before penetration; the tip is pinched shut and should extend about 1 cm beyond the penis to collect the ejaculate.

The female condom is a pouch with an inner and an outer ring; the inner ring is inserted into the vagina, and the outer ring remains outside and covers the perineum. The female condom should be placed no more than 8 h before intercourse and should be left in the vagina for 6 h after intercourse. The penis should be carefully guided through the external ring to make sure that the ejaculate is collected in the pouch.

When the penis is removed after intercourse, care must be taken to avoid spilling condom contents. Emergency contraception should be used if contents spill, the condom slips, or the condom breaks. A new condom should be used for each coital act.

Pregnancy rates at 1 yr are 2% with perfect use and 18% with typical use for the male condom and 5% with perfect use and 21% with typical use for the female condom.

Diaphragm: The diaphragm is a dome-shaped rubber cup with a flexible rim that fits over the cervix and upper part and lateral wall of the vagina. Diaphragms are made in various sizes. They are usually used with a spermicide and, together, provide an effective barrier to sperm. Spermicide is applied to the diaphragm before insertion. After the first coital act, additional spermicide should be inserted into the vagina before each subsequent act. Diaphragms can be washed and reused.

A health care practitioner fits a diaphragm for a woman so that it is comfortable for her and her partner. After childbirth or a significant weight change, the woman needs to be refitted. The diaphragm should remain in place for at least 6 to 8 h but not more than 24 h after intercourse. Pregnancy rates in the first year are about 6% with perfect use but about 12% with typical use.

Diaphragms were once widely used (one third of women in 1940), but by 2002, only 0.2% of women in the US reportedly used them. This decline in use is largely due to the development of many other more effective contraceptive methods. Also, the need for a physician visit for fitting and adverse effects (eg. discomfort, vaginal irritation) may have contributed to the decline.

A new diaphragm is being developed. This diaphragm is considered to be one size fits most. It is made of silicone and reportedly softer and more durable than traditional latex diaphragms. This diaphragm may be useful in developing nations where access to medical care is limited.

Cervical cap: The cervical cap resembles the diaphragm but is smaller and more rigid. It must be inserted before intercourse; it should remain in place for at least 6 h after intercourse and not more than 48 h. Pregnancy rates are 8% with typical use in the first year; rates are higher among parous women because obtaining a secure fit after childbirth is difficult.

Only one cervical cap is available in the US. It comes in 3 sizes (small, medium, large); size is chosen based on a woman's pregnancy history. A health care practitioner must write a prescription before the cervical cap can be used, but it does not require a custom fitting.

Contraceptive sponge: The contraceptive sponge acts as both a barrier device and a spermicidal agent. It can be purchased without a prescription and can be inserted up to 24 h before intercourse. It should be left in place for at least 6 h after intercourse. Maximum wear time should not exceed 30 h. Pregnancy rates with typical use are 12% for nulliparous women and 24% for parous women.

INTRAUTERINE DEVICES

In the US, 5.5% of women use intrauterine devices (IUDs); IUDs are becoming more popular because of their advantages over oral contraceptives:

- IUDs are highly effective.
- IUDs have minimal systemic effects.
- Only one contraceptive decision every 3, 5, or 10 yr is required.

In the US, 3 IUDs are currently available. There are 2 types of levonorgestrel-releasing IUDs; one is effective for 3 yr and has a 3-yr cumulative pregnancy rate of 0.9%. The other is effective for 5 yr and has a cumulative 5- yr pregnancy rate of 0.5%. The 3rd IUD is a copper-bearing T380A IUD. It is effective for 10 yr; it has a cumulative 12-yr pregnancy rate of < 2% (see Table 268–2).

Clinicians do not need to do a Papanicolaou (Pap) test before they insert an IUD unless they suspect cervical lesions are present. Then, a Pap test or cervical biopsy should be done. Also, clinicians do not need to wait for results of STD testing

Table 268–2. COMPARISON OF INTRAUTERINE DEVICES

	LEVONORGESTREL		
FEATURE	3-YR IUD	5-YR IUD	COPPER-T380A
Efficacy (1st-yr pregnancy rate with typical use)	0.3–0.5%	0.2%	0.8%
Reversibility	Rapid	Rapid	Rapid
Maximum duration	3 yr	5 yr	10 yr
Changes in bleeding	Irregular bleeding Amenorrhea at 1 yr: 6%	Irregular bleeding Amenorrhea at 1 yr: 20%	No change in cyclical nature of cycles
Mean monthly blood loss	—	5 mL	50–80 mL
Additional benefits	—	May be used to treat heavy menstrual bleeding, chronic pelvic pain, or endometriosis	May be used as emergency contraception Nonhormonal
Adverse effects	Minimal: Headache, spotting, breast tenderness, nausea (which usually resolves within 6 mo)	Same as for 3-yr IUD	More severe menstrual cramps (usually relieved by NSAIDs) and heavier flow
Primary mechanism of action	Thickens cervical mucus and prevents fertilization	Same as for 3-yr IUD	Use of copper ions to produce a sterile inflammatory response that is toxic to sperm, thus preventing fertilization

(for gonorrhea and chlamydial infection) before they insert an IUD. However, STD testing should be done just before the IUD is inserted, and if results are positive, patients should be treated with appropriate antibiotics; the IUD is left in place. If purulent discharge is observed at the time of IUD insertion, the IUD is not inserted, STD testing is done, and empiric treatment with antibiotics is started before test results are available.

When IUDs are inserted, sterile technique is used as much as possible. Bimanual examination should be done to determine the position of the uterus, and a tenaculum should be placed on the anterior lip of the cervix to stabilize the uterus, straighten the uterine axis, and help ensure correct placement of the IUD. A uterine sound device or an endometrial aspirator (used for biopsy) is often used to measure the length of the uterine cavity before IUD insertion. The package insert for the IUD should be reviewed before insertion because the 3 types of IUDs are inserted differently.

Most women can use an IUD. Contraindications include the following:

- Current pelvic infection, usually pelvic inflammatory disease (PID), mucopurulent cervicitis with a suspected STD, pelvic TB, septic abortion, or puerperal endometritis or sepsis within the past 3 mo
- Anatomic abnormalities that distort the uterine cavity
- Gestational trophoblastic disease with persistently elevated serum β–human chorionic gonadotropin (β-hCG) levels (a relative contraindication because supporting data are lacking)
- Unexplained vaginal bleeding
- Known cervical or endometrial cancer
- Pregnancy
- For levonorgestrel-releasing IUDs, breast cancer or allergy to levonorgestrel
- For copper-bearing T380 IUDs, Wilson disease or allergy to copper

Conditions that do not contraindicate IUDs include the following:

- Religious beliefs that prohibit abortion because IUDs are not abortifacients (however, a copper IUD used for emergency contraception may prevent implantation of the blastocyst)
- A history of PID, STDs, or ectopic pregnancy
- Contraindications to contraceptives that contain estrogen (eg, history of venous thromboembolism, smoking > 15 cigarettes/day in women > 35, migraine with aura, migraine of any type in women > 35)
- Breastfeeding
- Adolescence

Vaginal bleeding stops completely within 1 yr in 6% of women using the 3-yr IUD and in 20% of women using the 5-yr IUD. A copper-bearing T380A IUD may cause heavier menstrual bleeding and more severe cramping, which can be relieved by NSAIDs (eg, ibuprofen). Women should be told about these effects before the IUD is inserted because this information may help them decide which type of IUD to choose.

An IUD may be inserted at any time during the menstrual cycle if a woman has not had unprotected intercourse during the past month.

If a woman has had unprotected intercourse within the past 7 days, a copper-bearing T380 IUD may be inserted as emergency contraception. The copper-bearing IUD may be left in place for long-term contraception if the woman desires. The resumption of menses plus a negative pregnancy test reliably excludes pregnancy; a pregnancy test should be done 2 to 3 wk after insertion to be sure that an unintended pregnancy has not occurred before insertion.

An IUD may be inserted immediately after an induced or a spontaneous abortion during the 1st or 2nd trimester and immediately after delivery of the placenta during a cesarean or vaginal delivery.

IUDs do not increase and may decrease the risk of uterine cancer.

Complications: Average IUD expulsion rates are usually < 5% within the first year after insertion; however, expulsion rates are higher if the IUD is inserted immediately (< 10 min) after a delivery. After insertion, a clinician confirms correct placement at 6 wk by looking for the strings attached to the IUD, which are typically trimmed to 3 cm from the external cervical os.

The uterus is perforated in about 1/1000 IUD insertions. Perforation occurs at the time of IUD insertion. Sometimes only the distal part of the IUD penetrates; then over the next few months, uterine contractions force the IUD into the peritoneal cavity. If the string is not visible during pelvic examination, the uterine cavity is probed with a sound or biopsy instrument (unless pregnancy is suspected) and/or ultrasonography is done. If the IUD is not seen, an abdominal x-ray is taken to exclude an intraperitoneal location. Intraperitoneal IUDs may cause intestinal adhesions. IUDs that have perforated the uterus are removed via laparoscopy.

If expulsion or perforation is suspected, a backup contraceptive method should be used.

Rarely, salpingitis (PID) develops during the first month after insertion because bacteria are displaced into the uterine cavity during insertion; however, this risk is low and routine antibiotic prophylaxis is not indicated. If PID develops, antibiotics should be given. The IUD need not be removed unless the infection persists despite antibiotics. IUD strings do not provide access for bacteria. Except during the first month after insertion, IUDs do not increase the risk of PID.

The incidence of ectopic pregnancy is much lower in IUD users than in women using no contraceptive method because IUDs effectively prevent pregnancy. However, if a women becomes pregnant while an IUD is in place, she should be told that risk of ectopic pregnancy is increased, and she should be evaluated promptly (see p. 2346).

KEY POINTS

- IUDs are highly effective, have minimal systemic effects, and involve only one contraceptive decision every 3, 5, or 10 yr depending on the IUD chosen.
- Types include levonorgestrel-releasing IUDs (effective for 3 yr or 5 yr, depending on the type) and a copper-bearing IUD (effective for 10 to 12 yr).
- A Pap test is not required before IUD insertion.
- Inform women that both types of IUDs can affect menstrual bleeding (amenorrhea within 1 yr in 6% of women using the 3-yr IUD and in 20% of those using the 5-yr IUD and possibly heavier menstrual bleeding and more severe cramping in women using the copper-bearing T380 IUD).
- Confirm correct placement of the IUD by checking the strings 6 wk after insertion.
- If the strings are not visible during the pelvic examination, probe the uterine cavity using a uterine sound or biopsy instrument (unless pregnancy is suspected), and if needed, do ultrasonography or take an abdominal x-ray to check for an intraperitoneal location.

FERTILITY AWARENESS–BASED METHODS OF CONTRACEPTION

(Periodic Abstinence)

Although the ovum can be fertilized for only about 12 h after ovulation, sperm can fertilize an ovum for up to 5 days after intercourse; as a result, intercourse almost 5 days before ovulation can result in pregnancy. Thus, fertility awareness–based methods require abstinence from intercourse starting 5 days before ovulation.

Several methods can be used to identify the time of ovulation and thus determine when abstinence is required. They include

- Standard days method
- Two-day (ovulation) method
- Symptothermal method

The **standard days method** is based on the calendar (the dates that menses occur) and is appropriate only for women who have regular menses. Ovulation occurs about 14 days before onset of menses. Thus, the interval of abstinence during the menstrual cycle is determined by subtracting 18 days from the shortest of the previous 12 cycles and 11 days from the longest. For example, if cycles vary between 26 and 29 days, abstinence is required from days 8 through 18 of each cycle. The greater the variance in cycle length, the longer abstinence is required. Cyclebeads (a string of color-coded beads that represent the days of a menstrual cycle) can be used to help women keep track of their fertile days.

The **2-day (ovulation) method** is based only on cervical mucus assessment. Cervical mucus may be absent for a few days after menses. After the mucus reappears, it tends to be cloudy, thick, and inelastic. Then the amount of mucus increases, and the mucus becomes thinner, clearer, and more elastic than usual. It resembles raw egg whites and stretches between the fingers. Intercourse is avoided completely during menses (because mucus cannot be checked). It is permitted during the days when mucus is completely absent, but during these days, intercourse is restricted to every other day (so that semen is not confused with mucus). Intercourse is avoided from the time mucus first appears after menses until 4 days after the amount peaks. Intercourse is permitted without restriction from 4 days after the amount of mucus peaks until menses begin. A change in cervical mucus indicates ovulation more accurately than body temperature.

The **symptothermal method** combines measurement of basal body temperature (which increases after ovulation), cervical mucus assessment, and the standard days method. Intercourse is avoided from the first day requiring abstinence according to the standard days method until 3 days after the amount of cervical mucus decreases and temperature increases.

The symptothermal method has a lower pregnancy rate with perfect use than the 2-day method (based on cervical mucus) or the standard days method (with or without cyclebeads). However, pregnancy rates with any of these methods are high with typical use, so these methods are not recommended for women who strongly want to avoid pregnancy.

The **lactational amenorrhea method** is another fertility-based awareness method. It is based on the natural postpartum infertility that occurs when women breastfeed exclusively (or almost exclusively) and menses has not resumed. The infant's suckling inhibits the release of hormones that are necessary to stimulate ovulation. Without ovulation, pregnancy cannot occur. This method can be 98% effective if the following criteria are met:

- The infant is < 6 mo.
- Breastfeeding is the primary source of infant feeding (supplementation with formula or solid food or pumping breast milk decreases efficacy).
- Breastfeeding is done at least every 4 h during the day and every 6 h at night.
- Menses have not resumed (amenorrhea).

EMERGENCY CONTRACEPTION

Commonly used emergency contraception (EC) regimens include

- Insertion of a copper-bearing T380A IUD within 5 days of unprotected intercourse
- Levonorgestrel 0.75 mg po in 2 doses 12 h apart within 120 h of unprotected intercourse
- Levonorgestrel 1.5 mg po once within 120 h of unprotected intercourse
- Ulipristal acetate 30 mg po once within 120 h of unprotected intercourse

For women who have regular menses, the risk of pregnancy after a single act of intercourse is about 5%. This risk is 20 to 30% if intercourse occurs at midcycle.

When a copper-bearing IUD is used for EC, it must be inserted within 5 days of unprotected intercourse or within 7 days of suspected ovulation. The pregnancy rate with this EC method is 0.1%. Also, the IUD can be left in place to be used for long-term contraception. As EC, the copper-bearing IUD may affect blastocyst implantation; however, it does not appear to disrupt an already established pregnancy.

EC with levonorgestrel prevents pregnancy by inhibiting or delaying ovulation. The probability of pregnancy is reduced by 85% after levonorgestrel EC, which has a pregnancy rate of 2 to 3%. However, overall risk reduction depends on the following:

- The woman's risk of pregnancy without EC
- The time in the menstrual cycle that EC is given
- The woman's BMI (levonorgestrel EC is less effective than ulipristal acetate in obese women with a body mass index [BMI] > 30)

Ulipristal acetate (a progestin-receptor modulator) has a pregnancy rate of about 1.5% and is thus more effective than levonorgestrel. Ulipristal acetate, like levonorgestrel, prevents pregnancy primarily by delaying or inhibiting ovulation. Although ulipristal acetate is more effective than levonorgestrel for women with a BMI > 30, its effectiveness also decreases as BMI increases. Thus, in obese women who strongly desire to avoid an unintended pregnancy, the copper-bearing IUD is the preferred method for EC.

There are no absolute contraindications to levonorgestrel or ulipristal acetate EC. Levonorgestrel EC is available behind pharmacy counters without a prescription. Ulipristal acetate is available by prescription only. Levonorgestrel and ulipristal EC should be taken as soon as possible and within 120 h of unprotected intercourse.

Another regimen (the Yuzpe method) consists of 2 tablets, each containing ethinyl estradiol 50 mcg and levonorgestrel 0.25 mg, followed by 2 more tablets taken 12 h later but within 72 h of unprotected intercourse. The high estrogen dose often causes nausea and may cause vomiting. This method is also less effective than other methods; thus, it is no longer recommended except when women do not have access to other methods.

EC can be given when another hormonal contraceptive is started as part of a quick-start protocol. A urine pregnancy test 2 wk after use of EC is recommended.

KEY POINTS

- Usually, hormones (eg, ulipristal acetate, levonorgestrel) are used for EC; they are taken as soon as possible within 120 h of unprotected intercourse.
- A copper-bearing IUD, inserted within 5 days of unprotected intercourse, is also effective and can be left in place for long-term contraception.
- Pregnancy rates are 1.5% with ulipristal acetate, 2 to 3% with levonorgestrel, and 0.1% with a copper-bearing IUD.
- Likelihood of pregnancy after hormonal EC depends on pregnancy risk without EC, time in the menstrual cycle that EC is taken, and the woman's BMI.

STERILIZATION

In the US, one-third of couples attempting to prevent pregnancy, particularly if the woman is > 30, choose sterilization with vasectomy or tubal ligation. Sterilization should be assumed to be permanent. However, if pregnancy is desired, reanastomosis may restore fertility in 45 to 60% of men after vasectomy and in 50 to 80% of women after tubal ligation. Also, in vitro fertilization may be used successfully.

Male Sterilization (Vasectomy)

For this procedure, the vasa deferentia are cut, and the cut ends are ligated or fulgurated. Vasectomy can be done in about 20 min; a local anesthetic is used. Sterility requires about 20 ejaculations after the operation and should be documented by 2 sperm-free ejaculates, usually obtained 3 mo after the operation. A back-up contraceptive method should be used until that time.

Mild discomfort for 2 to 3 days after the procedure is common. Taking NSAIDs and not attempting ejaculation are recommended during this period.

Complications of vasectomy include hematoma (≤ 5%), sperm granulomas (inflammatory responses to sperm leakage), and spontaneous reanastomosis, which usually occurs shortly after the procedure. The cumulative pregnancy rate is 1.1% at 5 yr.

Female Sterilization

In this procedure, the fallopian tubes are cut and a segment is excised or the tubes are closed by ligation, fulguration, or various mechanical devices (plastic bands, spring-loaded clips). Alternatively, the tubes can be occluded. Sterilization that uses mechanical devices causes less tissue damage and thus may be more reversible.

One of several methods may be used; they include

- Laparoscopy
- Hysteroscopy
- Minilaparotomy

Tubal ligation can be done during cesarean delivery or 1 to 2 days after vaginal delivery via a small periumbilical incision (via laparoscopy). Laparoscopic methods of tubal sterilization are traditionally done as an interval procedure (unrelated to pregnancy), usually > 6 wk after delivery and in the operating room; a general anesthetic is used. The cumulative failure rate of tubal sterilization is about 1.8% at 10 yr; however, certain techniques have higher failure rates than others. Postpartum procedures have a lower failure rate than some laparoscopic methods.

For hysteroscopic sterilization, clinicians, using hysteroscopic guidance, occlude the lumen of the fallopian tubes by inserting microinserts with coils. The coils consist of an outer layer of a nickel/titanium alloy and an inner layer of stainless steel and polyethylene terephthalate (PET). The PET fibers stimulate an ingrowth reaction that occludes the tubes.

Advantages of hysteroscopic sterilization over tubal ligation include the following:

- It can be done in a clinic as an outpatient procedure.
- It does not require incisions or cutting, clipping, or burning of the tubes.

A comparative disadvantage is that after microinserts are placed, sterility is delayed for up to 3 mo because the reaction that occludes the tubes takes several weeks. Often, clinicians recommend that women use another contraceptive method for 3 mo after the procedure. Women should choose a method (eg, depot medroxyprogesterone) that stabilizes the endometrium and allows visualization during hysteroscopy. This method can be used until tubal occlusion is confirmed by hysterosalpingography 3 mo after sterilization. If women are allergic to radiopaque dyes, ultrasonography can be used to confirm tubal occlusion.

Minilaparotomy is sometimes used instead of laparoscopic sterilization, usually when women want to be sterilized soon after delivery of a baby. It requires a general, regional, or local anesthetic. It involves a small abdominal incision (about 2.5 to 7.6 cm) and removal of a section of each fallopian tube. Compared with laparoscopy, minilaparotomy caused more pain, and recovery takes slightly longer.

After laparoscopic or minilaparotomy sterilization, clinicians recommend that women do not place anything in the vagina (eg, tampons, douches) and that they do not have sexual intercourse for about 2 wk.

Adverse effects of female sterilization are uncommon. Some of these complications include

- Death: 1 to 2/100,000 women
- Hemorrhage or intestinal injuries: About 0.5% of women
- Other complications (eg, infarction, failure of occlusion): Up to about 5% of women
- Ectopic pregnancy: About 30% of pregnancies that occur after tubal ligation

KEY POINTS

- Tell patients that sterilization should be considered permanent, although reanastomosis can restore fertility (if desired) in about half of men and even more women.
- For men, the vasa deferentia are cut, then ligated or fulgurated; sterility is confirmed after 2 ejaculations are sperm-free, usually after 3 mo.
- For women, the fallopian tubes are cut; then part of the tubes is excised, or the tubes are occluded using microinserts or closed by ligation, fulguration, or mechanical devices such as plastic bands or spring-loaded clips; procedures used include laparoscopy, hysteroscopy, and minilaparotomy.

INDUCED ABORTION

(Termination of Pregnancy)

In the US, abortion of a previable fetus is legal, although state-specific restrictions (eg, mandatory waiting periods, gestational age restrictions) have been recently implemented. In the US, about half of pregnancies are unintended. About 40% of unintended pregnancies are terminated by elective abortion; 90% of procedures are done during the 1st trimester.

In countries where abortion is legal, abortion is usually safe and complications are rare. Worldwide, 13% of maternal deaths are secondary to induced abortion, and the overwhelming majority of these deaths occur in countries where abortion is illegal.

Common methods of inducing abortion are

- Instrumental evacuation through the vagina
- Medical induction (stimulation of uterine contractions)

Uterine surgery (hysterotomy or hysterectomy) is a last resort, which is usually avoided because mortality rates are higher. Hysterotomy also results in a uterine scar, which may rupture in subsequent pregnancies.

Pregnancy should be confirmed before abortion is induced. Often, gestational age is established by ultrasonography, but sometimes history and physical examination can accurately confirm gestational age during the 1st trimester. Doppler ultrasonography should be considered if a woman is in the 2nd trimester and has placenta previa or an anterior placenta plus a history of a uterine scar.

Termination of the pregnancy can be confirmed by directly observing removal of uterine contents via ultrasonography used during the procedure. If ultrasonography is not used during the procedure, termination can be confirmed by measuring quantitative serum β–human chorionic gonadotropin (β-hCG) levels before and after the procedure; a decrease of > 50% after 1 wk confirms termination.

Antibiotics effective against reproductive tract organisms (including chlamydiae) should be given to the patient on the day of the abortion. Traditionally, doxycycline is used; 100 mg is given before the procedure and 200 mg is given afterward. After the procedure, Rh_0(D) immune globulin is given to women with Rh-negative blood.

First-trimester abortions often require only local anesthesia, but trained clinicians may offer sedation in addition. For later abortions, deeper sedation is usually required.

Contraception (all forms) can be started immediately after an induced abortion done at < 28 wk.

Instrumental evacuation: Typically at < 14 wk, dilation and curettage (D & C) is used, usually with a large-diameter suction cannula, inserted into the uterus.

At < 9 wk, manual vacuum aspiration (MVA) can be used. It produces enough pressure to evacuate the uterus. MVA devices are portable, do not require an electrical source, and are quieter than electrical vacuum aspiration (EVA) devices. MVA may also be used to manage spontaneous abortion during early pregnancy. After 9 wk, EVA is used; it involves attaching a cannula to an electrical vacuum source.

At 14 to 24 wk, dilation and evacuation (D & E) is usually used. Forceps are used to dismember and remove the fetus, and a suction cannula is used to aspirate the amniotic fluid, placenta, and fetal debris. D & E requires more skill and requires more training than do other methods of instrumental evacuation.

Often, progressively increasing sizes of tapered dilators are used to dilate the cervix before the procedure. However, depending on gestational age and parity, clinicians may need to use another type of dilator instead of or in addition to tapered dilators to minimize the cervical damage that tapered dilators can cause. Choices include the prostaglandin E_1 analog (misoprostol) and osmotic dilators such as laminaria (dried seaweed stems). Osmotic dilators can be inserted into the cervix and left for ≥ 4 h (often overnight if the pregnancy is >18 wk). Misoprostol dilates the cervix by stimulating prostaglandin release; osmotic dilators dilate the cervix by expanding. Osmotic dilators are usually used at > 16 wk. Misoprostol is usually given buccally 2 to 4 h before the procedure.

If patients wish to avoid pregnancy and the need for subsequent abortions, an intrauterine device (IUD) can be inserted as soon as pregnancy is terminated. This approach makes repeat abortion less likely.

Medical induction: Medical induction can be used for pregnancies of < 9 wk or > 15 wk. If patients have severe anemia, medical induction should be done only in a hospital so that blood transfusion is readily available.

In the US, medical abortion accounts for 25% of abortions done at < 9 wk. For pregnancies of < 9 wk, 2 regimens are effective; both include the progesterone-receptor blocker mifepristone (RU 486) and the prostaglandin E_1 analog misoprostol, as follows:

- Evidence-based regimen: Mifepristone 200 mg po, followed by misoprostol 800 mcg, self-administered vaginally at 6 to 72 h or buccally at 24 to 48 h (requiring only 2 visits)
- FDA-approved regimen: Mifepristone 600 mg po, followed by misoprostol 400 mcg po given by a clinician at about 48 h (requiring 3 visits)

The evidence-based regimen is about 98% effective in terminating pregnancies up to 9 wk; the FDA-approved regimen is 95% effective at < 7 wk.

After either regimen, a follow-up visit is required to confirm termination of the pregnancy and, if necessary, to provide contraception.

After 15 wk, pretreatment with mifepristone 200 mg 24 to 48 h before induction reduces induction times. Prostaglandins are used to induce abortion. Options include vaginal prostaglandin E_2 (dinoprostone) suppositories, vaginal and buccal misoprostol tablets, and IM injections of prostaglandin $F_{2\alpha}$ (dinoprost tromethamine). The typical dose of misoprostol is 600 to 800 mcg vaginally, followed by 400 mcg buccally q 3 h for up to 5 doses. Or, two 200-mcg vaginal tablets of misoprostol q 6 h can be used; abortion occurs within 48 h in almost 100% of cases.

Adverse effects of prostaglandins include nausea, vomiting, diarrhea, hyperthermia, facial flushing, vasovagal symptoms, bronchospasm, and decreased seizure threshold.

Complications

Complication rates with abortion (serious complications in < 1%; mortality in < 1 in 100,000) are higher than those with contraception; however, rates are 14 times lower than those after delivery of a full-term infant, and rates have decreased in the last few decades. Complication rates increase as gestational age increases.

Serious early complications include perforation of the uterus (0.1%) or, less often, of the intestine or another organ by an instrument. Major hemorrhage (0.06%) may result from trauma or an atonic uterus. Laceration of the cervix (0.1 to 1%) ranges from superficial tenaculum tears to cervicovaginal tears, rarely with fistulas. General or local anesthesia rarely causes serious complications.

The most common delayed complications include bleeding and significant infection (0.1 to 2%), which usually occur because placental fragments are retained. If bleeding occurs or infection is suspected, pelvic ultrasonography is done; retained placental fragments may be visible on an ultrasound scan. Mild inflammation is expected, but if infection is moderate or severe, peritonitis or sepsis may occur. Sterility may result from synechiae in the endometrial cavity or tubal fibrosis due to infection. Forceful dilation of the cervix in more advanced pregnancies may contribute to incompetent cervix. However, elective abortion probably does not increase risks for the fetus or woman during subsequent pregnancies.

Psychologic complications do not typically occur but may occur in women who

- Had psychologic symptoms before pregnancy
- Had significant emotional attachment to the pregnancy (eg, terminated a desired pregnancy for a maternal or fetal medical indication)
- Have conservative political views about abortion
- Have limited social support

KEY POINTS

- About 40% of unintended pregnancies are terminated by elective abortion.
- Common methods for abortion are instrumental evacuation through the vagina or medical induction (to induce uterine contractions).
- Before abortion is done, confirm that the woman is pregnant, and if so, determine gestational age based on history and physical examination and/or ultrasonography.
- For instrumental evacuation, usually use D & C at < 14 wk gestation and D & E at 14 to 24 wk, sometimes preceded by cervical dilation using misoprostol or osmotic dilators (eg, laminaria).
- For medical induction, give mifepristone, followed by misoprostol at < 9 wk gestation; after 15 wk gestation, pretreat with mifepristone, then give a prostaglandin (eg, dinoprostone vaginally, misoprostol vaginally and buccally, prostaglandin $F_{2\alpha}$ IM), or misoprostol vaginally.
- Serious complications (eg, uterine perforation, major bleeding, serious infection) occur in < 1% of abortions.
- Elective abortion probably does not increase risks in subsequent pregnancies.

269 Female Reproductive Endocrinology

Hormonal interaction between the hypothalamus, anterior pituitary gland, and ovaries regulates the female reproductive system.

The hypothalamus secretes a small peptide, gonadotropin-releasing hormone (GnRH), also known as luteinizing hormone–releasing hormone.

GnRH regulates release of the gonadotropins luteinizing hormone (LH) and follicle-stimulating hormone (FSH) from specialized cells (gonadotropes) in the anterior pituitary gland (see Fig. 269–1). These hormones are released in short bursts (pulses) every 1 to 4 h. LH and FSH promote ovulation and stimulate secretion of the sex hormones estradiol (an estrogen) and progesterone from the ovaries.

Estrogen and progesterone circulate in the bloodstream almost entirely bound to plasma proteins. Only unbound estrogen and progesterone appear to be biologically active. They stimulate the target organs of the reproductive system (eg, breasts, uterus, vagina). They usually inhibit but, in certain situations (eg, around the time of ovulation), may stimulate gonadotropin secretion.

Puberty

Puberty is the sequence of events in which a child acquires adult physical characteristics and capacity for reproduction. Circulating LH and FSH levels are elevated at birth but fall to

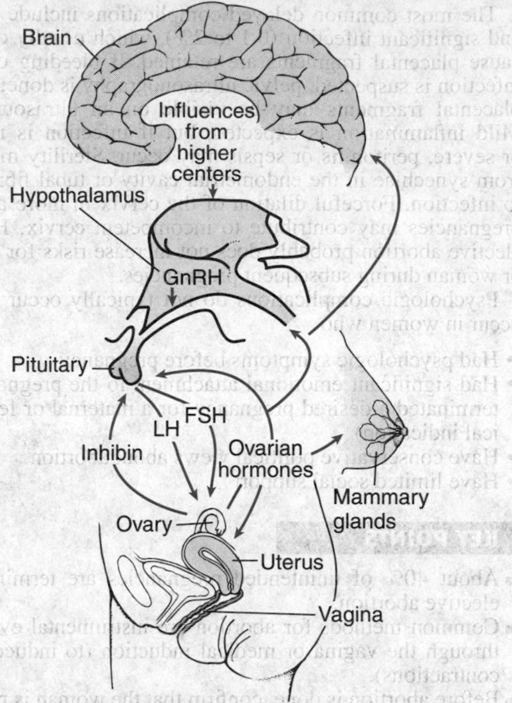

Fig. 269–1. The CNS-hypothalamic-pituitary-gonadal target organ axis. Ovarian hormones have direct and indirect effects on other tissues (eg, bone, skin, muscle). FSH = follicle-stimulating hormone; GnRH = gonadotropin-releasing hormone; LH = luteinizing hormone.

low levels within a few months and remain low until puberty. Until puberty, few qualitative changes occur in reproductive target organs.

Age of onset of puberty: The age of onset of puberty and the rate of development through different stages are influenced by different factors. Over the last 150 yr, the age at which puberty begins has been decreasing, primarily because of improved health and nutrition, but this trend has stabilized.

Puberty often occurs earlier than average in moderately obese girls and later than average in severely underweight and undernourished girls.[1] Such observations suggest that a critical body weight or amount of fat is necessary for puberty.

Many other factors can influence when puberty begins and how rapidly it progresses. For example, there is some evidence that intrauterine growth restriction, especially when followed by postnatal overfeeding, may contribute to earlier and more rapid development of puberty.

Puberty occurs earlier in girls whose mothers matured earlier and, for unknown reasons, in girls who live in urban areas or who are blind.

The age of onset of puberty also varies among ethnic groups (eg, tending to be earlier in blacks and Hispanics than in Asians and non-Hispanic whites).[2]

Physical changes of puberty: Physical changes of puberty occur sequentially during adolescence (see Fig. 269–2).

Breast budding (see Fig. 269–3)[3] and onset of the growth spurt are usually the first changes recognized.

Then, pubic and axillary hair appear (see Fig. 269–4), and the growth spurt peaks.

Menarche (the first menstrual period) occurs about 2 to 3 yr after breast budding. Menstrual cycles are usually irregular at menarche and can take up to 5 yr to become regular. The growth spurt is limited after menarche. Body habitus changes and the pelvis and hips widen. Body fat increases and accumulates in the hips and thighs.

Mechanisms initiating puberty: Mechanisms initiating puberty are unclear.

Central influences that regulate release of GnRH include neurotransmitters and peptides (eg, gamma-aminobutyric acid [GABA], kisspeptin). Such factors may inhibit release of GnRH during childhood, then initiate its release to induce puberty in early adolescence. Early in puberty, hypothalamic GnRH release becomes less sensitive to inhibition by estrogen and progesterone. The resulting increased release of GnRH promotes LH and FSH secretion, which stimulates production of sex hormones, primarily estrogen. Estrogen stimulates development of secondary sexual characteristics.

Pubic and axillary hair growth may be stimulated by the adrenal androgens dehydroepiandrosterone (DHEA) and DHEA sulfate; production of these androgens increases several years before puberty in a process called adrenarche.

1. Rosenfield RL, Lipton RB, Drum ML: Thelarche, pubarche, and menarche attainment in children with normal and elevated body mass index. *Pediatrics* 123(1):84–88, 2009. doi: 10.1542/peds.2008-0146.
2. Herman-Giddens ME, Slora EJ, Wasserman RC, et al: Secondary sexual characteristics and menses in young

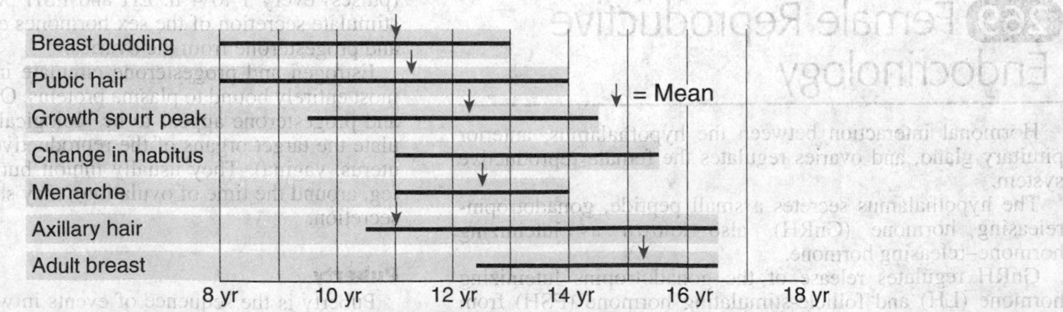

Fig. 269–2. Puberty—when female sexual characteristics develop. Bars indicate normal ranges.

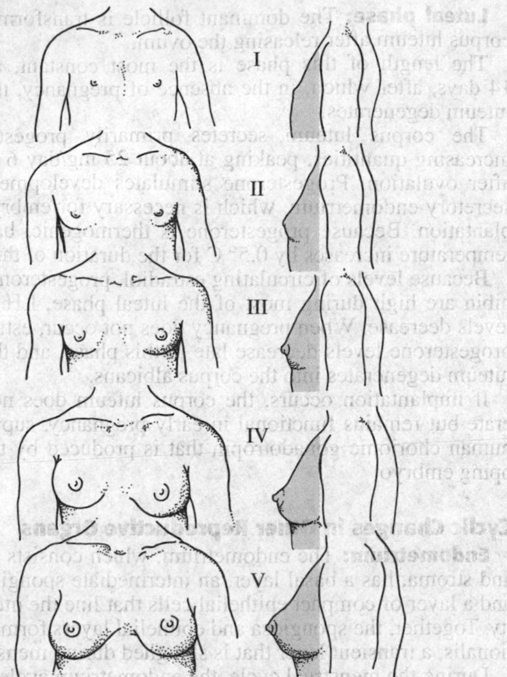

Fig. 269–3. Diagrammatic representation of Tanner stages I to V of human breast maturation. From Marshall WA, Tanner JM: Variations in patterns of pubertal changes in girls. *Archives of Disease in Childhood* 44:291–303, 1969; used with permission.

girls seen in office practice: A study from the Pediatric Research in Office Settings network. *Pediatrics* 99: 505–512, 1997.

3. Marshall WA, Tanner JM: Variations in patterns of pubertal changes in girls. *Arch Dis Child* 44:291–303, 1969.

Ovarian Follicular Development

A female is born with a finite number of egg precursors (germ cells). Germ cells begin as primordial oogonia that proliferate markedly by mitosis through the 4th mo of gestation. During the 3rd mo of gestation, some oogonia begin to undergo meiosis, which reduces the number of chromosomes by half.

By the 7th mo, all viable germ cells develop a surrounding layer of granulosa cells, forming a primordial follicle, and are arrested in meiotic prophase; these cells are primary oocytes. Beginning after the 4th mo of gestation, oogonia (and later oocytes) are lost spontaneously in a process called atresia; eventually, 99.9% are lost. In older mothers, the long time that surviving oocytes spend arrested in meiotic prophase may account for the increased incidence of genetically abnormal pregnancies.

FSH induces follicular growth in the ovaries. During each menstrual cycle, 3 to 30 follicles are recruited for accelerated growth. Usually in each cycle, only one follicle achieves ovulation. This dominant follicle releases its oocyte at ovulation and promotes atresia of the other recruited follicles.

Menstrual Cycle

Menstruation is the periodic discharge of blood and sloughed endometrium (collectively called menses or menstrual flow) from

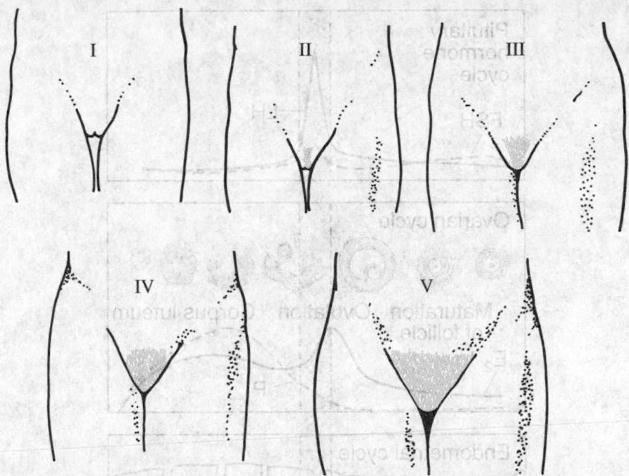

Fig. 269–4. Diagrammatic representation of Tanner stages I to V for development of pubic hair in girls. From Marshall WA, Tanner JM: Variations in patterns of pubertal changes in girls. *Archives of Disease in Childhood* 44:291–303, 1969; used with permission.

the uterus through the vagina. It is caused by the rapid decline in ovarian production of progesterone and estrogen that occurs each cycle in the absence of a pregnancy. Menstruation occurs throughout a woman's reproductive life in the absence of pregnancy.

Menopause is the permanent cessation of menses.

Average duration of menses is 5 (± 2) days. Blood loss per cycle averages 30 mL (normal range, 13 to 80 mL) and is usually greatest on the 2nd day. A saturated pad or tampon absorbs 5 to 15 mL. Menstrual blood does not usually clot (unless bleeding is very heavy), probably because fibrinolysin and other factors inhibit clotting.

The median menstrual cycle length is 28 days (usual range, about 25 to 36 days). Generally, variation is maximal and intermenstrual intervals are longest in the years immediately after menarche and immediately before menopause, when ovulation occurs less regularly. The menstrual cycle begins and ends with the first day of menses (day 1).

The menstrual cycle can be divided into phases, usually based on ovarian status. The ovary proceeds through the following phases:

- Follicular (preovulatory)
- Ovulatory
- Luteal (postovulatory—see Fig. 269–5)

The endometrium also cycles through phases.

Follicular phase: This phase varies in length more than other phases.

In the **early follicular phase** (first half of the follicular phase), the primary event is

- Growth of recruited follicles

At this time, the gonadotropes in the anterior pituitary contain little LH and FSH, and estrogen and progesterone production is low. As a result, overall FSH secretion increases slightly, stimulating growth of recruited follicles. Also, circulating LH levels increase slowly, beginning 1 to 2 days after the increase in FSH. The recruited ovarian follicles soon increase production of estradiol; estradiol stimulates LH and FSH synthesis but inhibits their secretion.

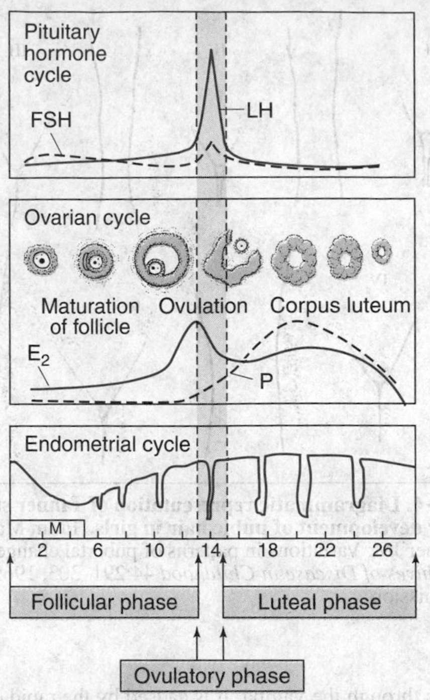

Fig. 269–5. The idealized cyclic changes in pituitary gonadotropins, estradiol (E_2), progesterone (P), and uterine endometrium during the normal menstrual cycle. Days of menstrual bleeding are indicated by M. FSH = follicle-stimulating hormone; LH = luteinizing hormone. (Adapted from Rebar RW: Normal physiology of the reproductive system. In *Endocrinology and Metabolism Continuing Education Program, American Association of Clinical Chemistry*, November 1982. Copyright 1982 by the American Association for Clinical Chemistry; reprinted with permission.)

During the **late follicular phase** (2nd half of the follicular phase), the follicle selected for ovulation matures and accumulates hormone-secreting granulosa cells; its antrum enlarges with follicular fluid, reaching 18 to 20 mm before ovulation. FSH levels decrease; LH levels are affected less. FSH and LH levels diverge partly because estradiol inhibits FSH secretion more than LH secretion. Also, developing follicles produce the hormone inhibin, which inhibits FSH secretion but not LH secretion. Other contributing factors may include disparate half-lives (20 to 30 min for LH; 2 to 3 h for FSH) and unknown factors. Levels of estrogen,particularly estradiol, increase exponentially.

Ovulatory phase: Ovulation (ovum release) occurs.

Estradiol levels usually peak as the ovulatory phase begins. Progesteronelevels also begin to increase.

Stored LH is released in massive amounts (LH surge), usually over 36 to 48 h, with a smaller increase in FSH. The LH surge occurs because at this time, high levels of estradiol trigger LH secretion by gonadotropes (positive feedback). The LH surge is also stimulated by GnRH and progesterone. During the LH surge, estradiol levels decrease, but progesterone levels continue to increase. The LH surge stimulates enzymes that initiate breakdown of the follicle wall and release of the now mature ovum within about 16 to 32 h. The LH surge also triggers completion of the first meiotic division of the oocyte within about 36 h.

Luteal phase: The dominant follicle is transformed into a corpus luteum after releasing the ovum.

The length of this phase is the most constant, averaging 14 days, after which, in the absence of pregnancy, the corpus luteum degenerates.

The corpus luteum secretes primarily progesterone in increasing quantities, peaking at about 25 mg/day 6 to 8 days after ovulation. Progesterone stimulates development of the secretory endometrium, which is necessary for embryonic implantation. Because progesterone is thermogenic, basal body temperature increases by 0.5° C for the duration of this phase.

Because levels of circulating estradiol, progesterone, and inhibin are high during most of the luteal phase, LH and FSH levels decrease. When pregnancy does not occur, estradiol and progesterone levels decrease late in this phase, and the corpus luteum degenerates into the corpus albicans.

If implantation occurs, the corpus luteum does not degenerate but remains functional in early pregnancy, supported by human chorionic gonadotropin that is produced by the developing embryo.

Cyclic Changes in Other Reproductive Organs

Endometrium: The endometrium, which consists of glands and stroma, has a basal layer, an intermediate spongiosa layer, and a layer of compact epithelial cells that line the uterine cavity. Together, the spongiosa and epithelial layers form the functionalis, a transient layer that is sloughed during menses.

During the menstrual cycle, the endometrium cycles through its own phases:

- Menstrual
- Proliferative
- Secretory

After menstruation, the endometrium is typically thin with dense stroma and narrow, straight, tubular glands lined with low columnar epithelium. As estradiol levels increase, the intact basal layer regenerates the endometrium to its maximum thickness late in the ovarian follicular phase (proliferative phase of the endometrial cycle). The mucosa thickens and the glands lengthen and coil, becoming tortuous.

Ovulation occurs at the beginning of the secretory phase of the endometrial cycle. During the ovarian luteal phase, progesterone stimulates the endometrial glands to dilate, fill with glycogen, and become secretory while stromal vascularity increases. As estradiol and progesterone levels decrease late in the luteal/secretory phase, the stroma becomes edematous, and the endometrium and its blood vessels necrose, leading to bleeding and menstrual flow (menstrual phase of the endometrial cycle). Fibrinolytic activity of the endometrium decreases blood clots in the menstrual blood.

Because histologic changes are specific to the phase of the menstrual cycle, the cycle phase or tissue response to sex hormones can be determined accurately by endometrial biopsy.

Cervix: The cervix acts as a barrier that limits access to the uterine cavity.

During the follicular phase, increasing estradiol levels increase cervical vascularity and edema and cervical mucus quantity, elasticity, and salt (sodium chloride or potassium chloride) concentration. The external os opens slightly and fills with mucus at ovulation.

During the luteal phase, increasing progesterone levels make the cervical mucus thicker and less elastic, decreasing success of sperm transport.

Menstrual cycle phase can sometimes be identified by microscopic examination of cervical mucus dried on a glass slide; ferning (palm leaf arborization of mucus) indicates increased salts in cervical mucus. Ferning becomes prominent just before ovulation, when estrogen levels are high; it is minimal or absent during the luteal phase. Spinnbarkeit, the stretchability (elasticity) of the mucus, increases as estrogen levels increase (eg, just before ovulation); this change can be used to identify the periovulatory (fertile) phase of the menstrual cycle.

Vagina: Early in the follicular phase, when estradiol levels are low, the vaginal epithelium is thin and pale. Later in the follicular phase, as estradiol levels increase, squamous cells mature and become cornified, causing epithelial thickening.

During the luteal phase, the number of precornified intermediate cells increases, and the number of leukocytes and amount of cellular debris increase as mature squamous cells are shed.

270 Gynecologic Tumors

Gynecologic cancers often involve the uterus, ovaries, cervix, vulva, vagina, fallopian tubes, or the peritoneum. The most common gynecologic cancer in the US is endometrial cancer, followed by ovarian cancer. Cervical cancer is not very common in developed countries because Papanicolaou (Pap) test screening is widely available and effective. Gestational trophoblastic disease is a gynecologic tumor that may behave aggressively whether malignant or not.

Many gynecologic cancers manifest as pelvic masses (for diagnostic approach to pelvic masses, see p. 2201).

CERVICAL CANCER

Cervical cancer is usually a squamous cell carcinoma caused by human papillomavirus (HPV) infection; less often, it is an adenocarcinoma. Cervical neoplasia is asymptomatic; the first symptom of early cervical cancer is usually irregular, often postcoital vaginal bleeding. Diagnosis is by a cervical Pap test and biopsy. Staging is clinical. Treatment usually involves surgical resection for early-stage disease or radiation therapy plus chemotherapy for locally advanced disease. If the cancer has widely metastasized, chemotherapy is often used alone.

Cervical cancer is the 3rd most common gynecologic cancer and the 8th most common cancer among women in the US. Mean age at diagnosis is 50, but the cancer can occur as early as age 20. In the US, it caused an estimated 12,990 new cases and 4,120 deaths in 2016.

Cervical cancer results from cervical intraepithelial neoplasia (CIN), which appears to be caused by infection with HPV type 16, 18, 31, 33, 35, or 39.

Risk factors for cervical cancer include

- Younger age at first intercourse
- A high lifetime number of sex partners
- Cigarette smoking
- Immunodeficiency

Regardless of sexual history, clinicians should assume that women have been exposed to someone with HPV because it is ubiquitous.

Pathology

CIN is graded as

- 1: Mild cervical dysplasia
- 2: Moderate dysplasia
- 3: Severe dysplasia and carcinoma in situ

CIN 3 is unlikely to regress spontaneously; if untreated, it may, over months or years, penetrate the basement membrane, becoming invasive carcinoma.

About 80 to 85% of all cervical cancers are squamous cell carcinoma; most of the rest are adenocarcinomas. Sarcomas and small cell neuroendocrine tumors are rare.

Invasive cervical cancer usually spreads by direct extension into surrounding tissues or via the lymphatics to the pelvic and para-aortic lymph nodes. Hematogenous spread is possible but rare.

If cervical cancer spreads to the pelvic or para-aortic lymph nodes, the prognosis is worse, and the location and size of the radiation therapy field is affected.

Symptoms and Signs

Early cervical cancer can be asymptomatic. When symptoms occur, they usually include irregular vaginal bleeding, which is most often postcoital but may occur spontaneously between menses. Larger cancers are more likely to bleed spontaneously and may cause a foul-smelling vaginal discharge or pelvic pain. More widespread cancer may cause obstructive uropathy, back pain, and leg swelling due to venous or lymphatic obstruction.

Pelvic examination may detect an exophytic necrotic tumor in the cervix.

Diagnosis

- Papanicolaou (Pap) test
- Biopsy
- Clinical staging, usually by biopsy, pelvic examination, and chest x-ray

Cervical cancer may be suspected during a routine gynecologic examination. It is considered in women with

- Visible cervical lesions
- Abnormal routine Pap test results
- Abnormal vaginal bleeding

Reporting of cervical cytology results is standardized (see Table 270–1).[1] Further evaluation is indicated if atypical or cancerous cells are found, particularly in women at risk. If cytology does not show any obvious cancer, colposcopy (examination of the vagina and cervix with a magnifying lens) can be used to identify areas that require biopsy. Colposcopy-directed biopsy with endocervical curettage is usually diagnostic. If not, cone biopsy (conization) is required; a cone of tissue is removed using a loop electrical excision procedure (LEEP), laser, or cold knife.

Staging: Cervical cancers are clinically staged based on biopsy, physical examination, and chest x-ray results (see Table 270–2). In the International Federation of Gynecology and Obstetrics (FIGO) staging system, stage does not include information about lymph node status. Although not included as staging, lymph node status is required for treatment planning

Table 270–1. BETHESDA CLASSIFICATION OF CERVICAL CYTOLOGY*

CATEGORY	SPECIFICS	COMMENTS
Specimen type	Conventional (Papanicolaou [Pap]), liquid-based preparation, or another	Type of test is noted.
Adequacy of the specimen	Satisfactory for evaluation	Any quality indicators (eg, presence or absence of endocervical or transformation zone component, partially obscuring blood, inflammation) are described.
	Unsatisfactory for evaluation (rejected and not processed)	Reason is specified.
	Unsatisfactory for evaluation but processed and evaluated	Reason is specified.
General categorization (optional)	Negative for intraepithelial lesion or cancer Epithelial cell abnormalities Other findings	Findings are stated or described under Interpretation, below.
Interpretation of negative (nonmalignant) abnormalities‡	Organisms	Possible findings include the following: • *Trichomonas vaginalis* • Fungi morphologically consistent with *Candida* sp • Shift in vaginal flora suggesting bacterial vaginosis • Bacteria morphologically consistent with *Actinomyces* sp • Cellular changes consistent with herpes simplex virus • Cellular changes consistent with cytomegalovirus
	Nonneoplastic findings (reporting is optional)	Possible findings include the following: • Nonneoplastic cellular variations (squamous metaplasia, keratotic changes, tubal metaplasia, atrophy, or pregnancy-associated changes) • Reactive cellular changes associated with inflammation (lymphocytic cervicitis), radiation, or IUD use • Glandular cell status after hysterectomy
Interpretation of epithelial cell abnormalities	Squamous cell	Possible findings include the following: • Atypical squamous cells of undetermined significance (ASC-US) • Atypical squamous cells for which a high-grade lesion cannot be excluded (ASC-H) • Low-grade squamous intraepithelial lesion encompassing HPV† infection or mild dysplasia (CIN 1) • High-grade squamous intraepithelial lesion encompassing moderate (CIN 2) and severe dysplasia (CIN 3/CIS), noting whether the lesion has features suggesting invasion • Squamous cell carcinoma
	Glandular cell	Possible findings include the following: • Atypical cells: Endocervical, endometrial, or glandular • Atypical cells likely to be cancerous: Endocervical or glandular • Adenocarcinoma in situ: Endocervical • Adenocarcinoma: Endocervical, endometrial, extrauterine, or NOS
Interpretation of other abnormalities	Endometrial cells (in a woman ≥ 45)*	Whether sample is negative for squamous intraepithelial lesion is specified.
Other cancers	———	Type is specified.

*Use of an automated device for scanning should be reported, as should adjunctive tests (eg, HPV) and their results.

†Cellular changes of HPV infection—previously called koilocytosis, koilocytotic atypia, and condylomatous atypia—are included in the category of low-grade squamous intraepithelial lesion.

‡If there is no cellular evidence of neoplasia, clinicians should state negative for intraepithelial lesion or malignancy here or in the general categorization.

CIN = cervical intraepithelial neoplasia; CIS = carcinoma in situ; HPV = human papillomavirus; IUD = intrauterine device; NOS = not otherwise specified.

Adapted from the Bethesda System 2014, National Institutes of Health.

and affects decisions about the size and location of the radiation therapy field.

If the stage is > IB1, CT or MRI of the abdomen and pelvis is typically done to identify metastases, although results are not used for staging. PET with CT (PET/CT) is being used more commonly to check for spread beyond the cervix. If PET/CT, MRI, or CT is not available, cystoscopy, sigmoidoscopy, and IV urography, when clinically indicated, may be used for staging.

The purpose of this staging system is to establish a large database for study; thus, the system uses worldwide uniform diagnostic criteria. The system excludes results of tests that are less likely to be available worldwide (eg, MRI) because most cases of cervical cancer occur in developing countries. Because such tests are not used, findings such as parametrial invasion and lymph node metastases are often missed, and thus understaging is possible.

When imaging tests suggest that pelvic or para-aortic lymph nodes are grossly enlarged (> 2 cm), surgical exploration, typically with a retroperitoneal approach, is occasionally indicated. Its sole purpose is to remove enlarged lymph nodes so that radiation therapy can be more precisely targeted and more effective.

1. Nayar R, Wilbur DC: The Pap test and Bethesda 2014. *Cancer Cytopathology* 123:271–281, 2015.

Prognosis

In squamous cell carcinoma, distant metastases usually occur only when the cancer is advanced or recurrent. The 5-yr survival rates are as follows:

- Stage I: 80 to 90%
- Stage II: 60 to 75%
- Stage III: 30 to 40%
- Stage IV: 0 to 15%

Nearly 80% of recurrences manifest within 2 yr.

Adverse prognostic factors include

- Lymph node involvement
- Large tumor size and volume
- Deep cervical stromal invasion
- Parametrial invasion
- Vascular space invasion
- Nonsquamous histology

Treatment

- Excision or curative radiation therapy if there is no spread to parametria or beyond
- Radiation therapy and chemotherapy if there is spread to parametria or beyond
- Chemotherapy for metastatic and recurrent cancer

Table 270–2. FIGO CLINICAL STAGING OF CERVICAL CARCINOMA

STAGE	DESCRIPTION
I	Carcinoma confined to the cervix
IA	Carcinoma diagnosed only by microscopy, with invasion of stroma ≤ 5 mm in depth and largest extension ≤ 7 mm in width*
IA1	Measured invasion of stroma ≤ 3 mm in depth and ≤ 7 mm in width
IA2	Measured invasion of stroma > 3 mm and ≤ 5 mm in depth and ≤ 7 mm in width
IB	Clinically visible lesions confined to the cervix or microscopic lesions larger than those in stage IA2
IB1	Clinically visible lesions ≤ 4 cm in largest dimension
IB2	Clinically visible lesions > 4sar cm in largest dimension
II	Extension beyond the cervix but not to the pelvic wall or to the lower third of the vagina
IIA	Involvement of up to the upper 2/3 of the vagina; no obvious parametrial involvement
IIA1	Clinically visible lesion ≤ 4.0 cm in largest dimension
IIA2	Clinically visible lesion > 4.0 cm in largest dimension
IIB	Parametrial involvement
III	Extension to the pelvic wall and/or involves the lower third of the vagina and/or causes hydronephrosis or a nonfunctioning kidney
IIIA	Extension to lower third of the vagina but not to the pelvic wall
IIIB	Extension to the pelvic wall and/or causes hydronephrosis or a nonfunctioning kidney
IV	Extension beyond the true pelvis or clinical involvement of the bladder or rectal mucosa (bullous edema does not signify stage IV)
IVA	Invades mucosa of bladder or rectum and/or extends beyond true pelvis
IVB	Spread to distant organs (including peritoneal spread)

*Depth of invasion should be measured from the base of the epithelium (surface or glandular) from which it originates. Vascular space involvement (venous or lymphatic) should not alter staging.

Based on staging established by the International Federation of Gynecology and Obstetrics (FIGO) and American Joint Committee on Cancer (AJCC), *AJCC Cancer Staging Manual*, ed. 7. New York, Springer, 2010.

Treatment of cervical cancer may include surgery, radiation therapy, and chemotherapy. If hysterectomy is indicated but patients cannot tolerate it, radiation therapy plus chemotherapy is used.

Cervical intraepithelial neoplasia (CIN) and squamous cell carcinoma stage IA1: Treatment involves

- Conization or simple hysterectomy

Microinvasive cervical cancer, defined as FIGO stage IA1 with no lymphovascular invasion, has a $< 1\%$ risk of lymph node metastases and may be managed conservatively with conization using LEEP, laser, or cold knife. Conization is indicated for patients who are interested in preserving fertility. Simple hysterectomy should be done if patients are not interested in preserving fertility or if margins are positive after conization.

In cases of stage IA1 with lymphovascular invasion, conization (with negative margins) and laparoscopic pelvic sentinel lymph node (SLN) mapping plus lymphadenectomy (lymph node dissection) is a reasonable strategy.

Stages IA2 to IIA: For **stage IA2 or IB1 cervical cancer,** the standard recommendation is

- Radical hysterectomy with bilateral pelvic lymphadenectomy (with or without SLN mapping)

Radical hysterectomy includes resection of the uterus (including the cervix), parts of the cardinal and uterosacral ligaments, the upper 1 to 2 cm of the vagina, and the pelvic lymph nodes. Radical hysterectomy can be done via laparotomy or minimally invasive surgery. Bilateral salpingo-oophorectomy is usually done concurrently.

The Querleu & Morrow classification system describes 4 basic types of radical hysterectomy, with a few subtypes that take nerve preservation and paracervical lymphadenectomy into account.[1]

For **stage IB2 to IIA cervical cancer,** the most common approach is

- Combined chemotherapy and pelvic radiation

Another treatment option is radical hysterectomy and bilateral pelvic lymphadenectomy, sometimes with radiation therapy (see Table 270–3).

With either treatment, the 5-yr cure rate in stage IB or IIA is 85 to 90%. With surgery, ovarian function can be preserved. Because ovarian metastases are less common in patients with squamous cell carcinoma (0.8%) than in those with adenocarcinoma (5%), the ovaries are typically preserved in patients with squamous cell carcinoma and more commonly removed in those with adenocarcinoma.

If extracervical spread is noted during surgery, radical hysterectomy is not done, and postoperative radiation therapy is recommended to prevent local recurrence.

In some patients who have early-stage cervical cancer and who wish to preserve fertility, a radical trachelectomy may be done. An abdominal, vaginal, laparoscopic, or robotic-assisted approach can be used. In this procedure, the cervix, parametria immediately adjacent to the cervix, upper 2 cm of the vagina, and pelvic lymph nodes are removed. The remaining uterus is reattached to the upper vagina, preserving the potential for fertility. Ideal candidates for this procedure are patients with the following:

- Histologic subtypes such as squamous cell carcinoma, adenocarcinoma, or adenosquamous carcinoma
- Stage IA1/grade 2 or 3 with vascular space invasion
- Stage IA2
- Stage IB1 with lesions < 2 cm in size

Invasion of the upper cervix and lower uterine segment should be excluded by MRI before surgery. Rates of recurrence and death are similar to those after radical hysterectomy. If patients who have this procedure plan to have children, delivery must be cesarean. After a radical trachelectomy, fertility rates range from 50 to 70%, and the recurrence rate is about 5 to 10%.

Stages IIB to IVA: For stages IIb to IVA cervical cancer, the standard therapy is

- Radiation therapy plus chemotherapy (eg, cisplatin)

Surgical staging should be considered to determine whether para-aortic lymph nodes are involved and thus whether extended-field radiation therapy is indicated, particularly in patients with positive pelvic lymph nodes identified during pretreatment imaging. A laparoscopic retroperitoneal approach is recommended.

When cancer is limited to the cervix and/or pelvic lymph nodes, the standard recommendation is

- External beam radiation therapy, followed by brachytherapy (local radioactive implants, usually using cesium) to the cervix

Radiation therapy may cause acute complications (eg, radiation proctitis and cystitis) and, occasionally, late complications (eg, vaginal stenosis, intestinal obstruction, rectovaginal and vesicovaginal fistula formation).

Chemotherapy is usually given with radiation therapy, often to sensitize the tumor to radiation.

Although stage IVA cancers are usually treated with radiation therapy initially, pelvic exenteration (excision of all pelvic organs) may be considered. If after radiation therapy, cancer remains but is confined to the central pelvis, exenteration is indicated and cures up to 40% of patients. The procedure may include continent or incontinent urostomy, low anterior rectal anastomosis without colostomy or with an end-descending colostomy, omental carpet to close the pelvic floor (J-flap), and vaginal reconstruction with gracilis or rectus abdominis myocutaneous flaps.

Stage IVB and recurrent cancer: Chemotherapy is the primary treatment, but only 15 to 25% of patients respond to it.

In a recent study, adding bevacizumab to combination chemotherapy (cisplatin plus paclitaxel or topotecan plus paclitaxel) resulted in an improvement of 3.7 mo in median overall survival in patients with recurrent, persistent, or metastatic cervical cancer.[2]

Metastases outside the radiation field appear to respond better to chemotherapy than does previously irradiated cancer or metastases in the pelvis.

SLN mapping for cervical cancer: SLN mapping is being evaluated as a potential tool to identify patients who do not need complete pelvic lymphadenectomy and to therefore decrease the number of these procedures, which can have adverse effects (eg, lymphedema, nerve damage).

For SLN mapping, blue dye or technetium-99 (^{99}Tc) is directly injected into the cervix, usually at 3 and 9 o'clock. A dye called indocyanine green (ICG) can be used when open or minimally invasive surgery is done. During surgery, SLNs are identified by direct visualization of blue dye, by a camera to detect the fluorescence of ICG, or by a gamma probe to detect ^{99}Tc. SLNs are commonly located medial to the external iliac vessels, ventral to the hypogastric vessels, or in the superior part of the obturator space.

Ultrastaging of all SLNs is done to detect micrometastasis. Any suspicious node must be removed regardless of mapping. If there is no mapping on a hemipelvis, a side-specific lymphadenectomy is done.

Detection rates for sentinel node lymph mapping are best for tumors < 2 cm.

Criteria for radiation therapy after radical hysterectomy: Criteria used to determine whether pelvic radiation should be done after radical hysterectomy include the following (see Table 270–3):

- Presence of lymphovascular space invasion
- Depth of invasion
- Tumor size

1. Querleu D, Morrow CP: Classification of radical hysterectomy. *Lancet Oncol* 9(3):297–303, 2008. doi: 10.1016/S1470-2045(08)70074-3.
2. Tewari KS, Sill MW, Long HJ III: Improved survival with bevacizumab in advanced cervical cancer. *N Engl J Med* 370(8):734-743, 2014. doi: 10.1056/NEJMoa1309748.

Prevention

Pap tests: Routine screening cervical Pap tests are recommended as follows:

- From age 21 to 30: Usually every 3 yr for the Pap test (HPV testing is not generally recommended)
- Age 30 to 65: Every 3 yr if only a Pap test is done or every 5 yr if a Pap test and an HPV test are done (more frequently in women at high risk of cervical cancer)
- After age 65: No more testing if test results have been normal in the preceding 10 yr

If women have had a hysterectomy for a disorder other than cancer and have not had abnormal Pap test results, screening is not indicated.

HPV testing is the preferred method of follow-up evaluation for all women with ASCUS (atypical squamous cells of undetermined significance), an inconclusive finding detected by Pap tests. If HPV testing shows that the woman does not have HPV, screening should continue at the routinely scheduled intervals. If HPV is present, colposcopy should be done.

HPV vaccine: Preventive HPV vaccines include

- A bivalent vaccine that protects against subtypes 16 and 18 (which cause most cervical cancers)
- A quadrivalent vaccine that protects against subtypes 16 and 18 plus 6 and 11
- A 9-valent vaccine that protects against the same subtypes as the quadrivalent plus subtypes 31, 33, 45, 52, and 58 (which cause about 15% of cervical cancers)

Table 270–3. SEDLIS CRITERIA FOR EXTERNAL PELVIC RADIATION AFTER RADICAL HYSTERECTOMY*

LYMPHOVASCULAR SPACE INVASION	STROMAL INVASION	TUMOR SIZE (cm)†
+	Deep third	Any
+	Middle third	≥ 2
+	Superficial third	≥ 5
–	Middle or deep third	≥ 4

*Criteria apply to node-negative, margin-negative, parametria-negative cases.
†Size is determined by clinical palpation.
Based on Sedlis A, Bundy BN, Rotman MZ, et al: A randomized trial of pelvic radiation therapy versus no further therapy in selected patients with stage IB carcinoma of the cervix after radical hysterectomy and pelvic lymphadenectomy: A gynecologic oncology group study. *Gynecol Oncol* 73, 177–183, 1999.

Subtypes 6 and 11 cause > 90% of visible genital warts.

The vaccines aim to prevent cervical cancer but do not treat it. For patients ≥ 15 yr, three doses are given over 6 mo (at 0, 1 to 2, and 6 mo). For patients < 15 yr, two doses are given 6 to 12 mo apart. The vaccine is recommended for boys and girls, ideally before they become sexually active. The standard recommendation is to vaccinate boys and girls beginning at age 11 to 12 yr, but vaccination can begin at age 9.

KEY POINTS

- Consider cervical cancer if women have abnormal Pap test results, visible cervical lesions, or abnormal, particularly postcoital vaginal bleeding.
- Do a biopsy to confirm the diagnosis.
- Stage cervical cancer clinically, using biopsy, pelvic examination, and chest x-ray, and if the stage is > IB1, use PET/CT, MRI, or CT to identify metastases.
- Treatment is surgical resection for early-stage cancer (usually stages IA to IB1), radiation therapy plus chemotherapy for locally advanced cancer (usually stages IB2 to IVA), and chemotherapy for metastatic cancer.
- Screen all women by doing Pap and HPV tests at regular intervals.
- Recommend HPV vaccination for girls and boys.

ENDOMETRIAL CANCER

(Uterine Cancer)

Endometrial cancer is usually endometrioid adenocarcinoma. Typically, postmenopausal vaginal bleeding occurs. Diagnosis is by biopsy. Staging is surgical. Treatment requires hysterectomy, bilateral salpingo-oophorectomy, and, in high-risk patients, usually pelvic and para-aortic lymphadenectomy. For advanced cancer, radiation, hormone, or cytotoxic therapy is usually indicated.

Endometrial cancer is more common in developed countries where the diet is high in fat. In the US, this cancer is the 4th most common cancer among women, affecting 1 in 50. The American Cancer Society estimates that in 2017, about 61,380 new cases of endometrial cancer will be diagnosed and that about 10,920 women will die of this cancer.

Endometrial cancer affects mainly postmenopausal women. Mean patient age at diagnosis is 61 yr. Most cases are diagnosed in women aged 50 to 60 yr; 92% of cases occur in women > 50 yr.

Etiology

Major risk factors for endometrial cancer are

- Unopposed estrogen
- Age > 50
- Obesity
- Diabetes

Other risk factors include

- Tamoxifen use for > 5 yr
- Previous pelvic radiation therapy
- A personal or family history of breast or ovarian cancer
- Family history of hereditary nonpolyposis colorectal cancer or possibly, among 1st-degree relatives, endometrial cancer
- Hypertension

Unopposed estrogen (high circulating levels of estrogenwith no or low levels of progesterone) may be associated with obesity, polycystic ovary syndrome, nulliparity, late menopause, estrogen-producing tumors, anovulation (ovulatory dysfunction), and estrogen therapy without progesterone.

Most endometrial cancer is caused by sporadic mutations. However, in about 5% of patients, inherited mutations cause endometrial cancer; endometrial cancer due to inherited mutations tends to occur earlier and is often diagnosed 10 to 20 yr earlier than sporadic cancer. About half of cases that involve heredity occur in families with hereditary nonpolyposis colorectal cancer (HNPCC; Lynch syndrome). Patients who have HNPCC have a high risk of developing a second cancer (eg, colorectal cancer, ovarian cancer).

Pathology

Endometrial cancer is usually preceded by endometrial hyperplasia. Endometrial carcinoma is commonly classified into 2 types.

Type I tumors are more common, are usually estrogen-responsive, and are usually diagnosed in younger, obese, or perimenopausal women. These tumors are usually low-grade. Endometrioid adenocarcinoma is the most common histology. These tumors may show microsatellite instability and have mutations in *PTEN*, *PIK3CA*, *KRAS*, and *CTNNBI*.

Type II tumors are usually high-grade (eg, serous or clear cell histology). They tend to occur in older women. About 10 to 30% have *p53* mutations. Up to 10% of endometrial carcinomas are type II.

Endometrioid adenocarcinomas account for about 75 to 80% of endometrial cancers.

Uterine papillary serous carcinomas, clear cell carcinomas, and carcinosarcomas are considered more aggressive, high-risk histologies and are thus associated with a higher incidence of extrauterine disease at presentation. Carcinosarcomas have been reclassified as high-risk malignant epithelial tumors.

Endometrial cancer may spread as follows:

- From the surface of the uterine cavity to the cervical canal
- Through the myometrium to the serosa and into the peritoneal cavity
- Via the lumen of the fallopian tube to the ovary, broad ligament, and peritoneal surfaces
- Via the bloodstream, leading to distant metastases
- Via the lymphatics

The higher (more undifferentiated) the grade of the tumor, the greater the likelihood of deep myometrial invasion, pelvic or para-aortic lymph node metastases, or extrauterine spread.

Symptoms and Signs

Most (> 90%) women with endometrial cancer have abnormal uterine bleeding (eg, postmenopausal bleeding, premenopausal recurrent metrorrhagia); one third of women with postmenopausal bleeding have endometrial cancer. A vaginal discharge may occur weeks or months before postmenopausal bleeding.

Diagnosis

- Endometrial biopsy
- Surgical staging

The following suggest endometrial cancer:

- Postmenopausal bleeding
- Abnormal bleeding in premenopausal women
- A routine Pap test showing endometrial cells in postmenopausal women
- A routine Pap test showing atypical endometrial cells in any woman

If endometrial cancer is suspected, outpatient endometrial biopsy is done; it is > 90% accurate. Endometrial sampling is also recommended for women with abnormal bleeding, particularly those > 40 yr. If results are inconclusive or suggest cancer (eg, complex hyperplasia with atypia), outpatient fractional D & C with hysteroscopy is done. An alternative is transvaginal ultrasonography; however, a histologic diagnosis is required.

Once endometrial cancer is diagnosed, pretreatment evaluation includes serum electrolytes, kidney and liver function tests, CBC, chest x-ray, and ECG.

Because endometrial cancer sometimes results from an inherited mutation, genetic counseling and/or testing should be considered if patients are < 50 yr or have a significant family history of endometrial cancer and/or HNPCC.

Pelvic and abdominal CT are also done to check for extrauterine or metastatic cancer in patients with any of the following:

- An abdominal mass or hepatomegaly detected during physical examination
- Abnormal liver function test results
- A high-risk histologic subtype of cancer (eg, papillary serous carcinoma, clear cell carcinoma, carcinosarcoma)

Staging: Staging of endometrial cancer is based on histologic differentiation (grade 1 [least aggressive] to 3 [most aggressive]) and extent of spread, including invasion depth, cervical involvement (glandular involvement vs stromal invasion), and extrauterine metastases (see Table 270–4).

Staging is surgical and includes exploration of the abdomen and pelvis, biopsy or excision of suspicious extrauterine lesions, total abdominal hysterectomy, and, in patients with high-risk features (grade 1 or 2 cancer plus deep myometrial invasion, grade 3 cancer, all cancers with high-risk histology), pelvic and para-aortic lymphadenectomy. Staging can be done via laparotomy, laparoscopy, or robotic-assisted surgery.

Prognosis

Prognosis is worse with higher-grade tumors, more extensive spread, and older patient age.

Average 5-yr survival rates are

- Stage I or II: 70 to 95%
- Stage III or IV: 10 to 60%

Overall, 63% of patients are cancer-free ≥ 5 yr after treatment.

Treatment

- Usually total hysterectomy and bilateral salpingo-oophorectomy
- Pelvic and para-aortic lymphadenectomy for grade 1 or 2 with deep (> 50%) myometrial invasion, for any grade 3, and for all cancers with high-risk histology
- Pelvic radiation therapy with or without chemotherapy for stage II or III
- Multimodal therapy usually recommended for stage IV

In patients with grade 1 or 2 endometrial cancer and < 50% invasion, the probability of lymph node metastasis is < 2%. In these patients, treatment is usually total hysterectomy and bilateral salpingo-oophorectomy via laparotomy, laparoscopy, or robotic-assisted surgery. However, for young women with stage IA or IB endometrioid adenocarcinoma, ovarian preservation is usually safe and recommended to preserve fertility.

Table 270–4. FIGO STAGING OF ENDOMETRIAL CARCINOMA

STAGE*,†	DEFINITION
I	Confined to the uterine corpus
IA	Limited to endometrium or involves less than half of the myometrium
IB	Invasion of half or more of the myometrium
II	Invasion of the cervical stroma but no extension outside the uterus
III	Local and/or regional spread of the tumor
IIIA	Invasion of serosa, adnexa, or both (direct extension or metastasis)
IIIB	Metastases or direct spread to the vagina and/or spread to the parametria
IIIC	Metastases to pelvic or para-aortic lymph nodes or to both
IIIC1	Metastases to pelvic lymph nodes
IIIC2	Metastases to para-aortic lymph nodes, with or without metastases to pelvic lymph nodes
IV	Involvement of the bladder and/or intestinal mucosa and/or distant metastases
IVA	Invasion of the bladder, intestinal mucosa, or both
IVB	Distant metastases, including to intra-abdominal or inguinal lymph nodes or both

*Endometrial cancer is usually surgically staged.

†For all but stage IVB, grade (G) indicates percentage of tumor with a nonsquamous or nonmorular solid growth pattern:

- G1: ≤ 5%
- G2: 6–50%
- G3: > 50%

Nuclear atypia excessive for the grade raises the grade of a G1 or G2 tumor by 1. In serous adenocarcinomas, clear cell adenocarcinomas, and squamous cell carcinomas, nuclear grading takes precedence. Adenocarcinomas with squamous differentiation are graded according to the nuclear grade of the glandular component.

*Based on staging established by the International Federation of Gynecology and Obstetrics (FIGO) and American Joint Committee on Cancer (AJCC), *AJCC Cancer Staging Manual*, ed. 7. New York, Springer, 2010.

If patients have any of the following, pelvic and para-aortic lymphadenectomy is also done:

- Grade 1 or 2 cancer with deep (> 50%) myometrial invasion
- Any grade 3 cancer
- All cancers with high-risk histology (papillary serous carcinoma, clear cell carcinoma, carcinosarcoma)

Whether the extent of para-aortic lymphadenectomy should reach the inferior mesenteric artery vs the renal vessels remains a topic of debate.

Stage II or III cancer requires pelvic radiation therapy with or without chemotherapy. Treatment of stage III cancer must be individualized, but surgery is an option; generally, patients who undergo combined surgery and radiation therapy have a better prognosis. Except in patients with bulky parametrial disease, a total abdominal hysterectomy and bilateral salpingo-oophorectomy should be done.

Treatment of stage IV is variable and patient-dependent but typically involves a combination of surgery, radiation therapy, and chemotherapy. Occasionally, hormonal therapy should also be considered.

Tumors respond to hormone therapy with a progestin in 20 to 25% of patients.

Several cytotoxic drugs (particularly carboplatin plus paclitaxel) are effective. They are given mainly to women with metastatic or recurrent cancer. Another option is doxorubicin.

SLN mapping in endometrial cancer: The role of sentinel lymph node (SLN) mapping in endometrial cancer is currently being evaluated. SLN mapping is done as for cervical cancer using the same tracers (blue dye, technetium-99 [^{99}Tc], ICG).

SLN mapping can be considered for the surgical staging of cancer that appears confined to the uterus. SLN mapping in cancers with high-risk histology (papillary serous carcinoma, clear cell carcinoma, carcinosarcomas) should be done with caution.

Where to inject the tracer in patients with endometrial carcinoma is controversial; however, injecting dye into the cervix is a useful and validated technique for identifying lymph nodes. Dye is usually injected into the cervix both superficially (1 to 3 mm) and deep (1 to 2 cm) at 3 and 9 o'clock. With this technique, dye penetrates to the uterine lymphatic trunks (which meet in the parametria) and appears in the broad ligament leading to pelvic and occasionally para-aortic SLNs.

The most common locations of pelvic SLNs are

- Medial to the external iliac blood vessels
- Ventral to the internal iliac blood vessels
- In the superior part of the obturator region

Less common locations are the iliac and/or presacral regions.

A complete pelvic lymphadenectomy should be done when any of the following occur:

- Mapping does not detect any SLNs.
- A hemipelvis cannot be mapped.
- There are any suspicious or grossly enlarged nodes, regardless of mapping.

Fertility preservation in endometrial hyperplasia and early endometrial cancer: Patients with complex endometrial hyperplasia and atypia have up to a 50% risk of having concurrent endometrial cancer. Treatment of endometrial hyperplasia consists of progestins or definitive surgery, depending on the complexity of the lesion and the patient's desire to preserve fertility.

If young patients with grade 1 tumors and no myometrial invasion (documented by MRI) wish to preserve fertility, progestin alone is an option. About 46 to 80% of patients have a complete response within 3 mo of initiation of therapy. After 3 mo, patients should be evaluated via D & C rather than endometrial biopsy.

Alternatively, use of a levonorgestrel-releasing intrauterine device (IUD) is being increasingly used to treat patients with complex atypical hyperplasia or grade 1 endometrial cancer.

Surgery is recommended if conservative treatment is not effective (endometrial cancer is still present after 6 to 9 mo of treatment) or if patients have completed childbearing. Fertility-sparing treatment is contraindicated in patients with high-grade endometrioid adenocarcinomas, uterine papillary serous carcinoma, clear cell carcinoma, or carcinosarcoma.

In young women with stage IA or IB endometrioid adenocarcinoma, ovarian preservation is safe and recommended.

General measures: Because obesity and hypertension increase the risk of endometrial cancer and because evidence suggests that certain lifestyle choices may help prevent endometrial cancer, patients should be counseled about the importance of exercise, weight loss, and an adequate diet.

High-risk histologies: Uterine papillary serous carcinoma, clear cell carcinomas, and carcinosarcomas (reclassified as high-risk malignant epithelial tumors) are considered histologically aggressive, high-risk cancers and are thus more likely to have spread outside the uterus at presentation.

Multimodality therapy is typically recommended for these histologically aggressive endometrial tumors. Primary treatment includes abdominal hysterectomy, bilateral salpingo-oophorectomy with pelvic and para-aortic lymphadenectomy, and omental and peritoneal biopsies.

In patients with gross extrauterine disease, cytoreduction should be done to reduce the bulk of the tumor to no gross residual disease.

Adjuvant therapy for papillary serous and clear cell carcinomas depends on the stage:

- Stage IA without myometrial invasion and without residual disease in the hysterectomy specimen: Observation and close follow-up (an acceptable approach)
- Other stage IA and IB or stage II cancers: Usually vaginal brachytherapy followed by systemic chemotherapy with carboplatin and paclitaxel
- More advanced disease: Chemotherapy

Adjuvant therapy for carcinosarcoma also depends on the stage:

- Stage IA without myometrial invasion and without residual disease in the hysterectomy specimen: Observation and close follow-up (an acceptable approach)
- All other stages: Usually systemic chemotherapy with ifosfamide plus paclitaxel

KEY POINTS

- Endometrial cancer is one of the most common cancers among women and, as prevalence of the metabolic syndrome increases, may become more common.
- Prognosis is better with type I tumors, which tend to be diagnosed in younger or perimenopausal women, to be estrogen-responsive, and to have more benign histologic features.
- Recommend endometrial sampling for women with abnormal bleeding, particularly those > 40 yr.
- Stage endometrial cancer surgically via laparotomy, laparoscopy, or a robotic-assisted surgery.
- Treatment is usually total hysterectomy, bilateral salpingo-oophorectomy, and lymphadenectomy and sometimes radiation therapy and/or chemotherapy.
- Consider SLN mapping for cancers that appear to be confined to the uterus.
- Consider fertility-sparing treatment for certain patients with grade 1 endometrioid adenocarcinoma or endometrial complex atypical hyperplasia.
- Consider genetic counseling and testing for patients < 50 yr and those with a significant family history of endometrial and/or colorectal cancer (HNPCC).

FALLOPIAN TUBE CANCER

Fallopian tube cancer is usually adenocarcinoma, manifesting as an adnexal mass or with vague symptoms. Diagnosis, staging, and primary treatment are surgical.

Primary fallopian tube cancer is rare. Patients are usually postmenopausal at the time of diagnosis.

Risk factors for fallopian tube cancer include

- Age
- Chronic salpingitis
- Infertility

Most (> 95%) fallopian tube cancers are papillary serous adenocarcinomas; a few are sarcomas.

Spread, like that of ovarian cancer, is as follows:

- By direct extension
- By peritoneal seeding
- Through the lymphatics

Symptoms and Signs

Most patients with fallopian tube cancer present with an adnexal mass or report vague abdominal or pelvic symptoms (eg, abdominal discomfort, bloating, pain). A few patients present with hydrops tubae profluens (a triad of pelvic pain, copious watery discharge, and adnexal mass), which is more specific for fallopian tube cancer.

Diagnosis

- CT
- Surgery to confirm diagnosis and to stage

Typically, CT is done. A distended solid adnexal mass and normal ovary suggest fallopian tube cancer. A pregnancy test is done to rule out ectopic pregnancy unless patients are postmenopausal.

If cancer is suspected, surgery is necessary for diagnosis, staging, and primary treatment. Surgical staging (similar to that for ovarian cancer) requires the following:

- Washings from the pelvis, abdominal gutters, and diaphragmatic recesses
- Multiple pelvic and abdominal peritoneal biopsies
- Pelvic and para-aortic lymph node dissection or lymph node sampling

Total abdominal hysterectomy, bilateral salpingo-oophorectomy, and supracolic omentectomy are usually done at the same time as surgical staging.

Treatment

- Total abdominal hysterectomy and bilateral salpingo-oophorectomy
- Supracolic omentectomy
- Sometimes cytoreductive surgery

Treatment of fallopian tube cancer includes total abdominal hysterectomy, bilateral salpingo-oophorectomy, and supracolic omentectomy. If cancer appears advanced, cytoreductive surgery is indicated. These procedures can be done during surgical staging.

As in ovarian cancer, clinicians must determine whether primary cytoreductive surgery (done during surgical staging) is likely to result in no gross residual disease or whether chemotherapy and interval surgery (usually 3 cycles of neoadjuvant chemotherapy followed by cytoreductive surgery and 3 cycles of adjuvant chemotherapy) is the best approach for the patient.

Laparoscopy may be done to determine the extent of the cancer and, in some cases, to treat the cancer. Laparoscopy enables clinicians to thoroughly evaluate the pelvis, small and large bowel, upper abdomen, diaphragmatic surface, and all other peritoneal surfaces.

As in ovarian cancer, a predictive index score such as the Fagotti score can be used (see Table 270–9 on p. 2264). In this scoring system, several sites in the abdomen and pelvis are evaluated and assigned a score based on the extent of cancer. If patients score ≥ 8, primary cytoreduction is not considered the best option for that patient, and chemotherapy is recommended as primary treatment.

Postoperative treatment is identical to postoperative treatment for ovarian cancer. External beam radiation is rarely indicated.

GESTATIONAL TROPHOBLASTIC DISEASE

Gestational trophoblastic disease is proliferation of trophoblastic tissue in pregnant or recently pregnant women. Manifestations may include excessive uterine enlargement, vomiting, vaginal bleeding, and preeclampsia, particularly during early pregnancy. Diagnosis includes measurement of the beta subunit of human chorionic gonadotropin, pelvic ultrasonography, and confirmation by biopsy. Tumors are removed by suction curettage. If disease persists after removal, chemotherapy is indicated.

Gestational trophoblastic disease is a tumor originating from the trophoblast, which surrounds the blastocyst and develops into the chorion and amnion (see p. 2318). This disease can occur during or after an intrauterine or ectopic pregnancy. If the disease occurs during a pregnancy, spontaneous abortion, eclampsia, or fetal death typically occurs; the fetus rarely survives.

Some forms of gestational trophoblastic disease are malignant; others are benign but behave aggressively.

Pathology

Gestational trophoblastic disease may be classified as

- Hydatidiform mole, which may be complete or partial
- Gestational trophoblastic neoplasia, which includes chorioadenoma destruens (invasive mole), choriocarcinoma, placental site trophoblastic tumor (very rare), and epithelioid trophoblastic tumor (extremely rare)

Gestational trophoblastic disease may also be classified morphologically:

- Hydatidiform mole: In this abnormal pregnancy, villi become edematous (hydropic), and trophoblastic tissue proliferates.
- Invasive mole: The myometrium is invaded locally by a hydatidiform mole.
- Choriocarcinoma: This invasive, usually widely metastatic tumor is composed of malignant trophoblastic cells and lacks hydropic villi; most of these tumors develop after a hydatidiform mole.
- Placental site trophoblastic tumor: This rare tumor consists of intermediate trophoblastic cells that persist after a term pregnancy; it may invade adjacent tissues or metastasize.
- Epithelioid trophoblastic tumor: This rare variant of placental site trophoblastic tumor consists of intermediate trophoblastic cells. Like placental site trophoblastic tumors, it may invade adjacent tissues or metastasize.

Hydatidiform moles are most common among women < 17 or > 35 and those who have previously had gestational trophoblastic disease. They occur in about 1/2000 gestations in the US. For unknown reasons, incidence in Asian countries approaches 1/200.

Most (> 80%) hydatidiform moles are benign. The rest may persist, tending to become invasive; 2 to 3% of hydatidiform moles are followed by choriocarcinoma.

Symptoms and Signs

Initial manifestations of a hydatidiform mole suggest early pregnancy, but the uterus often becomes larger than expected within 10 to 16 wk gestation. Commonly, women test positive for pregnancy and have vaginal bleeding and severe vomiting, and fetal movement and fetal heart sounds are absent. Passage of grapelike tissue strongly suggests the diagnosis.

Complications, such as the following, may occur during early pregnancy:

- Uterine infection
- Sepsis
- Hemorrhagic shock
- Preeclampsia

Placental site trophoblastic tumors tend to cause bleeding.

Choriocarcinoma usually manifests with symptoms due to metastases.

Gestational trophoblastic disease does not impair fertility or predispose to prenatal or perinatal complications (eg, congenital malformations, spontaneous abortions).

Diagnosis

- Serum beta subunit of human chorionic gonadotropin (beta-hCG)
- Pelvic ultrasonography
- Biopsy

Gestational trophoblastic disease is suspected in women with a positive pregnancy test and any of the following:

- Uterine size much larger than expected for dates
- Symptoms or signs of preeclampsia
- Passage of grapelike tissue
- Suggestive findings (eg, mass containing multiple cysts, absence of a fetus and amniotic fluid) seen during ultrasonography done to evaluate pregnancy
- Unexplained metastases in women of child-bearing age
- Unexpectedly high levels of beta-hCG detected during pregnancy testing (except for placental site trophoblastic tumor and epithelioid trophoblastic tumor, which result in low beta-hCG levels)
- Unexplained complications of pregnancy

PEARLS & PITFALLS

- Do ultrasonography during early pregnancy if uterine size is much larger than expected for dates, if women have symptoms or signs of preeclampsia, or if beta-hCG levels are unexpectedly high.

If gestational trophoblastic disease is suspected, testing includes measurement of serum beta-hCG and, if not previously done, pelvic ultrasonography. Findings (eg, very high beta-hCG levels, classic ultrasonographic findings) may suggest the diagnosis, but biopsy is required.

Invasive mole and choriocarcinoma are suspected if biopsy findings suggest invasive disease or if beta-hCG levels remain higher than expected after treatment for hydatidiform mole (see below).

Staging: The International FIGO has developed a staging system for gestational trophoblastic neoplasia (see Table 270–5).

Table 270–5. FIGO ANATOMIC STAGING OF GESTATIONAL TROPHOBLASTIC NEOPLASIA

STAGE	DESCRIPTION
I	Confined to the uterus
II	Extending outside the uterus but limited to genital structures (adnexa, vagina, broad ligament)
III	Extending to the lungs, with or without genital tract involvement
IV	Spread to all other distant sites (eg, brain, liver, kidneys, GI tract)

Based on the International Federation of Gynecology and Obstetrics (FIGO) Committee on Gynecologic Oncology: Current FIGO staging for cancer of the vagina, fallopian tube, ovary, and gestational trophoblastic neoplasia. *International Journal of Gynaecology and Obstetrics* 105(1):3–4, 2009.

Prognosis

In metastatic disease, the WHO prognostic scoring system for metastatic gestational trophoblastic disease can help predict prognosis, including risk of death (see Table 270–6).

Poor prognosis is also suggested by the following (National Institutes of Health [NIH] criteria):

- Urinary hCG excretion > 100,000 IU in 24 h
- Duration of disease > 4 mo (interval since prior pregnancy)
- Brain or liver metastases
- Disease after full-term pregnancy
- Serum hCG > 40,000 mIU/mL
- Unsuccessful prior chemotherapy
- WHO score ≥ 7

Treatment

- Tumor removal by suction curettage or hysterectomy
- Further evaluation for persistent disease and spread of tumor
- Chemotherapy for persistent disease
- Posttreatment contraception for persistent disease

Hydatidiform mole, invasive mole, placental site trophoblastic tumor, and epithelioid trophoblastic tumor are evacuated by suction curettage. Alternatively, if childbearing is not planned, hysterectomy may be done.

After tumor removal, gestational trophoblastic disease is classified clinically to determine whether additional treatment is needed. The clinical classification system does not correspond to the morphologic classification system. Invasive mole and choriocarcinoma are classified clinically as persistent disease. The clinical classification is used because invasive mole and choriocarcinoma are treated similarly and because exact histologic diagnosis may require hysterectomy.

A chest x-ray is taken, and serum beta-hCG is measured. If the beta-hCG level does not normalize within 10 wk, the disease is classified as persistent. Persistent disease requires CT of the brain, chest, abdomen, and pelvis. Results dictate whether disease is classified as nonmetastatic or metastatic.

Persistent disease is usually treated with chemotherapy. Treatment is considered successful if at least 3 consecutive serum beta-hCG measurements at 1-wk intervals are normal. Pregnancy should be prevented for 6 mo after treatment because pregnancy would increase beta-hCG levels, making it difficult to determine whether treatment has been successful. Typically, oral contraceptives (any is acceptable) are given for 6 mo; alternatively, any effective contraceptive method can be used.

Nonmetastatic disease can be treated with a single chemotherapy drug (methotrexate or dactinomycin). Alternatively, hysterectomy is considered for patients > 40 or those desiring sterilization and may be required for those with severe infection or uncontrolled bleeding. If single-drug chemotherapy is ineffective, hysterectomy or multidrug chemotherapy is indicated. Virtually 100% of patients with nonmetastatic disease can be cured.

Table 270–6. WHO SCORING SYSTEM IN METASTATIC GESTATIONAL TROPHOBLASTIC DISEASE*

PROGNOSTIC FACTOR	DESCRIPTION	SCORE†
Age (yr)	< 40	0
	≥ 40	1
Preceding pregnancy	Mole	0
	Abortion	1
	Term	2
Interval (mo)‡	< 4	0
	4–6	1
	7–12	2
	> 12	4
Pretreatment serum hCG (IU/mL)	< 1000	0
	1,000–< 10,000	1
	10,000–< 100,000	2
	≥ 100,000	4
Largest tumor, including any uterine tumors	3–< 5 cm	1
	≥ 5 cm	2
Site of metastases	Lungs	0
	Spleen, kidneys	1
	GI tract	2
	Brain, liver	4
Number of metastases identified	1–4	1
	5–8	2
	> 8	4
Number of chemotherapy drugs used unsuccessfully	1	2
	≥ 2	4

*Does not apply to placental site trophoblastic disease or epithelioid trophoblastic tumor.

†Total score obtained by adding the score for each prognostic factor:

- ≤ 6 = low risk
- ≥ 7 = high risk

‡Between the end of the preceding pregnancy and the start of chemotherapy.

hCG = human chorionic gonadotropin.

Adapted from the International Federation of Gynecology and Obstetrics (FIGO) Oncology Committee: FIGO staging for gestational trophoblastic neoplasia 2000. *International Journal of Gynaecology and Obstetrics* 77(3):285–287, 2002 and the American Joint Committee on Cancer (AJCC), *AJCC Cancer Staging Manual*, ed. 7. New York, Springer, 2010.

Low-risk metastatic disease is treated with single-drug or multidrug chemotherapy. High-risk metastatic disease requires aggressive multidrug chemotherapy. Cure rates are 90 to 95% for low-risk and 60 to 80% for high-risk disease.

Hydatidiform mole recurs in about 1% of subsequent pregnancies. Patients who have had a mole require ultrasonography early in subsequent pregnancies, and the placenta should be sent for pathologic evaluation.

KEY POINTS

- Suspect gestational trophoblastic disease if uterine size is much larger than expected for dates, if women have symptoms or signs of preeclampsia, if beta-hCG levels are unexpectedly high during early pregnancy, or if ultrasonographic findings suggest gestational trophoblastic disease.
- Measure beta-hCG level, do pelvic ultrasonography, and if findings suggest gestational trophoblastic disease, confirm the diagnosis by biopsy.
- Remove the tumor (eg, by suction curettage), then classify the tumor based on clinical criteria.
- If disease is persistent, treat patients with chemotherapy and prescribe posttreatment contraception for 6 mo.

OVARIAN CANCER

Ovarian cancer is often fatal because it is usually advanced when diagnosed. Symptoms are usually absent in early stages and nonspecific in advanced stages. Evaluation usually includes ultrasonography, CT or MRI, and measurement of tumor markers (eg, cancer antigen 125). Diagnosis is by histologic analysis. Staging is surgical. Treatment requires hysterectomy, bilateral salpingo-oophorectomy, excision of as much involved tissue as possible (cytoreduction), and, unless cancer is localized, chemotherapy.

In the US, ovarian cancer is the 2nd most common gynecologic cancer (affecting about 1/70 women). It is the 5th leading cause of cancer-related deaths in women and, in the US, will cause an estimated 22,440 new cases and 14,080 deaths in 2017. Incidence is higher in developed countries.

Etiology

Ovarian cancer affects mainly perimenopausal and postmenopausal women.

Risk of ovarian cancer is increased by

- A history of ovarian cancer in a 1st-degree relative
- Nulliparity
- Delayed childbearing
- Early menarche
- Delayed menopause
- A personal or family history of endometrial, breast, or colon cancer

Risk is decreased by

- Oral contraceptive use

Probably 5 to 10% of ovarian cancer cases are related to mutations in the autosomal dominant *BRCA* gene, which is associated with a 50 to 85% lifetime risk of developing breast cancer. Women with *BRCA1* mutations have a 20 to 40% lifetime risk of developing ovarian cancer; risk among women with *BRCA2* mutations is increased less. Incidence of these mutations is higher in Ashkenazi Jews than in the general population. Mutations in several other genes, including *TP53*, *PTEN*, *STK11/LKB1*, *CDH1*, *CHEK2*, *ATM*, *MLH1*, and *MSH2*, have been associated with hereditary breast and/or ovarian cancer.

XY gonadal dysgenesis predisposes to ovarian germ cell cancer.

Pathology

Ovarian cancers are histologically diverse (see Table 270–7).

At least 80% of ovarian cancers originate in the epithelium; 75% of these cancers are serous cystadenocarcinoma, and about 10% are invasive mucinous carcinoma. At presentation, nearly 27% of patients with stage I epithelial ovarian cancers have mucinous histology, but < 10% with stage III or IV do.

About 20% of ovarian cancers originate in primary ovarian germ cells or in sex cord and stromal cells or are metastases to the ovary (most commonly, from the breast or GI tract). Germ cell cancers usually occur in women < 30.

Ovarian cancer spreads by

- Direct extension
- Exfoliation of cells into the peritoneal cavity (peritoneal seeding)
- Lymphatic dissemination to the pelvis and around the aorta
- Less often, hematogenously to the liver or lungs

Symptoms and Signs

Early ovarian cancer is usually asymptomatic; an adnexal mass, often solid, irregular, and fixed, may be discovered incidentally. Pelvic and rectovaginal examinations typically detect diffuse nodularity. A few women present with severe abdominal pain secondary to torsion of the ovarian mass.

Most women with advanced cancer present with nonspecific symptoms (eg, dyspepsia, bloating, early satiety, gas pains, backache). Later, pelvic pain, anemia, cachexia, and abdominal swelling due to ovarian enlargement or ascites usually occur.

Germ cell or stromal tumors may have functional effects (eg, hyperthyroidism, feminization, virilization).

Table 270–7. TYPES OF OVARIAN CANCERS

ORIGIN	TYPES
Epithelium	Brenner tumor Clear cell carcinomas Endometrioid carcinomas Mucinous carcinomas Serous cystadenocarcinomas (most common overall) Transitional cell carcinomas Unclassified carcinomas
Primary germ cells	Choriocarcinomas Dysgerminomas Embryonal carcinomas Endodermal sinus tumors Immature teratomas Polyembryoma
Sex cord and stromal cells	Granulosa-theca cell tumors Sertoli-Leydig cell tumors
Metastases	Breast cancer Cancer of the GI tract

Diagnosis

- Ultrasonography (for suspected early cancers) or CT or MRI (for suspected advanced cancers)
- Tumor markers (eg, cancer antigen [CA] 125)
- Surgical staging

Ovarian cancer is suspected in women with the following:

- Unexplained adnexal masses
- Unexplained abdominal bloating
- Changes in bowel habits
- Unintended weight loss
- Unexplained abdominal pain

An ovarian mass is more likely to be cancer in older women. Benign functional cysts can simulate functional germ cell or stromal tumors in young women.

A pelvic mass plus ascites usually indicates ovarian cancer but sometimes indicates Meigs syndrome (a benign fibroma with ascites and right hydrothorax).

Imaging: If early cancer is suspected, ultrasonography is done first; the following findings suggest cancer:

- A solid component
- Surface excrescences
- Size > 6 cm
- Irregular shape
- Low vascular resistance detected by transvaginal Doppler flow studies

If advanced cancer is suspected (eg, based on ascites, abdominal distention, or nodularity or fixation detected during physical examination), CT or MRI is usually done before surgery to determine extent of the cancer.

Tumor markers: Tumor markers, including the beta subunit of human chorionic gonadotropin (beta-hCG), LDH, alpha-fetoprotein, inhibin, and CA 125, are typically measured in young patients, who are at higher risk of nonepithelial tumors (eg, germ cell tumors, stromal tumors). In perimenopausal and postmenopausal patients, only CA 125 is measured because most ovarian cancers in this age group are epithelial tumors. CA 125 is elevated in 80% of advanced epithelial ovarian cancers but may be mildly elevated in endometriosis, pelvic inflammatory disease, pregnancy, fibroids, peritoneal inflammation, or nonovarian peritoneal cancer.

A mixed solid and cystic pelvic mass in postmenopausal women, especially if CA 125 is elevated, suggests ovarian cancer.

Biopsy: A biopsy is not routinely recommended unless a patient is not a surgical candidate. In those rare cases, samples are obtained by needle biopsy for masses or by needle aspiration for ascitic fluid.

For masses that appear benign on ultrasonography, histologic analysis is not required, and ultrasonography is repeated after 6 wk. Such benign-appearing masses include benign cystic teratomas (dermoid cysts), follicular cysts, and endometriomas.

Staging: Suspected or confirmed ovarian cancer is staged surgically (see Table 270–8).

If early-stage cancer is suspected, staging may be done by laparoscopy or robotic-assisted laparoscopic surgery. Otherwise, an abdominal midline incision that allows adequate access to the upper abdomen is required. All peritoneal surfaces, hemidiaphragms, and abdominal and pelvic viscera are inspected and palpated. Washings from the pelvis, abdominal gutters, and diaphragmatic recesses are obtained, and multiple biopsies of the peritoneum in the central and lateral pelvis and in the abdomen are done. For early-stage cancer, the infracolic omentum is removed, and pelvic and para-aortic lymph nodes are sampled.

Cancers are also graded histologically from 1 (least aggressive) to 3 (most aggressive). The most recent classification distinguishes epithelial ovarian cancers as low-grade (grade 1) or high-grade (grade 2 or 3).

Screening: There is no screening test for ovarian cancer. However, women with a known hereditary risk, such as those with *BRCA* mutations, should be followed closely.

Although data from large trials indicate that CA 125 has a high specificity (up to 99.9% in one study), sensitivity is only moderate (71% in one study), and positive predictive value is low; thus, CA 125 is not recommended as a screening test for asymptomatic, average-risk women. Screening asymptomatic women using both ultrasonography and serum CA 125 measurements can detect some cases of ovarian cancer but has not been shown to improve outcome, even for high-risk subgroups (including women with *BRCA* mutations).

However, women should be screened for abnormalities in the *BRCA* gene if their family history includes any of the following:

- Diagnosis of ovarian cancer in a 1st-degree relative before age 40
- Diagnosis of breast and ovarian cancer in only one 1st-degree relative if one of the cancers was diagnosed before age 50
- Two cases of ovarian cancer among 1st- and 2nd-degree relatives of the same lineage
- Two cases of breast cancer and one case of ovarian cancer among 1st- or 2nd-degree relatives of the same lineage
- One case of breast and one case of ovarian cancer among 1st- or 2nd-degree relatives of the same lineage if breast cancer was diagnosed before age 40 or if ovarian cancer was diagnosed before age 50
- Two cases of breast cancer among 1st- or 2nd-degree relatives of the same lineage if both cases were diagnosed before age 50
- Two cases of breast cancer among 1st- or 2nd-degree relatives of the same lineage if one was diagnosed before age 40

Also, if Ashkenazi Jewish women have one family member with breast cancer diagnosed before age 50 or with ovarian cancer, screening for abnormalities in the *BRCA* gene should be considered.

Prognosis

The 5-yr survival rates with treatment are

- Stage I: 85 to 95%
- Stage II: 70 to 78%
- Stage III: 40 to 60%
- Stage IV: 15 to 20%

Prognosis is worse when tumor grade is higher or when surgery cannot remove all visibly involved tissue; in such cases, prognosis is best when the involved tissue can be reduced to < 1 cm in diameter or ideally to a microscopic residual amount (cytoreductive surgery).

With stages III and IV, recurrence rate is about 70%.

Treatment

- Usually hysterectomy and bilateral salpingo-oophorectomy
- Cytoreductive surgery
- Usually postoperative chemotherapy, often with carboplatin and paclitaxel

Hysterectomy and bilateral salpingo-oophorectomy are usually indicated except for stage I nonepithelial or low-grade unilateral epithelial cancers in young patients; fertility can be

Table 270–8. FIGO SURGICAL STAGING OF OVARIAN, FALLOPIAN TUBE, AND PERITONEAL CANCER

STAGE	DESCRIPTION
I	Tumor limited to the ovaries or fallopian tubes
IA	Tumor limited to one ovary (capsule intact) or fallopian tube; no tumor on the external surface of ovary or fallopian tube; and no malignant cells in ascitic fluid or in peritoneal washings*
IB	Tumor limited to both ovaries (capsule intact) or fallopian tubes; no tumor on the external surface of ovary or fallopian tube; and no malignant cells in ascitic fluid or in peritoneal washings*
IC	Tumor limited to one or both ovaries (stage IA or IB), plus any of the following:
IC1	• Surgical spill
IC2	• Capsule ruptured before surgery or tumor on the surface of the ovary or fallopian tube
IC3	• Malignant cells in ascitic fluid or in peritoneal washings*
II	Tumor involving one or both ovaries or fallopian tubes with pelvic extension (below pelvic brim) or primary peritoneal cancer
IIA	Extension and/or implants on the uterus, fallopian tubes, and/or ovaries
IIB	Extension to other pelvic intraperitoneal tissues
III	Tumor involving one or both ovaries or fallopian tubes or primary peritoneal cancer with cytologically or histologically confirmed peritoneal metastases outside the pelvis and/or metastasis to the retroperitoneal lymph nodes
IIIA	Positive retroperitoneal lymph nodes, with or without microscopic peritoneal metastases that extend beyond the pelvis
IIIA1	Positive retroperitoneal lymph nodes only (cytologically or histologically proved)
IIIA1(I)	Metastasis ≤ 10 mm in largest dimension
IIIA1(II)	Metastasis > 10 mm in largest dimension
IIIA2	Microscopic extrapelvic (beyond the pelvic brim) peritoneal involvement, with or without positive retroperitoneal lymph nodes
IIIB	Macroscopic peritoneal metastases that extend beyond the pelvis and that are ≤ 2 cm in largest dimension, with or without positive retroperitoneal lymph nodes
IIIC	Macroscopic peritoneal metastases that extend beyond the pelvis and are > 2 cm in largest dimension, with or without metastasis to retroperitoneal lymph nodes (includes extension of tumor to the capsule of the liver and spleen without parenchymal involvement of either organ)
IV	Distant metastases, excluding peritoneal metastases
IVA	Pleural effusion with positive cytology
IVB	Parenchymal metastasis and metastases to extra-abdominal organs (including inguinal lymph nodes and lymph nodes outside the abdominal cavity)

*For stages IC, knowing whether capsule rupture was spontaneous or caused by the surgeon and whether the source of malignant cells was ascites or peritoneal washings helps determine prognosis.

Based on staging established by the International Federation of Gynecology and Obstetrics (FIGO) in Prat J, FIGO Committee on Gynecologic Oncology. Staging classification for cancer of the ovary, fallopian tube, and peritoneum. *Int J Gynecol Obstet* 124(1):1–5, 2014. Copyright Elsevier (2013). (See also Prat J, FIGO Committee on Gynecologic Oncology: FIGO's staging classification for cancer of the ovary, fallopian tube, and peritoneum: Abridged republication. *Journal of Gynecologic Oncology* 26(2): 87–89, 2015.)

preserved by not removing the unaffected ovary and uterus. In patients with extensive spread, surgery is not indicated or can be deferred if they have one or more of the following:

- Multiple liver metastases
- Lymphadenopathy in the porta hepatis
- Suprarenal para-aortic lymph nodes
- Diffuse mesenteric disease
- Evidence of pleural or parenchymal lung disease

These patients are treated with neoadjuvant chemotherapy (eg, with carboplatin plus paclitaxel). Surgery can sometimes be done after initial chemotherapy.

When hysterectomy and bilateral salpingo-oophorectomy are done, all visibly involved tissue is surgically removed if possible (cytoreduction). Cytoreduction is associated with increased survival time; the volume of residual disease remaining after cytoreduction correlates inversely with survival time. Cytoreduction may be

- Complete: Cytoreduction to no grossly visible disease
- Optimal: Cytoreduction with residual disease that is ≤ 1 cm in maximum tumor diameter, as defined by the Gynecologic Oncology Group
- Suboptimal: Cytoreduction with tumor nodules > 1 cm remaining

Cytoreductive surgery usually includes

- Supracolic omentectomy, sometimes with rectosigmoid resection (usually with primary reanastomosis)
- Radical peritoneal stripping
- Resection of diaphragmatic peritoneum or splenectomy

Predicting feasibility of cytoreduction: Because cytoreduction is associated with increased survival, being able to predict when cytoreduction to no gross residual disease can be done is important, but doing so is difficult; there are no uniform criteria.

Optimal cytoreduction is less likely if patients have the following:

- Poor performance status
- Age > 60 yr
- American Society of Anesthesiologists physical status 3 or 4
- Medical comorbidities
- Poor nutritional status
- Extra-abdominal disease
- Large tumor bulk
- Involvement of large bowel
- Metastases to retroperitoneal lymph nodes above the renal vessels > 1 cm in largest dimension
- Parenchymal liver involvement
- A preoperative CA 125 > 500 U/mL

Algorithms based on results of preoperative imaging (eg, CT, MRI, PET/CT) to assess optimal cytoreduction have not been reliably reproducible.

Diagnostic laparoscopy before laparotomy could spare patients an unnecessary laparotomy resulting in suboptimal cytoreduction. Laparoscopy enables clinicians to do a tissue biopsy, make a definitive diagnosis, and analyze the biopsy sample. Thus, patients who are not candidates for cytoreduction can begin chemotherapy treatment earlier. Laparoscopic findings indicating that optimal cytoreduction is unlikely include

- Omental cake
- Extensive peritoneal or diaphragmatic carcinomatosis
- Mesenteric retraction
- Bowel and stomach infiltration
- Spleen and/or liver superficial metastasis

The Fagotti score, based on 7 laparoscopic findings, can help predict the likelihood of optimal cytoreduction in patients with advanced ovarian cancer (see Table 270–9). This scoring system assigns a value of 0 or 2 depending on whether disease is present in certain locations. If patients score ≥ 8, optimal cytoreduction is very unlikely. If they score < 8, they are considered candidates for cytoreductive surgery.

Postoperative treatment: Postoperative treatment depends on the stage and grade (see Table 270–10).

Even if chemotherapy results in a complete clinical response (ie, normal physical examination, normal serum CA 125, negative CT scan of the abdomen and pelvis), about 50% of patients with stage III or IV cancer have residual tumor. Of patients with persistent elevation of CA 125, 90 to 95% have residual tumor. Recurrence rate in patients with a complete clinical response after initial chemotherapy (6 courses of carboplatin and paclitaxel) is 60 to 70%.

If cancer recurs or progresses after effective chemotherapy, chemotherapy is restarted. Other useful drugs may include liposomal doxorubicin, docetaxel, paclitaxel, gemcitabine, bevacizumab, and a combination of cyclophosphamide plus bevacizumab or of gemcitabine plus cisplatin. Targeted therapy with biologic agents is under study.

Prevention

For patients with *BRCA1* or *BRCA2* gene mutations, risk of ovarian and, to a lesser degree, breast cancer is reduced if

Table 270–9. CALCULATING THE FAGOTTI SCORE TO PREDICT THE LIKELIHOOD OF OPTIMAL CYTOREDUCTION

	SCORE*	
LAPAROSCOPIC FEATURE	0	2
Peritoneal carcinomatosis	Carcinomatosis involving a limited area (along the paracolic gutter or the pelvic peritoneum) and surgically removable by peritonectomy	Unresectable massive peritoneal involvement with a miliary pattern of distribution
Diaphragmatic involvement	No infiltrating carcinomatosis and no nodules confluent with most of the diaphragmatic surface	Widespread infiltrating carcinomatosis or nodules confluent with most of the diaphragmatic surface
Mesenteric involvement	No large infiltrating nodules and no involvement of the root of the mesentery (ie, movement of intestinal segments is not limited)	Large infiltrating nodules or involvement of the root of the mesentery indicated by limited movement of intestinal segments
Omental involvement	No tumor diffusion observed along the omentum up to the greater curvature of the stomach	Tumor diffusion observed along the omentum up to the greater curvature of the stomach
Bowel infiltration	No bowel resection assumed and no miliary carcinomatosis observed on the bowel ansae	Bowel resection assumed or miliary carcinomatosis observed on the ansae
Stomach infiltration	No obvious neoplastic involvement of the gastric wall	Obvious neoplastic involvement of the gastric wall
Liver metastases	No surface lesions	Any surface lesion

*A value of 0 or 2 is assigned depending on whether disease is present in these locations. If patients score ≥ 8, optimal cytoreduction is very unlikely. If they score < 8, they are considered candidates for cytoreductive surgery.

Adapted from Fagotti A, Ferrandina G, Fanfani F, et al: Prospective validation of a laparoscopic predictive model for optimal cytoreduction in advanced ovarian carcinoma. *Am J Obstet Gynecol* 199:642, e1-642.e6, 2008. doi: 10.1016/j.ajog.2008.06.052.

Table 270–10. POSTOPERATIVE TREATMENT OF OVARIAN CANCER BY STAGE AND TYPE

STAGE AND TYPE	TREATMENT
Stage IA or B/grade 1 epithelial adenocarcinoma	No postoperative therapy
Stage IA or B/grade 2 or 3 cancers Stage II cancers	6 courses of chemotherapy (typically, paclitaxel and carboplatin)
Stage III cancer	6 courses of chemotherapy* as for stage IA or B/grade 2 or 3 Consideration of intraperitoneal cisplatin and paclitaxel
Stage IV cancer	Infrequently, radiation therapy
Germ cell tumors Stage II or III stromal tumors	Most often, combination chemotherapy, usually bleomycin, cisplatin, and etoposide

*Intraperitoneal chemotherapy with cisplatin plus paclitaxel results in longer survival than IV chemotherapy but may have a higher complication rate.

prophylactic bilateral salpingo-oophorectomy is done after childbearing is completed. Cancer risk appears to be lower with this approach than with surveillance. Patients with *BRCA1* or *BRCA2* gene mutations should be referred to a gynecologic oncologist for counseling.

KEY POINTS

- Ovarian cancer affects mostly postmenopausal and perimenopausal women; nulliparity, delayed childbearing, early menarche, delayed menopause, and certain genetic markers increase risk.
- Early symptoms (eg, dyspepsia, bloating, early satiety, gas pains, backache) are nonspecific.
- If cancer is being considered, do CT, measure tumor markers (eg, CA 125), and surgically stage tumors.
- Screening asymptomatic women with ultrasonography and/or CA 125 is not useful unless risk of *BRCA* mutations is high.
- Diagnostic laparoscopy before laparotomy could spare patients an unnecessary laparotomy that results in suboptimal cytoreduction.
- Typically, treatment is hysterectomy, bilateral salpingo-oophorectomy, and cytoreductive surgery followed by chemotherapy (eg, carboplatin and paclitaxel).

UTERINE SARCOMAS

Uterine sarcomas are a group of disparate, highly malignant cancers developing from the uterine corpus. Common manifestations include abnormal uterine bleeding and pelvic pain or mass. For suspected uterine sarcoma, endometrial biopsy or D & C can be done, but results are often falsely negative; most sarcomas are diagnosed histologically after hysterectomy or myomectomy. Treatment requires total abdominal hysterectomy and bilateral salpingo-oophorectomy; for advanced cancer, chemotherapy and sometimes radiation therapy are indicated.

In the US, an estimated 4910 cases of uterine sarcomas are will occur in 2017. Uterine sarcomas account for about 3% of all uterine cancers.

Risk factors for uterine sarcomas are

- Prior pelvic radiation
- Tamoxifen use

Uterine sarcomas include

- Leiomyosarcoma (the most common subtype [63%])
- Endometrial stromal sarcoma (21%)
- Undifferentiated uterine sarcoma

Rare uterine mesenchymal sarcoma subtypes include

- Adenosarcomas
- Perivascular epithelioid cell tumor (PEComas)
- Rhabdomyosarcoma

Carcinosarcomas used to be categorized as sarcomas but are now considered and treated as high-grade epithelial tumors (carcinomas).

High-grade uterine sarcomas tend metastasize hematogenously, most often to the lungs; lymph node metastases are uncommon.

Symptoms and Signs

Most sarcomas manifest as abnormal vaginal bleeding and, less commonly, as pelvic pain, a feeling of fullness in the abdomen, a mass in the vagina, frequent urination, or a palpable pelvic mass.

Diagnosis

- Histology, most often after surgical removal

Symptoms suggesting uterine sarcoma usually prompt transvaginal ultrasonography and endometrial biopsy or fractional D & C. However, these tests have limited sensitivity. Endometrial stromal sarcoma and uterine leiomyosarcoma are often incidentally diagnosed histologically after hysterectomy or myomectomy.

If cancer is identified preoperatively, CT or MRI is typically done. If uterine sarcoma is diagnosed after surgical removal, imaging is recommended, and surgical re-exploration can be considered.

Screening for HNPCC (Lynch syndrome) is not usually done when patients have uterine sarcoma; in contrast, such screening is done when patients have endometrial cancer.

Staging: Staging is done surgically (see Tables 270–11 and 270–12).

Prognosis

Prognosis is generally poorer than that with endometrial cancer of similar stage; survival is generally poor when the cancer has spread beyond the uterus. Histology is not an independent prognostic factor.

In one study, 5-yr survival rates were

- Stage I: 51%
- Stage II: 13%
- Stage III: 10%
- Stage IV: 3%

Most commonly, the cancer recurs locally, in the abdomen, or the lungs.

Treatment

- Total abdominal hysterectomy and bilateral salpingo-oophorectomy

Table 270–11. FIGO SURGICAL STAGING OF UTERINE SARCOMA: LEIOMYOSARCOMA AND ENDOMETRIAL STROMAL SARCOMA

STAGE	DESCRIPTION
I	Limited to the uterus
IA	Tumor ≤ 5 cm in largest dimension
IB	Tumor > 5 cm
II	Extending beyond the uterus but within the pelvis
IIA	Involving the adnexa
IIB	Involving other pelvic tissues
III	Infiltrating abdominal tissues
IIIA	In one site
IIIB	> 1 site
IIIC	Regional lymph node metastasis
IVA	Invading bladder or rectum
IVB	Distant metastases

Adapted from staging established by the International Federation of Gynecology and Obstetrics (FIGO) and American Joint Committee on Cancer (AJCC), *AJCC Cancer Staging Manual*, ed. 7. New York, Springer, 2010. (See also National Cancer Institute: Uterine Sarcoma Treatment.)

Table 270–12. FIGO SURGICAL STAGING OF UTERINE SARCOMA: ADENOSARCOMA

STAGE	DESCRIPTION
I	Limited to the uterus
IA	Limited to the endometrium and/or endocervix
IB	Invading less than half the myometrium
IC	Invading more than half the myometrium
II	Extending beyond the uterus but within the pelvis
IIA	Involving the adnexa
IIB	Involving other pelvic tissues
III	Infiltrating abdominal tissues
IIIA	In one site
IIIB	> 1 site
IIIC	Metastasis to regional lymph nodes
IVA	Invading the bladder or rectum
IVB	Distant metastases

*Based on staging established by the International Federation of Gynecology and Obstetrics (FIGO) and American Joint Committee on Cancer (AJCC), *AJCC Cancer Staging Manual*, ed. 7. New York, Springer, 2010. (See also National Cancer Institute: Uterine Sarcoma Treatment.)

Treatment of uterine sarcomas is total abdominal hysterectomy and bilateral salpingo-oophorectomy.

Uterine sarcomas should be removed en bloc; morcellation is contraindicated. If a specimen is fragmented during surgery, imaging is recommended, and re-exploration can be considered. Treatment with chemotherapy is also recommended.

The ovaries may be preserved in certain patients with early-stage uterine leiomyosarcoma if they wish to retain hormonal function. Additional surgical resection should be based on intraoperative findings.

The usefulness of lymphadenectomy in patients with leiomyosarcoma or endometrial stromal sarcoma is controversial; no therapeutic value has been shown.

For inoperable sarcomas, pelvic radiation therapy with or without brachytherapy and/or systemic therapy is recommended.

Adjuvant radiation therapy is typically used and appears to delay local recurrence but does not improve overall survival rate.

Chemotherapy drugs are typically used when tumors are advanced or recur; drugs vary by tumor type.

Combination chemotherapy regimens are recommended:

- Docetaxel/gemcitabine (preferred for leiomyosarcoma)
- Doxorubicin/ifosfamide
- Doxorubicin/dacarbazine
- Gemcitabine/dacarbazine
- Gemcitabine/vinorelbine

Overall, response to chemotherapy is poor.

Hormone therapy is used for patients with endometrial stromal sarcoma or hormone receptor–positive uterine leiomyosarcoma. Progestins are frequently effective. Hormone therapy includes

- Medroxyprogesterone acetate
- Megestrol acetate
- Aromatase inhibitors
- GnRH (gonadotropin-releasing hormone) agonists

KEY POINTS

- Uterine sarcomas are uncommon.
- Most sarcomas are asymptomatic; symptoms include abnormal vaginal bleeding, a mass in the vagina. pelvic pain, a feeling of fullness in the abdomen, and frequent urination.
- Prognosis is generally worse than that with endometrial cancer of similar stage.
- Treat most patients with total abdominal hysterectomy and bilateral salpingo-oophorectomy.
- Use hormone therapy for patients with endometrial stroma sarcoma and hormone receptor–positive leiomyosarcomas.
- Treat inoperable sarcomas with radiation therapy and/or chemotherapy.

VAGINAL CANCER

Vaginal cancer is usually a squamous cell carcinoma, most often occurring in women > 60. The most common symptom is abnormal vaginal bleeding. Diagnosis is by biopsy. Treatment for many small localized cancers is hysterectomy plus vaginectomy and lymph node dissection; for most others, radiation therapy is used.

Vaginal cancer accounts for 1% of gynecologic cancers in the US. Average age at diagnosis is 60 to 65.

Risk factors for vaginal cancer include

- HPV infection
- Cervical or vulvar cancer

Exposure to diethylstilbestrol in utero predisposes to clear cell adenocarcinoma of the vagina, which is rare; mean age at diagnosis is 19.

Most (95%) primary vaginal cancers are squamous cell carcinomas; others include primary and secondary adenocarcinomas, secondary squamous cell carcinomas (in older women), clear cell adenocarcinomas (in young women), and melanomas. The most common vaginal sarcoma is sarcoma botryoides (embryonal rhabdomyosarcoma); peak incidence is at age 3.

Most vaginal cancers occur in the upper third of the posterior vaginal wall. They may spread as follows:

- By direct extension (into the local paravaginal tissues, bladder, or rectum)
- Through inguinal lymph nodes from lesions in the lower vagina
- Through pelvic lymph nodes from lesions in the upper vagina
- Hematogenously

Symptoms and Signs

Most patients with vaginal cancer present with abnormal vaginal bleeding: postmenopausal, postcoital, or intermenstrual. Some also present with a watery vaginal discharge or dyspareunia. A few patients are asymptomatic, and the lesion is discovered during routine pelvic examination or evaluation of an abnormal Pap test.

Vesicovaginal or rectovaginal fistulas are manifestations of advanced disease.

Diagnosis

- Biopsy
- Clinical staging

Punch biopsy is usually diagnostic, but wide local excision is occasionally necessary.

Vaginal cancers are staged clinically (see Table 270–13), based primarily on physical examination, endoscopy (ie, cystoscopy, proctoscopy), chest x-ray (for pulmonary metastases), and usually CT (for abdominal or pelvic metastases). Survival rates depend on the stage.

Treatment

- Hysterectomy plus vaginectomy and lymph node dissection for tumors confined to the wall of the upper third of the vagina
- Radiation therapy for most others

Stage I tumors within the upper third of the vagina can be treated with radical hysterectomy, upper vaginectomy, and pelvic lymph node dissection, sometimes followed by radiation therapy.

Table 270–13. FIGO VAGINAL CANCER BY STAGE

STAGE	DESCRIPTION	5-YR SURVIVAL RATE*
I	Limited to the vaginal wall	65–70%
II	Invading subvaginal tissues	47%
III	Extending to the pelvic wall	30%
IV	Extending beyond the true pelvis or involving the bladder or rectal mucosa	15–20%

*Prognosis is worse if the primary tumor is large or poorly differentiated.

Based on staging established by the International Federation of Gynecology and Obstetrics (FIGO) and American Joint Committee on Cancer (AJCC), *AJCC Cancer Staging Manual*, ed. 7. New York, Springer, 2010.

Most other primary tumors are treated with radiation therapy, usually a combination of external beam radiation therapy and brachytherapy. If radiation therapy is contraindicated because of vesicovaginal or rectovaginal fistulas, pelvic exenteration is done.

KEY POINTS

- Risk factors for vaginal cancer include HPV infection and cervical or vulvar cancer.
- Most patients present with abnormal vaginal bleeding.
- Usually diagnose with punch biopsy; sometimes wide local excision is necessary.
- Treat tumors confined to the wall of the upper third of the vagina with hysterectomy plus vaginectomy and lymph node dissection, sometimes followed by radiation therapy, and treat most others with radiation therapy.

VULVAR CANCER

Vulvar cancer is usually a squamous cell skin cancer, most often occurring in elderly women. It usually manifests as a palpable lesion. Diagnosis is by biopsy. Treatment typically includes excision and lymph node dissection or sentinel lymph node (SLN) mapping.

Vulvar cancer is the 4th most common gynecologic cancer in the US; it accounts for 5% of cancers of the female genital tract. Vulvar cancer caused an estimated 5950 new cases and 1110 deaths in 2016.

Average age at diagnosis is about 70, and incidence increases with age. Incidence of vulvar cancer appears to be increasing in young women.

Risk factors for vulvar cancer include vulvar intraepithelial neoplasia (VIN), human papillomavirus (HPV) infection, heavy cigarette smoking, lichen sclerosus, squamous hyperplasia, squamous carcinoma of the vagina or cervix, and chronic granulomatous diseases.

Pathology

VIN is a precursor to vulvar cancer. VIN may be multifocal. Sometimes adenocarcinoma of the vulva, breast, or Bartholin glands also develops.

About 90% of vulvar cancers are squamous cell carcinomas; about 5% are melanomas. Others include adenocarcinomas and transitional cell, adenoid cystic, and adenosquamous carcinomas; all may originate in Bartholin glands. Sarcomas and basal cell carcinomas with underlying adenocarcinoma also occur.

Vulvar cancer may spread as follows:

- By direct extension (eg, into the urethra, bladder, vagina, perineum, anus, or rectum)
- Hematogenously
- To the inguinal lymph nodes
- From the inguinal lymph nodes to the pelvic and para-aortic lymph nodes

Symptoms and Signs

Most patients with vulvar cancer present with a palpable vulvar lesion, frequently noticed by the woman or by a clinician during pelvic examination. Women often have a long history of pruritus. They may not present until cancer is advanced. The lesion may become necrotic or ulcerated, sometimes resulting in bleeding or a watery vaginal discharge. Melanomas may appear bluish black, pigmented, or papillary.

Diagnosis

- Biopsy
- Surgical staging

Vulvar cancer may mimic sexually transmitted genital ulcers (see p. 1700) basal cell carcinoma, vulvar Paget disease (a pale eczematoid lesion), Bartholin gland cyst, or condyloma acuminatum. Clinicians should consider vulvar cancer if a vulvar lesion develops in women at low risk of sexually transmitted diseases (STDs) or if it does not respond to treatment for STDs.

A dermal punch biopsy using a local anesthetic is usually diagnostic. Occasionally, wide local excision is necessary to differentiate VIN from cancer. Subtle lesions may be delineated by staining the vulva with toluidine blue or by using colposcopy.

Table 270–14. VULVAR CANCER BY STAGE

STAGE	DESCRIPTION	5-YR SURVIVAL RATE*
I	Confined to the vulva or perineum and no lymph node metastases	> 90%
IA	≤ 2 cm in all dimensions and ≤ 1 mm of invasion	
IB	> 2 cm in any dimension or > 1 mm of invasion	
II	Tumor of any size with adjacent spread (lower third of the urethra, lower third of the vagina, or the anus) and no lymph node metastases	80%
III	Tumor of any size, with or without adjacent spread (lower third of the urethra, lower third of the vagina, or the anus), and with regional (inguinofemoral) lymph node metastases	50–60%
IIIA	1 or 2 lymph node metastases, each < 5 mm *or* 1 lymph node metastasis of ≥ 5 mm	
IIIB	3 or more lymph node metastases, each < 5 mm *or* 2 or more lymph node metastases, each ≥ 5 mm	
IIIC	Lymph node metastases with extracapsular spread	
IV	Invasion of other regional structures (upper two-thirds of the urethra, upper two-thirds of the vagina, bladder mucosa, or rectal mucosa), is fixed to the pelvic bone, or has fixed or ulcerated regional (inguinofemoral) lymph nodes or distant metastases	15%
IVA	Invasion of the upper two-thirds of the urethra, upper two-thirds of the vagina, bladder mucosa, or rectal mucosa; is fixed to pelvic bone; or has fixed or ulcerated regional lymph nodes	
IVB	Any distant metastases including in pelvic lymph nodes	

*Risk of lymph node spread is proportional to tumor size and invasion depth.

Based on staging established by the International Federation of Gynecology and Obstetrics (FIGO) and American Joint Committee on Cancer (AJCC), *AJCC Cancer Staging Manual*, ed. 7. New York, Springer, 2010.

PEARLS & PITFALLS

- If a vulvar lesion develops in a woman at low risk of STDs or does not respond to treatment for STDs, consider vulvar cancer.

Staging: Staging of vulvar cancer is based on tumor size and location and on regional lymph node spread as determined by lymph node dissection done as part of initial surgical treatment (see Table 270–14).

Prognosis

Overall 5-yr survival rates depend on stage. Risk of lymph node spread is proportional to the tumor size and invasion depth. Melanomas metastasize frequently, depending mostly on invasion depth but also on tumor size.

Treatment

- Wide excision and lymph node dissection except when stromal invasion is < 1 mm
- Radiation therapy, chemotherapy, or both for stage III or IV cancer

Wide (≥ 2-cm margin) radical excision of the local tumor is indicated in all cases. Lymph node dissection can be done when stromal invasion is > 1 mm but is unnecessary when stromal invasion is < 1 mm. Radical vulvectomy is usually reserved for Bartholin gland adenocarcinoma.

SLN biopsy is a reasonable alternative to lymph node dissection for some women with squamous cell vulvar carcinoma. SLN mapping should not be considered if clinical findings suggest cancer has spread to lymph nodes in the groin. For SLN mapping, a tracer (blue dye, technetium-99 [^{99}Tc], ICG) is injected intradermally around and in front of the leading edge of the vulvar carcinoma.

For lateralized lesions ≤ 2 cm, unilateral wide local excision and unilateral SLN dissection is recommended. Lesions near the midline and most lesions > 2 cm require bilateral SLN dissection.

For stage III, lymph node dissection followed by postoperative external beam radiation therapy, often with chemotherapy (eg, 5-fluorouracil, cisplatin), is usually done before wide radical excision. The alternative is more radical or exenterative surgery.

For stage IV, treatment is some combination of pelvic exenteration, radiation therapy, and systemic chemotherapy.

KEY POINTS

- Most vulvar cancers are skin cancers (eg, squamous cell carcinoma, melanoma).
- Consider vulvar cancers if vulvar lesions, including pruritic lesions and ulcers, do not respond to treatment for STDs or occur in women at low risk of STDs.
- Diagnose vulvar cancer by biopsy, and stage it surgically.
- For cancers without distant metastases, use wide excision, and unless stromal invasion is < 1 mm, do lymph node dissection or SLN biopsy.

271 Infertility

Infertility is usually defined as inability of a couple to conceive after 1 yr of unprotected intercourse.

Infertility is defined as a disease by the WHO.

Frequent, unprotected intercourse results in conception for 50% of couples within 3 mo, for 75% within 6 mo, and for 90% within 1 yr.

Infertility can be caused by the following:

- Sperm disorders (≥ 35% of couples)
- Ovulatory dysfunction or decreased ovarian reserve (about 20%)
- Tubal dysfunction and pelvic lesions (about 30%)
- Abnormal cervical mucus (≤ 5%)
- Unidentified factors (about 10%)

Inability to conceive often leads to feelings of frustration, anger, guilt, resentment, and inadequacy.

Couples wishing to conceive are encouraged to have frequent intercourse when conception is most likely—during the 6 days, and particularly the 3 days before ovulation. Ovulation is most likely to occur midway between menstrual periods.

Measuring morning basal body temperature (BBT) daily can help determine when ovulation is occurring in women with regular menstrual cycles. A decrease suggests impending ovulation; an increase of ≥ 0.5° C suggests ovulation has just occurred. However, commercially available luteinizing hormone (LH) prediction test kits, which identify the midcycle LH surge, are probably the best way for women to determine when ovulation occurs and are less disruptive than measuring BBT. BBT can be useful if women cannot afford or do not have access to LH prediction kits. There is no evidence that any test determining when ovulation occurs improves the likelihood of pregnancy in couples having regular intercourse.

Excessive use of caffeine and tobacco, which can impair fertility, is discouraged.

If these measures do not result in pregnancy after ≥ 1 yr, both partners are evaluated. Evaluation begins with history, examination, and counseling. Men are evaluated for sperm disorders, and women are evaluated for ovulatory and tubal dysfunction and pelvic lesions.

Evaluation is done sooner than 1 yr if

- The woman is > 35.
- The woman has infrequent menses.
- The woman has a known abnormality of the uterus, fallopian tubes, or ovaries.
- The man is known to be subfertile or is at risk of subfertility.

Support groups for couples (eg, Path2Parenthood, RESOLVE) may help. A clinician should mention adoption if the likelihood of conceiving is low (usually confirmed after 3 yr of infertility, even in women < 35, or after 2 yr of treatment).

SPERM DISORDERS

Sperm disorders include defects in quality or quantity of sperm produced and defects in sperm emission. Diagnosis is by semen and genetic testing. The most effective treatment is usually in vitro fertilization via intracytoplasmic sperm injection.

Pathophysiology

Spermatogenesis occurs continuously. Each germ cell requires about 72 to 74 days to mature fully. Spermatogenesis is most efficient at 34° C. Within the seminiferous tubules, Sertoli cells regulate maturation, and Leydig cells produce the necessary testosterone. Fructose is normally produced in the seminal vesicles and secreted through the ejaculatory ducts.

Sperm disorders may result in

- An inadequate quantity of sperm—too few (oligozoospermia) or none (azoospermia)
- Defects in sperm quality, such as abnormal motility or structure

Etiology

Impaired spermatogenesis: Spermatogenesis can be impaired (see Table 271–1) by the following, resulting in an inadequate quantity or defective quality of sperm:

- Heat
- Disorders (GU, endocrine, or genetic)
- Drugs
- Toxins

Impaired sperm emission: Sperm emission may be impaired because of retrograde ejaculation into the bladder.

Retrograde ejaculation is often due to

- Diabetes mellitus
- Neurologic dysfunction
- Retroperitoneal dissection (eg, for Hodgkin lymphoma)
- Transurethral resection of the prostate

Sperm emission can also be impaired by

- Obstruction of the vas deferens
- Congenital absence of both vasa deferentia or epididymides, often in men with mutations of the cystic fibrosis transmembrane conductance regulator (*CFTR*) gene
- Absence of both seminal vesicles

Almost all men with symptomatic cystic fibrosis have congenital bilateral absence of the vas deferens, but the vasa deferentia may also be absent in men with mutations of *CTFR* that do not cause symptomatic cystic fibrosis.

Other causes: Men with microdeletions affecting the Y chromosome, particularly in the AZFc (azoospermia factor c) region, can develop oligozoospermia via various mechanisms, depending on the specific deletion.

Another rare mechanism of infertility is destruction or inactivation of sperm by sperm antibodies, which are usually produced by the man.

Diagnosis

- Semen analysis
- Sometimes genetic testing

When couples are infertile, the man should always be evaluated for sperm disorders. History and physical examination focus on potential causes (eg, GU disorders). Volume of each testis should be determined; normal is 20 to 25 mL. Semen analysis should be done.

If oligozoospermia or azoospermia is detected, genetic testing should be done. These tests include

- Standard karyotyping
- PCR of tagged chromosomal sites (to detect microdeletions affecting the Y chromosome)
- Evaluation for mutations of the *CFTR* gene

Table 271–1. CAUSES OF IMPAIRED SPERMATOGENESIS

CONDITION	EXAMPLES
Endocrine disorders	Abnormalities of the hypothalamic-pituitary-gonadal axis Adrenal disorders Hyperprolactinemia Hypogonadism, sometimes related to obesity Hypothyroidism
Genetic disorders	Gonadal dysgenesis Klinefelter syndrome Microdeletions of sections of the Y chromosome (in 10–15% of men with severely impaired spermatogenesis)
GU disorders	Cryptorchidism Infections Injury Mumps orchitis Testicular atrophy Varicocele
Heat	Exposure to excessive heat within the last 3 mo Fever
Drugs and toxins	Anabolic steroids Androgens Antiandrogens (eg, bicalutamide, cyproterone, flutamide) Antimalarial drugs Aspirin when taken long term Caffeine in excessive amounts (possibly) Chlorambucil Cimetidine Colchicine Corticosteroids Cotrimoxazole Cyclophosphamide Ethanol Estrogens Gonadotropin-releasing hormone (GnRH) agonists (to treat prostate cancer) Ketoconazole Marijuana Medroxyprogesterone Methotrexate Monoamine oxidase inhibitors Nitrofurantoin Opioids Spironolactone Sulfasalazine Toxins

Before a man with a *CFTR* gene mutation and his partner attempt to conceive, the partner should also be tested to exclude cystic fibrosis carrier status.

Semen analysis: Before semen analysis, the man is typically asked to refrain from ejaculation for 2 to 3 days. However, data indicate that daily ejaculation does not reduce the sperm count in men unless there is a problem. Because sperm count varies, testing requires ≥ 2 specimens obtained ≥ 1 wk apart; each specimen is obtained by masturbation into a glass jar, preferably at the laboratory site. If this method is difficult, the man can use a condom at home; the condom must be free of lubricants and chemicals. After being at room temperature for 20 to 30 min, the ejaculate is evaluated (see Table 271–2).

Additional computer-assisted measures of sperm motility (eg, linear sperm velocity) are available; however, their correlation with fertility is unclear.

If a man without hypogonadism or congenital bilateral absence of the vas deferens has an ejaculate volume < 1 mL, urine is analyzed for sperm after ejaculation. A disproportionately large number of sperm in urine vs semen suggests retrograde ejaculation.

Other tests: Endocrine evaluation is warranted if the semen analysis is abnormal and especially if the sperm concentration is < 10 million/mL. Minimum initial testing should include

- Serum follicle-stimulating hormone (FSH) levels
- Testosterone levels

If testosteroneis low, serum LH and prolactin should also be measured. Men with abnormal spermatogenesis often have normal FSH levels, but any increase in FSH is a clear indication of abnormal spermatogenesis. Elevations in prolactin require evaluation for a tumor involving or impinging on the anterior pituitary or may indicate ingestion of various prescription or recreational drugs.

Specialized sperm tests, available at some infertility centers, may be considered if routine tests of both partners do not explain infertility and in vitro fertilization or gamete intrafallopian tube transfer is being contemplated. They include the following:

- The immunobead test detects sperm antibodies.
- The hypo-osmotic swelling test measures the structural integrity of sperm plasma membranes.
- The hemizona assay and sperm penetration assay determine the ability of sperm to fertilize the egg in vitro.

Table 271–2. SEMEN ANALYSIS

FACTOR	NORMAL	LOWER REFERENCE LIMITS (5TH PERCENTILE)
Volume	2 to 6 mL	1.5 mL
Viscosity	Beginning to liquefy within 30 min; completely liquefied within 1 h	—
Gross and microscopic appearance	Opaque, cream-colored, ≤ 1–3 WBC/high-power field	—
pH	7–8	—
Sperm count	> 20 million/mL	15 million/mL
Sperm motility at 1 and 3 h	> 50% motile	40% motile
Percentage of sperm with normal morphology	> 5.5% using 1999 WHO strict criteria	4% using 2010 WHO criteria
Fructose	Present (indicating at least one ejaculatory duct is patent)	—

The usefulness of these specialized tests is controversial and unproved.

If necessary, testicular biopsy can distinguish between obstructive and nonobstructive azoospermia.

Treatment

- Clomiphene
- Assisted reproductive techniques if clomiphene is ineffective

Underlying GU disorders are treated.

For men with sperm counts of 10 to 20 million/mL and no endocrine disorder, clomiphene citrate (25 to 50 mg po once/day taken 25 days/mo for 3 to 4 mo) can be tried. Clomiphene, an antiestrogen, may stimulate sperm production and increase sperm counts. However, whether it improves sperm motility or morphology is unclear, and it has not been proved to increase fertility.

If sperm count is < 10 million/mL or clomiphene is unsuccessful in men with normal sperm motility, the most effective treatment is usually in vitro fertilization with injection of a single sperm into a single egg (intracytoplasmic sperm injection). Alternatively, intrauterine insemination using washed semen samples and timed to coincide with ovulation is sometimes tried. If pregnancy is going to occur, it usually occurs by the 6th treatment cycle.

Decreased number and viability of sperm may not preclude pregnancy. In such cases, fertility may be enhanced by controlled ovarian stimulation of the woman plus artificial insemination or assisted reproductive techniques (eg, in vitro fertilization, intracytoplasmic sperm injection).

If the male partner cannot produce enough fertile sperm, a couple may consider insemination using donor sperm. Risk of AIDS and other sexually transmitted diseases is minimized by freezing donor sperm for ≥ 6 mo, after which donors are retested for infection before insemination proceeds. In the US, the CDC recommends postponing collection of semen for 6 mo if donors have been diagnosed with Zika virus infection or have lived in or traveled to an area with active Zika virus transmission.

KEY POINTS

- Impairment of spermatogenesis or impaired sperm emission can result in deficient sperm quantity or quality.
- Diagnose sperm disorders starting with semen analysis and sometimes genetic testing.
- Correct underlying GU disorders if present, or treat with clomiphene citrate or with in vitro fertilization and intracytoplasmic sperm injection.

ABNORMAL CERVICAL MUCUS

Abnormal cervical mucus may impair fertility by inhibiting penetration or increasing destruction of sperm.

Normally, cervical mucus is stimulated to change from thick and impenetrable to thin and stretchable by an increase in estradiol levels during the follicular phase of the menstrual cycle. Abnormal cervical mucus may

- Remain impenetrable to sperm around the time of ovulation
- Promote sperm destruction by facilitating influx of vaginal bacteria (eg, due to cervicitis)
- Contain antibodies to sperm (rarely)

Abnormal mucus rarely impairs fertility significantly, except in women with chronic cervicitis or cervical stenosis due to prior treatment for cervical intraepithelial neoplasia.

Diagnosis

- Examination to check for cervicitis and cervical stenosis

A pelvic examination is done to check for cervicitis and cervical stenosis. Cervicitis is diagnosed if women have cervical exudate (purulent or mucopurulent) or cervical friability. Complete cervical stenosis is diagnosed if a 1- to 2-mm diameter probe cannot be passed into the uterine cavity.

Postcoital testing of cervical mucus to determine whether viable sperm are present (which used to be routine during infertility evaluation) is no longer considered useful.

Treatment

- Assisted reproductive techniques (intrauterine insemination or in vitro fertilization)

Treatment may include intrauterine insemination and in vitro fertilization. However, whether either treatment is effective is unproved.

There is no evidence that using drugs to thin the mucus (eg, guaifenesin) improves fertility.

DECREASED OVARIAN RESERVE

Decreased ovarian reserve is a decrease in the quantity or quality of oocytes, leading to impaired fertility.

Ovarian reserve may begin to decrease at age 30 or even earlier and decreases rapidly after age 40. Ovarian lesions also decrease reserve. Although older age is a risk factor for decreased ovarian reserve, age and decreased ovarian reserve are each independent predictors of infertility and thus of a poorer response to fertility treatment.

Diagnosis

- Follicle-stimulating hormone (FSH) and estradiol levels for screening
- Antimüllerian hormone (AMH) level and antral follicle count (AFC)

Testing for decreased ovarian reserve is considered for women who

- Are ≥ 35
- Have had ovarian surgery
- Have responded poorly to treatments such as ovarian stimulation with exogenous gonadotropins

Measuring FSH or estradiol levels is useful as a screening test for decreased ovarian reserve. FSH levels > 10 mIU/mL or estradiol levels < 80 pg/mL on day 3 of the menstrual cycle suggest ovarian reserve is decreased. However, the AMH level and AFC are currently the best tests for diagnosing decreased ovarian reserve.

The **AMH level** is an early, reliable predictor of declining ovarian function. Increasingly, AMH measurement is used to assess ovarian reserve. A low AMH level predicts a lower chance of pregnancy after in vitro fertilization (IVF); pregnancy is rare when the level is too low to be detected.

The **AFC** is the total number of follicles that measure 2 to 10 mm (mean diameter) in both ovaries during the early follicular phase; AFC is determined by observation during transvaginal ultrasonography. If AFC is low (3 to 10), pregnancy after IVF is less likely.

Decreased ovarian reserve can also be measured using the clomiphene citrate challenge test; however, it is less reliable. For this test, the woman is given clomiphene 100 mg po once/day on days 5 to 9 of the menstrual cycle; then FSH and estradiol levels are measured again. A dramatic increase in FSH and estradiol levels from day 3 to day 10 of the cycle indicates decreased reserve.

Treatment

- Sometimes use of donor oocytes

Because pregnancy may still be possible, treatment of decreased ovarian reserve is individualized based on the woman's circumstances and age.

If women are > 42 or ovarian reserve is decreased, assisted reproduction using donor oocytes may be necessary.

OVULATORY DYSFUNCTION

Ovulatory dysfunction is abnormal, irregular (with ≤ 9 menses/yr), or absent ovulation. Menses are often irregular or absent. Diagnosis is often possible by history or can be confirmed by measurement of hormone levels or serial pelvic ultrasonography. Treatment is usually induction of ovulation with clomiphene or other drugs.

Etiology

Chronic ovulatory dysfunction in premenopausal women is most commonly caused by

- Polycystic ovary syndrome (PCOS—see p. 2290)

But it has many other causes, including

- Hyperprolactinemia
- Hypothalamic dysfunction (eg, hypothalamic amenorrhea)
- Other disorders that cause anovulation

Symptoms and Signs

Ovulatory dysfunction is suspected if menses are absent, irregular, or not preceded by symptoms, such as breast tenderness, lower abdominal bloating, or moodiness (collectively termed molimina).

Diagnosis

- Menstrual history
- Sometimes basal body temperature monitoring
- Measurement of urinary or serum hormones or ultrasonography

Anovulation is often apparent based on the menstrual history. Measuring morning body temperature daily can help determine whether and when ovulation is occurring. However, this method is often inaccurate.

More accurate methods include

- **Home testing kits,** which detect an increase in urinary LH excretion 24 to 36 h before ovulation (requiring daily testing for several days around midcycle, usually beginning about or after cycle day 9)
- **Pelvic ultrasonography,** which is used to monitor ovarian follicle diameter and rupture (and should also begin in the late follicular phase)
- **Measurement of serum progesterone and urinary pregnanediol glucuronide** (a urinary metabolite of progesterone)

Serum progesterone levels of ≥ 3 ng/mL (≥ 9.75 nmol/L) or elevated levels of pregnanediol glucuronide in urine (measured, if possible, 1 wk before onset of the next menstrual period) indicate that ovulation has occurred.

Intermittent or absent ovulation should prompt evaluation for disorders of the pituitary, hypothalamus, or ovaries (eg, PCOS).

Treatment

- Clomiphene or letrozole
- Possibly metformin if body mass index is ≥ 35
- Gonadotropins if clomiphene is ineffective

Ovulation can usually be induced with drugs.

Clomiphene: Commonly, chronic anovulation that is not due to hyperprolactinemia is initially treated with the antiestrogen clomiphene citrate.

Clomiphene is most effective when the cause is PCOS. Clomiphene 50 mg po once/day is started between the 3rd and 5th day after bleeding begins; bleeding may have occurred spontaneously or have been induced (eg, by progestin withdrawal). Clomiphene is continued for 5 days. Ovulation usually occurs 5 to 10 days (mean 7 days) after the last day of clomiphene; if ovulation occurs, menses follows within 35 days of the induced bleeding episode.

The daily dose can be increased by up to 50 mg every cycle to a maximum of 200 mg/dose as needed to induce ovulation. Treatment is continued as needed for up to 4 ovulatory cycles. Ovulation occurs in 75 to 80% of women treated with clomiphene, but the pregnancy rate is at most 40 to 50%.

Adverse effects of clomiphene include vasomotor flushes (10%), abdominal distention (6%), breast tenderness (2%), nausea (3%), visual symptoms (1 to 2%), and headaches (1 to 2%). Multifetal pregnancy (primarily twins) occurs in about 5%, and ovarian hyperstimulation syndrome occurs in ≤ 1%. Ovarian cysts are common. A previously suggested association between clomiphene taken for > 12 cycles and ovarian cancer has not been confirmed.

Clomiphene should not be given to women who are pregnant because theoretically, it may cause genital birth defects.

Letrozole: Evidence indicates that in obese women with PCOS, letrozole (an aromatase inhibitor) is more likely to induce ovulation than clomiphene.[1] Recent data indicate that this effect may also occur in thin women with PCOS. No evidence indicates that letrozole is more effective than clomiphene for causes of anovulation other than PCOS. Letrozole has a much shorter half-life than clomiphene.

Letrozole, like clomiphene, is started between the 3rd and 5th day after bleeding begins. Initially, women are given 2.5 mg po once/day for 5 days. If ovulation does not occur, the dose can be increased by 2.5 mg every cycle to a maximum of 7.5 mg/dose.

The **most common adverse effects** of letrozole are fatigue and dizziness.

Letrozole should not be given to women who are pregnant because theoretically, it may cause genital birth defects.

Metformin: For women with PCOS, metformin (750 to 1000 mg po bid) may be a useful adjunct in inducing ovulation, particularly if the patient is insulin-resistant, as are many patients with PCOS. However, clomiphene alone is more effective than metformin alone and is just as effective as metformin and clomiphene together. Metformin is not first-line therapy for women who have PCOS and want to become pregnant.

Metformin may be useful for women with a body mass index > 35 and should be considered for women with PCOS and glucose intolerance.

Exogenous gonadotropins: For all women with ovulatory dysfunction that does not respond to clomiphene (or letrozole, when used), human gonadotropins (ie, preparations that contain purified or recombinant FSH and variable amounts of LH) can be used. Several IM and sc preparations with similar efficacy are available; they typically contain 75 IU of FSH activity with or without LH activity. They are usually given once/day, beginning on the 3rd to 5th day after induced or spontaneous bleeding; ideally, they stimulate maturation of 1 to 3 follicles, determined ultrasonographically, within 7 to 14 days.

Ovulation is typically triggered with human chorionic gonadotropin (hCG) 5,000 to 10,000 IU IM after follicle maturation; criteria for using hCG may vary, but typically, at least one follicle should be > 16 mm in diameter. Alternatively, a gonadotropin-releasing hormone (GnRH) agonist can be used to trigger ovulation, especially in women at high risk of ovarian hyperstimulation syndrome.

Although risk of ovarian hyperstimulation syndrome in women at high risk is lower when a GnRH agonist is used to trigger ovulation, it is safer to not trigger ovulation if women are at high risk of ovarian hyperstimulation syndrome or multifetal pregnancy. Risk factors for these problems include

- Presence of > 3 follicles > 16 mm in diameter
- Preovulatory serum estradiol levels > 1500 pg/mL (or possibly > 1000 pg/mL) in women with several small ovarian follicles

When exogenous gonadotropins are used appropriately, > 95% of women treated with them ovulate, but the pregnancy rate is only 50 to 75%.

After gonadotropin therapy, 10 to 30% of successful pregnancies are multiple.

Ovarian hyperstimulation syndrome occurs in 10 to 20% of patients; ovaries can become massively enlarged, and intravascular fluid volume shifts into the peritoneal space, causing potentially life-threatening ascites and hypovolemia.

Treatment of the underlying disorder: Underlying disorders (eg, hyperprolactinemia) are treated.

If the cause is hypothalamic amenorrhea, gonadorelin acetate, a synthetic GnRH agonist given as a pulsatile IV infusion, can induce ovulation. Doses of 2.5- to 5.0-mcg boluses (pulse doses) regularly q 60 to 90 min are most effective. Gonadorelin acetate is unlikely to cause multifetal pregnancy.

Because gonadorelin is no longer available in the US, clomiphene citrate is the first drug used to treat hypothalamic amenorrhea, followed by exogenous gonadotropins, if ovulation induction with clomiphene is unsuccessful.

1. Legro RS, Brzyski RG, Diamond MP, et al: Letrozole versus clomiphene for infertility in the polycystic ovary syndrome. *N Engl J Med* 371:119–129, 2014.

KEY POINTS

- The most common cause of ovulatory dysfunction in premenopausal women is PCOS; other causes include hypothalamic and pituitary dysfunction.
- Diagnose ovulatory dysfunction based on menstrual history, results of pelvic ultrasonography, and/or measurement of serum progesterone and urinary pregnanediol glucuronide.
- Induce ovulation for most women, usually with clomiphene citrate or letrozole.

TUBAL DYSFUNCTION AND PELVIC LESIONS

Tubal dysfunction is fallopian tube obstruction or epithelial dysfunction that impairs oocyte, zygote, and/or sperm motility; pelvic lesions are structural abnormalities that can impede fertilization or implantation.

Etiology

Tubal dysfunction can result from

- Pelvic inflammatory disease
- Use of an intrauterine device (a rare cause of pelvic infection)
- Ruptured appendix
- Lower abdominal surgery leading to pelvic adhesions
- Inflammatory disorders (eg, TB)
- Ectopic pregnancy

Pelvic lesions that can impede fertility include

- Intrauterine adhesions (Asherman syndrome)
- Fibroids obstructing the fallopian tubes or distorting the uterine cavity
- Certain malformations
- Pelvic adhesions

Endometriosis can cause tubal, uterine, or other lesions that impair fertility.

Diagnosis

- Hysterosalpingography
- Sometimes sonohysterography or laparoscopy

All infertility evaluations include assessment of the fallopian tubes.

Most often, hysterosalpingography (fluoroscopic imaging of the uterus and fallopian tubes after injection of a radiopaque agent into the uterus) is done 2 to 5 days after cessation of menstrual flow. Hysterosalpingography rarely indicates tubal patency falsely but indicates tubal obstruction falsely in about 15% of cases. This test can also detect some pelvic and intrauterine lesions. For unexplained reasons, fertility in women appears to be enhanced after hysterosalpingography if the test result is normal. Thus, if hysterosalpingography results are normal, additional diagnostic tests of tubal function can be delayed for several cycles in young women.

Intrauterine and tubal lesions can be detected or further evaluated by sonohysterography (injection of isotonic fluid through the cervix into the uterus during ultrasonography). Tubal lesions can be further evaluated with laparoscopy, and intrauterine lesions with hysteroscopy. Diagnosis and treatment are often done simultaneously during laparoscopy or hysteroscopy.

Treatment

- Laparoscopy and/or hysteroscopy
- Assisted reproductive techniques

During laparoscopy, pelvic adhesions can be lysed, or pelvic endometriosis can be fulgurated or ablated by laser. During hysteroscopy, adhesions can be lysed, and submucous fibroids and intrauterine polyps can be removed. Pregnancy rates after laparoscopic treatment of pelvic abnormalities are low (typically no more than 25%), but hysteroscopic treatment of intrauterine abnormalities is often successful, with a pregnancy rate of about 60 to 70%. Assisted reproductive techniques are often necessary for women with pelvic abnormalities and are generally preferable.

UNEXPLAINED INFERTILITY

Infertility is usually considered unexplained when semen in the man is normal and ovulation and fallopian tubes are normal and ovulation is regular in the woman.

Some experts disagree with this definition and recommend continuing to test for other causes even when the man has normal semen and the woman has normal ovulation and fallopian tubes and ovulates regularly. Other experts, who accept the definition above, recommend starting empiric treatments.

Treatment

- Controlled ovarian stimulation

Controlled ovarian stimulation (COS) can be used to make pregnancy more likely and to achieve it sooner. This procedure stimulates development of multiple follicles; the goal is to induce ovulation of > 1 oocyte (superovulation). However, COS may result in multifetal pregnancy, which has increased risks and morbidity.

COS involves the following:

- Giving clomiphene, with hCG to trigger ovulation, for up to 3 menstrual cycles
- Intrauterine insemination within 2 days of hCG administration
- If pregnancy does not result, IVF or use of gonadotropins (preparations that contain purified or recombinant FSH and variable amounts of LH), followed by intrauterine insemination

Before using assisted reproductive techniques, some clinicians use gonadotropins, followed by hCG (as for ovulatory dysfunction), then intrauterine insemination within 2 days of hCG administration.

A progestogen may be needed during the luteal phase to maximize the chance of implantation. Gonadotropin dosage depends on the patient's age and ovarian reserve.

Prognosis

The pregnancy rate is the same (about 65%) whether IVF is used immediately after unsuccessful treatment with clomiphene plus hCG or whether gonadotropins with intrauterine insemination are used next before trying IVF.

However, when IVF is done immediately after unsuccessful treatment with clomiphene plus hCG, women become pregnant more quickly and high-order multifetal pregnancies (≥ 3 fetuses) are much less likely than when gonadotropins are used first. Thus, if clomiphene plus hCG is unsuccessful, more clinicians now recommend IVF as the next treatment. Recent data indicate that women > 38 with unexplained infertility conceive more quickly and costs are lower when IVF is done before COS is tried.[1]

1. Goldman MB, Thornton KL, Ryley D, et al: A randomized clinical trial to determine optimal infertility treatment in older couples: the forty and over treatment trial (FORT-T). *Fertil Steril* 101(6):1574–1581, 2014.

ASSISTED REPRODUCTIVE TECHNIQUES

Assisted reproductive techniques (ARTs) involve manipulation of sperm and ova or embryos in vitro with the goal of producing a pregnancy.

ARTs may result in multifetal pregnancy, but risk is much less than that with COS. If risk of genetic defects is high, the embryo can often be tested for defects before transfer and implantation (preimplantation genetic testing).

In vitro fertilization (IVF): IVF can be used to treat infertility due to oligospermia, sperm antibodies, tubal dysfunction, or endometriosis as well as unexplained infertility.

The procedure typically involves the following:

- **Controlled ovarian stimulation:** Clomiphene plus gonadotropins or gonadotropins alone can be used. A GnRH agonist or antagonist is often given to prevent premature ovulation. After sufficient follicular growth, hCG is given to trigger final follicular maturation and ovulation. Alternatively, a GnRH agonist can be used to trigger ovulation in women at high risk of ovarian hyperstimulation syndrome.
- **Oocyte retrieval:** About 34 h after hCG is given, oocytes are retrieved by direct needle puncture of the follicle, usually transvaginally with ultrasound guidance or less commonly laparoscopically. At some centers, natural cycle IVF (in which a single oocyte is retrieved) is offered as an alternative; pregnancy rates with this technique are lower than those with retrieval of multiple oocytes, but costs are lower and success rates are increasing.
- **Fertilization:** The oocytes are inseminated in vitro. The semen sample is typically washed several times with tissue culture medium and is concentrated for motile sperm, which are then added to the medium containing the oocytes. At this point, intracytoplasmic sperm injection—injection of a single sperm into each oocyte—may be done, particularly if spermatogenesis is abnormal in the male partner.
- **Embryo culture:** After sperm are added, the oocytes are cultured for about 2 to 5 days.
- **Embryo transfer:** Only 1 or a few of the resulting embryos are transferred to the uterine cavity, minimizing the chance of a multifetal pregnancy, the greatest risk of IVF. The number of embryos transferred is determined by the woman's age and likelihood of response to IVF. Some or all embryos (especially if women are at high risk of ovarian hyperstimulation syndrome) may be frozen in liquid nitrogen for transfer in a subsequent cycle.

Birth defects may be slightly more common after IVF, but experts are uncertain whether the increased risk is due to IVF or to factors contributing to infertility; infertility itself increases risk of birth defects. Still, as of early 2017, the overwhelming majority of the > 6 million children born after IVF have no birth defects.

Preimplantation genetic testing can be done using cells from the polar body of an oocyte or cells from an embryo (either a blastomere from a 3-day-old embryo or trophectoderm cells from a 5- or 6-day-old embryo). Testing may involve preimplantation genetic screening to rule out aneuploidy and/or preimplantation genetic diagnosis to check for specific serious hereditary disorders. If test results are delayed, the blastocyst can be frozen and transferred in a later cycle after the results are known.

Preliminary data for 2014 indicate that in the US, the cumulative chances of taking home a live baby for each oocyte retrieval (counting all transfers of the patient's own embryos—both fresh and frozen-thawed) was 48.7% for women < 35 and 12.3% for women aged 41 to 42.

Use of donor oocytes is usually recommended for women > 42.

Gamete intrafallopian tube transfer (GIFT): GIFT is an alternative to IVF but is being used less and less frequently because success rates for IVF have increased.

GIFT is used most often when women have one of the following:

- Unexplained infertility
- Normal tubal function plus endometriosis

Multiple oocytes and sperm are obtained as for IVF but are transferred—transvaginally with ultrasound guidance or laparoscopically—to the distal fallopian tubes, where fertilization occurs.

Live birth rates per cycle are about 25 to 35%.

Intracytoplasmic sperm injection: This technique is useful when

- Other techniques are not successful or are unlikely to be so.
- A severe sperm disorder is present.

Oocytes are obtained as for IVF. A single sperm is injected into each oocyte to avoid fertilization by abnormal sperm. The embryo is then cultured and transferred as for IVF.

In 2014, over two thirds of all ART cycles in the US involved intracytoplasmic sperm injection. There is no benefit to using intracytoplasmic sperm injection in couples with low oocyte yield or advanced maternal age. If a couple's infertility involves the woman, > 30 of these procedures must be done to make one additional pregnancy likely. Thus, the additional costs and risks of intracytoplasmic sperm injection must be considered when deciding whether to use it.

Risk of birth defects may be increased after intracytoplasmic sperm injection, possibly because of the following:

- The procedure itself can damage the sperm, egg, or embryo.
- Sperm from men who have mutations of the Y chromosome are used. Most reported birth defects involve the male reproductive tract.

Other techniques: Other techniques are sometimes used. They include the following:

- A combination of IVF and GIFT
- Zygote intrafallopian tube transfer
- Use of donor oocytes
- Transfer of frozen embryos to a surrogate mother

Some of these techniques raise moral and ethical issues (eg, rightful parentage in surrogate motherhood, selective reduction of the number of implanted embryos if multifetal pregnancy results).The use of IVF in postmenopausal women > 50 yr is controversial.

272 Menopause

Menopause is physiologic or iatrogenic cessation of menses (amenorrhea) due to decreased ovarian function. Manifestations may include hot flushes and vulvovaginal atrophy. Diagnosis is clinical: absence of menses for 1 yr. Manifestations may be treated (eg, with lifestyle modification, complementary and alternative medicine, and/or hormone therapy).

In the US, average age of physiologic menopause is 52. Factors such as smoking, living at high altitude, and undernutrition may lower the age.

Perimenopause refers to the several years (duration varies greatly) before and the 1 yr after the last menses. It is typically the most symptomatic phase.

The **menopausal transition** (the years in perimenopause that lead up to the last menses) is characterized by changes in the menstrual pattern.

Physiology

As ovaries age, their response to the pituitary gonadotropins follicle-stimulating hormone (FSH) and luteinizing hormone (LH) decreases, initially causing a shorter follicular phase (with shorter and less regular menstrual cycles), fewer ovulations, and decreased progesterone production (see Fig. 269–5 on p. 2250). Double ovulation and luteal out-of-phase (LOOP) events (ie, premature formation of a follicle due to the major surge in FSH during the luteal phase) occur and occasionally cause estradiol levels to be above normal. The number of viable follicles decreases; eventually, the few remaining follicles do not respond, and the ovaries produce very little estradiol. Estrogens are also produced by peripheral tissues (eg, fat, skin) from androgens (eg, androstenedione, testosterone). However, the total estrogen level is much lower, and estrone replaces estradiol as the most common estrogen.

Around menopause, androstenedione levels decrease by half. The decrease in testosterone, which begins in young adulthood, does not accelerate during menopause because the stroma of the postmenopausal ovary and adrenal gland continue to secrete substantial amounts.

Decreased levels of ovarian inhibin and estrogen, which inhibit pituitary release of LH and FSH, result in a substantial increase in circulating LH and FSH levels.

Rapid bone loss occurs during the first 2 yr after estrogen begins to decrease. After this period of rapid bone loss, the age-related rate of bone loss in women is similar to that in men.

Premature ovarian failure (primary ovarian insufficiency) is cessation of menses due to noniatrogenic ovarian failure before age 40. Contributory factors are thought to be primarily genetic.

Symptoms and Signs

Changes in the menstrual cycle usually begin during a woman's 40s, with variation in cycle length. A persistent difference in consecutive menstrual cycle length of ≥ 7 days defines early menopausal transition. Skipping ≥ 2 cycles defines late menopausal transition.

The marked fluctuations in estrogen levels may contribute to other perimenopausal symptoms and signs such as

- Breast tenderness
- Changes in menstrual flow
- Moodiness
- Exacerbation of menstrual migraines

Symptoms can last from 6 mo to > 10 yr and range from nonexistent to severe.

Vasomotor: Hot flushes (hot flashes, night sweats) due to vasomotor instability affect 75 to 85% of women and usually begin before menses stop. Hot flushes continue for

- > 1 yr in most women
- > 4 yr in 50%
- > 12 yr in 10%

Women feel warm or hot and may perspire, sometimes profusely; core temperature increases. The skin, especially of the face, head, and neck, may become red and warm. The episodic flush, which may last from 30 sec to 5 min, may be followed by chills. Flushes may manifest during the night as night sweats.

The mechanism of hot flushes is unknown, but they are thought to result from changes in the thermoregulatory center located in the hypothalamus. The range of core body temperatures that is comfortable to the woman decreases; as a result, a very small increase in core body temperature can trigger heat release as a hot flush.

Vaginal: These symptoms include dryness, dyspareunia, and occasionally irritation and itching. As estrogen production decreases, vulvar and vaginal mucosae become thinner, drier, more friable, and less elastic, and vaginal rugae are lost.

Genitourinary syndrome of menopause includes vaginal symptoms as well as symptoms related to the urethra and bladder, including urinary urgency, dysuria, and frequent UTIs.

Neuropsychiatric: Neuropsychiatric changes (eg, poor concentration, memory loss, depressive symptoms, anxiety) may transiently accompany menopause.

Recurrent night sweats can contribute to insomnia, fatigue, irritability, and poor concentration by disrupting sleep.

Other symptoms: Menopause is a normal, healthy phase in a woman's life, but each woman has a unique experience.

Quality of life may decrease if symptoms are severe or if less common symptoms of menopause, such as joint aches and pains, develop. For some women (eg, those with a history of endometriosis, dysmenorrhea, menorrhagia, premenstrual syndrome, or menstrual migraine), quality of life improves after menopause.

Diagnosis

- Clinical evaluation
- Rarely FSH levels

Diagnosis is clinical. Perimenopause is likely if the woman is in the appropriate age range and has some of the symptoms and signs of perimenopause. However, pregnancy should be considered. Menopause is confirmed when a woman has had no menses for 12 mo.

Pelvic examination is done; the presence of vulvovaginal atrophy supports the diagnosis. Any abnormal findings are evaluated (see p. 2201).

FSH levels may be measured, but this test is rarely necessary except perhaps in women who have had a hysterectomy and in women who are younger than the usual age of menopause. Consistently elevated levels confirm menopause.

Postmenopausal women who have a high risk of fracture (eg, based on the Fracture Risk Assessment Tool—FRAX) and all women > 65 should be screened for osteoporosis.

Treatment

- Lifestyle modification
- Complementary and alternative medicine
- Hormone therapy
- Other neuroactive drugs

Treatment is symptomatic (eg, to relieve hot flushes and symptoms due to vulvovaginal atrophy).

Hormone therapy (estrogen, a progestin, or both) is the most effective treatment for menopausal symptoms.

Discussing the physiologic causes of menopause and possible symptoms and signs with women helps them manage the changes that occur.

Lifestyle modification: For hot flushes, the following may help:

- Avoiding triggers (eg, bright lights, comforters, predictable emotional reactions)
- Cooling the environment (eg, lowering the thermostat, using fans)
- Wearing clothing in layers that can be removed as needed may help

OTC vaginal lubricants and moisturizers help relieve vaginal dryness. Regular sexual intercourse or other vaginal stimulation helps preserve vaginal function.

Complementary and alternative medicine: Black cohosh, other herbal preparations, and OTC products do not appear helpful. Soy protein has been studied with mixed results; however, one soy product, S-equol, has been reported to relieve hot flushes.

Dehydroepiandrosterone (DHEA) may relieve vaginal dryness and other symptoms of vaginal atrophy; it is under study as treatment for these symptoms.

Use of regular exercise, paced respirations (a type of slow, deep breathing), or relaxation techniques to reduce hot flushes has had mixed results, although exercise and relaxation techniques may improve sleep. Acupuncture has also had mixed results. In one study, hypnosis appeared to relieve hot flushes and may be recommended to women who want to try it.

Neuroactive drugs: In well-designed, randomized, controlled trials, selective serotonin reuptake inhibitors (SSRIs), serotonin-norepinephrine reuptake inhibitors (SNRIs), and gabapentin have been shown to be moderately effective in reducing hot flushes. A low dose of paroxetine can be used specifically for hot flushes. However, all of these drugs are less effective than hormone therapy.

Hormone Therapy

Hormone therapy (estrogen, a progestin, or both) is the most effective treatment for menopausal symptoms. It is used to relieve moderate to severe hot flushes and, when an estrogen is included, to relieve symptoms due to vulvovaginal atrophy.

Hormone therapy improves quality of life for many women by relieving their symptoms but does not improve quality of life for asymptomatic women and is thus not routinely given to postmenopausal women. If hormone therapy is needed to control menopausal symptoms, the lowest dose should be used for the shortest time period required. Also, hormone therapy is not recommended for prevention or treatment of chronic disorders (eg, coronary artery disease, dementia, osteoporosis).

Choice of hormonal therapy: For women who have had a hysterectomy, estrogen is used alone. Oral, transdermal (patch, lotion, spray, or gel), or vaginal forms may be used. Treatment should start with the lowest dose; the dose is increased every 2 to 4 wk as needed. Doses vary by preparation. Low doses include

- 0.3 mg po once/day (conjugated equine or synthetic estrogens)
- 0.5 mg po once/day (oral estradiol)
- 0.025 mg once/day (estradiol patch)

Women who have a uterus should be given a progestin in addition to estrogen because unopposed estrogen increases risk of endometrial cancer. The progestin is taken with estrogen continuously (ie, daily) or sequentially (12 to 14 consecutive days of every 4 wk). The dose is

- Medroxyprogesterone acetate: 2.5 mg for daily use and 5 mg for sequential use
- Micronized progesterone (a natural rather than synthetic progesterone): 100 mg for daily use and 200 mg for sequential use

Bleeding due to progestin withdrawal is less likely with continuous therapy. Combination products of estrogen and a progestin are available as pills (eg, 0.3 mg of conjugated equine estrogens plus 1.5 mg of medroxyprogesterone acetate once/day) or patches (eg, 0.045 mg of estradiol plus 0.015 mg of levonorgestrel once/day).

When the only symptoms are vaginal, low-dose vaginal estrogen therapy is preferred. Topical forms (eg, creams, vaginal tablets or rings) may be more effective for vaginal symptoms than oral forms. Vaginal tablets and rings that contain estradiol in low doses (eg, 10 mcg for tablets, 7.5 mcg for rings) deliver less estrogen to the systemic circulation. Vaginal estrogen should be used at the lowest recommended doses because higher doses can deliver as much estrogen as oral or transdermal therapy and, if given to women who still have a uterus, require the addition of a progestin.

Progestins (eg, medroxyprogesterone acetate 10 mg po once/day or depot 150 mg IM once/mo, megestrol acetate 10 to 20 mg po once/day) are sometimes used alone to relieve hot flushes when estrogen is contraindicated, but they are not as effective as estrogen for hot flushes and do not relieve vaginal dryness. Micronized progesterone can be taken in doses of 100 to 200 mg at bedtime. Drowsiness may occur. Micronized progesterone is contraindicated in women who are allergic to peanuts.

Estrogen therapy has beneficial effects on bone density and reduces the incidence of fractures in postmenopausal women (not particularly those with osteoporosis). Nonetheless, estrogen therapy (with or without a progestin) is not recommended as first-line treatment or as prophylaxis for osteoporosis. When osteoporosis is the only concern, clinicians should consider hormone therapy only if women who are at significant risk of osteoporosis cannot take first-line drugs for osteoporosis (see p. 326).

Risks and adverse effects: Risks with estrogen therapy or combined estrogen/progestin therapy include

- Endometrial cancer, mainly if women who have a uterus take estrogen without a progestin
- Deep vein thrombosis
- Pulmonary embolism
- Stroke
- Breast cancer
- Gallbladder disease
- Stress urinary incontinence

The risk of breast cancer begins to increase after 3 to 5 yr of combination therapy. When estrogenis used alone, risk of breast cancer may not increase until after 10 to 15 yr of use. Incidence of gallbladder disease and urinary incontinence may be increased. Risk of all these disorders is low in healthy women who take hormone therapy temporarily, during or shortly after perimenopause. Older postmenopausal women (> 10 yr past menopause) are at higher risk of most of these disorders and may be at risk of coronary artery disease when given combination therapy. The risk of venous thromboembolism may be lower when transdermal estrogen is used.

Estrogen therapy may be contraindicated in women who have had or are at high risk of breast cancer, stroke, coronary artery disease, or thrombosis.

Progestins may have adverse effects (eg, abdominal bloating, breast tenderness, increased breast density, headache, increased low-density lipoprotein, decreased high-density lipoprotein); micronized progesterone appears to have fewer adverse effects. Progestins may increase the risk of thrombosis. There are no long-term safety data for progestins.

Before prescribing hormone therapy, clinicians should discuss its risks and benefits with women.

Selective estrogen receptor modulators (SERMS): The SERMs tamoxifen and raloxifene have been used primarily for their antiestrogenic properties and not to relieve menopausal symptoms. However, ospemifene, a SERM, can be used to treat dyspareunia due to vaginal atrophy if women cannot use estrogen or a vaginal drug (eg, if they have severe arthritis) or if they prefer to use an oral drug other than estrogen; dose is 60 mg po once/day.

Bazedoxifene given with conjugated estrogens can relieve hot flushes and vaginal atrophy. Risk of venous thromboembolism is similar to that of estrogen, but the drug appears to protect the endometrium and potentially the breast. Bazedoxifene as a single drug is not yet available in the US.

KEY POINTS

- In the US, menopause occurs at an average age of 52.
- Symptoms of menopause tend to be maximal during the few years before and the year after menopause (during perimenopause), except for symptomatic vulvovaginal atrophy, which may worsen over time.
- Consider menopause confirmed if a woman who is an appropriate age and who is not pregnant has not had menses for 12 mo.
- For vaginal dryness, recommend vaginal stimulation and OTC vaginal lubricants and moisturizers, and if they are ineffective, prescribe low-dose vaginal estrogen creams, tablets, or rings.
- Before prescribing hormone therapy, talk to women about the risks (eg, deep vein thrombosis, pulmonary embolism, stroke, breast cancer; low risk of gallbladder disease and stress urinary incontinence).
- If women choose hormone therapy to relieve hot flushes, prescribe estrogen plus, for women with a uterus, a progestin.
- Consider SSRIs, SNRIs, and gabapentin as less effective alternatives to hormone therapy for relieving hot flushes.

273 Menstrual Abnormalities

(For a description of the menstrual cycle, see p. 2249.)

Menstrual abnormalities include

- Amenorrhea
- Dysfunctional uterine bleeding
- Dysmenorrhea
- Premenstrual syndrome

Irregular or absent menses and nonmenstrual vaginal bleeding have many causes, but in women of reproductive age, pregnancy should always be suspected.

Abnormal vaginal bleeding in nonpregnant women is evaluated differently from vaginal bleeding in pregnant women (see pp. 2326 and 2332).

Polycystic ovary syndrome can cause some of the same symptoms as menstrual abnormalities.

Pelvic congestion syndrome, a common cause of chronic pelvic pain, is often accompanied by abnormal menstrual bleeding.

AMENORRHEA

Amenorrhea (the absence of menstruation) can be primary or secondary.

Primary amenorrhea is failure of menses to occur by one of the following:

- Age 16 or 2 yr after the onset of puberty
- About age 14 in girls who have not gone through puberty (eg, growth spurt, development of secondary sexual characteristics)

If patients have had no menstrual periods by age 13 and have no signs of puberty (eg, any type of breast development), they should be evaluated for primary amenorrhea.

Secondary amenorrhea is cessation of menses after they have begun. Usually, patients should be evaluated for secondary amenorrhea if menses have been absent for ≥ 3 mo or ≥ 3 typical cycles because from menarche until perimenopause, a menstrual cycle lasting > 90 days is unusual.

Pathophysiology

Normally, the hypothalamus generates pulses of gonadotropin-releasing hormone (GnRH). GnRH stimulates the pituitary to produce gonadotropins (follicle-stimulating hormone [FSH] and luteinizing hormone [LH]—see p. 2249), which are released into the bloodstream. Gonadotropins stimulate the ovaries to produce estrogen (mainly estradiol), androgens (mainly testosterone), and progesterone. These hormones do the following:

- **FSH** stimulates tissues around the developing oocytes to convert testosterone to estradiol.
- Estrogen stimulates the endometrium, causing it to proliferate.
- **LH**, when it surges during the menstrual cycle, promotes maturation of the dominant oocyte, release of the oocyte, and formation of the corpus luteum, which produces progesterone.
- **Progesterone** changes the endometrium into a secretory structure and prepares it for egg implantation (endometrial decidualization).

If pregnancy does not occur, estrogen and progesterone production decreases, and the endometrium breaks down and is sloughed during menses. Menstruation occurs 14 days after ovulation in typical cycles.

When part of this system malfunctions, ovulatory dysfunction occurs; the cycle of gonadotropin-stimulated estrogen production and cyclic endometrial changes is disrupted, resulting in anovulatory amenorrhea, and menstrual flow may not occur. Most amenorrhea, particularly secondary amenorrhea, is anovulatory.

However, amenorrhea can occur when ovulation is normal, as occurs when genital anatomic abnormalities (eg, congenital anomalies causing outflow obstruction, intrauterine adhesions [Asherman syndrome]) prevent normal menstrual flow despite normal hormonal stimulation.

Etiology

Amenorrhea is usually classified as

- Anovulatory (see Table 273–1)
- Ovulatory (see Table 273–2)

Each type has many causes, but overall, the most common causes of amenorrhea include

- Pregnancy (the most common cause in women of reproductive age)
- Constitutional delay of puberty
- Functional hypothalamic anovulation (eg, due to excessive exercise, eating disorders, or stress)
- Use or abuse of drugs (eg, oral contraceptives, depoprogesterone, antidepressants, antipsychotics)
- Breastfeeding
- Polycystic ovary syndrome

Contraceptives can cause the endometrium to thin, sometimes resulting in amenorrhea; menses usually begin again about 3 mo after stopping oral contraceptives.

Antidepressants and antipsychotics can elevate prolactin, which stimulates the breasts to produce milk and can cause amenorrhea.

Some disorders can cause ovulatory or anovulatory amenorrhea. Congenital anatomic abnormalities cause only primary amenorrhea. All disorders that cause secondary amenorrhea can cause primary amenorrhea.

Anovulatory amenorrhea: The **most common causes** (see Table 273–1) involve a disruption of the hypothalamic-pituitary-ovarian axis. Thus, causes include

- Hypothalamic dysfunction (particularly functional hypothalamic anovulation)
- Pituitary dysfunction
- Primary ovarian insufficiency (premature ovarian failure)
- Endocrine disorders that cause androgen excess (particularly polycystic ovary syndrome)

Anovulatory amenorrhea is usually secondary but may be primary if ovulation never begins—eg, because of a genetic disorder. If ovulation never begins, puberty and development of secondary sexual characteristics are abnormal. Genetic disorders that confer a Y chromosome increase the risk of ovarian germ cell cancer.

Ovulatory amenorrhea: The **most common causes** (see Table 273–2) include

- Chromosomal abnormalities
- Congenital anatomic genital abnormalities that obstruct menstrual flow

Obstructive abnormalities are usually accompanied by normal hormonal function. Such obstruction may result in hematocolpos (accumulation of menstrual blood in the vagina), which can cause the vagina to bulge, or in hematometra (accumulation of blood in the uterus), which can cause uterine distention, a mass, or bulging of the cervix. Because ovarian function is normal, external genital organs and other secondary sexual characteristics develop normally. Some congenital disorders (eg, those accompanied by vaginal aplasia or a vaginal septum) also cause urinary tract and skeletal abnormalities.

Some acquired anatomic abnormalities, such as endometrial scarring after instrumentation for postpartum hemorrhage or infection (Asherman syndrome), cause secondary ovulatory amenorrhea.

Evaluation

Girls are evaluated if

- They have no signs of puberty (eg, breast development, growth spurt) by age 13.
- Pubic hair is absent at age 14.
- Menarche has not occurred by age 16 or by 2 yr after the onset of puberty (development of secondary sexual characteristics).

Women of reproductive age should have a pregnancy test after missing one menses. They are evaluated for amenorrhea if

- They are not pregnant and have missed menstrual cycles for ≥ 3 mo or ≥ 3 typical cycles.
- They have < 9 menses a year.
- They have a sudden change in menstrual pattern.

History: History of present illness includes the following:

- Whether menses have ever occurred (to distinguish primary from secondary amenorrhea) and, if so, how old patients were at menarche

Table 273–1. SOME CAUSES OF ANOVULATORY AMENORRHEA

CAUSE	EXAMPLES
Hypothalamic dysfunction, structural	Genetic disorders (eg, congenital gonadotropin-releasing hormone deficiency, GnRH receptor gene mutations that result in low FSH and estradiol levels and a high LH level, Prader-Willi syndrome) Infiltrative disorders of the hypothalamus (eg, Langerhans cell granulomatosis, lymphoma, sarcoidosis, TB) Irradiation to the hypothalamus Traumatic brain injury Tumors of the hypothalamus
Hypothalamic dysfunction, functional	Cachexia Chronic disorders, particularly respiratory, GI, hematologic, renal, or hepatic (eg, Crohn disease, cystic fibrosis, sickle cell disease, thalassemia major) Dieting Drug abuse (eg, of alcohol, cocaine, marijuana, or opioids) Eating disorders (eg, anorexia nervosa, bulimia) Exercise, if excessive HIV infection Immunodeficiency Psychiatric disorders (eg, stress, depression, obsessive-compulsive disorder, schizophrenia) Psychoactive drugs Undernutrition
Pituitary dysfunction	Aneurysms of the pituitary Hyperprolactinemia* Idiopathic hypogonadotropic hypogonadism Infiltrative disorders of the pituitary (eg, hemochromatosis, Langerhans cell granulomatosis, sarcoidosis, TB) Isolated gonadotropin deficiency Kallmann syndrome (hypogonadotropic hypogonadism with anosmia) Postpartum pituitary necrosis (Sheehan syndrome) Traumatic brain injury Tumors of the brain (eg, meningioma, craniopharyngioma, gliomas) Tumors of the pituitary (eg, microadenoma)
Ovarian dysfunction	Autoimmune disorders (eg, autoimmune oophoritis as may occur in myasthenia gravis, thyroiditis, or vitiligo) Chemotherapy (eg, high-dose alkylating drugs) Genetic abnormalities, including chromosomal abnormalities (eg, congenital thymic aplasia, Fragile X syndrome, Turner syndrome [45,X], idiopathic accelerated ovarian follicular atresia) Gonadal dysgenesis (incomplete ovarian development, sometimes secondary to genetic disorders) Irradiation to the pelvis Metabolic disorders (eg, Addison disease, diabetes mellitus, galactosemia) Viral infections (eg, mumps)
Other endocrine dysfunction	Androgen insensitivity syndrome (testicular feminization) Congenital adrenal virilism (congenital adrenal hyperplasia—eg, due to 17-hydroxylase deficiency or 17,20-lyase deficiency) or adult-onset adrenal virilism† Cushing syndrome†,‡ Drug-induced virilization (eg, by androgens, antidepressants, danazol, or high-dose progestins)† Hyperthyroidism Hypothyroidism Obesity (which causes excess extraglandular production of estrogen) Polycystic ovary syndrome† True hermaphroditism† Tumors producing androgens (usually ovarian or adrenal)† Tumors producing estrogens or tumors producing human chorionic gonadotropin (gestational trophoblastic disease)

*Hyperprolactinemia due to other conditions (eg, hypothyroidism, use of certain drugs) may also cause amenorrhea.
†Females with these disorders may have virilization or ambiguous genitals.
‡Virilization may occur in Cushing syndrome secondary to an adrenal tumor.

- Whether periods have ever been regular
- When the last normal menstrual period occurred
- How long and heavy menses is
- Whether patients have cyclic breast tenderness and mood changes
- When they reached certain growth and development milestones, including age at thelarche (development of breasts at puberty)

Review of systems should cover symptoms suggesting possible causes, including the following:

- Galactorrhea, headaches, and visual field defects: Pituitary disorders
- Fatigue, weight gain, and cold intolerance: Hypothyroidism
- Palpitations, nervousness, tremor, and heat intolerance: Hyperthyroidism

Table 273–2. SOME CAUSES OF OVULATORY AMENORRHEA

CAUSE	EXAMPLES
Congenital genital abnormalities	Cervical stenosis (rare) Imperforate hymen Pseudohermaphroditism Transverse vaginal septum Vaginal or uterine aplasia (eg, Müllerian agenesis)
Acquired uterine abnormalities	Asherman syndrome Endometrial TB Obstructive fibroids and polyps

- Acne, hirsutism, and deepening of the voice: Androgen excess
- For patients with secondary amenorrhea, hot flushes, vaginal dryness, sleep disturbance, fragility fractures, and decreased libido: Estrogen deficiency

Patients with primary amenorrhea are asked about symptoms of puberty (eg, breast development, growth spurt, presence of axillary and pubic hair) to help determine whether ovulation has occurred.

Past medical history should note risk factors for the following:

- Functional hypothalamic anovulation, such as stress; chronic illness; new drugs; and a recent change in weight, diet, or exercise intensity
- In patients with secondary amenorrhea, Asherman syndrome (eg, D & C, endometrial ablation, endometritis, obstetric injury, uterine surgery)

Drug history should include specific questions about use of drugs, such as the following:

- Drugs that affect dopamine (eg, antihypertensives, antipsychotics, opioids, tricyclic antidepressants)
- Cancer chemotherapy drugs (eg, busulfan, chlorambucil, cyclophosphamide)
- Sex hormones that can cause virilization (eg, androgens, estrogens, high-dose progestins, OTC anabolic steroids)
- Contraceptives, particularly recent use
- Systemic corticosteroids
- OTC products and supplements, some of which contain bovine hormones or interact with other drugs

Family history should include height of family members and any cases of delayed puberty or genetic disorders in family members, including Fragile X syndrome.

Physical examination: Clinicians should note vital signs and body composition and build, including height and weight, and should calculate body mass index (BMI). Secondary sexual characteristics are evaluated; breast and pubic hair development are staged using Tanner method. If axillary and pubic hair is present, adrenarche has occurred.

With the patient seated, clinicians should check for breast secretion by applying pressure to all sections of the breast, beginning at the base and moving toward the nipple. Galactorrhea (breast milk secretion not temporally associated with childbirth) may be observed; it can be distinguished from other types of nipple discharge by finding fat globules in the fluid using a low-power microscope.

Pelvic examination is done to detect anatomic genital abnormalities; a bulging hymen may be caused by hematocolpos, which suggests genital outflow obstruction. Pelvic examination findings also help determine whether estrogen has been deficient. In postpubertal females, thin, pale vaginal mucosa without rugae and pH > 6.0 indicate estrogen deficiency. The presence of cervical mucus with spinnbarkeit (a stringy, stretchy quality) usually indicates adequate estrogen.

General examination focuses on evidence of virilization, including hirsutism, temporal balding, acne, voice deepening, increased muscle mass, clitoromegaly (clitoral enlargement), and defeminization (a decrease in previously normal secondary sexual characteristics, such as decreased breast size and vaginal atrophy). Hypertrichosis (excessive growth of hair on the extremities, head, and back), which is common in some families, is differentiated from true hirsutism, which is characterized by excess hair on the upper lip and chin and between the breasts. Skin discoloration (eg, yellow due to jaundice or carotenemia, black patches due to acanthosis nigricans) should be noted.

Red flags: The following findings are of particular concern:

- Delayed puberty
- Virilization
- Visual field defects
- Impaired sense of smell

Interpretation of findings: Pregnancy should not be excluded based on history; a pregnancy test is required.

PEARLS & PITFALLS

- If amenorrhea occurs in girls with secondary sexual characteristics or in women of reproductive age, do a pregnancy test regardless of sexual and menstrual history.

In **primary amenorrhea,** the presence of normal secondary sexual characteristics usually reflects normal hormonal function; amenorrhea is usually ovulatory and typically due to a congenital anatomic genital tract obstruction. Primary amenorrhea accompanied by abnormal secondary sexual characteristics is usually anovulatory (eg, due to a genetic disorder).

In **secondary amenorrhea,** clinical findings sometimes suggest a mechanism (see Table 273–3):

- Galactorrhea suggests hyperprolactinemia (eg, pituitary dysfunction, use of certain drugs); if visual field defects and headaches are also present, pituitary tumors should be considered.
- Symptoms and signs of estrogen deficiency (eg, hot flushes, night sweats, vaginal dryness or atrophy) suggest primary ovarian insufficiency (premature ovarian failure) or functional hypothalamic anovulation (eg, due to excessive exercise, a low body weight, or low body fat)
- Virilization suggests androgen excess (eg, polycystic ovary syndrome, androgen-secreting tumor, Cushing syndrome, use of certain drugs). If patients have a high BMI, acanthosis nigricans, or both, polycystic ovary syndrome is likely.

Testing: History and physical examination help direct testing. If girls have secondary sexual characteristics, a pregnancy test should be done to exclude pregnancy and gestational trophoblastic disease as a cause of amenorrhea. Women of reproductive age should have a pregnancy test after missing one menses.

The approach to primary amenorrhea (see Fig. 273–1) differs from that to secondary amenorrhea (see Fig. 273–2), although no specific general approaches or algorithms are universally accepted.

If patients have primary amenorrhea and normal secondary sexual characteristics, testing should begin with pelvic ultrasonography to check for congenital anatomic genital tract obstruction.

Table 273–3. FINDINGS SUGGESTING POSSIBLE CAUSES OF AMENORRHEA

FINDING	OTHER POSSIBLE FINDINGS	POSSIBLE CAUSE
Use of certain drugs		
Drugs that affect dopamine (which helps regulate prolactin secretion): • Antihypertensives (eg, methyldopa, reserpine, verapamil) • Antipsychotics, 2nd generation (eg, molindone, olanzapine, risperidone) • Antipsychotics, conventional (eg, haloperidol, phenothiazines, pimozide) • Cocaine • Estrogens • GI drugs (eg, cimetidine, metoclopramide) • Hallucinogens • Opioids (eg, codeine, morphine) • Tricyclic antidepressants (eg, clomipramine, desipramine)s	Galactorrhea	Hyperprolactinemia
Hormones and certain other drugs that affect the balance of estrogenic and androgenic effects (eg, androgens, antidepressants, danazol, high-dose progestins)	Virilization	Drug-induced virilization
Body habitus		
High body mass index (eg, > 30 kg/m²)	—	Estrogen excess
	Virilization	Polycystic ovary syndrome
Low body mass index (eg, < 18.5 kg/m²)	Risk factors such as a chronic disorder, dieting, or an eating disorder	Functional hypothalamic anovulation
	Hypothermia, bradycardia, hypotension	Functional hypothalamic anovulation due to anorexia nervosa or starvation
	Reduced gag reflex, palatal lesions, subconjunctival hemorrhages	Functional hypothalamic anovulation due to bulimia with frequent vomiting
Short stature	Primary amenorrhea, webbed neck, widely spaced nipples	Turner syndrome
Skin abnormalities		
Warm, moist skin	Tachycardia, tremor	Hyperthyroidism
Coarse, thick skin; loss of eyebrow hair	Bradycardia, delayed deep tendon reflexes, weight gain, constipation	Hypothyroidism
Acne	Virilization	Androgen excess due to • Polycystic ovary syndrome • An androgen-secreting tumor • Cushing syndrome • Adrenal virilism • Drugs (eg, androgens, antidepressants, danazol, high-dose progestins)
Striae	Moon facies, buffalo hump, truncal obesity, thin extremities, virilization, hypertension	Cushing syndrome
Acanthosis nigricans	Obesity, virilization	Polycystic ovary syndrome
Vitiligo or hyperpigmentation of the palm	Orthostatic hypotension	Addison disease
General findings suggesting estrogenic or androgenic abnormalities		
Symptoms of estrogen deficiency (eg, hot flushes, night sweats, particularly with vaginal dryness or atrophy)	Risk factors such as oophorectomy, chemotherapy, or pelvic irradiation	Primary ovarian insufficiency Functional hypothalamic anovulation Pituitary tumors

Table continues on the following page.

Table 273–3. FINDINGS SUGGESTING POSSIBLE CAUSES OF AMENORRHEA (*Continued*)

FINDING	OTHER POSSIBLE FINDINGS	POSSIBLE CAUSE
Hirsutism with virilization	—	Androgen excess due to • Polycystic ovary syndrome • An androgen-secreting tumor • Cushing syndrome • Adrenal virilism • Drugs (eg, androgens, antidepressants, danazol, high-dose progestins)
	Primary amenorrhea	Androgen excess due to • True hermaphroditism • Pseudohermaphroditism • An androgen-secreting tumor • Adrenal virilism • Gonadal dysgenesis • A genetic disorder
	Enlarged ovaries	Androgen excess due to • 17-Hydroxylase deficiency • Polycystic ovary syndrome • An androgen-secreting ovarian tumor
Breast and genital abnormalities		
Galactorrhea	—	Hyperprolactinemia
	Nocturnal headache, visual field defects	Pituitary tumor
Absence or incomplete development of breasts (and of secondary sexual characteristics)	Normal adrenarche	Primary anovulatory amenorrhea due to isolated ovarian failure
	Absence of adrenarche	Primary anovulatory amenorrhea due to hypothalamic-pituitary dysfunction
	Absence of adrenarche with impaired sense of smell	Kallmann syndrome
Delay of breast development and secondary sexual characteristics	Family history of delayed menarche	Constitutional delay of growth and puberty
Normal breast development and secondary sexual characteristics with primary amenorrhea	Cyclic abdominal pain, bulging vagina, uterine distention	Genital outflow obstruction
Ambiguous genitals	—	True hermaphroditism Pseudohermaphroditism Virilization
Fused labia, clitoral enlargement at birth	—	Androgen exposure during the 1st trimester, possibly indicating • Congenital adrenal virilism • True hermaphroditism • Drug-induced virilization
Clitoral enlargement after birth	Virilization	Androgen-secreting tumor (usually ovarian) Adrenal virilism Use of anabolic steroids
Normal external genitals with incompletely developed secondary sexual characteristics (sometimes with breast development but minimal pubic hair)	Apparent absence of cervix and uterus	Androgen insensitivity syndrome
Ovarian enlargement (bilateral)	Symptoms of estrogen deficiency	Primary ovarian insufficiency due to autoimmune oophoritis
	Virilization	17-Hydroxylase deficiency Polycystic ovary syndrome
Lesions		
Pelvic mass (unilateral)	Pelvic pain	Pelvic tumors

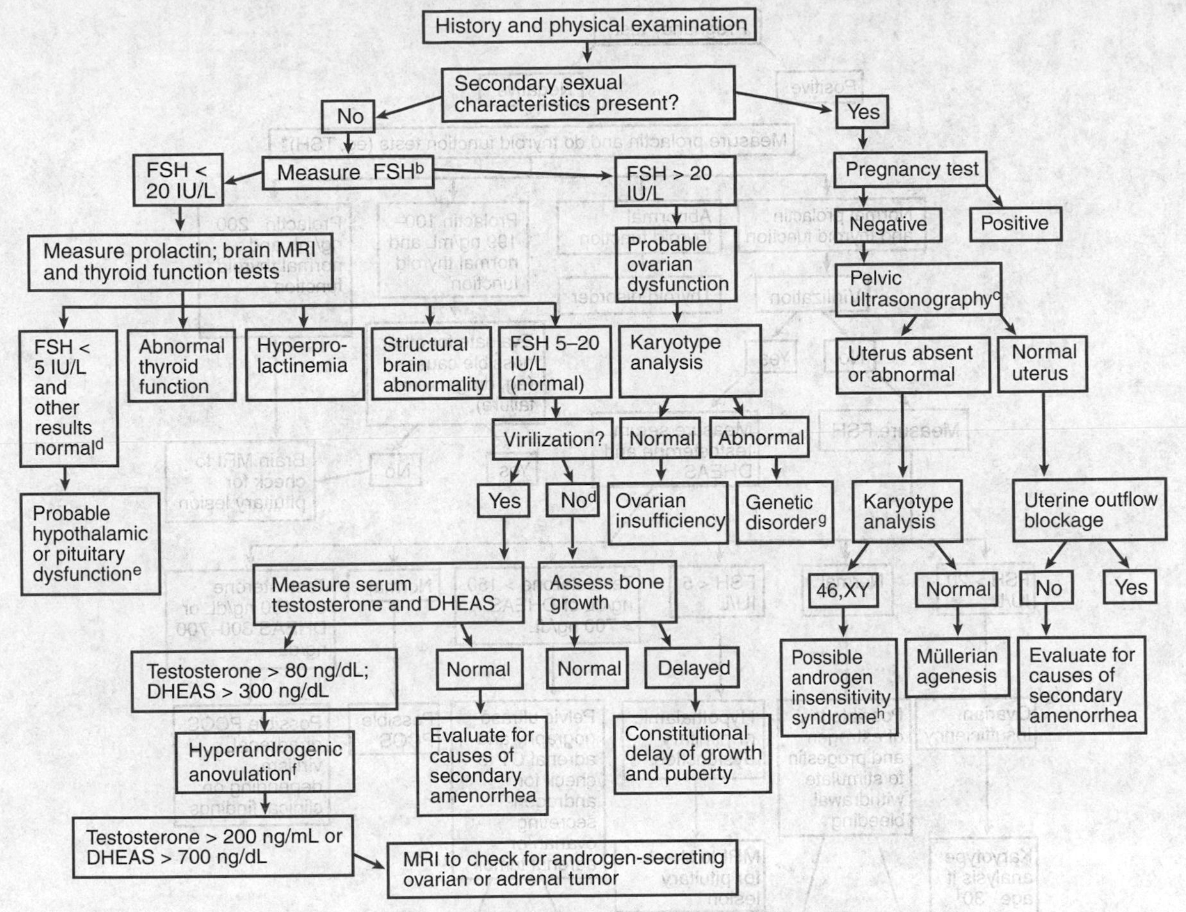

Fig. 273–1. Evaluation of primary amenorrhea[a].

[a]Normal values are

- DHEAS: 250–300 ng/dL (0.7–0.8 μmol/L)
- FSH: 5–20 IU/L
- LH: 5–40 IU/L
- Karyotype (female): 46,XX
- Prolactin: 100 ng/mL
- Testosterone: 20–80 ng/dL (0.7–2.8 nmol/L)

[b]Some clinicians measure LH levels when they measure FSH levels or when FSH levels are equivocal.

[c]If patients have primary amenorrhea and normal secondary sexual characteristics, testing should begin with pelvic ultrasonography to check for congenital anatomic genital tract obstruction.

[d]Constitutional delay of growth and puberty is possible.

[e]Possible diagnoses include functional hypothalamic chronic anovulation and genetic disorders (eg, congenital gonadotropin-releasing hormone deficiency, Prader-Willi syndrome).

[f]Possible diagnoses include Cushing syndrome, exogenous androgens, congenital adrenal virilism, and polycystic ovary syndrome.

[g]Possible diagnoses include Turner syndrome and disorders characterized by Y chromosome material.

[h]Public hair may be sparse.

DHEAS = dehydroepiandrosterone sulfate; FSH = follicle-stimulating hormone; LH = luteinizing hormone; TSH = thyroid-stimulating hormone.

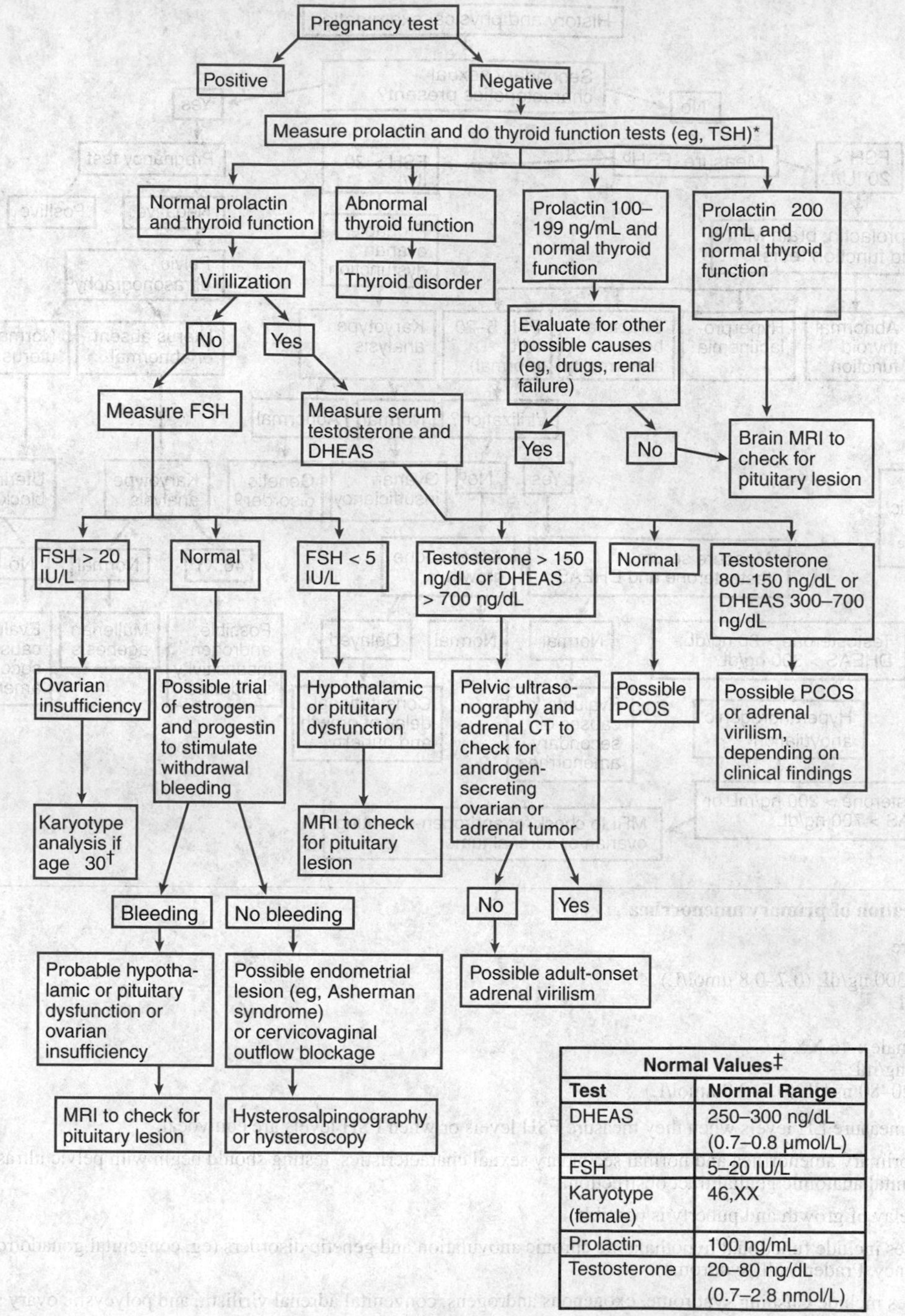

Normal Values‡

Test	Normal Range
DHEAS	250–300 ng/dL (0.7–0.8 μmol/L)
FSH	5–20 IU/L
Karyotype (female)	46,XX
Prolactin	100 ng/mL
Testosterone	20–80 ng/dL (0.7–2.8 nmol/L)

Fig. 273–2. Evaluation of secondary amenorrhea.

*Some clinicians simultaneously measure FSH and LH levels.

†Clinicians should check for the presence of Y chromosome and Fragile X syndrome.

‡Although these values are representative, normal ranges may vary between laboratories.

DHEAS = dehydroepiandrosterone sulfate; FSH = follicle-stimulating hormone; LH = luteinizing hormone; PCOS = polycystic ovary syndrome; TSH = thyroid-stimulating hormone.

If symptoms or signs suggest a specific disorder, specific tests may be indicated regardless of what an algorithm recommends. For example, patients with abdominal striae, moon facies, a buffalo hump, truncal obesity, and thin extremities should be tested for Cushing syndrome. Patients with headaches and visual field defects or evidence of pituitary dysfunction require brain MRI.

If clinical evaluation suggests a chronic disease, liver and kidney function tests are done, and ESR is determined.

Often, testing includes measurement of hormone levels; total serum testosterone or dehydroepiandrosterone sulfate (DHEAS) levels are measured only if signs of virilization are present. Certain hormone levels should be remeasured to confirm the results. For example, if serum prolactin is high, it should be remeasured; if serum FSH is high, it should be remeasured monthly at least twice. Amenorrhea with high FSH levels (hypergonadotropic hypogonadism) suggests ovarian dysfunction; amenorrhea with low FSH levels (hypogonadotropic hypogonadism) suggests hypothalamic or pituitary dysfunction.

If patients have secondary amenorrhea without virilization and have normal prolactin and FSH levels and normal thyroid function, a trial of estrogen and a progestogen to try to stimulate withdrawal bleeding can be done (progesterone challenge test).

The **progesterone challenge test** begins by giving medroxyprogesterone 5 to 10 mg po once/day or another progestin for 7 to 10 days.

- If bleeding occurs, amenorrhea is probably not caused by an endometrial lesion (eg, Asherman syndrome) or outflow tract obstruction, and the cause is probably hypothalamic-pituitary dysfunction, ovarian insufficiency, or estrogen excess.
- If bleeding does not occur, an estrogen (eg, conjugated equine estrogen 1.25 mg, estradiol 2 mg) once/day is given for 21 days, followed by medroxyprogesterone 10 mg po once/day or another progestin for 7 to 10 days. If bleeding does not occur after estrogen is given, patients may have an endometrial lesion or outflow tract obstruction. However, bleeding may not occur in patients who do not have these abnormalities (eg, because the uterus is insensitive to estrogen); thus, the trial using estrogen and progestin may be repeated for confirmation.

However, because this trial takes weeks and results can be inaccurate, diagnosis of some serious disorders may be delayed significantly; thus, brain MRI should be considered before or during the trial.

Mildly elevated levels of testosterone or DHEAS suggest polycystic ovary syndrome, but levels can be elevated in women with hypothalamic or pituitary dysfunction and are sometimes normal in hirsute women with polycystic ovary syndrome. The cause of elevated levels can sometimes be determined by measuring serum LH. In polycystic ovary syndrome, circulating LH levels are often increased, increasing the ratio of LH to FSH.

Treatment

Treatment is directed at the underlying disorder; with such treatment, menses sometimes resume. For example, most abnormalities obstructing the genital outflow tract are surgically repaired.

If a Y chromosome is present, bilateral oophorectomy is recommended because risk of ovarian germ cell cancer is increased.

Problems associated with amenorrhea may also require treatment, including

- Inducing ovulation if pregnancy is desired
- Treating symptoms and long-term effects of estrogen deficiency (eg, osteoporosis)
- Treating symptoms and managing long-term effects of estrogen excess (eg, prolonged bleeding, persistent or marked breast tenderness, risk of endometrial hyperplasia and cancer)
- Minimizing hirsutism and long-term effects of androgen excess (eg, cardiovascular disorders, hypertension)

KEY POINTS

- Primary amenorrhea in patients without normal secondary sexual characteristics is usually anovulatory (eg, due to a genetic disorder).
- Always exclude pregnancy by testing rather than by history.
- Primary amenorrhea is evaluated differently from secondary amenorrhea.
- If patients have primary amenorrhea and normal secondary sexual characteristics, begin testing with pelvic ultrasonography to check for congenital anatomic genital tract obstruction.
- If patients have signs of virilization, check for conditions that cause androgen excess (eg, polycystic ovary syndrome, an androgen-secreting tumor, Cushing syndrome, use of certain drugs).
- If patients have symptoms and signs of estrogen deficiency (eg, hot flushes, night sweats, vaginal dryness or atrophy), check for primary ovarian insufficiency and conditions that cause functional hypothalamic anovulation.
- If patients have galactorrhea, check for conditions that cause hyperprolactinemia (eg, pituitary dysfunction, use of certain drugs).

DYSFUNCTIONAL UTERINE BLEEDING

(Abnormal Uterine Bleeding; Functional Uterine Bleeding)

Dysfunctional uterine bleeding (DUB) is abnormal uterine bleeding that, after examination and ultrasonography, cannot be attributed to the usual causes (structural gynecologic abnormalities, cancer, inflammation, systemic disorders, pregnancy, complications of pregnancy, use of oral contraceptives or certain drugs). Treatment is usually with hormone therapy, such as oral contraceptives, or with NSAIDs.

DUB, the most common cause of abnormal uterine bleeding, occurs most often in women > 45 (> 50% of cases) and in adolescents (20% of cases).

About 90% of cases are anovulatory; 10% are ovulatory.

Pathophysiology

During an **anovulatory cycle,** the corpus luteum does not form. Thus, the normal cyclical secretion of progesterone does not occur, and estrogen stimulates the endometrium unopposed. Without progesterone, the endometrium continues to proliferate, eventually outgrowing its blood supply; it then sloughs incompletely and bleeds irregularly and sometimes profusely or for a long time. When this abnormal process occurs repeatedly, the endometrium can become hyperplastic, sometimes with atypical or cancerous cells.

In **ovulatory DUB,** progesterone secretion is prolonged; irregular shedding of the endometrium results, probably because estrogen levels remain low, near the threshold for bleeding (as occurs during menses). In obese women, ovulatory DUB can occur if estrogen levels are high, resulting in amenorrhea alternating with irregular or prolonged bleeding.

Complications: Chronic bleeding may cause iron deficiency anemia.

If DUB is due to chronic anovulation, infertility may also be present.

Etiology

Anovulatory DUB can result from any disorder or condition that causes anovulation (see Table 273–1). Anovulation is most often

- Secondary to polycystic ovary syndrome
- Idiopathic (sometimes occurring when gonadotropin levels are normal)

Sometimes anovulation results from hypothyroidism.

During perimenopause, DUB may be an early sign of ovarian insufficiency or failure; follicles are still developing but, despite increasing levels of follicle-stimulating hormone (FSH), do not produce enough estrogen to trigger ovulation. About 20% of women with endometriosis have anovulatory DUB due to unknown mechanisms.

Ovulatory DUB may occur in

- Polycystic ovary syndrome (because progesterone secretion is prolonged)
- Endometriosis, which does not affect ovulation

Other causes are a short follicular phase and luteal phase dysfunction (due to inadequate progesterone stimulation of the endometrium); a rapid decrease in estrogen before ovulation can cause spotting.

Symptoms and Signs

Compared with typical menses, bleeding may

- Occur more frequently (menses < 21 days apart—polymenorrhea)
- Involve more blood loss (> 7 days or > 80 mL) during menses (menorrhagia, or hypermenorrhea)
- Occur frequently and irregularly between menses (metrorrhagia)
- Involve more blood loss during menses and frequent and irregular bleeding between menses (menometrorrhagia)

Ovulatory DUB tends to cause excessive bleeding during regular menstrual cycles. Women may have other symptoms of ovulation, such as premenstrual symptoms, breast tenderness, midcycle cramping pain (mittelschmerz), a change in basal body temperature after ovulation (see p. 2272), and sometimes dysmenorrhea.

Anovulatory DUB occurs at unpredictable times and in unpredictable patterns and is not accompanied by cyclic changes in basal body temperature.

Diagnosis

- Exclusion of other potential causes
- CBC, pregnancy test, and hormone measurement (eg, thyroid-stimulating hormone [TSH], prolactin)
- Usually transvaginal ultrasonography and endometrial sampling
- Often sonohysterography and/or hysteroscopy

Women should be evaluated for DUB when the amount or timing of vaginal bleeding is inconsistent with normal menses.

DUB is a diagnosis of exclusion; other conditions that can cause similar bleeding must be excluded (see p. 2205). Pregnancy should be excluded, even in young adolescents and perimenopausal women. Coagulation disorders should be considered, particularly in adolescents who have anemia or require hospitalization for bleeding. Regular cycles with prolonged or excessive bleeding (possible ovulatory DUB) suggest structural abnormalities.

Laboratory testing: Several tests are typically done:

- A urine or blood pregnancy test
- CBC
- TSH, prolactin, and progesterone levels

All women of reproductive age should have a pregnancy test.

CBC is routinely done. However, Hct may be normal in women who report heavy bleeding, or anemia may be severe in women who regularly have heavy periods. The serum ferritin level, which reflects body iron stores, is measured if women have chronic, heavy bleeding.

Thyroid-stimulating hormone levels are usually measured, and prolactin levels are measured, even when galactorrhea is absent, because thyroid disorders and hyperprolactinemia are common causes of abnormal bleeding.

To determine whether bleeding is anovulatory or ovulatory, some clinicians measure serum progesterone levels during the luteal phase (after day 14 of a normal menstrual cycle or after basal body temperature increases, as occurs during this phase). A level of ≥ 3 ng/mL (≥ 9.75 nmol/L) suggests that ovulation has occurred.

Other tests are done depending on results of the history and physical examination and include the following:

- Coagulation tests if women have risk factors for coagulation disorders, bruising, or hemorrhage
- Liver function tests if a liver disorder is suspected
- Testosterone and DHEAS levels if polycystic ovary syndrome is suspected
- Follicle-stimulating hormone (FSH) and estradiol levels if primary ovarian insufficiency is possible
- A cervical cancer screening test (eg, Papanicolaou [Pap] test, HPV test) if results are out-of-date
- Testing for *Neisseria gonorrhea* and *Chlamydia* sp if pelvic inflammatory disease or cervicitis is suspected

If all clinically indicated tests are normal, the diagnosis is dysfunctional uterine bleeding.

Additional testing: Transvaginal ultrasonography is done if women have any of the following:

- Age ≥ 35
- Risk factors for endometrial cancer (eg, obesity, diabetes, hypertension, polycystic ovary syndrome, chronic eugonadal anovulation, hirsutism, other conditions associated with prolonged unopposed estrogen exposure)
- Bleeding that continues despite use of empiric hormone therapy
- Pelvic organs that cannot be examined adequately during the physical examination
- Clinical evidence that suggests abnormalities in the ovaries or uterus

These criteria include almost all women with dysfunctional uterine bleeding.

Transvaginal ultrasonography can detect structural abnormalities, including most polyps, fibroids, other masses, endometrial cancer, and any areas of focal thickening in the endometrium. If focal thickening is detected, further testing may be needed to identify smaller intrauterine masses (eg, small endometrial polyps, submucous myomas). Sonohysterography (ultrasonography after saline is infused into the uterus) is useful in evaluating such abnormalities; it can be used to determine whether hysteroscopy, a more invasive test, is indicated and to plan resection of intrauterine masses. Or hysteroscopy may be done without sonohysteroscopy.

In **endometrial sampling**, only about 25% of the endometrium is analyzed, but sensitivity for detecting abnormal cells is about 97%. This test is usually recommended to rule out hyperplasia or cancer in women with any of the following:

- Age > 35 yr with one or more risk factors for endometrial cancer (see above)
- Age < 35 yr with multiple risk factors for endometrial cancer (see above)
- Bleeding that is persistent, irregular, or heavy
- Irregular cycles that suggest chronic anovulatory bleeding
- Endometrial thickness that is > 4 mm, focal, or irregular, detected during transvaginal ultrasonography
- Inconclusive ultrasonography findings

Directed biopsy (with hysteroscopy) may be done to visualize the endometrial cavity directly and target the abnormal tissue. Most endometrial biopsy specimens contain proliferative or dyssynchronous endometrium, which confirms anovulation because no secretory endometrium is found.

Treatment

- Control of bleeding, usually with an NSAID, tranexamic acid, or hormone therapy
- In women with endometrial hyperplasia, prevention of endometrial cancer

Bleeding: Nonhormonal treatments have fewer risks and adverse effects than hormone therapy and can be given intermittently, when bleeding occurs. They are used mainly for heavy regular bleeding (menorrhagia). Choices include

- NSAIDs, which reduce bleeding by 25 to 35% and relieve dysmenorrhea by reducing prostaglandin levels
- Tranexamic acid, which inhibits plasminogen activator, reducing menstrual blood loss by 40 to 60%

Hormone therapy (eg, oral contraceptives, progestogens) is often tried first in perimenopausal women. This therapy does the following:

- Suppresses endometrial development
- Reestablishes predictable bleeding patterns
- Decreases menstrual flow

Hormone therapy is usually given until bleeding has been controlled for a few months.

Oral contraceptives (OCs) are commonly given. OCs, used cyclically or continuously, can control dysfunctional bleeding. Limited data suggest that they do the following:

- Decrease menstrual blood loss by 40 to 50%
- Decrease breast tenderness and dysmenorrhea
- Decrease risk of uterine and ovarian cancer

Combination formulations consisting of an estrogen and a progestin or a progestin alone may be used. Risks of an OC depend on the type of OC and on patient factors.

Progesterone or another progestin can be used alone in the following cases:

- Estrogen is contraindicated (eg, for patients with cardiovascular risk factors or prior deep vein thrombosis).
- Estrogen is declined by the patient.
- Combination OCs are ineffective after about 3 mo of use.

Withdrawal bleeding may be more predictable with cyclic progestin therapy (medroxyprogesterone acetate 10 mg/day po or norethindrone acetate 2.5 to 5 mg/day po) given for 21 days/mo than with a combination OC. Cyclic natural (micronized) progesterone 200 mg/day for 21 days/mo may be used, particularly if pregnancy is possible; however, it may cause drowsiness and does not decrease blood loss as much as a progestin.

If patients using cyclic progestins or progesterone wish to prevent pregnancy, contraception should be used. Contraceptive options include

- **A levonorgestrel-releasing intrauterine device (IUD):** It is effective in up to 97% by 6 mo, provides contraception, and relieves dysmenorrhea.
- **Depot medroxyprogesterone acetate injections:** They cause amenorrhea and provide contraception but may cause irregular spotting and reversible bone loss.

Other treatments that are occasionally used to treat DUB include

- **Danazol:** It reduces menstrual blood loss (by causing endometrial atrophy) but has many androgenic adverse effects, which may be lessened by using lower doses or a vaginal formulation. To be effective, danazol must be taken continuously, usually for about 3 mo. It is usually used when other forms of therapy are contraindicated.
- **Gonadotropin-releasing hormone (GnRH) agonists:** These drugs suppress ovarian hormone production and cause amenorrhea; they are used to shrink fibroids or the endometrium preoperatively. However, their hypoestrogenic adverse effects (eg, bone loss) limit their use.
- **Desmopressin:** It is used as a last resort to treat DUB in patients who have a coagulation disorder; it rapidly increases levels of von Willebrand factor and factor VIII for about 6 h.

Ergot derivatives are not recommended for treatment of DUB because they are rarely effective.

If pregnancy is desired and bleeding is not heavy, ovulation induction with clomiphene (50 mg po on days 5 through 9 of the menstrual cycle) can be tried.

Hysteroscopy with D & C may be therapeutic as well as diagnostic; it may be the treatment of choice when anovulatory bleeding is severe or when hormone therapy is ineffective. Structural causes such as polyps or fibroids may be identified or removed during hysteroscopy. This procedure may decrease bleeding but, in some women, causes amenorrhea due to endometrial scarring (Asherman syndrome).

Endometrial ablation (eg, laser, rollerball, resectoscopic, thermal, or freezing) may help control bleeding in 60 to 80%. Ablation is less invasive than hysterectomy, and the recovery time is shorter. Ablation may be repeated if heavy bleeding recurs after ablation is initially effective. If this treatment does not control bleeding or if bleeding continues to recur, the cause may be adenomyosis and thus is not DUB. Endometrial ablation does not prevent pregnancy. Pregnancy rates may be as high as 5% after ablation. Ablation causes scarring which may make sampling the endometrium difficult later.

Hysterectomy, abdominal or vaginal, may be recommended for patients who decline hormone therapy or who, despite other treatments, have symptomatic anemia or poor quality of life caused by persistent, irregular bleeding.

Emergency measures are needed only rarely, when bleeding is very heavy. Patients are stabilized hemodynamically with IV crystalloid fluid, blood products, and other measures as needed. If bleeding persists, a bladder catheter is inserted into the uterus and inflated with 30 to 60 mL of water to tamponade the bleeding. Once patients are stable, hormone therapy is used to control bleeding.

Very rarely, in patients with very heavy bleeding due to anovulatory DUB, conjugated estrogens 25 mg IV q 4 to 6 h for a total of 4 doses may be used. This therapy stops bleeding in about 70% of patients but increases risk of thrombosis. Immediately afterward, patients are given a combination OC, which may be continued until bleeding has been controlled for a few months.

Endometrial hyperplasia: In **postmenopausal women,** atypical adenomatous endometrial hyperplasia is usually treated with hysterectomy.

In **premenopausal women,** this disorder may be treated with medroxyprogesterone acetate 20 to 40 mg po once/day for 3 to 6 mo or a levonorgestrel-releasing IUD.[1] If repeat endometrial sampling indicates resolution of hyperplasia, women may be given cyclic medroxyprogesterone acetate (5 to 10 mg po once/day for 10 to 14 days each month) or, if pregnancy is desired, clomiphene. If sampling shows persistent or progressive atypical hyperplasia, hysterectomy is necessary.

More benign cystic or adenomatous hyperplasia can usually be treated with high-dose cyclic progestin therapy (eg, cyclic medroxyprogesterone acetate) or a progestin- or levonorgestrel-releasing IUD; sampling is repeated after about 3 mo.

1. Mentrikoski MJ, Shah AA, Hanley KZ, et al: Assessing endometrial hyperplasia and carcinoma treated with progestin therapy. *Am J Clin Pathol* 38(4): 524–534, 2012.

KEY POINTS

- Anovulatory DUB is the most common cause of abnormal uterine bleeding.
- Test for treatable causes of bleeding; tests may include a pregnancy test, CBC, measurement of hormone levels (TSH, prolactin, progesterone), and often ultrasonography and endometrial sampling.
- In women at risk, check for and treat endometrial hyperplasia.
- If drugs are needed to control bleeding, prescribe NSAIDs, tranexamic acid, OCs, or other hormones, which are usually effective.

DYSMENORRHEA

Dysmenorrhea is uterine pain around the time of menses. Pain may occur with menses or precede menses by 1 to 3 days. Pain tends to peak 24 h after onset of menses and subside after 2 to 3 days. It is usually sharp but may be cramping, throbbing, or a dull, constant ache; it may radiate to the legs.

Headache, nausea, constipation or diarrhea, lower back pain, and urinary frequency are common; vomiting occurs occasionally.

Symptoms of premenstrual syndrome may occur during part or all of menses.

Sometimes endometrial clots or casts are expelled.

Etiology

Dysmenorrhea can be

- Primary (more common)
- Secondary (due to pelvic abnormalities)

Primary dysmenorrhea: Symptoms cannot be explained by structural gynecologic disorders. Pain is thought to result from uterine contractions and ischemia, probably mediated by prostaglandins (eg, prostaglandin $F_{2\alpha}$, a potent myometrial stimulant and vasoconstrictor) and other inflammatory mediators produced in secretory endometrium and possibly associated with prolonged uterine contractions and decreased blood flow to the myometrium.

Contributing factors may include the following:

- Passage of menstrual tissue through the cervix
- A narrow cervical os
- A malpositioned uterus
- Lack of exercise
- Anxiety about menses

Primary dysmenorrhea begins within a year after menarche and occurs almost invariably in ovulatory cycles. The pain usually begins when menses start (or just before) and persists for the first 1 to 2 days; this pain, described as spasmodic, is superimposed over constant lower abdominal pain, which may radiate to the back or thigh. Patients may also have malaise, fatigue, nausea, vomiting, diarrhea, low back pain, or headache.

Risk factors for severe symptoms include the following:

- Early age at menarche
- Long or heavy menstrual periods
- Smoking
- A family history of dysmenorrhea

Symptoms tend to lessen with age and after pregnancy.

In about 5 to 15% of women with primary dysmenorrhea, cramps are severe enough to interfere with daily activities and may result in absence from school or work.

Secondary dysmenorrhea: Symptoms are due to pelvic abnormalities. Almost any abnormality or process that can affect the pelvic viscera can cause dysmenorrhea.

Common causes include

- Endometriosis (the most common cause)
- Uterine adenomyosis
- Fibroids

Less common causes include congenital malformations (eg, bicornuate uterus, subseptate uterus, transverse vaginal septum), ovarian cysts and tumors, pelvic inflammatory disease, pelvic congestion, intrauterine adhesions, psychogenic pain, and IUDs, particularly copper- or levonorgestrel-releasing IUDs. Levonorgestrel-releasing IUDs cause less cramping than copper-releasing IUDs.

In a few women, pain occurs when the uterus attempts to expel tissue through an extremely tight cervical os (secondary to conization, loop electrosurgical excision procedure [LEEP], cryocautery, or thermocautery). Pain occasionally results from a pedunculated submucosal fibroid or an endometrial polyp protruding through the cervix.

Risk factors for severe secondary dysmenorrhea are the same as those for primary.

Secondary dysmenorrhea usually begins during adulthood unless caused by congenital malformations.

Evaluation

History: History of present illness should cover complete menstrual history, including age at onset of menses, duration and amount of flow, time between menses, variability of timing, and relation of menses to symptoms. Clinicians should also ask about

- The age at which symptoms began
- Their nature and severity
- Factors that relieve or worsen symptoms (including the effects of contraceptives)
- Degree of disruption of daily life
- Effect on sexual activity
- Presence of pelvic pain unrelated to menses

Review of systems should include accompanying symptoms such as cyclic nausea, vomiting, bloating, diarrhea, and fatigue.

Past medical history should identify known causes, including endometriosis, uterine adenomyosis, or fibroids. Method of contraception should be ascertained, specifically asking about IUD use.

Sexual history should include prior or current history of sexual abuse.

Physical examination: Pelvic examination focuses on detecting causes of secondary dysmenorrhea. The vagina, vulva, and cervix are inspected for lesions and for masses protruding through the cervical os. Structures are palpated to check for a tight cervical os, prolapsed polyp or fibroid, uterine masses, adnexal masses, thickening of the rectovaginal septum, induration of the cul-de-sac, and nodularity of the uterosacral ligament.

The abdomen is examined for evidence of peritonitis.

Red flags: The following findings are of particular concern:

- New or sudden-onset pain
- Unremitting pain
- Fever
- Vaginal discharge
- Evidence of peritonitis

Interpretation of findings: Red flag findings suggest a cause of pelvic pain other than dysmenorrhea.

Primary dysmenorrhea is suspected if

- Symptoms begin soon after menarche or during adolescence.

Secondary dysmenorrhea is suspected if

- Symptoms begin after adolescence.
- Patients have known causes, including uterine adenomyosis, fibroids, a tight cervical os, a mass protruding from the cervical os, or, particularly, endometriosis.

Endometriosis is considered in patients with adnexal masses, thickening of the rectovaginal septum, induration of the cul-de-sac, nodularity of the uterosacral ligament, or, occasionally, nonspecific vaginal, vulvar, or cervical lesions.

Testing: Testing aims to exclude structural gynecologic disorders. Most patients should have

- Pregnancy testing
- Pelvic ultrasonography

Intrauterine and ectopic pregnancy are ruled out by pregnancy testing. If pelvic inflammatory disease is suspected, cervical cultures are done.

Pelvic ultrasonography is highly sensitive for pelvic masses (eg, ovarian cysts, fibroids, endometriosis, uterine adenomyosis) and can locate lost and abnormally located IUDs.

If these tests are inconclusive and symptoms persist, other tests are done, such as the following:

- Hysterosalpingography or sonohysterography to identify endometrial polyps, submucous fibroids, or congenital abnormalities
- MRI to identify other abnormalities, including congenital abnormalities, or, if surgery is planned, to further define previously identified abnormalities
- IV pyelography, but only if a uterine malformation has been identified as causing or contributing to the dysmenorrhea

If results of all other tests are inconclusive, hysteroscopy or laparoscopy can be done. Laparoscopy is the most definitive test because it enables clinicians to directly examine all of the pelvis and reproductive organs and to check for abnormalities.

Treatment

Underlying disorders are treated.

General measures: Symptomatic treatment begins with adequate rest and sleep and regular exercise. A low-fat diet and nutritional supplements such as ω-3 fatty acids, flaxseed, magnesium, vitamin E, zinc, and vitamin B_1 are suggested as potentially effective.

Women with primary dysmenorrhea are reassured about the absence of structural gynecologic disorders.

Drugs: If pain persists, NSAIDs (which relieve pain and inhibit prostaglandins) are typically tried. NSAIDs are usually started 24 to 48 h before and continued until 1 or 2 days after menses begin.

If the NSAID is ineffective, suppression of ovulation with a low-dose estrogen/progestin oral contraceptive may be tried.

Other hormone therapy, such as danazol, progestins (eg, levonorgestrel, etonogestrel, depot medroxyprogesterone acetate), GnRH agonists, or a levonorgestrel-releasing IUD, may decrease dysmenorrheal symptoms.

Periodic adjunctive use of analgesics may be needed.

Other treatments: Hypnosis is being evaluated as treatment. Other proposed nondrug therapies, including acupuncture, acupressure, chiropractic therapy, and transcutaneous electrical nerve stimulation, have not been well-studied but may benefit some patients.

For intractable pain of unknown origin, laparoscopic presacral neurectomy or uterosacral nerve ablation has been efficacious in some patients for as long as 12 mo.

KEY POINTS

- Most dysmenorrhea is primary.
- Check for underlying structural pelvic lesions.
- Usually, before doing other tests, do ultrasonography to check for structural gynecologic disorders.
- An NSAID or an NSAID plus a low-dose oral contraceptive is usually effective.

PELVIC CONGESTION SYNDROME

Pelvic congestion syndrome is chronic pain exacerbated by standing or sexual intercourse in women who have varicose veins in or near the ovaries.

Pelvic congestion syndrome is a common cause of chronic pelvic pain. Varicose veins and venous insufficiency are common in the ovarian veins but are often asymptomatic. Why some women develop symptoms is unknown.

Symptoms and Signs

Pelvic pain develops after pregnancy. Pain tends to worsen with each subsequent pregnancy.

Typically, the pain is a dull ache, but it may be sharp or throbbing. It is worse at the end of the day (after women have been sitting or standing a long time) and is relieved by lying down. The pain is also worse during or after sexual intercourse. It is often accompanied by low back pain, aches in the legs, and abnormal menstrual bleeding.

Some women occasionally have a clear or watery discharge from the vagina.

Other symptoms may include fatigue, mood swings, headaches, and abdominal bloating.

Pelvic examination detects tender ovaries and cervical motion tenderness.

Diagnosis

- Clinical criteria
- Ovarian varicosities, detected during imaging

Diagnosis requires that pain be present for > 6 mo and that ovaries be tender when examined.

Ultrasonography is done but may not show varicosities in women when they are recumbent.

Some experts recommend additional tests (eg, venography, CT, MRI, magnetic resonance venography) if necessary to confirm pelvic varicosities.

If pelvic pain is troublesome and the cause has not been identified, laparoscopy is done.

Treatment

- Usually NSAIDs

NSAIDs can be tried. If they are ineffective and if the pain is severe, embolization or sclerotherapy may be considered.

POLYCYSTIC OVARY SYNDROME

(Hyperandrogenic Chronic Anovulation; Stein-Leventhal Syndrome)

Polycystic ovary syndrom (PCOS) is a clinical syndrome characterized by mild obesity, irregular menses or amenorrhea, and signs of androgen excess (eg, hirsutism, acne).

- In most patients, the ovaries contain multiple cysts.
- Diagnosis is by pregnancy testing, hormone measurement, and imaging to exclude a virilizing tumor.
- Treatment is symptomatic.

PCOS occurs in 5 to 10% of women. In the US, it is the most common cause of infertility.

PCOS is usually defined as a clinical syndrome, not by the presence of ovarian cysts. But typically, ovaries contain many 2- to 6-mm follicular cysts and sometimes larger cysts containing atretic cells. Ovaries may be enlarged with smooth, thickened capsules or may be normal in size.

This syndrome involves anovulation or ovulatory dysfunction and androgen excess of unclear etiology. However, some evidence suggests that patients have a functional abnormality of cytochrome P450c17 affecting 17-hydroxylase (the rate-limiting enzyme in androgen production); as a result, androgen production increases.

Complications: PCOS has several serious complications.

Estrogen levels are elevated, increasing risk of endometrial hyperplasia and, eventually, endometrial cancer.

Androgen levels are often elevated, increasing the risk of metabolic syndrome and causing hirsutism. Hyperinsulinemia due to insulin resistance may be present and may contribute to increased ovarian production of androgens. Over the long term, androgen excess increases the risk of cardiovascular disorders, including hypertension. Risk of androgen excess and its complications may be just as high in women who are not overweight as in those who are.

Symptoms and Signs

Symptoms typically begin during puberty and worsen with time. Premature adrenarche, characterized by excess DHEAS and often early growth of axillary hair, body odor, and microcomedonal acne, is common.

Typical symptoms include mild obesity, slight hirsutism, and irregular menses or amenorrhea. However, in up to half of women with PCOS, weight is normal, and some women are underweight. Body hair may grow in a male pattern (eg, on the upper lip and chin, around the nipples, and along the linea alba of the lower abdomen). Some women have other signs of virilization, such as acne and temporal balding.

Areas of thickened, darkened skin (acanthosis nigricans) may appear in the axillae, on the nape of the neck, in skinfolds, and on knuckles and/or elbows; the cause is high insulin levels due to insulin resistance.

Diagnosis

- Clinical criteria
- Serum testosterone, FSH, prolactin, and TSH levels
- Pelvic ultrasonography

Ovulatory dysfunction is usually present at puberty, resulting in primary amenorrhea; thus, this syndrome is unlikely if regular menses occurred for a time after menarche.

Examination usually detects abundant cervical mucus, reflecting high estrogen levels. PCOS is suspected if women have at least two typical symptoms.

Testing includes pregnancy testing; measurement of serum total testosterone, FSH, prolactin, and TSH; and pelvic ultrasonography to exclude other possible causes of symptoms. Serum free testosterone is more sensitive than total testosterone but is technically more difficult to measure (see p. 2129). Normal to mildly increased testosterone and normal to mildly decreased FSH levels suggest PCOS.

The diagnosis requires at least 2 of the following 3 criteria:

- Ovulatory dysfunction causing menstrual irregularity
- Clinical or biochemical evidence of hyperandrogenism
- > 10 follicles per ovary (detected by pelvic ultrasonography), usually occurring in the periphery and resembling a string of pearls

In women meeting these criteria, serum cortisol is measured to exclude Cushing syndrome, and early-morning serum 17-hydroxyprogesterone is measured to exclude adrenal virilism. Serum DHEAS is measured. If DHEAS is abnormal, women are evaluated as for amenorrhea. Adult women with PCOS are evaluated for metabolic syndrome by measuring BP and usually serum glucose and lipids (lipid profile).

PEARLS & PITFALLS

- PCOS is unlikely if regular menses occurred for a time after menarche.

Treatment

- Intermittent progestogens or oral contraceptives
- Management of hirsutism and, in adult women, long-term risks of hormonal abnormalities
- Infertility treatments in women who desire pregnancy

Treatment aims to

- Correct hormonal abnormalities and thus reduce risks of estrogen excess (eg, endometrial hyperplasia) and androgen excess (eg, cardiovascular disorders)
- Relieve symptoms

Weight loss and regular exercise are encouraged. They may help induce ovulation, make menstrual cycles more regular, increase insulin sensitivity, and reduce acanthosis nigricans and hirsutism.

Metformin 500 to 1000 mg bid is used to help increase insulin sensitivity if weight loss is unsuccessful or menses do not resume. Metformin can also reduce free testosterone levels. When metformin is used, serum glucose should be measured, and kidney and liver function tests should be done periodically. Because metformin may induce ovulation, contraception is needed if pregnancy is not desired.

Women who do not desire pregnancy are usually given an intermittent progestin (eg, medroxyprogesterone 5 to 10 mg po once/day for 10 to 14 days every 1 to 2 mo) or oral contraceptives to reduce the risk of endometrial hyperplasia and cancer. These treatments also reduce circulating androgens and usually help make menstrual cycles more regular.

For women who desire pregnancy, infertility treatments (eg, clomiphene, metformin) are used. Weight loss may also be helpful. Hormone therapy that may have contraceptive effects is avoided.

For **hirsutism**, physical measures (eg, bleaching, electrolysis, plucking, waxing, depilation) can be used. Eflornithine cream 13.9% bid may help remove unwanted facial hair. In adult women who do not desire pregnancy, hormone therapy that decreases androgen levels or spironolactone can be tried.

Acne can be treated with the usual drugs (eg, benzoyl peroxide, tretinoin cream, topical and oral antibiotics).

KEY POINTS

- PCOS is a common cause of ovulatory dysfunction.
- Suspect PCOS in women who have irregular menses, are mildly obese, and are slightly hirsute, but be aware that weight is normal or low in many women with PCOS.
- Test for serious disorders (eg, Cushing syndrome, tumors) that can cause similar symptoms and for complications (eg, metabolic syndrome).

PRIMARY OVARIAN INSUFFICIENCY

(Hypergonadotropic Hypogonadism; Premature Menopause; Premature Ovarian Failure; Premature Ovarian Insufficiency)

In primary ovarian insufficiency, ovaries do not regularly release eggs and do not produce enough sex hormones despite high levels of circulating gonadotropins (especially FSH) in women < 40. Diagnosis is by measuring FSH and estradiol levels. Typically, treatment is with combined estrogen/progestogen therapy.

In primary ovarian insufficiency, the ovaries stop functioning normally in women who are < 40. This disorder used to be called premature ovarian failure or premature menopause; however, these terms are misleading because women with primary ovarian insufficiency do not always stop menstruating and their ovaries do not always completely stop functioning. Thus, a diagnosis of primary ovarian insufficiency does not always mean that pregnancy is impossible. Also, this disorder does not imply that a woman is aging prematurely; it means only that her ovaries are no longer functioning normally.

In primary ovarian insufficiency, the ovaries

- Stop releasing eggs or release them only intermittently
- Stop producing the hormones estrogen, progesterone, and testosterone or produce them only intermittently

Etiology

Primary ovarian insufficiency has various causes (see Table 273–4), including the following:

- The number of ovarian follicles present at birth is insufficient.
- The rate of follicular atresia is accelerated.
- The follicles are dysfunctional (as occurs in autoimmune ovarian dysfunction).
- Certain genetic disorders are present.

Genetic disorders that confer a Y chromosome can cause primary ovarian insufficiency. These disorders, which are usually evident by age 35, increase risk of ovarian germ cell cancer.

Symptoms and Signs

In women with occult or biochemical primary ovarian insufficiency (see Classification, below), the only sign may be unexplained infertility. Women with overt primary ovarian insufficiency or premature ovarian failure typically have amenorrhea or irregular bleeding and often symptoms or signs of estrogen deficiency (eg, osteoporosis, atrophic vaginitis, decreased libido).

Table 273–4. COMMON CAUSES OF PRIMARY OVARIAN INSUFFICIENCY

CAUSE	EXAMPLES
Enzyme defects	Galactosemia 17α-Hydroxylase deficiency 17,20-Lyase deficiency
Genetic defects	Accelerated ovarian follicular atresia (idiopathic) Certain autosomal defects *FMR1* premutation (Fragile X syndrome) Gonadal dysgenesis secondary to genetic defects (eg, Turner syndrome [45,X], pure [46,XX or 46,XY] or mixed gonadal dysgenesis) Idiopathic hypogonadotropic hypogonadism Kallmann syndrome Myotonic dystrophy Reduced germ cell number Trisomy X with or without chromosomal mosaicism
Immune-mediated disturbances	Autoimmune disorders (most commonly, thyroiditis, Addison disease, hypoparathyroidism, diabetes mellitus, myasthenia gravis, vitiligo, pernicious anemia, and mucocutaneous candidiasis) Congenital thymic aplasia Isolated ovarian failure Sarcoidosis
Other causes	Addison disease Adrenal insufficiency Chemotherapeutic (especially alkylating) drugs Cigarette smoking Diabetes Irradiation of the gonads Surgical extirpation of the gonads or adnexa Viral infections (eg, mumps)

The ovaries are usually small and barely palpable but occasionally are enlarged, usually when the cause is an immune disorder. Women may also have symptoms and signs of the causative disorder (eg, dysmorphic features due to Turner syndrome; intellectual disability, dysmorphic features, and autism due to Fragile X syndrome; rarely, orthostatic hypotension, hyperpigmentation, and decreased axillary and pubic hair due to adrenal insufficiency).

Unless women receive estrogen therapy, the risk of dementia, Parkinson disease, and coronary artery disease is increased.

If primary ovarian insufficiency is caused by an autoimmune disorder, women are at risk of potentially life-threatening primary adrenal insufficiency.

Diagnosis

- FSH and estradiol levels
- Thyroid function tests, fasting glucose, electrolytes, and creatinine
- Sometimes genetic testing

Primary ovarian insufficiency is suspected in women < 40 with unexplained infertility, menstrual abnormalities, or symptoms of estrogen deficiency.

A pregnancy test is done, and serum FSH and estradiol levels are measured weekly for 2 to 4 wk; if FSH levels are high (> 20 mIU/mL, but usually > 30 mIU/mL) and estradiol levels are low (usually < 20 pg/mL), ovarian insufficiency is confirmed. Then, further tests are done based on which cause is suspected.

Because antimüllerian hormone is produced only in small ovarian follicles, blood levels of this hormone have been used to attempt to diagnose decreased ovarian reserve. Normal levels are between 1.5 and 4.0 ng/ml. A very low level suggests decreased ovarian reserve.

Genetic counseling and testing for the *FMR1* premutation are indicated if women have a family history of primary ovarian insufficiency or have intellectual disability, tremor, or ataxia. Karyotype is determined if women with confirmed ovarian insufficiency or failure are < 35.

If karyotype is normal or if an autoimmune cause is suspected, tests for serum adrenal and anti-21 hydroxylase antibodies (adrenal autoantibodies) are done.

If an autoimmune cause is suspected, tests to check for autoimmune hypothyroidism are also done; they include measuring TSH, thyroxine (T4), and antithyroid–peroxidase and antithyroglobulin antibodies.

Bone density is measured if women have symptoms or signs of estrogen deficiency.

Ovarian biopsy is not indicated.

Classification: Primary ovarian insufficiency can be classified based on clinical findings and serum FSH levels:

- Occult primary ovarian insufficiency: Unexplained infertility and a normal basal serum FSH level
- Biochemical primary ovarian insufficiency: Unexplained infertility and an elevated basal serum FSH level
- Overt primary ovarian insufficiency: Irregular menstrual cycles and an elevated basal serum FSH level
- Premature ovarian failure: Irregular or occasional periods for years, the possibility of pregnancy, and an elevated basal serum FSH level
- Premature menopause: Amenorrhea, permanent infertility, and complete depletion of primordial follicles

Treatment

- Estrogen/progestogen therapy

Women who do not desire pregnancy are given cyclical estrogen/progestin therapy (combination hormone therapy) until about age 51 unless these hormones are contraindicated; this therapy relieves symptoms of estrogen deficiency, helps maintain bone density, and may help prevent coronary artery disease, Parkinson disease, and dementia.

For women who desire pregnancy, one option is in vitro fertilization of donated oocytes plus exogenous estrogen and a progestogen, which enable the endometrium to support the transferred embryo. The age of the oocyte donor is more important than the age of the recipient. This technique is fairly successful, but even without this technique, some women with diagnosed primary ovarian insufficiency become pregnant. No treatment has been proved to increase the ovulation rate or restore fertility in women with primary ovarian insufficiency.

Other options for women who desire pregnancy include cryopreservation of ovarian tissue, oocytes, or embryos and embryo or oocyte donation. These techniques may be used before or during ovarian failure, especially in cancer patients. Neonatal and adult ovaries possess a small number of oogonial stem cells that can stably proliferate for months and produce mature oocytes in vitro; these cells may be used to develop infertility treatments in the future.

To help prevent osteoporosis, women with primary ovarian insufficiency should consume an adequate amount of Ca and vitamin D (in the diet and/or as supplements).

Women with a Y chromosome require laparotomy or laparoscopy and bilateral oophorectomy because risk of ovarian germ cell cancer is increased.

KEY POINTS

- Suspect primary ovarian insufficiency in women with unexplained menstrual abnormalities, infertility, or symptoms of estrogen deficiency.
- Confirm the diagnosis by measuring FSH (which is high, usually > 30 mIU/mL) and estradiol (which is low, usually < 20 pg/mL).
- Unless contraindicated, prescribe cyclic estrogen/progestogen therapy to be taken until about age 51 to maintain bone density and relieve symptoms and complications of estrogen deficiency.

PREMENSTRUAL SYNDROME

(Premenstrual Tension)

Premenstrual syndrome (PMS) is characterized by irritability, anxiety, emotional lability, depression, edema, breast pain, and headaches, occurring during the 7 to 10 days before and usually ending a few hours after onset of menses. Diagnosis is clinical, often based on the patient's daily recording of symptoms. Treatment is symptomatic and includes diet, drugs, and counseling.

About 20 to 50% of women of reproductive age have PMS; about 5% have a severe form of PMS called premenstrual dysphoric disorder.

Etiology

The cause is unclear.

Possible causes or contributing factors include

- Multiple endocrine factors (eg, hypoglycemia, other changes in carbohydrate metabolism, hyperprolactinemia, fluctuations

in levels of circulating estrogen and progesterone, abnormal responses to estrogen and progesterone, excess aldosterone or ADH)
- A genetic predisposition
- Serotonin deficiency
- Possibly magnesium and calcium deficiencies

Estrogen and progesterone can cause transitory fluid retention, as can excess aldosterone or ADH.

Serotonin deficiency is thought to contribute because women who are most affected by PMS have lower serotonin levels and because SSRIs (which increase serotonin) sometimes relieve symptoms of PMS.

Magnesium and calcium deficiencies may contribute.

Symptoms and Signs

Type and intensity of symptoms vary from woman to woman and from cycle to cycle. Symptoms last a few hours to ≥ 10 days, usually ending when menses begins. Symptoms may become more severe during stress or perimenopause. In perimenopausal women, symptoms may persist until after menses.

The **most common symptoms** are irritability, anxiety, agitation, anger, insomnia, difficulty concentrating, lethargy, depression, and severe fatigue. Fluid retention causes edema, transient weight gain, and breast fullness and pain. Pelvic heaviness or pressure and backache may occur. Some women, particularly younger ones, have dysmenorrhea when menses begins.

Other nonspecific symptoms may include headache, vertigo, paresthesias of the extremities, syncope, palpitations, constipation, nausea, vomiting, and changes in appetite. Acne and neurodermatitis may also occur. Existing skin disorders may worsen, as may respiratory problems (eg, allergies, infection) and eye problems (eg, visual disturbances, conjunctivitis).

Premenstrual dysphoric disorder (PMDD): Some women have severe PMS symptoms that occur regularly and only during the 2nd half of the menstrual cycle; symptoms end with menses or shortly after. Mood is markedly depressed, and anxiety, irritability, and emotional lability are pronounced. Suicidal thoughts may be present. Interest in daily activities is greatly decreased.

In contrast to PMS, PMDD causes symptoms that are severe enough to interfere with routine daily activities or overall functioning. PMDD is a severely distressing, disabling, and often underdiagnosed.

PEARLS & PITFALLS

- Consider premenstrual dysphoric disorder if women have nonspecific but severe symptoms just before menses.

Diagnosis

- For PMS, patient's report of symptoms
- For PMDD, clinical criteria

PMS is diagnosed based on physical symptoms (eg, bloating, weight gain, breast tenderness, swelling of hands and feet). Women may be asked to record their symptoms daily. Physical examination and laboratory testing are not helpful.

If **PMDD** is suspected, women are asked to rate their symptoms daily for ≥ 2 cycles to determine whether severe symptoms occur regularly.

For PMDD to be diagnosed, women must have ≥ 5 of the following symptoms for most of the week before menses, and symptoms must become minimal or absent during the week after menstruation. Symptoms must include at least one of the following:

- Marked mood swings (eg, sudden sadness)
- Marked irritability or anger or increased interpersonal conflicts
- Marked depressed mood, feelings of hopelessness, or self-deprecating thoughts
- Marked anxiety, tension, or an on-edge feeling

In addition, ≥ 1 of the following must be present:

- Decreased interest in usual activities, possibly causing withdrawal
- Difficulty concentrating
- Low energy or fatigue
- Marked changes in appetite, overeating, or specific food cravings
- Insomnia or hyperinsomnia
- Feelings of being overwhelmed or out of control
- Physical symptoms associated with PMS (eg, breast tenderness, edema)

Also, the symptom pattern must have occurred for most of the previous 12 mo, and symptoms must be severe enough to interfere with daily activities and function.

Patients with symptoms of depression are evaluated using a depression inventory or are referred to a mental health care practitioner for formal evaluation.

Treatment

- General measures
- Sometimes SSRIs or hormonal manipulation

PMS can be difficult to treat. No single treatment has proven efficacy for all women, and few woman have complete relief with any single type of treatment. Treatment can thus require trial and error, as well as patience.

General measures: Treatment is symptomatic, beginning with adequate rest and sleep, regular exercise, and activities that are relaxing. Regular exercise may help alleviate bloating as well as irritability, anxiety, and insomnia. Yoga helps some women.

Dietary changes—increasing protein, decreasing sugar, consuming complex carbohydrates, and eating smaller meals more frequently—may help, as may counseling, avoiding stressful activities, relaxation training, light therapy, sleep adjustments, and cognitive-behavioral therapy. Other possible strategies include avoiding certain foods and drinks (eg, cola, coffee, hot dogs, potato chips, canned goods) and eating more of others (eg, fruits, vegetables, milk, high-fiber foods, low-fat meats, foods high in calcium and vitamin D). The beneficial effects of dietary supplements have not been substantiated.

Drugs: NSAIDs can help relieve aches, pains, and dysmenorrhea.

SSRIs (eg, fluoxetine 20 mg po once/day) are the drugs of choice for relief of anxiety, irritability, and other emotional symptoms, particularly if stress cannot be avoided. SSRIs effectively relieve symptoms of PMS and PMDD. Continuous dosing is more effective than intermittent dosing. No SSRI appears to be more effective than another.

Clomipramine, given for the full cycle or a half-cycle, effectively relieves emotional symptoms, as does nefazodone, a serotonin-norepinephrine reuptake inhibitor (SNRI).

Anxiolytics may help but are usually less desirable because dependence or addiction is possible. Buspirone, which may be given throughout the cycle or during the late luteal phase, helps relieve symptoms of PMS and PMDD. Adverse effects include nausea, headache, anxiety, and dizziness.

For some women, hormonal manipulation is effective. Options include

- Oral contraceptives
- Progesterone by vaginal suppository (200 to 400 mg once/day)
- An oral progestogen (eg, micronized progesterone 100 mg at bedtime) for 10 to 12 days before menses
- A long-acting progestin (eg, medroxyprogesterone 200 mg IM q 2 to 3 mo)

Women who choose to use an oral contraceptive for contraception can take drospirenone plus ethinyl estradiol. However, risk of venous thromboembolism may be increased.

Rarely, for very severe or refractory symptoms, a GnRH agonist (eg, leuprolide 3.75 mg IM, goserelin 3.6 mg sc q mo) with low-dose estrogen/progestin (eg, oral estradiol 0.5 mg once/day plus micronized progesterone 100 mg at bedtime) is given to minimize cyclic fluctuations.

Fluid retention may be relieved by reducing sodium intake and taking a diuretic (eg, spironolactone 100 mg po once/day) just before symptoms are expected. However, minimizing fluid retention and taking a diuretic do not relieve all symptoms and may have no effect.

Bromocriptine and monoamine oxidase inhibitors are not useful.

Surgery: In women with severe symptoms, bilateral oophorectomy may alleviate symptoms because it eliminates menstrual cycles; hormone replacement therapy is then indicated until about age 51 (when menopause usually occurs).

KEY POINTS

- Symptoms of PMS can be nonspecific and vary from woman to woman.
- PMS is diagnosed based on symptoms alone.
- If symptoms seem severe and disabling, consider PMDD (which is often underdiagnosed), and ask patients to record symptoms for ≥ 2 cycles; for a diagnosis of PMDD, clinical criteria must be met.
- Usually, treatment is a matter of trying various strategies to identify what helps a particular patient.

274 Pelvic Relaxation Syndromes

Pelvic relaxation syndromes result from laxities (similar to hernias) in the ligaments, fascia, and muscles supporting the pelvic organs (pelvic floor—see Fig. 274–1). About 9% of women require surgical repair for a pelvic relaxation syndrome.

Common contributing factors include

- Childbirth (particularly vaginal delivery)
- Obesity
- Aging
- Injury (eg, due to pelvic surgery)
- Chronic straining

Less common factors include congenital malformations, increased abdominal pressure (eg, due to ascites, abdominal tumors, or chronic respiratory disorders), sacral nerve disorders, and connective tissue disorders.

Pelvic relaxation syndromes involve various sites of prolapse and include cystocele, urethrocele, enterocele, rectocele, and uterine and vaginal prolapse. Usually, prolapse occurs in multiple sites.

CYSTOCELES, URETHROCELES, ENTEROCELES, AND RECTOCELES

These disorders involve protrusion of an organ into the vaginal canal: cystoceles (bladder), urethroceles (urethra), enteroceles (small intestine and peritoneum), and rectoceles (rectum). Symptoms include pelvic or vaginal fullness or pressure. Diagnosis is clinical. Treatment includes pessaries, pelvic muscle exercises, and surgery.

Cystocele, urethrocele, enterocele, and rectocele are particularly likely to occur together. Urethrocele is virtually always accompanied by cystocele (cystourethrocele).

Cystocele and cystourethrocele commonly develop when the pubocervical vesical fascia is weakened. Enterocele usually occurs after a hysterectomy. Weakness in the pubocervical fascia and rectovaginal fascia allows the apex of the vagina, which contains the peritoneum and small bowel, to descend. Rectocele results from disruption of the levator ani muscles.

Severity of these disorders can be graded based on level of protrusion:

- 1st degree: To the upper vagina
- 2nd degree: To the introitus
- 3rd degree: External to the introitus

Symptoms and Signs

Pelvic or vaginal fullness, pressure, and a sensation of organs falling out are common. Organs may bulge into the vaginal canal or through the vaginal opening (introitus), particularly during straining or coughing. Dyspareunia can occur.

Mild cases may not cause symptoms until women become older.

Stress incontinence often accompanies cystocele or cystourethrocele. When either of these disorders is severe, urinary retention and overflow incontinence can occur. When sacral nerves are damaged, urge incontinence may also develop.

Enteroceles may cause lower back pain. Rectoceles may cause constipation and incomplete defecation; patients may have to manually press the posterior vaginal wall to defecate.

Diagnosis

- Examination of the anterior or posterior vaginal wall while patients strain

Diagnosis is confirmed by examination.

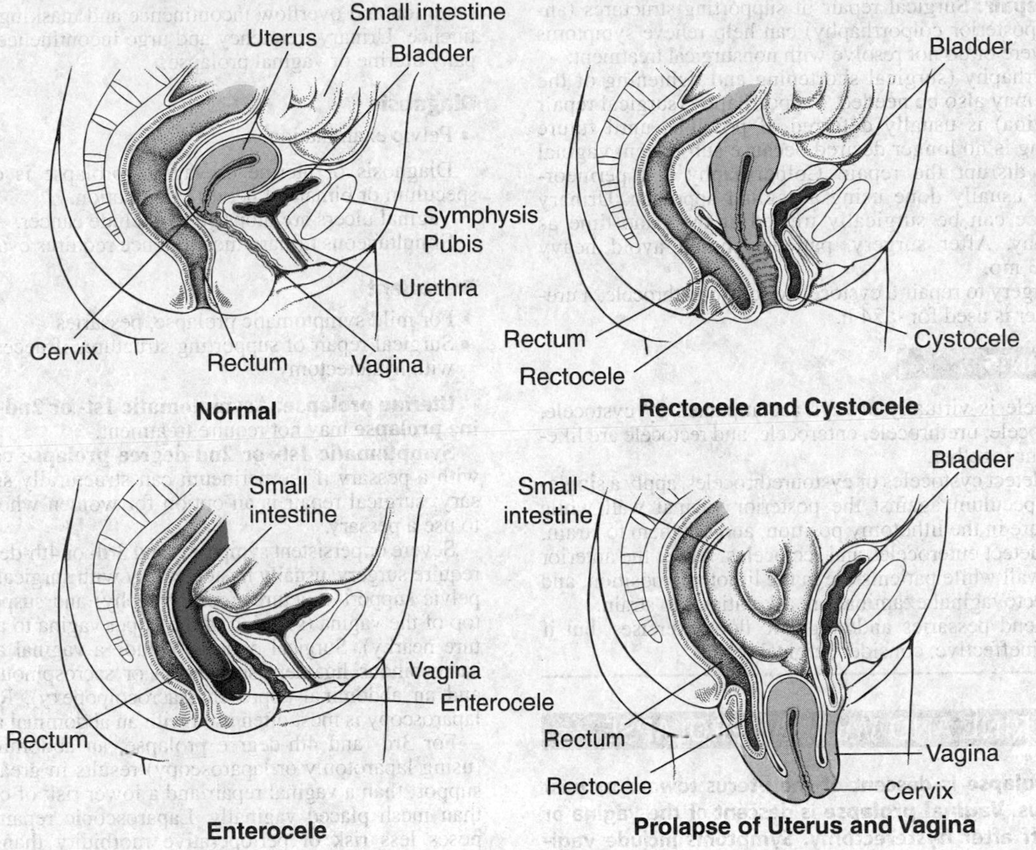

Fig. 274–1. Pelvic relaxation syndromes.

Cystoceles and **cystourethroceles** are detected by applying a single-bladed speculum against the posterior vaginal wall while patients are in the lithotomy position. Asking patients to strain makes cystoceles or cystourethroceles visible or palpable as soft reducible masses bulging into the anterior vaginal wall.

Inflamed paraurethral (Skene) glands are differentiated by their more anterior and lateral urethral location, tenderness, and occasionally expression of pus during palpation. Enlarged Bartholin glands can be differentiated because they develop in the medial labia majora and may be tender if infected.

Enteroceles and **rectoceles** are detected by retracting the anterior vaginal wall while patients are in the lithotomy position. Asking patients to strain can make enteroceles and rectoceles visible and palpable during rectovaginal examination. Patients are also examined while standing with one knee elevated (eg, on a stool) and straining; sometimes abnormalities are detected only by rectovaginal examination during this maneuver.

Urinary incontinence, if present, is also evaluated.

Treatment

- Pessary and pelvic floor exercises (eg, Kegel exercises)
- Surgical repair of supporting structures if necessary

Treatment may initially consist of a pessary and Kegel exercises.

Pessaries: Pessaries are prostheses inserted in the vagina to maintain reduction of the prolapsed structures. Pessaries are of varying shapes and sizes, and some are inflatable. They may cause vaginal ulceration if they are not correctly sized and routinely cleansed (at least monthly if not more frequently). Pessaries can be fitted by health care practitioners; in some countries, pessaries may be available over the counter.

Pelvic floor exercises: Pelvic floor exercises (including Kegel exercises) may be recommended. Kegel exercises involve isometric contractions of the pubococcygeus muscle. These muscles are contracted tightly for about 1 or 2 sec, then relaxed for about 10 sec. Gradually, contractions are held for about 10 sec each. The exercise is repeated about 10 times in a row. Doing the exercises several times a day is recommended.

Exercises can be facilitated by

- Use of weighted vaginal cones (which help patients focus on contracting the correct muscle)
- Biofeedback devices
- Electrical stimulation, which causes the muscle to contract

Pelvic floor exercises can lessen bothersome symptoms of prolapse and stress incontinence but do not appear to reduce the severity of prolapse.

Surgical repair: Surgical repair of supporting structures (anterior and posterior colporrhaphy) can help relieve symptoms that are severe or do not resolve with nonsurgical treatment.

Perineorrhaphy (surgical shortening and tightening of the perineum) may also be needed. Colporrhaphy (surgical repair of the vagina) is usually deferred, if possible, until future childbearing is no longer desired because subsequent vaginal birth may disrupt the repair. Colporrhaphy and perineorrhaphy are usually done using a vaginal approach. Urinary incontinence can be surgically treated at the same time as colporrhaphy. After surgery, patients should avoid heavy lifting for 3 mo.

After surgery to repair a cystocele or cystourethrocele, a urethral catheter is used for < 24 h.

KEY POINTS

- Urethrocele is virtually always accompanied by cystocele, and cystocele, urethrocele, enterocele, and rectocele are likely to occur together.
- To help detect cystoceles or cystourethroceles, apply a single-bladed speculum against the posterior vaginal wall while patients are in the lithotomy position, and ask them to strain.
- To help detect enteroceles and rectoceles, retract the anterior vaginal wall while patients are in the lithotomy position, and during rectovaginal examination, ask patients to strain.
- Recommend pessaries and/or pelvic floor exercises, but if they are ineffective, consider surgical repair.

UTERINE AND VAGINAL PROLAPSE

Uterine prolapse is descent of the uterus toward or past the introitus. Vaginal prolapse is descent of the vagina or vaginal cuff after hysterectomy. Symptoms include vaginal pressure and fullness. Diagnosis is clinical. Treatment includes reduction, pessaries, and surgery.

Uterine prolapse is graded based on level of descent:

- 1st degree: To the upper vagina
- 2nd degree: To the introitus
- 3rd degree: Cervix is outside the introitus
- 4th degree (sometimes referred to as procidentia): Uterus and cervix entirely outside the introitus

Vaginal prolapse may be 2nd or 3rd degree.

Symptoms and Signs

Symptoms tend to be minimal with 1st-degree uterine prolapse. In 2nd- or 3rd-degree uterine prolapse, fullness, pressure, dyspareunia, and a sensation of organs falling out are common. Lower back pain may develop. Incomplete emptying of the bladder and constipation are possible.

Third-degree uterine prolapse manifests as a bulge or protrusion of the cervix or vaginal cuff, although spontaneous reduction may occur before patients present. Vaginal mucosa may become dried, thickened, chronically inflamed, secondarily infected, and ulcerated. Ulcers may be painful or bleed and may resemble vaginal cancer. The cervix, if protruding, may also become ulcerated.

Symptoms of vaginal prolapse are similar. Cystocele or rectocele is usually present.

Urinary incontinence is common. The descending pelvic organs may intermittently obstruct urine flow, causing urinary retention and overflow incontinence and masking stress incontinence. Urinary frequency and urge incontinence may accompany uterine or vaginal prolapse.

Diagnosis

- Pelvic examination

Diagnosis of uterine or vaginal prolapse is confirmed by speculum or bimanual pelvic examination.

Vaginal ulcers are biopsied to exclude cancer.

Simultaneous urinary incontinence requires evaluation.

Treatment

- For mild symptomatic prolapse, pessaries
- Surgical repair of supporting structures if necessary, usually with hysterectomy

Uterine prolapse: Asymptomatic 1st- or 2nd-degree uterine prolapse may not require treatment.

Symptomatic 1st- or 2nd-degree prolapse can be treated with a pessary if the perineum can structurally support a pessary; surgical repair is an option for women who do not wish to use a pessary.

Severe or persistent symptoms and 3rd- or 4th-degree prolapse require surgery, usually hysterectomy with surgical repair of the pelvic support structures (colporrhaphy) and suspension of the top of the vagina (suturing of the upper vagina to a stable structure nearby). Surgical options include a vaginal approach (for sacrospinous ligament suspension or sacrospinous colpopexy) and an abdominal approach (sacrocolpopexy). Robot-assisted laparoscopy is most often used with an abdominal approach.

For 3rd- and 4th-degree prolapse, an abdominal approach (using laparotomy or laparoscopy) results in greater structural support than a vaginal repair and a lower risk of complications than mesh placed vaginally. Laparoscopic repair of prolapse poses less risk of perioperative morbidity than laparotomy. Using mesh may lower the risk of prolapse recurrence after a vaginal repair, but complications may occur more frequently. Patients should be advised that all mesh may not be removed completely so that they can make an informed decision.

Surgery is delayed until all ulcers, if present, have healed.

Vaginal prolapse: Vaginal prolapse is treated similarly to uterine prolapse.

The vagina may be obliterated if women are not good candidates for prolonged surgery (eg, if they have serious comorbidities). Advantages of vaginal obliteration include short duration of surgery, low risk of perioperative morbidity, and very low risk of prolapse recurrence. However, after vaginal obliteration, women are no longer able to have sexual intercourse.

Urinary incontinence requires concurrent treatment.

KEY POINTS

- The descending pelvic organs may intermittently obstruct urine flow, causing urinary retention and overflow incontinence and masking stress incontinence.
- Third-degree uterine prolapse (cervix outside the introitus) may spontaneously reduce before patients present.
- Confirm the diagnosis by examination, but biopsy vaginal or cervical ulcers to exclude cancer.
- Treat with a pessary if prolapse is 1st or 2nd degree and symptomatic and the perineum can support a pessary, or treat with surgery if women prefer it to a pessary.
- Treat surgically if prolapse is 3rd or 4th degree or if symptoms are severe or persistent.

275 Prenatal Genetic Counseling and Evaluation

PRENATAL GENETIC COUNSELING

Prenatal genetic counseling is provided for all prospective parents, ideally before conception, to assess risk factors for congenital disorders. Certain precautions to help prevent birth defects (eg, avoiding teratogens, taking supplemental folic acid—see p. 2323) are recommended for all women who are planning to become pregnant. Parents with risk factors are advised about possible outcomes and options for evaluation. If testing identifies a disorder, reproductive options are discussed.

Preconception options include

- Contraception
- Artificial insemination if the man is a carrier
- Oocyte donation if the woman is a carrier

Postconception options include

- Pregnancy termination
- Maternal antiarrhythmic drugs to treat a fetal arrhythmia
- Transfer care to tertiary center for delivery with more extensive neonatal services

Preimplantation genetic diagnosis is used to identify genetic defects in embryos created through in vitro fertilization before they are implanted. It may be done if a couple has or has a high risk of certain mendelian disorders or chromosomal abnormalities.

Information presented at genetic counseling should be as simple, nondirective, and jargon-free as possible to help anxious couples understand it. Frequent repetition may be necessary. Couples should be given time alone to formulate questions. Couples can be told about information that is available on the Internet (www.acog.org) for many common problems (eg, advanced maternal age, recurrent spontaneous abortions, previous offspring with neural tube defects, previous offspring with trisomy).

Many couples (eg, those with known or suspected risk factors) benefit from referral to genetic specialists for presentation of information and testing options. If a fetal abnormality is suspected, patients can be referred for ongoing care to a center that specializes in neonatal care.

Risk Factors

Some risk of genetic abnormality exists in all pregnancies. Among live births, incidence is

- 0.5% for numeric or structural chromosomal disorders
- 1% for single-gene (mendelian) disorders
- 1% for multiple-gene (polygenic) disorders

Among stillbirths, rates of abnormalities are higher. Most malformations involving a single organ system (eg, neural tube defects, most congenital heart defects) result from polygenic or multifactorial (ie, also influenced by environmental factors) inheritance.

Risk of having a fetus with a chromosomal disorder is increased for most couples who have had a previous fetus or infant with a chromosomal disorder (recognized or missed), except for a few specific types (eg, 45,X; triploidy; de novo chromosomal rearrangements). Chromosomal disorders are more likely to be present in the following:

- Fetuses that spontaneously abort during the 1st trimester (50 to 60%)
- Fetuses with a major malformation (30%; 35 to 38% if submicroscopic abnormalities are included)
- Stillborns (5%)

Rarely, a parent has a chromosomal disorder that increases risk of a chromosomal disorder in the fetus. Asymptomatic parental chromosomal disorders (eg, balanced abnormalities such as certain translocations and inversions) may not be suspected. A balanced parental chromosomal rearrangement should be suspected if couples have had recurrent spontaneous abortions, infertility, or a child with a malformation.

The chance of a fetal chromosomal disorder increases as maternal age increases because rates of nondisjunction (failure of chromosomes to separate normally) during meiosis increase. Among live births, the rate is about

- 0.2% at age 20
- 0.5% at age 35
- 1.5% at age 40
- 14% at age 49

Most chromosomal disorders due to older maternal age involve an extra chromosome (trisomy), particularly trisomy 21 (Down syndrome). Paternal age > 50 increases risk of some spontaneous dominant mutations, such as achondroplasia, in offspring.

Some chromosomal disorders are submicroscopic and thus not identified by traditional karyotyping. The submicroscopic chromosomal abnormalities, sometimes called copy number variants, occur independently of the age-related nondisjunction mechanisms. The precise incidence of these abnormalities is unclear, but incidence is higher in fetuses with structural abnormalities. A multicenter study sponsored by the Eunice Kennedy Shriver National Institute of Child Health and Human Development (NICHD) demonstrated a 1% incidence of clinically relevant copy number variants in fetuses with normal karyotypes independent of indication for testing and a 6% incidence in fetuses with structural abnormalities.[1]

An autosomal dominant disorder is suspected if there is a family history in more than one generation; autosomal disorders affect males and females equally. If one parent has an autosomal dominant disorder, risk is 50% that the disorder will be transmitted to an offspring.

For an autosomal recessive disorder to be expressed, an offspring must receive a mutant gene for that disorder from both parents. Parents may be heterozygous (carriers) and, if so, are usually clinically normal. If both parents are carriers, offspring (male or female) are at a 25% risk of being homozygous for the mutant gene and thus affected, 50% are likely to be heterozygous, and 25% are likely to be genetically normal. If only siblings and no other relatives are affected, an autosomal recessive disorder should be suspected. Likelihood that both parents carry the same autosomal recessive trait is increased if they are consanguineous.

Because females have 2 X chromosomes and males have only one, X-linked recessive disorders are expressed in all males who carry the mutation. Such disorders are usually transmitted through clinically normal, heterozygous (carrier) females. Thus, for each son of a carrier female, risk of having the disorder is 50%, and for each daughter, risk of being a carrier is 50%. Affected males do not transmit the gene to their sons, but they transmit it to all their daughters, who thus are carriers. Unaffected males do not transmit the gene.

1. Wapner RJ, Martin CL, Levy B: Chromosomal microarray versus karyotyping for prenatal diagnosis. *N Engl J Med* 367:2175–2184, 2012.

GENETIC EVALUATION

Genetic evaluation is part of routine prenatal care and is ideally done before conception. The extent of genetic evaluation a woman chooses is related to how the woman weighs factors such as

- The probability of a fetal abnormality based on risk factors and the results of any previous testing
- The probability of a complication from invasive fetal testing
- The importance of knowing the results (eg, would the pregnancy be terminated if an abnormality was diagnosed, would not knowing the results cause anxiety)

For these reasons, the decision is individual, and recommendations often cannot be generalized to all women, even those with similar risk.

A screening history is part of the evaluation. The history is summarized as a pedigree (see Fig. 380–1 on p. 3190). Information should include the health status and presence of genetic disorders or carrier status of both parents, of 1st-degree relatives (parents, siblings, offspring), and of 2nd-degree relatives (aunts, uncles, grandparents), as well as ethnic and racial background and consanguineous matings. Outcomes of previous pregnancies are noted. If genetic disorders are suspected, relevant medical records must be reviewed.

Genetic screening tests are best done before conception. Traditionally, tests are offered to parents at risk of being asymptomatic carriers for certain common mendelian disorders (see Table 275–1). Diagnostic tests for specific abnormalities are offered to parents when appropriate (see Table 275–2). Because parent ethnicity is more complex and less well-defined than previously thought and because prenatal genetic testing is becoming much less expensive and quicker, some clinicians are starting to screen all potential (and expectant) parents, regardless of ethnicity (called universal carrier screening). Consensus on which disorders should be tested for does not yet exist. Increasing the amount of testing and evaluation is expected to increase the complexity of pre-test counseling.

Pregnant women should be offered screening using multiple maternal serum markers (alpha-fetoprotein, beta-human chorionic gonadotropin [beta-hCG], estriol, inhibin A—see p. 2302) to detect neural tube defects, Down syndrome (and other chromosomal abnormalities), and some other birth defects. This screening is called analyte screening. It is done at 15 to 20 wk of pregnancy. An alternate form of screening for

Table 275–1. GENETIC SCREENING FOR SOME ETHNIC GROUPS

ETHNIC GROUP	DISORDER	PARENTAL SCREENING TESTS	PRENATAL DIAGNOSIS
All	Cystic fibrosis	DNA analysis of the 23 most common *CFTR* mutations, each of which is present in ≥ 0.1% of the US population	CVS or amniocentesis for genotype determination*
Ashkenazi Jews[†]	Canavan disease	DNA analysis to detect the most common mutations	CVS or amniocentesis for DNA analysis
	Familial dysautonomia	DNA analysis to detect the most common mutations	CVS or amniocentesis for DNA analysis
	Tay-Sachs disease	Measurement of serum hexosaminidase A to check for deficiency; possibly DNA analysis	CVS or amniocentesis for enzymatic assays or molecular analysis to check for hexosaminidase A; DNA analysis
Blacks	Sickle cell anemia	Hemoglobin electrophoresis	CVS or amniocentesis for genotype determination (direct DNA analysis)
Cajuns	Tay-Sachs disease	Measurement of serum hexosaminidase A to check for deficiency; possibly DNA analysis	CVS or amniocentesis for enzymatic assays or molecular analysis to check for hexosaminidase A
Southeast Asians, Asian Indians, Africans, people from the Mediterranean region and the Middle East	Beta-thalassemia	CBC; if MCV is < 80 fL, hemoglobin electrophoresis	CVS or amniocentesis for genotype determination (direct DNA analysis or linkage analysis)
Southeast Asians, Cambodians, Chinese, Filipinos, Laotians, Vietnamese	Alpha-thalassemia	CBC; if MCV is < 80 fL, hemoglobin electrophoresis	CVS or amniocentesis for genotype determination (direct DNA analysis or linkage analysis)

*Definitive diagnosis is not always possible; sensitivity varies by ethnic group.

[†]For Ashkenazi Jews, some experts also recommend screening for Gaucher disease, Niemann-Pick disease type A, Fanconi syndrome group C, Bloom syndrome, and mucolipidosis IV. Most (90%) Jews are Ashkenazi; thus, Jews who do not know whether they are Ashkenazi should be screened.

CFTR = cystic fibrosis transmembrane conductance regulator; CVS = chorionic villus sampling; MCV = mean corpuscular volume.

Table 275–2. INDICATIONS FOR FETAL GENETIC DIAGNOSTIC TESTS

INDICATION	COMMENTS
Desire for testing	Testing should be offered to all pregnant women, regardless of risk.
Maternal age > 35 at expected delivery	ACOG recommends that all pregnant women be offered invasive testing to assess fetal karyotype, regardless of maternal age.
Recurrent previous spontaneous abortions	Chromosome analysis may be indicated for both parents.
Chromosomal abnormality in a previous child	Chromosome analysis may be indicated for both parents.
Paternal age > 50	Need for testing is controversial.
Parental chromosomal disorder	Not all parental chromosomal rearrangements are associated with risks to offspring.
Suspected parental sex-linked mendelian disorder	—
Autosomal recessive mendelian disorder diagnosed or suspected in both parents	—
Levels of maternal serum markers* suggesting trisomy 21 or trisomy 18	Chorionic villus sampling during the 1st trimester or amniocentesis during the 2nd trimester is done.
Abnormal cell-free DNA analysis from maternal plasma	Chorionic villus sampling during the 1st trimester or amniocentesis during the 2nd trimester is done.
Elevated maternal alpha-fetoprotein and indeterminate ultrasound results	Amniocentesis is done.
Structural abnormalities in the fetus (including increased nuchal translucency in the 1st trimester) noted during ultrasonography	Risk of fetal chromosomal abnormality depends on specific anatomic findings.

*Measured during the 1st or 2nd trimester.
ACOG = American College of Obstetricians and Gynecologists.

fetal Down syndrome or trisomy 18 is with analysis of cell-free DNA (cfDNA) in maternal plasma.

Fetal genetic diagnostic tests: These tests are usually done via chorionic villus sampling, amniocentesis, or, rarely, percutaneous umbilical blood sampling. They can detect all trisomies, many other chromosomal abnormalities, and several hundred mendelian abnormalities. Submicroscopic chromosomal abnormalities are missed by traditional karyotype testing and can be identified only by microarray technologies, such as array comparative genomic hybridization and single nucleotide polymorphism (SNP)–based arrays.

Tests are usually recommended if risk of a fetal chromosomal abnormality is increased (see Table 275–2). Fetal genetic diagnostic tests, unlike screening tests, are usually invasive and involve fetal risk. Thus, in the past, these tests were not routinely recommended for women without risk factors. However, because fetal genetic diagnostic tests are now more widely available and safety has improved, offering fetal genetic testing to all pregnant women, regardless of risk, is recommended. The role of array comparative genomic hybridization in prenatal testing is under study; it is most frequently used to evaluate fetuses with structural abnormalities.

Preimplantation genetic diagnosis may be available for couples who are using in vitro fertilization.

Procedures

All procedures used to diagnose genetic disorders, except ultrasonography, are invasive and involve slight fetal risk. If testing detects a serious abnormality, the pregnancy can be terminated, or in some cases, a disorder can be treated (eg, fetal surgery to repair spina bifida). Even if neither of these possibilities is anticipated, some women prefer to know of fetal abnormalities before birth.

Prenatal Ultrasonography

Some experts recommend ultrasonography routinely for all pregnant women. Others use ultrasonography only for specific indications, such as checking for suspected genetic or obstetric abnormalities or helping interpret abnormal maternal serum marker levels. If ultrasonography is done by skilled operators, sensitivity for major congenital malformations is high. However, some conditions (eg, oligohydramnios, maternal obesity, fetal position) interfere with obtaining optimal images. Ultrasonography is noninvasive and has no known risks to the woman or fetus.

Basic ultrasonography is done to

- Confirm gestational age
- Determine fetal viability
- Detect a multifetal pregnancy
- During the 2nd or 3rd trimester, possibly identify major malformations in the fetal intracranial structures, spine, heart, bladder, kidneys, stomach, thorax, abdominal wall, long bones, and umbilical cord

Although ultrasonography provides only structural information, some structural abnormalities strongly suggest genetic abnormalities. Multiple malformations may suggest a chromosomal disorder.

Targeted ultrasonography, with high-resolution ultrasonography equipment, is available at certain referral centers and provides more detailed images than basic ultrasonography. This test may be indicated for couples with a family history of a congenital malformation (eg, congenital heart defects, cleft lip and palate, pyloric stenosis), particularly one that may be treated effectively before birth (eg, posterior urethral valves with megacystis) or at delivery (eg, diaphragmatic hernia). High-resolution ultrasonography may also be used if maternal serum marker levels are abnormal. High-resolution ultrasonography may allow detection of the following:

- Renal malformations (eg, renal agenesis [Potter syndrome], polycystic kidney disease)
- Lethal forms of short-limbed skeletal dysplasias (eg, thanatophoric skeletal dysplasia, achondrogenesis)
- Gut malformations (eg, obstruction)
- Diaphragmatic hernia
- Microcephalus
- Hydrocephalus

During the 2nd trimester, identifying structures that are statistically associated with increased risk of fetal chromosomal abnormalities helps refine risk estimate.

Amniocentesis

In amniocentesis, a needle is inserted transabdominally, using ultrasonographic guidance, into the amniotic sac to withdraw amniotic fluid and fetal cells for testing, including measurement of chemical markers (eg, alpha-fetoprotein, acetylcholinesterase). The safest time for amniocentesis is after 14 wk gestation. Immediately before amniocentesis, ultrasonography is done to assess fetal cardiac motion and determine gestational age, placental position, amniotic fluid location, and fetal number. If the mother has Rh-negative blood and is unsensitized, Rh_0 (D) immune globulin 300 mcg is given after the procedure to reduce the likelihood of sensitization (see p. 2348).

Amniocentesis has traditionally been offered to pregnant women > 35 because their risk of having an infant with Down syndrome or another chromosomal abnormality is increased. However, with the widespread availability and improved safety of amniocentesis, the American College of Obstetricians and Gynecologists recommends all pregnant women be offered amniocentesis to assess the risk of fetal chromosomal disorders.

Occasionally, the amniotic fluid obtained is bloody. Usually, the blood is maternal, and amniotic cell growth is not affected; however, if the blood is fetal, it may falsely elevate amniotic fluid alpha-fetoprotein level. Dark red or brown fluid indicates previous intra-amniotic bleeding and an increased risk of fetal loss. Green fluid, which usually results from meconium staining, does not appear to indicate increased risk of fetal loss.

Amniocentesis rarely results in significant maternal morbidity (eg, symptomatic amnionitis). With experienced operators, risk of fetal loss is about 0.1 to 0.2%. Vaginal spotting or amniotic fluid leakage, usually self-limited, occurs in 1 to 2% of women tested. Amniocentesis done before 14 wk gestation, particularly before 13 wk, results in a higher rate of fetal loss and an increased risk of talipes equinovarus (clubbed feet).

Chorionic Villus Sampling

In chorionic villus sampling (CVS), chorionic villi are aspirated into a syringe and cultured. CVS provides the same information about fetal genetic and chromosomal status as amniocentesis and has similar accuracy. However, CVS is done between 10 wk gestation and the end of the 1st trimester and thus provides earlier results. Therefore, if needed, pregnancy may be terminated earlier (and more safely and simply), or if results are normal, parental anxiety may be relieved earlier. Unlike amniocentesis, CVS does not enable clinicians to obtain amniotic fluid, and alpha-fetoprotein cannot be measured. Thus, women who have CVS should be offered maternal screening for serum alpha-fetoprotein at 16 to 18 wk to assess risk of fetal neural tube defects.

Depending on placental location (identified by ultrasonography), CVS can be done by passing a catheter through the cervix or by inserting a needle through the woman's abdominal wall. After CVS, Rh_0 (D) immune globulin 300 mcg is given to Rh-negative unsensitized women.

Errors in diagnosis due to maternal cell contamination are rare. Detection of certain chromosomal abnormalities (eg, tetraploidy) may not reflect true fetal status but rather mosaicism confined to the placenta. Confined placental mosaicism is detected in about 1% of CVS specimens. Consultation with experts familiar with these abnormalities is advised. Rarely, subsequent amniocentesis is required to obtain additional information.

Rate of fetal loss due to CVS is similar to that of amniocentesis (ie, about 0.2%). Transverse limb defects and oromandibular-limb hypogenesis have been attributed to CVS but are exceedingly rare if CVS is done after 10 wk gestation by an experienced operator.

Percutaneous Umbilical Blood Sampling

Fetal blood samples can be obtained by percutaneous puncture of the umbilical cord vein (funipuncture) using ultrasound guidance. Chromosome analysis can be completed in 48 to 72 h. For this reason, percutaneous umbilical blood sampling (PUBS) was formerly often done when results were needed rapidly. This test was especially useful late in the 3rd trimester, particularly if fetal abnormalities were first suspected at that time. Now, genetic analysis of amniotic fluid cells or chorionic villi via interphase fluorescent in situ hybridization (FISH) allows preliminary diagnosis (or exclusion) of more common chromosomal abnormalities within 24 to 48 h, and PUBS is rarely done for genetic indications.

Procedure-related fetal loss rate with PUBS is about 1%.

Preimplantation Genetic Testing

Preimplantation genetic testing (PGT) is sometimes possible before implantation when in vitro fertilization is done; polar bodies from oocytes, blastomeres from 6- to 8-cell embryos, or a trophectoderm sample from the blastocyst is used. These tests are available only in specialized centers and are expensive. However, newer techniques may reduce costs and make such tests more widely available. Preimplantation genetic diagnosis (PGD) which checks for specific hereditary disorders is used primarily for couples with a high risk of certain mendelian disorders (eg, cystic fibrosis) or chromosomal abnormalities. Preimplantation genetic screening (PGS) which screens for aneuploidy is used primarily for embryos from older women but does not appear to increase the chance of successful pregnancy.

Noninvasive Maternal Screening Strategies

Noninvasive maternal screening, unlike invasive testing, has no risk of test-related complications. By more precisely assessing the risk of fetal abnormalities, noninvasive maternal screening can help women decide whether to have invasive testing. Noninvasive maternal screening for fetal chromosomal abnormalities should be offered to all pregnant women who have not already decided to have amniocentesis or CVS. However, even if CVS is to be done, maternal serum screening should still be offered to check for fetal neural tube defects.

Normal values vary with gestational age. Corrections for maternal weight, diabetes mellitus, race, and other factors may be necessary. Screening can be done during the 1st trimester, 2nd trimester, or both (called sequential or integrated screening). Any of the 3 approaches is acceptable. Maternal levels of alpha-fetoprotein should be measured during the 2nd trimester to check for neural tube defects.

PEARLS & PITFALLS

- Measure maternal levels of alpha-fetoprotein during the 2nd trimester to check for neural tube defects regardless of other tests planned and the timing of those tests.

1st-Trimester Screening

Traditionally, 1st-trimester combined screening includes measurement of

- Maternal serum beta-hCG (total or free)
- Pregnancy-associated plasma protein A (PAPP-A)
- Fetal nuchal translucency (by ultrasonography)

Fetal Down syndrome is typically associated with high levels of beta-hCG, low levels of PAPP-A, and enlarged fetal nuchal translucency (NT). Although enlarged NT is associated with increased risk of fetal Down syndrome, no threshold NT value is considered diagnostic.

In large prospective US trials involving women of various ages, overall sensitivity for detection of Down syndrome was about 85%, with a false-positive rate of 5%. Specialized ultrasound training and adherence to rigorous quality-assurance monitoring of NT measurements are necessary to achieve this level of screening accuracy.

First-trimester screening should be offered to all pregnant women. It provides information early so that a definitive diagnosis can be made with CVS. An important advantage of 1st-trimester screening is that termination of pregnancy is safer during the 1st rather than the 2nd trimester.

Cell-free fetal nucleic acid testing: An increasingly used approach, called noninvasive prenatal screening or cfDNA screening, can identify fetal chromosomal abnormalities in singleton pregnancies by analyzing circulating cell-free fetal nucleic acids in a maternal blood sample. This test can be done as early as 10 gestational wk and may replace traditional 1st- and 2nd-trimester noninvasive screening.

Cell-free fetal nucleic acids, most commonly DNA fragments, are shed into the maternal circulation during normal breakdown of placental trophoblast cells. Variation in amounts of fragments from particular chromosomes predicts fetal chromosomal abnormalities with higher accuracy than traditional 1st- and 2nd-trimester combined screening using serum analytes and ultrasound. Also, sex chromosomal abnormalities (X, XXX, XYY, and XXY) can be identified in singleton pregnancies, although with somewhat lower accuracy. Early validation trials reported > 99% sensitivity and specificity for the identification of Down syndrome (trisomy 21) and trisomy 18 in high-risk pregnancies. Trisomy 13 can also be detected, although the sensitivity and specificity have not been precisely determined.[1]

Cell-free DNA (cfDNA) screening is currently recommended for women with pre-existing risk factors for fetal trisomy. However, in a recent large multicenter trial that studied the effectiveness of cfDNA screening in a low-risk population, sensitivity for detection of fetal Down syndrome was equivalent to that in a high-risk population. Given the lower incidence of fetal Down syndrome in younger pregnant women, the specificity and positive predictive value were lower than if screening only high-risk women. However, cfDNA screening was superior to traditional analyte screening in low-risk women in overall performance. Cell-free DNA screening has largely replaced serum analyte screening in high-risk women, but screening approaches in low-risk women still rely primarily on traditional, and less expensive, 1st- and 2nd-trimester combined screening with serum analytes and ultrasound.[1]

Abnormal results from cfDNA screening should be confirmed with diagnostic karyotyping using fetal specimens obtained through invasive techniques. Negative results from cfDNA screening will likely reduce the use of routine invasive testing.

1. Norton ME, Jacobsson B, Swamy GK, et al: Cell-free DNA analysis for noninvasive examination of trisomy. *N Engl J Med* 372(17):1589–1597, 2015.

2nd-Trimester Screening

Second-trimester screening may include cfDNA or the multiple marker screening approach, which includes

- Maternal levels of serum alpha-fetoprotein (MSAFP): MSAFP may be used independently as a screen for neural tube defects only, not for risk of Down syndrome. An elevated level suggests open spina bifida, anencephaly, or abdominal wall defects. Unexplained elevations in MSAFP may be associated with increased risk of later pregnancy complications, such as stillbirth or intrauterine growth retardation.
- Maternal levels of beta-hCG, unconjugated estriol, alpha-fetoprotein, and sometimes inhibin A: This screening may be used as an alternative or adjunct to 1st-trimester screening.

Second-trimester multiple marker screening is used to help assess the risk of Down syndrome, trisomy 18, and a few rarer single-gene syndromes (eg, Smith-Lemli-Opitz syndrome). Maternal serum tests are widely available, but detection rates for Down syndrome are not as high as those obtained with 1st-trimester screening or with cfDNA. Also, termination of pregnancy is riskier in the 2nd trimester than in the 1st trimester.

Second-trimester screening may also include

- Targeted ultrasonography

Maternal serum screening for neural tube defects: An elevated level of MSAFP may indicate a fetal malformation such as open spina bifida. Results are most accurate when the initial sample is obtained between 16 and 18 wk gestation, although screening can be done from about 15 to 20 wk. Designating a cutoff value to determine whether further testing is warranted involves weighing the risk of missed abnormalities against the risk of complications from unnecessary testing. Usually, a cutoff value in the 95th to 98th percentile, or 2.0 to 2.5 times the normal pregnancy median (multiples of the median, or MOM), is used. This value is about 80% sensitive for open spina bifida and 90% sensitive for anencephaly. Closed spina bifida is usually not detected. Amniocentesis is eventually required in 1 to 2% of women originally screened. Lower cutoff values of MSAFP increase sensitivity but decrease specificity, resulting in more amniocenteses. Women who have been screened for fetal chromosome disorders by cfDNA should have serum screening with MSAFP alone, not with multiple marker screening.

Ultrasonography is the next step if further testing is warranted. Targeted ultrasonography with or without amniocentesis is done if no explanation can be determined with basic ultrasonography. Ultrasonography can confirm gestational age (which may be underestimated) or detect multifetal pregnancy, fetal death, or congenital malformations. In some women, ultrasonography cannot identify a cause for elevated alpha-fetoprotein levels. Some experts believe that if high-resolution ultrasonography done by an experienced operator is normal, further testing is unnecessary. However, because this test occasionally misses neural tube defects, many experts recommend further testing by amniocentesis regardless of ultrasonography results.

Amniocentesis with measurement of alpha-fetoprotein and acetylcholinesterase levels in amniotic fluid is done if further testing is needed. Elevated alpha-fetoprotein in amniotic fluid suggests

- A neural tube defect
- Another malformation (eg, omphalocele, congenital nephrosis, cystic hygroma, gastroschisis, upper GI atresia)
- Contamination of the sample with fetal blood

Presence of acetylcholinesterase in amniotic fluid suggests

- A neural tube defect
- Another malformation

Elevated alpha-fetoprotein plus presence of acetylcholinesterase in amniotic fluid is virtually 100% sensitive for anencephaly and 90 to 95% sensitive for open spina bifida. Abnormal amniotic fluid markers indicate that a malformation is likely even if high-resolution ultrasonography (which can detect most of these malformations) does not detect a malformation, and parents should be informed.

Maternal serum screening for chromosomal abnormalities: During the 2nd trimester, the most common approach to screening is with cfDNA or multiple serum markers. These markers, adjusted for gestational age, are used mainly to refine estimates of Down syndrome risk beyond that associated with maternal age. With triple screening (ie, alpha-fetoprotein, hCG, and unconjugated estriol), sensitivity for Down syndrome is about 65 to 70%, with a false-positive rate of about 5%.

Quad screening is triple screening plus measurement of inhibin A. Quad screening increases sensitivity to about 80%, with a 5% false-positive rate.

If maternal serum screening suggests Down syndrome, ultrasonography is done to confirm gestational age, and risk is recalculated if the presumed gestational age is incorrect. If the original sample was drawn too early, another one must be drawn at the appropriate time. Amniocentesis is offered particularly if risk exceeds a specific prespecified threshold (usually 1 in 270, which is about the same as risk when maternal age is > 35).

Triple screening can also assess risk of trisomy 18, indicated by low levels of all 3 serum markers. Sensitivity for trisomy 18 is 60 to 70%; the false-positive rate is about 0.5%. Combining ultrasonography and serum screening increases sensitivity to about 80%.

Analysis of cfDNA does not depend on gestational age and thus is not prone to dating errors.

Targeted ultrasonography: Targeted ultrasonography is offered at some perinatal centers and is used to assess risk of chromosomal abnormalities by searching for structural features associated with fetal aneuploidy (so-called soft markers). However, no structural finding is diagnostic for a given chromosomal abnormality, and all soft markers may also be seen in fetuses that are chromosomally normal. Nonetheless, the discovery of such a marker may lead to offering the woman amniocentesis to confirm or exclude a chromosomal abnormality. If a major structural malformation is present, a fetal chromosomal abnormality is more likely.

Disadvantages include unnecessary anxiety if a soft marker is detected and unnecessary amniocentesis. Several experienced centers report high sensitivity, but whether a normal ultrasound indicates a substantially reduced risk of fetal chromosomal abnormalities is unclear.

Sequential 1st- and 2nd-Trimester Screening

Noninvasive 1st-trimester and 2nd-trimester quad screening can be combined sequentially, with invasive fetal genetic testing withheld until results of 2nd-trimester screening are available—whether 1st-trimester test results are abnormal or not. Sequential screening followed by amniocentesis for high-risk patterns increases sensitivity for Down syndrome to 95%, with a false-positive rate of only 5%.

A variation of sequential screening, called contingent sequential screening, is based on the level of risk indicated by 1st-trimester screening:

- High risk: Invasive testing is offered without doing 2nd-trimester screening.
- Intermediate risk: 2nd-trimester screening is offered.
- Low risk (eg, < 1 in 1500): 2nd-trimester screening for Down syndrome is not offered because the 1st-trimester risk is so low.

Patients with abnormal 1st-trimester, 2nd-trimester, or sequential screening may choose to pursue further testing for fetal trisomy with cfDNA (cell free DNA) analysis. Results of cfDNA testing may indicate low risk and be reassuring but are not definitive. Also, cfDNA testing may be inordinately expensive, and awaiting results of cfDNA testing delays definitive testing such as CVS or amniocentesis.[1]

1. Norton ME, Jacobsson B, Swamy GK, et al: Cell-free DNA analysis for noninvasive examination of trisomy. *N Engl J Med* 372(17):1589–1597, 2015.

276 Sexual Dysfunction in Women

Men and women initiate or agree to sexual activity for many reasons, including sharing sexual excitement and physical pleasure and experiencing affection, love, romance, or intimacy. However, women are more likely to report emotional motivations such as

- To experience and encourage emotional intimacy
- To increase their sense of well-being
- To confirm their desirability
- To please or placate a partner

Especially in established relationships, women often have little or no initial sense of sexual desire, but they access sexual desire (responsive desire) once sexual stimulation triggers excitement and pleasure (subjective arousal) and genital congestion (physical genital arousal). Desire for sexual satisfaction, which may or may not include one or multiple orgasms, builds as sexual activity and intimacy continue, and a physically and emotionally rewarding experience fulfills and reinforces the woman's original motivations.

A woman's sexual response cycle is strongly influenced by her mental health and by the quality of her relationship with her partner. Initial desire typically lessens with age but increases with a new partner at any age.

Physiology

Sexual response includes the following:

- Motivation (including desire)
- Subjective arousal
- Genital congestion
- Orgasm
- Resolution

Physiology of the female sexual response is incompletely understood but involves hormonal and CNS factors.

Estrogens influence sexual response. It is suspected but not proved that androgens are involved and act via androgen receptors and estrogen receptors (after intracellular conversion of testosterone to estradiol).

After menopause, ovarian estrogen production ceases, while ovarian androgen production varies. However, adrenal production of prohormones (eg, dehydroepiandrosterone sulfate [DHEAS]) that are converted to both androgens and estrogens in peripheral cells decreases starting in a woman's 30s. Ovarian production of prohormones also declines after menopause. Whether this decrease plays any role in diminishing sexual desire, interest, or subjective arousal is unclear.

The brain produces sex hormones (neurosteroids) from cholesterol, and production may increase after menopause. Whether this documented increase is universal, whether it facilitates arousal as peripheral production decreases, and whether it is affected by exogenous hormone administration are all unknown.

Motivation: Motivation is the wish to engage in sexual activity. There are many reasons for wanting sexual activity, including sexual desire. Desire may be triggered by thoughts, words, sights, smells, or touch. Desire may be obvious at the outset or may build once the woman is aroused.

Arousal: Brain areas involved in cognition, emotion, motivation, and organization of genital congestion are activated. Neurotransmitters acting on specific receptors are involved. Based on known actions of drugs and on animal studies, some neurotransmitters appear to be prosexual; they include dopamine, norepinephrine, and melanocortin. Serotonin is usually sexually inhibitory, as are prolactin and γ-aminobutyric acid (GABA).

Genital congestion: This reflexive autonomic response occurs within seconds of a sexual stimulus and causes genital engorgement and lubrication. The brain's appraisal of the stimulus as biologically sexual, not necessarily as erotic or subjectively arousing, triggers this response. Smooth muscle cells around blood spaces in the vulva, clitoris, and vaginal arterioles dilate, increasing blood flow (engorgement) and transudation of interstitial fluid across the vaginal epithelium (lubrication). Women are not always aware of congestion; genital tingling and throbbing are more typically reported by younger women. As women age, basal genital blood flow decreases, but genital congestion in response to sexual stimuli (eg, erotic videos) may not.

Orgasm: Peak excitement occurs; it is accompanied by contractions of pelvic muscles every 0.8 sec and is followed by slow release of genital congestion. Thoracolumbar sympathetic outflow tracts appear to be involved, but orgasm is possible even after complete spinal cord transection (when a vibrator is used to stimulate the cervix). Prolactin, ADH, and oxytocin are released at orgasm and may contribute to the sense of well-being, relaxation, or fatigue that follows (resolution). However, many women experience a sense of well-being and relaxation without experiencing any definite orgasm.

Resolution: Resolution is a sense of well-being, widespread muscular relaxation, or fatigue that typically follows orgasm. However, resolution can occur slowly after highly arousing sexual activity without orgasm. Many women can respond to additional stimulation almost immediately after resolution.

Classification

Female sexual dysfunction may involve decreased or increased sexual responsiveness. Classification is determined by symptoms. There are 5 major categories of decreased responsiveness and one of increased responsiveness (persistent genital arousal disorder).

Sexual desire/interest disorder is absence of or a decrease in sexual interest, desire, sexual thoughts, and fantasies and an absence of responsive desire.

Sexual arousal disorder is lack of subjective or genital arousal or both.

Orgasmic disorder involves orgasm that is absent, markedly diminished in intensity, or markedly delayed in response to stimulation despite high levels of subjective arousal.

Vaginismus is reflexive tightening around the vagina when vaginal entry is attempted or completed despite women's expressed desire for penetration and when no structural or other physical abnormalities are present.

Dyspareunia is pain during attempted or completed vaginal penetration or intercourse. Provoked vestibulodynia (PVD, formerly called vulvar vestibulitis), the most common type of superficial (introital) dyspareunia, is a chronic pain syndrome associated with altered immune function and sensitization of the nervous system.

Persistent genital arousal disorder involves excessive genital arousal.

A disorder is diagnosed when symptoms cause distress. Some women may not be distressed or bothered by decreased or absent sexual desire, interest, arousal, or orgasm.

Almost all women with sexual dysfunction have features of more than one disorder. For example, the chronic dyspareunia of PVD often leads to sexual desire/interest and arousal disorders; impaired arousal may make sex less enjoyable or even painful, decreasing the likelihood of orgasm and subsequent sexual motivation. However, dyspareunia due to impaired lubrication may occur as an isolated symptom in women with a high level of sexual desire, interest, and subjective arousal.

Female sexual disorders may be secondarily categorized as lifelong or acquired; situation-specific or generalized; and mild, moderate, or severe based on the degree of distress it causes the woman.

Although research is limited, these disorders probably apply equally to women in heterosexual and homosexual relationships.

Etiology

The traditional separation of psychologic and physical etiologies is artificial; psychologic distress causes changes in hormonal and neurologic physiology, and physical changes may generate psychologic reactions that compound the dysfunction. There are often several causes of symptoms within and between categories of dysfunction, and the cause is often unclear.

Primarily psychologic factors: Mood disorders are closely correlated with low desire and arousal. In up to 80% of women with major depression and sexual dysfunction, sexual dysfunction becomes less severe when antidepressants effectively treat the depression. However, sexual dysfunction persists or worsens when antidepressants are ineffective. Women with an anxiety disorder are also more likely to have sexual dysfunction involving desire, arousal, and/or orgasm and to have PVD. Various fears—of letting go, of being vulnerable, of being rejected, or of losing control—and low self-esteem can contribute.

Previous experiences can affect a woman's psychosexual development, as in the following:

- Past negative sexual or other experiences may lead to low self-esteem, shame, or guilt.
- Emotional, physical, or sexual abuse during childhood or adolescence can teach children to control and hide emotions—a useful defense mechanism—but such inhibition can make expressing sexual feelings difficult later.
- Early traumatic loss of a parent or another loved one may inhibit intimacy with a sex partner for fear of similar loss.

Concerns about a negative outcome (eg, unwanted pregnancy, sexually transmitted diseases [STDs], inability to have an orgasm, sexual dysfunction in a partner) can also impair sexual response.

Contextual causes (those specific to a woman's current circumstances) include the following:

- Intrapersonal context: Low sexual self-image (eg, due to infertility, premature menopause, or surgical removal of a breast, the uterus, or another body part associated with sex)
- Relationship context: Lack of trust, negative feelings, or reduced attraction toward a sex partner (eg, due to the partner's behavior or to a growing awareness of a change in sexual orientation)
- Sexual context: For example, surroundings that are not sufficiently erotic, private, or safe
- Cultural context: For example, cultural restrictions on sexual activity

Distractions (eg, from family, work, or finances) can interfere with arousal.

Primarily physical factors: Various genital lesions, systemic and hormonal factors, and drugs may lead or contribute to dysfunction (see Table 276–1).

SSRIs are a particularly common drug cause.

Although in the future, androgens may be shown to influence women's sexual response, current evidence is weak. Some evidence suggests that testosterone supplementation may modestly benefit women who have low desire but are able to have satisfactory sexual experiences. Total androgen activity (measured as metabolites) is similar in women with or without desire.

Alcohol dependence can cause sexual dysfunction.

Table 276–1. SOME PHYSICAL FACTORS CONTRIBUTING TO FEMALE SEXUAL DYSFUNCTION

CATEGORY	FACTOR
Genital lesions	Atrophic vaginitis Congenital malformations Genital herpes simplex Lichen sclerosus Postsurgical introital narrowing Radiation fibrosis Recurrent tearing of the posterior fourchette Vaginal infections Vulvar dystrophies
Other physical factors	Bilateral oophorectomy in premenopausal women Debility Fatigue Hyperprolactinemia Thyroid disorders, hypoadrenal states, hypopituitary states Nerve damage (eg, due to diabetes, multiple sclerosis, or spinal cord dysfunction)
Drugs	Alcohol Gonadotropin-releasing hormone agonists Anticonvulsants β-Blockers Certain antidepressants, particularly SSRIs

Diagnosis

- Interview with both partners, separately and together
- Pelvic examination, primarily to identify causes of dyspareunia

Diagnosis of sexual dysfunction and its causes is based on history and physical examination. Ideally, history is taken from both partners, interviewed separately and together; it begins by asking the woman to describe the problem in her own words and should include specific elements (see Table 276–2). Problematic areas (eg, past negative sexual experiences, negative sexual self-image) identified at the first visit can be investigated more fully at a follow-up visit.

Physical examination is most important for determining causes of dyspareunia; the technique may differ slightly from that used in a routine gynecologic examination. Explaining what will occur during the examination helps the woman relax and should be continued throughout the examination. The woman should be asked whether she wants to sit up and view her genitals in a mirror during the examination; doing so may impart a sense of control.

Wet-preparation examination of vaginal discharge and Gram stain with culture or DNA probe to detect *Neisseria gonorrhoeae* and chlamydiae are indicated when history or examination suggests vulvitis, vaginitis, or pelvic inflammatory disease.

Although low estrogen activity may contribute to sexual dysfunction, measuring levels is rarely indicated. Low estrogen is detected clinically. Sexual function does not correlate with testosterone levels, regardless of how they are measured. If hyperprolactinemia is clinically suspected, the prolactin level is measured. If a thyroid disorder is clinically suspected, appropriate testing is done; it includes TSH if hypothyroidism is suspected, thyroxine (T_4) if hyperthyroidism is suspected, and sometimes other thyroid function tests.

Treatment

- Explanation of the female sexual response to the couple
- Correction of contributing factors
- Substitution of other antidepressants for SSRIs or addition of bupropion
- Psychologic therapies

Treatment varies by disorder and cause; often, more than one treatment is required because disorders overlap. Sympathetic understanding of the patient and careful evaluation may themselves be therapeutic. Contributing factors are corrected if possible. Mood disorders are treated. Explaining what is involved in the female sexual response may also help.

Because SSRIs may contribute to several categories of sexual dysfunction, switching to an antidepressant that has fewer sexual adverse effects (eg, bupropion, moclobemide, mirtazapine, duloxetine) may be considered. Alternatively, some evidence suggests that adding bupropion to an SSRI may help.

Psychologic therapies are the mainstay of treatment. Cognitive-behavioral therapy targets the negative and often

Table 276–2. COMPONENTS OF THE SEXUAL HISTORY FOR ASSESSMENT OF FEMALE SEXUAL DYSFUNCTION

AREA	SPECIFIC ELEMENTS
Medical history (past and current)	General health (including physical energy, level of stress and anxiety, psychiatric history, and mood), drugs, pregnancies, pregnancy terminations, STDs, contraception, use of safe sex practices
Relationship with partner	Sexual orientation, emotional intimacy, trust, respect, attraction, communication, fidelity, anger, hostility, resentment
Current sexual context	Sexual function of partner, activities and behaviors during the hours before attempts at sexual activity, adequacy of sexual stimulation, adequacy of sexual communication, timing (eg, too late at night, too hurried), degree of privacy
Triggers of desire and arousal	Setting; visual, written and spoken sexual cues; activities (eg, showering together, dancing, listening to music); types of stimulation (nonphysical, physical nongenital, nonpenetrative genital)
Inhibitors of arousal	Fatigue, stress, anxiety, depression, negative past sexual experiences, fears about outcome (including loss of control, pain, unwanted pregnancy, and infertility), day-to-day distractions
Orgasms	Presence or absence, response to absence (whether the woman is distressed or not), differences in responses with partner and with self-stimulation
Outcome	Emotional and physical satisfaction or dissatisfaction
Quality and location of pain in dyspareunia	Burning, tearing, rubbing, stretching, or dull Superficial (introital) or deeper in pelvis
Timing of pain in dyspareunia	During partial or full entry, deep thrusting, penile movement, or the man's ejaculation; immediately after penetration; or during urination after vaginal penetration
Self-image	Self-confidence; feelings about desirability, body, genitals, or sexual competence
Developmental history	Relationship with caregivers and siblings, traumas, loss of a loved one, abuse (emotional, physical, or sexual), consequences of expressing emotions as a child, cultural or religious restrictions
Past sexual experiences	Type (whether desired, coercive, abusive, or a combination), subjective experience (how rewarding, varied, and pleasing), outcomes (positive or negative—eg, unplanned pregnancy, STDs, parental or societal disapproval, guilt due to religious teachings)
Personality factors	Ability to trust, comfort level with being vulnerable, suppressed anger causing suppression of sexual emotions, need to feel in control, unreasonable expectations of self, hypervigilance to self-harm (ie, worry about pain, which inhibits enjoyment), obsessiveness, anxiety, depressive tendencies

STDs = sexually transmitted diseases.

catastrophic self-view resulting from illness (including gynecologic disorders) or from infertility.

Mindfulness, an eastern practice with roots in Buddhist meditation, may help. It focuses on nonjudgmental awareness of the present moment. Its practice helps free women from distractions that interfere with attention to sexual sensations. Mindfulness lessens sexual dysfunction in healthy women and in women who have pelvic cancer or PVD. Women can be referred to community or Internet resources to learn how to practice mindfulness. Mindfulness-based cognitive therapy (MBCT) combines an adapted form of cognitive-behavioral therapy with mindfulness. As in cognitive-behavioral therapy, women are encouraged to identify maladaptive thoughts, but then to simply observe their presence, realizing that they are just mental events and may not reflect reality. This approach can make such thoughts less distracting. MBCT is used to prevent recurrent depression and can be adapted to treat sexual arousal disorder and sexual desire/interest disorder as well as the chronic pain of PVD.

KEY POINTS

- Psychologic and physical factors usually contribute to female sexual dysfunction; they may interact, worsening dysfunction.
- Psychologic factors include mood disorders, effects of past experiences, concerns about a negative outcome, the woman's specific circumstances (eg, low sexual self-image), and distractions.
- Physical factors include genital lesions, systemic and hormonal factors, and drugs (particularly SSRIs).
- Interview both partners, separately and together.
- Usually, use psychologic therapies (eg, cognitive-behavioral therapy, mindfulness, a combination of the two [MBCT]).

SEXUAL DESIRE/INTEREST DISORDER

Sexual desire/interest disorder is absence of or a decrease in sexual interest, desire, sexual thoughts, and fantasies and absence of responsive desire.

In sexual desire/interest disorder, motivations to become sexually aroused are scarce or absent. The decrease is greater than what might be expected based on a woman's age and the relationship duration.

Causes often involve primarily psychologic factors (eg, depression, anxiety, stress, relationship problems) and/or unrewarding experiences (eg, due to lack of sexual skills or poor communication of needs). Use of certain drugs, such as SSRIs (particularly), some anticonvulsants, and β-blockers, can reduce sexual desire, as can drinking excessive amounts of alcohol. Fluctuations and changes in hormone levels (eg, at menopause, during pregnancy, with the menstrual cycle) can affect sexual desire. For example, atrophic vaginitis and hyperprolactinemia may contribute.

Women with sexual desire/interest disorder tend to be anxious, to have a low self-image, and to have mood lability even if they do not have a clinical mood disorder.

Diagnosis is clinical (see p. 2304).

Treatment

- Education
- Psychologic therapies
- Hormonal therapy

If factors that limit trust, respect, attraction, and emotional intimacy between partners are the cause, the couple should be counseled that emotional intimacy is a normal requirement for female sexual response and needs to be enhanced with or without professional help. Education about sufficient and appropriate stimuli may help; women may need to remind their partner of their need for nonphysical, physical nongenital, and nonpenetrative genital stimulation. Recommendations for more intensely erotic stimuli and fantasies may help eliminate distractions; practical suggestions to improve privacy and a sense of security can help when fear of unwanted outcomes (eg, discovery, pregnancy, sexually transmitted diseases) inhibits arousability.

For patient-specific psychologic factors, psychologic therapies (eg, cognitive-behavioral therapy) may be required, although simple awareness of the importance of psychologic factors may be sufficient for women to change patterns of thinking and behavior. MBCT (see p. 2304), typically used in small groups of women, can improve arousal, orgasm, and subsequent desire and motivation.

Hormonal causes require targeted treatment—eg, topical estrogen for atrophic vaginitis or bromocriptine for hyperprolactinemia.

Systemic estrogen therapy: Systemic estrogen therapy (see p. 2276) initiated at menopause or within the next few years may improve mood and help maintain skin and genital sexual sensitivity and vaginal lubrication. These benefits may enhance sexual desire and arousal. Transdermal preparations of estrogen are usually preferred after menopause, but no studies identify which preparations available in the US are the most beneficial sexually. Progestins or progesterone is also given to women who have not had a hysterectomy.

Testosterone therapy: Benefits and risks of postmenopausal testosterone supplementation continue to be studied. Early studies in sexually healthy postmenopausal women who had some sexually satisfying experiences before treatment—most of whom were taking estrogen—showed modest efficacy. Thus, when no interpersonal, contextual, and intrapersonal factors were evident, some experienced clinicians have considered supplementation (eg, with methyltestosterone 1.5 mg po once/day or transdermal testosterone 300 mcg daily; transdermal preparations formulated for men are used). However, recent studies in sexually healthy postmenopausal women who were not depressed and who did not have relationship problems—about half of whom were taking estrogen—show no benefit with testosterone.

Taking testosterone might benefit some women who are taking estrogen and who have premature ovarian failure due to other conditions (eg, adrenal or pituitary dysfunction, chemotherapy, idiopathic). Taking testosterone might also benefit postmenopausal women who are taking estrogen therapy, who can no longer be aroused by previously effective stimuli and contexts, and who, as a result, have unsatisfactory sexual experiences. However, these groups have not been studied, so no recommendations can be given.

Too little is known about the long-term safety and efficacy of testosterone therapy to recommend it. However, if it is prescribed, full explanation of conflicting efficacy data and lack of long-term safety data, as well as periodic follow-up is essential. Periodically, the free testosterone level should be calculated or the bioavailable testosterone level should be measured (see p. 2129); if either is above the normal range for premenopausal women, the testosterone dose is decreased. Women should also be checked for hirsutism. Mammography should be done to check for breast changes because the evidence concerning testosterone's effect on the risk of breast cancer is conflicting. Tests should also be done to check for hyperlipidemia and impaired glucose tolerance.

SEXUAL AROUSAL DISORDERS

Sexual arousal disorders involve a lack of subjective arousal or of physical genital response to sexual stimulation—nongenital, genital, or both.

Sexual arousal disorders can be categorized as subjective, genital, or combined. All definitions are clinically based, distinguished in part by the woman's response to genital and nongenital stimulation, as follows:

- **Subjective:** Women do not feel aroused by any type of sexual genital or nongenital stimulation (eg, kissing, dancing, watching an erotic video, physical stimulation), despite the occurrence of physical genital response (eg, genital congestion).
- **Genital:** Subjective arousal occurs in response to nongenital stimulation (eg, an erotic video) but not in response to genital stimulation. This disorder typically affects postmenopausal women and is often described as genital deadness. Vaginal lubrication and/or genital sexual sensitivity is reduced.
- **Combined:** Subjective arousal in response to any type of sexual stimulation is absent or low, and women report absence of physical genital arousal (ie, they report the need of external lubricants and may state they know that swelling of the clitoris no longer occurs).

Etiology

Causes may involve psychologic (eg, depression, low self-esteem, anxiety, stress, distractibility) or physical factors or both (see p. 2303). Inadequate sexual stimulation or the wrong setting for sexual activity can also contribute.

Genital arousal disorder may result from a low level of estrogen after menopause or postpartum. Age-related reduction of testosterone or vulval dystrophy (eg, lichen sclerosus) may contribute. Certain chronic disorders (eg, diabetes, multiple sclerosis) can damage autonomic or somatic nerves, leading to decreased congestion or sensation in the genital area.

Diagnosis

Diagnosis is clinical (see p. 2304).

Treatment

Subjective arousal disorder: Treatment is similar to that of sexual desire/interest disorder.

Genital arousal disorder: When estrogen is deficient, initial treatment is vaginal estrogen (or systemic estrogen if indicated for other postmenopausal symptoms). Other investigational therapy includes vaginal dehydroepiandrosterone (DHEA) 13 mg at night. This drug may increase lubrication and lessen vulvovaginal atrophy in 2 wk and improve genital sensitivity and orgasm in 12 wk. This drug does not appear to increase serum testosterone or estrogen. It modestly increases serum DHEA, but levels are still considerably lower than those in younger women.

ORGASMIC DISORDER

Orgasmic disorder involves orgasm that is absent, markedly diminished in intensity, or markedly delayed in response to stimulation despite high levels of subjective arousal.

Women with orgasmic disorder often have difficulty relinquishing control in nonsexual circumstances.

Contextual factors (eg, consistently insufficient foreplay, early ejaculation by the partner, poor communication about sexual preferences), psychologic factors (eg, anxiety, stress, lack of trust in a partner, fear of not being in control), and drugs can contribute to orgasmic disorder (see p. 2303). Lack of knowledge about sexual function may also contribute.

Damage to genital sensory or autonomic nerves (eg, due to diabetes or multiple sclerosis), vulval dystrophy (eg, lichen sclerosus), or, much more commonly, use of SSRIs may lead to orgasmic disorder.

Treatment

- Self-stimulation
- Psychologic therapies

Data support encouraging self-stimulation. A vibrator placed on the mons pubis close to the clitoris may help, as may increasing the number and intensity of stimuli (mental, visual, tactile, auditory, written), simultaneously if necessary. Education about sexual function (eg, need to stimulate other areas of the body before the clitoris) may help.

Psychologic therapies, including cognitive-behavioral therapy and psychotherapy, may help women identify and manage fear of relinquishing control, fear of vulnerability, or issues of trust with a partner. Recommending the practice of mindfulness and using MBCT (see p. 2304) can help women pay attention to sexual sensations (by staying in the moment) and not judge or monitor these sensations.

In women taking an SSRI, symptoms may decrease when bupropion is added. One study supports the use of sildenafil.

VAGINISMUS

Vaginismus is reflexive tightening around the vagina when vaginal entry is attempted or completed (eg, using a penis, finger, or dildo) despite women's expressed desire for penetration and despite the absence of any structural or other physical abnormalities.

Vaginismus usually results from fear that intercourse will be painful; it usually begins with the first attempt at sexual intercourse but may develop later after periods of stress. Women may develop a phobia-like avoidance of penetration. Most women with vaginismus thus cannot tolerate full or often even partial penetration. Some cannot tolerate insertion of a tampon or have never wanted to try. However, most women with vaginismus enjoy nonpenetrative sexual activity.

Reflex muscle tightening can also accompany dyspareunia of any cause, thereby adding to the pain and difficulty with entry. Women anticipate a recurrence of pain when intercourse is initiated, and muscles tighten, making attempts at sexual intercourse even more painful.

Diagnosis

- Clinical evaluation

Diagnosis is suspected based on symptoms. Physical abnormalities that cause pain, such as those that cause dyspareunia should be excluded by physical examination. However, the condition itself makes examination difficult. One strategy is to initiate treatment as described below and defer the confirmatory examination. When the examination is done, the physician can give the patient a sense of control by having her sit up and view her genitals using a mirror. The woman then spreads her labia and inserts her or the examiner's gloved finger past the hymen as she bears down. This simple digital examination can simultaneously confirm a normal vagina and the presumed diagnosis of vaginismus.

Treatment

- Progressive desensitization

In progressive desensitization, women progressively accustom themselves to self-touch near, on, and then through the introitus.

- The woman first touches herself daily as close to the introitus as possible, separating the labia with her fingers.
- Once her fear and anxiety due to introital self-touch has diminished, the woman will be more able to tolerate the physical examination.
- The next stage is to insert her finger past her hymen; pushing or bearing down during insertion enlarges the opening and eases entry.
- Once finger insertion causes no discomfort, vaginal cones in gradually increasing sizes are inserted progressively; leaving a cone inside for 10 to 15 min helps perivaginal muscles become accustomed to gently increasing pressure without reflex contraction. The woman first inserts a cone herself; when comfortable with the cone, she then allows her partner to help her insert one during a sexual encounter to confirm that it can go in comfortably when she is sexually excited.
- Once insertion in this context is comfortable, the couple should include penile vulvar stimulation during sexual play so that the woman becomes accustomed to feeling the penis on her vulva.
- Ultimately, the woman inserts her partner's penis partially or fully, holding it like an insert. She may feel more confident in the woman superior position.

Some men experience situational erectile dysfunction in this process and may benefit from a phosphodiesterase inhibitor.

DYSPAREUNIA

Dyspareunia is pain during attempted or completed vaginal penetration.

Dyspareunia may occur at the moment of penetration (superficial or introital), with deeper entry, with penile movement, or postcoitally. Some pelvic muscle hypertonicity, manifested as both voluntary guarding and involuntary high muscle tension, is common in all types of chronic dyspareunia.

Etiology

Causes may involve psychologic and physical factors (see p. 2303).

Superficial dyspareunia may result from provoked vestibulodynia (PVD), atrophic vaginitis, vulvar disorders (eg, lichen sclerosus, vulvar dystrophies), congenital malformations, genital herpes simplex, radiation fibrosis, postsurgical introital narrowing, or recurrent tearing of the posterior fourchette.

Deep dyspareunia may result from pelvic muscle hypertonicity or uterine or ovarian disorders (eg, fibroids, chronic pelvic inflammatory disease, endometriosis).

Penile size and depth of penetration influence presence and severity of symptoms.

Women with dyspareunia due to PVD tend to have high self-expectations, fear of negative evaluation by other people, increased somatization, catastrophizing (gross exaggeration of possible consequences), low pain thresholds in general, hypervigilance to pain, and often other chronic pain syndromes (eg, irritable bowel syndrome, temporomandibular joint disorder, interstitial cystitis).

Diagnosis

- Clinical evaluation

Diagnosis is based on symptoms and a pelvic examination.

For superficial dyspareunia, evaluation focuses on inspecting all the vulvar skin, including the creases between the labia minora and majora (eg, for fissures typical of chronic candidiasis), and the clitoral hood, urethral meatus, hymen, and openings of major vestibular gland ducts (for atrophy, signs of inflammation, and abnormal skin lesions requiring biopsy. PVD can be diagnosed using a cotton swab to elicit allodynia (pain caused by a nonnoxious stimulus); nonpainful external areas are touched before moving to more typically painful areas (ie, outer edge of the hymenal ring, clefts adjacent to the urethral meatus). Pelvic muscle hypertonicity may be suspected if pain similar to the pain that occurs during intercourse can be elicited by palpating the deep levator ani muscles, particularly around the ischial spines. Palpating the urethra and bladder may identify abnormal tenderness.

For deep dyspareunia, evaluation requires a careful bimanual examination to determine whether cervical motion or uterine or adnexal palpation causes pain and to check for nodules in the cul-de-sac or vaginal fornices. A rectovaginal examination is usually indicated to check the rectovaginal septum and posterior surface of the uterus and adnexa. Suspected uterine and ovarian disorders are evaluated with imaging studies as clinically indicated.

Treatment

- Treatment of cause when possible (eg, topical estrogen for atrophic vaginitis, pelvic physical therapy for pelvic muscle hypertonicity)
- Education about chronic pain and its effects on sexuality
- Psychologic therapies

Management frequently includes the following:

- Encouraging and teaching the couple to develop satisfying forms of nonpenetrative sex
- Discussing psychologic issues contributing to and caused by the chronic pain
- When possible, treating the primarily physical abnormality that contributes to pain (eg, endometriosis, lichen sclerosus, vulvar dystrophies, vaginal infections, congenital malformations, radiation fibrosis—see elsewhere in The Manual).
- Treating coexisting pelvic muscle hypertonicity
- Treating comorbid sexual desire/interest or arousal disorders

Topical estrogen is helpful for atrophic vaginitis (see p. 2276) and recurrent posterior fourchette tearing. A topical anesthetic or sitz baths may help relieve superficial dyspareunia.

Psychologic therapies such as cognitive-behavioral therapy, mindfulness, and mindfulness-based cognitive therapy (see p. 2305) can often help.

Women with pelvic muscle hypertonicity, including some with PVD, may benefit from pelvic physical therapy using pelvic floor muscle training, possibly with biofeedback, to teach pelvic muscle relaxation.

PROVOKED VESTIBULODYNIA

Provoked vestibulodynia (PVD—formerly called vulvar vestibulitis, localized vulvar dysesthesia) is the most common type of superficial (introital) dyspareunia. Pain results from introital pressure. Treatment includes psychologic therapies used in chronic pain syndromes. Adjunctive therapies include topical lidocaine or cromoglycate, but when they are used alone, their efficacy is unproved.

PVD develops when the nervous system—from peripheral receptors to the cerebral cortex—is sensitized and remodeled. With sensitization, discomfort due to a stimulus that might otherwise be perceived as mild or trivial (eg, touch) is instead perceived as significant pain (allodynia). This disorder is considered to probably be a chronic pain syndrome (see p. 1973). The peripheral sensitization leads to a neurogenic inflammatory response. A small group of women have PVD and vulvovaginal candidiasis, which appears to contribute to PVD.

Symptoms and Signs

In vestibulodynia, introital pressure, penile movement, or a man's ejaculation typically causes immediate pain. Pain typically lessens when penile (or dildo) movement stops and resumes when it starts again. Vestibulodynia may also cause postcoital vulvar burning and dysuria.

Diagnosis

- Clinical evaluation

Diagnosis is based on symptoms and confirmed by the Q-tip test for allodynia. Vaginismus causes similar pain during introital pressure and penile containment and movement. However, vaginismus, unlike vestibulodynia, classically does not cause allodynia or postcoital symptoms. Some women who have allodynia have a history that strongly suggests vaginismus (ie, phobia-like avoidance of vaginal penetration), suggesting that vestibulodynia can develop secondary to vaginismus and that allodynia and vaginismus overlap.

Treatment

- Psychologic therapies used in chronic pain management
- Treating sexual dysfunction secondary to the pain
- Pelvic physical therapy
- Adjunctive drugs to treat chronic pain
- Possibly topical lidocaine or cromoglycate before penetration

Optimal treatment of PVD is unclear; many approaches are currently used, and there are probably still undefined subtypes that require different treatment. Because this disorder involves chronic pain, treatments are becoming more comprehensive, including management of stress and therapies to target the thoughts and emotions that accompany the pain.

Small-group therapy that combines mindfulness-based cognitive therapy or cognitive-behavioral therapy (see p. 2305) with education about chronic pain, PVD, sexuality, and stress appears to be beneficial. Adjunctive drug therapy (eg, with tricyclic antidepressants or anticonvulsants) is also sometimes used.

Once penetration seems worth trying, topical drugs (eg, 2% cromoglycate or 2% or 5% lidocaine in glaxal base) can be used to interrupt chronic pain circuits. Cromoglycate stabilizes WBC membranes, including those of mast cells, interrupting neurogenic inflammation due to PVD. Cromoglycate or lidocaine must be placed precisely on the area of allodynia using a 1-mL syringe without a needle. Physician supervision and use of a mirror (at least initially) are helpful.

Women with pelvic muscle hypertonicity may benefit from pelvic physical therapy using pelvic floor muscle training, possibly with biofeedback.

Surgery, consisting of excision of the hymen, proximal edge of the lower vagina, and innermost portion of the labia minora, is sometimes offered, usually to women who do not have depression, anxiety, or involvement of the introital rim next to the urethral meatus if they previously had pain-free intercourse and are willing to also participate in psychologic therapy. However, pain may recur as nerves regenerate.

Some women with PVD and vaginal candidiasis benefit from long-term candidal prophylaxis (eg, weekly vaginal boric acid capsules).

KEY POINTS

- PVD (a chronic pain syndrome) is local pain that results from nonnoxious introital pressure.
- Introital pressure (eg, due to penile or dildo movement or ejaculation) immediately causes pain, which usually lessens when the pressure stops.
- Confirm the diagnosis by provocation of pain with a Q-tip.
- Use psychologic therapies, sometimes supplemented with drugs and/or pelvic physical therapy.

PERSISTENT GENITAL AROUSAL DISORDER

Persistent genital arousal disorder is excessive unwanted unprovoked genital arousal.

Cause is unknown. Anxiety and hypervigilance for recurrence of pain episodes may perpetuate the syndrome. Symptoms are currently thought to result from pelvic muscle hypertonicity.

Unwanted, intrusive, spontaneous genital arousal (eg, tingling, throbbing) occurs, without any sexual desire or subjective arousal. The sensations persist for hours or days and typically cause great distress. Older women, especially, may be very embarrassed by the symptoms.

Treatment

Treatment is unclear. Self-stimulation to orgasm may provide relief initially, but this treatment usually becomes less effective over time, and most women find this treatment distressing.

Pelvic muscle physical therapy with biofeedback may help, especially when it is combined with mindfulness-based cognitive therapy (see p. 2304). High-dose SSRI therapy has been reported effective, but data are few.

Simple recognition of the existence of this disorder, with reassurance that it can spontaneously remit, may help some patients.

277 Uterine Fibroids

(Leiomyomas; Myomas)

Uterine fibroids are benign uterine tumors of smooth muscle origin. Fibroids frequently cause abnormal uterine bleeding, pelvic pain and pressure, urinary and intestinal symptoms, and pregnancy complications. Diagnosis is by pelvic examination, ultrasonography, or other imaging. Treatment of symptomatic patients depends on the patient's desire for fertility and her desire to keep her uterus. Treatment may include oral contraceptives, brief presurgical gonadotropin-releasing hormone therapy to shrink fibroids, progestin therapy, and more definitive surgical procedures (eg, hysterectomy, myomectomy).

Uterine fibroids are the most common pelvic tumor, occurring in about 70% of women by age 45. However, many fibroids are small and asymptomatic. About 25% of white and 50% of black women eventually develop symptomatic fibroids. Fibroids are more common among women who have a high body mass index. Potentially protective factors include parturition and cigarette smoking.

Most fibroids in the uterus are subserosal, followed by intramural, then submucosal (see Fig. 277–1). Occasionally, fibroids occur in the broad ligaments (intraligamentous), fallopian tubes, or cervix.

Some fibroids are pedunculated. Most fibroids are multiple, and each develops from a single smooth muscle cell, making them monoclonal in origin. Because they respond to estrogen, fibroids tend to enlarge during the reproductive years and decrease in size after menopause.

Fibroids may outgrow their blood supply and degenerate. Degeneration is described as hyaline, myxomatous, calcific, cystic, fatty, red (usually only during pregnancy), or necrotic. Although patients are often concerned about cancer in fibroids, sarcomatous change occurs in < 1% of patients.

Symptoms and Signs

Fibroids can cause abnormal uterine bleeding (eg, menorrhagia, menometrorrhagia).

If fibroids grow and degenerate or if pedunculated fibroids twist, severe acute or chronic pressure or pain can result.

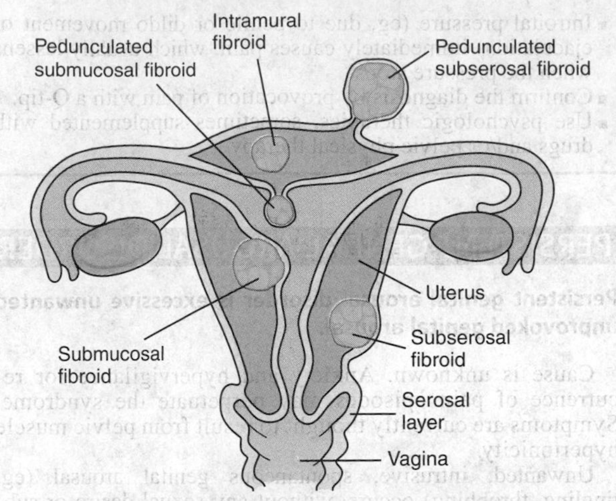

Fig. 277–1. Where fibroids grow. Fibroids may be

- Intramural (in the wall of the uterus)
- Submucosal (under the lining of the uterus)
- Subserosal (under the outer surface of the uterus)
- Pedunculated (growing on a stalk)

Urinary symptoms (eg, urinary frequency or urgency) can result from bladder compression, and intestinal symptoms (eg, constipation) can result from intestinal compression.

Fibroids may increase risk of infertility. During pregnancy, they may cause recurrent spontaneous abortion, premature contractions, or abnormal fetal presentation or make cesarean delivery necessary.

Diagnosis

- Imaging (ultrasonography, saline infusion sonography, or MRI)

The diagnosis of uterine fibroids is likely if bimanual pelvic examination detects an enlarged, mobile, irregular uterus that is palpable. Confirmation requires imaging, which is usually indicated if

- Fibroids are a new finding.
- They have increased in size.
- They are causing symptoms.
- They need to be differentiated from other abnormalities (eg, ovarian masses).

When imaging is indicated, ultrasonography (usually transvaginal) or saline infusion sonography (sonohysterography) is typically done. In saline infusion sonography, saline is instilled into the uterus, enabling the sonographer to more specifically locate the fibroid in the uterus.

If ultrasonography, including saline infusion sonography (if done), is inconclusive, MRI, the most accurate imaging test, is usually done.

Treatment

- Sometimes gonadotropin-releasing hormone (GnRH) agonists (analogs) or other drugs for temporary relief of minor symptoms
- Myomectomy (to preserve fertility) or hysterectomy for symptomatic fibroids

Asymptomatic fibroids do not require treatment. Patients should be reevaluated periodically (eg, every 6 to 12 mo).

For **symptomatic fibroids**, medical options, including suppression of ovarian hormones to stop the bleeding, are suboptimal and limited. However, clinicians should consider first trying medical treatment before doing surgery. GnRH agonists can be given before surgery to shrink fibroid tissues; these drugs often stop menses and allow blood counts to increase. In perimenopausal women, expectant management can usually be tried because symptoms may resolve as fibroids decrease in size after menopause.

Drugs for fibroids: Several drugs are used to relieve symptoms, reduce fibroid growth, or both:

- GnRH agonists
- Exogenous progestins
- Antiprogestins
- Selective estrogenreceptor modulators (SERMs)
- Danazol
- NSAIDs
- Tranexamic acid

GnRH agonists are often the drugs of choice. They can reduce fibroid size and bleeding. They may be given as follows:

- IM or sc (eg, leuprolide 3.75 mg IM q mo, goserelin 3.6 mg sc q 28 days)
- As a subdermal pellet
- As nasal spray (eg, nafarelin)

These drugs can decrease estrogen production. GnRH agonists are most helpful when given preoperatively to reduce fibroid and uterine volume, making surgery technically more feasible and reducing blood loss during surgery. In general, these drugs should not be used in the long term because rebound growth to pretreatment size within 6 mo is common and bone demineralization may occur. To prevent bone demineralization when these drugs are used long term, clinicians should give patients supplemental estrogen (add-back therapy), such as a low-dose estrogen-progestin combination.

Exogenous progestins can partially suppress estrogen stimulation of uterine fibroid growth. Progestins can decrease uterine bleeding but may not shrink fibroids as much as GnRH agonists. Medroxyprogesterone acetate 5 to 10 mg po once/day or megestrol acetate 40 mg po once/day taken 10 to 14 days each menstrual cycle can limit heavy bleeding, beginning after 1 or 2 treatment cycles. Alternatively, these drugs may be taken every day of the month (continuous therapy); this therapy often reduces bleeding and provides contraception. Depot medroxyprogesterone acetate 150 mg IM q 3 mo has effects similar to those of continuous oral therapy. Before IM therapy, oral progestins should be tried to determine whether patients can tolerate the adverse effects (eg, weight gain, depression, irregular bleeding). Progestin therapy causes fibroids to grow in some women. Alternatively, a levonorgestrel-releasing intrauterine device (IUD) may be used to reduce uterine bleeding.

For **antiprogestins** (eg, mifepristone), the dosage is 5 to 50 mg once/day for 3 to 6 mo. This dose is lower than the 200-mg dose used for termination of pregnancy; thus, this dose must be mixed specially by a pharmacist and may not always be available.

SERMS (eg, raloxifene) may help reduce fibroid growth, but whether they can relieve symptoms as well as other drugs is unclear.

Danazol, an androgenic agonist, can suppress fibroid growth but has a high rate of adverse effects (eg, weight gain, acne, hirsutism, edema, hair loss, deepening of the voice, flushing, sweating, vaginal dryness) and is thus often less acceptable to patients.

NSAIDs can be used to treat pain but probably do not decrease bleeding.

Tranexamic acid (an antifibrinolytic drug) can reduce uterine bleeding by up to 40%. The dosage is 1300 mg q 8 h for up to 5 days. Its role is evolving.

Surgery for fibroids: Surgery is usually reserved for women with any of the following:

- A rapidly enlarging pelvic mass
- Recurrent uterine bleeding refractory to drug therapy
- Severe or persistent pain or pressure (eg, that requires opioids for control or that is intolerable to the patient)
- A large uterus that has a mass effect in the abdomen, causing urinary or intestinal symptoms or compressing other organs and causing dysfunction (eg, hydronephrosis, urinary frequency, dyspareunia)
- Infertility (if pregnancy is desired)
- Recurrent spontaneous abortions (if pregnancy is desired)

Other factors favoring surgery are completion of childbearing and the patient's desire for definitive treatment.

Myomectomy is usually done laparoscopically or hysteroscopically (using an instrument with a wide-angle telescope and electrical wire loop for excision), with or without robotic techniques.

Hysterectomy can also be done laparoscopically, vaginally or by laparotomy.

Most indications for these procedures are similar. Patient choice is important, but patients must be fully informed about anticipated difficulties and sequelae of myomectomy vs hysterectomy.

If women desire pregnancy or want to keep their uterus, myomectomy is used. In about 55% of women with infertility due to fibroids alone, myomectomy can restore fertility, resulting in pregnancy after about 15 mo. However, hysterectomy is often necessary or preferred by the patient.

Factors that favor hysterectomy include

- It is more definitive treatment. After myomectomy, new fibroids may begin to grow again, and about 25% of women who have a myomectomy have a hysterectomy about 4 to 8 yr later.
- Multiple myomectomy can be much more difficult to do than hysterectomy.
- Other, less invasive treatments have been ineffective.
- Patients have other abnormalities that make surgery more complicated (eg, extensive adhesions, endometriosis).
- Hysterectomy would decrease the risk of another disorder (eg, cervical intraepithelial neoplasia, endometrial hyperplasia, endometriosis, ovarian cancer in women with a *BRCA* mutation).

Newer procedures may relieve symptoms, but duration of symptom relief and efficacy of the procedures in restoring fertility have not been evaluated. Such procedures include

- High-intensity focused sonography
- Cryotherapy
- Radiofrequency ablation
- Magnetic resonance-guided focused ultrasound surgery
- Uterine artery embolization

Uterine artery embolization aims to cause infarction of fibroids throughout the uterus while preserving normal uterine tissue. After this procedure, women recover more quickly than after hysterectomy or myomectomy, but rates of complications and return visits tend to be higher.

Choice of treatment: Treatment of uterine fibroids should be individualized, but some factors can help with the decision:

- Asymptomatic fibroids: No treatment
- Postmenopausal women: Trial of expectant management (because symptoms tend to remit as fibroids decrease in size after menopause)
- Symptomatic fibroids, particularly if pregnancy is desired: Uterine artery embolization, another new technique (eg, high-intensity focused sonography), or myomectomy
- Severe symptoms when other treatments were ineffective, particularly if pregnancy is not desired: Hysterectomy, possibly preceded by drug therapy (eg, with GnRH agonists)

KEY POINTS

- Fibroids occur in about 70% of women by age 45 but do not always cause symptoms.
- If necessary, confirm the diagnosis with imaging, usually ultrasonography (sometimes with saline infusion sonography) or MRI.
- For temporary relief of minor symptoms, consider drugs (eg, GnRH agonists, progestins, SERMs, mifepristone, tranexamic acid, danazol).
- For more lasting relief, consider surgery (eg, newer procedures or myomectomy, particularly if fertility may be desired; hysterectomy for definitive therapy).

278 Vaginitis, Cervicitis, and Pelvic Inflammatory Disease

The lower and upper female genital tracts are separated by the cervix. Inflammation of the lower tract may involve the vagina (vaginitis), vulva (vulvitis), or both (vulvovaginitis).

Pelvic inflammatory disease is infection of the upper tract: uterus, fallopian tubes, and, if infection is severe, ovaries (one or both). The cervix may also be inflamed (cervicitis).

OVERVIEW OF VAGINITIS

Vaginitis is infectious or noninfectious inflammation of the vaginal mucosa, sometimes with inflammation of the vulva. Symptoms include vaginal discharge, irritation, pruritus, and erythema. Diagnosis is by in-office testing of vaginal secretions. Treatment is directed at the cause and at any severe symptoms.

Vaginitis is one of the most common gynecologic disorders. Some of its causes affect the vulva alone (vulvitis) or in addition (vulvovaginitis).

Etiology

The most common causes vary by patient age.

Children: In children, vaginitis usually involves infection with GI tract flora (nonspecific vulvovaginitis). A common contributing factor in girls aged 2 to 6 yr is poor perineal hygiene (eg, wiping from back to front after bowel movements; not washing hands after bowel movements; fingering, particularly in response to pruritus).

Chemicals in bubble baths or soaps may cause inflammation.

Foreign bodies (eg, tissue paper) may cause nonspecific vaginitis with a bloody discharge.

Sometimes childhood vulvovaginitis is due to infection with a specific pathogen (eg, streptococci, staphylococci, *Candida* sp; occasionally, pinworm).

Women of reproductive age: In these women, vaginitis is usually infectious. The most common types are

- Bacterial vaginosis (see p. 2313)
- Candidal vaginitis (see p. 2314)
- Trichomonal vaginitis (see p. 1712), which is sexually transmitted

Normally in women of reproductive age, *Lactobacillus* sp is the predominant constituent of normal vaginal flora. Colonization by these bacteria keeps vaginal pH in the normal range (3.8 to 4.2), thereby preventing overgrowth of pathogenic bacteria. Also, high estrogen levels maintain vaginal thickness, bolstering local defenses.

Factors that predispose to overgrowth of bacterial vaginal pathogens may include the following:

- An alkaline vaginal pH due to menstrual blood, semen, or a decrease in lactobacilli
- Poor hygiene
- Frequent douching

Vaginitis may result from foreign bodies (eg, forgotten tampons). Inflammatory vaginitis, which is noninfectious, is uncommon.

Postmenopausal women: Usually, a marked decrease in estrogen causes vaginal thinning, increasing vulnerability to infection and inflammation. Some treatments (eg, oophorectomy, pelvic radiation, certain chemotherapy drugs) also result in loss of estrogen. Decreased estrogen predisposes to inflammatory (particularly atrophic) vaginitis.

Poor hygiene (eg, in patients who are incontinent or bedbound) can lead to chronic vulvar inflammation due to chemical irritation from urine or feces or due to nonspecific infection.

Bacterial vaginosis, candidal vaginitis, and trichomonal vaginitis are uncommon among postmenopausal women but may occur in those with risk factors.

Women of all ages: At any age, conditions that predispose to vaginal or vulvar infection include

- Fistulas between the intestine and genital tract, which allow intestinal flora to seed the genital tract
- Pelvic radiation or tumors, which break down tissue and thus compromise normal host defenses

Noninfectious vulvitis accounts for up to 30% of vulvovaginitis cases. It may result from hypersensitivity or irritant reactions to hygiene sprays or perfumes, menstrual pads, laundry soaps, bleaches, fabric softeners, fabric dyes, synthetic fibers, bathwater additives, toilet tissue, or, occasionally, spermicides, vaginal lubricants or creams, latex condoms, vaginal contraceptive rings, or diaphragms.

Symptoms and Signs

Vaginitis causes vaginal discharge, which must be distinguished from normal discharge. Normal discharge is common when estrogen levels are high—eg, during the first 2 wk of life because maternal estrogen is transferred before birth (slight bleeding often occurs when estrogen levels abruptly decrease) and during the few months before menarche, when estrogen production increases.

Normal vaginal discharge is commonly milky white or mucoid, odorless, and nonirritating; it can result in vaginal wetness that dampens underwear. Discharge due to vaginitis is accompanied by pruritus, erythema, and sometimes burning, pain, or mild bleeding. Pruritus may interfere with sleep. Dysuria or dyspareunia may occur. In atrophic vaginitis, discharge is scant, dyspareunia is common, and vaginal tissue appears thin and dry. Although symptoms vary among particular types of vaginitis, there is much overlap (see Table 278–1).

Table 278–1. COMMON TYPES OF VAGINITIS

DISORDER	TYPICAL SYMPTOMS AND SIGNS	CRITERIA FOR DIAGNOSIS	MICROSCOPIC FINDINGS	DIFFERENTIAL DIAGNOSIS
Bacterial vaginosis	Gray, thin, fishy-smelling discharge, often with pruritus and irritation; no dyspareunia	Three of the following: Gray discharge, pH > 4.5, fishy odor, and clue cells	Clue cells, decreased lactobacilli, increased coccobacilli	Trichomonal vaginitis
Candidal vaginitis	Thick, white discharge; vaginal and sometimes vulvar pruritus with or without burning, irritation, or dyspareunia	Typical discharge, pH < 4.5, and microscopic findings*	Budding yeast, pseudohyphae, or mycelia; best examined with 10% K hydroxide diluent	Contact irritant or allergic vulvitis Chemical irritation Vulvodynia
Trichomonal vaginitis	Profuse, malodorous, yellow-green discharge; dysuria; dyspareunia; erythema	Identification of causative organism by microscopy* (occasionally by culture)	Motile, flagellated protozoa, increased PMNs	Bacterial vaginosis Inflammatory vaginitis
Inflammatory vaginitis	Purulent discharge, vaginal dryness and thinning, dyspareunia, dysuria; usually in postmenopausal women	pH > 6, negative whiff test, and characteristic microscopy findings	Increased PMNs, parabasal cells, and cocci; decreased bacilli	Erosive lichen planus

*Culture is needed if microscopic findings are negative or symptoms persist.

Vulvitis can cause erythema, pruritus, and sometimes tenderness and discharge from the vulva.

Diagnosis

- Clinical evaluation
- Vaginal pH and saline and KOH wet mounts

Vaginitis is diagnosed using clinical criteria and in-office testing. First, vaginal secretions are obtained with a water-lubricated speculum, and pH paper is used to measure pH in 0.2 intervals from 4.0 to 6.0. Then, secretions are placed on 2 slides with a cotton swab and diluted with 0.9% NaCl on one slide (saline wet mount) and with 10% K hydroxide on the other (KOH wet mount). The KOH wet mount is checked for a fishy odor (whiff test), which results from amines produced in trichomonal vaginitis or bacterial vaginosis. The saline wet mount is examined microscopically as soon as possible to detect trichomonads, which can become immotile and more difficult to recognize within minutes after slide preparation. The KOH dissolves most cellular material except for yeast hyphae, making identification easier.

If clinical criteria and in-office test results are inconclusive, the discharge may be cultured for fungi or trichomonads.

Other causes of discharge are ruled out. If children have vaginal discharge, a vaginal foreign body is suspected. Cervical discharge due to cervicitis (see p. 2315) can resemble that of vaginitis. Abdominal pain, cervical motion tenderness, or cervical inflammation suggests PID (see p. 2315). Discharge that is watery, bloody, or both may result from vulvar, vaginal, or cervical cancer; cancers can be differentiated from vaginitis by examination and Papanicolaou (Pap) tests. Vaginal pruritus and discharge may result from skin disorders (eg, psoriasis, tinea versicolor), which can usually be differentiated by history and skin findings.

If children have trichomonal vaginitis, evaluation for sexual abuse is required. If they have unexplained vaginal discharge, cervicitis, which may be due to a sexually transmitted disease, should be considered. If women have bacterial vaginosis or trichomonal vaginitis (and thus are at increased risk of sexually transmitted diseases), cervical tests for *Neisseria gonorrhoeae* and *Chlamydia trachomatis*, common causes of sexually transmitted PID, are done.

Treatment

- Hygienic measures
- Symptomatic treatment
- Treatment of cause

The vulva should be kept as clean as possible. Soaps and unnecessary topical preparations (eg, feminine hygiene sprays) should be avoided. Intermittent use of ice packs or warm sitz baths with or without baking soda may reduce soreness and pruritus.

If symptoms are moderate or severe or do not respond to other measures, drugs may be needed. For pruritus, topical corticosteroids (eg, topical 1% hydrocortisone bid prn) can be applied to the vulva but not in the vagina. Oral antihistamines decrease pruritus and cause drowsiness, helping patients sleep.

Any infection or other cause is treated. Foreign bodies are removed. Prepubertal girls are taught good perineal hygiene (eg, wiping front to back after bowel movements and voiding, washing hands, avoiding fingering the perineum). If chronic vulvar inflammation is due to being bedbound or incontinent, better vulvar hygiene may help.

KEY POINTS

- Common age-related causes of vaginitis include nonspecific (often hygiene-related) vaginitis and chemical irritation in children; bacterial vaginosis and candidal and trichomonal vaginitis in women of reproductive age; and atrophic vaginitis in postmenopausal women.
- Diagnose vaginitis based mainly on clinical findings, measurement of vaginal pH, and examination of saline and KOH wet mounts.
- Treat infectious and other specific causes, treat symptoms, and discuss ways to improve hygiene as appropriate with patients.

BACTERIAL VAGINOSIS

Bacterial vaginosis (BV) is vaginitis due to a complex alteration of vaginal flora in which lactobacilli decrease and anaerobic pathogens overgrow. Symptoms include a gray, thin, fishy-smelling vaginal discharge and itching. Diagnosis is confirmed by testing vaginal secretions. Treatment is usually with oral or topical metronidazole or topical clindamycin.

BV is the most common infectious vaginitis. The cause is unknown. Anaerobic pathogens that overgrow include *Prevotella* sp, *Peptostreptococcus* sp, *Gardnerella vaginalis*, *Mobiluncus* sp, and *Mycoplasma hominis*, which increase in concentration by 10- to 100-fold and replace the normally protective lactobacilli.

Risk factors include those for sexually transmitted diseases (see p. 1699). In women who have sex with women, risk increases as the number of sex partners increases. However, BV can occur in virgins, and treating the male sex partner does not appear to affect subsequent incidence in sexually active heterosexual women. Use of an intrauterine device is also a risk factor.

BV appears to increase the risk of pelvic inflammatory disease, postabortion and postpartum endometritis, posthysterectomy vaginal cuff infection, chorioamnionitis, premature rupture of membranes, preterm labor, and preterm birth.

Symptoms and Signs

Vaginal discharge is malodorous, gray, and thin. Usually, a fishy odor is present, often becoming stronger when the discharge is more alkaline—after coitus and menses. Pruritus and irritation are common. Erythema and edema are uncommon.

Diagnosis

- Clinical criteria
- Vaginal pH and wet mount

For the diagnosis, 3 of 4 criteria must be present:

- Gray discharge
- Vaginal secretion pH > 4.5
- Fishy odor on the whiff test
- Clue cells

Clue cells (bacteria adhering to epithelial cells and sometimes obscuring their cell margins—see Plate 89) are identified by microscopic examination of a saline wet mount. Presence of WBCs on a saline wet mount suggests a concomitant infection (possibly trichomonal, gonorrheal, or chlamydial cervicitis) and the need for additional testing.

Treatment

- Metronidazole or clindamycin

The following treatments are equally effective:

- Metronidazole 0.75% vaginal gel bid for 5 days
- 2% clindamycin vaginal cream once/day for 7 days
- Oral metronidazole 500 mg bid for 7 days or 2 g once

Oral metronidazole 500 mg bid for 7 days is the treatment of choice for patients who are not pregnant, but because systemic effects are possible with oral drugs, topical regimens are preferred for pregnant patients. Women who use clindamycin cream cannot use latex products (ie, condoms or diaphragms) for contraception because the drug weakens latex.

Treatment of asymptomatic sex partners is unnecessary.

For vaginitis during the 1st trimester of pregnancy, metronidazole vaginal gel should be used, although treatment during pregnancy has not been shown to lower the risk of pregnancy complications. To prevent endometritis, clinicians may give oral metronidazole prophylactically before elective abortion to all patients or only to those who test positive for BV.

CANDIDAL VAGINITIS

Candidal vaginitis is vaginal infection with *Candida* sp, usually *C. albicans*.

Most fungal vaginitis is caused by *C. albicans* (see also p. 1031), which colonizes 15 to 20% of nonpregnant and 20 to 40% of pregnant women.

Risk factors for candidal vaginitis include the following:

- Diabetes
- Use of a broad-spectrum antibiotic or corticosteroids
- Pregnancy
- Constrictive nonporous undergarments
- Immunocompromise
- Use of an intrauterine device

Candidal vaginitis is uncommon among postmenopausal women except among those taking systemic hormone therapy.

Symptoms and Signs

Vaginal vulvar pruritus, burning, or irritation (which may be worse during intercourse) and dyspareunia are common, as is a thick, white, cottage cheese–like vaginal discharge that adheres to the vaginal walls. Symptoms and signs increase the week before menses. Erythema, edema, and excoriation are common.

Infection in male sex partners is rare.

Recurrences after treatment are uncommon.

Diagnosis

- Vaginal pH and wet mount

Vaginal pH is < 4.5; budding yeast, pseudohyphae, or mycelia are visible on a wet mount, especially with KOH (see Plate 90). If symptoms suggest candidal vaginitis but signs (including vulvar irritation) are absent and microscopy does not detect fungal elements, fungal culture is done. Women with frequent recurrences require culture to confirm the diagnosis and to rule out non-albicans *Candida*.

Treatment

- Antifungal drugs (oral fluconazole in a single dose preferred)
- Avoidance of excess moisture accumulation

Keeping the vulva clean and wearing loose, absorbent cotton clothing that allows air to circulate can reduce vulvar moisture and fungal growth.

Topical or oral drugs are highly effective (see Table 278–2). Adherence to treatment is better when a one-dose oral regimen of fluconazole 150 mg is used. Topical butoconazole, clotrimazole, miconazole, and tioconazole are available OTC. However, patients should be warned that topical creams and ointments containing mineral oil or vegetable oil weaken latex-based condoms. If symptoms persist or worsen during topical therapy, hypersensitivity to topical antifungals should be considered.

Frequent recurrences require long-term suppression with oral drugs (fluconazole 150 mg weekly to monthly or ketoconazole 100 mg once/day for 6 mo). Suppression is effective only while the drugs are being taken. These drugs may be contraindicated in patients with liver disorders. Patients taking ketoconazole should be monitored periodically with liver function tests.

INFLAMMATORY VAGINITIS

Inflammatory vaginitis is vaginal inflammation without evidence of the usual infectious causes of vaginitis.

Etiology may be autoimmune. Vaginal epithelial cells slough superficially, and streptococci overgrow.

The major risk factor is

- Estrogen loss, which can result from menopause or premature ovarian failure (eg, due to oophorectomy, pelvic radiation, or chemotherapy)

Genital atrophy predisposes to inflammatory vaginitis and increases risk of recurrence.

Symptoms and Signs

Purulent vaginal discharge, dyspareunia, dysuria, and vaginal irritation are common. Vaginal pruritus and erythema may

Table 278–2. DRUGS FOR CANDIDAL VAGINITIS

DRUG	DOSAGE
Topical or vaginal	
Butoconazole	Sustained-release preparation of 2% cream 5 g as a single application
Clotrimazole	1% cream 5 g once/day for 7 to 14 days *or* 2% cream 5 g for 3 days
Miconazole	2% cream 5 g once/day for 7 days *or* 4% cream 5 g for 3 days Vaginal suppository 100 mg once/day for 7 days *or* 200 mg once/day for 3 days *or* 1200 mg, only once
Terconazole	0.4% cream 5 g once/day for 7 days *or* 0.8% cream 5 g once/day for 3 days Vaginal suppository 80 mg once/day for 3 days
Tioconazole	6.5% ointment 5 g once
Oral	
Fluconazole	150 mg in a single dose

occur. Burning, pain, or mild bleeding occurs less often. Vaginal tissue may appear thin and dry. Vaginitis may recur.

Diagnosis

- Vaginal pH and wet mount

Because symptoms overlap with other forms of vaginitis, testing (eg, vaginal fluid pH measurement, microscopy, whiff test) is necessary. The diagnosis is made if vaginal fluid pH is > 6, whiff test is negative, and microscopy shows predominantly WBCs and parabasal cells.

Treatment

- Clindamycin vaginal cream

Treatment is with clindamycin vaginal cream 5 g every evening for 1 wk. After treatment with clindamycin, women are evaluated for genital atrophy. Genital atrophy, if present, can be treated with topical estrogens (eg, 0.01% estradiol vaginal cream 2 to 4 g once/day for 1 to 2 wk, followed by 1 to 2 g once/day for 1 to 2 wk, then 1 g 1 to 3 times weekly; estradiol hemihydrate vaginal tablets 10 mcg twice/wk; estradiol rings q 3 mo). Topical therapy is usually preferred because of concerns about the safety of oral hormonal therapy; topical therapy may have fewer systemic effects.

CERVICITIS

Cervicitis is infectious or noninfectious inflammation of the cervix. Findings may include vaginal discharge, vaginal bleeding, and cervical erythema and friability. Women are tested for infectious causes of vaginitis and pelvic inflammatory disease and are usually treated empirically for chlamydial infection and gonorrhea.

Acute cervicitis is usually caused by an infection; chronic cervicitis is usually not caused by an infection. Cervicitis may ascend and cause endometritis and pelvic inflammatory disease (PID).

The most common infectious cause of cervicitis is *Chlamydia trachomatis*, followed by *Neisseria gonorrhea*. Other causes include herpes simplex virus (HSV), *Trichomonas vaginalis*, and *Mycoplasma genitalium*. Often, a pathogen cannot be identified. The cervix may also be inflamed as part of vaginitis (eg, bacterial vaginosis, trichomoniasis).

Noninfectious causes of cervicitis include gynecologic procedures, foreign bodies (eg, pessaries, barrier contraceptive devices), chemicals (eg, in douches or contraceptive creams), and allergens (eg, latex).

Symptoms and Signs

Cervicitis may not cause symptoms. The most common symptoms are vaginal discharge and vaginal bleeding between menstrual periods or after coitus. Some women have dyspareunia, vulvar and/or vaginal irritation, and/or dysuria.

Examination findings can include purulent or mucopurulent discharge, cervical friability (eg, bleeding after touching the cervix with a swab), and cervical erythema and edema.

Diagnosis

- Clinical findings
- Testing for vaginitis and STDs

Cervicitis is diagnosed if women have cervical exudate (purulent or mucopurulent) or cervical friability.

Findings that suggest a specific cause or other disorders include the following:

- Fever: PID or HSV infection
- Cervical motion tenderness: PID
- Vesicles, vulvar or vaginal pain, and/or ulceration: HSV infection
- Punctate hemorrhages (strawberry spots): Trichomoniasis

Women should be evaluated clinically for PID and tested for chlamydial infection (see p. 1701) and gonorrhea (eg, with PCR or culture—see p. 1705), bacterial vaginosis (see p. 2313), and trichomoniasis (see p. 1712).

Treatment

- Usually empiric treatment for chlamydial infection and gonorrhea

At the first visit, most women with acute cervicitis should be treated for chlamydial infection empirically, particularly if they have risk factors for STDs (eg, age < 25, new or multiple sex partners, unprotected sex) or if follow-up cannot be ensured. Women should also be treated empirically for gonorrhea if they have risk factors for STDs, if local prevalence is high (eg, > 5%), or if follow-up cannot be ensured.

Treatment consists of the following:

- Chlamydial infection: Azithromycin 1 g po once or with doxycycline 100 mg po bid for 7 days
- Gonorrhea: Ceftriaxone 250 mg IM once plus azithromycin 1 g po once (due to emerging resistance of *N. gonorrhoeae* to cephalosporins)

Once the cause or causes are identified based on the results of microbiologic testing, subsequent treatment is adjusted accordingly.

If cervicitis persists despite this treatment, reinfection with chlamydiae and *N. gonorrhoeae* should be ruled out, and empiric treatment with moxifloxacin 400 mg po once/day for 7 to 14 days (eg, for 10 days) should be started to cover possible *M. genitalium* infection.

If the cause is a bacterial STD, sex partners should be tested and treated simultaneously. Women should abstain from sexual intercourse until the infection has been eliminated from them and their sex partners.

All women with confirmed chlamydial infection or gonorrhea should be tested between 3 and 6 mo after treatment because reinfection is common.

KEY POINTS

- Acute cervicitis is usually caused by an STD and can presage PID.
- Infection may be asymptomatic.
- Test women for chlamydial infection, gonorrhea, BV, and trichomoniasis.
- Treat most women for chlamydial infection and gonorrhea at the first visit.

PELVIC INFLAMMATORY DISEASE

Pelvic inflammatory disease (PID) is infection of the upper female genital tract: the cervix, uterus, fallopian tubes, and ovaries; abscesses may occur. Common symptoms and signs include lower abdominal pain, cervical discharge, and irregular vaginal bleeding. Long-term complications

include infertility, chronic pelvic pain, and ectopic pregnancy. Diagnosis includes PCR of cervical specimens for *Neisseria gonorrhoeae* and chlamydiae, microscopic examination of cervical discharge (usually), and ultrasonography or laparoscopy (occasionally). Treatment is with antibiotics.

Infection of the cervix (cervicitis—see p. 2315) causes mucopurulent discharge. Infection of the fallopian tubes (salpingitis) and uterus (endometritis) tend to occur together. If severe, infection can spread to the ovaries (oophoritis) and then the peritoneum (peritonitis). Salpingitis with endometritis and oophoritis, with or without peritonitis, is often called salpingitis even though other structures are involved. Pus may collect in the tubes (pyosalpinx), and an abscess may form (tubo-ovarian abscess).

Etiology

PID results from microorganisms ascending from the vagina and cervix into the endometrium and fallopian tubes. *Neisseria gonorrhoeae* and *Chlamydia trachomatis* are common causes of PID; they are transmitted sexually. *Mycoplasma genitalium*, which is also sexually transmitted, can also cause or contribute to PID.

PID usually also involves other aerobic and anaerobic bacteria, including pathogens that are associated with bacterial vaginosis (BV—see p. 2313).

Risk factors: PID commonly occurs in women < 35. It is rare before menarche, after menopause, and during pregnancy.

Risk factors include

- Previous PID
- Presence of BV or any sexually transmitted disease

Other risk factors, particularly for gonorrheal or chlamydial PID, include

- Younger age
- Nonwhite race
- Low socioeconomic status
- Multiple or new sex partners

Symptoms and Signs

Lower abdominal pain, fever, cervical discharge, and abnormal uterine bleeding are common, particularly during or after menses.

Cervicitis: The cervix appears red and bleeds easily (see p. 2315). Mucopurulent discharge is common; usually, it is yellow-green and can be seen exuding from the endocervical canal.

Acute salpingitis: Lower abdominal pain is usually present and bilateral but may be unilateral, even when both tubes are involved. Pain can also occur in the upper abdomen. Nausea and vomiting are common when pain is severe. Irregular bleeding (caused by endometritis) and fever each occur in up to one-third of patients.

In the early stages, signs may be mild or absent. Later, cervical motion tenderness, guarding, and rebound tenderness are common.

Occasionally, dyspareunia or dysuria occurs.

Many women with inflammation that is severe enough to cause scarring have minimal or no symptoms.

PID due to *N. gonorrhoeae* is usually more acute and causes more severe symptoms than that due to *C. trachomatis*, which can be indolent. PID due to *M. genitalium*, like that due to *C. trachomatis*, is also mild and should be considered in women who do not respond to first-line therapy for PID.

Complications: Acute gonococcal or chlamydial salpingitis may lead to the Fitz-Hugh-Curtis syndrome (perihepatitis that causes upper right quadrant pain). Infection may become chronic, characterized by intermittent exacerbations and remissions.

A tubo-ovarian abscess (collection of pus in the adnexa) develops in about 15% of women with salpingitis. It can accompany acute or chronic infection and is more likely if treatment is late or incomplete. Pain, fever, and peritoneal signs are usually present and may be severe. An adnexal mass may be palpable, although extreme tenderness may limit the examination. The abscess may rupture, causing progressively severe symptoms and possibly septic shock.

Hydrosalpinx is fimbrial obstruction and tubal distention with nonpurulent fluid; it is usually asymptomatic but can cause pelvic pressure, chronic pelvic pain, dyspareunia, and/or infertility.

Salpingitis may cause tubal scarring and adhesions, which commonly result in chronic pelvic pain, infertility, and increased risk of ectopic pregnancy.

Diagnosis

- High index of suspicion
- PCR
- Pregnancy test

PID is suspected when women of reproductive age, particularly those with risk factors, have lower abdominal pain or cervical or unexplained vaginal discharge. PID is considered when irregular vaginal bleeding, dyspareunia, or dysuria is unexplained. PID is more likely if lower abdominal, unilateral or bilateral adnexal, and cervical motion tenderness are present. A palpable adnexal mass suggests tubo-ovarian abscess. Because even minimally symptomatic infection may have severe sequelae, index of suspicion should be high.

If PID is suspected, PCR of cervical specimens for *N. gonorrhoeae* and *C. trachomatis* (which is about 99% sensitive and specific) and a pregnancy test are done. If PCR is unavailable, cultures are done. However, upper tract infection is possible even if cervical specimens are negative. At the point of care, cervical discharge is usually examined to confirm purulence; a Gram stain or saline wet mount is used, but these tests are neither sensitive nor specific.

If a patient cannot be adequately examined because of tenderness, ultrasonography is done as soon as possible.

WBC count may be elevated but is not helpful diagnostically.

If the pregnancy test is positive, ectopic pregnancy, which can produce similar findings, should be considered.

Other common causes of pelvic pain include endometriosis, adnexal torsion, ovarian cyst rupture, and appendicitis. Differentiating features of these disorders are discussed elsewhere (see p. 2202).

Fitz-Hugh-Curtis syndrome may mimic acute cholecystitis but can usually be differentiated by evidence of salpingitis during pelvic examination or, if necessary, with ultrasonography.

PEARLS & PITFALLS

- If clinical findings suggest PID but the pregnancy test is positive, test for ectopic pregnancy.

If an adnexal or pelvic mass is suspected clinically or if patients do not respond to antibiotics within 48 to 72 h, ultrasonography is done as soon as possible to exclude tubo-ovarian abscess, pyosalpinx, and disorders unrelated to PID (eg, ectopic pregnancy, adnexal torsion). If the diagnosis is uncertain after ultrasonography, laparoscopy should be done; purulent peritoneal material noted during laparoscopy is the diagnostic gold standard.

Treatment

- Antibiotics to cover *N. gonorrhoeae*, *C. trachomatis*, and sometimes other organisms

Antibiotics are given empirically to cover *N. gonorrhoeae* and *C. trachomatis* and are modified based on laboratory test results. Empirical treatment is needed whenever the diagnosis is in question for several reasons:

- Testing (particularly point-of-care testing) is not conclusive.
- Diagnosis based on clinical criteria can be inaccurate.
- Not treating minimally symptomatic PID can result in serious complications.

PEARLS & PITFALLS

- Treat empirically whenever the diagnosis is in question because testing (particularly point-of-care testing) is not conclusive, diagnosis based on clinical criteria can be inaccurate, and not treating minimally symptomatic PID can result in serious complications.

Patients with cervicitis or clinically mild to moderate PID do not require hospitalization. Outpatient treatment regimens (see Table 278–3) usually also aim to eradicate BV, which often coexists.

Sex partners of patients with *N. gonorrhoeae* or *C. trachomatis* infection should be treated.

If patients do not improve after treatment that covers the usual pathogens, PID due to *M. genitalium* should be considered. Patients can be treated empirically with moxifloxacin 400 mg po once/day for 7 to 14 days (eg, for 10 days).

Women with PID are usually hospitalized if any of the following are present:

- Uncertain diagnosis, with inability to exclude a disorder requiring surgical treatment (eg, appendicitis)
- Pregnancy
- Severe symptoms or high fever
- Tubo-ovarian abscess

Table 278–3. REGIMENS FOR TREATMENT OF PELVIC INFLAMMATORY DISEASE*

TREATMENT	REGIMEN	ALTERNATIVE REGIMENS
Parenteral†	**Regimen A:** Cefotetan 2 g IV q 12 h *or* Cefoxitin 2 g IV q 6 h *plus* Doxycycline 100 mg po or IV q 12 h	Ampicillin/sulbactam 3 g IV q 6 h *plus* Doxycycline 100 mg po or IV q 12 h
	Regimen B: Clindamycin 900 mg IV q 8 h *plus* Gentamicin 2 mg/kg (loading dose) IV or IM, followed by a maintenance dose (1.5 mg/kg) q 8 h; possibly substitution of single daily dosing (3–5 mg/kg once/day)	
Oral and IM‡	**Regimen A:** Ceftriaxone 250 mg IM in a single dose *plus* Doxycycline 100 mg po bid for 14 days *with or without* Metronidazole 500 mg po bid for 14 days	**Regimen D:** Azithromycin 500 mg IV once/day in 1 or 2 doses, followed by 250 mg po once/day for 12–14 days *with or without* Metronidazole 500 mg po bid for 14 days
	Regimen B: Cefoxitin 2 g IM in a single dose with probenecid 1 g po given concurrently in a single dose *plus* Doxycycline 100 mg po bid for 14 days *with or without* Metronidazole 500 mg po bid for 14 days	**Regimen E:** Azithromycin 1 g po once/wk for 2 wk *plus* Ceftriaxone 250 mg IM in a single dose *with or without* Metronidazole 500 mg po bid for 14 days
	Regimen C: Another parenteral 3rd-generation cephalosporin (eg, ceftizoxime, cefotaxime) *plus* Doxycycline 100 mg po bid for 14 days *with or without* Metronidazole 500 mg po bid for 14 days	**Regimen F:** §A fluoroquinolone (eg, levofloxacin 500 mg po once/day or ofloxacin 400 mg po bid, or moxifloxacin 400 mg po once/day for 14 days) *plus* Metronidazole 500 mg po bid for 14 days‖

*Recommendations are from the Centers for Disease Control and Prevention: Sexually Transmitted Diseases Treatment Guidelines, 2015. MMWR 64 (RR3):1–137, 2015. Available at www.cdc.gov/std/treatment.

†Clinical efficacy of parenteral and oral therapy for mild to moderately severe pelvic inflammatory disease (PID) appears similar. Clinical experience should guide the transition to oral therapy, which can usually be started within 24–48 h of clinical improvement.

‡Oral therapy can be considered for mild to moderately severe acute PID because the clinical outcomes with oral and parenteral therapy are similar. If patients do not respond to oral therapy within 72 h, they should be reevaluated to confirm the diagnosis, and parenteral therapy should be given on an outpatient or inpatient basis.

§This regimen may be considered if parenteral cephalosporin is not feasible, if community prevalence and individual risk of gonorrhea are low, and if follow-up is likely. Tests for gonorrhea must be done before therapy is started; if results are positive, the following is recommended:

- Positive culture for gonorrhea: Treatment based on results of antimicrobial susceptibility.
- Identification of quinolone-resistant *Neisseria gonorrhoeae* or antimicrobial susceptibility that cannot be assessed: Consultation with an infectious disease specialist.

- Inability to tolerate or follow outpatient therapy (eg, due to vomiting)
- Lack of response to outpatient (oral) treatment

In these cases, IV antibiotics (see Table 278–3) are started as soon as cultures are obtained and are continued until patients have been afebrile for 24 h.

Tubo-ovarian abscess may require more prolonged IV antibiotic treatment. Treatment with ultrasound- or CT-guided percutaneous or transvaginal drainage can be considered if response to antibiotics alone is incomplete. Laparoscopy or laparotomy is sometimes required for drainage. Suspicion of a ruptured tubo-ovarian abscess requires immediate laparotomy. In women of reproductive age, surgery should aim to preserve the pelvic organs (with the hope of preserving fertility).

KEY POINTS

- The sexually transmitted pathogens *Neisseria gonorrhoeae* and *Chlamydia trachomatis* are common causes of PID, but infection is often polymicrobial.
- PID can cause tubal scarring and adhesions, which commonly result in chronic pelvic pain, infertility, and increased risk of ectopic pregnancy.
- Because even minimally symptomatic infection may have severe sequelae, index of suspicion should be high.
- PCR and cultures are accurate tests; however, if results are not available at the point of care, empiric treatment is usually recommended.
- Hospitalize women with PID based on clinical criteria (see above).

279 Approach to the Pregnant Woman and Prenatal Care

CONCEPTION AND PRENATAL DEVELOPMENT

For conception (fertilization), a live sperm must unite with an ovum in a fallopian tube with normally functioning epithelium. Conception occurs just after ovulation, about 14 days after a menstrual period. At ovulation, cervical mucus becomes less viscid, facilitating rapid movement of sperm to the ovum, usually near the fimbriated end of the tube. Sperm may remain alive in the vagina for about 3 days after intercourse.

The fertilized egg (zygote) divides repeatedly as it travels to the implantation site in the endometrium (usually near the fundus) over a period of 5 to 8 days. By the time of implantation, the zygote has become a layer of cells around a cavity, called a blastocyst. The blastocyst wall is 1 cell thick except for the embryonic pole, which is 3 or 4 cells thick. The embryonic pole, which becomes the embryo, implants first.

Amniotic sac and placenta: Within 1 or 2 days of implantation, a layer of cells (trophoblast cells) develops around the blastocyst. The progenitor villous trophoblast cell, the stem cell of the placenta, develops along 2 cell lines:

- Nonproliferative extravillous trophoblast: These cells penetrate the endometrium, facilitating implantation and anchoring of the placenta.
- Syncytiotrophoblast: These cells produce chorionic gonadotropin by day 10 and other trophic hormones shortly thereafter.

An inner layer (amnion) and outer layer (chorion) of membranes develop from the trophoblast; these membranes form the amniotic sac, which contains the conceptus (term used for derivatives of the zygote at any stage—see Fig. 279–1). When the sac is formed and the blastocyst cavity closes (by about 10 days), the conceptus is considered an embryo. The amniotic sac fills with fluid and expands with the growing embryo, filling the endometrial cavity by about 12 wk after conception; then, the amniotic sac is the only cavity remaining in the uterus.

Trophoblast cells develop into cells that form the placenta. The extravillous trophoblast forms villi, which penetrate the uterus. The syncytiotrophoblast covers the villi. The syncytiotrophoblast synthesizes trophic hormones and provides arterial and venous exchange between the circulation of the conceptus and that of the mother.

The placenta is fully formed by wk 18 to 20 but continues to grow, weighing about 500 g by term.

Embryo: Around day 10, 3 germ layers (ectoderm, mesoderm, endoderm) are usually distinct in the embryo. Then the primitive streak, which becomes the neural tube, begins to develop.

Around day 16, the cephalad portion of the mesoderm thickens, forming a central channel that develops into the heart and great vessels. The heart begins to pump plasma around day 20, and on the next day, fetal RBCs, which are immature and nucleated, appear. Fetal RBCs are soon replaced by mature RBCs, and blood vessels develop throughout the embryo. Eventually,

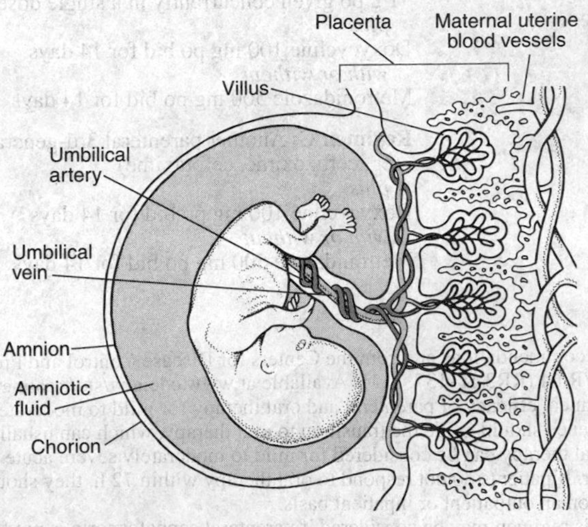

Fig. 279–1. Placenta and embryo at about 11 $^4/_7$ wk gestation. The embryo measures 4.2 cm.

the umbilical artery and vein develop, connecting the embryonic vessels with the placenta.

Most organs form between 21 and 57 days after fertilization (between 5 and 10 wk gestation); however, the CNS continues to develop throughout pregnancy. Susceptibility to malformations induced by teratogens is highest when organs are forming.

PHYSIOLOGY OF PREGNANCY

The earliest sign of pregnancy and the reason most pregnant women initially see a physician is missing a menstrual period. For sexually active women who are of reproductive age and have regular periods, a period that is ≥ 1 wk late is presumptive evidence of pregnancy.

Pregnancy is considered to last 266 days from the time of conception or 280 days from the first day of the last menstrual period if periods occur regularly every 28 days. Delivery date is estimated based on the last menstrual period. Delivery up to 2 wk earlier or later than the estimated date is normal.

Physiology

Pregnancy causes physiologic changes in all maternal organ systems; most return to normal after delivery. In general, the changes are more dramatic in multifetal than in single pregnancies.

Cardiovascular: Cardiac output (CO) increases 30 to 50%, beginning by 6 wk gestation and peaking between 16 and 28 wk (usually at about 24 wk). It remains near peak levels until after 30 wk. Then, CO becomes sensitive to body position. Positions that cause the enlarging uterus to obstruct the vena cava the most (eg, the recumbent position) cause CO to decrease the most. On average, CO usually decreases slightly from 30 wk until labor begins. During labor, CO increases another 30%. After delivery, the uterus contracts, and CO drops rapidly to about 15 to 25% above normal, then gradually decreases (mostly over the next 3 to 4 wk) until it reaches the prepregnancy level at about 6 wk postpartum.

The increase in CO during pregnancy is due mainly to demands of the uteroplacental circulation; volume of the uteroplacental circulation increases markedly, and circulation within the intervillous space acts partly as an arteriovenous shunt. As the placenta and fetus develop, blood flow to the uterus must increase to about 1 L/min (20% of normal CO) at term. Increased needs of the skin (to regulate temperature) and kidneys (to excrete fetal wastes) account for some of the increased CO.

To increase CO, heart rate increases from the normal 70 to as high as 90 beats/min, and stroke volume increases. During the 2nd trimester, BP usually drops (and pulse pressure widens), even though CO and renin and angiotensin levels increase, because uteroplacental circulation expands (the placental intervillous space develops) and systemic vascular resistance decreases. Resistance decreases because blood viscosity and sensitivity to angiotensin decrease. During the 3rd trimester, BP may return to normal. With twins, CO increases more and diastolic BP is lower at 20 wk than with a single fetus.

Exercise increases CO, heart rate, O_2 consumption, and respiratory volume/min more during pregnancy than at other times.

The hyperdynamic circulation of pregnancy increases frequency of functional murmurs and accentuates heart sounds. X-ray or ECG may show the heart displaced into a horizontal position, rotating to the left, with increased transverse diameter. Premature atrial and ventricular beats are common during pregnancy. All these changes are normal and should not be erroneously diagnosed as a heart disorder; they can usually be managed with reassurance alone. However, paroxysms of atrial tachycardia occur more frequently in pregnant women and may require prophylactic digitalization or other antiarrhythmic drugs. Pregnancy does not affect the indications for or safety of cardioversion.

Hematologic: Total blood volume increases proportionally with CO, but the increase in plasma volume is greater (close to 50%, usually by about 1600 mL for a total of 5200 mL) than that in RBC mass (about 25%); thus, Hb is lowered by dilution, from about 13.3 to 12.1 g/dL. This dilutional anemia decreases blood viscosity. With twins, total maternal blood volume increases more (closer to 60%).

WBC count increases slightly to 9,000 to 12,000/μL. Marked leukocytosis (≥ 20,000/μL) occurs during labor and the first few days postpartum.

Iron requirements increase by a total of about 1 g during the entire pregnancy and are higher during the 2nd half of pregnancy—6 to 7 mg/day. The fetus and placenta use about 300 mg of iron, and the increased maternal RBC mass requires an additional 500 mg. Excretion accounts for 200 mg. Iron supplements are needed to prevent a further decrease in Hb levels because the amount absorbed from the diet and recruited from iron stores (average total of 300 to 500 mg) is usually insufficient to meet the demands of pregnancy.

Urinary: Changes in renal function roughly parallel those in cardiac function. GFR increases 30 to 50%, peaks between 16 and 24 wk gestation, and remains at that level until nearly term, when it may decrease slightly because uterine pressure on the vena cava often causes venous stasis in the lower extremities. Renal plasma flow increases in proportion to GFR. As a result, BUN decreases, usually to < 10 mg/dL (< 3.6 mmol urea/L), and creatinine levels decrease proportionally to 0.5 to 0.7 mg/dL (44 to 62 μmol/L). Marked dilation of the ureters (hydroureter) is caused by hormonal influences (predominantly progesterone) and by backup due to pressure from the enlarged uterus on the ureters, which can also cause hydronephrosis. Postpartum, the urinary collecting system may take as long as 12 wk to return to normal.

Postural changes affect renal function more during pregnancy than at other times; ie, the supine position increases renal function more, and upright positions decrease renal function more. Renal function also markedly increases in the lateral position, particularly when lying on the left side; this position relieves the pressure that the enlarged uterus puts on the great vessels when pregnant women are supine. This positional increase in renal function is one reason pregnant women need to urinate frequently when trying to sleep.

Respiratory: Lung function changes partly because progesterone increases and partly because the enlarging uterus interferes with lung expansion. Progesterone signals the brain to lower CO_2 levels. To lower CO_2 levels, tidal and minute volume and respiratory rate increase, thus increasing plasma pH. O_2 consumption increases by about 20% to meet the increased metabolic needs of the fetus, placenta, and several maternal organs. Inspiratory and expiratory reserve, residual volume and capacity, and plasma P_{CO_2} decrease. Vital capacity and plasma P_{O_2} do not change. Thoracic circumference increases by about 10 cm.

Considerable hyperemia and edema of the respiratory tract occur. Occasionally, symptomatic nasopharyngeal obstruction and nasal stuffiness occur, eustachian tubes are transiently blocked, and tone and quality of voice change.

Mild dyspnea during exertion is common, and deep respirations are more frequent.

GI and hepatobiliary: As pregnancy progresses, pressure from the enlarging uterus on the rectum and lower portion of the colon may cause constipation. GI motility decreases because elevated progesterone levels relax smooth muscle. Heartburn and belching are common, possibly resulting from delayed gastric emptying and gastroesophageal reflux due to relaxation of the lower esophageal sphincter and diaphragmatic hiatus. HCl production decreases; thus, peptic ulcer disease is uncommon during pregnancy, and preexisting ulcers often become less severe.

Incidence of gallbladder disorders increases somewhat. Pregnancy subtly affects hepatic function, especially bile transport. Routine liver function test values are normal, except for alkaline phosphatase levels, which increase progressively during the 3rd trimester and may be 2 to 3 times normal at term; the increase is due to placental production of this enzyme rather than hepatic dysfunction.

Endocrine: Pregnancy alters the function of most endocrine glands, partly because the placenta produces hormones and partly because most hormones circulate in protein-bound forms and protein binding increases during pregnancy.

The placenta produces the beta subunit of human chorionic gonadotropin (beta-hCG), a trophic hormone that, like follicle-stimulating and luteinizing hormones, maintains the corpus luteum and thereby prevents ovulation. Levels of estrogen and progesterone increase early during pregnancy because beta-hCG stimulates the ovaries to continuously produce them. After 9 to 10 wk of pregnancy, the placenta itself produces large amounts of estrogen and progesterone to help maintain the pregnancy.

The placenta produces a hormone (similar to thyroid-stimulating hormone) that stimulates the thyroid, causing hyperplasia, increased vascularity, and moderate enlargement. Estrogen stimulates hepatocytes, causing increased thyroid-binding globulin levels; thus, although total thyroxine levels may increase, levels of free thyroid hormones remain normal. Effects of thyroid hormone tend to increase and may resemble hyperthyroidism, with tachycardia, palpitations, excessive perspiration, and emotional instability. However, true hyperthyroidism occurs in only 0.08% of pregnancies.

The placenta produces corticotropin-releasing hormone (CRH), which stimulates maternal ACTH production. Increased ACTH levels increase levels of adrenal hormones, especially aldosterone and cortisol, and thus contribute to edema. Increased production of corticosteroids and increased placental production of progesterone lead to insulin resistance and an increased need for insulin, as does the stress of pregnancy and possibly the increased level of human placental lactogen. Insulinase, produced by the placenta, may also increase insulin requirements, so that many women with gestational diabetes develop more overt forms of diabetes.

The placenta produces melanocyte-stimulating hormone (MSH), which increases skin pigmentation late in pregnancy.

The pituitary gland enlarges by about 135% during pregnancy. The maternal plasma prolactin level increases by 10-fold. Increased prolactin is related to an increase in thyrotropin-releasing hormone production, stimulated by estrogen. The primary function of increased prolactin is to ensure lactation. The level returns to normal postpartum, even in women who breastfeed.

Dermatologic: Increased levels of estrogens, progesterone, and MSH contribute to pigmentary changes, although exact pathogenesis is unknown. These changes include

- Melasma (mask of pregnancy), which is a blotchy, brownish pigment over the forehead and malar eminences
- Darkening of the mammary areolae, axilla, and genitals
- Linea nigra, a dark line that appears down the midabdomen

Melasma due to pregnancy usually regresses within a year.

Incidence of spider angiomas, usually only above the waist, and of thin-walled, dilated capillaries, especially in the lower legs, increases.

Symptoms and Signs

Pregnancy may cause breasts to be engorged because of increased levels of estrogen (primarily) and progesterone—an extension of premenstrual breast engorgement. Nausea, occasionally with vomiting, may occur because of increased secretion of estrogen and the beta subunit of human chorionic gonadotropin (beta-hCG) by syncytial cells of the placenta, beginning 10 days after fertilization (see p. 2318). The corpus luteum in the ovary, stimulated by beta-hCG, continues secreting large amounts of estrogen and progesterone to maintain the pregnancy. Many women become fatigued at this time, and a few women notice abdominal bloating very early.

Women usually begin to feel fetal movement between 16 and 20 wk.

During late pregnancy, lower-extremity edema and varicose veins are common; the main cause is compression of the inferior vena cava by the enlarged uterus.

Pelvic examination findings include a softer cervix and an irregularly softened, enlarged uterus. The cervix usually becomes bluish to purple, probably because blood supply to the uterus is increased. Around 12 wk gestation, the uterus extends above the true pelvis into the abdomen; at 20 wk, it reaches the umbilicus; and by 36 wk, the upper pole almost reaches the xiphoid process.

Diagnosis

- Urine beta-hCG test

Usually urine and occasionally blood tests are used to confirm or exclude pregnancy; results are usually accurate several days before a missed menstrual period and often as early as several days after conception.

Levels of beta-hCG, which correlate with gestational age in normal pregnancies, can be used to determine whether a fetus is growing normally. The best approach is to compare 2 serum beta-hCG values, obtained 48 to 72 h apart and measured by the same laboratory. In a normal single pregnancy, beta-hCG levels double about every 1.4 to 2.1 days during the first 60 days (7.5 wk), then begin to decrease between 10 and 18 wk. Regular doubling of the beta-hCG level during the 1st trimester strongly suggests normal growth.

Other accepted signs of pregnancy include the following:

- Presence of a gestational sac in the uterus, seen with ultrasonography typically at about 4 to 5 wk and typically corresponding to a serum beta-hCG level of about 1500 mIU/mL (a yolk sac can usually be seen in the gestational sac by 5 wk)
- Fetal heart motion, seen with real-time ultrasonography as early as 5 to 6 wk
- Fetal heart sounds, heard with Doppler ultrasonography as early as 8 to 10 wk if the uterus is accessible abdominally
- Fetal movements felt by the examining physician after 20 wk

EVALUATION OF THE OBSTETRIC PATIENT

Ideally, women who are planning to become pregnant should see a physician before conception; then they can learn about pregnancy risks and ways to reduce risks. As part of preconception care, primary care clinicians should advise all women of reproductive age to take a vitamin that contains folate 400 mcg (0.4 mg) once/day. Folate reduces risk of neural tube defects.

If women have had a fetus or infant with a neural tube defect, the recommended daily dose is 4000 mcg (4 mg). Taking folate before and after conception may also reduce the risk of other birth defects.[1]

Once pregnant, women require routine prenatal care to help safeguard their health and the health of the fetus. Also, evaluation is often required for symptoms and signs of illness. Common symptoms that are often pregnancy-related include

- Vaginal bleeding
- Pelvic pain
- Vomiting
- Lower-extremity edema

For specific obstetric disorders, see p. 2343; for nonobstetric disorders in pregnant women, see p. 2386.

The **initial routine prenatal visit** should occur between 6 and 8 wk gestation.

Follow-up visits should occur at

- About 4-wk intervals until 28 wk
- 2-wk intervals from 28 to 36 wk
- Weekly thereafter until delivery

Prenatal visits may be scheduled more frequently if risk of a poor pregnancy outcome is high or less frequently if risk is very low.

Prenatal care includes

- Screening for disorders
- Taking measures to reduce fetal and maternal risks
- Counseling

1. Shaw GM, O'Malley CD, Wasserman CR, et al: Maternal periconceptional use of multivitamins and reduced risk for conotruncal heart defects and limb deficiencies among offspring. *Am J Med Genet* 59:536–545, 1995. doi:10.1002/ajmg.1320590428.

History

During the initial visit, clinicians should obtain a full medical history, including

- Previous and current disorders
- Drug use (therapeutic, social, and illicit)
- Risk factors for complications of pregnancy (see Table 284–1 on p. 2368)
- Obstetric history, with the outcome of all previous pregnancies, including maternal and fetal complications (eg, gestational diabetes, preeclampsia, congenital malformations, stillbirth)

Family history should include all chronic disorders in family members to identify possible hereditary disorders (see p. 2298).

During subsequent visits, queries focus on interim developments, particularly vaginal bleeding or fluid discharge, headache, changes in vision, edema of face or fingers, and changes in frequency or intensity of fetal movement.

Gravidity and parity: Gravidity is the number of confirmed pregnancies; a pregnant woman is a gravida. Parity is the number of deliveries after 20 wk. Multifetal pregnancy is counted as one in terms of gravidity and parity. Abortus is the number of pregnancy losses (abortions) before 20 wk regardless of cause (eg, spontaneous, therapeutic, or elective abortion; ectopic pregnancy). Sum of parity and abortus equals gravidity.

Parity is often recorded as 4 numbers:

- Number of term deliveries (after 37 wk)
- Number of premature deliveries (> 20 and < 37 wk)
- Number of abortions
- Number of living children

Thus, a woman who is pregnant and has had one term delivery, one set of twins born at 32 wk, and 2 abortions is gravida 5, para 1-1-2-3.

Physical Examination

A full general examination, including height and weight, is done first. BMI should be calculated and recorded.

In the initial obstetric examination, speculum and bimanual pelvic examination is done for the following reasons:

- To check for lesions or discharge
- To note the color and consistency of the cervix
- To obtain cervical samples for testing

Also, fetal heart rate and, in patients presenting later in pregnancy, lie of the fetus are assessed (see Fig. 285–1 on p. 2375).

Pelvic capacity can be estimated clinically by evaluating various measurements with the middle finger during bimanual examination. If the distance from the underside of the pubic symphysis to the sacral promontory is > 11.5 cm, the pelvic inlet is almost certainly adequate. Normally, distance between the ischial spines is ≥ 9 cm, length of the sacrospinous ligaments is 4 to ≥ 5 cm, and the subpubic arch is ≥ 90°.

During subsequent visits, BP and weight assessment is important. Obstetric examination focuses on uterine size, fundal height (in cm above the symphysis pubis), fetal heart rate and activity, and maternal diet, weight gain, and overall well-being. Speculum and bimanual examination is usually not needed unless vaginal discharge or bleeding, leakage of fluid, or pain is present.

Testing

Laboratory testing: Prenatal evaluation involves urine tests and blood tests. Initial laboratory evaluation is thorough; some components are repeated during follow-up visits (see Table 279–1).

If a woman has Rh-negative blood, she may be at risk of developing Rh_0(D) antibodies, and if the father has Rh-positive blood, the fetus may be at risk of developing erythroblastosis fetalis. Rh_0(D) antibody levels should be measured in pregnant women at the initial prenatal visit and again at about 26 to 28 wk. At that time, women who have Rh-negative blood are given a prophylactic dose of Rh_0(D) immune globulin. Additional measures may be necessary to prevent development of maternal Rh antibodies.

Generally, women are routinely screened for gestational diabetes between 24 and 28 wk using a 50-g, 1-h glucose tolerance test. However, if women have significant risk factors for gestational diabetes, they are screened during the 1st trimester. These risk factors include

- Gestational diabetes or a macrosomic neonate (weight > 4500 g at birth) in a previous pregnancy
- Unexplained fetal losses
- A strong family history of diabetes in 1st-degree relatives
- A history of persistent glucosuria
- Body mass index (BMI) > 30 kg/m^2
- Polycystic ovary syndrome with insulin resistance

If the 1st-trimester test is normal, the 50-g test should be repeated at 24 to 28 wk, followed, if abnormal, by a 3-h test. Abnormal results on both tests confirms the diagnosis of gestational diabetes.

Women at high risk of aneuploidy (eg, those > 35 yr, those who have had a child with Down syndrome) should be offered screening with maternal serum cell-free DNA.

Table 279–1. COMPONENTS OF ROUTINE PRENATAL EVALUATION

TYPE	INITIAL VISIT	FOLLOW-UP VISITS
Physical examination	Height measurement	
	Weight and BP measurement	X
	Examination of thyroid, heart, lungs, breasts, abdomen, extremities, and optic fundus	
	Examination of ankles for edema	X
	Complete pelvic examination	
	Examination to determine pelvic capacity	
	Examination of uterus to determine size and fetal position[a]	X
	Evaluation for fetal heart sounds[a]	X
Blood tests[b]	CBC[c]	
	Blood typing and $Rh_0(D)$ antibody levels[d]	
	Hepatitis B serologic test	
	Human immunodeficiency virus (HIV)	
	Rubella and varicella immunity[e]	
	Serologic test for syphilis	
Cervical tests	Cervical cultures for gonorrhea and chlamydial infection[f]	
	Cervical Papanicolaou (Pap) test	
Urine tests	Urine culture	
	Urine protein and glucose determination	X
Other tests	Screening for TB (if at risk)	
	Genetic screening, including 1st-trimester screening for aneuploidy	
	Pelvic ultrasonography[g]	

[a]Component may not be detectable depending on the stage of pregnancy at presentation.
[b]Diabetes screening is done only once—routinely at 24–28 wk but earlier in women at risk.
[c]Hct is repeated in the 3rd trimester.
[d]$Rh_0(D)$ antibody levels are remeasured at 26–28 wk in Rh-negative women.
[e]Rubella and varicella titers are measured unless women have been vaccinated or have had a documented previous infection, thus confirming immunity.
[f]For women at high risk, cervical cultures for gonorrhea and chlamydial infection are repeated at 36 wk.
[g]Ideally, pelvic ultrasonography is done in the 2nd trimester, between 16 and 20 wk; it is not obtained routinely by all practitioners.
X = repeated at follow-up visits.

In some pregnant women, blood tests to screen for thyroid disorders (measurement of thyroid-stimulating hormone [TSH]) are done. These women may include those who

- Have symptoms
- Come from an area where moderate to severe iodine insufficiency occurs
- Have a family or personal history of thyroid disorders
- Have type 1 diabetes
- Have a history of infertility, preterm delivery, or miscarriage
- Have had head or neck radiation therapy
- Are morbidly obese (BMI > 40 kg/m²)
- Are > 30 yr

Ultrasonography: Most obstetricians recommend at least one ultrasound examination during each pregnancy, ideally between 16 and 20 wk, when estimated delivery date (EDD) can still be confirmed fairly accurately and when placental location and fetal anatomy can be evaluated. Estimates of gestational age are based on measurements of fetal head circumference, biparietal diameter, abdominal circumference, and femur length. Measurement of fetal crown-rump length during the 1st trimester is particularly accurate in predicting EDD: to within about 5 days when measurements are made at < 12 wk gestation and to within about 7 days at 12 to 15 wk. Ultrasonography during the 3rd trimester is accurate for predicting EDD to within about 2 to 3 wk.

Specific indications for ultrasonography include

- Investigation of abnormalities during the 1st trimester (eg, indicated by abnormal results of noninvasive maternal screening tests)
- Risk assessment for chromosomal abnormalities (eg, Down syndrome) including nuchal translucency measurement
- Need for detailed assessment of fetal anatomy (usually at about 16 to 20 wk), possibly including fetal echocardiography at 20 wk if risk of congenital heart defects is high (eg, in women who have type 1 diabetes or have had a child with a congenital heart defect)

- Detection of multifetal pregnancy, hydatidiform mole, polyhydramnios, placenta previa, or ectopic pregnancy
- Determination of placental location, fetal position and size, and size of the uterus in relation to given gestational dates (too small or too large)

Ultrasonography is also used for needle guidance during chorionic villus sampling, amniocentesis, and fetal transfusion. High-resolution ultrasonography includes techniques that maximize sensitivity for detecting fetal malformations.

If ultrasonography is needed during the 1st trimester (eg, to evaluate pain, bleeding, or viability of pregnancy), use of an endovaginal transducer maximizes diagnostic accuracy; evidence of an intrauterine pregnancy (gestational sac or fetal pole) can be seen as early as 4 to 5 wk and is seen at 7 to 8 wk in > 95% of cases. With real-time ultrasonography, fetal movements and heart motion can be directly observed as early as 5 to 6 wk.

Other imaging: Conventional x-rays can induce spontaneous abortion or congenital malformations, particularly during early pregnancy. Risk is remote (up to about 1/million) with each x-ray of an extremity or of the neck, head, or chest if the uterus is shielded. Risk is higher with abdominal, pelvic, and lower back x-rays. Thus, for all women of childbearing age, an imaging test with less ionizing radiation (eg, ultrasonography) should be substituted when possible, or if x-rays are needed, the uterus should be shielded (because pregnancy is possible).

Medically necessary x-rays or other imaging should not be postponed because of pregnancy. However, elective x-rays are postponed until after pregnancy.

Treatment

Problems identified during evaluation arc managed.

Women are counseled about exercise and diet and advised to follow the Institute of Medicine guidelines for weight gain, which are based on prepregnancy body mass index (BMI—see Table 279–2). Nutritional supplements are prescribed.

What to avoid, what to expect, and when to obtain further evaluation are explained. Couples are encouraged to attend childbirth classes.

Diet and supplements: To provide nutrition for the fetus, most women require about 250 kcal extra daily; most calories should come from protein. If maternal weight gain is excessive (> 1.4 kg/mo during the early months) or inadequate (< 0.9 kg/mo), diet must be modified further. Weight-loss dieting during pregnancy is not recommended, even for morbidly obese women.

Most pregnant women need a daily oral iron supplement of ferrous sulfate 300 mg or ferrous gluconate 450 mg, which may be better tolerated. Woman with anemia should take the supplements bid.

All women should be given oral prenatal vitamins that contain folate 400 mcg (0.4 mg), taken once/day; folate reduces risk of neural tube defects. For women who have had a fetus or infant with a neural tube defect, the recommended daily dose is 4000 mcg (4 mg).

Physical activity: Pregnant women can continue to do moderate physical activities and exercise but should take care not to injure the abdomen.

Sexual intercourse can be continued throughout pregnancy unless vaginal bleeding, pain, leakage of amniotic fluid, or uterine contractions occur.

Travel: The safest time to travel during pregnancy is between 14 and 28 wk, but there is no absolute contraindication to travel at any time during pregnancy. Pregnant women should wear seat belts regardless of gestational age and type of vehicle.

Travel on airplanes is safe until 36 wk gestation. The primary reason for this restriction is the risk of labor and delivery in an unfamiliar environment.

During any kind of travel, pregnant women should stretch and straighten their legs and ankles periodically to prevent venous stasis and the possibility of thrombosis. For example, on long flights, they should walk or stretch every 2 to 3 h. In some cases, the clinician may recommend thromboprophylaxis for prolonged travel.

Immunizations: Vaccines for measles, mumps, rubella, and varicella should not be used during pregnancy. The hepatitis B vaccine can be safely used if indicated, and the influenza vaccine is strongly recommended for women who are pregnant or postpartum during influenza season. Booster immunization for diphtheria, tetanus, and pertussis (Tdap) after 20 wk gestation or postpartum is recommended, even if women have been fully vaccinated.

Because pregnant women with Rh-negative blood are at risk of developing Rh_0(D) antibodies, they are given Rh_0(D) immune globulin 300 mcg IM in any of the following situations:

- After any significant vaginal bleeding or other sign of placental hemorrhage or separation (abruptio placentae)

Table 279–2. GUIDELINES FOR WEIGHT GAIN DURING PREGNANCY*

PREPREGNANCY WEIGHT CATEGORY	BMI	TOTAL WEIGHT GAIN†	APPROXIMATE WEIGHT GAIN DURING THE 2ND AND 3RD TRIMESTERS‡
Underweight	< 18.5	12.5–18 kg (28–40 lb)	0.4 kg/wk (1 lb/wk)
Normal weight	18.5–24.9	11.5–16 kg (25–35 lb)	0.4 kg/wk (1 lb/wk)
Overweight (0.5–0.7)	25.0–29.9	6.8–11.3 kg (15–25 lb)	0.27 kg/wk (0.6 lb/wk)
Obese (includes all classes)	≥ 30.0	5–9 kg (11–20 lb)	0.23 kg/wk (0.5 lb/wk)

*Recommendations for weight gain are based on prepregnancy BMI.

†For women who are pregnant with twins, provisional recommendations for total weight gain are as follows:

- Normal weight: 16.8–24.5 kg (37–54 lb)
- Overweight: 14.1–22.7 kg (31–50 lb)
- Obese women: 11.5–19.1 kg (25–42 lb)

‡A weight gain of 0.5–2 kg (1.1–4.4 lb) during the 1st trimester is assumed.

BMI = body mass index (kg/m^2)

Adapted from Institute of Medicine: Report Brief: Weight Gain During Pregnancy: Reexamining the Guidelines. 2009. Accessed 9/16.

- After a spontaneous or therapeutic abortion
- After amniocentesis or chorionic villus sampling
- Prophylactically at 28 wk
- If the neonate has Rh_0(D)-positive blood, after delivery

Modifiable risk factors: Pregnant women should not use alcohol and tobacco and should avoid exposure to secondhand smoke. They should also avoid the following:

- Exposure to chemicals or paint fumes
- Direct handling of cat litter (due to risk of toxoplasmosis)
- Prolonged temperature elevation (eg, in a hot tub or sauna)
- Exposure to people with active viral infections (eg, rubella, parvovirus infection [fifth disease], varicella)

Women with substance abuse problems should be monitored by a specialist in high-risk pregnancy. Screening for domestic violence and depression should be done.

Drugs and vitamins that are not medically indicated should be discouraged (see p. 2359).

Symptoms requiring evaluation: Women should be advised to seek evaluation for unusual headaches, visual disturbances, pelvic pain or cramping, vaginal bleeding, rupture of membranes, extreme swelling of the hands or face, diminished urine volume, any prolonged illness or infection, or persistent symptoms of labor.

Multiparous women with a history of rapid labor should notify the physician at the first symptom of labor.

280 Symptoms During Pregnancy

PELVIC PAIN DURING EARLY PREGNANCY

Pelvic pain is common during early pregnancy and may accompany serious or minor disorders. Some conditions causing pelvic pain also cause vaginal bleeding. In some of these disorders (eg, ruptured ectopic pregnancy, ruptured hemorrhagic corpus luteum cyst), bleeding may be severe, sometimes leading to hemorrhagic shock.

Causes of upper and generalized abdominal pain are similar to those in nonpregnant patients.

Etiology

Causes of pelvic pain during early pregnancy (see Table 280–1) may be

- Obstetric
- Gynecologic, nonobstetric
- Nongynecologic

Sometimes no particular disorder is identified.

The most common obstetric cause is

- Spontaneous abortion (threatened, inevitable, incomplete, complete, septic, or missed)

The most common serious obstetric cause is

- Ruptured ectopic pregnancy

Nonobstetric gynecologic causes include adnexal torsion, which is more common during pregnancy because during pregnancy, the corpus luteum causes the ovaries to enlarge, increasing the risk of the ovary twisting around the pedicle.

Common nongynecologic causes include various common GI and GU disorders:

- Viral gastroenteritis
- Irritable bowel syndrome
- Appendicitis
- Inflammatory bowel disease
- UTI
- Nephrolithiasis

Pelvic pain during late pregnancy may result from labor or one of the many nonobstetric causes of pelvic pain.

Evaluation

Evaluation should exclude potentially serious treatable causes (eg, ruptured or unruptured ectopic pregnancy, septic abortion, appendicitis).

History: History of present illness should include the patient's gravidity and parity as well as the pain's onset (sudden or gradual), location (localized or diffuse), and character (crampy or colicky). A history of illicitly attempted termination of pregnancy suggests septic abortion, but absence of this history does not exclude this diagnosis.

Review of systems should seek GU and GI symptoms that suggest a cause. Important GU symptoms include vaginal bleeding (ectopic pregnancy or abortion); syncope or near syncope (ectopic pregnancy); urinary frequency, urgency, or dysuria (UTI); and vaginal discharge and history of unprotected intercourse (pelvic inflammatory disease). Important GI symptoms include diarrhea (gastroenteritis, inflammatory bowel disease, or irritable bowel syndrome), vomiting (due to many disorders, including gastroenteritis and bowel obstruction), and obstipation (bowel obstruction, irritable bowel, or a functional disorder).

Past medical history should seek disorders known to cause pelvic pain (eg, inflammatory bowel disease, irritable bowel syndrome, nephrolithiasis, ectopic pregnancy, spontaneous abortion). Risk factors for these disorders should be identified.

Risk factors for ectopic pregnancy include

- History of sexually transmitted disease or pelvic inflammatory disease
- Cigarette smoking
- Use of intrauterine device
- Age > 35
- Previous abdominal surgery (especially tubal surgery)
- Use of fertility drugs or assisted reproductive techniques
- Previous ectopic pregnancy (the most important)
- Multiple sex partners
- Douching

Risk factors for spontaneous abortion include

- Age > 35
- History of spontaneous abortion
- Cigarette smoking
- Drugs (eg, cocaine, alcohol, high doses of caffeine)
- Uterine abnormalities (eg, leiomyoma, adhesions)

Risk factors for bowel obstruction include

- Previous abdominal surgery
- Hernia

Table 280–1. SOME CAUSES OF PELVIC PAIN DURING EARLY PREGNANCY

CAUSE	SUGGESTIVE FINDINGS	DIAGNOSTIC APPROACH
Obstetric disorders		
Ectopic pregnancy	Abdominal or pelvic pain, which is often sudden, localized, and constant (not crampy), with or without vaginal bleeding Closed cervical os No fetal heart sounds Possibly hemodynamic instability if ectopic pregnancy has ruptured	Quantitative β-hCG measurement CBC Blood type and Rh typing Pelvic ultrasonography
Spontaneous abortion (threatened, inevitable, incomplete, complete, missed)	Crampy, diffuse abdominal pain, often with vaginal bleeding Open or closed cervical os depending on the type of abortion (see Table 280–2)	Evaluation as for ectopic pregnancy
Septic abortion	Usually, apparent history of recent instrumentation of the uterus or induced abortion (often illegal or self-induced) Fever, chills, constant abdominal or pelvic pain with a purulent vaginal discharge Open cervical os	Evaluation as for ectopic pregnancy plus cervical cultures
Normal changes of pregnancy, including those due to stretching and growth of the uterus during early pregnancy	Crampy or burning sensation in the lower abdomen, pelvis, lower back, or a combination	Evaluation as for ectopic pregnancy Diagnosis of exclusion
Nonobstetric gynecologic disorders		
Uterine fibroid degeneration	Sudden onset of pelvic pain, often with nausea, vomiting, and fever Sometimes vaginal bleeding	Evaluation as for ectopic pregnancy
Adnexal (ovarian) torsion	Sudden onset of localized pelvic pain, which may be colicky and often mild if torsion spontaneously resolves Often, nausea, vomiting	Evaluation as for ectopic pregnancy plus Doppler ultrasonography
Ruptured corpus luteum cyst	Localized abdominal or pelvic pain, sometimes mimicking adnexal torsion Vaginal bleeding Usually, sudden onset	Evaluation as for ectopic pregnancy plus Doppler ultrasonography
Pelvic inflammatory disease (uncommon during pregnancy)	Cervical discharge, significant adnexal tenderness	Evaluation as for ectopic pregnancy plus cervical cultures
Nongynecologic disorders		
Appendicitis	Usually, continuous pain, tenderness Possibly atypical location (eg, right upper quadrant) or qualities (milder, crampy, no peritoneal signs) compared with pain in nonpregnant patients	Evaluation as for ectopic pregnancy plus cervical cultures Pelvic/abdominal ultrasonography Consideration of CT if ultrasonography is inconclusive
UTI	Suprapubic discomfort, often with bladder symptoms (eg, burning, frequency, urgency)	Urinalysis and culture
Inflammatory bowel disease	Variable pains (crampy or constant) in no consistent location, often with diarrhea and sometimes with mucus or blood Usually, a known history	Clinical evaluation Sometimes endoscopy
Bowel obstruction	Colicky pain, vomiting, no bowel movements or flatus Distended, tympanitic abdomen Usually, history of abdominal surgery (causing adhesions) or sometimes an incarcerated hernia detected during examination	Evaluation as for ectopic pregnancy plus cervical cultures Pelvic/abdominal ultrasonography Consideration of CT if ultrasonography is inconclusive
Gastroenteritis	Usually, vomiting, diarrhea No peritoneal signs	Clinical evaluation

β-hCG = β subunit of human chorionic gonadotropin.

Physical examination: Physical examination begins with a review of vital signs, particularly for fever and signs of hypovolemia (hypotension, tachycardia).

Evaluation focuses on abdominal and pelvic examinations. The abdomen is palpated for tenderness, peritoneal signs (rebound, rigidity, guarding), and uterine size and is percussed for tympany. Fetal heart sounds are checked using a Doppler probe.

Pelvic examination includes inspection of the cervix for discharge, dilation, and bleeding. Discharge, if present, should be sampled and sent for culture. Any blood or clots in the vaginal vault are gently removed. Bimanual examination should check for cervical motion tenderness, adnexal masses or tenderness, and uterine size.

Red flags: The following findings are of particular concern:

- Hemodynamic instability (hypotension, tachycardia, or both)
- Syncope or near syncope
- Peritoneal signs (rebound, rigidity, guarding)
- Fever, chills, and purulent vaginal discharge
- Vaginal bleeding

Interpretation of findings: Certain findings suggest causes of pelvic pain but are not always diagnostic (see Table 280–1).

For all women who present with pelvic pain during early pregnancy, the most serious cause—ectopic pregnancy—must be excluded, regardless of any other findings. Nonobstetric causes of pelvic pain (eg, acute appendicitis) must always be considered and investigated as in nonpregnant women.

As in any patient, findings of peritoneal irritation (eg, focal tenderness, guarding, rebound, rigidity) are a concern. Common causes include appendicitis, ruptured ectopic pregnancy, and, less often, ruptured ovarian cyst. However, absence of peritoneal irritation does not rule out such disorders, and index of suspicion must be high.

Vaginal bleeding accompanying the pain suggests spontaneous abortion or ectopic pregnancy. An open cervical os or tissue passed through the cervix strongly suggests an inevitable, incomplete, or complete abortion. The presence of fever, chills, and a purulent vaginal discharge suggests a septic abortion (particularly in patients with a history of instrumentation of the uterus or illicitly attempted termination of pregnancy). Pelvic inflammatory disease is rare during pregnancy but may occur.

Testing: If an obstetric cause of pelvic pain is suspected, quantitative measurement of β-hCG, CBC, blood type, and Rh typing should be done. If the patient is hemodynamically unstable (with hypotension, persistent tachycardia, or both), blood should be cross-matched, and fibrinogen level, fibrin split products, and PT/ PTT are determined.

Pelvic ultrasonography is done to confirm an intrauterine pregnancy. However, ultrasonography can and should be deferred in the hemodynamically unstable patient with a positive pregnancy test, given the very high likelihood of either ectopic pregnancy or spontaneous abortion with hemorrhage. Both transabdominal and transvaginal ultrasonography should be used as necessary. If the uterus is empty and tissue has not been passed, ectopic pregnancy is suspected. If Doppler ultrasonography shows that blood flow to the adnexa is absent or decreased, adnexal (ovarian) torsion is suspected. However, this finding is not always present because spontaneous detorsion can occur.

Treatment

Treatment is directed at the cause. If ectopic pregnancy is confirmed and is not ruptured, methotrexate can often be considered, or surgical salpingotomy or salpingectomy may be done. If the ectopic pregnancy is ruptured or leaking, treatment is immediate laparoscopy or laparotomy.

Treatment of spontaneous abortions depends on the type of abortion and the patient's hemodynamic stability. Threatened abortions are treated conservatively with oral analgesics. Inevitable, incomplete, or missed abortions are treated medically with misoprostol or surgically with uterine evacuation via D & C. Septic abortions are treated with uterine evacuation plus IV antibiotics.

Women who have Rh-negative blood should be given $Rh_0(D)$ immune globulin if they have vaginal bleeding or an ectopic pregnancy.

Ruptured corpus luteum cysts and degeneration of a uterine fibroid are treated conservatively with oral analgesics.

Treatment of adnexal torsion is surgical: manual detorsion if the ovary is viable; oophorectomy or salpingectomy if the ovary is infarcted and nonviable.

KEY POINTS

- Clinicians should always be alert for ectopic pregnancy.
- Nonobstetric causes should be considered; acute abdomen may develop during pregnancy.
- If no clear nonobstetric cause is identified, ultrasonography is usually necessary.
- A septic abortion is suspected when there is a history of recent uterine instrumentation or induced abortion.
- If vaginal bleeding occurred, Rh status is determined, and all women with Rh-negative blood are given $Rh_0(D)$ immune globulin.

VAGINAL BLEEDING DURING EARLY PREGNANCY

Vaginal bleeding occurs in 20 to 30% of confirmed pregnancies during the first 20 wk of gestation; about half of these cases end in spontaneous abortion. Vaginal bleeding is also associated with other adverse pregnancy outcomes such as low birth weight, preterm birth, stillbirth, and perinatal death.

Etiology

Obstetric or nonobstetric disorders may cause vaginal bleeding during early pregnancy (see Table 280–2).

The most dangerous cause is

- Ruptured ectopic pregnancy

The most common cause is

- Spontaneous abortion (threatened, inevitable, incomplete, complete, septic, missed)

Evaluation

A pregnant woman with vaginal bleeding must be evaluated promptly.

Ectopic pregnancy or other causes of copious vaginal bleeding (eg, inevitable abortion, ruptured hemorrhagic corpus luteum cyst) can lead to hemorrhagic shock. IV access should be established early during evaluation in case such complications occur.

History: History of present illness should include the patient's gravidity (number of confirmed pregnancies), parity (number of deliveries after 20 wk), and number of abortions (spontaneous or induced); description and amount of bleeding, including how many pads were soaked and whether clots or tissue were passed; and presence or absence of pain. If pain is present, onset, location, duration, and character should be determined.

Table 280–2. SOME CAUSES OF VAGINAL BLEEDING DURING EARLY PREGNANCY

CAUSE	SUGGESTIVE FINDINGS	DIAGNOSTIC APPROACH
Obstetric disorders		
Ectopic pregnancy	Vaginal bleeding, abdominal pain (often sudden, localized, and constant, not crampy), or both Closed cervical os Sometimes a palpable, tender adnexal mass Possible hemodynamic instability if ectopic pregnancy is ruptured	Quantitative β-hCG measurement CBC Blood typing Pelvic ultrasonography
Threatened abortion	Vaginal bleeding with or without crampy abdominal pain Closed cervical os, nontender adnexa Most common during the first 12 wk of pregnancy	Evaluation as for ectopic pregnancy
Inevitable abortion	Crampy abdominal pain, vaginal bleeding Open cervical os (dilated cervix) Products of conception often seen or felt through os	Evaluation as for ectopic pregnancy
Incomplete abortion	Vaginal bleeding, abdominal pain Open or closed cervical os Products of conception often seen or felt through os	Evaluation as for ectopic pregnancy
Complete abortion	Mild vaginal bleeding at presentation but usually a history of significant vaginal bleeding immediately preceding visit; some abdominal pain Closed cervical os, small and contracted uterus	Evaluation as for ectopic pregnancy
Septic abortion	Fever, chills, continuous abdominal pain, vaginal bleeding, purulent vaginal discharge Usually, apparent history of recent induced abortion or instrumentation of the uterus (often illegal or self-induced) Open cervical os	Evaluation as for ectopic pregnancy plus cervical cultures
Missed abortion	Vaginal bleeding, symptoms of early pregnancy (nausea, fatigue, breast tenderness) that decrease with time Closed cervical os	Evaluation as for ectopic pregnancy
Gestational trophoblastic disease	Larger-than-expected uterine size, often elevated BP, severe vomiting, sometimes passage of grapelike tissue	Evaluation as for ectopic pregnancy
Ruptured corpus luteum cyst	Localized abdominal pain, vaginal bleeding Most common during the first 12 wk of pregnancy	Evaluation as for ectopic pregnancy
Nonobstetric disorders		
Trauma	Apparent from history (eg, laceration of the cervix or vagina due to instrumentation or abuse, sometimes a complication of chorionic villus sampling or amniocentesis)	Clinical evaluation Questions about possible domestic violence if appropriate
Vaginitis	Only spotting or scant bleeding with vaginal discharge Sometimes dyspareunia, pelvic pain, or both	Diagnosis of exclusion Cervical cultures
Cervicitis	Only spotting or scant bleeding Sometimes cervical motion tenderness, abdominal pain, or both	Diagnosis of exclusion Cervical cultures
Cervical polyps (usually benign)	Scant bleeding, no pain Polypoid mass protruding from cervix	Clinical evaluation Obstetric follow-up for further evaluation and removal

β-hCG = β subunit of human chorionic gonadotropin.

Review of symptoms should note fever, chills, abdominal or pelvic pain, vaginal discharge, and neurologic symptoms such as dizziness, light-headedness, syncope, or near syncope.

Past medical history should include risk factors for ectopic pregnancy and spontaneous abortion (see p. 2324).

Physical examination: Physical examination includes review of vital signs for fever and signs of hypovolemia (tachycardia, hypotension).

Evaluation focuses on abdominal and pelvic examinations. The abdomen is palpated for tenderness, peritoneal signs (rebound, rigidity, guarding), and uterine size. Fetal heart sounds should be checked with a Doppler ultrasound probe.

Pelvic examination includes inspection of external genitals, speculum examination, and bimanual examination. Blood or products of conception in the vaginal vault, if present, are removed; products of conception are sent to a laboratory for confirmation. The cervix should be inspected for discharge, dilation, lesions, polyps, and tissue in the os. If the pregnancy is < 14 wk, the cervical os may be gently probed (but no more than fingertip depth) using ringed forceps to determine the integrity of the internal cervical os. If the pregnancy is ≥ 14 wk, the cervix should not be probed because the vascular placenta may tear, especially if it covers the internal os (placenta previa). Bimanual examination should check for cervical motion tenderness, adnexal masses or tenderness, and uterine size.

Red flags: The following findings are of particular concern:

- Hemodynamic instability (hypotension, tachycardia, or both)
- Orthostatic changes in pulse or BP
- Syncope or near-syncope
- Peritoneal signs (rebound, rigidity, guarding)
- Fever, chills, and mucopurulent vaginal discharge

Interpretation of findings: Clinical findings help suggest a cause but are rarely diagnostic (see Table 280–2). However, a dilated cervix plus passage of fetal tissue and crampy abdominal pain strongly suggests spontaneous abortion, and septic abortion is usually apparent from the circumstances and signs of severe infection (fever, toxic appearance, purulent or bloody discharge). Even if these classic manifestations are not present, threatened or missed abortion is possible, and the most serious cause—ruptured ectopic pregnancy—must be excluded. Although the classic description of ectopic pregnancy includes severe pain, peritoneal signs, and a tender adnexal mass, ectopic pregnancy can manifest in many ways and should always be considered, even when bleeding appears scant and pain appears minimal.

Testing: A self-diagnosed pregnancy is verified with a urine test. For women with a documented pregnancy, several tests are done:

- Quantitative β-hCG level
- Blood typing and Rh testing
- Usually ultrasonography

Rh testing is done to determine whether Rh_0(D) immune globulin is needed to prevent maternal sensitization. If bleeding is substantial, testing should also include CBC and either type and screen (for abnormal antibodies) or cross-matching. For major hemorrhage or shock, PT/PTT is also determined.

Transvaginal pelvic ultrasonography is done to confirm an intrauterine pregnancy unless products of conception have been obtained intact (indicating completed abortion). If patients are in shock or bleeding is substantial, ultrasonography should be done at the bedside. The quantitative β-hCG level helps interpret ultrasound results. If the level is ≥ 1500 mIU/mL and ultrasonography does not confirm an intrauterine pregnancy (a live or dead fetus), ectopic pregnancy is likely. If the level is < 1500 mIU/mL and no intrauterine pregnancy is seen, intrauterine pregnancy is still possible.

If the patient is stable and clinical suspicion for ectopic pregnancy is low, serial β-hCG levels may be done on an outpatient basis. Normally, the level doubles every 1.4 to 2.1 days up to 41 days gestation; in ectopic pregnancy (and in abortions), levels may be lower than expected by dates and usually do not double as rapidly. If clinical suspicion for ectopic pregnancy is moderate or high (eg, because of substantial blood loss, adnexal tenderness, or both), diagnostic uterine evacuation or D & C and possibly diagnostic laparoscopy should be done.

Ultrasonography can also help identify a ruptured corpus luteum cyst and gestational trophoblastic disease. It can show products of conception in the uterus, which are present in patients with incomplete, septic, or missed abortion.

Treatment

Treatment is directed at the underlying disorder:

- Ruptured ectopic pregnancy: Immediate laparoscopy or laparotomy
- Unruptured ectopic pregnancy: Methotrexate or salpingotomy or salpingectomy via laparoscopy or laparotomy
- Threatened abortion: Expectant management for hemodynamically stable patients
- Inevitable, incomplete, or missed abortions: D & C or uterine evacuation
- Septic abortion: IV antibiotics and urgent uterine evacuation if retained products of conception are identified during ultrasonography
- Complete abortion: Obstetric follow-up

KEY POINTS

- Clinicians should always be alert for ectopic pregnancy; symptoms can be mild or severe.
- Spontaneous abortion is the most common cause of bleeding during early pregnancy.
- Rh testing is required for all women who present with vaginal bleeding during early pregnancy to determine whether Rh_0(D) immune globulin is needed.

NAUSEA AND VOMITING DURING EARLY PREGNANCY

Nausea and vomiting affect up to 80% of pregnant women. Symptoms are most common and most severe during the 1st trimester. Although common usage refers to morning sickness, nausea, vomiting, or both typically may occur at any point during the day. Symptoms vary from mild to severe (hyperemesis gravidarum).

Hyperemesis gravidarum is persistent, severe pregnancy-induced vomiting that causes significant dehydration, often with electrolyte abnormalities, ketosis, and weight loss (see p. 2349).

Pathophysiology

The pathophysiology of nausea and vomiting during early pregnancy is unknown, although metabolic, endocrine, GI, and psychologic factors probably all play a role. Estrogen may contribute because estrogen levels are elevated in patients with hyperemesis gravidarum.

Etiology

The most common causes of uncomplicated nausea and vomiting during early pregnancy (see Table 280–3) are

- Morning sickness (most common)
- Hyperemesis gravidarum
- Gastroenteritis

Occasionally, prenatal vitamin preparations with iron cause nausea. Rarely, severe, persistent vomiting results from a hydatidiform mole.

Vomiting can also result from many nonobstetric disorders. Common causes of acute abdomen (eg, appendicitis, cholecystitis) may occur during pregnancy and may be accompanied by vomiting, but the chief complaint is typically pain rather than vomiting. Similarly, some CNS disorders (eg, migraine, CNS hemorrhage, increased intracranial pressure) may be accompanied by vomiting, but headache or other neurologic symptoms are typically the chief complaint.

Table 280–3. SOME CAUSES OF NAUSEA AND VOMITING DURING EARLY PREGNANCY

CAUSE	SUGGESTIVE FINDINGS	DIAGNOSTIC APPROACH
Obstetric		
Morning sickness (uncomplicated nausea and vomiting)	Mild, intermittent symptoms at varying times throughout the day, primarily during the 1st trimester Normal vital signs and physical examination	Diagnosis of exclusion
Hyperemesis gravidarum	Frequent, persistent nausea and vomiting with inability to maintain adequate oral intake of fluids, food, or both Usually, signs of dehydration (eg, tachycardia, dry mouth, thirst), weight loss	Urine ketones, serum electrolytes, Mg, BUN, creatinine If the condition persists, possibly liver function tests, pelvic ultrasonography
Hydatidiform mole	Larger-than-expected uterine size, absent fetal heart sounds and movement Sometimes elevated BP, vaginal bleeding, grapelike tissue from the cervix	BP measurement, quantitative hCG, pelvic ultrasonography, biopsy
Nonobstetric		
Gastroenteritis	Acute, not chronic; usually accompanied by diarrhea Normal (benign) abdomen (soft, nontender, not distended)	Clinical evaluation
Bowel obstruction	Acute, usually in patients who have had abdominal surgery Colicky pain, with obstipation and distended, tympanitic abdomen May be caused by or occur in patients with appendicitis	Abdominal imaging with flat and upright x-rays, ultrasonography, and possibly CT (if x-ray and ultrasound results are equivocal)
UTI or pyelonephritis	Urinary frequency, urgency, or hesitancy, with or without flank pain and fever	Urinalysis and culture

hCG = human chorionic gonadotropin.

Evaluation

Evaluation aims to exclude serious or life-threatening causes of nausea and vomiting. Morning sickness (uncomplicated nausea and vomiting) and hyperemesis gravidarum are diagnoses of exclusion.

History: History of present illness should particularly note the following:

- Onset and duration of vomiting
- Exacerbating and relieving factors
- Type (eg, bloody, watery, bilious) and amount of emesis
- Frequency (intermittent or persistent)

Important associated symptoms include diarrhea, constipation, and abdominal pain. If pain is present, the location, radiation, and severity should be queried. The examiner should also ask what social effects the symptoms have had on the patient and her family (eg, whether she is able to work or to care for her children).

Review of systems should seek symptoms of nonobstetric causes of nausea and vomiting, including fever or chills, particularly if accompanied by flank pain or voiding symptoms (UTI or pyelonephritis), and neurologic symptoms such as headache, weakness, focal deficits, and confusion (migraine or CNS hemorrhage).

Past medical history includes questions about morning sickness or hyperemesis in past pregnancies. Past surgical history should include questions about any prior abdominal surgery, which would predispose a patient to mechanical bowel obstruction.

Drugs taken by the patient are reviewed for drugs that could contribute (eg, iron-containing compounds, hormonal therapy) and for safety during pregnancy.

Physical examination: Examination begins with review of vital signs for fever, tachycardia, and abnormal BP (too low or too high).

A general assessment is done to look for signs of toxicity (eg, lethargy, confusion, agitation). A complete physical examination, including pelvic examination, is done to check for findings suggesting serious or potentially life-threatening causes of nausea and vomiting (see Table 280–4).

Red flags: The following findings are of particular concern:

- Abdominal pain
- Signs of dehydration (eg, orthostatic hypotension, tachycardia)
- Fever
- Bloody or bilious emesis

Table 280–4. RELEVANT PHYSICAL EXAMINATION FINDINGS IN A PREGNANT PATIENT WITH VOMITING

SYSTEM	FINDINGS
General	Lethargy, agitation
HEENT	Dry mucosa, icteric sclera
Neck	Stiffness to passive flexion (meningismus)
GI	Distention with tympany Absent or high-pitched tinkling bowel sounds Focal tenderness Peritoneal signs (guarding, rigidity, rebound)
GU	Flank tenderness to percussion Uterus too large for dates Absent fetal heart sounds Grapelike tissue from the cervix
Neurologic	Confusion, photophobia, focal weakness, nystagmus

HEENT = head, eyes, ears, nose, and throat.

- No fetal motion or heart sounds
- Abnormal neurologic examination
- Persistent or worsening symptoms

Interpretation of findings: Distinguishing pregnancy-related vomiting from vomiting due to other causes is important. Clinical manifestations help (see Table 280–3).

Vomiting is less likely to be due to pregnancy if it begins after the 1st trimester or is accompanied by abdominal pain, diarrhea, or both. Abdominal tenderness may suggest acute abdomen. Meningismus, neurologic abnormalities, or both suggest a neurologic cause.

Vomiting is more likely to be due to pregnancy if it begins during the 1st trimester, it lasts or recurs over several days to weeks, abdominal pain is absent, and there are no symptoms or signs involving other organ systems.

If vomiting appears to be pregnancy-related and is severe (ie, frequent, prolonged, accompanied by dehydration), hyperemesis gravidarum and hydatidiform mole should be considered.

Testing: Patients with significant vomiting, signs of dehydration, or both usually require testing. If hyperemesis gravidarum is suspected, urine ketones are measured; if symptoms are particularly severe or persistent, serum electrolytes are measured. If fetal heart sounds are not clearly audible or detected by fetal Doppler, pelvic ultrasonography should be done to rule out hydatidiform mole. Other tests are done based on clinically suspected nonobstetric disorders (see Table 280–3).

Treatment

Pregnancy-induced vomiting may be relieved by drinking or eating frequently (5 or 6 small meals/day), but only bland foods (eg, crackers, soft drinks, BRAT diet [bananas, rice, applesauce, dry toast]) should be eaten. Eating before rising may help. If dehydration (eg, due to hyperemesis gravidarum) is suspected, 1 to 2 L of normal saline or Ringer's lactate is given IV, and any identified electrolyte abnormalities are corrected.

Certain drugs (see Table 280–5) can be used to relieve nausea and vomiting during the 1st trimester without evidence of adverse effects on the fetus.

Table 280–5. SUGGESTED DRUGS FOR NAUSEA AND VOMITING DURING EARLY PREGNANCY

DRUG	DOSE
Vitamin B_6 (pyridoxine)	25 mg po tid
Doxylamine	25 mg po at bedtime
Promethazine	12.5–25 mg po, IM, or rectally q 6 h as needed
Metoclopramide	5–10 mg q 8 h po or IM
Ondansetron	8 mg po or IM q 12 h as needed

Vitamin B_6 is used as monotherapy; other drugs are added if symptoms are not relieved.

Ginger (eg, ginger capsules 250 mg po tid or qid, ginger lollipops), acupuncture, motion sickness bands, and hypnosis may help, as may switching from prenatal vitamins to a children's chewable vitamin with folate.

KEY POINTS

- Vomiting during pregnancy is usually self-limited and responds to dietary modification.
- Hyperemesis gravidarum is less common but is severe, leading to dehydration, ketosis, and weight loss.
- Nonobstetric causes should be considered.

LOWER-EXTREMITY EDEMA DURING LATE PREGNANCY

Edema is common during late pregnancy. It typically involves the lower extremities but occasionally appears as swelling or puffiness in the face or hands.

Etiology

The most common cause of edema in pregnancy is

- Physiologic edema

Physiologic edema results from hormone-induced Na retention. Edema may also occur when the enlarged uterus intermittently compresses the inferior vena cava during recumbency, obstructing outflow from both femoral veins.

Pathologic causes of edema are less common but often dangerous. They include deep venous thrombosis (DVT) and preeclampsia (see Table 280–6). DVT is more common during pregnancy because pregnancy is a hypercoagulable state, and women may be less mobile. Preeclampsia results from pregnancy-induced hypertension; however, not all women with preeclampsia develop edema. When extensive, cellulitis, which usually causes focal erythema, may resemble general edema.

Evaluation

Evaluation aims to exclude DVT and preeclampsia. Physiologic edema is a diagnosis of exclusion.

History: History of present illness should include symptom onset and duration, exacerbating and relieving factors (physiologic edema is reduced by lying in the left lateral decubitus position), and risk factors for DVT and preeclampsia. Risk factors for DVT include

- Venous insufficiency
- Trauma
- Hypercoagulability disorder
- Thrombotic disorders
- Cigarette smoking
- Immobility
- Cancer

Risk factors for preeclampsia include

- Chronic hypertension
- Personal or family history of preeclampsia
- Age < 17 or > 35
- First pregnancy
- Multifetal pregnancy
- Diabetes
- Vascular disorders
- Hydatidiform mole
- Abnormal maternal serum screening results

Review of symptoms should seek symptoms of possible causes, including nausea and vomiting, abdominal pain, and jaundice (preeclampsia); pain, redness, or warmth in an extremity (DVT or cellulitis); dyspnea (pulmonary edema or preeclampsia); sudden increase in weight or edema of the hands and face (preeclampsia); and headache, confusion, mental status changes, blurry vision, or seizures (preeclampsia).

Past medical history should include history of DVT, pulmonary embolism, preeclampsia, and hypertension.

Table 280–6. SOME CAUSES OF EDEMA DURING LATE PREGNANCY

CAUSE	SUGGESTIVE FINDINGS	DIAGNOSTIC APPROACH
Physiologic edema	Symmetric, bilateral leg edema that lessens with recumbency	Diagnosis of exclusion
DVT	Tender unilateral swelling of a leg or calf, erythema, and warmth Sometimes presence of risk factors for DVT	Lower-extremity duplex ultrasonography
Preeclampsia	Hypertension and proteinuria, with or without significant nondependent edema (eg, in face or hands), which, when present, is not red, warm, or tender Sometimes presence of risk factors for preeclampsia When preeclampsia is severe, possibly additional symptoms of headache; pain in the right upper quadrant, epigastric region, or both; and visual disturbances Possibly papilledema, visual field deficits, and lung crackles (in addition to edema), detected during physical examination	BP measurement Urine protein measurement CBC, electrolytes, BUN, glucose, creatinine, liver function tests
Cellulitis	Tender unilateral swelling in a leg or calf, erythema (asymmetric), warmth, and sometimes fever Manifestations often more circumscribed than in DVT	Ultrasonography to rule out DVT unless swelling is clearly localized Examination for source of infection

DVT = deep venous thrombosis.

Physical examination: Examination begins with review of vital signs, particularly BP.

Areas of edema are evaluated for distribution (ie, whether bilateral and symmetric or unilateral) and presence of redness, warmth, and tenderness.

General examination focuses on systems that may show findings of preeclampsia. Eye examination includes testing visual fields for deficits, and funduscopic examination should check for papilledema.

Cardiovascular examination includes auscultation of the heart and lungs for evidence of fluid overload (eg, audible S_3 or S_4 heart sounds, tachypnea, rales, crackles) and inspection of neck veins for jugular venous distention. The abdomen should be palpated for tenderness, especially in the epigastric or right upper quadrant region. Neurologic examination should assess mental status for confusion and seek focal neurologic deficits.

Red flags: The following findings are of particular concern:

- BP ≥ 140/90 mm Hg
- Unilateral leg or calf warmth, redness, or tenderness, with or without fever
- Hypertension and any systemic symptoms or signs, particularly mental status changes

Interpretation of findings: Although edema is common during pregnancy, considering and ruling out the most dangerous causes (preeclampsia and DVT) are important:

- If BP is > 140/90 mm Hg, preeclampsia should be considered.
- If edema involves only one leg, particularly when redness, warmth, and tenderness are present, DVT and cellulitis should be considered.
- Bilateral leg edema suggests a physiologic process or preeclampsia as the cause.

Clinical findings help suggest a cause (see Table 280–6). Additional findings may suggest preeclampsia (see Table 280–7).

Testing: If preeclampsia is suspected, urine protein is measured; hypertension plus proteinuria indicates preeclampsia. Urine dipstick testing is used routinely, but if diagnosis is unclear, urine protein may be measured in a 24-h collection. Many laboratories can more rapidly assess urine protein by measuring and calculating the urine protein:urine creatinine ratio.

If DVT is suspected, lower-extremity duplex ultrasonography is done.

Treatment

Specific causes are treated.

Table 280–7. SOME FINDINGS THAT SUGGEST PREECLAMPSIA

SYSTEM OR BODY PART	SYMPTOMS	CLINICAL FINDINGS
Eyes	Blurry vision	Visual field deficits, papilledema
Cardiovascular	Dyspnea	Increased S_3 or audible S_4 heart sound Tachypnea, rales, crackles
GI	Nausea, vomiting, jaundice	Epigastric or right upper quadrant tenderness
GU	Decreased urine output	Oliguria
Neurologic	Confusion, headache	Abnormal mental status
Extremities	Weight gain that is sudden and dramatic	Edema of legs, face, and hands
Skin	Rash	Petechiae, purpura

Physiologic edema can be reduced by intermittently lying on the left side (which moves the uterus off the inferior vena cava), by intermittently elevating the lower extremities, and by wearing elastic compression stockings.

KEY POINTS

- Edema is common and usually benign (physiologic) during late pregnancy.
- Physiologic edema is reduced by lying in the left lateral decubitus position, elevating the lower extremities, and using compression stockings.
- Hypertension and proteinuria indicate preeclampsia.
- Unilateral leg edema, redness, warmth, and tenderness require evaluation for DVT.

VAGINAL BLEEDING DURING LATE PREGNANCY

Bleeding during late pregnancy (≥ 20 wk gestation, but before birth) occurs in 3 to 4% of pregnancies.

Pathophysiology

Some disorders can cause substantial blood loss, occasionally enough to cause hemorrhagic shock or disseminated intravascular coagulation.

Etiology

The most common cause of bleeding during late pregnancy is

- Bloody show of labor

Bloody show heralds onset of labor, is scant and mixed with mucus, and results from tearing of small veins as the cervix dilates and effaces at the start of labor.

More serious but less common causes (see Table 280–8) include

- Abruptio placentae (placental abruption)
- Placenta previa
- Vasa previa
- Uterine rupture (rare)

Abruptio placentae is premature separation of a normally implanted placenta from the uterine wall. The mechanism is unclear, but it is probably a late consequence of chronic uteroplacental vascular insufficiency. Some cases follow trauma (eg, assault, motor vehicle crash). Because some or most of the bleeding may be concealed between the placenta and uterine wall, the amount of external (ie, vaginal) bleeding does not necessarily reflect the extent of blood loss or placental separation. Abruptio placentae is the most common life-threatening cause of bleeding during late pregnancy, accounting for about 30% of cases. It may occur at any time but is most common during the 3rd trimester.

Placenta previa is abnormal implantation of the placenta over or near the internal cervical os. It results from various risk factors. Bleeding may be spontaneous or triggered by digital examination or by onset of labor. Placenta previa accounts for about 20% of bleeding during late pregnancy and is most common during the 3rd trimester.

In **vasa previa**, the fetal blood vessels connecting the cord and placenta overlie the internal cervical os and are in front of the fetal presenting part. Usually, this abnormal connection occurs when vessels from the cord run through part of the chorionic membrane rather than directly into the placenta (velamentous insertion). The mechanical forces of labor can disrupt these small blood vessels, causing them to rupture. Because of the relatively small fetal blood volume, even a small blood loss due to vasa previa can represent catastrophic hemorrhage for the fetus and cause fetal death.

Uterine rupture may occur during labor—almost always in women who have had scarring of the uterus (eg, due to cesarean delivery, uterine surgery, or uterine infection)—or after severe abdominal trauma.

Table 280–8. SOME CAUSES OF BLEEDING DURING LATE PREGNANCY

CAUSE	SUGGESTIVE FINDINGS	DIAGNOSTIC APPROACH
Labor	Passage of blood-tinged mucus plug, not active bleeding Painful, regular uterine contractions with cervical dilation and effacement Normal fetal and maternal signs	Diagnosis of exclusion
Abruptio placentae	Painful, tender uterus, often tense with contractions Dark or clotted blood Sometimes maternal hypotension Signs of fetal distress (eg, bradycardia or prolonged deceleration, repetitive late decelerations, sinusoidal pattern)	Clinical suspicion Often, ultrasonography, although it is not very sensitive
Placenta previa	Sudden onset of painless vaginal bleeding with bright red blood and minimal or no uterine tenderness	Sometimes suspected based on findings during routine screening ultrasonography Transvaginal ultrasonography
Vasa previa	Painless vaginal bleeding with fetal instability but normal maternal signs Often, symptoms of labor	Sometimes suspected based on findings during routine screening ultrasonography Transvaginal ultrasonography with color Doppler studies
Uterine rupture	Severe abdominal pain, tenderness, cessation of contractions, often loss of uterine tone Mild to moderate vaginal bleeding Fetal bradycardia or loss of heart sounds	Clinical suspicion, usually history of prior uterine surgery Laparotomy

Evaluation

The evaluation aims to exclude potentially serious causes of bleeding (abruptio placentae, placenta previa, vasa previa, uterine rupture). Bloody show of labor and abruptio placentae are diagnoses of exclusion.

History: History of present illness should include the patient's gravidity (number of confirmed pregnancies), parity (number of deliveries after 20 wk), and number of abortions (spontaneous or induced); duration of bleeding; and amount and color (bright red vs dark) of blood. Important associated symptoms include abdominal pain and rupture of membranes. Clinicians should note whether these symptoms are present or not and describe them (eg, whether pain is intermittent and crampy, as in labor, or constant and severe, suggesting abruptio placentae or uterine rupture).

Review of systems should elicit any history of syncope or near syncope (suggesting major hemorrhage).

Past medical history should note risk factors for major causes of bleeding (see Table 280–9), particularly previous cesarean delivery. Clinicians should determine whether patients have a history of hypertension, cigarette smoking, in vitro fertilization, or any illicit drug use (particularly cocaine).

Physical examination: Examination starts with review of vital signs, particularly BP, for signs of hypovolemia. Fetal heart rate is assessed, and continuous fetal monitoring is started if possible.

The abdomen is palpated for uterine size, tenderness, and tonicity (normal, increased, or decreased).

A digital cervical examination is contraindicated when bleeding occurs during late pregnancy until ultrasonography confirms normal placental and vessel location (and excludes placenta previa and vasa previa). Careful speculum examination can be done. If ultrasonography is normal, clinicians may procced with a digital examination to determine cervical dilation and effacement.

Table 280–9. SOME RISK FACTORS FOR MAJOR CAUSES OF BLEEDING DURING LATE PREGNANCY

CAUSE	RISK FACTORS
Abruptio placentae	Hypertension Age > 35 Multiparity Cigarette smoking Cocaine Previous abruptio placentae Trauma
Placenta previa	Previous cesarean delivery Multiparity Multiple gestations Previous placenta previa Age > 35 Cigarette smoking
Vasa previa	Low-lying placenta Bilobed or succenturiate-lobed placenta Multiple gestations In vitro fertilization
Uterine rupture	Previous cesarean delivery Any uterine surgery Age > 30 History of uterine infection Induction of labor Trauma (eg, gunshot wound)

Red flags: The following findings are of particular concern:

- Hypotension
- Tense, tender uterus
- Fetal distress (loss of heart sounds, bradycardia, variable or late decelerations detected during monitoring)
- Cessation of labor and atonic uterus

Interpretation of findings: If more than a few drops of blood are observed or there are signs of fetal distress, the more serious causes must be ruled out: abruptio placentae, placenta previa, vasa previa, and uterine rupture. However, some patients with abruptio placentae or uterine rupture have minimal visible bleeding despite major intra-abdominal or intrauterine hemorrhage.

Clinical findings help suggest a cause (see also Table 280–8). Light bleeding with mucus suggests bloody show of labor. Sudden, painless bleeding with bright red blood suggests placenta previa or vasa previa. Dark red clotted blood suggests abruptio placentae or uterine rupture. A tense, contracted, tender uterus suggests abruptio placentae; an atonic or abnormally shaped uterus with abdominal tenderness suggests uterine rupture.

Testing: The tests should include the following:

- Ultrasonography
- CBC and type and screen
- Possibly Kleihauer-Betke testing

All women with bleeding during late pregnancy require transvaginal ultrasonography, done at the bedside if the patient is unstable. A normal placenta and normal cord and vessel insertion exclude placenta previa and vasa previa. Although ultrasonography sometimes shows abruptio placentae, this test is not sufficiently reliable to distinguish abruptio placentae from uterine rupture. These diagnoses are made clinically, based on risk factors and examination findings (a tense uterus is more common in abruptio placentae; loss of tone is more common in rupture). Rupture is confirmed during laparotomy.

In addition, CBC and type and screen (blood typing and screening for abnormal antibodies) should be done. If bleeding is severe, if moderate to severe abruptio placentae is suspected, or if maternal hypotension is present, several units of blood are cross-matched and tests for disseminated intravascular coagulation (PT/PTT, fibrinogen level, D-dimer level) are done.

The Kleihauer-Betke test can be done to measure the amount of fetal blood in the maternal circulation and determine the need for additional doses of $Rh_O(D)$ immune globulin to prevent maternal sensitization.

Treatment

Treatment is aimed at the specific cause. Patients with signs of hypovolemia require IV fluid resuscitation, starting with 20 mL/kg of normal saline solution. Blood transfusion should be considered for patients not responding to 2 L of saline.

KEY POINTS

- All patients require IV access for fluid or blood resuscitation, as well as continuous maternal and fetal monitoring.
- A digital cervical examination is contraindicated in evaluation of bleeding during late pregnancy until placenta previa and vasa previa are excluded.
- In abruptio placentae, vaginal bleeding may be absent if blood is concealed between the placenta and uterine wall.
- Uterine rupture is suspected in women with a history of cesarean delivery or other uterine surgery.
- Vaginal bleeding may be mild despite maternal hypotension.

281 Abnormalities and Complications of Labor and Delivery

Abnormalities and complications of labor and delivery should be diagnosed and managed as early as possible.

Most of the following complications are evident before onset of labor:

- Multifetal pregnancy
- Postterm pregnancy
- Premature rupture of membranes
- Abnormal fetal presentation

Some of the following complications develop or become evident during labor or delivery:

- Amniotic fluid embolism
- Shoulder dystocia
- Fetopelvic disproportion
- Preterm labor
- Protracted labor
- Umbilical cord prolapse
- Uterine rupture (rare)

Some complications may require alternatives to spontaneous labor and vaginal delivery. Alternatives include

- Induction of labor
- Operative vaginal delivery
- Cesarean delivery

The neonatal care team should be informed when alternative delivery methods are used so they can be ready to treat any neonatal complications.

Some complications (eg, postpartum hemorrhage, inverted uterus) occur immediately after delivery of the fetus and around the time the placenta is delivered.

Some placental abnormalities, such as placenta accreta, may be discovered during pregnancy or only after delivery.

For neonatal resuscitation and disorders of the birth process, see p. 2791; for meconium aspiration syndrome, see p. 2814. For preeclampsia and eclampsia, see p. 2353.

OPERATIVE VAGINAL DELIVERY

Operative vaginal delivery involves application of forceps or a vacuum extractor to the fetal head to assist during the 2nd stage of labor and facilitate delivery.

Indications for forceps delivery and vacuum extraction are essentially the same:

- Prolonged 2nd stage of labor (from full cervical dilation until delivery of the fetus)
- Suspicion of fetal compromise (eg, abnormal heart rate pattern)
- Need to shorten the 2nd stage for maternal benefit—eg, if maternal cardiac dysfunction (eg, left-to-right shunting) or neurologic disorders (eg, spinal cord trauma) contraindicate pushing or maternal exhaustion prevents effective pushing

A prolonged 2nd stage is defined as follows:

- In nulliparous women: Lack of continuing progress for 3 h with a regional anesthetic or 2 h without a regional anesthetic
- In multiparous women: Lack of continuing progress for 2 h with a regional anesthetic or 1 h without a regional anesthetic

Choice of device depends largely on user preference and operator experience and varies greatly. These procedures are used when the station of the fetal head is low (2 cm below the maternal ischial spines [station +2] or lower); then, minimal traction or rotation is required to deliver the head.

Before starting an operative vaginal delivery, the clinician should do the following:

- Confirm complete cervical dilation
- Confirm an engaged fetal vertex at station +2 or lower
- Confirm rupture of membranes
- Confirm that fetal position is compatible with operative vaginal delivery
- Drain the maternal bladder
- Clinically assess pelvic dimensions (clinical pelvimetry) to determine whether the pelvis is adequate

Also required are informed consent, adequate support and personnel, and adequate analgesia or anesthesia. Neonatal care providers should be alerted to the mode of delivery so they can be ready to treat any neonatal complications.

Contraindications include unengaged fetal head, unknown fetal position, and certain fetal disorders such as hemophilia. Vacuum extraction is typically considered contraindicated in preterm pregnancies of < 34 wk because risk of intraventricular hemorrhage is increased.

Major complications are maternal and fetal injuries and hemorrhage, particularly if the operator is inexperienced or if candidates are not appropriately chosen. Significant perineal trauma and neonatal bruising are more common with forceps delivery; shoulder dystocia, cephalohematoma, jaundice, and retinal bleeding are more common with vacuum-assisted delivery.

INDUCTION OF LABOR

Induction of labor is stimulation of uterine contractions before spontaneous labor to achieve vaginal delivery.

Indications: Induction of labor can be

- Medically indicated (eg, for preeclampsia or fetal compromise)
- Elective (to control when delivery occurs)

Before elective induction, gestational age must be determined. Elective induction is not recommended before 39 wk.

Contraindications to induction include having or having had the following:

- Fundal uterine surgery
- Open fetal surgery (eg, myelomeningocele repair)
- Myomectomy involving entry into the uterine cavity
- Prior classic or vertical cesarean incision in the thickened, muscular portion of the uterus
- Active genital herpes
- Placenta or vasa previa
- Abnormal fetal presentation (eg, transverse lie, umbilical cord presentation, certain types of fetopelvic disproportion)

Multiple prior uterine scars and breech presentation are relative contraindications.

Technique: If the cervix is closed, long, and firm (unfavorable), the goal is to cause the cervix to open and become effaced (favorable). Various pharmacologic or mechanical methods can be used. They include

- Misoprostol 25 mcg vaginally q 3 to 6 h
- Prostaglandin E_2 given intracervically (0.5 mg) or as an intravaginal pessary (10 mg) (Prostaglandins are contraindicated in women with prior cesarean delivery or uterine surgery because these drugs increase the risk of uterine rupture.)
- Oxytocin in low or high doses
- Use of laminaria and transcervical balloon catheters, which may be useful when other methods are ineffective or contraindications exist

Once the cervix is favorable, labor is induced.

Constant IV infusion of oxytocin is the most commonly used method; it is safe and cost-effective. Low-dose oxytocin is given at 0.5 to 2 milliunits/min, increased by 1 to 2 milliunits/min, usually q 15 to 60 min. High-dose oxytocin is given at 6 milliunits/min, increased by 1 to 6 milliunits/min q 15 to 40 min to a maximum of 40 milliunits/min. With doses > 40 milliunits/min, excessive water retention may lead to water intoxication. Use of oxytocin must be supervised to prevent uterine tachysystole (> 5 contractions in 10 min averaged over 30 min), which may compromise the fetus.

External fetal monitoring is routine; after amniotomy (deliberate rupture of the membranes), internal monitoring may be indicated if fetal status cannot be assessed externally. Amniotomy can be done to augment labor when the fetal head is applied to a favorable cervix and not ballotable (not floating).

CESAREAN DELIVERY

Cesarean delivery is surgical delivery by incision into the uterus.

Up to 30% of deliveries in the US are cesarean. The rate of cesarean delivery fluctuates. It has recently increased, partly because of concern about increased risk of uterine rupture in women attempting vaginal birth after cesarean (VBAC) delivery.

Indications: Although morbidity and mortality rates of cesarean delivery are low, they are still several times higher than those of vaginal delivery; thus, cesarean delivery should be done only when it is safer for the woman or fetus than vaginal delivery.

The **most common specific indications** for cesarean delivery are

- Previous cesarean delivery
- Protracted labor
- Fetal dystocia (particularly breech presentation)
- A nonreassuring fetal heart rate pattern, which requires rapid delivery

Many women are interested in elective cesarean delivery on demand. The rationale includes avoiding damage to the pelvic floor (and subsequent incontinence) and serious intrapartum fetal complications. However, such use is controversial, has limited supporting data, and requires discussion between the woman and her physician; the discussion should include immediate risks and long-term reproductive planning (eg, how many children the woman intends to have).

Many cesarean deliveries are done in women with previous cesarean deliveries because for them, vaginal delivery increases risk of uterine rupture; however, risk of rupture with vaginal delivery is only about 1% overall (risk is higher for women who have had multiple cesarean deliveries or a vertical incision, particularly if it extends through the thickened, muscular portion of the uterus).

Vaginal birth is successful in about 60 to 80% of women who have had a single prior cesarean delivery and should be offered to those who have had a single prior cesarean delivery by low transverse uterine incision. Success of VBAC depends on the indication for the initial cesarean delivery. VBAC should be done in a facility where an obstetrician, anesthesiologist, and surgical team are immediately available, which makes VBAC impractical in some situations.

Technique: During cesarean delivery, practitioners skilled in neonatal resuscitation should be readily available.

The uterine incision can be classic or lower segment.

- **Classic:** The incision is made vertically in the anterior wall of the uterus, ascending to the upper uterine segment or fundus. This incision typically results in more blood loss than a lower-segment incision and is usually done only when placenta previa is present, fetal position is transverse with the back down, the fetus is preterm, the lower uterine segment is poorly developed, or a fetal anomaly is present.
- **Lower segment:** Lower-segment incisions are done most often. A low transverse incision is made in the thinned, elongated lower portion of the uterine body, and the bladder reflection is dissected off the uterus. A vertical lower-segment incision is used only for certain abnormal presentations and for excessively large fetuses. In such cases, a transverse incision is not used because it can extend laterally into the uterine arteries, sometimes causing excessive blood loss. Women who have had deliveries by a low transverse uterine incision are advised about the safety of a trial of labor in subsequent pregnancies.

AMNIOTIC FLUID EMBOLISM

Amniotic fluid embolism is a clinical syndrome of hypoxia, hypotension, and coagulopathy that results from entry of fetal antigens into the maternal circulation.

Amniotic fluid embolism is a rare obstetric emergency, estimated to occur in 2 to 6/100,000 pregnancies. It usually occurs during late pregnancy but may occur during termination of a 1st- or 2nd-trimester pregnancy.

Although mortality estimates vary widely (from about 20 to 90%), the syndrome clearly poses a significant risk, and of women who die suddenly during labor, amniotic fluid embolism is one of the most likely causes.[1] Survival depends on early recognition and immediate institution of treatment.

1. Clark SL: Amniotic fluid embolism. *Obstet Gynecol* 123:337–348, 2014.

Pathophysiology

The long-standing term amniotic fluid "embolism" implies a primarily mechanical, obstructive disorder, as occurs in thromboembolism or air embolism. However, because amniotic fluid is completely soluble in blood, it cannot cause obstruction. Furthermore, the minor amounts of fetal cells and tissue debris that may accompany the amniotic fluid into the maternal circulation are too small to mechanically obstruct enough of the pulmonary vascular tree to cause the marked hemodynamic changes that occur in this syndrome. Instead, it is currently thought that exposure to fetal antigens during delivery activates proinflammatory mediators, which trigger an overwhelming inflammatory cascade and release of vasoactive substances (eg, norepinephrine) similar to the systemic inflammatory response syndrome (SIRS) that occurs in sepsis and septic shock.

The inflammatory response causes organ damage, particularly to the lungs and heart, and triggers the coagulation cascade, resulting in disseminated intravascular coagulation (DIC). The resulting maternal hypoxia and hypotension have profound adverse effects on the fetus.

Because maternal exposure to fetal antigens is likely fairly common during labor and delivery, it is not clear why only a few women develop amniotic fluid embolism. It is thought that different fetal antigens in varying amounts probably interact with unknown maternal susceptibility factors.

Risk factors: Many factors are associated with increased risk, but evidence is inconsistent. As with exposure to fetal antigens, many of the risk factors are commonplace or at least much more likely than amniotic fluid embolism, and there is no good pathophysiologic understanding of why only a few women with risk factors develop the syndrome. Nonetheless, risk is generally thought to be increased by the following:

- Cesarean delivery
- Advanced maternal age
- Multifetal pregnancy
- Abruptio placentae
- Abdominal trauma
- Placenta previa
- Uterine rupture
- Cervical lacerations
- Forceps delivery
- Polyhydramnios
- Induction of labor

Symptoms and Signs

Amniotic fluid embolism usually manifests during and shortly after labor and delivery. The first sign may be sudden cardiac arrest. Other patients suddenly develop dyspnea and have tachycardia, tachypnea, and hypotension. Respiratory failure, with significant cyanosis, hypoxia and pulmonary crackles, often quickly follows.

Coagulopathy manifests as bleeding from the uterus and/or sites of incisions and venipuncture.

Uterine hypoperfusion causes uterine atony and fetal distress.

Diagnosis

- Clinical evaluation
- Exclusion of other causes

Diagnosis of amniotic fluid embolism is suspected when the classic triad develops during labor or immediately after delivery:

- Sudden hypoxia
- Hypotension
- Coagulopathy

Diagnosis is clinical and by excluding other causes of the following:

- Sudden cardiac arrest in young women (eg, coronary artery dissection, congenital heart disease)
- Acute respiratory failure (pulmonary embolism, pneumonia)
- Coagulopathy (eg, sepsis, postpartum hemorrhage, uterine atony)

Autopsy may detect fetal squamous cells and hair in the pulmonary circulation, but this finding does not confirm the diagnosis. Fetal cells are sometimes detected in patients who do not have the amniotic fluid embolism syndrome.

Treatment

- Supportive care

Treatment of amniotic fluid embolism is supportive. It includes transfusion of RBCs (as needed to replace lost blood) and fresh frozen plasma and clotting factors (as needed to reverse the coagulopathy) plus ventilatory and circulatory support, with inotropic drugs as needed. Recombinant factor VIIa should not be used routinely but may be given to women who continue to bleed heavily despite use of other clotting factors.

Immediate operative delivery does not appear to improve or worsen maternal outcome but can be critical for fetal survival.

KEY POINTS

- Amniotic fluid embolism typically occurs during labor and delivery and causes a triad of hypoxia, hypotension and coagulopathy.
- The disorder is not a mechanical embolic phenomenon but is probably a biochemical response in which exposure to fetal antigens triggers an overwhelming inflammatory response in the mother.
- Mortality is high, and patients require immediate aggressive respiratory and hemodynamic support and replacement of clotting factors.
- Immediate delivery is necessary for fetal survival but does not seem to improve or worsen maternal outcome.

FETAL DYSTOCIA

Fetal dystocia is abnormal fetal size or position resulting in difficult delivery. Diagnosis is by examination, ultrasonography, or response to augmentation of labor. Treatment is with physical maneuvers to reposition the fetus, operative vaginal delivery, or cesarean delivery.

Fetal dystocia may occur when the fetus is too large for the pelvic opening (fetopelvic disproportion) or is abnormally positioned (eg, breech presentation). Normal fetal presentation is vertex, with the occiput anterior.

Fetopelvic disproportion: Diagnosis is suggested by prenatal clinical estimates of pelvic dimensions, ultrasonography, and protracted labor.

If augmentation of labor restores normal progress and fetal weight is < 5000 g in women without diabetes or < 4500 g in women with diabetes, labor can safely continue.

If progress is slower than expected in the 2nd stage of labor, women are evaluated to determine whether operative vaginal delivery (by forceps or vacuum extractor) is safe and appropriate.

Occiput posterior presentation: The most common abnormal presentation is occiput posterior.

The fetal neck is usually somewhat deflexed; thus, a larger diameter of the head must pass through the pelvis.

Many occiput posterior presentations require operative vaginal delivery or cesarean delivery.

Face or brow presentation: In face presentation, the head is hyperextended, and position is designated by the position of the chin (mentum). When the chin is posterior, the head is less likely to rotate and less likely to deliver vaginally, necessitating cesarean delivery.

Brow presentation usually converts spontaneously to vertex or face presentation.

Breech presentation: The 2nd most common abnormal presentation is breech (buttocks before the head). There are several types:

- **Frank breech:** The fetal hips are flexed, and the knees extended (pike position).
- **Complete breech:** The fetus seems to be sitting with hips and knees flexed.
- **Single or double footling presentation:** One or both legs are completely extended and present before the buttocks.

Breech presentation is a problem primarily because the presenting part is a poor dilating wedge, which can cause the head, which follows, to be trapped during delivery, often compressing the umbilical cord.

Umbilical cord compression may cause fetal hypoxemia. The fetal head can compress the umbilical cord if the fetal umbilicus is visible at the introitus, particularly in primiparas whose pelvic tissues have not been dilated by previous deliveries.

Predisposing factors for breech presentation include

- Preterm labor
- Uterine abnormalities
- Fetal anomalies

If delivery is vaginal, breech presentation may increase risk of

- Birth trauma
- Dystocia
- Perinatal death

Preventing complications is more effective and easier than treating them, so abnormal presentation must be identified before delivery. Cesarean delivery is usually done at 39 wk or when the woman presents in labor, although external cephalic version can sometimes move the fetus to vertex presentation before labor, usually at 37 or 38 wk. This technique involves gently pressing on the maternal abdomen to reposition the fetus. A dose of a short-acting tocolytic (terbutaline 0.25 mg sc) may help some women. The success rate is about 50 to 75%.

Transverse lie: Fetal position is transverse, with the fetal long axis oblique or perpendicular rather than parallel to the maternal long axis. Shoulder-first presentation requires cesarean delivery unless the fetus is a 2nd twin.

Shoulder dystocia: In this infrequent condition, presentation is vertex, but the anterior fetal shoulder becomes lodged behind the symphysis pubis after delivery of the fetal head, preventing vaginal delivery. Shoulder dystocia is recognized when the fetal head is delivered onto the perineum but appears to be pulled back tightly against the perineum (turtle sign).

Risk factors include a large fetus, maternal obesity, diabetes mellitus, prior shoulder dystocia, operative vaginal delivery, rapid labor, and prolonged labor. Risk of neonatal morbidity (eg, brachial plexus injury, bone fractures) and mortality is increased.

Once shoulder dystocia is recognized, extra personnel are summoned to the room, and various maneuvers are tried sequentially to disengage the anterior shoulder:

- The woman's thighs are hyperflexed to widen the pelvic outlet (McRoberts maneuver), and suprapubic pressure is applied to rotate and dislodge the anterior shoulder. Fundal pressure is avoided because it may worsen the condition or cause uterine rupture.
- The obstetrician inserts a hand into the posterior vagina and presses the posterior shoulder to rotate the fetus in whichever direction is easier (Wood screw maneuver).
- The obstetrician inserts a hand, flexes the posterior elbow, and sweeps the arm and hand across the fetal chest to deliver the infant's entire posterior arm.

These maneuvers increase risk of fracture of the humerus or clavicle. Sometimes the clavicle is intentionally fractured in a direction away from fetal lung to disengage the shoulder. An episiotomy can be done at any time to facilitate the maneuvers.

If all maneuvers are ineffective, the obstetrician flexes the infant's head and reverses the cardinal movements of labor, replacing the fetal head back into the vagina or uterus; the infant is then delivered by cesarean (Zavanelli maneuver).

INVERTED UTERUS

Inverted uterus is a rare medical emergency in which the corpus turns inside out and protrudes into the vagina or beyond the introitus.

The uterus is most commonly inverted when too much traction is applied to the umbilical cord in an attempt to deliver the placenta. Excessive pressure on the fundus during delivery of the placenta, a flaccid uterus, or placenta accreta (abnormally adherent placenta) can contribute.

Diagnosis of an inverted uterus is clinical.

Treatment

- Manual reduction

Treatment of an inverted uterus is immediate manual reduction by pushing up on the fundus until the uterus is returned to its normal position. If the placenta is still attached, the uterus should be replaced before the placenta is removed.

Because of discomfort, IV analgesics and sedatives or a general anesthetic is sometimes needed. Terbutaline 0.25 mg IV or nitroglycerin 50 mcg IV may also be needed.

If attempts to return the uterus are unsuccessful, a laparotomy may be necessary; the fundus is manipulated vaginally and abdominally to return it to its normal position. Once the uterus is in place, an oxytocin infusion should be started.

MULTIFETAL PREGNANCY

Multifetal pregnancy is presence of > 1 fetus in the uterus.

Multifetal (multiple) pregnancy occurs in 1 of 70 to 80 deliveries. Risk factors include

- Ovarian stimulation (usually with clomiphene or gonadotropins)
- Assisted reproduction (eg, in vitro fertilization)
- Prior multifetal pregnancy
- Advanced maternal age

The overdistended uterus tends to stimulate early labor, causing preterm delivery (average gestation is 35 to 36 wk with twins, 32 wk with triplets, and 30 wk with quadruplets). Fetal presentation may be abnormal. The uterus may contract after delivery of the first child, shearing away the placenta and increasing risk for the remaining fetuses. Sometimes uterine distention impairs postpartum uterine contraction, leading to atony and maternal hemorrhage.

Complications: Multifetal pregnancy increases the risk of preeclampsia, gestational diabetes, postpartum hemorrhage, cesarean delivery, preterm delivery, and growth restriction.

Some complications develop only in multifetal pregnancies. An example is twin-twin transfusion syndrome (when twins share the same placenta; this syndrome results in vascular communication between the two, which can lead to unequal sharing of blood).

Diagnosis

- Prenatal ultrasonography

Multifetal pregnancy is suspected if the uterus is large for dates; it is evident on prenatal ultrasonography.

Treatment

- Cesarean delivery when indicated

Cesarean delivery is done when indicated. Cesarean delivery is recommended for twins unless the presenting twin is in vertex presentation. Higher-order multiples are typically delivered by cesarean regardless of presentation.

PLACENTA ACCRETA

Placenta accreta is an abnormally adherent placenta, resulting in delayed delivery of the placenta. Placental function is normal, but trophoblastic invasion extends beyond the normal boundary (called Nitabuch layer). In such cases, manual removal of the placenta, unless scrupulously done, results in massive postpartum hemorrhage. Prenatal diagnosis is by ultrasonography. Treatment is usually with scheduled cesarean hysterectomy.

In placenta accreta, the placental villi are not contained by uterine decidual cells, as occurs normally, but extend to the myometrium.

Related abnormalities include

- Placenta increta (invasion of chorionic villi into the myometrium)
- Placenta percreta (penetration of chorionic villi into or through the uterine serosa)

All 3 abnormalities cause similar problems.

Etiology

The **main risk factor** for placenta accreta is

- Prior uterine surgery

In the US, placenta accreta most commonly occurs in women who have placenta previa and have had a cesarean delivery in a previous pregnancy. Incidence of placenta accreta has increased from about 1/30,000 in the 1950s, to about 1/500 to 2000 in the 1980s and 1990s, and to 3/1000 by the 2000s; it remains in the range of about 2/1000. Risk in women who have placenta previa increases from about 10% if they have had one cesarean delivery to > 60% if they have had > 4 cesarean deliveries. For women without placenta previa, having had a previous cesarean delivery increases risk very slightly (< 1% for up to 4 cesarean deliveries).

Other **risk factors** include the following:

- Maternal age > 35
- Multiparity (risk increases as parity increases)
- Submucosal fibroids
- Prior uterine surgery, including myomectomy
- Endometrial lesions such as Asherman syndrome

Symptoms and Signs

Usually, vaginal bleeding is profuse during manual separation of the placenta after delivery of the fetus. However, bleeding may be minimal or absent, but the placenta is not delivered within 30 min after delivery of the fetus.

Diagnosis

- Ultrasonography for women at risk

Thorough evaluation of the uteroplacental interface by ultrasonography (transvaginal or transabdominal) is warranted in women at risk; it can be done periodically, beginning at 20 to 24 wk gestation. If B-mode (gray-scale) ultrasonography is inconclusive, MRI or Doppler flow studies may help.

During delivery, placenta accreta is suspected if

- The placenta has not been delivered within 30 min of the infant's delivery.
- Attempts at manual removal cannot create a plane of separation.
- Placental traction causes large-volume hemorrhage.

When placenta accreta is suspected, laparotomy with preparation for large-volume hemorrhage is required.

Treatment

- Scheduled cesarean hysterectomy

Preparation for delivery is best. Usually, unless the woman objects, cesarean hysterectomy is done at 34 wk; this approach tends to result in the best balance of maternal and fetal outcomes.

If cesarean hysterectomy is done (preferably by an experienced pelvic surgeon), a fundal incision followed by immediate clamping of the cord after delivery can help minimize blood loss. The placenta is left in situ while hysterectomy is done. Balloon occlusion of the aorta or internal iliac vessels may be done preoperatively but requires a skilled angiographer and may cause serious thromboembolic complications.

Rarely (eg, when placenta accreta is focal, fundal, or posterior), clinicians can attempt to save the uterus, but only if acute hemorrhage is absent; for example, the uterus can be left in place, and a high dose of methotrexate can be given to dissolve the placenta. Uterine artery embolization, arterial ligation, and balloon tamponade are also sometimes used.

KEY POINTS

- In the US, placenta accreta is becoming increasingly common, occurring most often in women who have placenta previa and have had a cesarean delivery in a previous pregnancy.
- Consider using periodic ultrasonography to screen women who are > 35 yr of age or are multiparous (particularly if placenta previa developed previously or they have had a prior cesarean delivery), who have submucosal fibroids or endometrial lesions, or who have had prior uterine surgery.
- Suspect placenta accreta if the placenta has not been delivered within 30 min of the infant's delivery, if attempts at manual removal cannot create a plane of separation, or if placental traction causes large-volume hemorrhage.
- If placenta accreta is diagnosed, do cesarean hysterectomy at 34 wk.

POSTPARTUM HEMORRHAGE

Postpartum hemorrhage is blood loss of > 500 mL during or immediately after the 3rd stage of labor in a vaginal delivery or > 1000 mL in a cesarean delivery. Diagnosis is clinical. Treatment depends on etiology of the hemorrhage.

Causes

The **most common cause of postpartum hemorrhage** is

- Uterine atony

Risk factors for uterine atony include

- Uterine overdistention (caused by multifetal pregnancy, polyhydramnios, or an abnormally large fetus)
- Prolonged or dysfunctional labor
- Grand multiparity (delivery of ≥ 5 viable fetuses)
- Relaxant anesthetics
- Rapid labor
- Chorioamnionitis

Other causes of postpartum hemorrhage include

- Lacerations of the genital tract
- Extension of an episiotomy
- Uterine rupture
- Bleeding disorders
- Retained placental tissues
- Hematoma
- Uterine inversion
- Chorioamnionitis
- Subinvolution (incomplete involution) of the placental site (which usually occurs early but may occur as late as 1 mo after delivery)

Uterine fibroids may contribute to postpartum hemorrhage. A history of prior postpartum hemorrhage may indicate increased risk.

Diagnosis

- Clinical evaluation

Diagnosis of postpartum hemorrhage is clinical.

Treatment

- Removal of retained placental tissues and repair of genital lacerations
- Uterotonics (eg, oxytocin, prostaglandins, methylergonovine)
- Fluid resuscitation and sometimes transfusion
- Sometimes surgical procedures

Intravascular volume is replenished with 0.9% saline up to 2 L IV; blood transfusion is used if this volume of saline is inadequate.

Hemostasis is attempted by bimanual uterine massage and IV oxytocin infusion. A dilute oxytocin IV infusion (10 or 20 [up to 80] units/1000 mL of IV fluid) at 125 to 200 mL/h is given immediately after delivery of the placenta. The drug is continued until the uterus is firm; then it is decreased or stopped. Oxytocin should not be given as an IV bolus because severe hypotension may occur. In addition, the uterus is explored for lacerations and retained placental tissues. The cervix and vagina are also examined; lacerations are repaired. Bladder drainage via catheter can sometimes reduce uterine atony.

15-Methyl prostaglandin $F_2\alpha$ 250 mcg IM q 15 to 90 min up to 8 doses or methylergonovine 0.2 mg IM q 2 to 4 h (which may be followed by 0.2 mg po tid to qid for 1 wk) should be tried if excessive bleeding continues during oxytocin infusion; during cesarean delivery, these drugs may be injected directly into the myometrium. Oxytocin 10 units can also be directly injected into the myometrium. Prostaglandins should be avoided in women with asthma; methylergonovine should be avoided in women with hypertension. Sometimes misoprostol 800 to 1000 mcg rectally can be used to increase uterine tone.

Uterine packing or placement of a Bakri balloon can sometimes provide tamponade. This silicone balloon can hold up to 500 mL and withstand internal and external pressures of up to 300 mm Hg. If hemostasis cannot be achieved, surgical placement of a B-Lynch suture (a suture used to compress the lower uterine segment via multiple insertions), hypogastric artery ligation, or hysterectomy may be required. Uterine rupture requires surgical repair.

Blood products are transfused as necessary, depending on the degree of blood loss and clinical evidence of shock. Infusion of factor VIIa (50 to 100 mcg/kg, as a slow IV bolus over 2 to 5 min) can produce hemostasis in women with severe life-threatening hemorrhage. The dose is given q 2 to 3 h until hemostasis occurs.

Prevention

Predisposing conditions (eg, uterine fibroids, polyhydramnios, multifetal pregnancy, a maternal bleeding disorder, history of puerperal hemorrhage or postpartum hemorrhage) are identified antepartum and, when possible, corrected.

If women have an unusual blood type, that blood type is made available ahead of time. Careful, unhurried delivery with a minimum of intervention is always wise.

After placental separation, oxytocin 10 units IM or dilute oxytocin infusion (10 or 20 units in 1000 mL of an IV solution at 125 to 200 mL/h for 1 to 2 h) usually ensures uterine contraction and reduces blood loss.

After the placenta is delivered, it is thoroughly examined for completeness; if it is incomplete, the uterus is manually explored and retained fragments are removed. Rarely, curettage is required.

Uterine contraction and amount of vaginal bleeding must be observed for 1 h after completion of the 3rd stage of labor.

KEY POINTS

- Before delivery, assess risk of postpartum hemorrhage, including identification of antenatal risk factors (eg, bleeding disorders, multifetal pregnancy, polyhydramnios, an abnormally large fetus, grand multiparity).
- Replenish intravascular volume, repair genital lacerations, and remove retained placental tissues.
- Massage the uterus and use uterotonics (eg, oxytocin, prostaglandins, methylergonovine) if necessary.
- If hemorrhage persists, consider packing, surgical procedures, and transfusion of blood products.
- For women at risk, deliver slowly and without unnecessary interventions.

POSTTERM PREGNANCY

Postterm pregnancy refers to gestation that lasts ≥ 42 wk. Antenatal surveillance should be considered at 41 wk. Induction of labor should be considered after 41 wk and is recommended after 42 wk.

Accurate gestational age estimation is essential in making a diagnosis of postterm pregnancy. In women with regular, normal menstrual cycles, gestational age can be estimated based on the first day of the last normal menstrual period. If dating is uncertain or inconsistent with menstrual dating, ultrasonography early in gestation (up to 20 wk) is the most accurate with accepted variation of +/– 7 days. Later in gestation, the variation increases to +/– 14 days at 20 to 30 wk gestation and +/– 21 days after 30 wk.

Postterm pregnancy increases risks for the woman and fetus. Risks include

- Abnormal fetal growth (macrosomia and dysmaturity syndrome)
- Oligohydramnios
- Meconium-stained amniotic fluid
- Nonreassuring fetal test results
- Fetal and neonatal death
- Need for neonatal intensive care
- Dystocia (abnormal or difficult labor)
- Cesarean delivery
- Perineal lacerations
- Postpartum hemorrhage

Postmaturity refers to the condition of the fetus that results when the placenta can no longer maintain a healthy environment for growth and development, usually because the pregnancy has lasted too long. The fetus may have dry, peeling skin, overgrown nails, a large amount of scalp hair, marked creases on the palms and soles, lack of fat deposition, and skin that is stained green or yellow by meconium. Meconium aspiration is a risk.

Antenatal surveillance should be considered at 41 wk; it involves one of the following:

- Nonstress testing
- Modified biophysical profile (nonstress testing and assessment of amniotic fluid volume)
- A full biophysical profile (assessment of amniotic fluid volume and fetal movement, tone, breathing, and heart rate)

Treatment

- Induction of labor and delivery

If there is evidence of fetal compromise or oligohydramnios, delivery is required. Induction of labor can be considered at 41 to 42 wk, particularly if the cervix is favorable, and is recommended after 42 wk.

PREMATURE RUPTURE OF MEMBRANES

Rupture of membranes before onset of labor is considered premature. Diagnosis is clinical. Delivery is recommended when gestational age is ≥ 34 wk and is generally indicated for infection or fetal compromise regardless of gestational age.

Premature rupture of membranes (PROM) may occur at term (≥ 37 wk) or earlier (called preterm PROM if < 37 wk).

Preterm PROM predisposes to preterm delivery.

PROM at any time increases risk of infection in the woman (chorioamnionitis), neonate (sepsis), or both, as well as risk of abnormal fetal presentation and abruptio placentae. Group B streptococci and *Escherichia coli* are common causes of infection. Other organisms in the vagina may also cause infection.

PROM can increase risk of intraventricular hemorrhage in neonates; intraventricular hemorrhage may result in neurodevelopmental disability (eg, cerebral palsy).

Prolonged preterm PROM before viability (at < 24 wk) increases risk of limb deformities (eg, abnormal joint positioning) and pulmonary hypoplasia due to leakage of amniotic fluid (called Potter sequence or syndrome).

The interval between PROM and onset of spontaneous labor (latent period) and delivery varies inversely with gestational age. At term, > 90% of women with PROM begin labor within 24 h; at 32 to 34 wk, mean latency period is about 4 days.

Symptoms and Signs

Typically, unless complications occur, the only symptom of PROM is leakage or a sudden gush of fluid from the vagina.

Fever, heavy or foul-smelling vaginal discharge, abdominal pain, and fetal tachycardia, particularly if out of proportion to maternal temperature, strongly suggest chorioamnionitis.

Diagnosis

- Vaginal pooling of amniotic fluid or visible vernix or meconium
- Evaluation of vaginal fluid showing ferning or alkalinity (blue color) on Nitrazine paper
- Sometimes ultrasound-guided amniocentesis with dye for confirmation

Sterile speculum examination is done to verify PROM, estimate cervical dilation, collect amniotic fluid for fetal lung maturity tests, and obtain samples for cervical cultures. Digital pelvic examination, particularly multiple examinations, increases risk of infection and is best avoided unless imminent delivery is anticipated.

Fetal position should be assessed. If subclinical intra-amniotic infection is a concern, amniocentesis (obtaining amniotic fluid using sterile technique) can confirm this infection.

PEARLS & PITFALLS

- If premature rupture of membranes is suspected, avoid doing digital pelvic examinations unless delivery seems imminent.

Diagnosis is assumed if amniotic fluid appears to be escaping from the cervix or if vernix or meconium is visible. Other less accurate indicators include vaginal fluid that ferns when dried on a glass slide or turns Nitrazine paper blue, indicating alkalinity and hence amniotic fluid; normal vaginal fluid is acidic. Nitrazine test results may be false positive if blood, semen, alkaline antiseptics, or urine contaminate the specimen or if the woman has bacterial vaginosis. Oligohydramnios, detected by ultrasonography, suggests the diagnosis.

If the diagnosis is questionable, indigo carmine dye can be instilled using ultrasound-guided amniocentesis. Appearance of the blue dye on a vaginal tampon or peripad confirms the diagnosis.

If the fetus is viable, women are typically admitted to the hospital for serial fetal assessment.

Treatment

- Delivery if there is fetal compromise, infection, or gestational age > 34 wk
- Otherwise, pelvic rest, close monitoring, antibiotics, and sometimes corticosteroids

PROM management requires balancing risk of infection when delivery is delayed with risks due to fetal immaturity when delivery is immediate. No one strategy is correct, but generally, signs of fetal compromise or infection (eg, persistently nonreassuring fetal testing results, uterine tenderness plus fever) should prompt delivery. Otherwise, delivery can be delayed for a variable period if fetal lungs are still immature or if labor could start spontaneously (ie, later in the pregnancy).

Induction of labor is recommended when gestational age is > 34 wk.

When appropriate management is unclear, amniotic fluid tests can be done to assess fetal lung maturity and thus guide management; the sample may be obtained from the vagina or by amniocentesis.

Expectant management: When expectant management is used, the woman's activity is limited to modified bed rest and complete pelvic rest. BP, heart rate, and temperature must be measured ≥ 3 times/day.

Antibiotics (usually 48 h of IV ampicillin and erythromycin, followed by 5 days of oral amoxicillin and erythromycin) are given; they lengthen the latency period and reduce risk of neonatal morbidity.

In pregnancies of < 34 wk, corticosteroids should be given to accelerate fetal lung maturity (see p. 2342).

IV magnesium sulfate should be considered in pregnancies < 32 wk; in utero exposure to this drug appears to reduce the risk of severe neurologic dysfunction (eg, due to intraventricular hemorrhage), including cerebral palsy, in neonates.

Use of tocolytics (drugs that stop uterine contractions) to manage preterm PROM is controversial; their use must be determined case by case.

KEY POINTS

- Assume that membranes are ruptured if amniotic fluid pools in the vagina or if vernix or meconium is visible.
- Less specific indicators of PROM are ferning of vaginal fluid, alkaline vaginal fluid (detected by Nitrazine paper), and oligohydramnios.
- Consider inducing delivery if there is fetal compromise, infection, or evidence of fetal lung maturity or if gestational age is > 34 wk.
- If delivery is not indicated, treat with bed rest and antibiotics.
- If pregnancies are < 34 wk, give corticosteroids to accelerate fetal lung maturity, and if pregnancies are < 32 wk, consider magnesium sulfate to reduce risk of severe neurologic dysfunction.

PRETERM LABOR

Labor (contractions resulting in cervical change) that begins before 37 wk gestation is considered preterm. Risk factors include premature rupture of membranes, uterine abnormalities, infection, cervical incompetence, prior preterm birth, multifetal pregnancy, and placental abnormalities. Diagnosis is clinical. Causes are identified and treated if possible. Management typically includes bed rest, tocolytics (if labor persists), corticosteroids (if gestational age is < 34 wk), and possibly magnesium sulfate (if gestational age is < 32 wk). Antistreptococcal antibiotics are given pending negative anovaginal culture results.

Preterm labor may be triggered by

- Premature rupture of membranes
- Chorioamnionitis
- Another ascending uterine infection (commonly due to group B streptococci)
- Multifetal pregnancy
- Fetal or placental abnormalities
- Uterine abnormalities
- Pyelonephritis
- Some sexually transmitted diseases (STDs)

A cause may not be evident.

Prior preterm delivery and cervical incompetence increase the risk.

Premature labor can increase risk of intraventricular hemorrhage in neonates; intraventricular hemorrhage may result in neurodevelopmental disability (eg, cerebral palsy).

Diagnosis

- Clinical evaluation

Diagnosis of preterm labor is based on signs of labor and length of the pregnancy.

Anovaginal cultures for group B streptococci are done, and prophylaxis is appropriately initiated. Urinalysis and urine culture are done to check for cystitis and pyelonephritis. Cervical cultures are done to check for STDs if suggested by clinical findings.

Most women with a presumptive diagnosis of preterm labor do not progress to delivery.

Treatment

- Antibiotics for group B streptococci, pending anovaginal culture results
- Tocolytics
- Corticosteroids if gestational age is < 34 wk
- Magnesium sulfate if gestational age is < 32 wk

Bed rest and hydration are commonly used initially.

Antibiotics: Antibiotics effective against group B streptococci are given pending negative anovaginal cultures. Choices include the following:

- For women without penicillin allergy: Penicillin G 5 million units IV followed by 2.5 million units q 4 h or ampicillin 2 g IV followed by 1 g q 4 h
- For women with penicillin allergy but a low risk of anaphylaxis (eg, maculopapular rash with prior use): Cefazolin 2 g IV followed by 1 g q 8 h
- For women with penicillin allergy and an increased risk of anaphylaxis (eg, bronchospasm, angioneurotic edema, or hypotension with prior use, particularly within 30 min of exposure): Clindamycin 900 mg IV q 8 h or erythromycin 500 mg IV q 6 h if anovaginal cultures show susceptibility; if cultures document resistance or results are unavailable, vancomycin 1 g IV q 12 h

Tocolytics: If the cervix dilates, tocolytics (drugs that stop uterine contractions) can usually delay labor for at least 48 h so that corticosteroids can be given to reduce risks to the fetus. Tocolytics include

- Magnesium sulfate
- A calcium channel blocker
- Prostaglandin inhibitors

No tocolytic is clearly the first-line choice; choice should be individualized to minimize adverse effects.

Magnesium sulfate is commonly used and is typically well-tolerated.

Prostaglandin inhibitors may cause transient oligohydramnios. They are contraindicated after 32 wk gestation because they may cause premature narrowing or closure of the ductus arteriosus.

IV magnesium sulfate should be considered in pregnancies < 32 wk. In utero exposure to the drug appears to reduce the risk of severe neurologic dysfunction (eg, due to intraventricular hemorrhage), including cerebral palsy, in neonates.

Corticosteroids: If the fetus is < 34 wk, women are given corticosteroids unless delivery is imminent. One of the following may be used:

- Betamethasone 12 mg IM q 24 h for 2 doses
- Dexamethasone 6 mg IM q 12 h for 4 doses

These corticosteroids accelerate maturation of fetal lungs and decrease risk of neonatal respiratory distress syndrome, intracranial bleeding, and mortality.

Progestins: A progestin may be recommended in future pregnancies for women who have a preterm delivery to reduce the risk of recurrence. This treatment is initiated during the 2nd trimester and continued until just before delivery.

KEY POINTS

- Do anovaginal cultures for group B streptococci and cultures to check for any clinically suspected infections that could have triggered preterm labor (eg, pyelonephritis, STDs).
- Treat with antibiotics effective against group B streptococci pending culture results.
- If the cervix dilates, consider tocolysis with magnesium sulfate, a Ca channel blocker, or, if the fetus is ≤ 32 wk, a prostaglandin inhibitor.
- Give a corticosteroid if the fetus is < 34 wk.
- Consider magnesium sulfate if the fetus is < 32 wk.
- In future pregnancies, consider giving a progestin to prevent recurrence.

PROTRACTED LABOR

Protracted labor is abnormally slow cervical dilation orfetal descent during active labor. Diagnosis is clinical. Treatment is with oxytocin, operative vaginal delivery, or cesarean delivery.

Active labor usually occurs after the cervix dilates to ≥ 4 cm. Normally, cervical dilation and descent of the head into the pelvis proceed at a rate of at least 1 cm/h and more quickly in multiparous women.

Etiology

Protracted labor may result from fetopelvic disproportion (the fetus cannot fit through the maternal pelvis), which can occur because the maternal pelvis is abnormally small or because the fetus is abnormally large or abnormally positioned (fetal dystocia).

Another cause of protracted labor is uterine contractions that are too weak or infrequent (hypotonic uterine dysfunction) or, occasionally, too strong or close together (hypertonic uterine dysfunction).

Diagnosis

- Assessment of pelvic dimensions, fetal size and position, and uterine contractions
- Often response to treatment

Diagnosis of protracted labor is clinical.

The cause must be identified because it determines treatment. Assessing fetal and pelvic dimensions and fetal position (see p. 2321) can sometimes determine whether the cause is fetopelvic disproportion. For example, fetal weight > 5000 g (> 4500 g in diabetic women) suggests fetopelvic disproportion.

Uterine dysfunction is diagnosed by evaluating the strength and frequency of contractions via palpation of the uterus or use of an intrauterine pressure catheter.

Diagnosis is often based on response to treatment.

Treatment

- Oxytocin
- Cesarean delivery for fetopelvic disproportion or intractable hypotonic dysfunction
- Sometimes operative delivery during the 2nd stage of labor

If the 1st or 2nd stage of labor proceeds too slowly and fetal weight is < 5000 g (< 4500 g in diabetic women), labor can be augmented with oxytocin, which is the treatment for hypotonic dysfunction. If normal progress is restored, labor can then proceed. If not, fetopelvic disproportion or intractable hypotonic dysfunction may be present, and cesarean delivery may be required.

In the 2nd stage of labor, forceps or vacuum extraction may be appropriate after evaluation of fetal size, presentation, and station (2 cm below the maternal ischial spines [+2] or lower) and evaluation of the maternal pelvis.

Hypertonic uterine dysfunction is difficult to treat, but repositioning, short-acting tocolytics (eg, terbutaline 0.25 mg IV once), discontinuation of oxytocin if it is being used, and analgesics may help.

UMBILICAL CORD PROLAPSE

Umbilical cord prolapse is abnormal position of the cord in front of the fetal presenting part, so that the fetus compresses the cord during labor, causing fetal hypoxemia.

The prolapsed umbilical cord may be

- Occult: Contained within the uterus
- Overt: Protruding from the vagina

Both are uncommon.

Occult prolapse: In occult prolapse, the cord is often compressed by a shoulder or the head. A fetal heart rate pattern (see p. 2376) that suggests cord compression and progression to hypoxemia (eg, severe bradycardia, severe variable decelerations) may be the only clue.

Changing the woman's position may relieve pressure on the cord; however, if the abnormal fetal heart rate pattern persists, immediate cesarean delivery is necessary.

Overt prolapse: Overt prolapse occurs with ruptured membranes and is more common with breech presentation or a transverse lie. Overt prolapse can also occur with vertex presentation, particularly if membranes rupture (spontaneously or iatrogenically) before the head is engaged.

Treatment of overt prolapse begins with gently lifting the presenting part and continuously holding it off the prolapsed cord to restore fetal blood flow while immediate cesarean delivery is done. Placing the woman in the knee-to-chest position and giving her terbutaline 0.25 mg IV once may help by reducing contractions.

UTERINE RUPTURE

Uterine rupture is spontaneous tearing of the uterus that may result in the fetus being expelled into the peritoneal cavity.

Uterine rupture is rare. It can occur during late pregnancy or active labor.

Uterine rupture occurs most often along healed scar lines in women who have had prior cesarean deliveries. Other predisposing factors include congenital uterine abnormalities, trauma, and other uterine surgical procedures such as myomectomies or open fetal surgery.

Causes of uterine rupture include

- Uterine overdistention (multiple gestation, polyhydramnios, fetal anomalies)
- External or internal fetal version
- Iatrogenic perforation
- Excessive use of uterotonics
- Failure to recognize labor dystocia with excessive uterine contractions against a lower uterine restriction ring

If women who have had a prior cesarean delivery wish to try vaginal delivery, prostaglandins should not be used because they increase risk of uterine rupture.

Symptoms and signs of uterine rupture include fetal bradycardia, variable decelerations, evidence of hypovolemia, loss of fetal station (detected during cervical examination), and severe or constant abdominal pain. If the fetus has been expelled from the uterus and is located within the peritoneal cavity, morbidity and mortality increase significantly.

Diagnosis is confirmed by laparotomy.

Treatment of uterine rupture is immediate laparotomy with cesarean delivery and, if necessary, hysterectomy.

282 Abnormalities of Pregnancy

Abnormalities that develop during pregnancy may be directly related to the pregnancy or not (for nonobstetric disorders, see p. 2386). Obstetric abnormalities increase the risk of morbidity or mortality for the woman, fetus, or neonate, as do such factors as maternal characteristics, problems in previous pregnancies, and drug use (see p. 2366).

ABRUPTIO PLACENTAE

Abruptio placentae is premature separation of a normally implanted placenta from the uterus, usually after 20 wk gestation. It can be an obstetric emergency. Manifestations may include vaginal bleeding, uterine pain and tenderness, hemorrhagic shock, and disseminated intravascular coagulation. Diagnosis is clinical and sometimes by ultrasonography. Treatment is modified activity (eg, a trial of bed rest) for mild symptoms and prompt delivery for maternal or fetal instability or a near-term pregnancy.

Abruptio placentae occurs in 0.4 to 1.5% of all pregnancies; incidence peaks at 24 to 26 wk gestation.

Abruptio placentae may involve any degree of placental separation, from a few millimeters to complete detachment. Separation can be acute or chronic. Separation results in bleeding into the decidua basalis behind the placenta (retroplacentally). Most often, etiology is unknown.

Risk factors: Risk factors include the following:

- Older maternal age
- Hypertension (pregnancy-induced or chronic)
- Placental ischemia (ischemic placental disease) manifesting as intrauterine growth restriction
- Polyhydramnios
- Intra-amniotic infection (chorioamnionitis)
- Vasculitis
- Other vascular disorders
- Prior abruptio placentae
- Abdominal trauma
- Acquired maternal thrombotic disorders
- Tobacco use
- Premature rupture of membranes
- Cocaine use (risk of up to 10%)

Complications: Complications include the following:

- Maternal blood loss that may result in hemodynamic instability, with or without shock, and/or disseminated intravascular coagulation (DIC)
- Fetal compromise (eg, fetal distress, death) or, if abruptio placentae is chronic (usually), growth restriction
- Sometimes fetomaternal transfusion and alloimmunization (eg, due to Rh sensitization).

Symptoms and Signs

Acute abruptio placentae may result in bright or dark red blood exiting through the cervix (external hemorrhage). Blood may also remain behind the placenta (concealed hemorrhage). Severity of symptoms and signs depends on degree of separation and blood loss. As separation continues, the uterus may be painful, tender, and irritable to palpation. Hemorrhagic shock may occur, as may signs of DIC. Chronic abruptio placentae may cause continued or intermittent dark brown spotting.

Abruptio placentae may cause no or minimal symptoms and signs.

Diagnosis

- Combination of clinical, laboratory, and ultrasonographic findings

Diagnosis is suggested if any of the following occur during late pregnancy:

- Vaginal bleeding (painful or painless)
- Uterine pain and tenderness
- Fetal distress or death
- Hemorrhagic shock
- DIC
- Tenderness or shock disproportionate to the degree of vaginal bleeding

The diagnosis should also be considered in women who have had abdominal trauma. If bleeding occurs during late pregnancy, placenta previa, which has similar symptoms, must be ruled out before pelvic examination is done; if placenta previa is present, examination may increase bleeding.

Evaluation includes the following:

- Fetal heart monitoring
- CBC
- Blood and Rh typing
- PT/PTT
- Serum fibrinogen and fibrin-split products (the most sensitive indicator)
- Transabdominal or pelvic ultrasonography
- Kleihauer-Betke test if the patient has Rh-negative blood—to calculate the dose of Rh_0(D) immune globulin needed

Fetal heart monitoring may detect a nonreassuring pattern or fetal death.

Transvaginal ultrasonography is necessary if placenta previa is suspected based on transabdominal ultrasonography. However, findings with either type of ultrasonography may be normal in abruptio placentae.

PEARLS & PITFALLS

- Normal ultrasonographic findings do not rule out abruptio placentae.

Treatment

- Sometimes prompt delivery and aggressive supportive measures (eg, in a near-term pregnancy or for maternal or possible fetal instability)
- Trial of hospitalization and modified rest if the pregnancy is not near term and if mother and fetus are stable

Prompt cesarean delivery is usually indicated if any of the following is present, particularly if vaginal delivery is contraindicated:

- Maternal hemodynamic instability
- Nonreassuring fetal heart rate pattern
- Near-term pregnancy (eg, > 36 wk)

Once delivery is deemed necessary, vaginal delivery can be attempted if the mother is hemodynamically stable, fetal heart rate pattern is reassuring, and vaginal delivery is not contraindicated (eg, by placenta previa or vasa previa); labor can be carefully induced or augmented (eg, using oxytocin and/or amniotomy). Preparations for postpartum hemorrhage should be made.

Hospitalization and modified rest are advised if all of the following are present:

- Bleeding does not threaten the life of the mother or fetus.
- The fetal heart rate pattern is reassuring.
- The pregnancy is not near term.

This approach ensures that mother and fetus can be closely monitored and, if needed, rapidly treated. (Modified rest involves refraining from any activity that increases intra-abdominal pressure for a long period of time—eg, women should stay off their feet most of the day.) Corticosteroids should be considered (to accelerate fetal lung maturity) if gestational age is < 34 wk. If bleeding resolves and maternal and fetal status remains stable, ambulation and usually hospital discharge are allowed. If bleeding continues or if status deteriorates, prompt cesarean delivery may be indicated.

Complications (eg, shock, DIC) are managed with aggressive replacement of blood and blood products.

KEY POINTS

- Bleeding in abruptio placentae may be external or concealed.
- Sometimes abruptio placenta causes only minimal symptoms and signs.
- Do not exclude the diagnosis because a test result (including ultrasonographic) is normal.
- Consider prompt cesarean delivery if maternal of fetal stability is threatened or if pregnancy is near term.
- Consider vaginal delivery if mother and fetus are stable and pregnancy is near term.

CERVICAL INSUFFICIENCY

Cervical insufficiency (formerly called cervical incompetence) is painless cervical dilation resulting in delivery of a live fetus during the 2nd trimester. Transvaginal cervical ultrasonography during the 2nd trimester may help assess risk. Treatment is reinforcement of the cervical ring with suture material (cerclage) or use of vaginal progesterone.

Cervical insufficiency refers to presumed weakness of cervical tissue that contributes to or causes premature delivery not explained by another abnormality. Estimated incidence varies greatly (1/100 to 1/2000).

Etiology

The cause is not well-understood but seems to involve some combination of structural abnormalities and biochemical factors (eg, inflammation, infection); these factors may be acquired or genetic.

Risk factors: Most women with cervical insufficiency do not have risk factors; however, the following risk factors have been identified:

- Congenital disorders of collagen synthesis (eg, Ehlers-Danlos syndrome)
- Prior cone biopsies (particularly when ≥ 1.7 to 2.0 cm of the cervix was removed)
- Prior deep cervical lacerations (usually secondary to vaginal or cesarean delivery)
- Prior excessive or rapid dilation with instruments (now uncommon)
- Müllerian duct defects (eg, bicornuate or septate uterus)
- ≥ 3 prior fetal losses during the 2nd trimester

Recurrence: Overall risk of recurrence of fetal loss due to cervical insufficiency is probably ≤ 30%, leading to the question of how large a role fixed structural abnormalities have. Risk is greatest for women with ≥ 3 prior 2nd-trimester fetal losses.

Symptoms and Signs

Cervical insufficiency is often asymptomatic until premature delivery occurs. Some women have earlier symptoms, such as vaginal pressure, vaginal bleeding or spotting, nonspecific abdominal or lower back pain, or vaginal discharge. The cervix may be soft, effaced, or dilated.

Diagnosis

- Transvaginal ultrasonography at > 16 wk for women with symptoms or risk factors

Usually, cervical insufficiency is not identified until after preterm delivery occurs for the first time.

The diagnosis is suspected in women with risk factors or characteristic symptoms or signs. Then, transvaginal ultrasonography is done. Results are most accurate after 16 wk gestation. Suggestive ultrasonographic findings include cervical shortening to < 2.5 cm, cervical dilation, and protrusion of fetal membranes into the cervical canal.

Ultrasonography of women without symptoms or risk factors is not recommended because results do not accurately predict preterm delivery.

Treatment

- Cerclage
- Vaginal progesterone

Cerclage (reinforcement of the cervical ring with nonabsorbable suture material) may be indicated based on history alone (history-indicated cerclage) or based on ultrasonographic findings plus history (ultrasound-indicated cerclage). Cerclage appears to prevent preterm delivery in patients with ≥ 3 prior 2nd-trimester fetal losses. For other patients, the procedure should probably be done only if they have a history that strongly suggests cervical insufficiency and if cervical shortening is detected by ultrasonography before 22 to 24 wk gestation; restricting cerclage to such patients does not appear to increase risk of preterm delivery and reduces the number of cerclages currently being done by two thirds. Recent evidence suggests that cerclage may help prevent preterm delivery in women who have a history of idiopathic preterm delivery and whose cervix is < 2.0 cm long.

Vaginal progesterone (200 mg every night) can reduce risk of preterm delivery in certain women. It can be offered to women who have a history of idiopathic prior preterm delivery or cervical shortening (detected by ultrasonography) in the current pregnancy, particularly women who do not meet the criteria for cerclage. Whether vaginal progesterone further reduces risk in women treated with cerclage is unclear.

If preterm labor is suspected after 22 to 23 wk, corticosteroids (to accelerate fetal lung maturation) and modified rest may also be indicated.

KEY POINTS

- Usually, risk of cervical insufficiency cannot be predicted before premature delivery occurs for the first time.
- Do transvaginal ultrasonography after 16 wk if women have risk factors or symptoms.
- Treat at-risk women with cerclage or vaginal progesterone.

INTRA–AMNIOTIC INFECTION

(Chorioamnionitis)

Intra-amniotic infection is infection of the chorion, amnion, amniotic fluid, placenta, or a combination. Infection increases risk of obstetric complications and problems in the fetus and neonate. Symptoms include fever, uterine tenderness, foul-smelling vaginal discharge, and maternal and fetal tachycardia. Diagnosis is by specific clinical criteria or, for subclinical infection, analysis of amniotic fluid. Treatment includes broad-spectrum antibiotics and delivery.

Intra-amniotic infection typically results from an infection that ascends through the genital tract.

Risk factors: Risk factors include the following:

- Preterm labor
- Nulliparity
- Meconium-stained amniotic fluid
- Internal fetal or uterine monitoring
- Presence of genital tract pathogens (eg, those that cause sexually transmitted diseases or bacterial vaginosis, group B streptococci)
- Multiple digital examinations during labor in women with ruptured membranes
- Long labor
- Preterm premature rupture of membranes

Complications: Intra-amniotic infection can cause as well as result from preterm premature rupture of membranes or preterm delivery. This infection accounts for 50% of deliveries before 30 wk gestation. It occurs in 33% of women who have preterm labor with intact membranes, 40% who have premature rupture of membranes (PROM) and are having contractions when admitted, and 75% who go into labor after admission for PROM.

Fetal complications include increased risk of the following:

- Preterm delivery
- Apgar score < 3
- Neonatal infection (eg, sepsis, pneumonia, meningitis)
- Seizures
- Cerebral palsy
- Death

Maternal complications include increased risk of the following:

- Bacteremia
- Need for cesarean delivery
- Uterine atony
- Postpartum hemorrhage
- Pelvic abscess
- Thromboembolism
- Wound complications

Septic shock, coagulopathy, and adult respiratory distress syndrome are also risks but are uncommon if infection is treated.

Symptoms and Signs

Intra-amniotic infection typically causes fever. Other findings can include maternal tachycardia, fetal tachycardia, uterine tenderness, and foul-smelling amniotic fluid and/or vaginal discharge. However, infection may not cause typical symptoms (ie, subclinical infection).

Diagnosis

- Clinical criteria
- Amniocentesis for suspected subclinical infection

Diagnosis usually requires a maternal temperature of > 38° C (> 100.4° F) plus ≥ 2 of the following:

- Maternal WBC count > 15,000 cells/μL
- Maternal tachycardia (heart rate > 100 beats/min)
- Fetal tachycardia (heart rate > 160 beats/min)
- Uterine tenderness
- Foul-smelling amniotic fluid or vaginal discharge

Presence of a single symptom or sign, which may have other causes, is less reliable. For example, uterine pain and tenderness may result from abruptio placentae. Maternal tachycardia may be due to pain, epidural anesthesia, or drugs (eg, ephedrine); fetal tachycardia may be due to maternal use of drugs or fetal hypoxemia. Maternal and fetal heart rates also increase during fever. However, if intra-amniotic infection is absent, heart rates return to baseline as these conditions resolve. If fetal or maternal tachycardia is disproportionate to or occurs without such conditions or if it persists despite resolution of these conditions, intra-amniotic infection is suspected.

Subclinical infection: Refractory preterm labor (persisting despite tocolysis) may suggest subclinical infection. If membranes rupture prematurely before term, clinicians should also consider subclinical infection so that they can determine whether induction of labor is indicated.

Amniocentesis with culture of amniotic fluid is the best way to diagnose subclinical infection. The following fluid findings suggest infection:

- Presence of any bacteria or leukocytes using Gram staining
- Positive culture
- Glucose level < 15 mg/dL
- WBC count > 30 cells/μL
- Leukocyte esterase level at trace or higher levels

Other diagnostic tests for subclinical infection are under study.

Treatment

- Broad-spectrum antibiotics plus delivery

Treatment is broad-spectrum IV antibiotics plus delivery. A typical intrapartum antibiotic regimen is ampicillin 2 g IV q 6 h plus gentamicin 1.5 mg/kg IV q 8 h. How long antibiotics are given varies, depending on individual circumstances (eg, how high the fever was, when the fever last spiked in relation to delivery). The antibiotics reduce risk of morbidity due to infection for mother and neonate.

Prevention

Risk of intra-amniotic infection is decreased by avoiding or minimizing digital pelvic examinations in women with preterm PROM (see p. 2340). Broad-spectrum antibiotics are also given to women with preterm PROM to prolong latency until delivery and decrease risk of infant morbidity and mortality.

KEY POINTS

- Intra-amniotic infection can be subclinical and relatively asymptomatic.
- Consider the diagnosis when fetal or maternal tachycardia or refractory preterm labor is present, as well as when women have the more classic symptoms of infection (eg, fever, discharge, pain, tenderness).
- Consider analyzing and culturing amniotic fluid if women have refractory preterm labor or preterm PROM.
- Treat intra-amniotic infection with broad-spectrum antibiotics plus delivery.

ECTOPIC PREGNANCY

In ectopic pregnancy, implantation occurs in a site other than the endometrial lining of the uterine cavity—in the fallopian tube, uterine cornua, cervix, ovary, or abdominal or pelvic cavity. Ectopic pregnancies cannot be carried to term and eventually rupture or involute. Early symptoms and signs include pelvic pain, vaginal bleeding, and cervical motion tenderness. Syncope or hemorrhagic shock can occur with rupture. Diagnosis is by measurement of the β subunit of human chorionic gonadotropin and ultrasonography. Treatment is with laparoscopic or open surgical resection or with IM methotrexate.

Incidence of ectopic pregnancy is about 2/100 diagnosed pregnancies.

Etiology

Tubal lesions increase risk. Factors that particularly increase risk include

- Prior ectopic pregnancy (10 to 25% risk of recurrence)
- History of pelvic inflammatory disease (particularly due to *Chlamydia trachomatis*)
- Prior abdominal or particularly tubal surgery, including tubal ligation

Other specific risk factors include

- Intrauterine device (IUD) use
- Infertility
- Multiple sex partners
- Cigarette smoking
- Exposure to diethylstilbestrol
- Prior induced abortion

Pregnancy is less likely to occur when an IUD is in place; however, about 5% of such pregnancies are ectopic.

Pathophysiology

The most common site of ectopic implantation is a fallopian tube, followed by the uterine cornua. Pregnancies in the cervix, a cesarean delivery scar, an ovary, the abdomen, or fallopian tube interstitium are rare.

Heterotopic pregnancy (simultaneous ectopic and intrauterine pregnancies) occurs in only 1/10,000 to 30,000 pregnancies but may be more common among women who have had ovulation induction or used assisted reproductive techniques such as in vitro fertilization and gamete intrafallopian tube transfer (GIFT); in these women, the overall reported ectopic pregnancy rate is ≤ 1%.

The structure containing the fetus usually ruptures after about 6 to 16 wk. Rupture results in bleeding that can be gradual or rapid enough to cause hemorrhagic shock. Intraperitoneal blood irritates the peritoneum. The later the rupture, the more rapidly blood is lost and the higher the risk of death.

Symptoms and Signs

Symptoms vary and are often absent until rupture occurs. Most patients have pelvic pain (which is sometimes crampy), vaginal bleeding, or both. Menses may or may not be delayed or missed, and patients may not be aware that they are pregnant.

Rupture may be heralded by sudden, severe pain, followed by syncope or by symptoms and signs of hemorrhagic shock or peritonitis. Rapid hemorrhage is more likely in ruptured cornual pregnancies.

Cervical motion tenderness, unilateral or bilateral adnexal tenderness, or an adnexal mass may be present. The uterus may be slightly enlarged (but often less than anticipated based on date of the last menstrual period).

Diagnosis

- Quantitative serum β–human chorionic gonadotropin (β-hCG)
- Pelvic ultrasonography
- Sometimes laparoscopy

Ectopic pregnancy is suspected in any female of reproductive age with pelvic pain, vaginal bleeding, or unexplained syncope or hemorrhagic shock, regardless of sexual, contraceptive, and menstrual history. Findings of physical (including pelvic) examination are neither sensitive nor specific.

PEARLS & PITFALLS

- Suspect ectopic pregnancy in any female of reproductive age with pelvic pain, vaginal bleeding, or unexplained syncope or hemorrhagic shock, regardless of sexual, contraceptive, and menstrual history and examination findings.

The first step is doing a urine pregnancy test, which is about 99% sensitive for pregnancy (ectopic and otherwise). If urine β-hCG is negative and if clinical findings do not strongly suggest ectopic pregnancy, further evaluation is unnecessary unless symptoms recur or worsen. If urine β-hCG is positive or if clinical findings strongly suggest ectopic pregnancy, quantitative serum β-hCG and pelvic ultrasonography are indicated.

If quantitative serum β-hCG is < 5 mIU/mL, ectopic pregnancy is excluded. If ultrasonography detects an intrauterine gestational sac, ectopic pregnancy is extremely unlikely except in women who have used assisted reproductive techniques (which increase risk of heterotopic pregnancy); however, cornual and intra-abdominal pregnancies may appear to be intrauterine pregnancies. Ultrasonographic findings suggesting ectopic pregnancy (noted in 16 to 32%) include complex (mixed solid and cystic) masses, particularly in the adnexa, and free fluid in the cul-de-sac.

If serum β-hCG is above a certain level (called the discriminatory zone), ultrasonography should detect a gestational sac in patients with an intrauterine pregnancy. This level is usually about 2000 mIU/mL. If the β-hCG level is higher than the discriminatory zone and an intrauterine gestational sac is not detected, an ectopic pregnancy is likely. Use of transvaginal and color Doppler ultrasonography may improve detection rates.

If the β-hCG level is below the discriminatory zone and ultrasonography is unremarkable, patients may have an early intrauterine pregnancy or an ectopic pregnancy. If clinical evaluation suggests ectopic pregnancy (eg, signs of significant hemorrhage or peritoneal irritation), diagnostic laparoscopy may be necessary for confirmation. If ectopic pregnancy appears unlikely and patients are stable, serum levels of β-hCG can be measured serially on an outpatient basis (typically every 2 days). Normally, the level doubles every 1.4 to 2.1 days up to 41 days; in ectopic pregnancy (and in abortions), levels may be lower than expected by dates and usually do not double as rapidly. If β-hCG levels do not increase as expected or if they decrease, the diagnoses of spontaneous abortion and ectopic pregnancy are reconsidered.

Prognosis

Ectopic pregnancy is fatal to the fetus, but if treatment occurs before rupture, maternal death is very rare. In the US, ectopic pregnancy probably accounts for 9% of pregnancy-related maternal deaths.

Treatment

- Surgical resection (usually)
- Methotrexate for some small, unruptured ectopic pregnancies

Surgical resection: Hemodynamically unstable patients require immediate laparotomy and treatment of hemorrhagic shock (see p. 575). For stable patients, treatment is usually laparoscopic surgery; sometimes laparotomy is required. If possible, salpingotomy, usually using cautery, high-frequency (harmonic) ultrasound devices, or a laser, is done to conserve the tube, and the products of conception are evacuated.

Salpingectomy is indicated in any of the following cases:

- When ectopic pregnancies recur or are > 5 cm
- When the tubes are severely damaged
- When no future childbearing is planned

Only the irreversibly damaged portion of the tube is removed, maximizing the chance that tubal repair can restore fertility. The tube may or may not be repaired. After a cornual pregnancy, the tube and ovary involved can usually be salvaged, but occasionally repair is impossible, making hysterectomy necessary.

Methotrexate: If unruptured tubal pregnancies are < 3 cm in diameter, no fetal heart activity is detected, and the β-hCG level is < 5,000 mIU/mL ideally but up to 15,000 mIU/mL, women can be given a single dose of methotrexate 50 mg/m^2 IM. β-hCG measurement is repeated on about days 4 and 7. If the β-hCG level does not decrease by 15%, a 2nd dose of methotrexate or surgery is needed. Alternatively, other protocols can be used. For example, the β-hCG level can be measured on days 1 and 7, and a 2nd dose of methotrexate can be given if the level does not decrease by 25%. About 15 to 20% of women treated with methotrexate eventually require a 2nd dose.

The β-hCG level is measured weekly until it is undetectable. Success rates with methotrexate are about 87%; 7% of women have serious complications (eg, rupture). Surgery is indicated when methotrexate is ineffective.

KEY POINTS

- The most common site for ectopic pregnancies is a fallopian tube.
- Symptoms can include pelvic pain, vaginal bleeding, and/or missed menses, but symptoms may be absent until rupture occurs, sometimes with catastrophic results.
- Suspect ectopic pregnancy in any female of reproductive age with pelvic pain, vaginal bleeding, or unexplained syncope or hemorrhagic shock, regardless of history and examination findings.
- If a urine pregnancy test is positive or clinical findings suggest ectopic pregnancy, determine quantitative serum β-hCG and do pelvic ultrasonography.
- Treatment usually involves surgical resection.

ERYTHROBLASTOSIS FETALIS

Erythroblastosis fetalis is hemolytic anemia in the fetus (or neonate, as erythroblastosis neonatorum) caused by transplacental transmission of maternal antibodies to fetal RBCs. The disorder usually results from incompatibility between maternal and fetal blood groups, often Rh_0(D) antigens. Diagnosis begins with prenatal maternal antigenic and antibody screening and may require paternal screening, serial measurement of maternal antibody titers, and fetal testing. Treatment may involve intrauterine fetal transfusion or neonatal exchange transfusion. Prevention is Rh_0(D) immune globulin injection for women at risk.

Erythroblastosis fetalis classically results from Rh_0(D) incompatibility, which may develop when a woman with Rh-negative blood is impregnated by a man with Rh-positive blood and conceives a fetus with Rh-positive blood (see also p. 2786). Other fetomaternal incompatibilities that can cause erythroblastosis fetalis involve the Kell, Duffy, Kidd, MNSs, Lutheran, Diego, Xg, P, Ee, and Cc antigen systems, as well as other antigens. Incompatibilities of ABO blood types do not cause erythroblastosis fetalis.

Pathophysiology

Fetal RBCs normally move across the placenta to the maternal circulation throughout pregnancy. Movement is greatest at delivery or termination of pregnancy. Movement of large volumes (eg, 10 to 150 mL) is considered significant fetomaternal hemorrhage; it can occur after trauma and sometimes after delivery or termination of pregnancy. In women who have Rh-negative blood and who are carrying a fetus with Rh-positive blood, fetal RBCs stimulate maternal antibody production against the Rh antigens. The larger the fetomaternal hemorrhage, the more antibodies produced. The mechanism is the same when other antigen systems are involved; however, Kell antibody incompatibility also directly suppresses RBC production in bone marrow.

Other causes of maternal anti-Rh antibody production include injection with needles contaminated with Rh-positive blood and inadvertent transfusion of Rh-positive blood.

No complications develop during the initial sensitizing pregnancy; however, in subsequent pregnancies, maternal antibodies cross the placenta and lyse fetal RBCs, causing anemia, hypoalbuminemia, and possibly high-output heart failure or fetal death. Anemia stimulates fetal bone marrow to produce and release immature RBCs (erythroblasts) into fetal peripheral circulation (erythroblastosis fetalis). Hemolysis results in elevated indirect bilirubin levels in neonates, causing kernicterus (see p. 2730). Usually, isoimmunization does not cause symptoms in pregnant women.

Diagnosis

- Maternal blood and Rh typing and reflex antibody screening
- Serial antibody level measurements and middle cerebral artery blood flow measurements for pregnancies considered at risk

At the first prenatal visit, all women are screened for blood type, Rh type, and anti-Rh_0(D) and other antibodies that are formed in response to antigens and that can cause erythroblastosis fetalis (reflex antibody screening). If women have Rh-negative blood and test positive for anti-Rh_0(D) or they test positive for another antibody that can cause erythroblastosis fetalis, the father's blood type and zygosity (if paternity is certain) are determined. If he has Rh-negative blood and is negative for the antigen corresponding to the antibody identified in the mother, no further testing is necessary. If he has Rh-positive blood or has the antigen, maternal anti-Rh antibody titers are measured. If titers are positive but less than a laboratory-specific critical value (usually 1:8 to 1:32), they are measured every 2 to 4 wk after 20 wk. If the critical value is exceeded, fetal middle cerebral artery blood flow is measured at intervals of 1 to 2 wk depending on the initial blood flow result and patient history; the purpose is to detect high-output heart failure, indicating high risk of anemia. Elevated blood flow for gestational age should prompt consideration of percutaneous umbilical blood sampling to obtain a sample of fetal blood; however, because this procedure can cause complications, treatment is sometimes decided without doing such sampling. If paternity is reasonably certain and the father is likely to be heterozygous for Rh_0(D), the fetus's Rh type is determined. If fetal blood is Rh positive or status is unknown and if middle cerebral artery flow is elevated, fetal anemia is likely.

Treatment

- Fetal blood transfusions
- Delivery at 32 to 35 wk

If fetal blood is Rh negative or if middle cerebral artery blood flow remains normal, pregnancy can continue to term untreated. If fetal anemia is likely, the fetus can be given intravascular intrauterine blood transfusions by a specialist at an institution equipped to care for high-risk pregnancies. Transfusions occur every 1 to 2 wk until fetal lung maturity is confirmed (usually at 32 to 35 wk), when delivery should be done. Corticosteroids should be given before the first transfusion if the pregnancy is > 24 wk, possibly > 23 wk.

Neonates with erythroblastosis are immediately evaluated by a pediatrician to determine need for exchange transfusion (see p. 2787).

Prevention

Prevention involves giving the Rh-negative mother

- Rh_0(D) immune globulin at 28 wk gestation and within 72 h of pregnancy termination

Delivery should be as atraumatic as possible. Manual removal of the placenta should be avoided because it may force fetal cells into maternal circulation.

Maternal sensitization and antibody production due to Rh incompatibility can be prevented by giving the woman Rh_0(D) immune globulin. This preparation contains high titers of anti-Rh antibodies, which neutralize Rh-positive fetal RBCs. Because fetomaternal transfer and likelihood of sensitization is greatest at termination of pregnancy, the preparation is given within 72 h after termination of each pregnancy, whether by delivery, abortion, or treatment of ectopic pregnancy. The standard dose is 300 mcg IM. A rosette test can be used to rule out significant fetomaternal hemorrhage, and if results are positive, a Kleihauer-Betke (acid elution) test can measure the amount of fetal blood in the maternal circulation. If test results indicate fetomaternal hemorrhage is massive (> 30 mL whole blood), additional injections (300 mcg for every 30 mL of fetal whole blood, up to 5 doses within 24 h) are necessary.

If given only after delivery or termination of pregnancy, treatment is occasionally ineffective because sensitization can occur earlier during pregnancy. Therefore, at about 28 wk, all pregnant women with Rh-negative blood and no known prior sensitization are given a dose. Some experts recommend a 2nd dose if delivery has not occurred by 40 wk. Rh_0(D) immune globulin should also be given after any episode of vaginal bleeding and after amniocentesis or chorionic villus sampling. Anti-Rh antibodies persist for > 3 mo after one dose.

KEY POINTS

- The largest number of fetal RBCs move to the maternal circulation (resulting in the greatest risk of maternal sensitization) after delivery or termination of pregnancy.
- Screen all pregnant women for blood type, Rh type, anti-Rh_0(D), and other antibodies that can cause erythroblastosis fetalis.
- If women are at risk, measure antibody levels and middle cerebral artery blood flow periodically.
- Treat erythroblastosis fetalis with intrauterine fetal blood transfusions as needed and delivery as soon as fetal lung maturity is confirmed.
- Give Rh_0(D) immune globulin at 28 wk gestation and within 72 h of pregnancy termination to women at risk of sensitization.

PEMPHIGOID GESTATIONIS

(Herpes Gestationis)

Pemphigoid gestationis is a pruritic papular and vesicobullous eruption that occurs during pregnancy or postpartum. Diagnosis is clinical or by skin biopsy. Treatment is with topical or systemic corticosteroids.

Pemphigoid gestationis appears to be an autoimmune phenomenon, probably caused by an IgG antibody to a 180-kD antigen in the basement membrane zone of the epidermis. Although previously called herpes gestationis, this disorder is not caused by herpesvirus.

Pemphigoid gestationis occurs in 1/2,000 to 50,000 pregnancies; it usually begins during the 2nd or 3rd trimester but may begin during the 1st trimester or immediately postpartum. It usually recurs with subsequent pregnancies and occurs after oral contraceptive use in about 25% of women. Flare-ups are common 24 to 48 h postpartum and can occur during subsequent menses or ovulation.

Most fetuses are unaffected; however, transient lesions occur in < 5% of neonates born to mothers with pemphigoid gestationis. Risks, including infant mortality, are increased after premature delivery and in infants who are small for gestational age.

Symptoms and Signs

The rash is very pruritic. Lesions often start around the umbilicus, then become widespread. Vesicles and bullae are the most specific lesions; erythematous plaques may develop. The palms, soles, trunk, buttocks, and extremities may be affected but usually not the face or mucous membranes.

The rash worsens during labor or immediately postpartum in up to 75% of women, typically remitting within a few weeks or months.

Neonates may have erythematous plaques or vesicles that resolve spontaneously in a few weeks.

Diagnosis

- Clinical evaluation
- Sometimes biopsy with direct immunofluorescence

Pemphigoid gestationis may be confused clinically with several other pruritic eruptions of pregnancy, particularly pruritic urticarial papules and plaques of pregnancy. Pemphigoid gestationis can often be distinguished because it usually begins in the periumbilical area; pruritic urticarial papules and plaques of pregnancy usually begin in the striae.

Direct immunofluorescence examination of perilesional skin is diagnostic. It detects a linear band of C3 at the basement membrane zone.

Because fetal risks are increased, antenatal testing (eg, nonstress testing) is recommended.

Treatment

- Corticosteroids topically or, for severe symptoms, orally

For mild symptoms, topical corticosteroids (eg, 0.1% triamcinolone acetonide cream up to 6 times/day) may be effective. Prednisone (eg, 40 mg po once/day) relieves moderate or severe pruritus and prevents new lesions; dose is tapered until few new lesions erupt, but it may need to be increased if symptoms become more severe (eg, during labor). Systemic corticosteroids given late in pregnancy do not seem to harm the fetus.

Nonsedating oral antihistamines can also be used to relieve pruritus.

KEY POINTS

- Pemphigoid gestationis probably has an autoimmune etiology, even though the rash resembles the vesicobullous rash due to herpes simplex virus infection.
- Most fetuses are unaffected.
- Try to differentiate the rash based on clinical criteria (eg, its initial appearance in the periumbilical area).
- Treat women with topical corticosteroids or, if symptoms are severe, oral corticosteroids.

HYPEREMESIS GRAVIDARUM

Hyperemesis gravidarum is uncontrollable vomiting during pregnancy that results in dehydration, weight loss, and ketosis. Diagnosis is clinical and by measurement of urine ketones, serum electrolytes, and renal function. Treatment is with temporary suspension of oral intake and with IV fluids, antiemetics if needed, and vitamin and electrolyte repletion.

Pregnancy frequently causes nausea and vomiting; the cause appears to be rapidly increasing levels of estrogens or the β subunit of human chorionic gonadotropin (β-hCG). Vomiting usually develops at about 5 wk gestation, peaks at about 9 wk, and disappears by about 16 or 18 wk. It usually occurs in the morning (as so-called morning sickness), although it can occur any time of day. Women with morning sickness continue to gain weight and do not become dehydrated. Hyperemesis gravidarum is probably an extreme form of normal nausea and vomiting during pregnancy. It can be distinguished because it causes the following:

- Weight loss (> 5% of weight)
- Dehydration
- Ketosis
- Electrolyte abnormalities (in many women)

Hyperemesis gravidarum may cause mild, transient hyperthyroidism. Hyperemesis gravidarum that persists past 16 to 18 wk is uncommon but may seriously damage the liver, causing severe centrilobular necrosis or widespread fatty degeneration, and may cause Wernicke encephalopathy or esophageal rupture.

Diagnosis

- Clinical evaluation (sometimes including serial weight measurements)
- Urine ketones
- Serum electrolytes and renal function tests
- Exclusion of other causes (eg, acute abdomen)

If hyperemesis gravidarum is suspected, urine ketones, thyroid-stimulating hormone, serum electrolytes, BUN, creatinine, AST, ALT, Mg, P, and sometimes body weight are measured. Obstetric ultrasonography should be done to rule out hydatidiform mole and multifetal pregnancy.

Other disorders that can cause vomiting must be excluded; they include gastroenteritis, hepatitis, appendicitis, cholecystitis, other biliary tract disorders, peptic ulcer disease, intestinal obstruction, hyperthyroidism not caused by hyperemesis gravidarum (eg, caused by Graves disease), gestational trophoblastic disease, nephrolithiasis, pyelonephritis, diabetic ketoacidosis or gastroparesis, benign intracranial hypertension, and migraine headaches. Prominent symptoms in addition to nausea and vomiting often suggest another cause. Tests for alternative diagnoses are done based on laboratory, clinical, or ultrasound findings.

Treatment

- Temporary suspension of oral intake, followed by gradual resumption
- Fluids, thiamin, multivitamins, and electrolytes as needed
- Antiemetics if needed

At first, patients are given nothing by mouth. Initial treatment is IV fluid resuscitation, beginning with 2 L of Ringer's lactate infused over 3 h to maintain a urine output of > 100 mL/h. If dextrose is given, thiamin 100 mg should be given IV first, to prevent Wernicke encephalopathy. This dose of thiamin should be given daily for 3 days.

Subsequent fluid requirements vary with patient response but may be as much as 1 L q 4 h or so for up to 3 days. Electrolyte deficiencies are treated; K, Mg, and P are replaced as needed. Care must be taken not to correct low plasma Na levels too quickly because too rapid correction can cause osmotic demyelination syndrome.

Vomiting that persists after initial fluid and electrolyte replacement is treated with an antiemetic taken as needed; antiemetics include

- Vitamin B_6 10 to 25 mg po q 8 h or q 6 h
- Doxylamine 12.5 mg po q 8 h or q 6 h (can be taken in addition to vitamin B_6)
- Promethazine 12.5 to 25 mg po, IM, or rectally q 4 to 8 h
- Metoclopramide 5 to 10 mg IV or po q 8 h
- Ondansetron 8 mg po or IM q 12 h
- Prochlorperazine 5 to 10 mg po or IM q 3 to 4 h

After dehydration and acute vomiting resolve, small amounts of oral fluids are given. Patients who cannot tolerate any oral fluids after IV rehydration and antiemetics may need to be hospitalized or given IV therapy at home and take nothing by mouth for a longer period (sometimes several days or more). Once patients tolerate fluids, they can eat small, bland meals, and diet is expanded as tolerated. IV vitamin therapy is required initially and until vitamins can be taken by mouth.

If treatment is ineffective, TPN may be necessary, and corticosteroids, although controversial, can be tried; eg, methylprednisolone 16 mg q 8 h po or IV may be given for 3 days, then tapered over 2 wk to the lowest effective dose. Corticosteroids should be used for < 6 wk and with extreme caution. They should not be used during fetal organogenesis (between 20 and 56 days after fertilization); use of these drugs during the 1st trimester is weakly associated with facial clefting. The mechanism for corticosteroids' effect on nausea is unclear.

If progressive weight loss, jaundice, or persistent tachycardia occurs despite treatment, termination of the pregnancy can be offered.

KEY POINTS

- Hyperemesis gravidarum, unlike morning sickness, can cause weight loss, ketosis, dehydration, and sometimes electrolyte abnormalities.
- Exclude other disorders that can cause vomiting based on the woman's symptoms.
- Determine severity by measuring serum electrolytes, urine ketones, BUN, creatinine, and body weight.
- Suspend oral intake at first, give fluids and nutrients IV, restore oral intake gradually, and give antiemetics as needed.

POLYHYDRAMNIOS

Polyhydramnios is excessive amniotic fluid; it is associated with maternal and fetal complications. Diagnosis is by ultrasonographic measurement of amniotic fluid. Maternal disorders contributing to polyhydramnios are treated. If symptoms are severe or if painful preterm contractions occur, treatment may also include manual reduction of amniotic fluid volume.

The volume of amniotic fluid cannot be safely measured directly, except perhaps during cesarean delivery. Thus, excessive fluid is defined indirectly using ultrasonographic criteria, typically the amniotic fluid index (AFI). The AFI is the sum of the vertical depth of fluid measured in each quadrant of the uterus. The normal AFI ranges from 5 to 25 cm; values > 25 cm indicate polyhydramnios.

Causes of polyhydramnios include the following:

- Fetal malformations (eg, GI or urinary tract obstruction, brain and spinal cord defects)
- Multiple gestation
- Maternal diabetes
- Fetal anemia, including hemolytic anemia due to Rh incompatibility
- Other fetal disorders (eg, infections) or genetic abnormalities
- Idiopathic

Complications: With polyhydramnios, risk of the following complications is increased:

- Preterm contractions and possibly preterm labor
- Premature rupture of membranes
- Fetal malposition
- Maternal respiratory compromise
- Umbilical cord prolapse
- Uterine atony
- Abruptio placentae
- Fetal death (risk is increased even when polyhydramnios is idiopathic)

Risks tend to be proportional to the degree of fluid accumulation and vary with the cause. Other problems (eg, low Apgar score, fetal distress, nuchal cord, need for cesarean delivery) may occur. Women with polyhydramnios may have pregnancy-induced hypertension.

Symptoms and Signs

Polyhydramnios is often asymptomatic. However, some women, especially when polyhydramnios is severe, have difficulty breathing, and/or painful preterm contractions. Sometimes the uterus is larger than expected for dates.

Diagnosis

- Ultrasonographic measurement of AFI
- Comprehensive ultrasonographic examination, including evaluation for fetal malformations
- Maternal testing for causes suspected based on history

Polyhydramnios is usually suspected based on ultrasonographic findings or uterine size that is larger than expected for dates. However, qualitative estimates of amniotic fluid volume tend to be subjective. So if polyhydramnios is suspected, amniotic fluid should be assessed quantitatively using the AFI.

Identification of cause: If polyhydramnios is present, further testing is recommended to determine the cause. Which tests are done may depend on which causes are suspected clinically (usually based on history). Tests may include

- Comprehensive ultrasonographic examination for fetal malformations (always recommended)
- Maternal glucose tolerance test
- Kleihauer-Betke test (for fetomaternal hemorrhage)
- Maternal serologic tests (eg, for syphilis, parvovirus, cytomegalovirus, toxoplasmosis, and rubella)
- Amniocentesis and fetal karyotyping
- Tests for clinically suspected hereditary disorders, such as anemias

Treatment

- Possibly manual withdrawal of amniotic fluid (amnioreduction)

Because polyhydramnios increases risk of fetal death, prenatal monitoring should begin at 32 wk and should include nonstress testing at least once/wk. However, such monitoring has not been proved to decrease the fetal death rate. Delivery at about 39 wk should be planned. Mode of delivery should be based on the usual obstetrical indications (eg, presenting part).

Reducing amniotic fluid volume (eg, by amnioreduction) or reducing its production should be considered only if preterm labor occurs or if polyhydramnios causes severe symptoms; however, there is no evidence that this approach improves outcomes. Also, there is no consensus on how much fluid to remove and how rapidly it should be removed, although removal of about 1 L over 20 min has been suggested.

Disorders that could be contributing to polyhydramnios (eg, maternal diabetes) should be controlled.

KEY POINTS

- Polyhydramnios can be caused by fetal malformations, multiple gestation, maternal diabetes, and various fetal disorders.
- It is associated with increased risk of preterm contractions, premature rupture of membranes, maternal respiratory compromise, fetal malposition or death, and various problems during labor and delivery.
- If polyhydramnios is suspected, determine amniotic fluid index and test for possible causes (including a comprehensive ultrasonographic evaluation).
- Consider reducing amniotic fluid volume only if preterm labor occurs or if polyhydramnios causes severe symptoms.
- Begin prenatal monitoring with weekly nonstress tests at 32 wk.

OLIGOHYDRAMNIOS

Oligohydramnios is a deficient volume of amniotic fluid; it is associated with maternal and fetal complications. Diagnosis is by ultrasonographic measurement of amniotic fluid volume. Management involves close monitoring and serial ultrasonographic assessments.

The volume of amniotic fluid cannot be safely measured directly, except perhaps during cesarean delivery. Thus, deficient fluid is defined indirectly using ultrasonographic criteria, typically the amniotic fluid index (AFI). The AFI is the sum of the vertical depth of fluid measured in each quadrant of the uterus. The normal AFI ranges from 5 to 25 cm; values < 5 cm indicate oligohydramnios.

Causes of oligohydramnios include the following:

- Uteroplacental insufficiency (eg, due to preeclampsia, chronic hypertension, abruptio placentae, a thrombotic disorder, or another maternal disorder)
- Drugs (eg, ACE inhibitors, NSAIDs)
- Postterm pregnancy
- Fetal malformations, particularly those that decrease urine production
- Fetal growth restriction
- Fetal demise
- Fetal chromosomal abnormalities (eg, aneuploidy)
- Premature rupture of membranes
- Idiopathic

Complications: Complications of oligohydramnios include the following:

- Fetal death
- Fetal growth restriction
- Limb contractures (if oligohydramnios begins early in the pregnancy)
- Delayed lung maturation (if oligohydramnios begins early in the pregnancy)
- Inability of the fetus to tolerate labor, leading to the need for cesarean delivery

Risk of complications depends on how much amniotic is present and what the cause is.

Symptoms and Signs

Oligohydramnios itself tends not to cause maternal symptoms other than a sense of decreased fetal movement. Uterine size may be less than expected based on dates. Disorders causing or contributing to oligohydramnios may cause symptoms.

Diagnosis

- Ultrasonographic measurement of amniotic fluid volume
- Comprehensive ultrasonographic examination, including evaluation for fetal malformations
- Testing for clinically suspected maternal causes
- Sometimes Doppler ultrasonography of the umbilical artery

Oligohydramnios may be suspected if uterine size is less than expected for dates or if fetal movements are decreased; it may also be suspected based on incidental ultrasonographic findings. However, qualitative estimates of amniotic fluid volume tend to be subjective. If oligohydramnios is suspected, amniotic fluid should be assessed quantitatively using the AFI.

Identification of cause: If oligohydramnios is diagnosed, clinicians should check for possible causes, including premature rupture of membranes. Comprehensive ultrasonographic examination is done to check for fetal malformations and any evident placental causes (eg, abruptio placentae).

Clinicians can offer amniocentesis and fetal karyotyping, particularly if ultrasonography suggests fetal malformations or aneuploidy.

If uteroplacental insufficiency is suspected, the umbilical artery is assessed using Doppler ultrasonography.

Treatment

- Serial ultrasonography to determine AFI and monitor fetal growth
- Possibly for nonstress testing or biophysical profile

Ultrasonography should be done at least once every 4 wk (every 2 wk if growth is restricted) to monitor fetal growth. The AFI should be measured at least once/wk. Most experts recommend fetal monitoring with nonstress testing or biophysical profile at least once/wk and delivery at term. However, this approach has not been proved to prevent fetal death. Also, optimal time for delivery is controversial and can vary based on patient characteristics.

KEY POINTS

- Oligohydramnios can be caused by uteroplacental insufficiency, drugs, fetal abnormalities, or premature rupture of membranes.
- It can cause problems in the fetus (eg, growth restriction, limb contractures, death, delayed lung maturation, inability to tolerate labor).
- If oligohydramnios is suspected, determine the amniotic fluid index and test for possible causes (including doing a comprehensive ultrasonographic evaluation).
- Do ultrasonography a least once every 4 wk, and consider fetal monitoring at least once/wk and delivery at term (although optimal time for delivery varies).

PLACENTA PREVIA

Placenta previa is implantation of the placenta over or near the internal os of the cervix. Typically, painless vaginal bleeding with bright red blood occurs after 20 wk gestation. Diagnosis is by transvaginal or abdominal ultrasonography. Treatment is bed rest for minor vaginal bleeding before 36 wk gestation, with cesarean delivery at 36 wk if fetal lung maturity is documented. If bleeding is severe or refractory or if fetal status is nonreassuring, immediate delivery, usually cesarean, is indicated.

Placenta previa may be total (covering the internal os completely), partial (covering part of the os), or marginal (at the edge of the os), or the placenta may be low-lying (within 2 cm of the internal os but not reaching it). Incidence of placenta previa is 1/200 deliveries. If placenta previa occurs during early pregnancy, it usually resolves by 28 wk as the uterus enlarges.

Risk factors: Risk factors include the following:

- Multiparity
- Prior cesarean delivery
- Uterine abnormalities that inhibit normal implantation (eg, fibroids, prior curettage)
- Smoking
- Multifetal pregnancy
- Older maternal age

Complications: For patients with placenta previa or a low-lying placenta, risks include fetal malpresentation, preterm premature rupture of the membranes, fetal growth restriction, vasa previa, and velamentous insertion of the umbilical cord (in which the placental end of the cord consists of divergent umbilical vessels surrounded only by fetal membranes). In women who have had a prior cesarean delivery, placenta previa increases the risk of placenta accreta (see p. 2338); risk increases significantly as the number of prior cesarean deliveries increases (from about 10% if they have had one cesarean delivery to > 60% if they have had > 4).

Symptoms and Signs

Symptoms usually begin during late pregnancy. Then, sudden, painless vaginal bleeding often begins; the blood may be bright red, and bleeding may be heavy, sometimes resulting in hemorrhagic shock. In some patients, uterine contractions accompany bleeding.

Diagnosis

- Transvaginal ultrasonography

Placenta previa is considered in all women with vaginal bleeding after 20 wk. If placenta previa is present, digital pelvic examination may increase bleeding, sometimes causing sudden, massive bleeding; thus, if vaginal bleeding occurs after 20 wk, digital pelvic examination is contraindicated unless placenta previa is first ruled out by ultrasonography.

Although placenta previa is more likely to cause heavy, painless bleeding with bright red blood than abruptio placentae, clinical differentiation is still not possible. Thus, ultrasonography is frequently needed to distinguish the two. Transvaginal ultrasonography is an accurate, safe way to diagnose placenta previa.

PEARLS & PITFALLS

- If vaginal bleeding occurs after 20 wk gestation, exclude placenta previa by ultrasonography before doing a digital examination.

In all women with suspected symptomatic placenta previa, fetal heart rate monitoring is indicated. Unless the case is an emergency (requiring immediate delivery), amniotic fluid is tested at 36 wk to assess fetal lung maturity and thus document whether delivery at this time is safe.

Treatment

- Hospitalization and bed rest for a first episode of bleeding before 36 wk
- Delivery if mother or fetus is unstable or if fetal lungs are mature

For a first (sentinel) episode of vaginal bleeding before 36 wk, management consists of hospitalization, modified rest, and avoidance of sexual intercourse, which can cause bleeding by initiating contractions or causing direct trauma. (Modified rest involves refraining from any activity that increases intra-abdominal pressure for a long period of time—eg, women should stay off their feet most of the day.) If bleeding stops, ambulation and usually hospital discharge are allowed.

Some experts recommend giving corticosteroids to accelerate fetal lung maturity when early delivery may become necessary and gestational age is < 34 wk. Typically for a 2nd bleeding episode, patients are readmitted and kept for observation until delivery.

Delivery is indicated for any of the following:

- Heavy or uncontrolled bleeding
- Nonreassuring results of fetal heart monitoring
- Maternal hemodynamic instability
- Fetal lung maturity (usually at 36 wk)

Delivery is almost always cesarean, but vaginal delivery may be possible for women with a low-lying placenta if the fetal head effectively compresses the placenta and labor is already advanced or if the pregnancy is < 23 wk and rapid delivery is expected.

Hemorrhagic shock is treated (see p. 575). Prophylactic Rh_0(D) immune globulin should be given if the mother has Rh-negative blood (see p. 2348).

KEY POINTS

- Placenta previa is more likely to result in heavy, painless bleeding with bright red blood than abruptio placentae, but clinical differentiation is still not possible.
- Determine how urgently delivery is needed by monitoring fetal heart rate (to detect fetal distress) and testing amniotic fluid (to assess fetal lung maturity).
- For most first bleeding episodes before 36 wk, recommend hospitalization, modified rest, and abstinence from sexual intercourse.
- Consider corticosteroids to accelerate fetal lung maturity if delivery may be needed before about 34 wk.
- Delivery is indicated when bleeding is severe, the mother or fetus is unstable, or fetal lung maturity is confirmed.

PREECLAMPSIA AND ECLAMPSIA

Preeclampsia is new-onset hypertension and proteinuria after 20 wk gestation. Eclampsia is unexplained generalized seizures in patients with preeclampsia. Diagnosis is clinical and by urine protein measurement. Treatment is usually with IV Mg sulfate and delivery at term.

Preeclampsia affects 3 to 7% of pregnant women. Preeclampsia and eclampsia develop after 20 wk gestation; up to 25% of cases develop postpartum, most often within the first 4 days but sometimes up to 6 wk postpartum.

Untreated preeclampsia usually smolders for a variable time, then suddenly progresses to eclampsia, which occurs in 1/200 patients with preeclampsia. Untreated eclampsia is usually fatal.

Etiology

Etiology is unknown; however, risk factors include the following:

- Nulliparity
- Preexisting chronic hypertension
- Vascular disorders (eg, renal disorders, diabetic vasculopathy)
- Preexisting or gestational diabetes
- Older (> 35) or very young (eg, < 17) maternal age
- Family history of preeclampsia
- Preeclampsia or poor outcome in previous pregnancies
- Multifetal pregnancy
- Obesity
- Thrombotic disorders (eg, antiphospholipid antibody syndrome—see p. 1207)

Pathophysiology

Pathophysiology of preeclampsia and eclampsia is poorly understood. Factors may include poorly developed uterine placental spiral arterioles (which decrease uteroplacental blood flow during late pregnancy), a genetic abnormality on chromosome 13, immunologic abnormalities, and placental ischemia or infarction. Lipid peroxidation of cell membranes induced by free radicals may contribute to preeclampsia.

Complications: Fetal growth restriction or death may result. Diffuse or multifocal vasospasm can result in maternal ischemia, eventually damaging multiple organs, particularly the brain, kidneys, and liver. Factors that may contribute to vasospasm include decreased prostacyclin (an endothelium-derived vasodilator), increased endothelin (an endothelium-derived vasoconstrictor), and increased soluble Flt-1 (a circulating receptor for vascular endothelial growth factor). Women who have preeclampsia are at risk of abruptio placentae in the current and in future pregnancies, possibly because both disorders are related to uteroplacental insufficiency.

The coagulation system is activated, possibly secondary to endothelial cell dysfunction, leading to platelet activation. The HELLP syndrome (hemolysis, elevated liver function tests, and low platelet count) develops in 10 to 20% of women with severe preeclampsia or eclampsia; this incidence is about 100 times that for all pregnancies (1 to 2/1000). Most pregnant women with this syndrome have hypertension and proteinuria, but some have neither.

Symptoms and Signs

Preeclampsia may be asymptomatic or may cause edema or excessive weight gain. Nondependent edema, such as facial or hand swelling (the patient's ring may no longer fit her finger), is more specific than dependent edema. Reflex reactivity may be increased, indicating neuromuscular irritability, which can progress to seizures (eclampsia). Petechiae may develop, as may other signs of coagulopathy.

PEARLS & PITFALLS

- Check for swelling in the hands (eg, a ring that no longer fits) or face and hyperreflexia, which may be among the more specific findings in preeclampsia.

Severe preeclampsia may cause organ damage; manifestations may include headache, visual disturbances, confusion, epigastric or right upper quadrant abdominal pain (reflecting hepatic ischemia or capsular distention), nausea, vomiting, dyspnea (reflecting pulmonary edema, acute respiratory distress syndrome [ARDS], or cardiac dysfunction secondary to increased afterload), stroke (rarely), and oliguria (reflecting decreased plasma volume or ischemic acute tubular necrosis).

Diagnosis

- New-onset hypertension (BP > 140/90 mm Hg) plus new unexplained proteinuria > 300 mg/24 h after 20 wk

Diagnosis is suggested by symptoms or presence of hypertension, defined as systolic BP > 140 mm Hg, diastolic BP > 90 mm Hg, or both. Except in emergencies, hypertension should be documented in > 2 measurements taken at least 4 h apart. Urine protein excretion is measured in a 24-h collection. Proteinuria is defined as > 300 mg/24 h. Alternatively, proteinuria is diagnosed based on a protein:creatinine ratio ≥ 0.3 or a dipstick reading of 1+ (used only if other quantitative methods are not available). Absence of proteinuria on less accurate tests (eg, urine dipstick testing, routine urinalysis) does not rule out preeclampsia.

In the absence of proteinuria, preeclampsia is also diagnosed if pregnant women have new-onset hypertension plus new onset of any of the following:

- Thrombocytopenia (platelets < 100,000/μL)
- Renal insufficiency (serum creatinine > 1.1 mg/dL or doubling of serum creatinine in women without renal disease)
- Impaired liver function (aminotransferases > 2 times normal)
- Pulmonary edema
- Cerebral or visual symptoms

The following points help differentiate among hypertensive disorders in pregnant women:

- **Chronic hypertension** is identified if hypertension precedes pregnancy, is present at < 20 wk gestation, or persists for > 6 wk (usually > 12 wk) postpartum (even if hypertension is first documented at > 20 wk gestation). Chronic hypertension may be masked during early pregnancy by the physiologic decrease in BP.

- **Gestational hypertension** is hypertension without proteinuria or other findings of preeclampsia; it first occurs at > 20 wk gestation in women known not to have hypertension before pregnancy and resolves by 12 wk (usually by 6 wk) postpartum.
- **Preeclampsia** is new-onset hypertension (BP > 140/90 mm Hg) plus new unexplained proteinuria (> 300 mg/24 h) after 20 wk or other criteria (see above).
- **Preeclampsia superimposed on chronic hypertension** is diagnosed when new unexplained proteinuria develops after 20 wk in a woman known to have hypertension or when BP increases or signs of severe preeclampsia develop after 20 wk in a woman known to have hypertension and proteinuria.

Further evaluation: If preeclampsia is diagnosed, tests include urinalysis, CBC, platelet count, uric acid, liver function tests, and measurement of serum electrolytes, BUN, creatinine, and creatine clearance. The fetus is assessed using a nonstress test or biophysical profile (including assessment of amniotic fluid volume) and tests that estimate fetal weight.

HELLP syndrome is suggested by microangiopathic findings (eg, schistocytes, helmet cells) on peripheral blood smears, elevated liver enzymes, and a low platelet count.

Severe preeclampsia is differentiated from mild by one or more of the following:

- CNS dysfunction (eg, blurred vision, scotomata, altered mental status, severe headache unrelieved by acetaminophen)
- Symptoms of liver capsule distention (eg, right upper quadrant or epigastric pain)
- Nausea and vomiting
- Serum AST or ALT > 2 times normal
- Systolic BP > 160 mm Hg or diastolic BP > 110 mm Hg on 2 occasions ≥ 4 h apart
- Platelet count < 100,000/μL
- Urine output < 500 mL/24 h
- Pulmonary edema or cyanosis
- Stroke
- Progressive renal insufficiency (serum creatinine > 1.1 mg/dL or doubling of serum creatinine in women without renal disease)

Treatment

- Usually hospitalization and sometimes antihypertensive treatment
- Delivery, depending on factors such as gestational age, evidence of fetal maturity, and severity of preeclampsia
- Mg sulfate for prevention or treatment of seizures

General approach: Definitive treatment is delivery. However, risk of early delivery is balanced against gestational age, severity of preeclampsia, and response to other treatments. Usually, immediate delivery after maternal stabilization (eg, controlling seizures, beginning to control BP) is indicated for the following:

- Pregnancy of ≥ 37 wk
- Eclampsia
- Severe preeclampsia if pregnancy is ≥ 34 wk or if fetal lung maturity is documented
- Deteriorating renal, pulmonary, cardiac, or hepatic function
- Nonreassuring results of fetal monitoring or testing

Other treatments aim to optimize maternal health, which usually optimizes fetal health. If delivery can be delayed in pregnancies of about 32 to 34 wk, corticosteroids are given for 48 h to accelerate fetal lung maturity.

Most patients are hospitalized. Patients with eclampsia or severe preeclampsia are often admitted to a maternal special care unit or an ICU.

Mild preeclampsia: If preeclampsia is mild, outpatient treatment is possible; it includes strict bed rest, lying on the left side whenever possible, and BP measurements, laboratory monitoring, and physician visits 2 to 3 times/wk.

However, most patients with mild preeclampsia require hospitalization, at least initially; some also need drug treatment for a few hours to stabilize them and to lower systolic BP to 140 to 155 mm Hg and diastolic BP to 90 to 105 mm Hg. Hypertension can be treated with oral drugs as needed. As long as no criteria for severe preeclampsia are met, delivery can occur (eg, by induction) at 37 wk.

Monitoring: Outpatients are usually evaluated once every 2 or 3 days for evidence of seizures, symptoms of severe preeclampsia, and vaginal bleeding; BP, reflexes, and fetal heart status (with nonstress testing or a biophysical profile) are also checked. Platelet count, serum creatinine, and serum liver enzymes are measured frequently until stable, then at least weekly.

All hospitalized patients are followed by an obstetrician or a maternal-fetal medicine specialist and evaluated as for outpatients (described above); evaluation is more frequent if severe preeclampsia is diagnosed or if gestational age is < 34 wk.

Mg sulfate: As soon as eclampsia or severe preeclampsia is diagnosed, Mg sulfate must be given to stop or prevent seizures and reduce reflex reactivity. Whether patients with mild preeclampsia always require Mg sulfate before delivery is controversial.

Mg sulfate 4 g IV over 20 min is given, followed by a constant IV infusion of about 1 to 3 g/h, with supplemental doses as necessary. Dose is adjusted based on the patient's reflexes. Patients with abnormally high Mg levels (eg, with Mg levels > 10 mEq/L or a sudden decrease in reflex reactivity), cardiac dysfunction (eg, with dyspnea or chest pain), or hypoventilation after treatment with Mg sulfate can be treated with Ca gluconate 1 g IV.

IV Mg sulfate may cause lethargy, hypotonia, and transient respiratory depression in neonates. However, serious neonatal complications are uncommon.

Supportive treatments: Hospitalized patients are given IV Ringer lactate or 0.9% normal saline solution, beginning at about 125 mL/h (to increase urine output). Persistent oliguria is treated with a carefully monitored fluid challenge. Diuretics are usually not used. Monitoring with a pulmonary artery catheter is rarely necessary and, if needed, is done in consultation with a critical care specialist and in an ICU. Anuric patients with normovolemia may require renal vasodilators or dialysis.

If seizures occur despite Mg therapy, diazepam or lorazepam can be given IV to stop seizures, and IV hydralazine or labetalol is given in a dose titrated to lower systolic BP to 140 to 155 mm Hg and diastolic BP to 90 to 105 mm Hg.

Delivery method: The most efficient method of delivery should be used. If the cervix is favorable and rapid vaginal delivery seems feasible, a dilute IV infusion of oxytocin is given to accelerate labor; if labor is active, the membranes are ruptured. If the cervix is unfavorable and prompt vaginal delivery is unlikely, cesarean delivery can be considered. Preeclampsia and eclampsia, if not resolved before delivery, usually resolve rapidly afterward, beginning within 6 to 12 h.

All patients are typically given Mg sulfate for 24 h postpartum.

Follow-up: Patients should be evaluated every 1 to 2 wk postpartum with periodic BP measurement. If BP remains high after 6 wk postpartum, patients may have chronic hypertension and should be referred to their primary care physician for management.

KEY POINTS

- Preeclampsia develops after 20 wk gestation; it develops postpartum in 25% of cases.
- Swelling of the face or hands and hyperreflexia are relatively specific findings for preeclampsia.
- Preeclampsia is severe if it causes significant organ dysfunction (detected clinically or by testing).
- HELLP syndrome occurs in 10 to 20% of women with severe preeclampsia or eclampsia.
- Monitor the mother and fetus closely, usually in a hospital or ICU.
- As soon as severe preeclampsia or eclampsia is diagnosed, treat with high doses of Mg sulfate; for mild preeclampsia, use of Mg sulfate is less clear.
- Delivery is usually indicated when the pregnancy is ≥ 37 wk, severe problems develop, or the fetal lungs are mature.

PRURITIC URTICARIAL PAPULES AND PLAQUES OF PREGNANCY

Pruritic urticarial papules and plaques of pregnancy are pruritic eruptions of unknown cause that develop during pregnancy.

Most cases occur during a first pregnancy. Overall incidence is 1/160 to 300 pregnancies; however, with multiple gestation, risk is 8 to 12 times higher.

Symptoms and Signs

Lesions are intensely itchy, erythematous, solid, superficial, and elevated; some are surrounded by blanching, and some have minute vesicles in the center. Itching keeps most patients awake, but excoriation is uncommon. Lesions begin on the abdomen, frequently on striae atrophicae (stretch marks), and spread to the thighs, buttocks, and occasionally the arms. The palms, soles, and face arc usually spared. Most patients have hundreds of lesions.

Lesions develop during the 3rd trimester, most often in the last 2 to 3 wk and occasionally in the last few days or postpartum. They usually resolve within 15 days after delivery but can take longer. They may recur in up to 5% of subsequent pregnancies.

Diagnosis

Diagnosis is clinical. Differentiation from other pruritic eruptions may be difficult.

Treatment

- Corticosteroids

Mild symptoms are treated with topical corticosteroids (eg, 0.1% triamcinolone acetonide cream up to 6 times/day). Rarely, more severe symptoms require systemic corticosteroids (eg, prednisone 40 mg po once/day, tapered as tolerated). Short courses of systemic corticosteroids given late in pregnancy do not seem to have adverse effects on the fetus.

SPONTANEOUS ABORTION

(Miscarriage)

Spontaneous abortion is noninduced embryonic or fetal death or passage of products of conception before 20 wk gestation. Threatened abortion is vaginal bleeding without cervical dilation occurring during this time frame and indicating that spontaneous abortion may occur in a woman with a confirmed viable intrauterine pregnancy. Diagnosis is by clinical criteria and ultrasonography. Treatment is usually expectant observation for threatened abortion and, if spontaneous abortion has occurred or appears unavoidable, observation or uterine evacuation.

Fetal death and early delivery are classified as follows:

- Abortion: Death of the fetus or passage of products of conception (fetus and placenta) before 20 wk gestation
- Fetal demise (stillbirth): Fetal death after 20 wk
- Preterm delivery: Passage of a live fetus between 20 and 37 wk (see p. 2341)

Abortions may be classified as early or late, spontaneous or induced for therapeutic or elective reasons (see p. 2246), threatened or inevitable, incomplete or complete, recurrent (also called recurrent pregnancy loss—see p. 2357), missed, or septic (see Table 282–1).

About 20 to 30% of women with confirmed pregnancies bleed during the first 20 wk of pregnancy; half of these women spontaneously abort. Thus, incidence of spontaneous abortion is about 10 to 15% in confirmed pregnancies. Incidence in all pregnancies is probably higher because some very early abortions are mistaken for a late menstrual period.

Table 282–1. CLASSIFICATION OF ABORTION

TYPE	DEFINITION
Early	Abortion before 12 wk gestation
Late	Abortion between 12 and 20 wk gestation
Spontaneous	Noninduced abortion
Induced	Termination of pregnancy for medical or elective reasons
Therapeutic	Termination of pregnancy because the woman's life or health is endangered or because the fetus is dead or has malformations incompatible with life
Threatened	Vaginal bleeding occurring before 20 wk gestation without cervical dilation and indicating that spontaneous abortion may occur
Inevitable	Vaginal bleeding or rupture of the membranes accompanied by dilation of the cervix
Incomplete	Expulsion of some products of conception
Complete	Expulsion of all products of conception
Recurrent or habitual	≥ 3 consecutive spontaneous abortions
Missed	Undetected death of an embryo or a fetus that is not expelled and that causes no bleeding (also called blighted ovum, anembryonic pregnancy, or intrauterine embryonic demise)
Septic	Serious infection of the uterine contents during or shortly before or after an abortion

Table 282–2. CHARACTERISTIC SYMPTOMS AND SIGNS IN SPONTANEOUS ABORTIONS

TYPE OF ABORTION	VAGINAL BLEEDING	CERVICAL DILATION*	PASSAGE OF PRODUCTS OF CONCEPTION†
Threatened	Y	N	N
Inevitable	Y	Y	N
Incomplete	Y	Y	Y
Complete	Y	Y or N	Y
Missed	Y or N	N	N

*Internal cervical os is open enough to admit a fingertip during digital examination.
†Products of conception may be visible in the vagina. Tissue examination is sometimes required to differentiate blood clots from tissue products of conception. Before the evaluation, products of conception may have been expelled without the patient recognizing them.

Etiology

Isolated spontaneous abortions may result from certain viruses—most notably cytomegalovirus, herpesvirus, parvovirus, and rubella virus—or from disorders that can cause sporadic abortions or recurrent pregnancy loss (eg, chromosomal or mendelian abnormalities, luteal phase defects). Other causes include immunologic abnormalities, major trauma, and uterine abnormalities (eg, fibroids, adhesions). Most often, the cause is unknown.

Risk factors include

- Age > 35
- History of spontaneous abortion
- Cigarette smoking
- Use of certain drugs (eg, cocaine, alcohol, high doses of caffeine)
- A poorly controlled chronic disorder (eg, diabetes, hypertension, overt thyroid disorders) in the mother

Subclinical thyroid disorders, a retroverted uterus, and minor trauma have not been shown to cause spontaneous abortions.

Symptoms and Signs

Symptoms include crampy pelvic pain, bleeding, and eventually expulsion of tissue. Late spontaneous abortion may begin with a gush of fluid when the membranes rupture. Hemorrhage is rarely massive. A dilated cervix indicates that abortion is inevitable.

If products of conception remain in the uterus after spontaneous abortion, vaginal bleeding may occur, sometimes after a delay of hours to days. Infection may also develop, causing fever, pain, and sometimes sepsis.

Diagnosis

- Clinical criteria
- Usually ultrasonography and quantitative β subunit of human chorionic gonadotropin (β-hCG)

Diagnosis of threatened, inevitable, incomplete, or complete abortion is often possible based on clinical criteria (see Table 282–2) and a positive urine pregnancy test. However, ultrasonography and quantitative measurement of serum β-hCG are usually done to exclude ectopic pregnancy and to determine whether products of conception remain in the uterus (suggesting that abortion is incomplete rather than complete). However, results may be inconclusive, particularly during early pregnancy.

Missed abortion is suspected if the uterus does not progressively enlarge or if quantitative β-hCG is low for gestational age or does not double within 48 to 72 h. Missed abortion is confirmed if ultrasonography shows any of the following:

- Disappearance of previously detected embryonic cardiac activity
- Absence of such activity when the fetal crown-rump length is > 5 mm (determined by transvaginal ultrasonography)
- Absence of a fetal pole (determined by transvaginal ultrasonography) when the mean sac diameter (average of diameters measured in 3 orthogonal planes) is > 18 mm

For **recurrent pregnancy loss**, testing to determine the cause of abortion is necessary (see p. 2357).

Treatment

- Observation for threatened abortion
- Uterine evacuation for inevitable, incomplete, or missed abortions
- Emotional support

For **threatened abortion**, treatment is observation. No evidence suggests that bed rest decreases risk of subsequent completed abortion.

For **inevitable, incomplete, or missed abortions,** treatment is uterine evacuation or waiting for spontaneous passage of the products of conception. Evacuation usually involves suction curettage at < 12 wk, dilation and evacuation at 12 to 23 wk, or medical induction (for women without prior uterine surgery) at > 16 to 23 wk (for treatment of late fetal death, see Stillbirth on p. 2358). The later the uterus is evacuated, the greater the likelihood of placental bleeding, uterine perforation by long bones of the fetus, and difficulty dilating the cervix. These complications are reduced by preoperative use of osmotic cervical dilators (eg, laminaria), misoprostol, or mifepristone (RU 486).

If **complete abortion** is suspected, uterine evacuation need not be done routinely. Uterine evacuation can be done if bleeding occurs and/or if other signs indicate that products of conception may be retained.

After an **induced or spontaneous abortion,** parents may feel grief and guilt. They should be given emotional support and, in the case of spontaneous abortions, reassured that their actions were not the cause. Formal counseling is rarely indicated but should be made available.

KEY POINTS

- Spontaneous abortion probably occurs in about 10 to 15% of pregnancies.
- The cause of an isolated spontaneous abortion is usually unknown.

- A dilated cervix means that abortion is inevitable.
- Confirm spontaneous abortion and determine its type based on clinical criteria, ultrasonography, and quantitative β-hCG.
- Uterine evacuation is eventually necessary for inevitable, incomplete, or missed abortions.
- Often, uterine evacuation is not needed for threatened and complete abortions.
- After spontaneous abortion, provide emotional support to the parents.

Recurrent Pregnancy Loss

(Recurrent or Habitual Abortion)

Recurrent pregnancy loss is ≥ 3 consecutive spontaneous abortions. Determining the cause may require extensive evaluation of both parents. Some causes can be treated.

Etiology

Causes of recurrent pregnancy loss may be maternal, fetal, or placental.

Common **maternal** causes include

- Uterine or cervical abnormalities (eg, polyps, myomas, adhesions, cervical insufficiency)
- Maternal (or paternal) chromosomal abnormalities (eg, balanced translocations)
- Luteal phase defects (particularly at < 6 wk)
- Overt and poorly controlled endocrine disorders (eg, hypothyroidism, hyperthyroidism, diabetes mellitus)
- Chronic renal disorders

Acquired thrombotic disorders (eg, related to antiphospholipid antibody syndrome with lupus anticoagulant, anticardiolipin [IgG or IgM], or anti-β_2 glycoprotein I [IgG or IgM]) are associated with recurrent losses after 10 wk. The association with hereditary thrombotic disorders is less clear but does not appear to be strong, except for possibly factor V Leiden mutation.

Placental causes include preexisting chronic disorders that are poorly controlled (eg, SLE, chronic hypertension).

Fetal causes are usually

- Chromosomal or genetic abnormalities
- Anatomic malformations

Chromosomal abnormalities may cause 50% of recurrent pregnancy losses; losses due to chromosomal abnormalities are more common during early pregnancy. Aneuploidy is involved in up to 80% of all spontaneous abortions occurring at < 10 wk gestation but in < 15% of those occurring at ≥ 20 wk.

Whether a history of recurrent pregnancy loss increases risk of fetal growth restriction and premature delivery in subsequent pregnancies depends on the cause of the losses.

Diagnosis

Evaluation should include the following to help determine the cause:

- Genetic evaluation (karyotyping) of both parents and any products of conception as clinically indicated to exclude possible genetic causes (see p. 2298)
- Screening for acquired thrombotic disorders: Anticardiolipin antibodies (IgG and IgM), anti-β_2 glycoprotein I (IgG and IgM), and lupus anticoagulant
- Thyroid-stimulating hormone
- Diabetes testing
- Evaluation of ovarian reserve including measuring follicle-stimulating hormone level on day 3 of the menstrual cycle
- Hysterosalpingography or sonohysterography to check for structural uterine abnormalities

Cause cannot be determined in up to 50% of women. Screening for hereditary thrombotic disorders is no longer routinely recommended unless supervised by a maternal-fetal medicine specialist.

Treatment

Some causes can be treated. If the cause cannot be identified, the chance of a live birth in the next pregnancy is 35 to 85%.

SEPTIC ABORTION

Septic abortion is serious uterine infection during or shortly before or after an abortion.

Septic abortions usually result from induced abortions done by untrained practitioners using nonsterile techniques; they are much more common when induced abortion is illegal. Infection is less common after spontaneous abortion (see p. 2355).

Typical causative organisms include *Escherichia coli, Enterobacter aerogenes, Proteus vulgaris*, hemolytic streptococci, staphylococci, and some anaerobic organisms (eg, *Clostridium perfringens*). One or more organisms may be involved.

Symptoms and Signs

Symptoms and signs typically appear within 24 to 48 h after abortion and are similar to those of pelvic inflammatory disease (eg, chills, fever, vaginal discharge, often peritonitis) and often those of threatened or incomplete abortion (eg, vaginal bleeding, cervical dilation, passage of products of conception). Perforation of the uterus during the procedure typically causes severe abdominal pain.

Septic shock may result, causing hypothermia, hypotension, oliguria, and respiratory distress. Sepsis due to *C. perfringens* may result in thrombocytopenia, ecchymoses, and findings of intravascular hemolysis (eg, anuria, anemia, jaundice, hemoglobinuria, hemosiderinuria).

Diagnosis

- Clinical evaluation
- Cultures to guide antibiotic therapy
- Ultrasonography

Septic abortion is usually obvious clinically, typically based on finding severe infection in women who are pregnant. Ultrasonography should be done to check for retained products of conception as a possible cause. Uterine perforation is most obvious during the procedure; it should be suspected when women have unexplained severe abdominal pain and peritonitis. Ultrasonography is insensitive for perforation.

When septic abortion is suspected, aerobic and anaerobic cultures of blood are done to help direct antibiotic therapy. Laboratory tests should include CBC with differential, liver function tests, electrolyte levels, glucose, BUN, and creatinine. PT and PTT are done if liver function test results are abnormal or if women have excessive bleeding.

Treatment

- Intensive antibiotic therapy (eg, clindamycin plus gentamicin with or without ampicillin)
- Uterine evacuation

Treatment is intensive antibiotic therapy plus uterine evacuation as soon as possible. A typical antibiotic regimen includes clindamycin 900 mg IV q 8 h plus gentamicin 5 mg/kg IV once/day, with or without ampicillin 2 g IV q 4 h. Alternatively, a combination of ampicillin, gentamicin, and metronidazole 500 mg IV q 8 h can be used.

STILLBIRTH

(Fetal Demise)

Stillbirth is delivery of a dead fetus at > 20 wk gestation. Maternal and fetal testing is done to determine the cause. Management is as for routine care after live delivery.

Etiology

Fetal death during late pregnancy may have maternal, placental, or fetal anatomic or genetic causes (see Table 282–3). Overall, the most common cause is

- Abruptio placentae

Complications: If a fetus dies during late pregnancy or near term but remains in the uterus for weeks, disseminated intravascular coagulation (DIC) may occur.

Diagnosis

Tests to determine cause include the following:

- Fetal karyotype and autopsy
- Maternal CBC (for evidence of anemia or leukocytosis)
- Kleihauer-Betke test
- Directed screening for hereditary and acquired thrombotic disorders, including tests for prothrombin G20210A mutation, protein C and S levels, activated protein C resistance (if positive, factor V Leiden mutation testing), antithrombin activity, fasting homocysteine level, and antiphospholipid antibodies (lupus anticoagulant, anticardiolipin [IgG and IgM], anti-β_2 glycoprotein I[IgG and IgM])
- TORCH test (toxoplasmosis [with IgG and IgM], other pathogens [eg, human parvovirus B19, varicella-zoster viruses], rubella, cytomegalovirus, herpes simplex)

Table 282–3. COMMON CAUSES OF STILLBIRTH

TYPE	EXAMPLES
Maternal	Diabetes mellitus if uncontrolled Hereditary thrombotic disorders Preeclampsia or eclampsia Sepsis Substance abuse Trauma
Placental	Abruptio placentae Chorioamnionitis Fetomaternal hemorrhage Twin-twin transfusion Umbilical cord accidents (eg, prolapse, knots) Uteroplacental vascular insufficiency Vasa previa
Fetal	Alloimmune thrombocytopenia Chromosomal abnormalities Fetal alloimmune or inherited anemia Infection Major congenital malformations (eg, of the heart or brain) Nonimmune hydrops fetalis Single-gene disorders

- Rapid plasma reagin (RPR)
- TSH (and if abnormal, free T_4)
- Diabetes testing (HbA_{1C})
- Examination of the placenta

Often, cause cannot be determined.

Treatment

- Uterine evacuation if required
- Routine postdelivery care
- Emotional support

Uterine evacuation may have spontaneously occurred. If not, evacuation should be done using drugs (eg, oxytocin) or a surgical procedure (eg, dilation and evacuation [D & E], preceded by preabortion osmotic dilators to prepare the cervix, with or without misoprostol). Postdelivery management is similar to that for live birth.

If DIC develops, coagulopathy should be promptly and aggressively managed by replacing blood or blood products as needed.

After the products of conception are expelled, curettage may be needed to remove any retained placental fragments. Fragments are more likely to remain when stillbirth occurs very early in the pregnancy.

Parents typically feel significant grief and require emotional support and sometimes require formal counseling. Risks with future pregnancies, which are related to the presumed cause, should be discussed with patients.

KEY POINTS

- Abruptio placentae is the most common cause of stillbirth, but there are many other causes (maternal, fetal, or placental).
- DIC may develop secondarily.
- Do tests to determine the cause; however, the cause often cannot be determined.
- Evacuate the uterus using drugs or D & E, and provide emotional support to the parents.

VASA PREVIA

Vasa previa occurs when membranes that contain fetal blood vessels connecting the umbilical cord and placenta overlie the internal cervical os.

Vasa previa can occur on its own or with placental abnormalities, such as a velamentous cord insertion. In velamentous cord insertion, vessels from the umbilical cord run through part of the chorionic membrane rather than directly into the placenta (see Fig. 282–1). Thus, the blood vessels are not protected by Wharton jelly within the cord, making fetal hemorrhage more likely to occur when the fetal membranes rupture.

Prevalence is about 1/2500 to 5000 deliveries. Fetal mortality rate may approach 60% if vasa previa is not diagnosed before birth.

Symptoms and Signs

The classic presentation is painless vaginal bleeding, rupture of membranes, and fetal bradycardia.

Diagnosis

- Transvaginal ultrasonography

The diagnosis should be suspected based on presentation or results of routine prenatal ultrasonography. At presentation, the fetal heart rate pattern, commonly sinusoidal, is usually nonreassuring. The diagnosis is typically confirmed by transvaginal

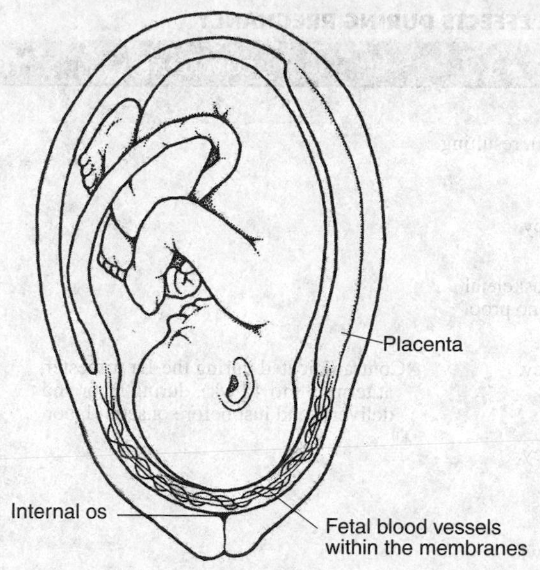

Fig. 282–1. Vasa previa.

ultrasonography. Fetal vessels can be seen within the membranes passing directly over the internal cervical os. Doppler color flow mapping can be used as an adjunct. Vasa previa must be distinguished from funic presentation (prolapse with the umbilical cord between the presenting part and the internal cervical os), in which fetal blood vessels wrapped with Wharton jelly can be seen covering the cervix.

Treatment

- Antenatal nonstress testing to detect cord compression
- Cesarean delivery

Antenatal management of vasa previa is controversial, partly because randomized clinical trials are lacking. At most centers, nonstress testing is done twice a week beginning at 28 to 30 wk. The purpose is to detect compression of the umbilical cord. Admission for continuous monitoring or for nonstress testing every 6 to 8 h at about 30 to 32 wk is often offered. Corticosteroids may be used to accelerate fetal lung maturity.

If premature rupture of the membranes occurs, vaginal bleeding continues, or fetal status is nonreassuring, emergency cesarean delivery is usually indicated. If none of these problems are present and labor has not occurred, clinicians can offer to schedule cesarean delivery; tests to assess fetal lung maturity (which usually occurs between 32 and 35 wk) may be done to determine the timing of delivery.

283 Drugs in Pregnancy

Drugs are used in over half of all pregnancies, and prevalence of use is increasing. The most commonly used drugs include antiemetics, antacids, antihistamines, analgesics, antimicrobials, diuretics, hypnotics, tranquilizers, and social and illicit drugs. Despite this trend, firm evidence-based guidelines for drug use during pregnancy are still lacking.

Regulatory information about drug safety during pregnancy: Until recently, the FDA classified OTC and prescription drugs into 5 categories of safety for use during pregnancy (A, B, C, D, X). However, few well-controlled studies of therapeutic drugs have been done in pregnant women. Most information about drug safety during pregnancy is derived from animal studies, uncontrolled studies, and postmarketing surveillance. Consequently, the FDA classification system led to confusion and difficulty applying available information to clinical decisions. In December 2014, the FDA responded by requiring that the pregnancy categories A, B, C, D, and X be removed from the labeling of all drugs.

Instead of categories, the FDA now requires that labeling provide information about the specific drug in a consistent format (called the final rule; for more information, see the FDA's announcement).

The information required by the FDA has 3 subsections:

- **Pregnancy:** Information relevant to the use of the drug in pregnant women (eg, dosing, fetal risks) and information about whether there is a registry that collects and maintains data on how pregnant women are affected
- **Lactation:** Information about using the drug while breastfeeding (eg, the amount of drug in breast milk, potential effects on the breastfed child)
- **Females and males of reproductive potential:** Information about pregnancy testing, contraception, and infertility as it relates to the drug

The pregnancy and lactation subsections each include 3 subheadings (risk summary, clinical considerations, and data) that provide more detail.

Effects of drug use during pregnancy: During pregnancy, drugs are often required to treat certain disorders. In general, when potential benefit outweighs known risks, drugs may be considered for treatment of disorders during pregnancy.

Not all maternal drugs cross the placenta to the fetus. Drugs that cross the placenta may have a direct toxic effect or a teratogenic effect. Drugs that do not cross the placenta may still harm the fetus by

- Constricting placental vessels and thus impairing gas and nutrient exchange
- Producing severe uterine hypertonia that results in anoxic injury
- Altering maternal physiology (eg, causing hypotension)

For a list of some drugs with adverse effects during pregnancy, see Table 283–1.

Drugs diffuse across the placenta similarly to the way they cross other epithelial barriers (see p. 2914). Whether and how quickly a drug crosses the placenta depend on the drug's molecular weight, extent of its binding to another substance (eg, carrier protein), area available for exchange across the placental villi, and amount of drug metabolized by the placenta. Most drugs with a molecular weight of < 500 daltons readily cross the placenta and enter the fetal circulation. Substances with a high molecular weight (eg, protein-bound drugs) usually do not cross the placenta. The exception is immune globulin G, which is occasionally used to treat disorders such as fetal alloimmune thrombocytopenia. Generally, equilibration between maternal blood and fetal tissues takes at least 30 to 60 min.

Table 283–1. SOME DRUGS WITH ADVERSE EFFECTS DURING PREGNANCY

EXAMPLES	ADVERSE EFFECTS	COMMENTS
Antibacterials		
Aminoglycosides	Ototoxicity (eg, damage to fetal labyrinth), resulting in deafness	—
Chloramphenicol	Gray baby syndrome In women or fetuses with G6PD deficiency, hemolysis	—
Fluoroquinolones	Possibly arthralgia; theoretically, musculoskeletal defects (eg, impaired bone growth), but no proof of this effect	—
Nitrofurantoin	In women or fetuses with G6PD deficiency, hemolysis	Contraindicated during the 1st trimester, at term (38 to 42 wk), during labor and delivery, and just before onset of labor
Primaquine	In women or fetuses with G6PD deficiency, hemolysis	—
Streptomycin	Ototoxicity	—
Sulfonamides (except sulfasalazine, which has minimal fetal risk)	When the drugs are given after about 34 wk gestation, neonatal jaundice and, without treatment, kernicterus In women or fetuses with G6PD deficiency, hemolysis	—
Tetracycline	Slowed bone growth, enamel hypoplasia, permanent yellowing of the teeth, and increased susceptibility to cavities in offspring Occasionally, liver failure in pregnant women	—
Trimethoprim	Increased risk of neural tube defects due to folate antagonism	—
Anticoagulants		
Low molecular weight heparin	Thrombocytopenia and maternal bleeding	Compatible with pregnancy
Unfractionated heparin	Thrombocytopenia and maternal bleeding	—
Warfarin	When warfarin is given during the 1st trimester, fetal warfarin syndrome (eg, nasal hypoplasia, bone stippling, bilateral optic atrophy, various degrees of intellectual disability) When the drug is given during the 2nd or 3rd trimester, optic atrophy, cataracts, intellectual disability, microcephaly, microphthalmia, and fetal and maternal hemorrhage	Absolutely contraindicated during 1st trimester of pregnancy
Anticonvulsants		
Carbamazepine	Hemorrhagic disease of the newborn Some risk of congenital malformations including neural tube defects	—
Lamotrigine	No appreciable increased risk with dosage up to 600 mg/day	Compatible with pregnancy
Levetiracetam	Minor skeletal malformations in animal studies, but no appreciable increased risk in humans	Compatible with pregnancy
Phenobarbital	Hemorrhagic disease of the newborn Some risk of congenital malformations	—
Phenytoin	Congenital malformations (eg, cleft lip, GU defects such as hypospadias, cardiovascular defects Hemorrhagic disease of the newborn	Persistent risk of congenital malformations despite folic acid supplementation

Table 283–1. SOME DRUGS WITH ADVERSE EFFECTS DURING PREGNANCY (*Continued*)

EXAMPLES	ADVERSE EFFECTS	COMMENTS
Trimethadione	High risk of congenital malformations (eg, cleft palate; cardiac, craniofacial, hand, and abdominal defects) and risk of spontaneous abortion	Almost always contraindicated during pregnancy
Valproate	Major congenital malformations (eg, neural tube defects such as meningomyelocele; cardiac, craniofacial, and limb defects)	Persistent risk of congenital malformations despite folic acid supplementation
Antidepressants		
Bupropion	Conflicting data on risk of congenital malformations from first trimester exposure	Dosing affected by hepatic or renal impairment
Citalopram	When citalopram is given during the 1st trimester, increased risk of congenital malformations (particularly cardiac) When the drug is given during the 3rd trimester, discontinuation syndrome and persistent pulmonary hypertension of the newborn	Consideration of dose tapering during the 3rd trimester in consultation with a mental health practitioner
Escitalopram	When escitalopram is given during the 3rd trimester, discontinuation syndrome and persistent pulmonary hypertension of the newborn	Consideration of dose tapering during the 3rd trimester in consultation with a mental health practitioner
Fluoxetine	When fluoxetine is given during the 3rd trimester, discontinuation syndrome and persistent pulmonary hypertension of the newborn	Long half-life; drug-drug interactions possibly occurring for weeks after the drug is stopped Consideration of dose tapering during the 3rd trimester in consultation with a mental health practitioner
Paroxetine	When paroxetine is given during the 1st trimester, increased risk of congenital malformations (particularly cardiac) When the drug is given during the 3rd trimester, discontinuation syndrome and persistent pulmonary hypertension of the newborn	Use during pregnancy not recommended by some experts* Consideration of dose tapering during the 3rd trimester in consultation with a mental health practitioner
Sertraline	When sertraline is given during the 3rd trimester, discontinuation syndrome and persistent pulmonary hypertension of the newborn	Consideration of dose tapering during the 3rd trimester in consultation with a mental health practitioner
Venlafaxine	When venlafaxine is given during the 3rd trimester, discontinuation syndrome	Dosing greatly affected by hepatic or renal impairment Consideration of dose tapering during the 3rd trimester in consultation with a mental health practitioner
Antiemetics		
Doxylamine and pyridoxine (vitamin B_6)	No evidence of increased risk of congenital malformations	—
Ondansetron	No significant teratogenic risk in animal studies When ondansetron is given during the 1st trimester, possible risk of congenital heart disease (evidence is weak)	Used during pregnancy only for hyperemesis gravidarum when other treatments are ineffective
Promethazine	No significant teratogenic risk in animal studies Generally no increased risk of congenital malformations Possibly decreased platelet aggregation in neonates	—
Antifungals		
Amphotericin B	No significant teratogenic risk in animal studies	Monitoring recommended for systemic toxicities (electrolyte imbalance, renal dysfunction) in the mother

Table continues on the following page.

Table 283–1. SOME DRUGS WITH ADVERSE EFFECTS DURING PREGNANCY (*Continued*)

EXAMPLES	ADVERSE EFFECTS	COMMENTS
Fluconazole	Teratogenic at high doses in animal studies No apparent increased risk of congenital malformations after a single dose of 150 mg/day After higher doses (> 400 mg/day) taken for most or all of the 1st trimester, increased risk of various malformations	—
Miconazole	With oral use, adverse effects in animal studies When applied to the skin, no significant risk of congenital malformations	Not to be used intravaginally during the 1st trimester unless essential to the mother's welfare
Terconazole	Adverse effects in animal studies No significant risk of congenital malformations	Not to be used intravaginally during the 1st trimester unless benefit to the mother outweighs risk to the fetus
Antihistamine/anticholinergic drug		
Meclizine	Teratogenic in rodents, but no proof of this effect in humans	—
Antihypertensives		
ACE inhibitors (see Table 84–7 on p. 734)	When the drugs are given during the 2nd or 3rd trimester, fetal hypocalvaria and hypoperfusion (which can cause renal defects), renal failure, and the oligohydramnios sequence (oligohydramnios, craniofacial deformities, limb contractures, and hypoplastic lung development)	—
Beta-blockers	Fetal bradycardia, hypoglycemia, and possibly fetal growth restriction and preterm birth	—
Calcium channel blockers	When the drugs are given during the 1st trimester, possibly phalangeal deformities When the drugs are given during the 2nd or 3rd trimester, fetal growth restriction	—
Thiazide diuretics	Prevention of normal maternal volume expansion, reducing placental perfusion and contributing to fetal growth restriction Neonatal hyponatremia, hypokalemia, and thrombocytopenia	—
Antineoplastic drugs[†]		
Actinomycin	Teratogenic in animals, but no proof of this effect in humans	—
Busulfan	Congenital malformations (eg, fetal growth restriction, mandibular hypoplasia, cleft palate, cranial dysostosis, spinal defects, ear defects, clubfoot)	—
Chlorambucil	Same as those for busulfan	—
Colchicine	Possibly congenital malformations and sperm abnormalities	—
Cyclophosphamide	Same as those for busulfan	—
Doxorubicin	Teratogenic in animals and humans Potential for dose-dependent cardiac dysfunction	Use during pregnancy not recommended Effective contraception recommended during pregnancy and for 6 mo after treatment of male or female partner
Mercaptopurine	Same as those for busulfan	—
Methotrexate	Same as those for busulfan	Contraindicated during pregnancy Effective contraception recommended for 8 wk after the last dose
Vinblastine	Teratogenic in animals, but no proof of this effect in humans	—
Vincristine	Teratogenic in animals, but no proof of this effect in humans	—

Table 283–1. SOME DRUGS WITH ADVERSE EFFECTS DURING PREGNANCY (*Continued*)

EXAMPLES	ADVERSE EFFECTS	COMMENTS
Antipsychotics and mood stabilizers		
Haloperidol	Adverse effects in animal studies When haloperidol is given during the 1st trimester, possibly limb malformations When haloperidol is given during the 3rd trimester, increased risk of extrapyramidal symptoms or withdrawal symptoms in the neonate	—
Lurasidone	No evidence of adverse effects in animal studies When lurasidone is given during the 3rd trimester, increased risk of extrapyramidal symptoms or withdrawal symptoms in the neonate	—
Lithium	Adverse effects in animal studies When lithium is given during the 1st trimester, teratogenic (cardiac malformations) When lithium is given later in pregnancy, lethargy, hypotonia, poor feeding, hypothyroidism, goiter, and nephrogenic diabetes insipidus in the neonate	—
Olanzapine	Adverse effects in animal studies When olanzapine is given during the 3rd trimester, increased risk of extrapyramidal symptoms or withdrawal symptoms in the neonate	—
Risperidone	Adverse effects in animal studies Based on limited data, no increased teratogenic risk When risperidone is given during the 3rd trimester, increased risk of extrapyramidal symptoms or withdrawal symptoms in the neonate	—
Anxiolytics		
Benzodiazepines	When benzodiazepines are given late in pregnancy, respiratory depression or a neonatal withdrawal syndrome that can cause irritability, tremors, and hyperreflexia	—
Hypoglycemic drugs (oral)		
Chlorpropamide	Neonatal hypoglycemia	—
Glyburide	Neonatal hypoglycemia	—
Metformin	Neonatal hypoglycemia	—
Tolbutamide	Neonatal hypoglycemia	—
NSAIDs		
Aspirin and other salicylates	Fetal kernicterus With high doses, possibly 1st-trimester spontaneous abortions, delayed onset of labor, premature closing of the fetal ductus arteriosus, jaundice, occasionally maternal (intrapartum and postpartum) and/or neonatal hemorrhage, necrotizing enterocolitis, and oligohydramnios With low doses (81 mg) of aspirin, no significant teratogenic risk	—
Nonsalicylate NSAIDs	Same as those for salicylate NSAIDs	Contraindicated in the 3rd trimester
Opioids and partial agonists		
Buprenorphine	Adverse effects but no teratogenicity in animal studies Risk of a neonatal opioid withdrawal syndrome (neonatal abstinence syndrome)	Improved fetal outcomes compared with those when pregnant women use illicit substances

Table continues on the following page.

Table 283–1. SOME DRUGS WITH ADVERSE EFFECTS DURING PREGNANCY (*Continued*)

EXAMPLES	ADVERSE EFFECTS	COMMENTS
Codeine Hydrocodone Hydromorphone Meperidine Morphine	In neonates of women addicted to opioids, withdrawal symptoms possibly occurring 6 h to 8 days after birth With high doses given in the hour before delivery, possibly neonatal CNS depression and bradycardia	—
Methadone	Adverse effects in animal studies Specific effects of methadone in pregnant women possibly difficult to differentiate from effects of concomitant drugs (eg, illicit drugs) Risk of a neonatal opioid withdrawal syndrome	Improved fetal outcomes compared with those when pregnant women use illicit substances Possible need for acute short-acting analgesics to supplement maintenance dosing during labor and delivery
Retinoids		
Isotretinoin	High teratogenic risk (eg, multiple congenital malformations), spontaneous abortion, and intellectual disability	Contraindicated during pregnancy and in women who may become pregnant
Sex hormones		
Danazol	When these drugs are given during the first 14 wk, masculinization of a female fetus's genitals (eg, pseudohermaphroditism)	Contraindicated during pregnancy
Synthetic progestins (but not the low doses used in oral contraceptives)	Same as those for danazol	Contraindicated during pregnancy
Thyroid drugs		
Methimazole	Fetal goiter and neonatal scalp defects (aplasia cutis)	To be avoided during the 1st trimester of pregnancy
Propylthiouracil	Fetal goiter and maternal hepatotoxicity and agranulocytosis	—
Radioactive iodine (^{131}I)	Destruction of the fetal thyroid gland or, when the drug is given near the end of the 1st trimester, severe fetal hyperthyroidism	Contraindicated during pregnancy
Saturated solution of K iodide	Large fetal goiter, which may obstruct breathing in neonates	—
Triiodothyronine	Fetal goiter	—
Vaccines		
Live-virus vaccines such as those for measles, mumps, rubella, polio, chickenpox, and yellow fever	With rubella and varicella vaccines, potential infection of the placenta and developing fetus With other vaccines, potential but unknown risks	Not given to women who are or may be pregnant
Others		
Corticosteroids	When these drugs are used during the 1st trimester, possibly orofacial clefts	—
Hydroxychloroquine	No increased risk at usual doses	—
Loratadine	Possible hypospadias	—
Pseudoephedrine	Placental vasoconstriction and possible risk of gastroschisis	—
Vitamin K	In women or fetuses with G6PD deficiency, hemolysis	—

*The American College of Obstetricians and Gynecologists (ACOG) recommends avoiding paroxetine use during pregnancy.

†The European Society for Medical Oncology (ESMO) has published guidelines for diagnosis, treatment, and follow-up of cancer during pregnancy. Generally, if chemotherapy is indicated, it should not be given during the1st trimester but may begin during the 2nd trimester; the last chemotherapy dose should be given ≥ 3 wk before anticipated delivery, and chemotherapy should not be given after wk 33 of gestation.

G6PD = glucose-6-phosphate dehydrogenase.

A drug's effect on the fetus is determined largely by fetal age at exposure, drug potency, and drug dosage. Fetal age affects the type of drug effect:

- **Before the 20th day after fertilization:** Drugs given at this time typically have an all-or-nothing effect, killing the embryo or not affecting it at all. Teratogenesis is unlikely during this stage.
- **During organogenesis (between 20 and 56 days after fertilization):** Teratogenesis is most likely at this stage. Drugs reaching the embryo during this stage may result in spontaneous abortion, a sublethal gross anatomic defect (true teratogenic effect), or covert embryopathy (a permanent subtle metabolic or functional defect that may manifest later in life), or the drugs may have no measurable effect.
- **After organogenesis (in the 2nd and 3rd trimesters):** Teratogenesis is unlikely, but drugs may alter growth and function of normally formed fetal organs and tissues. As placental metabolism increases, doses must be higher for fetal toxicity to occur.

Despite widespread concern about drug safety, exposure to therapeutic drugs accounts for only 2 to 3% of all fetal congenital malformations; most malformations result from genetic, environmental, or unknown causes.

Vaccines During Pregnancy

Immunization is as effective in women who are pregnant as in those who are not.

Influenza vaccine is recommended for all pregnant women in the 2nd or 3rd trimester during influenza season.

Other vaccines should be reserved for situations in which the woman or fetus is at significant risk of exposure to a hazardous infection and risk of adverse effects from the vaccine is low. Vaccinations for cholera, hepatitis A and B, measles, mumps, plague, poliomyelitis, rabies, tetanus-diphtheria, typhoid, and yellow fever may be given during pregnancy if risk of infection is substantial.

Live-virus vaccines should not be given to women who are or may be pregnant. Rubella vaccine, an attenuated live-virus vaccine, may cause subclinical placental and fetal infection. However, no defects in neonates have been attributed to rubella vaccine, and women vaccinated inadvertently during early pregnancy need not be advised to terminate pregnancy based solely on theoretical risk from the vaccine. Varicella vaccine is another attenuated live-virus vaccine that can potentially infect the fetus; risk is highest between 13 wk and 22 wk gestation. This vaccine is contraindicated during pregnancy.

Vitamin A During Pregnancy

In the amount typically present in prenatal vitamins (5000 IU/day), vitamin A has not been associated with teratogenic risk. However, doses > 10,000 IU/day during early pregnancy may increase risk of congenital malformations.

Antidepressants During Pregnancy

Antidepressants, particularly SSRIs, are commonly used during pregnancy because an estimated 7 to 23% of pregnant women have perinatal depression. Physiologic and psychosocial changes during pregnancy can affect depression (possibly worsening it) and possibly reduce the response to antidepressants. Ideally, a multidisciplinary team that includes an obstetrician and a psychiatric specialist should manage depression during pregnancy.

Pregnant women who are taking antidepressants should be asked about depressive symptoms at each prenatal visit, and appropriate fetal testing should be done. It may include the following:

- A detailed evaluation of fetal anatomy during the 2nd trimester
- If a pregnant woman takes paroxetine, echocardiography to evaluate the fetus's heart because paroxetine appears to increase the risk of congenital cardiac anomalies

Clinicians should consider tapering the dose of all antidepressants during the 3rd trimester to reduce the risk of withdrawal symptoms in the neonate. However, the benefits of tapering must be carefully balanced against the risk of symptom recurrence and postpartum depression. Postpartum depression is common, often unrecognized, and should be treated promptly. Periodic visits with a psychiatrist and/or social workers may be helpful.

Social and Illicit Drugs During Pregnancy

Cigarette smoking is the most common addiction among pregnant women. Also, percentages of women who smoke and of those who smoke heavily appear to be increasing. Only 20% of smokers quit during pregnancy. Carbon monoxide and nicotine in cigarettes cause hypoxia and vasoconstriction, increasing risk of the following:

- Spontaneous abortion (fetal loss or delivery < 20 wk)
- Fetal growth restriction
- Abruptio placentae
- Placenta previa
- Premature rupture of the membranes
- Preterm birth
- Chorioamnionitis
- Stillbirth

Neonates whose mothers smoke are also more likely to have anencephaly, congenital heart defects, orofacial clefts, sudden infant death syndrome, deficiencies in physical growth and intelligence, and behavioral problems. Smoking cessation or limitation reduces risks.

Alcohol is the most commonly used teratogen. Drinking alcohol during pregnancy increases risk of spontaneous abortion. Risk is probably related to amount of alcohol consumed, but no amount is known to be risk-free. Regular drinking decreases birth weight by about 1 to 1.3 kg. Binge drinking in particular, possibly as little as 45 mL of pure alcohol (equivalent to about 3 drinks) a day, can cause fetal alcohol syndrome. This syndrome occurs in 2.2/1000 live births; it includes fetal growth restriction, facial and cardiovascular defects, and neurologic dysfunction. It is a leading cause of intellectual disability and can cause neonatal death due to failure to thrive.

Cocaine use has indirect fetal risks (eg, maternal stroke or death during pregnancy). Its use probably also results in fetal vasoconstriction and hypoxia. Repeated use increases risk of the following:

- Spontaneous abortion
- Fetal growth restriction
- Abruptio placentae
- Preterm birth
- Stillbirth
- Congenital malformations (eg, CNS, GU, and skeletal malformations; isolated atresias)

Although **marijuana's** main metabolite can cross the placenta, recreational use of marijuana use does not consistently appear to increase risk of congenital malformations, fetal growth restriction, or postnatal neurobehavioral abnormalities.

Bath salts refers to a group of designer drugs made from a variety of amphetamine-like substances; these drugs are being increasingly used during pregnancy. Although effects are poorly understood, fetal vasoconstriction and hypoxia are likely, and there is a risk of stillbirth, abruptio placentae, and possibly congenital malformations.

Hallucinogens may, depending on the drug, increase risk of the following:

- Spontaneous miscarriage
- Premature delivery
- Withdrawal syndrome in the fetus or neonate

Hallucinogens include methylenedioxymethamphetamine (MDMA, or Ecstasy), rohypnol, ketamine, methamphetamine, and LSD (lysergic acid diethylamide).

Whether consuming **caffeine** in large amounts can increase perinatal risk is unclear. Consuming caffeine in small amounts (eg, 1 cup of coffee/day) appears to pose little or no risk to the fetus, but some data, which did not account for tobacco or alcohol use, suggest that consuming large amounts (> 7 cups of coffee/day) increases risk of stillbirths, preterm deliveries, low birth weight, and spontaneous abortions. Decaffeinated beverages theoretically pose little risk to the fetus.

Use of **aspartame** (a dietary sugar substitute) during pregnancy is often questioned. The most common metabolite of aspartame, phenylalanine, is concentrated in the fetus by active placental transport; toxic levels may cause intellectual disability. However, when ingestion is within the usual range, fetal phenylalanine levels are far below toxic levels. Thus, moderate ingestion of aspartame (eg, no more than 1 liter of diet soda per day) during pregnancy appears to pose little risk of fetal toxicity. However, in pregnant women with phenylketonuria, intake of phenylalanine and thus aspartame is prohibited.

284 High-Risk Pregnancy

In a high-risk (at-risk) pregnancy, the mother, fetus, or neonate is at increased risk of morbidity or mortality before or after delivery.

In 2015, **overall maternal mortality rate** in the US was 14/100,000 deliveries, as estimated by the WHO; incidence is 3 to 4 times higher in nonwhite women. The maternal mortality rate is higher in the US than in other Western countries (eg, Germany, Netherlands, Poland, Spain, Sweden, Switzerland, United Kingdom).

The most common causes of maternal death worldwide are

- Hemorrhage
- Preeclampsia
- Sepsis
- Abortion (including induced abortion, miscarriage, and ectopic pregnancy)
- Pulmonary embolism
- Obstetric complications
- Other disorders (eg, preexisting disorders such as HIV infection[1]

Nearly half of maternal deaths are preventable.

Perinatal mortality rate in offspring in the US is about 6 to 7/1000 deliveries; deaths are divided about equally between those during the late fetal period (gestational age > 28 wk) and those during the early neonatal period (< 7 days after birth).

The most common causes of perinatal death are

- Obstetric complications
- Maternal disorders (eg, hypertension, diabetes mellitus, obesity, autoimmune disorders)
- Infection
- Placental abnormalities
- Congenital malformations
- Preterm delivery

Other maternal characteristics that increase the risk of perinatal mortality include maternal age (much younger or older than average), unmarried status, smoking, and multiple gestations.

1. Say L, Chou D, Gemmill A, et al: Global causes of maternal death: A WHO systematic analysis. *Lancet Glob Health* 2(6):e323–33, 2014. doi: 10.1016/S2214-109X(14)70227-X.

Risk Assessment During Pregnancy

Risk assessment is part of routine prenatal care. Risk is also assessed during or shortly after labor and at any time that events may modify risk status. Risk factors (see Table 284–1) are assessed systematically because each risk factor present increases overall risk.

Several pregnancy monitoring and risk assessment systems are available. The most widely used system is the Pregnancy Assessment Monitoring System (PRAMS), which is a project of the CDC and state health departments. PRAMS provides information for state health departments to use to improve the health of mothers and infants. PRAMS also enables the CDC and states to monitor changes in health indicators (eg, unintended pregnancy, prenatal care, breastfeeding, smoking, drinking, infant health).

High-risk pregnancies require close monitoring and sometimes referral to a perinatal center. When referral is needed, transfer before rather than after delivery results in lower neonatal morbidity and mortality rates.

The **most common reasons for referral before delivery** are

- Preterm labor (often due to premature rupture of the membranes)
- Preeclampsia
- Hemorrhage

RISK FACTORS FOR COMPLICATIONS DURING PREGNANCY

Risk factors for complications during pregnancy include

- Preexisting maternal disorders
- Physical and social characteristics
- Age

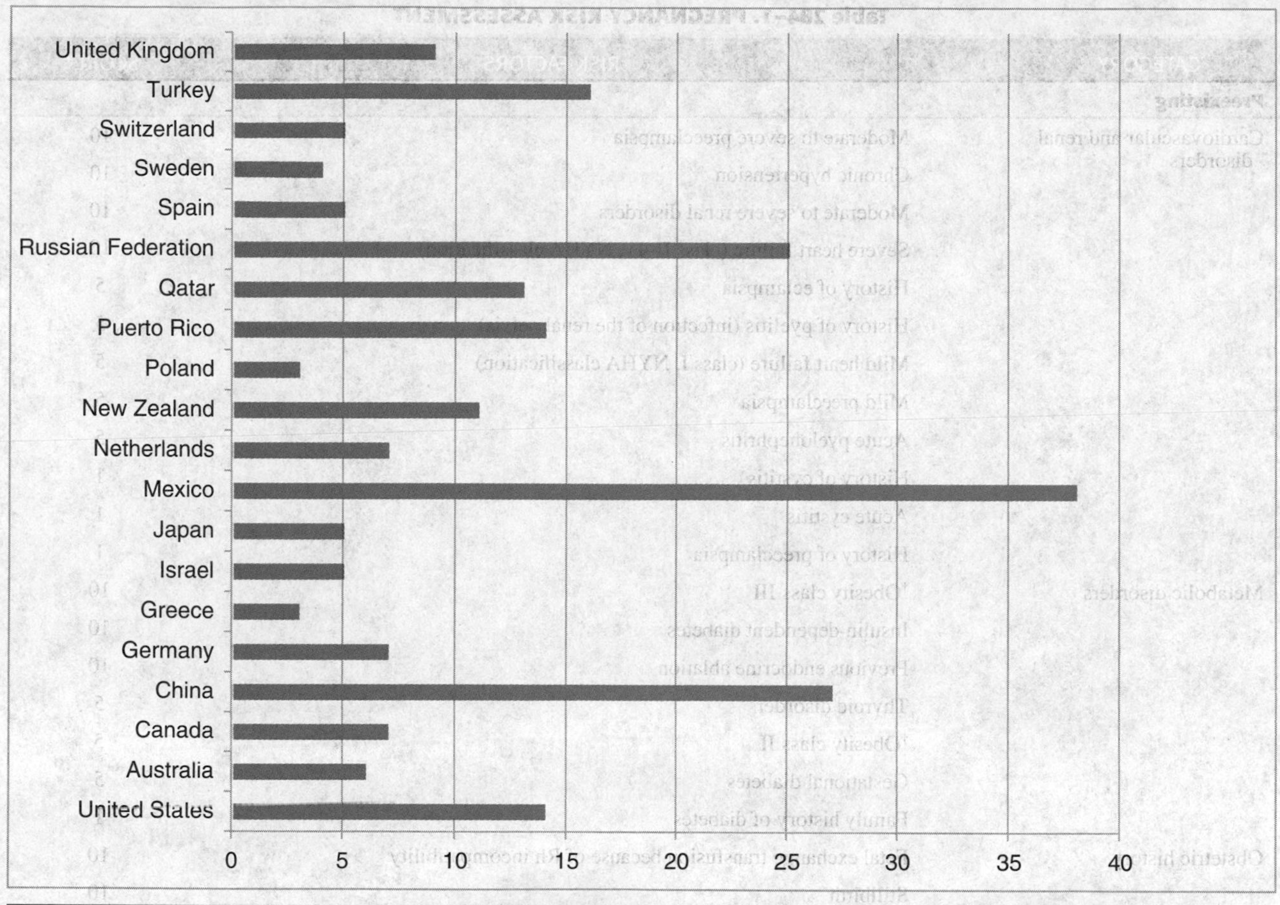

Fig. 284–1. Maternal mortality ratios in selected countries. Maternal mortality ratio refers to the number of women who die from pregnancy-related causes during pregnancy or within 42 days of the end of the pregnancy per 100,000 live births. In 2015, ratios ranged from 3 (Finland) to 1360 (Sierra Leone) per 100,000 live births (countries not shown). The maternal mortality ratio is higher in the US than in other Western countries. Data from WHO, UNICEF, UNFPA, The World Bank, and the United Nations Population Division. Trends in Maternal Mortality: 1990 to 2015. Geneva, World Health Organization, 2015.

- Problems in previous pregnancies (eg, spontaneous abortions)
- Problems that develop during pregnancy
- Problems that develop during labor and delivery

Hypertension

Pregnant women are considered to have chronic hypertension (CHTN) if

- Hypertension was present before the pregnancy
- Hypertension develops before 20 wk of pregnancy

CHTN is differentiated from gestational hypertension, which develops after 20 wk of pregnancy. In either case, hypertension is defined as systolic BP > 140 mm Hg or diastolic BP > 90 mm Hg on 2 occasions > 24 h apart.

Hypertension increases risk of the following:

- Fetal growth restriction (by decreasing uteroplacental blood flow)
- Adverse fetal and maternal outcomes

Before attempting to conceive, women with hypertension should be counseled about the risks of pregnancy. If they become pregnant, prenatal care begins as early as possible and includes measurements of baseline renal function (eg, serum creatinine, BUN), funduscopic examination, and directed cardiovascular evaluation (auscultation and sometimes ECG, echocardiography, or both). Each trimester, 24-h urine protein, serum uric acid, serum creatinine, and Hct are measured. Ultrasonography to monitor fetal growth is done at 28 wk and every 4 wk thereafter. Delayed growth is evaluated with multivessel Doppler testing by a maternal-fetal medicine specialist (for management of hypertension during pregnancy, see p. 2397).

Diabetes

Overt diabetes mellitus occurs in ≥ 6% of pregnancies, and gestational diabetes occurs in about 8.5% of pregnancies. Incidence is increasing as the incidence of obesity increases.

Table 284–1. PREGNANCY RISK ASSESSMENT

CATEGORY	RISK FACTORS	SCORE*
Preexisting		
Cardiovascular and renal disorders	Moderate to severe preeclampsia	10
	Chronic hypertension	10
	Moderate to severe renal disorders	10
	Severe heart failure (class II–IV, NYHA classification)	10
	History of eclampsia	5
	History of pyelitis (infection of the renal pelvis)	5
	Mild heart failure (class I, NYHA classification)	5
	Mild preeclampsia	5
	Acute pyelonephritis	5
	History of cystitis	1
	Acute cystitis	1
	History of preeclampsia	1
Metabolic disorders	†Obesity class III	10
	Insulin-dependent diabetes	10
	Previous endocrine ablation	10
	Thyroid disorders	5
	†Obesity class II	5
	Gestational diabetes	5
	Family history of diabetes	1
Obstetric history	Fetal exchange transfusion because of Rh incompatibility	10
	Stillbirth	10
	Late abortion (16–20 wk)	10
	Postterm pregnancy (> 42 wk)	10
	Preterm newborn (< 37 wk and < 2500 g)	10
	Intrauterine growth restriction (weight < 10th percentile for estimated gestational age)	10
	Abnormal fetal position	10
	Polyhydramnios (hydramnios)	10
	Multifetal pregnancy	10
	Previous brachial plexus injury	10
	Neonatal death	5
	Cesarean delivery	5
	Habitual (≥ 3) abortion	5
	Neonate > 4.5 kg	5
	Shoulder dystocia	5
	Multiparity of > 5	5
	Seizure disorders or cerebral palsy	5
	Fetal malformations	1

Table 284–1. PREGNANCY RISK ASSESSMENT (*Continued*)

CATEGORY	RISK FACTORS	SCORE*
Other disorders	Abnormal cervical cytologic findings	10
	Sickle cell disease	10
	Thrombophilia	10
	Autoimmune disorders	10
	Positive serologic results for STDs	5
	Severe anemia (Hb < 9 g/dL)	5
	History of TB or purified protein derivative injection site induration ≥ 10 mm	5
	Pulmonary disorders	5
	Mild anemia (Hb 9.0–10.9 g/dL)	1
Anatomic abnormalities	Uterine malformation	10
	Insufficient (incompetent) cervix	10
	Small pelvis	5
Maternal characteristics	Age ≥ 35 or ≤ 15 yr	5
	Weight < 45.5 or > 91 kg (obesity class III)	5
	Psychiatric disorder or intellectual disability	1
Antepartum		
Exposure to teratogens	Group B streptococcal infections	10
	Smoking > 10 cigarettes/day (associated with premature rupture of membranes)	10
	Certain viral infections (eg, rubella, cytomegalovirus infections)	5
	Flu syndrome (severe)	5
	Alcohol (moderate to severe)	1
Pregnancy complications	Preterm labor at < 37 wk	10
	Preterm premature rupture of membranes	10
	Rh sensitization only (not requiring an exchange transfusion)	5
	Vaginal spotting	5
Intrapartum		
Maternal	Moderate to severe preeclampsia	10
	Polyhydramnios (hydramnios) or oligohydramnios	10
	Uterine rupture	10
	Postterm (> 42 wk)	10
	Mild preeclampsia	5
	Premature rupture of membranes > 12 h	5
	Preterm labor at ≥ 37 wk	5
	Primary dysfunctional labor	5
	Secondary arrest of dilation	5
	Labor > 20 h	5
	Second stage > 2.5 h	5
	Medical induction of labor	5
	Precipitous labor (< 3 h)	5
	Primary cesarean delivery	5
	Repeat cesarean delivery	5
	Elective induction of labor	1
	Prolonged latent phase	1
	Oxytocin augmentation	1

Table continues on the following page.

Table 284–1. PREGNANCY RISK ASSESSMENT (*Continued*)

CATEGORY	RISK FACTORS	SCORE*
Placental	Placenta previa	10
	Abruptio placentae	10
	Chorioamnionitis	10
Fetal	Abnormal presentation (breech, brow, face) or transverse lie	10
	Multifetal pregnancy	10
	Fetal bradycardia > 30 min	10
	Prolapsed cord	10
	Fetal weight < 2.5 kg	10
	Fetal weight > 4 kg	10
	Fetal acidosis pH ≤7	10
	Fetal tachycardia > 30 min	10
	Operative delivery using vacuum extractor or forceps	5
	Breech delivery, spontaneous or assisted	5

*A score of 10 or more indicates a high risk.
†National Institutes of Health's obesity classes based on BMI:

- Class I: 30–34.9
- Class II: 35–39.9
- Class III: > 40

NYHA = New York Heart Association; STDs = sexually transmitted diseases.

Preexisting insulin-dependent diabetes increases the risk of the following:

- Pyelonephritis
- Ketoacidosis
- Preeclampsia
- Fetal death
- Major fetal malformations
- Fetal macrosomia (fetal weight > 4.5 kg)
- If vasculopathy is present, fetal growth restriction

Insulin requirements usually increase during pregnancy.

Gestational diabetes increases the risk of the following:

- Hypertensive disorders
- Fetal macrosomia
- The need for cesarean section

Gestational diabetes is routinely screened for at 24 to 28 wk and, if women have risk factors, during the 1st trimester. Risk factors include the following:

- Previous gestational diabetes
- A macrosomic infant in a previous pregnancy
- Family history of non-insulin-dependent diabetes
- Unexplained fetal losses
- Body mass index (BMI) > 30 kg/m^2
- Certain ethnicities (eg, Mexican Americans, American Indians, Asians, Pacific Islanders) in whom diabetes is prevalent

Some practitioners first do a random plasma glucose test to check whether gestational diabetes is possible. However, screening and confirmation of the diagnosis of gestational diabetes is best based on results of the oral glucose tolerance test (OGTT—see Table 284–2). Based on a recommendation from the 2013 National Institutes of Health (NIH) consensus development conference, screening begins with a 1-h 50-g glucose load test (GLT); if results are positive (plasma glucose > 130 to 140 mg/dL), a 3-h 100-g OGTT is done (Table 284–3).

Optimal treatment of gestational diabetes (with dietary modification, exercise, and close monitoring of blood glucose levels and insulin when necessary) reduces risk of adverse maternal, fetal, and neonatal outcomes.

Women with gestational diabetes mellitus may have had undiagnosed diabetes mellitus before pregnancy. Thus, they should be screened for diabetes mellitus 6 to 12 wk postpartum, using the same testing and criteria used for patients who are not pregnant.

Sexually Transmitted Diseases (STDs)

(See also Sexually Transmitted Diseases on p. 1699 and Infectious Disease in Pregnancy on p. 2398.)

Fetal syphilis in utero can cause fetal death, congenital malformations, and severe disability.

Without treatment, risk of transmission of HIV from woman to offspring is about 30% prepartum and about 25% intrapartum. Neonates are given antiretroviral treatment within 6 h of birth to minimize risk of transmission intrapartum.

During pregnancy, bacterial vaginosis, gonorrhea, and genital chlamydial infection increase risk of preterm labor and premature rupture of the membranes.

Routine prenatal care includes screening tests for these infections at the first prenatal visit. Syphilis testing is repeated during pregnancy if risk continues and at delivery for all women. Pregnant women who have any of these infections are treated with antimicrobials.

Table 284–2. THRESHOLD VALUES OF PLASMA GLUCOSE FOR DIAGNOSING* GESTATIONAL DIABETES MELLITUS USING THE 100-G ORAL GLUCOSE TOLERANCE TEST

100-g OGTT TIMING	PLASMA GLUCOSE (mg/dL) PER NDDG	PLASMA GLUCOSE (mg/dL) PER CARPENTER AND COUSTAN†
Fasting‡	105	95
1-h	190	180
2-h	165	155
3-h	145	140

*Gestational diabetes is diagnosed when at least 2 threshold values are met or exceeded.
†Vandorsten JP, Dodson WC, Espeland MA, et al: National Institutes of Health (NIH) Consensus Development Conference Statement: Diagnosing gestational diabetes mellitus. NIH Consensus State-of-the-Science Statements 29:1–31, 2013.
‡Fasting is required whenever clinicians suspect that patients have undiagnosed diabetes to avoid giving them an unnecessary load of glucose.
NDDG = National Diabetes Data Group; OGTT = oral glucose tolerance test.

Treatment of bacterial vaginosis, gonorrhea, or chlamydial infection may prolong the interval from rupture of the membranes to delivery and may improve fetal outcome by decreasing fetal inflammation.

Giving zidovudine or nevirapine to pregnant women with HIV infection reduces risk of transmission by two thirds; risk is probably lower (< 2%) with a combination of 2 or 3 antivirals (see p. 2612). These drugs are recommended despite potential toxic effects in the fetus and woman.

Pyelonephritis

Pyelonephritis increases risk of the following:

- Premature rupture of the membranes
- Preterm labor
- Infant respiratory distress syndrome

Pyelonephritis is the most common nonobstetric cause of hospitalization during pregnancy.

Pregnant women with pyelonephritis are hospitalized for evaluation and treatment, primarily with urine culture plus sensitivities, IV antibiotics (eg, a 3rd-generation cephalosporin with or without an aminoglycoside), antipyretics, and hydration. Oral antibiotics specific to the causative organism are begun 24 to 48 h after fever resolves and continued to complete the whole course of antibiotic therapy, usually 7 to 10 days.

Prophylactic antibiotics (eg, nitrofurantoin, trimethoprim/sulfamethoxazole) with periodic urine cultures are continued for the rest of the pregnancy.

Table 284–3. THRESHOLD VALUES FOR DIAGNOSING OVERT DIABETES IN PREGNANCY

TEST*	THRESHOLD VALUE
Fasting plasma glucose	126 mg/dL
HbA_{1C}	6.5%
Random plasma glucose	200 mg/dL on > 1 occasion

*Fasting plasma glucose and HbA_{1C} are measured if clinicians suspect diabetes (eg, in patients with risk factors, such as obesity, a strong family history of diabetes, or a history of gestational diabetes in a previous pregnancy).
HbA_{1c} = glycosylated Hb.

Acute Surgical Problems

Major surgery, particularly intra-abdominal, increases risk of the following:

- Preterm labor
- Fetal death

However, surgery is usually tolerated well by pregnant women and the fetus when appropriate supportive care and anesthesia (maintaining BP and oxygenation at normal levels) are provided, so physicians should not be reluctant to operate; delaying treatment of an abdominal emergency is far more dangerous.

After surgery, antibiotics and tocolytic drugs are given for 12 to 24 h.

If nonemergency surgery is necessary during pregnancy, it is most safely done during the 2nd trimester.

Genital Tract Abnormalities

Structural abnormalities of the uterus and cervix (eg, uterine septum, bicornuate uterus) make the following more likely:

- Fetal malpresentation
- Dysfunctional labor
- The need for cesarean delivery

Uterine fibroids uncommonly cause placental abnormalities (eg, placenta previa), preterm labor, and recurrent spontaneous abortion. Fibroids may grow rapidly or degenerate during pregnancy; degeneration often causes severe pain and peritoneal signs.

Cervical insufficiency (incompetence) makes preterm delivery more likely. Cervical insufficiency can be treated with surgical intervention (cerclage), vaginal progesterone, or sometimes a vaginal pessary.

If, before pregnancy, women have had a myomectomy in which the uterine cavity was entered, cesarean delivery is required because uterine rupture is a risk during subsequent vaginal delivery.

Uterine abnormalities that lead to poor obstetric outcomes often require surgical correction, which is done after delivery.

Maternal Age

Teenagers, who account for 13% of all pregnancies, have an increased incidence of preeclampsia, preterm labor, and anemia, which often leads to fetal growth restriction. The cause, at least in part, is that teenagers tend to neglect prenatal care, frequently smoke, and have higher rates of sexually transmitted diseases.

In women > 35, the incidence of preeclampsia is increased, as is that of gestational diabetes, dysfunctional labor, abruptio placentae, stillbirth, and placenta previa. These women are also more likely to have preexisting disorders (eg, CHTN, diabetes). Because risk of fetal chromosomal abnormalities increases as maternal age increases, genetic testing should be offered.

Maternal Weight

Pregnant women whose BMI was < 19.8 kg/m^2 before pregnancy are considered underweight, which predisposes to low birth weight (< 2.5 kg) in neonates. Such women are encouraged to gain at least 12.5 kg during pregnancy.

Pregnant women whose BMI was 25 to 29.9 kg/m^2 (overweight) or ≥ 30 (obese) before pregnancy are at risk of maternal hypertension and diabetes, postterm pregnancy, pregnancy loss, fetal macrosomia, congenital malformations, intrauterine growth restriction, preeclampsia, and the need for cesarean delivery. Ideally, weight loss should begin before pregnancy, first by trying lifestyle modifications (eg, increased physical activity, dietary changes). Women who are overweight or obese are encouraged to limit weight gain during pregnancy, ideally by modifying their lifestyle. The Institute of Medicine (IOM) uses the following guidelines:

- Overweight: Weight gain limited to < 6.8 to 11.3 kg (< 15 to 25 lb)
- Obese: Weight gain limited to < 5 to 9.1 kg (< 11 to 20 lb)

However, not all experts agree with IOM recommendations. Many experts recommend an individualized approach that can include more limited weight gain plus lifestyle modifications (eg, increased physical activity, dietary changes), particularly for obese women.[1]

For overweight and obese pregnant women, lifestyle modifications during pregnancy reduce the risk of gestational diabetes and preeclampsia.

Discussing appropriate weight gain, diet, and exercise at the initial visit and periodically throughout the pregnancy is important.

1. Artal R, Lockwood CJ, Brown HL: Weight gain recommendations in pregnancy and the obesity epidemic. *Obstet Gynecol* 115(1):152–155, 2010. doi: 10.1097/AOG.0b013e3181c51908.

Maternal Height

Short (about < 152 cm) women are more likely to have a small pelvis, which can lead to dystocia with fetopelvic disproportion or shoulder dystocia. For short women, preterm labor and intrauterine growth restriction are also more likely.

Exposure to Teratogens

Common teratogens (agents that cause fetal malformation) include infections, drugs, and physical agents. Malformations are most likely to result if exposure occurs between the 2nd and 8th wk after conception (the 4th to 10th wk after the last menstrual period), when organs are forming. Other adverse pregnancy outcomes are also more likely. Pregnant women exposed to teratogens are counseled about increased risks and referred for detailed ultrasound evaluation to detect malformations.

Common infections that may be teratogenic include herpes simplex, viral hepatitis, rubella, varicella, syphilis, toxoplasmosis, and cytomegalovirus, coxsackievirus, and Zika infections.

Commonly used drugs that may be teratogenic include alcohol, tobacco, and cocaine (see p. 2365) and some prescription drugs (see Table 283–1 on p. 2360).

Hyperthermia or exposure to temperatures > 39° C (eg, in a sauna) during the 1st trimester has been associated with spina bifida.

Exposure to Mercury

Mercury in seafood can be toxic to the fetus. The FDA recommends the following:

- Avoiding tilefish from the Gulf of Mexico, shark, swordfish, big-eye tuna, marlin, orange roughy, and king mackerel
- Limiting albacore tuna to 4 oz (one average meal)/wk
- Before eating fish caught in local lakes, rivers, and coastal areas, checking local advisories about the safety of such fish and, if levels of mercury are not known to be low, limiting consumption to 4 oz/wk while avoiding other seafood that week

Experts recommend that women who are pregnant or breastfeeding eat 8 to 12 oz (2 or 3 average meals)/wk of a variety of seafood that is lower in mercury. Such seafood includes flounder, shrimp, canned light tuna, salmon, pollock, tilapia, cod, and catfish. Fish has nutrients that are important for fetal growth and development.

Prior Stillbirth

Stillbirth is delivery of a dead fetus at > 20 wk gestation. Fetal death during late pregnancy may have maternal, placental, or fetal anatomic or genetic causes (see Table 282–3 on p. 2358). Having had a stillbirth or late abortion (ie, at 16 to 20 wk) increases risk of fetal death in subsequent pregnancies. Degree of risk varies depending on the cause of a previous stillbirth. Fetal surveillance using antepartum testing (eg, nonstress testing, biophysical profile) is recommended.

Treatment of maternal disorders (eg, CHTN, diabetes, infections) may lower risk of stillbirth in a current pregnancy.

Prior Preterm Delivery

Preterm delivery is delivery before 37 wk. Previous preterm delivery due to preterm labor increases risk of future preterm deliveries; if the previous preterm neonate weighed < 1.5 kg, risk of preterm delivery in the next pregnancy is 50%.

Women with prior preterm delivery due to preterm labor should be closely monitored at 2-wk intervals after 20 wk. Monitoring includes

- Ultrasound evaluation, including measurement of cervical length and shape, at 16 to 18 wk
- Uterine contraction monitoring
- Testing for bacterial vaginosis
- Measurement of fetal fibronectin

Women with a prior preterm birth due to preterm labor or with shortening (< 25 mm) or funneling of the cervix should be given 17 alpha-hydroxyprogesterone 250 mg IM once/wk.

Prior Neonate With a Genetic or Congenital Disorder

Risk of having a fetus with a chromosomal disorder is increased for most couples who have had a fetus or neonate with a chromosomal disorder (recognized or missed—see p. 2297). Recurrence risk for most genetic disorders is unknown. Most congenital malformations are multifactorial; risk of having a subsequent fetus with malformations is ≤ 1%.

If couples have had a neonate with a genetic or chromosomal disorder, genetic screening is recommended. If couples have had a neonate with a congenital malformation, genetic screening, high-resolution ultrasonography, and evaluation by a maternal-fetal medicine specialist is recommended.

Polyhydramnios (Hydramnios) and Oligohydramnios

Polyhydramnios (excess amniotic fluid) can lead to severe maternal shortness of breath and preterm labor. Risk factors include

- Uncontrolled maternal diabetes
- Multifetal pregnancy
- Isoimmunization
- Fetal malformations (eg, esophageal atresia, anencephaly, spina bifida)

Oligohydramnios (deficient amniotic fluid) often accompanies congenital malformations of the fetal urinary tract and severe fetal growth restriction (< 3rd percentile). Also, Potter syndrome with pulmonary hypoplasia or fetal surface compression abnormalities may result, usually in the 2nd trimester, and cause fetal death.

Polyhydramnios or oligohydramnios is suspected if uterine size does not correspond to gestational date or may be discovered incidentally via ultrasonography, which is diagnostic.

Multifetal (Multiple) Pregnancy

Multifetal pregnancy increases risk of the following:

- Fetal growth restriction
- Preterm labor
- Abruptio placentae
- Congenital malformations
- Perinatal morbidity and mortality
- After delivery, uterine atony and hemorrhage

Multifetal pregnancy is detected during routine ultrasonography at 16 to 20 wk.

Prior Birth Injury

Most cerebral palsy and neurodevelopmental disorders are caused by factors unrelated to a birth injury. Injuries such as brachial plexus damage can result from procedures such as forceps or vacuum extractor delivery but often result from intrauterine forces during labor or malposition during the last weeks of pregnancy.

Previous shoulder dystocia is a risk factor for future dystocia, and the delivery records should be reviewed for potentially modifiable risk factors (eg, fetal macrosomia, operative vaginal delivery) that may have predisposed to the injury.

285 Normal Labor and Delivery

MANAGEMENT OF NORMAL LABOR

Labor consists of a series of rhythmic, involuntary, progressive contractions of the uterus that cause effacement (thinning and shortening) and dilation of the uterine cervix. The stimulus for labor is unknown, but digitally manipulating or mechanically stretching the cervix during examination enhances uterine contractile activity, most likely by stimulating release of oxytocin by the posterior pituitary gland.

Normal labor usually begins within 2 wk (before or after) the estimated delivery date. In a first pregnancy, labor usually lasts 12 to 18 h on average; subsequent labors are often shorter, averaging 6 to 8 h.

Management of complications during labor requires additional measures (eg, induction of labor, forceps or a vacuum extractor, cesarean delivery).

Beginning of labor: Bloody show (a small amount of blood with mucous discharge from the cervix) may precede onset of labor by as much as 72 h. Bloody show can be differentiated from abnormal 3rd-trimester vaginal bleeding because the amount is small, bloody show is typically mixed with mucus, and the pain due to abruptio placentae (premature separation) is absent. In most pregnant women, previous ultrasonography has been done and ruled out placenta previa. However, if ultrasonography has not ruled out placenta previa and vaginal bleeding occurs, placenta previa is assumed to be present until it is ruled out. Digital vaginal examination is contraindicated, and ultrasonography is done as soon as possible.

Labor begins with irregular uterine contractions of varying intensity; they apparently soften (ripen) the cervix, which begins to efface and dilate. As labor progresses, contractions increase in duration, intensity, and frequency.

Stages of labor: There are 3 stages of labor.

The **1st stage**—from onset of labor to full dilation of the cervix (about 10 cm)—has 2 phases, latent and active.

During the **latent phase**, irregular contractions become progressively better coordinated, discomfort is minimal, and the cervix effaces and dilates to 4 cm. The latent phase is difficult to time precisely, and duration varies, averaging 8 h in nulliparas and 5 h in multiparas; duration is considered abnormal if it lasts > 20 h in nulliparas or > 12 h in multiparas.

During the **active phase**, the cervix becomes fully dilated, and the presenting part descends well into the midpelvis. On average, the active phase lasts 5 to 7 h in nulliparas and 2 to 4 h in multiparas. Traditionally, the cervix was expected to dilate about 1.2 cm/h in nulliparas and 1.5 cm/h in multiparas. However, recent data suggest that slower progression of cervical dilation from 4 to 6 cm may be normal.[1] Pelvic examinations are done every 2 to 3 h to evaluate labor progress. Lack of progress in dilation and descent of the presenting part may indicate dystocia (fetopelvic disproportion).

If the membranes have not spontaneously ruptured, some clinicians use amniotomy (artificial rupture of membranes) routinely during the active phase. As a result, labor may progress more rapidly, and meconium-stained amniotic fluid may be detected earlier. Amniotomy during this stage may be necessary for specific indications, such as facilitating internal fetal monitoring to confirm fetal well-being. Amniotomy should be avoided in women with HIV infection or hepatitis B or C, so that the fetus is not exposed to these organisms.

During the 1st stage of labor, maternal heart rate and BP and fetal heart rate should be checked continuously by electronic monitoring or intermittently by auscultation, usually with a portable Doppler ultrasound device (see p. 2376). Women may begin to feel the urge to bear down as the presenting part descends into the pelvis. However, they should be discouraged from bearing down until the cervix is fully dilated so that they do not tear the cervix or waste energy.

The **2nd stage** is the time from full cervical dilation to delivery of the fetus. On average, it lasts 2 h in nulliparas (median 50 min) and 1 h in multiparas (median 20 min). It may last another hour or more if conduction (epidural) analgesia or intense opioid sedation is used. For spontaneous delivery, women must supplement uterine contractions by expulsively bearing down. In the 2nd stage, women should be attended constantly, and fetal heart sounds should be checked continuously or after every contraction. Contractions may be monitored by palpation or electronically.

The **3rd stage** of labor begins after delivery of the infant and ends with delivery of the placenta. This stage usually lasts only a few minutes but may last up to 30 min.

Rupture of membranes: Occasionally, the membranes (amniotic and chorionic sac) rupture before labor begins, and amniotic fluid leaks through the cervix and vagina. Rupture of membranes at any stage before the onset of labor is called premature rupture of membranes (PROM—see p. 2340). Some women with PROM feel a gush of fluid from the vagina, followed by steady leaking.

Further confirmation is not needed if, during examination, fluid is seen leaking from the cervix. Confirmation of more subtle cases may require testing. For example, the pH of vaginal fluid may be tested with Nitrazine paper, which turns deep blue at a pH > 6.5 (pH of amniotic fluid: 7.0 to 7.6); false-positive results can occur if vaginal fluid contains blood or semen or if certain infections are present. A sample of the secretions from the posterior vaginal fornix or cervix may be obtained, placed on a slide, air dried, and viewed microscopically for ferning. Ferning (crystallization of sodium chloride in a palm leaf pattern in amniotic fluid) usually confirms rupture of membranes.

If rupture is still unconfirmed, ultrasonography showing oligohydramnios (deficient amniotic fluid) provides further evidence suggesting rupture. Rarely, amniocentesis with instillation of dye is done to confirm rupture; dye detected in the vagina or on a tampon confirms rupture.

When a woman's membranes rupture, she should contact her physician immediately. About 80 to 90% of women with PROM at term and about 50% of women with PROM preterm go into labor spontaneously within 24 h; > 90% of women with PROM go into labor within 2 wk. The earlier the membranes rupture before 37 wk, the longer the delay between rupture and labor onset. If membranes rupture at term but labor does not start within several hours, labor is typically induced to lower risk of maternal and fetal infection.

Birthing options: Most women prefer hospital delivery, and most health care practitioners recommend it because unexpected maternal and fetal complications may occur during labor and delivery or postpartum, even in women without risk factors. About 30% of hospital deliveries involve an obstetric complication (eg, laceration, postpartum hemorrhage). Other complications include abruptio placentae, abnormal fetal heart rate pattern, shoulder dystocia, need for emergency cesarean delivery, and neonatal depression or abnormality.

Nonetheless, many women want a more homelike environment for delivery; in response, some hospitals provide birthing facilities with fewer formalities and rigid regulations but with emergency equipment and personnel available. Birthing centers may be freestanding or located in hospitals; care at either site is similar or identical. In some hospitals, certified nurse-midwives provide much of the care for low-risk pregnancies. Midwives work with a physician, who is continuously available for consultation and operative deliveries (eg, by forceps, vacuum extractor, or cesarean). All birthing options should be discussed.

For many women, presence of the their partner or another support person during labor is helpful and should be encouraged. Moral support, encouragement, and expressions of affection decrease anxiety and make labor less frightening and unpleasant. Childbirth education classes can prepare parents for a normal or complicated labor and delivery. Sharing the stresses of labor and the sight and sound of their own child tends to create strong bonds between the parents and between parents and child. The parents should be fully informed of any complications.

Admission: Typically, pregnant women are advised to go to the hospital if they believe their membranes have ruptured or if they are experiencing contractions lasting at least 30 sec and occurring regularly at intervals of about 6 min or less. Within an hour after presentation at a hospital, whether a woman is in labor can usually be determined based on the following:

- Occurrence of regular and sustained painful uterine contractions
- Bloody show
- Membrane rupture
- Complete cervical effacement

If these criteria are not met, false labor may be tentatively diagnosed, and the pregnant woman is typically observed for a time and, if labor does not begin within several hours, is sent home.

When pregnant women are admitted, their blood pressure, heart and respiratory rates, temperature, and weight are recorded, and presence or absence of edema is noted. A urine specimen is collected for protein and glucose analysis, and blood is drawn for a CBC and blood typing. A physical examination is done. While examining the abdomen, the clinician estimates size, position, and presentation of the fetus, using Leopold maneuvers (see Fig. 285–1). The clinician notes the presence and rate of fetal heart sounds, as well as location for auscultation. Preliminary estimates of the strength, frequency, and duration of contractions are also recorded.

A helpful mnemonic device for evaluation is the 3 Ps:

- Powers (contraction strength, frequency, and duration)
- Passage (pelvic measurements)
- Passenger (eg, fetal size, position, heart rate pattern)

If labor is active and the pregnancy is at term, a clinician examines the vagina with 2 fingers of a gloved hand to evaluate progress of labor. If bleeding (particularly if heavy) is present, the examination is delayed until placental location is confirmed by ultrasonography. If bleeding results from placenta previa, vaginal examination can initiate severe hemorrhage.

If labor is not active but membranes are ruptured, a speculum examination is done initially to document cervical dilation and effacement and to estimate station (location of the presenting part); however, digital examinations are delayed until the active phase of labor or problems (eg, decreased fetal heart sounds) occur. If the membranes have ruptured, any fetal meconium (producing greenish-brown discoloration) should be noted because it may be a sign of fetal stress. If labor is preterm (< 37 wk) or has not begun, only a sterile speculum examination should be done, and a culture should be taken for gonococci, chlamydiae, and group B streptococci.

Cervical dilation is recorded in centimeters as the diameter of a circle; 10 cm is considered complete.

Effacement is estimated in percentages, from zero to 100%. Because effacement involves cervical shortening as well as thinning, it may be recorded in centimeters using the normal, uneffaced average cervical length of 3.5 to 4.0 cm as a guide.

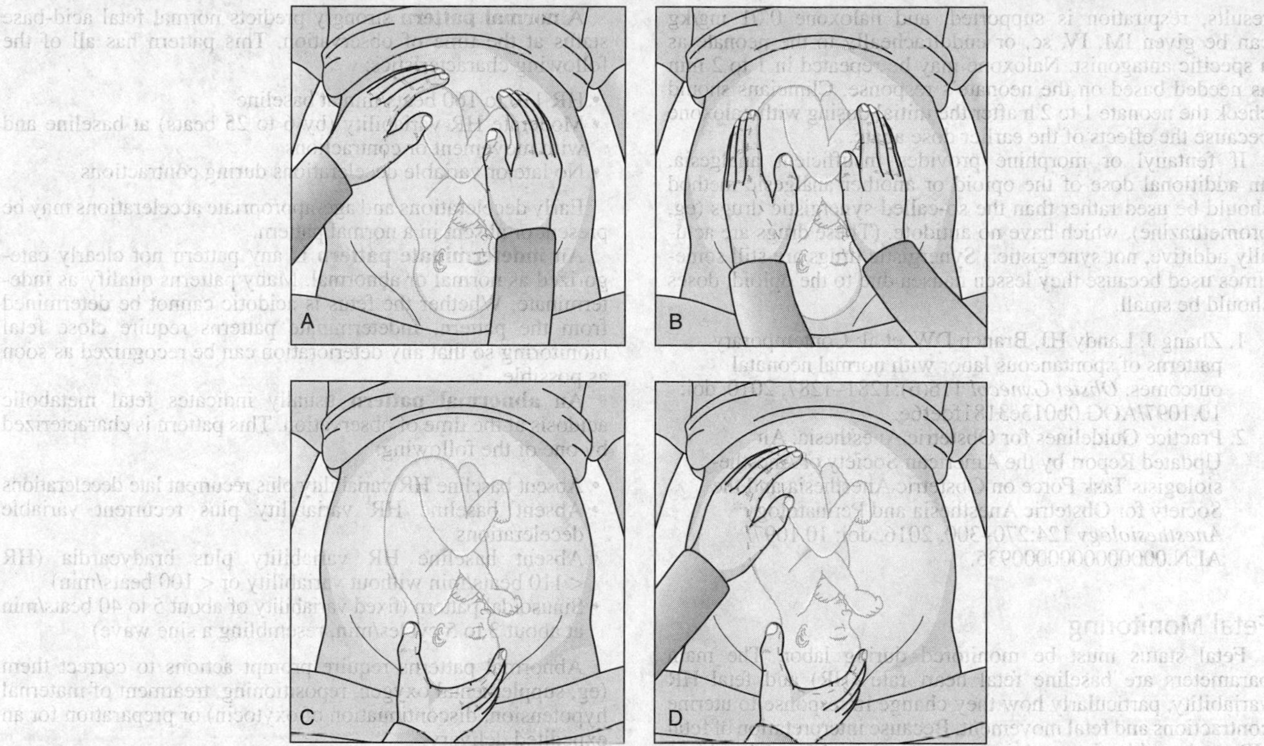

Fig. 285–1. Leopold maneuver. (A) The uterine fundus is palpated to determine which fetal part occupies the fundus. (B) Each side of the maternal abdomen is palpated to determine which side is fetal spine and which is the extremities. (C) The area above the symphysis pubis is palpated to locate the fetal presenting part and thus determine how far the fetus has descended and whether the fetus is engaged. (D) One hand applies pressure on the fundus while the index finger and thumb of the other hand palpate the presenting part to confirm presentation and engagement.

Station is expressed in centimeters above or below the level of the maternal ischial spines. Level with the ischial spines corresponds to 0 station; levels above (+) or below (–) the spines are recorded in cm increments. Fetal lie, position, and presentation are noted.

- **Lie** describes the relationship of the long axis of the fetus to that of the mother (longitudinal, oblique, transverse).
- **Position** describes the relationship of the presenting part to the maternal pelvis (eg, occiput left anterior [OLA] for cephalic, sacrum right posterior [SRP] for breech).
- **Presentation** describes the part of the fetus at the cervical opening (eg, breech, vertex, shoulder).

Preparation for delivery: Women are admitted to the labor suite for frequent observation until delivery. If labor is active, they should receive little or nothing by mouth to prevent possible vomiting and aspiration during delivery or in case emergency delivery with general anesthesia is necessary. Shaving or clipping of vulvar and pubic hair is not indicated; it increases the risk of wound infections.

An IV infusion of Ringer's lactate may be started, preferably using a large-bore indwelling catheter inserted into a vein in the hand or forearm. During a normal labor of 6 to 10 h, women should be given 500 to 1000 mL of this solution. The infusion prevents dehydration during labor and subsequent hemoconcentration and maintains an adequate circulating blood volume. The catheter also provides immediate access for drugs or blood if needed. Fluid preloading is valuable if epidural or spinal anesthesia is planned.

Analgesia: Analgesics may be given during labor as needed, but only the minimum amount required for maternal comfort should be given because analgesics cross the placenta and may depress the neonate's breathing. Neonatal toxicity can occur because after the umbilical cord is cut, the neonate, whose metabolic and excretory processes are immature, clears the transferred drug much more slowly by liver metabolism or by urinary excretion. Preparation for and education about childbirth lessen anxiety.

Physicians are increasingly offering epidural injection (providing regional anesthesia) as the first choice for analgesia during labor. Typically, a local anesthetic (eg, 0.2% ropivacaine, 0.125% bupivacaine) is continuously infused, often with an opioid (eg, fentanyl, sufentanil), into the lumbar epidural space. Initially, the anesthetic is given cautiously to avoid masking the awareness of pressure that helps stimulate pushing and to avoid motor block. Women should be reassured that epidural analgesia does not increase the risk of cesarean delivery.[2]

If epidural injection is inadequate or if IV administration is preferred, fentanyl (100 mcg) or morphine sulfate (up to 10 mg) given IV q 60 to 90 min is commonly used. These opioids provide good analgesia with only a small total dose. If toxicity results, respiration is supported, and naloxone 0.01 mg/kg can be given IM, IV, sc, or endotracheally to the neonate as a specific antagonist. Naloxone may be repeated in 1 to 2 min as needed based on the neonate's response. Clinicians should check the neonate 1 to 2 h after the initial dosing with naloxone because the effects of the earlier dose abate.

If fentanyl or morphine provides insufficient analgesia, an additional dose of the opioid or another analgesic method should be used rather than the so-called synergistic drugs (eg, promethazine), which have no antidote. (These drugs are actually additive, not synergistic.) Synergistic drugs are still sometimes used because they lessen nausea due to the opioid; doses should be small.

1. Zhang J, Landy HJ, Branch DW, et al: Contemporary patterns of spontaneous labor with normal neonatal outcomes. *Obstet Gynecol* 116(6):1281–1287, 2010. doi: 10.1097/AOG.0b013e3181fdef6e.
2. Practice Guidelines for Obstetric Anesthesia: An Updated Report by the American Society of Anesthesiologists Task Force on Obstetric Anesthesia and the Society for Obstetric Anesthesia and Perinatology*. *Anesthesiology* 124:270–300, 2016. doi: 10.1097/ALN.0000000000000935.

Fetal Monitoring

Fetal status must be monitored during labor. The main parameters are baseline fetal heart rate (HR) and fetal HR variability, particularly how they change in response to uterine contractions and fetal movement. Because interpretation of fetal HR can be subjective, certain parameters have been defined (see Table 285–1).

Several patterns are recognized; they are classified into 3 tiers (categories),[1] which usually correlate with the acid–base status of the fetus:

- Category I: Normal
- Category II: Indeterminate
- Category III: Abnormal

A **normal pattern** strongly predicts normal fetal acid-base status at the time of observation. This pattern has all of the following characteristics:

- HR 110 to 160 beats/min at baseline
- Moderate HR variability (by 6 to 25 beats) at baseline and with movement or contractions
- No late or variable decelerations during contractions

Early decelerations and age-appropriate accelerations may be present or absent in a normal pattern.

An **indeterminate pattern** is any pattern not clearly categorized as normal or abnormal. Many patterns qualify as indeterminate. Whether the fetus is acidotic cannot be determined from the pattern. Indeterminate patterns require close fetal monitoring so that any deterioration can be recognized as soon as possible.

An **abnormal pattern** usually indicates fetal metabolic acidosis at the time of observation. This pattern is characterized by one of the following:

- Absent baseline HR variability plus recurrent late decelerations
- Absent baseline HR variability plus recurrent variable decelerations
- Absent baseline HR variability plus bradycardia (HR < 110 beats/min without variability or < 100 beats/min)
- Sinusoidal pattern (fixed variability of about 5 to 40 beats/min at about 3 to 5 cycles/min, resembling a sine wave)

Abnormal patterns require prompt actions to correct them (eg, supplemental oxygen, repositioning, treatment of maternal hypotension, discontinuation of oxytocin) or preparation for an expedited delivery.

Patterns reflect fetal status at a particular point in time; patterns can and do change.

Monitoring can be manual and intermittent, using a fetoscope for auscultation of fetal HR. However, in the US, electronic fetal HR monitoring (external or internal) has become standard of care for high-risk pregnancies, and many clinicians use it for all pregnancies. The value of routine use of electronic monitoring in low-risk deliveries is often debated. However, electronic

Table 285–1. FETAL MONITORING DEFINITIONS

PARAMETER	DEFINITION
Heart rate: Baseline	Mean HR over a 10-min period, excluding periods of large variability, rounded to closest 0 or 5 Must be identified for ≥ 2 min (but not necessarily 2 consecutive min)
Heart rate: Variability	Difference between highest and lowest HR values in a 10-min period
Acceleration: Age-appropriate	< 32 wk EGA: ≥ 10 bpm > baseline HR for ≥ 10 sec ≥ 32 wk EGA: ≥ 15 bpm > baseline HR for ≥ 15 sec
Deceleration: Relation to uterine contractions	**Early:** Temporary, gradual decrease in HR that begins near the start of a uterine contraction and takes ≥ 30 sec to reach its nadir, which occurs near peak of uterine contraction Onset, peak, and end of deceleration usually near the onset, peak, and end of contraction **Late:** Temporary, gradual decrease in HR that begins after the start of a uterine contraction and takes ≥ 30 sec to reach its nadir, which occurs after peak of contraction Onset, peak, and end of deceleration usually later than the onset, peak, and end of contraction **Variable:** Temporary, abrupt decrease of ≥ 15 bpm in HR that reaches its nadir < 30 sec after deceleration begins and lasts between 15 sec and 2 min; decelerations that may or may not be associated with uterine contractions Onset, depth, and duration commonly varying between successive uterine contractions

EGA = estimated gestational age.

fetal monitoring has not been shown to reduce overall mortality rates in large clinical trials and has been shown to increase rates of cesarean delivery, probably because many apparent abnormalities are false positives. Rate of cesarean delivery is higher among women monitored electronically than among those monitored by auscultation.

Fetal pulse oximetry has been studied as a way to confirm abnormal or equivocal results of electronic monitoring; status of fetal oxygenation may help determine whether cesarean delivery is needed.

Fetal ST-segment and T-wave analysis in labor (STAN) can be used to check the fetal ECG for ST-segment elevation or depression; either finding presumably indicates fetal hypoxemia and has a high sensitivity and specificity for fetal acidosis. For STAN, an electrode must be attached to the fetal scalp; then changes in the T wave and ST segment of the fetal ECG are automatically identified and analyzed.

If manual auscultation of fetal HR is used, it must be done throughout labor according to specific guidelines, and one-on-one nursing care is needed.

- For low-risk pregnancies with normal labor, fetal HR must be checked after each contraction or at least every 30 min during the 1st stage of labor and every 15 min during the 2nd stage.
- For high-risk pregnancies, fetal HR must be checked every 15 min during the 1st stage and every 3 to 5 min during the 2nd stage.

Listening for at least 1 to 2 min beginning at a contraction's peak is recommended to check for late deceleration. Periodic auscultation has a lower false-positive rate for abnormalities and incidence of intervention than continuous electronic monitoring, and it provides opportunities for more personal contact with women during labor. However, following the standard guidelines for auscultation is often difficult and may not be cost-effective. Also, unless done accurately, auscultation may not detect abnormalities.

Electronic fetal HR monitoring may be

- External: Devices are applied to the maternal abdomen to record fetal heart sounds and uterine contractions.
- Internal: Amniotic membranes must be ruptured. Then, leads are inserted through the cervix; an electrode is attached to the fetal scalp to monitor HR, and a catheter is placed in the uterine cavity to measure intrauterine pressure.

Usually, external and internal monitoring are similarly reliable. External devices are used for women in normal labor; internal methods are used when external monitoring does not supply enough information about fetal well-being or uterine contraction intensity (eg, if the external device is not functioning correctly).

External electronic fetal monitoring can be used during labor or electively to continuously record fetal HR and correlate it with fetal movements (called a nonstress test). A nonstress test is typically done for 20 min (occasionally for 40 min). Results are considered reactive (reassuring) if there are 2 accelerations of 15 beats/min over 20 min. Absence of accelerations is considered nonreactive (nonreassuring). Presence of late decelerations suggests hypoxemia, potential for fetal acidosis, and the need for intervention.

A nonreassuring nonstress test is usually followed by a biophysical profile (adding assessment of amniotic fluid volume and sometimes assessment of fetal movement, tone, breathing, and heart rate, to the nonstress test). A nonstress test and biophysical profile are frequently used to monitor complicated or high-risk pregnancies (eg, complicated by maternal diabetes or hypertension or by stillbirth or fetal growth restriction in a previous pregnancy).

External monitoring can be used with a contraction stress test as well as a nonstress test; fetal movements and HR are monitored during contractions induced by oxytocin (oxytocin challenge test). However, contraction stress testing is now rarely done and, when done, must be done in a hospital.

If a problem (eg, fetal HR decelerations, lack of normal HR variability) is detected during labor, intrauterine fetal resuscitation is tried; women may be given oxygen by a tight nonrebreather face mask or rapid IV fluid infusion or may be positioned laterally. If fetal heart pattern does not improve in a reasonable period and delivery is not imminent, urgent delivery by cesarean is needed.

1. Macones GA, Hankins GD, Spong CY, et al: The 2008 National Institute of Child Health and Human Development workshop report on electronic fetal monitoring: Update on definitions, interpretation, and research guidelines. *J Obstet Gynecol Neonatal Nurs* 37(5):510–515, 2008. doi: 10.1111/j.1552-6909.2008.00284.x.

MANAGEMENT OF NORMAL DELIVERY

Many obstetric units now use a combined labor, delivery, recovery, and postpartum (LDRP) room, so that the woman, support person, and neonate remain in the same room throughout their stay. Some units use a traditional labor room and separate delivery suite, to which the woman is transferred when delivery is imminent. The woman's partner or other support person should be offered the opportunity to accompany her. In the delivery room, the perineum is washed and draped, and the neonate is delivered. After delivery, the woman may remain there or be transferred to a postpartum unit.

Management of complications during delivery requires additional measures (such as induction of labor).

Anesthesia

Options include regional, local, and general anesthesia. Local anesthetics and opioids are commonly used. These drugs pass through the placenta; thus, during the hour before delivery, such drugs should be given in small doses to avoid toxicity (eg, CNS depression, bradycardia) in the neonate.

Opioids used alone do not provide adequate analgesia and so are most often used with anesthetics.

Regional anesthesia: Several methods are available.

Lumbar epidural injection of a local anesthetic is the most commonly used method. Epidural analgesia is being increasingly used for delivery, including cesarean delivery, and has essentially replaced pudendal and paracervical blocks. When epidural analgesia is used, drugs can be titrated as needed during the course of labor. The local anesthetics often used for epidural injection (eg, bupivacaine) have a longer duration of action and slower onset than those used for pudendal block (eg, lidocaine).

Spinal injection (into the paraspinal subarachnoid space) may be used for cesarean delivery, but it is used less often for vaginal deliveries because it is short-lasting (preventing its use during labor) and has a small risk of spinal headache afterward. When spinal injection is used, patients must be constantly attended, and vital signs must be checked every 5 min to detect and treat possible hypotension.

Local anesthesia: Methods include pudendal block, perineal infiltration, and paracervical block.

Pudendal block, rarely used because epidural injections are used instead, involves injecting a local anesthetic through the vaginal wall so that the anesthetic bathes the pudendal nerve as it crosses the ischial spine. This block anesthetizes the lower vagina, perineum, and posterior vulva; the anterior vulva, innervated by lumbar dermatomes, is not anesthetized. Pudendal block is a safe, simple method for uncomplicated spontaneous vaginal deliveries if women wish to bear down and push or if labor is advanced and there is no time for epidural injection. Complications of pudendal block include intravascular injection of anesthetics, hematoma, and infection.

Infiltration of the perineum with an anesthetic is commonly used, although this method is not as effective as a well-administered pudendal block.

Paracervical block is rarely appropriate for delivery because incidence of fetal bradycardia is > 10%.[1] It is used mainly for 1st- or early 2nd-trimester abortion. The technique involves injecting 5 to 10 mL of 1% lidocaine or chloroprocaine (which has a shorter half-life) at the 3 and 9 o'clock positions; the analgesic response is short-lasting.

General anesthesia: Because potent and volatile inhalation drugs (eg, isoflurane) can cause marked depression in the fetus, general anesthesia is not recommended for routine delivery.

Rarely, nitrous oxide 40% with oxygen may be used for analgesia during vaginal delivery as long as verbal contact with the woman is maintained.

Thiopental, a sedative-hypnotic, is commonly given IV with other drugs (eg, succinylcholine, nitrous oxide plus oxygen) for induction of general anesthesia during cesarean delivery; used alone, thiopental provides inadequate analgesia. With thiopental, induction is rapid and recovery is prompt. It becomes concentrated in the fetal liver, preventing levels from becoming high in the CNS; high levels in the CNS may cause neonatal depression.

Epidural analgesia, which can be rapidly converted to epidural anesthesia, has reduced the need for general anesthesia except for cesarean delivery.

1. LeFevre ML: Fetal heart rate pattern and postparacervical fetal bradycardia. *Obstet Gynecol* 64(3):343–346, 1984.

Delivery of the Fetus

A vaginal examination is done to determine position and station of the fetal head; the head is usually the presenting part (see Fig. 285–2). When effacement is complete and the cervix is fully dilated, the woman is told to bear down and strain with each contraction to move the head through the pelvis and progressively dilate the vaginal introitus so that more and more of the head appears. When about 3 or 4 cm of the head is visible during a contraction in nulliparas (somewhat less in multiparas), the following maneuvers can facilitate delivery and reduce risk of perineal laceration:

- The clinician, if right-handed, places the left palm over the infant's head during a contraction to control and, if necessary, slightly slow progress.
- Simultaneously, the clinician places the curved fingers of the right hand against the dilating perineum, through which the infant's brow or chin is felt.
- To advance the head, the clinician can wrap a hand in a towel and, with curved fingers, apply pressure against the underside of the brow or chin (modified Ritgen maneuver).

Thus, the clinician controls the progress of the head to effect a slow, safe delivery.

Forceps or a vacuum extractor is often used for vaginal delivery when

- The 2nd stage of labor is likely to be prolonged (eg, because the mother is too exhausted to bear down adequately or because regional epidural anesthesia precludes vigorous bearing down).
- The woman has a disorder such as a heart disorder and must avoid pushing during the 2nd stage of labor.

If anesthesia is local (pudendal block or infiltration of the perineum), forceps or a vacuum extractor is usually not needed unless complications develop; local anesthesia may not interfere with bearing down.

Indications for forceps and vacuum extractor are essentially the same.

Both procedures have risks. Third- and 4th-degree perineal tears[1] and anal sphincter injuries[2] tend to be more common after forceps delivery than after vacuum extraction. Other fetal risks with forceps include facial lacerations and facial nerve palsy, corneal abrasions, external ocular trauma, skull fracture, and intracranial hemorrhage.[3,4]

Fetal risks with vacuum extraction include scalp laceration, cephalohematoma formation, and subgaleal or intracranial hemorrhage; retinal hemorrhages and increased rates of hyperbilirubinemia have been reported.

An **episiotomy** is not routinely done for most normal deliveries; it is done only if the perineum does not stretch adequately and is obstructing delivery. A local anesthetic can be infiltrated if epidural analgesia is inadequate. Episiotomy prevents excessive stretching and possible irregular tearing of the perineal tissues, including anterior tears. An episiotomy incision that extends only through skin and perineal body without disruption of the anal sphincter muscles (2nd-degree episiotomy) is usually easier to repair than a perineal tear.

The most common episiotomy is a midline incision made from the midpoint of the fourchette directly back toward the rectum. Extension into the rectal sphincter or rectum is a risk with midline episiotomy, but if recognized promptly, the extension can be repaired successfully and heals well. Tears or extensions into the rectum can usually be prevented by keeping the infant's head well flexed until the occipital prominence passes under the symphysis pubis.

Another type of episiotomy is a mediolateral incision made from the midpoint of the fourchette at a 45° angle laterally on either side. This type usually does not extend into the sphincter or rectum,[5] but it causes greater postoperative pain, is more difficult to repair, has increased blood loss, and takes longer to heal than midline episiotomy.[6] Thus, for episiotomy, a midline cut is often preferred.

However, use of episiotomy is decreasing because extension or tearing into the sphincter or rectum is a concern. Episioproctotomy (intentionally cutting into the rectum) is not recommended because rectovaginal fistula is a risk.

About 35% of women have dyspareunia after episiotomy.[7]

When the head is delivered, the clinician determines whether the umbilical cord is wrapped around the neck. If it is, the clinician should try to unwrap the cord; if the cord cannot be rapidly removed this way, the cord may be clamped and cut.

After delivery of the head, the infant's body rotates so that the shoulders are in an anteroposterior position; gentle downward pressure on the head delivers the anterior shoulder under the symphysis. The head is gently lifted, the posterior shoulder slides over the perineum, and the rest of the body follows without difficulty. The nose, mouth, and pharynx are aspirated with a bulb syringe to remove mucus and fluids and help start respirations. If appropriate traction and maternal pushing do not deliver the anterior shoulder, the clinician should explain to the woman what must be done next and begin delivery of a fetus with shoulder dystocia.

The cord should be double-clamped and cut between the clamps, and a plastic cord clip should be applied about

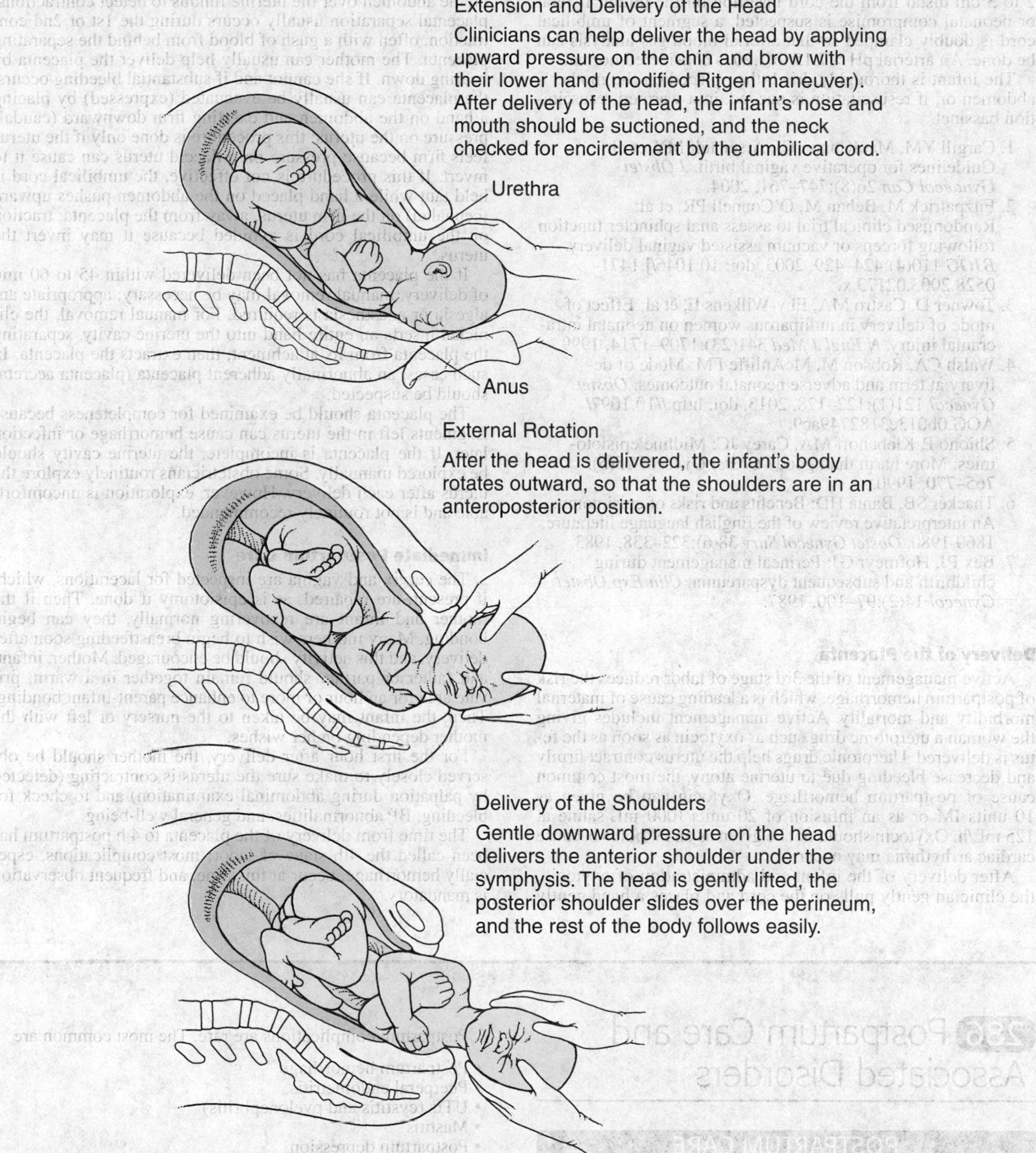

Extension and Delivery of the Head
Clinicians can help deliver the head by applying upward pressure on the chin and brow with their lower hand (modified Ritgen maneuver). After delivery of the head, the infant's nose and mouth should be suctioned, and the neck checked for encirclement by the umbilical cord.
Urethra
Anus
External Rotation
After the head is delivered, the infant's body rotates outward, so that the shoulders are in an anteroposterior position.
Delivery of the Shoulders
Gentle downward pressure on the head delivers the anterior shoulder under the symphysis. The head is gently lifted, the posterior shoulder slides over the perineum, and the rest of the body follows easily.

Fig. 285–2. Sequence of events in delivery for vertex presentations.

2 to 3 cm distal from the cord insertion on the infant. If fetal or neonatal compromise is suspected, a segment of umbilical cord is doubly clamped so that arterial blood gas analysis can be done. An arterial pH > 7.15 to 7.20 is considered normal.

The infant is thoroughly dried, then placed on the mother's abdomen or, if resuscitation is needed, in a warmed resuscitation bassinet.

1. Cargill YM, MacKinnon CJ, Arsenault MY, et al: Guidelines for operative vaginal birth. *J Obstet Gynaecol Can* 26(8):747–761, 2004.
2. Fitzpatrick M, Behan M, O'Connell PR, et al: Randomised clinical trial to assess anal sphincter function following forceps or vacuum assisted vaginal delivery. *BJOG* 110(4):424–429, 2003. doi: 10.1046/j.1471-0528.2003.02173.x.
3. Towner D, Castro MA, Eby-Wilkens E, et al: Effect of mode of delivery in nulliparous women on neonatal intracranial injury. *N Engl J Med* 341(23):1709–1714, 1999.
4. Walsh CA, Robson M, McAuliffe FM: Mode of delivery at term and adverse neonatal outcomes. *Obstet Gynecol* 121(1):122–128, 2013. doi: http://10.1097/AOG.0b013e3182749ac9.
5. Shiono P, Klebanoff MA, Carey JC: Midline episiotomies: More harm than good? *Obstet Gynecol* 75(5):765–770, 1990.
6. Thacker SB, Banta HD: Benefits and risks of episiotomy: An interpretative review of the English language literature, 1860-1980. *Obstet Gynecol Surv* 38(6):322–338, 1983.
7. Bex PJ, Hofmeyr GJ: Perineal management during childbirth and subsequent dyspareunia. *Clin Exp Obstet Gynecol* 14(2):97–100, 1987.

Delivery of the Placenta

Active management of the 3rd stage of labor reduces the risk of postpartum hemorrhage, which is a leading cause of maternal morbidity and mortality. Active management includes giving the woman a uterotonic drug such as oxytocin as soon as the fetus is delivered. Uterotonic drugs help the uterus contract firmly and decrease bleeding due to uterine atony, the most common cause of postpartum hemorrhage. Oxytocin can be given as 10 units IM or as an infusion of 20 units/1000 mL saline at 125 mL/h. Oxytocin should not be given as an IV bolus because cardiac arrhythmia may occur.

After delivery of the infant and administration of oxytocin, the clinician gently pulls on the cord and places a hand gently on the abdomen over the uterine fundus to detect contractions; placental separation usually occurs during the 1st or 2nd contraction, often with a gush of blood from behind the separating placenta. The mother can usually help deliver the placenta by bearing down. If she cannot and if substantial bleeding occurs, the placenta can usually be evacuated (expressed) by placing a hand on the abdomen and exerting firm downward (caudal) pressure on the uterus; this procedure is done only if the uterus feels firm because pressure on a flaccid uterus can cause it to invert. If this procedure is not effective, the umbilical cord is held taut while a hand placed on the abdomen pushes upward (cephalad) on the firm uterus, away from the placenta; traction on the umbilical cord is avoided because it may invert the uterus.

If the placenta has not been delivered within 45 to 60 min of delivery, manual removal may be necessary; appropriate analgesia or anesthesia is required. For manual removal, the clinician inserts an entire hand into the uterine cavity, separating the placenta from its attachment, then extracts the placenta. In such cases, an abnormally adherent placenta (placenta accreta) should be suspected.

The placenta should be examined for completeness because fragments left in the uterus can cause hemorrhage or infection later. If the placenta is incomplete, the uterine cavity should be explored manually. Some obstetricians routinely explore the uterus after each delivery. However, exploration is uncomfortable and is not routinely recommended.

Immediate Postpartum Care

The cervix and vagina are inspected for lacerations, which, if present, are repaired, as is episiotomy if done. Then if the mother and infant are recovering normally, they can begin bonding. Many mothers wish to begin breastfeeding soon after delivery, and this activity should be encouraged. Mother, infant, and father or partner should remain together in a warm, private area for an hour or more to enhance parent-infant bonding. Then, the infant may be taken to the nursery or left with the mother depending on her wishes.

For the first hour after delivery, the mother should be observed closely to make sure the uterus is contracting (detected by palpation during abdominal examination) and to check for bleeding, BP abnormalities, and general well-being.

The time from delivery of the placenta to 4 h postpartum has been called the 4th stage of labor; most complications, especially hemorrhage, occur at this time, and frequent observation is mandatory.

286 Postpartum Care and Associated Disorders

POSTPARTUM CARE

Clinical manifestations during the puerperium (6-wk period after delivery) generally reflect reversal of the physiologic changes that occurred during pregnancy (see Table 286–1). These changes are mild and temporary and should not be confused with pathologic conditions.

Postpartum complications are rare. The most common are

- Postpartum hemorrhage
- Puerperal endometritis
- UTIs (cystitis and pyelonephritis)
- Mastitis
- Postpartum depression

Clinical parameters: Within the first 24 h, the woman's pulse rate begins to drop, and her temperature may be slightly elevated.

Vaginal discharge is grossly bloody (lochia rubra) for 3 to 4 days, then becomes pale brown (lochia serosa), and

Table 286–1. NORMAL POSTPARTUM CHANGES

PARAMETER	FIRST 24 H	FIRST 3–4 DAYS	5 DAYS–2 WK	AFTER 2 WK	AFTER 4 WK
Clinical					
Heart rate	Starts decreasing	Decreased to baseline	Baseline	Baseline	Baseline
Temperature	Slightly elevated	Usually baseline	Baseline	Baseline	Baseline
Vaginal discharge	Bloody (lochia rubra)	Bloody (lochia rubra)	Pale brown (lochia serosa)*	Pale brown to yellowish white (lochia alba)	Yellowish white to normal
Urine volume	Increased	Increased	Decreasing to baseline	Baseline	Baseline
Uterus	Begins involution	Continues involution	Firm, no longer tender Located about midway between the symphysis and umbilicus	Not palpable in the abdomen	Prepregnancy size
Mood	Baby blues	Baby blues	Normal by 7 to 10 days	Baseline	Baseline
Breasts (if not breastfeeding)	Slightly enlarged	Engorged	Decreasing	Baseline	Baseline
Ovulation (if not breastfeeding)	Unlikely	Unlikely	Unlikely	Unlikely but possible	Possible
Laboratory					
WBC count	Up to 20,000–30,000/μL	Decreasing	Decreasing to baseline	Baseline	Baseline
Plasma fibrinogen and ESR	Elevated	Elevated	Decreasing to normal after 7 days	Baseline	Baseline

*Placental site sloughing may result in blood loss of about 250 mL at 7–14 days.

after the next 10 to 12 days, it changes to yellowish white (lochia alba).

About 1 to 2 wk after delivery, eschar from the placental site sloughs off and bleeding occurs; bleeding is usually self-limited. Total blood loss is about 250 mL; comfortably fitting intravaginal tampons (changed frequently) or external pads may be used to absorb it. Tampons should not be used if they might inhibit healing of perineal or vaginal lacerations. Prolonged bleeding (postpartum hemorrhage) may be a sign of infection or retained placenta and should be investigated.

The uterus involutes progressively; after 5 to 7 days, it is firm and no longer tender, extending midway between the symphysis and umbilicus. By 2 wk, it is no longer palpable abdominally and typically by 4 to 6 wk returns to a prepregancy size. Contractions of the involuting uterus, if painful (afterpains), may require analgesics.

Laboratory parameters: During the first week, urine temporarily increases in volume; care must be taken when interpreting urinalysis results as lochia can interfere.

Because blood volume is redistributed, Hct may fluctuate, although it tends to remain in the prepregnancy range if women do not hemorrhage. Because WBC count increases during labor, marked leukocytosis (up to 20,000 to 30,000/μL) occurs in the first 24 h postpartum; WBC count returns to normal within 1 wk. Plasma fibrinogen and ESR remain elevated during the first week postpartum.

Initial Management

Risk of infection, hemorrhage, and pain must be minimized. Women are typically observed for at least 1 to 2 h after the 3rd stage of labor and for several hours longer if regional or general anesthesia was used during delivery (eg, by forceps, vacuum extractor, or cesarean) or if the delivery was not completely routine.

Hemorrhage: (See also Postpartum Hemorrhage on p. 2339.) Minimizing bleeding is the first priority; measures include

- Uterine massage
- Sometimes parenteral oxytocin

During the first hour after the 3rd stage of labor, the uterus is massaged periodically to ensure that it contracts, preventing excessive bleeding.

If the uterus does not contract after massage alone, oxytocin 10 units IM or a dilute oxytocin IV infusion (10 or 20 [up to 80] units/1000 mL of IV fluid) at 125 to 200 mL/h is given immediately after delivery of the placenta. The drug is continued until the uterus is firm; then it is decreased or stopped. Oxytocin should not be given as an IV bolus because severe hypotension may occur.

If bleeding increases, methergine 0.2 mg IM h or misoprostol 800 mcg given rectally once can be used to increase uterine tone. Methergine 0.2 mg po q 6 to 8 h can be continued for up to 7 days if needed.

For all women, the following must be available during the recovery period

- O_2
- Type O-negative blood or blood tested for compatibility
- IV fluids

If blood loss was excessive, a CBC to verify that women are not anemic is required before discharge. If blood loss was not excessive, CBC is not required.

Diet and activity: After the first 24 h, recovery is rapid. A regular diet should be offered as soon as women desire food. Full ambulation is encouraged as soon as possible.

Exercise recommendations are individualized depending on the presence of other maternal disorders or complications. Usually, exercises to strengthen abdominal muscles can be started once the discomfort of delivery has subsided, typically within 1 day for women who deliver vaginally and later for those who deliver by cesarean. Curl-ups, done in bed with the hips and knees flexed, tighten only abdominal muscles, usually without causing backache. Whether pelvic floor (eg, Kegel) exercises are helpful is unclear, but these exercises can begin as soon as the patient is ready.

Perineal care: If delivery was uncomplicated, showering and bathing are allowed, but vaginal douching is prohibited in the early puerperium. The vulva should be cleaned from front to back.

Immediately after delivery, ice packs may help reduce pain and edema at the site of an episiotomy or repaired laceration; sometimes lidocaine cream or spray can be used to relieve pain.

Later, warm sitz baths can be used several times a day.

Discomfort and pain: NSAIDs, such as ibuprofen 400 mg po q 4 to 6 h, work effectively on both perineal discomfort and uterine cramping. Acetaminophen 500 to 1000 mg po q 4 to 6 h can also be used. Acetaminophen and ibuprofen appear to be relatively safe during breastfeeding. Many other analgesics are secreted in breast milk. After surgery or repair of significant laceration, women may require opioids to relieve discomfort.

If pain is significantly worsening, women should be evaluated for complications such as vulvar hematoma.

Bladder and bowel function: Urine retention, bladder overdistention, and catheterization should be avoided if possible. Rapid diuresis may occur, especially when oxytocin is stopped. Voiding must be encouraged and monitored to prevent asymptomatic bladder overfilling. A midline mass palpable in the suprapubic region or elevation of the uterine fundus above the umbilicus suggests bladder overdistention. If overdistention occurs, catheterization is necessary to promptly relieve discomfort and to prevent long-term urinary dysfunction. If overdistention recurs, an indwelling or intermittent catheter may be needed.

Women are encouraged to defecate before leaving the hospital, although with early discharge, this recommendation is often impractical. If defecation has not occurred within 3 days, a mild cathartic (eg, psyllium, docusate, bisacodyl) can be given. Avoiding constipation can prevent or help relieve existing hemorrhoids, which can also be treated with warm sitz baths. Women with an extensive perineal laceration repair involving the rectum or anal sphincter can be given stool softeners (eg, docusate).

Regional (spinal or epidural) or general anesthesia may delay defecation and spontaneous urination, in part by delaying ambulation.

Vaccination and Rh desensitization: Women who are seronegative for rubella should be vaccinated against rubella on the day of discharge.

If women have not yet received tetanus-diphtheria-acellular pertussis (Tdap) vaccination (ideally given between wk 27 and 36 of each pregnancy) and have not had a tetanus and diphtheria toxoids (Td) booster in ≥ 2 yr, they should be given Tdap before discharge from the hospital or birthing center, regardless of their breastfeeding status. If family members who anticipate having contact with the neonate have not previously received Tdap, they should be given Tdap to immunize them against pertussis.

If women with Rh-negative blood have an infant with Rh-positive blood but are not sensitized, they should be given Rh_0(D) immune globulin 300 mcg IM within 72 h of delivery to prevent sensitization (see p. 2348).

Breast engorgement: Milk accumulation may cause painful breast engorgement during early lactation. Breastfeeding helps reduce engorgement.

For **women who are going to breastfeed,** the following are recommended until milk production adjusts to the infant's needs:

- Expressing milk by hand in a warm shower or using a breast pump between feedings to relieve pressure temporarily (however, doing so tends to encourage lactation, so it should be done only when necessary)
- Breastfeeding the infant on a regular schedule
- Wearing a comfortable nursing bra 24 h/day

For **women who are not going to breastfeed,** the following are recommended:

- Firm support of the breasts to suppress lactation because gravity stimulates the let-down reflex and encourages milk flow
- Refraining from nipple stimulation and manual expression, which can increase milk production
- Tight binding of the breasts (eg, with a snug-fitting bra), cold packs, and analgesics as needed, followed by firm support, to control temporary symptoms while lactation is being suppressed

Suppression of lactation with drugs is not recommended.

Mental disorders: Transient depression (baby blues) is very common during the first week after delivery. Symptoms (eg, mood swings, irritability, anxiety, difficulty concentrating, insomnia, crying spells) are typically mild and usually subside by 7 to 10 days.

Physicians should ask women about symptoms of depression before and after delivery and be alert to recognizing symptoms of depression, which may resemble the normal effects of new motherhood (eg, fatigue, difficulty concentrating). They should also advise women to contact them if depressive symptoms continue for > 2 wk or interfere with daily activities or if women have suicidal or homicidal thoughts. In such cases, postpartum depression or another mental disorder may be present.

A preexisting mental disorder, including prior postpartum depression, is likely to recur or worsen during the puerperium, so affected women should be monitored closely.

Management at Home

The woman and infant can be discharged within 24 to 48 h postpartum; many family-centered obstetric units discharge them as early as 6 h postpartum if major anesthesia was not used and no complications occurred.

Serious problems are rare, but a home visit, office visit, or phone call within 24 to 48 h is necessary. A routine postpartum visit is usually scheduled at 6 wk for women with an uncomplicated vaginal delivery. If delivery was cesarean or if other complications occurred, follow-up may be scheduled sooner.

Normal activities may be resumed as soon as the woman feels ready.

Intercourse after vaginal delivery may be resumed as soon as desired and comfortable; however, a laceration or episiotomy repair must be allowed to heal first. Intercourse after cesarean delivery should be delayed until the surgical wound has healed.

Family planning: Pregnancy must be delayed for 1 mo if women were vaccinated against rubella or varicella. Also, subsequent obstetric outcomes are improved by delaying conception for at least 6 mo but preferably 18 mo after delivery.

To minimize the chance of pregnancy, women should start using contraception as soon as they are discharged. If women are not breastfeeding, ovulation usually occurs about 4 to 6 wk postpartum, 2 wk before the first menses. However, ovulation can occur earlier; women have conceived as early as 2 wk postpartum. Women who are breastfeeding tend to ovulate and menstruate later, usually closer to 6 mo postpartum, although a few ovulate and menstruate (and become pregnant) as quickly as those who are not breastfeeding.

Women should choose a method of contraception based on the specific risks and benefits of various options. Breastfeeding status affects choice of contraceptive. For breastfeeding women, nonhormonal methods are usually preferred; among hormonal methods, progestin-only oral contraceptives, depot medroxyprogesterone acetate injections, and progestin implants are preferred because they do not affect milk production. Estrogen-progesterone contraceptives can interfere with milk production and should not be initiated until milk production is well established. Combined estrogen-progestin vaginal rings can be used after 4 wk postpartum if women are not breastfeeding.

A diaphragm should be fitted only after complete involution of the uterus, at 6 to 8 wk; meanwhile, foams, jellies, and condoms should be used.

Intrauterine devices are typically best placed after 4 to 6 wk postpartum to minimize risk of expulsion.

MASTITIS

Mastitis is painful inflammation of the breast, usually accompanied by infection.

Fever later in the puerperium is frequently due to mastitis. Staphylococcal species are the most common causes.

Breast abscesses are very rare and occasionally caused by methicillin-resistant *Staphylococcus aureus*.

Mastitis symptoms may include high fever and breast symptoms: erythema, induration, tenderness, pain, swelling, and warmth to the touch. Mastitis is different from the pain and cracking of nipples that frequently accompanies the start of breastfeeding.

Diagnosis of mastitis is clinical.

Treatment

- Antistaphylococcal antibiotics

Treatment of mastitis includes encouragement of fluid intake and antibiotics aimed at *Staphylococcus aureus,* the most common causative pathogen. Examples are

- Dicloxacillin 500 mg po q 6 h for 7 to 10 days
- For women allergic to penicillin, cephalexin 500 mg po qid or clindamycin 300 mg po tid for 10 to 14 days

Erythromycin 250 mg po q 6 h is used less frequently.

If women do not improve and do not have an abscess, vancomycin 1 g IV q 12 h or cefotetan 1 to 2 g IV q 12 h to cover resistant organisms should be considered. Breastfeeding should be continued during treatment because treatment includes emptying the affected breast.

Breast abscesses are treated mainly with incision and drainage. Antibiotics aimed at *S. aureus* are often used.

It is not clear whether antibiotics aimed at methicillin-resistant *S. aureus* are necessary for treatment of mastitis or breast abscess.

PUERPERAL ENDOMETRITIS

Puerperal endometritis is uterine infection, typically caused by bacteria ascending from the lower genital or GI tract. Symptoms are uterine tenderness, abdominal or pelvic pain, fever, malaise, and sometimes discharge. Diagnosis is clinical, rarely aided by culture. Treatment is with broad-spectrum antibiotics (eg, clindamycin plus gentamicin).

Incidence of postpartum endometritis is affected mainly by the mode of delivery:

- Vaginal deliveries: 1 to 3%
- Scheduled caesarean deliveries (done before labor starts): 5 to 15%
- Unscheduled caesarean deliveries (done after labor starts): 15 to 20%

Patient characteristics also affect incidence.

Etiology

Endometritis may develop after chorioamnionitis during labor or postpartum. Predisposing conditions include

- Prolonged rupture of the membranes
- Internal fetal monitoring
- Prolonged labor
- Cesarean delivery
- Repeated digital examination
- Retention of placental fragments in the uterus
- Postpartum hemorrhage
- Colonization of the lower genital tract
- Anemia
- Bacterial vaginosis
- Young maternal age
- Low socioeconomic status

Infection tends to be polymicrobial; the most common pathogens include

- Gram-positive cocci (predominantly group B streptococci, *Staphylococcus epidermidis*, and *Enterococcus* sp)
- Anaerobes (predominantly peptostreptococci, *Bacteroides* sp, and *Prevotella* sp)
- Gram-negative bacteria (predominantly *Gardnerella vaginalis, Escherichia coli, Klebsiella pneumoniae,* and *Proteus mirabilis)*

Uncommonly, peritonitis, pelvic abscess, pelvic thrombophlebitis (with risk of pulmonary embolism), or a combination develops. Rarely, septic shock and its sequelae, including death, occur.

Symptoms and Signs

Typically, the first symptoms are lower abdominal pain and uterine tenderness, followed by fever—most commonly within the first 24 to 72 h postpartum. Chills, headache, malaise, and anorexia are common. Sometimes the only symptom is a low-grade fever.

Pallor, tachycardia, and leukocytosis usually occur, and the uterus is soft, large, and tender. Discharge may be decreased or profuse and malodorous, with or without blood. When parametria are affected, pain and fever are severe; the large, tender uterus is indurated at the base of the broad ligaments, extending to the pelvic walls or posterior cul-de-sac.

Pelvic abscess may manifest as a palpable mass separate from and adjacent to the uterus.

Diagnosis

- Clinical evaluation
- Usually tests to exclude other causes (eg, urinalysis and urine culture)

Diagnosis within 24 h of delivery is based on clinical findings of pain, tenderness, and temperature > 38° C after delivery.

After the first 24 h, puerperal endometritis is presumed present if no other cause is apparent in patients with temperature ≥ 38° C on 2 successive days. Other causes of fever and lower abdominal symptoms include UTI, wound infection, septic pelvic thrombophlebitis, and perineal infection. Uterine tenderness is often difficult to distinguish from incisional tenderness in patients who have had a cesarean delivery.

Patients with low-grade fever and no abdominal pain are evaluated for other occult causes, such as atelectasis, breast engorgement or infection, UTI, and leg thrombophlebitis. Fever due to breast engorgement tends to remain ≤ 39° C. If temperature abruptly rises after 2 or 3 days of low-grade fever, the cause is probably an infection rather than breast engorgement.

Urinalysis and urine culture are usually done.

Endometrial cultures are rarely indicated because specimens collected through the cervix are almost always contaminated by vaginal and cervical flora. Endometrial cultures should be done only when endometritis is refractory to routine antibiotic regimens and no other cause of infection is obvious; sterile technique with a speculum is used to avoid vaginal contamination, and the sample is sent for aerobic and anaerobic cultures.

Blood cultures are rarely indicated and should be done only when endometritis is refractory to routine antibiotic regimens or clinical findings suggest septicemia.

If despite adequate treatment of endometritis, fever persists for > 48 h (some clinicians use a 72-h cutoff) without a downward trend in peak temperature, other causes such as pelvic abscess and pelvic thrombophlebitis (particularly if no abscess is evident on scans) should be considered. Abdominal and pelvic imaging, usually by CT, is sensitive for abscess but detects pelvic thrombophlebitis only if the clots are large. If imaging shows neither abnormality, a trial of heparin is typically begun to treat presumed pelvic thrombophlebitis, usually a diagnosis of exclusion. A therapeutic response confirms the diagnosis.

PEARLS & PITFALLS

- If adequate treatment of puerperal endometritis does not result in a downward trend in peak temperature after 48 to 72 h, consider pelvic abscess and, particularly if no abscess is evident on scans, septic pelvic thrombophlebitis.

Treatment

- Clindamycin plus gentamicin, with or without ampicillin

Treatment is a broad-spectrum antibiotic regimen given IV until women are afebrile for 48 h. The first-line choice is clindamycin 900 mg q 8 h plus gentamicin 1.5 mg/kg q 8 h or 5 mg/kg once/day; ampicillin 1 g q 6 h is added if enterococcal infection is suspected or if no improvement occurs by 48 h. Continuing treatment with oral antibiotics is not necessary.

Prevention

Preventing or minimizing predisposing factors is essential. Appropriate hand washing should be encouraged. Vaginal delivery cannot be sterile, but aseptic techniques are used.

When delivery is cesarean, prophylactic antibiotics given within 60 min before surgery can reduce risk of endometritis by up to 75%.

KEY POINTS

- Puerperal endometritis is more common after cesarean delivery, particularly if unscheduled.
- The infection is usually polymicrobial.
- Treat based on clinical findings (eg, postpartum pain, fundal tenderness, or unexplained fever), using broad-spectrum antibiotics.
- Endometrial and blood cultures are not routinely done.
- For cesarean delivery, give prophylactic antibiotics within 60 min before surgery.

POSTPARTUM PYELONEPHRITIS

Pyelonephritis is bacterial infection of the renal parenchyma.

Pyelonephritis may occur postpartum if bacteria ascend from the bladder. The infection may begin as asymptomatic bacteriuria during pregnancy and is sometimes associated with bladder catheterization to relieve urinary distention during or after labor. The causative organism is usually a type of coliform bacteria (eg, *Escherichia coli*).

Symptoms include fever, flank pain, general malaise, and, occasionally, painful urination.

Diagnosis

- Urinalysis and urine culture

Diagnosis is based on urinalysis, urine culture, and clinical findings (see p. 2178).

Treatment

- Ceftriaxone alone or ampicillin plus gentamicin

Initial treatment is ceftriaxone 1 to 2 g IV q 12 to 24 h alone or ampicillin 1 g IV q 6 h plus gentamicin 1.5 mg/kg IV q 8 h until women are afebrile for 48 h. Sensitivities with culture should be checked. Treatment is adjusted accordingly and continued for a total of 7 to 14 days; oral antibiotics are used after the initial IV antibiotics. Women should be encouraged to consume large amounts of liquids.

A urine culture should be repeated 6 to 8 wk after delivery to verify cure. If episodes of pyelonephritis recur, imaging should be considered to look for calculi or congenital malformations. Imaging during pregnancy is usually with ultrasonography; imaging after pregnancy is usually with contrast CT.

POSTPARTUM DEPRESSION

Postpartum depression is depressive symptoms that last > 2 wk after delivery and that interfere with activities of daily living.

Postpartum depression occurs in 10 to 15% of women after delivery. Although every woman is at risk, women with the following are at higher risk:

- Baby blues (eg, rapid mood swings, irritability, anxiety, decreased concentration, insomnia, crying spells)
- Prior episode of postpartum depression
- Prior diagnosis of depression
- Family history of depression
- Significant life stressors (eg, marital conflict, stressful events in the last year, unemployment of partner, no partner, partner with depression)
- Lack of support from partner or family members (eg, financial or child care support)
- History of mood changes temporally associated with menstrual cycles or oral contraceptive use
- Prior or current poor obstetric outcomes (eg, previous miscarriage, an infant with a congenital malformation)
- Prior or continuing ambivalence about the current pregnancy (eg, because it was unplanned or termination was considered)

The exact etiology is unknown; however, prior depression is the major risk, and hormonal changes during the puerperium, sleep deprivation, and genetic susceptibility may contribute.

Transient depression (baby blues) is very common during the first week after delivery. Baby blues differs from postpartum depression because baby blues typically lasts 2 to 3 days (up to 2 wk) and is relatively mild; in contrast, postpartum depression lasts > 2 wk and is disabling, interfering with activities of daily living.

Symptoms and Signs

Symptoms of postpartum depression may be similar to those of major depression and may include

- Extreme sadness
- Guilt
- Uncontrollable crying
- Insomnia or increased sleep
- Loss of appetite or overeating
- Irritability and anger
- Headaches and body aches and pains
- Extreme fatigue
- Unrealistic worries about or disinterest in the baby
- A feeling of being incapable of caring for the baby or of being inadequate as a mother
- Fear of harming the baby
- Suicidal ideation
- Anxiety or panic attacks

Typically, symptoms develop insidiously over 3 mo, but onset can be more sudden. Postpartum depression interferes with women's ability to care for themselves and the baby.

Psychosis rarely develops, but postpartum depression increases the risk of suicide and infanticide, which are the most severe complications.

Women may not bond with their infant, resulting in emotional, social, and cognitive problems in the child later.

Fathers are at increased risk of depression, and marital stress is increased.

Without treatment, postpartum depression can resolve spontaneously or become chronic depression. Risk of recurrence is about 1 in 3 to 4.

Diagnosis

- Clinical evaluation
- Sometimes formal depression scales

Early diagnosis and treatment substantially improve outcomes for women and their infant.

Postpartum depression (or other serious mental disorders) should be suspected if women have the following:

- Symptoms for > 2 wk
- Symptoms that interfere with daily activities
- Suicidal or homicidal thoughts (women should be asked specifically about such thoughts)
- Hallucinations, delusions, or psychotic behavior

Because of cultural and social factors, women may not volunteer symptoms of depression, so health care providers should ask women about such symptoms before and after delivery. Also, women should be taught to recognize symptoms of depression, which they may mistake for the normal effects of new motherhood (eg, fatigue, difficulty concentrating).

Women can be screened at the postpartum visit for postpartum depression using various depression scales. Such tools, including the Edinburgh Postnatal Depression Scale and Postpartum Depression Screening Scale, are available at MedEdPPD (www.mededppd.org/screening_tools.asp).

Treatment

- Antidepressants
- Psychotherapy

Treatment of postpartum depression includes antidepressants and psychotherapy.

Exercise therapy, light therapy, massage therapy, acupuncture, and ω-3 fatty acid supplementation have shown some benefit in small studies.

Women who have postpartum psychosis may need to be hospitalized, preferably in a supervised unit that allows the infant to remain with them. Antipsychotic drugs may be needed as well as antidepressants.

KEY POINTS

- Baby blues is very common during the first week after delivery, typically lasts 2 to 3 days (up to 2 weeks), and is relatively mild.
- Postpartum depression occurs in 10 to 15% of women, lasts > 2 wk, and is disabling (in contrast to baby blues).
- Symptoms may be similar to those of major depression and can also include worries and fears about being a mother.
- Postpartum depression typically also affects other family members, often resulting in marital stress, depression in the father, and subsequent problems in the child.
- Teach all women to recognize the symptoms of postpartum depression, and ask them about symptoms of depression before and after delivery.
- For the best possible outcomes, identify and treat postpartum depression as early as possible.

287 Pregnancy Complicated by Disease

ANEMIA IN PREGNANCY

Normally during pregnancy, erythroid hyperplasia of the marrow occurs, and RBC mass increases. However, a disproportionate increase in plasma volume results in hemodilution (hydremia of pregnancy): Hct decreases from between 38 and 45% in healthy women who are not pregnant to about 34% during late single pregnancy and to 30% during late multifetal pregnancy. Thus during pregnancy, anemia is defined as Hb < 10 g/dL (Hct < 30%). If Hb is < 11.5 g/dL at the onset of pregnancy, women may be treated prophylactically because subsequent hemodilution usually reduces Hb to < 10 g/dL. Despite hemodilution, oxygen-carrying capacity remains normal throughout pregnancy. Hct normally increases immediately after birth.

Anemia occurs in up to one-third of women during the 3rd trimester. The most common causes are

- Iron deficiency
- Folate deficiency

Obstetricians, in consultation with a perinatologist, should evaluate anemia in pregnant Jehovah's Witness patients (who are likely to refuse blood transfusions) as soon as possible.

Symptoms and Signs

Early symptoms of anemia are usually nonexistent or nonspecific (eg, fatigue, weakness, light-headedness, mild dyspnea during exertion). Other symptoms and signs may include pallor and, if anemia is severe, tachycardia or hypotension.

Anemia increases risk of

- Preterm delivery
- Postpartum maternal infections

Diagnosis

- CBC, followed by testing based on MCV value

Diagnosis of anemia begins with CBC; usually, if women have anemia, subsequent testing is based on whether the MCV is low (< 79 fL) or high (> 100 fL):

- For **microcytic anemias:** Evaluation includes testing for iron deficiency (measuring serum ferritin) and hemoglobinopathies (using hemoglobin electrophoresis). If these tests are nondiagnostic and there is no response to empiric treatment, consultation with a hematologist is usually warranted.
- For **macrocytic anemias:** Evaluation includes serum folate and B_{12} levels.
- For **anemia with mixed causes:** Evaluation for both types is required.

Treatment

- Treatment to reverse the anemia
- Transfusion as needed for severe symptoms

Treatment of anemia during pregnancy is directed at reversing the anemia (see below).

Transfusion is usually indicated for any anemia if severe constitutional symptoms (eg, light-headedness, weakness, fatigue) or cardiopulmonary symptoms or signs (eg, dyspnea, tachycardia, tachypnea) are present; the decision is not based on the Hct.

PEARLS & PITFALLS

- Transfusion decisions are not based on the Hct but on the severity of symptoms.

KEY POINTS

- Hemodilution occurs during pregnancy, but oxygen-carrying capacity remains normal throughout pregnancy.
- The most common causes of anemia during pregnancy are iron deficiency and folate acid deficiency.
- Anemia increases risk of preterm delivery and postpartum maternal infections.
- If Hb is < 11.5 g/dL at the onset of pregnancy, consider treating women prophylactically.
- Treat the cause of the anemia if possible, but if patients have severe symptoms, transfusion is usually indicated.

Iron Deficiency Anemia in Pregnancy

About 95% of anemia cases during pregnancy are iron deficiency anemia (see p. 1095). The cause is usually

- Inadequate dietary intake (especially in adolescent girls)
- A previous pregnancy
- The normal recurrent loss of iron in menstrual blood (which approximates the amount normally ingested each month and thus prevents iron stores from building up)

Diagnosis

- Measurement of serum iron, ferritin, and transferrin

Typically, Hct is ≤ 30%, and MCV is < 79 fL. Decreased serum iron and ferritin and increased serum transferrin levels confirm the diagnosis of iron deficiency anemia.

Treatment

- Usually ferrous sulfate 325 mg po once/day

One 325-mg ferrous sulfate tablet taken midmorning is usually effective. Higher or more frequent doses increase GI adverse effects, especially constipation, and one dose blocks absorption of the next dose, thereby reducing percentage intake.

About 20% of pregnant women do not absorb enough supplemental oral iron; a few of them require parenteral therapy, usually iron dextran 100 mg IM every other day for a total of ≥ 1000 mg over 3 wk. Hct or Hb is measured weekly to determine response. If iron supplements are ineffective, concomitant folate deficiency should be suspected.

Neonates of mothers with iron deficiency anemia usually have a normal Hct but decreased total iron stores and a need for early dietary iron supplements.

Prevention

Although the practice is controversial, iron supplements (usually ferrous sulfate 325 mg po once/day) are usually given routinely to pregnant women to prevent depletion of body iron stores and prevent the anemia that may result from abnormal bleeding or a subsequent pregnancy.

Folate Deficiency Anemia in Pregnancy

Folate deficiency (see also p. 1101) increases risk of neural tube defects and possibly fetal alcohol syndrome. Deficiency occurs in 0.5 to 1.5% of pregnant women; macrocytic megaloblastic anemia is present if deficiency is moderate or severe.

Rarely, severe anemia and glossitis occur.

Diagnosis

- Measurement of serum folate

Folate deficiency is suspected if CBC shows anemia with macrocytic indices or high RBC distribution width (RDW). Low serum folate levels confirm the diagnosis.

Treatment

- Folic acid 1 mg po bid

Treatment is folic acid 1 mg po bid.

Severe megaloblastic anemia may warrant bone marrow examination and further treatment in a hospital.

Prevention

For prevention, all pregnant women and women who are trying to conceive are given folic acid 0.4 to 0.8 mg po once/day. Women who have had a fetus with spina bifida should take 4 mg once/day, starting before conception.

Hemoglobinopathies in Pregnancy

During pregnancy, hemoglobinopathies, particularly sickle cell disease, Hb S-C disease, and beta- and alpha-thalassemia, can worsen maternal and perinatal outcomes (for genetic screening for some of these disorders, see Table 275–1 on p. 2298).

Preexisting **sickle cell disease,** particularly if severe, increases risk of the following:

- Maternal infection (most often, pneumonia, UTIs, and endometritis)
- Pregnancy-induced hypertension
- Heart failure
- Pulmonary infarction
- Fetal growth restriction
- Preterm delivery
- Low birth weight

Anemia almost always becomes more severe as pregnancy progresses. Sickle cell trait increases the risk of UTIs but is not associated with severe pregnancy-related complications.

Treatment of sickle cell disease during pregnancy is complex. Painful crises should be treated aggressively. Prophylactic exchange transfusions to keep Hb A at ≥ 60% reduce risk of hemolytic crises and pulmonary complications, but they are not routinely recommended because they increase risk of transfusion reactions, hepatitis, HIV transmission, and blood group isoimmunization. Prophylactic transfusion does not appear to decrease perinatal risk. Therapeutic transfusion is indicated for the following:

- Symptomatic anemia
- Heart failure
- Severe bacterial infection
- Severe complications of labor and delivery (eg, bleeding, sepsis)

Hb S-C disease may first cause symptoms during pregnancy. The disease increases risk of pulmonary infarction by occasionally causing bony spicule embolization. Effects on the fetus are uncommon but, if they occur, often include fetal growth restriction.

Sickle cell–beta-thalassemia is similar to Hb S-C disease but is less common and more benign.

Alpha-thalassemia does not cause maternal morbidity, but if the fetus is homozygous, hydrops and fetal death occur during the 2nd or early 3rd trimester.

ASTHMA IN PREGNANCY

The effect of pregnancy on asthma varies; deterioration is slightly more common than improvement, but most pregnant women do not have severe attacks.

The effect of asthma on pregnancy also varies, but severe, poorly controlled asthma increases risk of

- Prematurity
- Preeclampsia
- Growth restriction
- Maternal morbidity and mortality

Also, cesarean delivery is required more often.

Treatment

- Inhaled bronchodilators and corticosteroids
- For an acute exacerbation, addition of IV methylprednisolone, followed by oral prednisone

Pregnancy does not usually change treatment of asthma (see also p. 404). Women are taught strategies to help manage asthma, including how to minimize exposure to triggers and how to serially measure pulmonary function (usually with a handheld peak flow meter).

Inhaled bronchodilators and corticosteroids are first-line maintenance therapy for asthma in pregnant women. Budesonide is the preferred inhaled corticosteroid. Based on available data, inhaled budesonide does not appear to increase the risk of congenital malformations in humans. Theophylline is no longer recommended routinely during pregnancy.

For an acute exacerbation, in addition to bronchodilators, methylprednisolone 60 mg IV q 6 h for 24 to 48 h may be used, followed by oral prednisone in a tapering dose.

AUTOIMMUNE DISORDERS IN PREGNANCY

Autoimmune disorders are 5 times more common among women, and incidence tends to peak during reproductive years. Thus, these disorders commonly occur in pregnant women.

Antiphospholipid Antibody Syndrome in Pregnancy

Antiphospholipid antibody syndrome (APS) is an autoimmune disorder that predisposes patients to thrombosis (see p. 1207) and, during pregnancy, increases risk of fetal demise, pregnancy-induced hypertension, preeclampsia, and intrauterine growth restriction.

APS is caused by autoantibodies to certain phospholipid-binding proteins that would otherwise protect against excessive coagulation activation.

Diagnosis

- Measurement of circulating antiphospholipid antibodies
- Clinical criteria

APS is suspected in women with a history of any of the following:

- ≥ 1 unexplained fetal losses or ≥ 3 unexplained embryonic losses
- Prior unexplained arterial or venous thromboembolism
- New arterial or venous thromboembolism during pregnancy

APS is diagnosed by measuring levels of circulating antiphospholipid antibodies (anticardiolipin, beta-2 glycoprotein I, lupus anticoagulant) with positive results on ≥ 2 occasions 12 wk apart.

Diagnosis of APS requires at ≥ 1 clinical criterion in addition to ≥ 1 of the laboratory criteria above. Clinical criteria can be vascular (prior unexplained arterial or venous thromboembolism in any tissue) or pregnancy-related. Pregnancy-related criteria include the following:

- ≥ 1 unexplained deaths of a morphologically normal (via ultrasonography or direct examination) fetus at ≥ 10 wk gestation
- ≥ 1 premature births of a morphologically normal neonate at ≤ 34 wk gestation because of eclampsia or severe preeclampsia or with features of placental insufficiency
- ≥ 3 unexplained consecutive spontaneous pregnancy losses at ≤ 10 wk gestation, with maternal anatomic and hormonal abnormalities and paternal and maternal chromosomal causes excluded

Treatment

- Prophylaxis with anticoagulants and low-dose aspirin

Women with APS are usually treated prophylactically with anticoagulants and with low-dose aspirin during pregnancy and for 6 wk postpartum.

Immune Thrombocytopenia in Pregnancy

Immune thrombocytopenia (ITP), mediated by maternal antiplatelet IgG, tends to worsen during pregnancy and increases risk of maternal morbidity.

Corticosteroids reduce IgG levels and cause remission in most women, but improvement is sustained in only 50%. Immunosuppressive therapy and plasma exchange further reduce IgG, increasing platelet counts. Rarely, splenectomy is required for refractory cases; it is best done during the 2nd trimester, when it causes sustained remission in about 80%.

IV immune globulin increases platelet count significantly but briefly, so that labor can be induced in women with low platelet counts. Platelet transfusions are indicated only when

- Cesarean delivery is required and maternal platelet counts are < 50,000 μL.
- Vaginal delivery is expected and maternal platelet counts are < 10,000/μL.

Although antiplatelet IgG can cross the placenta, it only very rarely causes fetal or neonatal thrombocytopenia. Maternal antiplatelet antibody levels (measured by direct or indirect assay) cannot predict fetal involvement. Risk of neonatal intracranial hemorrhage due to maternal ITP is not affected by the mode of delivery nor by birth trauma. Accordingly, the current accepted practice is vaginal delivery, without routinely determining the fetal platelet count, and cesarean delivery only for obstetric indications.

Myasthenia Gravis in Pregnancy

Myasthenia gravis varies in its course during pregnancy. Frequent acute myasthenic episodes may require increasing doses of anticholinesterase drugs (eg, neostigmine), which may cause symptoms of cholinergic excess (eg, abdominal pain, diarrhea, vomiting, increasing weakness); atropine may then be required. Sometimes myasthenia becomes refractory to standard therapy and requires corticosteroids or immunosuppressants.

During labor, women may need assisted ventilation and are extremely sensitive to drugs that depress respiration (eg, sedatives, opioids, magnesium sulfate). Because the IgG responsible for myasthenia crosses the placenta, transient myasthenia occurs in 20% of neonates, even more if mothers have not had a thymectomy.

Rheumatoid Arthritis in Pregnancy

RA may begin during pregnancy or, even more often, during the postpartum period. Preexisting RA generally abates temporarily during pregnancy. The fetus is not specifically affected, but delivery may be difficult if the woman's hip joints or lumbar spine is affected.

If a woman develops an RA flare during pregnancy, first-line treatment usually begins with prednisone. For refractory cases, other immunosuppressants may be required (see also p. 306).

Systemic Lupus Erythematosus in Pregnancy

SLE may first appear during pregnancy; women who have had an unexplained 2nd-trimester stillbirth, a fetus with growth restriction, preterm delivery, or recurrent spontaneous abortions are often later diagnosed with SLE.

The course of preexisting SLE during pregnancy cannot be predicted, but SLE may worsen, particularly immediately postpartum. Outcomes are better if conception can be delayed until the disorder has been inactive for at least 6 mo, the drug regimen has been adjusted in advance, and hypertension and renal function are normal.

Complications may include

- Fetal growth restriction
- Preterm delivery due to preeclampsia
- Congenital heart block due to maternal antibodies that cross the placenta

Significant preexisting renal or cardiac complications increase risk of maternal morbidity and mortality. Diffuse nephritis, hypertension, or the presence of circulating antiphospholipid antibodies (usually anticardiolipin antibody or lupus anticoagulant) increases risk of perinatal mortality. Neonates may have anemia, thrombocytopenia, or leukopenia; these disorders tend to resolve during the first weeks after birth when maternal antibodies disappear.

If hydroxychloroquine was used before conception, it may be continued throughout pregnancy. SLE flares are usually treated with low-dose prednisone, IV pulse methylprednisolone, hydroxychloroquine, and/or azathioprine (see also p. 265). High-dose prednisone and cyclophosphamide increase obstetric risks and are thus reserved for severe lupus complications.

CANCER IN PREGNANCY

Pregnancy should not delay treatment of cancer. Treatment is similar to that in nonpregnant women except for rectal and gynecologic cancers.

Because embryonic tissues grow rapidly and have a high DNA turnover rate, they resemble cancer tissues and are thus very vulnerable to antineoplastic drugs. Many antimetabolites and alkylating drugs (eg, busulfan, chlorambucil, cyclophosphamide, 6-mercaptopurine, methotrexate) can cause fetal abnormalities. Methotrexate is particularly problematic; use during the 1st trimester increases risk of spontaneous abortion and, if the pregnancy continues, multiple congenital malformations. Although pregnancy often concludes successfully despite cancer treatment, risk of fetal injury due to treatment leads some women to choose abortion.

Rectal cancer: Rectal cancers may require hysterectomy to ensure complete tumor removal. Cesarean delivery may be done as early as 28 wk, followed by hysterectomy so that aggressive cancer treatment can be started.

Cervical cancer: Pregnancy does not appear to worsen cervical cancer. Cervical cancer can develop during pregnancy, and an abnormal Papanicolaou (Pap) test should not be attributed to pregnancy. Abnormal Pap tests are followed by colposcopy and directed biopsies when indicated. Colposcopy does not increase risk of an adverse pregnancy outcome. Expert colposcopic evaluation and consultation with the pathologist are recommended before doing a cervical biopsy because the biopsy may cause hemorrhage and preterm labor. If the examination suggests that lesions are low-grade, a biopsy may not be done, particularly if cervical cytology also suggests that lesions are low-grade.

For **carcinoma in situ** (Federation of Gynecology and Obstetrics [FIGO] stage 0—see Table 270–2 on p. 2253) and microinvasive cancer (stage IA1), treatment is often deferred until after delivery because at these stages, cancer progresses very slowly and pregnancy can be completed safely without affecting the woman's prognosis.

If **invasive cancer** (FIGO stage IA2 or higher) is diagnosed, pregnancy should be managed in consultation with a gynecologic oncologist. If invasive cancer is diagnosed during early pregnancy, immediate therapy appropriate for the cancer is traditionally recommended. If invasive cancer is diagnosed after 20 wk and if the woman accepts the unquantified increase in risk, treatment can be deferred until into the 3rd trimester (eg, 32 wk) to maximize fetal maturity but not delay treatment too long. For patients with invasive cancer, cesarean delivery with radical hysterectomy is done; vaginal delivery is avoided.

Other gynecologic cancers: After 12 wk gestation, ovarian cancer is easily missed; then, the ovaries, with the uterus, rise out of the pelvis and are no longer easily palpable. If very advanced, ovarian cancer during pregnancy may be fatal before completion of the pregnancy. Affected women require bilateral oophorectomy as soon as possible.

Endometrial cancer and fallopian tube cancer rarely occur during pregnancy.

Leukemia and Hodgkin lymphoma: Leukemia and Hodgkin lymphoma are uncommon during pregnancy.

Antineoplastic drugs typically used increase risk of fetal loss and congenital malformations.

Because leukemias can become fatal rapidly, treatment is given as soon as possible, without any significant delay to allow the fetus to mature.

If Hodgkin lymphoma is confined to above the diaphragm, radiation therapy may be used; the abdomen must be shielded. If lymphoma is below the diaphragm, abortion may be recommended.

Breast cancer: Breast engorgement during pregnancy may make recognizing breast cancer difficult. Any solid or cystic breast mass should be evaluated (see p. 2226).

DIABETES MELLITUS IN PREGNANCY

(Gestational Diabetes; Pregestational Diabetes)

(See also Ch. 165 on p. 1253).

Pregnancy aggravates preexisting type 1 (insulin-dependent) and type 2 (non–insulin-dependent) diabetes but does not appear to exacerbate diabetic retinopathy, nephropathy, or neuropathy.[1]

Gestational diabetes (diabetes that begins during pregnancy)[2] can develop in overweight, hyperinsulinemic, insulin-resistant women or in thin, relatively insulin-deficient women. Gestational diabetes occurs in at least 5% of all pregnancies, but the rate may be much higher in certain groups (eg, Mexican Americans, American Indians, Asians, Indians, Pacific Islanders). Women with gestational diabetes are at increased risk of type 2 diabetes in the future.

Diabetes during pregnancy increases fetal and maternal morbidity and mortality. Neonates are at risk of respiratory distress, hypoglycemia, hypocalcemia, hyperbilirubinemia, polycythemia, and hyperviscosity.

Poor control of preexisting (pregestational) or gestational diabetes during organogenesis (up to about 10 wk gestation) increases risk of the following:

- Major congenital malformations
- Spontaneous abortion

Poor control of diabetes later in pregnancy increases risk of the following:

- Fetal macrosomia (usually defined as fetal weight > 4000 g or > 4500 g at birth)
- Preeclampsia
- Shoulder dystocia
- Cesarean delivery
- Stillbirth

However, gestational diabetes can result in fetal macrosomia even if blood glucose is kept nearly normal.

Guidelines for managing diabetes mellitus during pregnancy are available from the American College of Obstetricians and Gynecologists (ACOG).[1,2]

1. Committee on Practice Bulletins—Obstetrics: ACOG Practice Bulletin No. 60: Clinical management guidelines for obstetrician-gynecologists: Pregestational diabetes mellitus. *Obstet Gynecol* 105(3):675–685, 2005.
2. Committee on Practice Bulletins—Obstetrics: Practice Bulletin No. 137: Gestational diabetes mellitus. *Obstet Gynecol* 122(2 Pt 1):406–416, 2013. doi: 10.1097/01.AOG.0000433006.09219.f1.

Diagnosis

- Oral glucose tolerance test (OGTT) or a single plasma glucose measurement (fasting or random)

Most experts recommend that all pregnant women be screened for gestational diabetes. An OGTT is usually recommended, but the diagnosis can probably be made based on a fasting plasma glucose of > 126 mg/dL (> 6.9 mmol/L) or a random plasma glucose of > 200 mg/dL (> 11 mmol/L).

The recommended screening method has 2 steps. The first is a screening test with a 50-g oral glucose load and a single measurement of the glucose level at 1 h. If the 1-h glucose level is > 130 to 140 mg/dL (> 7.2 to 7.8 mmol/L), a second, confirmatory 3-h test is done using a 100-g glucose load (see Table 287–1).

Most organizations outside the US recommend a single-step, 2-h test.

Treatment

- Close monitoring
- Tight control of blood glucose
- Management of complications

Preconception counseling and optimal control of diabetes before, during, and after pregnancy minimize maternal and fetal risks, including congenital malformations. Because malformations may develop before pregnancy is diagnosed, the need for

Table 287–1. GLUCOSE THRESHOLDS FOR GESTATIONAL DIABETES USING A 3-H ORAL GLUCOSE TOLERANCE TEST*

ORGANIZATION	FASTING mg/dL (mmol/L)	1-H mg/dL (mmol/L)	2-H mg/dL (mmol/L)	3-H mg/dL (mmol/L)
Carpenter and Coustan	95 (5.3)	180 (10)	155 (8.6)	140 (7.8)
National Diabetes Data Group	105 (5.8)	190 (10.5)	165 (9.1)	145 (8)

*A 100-g glucose load is used.

constant, strict control of glucose levels is stressed to women who have diabetes and who are considering pregnancy (or who are not using contraception).

To minimize risks, clinicians should do all of the following:

- Involve a diabetes team (eg, physicians, nurses, nutritionists, social workers) and a pediatrician
- Promptly diagnose and treat complications of pregnancy, no matter how trivial
- Plan for delivery and have an experienced pediatrician present
- Ensure that neonatal intensive care is available

In regional perinatal centers, specialists in management of diabetic complications are available.

During pregnancy: Treatment can vary, but some general management guidelines are useful (see Tables 287–2, 287–3, and 287–4).

Table 287–2. MANAGEMENT OF TYPE 1 DIABETES MELLITUS* DURING PREGNANCY

TIME FRAME	MEASURES
Before conception	Diabetes is controlled. Risk is lowest if HbA_{1c} levels are ≤ 6.5% at conception.† Evaluation includes • 24-h urine collection (protein excretion and creatinine clearance) or spot urine protein:creatinine ratio to check for renal complications • Ophthalmologic examination to check for retinal complications • ECG to check for cardiac complications
Prenatal	Prenatal visits begin as soon as pregnancy is recognized. Frequency of visits is determined by degree of glycemic control. Diet should be individualized according to ADA guidelines and coordinated with insulin administration. Three meals and 3 snacks/day are recommended, with emphasis on consistent timing. Women are instructed in and should do blood glucose self-monitoring. Women should be cautioned about the dangers of hypoglycemia during exercise and at night. Women and their family members should be instructed in glucagon administration. HbA_{1c} level should be checked every trimester. Antenatal testing with the following should be done from 32 wk to delivery (or earlier if indicated): • Nonstress tests (weekly) • Biophysical profiles (weekly) • Kick counts (daily) Amount and type of insulin should be individualized. In the AM; two thirds of the total dose (60% NPH, 40% regular) is taken; in the PM; one third (50% NPH, 50% regular) is taken. Or, women can take long-acting insulin once/day or bid and insulin aspart immediately before breakfast, lunch, and dinner.‡
During labor and delivery	Vaginal delivery at term is possible if women have documented dating criteria and good glycemic control. Amniocentesis is not done unless indicated for another problem or requested by the couple. Cesarean delivery should be reserved for obstetric indications or fetal macrosomia (> 4500 g), which increases risk of shoulder dystocia. Delivery should occur by 39 wk. During delivery, a constant low-dose insulin infusion is usually preferred, and the usual sc administration of insulin is stopped. If induction is planned, the usual PM NPH insulin dose is given on the day before induction. Postpartum and continuing diabetes care should be arranged. Postpartum insulin requirements may decrease by up to 50%.

*Guidelines are only suggested; marked individual variations require appropriate adjustments.
†Normal values may differ depending on laboratory methods used.
‡Some hospital programs recommend up to 4 insulin injections daily. Continuous sc insulin infusion, which is labor-intensive, can sometimes be given in specialized diabetes clinics.
ADA = American Diabetes Association; HbA_{1c} = glycosylated Hb; NPH = neutral protamine Hagedorn.

Table 287–3. MANAGEMENT OF TYPE 2 DIABETES MELLITUS* DURING PREGNANCY

TIME FRAME	MEASURES
Before conception	Hyperglycemia is controlled. Risk is lowest if Hb A_{1c} levels are ≤ 6.5% at conception.† Weight loss is encouraged if BMI is >27 kg/m^2. The diet should be low in fat, relatively high in complex carbohydrates, and high in fiber. Exercise is encouraged.
Prenatal	For overweight women, diet and caloric intake are individualized and monitored to avoid weight gain of more than about 6.8–11.3 kg (> 15–25 lb) or, if they are obese, more than about 5–9.1 kg (> 11–20 lb). Moderate walking after meals is recommended. Women are instructed in and should do blood glucose self-monitoring. The 2-h postbreakfast blood glucose level is checked weekly at clinic visits if possible. HbA_{1c} level should be checked every trimester. Antenatal testing with the following should be done from 32 wk to delivery (or earlier if indicated): • Nonstress tests (weekly) • Biophysical profiles (weekly) • Kick counts (daily) Amount and type of insulin is individualized. For obese women, short-acting insulin is taken before each meal. For women who are not obese, two thirds of the total dose (60% NPH, 40% regular) is taken in the AM; one third (50% NPH, 50% regular) is taken in the PM. Or, women can take long-acting insulin once/day or bid and insulin aspart immediately before breakfast, lunch, and dinner.
During labor and delivery	Management is the same as for type 1 (see Table 287–2).

*Guidelines are only suggested; marked individual variations require appropriate adjustments.
†Normal values may differ depending on laboratory methods used.
BMI = body mass index; HbA_{1c} = glycosylated Hb; NPH = neutral protamine Hagedorn.

Women with type 1 or 2 should monitor their blood glucose levels at home. During pregnancy, normal fasting blood glucose levels are about 76 mg/dL (4.2 mmol/L).

Goals of treatment are

- Fasting blood glucose levels at < 95 mg/dL (< 5.3 mmol/L)
- 2-h postprandial levels at ≤ 120 mg/dL (≤ 6.6 mmol/L)
- No wide blood glucose fluctuations
- Glycosylated Hb (HbA_{1c}) levels at < 6.5%

Insulin is the traditional drug of choice because it cannot cross the placenta and provides more predictable glucose control; it is used for types 1 and 2 diabetes and for some women with gestational diabetes. Human insulin is used if possible because it minimizes antibody formation. Insulin antibodies cross the placenta, but their effect on the fetus is unknown. In some women with long-standing type 1 diabetes, hypoglycemia does not trigger the normal release of counterregulatory hormones (catecholamines, glucagon, cortisol, and growth hormone); thus, too much insulin can trigger hypoglycemic coma without premonitory symptoms. All pregnant women with type 1 should have glucagon kits and be instructed (as should family members) in giving glucagon if severe hypoglycemia (indicated by unconsciousness, confusion, or blood glucose levels < 40 mg/dL [< 2.2 mmol/L]) occurs.

PEARLS & PITFALLS

- All pregnant women with type 1 should have glucagon kits and be instructed (as should their family members) in giving glucagon if severe hypoglycemia occurs.

Oral hypoglycemic drugs (eg, glyburide) are being increasingly used to manage diabetes in pregnant women because of the ease of administration (pills compared to injections), low cost, and single daily dosing. Several studies have shown that glyburide is safe during pregnancy and that it provides control equivalent to that of insulin for women with gestational diabetes. For women with type 2 diabetes before pregnancy, data for use of oral drugs during pregnancy are scant; insulin is most often preferred. Oral hypoglycemics taken during pregnancy may be continued postpartum during breastfeeding, but the infant should be closely monitored for signs of hypoglycemia.

Management of complications: Although diabetic retinopathy, nephropathy, and mild neuropathy are not contraindications to pregnancy, they require preconception counseling and close management before and during pregnancy.

Retinopathy requires that an ophthalmologic examination be done every trimester. If proliferative retinopathy is noted at the first prenatal visit, photocoagulation should be used as soon as possible to prevent progressive deterioration.

Nephropathy, particularly in women with renal transplants, predisposes to pregnancy-induced hypertension. Risk of preterm delivery is higher if maternal renal function is impaired or if transplantation was recent. Prognosis is best if delivery occurs ≥ 2 yr after transplantation.

Congenital malformations of major organs are predicted by elevated HbA_{1c} levels at conception and during the first 8 wk of pregnancy. If the level is ≥ 8.5% during the 1st trimester, risk of congenital malformations is significantly increased, and targeted ultrasonography and fetal echocardiography are done during the 2nd trimester to check for malformations.[1] If women with type 2 diabetes take oral hypoglycemic drugs during the 1st trimester, fetal risk of congenital malformations is unknown (see Table 283–1 on p. 2360).

Labor and delivery: Certain precautions are required to ensure an optimal outcome.

Timing of delivery depends on fetal well-being. Women are told to count fetal movements during a 60-min period daily (fetal kick count) and to report any sudden decreases to the

Table 287–4. MANAGEMENT OF GESTATIONAL DIABETES DURING PREGNANCY

TIME FRAME	MEASURES
Before conception	Women who have had gestational diabetes in previous pregnancies should try to reach a normal weight and engage in modest exercise. The diet should be low in fat, relatively high in complex carbohydrates, and high in fiber. Fasting plasma glucose and HbA_{1c} levels should be checked.
Prenatal	Diet and caloric intake are individualized and monitored to prevent weight gain of more than about 6.8–11.3 kg (> 15–25 lb) or, if women are obese, more than about 5–9.1 kg (> 11–20 lb). Moderate exercise after meals is recommended. Antenatal testing with the following should be done from 32 wk to delivery (or earlier if indicated): • Nonstress tests (weekly) • Biophysical profiles (weekly) • Kick counts (daily) Insulin therapy is reserved for persistent hyperglycemia (fasting plasma glucose > 95 mg/dL or 2-h postprandial plasma glucose > 120 mg/dL) despite a trial of dietary therapy for ≥ 2 wk. Amount and type of insulin should be individualized. For obese women, short-acting insulin is taken before each meal. For women who are not obese, two thirds of the total dose (60% NPH, 40% regular) is taken in the AM; one third (50% NPH, 50% regular) is taken in the PM. Or, women can take long-acting insulin once/day or bid and insulin aspart immediately before breakfast, lunch, and dinner.
During labor and delivery	Vaginal delivery at term is possible if women have a well-documented delivery date and good diabetic control. Amniocentesis is not usually required. Cesarean delivery should be reserved for obstetric indications or fetal macrosomia (> 4500 g), which increases risk of shoulder dystocia. Delivery should occur by 39 wk.

HbA_{1c} = glycosylated Hb; NPH = neutral protamine Hagedorn.

obstetrician immediately. Antenatal testing is begun at 32 wk; it is done earlier if women have severe hypertension or a renal disorder or if fetal growth restriction is suspected. Amniocentesis to assess fetal lung maturity may be necessary for women with the following:

- Obstetric complications in past pregnancies
- Inadequate prenatal care
- Uncertain delivery date
- Poor glucose control
- Poor adherence to therapy

Type of delivery is usually spontaneous vaginal delivery at term. Risk of stillbirth and shoulder dystocia increases near term. Thus, if labor does not begin spontaneously by 39 wk, induction is often necessary; also, delivery may be induced between 37 to 39 wk without amniocentesis if adherence to therapy is poor or if blood glucose is poorly controlled. Dysfunctional labor, fetopelvic disproportion, or risk of shoulder dystocia may make cesarean delivery necessary.

Blood glucose levels are best controlled during labor and delivery by a continuous low-dose insulin infusion. If induction is planned, women eat their usual diet the day before and take their usual insulin dose. On the morning of labor induction, breakfast and insulin are withheld, baseline fasting plasma glucose is measured, and an IV infusion of 5% dextrose in 0.45% saline solution is started at 125 mL/h, using an infusion pump. Initial insulin infusion rate is determined by capillary glucose level. Insulin dose is determined as follows:

- Initially: 0 units for a capillary level of < 80 mg/dL (< 4.4 mmol/L) or 0.5 units/h for a level of 80 to 100 mg/dL (4.4 to 5.5 mmol/L)
- Thereafter: Increased by 0.5 units/h for each 40-mg/dL (2.2-mmol/L) increase in glucose level over 100 mg/dL up to 2.5 units/h for levels > 220 mg/dL (> 12.2 mmol/L)
- Every hour during labor: Measurement of glucose level at bedside and adjustment of dose to keep the level at 70 to 120 mg/dL (3.8 to 6.6 mmol/L)
- If the glucose level is significantly elevated: Possibly additional bolus doses

For spontaneous labor, the procedure is the same, except that if intermediate-acting insulin was taken in the previous 12 h, the insulin dose is decreased. For women who have fever, infection, or other complications and for obese women who have type 2 and have required > 100 units of insulin/day before pregnancy, the insulin dose is increased.

Postpartum: After delivery, loss of the placenta, which synthesizes large amounts of insulin antagonist hormones throughout pregnancy, decreases the insulin requirement immediately. Thus, women with gestational diabetes and many of those with type 2 require no insulin postpartum. For women with type 1, insulin requirements decrease dramatically but then gradually increase after about 72 h.

During the first 6 wk postpartum, the goal is tight glucose control. Glucose levels are checked before meals and at bedtime. Breastfeeding is not contraindicated but may result in neonatal hypoglycemia if oral hypoglycemics are taken. Women who have had gestational diabetes should have a 2-h OGTT with 75 g of glucose at 6 to 12 wk postpartum to determine whether diabetes has resolved.

1. Miller E, Hare JW, Cloherty JP, et al: Elevated maternal hemaglogin A1c in early pregnancy and major congenital anomalies in infants of diabetic mothers. *N Engl J Med* 304(22):1331–1334, 1981. doi: 10.1056/NEJM198105283042204.

KEY POINTS

- Diabetes in pregnancy increases risk of fetal macrosomia, shoulder dystocia, preeclampsia, cesarean delivery, stillbirth, and, if preexisting or gestational diabetes is poorly controlled during organogenesis, major congenital malformations and spontaneous abortion.
- Screen all pregnant women for gestational diabetes using an OGTT.
- Involve a diabetes team if available, and aim to keep fasting blood glucose levels at < 95 mg/dL (< 5.3 mmol/L) and 2-h postprandial levels at ≤ 120 mg/dL (≤ 6.6 mmol/L).
- Begin antenatal testing at 32 wk and deliver by 39 wk.
- Adjust insulin dose immediately after delivery of the placenta.

FEVERS DURING PREGNANCY

A temperature of > 39.5° C (> 103° F) during the 1st trimester increases risk of

- Spontaneous abortion
- Fetal brain or spinal cord defects

Fever late in pregnancy increases risk of

- Preterm labor

Treatment of fever is directed at the cause, but antipyretics are indicated to decrease maternal temperature. In women with severe hyperthermia, cooling blankets may be used.

FIBROIDS IN PREGNANCY

(See also Ch. 277 on p. 2309).

Fibroids may increase risk of

- Preterm labor
- Abnormal fetal presentation
- Placenta previa
- Recurrent spontaneous abortions
- Postpartum hemorrhage

Rarely, fibroids partially obstruct the birth canal.

Preconception evaluation is recommended for women who have very large fibroids or who have fibroids and have had a spontaneous abortion.

HEART DISORDERS IN PREGNANCY

Heart disorders account for about 10% of maternal obstetric deaths. In the US, because incidence of rheumatic heart disease has markedly declined, most heart problems during pregnancy result from congenital heart disease. However, in Southeast Asia, Africa, India, the Middle East, and parts of Australia and New Zealand, rheumatic heart disease is still common.

Despite dramatic improvements in survival and quality of life for patients with severe congenital heart defects and other heart disorders, pregnancy remains inadvisable for women with certain high-risk disorders such as the following:[1]

- Pulmonary hypertension (pulmonary artery systolic pressure > 25 mm Hg) caused by any condition, including Eisenmenger syndrome
- Coarctation of the aorta if uncorrected or if accompanied by an aneurysm
- Marfan syndrome with aortic root diameter of > 4.5 cm
- Severe symptomatic aortic stenosis or severe mitral stenosis
- Bicuspid aortic valve with ascending aorta diameter > 50 mm
- A single ventricle and impaired systolic function (whether treated with the Fontan procedure or not)
- Cardiomyopathy with ejection fraction < 30% or New York Heart Association (NYHA) class III or IV heart failure (see Table 83–2 on p. 716)

1. European Society of Gynecology (ESG); Association for European Paediatric Cardiology (AEPC); German Society for Gender Medicine (DGesGM): ESC Guidelines on the management of cardiovascular diseases during pregnancy: the Task Force on the Management of Cardiovascular Diseases During Pregnancy of the European Society of Cardiology (ESC). *Eur Heart J* 32(24):3147–3197, 2011. doi: 10.1093/eurheartj/ehr218.

Pathophysiology

Pregnancy stresses the cardiovascular system, often worsening known heart disorders; mild heart disorders may first become evident during pregnancy.

Stresses include decreased Hb and increased blood volume, stroke volume, and eventually heart rate. Cardiac output increases by 30 to 50%. These changes become maximal between 28 and 34 wk gestation.

During labor, cardiac output increases about 20% with each uterine contraction; other stresses include straining during the 2nd stage of labor and the increase in venous blood returning to the heart from the contracting uterus. Cardiovascular stresses do not return to prepregnancy levels until several weeks after delivery.

Symptoms and Signs

Findings resembling heart failure (eg, mild dyspnea, systolic murmurs, jugular venous distention, tachycardia, dependent edema, mild cardiomegaly seen on chest x-ray) typically occur during normal pregnancy or may result from a heart disorder. Diastolic or presystolic murmurs are more specific for heart disorders.

Heart failure can cause premature labor or arrhythmias. Risk of maternal or fetal death correlates with NYHA functional classification, which is based on the amount of physical activity that causes symptoms of heart failure.

Risk is increased only if symptoms

- Occur during mild exertion (NYHA class III)
- Occur during minimal or no exertion (NYHA class IV)

Diagnosis

- Clinical evaluation
- Usually echocardiography

Diagnosis of a heart disorder during pregnancy is usually based on clinical evaluation and echocardiography.

Because genetics can contribute to the risk of heart disorders, genetic counseling and fetal echocardiography should be offered to women with congenital heart disease.

Treatment

- Avoidance of warfarin, ACE inhibitors, angiotensin II receptor blockers (ARBs), aldosterone antagonists, thiazide diuretics, and certain antiarrhythmics (eg, amiodarone)
- For NYHA class III or IV, activity restriction and possibly bed rest after 20 wk
- Most other usual treatments for heart failure and arrhythmias

Frequent prenatal visits, ample rest, avoidance of excessive weight gain and stress, and treatment of anemia are required. An anesthesiologist familiar with heart disorders in pregnancy should attend the labor and ideally should be consulted prenatally. During labor, pain and anxiety are treated aggressively to minimize tachycardia. Women are closely monitored immediately postpartum and are followed for several weeks postpartum by a cardiologist.

Before women with NYHA class III or IV status conceive, the disorder should be optimally treated medically and, if indicated (eg, if due to a valvular heart disorder), treated surgically. Women with class III or IV heart failure or another high-risk disorders (listed above) may be advised to obtain an early therapeutic abortion.

Some women with a heart disorder and poor cardiac function require digoxin 0.25 mg po once/day plus bed rest, beginning at 20 wk. Cardiac glycosides (eg, digoxin, digitoxin) cross the placenta, but neonates (and children) are relatively resistant to their toxicity. ACE inhibitors and ARBs are contraindicated because they may cause fetal renal damage. Aldosterone antagonists (spironolactone, eplerenone) should be avoided because they may cause feminization of a male fetus. Other treatments for heart failure (eg, nonthiazide diuretics, nitrates, inotropes) may be continued during pregnancy depending on disease severity and fetal risk, as determined by a cardiologist and a perinatologist.

Arrhythmias: Atrial fibrillation may accompany cardiomyopathy or valvular lesions. Rate control is usually similar to that in nonpregnant patients, with beta-blockers, calcium channel blockers, or digoxin (see p. 623). Certain antiarrhythmics (eg, amiodarone) should be avoided. If pregnant patients have new-onset atrial fibrillation or hemodynamic instability or if drugs do not control ventricular rate, cardioversion may be used to restore sinus rhythm.

Anticoagulation may be required because the relative hypercoagulability during pregnancy makes atrial thrombi (and subsequent systemic or pulmonary embolization) more likely. Standard or low molecular weight heparin is used. Neither standard heparin nor low molecular weight heparins cross the placenta, but low molecular weight heparins may have less risk of thrombocytopenia. Warfarin crosses the placenta and may cause fetal abnormalities (see Table 283–1 on p. 2360), particularly during the 1st trimester. However, risk is dose-dependent, and incidence is very low if the dose is ≤ 5 mg per day. Warfarin use during the last month of pregnancy has risks. Rapid reversal of warfarin's anticoagulant effects may be difficult and may be required because of fetal or neonatal intracranial hemorrhage resulting from birth trauma or because of maternal bleeding (eg, resulting from trauma or emergency cesarean delivery).

Management of acute supraventricular tachycardia or ventricular tachycardia is the same as for nonpregnant patients.

Endocarditis prophylaxis: For pregnant patients with a structural heart disorder, indications and use of endocarditis prophylaxis for nonobstetric events are the same as those for nonpregnant patients. The American Heart Association guidelines do not recommend endocarditis prophylaxis for vaginal and cesarean deliveries because the rate of bacteremia is low. However, in the highest-risk patients (eg, those with prosthetic heart materials, a history of endocarditis, an unrepaired congenital cyanotic heart lesion, or a heart transplant with a valvulopathy), prophylaxis is often considered when the membranes rupture, even though no evidence indicates any benefit.

If patients with a structural heart disorder develop chorioamnionitis or another infection (eg, pyelonephritis) requiring hospital admission, the antibiotics used to treat the infection should cover the pathogens most likely to cause endocarditis.

KEY POINTS

- Pregnancy may not be advisable for women with certain high-risk heart disorders (eg, pulmonary hypertension, coarctation of the aorta if uncorrected or accompanied by an aneurysm, Marfan syndrome with aortic root diameter of > 4.5 cm, severe symptomatic aortic stenosis, severe mitral stenosis, bicuspid aortic valve with ascending aorta > 50 mm, a single ventricle with impaired systolic function, cardiomyopathy, NYHA class III or IV heart failure).
- Treat heart failure and arrhythmias during pregnancy as for nonpregnant patients, except avoid certain drugs (eg, warfarin, ACE inhibitors, ARBs, aldosterone antagonists, thiazide diuretics, certain antiarrhythmics such as amiodarone).
- Treat most pregnant patients who have atrial fibrillation with standard or low molecular weight heparin.
- Indications for endocarditis prophylaxis for pregnant patients with a structural heart disorder are the same as those for other patients.

Valvular Stenosis and Insufficiency in Pregnancy

During pregnancy, stenosis and regurgitation (insufficiency) most often affect the mitral and aortic valves. Mitral stenosis is the most common valvular disorder during pregnancy.

Pregnancy amplifies the murmurs of mitral and aortic stenosis but diminishes those of mitral and aortic regurgitation. During pregnancy, mild mitral or aortic regurgitation is usually easy to tolerate; stenosis is more difficult to tolerate and predisposes to maternal and fetal complications. Mitral stenosis is especially dangerous; the tachycardia, increased blood volume, and increased cardiac output during pregnancy interact with this disorder to rapidly increase pulmonary capillary pressure, causing pulmonary edema. Atrial fibrillation is also common.

Treatment

- For mitral stenosis, prevention of tachycardia, treatment of pulmonary edema and atrial fibrillation, and sometimes valvotomy
- For aortic stenosis, surgical correction before pregnancy if possible

Ideally, valvular disorders are diagnosed and treated medically before conception; surgical correction is often recommended for severe disorders. Prophylactic antibiotics are required in certain situations (eg, for endocarditis).

Mitral stenosis: Patients must be closely observed throughout pregnancy because mitral stenosis may rapidly become more severe. If required, valvotomy is relatively safe during pregnancy; however, open heart surgery increases fetal risk. Tachycardia should be prevented so that diastolic flow through the stenotic mitral valve can be maximized.

If pulmonary edema occurs, loop diuretics can be used.

If atrial fibrillation occurs, anticoagulation and control of heart rate are necessary. Control of heart rate is usually similar to that in nonpregnant patients and involves beta-blockers, calcium channel blockers, or digoxin (see p. 623).

During labor, conduction anesthesia (eg, slow epidural infusion) is usually preferred.

Aortic stenosis: Aortic stenosis should be corrected before pregnancy if possible because surgical repair during pregnancy has more risks and catheter valvuloplasty is not very effective.

During labor, local anesthesia is preferred, but if necessary, general anesthesia is used. Conduction anesthesia should be avoided because it decreases filling pressures (preload), which may already be decreased by aortic stenosis.

Straining, which can suddenly reduce filling pressures and impair cardiac output, is discouraged during the 2nd stage of labor; operative vaginal delivery is preferred. Cesarean delivery is done if indicated for obstetric reasons.

Other Heart Disorders in Pregnancy

Mitral valve prolapse: Mitral valve prolapse (MVP) occurs more frequently in younger women and tends to be familial (see also p. 777). MVP is usually an isolated abnormality that has no clinical consequences; however, patients may also have some degree of mitral regurgitation. Rarely, MVP occurs with Marfan syndrome or an atrial septal defect.

Women with MVP and resulting mitral regurgitation generally tolerate pregnancy well. The relative increase in ventricular size during normal pregnancy reduces the discrepancy between the disproportionately large mitral valve and the ventricle.

Beta-blockers are indicated for recurrent arrhythmias. Rarely, thrombi and systemic emboli (due to concomitant atrial fibrillation) develop and require anticoagulation.

Congenital heart disease: For most asymptomatic patients, risk is not increased during pregnancy. However, patients with Eisenmenger syndrome (now rare), primary pulmonary hypertension, or perhaps isolated pulmonary stenosis are predisposed, for unknown reasons, to sudden death during labor, during the postpartum period (the 6 wk after delivery), or after abortion at > 20 wk gestation.

Thus, pregnancy is inadvisable. If these patients become pregnant, they should be closely monitored with a pulmonary artery catheter and/or an arterial line during delivery.

For patients with intracardiac shunts, the goal is to prevent right-to-left shunting by maintaining peripheral vascular resistance and by minimizing pulmonary vascular resistance.

Patients with Marfan syndrome are at increased risk of aortic dissection and rupture of aortic aneurysms during pregnancy. Bed rest, beta-blockers, avoidance of Valsalva maneuvers, and measurement of aortic diameter with echocardiography are required.

Peripartum cardiomyopathy: Heart failure with no identifiable cause (eg, MI, valvular disorder) can develop between the last month of pregnancy and 6 mo postpartum in patients without a previous heart disorder.[1] Risk factors include

- Multiparity
- Age ≥ 30
- Multifetal pregnancy
- Preeclampsia

The 5-yr mortality rate is 50%. Recurrence is likely in subsequent pregnancies, particularly in patients with residual cardiac dysfunction; future pregnancies are therefore not recommended.

Treatment is as for heart failure. ACE inhibitors and aldosterone are relatively contraindicated but may be used when the expected benefit clearly exceeds the potential risks.

1. Sliwa K, Hilfiker-Kleiner D, Petrie MC, et al: Current state of knowledge on aetiology, diagnosis, management, and therapy of peripartum cardiomyopathy: A position statement from the Heart Failure Association of the European Society of Cardiology Working Group on peripartum cardiomyopathy. *Eur J Heart Fail* 12(8):767–778, 2010. doi: 10.1093/eurjhf/hfq120.

HEPATIC DISORDERS IN PREGNANCY

Hepatic disorders in pregnancy may be

- Unique to pregnancy
- Preexisting
- Coincident with pregnancy and possibly exacerbated by pregnancy

Jaundice: Jaundice may result from nonobstetric or obstetric conditions.

Nonobstetric causes of jaundice include

- Acute viral hepatitis (most common)
- Drugs
- Acute cholecystitis
- Biliary obstruction by gallstones

Gallstones appear to be more common during pregnancy, probably because bile lithogenicity is increased and gallbladder contractility is impaired.

Obstetric causes of jaundice include

- Hyperemesis gravidarum (usually causing mild jaundice)
- Septic abortion

Both cause hepatocellular injury and hemolysis.

Acute viral hepatitis: The most common cause of jaundice during pregnancy is acute viral hepatitis. Pregnancy does not affect the course of most types of viral hepatitis (A, B, C, D); however, hepatitis E may be more severe during pregnancy.

Acute viral hepatitis may predispose to preterm delivery but does not appear to be teratogenic.

Hepatitis B virus may be transmitted to the neonate immediately after delivery or, less often, to the fetus transplacentally. Transmission is particularly likely if women are e-antigen–positive and are chronic carriers of hepatitis B surface antigen (HBsAg) or if they contract hepatitis during the 3rd trimester. Affected neonates are more likely to develop subclinical hepatic dysfunction and become carriers than to develop clinical hepatitis. All pregnant women are tested for HBsAg to determine whether precautions against vertical transmission are needed (for prenatal prophylaxis with immune globulin and vaccination for neonates exposed to hepatitis B virus).

Chronic hepatitis: Chronic hepatitis, especially with cirrhosis, impairs fertility. When pregnancy occurs, risk of spontaneous abortion and prematurity is increased, but risk of maternal mortality is not.

Despite standard immunoprophylaxis, many neonates of women with a high viral load are infected with hepatitis B virus. Data suggest that antiviral drugs given during the 3rd trimester may prevent immunoprophylaxis failure. Fetal exposure should be minimized by using antiviral drugs only when women have advanced hepatitis or hepatic decompensation is a risk. Lamivudine, telbivudine, or tenofovir are most commonly used.

Corticosteroids given to treat chronic autoimmune hepatitis before pregnancy can be continued during pregnancy because fetal risks due to corticosteroids have not been proved to exceed those due to maternal chronic hepatitis. Azathioprine and other immunosuppressants, despite fetal risks, are sometimes indicated for severe disease.

Intrahepatic cholestasis (pruritus) of pregnancy: This relatively common disorder apparently results from idiosyncratic exaggeration of normal bile stasis due to hormonal changes. Incidence varies based on ethnicity and is highest in Bolivia and Chile.

Consequences of intrahepatic cholestasis include increased risk of

- Fetal prematurity
- Stillbirth
- Respiratory distress syndrome

Intense pruritus, the earliest symptom, develops during the 2nd or 3rd trimester; dark urine and jaundice sometimes follow. Acute pain and systemic symptoms are absent. Intrahepatic cholestasis usually resolves after delivery but tends to recur with each pregnancy or with use of oral contraceptives.

Intrahepatic cholestasis is suspected based on symptoms. The most sensitive and specific laboratory finding is a fasting total serum bile acid level of > 10 mmol/L. This finding may be the only biochemical abnormality present. Fetal demise is more likely when the fasting total bile acid level is > 40 mmol/L.

Ursodeoxycholic acid (UDCA) 5 mg/kg po bid or tid (or up to 7.5 mg/kg bid) is the drug of choice. It helps lessen the severity of symptoms and normalize biochemical markers of liver function; however, it does not decrease the incidence of fetal complications.

Fatty liver of pregnancy: This rare, poorly understood disorder occurs near term, sometimes with preeclampsia. Patients may have an inherited defect in mitochondrial fatty acid beta-oxidation (which provides energy for skeletal and cardiac muscle); risk of fatty liver of pregnancy is 20 times higher in women with a mutation affecting long-chain 3-hydroxyacyl-CoA dehydrogenase (LCHAD), particularly the G1528C mutation on one or both alleles (autosomally inherited).

Symptoms of fatty liver include acute nausea and vomiting, abdominal discomfort, and jaundice, followed in severe cases by rapidly progressive hepatocellular failure. Maternal and fetal mortality rates are high in severe cases.

A seemingly identical disorder may develop at any stage of pregnancy if high doses of tetracyclines are given IV.

Clinical and laboratory findings resemble those of fulminant viral hepatitis except that aminotransferase levels may be < 500 units/L and hyperuricemia may be present.

Diagnosis of fatty liver of pregnancy is based on

- Clinical criteria
- Liver function tests
- Hepatitis serologic tests
- Liver biopsy

Biopsy shows diffuse small droplets of fat in hepatocytes, usually with minimal apparent necrosis, but in some cases, findings are indistinguishable from viral hepatitis.

Affected women and their infants should be tested for known genetic variants of LCHAD.

Depending on gestational age, prompt delivery or termination of pregnancy is usually advised, although whether either alters maternal outcome is unclear. Survivors recover completely and have no recurrences.

Preeclampsia: Severe preeclampsia can cause liver problems with hepatic fibrin deposition, necrosis, and hemorrhage that can result in abdominal pain, nausea, vomiting, and mild jaundice.

Subcapsular hematoma with intra-abdominal hemorrhage occasionally occurs, most often in women with preeclampsia that progresses to the HELLP syndrome (hemolysis, elevated liver enzymes, and low platelet count). Rarely, the hematoma causes the liver to rupture spontaneously; rupture is life threatening, and pathogenesis is unknown.

Chronic hepatic disorders: Pregnancy may temporarily worsen cholestasis in primary biliary cirrhosis and other chronic cholestatic disorders, and the increased plasma volume during the 3rd trimester slightly increases risk of variceal hemorrhage in women with cirrhosis. However, pregnancy usually does not harm women with a chronic hepatic disorder.

Cesarean delivery is reserved for the usual obstetric indications.

KEY POINTS

- In pregnant women, hepatic disorders may be related or unrelated to the pregnancy.
- The most common cause of jaundice during pregnancy is acute viral hepatitis; pregnancy does not affect the course of most types of viral hepatitis (A, B, C, D), but hepatitis E may be more severe during pregnancy.
- Hepatitis B virus may be transmitted to the neonate immediately after delivery or, less often, to the fetus transplacentally; test all pregnant women for HBsAg to determine whether precautions against vertical transmission are needed.
- Intrahepatic cholestasis of pregnancy causes intense pruritus and increases risk of fetal prematurity, stillbirth, and respiratory distress syndrome.
- Fatty liver of pregnancy occurs near term, sometimes with preeclampsia; because maternal and fetal mortality rates can be high in severe cases, prompt delivery or termination of pregnancy is usually advised.
- Usually, pregnancy does not harm women with a chronic hepatic disorder.

HYPERTENSION IN PREGNANCY

(See also Ch. 84 on p. 726).

Recommendations regarding classification, diagnosis, and management of hypertensive disorders (including preeclampsia) are available from the American College of Obstetricians and Gynecologists (ACOG).[1]

Hypertension (systolic BP ≥ 140 mm Hg, diastolic BP ≥ 90 mm Hg, or both) during pregnancy can be classified as one of the following:

- **Chronic:** BP is high before pregnancy or before 20 wk gestation. Chronic hypertension complicates about 1 to 5% of all pregnancies.
- **Gestational:** Hypertension develops after 20 wk gestation (typically after 37 wk) and remits by 6 wk postpartum; it occurs in about 5 to 10% of pregnancies, more commonly in multifetal pregnancy.

Both types of hypertension increase risk of preeclampsia and eclampsia and of other causes of maternal mortality or morbidity, including hypertensive encephalopathy, stroke, renal failure, left ventricular failure, and the HELLP syndrome (hemolysis, elevated liver enzymes, and low platelet count).

Risk of fetal mortality or morbidity increases because of decreased uteroplacental blood flow, which can cause vasospasm, growth restriction, hypoxia, and abruptio placentae. Outcomes are worse if hypertension is severe (systolic BP ≥ 160, diastolic BP ≥ 110 mm Hg, or both) or accompanied by renal insufficiency (eg, creatinine clearance < 60 mL/min, serum creatinine > 2 mg/dL [> 180 μmol/L]).

1. American College of Obstetricians and Gynecologists, Task Force on Hypertension in Pregnancy: Hypertension in pregnancy. Report of the American College of Obstetricians and Gynecologists' Task Force on Hypertension in Pregnancy. *Obstet Gynecol* 122(5):1122–1131, 2013. doi: 10.1097/01.AOG.0000437382.03963.88.

Diagnosis

- Tests to rule out other causes of hypertension

BP is measured routinely at prenatal visits. If severe hypertension occurs for the first time in pregnant women who do not have a multifetal pregnancy or gestational trophoblastic disease, tests to rule out other causes of hypertension (eg, renal artery stenosis, coarctation of the aorta, Cushing syndrome, SLE, pheochromocytoma) should be considered.

Treatment

- For mild hypertension, conservative measures followed by antihypertensives if needed
- Methyldopa, beta-blockers, or calcium channel blockers tried first
- Avoidance of ACE inhibitors, ARBs, and aldosterone antagonists
- For moderate or severe hypertension, antihypertensive therapy, close monitoring, and, if condition worsens, possibly termination of pregnancy or delivery, depending on gestational age

Recommendations for chronic and gestational hypertension are similar and depend on severity. However, chronic hypertension may be more severe. In gestational hypertension, the increases in BP often occur only late in gestation and may not require treatment.

Treatment of mild to moderate hypertension without renal insufficiency during pregnancy is controversial; the issues are whether treatment improves outcome and whether the risks of drug treatment outweigh risks of untreated disease. Because the uteroplacental circulation is maximally dilated and cannot autoregulate, decreasing maternal BP with drugs may abruptly decrease uteroplacental blood flow. Diuretics reduce effective maternal circulating blood volume; consistent reduction increases risk of fetal growth restriction. However, hypertension with renal insufficiency is treated even if hypertension is mild or moderate.

For **mild to moderate hypertension** (systolic BP 140 to 159 mm Hg or diastolic BP 90 to 109 mm Hg) with labile BP, reduced physical activity may decrease BP and improve fetal growth, making perinatal risks similar to those for women without hypertension. However, if this conservative measure does not decrease BP, many experts recommend drug therapy. Women who were taking methyldopa, a beta-blocker, a calcium channel blocker, or a combination before pregnancy may continue to take these drugs. However, ACE inhibitors and ARBs should be stopped once pregnancy is confirmed.

For **severe hypertension** (systolic BP ≥ 160 mm Hg or diastolic BP ≥ 110 mm Hg), drug therapy is indicated. Risk of complications—maternal (progression of end-organ dysfunction, preeclampsia) and fetal (prematurity, growth restriction, stillbirth)—is increased significantly. Several antihypertensives may be required.

For systolic BP > 180 mm Hg or diastolic BP > 110 mm Hg, immediate evaluation is required. Multiple drugs are often required. Also, hospitalization may be necessary for much of the latter part of pregnancy. If the woman's condition worsens, pregnancy termination may be recommended.

All women with chronic hypertension during pregnancy should be taught to self-monitor BP, and they should be evaluated for target organ damage. Evaluation, done at baseline and periodically thereafter, includes

- Serum creatinine, electrolytes, and uric acid levels
- Liver function tests
- Platelet count
- Urine protein assessment
- Usually funduscopy

Maternal echocardiography should be considered if women have had hypertension for > 4 yr. After initial ultrasonography to evaluate fetal anatomy, ultrasonography is done monthly starting at about 28 wk to monitor fetal growth; antenatal testing often begins at 32 wk. Ultrasonography to monitor fetal growth and antenatal testing may start sooner if women have additional complications (eg, renal disorders) or if complications (eg, growth restriction) occur in the fetus. Delivery should occur by 37 to 39 wk but may be induced earlier if preeclampsia or fetal growth restriction is detected or if fetal test results are nonreassuring.

Drugs: First-line drugs for hypertension during pregnancy include

- Methyldopa
- Beta-blockers
- Calcium channel blockers

Initial methyldopa dose is 250 mg po bid, increased as needed to a total of 2 g/day unless excessive somnolence, depression, or symptomatic orthostatic hypotension occurs.

The most commonly used beta-blocker is labetalol (a beta-blocker with some alpha-1 blocking effects), which can be used alone or with methyldopa when the maximum daily dose of methyldopa has been reached. Usual dose of labetalol is 100 mg bid to tid, increased as needed to a total maximum daily dose of 2400 mg. Adverse effects of beta-blockers include increased risk of fetal growth restriction, decreased maternal energy levels, and maternal depression.

Extended-release nifedipine, a calcium channel blocker, may be preferred because it is given once/day (initial dose of 30 mg; maximum daily dose of 120 mg); adverse effects include headaches and pretibial edema. Thiazide diuretics are only used to treat chronic hypertension during pregnancy if the potential benefit outweighs the potential risk to the fetus. Dose may be adjusted to minimize adverse effects such as hypokalemia.

Several classes of antihypertensives are usually avoided during pregnancy:

- **ACE inhibitors** are contraindicated because risk of fetal urinary tract abnormalities is increased.
- **ARBs** are contraindicated because they increase risk of fetal renal dysfunction, lung hypoplasia, skeletal malformations, and death.
- **Aldosterone antagonists** (spironolactone and eplerenone) should be avoided because they may cause feminization of a male fetus.

KEY POINTS

- Both chronic and gestational hypertension increase risk of preeclampsia, eclampsia, other causes of maternal mortality or morbidity (eg, hypertensive encephalopathy, stroke, renal failure, left ventricular failure, HELLP syndrome), and uteroplacental insufficiency.
- Check for other causes of hypertension if severe hypertension occurs for the first time in a pregnant woman who does not have a multifetal pregnancy or gestational trophoblastic disease.
- If drug therapy is necessary, start with methyldopa, a beta-blocker, or a calcium channel blocker.
- Do not use ACE inhibitors, ARBs, or aldosterone antagonists.
- Consider hospitalization or termination of pregnancy if BP is > 180/110 mm Hg.

INFECTIOUS DISEASE IN PREGNANCY

Most common maternal infections (eg, UTIs, skin and respiratory tract infections) are usually not serious problems during pregnancy, although some genital infections (bacterial vaginosis and genital herpes) affect labor or choice of delivery method. Thus, the main issue is usually use and safety of antimicrobial drugs.

However, certain maternal infections can damage the fetus, as may occur in the following:

- Congenital cytomegalovirus infection
- Neonatal herpes simplex virus infection
- Congenital rubella
- Congenital toxoplasmosis
- Neonatal hepatitis B
- Congenital syphilis

HIV infection can be transmitted from mother to child transplacentally or perinatally. When the mother is not treated, risk of transmission at birth is about 25 to 35%.

Listeriosis is more common during pregnancy. Listeriosis increases risk of

- Spontaneous abortion
- Preterm labor
- Stillbirth

Neonatal transmission of listeriosis is possible.

Bacterial vaginosis and possibly **genital chlamydial infection** predispose to

- Premature rupture of the membranes
- Preterm labor

Tests for these infections are done during routine prenatal evaluations or if symptoms develop.

Genital herpes can be transmitted to the neonate during delivery. Risk is high enough that cesarean delivery is preferred in the following situations:

- When women have visible herpetic lesions
- When women who have a known history of infection develop prodromal symptoms before labor
- When herpes infection first occurs during the late 3rd trimester (when cervical viral shedding at delivery is likely)

If visible lesions or prodrome is absent, even in women with recurrent infections, risk is low, and vaginal delivery is possible. If women are asymptomatic, serial antepartum cultures do not help identify those at risk of transmission. If women have recurrent herpes infections during pregnancy but no other risk factors for transmission, labor can sometimes be induced so that delivery occurs between recurrences. When delivery is vaginal, cervical and neonatal herpesvirus cultures are done. Acyclovir (oral and topical) appears to be safe during pregnancy.

Antibacterials: It is important to avoid giving antibacterials to pregnant patients unless there is strong evidence of a bacterial infection. Use of any antibacterial during pregnancy should be based on whether benefits outweigh risk, which varies by trimester (see Table 283–1 on p. 2360 for specific adverse effects). Severity of the infection and other options for treatment are also considered.

Aminoglycosides may be used during pregnancy to treat pyelonephritis and chorioamnionitis, but treatment should be carefully monitored to avoid maternal or fetal damage.

Cephalosporins are generally considered safe.

Chloramphenicol, even in large doses, does not harm the fetus; however, neonates cannot adequately metabolize chloramphenicol, and the resulting high blood levels may lead to circulatory collapse (gray baby syndrome). Chloramphenicol is rarely used in the US.

Fluoroquinolones are not used during pregnancy; they tend to have a high affinity for bone and cartilage and thus may have adverse musculoskeletal effects.

Macrolides are generally considered safe.

Metronidazole use during the 1st trimester used to be considered controversial; however, in multiple studies, no teratogenic or mutagenic effects were seen.

Nitrofurantoin is not known to cause congenital malformations. It is contraindicated near term because it can cause hemolytic anemia in neonates.

Penicillins are generally considered safe.

Sulfonamides are usually safe during pregnancy. However, long-acting sulfonamides cross the placenta and can displace bilirubin from binding sites. These drugs are often avoided after 34 wk gestation because neonatal kernicterus is a risk.

Tetracyclines cross the placenta and are concentrated and deposited in fetal bones and teeth, where they combine with calcium and impair development (see Table 283–1 on p. 2360); they are not used from the middle to the end of pregnancy.

KEY POINTS

- Most common maternal infections (eg, UTIs, skin and respiratory tract infections) are usually not serious problems during pregnancy.
- Maternal infections that can damage the fetus include cytomegalovirus infection, herpes simplex virus infection, rubella, toxoplasmosis, hepatitis B, and syphilis.
- Give antibacterials to pregnant patients only when there is strong evidence of a bacterial infection and only if benefits of treatment outweigh risk, which varies by trimester.

RENAL INSUFFICIENCY IN PREGNANCY

Pregnancy often does not worsen renal disorders; it seems to exacerbate noninfectious renal disorders only when uncontrolled hypertension coexists. However, significant renal insufficiency (serum creatinine > 3 mg/dL [> 270 μmol/L] or BUN > 30 mg/dL [> 10.5 mmol urea/L]) before pregnancy usually prevents women from maintaining a pregnancy to term.

Maternal renal insufficiency may cause

- Fetal growth restriction
- Stillbirth

After kidney transplantation, full-term, uncomplicated pregnancy is often possible if women have all of the following:

- A transplanted kidney that has been in place for > 2 yr
- Normal renal function
- No episodes of rejection
- Normal BP

Treatment of renal insufficiency during pregnancy requires close consultation with a nephrologist. BP and weight are measured every 2 wk; BUN and creatinine levels plus creatinine clearance are measured often, at intervals dictated by severity and progression of disease. Furosemide is given only as needed to control BP or excessive edema; some women require other drugs to control BP. Women with severe renal insufficiency may require hospitalization after 28 wk gestation for bed rest, BP control, and close fetal monitoring. If results of antenatal testing remain normal and reassuring, the pregnancy continues.

Delivery is usually required before term because preeclampsia, fetal growth restriction, or uteroplacental insufficiency develop. Sometimes amniocentesis to check fetal lung maturity can help determine when delivery should be done; a lecithin/sphingomyelin ratio of > 2:1 or presence of phosphatidylglycerol indicates maturity. Cesarean delivery is very common, although vaginal delivery may be possible if the cervix is ripe and no impediments to vaginal delivery are evident.

End-stage renal disease: Advances in dialysis treatment have increased life expectancy for patients with end-stage renal disease, improved pregnancy outcomes, and increased fertility. The survival rate for fetuses of pregnant women receiving hemodialysis has improved from 23% (in about 1980) to almost 90% currently. The reason is probably the substantial increase in hemodialysis dose used during pregnancy; now, high-flux, high-efficiency hemodialysis is typically done 6 times/wk. Dialysis can be adjusted based on laboratory, ultrasonographic, and clinical findings (eg, severe hypertension, nausea or vomiting, edema, excessive weight gain, persistent polyhydramnios).

Although pregnancy outcomes have improved, complication rates for patients with end-stage renal disease remain high.

KEY POINTS

- Women who have significant renal insufficiency before pregnancy usually cannot maintain a pregnancy to term.
- In pregnant women with renal insufficiency, measure BP and weight every 2 wk, and measure BUN and creatinine levels plus creatinine clearance often, as indicated by severity and progression of disease.
- Consult closely with a nephrologist when treating renal insufficiency in a pregnant woman; delivery is usually required before term.
- Advances in dialysis treatment have increased life expectancy for patients with end-stage renal disease, improved pregnancy outcomes, and increased fertility, but complication rates for these patients remain high.

SEIZURE DISORDERS IN PREGNANCY

(See also Ch. 238 on p. 2001).

Seizure disorders may impair fertility. But certain anticonvulsants may make oral contraceptives less effective, resulting in unintentional pregnancy.

The dose of anticonvulsant drugs may have to be increased during pregnancy to maintain therapeutic levels. If women get enough sleep and anticonvulsant levels are kept in the therapeutic range, seizure frequency does not usually increase during pregnancy, and pregnancy outcome is good; however, risks of preeclampsia, fetal growth restriction, and stillbirth are slightly increased.

Generally, uncontrolled seizures are more harmful during pregnancy than is use of anticonvulsants; thus, the top priority of treatment during pregnancy is to control seizures. Preconception consultation with a neurologist is recommended to stabilize maternal seizures before pregnancy. Clinicians should use the lowest possible dose of anticonvulsants and as few different anticonvulsants as possible.

Congenital malformations are more frequent in the fetuses of women with a seizure disorder (6 to 8%) than in fetuses of women in the general population (2 to 3%). Risk of intellectual disability may also be increased. These risks may be related to the seizure disorder as well as anticonvulsant use. Risk of hemorrhagic disease of the newborn (erythroblastosis neonatorum) may be increased by in utero exposure to certain anticonvulsants (eg, phenytoin, carbamazepine, phenobarbital); however, if prenatal vitamins with vitamin D are taken and vitamin K is given to the neonate, hemorrhagic disease is rare.

Taken during pregnancy, phenobarbital may reduce the physiologic jaundice neonates commonly have, perhaps because the drug induces neonatal hepatic conjugating enzymes. Phenytoin is generally preferred.

All anticonvulsants increase the need for supplemental folic acid; 4 mg po is given once/day. Ideally, it is started before conception.

Vaginal delivery is usually preferred, but if women have repeated seizures during labor, cesarean delivery is indicated.

Anticonvulsant levels can rapidly change postpartum and should be closely monitored then.

DISORDERS REQUIRING SURGERY DURING PREGNANCY

Certain disorders treated with surgery are difficult to diagnose during pregnancy. A high level of suspicion is required; assuming that all abdominal symptoms are pregnancy-related is an error.

Major surgery, particularly intra-abdominal, increases risk of preterm labor and fetal death. However, surgery is tolerated well by pregnant women and the fetus when appropriate supportive care and anesthesia (maintaining BP and oxygenation at normal levels) are provided, so physicians should not be reluctant to operate; delaying treatment of a surgical emergency is far more dangerous.

PEARLS & PITFALLS

- Surgery is tolerated well by pregnant women and the fetus when appropriate supportive care and anesthesia are provided; delaying treatment of a surgical emergency is far more dangerous than operating.

Appendicitis: Appendicitis may occur during pregnancy but is more common immediately postpartum. Because the appendix rises in the abdomen as pregnancy progresses, pain and tenderness may not occur in the classic right lower quadrant location, and pain may be mild and cramping, mimicking pregnancy-related symptoms. Also, WBC count is normally somewhat elevated during pregnancy, making WBC count even less useful than usual. Serial clinical assessment and compression-graded ultrasonography are useful.

Because diagnosis is often delayed, mortality rate from ruptured appendix is increased during pregnancy and particularly postpartum. Thus, if appendicitis is suspected, surgical evaluation (laparoscopy or laparotomy depending on the stage of pregnancy) should proceed without delay.

Benign ovarian cysts: These cysts are common during pregnancy. Cysts that occur during the first 14 to 16 wk are often corpus luteal cysts, which spontaneously resolve. Adnexal torsion may occur. If adnexal torsion does not resolve, surgical therapy to unwind the adnexa or removal may be required. After 12 wk, cysts become difficult to palpate because the ovaries, with the uterus, rise out of the pelvis.

Ovarian masses are evaluated first by ultrasonography. Definitive evaluation (eg, excision) is delayed, if possible, until after 14 wk unless any of the following occur:

- The cyst enlarges continuously.
- The cyst is tender.
- The cyst has radiographic characteristics of cancer (eg, a solid component, surface excrescences, size > 6 cm, irregular shape).

Gallbladder disease: This disease occurs occasionally during pregnancy. If possible, treatment is expectant; if women do not improve, surgery is needed.

Intestinal obstruction: During pregnancy, intestinal obstruction may cause intestinal gangrene with peritonitis and maternal or fetal morbidity or mortality. If pregnant women have symptoms and signs of intestinal obstruction and risk factors (eg, previous abdominal surgery, intra-abdominal infection), prompt exploratory laparotomy is indicated.

THROMBOEMBOLIC DISORDERS IN PREGNANCY

In the US, thromboembolic disorders—deep venous thrombosis (DVT) or pulmonary embolism (PE)—are a leading cause of maternal mortality.

During pregnancy, risk is increased because

- Venous capacitance and venous pressure in the legs are increased, resulting in stasis.
- Pregnancy causes a degree of hypercoagulability.

However, most thromboemboli develop postpartum and result from vascular trauma during delivery. Cesarean delivery also increases risk.

Symptoms of thrombophlebitis or their absence does not accurately predict the diagnosis, disease severity, or risk of embolization. Thromboembolic disorders can occur without symptoms, with only minimal symptoms, or with significant symptoms. Also, calf edema, cramping, and tenderness, which may occur normally during pregnancy, may simulate Homans sign.

Diagnosis

- Doppler ultrasonography or sometimes CT with contrast for DVT
- Helical CT for PE

Diagnosis of DVT is usually by Doppler ultrasonography. In the postpartum period, if Doppler ultrasonography and plethysmography are normal but iliac, ovarian, or other pelvic venous thrombosis is suspected, CT with contrast is used.

Diagnosis of PE is increasingly being made by helical CT rather than ventilation-perfusion scanning because CT involves less radiation and is equally sensitive. If the diagnosis of PE is uncertain, pulmonary angiography is required.

Treatment

- Similar to that in nonpregnant patients, except for avoidance of warfarin
- For women with increased risk, prophylactic low molecular weight heparin throughout pregnancy and for 6 wk postpartum

If DVT or PE is detected during pregnancy, the anticoagulant of choice is a low molecular weight heparin (LMWH). LMWH, because of its molecular size, does not cross the placenta. It does not cause maternal osteoporosis and may be less likely to cause thrombocytopenia, which can result from prolonged (≥ 6 mo) use of unfractionated heparin. Warfarin crosses the placenta and may cause fetal abnormalities or death (see Table 283–1 on p. 2360).

Indications for thrombolysis during pregnancy are the same as for patients who are not pregnant.

If PE recurs despite effective anticoagulation, surgery, usually placement of an inferior vena cava filter just distal to the renal vessels, is indicated.

If women developed DVT or PE during a previous pregnancy or have an underlying thrombophilic disorder, they are treated with prophylactic LMWH (eg, enoxaparin 40 mg sc once/day) beginning when pregnancy is first diagnosed and continuing until 6 wk postpartum.

KEY POINTS

- During pregnancy, risk of thromboembolic disorders is increased, but most thromboemboli develop postpartum and result from vascular trauma during delivery.
- Symptoms of thrombophlebitis or their absence does not accurately predict the diagnosis, disease severity, or risk of embolization.
- Diagnose deep vein thrombosis using Doppler ultrasonography, but postpartum, if Doppler ultrasonography and plethysmography findings are normal but pelvic venous thrombosis is suspected, do CT with contrast.
- Diagnose pulmonary embolism using helical CT or, if needed, pulmonary angiography.
- LMWH is the treatment of choice; warfarin should be avoided.
- Treat high-risk women prophylactically with LMWH as soon as pregnancy is diagnosed and continue until 6 wk postpartum.

THYROID DISORDERS IN PREGNANCY

(See also Ch. 173 on p. 1342).

Thyroid disorders may predate or develop during pregnancy. Pregnancy does not change the symptoms of hypothyroidism and hyperthyroidism or the normal values and ranges of free serum thyroxine (T_4) and thyroid-stimulating hormone (TSH).

Fetal effects vary with the disorder and the drugs used for treatment. But generally, untreated or inadequately treated hyperthyroidism can result in

- Fetal growth restriction
- Preeclampsia
- Stillbirth

Untreated hypothyroidism can cause

- Intellectual deficits in offspring
- Miscarriage

The most common causes of maternal hypothyroidism are Hashimoto thyroiditis and treatment of Graves disease.

If women have or have had a thyroid disorder, thyroid status should be closely monitored during and after pregnancy in the women and in their offspring. Goiters and thyroid nodules discovered during pregnancy should be evaluated as they are in other patients (see pp. 1344 and 1353).

Graves disease: Maternal Graves disease is monitored clinically and with free T_4 and high-sensitivity TSH assays.

Treatment varies. Usually, pregnant women are given the lowest possible dose of oral propylthiouracil (50 to 100 mg q 8 h). Therapeutic response occurs over 3 to 4 wk; then the dose is changed if needed. Propylthiouracil crosses the placenta and may cause goiter and hypothyroidism in the fetus. Simultaneous use of L-thyroxine or L-triiodothyronine is contraindicated because these hormones may mask the effects of excessive propylthiouracil in pregnant women and result in hypothyroidism in the fetus. Methimazole is an alternative to propylthiouracil. Graves disease commonly abates during the 3rd trimester, often allowing dose reduction or discontinuation of the drug.

In centers with experienced thyroid surgeons, a 2nd-trimester thyroidectomy, although very uncommon, may be considered after drug treatment restores euthyroidism. After thyroidectomy, women are given full replacement of L-thyroxine (0.15 to 0.2 mg po once/day), beginning 24 h later.

Radioactive iodine (diagnostic or therapeutic) and iodide solutions are contraindicated during pregnancy because of adverse effects on the fetal thyroid gland. Beta-blockers are used only for thyroid storm or severe maternal symptoms.

If pregnant women have or have had Graves disease, fetal hyperthyroidism may develop. Whether these women are clinically euthyroid, hyperthyroid, or hypothyroid, thyroid-stimulating immunoglobulins (Igs) and thyroid-blocking Igs (if present) cross the placenta. Fetal thyroid function reflects the relative fetal levels of these stimulating and blocking Igs. Hyperthyroidism can cause fetal tachycardia (> 160 beats/min), growth restriction, and goiter; rarely, goiter leads to decreased fetal swallowing, polyhydramnios, and preterm labor. Ultrasonography is used to evaluate fetal growth, thyroid gland, and heart.

Congenital Graves disease: If pregnant women have taken propylthiouracil, congenital Graves disease in the fetus may be masked until 7 to 10 days after birth, when the drug's effect subsides.

Maternal hypothyroidism: Women with mild to moderate hypothyroidism frequently have normal menstrual cycles and can become pregnant.

During pregnancy, the usual dose of L-thyroxine is continued. As pregnancy progresses, minor dose adjustments may be necessary, ideally based on TSH measurement after several weeks.

If hypothyroidism is first diagnosed during pregnancy, L-thyroxine is started; dosing is based on weight. Usually, pregnant women require a higher dose than nonpregnant women.

Hashimoto thyroiditis: Maternal immune suppression during pregnancy often ameliorates Hashimoto thyroiditis; however, hypothyroidism or hyperthyroidism that requires treatment sometimes develops.

Acute (subacute) thyroiditis: Common during pregnancy, acute thyroiditis usually produces a tender goiter during or after a respiratory infection. Transient, symptomatic hyperthyroidism with elevated T_4 can occur, often resulting in misdiagnosis as Graves disease.

Usually, treatment is unnecessary.

Postpartum maternal thyroid dysfunction: Hypothyroid or hyperthyroid dysfunction occurs in 4 to 7% of women during the first 6 mo after delivery. Incidence seems to be higher among pregnant women with any of the following:

- Goiter
- Hashimoto thyroiditis
- A strong family history of autoimmune thyroid disorders
- Type 1 (insulin-dependent) diabetes mellitus

In women with any of these risk factors, TSH and free serum T_4 levels should be checked during the 1st trimester and postpartum. Dysfunction is usually transient but may require treatment. After delivery, Graves disease may recur transiently or persistently.

Painless thyroiditis with transient hyperthyroidism is a recently recognized postpartum, probably autoimmune disorder. It occurs abruptly in the first few weeks postpartum, results in a low radioactive iodine uptake, and is characterized by lymphocytic infiltration. Diagnosis is based on symptoms, thyroid function tests, and exclusion of other conditions. This disorder may persist, recur transiently, or progress.

URINARY TRACT INFECTION IN PREGNANCY

(See also Ch. 260 on p. 2175).

UTI is common during pregnancy, apparently because of urinary stasis, which results from hormonal ureteral dilation, hormonal ureteral hypoperistalsis, and pressure of the expanding uterus against the ureters. Asymptomatic bacteriuria occurs in about 15% of pregnancies and sometimes progresses to symptomatic cystitis or pyelonephritis. Frank UTI is not always preceded by asymptomatic bacteriuria.

Asymptomatic bacteriuria, UTI, and pyelonephritis increase risk of

- Preterm labor
- Premature rupture of the membranes

Diagnosis

- Urinalysis and culture

Urinalysis and culture are routinely done at initial evaluation to check for asymptomatic bacteriuria. Diagnosis of symptomatic UTI is not changed by pregnancy.

Treatment

- Antibacterial drugs such as cephalexin, nitrofurantoin, or trimethoprim/sulfamethoxazole
- Proof-of-cure cultures and sometimes suppressive therapy

Treatment of symptomatic UTI is not changed by pregnancy, except drugs that may harm the fetus are avoided (see Table 283–1 on p. 2360). Because asymptomatic bacteriuria may lead to pyelonephritis, it should be treated with antibiotics similar to an acute UTI.

Antibacterial drug selection is based on individual and local susceptibility and resistance patterns, but good initial empiric choices include the following:

- Cephalexin
- Nitrofurantoin
- Trimethoprim/sulfamethoxazole

After treatment, proof-of-cure cultures are required.

Women who have pyelonephritis or have had more than one UTI may require suppressive therapy, usually with trimethoprim/sulfamethoxazole (before 34 wk) or nitrofurantoin, for the rest of the pregnancy.

In women who have bacteriuria with or without UTI or pyelonephritis, urine should be cultured monthly.

KEY POINTS

- Asymptomatic bacteriuria, UTI, and pyelonephritis increase risk of preterm labor and premature rupture of the membranes.
- Initially treat with cephalexin, nitrofurantoin, or trimethoprim/sulfamethoxazole.
- Obtain proof-of-cure cultures after treatment.
- For women who have had pyelonephritis or more than one UTI, consider suppressive therapy, usually with trimethoprim/sulfamethoxazole (before 34 wk) or nitrofurantoin.

SECTION 20

Pediatrics

288 Care of Newborns and Infants

EVALUATION AND CARE OF THE NORMAL NEONATE

Hand washing is critical for all personnel to prevent transmission of infection.

Active participation in the birth by the mother and her partner helps them adapt to parenting.

The First Few Hours

Immediately at delivery, the neonate's respiratory effort, heart rate, color, tone, and reflex irritability should be assessed; all are key components of the Apgar score assigned at 1 min and 5 min after birth (see Table 288–1). Apgar scores between 8 and 10 indicate that the neonate is making a smooth transition to extrauterine life; scores ≤ 7 at 5 min (particularly if sustained beyond 10 min) are linked to higher neonatal morbidity and mortality rates. Many normal neonates have cyanosis 1 min after birth that clears by 5 min. Cyanosis that does not clear may indicate congenital cardiopulmonary anomalies or CNS depression.

In addition to Apgar scoring, neonates should be evaluated for gross deformities (eg, clubfoot, polydactyly) and other important abnormalities (eg, heart murmurs). The evaluation should ideally be done under a radiant warmer with the family close by.

Preventive interventions include administration into both eyes of an antimicrobial agent (eg, 0.5% erythromycin 1 cm ribbon, 1% tetracycline 1 cm ribbon, 1% silver nitrate solution 2 drops; in some countries, 2.5% povidone iodine drops) to prevent gonococcal and chlamydial ophthalmia and administration of vitamin K 1 mg IM to prevent hemorrhagic disease of the newborn (see Vitamin K Deficiency on p. 53).

Subsequently, the neonate is bathed, wrapped, and brought to the family. The head should be covered with a cap to prevent heat loss. Rooming-in and early breastfeeding should be encouraged so the family can get to know the infant and can receive guidance from staff members during the hospital stay. Breastfeeding is more likely to be successful when the family is given frequent and adequate support.

The First Few Days

Physical Examination of the Newborn

A thorough physical examination should be done within 24 h. Doing the examination with the mother and other family members present allows them to ask questions and the clinician to point out physical findings and provide anticipatory guidance.

Basic measurements include length, weight, and head circumference (see also Growth Parameters in Neonates on p. 2791). Length is measured from crown to heel; normal values are based on gestational age and should be plotted on a standard growth chart. When gestational age is uncertain or when the infant seems large for gestational age or small for gestational age, the gestational age can be precisely determined using physical and neuromuscular findings (see Fig. 288–1). These methods are typically accurate to ± 2 wk.

Many clinicians begin with examination of the heart and lungs, followed by a systematic head-to-toe examination, looking particularly for signs of birth trauma and congenital abnormalities.

Cardiorespiratory system: The heart and lungs are evaluated when the infant is quiet.

The clinician should identify where the heart sounds are loudest to exclude dextrocardia. Heart rate (normal: 100 to 160 beats/min) and rhythm are checked. Rhythm should be regular, although an irregular rhythm from premature atrial or ventricular contractions is not uncommon. A murmur heard in the first 24 h is most commonly caused by a patent ductus arteriosus. Daily heart examination confirms the disappearance of this murmur, usually within 3 days.

Femoral pulses are checked and compared with brachial pulses. A weak or delayed femoral pulse suggests aortic coarctation or other left ventricular outflow tract obstruction. Central cyanosis suggests congenital heart disease, pulmonary disease, or sepsis.

The respiratory system is evaluated by counting respirations over a full minute because breathing in neonates is irregular; normal rate is 40 to 60 breaths/min. The chest wall should be examined for symmetry, and lung sounds should be equal throughout. Grunting, nasal flaring, and retractions are signs of respiratory distress.

Table 288–1. APGAR SCORE

CRITERIA	MNEMONIC	SCORE* 0	1	2+
Color	Appearance	All blue, pale	Pink body, blue extremities	All pink
Heart rate	Pulse	Absent	< 100 beats/min	> 100 beats/min
Reflex response to nasal catheter/tactile stimulation	Grimace	None	Grimace	Sneeze, cough
Muscle tone	Activity	Limp	Some flexion of extremities	Active
Respiration	Respiration	Absent	Irregular, slow	Good, crying

*A total score of 7–10 at 5 min is considered normal; 4–6, intermediate; and 0–3, low.

Neuromuscular Maturity

Score	–1	0	1	2	3	4	5
Posture							
Square window (wrist)	>90°	90°	60°	45°	30°	0°	
Arm recoil		180°	140–180°	110–140°	90–110°	<90°	
Popliteal angle	180°	160°	140°	120°	100°	90°	<90°
Scarf sign							
Heel to ear							

Physical Maturity

Skin	Sticky, friable, transparent	Gelatinous, red, translucent	Smooth, pink; visible veins	Superficial peeling and/or rash; few veins	Cracking, pale areas; rare veins	Parchment, deep cracking; no vessels	Leathery, cracked, wrinkled
Lanugo	None	Sparse	Abundant	Thinning	Bald areas	Mostly bald	
Plantar surface	Heel-toe 40–50 mm: –1 <40 mm: –2	>50 mm, no crease	Faint red marks	Anterior transverse crease only	Creases, anterior 2/3	Creases over entire sole	
Breast	Imperceptible	Barely perceptible	Flat areola, no bud	Stippled areola, 1–2 mm bud	Raised areola, 3–4 mm bud	Full areola, 5–10 mm bud	
Eye/Ear	Lids fused loosely: –1 tightly: –2	Lids open; pinna flat; stays folded	Slightly curved pinna; soft; slow recoil	Well curved pinna; soft but ready recoil	Formed and firm, instant recoil	Thick cartilage, ear stiff	
Genitals (male)	Scrotum flat, smooth	Scrotum empty, faint rugae	Testes in upper canal, rare rugae	Testes descending, few rugae	Testes down, good rugae	Testes pendulous, deep rugae	
Genitals (female)	Clitoris prominent, labia flat	Clitoris prominent, small labia minora	Clitoris prominent, enlarging minora	Majora and minora equally prominent	Majora large, minora small	Majora cover clitoris and minora	

Maturity Rating

Score	Weeks
–10	20
–5	22
0	24
5	26
10	28
15	30
20	32
25	34
30	36
35	38
40	40
45	42
50	44

Fig. 288–1. Assessment of gestational age—new Ballard score. Scores from neuromuscular and physical domains are added to obtain total score. (Adapted from Ballard JL, Khoury JC, Wedig K, et al: New Ballard score, expanded to include extremely premature infants. *The Journal of Pediatrics* 119(3):417–423, 1991; used with permission of the CV Mosby Company.)

Head and neck: In a vertex delivery, the head is commonly molded with overriding of the cranial bones at the sutures and some swelling and ecchymosis of the scalp (caput succedaneum). In a breech delivery, the head has less molding, with swelling and ecchymosis occurring in the presenting part (ie, buttocks, genitals, or feet). The fontanelles vary in diameter from a fingertip breadth to several centimeters. A large anterior fontanelle may be a sign of hypothyroidism.

A cephalohematoma is a common finding (see p. 2794); blood accumulates between the periosteum and the bone, producing a swelling that does not cross suture lines. It may occur over one or both parietal bones and occasionally over the occiput. Cephalohematomas usually are not evident until soft-tissue edema subsides; they gradually disappear over several months.

Head size and shape are inspected to detect congenital hydrocephalus.

Numerous genetic syndromes cause craniofacial abnormalities. The face is inspected for symmetry and normal development, particularly of the mandible, palate, pinnae, and external auditory canals.

The eyes may be easier to examine the day after birth because the birth process causes swelling around the eyelids. Eyes should be examined for the red reflex; its absence may indicate glaucoma, cataracts, or retinoblastoma. Subconjunctival hemorrhages are common and caused by forces exerted during delivery.

Low-set ears may indicate genetic anomalies, including trisomy 21 (Down syndrome). Malformed ears, external auditory canals, or both may be present in many genetic syndromes. Clinicians should look for external ear pits or tags, which are sometimes associated with hearing loss and kidney abnormalities.

The clinician should inspect and palpate the palate to check for soft or hard palate defects. Orofacial clefts are among the most common congenital defects. Some neonates are born with an epulis (a benign hamartoma of the gum), which, if large enough, can cause feeding difficulties and may obstruct the airway. These lesions can be removed; they do not recur. Some neonates are born with primary or natal teeth. Natal teeth do not have roots and may need to be removed to prevent them from falling out and being aspirated. Inclusion cysts called Epstein pearls may occur on the roof of the mouth.

When examining the neck, the clinician must lift the chin to look for abnormalities such as cystic hygromas, goiters, and branchial arch remnants. Torticollis can be caused by a sternocleidomastoid hematoma due to birth trauma.

Abdomen and pelvis: The abdomen should be round and symmetric. A scaphoid abdomen may indicate a diaphragmatic hernia (see p. 2523), allowing the intestine to migrate through it to the chest cavity in utero; pulmonary hypoplasia and postnatal respiratory distress may result. An asymmetric abdomen suggests an abdominal mass.

Splenomegaly suggests congenital infection or hemolytic anemia.

The kidneys may be palpable with deep palpation; the left is more easily palpated than the right. Large kidneys may indicate obstruction, tumor, or cystic disease.

The liver is normally palpable 1 to 2 cm below the costal margin. An umbilical hernia, due to a weakness of the umbilical ring musculature, is common but rarely significant. The presence of a normally placed, patent anus should be confirmed.

In boys, the penis should be examined for hypospadias or epispadias. In term boys, the testes should be in the scrotum. Scrotal swelling may signify hydrocele, inguinal hernia, or, more rarely, testicular torsion. With hydrocele, the scrotum transilluminates. Torsion, a surgical emergency, causes ecchymosis and firmness.

In term girls, the labia are prominent. Mucoid vaginal and serosanguineous secretions (pseudomenses) are normal; they result from exposure to maternal hormones in utero and withdrawal at birth. A small tag of hymenal tissue at the posterior fourchette, believed to be due to maternal hormonal stimulation, is sometimes present but disappears over a few weeks.

Ambiguous genitals (intersex) may indicate several uncommon disorders (eg, congenital adrenal hyperplasia; 5 alpha-reductase deficiency; Klinefelter syndrome, Turner syndrome, or Swyer syndrome). Referral to an endocrinologist is indicated for evaluation as is a discussion with the family about benefits and risks of immediate vs delayed sex assignment.

Musculoskeletal system: The extremities are examined for deformities, amputations (incomplete or missing limbs), contractures, and maldevelopment. Brachial nerve palsy due to birth trauma may manifest as limited or no spontaneous arm movement on the affected side, sometimes with adduction and internal rotation of the shoulder and pronation of the forearm.

The spine is inspected for signs of spina bifida, particularly exposure of the meninges, spinal cord, or both (meningomyelocele).

Orthopedic examination includes palpation of long bones for birth trauma (particularly clavicle fracture) but focuses on detection of hip dysplasia. Risk factors for dysplasia include female sex, breech position in utero, twin gestation, and family history. The Barlow and Ortolani maneuvers are used to check for dysplasia. These maneuvers must be done when neonates are quiet. The starting position is the same for both: Neonates are placed on their back with their hips and knees flexed to 90° (the feet will be off the bed), feet facing the clinician, who places an index finger on the greater trochanter and a thumb on the lesser trochanter.

For the **Barlow maneuver,** the clinician adducts the hip (ie, the knee is drawn across the body) while pushing the thigh posteriorly. A clunk indicates that the head of the femur has moved out of the acetabulum; the Ortolani maneuver then relocates it and confirms the diagnosis.

For the **Ortolani maneuver,** the hip is returned to the starting position; then the hip being tested is abducted (ie, the knee is moved away from the midline toward the examining table into a frog-leg position) and gently pulled anteriorly. A palpable clunk of the femoral head with abduction signifies movement of an already dislocated femoral head into the acetabulum and constitutes a positive test for hip dysplasia.

The maneuvers may be falsely negative in infants > 3 mo because of tighter hip muscles and ligaments. If the examination is equivocal or the infant is at high risk (eg, girls who were in the breech position), hip ultrasonography should be done at 4 to 6 wk; some experts recommend screening ultrasonography at 4 to 6 wk for all infants with risk factors.

Neurologic system: The neonate's tone, level of alertness, movement of extremities, and reflexes are evaluated. Typically, neonatal reflexes, including the Moro, suck, and rooting reflexes, are elicited:

- Moro reflex: The neonate's response to startle is elicited by pulling the arms slightly off the bed and releasing suddenly. In response, the neonate extends the arms with fingers extended, flexes the hips, and cries.
- Rooting reflex: Stroking the neonate's cheek or lateral lip prompts the neonate to turn the head toward the touch and open the mouth.
- Suck reflex: A pacifier or gloved finger is used to elicit this reflex.

These reflexes are present for several months after birth and are markers of a normal peripheral nervous system.

Skin: A neonate's skin is usually ruddy; cyanosis of fingers and toes is common in the first few hours. Vernix caseosa covers most neonates > 24 wk gestation. Dryness and peeling often develop within days, especially at wrist and ankle creases.

Petechiae may occur in areas traumatized during delivery, such as the face when the face is the presenting part; however, neonates with diffuse petechiae should be evaluated for thrombocytopenia.

Many neonates have erythema toxicum, a benign rash with an erythematous base and a white or yellow papule. This rash, which usually appears 24 h after birth, is scattered over the body and can last for up to 2 wk.

Screening Tests for Newborns

Screening recommendations vary by clinical context and state requirements.

Blood typing is indicated when the mother has type O or Rh-negative blood or when minor blood antigens are present because hemolytic disease of the newborn (see p. 2347) is a risk.

All neonates are evaluated for jaundice throughout the hospital stay and before discharge. The risk of hyperbilirubinemia is assessed using risk criteria, measurement of bilirubin, or both. Bilirubin can be measured transcutaneously or in serum. Many hospitals screen all neonates and use a predictive nomogram to determine the risk of extreme hyperbilirubinemia. Follow-up is based on age at discharge, predischarge bilirubin level, and risk of developing jaundice.

Most states test for specific inherited diseases, including phenylketonuria, tyrosinemia, biotinidase deficiency, homocystinuria, maple syrup urine disease, galactosemia, congenital adrenal hyperplasia, sickle cell disease, and hypothyroidism. Some states also include testing for cystic fibrosis, disorders of fatty acid oxidation, other organic acidemias, and severe combined immunodeficiency.

HIV screening is required by some states and is indicated for children of mothers known to be HIV-positive or those engaging in HIV high-risk behaviors.

Toxicology screening is indicated when any of the following are present: maternal history of drug use, unexplained placental abruption, unexplained premature labor, poor prenatal care, or evidence of drug withdrawal in the neonate.

Screening for critical congenital heart disease (CCHD) using pulse oximetry is now part of routine newborn assessment. Previously, newborns were screened for CCHD by prenatal ultrasonography and by physical examination, but this approach failed to identify many cases of CCHD, which led to increased morbidity and mortality. The screening is done when infants are ≥ 24 h old and is considered positive if

- Any oxygen saturation measurement is < 90%.
- The oxygen saturation measurements in both the right hand and foot are < 95% on 3 separate measurements taken 1 h apart.
- There is > 3% absolute difference between the oxygen saturation in the right hand (preductal) and foot (postductal) on 3 separate measurements taken 1 h apart.

Any infant with a positive screen should have additional testing, including chest x-ray, ECG, and echocardiography. The infant's pediatrician should be notified, and the infant may need to be evaluated by a cardiologist.

Hearing screening varies by state. Hearing loss is one of the most frequently occurring birth defects. About 3/1000 infants are born with moderate, profound, or severe hearing loss. Hearing loss is even more common among infants admitted to ICUs at birth. Currently, some states screen only high-risk neonates (see Table 288–2); others screen all neonates. Initial screening often involves using a handheld device to test for echoes produced by healthy ears in response to soft clicks (otoacoustic emissions); if this test is abnormal, auditory brain stem response (ABR) testing is done. Some institutions use ABR testing as an initial screening test. Further testing by an audiologist may be needed.

Table 288–2. HIGH-RISK FACTORS FOR HEARING DEFICITS IN NEONATES

FACTOR	SPECIFICS
Birth weight	< 1500 g
Apgar score	≤ 7 at 5 min
Serum bilirubin	> 22 mg/dL (> 376 μmol/L) in neonate whose birth weight is > 2000 g > 17 mg/dL (> 290 μmol/L) in neonate whose birth weight is < 2000 g
Disorders	Perinatal anoxia or hypoxia Neonatal sepsis or meningitis Craniofacial abnormalities Seizures or apneic spells
Congenital infections	Rubella Syphilis Herpes simplex infection Cytomegalovirus infection Toxoplasmosis
Maternal exposure	Aminoglycosides
Family history	Early hearing loss in a parent or close relative

Routine Infant Care and Observation

Neonates can be bathed (if the parents wish) once their temperature has stabilized at 37° C for 2 h.

The umbilical cord clamp can be removed when the cord appears dry, usually at 24 h. Umbilical cord care is aimed at reducing the risk of umbilical infection (omphalitis). The umbilical stump should be kept clean and dry; other care varies depending on the birth setting. In a hospital delivery (or properly managed home birth), where the cord is clamped and cut aseptically, dry cord care or cleansing with soap and water is adequate; topical agents do not decrease risk of infection. However, when cord clamping and/or cutting is not aseptic (eg, in some developing countries, precipitous out-of-hospital deliveries), applying a topical antiseptic (eg, chlorhexidine) to the cord reduces the risk of omphalitis and neonatal mortality. The cord should be observed daily for redness or drainage.

Circumcision, if desired by the family, can be safely done, using a local anesthetic, within the first few days of life. Circumcision should be delayed if the mother has taken anticoagulants or aspirin, if there is a family history of bleeding disorders, or if the neonate has displacement of the urethral meatus, hypospadias, or any other abnormality of the glans or penis (because the prepuce may be used later in plastic surgical repair). Circumcision should not be done if the neonate has hemophilia or another bleeding disorder.

Most neonates lose 5 to 7% of their birth weight during the first few days of life, primarily because fluid is lost in urine and insensibly and secondarily because meconium is passed, vernix caseosa is lost, and the umbilical cord dries.

In the first 2 days, urine may stain the diaper orange or pink because of urate crystals, which are a normal result of urine concentration. Most neonates void within 24 h after birth; the average time of first void is 7 to 9 h after birth, and most void at least 2 times in the 2nd 24 h of life. A delay in voiding is more common among male neonates and may result from a tight foreskin; a male neonate's inability to void may indicate posterior urethral valves. Circumcision is usually delayed until at least after the first void; not voiding within 12 h of the procedure may indicate a complication.

If meconium has not been passed within 24 h, the clinician should consider evaluating the neonate for anatomic abnormalities, such as imperforate anus, Hirschsprung disease, and cystic fibrosis (which can cause meconium ileus).

Hospital Discharge

Neonates discharged within 48 h should be evaluated within 2 to 3 days to assess feeding success (breast or formula), hydration, and jaundice (for those at increased risk). Follow-up for neonates discharged after 48 h should be based on risk factors, including those for jaundice and for breastfeeding difficulties, and any identified problems.

NUTRITION IN INFANTS

If the delivery was uncomplicated and the neonate is alert and healthy, the neonate can be brought to the mother for feeding immediately. Successful breastfeeding is enhanced by putting the neonate to the breast as soon as possible after delivery. Spitting mucus after feeding is common (because gastroesophageal

Table 288–3. CALORIE REQUIREMENTS AT DIFFERENT AGES*

	REQUIREMENT	
AGE	kcal/lb/day	kcal/kg/day
< 6 mo	50–55	110–120
1 yr	45	95–100
15 yr	20	44

*When protein and calories are provided by breast milk that is completely digested and absorbed, the requirements between 3 mo and 9 mo of age may be lower.

smooth muscle is lax) but should subside within 48 h. If spitting mucus or emesis persists past 48 h or if vomit is bilious, complete evaluation of the upper GI and respiratory tracts is needed to detect congenital GI anomalies.

Daily fluid and calorie requirements vary with age and are proportionately greater in neonates and infants than in older children and adults (see Table 288–3). Relative requirements for protein and energy (g or kcal/kg body weight) decline progressively from the end of infancy through adolescence (see Table 1–4 on p. 4), but absolute requirements increase. For example, protein requirements decrease from 1.2 g/kg/day at 1 yr to 0.9 g/kg/day at 18 yr, and mean relative energy requirements decrease from 100 kcal/kg at 1 yr to 40 kcal/kg in late adolescence.

Nutritional recommendations are generally not evidence-based. Requirements for vitamins depend on the source of nutrition (eg, breast milk vs standard infant formula), maternal dietary factors, and daily intake.

Feeding problems: Minor variations in day-to-day food intake are common and, although often of concern to parents, usually require only reassurance and guidance unless there are signs of disease or changes in growth parameters, particularly weight (changes in the child's percentile rank on standard growth charts are more significant than absolute changes).

Loss of > 5 to 7% of birth weight in the first week indicates undernutrition. Birth weight should be regained by 2 wk, and a subsequent gain of about 20 to 30 g/day (1 oz/day) is expected for the first few months. Infants should double their birth weight by about 6 mo.

BREASTFEEDING

Breast milk is the nutrition of choice. The American Academy of Pediatrics (AAP) recommends exclusive breastfeeding for a minimum of 6 mo and introduction of appropriate solid food from 6 mo to 1 yr. Beyond 1 yr, breastfeeding continues for as long as both infant and mother desire, although after 1 yr breastfeeding should complement a full diet of solid foods and fluids. To encourage breastfeeding, practitioners should begin discussions prenatally, mentioning the multiple advantages:

- For the child: Nutritional and cognitive advantages and protection against infection, allergies, obesity, Crohn disease, and diabetes
- For the mother: Reduced fertility during lactation, more rapid return to normal prepartum condition (eg, uterine involution, weight loss), and protection against osteoporosis, obesity, and ovarian and premenopausal breast cancers

Milk production is fully established in primiparas by 72 to 96 h and in less time in multiparas. The first milk produced is colostrum, a high-calorie, high-protein, thin yellow fluid that is immunoprotective because it is rich in antibodies, lymphocytes, and macrophages; colostrum also stimulates passage of meconium. Subsequent breast milk has the following characteristics:

- Has a high lactose content, providing a readily available energy source compatible with neonatal enzymes
- Contains large amounts of vitamin E, an important antioxidant that may help prevent anemia by increasing erythrocyte life span
- Has a calcium:phosphorus ratio of 2:1, which prevents calcium-deficiency tetany
- Favorably changes the pH of stools and the intestinal flora, thus protecting against bacterial diarrhea
- Transfers protective antibodies from mother to infant
- Contains cholesterol and taurine, which are important to brain growth, regardless of the mother's diet
- Is a natural source of omega-3 and omega-6 fatty acids

These fatty acids and their very long-chain polyunsaturated derivatives (LC-PUFAS), arachidonic acid (ARA) and docosahexaenoic acid (DHA), are believed to contribute to the enhanced visual and cognitive outcomes of breastfed compared with formula-fed infants. Most commercial formulas are now supplemented with ARA and DHA to more closely resemble breast milk and to reduce these potential developmental differences.

If the mother's diet is sufficiently diverse, no dietary or vitamin supplementation is needed for the mother or her term breastfed infant. However, to prevent vitamin D deficiency rickets, vitamin D 400 units once/day beginning in the first 2 mo is given to all infants who are exclusively breastfed. Premature and dark-skinned infants and infants with limited sunlight exposure (residence in northern climates) are especially at risk of vitamin D deficiency. After 6 mo, breastfed infants in homes where the water does not have adequate fluoride (supplemental or natural) should be given fluoride drops. Clinicians can obtain information about fluoride content from a local dentist or health department.

Infants < 6 mo should not be given additional water because hyponatremia is a risk.

Breastfeeding Technique

The mother should use whatever comfortable, relaxed position works best and should support her breast with her hand to ensure that it is centered in the infant's mouth, minimizing any soreness. The center of the infant's lower lip should be stimulated with the nipple so that rooting occurs and the mouth opens wide. The infant should be encouraged to take in as much of the breast and areola as possible, placing the lips 2.5 to 4 cm from the base of the nipple. The infant's tongue then compresses the nipple against the hard palate. Initially, it takes at least 2 min for the let-down reflex to occur.

Volume of milk increases as the infant grows and stimulation from suckling increases. Feeding duration is usually determined by the infant.

Some mothers require a breast pump to increase or maintain milk production; in most mothers, a total of 90 min/day of breast pumping divided into 6 to 8 sessions produces enough milk for an infant who is not directly breastfed.

The infant should nurse on one breast until the breast softens and suckling slows or stops. The mother can then break suction with a finger before removing the infant from one breast and offering the infant the other breast. In the first days after birth, infants may nurse on only one side; then the mother should alternate sides with each feeding. If the infant tends to fall asleep before adequately nursing, the mother can remove the infant when suckling slows, burp the infant, and move the infant to the other side. This switch keeps the infant awake for feedings and stimulates milk production in both breasts.

Mothers should be encouraged to feed on demand or about every 1½ to 3 h (8 to 12 feedings/day), a frequency that gradually decreases over time; some neonates < 2500 g may need to feed even more frequently to prevent hypoglycemia. In the first few days, neonates may need to be wakened and stimulated; small infants and late preterm infants should not be allowed to sleep long periods at night. Large full-term infants who are feeding well (as evidenced by stooling pattern) can sleep longer. Eventually, a schedule that allows infants to sleep as long as possible at night is usually best for the infant and family.

Mothers who work outside the home can pump breast milk to maintain milk production while they are separated from their infants. Frequency varies but should approximate the infant's feeding schedule. Pumped breast milk should be immediately refrigerated if it is to be used within 48 h and immediately frozen if it is to be used after 48 h. Refrigerated milk that is not used within 96 h should be discarded because risk of bacterial contamination is high. Frozen milk should be thawed by placing it in warm water; microwaving is not recommended.

Infant Breastfeeding Complications

The primary complication is underfeeding, which may lead to dehydration and hyperbilirubinemia. Risk factors for underfeeding include small or premature infants and mothers who are primiparous, who become ill, or who have had difficult or operative deliveries.

A rough assessment of feeding adequacy can be made by daily diaper counts. By age 5 days, a normal neonate wets at least 6 diapers/day and soils at least 4 diapers/day; lower numbers suggest underhydration and undernutrition. Also, stools should have changed from dark meconium at birth to light brown and then yellow. Weight is also a reasonable parameter to follow (see p. 2415); not attaining growth landmarks suggests undernutrition. Constant fussiness before age 6 wk (when colic may develop unrelated to hunger or thirst) may also indicate underfeeding.

Dehydration should be suspected if vigor of the infant's cry decreases or skin becomes turgid; lethargy and sleepiness are extreme signs of dehydration and should prompt testing for hypernatremia.

Maternal Breastfeeding Complications

Common maternal complications include breast engorgement, sore nipples, plugged ducts, mastitis, and anxiety.

Breast engorgement, which occurs during early lactation and may last 24 to 48 h, may be minimized by early frequent feeding. A comfortable nursing brassiere worn 24 h/day can help, as can applying cool compresses after breastfeeding and taking a mild analgesic (eg, ibuprofen). Just before breastfeeding, mothers may have to use massage and warm compresses and express breast milk manually to allow infants to get the swollen areola into their mouth. After breastfeeding, cool compresses reduce engorgement and provide further relief. Excessive expression of milk between feedings facilitates engorgement, so expression should be done only enough to relieve discomfort.

For **sore nipples,** the infant's position should be checked; sometimes the infant draws in a lip and sucks it, which irritates the nipple. The mother can ease the lip out with her thumb. After feedings, she can express a little milk, letting the milk dry on the nipples. After breastfeeding, cool compresses reduce engorgement and provide further relief.

Plugged ducts manifest as mildly tender lumps in the breasts of lactating women who have no other systemic signs of illness. Continued breastfeeding ensures adequate emptying of the breast. Warm compresses and massage of the affected area before breastfeeding may further aid emptying. Women may also alternate positions because different areas of the breast empty better depending on the infant's position at the breast. A good nursing brassiere is helpful because regular brassieres with wire stays or constricting straps may contribute to milk stasis in a compressed area.

Mastitis is common and manifests as a tender, warm, swollen, wedge-shaped area of breast. It is caused by engorgement, blocking, or plugging of an area of the breast; infection may occur secondarily, most often with penicillin-resistant *Staphylococcus aureus* and less commonly with *Streptococcus* sp or *Escherichia coli*. With infection, fever ≥ 38.5° C, chills, and flu-like aching may develop. Diagnosis of mastitis is by history and examination. Cell counts (WBCs > 10^6/mL) and cultures of breast milk (bacteria > 10^3/mL) may distinguish infectious from noninfectious mastitis. If symptoms are mild and present < 24 h, conservative management (milk removal via breastfeeding or pumping, compresses, analgesics, a supportive brassiere, and stress reduction) may be sufficient. If symptoms do not lessen in 12 to 24 h or if the woman is acutely ill, antibiotics that are safe for breastfeeding infants and effective against *S. aureus* (eg, dicloxacillin, cloxacillin, or cephalexin 500 mg po qid) should be started; duration of treatment is 7 to 14 days. Community-acquired methicillin-resistant *S. aureus* should be considered if cases do not respond promptly to these measures or if an abscess is present. Complications of delayed treatment are recurrence and abscess formation. Breastfeeding may continue during treatment.

Maternal anxiety, frustration, and feelings of inadequacy may result from lack of experience with breastfeeding, mechanical difficulties holding the infant and getting the infant to latch on and suck, fatigue, difficulty assessing whether nourishment is adequate, and postpartum physiologic changes. These factors and emotions are the most common reasons mothers stop breastfeeding. Early follow-up with a pediatrician or consultation with a lactation specialist is helpful and effective for preventing early breastfeeding termination.

Drugs and Breastfeeding

Breastfeeding mothers should avoid taking drugs if possible. When drug therapy is necessary, the mother should avoid contraindicated drugs and drugs that suppress lactation (eg, bromocriptine, levodopa, trazodone). The US National Library of Medicine maintains an extensive database regarding drugs and breastfeeding, which should be consulted regarding use of or exposure to specific drugs or classes of drugs. For some common drugs contraindicated for breastfeeding mothers, see Table 288–4.

When drug treatment is necessary, the safest known alternative should be used; when possible, most drugs should be taken immediately after breastfeeding or before the infant's longest sleep period, although this strategy is less helpful with neonates who nurse frequently and exclusively. Knowledge of the adverse effects of most drugs comes from case reports and small studies. Safety of some drugs (eg, acetaminophen, ibuprofen, cephalosporins, insulin) has been determined by extensive research, but others are considered safe only because there are no case reports of adverse effects. Drugs with a long history of use are generally safer than newer drugs for which few data exist.

Table 288–4. SOME DRUGS CONTRAINDICATED FOR BREASTFEEDING MOTHERS

DRUG CLASS	EXAMPLES	GENERAL CONCERNS AND SPECIFIC EFFECTS IN INFANTS
Anticoagulants	Dicumarol Warfarin	May be given cautiously but, in very large doses, may cause hemorrhage (heparin is not excreted in milk)
Cytotoxic drugs	Cyclophosphamide Cyclosporine Doxorubicin Methotrexate	May interfere with cellular metabolism of a breastfeeding infant, causing possible immunosuppression and neutropenia Unknown effect on growth and unknown association with carcinogenesis
Psychoactive drugs	Anxiolytics, including benzodiazepines (alprazolam, diazepam, lorazepam, midazolam, prazepam, quazepam, temazepam) and perphenazine Antidepressants (tricyclics, SSRIs, bupropion) Antipsychotics (chlorpromazine, chlorprothixene, clozapine, haloperidol, mesoridazine, trifluoperazine)	For most psychoactive drugs, unknown effect on infants, but because drugs and metabolites appear in breast milk and in infant plasma and tissues, possible alteration of short-term and long-term CNS function Fluoxetine: Linked to colic, irritability, feeding problems and sleep disorders, and slow weight gain Chlorpromazine: Possible drowsiness, lethargy, decline in developmental scores Haloperidol: Decline in developmental scores
Individual drugs that are detectable in breast milk and pose theoretical risk	Amiodarone	Possible hypothyroidism
	Chloramphenicol	Possible idiosyncratic bone marrow suppression
	Clofazimine	Potential for transfer of high percentage of maternal dose Possible increase in skin pigmentation
	Corticosteroids	With large maternal doses given for weeks or months, can produce high concentrations in milk and may suppress growth and interfere with endogenous corticosteroid production in the infant
	Lamotrigine	Potential for therapeutic serum concentrations in the infant
	Metoclopramide	None described
	Metronidazole Tinidazole	In vitro mutagens May stop breastfeeding for 12–24 h to allow excretion of dose when a mother is given a single dose of 2 g Safe after the infant is 6 mo
	Sulfapyridine Sulfisoxazole	Caution required if infants have jaundice or G6PD deficiency or are ill, stressed, or premature
Individual drugs that are detectable in breast milk and have documented risk	Acebutolol	Hypotension, bradycardia, tachypnea
	Aminosalicylic acid	Diarrhea
	Atenolol	Cyanosis, bradycardia
	Bromocriptine	Suppresses lactation May be hazardous to the mother
	Aspirin (salicylates)	Metabolic acidosis With large maternal doses and sustained use, may produce plasma concentrations that increase risk of hyperbilirubinemia (salicylates compete for albumin-binding sites) and hemolysis only in G6PD-deficient infants who are < 1 mo
	Clemastine	Drowsiness, irritability, refusal to feed, high-pitched cry, neck stiffness
	Ergotamine	Vomiting, diarrhea, seizures (with doses used in migraine drugs)
	Estradiol	Withdrawal vaginal bleeding
	Iodides Iodine	Goiter
	Lithium	$^1/_3$ to $^1/_2$ therapeutic blood concentration in infants
	Phenobarbital	Sedation, infantile spasms after weaning, methemoglobinemia
	Phenytoin	Methemoglobinemia
	Primidone	Sedation, feeding problems
	Sulfasalazine (salicylazosulfapyridine)	Bloody diarrhea
	Nitrofurantoin, sulfapyridine, sulfisoxazole	Hemolysis in infants with G6PD deficiency; safe in others

Table continues on the following page.

Table 288–4. SOME DRUGS CONTRAINDICATED FOR BREASTFEEDING MOTHERS (*Continued*)

DRUG CLASS	EXAMPLES	GENERAL CONCERNS AND SPECIFIC EFFECTS IN INFANTS
Drugs of abuse*	Amphetamine	Irritability, poor sleeping pattern
	Alcohol	With < 1 g/kg daily, decreased milk ejection reflex With large amounts, drowsiness, diaphoresis, deep sleep, weakness, decrease in linear growth, abnormal weight gain in the infant
	Cocaine	Cocaine intoxication: Irritability, vomiting, diarrhea, tremulousness, seizures
	Heroin	Tremors, restlessness, vomiting, poor feeding
	Marijuana	Components detectable in breast milk but effects uncertain
	Phencyclidine	Hallucinogen

*Effects of smoking are unclear; nicotine is detectable in breast milk, and smoking decreases breast milk production and infant weight gain but may decrease incidence of respiratory illness.

Data from Committee on Drugs of the American Pediatric Association: The transfer of drugs and other chemicals into human milk. *Pediatrics* 108(3):776–789, 2001.

Weaning

Weaning can occur whenever the mother and infant mutually desire, although preferably not until the infant is at least 12 mo old. Gradual weaning over weeks or months during the time solid food is introduced is most common; some mothers and infants stop abruptly without problems, but others continue breastfeeding 1 or 2 times/day for 18 to 24 mo or longer. There is no correct schedule.

FORMULA FEEDING

The only acceptable alternative to breastfeeding during the first year is formula; water can cause hyponatremia, and whole cow's milk is not nutritionally complete. Advantages of formula feeding include the ability to quantify the amount of nourishment and the ability of family members to participate in feedings. But all other factors being equal, these advantages are outweighed by the undisputed health benefits of breastfeeding.

Commercial infant formulas are available as powders, concentrated liquids, and prediluted (ready-to-feed) liquids; each contains vitamins, and most are supplemented with iron. Formula should be prepared with fluoridated water; fluoride drops (0.25 mg/day po) should be given after age 6 mo in areas where fluoridated water is unavailable and when using prediluted liquid formula, which is prepared with nonfluoridated water.

Choice of formula is based on infant need. Cow's milk–based formula is the standard choice unless spitting up, diarrhea (with or without blood), rash (hives), or poor weight gain suggests sensitivity to cow's milk protein or lactose intolerance (extremely rare in neonates); then, a change in formula may be recommended. All soy formulas in the US are lactose free, but some infants allergic to cow's milk protein may also be allergic to soy protein; then, a hydrolyzed formula is indicated. Hydrolyzed formulas are derived from cow's milk, but the proteins are broken down into smaller chains, making them less allergenic. True elemental formulas made from free amino acids are available for the few infants who have allergic reactions to hydrolyzed formula.

Bottle-fed infants are fed on demand, but because formula is digested more slowly than breast milk, they typically can go longer between feedings, initially every 3 to 4 h. Initial volumes of 15 to 60 mL (0.5 to 2 oz) can be increased gradually during the first week of life up to 90 mL (3 oz) about 6 times/day, which supplies about 120 kcal/kg at 1 wk for a 3-kg infant.

SOLID FOODS IN INFANCY

The WHO recommends exclusive breastfeeding for about 6 mo, with introduction of solid foods thereafter. Other organizations suggest introducing solid food between age 4 mo and 6 mo while continuing breastfeeding or bottle-feeding. Before 4 mo, solid food is not needed nutritionally and may be associated with an increased risk of food allergies, and the extrusion reflex, in which the tongue pushes out anything placed in the mouth, makes feeding of solids difficult.

Some evidence suggests that the early introduction of some foods (eg, egg, peanuts, wheat) might actually be protective against the development of food allergies.[1] In 2008, the American Academy of Pediatrics released guidelines stating there is no current evidence that delaying the introduction of solid food (including egg and peanuts) beyond 4 to 6 mo is protective against the development of food allergies.[2] However, there is still insufficient data to definitively show that early introduction of these foods *prevents* the development of a food allergy. Thus, the introduction of any specific solid food need not be delayed beyond 4 to 6 mo in most children. Exceptions may be children who have older siblings who have a peanut allergy because these younger children have an almost 7-fold increased risk of developing a peanut allergy. Skin testing of these younger children should be considered before introducing peanuts.[3]

Initially, solid foods should be introduced after breastfeeding or bottle-feeding to ensure adequate nourishment. Iron-fortified rice cereal is traditionally the first food introduced because it is nonallergenic, easily digested, and a needed source of iron.

It is generally recommended that only one new, single-ingredient food be introduced per week so that food allergies can be identified. Foods need not be introduced in any specific order, although in general they can gradually be introduced by increasingly coarser textures—eg, from rice cereal to soft table food to chopped table food.

Meat, pureed to prevent aspiration, is a good source of iron and zinc (both of which can be limited in the diet of an exclusively breastfed infant) and is therefore a good early complementary food.

Vegetarian infants can get adequate iron from iron-fortified cereals and grains, green leafy vegetables, and dried beans and adequate zinc from yeast-fermented whole-grain breads and fortified infant cereals.

Home preparations are equivalent to commercial foods, but commercial preparations of carrots, beets, turnips, collard greens, and spinach are preferable before 1 yr if available because they are screened for nitrates. High nitrate levels, which can induce methemoglobinemia in young children, are present when vegetables are grown using water supplies contaminated by fertilizer.

Foods to avoid include

- Honey until 1 yr because infant botulism is a risk
- Foods that, if aspirated, could obstruct the child's airway (eg, whole nuts, round candies, popcorn, hot dogs, meat unless it is pureed, grapes unless they are cut into small pieces)

Whole nuts should be avoided until age 2 or 3 yr because they do not fully dissolve with mastication and small pieces can be aspirated whether bronchial obstruction is present or not, causing pneumonia and other complications.

At or after 1 yr, children can begin drinking whole cow's milk; reduced-fat milk is avoided until 2 yr, when their diet essentially resembles that of the rest of the family. Parents should be advised to limit milk intake to 16 to 24 oz/day in young children; higher intake can reduce intake of other important sources of nutrition and contribute to iron deficiency.

Juice is a poor source of nutrition, contributes to dental caries, and should be limited to 4 to 6 oz/day or avoided altogether.

By about 1 yr, growth rate usually slows. Children require less food and may refuse it at some meals. Parents should be reassured and advised to assess a child's intake over a week rather than at a single meal or during a day. Underfeeding of solid food is only a concern when children do not achieve expected weights at an appropriate rate.

1. Du Toit G, Katz Y, Sasieni P, et al: Early consumption of peanuts in infancy is associated with a low prevalence of peanut allergy. *J Allergy Clin Immunol* 122:984–991, 2008. doi: 10.1016/j.jaci.2008.08.039.
2. Greer FR, Sicherer SH, Burks AW, American Academy of Pediatrics Committee on Nutrition; American Academy of Pediatrics Section on Allergy and Immunology: Effects of early nutritional interventions on the development of atopic disease in infants and children: The role of maternal dietary restriction, breastfeeding, timing of introduction of complementary foods, and hydrolyzed formulas. *Pediatrics* 121:183–191, 2008. doi: 10.1542/peds.2007-3022.
3. Liem JJ, Huq S, Kozyrskyj AL, Becker AB: Should younger siblings of peanut-allergic children be assessed by an allergist before being fed peanut? *Allergy Asthma Clin Immunol* 4:144–1499, 2008. doi: 10.1186/1710-1492-4-4-144.

SLEEPING IN INFANTS AND CHILDREN

Sleep behaviors are culturally determined, and problems tend to be defined as behaviors that vary from accepted customs or norms. In cultures where children sleep separately from their parents in the same house, sleep problems are among the most common that parents and children face.

The supine sleep position is recommended for every sleep period for all infants to reduce the risk of sudden infant death syndrome (SIDS). Prone or side sleep positions place infants at high risk of SIDS, particularly for those who are placed on their side and found on their stomach.

Co-sleeping is when parent and infant sleep in close proximity (on the same surface or different surfaces) so as to be able to see, hear, and/or touch each other. Co-sleeping arrangements can include

- Bed-sharing (the infant sleeps on the same surface as the parent)
- Room-sharing (the infant sleeps in the same room as the parent in close proximity)

Parent-infant bed-sharing is common but controversial. There are often cultural and personal reasons why parents choose to bed-share, including convenience for feeding, bonding, believing their own vigilance is the only way to keep their infant safe, and believing that bed-sharing allows them to maintain vigilance even while sleeping. However, bed-sharing has been associated with an increased risk of SIDS as well as infant injury or death resulting from suffocation, strangulation, and entrapment.

Room-sharing without bed-sharing allows for close proximity to the infant and for the facilitation of feeding, comforting, and monitoring; is safer than bed-sharing or solitary sleeping (the infant sleeps in a separate room); and is associated with a decreased risk of SIDS. For these reasons, room-sharing without bed-sharing is the recommended sleeping arrangement for parents and infants in the first few months of life.

Infants usually adapt to a day-night sleep schedule between 4 and 6 mo. Sleep problems beyond these ages take many forms, including difficulty falling asleep at night, frequent nighttime awakening, atypical daytime napping, and dependence on feeding or on being held before being able to go to sleep. These problems are related to parental expectations, the child's temperament and biologic rhythms, and child-parent interactions.

Factors that influence sleep patterns vary by age. For infants, inborn biologic patterns are central. At 9 mo and again around 18 mo, sleep disturbances become common because

- Separation anxiety develops.
- Children can move independently and control their environment.
- They may take long late-afternoon naps.
- They may become overstimulated while playing before bedtime.
- Nightmares tend to become more common.

In toddlers and older children, emotional factors and established habits become more important. Stressful events (eg, moving, illness) may cause acute sleep problems in older children.

Evaluation

History: History focuses on the child's sleeping environment, consistency of bedtime, bedtime routines, and parental expectations. A detailed description of the child's average day can be useful. The history should probe for stressors in the child's life, such as difficulties in school, as well as exposure to unsettling television programs and caffeinated beverages (eg, sodas). Reports of inconsistent bedtimes, a noisy or chaotic environment, or frequent attempts by the child to manipulate parents by using sleep behaviors suggest the need for lifestyle changes. Extreme parental frustration suggests tension within the family or parents who are having difficulty being consistent and firm.

A sleep diary compiled over several nights may help identify unusual sleep patterns and sleep disorders (eg, sleepwalking, night terrors). Careful questioning of older children and adolescents about school, friends, anxieties, depressive symptoms, and overall state of mind often reveals a source for a sleep problem.

Physical examination and testing: Examination and diagnostic testing generally yield little useful information.

Treatment

- Options for parents
- Measures to help children fall asleep on their own

The clinician's role in treatment is to present explanations and options to parents, who must implement changes to get the child on an acceptable sleep schedule. Approaches vary with age and circumstances. Infants are often comforted by swaddling, ambient noise, and movement. However, always rocking infants to sleep does not allow them to learn how to fall asleep on their own, which is an important developmental task. As a substitute for rocking, the parent can sit quietly by the crib until the infant falls asleep; the infant eventually learns to be comforted and to fall asleep without being held.

All children awaken during the night, but children who have been taught to fall asleep by themselves usually settle themselves back to sleep. When children cannot get back to sleep, parents can check on them to make sure they are safe and to reassure them, but children should then be allowed to settle themselves back to sleep.

In older children, a period of winding down with quiet activities such as reading at bedtime facilitates sleep. A consistent bedtime is important, and a fixed ritual is helpful for young children. Asking fully verbal children to recount the events of the day often eliminates nightmares and waking. Encouraging exercise in the daytime, avoiding scary television programs and movies, and refusing to allow bedtime to become an element of manipulation can also help prevent sleep problems.

If stressful events are the cause, reassurance and encouragement are always ultimately effective. Allowing children to sleep in their parents' bed in such instances almost always prolongs rather than resolves the problem.

289 Health Supervision of the Well Child

Well-child visits aim to do the following:

- Promote health
- Prevent disease through routine vaccinations and education
- Detect and treat disease early
- Guide parents to optimize the child's emotional and intellectual development

The American Academy of Pediatrics (AAP) has recommended preventive health care schedules (see Tables 289–1, 289–2, and 289–3) for children who have no significant health problems and who are growing and developing satisfactorily. Those who do not meet these criteria should have more frequent and intensive visits. If children come under care for the first time late on the schedule or if any items are not done at the suggested age, children should be brought up to date as soon as possible.

Children who have developmental delay, psychosocial problems, or chronic disease may require more frequent counseling and treatment visits that are separate from preventive care visits.

If the pregnancy is high risk (see p. 2366) or if the parents are first time parents or wish to have a conference, a prenatal visit with the pediatrician is appropriate.

In addition to physical examination, practitioners should evaluate the child's motor, cognitive, and social development and parent-child interactions. These assessments can be made by

- Taking a thorough history from parents and child
- Making direct observations
- Sometimes seeking information from outside sources such as teachers and child care providers

Tools are available for office use to facilitate evaluation of cognitive and social development.

Both physical examination and screening are important parts of preventive health care in infants and children. Most parameters, such as weight, are included for all children; others are applicable to selected patients, such as lead screening in 1- and 2-yr-olds.

Table 289–1. RECOMMENDATIONS FOR PREVENTIVE CARE DURING INFANCY[a]

ITEM	NEONATE	AGE 3–5 DAYS	BY AGE 1 MO	AGE 2 MO	AGE 4 MO	AGE 6 MO	AGE 9 MO
History (initial or interval)							
—	X	X	X	X	X	X	X
Measurements							
Length or height and weight	X	X	X	X	X	X	X
Head circumference	X	X	X	X	X	X	X
Weight for length	X	X	X	X	X	X	X
Blood pressure[b]	RA	RA	RA	RA	RA	RA	RA

Table 289–1. RECOMMENDATIONS FOR PREVENTIVE CARE DURING INFANCY[a] (*Continued*)

ITEM	NEONATE	AGE 3–5 DAYS	BY AGE 1 MO	AGE 2 MO	AGE 4 MO	AGE 6 MO	AGE 9 MO
Sensory screening							
Vision	RA	RA	RA	RA	RA	RA	RA
Hearing	X	RA	RA	RA	RA	RA	RA
Developmental and behavioral assessment							
Developmental surveillance[c]	X	X	X	X	X	X	
Developmental screening[d]							X
Psychosocial and behavioral assessment	X	X	X	X	X	X	X
Physical examination							
—	X	X	X	X	X	X	X
Laboratory testing[e]							
Neonatal metabolic and hemoglobinopathy screening[f]	←———	———	X	———→			
Critical congenital heart defect screening[g]	X						
Hematocrit or hemoglobin					RA		
Lead screening[h]						RA	RA
Tuberculin test[i]			RA			RA	
Other							
Immunization[j] (see Tables 291–2 on p. 2462 and 291–4 on p. 2469)	X	X	X	X	X	X	X
Oral health[k]						RA	RA
Fluoride varnish[l]						X	X
Anticipatory guidance	X	X	X	X	X	X	X

[a]These guidelines are based on a consensus by the American Academy of Pediatrics (AAP) and Bright Futures.

[b]If infants and children have certain high-risk conditions, BP should be measured at visits before age 3 yr.

[c]Developmental surveillance is an ongoing process. It involves determining what concerns parents have about their child's development, accurately observing the child, identifying risk and protective factors, and recording the process (child's developmental history, methods used, findings).

[d]Developmental screening involves using a standardized test and is routinely done at 9, 18, and 30 mo. However, screening is also done when risk factors are identified or when developmental surveillance detects a problem; in such cases, screening focuses on the area of concern.

[e]Testing may be modified, depending on when the child enters the schedule and what the child's needs are.

[f]For metabolic and hemoglobinopathy screening, state law should be followed. Clinicians should review results at visits and retest or refer as needed.

[g]Clinicians should screen newborns for critical congenital heart disease using pulse oximetry, waiting at least 24 h after birth, but screening should be done before newborns are discharged from the hospital, as recommended in the 2011 AAP statement: Endorsement of Health and Human Services recommendation for pulse oximetry screening for critical congenital heart disease.

[h]If children are at risk of lead exposure, clinicians should consult the CDC's statement Low Level Lead Exposure Harms Children: A Renewed Call for Primary Prevention; Report of the Advisory Committee on Childhood Lead Poisoning Prevention (2012) and should screen children according to state law where applicable.

[i]For tuberculosis testing, recommendations of the Committee on Infectious Diseases, published in the current edition of *Red Book:* 2012 Report of the Committee on Infectious Diseases, 29th ed., should be followed. As soon as high-risk children are identified, they should be tested.

[j]Clinicians should follow schedules recommended by the Committee on Infectious Diseases, which are published annually in the January issue of *Pediatrics*. Every visit should be used as an opportunity to update and complete a child's immunizations (see also CDC: Recommended Immunization Schedule for Persons Aged 0 Through 18 Years).

[k]Children should be referred to a dentist, if available. Otherwise, clinicians should assess oral health risk. If the primary water source is fluoride-deficient, oral fluoride supplementation should be considered.

[l]Once teeth are present, fluoride varnish may be applied to all children every 3 to 6 mo in the primary care or dental office. For indications for fluoride use, see the 2014 AAP clinical report: Fluoride Use in Caries Prevention in the Primary Care Setting.

RA = age at which risk assessment should be done, followed, if results are positive, by appropriate examination or testing; X = age at which evaluation should be done; ←X→ = range during which evaluation may be done, with X indicating the preferred age.

Adapted from the Bright Futures/Academy of Pediatrics: Recommendations for preventive pediatric health care, 2016.

Table 289–2. RECOMMENDATIONS FOR PREVENTIVE CARE DURING EARLY AND MIDDLE CHILDHOOD[a]

ITEM	AGE 12 MO	AGE 15 MO	AGE 18 MO	AGE 24 MO	AGE 30 MO	AGE 3 YR	AGE 4 YR	AGE 5 YR	AGE 6 YR	AGE 7 YR	AGE 8 YR	AGE 9 YR	AGE 10 YR
History (initial or interval)													
—	X	X	X	X	X	X	X	X	X	X	X	X	X
Measurements													
Height and weight	X	X	X	X	X	X	X	X	X	X	X	X	X
Head circumference	X	X	X	X									
Weight for length	X	X	X										
Body mass index				X	X	X	X	X	X	X	X	X	X
Blood pressure[b]	RA	RA	RA	RA	RA	X	X	X	X	X	X	X	X
Sensory screening													
Vision	RA	RA	RA	RA	RA	X[c]	X	X	X	RA	X	RA	X
Hearing	RA	RA	RA	RA	RA	RA	X	X	X	RA	X	RA	X
Developmental and behavioral assessment													
Developmental surveillance[d]	X	X		X		X	X	X	X	X	X	X	X
Developmental screening[e]			X		X								
Autism[f]			X	X									
Psychosocial and behavioral assessment	X	X	X	X	X	X	X	X	X	X	X	X	X
Physical examination													
—	X	X	X	X	X	X	X	X	X	X	X	X	X
Laboratory testing[g]													
Hematocrit or hemoglobin	X	RA	RA	RA	RA	RA	RA	RA	RA	RA	RA	RA	RA
Lead screening[h]	X or RA		RA	X or RA		RA	RA	RA	RA				
Tuberculin test[i]	RA			RA		RA	RA	RA	RA	RA	RA	RA	RA
Dyslipidemia screening[j]				RA			RA		RA		RA	←— X —→	

Table 289–2. RECOMMENDATIONS FOR PREVENTIVE CARE DURING EARLY AND MIDDLE CHILDHOOD[a] (*Continued*)

ITEM	AGE 12 MO	AGE 15 MO	AGE 18 MO	AGE 24 MO	AGE 30 MO	AGE 3 YR	AGE 4 YR	AGE 5 YR	AGE 6 YR	AGE 7 YR	AGE 8 YR	AGE 9 YR	AGE 10 YR
Other													
Immunization[k] (see Tables 291–2, 291–3, and 291–4)	X	X	X	X	X	X	X	X	X	X	X	X	X
Oral health[l]	X or RA		X or RA	X or RA	X or RA	X			X				
Fluoride varnish[m]	←	—	—	X	—	—	—	→					
Anticipatory guidance	X	X	X	X	X	X	X	X	X	X	X	X	X

[a]These guidelines are based on a consensus by the American Academy of Pediatrics (AAP) and Bright Futures.

[b]If infants and children have certain high-risk conditions, BP should be measured at visits before age 3 yr.

[c]If children are uncooperative, they can be rescreened within 6 mo.

[d]Developmental surveillance is an ongoing process. It involves determining what concerns parents have about their child's development, accurately observing the child, identifying risk and protective factors, and recording the process (child's developmental history, methods used, findings).

[e]Developmental screening involves using a standardized test and is routinely done at 9, 18, and 30 mo. However, screening is also done when risk factors are identified or when developmental surveillance detects a problem; in such cases, screening focuses on the area of concern.

[f]Screening with an autism-specific tool at age 18 mo is recommended. Screening is repeated at age 24 mo because parents may not notice problems by age 18 mo (the mean age that parents report autistic regression is 20 mo). See Gupta VB, Hyman SL, Johnson CP, et al: Identifying children with autism early? *Pediatrics* 2007;119:152–153.

[g]Testing may be modified, depending on when the child enters the schedule and what the child's needs are.

[h]If children are at risk of lead exposure, clinicians should consult the CDC's statement: Low Level Lead Exposure Harms Children: A Renewed Call for Primary Prevention; Report of the Advisory Committee on Childhood Lead Poisoning Prevention (2012) and should screen children according to state law where applicable. Risk is assessed or screening is done based on universal screening requirements for patients with Medicaid or in high-prevalence areas.

[i]For tuberculosis testing, recommendations of the Committee on Infectious Diseases, published in the current edition of *Red Book:* 2012 Report of the Committee on Infectious Diseases, 29th ed, should be followed. As soon as high-risk children are identified, they should be tested.

[j]The AAP recommends screening children between ages 1 and 8 yr and between ages 12 and 17 yr only if they have a family history of high cholesterol or coronary artery disease or risk factors for coronary artery disease (eg, diabetes, obesity, hypertension). Most useful is a fasting lipid profile. A lipid profile is also recommended for all children between ages 9 and 11 yr and again between ages 18 and 21 yr (see the AAP-endorsed 2011 guidelines from the National Heart, Blood, and Lung Institute: Integrated guidelines for cardiovascular health and risk reduction in children and adolescents).

[k]Clinicians should follow schedules recommended by the Committee on Infectious Diseases, which are published annually in the January issue of *Pediatrics.* Every visit should be used as an opportunity to update and complete a child's immunizations.

[l]Children should be referred to a dentist, if available. Otherwise, clinicians should assess oral health risk. If the primary water source is fluoride-deficient, oral fluoride supplementation should be considered. At the 3-yr and 6-yr visits, the clinician should determine whether the child has a dental home and, if not, should refer the child to one.

[m]Once teeth are present, fluoride varnish may be applied to all children every 3 to 6 mo in the primary care or dental office. For indications for fluoride use, see the 2014 AAP clinical report: Fluoride Use in Caries Prevention in the Primary Care Setting.

RA = age at which risk assessment should be done, followed, if results are positive, by appropriate examination or testing; X = age at which evaluation should be done.

Adapted from the Bright Futures/Academy of Pediatrics: Recommendations for preventive pediatric health care, 2016.

Table 289–3. RECOMMENDATIONS FOR PREVENTIVE CARE DURING ADOLESCENCE[a]

ITEM	AGE 11 YR	AGE 12 YR	AGE 13 YR	AGE 14 YR	AGE 15 YR	AGE 16 YR	AGE 17 YR	AGE 18 YR	AGE 19 YR	AGE 20 YR	AGE 21 YR
History (initial or interval)											
—	X	X	X	X	X	X	X	X	X	X	X
Measurements											
Height and weight	X	X	X	X	X	X	X	X	X	X	X
Body mass index	X	X	X	X	X	X	X	X	X	X	X
Blood pressure	X	X	X	X	X	X	X	X	X	X	X
Sensory screening											
Vision	RA	X	RA	RA	X	RA	RA	RA	RA	RA	RA
Hearing	RA	RA	RA	RA	RA	RA	RA	RA	RA	RA	RA
Developmental/behavioral assessment											
Developmental surveillance[b]	X	X	X	X	X	X	X	X	X	X	X
Psychosocial and behavioral assessment	X	X	X	X	X	X	X	X	X	X	X
Alcohol and drug use assessment[c]	RA	RA	RA	RA	RA	RA	RA	RA	RA	RA	RA
Depression screening[d]	X	X	X	X	X	X	X	X	X	X	X
Physical examination											
—	X	X	X	X	X	X	X	X	X	X	X
Testing[e]											
Hematocrit or hemoglobin	RA	RA	RA	RA	RA	RA	RA	RA	RA	RA	RA
Tuberculin test[f]	RA	RA	RA	RA	RA	RA	RA	RA	RA	RA	RA
Dyslipidemia screening[g]	X	RA	RA	RA	RA	RA	RA	←	— X	—	→
STD/HIV screening[h]	RA	RA	RA	RA	RA	←	X	→	RA	RA	RA
Cervical dysplasia screening[i]											X

Table 289–3. RECOMMENDATIONS FOR PREVENTIVE CARE DURING ADOLESCENCE[a] (*Continued*)

ITEM	AGE 11 YR	AGE 12 YR	AGE 13 YR	AGE 14 YR	AGE 15 YR	AGE 16 YR	AGE 17 YR	AGE 18 YR	AGE 19 YR	AGE 20 YR	AGE 21 YR
Other											
Immunization[j] (see Tables 291–3 and 91–4)	X	X	X	X	X	X	X	X	X	X	X
Anticipatory guidance	X	X	X	X	X	X	X	X	X	X	X

[a]These guidelines represent a consensus by the American Academy of Pediatrics (AAP) and Bright Futures.

[b]Developmental surveillance is an ongoing process. It involves determining what concerns parents have about their child's development, accurately observing the child, identifying risk and protective factors, and recording the process (child's developmental history, methods used, findings).

[c]Validated screening tools for use of alcohol and other drugs in children < 21 yr are available (see Levy SJ, Williams JF, Committee on Substance Use and Prevention: Substance use screening, brief intervention, and referral to treatment. *Pediatrics* 138 (1). 2016. pii: e20161211. doi: 10.1542/peds.2016-1211).

[d] For a list of available mental health screening tools, see the AAP's list: Mental health screening and assessment tools for primary care.

[e]Testing may be modified, depending on when the child enters the schedule and what the child's needs are.

[f]For tuberculosis testing, recommendations of the Committee on Infectious Diseases, published in the current edition of the *Red Book:* 2012 Report of the Committee on Infectious Diseases, should be followed. As soon as high-risk children are identified, they should be tested.

[g]The AAP recommends screening between ages 12 and 17 yr only if they have a family history of high cholesterol or coronary artery disease or risk factors for coronary artery disease (eg, diabetes, obesity, hypertension). Most useful is a fasting lipid profile. A lipid profile is also recommended for all children between ages 9 and 11 yr and again between ages 18 and 21 yr (see the AAP-endorsed 2011 guidelines from the National Heart, Blood, and Lung Institute: Integrated guidelines for cardiovascular health and risk reduction in children and adolescents).

[h]All sexually active patients should be screened for STDs as recommended in the current edition of the AAP Red Book: Report of the Committee on Infectious Diseases. Also, all adolescents should be offered HIV screening in appropriate settings at least once by age 16 to 18 yr, as recommended in the 2011 AAP statement: Adolescents and HIV infection: The pediatrician's role in promoting routine testing; every effort should be made to preserve the confidentiality of the adolescent. Adolescents at increased risk of HIV infection (eg, because they are sexually active, use injection drugs, or have another STD) should be tested yearly.

[i]Adolescents should not be routinely screened for cervical dysplasia until they are age 21. In certain circumstances, pelvic examinations are indicated before age 21 (see the 2010 AAP statement: Gynecologic examination for adolescents in the pediatric office setting).

[j]Clinicians should follow schedules recommended by the Committee on Infectious Diseases, which are published annually in the January issue of *Pediatrics*. Every visit should be used as an opportunity to update and complete a child's immunizations.

RA = age at which risk assessment should be done, followed, if results are positive, by appropriate examination or testing; STDs = sexually transmitted diseases; X = age at which evaluation should be done; ←X→ = range during which evaluation may be done, with X indicating the preferred age.

Adapted from the Bright Futures/Academy of Pediatrics: Recommendations for preventive pediatric health care, 2016.

Anticipatory guidance is also important to preventive health care. It includes

- Obtaining information about the child and parents (eg, via questionnaire, interview, or evaluation)
- Working with parents to promote health (forming a therapeutic alliance)
- Teaching parents what to expect in their child's development, how they can help enhance development (eg, by establishing a healthy lifestyle), and what the benefits of a healthy lifestyle are

Physical Examination

Growth: Length (crown-heel) or height (once children can stand) and weight should be measured at each visit. Head circumference should be measured at each visit through 36 mo. Growth rate should be monitored using a growth curve with percentiles; deviations in these parameters should be evaluated (see p. 2589).

Blood pressure: Starting at age 3 yr, BP should be routinely checked by using an appropriate-sized cuff. The cuff should cover at least two thirds of the upper arm, and the bladder should encircle 80 to 100% of the circumference of the arm. If no available cuff fits the criteria, using the larger cuff is better.

Systolic and diastolic BPs are considered normal if they are < 90th percentile; actual values for each percentile vary by sex, age, and size (as height percentile), so reference to published tables is essential (see Tables 289–4 and 289–5). Systolic and diastolic BP measurements between the 90th and 95th percentiles should prompt continued observation and assessment of hypertensive risk factors. If measurements are consistently ≥ 95th percentile, children should be considered hypertensive, and a cause should be determined.

Head: The most common abnormality is fluid in the middle ear (otitis media with effusion), manifesting as a change in the appearance of the tympanic membrane. Clinicians should screen for hearing deficits.

Eyes should be assessed at each visit. Clinicians should check for all of the following:

- Esotropia or exotropia
- Abnormalities in globe size: Suggesting congenital glaucoma
- A difference in pupil size, iris color, or both: Suggesting Horner syndrome, trauma, or neuroblastoma (asymmetric pupils may be normal or represent an ocular, autonomic, or intracranial disorder)
- Absence or distortion of the red reflex: Suggesting cataract or retinoblastoma

Ptosis and eyelid hemangioma obscure vision and require attention. Infants born at < 32 wk gestation should be assessed by an ophthalmologist for evidence of retinopathy of prematurity and for refractive errors, which are more common. By age 3 or 4 yr, vision testing by Snellen charts or newer testing machines can be used. E charts are better than pictures; visual acuity of < 20/30 should be evaluated by an ophthalmologist.

Detection of dental caries is important, and referral to a dentist should be made if cavities are present, even in children who have only deciduous teeth. If the primary water source is deficient in fluoride, oral fluoride supplementation should begin when a child is 6 mo old and be continued daily until the child is 16 yr (see Table 289–6). Brushing with fluoride toothpaste in the appropriate dosage for age should be recommended. Once teeth are present, fluoride varnish may be applied to all children every 3 to 6 mo in the primary care setting or dental office.

Thrush is common among infants and not usually a sign of immunosuppression.

Heart: Auscultation is done to identify new murmurs, heart rate abnormalities, or rhythm disturbances; benign flow murmurs are common and need to be distinguished from pathologic murmurs. The chest wall is palpated for the apical impulse to check for cardiomegaly; femoral pulses are palpated to check for asymmetry, which suggests aortic coarctation.

Abdomen: Palpation is repeated at every visit because many masses, particularly Wilms tumor and neuroblastoma, may be apparent only as children grow.

Stool is often palpable in the left lower quadrant.

Spine and extremities: Children old enough to stand should be screened for scoliosis by observing posture, shoulder tip and scapular symmetry, torso list, and especially paraspinal asymmetry when children bend forward.

At each visit before children start to walk, evaluation for developmental dysplasia of the hip should be done. The Barlow and Ortolani maneuvers are used until about age 4 mo. After that, dysplasia may be suggested by unequal leg length, adductor tightness, or asymmetry of abduction or leg creases.

Toeing-in can result from adduction of the forefoot, tibial torsion, or femoral torsion. Only pronounced cases require therapy and referral to an orthopedist. Asymmetric toeing (toeing-in on one side and toeing-out on the other—windswept appearance) typically requires orthopedic evaluation.

Genital examination: Girls should be offered a pelvic examination and Papanicolaou (Pap) testing at age 21. All sexually active patients should be screened for sexually transmitted diseases.

Testicular and inguinal evaluation should be done at every visit, specifically looking for undescended testes in infants and young boys, testicular masses in older adolescents, and inguinal hernia in boys of all ages. Adolescent boys should be taught how to do testicular self-examination to check for masses, and adolescent girls should be taught how to do breast self-examination.

Prevention

Preventive counseling is part of every well-child visit and covers a broad spectrum of topics, such as recommendations to have infants sleep on their backs, injury prevention, nutritional and exercise advice, and discussions of violence, firearms, and substance abuse.

Safety: Recommendations for injury prevention vary by age. Some examples follow.

For infants from birth to 6 mo:

- Using a rear-facing car seat
- Reducing home water temperature to < 49° C (< 120° F)
- Preventing falls
- Using sleeping precautions: Placing infants on their back, not sharing a bed, using a firm mattress, and not allowing stuffed animals, pillows, and blankets in the crib
- Avoiding foods and objects that children can aspirate

For infants from 6 to 12 mo:

- Continuing to use a rear-facing car seat
- Continuing to place infants on their back to sleep
- Not using baby walkers
- Using safety latches on cabinets
- Preventing falls from changing tables and around stairs
- Vigilantly supervising children when in bathtubs and while learning to walk

Table 289–4. BP LEVELS FOR THE 50TH TO 99TH PERCENTILES OF BP FOR BOYS AGED 1 TO 17 YR BY PERCENTILES OF HEIGHT

		SBP (MM HG)/PERCENTILE OF HEIGHT							DBP (MM HG)/PERCENTILE OF HEIGHT						
Age	BP Percentile	5th	10th	25th	50th	75th	90th	95th	5th	10th	25th	50th	75th	90th	95th
1	50th	80	81	83	85	87	88	89	34	35	36	37	38	39	39
	90th	94	95	97	99	100	102	103	49	50	51	52	53	53	54
	95th	98	99	101	103	104	106	106	54	54	55	56	57	58	58
	99th	105	106	108	110	112	113	114	61	62	63	64	65	66	66
2	50th	84	85	87	88	90	92	92	39	40	41	42	43	44	44
	90th	97	99	100	102	104	105	106	54	55	56	57	58	58	59
	95th	101	102	104	106	108	109	110	59	59	60	61	62	63	63
	99th	109	110	111	113	115	117	117	66	67	68	69	70	71	71
3	50th	86	87	89	91	93	94	95	44	44	45	46	47	48	48
	90th	100	101	103	105	107	108	109	59	59	60	61	62	63	63
	95th	104	105	107	109	110	112	113	63	63	64	65	66	67	67
	99th	111	112	114	116	118	119	120	71	71	72	73	74	75	75
4	50th	88	89	91	93	95	96	97	47	48	49	50	51	51	52
	90th	102	103	105	107	109	110	111	62	63	64	65	66	66	67
	95th	106	107	109	111	112	114	115	66	67	68	69	70	71	71
	99th	113	114	116	118	120	121	122	74	75	76	77	78	78	79
5	50th	90	91	93	95	96	98	98	50	51	52	53	54	55	55
	90th	104	105	106	108	110	111	112	65	66	67	68	69	69	70
	95th	108	109	110	112	114	115	116	69	70	71	72	73	74	74
	99th	115	116	118	120	121	123	123	77	78	79	80	81	81	82
6	50th	91	92	94	96	98	99	100	53	53	54	55	56	57	57
	90th	105	106	108	110	111	113	113	68	68	69	70	71	72	72
	95th	109	110	112	114	115	117	117	72	72	73	74	75	76	76
	99th	116	117	119	121	123	124	125	80	80	81	82	83	84	84
7	50th	92	94	95	97	99	100	101	55	55	56	57	58	59	59
	90th	106	107	109	111	113	114	115	70	70	71	72	73	74	74
	95th	110	111	113	115	117	118	119	74	74	75	76	77	78	78
	99th	117	118	120	122	124	125	126	82	82	83	84	85	86	86
8	50th	94	95	97	99	100	102	102	56	57	58	59	60	60	61
	90th	107	109	110	112	114	115	116	71	72	72	73	74	75	76
	95th	111	112	114	116	118	119	120	75	76	77	78	79	79	80
	99th	119	120	122	123	125	127	127	83	84	85	86	87	87	88
9	50th	95	96	98	100	102	103	104	57	58	59	60	61	61	62
	90th	109	110	112	114	115	117	118	72	73	74	75	76	76	77
	95th	113	114	116	118	119	121	121	76	77	78	79	80	81	81
	99th	120	121	123	125	127	128	129	84	85	86	87	88	88	89

Table continues on the following page.

Table 289–4. BP LEVELS FOR THE 50TH TO 99TH PERCENTILES OF BP FOR BOYS AGED 1 TO 17 YR BY PERCENTILES OF HEIGHT (*Continued*)

		SBP (MM HG)/PERCENTILE OF HEIGHT							DBP (MM HG)/PERCENTILE OF HEIGHT						
Age	BP Percentile	5th	10th	25th	50th	75th	90th	95th	5th	10th	25th	50th	75th	90th	95th
10	50th	97	98	100	102	103	105	106	58	59	60	61	61	62	63
	90th	111	112	114	115	117	119	119	73	73	74	75	76	77	78
	95th	115	116	117	119	121	122	123	77	78	79	80	81	81	82
	99th	122	123	125	127	128	130	130	85	86	86	88	88	89	90
11	50th	99	100	102	104	105	107	107	59	59	60	61	62	63	63
	90th	113	114	115	117	119	120	121	74	74	75	76	77	78	78
	95th	117	118	119	121	123	124	125	78	78	79	80	81	82	82
	99th	124	125	127	129	130	132	132	86	86	87	88	89	90	90
12	50th	101	102	104	106	108	109	110	59	60	61	62	63	63	64
	90th	115	116	118	120	121	123	123	74	75	75	76	77	78	79
	95th	119	120	122	123	125	127	127	78	79	80	81	82	82	83
	99th	126	127	129	131	133	134	135	86	87	88	89	90	90	91
13	50th	104	105	106	108	110	111	112	60	60	61	62	63	64	64
	90th	117	118	120	122	124	125	126	75	75	76	77	78	79	79
	95th	121	122	124	126	128	129	130	79	79	80	81	82	83	83
	99th	128	130	131	133	135	136	137	87	87	88	89	90	91	91
14	50th	106	107	109	111	113	114	115	60	61	62	63	64	65	65
	90th	120	121	123	125	126	128	128	75	76	77	78	79	79	80
	95th	124	125	127	128	130	132	132	80	80	81	82	83	84	84
	99th	131	132	134	136	138	139	140	87	88	89	90	91	92	92
15	50th	109	110	112	113	115	117	117	61	62	63	64	65	66	66
	90th	122	124	125	127	129	130	131	76	77	78	79	80	80	81
	95th	126	127	129	131	133	134	135	81	81	82	83	84	85	85
	99th	134	135	136	138	140	142	142	88	89	90	91	92	93	93
16	50th	111	112	114	116	118	119	120	63	63	64	65	66	67	67
	90th	125	126	128	130	131	133	134	78	78	79	80	81	82	82
	95th	129	130	132	134	135	137	137	82	83	83	84	85	86	87
	99th	136	137	139	141	143	144	145	90	90	91	92	93	94	94
17	50th	114	115	116	118	120	121	122	65	66	66	67	68	69	70
	90th	127	128	130	132	134	135	136	80	80	81	82	83	84	84
	95th	131	132	134	136	138	139	140	84	85	86	87	87	88	89
	99th	139	140	141	143	145	146	147	92	93	93	94	95	96	97

The 90th percentile is 1.28 standard deviations (SDs), the 95th percentile is 1.645 SDs, and the 99th percentile is 2.326 SDs over the mean.

Table 289–5. BP LEVELS FOR THE 50TH TO 99TH PERCENTILES OF BP FOR GIRLS AGED 1 TO 17 YR BY PERCENTILES OF HEIGHT

		SBP (MM HG)/PERCENTILE OF HEIGHT							DBP (MM HG)/PERCENTILE OF HEIGHT						
1	50th	83	84	85	86	88	89	90	38	39	39	40	41	41	42
	90th	97	97	98	100	101	102	103	52	53	53	54	55	55	56
	95th	100	101	102	104	105	106	107	56	57	57	58	59	59	60
	99th	108	108	109	111	112	113	114	64	64	65	65	66	67	67
2	50th	85	85	87	88	89	91	91	43	44	44	45	46	46	47
	90th	98	99	100	101	103	104	105	57	58	58	59	60	61	61
	95th	102	103	104	105	107	108	109	61	62	62	63	64	65	65
	99th	109	110	111	112	114	115	116	69	69	70	70	71	72	72
3	50th	86	87	88	89	91	92	93	47	48	48	49	50	50	51
	90th	100	100	102	103	104	106	106	61	62	62	63	64	64	65
	95th	104	104	105	107	108	109	110	65	66	66	67	68	68	69
	99th	111	111	113	114	115	116	117	73	73	74	74	75	76	76
4	50th	88	88	90	91	92	94	94	50	50	51	52	52	53	54
	90th	101	102	103	104	106	107	108	64	64	65	66	67	67	68
	95th	105	106	107	108	110	111	112	68	68	69	70	71	71	72
	99th	112	113	114	115	117	118	119	76	76	76	77	78	79	79
5	50th	89	90	91	93	94	95	96	52	53	53	54	55	55	56
	90th	103	103	105	106	107	109	109	66	67	67	68	69	69	70
	95th	107	107	108	110	111	112	113	70	71	71	72	73	73	74
	99th	114	114	116	117	118	120	120	78	78	79	79	80	81	81
6	50th	91	92	93	94	96	97	98	54	54	55	56	56	57	58
	90th	104	105	106	108	109	110	111	68	68	69	70	70	71	72
	95th	108	109	110	111	113	114	115	72	72	73	74	74	75	76
	99th	115	116	117	119	120	121	122	80	80	80	81	82	83	83
7	50th	93	93	95	96	97	99	99	55	56	56	57	58	58	59
	90th	106	107	108	109	111	112	113	69	70	70	71	72	72	73
	95th	110	111	112	113	115	116	116	73	74	74	75	76	76	77
	99th	117	118	119	120	122	123	124	81	81	82	82	83	84	84
8	50th	95	95	96	98	99	100	101	57	57	57	58	59	60	60
	90th	108	109	110	111	113	114	114	71	71	71	72	73	74	74
	95th	112	112	114	115	116	118	118	75	75	75	76	77	78	78
	99th	119	120	121	122	123	125	125	82	82	83	83	84	85	86
9	50th	96	97	98	100	101	102	103	58	58	58	59	60	61	61
	90th	110	110	112	113	114	116	116	72	72	72	73	74	75	75
	95th	114	114	115	117	118	119	120	76	76	76	77	78	79	79
	99th	121	121	123	124	125	127	127	83	83	84	84	85	86	87

Table continues on the following page.

Table 289–5. BP LEVELS FOR THE 50TH TO 99TH PERCENTILES OF BP FOR GIRLS AGED 1 TO 17 YR BY PERCENTILES OF HEIGHT (*Continued*)

		SBP (MM HG)/PERCENTILE OF HEIGHT							DBP (MM HG)/PERCENTILE OF HEIGHT						
10	50th	98	99	100	102	103	104	105	59	59	59	60	61	62	62
	90th	112	112	114	115	116	118	118	73	73	73	74	75	76	76
	95th	116	116	117	119	120	121	122	77	77	77	78	79	80	80
	99th	123	123	125	126	127	129	129	84	84	85	86	86	87	88
11	50th	100	101	102	103	105	106	107	60	60	60	61	62	63	63
	90th	114	114	116	117	118	119	120	74	74	74	75	76	77	77
	95th	118	118	119	121	122	123	124	78	78	78	79	80	81	81
	99th	125	125	126	128	129	130	131	85	85	86	87	87	88	89
12	50th	102	103	104	105	107	108	109	61	61	61	62	63	64	64
	90th	116	116	117	119	120	121	122	75	75	75	76	77	78	78
	95th	119	120	121	123	124	125	126	79	79	79	80	81	82	82
	99th	127	127	128	130	131	132	133	86	86	87	88	88	89	90
13	50th	104	105	106	107	109	110	110	62	62	62	63	64	65	65
	90th	117	118	119	121	122	123	124	76	76	76	77	78	79	79
	95th	121	122	123	124	126	127	128	80	80	80	81	82	83	83
	99th	128	129	130	132	133	134	135	87	87	88	89	89	90	91
14	50th	106	106	107	109	110	111	112	63	63	63	64	65	66	66
	90th	119	120	121	122	124	125	125	77	77	77	78	79	80	80
	95th	123	123	125	126	127	129	129	81	81	81	82	83	84	84
	99th	130	131	132	133	135	136	136	88	88	89	90	90	91	92
15	50th	107	108	109	110	111	113	113	64	64	64	65	66	67	67
	90th	120	121	122	123	125	126	127	78	78	78	79	80	81	81
	95th	124	125	126	127	129	130	131	82	82	82	83	84	85	85
	99th	131	132	133	134	136	137	138	89	89	90	91	91	92	93
16	50th	108	108	110	111	112	114	114	64	64	65	66	66	67	68
	90th	121	122	123	124	126	127	128	78	78	79	80	81	81	82
	95th	125	126	127	128	130	131	132	82	82	83	84	85	85	86
	99th	132	133	134	135	137	138	139	90	90	90	91	92	93	93
17	50th	108	109	110	111	113	114	115	64	65	65	66	67	67	68
	90th	122	122	123	125	126	127	128	78	79	79	80	81	81	82
	95th	125	126	127	129	130	131	132	82	83	83	84	85	85	86
	99th	133	133	134	136	137	138	139	90	90	91	91	92	93	93

The 90th percentile is 1.28 standard deviations (SDs), the 95th percentile is 1.645 SDs, and the 99th percentile is 2.326 SDs over the mean.

Table 289–6. FLUORIDE SUPPLEMENTATION BASED ON FLUORIDE CONTENT IN DRINKING WATER

AGE	FLUORIDE < 0.3 ppm	FLUORIDE 0.3–0.6 ppm	FLUORIDE > 0.6 ppm
6 mo–3 yr	0.25 mg/day	None	None
3–6 yr	0.5 mg/day	0.2 mg/day	None
6–16 yr	1.0 mg/day	0.5 mg/day	None

For children aged 1 to 4 yr:

- Using an age- and weight-appropriate car seat (infants and toddlers should use a rear-facing car seat until they are at least 2 yr of age or until they exceed the rear-facing weight or height limits for their convertible child safety seat)
- Reviewing automobile safety both as passenger and pedestrian
- Tying window cords
- Using safety caps and latches
- Preventing falls
- Removing handguns from the home

For children ≥ 5 yr:

- All of the recommendations for children aged 1 to 4 yr
- Using a bicycle helmet and protective sports gear
- Instructing children about safe street crossing
- Closely supervising swimming and sometimes requiring the use of life jackets during swimming

Nutrition: Excessive caloric intake underlies the epidemic of obesity in children. Recommendations for calorie intake vary by age; for children up to 2 yr, see p. 2415.

As children grow older, parents can allow them some discretion in food choices, while keeping the diet within healthy parameters. Children should be guided away from frequent snacking and foods that are high in calories, salt, and sugar. Soda and excessive fruit juice consumption have been implicated as major contributors to obesity.

Exercise: Physical inactivity also underlies the epidemic of obesity in children, and the benefits of exercise in maintaining good physical and emotional health should induce parents to make sure their children develop good habits early in life. During infancy and early childhood, children should be allowed to roam and explore in a safe environment under close supervision. Outdoor play should be encouraged from infancy.

As children grow older, play becomes more complex, often evolving to formal school-based athletics. Parents should set good examples and encourage both informal and formal play, always keeping safety issues in mind and promoting healthy attitudes about sportsmanship and competition. Participation in sports and activities as a family provides children with exercise and has important psychologic and developmental benefits. Screening of children before sports participation is recommended.

Limits to television watching, which is linked directly to inactivity and obesity, should start at birth and be maintained throughout adolescence. Similar limits should be set for video games and noneducational computer time as children grow older.

SCREENING TESTS FOR INFANTS AND CHILDREN

Screening (along with physical examination) is an important part of preventive health care in infants and children.

Blood tests: To detect iron deficiency, clinicians should determine Hct or Hb as follows:

- In term infants: At age 9 to 12 mo
- In premature infants: At age 5 to 6 mo
- In menstruating adolescents: Annually if they have any of the following risk factors: moderate to heavy menses, chronic weight loss, a nutritional deficit, or participation in athletic activity

Testing for Hb S can be done at age 6 to 9 mo if not done as part of neonatal screening.

Recommendations for blood testing for lead exposure vary by state. In general, testing should be done between ages 9 mo and 1 yr in children at risk of exposure (those living in housing built before 1980) and should be repeated at 24 mo. If the clinician is not sure of a child's risk, testing should be done. Levels > 10 μg/dL (> 0.48 μmol/L) pose a risk of neurologic damage, although some experts question this threshold because they believe that any lead in the system can be toxic.

Cholesterol screening is indicated for all children between ages 9 and 11 yr and again between ages 18 and 21 yr. Most useful is a fasting lipid profile. Cholesterol screening is indicated for children between ages 1 and 8 yr and between ages 12 and 17 yr only if they have a family history of high cholesterol or coronary artery disease or risk factors for coronary artery disease (eg, diabetes, obesity, hypertension).

Hearing tests: Parents may suspect a hearing deficit if their child ceases responding appropriately to noises or voices or does not understand or develop speech (see Table 289–7).

Because hearing deficits impair language development, hearing problems must be remedied as early as possible. The clinician therefore should seek parental input about hearing at every visit during early childhood and be prepared to do formal testing or refer to an audiologist whenever there is any question of the child's ability to hear.

Audiometry can be done in the primary care setting; most other audiologic procedures (eg, otoacoustic emission testing, brain stem auditory evoked response) should be done by an audiologist. Conventional audiometry can be used for children beginning at about age 3 yr; young children can also be tested by observing their responses to sounds made through headphones, watching their attempts to localize the sound or complete a simple task.

Table 289–7. NORMAL HEARING IN VERY YOUNG CHILDREN*

AGE	EXPECTED RESPONSE
3 mo	Startles to a nearby loud sound Stirs or awakens from sleep when someone talks or makes a sound Is soothed by mother's voice
6 mo	Looks toward an interesting sound Turns when name is called Makes "moo," "ma," "da," "di" sounds to toys Coos when listening to music
10 mo	Makes own sounds Imitates some sounds Understands "no" and "bye-bye"
18 mo	Understands many single words or commands Babbles in sentence-like patterns

*If a child does not pass these minimal performance standards or if parents suspect a hearing loss in their child at any age, the child should be referred for testing.

Tympanometry, another in-office procedure, can be used with children of any age and is useful for evaluating middle ear function. Abnormal tympanograms often denote eustachian tube dysfunction or the presence of middle ear fluid that cannot be detected during otoscopic examination.

Pneumatic otoscopy is helpful in evaluating middle ear status, but combining it with tympanometry is more informative than either procedure alone.

Tuberculin testing: Tuberculin testing should be done if

- Children have been exposed to TB (eg, to an infected family member or close contact).
- They have had a family member with a positive tuberculin test.
- They were born in a developing country.
- Their parents are new immigrants from those countries or have been recently incarcerated.

Screening for sexually transmitted diseases: Routine laboratory screening for common sexually transmitted diseases (STDs) is indicated for sexually active adolescents (see also p. 1702).

Screening is also recommended for the following:

- All sexually active females aged ≤ 25 yr and those who are no longer active but have a history of an STD: Annual screening for *Chlamydia trachomatis* and *Neisseria gonorrhoeae*
- Pregnant women ≤ 25 yr: Screening during their initial prenatal visit and again during the 3rd trimester
- Heterosexually active young men: If seen in clinical settings associated with high prevalence of STDs (eg, in adolescent and STD clinics, at entrance into correctional facilities)
- Men who have sex with men: If they have been sexually active within the previous year

Nucleic acid amplification tests (NAATs) are the most sensitive tests for detecting *C. trachomatis* and *N. gonorrhoeae* infection. NAATs using urine, cervical, and urethral specimens are available.

All adolescents should be offered HIV screening at least once by age 16 to 18 yr; every effort should be made to preserve the confidentiality of the adolescent. Adolescents at increased risk of HIV infection (eg, because they are sexually active, use injection drugs, or have another STD) should be tested yearly.

Adolescents should not be routinely screened for cervical dysplasia until they are age 21.

TOILET TRAINING

Toilet training involves recognition of readiness for and implementation of the separate steps of toileting: discussion, undressing, eliminating, dressing again, flushing, and hand washing.

Most children can be trained for bowel control between age 2 yr and 3 yr and for urinary control between age 3 yr and 4 yr. By age 5 yr, the average child can go to the toilet alone. For children ≥ 4 yr, see p. 2613 for incontinence of urine (enuresis) and p. 2618 for incontinence of stool (encopresis).

The key to successful toilet training is recognizing signs of readiness to train (usually at age 18 to 24 mo):

- Children can remain dry for several hours.
- They show interest in sitting on a potty chair and express visible signs of preparing to urinate or defecate.
- They want to be changed after either.
- They can place things where they belong and can understand and carry out simple verbal commands.

Approaches to toilet training must be consistent among all caregivers.

The **timing method** is the most common approach. Once children have demonstrated readiness, the parent discusses with them what will be happening, selecting words that they can readily understand and say. Children are gradually introduced to the potty chair and briefly sit on it fully clothed; they then practice taking their pants down, sitting on the potty chair for ≤ 5 or 10 min, and redressing. The purpose of the exercise is explained repeatedly and emphasized by placing wet or dirty diapers in the potty. Once this connection between the potty and elimination has been made, the parent should try to anticipate children's need to eliminate and provide positive reinforcement for successful elimination. Children are also encouraged to practice using the potty whenever the need to eliminate is sensed. They should be taught about flushing and hand washing after each elimination. For children with an unpredictable schedule, this type of plan is difficult, and training must be delayed until they can anticipate elimination themselves. Anger or punishment for accidents or lack of success is counterproductive.

Children who resist sitting on the potty should try again after a meal. If resistance continues for days, postponing toilet training for at least several weeks is the best strategy. Behavior modification with a reward given for successful toileting is one option; once the pattern is established, rewards are gradually withdrawn.

Power struggles must be avoided because they often cause regression from any progress that has been made and may strain the parent-child relationship. Toilet-trained children may also regress when they are ill or emotionally upset or when they feel the need for more attention, as when a new sibling arrives. Refusal to use the potty may also represent manipulation. In these situations, parents are advised to avoid pressuring children, offer incentives, and, if possible, give children more care and attention at times other than when toileting is involved.

290 Symptoms in Infants and Children

COLIC

Colic is frequent and extended periods of crying for no discernible reason in an otherwise healthy infant.

Although the term colic suggests an intestinal origin, etiology is unknown.

Colic typically appears within the first month of life, peaks at about age 6 wk, and reliably and spontaneously ends by age 3 to 4 mo. Paroxysms of crying and fussiness often occur at about the same time of day or night and continue for hours for no apparent reason. A few infants cry almost incessantly. Excessive crying may cause aerophagia, which results in flatulence and abdominal distention. Typically, colicky infants eat and gain weight well, although vigorous nonnutritive sucking may suggest excessive hunger. Colic probably has no relation to development of an insistent, impatient personality.

Evaluation

The goal is to distinguish colic from other causes of excessive crying, particularly serious and/or treatable medical disorders such as

- Ear infection
- UTI
- Meningitis
- Appendicitis
- Food allergy
- Acid reflux
- Constipation
- Intestinal obstruction
- Increased intracranial pressure
- Hair tourniquet
- Corneal abrasion
- Glaucoma
- Nonaccidental injury

History: History of present illness should establish the onset and duration of crying and response to attempts to console and thus determine whether the infant's crying is outside the normal range (up to 3 h/day in a 6-wk-old infant).

Review of systems should seek symptoms of causative disorders, including constipation, diarrhea, and vomiting (GI disorders) and cough, wheezing, and nasal congestion (respiratory infection).

Past medical history involves thorough questioning, which may reveal that crying is not the chief concern but a symptom that the parents have used to justify their visiting the physician to present another problem—eg, concern over the death of a previous child or over their feelings of inability to cope with a new infant.

Physical examination: Physical examination begins with review of vital signs and then a thorough examination for signs of trauma or medical illness. The examination in children with colic typically detects no abnormalities but reassures parents.

Red flags: The following findings are of particular concern:

- Vomiting (especially if vomit is green or bloody or occurs > 5 times a day
- Constipation or diarrhea, especially with blood or mucus
- Fever
- Respiratory distress
- Lethargy
- Poor weight gain

Interpretation of findings: Often, infants with colic present after days or weeks of repetitive, daily crying; an otherwise normal history and examination at this point is more reassuring than in infants with acute (1 to 2 days) crying.

Testing: No testing is necessary unless specific abnormalities are detected by history and examination.

Treatment

Parents should be reassured that the infant is healthy, that the irritability is not due to poor parenting, and that colic will resolve on its own with no long-term adverse effects. Physicians should also offer reassurance that they understand how stressful a colicky infant can be for parents.

The following measures may help:

- For infants who cry for short periods: Being held, rocked, or patted gently
- For infants who have a strong sucking urge and who fuss soon after a feeding: Opportunity to suck more (eg, a pacifier)
- If bottle-feeding takes < 15 to 20 min: Nipples with smaller holes, a pacifier, or both
- For very active, restless infants: Paradoxically, being swaddled tightly

An infant swing, music, and white noise (eg, from a vacuum cleaner, car engine, or clothes or hair dryer) may also be calming. Because fatigue often contributes to excessive crying, parents should also be instructed to routinely lay the infant in the crib while the infant is awake to encourage self-soothing and good sleep habits and to prevent the infant from becoming dependent on the parents, rocking, a pacifier, a specific noise, or something else to fall asleep.

A hypoallergenic formula may be tried briefly to determine whether infants have cow's milk protein intolerance, but frequent formula switching should be avoided. Sometimes in breastfed infants, removing cow's milk or another food (particularly stimulant foods [eg, coffee, tea, cola, chocolate, diet supplements]) from the mother's diet brings relief, as may stopping drugs that contain stimulants (eg, decongestants).

KEY POINTS

- Colic is excessive crying for no discernible reason in an otherwise healthy infant.
- Colic should end by age 3 to 4 mo.
- Rule out medical causes of crying by history and physical examination; testing is unnecessary unless there are specific findings.
- Physical measures (eg, rocking, swinging, swaddling) can be tried, as may dietary changes; response to these measures varies, and often colic resolves only with time.

CONSTIPATION IN CHILDREN

Constipation is responsible for up to 5% of pediatric office visits. It is defined as delay or difficulty in defecation.

Normal frequency and consistency of stool varies with children's age, and diet; there is also considerable variation from child to child.

Most (90%) normal neonates pass meconium within the first 24 h of life. During the first week of life, infants pass an average of 4 to 8 stools/day; breastfed infants typically have more stools than formula-fed infants. During the first few months of life, breastfed infants pass a mean of 3 stools/day, vs about 2 stools/day for formula-fed infants. By age 2 yr, the number of bowel movements has decreased to slightly < 2/day. After age 4 yr, it is slightly > 1/day.

In general, signs of effort (eg, straining) in a young infant do not signify constipation. Infants only gradually develop the muscles to assist a bowel movement.

Etiology

Constipation in children is divided into 2 main types:

- Organic (5%)
- Functional (95%)

Organic: Organic causes of constipation involve specific structural, neurologic, toxic/metabolic, or intestinal disorders. They are rare but important to recognize (see Table 290–1).

The most common organic cause is

- Hirschsprung disease

Table 290–1. ORGANIC CAUSES OF CONSTIPATION IN INFANTS AND CHILDREN

CAUSE	SUGGESTIVE FINDINGS	DIAGNOSTIC APPROACH
Anatomic		
Anal stenosis	Delayed passage of stool in the first 24–48 h of life Explosive and painful stools Abdominal distention Abnormal appearance or position of the anus Tight anal canal detected by digital examination	Clinical evaluation
Anteriorly displaced anus	Severe chronic constipation with marked straining and pain when stool is passed Typically no response to aggressive use of stool softeners and cathartics Anal opening not located in the center of the pigmented area of the perineum	Calculation of API* indicating anterior placement, which varies by sex: • Girls: < 0.29 • Boys: < 0.49
Imperforate anus	Abdominal distention No passage of stool Abnormal appearance or position of the anus or possibly no anus	Clinical examination
Endocrine or metabolic disorders		
Diabetes insipidus	Polydipsia Polyuria Excessive crying quieted with water intake Weight loss Vomiting	Urine and serum osmolality ADH levels Serum sodium Sometimes water deprivation test
Hypercalcemia	Nausea, vomiting Muscle weakness Abdominal pain Anorexia, weight loss Polydipsia Polyuria	Serum calcium
Hypokalemia	Muscular weakness Polyuria, dehydration History of growth failure Possibly history of aminoglycoside, diuretics, cisplatin, or amphotericin use	Electrolyte panel
Hypothyroidism	Poor feeding Bradycardia Large fontanelles and hypotonia in neonates Cold intolerance, dry skin, fatigue, prolonged jaundice	Thyroid-stimulating hormone (TSH) Thyroxine (T_4)
Spinal cord defects		
Myelomeningocele	Grossly visible lesion in vertebral spine at birth Decrease in lower-extremity reflexes or muscular tone Absence of anal wink	Plain x-rays of lumbosacral spine Spinal MRI
Occult spina bifida	Sacral hair tuft or pit	Spinal MRI
Tethered cord	Change in gait Pain or weakness in lower extremities Urinary incontinence Back pain	Spinal MRI
Spinal cord tumor or infection	Back pain Pain or weakness in lower extremities Decrease in lower-extremity reflexes Change in gait Urinary incontinence	Spinal MRI
Intestinal disorders		
Celiac disease (gluten enteropathy)	Symptom onset after introduction of wheat into diet (typically after age 4–6 mo) Failure to thrive Recurrent abdominal pain Bloating Diarrhea or constipation	CBC Serologic screening for celiac disease (IgA antibody to tissue transglutaminase) Endoscopy for duodenal biopsy

Table 290–1. ORGANIC CAUSES OF CONSTIPATION IN INFANTS AND CHILDREN (*Continued*)

CAUSE	SUGGESTIVE FINDINGS	DIAGNOSTIC APPROACH
Cow's milk protein intolerance (milk protein allergy)	Vomiting Diarrhea or constipation Hematochezia Anal fissures Failure to thrive	Symptom resolution with elimination of cow's milk protein Sometimes endoscopy or colonoscopy
Cystic fibrosis	Delayed passage of meconium or meconium ileus in the neonate Possible repeated episodes of small-bowel obstruction (meconium ileus equivalent) in older children Failure to thrive Repeated episodes of pneumonia or wheezing	Sweat test Genetic testing
Hirschsprung disease	Delayed passage of meconium Abdominal distention Tight anal canal detected by digital examination	Barium enema Anorectal manometry and rectal biopsy for confirmation
Irritable bowel syndrome	Chronic recurrent abdominal pain Often alternating diarrhea and constipation Feeling of incomplete evacuation Passage of mucus No anorexia or weight loss	Clinical evaluation
Intestinal pseudo-obstruction	Nausea, vomiting Abdominal pain and distention	Abdominal x-ray Colonic transit time Antroduodenal manometry
Intestinal tumor	Weight loss Night sweats Fever Abdominal pain and/or distention Palpable abdominal mass Bowel obstruction	MRI
Cerebral palsy and other severe neurologic deficits	In most children with cerebral palsy, which causes intestinal hypotonia and motor paralysis Tube feedings with low-fiber formulas	Clinical evaluation
Drug adverse effects		
Use of anticholinergics, antidepressants, chemotherapeutics, or opioids	Suggestive history	Clinical evaluation
Toxins		
Infant botulism	New onset of poor suck, feeding difficulties, anorexia, drooling Weak cry Irritability Ptosis Descending or global hypotonia and weakness Possible history of ingestion of honey before age 12 mo	Test for botulinum toxin in stool
Lead toxicity	Most likely asymptomatic Possible intermittent abdominal pain, sporadic vomiting, fatigue, irritability Loss of developmental milestones	Blood lead level

*API (anal position index) is calculated as follows:

- Girls: Distance from anus to fourchette/distance from coccyx to fourchette (normal mean ± SD 0.45 ± 0.08)
- Boys: Distance from anus to scrotum/distance from coccyx to scrotum (normal mean ± SD 0.54 ± 0.07)

SD = standard deviation.

Other organic causes that may manifest in the neonatal period or later include

- Anorectal malformations
- Cystic fibrosis
- Metabolic disorders (eg, hypothyroidism, hypercalcemia, hyperkalemia)
- Spinal cord abnormalities

Functional: Functional constipation is difficulty passing stools for reasons other than organic causes.

Children are prone to develop functional constipation during 3 periods:

- After the introduction of cereals and solid food
- During toilet training
- During the start of school

Each of these milestones has the potential to convert defecation into an unpleasant experience.

Children may put off having bowel movements because the stools are hard and uncomfortable to pass or because they do not want to interrupt play. To avoid having a bowel movement, children may tighten the external sphincter muscles, pushing the stool higher in the rectal vault. If this behavior is repeated, the rectum stretches to accommodate the retained stool. The urge to defecate is then decreased, and the stool becomes harder, leading to a vicious circle of painful defecation and worsened constipation. Occasionally, soft stool passes around the impacted stool and leads to stool incontinence.

In older children, diets low in fiber and high in dairy may lead to hard stools that are uncomfortable to pass and can cause anal fissures. Anal fissures cause pain with stool passage, leading to a similar vicious circle of delayed bowel movements, resulting in harder stool that is more painful to pass.

Stress, desire for control, and sexual abuse are also some of the functional causes of stool retention and subsequent constipation.

Evaluation

Evaluation should focus on differentiating functional constipation from constipation with an organic cause.

History: History of present illness in neonates should determine whether meconium has been passed at all and, if so, when. For older infants and children, history should note onset and duration of constipation, frequency and consistency of stools, and timing of symptoms—whether they began after a specific event, such as introduction of certain foods or a stressor that could lead to stool retention (eg, introduction of toilet training). Important associated symptoms include soiling (stool incontinence), discomfort during defecation, and blood on or in the stool. The composition of the diet, especially the amount of fluids and fiber, should be noted.

Review of systems should ask about symptoms that suggest an organic cause, including new onset of poor suck, hypotonia, and ingestion of honey before age 12 mo (infantile botulism); cold intolerance, dry skin, fatigue, hypotonia, prolonged neonatal hyperbilirubinemia, urinary frequency, and excessive thirst (endocrinopathies); change in gait, pain or weakness in lower extremities, and urinary incontinence (spinal cord defects); night sweats, fever, and weight loss (cancer); and vomiting, abdominal pain, poor growth, and intermittent diarrhea (intestinal disorders).

Past medical history should ask about known disorders that can cause constipation, including cystic fibrosis and celiac disease. Exposure to constipating drugs or lead paint dust should be noted. Clinicians should ask about delayed passage of meconium within the first 24 to 48 h of life, as well as previous episodes of constipation and family history of constipation.

Physical examination: The physical examination begins with general assessment of the child's level of comfort or distress and overall appearance (including skin and hair condition). Height and weight should be measured and plotted on growth charts.

Examination should focus on the abdomen and anus and on the neurologic examination.

The abdomen is inspected for distention, auscultated for bowel sounds, and palpated for masses and tenderness. The anus is inspected for a fissure (taking care not to spread the buttocks so forcefully as to cause one). A digital rectal examination is done gently to check stool consistency and to obtain a sample for occult blood testing. Rectal examination should note the tightness of the rectal opening and presence or absence of stool in the rectal vault. Examination includes placement of the anus and presence of any hair tuft or pit superior to the sacrum.

In infants, neurologic examination focuses on tone and muscle strength. In older children, the focus is on gait, deep tendon reflexes, and signs of weakness in the lower extremities.

Red flags: The following findings are of particular concern:

- Delayed passage of meconium (> 24 to 48 h after birth)
- Hypotonia and poor suck (suggesting infant botulism)
- Abnormal gait and deep tendon reflexes (suggesting spinal cord involvement)

Interpretation of findings: A primary finding that suggests an organic cause in neonates is constipation from birth; those who have had a normal bowel movement are unlikely to have a significant structural disorder.

In older children, clues to an organic cause include constitutional symptoms (particularly weight loss, fever, or vomiting), poor growth (decreasing percentile on growth charts), an overall ill appearance, and any focal abnormalities detected during examination (see Table 290–1). A well-appearing child who has no other complaints besides constipation, who is not taking any constipating drugs, and who has a normal examination likely has a functional disorder.

A distended rectum filled with stool or the presence of an anal fissure is consistent with functional constipation in an otherwise normal child. Constipation that began after starting a constipating drug or that coincides with a dietary change can be attributed to that drug or food. Foods that are known to be constipating include dairy (eg, milk, cheese, yogurt) and starches and processed foods that do not contain fiber. However, if constipation complaints begin after ingestion of wheat, celiac disease should be considered. History of a new stress (eg, a new sibling) or other potential causes of stool retention behavior, with normal physical findings, support a functional etiology.

Testing: For patients whose histories are consistent with functional constipation, no tests are needed unless there is no response to conventional treatment of constipation. An abdominal x-ray should be done if patients have been unresponsive to treatment or an organic cause is suspected. Tests for organic causes should be done based on the history and physical examination (see Table 290–1):

- Barium enema, rectal manometry, and biopsy (Hirschsprung disease)
- Plain x-rays of lumbosacral spine; MRI considered (tethered spinal cord or tumor)
- Thyroid-stimulating hormone and thyroxine (hypothyroidism)
- Blood lead level (lead poisoning)
- Stool for botulinum toxin (infant botulism)
- Sweat test and genetic testing (cystic fibrosis)
- Calcium and other electrolytes (metabolic derangement)
- Serologic screening usually for IgA antibodies to tissue transglutaminase (celiac disease)

Treatment

Specific organic causes of constipation should be treated. Functional constipation is ideally initially treated with

- Dietary changes
- Behavior modification

Dietary changes include adding prune juice to formula for infants; increasing fruits, vegetables, and other sources of fiber for older infants and children; increasing water intake; and decreasing the amount of constipating foods (eg, milk, cheese).

Table 290–2. TREATMENT OF CONSTIPATION

TYPE OF THERAPY	AGENT	DOSE	SELECTED ADVERSE EFFECTS
Disimpaction			
Oral	Oral high-dose mineral oil (should not be used in infants < 1 yr or in neurologically impaired children to avoid aspiration)	15–20 mL/yr of age (maximum 240 mL/day) for 3 days or until stool appears	Fecal incontinence, malabsorption of fat-soluble vitamins (if treatments are repeated)
	Oral polyethylene glycol–electrolyte solution	25 mL/kg/h (maximum 1000 mL/h) by NGT until stool appears or 20 mL/kg/h for 4 h/day	Nausea, vomiting, cramping, bloating
	Oral polyethylene glycol without electrolytes	1–1.5 g/kg dissolved in 10 mL/kg water once/day for 3 days	Fecal incontinence
Rectal	Glycerin suppositories	**Infants and older children:** 1/2–1 suppository once/day for 3 days or until stool appears	None
	Rectal mineral oil enema	**2–11 yr:** 2.25 oz once/day for 3 days or until stool appears **≥ 12 yr:** 4.5 oz once/day for 3 days or until stool appears	Fecal incontinence, mechanical trauma
	Rectal phosphate sodium enema	**2– 4 yr:** 1.13 oz once/day for 3 days or until stool appears **5–11 yr:** 2.25 oz once/day for 3 days or until stool appears **≥ 12 yr:** 4.5 oz once/day for 3 days or until stool appears	Mechanical trauma, hyperphosphatemia
Maintenance agents			
Oral osmotic and lubricant laxatives	Lactulose (70% solution)	1 mL/kg once/day or bid (maximum 60 mL/day)	Abdominal cramping, flatus
	Magnesium hydroxide (400 mg/5 mL solution)	1–2 mL/kg once/day	If overdose, risk of hypermagnesemia, hypophosphatemia, or secondary hypocalcemia
	Mineral oil	1–3 mL/kg once/day	Fecal incontinence
	Polyethylene glycol 3350 powder dissolved in water	**1–18 mo:** 1 tsp powder in 60 mL (2 oz) water once/day **> 18 mo–3 yr:** 1/2 packet powder (8.5 g) in 120 mL (4 oz) water once/day **≥ 3 yr:** 1 packet (17 g) in 240 mL (8 oz) water once/day	Fecal incontinence
Oral stimulant laxatives (to be used for a limited period of time)	Bisacodyl (5 mg tablets)	**2–11 yr:** 1–2 tablets once/day **≥ 12 yr:** 1–3 tablets once/day	Fecal incontinence, hypokalemia, abdominal cramps
	Senna syrup: 8.8 mg sennosides/5 mL Senna tablets: 8.6 mg sennosides/tablet	**> 1 yr:** 1.25 mL once/day up to 2.25 mL bid **2–5 yr:** 2.5 mL once/day up to 3.75 mL bid **6–11 yr:** 5 mL once/day up to 7.5 mL bid **≥ 12 yr:** 1 tablet once/day up to 2 tablets bid	Abdominal cramping, melanosis coli
Maintenance diet supplements			
Dietary fiber supplements	Methylcellulose*	**< 6 yr:** 0.5–1 g once/day **6–11 yr:** 1 g 1–3 times/day **≥ 12 yr:** 2 g 1–3 times/day	Less bloating than other fiber supplements
	Psyllium*	**6–11 yr:** 1.25–15 g 1–3 times/day **≥12 yr:** 2.5–30 g 1–3 times/day	Bloating, flatus
	Sorbitol-containing fruit juices (eg, prune, pear, apple)	**Infants and older children:** 30 to 120 mL (1–4 oz)/day	Flatus
	Wheat dextrin*	**2–20 yr:** 5 g plus 1 g for each yr of age once/day	Bloating, flatus

*Numerous commercial products and preparations are available in differing concentrations, so doses are given in terms of grams of fiber.

Behavior modification for older children involves encouraging regular stool passage after meals if they are toilet trained and providing a reinforcement chart and encouragement to them. For children who are in the process of toilet training, it is sometimes worthwhile to give them a break from training until the constipation concern has passed.

Unresponsive constipation is treated by disimpacting the bowel and maintaining a regular diet and stool routine. Disimpaction can occur through oral or rectal agents. Oral agents require consumption of large volumes of liquid. Rectal agents can feel invasive and can be difficult to give. Both methods can be done by parents under medical supervision; however, disimpaction sometimes requires hospitalization if outpatient management is unsuccessful. Usually, infants do not require extreme measures, but if intervention is required, a glycerin suppository is typically adequate. For maintenance of healthy bowels, some children may require OTC dietary fiber supplements. These supplements require consuming 32 to 64 oz of water/day to be effective (see Table 290–2).

KEY POINTS

- Functional constipation accounts for about 95% of cases.
- Organic causes are rare but need to be considered.
- Delayed passage of meconium for > 24 to 48 h after birth raises suspicion of structural disorders, especially Hirschsprung disease.
- Early intervention with dietary and behavior changes can successfully treat functional constipation.

COUGH IN CHILDREN

Cough is a reflex that helps clear the airways of secretions, protects the airway from foreign body aspiration, and can be the manifesting symptom of a disease. Cough is one of the most common complaints for which parents bring their children to a health care practitioner.

Etiology

Causes of cough differ depending on whether the symptoms are acute (< 4 wk) or chronic (see Table 290–3).

For **acute cough,** the most common cause is

- Viral URI

For **chronic cough,** the most common causes are

- Asthma (most common)
- Gastroesophageal reflux disorder (GERD)
- Postnasal drip

Foreign body aspiration and diseases such as cystic fibrosis and primary ciliary dyskinesia are less common, although they can all result in persistent cough.

Evaluation

History: History of present illness should cover duration and quality of cough (barky, staccato, paroxysmal) and onset (sudden or indolent). The physician should ask about associated symptoms. Some of these symptoms are ubiquitous (eg, runny nose, sore throat, fever); others may suggest a specific cause: headache, itchy eyes, and sore throat (postnasal drip); wheezing and cough with exertion (asthma); night sweats (TB); and spitting up, irritability, or arching of the back after feedings in infants (gastroesophageal reflux). For children 6 mo to 6 yr, the parents should be asked about potential for foreign body aspiration, including older siblings or visitors with small toys, access to small objects, and consumption of small, smooth foods (eg, peanuts, grapes).

Review of systems should note symptoms of possible causes, including abdominal pain (some bacterial pneumonias), weight loss or poor weight gain and foul-smelling stools (cystic fibrosis), and muscle soreness (possible association with viral illness or atypical pneumonia but usually not with bacterial pneumonia).

Past medical history should cover recent respiratory infections, repeated pneumonias, history of known allergies or asthma, risk factors for TB (eg, exposure to a person who has known or suspected TB infection, exposure to prisons, HIV infection, travel to or immigration from countries that have endemic infection), and exposure to respiratory irritants.

Physical examination: Vital signs, including respiratory rate, temperature, and oxygen saturation, should be noted. Signs of respiratory distress (eg, nasal flaring, intercostal retractions, cyanosis, grunting, stridor, marked anxiety) should be noted.

Head and neck examination should focus on presence and amount of nasal discharge and the condition of the nasal turbinates (pale, boggy, or inflamed). The pharynx should be checked for postnasal drip.

The cervical and supraclavicular areas should be inspected and palpated for lymphadenopathy.

Lung examination focuses on presence of stridor, wheezing, crackles, rhonchi, decreased breath sounds, and signs of consolidation (eg, egophony, E to A change, dullness to percussion).

Abdominal examination should focus on presence of abdominal pain, especially in the upper quadrants (indicating possible left or right lower lobe pneumonia).

Examination of extremities should note clubbing or cyanosis of nail beds (cystic fibrosis).

Red flags: The following findings are of particular concern:

- Cyanosis or hypoxia on pulse oximetry
- Stridor
- Respiratory distress
- Toxic appearance
- Abnormal lung examination

Interpretation of findings: Clinical findings frequently indicate a specific cause (see Table 290–3); the distinction between acute and chronic cough is particularly helpful although it is important to note that many disorders that cause chronic cough begin acutely and patients may present before 4 wk have passed.

Other characteristics of the cough are helpful but less specific. A barky cough suggests croup or tracheitis; it can also be characteristic of psychogenic cough or a postrespiratory tract infection cough. A staccato cough is consistent with a viral or atypical pneumonia. A paroxysmal cough is characteristic of pertussis or certain viral pneumonias (adenovirus). Failure to thrive or weight loss can occur with TB or cystic fibrosis. Nighttime cough can indicate postnasal drip or asthma. Coughing at the beginning of sleep and in the morning with waking usually indicates sinusitis; coughing in the middle of the night is more consistent with asthma. In young children with sudden cough and no fever or URI symptoms, the examiner should have a high index of suspicion for foreign body aspiration.

Testing: Children with red flag findings should have pulse oximetry and chest x-ray. All children with chronic cough require a chest x-ray.

Children with stridor, drooling, fever, and marked anxiety need to be evaluated for epiglottitis, typically in the operating room by an ENT specialist prepared to immediately place an endotracheal or tracheostomy tube. If foreign body aspiration

Table 290–3. SOME CAUSES OF COUGH IN CHILDREN

CAUSE	SUGGESTIVE FINDINGS	DIAGNOSTIC APPROACH
Acute		
Bacterial tracheitis (rare)	URI-like prodrome, stridor, barky cough, high fever, respiratory distress, toxic appearance, purulent secretions	Anteroposterior and lateral neck x-rays Possibly bronchoscopy
Bronchiolitis	Rhinorrhea, tachypnea, wheezing, crackles, retractions, nasal flaring, possible posttussive emesis In infants up to 24 mo; most common among those 3–6 mo	Clinical evaluation Sometimes chest x-ray Sometimes nasal swab for rapid viral antigen assays or viral culture
Croup	URI-like prodrome, barky cough (worsening at night), stridor, nasal flaring, retractions, tachypnea	Clinical evaluation Sometimes anteroposterior and lateral neck x-rays
Environmental pulmonary toxicants	Exposure to tobacco smoke, perfume, or ambient pollutants	Clinical evaluation
Epiglottitis (rare)	Abrupt onset, high fever, irritability, marked anxiety, stridor, respiratory distress, drooling, toxic appearance	If patient is stable and clinical suspicion is low, lateral neck x-ray Otherwise, examination in operating room with direct laryngoscopy
Foreign body	Sudden onset of cough and/or choking No fever initially No URI prodrome	Chest x-ray (inspiratory and expiratory views) Sometimes bronchoscopy
Pneumonia (viral, bacterial)	**Viral:** URI prodrome, fever, wheezing, staccato-like or paroxysmal cough, possible muscle soreness or pleuritic chest pain Possible increased work of breathing, diffuse crackles, rhonchi, or wheezing **Bacterial:** Fever, ill appearance, chest pain, shortness of breath, possible stomach pain or vomiting Signs of focal consolidation including localized crackles, rhonchi, decreased breath sounds, egophony, and dullness to percussion	Chest x-ray
Sinusitis	Coughing at the beginning of sleep or in the morning with waking Sometimes nasal discharge, congestion; pain on either side of the nose; pain in the forehead, upper jaw, teeth, or between the eyes; headache and sore throat	Clinical evaluation Sometimes CT
URI	Rhinorrhea, red swollen nasal mucosa, possible fever and sore throat, shotty cervical adenopathy (many small nontender nodes)	Clinical evaluation
Chronic*		
Airway lesions (tracheomalacia, TEF)	**Tracheomalacia:** Congenital stridor or barky cough, possible respiratory distress **TEF:** History of polyhydramnios (if accompanied by esophageal atresia), cough or respiratory distress with feeding, recurrent pneumonia	**Tracheomalacia:** Airway fluoroscopy and/or bronchoscopy **TEF:** Attempt passage of a catheter into the stomach (helps in diagnosis of TEF with esophageal atresia) Chest x-ray Contrast swallowing study, including esophagography Bronchoscopy and endoscopy
Asthma	Intermittent episodes of cough with exercise, allergens, weather changes, or URIs Nighttime cough Family history of asthma History of eczema or allergic rhinitis	Clinical evaluation Trial of asthma drugs Pulmonary function tests
Atypical pneumonia (mycoplasma, *Chlamydia*)	Gradual onset of illness Headache, malaise, muscle soreness Possible ear pain, rhinitis, and sore throat Possible wheezing and crackles Persistent staccato cough	Chest x-ray PCR testing

Table continues on the following page.

Table 290–3. SOME CAUSES OF COUGH IN CHILDREN (*Continued*)

CAUSE	SUGGESTIVE FINDINGS	DIAGNOSTIC APPROACH
Birth defects of the lungs (eg, congenital adenomatoid malformation)	Several episodes of pneumonia in the same part of the lungs	Chest x-ray Sometimes CT or MRI
Cystic fibrosis	History of meconium ileus, recurrent pneumonia or wheezing, failure to thrive, foul-smelling stools, clubbing or cyanosis of nail beds	Sweat chloride test Molecular diagnosis with direct mutation analysis
Foreign body	History of acute onset of cough and choking followed by a period of persistent cough Possible development of fever **Infants and toddlers:** No URI prodrome Presence of small objects or toys near child	Chest x-ray (inspiratory and expiratory views) Bronchoscopy
Gastroesophageal reflux	History of spitting up after feedings, irritability with feeding, stiffening and arching of the back (Sandifer syndrome), failure to thrive, recurrent wheezing or pneumonia (see Gastroesophageal Reflux in Infants on p. 2582) **Older children and adolescents:** Chest pain or heartburn after meals and lying down, nighttime cough, wheezing, hoarseness, halitosis, water brash, nausea, abdominal pain, regurgitation (see Gastroesophageal Reflux Disease on p. 113)	**Infants:** Clinical evaluation Sometimes upper GI study for determination of anatomy Trial of H_2 blockers or a proton pump inhibitor Possible esophageal pH or impedance probe study **Older children:** Clinical evaluation Trial of H_2 blockers or proton pump inhibitors Possible endoscopy
Pertussis or parapertussis	1–2 wk catarrhal phase of mild URI symptoms, progression to paroxysmal cough, difficulty eating, apneic episodes in infants, inspiratory whoop in older children, posttussive emesis	Intranasal specimen for bacterial culture and PCR
Allergic rhinitis with postnasal drip	Headache, itchy eyes, sore throat, pale nasal turbinates, cobblestoning of posterior oropharynx, history of allergies, nighttime cough	Trial of antihistamine and/or intranasal steroids Possible trial of a leukotriene inhibitor
Postrespiratory tract infection	History of respiratory infection followed by a persistent, staccato cough	Clinical evaluation
Primary ciliary dyskinesia	History of repeated upper (otitis media, sinusitis) and lower (pneumonia) respiratory tract infections	Chest x-ray Sinus x-ray or CT Chest CT Microscopic examination of living tissue (typically from sinus or airway mucosa) for cilia abnormalities
Psychogenic cough	Persistent barky cough, possibly prominent during classes and absent during play and at night No fevers or other symptoms	Clinical evaluation
Tuberculosis (TB)	History or risk of exposure Immunocompromise Sometimes fever, chills, night sweats, lymphadenopathy, weight loss	PPD Sputum culture (or morning gastric aspirate culture for children < 5 yr) Interferon-gamma release assay (especially if there is a history of BCG vaccination) Chest x-ray

*All patients require a chest x-ray when they present for the first time with chronic cough.
TEF = tracheoesophageal fistula.

is suspected, chest x-ray with inspiratory and expiratory views should be done.

Children with TB risk factors or weight loss should have a chest x-ray and PPD testing for TB.

Children with repeated episodes of pneumonia, poor growth, or foul-smelling stools should have a chest x-ray and sweat testing for cystic fibrosis.

Acute cough in children with URI symptoms and no red flag findings is usually caused by a viral infection, and testing is rarely indicated. Many other children without red flag findings have a presumptive diagnosis after the history and physical examination. Testing is not necessary in such cases; however, if empiric treatment has been instituted and has not been successful, testing may be necessary. For example, if allergic sinusitis is suspected and treated with an antihistamine that does not alleviate symptoms, a head CT may be necessary for further evaluation. Suspected GERD unsuccessfully treated with an H_2 blocker and/or proton pump inhibitor may require evaluation with a pH or impedance probe study or endoscopy.

Treatment

Treatment of cough is management of the underlying disorder. For example, antibiotics should be given for bacterial pneumonia; bronchodilators and anti-inflammatory drugs should be given for asthma. Children with viral infections should receive supportive care, including oxygen and/or bronchodilators as needed.

Little evidence exists to support the use of cough suppressants and mucolytic agents. Coughing is an important mechanism for clearing secretions from the airways and can assist in recovery from respiratory infections. Use of nonspecific drugs for cough suppression is discouraged in children.

KEY POINTS

- Clinical diagnosis is often adequate.
- A high index of suspicion for foreign body aspiration is needed if children are age 6 mo to 6 yr.
- Antitussives and expectorants lack proof of effect in most cases.
- Obtain a chest x-ray if patients have red flag findings or chronic cough.

CRYING

All infants and young children cry as a form of communication; it is the only means they have to express a need. Thus, most crying is in response to hunger, discomfort (eg, a wet diaper), or separation, and it ceases when the needs are met (eg, by feeding, changing, cuddling). This crying is normal and tends to lessen in duration and frequency after 3 mo of age. However, crying that persists after attempts to address routine needs and efforts to console or that is prolonged in relation to the child's baseline should be investigated to identify a specific cause.

Etiology

Cause of crying is

- Organic in < 5%
- Functional in 95%

Organic: Organic causes, although rare, must always be considered. Causes to consider are classified as cardiac, GI, infectious, and traumatic (see Table 290–4). Of these, potential life threats include heart failure, intussusception, volvulus, meningitis, and intracranial bleeding due to head trauma.

Colic is excessive crying that occurs in infants ≤ 4 mo of age, that has no identifiable organic cause, and that occurs at least 3 h/day > 3 days/wk for > 3 wk.

Evaluation

History: History of present illness focuses on onset of crying, duration, response to attempts to console, and frequency or uniqueness of episodes. Parents should be asked about associated events or conditions, including recent immunizations, trauma (eg, falls), interaction with a sibling, infections, drug use, and relationship of crying with feedings and bowel movements.

Review of systems focuses on symptoms of causative disorders, including constipation, diarrhea, vomiting, arching of back, explosive stools, and bloody stools (GI disorders); fever, cough, wheezing, nasal congestion, and difficulty breathing (respiratory infection); and apparent pain during bathing or changing (trauma).

Past medical history should note previous episodes of crying and conditions that can potentially predispose to crying (eg, history of heart disease, developmental delay).

Physical examination: Examination begins with a review of vital signs, particularly for fever and tachypnea. Initial observation assesses the infant or child for signs of lethargy or distress and notes how the parents are interacting with the child.

The infant or child is undressed and observed for signs of respiratory distress (eg, superclavicular and subcostal retractions, cyanosis). The entire body surface is inspected for swelling, bruising, and abrasions.

Auscultatory examination focuses on signs of respiratory infection (eg, wheezing, crackles, decreased breath sounds) and cardiac compromise (eg, tachycardia, gallop, holosystolic murmur, systolic click). The abdomen is palpated for signs of tenderness. The diaper is removed for examination of the genitals and anus to look for signs of testicular torsion (eg, red-ecchymotic scrotum, pain on palpation), hair tourniquet on the penis, inguinal hernia (eg, swelling in the inguinal region or scrotum), and anal fissures.

Extremities are examined for signs of fracture (eg, swelling, erythema, tenderness, pain with passive motion). Fingers and toes are checked for hair tourniquets.

The ears are examined for signs of trauma (eg, blood in the canal or behind the tympanic membrane) or infection (eg, red, bulging tympanic membrane). The corneas are stained with fluorescein and examined with a blue light to rule out corneal abrasion, and the fundi are examined with an ophthalmoscope for signs of hemorrhage. (If retinal hemorrhages are suspected, examination by an ophthalmologist is advised.) The oropharynx is examined for signs of thrush or oral abrasions. The skull is gently palpated for signs of fracture.

Red flags: The following findings are of particular concern:

- Respiratory distress
- Bruising and abrasions
- Extreme irritability
- Fever and inconsolability
- Fever in an infant ≤ 8 wk of age

Interpretation of findings: A high index of suspicion is warranted when evaluating crying. Parental concern is an important variable. When concern is high, the clinician should be wary even when there are no conclusive findings because the parents may be reacting subconsciously to subtle but significant changes. Conversely, a very low level of concern, particularly if there is lack of parental interaction with the infant or child, can indicate a bonding problem or an inability to assess and manage the child's needs. Inconsistency of the history and the child's clinical presentation should raise concerns about possible abuse.

It is helpful to distinguish the general area of concern. For example, with fever, the most likely etiology is infectious; respiratory distress without fever indicates possible cardiac etiology or pain. Abnormalities in stool history or abdominal pain during examination is consistent with a GI etiology. Specific findings often suggest certain causes (see Table 290–4).

Table 290–4. SOME CAUSES OF CRYING

CAUSE	SUGGESTIVE FINDINGS	DIAGNOSTIC APPROACH
Cardiac		
Coarctation of the aorta	Delayed or absent femoral pulses Tachypnea Cough Diaphoresis Poor feeding Systolic ejection murmur, systolic click	Chest x-ray ECG Ultrasonography
Heart failure	Tachypnea Cough Diaphoresis Poor feeding S_3 gallop	Chest x-ray ECG Echocardiography
Supraventricular tachycardia	Tachypnea Cough Diaphoresis Poor feeding Heart rate > 180 beats/min (usually 220–280 beats/min in infants; 180–220 beats/min in older children)	Chest x-ray ECG
GI		
Constipation	Anal tears or fissures History of decreased stool frequency and hard pellet stools Distended abdomen	Clinical evaluation
Gastroenteritis	Hyperactive bowel sounds Loose, frequent stools	Clinical evaluation
Gastroesophageal reflux	History of spitting up, arching, or crying after feedings	Swallowing study Esophageal pH or impedance probe study
Intussusception	Severe colicky abdominal pain alternating with calm, pain-free periods Lethargy Vomiting Currant-jelly stools	Abdominal x-ray Air enema
Cow's milk protein intolerance (milk protein allergy)	Vomiting Diarrhea or constipation Poor feeding Failure to thrive	Stool heme test
Volvulus	Bilious vomiting Tender, distended abdomen Bloody stools Absent bowel sounds	Abdominal x-ray Barium enema
Incarcerated hernia	Tender, erythematous mass in groin	Clinical evaluation
Infection		
Meningitis	Fever Inconsolability, irritability Lethargy Bulging anterior fontanelle in infants Nuchal rigidity (meningismus) in older children	Lumbar puncture for CSF testing
Otitis media	Fever Pulling at ears or complaints of ear pain Erythematous, opaque, bulging tympanic membrane	Clinical evaluation

Table 290–4. SOME CAUSES OF CRYING (*Continued*)

CAUSE	SUGGESTIVE FINDINGS	DIAGNOSTIC APPROACH
Respiratory infection (bronchiolitis, pneumonia)	Fever Tachypnea Sometimes hypoxia Sometimes wheezing, crackles, or decreased breath sounds on auscultation	Chest x-ray
Urinary tract infection (UTI)	Fever Possible vomiting	Urinalysis and culture
Trauma		
Corneal abrasion	Crying with no other symptoms	Fluorescein test
Fracture (abuse)	Area of swelling and/or ecchymoses Favoring of a limb	Skeletal survey x-rays to check for current and old fractures
Hair tourniquet	Swollen tip of a toe, finger, or penis with hair wrapped around the appendage proximal to the swelling	Clinical evaluation
Head trauma with intracranial bleeding	Inconsolable, high-pitched cry Localized swelling on skull with underlying deformity	Head CT
Abusive head trauma (shaken baby syndrome)	Inconsolable, high-pitched cry Lethargy Seizure activity	Head CT Retinal examination Skeletal survey
Other		
Cold drugs	History of recent cold drug therapy	Clinical evaluation
Testicular torsion	Swollen erythematous asymmetric scrotum, absent cremasteric reflex	Doppler ultrasonography or nuclear scanning of the scrotum
Vaccine reaction	History of recent immunization	Clinical evaluation

S_3 = 3rd heart sound.

The time frame is also helpful. Crying that has been intermittent over a number of days is of less concern than sudden, constant crying. Whether the cry is exclusive to a time of day or night is helpful. For example, recent onset of crying at night in an otherwise happy, healthy infant or child may be consistent with separation anxiety or sleep association issues.

The character of the cry is also revealing. Parents frequently can distinguish a cry that is painful in character from a frantic or scared cry. It is also important to determine the level of acuity. An inconsolable infant or child is of more concern than an infant or child who is well-appearing and consolable in the office.

Testing: Testing is targeted at the suspected cause (see Table 290–4) and particular attention is paid to potential life threats, unless the history and physical examination are sufficient for diagnosis. When there are few or no specific clinical findings and no testing is immediately indicated, close follow-up and reevaluation are appropriate.

Treatment

The underlying organic disorder should be treated. Support and encouragement are important for parents when the infant or child has no apparent underlying disorder. Swaddling an infant in the first month of life can be helpful. Holding an infant or child is helpful in decreasing the duration of crying. It is also valuable to encourage parents, if they are feeling frustrated, to take a break from a crying baby and put the infant or child down in a safe environment for a few minutes. Educating parents and "giving permission" to take a break are helpful in preventing abuse. Supplying resources for support services to parents who seem overwhelmed may prevent future concerns.

KEY POINTS

- Crying is part of normal development and is most prevalent during the first 3 mo of life.
- Excessive crying with organic causes needs to be differentiated from colic.
- Less than 5% of crying has an organic cause.
- When no organic cause is identified, parents may need support.

DIARRHEA IN CHILDREN

Diarrhea is frequent loose or watery bowel movements that deviate from a child's normal pattern.

Diarrhea may be accompanied by anorexia, vomiting, acute weight loss, abdominal pain, fever, or passage of blood. If diarrhea is severe or prolonged, dehydration is likely. Even in the absence of dehydration, chronic diarrhea usually results in weight loss or failure to gain weight.

Diarrhea is a very common pediatric concern and causes about 1.5 million deaths/yr worldwide. It accounts for about 9% of hospitalizations in the US among children aged < 5 yr.

Diarrhea in adults is discussed on p. 73.

Pathophysiology

Mechanisms of diarrhea may include the following:

- Osmotic
- Secretory
- Inflammatory
- Malabsorptive

Osmotic diarrhea results from the presence of nonabsorbable solutes in the GI tract, as with lactose intolerance. Fasting for 2 to 3 days stops osmotic diarrhea.

Secretory diarrhea results from substances (eg, bacterial toxins) that increase secretion of chloride ions and water into the intestinal lumen. Secretory diarrhea does not stop with fasting.

Inflammatory diarrhea is associated with conditions that cause inflammation or ulceration of the intestinal mucosa (eg, Crohn disease, ulcerative colitis). The resultant outpouring of plasma, serum proteins, blood, and mucous increases fecal bulk and fluid content.

Malabsorption may result from osmotic or secretory mechanisms or conditions that lead to less surface area in the bowel. Conditions such as pancreatic insufficiency and short bowel syndrome and conditions that speed up transit time cause diarrhea due to decreased absorption.

Etiology

The causes and significance of diarrhea (see Table 290–5) differ depending on whether it is acute (< 2 wk) or chronic (> 2 wk). Most cases of diarrhea are acute.

Acute diarrhea usually is caused by

- Gastroenteritis
- Antibiotic use
- Food allergies
- Food poisoning

Most gastroenteritis is caused by a virus; however, any enteric pathogen can cause acute diarrhea.

Chronic diarrhea usually is caused by

- Dietary factors
- Infection
- Celiac disease
- Inflammatory bowel disease

Chronic diarrhea can also be caused by anatomic disorders and disorders that interfere with absorption or digestion.

Evaluation

History: History of present illness focuses on quality, frequency, and duration of stools, as well as on any accompanying fever, vomiting, abdominal pain, or blood in the stool. Parents are asked about current or recent (within 2 mo) antibiotic use. Clinicians should establish elements of the diet (eg, amounts of juice, foods high in sugars or sorbitol). Any history of hard stools or constipation should be noted. Clinicians should also assess risk factors for infection (eg, recent travel; exposure to questionable food sources; recent contact with animals at a petting zoo, reptiles, or someone with similar symptoms).

Review of systems should seek symptoms of both complications and causes of diarrhea. Symptoms of complications include weight loss and decreased frequency of urination and fluid intake (dehydration). Symptoms of causes include urticarial rash associated with food intake (food allergy); nasal polyps, sinusitis, and poor growth (cystic fibrosis); and arthritis, skin lesions, and anal fissures (inflammatory bowel disease).

Past medical history should assess known causative disorders (eg, immunocompromise, cystic fibrosis, celiac disease, inflammatory bowel disease) in the patient and family members.

Physical examination: Vital signs should be reviewed for indications of dehydration (eg, tachycardia, hypotension) and fever.

General assessment includes checking for signs of lethargy or distress. Growth parameters should be noted.

Because the abdominal examination may elicit discomfort, it is advisable to begin the examination with the head. Examination should focus on the mucous membranes to assess whether they are moist or dry. Nasal polyps; psoriasiform dermatitis around the eyes, nose, and mouth; and oral ulcerations should be noted.

Examination of the extremities focuses on skin turgor, capillary refill time, and the presence of petechiae, purpura, other skin lesions (eg, erythema nodosum, pyoderma gangrenosum), rashes, and erythematous, swollen joints.

Abdominal examination focuses on distention, tenderness, and quality of bowel sounds (eg, high-pitched, normal, absent). Examination of the genitals focuses on presence of rashes and signs of anal fissures or ulcerative lesions.

Red flags: The following findings are of particular concern:

- Tachycardia, hypotension, and lethargy (significant dehydration)
- Bloody stools
- Bilious vomiting
- Extreme abdominal tenderness and/or distention
- Petechiae and/or pallor

Interpretation of findings: Antibiotic-related, postinfectious, and anatomic-related causes of diarrhea are typically clear from the history. Determination of the time frame helps establish whether diarrhea is acute or chronic. Establishing the level of acuity is also important. Most cases of acute diarrhea have a viral etiology, are low acuity, and cause fever and nonbloody diarrhea. However, bacterial diarrhea can lead to serious consequences; manifestations include fever, bloody diarrhea, and possibly a petechial or purpuric rash.

Symptoms associated with chronic diarrhea can vary and those of different conditions can overlap. For example, Crohn disease and celiac disease can cause oral ulcerations, a number of conditions can cause rashes, and any condition can lead to a poor growth pattern. If the cause is unclear, further tests are done based on clinical findings (see Table 290–5).

Testing: Testing is unnecessary in most cases of acute self-limited diarrhea. However, if the evaluation suggests an etiology other than viral gastroenteritis, testing should be directed by the suspected etiology (see Table 290–5).

Treatment

Specific causes of diarrhea are treated (eg, gluten-free diet for children with celiac disease).

General treatment focuses on hydration, which can usually be done orally. IV hydration is rarely essential. (Caution: Antidiarrheal drugs [eg, loperamide] are not recommended for infants and young children.)

Rehydration: Oral rehydration solution (ORS) should contain complex carbohydrate or 2% glucose and 50 to 90 mEq/L sodium. Sports drinks, sodas, juices, and similar drinks do not meet these criteria and should not be used. They generally have too little sodium and too much carbohydrate to take advantage of sodium/glucose cotransport, and the osmotic effect of the excess carbohydrate may result in additional fluid loss.

ORS is recommended by the WHO and is widely available in the US without a prescription. Premixed solutions are also available at most pharmacies and supermarkets.

If the child is also vomiting, small, frequent amounts are used, starting with 5 mL q 5 min and increasing gradually as tolerated (see Oral Rehydration on p. 2557). If the child is not vomiting, the initial amount is not restricted. In either case, generally 50 mL/kg is given over 4 h for mild dehydration, and

Table 290–5. SOME CAUSES OF DIARRHEA

CAUSE	SUGGESTIVE FINDINGS	DIAGNOSTIC APPROACH
Acute		
Antibiotics (eg, broad-spectrum antibiotics, multiple concomitant antibiotics)	Temporal relationship of onset of diarrhea with taking of antibiotics	Clinical evaluation
Bacteria (eg, *Campylobacter sp*, *Clostridium difficile*, *Escherichia coli* [can cause hemolytic-uremic syndrome], *Salmonella sp*, *Shigella sp*, *Yersinia enterocolitica*)*	Fever, bloody stool, abdominal pain	Stool culture
	Possibly petechiae or pallor (in patients with hemolytic uremic syndrome)	Fecal leukocytes
	History of contact with animals (*E. coli*) or reptiles (*Salmonella*)	If patients appear ill, CBC, renal function tests, and blood culture
	History of eating undercooked food (Salmonella)	If patient has recently been given antibiotics, stool testing for *C. difficile* toxin
	Recent (< 2 mo) antibiotic use (*C. difficile*)	
	Day care center outbreak	
Food allergy or food poisoning	**Allergy:** Urticarial rash, lip swelling, abdominal pain, vomiting, diarrhea, difficulty breathing within minutes to several hours after eating	Clinical evaluation
	Poisoning: Nausea, vomiting, abdominal pain, diarrhea several hours after ingestion of contaminated food	
Parasites (eg, *Giardia intestinalis [lamblia]*, *Cryptosporidium parvum*)*	Abdominal bloating and cramping, foul-smelling stools, anorexia	
	Possibly history of travel, use of contaminated water source	Stool antigen tests
Viruses (eg, astrovirus, calicivirus, enteric adenovirus, rotavirus)*	< 5 days of diarrhea with no blood	Clinical evaluation
	Often vomiting	
	Possibly fever	
	Contact with infected people	
	Appropriate season for the infection	
Chronic		
Hirschsprung enterocolitis	Delayed passage of stool > 48 h after birth	Abdominal x-ray
	Possibly long-standing history of constipation	Barium enema
	Bilious vomiting, abdominal distention, ill appearance	Rectal biopsy
Short bowel syndrome	History of bowel resection (eg, for necrotizing enterocolitis, volvulus, or Hirschsprung disease)	Clinical evaluation

Table continues on the following page.

Table 290–5. SOME CAUSES OF DIARRHEA (*Continued*)

CAUSE	SUGGESTIVE FINDINGS	DIAGNOSTIC APPROACH
Lactose intolerance	Abdominal bloating, flatus, explosive diarrhea Diarrhea after ingestion of dairy products	Clinical evaluation Sometimes hydrogen breath test Sometimes test for reducing substances in stool (to check for carbohydrates) and stool pH (< 6.0 indicates carbohydrates in stool)
Cow's milk protein intolerance (milk protein allergy)	Vomiting Diarrhea or constipation Hematochezia Anal fissures Failure to thrive	Symptom resolution when cow's milk protein is eliminated Sometimes endoscopy or colonoscopy
Excessive juice intake	History of excessive juice or sugary drink intake (4–6 oz/day)	Clinical evaluation
Chronic nonspecific diarrhea of childhood (toddler's diarrhea)	Age 6 mo–5 yr 3–10 loose stools/day typically during the day while awake and sometimes immediately after eating Sometimes undigested food visible in stool Normal growth, weight gain, activity, and appetite	Clinical evaluation
Immunodeficiency (eg, HIV infection, IgA deficiency, or IgG deficiency)	History of recurrent skin, respiratory tract, or intestinal infections Weight loss or poor weight gain	HIV test CBC Immunoglobulin levels
Eosinophilic gastroenteritis	Abdominal pain, nausea, vomiting, weight loss	CBC for peripheral blood eosinophilia Sometimes IgE level Endoscopy and/or colonoscopy
Inflammatory bowel disease (eg, Crohn disease, ulcerative colitis)	Bloody stools, crampy abdominal pain, weight loss, anorexia Possibly arthritis, oral ulcerations, skin lesions, rectal fissures	Colonoscopy
Celiac disease (gluten enteropathy)	Symptom onset after introduction of wheat into diet (typically after age 4–6 mo) Failure to thrive Recurrent abdominal pain Bloating Diarrhea or constipation	CBC Serologic screening for celiac disease (IgA antibody to tissue transglutaminase) Endoscopy for duodenal biopsy
Cystic fibrosis	Failure to thrive Repeated episodes of pneumonia or wheezing Fatty and foul-smelling stools Bloating, flatus	72-h fecal fat excretion Sweat test Genetic testing
Acrodermatitis enteropathica	Sometimes psoriasiform rash, angular stomatitis	Zinc levels
Constipation with encopresis	History of hard stools Fecal incontinence	Abdominal x-ray

*Can also cause chronic diarrhea.

100 mL/kg is given over 4 h for moderate dehydration. For each diarrheal stool, an additional 10 mL/kg (up to 240 mL) is given. After 4 h, the patient is reassessed. If signs of dehydration persist, the same volume is repeated.

Diet and nutrition: Children with an acute diarrheal illness should eat an age-appropriate diet as soon as they have been rehydrated and are not vomiting. Infants may resume breast milk or formula.

For chronic nonspecific diarrhea of childhood (toddler's diarrhea), dietary fat and fiber should be increased, and fluid intake (especially fruit juices) should be decreased.

For other causes of chronic diarrhea, adequate nutrition must be maintained, particularly of fat-soluble vitamins.

KEY POINTS

- Diarrhea is a common pediatric concern.
- Gastroenteritis is the most common cause.
- Testing is rarely necessary in children with acute diarrheal illnesses.
- Dehydration is likely if diarrhea is severe or prolonged.
- Oral rehydration is effective in most cases.
- Antidiarrheal drugs (eg, loperamide) are not recommended for infants and young children.

FEVER IN INFANTS AND CHILDREN

Normal body temperature varies from person to person and throughout the day. Normal body temperature is highest in children who are preschool aged. Several studies have documented that peak temperature tends to be in the afternoon and is highest at about 18 to 24 mo of age when many normal healthy children have a temperature of 101° F. However, fever usually is defined as a core body (rectal) temperature ≥ 38.0° C (100.4° F).

Significance of fever depends on clinical context rather than peak temperature; some minor illnesses cause high fever, whereas some serious illnesses cause only a mild temperature elevation. Although parental assessment is frequently clouded by fear of fever, the history of a temperature taken at home should be considered equivalent to a temperature taken in the office.

Pathophysiology

Fever occurs in response to the release of endogenous pyogenic mediators called cytokines. Cytokines stimulate the production of prostaglandins by the hypothalamus; prostaglandins readjust and elevate the temperature set point.

Fever plays an integral role in fighting infection and, although it may be uncomfortable, does not necessitate treatment in an otherwise healthy child. Some studies even indicate that lowering the temperature can prolong some illnesses. However, fever increases the metabolic rate and the demands on the cardiopulmonary system. Therefore, fever can be detrimental to children with pulmonary or cardiac compromise or neurologic impairment. It can also be the catalyst for febrile seizures, a typically benign childhood condition.

Etiology

Causes of fever (see Table 290–6) differ based on whether the fever is acute (≤ 14 days), acute recurrent or periodic (episodic fever separated by afebrile periods), or chronic (> 14 days), which is more commonly referred to as fever of unknown origin (FUO—see p. 1437). Response to antipyretics and height of the temperature have no direct relationship to the etiology or its seriousness.

Acute: Most acute fevers in infants and young children are caused by infection. The most common are

- Viral respiratory or GI infections (most common causes overall)
- Certain bacterial infections (otitis media, pneumonia, UTIs)

However, potential infectious causes of acute fever vary with the child's age. Neonates (infants < 28 days) are considered functionally immunocompromised because they often fail to contain infection locally and, as a result, are at higher risk of serious invasive bacterial infections most commonly caused by organisms acquired during the perinatal period. The most common perinatal pathogens in neonates are group B streptococci, *Escherichia coli* (and other gram-negative enteric organisms), *Listeria monocytogenes*, and herpes simplex virus. These organisms can cause bacteremia, pneumonia, pyelonephritis, meningitis, and/or sepsis.

Most febrile children 1 mo to 2 years of age without an obvious focus of infection on examination (fever without source [FWS]) have self-limited viral disease. However, a small number (perhaps < 1% in the post–conjugate vaccine era) of such patients are early in the course of a serious infection (eg, bacterial meningitis). Thus, the main concern in a patient with FWS is whether occult bacteremia (pathogenic bacteria in the bloodstream without focal symptoms or signs on examination) is present. The most common causative organisms of occult bacteremia are *Streptococcus pneumoniae* and *Haemophilus influenzae*. The widespread use of vaccinations against both of these organisms has made occult bacteremia much less common.

Noninfectious causes of acute fevers include Kawasaki disease, heatstroke, and toxic ingestions (eg, of drugs with anticholinergic effects). Some vaccinations can cause fever either in the first 24 to 48 h after the vaccine is given (eg, with pertussis vaccination) or 1 to 2 wk after the vaccine is given (eg, with measles vaccination). These fevers typically last from a few hours to a day. If the child is otherwise well, no evaluation is necessary. Teething does not cause significant or prolonged fevers.

Acute recurrent/periodic: Acute recurrent or periodic fever is episodes of fever alternating with periods of normal temperature (see Table 290–6).

Chronic: Fever that occurs daily for ≥ 2 wk and for which initial cultures and other investigations fail to yield a diagnosis is considered FUO.

Potential categories of causes (see Table 290–6) include localized or generalized infection, connective tissue disease, and cancer. Miscellaneous specific causes include inflammatory bowel disease, diabetes insipidus with dehydration, and disordered thermoregulation. Pseudo FUO is likely much more common than true FUO because frequent, minor viral illness may be overinterpreted. In children, despite the numerous possible causes, true FUO is more likely to be an uncommon manifestation of a common disease rather than an uncommon disease; respiratory infections account for almost one half of cases of infection-associated FUO.

Evaluation

History: **History of present illness** should note degree and duration of fever, method of measurement, and the dose and frequency of antipyretics (if any). Important associated symptoms that suggest serious illness include poor appetite, irritability, lethargy, and change in crying (eg, duration, character). Associated

Table 290–6. SOME COMMON CAUSES OF FEVER IN CHILDREN

TYPE	EXAMPLES
Acute	
Viral infections	**< 1 mo:** TORCH infections (toxoplasmosis, syphilis, varicella, coxsackievirus, HIV, parvovirus B19), rubella, cytomegalovirus (CMV), herpes simplex virus (HSV) **≥ 1 mo:** Enterovirus and respiratory viruses (eg, respiratory syncytial virus, parainfluenza, adenovirus, influenza, rhinovirus, metapneumovirus), CMV, Epstein-Barr virus (EBV), HSV, human herpesvirus 6
Bacterial infections (most common pathogens vary by age)	**< 1 mo:** Group B streptococci, Escherichia coli and other enteric pathogens, Listeria monocytogenes (these organisms can cause bacteremia, pneumonia, pyelonephritis, meningitis, and/or sepsis; also, *Salmonella* sp and *Staphylococcus aureus* [eg, in nursery outbreaks], which in addition to bacteremia and sepsis, can cause soft-tissue, bone, and joint infections) **1–3 mo:** *Streptococcus pneumoniae,* group B streptococci, *Neisseria meningitidis, L. monocytogenes* (these organisms can cause bacteremia, pneumonia, meningitis, and/or sepsis; other common infections include otitis media [*S. pneumoniae, Haemophilus influenzae, Moraxella catarrhalis*], UTI [*E. coli* and other enteric pathogens], enteritis [*Salmonella* sp, *Shigella* and others], skin and soft-tissue infections [*S. aureus*, group A and B streptococci], bone and joint infections [*S. aureus, Salmonella* sp]) **3–24 mo:** *S. pneumoniae, N. meningitidis* (these organisms can cause bacteremia, meningitis, and/or sepsis; other common infections include otitis media and pneumonia [*S. pneumoniae, H. influenzae, M. catarrhalis*], UTI [*E. coli* and other enteric pathogens], enteritis [*Salmonella* sp, *Shigella* and others], skin and soft-tissue infections [*S. aureus*, group A streptococci], bone and joint infections [*S. aureus, Salmonella* sp, *Kingella kingae*]) **> 24 mo:** *S. pneumoniae*, *N. meningitidis* (these organisms can cause bacteremia, meningitis, and/or sepsis; other common infections include otitis media, sinusitis, and pneumonia [*S. pneumoniae, H. influenzae, M. catarrhalis,* mycoplasma], pharyngitis or scarlet fever [group A streptococci], UTI [*E. coli* and other enteric pathogens], enteritis [*Salmonella* sp, *Shigella* and others], skin and soft-tissue infections [*S. aureus,* group A streptococci], bone and joint infections [*S. aureus, Salmonella* sp, *K. kingae*]) Mycobacterium tuberculosis in exposed or at risk populations Rickettsial infections in appropriate geographic locations Other vector-transmitted infection (eg, Lyme disease)
Noninfectious	Kawasaki disease Acute rheumatic fever Heatstroke Thermoregulatory disorders (eg, dysautonomia, diabetes insipidus, anhidrosis) Toxic ingestions (eg, anticholinergics) Vaccines Drugs
Fungal infections	**Neonates or immunocompromised hosts:** Candida sp most common (UTI, meningitis, and/or sepsis)
Acute recurrent	
Viral infections	Frequent or back-to-back minor viral illnesses in a young child
Periodic fever syndromes	Cyclic neutropenia Periodic fever with aphthous stomatitis, pharyngitis, adenitis (PFAPA) syndrome Familial Mediterranean fever (FMF) TNF receptor–associated periodic syndrome (TRAPS) Hyperimmunoglobulinemia D syndrome (HIDS)
Chronic (fever of unknown origin)	
Infectious*	Viral infections (eg, EBV, CMV, hepatitis viruses, arboviruses) Sinusitis Pneumonia Enteric infections (eg, Salmonella) Abscesses (intra-abdominal, hepatic, nephric) Bone and joint infections (eg, osteomyelitis, septic arthritis) Endocarditis HIV infection (uncommon) TB (uncommon) Parasitic infections (eg, malaria—uncommon) Cat-scratch disease Lyme disease (rarely causes chronic fever)

Table 290–6. SOME COMMON CAUSES OF FEVER IN CHILDREN (*Continued*)

TYPE	EXAMPLES
Noninfectious	Inflammatory bowel disease Connective tissue disorders (eg, juvenile idiopathic arthritis, SLE, acute rheumatic fever) Cancer (most commonly lymphoreticular malignancies such as lymphoma or leukemia but also neuroblastoma or sarcomas) Drugs Thermoregulatory disorders (eg, dysautonomia, diabetes insipidus, anhidrosis) Pseudo FUO Factitious fever (eg, factitious disorder imposed on another)

*There are many infectious causes of chronic fever. This list is not exhaustive.

symptoms that may suggest the cause include vomiting, diarrhea (including presence of blood or mucus), cough, difficulty breathing, favoring of an extremity or joint, and strong or foul-smelling urine. Drug history should be reviewed for indications of drug-induced fever.

Factors that predispose to infection are identified. In neonates, these factors include prematurity, prolonged rupture of membranes, maternal fever, and positive prenatal tests (usually for group B streptococcal infections, cytomegalovirus infections, or sexually transmitted diseases). For all children, predisposing factors include recent exposures to infection (including family and caregiver infection), indwelling medical devices (eg, catheters, ventriculoperitoneal shunts), recent surgery, travel and environmental exposures (eg, to endemic areas, to ticks, mosquitoes, cats, farm animals, or reptiles), and known or suspected immune deficiencies.

Review of systems should note symptoms suggesting possible causes, including runny nose and congestion (viral URI), headache (sinusitis, Lyme disease, meningitis), ear pain or waking in the night with signs of discomfort (otitis media), cough or wheezing (pneumonia, bronchiolitis), abdominal pain (pneumonia, strep pharyngitis, gastroenteritis, UTI, abdominal abscess), back pain (pyelonephritis), and any history of joint swelling or redness (Lyme disease, osteomyelitis). A history of repeated infections (immunodeficiency) or symptoms that suggest a chronic illness, such as poor weight gain or weight loss (TB, cancer), is identified. Certain symptoms can help direct the evaluation toward noninfectious causes; they include heart palpitations, sweating, and heat intolerance (hyperthyroidism) and recurrent or cyclic symptoms (a rheumatoid, inflammatory, or hereditary disorder).

Past medical history should note previous fevers or infections and known conditions predisposing to infection (eg, congenital heart disease, sickle cell anemia, cancer, immunodeficiency). A family history of an autoimmune disorder or other hereditary conditions (eg, familial dysautonomia, familial Mediterranean fever) is sought. Vaccination history is reviewed to identify patients at risk of infections that can be prevented by a vaccine.

Physical examination: Vital signs are reviewed, noting abnormalities in temperature and respiratory rate. In ill-appearing children, BP should also be measured. Temperature should be measured rectally in infants for accuracy. Any child with cough, tachypnea, or labored breathing requires pulse oximetry.

The child's overall appearance and response to the examination are important. A febrile child who is overly compliant or listless is of more concern than one who is uncooperative. However, an irritable infant or child who is inconsolable is also of concern. The febrile child who looks quite ill, especially when the temperature has come down, is of great concern and requires in-depth evaluation and continued observation. However, children who appear more comfortable after antipyretic therapy do not always have a benign disorder.

The remainder of the physical examination seeks signs of causative disorders (see Table 290–7).

Red flags: The following findings are of particular concern:

- Age < 1 mo
- Lethargy, listlessness, or toxic appearance
- Respiratory distress
- Petechiae or purpura
- Inconsolability

Interpretation of findings: Although serious illness does not always cause high fever and many high fevers result from self-limited viral infections, a temperature of ≥ 39° C in children < 2 yr indicates higher risk of occult bacteremia.

Other vital signs also are significant. Hypotension should raise concern about hypovolemia, sepsis, or myocardial dysfunction. Tachycardia in the absence of hypotension may be caused by fever (10 to 20 beats/min increase for each degree above normal) or hypovolemia. An increased respiratory rate may be a response to fever, indicate a pulmonary source of the illness, or be respiratory compensation for metabolic acidosis.

Acute fever is infectious in most cases, and of these, most are viral. History and examination are adequate to make a diagnosis in children > 2 yr who are otherwise well and not toxic-appearing. Typically, they have a viral respiratory illness (recent ill contact, runny nose, wheeze, or cough) or GI illness (ill contact, diarrhea, and vomiting). Other findings also suggest specific causes (see Table 290–7).

However, in infants < 24 mo, the possibility of occult bacteremia, plus the frequent absence of focal findings in neonates and young infants with serious bacterial infection, necessitates a different approach. Evaluation varies by age group. Accepted categories are neonates (≤ 28 days), young infants (1 to 3 mo), and older infants and children (3 to 24 mo). Regardless of clinical findings, a neonate with fever requires immediate hospitalization and testing to rule out a dangerous infection. Young infants may require hospitalization depending on screening laboratory results and the likelihood that they will be brought in for follow-up.

Acute recurrent or periodic fever and chronic fever (FUO) require a high index of suspicion for the many potential causes. However, certain findings can suggest the disorder: aphthous stomatitis, pharyngitis and adenitis (PFAPA syndrome); intermittent headaches with runny nose or congestion (sinusitis); weight loss, high-risk exposure, and night sweats (TB); weight loss or difficulty gaining weight, heart palpitations, and sweating (hyperthyroidism); and weight loss, anorexia, and night sweats (cancer).

Table 290–7. EXAMINATION OF THE FEBRILE CHILD

AREA	FINDING	POSSIBLE CAUSE
Skin	Nonblanching rash (ie, petechiae or purpura)	Variety of infections including enterovirus, meningococcemia, and Rocky Mountain spotted fever Disseminated intravascular coagulation due to sepsis
	Vesicular lesions	Varicella virus, herpes simplex virus
	Lacelike maculopapular rash on trunk and extremities with slapped-cheek appearance	Erythema infectiosum
	Focal erythema with swelling, induration, and tenderness	Cellulitis, skin abscess
	Evanescent erythematous morbilliform rash on trunk and proximal extremities	Juvenile idiopathic arthritis
	Bull's-eye erythematous rash, single or multiple lesions	Lyme disease
	Erythematous, sandpaper-like rash	Scarlet fever (group A streptococcal infection)
	Erythroderma	Toxic shock syndrome, toxin-mediated disease
Fontanelle (infants)	Bulging	Meningitis or encephalitis
Ears	Red, bulging tympanic membrane, loss of landmarks and mobility	Otitis media
Nose	Congestion, discharge	URI Sinusitis
	Nostril flaring with inspiration	Lower respiratory infection
Throat	Redness Sometimes exudate or swelling Sometimes drooling	Pharyngitis (URI or strep infection) Retropharyngeal abscess Peritonsillar abscess
Neck	Focal adenopathy with overlying redness, warmth, and tenderness; possible torticollis	Lymphadenitis secondary to *Staphylococcus aureus* or group A streptococcal infection
	Focal adenopathy with limited or no redness, warmth, or tenderness	Cat-scratch disease
	Generalized cervical adenopathy	Lymphoma Viral infection (particularly Epstein-Barr virus)
	Pain or resistance to flexion (meningismus*)	Meningitis
Lungs	Coughing, tachypnea, crackles, rhonchi, decreased breath sounds, wheezing	Lower respiratory infection (eg, pneumonia, bronchiolitis, chronic foreign body aspiration)
Heart	New murmur, particularly mitral or aortic regurgitant	Acute rheumatic fever Endocarditis
Abdomen	Tenderness, distention Absent bowel sounds	Gastroenteritis Appendicitis Pancreatitis Abdominal abscess
	Mass	Tumor
	Hepatomegaly	Hepatitis
	Splenomegaly	In neonate, Epstein-Barr virus infection, TORCH infections (toxoplasmosis, syphilis, varicella, coxsackievirus, HIV, parvovirus B19) Leukemia, lymphoma
Genitourinary	Costovertebral tenderness (less reliable in younger children)	Pyelonephritis
	Testicular tenderness	Epididymitis, orchitis
Extremities	Joint swelling, erythema, warmth, tenderness, decreased range of motion	Septic arthritis (very tender) Lyme arthritis Rheumatoid or inflammatory disorder
	Focal bone tenderness	Osteomyelitis
	Swelling of the hands or feet	Kawasaki disease

*Meningismus is not consistently present in children < 2 yr with meningitis.

Testing: Testing depends on age, appearance of the child and whether the fever is acute or chronic.

For **acute fever,** testing for infectious causes is directed by the age of the child. Typically, children < 36 mo, even those who do not appear very ill and those who have an apparent source of infection (eg, otitis media), require a thorough search to rule out serious bacterial infections (eg, meningitis, sepsis). In this age group, early follow-up (by phone and/or outpatient visit) is important for all those managed at home.

All febrile children < 1 mo require a WBC count with a manual differential, blood cultures, urinalysis and urine culture (obtained by catheterization, not an external bag) and CSF evaluation with culture and appropriate PCR testing (eg, for herpes simplex, enterovirus) as indicated by historical risk factors. Chest x-ray is done in those with respiratory manifestations, and stool swabs for WBCs and stool cultures are done in those with diarrhea. Neonates are hospitalized and given empiric IV antibiotic coverage for the most common neonatal pathogens (eg, using ampicillin and gentamycin or ampicillin and cefotaxime); antibiotics are continued until blood, urine, and CSF cultures have been negative for 48 to 72 h. Acyclovir also should be given if neonates are ill-appearing, have mucocutaneous vesicles, have a maternal history of genital herpesvirus (HSV) infection, or have seizures; acyclovir is stopped if results of CSF HSV PCR testing are negative.

Febrile children between 1 and 3 mo are differentiated based on their temperature, clinical appearance, and laboratory results. Typically, all should have a WBC count with a manual differential, blood cultures, and urinalysis and urine culture (obtained by catheterization, not an external bag). Chest x-ray is done in those with respiratory manifestations, and stool swabs for WBCs and stool culture are done in those with diarrhea. Lumbar puncture with CSF evaluation, including culture, is also done *except* in infants aged 61 to 90 days who appear well, have a rectal temperature < 38.5° C, have a normal urinalysis and a normal WBC count (5,000 to 15,000/μL), and who have knowledgeable caregivers, reliable transportation, and well-established follow-up; some experts also defer CSF testing in similar well-appearing infants aged 29 to 60 days, although there are no firm guidelines regarding minimum necessary testing in this age group.

Febrile infants between 1 and 3 mo who are ill-appearing, have an abnormal cry, or have rectal temperature ≥ 38.5° C have a high risk of serious bacterial infection (SBI) regardless of initial laboratory results. Such infants should be hospitalized and given empiric antibiotic therapy using ampicillin and cefotaxime in those aged 29 to 60 days or ceftriaxone in those aged 61 to 90 days, pending the results of blood, urine and CSF cultures.

Well-appearing infants between 1 and 3 mo with CSF pleocytosis, an abnormal urinalysis or chest x-ray, or a peripheral WBC ≤ 5000/μL or ≥ 15,000/μL should be admitted to the hospital for treatment with age-specific empiric antibiotics as described above. If empiric antibiotics are to be given, CSF analysis should be done (if not already done).

Well-appearing febrile infants between 1 and 3 mo with a rectal temperature < 38.5° C, and a normal WBC count and urinalysis (and CSF analysis and chest x-ray, if done) are at low risk of SBI. Such infants can be managed as outpatients if reliable follow-up is arranged within 24 h either by telephone or by return visit, at which time preliminary culture results are reviewed. If the family's social situation suggests that follow-up within 24 h is problematic, infants should be admitted to the hospital and observed. If infants are sent home, any deterioration in clinical status or worsening of fever, a positive blood culture not thought to be a contaminant, or a positive urine culture in an infant who remains febrile warrants immediate hospitalization with repeat cultures and age-specific empiric antibiotic therapy as described above.

Febrile children between 3 mo and 36 mo who have an apparent source of fever on examination and who do not appear ill or toxic can be managed based on this clinical diagnosis. Children who are ill-appearing should be fully evaluated for SBI with WBC count, cultures of blood, urine, and, when meningitis is suspected, CSF. Those with tachypnea or a WBC count > 20,000/μL should have a chest x-ray. These children should be given parenteral antibiotic therapy (usually using ceftriaxone) targeting the likely pathogens in this age group (*S. pneumoniae*, *Staphylococcus aureus*, *Neisseria meningitidis*, *H. influenzae* type b) and be admitted to the hospital pending culture results.

Well-appearing children in this age group who have a temperature > 39° C and no identifiable source on examination (fever without source [FWS]) and who are not fully immunized have a risk of occult bacteremia as high as 5% (equal to the risk before the pneumococcal and *H. influenzae* conjugate vaccines came into use). These children should have a CBC with differential, blood culture, and urinalysis and urine culture. A chest x-ray should be done if the WBC count is ≥ 20,000/μL. Children who have a WBC count ≥ 15,000/μL should be given parenteral antibiotics pending blood and urine culture results. Ceftriaxone (50 mg/kg IM) is preferred because of its broad antimicrobial spectrum and prolonged duration of action. Children who received parenteral antibiotics should have follow-up within 24 h by telephone or by return visit, at which time preliminary culture results are reviewed. If the social situation suggests that follow-up within 24 h is problematic, children should be admitted to the hospital. Children who are not treated with antibiotics should be brought for reevaluation if they are still febrile (≥ 38° C) after 48 h (or earlier if they become sicker or if new symptoms or signs develop).

For well-appearing children who have a temperature > 39° C and FWS and who are completely immunized, risk of bacteremia is < 0.5%. At this low-risk level, most laboratory testing and empiric antibiotic therapy are not indicated or cost-effective. However, UTI can be an occult source of infection in fully immunized children in this age group. Girls < 24 mo, circumcised boys < 6 mo, and uncircumcised boys < 12 mo should have a urinalysis and urine culture (obtained by catheterization, not an external bag) and be appropriately treated if UTI is detected. For other completely immunized children, urine testing is done only when they have symptoms or signs of UTI, they have a prior history of UTI or urogenital anomalies, or fever has lasted > 48 h. For all children, caregivers are instructed to return immediately if fever becomes higher, the child looks sicker, or new symptoms or signs develop.

For **febrile children** > 36 mo, testing is directed by history and examination. In this age group, a child's response to serious illnesses is sufficiently developed to be recognized clinically (eg, nuchal rigidity is a reliable finding of meningeal irritation), so empiric testing (eg screening WBC counts, urine and blood cultures) is not indicated.

For **acute recurrent or periodic fever,** laboratory tests and imaging should be directed toward likely causes based on findings from the history and physical examination. PFAPA should be considered in young children who have periodic high fever at intervals of about 3 to 5 wk with aphthous ulcers, pharyngitis, and/or adenitis. Between episodes and even during the episodes, the children appear healthy. Diagnosis requires 6 mo of stereotypic episodes, negative throat cultures during episodes, and exclusion of other causes (eg, specific viral infections). In patients with attacks of fever, arthralgia, skin lesions, mouth ulcers, and diarrhea, IgD levels should be measured to look for hyperimmunoglobulinemia D syndrome (HIDS). Laboratory features of HIDS include elevated C-reactive protein (CRP) and ESR and markedly elevated IgD (and often IgA). Genetic testing is available for the hereditary periodic fever syndromes including familial Mediterranean fever (FMF), TNF receptor–associated periodic syndrome (TRAPS) and HIDS.

For chronic fever (FUO), laboratory tests and imaging should be directed toward likely causes of fever based on the patient's age and findings from the history and physical examination. Indiscriminate ordering of laboratory tests is unlikely to be helpful and can be harmful (ie, because of adverse effects of unnecessary confirmatory testing of false positives). The pace of the evaluation is dictated by the appearance of the child. The pace should be rapid if the child is ill-appearing, but can be more deliberate if the child appears well.

All children with FUO should have

- CBC with manual differential
- ESR and CRP
- Blood cultures
- Urinalysis and urine culture
- Chest x-ray
- Serum electrolytes, BUN, creatinine, albumin, and hepatic enzymes
- HIV serology
- PPD testing

The results of these studies in conjunction with findings from the history and physical examination can focus further diagnostic tests.

Anemia may be a clue to malaria, infective endocarditis, inflammatory bowel disease, SLE, or TB. Thrombocytosis is a nonspecific acute-phase reactant. The total WBC and the differential generally are less helpful, although children with an absolute neutrophil count > 10,000 have a higher risk of SBI. If atypical lymphocytes are present, a viral infection is likely. Immature white cells should prompt further evaluation for leukemia. Eosinophilia may be a clue to parasitic, fungal, neoplastic, allergic, or immunodeficiency disorders.

The ESR and CRP are nonspecific acute-phase reactants that are general indicators of inflammation; an elevated ESR or CRP makes factitious fever less likely. A normal ESR or CRP can slow the pace of the evaluation. However, ESR or CRP may be normal in noninflammatory causes of FUO (see Table 178–2 on p. 1438).

Blood cultures should be done in all patients with FUO at least once and more often if suspicion of SBI is high. Three blood cultures should be done over 24 h in patients who have any manifestations of infective endocarditis. A positive blood culture, particularly for *S. aureus*, should raise suspicion for occult skeletal or visceral infection or endocarditis and lead to performance of a bone scan and/or echocardiography.

Urinalysis and urine culture are important because UTI is among the most frequent causes of FUO in children. Patients with FUO should have a chest x-ray to check for infiltrates and lymphadenopathy even if lung examination is normal. Serum electrolytes, BUN, creatinine, and hepatic enzymes are measured to check for renal or hepatic involvement. HIV serologic tests and PPD testing are done because primary HIV infection or TB can manifest as FUO.

Other tests are done selectively based on findings:

- Stool testing
- Bone marrow examination
- Serologic testing for specific infections
- Testing for connective tissue and immunodeficiency disorders
- Imaging

Stool cultures or examination for ova and parasites may be warranted in patients with loose stools or recent travel. *Salmonella* enteritis can infrequently manifest as FUO without diarrhea.

Bone marrow examination in children is most useful in diagnosing cancer (especially leukemia) or other hematologic disorders (eg, hemophagocytic disease) and may be warranted in children with otherwise unexplained hepatosplenomegaly, lymphadenopathy or cytopenias.

Serologic testing that may be warranted, depending on the case, include but are not limited to Epstein-Barr virus infection, cytomegalovirus infection, toxoplasmosis, bartonellosis (cat-scratch disease), syphilis, and certain fungal or parasitic infections.

An antinuclear antibody (ANA) test should be done in children > 5 yr with a strong family history of rheumatologic disease. A positive ANA test suggests an underlying connective tissue disorder, particularly SLE. Immunoglobulin levels (IgG, IgA, and IgM) should be measured in children with a negative initial evaluation. Low levels may indicate an immunodeficiency. Elevated levels can occur in chronic infection or an autoimmune disorder.

Imaging of the nasal sinuses, mastoids, and GI tract should be done initially only when children have symptoms or signs related to those areas but may be warranted in children in whom FUO remains undiagnosed after initial testing. Children with elevated ESR or CRP, anorexia, and weight loss should have studies to exclude inflammatory bowel disease, particularly if they also have abdominal complaints with or without anemia. However, imaging of the GI tract should be done eventually in children whose fevers persist without other explanation and may be caused by disorders such as psoas abscess or cat-scratch disease. Ultrasonography, CT, and MRI can be useful in evaluating the abdomen and can detect abscesses, tumors, and lymphadenopathy. Imaging of the CNS is generally not helpful in the evaluation of children with FUO. Lumbar puncture may be warranted in children with persistent headache, neurologic signs, or an indwelling ventriculoperitoneal shunt. Other imaging techniques, including bone scan or tagged WBC scan, can be helpful in selected children whose fevers persist without other explanation when suspicion for a source that could be detected by these tests exists. Ophthalmologic examination by slit lamp is useful in some patients with FUO to look for uveitis (eg, as occurs in juvenile idiopathic arthritis [JIA]) or leukemic infiltration. Biopsy (eg, of lymph nodes or liver) should be reserved for children with evidence of involvement of specific organs.

Empiric treatment with anti-inflammatory drugs or antibiotics should not be used as diagnostic measures except when JIA is suspected; in such cases, a trial of NSAIDs is the recommended first-line therapy. Response to anti-inflammatory drugs or antibiotics does not help distinguish infectious from noninfectious causes. Also, antibiotics can cause false-negative cultures and mask or delay the diagnosis of important infections (eg, meningitis, parameningeal infection, endocarditis, osteomyelitis).

Treatment

Treatment is directed at the underlying disorder.

Fever in an otherwise healthy child does not necessarily require treatment. Although antipyretics can provide comfort, they do not change the course of an infection. In fact, fever is an integral part of the inflammatory response to infection and can help the child fight the infection. However, most clinicians use antipyretics to help alleviate discomfort and to reduce physiologic stresses in children who have cardiopulmonary disorders, neurologic disorders, or a history of febrile seizures.

Antipyretic drugs that are typically used include

- Acetaminophen
- Ibuprofen

Acetaminophen tends to be preferred because ibuprofen decreases the protective effect of prostaglandins in the stomach and, if used chronically, can lead to gastritis. However, recent epidemiologic studies have found an association between the use of acetaminophen and the prevalence of asthma in children and adults; so some clinicians suggest that children with asthma or a strong family history of asthma should avoid using acetaminophen. The dosage of acetaminophen is 10 to 15 mg/kg po, IV, or rectally q 4 to 6 h. Ibuprofen dosage is 10 mg/kg po q 6 h. Use of one antipyretic at a time is preferred. Some clinicians alternate the 2 drugs to treat high fever (eg, acetaminophen at 6 AM, 12 PM, and 6 PM and ibuprofen at 9 AM, 3 PM, and 9 PM); this approach is not encouraged because caregivers may become confused and inadvertently exceed the recommended daily dose. Aspirin should be avoided in children because it increases the risk of Reye syndrome if certain viral illnesses such as influenza and varicella are present.

Nondrug approaches to fever include putting the child in a warm or tepid bath, using cool compresses, and undressing the child. Caregivers should be cautioned not to use a cold water bath, which is uncomfortable and which, by inducing shivering, may paradoxically elevate body temperature. As long as the temperature of the water is slightly cooler than the temperature of the child, a bath provides temporary relief.

Things to avoid: Wiping the body down with isopropyl alcohol should be strongly discouraged because alcohol can be absorbed through the skin and cause toxicity. Numerous folk remedies exist, ranging from the harmless (eg, putting onions or potatoes in socks) to the uncomfortable (eg, coining, cupping).

KEY POINTS

- Most acute fever is caused by viral infections.
- Causes and evaluation of acute fever differ depending on the age of a child.
- A rare but real number of children < 24 mo with fever without localizing signs (primarily those who are incompletely immunized) can have pathogenic bacteria in their bloodstream (occult bacteremia) and be early in the course of a potentially life-threatening infection.
- Teething does not cause significant fever.
- Antipyretics do not alter the outcome but may make children feel better.

NAUSEA AND VOMITING IN INFANTS AND CHILDREN

Nausea is the sensation of impending emesis and is frequently accompanied by autonomic changes, such as increased heart rate and salivation. Nausea and vomiting typically occur in sequence; however, they can occur separately (eg, vomiting can occur without preceding nausea as a result of increased intracranial pressure).

Vomiting is uncomfortable and can cause dehydration because fluid is lost and because the ability to rehydrate by drinking is limited.

Pathophysiology

Vomiting is the final part of a sequence of events coordinated by the emetic center located in the medulla. The emetic center can be activated by afferent neural pathways from digestive (eg, pharynx, stomach, small bowel) and nondigestive (eg, heart, testes) organs, the chemoreceptor trigger zone located in the area postrema on the floor of the 4th ventricle (containing dopamine and serotonin receptors), and other CNS centers (eg, brain stem, vestibular system).

Etiology

The causes of vomiting vary with age and range from relatively benign to potentially life threatening (see Table 290–8). Vomiting is a protective mechanism that provides a means to expel potential toxins; however, it can also indicate serious disease (eg, intestinal obstruction). Bilious vomiting indicates a high intestinal obstruction and, especially in an infant, requires immediate evaluation.

Infants: Infants normally spit up small amounts (usually < 5 to 10 mL) during or soon after feedings, often when being burped. Rapid feeding, air swallowing, and overfeeding may be causes, although spitting up occurs even without these factors. Occasional vomiting may also be normal, but repeated vomiting is abnormal.

The most common causes of vomiting in infants and neonates include the following:

- Acute viral gastroenteritis
- Gastroesophageal reflux disease

Other important causes in infants and neonates include the following:

- Pyloric stenosis
- Intestinal obstruction (eg, meconium ileus, volvulus, intestinal atresia, stenosis)
- Intussusception (typically in infants aged 3 to 36 mo)

Less common causes of recurrent vomiting include sepsis and food intolerance. Metabolic disorders (eg, urea cycle disorders, organic acidemias) are uncommon but can manifest with vomiting.

Older children: The most common cause is

- Acute viral gastroenteritis

Non-GI infections may cause a few episodes of vomiting. Other causes to consider include serious infection (eg, meningitis, pyelonephritis), acute abdomen (eg, appendicitis), increased intracranial pressure secondary to a space-occupying lesion (eg, caused by trauma or tumor), and cyclic vomiting.

In adolescents, causes of vomiting also include pregnancy, eating disorders, and toxic ingestions (eg, acetaminophen, iron, ethanol).

Evaluation

Evaluation includes assessment of severity (eg, presence of dehydration, surgical or other life-threatening disorder) and diagnosis of cause.

History: History of present illness should determine when vomiting episodes started, frequency, and character of episodes (particularly whether vomiting is projectile, bilious, or small in amount and more consistent with spitting up). Any pattern to the vomiting (eg, after feeding, only with certain foods, primarily in the morning or in recurrent cyclic episodes) should be established. Important associated symptoms include diarrhea (with or without blood), fever, anorexia, and abdominal pain, distention, or both. Stool frequency and consistency and urinary output should be noted.

Review of systems should seek symptoms of causative disorders, including weakness, poor suck, and failure to thrive (metabolic disorders); delay in passage of meconium,

Table 290–8. SOME CAUSES OF VOMITING IN INFANTS, CHILDREN, AND ADOLESCENTS

CAUSE*	SUGGESTIVE FINDINGS	DIAGNOSTIC APPROACH
Vomiting in infants		
Viral gastroenteritis	Usually with diarrhea Sometimes fever and/or contact with a person who has similar symptoms	Clinical evaluation Sometimes rapid immunoassays for viral antigens (eg, rotavirus, adenovirus)
Gastroesophageal reflux disease	Recurrent fussiness during or after feedings Possibly poor weight gain, arching of the back, recurrent respiratory symptoms (eg, cough, stridor, wheezing)	Empiric trial of acid suppression Sometimes upper GI contrast study, a milk scan, esophageal pH monitoring and/or impedance study, or endoscopy
Bacterial enteritis or colitis	Usually with diarrhea (often bloody), fever, crampy abdominal pain, distention Often contact with a person who has similar symptoms	Clinical evaluation Sometimes stool examination for WBC and culture
Pyloric stenosis	Recurrent projectile vomiting immediately after feeding in neonates aged 2–12 wk, infrequent stools May be emaciated and dehydrated Sometimes palpable "olive" in right upper quadrant	Ultrasonography of pylorus Upper GI contrast study if ultrasonography is unavailable or uncertain
Congenital atresias or stenoses	Abdominal distention Bilious emesis in first 24–48 h of life (with lesser degrees of stenosis, vomiting can be delayed) Sometimes polyhydramnios during pregnancy, Down syndrome, jaundice	Abdominal x-ray Upper GI series or contrast enema depending on findings
Intussusception	Colicky abdominal pain, inconsolable crying, lethargy, drawing of legs up to chest Later, bloody ("current jelly") stool Typically age 3–36 mo, but can be outside this range	Abdominal ultrasonography If ultrasonography is positive or nondiagnostic, air or contrast enema (unless patient has signs of peritonitis or perforation)
Hirschsprung disease	In neonates, delayed passage of meconium, abdominal distention, bilious emesis	Abdominal x-ray Contrast enema Rectal biopsy
Malrotation with volvulus	In neonates, bilious emesis, abdominal distention and pain Bloody stool	Abdominal x-ray Contrast enema or upper GI series
Sepsis	Fever, lethargy, tachycardia, tachypnea Widened pulse pressure, hypotension	Cell counts and cultures (blood, urine, CSF) Chest x-ray if pulmonary symptoms are present
Food intolerance	Abdominal pain, diarrhea Possibly eczematous rash or urticaria	Elimination diet Sometimes skin testing and/or radioallergosorbent testing (RAST)
Metabolic disorders	Poor feeding, failure to thrive, lethargy, hepatosplenomegaly, jaundice Sometimes unusual odor, cataracts	Electrolytes, ammonia, liver function tests, BUN, creatinine, serum glucose, total and direct bilirubin, CBC, PT/PTT Neonatal metabolic screening Further specific tests based on findings
Vomiting in children and adolescents		
Viral gastroenteritis	Usually with diarrhea Sometimes fever, contact with a person who has similar symptoms, or history of travel	Clinical evaluation Sometimes rapid immunoassays for viral antigens (eg, rotavirus, adenovirus)
Bacterial enteritis or colitis	Usually with diarrhea (often bloody), fever, crampy abdominal pain, distention, fecal urgency Often contact with a person who has similar symptoms or history of travel	Clinical evaluation Sometimes stool for WBC, culture
Non-GI infection	Fever Often localizing findings (eg, headache, ear pain, sore throat, cervical adenopathy, dysuria, flank pain, nasal discharge) depending on cause	Clinical evaluation Testing as needed for suspected cause

Table 290–8. SOME CAUSES OF VOMITING IN INFANTS, CHILDREN, AND ADOLESCENTS (*Continued*)

CAUSE*	SUGGESTIVE FINDINGS	DIAGNOSTIC APPROACH
Appendicitis	Initial general malaise and periumbilical discomfort followed by pain localizing to right lower quadrant, vomiting *after* pain manifestation, anorexia, fever, tenderness at McBurney point, decreased bowel sounds	Ultrasonography (preferred over CT to limit radiation exposure)
Serious infection	Fever, toxic appearance, back pain, dysuria (pyelonephritis) Nuchal rigidity, photophobia (meningitis) Listlessness, hypotension, tachycardia (sepsis)	Cell counts and cultures (blood, urine, CSF) as indicated by findings
Cyclic vomiting	≥ 3 episodes of intense acute nausea and unremitting vomiting and sometimes abdominal pain or headache lasting hours to days Intervening symptom-free intervals lasting weeks to months	Exclusion of metabolic, GI (eg, malrotation), or CNS (eg, brain tumor) disorders
Intracranial hypertension (caused by tumor or trauma)	Chronic, progressive headache; nocturnal awakenings; morning vomiting; headache worsened by coughing or Valsalva maneuver; vision changes	Brain CT (without contrast)
Eating disorders	Binge and purge cycles, erosion of tooth enamel, weight loss or gain Sometimes skin lesions on hand from inducing vomiting (Russell sign)	Clinical evaluation
Pregnancy	Amenorrhea, morning sickness, bloating, breast tenderness History of unprotected sexual activity†	Urine pregnancy test
Toxic ingestions (eg, acetaminophen, iron, ethanol)	Often history of ingestion Various findings depending on ingested substance	Qualitative and sometimes quantitative serum drug levels (depending on substance)
Adverse drug reaction (eg, to chemotherapeutic drugs)	Exposure to a specific drug	Clinical evaluation

*Causes are listed in order of frequency.
†Many adolescents do not admit to sexual activity.

abdominal distention, and lethargy (intestinal obstruction); headache, nuchal rigidity, and vision changes (intracranial disorders); food bingeing or signs of distorted body image (eating disorders); missed periods and breast swelling (pregnancy); rashes (eczema or urticaria in food allergies, petechiae in sepsis or meningitis); ear pain or sore throat (focal non-GI infection); and fever with headache, neck or back pain, or abdominal pain (meningitis, pyelonephritis, or appendicitis).

Past medical history should note history of travel (possible infectious gastroenteritis), any recent head trauma, and unprotected sex (pregnancy).

Physical examination: Vital signs are reviewed for indicators of infection (eg, fever) and volume depletion (eg, tachycardia, hypotension).

During the general examination, signs of distress (eg, lethargy, irritability, inconsolable crying) and signs of weight loss (cachexia) or gain are noted.

Because the abdominal examination may cause discomfort, the physical examination should begin with the head. The head and neck examination should focus on signs of infection (eg, red, bulging tympanic membrane; bulging anterior fontanelle; erythematous tonsils) and dehydration (eg, dry mucous membranes, lack of tears). The neck should be passively flexed to detect resistance or discomfort, suggesting meningeal irritation.

Cardiac examination should note presence of tachycardia (eg, dehydration, fever, distress). Abdominal examination should note distention; presence and quality of bowel sounds (eg, high-pitched, normal, absent); tenderness and any associated guarding, rigidity, or rebound (peritoneal signs); and presence of organomegaly or mass.

The skin and extremities are examined for petechiae or purpura (severe infection) or other rashes (possible viral infection or signs of atopy), jaundice (possible metabolic disorder), and signs of dehydration (eg, poor skin turgor, delayed capillary refill).

Growth parameters and signs of developmental progress should be noted.

Red flags: The following findings are of particular concern:

- Bilious emesis
- Lethargy or listlessness
- Inconsolability and bulging fontanelle in infant
- Nuchal rigidity, photophobia, and fever in older child
- Peritoneal signs or abdominal distention (surgical abdomen)
- Persistent vomiting with poor growth or development

Interpretation of findings: Initial findings help determine severity of diagnosis and need for immediate intervention.

- Any neonate or infant with recurrent or bilious (yellow or green) emesis or projectile vomiting most likely has a GI obstruction and probably requires surgical intervention.
- An infant or young child with colicky abdominal pain, signs of intermittent pain or listlessness, and absent or bloody stools needs to be evaluated for an intussusception.
- A child or adolescent with fever, nuchal rigidity, and photophobia should be evaluated for meningitis.

- A child or adolescent with fever and abdominal pain followed by vomiting, anorexia, and decreased bowel sounds should be evaluated for appendicitis.
- Recent history of head trauma or chronic progressive headaches with morning vomiting and vision changes indicate intracranial hypertension.

Other findings can be interpreted primarily depending on age (see Table 290–8).

In **infants,** irritability, choking, and respiratory signs (eg, stridor) may be manifestations of gastroesophageal reflux. A history of poor development or neurologic manifestations suggests a CNS or metabolic disorder. Delayed passage of meconium, later onset of vomiting, or both may indicate Hirschsprung disease or intestinal stenosis.

In **children and adolescents,** fever suggests infection; the combination of vomiting and diarrhea suggests acute gastroenteritis. Lesions on fingers and erosion of tooth enamel or an adolescent unconcerned about weight loss or with distorted body image suggests an eating disorder. Morning nausea and vomiting, amenorrhea, and possibly weight gain suggest pregnancy. Vomiting that has occurred in the past and is episodic, short-lived, and has no other accompanying symptoms suggests cyclic vomiting.

Testing: Testing should be directed by suspected causative disorders (see Table 290–8). Imaging studies are typically done to evaluate abdominal or CNS pathology. Various specific blood tests or cultures are done to diagnose inherited metabolic disorders or serious infection.

If dehydration is suspected, serum electrolytes should be measured.

Treatment

Treatment of nausea and vomiting is targeted at the causative disorder. Rehydration is important.

Drugs frequently used in adults to decrease nausea and vomiting are used less often in children because the usefulness of treatment has not been proved and because these drugs have potential risks of adverse effects and of masking an underlying condition. However, if nausea or vomiting is severe or unremitting, antiemetic drugs can be used cautiously in children > 2 yr. Useful drugs include

- Promethazine: For children > 2 yr, 0.25 to 1 mg/kg (maximum 25 mg) po, IM, IV, or rectally q 4 to 6 h
- Prochlorperazine: For children > 2 yr and weighing 9 to 13 kg, 2.5 mg po q 12 to 24 h; for those 13 to 18 kg, 2.5 mg po q 8 to 12 h; for those 18 to 39 kg, 2.5 mg po q 8 h; for those > 39 kg, 5 to 10 mg po q 6 to 8 h
- Metoclopramide: 0.1 mg/kg po or IV q 6 h (maximum 10 mg/dose)
- Ondansetron: 0.15 mg/kg (maximum 8 mg) IV q 8 h or, if the oral form is used, for children 2 to 4 yr, 2 mg q 8 h; for those 4 to 11 yr, 4 mg q 8 h; for those ≥ 12 yr, 8 mg q 8 h

Promethazine is an H_1 receptor blocker (antihistamine) that inhibits the emetic center response to peripheral stimulants. The most common adverse effect is respiratory depression and sedation; the drug is contraindicated in children < 2 yr. Therapeutic doses of promethazine can cause extrapyramidal adverse effects, including torticollis.

Prochlorperazine is a weak dopamine receptor blocker that depresses the chemoreceptor trigger zone. Akathisia and dystonia are the most common adverse effects, occurring in up to 44% of patients.

Metoclopramide is a dopamine receptor antagonist that acts both centrally and peripherally by increasing gastric motility and decreasing afferent impulses to the chemoreceptor trigger zone. Akathisia and dystonia occur in up to 25% of children.

Ondansetron is a selective serotonin (5-HT_3) receptor blocker that inhibits the initiation of the vomiting reflex in the periphery. A single dose of ondansetron is safe and effective in children who have acute gastroenteritis and do not respond to oral rehydration therapy (ORT). By facilitating ORT, this drug may prevent the need for IV fluids or, in children given IV fluids, may help prevent hospitalization. Typically, only a single dose is used because repeated doses can cause persistent diarrhea.

KEY POINTS

- In general, the most common cause of vomiting is acute viral gastroenteritis.
- Associated diarrhea suggests an infectious GI cause.
- Bilious emesis, bloody stools, or lack of bowel movements suggests an obstructive cause.
- Persistent vomiting (especially in an infant) requires immediate evaluation.

RASH IN INFANTS AND YOUNG CHILDREN

Rash is a common complaint, particularly during infancy. Most rashes are not serious.

Etiology

Rashes can be caused by infection (viral, fungal, or bacterial), contact with irritants, atopy, drug hypersensitivity, other allergic reactions, inflammatory conditions, or vasculitides (see Table 290–9).

Overall, the **most common causes** of rash in infants and young children include

- Diaper rash (with or without candidal infection)
- Seborrhea
- Atopic dermatitis (eczema)
- Viral exanthem

Numerous viral infections cause rash. Some (eg, chickenpox, erythema infectiosum, measles) have a fairly typical appearance and clinical manifestation; others are nonspecific. Cutaneous drug reactions are usually self-limited maculopapular exanthems, but sometimes more serious reactions occur.

Uncommon but serious causes of rash include

- Staphylococcal scalded skin syndrome
- Meningococcemia
- Kawasaki disease
- Stevens-Johnson syndrome

Evaluation

History: History of present illness focuses on the time course of illness, particularly the relationship between the rash and other symptoms.

Review of systems focuses on symptoms of causative disorders, including GI symptoms (suggesting immunoglobulin A–associated vasculitis [formerly called Henoch-Schönlein purpura] or hemolytic-uremic syndrome), joint symptoms (suggesting immunoglobulin A–associated vasculitis or Lyme disease), headache or neurologic symptoms (suggesting meningitis or Lyme disease).

Past medical history should note any drugs recently used, particularly antibiotics and anticonvulsants. Family history of atopy is noted.

Physical examination: Examination begins with a review of vital signs, particularly to check for fever. Initial observa-

Table 290–9. SOME CAUSES OF RASH IN INFANTS AND CHILDREN

CAUSE	SUGGESTIVE FINDINGS	DIAGNOSTIC APPROACH
Infections		
Candidal infections	Beefy red rash with adjacent satellite lesions in the diaper area, including skin creases Often fluffy white plaques on the tongue or oral mucosa Sometimes history of recent antibiotic use	Clinical evaluation Sometimes scrapings of lesions for KOH wet mount
Chickenpox*	Red dots on the face, scalp, torso and proximal extremities that progress over 10–12 h to small bumps, vesicles, and then umbilicated pustules, which form crusts Intensely itchy blisters, which may also occur on the palms, soles, scalp, and mucous membranes, as well as in the diaper area	Clinical evaluation
Erythema infectiosum	Confluent erythema on cheeks (slapped cheek appearance) Sometimes fever, malaise	Clinical evaluation
Impetigo	Nonbullous impetigo: Painless but itchy red sore near the nose or mouth that soon leaks pus or fluid and forms a honey-colored scab Bullous impetigo: Occurs mainly in children < 2 yr Painless, fluid-filled blisters—mostly on the arms, legs, and trunk, surrounded by red and itchy skin—which, after breaking, form yellow or silvery scabs	Clinical evaluation
Lyme disease	Erythema migrans rash; an enlarging (to about 5–7 cm) erythematous lesion sometimes with central clearing or rarely purpura (2%) Often fatigue, headache, joint or body aches Usually in endemic area with risk of exposure to ticks, with or without a known tick bite	Clinical evaluation Sometimes serologic testing
Measles*	Maculopapular rash beginning on the face and spreading to the trunk and extremities Often Koplik spots (white spots on buccal mucosa) Fever, cough, coryza, conjunctival injection	Clinical evaluation Serologic testing (for public health reasons)
Meningococcemia	Petechial rash, sometimes with purpura fulminans Fever, lethargy, irritability In older children, meningeal signs Tachycardia, sometimes hypotension	Gram stain and culture of blood and CSF
Molluscum contagiosum	Clusters of flesh-colored, umbilicated papules No itching or discomfort	Clinical evaluation
Roseola infantum	Maculopapular rash that appears suddenly after 4 or 5 days of high fever, typically as fever resolves	Clinical evaluation
Rubella*	Sometimes itchy rash that begins on the face and spreads downward, appears as pink or light red spots (which may merge to form evenly colored patches), and usually clears on the face as it spreads Lasts up to 3 days Often lymphadenopathy (occipital, postauricular, posterior cervical), mild fever	Clinical evaluation Serologic testing (for public health reasons)
Scarlet fever (scarlatina)	Fever, sometimes sore throat Generalized fine, red, rough-textured, blanching rash that typically appears 12–72 h after the fever and starts on the chest, in the armpits, and on the groin Characteristic pale area around the mouth (circumoral pallor) and accentuation in the skinfolds (Pastia lines), strawberry tongue Often followed by extensive desquamation of the palms and soles, tips of fingers and toes, and groin	Clinical evaluation Sometimes rapid streptococcal assay or throat culture
Staphylococcal scalded skin syndrome	Widespread areas of painful erythema that develop large, flaccid blisters, which are easily ruptured, leaving large areas of desquamation Lateral extension of blisters with gentle pressure (positive Nikolsky sign) Spares the mucous membranes Usually in children < 5 yr	Clinical evaluation Sometimes confirmed by biopsy and/or cultures

Table continues on the following page.

Table 290–9. SOME CAUSES OF RASH IN INFANTS AND CHILDREN (*Continued*)

CAUSE	SUGGESTIVE FINDINGS	DIAGNOSTIC APPROACH
Tinea	Scaly, oval lesions with a slightly raised border and central clearing Mild itching	Clinical evaluation Sometimes scrapings of lesions for KOH wet mount
Viral infection (systemic)	Maculopapular rash Often viral respiratory prodrome	Clinical evaluation
Hypersensitivity reactions		
Atopic dermatitis (eczema)	Chronic or recurrent red, scaly patches, often in flexor creases Sometimes family history	Clinical evaluation
Contact dermatitis	Intensely itchy erythema, sometimes with vesicles No systemic manifestations	Clinical evaluation
Drug reaction	Diffuse maculopapular rash History of current or recent (within 1 wk) drug use	Clinical evaluation
Stevens-Johnson syndrome Toxic epidermal necrolysis	Prodrome of fever, malaise, cough, sore throat, and conjunctivitis Painful mucosal ulcers, almost always in the mouth and lips but sometimes in the genital and anal regions Widespread areas of painful erythema that develop large, flaccid blisters, which are easily ruptured, leaving large areas of desquamation; possibly affecting the soles but usually not the scalp Lateral extension of blisters with gentle pressure (positive Nikolsky sign) Sometimes use of a causative drug (eg, sulfonamides, penicillins, anticonvulsants)	Clinical evaluation Sometimes biopsy
Urticaria	Well-circumscribed, pruritic, red, raised lesions With or without history of exposure to known or potential allergens	Clinical evaluation
Vasculitides		
Immunoglobulin A–associated vasculitis (formerly called Henoch-Schönlein purpura)	Palpable purpura appearing in crops over days to weeks, typically in dependent areas (eg, legs, buttocks) Often arthritis, abdominal pain Sometimes hematuria, heme-positive stool, and/or intussusception Usually in children < 10 yr	Clinical evaluation Sometimes skin biopsy
Kawasaki disease	Diffuse erythematous maculopapular rash that can vary in appearance (eg, urticarial, target-like, purpuric) but never bullous or vesicular; may involve the palms and/or soles Fever (often > 39° C) for > 5 days Red, cracked lips, strawberry tongue, conjunctivitis, cervical lymphadenopathy Edema of hands and feet Later desquamation of fingers and toes extending to palms and soles	Clinical criteria Testing to exclude other disorders
Other		
Seborrheic dermatitis	Red and yellow scaling on the scalp (cradle cap) and sometimes in skinfolds	Clinical evaluation
Diaper rash (noncandidal)	Bright red rash in the diaper area, sparing creases	Clinical evaluation
Hemolytic-uremic syndrome	Petechial rash, pallor Usually during or after infectious colitis manifesting with abdominal pain, vomiting, and bloody diarrhea Oliguria or anuria Hypertension	CBC with platelets and peripheral smear to check for evidence of microangiopathic anemia and thrombocytopenia Renal function tests Stool testing (Shiga toxin assay or specific culture for *E. coli* O157:H7)
Milia	Small pearly cysts on a neonate's face	Clinical evaluation
Erythema multiforme	Pink-red blotches, symmetrically arranged and starting on the extremities, then evolving into the classic target-like lesion with a pink-red ring around a pale center Sometimes oral mucosal lesions, pruritis	Clinical evaluation

Table 290–9. SOME CAUSES OF RASH IN INFANTS AND CHILDREN (*Continued*)

CAUSE	SUGGESTIVE FINDINGS	DIAGNOSTIC APPROACH
Miliaria (heat rash)	Small red bumps or occasionally small blisters Most common in very young children but can occur at any age, particularly during hot and humid weather	Clinical evaluation
Erythema toxicum	Flat red splotches (usually with a white, pimple-like bump in the middle), which appear in up to half of all babies Rarely appears after 5 days of age and is usually gone in 7–14 days	Clinical evaluation
Neonatal acne	Red bumps, sometimes with white dots in the center on a neonate's face Usually occurs between 2 and 4 wk after birth but may appear up to 4 mo after birth and can last for 12–18 mo	Clinical evaluation
Pityriasis rosea	Sometimes URI prodrome Typically begins as a single, pruritic 2- to 10-cm oval red herald patch on the trunk or proximal limbs 7–14 days after the herald patch, appearance of large patches of pink or red, flaky, oval-shaped rash on the torso, sometimes in a characteristic Christmas tree–like distribution	Clinical evaluation

*This cause is currently uncommon because of vaccination but should be considered in unvaccinated children.
KOH = potassium hydroxide.

tion assesses the infant or child for signs of lethargy, irritability, or distress. A full physical examination is done, with particular attention to the characteristics of the skin lesions, including the presence of blistering, vesicles, petechiae, purpura, or urticaria and mucosal involvement. Children are evaluated for meningeal signs (neck stiffness, Kernig and Brudzinski signs) although these signs are often absent in children < 2 yr.

Red flags: The following findings are of particular concern:

- Blistering or skin sloughing
- Diarrhea and/or abdominal pain
- Fever and inconsolability or extreme irritability
- Mucosal inflammation
- Petechiae and/or purpura
- Urticaria with respiratory distress

Interpretation of findings: Well-appearing children without systemic symptoms or signs are unlikely to have a dangerous disorder. The appearance of the rash typically narrows the differential diagnosis. The associated symptoms and signs help identify patients with a serious disorder and often suggest the diagnosis (see Table 290–9).

Bullae and/or sloughing suggest staphylococcal scalded skin syndrome or Stevens-Johnson syndrome and are considered dermatologic emergencies. Conjunctival inflammation may occur in Kawasaki disease, measles, staphylococcal scalded skin syndrome, and Stevens-Johnson syndrome. Any child presenting with fever and petechiae or purpura must be evaluated carefully for the possibility of meningococcemia. Bloody diarrhea with pallor and petechiae should raise concern about the possibility of hemolytic uremic syndrome. Fever for > 5 days with evidence of mucosal inflammation and rash should prompt consideration of and further evaluation for Kawasaki disease.

Testing: For most children, the history and physical examination are sufficient for diagnosis. Testing is targeted at potential life threats; it includes Gram stain and cultures of blood and CSF for meningococcemia; CBC, renal function tests, and stool tests for hemolytic uremic syndrome).

Treatment

Treatment of rash is directed at the cause (eg, antifungal cream for candidal infection).

For diaper rash, the goal is to keep the diaper area clean and dry, primarily by changing diapers more frequently and gently washing the area with mild soap and water. Sometimes a barrier ointment containing zinc oxide or vitamins A and D may help.

Pruritus in infants and children can be lessened by oral antihistamines:

- Diphenhydramine: For children > 6 mo, 1.25 mg/kg q 6 h (maximum 50 mg q 6 h)
- Hydroxyzine: For children > 6 mo, 0.5 mg/kg q 6 h (maximum for children < 6 yr, 12.5 mg q 6 h; for those ≥ 6 yr, 25 mg q 6 h)
- Cetirizine: For children 6 to 23 mo, 2.5 mg once/day; for those 2 to 5 yr, 2.5 to 5 mg once/day; for those > 6 yr, 5 to 10 mg once/day
- Loratadine: For children 2 to 5 yr, 5 mg once/day; for those > 6 yr, 10 mg once/day

KEY POINTS

- Most rashes in children are benign.
- For most rashes in infants and children, the history and physical examination are sufficient for diagnosis.
- Children with rash due to serious illness typically have systemic manifestations of disease.

SEPARATION ANXIETY AND STRANGER ANXIETY

Separation anxiety: Separation anxiety is fussing and crying when a parent leaves the room. Some children scream and have tantrums, refuse to leave their parents' side, and/or have nighttime awakenings.

Separation anxiety is a normal stage of development and typically begins at about 8 mo, peaks in intensity between 10 and 18 mo, and generally resolves by 24 mo. It should be distinguished from separation anxiety disorder (see p. 2712), which occurs at an older age, when such a reaction is developmentally inappropriate; refusal to go to school (or preschool) is a common manifestation of separation anxiety disorder.

Separation anxiety occurs when infants begin to understand that they are a separate person from their primary caregiver but still have not mastered the concept of object permanence—the idea that something still exists when it is not seen or heard. Thus, when infants are separated from their primary caregiver, they do not understand that the caregiver will return. Because infants do not have a concept of time, they fear that the departure of their parents is permanent. Separation anxiety resolves as children develop a sense of memory. They can keep an image of their parents in mind when the parents are gone and can recall that in the past, the parents returned.

Parents should be advised not to limit or forego separations in response to separation anxiety; this response could compromise the child's maturation and development. When parents leave the home (or leave the child at a child care center), they can try the following strategies:

- Encouraging the person caring for the child to create distractions
- Leaving without responding at length to a child's crying
- Remaining calm and reassuring
- Establishing routines at separations to ease the child's anxiety
- Feeding the child and letting the child nap before parents leave (because separation anxiety may be worse when a child is hungry or tired)

If the parents must momentarily go to another room in the home, they should call to the child while in the other room to reassure the child. This strategy gradually teaches the child that parents are still present even though the child cannot see them.

Separation anxiety causes no long-term harm to children if it resolves by age 2 yr. If it persists beyond age 2, separation anxiety may or may not be a problem depending how much it interferes with the child's development.

For children, feeling some fear when they leave for preschool or kindergarten is normal. This feeling should diminish with time. Rarely, excessive fear of separations inhibits children from attending child care or preschool or keeps them from playing normally with peers. This anxiety is probably abnormal (separation anxiety disorder). In such cases, children require medical attention.

Stranger anxiety: Stranger anxiety is manifested by crying when an unfamiliar person approaches. It is normal when it starts at about 8 to 9 mo and usually abates by age 2 yr. Stranger anxiety is linked with the infant's developmental task of distinguishing the familiar from the unfamiliar. Both the duration and intensity of the anxiety vary greatly among children.

Some infants and young children show a strong preference for one parent over another at a given age, and grandparents may suddenly be viewed as strangers. Anticipating these occurrences during well-child visits helps prevent misinterpretation of the behavior. Comforting the child and avoiding overreaction to the behavior are usually the only therapy needed.

Common sense should dictate management. If a new sitter is coming, having that person spend some time with the family before the actual day makes sense. When the event arrives, having parents spend some time with the child and sitter before they leave is prudent. If grandparents are coming to watch the child for a few days while parents go away, they should arrive a day or two early. Similar techniques can be used in anticipation of hospitalization.

Stranger anxiety of pronounced intensity or extended duration may be a sign of more generalized anxiety and should prompt evaluation of the family situation, parenting techniques, and the child's overall emotional state.

291 Childhood Vaccination

EFFECTIVENESS AND SAFETY OF CHILDHOOD VACCINATION

Vaccination has been profoundly effective in preventing serious disease (see Table 291–1). Given their modest cost (particularly in comparison to drugs that must be taken long-term), vaccines are one of the most cost-effective pharmaceutical products. Vaccines have been so effective that many health care practitioners currently in practice have seen few or no cases of diseases that were once extremely common and fatal. Because the diseases that vaccines prevent have typically become so rare in the US and because vaccines are given to otherwise healthy children, vaccines must have a high safety profile.

Before licensure, vaccines (like any medical product) are tested in randomized controlled trials (RCTs) that compare the new vaccine to placebo (or a previously existing vaccine if one exists). Such prelicensing RCTs are designed primarily to assess vaccine efficacy and to identify common adverse events (eg, fever; local reactions such as injection site redness, swelling, and pain). However, some adverse events occur too rarely to be detected in an RCT of any practical size and may not appear until after a vaccine enters routine use. Thus, two surveillance systems, the Vaccine Adverse Event Reporting System (VAERS) and the Vaccine Safety Datalink (VSD), were created to monitor vaccine safety postlicensure.

VAERS is a safety program cosponsored by the FDA and the Centers for Disease Control and Prevention (CDC); VAERS collects reports from individual patients who believe that they had an adverse event after a recent vaccination. Health care practitioners are also required to report certain events after vaccination and may report events even if they are unsure the events are vaccine-related. VAERS reports originate all across the country and provide a rapid assessment of potential safety issues. However, VAERS reports can show only temporal associations between vaccination and the suspected adverse event; they do not prove causation. Thus, VAERS reports must be further evaluated using other methods. One such method uses the VSD, which uses data from 9 large managed care organizations (MCOs) representing more than 9 million people. The data include vaccine administration (noted in the medical record as part of routine care), as well as subsequent medical history, including adverse events. Unlike VAERS, the VSD includes data from patients who have not received a given vaccine as well as those who have. As a result, the VSD can help distinguish actual adverse events from symptoms and disorders that occurred coincidentally after vaccination and thus determine the actual incidence of adverse events.

For adverse effects of specific vaccines, see pp. 1451–1460.

Table 291–1. CASE RATES OF SOME DISEASES PREVENTABLE BY VACCINES

DISEASE	AVERAGE CASES/ YR BEFORE VACCINE DEVELOPMENT (20TH CENTURY)	CASES IN 2010 (2008)
Diphtheria	21,053	0
Haemophilus influenzae type b	20,000 (estimated)	270
Hepatitis A (HepA)	117,333	(11,049)
Hepatitis B (HepB; acute)	66,232	(11,269)
Measles	503,217	61
Mumps	162,344	2,528
Pertussis	200,752	21,291
Pneumococcus (invasive, all ages)	63,067	(44,000)
Pneumococcus (invasive, < 5 yr)	16,069	(4,167)
Polio (paralytic)	16,316	0
Rotavirus (hospitalizations < 5 yr)	62,500	(7,500)
Rubella	47,745	6
Smallpox	29,005	0
Tetanus	580	8
Varicella	4,085,120	(449,363)

Adapted from Appendix G: Data and statistics: Impact of vaccines in the 20th and 21st centuries. In *Epidemiology and Prevention of Vaccine-Preventable Diseases: The Pink Book*, ed. 12. Centers for Disease Control and Prevention, 2012. Available at http://www.cdc.gov/vaccines/pubs/pinkbook/downloads/appendices/G/impact-of-vaccines.pdf.

ANTI-VACCINATION MOVEMENT

Despite the rigorous vaccine safety systems in place in the US, many parents remain concerned about the safety of the childhood vaccines and immunization schedule. These concerns have led some parents to not allow their children to receive some or all of the recommended vaccines. In the US, rates of vaccine exemptions increased from 1% in 2006 to 2% in 2011; some states reported that 6% of children received exemptions. The rate of vaccine-preventable diseases is higher in children whose parents have refused ≥ 1 vaccines for nonmedical reasons. Specifically, they are[1] 23 times more likely to contract pertussis,[2] 8.6 times more likely to contract varicella,[3] and 6.5 times more likely to contract pneumococcal disease. Children in the US still die from vaccine-preventable diseases.[4] In 2008, there were 5 cases (one fatal) of invasive *Haemophilus influenza* type B infection in Minnesota, the most since 1992. Three of the infected children, including the child who died, had received no vaccines because their parents had deferred or refused the vaccine.

The decision to defer or refuse vaccines also affects public health. When the proportion of the overall population that is immune to a disease (herd immunity) decreases, disease prevalence increases, increasing the possibility of disease in people at risk. People may be at risk because

- They were previously vaccinated, but the vaccine did not induce immunity (eg, 2 to 5% of recipients do not respond to the first dose of measles vaccine).
- Immunity may wane over time (eg, in the elderly).
- They (ie, some immunocompromised patients) cannot receive live-virus vaccines (eg, measles-mumps-rubella, varicella) and rely on herd immunity for protection against such diseases.

Parents hesitate to vaccinate their children for many reasons. Two of the more prominent parental concerns over the past decade have been that

- Vaccines may cause autism.
- Children receive too many vaccines.

Conversations with reluctant parents typically require more than presenting evidence. Finding common ground with parents' goals and hopes for their children and sharing compelling individual accounts can help.[5]

1. Glanz JM, et al: Parental refusal of pertussis vaccination is associated with an increased risk of pertussis infection in children. *Pediatrics* 123(6):1446–1451, 2009.
2. Glanz JM, et al: Parental refusal of varicella (VAR) vaccination and the associated risk of VAR infection in children. *Arch Pediatr Adolesc Med* 164(1):66–70, 2010.
3. Glanz JM, et al: Parental decline of pneumococcal vaccination and risk of pneumococcal related disease in children. *Vaccine* 29(5):994–999, 2011.
4. Invasive Haemophilus influenzae type B disease in five young children—Minnesota, 2008. *MMWR Morb Mortal Wkly Rep* 58(3):58–60, 2009.
5. Politi MC, Jones KM, Philpott SE: The role of patient engagement in addressing parents' perceptions about immunizations. *JAMA*. Published online June 22, 2017. doi:10.1001/jama.2017.7168.

MMR vaccine and autism: In 1998, Andrew Wakefield and colleagues published a brief report in *The Lancet*. This report concerned 12 children with developmental disorders and GI problems; 9 of them also had autism. According to the report, parents claimed that 8 of the 12 children had received the combined measles-mumps-rubella (MMR) vaccine within 1 mo before the development of symptoms. Wakefield postulated that the measles virus in the MMR vaccine traveled to the intestine where it caused inflammation, enabling proteins from the GI tract to enter the bloodstream, travel to the brain, and cause autism. This study received significant media attention worldwide, and many parents began to doubt the safety of the MMR vaccine. In another study, Wakefield claimed to find the measles virus in intestinal biopsy specimens of 75 of 90 children with autism and in only 5 of 70 control patients, leading to speculation that the live measles virus in the MMR vaccine was somehow implicated in autism.

Because Wakefield's methodology could show only a temporal association rather than a cause-and-effect relationship, numerous other researchers studied the possible connection between the MMR vaccine and autism. Gerber and Offit[1] reviewed at least 13 large epidemiologic studies, all of which failed to support an association between MMR vaccine and

Table 291–2. RECOMMENDED IMMUNIZATION SCHEDULE FOR AGES 0–6 YR

VACCINE	BIRTH	1 MO	2 MO	4 MO	6 MO	9 MO	12 MO	15 MO	18 MO	19–23 MO	2–3 YR	4–6 YR
Hepatitis B (HepB)[a]	1st dose	2nd dose		*	3rd dose							
Rotavirus (RV)[b]			1st dose	2nd dose	See footnote b							
Diphtheria, tetanus, pertussis (DTaP, < 7 yr)[c]			1st dose	2nd dose	3rd dose	*	4th dose		*		5th dose	
Haemophilus influenzae type b (Hib)[d]			1st dose	2nd dose	See footnote d	*	3rd or 4th dose[d]		*			†
Pneumococcal conjugate vaccine (PCV13)[e]			1st dose	2nd dose	3rd dose	*	4th dose		*			†
Inactivated polio virus (IPV)[f]			1st dose	2nd dose	3rd dose						4th dose	
Influenza (inactivated influenza vaccine [IIV] or LAIV[g]					Yearly (IIV)							
Measles, mumps, rubella (MMR)[h]							1st dose		*			2nd dose
Varicella (VAR)[i]							1st dose		*			2nd dose
Hepatitis A (HepA)[j]							2-dose series[j]				‡	
Meningococcal conjugate vaccines (Hib-Men-CY, MenACWY-D, and MenACWY-CRM)[k]			†See footnote k									
Pneumococcal polysaccharide vaccine (PPSV23)[e]											†	

* = Range of recommended ages for catch-up immunization.

† = Range of recommended ages for certain high-risk groups.

‡ = Range of recommended ages for catch-up and for certain high-risk groups.

This schedule includes recommendations in effect as of February 1, 2016. Any dose not administered at the recommended age should be administered at a subsequent visit, when indicated and feasible. The use of a combination vaccine is generally preferred over separate injections of its equivalent component vaccines. Considerations should include provider assessment, patient preference, and the potential for adverse events. Providers should consult the relevant ACIP statement for detailed recommendations. Clinically significant adverse events that follow immunization should be reported to the Vaccine Adverse Event Reporting System (VAERS) at http://www.vaers.hhs.gov or by telephone, **800-822-7967**. Suspected cases of vaccine-preventable diseases should be reported to the state or local health department. If children fall behind or start late, a catch-up schedule should be followed.

For calculating intervals between doses, 4 wk = 28 days. Intervals of ≥ 4 mo are determined by calendar months.

For information about travel vaccine requirements, see the CDC's web site For Travelers.

[a]**HepB vaccine.** Minimum age is at birth.

Table 291–2. RECOMMENDED IMMUNIZATION SCHEDULE FOR AGES 0–6 YR (*Continued*)

At birth:

- Administer monovalent HepB to all newborns before hospital discharge.
- If the mother is HepB surface antigen (HBsAg)–positive, administer HepB and 0.5 mL of HepB immune globulin (HBIG) within 12 h of birth. These infants should be tested for HBsAg and antibody to HBsAg (anti-HBs) at age 9–18 mo (preferably at the next well-child visit) or 1–2 mo after completion of the HepB series. The Centers for Disease Control and Prevention (CDC) recently recommended that testing occur at age 9–12 mo (Update: Shortened Interval for Postvaccination Serologic Testing of Infants Born to HepB-Infected Mothers).
- If the mother's HBsAg status is unknown, administer HepB vaccine to all infants within 12 h of birth, regardless of birth weight. If infants weigh < 2000 g, administer HBIG in addition to HepB vaccine within 12 h of birth. Determine the mother's HBsAg status as soon as possible, and if she is HBsAg-positive, administer HBIG to infants weighing ≥ 2000 g (no later than age 7 days).

After the birth dose:

- The 2nd dose should be administered at age 1–2 mo. Monovalent HepB vaccine should be used for doses administered before age 6 wk.
- Administration of a total of 4 doses of HepB vaccine is permissible when a combination vaccine containing HepB is administered after the birth dose.
- Infants who did not receive a birth dose should receive 3 doses of a HepB-containing vaccine on a schedule of 0 mo, 1–2 mo, and 6 mo starting as soon as feasible (see Table 291–4).
- The minimum interval between dose 1 and dose 2 is 4 wk, and between dose 2 and 3, it is 8 wk. The final (3rd or 4th) dose in the HepB vaccine series should be administered no earlier than age 24 wk and at least 16 wk after the first dose.

[b]**RV vaccines.** Minimum age is 6 wk for RV-1 (Rotarix®) and RV-5 (RotaTeq®).

- If RV-1 (Rotarix®) is used, administer 2 doses: at ages 2 mo and 4 mo.
- If RV-5 (RotaTeq®) is used, administer 3 doses: at ages 2 mo, 4 mo, and 6 mo.
- If any dose in a series was RV-5 (RotaTeq®) or is unknown, 3 doses should be administered.
- The maximum age is 14 wk, 6 days for the first dose in the series and is 8 mo, 0 days for the final dose in the series. Vaccination should not be initiated for infants aged 15 wk, 0 days or older.
- If RV-1 (Rotarix®) is administered for the first and 2nd doses, a 3rd dose is not indicated.

[c]**Diphtheria and tetanus toxoids and acellular pertussis (DTaP) vaccine.** Minimum age is 6 wk, except for DTaP-IPV (Kinrix®), which has a minimum age of 4 yr.

- Administer a 5-dose DTaP series at ages 2, 4, 6, 15–18 mo, and 4–6 yr. The 4th dose may be administered as early as age 12 mo, provided at least 6 mo have elapsed since the 3rd dose.
- If the 4th dose is administered at least 4 mo but < 6 mo after the 3rd dose, it does not need to be repeated.
- A 5th dose of DTaP vaccine is not needed if the 4th dose was administered at age ≥ 4 yr.

[d]***Haemophilus influenzae* type b (Hib) conjugate vaccine.** Minimum age is 6 wk for PRP-T (ActHIB®, DTaP-IPV/Hib [Pentacel®], and Hib-MenCY [MenHibrix®]) and PRP-OMP (PedvaxHIB® or COMVAX) and 12 mo for PRP-T (Hiberix).

- Administer a 2- or 3-dose Hib vaccine primary series with a booster dose (dose 3 or 4 depending on the vaccine used in the primary series) at age 12–15 mo to complete the full Hib series. The primary series consists of 3 doses given at ages 2, 4, and 6 mo for PRP-T and consists of 2 doses given at ages 2 and 4 mo for PRP-OMP.
- If PRP-OMP (PedvaxHIB or ComVax [HepB-Hib]) is administered at ages 2 and 4 mo, a dose at age 6 mo is not indicated.
- One booster dose (dose 3 or 4 depending on the vaccine used in the primary series) should be given at age 12–15 mo. An exception is Hiberix, which should only be used for the booster (final) dose in children aged 12 mo–4 yr who have received at least 1 dose of Hib.
- Hib vaccine is not routinely given to patients > 5 yr. However, 1 dose should be administered to unimmunized patients aged ≥ 5 yr if they have anatomic or functional asplenia (including sickle cell disease) and to unvaccinated patients aged 5–18 yr with HIV infection. Patients are considered unimmunized if they have not been given a primary series and booster dose or at least 1 dose of Hib vaccine after age 14 mo.
- Administer only 1 dose to unvaccinated children aged ≥ 15 mo. For other catch-up recommendations, see Table 291–4.

The following are recommendations for children at increased risk of Hib infection:

- If children aged 12–59 mo are at increased risk for Hib infection (including chemotherapy recipients and those with anatomic or functional asplenia [eg, with sickle cell disease], HIV infection, immunoglobulin deficiency, or early component complement deficiency) and have received no doses or only 1 dose of Hib vaccine before age 12 mo, they should be given 2 additional doses of Hib vaccine 8 wk apart. Children who were given ≥ 2 doses of Hib vaccine before age 12 mo should be given 1 additional dose.
- If patients < 5 yr who are having chemotherapy or radiation therapy were given ≥ 1 Hib vaccine doses within 14 days of starting therapy or during therapy, the doses should be repeated at least 3 mo after therapy is completed.
- Recipients of a hematopoietic stem cell transplant should be revaccinated with a 3-dose regimen of Hib vaccine starting 6–12 mo after successful transplantation, regardless of vaccination history; doses should be given at least 4 wk apart.
- A single dose of any vaccine that contains Hib should be given to unimmunized children and adolescents aged ≥15 mo if they are having elective splenectomy; if possible, the vaccine should be given at least 14 days before the procedure.

Table continues on the following page.

Table 291–2. RECOMMENDED IMMUNIZATION SCHEDULE FOR AGES 0–6 YR (*Continued*)

[e]**Pneumococcal vaccines.** Minimum age is 6 wk for 13-valent pneumococcal conjugate vaccine (PCV13) and 2 yr for 23-valent pneumococcal polysaccharide vaccine (PPSV23).

- Administer 1 dose of PCV13 to all healthy children aged 24–59 mo who are not completely vaccinated for their age.
- For all children aged 14–59 mo who have received an age-appropriate series of 7-valent PCV (PCV7), administer a single supplemental dose of PCV13.
- For children aged 2–5 yr with certain medical conditions, administer 1 dose of PCV13 if they have received 3 doses of PCV (PCV7 and/or PCV13) previously, or administer 2 doses ≥ 8 wk apart if they have received < 3 doses of PCV (PCV7 and/or PCV13). Administer 1 supplemental dose of PCV13 to children who have received 4 doses of PCV7 or completed another age-appropriate PCV7 series.
- If children aged 6–18 yr with certain medical conditions (including a cochlear implant) have not received PCV13 nor PPSV23, administer 1 dose of PCV13, followed by 1 dose of PPSV23 at least 8 wk later (see *MMWR* 59 [RR-11]:1–19, 2010).
- Administer PPSV23 at least 8 wk after the last dose of PCV13 to children aged ≥ 2 yr with certain medical conditions, including a cochlear implant. A single revaccination with PPSV23 should be administered 5 yr after the first dose to children with anatomic or functional asplenia or an immunocompromising condition.

[f]**Inactivated poliovirus vaccine (IPV).** Minimum age is 6 wk.

- Administer a 4-dose IPV series at ages 2, 4, 6–18 mo, and 4–6 yr. The final dose in the series should be administered on or after the 4th birthday and at least 6 mo after the previous dose.
- During the first 6 mo of life, minimum age and minimum intervals are recommended only if the infant is at risk of imminent exposure to circulating poliovirus (eg, traveling to a polio-endemic region, during an outbreak).
- If ≥ 4 doses are administered before age 4 yr, an additional dose should be administered at age 4–6 yr and at least 6 mo after the previous dose.
- A 4th dose is not necessary if the 3rd dose was administered at age ≥ 4 yr and at least 6 mo after the previous dose.
- If both oral polio vaccine (OPV) and IPV were administered as part of a series, a total of 4 doses should be administered regardless of the child's current age. If only OPC was administered and all the doses were given before age 4 yr, one dose of IPV should be given at age ≥ 4 yr and at least 4 wk after the last OPV dose.

[g]**Influenza vaccine (seasonal).** Minimum age is 6 mo for IIV and 2 yr for LAIV.

- For most healthy children aged ≥ 2 yr, either LAIV or IIV may be used. However, LAIV should not be administered to some children, including children with asthma, children aged 2–4 yr who have had wheezing in the past 12 mo, and children who have any other medical conditions that predispose them to influenza complications. For all other contraindications to use of LAIV, see *MMWR* 62 (RR-7)1–43, 2013.
- For children aged 6 mo–8 yr:
  - For the 2015–16 season, administer 2 doses (separated by at least 4 wk) to children who are receiving the influenza vaccine for the first time. Some children who have been previously vaccinated also need 2 doses. For additional guidance, see the dosing guidelines in the 2015–16 ACIP recommendations for influenza vaccine in *MMWR* 64 (30):818–25, 2015.
  - For more information, see Influenza ACIP Vaccine Recommendations.

[g]**Influenza vaccine (seasonal).** Minimum age is 6 mo for IIV and 2 yr for LAIV.

- For most healthy children aged ≥ 2 yr, either LAIV or IIV may be used. However, LAIV should not be administered to some children, including children with asthma, children aged 2–4 yr who have had wheezing in the past 12 mo, and children who have any other medical conditions that predispose them to influenza complications. For all other contraindications to use of LAIV, see *MMWR* 62 (RR-7)1–43, 2013.
- For children aged 6 mo–8 yr:
  - For the 2015–16 season, administer 2 doses (separated by at least 4 wk) to children who are receiving the influenza vaccine for the first time. Some children who have been previously vaccinated also need 2 doses. For additional guidance, see the dosing guidelines in the 2015–16 ACIP recommendations for influenza vaccine in *MMWR* 64 (30):818–25, 2015.
  - For more information, see the ACIP recommendations for influenza vaccine

[h]**Measles, mumps, and rubella (MMR) vaccine.** Minimum age is 12 mo.

- The 2nd dose may be administered before age 4, provided at least 4 wk have elapsed since the first dose.
- Administer 1 dose of MMR vaccine to infants aged 6–11 mo who are traveling internationally. These children should be revaccinated with 2 doses of MMR vaccine: the first dose at age 12–15 mo (at age 12 mo if the child remains in a high-risk area) and the 2nd dose at least 4 wk after the previous dose.
- Administer 2 doses of MMR vaccine to children aged ≥ 12 mo who are traveling internationally; the first dose is given at or after age 12 mo, and the 2nd dose is given at least 4 wk after the previous dose.

Table 291–2. RECOMMENDED IMMUNIZATION SCHEDULE FOR AGES 0–6 YR (*Continued*)

[i]**VAR vaccine.** Minimum age is 12 mo.

- The 2nd dose may be administered before age 4, provided at least 3 mo have elapsed since the first dose. If the 2nd dose was administered at least 4 wk after the first dose, it can be accepted as valid.

[j]**HepA vaccine.** Minimum age is 12 mo.

- Administer the 2nd (final) dose 6–18 mo after the first.
- If children have received 1 dose of HepA before age 24 mo, administer a 2nd dose 6–18 mo after the first.
- Unvaccinated children who are at high risk or who live in areas where vaccination programs target older children should be vaccinated. See *MMWR* 55 [RR-7], 2006.
- A 2-dose HepA vaccine series is recommended for any people aged ≥ 2 yr if they have not been previously vaccinated and if immunity against HepA is desired for them.

[k]**Meningococcal conjugate vaccines, quadrivalent.** Minimum age is 6 wk for Hib-MenCY (MenHibrix; for *H. influenzae* type b and *Neisseria meningitidis* serogroups C and Y), 9 mo for MenACWY-D (Menactra®), 2 mo for MenACWY-CRM (Menveo®), and 10 yr for serogroup B meningococcal (MenB) vaccines (Men B-4C [Bexsero®],
MenB-FHbp [Trumenbal®]).

- For children aged 2–18 mo who have persistent complement component deficiency (including patients with inherited or chronic deficiencies in C3, C5–9, properdin, factor D, or factor H and those taking eculizumab) or anatomic or functional asplenia (including sickle cell anemia), administer a 4-dose infant series of Hib-MenCY at age 2, 4, 6, and 12–15 mo or MenACWY-CRM at age 2, 4, 6, and 12 mo.
- For children aged 7–23 mo who have persistent complement component deficiency and who have not initiated vaccination, there are two options. MenACWY-CRM may be given at age 7–23 mo in a 2-doses series, with the 2nd dose given after age 12 mo and at least 12 wk after the first dose. Or MenACWY-D may be given at age 9–23 mo given in a 2-dose series, with the doses given at least 12 wk apart.
- For children aged 19–23 mo who have anatomic or functional asplenia and who have not been completely vaccinated with Hib-MenCY or MenACWY-CRM, administer 2 primary doses of Men-ACWY-CRM at least 12 wk apart.
- For children aged ≥ 24 mo who have persistent complement component deficiency or anatomic or functional asplenia and who have not been completely vaccinated, administer 2 primary doses of either MenACWY-D or MenACWY-CRM vaccine at least 8 wk apart.
- If MenACWY-D is used in children with anatomic or functional asplenia, administer at a minimum age of 2 yr and at least 4 wk after completion of all PCV13 doses.
- If children with a high-risk condition live in or are traveling to countries where meningococcal disease is hyperendemic or epidemic (eg, the African meningitis belt, the Hajj), administer at age-appropriate formulation and series of MenACWY-D or MenACWY-CRM for protection against serogroups A and W. Prior vaccination with Hib-MenCY is not sufficient for children traveling to these areas (see *MMWR* 62 (RR2):1–22, 2013.
- If children with a high-risk condition are present during outbreaks caused by a vaccine serogroup, administer or complete an age- and formula-appropriate series of Hib-MenCY, MenACWY-D, MenACWY-CRM, MenB-4C, or MenB-FHbp.
- If children with a high-risk condition receive the first dose of Hib-MenCY at or after age 12 mo, administer a total of 2 doses at least 8 wk apart to ensure protection against serogroups C and Y meningococcal disease.
- If children with a high-risk condition receive the first dose of MenACWY-CRM at age 7–9 mo, administer a 2-dose series, with the 2nd dose given after age 12 mo and at least 3 mo after the first dose.
- If patients ≥ 10 yr have persistent complement component deficiency or anatomic or functional asplenia and have not received a complete meningococcal vaccine series, they may be given 2 doses of Men B-4C at least 1 mo apart or 3 doses of Men B-FHbp, with the 2nd dose at least 2 mo after the first and the 3rd dose at least 6 mo after the first. The two MenB vaccines are not interchangeable; the same vaccine product must be used for all doses.
- For further guidance, including revaccination guidelines, see *MMWR* 62 (RR2):1–22, 2013, *MMWR* 64 (41):1171–76, 2015 and Meningococcal ACIP Vaccine Recommendations.

ACIP = Advisory Committee on Immunization Practices; MMWR = *Morbidity and Mortality Weekly Review*; PRP-OMP = *Neisseria meningitidis* polyribosyl ribitol phosphate/outer membrane protein.
Adapted from the Centers for Disease Control and Prevention: Recommended Immunization Schedule for Persons Aged 0 Through 18 Years, United States—2016.

autism. Many of these studies showed that national trends of MMR vaccination were not directly associated with national trends in the diagnosis of autism. For example, in the UK between 1988 and 1999, the rate of MMR vaccination did not change, but the rate of autism increased.

Other studies compared the risk of autism in individual children who did or did not receive the MMR vaccine. In the largest and most compelling of these studies, Madsen et al[2] assessed 537,303 Danish children born between 1991 and 1998, 82% of whom had received MMR vaccine. After controlling for possible confounders, they found no difference in relative risk of autism or other autism-spectrum disorders in vaccinated and unvaccinated children. Overall incidence of autism or an autistic-spectrum disorder was 608 of 440,655 (0.138%) in the vaccinated group and 130 of 96,648 (0.135%) in the unvaccinated group. Other population-based studies from across the world have reached similar conclusions.

In response to Wakefield's increased detection of measles virus in intestinal biopsy specimens from autistic children, Hornig et al[3] searched for the measles virus in biopsy samples taken from 38 children who had GI symptoms and were having a colonoscopy; 25 children had autism, and 13 did not. The measles virus was not detected more often in the children with autism than in those without.

1. Gerber JS, Offit PA: Vaccines and autism: A tale of shifting hypotheses, *Clin Infect Dis* 48(4):456–461, 2009.
2. Madsen KM, et al: A population-based study of measles, mumps, and rubella vaccination and autism. *N Engl J Med* 347(19):1477–482, 2002.
3. Hornig M, et al: Lack of association between measles virus vaccine and autism with enteropathy: A case-control study. *PLoS ONE*, 3(9):e3140, 2008.

Thimerosal and autism: Thimerosal is a mercury compound previously used as a preservative in many multidose vaccine vials; preservatives are not needed in single-dose vials and cannot be used in live-virus vaccines. Thimerosal is metabolized to ethylmercury, which is eliminated quickly from the body. Because environmental methylmercury (which is a different compound that is *not* eliminated from the body quickly) is toxic to humans, there was concern that the very small amounts of thimerosal used in vaccines might cause neurologic problems, particularly autism, in children. Because of these theoretical concerns, although no studies had shown evidence of harm, thimerosal was removed from routine childhood vaccines in the US, Europe, and several other countries by 2001. However, in these countries, thimerosal continues to be used in certain influenza vaccines and in several other vaccines intended for use in adults. It is also used in many vaccines produced in developing countries; the WHO has not recommended its removal because there is no clinical evidence of toxicity due to routine use.

Despite the removal of thimerosal, rates of autism have continued to increase, strongly suggesting that thimerosal in vaccines does not cause autism. Also, 2 separate Vaccine Safety Datalink (VSD) studies have concluded that there is no association between thimerosal and autism. In a cohort study of 124,170 children in 3 managed care organizations (MCOs); Verstraeten et al[1] found no association between thimerosal and autism or other developmental conditions, although inconsistent associations (ie, seen in one MCO but not another) were seen between thimerosal and certain language disorders. In a case-control study of 1000 children (256 with an autism-spectrum disorder and 752 matched controls without autism), Price et al.,[2] using regression analysis, found no association between exposure to thimerosal and autism.

Practitioners who work with parents who are still concerned about thimerosal in the influenza vaccine may use single-dose vials or give live-attenuated influenza vaccine (LAIV); neither of them contains thimerosal.

1. Verstraeten T, et al: Safety of thimerosal-containing vaccines: A two-phased study of computerized health maintenance organization databases. *Pediatrics* 112: 1039–1048, 2003.
2. Price CS, et al: Prenatal and infant exposure to thimerosal from vaccines and immunoglobulins and risk of autism. *Pediatrics* 126(4):656–664, 2010.

Use of multiple, simultaneous vaccines: A nationally representative survey done in the late 1990s revealed that nearly one fourth of all parents felt that their children receive more immunizations than they should. Since then, additional vaccines have been added to the immunization schedule so that by age 6, children are now recommended to receive multiple doses of vaccines for 15 different infections (see Table 291–2). To minimize the number of injections and visits, practitioners give many vaccines as combination products (eg, diphtheria-tetanus-pertussis, measles-mumps-rubella). However, some parents have become concerned that children's (particularly infants') immune system cannot handle multiple simultaneously presented antigens. This concern has caused some parents to request alternative immunization schedules that delay and sometimes completely exclude certain vaccines. A recent nationally representative survey found that 13% of parents use such a schedule.

The use of alternative schedules is risky and scientifically unfounded. The official schedule is designed to protect children against diseases when they are most susceptible. Delaying vaccination increases the amount of time children are at risk of acquiring these diseases. In addition, although parents may plan to only delay vaccination, the increased number of visits needed for alternative schedules increases the difficulty of adherence and thus the risk that children will not receive a full series of vaccines. Regarding the immunologic challenges, parents should be informed that the amount and number of antigens contained in vaccines is miniscule compared with that encountered in everyday life. Even at birth, an infant's immune system is prepared to respond to the hundreds of antigens the infant is exposed to while passing through the birth canal and being handled by the (unsterile) mother. Children typically encounter and respond immunologically to dozens and perhaps hundreds of antigens during an ordinary day without difficulty. A typical infection with a single organism stimulates an immune response to multiple antigens of that organism (perhaps 4 to 10 in a typical URI). Furthermore, because current vaccines contain fewer antigens overall (ie, because key antigens have been better identified and purified), children are exposed to fewer vaccine antigens today than they were for most of the 20th century.

In summary, alternative vaccine schedules are not evidence-based and put children at increased risk of infectious diseases. More importantly, they offer no advantage. Using data from the VSD, Smith and Woods[1] compared neurodevelopmental outcomes in a group of children who received all vaccines on

Table 291–3. RECOMMENDED IMMUNIZATION SCHEDULE FOR AGES 7–18 YR

VACCINE	7–10 YR	11–12 YR	13–18 YR
Hepatitis B (HepB)[a]	*Complete 3-dose series		
Haemophilus influenzae type b (Hib)[b]	†See footnote b.		
Pneumococcal conjugate vaccine (PCV13) and pneumococcal polysaccharide vaccine (PPSV23)[c]	†See footnote c.		
Inactivated poliovirus (IPV)[d]	*See footnote d.		
Influenza[e]	Yearly (IIV or LAIV)		
Measles, mumps, rubella (MMR)[f]	*Complete 2-dose series		
Varicella (VAR)[g]	*Complete 2-dose series		
Hepatitis A (HepA)[h]	‡Complete 2-dose series		
Meningococcal conjugate vaccines, quadrivalent (Hib-Men-CY, MenACWY-D, and MenACWY-CRM)[i]	†	1st dose	*Booster at age 16 yr
Tetanus, diphtheria, pertussis (Tdap)[j]	*	Tdap	*
Human papillomavirus (HPV)[k]	See footnote k.	3 doses	*
Meningococcal B vaccine[i]	†See footnote i.		

* = Range of recommended ages for catch-up immunization.

† = Range of recommended ages for certain high-risk groups.

‡ = Range of recommended ages for catch-up and for certain high-risk groups.

This schedule includes recommendations in effect as of January 1, 2014. Any dose not administered at the recommended age should be administered at a subsequent visit, when indicated and feasible. The use of a combination vaccine is generally preferred over separate injections of its equivalent component vaccines. Vaccination providers should consult the relevant ACIP statement for detailed recom mendations available at http://www.cdc.gov/vaccines/pubs/acip-list.htm. Clinically significant adverse events that follow immunization should be reported to the Vaccine Adverse Event Reporting System (VAERS) at **http://www.vaers.hhs.gov** or by telephone, **800-822-7967**. Suspected cases of vaccine-preventable diseases should be reported to the state or local health department. If children fall behind or start late, a catch-up schedule should be followed.

For calculating intervals between doses, 4 wk = 28 days. Intervals of ≥ 4 mo are determined by calendar months.

For information about travel vaccine requirements, see the CDC's web site For Travelers.

[a]**HepB vaccine.**

- Administer the 3-dose series to children not previously vaccinated.
- For children with incomplete vaccination, follow the catch-up recommendations (see Table 291–4).
- A 2-dose series (doses separated by at least 4 mo) of adult formulation Recombivax HB® is licensed for use in children aged 11–15 yr.

[b]***Haemophilus influenzae* type b (Hib) conjugate vaccine.**

- Hib vaccine is not routinely given to patients > 5 yr. However, 1 dose should be administered to unimmunized patients aged ≥ 5 yr if they have anatomic or functional asplenia (including sickle cell disease) and to unvaccinated patients aged 5–18 yr with HIV infection. Patients are considered unimmunized if they have not received a primary series and booster dose or at least 1 dose of Hib vaccine after age 14 mo.
- A single dose of any vaccine that contains Hib should be given to unimmunized children and adolescents aged ≥15 mo if they are having an elective splenectomy; if possible, the vaccine should be given at least 14 days before procedure.

[c]**Pneumococcal vaccines (13-valent pneumococcal conjugate vaccine [PCV13] and 23-valent pneumococcal polysaccharide vaccine [PPSV23]).**

- If children aged 6–18 yr with certain medical conditions (including a cochlear implant) have not received PCV13 nor PPSV23, administer 1 dose of PCV13, followed by 1 dose of PPSV23 at least 8 wk later (see MMWR 59 [RR-11]:1–19, 2010).
- Administer PPSV23 at least 8 wk after the last dose of PCV13 to children aged ≥ 2 yr with certain medical conditions, including a cochlear implant. A single revaccination with PPSV23 should be administered 5 yr after the first dose to children with anatomic or functional asplenia or an immunocompromising condition.

[d]**Inactivated poliovirus vaccine (IPV).**

- The final dose in the series should be administered at least 6 mo after the previous dose.
- If both oral poliovirus (OPV) and IPV were administered as part of a series, a total of 4 doses should be administered, regardless of the child's current age. If only OPC was administered and all the doses were given before age 4 yr, one dose of IPV should be given at age ≥ 4 yr and at least 4 wk after the last OPV dose.
- IPV is not routinely recommended for US residents aged ≥ 18 yr.

Table continues on the following page.

Table 291–3. RECOMMENDED IMMUNIZATION SCHEDULE FOR AGES 7–18 YR (*Continued*)

[e]**Influenza vaccines IIV and LAIV).**

- For most healthy, nonpregnant people aged 2–49 yr, either LAIV or IIV may be used. However, LAIV should not be administered to some people, including those with asthma or any other medical conditions that predispose them to influenza complications. For all other contraindications to use of LAIV, see *MMWR* 62 (RR-7):1–43, 2013.
- Administer 1 dose to people aged ≥ 9 yr.
- For children aged 6 mo–8 yr:
  - For the 2015–16 season, administer 2 doses (separated by at least 4 wk) to children who are receiving the influenza vaccine for the first time. Some children who have been previously vaccinated also need 2 doses. For additional guidance, see the dosing guidelines in the 2015–16 ACIP recommendations for influenza vaccine in *MMWR* 64 (30):818–25, 2015.
  - For more information, see the ACIP recommendations for influenza vaccine.

[f]**Measles, mumps, and rubella (MMR) vaccine.**

- The minimum interval between 2 doses of MMR vaccine is 4 wk.
- Make sure all school-aged children and adolescents have had 2 doses of MMR vaccine.

[g]**VAR vaccine.**

- For people aged 7–18 yr without evidence of immunity (see *MMWR* 56 [RR-4], 2007, and ACIP recommendations), administer 2 doses if they were not previously vaccinated or the 2nd dose if only 1 dose has been administered.
- For children aged 7–12 years, the recommended minimum interval between doses is 3 mo. However, if the 2nd dose was administered at least 4 wk after the first dose, it can be accepted as valid.
- For children aged ≥ 13 yr, the minimum interval between doses is 4 wk.

[h]**HepA vaccine.**

- A 2-dose HepA vaccine series is recommended for previously unvaccinated children if they live in areas where vaccination programs target older children, if they are at increased risk of infection, or if immunity against HepA is desired for them.
- Administer 2 doses at least 6 mo apart to unvaccinated people.

[i]**Meningococcal conjugate vaccines, quadrivalent (Hib-MenCY [MenHibrix®], MenACWY-D [Menactra®], and MenACWY-CRM [Menveo®])**, serogroup B meningococcal (MenB) vaccines (Men B-4C [Bexsero®], MenB-FHbp [Trumenbal®]).

- Administer MenACWY-D or MenACWY-CRM at age 11–12 yr with a booster dose at age 16 yr.
- Administer MenACWY-D or MenACWY-CRM at age 13–18 yr if patients have not been previously vaccinated.
- If the first dose is administered at age 13–15 yr, a booster dose should be administered at age 16–18 yr with a minimum interval of at least 8 wk after the preceding dose.
- If the first dose is administered at age ≥ 16 yr, a booster dose is not needed.
- If patients have persistent complement component deficiency (including patients with inherited or chronic deficiencies in C3, C5–9, properdin, factor D, or factor H and those taking eculizumab) or anatomic or functional asplenia and have not been completely vaccinated, administer 2 primary doses either MenACWY-D or MenACWY-CRM vaccine at least 2 mo apart and 1 dose every 5 yr thereafter. Children who receive the primary series before their 7th birthday should receive the first booster dose in 3 yr and subsequent doses every 5 yr (for additional information, see Prevention and Control of Meningococcal Disease: Recommendations of the Advisory Committee on Immunization Practices [ACIP]).
- Adolescents aged 11–18 yr with HIV infection should receive a 2-dose primary series of MenACWY-D or MenACWY-CRM with at least 8 wk between doses.
- Young adults aged 16–23 yr (preferred age range: 16–18 yr) may be vaccinated with either a 2-dose series of Men B-4C or a 3-dose series of MenB-FHbp to provide short-term protection against most strains of serogroup B meningococcal disease (at the clinician's discretion). The two MenB vaccines are not interchangeable; the same vaccine product must be used for all doses.
- If patients ≥ 10 yr have persistent complement component deficiency or anatomic or functional asplenia and have not received a complete meningococcal vaccine series, they may be given 2 doses of Men B-4C at least 1 mo apart or 3 doses of Men B-FHbp, with the 2nd dose at least 2 mo after the first and the 3rd dose at least 6 mo after the first. The two Men B vaccines are not interchangeable; the same vaccine product must be used for all doses.
- For further guidance, including revaccination guidelines, see *MMWR* 62 (RR2):1–22, 2013, *MMWR* 64 (41):1171–76, 2015 and Meningococcal ACIP Vaccine Recommendations.

[j]**Tetanus and diphtheria toxoids and acellular pertussis (Tdap) vaccine.** Minimum age is 10 yr for Boostrix® and 11 yr for Adacel®.

- People aged 11–18 yr who have not received Tdap vaccine should receive a dose followed by tetanus and diphtheria toxoids (Td) booster doses every 10 yr thereafter.
- Children aged 7–10 yr who are not fully immunized with the childhood DTaP vaccine series should be given Tdap vaccine as the first dose of Td in the catch-up series. If additional doses are needed, Td vaccine is used. These children should not be given adolescent Tdap vaccine.
- An inadvertent dose of DTaP vaccine administered to children aged 7–10 yr can count as part of the catch-up series. This dose can count as the adolescent Tdap dose, or the child can later receive a Tdap booster dose at age 11–12 yr.
- An inadvertent dose of DTaP vaccine administered to adolescents aged 11–18 yr should be counted as the adolescent Tdap dose.
- Tdap vaccine can be administered regardless of the interval since the last tetanus and diphtheria toxoid–containing vaccine.

Table 291–3. RECOMMENDED IMMUNIZATION SCHEDULE FOR AGES 7–18 YR (*Continued*)

[k]**HPV vaccines (HPV4 [Gardasil®], HPV2 [Cervarix®], HPV9 [Gardasil® 9]).** Minimum age is 9 yr.

- Either HPV4, HPV2, or HPV9 is recommended in a 3-dose series for females aged 11 or 12 yr. HPV4 or HPV9 is recommended in a 3-dose series for males aged 11 or 12 yr. The doses are given on a schedule of 0, 1–2, and 6 mo.
- The vaccine series can be started beginning at age 9 yr. It should be given at age 9 yr if children have any history of sexual abuse or assault and have not completed the 3-dose series.
- Administer the 2nd dose 1–2 mo after the first dose (minimum interval of 4 wk) and the 3rd dose 24 wk after the first dose and 16 wk after the 2nd dose (minimum interval of 12 wk).
- Administer the vaccine series to previously unvaccinated females (HPV4, HPV2, or HPV9) and males (HPV4 or HPV9) at age 13–18 yr.

ACIP = Advisory Committee on Immunization Practices; MMWR = *Morbidity and Mortality Weekly Review*.
Adapted from the Centers for Disease Control and Prevention: Recommended Immunization Schedule for Persons Aged 0 Through 18 Years, United States—2016.

time with those who did not. The children in the delayed group did not do better on any of the 42 outcomes tested. These results should reassure parents who are concerned that children receive too many vaccines too soon.

1. Smith MJ, Woods CR: On-time vaccine receipt in the first year does not adversely affect neuropsychological outcomes. *Pediatrics* 125(6): 1134–1141, 2010.

CHILDHOOD VACCINATION SCHEDULE

Vaccination follows a schedule recommended by the Centers for Disease Control and Prevention, the American Academy of Pediatrics, and the American Academy of Family Physicians (see Tables 291–2, 291–3, and 291–4). The latest recommendations can be obtained at www.cdc.gov/vaccines and are available as a free mobile app; vaccination status should be reassessed at every visit. For adverse effects and details of administration of specific vaccines, see pp. 1451–1460.

Table 291–4. CATCH-UP IMMUNIZATION SCHEDULE FOR AGES 4 MO–18 YR

VACCINE	MINIMUM AGE FOR DOSE 1	MINIMUM INTERVAL BETWEEN DOSES 1 AND 2	MINIMUM INTERVAL BETWEEN DOSES 2 AND 3	MINIMUM INTERVAL BETWEEN DOSES 3 AND 4	MINIMUM INTERVAL BETWEEN DOSES 4 AND 5
For ages 4 mo–6 yr					
Hepatitis B (HepB)[a]	Birth	4 wk	8 wk and at least 16 wk after the first dose Minimum age for the final dose: 24 wk	—	—
Rotavirus (RV)[b]	6 wk	4 wk	4 wk[a]	—	
Diphtheria, tetanus, pertussis (DTaP)[c]	6 wk	4 wk	4 wk	6 mo	6 mo[b]
Haemophilus influenzae type b (Hib)[d]	6 wk	4 wk if the first dose is administered at age < 12 mo 8 wk (as the final dose) if the first dose is administered at age 12–14 mo No further doses needed if the first dose is administered at age ≥ 15 mo	4 wk[c] if the current age is < 12 mo and the first dose is administered at age < 7 mo 8 wk and age 12–59 mo (as the final dose)[c] if the current age is < 12 mo and the first dose was administered at age 7–11 mo (regardless of Hib vaccine used for the first dose), if the current age is 12–59 mo and the first dose was administered at age < 12 mo, or if the first 2 doses were PRP-OMP and administered at age < 12 mo No further doses needed if the previous dose is administered at age ≥ 15 mo	8 wk (as the final dose) Only necessary for children aged 12–59 mo who received 3 doses (PRP-T) before age 12 mo and started the primary series before age 7 mo	—

Table continues on the following page.

Table 291–4. CATCH-UP IMMUNIZATION SCHEDULE FOR AGES 4 MO–18 YR (*Continued*)

VACCINE	MINIMUM AGE FOR DOSE 1	MINIMUM INTERVAL BETWEEN DOSES 1 AND 2	MINIMUM INTERVAL BETWEEN DOSES 2 AND 3	MINIMUM INTERVAL BETWEEN DOSES 3 AND 4	MINIMUM INTERVAL BETWEEN DOSES 4 AND 5
Pneumococcal vaccine[e]	6 wk	4 wk if the first dose is administered at age < 12 mo 8 wk (as the final dose for healthy children) if the first dose is administered at age ≥ 12 mo No further doses needed for healthy children if the first dose is administered at age ≥ 24 mo	4 wk if the current age is < 12 mo 8 wk (as the final dose for healthy children) if the current age is ≥ 12 mo No further doses needed for healthy children if the previous dose is administered at age ≥ 24 mo	8 wk (as the final dose) Only necessary for children aged 12–59 mo who received 3 doses before age 12 mo or for high-risk children who received 3 doses at any age	
Inactivated polio virus (IPV)[f]	6 wk	4 wk	4 wk	6 mo[e] Minimum age: 4 yr for the final dose	—
Meningococcal[g]	6 wk	8 wk[f]	See footnote f	See footnote f	
Measles, mumps, rubella (MMR)[h]	12 mo	4 wk	—	—	—
Varicella (VAR)[i]	12 mo	3 mo	—	—	—
Hepatitis A (HepA)[j]	12 mo	6 mo	—	—	—
For ages 7–18 yr					
Tetanus, diphtheria (Td) Tetanus, diphtheria, pertussis (Tdap)[k]	7 yr[j]	4 wk	4 wk if the first dose of DTaP/DT is administered at age < 12 mo 6 mo if the first dose of DTaP/DT is administered at age ≥ 12 mo	6 mo if the first dose of DTaP/DT is administered at age < 12 mo	—
Human papillomavirus (HPV)[l]	9 yr	Routine dosing intervals recommended[k]			
HepA[j]	12 mo	6 mo	—	—	—
Hepatitis B (HepB)[b]	Birth	4 wk	8 wk and at least 16 wk after the first dose	—	—
Inactivated polio virus (IPV)[f]	6 wk	4 wk	4 wk[e]	6 mo[e]	—
Meningococcal[g]	6 wk	8 wk[f]	—	—	—
Measles, mumps, rubella (MMR)[h]	12 mo	4 wk	—	—	—
Varicella (VAR)[i]	12 mo	3 mo if age is < 13 yr 4 wk if age is ≥ 13 yr	—	—	—

NOTE: For children whose vaccinations were started late or are > 1 mo behind, the table provides catch-up schedules and minimum intervals between doses. A vaccine series does not need to be restarted, regardless of the time that has elapsed between doses. Use the section appropriate for the child's age. Always use this table in conjunction with the childhood and adolescent immunization schedules, including their footnotes (see Table 291–2 and 291–3). Information about reporting reactions after immunization is available online at http://ww0w.vaers.hhs.gov or by telephone, **800-822-7967**. Suspected cases of vaccine-preventable diseases should be reported. Additional information, including precautions and contraindications for vaccination, is available from the Centers for Disease Control and Prevention (CDC) at www.cdc.gov/vaccines or by telephone (800-232-4636 [800-CDC-INFO]).

For calculating intervals between doses, 4 wk = 28 days. Intervals of ≥ 4 mo are determined by calendar months.

For information about travel vaccine requirements, see the CDC's web site For Travelers.

For contraindications and precautions to use of a vaccine and for additional information, see ACIP recommendations.

Table 291–4. CATCH-UP IMMUNIZATION SCHEDULE FOR AGES 4 MO–18 YR (*Continued*)

[a]**HepB vaccine.**

- Administer the 3-dose series to children not previously vaccinated.
- A 2-dose series (with doses separated by at least 4 mo) of adult formulation Recombivax HB® can be used in children aged 11–15 yr.

[b]**RV vaccines (RV-1 [Rotarix®] and RV-5 [RotaTeq®]).**

- The maximum age is 14 wk 6 days for the first dose in the series and 8 mo 0 days for the final dose in the series. Vaccination should not be initiated for infants aged ≥ 15 wk 0 days.
- If RV-1 was administered for the first and 2nd doses, a 3rd dose is not indicated.

[c]**Diphtheria and tetanus toxoids and acellular pertussis (DTaP) vaccine.**

- The 5th dose is not necessary if the 4th dose was administered at age ≥ 4 yr.

[d]**Type b (Hib) conjugate vaccine.**

- One dose of Hib vaccine should be administered to unvaccinated or partially vaccinated children aged ≥ 5 yr who have sickle cell disease, leukemia, HIV infection, anatomic or functional asplenia, or another immunocompromising condition.
- If the first 2 doses were PRP-OMP (PedvaxHIB® or ComVax® [HepB-Hib]) and were administered at age ≤ 11 mo, the 3rd (and final) dose should be administered at age 12–15 mo and at least 8 wk after the 2nd dose.
- If the first dose was administered at age 12–14 mo, administer the 2nd dose at least 8 wk after the first dose.
- If the first dose was administered at age 7–11 mo, administer the 2nd dose at least 4 wk later and a final dose at age 12–15 mo regardless of the Hib vaccine used for the first dose.
- Administer only 1 dose to unvaccinated children aged ≥ 15 mo.

[e]**Pneumococcal vaccines.** Minimum age is 6 wk for 13-valent pneumococcal conjugate vaccine (PCV13) and 2 yr for 23-valent pneumococcal polysaccharide vaccine (PPSV23).

- For children aged 24–71 mo with certain medical conditions, administer 1 dose of PCV if 3 doses were received previously, or administer 2 doses of PCV at least 8 wk apart if < 3 doses were received previously.
- A single dose of PCV may be administered to previously unvaccinated children aged 6–18 yr with certain medical conditions (see Tables 291–2 and 291–3 for details).
- Administer PPSV23 at least 8 wk after the last dose of PCV to children aged ≥ 2 yr with certain medical conditions. A single revaccination with PPSV23 should be administered after 5 yr to children with anatomic or functional asplenia or an immunocompromising condition. See *MMWR* 59 [RR-11], 2010.

[f]**Inactivated poliovirus vaccine (IPV).**

- A 4th dose is not necessary if the 3rd dose was administered at age ≥ 4 yr and at least 6 mo after the previous dose.
- A ≥ 4 doses are administered before age 4 yr, an additional dose should be administered at age 4–6 yr.
- In the first 6 mo of life, minimum age and minimum intervals are recommended only if the infant is at risk of imminent exposure to circulating poliovirus (eg, traveling to a polio-endemic region, during an outbreak).
- IPV is not routinely recommended for US residents age ≥ 18 yr.
- If both oral polio vaccine (OPV) and IPV were administered as part of a series, a total of 4 doses should be administered regardless of the child's current age. If only OPC was administered and all the doses were given before age 4 yr, one dose of IPV should be given at age ≥ 4 yr and at least 4 wk after the last OPV dose.

[g]**Meningococcal conjugate vaccine, quadrivalent (MCV4).** Minimum age is 6 wk for Hib-MenCY (for *H. influenzae* type b and *Neisseria meningitidis* serogroups C and Y), 9 mo for MCV4-D (Menactra®), and 2 yr for MCV4-CRM (Menveo®).

- Administer MCV4 vaccine at age 13–18 yr to unvaccinated children.
- If the first dose is administered at age 13–15 yr, a booster dose is administered at age 16–18 yr at least 8 wk after the first dose. If the first dose is administered at age ≥ 16 yr, a booster dose is not needed.
- For further guidance, see Table 291–2 and 291–3.

[h]**Measles, mumps, and rubella (MMR) vaccine.**

- Administer the 2nd dose routinely at age 4–6 yr.
- Make sure all school-aged children and adolescents have had 2 doses of MMR vaccine. The minimal interval between doses is 4 wk.

[i]**VAR vaccine.**

- Administer the 2nd dose routinely at age 4–6 yr. If the 2nd dose was administered at least 4 wk after the first dose, it can be accepted as valid.
- For people aged 7–18 yr without evidence of immunity (see Prevention of Varicella. *MMWR* 56 [RR-4], 2007), administer 2 doses if they were not previously vaccinated or the 2nd dose if only 1 dose has been administered.
- For children aged 7–12 yr, the recommended minimum interval between doses is 3 mo. However, if the 2nd dose was administered at least 4 wk after the first dose, it can be accepted as valid. For people aged ≥ 13 yr, the minimum interval between doses is 4 wk.

[j]**HepA vaccine.**

- For people ≥ 2 yr who have not received the HepA vaccine series, administer 2 doses separated by 6–18 mo if immunity against HepA is desired for them.

Table continues on the following page.

Table 291–4. CATCH-UP IMMUNIZATION SCHEDULE FOR AGES 4 MO–18 YR (*Continued*)

[k]**Tetanus and diphtheria toxoids (Td) and tetanus and diphtheria toxoids and acellular pertussis (Tdap) vaccines.**

- People aged 11–18 yr who have not received Tdap vaccine should receive a dose followed by tetanus and diphtheria toxoids (Td) booster doses every 10 yr thereafter.
- Children aged 7–10 yr who are not fully immunized with the childhood DTaP vaccine series, should receive Tdap vaccine as the first dose in the catch-up series; if additional doses are needed, use Td vaccine. An adolescent Tdap vaccine dose should not be given to these children.
- An inadvertent dose of DTaP vaccine administered to children aged 7–10 yr can count as part of the catch-up series. This dose can count as the adolescent Tdap dose, or the child can later receive a Tdap booster dose at age 11–12 yr.
- An inadvertent dose of DTaP vaccine administered to adolescents aged 11–18 yr should be counted as the adolescent Tdap dose.

[l]**HPV vaccines (HPV4 [Gardasil®] and HPV2 [Cervarix®]).**

- Administer the vaccine series to previously unvaccinated females (either HPV2 or HPV4) and males (HPV4) at age 13–18 yr.
- Use recommended routine dosing intervals for vaccine series catch-up (see Table 291–3).

MMWR = Morbidity and Mortality Weekly Review.
Adapted from the Centers for Disease Control and Prevention: Recommended Immunization Schedule for Persons Aged 0 Through 18 Years, United States—2016.

292 Behavioral Concerns and Problems in Children

Many behaviors exhibited by children or adolescents concern parents or other adults. Behaviors or behavioral patterns become clinically significant if they are frequent or persistent and maladaptive (eg, interfere with emotional maturation or social and cognitive functioning). Severe behavioral problems may be classified as mental disorders (eg, oppositional defiant disorder [see p. 2720], conduct disorder [see p. 2716]). Prevalence rates vary according to how behavioral problems are defined and measured.

Evaluation

Diagnosis consists of a multistep behavioral assessment. Concerns with infants and young children often involve bodily functions (eg, eating, eliminating, sleeping), whereas in older children and adolescents interpersonal behavioral concerns (eg, activity level, disobedience, aggression) predominate.

Problem identification: A behavioral problem may manifest alarmingly and abruptly as a single incident (eg, setting a fire, fighting at school). More often, problems manifest gradually, and identification involves gathering information over time. Behavior is best assessed in the context of the child's

- Physical and mental development
- General health
- Temperament (eg, difficult, easygoing)
- Relationships with parents and caregivers

Direct observation of parent-child interaction during an office visit provides valuable clues, including parental response to behaviors. These observations are supplemented, whenever possible, by information from others, including relatives, teachers, and school nurses.

Interviewing parents or caregivers provides a chronology of the child's activities during a typical day. Parents are asked to provide examples of events that precede and follow the specific behavior. Parents also are asked for their interpretation of

- Typical age-related behaviors
- Expectations for the child
- Their parenting style
- Support (eg, social, emotional, financial) for fulfilling their parenting role
- The child's relationship with the rest of the family

Problem interpretation: The child's history may include factors thought to increase the likelihood of developing behavioral problems, such as exposure to toxins, complications during pregnancy, or occurrence of a serious illness or death in the family.

Some problems may involve the parent-child relationship and can be interpreted in a number of ways:

- Unrealistic parental expectations: For example, some parents may expect that a 2-yr-old will pick up toys without help. Parents may misinterpret other normal, age-related behaviors, such as oppositional behavior (eg, refusal of a 2-yr old to follow an adult's request or rule) as problematic.
- Poor quality of parent-child interactions: For example, children of less attentive parents may have behavioral problems.
- Over-indulgent parenting: Well-meaning parental reactions to a problem may worsen it (eg, overprotecting a fearful, clinging child, giving in to a manipulative child).
- Circular behavioral pattern: In young children, some problems represent a circular behavioral pattern in which negative parental reaction to a child's behavior causes an adverse response from the child, which in turn leads to continued negative parental reaction. In this pattern, children often respond to stress and emotional discomfort with stubbornness, back talk, aggressiveness, and temper outbursts rather than with crying. Most commonly, a parent reacts to an aggressive and resistant child by scolding, yelling, and spanking; the child then escalates the behaviors that led to the parent's initial response, and the parent reacts more forcefully.

In older children and adolescents, behavioral problems may arise as independence is sought from parental rules and supervision. Such problems must be distinguished from occasional errors in judgment.

Treatment

Once a behavioral problem has been identified and its etiology has been investigated, early intervention is desirable because behaviors are more difficult to change the longer they exist.

The clinician reassures parents that the child is physically well (ie, that the child's misbehavior is not a manifestation of physical illness). By identifying with parental frustrations and pointing out the prevalence of behavioral problems, the clinician often can allay parental guilt and facilitate exploration of possible sources and treatment of problems. For simple problems, parental education, reassurance, and a few specific suggestions often are sufficient. Parents should be reminded of the importance of spending at least 15 to 20 min/day in a pleasurable activity with the child and to calling attention to desirable behaviors when the child exhibits them ("catching the child being good"). Parents also can be encouraged to regularly spend time away from the child.

For some problems, however, parents benefit from additional strategies for disciplining children and modifying behavior.

- Parents can limit the child's dependency-seeking and manipulative behavior so that mutual respect is reestablished.
- Desired and undesired behavior should be clearly defined.
- Consistent rules and limits should be established.
- Parents need to track compliance on an ongoing basis and provide appropriate rewards for success and consequences for inappropriate behavior.
- Parents should try to minimize anger when enforcing rules and increase positive contact with the child.

PEARLS & PITFALLS

- Positive reinforcement for appropriate behavior is a powerful tool with no adverse effects.

Helping parents to understand that "discipline" implies structure and not just punishment allows them to provide the structure and clear expectations that children need. Ineffective discipline may result in inappropriate behavior. Scolding or physical punishment may briefly control a child's behavior but eventually may decrease the child's sense of security and self-esteem. Threats to leave or send the child away are damaging.

A time-out technique (see Table 292–1), in which the child must sit alone in a dull place (a corner or room [other than the child's bedroom] that is not dark or scary and has no television or toys) for a brief period, is a good approach to altering unacceptable behavior. Time-outs are learning processes for the child and are best used for one inappropriate behavior or a few at one time. Physical restraint should be avoided. For children who escalate in the intensity of their reactions when put in time-out, parents may prefer to move more rapidly to redirection once they recognize the children have registered the reprimand for inappropriate behavior.

The circular behavioral pattern may be interrupted if parents ignore behavior that does not disturb others (eg, refusal to eat) and use distraction or temporary isolation to limit behavior that cannot be ignored (public tantrums).

A behavioral problem that does not change in 3 to 4 mo should be reevaluated; mental health consultation may be indicated.

BREATH-HOLDING SPELLS

A breath-holding spell is an episode in which the child stops breathing involuntarily and loses consciousness for a short period immediately after a frightening or emotionally upsetting event or after a painful experience.

Breath-holding spells occur in 5% of otherwise healthy children. They usually begin in the first year of life and peak at age 2. They disappear by age 4 in 50% of children and by age 8 in about 83% of children. The remainder may continue to have spells into adulthood. Breath-holding spells do not appear to be risk factors for true epilepsy but may be associated with an increased risk of fainting spells in adulthood. There are 2 forms of breath-holding spells:

- **Cyanotic form:** This form is the most common and often occurs as part of a temper tantrum or in response to a scolding or other upsetting event.
- **Pallid form:** This form typically follows a painful experience, such as falling and banging the head, but can follow frightening or startling events.

Both forms are involuntary and readily distinguished from uncommon brief periods of voluntary breath-holding by stubborn children, who invariably resume normal breathing after getting what they want or after becoming uncomfortable when they fail to get what they want.

During a **cyanotic breath-holding spell,** children hold their breath (without necessarily being aware they are doing so) until they lose consciousness. Typically, the child cries out, exhales, and stops breathing. Shortly afterward, the child begins to turn blue and unconsciousness ensues. A brief seizure may occur. After a few seconds, breathing resumes and normal skin color and consciousness return. It may be possible to interrupt a spell by placing a cold rag on the child's face at onset. Despite the

Table 292–1. TIME-OUT TECHNIQUE

This disciplinary technique is best used when children are aware that their actions are incorrect or unacceptable and when they perceive withholding of attention as a punishment; typically this is not the case until age 2 yr. Care should be taken when this technique is used in group settings like day care because it can result in harmful humiliation.

The technique can be applied when a child misbehaves in a way that is known to result in a time-out. Usually, verbal reprimands and reminders should precede the time-out.

- The misbehavior is explained to the child, who is told to sit in the time-out chair or is led there if necessary.
- The child should sit in the chair 1 min for each year of age (maximum, 5 min).
- A child who gets up from the chair before the allotted time is returned to the chair, and the time-out is restarted. Talking and eye contact are avoided.
- When it is time for the child to get up, the caregiver asks the reason for the time-out without anger and nagging. A child who does not recall the correct reason is briefly reminded. The child does not need to express remorse for the inappropriate behavior as long as it is clear that the child understands the reason for the time-out.

As soon as possible after the time-out, the caregiver should praise the child's good behavior, which may be easier to achieve if the child is redirected to a new activity far from the scene of the inappropriate behavior.

spell's frightening nature, parents must try to avoid reinforcing the initiating behavior. As the child recovers, parents should continue to enforce household rules. Distracting the child and avoiding situations that lead to tantrums are good strategies. Cyanotic breath-holding has been found to respond to iron therapy, even in the absence of anemia, and to treatment for obstructive sleep apnea (when present).

During a **pallid breath-holding spell,** vagal stimulation severely slows the heart rate. The child stops breathing, rapidly loses consciousness, and becomes pale and limp. If the spell lasts more than a few seconds, muscle tone increases, and a seizure and incontinence may occur. After the spell, the heart speeds up again, breathing restarts, and consciousness returns without any treatment. Because this form is rare, further diagnostic evaluation and treatment may be needed if the spells occur often. Simultaneous ECG and EEG can help to differentiate cardiac and neurologic causes.

EATING PROBLEMS

Eating problems range from age-appropriate variability in appetite to serious or even life-threatening eating disorders (see p. 1753) such as anorexia nervosa, bulimia nervosa, and binge eating. Eating problems also can result in overeating and obesity (see p. 19). Parents of young children are often concerned that a child is not eating enough or eating too much, eating the wrong foods, refusing to eat certain foods, or engaging in inappropriate mealtime behavior (eg, sneaking food to a pet, throwing or intentionally dropping food).

Assessment includes problem frequency, duration, and intensity. Height and weight are measured and plotted on appropriate charts. Often, when parents are shown charts that show the child is growing at a normal rate, their concerns about eating often diminish. Children should be assessed more thoroughly for serious eating disorders if

- They voice persistent concerns about their appearance or weight
- Their weight decreases
- Their weight begins to increase at a noticeably faster rate than their previous growth rate

However, most eating problems do not persist long enough to interfere with growth and development. If children appear well and growth is within an acceptable range, parents should be reassured and encouraged to minimize conflict and coercion related to eating. Prolonged and excessive parental concern may in fact contribute to subsequent eating disorders. Attempts to force-feed are unlikely to increase intake; children may hold food in their mouth or vomit. Parents should offer meals while sitting at a table with the family, without distractions such as television or pets, and show little emotion when putting the food in front of children. Food should be removed in 20 to 30 min without comment about what is or is not eaten. Children should participate in cleaning up any food that is thrown or intentionally dropped on the floor. These techniques, along with restricting between-meal eating to one morning and one afternoon snack, usually restore the relationship between appetite, the amount eaten, and children's nutritional needs.

SCHOOL AVOIDANCE

School avoidance occurs in about 5% of all school-aged children and affects girls and boys equally. It usually occurs between the ages of 5 and 11.

The cause is often unclear, but psychologic factors (eg, anxiety, depression) and social factors (eg, having no friends, feeling rejected by peers, being bullied) may contribute. If school avoidance behaviors escalate to the point at which a child is missing a lot of school, the behaviors may be an indication of more serious problems (see p. 2708). A sensitive child may be overreacting with fear to a teacher's strictness or rebukes. Changes in classroom staffing or curriculum can precipitate school resistance in children with special educational needs. Younger children tend to manifest somatic complaints (eg, stomachache, nausea) or make excuses to avoid school. Some children directly refuse to go to school. Alternatively, children may go to school without difficulty but become anxious or develop physical symptoms during the school day, often going regularly to the nurse's office. This behavior is unlike that of adolescents, who may decide not to attend school (truancy).

School avoidance tends to result from

- Poor academic performance
- Family difficulties
- Difficulties with peers

Most children recover from school avoidance, although some develop it again after a real illness or a vacation.

Home tutoring generally is not a solution. Children with school avoidance should return to school immediately, so that they do not fall behind in their schoolwork. If school avoidance is so intense that it interferes with the child's activity and if the child does not respond to simple reassurance by parents or teachers, referral to a mental health practitioner may be warranted.

Treatment should include communication between parents and school personnel, regular attendance at school, and sometimes therapy involving the family and child with a psychologist. Therapy includes treatment of underlying disorders as well as behavioral techniques to cope with the stresses at school.

SLEEP PROBLEMS

For most children, sleep problems are intermittent or temporary and often do not require treatment.

Normal sleep: Most children sleep for a stretch of at least 5 h by age 3 mo but then experience periods of night waking later in the first years of life, often associated with illness. With maturation, the amount of rapid eye movement (REM) sleep increases, with increasingly complex transitions between sleep stages. For most people, non-REM sleep predominates early in the night, with increasing REM as the night progresses. Thus, non-REM phenomena cluster early in the night, and REM-related phenomena occur later. Differentiating between true sleep (REM or non-REM)–related phenomena and awake behaviors can help to direct treatment.

It is important to determine whether parents view the child sleeping with them as a problem, because there is much cultural variation among sleep habits.

Nightmares: Nightmares are frightening dreams that occur during REM sleep. A child having a nightmare can awaken fully and vividly recall the details of the dream. Nightmares are not a cause for alarm, unless they occur very often. They can occur more often during times of stress or even when the child has seen a movie or television program containing frightening content. If nightmares occur often, parents can keep a diary to see whether they can identify the cause.

Night terrors and sleepwalking: Night terrors are non-REM episodes of incomplete awakening with extreme anxiety shortly after falling asleep; they are most common between the ages of 3 and 8. The child screams and appears frightened, with a rapid heart rate and rapid breathing. The child seems unaware of the parents' presence, may thrash around violently, and does not respond to comforting. The child may talk but is unable to answer questions. Usually, the child returns to sleep after a few minutes. Unlike with nightmares, the child cannot recall these episodes. Night terrors are dramatic because the child screams and is inconsolable during the episodes. About one third of children with night terrors also sleepwalk (the act of rising from bed and walking around while apparently asleep, also called somnambulism). About 15% of children between the ages of 5 and 12 have at least one episode of sleepwalking.

Night terrors and sleepwalking almost always stop on their own, although occasional episodes may occur for years. Usually, no treatment is needed, but if a disorder persists into adolescence or adulthood and is severe, treatment may be necessary. In children who need treatment, night terrors may sometimes respond to a sedative or certain antidepressants. There is some evidence that disrupted sleep associated with periodic leg movements often responds to iron supplementation, even in the absence of anemia. If children snore and thrash, evaluation for obstructive sleep apnea also should be considered.

Resistance to going to bed: Children, particularly between the ages of 1 and 2, often resist going to bed due to separation anxiety, whereas older children may be attempting to control more aspects of their environment. Young children often cry when left alone in bed, or they climb out and seek their parents. Another common cause of bedtime resistance is delayed sleep onset time. These situations arise when children are allowed to stay up later and sleep later than usual for enough nights to reset their internal clock to a later sleep onset time. It can be difficult to move bedtime earlier, but brief treatment with an OTC antihistamine or melatonin can help children reset their clock.

Resistance to going to bed is not helped if parents stay in the room at length to provide comfort or let children get out of bed. In fact, these responses reinforce night waking, in which children attempt to reproduce the conditions under which they fell asleep. To avoid these problems, a parent may have to sit quietly in the hallway in sight of the child and make sure the child stays in bed. The child then establishes a sleep-onset routine of falling asleep alone and learns that getting out of bed is discouraged. The child also learns that the parents are available but will not provide more stories or play. Eventually, the child settles down and goes to sleep. Providing the child with an attachment object (like a teddy bear) often is helpful. A small night-light, white noise, or both also can be comforting.

If the child is accustomed to falling asleep while in physical contact with a parent, the first step in establishing a different bedtime routine is to gradually lessen the contact from full body to a hand touching the child to a parent sitting next to the child's bed. Once the child is regularly falling asleep with a parent next to the bed, the parent can leave the room for increasing durations.

Awakening during the night: Everyone awakens multiple times each night. Most people, however, usually fall back to sleep with no intervention. Children often experience repeated night awakening after a move, an illness, or another stressful event. Sleeping problems may be worsened when children take long naps late in the afternoon or are overstimulated by playing before bedtime.

Allowing the child to sleep with the parents because of the night awakening reinforces the behavior. Also counterproductive are playing with or feeding the child during the night, spanking, and scolding. Returning the child to bed with simple reassurance is usually more effective. A bedtime routine that includes reading a brief story, offering a favorite doll or blanket, and using a small night-light (for children > 3) is often helpful. To prevent arousal, it is important that the conditions under which the child awakens during the night are the same as those under which the child falls asleep. Parents and other caregivers should try to keep to a routine each night, so that the child learns what is expected. If children are physically healthy, allowing them to cry for a few minutes often allows them to settle down by themselves, which diminishes the night awakening. Extended crying is counterproductive, however, because parents then may feel the need to revert to a routine of close contact. Gentle reassurance while keeping the child in bed is usually effective.

TEMPER TANTRUMS

A temper tantrum is a violent emotional outburst, usually in response to frustration.

Temper tantrums usually appear toward the end of the first year, are most common at age 2 (terrible twos) to 4, and are infrequent after age 5. If tantrums are frequent after age 5, they may persist throughout childhood.

Causes include frustration, tiredness, and hunger. Children also may have temper tantrums to seek attention, obtain something, or avoid doing something. Parents often blame themselves (because of imagined poor parenting) when the actual cause is often a combination of the child's personality, immediate circumstances, and developmentally normal behavior. An underlying mental, physical, or social problem rarely may be the cause but is likely only if tantrums last > 15 min or occur multiple times each day.

Temper tantrums may involve

- Shouting
- Screaming
- Crying
- Thrashing about
- Rolling on the floor
- Stomping
- Throwing things

The child may become red in the face and hit or kick. Some children may voluntarily hold their breath for a few seconds and then resume normal breathing (unlike breath-holding spells, which also can follow crying bouts caused by frustration—see p. 2473).

Although providing a safe setting for children to compose themselves (eg, a time-out—Table 292–1) is often effective, many children have difficulty stopping tantrums on their own. In most cases, addressing the source of the tantrum only prolongs it. It is therefore preferable to redirect the child by providing an alternative activity on which to focus. The child may benefit from being removed physically from the situation.

VIOLENCE IN CHILDREN AND ADOLESCENTS

Children and adolescents may engage in occasional physical confrontations, but most do not develop a sustained pattern of violent behavior or engage in violent crime. Children and adolescents who become violent before puberty may be at higher risk of committing crimes.

Violent behavior is increasingly common among children and adolescents. Up to one-third of children may be involved in bullying as bullies, victims, or both. Social stresses (eg, low family income, low parental education levels) are risk factors for bullying. In 2015, nearly 25% of male high school students in the US reported carrying a weapon at least once during the month before they were surveyed as part of a study on youth risks.

Despite ongoing interest in the possibility of a relationship between violent behavior and genetic defects or chromosomal anomalies, there is minimal evidence for such a relationship. However, several risk factors have been associated with violent behavior, including

- Intense corporal punishment
- Alcohol and drug abuse
- Gang involvement
- Developmental issues
- Poverty
- Access to firearms

There seems to be a relationship between violence and access to firearms, exposure to violence through media, and exposure to child abuse and domestic violence. Children who are bullied may reach a breaking point, at which time they strike back with potentially dangerous or catastrophic results.

Bullying: Bullying is intentional infliction of psychologic or physical damage on less powerful children. Bullying can take several forms, including

- Persistent teasing
- Threats
- Intimidation
- Harassment
- Violent assaults
- Cyber-bullying (use of e-mail, texting, social media, and other digital communication tools to convey threats and/or spread hurtful information)

Bullies act to inflate their sense of self-worth. Bullies often report that bullying creates feelings of power and control. Both bullies and their victims are at risk of poor outcomes. Victims often tell no one about being bullied because of feelings of helplessness and shame and fear of retaliation. Victims are at risk of physical injury, poor self-esteem, anxiety, depression, and school absence. Many victims of bullying become bullies themselves. Bullies are more likely to be incarcerated in later life; they are less likely to remain in school, be employed, or have stable relationships as adults.

Gang involvement: Participation in gangs has been linked with violent behavior. Youth gangs are self-formed associations of ≥ 3 members, typically ages 13 to 24. Gangs usually adopt a name and identifying symbols, such as a particular style of clothing, the use of certain hand signs, tattoos, or graffiti. Some gangs require prospective members to perform random acts of violence before membership is granted. Increasing youth gang violence has been blamed at least in part on gang involvement in drug distribution and drug use, particularly methamphetamines and heroin. Use of firearms is a frequent feature of gang violence.

Prevention

Violence prevention should begin in early childhood. Strategies include

- Violence-free discipline in young children
- Limiting access to weapons and exposure to violence through media and video games
- Creating and maintaining a safe school environment for school-age children
- Encouraging victims to discuss problems with parents, school authorities, and their doctor
- Teaching older children and adolescents strategies for avoiding high-risk situations (eg, places or settings where others have weapons or are using alcohol or drugs) and for reacting to or defusing tense situations

293 Bone Disorders in Children

CONGENITAL HYPOPHOSPHATASIA

Congenital hypophosphatasia is absence or low levels of serum alkaline phosphatase due to mutations in the gene encoding tissue nonspecific alkaline phosphatase (TNSALP).

Because serum alkaline phosphatase is absent or decreased, calcium is not diffusely deposited in bones, causing low bone density and hypercalcemia. Alkaline phosphatase deficiency also causes intracellular pyridoxine deficiency (vitamin B6 deficiency), which can cause generalized seizures. Vomiting, inability to gain weight, and enlargement of the epiphyses (similar to that in rickets) usually occur. Patients who survive infancy have bony deformities and short stature, but mental development is normal.

Until recently, no treatment was effective, but in 2015, asfotase alfa (a recombinant protein carrying the catalytic domain of tissue nonspecific alkaline phosphatase) subcutaneous injection was approved for treatment of congenital hypophosphatasia. Vitamin B6 in high doses may reduce seizures; 50 to 100 mg IV is given once for an active seizure, followed by 50 to 100 mg po once/day. NSAIDs reduce bone pain. Infusions of alkaline phosphatase and bone marrow transplantation have limited roles.

IDIOPATHIC SCOLIOSIS

Idiopathic scoliosis is lateral curvature of the spine.

Idiopathic scoliosis is the most common form of scoliosis and is present in 2 to 4% of children aged 10 to 16 yr. Boys and girls are equally affected; however, it is 10 times more likely to progress and require treatment in girls.

Genetic factors contribute about one third of the risk of disease development. Mutations in the *CHD7* and *MATN1* genes have been implicated in some cases.

Symptoms and Signs

Scoliosis may first be suspected when one shoulder seems higher than the other or when clothes do not hang straight, but it is often detected during routine physical examination. Other findings include apparent leg-length discrepancy and asymmetry of the chest wall. Patients may initially report fatigue in the lumbar region after prolonged sitting or standing. Muscular backaches in areas of strain (eg, in the lumbosacral angle) may follow.

Diagnosis

- X-ray of the spine

The curve is most pronounced when patients bend forward. Most curves are convex to the right in the thoracic area and to the left in the lumbar area, so that the right shoulder is higher than the left. X-ray examination should include standing anteroposterior and lateral views of the spine.

The greater the curve, the greater the likelihood that it will progress after the skeleton matures. Curves > 10° are considered significant. Prognosis depends on site and severity of the curve and age at symptom onset. Significant intervention is required in < 10% of patients.

Treatment

- Physical therapy and bracing
- Sometimes surgery

Prompt referral to an orthopedist is indicated when progression is of concern or the curve is significant. Likelihood of progression is greatest around puberty. Moderate curves (20 to 40°) are treated conservatively (eg, physical therapy and bracing) to prevent further deformity.

Severe curves (> 40°) may be ameliorated surgically (eg, spinal fusion with rod placement).

Scoliosis and its treatment often interfere with an adolescent's self-image and self-esteem. Counseling or psychotherapy may be needed.

OVERVIEW OF OSTEOCHONDROSES

Osteochondroses are noninflammatory, noninfectious derangements of bony growth at various ossification centers. These derangements occur during the period of greatest developmental activity and affect the epiphyses.

Etiology of osteochondroses is typically unknown; some of the disorders have a familial component, but inheritance is complex. Osteochondroses differ in their anatomic distribution, course, and prognosis; they typically cause pain and have important orthopedic implications. Common examples include

- Köhler bone disease
- Legg-Calvé-Perthes disease
- Osgood-Schlatter disease
- Scheuermann disease

Rare osteochondroses and the involved bones include Freiberg disease (head of 2nd metatarsal), Panner disease (capitulum), and Blount disease (proximal tibia). Sever disease (calcaneal apophysitis) is a more common osteochondrosis.

KÖHLER BONE DISEASE

Köhler bone disease is osteochondrosis of the tarsal navicular bone.

Osteochondroses are noninflammatory, noninfectious derangements of bony growth at various ossification centers.

Köhler bone disease usually affects children aged 3 to 5 yr (more commonly boys) and is unilateral. The foot becomes swollen and painful; tenderness is maximal over the medial longitudinal arch. Weight bearing and walking increase discomfort, and gait is disturbed.

On x-ray, the navicular bone is initially flattened and sclerotic and later becomes fragmented, before reossification. X-rays comparing the affected side with the unaffected side help assess progression.

The course is chronic, but the disease rarely persists ≥ 2 yr. Rest, pain relief, and avoiding excessive weight bearing are required. The condition usually resolves spontaneously with no long-term sequelae. In acute cases, a few weeks of wearing a below-knee walking plaster cast, well molded under the longitudinal arch, may help.

LEGG-CALVÉ-PERTHES DISEASE

Legg-Calvé-Perthes disease is an osteochondrosis that involves idiopathic aseptic necrosis of the femoral capital epiphysis.

Legg-Calvé-Perthes disease has a maximum incidence at age 5 to 10 yr, is more common among boys, and is usually unilateral. About 10% of cases are familial, but contributing gene defects have not been identified.

Characteristic symptoms of Legg-Calvé-Perthes disease are pain in the hip joint and gait disturbance (eg, limping); some children complain of pain in the knee. Onset is gradual, and progression is slow. Joint movements are limited, and thigh muscles may become wasted.

Diagnosis

- X-rays
- Usually MRI

Diagnosis of Legg-Calvé-Perthes disease is suspected based on symptoms. X-rays are usually obtained and, if needed, an MRI is done to confirm the diagnosis and extent of the lesion. X-rays initially may not be diagnostic, because they can be normal or show minimal flattening. Later x-rays can show fragmentation of the femoral head, which contains areas of lucency and sclerosis.

In bilateral or familial cases, an x-ray skeletal survey to exclude hereditary skeletal disorders, particularly multiple epiphyseal dysplasia, is mandatory because prognosis and optimal management differ. Hypothyroidism, sickle cell anemia, and trauma must also be excluded.

Treatment

- Rest and immobilization
- Sometimes surgery

Orthopedic treatment of Legg-Calvé-Perthes disease includes prolonged bed rest, mobile traction, slings, and abduction plaster casts and splints to contain the femoral head. Some experts advocate subtrochanteric osteotomy with internal fixation and early ambulation. Bisphosphonates have been effective in initial trials, but further studies are needed.

Without treatment, the course is usually prolonged but self-limited (usually 2 to 3 yr). When the disease eventually becomes quiescent, residual distortion of the femoral head and acetabulum predisposes to secondary degenerative osteoarthritis. With treatment, sequelae are less severe. Young children and children with less femoral head destruction when diagnosed have the best outcome.

OSGOOD-SCHLATTER DISEASE

Osgood-Schlatter disease is osteochondrosis of the tibial tubercle.

Osgood-Schlatter disease occurs between ages 10 yr and 15 yr and is usually unilateral. Although the disease is more common among boys, this status is changing as girls become more active in sports programs.

Etiology of Osgood-Schlatter disease is thought to be trauma due to excessive traction by the patellar tendon on its immature epiphyseal insertion, leading to microavulsion fractures.

Characteristic symptoms of Osgood-Schlatter disease are pain, swelling, and tenderness over the tibial tubercle at the patellar tendon insertion. There is no systemic disturbance.

Diagnosis

- Clinical evaluation
- Sometimes x-rays

Diagnosis of Osgood-Schlatter disease is by characteristic findings isolated over the tibial tubercle on examination.

Lateral knee x-rays may show fragmentation of the tibial tubercle. However, x-rays are not needed unless other disorders (eg, injury, joint inflammation) are suggested by pain and swelling extending beyond the area over the tibial tubercle or pain is accompanied by redness and warmth.

Treatment

- Analgesics
- Rest
- Rarely immobilization, corticosteroid injection, and surgery

Resolution is usually spontaneous within weeks or months. Usually, taking analgesics and avoiding excessive exercise, especially deep knee bending, are the only necessary measures. Complete avoidance of sports is unnecessary.

Rarely, immobilization in plaster, intralesional injection of hydrocortisone, surgical removal of loose bodies (eg, ossicles, avulsed fragments of bone), drilling, and grafting are required.

SCHEUERMANN DISEASE

Scheuermann disease is an osteochondrosis that causes localized changes in vertebral bodies, leading to backache and kyphosis.

Scheuermann disease manifests in adolescence and is slightly more common among boys. It probably represents a group of diseases with similar symptoms, but etiology and pathogenesis are uncertain. It may result from osteochondritis of the upper and lower cartilaginous vertebral end plates or trauma. Some cases are familial.

Most patients present with a round-shouldered posture and they may have persistent low-grade backache. Some have an appearance similar to people with Marfan syndrome; trunk and limb length are disproportionate. Normal thoracic kyphosis is increased diffusely or locally.

Diagnosis

- X-rays

Some cases are recognized during routine screening for spinal deformity at school. Lateral spinal x-rays confirm the diagnosis of Scheuermann disease by showing anterior wedging of ≥ 5° of 3 or more consecutive vertebral bodies, usually in the lower thoracic and upper lumbar regions. Later, the end plates become irregular and sclerotic. Spinal misalignment is predominantly kyphotic but is sometimes partly scoliotic. In atypical cases, generalized skeletal dysplasia must be excluded by x-ray skeletal survey, and, if suspected on clinical grounds, spinal TB must be excluded by CT or MRI.

Treatment

- Reducing weight-bearing, strenuous activity, or both
- Rarely spinal brace or surgery

The course is mild but long, often lasting several years (although duration varies greatly). Trivial spinal misalignment often persists after the disorder has become quiescent.

Mild, nonprogressive disease can be treated by reducing weight-bearing stress and by avoiding strenuous activity. Occasionally, when kyphosis is more severe, a spinal brace or rest with recumbency on a rigid bed is indicated. Rarely, progressive cases require surgical stabilization and correction of misalignment.

OVERVIEW OF OSTEOPETROSES

(Marble Bones)

Osteopetroses are familial disorders characterized by increased bone density and skeletal modeling abnormalities.

Osteopetroses can be categorized based on whether sclerosis or defective skeletal modeling predominates. There are a number of different types, including

- Craniotubular dysplasias
- Craniotubular hyperostoses
- Osteosclerosis

They are all familial but have different inheritance patterns. Some types are comparatively benign; others are progressive and fatal.

Bony overgrowth sometimes severely distorts the face. Malocclusion of the teeth may require specialized orthodontic measures. Plain x-rays typically are diagnostic.

Surgical decompression may be required to relieve elevated intracranial pressure or to release a trapped facial or auditory nerve.

CRANIOTUBULAR DYSPLASIAS

Craniotubular dysplasias are osteopetroses that involve minor osteosclerosis with normal skeletal modeling.

Osteopetroses are familial disorders characterized by increased bone density and abnormal skeletal modeling.

Craniometaphyseal dysplasia: This autosomal dominant disorder is caused by mutations in the *ANKH* gene. Paranasal bossing develops during infancy, and progressive expansion and thickening of the skull and mandible distort the jaw and face. The encroaching bone entraps cranial nerves, causing dysfunction. Malocclusion of the teeth may be troublesome; partial sinus obliteration predisposes to recurrent nasorespiratory infection. Height and general health are normal, but progressive elevation of intracranial pressure is a rare, serious complication.

Diagnosis of craniometaphyseal dysplasia is suspected by typical craniofacial abnormalities, which are at times coupled with increased susceptibility to URI, or the disorder may be found during an evaluation for cranial nerve dysfunction that may result from entrapment at the skull base. Typically, plain x-rays are done. X-ray changes are age-related and usually evident by age 5 yr. Sclerosis is the main feature in the skull. Long bones have widened metaphyses, appearing club-shaped, particularly at the distal femur. However, these changes are much less severe than those in Pyle disease. The spine and pelvis are unaffected.

Treatment of craniometaphyseal dysplasia consists of surgical decompression of entrapped nerves and remodeling of severe bony abnormalities; however, regrowth does occur.

Frontometaphyseal dysplasia: This disorder has distinct autosomal dominant and X-linked forms and is caused by mutations in the *FLNA* and *MAP3K7* genes; however, these mutations are not present in all cases.

The disorder becomes evident during early childhood. The supraorbital ridge is prominent, resembling a knight's visor. The mandible is hypoplastic with anterior constriction; dental anomalies are common. Deafness develops during adulthood because sclerosis narrows the internal acoustic foramina and middle ear or may cause deformities of the ossicles. Long leg bones are moderately bowed. Progressive contractures in the digits may simulate arthritis. Height and general health are normal.

Diagnosis of frontometaphyseal dysplasia is suspected by hearing loss in a patient with features of the skeletal abnormalities described previously. Typically, plain x-rays are done. On x-ray examination, bony overgrowth of the frontal region is obvious; patchy sclerosis is seen in the cranial vault. Vertebral bodies are dysplastic but not sclerotic. Iliac crests are abruptly flared, and pelvic inlet is distorted. Femoral capital epiphyses are flattened, with expansion of the femoral heads and coxa valga (hip deformity). Finger bones are undermodeled, with erosion and loss of joint space.

Corrective surgery is indicated for severely disfiguring deformities, including severe micrognathia, or those causing orthopedic problems. Hearing loss is treated with hearing aids.

Metaphyseal dysplasia (Pyle disease): This rare, autosomal recessive disorder is often confused semantically with craniometaphyseal dysplasia. Affected people are clinically normal, apart from genu valgum, although scoliosis and bone fragility occasionally occur.

The diagnosis of metaphyseal dysplasia is usually made when x-rays are done for an unrelated reason. X-ray changes are striking. Long bones are undermodeled, and bony cortices are generally thin. Tubular leg bones have gross Erlenmeyer flask flaring, particularly in the distal femur. Pelvic bones and thoracic cage are expanded. However, the skull is essentially spared.

Treatment of metaphyseal dysplasia is often not necessary but may involve orthodontic treatments for dental malformations or orthopedic surgery for clinically significant skeletal deformities.

CRANIOTUBULAR HYPEROSTOSES

Craniotubular hyperostoses are osteopetroses that involve bony overgrowths that alter contour and increase skeletal density.

Diaphyseal dysplasia (Camurati-Engelmann disease): This autosomal dominant disorder is caused by mutations in the *TGFB1* gene. It manifests during mid-childhood with muscular pain, weakness, and wasting, typically in the legs. These symptoms usually resolve by age 30. Hyperostoses affect the long bones and skull. Cranial nerve compression and elevated intracranial pressure occur occasionally. Some patients are severely handicapped; others are virtually asymptomatic.

Diagnosis of diaphyseal dysplasia is suspected by the combination of muscular deficits and hyperostoses of the long bones and skull. Typically, plain x-rays are done. The predominant x-ray feature is marked thickening of the periosteal and medullary surfaces of the diaphyseal cortices of the long bones, but findings vary. Medullary canals and external bone contours are irregular. The extremities and axial skeleton usually are spared. Rarely, the skull is involved, with calvarial widening and basal sclerosis.

Corticosteroids may help relieve bone pain and improve muscle strength.

Endosteal hyperostosis (van Buchem syndrome): This disorder is usually autosomal recessive. Overgrowth and distortion of the mandible and brow become evident during mid-childhood. Subsequently, cranial nerves become entrapped, leading to facial palsy and deafness. Life span is not compromised, stature is normal, and bones are not fragile. X-rays show widening and sclerosis of the calvaria, cranial base, and mandible. Diaphyseal endosteum in the tubular bones is thickened.

Surgical decompression of entrapped nerves may be helpful.

Sclerosteosis: This autosomal recessive disorder is caused by a mutation in the *SOST* gene, which codes for the protein sclerostin. Sclerosteosis is most common among Afrikaners of South Africa. Overgrowth and sclerosis of the skeleton, particularly of the skull, develop during early childhood. Height and weight are often excessive. Initial symptoms and signs may include deafness and facial palsy due to cranial nerve entrapment. Distortion of facies, apparent by age 10 yr, eventually becomes severe. Cutaneous or bony syndactyly of the 2nd and 3rd fingers distinguishes sclerosteosis from other forms of craniotubular hyperostoses.

Diagnosis of sclerosteosis is suspected by characteristic skeletal abnormalities, particularly when the patient also has syndactyly. Typically, plain x-rays are done. Predominant x-ray features are gross widening and sclerosis of the calvaria and mandible. Vertebral bodies are spared, although their pedicles are dense. Pelvic bones are sclerotic but have normal contours. Long bones have sclerosed, hyperostotic cortices and undermodeled shafts. A diagnostic genetic test is available.

Surgery to relieve intracranial pressure or to decompress entrapped nerves may help.

OSTEOSCLEROSIS

Osteosclerosis is a type of osteopetrosis that involves abnormal hardening of bone that involves increased skeletal density with little disturbance of modeling; in some types, bony encroachment on the marrow cavity causes cytopenias.

Osteopetrosis with delayed manifestations (Albers-Schönberg disease): This type of osteopetrosis is autosomal dominant, benign, and delayed (tarda), manifesting during childhood, adolescence, or young adulthood. The defective *CLCN7* gene encodes a chloride channel that is apparently important in osteoclast function. This type is relatively common and has a wide geographic and ethnic distribution. Affected people may be asymptomatic; general health is usually unimpaired. However, facial palsy and deafness may occur due to cranial nerve entrapment. Bony overgrowths may narrow the marrow cavity and cause cytopenias ranging from anemia to pancytopenia. Extramedullary hematopoiesis may occur, resulting in hepatosplenomegaly; consequent hypersplenism may worsen anemia.

The skeleton usually is radiologically normal at birth. However, bone sclerosis becomes increasingly apparent as children age, and diagnosis is typically based on x-rays done for unrelated reasons. Bony involvement is widespread but patchy. The calvaria is dense, and sinuses may be obliterated. Sclerosis of the vertebral end plate causes the characteristic rugby-shirt appearance (horizontal banding).

Some patients require transfusion or splenectomy to treat anemia.

Osteopetrosis with precocious manifestations: This type of osteopetrosis is autosomal recessive, malignant, and congenital, manifesting during infancy. It is uncommon, frequently lethal, and often due to a mutation in the osteoclast-associated gene *TCIRG1*. Bony overgrowth progressively obliterates the marrow cavity, causing severe pancytopenia. Initial symptoms include failure to thrive, spontaneous bruising, abnormal bleeding, and anemia. Palsies of the 2nd, 3rd, and 7th cranial nerves and hepatosplenomegaly occur later. Bone marrow failure (anemia, overwhelming infection, or hemorrhage) usually causes death in the first year of life.

Diagnosis of osteopetrosis with precocious manifestations is suspected by the presence of bony overgrowths in the context of anemia, unusual bleeding, and poor growth. Typically, plain x-rays are done, along with CBC and coagulation tests. General increased bone density is the predominant feature on x-ray. Penetrated x-rays of long bones show transverse bands in the metaphyseal regions and longitudinal striations in the shafts. As the disorder progresses, the ends of the long bones, particularly the proximal humerus and distal femur, become flask-shaped. Characteristic endobones (bone within a bone) form in the vertebrae, pelvis, and tubular bones. The skull becomes thickened, and the spine has a rugby-shirt appearance.

Bone marrow transplantation with HLA-identical sibling grafts has had excellent results. However, prognosis is poor with HLA-mismatched grafts. Prednisone, calcitriol, and interferon gamma are effective in some cases.

Osteopetrosis with renal tubular acidosis: This type of osteopetrosis is autosomal recessive. The genetic defect involves mutations of the gene encoding carbonic anhydrase II. It causes weakness, stunted stature, and failure to thrive.

Bones appear dense on x-rays, and cerebral calcifications are seen; renal tubular acidosis (RTA) is present, and RBC carbonic anhydrase activity is decreased.

Bone marrow transplantation cures the osteopetrosis but has no effect on the RTA. Maintenance therapy consists of bicarbonate and electrolyte supplementation to correct renal losses.

Pyknodysostosis: This autosomal recessive disorder is caused by loss of function mutations in the gene encoding cathepsin K, an osteoclast-derived protease important in degradation of extracellular bone matrix. Short stature becomes evident in early childhood; adult height is ≤ 150 cm (5 ft). Other manifestations include an enlarged skull, short and broad hands and feet, short sclerotic terminal phalanges, dystrophic nails, and retention of primary teeth. Blue sclerae (due to a deficiency in connective tissue allowing the underlying vessels to show through) are usually recognized during infancy. Affected people resemble each other closely; they have a small face, a receding chin, and carious, misplaced teeth. The cranium bulges, and the anterior fontanelle remains patent. Pathologic fractures are a complication.

Diagnosis of pyknodysostosis is suspected by the presence of blue sclerae, short stature, and characteristic skeletal features. Typically, plain x-rays are done. Bone sclerosis appears on x-rays during childhood, but neither bone striations nor endobones (bone within bone) are seen. Facial bones and paranasal sinuses are hypoplastic, and the mandibular angle is obtuse. Clavicles may be gracile, and their lateral portions may be underdeveloped; distal phalanges are rudimentary.

Plastic surgery has been used to correct severe deformities of the face and jaw.

SLIPPED CAPITAL FEMORAL EPIPHYSIS

Slipped capital femoral epiphysis (SCFE) is movement of the femoral neck upward and forward on the femoral epiphysis.

SCFE usually occurs in early adolescence and preferentially affects boys. Obesity is a significant risk factor. Genetic factors also contribute. SCFE is bilateral in one fifth of patients, and unilateral SCFE becomes bilateral in up to two thirds of patients. The exact cause is unknown but probably relates to weakening of the physis (growth plate), which can result from trauma, hormonal changes, inflammation, or increased shearing forces due to obesity.

Symptoms and Signs

Onset is usually insidious, and symptoms of SCFE are associated with stage of slippage. The first symptom SCFE may be hip stiffness that abates with rest; it is followed by a limp, then hip pain that radiates down the anteromedial thigh to the knee. Up to 15% of patients present with knee or thigh pain, and the true problem (hip) may be missed until slippage worsens. Early hip examination may detect neither pain nor limitation of movement.

In more advanced stages, findings may include pain during movement of the affected hip, with limited flexion, abduction, and medial rotation; knee pain without specific knee abnormalities; and a limp or Trendelenburg gait. The affected leg is externally rotated. If blood supply to the area is compromised, avascular necrosis and collapse of the epiphysis may occur.

Diagnosis

- Plain x-rays
- Sometimes MRI or ultrasonography

Because treatment of advanced slippage is difficult, early diagnosis of SCFE is vital. Anteroposterior and frog-leg lateral x-rays of both hips are taken. X-rays show widening of the epiphyseal line or apparent posterior and inferior displacement of the femoral head. Ultrasonography and MRI are also useful, especially if x-rays are normal.

Treatment

- Surgical repair

SCFE usually progresses; it requires surgery as soon as it is diagnosed. Patients should not bear weight on the affected leg until SCFE has been ruled out or treated. Surgical treatment consists of screw fixation through the physis.

294 Caring for Sick Children and Their Families

Illness and death cause emotional stresses in children and their families.

CARING FOR SICK NEONATES

Difficulties arise when a sick or premature infant must be taken away from the family after birth because of illness. The parents may not be able to see a critically ill infant during stabilization and may be separated from the infant because of transport to a different hospital. Some infants require prolonged separation from their families because of lengthy hospitalizations and treatments. Experts now recommend that neonatal transport teams encourage physical contact between parents and their sick infant before moving the infant to the specialty care center.

Many hospitals have recognized the importance of encouraging contact between infants and their families. In most places, parents are encouraged to visit, taking precautions to minimize the risk of spreading infections. Many hospitals have unlimited visiting hours for parents. Some hospitals have areas in which parents can stay for prolonged periods to be near their infant.

In most hospitals, parents are encouraged to interact with their sick infant as much as possible. *No infant, even one on a respirator, is too ill for the parents to see and touch.*

Parents are also encouraged to provide direct care for the infant as a way to get to know the infant and to prepare for taking the infant home. Some hospitals increase contact between parents and premature or sick infants by encouraging skin-to-skin contact; this may help parents feel more confident about taking care of their infant at home. Infants who experience skin-to-skin contact gain weight faster when compared with those who do not receive such care. Mothers can also provide breast milk directly or pumped to be given through a feeding tube.

When an infant has a birth defect, the parents should see the infant as soon after birth as possible, regardless of the medical condition. Otherwise, they may imagine the appearance and condition to be much worse than the reality. Intensive parental support is essential, with as many counseling sessions as are needed for parents to understand their infant's condition and recommended treatment and to accept the infant psychologically. To balance discussion of abnormalities, the physician should emphasize what is normal about the infant and the infant's potential.

When neonates die without having been seen or touched by their parents, the parents may later feel as though they never really had a child. Such parents have reported exaggerated feelings of emptiness and may develop prolonged depression because they could not mourn the loss of a "real" child. Parents who have not been able to see or hold their infant while alive will usually be helped in the long term if allowed to do so after the infant has died. In all cases, follow-up visits with the physician and a social worker are helpful to review the circumstances of the infant's illness and death, answer questions that often arise later, and assess and alleviate feelings of guilt. The physician can also evaluate the parents' grieving process and provide appropriate guidance or a referral for more extensive support if necessary.

CHILDREN WITH CHRONIC HEALTH CONDITIONS

Chronic health conditions (both chronic illnesses and chronic physical disabilities) are generally defined as those conditions that last > 12 mo and are severe enough to create some limitations in usual activity. It has been estimated that chronic health conditions affect 10 to 30% of children, depending on the criteria. Examples of chronic illnesses include asthma, cystic fibrosis, congenital heart disease, diabetes mellitus, attention-deficit/hyperactivity disorder, and depression. Examples of chronic physical disabilities include meningomyelocele, hearing or visual impairments, cerebral palsy, and loss of limb function.

Effects on the children: Children with chronic health conditions may have some activity limitations, frequent pain or discomfort, abnormal growth and development, and more hospitalizations, outpatient visits, and medical treatments. Children with severe disabilities may be unable at times to participate in school and peer activities.

Children's response to a chronic health condition largely depends on their developmental stage when the condition occurs. Children with chronic conditions that appear in infancy will respond differently than children who develop conditions during adolescence. School-aged children may be most affected by the inability to attend school and form relationships with peers. Adolescents may struggle with their inability to achieve independence if they require assistance from parents and others for many of their daily needs; parents should encourage self reliance within the adolescent's capability and avoid overprotection. Adolescents also find it particularly difficult to be viewed as different from their peers.

Health care practitioners can be advocates for appropriate hospital services for children with chronic health conditions. Age-appropriate playrooms can be set up and a school program can be initiated with the oversight of a trained child life specialist. Children can be encouraged to interact with peers whenever possible. All procedures and plans should be explained to families and children whenever possible so the families know what to expect during the hospitalization, thus relieving the anxiety that can be created by uncertainty.

Effects on the family: For families, having a child who has a chronic health condition can lead to loss of their hope for an "ideal" child, neglected siblings, major expense and time commitment, confusion caused by conflicting systems of health care management, lost opportunities (eg, family members providing primary care to the child are therefore unable to return to work), and social isolation. Siblings may resent the extra attention the ill child receives. Such stress may cause family breakup, especially when there are preexisting difficulties with family function.

Conditions that affect the physical appearance of an infant (eg, cleft lip and palate, hydrocephalus) can affect the bond between the infant and family members or caretakers. Once the diagnosis of abnormality is made, parents may react with shock, denial, anger, sadness or depression, guilt, and anxiety. These reactions may occur at any time in the child's development, and each parent may be at a different stage of acceptance, making communication between them difficult. Parents may express their anger at the health care practitioner, or their denial may cause them to seek many opinions about their child's condition.

Care coordination: Without coordination of services, care is crisis-oriented. Some services will be duplicated, whereas others will be neglected. Care coordination requires knowledge of the children's condition, their family and support systems, and the community in which they function.

All professionals who care for children with chronic health conditions must ensure that someone is coordinating care. Sometimes the coordinator can be the child's parent. However, the systems that must be negotiated are often so complex that even the most capable parents need assistance. Other possible coordinators include the primary care physician, the subspecialty program staff, the community health nurse, and staff of the 3rd-party payer. Regardless of who coordinates services, families and children must be partners in the process. In general, children from low-income families who have chronic conditions fare worse than others, in part because of lack of access to health care and care coordination services. Some children with terminal illness benefit from hospice care.

DEATH AND DYING IN CHILDREN

Families often have difficulty dealing with an ill and dying child. Children who are trying to make sense of the death of a friend or family member may have particular difficulty.

Death of a child: Most often the death of a child happens in the hospital or emergency department. Death can occur after a prolonged illness, such as cancer, or suddenly and unexpectedly, such as after an injury or sudden infant death. The death of a child can be difficult for families to comprehend and accept. For parents, the death of a child means that they must give up their dreams and hopes for their child. The grieving process may also mean that they are unable to attend to the needs of other family members, including other children. Health care practitioners can help in the process by being available to the family for consultation and to provide comfort whenever possible. In some circumstances, referral to specialists skilled in working with families who have experienced the death of a child is appropriate.

Some parents respond to the death of a child by quickly planning another pregnancy, perhaps in an attempt to create a "replacement" child. Health care providers who have a supportive relationship with the grieving parents should dissuade such a quick pregnancy. As parents embark on a subsequent pregnancy, anxiety and fear of another loss may make it difficult for them to form an attachment to the new child. A child who is born after another child has died is at risk of replacement child syndrome or vulnerable child syndrome. In replacement child syndrome, feelings and expectations for the "ideal" child who died are overlaid on feelings for the next child. In vulnerable child syndrome, because of their previous loss, parents mistakenly perceive the new child to be at risk of behavioral, developmental, or medical problems and think the child needs special care and protection from potential harm. Parents who are grieving the loss of a dead child and who are also struggling with an inability to attach to a new child need to know their feelings are normal. If their feelings are not acknowledged as normal, the parents and child are at risk of mental health disorders. The next pregnancy, when and if it occurs, should be forward-looking and not backward-looking.

Death of a family member or friend: Many children experience the death of a loved one. The way children perceive the event (and hence the best response by parents and health care practitioners) is affected by their developmental level. Preschool children may have limited understanding of death. Relating the event to previous experience with a beloved pet may be helpful. Older children may be able to understand the event more easily. Death should never be equated with going to sleep and never waking up because children may become fearful of sleeping.

Parents should discuss with health care practitioners whether to have children visit severely ill children or adults. Some children may express a specific desire to visit family members or friends who are dying. Children should be adequately prepared for such a visit so they will know what to expect. In the same way, adults often wonder whether to bring children to a funeral. This decision should be made individually, in consultation with the children whenever possible. When children attend a funeral, a close friend or relative should accompany them to provide support throughout, and children should be allowed to leave if necessary.

295 Child Maltreatment

(Child Abuse)

Child maltreatment is behavior toward a child that is outside the norms of conduct and entails substantial risk of causing physical or emotional harm. Four types of maltreatment are generally recognized: physical abuse, sexual abuse, emotional abuse (psychologic abuse), and neglect. The causes of child maltreatment are varied and not well understood. Abuse and neglect are often associated with physical injuries, delayed growth and development, and mental problems. Diagnosis is based on history, physical examination, and sometimes laboratory tests and diagnostic imaging. Management includes documentation and treatment of any injuries and urgent physical and mental conditions, mandatory reporting to appropriate state agencies, and sometimes hospitalization and/or foster care to keep the child safe.

In 2015, 4 million reports of alleged child maltreatment were made to Child Protective Services in the US involving 7.2 million children. About 2.2 million of these reports were investigated in detail and about 683,000 maltreated children were identified. Both sexes are affected equally; the younger the child, the higher the rate of victimization.

About three fifths of all reports to Child Protective Services were made by professionals who are mandated to report maltreatment (eg, educators, law enforcement personnel, social services personnel, legal professionals, day care providers, medical or mental health personnel, foster care providers).

Of substantiated cases in the US in 2015, 75.3% involved neglect (including medical neglect), 17.2% involved physical abuse, and 8.4% involved sexual abuse. In addition, 6.9% involved other types of maltreatment. Many children were victims of multiple types of maltreatment.

About 1670 children died in the US from maltreatment in 2015, about three quarters of whom were < 3 yr. Over 70% of these children were victims of neglect and about 44% were victims of physical abuse with or without other forms of maltreatment. Over 90% of perpetrators were parents acting alone or with another parent, and 26.7% of child abuse fatalities were perpetrated by the mother acting alone.

Classification

Different forms of maltreatment often coexist, and overlap is considerable.

Physical abuse: Physical abuse involves a caregiver inflicting physical harm or engaging in actions that create a high risk of harm. Specific forms include shaking, dropping, striking, biting, and burning (eg, by scalding or touching with cigarettes). Abuse is the most common cause of serious head injury in infants. In toddlers, abdominal injury is common.

Infants and toddlers are the most vulnerable because the developmental stages that they may go through (eg, colic, inconsistent sleep patterns, temper tantrums, toilet training) may frustrate caregivers. This age group is also at increased risk because they cannot report their abuse. The risk declines in the early school years and increases again in adolescence.

Sexual abuse: Any action with a child that is done for the sexual gratification of an adult or significantly older child constitutes sexual abuse (see p. 1802). Forms of sexual abuse include intercourse, which is oral, anal, or vaginal penetration; molestation, which is genital contact without intercourse; and forms that do not involve physical contact, including exposure of the perpetrator's genitals, showing sexually explicit material to a child, and forcing a child to participate in a sex act with another child or to participate in the production of sexual material.

Sexual abuse does not include sexual play, in which children close in age view or touch each other's genital area without force or coercion. The guidelines that determine sexual abuse from play vary from state to state, but in general a difference of > 4 yr (chronologically, or in mental or physical development) is considered to be abuse.

Emotional abuse: Emotional abuse is inflicting emotional harm through the use of words or actions. Specific forms include berating a child by yelling or screaming, spurning by belittling the child's abilities and achievements, intimidating and terrorizing with threats, and exploiting or corrupting by encouraging deviant or criminal behavior. Emotional abuse can also occur when words or actions are omitted or withheld, in essence becoming emotional neglect (eg, ignoring or rejecting children or isolating them from interaction with other children or adults).

Abuse in a medical setting: Child abuse in a medical setting (fictitious disorder imposed on another, previously called Munchausen syndrome by proxy—see p. 1804) occurs when caregivers intentionally produce or falsify physical or psychologic symptoms or signs in a child. Caregivers may injure the child with drugs or other agents or add blood or bacterial contaminants to urine specimens to simulate disease. Many children receive unnecessary and harmful or potentially harmful tests and treatments.

Neglect: Neglect is the failure to provide for or meet a child's basic physical, emotional, educational, and medical needs. Neglect differs from abuse in that it usually occurs without intent to harm. Physical neglect includes failure to provide adequate food, clothing, shelter, supervision, and protection from potential harm. Emotional neglect is failure to provide affection or love or other kinds of emotional support. Educational neglect is failure to enroll a child in school, ensure attendance at school, or provide home schooling. Medical neglect is failure to ensure that a child receives appropriate preventive care (eg, vaccinations, routine dental examinations) or needed treatment for injuries or physical or mental disorders.

Cultural factors: Severe corporal punishment (eg, whipping, burning, scalding) clearly constitutes physical abuse, but for lesser degrees of physical and emotional chastisement, the boundary between socially accepted behavior and abuse varies among different cultures. Likewise, certain cultural practices (eg, female genital mutilation—see p. 2486) are so extreme as to constitute abuse. However, certain folk remedies (eg, coining, cupping, irritant poultices) often create lesions (eg, bruises, petechiae, minor burns) that can blur the line between acceptable cultural practices and abuse.

Members of certain religious and cultural groups have sometimes failed to obtain life-saving treatment (eg, for diabetic ketoacidosis or meningitis), resulting in a child's death. Such failure is typically considered neglect regardless of the parents' or caregivers' intent. Additionally, in the US, certain people and cultural groups have increasingly been declining to have their children vaccinated, citing safety concerns (see p. 2461). It is not clear whether this refusal of vaccination is true medical neglect. However, in the face of illness, refusal of scientifically and medically accepted treatment often requires further investigation and sometimes legal intervention.

Etiology

Abuse: Generally, abuse can be attributed to a breakdown of impulse control in the parent or caregiver. Several factors contribute.

Parental characteristics and personality features can play a role. The parent's own childhood may have lacked affection and warmth, may not have been conducive to the development of adequate self-esteem or emotional maturity, and, in most cases, also included other forms of maltreatment. Abusive parents may see their children as a source of unlimited and unconditional affection and look to them for the support that they never received. As a result, they may have unrealistic expectations of what their children can supply for them, they are frustrated easily and have poor impulse control, and they may be unable to give what they never experienced. Drug or alcohol use may provoke impulsive and uncontrolled behaviors toward their children. Parental mental disorders also increase the risk of maltreatment.

Irritable, demanding, or hyperactive children may provoke parents' tempers, as may developmentally or physically disabled children, who often are more dependent than a typically developing child. Sometimes strong emotional bonds do not develop between parents and children. This lack of bonding occurs more commonly with premature or sick infants separated from parents early in infancy or with biologically unrelated children (eg, stepchildren), increasing the risk of abuse.

Situational stress may precipitate abuse, particularly when emotional support of relatives, friends, neighbors, or peers is unavailable.

Physical abuse, emotional abuse, and neglect are associated with poverty and lower socioeconomic status. However, all types of abuse, including sexual abuse, occur across the spectrum of socioeconomic groups. The risk of sexual abuse is increased in children who have several caregivers or a caregiver who has several sex partners.

Neglect: Neglect usually results from a combination of factors such as poor parenting, poor stress-coping skills, unsupportive family systems, and stressful life circumstances. Neglect often occurs in impoverished families experiencing financial and environmental stresses, particularly those in which parents also have mental disorders (typically depression, bipolar disorder, or schizophrenia), abuse drugs or alcohol, or have limited intellectual capacity. Children in single-parent families may be at risk of neglect due to a lower income and fewer available resources.

Symptoms and Signs

Symptoms and signs depend on the nature and duration of the abuse or neglect.

Physical abuse: Skin lesions are common and may include

- Handprints or oval fingertip marks caused by slapping or grabbing and shaking
- Long, bandlike ecchymoses caused by belt whipping
- Narrow arcuate bruises caused by extension cord whipping
- Multiple small round burns caused by cigarettes
- Symmetric scald burns of upper or lower extremities or buttocks caused by intentional immersion
- Bite marks
- Thickened skin or scarring at the corners of the mouth caused by being gagged
- Patchy alopecia, with varying hair lengths, caused by hair pulling

However, more commonly, skin findings are subtle (eg, a small bruise, petechiae on the face and/or neck).

Fractures frequently associated with physical abuse include rib fractures, vertebral fractures, long bone and digit fractures in nonambulatory children, and metaphyseal fractures; in children < 1 yr, about 75% of fractures are inflicted by others.

Confusion and localizing neurologic abnormalities can occur with CNS injuries. Lack of visible head lesions does not exclude traumatic brain injury, particularly in infants subjected to violent shaking. These infants may be comatose or stuporous from brain injury yet lack visible signs of injury (with the common exception of retinal hemorrhage) or they may present with nonspecific signs such as fussiness and vomiting. Traumatic injury to organs within the chest or abdominal/pelvic region may also occur without visible signs.

Children who are frequently abused are often fearful and irritable and sleep poorly. They may have symptoms of depression (see p. 2716), posttraumatic stress reactions (see p. 2713), or anxiety (see p. 2708). Violent or suicidal behavior may occur.

PEARLS & PITFALLS

- Lack of visible head lesions does not exclude traumatic brain injury.

Sexual abuse: In most cases, children do not spontaneously disclose sexual abuse and rarely exhibit behavioral or physical signs of sexual abuse. If a disclosure is made, it is generally delayed, sometimes days to years. In some cases, abrupt or extreme changes in behavior may occur. Aggressiveness or withdrawal may develop, as may phobias or sleep disturbances. Some sexually abused children act in ways that are sexually inappropriate for their age.

Physical signs of sexual abuse that involves penetration may include

- Difficulty in walking or sitting
- Bruises or tears around the genitals, anus, or mouth
- Vaginal discharge, bleeding, or pruritus

Other manifestations include a sexually transmitted infection, and pregnancy. Within a few days of the abuse, examination of the genitals, anus, and mouth may be normal or may show healed lesions or subtle changes.

Emotional abuse: In early infancy, emotional abuse may blunt emotional expressiveness and decrease interest in the environment. Emotional abuse commonly results in failure to thrive and is often misdiagnosed as intellectual disability or physical illness. Delayed development of social and language skills often results from inadequate parental stimulation and interaction. Emotionally abused children may be insecure, anxious, distrustful, superficial in interpersonal relationships, passive, and overly concerned with pleasing adults. Children who are spurned may have very low self-esteem. Children who are terrorized or threatened may seem fearful and withdrawn. The emotional effect on children usually becomes obvious at school age, when difficulties develop in forming relationships with teachers and peers. Often, emotional effects are appreciated only after the child has been placed in another environment or after aberrant behaviors abate and are replaced by more acceptable behaviors. Children who are exploited may commit crimes or abuse alcohol or drugs.

Neglect: Undernutrition, fatigue, poor hygiene, lack of appropriate clothing, and failure to thrive (see p. 2751) are common signs of inadequate provision of food, clothing, or shelter. Stunted growth and death resulting from starvation or exposure to extremes in temperature or weather may occur. Neglect that involves inadequate supervision may result in preventable illness or injury.

Diagnosis

- High index of suspicion (eg, for history that does not match physical findings or for atypical injury patterns)
- Supportive, open-ended questioning
- Sometimes imaging and laboratory tests
- Reporting to authorities for further investigation

Evaluation of injuries and nutritional deficiencies is discussed elsewhere in THE MANUAL. Recognizing maltreatment as the cause can be difficult, and a high index of suspicion must be maintained. Because of social biases, abuse is considered less often in children living in a 2-parent household with a median-level income; child abuse can occur regardless of family composition or socioeconomic status.

Sometimes direct questions provide answers. Children who have been maltreated may describe the events and the perpetrator, but some children, particularly those who have been sexually abused, may be sworn to secrecy, threatened, or so traumatized that they are reluctant to speak about the abuse (and may even deny abuse when specifically questioned). A medical history including a history of the events should be obtained from children and their caregivers in a relaxed environment. Open-ended questions (eg, "Can you tell me what happened?") are particularly important in these cases because yes-or-no questions (eg, "Did daddy do this?", "Did he touch you here?") can easily sculpt an untrue history in young children.

Examination includes observation of interactions between the child and the caregivers whenever possible. Documentation of the history and physical examination should be as comprehensive and accurate as possible, including recording of exact quotes from the history and photographs of injuries.

Often it is unclear after the initial evaluation whether abuse occurred. In such cases, the mandatory reporting requirement of *suspected* abuse allows appropriate authorities and social agencies to investigate; if their evaluation confirms abuse, appropriate legal and social interventions can be done.

Physical abuse: Both history and physical examination provide clues suggestive of maltreatment.

Features suggestive of abuse in the history are

- Parental reluctance or inability to give a history of injury
- History that is inconsistent with the injury (eg, bruises on the backs of the legs attributed to a fall) or apparent stage of resolution (eg, old injuries described as recent)
- History that varies depending on the information source or over time

- History of injury that is incompatible with the child's stage of development (eg, injuries ascribed to rolling off a bed in an infant too young to roll over, or to a fall down stairs in an infant too young to crawl)
- Inappropriate response by the parents to the severity of the injury—either overly concerned or unconcerned
- Delay in seeking care for the injury

Major indicators of abuse on examination are

- Atypical injuries
- Injuries incompatible with stated history

Childhood injuries resulting from falls are typically solitary and occur on the forehead, chin, or mouth or extensor surfaces of the extremities, particularly elbows, knees, forearms, and shins. Bruises on the back, buttocks, and the back of the legs are extremely rare from falls. Fractures, apart from clavicular fracture, tibial (toddler's) fractures, and distal radius (Colles) fracture, are less common in typical falls during play or down stairs. No fractures are pathognomonic of abuse, but classic metaphyseal lesions, rib fractures (especially posterior and 1st rib), and depressed or multiple skull fractures (caused by apparently minor trauma), scapular fractures, sternal fractures, and spinous processes fractures should raise concern for abuse.

Physical abuse should be considered when an infant who is not walking has a serious injury. Young infants with minor injuries to the face also should be further evaluated. The younger infant may appear to be normal despite significant brain trauma, and inflicted acute head trauma should be part of the differential diagnosis of every lethargic infant. Other hints are multiple injuries at different stages of resolution or development; cutaneous lesions with patterns suggestive of particular sources of injury (see p. 2484); and repeated injury, which is suggestive of abuse or inadequate supervision.

A dilated eye examination and neuroimaging are recommended for all children < 1 yr with suspected abuse. Retinal hemorrhages occur in 85 to 90% of cases of abusive head trauma vs < 10% of cases of accidental head trauma. They also may result from childbirth and persist for up to 4 wk. When retinal hemorrhages result from accidental trauma, the mechanism is usually obvious and life-threatening (eg, major motor vehicle crash), and the hemorrhages are typically few in number and confined to the posterior poles.

Children < 36 mo (previous recommendation 24 mo) with possible physical abuse should undergo a skeletal survey for evidence of previous bony injuries (fractures in various stages of healing or subperiosteal elevations in long bones). Surveys are sometimes done on children aged 3 to 5 yr but are generally not helpful for those > 5 yr. The standard survey includes images of the

- Appendicular skeleton: Humeri, forearms, hands, femurs, lower legs and feet
- Axial skeleton: Thorax (including oblique views), pelvis, lumbosacral spine, cervical spine, and skull

Physical disorders causing multiple fractures include osteogenesis imperfecta (see p. 2548) and congenital syphilis (see p. 2625).

Sexual abuse: Sexually transmitted infections in a child < 12 yr should make practitioners extremely suspicious about the possibility of sexual abuse. When a child has been sexually abused, behavioral changes (eg, irritability, fearfulness, insomnia) may be the only clues initially. If sexual abuse is suspected, the perioral and anal areas and the external genitals must be examined for evidence of injury. If the suspected abuse is thought to have occurred recently (≤ 96 h), forensic evidence should be gathered using an appropriate kit and handled according to required legal standards (see p. 2230). An examination involving use of a magnifying light source with a camera, such as with a specially equipped colposcope, may be helpful to the examiner as well as for documentation for legal purposes.

Emotional abuse and neglect: Evaluation focuses on general appearance and behavior to determine whether the child is failing to develop normally. Teachers and social workers are often the first to recognize neglect. The physician may notice a pattern of missed appointments and vaccinations that are not up-to-date. Medical neglect of life-threatening, chronic diseases, such as asthma or diabetes, can lead to a subsequent increase in office or emergency department visits and poor adherence with recommended treatment regimens.

Treatment

- Treatment of injuries
- Creation of a safety plan
- Family counseling and support
- Sometimes removal from the home

Treatment first addresses urgent medical needs (including possible sexually transmitted infections) and the child's immediate safety. Referral to a pediatrician specializing in child abuse should be considered. In both abuse and neglect situations, families should be approached in a helping rather than a punitive manner.

Immediate safety: Physicians and other professionals in contact with children (eg, nurses, teachers, day care workers, police) are mandated reporters who are required by law in all states to report incidents of suspected abuse or neglect (see US Dept of Health and Human Services, Mandated Reporting at www.childwelfare.gov). Every state has its own laws. Members of the general public are encouraged, but not mandated, to report suspected abuse. Any person who makes a report of abuse based on reasonable cause and in good faith is immune from criminal and civil liability. A mandated reporter who fails to make a report can be subject to criminal and civil penalties. The reports are made to Child Protective Services or another appropriate child protection agency. In most situations, it is appropriate for professionals to tell caregivers that a report is being made pursuant to the law and that they will be contacted, interviewed, and likely visited at their home. In some cases, the professional may determine that informing the parent or caregiver before police or other agency assistance is available creates greater risk of injury to the child and/or themselves. Under those circumstances, the professional may choose to delay informing the parent or caregiver.

Representatives of child protective agencies and social workers can help the physician determine likelihood of subsequent harm and thus identify the best immediate disposition for the child. Options include

- Protective hospitalization
- Placement with relatives or in temporary housing (sometimes a whole family is moved out of an abusive partner's home)
- Temporary foster care
- Going home with prompt social service and medical follow-up

The physician plays an important role in working with community agencies to advocate for the best and safest disposition for the child. Healthcare professionals in the US are often asked to write an impact statement, which is a letter typically addressed to a Child Protective Services worker (who can then bring it to the attention of the judicial system), about a child who is suspected to be the victim of maltreatment. The letter should contain a clear explanation of the history and physical examination findings (in layman's terms) and an opinion as to the likelihood that the child was maltreated.

Follow-up: A source of primary medical care is fundamental. However, the families of abused and neglected children frequently relocate, making continuity of care difficult. Broken appointments are common; outreach and home visits by social workers and/or public health nurses may be helpful A local child advocacy center can help community agencies, health care practitioners, and the legal system work together as a multidisciplinary team in a more coordinated, child-friendly, and effective manner.

A close review of the family setting, prior contacts with various community service agencies, and the caregivers' needs is essential. A social worker can conduct such reviews and help with interviews and family counseling. Social workers also provide tangible assistance to the caregivers by helping them obtain public assistance, child care, and respite services (which can decrease stress for caregivers). They can also help to coordinate mental health services for caregivers. Periodic or ongoing social work contact usually is needed.

Parent-aide programs, which employ trained nonprofessionals to support abusive and negligent parents and provide an example of appropriate parenting, are available in some communities. Other parent support groups also have been successful.

Sexual abuse may have lasting effects on the child's development and sexual adaptation, particularly among older children and adolescents. Counseling or psychotherapy for the child and the adults concerned may lessen these effects. Physical abuse, particularly significant head trauma, also can have long-lasting effects on development. If physicians or caregivers are concerned that children have a disability or delayed development, they may request an evaluation from their state's Early Intervention system (see National Dissemination Center for Children with Disabilities), which is a program to evaluate and treat children with suspected disabilities or developmental delays.

Removal from the home: Although emergency temporary removal from the home until evaluation is complete and safety is ensured is sometimes done, the ultimate goal of Child Protective Services is to keep children with their family in a safe, healthy environment. Often, families are offered services to rehabilitate the caregivers so that children who have been removed may be reunited with their family. If the previously described interventions do not ensure safety, consideration must be made for long-term removal and possibly termination of parental rights. This significant step requires a court petition, presented by the legal counsel of the appropriate welfare department. The specific procedure varies from state to state but usually entails family court testimony by a physician. When the court decides in favor of removing the child from the home, a disposition is arranged, typically to a temporary placement, such as foster care. While the child is in temporary placement, the child's own physician or a medical team that specializes in children in foster care should, if possible, maintain contact with the parents and ensure that adequate efforts are being made to help them. Occasionally, children are re-abused while in foster care. The physician should be alert to this possibility. As the dynamics of the family setting improve, the child may be able to return to the original caregivers. However, recurrences of maltreatment are common.

Prevention

Prevention of maltreatment should be a part of every well-child office visit through education of parents, caregivers, and children and identification of risk factors. At-risk families should be referred to appropriate community services.

Parents who were victims of maltreatment are at increased risk of abusing their own children. These parents often verbalize anxiety about their abusive background and are amenable to assistance. First-time parents and teenage parents as well as parents with several children < 5 yr are also at increased risk of abusing their children. Often, maternal risk factors for abuse are identified prenatally (eg, a mother who does not seek prenatal care, smokes, abuses drugs, or has a history of domestic violence). Medical problems during pregnancy, delivery, or early infancy that may affect the mother's and/or infant's health can weaken parent-infant bonding (see also p. 2481). During such times it is important to elicit the parents' feelings about themselves and the infant's well-being. How well can they tolerate an infant with many needs or health demands? Do the parents give moral and physical support to each other? Are there relatives or friends to help in times of need? The health care practitioner who is alert to clues and able to provide support can make a major impact on the family and possibly prevent child maltreatment.

FEMALE GENITAL MUTILATION

Female genital mutilation is practiced routinely in parts of Africa (usually northern or central Africa), where it is deeply ingrained as part of some cultures. It is also done in some parts of the Middle East. It is reportedly done because women who experience sexual pleasure are considered impossible to control, are shunned, and cannot be married.

The average age of girls who undergo mutilation is 7 yr, and mutilation is done without anesthesia. There are four main types of female genital mutilation defined by the WHO:

- Type I: Clitoridectomy—Partial or total removal of the clitoris and, in very rare cases, only the fold of skin surrounding the clitoris (the prepuce)
- Type II: Excision—Partial or total removal of the clitoris and the labia minora, with or without removal of the labia majora
- Type III: Infibulation—Narrowing of the vaginal opening by cutting and repositioning the labia to create a seal except for a small opening for menses and urine
- Type IV: Other—All other harmful procedures done to the female genitals for nonmedical purposes (such as pricking, piercing, carving [incising], scraping, and cauterizing the genital area)

With infibulation, the legs are often bound together for weeks afterward. Traditionally, infibulated females are cut open on their wedding night.

Sequelae of genital mutilation may include operative or postoperative bleeding and infection (including tetanus). For infibulated females, recurrent urinary and/or gynecologic infection and scarring are possible. Females who become pregnant after female genital mutilation may have significant hemorrhage during childbirth. Psychologic sequelae may be severe.

Female genital mutilation may be decreasing due to the influence of religious leaders who have spoken out against the practice and growing opposition in some communities.

296 Chromosome and Gene Anomalies

Chromosomal anomalies cause various disorders. Anomalies that affect autosomes (the 22 paired chromosomes that are alike in males and females) are more common than those that affect sex chromosomes (X and Y).

Chromosomal abnormalities fit into several categories but broadly may be considered as numerical or structural.

Numerical abnormalities include

- Trisomy (an extra chromosome)
- Monosomy (a missing chromosome)

Structural abnormalities include

- Translocations (anomalies in which a whole chromosome or segments of chromosomes inappropriately join with other chromosomes)
- Deletions and duplications of various chromosomes or parts of chromosomes

Terminology: Some specific terms from the field of genetics are important for describing chromosomal anomalies:

- Aneuploidy: The most common chromosomal abnormality caused by an extra or missing chromosome.
- Karyotype: The full set of chromosomes in a person's cells.
- Genotype: The genetic constitution determined by the karyotype.
- Phenotype: The person's clinical findings including outward appearance—the biochemical, physiologic, and physical makeup as determined by the genotype and environmental factors (see p. 3188).
- Mosaicism: The presence of ≥ 2 cell lines differing in genotype in a person who has developed from a single fertilized egg.

Diagnosis

- Chromosomal analysis
- Banding
- Karyotype analysis
- Chromosomal microarray analysis (CMA)

Lymphocytes are typically used for chromosomal analysis, except prenatally, when amniocytes or cells from placental chorionic villi are used (see Amniocentesis on p. 2300). A karyotype analysis involves blocking cells in mitosis during metaphase and staining the condensed chromosomes. Chromosomes from single cells are photographed, and their images are arranged, forming a karyotype.

Several techniques are used to better delineate the chromosomes:

- In classical banding (eg, G [Giemsa]-, Q [fluorescent]-, and C-banding), a dye is used to stain bands on the chromosomes.
- High-resolution chromosome analysis uses special culture methods to obtain a high percentage of prophase and prometaphase spreads. The chromosomes are less condensed than in routine metaphase analysis, and the number of identifiable bands is expanded, allowing a more sensitive karyotype analysis.
- Spectral karyotyping analysis (also called chromosome painting) uses chromosome-specific multicolor fluorescent in situ hybridization (FISH) techniques that improve the visibility of certain defects, including translocations and inversions.
- CMA (also called array comparative genomic hybridization) is a single-step technique that allows the entire genome to be scanned for chromosome dosage abnormalities, including increases (duplications) or decreases (deletions), which may be suggestive of an unbalanced translocation. Single nucleotide polymorphism (SNP) microarray analysis has the additional ability to detect regions of homozygosity, which may be seen in cases where parents share common ancestry (consanguinity), and also when there is uniparental disomy (UPD, ie, both of a pair of chromosomes inherited from one parent). It is important to note that CMA does not detect balanced rearrangements (eg, translocations, inversions) that are not associated with deletions and duplications.

Screening: Recently, noninvasive prenatal screening (NIPS) methods have been developed in which cell-free fetal DNA sequences obtained from a maternal blood sample are used for prenatal screening for trisomy 21 (Down syndrome), trisomy 13, and trisomy 18 and sex chromosome aneuploidy. Although NIPS has good sensitivity and specificity for some chromosomal abnormalities, it is recommended that the results be confirmed using a diagnostic test. More recently, NIPS has been used as a screening test for common microdeletion syndromes (eg, 22q11 deletion); however, the sensitivity and specificity are still relatively low.

DOWN SYNDROME

(Trisomy 21; Trisomy G)

Down syndrome is an anomaly of chromosome 21 that can cause intellectual disability, microcephaly, short stature, and characteristic facies. Diagnosis is suggested by physical anomalies and abnormal development and confirmed by cytogenetic analysis. Treatment depends on specific manifestations and anomalies.

Overall incidence among live births is about 1/700, but the risk increases with increasing maternal age. At 20 yr of maternal age, the risk is 1/2000 births; at 35, it is 1/365; and at 40, it is 1/100. However, because most births occur among younger women, the majority of children with Down syndrome are born to women < 35 yr; only about 20% of infants with Down syndrome are born to mothers > 35 yr.

Etiology

In about 95% of cases, there is an extra whole chromosome 21 (trisomy 21), which is almost always maternally derived. Such people have 47 chromosomes.

The remaining 5% of people with Down syndrome have the normal count of 46 chromosomes but have an extra chromosome 21 translocated to another chromosome (the resulting abnormal chromosome is still counted only as 1).

The most common translocation is t(14;21), in which a piece of an additional chromosome 21 is attached to chromosome 14. In about half of people with the t(14;21) translocation, both parents have normal karyotypes, indicating a de novo translocation. In the other half, one parent (almost always the mother), although phenotypically normal, has only 45 chromosomes, one of which is t(14;21). Theoretically, the chance that a carrier mother will have a child with Down syndrome is 1:3, but the actual risk is lower (about 1:10). If the father is the carrier, the risk is only 1:20.

The next most common translocation is t(21;22). In these cases, carrier mothers have about a 1:10 risk of having a child with Down syndrome; the risk is smaller for carrier fathers.

A 21q21q translocation chromosome, which occurs when the extra chromosome 21 is attached to another chromosome 21, is much less common. It is particularly important to determine whether a parent is a carrier of, or mosaic for, translocation 21q21q (such mosaics have some normal cells and some 45 chromosome cells with the 21q21q translocation). In such cases, each offspring of a carrier of the translocation will either have Down syndrome or monosomy 21 (the latter is not typically compatible with life). If the parent is mosaic, the risk is similar, although these people may also have offspring with normal chromosomes.

Down syndrome mosaicism presumably results from nondisjunction (when chromosomes fail to pass to separate cells) during cell division in the embryo. People with mosaic Down syndrome have two cell lines, one with the normal 46 chromosomes and another with 47 chromosomes, including an extra chromosome 21. The prognosis for intelligence and risk of medical complications probably depends on the proportion of trisomy 21 cells in each different tissue, including the brain. However, in practice, risk cannot be predicted because it is not feasible to determine the karyotype in every single cell in the body. Some people with mosaic Down syndrome have very subtle clinical signs and may have normal intelligence; however, even people with no detectable mosaicism can have very variable findings. If a parent has germline mosaicism for trisomy 21, an increased risk exists for a second affected child.

Pathophysiology

As with most conditions that result from chromosome imbalance, Down syndrome affects multiple systems and causes both structural and functional defects (see Table 296–1). Not all defects are present in each person.

Most affected people have some degree of cognitive impairment, ranging from severe (IQ 20 to 35) to mild (IQ 50 to 75). Gross motor and language delays also are evident early in life. Height is often reduced, and there is an increased risk of obesity. About 50% of affected neonates have congenital heart disease; ventricular septal defect and atrioventricular canal (endocardial cushion) defect are most common. About 5% of affected people have GI anomalies, particularly duodenal atresia, sometimes along with annular pancreas. Hirschsprung disease and celiac disease also are more common. Many people develop endocrinopathies, including thyroid disease (most often hypothyroidism) and diabetes. Atlanto-occipital and atlantoaxial hypermobility, as well as bony anomalies of the cervical spine, can cause atlanto-occipital and cervical instability; weakness and paralysis may result. About 60% of people have eye problems, including congenital cataracts, glaucoma, strabismus, and refractive errors. Most people have hearing loss, and ear infections are very common.

The aging process seems to be accelerated. The average life expectancy is about 55 yr; however, more recently, some affected people have been living into their 70s and 80s. Life expectancy is decreased primarily by heart disease and, to a lesser degree, by increased susceptibility to infections and acute myelogenous leukemia. There is an increased risk of Alzheimer disease at an early age, and at autopsy, brains of adults with Down syndrome show typical microscopic findings. The results of recent research indicate that blacks with Down syndrome have a substantially shorter life span than whites. This finding may be the result of poor access to medical, educational, and other support services.

Affected women have a 50% chance of having a fetus that also has Down syndrome. However, many affected fetuses abort spontaneously. Men with Down syndrome are infertile, except for those with mosaicism.

Table 296–1. SOME COMPLICATIONS OF DOWN SYNDROME*

SYSTEM	DEFICIT
Cardiac	Congenital heart disease, most often VSD and AV canal Increased risk of mitral valve prolapse and aortic regurgitation (more frequently seen in adults)
CNS	Cognitive impairment (mild to severe) Motor and language delay Autistic behavior Alzheimer disease
GI	Duodenal atresia or stenosis Hirschsprung disease Celiac disease
Endocrine	Hypothyroidism Diabetes
EENT	Ophthalmic disorders (eg, congenital cataracts, glaucoma, strabismus, refractive errors) Hearing loss Increased incidence of otitis media
Growth	Short stature Obesity
Hematologic	Thrombocytopenia Neonatal polycythemia Transient myelodysplastic disorder Acute megakaryoblastic leukemia Acute lymphocytic leukemia
Musculoskeletal	Atlantoaxial and atlanto-occipital instability Joint laxity

*Not all complications are present in a given patient, but incidence is increased compared with unaffected population.

AV = atrioventricular; EENT = eyes, ears, nose, and throat; VSD = ventricular septal defect.

Symptoms and Signs

General appearance: Affected neonates tend to be placid, rarely cry, and have hypotonia. Most have a flat facial profile (particularly flattening of the bridge of the nose), but some do not have obviously unusual physical characteristics at birth and then develop more noticeable characteristic facial features during infancy. A flattened occiput, microcephaly, and extra skin around the back of the neck are common. The eyes are slanted upward, and epicanthal folds at the inner corners usually are present. Brushfield spots (gray to white spots resembling grains of salt around the periphery of the iris) may be visible. The mouth is often held open with a protruding, furrowed tongue that lacks the central fissure. The ears are often small and rounded.

The hands are short and broad and often have a simian crease (a single, palmar crease). The fingers are often short, with clinodactyly (incurving) of the 5th digit, which often has only 2 phalanges. The feet may have a wide gap between the 1st and 2nd toes, and a plantar furrow often extends backward on the foot. Hands and feet show characteristic dermatoglyphics.

Growth and development: As affected children grow, delay of physical and mental development quickly becomes apparent. Stature is short, and the mean IQ is about 50. Behavior suggestive of attention-deficit/hyperactivity disorder is often present in childhood, and the incidence of autistic behavior is increased (particularly in children with profound intellectual disability). Depression is common among children and adults.

Cardiac manifestations: Symptoms of heart disease are determined by the type and extent of the cardiac anomaly. Infants with ventricular septal defects can either be asymptomatic or show signs of heart failure (eg, labored breathing, fast respiratory rate, difficulty with feeding, sweating, poor weight gain). A high-frequency, 2/6 or louder systolic murmur may be present depending on the size of the defect. Infants with atrioventricular canal defects can show signs of heart failure or be asymptomatic initially. Characteristic heart sounds include a wide fixed splitting of the second sound. Murmurs may not be appreciated; however, a number of different murmurs are possible.

GI manifestations: Infants with Hirschsprung disease usually have delay in passage of meconium for 48 h after birth. Severely affected infants may have signs of intestinal obstruction (eg, bilious vomiting, failure to pass stool, abdominal distention). Duodenal atresia or stenosis can manifest with bilious vomiting or with no symptoms, depending on the extent of the stenosis.

Diagnosis

- Prenatal chorionic villus sampling and/or amniocentesis with karyotype analysis and/or CMA
- Neonatal karyotype analysis (if prenatal karyotype analysis not done)

Diagnosis of Down syndrome may be suspected prenatally based on physical anomalies detected by fetal ultrasonography (eg, increased nuchal translucency) or based on abnormal levels of plasma protein A in late 1st trimester and alpha-fetoprotein, beta-hCG (human chorionic gonadotropin), unconjugated estriol, and inhibin in early 2nd trimester (15 to 16 wk gestation) on maternal serum screening. More recently, NIPS, in which fetal DNA obtained from the maternal circulation is tested, has become a screening option for trisomy 21.

If Down syndrome was suspected based on maternal serum screening tests or ultrasonography, fetal or neonatal confirmatory testing is recommended. Confirmatory methods include chorionic villus sampling and/or amniocentesis with testing by karyotype analysis and/or CMA. Confirmatory testing is done particularly in cases where the screening result is indeterminate or unclear; in younger women, in whom the positive predictive value of NIPS is lower; and to diagnose other fetal chromosomal disorders. Management decisions, including termination of pregnancy, should not be made based on NIPS testing alone. Karyotyping can also be used to diagnose an associated translocation so parents can receive appropriate genetic counseling regarding recurrence risk.

Maternal serum screening and diagnostic testing for Down syndrome are recommended for all women who present for prenatal care before 20 wk gestation regardless of maternal age.

The American College of Obstetricians and Gynecologists Committee on Genetics and the Society for Maternal–Fetal Medicine committee opinion advises that cell-free fetal DNA testing be offered to patients at increased risk of aneuploidy. At-risk patients include women ≥ 35 yr and in cases where fetal ultrasonographic findings indicate an increased risk. The committee advises that cell-free fetal DNA does not replace the accuracy and diagnostic precision of prenatal diagnosis with chorionic villus sampling or amniocentesis.

If diagnosis is not made prenatally, then neonatal diagnosis is based on physical anomalies and confirmed by cytogenetic testing.

Concomitant medical conditions: Certain age-specific routine screening helps identify conditions associated with Down syndrome (see also the American Academy of Pediatrics Guidelines on Health Supervision for Children with Down Syndrome at http://pediatrics.aappublications.org):

- Echocardiography: At prenatal visit or at birth
- Thyroid screening (thyroid-stimulating hormone [TSH] levels): At birth, 6 mo, 12 mo, and annually thereafter
- Hearing evaluations: At birth, every 6 mo thereafter until normal hearing established (about age 4 yr), then annually
- Ophthalmology evaluation: By 6 mo, then annually until age 5; then every 2 yr until age 13 and every 3 yr until age 21 (more frequently as indicated)
- Growth: Height, weight, and head circumference plotted at each health supervision visit using a Down syndrome growth chart
- Evaluation for obstructive sleep apnea completed by age 4 yr

Routine screening for atlantoaxial instability and celiac disease is no longer recommended. Children are tested based on clinical suspicion, and it is recommended that patients with a history of neck pain, radicular pain, weakness, or any other neurologic symptoms that suggest myelopathy have x-rays of the cervical spine in the neutral position; if no suspicious abnormalities are seen, they should have x-rays done in flexion and extension positions.

Treatment

- Specific manifestations treated
- Genetic counseling

The underlying disorder cannot be cured. Management depends on specific manifestations. Some congenital cardiac anomalies are repaired surgically. Hypothyroidism is treated with thyroid hormone replacement.

Care should also include genetic counseling for the family, social support, and educational programming appropriate for the level of intellectual functioning (see Intellectual Disability on p. 2700).

KEY POINTS

- Down syndrome involves an extra chromosome 21, either a separate chromosome or a translocation onto another chromosome.
- Diagnosis may be suspected prenatally based on anomalies detected by fetal ultrasonography (eg, increased nuchal translucency) or based on cell-free fetal DNA analysis of maternal blood or maternal multiple marker screening for levels of plasma protein A in late 1st trimester and levels of alpha-fetoprotein, beta-human chorionic gonadotropin (beta-hCG), unconjugated estriol, and inhibin in early 2nd trimester.
- Diagnosis should be confirmed by karyotype analysis, or CMA from chorionic villus sampling in the 1st trimester or

amniocentesis in the 2nd trimester, or postnatally by cytogenetic testing of a blood sample.
- Life expectancy is decreased primarily by heart disease and, to a lesser degree, by increased susceptibility to infections, acute myelocytic leukemia, and early-onset Alzheimer disease.
- Do routine age-specific screening to detect associated medical conditions (eg, cardiac anomalies, hypothyroidism).
- Treat specific manifestations, and provide social and educational support and genetic counseling.

TRISOMY 18

(Edwards Syndrome; Trisomy E)

Trisomy 18 is caused by an extra chromosome 18 and is usually associated with intellectual disability, small birth size, and various congenital anomalies, including severe microcephaly, heart defects, prominent occiput, low-set malformed ears, and a characteristic pinched facial appearance.

Trisomy 18 occurs in 1/6000 live births, but spontaneous abortions are common. More than 95% of affected children have complete trisomy 18. The extra chromosome is almost always maternally derived, and advanced maternal age increases risk. The female:male ratio is 3:1.

Symptoms and Signs

A prenatal history of feeble fetal activity, polyhydramnios, a small placenta, and a single umbilical artery often exist. Size at birth is markedly small for gestational age, with hypotonia and marked hypoplasia of skeletal muscle and subcutaneous fat. The cry is weak, and response to sound is decreased. The orbital ridges are hypoplastic, the palpebral fissures are short, and the mouth and jaw are small; all of these characteristics give the face a pinched appearance. Microcephaly, prominent occiput, low-set malformed ears, narrow pelvis, and a short sternum are common.

A clenched fist with the index finger overlapping the 3rd and 4th fingers usually occurs. The distal crease on the 5th finger is often absent, and there is a low-arch dermal ridge pattern on the fingertips. Redundant skinfolds, especially over the back of the neck, are common. The fingernails are hypoplastic, and the big toe is shortened and frequently dorsiflexed. Clubfeet and rocker-bottom feet are common. Severe congenital heart disease is common, especially patent ductus arteriosus and ventricular septal defects. Anomalies of lungs, diaphragm, GI tract, abdominal wall, kidneys, and ureters are frequent. Boys may have undescended testes. Common muscular manifestations include hernias, separation of the rectus muscles of the abdominal wall, or both.

Diagnosis

- Prenatal chorionic villus sampling and/or amniocentesis with cytogenetic testing by karyotype analysis, FISH, and/or CMA

Diagnosis of trisomy 18 may be suspected postnatally by appearance, or prenatally on ultrasonography (eg, with abnormalities of extremities and fetal growth restriction), or by multiple marker screening or NIPS using cell-free fetal DNA sequences obtained from a maternal blood sample.

Confirmation in all cases is by cytogenetic testing (karyotyping, fluorescent in situ hybridization [FISH] analysis, and/or CMA) of samples obtained by amniocentesis or chorionic villus sampling. Trisomy 18 detected on chorionic villus sampling may warrant further investigation either by amniocentesis or postnatal testing because the trisomy may represent confined placental mosaicism, in which aneuploidy is present in the placenta but undetectable in the fetus.

Confirmatory testing also is done in cases suspected based on NIPS, particularly when the screening result is indeterminate or unclear; in younger women, in whom the positive predictive value of NIPS is lower; and to diagnose other fetal chromosomal disorders. Management decisions, including termination of pregnancy, should not be made based on NIPS testing alone. See also The American College of Obstetricians and Gynecologists Committee on Genetics and the Society for Maternal–Fetal Medicine committee opinion regarding cell-free fetal DNA testing at www.acog.org.

Treatment

- Supportive care

No specific trisomy 18 treatment is available. More than 50% of children die within the first week; < 10% are still alive at age 1 yr. Children who survive have marked developmental delay and disability. Support for the family is critical.

TRISOMY 13

(Patau Syndrome; Trisomy D)

Trisomy 13 is caused by an extra chromosome 13 and causes abnormal forebrain, midface, and eye development; severe intellectual disability; heart defects; and small birth size.

Trisomy 13 occurs in about 1/10,000 live births; about 80% of cases are complete trisomy 13. Advanced maternal age increases the likelihood, and the extra chromosome is usually maternally derived.

Infants tend to be small for gestational age. Midline anomalies are common and include holoprosencephaly (failure of the forebrain to divide properly), facial anomalies such as cleft lip and cleft palate, microphthalmia, colobomas (fissures) of the iris, and retinal dysplasia. Supraorbital ridges are shallow, and palpebral fissures usually are slanted. The ears are abnormally shaped and usually low-set. Deafness is common. Scalp defects and dermal sinuses are also common. Loose folds of skin often are present over the back of the neck.

Simian crease (a single, palmar crease), polydactyly, and hyperconvex narrow fingernails are also common. About 80% of cases have severe congenital cardiovascular anomalies; dextrocardia is common. Genitals are frequently abnormal in both sexes; cryptorchidism and an abnormal scrotum occur in boys, and a bicornuate uterus occurs in girls. Apneic spells in early infancy are frequent. Intellectual disability is severe.

Diagnosis

- Cytogenetic testing by karyotyping, FISH analysis, and/or CMA

Diagnosis of trisomy 13 may be suspected postnatally by appearance or prenatally by abnormalities on ultrasonography (eg, intrauterine growth restriction), or by increased risk noted on multiple marker screening or NIPS using cell-free fetal DNA sequences obtained from a maternal blood sample.

Confirmation in all cases is by cytogenetic testing (karyotyping, fluorescent in situ hybridization [FISH] analysis, and/or CMA) of samples obtained by chorionic villus sampling or amniocentesis. Postnatally, confirmation is by cytogenetic testing of a blood sample.

Confirmatory testing also is done in cases suspected based on NIPS, particularly when the screening result is indeterminate or unclear; in younger women, in whom the positive predictive value of NIPS is lower; and to diagnose other fetal chromosomal disorders. Management decisions, including termination of pregnancy, should not be made based on NIPS testing alone. See also The American College of Obstetricians and Gynecologists Committee on Genetics and the Society for Maternal–Fetal Medicine committee opinion regarding cell-free fetal DNA testing at www.acog.org.

Treatment

- Supportive care

Most patients (80%) are so severely affected that they die before age 1 mo; < 10% survive longer than 1 yr. Support for the family is critical.

CHROMOSOMAL DELETION SYNDROMES

Chromosomal deletion syndromes result from loss of parts of chromosomes. They may cause severe congenital anomalies and significant intellectual and physical disability. Chromosomal deletion syndromes are rarely suspected prenatally but may be incidentally discovered at that time if karyotyping is done for other reasons. Postnatal diagnosis is suspected by clinical appearance and is confirmed by karyotyping, if the deletion is relatively large, or by other cytogenetic techniques such as fluorescent in situ hybridization or microarray analysis.

Chromosomal deletion syndromes typically involve larger deletions, that are typically visible on karyotyping. Syndromes involving smaller deletions (and additions) that affect one or more contiguous genes on a chromosome and are not visible on karyotyping are considered microdeletion and duplication syndromes.

5p-Deletion (cri du chat syndrome): Deletion of the end of the short arm of chromosome 5 (5p—usually paternal) is characterized by a high-pitched, mewing cry, closely resembling the cry of a kitten, which is typically heard in the immediate neonatal period, lasts several weeks, and then disappears. Affected neonates are hypotonic and have low birth weight, microcephaly, a round face with wide-set eyes, downward slanting of the palpebral fissures (with or without epicanthal folds), strabismus, and a broad-based nose. The ears are low-set, abnormally shaped, and frequently have narrow external auditory canals and preauricular tags. Syndactyly, hypertelorism, and cardiac anomalies occur often. Mental and physical development is markedly retarded. Many affected children survive into adulthood but have significant disability.

4p-Deletion (Wolf-Hirschhorn syndrome): Deletion of the short arm of chromosome 4 (4p) results in variable intellectual disability; individuals with larger deletions are usually more severely affected. Manifestations also may include epilepsy, a broad or beaked nose, midline scalp defects, ptosis and colobomas, cleft palate, delayed bone development, and, in boys, hypospadias and cryptorchidism. Some patients with Wolf-Hirschhorn syndrome also have immune deficiency. Many affected children die during infancy; those who survive into their 20s often have severe disability.

Subtelomeric deletions: These deletions may be visible on karyotyping but are also sometimes small and submicroscopic and may occur at either telomere (the end of a chromosome). Phenotypic changes may be subtle. Subtelomeric deletions may be present in people with nonspecific intellectual disability and mildly dysmorphic features as well in more severely affected people with multiple congenital anomalies.

MICRODELETION GENE SYNDROMES

Microdeletion syndromes are disorders caused by microscopic and submicroscopic deletions or duplications of contiguous genes on particular parts of chromosomes. Postnatal diagnosis is suspected by clinical appearance and confirmed by fluorescent in situ hybridization and CMA.

Microdeletion syndromes differ from chromosomal deletion syndromes in that deletion syndromes are usually visible on karyotyping because of their larger size (typically > 5 megabases), whereas the abnormalities in microdeletion syndromes involve smaller segments (typically 1 to 3 megabases) and are detectable only with fluorescent probes (fluorescent in situ hybridization) and microarray analysis. A given gene segment can be deleted or duplicated (termed a reciprocal duplication). The clinical effects of microscopic reciprocal duplications tend to be similar but less severe than those of deletions involving the same segment. The term contiguous gene syndrome encompasses both microdeletion syndromes and contiguous abnormalities visible on karyotyping.

Most clinically significant microdeletions and duplications seem to occur sporadically; however, mildly affected parents may be diagnosed when parental testing is done after a child is found to have an abnormality. Numerous syndromes have been identified, with widely varying manifestations (see Table 296–2).

OVERVIEW OF SEX CHROMOSOME ANOMALIES

Sex chromosome anomalies may involve aneuploidy, partial deletions or duplications of sex chromosomes, or mosaicism.

Sex chromosome anomalies are common and cause syndromes that are associated with a range of congenital and developmental anomalies. The majority are not suspected prenatally but may be incidentally discovered if karyotyping is done for other reasons, such as advanced maternal age. The anomalies are often hard to recognize at birth and may not be diagnosed until puberty.

The effects of X chromosome anomalies are not as severe as those from analogous autosomal anomalies. Females with 3 X chromosomes often appear normal physically and mentally and are fertile. In contrast, all known autosomal trisomies have devastating effects. Similarly, whereas the absence of 1 X chromosome leads to a specific syndrome (Turner syndrome), the absence of an autosome is invariably lethal.

Lyon hypothesis (X-inactivation): By virtue of having 2 X chromosomes, females have 2 loci for every X-linked gene, as compared with a single locus in males. This imbalance would seem to cause a genetic "dosage" problem. However, according to the Lyon hypothesis, 1 of the 2 X chromosomes in each female somatic cell is inactivated genetically early in embryonic life (on or about day 16). In fact, no matter how many X chromosomes are present, all but 1 are inactivated. However, molecular genetic studies have shown that some genes on the inactivated X chromosome (or chromosomes) remain functional, and these few are essential to normal female development. *XIST* is the gene responsible for inactivating the genes of the X chromosome, producing RNA that triggers inactivation.

Table 296–2. EXAMPLES OF MICRODELETION SYNDROMES

SYNDROME	CHROMOSOMAL DELETION	DESCRIPTION
Alagille syndrome	20p.12	Cholestasis, bile duct paucity, cardiac anomalies, pulmonary artery stenosis, butterfly vertebrae, posterior embryotoxon of the eye
Angelman syndrome	Maternal chromosome at 15q11	Seizures, puppet-like ataxia, frequent laughter, hand flapping, severe intellectual disability
DiGeorge syndrome (DiGeorge anomaly, velocardiofacial syndrome, pharyngeal pouch syndrome, thymic aplasia)	22q11.21	Hypoplasia or lack of thymus and parathyroids, cardiac anomalies, cleft palate, intellectual disability, psychiatric problems
Langer-Giedion syndrome (trichorhinophalangeal syndrome type II)	8q24.1	Exostosis, cone epiphyses, sparse hair, bulbous nose, hearing loss, intellectual disability
Miller-Dieker syndrome	17p13.3	Lissencephaly; short, upturned nose; severe growth retardation; seizures; severe intellectual disability
Prader-Willi syndrome	Paternal chromosome at 15q11	In infancy: Hypotonia, poor feeding, failure to thrive In childhood and adolescence: Obesity, hypogonadism, small hands and feet, intellectual disability, obsessive-compulsive behaviors
Rubinstein-Taybi syndrome	16p13–	Broad thumbs and large toes, prominent nose and columella, intellectual disability
Smith-Magenis syndrome	17p11.2	Brachycephaly, midfacial hypoplasia, prognathism, hoarse voice, short stature, intellectual disability
Williams syndrome	7q11.23	Aortic stenosis, intellectual disability, elfin facies, transient hypercalcemia in infants

Whether the maternal or paternal X is inactivated usually is a random event within each cell at the time of inactivation; that same X then remains inactive in all descendant cells. Thus, all females are mosaics, with some cells having an active maternal X and others having an active paternal X.

Sometimes, random statistical distribution of inactivation in the relatively small number of cells present at the time of inactivation results in a particular descendant tissue having a preponderance of active maternal or paternal X chromosomes (skewed inactivation). Skewed inactivation may account for the occasional manifestation of minor symptoms in females who are heterozygous for X-linked disorders such as hemophilia and muscular dystrophy (all would presumably be asymptomatic if they had a 50:50 distribution of active X chromosomes). Skewed inactivation also may occur by postinactivation selection.

TURNER SYNDROME

(Gonadal Dysgenesis; Monosomy X)

In Turner syndrome, girls are born with one of their two X chromosomes partly or completely missing. Diagnosis is based on clinical findings and is confirmed by karyotype analysis. Treatment depends on manifestations and may include surgery for cardiac anomalies and often growth hormone therapy for short stature and estrogen replacement for pubertal failure.

Turner syndrome occurs in about 1/2500 live female births worldwide. However, 99% of 45,X conceptions abort spontaneously.

About 50% of affected girls have a 45,X karyotype; about 80% have lost the paternal X. Most of the other 50% are mosaics (eg, 45,X/46,XX or 45,X/47,XXX). Among mosaic girls, phenotype may vary from that of typical Turner syndrome to normal. Occasionally, affected girls have one normal X and one X that has formed a ring chromosome. Some affected girls have one normal X and one long-arm isochromosome formed by the loss of short arms and development of a chromosome consisting of two long arms of the X chromosome. These girls tend to have many of the phenotypic features of Turner syndrome; thus, deletion of the X chromosome's short arm seems to play an important role in producing the phenotype.

Pathophysiology

Common cardiac anomalies include coarctation of the aorta and bicuspid aortic valve. Hypertension frequently occurs with aging, even without coarctation. Renal anomalies and hemangiomas are frequent. Occasionally, telangiectasia occurs in the GI tract, with resultant GI bleeding or protein loss. Hearing loss occurs; strabismus and hyperopia (farsightedness) are common and increase the risk of amblyopia. Thyroiditis, diabetes mellitus, and celiac disease are more common than among the general population.

Infants are at a higher risk of developmental dysplasia of the hip. Of adolescents, 10% have scoliosis. Osteoporosis and fractures are fairly common among women with Turner syndrome. Gonadal dysgenesis (ovaries replaced by bilateral streaks of fibrous stroma and devoid of developing ova) occurs in 90% of females. Between 15% and 40% of adolescents with Turner syndrome undergo spontaneous puberty, but only 2 to 10% undergo spontaneous menarche.

Intellectual disability is rare, but many girls have nonverbal learning disability, attention-deficit/hyperactivity disorder, or both and thus score poorly on performance tests and in mathematics, even though they score average or above in the verbal components of intelligence tests.

Symptoms and Signs

Many neonates are very mildly affected; however, some present with marked dorsal lymphedema of the hands and feet and with lymphedema or loose folds of skin over the back of the neck. Other frequent anomalies include a webbed neck and a broad chest with widely spaced and inverted nipples. Affected girls have short stature compared with family members.

Less common findings include a low hairline on the back of the neck, ptosis, multiple pigmented nevi, short 4th metacarpals and metatarsals, prominent finger pads with whorls in the dermatoglyphics on the ends of the fingers, and hypoplasia of the nails. Increased carrying angle at the elbow occurs.

Symptoms of cardiac anomalies depend on severity. Coarctation of the aorta can cause high BP in the upper extremities, diminished femoral pulses, and low or absent BP in the lower extremities. Gonadal dysgenesis results in the inability to undergo puberty, develop breast tissue, or begin menses. Other medical problems that are associated with Turner syndrome develop with aging and may not be evident without screening.

Diagnosis

- Clinical appearance
- Cytogenetic testing by karyotyping, FISH analysis and/or CMA
- Testing for associated conditions

In neonates, the diagnosis of Turner syndrome may be suspected based on the presence of lymphedema or a webbed neck. In the absence of these findings, some children are diagnosed later, based on short stature, lack of pubertal development, and amenorrhea.

Diagnosis is confirmed by cytogenetic analysis (karyotyping, fluorescent in situ hybridization [FISH] analysis, and CMA).

Echocardiography or MRI is indicated to detect cardiac anomalies.

Cytogenetic analysis and Y-specific probe studies are done for all people with gonadal dysgenesis to rule out mosaicism with a Y-bearing cell line (eg, 45,X/46,XY). These people are usually phenotypic females who have variable features of Turner syndrome. They are at an increased risk of gonadal cancer, especially gonadoblastoma, and, although controversial, it is often recommended that the gonads be removed prophylactically.

Concomitant medical conditions: Certain routine evaluations help identify problems that may be associated with Turner syndrome:

- Cardiovascular evaluation by a specialist; MRI and echocardiography at time of diagnosis to rule out coarctation and bicuspid aortic valve and every 3 to 5 yr thereafter to evaluate aortic root diameter
- Renal ultrasonography at time of diagnosis, annual urinalysis, BUN, and creatinine for patients with renal system anomalies
- Hearing evaluation by an audiologist and audiogram every 3 to 5 yr
- Evaluation for scoliosis/kyphosis annually during childhood and adolescence
- Evaluation for hip dislocation
- Eye examination by pediatric ophthalmologist
- Thyroid function tests at diagnosis and every 1 to 2 yr thereafter
- Celiac screen (eg, endomysial antibody levels)
- Glucose tolerance test may be abnormal; fasting blood sugar and lipid profile annually during adulthood (started earlier if indicated)

Treatment

- Management of comorbid conditions
- Possible surgical repair of cardiac abnormalities

There is no specific treatment for the underlying genetic condition and management is based on an individual's findings.

Coarctation of the aorta is usually repaired surgically. Other cardiac anomalies are monitored and repaired as needed.

Lymphedema can usually be controlled with support hosiery and other techniques such as massage.

Treatment with growth hormone can stimulate growth. Estrogen replacement is usually needed to initiate puberty and is typically given at age 12 to 13 yr. Thereafter, birth control pills with a progestin are given to maintain secondary sexual characteristics. Growth hormone can be given with estrogen replacement until epiphyses are fused, at which time growth hormone is stopped. Continuation of estrogen replacement helps establish optimal bone density and skeletal development.

KEY POINTS

- Girls are missing all or part of one of their two X chromosomes.
- Manifestations vary, but short stature, webbed neck, broad chest, gonadal dysgenesis, and cardiac anomalies (commonly coarctation of the aorta and bicuspid aortic valve) are common; intellectual disability is rare.
- Risk of gonadal cancer is increased; it is often recommended to remove the gonads prophylactically, although this is controversial.
- Do routine age-specific screening to detect associated medical conditions (eg, cardiac and renal anomalies).
- Give estrogen to initiate puberty, followed by use of birth control pills with progestin to maintain secondary sexual characteristics.
- Treat specific manifestations, and provide social and educational support and genetic counseling.

KLINEFELTER SYNDROME

(47,XXY)

Klinefelter syndrome is ≥ two X chromosomes plus one Y, resulting in a phenotypic male.

Klinefelter syndrome is the most common sex chromosome disorder, occurring in about 1/500 live male births. The extra X chromosome is maternally derived in 60% of cases. Germ cells do not survive in the testes, leading to decreased sperm and androgens.

Affected boys tend to be tall with disproportionately long arms and legs. They often have small, firm testes, and about 30% develop gynecomastia.

Puberty usually occurs at the normal age, but often facial hair growth is light. There is a predisposition for verbal learning disorders. Clinical variation is great, and many 47,XXY males have normal appearance and intellect. Testicular development varies from hyalinized nonfunctional tubules to some production of spermatozoa; urinary excretion of follicle-stimulating hormone is frequently increased.

Mosaicism occurs in about 15% of cases. These men may be fertile. Some affected men have 3, 4, and even 5 X chromosomes along with the Y. As the number of X chromosomes increases, the severity of intellectual disability and of malformations also increases. Each extra X is associated with a 15- to 16-point reduction in IQ, with language most affected, particularly expressive language skills.

Diagnosis

- Prenatal diagnosis often when cytogenetic testing is done for other reasons such as advanced maternal age
- Detected postnatally on clinical appearance
- Cytogenetic testing by karyotyping, FISH analysis, and/or CMA

The diagnosis of Klinefelter syndrome is suspected on physical examination of an adolescent with small testes and gynecomastia. Many men are diagnosed during an infertility evaluation (probably all nonmosaic 47,XXY males are infertile).

Diagnosis is confirmed by cytogenetic analysis (karyotyping, fluorescent in situ hybridization [FISH] analysis, and/or CMA).

Treatment

- Testosterone supplementation
- Fertility preservation counseling just after onset of puberty

Males with Klinefelter syndrome should have lifelong testosterone supplementation beginning at puberty to ensure the development of male sexual characteristics, muscle bulk, bone structure, and better psychosocial functioning.

Boys with Klinefelter syndrome usually benefit from speech and language therapy and neuropsychologic testing for language comprehension, reading, and cognitive deficits.

After the onset of puberty, boys should receive counseling regarding fertility preservation.

47,XYY SYNDROME

47,XYY syndrome is two Y chromosomes and one X, resulting in a phenotypic male.

The 47,XYY syndrome occurs in about 1/1000 live male births.

Affected boys tend to be taller than average and have a 10- to 15-point IQ reduction compared with family members. There are few physical problems. Minor behavior disorders, hyperactivity, attention-deficit disorder, and learning disorders are more common.

OTHER X CHROMOSOME ANOMALIES

About 1/1000 apparently normal females have a 47,XXX (trisomy X) karyotype. Physical anomalies are rare. Menstrual irregularity and infertility sometimes occur. Affected girls may have mildly impaired intellect and may have more school problems than siblings. Advanced maternal age increases risk of the triple X anomaly, and the extra X chromosome is usually maternally derived.

Although rare, 48,XXXX and 49,XXXXX females exist. There is no consistent phenotype. The risk of intellectual disability and congenital anomalies increases markedly when there are > 3 X chromosomes. The genetic imbalance in early embryonic life may cause anomalous development.

FRAGILE X SYNDROME

Fragile X syndrome is a genetic abnormality in an X chromosome that leads to intellectual disability and behavioral disorders.

Fragile X syndrome is the most common inherited cause of moderate intellectual disability, with males being more commonly affected than females. (Down syndrome is the most common cause of intellectual disability in males; although it is a genetic disorder, most cases occur sporadically and are not inherited.) For more information, see the National Fragile X Foundation (https://fragilex.org/).

The symptoms of fragile X syndrome are caused by an abnormality of the *FMR1* gene on the X chromosome. The abnormality is an unstable triplet repeat expansion; normal people have < 60 CGG repeats and people with fragile X syndrome have > 200. People with 60 to 200 CGG repeats are considered to have a premutation because the increased number of repeats increases the likelihood that further mutation will result in > 200 repeats in a subsequent generation. Because of the relatively small number of base pairs involved, Fragile X syndrome is not considered a chromosome abnormality.

Fragile X syndrome affects about 1/4000 males and 1/8000 females. The premutation is more common. Females with the disorder are typically less impaired than males. Fragile X is inherited in an X-linked pattern and does not always cause clinical symptoms.

In the past, examination of the karyotype revealed a constriction at the end of the long arm of the X chromosome, followed by a thin strand of genetic material, which was why the syndrome was considered a chromosomal anomaly. However, this structural defect does not appear when modern cytogenetic techniques are used, and this is the reason why fragile X syndrome is now considered a single-gene disorder and not a chromosomal anomaly.

Symptoms and Signs

People with fragile X syndrome may have physical, cognitive, and behavioral abnormalities. Typical features include large, protuberant ears, a prominent chin and forehead, a high arched palate, and, in postpubertal males, macroorchidism. The joints may be hyperextensible, and heart disease (mitral valve prolapse) may occur.

Cognitive abnormalities may include mild to moderate intellectual disability. Features of autism may develop, including perseverative speech and behavior, poor eye contact, and social anxiety.

Women with the premutation may have premature ovarian failure; sometimes menopause occurs in the mid-30s.

Diagnosis

- DNA testing

Fragile X syndrome is frequently not suspected until school age or adolescence, depending on the severity of the symptoms. Boys with autism and intellectual disability should be tested for fragile X syndrome. Molecular DNA analysis is done to detect the increased number of CGG repeats.

Treatment

- Supportive measures

Early intervention, including speech and language therapy and occupational therapy, can help children with fragile X syndrome maximize their abilities.

Stimulants, antidepressants, and antianxiety drugs may be beneficial for some children.

297 Congenital Cardiovascular Anomalies

Congenital heart disease (CHD) is the most common congenital anomaly, occurring in almost 1% of live births. Among birth defects, CHD is the leading cause of infant mortality.

Etiology

Environmental and genetic factors contribute to the development of CHD.

Common environmental factors include maternal illness (eg, diabetes, rubella, systemic lupus erythematosus) or maternal intake of teratogenic agents (eg, lithium, isotretinoin, anticonvulsants). Paternal age may also be a risk factor.

Certain numerical chromosomal abnormalities, such as Down syndrome (trisomy 21), trisomy 18, trisomy 13, and monosomy X (Turner syndrome), are strongly associated with CHD. However, these abnormalities account for only about 5% of patients with CHD. Many other cases involve microscopic deletions on chromosomes or single-gene mutations. Often, the microscopic deletions and mutations cause congenital syndromes affecting multiple organs in addition to the heart. Examples include DiGeorge syndrome (microdeletion in 22q11.2) and Williams-Beuren syndrome (microdeletion in 7p11.23). Single-gene defects that cause syndromes associated with CHD include mutations in fibrillin-1 (Marfan syndrome), *TXB5* (Holt-Oram syndrome), and possibly *PTPN11* (Noonan syndrome). Single-gene defects can also cause isolated (ie, nonsyndromic) congenital heart defects.

The recurrence risk of CHD in a family varies depending on the cause. Risk is negligible in de novo mutations, 2 to 5% in nonsyndromic multifactorial CHD, and 50% when an autosomal dominant mutation is the cause. It is important to identify genetic factors because more patients with CHD are surviving into adulthood and potentially starting families.

Pathophysiology

Congenital heart anomalies are classified (see Table 297–1) as

- Cyanotic
- Acyanotic (left-to-right shunts or obstructive lesions)

The physiologic consequences of congenital heart anomalies vary greatly, ranging from a heart murmur or discrepancy in pulses in an asymptomatic child to severe cyanosis, heart failure (HF), or circulatory collapse.

Left-to-right shunts: Oxygenated blood from the left heart (left atrium or left ventricle) or the aorta shunts to the right heart (right atrium or right ventricle) or the pulmonary artery through an opening or communication between the 2 sides. Immediately after birth, pulmonary vascular resistance is high and flow through this communication may be minimal or bidirectional. Within the first 24 to 48 h of life, however, the pulmonary vascular resistance progressively falls, at which point blood will increasingly flow from left to right. The additional blood flow to the right side increases pulmonary blood flow and pulmonary artery pressure to a varying degree. The greater the increase, the more severe the symptoms; a small left-to-right shunt typically does not cause symptoms or signs.

High-pressure shunts (those at the ventricular or great artery level) become apparent several days to a few weeks after birth; low-pressure shunts (atrial septal defects) become apparent considerably later. If untreated, elevated pulmonary blood flow and pulmonary artery pressure may lead to pulmonary vascular disease and eventually Eisenmenger syndrome. Large left-to-right shunts (eg, large ventricular septal defect [VSD], patent ductus arteriosus [PDA]) cause excess pulmonary blood flow and volume overload, which may lead to signs of HF and during infancy often result in failure to thrive. A large left-to-right shunt also decreases lung compliance, leading to frequent lower respiratory tract infections.

Obstructive lesions: Blood flow is obstructed, causing a pressure gradient across the obstruction. The resulting pressure overload proximal to the obstruction may cause ventricular hypertrophy and HF. The most obvious manifestation is a heart murmur, which results from turbulent flow through the obstructed (stenotic) point. Examples are congenital aortic stenosis, which accounts for 3 to 6% of congenital heart anomalies, and congenital pulmonic stenosis, which accounts for 8 to 12%.

Cyanotic heart anomalies: Varying amounts of deoxygenated venous blood are shunted to the left heart (right-to-left shunt), reducing systemic arterial oxygen saturation. If there is > 5 g/dL of deoxygenated Hb, cyanosis results. Detection of cyanosis may be delayed in infants with dark pigmentation. Complications of persistent cyanosis include polycythemia, clubbing, thromboembolism (including stroke), bleeding disorders, brain abscess, and hyperuricemia. Hypercyanotic spells can occur in infants with unrepaired tetralogy of Fallot.

Depending on the anomaly, pulmonary blood flow may be reduced, normal, or increased (often resulting in HF in addition to cyanosis), resulting in cyanosis of variable severity. Heart murmurs are variably audible and are not specific.

Heart failure: Some congenital heart anomalies (eg, bicuspid aortic valve, mild aortic stenosis) do not significantly alter hemodynamics. Other anomalies cause pressure or volume

Table 297–1. CLASSIFICATION OF CONGENITAL HEART ANOMALIES*

CLASSIFICATION	EXAMPLES
Cyanotic	
—	Tetralogy of Fallot Transposition of the great arteries Tricuspid atresia Pulmonary atresia Persistent truncus arteriosus Total anomalous pulmonary venous return
Acyanotic	
Left-to-right shunt	Ventricular septal defect Atrial septal defect Patent ductus arteriosus Atrioventricular septal defect
Obstructive	Pulmonic stenosis Aortic stenosis Aortic coarctation Hypoplastic left heart syndrome (often also manifests with cyanosis, which may be mild)

*In decreasing order of frequency.

overload, sometimes causing HF. HF occurs when cardiac output is insufficient to meet the body's metabolic needs or when the heart cannot adequately handle venous return, causing pulmonary congestion (in left ventricular failure), edema primarily in dependent tissues and abdominal viscera (in right ventricular failure), or both. HF in infants and children has many causes other than congenital heart anomalies (see Table 297–2).

Symptoms and Signs

Manifestations of CHD are varied but commonly include

- Murmurs
- Cyanosis
- Heart failure
- Diminished or nonpalpable pulses

Other physical examination abnormalities may include circulatory shock, poor perfusion, abnormal 2nd heart sound (S_2—single or widely split), systolic click, gallop, or irregular rhythm.

Murmurs: Most left-to-right shunts and obstructive lesions cause systolic murmurs. Systolic murmurs and thrills are most prominent at the surface closest to their point of origin, making location diagnostically helpful. Increased flow across the pulmonary or aortic valve causes a midsystolic crescendo-decrescendo (ejection systolic) murmur. Regurgitant flow through an atrioventricular (AV) valve or flow across a VSD causes a holosystolic (pansystolic) murmur, often obscuring heart sounds as its intensity increases.

PDA typically causes a continuous murmur that is uninterrupted by the S_2 because blood flows through the ductus during systole and diastole. This murmur is 2-toned, having a different sound during systole (when driven by higher pressure) than during diastole.

Cyanosis: Central cyanosis is characterized by bluish discoloration of the lips and tongue and/or nail beds; it implies a low blood oxygen level (usually oxygen saturation < 90%). Perioral cyanosis and acrocyanosis (cyanosis of the hands and feet) without lip or nail bed cyanosis is caused by peripheral

Table 297–2. COMMON CAUSES OF HEART FAILURE IN CHILDREN

AGE AT ONSET	CAUSES
In utero	Chronic anemia with subsequent high-output heart failure Large systemic arteriovenous fistulas (eg, cerebral vein of Galen shunt) Myocardial dysfunction secondary to myocarditis Sustained intrauterine tachycardia
Birth through first few days	Any of the above Critical aortic stenosis or critical coarctation Ebstein anomaly with severe tricuspid and/or pulmonary insufficiency Hypoplastic left heart syndrome Intrauterine or neonatal paroxysmal supraventricular tachycardia Metabolic disorders (eg, hypoglycemia, hypothermia, severe metabolic acidosis) Perinatal asphyxia with myocardial damage Severe intrauterine anemia (hydrops fetalis) Total anomalous pulmonary venous return with severe obstruction (usually infracardiac type)
Up to 1 mo	Any of the above Anomalous pulmonary venous drainage (with less severe obstruction) Coarctation of the aorta, with or without associated abnormalities Complete heart block associated with structural heart anomalies Large left-to-right shunts in premature infants (eg, patent ductus arteriosus) Transposition of the great arteries with a large ventricular septal defect
Infancy (especially 6 to 8 wk)	Anomalous pulmonary venous return (unobstructed) Bronchopulmonary dysplasia (right ventricular failure) Complete atrioventricular septal defects Patent ductus arteriosus Persistent truncus arteriosus Rare metabolic disorders (eg, glycogen storage disease) Single ventricle Supraventricular tachycardia Ventricular septal defect
Childhood	Acute cor pulmonale (caused by upper airway obstructions such as large tonsils) Acute rheumatic fever with carditis Acute severe hypertension (with acute glomerulonephritis) Bacterial endocarditis Chronic anemia (severe) Dilated congestive cardiomyopathy Iron overload due to altered iron metabolism (hereditary hemachromatosis) or due to frequent transfusions (eg, for thalassemia major) Nutritional deficiencies Valvular heart disorders due to congenital or acquired cardiac disease (eg, rheumatic fever) Viral myocarditis Volume overload in a noncardiac disorder

vasoconstriction rather than hypoxemia and is a common, normal finding in neonates. Older children with longstanding cyanosis often develop clubbing of the nail beds.

Heart failure: In infants, symptoms or signs of HF include

- Tachycardia
- Tachypnea
- Dyspnea with feeding
- Diaphoresis, especially with feeding
- Restlessness, irritability
- Hepatomegaly

Dyspnea with feeding causes inadequate intake and poor growth, which may be worsened by increased metabolic demands in HF and frequent respiratory tract infections. In contrast to adults and older children, most infants do not have distended neck veins and dependent edema; however, they occasionally have edema in the periorbital area. Findings in older children with HF are similar to those in adults.

Other manifestations: In neonates, circulatory shock may be the first manifestation of certain anomalies (eg, hypoplastic left heart syndrome, critical aortic stenosis, interrupted aortic arch, coarctation of the aorta). Neonates appear extremely ill and have cold extremities, diminished pulses, low BP, and reduced response to stimuli.

Chest pain in children is usually noncardiac. In infants, chest pain may be manifested by unexplained marked irritability, particularly during or after feeding, and can be caused by anomalous origin of the left coronary artery from the pulmonary artery. In older children and adolescents, chest pain due to a cardiac etiology is usually associated with exertion and may be caused by a coronary anomaly, myocarditis, or severe aortic stenosis.

Syncope, typically without warning symptoms and often in association with exertion, may occur with certain anomalies including cardiomyopathy, anomalous origin of a coronary artery, or inherited arrhythmia syndromes (eg, long QT syndrome, Brugada syndrome). High school–age athletes are most commonly affected.

Diagnosis

- Screening by pulse oximetry
- ECG and chest x-ray
- Echocardiography
- Sometimes cardiac MRI or CT angiography, cardiac catheterization with angiocardiography

When present, heart murmurs, cyanosis, abnormal pulses, or manifestations of HF suggest CHD. In such neonates, echocardiography is done to confirm the diagnosis of CHD. If the only abnormality is cyanosis, methemoglobinemia also should be ruled out.

Although echocardiography is typically diagnostic, in select cases, cardiac MRI or CT angiography may clarify important anatomic details. Cardiac catheterization with angiocardiography is occasionally needed to confirm the diagnosis or to assess severity of the anomaly; it is done more often for therapeutic purposes.

Newborn screening: Manifestations of CHD may be subtle or absent in neonates, and failure or delay in detecting CHD, particularly in the 10 to 15% of neonates who require surgical or inpatient medical treatment in the first month of life (termed critical congenital heart disease [CCHD]), may lead to neonatal mortality or significant morbidity. Thus, universal screening for CCHD using pulse oximetry is recommended for all neonates before hospital discharge. The screening is done when infants are ≥ 24 h old and is considered positive if ≥ 1 of the following is present:

- Any oxygen saturation measurement is < 90%.
- The oxygen saturation measurements in both the right hand and foot are < 95% on 3 separate measurements taken 1 h apart.
- There is > 3% absolute difference between the oxygen saturation in the right hand (preductal) and foot (postductal) on 3 separate measurements taken 1 h apart.

All neonates with a positive screen should undergo a comprehensive evaluation for CHD and other causes of hypoxemia (eg, various respiratory disorders, CNS depression, sepsis) typically including a chest x-ray, ECG, echocardiography, and often blood testing. Sensitivity of pulse oximetry screening is slightly > 75%; the CHD lesions most often missed are left heart obstructive lesions (eg, coarctation of the aorta).

Treatment

- Medical stabilization of HF (eg, with oxygen, diuretics, ACE inhibitors, digoxin, and salt restriction)
- Surgical repair or transcatheter intervention

After medical stabilization of acute HF symptoms or cyanosis, most children require surgical or transcatheter repair; the exceptions are certain VSDs that are likely to become smaller or close with time or mild valve dysfunction. Transcatheter procedures include

- Balloon atrial septostomy for palliation of severely cyanotic neonates with transposition of the great arteries (TGA)
- Balloon dilation of severe aortic or pulmonary valve stenosis
- Transcatheter closure of cardiac shunts (most often atrial septal defect and PDA)

Heart failure in neonates: Acute, severe HF or cyanosis in the first week of life is a medical emergency. Secure vascular access should be established, preferably via an umbilical venous catheter.

When CCHD is suspected or confirmed, an IV infusion of prostaglandin E_1 should be started at an initial dose of 0.01 mcg/kg/min. Occasional infants will require higher doses, such as 0.05 to 0.1 mcg/kg/min, to reopen or maintain patency of the ductus arteriosus. Keeping the ductus open is important because most cardiac lesions manifesting at this age are ductal-dependent for either systemic blood flow (eg, hypoplastic left heart syndrome, critical aortic stenosis, coarctation of the aorta) or pulmonary blood flow (cyanotic lesions such as pulmonary atresia or severe tetralogy of Fallot).

Mechanical ventilation is often necessary in critically ill neonates. Supplemental oxygen should be given judiciously or even withheld because oxygen can decrease pulmonary vascular resistance, which is harmful to infants with certain defects (eg, hypoplastic left heart syndrome).

Other therapies for neonatal HF include diuretics, inotropic drugs, and drugs to reduce afterload. The diuretic furosemide is given as an initial bolus of 1 mg/kg IV and titrated based on urine output. Infusions of the inotropes dopamine or dobutamine can support BP but have the disadvantage of increasing heart rate and afterload, thus increasing myocardial oxygen consumption. Milrinone, frequently used in postoperative patients with CHD, is both a positive inotrope and a vasodilator. Dopamine, dobutamine, and milrinone all have the potential to increase the risk of arrhythmias. Nitroprusside, a pure vasodilator, is often used for postoperative hypertension. It is started at 0.3 to 0.5 mcg/kg/min and titrated to desired effect (usual maintenance dose is about 3 mcg/kg/min).

Heart failure in older infants and children: Therapies often include a diuretic (eg, furosemide 0.5 to 1.0 mg/kg IV or 1 to 3 mg/kg po q 8 to 24 h, titrated upward as needed) and an ACE inhibitor (eg, captopril 0.1 to 0.3 mg/kg po tid). A potassium-sparing diuretic (eg, spironolactone 1 mg/kg po once/day or bid, titrated up to 2 mg/kg/dose if needed) may be useful, particularly if high-dose furosemide is required. Beta-blockers (eg, carvedilol, metoprolol) are often added for children with chronic congestive HF. Digoxin is used less often than in the past but may still have a role in children with HF who have large left-to-right shunts, in certain postoperative patients with CHD, and in some infants with supraventricular tachycardia (SVT; dose varies by age; see Table 297–3).

Supplemental oxygen may lessen hypoxemia and alleviate respiratory distress in HF; when possible, fractional inspired oxygen (FIO_2) should be kept < 40% to minimize the risk of pulmonary epithelial damage. Supplemental oxygen must be used with caution, if at all, in patients with left-to-right shunt lesions or left heart obstructive disease because it may exacerbate pulmonary overcirculation.

In general, a healthy diet, including salt restriction, is recommended, although dietary modifications may be needed depending on the specific disorder and manifestations. HF increases metabolic demands and the associated dyspnea makes feeding more difficult. In infants with CCHD, particularly those with left heart obstructive lesions, feedings may be withheld to minimize the risk of necrotizing enterocolitis. In infants with HF due to left-to-right-shunt lesions, enhanced caloric content feedings are recommended; these feedings increase calories supplied and do so with less risk of volume overload. Some children require tube feedings to maintain growth. If these measures do not result in weight gain, surgical repair of the anomaly is indicated.

Endocarditis prophylaxis: Current guidelines of the American Heart Association for prevention of endocarditis state that antibiotic prophylaxis is required for children with CHD who have the following:

- Unrepaired cyanotic CHD (including children with palliative shunts and conduits)
- Completely repaired CHD during the first 6 mo after surgery if prosthetic material or a device was used
- Repaired CHD with residual defects at or adjacent to the site of a prosthetic patch or prosthetic device

Table 297–3. ORAL DIGOXIN DOSAGE IN CHILDREN*

AGE	TOTAL DIGITALIZING DOSE† (mcg/kg)	MAINTENANCE DOSE‡ (mcg/kg bid)
Preterm neonates	20	2.5
Term neonates	30	5
1 mo–2 yr	30–50	5–6
2–5 yr	30–40	4–5
6–10 yr	20–35	2.5–4
> 10 yr§	10–15	1.25–2.5

*All doses are based on ideal body weight for children with normal renal function. The IV dose is 75% of the oral dose.

†The digitalizing dose is usually only necessary when treating arrhythmias or acute congestive heart failure. The total digitalizing dose is usually given over 24 h with half of the dose given initially, followed by one fourth of the dose given twice, separated by 8- to 12-h intervals; ECG monitoring is necessary.

‡The maintenance dose is 25% of the digitalizing dose, given in 2 divided doses.

§Not to exceed adult digitalizing/maintenance doses of 1–1.5 mg/0.125–0.250 mg/day (once/day dosing acceptable after age 10 yr).

ATRIAL SEPTAL DEFECT

An atrial septal defect (ASD) is an opening in the interatrial septum, causing a left-to-right shunt and volume overload of the right atrium and right ventricle. Children are rarely symptomatic, but long-term complications after age 20 yr include pulmonary hypertension, heart failure, and atrial arrhythmias. Adults and, rarely, adolescents may present with exercise intolerance, dyspnea, fatigue, and atrial arrhythmias. A soft midsystolic murmur at the upper left sternal border with wide and fixed splitting of the 2nd heart sound (S2) is common. Diagnosis is by echocardiography. Treatment is transcatheter device closure or surgical repair.

ASDs account for about 6 to 10% of cases of CHD. Most cases are isolated and sporadic, but some are part of a genetic syndrome (eg, mutations of chromosome 5, Holt-Oram syndrome).

Classification: ASDs can be classified by location:

- Ostium secundum: A defect in the fossa ovalis—in the center (or middle) part of the atrial septum
- Sinus venosus: A defect in the posterior aspect of the septum, near the superior vena cava or inferior vena cava, and frequently associated with anomalous return of the right upper or lower pulmonary veins to the right atrium or vena cava
- Ostium primum: A defect in the anteroinferior aspect of the septum, a form of atrioventricular septal (endocardial cushion) defect

Pathophysiology

To understand hemodynamic changes that occur in ASD (and other anomalies), see Fig. 297–1 for normal hemodynamic data.

In ASD, shunting is left to right initially (see Fig. 297–2). Some small ASDs, often just a stretched patent foramen ovale, close spontaneously during the first few years of life. Persistent moderate-to-large ASDs result in large shunts, leading to right atrial and right ventricular volume overload. If unrepaired, these large shunts may lead to pulmonary artery hypertension, elevated pulmonary vascular resistance, and right ventricular hypertrophy by the time people are in their 20s. Atrial arrhythmias, such as supraventricular tachycardia (SVT), atrial flutter, or atrial fibrillation may also occur later. Ultimately, the increase in the pulmonary artery pressure and vascular resistance may result in a bidirectional atrial shunt with cyanosis during adulthood (Eisenmenger reaction).

Symptoms and Signs

Most patients with small or moderate-sized ASDs are asymptomatic. Even large ASDs may not cause symptoms in young children. Larger shunts may cause slow weight gain in early childhood and exercise intolerance, dyspnea during exertion, fatigue, and/or palpitations in older patients. Passage of microemboli from the venous circulation across the ASD (paradoxical embolization), often associated with arrhythmias, may lead to cerebral or systemic thromboembolic events, such as stroke. Rarely, when an ASD is undiagnosed or untreated for decades, Eisenmenger syndrome develops.

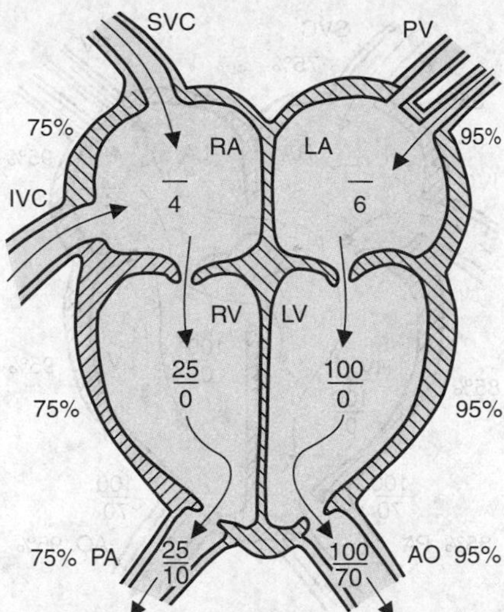

Fig. 297–1. Normal circulation with representative right and left cardiac pressures (in mm Hg). Representative right heart oxygen saturation = 75%; representative left heart oxygen saturation = 95%. Atrial pressures are mean pressures. AO = aorta; IVC = inferior vena cava; LA = left atrium; LV = left ventricle; PA = pulmonary artery; PV = pulmonary veins; RA = right atrium; RV = right ventricle; SVC = superior vena cava.

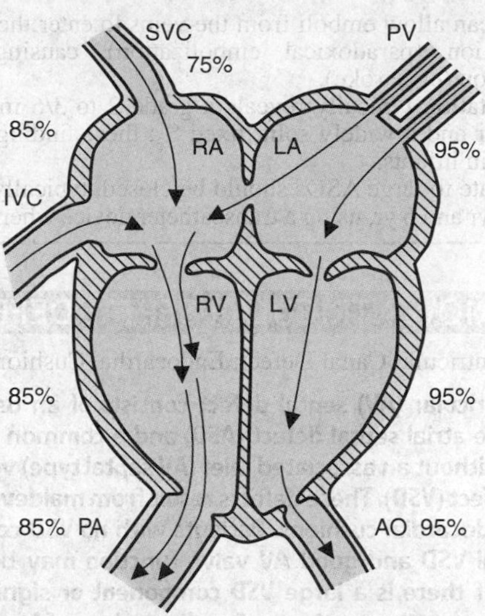

Fig. 297–2. Atrial septal defect. Pulmonary blood flow and RA and RV volume are increased. (NOTE: Intracardiac pressures generally remain in the normal range throughout childhood.) With a large defect, RA and LA pressures are equal. AO = aorta; IVC = inferior vena cava; LA = left atrium; LV =left ventricle; PA = pulmonary artery; PV = pulmonary veins; RA = right atrium; RV = right ventricle; SVC = superior vena cava.

Auscultation typically reveals a grade 2 to 3/6 midsystolic (ejection systolic) murmur (see Table 73–3 on p. 584) and a widely split, fixed S_2 at the upper left sternal border in children. A large left-to-right atrial shunt may produce a rumbling low-pitched diastolic murmur (due to increased tricuspid flow) at the lower sternal borders. These findings may be absent in infants, even those who have a large defect. A prominent right ventricular cardiac impulse, manifested as a parasternal heave or lift, may be present.

Diagnosis

- Chest x-ray and ECG
- Echocardiography

Diagnosis of an ASD is suggested by cardiac examination, chest x-ray, and ECG and is confirmed by 2-dimensional echocardiography with color flow and Doppler studies.

With a significant shunt, ECG may show right axis deviation, right ventricular hypertrophy, or right ventricular conduction delay (an rSR′ pattern in V_1 with a tall R'). Chest x-ray shows cardiomegaly with dilation of the right atrium and right ventricle, a prominent main pulmonary artery segment, and increased pulmonary vascular markings.

Cardiac catheterization is rarely necessary unless transcatheter closure of the defect is planned.

Treatment

- Observation, transcatheter closure, or surgical repair

Most small centrally located ASDs (< 3 mm) close spontaneously; many defects between 3 mm and 8 mm close spontaneously by age 3 yr. These defects probably represent a stretched patent foramen ovale rather than true secundum ASDs. Ostium primum ASDs and sinus venosus ASDs do not close spontaneously.

Asymptomatic children with a small shunt require only observation and periodic echocardiography. Although these children are theoretically at risk of paradoxical systemic embolization, this event is rare in childhood. Thus, it is not standard practice to close a small, hemodynamically insignificant defect.

Moderate to large ASDs (evidence of right ventricular volume overload on echocardiography) should be closed, typically between ages 2 yr and 6 yr. Repair may be considered earlier in children with chronic lung disease. Transcatheter closure with various commercial devices (eg, Amplatzer® or Gore HELEX® septal occluder) is preferred when appropriate anatomic characteristics, such as adequate rims of septal tissue and distance from vital structures (eg, aortic root, pulmonary veins, tricuspid annulus), are present. Otherwise, surgical repair is indicated. Sinus venosus and ostium primum (AV septal type) defects are not amenable to device closure. If ASDs are repaired during childhood, perioperative mortality rate approaches 0, and long-term survival rates approach those of the general population.

Endocarditis prophylaxis is not needed preoperatively and is required only for the first 6 mo after repair or if there is a residual defect adjacent to a surgical patch.

KEY POINTS

- An ASD is an opening in one of several parts of the interatrial septum, causing a left-to-right shunt.
- Small atrial communications often close spontaneously, but larger ones do not, causing right atrial and ventricular overload and ultimately pulmonary artery hypertension, elevated pulmonary vascular resistance, and right ventricular hypertrophy; SVT, atrial flutter, or atrial fibrillation may also occur.

- ASDs can allow emboli from the veins to enter the systemic circulation (paradoxical embolization), causing arterial occlusion (eg, stroke).
- Auscultation typically reveals a grade 2 to 3/6 midsystolic murmur and a widely split, fixed S_2; these findings may be absent in infants.
- Moderate to large ASDs should be closed, typically between ages 2 yr and 6 yr, using a transcatheter device when possible.

ATRIOVENTRICULAR SEPTAL DEFECT

(Atrioventricular Canal Defect; Endocardial Cushion Defect)

Atrioventricular (AV) septal defect consists of an ostium primum type atrial septal defect (ASD) and a common AV valve, with or without an associated inlet (AV septal type) ventricular septal defect (VSD). These defects result from maldevelopment of the endocardial cushions. Patients with no VSD component or a small VSD and good AV valve function may be asymptomatic. If there is a large VSD component or significant AV valve regurgitation, patients often have signs of heart failure, including dyspnea with feeding, poor growth, tachypnea, and diaphoresis. Heart murmurs, tachypnea, tachycardia, and hepatomegaly are common. Diagnosis is by echocardiography. Treatment is surgical repair for all but the smallest defects.

AV septal defect accounts for about 5% of congenital heart anomalies. An AV septal defect may be

- Complete, with a large (nonrestrictive) inlet VSD
- Transitional, with a small or moderate-sized (restrictive) VSD
- Partial, with no VSD

The majority of patients with the complete form have Down syndrome. AV septal defect is also common among patients with asplenia or polysplenia (heterotaxy) syndromes.

Complete AV septal defect: A complete AV septal defect (see Fig. 297–3) consists of a large ostium primum ASD in the anteroinferior aspect of the septum, a nonrestrictive inlet VSD, and a common AV valve orifice. This defect is also called a complete common AV canal defect. A left-to-right shunt occurs at the atrial and ventricular levels and is often large; AV valve regurgitation may be significant, sometimes causing a direct left ventricle-to-right atrial shunt. These abnormalities result in enlargement of all 4 cardiac chambers. Hemodynamic findings are similar to those of a large VSD.

If a complete AV septal defect is unrepaired, over time, the increase in pulmonary blood flow, pulmonary artery pressure, and pulmonary vascular resistance may lead to reversal of shunt direction with cyanosis and Eisenmenger syndrome.

Transitional AV septal defect: A transitional AV septal defect consists of an ostium primum ASD; a restrictive inlet VSD, which may be small or moderate in size; and a common AV valve. This defect is also called transitional AV canal defect. The shunt at the atrial level is usually large. The shunt at the ventricular level is smaller than in complete AV septal defect, and right ventricular pressure is lower than left ventricular pressure. The hemodynamics depend largely on the size of the VSD and whether there is significant AV valve regurgitation.

Partial AV septal defect: A partial AV septal defect consists of an ostium primum ASD and partitioning of the common AV valve into 2 separate AV orifices, resulting in a so-called cleft in the mitral valve (left AV orifice). The ventricular septum is intact. Hemodynamic abnormalities are similar to those of ostium secundum ASD (eg, left-to-right shunt at the atrial level, enlarged right heart chambers, increased pulmonary blood flow) with the additional finding of variable degrees of AV valve regurgitation.

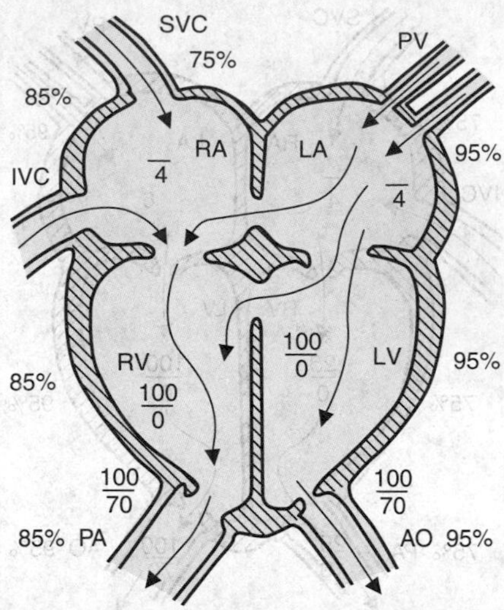

Fig. 297–3. Atrioventricular septal defect (complete form). Pulmonary blood flow, all chamber volumes, and often pulmonary vascular resistance are increased. Atrial pressures are mean pressures. AO = aorta; IVC = inferior vena cava; LA = left atrium; LV = left ventricle; PA = pulmonary artery; PV = pulmonary veins; RA = right atrium; RV = right ventricle; SVC = superior vena cava.

Symptoms and Signs

Complete AV septal defect with a large left-to-right shunt causes signs of heart failure (eg, tachypnea, dyspnea during feeding, poor weight gain, diaphoresis) by age 4 to 6 wk. Pulmonary vascular obstructive disease (Eisenmenger syndrome) is usually a late complication but may occur earlier, especially in children with Down syndrome.

Partial AV septal defects do not usually cause symptoms during childhood if left AV valve regurgitation is mild or absent. However, symptoms (eg, exercise intolerance, fatigue, palpitations) may develop during adolescence or early adulthood. Infants with moderate or severe left AV valve regurgitation often have signs of heart failure. Patients with transitional AV septal defects may have signs of heart failure if the VSD is only mildly restrictive or may be asymptomatic if the VSD is highly restrictive (small).

Physical examination in children with complete AV septal defects shows an active precordium due to volume and pressure overload of the right ventricle; a single, loud 2nd heart sound (S_2) due to pulmonary hypertension; a grade 3 to 4/6 systolic murmur; and sometimes a diastolic murmur at the apex and low left sternal border (see Table 73–3 on p. 584).

Most children with a partial defect have wide splitting of the S_2 and a midsystolic (eg, ejection systolic) murmur audible at the upper left sternal border. A mid-diastolic rumble may be present at the lower left sternal border when the atrial shunt is large. A cleft in the left AV valve results in a blowing apical systolic murmur of mitral regurgitation.

Cardiac findings in children with the partial form are the same as those described for secundum ASD; if mitral regurgitation coexists, there is also a high-pitched holosystolic murmur at the apex.

Diagnosis

- Chest x-ray and ECG
- Echocardiography

Diagnosis of AV septal defects is suggested by clinical examination, supported by chest x-ray and ECG, and established by 2-dimensional echocardiography with color flow and Doppler studies.

Chest x-ray shows cardiomegaly with right atrial enlargement, biventricular enlargement, a prominent main pulmonary artery segment, and increased pulmonary vascular markings.

ECG shows a superiorly directed QRS axis (eg, left axis deviation or northwest axis), frequent 1st-degree AV block, left or right ventricular hypertrophy or both, and occasional right atrial enlargement and right bundle branch block.

Two-dimensional echocardiography with color flow and Doppler studies establishes the diagnosis and can provide important anatomic and hemodynamic information. Cardiac catheterization is not usually necessary unless hemodynamics must be further characterized before surgical repair (for example, to assess pulmonary vascular resistance in a patient presenting at an older age).

Treatment

- Surgical repair
- For heart failure (HF), medical therapy (eg, diuretics, digoxin, ACE inhibitors) before surgery

Complete AV septal defect should be repaired by age 2 to 4 mo because most infants have HF and failure to thrive. Even if infants are growing well without significant symptoms, repair should be done before 6 mo to prevent development of pulmonary vascular disease, especially in infants with Down syndrome.

In patients with 2 adequately sized ventricles and no additional defects, the large central defect (combination of the primum ASD and inlet VSD) is closed and the common AV valve is reconstructed into 2 separate valves. Surgical mortality rate was 5 to 10% in older series but more recently was as low as 3 to 4%. Surgical complications include complete heart block (3%), residual VSD, and/or left AV valve regurgitation.

Pulmonary artery banding may be used, particularly in premature infants or those with associated abnormalities that make complete repair higher risk.

For asymptomatic patients with a partial defect, elective surgery is done at age 1 to 3 yr. Surgical mortality rate should be very low.

In a subset of patients with AV septal defect, the common AV valve is positioned more over one ventricle than the other. This condition, referred to as unbalanced AV septal defect, results in one ventricle receiving more blood flow and underdevelopment of the other ventricle. Surgical intervention for patients with unbalanced AV septal defect, particularly those with a hypoplastic left ventricle, may be a single ventricle type repair.

For patients with large shunts and HF, diuretics, digoxin, and ACE inhibitors may help to manage symptoms before surgery.

Endocarditis prophylaxis is not needed preoperatively and is required only for the first 6 mo after repair or if there is a residual defect adjacent to a surgical patch.

KEY POINTS

- An AV septal defect may be complete, transitional, or partial; the majority of patients with the complete form have Down syndrome.
- A complete AV septal defect involves a large ostium primum ASD, a VSD, and a common AV valve (often with significant regurgitation), all resulting in a large left-to-right shunt at both atrial and ventricular levels and enlargement of all 4 cardiac chambers.
- A partial AV septal defect also involves an ASD, but the common AV valve is partitioned into 2 separate AV orifices and there is no VSD, resulting in enlargement of the right heart chambers because of a large atrial shunt but no ventricular shunt.
- A transitional AV septal defect involves an ostium primum ASD, a common AV valve, and a small- or moderate-size VSD.
- Complete AV septal defect with a large left-to-right shunt causes signs of HF by age 4 to 6 wk.
- Symptoms in partial AV septal defects vary with the degree of mitral regurgitation; if mild or absent, symptoms may develop during adolescence or early adulthood, but infants with moderate or severe mitral regurgitation often have manifestations of HF.
- Symptoms in transitional AV septal defect fall on a spectrum, depending on the size of the VSD.
- Defects are repaired surgically between age 2 to 4 mo and 1 to 3 yr depending on the specific defect and severity of symptoms.

COARCTATION OF THE AORTA

Coarctation of the aorta is a localized narrowing of the aortic lumen that results in upper-extremity hypertension, left ventricular hypertrophy, and malperfusion of the abdominal organs and lower extremities. Symptoms vary with the anomaly's severity and range from headache, chest pain, cold extremities, fatigue, and leg claudication to fulminant heart failure and shock. A soft bruit may be heard over the coarctation site. Diagnosis is by echocardiography or by CT or MR angiography. Treatment is balloon angioplasty with stent placement, or surgical correction.

Coarctation of the aorta accounts for 6 to 8% of congenital heart anomalies. It occurs in 10 to 20% of patients with Turner syndrome. The male:female ratio is 2:1.

Pathophysiology

Coarctation of the aorta usually occurs at the proximal thoracic aorta just beyond the left subclavian artery and before the opening of the ductus arteriosus. Coarctation rarely involves the abdominal aorta. Thus, in utero and before the patent ductus arteriosus (PDA) closes, much of the cardiac output bypasses the coarctation via the PDA. Coarctation may occur alone or with various other congenital anomalies (eg, bicuspid aortic valve, ventricular septal defect, aortic stenosis, PDA, mitral valve disorders, intracerebral aneurysms).

Physiologic consequences involve 2 phenomena:

- Pressure overload in the arterial circulation proximal to the coarctation
- Hypoperfusion distal to the coarctation

Pressure overload causes left ventricular hypertrophy and hypertension in the upper part of the body including the brain.

Hypoperfusion affects the abdominal organs and lower extremities. Malperfusion of the intestine increases the risk of sepsis due to enteric organisms.

Ultimately, the pressure gradient increases collateral circulation to the abdomen and lower extremities via intercostal, internal mammary, scapular, and other arteries.

Untreated coarctation may result in left ventricular hypertrophy, heart failure (HF), collateral vessel formation, bacterial endocarditis, intracranial hemorrhage, hypertensive encephalopathy, and hypertensive cardiovascular disease during adulthood. Patients with untreated coarctation are at increased risk of aortic dissection or rupture later in life or in association with pregnancy. The ascending aorta is the area most frequently involved in dissection or rupture. Current data suggest that this risk is less likely a direct consequence of the coarctation and more likely related to a bicuspid aortic valve and associated aortopathy.

Symptoms and Signs

If coarctation is significant, circulatory shock with renal insufficiency (oliguria or anuria) and metabolic acidosis may develop in the first 7 to 10 days of life and may mimic findings of other systemic disorders such as sepsis. Infants with critical (severe) coarctation are likely to become acutely ill as soon as the ductus arteriosus constricts or closes.

Less severe coarctation may be asymptomatic during infancy. Subtle symptoms (eg, headache; chest pain, fatigue, and leg claudication during physical activities) may be present as children age. Upper-extremity hypertension is often present, but HF rarely develops after the neonatal period. Rarely, intracerebral aneurysms rupture, resulting in subarachnoid or intracerebral hemorrhage.

Typical physical examination findings include strong pulses and hypertension in the upper extremities, diminished or delayed femoral pulses, and a BP gradient, with low or unobtainable arterial BP in the lower extremities.

A grade 2 to 3/6 ejection systolic murmur is often present at the upper left sternal border, left axilla, and sometimes most prominently in the left interscapular area (see Table 73–3 on p. 584). An apical systolic ejection click is present if a bicuspid aortic valve is also present. Dilated intercostal collateral arteries may cause a continuous murmur in the intercostal spaces.

Affected females may have Turner syndrome, a congenital disorder causing lymphedema of the feet, webbed neck, squarely shaped chest, cubitus valgus, and widely spaced nipples.

Diagnosis

- Chest x-ray and ECG
- Echocardiography or CT or MR angiography

Diagnosis is suggested by clinical examination (including BP measurement in all 4 extremities), supported by chest x-ray and ECG, and established by 2-dimensional echocardiography with color flow and Doppler studies or, in older patients with a suboptimal echocardiographic window, with CT or MR angiography.

Chest x-ray shows coarctation as a "3" sign in the upper left mediastinal shadow. Heart size is normal unless HF supervenes. Dilated intercostal collateral arteries may erode the 3rd to 8th ribs, causing rib notching, but this is seldom seen before age 5 yr.

ECG usually shows left ventricular hypertrophy but may be normal. In neonates and small infants, ECG usually shows right ventricular hypertrophy rather than left ventricular hypertrophy.

Treatment

- For symptomatic neonates, prostaglandin E_1 infusion
- For hypertension, beta-blockers
- Surgical correction or balloon angioplasty (sometimes with stent placement)

Symptomatic neonates are treated promptly. In infants who do not have symptoms, the condition is monitored until definitive repair is done.

Medical management of coarctation: Symptomatic neonates require cardiopulmonary stabilization with infusion of prostaglandin E_1 (0.01 to 0.10 mcg/kg/min—titrate to the lowest effective dose) to reopen the constricted ductus arteriosus. Opening the ductus and its aortic ampulla provides some relief by allowing pulmonary artery blood to bypass the aortic obstruction via the ductus and increase perfusion of the descending aorta, improving systemic perfusion and reversing metabolic acidosis.

Diuretics can help treat HF symptoms. IV cardioactive drugs (eg, milrinone, dopamine, dobutamine) can be useful in select circumstances (eg, infants with HF and significant left ventricle dysfunction).

In nonemergent situations, patients with hypertension may be treated with beta-blockers; ACE inhibitors may adversely affect renal function. After repair of the coarctation, hypertension may persist or develop years after repair and can be treated with beta-blockers, ACE inhibitors, angiotensin II receptor blockers, or calcium channel blockers.

Supplemental oxygen should be used with caution in neonates because the resulting decrease in pulmonary vascular resistance may increase pulmonary blood flow at the expense of systemic blood flow.

Surgical management: The preferred definitive treatment is controversial. Some centers prefer balloon angioplasty with or without stent placement, but most prefer surgical correction and reserve the balloon procedure for recoarctation after surgical correction or for primary treatment of discrete coarctation in older children or adolescents. Initial success rate after balloon angioplasty is about 73% in patients with native coarctation and about 80% in patients with recurrent coarctation. Subsequent catheterization can dilate the stent as children grow.

Surgical options include resection and end-to-end anastomosis, patch aortoplasty, and left subclavian flap aortoplasty. In severe coarctation manifesting early in life, the transverse aorta and isthmus are often hypoplastic, and this region of the aorta may need to be surgically enlarged.

Choice of surgical technique depends on anatomy and center preference. Surgical mortality rate is < 5% for symptomatic infants and < 1% for older children. Residual coarctation is common (6 to 33%). Rarely, paraplegia results from cross-clamping of the aorta during surgery.

Endocarditis prophylaxis is not needed preoperatively and is required only for the first 6 mo after repair.

KEY POINTS

- Coarctation of the aorta is a localized narrowing of the lumen, typically in the proximal thoracic aorta just beyond the left subclavian artery and before the opening of the ductus arteriosus.
- Manifestations depend on severity of coarctation but typically involve pressure overload proximal to the coarctation, leading to HF, and hypoperfusion distal to the coarctation.
- Severe coarctation can manifest in the neonatal period with acidosis, renal insufficiency, and shock, but mild coarctation may not be apparent until an adolescent or adult is evaluated for hypertension.
- There is typically a BP gradient between upper and lower extremities and a grade 2 to 3/6 ejection systolic murmur, sometimes most prominent in the left interscapular area.
- For symptomatic neonates, infuse prostaglandin E_1 to reopen the constricted ductus arteriosus.
- Correct coarctation surgically or using balloon angioplasty with or without stent placement.

EISENMENGER SYNDROME

(Pulmonary Vascular Obstructive Disease)

Eisenmenger syndrome is a complication of uncorrected large intracardiac left-to-right shunts. Increased pulmonary resistance may develop over time, eventually leading to bidirectional shunting and then to right-to-left shunting. Deoxygenated blood enters the systemic circulation, causing symptoms of hypoxia. Murmurs and heart sounds depend on the underlying anomaly. Diagnosis is by echocardiography or cardiac catheterization. Treatment is generally supportive, but heart and lung transplantation may be an option when symptoms are severe. Endocarditis prophylaxis is recommended.

Congenital heart anomalies that, if untreated, may result in Eisenmenger syndrome include

- Ventricular septal defect (VSD)
- Atrioventricular (AV) septal defect
- Atrial septal defect (ASD)
- Patent ductus arteriosus (PDA)
- Truncus arteriosus
- Transposition of the great arteries (TGA)

In the US, the incidence has markedly decreased because of early diagnosis and definitive repair of the causative anomaly.

Right-to-left shunting due to Eisenmenger syndrome results in cyanosis and its complications. Systemic oxygen desaturation leads to clubbing of fingers and toes, secondary polycythemia, hyperviscosity, hemoptysis, CNS events (eg, brain abscess or cerebrovascular accident), and sequelae of increased RBC turnover (eg, hyperuricemia causing gout, hyperbilirubinemia causing cholelithiasis, iron deficiency with or without anemia).

Symptoms and Signs

Symptoms of Eisenmenger syndrome usually do not occur until age 20 to 40 yr; they include cyanosis, syncope, dyspnea during exertion, fatigue, chest pain, palpitations, atrial and ventricular arrhythmias, and rarely right heart failure (eg, hepatomegaly, peripheral edema, jugular venous distention).

Hemoptysis is a late symptom. Signs of cerebral embolic phenomena, brain abscess, or endocarditis may develop.

Secondary polycythemia commonly causes symptoms (eg, transient ischemic attacks with slurred speech or other neurologic symptoms, visual problems, headaches, increased fatigue, signs of thromboembolism). Abdominal pain may result from cholelithiasis.

Physical examination detects central cyanosis and digital clubbing. Rarely, signs of right ventricular failure may be present. A holosystolic murmur of tricuspid regurgitation may be present at the lower left sternal border. An early diastolic, decrescendo, high-pitched murmur of pulmonary insufficiency may be audible along the left sternal border. A loud, single 2nd heart sound (S_2) is a constant finding; an ejection click is common. Scoliosis is present in about one third of patients.

Diagnosis

- Chest x-ray and ECG
- Echocardiography or cardiac catheterization

Diagnosis of Eisenmenger syndrome is suspected by history of uncorrected cardiac anomalies, supported by chest x-ray and ECG, and established by 2-dimensional echocardiography with color flow and Doppler studies. Cardiac catheterization is often done to measure pulmonary artery pressure, pulmonary vascular resistance, and response to pulmonary vasodilators.

Laboratory testing shows polycythemia with Hct > 55%. Increased RBC turnover may be reflected as an iron deficiency state (eg, microcythemia), hyperuricemia, and hyperbilirubinemia.

Chest x-ray usually shows prominent central pulmonary arteries, peripheral pulmonary vessel pruning, and right heart enlargement. ECG shows right ventricular hypertrophy, right axis deviation, and, occasionally, right atrial enlargement.

Treatment

- Drugs to treat pulmonary arterial hypertension (eg, prostacyclin analogs, endothelin antagonists, nitric oxide enhancers)
- "Treat and repair" approach
- Supportive care
- Heart and lung transplantation

Ideally, corrective operations should have been done earlier to prevent Eisenmenger syndrome. There is no specific treatment once the syndrome develops, other than heart and lung transplantation, but drugs that may lower pulmonary artery pressure are being studied.

Prostacyclin analogs (eg, treprostinil, epoprostenol), endothelin antagonists (eg, bosentan), and nitric oxide enhancers (eg, sildenafil) have been shown to improve performance on 6-min walk tests and to reduce N-terminal pro-brain natriuretic peptide (NT-proBNP). In a small number of patients, aggressive therapy with advanced pulmonary vasodilating drugs has resulted in net left-to-right shunt, allowing surgical repair of the underlying cardiac defect and significant reduction in mean pulmonary artery pressure. This has been called the treat and repair approach.

Supportive treatment includes avoidance of conditions that may exacerbate the syndrome (eg, pregnancy, volume depletion, isometric exercise, high altitudes) and use of supplemental oxygen.

Symptomatic polycythemia can be treated by cautious phlebotomy to lower Hct to 55 to 65% plus simultaneous volume replacement with normal saline. However, compensated and asymptomatic polycythemia does not require phlebotomy, regardless of Hct; phlebotomy eventually leads to iron deficiency and does not change the natural history.

Hyperuricemia can be treated with allopurinol 300 mg po once/day. Anticoagulation therapy with warfarin is potentially harmful and its use should be individualized, but aspirin 81 mg po once/day is indicated to prevent thrombotic complications.

Life expectancy depends on type and severity of the underlying congenital anomaly and ranges from 20 to 50 yr; median age at death is 37 yr. However, low exercise tolerance and secondary complications severely limit quality of life.

Heart transplantation and lung transplantation may be an option but is reserved for patients with severe symptoms and unacceptable quality of life. Long-term survival after transplantation is not promising.

All patients should be given endocarditis prophylaxis before dental or surgical procedures that are likely to cause bacteremia.

KEY POINTS

- Cardiac anomalies that involve large intracardiac left-to-right shunts often eventually cause increased pulmonary resistance, which first causes bidirectional shunting and ultimately right-to-left shunting (shunt reversal).

- With shunt reversal, deoxygenated blood enters the systemic circulation, causing hypoxia and its complications (eg, clubbing of fingers and toes, secondary polycythemia); polycythemia may cause hyperviscosity, stroke or other thromboembolic disorders, and/or hyperuricemia.
- Symptoms usually do not occur until age 20 to 40 yr; they include cyanosis, syncope, dyspnea during exertion, fatigue, chest pain, palpitations, atrial and ventricular arrhythmias, and rarely right heart failure.
- Doing a corrective operation for the underlying cardiac anomaly at the appropriate age should prevent Eisenmenger syndrome.
- There is no specific treatment once the syndrome develops, other than heart and lung transplantation, but drugs that may lower pulmonary artery pressure (eg, prostacyclin analogs, endothelin antagonists, nitric oxide enhancers) are being studied.

HYPOPLASTIC LEFT HEART SYNDROME

Hypoplastic left heart syndrome consists of hypoplasia of the left ventricle and ascending aorta, maldevelopment and hypoplasia of the aortic and mitral valves (frequently aortic atresia is present), an atrial septal defect (ASD), and a patent ductus arteriosus (PDA). Unless normal closure of the PDA is prevented with prostaglandin infusion, cardiogenic shock and death ensue. A loud, single 2nd heart sound (S_2) and nonspecific systolic murmur are common. Diagnosis is by emergency echocardiography. Definitive treatment is staged surgical correction or heart transplantation.

Hypoplastic left heart syndrome (HLHS) accounts for 2% of congenital heart anomalies. Because the mitral valve, left ventricle, and aortic valve are hypoplastic (often with aortic atresia), oxygenated blood coming into the left atrium from the lungs is diverted across the atrial communication into the right heart, where it mixes with desaturated systemic venous return (see Fig. 297–4). This relatively desaturated blood exits the right ventricle through the pulmonary artery to the lungs and through the ductus arteriosus to the systemic circulation. Systemic blood flow is maintained only through the right-to-left ductal shunt; thus immediate survival depends on patency of the ductus arteriosus.

Symptoms and Signs

Symptoms appear when the ductus arteriosus begins to close during the first 24 to 48 h of life. Subsequently, the clinical picture of cardiogenic shock (eg, tachypnea, dyspnea, weak pulse, pallor, cyanosis, hypothermia, metabolic acidosis, lethargy, oliguria or anuria) rapidly develops. When systemic circulation is compromised, coronary and cerebral perfusion may be reduced, leading to symptoms of myocardial or cerebral ischemia. Perfusion of the kidneys, liver, and mesentery is also inadequate and oliguria or anuria are common. If the ductus arteriosus is not reopened, death rapidly ensues.

The patient often presents with a history of poor feeding, increased work of breathing, pale or gray coloration, and lethargy. Physical examination shows a very active precordium with a marked parasternal lift associated with very poor peripheral perfusion, cool extremities, bluish gray skin color, and absent or barely palpable pulses. The 2nd heart sound (S_2) is loud and single. A soft, nonspecific systolic murmur is often present, as is hepatomegaly. Severe metabolic acidosis is typical, often

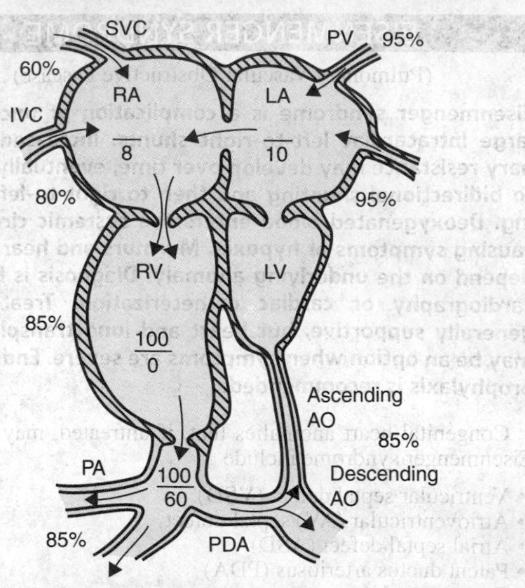

Fig. 297–4. Hypoplastic left heart. The left ventricle, ascending aorta, and aortic and mitral valves are hypoplastic; an ASD and a large PDA are also present. AO = aorta; IVC = inferior vena cava; LA = left atrium; LV = left ventricle; PA = pulmonary artery; PDA = patent ductus arteriosus; PV = pulmonary veins; RA = right atrium; RV = right ventricle; SVC = superior vena cava.

worsening if supplemental oxygen is administered, which is characteristic of hypoplastic left heart syndrome.

Diagnosis

- Chest x-ray and ECG
- Echocardiography

Diagnosis of hypoplastic left heart syndrome is suspected clinically, particularly in neonates with metabolic acidosis that worsens after receiving oxygen; oxygen lowers pulmonary vascular resistance and thus increases the relative proportion of the right ventricle output that flows to the lungs rather than through the PDA to the body. Diagnosis is confirmed by emergency echocardiography.

PEARLS & PITFALLS

- Metabolic acidosis that worsens when supplemental oxygen is administered is characteristic of hypoplastic left heart syndrome.

Cardiac catheterization is rarely required.

Chest x-ray shows cardiomegaly and pulmonary venous congestion or pulmonary edema. ECG shows right ventricular hypertrophy and diminished left ventricular forces, though it may be within normal limits for a neonate.

Treatment

- Prostaglandin E_1 (PGE_1) infusion
- Staged surgical repair
- Sometimes heart transplantation

Fortunately, most patients with hypoplastic left heart syndrome are now diagnosed with prenatal ultrasonography or fetal echocardiography, allowing initiation of prostaglandin E_1 and other appropriate therapies immediately after birth and before organ hypoperfusion can occur.

Medical management: All infants with hypoplastic left heart syndrome should be stabilized immediately in a neonatal ICU or pediatric cardiac ICU. Vascular access should be established rapidly via an umbilical venous catheter and/or peripheral IV, whichever is quicker. PGE_1 (beginning at 0.01 to 0.1 mcg/kg/min IV) is infused to prevent closure of the ductus arteriosus or to reopen a constricted ductus. Neonates, particularly those that are critically ill at presentation, usually require tracheal intubation and mechanical ventilation. Metabolic acidosis is corrected via infusion of sodium bicarbonate. Severely ill neonates with cardiogenic shock may require inotropic drugs (eg, milrinone) and diuretics to improve cardiac function and control volume status.

It is critical to keep pulmonary vascular resistance relatively high and systemic vascular resistance low to prevent marked pulmonary overcirculation at the expense of systemic perfusion. These resistance ranges are maintained by avoiding hyperoxia, alkalosis, and hypocarbia, all of which may lead to pulmonary vasodilation. Because oxygen is one of the most potent pulmonary vasodilators, infants are ventilated with room air or even hypoxic gas mixtures to aim for systemic saturations of 70 to 80%. If the infant requires mechanical ventilation, Pco_2 can be controlled in the high normal or mildly elevated range. Systemic vascular resistance is managed by avoiding, or minimizing, the use of vasoconstricting drugs (eg, epinephrine or high-dose dopamine). Milrinone may be beneficial because it can cause systemic vasodilation.

PEARLS & PITFALLS

- Keep pulmonary vascular resistance relatively high and systemic vascular resistance low to avoid increasing pulmonary circulation at the expense of systemic perfusion.
- Thus, avoid hyperoxia, alkalosis, and hypocarbia (which cause pulmonary vasodilation) and minimize use of vasoconstrictors.

Surgical procedures: Survival ultimately requires staged surgical procedures that enable the right ventricle to function as the systemic ventricle and control pulmonary blood flow.

Stage 1, done during the first week of life, is the Norwood procedure. The main pulmonary artery is divided, the distal stump is closed with a patch, and the hypoplastic aorta and proximal pulmonary artery are combined into a neoaorta. The ductus arteriosus is ligated. Pulmonary blood flow is reestablished by inserting a right-sided modified Blalock-Taussig shunt or a right ventricular-pulmonary artery conduit (Sano modification). Finally, the atrial septal communication is enlarged. An alternative hybrid procedure, often a joint effort of heart surgeons and interventional cardiologists, involves inserting a stent into the ductus arteriosus (to maintain systemic blood flow) and placing bilateral branch pulmonary artery bands (to limit pulmonary blood flow). In some centers, the hybrid procedure is reserved for higher risk patients (eg, premature infants, those with multisystem organ dysfunction).

Stage 2, done at 3 to 6 mo of age, consists of a bidirectional Glenn or hemi-Fontan procedure (connection of the superior vena cava to the right pulmonary artery). The 3rd stage, done at 18 to 36 mo, is a modified Fontan procedure.

Survival rate is 75% for stage 1, 95% for stage 2, and 90% for stage 3. Overall survival rate is about 70% at 5 yr after surgical correction. As with other children with complex congenital heart disease, survivors may have some degree of neurodevelopmental disability, which may be due to preexisting developmental abnormalities of the CNS or to overt or occult CNS hypoperfusion or thromboemboli occurring during the multistage procedures.

In some centers, **heart transplantation** is considered the procedure of choice for hypoplastic left heart syndrome; however, PGE_1 infusion must be continued along with careful management of pulmonary and systemic vascular resistance until a donor heart is available. Because availability of donor hearts is very limited, about 20% of infants die while awaiting transplant. The 5-yr survival rates after transplantation and after multistage surgery are similar. After heart transplantation, immunosuppressants are required. These drugs make patients more susceptible to infections and cause pathologic changes in the coronary arteries of the transplanted heart in a significant percentage of patients over a 5-yr period. The only known treatment for allograft coronary artery disease is retransplantation.

Endocarditis prophylaxis is recommended preoperatively and for at least 6 mo after each surgical intervention and subsequently for as long as the patient remains cyanotic or has a residual defect adjacent to a surgical patch or prosthetic material.

KEY POINTS

- In hypoplastic left heart syndrome, there is hypoplasia of the left ventricle and ascending aorta and maldevelopment and hypoplasia of the aortic and mitral valves; an ASD and a PDA are necessary for systemic blood flow (and thus immediate survival).
- Symptoms of cardiogenic shock (eg, tachypnea, dyspnea, weak pulse, pallor, cyanosis, hypothermia, metabolic acidosis, lethargy, oliguria or anuria) appear when the ductus arteriosus begins to close during the first 24 to 48 h of life, becoming more pronounced if supplemental oxygen is given.
- Initially, give PGE_1 to keep the ductus arteriosus open, give as little oxygen as possible (to avoid increasing pulmonary flow at the expense of systemic flow), and avoid vasoconstrictors; give sodium bicarbonate as needed.
- Definitive treatment requires staged operations.

OTHER CONGENITAL CARDIAC ANOMALIES

Other structural congenital cardiac anomalies include the following:

- Single ventricle with or without pulmonary stenosis
- Pulmonary atresia with an intact ventricular septum
- Double outlet right ventricle
- Ebstein anomaly
- Congenitally corrected transposition

Rare nonstructural cardiac anomalies include

- Congenital complete heart block
- Congenital metabolic errors leading to cardiomyopathy

Long QT syndrome and other genetic arrhythmia syndromes with risks of severe and possibly fatal ventricular arrhythmias are discussed elsewhere.

Single ventricle spectrum: These anomalies include any complex lesion with only one functional ventricle and include hypoplastic right ventricle (RV) and left ventricle (LV) and, less commonly, a true undifferentiated single ventricular chamber. Surgical management involves ensuring adequate pulmonary blood flow via a systemic-to-pulmonary artery anastomosis (eg, modified Blalock-Taussig shunt [see p. 2510]) for patients with decreased pulmonary blood flow or protecting the pulmonary vascular bed via pulmonary artery banding if pulmonary overcirculation exists. Later, the Fontan procedure (see p. 2513) can be used as definitive treatment to make the functioning single ventricle solely a systemic ventricle.

Pulmonary atresia with intact septum: This anomaly is most frequently associated with hypoplasia of the tricuspid valve and right ventricle. Coronary arterial abnormalities, particularly fistulous connections of the coronary arteries to the hypoplastic right ventricle and coronary artery stenoses, are common and have a major impact on prognosis and surgical options.

Double outlet right ventricle: This anomaly is associated with a very wide spectrum of anatomy and physiology depending on the size and location of the ventricular septal defect (VSD), as well as the presence and degree of pulmonic stenosis. In the most common variety with a subaortic VSD, a complete repair is possible with closure of the VSD in such a way as to direct left ventricular outflow to the aorta.

Ebstein anomaly: This anomaly consists of variable apical displacement and dysplasia of the septal and inferior leaflets of the tricuspid valve with dysplasia, but normal origin, of the anterior leaflet as well. These abnormalities displace the effective valve orifice downward, resulting in compromise of the function of the right ventricle with an atrialized portion that is proximal to the valve opening. This anomaly has been associated with maternal use of lithium during pregnancy. Associated abnormalities include atrial septal defect (ASD), pulmonic stenosis, and Wolff-Parkinson-White syndrome.

There is a remarkably wide spectrum of presentation, ranging from severely cyanotic newborns to cardiomegaly with mild cyanosis in childhood to a previously asymptomatic adult presenting with atrial arrhythmias or reentry supraventricular tachycardia. The onset of symptoms depends on the degree of tricuspid valve anatomic and functional derangement and presence of accessory pathways (eg, Wolff-Parkinson-White syndrome). When symptoms result from a severely dysfunctional tricuspid valve, surgical repair should be considered.

Congenitally corrected transposition (Levo-transposition): This anomaly is relatively rare and accounts for about 0.5% of congenital cardiac anomalies. The normal embryologic looping of the fetal heart tube is reversed, resulting in atrioventricular and ventriculoarterial discordance. The result is the right atrium connects to a right-sided morphologic left ventricle (LV) and the left atrium connects to a left-sided morphologic right ventricle (RV). In almost all cases, the morphologic LV connects to the pulmonary artery and the morphologic RV connects to the aorta. The circulation is thus physiologically "corrected," but associated anomalies are present in the majority of patients, including VSD, pulmonic stenosis, Ebstein anomaly or other dysplasia of the left-sided tricuspid valve, congenital atrioventricular block, mesocardia or dextrocardia, and heterotaxy syndromes.

These anomalies result in a wide range of clinical manifestations. As patients reach adulthood, a common concern is the development of dysfunction of the morphologic RV, which serves as the systemic ventricle. This dysfunction may be subclinical or manifest as severe cardiomyopathy and heart failure, leading to consideration of heart transplantation.

PATENT DUCTUS ARTERIOSUS

(Persistent Ductus Arteriosus)

Patent ductus arteriosis (PDA) is a persistence of the fetal connection (ductus arteriosus) between the aorta and pulmonary artery after birth. In the absence of other structural heart abnormalities or elevated pulmonary vascular resistance, shunting in the PDA will be left to right (from aorta to pulmonary artery). Symptoms may include failure to thrive, poor feeding, tachycardia, and tachypnea. A continuous murmur at the upper left sternal border is common. Diagnosis is by echocardiography. Administration of a cyclo-oxygenase (COX) inhibitor (ibuprofen lysine or indomethacin) with or without fluid restriction may be tried in premature infants with a significant shunt, but this therapy is not effective in term infants or older children with PDA. If the connection persists, surgical or catheter-based correction is indicated.

PDA accounts for 5 to 10% of congenital heart anomalies; the male:female ratio is 1:3. PDA is very common among premature infants (present in about 45% with birth weight < 1750 g and in 70 to 80% with birth weight < 1200 g). About one third of PDAs will close spontaneously, even in extremely low birth weight infants. When persistent in premature infants, a significant PDA can result in heart failure, pulmonary hemorrhage, renal insufficiency, feeding intolerance, necrotizing enterocolitis, and even death.

Pathophysiology

The ductus arteriosus is a normal connection between the pulmonary artery and aorta; it is necessary for proper fetal circulation. At birth, the rise in Pao_2 and decline in prostaglandin concentration cause closure of the ductus arteriosus, typically beginning within the first 10 to 15 h of life. If this normal process does not occur, the ductus arteriosus will remain patent (see Fig. 297–5).

Physiologic consequences depend on ductal size. A small ductus rarely causes symptoms. A large ductus causes a large left-to-right shunt. Over time, a large shunt results in left heart enlargement, pulmonary artery hypertension, and elevated pulmonary vascular resistance, ultimately leading to Eisenmenger syndrome.

Symptoms and Signs

Clinical presentation depends on PDA size and gestational age at delivery. Infants and children with a small PDA are generally asymptomatic; infants with a large PDA present with signs of heart failure (eg, failure to thrive, poor feeding, tachypnea,

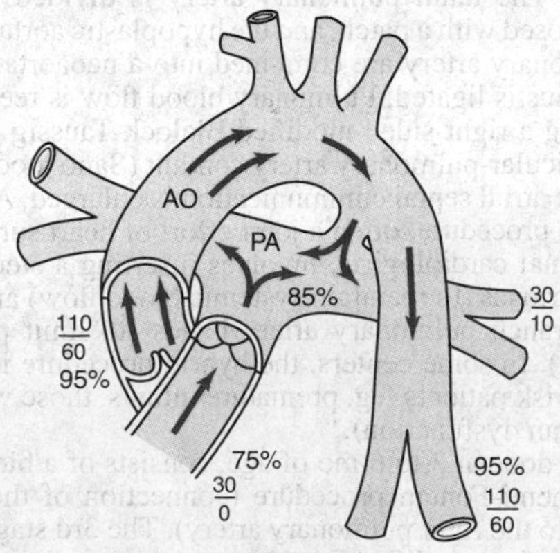

Fig. 297–5. Patent ductus arteriosis. Pulmonary blood flow, LA and LV volumes, and ascending AO volume are increased. AO = aorta; LA = left atrium; LV = left ventricle; PA = pulmonary artery.

dyspnea with feeding, tachycardia). Premature infants may present with respiratory distress, apnea, worsening mechanical ventilation requirements, or other serious complications (eg, necrotizing enterocolitis). Signs of heart failure occur earlier in premature infants than in full-term infants and may be more severe. A large ductal shunt in a premature infant often is a major contributor to the severity of the lung disease of prematurity.

Most children with a small PDA have normal heart sounds and peripheral pulses. A grade 1 to 3/6 continuous murmur is heard best in the upper left sternal border (see Table 73–3 on p. 584). The murmur extends from systole to beyond the 2nd heart sound (S_2) into diastole and typically has a different pitch in systole and diastole.

Full-term infants with a significant PDA shunt have full or bounding peripheral pulses with a wide pulse pressure. A grade 1 to 4/6 continuous murmur is characteristic. If the murmur is loud, it has a "machinery-sounding" quality. An apical diastolic rumble (due to high flow across the mitral valve) or gallop rhythm may be audible if there is a large left-to-right shunt or heart failure develops.

Premature infants with a significant shunt have bounding pulses and a hyperdynamic precordium. A heart murmur occurs in the pulmonary area; the murmur may be continuous, systolic with a short diastolic component, or only systolic, depending on the pulmonary artery pressure. Some infants have no audible heart murmur.

Diagnosis

- Chest x-ray and ECG
- Echocardiography

Diagnosis is suggested by clinical examination, supported by chest x-ray and ECG, and established by 2-dimensional echocardiography with color flow and Doppler studies.

Chest x-ray and ECG are typically normal if the PDA is small. If the shunt is significant, chest x-ray shows prominence of the left atrium, left ventricle, and ascending aorta and increased pulmonary vascular markings; ECG may show left ventricular hypertrophy.

Echocardiography provides important information about the hemodynamic significance of a PDA by assessing a number of parameters, including the

- Size of the PDA (often compared to the left pulmonary artery size)
- Flow velocity in the PDA
- Presence of left heart enlargement
- Presence of diastolic reversal of flow in the descending aorta
- Presence of diastolic antegrade flow in the left pulmonary artery

Cardiac catheterization is not necessary unless used for therapy.

Treatment

- Supportive medical therapy
- In symptomatic premature infants, COX inhibitor therapy (eg, indomethacin, ibuprofen lysine)
- Sometimes transcatheter closure or surgical repair

Typical medical management of PDA includes fluid restriction, a diuretic (usually a thiazide), maintenance of hematocrit ≥ 35, providing a neutral thermal environment, and, for ventilated patients, use of positive end-expiratory pressure (PEEP) to improve gas exchange.

Treatment differs depending on whether the infant is premature or full term.

PDA treatment in premature infants: Fluid restriction may facilitate ductal closure.

In premature infants without respiratory or other compromise, a PDA is typically not treated.

In premature infants with a hemodynamically significant PDA and compromised respiratory status, the PDA can sometimes be closed by using a COX inhibitor (either ibuprofen lysine or indomethacin [see Table 297–4 for doses]). COX inhibitors work by blocking the production of prostaglandins. Three doses of indomethacin are given IV q 12 to 24 h based on urine output; doses are withheld if urine output is < 0.6 mL/kg/h. An alternative is ibuprofen lysine 10 mg/kg po followed by 2 doses of 5 mg/kg at 24-h intervals.

In the past, if fluid restriction and/or COX inhibitor was unsuccessful, the PDA was ligated surgically. Over the past decade, it has been recognized that this nonselective approach to PDA therapy has not resulted in better long-term outcomes. More recent efforts have focused on better defining the subgroup of patients with a hemodynamically significant PDA in whom surgery is more likely to be beneficial. Echocardiography plays an important role in this determination of hemodynamic significance.

A few centers have successfully used transcatheter closure of PDAs in preterm infants < 2 kg.

PDA treatment in full-term infants: In full-term infants, COX inhibitors are usually ineffective.

Transcatheter closure has become the treatment of choice for PDA in children > 1 yr, and some authors consider transcatheter closure to be the preferred route in term neonates and young infants as well. A variety of catheter-delivered occlusion devices are available (eg, coils, septal duct occluder).

In infants < 1 yr who have ductal anatomy unfavorable for transcatheter closure, surgical division and ligation may be preferred over the transcatheter approach. For a PDA with a shunt large enough to cause symptoms of heart failure or pulmonary hypertension, closure should be done after medical stabilization. For a persistent PDA without heart failure or pulmonary hypertension, closure can be done electively any time after 1 yr. Delaying the procedure minimizes the risk of a vascular complication and allows time for spontaneous closure.

Outcomes after PDA closure are excellent.

Endocarditis prophylaxis is not needed preoperatively and is required only for the first 6 mo after closure or if there is a residual defect adjacent to a transcatheter-placed device or surgical material.

KEY POINTS

- PDA is a persistence after birth of the normal fetal connection (ductus arteriosus) between the aorta and pulmonary artery, resulting in a left-to-right shunt.
- Manifestations depend on the size of the PDA and the age of the child, but a continuous murmur is characteristic and, if loud, has a "machinery-sounding" quality.
- Premature infants may have respiratory distress or other serious complications (eg, necrotizing enterocolitis).

Table 297–4. INDOMETHACIN DOSING GUIDELINES (MG/KG)*

AGE AT DOSE 1	DOSE 1	DOSE 2	DOSE 3
< 48 h	0.2	0.1	0.1
2–7 days	0.2	0.2	0.2
> 7 days	0.2	0.25	0.25

*Dose intervals are based on urine output (see text).

- Over time, a large shunt causes left heart enlargement, pulmonary artery hypertension, and elevated pulmonary vascular resistance, ultimately leading to Eisenmenger syndrome if untreated.
- For premature infants with hemodynamically significant PDA, give a COX inhibitor (eg. ibuprofen lysine or indomethacin). Surgical closure may benefit patients with a hemodynamically significant PDA in whom medical therapy has failed.
- For full-term infants and older children, COX inhibitors are usually ineffective but catheter-delivered occlusion devices or surgery is typically beneficial.

PERSISTENT TRUNCUS ARTERIOSUS

Persistent truncus arteriosus occurs when, during fetal development, the primitive truncus does not divide into the pulmonary artery and aorta, resulting in a single, large, arterial trunk that overlies a large, malaligned, perimembranous ventricular septal defect (VSD). Consequently, a mixture of oxygenated and deoxygenated blood enters systemic, pulmonary, and coronary circulations. Symptoms include cyanosis and heart failure, with poor feeding, diaphoresis, and tachypnea. A normal 1st heart sound (S_1) and a loud, single 2nd heart sound (S_2) are common; murmurs may vary. Diagnosis is by echocardiography or cardiac catheterization. Medical treatment for heart failure is typically followed by early surgical repair.

Persistent truncus arteriosus (see Fig. 297–6) accounts for 1 to 2% of congenital heart anomalies. About 35% of patients have 22q11 deletion syndrome, which includes DiGeorge syndrome and velocardiofacial syndromes.

Classification: There are several classification systems in use.

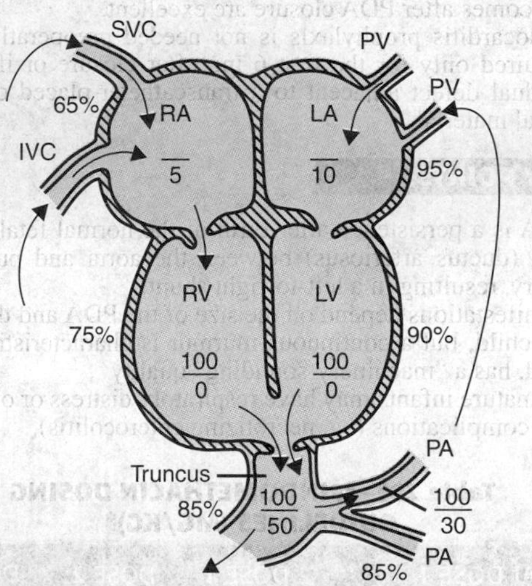

Fig. 297–6. Truncus arteriosus. The primitive truncus does not divide into the pulmonary artery and aorta, resulting in a single large arterial trunk that overlies a large VSD. IVC = inferior vena cava; LA = left atrium; LV = left ventricle; PA = pulmonary artery; PV = pulmonary veins; RA = right atrium; RV = right ventricle; SVC = superior vena cava.

The first classification, by Collett and Edwards, is

- Type I: The main pulmonary artery arises from the truncus and then divides into the right and left pulmonary arteries.
- Type II: The right and left pulmonary arteries arise separately (but adjacent to each other) from the posterior aspect of the truncus.
- Type III: The right and left pulmonary arteries arise from the lateral aspects of the truncal root reasonably distant from each other.
- Type IV: Both pulmonary arteries are supplied by collateral vessels from the descending aorta. (Type IV is now reclassified as tetralogy of Fallot with pulmonary atresia.)

An updated classification by Van Praagh consists of type A (truncus arteriosus *with* VSD) and the very rare type B (truncus arteriosus *without* VSD). Type A is subdivided into 4 types:

- Type A1: The main pulmonary artery arises from the truncus and then divides into right and left pulmonary arteries.
- Type A2: The right and left pulmonary arteries arise separately from the posterior aspect of the truncus.
- Type A3: One lung is supplied by a pulmonary artery branch that arises from the truncus and the other lung (usually the left) is supplied by a ductus-like collateral artery
- Type A4: The truncus is a large pulmonary artery and the aortic arch is interrupted or coarctation is present.

The truncal valve may be quite abnormal and manifest with stenosis, insufficiency, or both. Other anomalies (eg, right aortic arch, interrupted aortic arch, coronary artery anomalies, AV septal defect) may be present and may contribute to the high surgical mortality rate.

Physiologic consequences of truncus arteriosus include mild cyanosis, significant pulmonary overcirculation, and heart failure.

Symptoms and Signs

Infants usually present with mild cyanosis and symptoms and signs of heart failure (eg, tachypnea, poor feeding, diaphoresis) in the first few weeks of life. Physical examination may detect a hyperdynamic precordium, increased pulse pressure with bounding pulses, a loud and single 2nd heart sound (S_2), and an ejection click. A grade 2 to 4/6 systolic murmur is audible along the left sternal border (see Table 73–3 on p. 584). A mid-diastolic mitral flow murmur may be audible at the apex when pulmonary blood flow is increased. With truncal valve insufficiency, a high-pitched diastolic decrescendo murmur is audible over the mid left sternal border.

Diagnosis

- Chest x-ray and ECG
- Echocardiography
- Occasionally cardiac catheterization, cardiac MRI, or CT angiography

Diagnosis is suspected clinically, supported by chest x-ray and ECG, and established by 2-dimensional echocardiography with color flow and Doppler studies. Cardiac catheterization is occasionally necessary to delineate associated anomalies before surgery, but cardiac MRI or CT angiography may supplant the need for catheterization.

Chest x-ray shows varying degrees of cardiomegaly with increased pulmonary vascular markings, right aortic arch (in about 30%), and relatively high position of pulmonary arteries. ECG commonly shows combined ventricular hypertrophy. Substantial pulmonary overcirculation may produce evidence of left atrial enlargement.

Treatment

- Medical treatment of heart failure (eg, diuretics, digoxin, ACE inhibitors) before surgery
- Surgical repair

Heart failure is treated vigorously with diuretics, digoxin, and ACE inhibitors, followed by early surgical repair. Prostaglandin infusion is not beneficial unless there is interruption or coarctation of the aortic arch, in which case right-to-left shunt through the ductus provides systemic blood flow.

Surgical management consists of complete repair. The VSD is closed so that the left ventricle ejects into the truncal root. Usually, continuity between the right ventricle and the confluence of the pulmonary arteries is achieved using a conduit with or without a valve. Some centers have reported good success using a nonconduit approach, in which the left atrial appendage is used as the posterior wall of the pulmonary outflow and a patch is used as the anterior wall, with or without the insertion of a monocusp valve.

When a conduit is placed during early infancy, its size becomes inadequate as children grow, and the conduit must be revised during childhood. When the patient's own tissue is used for part of this outflow tract, there is the potential for growth as the child grows.

Branch pulmonary artery stenosis is a common sequela. Surgical mortality rates have decreased to as low as 10% in recent years.

Endocarditis prophylaxis is recommended preoperatively but is required only for the first 6 mo after repair unless there is a residual defect adjacent to a surgical patch or prosthetic material.

KEY POINTS

- In persistent truncus arteriosus, the primitive truncus does not divide into the pulmonary artery and aorta, resulting in a single large arterial trunk that overlies a large VSD.
- Different types are distinguished based on the origin of the pulmonary arteries and associated defects.
- Patients present with mild cyanosis, significant pulmonary overcirculation, and heart failure; a grade 2 to 4/6 systolic murmur is audible along the left sternal border and a mid-diastolic mitral flow murmur may be audible at the apex.
- Treat heart failure with diuretics, digoxin, and ACE inhibitors; prostaglandin infusion is beneficial only in patients with type A4 truncus with interrupted aortic arch or coarctation.
- Do surgical repair early; one or more revisions are usually needed as children grow.

TETRALOGY OF FALLOT

Tetralogy of Fallot consists of 4 features: a large ventricular septal defect (VSD), right ventricular outflow tract and pulmonary valve obstruction, right ventricular hypertrophy, and over-riding of the aorta. Symptoms include cyanosis, dyspnea with feeding, poor growth, and hypercyanotic "tet" spells (sudden, potentially lethal episodes of severe cyanosis). A harsh systolic murmur at the left upper sternal border with a single 2nd heart sound (S2) is common. Diagnosis is by echocardiography. Cardiac catheterization may be done. Definitive treatment is surgical repair.

Tetralogy of Fallot (see Fig. 297–7) accounts for 7 to 10% of congenital heart anomalies. Associated anomalies include right

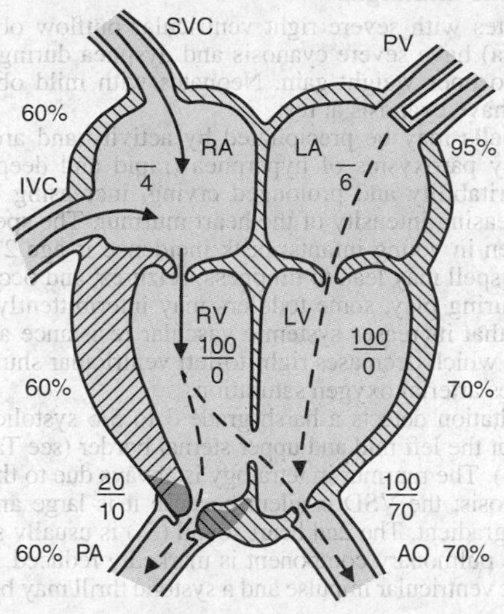

Fig. 297–7. Tetralogy of Fallot. Pulmonary blood flow is decreased, the RV is hypertrophied, and unoxygenated blood enters the AO. Systolic pressures in the RV, LV, and AO are identical. Level of arterial desaturation is related to severity of the RV outflow tract obstruction. Atrial pressures are mean pressures. AO = aorta; IVC = inferior vena cava; LA =left atrium; LV = left ventricle; PA = pulmonary artery; PV = pulmonary veins; RA = right atrium; RV = right ventricle; SVC = superior vena cava.

aortic arch (25%), abnormal coronary artery anatomy (5%), stenosis of the pulmonary artery branches, presence of aorticopulmonary collateral vessels, patent ductus arteriosus (PDA), complete atrioventricular (AV) septal defect, atrial septal defect (ASD), additional muscular VSDs, and aortic valve regurgitation.

Pathophysiology

The VSD is typically large; thus, systolic pressures in the right and left ventricles (and in the aorta) are the same. Pathophysiology depends on the degree of right ventricular outflow obstruction. A mild obstruction may result in a net left-to-right shunt through the VSD; a severe obstruction causes a right-to-left shunt, resulting in low systemic arterial saturation (cyanosis) that is unresponsive to supplemental oxygen.

Tet spells: In some children with unrepaired tetralogy of Fallot, most often those several months up to 2 yr of age, sudden episodes of profound cyanosis and hypoxia (tet spell) may occur, which may be lethal. A spell may be triggered by any event that slightly decreases oxygen saturation (eg, crying, defecating) or that suddenly decreases systemic vascular resistance (eg, playing, kicking legs when awakening) or by sudden onset of tachycardia or hypovolemia.

The mechanism of a tet spell remains uncertain, but several factors are probably important in causing an increase in right-to-left shunting and a fall in arterial saturation. Factors include an increase in right ventricular outflow tract obstruction, an increase in pulmonary vascular resistance, and/or a decrease in systemic resistance—a vicious circle caused by the initial fall in arterial Po_2, which stimulates the respiratory center and causes hyperpnea and increased adrenergic tone. The increased circulating catecholamines then stimulate increased contractility, which increases outflow tract obstruction.

Symptoms and Signs

Neonates with severe right ventricular outflow obstruction (or atresia) have severe cyanosis and dyspnea during feeding, leading to poor weight gain. Neonates with mild obstruction may not have cyanosis at rest.

Tet spells may be precipitated by activity and are characterized by paroxysms of hyperpnea (rapid and deep respirations), irritability and prolonged crying, increasing cyanosis, and decreasing intensity of the heart murmur. The spells occur most often in young infants; peak incidence is age 2 to 4 mo. A severe spell may lead to limpness, seizures, and occasionally death. During play, some toddlers may intermittently squat, a position that increases systemic vascular resistance and aortic pressure, which decreases right-to-left ventricular shunting and thus raises arterial oxygen saturation.

Auscultation detects a harsh grade 3 to 5/6 systolic ejection murmur at the left mid and upper sternal border (see Table 73–3 on p. 584). The murmur in tetralogy is always due to the pulmonary stenosis; the VSD is silent because it is large and has no pressure gradient. The 2nd heart sound (S_2) is usually single because the pulmonary component is markedly reduced. A prominent right ventricular impulse and a systolic thrill may be present.

Diagnosis

- Chest x-ray and ECG
- Echocardiography

Diagnosis of tetralogy of Fallot is suggested by history and clinical examination, supported by chest x-ray and ECG, and established by 2-dimensional echocardiography with color flow and Doppler studies. Chest x-ray shows a boot-shaped heart with a concave main pulmonary artery segment and diminished pulmonary vascular markings. A right aortic arch is present in 25%.

ECG shows right ventricular hypertrophy and may also show right atrial hypertrophy.

Cardiac catheterization is rarely needed, unless there is suspicion of a coronary anomaly that might affect the surgical approach (eg, anterior descending arising from the right coronary artery) that cannot be clarified with echocardiography.

Treatment

- For symptomatic neonates, prostaglandin E_1 infusion
- For tet spells, knee-chest positioning, calming, oxygen, and sometimes drugs
- Surgical repair

Neonates with severe cyanosis may be palliated with an infusion of prostaglandin E_1 (0.01 to 0.1 mcg/kg/min IV) to open the ductus arteriosus and thereby increase pulmonary blood flow.

Tet spells: Tet spells require immediate intervention. The first steps are to place infants in a knee-chest position (older children usually squat spontaneously and do not develop tet spells), establish a calm environment, and give supplemental oxygen. If the spell persists, standard medical therapy includes morphine 0.1 to 0.2 mg/kg IV or IM, IV fluids for volume expansion and, if metabolic acidosis is present, sodium bicarbonate 1 mEq/kg IV.

Intranasal midazolam and intranasal fentanyl are alternatives to morphine and have the advantage of not requiring IV access.

Other options for more severe or prolonged tet spells include phenylephrine starting at 5 to 20 mcg/kg IV every 10 to 15 min as needed (to a maximum of 500 mg) followed by an infusion of 0.1 mcg/kg/min (to a maximum of 5 mcg/kg/min) if needed and beta-blockers (propranolol 0.015 mg/kg IV infused over 10 min (to a maximum of 1mg) or esmolol 0.1 to 0.5 mg/kg IV over 1 min followed by an infusion of 25 to 100 mcg/kg/min if needed. If these measures do not control the spell, systemic BP can be increased with ketamine 0.5 to 3 mg/kg IV or 2 to 3 mg/kg IM (ketamine also has a beneficial sedating effect).

Ultimately, if the preceding steps do not relieve the spell or if the infant is rapidly deteriorating, tracheal intubation with muscle paralysis and general anesthesia, extracorporeal membrane oxygenation (ECMO), or urgent surgical intervention may be necessary. Propranolol 0.25 to 1 mg/kg po q 6 h may prevent recurrences, but most experts feel that even one significant spell indicates the need for expeditious surgical repair.

Definitive management: Complete repair of tetralogy of Fallot consists of patch closure of the VSD, widening of the right ventricular outflow tract with muscle resection and pulmonary valvuloplasty, and a limited patch across the pulmonic annulus or main pulmonary artery if necessary. Surgery is usually done electively at age 3 to 6 mo but can be done at any time if symptoms are present.

In some neonates with low birth weight or complex anatomy, initial palliation may be preferred to complete repair; the usual procedure is a modified Blalock-Taussig shunt, in which the subclavian artery is connected to the ipsilateral pulmonary artery with a synthetic graft.

Perioperative mortality rate for complete repair is < 5% for uncomplicated tetralogy of Fallot. For untreated patients, survival rates are 55% at 5 yr and 30% at 10 yr.

Endocarditis prophylaxis is recommended preoperatively but is required only for the first 6 mo after repair unless there is a residual defect adjacent to a surgical patch or prosthetic material.

KEY POINTS

- Tetralogy of Fallot involves a large VSD, right ventricular outflow tract and pulmonary valve obstruction, and overriding of the aorta.
- Pulmonary blood flow is decreased, the right ventricle hypertrophies, and unoxygenated blood enters the aorta via the VSD.
- Manifestations depend on the degree of right ventricle outflow obstruction; severely affected neonates have marked cyanosis, dyspnea with feeding, poor weight gain, and a harsh grade 3 to 5/6 systolic ejection murmur.
- Tet spells are sudden episodes of profound cyanosis and hypoxia that may be triggered by a fall in oxygen saturation (eg, during crying, defecating), decreased systemic vascular resistance (eg, during playing, kicking legs), or sudden tachycardia or hypovolemia.
- Give neonates with severe cyanosis an infusion of prostaglandin E_1 to open the ductus arteriosus.
- Place infants with tet spells in the knee-chest position and give oxygen; sometimes, opioids (morphine or fentanyl), volume expansion, sodium bicarbonate, beta-blockers (propranolol or esmolol), or phenylephrine may help.
- Repair surgically at 3 to 6 mo or earlier if symptoms are severe.

TOTAL ANOMALOUS PULMONARY VENOUS RETURN

In total anomalous pulmonary venous return (TAPVR), the pulmonary veins do not connect to the left atrium. Instead, the entire pulmonary venous return enters the systemic venous circulation through one or more persistent

embryologic connections. If there is no obstruction to pulmonary venous return, cyanosis is mild and patients may be minimally symptomatic. Severe obstruction of the pulmonary venous return may occur, resulting in severe neonatal cyanosis, pulmonary edema, and pulmonary hypertension. Diagnosis is by echocardiography. Surgical repair is required.

TAPVR (see Fig. 297–8) accounts for 1 to 2% of congenital heart anomalies. The clinical manifestation depends on the connection between the pulmonary venous confluence and the right side of the circulation. The most common types include

- Return via an ascending left vertical vein that drains to the innominate vein or to the superior vena cava (supracardiac TAPVR)
- A descending vein that drains infradiaphragmatically to the portal circulation (infracardiac TAPVR)
- Connection of the pulmonary vein confluence to the coronary sinus (cardiac TAPVR)

The infradiaphragmatic drainage type is invariably severely obstructed, leading to dramatic pulmonary edema and cyanosis unresponsive to supplemental oxygen. The other 2 types do not typically involve obstruction and lead to mild signs of heart failure (HF) and mild cyanosis in the first month of life.

Symptoms and Signs

Neonates with obstructed pulmonary venous return present with respiratory distress, pulmonary edema, and marked cyanosis. Physical examination usually shows a parasternal lift and a single, loud 2nd heart sound (S_2), with no significant murmur.

If pulmonary venous return is not obstructed, subtle symptoms of heart failure may be present. Some infants with unobstructed supracardiac or cardiac TAPVR may be asymptomatic. Physical examination detects a hyperdynamic precordium, a widely split S_2 sometimes with a loud pulmonary component, and a grade 2 to 3/6 systolic ejection murmur audible along the left sternal border (see Table 73–3 on p. 584). A mid-diastolic tricuspid flow murmur may be audible at the lower left sternal border.

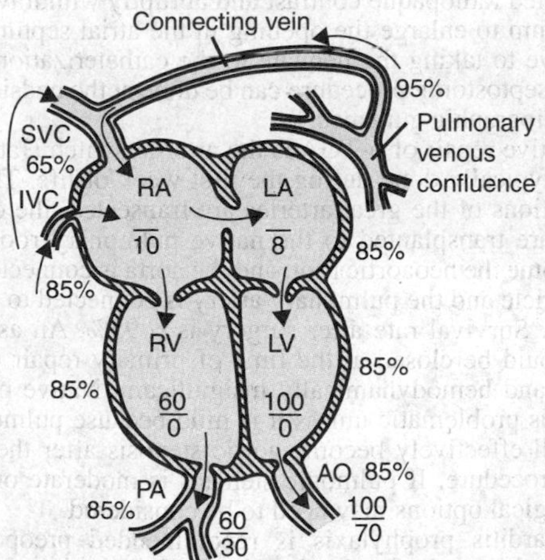

Fig. 297–8. Total anomalous pulmonary venous return. The pulmonary veins do not connect to the left atrium; instead, the entire pulmonary venous return enters systemic venous circulation through various connections. Systemic blood flow depends on right-to-left atrial shunting. AO = aorta; IVC = inferior vena cava; LA = left atrium; LV = left ventricle; PA = pulmonary artery; PV = pulmonary veins; RA = right atrium; RV = right ventricle; SVC = superior vena cava.

Diagnosis

- Chest x-ray and ECG
- Echocardiography

Diagnosis of TAPVR is suspected by chest x-ray and established by echocardiography. Cardiac catheterization is rarely necessary; occasionally, cardiac MRI or CT angiography may need to be done to better delineate the anatomy of pulmonary venous return.

Chest x-ray shows a small heart and severe diffuse pulmonary edema when there is pulmonary venous obstruction; otherwise, there is cardiomegaly with increased pulmonary vascular markings. ECG shows right axis deviation, right ventricular hypertrophy, and occasionally right atrial enlargement.

Treatment

- Surgical repair
- Medical treatment of HF (eg, diuretics, digoxin, ACE inhibitors) before surgery

Neonates with TAPVR with obstruction require emergent surgical repair. In older infants, HF should be treated, followed by surgical repair as soon as the infant is stabilized.

Surgical repair consists of creating a wide anastomosis between the pulmonary venous confluence and the posterior wall of the left atrium, along with ligation of the vein decompressing the confluence into the systemic venous circulation. The repair is different for return to the coronary sinus, in which case the coronary sinus is unroofed into the left atrium and its opening to the right atrium is closed.

Endocarditis prophylaxis is recommended preoperatively but is required only for the first 6 mo after repair unless there is a residual defect adjacent to a surgical patch or prosthetic material.

TRANSPOSITION OF THE GREAT ARTERIES

Transposition of the great arteries (in this case dextro-transposition) occurs when the aorta arises directly from the right ventricle and the pulmonary artery arises from the left ventricle, resulting in independent, parallel pulmonary and systemic circulations; oxygenated blood cannot reach the body except through openings connecting the right and left sides (eg, patent foramen ovale, ventricular septal defect [VSD]). Symptoms are primarily severe neonatal cyanosis and occasionally heart failure, if there is an associated VSD. Heart sounds and murmurs vary depending on the presence of associated congenital anomalies. Diagnosis is by echocardiography. Definitive treatment is surgical repair.

TGA is a broad term that includes both dextro-TGA (D-TGA) and a rarer defect called levo-TGA (L-TGA). D-TGA refers to a variation in which the aorta is positioned to the right and front of the pulmonary artery arising from the right ventricle rather than the left. In L-TGA, the aorta is positioned to the *left* and front of the pulmonary artery. Because D-TGA is by far the most common form, it is often simply called transposition. D-TGA is discussed in this topic, and L-TGA is discussed on p. 2506. There are also other rare variants of the TGA but D-TGA and L-TGA are the most common.

Dextro-TGA (see Fig. 297–9) accounts for 5 to 7% of congenital heart anomalies. About 30 to 40% of patients have a VSD; up to 25% have left ventricular outflow tract obstruction (either pulmonary or subpulmonary stenosis).

Pathophysiology

Systemic and pulmonary circulations are completely separated in TGA. After returning to the right heart, desaturated systemic venous blood is pumped into the systemic circulation without being oxygenated in the lungs; oxygenated blood entering the left heart goes back to the lungs rather than to the rest of the body. This anomaly is not compatible with life unless desaturated and oxygenated blood can mix through openings at one or more levels (eg, atrial, ventricular, or great artery level).

Symptoms and Signs

Severe cyanosis occurs within hours of birth, followed rapidly by metabolic acidosis secondary to poor tissue oxygenation. Patients with a moderate or large atrial septal defect, a large ventricular septal defect, a patent ductus arteriosus, or a combination of these tend to have less severe cyanosis, but symptoms and signs of heart failure (eg, tachypnea, dyspnea, tachycardia, diaphoresis, inability to gain weight) may develop during the first weeks of life.

Except for generalized cyanosis, physical examination is rather unremarkable. Heart murmurs may be absent unless associated anomalies are present. The 2nd heart sound (S_2) is single and loud.

Diagnosis

- Chest x-ray and ECG
- Echocardiography

Diagnosis of TGA is suspected clinically, supported by chest x-ray and ECG, and established by 2-dimensional echocardiography with color flow and Doppler studies.

On chest x-ray, the cardiac shadow may have the classic egg-on-a-string appearance with a narrow upper mediastinum. ECG shows right ventricular hypertrophy but may be normal for a neonate.

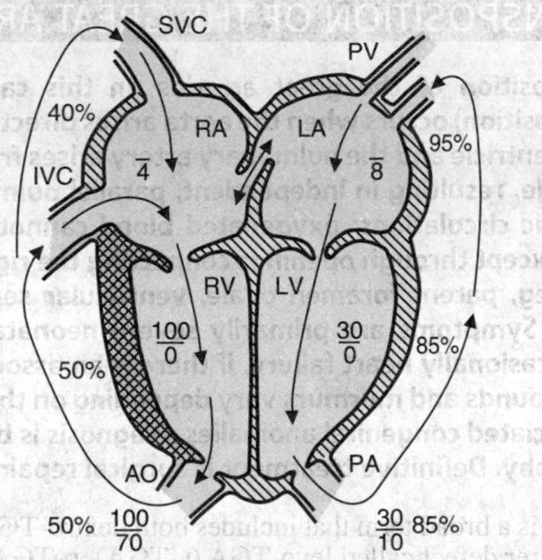

Fig. 297–9. Dextro-TGA. Unoxygenated blood returning to the right heart enters the AO, causing severe cyanosis. Oxygenated blood returning to the LA enters the pulmonary circulation again. The RV is hypertrophied, and mixing at the foramen ovale occurs but may be inadequate. Atrial pressures are mean pressures. AO = aorta; IVC = inferior vena cava; LA = left atrium; LV = left ventricle; PA = pulmonary artery; PV = pulmonary veins; RA = right atrium; RV = right ventricle; SVC = superior vena cava.

Cardiac catheterization is not usually necessary for diagnosis but may be done to enlarge the atrial communication (balloon atrial septostomy) or to further elucidate complex coronary artery anatomy.

Treatment

- Prostaglandin E_1 (PGE_1) infusion
- Sometimes balloon atrial septostomy
- Surgical repair

Unless arterial oxygen saturation is only mildly decreased and the atrial communication is adequate, a PGE_1 infusion (0.01 to 0.1 mcg/kg/min IV) may help by opening and maintaining patency of the ductus arteriosus; this infusion increases pulmonary blood flow, which may promote left-to-right atrial shunting, leading to improved systemic oxygenation. However, if the patent foramen ovale has a small opening, PGE_1 may have the opposite effect because the increased blood return to the left atrium may close the flap of the foramen ovale, leading to *decreased* mixing. Also, opening the ductus may decrease systemic blood flow. Thus, PGE_1 must be used with caution and patients must be monitored closely.

Metabolic acidosis is treated with sodium bicarbonate. Pulmonary edema and respiratory failure may require mechanical ventilatory support.

PEARLS & PITFALLS

- PGE_1 infusion is usually helpful in D-TGA, but it can be harmful if the patent foramen ovale is small.

For severely hypoxemic neonates who do not immediately respond to PGE_1 or who have a very restrictive foramen ovale, cardiac catheterization and balloon atrial septostomy (Rashkind procedure) can immediately improve systemic arterial oxygen saturation. A balloon-tipped catheter is advanced into the left atrium through the patent foramen ovale. The balloon is inflated with diluted radiopaque contrast and abruptly withdrawn to the right atrium to enlarge the opening in the atrial septum. As an alternative to taking the neonate to the catheterization laboratory, the septostomy procedure can be done at the bedside under echocardiographic guidance.

Definitive repair of D-TGA is the arterial switch (Jatene) operation, typically done during the first week of life. The proximal portions of the great arteries are transected, the coronary arteries are transplanted to the native pulmonary root, which will become the neoaortic root, and the aorta is connected to the left ventricle and the pulmonary artery is connected to the right ventricle. Survival rate after surgery is > 95%. An associated VSD should be closed at the time of primary repair unless it is small and hemodynamically insignificant. Native pulmonic stenosis is problematic unless it is mild because pulmonic stenosis will effectively become aortic stenosis after the arterial switch procedure. If pulmonic stenosis is moderate or severe, other surgical options may need to be considered.

Endocarditis prophylaxis is recommended preoperatively but is required only for the first 6 mo after repair unless there is a residual defect adjacent to a surgical patch or prosthetic material.

KEY POINTS

- In dextro-TGA (D-TGA), the aorta arises from the right ventricle and the pulmonary artery arises from the left ventricle, resulting in independent pulmonary and systemic circulations.

- D-TGA is incompatible with life unless mixing of the circulations occurs through an atrial and/or ventricular septal opening, or a patent ductus.
- Severe cyanosis occurs within hours of birth, followed rapidly by metabolic acidosis; there are no murmurs unless other anomalies are present.
- Relieve cyanosis by giving PGE_1 infusion to keep the ductus arteriosus open and sometimes by using a balloon catheter to enlarge the foramen ovale.
- Do definitive surgical repair during the first week of life.

TRICUSPID ATRESIA

Tricuspid atresia is absence of the tricuspid valve accompanied by a hypoplastic right ventricle. Associated anomalies are common and include atrial septal defect (ASD), ventricular septal defect (VSD), patent ductus arteriosus (PDA), pulmonic valve stenosis, and transposition of the great arteries (TGA). Presenting signs include cyanosis or signs of heart failure. The first heart sound (S1) is single and may be accentuated. The 2nd heart sound (S2) can be split or single. Most infants have a murmur, the nature of which depends on the presence of associated anomalies. Diagnosis is by echocardiography. Cardiac catheterization may be needed. Definitive treatment is surgical repair.

Tricuspid atresia accounts for 1 to 3% of congenital heart anomalies. The most common type (sometimes referred to as classic tricuspid atresia) includes a VSD and pulmonic stenosis, which results in decreased pulmonary blood flow, elevated right atrial pressure, and an obligatory right-to-left shunt at the atrial level through a stretched patent foramen ovale or an ASD, causing cyanosis (see Fig. 297–10). In 12 to 25% of cases, the

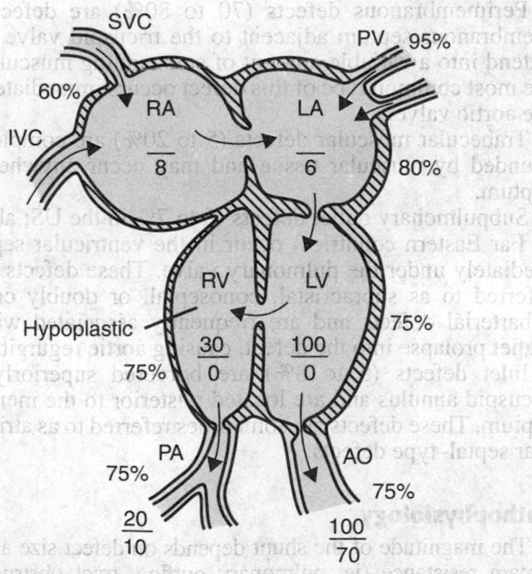

Fig. 297–10. Tricuspid atresia with normally related great vessels. The tricuspid valve is absent, and the right ventricle is hypoplastic. An atrial communication must be present. AO = aorta; IVC = inferior vena cava; LA = left atrium; LV = left ventricle; PA = pulmonary artery; PV = pulmonary veins; RA = right atrium; RV = right ventricle; SVC = superior vena cava.

great arteries are transposed with a VSD and a normal pulmonary valve, with unrestricted pulmonary blood flow coming directly from the left ventricle, typically resulting in heart failure and pulmonary hypertension. Thus, pulmonary blood flow may be increased or decreased.

Symptoms and Signs

Infants with decreased pulmonary blood flow usually have mild to moderate cyanosis at birth, which increases, sometimes dramatically, over the first several months of life. Infants with increased pulmonary blood flow usually show signs of heart failure (eg, tachypnea, dyspnea with feeding, poor weight gain, diaphoresis) by age 4 to 6 wk.

Physical examination usually detects a single prominent 1st heart sound (S_1), a single 2nd heart sound (S_2—in patients with marked pulmonic valve stenosis or transposed great vessels), and a grade 2 to 3/6 holosystolic or early systolic murmur of a VSD at the lower left sternal border (see Table 73–3 on p. 584). A systolic ejection murmur of pulmonic stenosis or a continuous murmur of PDA may be present at the upper left sternal border. A systolic thrill is rarely palpable. An apical diastolic rumble may be audible if pulmonary blood flow is markedly increased. Cyanosis, when present for > 6 mo, may result in clubbing.

Diagnosis

- Chest x-ray and ECG
- Echocardiography
- Usually cardiac catheterization

Diagnosis of tricuspid atresia is suspected clinically, supported by chest x-ray and ECG, and established by 2-dimensional echocardiography with color flow and Doppler studies.

In the most common form, chest x-ray shows normal or slightly increased heart size, right atrial enlargement, and decreased pulmonary vascular markings. Occasionally, the cardiac silhouette resembles that of tetralogy of Fallot (with a boot-shaped heart and concave pulmonary artery segment). Pulmonary vascular markings may be increased and cardiomegaly may be present in infants with associated TGA. ECG characteristically shows left axis deviation (between 0° and –90°) and left ventricular hypertrophy. Left axis deviation is not usually present if there is associated TGA. Right atrial or combined atrial enlargement is also common.

Cardiac catheterization may be necessary (particularly in older children) before the first palliative procedure to define hemodynamics and pulmonary artery anatomy unless echocardiography or other modalities clearly show the pulmonary vascular anatomy and confidently predict normal pulmonary artery pressures.

Treatment

- For severely cyanotic neonates, prostaglandin E_1 infusion
- Sometimes balloon atrial septostomy
- Staged surgical repair

Most neonates with tricuspid atresia, although cyanotic, are well compensated in the first several weeks of life. In severely cyanotic neonates, prostaglandin E_1 (beginning at 0.01 to 0.1 mcg/kg/min IV) is infused to prevent closure of the ductus arteriosus or to reopen the constricted ductus before cardiac catheterization or surgical repair.

Although not usually required, balloon atrial septostomy (Rashkind procedure) may be done as part of the initial catheterization to decompress the right atrium and facilitate unrestricted right-to-left atrial shunting when the interatrial communication is inadequate.

Some infants with TGA and signs of heart failure require medical treatment (eg, diuretics, digoxin, ACE inhibitors).

Definitive repair requires staged operations. If intervention is needed for hypoxemia within the first 4 to 8 wk of life, a modified Blalock-Taussig shunt (connection of a systemic and a pulmonary artery by a synthetic tube) is done.

In infants with excess pulmonary blood flow and signs of heart failure, a pulmonary artery band may be placed to limit pulmonary blood flow. Otherwise, if the infant remains stable with good growth, the first procedure would be a bidirectional Glenn or hemi-Fontan procedure (anastomosis between the superior vena cava and right pulmonary artery) at 3 to 6 mo of age. A modified Fontan procedure is then done, usually between 1 yr and 2 yr.

The Fontan procedure involves diverting the inferior vena cava flow directly to the pulmonary artery using either a baffle created within the right atrium (lateral tunnel) or an extracardiac conduit that completely bypasses the right atrium. The proximal pulmonary root is ligated, which prevents anterograde flow across the pulmonary outflow tract, and an adequate interatrial opening is created, if not already present, to allow equalization of right and left atrial pressures and free communication between these chambers. A fenestration (small opening) is frequently made between the Fontan pathway and the right atrium. Right-to-left shunting from the Fontan pathway to the atria and left ventricle allows decompression of the systemic venous pressure and improvement in cardiac output, albeit at the expense of mild arterial desaturation. This approach has increased early survival rates to > 90%, 5-yr survival rates to > 80%, and 10-yr survival rates to > 70%.

Endocarditis prophylaxis is recommended preoperatively and for at least 6 mo after each surgical intervention and for as long as the patient remains cyanotic or has a residual defect adjacent to a surgical patch or prosthetic material.

KEY POINTS

- The tricuspid valve is absent, and the right ventricle is hypoplastic; these defects are fatal unless there is an opening between the atria along with a VSD and/or PDA.
- Infants with decreased pulmonary blood flow have progressively worsening cyanosis; infants with increased pulmonary blood flow usually have heart failure (eg, tachypnea, dyspnea with feeding, poor weight gain, diaphoresis).
- Relieve severe cyanosis by giving prostaglandin E_1 infusion to keep the ductus arteriosus open.
- Definitive treatment requires staged operations.

VENTRICULAR SEPTAL DEFECT

A ventricular septal defect (VSD) is an opening in the interventricular septum, causing a shunt between ventricles. Large defects result in a significant left-to-right shunt and cause dyspnea with feeding and poor growth during infancy. A loud, harsh, holosystolic murmur at the lower left sternal border is common. Recurrent respiratory infections and heart failure may develop. Diagnosis is by echocardiography. Defects may close spontaneously during infancy or require surgical repair.

VSD (see Fig. 297–11) is the 2nd most common congenital heart anomaly after bicuspid aortic valve, accounting for 20% of all defects. It can occur alone or with other congenital anomalies (eg, tetralogy of Fallot, complete atrioventricular septal defects, transposition of the great arteries).

Classification: VSDs are classified by location:

- Perimembranous (also called conoventricular)
- Trabecular muscular

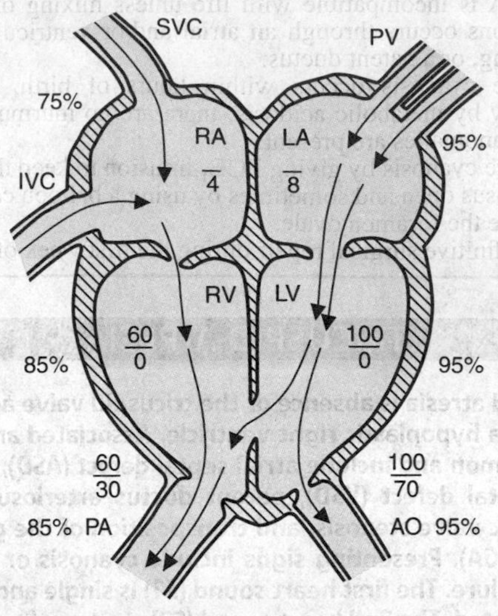

Fig. 297–11. Ventricular septal defect. Pulmonary blood flow and LA and LV volumes are increased. Atrial pressures are mean pressures. RV pressure and oxygen saturation are variably elevated, positively related to defect size. AO = aorta; IVC = inferior vena cava; LA = left atrium; LV = left ventricle; PA = pulmonary artery; PV = pulmonary veins; RA = right atrium; RV = right ventricle; SVC = superior vena cava.

- Subpulmonary outlet (supracristal, conoseptal, doubly committed subarterial)
- Inlet (atrioventricular septal type, atrioventricular canal type)

Perimembranous defects (70 to 80%) are defects in the membranous septum adjacent to the tricuspid valve and they extend into a variable amount of surrounding muscular tissue; the most common type of this defect occurs immediately below the aortic valve.

Trabecular muscular defects (5 to 20%) are completely surrounded by muscular tissue and may occur anywhere in the septum.

Subpulmonary outlet defects (5 to 7% in the US; about 30% in Far Eastern countries) occur in the ventricular septum immediately under the pulmonary valve. These defects are often referred to as supracristal, conoseptal, or doubly committed subarterial defects and are frequently associated with aortic leaflet prolapse into the defect, causing aortic regurgitation.

Inlet defects (5 to 8%) are bordered superiorly by the tricuspid annulus and are located posterior to the membranous septum. These defects are sometimes referred to as atrioventricular septal–type defects.

Pathophysiology

The magnitude of the shunt depends on defect size and downstream resistance (ie, pulmonary outflow tract obstruction and pulmonary vascular resistance). Blood flows easily across larger defects, which are thus called nonrestrictive; pressure equalizes between the right and left ventricles and there is a large left-to-right shunt. Assuming there is no pulmonic stenosis, over time, a large shunt causes pulmonary artery hypertension, elevated pulmonary artery vascular resistance, right ventricular pressure overload, and right ventricular hypertrophy. Ultimately, the increased pulmonary vascular resistance causes shunt direction to reverse (from the right to the left ventricle), leading to Eisenmenger syndrome.

Smaller defects, also referred to as restrictive VSDs, limit the flow of blood and the transmission of high pressure to the right heart. Small VSDs result in a relatively small left-to-right shunt, and pulmonary artery pressure is normal or minimally elevated. Heart failure, pulmonary hypertension, and Eisenmenger syndrome do not develop. Moderate VSDs result in intermediate manifestations.

Symptoms and Signs

Symptoms depend on defect size and magnitude of the left-to-right shunt. Children with a small VSD are typically asymptomatic and grow and develop normally. In children with a larger defect, symptoms of heart failure (eg, respiratory distress, poor weight gain, fatigue after feeding) appear at age 4 to 6 wk when pulmonary vascular resistance falls. Frequent lower respiratory tract infections may occur. Eventually, untreated patients may develop symptoms of Eisenmenger syndrome.

Auscultatory findings vary with the size of the defect. Small VSDs typically produce murmurs ranging from a grade 1 to 2/6 high-pitched, short systolic murmur (due to tiny defects that actually close during late systole) to a grade 3 to 4/6 holosystolic murmur (with or without thrill) at the lower left sternal border; this murmur is usually audible within the first few days of life (see Table 73–3 on p. 584). The precordium is not hyperactive, and the 2nd heart sound (S_2) is normally split and has normal intensity.

Moderate to large VSDs produce a holosystolic murmur that is present by age 2 to 3 wk; S_2 is usually narrowly split with an accentuated pulmonary component. An apical diastolic rumble (due to increased flow through the mitral valve) and findings of heart failure (eg, tachypnea, dyspnea with feeding, failure to thrive, gallop, crackles, hepatomegaly) may be present. In moderate high-flow VSDs, the murmur is often very loud and accompanied by a thrill (grade 4 or 5 murmur). With large defects allowing equalization of left ventricular and right ventricular pressures, the systolic murmur is often attenuated.

Diagnosis

- Chest x-ray and ECG
- Echocardiography

Diagnosis of VSD is suggested by clinical examination, supported by chest x-ray and ECG, and established by echocardiography.

If the VSD is large, chest x-ray shows cardiomegaly and increased pulmonary vascular markings. ECG shows right ventricular hypertrophy or combined ventricular hypertrophy and, occasionally, left atrial enlargement. ECG and chest x-ray are typically normal if the VSD is small.

Two-dimensional echocardiography with color flow and Doppler studies establishes the diagnosis and can provide important anatomic and hemodynamic information, including the defect's location and size and right ventricular pressure. Cardiac catheterization is rarely necessary for diagnosis.

Treatment

- For heart failure, medical therapy (eg, diuretics, digoxin, ACE inhibitors)
- Sometimes surgical repair

Small VSDs, particularly muscular septal defects, often close spontaneously during the first few years of life. A small defect that remains open does not require medical or surgical therapy. Larger defects are less likely to close spontaneously.

Diuretics, digoxin, and ACE inhibitors may be useful to control symptoms of heart failure before cardiac surgery or to temporize in infants with moderate VSDs that seem likely to close spontaneously over time. If infants do not respond to medical treatment or have poor growth, surgical repair is often recommended during the first few months of life. Even in asymptomatic children large VSDs should be repaired, usually within the first year of life, to prevent later complications. Current surgical mortality rate is < 2%. Surgical complications may include residual ventricular shunt and/or complete heart block.

Endocarditis prophylaxis is not needed preoperatively and is required only for the first 6 mo after repair or if there is a residual defect adjacent to a surgical patch.

KEY POINTS

- A VSD is an opening in the interventricular septum, causing a left-to-right shunt.
- Over time, large left-to-right shunts cause pulmonary artery hypertension, elevated pulmonary artery vascular resistance, right ventricular pressure overload, and right ventricular hypertrophy, which ultimately cause shunt direction to reverse, leading to Eisenmenger syndrome.
- Larger defects cause symptoms of heart failure at age 4 to 6 wk.
- Typically, a grade 3 to 4/6 holosystolic murmur at the lower left sternal border is audible shortly after birth.
- Infants who do not respond to medical treatment of heart failure or have poor growth should have surgical repair during the first few months of life; even asymptomatic children should have repair during the first year of life.

298 Congenital Craniofacial and Musculoskeletal Abnormalities

Craniofacial and musculoskeletal abnormalities are common among children. They may involve only a single, specific site (eg, cleft lip, cleft palate, clubfoot) or be part of a syndrome of multiple congenital anomalies (eg, velocardiofacial syndrome, Treacher Collins syndrome). Careful clinical assessment may be necessary to distinguish an isolated abnormality from an atypical or mildly manifested syndrome.

Congenital abnormalities may be classified as deformities or malformations.

A **deformity** is an alteration in shape due to unusual pressure and/or positioning in utero during late pregnancy. Deformities are present in about 2% of births; some resolve spontaneously within a few days, but others persist and require treatment.

A **malformation** is an error in normal organ or tissue development. Causes include chromosomal abnormalities, single-gene defects, teratogenic agents, or a combination of genetic and environmental factors; a decreasing number of cases are idiopathic. Congenital malformations are present in about 3 to 5% of births. A clinical geneticist should assess affected patients to establish a definitive diagnosis, which is essential for formulating an optimal treatment plan, providing anticipatory guidance and genetic counseling, and identifying relatives at risk of similar abnormalities.

ARTHROGRYPOSIS MULTIPLEX CONGENITA

(Multiple Congenital Contractures)

Arthrogryposis multiplex congenita (AMC) refers to a variety of conditions that involve congenital limitation of joint movement. Intelligence is relatively normal except when the arthrogryposis is caused by a disorder or syndrome that also affects intelligence.

Arthrogryposis is not a specific diagnosis but rather a clinical finding of congenital contractures; these may be present in > 300 different disorders. Prevalence varies in different studies between about 1/3,000 to 1/12,000 live births. The perinatal mortality for some of the underlying conditions is as high as 32%, so establishing a specific diagnosis is important for prognosis and genetic counseling.

There are two major types of AMC:

- **Amyoplasia (classic arthrogryposis):** Multiple symmetric contractures occur in the limbs. Affected muscles are hypoplastic and have fibrous and fatty degeneration. Usually intelligence is normal. About 10% of patients have abdominal abnormalities (eg, gastroschisis, bowel atresia) due to a lack of muscle formation. Nearly all cases are sporadic.
- **Distal arthrogryposis:** The hands and feet are involved, but the large joints are typically spared. Distal arthrogryposes are a heterogeneous group of disorders, many of which are associated with a specific gene defect in one of a number of genes that encode components of the contractile apparatus. Many distal arthrogryposes are transmitted as autosomal dominant disorders, but x-linked mutations are known.

Etiology

Any condition that impairs in utero movement for > 3 wk can result in AMC. Causes may involve

- Physical limitation of movement (eg, due to uterine malformations, multiple gestations, or oligohydramnios) causing fetal akinesia/hypokinesia syndrome (Pena-Shokeir syndrome), frequently associated with pulmonary hypoplasia
- Maternal disorders (eg, multiple sclerosis, impaired uterine vascularity)
- Genetic disorders affecting the fetus (eg, neuropathies; myopathies, including muscular dystrophies; connective tissue abnormalities; impaired fetal vascularity; anterior horn cell disease)

More than 35 specific genetic disorders (eg, spinal muscular atrophy type I, trisomy 18) have been linked to AMC.

Symptoms and Signs

Deformities are prominent at birth. AMC is not progressive; however, the condition that causes it (eg, muscular dystrophy) may be. Affected joints are contracted in flexion or extension. In the classic manifestations of AMC, shoulders are sloped, adducted, and internally rotated, the elbows are extended, and the wrists and digits are flexed. Hips may be dislocated and are usually slightly flexed. Knees are extended; feet are often in the equinovarus position. Leg muscles are usually hypoplastic, and limbs tend to be tubular and featureless. Soft-tissue webbing sometimes occurs over ventral aspects of the flexed joints. The spine may be scoliotic. Except for slenderness of the long bones, the skeleton appears normal on x-rays. Physical disabilities may be severe. As noted, some children may have primary CNS dysfunction, but intelligence is usually unimpaired.

Endotracheal intubation during surgery may be difficult because children have small immobile jaws. Other abnormalities that rarely accompany arthrogryposis include microcephaly, cleft palate, cryptorchidism, and cardiac and urinary tract abnormalities; these findings raise suspicion for an underlying chromosomal defect or genetic syndrome.

Diagnosis

- Clinical evaluation
- Testing for cause

If a newborn has multiple contractures, the initial evaluation should determine whether the condition is amyoplasia, distal arthrogryposis, or another syndrome where multiple contractures are associated with unrelated congenital anomalies and/or metabolic disorders. When available, a clinical geneticist should coordinate the assessment and management; typically, practitioners from many specialties are involved. A syndromic form of AMC is suspected when developmental delays and/or other congenital anomalies are present, and such patients should be evaluated for CNS disorders and monitored for progressive neurologic symptoms.

Evaluation should also include a thorough assessment for associated physical, chromosomal, and genetic abnormalities. Specific disorders to be sought include Freeman-Sheldon syndrome, Holt-Oram syndrome, Larsen syndrome, Miller syndrome, multiple pterygium syndrome, and DiGeorge syndrome (22q11 deletion syndrome). Testing typically starts with a chromosomal microarray analysis and followed by specific gene tests that are done individually or as a standard panel by many genetic laboratories. Electromyography and muscle biopsy are useful to diagnose neuropathic and myopathic disorders. In classic AMC, muscle biopsy typically shows amyoplasia, with fatty and fibrous replacement of tissues.

Treatment

- Joint manipulation and casting
- Sometimes surgical procedures

Early orthopedic and physical therapy evaluations are indicated. Joint manipulation and casting during the first few months of life may produce considerable improvement. Orthotics may help. Surgery may be needed later to align the angle of ankylosis, but mobility is rarely enhanced. Muscle transfers (eg, surgically moving the triceps so that it can flex the elbow) may improve function. Many children do remarkably well; two thirds are ambulatory after treatment.

COMMON CONGENITAL LIMB DEFECTS

Congenital limb defects involve missing, incomplete, supernumerary, or abnormally developed limbs present at birth.

Limb deficiencies: Congenital limb amputations and deficiencies are missing or incomplete limbs at birth. The overall prevalence is 7.9/10,000 live births. Most are due to primary intrauterine growth inhibition, or disruptions secondary to intrauterine destruction of normal embryonic tissues. The upper extremities are more commonly affected.

Congenital limb deficiencies have many causes and often occur as a component of various congenital syndromes. Teratogenic agents (eg, thalidomide, vitamin A) are known causes of hypoplastic/absent limbs. The most common cause of congenital limb amputations are vascular disruption defects, such as amniotic band-related limb deficiency, in which loose strands of amnion entangle or fuse with fetal tissue.

Limb deficiencies can be

- Longitudinal (more common)
- Transverse

Longitudinal deficiencies involve specific maldevelopments (eg, complete or partial absence of the radius, fibula, or tibia). Radial ray deficiency is the most common upper-limb deficiency, and hypoplasia of the fibula is the most common lower-limb deficiency. About two thirds of cases are associated with other congenital disorders, including Adams-Oliver syndrome (aplasia cutis congenita with partial aplasia of the skull bones and terminal transverse limb malformations), Holt-Oram syndrome, TAR syndrome (*t*hrombocytopenia-*a*bsent *r*adius), and VACTERL (*v*ertebral anomalies, *a*nal atresia, *c*ardiac malformations, *t*racheo*e*sophageal fistula, *r*enal anomalies and *r*adial aplasia, and *l*imb anomalies).

In **transverse deficiencies,** all elements beyond a certain level are absent, and the limb resembles an amputation stump. Amniotic bands are the most common cause; the degree of deficiency varies based on the location of the band, and typically, there are no other defects or anomalies. The remaining cases are mostly due to underlying genetic syndromes such as Adams-Oliver syndrome or chromosomal abnormalities.

With transverse or longitudinal deficiency, depending on the etiology, infants may also have hypoplastic or bifid bones, synostoses, duplications, dislocations, or other bony defects; eg, in proximal femoral focal deficiency, the proximal femur and acetabulum do not develop. One or more limbs may be affected, and the type of defect may be different in each limb. CNS abnormalities are rare.

Polydactyly: Polydactyly is supernumerary digits and is the most frequent congenital limb deformity. This deformity is classified as preaxial, central, and postaxial.

Preaxial polydactyly is an extra thumb or great toe. The manifestations range from a broad or duplicated distal phalange to complete duplication of the digit. It may occur in isolation, possibly with autosomal dominant inheritance, or it may be part of certain genetic syndromes, including acrocallosal syndrome (with developmental delay and corpus callosum defects), Carpenter and Pfeiffer syndromes (with craniosynostosis), Fanconi and Diamond-Blackfan anemias, and Holt-Oram syndrome (with congenital heart defects).

Central polydactyly is rare and involves duplication of the ring, middle, index fingers. It can be associated with syndactyly and cleft hand. The majority of cases are syndromic.

Postaxial polydactyly is most common and involves an extra digit on the ulnar/fibular side of the limb. Most commonly, the extra finger is rudimentary, but it can be completely developed. In people of African descent, this type of polydactyly is usually an isolated defect. In other populations, it is more often associated with a syndrome of multiple congenital anomalies or chromosomal defects. Among the syndromes to be considered are Greig cephalopolysyndactyly syndrome, Meckel syndrome, Ellis-van Creveld syndrome, McKusick-Kaufman syndrome, Down syndrome, and Bardet-Biedl syndrome.

Syndactyly: Syndactyly is webbing or fusion of fingers or toes. Several different types are defined, and the majority follow an autosomal dominant inheritance pattern. Simple syndactyly involves only fusion of the soft tissue, whereas complex syndactyly also involves fusion of the bones. Complex syndactyly is present in Apert syndrome (with craniosynostosis). Syndactyly of the ring and the small fingers is common in oculo-dento-digital dysplasia. Smith-Lemli-Opitz syndrome manifests with syndactyly of the 2nd and 3rd toes along with multiple other congenital anomalies.

Diagnosis

- Usually x-rays
- Sometimes genetic testing

Typically, x-rays are done to determine which bones are involved. When defects appear to be familial or if a genetic syndrome is suspected, evaluation should also include a thorough assessment for other physical, chromosomal, and genetic abnormalities. When available, assessment by a clinical geneticist is useful.

Treatment

- Prosthetic devices

Treatment consists mainly of prosthetic devices, which are most valuable for lower-limb deficiencies and for completely or almost completely absent upper limbs. If any activity in an arm or hand exists, no matter how great the malformation, functioning capacity must be thoroughly assessed before a prosthesis or surgical procedure is recommended. Therapeutic amputation of any limb or portion of a limb should be considered only after evaluating the functional and psychologic implications of the loss and when amputation is essential for fitting a prosthesis.

An upper-limb prosthesis should be designed to serve as many needs as possible so that the number of devices is kept to a minimum. Children use a prosthesis most successfully when it is fitted early and becomes an integral part of their body and body image during the developmental years. Devices used during infancy should be as simple and durable as possible; eg, a hook rather than a bioelectric arm. With effective orthopedic and ancillary support, most children with congenital amputations lead normal lives.

CONGENITAL CRANIOFACIAL ABNORMALITIES

Congenital craniofacial abnormalities are a group of defects caused by abnormal growth and/or development of the head and facial bones.

Various craniofacial abnormalities (CFA) result from maldevelopment of the 1st and 2nd visceral arches, which form the facial bones and ears during the 2nd month of gestation. Causes include several thousand genetic syndromes as well as prenatal environmental factors (eg, use of vitamin A, valproic acid).

Each of the specific congenital anomalies discussed here typically can be associated with many different genetic syndromes, some of which are named (eg, Treacher Collins syndrome). Because of the large number of syndromes, the discussions focus on the different structural manifestations. Detailed information on many of the specific syndromes is available from the Online Mendelian Inheritance in Man® (OMIM®) catalog of genetic disorders (see www.omim.org).

In general, children with CFA should be evaluated for other associated physical anomalies and developmental delays that may require treatment and/or help identify specific syndromes and causes. Identification of the underlying syndrome is important for prognosis and family counseling; a clinical geneticist, when available, can help guide the evaluation.

Macrocephaly: Macrocephaly (megacephaly) is a head circumference > 3 standard deviations above the mean for age. There are two types.

In **disproportionate macrocephaly,** the head is larger than appropriate for the child's size; affected children are at risk of autism spectrum disorders, developmental disability, and seizures.

In **proportionate macrocephaly,** the head appears appropriately sized for the body (ie, the large head is associated with a large stature), and an overgrowth syndrome (eg, growth hormone excess) should be considered.

Evaluation should include a 3-generation family history, developmental and neurologic assessment, examination for limb asymmetry and cutaneous lesions, and brain MRI. Sometimes disproportionate macrocephaly is familial and not associated with other anomalies, complications, or developmental delays; this form is transmitted in an autosomal dominant pattern, so at least one parent has a large head circumference. The diagnoses to be considered include neurofibromatosis type I, Fragile X syndrome, Sotos syndrome, and lysosomal storage disorders.

Microcephaly: Microcephaly is a head circumference < 2 standard deviations below the mean for age. In microcephaly, the head is disproportionately small in relation to the rest of the body. Microcephaly has many chromosomal or environmental causes, including prenatal drug, alcohol, or radiation exposure, prenatal infections (eg, TORCH [toxoplasmosis, other pathogens, rubella, cytomegalovirus, and herpes simplex] and Zika virus), and poorly controlled maternal phenylketonuria. Microcephaly also is a feature of > 400 genetic syndromes. The consequences of microcephaly itself include neurologic and developmental disorders (eg, seizure disorders, intellectual disability, spasticity).

Evaluation should include detailed prenatal history to identify risk factors, developmental and neurologic assessment, and brain MRI. Primary autosomal recessive microcephaly may involve a defect in one or more of at least four genes.

Among the genetic syndromes to be considered are Seckel syndrome, Smith-Lemli-Opitz syndrome, syndromes due to defective DNA repair (eg, Fanconi and Cockayne syndromes), and Angelman syndrome. For parents of an affected child, risk of the disorder appearing in subsequent offspring may be as high as 25%, depending on which syndrome is present, and thus clinical genetic assessment is necessary.

Craniosynostosis: Craniosynostosis is premature fusion of one or more calvarial sutures, which causes a characteristic skull deformity due to decreased growth in a direction perpendicular to the closed suture. It occurs in 1 of 2500 live births. There are several types, depending on which suture is fused.

Sagittal craniosynostosis is the most common type and causes a narrow and long skull (dolichocephaly). Most cases are isolated and sporadic, with risk of transmission to offspring < 3%. Learning disability may be present in up to 40 to 50% of patients.

Coronal craniosynostosis is the second most common type and can be bilateral, causing a short and broad skull (brachycephaly), or unilateral, causing a diagonal skull deformity (plagiocephaly). True plagiocephaly (ie, caused by craniosynostosis) often results in asymmetric orbits and is to be differentiated from positional plagiocephaly, which is due to torticollis or positioning the infant predominantly on one side and does not result in asymmetric orbits. In positional plagiocephaly, the back of the skull is flattened on one side, there is frontal bossing on the same side, and the ear on the flattened side may be pushed forward, but the orbits remain symmetrical. About 25% of coronal craniosynostosis cases are syndromic and due to single-gene mutations or chromosomal defects. Coronal craniosynostosis is commonly associated with facial and extracranial anomalies within the context of Crouzon, Muenke, Pfeiffer, Saethre-Chotzen, Carpenter, or Apert syndromes.

Eye anomalies: Hypertelorism is widely spaced eyes, as determined by increased interpupillary distance, and can occur in several congenital syndromes, including frontonasal dysplasia (with midline facial cleft, and brain abnormalities), craniofrontonasal dysplasia (with craniosynostosis), and Aarskog syndrome (with limb and genital anomalies).

Hypotelorism is closely spaced eyes, as determined by decreased interpupillary distance. This anomaly should raise suspicion of holoprosencephaly (a midline brain abnormality).

Coloboma is a gap in the structure of the eye that may affect the eyelid, iris, retina, or optic nerve of one or both eyes. Coloboma of the eyelid is frequently associated with epibulbar dermoid cysts and is common in Treacher Collins syndrome, Nager syndrome, and Goldenhar syndrome. Coloboma of the iris raises the possibility of CHARGE association (*c*oloboma, *h*eart defects, *a*tresia of the choanae, *r*etardation of mental and/or physical development, *g*enital hypoplasia, and *e*ar abnormalities), cat eye syndrome, Kabuki syndrome, or Aicardi syndrome.

Microphthalmia is a small eye globe, which may be unilateral or bilateral. Even when unilateral, mild abnormalities (eg, microcornea, colobomas, congenital cataract) of the other eye are frequently present. It causes sight-threatening complications such as angle-closure glaucoma, chorioretinal pathology (eg, uveal effusion), strabismus, and amblyopia. Causes include prenatal exposure to teratogens, alcohol, and infections (TORCH), and numerous chromosomal or genetic disorders, some of which are suggested by other clinical features. Growth and developmental delays are frequently present in microphthalmia that is caused by a chromosomal disorder. Facial asymmetry suggests Goldenhar syndrome or Treacher Collins syndrome; hand abnormalities suggest trisomy 13, oculo-dental-digital syndrome, or fetal alcohol syndrome; and genital abnormalities may suggest chromosomal defects, Fraser syndrome, or CHARGE association.

Anophthalmia is complete absence of the eye globe and occurs in > 50 genetic syndromes caused by chromosomal anomalies or mutations in one of several genes (eg, *SOX2*, *OTX2*, *BMP4*). When skin covers the orbit, the anomaly is called cryptophthalmos, which suggests Fraser syndrome, Nager syndrome, or ophthalmia-mental retardation.

Cleft palate and cleft lip: Cleft lip, cleft lip and palate, and isolated cleft palate, are collectively termed oral clefts (OCs). OCs are the most common congenital anomalies of the head and the neck with a total prevalence of 2.1 per 1000 live births. Both environmental and genetic factors have been implicated as causes. Prenatal maternal use of tobacco and alcohol may increase risk. Having one affected child increases risk of having a second affected child. Folate, taken just before becoming pregnant and through the 1st trimester, decreases the risk.

Oral clefts are divided into 2 groups:

- Syndromic (30%)
- Nonsyndromic (70%)

Syndromic OCs are those present in patients with recognized congenital syndromes or with multiple congenital anomalies. These OCs are typically caused by chromosome abnormalities and defined monogenic syndromes.

Nonsyndromic (isolated) OCs are those present in patients without associated anomalies or developmental delays. A number of different gene mutations can cause the phenotype, including mutations of some of the genes that are involved with syndromic OCs, which suggests there is significant overlap between syndromic and nonsyndromic OCs.

The cleft may vary from involvement of only the soft palate to a complete fissure of the soft and hard palates, the alveolar process of the maxilla, and the lip. The mildest form is a bifid uvula. An isolated cleft lip can occur.

A cleft palate interferes with feeding and speech development and increases the risk of ear infections. Goals of treatment are to ensure normal feeding, speech, and maxillofacial growth and to avoid formation of fistulas.

Early treatment, pending surgical repair, depends on the specific abnormality but may include specially designed bottle nipples (to facilitate flow), dental appliances (to occlude the cleft so suckling can occur), a feeder that can be squeezed to deliver formula, taping, and an artificial palate molded to the child's own palate. The frequent episodes of acute otitis media must be recognized and treated.

Ultimate treatment is surgical closure; however, timing of surgery, which may interfere with growth centers around the premaxilla, is somewhat controversial. For a cleft palate, a 2-stage procedure is often done. The cleft lip, nose, and soft palate are repaired during infancy (at age 3 to 6 mo). Then, the residual hard palate cleft is repaired at age 15 to 18 mo. Surgery can result in significant improvement, but if deformities are severe or treatment is inadequate, patients may be left with a nasal voice, compromised appearance, and a tendency to regurgitate. Dental and orthodontic treatment, speech therapy, and counseling may be required.

Micrognathia (small mandible): Micrognathia may occur in > 700 genetic syndromes.

Pierre Robin sequence is a common manifestation of micrognathia characterized by a U-shaped cleft soft palate and upper airway obstruction caused by glossoptosis (a tongue that falls to the back of the throat); conductive hearing loss may also be present. Feeding can be difficult, and sometimes cyanosis develops because the tongue is posterior and may obstruct the pharynx. Prone positioning during feeding may help, but uncoordinated swallowing may require nasogastric gavage feedings or a gastrostomy tube. If cyanosis or respiratory problems persist, tracheostomy or surgery to affix the tongue in a forward position (eg, sewing it to the inner lower lip) may be required. Otologic evaluation is indicated.

About one-third of patients with micrognathia have associated anomalies that suggest an underlying chromosomal defect or genetic syndrome. When other anomalies are present, a clinical geneticist can help guide the evaluation because identification of the underlying syndrome is important for prognosis and family counseling. Some of the diagnoses to be considered include Treacher Collins syndrome (associated with downward slant of the eyes, coloboma of the eyelid, malformed pinna [microtia], and hearing loss), Nager syndrome, Goldenhar (oculoauriculovertebral) syndrome, and cerebrocostomandibular syndrome.

Surgical extension of the mandible can improve appearance and function. In the typical procedure, called distraction osteogenesis, an osteotomy is done and a distraction (separator) device is attached to both pieces. Over time, the distance between the two pieces is widened, and new bone grows in between to enlarge the mandible.

Agnathia: Congenital absence of the condyloid process (and sometimes the coronoid process, the ramus, and parts of the mandibular body) is a severe malformation. The mandible deviates to the affected side, resulting in severe malocclusion; the unaffected side is elongated and flattened. Abnormalities of the external, middle, and inner ears, temporal bone, parotid gland, masticatory muscles, and facial nerve often coexist. Syndromes to be considered include agnathia-holoprosencephaly, otocephaly, a severe form of cerebrocostomandibular syndrome, and Ivemark syndrome.

X-rays or facial CT of the mandible and temporomandibular joint show the degree of underdevelopment and distinguish agenesis from other conditions that result in similar facial deformities but do not involve severe structural loss. Facial CT is usually done before surgery.

Treatment consists of prompt reconstruction with autogenous bone grafting (costochondral graft) to limit progression of facial deformity. Often, mentoplasty, onlay grafts of bone and cartilage, and soft-tissue flaps and grafts further improve facial symmetry. Distraction osteogenesis is being increasingly used. Orthodontic treatment in early adolescence helps correct malocclusion.

Congenital ear malformations: Microtia and external auditory canal atresia (which causes conductive hearing loss) involve the external ear. These malformations, which frequently coexist, are often identified at or soon after birth. Occasionally, school-based screening tests identify a partially occluded external auditory canal in children with a normal pinna.

Hearing tests (see p. 810) and CT of the temporal bone are necessary to evaluate possible additional bony malformations.

Treatment can include surgery and a bone-conduction hearing aid, depending on whether the malformation is unilateral or bilateral; whether it affects hearing, learning, and social development; and whether complications (eg, facial nerve involvement, cholesteatoma, otitis media) are present. Surgery may include pinna reconstruction and the creation of an external auditory canal, tympanic membrane, and ossicles.

CONGENITAL HIP, LEG, AND FOOT ABNORMALITIES

Orthopedic abnormalities of the hip, leg, and foot are sometimes not apparent at birth. Causes include in utero positioning, ligamentous laxity, and skeletal deformities. Some abnormalities resolve without intervention; however, others require treatment.

Developmental dysplasia of the hip (DDH—formerly congenital dislocation of the hip): DDH is abnormal development of the hip joint, leading to subluxation or dislocation; it can be unilateral or bilateral. High risk factors include

- Breech presentation
- Presence of other deformities (eg, torticollis, congenital foot deformity)
- Positive family history (particularly for girls)

DDH seems to result from laxity of the ligaments around the joint or from in utero positioning. Asymmetric skin creases in the thigh and groin are common, but such creases also occur in infants without DDH. If DDH remains undetected and untreated, the affected leg eventually becomes shorter, and the hip may become painful. Abduction of the hip is often impaired due to adductor spasm.

All infants are screened by physical examination. Because physical examination has limited sensitivity, high-risk infants and those with abnormalities found during physical examination typically should have an imaging study.

Two screening maneuvers commonly are used. The Ortolani maneuver detects the hip sliding back *into* the acetabulum, and the Barlow maneuver detects the hip sliding *out of* the acetabulum. Each hip is examined separately. Both maneuvers begin with the infant supine and the hips and knees flexed to 90° (the feet will be off the bed). To do the Ortolani maneuver, the thigh of the hip being tested is abducted (ie, the knee is moved away from the midline into a frog-leg position) and gently pulled anteriorly. Instability is indicated by the palpable, sometimes audible, clunk of the femoral head moving over the posterior rim of the acetabulum and relocating in the cavity. Next, in the Barlow maneuver, the hip is returned to the starting position and then slightly adducted (ie, the knee is drawn across the body) and the thigh is pushed posteriorly. A clunk indicates that the head of the femur is moving out of the acetabulum. Also, a difference in knee height when the child is supine with hips flexed, knees bent, and feet on the examining table (Galeazzi sign—see Fig. 298–1) suggests dysplasia, especially unilateral. Somewhat later (eg, by 3 or 4 mo of age), subluxation or dislocation is indicated by inability to completely abduct the thigh when the hip and knee are flexed; abduction is impeded by adductor spasm, which is often present even if the hip is not actually dislocated at the time of examination. Minor benign clicks are commonly detected. Although clicks usually disappear within 1 or 2 mo, they should be checked regularly. Because bilateral dysplasia may be difficult to detect at birth, periodic testing for limited hip abduction during the first year of life is advised.

Ultrasonography of the hips is recommended at 6 wk of age for infants at high risk, including those with a breech presentation, those born with other deformities (eg, torticollis, congenital foot deformity), and girls with a positive family history of DDH.

Imaging is also required when any abnormality is suspected during examination. Hip ultrasonography can accurately establish the diagnosis earlier in life. Hip x-rays are helpful after the bones have started to ossify, typically after age 4 mo.

Early treatment is critical. With any delay, the potential for correction without surgery decreases steadily. The hip usually can be reduced immediately after birth, and with growth, the acetabulum can form a nearly normal joint. Treatment is with devices, most commonly the Pavlik harness, which hold the affected hips abducted and externally rotated. The Frejka pillow and other splints may help. Padded diapers and double or triple diapering are not effective and should not be done to correct DDH.

Femoral torsion (twisting): The femoral head may be twisted. Torsion may be either internal (femoral anteversion—knees pointing toward each other with toes in) or external (femoral retroversion—knees pointing in opposite directions) and is common among neonates. At birth, internal torsion can be as much as 40° and still be normal. External torsion can also be prominent at birth and still be normal. Torsion is recognized by laying the child prone on the examining table. The hips are rotated externally and internally. Limitation of internal rotation indicates femoral anteversion, whereas limitation of external rotation indicates femoral retroversion.

Children with **internal torsion** may regularly sit in the W position (ie, knees are together and feet are spread apart) or sleep prone with legs extended or flexed and internally rotated. These children probably assume this position because it is more comfortable. The W sitting position was thought to worsen torsion, but there is little evidence that the position should be discouraged or avoided. By adolescence, internal torsion tends to gradually decrease to about 15° without intervention. Orthopedic referral and treatment, which includes derotational osteotomy (in which the bone is broken, rotated into normal alignment, and casted), is reserved for children who have a neurologic deficit such as spina bifida or those in whom torsion interferes with ambulation.

External torsion may occur if in utero forces result in an abduction or external rotation of the lower extremity. If external torsion is prominent at birth, a thorough evaluation (including x-rays or ultrasonography) for hip dislocation is indicated. External torsion typically corrects spontaneously, especially after children begin to stand and walk, but orthopedic referral is needed when excessive torsion persists after 8 yr. Treatment includes derotational osteotomy.

Genu varum and genu valgum: The 2 major types of knee or femoral-tibial angular deformities are genu varum (bowlegs) and genu valgum (knock-knees). Untreated, both can cause osteoarthritis of the knee in adulthood.

Genu varum is common among toddlers and usually resolves spontaneously by age 18 mo. If it persists or becomes more severe, Blount disease (tibia vara) should be suspected, and rickets and other metabolic bone diseases should also be ruled out (see p. 2543). Blount disease is due to a growth distur-

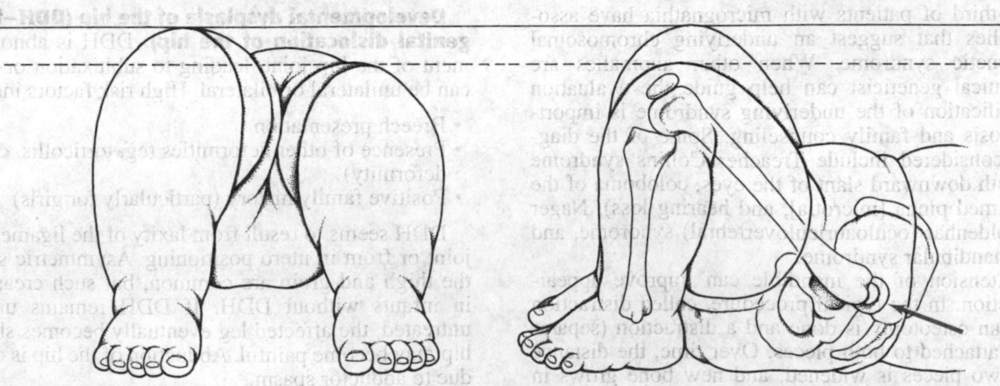

Fig. 298–1. Galeazzi sign. The child is positioned as shown. The knee is lower on the affected side because of posterior displacement in the developmentally dysplastic hip (arrow).

bance of the medial aspect of the proximal tibial growth plate; genu varum and tibial torsion may occur. Blount disease may occur in early childhood or in adolescence (when it is associated with overweight). Early diagnosis of Blount disease is difficult because x-rays may be normal; the classic x-ray finding is angulation (beaking) of the medial metaphysis. Early use of splints or braces can be effective, but surgery with or without an external fixator is often needed.

Genu valgum is less common and, even if severe, usually resolves spontaneously by age 9 yr. Skeletal dysplasia or hypophosphatasia should be excluded. If marked deformity persists after age 10 yr, surgical stapling of the medial distal femoral epiphysis is indicated.

Knee dislocation: Anterior knee dislocation with hyperextension is rare at birth but requires emergency treatment. It may occur with Larsen syndrome, which consists of multiple congenital dislocations (eg, elbows, hips, knees), clubfoot, and characteristic facies (eg, prominent forehead, depressed nasal bridge, wide-spaced eyes), or with arthrogryposis (see p. 2516). The dislocation may be related to muscle imbalance (if myelodysplasia or arthrogryposis is present) or intrauterine positioning. Ipsilateral hip dislocation often coexists.

On examination the leg is extended and cannot be flexed more than a few degrees.

If the infant is otherwise normal, immediate treatment with daily passive flexion movements and splinting in flexion usually results in a functional knee.

Tibial torsion: Tibial torsion can be external (lateral) or internal (medial) twisting. External torsion occurs normally with growth: from 0° at birth to 20° by adulthood. External torsion is rarely a problem.

Internal torsion is common at birth, but it typically resolves with growth. However, an excessive degree of torsion may indicate a neuromuscular problem. Torsion also occurs with Blount disease (see p. 2520). Persistent, excessive torsion can lead to toeing-in and bowlegs.

To evaluate for tibial torsion, the angle between the axis of the foot and the axis of the thigh is measured with the child prone and the knees flexed to 90°. Typically the foot axis is 10° lateral relative to the thigh axis. This angle can also be measured by seating the child and drawing an imaginary line connecting the lateral and medial malleoli.

Talipes equinovarus: Sometimes called clubfoot, talipes equinovarus is characterized by plantar flexion, inward tilting of the heel (from the midline of the leg), and adduction of the forefoot (medial deviation away from the leg's vertical axis). It results from an abnormality of the talus. It occurs in about 2/1000 live births, is bilateral in up to 50% of affected children, and may occur alone or as part of a syndrome. Developmental dysplasia of the hip is more common among these children. Similar deformities that result from in utero positioning can be distinguished from talipes equinovarus because they can be easily corrected passively.

Treatment requires orthopedic care, which consists initially of repeated cast applications, taping, or use of malleable splints to normalize the foot's position. If casting is not successful and the abnormality is severe, surgery may be required. Optimally, surgery is done before 12 mo, while the tarsal bones are still cartilaginous. Talipes equinovarus may recur as children grow.

Talipes calcaneovalgus: The foot is flat or convex and dorsiflexed with the heel turned outward. The foot can easily be approximated against the lower tibia. Developmental dysplasia of the hip is more common among these children. Early treatment with a cast (to place the foot in the equinovarus position) or with corrective braces is usually successful.

Metatarsus adductus: The forefoot turns toward the midline. The foot may be supinated at rest. Usually, the foot can be passively abducted and everted beyond the neutral position when the sole is stimulated. Occasionally, an affected foot is rigid, not correcting to neutral. Developmental dysplasia of the hip is more common among these children.

The deformity usually resolves without treatment during the first year of life. If it does not, casting or surgery (abductory midfoot osteotomy) is required.

Metatarsus varus: The plantar surface of the foot is turned inward, so that the arch is raised. This deformity usually results from in utero positioning. It typically does not resolve after birth and may require corrective casting.

CONGENITAL MUSCLE ABNORMALITIES

Individual muscles or groups of muscles may be absent or incompletely developed at birth. Muscle abnormalities can occur alone or as part of a syndrome.

Partial or complete agenesis of the pectoralis major is common and occurs alone or with ipsilateral hand abnormalities and various degrees of breast and nipple aplasia, as in Poland syndrome. Poland syndrome may be associated with Möbius syndrome (paralysis of the lower cranial nerves, especially the 6th, 7th, and 12th), which has been linked to autism.

In prune-belly syndrome (see p. 2536), ≥ 1 layers of the abdominal musculature are absent at birth; this often occurs with severe GU abnormalities, particularly hydronephrosis. Incidence is higher in males who often also have bilateral undescended testes. Malformations involving the feet and rectum also often coexist. Prognosis is guarded, even with early relief of urinary tract obstruction.

Treatment depends on severity of the condition and can range from minimal intervention to reconstructive surgery.

CONGENITAL NECK AND BACK ABNORMALITIES

Neck and back abnormalities can be caused by soft-tissue or bony injuries or by vertebral anomalies. Vertebral anomalies can be singular or part of a syndrome.

Congenital torticollis: The head becomes tilted at or soon after birth. The most common cause is neck injury during delivery. Torticollis that develops within the first few days or weeks of life may result from hematoma, fibrosis, and contracture of the sternocleidomastoid (SCM) muscle. A nontender mass may be noted in the SCM, usually in the midsegment. Torticollis is a frequent cause of plagiocephaly (flattening of one side of the head) and asymmetric facies (see p. 1932).

Other causes include spinal abnormalities, such as Klippel-Feil syndrome (fusion of the cervical vertebrae, short neck, and low hairline, often with urinary tract abnormalities) or atlanto-occipital fusion. CNS tumors, bulbar palsies, and ocular dysfunction are common neurologic causes but are rarely present at birth. Fractures, dislocations, or subluxations of the cervical spine (especially C1 and C2) or odontoid abnormalities are rare but serious causes; permanent neurologic damage may result from spinal cord injury.

Cervical imaging should be done to exclude bony causes, which may require stabilization.

When torticollis is due to birth trauma, frequent passive SCM stretching (rotating the head and stretching the neck laterally to the opposite side) is indicated. Injections of botulinum toxin into the SCM may help in refractory cases.

Congenital vertebral defects: Examples are idiopathic scoliosis (see p. 2476), which is rarely apparent at birth, and isolated vertebral defects (eg, hemivertebrae, wedge or butterfly vertebrae), which are more likely to be diagnosed at birth. Vertebral defects should be suspected when posterior midline cutaneous, renal, or congenital lower-limb abnormalities exist. Some syndromes or associations such as VACTERL (*v*ertebral anomalies, *a*nal atresia, *c*ardiac malformations, *t*racheo*e*sophageal fistula, *r*enal anomalies and *r*adial aplasia, and *l*imb anomalies) include vertebral defects. Alagille syndrome manifests with butterfly vertebrae, jaundice due to hypoplastic bile ducts, and congenital heart defects. Ovoid vertebrae are present in mucopolysaccharidosis and several other storage disorders.

As children grow, the spinal curve caused by a vertebral defect or defects can progress rapidly; therefore, the spine should be monitored closely. Braces or body jackets, which may have to be worn 18 h/day, are often necessary initially. Surgery may be needed if the curvature progresses. Because renal abnormalities commonly coexist, renal ultrasonography is indicated for initial screening.

299 Congenital Gastrointestinal Anomalies

Most congenital GI anomalies result in some type of intestinal obstruction, frequently manifesting with feeding difficulties, distention, and emesis at birth or within 1 or 2 days. Some congenital GI malformations, such as malrotation, have a very good outcome, whereas others, such as congenital diaphragmatic hernia, have a poor outcome, with a relatively high mortality rate of 10 to 30%.

A common type of anomaly is atresia, in which a segment of the GI tract fails to form or develop normally. The most common type is esophageal atresia, followed by atresia in the jejunoileal region and in the duodenum.

Immediate management includes bowel decompression (by continuous nasogastric suction to prevent emesis, which can lead to aspiration pneumonia or further abdominal distention with respiratory embarrassment) and referral to a center for neonatal surgery. Also vital are maintenance of body temperature, prevention of hypoglycemia with IV 10% dextrose and electrolytes, and prevention or treatment of acidosis and infections so that the infant is in optimal condition for surgery.

Because about one third of infants with a GI malformation have another congenital anomaly (up to 50% in those with congenital diaphragmatic hernia and up to 70% in those with omphalocele), they should be evaluated for malformations of other organ systems, especially of the CNS, heart, and kidneys.

High Alimentary Tract Obstruction

Esophageal, gastric, duodenal, and sometimes jejunal obstruction should be considered when excess amniotic fluid (polyhydramnios) is diagnosed, because such obstructions prevent the fetus from swallowing and absorbing amniotic fluid.

An orogastric tube should be passed into the neonate's stomach immediately after cardiovascular stability has been attained after delivery. Finding large amounts of fluid in the stomach, especially if bile-stained, supports the diagnosis of upper GI obstruction, whereas inability to pass the tube into the stomach suggests esophageal atresia (or nasal obstruction [eg, choanal atresia]).

Jejunoileal and Large-Bowel Obstruction

Obstruction of the jejunum and ileum can occur as the result of jejunoileal atresia, malrotation, or meconium ileus. Large-bowel obstruction is typically caused by meconium plug syndrome, or colonic or anal atresia.

In 75% of cases, no history of maternal polyhydramnios exists because much of the swallowed amniotic fluid can be absorbed from the intestine proximal to the obstruction. These disorders, other than malrotation, intestinal duplication, and Hirschsprung disease, typically manifest in the first few days of life with feeding problems, abdominal distention, and emesis that may be bilious or fecal. The neonate may pass a small amount of meconium initially but thereafter does not pass stools. Malrotation, intestinal duplication, and Hirschsprung disease can manifest in the first several days of life or years later.

General diagnostic approach and preoperative management include giving nothing by mouth, placing an NGT to prevent further bowel distention or possible aspiration of vomitus, correcting fluid and electrolyte disturbances, taking a plain abdominal x-ray, and then doing a contrast enema to delineate the anatomy (the enema may also relieve obstruction in meconium plug syndrome or meconium ileus). For Hirschsprung disease, a rectal biopsy is needed.

Defects in Abdominal Wall Closure

Several congenital defects involve the abdominal wall, allowing protrusion of the viscera (see Gastroschisis on p. 2526 and Omphalocele on p. 2529).

ANAL ATRESIA

(Imperforate Anus)

Anal atresia is an imperforate anus.

In anal atresia, the tissue closing the anus may be several centimeters thick or just a thin membrane of skin. A fistula often extends from the anal pouch to the perineum or the urethra in males and to the vagina, the fourchette, or, rarely, the bladder in females.

The incidence of anal atresia is 1 in 5000 live births. This disorder is frequently associated with other congenital anomalies such as VACTERL (*v*ertebral anomalies, *a*nal atresia, *c*ardiac malformations, *t*racheo*e*sophageal fistula, *e*sophageal atresia, *r*enal anomalies and *r*adial aplasia, and *l*imb anomalies). Before surgery, neonates with anal atresia should be evaluated for other congenital anomalies.

Anal atresia is obvious on routine physical examination of the neonate because the anus is not patent. If the diagnosis of anal atresia is missed and the neonate is fed, signs of distal bowel obstruction soon develop.

The urine should be filtered and examined for meconium, indicating the presence of a fistula to the urinary tract. Plain x-rays and fistulograms with the neonate in a lateral prone position can define the level of the lesion. A cutaneous fistula generally indicates low atresia. In such cases, definitive repair using a perineal approach is possible. If no perineal fistula exists, a high lesion is likely.

Neonates with a cutaneous fistula and a low lesion can undergo primary repair. Neonates with a high lesion should have a temporary colostomy; definitive repair is deferred until the infant is older and the structures to be repaired are larger.

DIAPHRAGMATIC HERNIA

Diaphragmatic hernia is protrusion of abdominal contents into the thorax through a defect in the diaphragm. Lung compression may cause persistent pulmonary hypertension. Diagnosis is by chest x-ray. Treatment is surgical repair.

Diaphragmatic hernia usually occurs in the posterolateral portion of the diaphragm (Bochdalek hernia) and is on the left side in 90% of cases; in 2% of cases it is bilateral. The estimated incidence is 1 to 4 in 10,000 live births. Anterior hernias (Morgagni hernia) are far less common. Other congenital anomalies are present in about 50% of cases, and adrenal insufficiency is relatively common.

Loops of small and large bowel, stomach, liver, and spleen may protrude into the hemithorax on the involved side. If the hernia is large and the amount of herniated abdominal contents is substantial, the lung on the affected side is hypoplastic. Other pulmonary consequences include underdevelopment of the pulmonary vasculature, resulting in an elevation of pulmonary vascular resistance and hence pulmonary hypertension. Persistent pulmonary hypertension leads to right-to-left shunting at the level of the foramen ovale or through a patent ductus arteriosus, which prevents adequate oxygenation even with oxygen supplementation or mechanical ventilation. Persistent pulmonary hypertension is the major cause of death among infants with congenital diaphragmatic hernia.

Symptoms and Signs

Respiratory distress typically occurs in the first several hours after birth and occurs immediately after delivery in severe cases. After delivery, as the neonate cries and swallows air, the stomach and the loops of intestine quickly fill with air and rapidly enlarge, causing acute respiratory embarrassment as the heart and mediastinal structures are pushed to the right, compressing the more normal right lung. A scaphoid abdomen (due to displacement of abdominal viscera into the chest) is likely. Bowel sounds (and an absence of breath sounds) may be heard over the involved hemithorax.

In less severe cases, mild respiratory difficulty develops a few hours or days later as abdominal contents progressively herniate through a smaller diaphragmatic defect. Rarely, presentation is delayed until later in childhood, sometimes after a bout of infectious enteritis, which causes sudden herniation of bowel into the chest.

Diagnosis

- Sometimes prenatal ultrasonography
- Chest x-ray

Sometimes diagnosis of diaphragmatic hernia is by prenatal ultrasonography.

After delivery, diagnosis is by chest x-ray showing the stomach and intestine protruding into the chest. In a large defect, there are numerous air-filled loops of intestine filling the hemithorax and contralateral displacement of the heart and mediastinal structures. If the x-ray is taken immediately after delivery before the neonate has swallowed air, the abdominal contents appear as an opaque airless mass in the hemithorax.

Treatment

- Surgical repair

The neonate should be immediately endotracheally intubated and ventilated in the delivery room. Bag-and-mask ventilation should be avoided because it may fill the intrathoracic viscera with air and worsen respiratory compromise. Continuous nasogastric suction with a double-lumen NGT prevents swallowed air from progressing through the GI tract and causing further lung compression.

Surgery is required to replace the intestine in the abdomen and to close the diaphragmatic defect after the neonate's lung function, acid-base balance, and BP have been optimally managed.

PEARLS & PITFALLS

- Avoid bag-and-mask ventilation in neonates with respiratory distress due to diaphragmatic hernia because it may further inflate the intrathoracic viscera.

Severe persistent pulmonary hypertension requires stabilization before surgery with inhaled nitric oxide, which may help dilate the pulmonary arteries and improve systemic oxygenation. Recent studies show improved outcome with use of extracorporeal membrane oxygenation (ECMO); however, neonates with extreme pulmonary hypoplasia still do not survive. Successful transport of a critically ill neonate with congenital diaphragmatic hernia and persistent pulmonary hypertension is very difficult. Therefore, if diaphragmatic hernia is diagnosed by prenatal ultrasonography, delivery at a pediatric center with ECMO facilities is prudent.

KEY POINTS

- A congenital diaphragmatic hernia can allow abdominal contents to enter the chest cavity, compressing the lung and causing neonatal respiratory distress.
- Diagnose by chest x-ray.
- Treat with endotracheal intubation followed by surgical repair.

DUODENAL OBSTRUCTION

The duodenum can be obstructed by atresia, stenosis, and pressure due to an extrinsic mass.

Duodenal atresia: This anomaly is the 3rd most common atresia of the GI tract. The estimated incidence is 1 in, 5,000 to 10,000 live births. Duodenal atresia is due to the failure of canalization of the embryonic duodenum. This failure may be related to an ischemic event or genetic factors.

Duodenal atresia, unlike other intestinal atresias, is commonly associated with other congenital anomalies such as Down syndrome, which is present in 25 to 40% of cases. Other associated anomalies include VACTERL (*v*ertebral anomalies, *a*nal atresia, *c*ardiac malformations, *t*racheoesophageal fistula, *e*sophageal atresia, *r*enal anomalies and *r*adial aplasia, and *l*imb anomalies), malrotation, annular pancreas, biliary tract abnormalities, and mandibulofacial anomalies.

Diagnosis of duodenal atresia can be suspected prenatally if there is polyhydramnios, dilated bowel, ascites, or a combination.

Postnatally, infants with duodenal atresia present with polyhydramnios, feeding difficulties, and emesis that may be bilious. The diagnosis is suspected by symptoms and classic double-bubble x-ray findings—one bubble is in the stomach and the other is in the proximal duodenum; little to no air is in the distal gut. Although an upper GI series provides definitive diagnosis, it must be done carefully by a radiologist experienced with doing this procedure on children to avoid aspiration and is not typically necessary if surgery is to be done immediately. If surgery is to be delayed (eg, because other medical issues, such as respiratory distress syndrome, need to be stabilized), a contrast enema should be done to confirm that the double-bubble sign is not due to malrotation. Once the disorder is suspected, infants should receive nothing by mouth, and an NGT should be placed to decompress the stomach.

Surgery is the definitive therapy.

Duodenal stenosis: This anomaly occurs less commonly than duodenal atresia but manifests in a similar fashion and requires surgery. It too is frequently associated with Down syndrome.

Choledochal cyst: A choledochal cyst may obstruct the duodenum by extrinsic pressure. There is some evidence that the incidence of choledochal cysts is increasing.

Infants with choledochal cyst classically present with a triad of abdominal pain (a very difficult finding to infer in the neonate), right upper quadrant mass, and jaundice. If the cyst is large, it may also manifest with variable degrees of duodenal obstruction. Neonates can present with cholestasis. These cases are relatively rare and occur most commonly in neonates of Asian descent.

Choledochal cyst is most commonly diagnosed by ultrasonography. These cysts can be further defined by using magnetic resonance cholangiopancreatography, ERCP, or endoscopic ultrasonography.

Treatment of choledochal cyst is surgical and requires complete excision of the cyst because of the high risk (20 to 30%) of developing cancer in the cyst remnants. The surgical procedure most commonly used is a Roux-en-Y hepaticojejunostomy.

Annular pancreas: Annular pancreas is a rare congenital anomaly (5 to 15 per 100,000 live births), often associated with Down syndrome, in which pancreatic tissue encircles the 2nd portion of the duodenum, causing duodenal obstruction.

About two thirds of affected individuals remain asymptomatic. Of those who do develop symptoms, most present in the neonatal period, but manifestation may be delayed until adulthood. Neonates present with polyhydramnios, feeding problems, and emesis that may be bilious.

The diagnosis of annular pancreas can be suggested by an x-ray of the abdomen showing the same double-bubble sign seen in duodenal atresia. The diagnosis can also be made by an upper GI series and is more definitively made with CT or magnetic resonance cholangiopancreatography. ERCP can be done in older children.

Treatment of annular pancreas is surgical bypass of the annular pancreas with duodenoduodenostomy, duodenojejunostomy, or gastrojejunostomy. Resection of the pancreas should be avoided because of the potential complications of pancreatitis and pancreatic fistula development.

ESOPHAGEAL ATRESIA

Esophageal atresia is incomplete formation of the esophagus, frequently associated with tracheoesophageal fistula. Diagnosis is suspected by failure to pass a nasogastric or orogastric tube. Treatment is surgical repair.

Esophageal atresia is the most common GI atresia. The estimated incidence is 1 in 3500 live births. Other congenital malformations are present in up to 50% of cases. Two syndromes in particular are associated with esophageal atresia:

- VACTERL (*v*ertebral anomalies, *a*nal atresia, *c*ardiac malformations, *t*racheoesophageal fistula, *e*sophageal atresia, *r*enal anomalies and *r*adial aplasia, and *l*imb anomalies)
- CHARGE (*c*oloboma, *h*eart defects, *a*tresia of the choanae, *r*etardation of mental and/or physical development, *g*enital hypoplasia, and *e*ar abnormalities)

About 19% of infants with esophageal atresia meet criteria for VACTERL.

There are 5 major types of esophageal atresia (see Fig. 299–1). Most of the types also involve a fistula between the trachea and esophagus.

Most infants present during the neonatal period, but infants with the H type fistula may not present until later in life.

Characteristic signs are excessive secretions, coughing and cyanosis after attempts at feeding, and aspiration pneumonia. Esophageal atresia with a distal fistula leads to abdominal distention because, as the infant cries, air from the trachea is forced through the fistula into the lower esophagus and stomach.

Diagnosis

- Prenatal: Ultrasonography
- Postnatal: NGT or orogastric tube placement and x-ray

Routine prenatal ultrasonography may suggest esophageal atresia. Polyhydramnios may be present but is not diagnostic because it can occur with many other disorders. The fetal stomach bubble may be absent but only in < 50% of cases. Less commonly, there is a dilated upper esophageal pouch, but this is typically looked for only in fetuses with polyhydramnios and no stomach bubble.

After delivery, an NGT or an orogastric tube is inserted if esophageal atresia is suspected by prenatal ultrasonography or clinical findings; diagnosis of esophageal atresia is suggested by inability to pass the tube into the stomach. A radiopaque catheter determines the location of the atresia on x-ray. In atypical cases, a small amount of water-soluble contrast material may be needed to define the anatomy under fluoroscopy. The contrast material should be quickly aspirated back because it can cause a chemical pneumonitis if it enters the lungs. This procedure should be done only by an experienced radiologist at the center where neonatal surgery will be done.

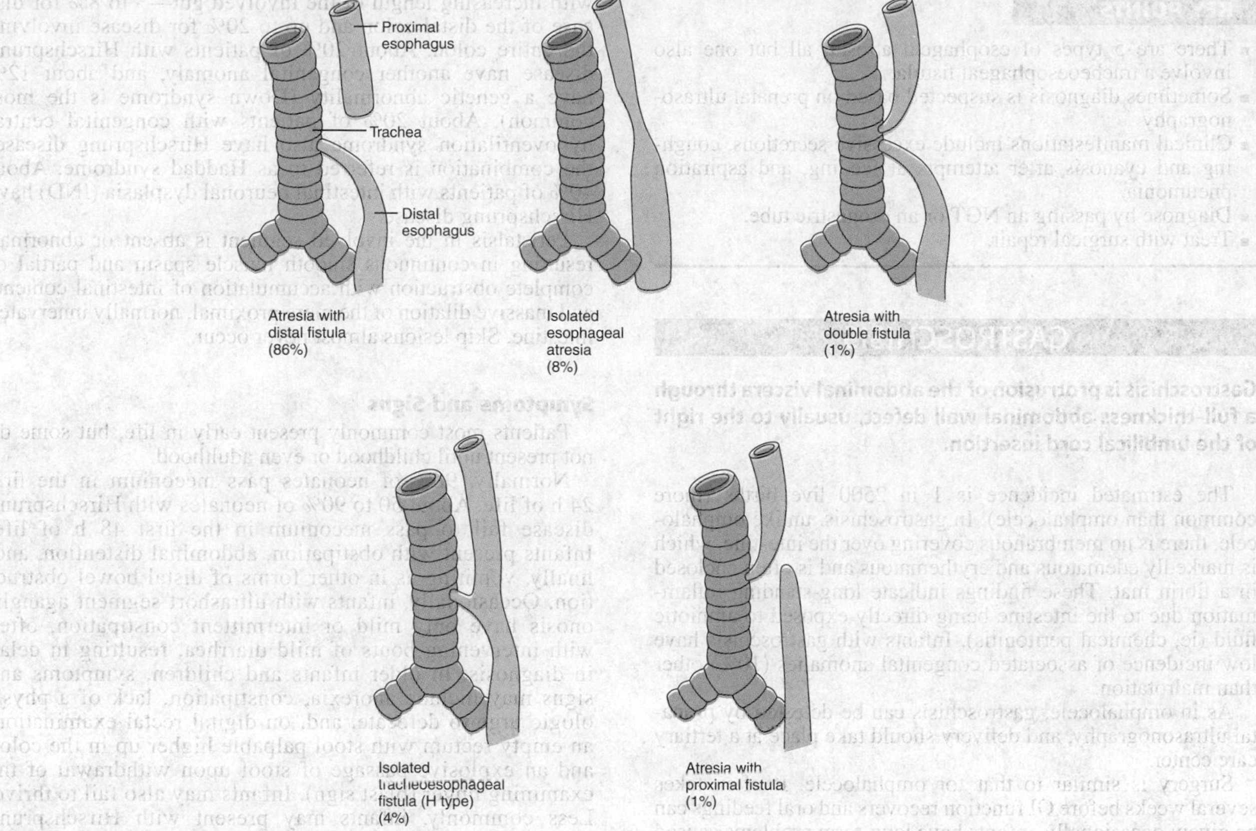

Fig. 299–1. Types and relative frequencies of esophageal atresia and tracheoesophageal fistula. Relative frequencies are based on a compilation of various sources.

Treatment

- Surgical repair

Preoperative management aims to get the infant into optimal condition for surgery and prevent aspiration pneumonia, which makes surgical correction more hazardous. Oral feedings are withheld. Continuous suction with an NGT in the upper esophageal pouch prevents aspiration of swallowed saliva. The infant should be positioned prone with the head elevated 30 to 40° and with the right side down to facilitate gastric emptying and minimize the risk of aspirating gastric acid through the fistula. If definitive repair must be deferred because of extreme prematurity, aspiration pneumonia, or other congenital malformations, a gastrostomy tube is placed to decompress the stomach. Suction through the gastrostomy tube then reduces the risk that gastric contents will reflux through the fistula into the tracheobronchial tree.

Surgical repair: When the infant's condition is stable, extrapleural surgical repair of the esophageal atresia and closure of the tracheoesophageal fistula can be done. If a fistula is noted, it needs to be ligated. In about 90% of cases, primary anastomosis of the esophagus can be done. In the remaining cases, where an extremely long gap exists, options are to do a gastric transposition procedure or a colonic interposition procedure.

Some pediatric surgeons do a Foker procedure. In this procedure, traction sutures are placed in the ends of the esophageal pouches, brought out through the skin, and fixed with silastic buttons. Traction is gradually applied to the sutures, which stimulates elongation of the esophagus by as much as 1 to 2 mm/day. Once the ends of the esophagus have come together, or are in close proximity, a primary anastomosis is done.[1]

The most common acute complications are leakage at the anastomosis site and stricture formation. Feeding difficulties are common after successful surgical repair because of poor motility of the distal esophageal segment, which occurs in up to 85% of cases. This poor motility predisposes the infant to gastroesophageal reflux. If medical management for reflux fails, a Nissen fundoplication may be required.

1. Bairdain S, Ricca R, Riehle K, et al: Early results of an objective feedback-directed system for the staged traction repair of long-gap esophageal atresia. *J Pediatr Surg* 48(10):2027–2031, 2013. doi: 10.1016/j.jpedsurg.2013.05.008.

KEY POINTS

- There are 5 types of esophageal atresia; all but one also involve a tracheoesophageal fistula.
- Sometimes diagnosis is suspected based on prenatal ultrasonography.
- Clinical manifestations include excessive secretions, coughing and cyanosis after attempts at feeding, and aspiration pneumonia.
- Diagnose by passing an NGT or an orogastric tube.
- Treat with surgical repair.

GASTROSCHISIS

Gastroschisis is protrusion of the abdominal viscera through a full-thickness abdominal wall defect, usually to the right of the umbilical cord insertion.

The estimated incidence is 1 in 2500 live births (more common than omphalocele). In gastroschisis, unlike omphalocele, there is no membranous covering over the intestine, which is markedly edematous and erythematous and is often enclosed in a fibrin mat. These findings indicate long-standing inflammation due to the intestine being directly exposed to amniotic fluid (ie, chemical peritonitis). Infants with gastroschisis have low incidence of associated congenital anomalies (10%) other than malrotation.

As in omphalocele, gastroschisis can be detected by prenatal ultrasonography, and delivery should take place at a tertiary care center.

Surgery is similar to that for omphalocele. It often takes several weeks before GI function recovers and oral feedings can be given; occasionally, infants have long-term problems caused by abnormal intestinal motility.

HIRSCHSPRUNG DISEASE

(Congenital Megacolon)

Hirschsprung disease is a congenital anomaly of innervation of the lower intestine, usually limited to the colon, resulting in partial or total functional obstruction. Symptoms are obstipation and distention. Diagnosis is by barium enema and rectal biopsy. Anal manometry can help in the evaluation and reveals lack of relaxation of the internal anal sphincter. Treatment is surgical.

Hirschsprung disease is caused by congenital absence of the Meissner and Auerbach autonomic plexus (aganglionosis) in the intestinal wall. The estimated incidence is 1 in 5000 live births. Disease is usually limited to the distal colon (75% of cases) but can involve the entire colon or even the entire large and small bowels; the denervated area is always contiguous. Males are more commonly affected (male:female ratio 4:1) unless the entire colon is involved, in which case there is no gender difference.

The etiology of the aganglionosis is thought to be the failure of migration of neuroblasts from the neural crest. There is a significant genetic component to this disorder and at least 12 different genetic mutations are associated with Hirschsprung. The likelihood of disease among family members increases with increasing length of the involved gut—3 to 8% for disease of the distal colon and up to 20% for disease involving the entire colon. About 20% of patients with Hirschsprung disease have another congenital anomaly, and about 12% have a genetic abnormality (Down syndrome is the most common). About 20% of patients with congenital central hypoventilation syndrome also have Hirschsprung disease; the combination is referred to as Haddad syndrome. About 40% of patients with intestinal neuronal dysplasia (IND) have Hirschsprung disease.

Peristalsis in the involved segment is absent or abnormal, resulting in continuous smooth muscle spasm and partial or complete obstruction with accumulation of intestinal contents and massive dilation of the more proximal, normally innervated intestine. Skip lesions almost never occur.

Symptoms and Signs

Patients most commonly present early in life, but some do not present until childhood or even adulthood.

Normally, 98% of neonates pass meconium in the first 24 h of life. About 50 to 90% of neonates with Hirschsprung disease fail to pass meconium in the first 48 h of life. Infants present with obstipation, abdominal distention, and, finally, vomiting as in other forms of distal bowel obstruction. Occasionally, infants with ultrashort segment aganglionosis have only mild or intermittent constipation, often with intervening bouts of mild diarrhea, resulting in delay in diagnosis. In older infants and children, symptoms and signs may include anorexia, constipation, lack of a physiologic urge to defecate, and, on digital rectal examination, an empty rectum with stool palpable higher up in the colon and an explosive passage of stool upon withdrawal of the examining finger (blast sign). Infants may also fail to thrive. Less commonly, infants may present with Hirschsprung enterocolitis.

Diagnosis

- Barium enema
- Rectal biopsy
- Sometimes rectal manometry

Diagnosis of Hirschsprung disease should be made as soon as possible. The longer the disease goes untreated, the greater the chance of developing Hirschsprung enterocolitis (toxic megacolon), which may be fulminant and fatal. Most patients can be diagnosed in early infancy.

Initial approach is typically with barium enema and/or rectal suction biopsy. Barium enema may show a transition in diameter between the dilated, normally innervated colon proximal to the narrowed distal segment (which lacks normal innervation). Barium enema should be done without prior preparation, which can dilate the abnormal segment, rendering the test nondiagnostic. Because characteristic findings may not be present in the neonatal period, a 24-h postevacuation x-ray should be taken; if the colon is still filled with barium, Hirschsprung disease is likely. A rectal suction biopsy can disclose the absence of ganglion cells. Acetylcholinesterase staining can be done to highlight the enlarged nerve trunks. Some centers also can do rectal manometrics, which can reveal lack of relaxation of the internal anal sphincter that is characteristic of the abnormal innervation. Definitive diagnosis requires a full-thickness biopsy of the rectum or colon to identify the full extent of the disease and thus plan surgical treatment.

PEARLS & PITFALLS

- Barium enema for Hirschsprung disease should be done without prior bowel preparation.

Treatment

- Surgical repair

Treatment of Hirschsprung disease is surgical repair by bringing normally innervated bowel to the anus with preservation of the anal sphincters. In the neonate, this procedure typically involved a colostomy proximal to the aganglionic segment to decompress the colon and allow the neonate to grow before the 2nd stage of the procedure. Later resection of the entire aganglionic portion of the colon and a pull-through procedure is done. However, a number of centers now do a 1-stage procedure in the neonatal period for short-segment disease. Results using laparoscopic technique are similar to those of the open method and are associated with shorter hospitalizations, earlier initiation of feeding, and less pain.

After definitive repair, the prognosis is good, although a number of infants have chronic dysmotility with constipation, obstructive problems, or both.

KEY POINTS

- Congenital denervation affects the distal colon and less often larger regions of the colon and sometimes even the small bowel.
- Infants typically present with findings of distal bowel obstruction, such as obstipation, abdominal distention, and vomiting.
- Barium enema findings (done without prior preparation) and rectal manometry are highly suggestive; diagnosis is confirmed by rectal biopsy.
- The affected segment is resected surgically.

Hirschsprung Enterocolitis

(Toxic Megacolon)

Hirschsprung enterocolitis is a life-threatening complication of Hirschsprung disease resulting in a grossly enlarged colon, often followed by sepsis and shock.

The etiology of Hirschsprung enterocolitis seems to be marked proximal dilation secondary to obstruction, with thinning of the colonic wall, bacterial overgrowth, and translocation of gut bacteria. Sepsis or shock can develop (more often when the entire colon is affected by Hirschsprung), and death can follow rapidly; mortality rate is about 1%. Close monitoring of infants with Hirschsprung disease is therefore essential.

Hirschsprung enterocolitis occurs most commonly in the first several months of life before surgical correction but can occur postoperatively, typically in the first year after surgery. Infants present with fever, abdominal distention, diarrhea (which may be bloody), and, subsequently, obstipation.

Initial treatment of Hirschsprung enterocolitis is supportive with fluid resuscitation, decompression with an NGT and rectal tube, and broad-spectrum antibiotics to include anaerobic coverage (eg, a combination of ampicillin, gentamicin, and clindamycin). Some experts advocate saline enemas to clean out the colon, but this must be done carefully so as not to increase colonic pressure and cause perforation. Surgery is the definitive treatment for infants who have not yet undergone surgical repair, as well as for infants with perforation or necrotic gut.

INTESTINAL DUPLICATION

Intestinal duplications are tubular structures attached to the intestines that share a common blood supply; their lining resembles that of the GI tract.

Duplications can be cystic or tubular depending on their length.

Intestinal duplications are rare, occurring in just 1 in 100,000 live births. Males appear to be more commonly affected (60 to 80% of cases). About one-third of affected children have associated congenital anomalies.

The **etiology** of intestinal duplications is unknown. Theories include abnormalities in recanalization, a vascular insult, persistence of embryonic diverticula, and partial twinning.

The **most common site** of duplication is the jejunum and ileum followed by the colon, stomach, duodenum, and esophagus. Colonic duplication is often associated with anomalies of the urogenital system. Intestinal duplications usually manifest in the 1st or 2nd yr of life.

Duplications can be asymptomatic or cause obstructive symptoms, chronic pain, GI bleeding, or abdominal mass.

If they are detected, treatment of intestinal duplications is surgical with complete resection of the duplicated portion. For proximal lesions, an endoscopic approach can be considered when a highly skilled endoscopist is available.[1-3]

1. Arantes V, Nery SR, Starling SV, et al: Duodenal duplication cyst causing acute recurrent pancreatitis, managed curatively by endoscopic marsupialization. *Endoscopy* 44(supplement 2):E117–E118, 2012. doi: 10.1055/s-0031-1291674.
2. Meier AH, Mellinger JD: Endoscopic management of a duodenal duplication cyst. *J Pediatr Surg* 47:e33–e35, 2012. doi: 10.1016/j.jpedsurg.2012.07.035.
3. Ballehaninna UK, Nguyen T, Burjonrappa SC: Laparoscopic resection of antenatally identified duodenal duplication cyst. *JSLS* 17:454–458, 2013. doi: 10.4293/108680813X13693422521151.

JEJUNOILEAL ATRESIA

Jejunoileal atresia is incomplete formation of part of the small intestine. Diagnosis is by abdominal x-ray. Treatment is surgical repair.

Neonates with jejunoileal atresia usually present late during day 1 or on day 2 with increasing abdominal distention, failure to pass stools, emesis, and feeding problems.

Etiology

Jejunoileal atresias occur as a result of an ischemic insult during pregnancy. The ischemic insult can be due to intussusception, perforation, volvulus, intestinal strangulation via a hernia, or thromboembolism. Maternal smoking and cocaine use have been associated with intestinal atresia. There is an estimated incidence of about 1 to 3 in 10,000 live births. This disorder affects both sexes equally. Jejunoileal atresias are equally distributed between the jejunum and ileum.

Associated congenital anomalies are less common with jejunoileal atresia than duodenal atresia. The most common associated conditions are cystic fibrosis, malrotation, and gastroschisis, all of which are present in about 10% of cases. Peritoneal calcifications suggest the presence of meconium peritonitis, which is a sign of intrauterine intestinal perforation and can be seen in about 10% of cases. The presence of meconium peritonitis should raise suspicion of meconium ileus and cystic fibrosis.

Classification

There are 5 major types of jejunoileal atresia:

- Type I consists of a membrane completely occluding the lumen with the intestine intact.
- Type II is a gap in the intestine with a fibrous cord between the proximal and distal segments of intestine.
- Type IIIA is a mesenteric gap without any connection between the segments.
- Type IIIB is jejunal atresia with absence of the distal superior mesenteric artery; the distal small bowel is coiled like an apple peel, and the gut is short.
- Type IV consists of multiple atretic segments (resembling a string of sausages).

Diagnosis

- Abdominal x-rays

Plain abdominal x-rays are done; they may reveal dilated loops of small bowel with air-fluid levels and a paucity of air in the colon and rectum. A barium enema reveals a microcolon (due to disuse).

Because about 10% of patients also have cystic fibrosis (nearly 100% if meconium ileus is also present), testing for cystic fibrosis should be done.

Treatment

- Surgical repair

Preoperative management of jejunoileal atresia consists of placing an NGT, giving nothing by mouth, and providing IV fluids.

Surgical repair is the definitive therapy. During surgery, the entire intestine should be inspected for multiple areas of atresia. The atretic portion is resected, usually with a primary anastomosis. If the proximal portion of the ileum is extremely dilated and difficult to anastomose to the distal, unused part of the intestine, it is sometimes safer to do a double-barreled ileostomy and defer anastomosis until the caliber of the distended proximal intestine has diminished.

The prognosis for infants with jejunoileal atresia is very good with > 90% survival. Prognosis is based on the length of remaining small bowel and the presence of the ileocecal valve. Infants who subsequently develop short bowel syndrome require TPN for extended periods. They should be provided continuous enteral feedings to promote gut adaptation, maximize absorption, and minimize the use of TPN. Infants should also be provided small amounts of nutrition by mouth to maintain sucking and swallowing. Prognosis for infants with ultrashort bowel syndrome has improved significantly because of newer surgical techniques including bowel-lengthening procedures (eg, serial transverse enteroplasty procedure or STEP), improved medical care, and the ability to do small bowel transplantation.[1-3]

1. Thompson JS, Rochling FA, Weseman RA, Mercer DF: Current management of short bowel syndrome. *Curr Probl Surg* 49:52–115, 2012. doi: 10.1067/j.cpsurg.2011.10.002.
2. Infantino BJ, Mercer DF, Hobson BD, et al: Successful rehabilitation in pediatric ultrashort small bowel syndrome. *J Pediatr* 163:1361–1366, 2013. doi: 10.1016/j.jpeds.2013.05.062.
3. Squires RH, Duggan C, Teitelbaum DH, et al: Natural history of pediatric intestinal failure: Initial report from the Pediatric Intestinal Failure Consortium. *J Pediatr* 161:723–728, 2012. doi: 10.1016/j.jpeds.2012.03.062.

MALROTATION OF THE BOWEL

Malrotation of the bowel is failure of the bowel to assume its normal place in the abdomen during intrauterine development. Diagnosis is by abdominal x-ray. Treatment is surgical repair.

Malrotation is the most common congenital anomaly of the small intestine. It is estimated that 1 in 200 live births has an asymptomatic rotational anomaly; however, symptomatic malrotation occurs less frequently (1 in 6000 live births).

During embryonic development, the primitive bowel protrudes from the abdominal cavity. As it returns to the abdomen, the large bowel normally rotates counterclockwise, with the cecum coming to rest in the right lower quadrant. Incomplete rotation, in which the cecum ends up elsewhere (usually in the right upper quadrant or midepigastrium), may cause bowel obstruction due to retroperitoneal bands (Ladd bands) that stretch across the duodenum or due to a volvulus of the small bowel, which, lacking its normal peritoneal attachment, twists on its narrow, stalk-like mesentery. Other malformations occur in 30 to 60% of patients, most commonly other GI malformations (eg, gastroschisis, omphalocele, diaphragmatic hernia, intestinal atresia, Meckel diverticulum).

Patients with malrotation can present in infancy or in adulthood with acute abdominal pain and bilious emesis, with an acute volvulus, with typical reflux symptoms, or with chronic abdominal pain. Bilious emesis in an infant is an emergency and should be evaluated immediately to make sure the infant does not have malrotation and a midgut volvulus; untreated, the risk of bowel infarction and subsequent short bowel syndrome or death is high.

Diagnosis

- Abdominal x-rays
- Upper GI series

In infants with bilious emesis, plain x-rays of the abdomen should be done immediately. If they show a dilated stomach and proximal small bowel (double-bubble sign), a paucity of bowel gas distal to the duodenum, or both (suggesting a midgut volvulus), further diagnosis and treatment must be done emergently. Barium enema typically identifies malrotation by showing the cecum outside the right lower quadrant. If the diagnosis remains uncertain, an upper GI series can be done cautiously.

In nonemergent situations, the definitive imaging for malrotation is an upper GI series. Studies have investigated the use of ultrasonography to diagnose malrotation by looking for retromesenteric localization of the third portion of the duodenum, or reversed mesenteric vessel position and the whirlpool sign (bowel wrapped around the superior mesenteric artery in a whirlpool-like pattern). The use of ultrasonography depends on the availability of an experienced radiologist or radiology technician. For now, an upper GI series is the standard diagnostic technique for malrotation with or without volvulus.[1,2]

1. Graziano K, Islam S, Dasgupta R, et al: Asymptomatic malrotation: Diagnosis and surgical management: An American Pediatric Surgical Association outcomes and evidence based practice committee systematic review. *J Pediatr Surg* 50:1783–1790, 2015. doi: 10.1016/j.jpedsurg.2015.06.019.
2. Zhou LY, Li SR, Wang W, et al: Usefulness of sonography in evaluating children suspected of malrotation: Comparison with an upper gastrointestinal contrast study. *J Ultrasound Med* 34:1825–1832, 2015. doi: 10.7863/ultra.14.10017.

Treatment

- Surgical repair

The presence of malrotation and midgut volvulus is an emergency requiring immediate surgery, which is a Ladd procedure with lysis of the retroperitoneal bands and relief of the midgut volvulus. The Ladd procedure can be done laparoscopically or as an open procedure.

When malrotation is found incidentally in an asymptomatic child, the Ladd procedure should be considered given the potentially devastating outcome of a volvulus; however, doing this procedure in this situation is controversial. Doing the Ladd procedure laparoscopically for malrotation without volvulus may decrease the time until enteral nutrition is reintroduced and reduce the length of hospital stay compared to an open procedure.[1]

1. Ooms N, Matthyssens LE, Draaisma JM, et al: Laparoscopic treatment of intestinal malrotation in children. *Eur J Pediatr Surg* 26:376–381, 2016. doi: 10.1055/s-0035-1554914.

OMPHALOCELE

An omphalocele is a protrusion of abdominal viscera from a midline defect at the base of the umbilicus.

In omphalocele, the herniated viscera are covered by a thin membrane and may be small (only a few loops of intestine) or may contain most of the abdominal viscera (intestine, stomach, liver). Immediate dangers are drying of the viscera, hypothermia and dehydration due to evaporation of water from the exposed viscera, and infection of the peritoneal surfaces. The estimated incidence is 1 in 3000 live births. Infants with omphalocele have a very high incidence of other congenital anomalies (up to 70%), including

- Bowel atresia
- Chromosomal abnormalities (eg, Down syndrome)
- Cardiac anomalies and renal anomalies

Omphalocele can be detected by routine prenatal ultrasonography; if the disorder is present, delivery should be at a tertiary care center by personnel experienced in dealing with this disorder and the other associated congenital anomalies.

At delivery, the exposed viscera should be immediately covered with a sterile, moist, nonadherent dressing (eg, medicated petrolatum gauze that can then be covered with plastic wrap) to maintain sterility and prevent evaporation. The infant should then be given IV fluids and antibiotics.

The infant is evaluated for associated anomalies before surgical repair of the omphalocele. Primary closure is done when feasible. With a large omphalocele, the abdominal cavity may be too small to accommodate the viscera. In this case, the viscera are covered by a pouch or silo of polymeric silicone sheeting, which is progressively reduced in size over several days as the abdominal capacity slowly increases, until all the viscera are enclosed within the abdominal cavity.

300 Congenital Neurologic Anomalies

Congenital brain anomalies usually cause severe neurologic deficits; some may be fatal.

Some of the most serious neurologic anomalies (eg, anencephaly, encephalocele, spina bifida) develop in the first 2 mo of gestation and represent defects in neural tube formation (dysraphism). Others, such as lissencephaly, result from problems with neuronal migration, which occurs between 9 wk and 24 wk of gestation. Hydranencephaly and porencephaly are secondary to destructive processes that occur after the brain has formed. Some anomalies (eg, meningocele) are relatively benign.

Amniocentesis and ultrasonography permit accurate in utero detection of many malformations. Parents need psychologic support when a malformation is detected and also genetic counseling, because the risk of having a subsequent child with such a malformation is high.

Prevention

Women who *have* had a fetus or infant with a neural tube defect are at high risk and should take folate supplementation 4 mg (4000 mcg) po once/day beginning 3 mo before conception and continuing through the 1st trimester. Folate supplementation reduces the risk of neural tube defects in future pregnancies by 75%.

All women of childbearing age who *have not* had a fetus or infant with a neural tube defect should consume at least 400 mcg/day of folate through diet or by taking a supplement (some experts recommend 800 mcg/day to further reduce risk) and continue doing so through the 1st trimester. Although folate supplementation reduces the risk of having a child with a neural tube defect, risk reduction is less than in women who previously had a fetus or infant with a neural tube defect (ie, risk reduction is < 75%).

HYDROCEPHALUS

Hydrocephalus is accumulation of excessive amounts of CSF, causing cerebral ventricular enlargement and/or increased intracranial pressure. Manifestations can include enlarged head, bulging fontanelle, irritability, lethargy, vomiting, and seizures. Diagnosis is by ultrasonography in neonates and young infants with an open fontanelle and by CT or MRI in older infants and children. Treatment ranges from observation to surgical intervention, depending on severity and progression of symptoms.

Hydrocephalus is the most common cause of abnormally large heads in neonates. Hydrocephalus that develops only after the fontanelles have closed does not increase head circumference or cause the fontanelle to bulge but can markedly and rapidly increase intracranial pressure.

Etiology

Hydrocephalus can result from

- Obstruction of CSF flow (obstructive hydrocephalus)
- Impaired resorption of CSF (communicating hydrocephalus)

It can be either congenital or acquired from events during or after birth.

Obstruction most often occurs in the aqueduct of Sylvius but sometimes at the outlets of the 4th ventricle (Luschka and Magendie foramina). The most common causes of obstructive hydrocephalus are

- Aqueductal stenosis
- Dandy-Walker malformation
- Chiari II type malformation

Aqueductal stenosis is narrowing of the outflow pathway for CSF from the 3rd ventricle to the 4th ventricle. It may be either primary, or secondary to scarring or narrowing of the aqueduct resulting from a tumor, hemorrhage, or infection. Primary aqueductal stenosis may involve true stenosis (forking of the aqueduct into smaller, poorly functioning channels) or presence of a septum in the aqueduct. Primary aqueductal stenosis may be inheritable; there are many genetic syndromes, some which are x-linked (thus male infants inherit the condition from otherwise unaffected mothers).

Dandy-Walker malformation is progressive cystic enlargement of the 4th ventricle.

In Chiari II type (formerly Arnold-Chiari) malformation, hydrocephalus occurs with spina bifida (see p. 2532) and syringomyelia (see p. 2033). Significant elongation of the cerebellar tonsils in Chiari type I or midline vermis in Chiari type II causes them to protrude through the foramen magnum, with beaking of the colliculi and thickening of the upper cervical spinal cord.

Impaired resorption in the subarachnoid spaces usually results from meningeal inflammation, secondary either to infection or to blood in the subarachnoid space, resulting from either subarachnoid or intraventricular hemorrhages, which are complications of delivery, particularly in premature infants (see p. 2797).

Symptoms and Signs

Neurologic findings depend on whether intracranial pressure is increased, symptoms of which in infants include irritability, high-pitched cry, vomiting, lethargy, strabismus, and bulging fontanelle. Older, verbal children may complain of headache, decreased vision, or both. Papilledema is a late sign of increased intracranial pressure; its initial absence does not exclude hydrocephalus.

Consequences of chronic hydrocephalus may include precocious puberty in girls, learning disorders (eg, difficulties with attention, information processing, and memory), loss of vision, and impaired executive function (eg, problems with conceptualizing, abstracting, generalizing, reasoning, and organizing and planning information for problem-solving).

Diagnosis

- Prenatal ultrasonography
- Neonates: Cranial ultrasonography
- Older infants and children: CT or MRI

Diagnosis is often made by routine prenatal ultrasonography. After birth, diagnosis is suspected if routine examination reveals an increased head circumference; infants may have a bulging fontanelle or widely separated cranial sutures. Similar findings can result from intracranial, space-occupying lesions (eg, subdural hematomas, porencephalic cysts, tumors). Macrocephaly may result from an underlying brain problem (eg, Alexander disease or Canavan disease), or it may be a benign, sometimes inherited, feature characterized by an increased amount of CSF surrounding a normal brain. Children suspected of having hydrocephalus require cranial imaging by CT, MRI, or ultrasonography (if the anterior fontanelle is open). Cranial CT or ultrasonography is used to monitor progression of hydrocephalus once an anatomic diagnosis has been made. If seizures occur, an EEG may be helpful.

Treatment

- Sometimes observation or serial lumbar punctures
- For severe cases, a ventricular shunt procedure

Treatment depends on etiology, severity, and whether hydrocephalus is progressive (ie, size of the ventricles increases over time relative to the size of the brain). Mild, nonprogressive cases may be observed with serial imaging studies and measurement of head size. To temporarily reduce CSF pressure in infants, ventricular taps or serial lumbar punctures (if the hydrocephalus is communicating) may be used.

Progressive hydrocephalus usually requires a ventricular shunt. Shunts typically connect the right lateral ventricle to the peritoneal cavity or, rarely, to the right atrium via a plastic tube with a one-way, pressure-relief valve. When a shunt is first placed in an infant or older child whose fontanelle is closed, rapid withdrawal of fluid can cause subdural bleeding as the brain shrinks away from the skull. When the fontanelles are open, the skull can decrease in circumference to match the decrease in brain size; thus, some clinicians recommend an early decision regarding shunt placement so that it can be done before fontanelle closure.

In a third ventriculostomy, an opening is created endoscopically between the 3rd ventricle and the subarachnoid space, allowing CSF to drain. This procedure is often combined with ablation of the choroid plexus and is becoming more commonly used in the US. It is particularly useful in less developed countries where access to consistent neurosurgical care is often limited. In certain cases (eg, hydrocephalus caused by primary aqueductal stenosis), third ventriculostomy may be adequate primary treatment.

A ventricular shunt that goes to the subgaleal space may be used in infants as a temporary measure for patients who may not require a more permanent shunt.

Although some children do not need the shunt as they age, shunts are rarely removed because of the risk of bleeding and trauma. Fetal surgery to treat congenital hydrocephalus has not been successful.

Shunt complications: The type of ventricular shunt used depends on the neurosurgeon's experience, although ventriculoperitoneal shunts cause fewer complications than ventriculoatrial shunts. Shunt complications include

- Infection
- Malfunction

Any shunt has a risk of infection. Manifestations include chronic fever, lethargy, irritability, headache, or a combination and other symptoms and signs of increased intracranial pressure; sometimes redness becomes apparent over the shunt tubing. Antibiotics effective against the organism infecting the shunt, which may include skin flora, are given, and typically the shunt must be removed and replaced.

Shunts can malfunction because of a mechanical obstruction (typically blockage at the ventricular end) or because of fracture of the tubing. In either case, intracranial pressure can increase, which, if sudden, can be a medical emergency. Children present with headache, vomiting, lethargy, irritability, esotropia, or paralysis of upward gaze. Seizures may occur. If the obstruction is gradual, more subtle symptoms and signs can occur, such as irritability, poor school performance, and lethargy, which may be mistaken for depression. To assess shunt function, a shunt series (x-rays of the shunt tubing) and neuroimaging studies are done. The ability to compress the bulb that is present on many shunt systems is not a reliable sign of shunt function.

After the shunt is placed, head circumference and development are assessed, and imaging is done periodically.

KEY POINTS

- Hydrocephalus is usually caused by obstruction to the normal flow of CSF but can be due to impaired resorption of CSF.
- If the disorder occurs before the cranial sutures have fused, the head may be enlarged, with bulging fontanelles.
- Neurologic symptoms develop mainly if intracranial pressure increases; infants may have irritability, high-pitched cry, vomiting, lethargy, and strabismus.
- Diagnose using ultrasonography prenatally and in neonates; use MRI or CT for older children.
- Treat with observation or serial lumbar punctures or a ventricular shunt procedure depending on the etiology and severity and progression of symptoms.

ANENCEPHALY

Anencephaly is absence of the cerebral hemispheres.

The absent brain is sometimes replaced by malformed cystic neural tissue, which may be exposed or covered with skin. Parts of the brain stem and spinal cord may be missing or malformed. Infants are stillborn or die within days or weeks.

Treatment is palliative only.

ENCEPHALOCELE

An encephalocele is a protrusion of nervous tissue and meninges through a skull defect.

The defect is caused by incomplete closure of the cranial vault (cranium bifidum). Encephaloceles usually occur in the midline and protrude anywhere along a line from the occiput to the nasal passages but can be present asymmetrically in the frontal or parietal regions. Small encephaloceles may resemble cephalhematomas, but x-rays show a bony skull defect at their base. Hydrocephalus (see p. 2529) often occurs with encephalocele. About 50% of affected infants have other congenital anomalies. Symptoms and signs include the visible defect, seizures, and impaired cognition, including intellectual and developmental disability.

Prognosis depends on the location and size of the lesion. Most encephaloceles can be repaired. Even large ones often contain mostly heterotopic nervous tissue, which can be removed without worsening functional ability. When other serious malformations coexist, the decision to repair may be more difficult.

MALFORMED CEREBRAL HEMISPHERES

Cerebral hemispheres may be large, small, or asymmetric; the gyri may be absent, unusually large, or multiple and small.

In addition to the grossly visible malformations, microscopic sections of normal-appearing brain may show disorganization of the normal laminar neuronal arrangement. Localized deposits of gray matter may be present in regions normally occupied only by white matter (heterotopic gray matter).

Malformations of the cerebral hemispheres may be due to genetic or acquired causes. Acquired causes include infections (eg, cytomegalovirus), and vascular events that interrupt the blood supply to the developing brain.

Microcephaly or macrocephaly, moderate to severe motor and intellectual disability, and epilepsy often occur with these defects.

Treatment is supportive, including anticonvulsants, if needed.

Holoprosencephaly: Holoprosencephaly occurs when the embryonic prosencephalon does not undergo segmentation and cleavage. The anterior midline brain, cranium, and face are abnormal. This malformation may be caused by defects of the protein produced by the *sonic hedgehog* gene. Severely affected fetuses may die before birth.

Treatment is supportive.

Lissencephaly: Lissencephaly consists of an abnormally thick cortex, diminished or absent gyral pattern on the surface of the brain, reduced or abnormal lamination of the cerebral cortex, and often diffuse neuronal heterotopias. This malformation is caused by abnormal neuronal migration, the process by which immature neurons attach to radial glia and move from their points of origin near the ventricle to the cerebral surface. Several single-gene defects may cause this anomaly (eg, *LIS1*).

Affected infants may have intellectual disability and seizures (often infantile spasms—see p. 2773).

Treatment is supportive; survival depends on seizure severity and the presence of other complications including swallowing dysfunction, apnea, and difficulty clearing oropharyngeal secretions.

Polymicrogyria: Polymicrogyria, in which the gyri are small and overabundant, also involves abnormal neuronal migration. Other common findings include simplified or absent cortical lamination in affected regions, heterotopic gray matter, a hypoplastic or absent corpus callosum and septum pellucidum, and malformations of the brain stem and/or cerebellum. The structural abnormalities may be diffuse or focal. The most common area of focal involvement is the perisylvian fissure (bilaterally or unilaterally).

Polymicrogyria is highly associated with schizencephaly (see p. 2532), in which there are abnormal slits, or clefts, in the cerebral hemispheres. Numerous causes of polymicrogyria have been identified, including a number of single-gene mutations (eg, of *SRPX2*), and primary maternal infection with cytomegalovirus (ie, in which the mother has no prior immunity—see p. 2619). The most common clinical manifestations are seizures, intellectual disability, and spastic hemiplegia or diplegia.

Treatment is supportive.

PORENCEPHALY

Porencephaly is a cavity that may develop prenatally or postnatally in a cerebral hemisphere.

Cavities often communicate with a ventricle, but they may also be enclosed (ie, noncommunicating) fluid-filled cysts. Increased intracranial pressure and progressive hydrocephalus (see p. 2529) can occur with porencephaly, especially with noncommunicating forms, but is uncommon.

Causes of porencephaly include

- Genetic anomalies
- Inflammatory diseases
- Disorders that interrupt regional cerebral blood flow (eg, intraventricular hemorrhage with parenchymal extension)

Neurologic examination is usually abnormal, with manifestations including either low or increased muscle tone, developmental delays, hemiparesis, or impairment of visual attention. However, a few children develop only minor neurologic signs and have normal intelligence. Diagnosis is confirmed by cranial CT, MRI, or ultrasonography. Prognosis is variable. Treatment is supportive.

Hydranencephaly: Hydranencephaly is an extreme form of porencephaly in which the cerebral hemispheres are almost totally absent. Usually, the cerebellum and brain stem are formed normally, and the basal ganglia are intact. The meninges, bones, and skin over the cranial vault are normal. Often hydranencephaly is diagnosed by prenatal ultrasonography.

Neurologic examination is usually abnormal, and the infant does not develop normally; children often have seizures and intellectual disability. Externally, the head may appear normal, but when transilluminated, light shines completely through.

CT or ultrasonography confirms the diagnosis.

Treatment is supportive, with shunting if head growth is excessive.

Schizencephaly: Schizencephaly, which some experts classify as a form of porencephaly, involves the presence of abnormal slits, or clefts, in the cerebral hemispheres. These clefts extend from the cortical surface to the ventricles and, unlike in other porencephalies, are lined with heterotopic gray matter. This gray matter bears some of the structural features of polymicrogyria (see p. 2531), ie, there are miniature folds and abnormal lamination, resembling abnormally formed gyri. If the walls of the cleft are tightly opposed, so that MRI does not show a clear channel of CSF from the ventricle to the subarachnoid space, the defect is called closed-lip schizencephaly; if a CSF channel is visible, the defect is called open-lip schizencephaly. Open-lip schizencephaly may lead to hydrocephalus.

Unlike other porencephalies, many of which are thought to result from brain injury, schizencephaly represents a defect in neuronal migration and is thus more often a genetically determined malformation. Affected infants often have developmental delay and, depending on the location of the defect, may have focal neurologic findings such as hemiparetic weakness or spasticity. Seizures are common in both types of schizencephaly.

Treatment is supportive.

SEPTO-OPTIC DYSPLASIA

(de Morsier Syndrome)

Septo-optic dysplasia is a malformation of the front of the brain that occurs toward the end of the first month of gestation and includes optic nerve hypoplasia, absence of the septum pellucidum (the membranes that separate the front of the 2 lateral ventricles), and pituitary deficiencies.

Although the cause may be multiple, abnormalities of one particular gene (*HESX1*) have been found in some children with septo-optic dysplasia.

Symptoms may include decreased visual acuity in one or both eyes, nystagmus, strabismus, and endocrine dysfunction (including growth hormone deficiency, hypothyroidism, adrenal insufficiency, diabetes insipidus, and hypogonadism). Seizures may occur. Although some children have normal intelligence, many have learning disabilities, intellectual disability, cerebral palsy, or other developmental delay.

Diagnosis

- MRI

Diagnosis is by MRI. All children diagnosed with this anomaly should be screened for endocrine and developmental dysfunction.

Treatment

- Supportive care
- Pituitary hormone replacement

Treatment is supportive, including replacement of any deficient pituitary hormones.

SPINA BIFIDA

Spina bifida is defective closure of the vertebral column. Although the cause is not known, low folate levels during pregnancy increase risk. Some children are asymptomatic, and others have severe neurologic dysfunction below the lesion. Open spina bifida can be diagnosed prenatally by ultrasonography or suggested by elevated α-fetoprotein levels in maternal serum and amniotic fluid. After birth, a lesion is typically visible on the back. Treatment is usually surgical.

Spina bifida is one of the most serious neural tube defects compatible with prolonged life. This defect is one of the more common congenital anomalies overall, with an incidence in the US of about 1/1500. It is most common in the lower thoracic, lumbar, or sacral region and usually extends for 3 to 6 vertebral segments. Severity ranges from occult, in which there are no apparent anomalies, to protruding sacs (spina bifida cystica), to a completely open spine (rachischisis) with severe neurologic disability and death.

In **occult spinal dysraphism** (OSD), anomalies of the skin overlying the lower back (typically in the lumbosacral area) occur; these include sinus tracts that have no visible bottom, are above the lower sacral area, or are not in the midline; hyperpigmented areas; asymmetry of the gluteal cleft with the upper margin deviated to one side; and tufts of hair. These children often have anomalies in the underlying portion of the spinal cord, such as lipomas and tethering (in which the cord has an abnormal attachment—see Fig. 300–1).

In **spina bifida cystica,** the protruding sac can contain meninges (meningocele), spinal cord (myelocele), or both (myelomeningocele). In a myelomeningocele, the sac usually consists of meninges with a central neural plaque. If not well covered with skin, the sac can easily rupture, increasing the risk of meningitis.

Hydrocephalus is common because many children have a Chiari II type malformation (see p. 2529).

Syringomyelia (a dilation of the normally small fluid-filled central canal of the spinal cord—see p. 2033) and other congenital anomalies and soft-tissue masses around the spinal cord may be present.

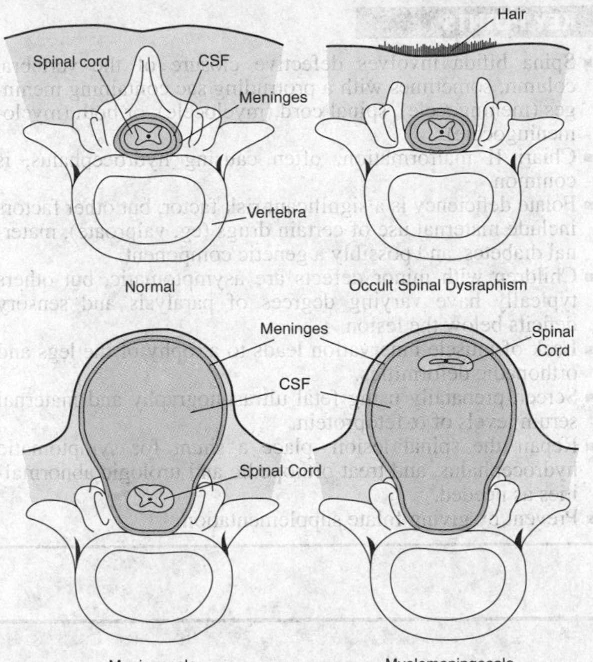

Fig. 300–1. Forms of spina bifida. In **occult spinal dysraphism,** ≥ 1 vertebrae do not form normally, and the spinal cord and meninges may also be affected. In **spina bifida cystica,** the protruding sac can contain meninges (meningocele), spinal cord (myelocele), or both (meningomyelocele).

Etiology

Causes seem multifactorial. Folate deficiency is a significant factor, and there seems to be a genetic component. Other risk factors include maternal use of certain drugs (eg, valproate) and maternal diabetes.

Symptoms and Signs

Many children with minor defects are asymptomatic.

Neurologic: When the spinal cord or lumbosacral nerve roots are involved, as is usual, varying degrees of paralysis and sensory deficits are present below the lesion. Rectal tone is usually decreased.

Hydrocephalus (see p. 2529) may cause minimal symptoms or signs of increased intracranial pressure. Brain stem involvement may cause manifestations such as stridor, swallowing difficulties, and intermittent apnea.

Orthopedic: Lack of muscle innervation leads to atrophy of the legs. Because paralysis occurs in the fetus, orthopedic problems may be present at birth (eg, clubfoot, arthrogryposis of the legs, dislocated hip—see p. 2519). Kyphosis is sometimes present and can hinder surgical closure and prevent the child from lying supine. Scoliosis may develop later and is more common among children with higher lesions (ie, above L3).

Urologic: Paralysis also impairs bladder function, occasionally leading to a neurogenic bladder and, consequently, urinary reflux, which can cause hydronephrosis, frequent UTIs, and, ultimately, kidney damage.

Diagnosis

- Ultrasonography or MRI

Spinal cord imaging, with ultrasonography or MRI, is essential in children with OSD; even children with minimal cutaneous findings may have underlying spinal abnormalities (those with overt defects do not require spinal cord imaging because the anatomy is known). Plain x-rays of the spine, hips, and, if they are malformed, lower extremities are done. Cranial imaging using ultrasonography, CT, or MRI is done to look for hydrocephalus and syringomyelia.

Once the diagnosis of spina bifida is made, urinary tract evaluation is essential and includes urinalysis, urine culture, BUN and creatinine determination, and ultrasonography. Measurement of bladder capacity and pressure at which urine exits into the urethra can determine prognosis and intervention. Need for further testing, such as urodynamics and voiding cystourethrogram, depends on previous findings and associated anomalies.

Screening: Prenatal screening can be done by doing fetal ultrasonography and by measuring maternal serum levels of α-fetoprotein (see p. 2301), ideally between 16 wk and 18 wk gestation; levels can also be done on amniotic fluid samples if previous testing suggests an increased risk. Elevated levels suggest increased risk of spina bifida cystica (OSD rarely causes elevated levels).

Prognosis

Prognosis varies by the level of cord involvement and the number and severity of associated anomalies. Prognosis is worse for children with higher cord level (eg, thoracic) lesions or who have kyphosis, hydrocephalus, early hydronephrosis, and associated congenital anomalies. With proper care, however, most children do well. Loss of renal function and ventricular shunt complications are the usual causes of death in older children.

Treatment

- Surgical repair of the spinal lesion
- Sometimes a ventricular shunt
- Various measures for orthopedic and urologic complications

Without early surgical treatment, neurologic damage can progress in OSD. Treatment for all spina bifida requires a united effort by specialists from several disciplines; neurosurgical, urologic, orthopedic, pediatric, psychiatric/psychologic, and social service evaluations are important. It is important to assess the type, vertebral segment, and extent of the lesion; the infant's health status; and associated anomalies. Discussion with the family should ascertain the family's strengths, desires, and resources, and community resources, including availability of ongoing care.

A **myelomeningocele** identified at birth is covered immediately with a sterile dressing. If the myelomeningocele is leaking CSF, antibiotics are started to prevent meningitis. Neurosurgical repair of a myelomeningocele or an open spine typically is done within the first 72 h after birth to reduce the risk of meningeal or ventricular infection. If the lesion is large or is in a difficult location, plastic surgeons may be consulted to ensure adequate closure.

Hydrocephalus may require a shunt procedure in the neonatal period; sometimes a ventricular shunt is inserted when the back is repaired (see p. 2530).

Kidney function must be monitored closely, and UTI should be treated promptly. Obstructive uropathy at either the bladder outlet or ureteral level must be treated vigorously to prevent infection. When children are between 2 and 3 yr of age, or at any time if they have elevated pressure in the bladder with vesicoureteral reflux, clean intermittent catheterization is done to empty the bladder on a regular basis. Catheterization increases continence and maintains bladder and kidney health.

At around the same time, children are placed on the commode or toilet after meals to encourage fecal continence. Well-balanced diets are encouraged; stool softeners, laxatives, or a combination may be helpful to ensure regular bowel movements and to increase continence (see p. 2618). In older children, an antegrade colonic enema procedure, in which a hole is placed through the abdominal wall into the colon to allow infusion of liquids, can improve continence. The hole is kept open by a tube (eg, a gastrostomy feeding tube).

Orthopedic care should begin early. If a clubfoot is present, a cast is applied; surgery is often necessary after casting (see p. 2521). Hip joints are checked for dislocation. Affected children should be monitored for development of scoliosis, pathologic fractures, pressure sores, and muscle weakness and spasm.

Prevention

Folate supplementation (400 to 800 mcg po once/day) in women beginning 3 mo before conception and continuing through the 1st trimester reduces the risk of neural tube defects (see p. 2529). Women who are considered at high risk of neural tube defects, ie, women who *have* had a fetus or infant with a neural tube defect, should take folate 4 mg (4000 mcg) po once/day.

KEY POINTS

- Spina bifida involves defective closure of the vertebral column, sometimes with a protruding sac containing meninges (meningocele), spinal cord (myelocele), or both (myelomeningocele).
- Chiari II malformation, often causing hydrocephalus, is common.
- Folate deficiency is a significant risk factor, but other factors include maternal use of certain drugs (eg, valproate), maternal diabetes, and possibly a genetic component.
- Children with minor defects are asymptomatic, but others typically have varying degrees of paralysis and sensory deficits below the lesion.
- Lack of muscle innervation leads to atrophy of the legs and orthopedic deformities.
- Screen prenatally using fetal ultrasonography and maternal serum levels of α-fetoprotein.
- Repair the spinal lesion, place a shunt for symptomatic hydrocephalus, and treat orthopedic and urologic abnormalities as needed.
- Prevent by giving folate supplementation.

301 Congenital Renal and Genitourinary Anomalies

Congenital anatomic anomalies of the GU tract are more common than those of any other organ system.

Urinary tract anomalies predispose patients to many complications, including urinary tract infection, obstruction, stasis, calculus formation, and impaired renal function.

Genital anomalies may cause voiding or sexual dysfunction, impaired fertility, psychosocial difficulties, or a combination.

GU anomalies frequently require surgical reconstruction.

Many GU anomalies are diagnosed in utero via routine prenatal ultrasonography. Some congenital renal anomalies (eg, autosomal dominant polycystic kidney disease, medullary sponge kidney, hereditary nephritis) typically do not manifest until adulthood.

BLADDER ANOMALIES

Congenital urinary bladder anomalies often occur without other GU abnormalities. They may cause infection, retention, incontinence, and reflux. Symptomatic anomalies may require surgery.

Bladder diverticulum: A bladder diverticulum is a herniation of the bladder mucosa through a defect in bladder muscle. It predisposes to UTIs and may coexist with vesicoureteral reflux (VUR). It is usually discovered during evaluation of recurrent UTIs in young children.

Diagnosis of bladder diverticulum is by voiding cystourethrography.

Surgical removal of the diverticulum and reconstruction of the bladder wall may be necessary.

Bladder exstrophy: In exstrophy, there is a failure of midline closure from the umbilicus to the perineum, resulting in bladder mucosa continuity with the abdominal skin, separation of the pubic symphysis, and epispadias or bifid genitalia. The bladder is open suprapubically, and urine drips from the open bladder rather than through the urethra. Despite the seriousness of the deformity, normal renal function usually is maintained.

The bladder can usually be reconstructed and returned to the pelvis, although VUR invariably occurs and is managed as needed. Additional surgical intervention may be necessary to treat a bladder reservoir that fails to expand sufficiently or has sphincter insufficiency. Reconstruction of the genitals is required.

Megacystis syndrome: In this syndrome, a large, thin-walled, smooth bladder without evident outlet obstruction develops, usually in girls. Megacystis syndrome is poorly understood. The syndrome may be a manifestation of a primary myoneural defect, especially when intestinal obstruction (eg, megacystis-microcolon, intestinal hypoperistalsis syndrome) is also present.

Symptoms are related to UTIs, and VUR is common.

Ultrasonography with the bladder empty may disclose normal-appearing upper tracts, but voiding cystourethrography may show reflux with massive upper tract dilation.

Ureteral reimplantation may be effective, although some patients benefit from antibacterial prophylaxis, timed voiding with behavioral modification, intermittent catheterization, or a combination.

Neurogenic bladder: Neurogenic bladder is bladder dysfunction caused by neurologic disorders, including spinal cord or CNS abnormalities, trauma, or the sequelae of pelvic surgery (eg, for sacrococcygeal teratoma or imperforate anus). The bladder may be flaccid, spastic, or a combination. A flaccid bladder has high-volume, low-pressure, and minimal contractions. A spastic bladder has normal or low-volume, high-pressure, and involuntary contractions. When present, chronically elevated bladder pressure (> 40 cm H_2O) often causes progressive kidney damage, even without infection or reflux.

Manifestations include recurrent UTIs and urinary retention and/or incontinence.

The underlying neurologic abnormality is usually readily apparent. Usually, postvoid residual volume is measured, renal ultrasonography is done to detect hydronephrosis, and serum creatinine is measured to assess renal function. Urodynamic testing is often done to confirm diagnosis and to monitor bladder pressures and function.

Management goals include lowering risk of infection, maintaining adequate bladder storage pressure and volume, effective bladder emptying, and achieving social continence. Treatment of neurogenic bladder includes drugs (eg, anticholinergics, prophylactic antibiotics), intermittent catheterization, and/or surgical intervention (eg, augmentation cystoplasty, appendicovesicostomy, botulinum toxin injections, neurostimulation). Children with neurogenic bladder often also have a neurogenic bowel with constipation and stool incontinence that also require proper management.

CRYPTORCHIDISM

(Undescended Testes)

Cryptorchidism is failure of one or both testes to descend into the scrotum; it is typically accompanied by inguinal hernia. Diagnosis is by examination, sometimes followed by laparoscopy. Treatment is surgical orchiopexy.

Cryptorchidism affects about 3% of term infants and up to 30% of preterm infants; two thirds of undescended testes spontaneously descend within the first 4 mo of life. Thus, about 0.8% of male infants require treatment.

Eighty percent of undescended testes are diagnosed at birth. The remainder are diagnosed during childhood or early adolescence; these are usually caused by an ectopic gubernacular attachment and become apparent after a somatic growth spurt.

Pathophysiology

Normally, the testes develop at 7 to 8 wk gestation and remain cephalad to the internal inguinal ring until about 28 wk, when they begin their descent into the scrotum guided by condensed mesenchyme (the gubernaculum). Onset of descent is mediated by hormonal (eg, androgens, müllerian-inhibiting factor), physical (eg, gubernacular regression, intra-abdominal pressure), and environmental (eg, maternal exposure to estrogenic or antiandrogenic substances) factors.

A true undescended testis remains in the inguinal canal along the path of descent or is less commonly present in the abdominal cavity or retroperitoneum. An ectopic testis is one that descends normally through the external ring but diverts to an abnormal location and lies outside the normal course of descent (eg, suprapubically, in the superficial inguinal pouch, within the perineum, or along the inner aspect of the thigh).

Complications: Undescended testes may cause subfertility and are associated with testicular carcinoma, mainly in the undescended testis and particularly with intra-abdominal malposition. However, in patients with one undescended testis, 10% of cancers develop on the normal side. In untreated cases of intra-abdominal testes, testicular torsion may occur, manifesting as an acute abdomen. Almost all neonates who present with an undescended testis at birth also have an inguinal hernia (patent processus).

Etiology

Undescended testes are almost always idiopathic. About 10% of cases are bilateral; suspicion should be high for female virilization caused by congenital adrenal hyperplasia in phenotypic boys with bilateral, nonpalpable testes at birth (especially if associated with hypospadias).

Symptoms and Signs

In about 80% of cases, the scrotum is empty at birth; in the remainder of cases, a testis is palpable in the scrotum at birth but appears to ascend with linear growth because of an ectopic gubernacular attachment that restrains it from following the normal "descent" of the scrotum. Inguinal hernia rarely causes a palpable mass lesion, but the patent process is often detectable, especially in infants (but less commonly in those with ectopic undescended testes).

Diagnosis

- Clinical evaluation
- Sometimes laparoscopy
- Rarely ultrasonography or MRI

All boys should have a testicular examination at birth and annually thereafter to assess testicular location and growth.

Undescended and ectopic testes must be distinguished from hypermobile (retractile) testes, which are present in the scrotum but easily retract into the inguinal canal via the cremasteric reflex. Diagnosis of cryptorchidism is by physical examination; a warm environment, warm examiner's hands, and a relaxed patient are important to avoid stimulating testicular retraction.

In patients with a unilateral nonpalpable testis, a descended testis that is larger than expected suggests an atrophic undescended testis; confirmation requires surgical intervention typically via diagnostic laparoscopy to seek an intra-abdominal testis or confirm testicular agenesis. However, scrotal or inguinal exploration is sometimes done if a testicular remnant distal to the internal inguinal ring is suspected.

For bilateral nonpalpable testes, patients in the immediate neonatal period should be evaluated for a possible disorder of sexual differentiation (consultation with a pediatric endocrinologist should be considered). If a disorder of sexual differentiation has been ruled out, laparoscopy is often necessary to identify testes located in the abdomen and then bilateral orchiopexy may be done.

Treatment

- Surgical repair

For a palpable undescended testis, treatment is surgical orchiopexy, in which the testis is brought into the scrotum and sutured into place; the associated inguinal hernia also is repaired. For a nonpalpable undescended testis, abdominal laparoscopy is done; if the testis is present, it is moved into the scrotum. If it is atrophic, the tissue is removed. Surgery should be done at about 6 mo of age because early intervention improves fertility potential and may reduce cancer risk. Also, the shorter the child, the shorter the distance necessary to place the testis into the scrotum. Atrophic undescended testes are likely the result of prenatal testicular torsion.

No intervention is needed for a retractile testis as long as the spermatic cord length is sufficient to allow the testis to rest in a dependent scrotal position without traction when the cremasteric reflex is not stimulated. Hypermobility usually resolves without treatment by puberty when increased testicular size makes retraction more difficult.

KEY POINTS

- Cryptorchidism affects about 3% of term infants and up to 30% of preterm infants; two-thirds of undescended testes descend spontaneously.
- Undescended testes may cause subfertility and increase risk of testicular carcinoma (including in a descended testis).

- Clinical evaluation is usually adequate, but some patients should have laparoscopy.
- Treatment is surgical orchiopexy.

PENILE AND URETHRAL ANOMALIES

Congenital anomalies of the urethra in boys usually involve anatomic abnormalities of the penis and vice versa. In girls, urethral anomalies may exist without other external genital abnormalities. Surgical repair is needed when function is impaired or cosmetic correction is desired.

Chordee: This anomaly is ventral, lateral, and/or rotational curvature of the penis, which is most apparent with erection and is caused by fibrous tissue along the usual course of the corpus spongiosum, or by a size difference between the two corpora. Chordee may be associated with hypospadias. Severe deformity may require surgical correction.

Epispadias: The urethra opens on the dorsum of the glans or penile shaft, or at the penopubic junction. In girls, the urethra opens between the clitoris and labia or in the abdomen. Epispadias can be partial (in 15%) or complete; the most severe form occurs with bladder exstrophy. Symptoms and signs of epispadias are incontinence, reflux, and UTIs.

Treatment of epispadias is surgical. In partial epispadias, prognosis for continence with treatment is good. In complete epispadias, surgical reconstruction of the penis alone may lead to persistent incontinence; bladder outlet reconstruction is required to achieve complete urinary control.

Hypospadias: This anomaly is caused by failure of tubularization and fusion of the urethral groove. It almost always occurs in boys, in whom the urethra opens onto the underside of the penile shaft, at the penoscrotal junction, between the scrotal folds, or in the perineum. The foreskin fails to become circumferential and appears as a dorsal hood. Hypospadias is frequently associated with chordee.

Prognosis for functional and cosmetic correction is good. Outpatient surgery at about 6 mo of age involves construction of a neourethra using penile shaft skin or foreskin and repair of the chordee.

Hypospadias is extremely rare in girls; the urethra opens into the vaginal introitus.

Phimosis and paraphimosis: Phimosis, the most common penile abnormality, is constriction of the foreskin with inability to retract over the glans; it may be congenital or acquired.

Paraphimosis is inability of the retracted constricting foreskin to be reduced distally over the glans.

Phimosis may respond to topical corticosteroids and gentle stretching; some boys require circumcision.

Paraphimosis should be reduced immediately because the constricting foreskin functions as a tourniquet, causing edema and pain. Firm circumferential compression of the edematous foreskin with the fingers may reduce edema sufficiently to allow the foreskin to be restored to its normal position by pushing the glans back through the tight foreskin using both thumbs. If this technique is ineffective, a dorsal slit done using a local anesthetic relieves the condition temporarily. When edema has resolved, the phimosis may be treated with circumcision or topical corticosteroids.

Other penile anomalies: A very tight frenulum may prevent complete retraction of the foreskin or cause pain or bleeding with foreskin retraction or erection. Frenulectomy may be sufficient to resolve symptoms if patients do not want circumcision.

Less common anomalies include penile agenesis, duplication, and lymphedema. Many anomalies also involve urethral abnormality, or other anomalies, such as exstrophy. Treatment of most anomalies is surgical.

Microphallus results from androgen deficiency or insensitivity; in boys with deficiency, treatment is testosterone supplementation.

Urethral meatal stenosis: Most commonly acquired after circumcision in newborn boys, urethral meatal stenosis is occasionally congenital and associated with hypospadias. Meatotomy is needed for a significantly deflected stream or for a pinpoint stream.

Urethral stricture: Urethral stricture causes obstruction along some part of the length of the urethra. It almost always occurs in boys, is usually acquired, and typically results from a crush injury after straddle trauma. Congenital urethral stricture may manifest similarly to urethral valves and may be diagnosed by prenatal ultrasonography, or postnatally by symptoms and signs of outlet obstruction or patent urachus and is confirmed by retrograde urethrography. Initial management is often with endoscopic urethrotomy, although open urethroplasty may be necessary.

Urethral duplications and triplications are urethral anomalies. The patent urethra is the most ventral channel. Voiding cystourethrography (VCUG) should be done to determine patency and detect connection between the channels and the bladder. Surgical intervention is almost always necessary.

Urethral valves: In boys, folds in the posterior urethra may act as valves impairing urine flow. Urologic sequelae of urethral valves include urinary hesitancy, decreased urinary stream, UTI, overflow incontinence, myogenic bladder malfunction, vesicoureteral reflux, upper urinary tract damage, and renal insufficiency. The valves occasionally occur with a patent urachus. Because fetal urine excretion contributes to the amniotic fluid, severe urethral obstruction can cause decreased amniotic fluid (oligohydramnios), which can cause lung hypoplasia and consequent pulmonary hypertension, pulmonary hypoplasia, and/or respiratory failure. Pulmonary hypertension can then cause systemic hypertension. Severe cases may result in perinatal demise.

Diagnosis is often made by findings on routine prenatal ultrasonography, including severe bilateral hydroureteronephrosis or oligohydramnios. Cases suspected postnatally (often because of history of an abnormal urine stream) are confirmed by immediate voiding cystourethrography.

Surgery (usually via endoscopy) is done at time of diagnosis to prevent progressive renal deterioration.

A much less common anomaly, diverticulum of the anterior urethra, may act as a valve (anterior urethral valve) and is also treated endoscopically.

PRUNE-BELLY SYNDROME

(Triad Syndrome)

Prune-belly syndrome consists of abdominal muscle deficiency, urinary tract abnormalities, and intra-abdominal undescended testes.

The name prune-belly syndrome derives from the characteristic wrinkled appearance of the abdominal wall in neonates. The cause of this congenital syndrome, which occurs primarily but not exclusively in males, is unclear. Urinary abnormalities may include hydronephrosis, megaureters, vesicoureteral reflux, and urethral abnormalities. Severe cases may involve renal failure, bronchopulmonary dysplasia, and fetal demise.

Diagnosis of prune-belly syndrome is often made during routine prenatal ultrasonography. In addition to postnatal ultrasonography, further evaluation may include voiding cystourethrography and/or an isotope renography.

Urinary tract abnormalities may require open surgical reconstruction. If no urinary intervention is necessary, orchiopexy is done in conjunction with an abdominoplasty.

RENAL ANOMALIES

(See also Congenital Renal Cystic Dysplasia on p. 2092.)

The urinary tract is a common location for congenital anomalies of varying significance. Many anomalies are asymptomatic and diagnosed via prenatal ultrasonography or part of a routine evaluation for other congenital anomalies. Other anomalies are diagnosed secondary to urinary tract obstruction, UTI, or trauma.

Autosomal recessive polycystic kidney disease: Incidence of autosomal recessive polycystic kidney disease is about 1/10,000 to 1/20,000 births; it is caused by a mutation in the *PKHD1* gene, located in chromosome 6p21. In contrast, autosomal dominant polycystic kidney disease (see p. 2088) is much more common, occurring in about 1/500 to 1/1000 live births. Symptoms of autosomal dominant polycystic kidney disease are usually not present until adulthood. Rarely, symptoms manifest in infancy in the more aggressive form. Children may be diagnosed earlier when a cyst is found incidentally or via family history.

Autosomal recessive polycystic kidney disease affects

- Kidneys
- Liver

The kidneys are usually greatly enlarged and contain small cysts; renal failure is common in childhood.

The liver is enlarged and has periportal fibrosis, bile duct proliferation, and scattered cysts; the remainder of the hepatic parenchyma is normal. Fibrosis causes portal hypertension by age 5 to 10 yr, but hepatic function is normal or minimally impaired.

Disease severity and progression vary. Severe disease may manifest prenatally or soon after birth or in early childhood with renal-related symptoms; less severely affected patients present in late childhood or adolescence with hepatic-related symptoms.

Affected neonates have a protuberant abdomen with huge, firm, smooth, symmetric kidneys. Severely affected neonates commonly have pulmonary hypoplasia secondary to the in utero effects of renal dysfunction and oligohydramnios.

In patients aged 5 to 10 yr, signs of portal hypertension, such as esophageal and gastric varices and hypersplenism, occur. If the patient presents in adolescence, nephromegaly is less marked, renal insufficiency may be mild to moderate, and the major symptoms are those related to portal hypertension.

Diagnosis of autosomal recessive polycystic kidney disease may be difficult, especially without a family history. Ultrasonography may show renal or hepatic cysts; definitive diagnosis may require biopsy. Ultrasonography in late pregnancy usually allows presumptive in utero diagnosis. If postnatal ultrasonography is not definitive, MRI or CT may be diagnostic. If needed, molecular testing for *PKHD1* can be done when clinical criteria is not met.

Many neonates die in the first few days or weeks of life from pulmonary insufficiency. Most who survive develop progressive renal failure often requiring renal replacement therapy. Experience with renal transplantation with or without hepatic transplantation is limited. When transplantation is done, hypersplenism must be controlled to obviate difficulty with hypersplenism-induced leukopenia, which increases the risk of systemic infection. Portal hypertension may be treated by portacaval or splenorenal shunts, which reduce morbidity but not mortality.

Duplication anomalies: Supernumerary collecting systems may be unilateral or bilateral and may involve the renal pelvis and ureters (accessory renal pelvis, double or triple pelvis and ureter), calyx, or ureteral orifice. Duplex kidneys have a single renal unit with more than one collecting system. This anomaly differs from fused kidneys, which involves fusion of two renal parenchymal units maintaining their respective individual collecting systems. Some duplication anomalies have ureteral ectopy with or without ureterocele and/or vesicoureteral reflux (VUR).

Management depends on the anatomy and function of each separately drained segment. Surgery may be necessary to correct obstruction or VUR.

Fusion anomalies: With fusion anomalies, the kidneys are joined, but the ureters enter the bladder on each side. These anomalies increase the risk of ureteropelvic junction obstruction, VUR, congenital renal cystic dysplasia, and injury caused by anterior abdominal trauma.

Horseshoe kidney, the most common fusion anomaly, occurs when renal parenchyma on each side of the vertebral column is joined at the corresponding (usually lower) poles; an isthmus of renal parenchyma or fibrous tissue joins at the midline. The ureters course medially and anteriorly over this isthmus and generally drain well. Obstruction, if present, is usually secondary to insertion of the ureters high in the renal pelvis. Pyeloplasty relieves the obstruction and can be done without resecting the isthmus.

Crossed fused renal ectopia is the 2nd most common fusion anomaly. The renal parenchyma (representing both kidneys) is on one side of the vertebral column. One of the ureters crosses the midline and enters the bladder on the side opposite the fused kidneys. When ureteropelvic junction obstruction is present, pyeloplasty is the treatment of choice.

Fused pelvic kidney (pancake kidney) is much less common. A single pelvic kidney is served by two collecting systems and ureters. If obstruction is present, reconstruction is needed.

Malrotation: Malrotation is usually of little clinical significance. Ultrasonography often shows hydronephrosis. Further evaluation with a magnetic resonance urogram or renal scan may be done when clinicians are concerned about possible obstruction.

Multicystic dysplastic kidney (MCDK): In this condition, there is a nonfunctioning renal unit consisting of noncommunicating cysts with intervening solid tissue composed of fibrosis, primitive tubules, and foci of cartilage. Usually, ureteral atresia is also present. The contralateral kidney is usually normal, but up to 10% of patients may have VUR or ureteropelvic junction obstruction. Frequently, the kidney progressively involutes and eventually is no longer visible on ultrasonography. Development of tumors, infection, and/or hypertension is rare.

Most experts recommend observation to monitor for involution. Nephrectomy may be considered for the presence of solid tissue, progressive enlargement, or rarely hypertension or a ruptured cyst that is causing pain.

Renal agenesis: Bilateral renal agenesis as part of a syndrome of oligohydramnios, pulmonary hypoplasia, and extremity and facial anomalies (classic Potter syndrome) is fatal within minutes to hours. Fetal demise is common.

Unilateral renal agenesis accounts for about 5% of renal anomalies. Many cases result from complete involution in utero of a multicystic dysplastic kidney. It usually is accompanied by ureteral agenesis with absence of the ipsilateral trigone and ureteral orifice. However, the ipsilateral adrenal gland is unaffected. No treatment is necessary; compensatory hypertrophy of the solitary kidney maintains normal renal function. Because the kidneys share a common embryologic origin with the vas deferens and uterus, boys may have agenesis of the vas deferens and girls may have uterine anomalies.

Renal dysplasia: In renal dysplasia (a histologic diagnosis), the renal vasculature, tubules, collecting ducts, or drainage apparatus develops abnormally. Diagnosis of renal dysplasia is by biopsy.

If dysplasia is segmental, treatment of renal dysplasia is often unnecessary. If dysplasia is extensive, renal dysfunction may necessitate nephrologic care, including renal replacement therapy.

Renal ectopia: Renal ectopia (abnormal renal location) usually results when a kidney fails to ascend from its origin in the true pelvis; a rare exception occurs with a superiorly ascended (thoracic) kidney. Pelvic ectopia increases the incidence of ureteropelvic junction obstruction, VUR, and multicystic renal dysplasia.

Obstruction and severe reflux may be corrected surgically when indicated (if causing hypertension, recurrent infections, or renal growth retardation).

Renal hypoplasia: Hypoplasia usually occurs because inadequate ureteral bud branching causes an underdeveloped, small kidney with histologically normal nephrons. If hypoplasia is segmental, hypertension can occur, and ablative surgery may be needed. Patients should be evaluated for VUR.

TESTICULAR AND SCROTAL ANOMALIES

The most common anomalies are

- Congenital hydrocele
- Undescended testes (cryptorchidism)
- Testicular torsion

Rare anomalies include scrotal agenesis, hypoplasia, ectopia, or hemangioma; penoscrotal transposition; and bifid scrotum.

Congenital hydrocele: A congenital hydrocele is a collection of fluid in the scrotum between layers of the tunica vaginalis (see Fig. 301–1). It may be isolated (noncommunicating) or may communicate with the abdominal cavity through a patent processus vaginalis (a potential hernia space). Hydrocele manifests as a painless, enlarged scrotum. The condition may resolve spontaneously but usually requires repair if it persists after 12 mo or if it enlarges.

URETERAL ANOMALIES

Ureteral anomalies frequently occur with renal anomalies but may occur independently. Complications include

- Obstruction, vesicoureteral reflux (VUR), infection, and calculus formation (due to urinary stasis)
- Urinary incontinence (due to abnormal termination of the ureter in the urethra, perineum, or vagina)

Diagnosis of ureteral anomalies may be suggested by abnormalities on routine prenatal ultrasonography (eg, hydronephrosis) and occasionally by physical examination (eg, finding an external ectopic ureteral orifice or a palpable mass). Ureteral anomalies should be suspected in children with an episode of pyelonephritis or recurrent UTIs. Testing typically involves ultrasonography of the kidneys, ureters, and bladder before and after voiding, and then fluoroscopic voiding cystourethrography.

Ureteral anomaly treatments are surgical.

Ectopic ureteral orifices: Openings of single or duplicated ureters may be malpositioned on the lateral bladder wall, distally along the trigone, in the bladder neck, in the female urethra distal to the sphincter (leading to continuous incontinence despite a normal voiding pattern), in the genital system (prostate and seminal vesicle in the male, uterus or vagina in the female), or externally. Lateral ectopic orifices frequently lead to VUR, whereas distal ectopic orifices more often cause obstruction and incontinence. Surgery is needed for obstruction and incontinence and sometimes for VUR.

Retrocaval ureter: Anomalous development of the vena cava (pre-ureteric vena cava) allows the infrarenal vena cava to form anterior to the ureter (usually the right); a retrocaval ureter on the left occurs only with persistence of the left cardinal vein system or with complete situs inversus. Retrocaval ureter can cause ureteral obstruction. For significant ureteral obstruction,

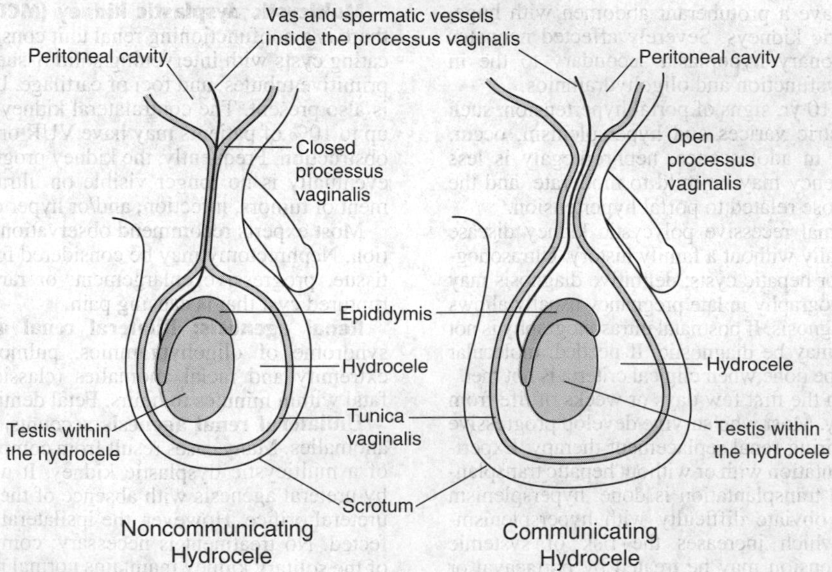

Fig. 301–1. Congenital hydrocele.

the ureter is surgically divided with uretero-ureteral anastomosis anterior to the vena cava or iliac vessel.

Ureter duplication anomalies: Partial or complete duplication of one or both ureters may occur with duplication of the ipsilateral renal pelvis. In complete duplication, the ureter from the upper pole of the kidney opens at a more caudal location than the orifice of the lower pole ureter. As a result, the lower pole tends to reflux and the upper pole tends to obstruct when pathology is present. Ectopia or stenosis of one or both orifices, VUR into the lower ureter or both ureters, and ureterocele may occur. Surgery may be necessary if there is obstruction, VUR, or urinary incontinence. Incomplete duplication is rarely of clinical significance.

Ureteral stenosis: Narrowing may occur at any location in the ureter, most frequently at the ureteropelvic junction and less commonly at the ureterovesical junction (primary megaureter). Consequences include infection, hematuria, and obstruction. Stenoses often diminish as the child grows.

In primary megaureter, ureteral tapering and reimplantation may be needed when dilation increases or infection or obstruction occurs. In ureteropelvic junction obstruction, pyeloplasty (excision of the obstructed segment and reanastomosis) may be done by open, laparoscopic, or robotic techniques.

Ureterocele: Prolapse of the lower end of the ureter into the bladder with pinpoint obstruction may cause progressive ureterectasis, hydronephrosis, infection, occasional calculus formation, and impaired renal function. Ureterocele treatment options include endoscopic transurethral incision and open repair.

When a ureterocele involves the upper pole of duplex ureters, treatment depends on function in that renal segment, because of the significant incidence of renal dysplasia. Removal of the affected renal segment and ureter may be preferable to obstruction repair if no segmental renal function is found or if significant renal dysplasia is suspected.

In rare instances, the ureterocele may prolapse beyond the bladder neck, causing a bladder outlet obstruction. In girls, this may manifest as an interlabial mass.

VAGINAL ANOMALIES

Most congenital anomalies of the vagina are rare. Vaginal anomalies include vaginal agenesis, obstruction, duplication, and fusion.

Duplication and fusion anomalies have numerous manifestations (eg, as 2 uteri, 2 cervices, and 2 vaginas, or 2 uteri with 1 cervix and 1 vagina). Girls may also have urogenital sinus anomalies, in which urinary and genital tracts open into a common channel, and cloacal anomalies, in which urinary, genital, and anorectal tracts open into a common channel.

Imperforate hymen manifests as a bulge at the location of the vaginal opening due to collection of uterine and vaginal secretions caused by maternal estrogens. Treatment of imperforate hymen is surgical drainage.

Diagnosis of most congenital anomalies of the vagina is by physical examination, ultrasonography, and retrograde contrast studies.

Duplication and fusion anomalies may not require treatment, but others require surgical correction.

VESICOURETERAL REFLUX

Vesicoureteral reflux (VUR) is retrograde passage of urine from the bladder back into the ureter and sometimes also into the renal collecting system, depending on severity.

Etiology

VUR is most often due to congenital anomalous development of the ureterovesical junction. Incomplete development of the intramural ureteral tunnel causes failure of the normal flap valve mechanism at the ureterovesical junction that permits reflux of bladder urine into the ureter and renal pelvis. Reflux can occur even when the tunnel is ordinarily sufficient if bladder pressure increases due to bladder outlet obstruction or dysfunctional voiding. Dysfunctional voiding includes infrequent voiding, constipation, or both, which may prolong resolution of VUR.

Pathophysiology

Reflux of urine from the bladder into the ureter may damage the upper urinary tract by bacterial infection and occasionally by increased hydrostatic pressure. Bacteria in the lower urinary tract can easily be transmitted by reflux to the upper tract, leading to recurrent parenchymal infection with potential scarring. Renal scarring can eventually cause hypertension and sometimes renal dysfunction. VUR is a common cause of UTI in children; about 30 to 40% of infants and toddlers with UTI have VUR.

Symptoms and Signs

Children typically present with a history of fetal hydronephrosis or with a UTI or appear as part of a sibling screening. Rarely, children present with hypertension, which is more commonly a long-term consequence of renal scarring. Children with UTI may have fever, abdominal or flank pain, dysuria, frequency, urgency, wetting accidents, or rarely hematuria.

Diagnosis

- Ultrasonography
- Voiding cystourethrography (VCUG)
- Sometimes radioisotope scan

Urinalysis and culture are done to detect infection. In infants and young children, a catheterized specimen is usually required.

Evaluation includes ultrasonography of the kidneys, ureters, and bladder before and after voiding, and then fluoroscopic VCUG. Renal ultrasonography is used to evaluate kidneys for size, hydronephrosis, and scarring. VCUG is used to diagnose VUR and to evaluate for other bladder abnormalities. A radioisotope cystogram (radionuclide cystography) may be used to monitor reflux. Renal cortical involvement with acute infection or scarring is best diagnosed with succimer (dimercaptosuccinic acid) nuclear scans when indicated. Urodynamic studies, when appropriate, may show elevated intravesical pressure.

Reflux findings on VCUG are graded on a scale from I to V (see Table 301–1). The degree of reflux can be affected by bladder capacity and bladder dynamics.

- Mild: Grades I and II
- Moderate: Grade III
- Severe: Grades IV and V

Treatment

- Sometimes antibiotic prophylaxis
- Sometimes injection of a bulking agent or ureteral reimplantation

Mild to moderate VUR often resolves spontaneously over months to several years. It is very important to keep children free of infection. Previously, children with mild to moderate VUR were given daily antibacterial prophylaxis, but there is currently no consensus on this practice. Most pediatric urologists recommend antibiotics for severe VUR at all ages

Table 301–1. GRADES OF VESICOURETERAL REFLUX*

GRADE	CHARACTERISTICS
I	Only the ureters are involved, but not the renal pelvis.
II	Reflux reaches the renal pelvis, but the calyces are not dilated.
III	The ureter and renal pelvis are dilated, with minimal or no blunting of calyces.
IV	Dilation increases, and the sharp angle of the calyceal fornices is obliterated.
V	The ureter, pelvis, and calices are grossly dilated. Papillary impressions frequently are absent.

*As defined by the International Reflux Study Committee.

and for VUR grades II to V in children < 2 yr. However, the American Academy of Pediatrics does not recommend prophylaxis for children with VUR grades I to IV after the first febrile UTI. There are multiple age- and weight-based recommendations for antibiotics, but, typically, children are given trimethoprim/sulfamethoxazole at bedtime, nitrofurantoin at dinnertime, or cephalexin twice daily.

Severe VUR accompanied by high intravesical pressures is treated with anticholinergic drugs (eg, oxybutynin, solifenacin succinate) and rarely surgery (such as botulinum toxin or bladder augmentation). Patients with bowel and bladder dysfunction benefit from behavioral modification with or without biofeedback.

Symptomatic reflux (recurrent infections, impaired renal growth, renal scarring) is treated with endoscopic injection of a bulking agent (eg, dextranomer/hyaluronic acid) or ureteral reimplantation.

Monitoring: History, physical examination (including BP measurement), laboratory testing with urinalysis and serum creatinine, and imaging using VCUG and ultrasonography are done at regular intervals depending on the child's age and the severity of the reflux and associated complications. Typically, children < 2 yr have ultrasonography every 4 to 6 mo (more frequently in children with significant nephropathy visible on ultrasonography); older children have ultrasonography every 6 to 12 mo. VCUGs are repeated every 1 to 2 yr (longer intervals for higher grade VUR, bilateral VUR, and/or older children).

In addition, toilet-trained children should be assessed at each visit for constipation and infrequent voiding, incontinence, urinary urgency, and nocturnal enuresis, which are common signs of elimination dysfunction, and treated as needed with behavioral modification and/or drug therapy.

KEY POINTS

- VUR is most often due to congenital anomalous development of the ureterovesical junction.
- Reflux of urine from the bladder into the ureter may cause bacterial infection of the upper urinary tract; about 30 to 40% of infants and toddlers with UTI have VUR.
- Diagnose by using VCUG.
- Monitor by using serial ultrasonography and VCUGs.
- Mild to moderate VUR often resolves spontaneously, but more serious disease may require surgical intervention.
- Children with newly diagnosed VUR are given prophylactic antibiotics depending on their clinical course.
- Assess toilet-trained children for dysfunctional elimination and treat them appropriately.

302 Congenital Renal Transport Abnormalities

BARTTER SYNDROME AND GITELMAN SYNDROME

Bartter syndrome and Gitelman syndrome are characterized by fluid, electrolyte, urinary, and hormonal abnormalities, including renal potassium, sodium, chloride, and hydrogen wasting; hypokalemia; hyperreninemia and hyperaldosteronism without hypertension; and metabolic alkalosis. Findings include electrolyte, growth, and sometimes neuromuscular abnormalities. Diagnosis is assisted by urine electrolyte measurements and hormone assays but is typically a diagnosis of exclusion. Treatment consists of NSAIDs, potassium-sparing diuretics, low-dose ACE inhibitors, and electrolyte replacement.

Pathophysiology

Bartter syndrome and the more common Gitelman syndrome result from deranged sodium chloride reabsorption. In Bartter syndrome, the defect is in the ascending thick limb of the loop of Henle. In Gitelman syndrome, the defect is in the distal tubule. In both syndromes, the impairment of sodium chloride reabsorption causes mild volume depletion, which leads to increases in renin and aldosterone release, resulting in potassium and hydrogen losses. In Bartter syndrome, there is increased prostaglandin secretion as well as a urinary concentrating defect due to impaired generation of the medullary concentration gradient. In Gitelman syndrome, hypomagnesemia and a low urinary calcium excretion are common. In both disorders, sodium wasting contributes to a chronic mild plasma volume contraction reflected by a normal to low BP despite high renin and angiotensin levels.

The features at clinical presentation vary (see Table 302–1).

Etiology

Both syndromes are usually autosomal recessive, although sporadic cases and other types of familial patterns can occur. There are several genotypes of both syndromes; different genotypes can have different manifestations.

Symptoms and Signs

Bartter syndrome tends to manifest prenatally or during infancy or early childhood. Gitelman syndrome tends to manifest during late childhood to adulthood. Bartter syndrome can manifest prenatally with intrauterine growth restriction and

Table 302–1. SOME DIFFERENCES BETWEEN BARTTER SYNDROME AND GITELMAN SYNDROME

FEATURE	BARTTER SYNDROME	GITELMAN SYNDROME
Location of kidney defect	Ascending loop of Henle (mimics effects of loop diuretics)	Distal tubule (mimics effects of thiazides)
Urinary calcium excretion	Normal or increased, commonly with nephrocalcinosis	Decreased
Serum magnesium level	Normal or decreased	Decreased, sometimes greatly
Renal prostaglandin E2 production	Increased	Normal
Usual age at presentation	Before birth to early childhood, often with intellectual disability and growth disturbance	Late childhood to adulthood
Neuromuscular symptoms (eg, muscle spasms, weakness)	Uncommon or mild	Common

polyhydramnios. Different forms of Bartter syndrome can have specific manifestations, including hearing loss, hypocalcemia, and nephrocalcinosis, depending on the underlying genetic defect. Children with Bartter syndrome, more so than those with Gitelman syndrome, may be born prematurely and may have poor growth and development postnatally, and some children have intellectual disability.

Most patients have low or low-normal BP and may have signs of volume depletion. Inability to retain potassium, calcium, or magnesium can lead to muscle weakness, cramping, spasms, tetany, or fatigue, particularly in Gitelman syndrome. Polydipsia, polyuria, and vomiting may be present.

In general, neither Bartter syndrome nor Gitelman syndrome typically leads to chronic renal insufficiency.

Diagnosis

- Serum and urine electrolyte levels
- Exclusion of similar disorders

Bartter syndrome and Gitelman syndrome should be suspected in children with characteristic symptoms or incidentally noted laboratory abnormalities, such as metabolic alkalosis and hypokalemia. Measurement of urine electrolytes shows high levels of sodium, potassium, and chloride that are inappropriate for the euvolemic or hypovolemic state of the patient. Diagnosis is by exclusion of other disorders:

- Primary and secondary aldosteronism can often be distinguished by the presence of hypertension and normal or low plasma levels of renin (see Table 178–2 on p. 1438).
- Surreptitious vomiting or laxative abuse can often be distinguished by low levels of urinary chloride (usually < 20 mmol/L).
- Surreptitious diuretic abuse can often be distinguished by low levels of urinary chloride and by a urine assay for diuretics.

Definitive diagnosis is through genetic testing, which is rarely done because of factors such as the large number of known mutations, large gene size, and prohibitive cost.

A 24-h measurement of urinary calcium or the urine calcium/creatinine ratio may help distinguish the two syndromes; the levels are typically normal to increased in Bartter syndrome and low in Gitelman syndrome.

Treatment

- NSAIDs (for Bartter syndrome)
- Spironolactone or amiloride
- Low-dose ACE inhibitors
- Potassium, magnesium, and calcium supplements

Because renal prostaglandin E2 secretion contributes to the pathogenesis in Bartter syndrome, NSAIDs (eg, indomethacin 1 to 2 mg/kg po once/day) are helpful; patients are also given potassium-sparing diuretics (eg, spironolactone 150 mg po bid or amiloride 10 to 20 mg po bid). Potassium-sparing diuretics alone are used in Gitelman syndrome. Low-dose ACE inhibitors can help limit the aldosterone-mediated electrolyte derangements. However, no therapy can completely eliminate potassium wasting, and potassium supplementation (KCl 20 to 40 mEq po once/day or bid) is often necessary. Magnesium and calcium supplements may also be needed.

Exogenous growth hormone can be considered to treat short stature.

KEY POINTS

- Both syndromes have impaired sodium chloride reabsorption, which causes mild volume depletion, leading to increases in renin and aldosterone release, resulting in urinary potassium and hydrogen losses.
- Manifestations vary depending on genotype, but growth and development may be affected and electrolyte abnormalities may cause muscle weakness, cramping, spasms, tetany, or fatigue.
- Diagnosis involves serum and urinary electrolyte measurement; genetic testing is rarely done.
- Treatment involves potassium and sometimes magnesium replacement. Potassium-sparing diuretics and low-dose ACE inhibitors may be used; for Bartter syndrome, NSAIDs may be added.

CYSTINURIA

Cystinuria is an inherited defect of the renal tubules in which resorption of the amino acid cystine is impaired, urinary excretion is increased, and cystine stones form in the urinary tract. Symptoms are colic caused by stones and perhaps urinary infection or the sequela of renal failure. Diagnosis is by measurement of cystine excretion in the urine. Treatment is with increased fluid intake and alkalinization of the urine.

Cystinuria was originally classified according to urinary excretion of cystine and dibasic amino acids in obligate carriers. In this classification, parents of affected children were assessed as having either normal (Type I), moderate (Type III), or significant (Type II) increases in cystine excretion.

A newer classification is based on genotype: Type A patients have homozygous mutations in the gene SLC3A1 and type B patients have homozygous mutations in SLC7A9. These genes encode proteins that together form a heterodimer responsible for cystine and dibasic amino acid transport in the proximal tubule. Cystinuria should not be confused with cystinosis (see p. 2151).

Pathophysiology

The primary defect results in diminished renal proximal tubular resorption of cystine and increased urinary cystine concentration. Cystine is poorly soluble in acidic urine, so when its urinary concentration exceeds its solubility, crystals precipitate and cystine kidney stones form.

Resorption of other dibasic amino acids (lysine, ornithine, arginine) is also impaired but causes no problems because these amino acids have an alternative transport system separate from that shared with cystine. Furthermore, they are more soluble than cystine in urine, and their increased excretion does not result in crystal or stone formation. Their absorption (and that of cystine) is also decreased in the small bowel.

Symptoms and Signs

Symptoms, most commonly renal colic, may occur in infants but usually appear between ages 10 and 30. UTI and renal failure due to urinary tract obstruction may develop.

Diagnosis

- Microscopic examination of urinary sediment
- Measurement of urinary cystine excretion
- Analysis of collected kidney stones

Radiopaque cystine stones form in the renal pelvis or bladder. Staghorn stones are common. Cystine may appear in the urine as yellow-brown hexagonal crystals, which are diagnostic. Excessive cystine in the urine may be detected with the nitroprusside cyanide test. Quantitative cystine excretion is typically > 400 mg/day in cystinuria (normal is < 30 mg/day).

Treatment

- High fluid intake
- Alkalinization of the urine
- Dietary sodium restriction
- Dietary protein restriction (when possible)

End-stage renal disease may develop. Decreasing urinary cystine excretion decreases renal toxicity and is accomplished by increasing urine volume with fluid intake sufficient to provide a urine flow rate of 3 to 4 L/day. Hydration is particularly important at night when urinary pH drops. Alkalinization of the urine to pH > 7.0 with potassium citrate or potassium bicarbonate 1 mEq/kg po tid to qid and in some cases acetazolamide 5 mg/kg (up to 250 mg) po at bedtime increases the solubility of cystine significantly. Mild restrictions of dietary sodium (100 mEq/day) and protein (0.8 to 1.0 g/kg/day) may help reduce cystine excretion.

When high fluid intake and alkalinization do not reduce stone formation, other drugs may be tried. Penicillamine (7.5 mg/kg po qid in young children and 125 mg to 0.5 g po qid in older children) improves cystine solubility, but toxicity limits its usefulness. About half of all patients develop some toxic manifestation, such as fever, rash, arthralgias, or, less commonly, nephrotic syndrome, pancytopenia, or SLE-like reaction. Pyridoxine supplements (50 mg po once/day) should be given with penicillamine. Tiopronin (100 mg to 300 mg po qid) can be used instead of penicillamine to treat some children because it has a lower frequency of adverse effects. Captopril (0.3 mg/kg po tid) is not as effective as penicillamine but is less toxic. Close monitoring of response to therapy is very important.

KEY POINTS

- Defective urinary resorption of cystine increases urinary cystine levels, leading to cystine kidney stones and sometimes chronic kidney disease.
- Yellow-brown hexagonal crystals in the urine are pathognomonic; quantitative cystine excretion is typically > 400 mg/day.
- Treat with increased fluid intake to give urine output 3 to 4 L/day, and alkalinize urine with potassium citrate or potassium bicarbonate.
- Restrict dietary sodium and protein.
- Drugs such as penicillamine, tiopronin, or captopril may be necessary, but adverse effects are a concern.

HARTNUP DISEASE

Hartnup disease is a rare disease due to abnormal absorption and excretion of tryptophan and other amino acids. Symptoms are rash, CNS abnormalities, short stature, headache, and collapsing or fainting. Diagnosis is by high urinary content of tryptophan and other amino acids. Prevention is with niacinamide or niacin, and attacks are treated with nicotinamide.

Hartnup disease is caused by a mutation in the sodium-dependent neutral amino acid transporter gene that is expressed in kidney and intestinal epithelia. It is inherited as an autosomal recessive trait.

Small-bowel malabsorption of tryptophan, phenylalanine, methionine, and other monoamino monocarboxylic amino acids occurs. Accumulation of unabsorbed amino acids in the GI tract increases their metabolism by bacterial flora. Some tryptophan degradation products, including indoles, kynurenine, and serotonin, are absorbed by the intestine and appear in the urine. Renal amino acid resorption is also defective, causing a generalized aminoaciduria involving all neutral amino acids except proline and hydroxyproline. Conversion of tryptophan to niacinamide is also defective.

Symptoms and Signs

Although the disorder is present from birth, symptoms of Hartnup disease may manifest in infancy, childhood, or early adulthood. Symptoms may be precipitated by sunlight, fever, drugs, or other stresses.

Poor nutritional intake nearly always precedes appearance of symptoms. Symptoms and signs are due to niacinamide deficiency and resemble those of pellagra, particularly the rash on parts of the body exposed to the sun; mucous membrane and neurologic symptoms also occur. Neurologic manifestations include cerebellar ataxia and mental abnormalities. Intellectual disability, short stature, headache, and collapsing or fainting are common.

Diagnosis

- Urine testing for amino acids

Diagnosis of Hartnup disease is made by showing the characteristic amino acid excretion pattern in the urine. Indoles and other tryptophan degradation products in the urine provide supplementary evidence of the disease.

Treatment

- Niacin or niacinamide supplements
- Nicotinamide for attacks

Prognosis is good, and frequency of attacks usually diminishes with age. The number and severity of attacks can be reduced by maintaining good nutrition and supplementing the diet with niacin or niacinamide 50 to 100 mg po tid. Attacks may be treated with nicotinamide 20 mg po once/day.

HYPOPHOSPHATEMIC RICKETS

(Vitamin D–Resistant Rickets)

Hypophosphatemic rickets is a disorder characterized by hypophosphatemia, defective intestinal absorption of calcium, and rickets or osteomalacia unresponsive to vitamin D. It is usually hereditary. Symptoms are bone pain, fractures, and growth abnormalities. Diagnosis is by serum phosphate, alkaline phosphatase, and 1,25-dihydroxyvitamin D3 levels. Treatment is oral phosphate plus calcitriol.

Familial hypophosphatemic rickets is usually inherited as an X-linked dominant trait; other familial patterns occur but are rarer.

Sporadic acquired cases sometimes are associated with benign mesenchymal tumors that produce a humoral factor that decreases proximal renal tubular resorption of phosphate (tumor-induced osteomalacia).

Pathophysiology

The observed abnormality is decreased proximal renal tubular resorption of phosphate, resulting in renal phosphate wasting and hypophosphatemia. This defect is due to circulating factors called phosphatonins. The principle phosphatonin in hereditary hypophosphatemic rickets is FGF-23. Decreased intestinal calcium and phosphate absorption also occurs. Deficient bone mineralization is due to low phosphate levels and osteoblast dysfunction rather than to the low calcium and elevated parathyroid hormone (PTH) levels as in calcipenic rickets (see p. 50). Because 1,25-dihydroxyvitamin D_3 levels are normal to slightly low, a defect in conversion is presumed; hypophosphatemia would normally cause elevated 1,25-dihydroxyvitamin D_3 levels.

A form of hereditary hypophosphatemic rickets with hypercalciuria (HHRH) is known to occur due to mutations in the proximal tubule type 2c sodium-phosphate cotransporter. Defective phosphate transport and hypophosphatemia in this case result in appropriately increased 1,25-dihydroxyvitamin D_3 levels, thus leading to hypercalciuria.

Symptoms and Signs

The disease manifests as a spectrum of abnormalities, from hypophosphatemia alone to growth retardation and short stature to severe rickets or osteomalacia. Children usually present after they begin walking, with bowing of the legs and other bone deformities, pseudofractures (ie, x-ray findings in osteomalacia that may represent areas of prior stress fractures that have been replaced by inadequately mineralized osteoid vs areas of bony erosions), bone pain, and short stature. Bony outgrowth at muscle attachments may limit motion.

Rickets of the spine or pelvis, dental enamel defects, and tetany that occur in dietary vitamin D deficiency are rarely present in hypophosphatemic rickets.

Patients with HHRH may present with nephrolithiasis and/or nephrocalcinosis.

Diagnosis

- Serum levels of calcium, phosphate, alkaline phosphatase, 1,25-dihydroxyvitamin D_3, PTH, FGF-23, and creatinine
- Urinary phosphate and creatinine levels (for calculation of the tubular reabsorption of phosphate)
- Bone x-rays

Serum phosphate levels are depressed, but urinary phosphate excretion is large. Serum calcium and PTH are normal, and alkaline phosphatase often is elevated. Hypophosphatemia-induced stimulation of calcitriol production does not occur. Typically, calcidiol levels are normal, whereas calcitriol levels are normal to low. In calcipenic rickets, hypocalcemia is present, hypophosphatemia is mild or absent, and urinary phosphate is not elevated.

Treatment

- Oral phosphate and calcitriol

Treatment of hypophosphatemic rickets consists of neutral phosphate solution or tablets. Starting dose in children is 10 mg/kg (based on elemental phosphorus) po qid. Phosphate supplementation lowers ionized calcium concentrations and further inhibits calcitriol conversion, leading to secondary hyperparathyroidism and exacerbating urinary phosphate wasting. Therefore, vitamin D is given as calcitriol, initially 5 to 10 ng/kg po bid. This, however, is not the case with HHRH, where 1,25-dihydroxyvitamin D3 levels are elevated and dosing with calcitriol can be detrimental.

Phosphate dose may need to be increased to achieve bone growth or relieve bone pain. Diarrhea may limit oral phosphate dosage. Increase in plasma phosphate and decrease in alkaline phosphatase concentrations, healing of rickets, and improvement of growth rate occur. Hypercalcemia, hypercalciuria, and nephrocalcinosis with reduced renal function may complicate treatment. Patients undergoing treatment need frequent follow-up evaluations.

Adults with oncogenic rickets may dramatically improve once the mesenchymal tumor that causes the disorder is removed. Otherwise, oncogenic rickets is treated with calcitriol 5 to 10 ng/kg po bid and elemental phosphorus 250 mg to 1 g po tid or qid.

KEY POINTS

- Decreased renal resorption of phosphate results in renal phosphate wasting and hypophosphatemia.
- There is deficient bone mineralization due to low phosphate levels and osteoblast dysfunction.
- Children have growth retardation, bone pain and deformities (eg, leg bowing), and short stature.
- Patients with hypophosphatemic rickets with hypercalciuria (HHRH) may present with nephrolithiasis and/or nephrocalcinosis.
- Diagnose by finding low serum phosphate levels, elevated urinary phosphate, and normal serum calcium and PTH.
- Treat with oral phosphate supplements and, except for HHRH, vitamin D (given as calcitriol).

303 Connective Tissue Disorders in Children

There are over 200 disorders that involve connective tissue. Certain disorders are characterized by overactivity of the immune system with resulting inflammation and systemic damage to the tissues (eg, systemic lupus erythematosus [SLE] and juvenile idiopathic arthritis [formerly known as juvenile rheumatoid arthritis]). Other disorders involve biochemical abnormalities or structural defects of the connective tissue. Some of these disorders are inherited, and some are of unknown etiology.

CHONDROMALACIA PATELLAE

(Patellofemoral Syndrome)

Chondromalacia patellae is softening of the cartilage underneath the patella.

Chondromalacia patellae often causes generalized knee pain especially when climbing or descending stairs, playing sports that exert an axial load on the knee, or sitting for a long time (theater sign). Usually the pain occurs without swelling. This disorder probably results from angular or rotational changes in the leg that unbalance elements of the quadriceps and cause patellar misalignment during movement.

Acute pain due to chondromalacia patellae is treated by doing physical therapy to improve the mechanics, applying ice, and taking analgesics. Children with chondromalacia patellae should avoid pain-causing activities (typically, those that involve bending the knee) for several days. Persistent or recurrent pain due to chondromalacia patellae may rarely require arthroscopic smoothing of the patella's undersurface.

CUTIS LAXA

Cutis laxa is characterized by lax skin hanging in loose folds. Diagnosis is clinical. There is no specific treatment, but plastic surgery is sometimes done.

Cutis laxa (CL) may be inherited or acquired. There are 4 hereditary forms:

- Autosomal dominant
- X-linked recessive
- 2 autosomal recessive

The autosomal recessive forms tend to be more common, and one of them causes potentially lethal cardiovascular, respiratory, and GI complications. The other inherited forms may be relatively benign.

Rarely, infants can acquire cutis laxa after a febrile illness or after exposure to a specific drug (eg, hypersensitivity reaction to penicillin, fetal exposure to penicillamine). In children or adolescents, cutis laxa usually develops after a severe illness involving fever, polyserositis, or erythema multiforme. In adults, it may develop insidiously or in association with a variety of disorders, particularly plasma cell dyscrasias. The underlying defect in these acquired cases is unknown, but fragmented elastin is present in all forms.

Pathophysiology

Cutis laxa is caused by abnormal elastin metabolism that results in reduced elasticity of the skin. The precise cause is unknown except in congenital cases where an underlying gene defect (eg, in the *ELN*, *FBLN4*, *FBLN5*, *ATP6V0A2*, or *ATP7A* genes) can be identified. Several factors, such as copper deficiency, elastin quantity and morphology, and elastases and elastase inhibitors, are implicated in the abnormal elastin degradation.

Symptoms and Signs

In hereditary forms, dermal laxity may be present at birth or develop later; it occurs wherever the skin is normally loose and hanging in folds, most obviously on the face. Affected children have mournful or Churchillian facies and a hooked nose. The benign autosomal recessive form also causes intellectual disability and joint laxity. GI tract hernias and diverticula are common. If the disorder is severe, progressive pulmonary emphysema may precipitate cor pulmonale. Bronchiectasis, heart failure, and aortic aneurysms can also occur.

Diagnosis

- Clinical evaluation
- Sometimes skin biopsy, testing for complications

Diagnosis of cutis laxa is clinical. There are no specific laboratory findings; however, a skin biopsy may be done. Certain tests (eg, echocardiography, chest x-ray) may be done to check for associated conditions (eg, emphysema, cardiomegaly, heart failure) in patients with cardiopulmonary symptoms. Genetic testing is indicated for patients with early-onset cutis laxa or a suggestive family history because test results may predict the risk of transmission to offspring and of extracutaneous organ involvement.

Typical cutis laxa can be distinguished from Ehlers-Danlos syndrome because dermal fragility and articular hypermobility are absent. Other disorders sometimes cause localized areas of loose skin. In Turner syndrome, lax skinfolds at the base of an affected girl's neck tighten and resemble webbing as she ages. In neurofibromatosis, unilateral pendular plexiform neuromas occasionally develop, but their configuration and texture distinguish them from cutis laxa.

Treatment

- Sometimes plastic surgery

There is no specific cutis laxa treatment. Physical therapy may sometimes help increase skin tone.

Plastic surgery considerably improves appearance in patients with hereditary cutis laxa but is less successful in those with acquired disease. Healing is usually uncomplicated, but dermal laxity may recur. Extracutaneous complications are treated appropriately.

EHLERS-DANLOS SYNDROME

Ehlers-Danlos syndrome is a hereditary collagen disorder characterized by articular hypermobility, dermal hyperelasticity, and widespread tissue fragility. Diagnosis is clinical. Treatment is supportive.

Inheritance is usually autosomal dominant, but Ehlers-Danlos syndrome is heterogeneous. Different gene mutations affect the amount, structure, or assembly of different collagens. Mutations can exist in the genes that encode collagens (eg, type I, III, or V) or collagen-modifying enzymes (eg, lysyl hydroxylase, a collagen-cleaving protease). There are 6 major types:

- Classic
- Hypermobility
- Vascular
- Kyphoscoliosis
- Arthrochalasis
- Dermatosparaxis

There are also several rare or hard-to-classify types.

Symptoms and Signs

Symptoms and signs of Ehlers-Danlos syndrome vary widely.

Predominant symptoms include hypermobile joints, abnormal scar formation and wound healing, fragile vessels, and velvety, hyperextensible skin. Skin can be stretched several centimeters but returns to normal when released.

Wide papyraceous scars often overlie bony prominences, particularly elbows, knees, and shins; scarring is less severe in the hypermobility type. Molluscoid pseudotumors (fleshy outgrowths) frequently form on top of scars or at pressure points.

Extent of joint hypermobility varies but may be marked in the arthrochalasis, classic, and hypermobility types.

Bleeding tendency is rare, although the vascular type is characterized by vascular rupture and bruising. Subcutaneous calcified spherules may be palpated or seen on x-rays.

Complications of Ehlers-Danlos syndrome: Minor trauma may cause wide gaping wounds but little bleeding; surgical wound closure may be difficult because sutures tend to tear out of the fragile tissue. Surgical complications occur because of deep tissue fragility. Sclera may be fragile, leading to perforation of the globe in the kyphoscoliosis type.

Bland synovial effusions, sprains, and dislocations occur frequently. Spinal kyphoscoliosis occurs in 25% of patients (especially in those with the kyphoscoliosis type), thoracic deformity in 20%, and talipes equinovarum in 5%. About 90% of affected adults have pes planus (flat feet). Congenital hip dislocation occurs in 1% (the arthrochalasis type is characterized by bilateral congenital hip dislocation).

GI hernias and diverticula are common. Rarely, portions of the GI tract spontaneously hemorrhage and perforate, and dissecting aortic aneurysm and large arteries spontaneously rupture.

Valvular prolapse is a common complication in the most severe type (vascular type).

In pregnant women, tissue extensibility may cause premature birth, cervical incompetence, and possibly uterine rupture; if the fetus is affected, fetal membrane is fragile, sometimes resulting in early rupture. Maternal tissue fragility may complicate episiotomy or cesarean delivery. Antenatal, perinatal, and postnatal bleeding may occur.

Other potentially serious complications include arteriovenous fistula, ruptured viscus, and pneumothorax or pneumohemothorax.

Diagnosis

- Clinical evaluation
- Echocardiography and/or other vascular imaging to screen for cardiovascular complications

Initial diagnosis of Ehlers-Danlos syndrome is largely clinical but should be confirmed by genetic testing, which is now available for most subtypes. Ultrastructural examination of skin biopsy can help in diagnosing the classic, hypermobility, and vascular types.

Echocardiography and other vascular imaging are done to check for heart disorders (eg, valvular prolapse, arterial aneurysm) that are associated with some of the types.

Prognosis

Life span is usually normal with most types. Potentially lethal complications occur in certain types (eg, arterial rupture in the vascular type).

Treatment

- Early recognition and treatment of complications

There is no specific treatment for Ehlers-Danlos syndrome. Trauma should be minimized. Protective clothing and padding may help. If surgery is done, hemostasis must be meticulous. Wounds are carefully sutured, and tissue tension is avoided.

Obstetric supervision during pregnancy and delivery is mandatory. Genetic counseling should be provided.

INFRAPATELLAR TENDINITIS

(Jumper's Knee; Sinding-Larsen-Johansson Syndrome)

Infrapatellar tendinitis is an overuse injury to the patellar tendon at the attachment to the lower pole of the patella.

Knee pain with infrapatellar tendon tenderness in physically active children is caused by an overuse syndrome that usually occurs in figure skaters and basketball or volleyball players. It typically affects children 10 to 13 yr. Pain is the most exaggerated when straightening the knee against force (eg, climbing stairs, jumping, doing knee bends).

Etiology of infrapatellar tendinitis is thought to be trauma due to excessive traction by the patellar tendon at its site of origin, leading to microavulsion fractures.

History and physical examination are usually sufficient for diagnosis of infrapatellar tendinitis; however, MRI can show the extent of the injury.

Pain is treated with modification of activities, NSAIDs, and physical therapy. Persistent pain may be treated with surgical repair; however, this is usually not necessary.

MARFAN SYNDROME

Marfan syndrome consists of connective tissue anomalies resulting in ocular, skeletal, and cardiovascular abnormalities (eg, dilation of ascending aorta, which can lead to aortic dissection). Diagnosis is clinical. Treatment may include prophylactic beta-blockers to slow dilation of the ascending aorta and prophylactic aortic surgery.

Inheritance of Marfan syndrome is autosomal dominant. The basic molecular defect results from mutations in the gene encoding the glycoprotein fibrillin-1 (*FBN1*), which is the main component of microfibrils and helps anchor cells to the extracellular matrix. The principal structural defect involves the cardiovascular, musculoskeletal, and ocular systems. The pulmonary system and CNS are also affected. There are many different manifestations of the genetic mutation that causes Marfan syndrome; however, it is typically recognized by the constellation of long limbs, aortic root dilation, and dislocated lenses.

Symptoms and Signs

Cardiovascular system: Major findings include

- Aortic aneurysm
- Valvular prolapse

Most severe complications result from pathologic changes in the aortic root and ascending aorta. The aortic media is affected preferentially in areas subject to the greatest hemodynamic stress. The aorta progressively dilates or acutely dissects, beginning in the coronary sinuses, sometimes before age 10 yr. The aortic root dilates in 50% of children and in 60 to 80% of adults and can cause aortic regurgitation, in which case a diastolic murmur may be heard over the aortic valve.

Redundant cusps and chordae tendineae may lead to mitral valve prolapse or regurgitation; mitral valve prolapse may cause a systolic click and a late systolic murmur or, in severe cases, a holosystolic murmur. Bacterial endocarditis may develop in affected valves.

Musculoskeletal system: Severity varies greatly. Patients are taller than average for age and family; arm span exceeds height. Arachnodactyly (disproportionately long, thin digits) is noticeable, often by the thumb sign (the distal phalanx of the thumb protrudes beyond the edge of the clenched fist). Sternum deformity—pectus carinatum (outward displacement) or pectus excavatum (inward displacement)—is common, as are joint hyperextensibility (but usually small flexion contractures to the elbows), genu recurvatum (backward curvature of the legs at the knees), pes planus (flat feet), kyphoscoliosis, and diaphragmatic and inguinal hernias. Subcutaneous fat usually is sparse. The palate is often high-arched.

Ocular system: Findings include ectopia lentis (subluxation or upward dislocation of the lens) and iridodonesis (tremulousness of the iris). The margin of the dislocated lens can often be seen through the undilated pupil. High-grade myopia may be present, and spontaneous retinal detachment may occur.

Pulmonary system: Cystic lung disease and recurrent spontaneous pneumothorax may occur. These disorders can cause pain and shortness of breath.

CNS: Dural ectasia (widening of the dural sac surrounding the spinal cord) is a common finding and most frequently occurs in the lumbosacral spine. It may cause headache, lower back pain, or neurologic deficits manifested by bowel or bladder weakness.

Diagnosis

- Clinical criteria
- Genetic testing
- Echocardiography/MRI (measurement of the aortic root, detection of valve prolapse)
- Slit-lamp examination (lens abnormalities)
- X-rays of skeletal system (hand, spine, pelvis, chest, foot, and skull for characteristic abnormalities)
- MRI of the lumbosacral spine (dural ectasia)

Diagnosis of Marfan syndrome can be difficult because many patients have only a few typical symptoms and signs and no specific histologic or biochemical changes. Considering this variability, diagnostic criteria are based on constellations of clinical findings and family and genetic history. (For more on diagnosis, see the revised Ghent nosology.) Nonetheless, diagnosis is uncertain in many partial cases of Marfan syndrome.

Homocystinuria can partially mimic Marfan syndrome but can be differentiated by detecting homocystine in the urine. Genetic testing for *FBN1* mutations can help establish the diagnosis in people who do not meet all clinical criteria, but *FBN1* mutation-negative cases exist. Prenatal diagnosis by analysis of the *FBN1* gene is hampered by poor genotype/phenotype correlation (> 1700 different mutations have been described). Standard imaging of the skeletal, cardiovascular, and ocular systems is done to detect any clinically relevant structural abnormalities and to provide information contributing to the diagnostic criteria (eg, echocardiography to identify aortic root enlargement). In addition to the criteria established within organ systems, family history (1st-degree relative with Marfan syndrome) and genetic history (presence of the *FBN1* mutation known to cause Marfan syndrome) are considered major criteria.

Prognosis

Advancements in therapy and regular monitoring have improved quality of life and reduced mortality. Median life expectancy increased from 48 yr in 1972 to near normal in people receiving appropriate medical care. However, life expectancy is still reduced for the average patient, primarily because of the cardiac and vascular complications. This decreased life expectancy can take an emotional toll on an adolescent and the family.

Treatment

- Induction of precocious puberty in tall girls
- Beta-blockers
- Elective aortic repair and valve repair
- Bracing and surgery for scoliosis

Treatment of Marfan syndrome focuses on prevention and treatment of complications.

For very tall girls, inducing precocious puberty by age 10 with estrogens and progesterone may reduce potential adult height.

All patients should routinely be given beta-blockers (eg, atenolol, propranolol) to help prevent cardiovascular complications. These drugs lower myocardial contractility and pulse pressure and reduce progression of aortic root dilation and risk of dissection.

Prophylactic surgery is offered if aortic diameter is > 5 cm (less in children). Pregnant women are at especially high risk of aortic complications; elective aortic repair before conception should be discussed. Severe valve regurgitation is also surgically repaired. Bacterial endocarditis prophylaxis before invasive procedures is not indicated except in patients who have prosthetic valves or who previously had infective endocarditis (see Tables 82–3 and 82–4 on p. 711).

Scoliosis is managed with bracing as long as possible, but surgical intervention is encouraged in patients with curves of 40 to 50°.

Cardiovascular, skeletal, and ocular findings (including echocardiography) should be reevaluated annually. Appropriate genetic counseling is indicated.

KEY POINTS

- Marfan syndrome results from an autosomal dominant mutation of the gene encoding the glycoprotein fibrillin-1, which is the main component of microfibrils, resulting in numerous possible deformities and defects.
- Manifestations vary widely, but the principal structural defects involve the cardiovascular, musculoskeletal, and ocular systems, causing a typical constellation of long limbs, aortic root dilation, and dislocated lenses.
- Aortic dissection is the most dangerous complication.
- Diagnose using clinical criteria; genetic testing is often done.

- Do imaging tests of the skeletal, cardiovascular, and ocular systems to detect structural abnormalities.
- Give all patients a beta-blocker to help prevent aortic complications; treat other complications as they arise.

NAIL-PATELLA SYNDROME

(Arthro-Onychodysplasia; Onycho-Osteodysplasia; Osteo-Onychodysplasia)

Nail-patella syndrome is a rare inherited disorder of mesenchymal tissue characterized by abnormalities of bones, joints, fingernails and toenails, and kidneys. Diagnosis is clinical. There is no specific treatment, but ACE inhibitors may be given for proteinuria and hypertension, and kidney transplantation is sometimes done.

Nail-patella syndrome is an autosomal dominant disorder caused by a mutation in the gene for the transcription factor *LMX1B*, which plays an important role in vertebrate limb and kidney development.

Symptoms and Signs

There is bilateral hypoplasia or absence of the patella, subluxation of the radial head at the elbows, and bilateral accessory iliac horns. Fingernails and toenails are absent or hypoplastic, with pitting and ridges.

Renal dysfunction occurs in up to 50% of patients due to focal segmental glomerular deposits of IgM and C3. Proteinuria, hypertension, and hematuria are the most common manifestations, but about 30% of patients with renal involvement slowly progress to renal failure.

Diagnosis

- Clinical evaluation

Diagnosis of nail-patella syndrome is suggested clinically; sometimes renal biopsy and bone x-rays are indicated, which are diagnostic.

LMX1B mutation analysis is possible, including for prenatal diagnosis, but the type of mutation does not usually predict clinical severity. *LMXB1* mutations affecting only the kidney have been described.

Treatment

- ACE inhibitors for proteinuria and hypertension
- Sometimes kidney transplantation

There is no specific treatment for nail-patella syndrome, but proteinuria and hypertension can be treated with ACE inhibitors.

When indicated, kidney transplantation has been successful without evidence of recurrent disease in the graft.

OSTEOCHONDRODYSPLASIAS

(Genetic Skeletal Dysplasias; Osteochondrodysplastic Dwarfism)

Osteochondrodysplasias involve abnormal bone or cartilage growth, leading to skeletal maldevelopment, often short-limbed dwarfism. Diagnosis is by physical examination, x-rays, and, in some cases, genetic testing. Treatment is surgical.

The basic genetic defects have been identified in most of the osteochondrodysplasias. The mutations typically cause perturbation of function in proteins involved in growth and development of connective tissue, bone, or cartilage (see Table 303–1).

Dwarfism is markedly short stature (adult height < 4 ft 10 in) frequently associated with disproportionate growth of the trunk and extremities. Achondroplasia is the most common and best-known type of short-limbed dwarfism, but there are many other distinct types, which differ widely in genetic background, course, and prognosis (see Table 303–1). Lethal short-limbed dwarfism (thanatophoric dysplasia, caused by mutations in the same gene as achondroplasia) causes severe chest wall deformities and respiratory failure in neonates, resulting in death.

Diagnosis

- X-rays

Characteristic x-ray changes may be diagnostic. A whole-body x-ray of every affected neonate, even if stillborn, should be taken because diagnostic precision is essential for predicting prognosis.

Prenatal diagnosis by fetoscopy or ultrasonography is possible in some cases (eg, when fetal limb shortening is severe).

Standard laboratory tests do not help, but molecular diagnosis is feasible for chondrodysplasias with known molecular defects. Genetic testing is advised if a diagnosis cannot be made based on clinical grounds or if genetic counseling is desired.

Treatment

- Sometimes surgical limb-lengthening or joint replacement

In achondroplasia, treatment with human growth hormone is generally not effective. An increase in adult height may be achieved by surgical limb lengthening. In this and other nonlethal osteochondrodysplasias, surgery (eg, hip replacement) can help improve joint function. Hypoplasia of the odontoid process can predispose to subluxation of the 1st and 2nd cervical vertebrae and compression of the spinal cord. Therefore, the odontoid process should be evaluated preoperatively and, if it is abnormal, the patient's head should be carefully supported when hyperextended for endotracheal intubation during anesthesia.

Because the inheritance pattern and gene mutations in most types are known, genetic counseling can be effective. Organizations such as Little People of America provide resources for affected people and act as advocates on their behalf. Similar societies are active in other countries.

KEY POINTS

- Osteochondrodysplasias are inherited abnormalities of growth and development of connective tissue, bone, and/or cartilage.
- There are many types, which differ widely in genetic background, course, and prognosis, but all cause markedly short stature and often disproportionate growth of the trunk and extremities.
- Diagnosis is by clinical manifestations and identification of characteristic x-ray changes.
- Growth hormone treatments are typically ineffective.

Table 303–1. TYPES OF OSTEOCHONDRODYSPLASTIC DWARFISM

DISORDER	SYMPTOMS AND SIGNS	USUAL MODE OF INHERITANCE	DEFECTIVE GENE PRODUCT
Achondroplasia	Bulky forehead, saddle nose, lumbar lordosis, bowlegs	AD	Fibroblast growth factor receptor 3 (FGFR)
Chondrodysplasia punctata	Variable extraskeletal manifestations X-rays show epiphyseal stippling in infancy due to calcifications	See below	See below
Chondrodysplasia punctata (rhizomelic form)	Marked proximal limb shortening Death during infancy	AR	Peroxisomal type 2 targeting signal receptor (PTS2)
Chondrodysplasia punctata (Conradi-Hünermann form)	Mild, asymmetric limb shortening Benign	AD or XL dominant	Delta(8)-delta(7)-sterol isomerase mopamil-binding protein (EBP)
Chondroectodermal dysplasia (Ellis-van Creveld [EVC] syndrome)	Distal limb shortening, postaxial polydactyly, structural cardiac defects	AR	EVC, EVC2
Diastrophic dysplasia	Severe dwarfism with rigid hitchhiker thumb and fixed talipes equinovarum	AR	Solute carrier family 26 (sulfate transporter), member 2 (SLC26A2)
Hypochondroplasia	Symptoms of achondroplasia but milder	AD	Fibroblast growth factor receptor 3 (FGFR3—not all patients)
Mesomelic dysplasia*	Predominantly, shortening of the forearms and shanks Normal facies and spine	AD or AR	Not defined
Metaphyseal chondrodysplasia[†]	In some forms, malabsorption, neutropenia, thymolymphopenia	AR or AD	Parathyroid hormone receptor (PTHR), type X collagen (COL10A1)
Multiple epiphyseal dysplasia	Mild dwarfism, normal spine and facies, sometimes stubby digits, hip dysplasia (often as 1st symptom) Very heterogeneous	AR or AD	Solute carrier family 26 (sulfate transporter), member 2 (SLC26A2; AR form)
Pseudoachondroplasia	Normal facies, various degrees of dwarfism and kyphoscoliosis Heterogeneous	AD or AR	Cartilage oligomeric matrix protein (COMP)
Spondyloepiphyseal dysplasia	Predominantly, kyphoscoliosis Sometimes myopia and a flat facies Heterogeneous	AD, AR, or XL	Type II collagen (COL2A1), tracking protein particle complex, subunit 2 (TRAPPC2, also known as SEDL)

*There are several eponymous forms (eg, Nievergelt, Langer).
[†]There are many different eponymous forms (eg, Jansen, Schmid, McKusick).
AD = autosomal dominant; AR = autosomal recessive; XL =X-linked.

OSTEOGENESIS IMPERFECTA

Osteogenesis imperfecta is a hereditary collagen disorder causing diffuse abnormal fragility of bone and is sometimes accompanied by sensorineural hearing loss, blue sclerae, dentinogenesis imperfecta, and joint hypermobility. Diagnosis is usually clinical. Treatment includes growth hormone for some types and bisphosphonates.

There are 4 main types of osteogenesis imperfecta (OI):

- I (autosomal dominant)
- II (autosomal recessive)
- III (autosomal recessive)
- IV (autosomal dominant)

Ninety percent of people who have one of the major types have mutations in the genes encoding the pro-alpha chains of type I procollagen (a structural component of bones, ligaments, and tendons), *COL1A1* or *COL1A2*. Other types are rare and are caused by mutations in different genes.

Symptoms and Signs

Hearing loss is present in 50 to 65% of all patients with osteogenesis imperfecta and may occur in any of the 4 types.

Type I is the mildest. Symptoms and signs in some patients are limited to blue sclerae (due to a deficiency in connective tissue allowing the underlying vessels to show through) and musculoskeletal pain due to joint hypermobility. Recurrent fractures in childhood are possible.

Type II (neonatal lethal type or OI congenita) is the most severe and is lethal. Multiple congenital fractures result in shortened extremities. Sclerae are blue. The skull is soft and, when palpated, feels like a bag of bones. Because the skull is soft, trauma during delivery may cause intracranial hemorrhage and stillbirth, or neonates may die suddenly during the first few days or weeks of life.

Type III is the most severe nonlethal form of OI. Patients with type III have short stature, spinal curvature, and multiple, recurrent fractures. Macrocephaly with triangular facies and pectal deformities are common. Scleral hue varies.

Type IV is intermediate in severity. Survival rate is high. Bones fracture easily in childhood before adolescence. Sclera are typically normal in color. Height is moderate-short stature. Accurate diagnosis is important because these patients may benefit from treatment.

Diagnosis

- Clinical evaluation
- Sometimes analysis of type I procollagen or genetic testing

Diagnosis of osteogenesis imperfecta is usually clinical, but there are no standardized criteria.

Analysis of type I procollagen from cultured fibroblasts (from a skin biopsy) or sequence analysis of the *COL1A1* and *COL1A2* genes can be used when clinical diagnosis is unclear.

Severe osteogenesis imperfecta can be detected in utero by level II ultrasonography.

Treatment

- Growth hormone
- Bisphosphonates

Growth hormone helps growth-responsive children (types I and IV).

Treatment with bisphosphonates is aimed at increasing bone density and decreasing bone pain and fracture risk.[1] IV pamidronate (0.5 to 3 mg/kg once/day for 3 days, repeated as needed q 4 to 6 mo) or oral alendronate (1 mg/kg, 20 mg maximum, once/day) are used.

Orthopedic surgery, physical therapy, and occupational therapy help prevent fractures and improve function.

Cochlear implantation is indicated in selected cases of hearing loss.

1. Dwan K, Phillipi CA, Steiner RD, Basel D: Bisphosphonate therapy for osteogenesis imperfecta. *Cochrane Database Syst Rev* CD005088, 2016. 10.1002/14651858.CD005088.pub4

PSEUDOXANTHOMA ELASTICUM

Pseudoxanthoma elasticum is a rare genetic disorder characterized by calcification of the elastic fibers of the skin, retina, and cardiovascular system. Diagnosis is clinical. There is no specific treatment, but intravitreal injections of angiogenesis-blocking antibodies may be given for angioid streaks.

Pseudoxanthoma elasticum is caused by mutations in the *ABCC6* gene that are inherited in both autosomal dominant and recessive forms. The *ABCC6* gene product is a transmembrane transporter protein that probably plays roles in cellular detoxification. Characteristic cutaneous papular lesions begin in childhood and are primarily of cosmetic concern. They appear as small yellowish papules that typically occur on the neck and axillae and flexural surfaces. Elastic tissues become calcified and fragmented, leading to disruption of the involved organ systems:

- Ocular system: Angioid streaks of the retina, retinal hemorrhages, and gradual vision loss
- Cardiovascular system: Premature atherosclerosis with subsequent intermittent claudication, hypertension, angina, and MI
- Vascular fragility: GI hemorrhage and small-vessel bleeding with subsequent anemia

Diagnosis

- Clinical evaluation

Diagnosis of pseudoxanthoma elasticum is based on clinical and histologic findings.

Laboratory and imaging studies are done for associated conditions (eg, CBC, echocardiography, head CT).

Treatment

- Angiogenesis-blocking antibodies for angioid streaks

Treatment of retinal angioid streaks with intravitreal injections of angiogenesis-blocking antibodies (eg, bevacizumab) shows promise.

Otherwise, there is no specific treatment, and the aim is to prevent complications. People should avoid drugs that may cause stomach or intestinal bleeding, such as aspirin, other NSAIDs, and anticoagulants. People with pseudoxanthoma elasticum should avoid contact sports because of the risk of injury to the eye.

Complications may limit life span.

304 Cystic Fibrosis

Cystic fibrosis (CF) is an inherited disease of the exocrine glands affecting primarily the GI and respiratory systems. It leads to chronic lung disease, exocrine pancreatic insufficiency, hepatobiliary disease, and abnormally high sweat electrolytes. Diagnosis is by sweat test or identification of 2 CF-causing mutations in patients with a positive newborn screening test result or characteristic clinical features. Treatment is supportive through aggressive multidisciplinary care along with small-molecule correctors and potentiators targeting the CF transmembrane conductance regulator protein defect.

CF is the most common life-threatening genetic disease in the white population. In the US, it occurs in about 1/3,300 white births, 1/15,300 black births, and 1/32,000 Asian American births. Because of improved treatment and life expectancy, about 50% of patients in the US with CF are adults.

Etiology

CF is carried as an autosomal recessive trait by about 3% of the white population. The responsible gene has been localized on the long arm of chromosome 7. It encodes a membrane-associated protein called the CF transmembrane conductance regulator (CFTR). The most common gene mutation, F508del, occurs in about 86% of CF alleles; > 1900 less common CFTR mutations have been identified.

CFTR is a cAMP-regulated chloride channel, regulating chloride and sodium transport across epithelial membranes. A number of additional functions are considered likely. Disease manifests only in homozygotes. Heterozygotes may show subtle abnormalities of epithelial electrolyte transport but are clinically unaffected.

The CFTR mutations have been divided between five classes based on how the mutation affects the function or processing of the CFTR protein. Patients with class I, II, or III mutations are considered to have a more severe genotype that results in little or no CFTR function, whereas patients with 1 or 2 class IV or V mutations are considered to have a milder genotype that results in residual CFTR function. However, there is no strict relationship between specific mutations and disease manifestation, so clinical testing (ie, of organ function) rather than genotyping is a better guide to prognosis.

Pathophysiology

Nearly all exocrine glands are affected in varying distribution and degree of severity. Glands may

- Become obstructed by viscid or solid eosinophilic material in the lumen (pancreas, intestinal glands, intrahepatic bile ducts, gallbladder, and submaxillary glands)
- Appear histologically abnormal and produce excessive secretions (tracheobronchial and Brunner glands)
- Appear histologically normal but secrete excessive sodium and chloride (sweat, parotid, and small salivary glands)

Respiratory: Although the lungs are generally histologically normal at birth, most patients develop pulmonary disease beginning in infancy or early childhood. Mucus plugging and chronic bacterial infection, accompanied by a pronounced inflammatory response, damage the airways, ultimately leading to bronchiectasis and respiratory insufficiency. The course is characterized by episodic exacerbations with infection and progressive decline in pulmonary function.

Pulmonary damage is probably initiated by diffuse obstruction in the small airways by abnormally thick mucus secretions. Bronchiolitis and mucopurulent plugging of the airways occur secondary to obstruction and infection. Airway changes are more common than parenchymal changes, and emphysema is not prominent. About 50% of patients have bronchial hyperreactivity that responds to bronchodilators.

In patients with advanced pulmonary disease, chronic hypoxemia results in muscular hypertrophy of the pulmonary arteries, pulmonary hypertension, and right ventricular hypertrophy. Much of the pulmonary damage may be caused by inflammation secondary to the release of proteases and proinflammatory cytokines by cells in the airways.

The lungs of most patients are colonized by pathogenic bacteria. Early in the course, *Staphylococcus aureus* is the most common pathogen, but as the disease progresses, *Pseudomonas aeruginosa* is most frequently isolated. A mucoid variant of *P. aeruginosa* is uniquely associated with CF and results in a worse prognosis than nonmucoid *P. aeruginosa*.

The prevalence of methicillin-resistant *S. aureus* (MRSA) in the respiratory tract is now > 25%; patients who are infected with MRSA have lower survival rates than those who are not.

Colonization with *Burkholderia cepacia* complex occurs in about 2% of patients and may be associated with more rapid pulmonary deterioration.

Nontuberculous mycobacteria, including *Mycobacterium avium* complex and *M. abscessus*, are potential respiratory pathogens. Prevalence varies with age and geographic location and probably exceeds 10%. Differentiating infection from colonization can be challenging.

Other common respiratory pathogens include *Stenotrophomonas maltophilia, Achromobacter xylosoxidans,* and *Aspergillus* sp.

GI: The pancreas, intestines, and hepatobiliary system are frequently affected. Exocrine pancreatic function is compromised in 85 to 95% of patients. An exception is a subset of patients who have certain "mild" CF mutations, in whom pancreatic function is unaffected. Patients with pancreatic insufficiency have malabsorption of fats (and fat-soluble vitamins) and protein. Duodenal fluid is abnormally viscid and shows absence or diminution of enzyme activity and decreased HCO_3^- concentration; stool trypsin and chymotrypsin are absent or diminished. Endocrine pancreatic dysfunction is less common, but impaired glucose tolerance or diabetes mellitus is present in about 2% of children, 20% of adolescents, and up to 40% of adults.

Bile duct involvement with bile stasis and biliary plugging leads to asymptomatic hepatic fibrosis in 30% of patients. About 2 to 3% of patients progress to irreversible multinodular biliary cirrhosis with varices and portal hypertension, usually by 12 yr of age. Hepatocellular failure is a rare and late event. There is an increased incidence of cholelithiasis, which is usually asymptomatic.

Abnormally viscid intestinal secretions often cause meconium ileus in neonates and sometimes meconium plugging of the colon. Older children and adults also may have intermittent or chronic constipation and intestinal obstruction.

Other GI problems include intussusception, volvulus, rectal prolapse, periappendiceal abscess, pancreatitis, an increased risk of cancer of the hepatobiliary and GI tracts (including of the pancreas), gastroesophageal reflux, and esophagitis.

Other: Infertility occurs in 98% of adult men secondary to maldevelopment of the vas deferens or to other forms of obstructive azoospermia. In women, fertility is somewhat decreased secondary to viscid cervical secretions, although many women have carried pregnancies to term. Pregnancy outcome for both the mother and neonate is related to the mother's health.

Other complications include osteopenia/osteoporosis, depression, renal stones, dialysis-dependent chronic kidney disease (possibly related to treatments as well as to CF), iron deficiency anemia, and episodic arthralgias/arthritis.

Symptoms and Signs

Respiratory: Fifty percent of patients not diagnosed through newborn screening present with pulmonary manifestations, often beginning in infancy. Recurrent or chronic infections manifested by cough, sputum production, and wheezing are common. Cough is the most troublesome complaint, often accompanied by sputum, gagging, vomiting, and disturbed sleep. Intercostal retractions, use of accessory muscles of respiration, a barrel-chest deformity, digital clubbing, cyanosis, and a declining tolerance for exercise occur with disease progression. Upper respiratory tract involvement includes nasal polyposis and chronic or recurrent sinusitis.

Pulmonary complications include pneumothorax, infection with nontuberculous mycobacteria, hemoptysis, allergic bronchopulmonary aspergillosis, and right heart failure secondary to pulmonary hypertension.

GI: Meconium ileus due to obstruction of the ileum by viscid meconium may be the earliest sign and is present in 13 to 18% of CF-affected neonates. It typically manifests with abdominal distention, vomiting, and failure to pass meconium. Some infants have intestinal perforation, with signs of peritonitis and shock. Infants with meconium plug syndrome have a delayed passage of meconium. They can have similar signs of obstruction or very mild and transient symptoms that go unnoticed. Older patients may have episodes of constipation or develop recurrent and sometimes chronic episodes of partial or complete small- or large-bowel obstruction (distal intestinal obstruction syndrome). Symptoms include crampy abdominal pain, change in stooling pattern, decreased appetite, and sometimes vomiting.

In infants without meconium ileus, disease onset may be heralded by a delay in regaining birth weight and inadequate weight gain at 4 to 6 wk of age.

Occasionally, infants who are undernourished, especially if on hypoallergenic formula or soy formula, present with generalized edema secondary to protein malabsorption.

Pancreatic insufficiency is usually clinically apparent early in life and may be progressive. Manifestations include the frequent passage of bulky, foul-smelling, oily stools; abdominal protuberance; and poor growth pattern with decreased subcutaneous tissue and muscle mass despite a normal or voracious appetite. Clinical manifestations may occur secondary to deficiency of fat-soluble vitamins.

Rectal prolapse occurs in 20% of untreated infants and toddlers. Gastroesophageal reflux is relatively common among children and adults.

Other: Excessive sweating in hot weather or with fever may lead to episodes of hyponatremic/hypochloremic dehydration and circulatory failure. In arid climates, infants may present with chronic metabolic alkalosis. Salt crystal formation and a salty taste on the skin are highly suggestive of CF. Adolescents may have retarded growth and delayed onset of puberty.

Diagnosis

- Universal newborn screening when feasible
- May also be suggested by a positive prenatal screening test result, family history, or symptomatic presentation
- Confirmed by a sweat test showing elevated sweat chloride on ≥ 2 occasions
- Identifying 2 CF-causing mutations (1 on each chromosome) is consistent with the diagnosis
- May rarely be confirmed, in atypical cases, by demonstrating abnormal ion transport across the nasal epithelium

Universal newborn screening for CF is now standard in the US; > 90% of cases are first identified by newborn screening, but up to 10% are not diagnosed until adolescence or early adulthood. Despite advances in genetic testing, the sweat chloride test remains the standard for confirming a CF diagnosis in most cases because of its sensitivity and specificity, simplicity, and availability.

Sweat testing: In this test, localized sweating is stimulated with pilocarpine, the amount of sweat is measured, and the chloride concentration is determined (see Table 304–1). The results are valid after 48 h of life, but an adequate sweat sample (> 75 mg on filter paper or > 15 μL in microbore tubing) may be difficult to obtain before 2 wk of age. False-negative results are rare but may occur in the presence of edema and hypoproteinemia or an inadequate quantity of sweat. False-positive results are usually due to technical error. Transient elevation of sweat chloride concentration can result from psychosocial deprivation (eg, child abuse, neglect) and can occur in patients with anorexia nervosa. Although the sweat chloride concentration increases slightly with age, the sweat test is valid at all ages. A positive sweat test result should be confirmed by a 2nd sweat test or by identification of 2 CF-causing mutations.

Table 304–1. SWEAT CHLORIDE CONCENTRATION RANGES IN CYSTIC FIBROSIS

AGE	NORMAL (mmol/L)*	INTERMEDIATE (mmol/L)†	ABNORMAL (mmol/L)‡
≤ 6 mo	≤ 29	30–59	≥ 60
> 6 mo	≤ 39	40–59	≥ 60

*These concentrations indicate that CF is unlikely.
†These concentrations indicate that CF is possible.
‡These concentrations are consistent with CF.

Intermediate sweat test results: A small subset of patients have a mild or partial CF phenotype and sweat chloride values that are persistently in the intermediate or even normal range. In addition, there are patients who have single-organ manifestations such as pancreatitis, bronchiectasis, or congenital bilateral absence of the vas deferens that may be due to partial CFTR protein dysfunction. In some of these patients, the diagnosis of CF can be confirmed by the identification of 2 CF-causing mutations, 1 on each chromosome. If 2 CF-causing mutations are not identified, ancillary evaluations such as pancreatic function testing and pancreatic imaging, high-resolution chest CT, sinus CT, pulmonary function testing, urogenital evaluation in males, and bronchoalveolar lavage including assessment of microbial flora may be useful.

Additional potentially helpful diagnostic tests include expanded CFTR genetic analysis and measurement of nasal transepithelial potential difference (based on the observation of increased sodium reabsorption across epithelium that is relatively impermeable to chloride in patients with CF).

CFTR-related metabolic syndrome: Infants who have evidence of possible CFTR dysfunction but do not meet the diagnostic criteria for CF have CFTR-related metabolic syndrome (CRMS). CRMS is diagnosed in 3 to 4% of infants who have a positive newborn screen. To be diagnosed, infants must be asymptomatic and have *either* of the following:

- Sweat chloride concentrations in the intermediate range on at least 2 separate occasions and < 2 known CF-causing mutations
- Sweat chloride concentrations in the normal range and 2 CFTR mutations ≤ 1 of which may be a known CF-causing mutation

Some children with CRMS will develop symptoms of CF over time, but most remain healthy. Such patients should be evaluated and monitored regularly in a CF care center.

Pancreatic tests: Pancreatic function should be assessed at the time of diagnosis, usually by measuring 72-h fecal fat excretion or the concentration of human pancreatic elastase in stool. This latter test is valid even in the presence of exogenous pancreatic enzymes. Infants who are initially pancreatic sufficient and who carry 2 "severe" mutations should have serial measurements to detect progression to pancreatic insufficiency.

Respiratory assessment: Chest x-rays are done at times of pulmonary deterioration or exacerbations and routinely every 1 to 2 yr. High-resolution chest CT may be helpful to more precisely define the extent of lung damage and to detect subtle airway abnormalities. Both may show hyperinflation and bronchial wall thickening as the earliest findings. Subsequent changes include areas of infiltrate, atelectasis, and hilar adenopathy.

With advanced disease, segmental or lobar atelectasis, cyst formation, bronchiectasis, and pulmonary artery and right ventricular hypertrophy occur. Branching, fingerlike opacifications that represent mucoid impaction of dilated bronchi are characteristic.

Sinus CT studies are indicated in patients with significant sinus symptoms or nasal polyps in whom endoscopic sinus surgery is being considered. These studies almost always show persistent opacification of the paranasal sinuses.

Pulmonary function tests are the best indicators of clinical status and should be done routinely 4 times/yr and at times of clinical decline. Pulmonary function can now be evaluated in infants by using a raised volume rapid thoracoabdominal compression technique and in children age 3 to 5 yr by using impulse oscillometry or the multiple breath washout procedure.[1] Pulmonary function tests indicate

- A reduction in forced vital capacity (FVC), forced expiratory volume in 1 sec (FEV_1), forced expiratory flow between 25% and 75% expired volume (FEF_{25-75}), and FEV_1/FVC ratio
- An increase in residual volume and the ratio of residual volume to total lung capacity

Fifty percent of patients have evidence of reversible airway obstruction as shown by improvement in pulmonary function after administration of an inhaled bronchodilator.

Screening oropharyngeal or sputum cultures should be done at least 4 times/yr, especially in patients not yet colonized with *P. aeruginosa.* Bronchoscopy/bronchoalveolar lavage is indicated when it is important to precisely define the patient's lower airway microbial flora (eg, to direct antibiotic selection) or to remove inspissated mucus plugs.

Newborn screening: Newborn screening for CF is now universal in the US. Screening is based on detecting an elevated concentration of immunoreactive trypsinogen (IRT) in the blood. There are two methods of following up on an elevated IRT level. In one method, a second IRT test is done, which, if also elevated, is followed by a sweat test. In the other, more commonly used method, an elevated IRT level is followed by CFTR mutation testing and, if 1 or 2 mutations are identified, then a sweat test is done. For diagnosis, both strategies have about 90 to 95% sensitivity.

Carrier screening: CF carrier screening is available in the US and is recommended for couples who are planning a pregnancy or seeking prenatal care. If both potential parents carry a CFTR mutation, prenatal screening of the fetus can be done by chorionic villus sampling or amniocentesis. Prenatal counseling in such cases is complicated by the wide phenotypic variability of CF and incomplete information on the clinical consequences of many of the CFTR mutations that are identified through screening.

1. Aurora P, Gustafsson P, Bush A, et al: Multiple breath inert gas washout as a measure of ventilation distribution in children with CF. *Thorax* 59:1068–73, 2004.

Prognosis

The course is largely determined by the degree of pulmonary involvement. Deterioration is inevitable, leading to debilitation and eventual death, usually due to a combination of respiratory failure and cor pulmonale.

Prognosis has improved steadily over the past 5 decades, mainly because of aggressive treatment before the onset of irreversible pulmonary changes. Median survival in the US is to age 41 yr. Long-term survival is significantly better in patients without pancreatic insufficiency. Outcomes are also affected by CFTR mutation profile, modifier genes, airway microbiology, sex, ambient temperature, exposure to air pollutants (including tobacco smoke), adherence to prescribed therapies, and socioeconomic status. The FEV_1, adjusted for age and sex, is the best predictor of survival.

Treatment

- Comprehensive, multidisciplinary support
- Antibiotics, inhaled drugs to thin airway secretions, and physical maneuvers to clear airway secretions
- Inhaled bronchodilators and sometimes corticosteroids for responders
- Usually pancreatic enzyme supplementation
- High-calorie diet (sometimes requiring supplemental enteral tube feedings)
- In patients with specific mutations, a CFTR potentiator or combination of a CFTR corrector and potentiator

Comprehensive and intensive therapy should be directed by an experienced physician working with a multidisciplinary team that includes other physicians, nurses, dieticians, physical and respiratory therapists, counselors, pharmacists, and social workers. The goals of therapy are maintenance of normal nutritional status, prevention or aggressive treatment of pulmonary and other complications, encouragement of physical activity, and provision of psychosocial support. With appropriate support, most patients can make an age-appropriate adjustment at home and school. Despite myriad problems, the educational, occupational, and marital successes of patients are impressive.

Respiratory: Treatment of pulmonary problems centers on prevention of airway obstruction and prophylaxis against and control of pulmonary infection. Prophylaxis against pulmonary infections includes maintenance of pertussis, *Haemophilus influenzae,* varicella, *Streptococcus pneumoniae,* and measles immunity and annual influenza vaccination. In patients exposed to influenza, a neuraminidase inhibitor can be used prophylactically. Giving palivizumab to infants with CF for prevention of respiratory syncytial virus infection has been shown to be safe, but efficacy has not been documented.

Airway clearance measures consisting of postural drainage, percussion, vibration, and assisted coughing (chest physiotherapy) are recommended at the time of diagnosis and should be done on a regular basis. In older patients, alternative airway clearance measures, such as active cycle of breathing, autogenic drainage, positive expiratory pressure devices, and high-frequency chest wall oscillation, may be effective. Regular aerobic exercise is recommended; it may also help airway clearance.

For patients with reversible airway obstruction, bronchodilators may be given by inhalation. Corticosteroids by inhalation usually are not effective. O_2 therapy is indicated for patients with severe pulmonary insufficiency and hypoxemia.

Mechanical ventilation is typically not indicated for chronic respiratory failure. Its use should be restricted to patients with good baseline status in whom acute reversible respiratory complications develop, in association with pulmonary surgery, or to patients in whom lung transplantation is imminent. Noninvasive positive pressure ventilation nasally or by face mask also can be beneficial.

Oral expectorants are widely used, but few data support their efficacy. Cough suppressants should be discouraged.

Long-term daily inhalation therapy with dornase alfa (recombinant human deoxyribonuclease) as well as 7% hypertonic saline (in patients > 6 yr) has been shown to slow the rate of decline in pulmonary function and to decrease the frequency of respiratory tract exacerbations.

Pneumothorax can be treated with closed chest tube thoracostomy drainage. Open thoracotomy or thoracoscopy with resection of pleural blebs and mechanical abrasion of the pleural surfaces is effective in treating recurrent pneumothoraces.

Massive or recurrent hemoptysis is treated by embolizing involved bronchial arteries.

Oral corticosteroids are indicated in infants with prolonged bronchiolitis and in patients with refractory bronchospasm, allergic bronchopulmonary aspergillosis, and inflammatory complications (eg, arthritis, vasculitis). Long-term use of alternate-day corticosteroid therapy can slow the decline in pulmonary function, but because of corticosteroid-related complications, it is not recommended for routine use. Patients receiving corticosteroids must be closely monitored for evidence of diabetes and linear growth retardation.

Allergic bronchopulmonary aspergillosis is also treated with an oral antifungal drug.

Ibuprofen, when given over several years at a dose sufficient to achieve a peak plasma concentration between 50 and 100 μg/mL, has been shown to slow the rate of decline in pulmonary function, especially in children 5 to 13 yr. The appropriate dose must be individualized based on pharmacokinetic studies.

Ivacaftor is a drug that potentiates the CFTR ion channel in patients with the following CFTR mutations: *G551D*, *G178R*, *S549N*, *S549R*, *G551S*, *G1244E*, *S1251N*, *S1255P*, *G1349D*, or *R117H*; it is a small-molecule drug and the first drug to target a specific CF mutation. Ivacaftor may be used in patients ≥ 2 yr who carry 1 or 2 copies of that specific mutation. The drug is given orally twice a day and can improve pulmonary function, increase weight, decrease CF symptoms and pulmonary exacerbations, and reduce and sometimes normalize sweat chloride concentrations.

Lumacaftor is a small-molecule drug that partially corrects the defective CFTR (by altering protein misfolding) in patients who carry the F508del mutation. The combination of lumacaftor and ivacaftor is recommended for patients with CF age ≥ 6 yr who carry 2 copies of this mutation.

Other drugs that may correct defective CFTR or potentiate CFTR function in other CF mutations are under study.

Antibiotics: For **mild pulmonary exacerbations,** a short course of antibiotics should be given based on culture and sensitivity testing. A penicillinase-resistant penicillin (eg, cloxacillin or dicloxacillin), a cephalosporin (eg, cephalexin), or trimethoprim/sulfamethoxazole is the drug of choice for staphylococci. Erythromycin, amoxicillin/clavulanate, ampicillin, tetracycline, linezolid, or occasionally chloramphenicol may be used. For patients colonized with *P. aeruginosa,* a short course of inhaled tobramycin or aztreonam lysine (eg, 4 wk) and/or an oral fluoroquinolone (eg, 2 to 3 wk) may be effective. Fluoroquinolones have been used safely in young children.

For **moderate-to-severe pulmonary exacerbations,** especially in patients colonized with *P. aeruginosa,* IV antibiotic therapy is advised. Patients often require hospital admission, but carefully selected patients can safely receive the therapy at home. Combinations of an aminoglycoside (eg, tobramycin, gentamicin) and an antipseudomonal penicillin are given IV. IV administration of cephalosporins and monobactams with antipseudomonal activity may also be useful. The usual starting dose of tobramycin or gentamicin is 2.5 to 3.5 mg/kg tid, but higher doses (3.5 to 4 mg/kg tid) may be required to achieve acceptable serum concentrations (peak level 8 to 10 μg/mL [11 to 17 μmol/L], trough value of < 2 μg/mL [< 4 μmol/L]). Alternatively, tobramycin can be given safely and effectively in one daily dose (10 to 12 mg/kg). Because of enhanced renal clearance, large doses of some penicillins may be required to achieve adequate serum levels. For patients colonized with methicillin-resistant *S. aureus,* vancomycin or linezolid can be added to the IV regimen.

In patients who are chronically colonized with *P. aeruginosa,* antibiotics delivered by inhalation improve clinical parameters and possibly reduce the bacterial burden in the airways. The long-term use of alternate-month inhaled tobramycin or aztreonam lysine therapy along with continuous (every month) oral azithromycin given 3 times/wk may be effective in improving or stabilizing pulmonary function and decreasing the frequency of pulmonary exacerbations.

Eradication of chronic *Pseudomonas* colonization is not usually possible. It has been shown, however, that early antibiotic treatment around the time the airways are initially infected with *P. aeruginosa* may be effective in eradicating the organism for some period of time. Treatment strategies vary but usually consist of inhaled tobramycin or colistin sometimes along with an oral fluoroquinolone. Patients who have a clinically significant nontuberculous mycobacterium infection may require long-term therapy with a combination of oral, inhaled, and IV antibiotics.

GI: Neonatal intestinal obstruction can sometimes be relieved by enemas containing a hyperosmolar or iso-osmolar radiopaque contrast material; otherwise, surgical enterostomy to flush out the viscid meconium in the intestinal lumen may be necessary. After the neonatal period, episodes of partial intestinal obstruction (distal intestinal obstruction syndrome) can be treated with enemas containing a hyperosmolar or iso-osmolar radiopaque contrast material or acetylcysteine, or by oral administration of a balanced intestinal lavage solution. A stool softener such as dioctyl sodium sulfosuccinate or lactulose may help prevent such episodes. Ursodeoxycholic acid, a hydrophilic bile acid, is often used in patients with liver disease caused by CF, but there is little evidence to support its efficacy in preventing progression from bile stasis to cirrhosis.

Pancreatic enzyme replacement should be given with all meals and snacks to patients with pancreatic insufficiency. The most effective enzyme preparations contain pancrelipase in pH-sensitive, enteric-coated microspheres or microtablets. Infants are usually started at a dose of 2000 to 4000 IU lipase per 120 mL of formula or per breastfeeding session. For infants, the capsules are opened and the contents are mixed with acidic food. After infancy, weight-based dosing is used starting at 1000 IU lipase/kg/meal for children < 4 yr and at 500 IU lipase/kg/meal for those > 4 yr. Usually, half the standard dose is given with snacks. Doses > 2,500 IU lipase/kg/meal or > 10,000 IU lipase/kg/day should be avoided because high enzyme dosages have been associated with fibrosing colonopathy. In patients with high enzyme requirements, acid suppression with an H_2 blocker or proton pump inhibitor may improve enzyme effectiveness.

Diet therapy includes sufficient calories and protein to promote normal growth—30 to 50% more than the usual recommended dietary allowances may be required (see Table 1–4 on p. 4). Diet therapy also includes a normal-to-high total fat intake to increase the caloric density of the diet, a water-miscible multivitamin supplement in double the recommended daily allowance, supplementation with vitamin D_3 (cholecalciferol) in patients with vitamin D deficiency or insufficiency, and salt supplementation during infancy and periods of thermal stress and increased sweating. Infants receiving broad-spectrum antibiotics and patients with liver disease and hemoptysis should be given additional supplemental vitamin K. Formulas containing protein hydrolysates and medium-chain triglycerides may be used instead of modified whole-milk formulas for infants with severe malabsorption. Glucose polymers and medium-chain triglyceride supplements can be used to increase caloric intake.

In patients who fail to maintain adequate nutritional status, enteral supplementation via gastrostomy or jejunostomy may restore normal growth and stabilize pulmonary function (see p. 14). The use of appetite stimulants to enhance growth may be helpful in some patients.

Other: Cystic fibrosis-related diabetes (CFRD) is caused by insulin insufficiency and shares features of both type 1 and type 2 diabetes. Insulin is the only recommended treatment. Management includes an insulin regimen, nutrition counseling, a diabetes self-management education program, and monitoring for microvascular complications. The plan should be carried out in conjunction with an endocrinologist with experience in treating both CF and diabetes.

Patients with symptomatic **right heart failure** should be treated with diuretics, salt restriction, and O_2.

Recombinant human growth hormone (rhGH) may improve pulmonary function, increase height and weight and bone mineral content, and reduce the rate of hospitalization. However, because of the added cost and inconvenience, rhGH is not commonly used.

Surgery may be indicated for localized bronchiectasis or atelectasis that cannot be treated effectively with drugs, nasal polyps, chronic sinusitis, bleeding from esophageal varices secondary to portal hypertension, gallbladder disease, and intestinal obstruction due to a volvulus or an intussusception that cannot be medically reduced.

Liver transplantation has been done successfully in patients with end-stage liver disease.

Bilateral cadaveric lung and live donor lobar transplantation has been done successfully in patients with advanced pulmonary disease, as well as combined liver-lung transplantation for patients with end-stage liver and lung disease.

Bilateral lung transplantation for severe lung disease is becoming more routine and more successful with experience and improved techniques. About 50 to 60% of people are alive 5 yr after transplantation of both lungs, and their condition is much improved.

End-of-life care: The patient and family deserve sensitive discussions of prognosis and preferences for care throughout the course of illness, especially as the patient's pulmonary reserves become increasingly limited. Most people facing the end of life with CF will be older adolescents or adults and will be appropriately responsible for their own choices. Thus, they must know what is in store and what can be done.

One mark of respect for patients living with CF is to ensure that they are given the information and opportunity to make life choices, including having a substantial hand in determining how and when to accept dying. Often, discussion of transplantation is needed. In considering transplantation, patients need to weigh the merits of longer survival with a transplant against the uncertainty of getting a transplant and the ongoing (but different) burden of living with an organ transplant.

Deteriorating patients need to discuss the eventuality of dying. Patients and their families need to know that most often dying is actually gentle and not profoundly symptomatic. When appropriate, palliative care, including sufficient sedation, should be offered to ensure peaceful dying. A useful strategy for the patient to consider is to accept a time-limited trial of fully aggressive treatment when needed, but to agree in advance to parameters that indicate when to stop aggressive measures (see Do-Not-Resuscitate [DNR] Orders and Physician Orders for Life-Sustaining Treatment [POLST] on p. 3213).

KEY POINTS

- CF is caused by one of a large number of mutations of the gene for a protein called the CFTR, which regulates chloride and sodium transport across epithelial membranes.
- The main complications involve the lungs, with damage to the small and large airways and chronic and recurrent bacterial infections, particularly by *Pseudomonas aeruginosa*.
- Other major consequences include pancreatic malfunction, leading to malabsorption of nutrients and vitamins with consequent impaired growth and development, and, in older patients, diabetes.
- Airway clearance measures (eg, postural drainage, percussion, vibration, assisted coughing) are begun at diagnosis and done on a regular basis; regular aerobic exercise is recommended.
- Antibiotics are given early in any pulmonary exacerbation; drug selection may be based on culture and sensitivity testing.
- Diet should be supplemented with pancreatic enzymes, high-dose vitamins, and 30 to 50% more calories derived primarily from fat.

305 Dehydration and Fluid Therapy in Children

Unlike in adults, fluid management in children is based on weight and on specific guidelines, because children are more sensitive to fluid depletion (and excess). All guidelines are approximations; individualized adjustments based on close monitoring are essential.

DEHYDRATION IN CHILDREN

Dehydration is significant depletion of body water and, to varying degrees, electrolytes. Symptoms and signs include thirst, lethargy, dry mucosa, decreased urine output, and, as the degree of dehydration progresses, tachycardia, hypotension, and shock. Diagnosis is based on history and physical examination. Treatment is with oral or IV replacement of fluid and electrolytes.

Dehydration remains a major cause of morbidity and mortality in infants and young children worldwide. Dehydration is a symptom or sign of another disorder, most commonly diarrhea. Infants are particularly susceptible to the ill effects of dehydration because of their greater baseline fluid requirements (due to a higher metabolic rate), higher evaporative losses (due to a higher ratio of surface area to volume), and inability to communicate thirst or seek fluid.

Etiology

Dehydration results from

- Increased fluid loss
- Decreased fluid intake
- Both

The most common source of increased fluid loss is the GI tract—from vomiting, diarrhea, or both (eg, gastroenteritis—see p. 124). Other sources are renal (eg, diabetic ketoacidosis), cutaneous (eg, excessive sweating, burns), and 3rd-space losses (eg, into the intestinal lumen in bowel obstruction or ileus).

Decreased fluid intake is common during mild illnesses such as pharyngitis or during serious illnesses of any kind. Decreased fluid intake is particularly problematic when the child is vomiting or when fever, tachypnea, or both increase insensible losses. It may also be a sign of neglect.

Pathophysiology

All types of lost fluid contain electrolytes in varying concentrations, so fluid loss is always accompanied by some degree of electrolyte loss. The exact amount and type of electrolyte loss varies depending on the cause (eg, significant amounts of HCO_3^- may be lost with diarrhea but not with vomiting). However, fluid lost always contains a lower concentration of Na than the plasma. Thus, in the absence of any fluid replacement, serum Na rises (hypernatremia). Hypernatremia causes water to shift from the intracellular and interstitial space into the intravascular space, helping, at least temporarily, to maintain vascular volume. With hypotonic fluid replacement (eg, with plain water), serum Na may normalize but can also decrease (hyponatremia). Hyponatremia results in some fluid shifting out of the intravascular space into the interstitium at the expense of vascular volume.

Symptoms and Signs

Symptoms and signs vary according to degree of deficit (see Table 305–1) and by the serum Na level. Because of the fluid shift out of the interstitium *into* the vascular space, children with hypernatremia *appear* more ill (eg, with very dry mucous membranes, a doughy appearance to the skin) for a given degree of water loss than do children with hyponatremia. However, children with hypernatremia have better hemodynamics (eg, less tachycardia and better urine output) than do children with hyponatremia, in whom fluid has shifted *out* of the vascular space. Dehydrated children with hyponatremia may appear only mildly dehydrated until closer to cardiovascular collapse and hypotension.

Diagnosis

- Clinical evaluation

In general, dehydration is defined as follows:

- Mild: No hemodynamic changes (about 5% body wt in infants and 3% in adolescents)
- Moderate: Tachycardia (about 10% body wt in infants and 6% in adolescents)
- Severe: Hypotension with impaired perfusion (about 15% body wt in infants and 9% in adolescents)

However, using a combination of symptoms and signs to assess dehydration is a more accurate method than using only one sign. Another way to assess the degree of dehydration in children with acute dehydration is change in body weight; all short-term weight loss > 1%/day is presumed to represent fluid deficit. However, this method depends on knowing a precise, recent pre-illness weight. Parental estimates are usually inadequate; a 1-kg error in a 10-kg child causes a 10% error in the calculated percentage of dehydration—the difference between mild and severe dehydration.

Laboratory testing is usually reserved for moderately or severely ill children, in whom electrolyte disturbances (eg, hypernatremia, hypokalemia, metabolic acidosis or alkalosis) are more common, and for children who need IV fluid therapy. Other laboratory abnormalities in dehydration include relative polycythemia resulting from hemoconcentration, elevated BUN, and increased urine specific gravity.

Treatment

- Fluid replacement (oral if possible)

Treatment is best approached by considering separately the fluid resuscitation requirements, current deficit, ongoing losses, and maintenance requirements. The volume (eg, amount of fluid), composition, and rate of replacement differ for each. Formulas and estimates used to determine treatment parameters provide a starting place, but treatment requires ongoing monitoring of vital signs, clinical appearance, urine output, weight, and sometimes serum electrolyte levels.

The American Academy of Pediatrics and the WHO both recommend oral replacement therapy for mild and moderate dehydration. Children with severe dehydration (eg, evidence of circulatory compromise) should receive fluids IV. Children who are unable or unwilling to drink or who have repetitive vomiting can receive fluid replacement orally through frequently repeated small amounts, through an IV, or through an NGT (see p. 2557).

Resuscitation: Patients with signs of hypoperfusion should receive fluid resuscitation with boluses of isotonic fluid (eg, 0.9% saline or lactated Ringer solution). The goal is to restore adequate circulating volume to restore BP and perfusion. The resuscitation phase should reduce moderate or severe dehydration to a deficit of about 8% body wt. If dehydration is moderate,

Table 305–1. CLINICAL CORRELATES OF DEHYDRATION

	FLUID DEFICIT IN ML/KG (PERCENT BODY WT)*		
SEVERITY	INFANTS	ADOLESCENTS	SIGNS†
Mild	50 (5%)	30 (3%)	Typically minimal findings but may have slightly dry buccal mucous membranes, increased thirst, slightly decreased urine output
Moderate	100 (10%)	50–60 (5–6%)	Dry buccal mucous membranes, tachycardia, little or no urine output, lethargy, sunken eyes and fontanelles, loss of skin turgor
Severe	150 (15%)	70–90 (7–9%)	Same as moderate plus a rapid, thready pulse; no tears; cyanosis; rapid breathing; delayed capillary refill; hypotension; mottled skin; coma

*Standard estimates for children between infancy and adolescence have not been established. For children between these age ranges, clinicians must estimate values between those for infants and those for adolescents based on clinical judgment.

†These findings are for patients with a serum Na level in the normal range; clinical manifestations may differ with hyper- and hyponatremia.

Table 305–2. ESTIMATED ELECTROLYTE DEFICITS BY CAUSE

CAUSE	SODIUM (mEq/L)	POTASSIUM (mEq/L)
Diarrhea	—	—
Isotonic dehydration	80	80
Hypotonic dehydration	100	80
Hypertonic dehydration	20	10
Pyloric stenosis	80	100
Diabetic ketoacidosis	80	50

20 mL/kg (2% body wt) is given IV over 20 to 30 min, reducing a 10% deficit to 8%. If dehydration is severe, sometimes 3 boluses of 20 mL/kg will likely be required. The end point of the fluid resuscitation phase is reached when peripheral perfusion and BP are restored and the heart rate is returned to normal (in an afebrile child).

Deficit replacement: Total deficit volume is estimated clinically as described previously. Na deficits are usually about 60 mEq/L of fluid deficit, and K deficits are usually about 30 mEq/L of fluid deficit. The resuscitation phase should have reduced moderate or severe dehydration to a deficit of about 8% body wt; this remaining deficit can be replaced by providing 10 mL/kg (1% body wt)/h for 8 h. Because 0.45% saline has 77 mEq Na per liter, it is usually an appropriate fluid choice, particularly in children with diarrhea because the electrolyte content of diarrhea is typically 50 to 100 mEq/L (see Table 305–2). K replacement (usually by adding 20 to 40 mEq K per liter of replacement fluid) should not begin until adequate urine output is established.

Dehydration in neonates with significant hypernatremia (eg, serum Na > 160 mEq/L) or hyponatremia (eg, serum Na < 120 mEq/L) requires special consideration to avoid complications (see pp. 2733 and 2734).

Ongoing losses: Volume of ongoing losses should be measured directly (eg, NGT, catheter, stool measurements) or estimated (eg, 10 mL/kg per diarrheal stool). Replacement should be milliliter for milliliter in time intervals appropriate for the rapidity and extent of the loss. Ongoing electrolyte losses can be estimated by source or cause (see Table 305–2). Urinary electrolyte losses vary with intake and disease process but can be measured if deficits fail to respond to replacement therapy.

Maintenance requirements: Fluid and electrolyte needs from basal metabolism must also be accounted for. Maintenance requirements are related to metabolic rate and affected by body temperature. Insensible losses (evaporative free water losses from the skin and respiratory tract) account for about one third of total maintenance water (slightly more in infants and less in adolescents and adults).

Volume rarely must be exactly determined but generally should aim to provide an amount of water that does not require the kidney to significantly concentrate or dilute the urine. The most common estimate is the Holliday-Segar formula, which uses patient weight to calculate metabolic expenditure in kcal/24 h, which approximates fluid needs in mL/24 h (see Table 305–3). The Holliday-Segar formula uses 3 weight classes because metabolic expenditure changes are based on weight. More complex calculations (eg, those using body surface area) are rarely required. Maintenance fluid volumes can be given as a separate simultaneous infusion, so that the infusion rate for replacing deficits and ongoing losses can be set and adjusted independently of the maintenance infusion rate.

Baseline estimates are affected by fever (increasing by 12% for each degree > 37.8° C), hypothermia, and activity (eg, increased for hyperthyroidism or status epilepticus, decreased for coma).

Composition differs from solutions used to replace deficits and ongoing losses. According to the Holliday-Segar formula, patients require Na 3 mEq/100 kcal/24 h (3 mEq/100 mL/24 h) and K 2 mEq/100 kcal/24 h (2 mEq/100 mL/24 h). (NOTE: 2 to 3 mEq/100 mL/24 h is equivalent to a solution that is 20 to 30 mEq/L.) This need is met by using 0.2% to 0.3% saline with 20 mEq/L of K in a 5% dextrose solution. However, recent literature suggests that hospitalized dehydrated children receiving 0.2% saline for maintenance fluid sometimes develop hyponatremia, perhaps because they release significant amounts of antidiuretic hormone because of stimuli such as stress, vomiting, dehydration, and hypoglycemia, causing increased free water retention. Due to this possibility of iatrogenic hyponatremia, many centers are now using a more isotonic fluid such as 0.45% or 0.9% saline for maintenance in dehydrated children and reserving 0.2% saline for routine maintenance in nondehydrated children, eg, those who require IV fluids but can have nothing by mouth before a test or procedure. Iatrogenic hyponatremia may be a greater problem for more seriously ill children and those who are hospitalized after surgery. Although the appropriate fluid remains controversial, all clinicians agree the important point is to closely monitor dehydrated patients receiving IV fluids. Other electrolytes (eg, Mg, Ca) are not routinely added. It is inappropriate to replace deficits and ongoing losses solely by increasing the amount or rate of maintenance fluids.

Practical Example

A 7-mo-old infant has diarrhea for 3 days with weight loss from 10 kg to 9 kg. The infant is currently producing 1 diarrheal stool every 3 h and refusing to drink. Clinical findings of dry mucous membranes, poor skin turgor, markedly decreased urine output, and tachycardia with normal BP and capillary refill suggest 10% fluid deficit. Rectal temperature is 37° C; serum Na, 136 mEq/L; K, 4 mEq/L; Cl, 104 mEq/L; and HCO_3, 20 mEq/L.

Table 305–3. HOLLIDAY-SEGAR FORMULA FOR MAINTENANCE FLUID REQUIREMENTS BY WEIGHT

WT (kg)	WATER mL/day	WATER mL/h	ELECTROLYTES (mEq/L H_2O)
0–10 kg	100/kg	4/kg	Na 30, K 20
11–20 kg	1000 + 50/kg for each kg > 10	40 + 2/kg for each kg > 10	Na 30, K 20
> 20 kg	1500 + 20/kg for each kg > 20	60 + 1/kg for each kg > 20	Na 30, K 20

Fluid volume is estimated by deficits, ongoing losses, and maintenance requirements.

The total fluid deficit given 1 kg wt loss = 1 L.

Ongoing diarrheal losses are measured as they occur by weighing the infant's diaper before application and after the diarrheal stool.

Baseline maintenance requirements by the weight-based Holliday-Segar method are 100 mL/kg × 10 kg = 1000 mL/day = 1000/24 or 40 mL/h.

Electrolyte losses resulting from diarrhea in a eunatremic patient (see Table 305–2) are an estimated 80 mEq of Na and 80 mEq of K.

Procedure

Resuscitation: The patient is given an initial bolus of lactated Ringer solution 200 mL (20 mL/kg × 10 kg) over 30 min. This amount replaces 26 mEq of the estimated 80 mEq Na deficit.

Deficits: Residual fluid deficit is 800 mL (1000 initial − 200 mL resuscitation), and Na deficit is 54 mEq (80 − 26 mEq). This residual amount is given over the next 24 h. Typically, half (400 mL) is given over the first 8 h (400 ÷ 8 = 50 mL/h) and the other half is given over the next 16 h (25 mL/h). The fluid used is 5% dextrose/0.45% saline. This amount replaces the Na deficit (0.8 L × 77 mEq Na/L = 62 mEq Na). When urine output is established, K is added at a concentration of 20 mEq/L (for safety reasons, no attempt is made to replace complete K deficit acutely).

Ongoing losses: Five percent dextrose/0.45% saline also is used to replace ongoing losses; volume and rate are determined by the amount of diarrhea.

Maintenance fluid: Five percent dextrose/0.2% or 0.45% saline is given at 40 mL/h with 20 mEq/L of K added when urine output is established. Alternatively, the deficit could be replaced during the initial 8 h followed by the entire day's maintenance fluid in the next 16 h (ie, 60 mL/h); 24 h of maintenance fluid given in 16 h reduces mathematically to a rate of 1.5 times the usual maintenance rate and obviates the need for simultaneous infusions (which may require 2 rate-controlling pumps).

ORAL REHYDRATION

Oral fluid therapy is effective, safe, convenient, and inexpensive compared with IV therapy. Oral fluid therapy is recommended by the American Academy of Pediatrics and the WHO and should be used for children with mild to moderate dehydration who are accepting fluids orally unless prohibited by copious vomiting or underlying disorders (eg, surgical abdomen, intestinal obstruction).

Solutions

Oral rehydration solution (ORS) should contain complex carbohydrate or 2% glucose and 50 to 90 mEq/L of Na. Sports drinks, sodas, juices, and similar drinks do not meet these criteria and should not be used. They generally have too little Na and too much carbohydrate to take advantage of Na/glucose cotransport, and the osmotic effect of the excess carbohydrate may result in additional fluid loss. The Na/glucose cotransport in the gut is optimized with an Na:glucose ratio of 1:1.

ORS is recommended by the WHO and is widely available in the US without prescription. Most solutions come as powders that are mixed with tap water. An ORS packet is dissolved in 1 L of water to produce a solution containing (in mmol/L) Na 90, K 20, Cl 80, citrate 10, and glucose 111 (standard WHO ORS) or Na 75, K 20, Cl 65, citrate 10, and glucose 75 (WHO reduced-osmolarity ORS). It can also be made manually by adding 1 L of water to 3.5 g NaCl, 2.9 g trisodium citrate (or 2.5 g $NaHCO_3$), 1.5 g KCL, and 20 g glucose. ORS is effective in patients with dehydration regardless of age, cause, or type of electrolyte imbalance (hyponatremia, hypernatremia, or isonatremia) as long as their kidneys are functioning adequately.

Premixed commercial rehydration solutions are readily available in most pharmacies and supermarkets. These solutions are effective despite having an Na:glucose ratio of about 1:3 (45 mEq/L Na to 140 mmol/L glucose). After rehydration, this solution must be replaced by a lower-Na fluid to avoid hypernatremia.

Administration

Generally, 50 mL/kg is given over 4 h for mild dehydration and 100 mL/kg for moderate. For each diarrheal stool, an additional 10 mL/kg (up to 240 mL) is given. After 4 h, the patient is reassessed. If signs of dehydration persist, the same volume is repeated. Patients with cholera may require many liters of fluid/day.

Vomiting usually should not deter oral rehydration (unless there is bowel obstruction or other contraindication) because vomiting typically abates over time. Small, frequent amounts are used, starting with 5 mL every 5 min and increasing gradually as tolerated. The calculated volume required over a 4-h period can be divided into 4 separate aliquots. These 4 aliquots can then be divided into 12 smaller aliquots and given every 5 min over the course of an hour with a syringe if needed.

In children with diarrhea, oral intake often precipitates a diarrheal stool, so the same volume should be given in fewer aliquots.

Once the deficit has been replaced, an oral maintenance solution containing less Na should be used. Children should eat an age-appropriate diet as soon as they have been rehydrated and are not vomiting. Infants may resume breastfeeding or formula.

306 Some Ear, Nose, and Throat Disorders in Children

The common childhood ENT disorders acute otitis media, tonsillopharyngitis, sore throat, adenoid disorders, epistaxis, nasal congestion and rhinorrhea, sinusitis, and ear foreign bodies and nasal foreign bodies are discussed elsewhere in THE MANUAL.

The less common childhood ENT disorders retropharyngeal abscess, mastoiditis, and epiglottitis are also discussed elsewhere.

HEARING IMPAIRMENT IN CHILDREN

Common causes of hearing loss are genetic defects in neonates and ear infections and cerumen in children. Many cases are detected by screening, but hearing loss should be suspected if children do not respond to sounds or have

delayed speech development. Diagnosis is usually by electrodiagnostic testing (evoked otoacoustic emissions testing and auditory brain stem response) in neonates and by clinical examination and tympanometry in children. Treatment for irreversible hearing loss may include a hearing aid or cochlear implant.

In the US, permanent childhood hearing loss is detected in 1.1/1000 infants screened. On average, 1.9% of children reported "hearing trouble." Hearing impairment is slightly more common among boys than girls; the average male:female ratio is 1.24:1.

Etiology

The most common causes of hearing loss in neonates are

- Genetic defects

The most common causes in infants and children are

- Cerumen accumulations
- Middle ear effusions, including otitis media with effusion

Other causes in older children include head injuries, loud noises (including loud music), use of ototoxic drugs (eg, aminoglycosides, thiazides), viral infections (eg, mumps), tumors or injuries affecting the auditory nerve, foreign bodies of the ear canal, and, rarely, autoimmune disorders.

Risk factors for hearing loss in neonates include the following:

- Low birth weight (eg, < 1.5 kg)
- Apgar score < 5 (1 min) or 7 (5 min)
- Hypoxemia or seizures resulting from a difficult delivery
- Prenatal infection with rubella, syphilis, herpes, cytomegalovirus, or toxoplasmosis
- Craniofacial anomalies, particularly those that involve the external ear
- Hyperbilirubinemia
- Sepsis or meningitis
- Ventilator dependence
- Use of ototoxic drugs
- Family history of early hearing loss

Risk factors for hearing loss in children include those for neonates plus the following:

- Skull fracture or traumatic loss of consciousness
- Cholesteatoma
- Neurodegenerative disorders, including neurofibromatosis
- Noise exposure
- Tympanic membrane perforation

Symptoms and Signs

If hearing loss is severe, the infant or child may not respond to sounds or may have delayed speech or language comprehension. If hearing loss is less severe, children may intermittently ignore people talking to them. Children may appear to be developing well in certain settings but have problems in others. For example, because the background noise of a classroom can make speech discrimination difficult, the child may have problems hearing only at school.

Not recognizing and treating impairment can seriously impair language comprehension and speech. The impairment can lead to failure in school, teasing by peers, social isolation, and emotional difficulties.

Diagnosis

- Electrodiagnostic testing (neonates)
- Clinical examination and tympanometry (children)

Screening all infants before age 3 mo is often recommended and is legally mandated in most states.[1] The initial screening test is evoked otoacoustic emissions testing, using soft clicks made by a handheld device. If results are abnormal or equivocal, auditory brain stem evoked responses are tested, which can be done during sleep; abnormal results should be confirmed with repeat testing after 1 mo.

In children, other methods can be used. Speech and overall development are assessed clinically. The ears are examined, and tympanic membrane movement is tested in response to various frequencies to screen for middle ear effusions. In children age 6 mo to 2 yr, response to sounds is tested. At age > 2 yr, ability to follow simple auditory commands can be assessed, as can responses to sounds using earphones. Central auditory processing evaluation can be used for children > 7 yr without neurocognitive deficits who seem to hear but not comprehend.

Imaging is often indicated to identify the etiology and guide prognosis. For most cases, including when neurologic examination is abnormal, word recognition is poor, and/or hearing loss is asymmetric, gadolinium-enhanced MRI is done. If bone abnormalities are suspected, CT is done.

1. US Preventive Services Task Force: Universal screening for hearing loss in newborns: US Preventive Services Task Force recommendation statement. *Pediatrics* 122(1):143–148, 2008. doi: 10.1542/peds.2007-2210.

Treatment

- Hearing aids or cochlear implants for irreversible hearing loss
- Sometimes teaching a nonauditory language

Reversible causes are treated. If hearing loss is irreversible, a hearing aid can usually be used. They are available for infants as well as children. If hearing loss is mild or moderate or affects only one ear, a hearing aid or earphones can be used. In the classroom, an FM auditory trainer can be used. With an FM auditory trainer, the teacher speaks into a microphone that send signals to a hearing aid in the nonaffected ear.

If hearing loss is severe enough that it cannot be managed with hearing aids, a cochlear implant may be needed. Children may also require therapy to support their language development, such as being taught a visually based sign language.

KEY POINTS

- Common causes of hearing loss are genetic defects (in neonates) and cerumen accumulation and middle ear infusions (in children).
- Suspect hearing loss if a child's response to sounds or development of speech and language is abnormal.
- Screen infants for hearing loss, beginning with evoked otoacoustic emissions testing.
- Diagnose children based on results of clinical examination and tympanometry.
- Treat irreversible hearing loss with a hearing aid or cochlear implant and language support (eg, teaching sign language) as needed.

JUVENILE ANGIOFIBROMAS

Juvenile angiofibromas are rare and benign and can develop in the nasopharynx.

Juvenile angiofibromas are most common among adolescent boys. They are vascular and grow slowly. They can spread into the orbits or cranial vault or recur after treatment.

Symptoms and Signs

Common symptoms of juvenile angiofibromas include nasal obstruction and epistaxis (sometimes severe, usually unilateral). The tumor may cause facial swelling, eye bulging, or nasal disfigurement or mass.

Diagnosis

- CT and MRI

Diagnosis of juvenile angiofibromas usually requires CT and MRI.

Angiography is often done so that the tumor vessels can be embolized before surgery.

Because incising the tumor may cause severe bleeding, incisional biopsy is avoided.

Treatment

- Excision and sometimes radiation therapy

Treatment of juvenile angiofibromas is excision. Radiation therapy is sometimes used adjunctively, particularly if complete excision is difficult or impossible or if the tumor recurs.

RECURRENT RESPIRATORY PAPILLOMATOSIS

(Laryngeal Papillomas)

Recurrent respiratory papillomatosis is a rare, benign, viral airway tumor that is caused by the human papillomavirus. The most common way for patients to present is with laryngeal papillomas.

Recurrent respiratory papillomatosis most often occurs in the larynx as laryngeal papillomas. Laryngeal papillomas can occur at any age but are most common at ages 1 to 4 yr. They may reappear after treatment, undergo malignant transformation, and/or occasionally spread to the trachea or lungs.

Symptoms and Signs

Symptoms of recurrent respiratory papillomatosis can include weak cry, hoarseness, and, in severe cases, airway obstruction.

Diagnosis

- Biopsy

The tumor is identified by laryngoscopy. The diagnosis of recurrent respiratory papillomatosis is confirmed by biopsy.

Treatment

- Excision

Treatment of recurrent respiratory papillomatosis is excision. Because tumors may recur in weeks or months, multiple procedures may be required and surveillance by laryngoscopy and bronchoscopy is necessary. Surgery may involve pulsed-dye laser therapy or photodynamic therapy.

Antiviral drugs (eg, cidofovir) have been tried in severe cases. Lesions may regress at puberty in some patients. The quadrivalent human papillomavirus vaccine offers hope of prevention, but efficacy has not yet been proved.

COMMUNICATION DISORDERS IN CHILDREN

Communication in children can be disordered because of a problem with voice, hearing, speech, language, or a combination. Diagnosis involves evaluation of each of these components.

More than 10% of children have a communication disorder. A disorder in one component may affect another component. For example, hearing impairment impairs voice modulation and can lead to disordered voice. Hearing loss due to otitis media can interfere with language development. All communication disorders, including voice disorders, may interfere with academic performance and social relationships.

Voice Disorders

More than 6% of school-age children have a voice problem, most often hoarseness. The cause is often chronic overuse of the voice and/or speaking too loudly. The most common corresponding anatomic abnormality is vocal cord nodules. Other laryngeal lesions or endocrine abnormalities may also contribute. Hearing loss can contribute by impairing the ability to sense voice volume and thus modulate voice force. Nodules usually resolve with voice therapy and only rarely require surgery.

Hearing Disorders

For a discussion of hearing disorders, see p. 2557.

Speech Disorders

About 5% of children entering first grade have a speech disorder. In speech disorders, speech production is impaired. Speech disorders include the following:

- Hypernasal voice quality: Hypernasality is typically caused by a cleft palate or other structural abnormality that prevents normal closure of the soft palate with the pharyngeal wall (velopharyngeal insufficiency).
- Stuttering: Developmental stuttering, the usual form of stuttering, typically begins between age 2 yr and 5 yr and is more common among boys. The etiology of stuttering is unknown, but family clustering is common. Neurologic causes of stuttering are less common.
- Articulation disorders: Most children with disordered articulation have no detectable physical cause. Secondary dysarthria can result from neurologic disorders that impair innervation or coordination of speech muscles. Because swallowing muscles are also usually affected, dysphagia may be noticed before dysarthria is detected. Hearing disorders and structural abnormalities (eg, of the tongue, lip, or palate) can also impair articulation.

Speech therapy is helpful in many primary speech disorders. Children who have lesions that cause velopharyngeal insufficiency generally require surgery as well as speech therapy.

Language Disorders

About 5% of otherwise healthy children have difficulty with language comprehension or expression (called specific language impairment). Boys are more often affected, and genetic factors probably contribute. Alternatively, language problems can develop secondary to another disorder (eg, traumatic brain injury, intellectual disability, hearing loss, neglect or abuse, autism, attention-deficit/hyperactivity disorder).

Children may benefit from language therapy. Some children with specific language impairment recover spontaneously.

Diagnosis

Parents can be taught to seek medical attention if a child has impaired communication (eg, inability to say at least 2 words by the first birthday). Assessment should include neurologic and ENT examinations. Hearing and language are assessed; laryngoscopy should be considered if a voice disorder (eg, hoarseness, breathy voice) is suspected.

KEY POINTS

- Problems with voice, hearing, speech, and/or language (communication disorders) are common and have academic and social consequences.
- Evaluate children whose communication appears delayed (eg, who are unable to say at least 2 words by the first birthday).
- Assess hearing and language development and consider laryngoscopy in children with communication disorders.

307 Endocrine Disorders in Children

CONGENITAL GOITER

Congenital goiter is a diffuse or nodular enlargement of the thyroid gland present at birth. Thyroid hormone secretion may be decreased, increased, or normal. Diagnosis is by confirming thyroid size with ultrasonography. Treatment is thyroid hormone replacement when hypothyroidism is the cause. Surgery is indicated when breathing or swallowing is impaired.

Etiology

Congenital goiters may be caused by dyshormonogenesis (abnormal thyroid hormone production), transplacental passage of maternal antibodies, or transplacental passage of goitrogens. Some causes of congenital goiter are hereditary.

Dyshormonogenesis: Genetic defects in thyroid hormone production result in increased levels of thyroid-stimulating hormone (TSH), which in turn can cause congenital goiter. Goiter is present in about 15% of cases of congenital hypothyroidism. There are a number of gene abnormalities that cause dyshormonogenesis; they commonly have an autosomal recessive form of inheritance, and many are single-gene defects.

Dyshormonogenesis can result from a defect in any of the steps in thyroid hormone biosynthesis, including

- Failure to concentrate iodide
- Defective organification of iodide due to an abnormality in the thyroid peroxidase enzyme or in the hydrogen peroxide–generating system
- Defective thyroglobulin synthesis or transport
- Abnormal iodotyrosine deiodinase activity

Children with **Pendred syndrome** have mild hypothyroidism or euthyroidism, goiter, and sensorineural hearing loss due to a genetic abnormality of a protein (pendrin) involved in iodine transport and cochlear function. Although Pendred syndrome is caused by a genetic defect, it rarely manifests in the newborn period.

Transplacental passage of maternal antibodies: Women with an autoimmune thyroid disorder produce antibodies that may cross the placenta during the 3rd trimester. Depending on the disorder, the antibodies either block TSH receptors, causing hypothyroidism, or stimulate them, causing hyperthyroidism. Typically, in affected infants, the changes in hormone secretion and the associated goiter resolve spontaneously within 3 to 6 mo.

Transplacental passage of goitrogens: Goitrogens such as amiodarone or antithyroid drugs (eg, propylthiouracil, methimazole) can cross the placenta, sometimes causing hypothyroidism and rarely causing goiter.

Symptoms and Signs

The most common manifestation of congenital goiter is firm, nontender enlargement of the thyroid. Enlargement is most often diffuse but can be nodular. It may be noticeable at birth or detected later. In some patients, enlargement is not directly observable, but continued growth can cause deviation or compression of the trachea, compromising breathing and swallowing. Many children with goiters are euthyroid, but some present with hypothyroidism or hyperthyroidism.

Diagnosis

- Ultrasonography

If the diagnosis of congenital goiter is suspected, thyroid size is typically assessed by ultrasonography. Thyroxine (T_4) and TSH are measured.

Treatment

- Surgical treatment of symptomatic enlargement
- Sometimes thyroid hormone

Hypothyroidism is treated with thyroid hormone. Goiters that compromise breathing and swallowing can be treated surgically.

DELAYED PUBERTY

Delayed puberty is absence of sexual maturation at the expected time.

Delayed puberty may result from constitutional delay, which often occurs in adolescents with a family history of delayed growth. Prepubertal growth velocity is normal, but skeletal maturation and adolescent growth spurt are delayed; sexual maturation is delayed but normal. Other causes include Turner syndrome in girls, Klinefelter syndrome in boys, CNS disorders (eg, pituitary tumors that reduce gonadotropin secretion), CNS radiation, certain chronic disorders (eg, diabetes mellitus, inflammatory bowel disorders, renal disorders, cystic fibrosis), Kallman syndrome, and excess physical activity, especially in girls.

In girls, delayed puberty is diagnosed if one of the following occurs:

- No breast development by age 13
- > 5 yr elapse between the beginning of breast growth and menarche
- Menstruation does not occur by age 16

In boys, delayed puberty is diagnosed if one of the following occurs:

- No testicular enlargement by age 14
- > 5 yr elapse between initial and complete growth of the genitals

Short stature may indicate delayed puberty in either sex. Although many children seem to be starting puberty earlier than in past years, there are no indications that the criteria for delayed puberty should change.

Constitutional delay of puberty is more prevalent in boys. Girls with severe pubertal delay should be investigated for primary amenorrhea. If boys show no sign of pubertal development or of skeletal maturation beyond 11 to 12 yr by age 14, they may be given a 4- to 6-mo course of testosterone enanthate or cypionate 50 to 100 mg IM once/mo. These low doses induce puberty with some degree of virilization and do not jeopardize adult height potential.

Unless there are early physical signs of puberty, distinguishing constitutional delay of puberty from permanent causes of hypogonadotropic hypogonadism can be difficult. Chronic disorders can delay puberty by causing inadequate nutrition and impairing gonadotropin-releasing hormone release. Permanent forms of hypogonadotropic hypogonadism are more likely if there is a lack of response to 1 or 2 short courses of testosterone. When suspected, other pituitary hormones should be reevaluated, because hypogonadotropic hypogonadism can be isolated or associated with other hormone deficiencies. About one third of cases of idiopathic hypogonadotropic hypogonadism are genetic, and Kallman syndrome is the most common cause (see Secondary hypogonadism—p. 2572). If other pituitary hormone deficiencies are noted, specific genetic abnormalities can be identified (eg, *PROP1*).

DIABETES IN CHILDREN AND ADOLESCENTS

Diabetes mellitus involves absence of insulin secretion (type 1) or peripheral insulin resistance (type 2), causing hyperglycemia. Early symptoms are related to hyperglycemia and include polydipsia, polyphagia, polyuria, and weight loss. Diagnosis is by measuring plasma glucose levels. Treatment depends on type but includes drugs that reduce blood glucose levels, diet, and exercise.

The types of diabetes mellitus (DM) in children are similar to those in adults, but psychosocial problems are different and can complicate treatment.

Type 1 DM is the most common type in children, accounting for two thirds of new cases in children of all ethnic groups. It is one of the most common chronic childhood diseases, occurring in 1 in 350 children by age 18; the incidence has recently been increasing, particularly in children < 5 yr. Although type 1 can occur at any age, it typically manifests between age 4 yr and 6 yr and between 10 yr and 14 yr.

Type 2 DM, once rare in children, has been increasing in frequency in parallel with the increase in childhood obesity (see pp. 23 and 2823). It typically manifests after puberty, with the highest rate between age 15 yr and 19 yr.

Monogenic forms of diabetes, previously termed maturity-onset diabetes of youth (MODY), are not considered type 1 or type 2 (although they are sometimes mistaken for them) and are uncommon (1 to 4% of cases).

Prediabetes is impaired glucose regulation resulting in intermediate glucose levels that are too high to be normal but do not meet criteria for diabetes. In obese adolescents, prediabetes may be transient (with reversion to normal in 2 yr in 60%) or progress to diabetes, especially in adolescents who persistently gain weight. Prediabetes is associated with the metabolic syndrome (impaired glucose regulation, dyslipidemia, hypertension, obesity).

Etiology

There appears to be a familial component to all types of DM in children, although the incidence and mechanism vary.

In **type 1 DM,** the pancreas produces no insulin because of autoimmune destruction of pancreatic beta-cells, possibly triggered by an environmental exposure in genetically susceptible people. Close relatives are at increased risk of DM, with overall incidence 10 to 13% (30 to 50% in monozygotic twins). Children with type 1 DM are at higher risk of other autoimmune disorders, particularly thyroid disease and celiac disease. Inherited susceptibility to type 1 DM is determined by multiple genes (> 60 risk loci have been identified). Susceptibility genes are more common among some populations and explain the higher prevalence of type 1 DM in certain ethnic groups (eg, Scandinavians, Sardinians).

In **type 2 DM,** the pancreas produces insulin, but there are varying degrees of insulin resistance and insulin secretion is inadequate to meet the increased demand caused by insulin resistance (ie, there is *relative* insulin deficiency). Onset often coincides with the peak of physiologic pubertal insulin resistance, which may lead to symptoms of hyperglycemia in previously compensated adolescents. The cause is not autoimmune destruction of beta-cells but rather a complex interaction between many genes and environmental factors, which differ among different populations and patients. Risk factors include

- Obesity
- Native American, black, Hispanic, Asian American, and Pacific Islander heritage
- Positive family history (60 to 90% have a 1st- or 2nd-degree relative with type 2 DM)

Monogenic forms of diabetes are caused by genetic defects that are inherited in an autosomal dominant pattern, so patients typically have one or more affected family members. There is no insulin resistance or autoimmune destruction of beta-cells. Onset is usually before age 25 yr.

Pathophysiology

In **type 1 DM,** lack of insulin causes hyperglycemia and impaired glucose utilization in skeletal muscle. Muscle and fat are then broken down to provide energy. Fat breakdown produces ketones, which cause acidemia and sometimes a significant, life-threatening acidosis (diabetic ketoacidosis [DKA]).

In **type 2 DM,** there is usually enough insulin function to prevent DKA at diagnosis, but children can sometimes present with DKA (up to 25%) or, less commonly, hyperglycemic hyperosmolar state (HHS), in which severe hyperosmolar dehydration occurs. HHS most often occurs during a period of stress or infection, with nonadherence to treatment regimens, or when glucose metabolism is further impaired by drugs (eg, corticosteroids). Other metabolic derangements associated with insulin resistance include

- Dyslipidemia (leading to atherosclerosis)
- Hypertension
- Polycystic ovary syndrome
- Obstructive sleep apnea
- Nonalcoholic steatohepatitis (fatty liver)

Atherosclerosis begins in childhood and adolescence and markedly increases risk of cardiovascular disease.

In **monogenic forms of DM,** the underlying defect depends on the type. The most common types are caused by defects in transcription factors that regulate pancreatic beta-cell function (eg, hepatic nuclear factor 4-alpha [HNF-4-α] and hepatic nuclear factor 1-alpha [HNF-1-α]). In these types, insulin secretion is impaired but not absent, there is no insulin resistance, and hyperglycemia worsens with age. Another type of monogenic DM is caused by a defect in the glucose sensor, glucokinase. With glucokinase defects, insulin secretion is normal but glucose levels are regulated at a higher set point, causing fasting hyperglycemia that worsens minimally with age.

PEARLS & PITFALLS

- Despite the common misconception, DKA can occur in children with type 2 DM.

Symptoms and Signs

In **type 1 DM,** initial manifestations vary from asymptomatic hyperglycemia to life-threatening DKA. However, most commonly, children have symptomatic hyperglycemia without acidosis, with several days to weeks of urinary frequency, polydipsia, and polyuria. Polyuria may manifest as nocturia, bed-wetting, or daytime incontinence; in children who are not toilet-trained, parents may note an increased frequency of wet or heavy diapers. About half of children have weight loss as a result of increased catabolism and also have impaired growth. Fatigue, weakness, candidal rashes, blurry vision (due to the hyperosmolar state of the lens and vitreous humor), and/or nausea and vomiting (due to ketonemia) may also be present initially.

In **type 2 DM,** children are often asymptomatic and their condition may be detected only on routine testing. However, some children present with symptomatic hyperglycemia, HHS, or, despite the common misconception, DKA.

Complications of diabetes: DKA is common among patients with known type 1 DM; it develops in about 1 to 10% of patients each year, usually because they have not taken their insulin. Other risk factors for DKA include prior episodes of DKA, difficult social circumstances, depression or other psychiatric disturbances, intercurrent illness, and use of an insulin pump (because of a kinked or dislodged catheter, poor insulin absorption due to infusion site inflammation, or pump malfunction). Clinicians can help minimize the effects of risk factors by providing education, counseling, and support.

Psychosocial problems are very common among children with diabetes and their families. Up to half of children develop depression, anxiety, or other psychologic problems (see p. 2708). Eating disorders are a serious problem in adolescents, who sometimes also skip insulin doses in an effort to control weight. Psychosocial problems can also result in poor glycemic control by affecting children's ability to adhere to their dietary and/or drug regimens. Social workers and mental health professionals (as part of a multidisciplinary team) can help identify and alleviate psychosocial causes of poor glycemic control.

Vascular complications rarely are clinically evident in childhood. However, early pathologic changes and functional abnormalities may be present a few years after disease onset. Microvascular complications include diabetic nephropathy, retinopathy, and neuropathy. Macrovascular complications include coronary artery disease, peripheral vascular disease, and stroke. Although neuropathy is more common among children who have had diabetes for a long duration (≥ 5 yr) and poor control (glycosylated Hb [HbA_{1c}] > 10%), it can happen in young children who have had diabetes for a short duration and good control.

Diagnosis

- Fasting plasma glucose level ≥ 126 mg/dL (≥ 7.0 mmol/L)
- Random glucose level ≥ 200 mg/dL (≥ 11.1 mmol/L)
- Glycosylated Hb (HbA_{1c}) ≥ 6.5%
- Sometimes oral glucose tolerance testing

(For recommendations about diagnosis, see also the American Diabetes Association's standards in medical care in diabetes and the International Society for Pediatric and Adolescent Diabetes' (ISPAD) guidelines for type 2 diabetes in children and adolescents.)

Diagnosis of diabetes: Diagnosis of DM and prediabetes is similar to that in adults, typically using fasting or random plasma glucose levels and/or HbA_{1c} levels, and depends on the presence or absence of symptoms (see Table 165–2 on p. 1254). Diabetes may be diagnosed with the presence of classic symptoms of diabetes and blood glucose measurements (random plasma glucose ≥ 200 mg/dL (≥ 11.1 mmol/L) or fasting plasma glucose ≥ 126 mg/dL (≥ 7.0 mmol/L); fasting is defined as no caloric intake for 8 h).

An oral glucose tolerance test is not required and should not be done if diabetes can be diagnosed by other criteria. When needed, the test should be done using 1.75 g/kg (maximum 75 g) glucose dissolved in water. The test may be helpful in children without symptoms or with mild or atypical symptoms and may be helpful in suspected cases of type 2 or monogenic DM. The HbA_{1c} criterion is typically more useful to diagnose type 2 DM, and hyperglycemia should be confirmed.

Initial evaluation and testing: For patients suspected of having diabetes but who do not appear ill, initial testing should include a basic metabolic panel, including electrolytes and glucose, and urinalysis. For ill patients, testing also includes a venous or arterial blood gas, liver function tests, and calcium, magnesium, phosphorus, and Hct levels.

Diagnosis of diabetes type: Additional tests should be done to confirm the type of diabetes, including

- C-peptide and insulin (if not yet treated with insulin) levels
- HbA_{1c} levels (if not already done)
- Tests for autoantibodies against pancreatic islet cell proteins

Autoantibodies include glutamic acid decarboxylase, insulin, insulinoma-associated protein, and zinc transporter ZnT8. More than 90% of patients with newly diagnosed type 1 DM have ≥ 1 of these autoantibodies, whereas the absence of antibodies strongly suggests type 2 DM. However, about 10 to 20% of children with the type 2 DM phenotype have autoantibodies and are reclassified as type 1 DM, because such children are more likely to require insulin therapy and are at greater risk of developing other autoimmune disorders.

Monogenic diabetes is important to recognize because treatment differs from type 1 DM and type 2 DM. The diagnosis should be considered in children with a strong family history of diabetes but who lack typical features of type 2 DM; that is, they have only mild fasting (100 to 150 mg/dL) or postprandial hyperglycemia, are young and nonobese, and have no autoantibodies or signs of insulin resistance (eg, acanthosis nigricans). Genetic testing is available to confirm monogenic diabetes. This testing is important because some types of monogenic DM can progress with age.

Testing for complications and other disorders: Patients with **type 1 DM** should be tested for other autoimmune disorders by measuring celiac disease antibodies (see p. 150), TSH, thyroxine, and thyroid antibodies (see p. 1343).

Patients with **type 2 DM** should have liver function tests, fasting lipid profile, and urine microalbumin:creatinine ratio done at the time of diagnosis because such children (unlike those with type 1 DM, in whom complications develop over many years) often have comorbidities, such as fatty liver, hyperlipidemia, and hypertension, at diagnosis. Children with clinical findings suggestive of complications should also be tested:

- Obesity: Test for nonalcoholic steatohepatitis
- Daytime somnolence or snoring: Test for obstructive sleep apnea
- Hirsutism, acne, or menstrual irregularities: Test for polycystic ovary syndrome

Screening for diabetes: Asymptomatic children (≤ 18 yr) who are at risk should be screened for type 2 diabetes or prediabetes by measuring HbA_{1c}. This test should first be done at age 10 yr or at onset of puberty, if puberty occurred at a younger age, and should be repeated every 3 yr.

Children at risk include those who are overweight (BMI > 85th percentile for age and sex, weight for height > 85th percentile, or weight > 120% of ideal body weight) and who have any 2 of the following:

- Family history of type 2 DM in 1st- or 2nd-degree relative
- Native American, black, Hispanic, Asian American and Pacific Islander heritage
- Signs of insulin resistance or conditions associated with insulin resistance (eg, acanthosis nigricans, hypertension, dyslipidemia, polycystic ovary syndrome, or small-for-gestational-age birth weight)
- Maternal gestational diabetes or maternal history of diabetes

Treatment

- Diet and exercise
- For type 1 DM, insulin
- For type 2 DM, metformin and sometimes insulin

Intensive education and treatment in childhood and adolescence may help achieve treatment goals, which are to normalize blood glucose levels while minimizing the number of hypoglycemic episodes and to prevent or delay the onset and progression of complications. (For recommendations about treatment, see also the American Diabetes Association's standards in medical care in diabetes and the International Society for Pediatric and Adolescent Diabetes' [ISPAD] guidelines for type 2 diabetes in children and adolescents.)

Lifestyle modifications: Lifestyle modifications that benefit all patients include

- Eating regularly and in consistent amounts
- Limiting intake of refined carbohydrates and saturated fats
- Increasing physical activity

In general, the term *diet* should be avoided in favor of *meal plan* or *healthy food choices*. The main focus is on encouraging heart-healthy diets low in cholesterol and saturated fats.

In **type 1 DM,** the popularity of basal–bolus regimens and the use of carbohydrate counting (parents estimate the amount of carbohydrate in an upcoming meal and use that amount to calculate the preprandial insulin dose) has changed meal plan strategies. In this flexible approach, food intake is not rigidly specified. Instead, meal plans are based on the child's usual eating patterns rather than on a theoretically optimal diet to which the child is unlikely to adhere, and insulin dose is matched to actual carbohydrate intake. The insulin: carbohydrate ratio is individualized but varies with age. A good rule of thumb for age is

- Birth to 5 yr: 1 unit insulin per 30 g carbohydrate
- 6 to 12 yr: 1 unit insulin per 15 g carbohydrate
- Adolescence: 1 unit insulin per 8 to 10 g carbohydrate

In **type 2 DM,** patients should be encouraged to lose weight and thus increase insulin sensitivity. A good rule of thumb to determine the amount of calories needed by a child age 3 to 13 yr is 1000 calories + (100 × child's age in yr). Simple steps to improve the diet and manage caloric intake include

- Eliminating sugar-containing drinks and foods made of refined, simple sugars (eg, processed candies and high fructose corn syrups)
- Discouraging skipping meals
- Avoiding grazing on food throughout the day
- Controlling portion size
- Limiting high-fat, high-calorie foods in the home
- Increasing fiber intake by eating more fruits and vegetables

Type 1 diabetes Insulin regimens: Insulin is the cornerstone of management of type 1 DM. Available insulin formulations are similar to those used in adults (see Table 165–3 on p. 1262). Insulin should be given before a meal, except in young children whose consumption at any given meal is difficult to predict. Dosing requirements vary by age, activity level, pubertal status, and length of time from initial diagnosis. Within a few weeks of initial diagnosis, many patients have a temporary decrease in their insulin requirements because of residual beta-cell function (honeymoon phase). This honeymoon phase can last from a few months up to 2 yr, after which insulin requirements typically range from 0.7 to 1 unit/kg/day. During puberty, patients require higher doses (up to 1.5 units/kg/day) to counteract insulin resistance caused by increased pubertal hormone levels.

Types of insulin regimens include

- Basal–bolus regimen
- Multiple daily injections (MDI) regimen
- Premixed insulin regimen

A **basal–bolus regimen** is typically preferred. In this regimen, children are given a daily baseline dose of insulin that is then supplemented by doses of short-acting insulin before each meal based on anticipated carbohydrate intake and on measured glucose levels. The basal dose can be given as a once/day injection (sometimes q 12 h for younger children) of a long-acting insulin (glargine or detemir) or as a continuous infusion of rapid-acting insulin (usually aspart or lispro) using an insulin pump, which delivers insulin continuously through a catheter placed under the skin. The supplemental boluses are given as separate injections of rapid-acting insulin or by using the insulin pump. Glargine or detemir injections are typically given at dinner or bedtime and must not be mixed with short-acting insulin. The basal dose helps keep blood glucose levels in range between meals and at night. Using an insulin pump to deliver the basal dose allows for maximal flexibility; the pump can be programmed to give different rates at different times throughout the day and night. A basal–bolus regimen may not be an option if adequate supervision is not available, particularly if an adult is not available to give daytime injections at school or daycare.

An **MDI regimen** can be used if a basal–bolus regimen is not an option (eg, because the family needs a simpler regimen, the child or parents have a needle phobia, lunchtime injections cannot be given at school or daycare). In this regimen, children usually receive neutral protamine Hagedorn (NPH) insulin before eating breakfast and dinner and at bedtime and receive rapid-acting insulin before eating breakfast and dinner. Because NPH and rapid-acting insulin can be mixed, this regimen provides fewer injections than the basal–bolus regimen and may be preferred by younger children. However, this regimen provides less flexibility and requires a set daily schedule for meals and snack times.

Premixed insulin regimens use preparations of 70/30 (70% insulin aspart protamine/30% regular insulin) or 75/25 (75% insulin lispro protamine/25% insulin lispro). Premixed regimens are not a good choice but are simpler and may improve adherence because they require fewer injections. Children are given set doses twice daily, with two thirds of the total daily dose given at breakfast and one third at dinner. However, premixed regimens provide much less flexibility with respect to timing and amount of meals and are less precise than other regimens because of the fixed ratios.

Clinicians should use the most intensive management program children and their family can adhere to in order to maximize glycemic control and thus reduce the risk of long-term vascular complications.

Type 1 diabetes glucose and HbA_{1c} target levels: Plasma glucose targets (see Table 307–1) are established to balance the need to normalize glucose levels with the risk of hypoglycemia. Patients beyond the honeymoon phase should try to have ≥ 50% of blood glucose levels in the normal range (70 to 180 mg/dL [3.9 to 10 mmol/L]) and < 10% below range.

HbA_{1c} targets were previously higher for younger children (< 8.5%) but recently, a target of < 7.5% was recommended for all patients < 18 yr to reduce risk of harm from prolonged hyperglycemia in childhood. However, many children and adolescents do not meet this target. An increased frequency of self-monitoring of blood glucose levels is associated with improved HbA_{1c} levels because patients are better able to adjust insulin for meals, have an improved ability to correct hyperglycemic values, and are potentially able to detect hypoglycemia earlier, which prevents overcorrection (ie, excessive carbohydrate intake as treatment for hypoglycemia, resulting in hyperglycemia).

Treatment goals should be individualized based on patient age, diabetes duration, comorbid conditions, and psychosocial circumstances. The risk of hypoglycemia in children who have hypoglycemia unawareness or lack the maturity to recognize the symptoms of hypoglycemia can limit aggressive attempts to achieve treatment goals.

Type 1 diabetes management of complications: Hypoglycemia is a critical but common complication in children treated with an intensive insulin regimen. Most children have several mild hypoglycemic events per week and self-treat with 15 g of fast-acting carbohydrates (eg, 4 oz of juice, glucose tablets, hard candies, graham crackers, or glucose gel).

Severe hypoglycemia, defined as an episode requiring the assistance of another person to give carbohydrates or glucagon, occurs in about 30% of children each year, and most will have had such an episode by age 18. Oral carbohydrates may be tried, but glucagon 1 mg IM is usually used if neuroglycopenic symptoms (eg, behavioral changes, confusion, difficulty thinking) prevent eating or drinking. If untreated, severe hypoglycemia can cause seizures or even coma or death. Real-time continuous glucose monitoring (CGM) devices can help children with hypoglycemia unawareness because they sound an alarm when glucose is below a specified range or when glucose declines at a rapid rate (see Monitoring glucose and HbA_{1c} levels on p. 2565).

Ketonuria/ketonemia is most often caused by intercurrent illness but also can result from not taking enough insulin or from missing doses and can be a warning of impending DKA. Because early detection of ketones is crucial to prevent progression to DKA and minimize need for emergency department or hospital admission, children and families should be taught to check for ketones in the urine or capillary blood using ketone test strips. Blood ketone testing may be preferred in younger children, those with recurrent DKA, and insulin pump users or if a urine sample is difficult to obtain. Ketone testing should be done whenever the child become ill (regardless of the blood sugar level) or when the blood sugar is high (typically > 240 mg/dL [13.3 mmol/L]). The presence of moderate or large urine ketone levels or blood ketone levels > 1.5 mmol/L can suggest DKA, especially if children also have abdominal pain, vomiting, drowsiness, or rapid breathing. Small urine ketone levels or blood ketone levels 0.6 to 1.5 mmol/L also must be addressed.

When ketones are present, children are given additional short-acting insulin, typically 10 to 20% of the total daily dose, every 2 to 3 h until ketones are cleared. Also, additional

Table 307–1. GLUCOSE AND HBA_{1C} TARGET LEVELS

BLOOD TESTS	IDEAL TARGET	OPTIMAL TARGET	SUBOPTIMAL TARGET	HIGH-RISK TARGET
Self-monitoring of blood glucose (mg/dL [mmol/L])				
Morning fasting	65–100 (3.6–5.6)	70–145 (4–8)	> 145 (> 8)	> 162 (> 9)
Postprandial	80–126 (4.5–7.0)	90–180 (5–10)	180–250 (10–14)	> 250 (> 14)
Bedtime	80–100 (4.0–5.6)	120–180 (6.7–10)	< 75 or > 162 (< 4.2 or > 9)	< 80 or > 200 (< 4.4 or > 11)
Overnight	65–100 (3.6–5.6)	80–162 (4.5–9)	< 75 or > 162 (< 4.2 or > 9)	< 80 or > 200 (< 4.4 or > 11)
HbA_{1C}(%)				
—	< 6.5	< 7.5	7.5–9.0	> 9.0

HbA_{1c} = glycosylated hemoglobin.

Adapted from Rewers MJ, Pillay K, de Beaufort C, et al: Assessment and monitoring of glycemic control in children and adolescents with diabetes. *Pediatr Diabetes* 15 (supplement 20):S102–S114, 2014.

fluid should be given to prevent dehydration. This program of measuring ketones and giving additional fluid and insulin during illness and/or hyperglycemia is called sick-day management. Parents should be instructed to call their health care provider or go to the emergency department if ketones increase or do not clear after 4 to 6 h, or if the clinical status worsens (eg, respiratory distress, continued vomiting, change in mental status).

Type 2 diabetes treatment: As in type 1 DM, lifestyle modifications, with improved nutrition and increased physical activity, are important.

Insulin is started in children who present with more severe DM (HbA_{1c} > 9% or with DKA); glargine, detemir, or premixed insulin can be used. If acidosis is not present, metformin is usually started at the same time. Insulin requirements may decline rapidly during the initial weeks of treatment as endogenous insulin secretion increases; insulin often can be stopped several weeks after regaining acceptable metabolic control.

Metformin is an insulin sensitizer and is the only oral antihyperglycemic drug approved for patients < 18 yr. Other oral drugs used in adults may benefit some adolescents, but they are more expensive, and there is limited evidence for their use in youth. Metformin should be started at a low dose and taken with food to prevent nausea and abdominal pain. A typical starting dose is 500 mg once/day for 1 wk, which is increased weekly by 500 mg for 3 to 6 wk until reaching the maximal target dose of 1000 mg po bid. The goal of treatment is HbA_{1c} < 6.5%. If this cannot be achieved with metformin alone, insulin should be started. Unfortunately, about half of adolescents with type 2 DM ultimately fail metformin monotherapy and require insulin.

Monogenic diabetes treatment: Management of monogenic diabetes is individualized and depends on subtype. The glucokinase subtype generally does not require treatment because children are not at risk of long-term complications. Most patients with HNF-4-α and HNF-1-α types are sensitive to sulfonylureas, but some ultimately require insulin. Other oral hypoglycemics such as metformin are typically not effective.

Monitoring glucose and HbA_{1c} levels: Routine monitoring involves

- Multiple daily glucose checks by fingerstick
- HbA_{1c} measurements every 3 mo

In **type 1 DM,** blood glucose levels should be measured using a fingerstick sample before all meals and before a bedtime snack. Levels also should be checked during the night (around 2 to 3 AM) if nocturnal hypoglycemia is a concern (eg, because of hypoglycemia or vigorous exercise during the day, or when an insulin dose is increased). Because exercise can lower glucose levels for up to 24 h, levels should be checked more frequently on days when children exercise or are more active. To prevent hypoglycemia, children may increase carbohydrate intake or lower insulin dosing when they anticipate increased activity. Sick-day management should be used with hyperglycemia or illness.

Parents should keep detailed daily records of all factors that can affect glycemic control, including blood glucose levels; timing and amount of insulin doses, carbohydrate intake, and physical activity; and any other relevant factors (eg, illness, late snack, missed insulin dose).

CGM systems use a subcutaneous sensor to measure interstitial fluid glucose levels every 1 to 5 min. CGM systems are calibrated with fingerstick blood glucose levels and transmit results wirelessly to a monitoring and display device that may be built into an insulin pump or be a stand-alone device. By identifying times of consistent hyperglycemia and times of increased risk of hypoglycemia, CGM systems can help patients with type 1 DM more safely reach glycemic goals. All devices allow targets to be set; alarms will alert the user if glucose levels are above or below the target, and some CGMs integrated with a pump can also suspend the basal rate for up to 2 h when glucose level drops below a set threshold. Although CGM devices can be used with any regimen, they are typically worn by insulin pump users.

The so-called artificial pancreas (a closed-loop insulin delivery system) for patients ≥ 14 yr has been approved by the FDA. These systems automate blood glucose management through sophisticated computer algorithms that are on a smartphone or similar device. Artificial pancreas systems link to a CGM sensor and insulin pump to determine blood glucose levels and control insulin delivery. These systems help to more tightly control insulin dosing and limit hyperglycemic and hypoglycemic episodes.

In **type 2 DM,** blood glucose levels should be measured regularly but typically less often than in type 1 DM. The frequency of self-monitoring of blood glucose (SMBG) should be individualized based on the patient's fasting and postprandial glucose levels, the degree of glycemic control deemed achievable, and the available resources. The frequency of monitoring should increase if glycemic control targets are not being met, during illness, or when symptoms of hypoglycemia or hyperglycemia are felt. Once targets are achieved, home testing is limited to a few fasting and postprandial blood glucose measurements per week.

HbA_{1c} levels should be measured every 3 mo in type 1 DM and in type 2 DM if insulin is being used or metabolic control is suboptimal. Otherwise, in type 2 DM, levels can be measured twice a year, although every 3 mo is optimal.

Screening for complications of diabetes: Patients are screened regularly for complications depending on the type of diabetes (see Table 307–2). If complications are detected, subsequent testing is done more frequently.

Complications detected on examination or screening are treated first with lifestyle interventions: increased exercise, dietary changes (particularly limiting saturated fat intake), and cessation of smoking (if applicable). Children with microalbuminuria (albumin/creatinine ratio 30 to 300 mg/g) on repeat samples or with persistently elevated BP readings (> 90th to 95th percentiles for age or > 130/80 mm Hg for adolescents) who do not respond to lifestyle interventions typically require antihypertensive therapy, most commonly using an ACE inhibitor. For children with dyslipidemia, if LDL cholesterol remains > 160 mg/dL (or > 130 mg/dL plus one or more cardiovascular risk factors) despite lifestyle interventions, statins should be considered in children > 10 yr, although long-term safety is not established.

KEY POINTS

- Type 1 DM is caused by an autoimmune attack on pancreatic beta-cells, causing complete lack of insulin; it accounts for two thirds of new cases in children and can occur at any age.
- Type 2 DM is caused by insulin resistance and relative insulin deficiency due to a complex interaction among many genetic and environmental factors (particularly obesity); it is increasing in frequency in children and occurs after puberty.
- Most children have symptomatic hyperglycemia without acidosis, with several days to weeks of urinary frequency, polydipsia, and polyuria; children with type 1 DM and rarely type 2 DM may present with DKA.
- Screen asymptomatic, at-risk children for type 2 DM or prediabetes.
- All children with type 1 DM require insulin treatment; intensive glycemic control helps prevent long-term complications but increases risk of hypoglycemic episodes.

Table 307–2. SCREENING FOR COMPLICATIONS OF DIABETES

COMPLICATION	BEGIN SCREENING	SCREENING FREQUENCY	METHOD
Type 1 Diabetes			
Celiac disease	Upon diagnosis	1 to 2 yr	Celiac antibodies
Dyslipidemia	Upon diagnosis (once diabetes stabilized) in all children > 10 yr or if positive family history of early cardiovascular disease or hypercholesterolemia	5 yr	LDL, HDL, and triglyceride levels
Nephropathy	Age 10 yr, when pubertal, or after 5 yr of diabetes	1 yr	Urinary albumin:creatinine ratio, BP measurement
Neuropathy	*Upon diagnosis in all patients ≥ 8 yr	At regular visits, at least annually	Clinical assessment from history (eg, of numbness, persistent pain, paresthesia) and physical examination (eg, ankle reflexes, vibration, and light touch sensation)
Retinopathy	Baseline evaluation: Within 1st yr; Subsequent evaluations: Age 10 yr, when pubertal, or after 5 yr of diabetes	1 yr	Dilated examination by an ophthalmologist or other trained, experienced observer
Thyroid disease	Upon diagnosis	1 to 2 yr	TSH, and T_4 levels, thyroid antibodies
Type 2 Diabetes			
Dyslipidemia	Upon diagnosis	1 to 2 yr	Same as type 1
Nephropathy	Upon diagnosis	1 yr	Same as type 1
Neuropathy	Upon diagnosis	At regular visits, at least annually*	Same as type 1
Retinopathy	Upon diagnosis	1 yr	Same as type 1

*There are no firm guidelines on timing and methodology of screening children for neuropathy.

HDL = high-density lipoprotein; LDL = low-density lipoprotein; T_4 = thyroxine; TSH = thyroid-stimulating hormone.

- Children with type 2 DM are initially treated with metformin and/or insulin; although most children requiring insulin at diagnosis can be successfully transitioned to metformin monotherapy, about half eventually require insulin treatment.
- Psychosocial problems can lead to poor glycemic control through lack of adherence to dietary and drug regimens.
- Insulin doses are adjusted based on frequent glucose monitoring and anticipated carbohydrate intake and activity levels.
- Children are at risk of microvascular and macrovascular complications of DM, which must be sought by regular screening tests.

GROWTH HORMONE DEFICIENCY IN CHILDREN

(Pituitary Dwarfism)

Growth hormone (GH) deficiency is the most common pituitary hormone deficiency in children and can be isolated or accompanied by deficiency of other pituitary hormones. GH deficiency typically results in abnormally slow growth and short stature with normal proportions. Diagnosis involves measurement of pituitary hormone levels and CT or MRI to detect structural pituitary anomalies or brain tumors. Treatment usually involves specific hormone replacement and removal of any causative tumor.

Patients with GH deficiency associated with generalized hypopituitarism (panhypopituitarism) will also have deficiency of one or more other pituitary hormones (eg, follicle-stimulating hormone [FSH], luteinizing hormone [LH], adrenocorticotropic hormone [ACTH], TSH, antidiuretic hormone [ADH]). Hypopituitarism can be primary (a pituitary disorder) or secondary to interference with hypothalamic secretion of specific releasing hormones that control anterior pituitary hormone (GH, FSH, LH, ACTH, TSH) production.

Etiology

GH deficiency can occur in isolation or in association with generalized hypopituitarism. In both instances, GH deficiency may be acquired or congenital (including hereditary genetic causes). Rarely, GH is not deficient but the GH receptors are abnormal (GH insensitivity).

Isolated GH deficiency is estimated to occur in 1/4,000 to 1/10,000 children. It is usually idiopathic, but about 25% of patients have an identifiable etiology. Congenital causes include abnormalities of the GH-releasing hormone receptor and of the *GH1* gene and certain CNS malformations. Acquired causes include therapeutic radiation of the CNS (high-dose radiation can cause generalized hypopituitarism), meningitis, histiocytosis, and brain injury. Radiation of the spine, either prophylactic or therapeutic, may further impair the growth potential of the vertebrae and further jeopardize height gain.

Generalized hypopituitarism may have genetic causes, involving hereditary or sporadic mutations that affect cells of the pituitary. In such cases, there also may be anomalies of other organ systems, particularly midline defects, such as cleft palate, or septo-optic dysplasia (which involves absence of the septum pellucidum, optic nerve atrophy, and hypopituitarism). Generalized hypopituitarism also can be acquired from many types of lesions that affect the hypothalamus (impairing secretion of releasing hormones) or pituitary; examples include tumors (eg, most commonly craniopharyngioma), infections (eg, TB, toxoplasmosis, meningitis), and infiltrative disorders. The combination of lytic lesions of the bones or skull and diabetes insipidus suggests Langerhans cell histiocytosis.

Symptoms and Signs

Manifestations of GH deficiency depend on the patient's age, the underlying etiology, and the specific hormone deficiencies.

GH deficiency itself typically manifests as growth failure, sometimes along with delay in tooth development. Height is below the 3rd percentile, and growth velocity is < 6 cm/yr before age 4 yr, < 5 cm/yr from age 4 to 8 yr, and < 4 cm/yr before puberty. Although of small stature, a child with hypopituitarism retains normal proportionality between upper and lower body segments. Skeletal maturation, assessed by bone age determination, is > 2 yr behind chronologic age.

Other abnormalities may be present, depending on the underlying defect, and the child may have delayed or absent pubertal development. Weight gain may be out of proportion to growth, resulting in relative obesity. Neonates who have congenital defects of the pituitary or hypothalamus may have hypoglycemia (which also can occur in older children), midline defects (eg, cleft palate), or micropenis, as well as manifestations of other endocrine deficiencies.

Diagnosis

- Clinical evaluation, including growth criteria and other medical history
- Imaging studies
- Insulin-like growth factor 1 (IGF-1) levels and IGF binding protein type 3 (IGFBP-3) levels
- Usually confirmation by provocative testing
- Evaluation of other pituitary hormones and for other causes of poor growth

Current consensus guidelines for diagnosis of GH deficiency require integration of growth criteria, medical history, laboratory testing, and imaging results.

Growth is assessed; data for height and weight should be plotted on a growth chart (auxologic assessment) for all children. (For children 0 to 2 yr, see WHO Growth Charts; for children 2 yr and older, see CDC Growth Charts—both can be found at www.cdc.gov.)

Measurement of IGF-1 and IGFBP-3 levels begins the assessment of the GH/IGF-1 axis. IGF-1 reflects GH activity, and IGFBP-3 is the major carrier of IGF peptides. Levels of IGF-1 and IGFBP-3 are measured because GH levels are pulsatile, highly variable, and difficult to interpret.

IGF-1 levels vary by age and should be interpreted relative to bone age rather than to chronologic age. IGF-1 levels are lowest in infancy and early childhood (< 5 yr) and thus do not reliably discriminate between normal and subnormal in these age groups. However, IGFBP-3 levels, unlike IGF-1, are less affected by undernutrition and allow discrimination between normal and subnormal in younger children. At puberty, IGF-1 levels rise and normal levels help exclude GH deficiency. Low IGF-1 levels in older children suggest GH deficiency; however, IGF-1 levels are low in conditions other than GH deficiency (eg, psychosocial deprivation, undernutrition, celiac disease, hypothyroidism) and these disorders must be excluded.

In children with low levels of IGF-1 and IGFBP-3, GH deficiency is usually confirmed by measuring GH levels. Because basal GH levels are typically low or undetectable (except after the onset of sleep), random GH levels are not useful and assessment of GH levels requires provocative testing. However, provocative testing is nonphysiologic, subject to laboratory error, and poorly reproducible. Also, the definition of a normal response varies by age, sex, and testing center and is based on limited evidence.

Imaging studies are done when growth is abnormal; bone age should be determined from an x-ray of the left hand (by convention). In GH deficiency, skeletal maturation is usually delayed to the same extent as height. With GH deficiency, evaluating the pituitary gland and hypothalamus with CT or MRI is indicated to rule out calcifications, tumors, and structural anomalies.

Screening laboratory tests are done to look for other possible causes of poor growth, including

- Hypothyroidism (eg, TSH, thyroxine)
- Renal disorders (electrolytes, creatinine levels)
- Inflammatory and immune conditions (eg, tissue transglutaminase antibodies, ESR)
- Hematologic disorders (eg, CBC with differential)

Genetic testing for specific syndromes (eg, Turner syndrome) may be indicated by physical findings or if growth pattern differs significantly from family. If GH deficiency is highly suspected, additional tests of pituitary function are done (eg, ACTH, 8 AM serum cortisol level, LH, FSH, and prolactin levels).

PEARLS & PITFALLS

- Unlike in many endocrine deficiencies in which hormone levels are diagnostic, random GH levels are of little use in diagnosing GH deficiency.

Provocative testing: Because GH responses are typically abnormal in patients with diminished thyroid or adrenal function, provocative testing should be done in these patients only after adequate hormone replacement therapy.

The insulin tolerance test is the best provocative test for stimulating GH release but is rarely done because it is risky. Other provocative tests are less dangerous but also less reliable. These include tests using arginine infusion (500 mg/kg IV given over 30 min), clonidine (0.15 mg/m^2 po [maximum 0.25 mg]), levodopa (10 mg/kg po for children; 500 mg po for adults), and glucagon (0.03 mg/kg IV [maximum 1 mg]). GH levels are measured at different times after drug administration depending on the drug.

Because no single test is 100% effective in eliciting GH release, two GH provocation tests are done (typically on the same day). GH levels generally peak 30 to 90 min after administration of insulin or the onset of arginine infusion, 30 to 120 min after levodopa, 60 to 90 min after clonidine, and 120 to 180 min after glucagon. The GH response that is considered normal is somewhat arbitrary. Generally, any stimulated GH level > 10 ng/mL is sufficient to rule out GH deficiency. GH deficiency may be considered for responses < 10 ng/mL (some centers use a lower cutoff, eg, 7 ng/mL) to two pharmacologic stimuli, but results must be interpreted in the context of auxologic data. Because GH levels rise during puberty, many children who fail provocative GH stimulation testing before puberty may have normal results after puberty or when primed with gonadal steroids.

Provocative testing may not detect subtle defects in the regulation of GH release. For example, in children with short stature secondary to GH secretory dysfunction, results of provocative testing for GH release are usually normal. However, serial measurements of GH levels over 12 to 24 h indicate abnormally low 12- or 24-h integrated GH secretion. However, this test is expensive and uncomfortable and thus is not the test of choice for GH deficiency.

If diminished GH release is confirmed, tests of secretion of other pituitary hormones and (if abnormal) hormones of their target peripheral endocrine glands along with pituitary imaging studies must be done if not done previously.

Treatment

- Recombinant GH supplements
- Sometimes other pituitary hormone replacement

Recombinant GH is indicated for all children with short stature who have documented GH deficiency. Dosing is usually from 0.03 to 0.05 mg/kg sc once/day. With therapy, height velocity often increases to 10 to 12 cm/yr in the first year and, although it increases more slowly thereafter, remains above pretreatment rates. Therapy is continued until an acceptable height is reached or growth rate falls below 2.5 cm/yr.

Adverse effects of GH therapy are few but include idiopathic intracranial hypertension (pseudotumor cerebri), slipped capital femoral epiphysis, and transient mild peripheral edema. Before the advent of recombinant GH, GH extracted from pituitary glands was used. This preparation rarely led to Creutzfeldt-Jakob disease 20 to 40 yr after treatment. Pituitary-extracted GH was last used in the 1980s.

It is controversial whether short children with clinical features of GH deficiency but with normal GH secretion and normal IGF-1 levels should be treated with GH. Many experts recommend a trial of GH therapy for 6 to 12 mo, continuing GH only if there is a doubling of or an increase of 3 cm/yr over the pretreatment height velocity. Others object to this approach because it is expensive, is experimental, may lead to adverse effects, labels otherwise healthy children as abnormal, and raises ethical and psychosocial concerns that feed into the bias of "heightism."

When other pituitary hormone deficiencies accompany GH deficiency, additional hormone replacement is required. Cortisol (see p. 1239) and thyroid hormone (see p. 1351) should be replaced throughout childhood, adolescence, and adulthood when circulating levels of these hormones are low. Diabetes insipidus typically requires lifelong treatment with desmopressin in tablet or intranasal form (see p. 1319). When puberty fails to occur normally, treatment with gonadal sex steroids is indicated (see p. 2560).

GH therapy in children with short stature due to therapeutic radiation of the pituitary gland for cancer carries a theoretic risk of causing cancer recurrence. However, studies have not shown a greater-than-expected incidence of new cancers or a greater recurrence rate. GH replacement can probably be safely instituted at least 1 yr after the successful completion of anticancer therapy.

KEY POINTS

- GH deficiency can occur in isolation or in association with generalized hypopituitarism.
- Causes include congenital (including genetic) disorders and a number of acquired disorders of the hypothalamus and/or pituitary.
- GH deficiency causes short stature; numerous other manifestations may be present depending on the cause.
- Diagnosis is based on a combination of clinical findings, imaging studies, and laboratory testing, usually including provocative tests of GH release.
- Children with short stature and documented GH deficiency should receive recombinant GH; other manifestations of hypopituitarism are treated as needed.

HYPERTHYROIDISM IN INFANTS AND CHILDREN

Hyperthyroidism is excessive thyroid hormone production. Diagnosis is by thyroid function testing (eg, free serum thyroxine, TSH). Treatment is with methimazole and sometimes radioactive iodine or surgery.

Etiology

In infants, hyperthyroidism is rare but potentially life-threatening. It develops in fetuses of women with current or prior Graves disease. In Graves disease, patients have autoantibodies against the thyroid receptor for TSH, and these autoantibodies overstimulate thyroid hormone production by binding to TSH receptors in the thyroid gland. These antibodies cross the placenta and cause thyroid hyperfunction in the fetus (intrauterine Graves disease), which can result in fetal death or premature birth. Because infants clear the antibodies after birth, neonatal Graves disease is usually transient. However, because the clearance rate varies, duration of neonatal Graves disease varies.

In children and adolescents, Graves disease is the cause of hyperthyroidism in > 90%. Less common causes include autonomously functioning toxic nodules, transient hyperthyroidism during the early phase of Hashimoto thyroiditis followed by eventual hypothyroidism (hashitoxicosis), or adverse drug effects (eg, amiodarone-induced hyperthyroidism). Occasionally, transient hyperthyroidism can be caused by infections, including bacterial (acute thyroiditis) and viral (subacute thyroiditis) infections; bacterial causes include *Staphylococcus aureus, S. epidermis, Streptococcus pyogenes, S. pneumoniae, Escherichia coli,* and *Clostridium septicum*. Predisposing factors for acute thyroiditis in children include congenital anomalies (eg, persistent pyriform sinus fistula) and immunocompromised status. Prepubertal children with Graves disease commonly present with isolated triiodothyronine (T_3) toxicosis, but if diagnosis is delayed, they can have high levels of free serum thyroxine (T_4) and high antibody titers directed against the TSH receptor.

Symptoms and Signs

In infants, symptoms and signs of hyperthyroidism include irritability, feeding problems, hypertension, tachycardia, exophthalmos, goiter (see p. 2560), frontal bossing, and microcephaly. Other early findings are failure to thrive, vomiting, and diarrhea. Affected infants almost always recover within 6 mo; the course is rarely longer. The onset and severity of symptoms also vary depending on whether the mother is taking antithyroid drugs. If the mother is not taking drugs, infants are hyperthyroid at birth; if the mother is taking drugs, infants may not become hyperthyroid until the drugs are metabolized at about 3 to 7 days.

Signs of hyperthyroidism (eg, poor intrauterine growth, fetal tachycardia [> 160 beats/min], goiter) may be detected in the fetus as early as the 2nd trimester. If fetal hyperthyroidism is not detected until the neonatal period, the infant may be severely affected; possible manifestations include craniosynostosis (premature fusion of the cranial sutures), impaired intellect, growth failure, and short stature. Mortality rate may reach 10 to 15%.

In children and adolescents, symptoms of acquired Graves disease may include sleep difficulties, hyperactivity, emotional lability, marked decrease in concentration and school performance, heat intolerance, diaphoresis, fatigue, weight loss, increased frequency of bowel movements, tremor, and palpitations. Signs include diffuse goiter, tachycardia, and hypertension. Graves ophthalmopathy occurs in up to one-third of children. Although eye findings are less dramatic than in adults, children may have eyelid lag or red or prominent eyes, sometimes with proptosis (exophthalmos). Children and adolescents may present with alterations in growth, including growth acceleration and advanced bone age; however, puberty is often delayed rather than precocious.

Acute thyroiditis may manifest with sudden onset of symptoms of hyperthyroidism, tenderness over the thyroid gland, and fever. About 10% of patients with acute thyroiditis have hyperthyroidism. Many have leukocytosis with a left shift. In subacute thyroiditis these manifestations are present but less severe and may have been preceded by a viral illness; fever may last for several weeks.

Thyroid storm, a rare, severe complication in children with hyperthyroidism, may manifest with extreme tachycardia, hyperthermia, hypertension, congestive heart failure, and delirium, with progression to coma and death.

Diagnosis

- Thyroid function tests
- Sometimes thyroid ultrasonography or radionuclide scanning

In infants, diagnosis of hyperthyroidism is suspected if their mother has active Graves disease or a history of Graves disease and high titers of stimulatory antibodies (thyroid-stimulating immunoglobulins or TSIs) and is confirmed by measuring serum T4, free T4, T3, and TSH. TSH receptor antibodies may be used instead of TSIs because the newer assays are highly sensitive and have faster turnaround times for results.

Diagnosis in **older children and adolescents** is similar to that in adults and also includes thyroid function tests (see diagnosis of hyperthyroidism). In contrast to the evaluation of hypothyroidism, measurement of T_3 is essential because early in Graves disease, T_3 may rise before T_4 levels increase. Many clinicians do thyroid ultrasonography in older children with hyperthyroidism and thyroid gland asymmetry, negative TSIs/TSH receptor antibody testing, or a palpable nodule. Ultrasonography or CT can also help localize an abscess or identify a congenital anomaly. If a nodule is confirmed, fine-needle aspiration (FNA) biopsy should be considered as well as radionuclide scanning (either ^{99m}Tc pertechnetate or ^{123}I) to exclude an autonomously functioning toxic nodule or concurrent differentiated thyroid cancer. FNA biopsy can also help differentiate acute from subacute thyroiditis and provide bacterial sensitivities for proper antibiotic coverage.

Treatment

- Antithyroid drugs
- Sometimes radioactive iodine or surgery

Infants are given an antithyroid drug, typically methimazole 0.17 to 0.33 mg/kg po tid, sometimes with a beta-blocker (eg, propranolol 0.8 mg/kg po tid, atenolol 0.5 to 1.2 mg/kg po once/day to bid) to treat symptoms. Propylthiouracil, another antithyroid drug, has recently been found to sometimes cause severe liver failure and is no longer a first-line drug but may be used in special situations, such as thyroid storm. Treatment of hyperthyroidism must be monitored closely and stopped as soon as the disease has run its course. (For treatment of Graves disease during pregnancy, see p. 2400.)

For **older children and adolescents,** treatment is similar to that for adults and includes antithyroid drugs and sometimes definitive therapy with thyroid ablation using radioactive iodine or surgery. Beta-blockers, such as atenolol or propranolol, may be used to control hypertension and tachycardia. Children treated with antithyroid drugs have a 35% likelihood of remission, which is lower than that in adults (50%), and is defined as the lack of recurrence ≥ 12 mo after antithyroid drugs have been stopped.

Definitive therapy may be needed for patients who do not achieve remission with 18 to 24 mo of antithyroid drug therapy, who have drug adverse effects, or who are nonadherent. Characteristics associated with lower likelihood of remission include younger age at onset (eg, prepubertal vs pubertal), higher thyroid hormone levels at initial presentation, larger thyroid gland (> 2.5 times normal size for age), and persistent elevation in TSH receptor antibody titers. Both radioactive iodine and surgery are reliable options for definitive therapy, with the goal of producing hypothyroidism. However, radioactive iodine is usually not used in children who are under age 10 yr and is often not effective in larger thyroid glands. Therefore, surgery may be preferable for children and adolescents who have these factors.

If an autonomously functioning toxic nodule is detected, surgical excision is recommended in children and adolescents.

Treatment of **acute thyroiditis** involves oral or IV antibiotics (typically amoxicillin/clavulanic acid or cephalosporins for patients allergic to penicillin but ideally based on antibiotic sensitivities obtained from fine-needle aspiration biopsy specimen). Surgical treatment may be needed (eg, to drain an abscess or repair a fistula). Subacute thyroiditis is self-limiting, and nonsteroidal anti-inflammatory drugs are given for pain control. Antithyroid drugs are not indicated, but beta-blockers can be used if patients are symptomatic.

KEY POINTS

- Hyperthyroidism in infants is usually caused by transplacental thyroid-stimulating antibodies from mothers with Graves disease.
- Hyperthyroidism in older children and adolescents is usually caused by Graves disease.
- There are numerous manifestations of hyperthyroidism, including tachycardia, hypertension, weight loss, irritability, decreased concentration and school performance, and sleep difficulties.
- Diagnosis is with serum thyroxine (T_4), free T_4, triiodothyronine (T_3), and TSH; if there are significant palpable abnormalities of the thyroid, do ultrasonography.
- Treat with methimazole and, for symptoms, a beta-blocker; however, only about 35% of cases acquired outside the neonatal period resolve with antithyroid drugs and patients may need definitive therapy using radioactive iodine or surgery.

HYPOTHYROIDISM IN INFANTS AND CHILDREN

Hypothyroidism is thyroid hormone deficiency. Symptoms in infants include poor feeding and growth failure;

symptoms in older children and adolescents are similar to those of adults but also include growth failure, delayed puberty, or both. Diagnosis is by thyroid function testing (eg, serum thyroxine, TSH). Treatment is thyroid hormone replacement.

Etiology

Hypothyroidism in infants and young children may be congenital or acquired.

Congenital hypothyroidism: Congenital hypothyroidism occurs in about 1/2000 to 1/3000 live births. Most congenital cases are sporadic, but about 10 to 20% are inherited. The causes usually involve

- Dysgenesis of the gland (85% of cases)
- Dyshormonogenesis (abnormal thyroid hormone production, 10 to 15% of cases)

Dysgenesis may involve ectopy (two-thirds of cases), absence (agenesis), or underdevelopment (hypoplasia) of the thyroid gland.

Dyshormonogenesis has multiple types, which can result from a defect in any of the steps of thyroid hormone biosynthesis (see p. 2560).

Rarely in the US but commonly in certain developing countries, hypothyroidism results from maternal iodine deficiency. Rarely, transplacental transfer of antibodies, goitrogens (eg, amiodarone), or antithyroid drugs (eg, propylthiouracil, methimazole) causes transient hypothyroidism. Another rare cause is central hypothyroidism, which is caused by structural anomalies in pituitary development; patients usually also have other pituitary hormone deficiencies.

Acquired hypothyroidism: Acquired hypothyroidism is typically caused by autoimmune thyroiditis (Hashimoto thyroiditis) and occurs during later childhood and adolescence. About 50% of affected children have a family history of autoimmune thyroid disease.

Less commonly, hypothyroidism may occur after radiation therapy to the head and neck for certain cancers, after total body irradiation in preparation for bone marrow transplant, and secondary to certain drugs (eg, antiepileptic drugs, lithium, amiodarone, tyrosine kinase inhibitors). Permanent hypothyroidism is also the goal of therapy for patients undergoing definitive therapy for Graves disease (see treatment of hyperthyroidism in infants and children) or thyroid cancer.

Iodine deficiency remains the most common worldwide cause of hypothyroidism but is rare in the US.

Symptoms and Signs

Symptoms and signs of hypothyroidism in infants and young children differ from those in older children and adults. If iodine deficiency occurs very early during pregnancy, infants may present with severe growth failure, coarse facial features, intellectual disability, and spasticity. Most other hypothyroid infants initially have few if any symptoms or signs and are detected only through newborn screening.

Symptoms that do occur may be subtle or develop slowly because some maternal thyroid hormone crosses the placenta. However, after the maternal thyroid hormone is metabolized, if the underlying cause of hypothyroidism persists and hypothyroidism remains undiagnosed or untreated, it usually slows CNS development moderately to severely and may be accompanied by low muscle tone, sensorineural hearing loss, prolonged hyperbilirubinemia, umbilical hernia, respiratory distress, macroglossia, large fontanelles, poor feeding, and hoarse crying. Rarely, delayed diagnosis and treatment of severe hypothyroidism lead to intellectual disability and short stature.

Some symptoms and signs of hypothyroidism in older children and adolescents are similar to those of adults (eg, weight gain; fatigue; constipation; coarse, dry hair; sallow, cool, or mottled coarse skin—see p. 1350). Signs specific to children are growth retardation, delayed skeletal maturation, and usually delayed puberty.

Diagnosis

- Routine newborn screening
- Thyroid function tests
- Sometimes thyroid ultrasonography or radionuclide scan

(See also the European Society for Paediatric Endocrinology's consensus guidelines on screening, diagnosis, and management of congenital hypothyroidism at www.ncbi.nlm.nih.gov.)

Routine newborn screening detects hypothyroidism before clinical signs are evident. If screening is positive, confirmation is necessary with thyroid function tests, including measurement of free serum thyroxine (free T_4) and TSH. These tests are also done in older children and adolescents in whom hypothyroidism is suspected. Free T_4 is a better measure of thyroid function than total T_4 in these patients because the levels of thyroid-binding proteins (thyroid-binding globulin, transthyretin, and albumin) affect total T_4 levels. Triiodothyronine (T_3) and reverse T_3 levels are rarely helpful in the diagnosis of hypothyroidism and should not be done in most patients.

Severe congenital hypothyroidism, even when treated promptly, may still cause subtle developmental problems and sensorineural hearing loss. Hearing loss may be so mild that initial screening misses it, but it may still interfere with language acquisition. Retesting after infancy is advised to detect subtle hearing loss.

When congenital hypothyroidism is diagnosed, radionuclide scanning (either ^{99m}Tc pertechnetate or ^{123}I) or ultrasonography can be done to evaluate the size and location of the thyroid gland and thus help distinguish a structural abnormality (ie, thyroid dysgenesis) from dyshormonogenesis and transient abnormalities.

In older children and adolescents with suspected hypothyroidism (elevated TSH and low T_4/free T_4), thyroid antibody titers (to thyroid peroxidase and thyroglobulin) should be measured to evaluate for autoimmune thyroiditis. Thyroid ultrasonography is not necessary to establish the diagnosis of autoimmune thyroiditis and should be restricted to children with thyroid gland asymmetry or palpable thyroid nodules.

Central hypothyroidism manifests with a pattern of low free T_4 and non-elevated TSH levels. Children confirmed to have central hypothyroidism should have MRI of the brain and pituitary to rule out CNS lesions.

Treatment

- Thyroid hormone replacement

In most treated infants, motor and intellectual development is normal.

(See also the American Thyroid Association Task Force on Thyroid Hormone Replacement's guidelines for the treatment of hypothyroidism at www.ncbi.nlm.nih.gov.)

When to treat: Most cases of congenital hypothyroidism require lifelong thyroid hormone replacement. However, if the initial TSH level is < 40 mU/L, an organic basis is not established, and the disease is thought to be transient (based on a lack of dose increase since infancy), clinicians may try stopping therapy after age 3 yr, at which time the trial poses no danger to the developing CNS. If the TSH rises once therapy is stopped (typically allowing about 6 wk off treatment) and the free T_4 or T_4 is low, permanent congenital hypothyroidism is confirmed and treatment should be restarted. Thyroxine-binding globulin deficiency, detected by screening that relies primarily on total serum T_4 measurement, does not require treatment because affected infants have normal free T_4 and TSH levels and are thus euthyroid.

Older children who have only slight elevations in TSH (< 10 mU/L) and normal T_4 or free T_4 levels are considered to have subclinical hypothyroidism whether they have thyroid autoantibodies or not. Such children do not need thyroid replacement unless they develop symptoms of hypothyroidism or goiter or their levels of TSH increase.

Treatment regimens: In congenital hypothyroidism, treatment with L-thyroxine 10 to 15 mcg/kg po once/day must be started immediately and be closely monitored. This dosage is intended to rapidly (within 2 wk) bring the serum T_4 level into the upper half of the normal range for age (between 10 μg/dL and 15 μg/dL) and promptly (within 4 wk) reduce the TSH.

In acquired hypothyroidism, the usual starting dosage of L-thyroxine is based on body surface area (100 mcg/m^2 po once/day) or on age and weight as follows:

- For ages 1 to 3 yr: 4 to 6 mcg/kg once/day
- For ages 3 to 10 yr: 3 to 5 mcg/kg once/day
- For ages 10 to 16 yr: 2 to 4 mcg/kg once/day
- For ages ≥ 17 yr: 1.6 mcg/kg once/day

For both forms of hypothyroidism, the dose is titrated to maintain serum T_4 and TSH levels within the normal range for age.

Thyroid replacement should be given only as a tablet, which can be crushed and made into paste for infants; it should not be given simultaneously with soy formula, or iron or calcium supplements, all of which can decrease thyroid hormone absorption.

Monitoring: Children are monitored more frequently during the first few years of life:

- Every 1 to 2 mo during the 1st 6 mo
- Every 3 to 4 mo between age 6 mo and 3 yr
- Every 6 to 12 mo from age 3 yr to the end of growth

Older children can be monitored more frequently if there are concerns about adherence. After a dose adjustment in older children, TSH and T_4 levels are measured in 6 to 8 wk.

KEY POINTS

- Hypothyroidism in infants is usually congenital; acquired causes become more common with age.
- Most congenital causes involve dysgenesis of the gland, but genetic disorders affecting thyroid hormone synthesis may occur.
- Most hypothyroid infants are detected through routine newborn screening.
- Confirm diagnosis with free T_4 and TSH levels; if confirmed, do imaging tests to detect structural thyroid disorders.
- Treat with L-thyroxine, adjusting the dose to maintain T_4 and TSH levels within the normal range for age.

MALE HYPOGONADISM IN CHILDREN

Male hypogonadism is decreased production of testosterone, sperm, or both or, rarely, decreased response to testosterone, resulting in delayed puberty, reproductive insufficiency, or both. Diagnosis is by measurement of serum testosterone, luteinizing hormone (LH), and follicle-stimulating hormone (FSH) and by stimulation tests with human chorionic gonadotropin or gonadotropin-releasing hormone. Treatment depends on the cause.

Classification

There are 3 types of hypogonadism: primary, secondary, and a type caused by defective androgen action, primarily due to defective androgen receptor activity.

Primary hypogonadism: In primary (hypergonadotropic) hypogonadism, damage to the Leydig cells impairs testosterone production, damages the seminiferous tubules, or does both; oligospermia or azoospermia and elevated gonadotropins result.

The most common cause is Klinefelter syndrome; other causes are disorders of sexual development such as gonadal dysgenesis (rare), cryptorchidism, bilateral anorchia, Leydig cell aplasia, Noonan syndrome, and myotonic dystrophy. Rare causes include orchitis due to mumps, testicular torsion, chemotherapy with alkylating drugs, and trauma.

Klinefelter syndrome is seminiferous tubule dysgenesis associated with the 47,XXY karyotype, in which an extra X chromosome is acquired through maternal or, to a lesser extent, paternal meiotic nondisjunction. The syndrome is usually identified at puberty, when inadequate sexual development is noted, or later, when infertility is investigated. Diagnosis is based on elevated gonadotropin levels and low to low-normal testosterone levels.

Errors of sex determination and gonadal development, such as gonadal dysgenesis (46,XX or 46,XY) and testicular and ovotesticular disorders of sex development, represent rare forms of male hypogonadism. They may result in a male or undervirilized male phenotype, ambiguous genitals at birth, and some degree of testicular and spermatogenic failure.

In **cryptorchidism,** one or both testes are undescended. Etiology is usually unknown. Sperm counts may be slightly low if one testis is undescended but are almost always very low if both are undescended.

In **bilateral anorchia (vanishing testes syndrome),** the testes were presumably present but were resorbed before or after birth. External genitals and wolffian structures are normal, but müllerian duct structures are lacking. Thus, testicular tissue must have been present during the first 12 wk of embryogenesis because testicular differentiation occurred and testosterone and müllerian-inhibiting factor were produced.

Leydig cell aplasia occurs when congenital absence of Leydig cells causes partially developed or ambiguous external genitals. Although wolffian ducts develop to some extent, testosterone production is insufficient to induce normal male differentiation of the external genitals. Müllerian ducts are absent because of normal production of müllerian-inhibiting hormone by Sertoli cells. Gonadotropin levels are high with low testosterone levels.

Noonan syndrome may occur sporadically or as an autosomal dominant disorder. Phenotypic abnormalities include hyperelasticity of the skin, hypertelorism, ptosis, low-set ears, short stature, shortened 4th metacarpals, high-arched palate, and primarily right-sided cardiovascular abnormalities (eg, pulmonic valve stenosis, atrial septal defect). Testes are often small or cryptorchid. Testosterone levels may be low with high gonadotropin levels.

Defective androgen synthesis is caused by enzyme defects that impair androgen synthesis, which may occur in any of the pathways leading from cholesterol to dihydrotestosterone. These congenital problems may occur in congenital adrenal hyperplasia (eg, steroidogenic acute regulatory [StAR] protein deficiency, 17alpha-hydroxylase deficiency, 3beta-hydroxysteroid dehydrogenase deficiency) when the same enzyme defect occurs in the adrenal glands and the testes, resulting in defective androgen activity and ambiguous external genitals of varying degrees.

Secondary hypogonadism: Causes of secondary hypogonadism include panhypopituitarism, hypothalamic or pituitary tumors, isolated gonadotropin deficiency, Kallmann syndrome, Laurence-Moon syndrome, isolated LH deficiency, Prader-Willi syndrome, and functional and acquired disorders of the CNS (eg, trauma, infection). Causes of secondary hypogonadism must be differentiated from constitutional delay of puberty, which is a functional form of secondary hypogonadism. Several acute disorders and chronic systemic disorders (eg, chronic renal insufficiency, anorexia nervosa) may lead to hypogonadotropic hypogonadism, which resolves after recovery from the underlying disorder. Relative hypogonadism is becoming more common among long-term survivors of childhood cancers treated with craniospinal irradiation.

Panhypopituitarism may occur congenitally or anatomically (eg, in septo-optic dysplasia or Dandy-Walker malformation), causing deficiency of hypothalamic-releasing factors or pituitary hormones. Acquired hypopituitarism may result from tumors, neoplasia, or their treatment, vascular disorders, infiltrative disorders (eg, sarcoidosis, Langerhans cell histiocytosis), infections (eg, encephalitis, meningitis), or trauma. Hypopituitarism in childhood may cause delayed growth, hypothyroidism, diabetes insipidus, hypoadrenalism, and lack of sexual development when puberty is expected. Hormone deficiencies, whether originating in the anterior or posterior pituitary, may be varied and multiple.

Kallmann syndrome is characterized by anosmia due to aplasia or hypoplasia of the olfactory lobes and by hypogonadism due to deficiency of hypothalamic gonadotropin-releasing hormone (GnRH). It occurs when fetal GnRH neurosecretory neurons do not migrate from the olfactory placode to the hypothalamus. The genetic defect is known; inheritance is classically X-linked but can also be autosomal dominant or autosomal recessive. Other manifestations include microphallus, cryptorchidism, midline defects, and unilateral kidney agenesis. Presentation is clinically heterogeneous, and some patients have normosmia.

Laurence-Moon syndrome is characterized by obesity, intellectual disability, retinitis pigmentosa, and polydactyly.

Isolated LH deficiency (fertile eunuch syndrome) is a rare cause of hypogonadism due to monotropic loss of LH secretion in boys; FSH levels are normal. At puberty, growth of the testes is normal because most testicular volume consists of seminiferous tubules, which respond to FSH. Spermatogenesis may occur as tubular development proceeds. However, absence of LH results in Leydig cell atrophy and testosterone deficiency. Therefore, patients do not develop normal secondary sexual characteristics, but they continue to grow, reaching eunuchoidal proportions because the epiphyses do not close.

Prader-Willi syndrome is characterized by diminished fetal activity, muscular hypotonia, and failure to thrive during early childhood followed later by obesity, intellectual disability, and hypogonadotropic hypogonadism. The syndrome is caused by deletion or disruption of a gene or genes on the proximal long arm of paternal chromosome 15 or by uniparental disomy of maternal chromosome 15. Failure to thrive due to hypotonia and feeding difficulties during infancy usually resolves after age 6 to 12 mo. From 12 to 18 mo onward, uncontrollable hyperphagia causes excessive weight gain and psychologic problems; plethoric obesity becomes the most striking feature. Rapid weight gain continues into adulthood; stature remains short and may be caused by GH deficiency. Features include emotional lability, poor gross motor skills, facial abnormalities (eg, a narrow bitemporal dimension, almond-shaped eyes, a mouth with thin upper lips and down-turned corners), and skeletal abnormalities (eg, scoliosis, kyphosis, osteopenia). Hands and feet are small. Other features include cryptorchidism and a hypoplastic penis and scrotum.

Constitutional delay of puberty is absence of pubertal development before age 14 yr; it is more common in boys. By definition, children with constitutional delay show evidence of sexual maturation by age 18 yr, but pubertal delay and short stature may generate anxiety in adolescents and their families. Many children have a family history of delayed sexual development in a parent or sibling. Typically, stature is usually short during childhood, adolescence, or both but ultimately reaches the normal range. Growth velocity is nearly normal, and growth pattern parallels the lower percentile curves of the growth chart. The pubertal growth spurt is delayed, and at the expected time of puberty, height percentile begins to drop, which may contribute to psychosocial difficulties for some children. Skeletal age is delayed and is most consistent with the child's height age (age at which a child's height is at the 50th percentile) rather than chronologic age. Diagnosis is by exclusion of deficiency, hypothyroidism, systemic conditions that may interfere with puberty (eg, inflammatory bowel disease, eating disorders), and hypogonadism (whether primary or due to gonadotropin deficiency).

Symptoms and Signs

Clinical presentation depends on whether, when, and how testosterone and sperm production are affected. (For presentation in adulthood, see p. 2128.)

If androgen deficiency or defects in androgen activity occur during the 1st trimester (< 12 wk gestation), differentiation of internal wolffian ducts and external genitals is inadequate. Presentation may range from ambiguous external genitals to normal-appearing female external genitals. Androgen deficiency during the 2nd and 3rd trimesters may cause a microphallus and partially or completely undescended testes.

Androgen deficiency that develops early in childhood has few consequences, but if it occurs when puberty is expected, secondary sexual development is impaired. Such patients have poor muscle development, a high-pitched voice, inadequate phallic and testicular growth, a small scrotum, sparse pubic and axillary hair, and absent body hair. They may develop gynecomastia and grow to eunuchoidal body proportions (arm span exceeds height by 5 cm; pubic to floor length exceeds crown to pubic length by > 5 cm) because fusion of the epiphyses is delayed and long bone growth continues.

Diagnosis

- Measurement of testosterone, LH, and FSH
- Karyotyping (for primary hypogonadism)

Diagnosis of male hypogonadism in children is often suspected based on developmental abnormalities or delayed puberty but requires confirmation by testing, including measurement of testosterone, LH, and FSH. LH and FSH levels are more sensitive than testosterone levels, especially for detecting primary hypogonadism.

LH and FSH levels also help determine whether hypogonadism is primary or secondary:

- High levels, even with low-normal testosterone levels, indicate primary hypogonadism.
- Levels that are low or lower than expected for the testosterone level indicate secondary hypogonadism.

In boys with short stature, delayed pubertal development, low testosterone, and low FSH and LH levels may indicate constitutional delay. Elevated serum FSH levels with normal serum testosterone and LH levels typically indicate impaired spermatogenesis but not impaired testosterone production. In primary hypogonadism, it is important to determine the karyotype to investigate for Klinefelter syndrome.

Measurement of testosterone, FSH, and LH for diagnosis of hypogonadism requires an understanding of how the levels vary. Before puberty, serum testosterone levels are < 20 ng/dL (< 0.7 nmol/L) and in adulthood, levels are > 300 to 1200 ng/dL (12 to 42 nmol/L). Serum testosterone secretion is primarily circadian. In the 2nd half of puberty, levels are higher at night than during the latter part of the day. A single sample obtained in the morning can establish that circulating testosterone levels are normal. Because 98% of testosterone is bound to carrier proteins in serum (testosterone-binding globulin), alterations in these protein levels alter total testosterone levels. Measurement of total serum testosterone (protein bound and free) is usually the most accurate indicator of testosterone secretion.

Although serum LH and FSH levels are pulsatile, testing can be valuable. Puberty begins when GnRH secretion increases and serum LH rises disproportionately to FSH. Early in puberty, early morning levels are preferred. Serum LH levels are usually below 0.3 mIU/mL before puberty and range from 2 to 12 mIU/mL during later stages of puberty and into adulthood. Serum FSH levels are usually < 3 mIU/mL before puberty and fluctuate between 5 and 10 mIU/mL during the 2nd half of puberty and into adulthood.

The human chorionic gonadotropin (hCG) stimulation test is done to assess the presence and secretory ability of testicular tissue. Multiple protocols exist. In one protocol, a one-time dose of hCG 100 units/kg IM is given. hCG stimulates Leydig cells, as does LH, with which it shares a structural subunit, and stimulates testicular production of testosterone. Testosterone levels should double after 3 to 4 days.

Treatment

- Surgery as needed
- Hormone replacement

Cryptorchidism is corrected early to obviate concerns about cancer developing in later adulthood and to prevent testicular torsion.

For secondary hypogonadism, any underlying pituitary or hypothalamic disorder is treated. Overall, the goal is to provide androgen replacement starting with a low dose and progressively increasing the dose over 18 to 24 mo.

Adolescents with androgen deficiency should be given long-acting injectable testosterone enanthate or cypionate 50 mg q 2 to 4 wk; the dose is increased up to 200 mg over 18 to 24 mo. A transdermal patch or gel may be used instead.

Treatment of Kallmann syndrome with hCG can correct cryptorchidism and establish fertility. Puberty is typically induced using testosterone injectable or gel. GnRH therapy has been previously shown to help endogenous sex hormone secretion, progressive virilization, and even fertility.

In isolated LH deficiency, testosterone, via conversion to estrogen by aromatase, induces normal epiphyseal closure.

Constitutional delay of puberty can be treated with a 4- to 6-mo course of testosterone. After the course is complete, treatment is stopped and testosterone levels are measured several weeks or months later to differentiate temporary from permanent deficiency. If testosterone levels are not higher than the initial value and/or pubertal development does not proceed after completion of this treatment, a second course of low-dose treatment can be given. If endogenous puberty has not begun after two courses of treatment, the likelihood of permanent deficiency increases, and patients need to be reevaluated for other causes of hypogonadism.

KEY POINTS

- In primary hypogonadism, a congenital (or rarely acquired) testicular disorder impairs testosterone production and/or damages the seminiferous tubules.
- In secondary hypogonadism, congenital or acquired disorders of the hypothalamus or pituitary cause gonadotropin deficiency and failure to stimulate normal testicles.
- Manifestations and their timing vary widely depending on when testosterone production is affected.
- Prenatal androgen deficiency may result in manifestations ranging from partially undescended testes, microphallus, and ambiguous external genitals to normal-appearing female external genitals.
- Androgen deficiency that occurs when puberty is expected impairs secondary sexual development.
- Diagnose by measurement of testosterone, LH, and FSH levels.
- Treat with hormone replacement and surgery as needed.

PRECOCIOUS PUBERTY

Precocious puberty is onset of sexual maturation before age 8 in girls or age 9 in boys. Diagnosis is by comparison with population standards, x-rays of the left hand and wrist to assess skeletal maturation and check for accelerated bone growth, and measurement of serum levels of gonadotropins and gonadal and adrenal steroids. Treatment depends on the cause.

In girls, the first pubertal milestone is typically breast development (thelarche), followed soon after by appearance of pubic hair (pubarche) and axillary hair and later by the first menstrual period (menarche), which traditionally occurs 2 to 3 yr after thelarche (see Fig. 269–2 on p. 2248).

In boys, the first pubertal milestone is typically testicular growth, followed by penile growth and appearance of pubic and axillary hair (see Fig. 251–1 on p. 2128).

In both sexes, appearance of pubic and axillary hair is called adrenarche. Adrenarche may occur before gonadarche in about 10% of children (premature adrenarche). Although gonadarche and adrenarche may have overlapping signs, they are regulated independently.

The definition of precocious puberty depends on reliable population standards for onset of puberty (ie, when pubertal milestones occur); because onset seems to be occurring earlier in the US, especially in females, these traditional standards are being reevaluated. Breast development is increasingly occurring at younger ages and this trend is mirroring the obesity epidemic, with a higher body mass index (> 85th percentile) associated with earlier thelarche.

Almost 8 to 10% of white girls, 20 to 30% of black girls, and an intermediate percentage of Hispanic girls reach early puberty at age 8. The lower limit of normal puberty may be 7 yr for white girls and 6 yr for black girls. The mean age for early breast development is about 9.5 to 10 yr for white girls and 8.5 to 9 yr for black girls (range 8 to 13 yr). However, the age of menarche has not lowered as drastically, with a mean decrease of only 3 mo in the past 30 yr (mean age 11.5 yr in black girls and 12.5 yr in white girls). The mean age for pubic hair growth is 9 to 10.5 yr for both groups. These findings imply that guidelines for evaluating disorders that cause precocious puberty can be interpreted more leniently if children are otherwise healthy and are projected to reach their full adult height potential.

Classification

Precocious puberty can be divided into 2 types:

- Gonadotropin-releasing hormone (GnRH)–dependent (central precocious puberty)
- GnRH-independent (peripheral sex hormone effects)

GnRH-dependent precocious puberty is more common overall and 5 to 10 times more frequent in girls. In GnRH-dependent precocious puberty, the hypothalamic-pituitary axis is activated, resulting in enlargement and maturation of the gonads, development of secondary sexual characteristics, and oogenesis or spermatogenesis.

GnRH-independent precocious puberty is much less common. Secondary sexual characteristics result from high circulating levels of estrogens or androgens, without activation of the hypothalamic-pituitary axis.

Precocious puberty may also be classified by whether gonadarche or adrenarche occurs. In girls, gonadarche includes breast development, change in body habitus, growth of the uterus, and eventually menarche. In boys, gonadarche includes testicular enlargement; phallic growth; the initial appearance of pubic, facial, and axillary hair; adult body odor; and facial skin oiliness or acne. Adrenarche for both girls and boys involves the development of body hair, body odor, and acne.

Incomplete or unsustained pubertal development is common, most often as isolated premature thelarche or adrenarche. Girls with premature thelarche typically display breast development during the first 2 years of life, but this change is not accompanied by pubertal hormone levels, menarche, advanced bone age on x-ray, androgen effects, or growth acceleration. Isolated premature adrenarche is likewise not associated with progressive pubertal development.

Children with premature adrenarche may have signs of adrenal androgen production (eg, pubic hair, acne, body odor) that progress slowly without acceleration of linear growth. Premature adrenarche may be associated with later development of polycystic ovary syndrome in adolescence.

Etiology

GnRH-dependent precocious puberty: Physical changes are typically those of normal puberty for a child of that sex, with the exception of age of onset. In most affected girls, a specific cause cannot be identified. In the absence of specific symptoms or signs of CNS disease, the probability of an intracranial abnormality depends on younger age of onset of puberty (< 4 yr in girls) and sex of the child (more common among boys). Overall, affected boys are more likely (up to 60%) to have an identifiable underlying lesion. Such lesions include intracranial tumors, especially of the hypothalamus or pineal gland region, including hamartomas, gliomas, germinomas, and adenomas. Neurofibromatosis and a few other rare disorders have also been linked to precocious puberty. Central precocious puberty can also arise from iatrogenic causes (eg, surgery, radiation, or chemotherapy for cancer).

GnRH-independent precocious puberty: The etiology of GnRH-independent precocious puberty depends on the predominant sex hormone effect (estrogenic or androgenic), and physical changes are often markedly discordant from normal pubertal development. Estrogenic effects are most commonly caused by follicular ovarian cysts; other causes include granulosa-theca cell tumors and McCune-Albright syndrome (a triad of follicular cysts, polyostotic fibrous dysplasia, and café-au-lait spots). Adrenal enzyme defects, specifically congenital adrenal hyperplasia, are the most common pathologic form of androgen excess in children of either sex. Additional causes of GnRH-independent precocious puberty in boys include familial male gonadotropin-independent precocity (due to an activating mutation of the gene for luteinizing hormone [LH] receptors), testosterone-producing testicular tumors, and occasionally McCune-Albright syndrome.

Symptoms and Signs

In girls, breasts develop, and pubic hair, axillary hair, or both appear. Girls may begin to menstruate. In boys, facial, axillary, and pubic hair appears and the penis grows, with or without enlargement of testes, depending on the etiology. Body odor, acne, and behavior changes may develop in either sex.

Pubertal growth spurt is seen in both sexes (with early-mid puberty in females, mid-late puberty in males), but premature closure of the epiphyses results in short adult stature. Ovarian or testicular enlargement occurs in precocious puberty but is absent in isolated precocious adrenarche.

Diagnosis

- Bone age x-rays
- Serum hormone measurement
- Possibly pelvic ultrasonography and brain MRI

Diagnosis of precocious puberty is clinical. X-rays of the left hand and wrist are done to check for accelerated skeletal maturation as a result of sex hormone effect. Unless history and examination suggest an abnormality, no further evaluation is required for children with pubertal milestones that are within 1 yr of population standards. Girls and boys with isolated premature adrenarche and girls with premature thelarche also do not require further evaluation as long as x-rays confirm that skeletal maturation is not accelerated.

When further evaluation is necessary, blood tests should be chosen according to the features present. For patients who have mainly androgen effects, the most useful initial tests include measurements of total testosterone, dehydroepiandrosterone sulfate, 17-hydroxyprogesterone, and LH; all should be measured using high-sensitivity assays designed for pediatric patients. For patients who have only estrogen effects, the most useful screens for girls include ultrasensitive LH and follicle-stimulating hormone (FSH), and estradiol, and, for boys, LH, FSH, beta-human chorionic gonadotropin, and estradiol. Pelvic and adrenal ultrasonography may be useful if any of the steroid levels are elevated, and MRI of the brain may be done to rule out intracranial anomalies in younger patients or in males with central precocious puberty.

A GnRH stimulation test may be considered to confirm GnRH-dependent precocious puberty when initial tests are inconclusive. Previously, a 1-h stimulation test with the GnRH agonist gonadorelin was used, but because gonadorelin is no longer available, other GnRH agonists such as leuprolide are used. Leuprolide acetate 10 to 20 mcg/kg sc is given and LH, FSH, testosterone (in boys), and estradiol (in girls) are measured at 0, 1, and 2 h. At 24 h post-leuprolide, estradiol and testosterone may be measured to improve sensitivity of the test. In GnRH-dependent precocious puberty, gonadotropin responses are pubertal. In GnRH-independent precocious puberty, gonadotropin responses to leuprolide are prepubertal.

Treatment

- GnRH agonist therapy (GnRH-dependent precocious puberty)
- Androgen or estrogen antagonist therapy (GnRH-independent precocious puberty)
- Tumor excision as needed

If pubertal milestones are within 1 yr of population standards, reassurance and regular reexamination are sufficient. Treatment is not needed for premature adrenarche or thelarche, but regular reexamination is warranted to check for later development of precocious puberty. For GnRH-dependent precocious puberty, pituitary LH and FSH secretion can be suppressed with GnRH agonists, including leuprolide acetate 7.5 to 15 mg IM q 4 wk or 11.25 mg or 30 mg IM q 12 wk, or histrelin implants (changed annually). Responses to treatment must be monitored, and drug dosages modified accordingly. Treatment may be continued until age 11 yr in girls and age 12 yr in boys.

In girls with McCune-Albright syndrome, aromatase inhibitors, including older drugs such as testolactone and newer drugs such as letrozole and anastrozole, have been used with varying success to reduce estradiol; alternatively, tamoxifen, an estrogen antagonist, may be beneficial.

If GnRH-independent precocious puberty in boys is due to familial male gonadotropin-independent precocity or McCune-Albright syndrome, androgen antagonists (eg, spironolactone) ameliorate the effects of excess androgen. The antifungal drug ketoconazole reduces testosterone in boys with familial male gonadotropin-independent precocity.

If GnRH-independent precocious puberty is due to a hormone-producing tumor (eg, granulosa-theca cell tumors in girls, testicular tumors in boys), the tumor should be excised. However, girls require extended follow-up to check for recurrence in the contralateral ovary.

KEY POINTS

- Precocious puberty is the onset of sexual maturation before age 8 in girls or age 9 in boys; however, in recent years, puberty has been starting earlier, and traditional standards are being reevaluated.
- Most commonly, secondary sexual characteristics develop prematurely because the hypothalamic-pituitary axis is activated (GnRH-dependent precocious puberty); often the cause is idiopathic, but some children have a CNS tumor.
- Less commonly, the cause is high circulating levels of estrogens or androgens (GnRH-independent precocious puberty) caused by congenital adrenal hyperplasia or various gonadal tumors.
- Diagnosis is made by bone age x-rays and measurement of hormone levels.
- Treat GnRH-dependent precocious puberty with the GnRH agonists leuprolide or histrelin.
- Treat GnRH-independent precocious puberty based on the cause, including giving androgen or estrogen antagonists and removing tumors.

OVERVIEW OF CONGENITAL ADRENAL HYPERPLASIA

(Adrenal Virilism; Adrenogenital Syndrome)

Congenital adrenal hyperplasia is a group of genetic disorders, each characterized by inadequate synthesis of cortisol, aldosterone, or both. In the most common forms, accumulated hormone precursors are shunted into androgen production, causing androgen excess; in rarer forms, synthesis of androgens is also inadequate.

In the various forms of congenital adrenal hyperplasia, production of cortisol (a glucocorticoid), aldosterone (a mineralocorticoid), or both is impaired because of an autosomal recessive genetic defect in one of the adrenal enzymes involved in synthesizing adrenal steroid hormones from cholesterol. The enzyme may be absent or deficient, completely or partially disabling synthesis of cortisol, aldosterone, or both. In the forms in which cortisol synthesis is absent or decreased, ACTH (corticotropin) release, normally suppressed by cortisol, is excessive.

The most common forms of congenital adrenal hyperplasia are 21-hydroxylase deficiency and 11beta-hydroxylase deficiency. In these forms, precursors proximal to the enzyme block accumulate and are shunted into adrenal androgens. The consequent excess androgen secretion causes varying degrees of virilization in external genitals of affected females; no defects are discernible in external genitals of males.

In some less common forms affecting enzymes other than 21-hydroxylase and 11beta-hydroxylase, the enzyme block impairs androgen synthesis (dehydroepiandrosterone [DHEA] or androstenedione). As a result, virilization of males is inadequate, but no defect is discernible in females.

CONGENITAL ADRENAL HYPERPLASIA CAUSED BY 11BETA-HYDROXYLASE DEFICIENCY

11Beta-hydroxylase (CYP11B1) deficiency involves defective production of cortisol, with accumulation of mineralocorticoid precursors, resulting in hypernatremia, hypokalemia, and hypertension and increased production of adrenal androgens, leading to virilization. Diagnosis is by measurement of cortisol, its precursors, and adrenal androgens and sometimes by measuring 11-deoxycortisol after ACTH administration. Treatment is with a corticosteroid.

11Beta-hydroxylase deficiency causes about 5 to 8% of all cases of congenital adrenal hyperplasia. Conversion of 11-deoxycortisol to cortisol and deoxycorticosterone to corticosterone is partially blocked, leading to

- Increased levels of ACTH
- Accumulation of 11-deoxycortisol (which has limited biological activity) and deoxycorticosterone (which has mineralocorticoid activity)
- Overproduction of adrenal androgens (dehydroepiandrosterone [DHEA], androstenedione, and testosterone)

Symptoms and Signs

Female neonates may present with genital ambiguity, including clitoral enlargement, labial fusion, and a urogenital sinus. Male neonates usually appear normal, but some present with penile enlargement. Some children present later, with sexual precocity or, in females, menstrual irregularities and hirsutism. Salt retention with hypernatremia, hypertension, and hypokalemic alkalosis may result from increased mineralocorticoid activity due to increased deoxycorticosterone levels.

Diagnosis

- Plasma levels of 11-deoxycortisol and adrenal androgens

Prenatal diagnosis is not available. Diagnosis of 11beta-hydroxylase deficiency in neonates is established by increased plasma levels of 11-deoxycortisol and adrenal androgens (DHEA, androstenedione, and testosterone). Plasma renin activity is often suppressed because of increased mineralocorticoid activity; this test may be useful in older children but is less reliable in neonates. If the diagnosis is uncertain, levels of 11-deoxycortisol and adrenal androgens are measured before and 60 min after ACTH stimulation. In affected adolescents, basal plasma levels may be normal, so ACTH stimulation is recommended.

Hypertension occurs in about two thirds of patients with *CYP11B1* deficiency and distinguishes it from *CYP21A2* deficiency, which causes hypotension. Because both *CYP11B1* deficiency and *CYP21A2* deficiency can cause increased levels of 17-hydroxyprogesterone, which is measured during routine newborn screening, patients with mild to moderately increased levels of 17-hydroxyprogesterone should have 11-deoxycortisol levels measured. Hypokalemia may occur but not in all patients.

PEARLS & PITFALLS

- 11 Beta-hydroxylase deficiency causes hypertension and sometimes hypokalemia, in contrast to 21-hydroxylase deficiency, which causes hypotension and hyperkalemia.

Treatment

- Corticosteroid replacement
- Possibly antihypertensive therapy
- Possibly reconstructive surgery

Treatment is cortisol replacement, typically with hydrocortisone 3.5 to 5 mg/m^2 tid, with total daily dose typically ≤ 20 mg/m^2, which prevents further virilization and ameliorates hypertension by reducing levels of 11-deoxycortisol, deoxycorticosterone, and adrenal androgens that are stimulated by ACTH. Unlike *CYP21A2* deficiency, mineralocorticoid replacement is not required, because sodium and potassium homeostasis is maintained from mineralocorticoid effects of deoxycorticosterone.

Response to treatment should be monitored, typically by measuring serum 11-deoxycortisol and adrenal androgens and by assessing growth velocity and skeletal maturation. BP should be monitored closely in patients who presented with hypertension. Antihypertensives, such as potassium-sparing diuretics or calcium channel blockers, may be required.

Affected female infants may require surgical reconstruction with reduction clitoroplasty and construction of a vaginal opening. Often, further surgery is required in adulthood, but with appropriate care and attention to psychosexual issues, a normal sex life and fertility may be expected.

KEY POINTS

- Children with 11beta-hydroxylase deficiency have excess mineralocorticoid activity and increased adrenal androgens, which cause hypertension, hypokalemia, and virilization.
- In females, androgen excess usually manifests at birth with ambiguous external genitals (eg, clitoral enlargement, fusion of the labia majora, a urogenital sinus rather than distinct urethral and vaginal openings); later in life they may have hirsutism, oligomenorrhea, and acne.
- Male infants usually appear normal but may later have sexual precocity.
- Diagnose by steroid hormone levels and sometimes ACTH stimulation.
- Treat with corticosteroid replacement and sometimes antihypertensives; females may require reconstructive surgery.

CONGENITAL ADRENAL HYPERPLASIA CAUSED BY 21-HYDROXYLASE DEFICIENCY

21-Hydroxylase (CYP21A2) deficiency causes defective conversion of adrenal precursors to cortisol and, in some cases, to aldosterone, sometimes resulting in severe hyponatremia and hyperkalemia. Accumulated hormone precursors are shunted into androgen production, causing virilization. Diagnosis is by measurement of cortisol, its precursors, and adrenal androgens, sometimes after ACTH administration. Treatment is with a glucocorticoid plus, if needed, a mineralocorticoid and, for some female neonates with genital ambiguity, surgical reconstruction.

21-Hydroxylase deficiency causes 90% of all cases of congenital adrenal hyperplasia (see Fig. 307–1).). Incidence ranges from 1/10,000 to 1/15,000 live births. Disease severity depends on the specific *CYP21A2* mutation and degree of enzyme deficiency. The deficiency completely or partially blocks conversion of 17-hydroxyprogesterone to 11-deoxycortisol, a precursor of cortisol, and conversion of progesterone to deoxycorticosterone, a precursor of aldosterone. Because cortisol synthesis is decreased, ACTH levels increase, which stimulates the adrenal cortex, causing accumulation of cortisol precursors (eg, 17-hydroxyprogesterone) and excessive production of the adrenal androgens dehydroepiandrosterone (DHEA) and androstenedione. Aldosterone deficiency can lead to salt wasting, hyponatremia, and hyperkalemia.

Classic 21-hydroxylase deficiency: Classic 21-hydroxylase deficiency can be divided into 2 forms:

- Salt wasting
- Simple virilizing

In both forms, adrenal androgen levels are elevated, causing virilization.

The **salt-wasting form** is the most severe and accounts for 70% of classic 21-hydroxylase deficiency cases; there is complete deficiency of enzyme activity that leads to very low levels of cortisol and aldosterone. Because minimal aldosterone is secreted, salt is lost, leading to hyponatremia, hyperkalemia, and increased plasma renin activity.

In the **simple virilizing form,** cortisol synthesis is impaired, leading to increased androgen activity, but there is sufficient enzyme activity to maintain normal, or only slightly decreased, aldosterone production.

Nonclassic 21-hydroxylase deficiency: Nonclassic 21-hydroxylase deficiency is more common than classic 21-hydroxylase deficiency. Incidence ranges from 1/1000 to 1/2000 live births in white populations (0.1 to 0.2%) to 1 to 2% in certain ethnic groups (eg, Ashkenazi Jews). Nonclassic 21-hydroxylase deficiency causes a less severe form of the disorder in which there is 20 to 50% of 21-hydroxylase activity (compared to 0 to 5% activity in classic 21-hydroxylase deficiency). Salt wasting is absent because aldosterone and cortisol levels are normal, however, adrenal androgen levels are slightly elevated, resulting in mild androgen excess in childhood or adulthood.

Symptoms and Signs

The salt-wasting form causes hyponatremia (sometimes severe), hyperkalemia, and hypotension as well as virilization. If undiagnosed and untreated, this form can lead to life-threatening adrenal crisis, with vomiting, diarrhea, hypoglycemia, hypovolemia, and shock.

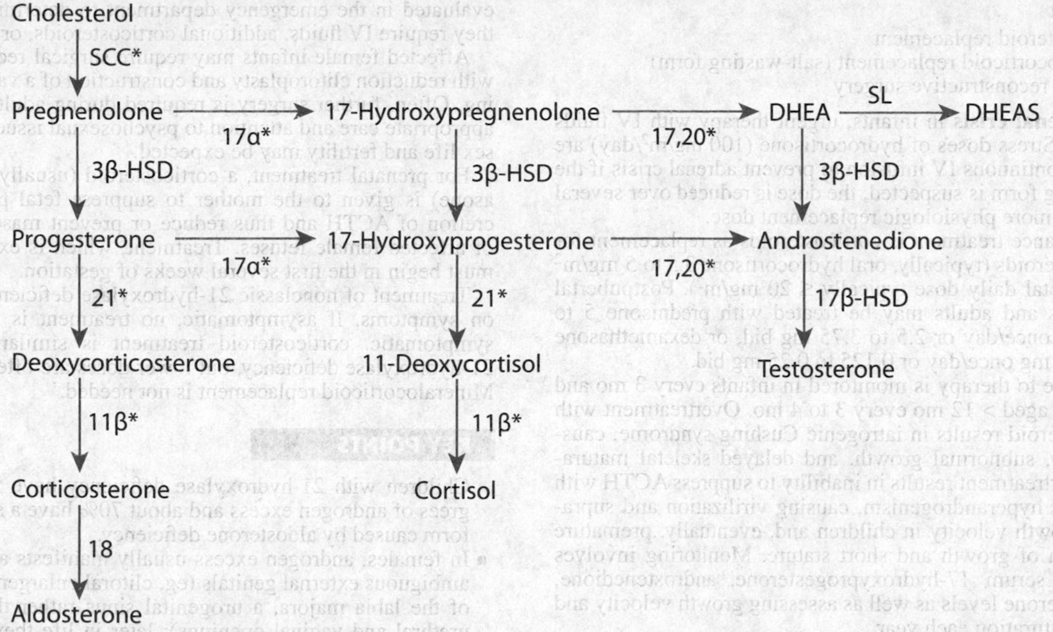

Fig. 307–1. Adrenal hormone synthesis.

*Enzymes stimulated by ACTH.
11β = 11β-hydroxylase (P-450c11); 17α = 17α-hydroxylase (P-450c17); 17,20 = 17,20 lyase (P-450c17); 18 = aldosterone synthase (P-450aldo); 21 = 21-hydroxylase (P-450c21); DHEA = dehydroepiandrosterone; DHEAS = DHEA sulfate; 3β-HSD = 3β-hydroxysteroid dehydrogenase (3β2 HSD); 17β-HSD = 17β-hydroxysteroid dehydrogenase (17β-HSD); SCC = side-chain cleavage (P-450scc); SL = sulfotransferase (SULT1A1, SULT1E1).

With either form of classic 21-hydroxylase deficiency, female neonates have ambiguous external genitals, with clitoral enlargement, fusion of the labia majora, and a urogenital sinus rather than distinct urethral and vaginal openings. Male infants typically have normal genital development, which can delay the diagnosis of the salt-wasting form; affected boys are often identified only through routine newborn screening. Unless detected by newborn screening, boys with the simple virilizing form may not be diagnosed for several years, when they develop signs of androgen excess. Signs of androgen excess may include early appearance of pubic hair and increase in growth velocity in both sexes, clitoral enlargement in girls, and penile enlargement and earlier deepening of voice in boys.

Children with nonclassic 21-hydroxylase deficiency do not have symptoms at birth and usually do not present until childhood or adolescence. Affected females may have early pubic hair development, advanced bone age, hirsutism, oligomenorrhea, and/or acne; these symptoms may resemble the manifestations of polycystic ovary syndrome. Affected males may have early pubic hair development, growth acceleration, and advanced bone age.

In affected females, especially those with the salt-wasting form, reproductive function may be impaired as they reach adulthood; they may have labial fusion and anovulatory cycles or amenorrhea. Some males with the salt-wasting form are fertile as adults, but others may develop testicular adrenal rest tumors (benign intratesticular masses composed of adrenal tissue that hypertrophies under chronic ACTH stimulation), Leydig cell dysfunction, decreased testosterone, and impaired spermatogenesis. Most affected males with the non–salt-wasting form, even if untreated, are fertile, but in some, spermatogenesis is impaired.

Diagnosis

- Blood tests
- Possibly ACTH stimulation test
- Possibly genotyping

Routine newborn screening typically includes measuring serum levels of 17-hydroxyprogesterone. If levels are elevated, the diagnosis of 21-hydroxylase deficiency is confirmed by identifying low blood levels of cortisol and by identifying high blood levels of dehydroepiandrosterone, androstenedione, and testosterone. Rarely, the diagnosis is uncertain, and levels of these hormones must be measured before and 60 min after ACTH is given (ACTH or cosyntropin stimulation test). In patients who develop symptoms later, ACTH stimulation testing may help, but genotyping may be required.

Children with the salt-wasting form have hyponatremia and hyperkalemia; low levels of deoxycorticosterone, corticosterone, and aldosterone; and high levels of renin.

Prenatal screening and diagnosis (and experimental treatment) are possible; *CYP21* genes are analyzed if risk is high (eg, the fetus has an affected sibling with the genetic defect). Carrier status (heterozygosity) can be determined in children and adults.

Treatment

- Corticosteroid replacement
- Mineralocorticoid replacement (salt-wasting form)
- Possibly reconstructive surgery

For **adrenal crisis** in infants, urgent therapy with IV fluids is needed. Stress doses of hydrocortisone (100 mg/m^2/day) are given by continuous IV infusion to prevent adrenal crisis if the salt-wasting form is suspected; the dose is reduced over several weeks to a more physiologic replacement dose.

Maintenance treatment is corticosteroids as replacement for deficient steroids (typically, oral hydrocortisone 3.5 to 5 mg/m^2 tid, with total daily dose typically ≤ 20 mg/m^2). Postpubertal adolescents and adults may be treated with prednisone 5 to 7.5 mg po once/day or 2.5 to 3.75 mg bid, or dexamethasone 0.25 to 0.5 mg once/day or 0.125 to 0.25 mg bid.

Response to therapy is monitored in infants every 3 mo and in children aged > 12 mo every 3 to 4 mo. Overtreatment with a corticosteroid results in iatrogenic Cushing syndrome, causing obesity, subnormal growth, and delayed skeletal maturation. Undertreatment results in inability to suppress ACTH with consequent hyperandrogenism, causing virilization and supranormal growth velocity in children and, eventually, premature termination of growth and short stature. Monitoring involves measuring serum 17-hydroxyprogesterone, androstenedione, and testosterone levels as well as assessing growth velocity and skeletal maturation each year.

Maintenance treatment for the salt-wasting form, in addition to corticosteroids, is mineralocorticoid replacement for restoration of sodium and potassium homeostasis. Oral fludrocortisone (usually 0.1 mg once/day, range 0.05 to 0.3 mg) is given if salt loss occurs. Infants often require supplemental oral salt for about 1 yr. Close monitoring during therapy is critical.

With illness, corticosteroid dosages are increased (typically doubled or tripled) to prevent adrenal crisis. Mineralocorticoid replacement is not adjusted. When oral therapy is unreliable (eg, severe vomiting or life-threatening situations), a single IM injection of hydrocortisone (50 to 100 mg/m^2) can be given. When the injection is given, children typically need to be evaluated in the emergency department to determine whether they require IV fluids, additional corticosteroids, or both.

Affected female infants may require surgical reconstruction with reduction clitoroplasty and construction of a vaginal opening. Often, further surgery is required during adulthood. With appropriate care and attention to psychosexual issues, a normal sex life and fertility may be expected.

For prenatal treatment, a corticosteroid (usually dexamethasone) is given to the mother to suppress fetal pituitary secretion of ACTH and thus reduce or prevent masculinization of affected female fetuses. Treatment, which is experimental, must begin in the first several weeks of gestation.

Treatment of nonclassic 21-hydroxylase deficiency depends on symptoms. If asymptomatic, no treatment is required. If symptomatic, corticosteroid treatment is similar to classic 21-hydroxylase deficiency, but lower doses are often effective. Mineralocorticoid replacement is not needed.

KEY POINTS

- Children with 21-hydroxylase deficiency have varying degrees of androgen excess and about 70% have a salt-wasting form caused by aldosterone deficiency.
- In females, androgen excess usually manifests at birth with ambiguous external genitals (eg, clitoral enlargement, fusion of the labia majora, a urogenital sinus rather than distinct urethral and vaginal openings); later in life they may have hirsutism, oligomenorrhea, and acne.
- In males, androgen excess may not be apparent or may manifest in childhood with increased growth velocity and early signs of puberty.
- In both sexes, salt wasting causes hyponatremia and hyperkalemia.
- Diagnose by steroid hormone levels and sometimes ACTH stimulation and/or genotyping.
- Treat with replacement of corticosteroids and sometimes mineralocorticoids; females may require reconstructive surgery.

308 Eye Defects and Conditions in Children

AMBLYOPIA

Amblyopia is functional reduction in visual acuity of an eye caused by disuse during visual development. Severe loss of vision can occur in the affected eye if amblyopia is not detected and treated before age 8. Diagnosis is based on detecting a difference in best corrected visual acuity between the two eyes that is not attributable to other pathology. Treatment depends on the cause.

Amblyopia affects about 2 to 3% of children and usually develops before age 2; however, any child under about age 8 can develop amblyopia.

The brain must simultaneously receive a clear, focused, properly aligned image from each eye for the visual system to develop properly. This development takes place mainly in the first 3 yr of life but is not complete until about 8 yr of age. Amblyopia results when there is persistent interference with the image from one eye but not the other. The visual cortex suppresses the image from the affected eye. If suppression persists long enough, vision loss can be permanent.

Etiology

There are 3 causes:

- Strabismus
- Anisometropia
- Obstruction of the visual axis

Strabismus can cause amblyopia because misalignment of the eyes results in different retinal images being sent to the visual cortex. When this misalignment occurs, a child's brain can pay attention to only one eye at a time, and the input from the other eye is suppressed. Because the visual pathways are already fully developed in adults, presentation of 2 different images results in diplopia rather than suppression of one image.

Anisometropia (inequality of refraction in the 2 eyes due to astigmatism, myopia, or hyperopia) can also cause amblyopia because it results in different focus of the retinal images, with the image from the eye with the greater refractive error being less well focused.

Obstruction of the visual axis at some point between the surface of the eye and the retina (eg, by a congenital cataract) interferes with or completely prevents formation of a retinal image in the affected eye. This obstruction can cause amblyopia.

Symptoms and Signs

Amblyopia is often asymptomatic and is commonly uncovered only on routine vision screening. Children rarely complain of unilateral vision loss, although they may squint or cover one eye. Very young children do not notice or are unable to express awareness that their vision differs in one eye compared with the other. Some older children may report impaired vision in the affected eye or exhibit poor depth perception. When strabismus is the cause, deviation of gaze may be noticeable to others. A cataract causing occlusion of the visual axis may go unnoticed.

Diagnosis

- Early screening
- Photoscreening
- Additional testing (eg, cover test, cover-uncover test, refraction, ophthalmoscopy, slit lamp)

Screening for amblyopia (and strabismus) is recommended for all children before starting school, optimally around age 3. Photoscreening is one approach for screening very young children who are unable to undergo subjective testing because of learning or developmental disorders. Photoscreening involves use of a camera to record images of pupillary reflexes during fixation on a visual target and red reflexes in response to light; the images are then compared for symmetry. Screening in older children consists of acuity testing with figures (eg, tumbling E figures, Allen cards, HOTV figures or characters) or Snellen eye charts.

Identifying the underlying cause requires additional testing. Strabismus can be confirmed with the alternate cover test or the cover-uncover test (see p. 2581). Ophthalmologists can confirm anisometropia by doing a refraction on each eye. Obstruction of the visual axis can be confirmed by ophthalmoscopy or slit-lamp examination.

Prognosis

Amblyopia may become irreversible if not diagnosed and treated before age 8, at which time the visual system has often matured. Most children identified and treated before age 5 have some vision improvement. Earlier treatment increases the likelihood of complete vision recovery. In certain circumstances, older children with amblyopia can still have vision improvement with treatment. Recurrence (recidivism) is possible in certain cases until the visual system matures. Some patients have a small decrease in visual acuity even after visual maturity has occurred.

Treatment

- Eyeglasses or contact lenses
- Cataract removal
- Patching
- Atropine drops
- Treatment of strabismus if present

Treatment of amblyopia should be directed by an ophthalmologist experienced in managing eye disorders in children. Any underlying causes must be treated (eg, eyeglasses or contact lenses to correct refractive error, removal of a cataract, treatment of strabismus). Use of the amblyopic eye is then encouraged by patching the better eye or by administering atropine drops into the better eye to provide a visual advantage to the amblyopic eye. Adherence to treatment is better with drop therapy. Maintenance treatment for prevention of recurrences may be recommended after improvement has stabilized, until a child is about age 8 to 10.

KEY POINTS

- Amblyopia is visual loss in one eye caused by lack of clearly focused, properly aligned input to the visual cortex from each eye during early childhood prior to maturation of the visual pathways.
- Diagnosis is mainly by screening tests, which should be done at about age 3 yr.
- Treatment is directed at the cause (eg, correcting refractive error, removing cataracts, treatment of strabismus) followed by patching or administering atropine drops into the better eye.

CONGENITAL CATARACT

(Infantile Cataract)

Congenital cataract is a lens opacity that is present at birth or shortly after birth.

Congenital cataracts may be sporadic, or they may be caused by chromosomal anomalies, metabolic disease (eg, galactosemia), or intrauterine infection (eg, rubella) or other maternal disease during pregnancy. Congenital cataracts may also be an isolated familial anomaly that is commonly autosomal dominantly inherited.

Cataracts may be located in the center of the lens (nuclear), or they may involve the lens material underneath the anterior or posterior lens capsule (subcapsular or cortical). They may be unilateral or bilateral. They may not be noticed unless the red reflex is checked or unless ophthalmoscopy is done at birth. As with other cataracts, the lens opacity obscures vision. Cataracts may obscure the view of the optic disc and vessels and should always be evaluated by an ophthalmologist.

Cataracts are removed by aspirating them through a small incision. In many children, an intraocular lens may be implanted. Postoperative visual correction with eyeglasses, contact lenses, or both is usually required to achieve the best outcome.

After a unilateral cataract is removed, the quality of the image in the treated eye is inferior to that of the other eye (assuming the other eye is normal). Because the better eye is preferred, the brain suppresses the poorer-quality image, and amblyopia develops. Thus, effective amblyopia therapy is necessary for the treated eye to develop normal sight. Some children are unable to attain good visual acuity because of accompanying structural defects. In contrast, children with bilateral cataract removal in which image quality is similar in both eyes more frequently develop equal vision in both eyes.

Some cataracts are partial (posterior lenticonus) and opacify during the first 10 yr of life. Eyes with partial cataracts will have a better visual outcome.

PRIMARY INFANTILE GLAUCOMA

(Infantile Glaucoma; Congenital Glaucoma; Buphthalmos)

Primary infantile glaucoma is a rare developmental defect in the iridocorneal filtration angle of the anterior chamber that prevents aqueous fluid from properly draining from the eye. This obstruction increases the intraocular pressure,

which, if untreated, damages the optic nerve. Infantile glaucoma can cause complete blindness if left untreated.

The disorder occurs in infants and young children and may be unilateral (40%) or bilateral (60%). Intraocular pressure increases above the normal range (10 to 22 mm Hg). Glaucoma can also occur in infants after trauma or intraocular surgery (eg, cataract extraction). Glaucoma associated with another ocular disorder, such as aniridia, Lowe syndrome, or Sturge-Weber syndrome, is called secondary glaucoma.

In primary infantile glaucoma or early childhood glaucoma, the affected eyes become enlarged because the collagen of the sclera and cornea can stretch because of the increased intraocular pressure. This enlargement does not occur in adult glaucoma. The large-diameter (> 12 mm) cornea is thinned and sometimes cloudy. The infant may have tearing and photophobia. If untreated, corneal clouding progresses, the optic nerve is damaged (as evidenced clinically by optic nerve cupping), and blindness can occur. Early surgical intervention (eg, goniotomy, trabeculotomy, trabeculectomy) is the mainstay of treatment.

STRABISMUS

Strabismus is misalignment of the eyes, which causes deviation from the parallelism of normal gaze. Diagnosis is clinical, including observation of the corneal light reflex and use of a cover test. Treatment may include correction of visual impairment with patching and corrective lenses, alignment by corrective lenses, and surgical repair.

Strabismus occurs in about 3% of children. Left untreated, about 50% of children with strabismus have some visual loss due to amblyopia.

Classification

Several varieties of strabismus have been described, based on direction of deviation, specific conditions under which deviation occurs, and whether deviation is constant or intermittent. Description of these varieties requires the definition of several terms.

The prefix "eso" refers to nasal deviations, and the prefix "exo" refers to temporal deviations. The prefix "hyper" refers to upward deviations, and the prefix "hypo" refers to downward deviations (see Fig. 308–1).

A **tropia** is a manifest deviation, detectable with both eyes open (so that vision is binocular). A tropia can be constant or intermittent and may involve one eye or both eyes.

A **phoria** is a latent deviation, detectable only when one eye is covered so that vision is monocular. The deviation in a phoria is latent because the brain, using the extraocular muscles, corrects the minor misalignment.

Deviations that are the same (amplitude or degree of misalignment remains the same) in all gaze directions are designated as comitant, whereas deviations that vary (amplitude or degree of misalignment changes) depending on gaze direction are referred to as incomitant.

Etiology

Most strabismus is caused by

- Refractive error
- Muscle imbalance

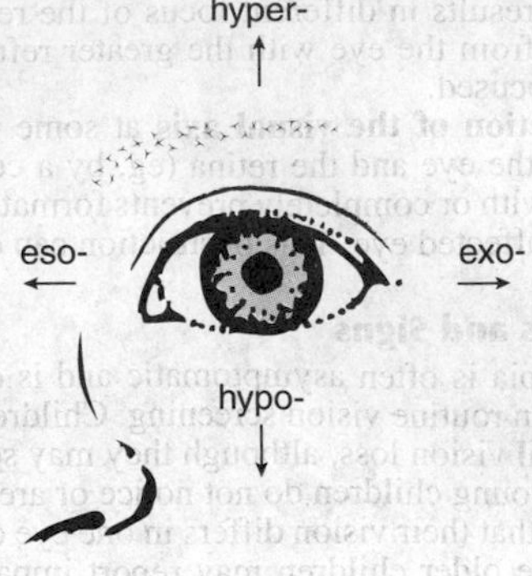
hyper-
eso-
exo-
hypo-
-tropia = manifest deviation
(visible when both eyes are open).
-phoria = latent deviation
(visible only when one eye is
covered).

Fig. 308–1. Ocular deviations in strabismus. Strabismus involves both eyes; the left eye is shown here. The direction of the deviation is designated by the prefixes eso-, exo-, hyper-, and hypo-. When the deviation is visible, it is indicated by the suffixes -tropia and -phoria.

Rare causes include retinoblastoma or other serious ocular defects and neurologic disease.

Strabismus may be infantile or acquired. The term infantile rather than congenital is preferred because the presence of true strabismus at birth is uncommon, and the term infantile permits inclusion of varieties that develop within the first 6 mo of life. The term acquired includes varieties that develop after 6 mo.

Risk factors for infantile strabismus include family history (1st- or 2nd-degree relative), genetic disorders (Down syndrome and Crouzon syndrome), prenatal drug exposure (including alcohol), prematurity or low birth weight, congenital eye defects, and cerebral palsy.

Acquired strabismus can develop acutely or gradually. Causes of acquired strabismus include refractive error (high hyperopia), tumors (eg, retinoblastoma), head trauma, neurologic conditions (eg, cerebral palsy; spina bifida; palsy of the 3rd cranial nerve, 4th cranial nerve, or 6th cranial nerve), viral infections (eg, encephalitis, meningitis), and acquired eye defects. Specific causes vary depending on the type of deviation.

Esotropia is commonly infantile. Infantile esotropia is considered idiopathic, although an anomaly of fusion is the suspected cause. Accommodative esotropia, a common variety of acquired esotropia, develops between 2 yr and 4 yr of age and is associated with hyperopia. Sensory esotropia occurs when severe visual loss (due to conditions such as cataracts, optic nerve anomalies, or tumors) interferes with the brain's effort to maintain ocular alignment.

Esotropia can be paralytic, so designated because the cause is a 6th (abducens) cranial nerve palsy, but it is an uncommon cause. Esotropia can also be a component of a syndrome. Duane syndrome (congenital absence of the abducens nucleus with anomalous innervation of the lateral rectus extraocular muscle by the 3rd [oculomotor] cranial nerve) and Möbius syndrome (anomalies of multiple cranial nerves) are specific examples.

Exotropia is most often intermittent and idiopathic. Less often, exotropia is constant and paralytic, as with infantile exotropia or 3rd (oculomotor) cranial nerve palsy.

Hypertropia can be paralytic, caused by 4th (trochlear) cranial nerve palsy that occurs congenitally or after head trauma or, less commonly, as a result of 3rd cranial nerve palsy.

Hypotropia can be restrictive, caused by mechanical restriction of full movement of the globe rather than neurologic interference with eye movement. For example, restrictive hypotropia can result from a blowout fracture of the orbit floor or walls. Less commonly, restrictive hypotropia can be caused by Graves ophthalmopathy (thyroid eye disease). Third cranial nerve palsy and Brown syndrome (congenital or acquired tightness and restriction of the superior oblique muscle tendon) are other uncommon causes.

Symptoms and Signs

Unless severe, phorias rarely cause symptoms of strabismus. If symptomatic, phorias typically cause asthenopia (eye strain).

Tropias sometimes result in symptoms. For example, torticollis may develop to compensate for the brain's difficulty in fusing images from misaligned eyes and to reduce diplopia. Some children with tropias have normal and equal visual acuity; however, amblyopia frequently develops with tropias and is due to cortical suppression of the image in the deviating eye to avoid confusion and diplopia.

Diagnosis

- Physical and neurologic examinations at well-child checkups
- Tests (eg, corneal light reflex, alternate cover, cover-uncover)
- Prisms

Strabismus can be detected during well-child checkups through the history and eye examination. Evaluation should include questions about family history of amblyopia or strabismus and, if family or caregivers have noticed deviation of gaze, questions about when the deviation began, when or how often it is present, and whether there is a preference for using one eye for fixation. Physical examination should include an assessment of visual acuity, pupil reactivity, and the extent of extraocular movements. Slit-lamp examination is done to detect signs of cataract, and funduscopic examination is done to detect signs of retinoblastoma. Neurologic examination, particularly of the cranial nerves, is important.

The corneal light reflex test is a good screening test, but it is not very sensitive for detecting small deviations. The child looks at a light and the light reflection (reflex) from the pupil is observed; normally, the reflex appears symmetric (ie, in the same location on each pupil). The light reflex for an exotropic eye is nasal to the pupillary center, whereas the reflex for an esotropic eye is temporal to the pupillary center. Vision screening machines operated by trained personnel are being introduced to identify children at risk.

When doing the cover test, the child is asked to fixate on an object. One eye is then covered while the other is observed for movement. No movement should be detected if the eyes are properly aligned, but manifest strabismus is present if the uncovered eye shifts to establish fixation once the other eye, which had fixed on the object, is covered. The test is then repeated on the other eye.

In a variation of the cover test, called the alternate uncover test, the child is asked to fixate on an object while the examiner alternately covers one eye and then the other, back and forth. An eye with a latent strabismus shifts position when it is uncovered. In exotropia, the eye that was covered turns *in* to fixate; in esotropia, it turns *out* to fixate. Deviations can be quantified by using prisms positioned such that the deviating eye need not move to fixate. The power of the prism is used to quantify the deviation and provide a measurement of the magnitude of misalignment of the visual axes. The unit of measurement used by ophthalmologists is the prism diopter. One prism diopter is a deviation of the visual axes of 1 cm at 1 m.

Strabismus should be distinguished from pseudostrabismus, which is the appearance of esotropia in a child with good visual acuity in both eyes but a wide nasal bridge or broad epicanthal folds that obscure much of the white sclera nasally when looking laterally. The light reflex and cover tests are normal in a child with pseudostrabismus.

Neuroimaging may be necessary to identify the cause of acquired cranial nerve palsies. In addition, genetics evaluation may be beneficial for certain ocular malformations.

Prognosis

Strabismus should not be ignored on the assumption that it will be outgrown. Permanent vision loss can occur if strabismus and its attendant amblyopia are not treated before age 4 to 6 yr; children treated later respond somewhat, but once the visual system has matured (typically by age 8), response is minimal. As a result, all children should have formal vision screening in the preschool years.

Treatment

- Patching or atropine drops for attendant amblyopia
- Contact lenses or eyeglasses (for refractive error)
- Eye exercises (for convergence insufficiency only)
- Surgical alignment of the eyes

Treatment of strabismus aims to equalize vision and then align the eyes. Treatment of children with amblyopia requires patching or penalization of the normal eye or atropine drops; improved vision offers a better prognosis for development of binocular vision and for stability if surgery is done. Patching is not, however, a treatment for strabismus. Eyeglasses or contact lenses are sometimes used if the amount of refractive error is significant enough to interfere with fusion, especially in children with accommodative esotropia. Orthoptic eye exercises can help correct intermittent exotropia with convergence insufficiency.

Surgical repair is generally done when nonsurgical methods are unsuccessful in aligning the eyes satisfactorily. Surgical repair consists of loosening (recession) and tightening (resection) procedures, most often involving the horizontal rectus muscles. Surgical repair is typically done in an outpatient setting. Rates for successful realignment can exceed 80%. The most common complications are overcorrection or undercorrection and recurrence of strabismus later in life. Rare complications include infection, excessive bleeding, and vision loss.

KEY POINTS

- Strabismus is misalignment of the eyes; it occurs in about 3% of children and causes some vision loss in about half of them.
- Most cases are caused by refractive error or muscle weakness but sometimes a serious disorder is involved (eg, retinoblastoma, cranial nerve palsy).
- Permanent vision loss can occur if strabismus and its attendant amblyopia are not treated before age 4 to 6 yr; the visual system often does not respond to treatment after age 8 yr.
- Physical examination can detect most strabismus.
- Treatment depends on cause, but surgery of the extraocular muscles is sometimes necessary.

309 Gastrointestinal Disorders in Neonates and Infants

Gastrointestinal disorders can affect neonates and infants:

- Gastroesophageal reflux
- Hypertrophic pyloric stenosis
- Intussusception
- Meconium ileus
- Meconium plug syndrome
- Necrotizing enterocolitis
- Neonatal cholestasis

Neonates are also susceptible to miscellaneous surgical emergencies (inguinal hernia, gastric perforation, ileal perforation, and mesenteric arterial occlusion).

Infectious gastroenteritis is the most common pediatric GI disorder. About 5 billion episodes occur worldwide each year, most commonly in developing countries among children < 5 yr. Death due to dehydration occurs in about 2 million cases/yr. In the US, 15 to 25 million cases occur annually, resulting in 300 to 400 deaths. About 2% of children in developed countries will require hospitalization at some time due to acute gastroenteritis and dehydration. In the US, acute gastroenteritis accounts for an estimated 200,000 hospitalizations and 3 to 5 million outpatient visits at a cost in excess of 1 billion dollars.

GASTROESOPHAGEAL REFLUX IN INFANTS

(Gastroesophageal Reflux Disease)

Gastroesophageal reflux (GER) is the movement of gastric contents into the esophagus. Gastroesophageal reflux disease (GERD) is reflux that causes complications such as irritability, respiratory problems, and poor growth. Diagnosis is often made clinically, including by trial of dietary change, but some infants require an upper GI series, use of esophageal pH and impedance probes, and sometimes endoscopy. GER requires only reassurance. Treatment of GERD begins with modification of feeding and positioning; some infants require acid-suppressing drugs such as ranitidine or lansoprazole. Antireflux surgery is rarely needed.

GER occurs in almost all infants, manifesting as wet burps after feeding. Incidence of GER increases between 2 mo and 6 mo of age (likely due to an increased volume of liquid at each feeding) and then starts to decrease after 7 mo. GER resolves in about 85% of infants by 12 mo and in 95% by 18 mo. GERD is much less common.

Etiology

The **most common cause** of GERD in infants is similar to that of GERD in older children and adults—the lower esophageal sphincter (LES) fails to prevent reflux of gastric contents into the esophagus. LES pressure may transiently decrease spontaneously (inappropriate relaxation), which is the most common cause of reflux, or after exposure to cigarette smoke and caffeine (in beverages or breast milk). The esophagus is normally at a negative pressure, whereas the stomach is at a positive pressure. The pressure in the LES has to exceed that pressure gradient to prevent reflux. Factors that increase this gradient or decrease the pressure in the LES predispose to reflux. The pressure gradient may increase in infants who are overfed (excessive food causes a higher gastric pressure) and in infants who have chronic lung disease (lower intrathoracic pressure increases the gradient across the LES) and by positioning (eg, sitting increases gastric pressure).

Other causes include food allergies, most commonly milk allergy. A less common cause is gastroparesis (delayed emptying of the stomach), in which food remains in the stomach for a longer period of time, maintaining a high gastric pressure that predisposes to reflux. Infrequently, an infant can have recurrent emesis that mimics GERD because of a metabolic disease (eg, urea cycle defects, galactosemia, hereditary fructose intolerance) or an anatomic abnormality (such as pyloric stenosis or malrotation).

Complications: Complications of GERD are due mainly to irritation caused by stomach acid and to caloric deficit caused by the frequent regurgitation of food.

Stomach acid may irritate the esophagus, larynx, and, if aspiration occurs, the airways. Esophageal irritation may decrease food intake as infants learn to avoid reflux by eating less. Significant esophageal irritation (esophagitis) may cause mild, chronic blood loss and esophageal stricture. Laryngeal and airway irritation may cause respiratory symptoms. Aspiration may cause recurrent pneumonia.

Symptoms and Signs

Frequent regurgitation (spitting up) is the main symptom of GER. Caregivers often refer to this spitting up as vomiting, but it is not because it is not due to peristaltic contractions. The spit ups appear effortless and not particularly forceful.

Infants with GERD may be irritable and/or have respiratory symptoms such as chronic recurrent coughing or wheezing and sometimes stridor. Much less commonly, infants have intermittent apnea or episodes of arching the back and turning the head to one side (Sandifer syndrome). Infants may fail to gain weight appropriately or, less often, lose weight.

Diagnosis

- Clinical evaluation
- Typically upper GI series
- Sometimes esophageal pH measurement or endoscopy

Infants who have effortless spit ups, who are growing normally, and who have no other symptoms (sometimes referred to as "happy spitters") have GER and require no further evaluation.

Because spitting up is so common, many infants with serious disorders also have a history of spitting up. Red flags that infants have something other than GERD include forceful emesis, emesis containing blood or bile, fever, poor weight gain, blood in the stools, persistent diarrhea, and abnormal development or neurologic symptoms. Infants with such findings require prompt evaluation as described elsewhere in THE MANUAL. Bilious emesis in an infant is a medical emergency because it may be a symptom of malrotation of the intestines and midgut volvulus.

Irritability has many causes, including serious infections and neurologic disorders, which should be ruled out before concluding that the irritability is caused by GERD.

Infants who have symptoms consistent with GERD and no severe complications may be given a therapeutic trial of medical therapy for GERD; improvement or elimination of symptoms suggests GERD is the diagnosis and that other testing is unnecessary. Infants can also be given an extensively hydrolyzed (hypoallergenic) formula for 7 to 10 days to see whether the symptoms are caused by a food allergy.

Infants who fail to respond to a therapeutic trial, or who present with signs of complications of GERD, may require further evaluation. Typically, an upper GI series is the first test; it may help diagnose reflux and also identify any anatomic GI disorders that cause regurgitation. Finding barium reflux into the mid or upper esophagus is much more significant than seeing reflux into only the distal esophagus. For infants with regurgitation hours after eating, who may have gastroparesis, a liquid gastric emptying scan, which uses a radiolabeled liquid, is an alternative to an upper GI series.

If the diagnosis remains unclear or there is still a question of whether reflux is actually the cause of symptoms such as coughing or wheezing, a pediatric gastroenterologist may do tests using esophageal pH or impedance probes (see p. 58). Caregivers record the occurrence of symptoms (manually or by using an event marker on the probe); the symptoms are then correlated with reflux events detected by the probe. A pH probe can also assess the effectiveness of acid-suppression therapy. An impedance probe has the ability to detect nonacid reflux as well as acid reflux.

Upper GI endoscopy and biopsy are sometimes done to help diagnose infection or food allergy and detect and quantify the degree of esophagitis. Laryngotracheobronchoscopy may be done to detect laryngeal inflammation, vocal cord nodules, and evidence of lipid-laden macrophages on bronchial aspirates in patients with significant respiratory symptoms.

Treatment

- Modifying feedings
- Positioning
- Sometimes acid-suppressive therapy
- Rarely surgery

For infants with GER, the only necessary treatment is to reassure caregivers that the symptoms are normal and will be outgrown. Infants with GERD require treatment, typically beginning with conservative measures.

Modifying feedings:

- Thickened feedings
- Smaller, more frequent feedings
- Sometimes a hypoallergenic formula

As a first step, most clinicians recommend thickening feedings, which can be done by adding 1/2 to 1 tbsp rice cereal/30 mL formula. Thickened formula seems to reflux less, particularly when the infant is kept in an upright position for 20 to 30 min after feeding. Thickened formula may not flow through the nipple properly, so the nipple orifice may need to be cross-cut to allow adequate flow.

Providing smaller, more frequent feedings helps keep the pressure in the stomach down and minimizes the amount of reflux. However, it is important to maintain an appropriate total amount of formula/24-h period to ensure adequate growth. In addition, burping the infant after every 1 to 2 oz can help decrease gastric pressure by expelling the air the infant is swallowing.

A hypoallergenic formula can be given to infants who may have a food allergy. Hypoallergenic formula can even be helpful for infants who do not have a food allergy by improving gastric emptying. All children should be kept away from caffeine and tobacco smoke.

Positioning: After feeding, infants are kept in an upright, nonseated position for 20 to 30 min (sitting, as in an infant seat, increases gastric pressure and is not helpful). For sleeping, the head of the crib can be raised about 15 cm (6 in); if the head of the crib is raised, infants should be secured in a sling fitted over the mattress or wedge to keep them from rolling or sliding down to a horizontal position on the lower end of the crib.

Drug treatment: Three classes of drugs can be used in infants who do not respond to feeding modification and positioning:

- Histamine-2 (H2) blockers
- Proton pump inhibitors (PPI)
- Promotility drugs

Typically, treatment of GERD is begun with an H2 blocker such as ranitidine 2 mg/kg po bid to tid. If the infant responds, the drug is continued for several months and then tapered and stopped (if possible). If infants fail to respond to H2 blockers, a PPI such as lansoprazole can be considered, although there are few data on PPI use in infants. PPIs are more effective at suppressing gastric acid than are H2 blockers and are given only once/day. For infants with GERD and an acute symptom such as irritability, a liquid antacid can be used.

Infants who have gastroparesis may benefit from a promotility drug in addition to acid-suppressive therapy. Erythromycin is one of the most commonly used promotility drugs for this situation. Metoclopramide was used previously but does not seem as effective and can have significant adverse effects. More recently, amoxicillin/clavulanate has also been used for its promotility properties.

Surgery: Infants with severe or life-threatening complications of reflux that are unresponsive to medical therapy can be considered for surgical therapy. The main type of antireflux surgery is fundoplication. During this procedure, the top of the stomach is wrapped around the distal esophagus to help tighten the LES. Fundoplication can be very effective at resolving reflux but has several complications. It can cause pain when infants vomit (eg, during acute gastroenteritis), and if the wrap is too tight, infants may have dysphagia. If dysphagia occurs, the wrap can be dilated endoscopically. Some anatomic causes of reflux also may have to be corrected surgically.

KEY POINTS

- Most reflux in infants does not cause other symptoms or complications and resolves spontaneously by age 12 to 18 mo.
- GERD is diagnosed when reflux causes complications such as esophagitis, respiratory symptoms (eg, cough, stridor, wheezing, apnea), or impaired growth.
- Prescribe a therapeutic trial of feeding modifications and positioning if GERD symptoms are mild.
- Consider testing with an upper GI series, gastric emptying scan, esophageal probes, or endoscopy for infants with more severe GERD symptoms or for whom a therapeutic trial is not helpful.
- Acid suppression with an H2 blocker or PPI may help infants with significant GERD.
- Most infants with GERD respond to medical therapy, but a few require surgical therapy.

HYPERTROPHIC PYLORIC STENOSIS

Hypertrophic pyloric stenosis is obstruction of the pyloric lumen due to pyloric muscular hypertrophy. Diagnosis is by abdominal ultrasonography. Treatment is surgical.

Hypertrophic pyloric stenosis may cause almost complete gastric outlet obstruction. It affects 2 to 3 out of 1000 infants and is more common among males by a 5:1 ratio, particularly firstborn males. It occurs most often between 3 wk and 6 wk of age and rarely after 12 wk.

Etiology

The exact etiology of hypertrophic pyloric stenosis is uncertain, but a genetic component is likely because siblings and offspring of affected people are at increased risk, particularly monozygotic twins. Maternal smoking during pregnancy also increases risk. Proposed mechanisms include lack of neuronal nitric oxide synthase, abnormal innervation of the muscular layer, and hypergastrinemia. Infants exposed to certain macrolide antibiotics (eg, erythromycin) in the first few weeks of life are at significantly increased risk.

Symptoms and Signs

Symptoms of hypertrophic pyloric stenosis typically develop between 3 wk and 6 wk of life. Projectile vomiting (without bile) occurs shortly after eating. Until dehydration sets in, children feed avidly and otherwise appear well, unlike many of those with vomiting caused by systemic illness. Gastric peristaltic waves may be visible, crossing the epigastrium from left to right. A discrete, 2- to 3-cm, firm, movable, and olive-like pyloric mass is sometimes palpable deep in the right side of the epigastrium. With progression of illness, children fail to gain weight, and dehydration develops.

Diagnosis

- Clinical evaluation
- Ultrasonography

Hypertrophic pyloric stenosis should be suspected in all infants in the first several months of life with projectile vomiting.

Diagnosis of hypertrophic pyloric stenosis is by abdominal ultrasonography showing increased thickness of the pylorus (typically to ≥ 4 mm; normal, < 2 mm) along with an elongated pylorus (> 16 mm).

If the diagnosis remains uncertain, ultrasonography can be repeated serially or an upper GI series can be done, which typically shows delayed gastric emptying and a string sign or railroad track sign of a markedly narrowed, elongated pyloric lumen. In rare cases, upper endoscopy is required for confirmation.

The classic electrolyte pattern of an infant with pyloric stenosis is that of hypochloremic metabolic alkalosis (due to loss of hydrochloric acid and simultaneous hypovolemia). About 5 to 14% of infants have jaundice, and about 5% have malrotation.

Treatment

- Surgery (pyloromyotomy)

Initial treatment of hypertrophic pyloric stenosis is directed at hydration and correcting electrolyte abnormalities.

Definitive treatment is a longitudinal pyloromyotomy, which leaves the mucosa intact and separates the incised muscle fibers. Postoperatively, the infant usually tolerates feeding within a day.

KEY POINTS

- Projectile vomiting occurs shortly after feeding in an infant < 3 mo old.
- Diagnosis is by ultrasonography.
- Treatment is surgical incision of the hypertrophied pyloric muscle.

INTUSSUSCEPTION

Intussusception is telescoping of one portion of the intestine (intussusceptum) into an adjacent segment (intussuscipiens), causing intestinal obstruction and sometimes intestinal ischemia. Diagnosis is by ultrasonography. Treatment is with an air enema and sometimes surgery.

Intussusception generally occurs between ages 6 mo and 3 yr, with 65% of cases occurring before age 1 and 80 to 90% occurring before age 2. It is the most common cause of intestinal obstruction in this age group.

The telescoping segment obstructs the intestine and ultimately impairs blood flow to the intussuscepting segment (see Fig. 309–1), causing ischemia, gangrene, and perforation.

Etiology

Most cases are idiopathic. However, there is a slight male predominance as well as a seasonal variation; peak incidence coincides with the viral enteritis season. An older rotavirus vaccine was associated with a marked increase in risk of intussusception and was taken off the market in the US. The newer vaccines, when given in the recommended sequence and timing, are not associated with any clinically significant increased risk.

In about 25% of children who have intussusception, typically very young and older children, a lead point (ie, a mass or other intestinal abnormality) triggers the telescoping. Examples include polyps, lymphoma, Meckel diverticulum, and immunoglobulin A–associated vasculitis (formerly called Henoch-Schönlein purpura) when purpura involve the bowel wall. Cystic fibrosis is also a risk factor.

Symptoms and Signs

The initial symptoms of intussusception are sudden onset of significant, colicky abdominal pain that recurs every 15 to 20 min, often with vomiting. The child appears relatively well between episodes. Later, as intestinal ischemia develops, pain becomes steady, the child becomes lethargic, and mucosal hemorrhage causes heme-positive stool on rectal examination and sometimes spontaneous passage of a currant-jelly stool. The latter, however, is a late occurrence, and physicians should not wait for this symptom to occur to suspect intussusception. A palpable abdominal mass, described as sausage-shaped, is sometimes present. Perforation results in signs of peritonitis, with significant tenderness, guarding, and rigidity. Pallor, tachycardia, and diaphoresis indicate shock.

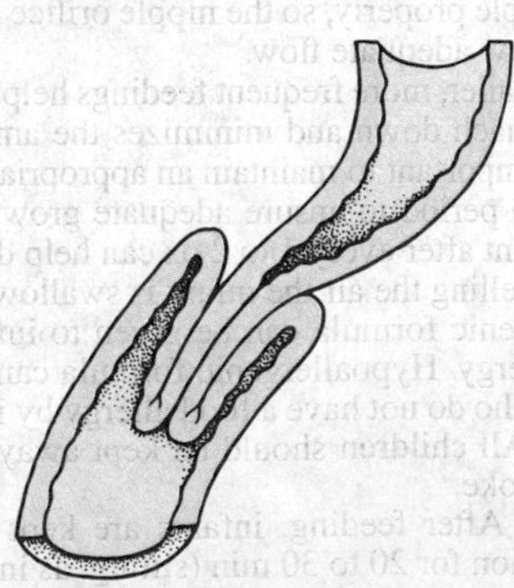

Fig. 309–1. Intussusception.

About 5 to 10% of children present without the colicky pain phase. Instead, they appear lethargic, as if drugged (atypical or apathetic presentation). In such cases, the diagnosis of intussusception is often missed until the currant-jelly stool appears or an abdominal mass is palpated.

Diagnosis

- Ultrasonography

Suspicion of the diagnosis must be high, particularly in children with atypical presentation, and studies and intervention must be done urgently, because survival and likelihood of nonoperative reduction decrease significantly with time. Approach depends on clinical findings. Ill children with signs of peritonitis require fluid resuscitation, broad-spectrum antibiotics (eg, ampicillin, gentamicin, clindamycin), nasogastric suction, and surgery. Clinically stable children require imaging studies to confirm the diagnosis and treat the disorder.

Barium enema was once the preferred initial study because it revealed the classic coiled-spring appearance around the intussusceptum. In addition to being diagnostic, barium enema was also usually therapeutic; the pressure of the barium often reduced the telescoped segments. However, barium occasionally enters the peritoneum through a clinically unsuspected perforation and causes significant peritonitis. Currently, ultrasonography is the preferred means of diagnosis; it is easily done, relatively inexpensive, and safe.

PEARLS & PITFALLS

- Physicians should not wait for passage of a currant-jelly stool to suspect intussusception because it is a late occurrence.

Treatment

- Air enema
- Surgery if enema unsuccessful or if perforation present

If intussusception is confirmed, an air enema is used for reduction, which lessens the likelihood and consequences of perforation. The intussusceptum can be successfully reduced in 75 to 95% of children. If the air enema is successful, children are observed overnight to rule out occult perforation. If reduction is unsuccessful or if the intestine has perforated, immediate surgery is required.

When reduction is achieved without surgery, the recurrence rate is 5 to 10%.

KEY POINTS

- Intussusception is telescoping of one segment of intestine into another, usually in children < 3 yr.
- Children typically present with colicky abdominal pain and vomiting, followed by passage of currant-jelly stool.
- Diagnosis is made by ultrasonography.
- Treatment is reduction by air enema and sometimes surgery.

MECONIUM ILEUS

Meconium ileus is obstruction of the terminal ileum by abnormally tenacious meconium; it most often occurs in neonates with cystic fibrosis. Meconium ileus accounts for up to 33% of neonatal small-bowel obstructions. Symptoms include emesis that may be bilious, abdominal distention, and failure to pass meconium in the first several days of life. Diagnosis is based on clinical presentation and x-rays. Treatment is enemas with dilute contrast under fluoroscopy and surgery if enemas fail.

Meconium ileus is most often an early manifestation of cystic fibrosis, which causes GI secretions to be extremely viscid and adherent to the intestinal mucosa. Meconium ileus is the presenting clinical manifestation of cystic fibrosis in 10 to 20% of cases. Of infants with meconium ileus, 80 to 90% have cystic fibrosis.

Obstruction occurs at the level of the terminal ileum (unlike the colonic obstruction caused by meconium plug syndrome) and may be diagnosed by prenatal ultrasonography. Distal to the obstruction, the colon is narrow and empty or contains small amounts of desiccated meconium pellets. The relatively empty, small-caliber colon is called a microcolon and is secondary to disuse.

Complications of meconium ileus: About 50% of cases are complicated by malrotation, intestinal atresia, or perforation. The distended loops of small bowel may twist to form a volvulus in utero. If the intestine loses its vascular supply and infarcts, sterile meconium peritonitis can result. The infarcted intestinal loop may be resorbed, leaving an area or areas of intestinal atresia. Infants with meconium ileus are also at increased risk of developing cholestasis.

Symptoms and Signs

After birth, unlike normal neonates, infants with meconium ileus fail to pass meconium in the first 12 to 24 h. They have signs of intestinal obstruction, including emesis that may be bilious and abdominal distention. Loops of distended small bowel somctimes can be palpated through the abdominal wall and may feel characteristically doughy. Meconium peritonitis with respiratory distress and ascites can occur secondary to perforation.

Diagnosis

- Plain x-rays
- If positive, tests for cystic fibrosis

Prenatal ultrasonography can detect changes in utero suggestive of cystic fibrosis and meconium ileus (eg, dilated bowel, polyhydramnios), but these changes are not specific.

Diagnosis of meconium ileus is suspected in a neonate with signs of intestinal obstruction, particularly if a family history of cystic fibrosis exists. Patients should undergo abdominal x-rays, which show dilated intestinal loops; however, fluid levels may be absent. A "soap bubble" or "ground glass" appearance due to small air bubbles mixed with the meconium is diagnostic of meconium ileus. If meconium peritonitis is present, calcified meconium flecks may line the peritoneal surfaces and even the scrotum. A water-soluble contrast enema reveals a microcolon with an obstruction in the terminal ileum.

Patients diagnosed with meconium ileus should be tested for cystic fibrosis.

Treatment

- Radiographic contrast enema
- Sometimes surgery

Obstruction may be relieved in uncomplicated cases (ie, without perforation, volvulus, or atresia) by giving ≥ 1 enema with a dilute radiographic contrast medium plus *N*-acetylcysteine under fluoroscopy; hypertonic contrast material may cause large GI water losses requiring IV rehydration.

If the enema does not relieve the obstruction, laparotomy is required. A double-barreled ileostomy with repeated *N*-acetylcysteine lavage of the proximal and distal loops is usually required to liquefy and remove the abnormal meconium.

MECONIUM PLUG SYNDROME

(Small Left Colon Syndrome)

Meconium plug syndrome is colonic obstruction caused by thick meconium. Diagnosis is based on radiographic contrast enema and sometimes testing for Hirschsprung disease. Treatment is radiographic contrast enema; surgical decompression is rarely required.

Meconium plug syndrome usually occurs in infants who are otherwise healthy. It is generally regarded as a functional immaturity of the colon, resulting in failure to pass the first stool.

Etiology

Meconium plug syndrome is more common among

- Premature infants
- Infants of diabetic mothers
- Infants of mothers treated with magnesium sulfate for eclampsia, preeclampsia, or preterm labor

One study noted that 16% of cases of meconium plug syndrome were associated with magnesium tocolysis and only 3% were associated with Hirschsprung disease; however, other reports have noted Hirschsprung in 10 to 30% of infants with meconium plug syndrome.

Symptoms and Signs

Infants present in the first few days of life with failure to pass stools, abdominal distention, and vomiting. Thick, inspissated, rubbery meconium forms a cast of the colon, resulting in complete obstruction.

Diagnosis

- Radiographic contrast enema
- Sometimes testing for Hirschsprung disease

Diagnosis of meconium plug syndrome is of exclusion and should be differentiated primarily from Hirschsprung disease.

Plain abdominal x-rays are nonspecific and can show signs of low intestinal obstruction. Conversely, contrast enema shows the characteristic appearance of the outline of the inspissated meconium against the wall of the colon, providing a double-contrast impression. Unlike meconium ileus, microcolon is not typically seen on x-ray with meconium plug syndrome.

Treatment

- Radiographic contrast enema

The water-soluble contrast enema can be therapeutic by separating the plug from the intestinal wall and expelling it. Occasionally, repeated enemas are required.

Rarely, surgical decompression is required. Although most infants are healthy thereafter, diagnostic studies may be needed to rule out Hirschsprung disease or cystic fibrosis.

NECROTIZING ENTEROCOLITIS

Necrotizing enterocolitis (NEC) is an acquired disease, primarily of preterm or sick neonates, characterized by mucosal or even deeper intestinal necrosis. It is the most common GI emergency among neonates. Symptoms and signs include feeding intolerance, lethargy, temperature instability, ileus, bloating, bilious emesis, hematochezia, reducing substances in the stool, apnea, and sometimes signs of sepsis. Diagnosis is clinical and is confirmed by imaging studies. Treatment is primarily supportive and includes nasogastric suction, parenteral fluids, TPN, antibiotics, isolation in cases of infection, and, often, surgery.

Over 85% of cases of NEC occur in premature infants. It occurs in about 1 to 8% of neonatal ICU admissions.

Risk factors: General risk factors for NEC in addition to prematurity include

- Prolonged rupture of the membranes with amnionitis
- Birth asphyxia
- Small-for-gestational-age infants
- Congenital heart disease
- Exchange transfusions

The incidence may also be higher in infants fed hypertonic formulas.

Three intestinal factors are usually present:

- A preceding ischemic insult
- Bacterial colonization
- Intraluminal substrate (ie, enteral feedings)

Etiology

The exact etiology of NEC is not clear. It is believed that an ischemic insult damages the intestinal lining, leading to increased intestinal permeability and leaving the intestine susceptible to bacterial invasion. NEC rarely occurs before enteral feedings have begun and is less common among breast-fed infants. However, once feedings are begun, ample substrate is present for proliferation of luminal bacteria, which can penetrate the damaged intestinal wall, producing hydrogen gas. The gas may collect within the intestinal wall (pneumatosis intestinalis) or enter the portal veins.

The initial ischemic insult may result from vasospasm of the mesenteric arteries, which can be caused by an anoxic insult triggering the primitive diving reflex that markedly diminishes intestinal blood flow. Intestinal ischemia may also result from low blood flow during an exchange transfusion, during sepsis, or from the use of hyperosmolar formulas. Similarly, congenital heart disease with reduced systemic blood flow or arterial oxygen desaturation may lead to intestinal hypoxia/ischemia and predispose to NEC.

NEC may occur as clusters of cases or as outbreaks in neonatal ICUs. Some clusters appear to be associated with specific organisms (eg, *Klebsiella, Escherichia coli,* coagulase-negative staphylococci), but often no specific pathogen is identified.

Complications of necrotizing enterocolitis: Necrosis begins in the mucosa and may progress to involve the full thickness of the intestinal wall, causing perforation with subsequent peritonitis and often free intra-abdominal air. Perforation occurs most commonly in the terminal ileum; the colon and the proximal small bowel are involved less frequently. Sepsis occurs in 33% of infants, and death may occur.

Symptoms and Signs

Infants may present with feeding difficulties and bloody or bilious gastric residuals (after feedings) that may progress to bilious emesis, ileus manifested by abdominal distention, or gross blood in stool. Sepsis may be manifested by lethargy, temperature instability, increased apneic spells, and metabolic acidosis.

Diagnosis

- Detection of blood in stool
- Abdominal x-rays

Early x-rays may be nonspecific and reveal only ileus. However, a fixed, dilated intestinal loop that does not change on repeated x-rays indicates NEC. X-ray signs diagnostic of NEC are pneumatosis intestinalis and portal vein gas. Pneumoperitoneum indicates bowel perforation and an urgent need for surgery.

Treatment

- Feedings stopped
- Nasogastric suction
- Fluid resuscitation
- Broad-spectrum antibiotics
- TPN
- Sometimes surgery

The mortality rate is 20 to 30%. Aggressive support and judicious timing of surgical intervention maximize the chance of survival.

Support: Nonsurgical support is sufficient in over 75% of cases. Feedings must be stopped immediately if NEC is suspected, and the intestine should be decompressed with a double-lumen NGT attached to intermittent suction. Appropriate colloid and crystalloid parenteral fluids must be given to support circulation, because extensive intestinal inflammation and peritonitis may lead to considerable 3rd-space fluid loss. TPN is needed for 14 to 21 days while the intestine heals.

Systemic antibiotics should be started at once with a beta-lactam antibiotic (eg, ampicillin, ticarcillin) and an aminoglycoside. Additional anaerobic coverage (eg, clindamycin, metronidazole) may also be considered and should continue for 10 days (for dosage, see Table 314–1 on p. 2620). Because some outbreaks may be infectious, patient isolation should be considered, particularly if several cases occur within a short time.

The infant requires close monitoring; frequent complete re-evaluation (eg, at least every 12 h); and serial abdominal x-rays, CBCs, platelet counts, and blood gases. Intestinal strictures are the most common long-term complication of NEC, occurring in 10 to 36% of infants who survive the initial event. Strictures typically manifest within 2 to 3 mo of an NEC episode. Strictures are most commonly noted in the colon, especially on the left side. Resection of the stricture is then required.

Surgery: Surgical intervention is needed in < 25% of infants. Absolute indications are intestinal perforation (pneumoperitoneum), signs of peritonitis (absent intestinal sounds and diffuse guarding and tenderness or erythema and edema of the abdominal wall), or aspiration of purulent material from the peritoneal cavity by paracentesis. Surgery should be considered for an infant with NEC whose clinical and laboratory condition worsens despite nonsurgical support.

During surgery, gangrenous bowel is resected, and ostomies are created. (Primary reanastomosis may be done if the remaining intestine shows no signs of ischemia.) With resolution of sepsis and peritonitis, intestinal continuity can be reestablished several weeks or months later.

Prevention

At-risk infants should be fed breast milk, and feedings should begin with small amounts that are gradually increased according to standardized protocols. (Preterm formula is an appropriate substitute if breast milk is not available.) Hypertonic formula, drugs, or contrast material should be avoided. Polycythemia should be treated promptly.

Probiotics (eg, *Bifidus infantis, Lactobacillus acidophilus*) help prevent NEC, but further studies to determine optimal dosing and appropriate strains are required.

KEY POINTS

- NEC is intestinal necrosis of uncertain etiology; it occurs mainly in preterm or sick neonates after enteral feedings have begun.
- Complications include intestinal perforation (most often in the terminal ileum) and peritonitis; sepsis occurs in 33%, and death may occur.
- Initial manifestations are feeding difficulties and bloody or bilious gastric residuals (after feedings) followed by bilious emesis, abdominal distention, and/or gross blood in stool.
- Diagnose using plain x-rays.
- Supportive treatment using fluid resuscitation, nasogastric suction, broad-spectrum antibiotics, and TPN is effective in > 75% of cases.
- Surgery to resect gangrenous bowel and treat perforation is needed in < 25% of infants.

NEONATAL CHOLESTASIS

Cholestasis is failure of bilirubin secretion, resulting in conjugated hyperbilirubinemia and jaundice. There are numerous causes, which are identified by laboratory testing, hepatobiliary scan, and, sometimes, liver biopsy and surgery. Treatment depends on cause.

Cholestasis occurs in 1/2500 full-term infants. It is defined as direct bilirubin > 1 mg/dL. Cholestasis is never normal and warrants evaluation.

Etiology

Cholestasis (see p. 186) may result from extrahepatic or intrahepatic disorders, although some conditions overlap.

Extrahepatic causes of cholestasis: The most common extrahepatic disorder is

- Biliary atresia (incidence in the US 1/12,000 live births)

Biliary atresia is obstruction of the biliary tree due to progressive sclerosis of the extrahepatic bile duct. In most cases, biliary atresia manifests several weeks after birth, probably after inflammation and scarring of the extrahepatic (and sometimes intrahepatic) bile ducts. It is rarely present in premature infants or in neonates at birth. The cause of the inflammatory response is unknown, but infectious organisms have been implicated.

Intrahepatic causes of cholestasis: Intrahepatic causes can be infectious, alloimmune, metabolic/genetic, or toxic.

Infections can cause cholestasis. Infections may be viral (eg, herpes simplex virus, cytomegalovirus, rubella), bacterial (eg, gram-positive and gram-negative bacteremia, UTI caused by *Escherichia coli*), or parasitic (eg, toxoplasmosis). Sepsis in neonates receiving parental nutrition can also cause cholestasis.

Gestational alloimmune liver disease involves transplacental passage of maternal IgG that induces a complement-mediated membrane attack complex that injures the fetal liver.

Metabolic causes include numerous inborn errors of metabolism such as galactosemia, tyrosinemia, alpha-1 antitrypsin deficiency, disorders of lipid metabolism, mitochondrial disorders, and fatty acid oxidation defects. Genetic defects include Alagille syndrome, cystic fibrosis, and arthrogryposis-renal dysfunction-cholestasis (ARC) syndrome. There are also a number of gene mutations that interfere with normal bile production and excretion and cause cholestasis; the resultant disorders are termed progressive familial intrahepatic cholestasis.

Toxic causes are due mainly to the use of prolonged parenteral nutrition in extremely preterm neonates or infants with short bowel syndrome.

Idiopathic neonatal hepatitis syndrome (giant cell hepatitis) is an inflammatory condition of the neonatal liver. Its incidence has decreased, and it is becoming rare as improved diagnostic studies allow identification of specific causes of cholestasis.

Pathophysiology

In cholestasis, the primary failure is of bilirubin excretion, resulting in excess conjugated bilirubin in the bloodstream and decreased bile salts in the GI tract. As a result of inadequate bile in the GI tract, there is malabsorption of fat and fat-soluble vitamins (A, D, E, and K), leading to vitamin deficiency, inadequate nutrition, and growth failure.

Symptoms and Signs

Cholestasis typically is noted in the first 2 wk of life. Infants are jaundiced and often have dark urine (containing conjugated bilirubin), acholic stools, and hepatomegaly. If cholestasis persists, chronic pruritus is common, as are symptoms and signs of fat-soluble vitamin deficiency; progression on growth charts may show a decline.

If the underlying disorder causes hepatic fibrosis and cirrhosis, portal hypertension with subsequent abdominal distention resulting from ascites, dilated abdominal veins, and upper GI bleeding resulting from esophageal varices may develop.

Diagnosis

- Total and direct bilirubin
- Liver function tests
- Tests for metabolic, infectious, and genetic causes
- Liver ultrasonography
- Hepatobiliary scan
- Occasionally biopsy of liver or other tissue (eg, lip), operative cholangiography, or genetic testing

Any infant who is jaundiced after age 2 wk should be evaluated for cholestasis including with total and direct bilirubin levels. Some experts advocate that breastfed infants who have jaundice do not need to be evaluated until age 3 wk. The initial approach should be directed at diagnosing treatable conditions (eg, extrahepatic biliary atresia, in which early surgical intervention improves short-term outcome).

Cholestasis is identified by an elevation in both total and direct bilirubin. Tests that are needed to further evaluate liver function include albumin, fractionated serum bilirubin, liver enzymes, PT/PTT, and ammonia level (see Tests for Cholestasis on p. 197). Once cholestasis is confirmed, testing is required to determine etiology (see Table 309–1) and evidence of malabsorption (eg, low levels of the fat-soluble vitamins E, D, and A, or prolonged PT, suggesting a low level of vitamin K).

Abdominal ultrasonography is often the first test; it is noninvasive and can assess liver size and certain abnormalities of the gallbladder and common bile duct. However, it is nonspecific. A hepatobiliary scan using hydroxy iminodiacetic acid (HIDA scan) should also be done; excretion of contrast into the intestine rules out biliary atresia, but lack of excretion can occur with both biliary atresia, severe neonatal hepatitis, and other causes of cholestasis. Infants with cholestasis are frequently given phenobarbital for 5 days prior to a HIDA scan in an attempt to enhance the excretion.

Table 309–1. DIAGNOSTIC EVALUATION FOR NEONATAL CHOLESTASIS

ETIOLOGY	TEST
Hepatic dysfunction	Albumin, ammonia, PT/PTT, AST, ALT, GGT, total and direct bilirubin (see Tests for Cholestasis)
Infections	Urine cultures, TORCH titers
Endocrinopathy	TSH, thyroxine
Cystic fibrosis	Sweat chloride test
Galactosemia	Neonatal screen, reducing substances (eg, galactose) in urine (see diagnosis of galactosemia)
Alpha-1 antitrypsin deficiency	Serum levels of alpha-1 antitrypsin, alpha-1 antitrypsin phenotype testing
Genetic errors in bile acid synthesis	Bile acid levels in urine and serum Genetic testing
Inborn errors of metabolism	Urine organic acids, serum ammonia, serum electrolytes (see testing of inherited disorders of metabolism)
Alloimmune liver disease	Alpha-1 antitrypsin, ferritin, lipid profile, tissue iron determined from either lip or liver, liver histology

GGT = gamma-glutamyl transpeptidase; TORCH = toxoplasmosis, other pathogens, rubella, cytomegalovirus, and herpes simplex; TSH = thyroid-stimulating hormone.

When no diagnosis has been made, a liver biopsy is generally done relatively early on, sometimes with operative cholangiography. Patients with biliary atresia typically have enlarged portal triads, bile duct proliferation, and increased fibrosis. Neonatal hepatitis is characterized by lobular disarray with multinucleated giant cells. Alloimmune liver disease is characterized by elevated hepatic iron stores (increased iron may also be demonstrated using lip biopsy if liver biopsy is not otherwise needed).

Prognosis

Biliary atresia is progressive and, if untreated, results in liver failure, cirrhosis with portal hypertension by several months of age, and death by 1 yr of age.

Prognosis of cholestasis due to specific disorders (eg, metabolic disease) is variable, ranging from a completely benign course to a progressive disease resulting in cirrhosis.

Idiopathic neonatal hepatitis syndrome usually resolves slowly, but permanent liver damage may result and lead to liver failure and death.

Alloimmune liver disease has a poor prognosis without early intervention.

Treatment

- Specific cause treated
- Vitamin A, D, E, and K supplements
- Medium-chain triglycerides
- Sometimes ursodeoxycholic acid

Specific treatment is directed at the cause. If there is no specific therapy, treatment is supportive and consists primarily of nutritional therapy, including supplements of vitamins A, D, E, and K. For formula-fed infants, a formula that is high in medium-chain triglycerides should be used because it is absorbed better in the presence of bile salt deficiency. Adequate calories are required; infants may need > 130 calories/kg day. In infants with some bile flow, ursodeoxycholic acid 10 to 15 mg/kg once/day or bid may relieve itching.

Infants with presumed biliary atresia require surgical exploration with an intraoperative cholangiogram. If biliary atresia is confirmed, a portoenterostomy (Kasai procedure) should be done. Ideally, this procedure should be done in the first 1 to 2 mo of life. After this period, the short-term prognosis significantly worsens. Postoperatively, many patients have significant chronic problems, including persistent cholestasis, recurrent ascending cholangitis, and failure to thrive. Prophylactic antibiotics (eg, trimethoprim/sulfamethoxazole) are frequently prescribed for a year postoperatively in an attempt to prevent ascending cholangitis. Even with optimal therapy, most infants develop cirrhosis and require liver transplantation.

Because alloimmune liver disease has no definitive marker and/or test, treatment with IV immune globulin (IVIG) or exchange transfusion needs to be considered early to reverse the ongoing liver injury if no definite diagnosis has been made.

KEY POINTS

- There are numerous inherited and acquired causes of neonatal cholestasis, resulting in failure of bilirubin excretion and thus excess conjugated bilirubin.
- Neonatal cholestasis typically is noted in the first 2 wk of life; infants are jaundiced and often have dark urine, acholic stools, and hepatomegaly.
- Begin with laboratory testing of liver function, ultrasonography, and hepatobiliary scan and do tests for causes, sometimes including liver biopsy.
- Treat specific cause and give supportive care, including supplementation of fat-soluble vitamins and a formula that is high in medium-chain triglycerides and contains sufficient calories.

MISCELLANEOUS SURGICAL EMERGENCIES IN NEONATES

Inguinal hernia in neonates: Inguinal hernias develop most often in male neonates, particularly if they are premature (in which case the incidence is about 10%). The right side is affected most commonly, and about 10% of inguinal hernias are bilateral. Because inguinal hernias can become incarcerated, repair should be done shortly after diagnosis. For premature infants, repair typically is not done until they have reached a weight of 2 kg. In contrast, umbilical hernias rarely become incarcerated, close spontaneously after several years, and do not ordinarily need surgical repair.

Gastric perforation in neonates: In neonates, gastric perforations are often spontaneous and typically occur in the first week of life. Although this is overall an uncommon occurrence, perforation is more common among premature than full-term infants. The etiology of gastric perforation is uncertain, but the perforation may be due to a congenital defect in the stomach wall, usually along the greater curvature. The abdomen suddenly becomes distended, infants develop respiratory distress, and massive pneumoperitoneum is seen on abdominal x-ray. This disorder has a high mortality rate (25%), which is even greater in premature infants (60%). Prognosis is usually good after surgical repair of the perforation.

Ileal perforation in neonates: Ileal perforation is another uncommon disorder that is most common among very low-birth-weight infants (< 1500 g) and during the first 2 wk of life. It has been associated with chorioamnionitis, postnatal glucocorticoid use, and indomethacin therapy to close a patent ductus arteriosis. The etiology of ileal perforation is uncertain but may be related to a muscular defect in the ileal wall or to a problem with nitric oxide synthase and local ischemia resulting from vasoconstriction. Treatment of ileal perforation is stabilization with IV fluids and antibiotics, followed by surgical repair.

Mesenteric arterial occlusion in neonates: Mural thrombi or emboli may occlude a mesenteric artery after high placement of an umbilical artery catheter. Such an occurrence is extremely rare but can cause extensive intestinal infarction requiring surgery and intestinal resection.

310 Growth and Development

Physical growth is an increase in size. Development is growth in function and capability. Both processes highly depend on genetic, nutritional, and environmental factors.

As children develop physiologically and emotionally, it is useful to define certain age-based groups. The following terminology is used:

- Neonate (newborn): Birth to 1 mo
- Infant: 1 mo to 1 yr
- Young child: 1 yr through 4 yr
- Older child: 5 yr through 10 yr
- Adolescent: 11 yr through 17 to 19 yr

PHYSICAL GROWTH OF INFANTS AND CHILDREN

Physical growth includes attainment of full height and appropriate weight and an increase in size of all organs (except lymphatic tissue, which decreases in size). Growth from birth to adolescence occurs in 2 distinct phases:

- Phase 1 (from birth to about age 1 to 2 yr): This phase is one of rapid growth, although the rate of growth decreases over that period.
- Phase 2 (from about 2 yr to the onset of puberty): In this phase, growth occurs in relatively constant annual increments.

Puberty is the process of physical maturation from child to adult. Adolescence defines an age group; puberty occurs during adolescence (see Physical Growth and Sexual Maturation of

Adolescents on p. 2594). At puberty, a 2nd growth spurt occurs, affecting boys and girls slightly differently.

From birth until age 2 yr, it is recommended that all growth parameters be charted using standard growth charts from the WHO. After age 2, growth parameters are charted using growth charts from the CDC.[1]

1. Grummer-Strawn LM, Reinold C, Krebs NF, Centers for Disease Control and Prevention (CDC): Use of World Health Organization and CDC growth charts for children aged 0–59 months in the United States. *MMWR Recomm Rep* 10(RR-9):1–15, 2010. Clarification and additional information. *MMWR Recomm Rep* 59(36): 1184, 2010.

Length

Length is measured in children too young to stand; height is measured once the child can stand. In general, length in normal-term infants increases about 30% by 5 mo and > 50% by 12 mo; infants grow 25 cm during the 1st yr, and height at 5 yr is about double the birth length. In most boys, half the adult height is attained by about age 2; in most girls, height at 19 mo is about half the adult height.

Rate of change in height (height velocity) is a more sensitive measure of growth than time-specific height measures. In general, healthy term infants and children grow about 2.5 cm/mo between birth and 6 mo, 1.3 cm/mo from 7 to 12 mo, and about 7.6 cm/yr between 12 mo and 10 yr.

Before 12 mo, height velocity varies and is due in part to perinatal factors (eg, prematurity). After 12 mo, height is mostly genetically determined, and height velocity stays nearly constant until puberty; a child's height relative to peers tends to remain the same.

Some small-for-gestational-age infants tend to be shorter throughout life than infants whose size is appropriate for their gestational age. Boys and girls show little difference in height and growth rate during infancy and childhood.

Extremities grow faster than the trunk, leading to a gradual change in relative proportions; the crown-to-pubis/pubis-to-heel ratio is 1.7 at birth, 1.5 at 12 mo, 1.2 at 5 yr, and 1.0 after 7 yr.

Weight

Weight follows a similar pattern. Normal-term neonates generally lose 5 to 8% of birth weight in the days after delivery but regain their birth weight within 2 wk. They then gain 14 to 28 g/day until 3 mo, then 4000 g between 3 and 12 mo, doubling their birth weight by 5 mo, tripling it by 12 mo, and almost quadrupling it by 2 yr. Between age 2 yr and puberty, weight increases 2 kg/yr. The recent epidemic of childhood obesity (see Table 4–1 on p. 19) has involved markedly greater weight gain, even among very young children. In general, boys are heavier and taller than girls when growth is complete because boys have a longer prepubertal growth period, increased peak velocity during the pubertal growth spurt, and a longer adolescent growth spurt.

Head Circumference

Head circumference reflects brain size and is routinely measured up to 36 mo. At birth, the brain is 25% of adult size, and head circumference averages 35 cm. Head circumference increases an average 1 cm/mo during the 1st yr; growth is more rapid in the 1st 8 mo, and by 12 mo, the brain has completed half its postnatal growth and is 75% of adult size. Head circumference increases 3.5 cm over the next 2 yr; the brain is 80% of adult size by age 3 yr and 90% by age 7 yr.

Body Composition

Body composition (proportions of body fat and water) changes and affects drug volume of distribution. Proportion of fat increases rapidly from 13% at birth to 20 to 25% by 12 mo, accounting for the chubby appearance of most infants. Subsequently, a slow fall occurs until preadolescence, when body fat returns to about 13%. There is a slow rise again until the onset of puberty, when body fat may again fall, especially in boys. After puberty, the percentage generally stays stable in girls, whereas in boys there tends to be a slight decline.

Body water measured as a percentage of body weight is 70% at birth, dropping to 61% at 12 mo (about equal to the adult percentage). This change is fundamentally due to a decrease in ECF from 45% to 28% of body weight. ICF stays relatively constant. After age 12 mo, there is a slow and variable fall in ECF to adult levels of about 20% and a rise in ICF to adult levels of about 40%. The relatively larger amount of body water, its high turnover rate, and the comparatively high surface losses (due to a proportionately large surface area) make infants more susceptible to fluid deprivation than older children and adults.

Tooth Eruption

Tooth eruption is variable (see Table 310–1), primarily because of genetic factors. On average, normal infants should have 6 teeth by 12 mo, 12 teeth by 18 mo, 16 teeth by 2 yr, and all teeth (20) by 2½ yr; deciduous teeth are replaced by permanent teeth between the ages of 5 yr and 13 yr. Eruption of deciduous teeth is similar in both sexes; permanent teeth tend to appear earlier in girls. Tooth eruption may be delayed by familial patterns or by conditions such as rickets, hypopituitarism, hypothyroidism, or Down syndrome. Supernumerary teeth and congenital absence of teeth are probably normal variants.

Table 310–1. TOOTH ERUPTION TIMES

TEETH	NO.	AGE AT ERUPTION*
Deciduous (20 total)		
Lower central incisors	2	5–9 mo
Upper central incisors	2	8–12 mo
Upper lateral incisors	2	10–12 mo
Lower lateral incisors	2	12–15 mo
1st molars†	4	10–16 mo
Canines	4	16–20 mo
2nd molars†	4	20–30 mo
Permanent (32 total)		
1st molars†	4	5–7 yr
Incisors	8	6–8 yr
Bicuspids	8	9–12 yr
Canines	4	10–13 yr
2nd molars†	4	11–13 yr
3rd molars†	4	17–25 yr

*Varies greatly.

†Molars are numbered from the front to the back of the mouth (see Fig. 101–1 on p. 858).

CHILDHOOD DEVELOPMENT

Development is often divided into specific domains, such as gross motor, fine motor, language, cognition, and social/emotional growth. These designations are useful, but substantial overlap exists. Studies have established average ages at which specific milestones are reached, as well as ranges of normality. In a normal child, progress within the different domains varies, as in the toddler who walks late but speaks in sentences early (see Table 310–2).

Environmental influences, ranging from nutrition to stimulation and from the impact of disease to the effects of psychologic factors, interact with genetic factors to determine the pace and pattern of development.

Assessment of development occurs constantly as parents, school personnel, and clinicians evaluate children. Many tools are available for monitoring development more specifically. The Denver Developmental Screening Test II facilitates evaluation in several domains. The scoring sheet indicates the average ages for achieving certain milestones and nicely shows the critical concept of a range of normality. Other tools can also be used (see Table 310–2).

Motor Development

Motor development includes fine motor (eg, picking up small objects, drawing) and gross motor (eg, walking, climbing stairs) skills. It is a continuous process that depends on familial patterns, environmental factors (eg, when activity is limited by prolonged illness), and specific disorders (eg, cerebral palsy, intellectual disability, muscular dystrophy). Children typically begin to walk at 12 mo, can climb stairs holding on at 18 mo,

Table 310–2. DEVELOPMENTAL MILESTONES*

AGE	BEHAVIOR
Birth	Sleeps much of the time Sucks Clears airway Responds with crying to discomforts and intrusions
4 wk	Brings hands toward eyes and mouth Moves head from side to side when lying on stomach Eyes follow an object moved in an arc about 15 cm above face to the midline Responds to a noise in some way (eg, startling, crying, quieting) May turn toward familiar sounds and voices Focuses on a face
6 wk	Regards objects in the line of vision Begins to smile when spoken to Lies flat on abdomen Head lags when pulled to a sitting position
3 mo	Holds head steady on sitting Raises head 45° when lying on stomach Opens and shuts hands Pushes down when feet are placed on a flat surface Swings at and reaches for dangling toys Follows an object moved in an arc above face from one side to the other Watches faces intently Smiles at sound of caretaker's voice Vocalizes sounds
5–6 mo	Holds head steady when upright Sits with support Rolls over, usually from stomach to back Reaches for objects Recognizes people at a distance Listens intently to human voices Smiles spontaneously Squeals in delight Babbles to toys
7 mo	Sits without support Bears some weight on legs when held upright Transfers objects from hand to hand Holds own bottle Looks for dropped object Responds to own name Responds to being told "no" Combines vowels and consonants to babble Moves body with excitement in anticipation of playing Plays peekaboo

Table continues on the following page.

Table 310–2. DEVELOPMENTAL MILESTONES* (*Continued*)

AGE	BEHAVIOR
9 mo	Sits well Crawls or creeps on hands and knees Pulls self up to standing position Works to get a toy that is out of reach; objects if toy is taken away Gets into a sitting position from stomach Stands holding on to someone or something Says "mama" or "dada" indiscriminately
12 mo	Walks by holding furniture ("cruising") or others' hands May walk 1 or 2 steps without support Stands for a few moments at a time Says "Dada" and "Mama" to the appropriate person Drinks from a cup Claps hands and waves bye-bye Speaks several words
18 mo	Walks well Can climb stairs holding on Draws a vertical stroke Makes a tower of 4 cubes Turns several book pages at a time Speaks about 10 words Pulls toys on strings Partially feeds self
2–2½ yr	Runs well/with coordination Climbs on furniture Jumps Climbs up and down stairs without help Handles a spoon well Turns single book pages Makes a tower of 7 cubes Opens doors Scribbles in a circular pattern Puts on simple clothing Makes 2- or 3-word sentences Verbalizes toilet needs
3 yr	Mature gait in walking Rides a tricycle Favors using one hand over the other Copies a circle Dresses well except for buttons and laces Counts to 10 and uses plurals Recognizes at least 3 colors Questions constantly Feeds self well Can take care of toilet needs (in about half of children)
4 yr	Alternates feet going up and down stairs Throws a ball overhand Hops on 1 foot Copies a cross Dresses self Washes hands and face
5 yr	Skips Catches a bounced ball Copies a triangle Draws a person in 6 parts Knows 4 colors Dresses and undresses without help
6 yr	Walks along a straight line from heel to toe Writes name

*The sequence is fairly consistent, but the timing of milestones varies; times above represent median values.

and run well at 2 yr, but the age at which these milestones are achieved by normal children varies widely. Motor development cannot be significantly accelerated by applying increased stimulation.

Language Development

The ability to understand language precedes the ability to speak; children with few words usually can understand a great deal. Although delays in expressive speech are typically not accompanied by other developmental delays, all children with excessive language delays should be evaluated for the presence of other delays in development. Children who have delays in both receptive and expressive speech more often have additional developmental problems. Evaluation of any delay should start with an assessment of hearing. Most children who experience speech delay have normal intelligence. In contrast, children with accelerated speech development are often of above-average intelligence.

Speech progresses from the utterance of vowel sounds (cooing) to the introduction of syllables that start with consonants (ba-ba-ba). Most children can say "Dada" and "Mama" specifically by 12 mo, use several words by 18 mo, and form 2- or 3-word phrases by 2 yr. The average 3-yr-old child can carry on a conversation. A 4-yr-old child can tell simple stories and can engage in conversation with adults or other children. A 5-yr-old child may have a vocabulary of several thousand words.

Even before age 18 mo, children can listen to and understand a story being read to them. By age 5, children are able to recite the alphabet and to recognize simple words in print. These skills are all fundamental to learning how to read simple words, phrases, and sentences. Depending on exposure to books and natural abilities, most children begin to read by age 6 or 7. These milestones are highly variable.

Cognitive Development

Cognitive development refers to the intellectual maturation of children. Increasingly, appropriate attachments and nurturing in infancy and early childhood are recognized as critical factors in cognitive growth and emotional health. For example, reading to children from an early age, providing intellectually stimulating experiences, and providing warm and nurturing relationships all have a major impact on growth in these domains.

Intellect is appraised in young children by observations of language skills, curiosity, and problem-solving abilities. As children become more verbal, intellectual functioning becomes easier to assess using a number of specialized clinical tools. Once children start school, they undergo constant monitoring as part of the academic process.

At age 2 yr, most children understand the concept of time in broad terms. Many 2- and 3-yr-old children believe that anything that happened in the past happened "yesterday," and anything that will happen in the future will happen "tomorrow." A child at this age has a vivid imagination but has difficulty distinguishing fantasy from reality.

By age 4 yr, most children have a more complicated understanding of time. They realize that the day is divided into morning, afternoon, and night. They can even appreciate the change in seasons.

By age 7 yr, children's intellectual capabilities become more complex. By this time, children become increasingly able to focus on more than one aspect of an event or situation at the same time. For example, school-aged children can appreciate that a tall, slender container can hold the same amount of water as a short, broad one. They can appreciate that medicine can taste bad but can make them feel better, or that their mother can be angry at them but can still love them. Children are increasingly able to understand another person's perspective and so learn the essentials of taking turns in games or conversations. In addition, school-aged children are able to follow agreed-upon rules of games. Children of this age are also increasingly able to reason using the powers of observation and multiple points of view.

Emotional and Behavioral Development

Emotion and behavior are based on the child's developmental stage and temperament. Every child has an individual temperament, or mood. Some children may be cheerful and adaptable and easily develop regular routines of sleeping, waking, eating, and other daily activities. These children tend to respond positively to new situations. Other children are not very adaptable and may have great irregularities in their routine. These children tend to respond negatively to new situations. Still other children are in between.

Emotional growth and the acquisition of social skills are assessed by watching children interact with others in everyday situations. When children acquire speech, the understanding of their emotional state becomes much more accurate. As with intellect, emotional functioning can be delineated more precisely with specialized tools.

Crying is infants' primary means of communication. Infants cry because they are hungry, uncomfortable, distressed, and for many other reasons that may not be obvious. Infants cry most—typically 3 h/day—at age 6 wk, usually decreasing to 1 h/day by age 3 mo. Parents typically offer crying infants food, change their diaper, and look for a source of pain or discomfort. If these measures do not work, holding or walking with the infant sometimes helps. Occasionally nothing works. Parents should not force food on crying infants, who will readily eat if hunger is the cause of their distress.

At about age 8 mo, infants normally become more anxious about being separated from their parents. Separations at bedtime and at places like child care centers may be difficult and can be marked by temper tantrums. This behavior can last for many months. For many older children, a special blanket or stuffed animal serves at this time as a transitional object that acts as a symbol for the absent parent.

At age 2 to 3 yr, children begin to test their limits and do what they have been forbidden to do, simply to see what will happen. The frequent "nos" that children hear from parents reflect the struggle for independence at this age. Although distressing to parents and children, tantrums are normal because they help children express their frustration during a time when they cannot verbalize their feelings well. Parents can help decrease the number of tantrums by not letting their children become overtired or unduly frustrated and by knowing their children's behavior patterns and avoiding situations that are likely to induce tantrums. Some young children have particular difficulty controlling their impulses and need their parents to set stricter limits around which there can be some safety and regularity in their world.

At age 18 mo to 2 yr, children typically begin to establish gender identity. During the preschool years, children also acquire a notion of gender role, of what boys and girls typically do. Exploration of the genitals is expected at this age and signals that children are beginning to make a connection between gender and body image.

Between age 2 yr and 3 yr, children begin to play more interactively with other children. Although they may still be possessive about toys, they may begin to share and even take turns in play. Asserting ownership of toys by saying, "That is mine!" helps establish the sense of self. Although children at this age strive for independence, they still need their parents nearby for security and support. For example, they may walk away from their parents when they feel curious only to later hide behind their parents when they are fearful.

At age 3 to 5 yr, many children become interested in fantasy play and imaginary friends. Fantasy play allows children to safely act out different roles and strong feelings in acceptable ways. Fantasy play also helps children grow socially. They learn to resolve conflicts with parents or other children in ways that help them vent frustrations and maintain self-esteem. Also at this time, typical childhood fears like that of "the monster in the closet" emerge. These fears are normal.

At age 7 to 12 yr, children work through numerous issues: self-concept, the foundation for which is laid by competency in the classroom; relationships with peers, which are determined by the ability to socialize and fit in well; and family relationships, which are determined in part by the approval children gain from parents and siblings. Although many children seem to place a high value on the peer group, they still look primarily to parents for support and guidance. Siblings can serve as role models and as valuable supports and critics regarding what can and cannot be done. This period of time is very active for children, who engage in many activities and are eager to explore new activities. At this age, children are eager learners and often respond well to advice about safety, healthy lifestyles, and avoidance of high-risk behaviors.

PHYSICAL GROWTH AND SEXUAL MATURATION OF ADOLESCENTS

During adolescence (usually considered age 10 to the late teens or early 20s), boys and girls reach adult height and weight and undergo puberty. For boys, see Sexual Differentiation, Adrenarche, and Puberty on p. 2127; for girls, see Puberty on p. 2247. The timing and speed with which these changes occur vary and are affected by both heredity and environment.

After age 2, growth parameters are charted using growth charts from the CDC.[1]

1. Grummer-Strawn LM, Reinold C, Krebs NF, Centers for Disease Control and Prevention (CDC): Use of World Health Organization and CDC growth charts for children aged 0–59 months in the United States. *MMWR Recomm Rep* 10(RR-9):1–15, 2010. Clarification and additional information. *MMWR Recomm Rep* 59(36): 1184, 2010.

Physical Growth

A growth spurt in boys occurs sometime between ages 12 and 17, with the peak typically between ages 13 and 15; a gain of > 10 cm can be expected in the year of peak velocity. A growth spurt in girls occurs sometime between ages 9½ and 14½, with the peak typically between ages 11 and 13½; gain may reach 9 cm in the year of peak velocity.

If puberty is delayed, growth in height may slow considerably. If the delay is not pathologic, the adolescent growth spurt occurs later and growth catches up, with height crossing percentile lines until the child reaches a genetically determined stature. At age 18, almost 2.5 cm of growth remains for boys and slightly less for girls, for whom growth is 99% complete. In girls with true precocious puberty (before age 8), an early growth spurt occurs along with menarche at a young age and, ultimately, short stature results because of early closure of growth plates. Although precocious puberty is defined as development starting before age 8, some girls who develop before age 8 may be normal.

All organ systems and the body as a whole undergo major growth during adolescence; breasts in girls and genitals and body hair in both sexes undergo the most obvious changes. Even when this process goes normally, substantial emotional adjustments are required. If the timing is atypical, particularly in a boy whose physical development is delayed or in a girl whose development occurs early, additional emotional stress is likely. Most boys who grow slowly have a constitutional delay and catch up eventually. Evaluation to exclude pathologic causes and reassurance are needed.

Guidance concerning nutrition, fitness, and lifestyle should be given to all adolescents, with special attention paid to the role of activities such as sports, the arts, social activities, and community service in the adolescent's life. Relative requirements for protein and energy (g or kcal/kg body weight) decline progressively from the end of infancy through adolescence (see Table 1–4 on p. 4), although absolute requirements increase. Protein requirements for boys age 15 to 18 yr are 0.9 g/kg/day and for girls of the same age are 0.8 g/kg/day; mean relative energy requirements for boys age 15 to 18 yr are 45.5 kcal/kg and for girls of the same age are 40 kcal/kg.

Sexual Maturation

Sexual maturation generally proceeds in an established sequence in both sexes. The age at onset and rapidity of sexual development vary and are influenced by genetic and environmental factors. Sexual maturity begins earlier today than a century ago, probably because of improvements in nutrition, general health, and living conditions—eg, the average age of menarche has decreased by about 3 yr over the past 100 yr. The physiologic changes that underlie sexual maturation are discussed in Chs. 251 and 269.

In boys, sexual changes begin with enlargement of the scrotum and testes, followed by lengthening of the penis and enlargement of the seminal vesicles and prostate. Next, pubic hair appears. Axillary and facial hair appears about 2 yr after pubic hair. The growth spurt usually begins a year after the testes start enlarging (see Fig. 251–1 on p. 2128). The median age for first ejaculation (between 12½ yr and 14 yr in the US) is affected by psychologic, cultural, and biologic factors. First ejaculation takes place about 1 yr after penis growth accelerates. Gynecomastia, usually in the form of breast buds, is common among young adolescent boys and usually resolves within several years.

In most girls, breast budding is the first visible sign of sexual maturation, followed closely by the initiation of the growth spurt. Shortly thereafter, pubic and axillary hair appears. Menarche generally occurs about 2 yr after onset of breast development and when growth in height slows after reaching its peak. Menarche occurs within a wide range, with most girls in the US starting their periods at 12 or 13 yr (see Fig. 269–2 on p. 2248). The stages of breast growth (see Fig. 269–3 on p. 2249) and pubic hair development (see Fig. 269–4 on p. 2249) can be detailed using the Tanner method.

If the order of sexual changes is disturbed, growth may be abnormal, and the physician should consider pathologic reasons.

ADOLESCENT DEVELOPMENT

Adolescence is a developmental period during which dependent children grow into independent adults. This period usually begins at about age 10 yr and lasts until the late teens or early 20s. During adolescence, children undergo striking physical, intellectual, and emotional growth. Guiding adolescents through this period is a challenge for parents as well as clinicians.

Intellectual and Behavioral Development

In early adolescence, children begin to develop the capacity for abstract, logical thought. This increased sophistication leads to an enhanced awareness of self and the ability to reflect on one's own being. Because of the many noticeable physical changes of adolescence, this self-awareness often turns into self-consciousness, with an accompanying feeling of awkwardness. The adolescent also has a preoccupation with physical appearance and attractiveness and a heightened sensitivity to differences from peers.

Adolescents also apply their new reflective capabilities to moral issues. Preadolescents understand right and wrong as fixed and absolute. Older adolescents often question standards of behavior and may reject traditions—to the consternation of parents. Ideally, this reflection culminates in the development and internalization of the adolescent's own moral code.

As adolescents encounter schoolwork that is more complex, they begin to identify areas of interest as well as relative strengths and weaknesses. Adolescence is a period during which young people begin to consider career options, although most do not have a clearly defined goal. Parents and clinicians must be aware of the adolescent's capabilities, help the adolescent formulate realistic expectations, and be prepared to identify impediments to learning that need remediation, such as learning disabilities, attention problems, behavior problems, or inappropriate learning environments. Parents and clinicians should facilitate apprenticeships and experiences that expose older adolescents to potential career opportunities either during school or during school vacations. These opportunities may help adolescents focus their career choices and future studies.

Many adolescents begin to engage in risky behaviors, such as fast driving. Many adolescents begin to experiment sexually, and some may engage in risky sexual practices. Some adolescents may engage in illegal activities, such as theft and alcohol and drug use. Experts speculate that these behaviors occur in part because adolescents tend to overestimate their own abilities in preparation for leaving their home. Recent studies of the nervous system also have shown that the parts of the brain that suppress impulses are not fully mature until early adulthood.

Emotional Development

During adolescence, the regions of the brain that control emotions develop and mature. This phase is characterized by seemingly spontaneous outbursts that can be challenging for parents and teachers who often receive the brunt. Adolescents gradually learn to suppress inappropriate thoughts and actions and replace them with goal-oriented behaviors.

The emotional aspect of growth is most trying, often taxing the patience of parents, teachers, and clinicians. Emotional lability is a direct result of neurologic development during this period, as the parts of the brain that control emotions mature. Frustration may also arise from growth in multiple domains.

A major area of conflict arises from the adolescent's desire for more freedom, which clashes with the parents' strong instincts to protect their children from harm. Parents may need help in renegotiating their role and slowly allowing their adolescents more privileges as well as expecting them to accept greater responsibility for themselves and within the family.

Communication within even stable families can be difficult and is worsened when families are divided or parents have emotional problems of their own. Clinicians can be of great help by offering adolescents and parents sensible, practical, concrete, supportive help while facilitating communication within the family.

Social and Psychologic Development

The family is the center of social life for children. During adolescence, the peer group begins to replace the family as the child's primary social focus. Peer groups are often established because of distinctions in dress, appearance, attitudes, hobbies, interests, and other characteristics that may seem profound or trivial to outsiders. Initially, peer groups are usually same-sex but typically become mixed later in adolescence. These groups assume an importance to adolescents because they provide validation for the adolescent's tentative choices and support in stressful situations.

Adolescents who find themselves without a peer group may develop intense feelings of being different and alienated. Although these feelings usually do not have permanent effects, they may worsen the potential for dysfunctional or antisocial behavior. At the other extreme, the peer group can assume too much importance, also resulting in antisocial behavior. Gang membership is more common when the home and social environments are unable to counterbalance the dysfunctional demands of a peer group.

Clinicians should screen all adolescents for mental health disorders, such as depression, bipolar disorder, and anxiety. Mental health disorders increase in incidence during this stage of life and may result in suicidal thinking or behavior. Psychotic disorders, such as schizophrenia, although rare, most often come to attention during late adolescence. Eating disorders, such as anorexia nervosa and bulimia nervosa, are relatively common among girls and may be difficult to detect because adolescents go to great lengths to hide the behaviors and weight changes.

Substance use typically begins during adolescence. More than 70% of adolescents in the United States try alcohol before they graduate high school. Binge drinking is common and leads to both acute and chronic health risks. Research has shown that adolescents who start drinking alcohol at a young age are more likely to develop an alcohol use disorder as an adult. For example, adolescents who start drinking at age 13 are 5 times more likely to develop an alcohol use disorder than those who start drinking at age 21.

Almost 50% of US adolescents try cigarettes and more than 40% try marijuana while they are in high school. Use of other drugs is much less common, although misuse of prescription drugs, including drugs for pain and stimulants, is on the rise.

Parents can have a strong positive influence on their children by setting a good example (eg, using alcohol in moderation, avoiding use of illicit drugs), sharing their values, and setting high expectations regarding staying away from drugs. Parents also should teach children that prescription drugs should be used only as directed by a physician. All adolescents should be confidentially screened for substance use. Appropriate advice should be given as part of routine health care because even very brief interventions by physicians and health care practitioners have been shown to decrease substance use by adolescents.

Sexuality

In addition to adapting to bodily changes, the adolescent must become comfortable with the role of adult and must put sexual urges, which can be very strong and sometimes frightening, into perspective.

Some adolescents struggle with the issue of sexual identity and may be afraid to reveal their sexual orientation to friends or family members. Homosexual adolescents may face unique challenges as their sexuality develops. Adolescents may feel unwanted or unaccepted by family or peers if they express homosexual desires. Such pressure (especially during a time when social acceptance is critically important) can cause severe stress. Fear of abandonment by parents, sometimes real, may lead to dishonest or at least incomplete communication between adolescents and their parents. These adolescents also can be taunted and bullied by their peers. Threats of physical violence should be taken seriously and reported to school officials. The emotional development of homosexual and heterosexual adolescents is best helped by supportive clinicians, friends, and family members.

Few elements of the human experience combine physical, intellectual, and emotional aspects as thoroughly as sexuality. Helping adolescents put sexuality into a healthy context through honest answers regarding reproduction and sexually transmitted diseases is extremely important. Adolescents and their parents should be encouraged to speak openly regarding their attitudes toward sex and sexuality; parents' opinions remain an important determinant of adolescent behavior.

311 Hereditary Periodic Fever Syndromes

Hereditary periodic fever syndromes are hereditary disorders characterized by recurrent fever and other symptoms that are not explained by other causes.

Most patients develop symptoms during childhood; < 10% develop symptoms after age 18. Disorders best characterized are

- Familial Mediterranean fever
- Hyper-IgD syndrome
- Tumor necrosis factor (TNF) receptor–associated periodic syndrome

Other disorders include

- The hereditary cryopyrin-associated periodic syndromes (CAPS; cryopyrinopathies): Familial cold autoinflammatory syndrome (FCAS), Muckle-Wells syndrome (MWS), and neonatal-onset multisystem inflammatory disease (NOMID)
- PAPA (pyogenic arthritis, pyoderma gangrenosum, and acne) syndrome
- PFAPA (periodic fever, aphthous stomatitis, pharyngitis, and cervical adenitis) syndrome, which may not be hereditary

FAMILIAL MEDITERRANEAN FEVER

Familial Mediterranean fever is an autosomal recessive disorder characterized by recurrent bouts of fever and peritonitis, sometimes with pleuritis, skin lesions, arthritis, and, very rarely, pericarditis. Renal amyloidosis may develop, sometimes leading to renal failure. People with genetic origins in the Mediterranean basin are more frequently affected than other ethnic groups. Diagnosis is largely clinical, although genetic testing is available. Treatment with prophylactic colchicine prevents acute attacks as well as amyloidosis in almost all patients. Prognosis is excellent with treatment.

Familial Mediterranean fever (FMF) is a disease of people with genetic origins in the Mediterranean basin, predominantly Sephardic Jews, North African Arabs, Armenians, Turks, Greeks, and Italians. However, cases have occurred among enough other groups (eg, Ashkenazi Jews, Cubans, Japanese) to caution against excluding the diagnosis solely on the basis of ancestry. Up to 50% of patients have a family history of the disorder, usually involving siblings.

Etiology

FMF is caused by mutations in the *MEFV* gene on the short arm of chromosome 16 and is inherited in an autosomal recessive manner. The *MEFV* gene normally codes a protein named pyrin, which is expressed in circulating neutrophils. Its presumed action is to blunt the inflammatory response, possibly by inhibiting neutrophil activation and chemotaxis. Gene mutations result in defective pyrin molecules; it is hypothesized that the altered pyrin cannot suppress minor, unknown triggers to inflammation that are normally checked by intact pyrin. The clinical consequence is spontaneous bouts of neutrophil-predominant inflammation in the abdominal cavity as well as in other sites.

Symptoms and Signs

Onset of familial Mediterranean fever is usually between the ages of 5 and 15 yr but may be much later or earlier, even during infancy. Attacks have no regular pattern of recurrence. They usually last 24 to 72 h but may last longer. Frequency ranges from 2 attacks/wk to 1 attack/yr (most commonly, once every 2 to 6 wk). Severity and frequency tend to decrease during pregnancy and in patients with amyloidosis. Spontaneous remissions may last years.

Fever as high as 40° C, usually accompanied by peritonitis, is the major manifestation. Abdominal pain (usually starting in one quadrant and spreading to the whole abdomen) occurs in about 95% of patients and can vary in severity with each attack. Decreased bowel sounds, distention, guarding, and rebound tenderness are likely to occur at the peak of an attack and cannot be differentiated from a perforated viscus by physical examination. Consequently, some patients have undergone urgent laparotomy before the correct diagnosis was made. With diaphragmatic involvement, splinting of the chest and pain in one or both shoulders may occur.

Other manifestations of FMF include acute pleurisy (in 30%); arthritis (in 25%), usually involving the knee, ankle, and hip; an erysipelas-like rash of the lower leg; and scrotal swelling and pain caused by inflammation of the tunica vaginalis of the testis. Pericarditis occurs very rarely. The pleural, synovial, and skin manifestations of FMF vary in frequency among different populations and are less frequently encountered in the US than elsewhere.

Despite the severity of symptoms during acute attacks, most patients recover swiftly and remain free of illness until their next attack.

Complications of FMF: The most significant long-term complication is

- Chronic renal failure caused by deposition of amyloid protein in the kidneys

Amyloid may also be deposited in the GI tract, liver, spleen, heart, testes, and thyroid.

FMF causes infertility or spontaneous abortion in about one third of women because peritoneal pelvic adhesions form, interfering with conception. In women with FMF, about 20 to 30% of pregnancies end in fetal loss.

Diagnosis

- Clinical evaluation
- Genetic testing

Diagnosis of FMF is mainly clinical, but genetic testing is available and is particularly useful in evaluation of atypical cases. However, current genetic testing is not infallible; some patients with phenotypically unmistakable FMF have only a single mutated gene or occasionally no evident pyrin mutations.

Nonspecific findings include elevations in WBCs with neutrophil predominance, ESR, C-reactive protein, and fibrinogen. Urinary excretion of > 0.5 g protein/24 h suggests renal amyloidosis.

Differential diagnosis includes acute intermittent porphyria, hereditary angioedema with abdominal attacks, relapsing pancreatitis, and other hereditary relapsing fevers.

Treatment

- Colchicine

Prophylactic colchicine 0.6 mg po bid (some patients require qid dosing; others a single daily dose) provides complete remission or distinct improvement in about 85% of patients. If attacks or subclinical inflammation persist, the colchicine dose should be increased. For patients with infrequent attacks that have a gradual onset, colchicine can be reserved until initial symptoms occur and then begun at 0.6 mg po q 1 h for 4 h, then q 2 h for 4 h, then q 12 h for 48 h. Initiation of colchicine at the peak of an attack is unlikely to be beneficial. Children often require adult dosages for effective prophylaxis. Widespread use of prophylactic colchicine has led to a dramatic reduction in the incidence of amyloidosis and subsequent renal failure.

Colchicine does not add to the increased risk of infertility and miscarriage among affected women; when taken during pregnancy, it does not increase the risk of teratogenic events. Lack of response to colchicine is often caused by poor adherence to the drug regimen, but a correlation has also been noted between poor response and diminished colchicine concentration in circulating monocytes. Alternative therapies for nonresponders include anakinra 100 mg sc once/day, rilonacept 2.2 mg/kg sc weekly, or canakinumab 150 mg sc q 4 wk.[1]

Opioids are sometimes needed for pain relief but should be used prudently to avoid addiction.

1. Ozen S, Demirkaya E, Erer B, et al: EULAR recommendations for the management of familial Mediterranean fever. *Ann Rheum Dis* 75(4):644–651, 2016. doi: 10.1136/annrheumdis-2015-208690.

KEY POINTS

- FMF is caused by an autosomal recessive mutation in a protein that helps modulate the inflammatory response in neutrophils.
- People with genetic origins in the Mediterranean basin are more commonly (but not exclusively) affected.
- Patients have brief episodes of fever, abdominal pain, and sometimes other symptoms such as pleuritis, arthritis, and rash.
- Renal amyloidosis, sometimes causing renal failure, is the most common complication, but prophylactic colchicine provides protection against amyloidosis.
- Diagnose clinically, but consider genetic testing for atypical cases.
- Daily colchicine results in significant protection against attacks in most patients, but a few require an immunomodulator such as anakinra, rilonacept, or canakinumab.

HYPER-IgD SYNDROME

Hyper-IgD syndrome is a rare autosomal recessive disorder in which recurring attacks of chills and fever begin during the first year of life. Episodes usually last 4 to 6 days and may be triggered by physiologic stress, such as vaccination or minor trauma. Diagnosis is mainly clinical but includes serum IgD level and possibly gene testing. Symptoms can be treated with NSAIDS, corticosteroids, and/or anakinra.

Hyper-IgD syndrome clusters in children of Dutch, French, and other Northern European ancestry and is caused by mutations in the gene coding mevalonate kinase, an enzyme important for cholesterol synthesis. Reduction in the synthesis of anti-inflammatory isoprenylated proteins may account for the clinical syndrome.

In addition to chills and fever, patients may have abdominal pain, vomiting or diarrhea, headache, and arthralgias. Signs of hyper-IgD syndrome include cervical lymphadenopathy, splenomegaly, arthritis, skin lesions (maculopapular rash, petechiae, or purpura), and orogenital aphthous ulcers.

Diagnosis of hyper-IgD syndrome is based on history, examination, and a serum IgD level of > 14 mg/mL; however, up to 20% of patients have normal serum IgD levels. Nonspecific abnormalities include leukocytosis and elevated acute-phase reactants during fever; elevated urinary mevalonic acid during attacks helps confirm the diagnosis. Gene testing is available but is negative in 25% of patients.

Treatment

- For attacks, anakinra

There are no proven treatments to prevent attacks. Patients can expect to have recurrent bouts of fever throughout their life, although episodes tend to become less frequent after adolescence. NSAIDs and corticosteroids may help relieve symptoms during attacks.

On-demand treatment of symptoms with anakinra has been used successfully.[1]

1. ter Haar NM, Oswald M, Jeyaratnam J, et al: Recommendations for the management of autoinflammatory diseases. *Ann Rheum Dis* 74(9):1636–1644, 2015. doi: 10.1136/annrheumdis-2015-207546.

TNF RECEPTOR–ASSOCIATED PERIODIC SYNDROME

(Familial Hibernian Fever)

TNF receptor–associated periodic syndrome is an autosomal dominant disorder causing recurrent fever and painful, migratory myalgias with tender overlying erythema. Levels of type 1 TNF receptors are low. Diagnosis is by genetic testing. Treatment is with corticosteroids, etanercept, anakinra, and canakinumab.

TNF receptor–associated periodic syndrome (TRAPS) was originally described in a family of Irish and Scottish pedigree but has been reported in many different ethnic groups. It results from mutations in the gene coding the TNF receptor 1 (TNFR1). The mutation leads to aberrant inflammation due to accumulation of misfolded TNFR1 in the endoplasmic reticulum which activates the unfolded protein response. This response is an attempt to correct the abnormal proteins, but it generates reactive oxygen species that trigger inflammation.[1]

Attacks of this rare disorder usually begin before age 20. In 70% of patients, attacks last 7 to 21 days (average of 10 days).[2] The most distinctive features of an attack are fever and migratory myalgia and swelling in the extremities. The overlying skin is red and tender. Other symptoms of TRAPS may include headache, abdominal pain, diarrhea or constipation, nausea, painful conjunctivitis, periorbital edema, joint pain, rash, and testicular pain. Males are prone to develop inguinal hernias. Amyloidosis involving the kidneys has been reported in 10% of patients; the median age of presentation is 43 yr.

With treatment, the prognosis is good, but it is more guarded in patients with renal amyloidosis.

1. Dickie LJ, Aziz AM, Savic S, et al: Involvement of X-box binding protein 1 and reactive oxygen species pathways in the pathogenesis of tumour necrosis factor receptor-associated periodic syndrome. *Ann Rheum Dis* 71(12):2035–2043, 2012. doi: 10.1136/annrheumdis-2011-201197.
2. Lachmann HJ, Papa R, Gerhold K, et al: The phenotype of TNF receptor-associated autoinflammatory syndrome (TRAPS) at presentation: A series of 158 cases from the Eurofever/EUROTRAPS international registry. *Ann Rheum Dis* 73(12):2160–2167, 2014. doi: 10.1136/annrheumdis-2013-204184.

Diagnosis

- Clinical evaluation
- Genetic testing

Diagnosis of TRAPS is based on history, examination, and genetic testing. Nonspecific findings include neutrophilia, elevated acute-phase reactants, and polyclonal gammopathy during attacks. Patients should be screened regularly for proteinuria.

Treatment

- Corticosteroids
- Anakinra and canakinumab

Short-term corticosteroids (prednisone at least 20 mg po once/day), with or without NSAIDs, are effective for terminating inflammatory attacks. Dosage may need to be increased over time and may, over time, lead to more prolonged flare-ups.

Other options include anakinra 100 mg sc once/day[3,4] and canakinumab 150 mg sc q 4 wk.[5] Etanercept has proved to be only partially effective.[6,7]

3. ter Haar NM, Oswald M, Jeyaratnam J, et al: Recommendations for the management of autoinflammatory diseases. *Ann Rheum Dis* 74(9):1636–1644, 2015. doi: 10.1136/annrheumdis-2015-207546.
4. Gattorno M, Pelagatti MA, Meini A, et al: Persistent efficacy of anakinra in patients with TNFreceptor-associated periodic syndrome. *Arthritis Rheum* 58:1516–1520, 2008. doi: 10.1002/art.23475.
5. Gattorno M, Obici L, Cattalini M, et al: Canakinumab treatment for patients with active recurrent or chronic TNF receptor-associated periodic syndrome (TRAPS): An open-label, phase II study. *Ann Rheum Dis* 76(1):173–178, 2016. doi: 10.1136/annrheumdis-2015-209031.
6. Drewe E, McDermott EM, Powell PT, et al: Prospective study of anti-tumour necrosis factor receptor superfamily 1B fusion protein, and case study of anti-tumour necrosis factor receptor superfamily 1A fusion protein, in tumour necrosis factor receptor associated periodic syndrome (TRAPS): Clinical and laboratory findings in a series of seven patients. *Rheumatology* 42:235–239, 2003. doi:10.1093/rheumatology/keg070.
7. Quillinan N, Mannion G, Mohammad A, et al: Failure of sustained response to etanercept and refractoriness to anakinra in patients with T50M TNF-receptor-associated periodic syndrome. *Ann Rheum Dis* 70(9):1692–1693, 2011. doi: 10.1136/ard.2010.144279.

HEREDITARY CRYOPYRIN-ASSOCIATED PERIODIC SYNDROMES

(Cryopyrinopathies)

The hereditary cryopyrin-associated periodic syndromes (CAPS) are a group of autoinflammatory conditions triggered by cold ambient temperatures; they include familial cold autoinflammatory syndrome, Muckle-Wells syndrome, and neonatal-onset multisystem autoinflammatory disease.

Hereditary CAPS represent a spectrum of progressively severe disease. They are due to mutations in the gene encoding the protein cryopyrin, which mediates inflammation and IL-1β processing. Cryopyrin activity is augmented, triggering increased release of IL-1β from the NLRP3 inflammasome; the result is inflammation and fever. The lack of a confirmed genetic mutation may not preclude the diagnosis of CAPS because 40% of patients who have neonatal-onset multisystem autoinflammatory disease, 25% who have Muckle-Wells syndrome, and 10% of who have familial cold autoinflammatory syndrome do not have identifiable mutations based on standard genetic testing. Many of these patients exhibit somatic mosaicism, causing their phenotype.

Typically, **familial cold autoinflammatory syndrome** causes a cold-induced urticarial rash accompanied by fever and sometimes arthralgias. The condition often appears in the first year of life.

Muckle-Wells syndrome causes intermittent fevers, urticarial rash, joint pain, and progressive deafness; 25% of patients develop renal amyloidosis.

Neonatal-onset multisystem autoinflammatory disease tends to cause joint and limb deformities, facial deformities, chronic aseptic meningitis, cerebral atrophy, uveitis, papillary edema, delayed development, and amyloidosis, in addition to fever and a migratory urticarial rash. As many as 20% of patients die by age 20 if untreated.

CAPS are inherited as autosomal dominant disorders. They are treated with anakinra or canakinumab.[1,2]

1. Lachmann HJ, Kone-Paut I, Kuemmerle-Deschner JB, et al: Use of canakinumab in the cryopyrin-associated periodic syndrome. *N Engl J Med* 360(23):2416–2425, 2009. doi: 10.1056/NEJMoa0810787.
2. Sibley CH, Plass N, Snow J, et al: Sustained response and prevention of damage progression in patients with neonatal-onset multisystem inflammatory disease treated with anakinra: A cohort study to determine three- and five-year outcomes. *Arthritis Rheum* 64(7):2375–2386, 2012. doi: 10.1002/art.34409.

PAPA SYNDROME

PAPA (pyogenic arthritis, pyoderma gangrenosum, and acne) syndrome is an autosomal dominant disorder that affects the skin and joints.

PAPA syndrome is caused by mutations in a gene on chromosome 15q. The mutated gene produces a hyperphosphorylated protein that binds excessively to pyrin, thus restricting pyrin's anti-inflammatory activity.

Arthritis begins in the first decade of life and is progressively destructive. Episodes of mild trauma may trigger the arthritis. Poorly healing ulcers with undermined edges may appear, often at sites of injury (eg, at vaccination sites). Acne is usually nodulocystic and, if untreated, causes scarring.

Diagnosis of PAPA is based on clinical findings and a family history. The ulcers may be biopsied. Biopsy shows superficial ulceration and neutrophilic inflammation.

Treatment with etanercept or anakinra may be useful. Acne is treated with oral tetracycline or isotretinoin.

PFAPA SYNDROME

PFAPA (periodic fevers with aphthous stomatitis, pharyngitis, and adenitis) syndrome is a periodic fever syndrome that typically manifests between ages 2 yr and 5 yr; it is characterized by febrile episodes lasting 3 to 6 days, pharyngitis, aphthous ulcers, and adenopathy. Etiology and pathophysiology are undefined. Diagnosis is clinical. Treatment can include glucocorticoids, cimetidine, and, rarely, tonsIllectomy.

PFAPA syndrome is a relatively common periodic fever among children. Although genetic causes have not been determined, this syndrome tends to be grouped with hereditary fever syndromes. It typically starts in early childhood (between ages 2 yr and 5 yr) and tends to be more common among males.

Febrile episodes last 3 to 6 days and recur about every 28 days. The syndrome causes fatigue, chills, and occasionally abdominal pain and headache, as well as fever, pharyngitis, aphthous ulcers, and lymphadenopathy. Patients are healthy between episodes, and growth is normal.

Diagnosis

- Clinical evaluation

Diagnosis of PFAPA syndrome is based on clinical findings, which include the following:

- ≥ 3 febrile episodes, lasting up to 5 days and occurring at regular intervals
- Pharyngitis plus adenopathy or aphthous ulcers
- Good health between episodes and normal growth

Acute-phase reactants (eg, C-reactive protein, ESR) are elevated during a febrile episode but not between episodes. Neutropenia or other symptoms (eg, diarrhea, rash, cough) are not present; their presence suggests a different disorder. Specifically, cyclic neutropenia needs to be ruled out.

Treatment

- Sometimes glucocorticoids, cimetidine, and/or tonsillectomy

Treatment of PFAPA syndrome is optional; it can include glucocorticoids, cimetidine, and, rarely, tonsillectomy. Other drugs such as anakinra have been tried with some success in refractory cases. Patients tend to outgrow this syndrome without sequelae.

312 Human Immunodeficiency Virus Infection in Infants and Children

Human immunodeficiency virus (HIV) infection is caused by the retrovirus HIV-1 (and less commonly by the related retrovirus HIV-2). Infection leads to progressive immunologic deterioration and opportunistic infections and cancers. The end stage is acquired immunodeficiency syndrome (AIDS). Diagnosis is by viral antibodies in children > 18 mo and virologic nucleic acid amplification tests (such as PCR) in children < 18 mo. Treatment is with combinations of antiretroviral drugs.

The general natural history and pathophysiology of pediatric HIV infection is similar to that in adults; however, the method of infection, clinical presentations, and treatments often differ. HIV-infected children also have unique social integration issues (see Sidebar 312–1).

Epidemiology

In the US, HIV probably occurred in children almost as early as in adults but was not clinically recognized for several years. Thus far, about 10,000 cases have been reported in children and young adolescents, representing only 1% of total cases. In 2013, fewer than 100 new cases were diagnosed in children < 13 yr.

More than 95% of HIV-infected US children acquired the infection from their mother, either before or around the time of birth (vertical transmission). Most of the remainder (including children with hemophilia or other coagulation disorders) received contaminated blood or blood products. A few cases are the result of sexual abuse. Vertical transmission has declined significantly in the US from about 25% in 1991 (resulting in > 1600 infected children annually) to 1% in 2013 (resulting in only about 70 to 100 infected children annually). Vertical transmission has been reduced by using comprehensive serologic screening and treating of infected pregnant women during both pregnancy and delivery and by providing short-term antiretroviral prophylaxis to exposed newborns.

However, the total number of HIV-infected US adolescents continues to increase despite the marked success in decreasing perinatal HIV infection. This paradoxical increase is a result of both greater survival among perinatally infected children and new cases of HIV infection acquired via sexual transmission among other adolescents (in particular, among young men who

Sidebar 312–1. Integration of HIV-Infected Children

HIV infection in a child affects the entire family. Serologic testing of siblings and parents is recommended. The physician must provide education and ongoing counseling.

The infected child should be taught good hygiene and behavior to reduce risk to others. How much and when the child is told about the illness depends on age and maturity. Older children and adolescents should be made aware of their diagnosis and the possibility of sexual transmission and should be counseled appropriately. Families may be unwilling to share the diagnosis with people outside the immediate family because it can create social isolation. Feelings of guilt are common. Family members, including children, can become clinically depressed and require counseling.

Because HIV infection is not acquired through the typical types of contact that occur among children (eg, through saliva or tears), HIV-infected children should be allowed to attend school without restrictions. Similarly, there are no inherent reasons to restrict foster care, adoptive placement, or child care of HIV-infected children. Conditions that may pose an increased risk to others (eg, aggressive biting or the presence of exudative, weeping skin lesions that cannot be covered) may require special precautions.

The number of school personnel aware of the child's condition should be kept to the minimum needed to ensure proper care. The family has the right to inform the school, but people involved in the care and education of an infected child must respect the child's right to privacy. Disclosures of information should be made only with the informed consent of the parents or legal guardians and age-appropriate assent of the child.

have sex with men). Reducing transmission of HIV among young men who have sex with men continues to be an important focus of domestic HIV control efforts as is continuing the reduction of vertical transmission.

Worldwide, about 2 million children have HIV infection (5% of the total caseload worldwide). Each year, about 150,000 more children are infected (7 to 10% of all new infections), and about 110,000 children die. Although these numbers represent a daunting amount of illness, new programs created to deliver antiretroviral therapy (ART) to pregnant women and children have reduced the annual number of new childhood infections and childhood deaths by 33% in the past few years. However, infected children still do not receive ART nearly as often as adults. Interrupting vertical transmission and providing treatment to HIV-infected children remain the two most important goals of global pediatric HIV medicine.

Transmission: The infection risk for an infant born to an HIV-positive mother who did not receive ART during pregnancy is estimated at 25% (range 13 to 39%). Risk factors for vertical transmission include

- Seroconversion during pregnancy or breastfeeding (major risk)
- High plasma viral RNA concentrations (major risk)
- Advanced disease
- Low peripheral CD4+ T-cell counts

Cesarean delivery before onset of active labor reduces the risk of mother-to-child transmission (MTCT). However, it is clear that MTCT is reduced most significantly by giving combination ART, usually including zidovudine (ZDV), to the mother and neonate (see p. 2611). ZDV monotherapy reduces MTCT from 25% to about 8%, and current combination ART reduces it to 1%.

HIV has been detected in both the cellular and cell-free fractions of human breast milk. The incidence of transmission by breastfeeding is about 6/100 breastfed children/yr. Estimates of the overall risk of transmission through breastfeeding are 12 to 14%, reflecting varying durations of breastfeeding. Transmission by breastfeeding is greatest in mothers with high plasma viral RNA concentrations (eg, women who become infected during pregnancy or during the period of breastfeeding).

Classification: HIV infection causes a broad spectrum of disease, of which AIDS is the most severe. Classification schemes established by the Centers for Disease Control and Prevention (CDC) define the progression of clinical and immunologic decline.

Clinical categories in children < 13 yr (Table 312–1) are defined by presence or absence of certain common opportunistic infections or cancers. These categories are

- N = Not symptomatic
- A = Mildly symptomatic
- B = Moderately symptomatic
- C = Severely symptomatic

Immunologic categories in children < 13 yr (see Table 312–2) reflect the degree of immune suppression based on the CD4+ T-cell count (absolute count and as percentage of total lymphocyte count):

- 1 = No evidence of immune suppression
- 2 = Moderate suppression
- 3 = Severe suppression

Thus, a child classified in stage B3 would have moderately advanced clinical symptoms and severe immunocompromise. Clinical and immunologic categories form a unidirectional hierarchy; once classified at a certain level, children cannot be reclassified at a less severe level, regardless of clinical or immunologic improvement.

These clinical and immunologic categories are becoming less relevant in the era of combination ART, which, when taken as prescribed, almost invariably leads to a decrease in symptoms and an increase in CD4+ T-cell counts. The categories are most useful for clinical research and for describing the severity of illness at the time of diagnosis. The classification system for adolescents > 13 yr and adults has been revised and now simply includes CD4+ T-cell counts as the major component of staging, unless AIDS-defining conditions (eg, opportunistic infections) are present (see Table 312–1).

Table 312–1. CLINICAL CATEGORIES FOR CHILDREN AGED < 13 YR WITH HIV INFECTION

Category N: Not symptomatic

Children who have no symptoms or signs considered to result from HIV infection or who have only 1 of the conditions listed in category A

Category A: Mildly symptomatic

Children with ≥ 2 of the conditions listed below but none of the conditions listed in category B or C:

Dermatitis
Hepatomegaly
Lymphadenopathy (≥ 0.5 cm at > 2 sites; bilateral = 1 site)
Parotitis
Recurrent or persistent upper respiratory tract infection, sinusitis, or otitis media
Splenomegaly

Category B: Moderately symptomatic

Children with symptomatic conditions attributed to HIV infection beyond those listed in category A but not among those listed in category C; conditions in category B include but are not limited to the following:

Anemia (Hb < 8 g/dL), neutropenia (< 1,000/μL), or thrombocytopenia (< 100,000/μL) persisting ≥ 30 days
Bacterial meningitis, pneumonia, or sepsis (single episode)
Candidiasis Cervical cancer, invasive, in a child or adolescent > 6 yr of age, oropharyngeal (thrush), persisting (> 2 mo) in children > 6 mo of age
Cardiomyopathy
Cytomegalovirus infection with onset before 1 mo of age
Diarrhea, recurrent or chronic
Hepatitis
Herpes zoster (shingles) involving ≥ 2 distinct episodes or > 1 dermatome
HSV stomatitis, recurrent (> 2 episodes within 1 yr)
HSV bronchitis, pneumonitis, or esophagitis with onset before 1 mo of age
Leiomyosarcoma
Lymphoid interstitial pneumonitis or pulmonary lymphoid hyperplasia complex
Nephropathy
Nocardiosis
Persistent fever (lasting > 1 mo)
Toxoplasmosis with onset before 1 mo of age
Varicella, disseminated (complicated chickenpox)

Category C: Severely symptomatic (Stage 3-defining opportunistic infections)

Children with ≥ 1 of the following conditions:

Serious bacterial infections, multiple or recurrent (ie, any combination of ≥ 2 culture-confirmed infections within a 2-yr period), of the following types: septicemia, pneumonia, meningitis, bone or joint infection, or abscess of an internal organ or body cavity (excluding otitis media, superficial skin or mucosal abscesses, and indwelling catheter-related infections)
Candidiasis, esophageal or pulmonary (bronchi, trachea, lungs)
Cervical cancer, invasive, in a child or adolescent > 6 yr of age
Coccidioidomycosis, disseminated (at a site other than or in addition to the lungs or cervical or hilar lymph nodes)
Cryptococcosis, extrapulmonary
Cryptosporidiosis or isosporiasis with diarrhea persisting > 1 mo
Cytomegalovirus disease with onset of symptoms at age > 1 mo (at a site other than the liver, spleen, or lymph nodes)
Cytomegalovirus retinitis (with loss of vision)
Encephalopathy (≥1 of the following progressive findings present for ≥ 2 mo in the absence of a concurrent illness other than HIV infection that could explain the findings):

- Failure to attain or loss of developmental milestones or loss of intellectual ability, verified by standard developmental scale or neuropsychologic tests
- Impaired brain growth or acquired microcephaly shown by head circumference measurements or presence of brain atrophy on CT or MRI (serial imaging is required for children < 2 yr)
- Acquired symmetric motor deficit manifested by ≥ 2 of the following: paresis, pathologic reflexes, ataxia, or gait disturbance

Histoplasmosis, disseminated (at a site other than or in addition to the lungs or cervical or hilar lymph nodes)
HSV infection causing a mucocutaneous ulcer persisting for > 1 mo or HSV bronchitis, pneumonitis, or esophagitis for any duration affecting a child > 1 mo of age
Kaposi sarcoma
Lymphoma, primary, in the brain
Lymphoma: Small, noncleaved cell lymphoma (Burkitt), or immunoblastic or large-cell lymphoma of B-cell or unknown immunologic phenotype

Table continues on the following page.

Table 312–1. CLINICAL CATEGORIES FOR CHILDREN AGED < 13 YR WITH HIV INFECTION (*Continued*)

Mycobacterium tuberculosis, of any site, pulmonary, disseminated, or extrapulmonary
Mycobacterium avium complex, *Mycobacterium kansaii*, or other species or unidentified species, disseminated or extrapulmonary
Pneumocystis jirovecii pneumonia
Pneumonia, recurrent, in children > 6 yr of age or in adolescents
Progressive multifocal leukoencephalopathy
Salmonella (nontyphoid) septicemia, recurrent
Toxoplasmosis of the brain with onset at > 1 mo of age
Wasting syndrome in the absence of a concurrent illness (other than HIV infection) that could explain any one of the following 3 findings:

- Persistent weight loss > 10% of baseline
- Downward crossing of ≥ 2 of the following percentile lines on the weight-for-age chart (eg, 95th, 75th, 50th, 25th, 5th) in a child ≥ 1 yr
- < 5th percentile on weight-for-height chart on 2 consecutive measurements ≥ 30 days apart

plus 1 of the following:

- Chronic diarrhea (ie, ≥ 2 loose stools/day for ≥ 30 days)
- Documented fever (for ≥ 30 days, intermittent or constant)

HSV = herpes simplex virus.
Adapted from Centers for Disease Control and Prevention: Revised surveillance case definitions for HIV infection among adults, adolescents, and children aged < 18 months and for HIV infection and AIDS among children aged 18 months to < 13 years of age—United States, 2008. *Morbidity and Mortality Weekly Report* 57(RR-10):1–13, 2008, and Centers for Disease Control and Prevention: Revised surveillance case definition for HIV infection---United States, 2014. *Morbidity and Mortality Weekly Report* 63(RR-3):1-10, 2014.

Symptoms and Signs

Natural history in untreated children: Infants infected perinatally usually are asymptomatic during the first few months of life, even if no combination ART is begun. Although the median age at symptom onset is about 3 yr, some children remain asymptomatic for > 5 yr and, with appropriate ART, are expected to survive to adulthood. In the pre-ART era, about 10 to 15% of children had rapid disease progression, with symptoms occurring in the first year of life and death occurring by 18 to 36 mo; these children were thought to have acquired HIV infection earlier in utero. However, most children probably acquire infection at or near birth and have slower disease progression (surviving beyond 5 yr even before ART was used routinely).

The most common manifestations of HIV infection in children not receiving ART include generalized lymphadenopathy, hepatomegaly, splenomegaly, failure to thrive, oral candidiasis, CNS disease (including developmental delay, which can be progressive), lymphoid interstitial pneumonitis, recurrent bacteremia, opportunistic infections, recurrent diarrhea, parotitis, cardiomyopathy, hepatitis, nephropathy, and cancers.

Complications: When complications occur, they typically involve opportunistic infections (and rarely cancer). Combination ART has made such infections uncommon, and they now occur mainly in undiagnosed children who have not yet received ART or in children who are not adherent to ART.

When opportunistic infections occur, *Pneumocystis jirovecii* pneumonia is the most common and serious and has high mortality. *Pneumocystis* pneumonia can occur as early as age 4 to 6 wk but occurs mostly in infants aged 3 to 6 mo who acquired infection before or at birth. Infants and older children with *Pneumocystis* pneumonia characteristically develop a subacute, diffuse pneumonitis with dyspnea at rest, tachypnea, O_2 desaturation, nonproductive cough, and fever (in contrast to non–HIV-infected immunocompromised children and adults, in whom onset is often more acute and fulminant).

Other opportunistic infections in immunosuppressed children include *Candida* esophagitis, disseminated cytomegalovirus infection, chronic or disseminated herpes simplex and varicella-zoster virus infections, and, less commonly, *Mycobacterium tuberculosis* and *M. avium* complex infections, chronic enteritis caused by *Cryptosporidium* or other organisms, and disseminated or CNS cryptococcal or *Toxoplasma gondii* infection.

Cancers in immunocompromised children with HIV infection are relatively uncommon, but leiomyosarcomas and certain lymphomas, including CNS lymphomas and non-Hodgkin B-cell lymphomas (Burkitt type), occur much more often than in immunocompetent children. Kaposi sarcoma is very rare in HIV-infected children.

Children receiving combination antiretroviral therapy: Combination ART has significantly changed the clinical manifestations of pediatric HIV infection. Although bacterial pneumonia and other bacterial infections (eg, bacteremia, recurrent otitis media) still occur more often in HIV-infected

Table 312–2. IMMUNOLOGIC CATEGORIES (HIV INFECTION STAGE) FOR CHILDREN < 13 YR WITH HIV INFECTION BASED ON AGE-SPECIFIC CD4+ T-CELL COUNT OR PERCENTAGE

IMMUNOLOGIC CATEGORY (STAGE*)	< 1 YR		1 to < 6 YR		≥ 6 YR	
	CELLS/μL	%	CELLS/μL	%	CELLS/μL	%
1	≥ 1500	≥ 34	≥ 1000	≥ 30	≥ 500	≥ 26
2	750–1499	26–33	500–999	22-29	200–499	14–25
3	< 750	< 26	< 500	< 22	< 200	< 14

*The stage is based primarily on the CD4 cell count; the CD4 cell count takes precedence over the CD4 percentage, and the percentage is considered only if the count is missing. If a Stage 3-defining opportunistic illness has been diagnosed, then the stage is 3 regardless of CD4 test results.
Adapted from Centers for Disease Control and Prevention: Revised surveillance case definitions for HIV infection—United States, 2014. *Morbidity and Mortality Weekly Report* 63(RR-3):1-10, 2014.

children, opportunistic infections and growth failure are much less frequent than in the pre-ART era. New problems, such as alterations in serum lipids, hyperglycemia, fat maldistribution (lipodystrophy and lipoatrophy), nephropathy, and osteonecrosis, are reported; however, the incidence is lower in children than in HIV-infected adults.

Although combination ART clearly improves neurodevelopmental outcome, there seems to be an increased rate of behavioral, developmental, and cognitive problems in treated HIV-infected children. It is unclear whether these problems are caused by HIV infection itself, therapeutic drugs, or other biopsychosocial factors among HIV-infected children. It is unknown whether any additional effects of HIV infection or ART during critical periods of growth and development will manifest later in life because the first wave of perinatally infected children is just now reaching adulthood. To detect such adverse effects, providers will need to monitor HIV-infected children over time.

Diagnosis

- Serum antibody tests
- Virologic nucleic acid tests (NATs; includes HIV DNA PCR or HIV RNA assays)

HIV-specific tests: In children > 18 mo, the diagnosis of HIV infection is made using serum 4th-generation HIV-1/2 antigen/antibody combination immunoassay followed by a 2nd-generation HIV-1/2 antibody differentiation assay and, if required, an HIV-1 qualitative RNA assay. This diagnostic algorithm has supplanted the previous sequential testing by serum immunoassay and Western blot confirmation. Only very rarely does an older HIV-infected child lack HIV antibody because of significant hypogammaglobulinemia.

Children < 18 mo retain maternal antibody, causing false-positive results even in the new 4th generation HIV-1/2 antigen/antibody combination immunoassay, so diagnosis is made by HIV virologic assays such as qualitative RNA assays (eg, transcription-mediated amplification of RNA) or DNA PCR assays (known collectively as NATs), which can diagnose about 30 to 50% of cases at birth and nearly 100% by 4 to 6 mo of age. HIV viral culture has acceptable sensitivity and specificity but is technically more demanding and hazardous and has been replaced by NATs.

Another type of NAT, the quantitative HIV RNA assay (ie, the viral load assay used for monitoring efficacy of treatment) is becoming more widely used for diagnostic testing of infants. Quantitative RNA assays are as sensitive as DNA PCR in infants not given ART, are less expensive, and are more widely available than are the other NATs. However, care must be taken when using RNA assays for infant diagnosis because test specificity is uncertain at very low RNA concentrations (< 5,000 copies/mL) and sensitivity is unknown in infants of mothers with complete treatment-mediated viral suppression at the time of delivery.

A virologic test (a NAT) should be done initially within the first 2 wk of life, at about 1 mo of age, and between 4 mo and 6 mo for all infants with perinatal HIV exposure (3 serial tests). A positive test should be confirmed immediately by using the same or another virologic test. If the serial HIV virologic tests are negative at ≥ 2 wk and ≥ 4 wk, the infant is considered uninfected with > 95% accuracy (in the absence of any AIDS-defining illness). If HIV virologic tests are also negative at ≥ 4 wk and ≥ 4 mo, the infant is considered uninfected with about 100% accuracy (in the absence of any AIDS-defining illness). Nevertheless, many experts continue to recommend follow-up antibody tests (1 antigen/antibody combination assay at > 18 mo or, alternatively, 2 such assays done between 6 mo and 18 mo) to definitively exclude HIV infection and confirm seroreversion (loss of passively acquired HIV antibodies). If an infant < 18 mo with a positive antibody test but negative virologic tests develops an AIDS-defining illness (category C—see Table 312–1), HIV infection is diagnosed.

Most experts perform additional NATs in infants judged to be at high risk of HIV transmission (increased or unknown maternal viral load at delivery; infants born to women not taking antiretroviral drugs; known highly antiretroviral drug-resistant virus in mother). These additional NAT assays are suggested to be done at birth and at 8 to 10 wk of age in addition to the 5 serial tests already mentioned.

Rapid immunoassay tests for HIV antibody provide results within minutes to hours. They can be done as point-of-care tests on oral secretions, whole blood, or serum. In the US, these tests are perhaps most useful in labor and delivery suites to test women of unknown HIV serostatus, thus allowing counseling, commencement of ART to prevent MTCT, and testing of the infant to be arranged during the birth visit. Similar advantages accrue in other episodic care settings (eg, emergency departments, adolescent medicine clinics, sexually transmitted disease clinics) and in the developing world. Rapid assays typically require confirmatory tests, such as a second antigen/antibody assay, HIV-1/2 antibody differentiation assay, or NAT. These confirmatory tests are especially important because in areas where the expected HIV prevalence is low, even a specific rapid assay yields mostly false positives (low positive predictive value by Bayes theorem. If the expected probability of HIV (or seroprevalence) is high, the positive predictive value increases.

As more laboratories are able to offer 4th generation antigen/antibody assays with same day turnaround, the comparatively less sensitive and less specific rapid immunoassays should not be needed for routine testing.

Before HIV testing of a child is done, the mother or primary caregiver (and the child, if old enough) should be counseled about the possible psychosocial risks and benefits of testing. Written or oral consent should be obtained and recorded in the patient's chart, consistent with state, local, and hospital laws and regulations. Counseling and consent requirements should not deter testing if it is medically indicated; refusal of a patient or guardian to give consent does not relieve physicians of their professional and legal responsibilities, and sometimes authorization for testing must be obtained by other means (eg, court order). Test results should be discussed in person with the family, the primary caregiver, and, if old enough, the child. If the child is HIV-positive, appropriate counseling and subsequent follow-up care must be provided. In all cases, maintaining confidentiality is essential.

Children and adolescents meeting the criteria for HIV infection or AIDS must be reported to the appropriate public health department.

Other tests: Once infection is diagnosed, other tests are done:

- CD4+ T-cell count
- CD8+ T-cell count
- Plasma viral RNA concentration

Infected children require measurement of CD4+ and CD8+ T-cell counts and plasma viral RNA concentration (viral load) to help determine their degree of illness, prognosis, and the effects of therapy. CD4+ counts may be normal (eg, above the age-specific cutoffs of category 1 in Table 312–2) initially but fall eventually. CD8+ counts usually increase initially and do not fall until late in the infection. These changes in cell populations result in a decrease in the CD4+:CD8+ cell ratio, a characteristic of HIV infection (although sometimes occurring in other infections). Plasma viral RNA concentrations in untreated children < 12 mo are typically very high (mean of about 200,000 RNA copies/mL). By 24 mo, viral concentrations in untreated children decrease (to a mean of about 40,000 RNA copies/mL). Although the wide range of HIV RNA concentrations in children make the data less predictive of morbidity and mortality than in adults, determining plasma viral concentrations in conjunction with CD4+ counts still yields more accurate prognostic information than does determining either marker alone. Less expensive alternative surrogate markers such as total lymphocyte counts and serum albumin levels may also predict AIDS mortality in children, which may be useful in developing nations.

Although not routinely measured, serum immunoglobulin concentrations, particularly IgG and IgA, often are markedly elevated, but occasionally some children develop panhypogammaglobulinemia. Patients may be anergic to skin test antigens.

Prognosis

In the pre-ART era, 10 to 15% of children from industrialized countries and perhaps 50 to 80% of children from developing countries died before age 4 yr; however, with appropriate combination ART regimens, most perinatally infected children survive well into adolescence. The majority of vertically infected children born during the past decade in the US is surviving into young adulthood; increasing numbers of these young adults have given birth to or fathered their own children.

Nevertheless, if opportunistic infections occur, particularly *Pneumocystis* pneumonia, progressive neurologic disease, or severe wasting, the prognosis is poor unless virologic and immunologic control is regained with combination ART. Mortality due to *Pneumocystis* pneumonia ranges from 5 to 40% if treated and is almost 100% if untreated. Prognosis is also poor for children in whom virus is detected early (ie, by 7 days of life) or who develop symptoms in the first year of life.

There has been only one well-documented case of an adult in whom replication-competent HIV was eradicated (ie, the person has been "cured" for > 5 yr). This person required a hematopoietic stem cell transplant for leukemia. The donor cells were homozygous for the CCR5-delta 32 mutation, which made the engrafted lymphocytes resistant to infection with CCR5-tropic HIV; subsequently, HIV has remained undetectable. It is likely that ART, bone marrow ablation, and graft-vs-host disease contributed to this person's cure. However, other HIV-infected transplant recipients have not experienced cure. One well-documented case of an infant with transient eradication of replication-competent HIV also has been reported. The infant was born to an HIV-infected mother who had not received prenatal care or prenatal (or intrapartum) ART. Beginning on the second day of life, the infant was given combination ART at high doses not yet known to be safe and effective for use in the first 2 wk of life. The ART was given for about 15 mo, after which time it was inadvertently interrupted. Nevertheless, at 24 mo of age the infant had no detectable replicating virus DNA (a "functional cure") but did have detectable proviral DNA. Subsequently, however, HIV replication ensued. Several similar cases of infants with temporary interruption of HIV replication have been reported; none have been "cured" of their HIV infection, and it is not yet known if cure is possible. What is known, however, is that HIV infection is a treatable infection that is already compatible with long-term survival if effective ART is given. Future research will undoubtedly uncover ways to improve ART tolerance and efficacy and perhaps help achieve the goal of curative therapy.

Treatment

- Antiretroviral (ARV) drugs: Combination ART most commonly includes 2 nucleoside reverse transcriptase inhibitors (NRTIs) plus either a protease inhibit or (PI) or an integrase strand transfer inhibitor (INSTI); sometimes a nonnucleoside reverse transcriptase inhibitor (NNRTI) given with 2 NRTIs
- Supportive care

Because of the success of combination ART, much of the current focus is on the management of HIV infection as a chronic disease, addressing both medical and social issues. Important long-term medical issues include the need to manage HIV-related and drug-related metabolic complications and to account for age-related changes in drug pharmacokinetics and pharmacodynamics. Social issues include the need to cope with peer pressure from noninfected adolescents, ensure school success and appropriate career choice, and educate children about transmission risk. Adolescents often have difficulty seeking and following health care advice and need particular help with treatment adherence. Children and adolescents should be managed in collaboration with specialists who have experience in the management of pediatric HIV infection.

ARV drugs: There are > 2 dozen ARV drugs (see Table 312–3), including multidrug combination products, available in the US, each of which may have adverse effects and drug interactions with other ARV drugs or commonly used antibiotics, anticonvulsants, and sedatives. New ARV drugs, immunomodulators, and vaccines are under evaluation. For current information on dosing, adverse effects, and drug interactions, see guidelines for the use of antiretroviral agents in pediatric HIV infection and guidelines for adults and adolescents available at www.aidsinfo.nih.gov. Useful treatment information is also available at www.hivguidelines.org and www.unaids.org/en/. Consultation regarding ART, especially for issues surrounding HIV postexposure prophylaxis and prevention of HIV mother to child transmission, are also available through the National HIV/AIDS Clinicians' Consultation Center located at the University of California San Francisco available at www.nccc.ucsf.edu.

Because expert opinions on therapeutic strategies change rapidly, consultation with specialists is strongly advised. Tablets containing fixed-dose combinations of ≥ 3 drugs are now widely used in older children and adolescents to simplify regimens and improve adherence; for young children, such combinations are unavailable in the US or difficult to use. The standard treatment is similar to that for adults, ie, combination ART to maximize viral suppression and minimize selection of drug-resistant strains. Preferred regimens vary somewhat by age (see Table 321–4).

Indications: Initiation of ART for children is similar to that in adults; essentially all children with HIV infection should be given ART. The urgency of initiating ART primarily depends on the child's age, immunologic and clinical criteria, and readiness of the caregivers to administer the drugs. The goal of therapy, is similar to that in adults: to suppress HIV replication (as measured by plasma HIV RNA PCR viral load) and maintain or achieve age-normal CD4+ counts and percentages with the least amount of drug toxicity. Before making the decision to initiate therapy, the practitioner should fully assess the readiness of the caregiver and child to adhere with ARV drug administration and discuss the potential benefits and risks of therapy. Because expert opinions on therapeutic strategies change rapidly, consultation with specialists is strongly advised.

Table 312–3. DOSAGE AND ADMINISTRATION OF SELECTED ANTIRETROVIRAL DRUGS FOR CHILDREN*

DRUG	PREPARATIONS	RECOMMENDED DOSAGE (ORAL)	SELECTED ADVERSE EFFECTS AND COMMENTS
Nucleoside reverse transcriptase inhibitors (NRTIs)			
Abacavir (ABC)	Syrup: 20 mg/mL Tablet: 300 mg (scored)	3 mo–18 yr: 8 mg/kg q 12 h (up to a maximum of 300 mg q 12 h); may give 600 mg q 24 h if > 25 kg	ABC may cause the following: • Possibly fatal hypersensitivity reaction—symptoms may include rash, nausea and vomiting, sore throat, cough, or shortness of breath The incidence of hypersensitivity reaction is about 5%. The reaction mostly occurs during the first 6 wk of use and primarily among patients with the HLA-B*5701 genotype (who should not receive ABC). There is risk of hypotension or death with rechallenge after a hypersensitivity reaction. Before prescribing ABC, clinicians should test for the HLA-B*5701 allele. ABC may be given without regard to food.
Emtricitabine (FTC)	Oral solution: 10 mg/mL Capsules: 200 mg	0– < 3 mo: 3 mg/kg q 24 h ≥ 3 mo–18 yr: 6 mg/kg q 24 h (maximum oral solution 240 mg q 24 h; maximum capsule 200 mg q 24 h)	FTC is well-tolerated; however, it may rarely cause the following: • Neutropenia, hyperpigmentation, lactic acidosis • Severe exacerbation of hepatitis in patients coinfected with hepatitis B infection if FTC suddenly discontinued FTC may be given without regard to food.
Lamivudine (3TC)	Oral solution: 10 mg/mL Tablets: 100, 150 (scored), and 300 mg	0–1 mo: 2 mg/kg q 12 h ≥ 1 mo–18 yr: 4 mg/kg q 12 h (up to 150 mg q 12 h) For those children ≥ 3 yr of age and weighing ≥ 25 kg, who have an undetectable viral load, a stable CD4 lymphocyte count, and good adherence, dose may be 8–10 mg/kg q 24 h not to exceed 300 mg q 24 h	3TC is well-tolerated; however, it may rarely cause the following: • Neutropenia, hyperpigmentation, lactic acidosis • Severe exacerbation of hepatitis in patients coinfected with hepatitis B infection if 3TC suddenly discontinued 3TC may be given without regard to food.
Tenofovir disoproxil fumarate (TDF)[†] See Fixed-dose combination products for tenofovir alafenamide (TAF)†	Oral powder: 40 mg/1 level scoop Tablets: 150, 200, 250, and 300 mg	< 2 yr: Not recommended 2–12 yr: 8 mg/kg q 24 h up to 300 mg q 24 h as follows: 10–11 kg: 2 scoops powder q 24 h 12–13 kg: 2.5 scoops powder q 24 h 14–16 kg: 3 scoops powder q 24 h 17–18 kg: 3.5 scoops powder or 1 × 150-mg tablet q 24 h 19–21 kg: 4 scoops powder or 1 × 150-mg tablet q 24 h 22–23 kg: 4.5 scoops powder or 1 × 200-mg tablet q 24 h 24–26 kg: 5 scoops powder or 1 × 200-mg tablet q 24 h 27–28 kg: 5.5 scoops powder or 1 × 250-mg tablet q 24 h 29–31 kg: 6 scoops powder or 1 × 250-mg tablet q 24 h 32–33 kg: 6.5 scoops powder or 1 × 250-mg tablet q 24 h 34 kg: 7 scoops powder or 1 × 250-mg tablet q 24 h ≥ 35 kg: 7.5 scoops powder or 1 × 300-mg tablet q 24 h ≥ 12 yr and ≥ 35 kg: 1 × 300-mg tablet q 24 h	TDF is usually well-tolerated; however, it may cause the following: • Occasional asthenia, headache, diarrhea, nausea, vomiting • Renal insufficiency (proximal tubular dysfunction including Fanconi syndrome) • Decreased bone mineral density • Severe exacerbation of hepatitis in patients coinfected with hepatitis B infection if TDF is discontinued The powder preparation is bitter and insoluble and should be given in soft food such as applesauce or yogurt rather than liquid. TDF may be given without regard to food. TDF powder should be measured only with the supplied 1-g scoop. Tenofovir alafenamide (TAF) is used for adolescents ≥ 6 yr of age weighing ≥ 25 kg as part of fixed-dose combination products. It is designed to have equivalent antiretroviral efficacy to TDF but with fewer renal and bone adverse effects.

Table continues on the following page.

Table 312–3. DOSAGE AND ADMINISTRATION OF SELECTED ANTIRETROVIRAL DRUGS FOR CHILDREN* (*Continued*)

DRUG	PREPARATIONS	RECOMMENDED DOSAGE (ORAL)	SELECTED ADVERSE EFFECTS AND COMMENTS
Zidovudine (ZDV)‡	Oral syrup: 10 mg/mL IV solution: 10 mg/mL Capsule: 100 mg Tablet: 300 mg	0–6 wk: 4 mg/kg q 12 h 6 wk–17 yr: 240 mg/m² q 12 h or weight-based dosing: 4–8 kg: 12 mg/kg q 12 h 9–29 kg: 9 mg/kg q 12 h ≥ 30 kg: 300 mg q 12 h ≥ 18 yr: 300 mg q 12 h	ZDV may cause the following: • Macrocytic anemia, granulocytopenia • Headache, malaise, anorexia, nausea, vomiting • Nail pigmentation • Hyperlipidemia, hyperglycemia • Lactic acidosis, hepatomegaly with hepatic steatosis • Myopathy ZDV may be given without regard to food.
Nonnucleoside reverse transcriptase inhibitors (NNRTIs)			
Nevirapine (NVP)	Suspension: 10 mg/mL Tablet: 200 mg Extended-release tablets: 100 and 400 mg Therapy initiation: Age-appropriate dose given once/day for 14 days then increased to twice/day if tolerated (to lessen incidence of adverse reactions)	< 4 wk (investigational dose, not FDA-approved): no lead-in, 6 mg/kg q 12 h 4 wk–8 yr: 200 mg/m² q 12 h ≥ 8 yr: 120–150 mg/m² q 12 h (up to 200 mg q 12 h or, if using extended-release tablets, 400 mg q 24 h) If an older child or adolescent has been taking NVP tablets twice daily without adverse effects, the extended-release tablets may be used as follows to convert to once-daily dosing: 0.58–0.83 m²: 200 mg once/day (2 × 100 mg) 0.84–1.16 m²: 300 mg once/day (3 × 100 mg) ≥1.17 m²: 400 mg once/day (1 x 400 mg)	NVP may cause the following: • Rash, including Stevens-Johnson syndrome • Symptomatic hepatitis, including fatal hepatic necrosis • Severe systemic hypersensitivity syndrome with potential for multisystem organ involvement and shock Rash is most common during first 6 wk of therapy; if rash occurs during 14-day regimen, the dose is not increased until rash resolves. Hepatic toxicity is most common during first 12 wk of therapy, and frequent clinical and laboratory monitoring should be done during this time and periodically thereafter; if clinical hepatitis is suspected, hepatic transaminase levels are obtained. If hepatitis or hypersensitivity reaction occurs, no rechallenge is done. If NVP therapy is interrupted for > 7 days, it should be restarted with a 14-day regimen. NVP may be given without regard to food.
Protease inhibitors (PIs)			
Atazanavir (ATV)	Capsules: 150, 200, and 300 mg Powder: 50 mg/packet Given with low-dose ritonavir (RTV) as a pharmacokinetic booster	< 3 mo: Not approved ≥ 3 mo-6 yr, weight-based dosing: 5–14 kg: ATV 200 mg (4 packets) + RTV 80 mg (1 mL oral solution) q 24 h 15–24 kg: ATV 250 mg (5 packets) + RTV 80 mg (1 mL oral solution) q 24 h > 6–17 yr, weight-based dosing: 15–19 kg: ATV 150 mg + RTV 100 mg q 24 h 20–39 kg: ATV 200 mg + RTV 100 mg q 24 h ≥ 40 kg: ATV 300 mg + RTV 100 mg q 24 h ≥ 18 yr: ATV 300 mg + RTV 100 mg q 24 h	ATV may cause the following: • Asymptomatic indirect hyperbilirubinemia (incidence 30%), jaundice (incidence 10%) • Hyperglycemia, hyperlipidemia, fat maldistribution • Prolongation of PR interval (see p. 621) on ECG • Nephrolithiasis (rare) ATV should be given with food to enhance absorption.

Table 312–3. DOSAGE AND ADMINISTRATION OF SELECTED ANTIRETROVIRAL DRUGS FOR CHILDREN* (*Continued*)

DRUG	PREPARATIONS	RECOMMENDED DOSAGE (ORAL)	SELECTED ADVERSE EFFECTS AND COMMENTS
Lopinavir/ ritonavir (LPV/r)	Oral solution: 80/20 mg/mL (contains 43% alcohol and 15% propylene glycol) Film-coated tablets: 100/25 and 200/50 mg	< 2 wk: Do not use 2 wk–12 mo: 300 mg (of LPV component) per m^2 of body surface area q 12 h 1–17 yr: 230–300 mg (of LPV component; many experts prefer the higher dosage) per m^2 of body surface area q 12 h (up to maximum of LPV 400 mg q 12 h) ≥ 18 yr: LPV 400 mg q 12 h	LPV/r may cause the following: • GI intolerance (diarrhea, nausea, vomiting) • Hyperglycemia, hyperlipidemia (especially triglycerides), fat maldistribution • Possible prolongation of PR and QT intervals • Rash, including Stevens-Johnson syndrome Do not give to premature or young neonates (ie, before 42 wk postmenstrual age or 14 days postnatal age) because of risk of life-threatening cardiotoxicity. Once-daily dosing is not recommended for children or adolescents because of greater clearance. A dose increase is required if patients are receiving concomitant NVP, EFV, FPV, or NFV. LPV/r tablets may be given without regard to food, but the oral solution should be given with food to increase absorption and mask taste (very poor palatability).
Ritonavir (RTV)	Oral solution: 80 mg/mL (contains 43% alcohol by volume) Capsule: 100 mg Tablet: 100 mg	Used only as a pharmacokinetic booster, 80-100 mg q 12-24 h	RTV may cause the following: • GI intolerance (diarrhea, nausea, vomiting) • Hyperglycemia, hyperlipidemia (especially triglycerides), fat maldistribution • Rash, including Stevens-Johnson syndrome RTV is very rarely used as a primary ARV drug because of GI intolerance at higher doses. RTV is best absorbed when given with food. Tablets may be more palatable than capsules, but both are superior to liquid, which is poorly palatable. The oral solution may be given with certain foods (eg, chocolate milk, ice cream, peanut butter) to mask its taste.
Entry inhibitor (CCR5 antagonist)			
Maraviroc (MVC)	Tablets: 150 and 300 mg	Approved for use in children > 2 yr weighing > 10 kg; consult pediatric HIV guidelines	MVC may cause the following: • Cough, fever, rash, abdominal pain • Hepatotoxicity (may be preceded by severe rash and/or significant allergic reaction) • Orthostatic hypotension (especially in patients with severe renal insufficiency) • Multiple drug interactions MVC is effective against only CCR5-tropic HIV; an HIV tropism assay is required before use. MVC should be given with food.
Fusion inhibitor			
Enfuvirtide (ENF, T20)	Lyophilized powder for injection: Delivers 90 mg/mL	6–15 yr: 2 mg/kg sc q 12 h (up to 90 mg sc q 12 h) ≥ 16 yr: 90 mg sc q 12 h	Not commonly used because of cost, twice-daily injections, local adverse effects ENF may cause the following: • Local injection site reaction (eg, pain, discomfort, induration, erythema, nodules, ecchymosis) in 88–98% of patients • Hypersensitivity reaction (< 1% incidence of fever, malaise, nausea, vomiting, chills, possibly elevated hepatic transaminases) • If hypersensitivity reaction occurs, no rechallenge is done. ENF may be given without regard to food.

Table continues on the following page.

Table 312–3. DOSAGE AND ADMINISTRATION OF SELECTED ANTIRETROVIRAL DRUGS FOR CHILDREN* (*Continued*)

DRUG	PREPARATIONS	RECOMMENDED DOSAGE (ORAL)	SELECTED ADVERSE EFFECTS AND COMMENTS
Integrase inhibitor			
Dolutegravir (DTG)	Tablet: 10, 25, and 50 mg	Infant/child < 30 kg: Not recommended Child 30–39 kg: 35 mg q 24 h Child/adolescent ≥ 40 kg: 50 mg q 24 h (may need to give q 12 h with certain UGT1A or CYP3A inducers or inhibitors; package insert should be consulted)	DTG may cause the following: • Insomnia • Headache DTG may be given without regard to food; however, it should be given 2 h before or 6 h after divalent cation-containing oral antacids, laxatives, sucralfate, iron supplements, Ca supplements, or buffered drugs.
Elvitegravir (EVG)	Available only as fixed-dose combination tablet with FTC, TDF, and cobicistat (COBI)	See Fixed-dose combination products	EVG may cause the following: • Diarrhea, nausea • Renal insufficiency, decreased bone mineral density (see TDF) • Severe exacerbation of hepatitis in patients coinfected with hepatitis B infection if coformulation containing FTC or TDF is discontinued suddenly EVG is coformulated with cobicistat (COBI), a pharmacokinetic booster. EVG should be given with food.
Raltegravir (RAL)	Chewable tablets: 25 and 100 mg Film-coated tablet: 400 mg Granules for oral suspension: Packet of 100 mg to be added to 5 mL of water to make 20 mg/mL	Infants and children ≥ 4 wk and weighing ≥ 3 kg–19 kg: Oral suspension 6 mg/kg q 12 h (see package insert) Children: 10–13 kg: 75 mg q 12 h (3 × 25-mg chewables) 14–19 kg: 100 mg q 12 h (1 × 100-mg chewable) 20–27 kg: 150 mg q 12 h (1.5 × 100-mg chewables) 28–39 kg: 200 mg q 12 h (2 × 100-mg chewables) ≥ 40 kg: 300 mg q 12 h (3 × 100-mg chewables) ≥ 12 yr: 400 mg q 12 h (1 × 400-mg film-coated)	RAL may cause the following: • Nausea, headache, diarrhea, fatigue • Rash, including Stevens-Johnson syndrome • Creatine phosphokinase elevation; rarely, rhabdomyolysis Chewable tablets may be chewed or swallowed whole but are not interchangeable with film-coated tablets because of different bioavailability. RAL may be given without regard to food.
Some fixed-dose combination products			
ZDV/3TC (Combivir®)	Combination tablets: ZDV 300 mg + 3TC 150 mg	≥ 30 kg: 1 tablet q 12 h	See individual drugs
3TC/ABC (Epzicom®)	Combination tablets: 3TC 300 mg + ABC 600 mg	> 25 kg: 1 tablet q 24 h	See individual drugs
FTC/TDF (Truvada®)	Combination tablets: FTC 200 mg + TDF 300 mg	≥ 12 yr and ≥ 35 kg: 1 tablet q 24 h	See individual drugs
ABC/DTG/3TC (Triumeq®)	Combination tablets: ABC 600 mg + DTG 50 mg + 3TC 300 mg	≥ 40 kg: 1 tablet q 24 h	See individual drugs
FTC/TDF/EVG/COBI (Stribild®)	Combination tablets: FTC 200 mg + TDF 300 mg + EVG 150 mg + COBI 150 mg	≥ 12 yr and > 35 kg: 1 tablet q 24 h	See individual drugs

Table 312–3. DOSAGE AND ADMINISTRATION OF SELECTED ANTIRETROVIRAL DRUGS FOR CHILDREN* (*Continued*)

DRUG	PREPARATIONS	RECOMMENDED DOSAGE (ORAL)	SELECTED ADVERSE EFFECTS AND COMMENTS
FTC/TAF/ EVG/COBI (Genvoya®)	Combination tablets: FTC 200 mg + TAF 10 mg + EVG 150 mg + COBI 150 mg	≥ 6 yr and ≥ 25 kg: 1 tablet q 24 h	See individual drugs

*Several alternative ARV drugs are not included here; consultation with an expert in pediatric HIV medicine is advised. For information on adverse effects, other doses (especially for information on fixed-dose combination products), and drug interactions, see the continually updated Department of Health and Human Services Panel on Antiretroviral Therapy and Medical Management of HIV-Infected Children, a Working Group of the Office of AIDS Research Council. Guidelines for the use of antiretroviral agents in pediatric HIV infection, April 27, 2017.

†Tenofovir disoproxil fumarate and tenofovir alafenamide are functionally grouped within the NRTIs but are actually nucleotide reverse transcriptase inhibitors by chemical structure.

‡The dosing for zidovudine should be reduced for premature infants < 35 wk gestation; see Department of Health and Human Services Panel on Antiretroviral Therapy and Medical Management of HIV-Infected Children, a Working Group of the Office of AIDS Research Council. Guidelines for the use of antiretroviral agents in pediatric HIV infection, April 27, 2017.

ARV = antiretroviral; COBI = cobicistat

Table 314-4. SELECTED ARV REGIMENS FOR INITIAL THERAPY OF HIV INFECTION IN CHILDREN

AGE GROUP	NRTI BACKBONE COMPONENT	NNRTI, PI OR INSTI COMPONENT
Infants, birth to < 14 days	Zidovudine **plus** lamivudine (or emtricitabine)	Nevirapine
Children ≥ 14 days to < 2 yr	Zidovudine **plus** lamivudine (or emtricitabine)	Lopinavir-ritonavir
Children ≥ 2 yr to < 3 yr	Zidovudine (or abacavir) **plus** lamivudine (or emtricitabine)	Atazanavir-ritonavir ***or*** raltegravir
Children ≥ 3 yr to < 6 yr	Abacavir (or zidovudine) **plus** lamivudine (or emtricitabine)	Atazanavir-ritonavir ***or*** raltegravir
Children ≥ 6 yr to < 12 yr	Abacavir (or zidovudine) **plus** lamivudine (or emtricitabine)	Atazanavir-ritonavir ***or*** dolutegravir
Adolescents ≥ 12 yr	One of the following regimens (includes fixed-dose combination tablets):	
	Tenofovir **plus** emtricitabine	Atazanavir-ritonavir
	Tenofovir **plus** emtricitabine	Elvitegravir-cobicistat
	Abacavir **plus** lamivudine	Dolutegravir

* **Each regimen is designed to contain 2 NRTI ARV agents plus either an NNRTI, PI, or INSTI component.** Several alternative ARV regimens exist; consultation with an expert in pediatric HIV medicine is advised. For information on adverse effects, other doses (especially for information on fixed-dose combination products), and drug interactions, see the continually updated Department of Health and Human Services Panel on Antiretroviral Therapy and Medical Management of HIV-Infected Children, a Working Group of the Office of AIDS Research Council. Guidelines for the use of antiretroviral agents in pediatric HIV infection, April 27, 2017. Available at www.aidsinfo.nih.gov.

ARV = antiretroviral; NRTI = nucleoside reverse transcriptase inhibitor; NNRTI = nonnucleoside reverse transcriptase inhibitor; PI = protease inhibitor; INSTI = integrase strand transfer inhibitor.

Table 312–5. INDICATIONS FOR INITIATION OF ANTIRETROVIRAL THERAPY IN HIV-INFECTED CHILDREN AND ADOLESCENTS

AGE	CRITERIA	RECOMMENDATION*
< 12 mo	Regardless of clinical symptoms, immune status, or viral load	Urgent treatment (within 1-2 wk, including expedited discussion on adherence)
1–6 yr	CDC Stage 3-defining opportunistic illnesses or CD4 count < 500 cells/μL (see Table 312–1)	Urgent treatment (within 1-2 wk, including expedited discussion on adherence)
	Moderate symptoms (Category B) or CD4 cell count 500-999 cells/μL	Treat
	Asymptomatic or mild symptoms (CDC clinical category A or N) and CD4 cell count ≥ 1000 cells/μL	Treat, but on a case-by-case basis, while fully assessing adherence, clinical, and/or psychosocial factors; may temporarily defer with close monitoring
≥ 6 yr	CDC Stage 3-defining opportunistic illnesses or CD4 count < 200 cells/μL (see Table 312–1)	Urgent treatment (within 1–2 wk, including expedited discussion on adherence)
	Moderate symptoms (Category B) or CD4 cell count 200–499 cells/μL	Treat
	Asymptomatic or mild symptoms (CDC clinical category A or N) and CD4 cell count ≥ 500 cells/μL	Treat; for adolescents aged ≥ 13 yr with sexual maturity ratings 4 or 5, many alternative fixed-dose ARV combinations are available; consultation with an expert in HIV medicine is advised

*Adherence should be assessed and discussed with children with HIV infection and their caregivers before initiation of therapy.

ARV = antiretroviral; ART = antiretroviral therapy; CDC = Centers for Disease Control and Prevention.

For information on adverse effects, other doses (especially for information on fixed-dose combination products), and drug interactions, see the continually updated Department of Health and Human Services Panel on Antiretroviral Therapy and Medical Management of HIV-Infected Children, a Working Group of the Office of AIDS Research Council. Guidelines for the Use of Antiretroviral Agents in Pediatric HIV Infection, April 27, 2017.

Treatment initiation criteria vary with age and clinical criteria (see Table 312–5).

Adherence: Therapy will be successful only if the family and child are able to adhere to a possibly complex medical regimen. Nonadherence not only leads to failure to control HIV but also selects drug-resistant HIV strains, which reduces future therapeutic choices. Barriers to adherence should be addressed before starting treatment. Barriers include availability and palatability of pills or suspensions, adverse effects (including those due to drug interactions with current therapy), pharmacokinetic factors such as the need to take some drugs with food or in a fasted state, and a child's dependence on others to give drugs (and HIV-infected parents may have problems with remembering to take their own drugs). Newer once- or twice-daily combination regimens and more palatable pediatric formulations may help improve adherence.

Adherence may be especially problematic in adolescents regardless of whether they have been infected perinatally or have acquired HIV infection later on through sexual activity or injection drug use. Adolescents have complex biopsychosocial issues, such as low self-esteem, chaotic and unstructured lifestyles, fear of being singled out because of illness, and sometimes a lack of family support, all of which may reduce drug adherence. In addition, adolescents may not be developmentally able to understand why drugs are necessary during periods of asymptomatic infection and they may worry greatly about adverse effects. Despite frequent contact with the medical system, perinatally infected adolescents may fear or deny their HIV infection, distrust information provided by the health care team, and poorly make the transition to the adult health care system (see p. 2611). Treatment regimens for adolescents must balance these issues. Although the goal is to have the adolescent adhere to a maximally potent regimen of ARV drugs, a realistic assessment of the adolescent's maturity and support systems may suggest that the treatment plan begin by focusing on avoidance of opportunistic illness and provide information about reproductive health services, housing, and how to succeed in school. Once care team members are confident the adolescent is receiving proper support, they can decide exactly which ARV drugs are best.

Monitoring: Clinical and laboratory monitoring are important for identifying drug toxicity and therapeutic failure.

- At entry into care and at initiation of ART (and if changing ART regimen): Physical examination, adherence evaluation, CBC, serum chemistry values, including electrolytes, liver and kidney function tests, HIV RNA viral load, and CD4+ lymphocyte counts
- HIV genotypic resistance testing should be performed at entry into care and upon ART changes due to presumed virologic failure
- If abacavir is to be administered, HLA-B*5701 status must be tested; abacavir should only be given to those who are HLA-B*5701-negative
- Every 3 to 4 mo: Physical examination, adherence evaluation, CBC, serum chemistry values, including electrolytes, liver and kidney function tests, HIV RNA viral load, and CD4+ lymphocyte counts
- Every 6 to 12 mo: Lipid profiles, urinalysis

If children have a stable treatment status, ie, nondetectable HIV RNA and normal age-adjusted CD4+ lymphocyte counts without clinical signs of toxicity for at least 12 mo, and a stable family support system, many clinicians will extend the interval of laboratory evaluations to every 6 mo. However, clinical care visits every 3 mo are valuable because clinicians have the opportunity to review adherence, monitor growth and clinical symptoms, and update weight-based dosing of ARV drugs as needed.

Vaccination: Routine pediatric vaccination protocols (see Tables 291–2 on p. 2462 and 291–3 on p. 2467) are recommended for children with HIV infection, with several exceptions. The main exception is that live-virus vaccines and live-bacteria vaccines (eg, BCG) should be avoided or used only in certain circumstances (see Table 312–6). In addition, 1 to 2 mo after the last dose of the hepatitis B vaccine series, HIV-infected children should be tested to determine whether the level of antibodies to hepatitis B surface antigen (anti-HBs) is protective (≥ 10 mIU/mL). HIV-infected children and adolescents < 18 yr of age should be immunized with 13-valent pneumococcal conjugate vaccine (PCV-13) as well as pneumococcal polysaccharide vaccine (PPSV). Certain postexposure treatment recommendations also differ. Recently, quadrivalent meningococcal conjugate immunization has been recommended for routine and catch-up use in HIV-infected children, adolescents, and adults.

Live oral poliovirus vaccine and live-attenuated influenza vaccine are not recommended; however, inactivated influenza vaccination should be given yearly.

The live measles-mumps-rubella (MMR) and varicella vaccines should not be given to children with manifestations of severe immunosuppression. However, the MMR and varicella-zoster virus (VZV) vaccines (separately; not combined as MMRV vaccine, which has a higher titer of attenuated varicella virus, the safety of which has not been shown in this population) *can* be given to asymptomatic patients following the routine schedule and to patients who have had HIV symptoms but who are not severely immunocompromised (ie, not in category 3 [see Table 312–2], including having a CD4+ T-cell percentage of ≥ 15%). If possible, the MMR and VZV vaccines should be given starting at age 12 mo in symptomatic patients to enhance the likelihood of an immune response, ie, before the immune system deteriorates. The 2nd dose of each may be given as soon as 4 wk later in an attempt to induce seroconversion as early as possible, although typically a 3-mo interval between varicella vaccine doses is preferred in noninfected children < 13 yr. If the risk of exposure to measles is increased, such as during an outbreak, the measles vaccine should be given at an earlier age, such as 6 to 9 mo.

The live oral rotavirus vaccine may be given to HIV-exposed or HIV-infected infants according to the routine schedule. Safety and efficacy data are limited in symptomatic infants but there very likely is overall benefit to immunization, particularly in areas where rotavirus causes significant mortality.

The BCG vaccine is not recommended in the US because it is an area of low TB prevalence. However, elsewhere in the world, especially in developing countries where TB prevalence is high, BCG is routinely used; many of these countries also have high HIV prevalence among childbearing women. BCG as a live bacterial vaccine has caused some harm in HIV-infected children but likely protects non–HIV-infected and even some HIV-infected children from acquiring TB. Thus, the WHO now recommends that children who are known to be HIV-infected, even if asymptomatic, should no longer be immunized with BCG vaccine. However, BCG may be given to asymptomatic infants of unknown HIV infection status born to HIV-infected women, depending on the relative incidence of TB and HIV in the particular area. BCG also may be given to asymptomatic infants born to women of unknown HIV infection status.

In some areas of the world, children are routinely given the yellow fever vaccine; it should be given only to those without severe immunosuppression.

Because children with symptomatic HIV infection generally have poor immunologic responses to vaccines, they should be considered susceptible when they are exposed to a vaccine-preventable disease (eg, measles, tetanus, varicella) regardless of their vaccination history. Such children should receive passive immunization with IV immune globulin. IV immune globulin also should be given to any nonimmunized household member who is exposed to measles.

Seronegative children living with a person with symptomatic HIV infection should receive inactivated poliovirus vaccine rather than oral polio vaccine. Influenza (inactivated or live), MMR, varicella, and rotavirus vaccines may be given normally because these vaccine viruses are not commonly transmitted by the vaccinee. Adult household contacts should receive annual influenza vaccination (inactivated or live) to reduce the risk of transmitting influenza to the HIV-infected person.

Transition to Adult Care

Transition of HIV-infected youth from the pediatric health care model to the adult health care model takes time and advance planning. This process is active and ongoing and does not simply involve a one-time referral to an adult care clinic or office. The pediatric health care model tends to be family-centered, and the care team includes a multidisciplinary team of physicians, nurses, social workers, and mental health professionals; perinatally infected youth may have been cared for by such a team for their entire life. In contrast, the typical adult health care model tends to be individual-centered, and the health care practitioners involved may be located in separate offices requiring multiple visits. Health care practitioners at adult care clinics and offices are often managing high patient volumes, and the consequences of lateness or missed appointments (which may be more common among adolescents) are stricter. Finally, changes in insurance coverage in adolescence or young adulthood can complicate transition of medical care as well. Planning transition over several months and having adolescents have discussions or joint visits with the pediatric and adult health care practitioners can lead to a smoother and more successful transition. Several resources for transition of HIV-infected youth into adult health care are now available from the American Academy of Pediatrics (see Policy Statement: Transitioning HIV-Infected Youth Into Adult Health Care at http://pediatrics.aappublications.org) and the New York State Department of Health AIDS Institute (www.hivguidelines.org).

Prevention

For postexposure prevention, see p. 1641.

Prevention of perinatal transmission: Appropriate prenatal ART attempts to optimize maternal health, interrupt MTCT, and minimize in utero drug toxicity. In the US and other countries where ARV drugs and HIV testing are readily available, treatment with ARV drugs is standard for all HIV-infected pregnant women (see p. 1641). Rapid HIV testing of pregnant women who present in labor without documentation of their HIV serostatus may allow immediate institution of such measures.

All HIV-infected pregnant women should initiate combination ART to prevent MTCT, as well as for their own health, as soon as the diagnosis of HIV infection is made and the woman is ready to adhere to ART. Pregnancy is not a contraindication to combination ARV regimens; the use of the ARV agent efavirenz (more common in adults than in children in the US) is no longer contraindicated during the 1st trimester. Most experts believe that HIV-infected women already receiving combination ART who become pregnant should continue that therapy, even during

Table 312–6. CONSIDERATIONS FOR USE OF LIVE VACCINES IN CHILDREN WITH HIV INFECTION

LIVE VACCINE	COMMENTS
BCG	Not recommended in US; internationally, may be given to HIV-exposed neonates of unknown HIV infection status (see p. 2611)
Oral poliovirus	Not recommended in US; inactivated polio vaccine given instead according to routine schedule*
Live-attenuated influenza (LAI)	Not recommended; inactivated vaccine given instead according to routine schedule*
Measles-mumps-rubella (MMR)	Can be given to children whose CD4+ T-cell percentage is ≥ 15% Administration at 12 mo of age followed by 2nd dose within 1–3 mo enhances likelihood of response before HIV-induced immunologic decline occurs MMR plus separate varicella-zoster virus (VZV) vaccine preferred over MMRV to minimize adverse effects If risk of exposure to measles is increased (eg, during an outbreak), given at a younger age (eg, 6–9 mo); however, this dose not considered part of routine schedule (ie, restart at 12 mo)
Rotavirus, live-attenuated	Limited evidence to date suggests that benefits of vaccine very likely outweigh its risks
Varicella-zoster virus (VZV)	Can be given to children whose CD4+ T-cell percentage is ≥ 15% Administration at 12 mo of age followed by 2nd dose within 1–3 mo enhances likelihood of response before HIV-induced immunologic decline occurs MMR plus separate VZV vaccine preferred over MMRV to minimize adverse effects

*Given according to the usual pediatric immunization schedule (see Tables 291–2 on p. 2462 and 291–3 on p. 2467).
AAP = American Academy of Pediatrics; ACIP = Advisory Committee on Immunization Practices; MMRV = measles-mumps-rubella-varicella.

the 1st trimester. An alternative is to stop all therapy until the beginning of the 2nd trimester and resume at that time.

Combination ARV oral therapy is continued throughout the pregnancy, and IV ZDV is given during labor, at 2 mg/kg IV for the first hour and then 1 mg/kg/h IV until delivery. Some experts now believe that IV ZDV is not required for women receiving combination ART who have achieved HIV plasma RNA viral loads < 400 copies/mL near delivery; others recommend its use regardless of the degree of virologic control. Ideally, combination ART is continued for all women post-partum, even for those not previously receiving ART before the pregnancy.

The full-term neonate born to a woman who has had good virologic control to her ART (as shown by a plasma HIV viral RNA of <400 copies/mL) is considered at low risk for HIV acquisition (< 0.5 to 1%) and should be given ZDV 4 mg/kg po q 12 h for the first 4 to 6 wk of life. This regimen is the backbone of infant prophylaxis, utilized for all infants born to HIV-infected women regardless of the woman's degree of virologic control. If virologic control is poor, however, additional interventions are considered.

Infants born to women who are not receiving ART, who have either unknown plasma viral loads or viral loads ≥ 400 copies/mL at the time of labor and delivery, or who are known to be infected with highly ARV-resistant HIV, are considered at high risk of HIV acquisition (1 to 25%). In this situation, elective cesarean delivery before onset of labor is recommended if the maternal viral load is > 1000 copies/mL. If labor has already begun, it is less certain whether cesarean delivery will contribute to further reduction of MTCT. Women and their high-risk infants are given zidovudine as described previously (ie, the women receive drugs IV during labor and delivery; the infants receive drugs by mouth). In addition, additional ARV drugs should be given to the infant. Unfortunately, very few ARV drugs (notably zidovudine, nevirapine, and lamivudine) are known to be safe and effective for infants < 14 days postnatal age, and fewer still have dosing data available for premature infants. Recent clinical trial data and expert opinion suggest that either a regimen of oral zidovudine given for 6 wk and supplemented with 3 separate doses of nevirapine given over the first several days of life, or a combination regimen of zidovudine, lamivudine, and nevirapine given for 6 weeks, can significantly reduce MTCT among infants judged to be at high risk of HIV acquisition born to women who did not receive any antepartum therapy. An expert in pediatric or maternal HIV infection should be immediately consulted.

Although the final decision to accept ART remains with the pregnant woman, it should be stressed that the proven benefits of therapy in preventing mother-to-child HIV transmission far outweigh the theoretical risks of any ARV fetal toxicity.

Breastfeeding (or donating to milk banks) is contraindicated for HIV-infected women in the US and other countries where safe and affordable alternative sources of feeding are readily available. Premastication of infant food by HIV-infected mothers is also contraindicated. However, in countries where infectious diseases and undernutrition are major causes of early childhood mortality and safe, affordable infant formula is not available, the protection breastfeeding offers against the mortality risks of any ARV respiratory and GI infections may counterbalance the risk of HIV transmission. In these developing countries, the WHO recommends that HIV-infected mothers continue to breastfeed for the first 6 mo of the infant's life and then rapidly wean the infant to food.

Prevention of adolescent transmission: Because adolescents are at special risk of HIV infection, they should receive education, have access to HIV testing, and know their serostatus. Education should include information about transmission, implications of infection, and strategies for prevention, including abstaining from high-risk behaviors and engaging in safe sex practices (eg, correct and consistent use of condoms [see p. 2242]) for those who are sexually active. Efforts should especially target adolescents at high risk of HIV infection, in particular, black and Hispanic adolescent men who have sex with other men because this is the fastest-growing US demographic of new HIV infections among youth; however, all adolescents should receive risk-reduction education.

In most US states, informed consent is necessary for testing and the release of information regarding HIV serostatus. Decisions regarding disclosure of HIV status to a sex partner without the patient's consent should be based on the possibility of domestic violence to the patient after disclosure to the partner, likelihood that the partner is at risk, whether the partner has reasonable cause to suspect the risk and to take precautions, and presence of a legal requirement to withhold or disclose such information. Pre-exposure prophylaxis (PrEP) with a fixed dose combination of TDF and FTC is being used more frequently for the HIV-negative partner of an HIV-infected adult. Older adolescents may also receive PrEP, although issues of confidentiality and cost (with possible lack of insurance reimbursement) are more complex than with adult PrEP. For further discussion, see www.hivguidelines.org or www.aidsinfo.nih.gov.

Prevention of opportunistic infections: Prophylactic drug treatment is recommended in certain HIV-infected children for prevention of *Pneumocystis* pneumonia and *M. avium* complex infections. Data are limited on the use of prophylaxis for opportunistic infection by other organisms, such as cytomegalovirus, fungi, and toxoplasma. Guidance on prophylaxis of these and other opportunistic infections is also available at www.aidsinfo.nih.gov.

Prophylaxis against *Pneumocystis* pneumonia is indicated for

- HIV-infected children ≥ 6 yr of age with CD4+ count < 200 cells/μL or CD4+ percentage < 14%
- HIV-infected children 1 to 6 yr of age with CD4+ count < 500 cells/μL or CD4+ percentage < 22%
- HIV-infected infants < 12 mo of age regardless of CD4+ count or percentage
- Infants born to HIV-infected women (beginning at 4 to 6 wk of age), until HIV infection is either presumptively excluded (by documentation of 2 negative virologic test results, 1 at ≥ 2 wk of age and 1 at ≥ 4 wk of age) or definitively excluded (by documentation of 2 negative virologic test results, 1 at ≥ 1 mo of age and 1 at ≥ 4 mo of age) (NOTE: For these definitions of HIV exclusion to be valid, the infant must not be breastfeeding.)

Once immune reconstitution with combination ART occurs, discontinuation of *Pneumocystis* pneumonia prophylaxis may be considered for HIV-infected children who have received combination ART for > 6 mo and whose CD4+ percentage and CD4+ count have remained higher than the previously described treatment thresholds for > 3 consecutive mo. Subsequently, the CD4+ percentage and count should be reevaluated at least every 3 mo, and prophylaxis should be reinstituted if the original criteria are reached.

The drug of choice for *Pneumocystis* prophylaxis at any age is trimethoprim/sulfamethoxazole (TMP/SMX) TMP 75 mg/SMX 375 mg/m^2 po bid on 3 consecutive days/wk (eg, Monday-Tuesday-Wednesday); alternative schedules include the same dose 2 times/day every day, the same dose 2 times/day on alternate days, or twice the dose (TMP 150 mg/SMX 750 mg/m^2) po once/day for 3 consecutive days/wk. Some experts find it easier to use weight-based dosing (TMP 2.5 to 5 mg/SMX 12.5 to 25 mg/kg po bid).

For patients who cannot tolerate TMP/SMX, dapsone 2 mg/kg (not to exceed 100 mg) po once/day is an alternative, especially for those < 5 yr of age. Oral atovaquone given daily or aerosolized pentamidine (300 mg via specially designed inhaler for children ≥ 5 yr) given once/mo is an additional alternative. IV pentamidine has also been used but is both less effective and more toxic.

Prophylaxis against *Mycobacterium avium* complex infection is indicated in

- Children ≥ 6 yr with CD4+ count < 50/μL
- Children 2 to 6 yr with CD4+ count < 75/μL
- Children 1 to 2 yr with CD4+ count < 500/μL
- Children < 1 yr with CD4+ count < 750/μL

Weekly azithromycin or daily clarithromycin is the drug of choice, and daily rifabutin is an alternative.

KEY POINTS

- Most HIV cases in infants and children result from MTCT before or during birth, or (in countries where safe and affordable infant formula is not available) from breastfeeding.
- Maternal antiretroviral treatment can reduce incidence of MTCT from about 25% to < 1%.
- Diagnose children < 18 mo using qualitative RNA assays (eg, transcription-mediated amplification of RNA) or DNA PCR assays.
- Diagnose children > 18 mo using a 4th-generation HIV-1/2 antigen/antibody combination immunoassay followed by a 2nd-generation HIV-1/2 antibody differentiation assay and, if required, an HIV-1 qualitative RNA assay.
- Urgently treat all HIV-infected infants < 12 mo of age; those 1 to < 6 yr of age who have Stage 3-defining opportunistic illnesses or CD4 counts < 500 cells/μL; and those ≥ 6 yr of age who have Stage 3-defining opportunistic illnesses or CD4 counts < 200 μL.
- Treat all other HIV-infected children and adolescents as soon as issues of adherence are more fully assessed and addressed with the children and their caretakers.
- Combination ART is given, preferably using a fixed-dose combination product if feasible, for increased adherence.
- Give prophylaxis for opportunistic infections based on age and CD4+ count.

313 Incontinence in Children

URINARY INCONTINENCE IN CHILDREN

(Enuresis)

Urinary incontinence is defined as involuntary voiding of urine ≥ 2 times/mo during the day or night. Daytime incontinence (diurnal enuresis) is usually not diagnosed until age 5 or 6. Nighttime incontinence (nocturnal enuresis, or bed-wetting) is usually not diagnosed until age 7. Before this time, nocturnal enuresis is typically referred to as nighttime wetting. These age limits are based on children who are developing typically and so may not be applicable to children with developmental delay. Both nocturnal and diurnal enuresis are symptoms—not diagnoses—and necessitate consideration of an underlying cause.

The age at which children attain urinary continence varies, but > 90% are continent during the day by age 5. Nighttime continence takes longer to achieve. Nocturnal enuresis affects about 30% of children at age 4, 10% at age 7, 3% at age 12, and 1% at age 18. About 0.5% of adults continue to have nocturnal wetting episodes. Nocturnal enuresis is more common among boys and when there is a family history.[1]

In primary enuresis, children have never achieved urinary continence for ≥ 6 mo. In secondary enuresis, children have developed incontinence after a period of at least 6 mo of urinary control. An organic cause is more likely in secondary enuresis. Even when there is no organic cause, appropriate treatment and parental education are essential because of the physical and psychologic impact of urine accidents.[2]

1. Horowitz M, Misseri R: Diurnal and nocturnal enuresis. In *Clinical Pediatric Urology,* ed. 5, edited by Docimo S, Canning D, Khoury A. London, Martin Dunitz Ltd., 2007, pp. 819–840.
2. Austin PF, Vricella GJ: Functional disorders of the lower urinary tract in children. In *Campbell-Walsh Urology,* ed. 11, edited by Wein A, Kavoussi L, Partin A, Peters C. Philadelphia, Elsevier, 2016, pp. 3297–3316.

Pathophysiology

Bladder function has a storage phase and a voiding phase. Abnormalities in either phase can cause primary or secondary enuresis.

In the **storage phase,** the bladder acts as a reservoir for urine. Storage capacity is affected by bladder size and compliance. Storage capacity increases as children grow. Compliance can be decreased by repeated infections or by outlet obstruction, with resulting bladder muscle hypertrophy.

In the **voiding phase,** bladder contraction synchronizes with the opening of the bladder neck and the external urinary sphincter. If there is dysfunction in the coordination or sequence of voiding, enuresis can occur. There are multiple reasons for dysfunction. One example is bladder irritation, which can lead to irregular contractions of the bladder and asynchrony of the voiding sequence, resulting in enuresis. Bladder irritation can result from a UTI or from anything that presses on the bladder (eg, a dilated rectum caused by constipation).

Etiology

Urinary incontinence in children has different causes and treatments than urinary incontinence in adults. Although some abnormalities cause both nocturnal and diurnal enuresis, etiology can vary depending on whether enuresis is nocturnal or diurnal, as well as primary or secondary. Most primary enuresis is nocturnal and not due to an organic disorder. Nocturnal enuresis can be divided into monosymptomatic (occurring only during sleep) and complex (other abnormalities are present, such as diurnal enuresis and/or urinary symptoms).

Nocturnal enuresis: Organic disorders account for about 30% of cases and are more common in complex compared to monosymptomatic enuresis. The remaining majority of cases are of unclear etiology but are thought to be due to a combination of factors, including

- Maturational delay
- Uncompleted toilet training
- Functionally small bladder capacity (the bladder is not actually small but contracts before it is completely full)
- Increased nighttime urine volume
- Difficulties in arousal from sleep
- Family history (if one parent had nocturnal enuresis, there is a 30% chance offspring will have it, increasing to 70% if both parents were affected)

The factors contributing to **organic causes of nocturnal enuresis** (see Table 313–1) include

- Conditions that increase urine volume (eg, diabetes mellitus, diabetes insipidus, chronic renal failure, excessive water intake, sickle cell disease, and sometimes sickle trait [hyposthenuria])
- Conditions that increase bladder irritability (eg, UTI, pressure on the bladder by the rectum and sigmoid colon [caused by constipation])
- Structural abnormalities (eg, ectopic ureter, which can cause both nocturnal and diurnal enuresis)
- Abnormal sphincter weakness (eg, spina bifida, which can cause both nocturnal and diurnal enuresis)

Diurnal enuresis: Common causes (see Table 313–2) include

- Bladder irritability
- Relative weakness of the detrusor muscle (making it difficult to inhibit incontinence)
- Constipation, urethrovaginal reflux, or vaginal voiding: girls who use an incorrect position during voiding (eg, with legs close together) or have redundant skinfolds may have reflux of urine into the vagina, which subsequently leaks out on standing
- Structural abnormalities (eg, ectopic ureter)
- Abnormal sphincter weakness (eg, spina bifida, tethered cord)

Evaluation

Evaluation should always include assessment for constipation (which can be a contributing factor to both nocturnal and diurnal enuresis).

History: History of present illness inquires about onset of symptoms (ie, primary vs secondary), timing of symptoms (eg, at night, during the day, only after voiding), and whether symptoms are continuous (ie, constant dribbling) or intermittent. Recording a voiding schedule (voiding diary), including timing, frequency, and volume of voids, can be helpful. Important associated symptoms include polydipsia, dysuria, urgency, frequency, dribbling, and straining. Position during voiding and strength of urine steam should be noted. To prevent leakage, children with enuresis may use holding maneuvers, such as crossing their legs or squatting (sometimes with their hand or heel pushed against their perineum). In some children, holding maneuvers can increase their risk of UTIs. Similar to the voiding diary, a stooling diary can help identify constipation.

Review of systems should seek symptoms suggesting a cause, including frequency and consistency of stools (constipation); fever, abdominal pain, dysuria, and hematuria (UTI); perianal itching and vaginitis (pinworm infection); polyuria and polydipsia (diabetes insipidus or diabetes mellitus); and snoring or breathing pauses during sleep (sleep apnea). Children should be screened for the possibility of sexual abuse, which, although an uncommon cause, is too important to miss.

Past medical history should identify known possible causes, including perinatal insults or birth defects (eg, spina bifida), neurologic disorders, renal disorders, and history of UTIs. Any current or previous treatments for enuresis and how they were actually instituted should be noted, as well as a list of current drugs.

Developmental history should note developmental delay or other developmental disorders related to voiding dysfunction (eg, attention-deficit/hyperactivity disorder, which increases the likelihood of enuresis).

Family history should note the presence of nocturnal enuresis and any urologic disorders.

Social history should note any stressors occurring near the onset of symptoms, including difficulties at school, with friends, or at home; although enuresis is not a psychologic disorder, a brief period of wetting may occur during stress.

Clinicians also should ask about the impact of enuresis on the child because it also affects treatment decisions.

Table 313–1. SOME FACTORS CONTRIBUTING TO NOCTURNAL ENURESIS

CAUSE	SUGGESTIVE FINDINGS	DIAGNOSTIC APPROACH
Constipation	Infrequent, hard-pebble stools Encopresis Abdominal discomfort History of a constipating diet (eg, excessive milk and dairy, few fruits and vegetables)	Clinical evaluation (including stooling diary) Sometimes abdominal x-ray
Increased urine output due to any cause (eg, diabetes mellitus, diabetes insipidus, excessive water intake, sickle cell disease or trait)	Vary by disorder	For diabetes mellitus, serum glucose For diabetes insipidus, serum and blood osmolality For sickle cell, sickle cell screen
Maturational delay	No diurnal enuresis More common among boys and heavy sleepers Possible family history of bed-wetting	Clinical evaluation
Sleep apnea	History of snoring with sounds of breathing pauses followed by loud snorts Excessive daytime sleepiness Enlarged tonsils	Polysomnography
Spinal dysraphism (eg, spina bifida, tethered cord, occult defects), leading to urinary retention	Obvious vertebral defects, protruding meningeal sac, lumbosacral dimple or hair tuft, lower-extremity weakness, decreased sensation in lower extremities Absence of ankle jerk reflex, cremasteric reflex, and anal wink	Lumbosacral x-rays For occult conditions, spinal MRI
Stress	School difficulties, social isolation or difficulties, family stress (eg, divorce, separation)	Clinical evaluation (including voiding diary)
UTI	Dysuria, hematuria, frequency, urgency Fever Abdominal pain	Urinalysis Urine culture For patients with pyelonephritis, ultrasonography and voiding cystourethrogram

Physical examination: Examination begins with review of vital signs for fever (UTI), signs of weight loss (diabetes), and hypertension (renal disorder). Examination of the head and neck should note enlarged tonsils, mouth breathing, or poor growth (sleep apnea). Abdominal examination should note any masses consistent with stool or a full bladder.

In girls, genital examination should note any labial adhesions, scarring, or lesions suspicious of sexual abuse. An ectopic ureteral orifice is often difficult to see but should be sought. In boys, examination should check for meatal irritation or any lesions on the glans or around the rectum. In either sex, perianal excoriations can suggest pinworms.

The spine should be examined for any midline defects (eg, deep sacral dimple, sacral hair patch). A complete neurologic evaluation is essential and should specifically target lower-extremity strength, sensation and deep tendon reflexes, sacral reflexes (eg, anal wink), and, in boys, cremasteric reflex to identify possible spinal dysraphism. A rectal examination may be useful to detect constipation or decreased rectal tone.

Red flags: Findings of particular concern are

- Signs or concerns of sexual abuse
- Excessive thirst, polyuria, and weight loss
- Prolonged primary diurnal enuresis (beyond age 6 yr)
- Any neurologic signs, especially in the lower extremities
- Physical signs of neurologic impairment

Interpretation of findings: Usually, primary **nocturnal enuresis** occurs in children with an otherwise unremarkable history and examination and probably represents maturational delay. A small percentage of children have a treatable medical disorder; sometimes findings suggest possible causes (see Table 313–1).

For children who are being evaluated for nocturnal enuresis, it is important to determine whether diurnal symptoms of urgency, frequency, body posturing or holding maneuvers, and incontinence are present. Children with these symptoms have complex nocturnal enuresis, and management should be directed primarily toward controlling the diurnal symptoms.

In **diurnal enuresis,** dysfunctional voiding is suggested by intermittent enuresis preceded by a sense of urgency, a history of being distracted by play, or a combination. Enuresis after urination (due to lack of total bladder emptying) can also be part of the history.

Enuresis caused by a UTI is likely a discrete episode rather than a chronic, intermittent problem and may be accompanied by typical symptoms (eg, urgency, frequency, pain on urination); however, other causes of enuresis can result in secondary UTI.

Constipation should be considered in the absence of other findings in children who have hard stools and difficulty with elimination (and sometimes palpable stool on examination).

Sleep apnea should be considered with a history of excessive daytime sleepiness and disrupted sleep; parents may provide a history of snoring or respiratory pauses.

Rectal itching (especially at night), vaginitis, urethritis, or a combination can be an indication of pinworms.

Excessive thirst, diurnal and nocturnal enuresis, and weight loss suggest a possible organic cause (eg, diabetes mellitus).

Stress or sexual abuse can be difficult to ascertain but should be considered.

Table 313–2. SOME ORGANIC CAUSES OF DIURNAL ENURESIS

CAUSE	SUGGESTIVE FINDINGS	DIAGNOSTIC APPROACH
Constipation	Infrequent, hard-pebble stools Sometimes encopresis, abdominal discomfort History of a constipating diet (eg, excessive milk and dairy, few fruits and vegetables)	Clinical evaluation (including stooling diary) Sometimes abdominal x-ray
Dysfunctional voiding secondary to lack of coordination of the detrusor muscle and urethral sphincter and not related to a neurologic cause	Often encopresis, VUR, and UTI Possibly nocturnal and diurnal enuresis	Urodynamic studies to show dyssynergy of bladder musculature Uroflow testing Sometimes VCUG
Giggle incontinence	Voiding during laughing, almost exclusively in girls At other times, completely normal voiding	Clinical evaluation
Increased urine output due to any cause (eg, diabetes mellitus, diabetes insipidus, excessive water intake, sickle cell disease or trait)	Vary by disorder	For diabetes mellitus, serum glucose For diabetes insipidus, serum and blood osmolality For sickle cell, sickle cell screen
Micturation deferral with overflow incontinence	In children, waiting to the last minute to void Common among preschool children when absorbed in playing	Consistent history Voiding diary
Neurogenic bladder secondary to spinal dysraphism (eg, spina bifida, tethered cord, occult defects) or nervous system defect	Obvious vertebral defects, protruding meningeal sac, lumbosacral dimple or hair tuft, lower-extremity weakness, decreased sensation in lower extremities	Lumbosacral x-rays For occult conditions, spinal MRI Ultrasonography of the kidneys and bladder Urodynamic studies
Overactive bladder	Urinary urgency (essential for diagnosis); frequency and nocturia also common Sometimes use of holding maneuvers or body posturing (eg, squatting or Vincent curtsy sign)	History consistent with symptoms or overactive bladder Consideration of voiding diary, urodynamic studies, uroflow testing
Sexual abuse	Sleep problems, school difficulties (eg, delinquency, poor grades) Seductive behavior, depression, unusual interest in or avoidance of all things sexual, inappropriate knowledge of sexual things for age	Evaluation by sexual abuse experts
Stress*	School difficulties, social isolation or difficulties, family stress (eg, divorce, separation)	Clinical evaluation
Structural abnormality (eg, ectopic ureter, posterior urethral valves)	In children, full diurnal continence never achieved Diurnal and nocturnal enuresis in girls, history of normal voiding but with continually wet underwear, vaginal discharge Possible history of UTIs, history of other urinary tract abnormalities	Ultrasonography of the kidneys Nuclear renal flow scan or IV urography CT of abdomen and pelvis or MRI urography
UTI	Dysuria, hematuria, frequency, urgency Fever Abdominal pain	Urinalysis Urine culture For patients with pyelonephritis, ultrasonography and VCUG
Vaginal reflux (urethrovaginal reflux, or vaginal voiding) due to any cause (including labial adhesions)	Dribbling when standing after urination	Clinical evaluation, including improvement with instruction on proper method of voiding to discourage retention of urine in vagina (eg, sitting backward on toilet or with knees wide apart)

*Stress is a cause primarily when incontinence is acute.
VCUG = voiding cystourethrogram; VUR = vesicoureteral reflux.

Testing: Diagnosis is often apparent after history and physical examination. Urinalysis and urine culture are appropriate for both sexes. Further testing is useful mainly when history, physical examination, or both suggest an organic cause (see Tables 313–1 and 313–2). Ultrasonography of the kidneys and bladder is often done to verify urinary tract anatomy is normal. Uroflow testing can show a staccato voiding pattern in patients with dysfunctional voiding.

Treatment

The most important part of treatment is family education about the cause and clinical course of enuresis. Education helps decrease the negative psychologic impact of urine accidents and results in increased adherence with treatment.

Treatment of urinary incontinence should be targeted toward any cause that is identified; however, frequently no cause is found. In such cases, the following treatments may be useful.

Nocturnal enuresis: The most effective long-term strategy is a bed-wetting alarm. Although labor intensive, the success rate can be as high as 70% when children are motivated to end the enuresis, and the family is able to adhere. It can take up to 4 mo of nightly use for complete resolution of symptoms. The alarm triggers when wetting occurs. Although children initially continue to have wetting episodes, over time, they learn to associate the sensation of a full bladder with the alarm and then wake up to void prior to an enuretic event. These alarms are readily available online without prescription. An alarm should not be used by children with complex nocturnal enuresis or children with reduced bladder capacity (as evidenced by voiding diary). These children should be treated the same as children with diurnal enuresis. It is essential to avoid punitive approaches because these undermine treatment and lead only to poor self-esteem.

Drugs such as desmopressin (DDAVP) and imipramine (see Table 313–3) can decrease nighttime wetting episodes. However, results are not sustained in most patients when the treatment is stopped; parents and children should be forewarned of this to help limit disappointment. DDAVP is preferable to imipramine because of the rare potential of sudden death with imipramine use.

Diurnal enuresis: It is important to treat any underlying constipation. Information from the voiding diary can help identify children with reduced functional bladder capacity, frequency and urgency of urination, and urinary infrequency, all of whom may present with urinary incontinence.

General measures may include

- Urgency containment exercises: Children are directed to go to the bathroom as soon as they feel the urge to urinate. They then hold the urine as long as they can and, when they can hold it no longer, start to urinate and then stop and start the urine stream. This exercise strengthens the sphincter and gives children confidence that they can make it to the bathroom before they have an accident.
- Gradual lengthening of voiding intervals (if detrusor instability or dysfunctional voiding is suspected)
- Changes in behaviors (eg, delayed urination) through positive reinforcement and scheduled urination (time voiding): Children are reminded to urinate by a clock that vibrates or sounds an alarm (preferable to having a parent in the reminder role).
- Use of correct voiding methods to discourage retention of urine in the vagina: In girls experiencing vaginal pooling of urine, treatment is to encourage sitting facing backward on the toilet or with the knees wide apart, which will spread the introitus and allow direct flow of urine into the toilet.

For labial adhesions, a conjugated estrogen or triamcinolone 0.5% cream may also be used.

Drug treatment (see Table 313–3) is sometimes helpful but is not typically first-line therapy. Anticholinergic drugs (oxybutynin and tolterodine) may benefit patients with diurnal enuresis due to voiding dysfunction when behavioral therapy or physiotherapy is unsuccessful. Drugs for nocturnal enuresis may be useful in decreasing nighttime wetting episodes and are sometimes useful to encourage dryness during overnight events such as sleepovers.

KEY POINTS

- Primary urinary incontinence most frequently manifests as nocturnal enuresis.
- Constipation should be considered as a contributing source.
- Most nocturnal enuresis abates with maturation (15%/yr resolve with no intervention), but at least 0.5% of adults have nighttime wetting episodes.
- Organic causes of enuresis are infrequent but should be considered.
- Alarms are the most effective treatment for nocturnal enuresis.
- Other treatments include behavioral interventions and sometimes drugs.
- Parental education is essential to the child's outcome and well-being.

Table 313–3. DRUGS USED FOR ENURESIS IN CHILDREN*

DRUG	DOSAGE	SOME ADVERSE EFFECTS
Voiding dysfunction in diurnal enuresis (bladder overactivity)		
Oxybutynin	For children > 5 yr, 5 mg po bid, may be increased to 5 mg tid Extended-release: For children > 6 yr, 5 mg po once/day, increased as tolerated by 5 mg/day to a maximum of 15 mg/day	Confusion, dizziness, increased temperature, flushing, constipation, dry mouth
Tolterodine	For children > 5 yr, 1 mg po bid Children who can swallow pills, extended-release capsules 2 mg to 4 mg once/day	Constipation, flushing, dry mouth
Nocturnal enuresis		
Desmopressin (DDAVP)	For children ≥ 6 yr, initially 0.2 mg po once/day 1 h before bedtime, increased prn to a maximum of 0.6 mg once/day	Intranasal DDAVP is no longer recommended because of the risk of dilutional hyponatremia
Imipramine	For children 6–8 yr, 25 mg po once/day at night) For children > 8 yr, 50 mg po once/day at night	Rarely, death† Possible nervousness, personality change, disordered sleep, cardiac arrhythmias‡

*These drugs are mostly used as 2nd-line therapy. Treatment of the underlying disorder and behavioral therapy should be used first.
†Sudden death of unclear etiology has been reported. This drug is now rarely used.
‡ECG should be done to identify prolongation of the QT interval and/or the corrected QT (QTc) interval, which contraindicate use of imipramine.

STOOL INCONTINENCE IN CHILDREN

(Encopresis)

Stool incontinence is the voluntary or involuntary passage of stool in inappropriate places in children > 4 yr (or developmental equivalent) who do not have an organic defect or illness with the exception of constipation.

Encopresis is a common childhood problem; it occurs in about 3 to 4% of 4-yr-old children and decreases in frequency with age.

Etiology

Encopresis is most commonly caused by constipation in children with behavioral and physical predisposing factors. It rarely occurs without retention or constipation, but when it does, other organic processes (eg, Hirschsprung disease, celiac disease) or psychologic problems should be considered.

Pathophysiology

Stool retention and constipation result in dilation of the rectum and sigmoid colon, which leads to changes in the reactivity of muscles and nerves of the bowel wall. These changes decrease the efficacy of bowel excretory function and lead to further retention. As stool remains in the bowel, water is absorbed, which hardens the stool, making passage more difficult and painful. Softer, looser stool may then leak around the hardened stool bolus, resulting in overflow. Both leakage and ineffective bowel control result in stool accidents.

Diagnosis

- Clinical evaluation

Any organic process that results in constipation[1] can result in encopresis and so should be considered. For most routine cases of encopresis, a thorough history and physical examination can help identify any physical cause. However, if further concerns arise, additional diagnostic tests (eg, abdominal x-rays, rarely rectal wall biopsy, and even more rarely bowel motility studies) can be considered.

1. Koyle MA, Lorenzo AJ: Management of defecation disorders. In *Campbell-Walsh Urology,* ed. 11, edited by Wein A, Kavoussi L, Partin A, Peters C. Philadelphia, Elsevier, 2016, pp. 3317–3329.

Treatment

- Education and demystification (for parents and child)
- Relief of stool impaction
- Maintenance (eg, behavioral and dietary interventions, laxative therapy)
- Slow withdrawal of laxatives with continued behavioral and dietary intervention (see Table 290–2 on p. 2437)

Any underlying disorders are treated. If there is no specific underlying pathology, symptoms are addressed. Initial treatment involves educating the parents and child about the physiology of encopresis, removing blame from the child, and diffusing the emotional reactions of those involved. Next the goal is to relieve any stool impaction.

Stool impaction can be relieved by a variety of regimens and drugs (see p. 2436); choice depends on the age of the child and other factors. A combination of polyethylene glycol (PEG) with electrolytes plus a stimulant laxative (eg, bisacodyl or senna), or a sequence of Na phosphate enemas plus a 2-wk regimen of oral drugs (eg, bisacodyl tablets) and suppositories are often used.

After evacuation, a follow-up visit should be held to assess whether the evacuation has been successful, make sure soiling has resolved, and establish a maintenance plan. This plan includes encouragement of maintenance of regular bowel movements (usually via ongoing laxative management) and behavioral interventions to encourage stool evacuation. There are many options for maintenance laxative therapy (see Table 290–2 on p. 2437), but PEG without electrolytes is used most often, typically 1 to 2 doses of 17 g/day titrated to effect. At times a stimulant laxative may also be continued on the weekends to encourage extra evacuation of stool.

Behavioral strategies include structured toilet-sitting times (eg, having children sit on the toilet for 5 to 10 min after each meal to take advantage of the gastrocolic reflex). If children have accidents during certain times of the day, they also should sit on the toilet immediately prior to those times. Small rewards are often useful incentives. For example, giving children stickers to place on a chart each time they sit on the toilet (even if there is no stool production) can increase adherence to a plan. Often a stepwise program is used in which children receive small tokens (eg, stickers) for sitting on the toilet and larger rewards for consistent adherence. Rewards may need to be changed over time to maintain children's interest in the plan.

In the maintenance phase, regular toilet sitting sessions still are needed to encourage evacuation of stool before the sensation is felt. This strategy decreases the likelihood of stool retention and allows the rectum to return to its normal size. During the maintenance phase, parent and child education about toilet sitting is instrumental to the success of the regimen.

Regular follow-up visits are necessary for ongoing guidance and support. Bowel retraining is a long process that may take months to years and includes slow withdrawal of laxatives once symptoms resolve and continued encouragement of toilet sitting. Relapses often occur during withdrawal of the maintenance regimen, so it is important to provide ongoing support and guidance during this phase.

Encopresis can recur in times of stress or transition, so family members must be prepared for this possibility. Success rates are affected by physical and psychosocial factors, but 1-yr cure rates are about 30 to 50% and 5-yr cure rates are about 48 to 75%. The mainstay of treatment is family education, bowel cleanout and maintenance, and ongoing support.

KEY POINTS

- Encopresis is most commonly caused by constipation in children with behavioral and physical predisposing factors.
- For most routine cases of encopresis, a thorough history and physical examination can help identify any physical cause.
- Any organic process that results in constipation can result in encopresis and so should be considered.
- Treatment is through education, relief of stool impaction, maintenance of proper stooling, and slow withdrawal of laxatives with continued behavioral and dietary intervention.
- Stool impaction can be relieved by a variety of regimens and drugs.
- Behavioral strategies include structured toilet-sitting times.
- Encopresis can recur in times of stress or transition, so family members must be prepared for this possibility.

314 Infections in Neonates

Neonatal infection can be acquired

- In utero transplacentally or through ruptured membranes
- In the birth canal during delivery (intrapartum)
- From external sources after birth (postpartum)

In utero infection, which can occur any time before birth, results from overt or subclinical maternal infection. Consequences depend on the agent and timing of infection in gestation and include spontaneous abortion, intrauterine growth restriction, premature birth, stillbirth, congenital malformation (eg, rubella), and symptomatic (eg, cytomegalovirus [CMV], toxoplasmosis, syphilis) or asymptomatic (eg, CMV) neonatal infection.

Common viral agents include herpes simplex viruses, HIV, CMV, and hepatitis B. Intrapartum infection with HIV or hepatitis B occurs from passage through an infected birth canal or by ascending infection if delivery is delayed after rupture of membranes; these viruses can less commonly be transmitted transplacentally. CMV is commonly transmitted transplacentally.

Bacterial agents include group B streptococci, enteric gram-negative organisms (primarily *Escherichia coli*), *Listeria monocytogenes,* gonococci, and chlamydiae.

Postpartum infections are acquired from contact with an infected mother directly (eg, TB, which also is sometimes transmitted in utero) or through breastfeeding (eg, HIV, CMV) or from contact with health care practitioners and the hospital environment (numerous organisms—see p. 2632).

In utero infection: In utero infection, which can occur any time before birth, results from overt or subclinical maternal infection. Consequences depend on the agent and timing of infection in gestation and include spontaneous abortion, intrauterine growth restriction, premature birth, stillbirth, congenital malformation (eg, rubella), and symptomatic (eg, CMV, toxoplasmosis, syphilis) or asymptomatic (eg, CMV) neonatal infection.

Common **infectious agents** transmitted transplacentally include rubella, toxoplasma, CMV, and syphilis. HIV and hepatitis B are less commonly transmitted transplacentally.

Intrapartum infection: Neonatal infections with herpes simplex viruses, HIV, hepatitis B, group B streptococci, enteric gram-negative organisms (primarily *Escherichia coli*), *Listeria monocytogenes,* gonococci, and chlamydiae usually occur from passage through an infected birth canal. Sometimes ascending infection can occur if delivery is delayed after rupture of membranes.

Postpartum infection: Postpartum infections are acquired from contact with an infected mother directly (eg, TB, which also is sometimes transmitted in utero) or through breastfeeding (eg, HIV, CMV) or from contact with family or visitors, health care practitioners, or the hospital environment (numerous organisms—see p. 2632).

Risk factors for neonatal infection: Risk of contracting intrapartum and postpartum infection is inversely proportional to gestational age. Neonates are immunologically immature, with decreased polymorphonuclear leukocyte, monocyte, and cell-mediated immune function; premature infants are particularly so (see p. 2790).

Maternal IgG antibodies are actively transported across the placenta, but effective levels for all organisms are not achieved until near term. IgM antibodies do not cross the placenta. Premature infants have decreased intrinsic antibody production and reduced complement activity. Premature infants are also more likely to require invasive procedures (eg, endotracheal intubation, prolonged IV access) that predispose to infection.

Symptoms and Signs

Symptoms and signs in neonates tend to be nonspecific (eg, vomiting or poor feeding, increased sleepiness or lethargy, fever or hypothermia, tachypnea, rashes, diarrhea, abdominal distention). Many congenital infections acquired before birth can cause or be accompanied by various symptoms or abnormalities (eg, growth restriction, deafness, microcephaly, anomalies, failure to thrive, hepatosplenomegaly, neurologic abnormalities).

Diagnosis

- Clinical evaluation

A wide variety of infections, including sepsis, should be considered in neonates who are ill at or shortly after birth, particularly those with risk factors. Infections such as congenital rubella, syphilis, toxoplasmosis, and CMV should be pursued in neonates with abnormalities such as growth restriction, deafness, microcephaly, anomalies, hepatosplenomegaly, or neurologic abnormalities.

Treatment

- Antimicrobial therapy

The primary treatment for presumed bacterial infection in the neonate is prompt empiric antimicrobial therapy with drugs such as ampicillin and gentamicin or ampicillin and cefotaxime. Final drug selection is based on culture results similar to the practice in adults, because infecting organisms and their sensitivities are not specific to neonates. However, drug dose and frequency are affected by numerous factors, including age and weight (see Tables 314–1 and 314–3).

ANTIBIOTICS IN NEONATES

In neonates, the ECF constitutes up to 45% of total body weight, requiring relatively larger doses of certain antibiotics (eg, aminoglycosides) compared with adults. Lower serum albumin concentrations in premature infants may reduce antibiotic protein binding. Drugs that displace bilirubin from albumin (eg, sulfonamides, ceftriaxone) increase the risk of kernicterus.

Absence or deficiency of certain enzymes in neonates may prolong the half-life of certain antibiotics (eg, chloramphenicol) and increase the risk of toxicity. Changes in GFR and renal tubular secretion during the first month of life necessitate dosing changes for renally excreted drugs (eg, penicillins, aminoglycosides, vancomycin).

CONGENITAL AND PERINATAL CYTOMEGALOVIRUS INFECTION

Cytomegalovirus (CMV) infection may be acquired prenatally or perinatally and is the most common congenital viral infection. Signs at birth, if present, are intrauterine growth restriction, prematurity, microcephaly, jaundice, petechiae, hepatosplenomegaly, periventricular calcifications, chorioretinitis, pneumonitis, hepatitis, and sensorineural hearing

Table 314–1. RECOMMENDED DOSAGES OF SELECTED PARENTERAL ANTIBIOTICS FOR NEONATES

ANTIBIOTIC	ROUTE OF ADMINISTRATION	INDIVIDUAL DOSE	INTERVAL OF ADMINISTRATION						COMMENTS
			BODY WEIGHT < 1200 G		BODY WEIGHT 1200–1999 G		BODY WEIGHT ≥ 2000 G		
			AGE		AGE		AGE		
			≤ 7 days	8–28 days	≤ 7 days	8–28 days	≤ 7 days	8–28 days	
	IV, IM	15 mg/kg	q 48 h	q 24–48 h	q 48 h	q 24–48 h	q 24 h	q 12–24 h	Monitoring of serum drug levels required (peak = 20–30 µg/mL; trough = < 10 µg/mL) Dose reduction required for impaired renal function For extended dosing intervals, may be given as a single dose of 15–20 mg/kg given once/day or once every 48 h
Amphotericin B deoxycholate	IV	0.25–1.5 mg/kg	After dilution in 5% or 10% D/W (saline solution should not be used), infusion of a test dose of 0.1 mg/kg (maximum 1 mg) over 1 h to assess patient's febrile and hemodynamic response;[†] if no serious adverse effects are observed, infusion of a therapeutic dose (usually 0.25–1.5 mg/kg over 2–6 h), which may be given the same day as the test dose After the patient improves, may give the dose every other day until therapy is complete Monitoring of K levels and hematologic and renal functions required						
Ampicillin									
For meningitis	IV	75 mg/kg	q 6 h	q 6 h	q 6 h	q 6 h	q 6 h	q 6 h	IV as 15- to 30-min infusion (≤ 10 mg/kg/min)
For other diseases	IV, IM	50 mg/kg	q 12 h	q 8 h	q 12 h	q 8 h	q 8 h	q 6 h	
Aztreonam	IV, IM	30 mg/kg	q 12 h	q 12 h	q 12 h	q 8–12 h	q 8–12 h	q 6–8 h	Limited data For gram-negative bacilli only
Cefazolin[‡]	IV, IM	20–25 mg/kg	q 12 h	q 12 h	q 12 h	q 12 h	q 12 h	q 8 h	Limited data No primary indication; not used as initial therapy for sepsis or meningitis
Cefepime	IV, IM	30–50 mg/kg	q 12 h	q 8–12 h	q 12 h	q 8–12 h	q 8–12 h	q 8–12 h	May be used for *Pseudomonas aeruginosa* infections (consider using 50 mg/kg every 8 h for *P. aeruginosa* and other serious gram-negative pathogens) Sometimes used for meningitis, although usually as a 2nd-line drug and not always recommended
Cefotaxime	IV, IM	50 mg/kg	q 12 h	q 8 h	q 12 h	q 8 h	q 12 h For meningitis, q 8–12 h	q 8 h For meningitis, q 6–8 h	Often a first-line therapy for neonatal meningitis

Table 314–1. RECOMMENDED DOSAGES OF SELECTED PARENTERAL ANTIBIOTICS FOR NEONATES (*Continued*)

			INTERVAL OF ADMINISTRATION						
			BODY WEIGHT < 1200 G		BODY WEIGHT 1200–1999 G		BODY WEIGHT ≥ 2000 G		
			AGE		AGE		AGE		
ANTIBIOTIC	ROUTE OF ADMINISTRATION	INDIVIDUAL DOSE	≤ 7 days	8–28 days	≤ 7 days	8–28 days	≤ 7 days	8–28 days	COMMENTS
Ceftazidime	IV, IM	50 mg/kg	q 12 h	q 8 h	q 12 h	q 8 h	q 12 h	q 8 h	Penetrates well into inflamed meninges 70–90% of drug excreted unchanged in urine
Ceftriaxone	IV, IM	50 mg/kg	q 24 h	q 24 h	q 24 h	q 24 h	q 24 h	q 24 h	Limited data May cause biliary pseudolithiasis and, in jaundiced premature infants, may increase risk of bilirubin encephalopathy via displacement of bilirubin from albumin Contraindicated in neonates receiving or expected to receive infusions of Ca-containing solutions 2nd-line drug for meningitis, after the first wk of life (40–50 mg/kg q 12 h or 80–100 mg/kg q 24 h)
Chloramphenicol	IV	25 mg/kg	q 24 h	q 24 h	q 24 h	q 12–24 h	q 24 h	q 12 h	Doses adjusted by monitoring serum drug levels and hematologic parameters For meningitis, desired peak serum levels = 15–25 µg/mL and trough levels = 5–15 µg/mL For other infections, dose adjusted to attain a peak level of 10–20 µg/mL and a trough level of 5–10 µg/mL Large variability in serum levels and serum half life, especially in preterm neonates
Clindamycin	IV, IM	5 mg/kg	q 12 h	q 12 h	q 12 h	q 8 h	q 8 h	q 6 h	For anaerobes and gram-positive cocci (not enterococci)
Gentamicin*/ tobramycin	IV, IM	4–5 mg/kg	q 48 h	q 24–48 h	q 36 h	q 24–48 h	q 24 h	q 12–24 h	Monitoring of serum drug levels required (peak = 5–12 µg/mL; trough = < 2 µg/mL) Dose reduction required for impaired renal function
Meropenem	IV	20–40 mg/kg	q 12 h	q 8 h	q 12 h	q 8 h	q 8 h	q 8 h	Higher doses used for meningitis

Table continues on the following page.

Table 314–1. RECOMMENDED DOSAGES OF SELECTED PARENTERAL ANTIBIOTICS FOR NEONATES (*Continued*)

ANTIBIOTIC	ROUTE OF ADMINISTRATION	INDIVIDUAL DOSE	INTERVAL OF ADMINISTRATION						COMMENTS
			BODY WEIGHT < 1200 G		BODY WEIGHT 1200–1999 G		BODY WEIGHT ≥ 2000 G		
			AGE		AGE		AGE		
			≤ 7 days	8–28 days	≤ 7 days	8–28 days	≤ 7 days	8–28 days	
Metronidazole	IV	15 mg/kg (7.5 mg/kg for neonates ≤ 7 days *and* < 1200 g)	q 24–48 h	q 24–48 h	q 24 h	q 24 h	q 24 h	q 12 h	Limited data Loading dose of 15 mg/kg, then a subsequent dose 48 h later in preterm infants
Nafcillin/ oxacillin									Monitoring of CBC and liver function required Excretion may be decreased due to renal and hepatic immaturity, leading to possible accumulation in serum, which may have adverse effects
For meningitis or endocarditis	IV	50 mg/kg	q 12 h	q 12 h	q 12 h	q 8 h	q 8 h	q 6 h	
For other diseases	IV, IM	25 mg/kg	q 12 h	q 8–12 h	q 12 h	q 8 h	q 8 h	q 6 h	
Oxacillin (see Nafcillin/oxacillin)	—	—	—	—	—	—	—	—	
Penicillin G, aqueous									
For meningitis	IV	50,000–75,000 units/kg	q 12 h	q 12 h	q 12 h	q 8 h	q 8 h	q 6 h	Maximum for group B streptococcal meningitis = 450,000 units/kg/day
For most other diseases	IV, IM	25,000 units/kg	q 12 h	q 12 h	q 12 h	q 8 h	q 8 h	q 6 h	
Penicillin G, procaine	IM	50,000 units/kg	Not recommended	Not recommended	q 24 h	q 24 h	q 24 h	q 24 h	CAUTION: *Sterile abscess and procaine toxicity*
Piperacillin/ tazobactam	IV (dose based on piperacillin component)	100 mg/kg	q 12 h	q 8 h	q 12 h	q 8 h	q 12 h	q 8 h	May be increased to 100 mg/kg q 6 h in infants > 28 days
Tobramycin (see Gentamicin/ tobramycin)	—	—	—	—	—	—	—	—	—
Vancomycin (see Table 314–2)	—	—	—	—	—	—	—	—	Dosing based on gestational age and serum creatinine (see Table 314–2)

*Sample should be obtained 30 min after a 30-min IV infusion.
†The need to administer a test dose of amphotericin B is controversial.
‡Cefazolin does not cross the blood-brain barrier.

Table 314–2. VANCOMYCIN DOSAGE FOR NEONATES

SERUM CREATININE (mg/dL)			
≤ 28 WK GESTATION	> 28 WK GESTATION	DOSE	INTERVAL OF ADMINISTRATION
< 0.5	< 0.7	15 mg/kg	q 12 h
0.5–0.7	0.7–0.9	20 mg/kg	q 24 h
0.8–1	1–1.2	15 mg/kg	q 24 h
1.1–1.4	1.3–1.6	10 mg/kg	q 24 h
> 1.4	> 1.6	15 mg/kg	q 48 h

*Dose is given by slow IV infusion, over at least 60 min. Monitoring of serum trough level is recommended (trough = 10–15 μg/mL).

loss. If acquired later in infancy, signs may include pneumonia, hepatosplenomegaly, hepatitis, thrombocytopenia, sepsis-like syndrome, and atypical lymphocytosis. Diagnosis of neonatal infection is best made by viral detection via culture or PCR. Treatment is mainly supportive. Parenteral ganciclovir or oral valganciclovir may prevent hearing deterioration and improve developmental outcomes and is given to infants with symptomatic disease identified in the neonatal period.

CMV is frequently isolated from neonates. Although most infants shedding this virus are asymptomatic, others have life-threatening illness and devastating long-term sequelae.

It is not known when a woman with primary CMV can safely conceive. Because risk to the fetus is difficult to assess, women who develop primary CMV during pregnancy should be counseled, but few experts recommend routine serologic testing for CMV before or during pregnancy in healthy women.

Etiology

Congenital CMV infection, which occurs in 0.2 to 1% of live births worldwide, may result from transplacental acquisition of either a primary or recurrent maternal infection. Clinically apparent disease in the neonate is much more likely to occur after a primary maternal exposure, particularly in the first half of pregnancy. In some higher socioeconomic groups in the

Table 314–3. RECOMMENDED DOSAGES OF SELECTED ORAL ANTIBIOTICS FOR NEONATES*

ANTIBIOTIC	DOSAGE	INTERVAL	COMMENTS
Amoxicillin	10–15 mg/kg	q 12 h	Limited data
Azithromycin	5–10 mg/kg	q 24 h	Preferred drug for treatment or prevention of pertussis in neonates < 1 mo For treatment or prevention of pertussis, 10 mg/kg given once/day for 5 days For most other infections, 10 mg/kg given on day 1 and then 5 mg/kg given on days 2–5
Clindamycin†	5 mg/kg	q 6–12 h	Limited data
Erythromycin ethylsuccinate	10–12.5 mg/kg	q 6–12 h	For chlamydial infections or pertussis in neonates > 1 mo Associated with idiopathic hypertrophic pyloric stenosis
Fluconazole	3–12 mg/kg	q 24–72 h	For minor candidal infections, 6 mg/kg on day 1, then 3 mg/kg/dose q 24–72 h For serious infections, 12 mg/kg once/day recommend for all gestational and postnatal ages A first (loading) dose of 25 mg/kg also possibly considered During the 1st 2 wk of life, adjustment of dosing interval possibly necessary if renal function is abnormal
Flucytosine	12.5–37.5 mg/kg	q 6 h	Limited data Used only with amphotericin B to slow emergence of resistance Monitoring of levels recommended For neonates < 2000 g and < 7 days, 25 mg/kg q 8 h
Linezolid	10 mg/kg	q 8–12 h	Can be given IV or orally Used for resistant gram-positive infections
Rifampin	10 mg/kg	q 24 h	For TB
	5 mg/kg	q 12 h	For meningococcus prophylaxis, given for 2 days
	10 mg/kg	q 24 h	For *Haemophilus influenzae* prophylaxis, given for 4 days

*Unless otherwise stated, doses are for neonates who are > 7 days and > 2000 g.
†The dose for neonates who are < 7 days and < 2000 g is 5 mg/kg q 12 h.

US, 50% of young women lack antibody to CMV, making them susceptible to primary infection.

Perinatal CMV infection is acquired by exposure to infected cervical secretions, breast milk, or blood products. Maternal antibody is thought to be protective, and most exposed term infants are asymptomatic or not infected. In contrast, preterm infants (who lack antibody to CMV) can develop serious infection or can die, particularly when transfused with CMV-positive blood. Efforts should be made to transfuse these infants with only CMV-negative blood or components or to use blood that has been filtered to remove leukocytes, which carry CMV. Such leukoreduced blood is considered by many experts to be CMV safe.

Symptoms and Signs

Many women who become infected with CMV during pregnancy are asymptomatic, but some develop a mononucleosis-like illness.

About 10% of infants with congenital CMV infection are symptomatic at birth. Manifestations include the following:

- Intrauterine growth restriction
- Prematurity
- Microcephaly
- Jaundice
- Petechiae
- Hepatosplenomegaly
- Periventricular calcifications
- Chorioretinitis
- Hepatitis
- Pneumonitis
- Sensorineural hearing loss

Infants who acquire CMV during or after birth, especially if they are premature, may develop a sepsis-like syndrome, pneumonia, hepatosplenomegaly, hepatitis (which can lead to liver failure), thrombocytopenia, and atypical lymphocytosis. However, if transmission is via breast milk, the risk of severe symptomatic disease and long-term sequelae is low.

Diagnosis

- Viral culture using urine, saliva, or tissue
- PCR using urine, saliva, blood, or tissue

Symptomatic congenital CMV infection must be distinguished from other congenital infections, including toxoplasmosis, rubella, lymphocytic choriomeningitis virus (LCMV), and syphilis.

In neonates, viral detection using culture or PCR of urine, saliva, or a tissue sample is the primary diagnostic tool; maternal diagnosis can also be made by serologic testing or PCR (see p. 1620). Culture specimens should be refrigerated until inoculation of fibroblast cells. Congenital CMV is diagnosed if the virus is identified in urine, saliva, or other body fluids obtained within the first 2 to 3 wk of life; urine and saliva have the highest sensitivity. After 3 wk, viral detection may indicate perinatal or congenital infection. Infants may shed CMV for several years after either type of infection.

A CBC with differential and liver function tests may be helpful but are not specific. Cranial ultrasonography or CT and an ophthalmologic evaluation should also be done. Periventricular calcifications are commonly found on CT. Hearing tests should be routinely done at birth in all infected neonates, and continued close monitoring is required because hearing loss may develop after the neonatal period and be progressive.

Prognosis

Symptomatic neonates have a mortality rate of up to 30%, and 40 to 90% of survivors have some neurologic impairment, including

- Hearing loss
- Intellectual disability
- Visual disturbances

Among asymptomatic neonates, 5 to 15% eventually develop neurologic sequelae; hearing loss is the most common.

Treatment

- Ganciclovir or valganciclovir for symptomatic neonates

Symptomatic neonates are given antiviral drugs. Oral valganciclovir 16 mg/kg bid for 6 mo decreases viral shedding in neonates with congenital CMV and modestly improves hearing and developmental outcomes at 12 and 24 mo of age. The main toxicity of treatment is neutropenia.

Prevention

Nonimmune pregnant women should attempt to limit exposure to the virus. For instance, because CMV infection is common among children attending day care centers, pregnant women should always wash their hands thoroughly after exposure to urine and oral or respiratory secretions from children.

Transfusion-associated perinatal CMV disease can be avoided by giving preterm neonates blood products from CMV-seronegative donors or leukoreduced products.

A vaccine to prevent congenital CMV is under development. A recent trial giving CMV hyper immune globulin to pregnant women with primary CMV infection did not show a reduction in congenital infection.

KEY POINTS

- CMV is the most common congenital viral infection and may be asymptomatic or symptomatic.
- Multiple organs can be affected, and risk of premature birth increases.
- Distinguish symptomatic congenital CMV infection from other congenital infections (eg, toxoplasmosis, rubella, lymphocytic choriomeningitis virus, syphilis) using PCR or viral culture.
- IV ganciclovir or oral valganciclovir may help prevent hearing loss and developmental delay in infants with symptomatic infection.

CONGENITAL RUBELLA

Congenital rubella is a viral infection acquired from the mother during pregnancy. Signs are multiple congenital anomalies that can result in fetal death. Diagnosis is by serology and viral culture. There is no specific treatment. Prevention is by routine vaccination.

Congenital rubella typically results from a primary maternal infection. Congenital rubella is rare in the US.

Rubella is believed to invade the upper respiratory tract, with subsequent viremia and dissemination of virus to different sites, including the placenta. The fetus is at highest risk of developmental abnormalities when infected during the first 16 wk of gestation, particularly the first 8 to 10 wk. Early in gestation, the virus is thought to establish a chronic intrauterine infection. Its effects include endothelial damage to blood vessels, direct cytolysis of cells, and disruption of cellular mitosis.

Symptoms and Signs

Rubella in a pregnant woman may be asymptomatic or characterized by upper respiratory tract symptoms, mild fever, conjunctivitis, lymphadenopathy (especially in the suboccipital and posterior auricular areas), and a maculopapular rash. This illness may be followed by joint symptoms.

In the fetus, there may be no effects, death in utero, or multiple anomalies referred to as congenital rubella syndrome (CRS). The most frequent abnormalities include

- Intrauterine growth restriction
- Microcephaly
- Meningoencephalitis
- Cataracts
- Retinopathy
- Hearing loss
- Cardiac defects (patent ductus arteriosus and pulmonary artery stenosis)
- Hepatosplenomegaly
- Bone radiolucencies

Less common manifestations include thrombocytopenia with purpura, dermal erythropoiesis resulting in bluish red skin lesions, adenopathy, hemolytic anemia, and interstitial pneumonia. Ongoing observation is needed to detect subsequent hearing loss, intellectual disability, abnormal behavior, endocrinopathies (eg, diabetes mellitus), or a rare progressive encephalitis. Infants with congenital rubella infections may develop immune deficiencies such as hypogammaglobulinemia.

Diagnosis

- Maternal serum rubella titers
- Viral detection in the mother via culture and/or reverse transcriptase–PCR (RT-PCR) of amniotic fluid, nose, throat (preferred), urine, CSF, or blood specimens
- Infant antibody titers (measured serially) and viral detection as above

Pregnant women routinely have a serum rubella IgG titer measured early in pregnancy. Titer is repeated in seronegative women who develop symptoms or signs of rubella; diagnosis is made by a positive serologic test for IgM antibody, IgG seroconversion, or a ≥ 4-fold rise between acute and convalescent IgG titers. Virus may be cultured from nasopharyngeal swabs but is difficult to cultivate. RT-PCR can be used to confirm culture results or detect viral RNA directly in patient specimens as well as allow for genotyping and epidemiological tracking of wild-type rubella infections.

Infants suspected of having CRS should have antibody titers and specimens obtained for viral detection. Persistence of rubella-specific IgG in the infant after 6 to 12 mo suggests congenital infection. Detection of rubella-specific IgM antibodies generally also indicates rubella infection, but false-positive IgM results can occur. Specimens from the nasopharynx, urine, CSF, buffy coat, and conjunctiva from infants with CRS usually contain virus; samples from the nasopharynx usually offer the best sensitivity for culture, and the laboratory should be notified that rubella virus is suspected. In a few centers, diagnoses can be made prenatally by detecting the virus in amniotic fluid, detecting rubella-specific IgM in fetal blood, or applying RT-PCR techniques to fetal blood or chorionic villus biopsy specimens.

Other tests include a CBC with differential, CSF analysis, and x-ray examination of the bones to detect characteristic radiolucencies. Thorough ophthalmologic and cardiac evaluations are also useful.

Treatment

- Counseling
- Possibly immune globulin for the mother

No specific therapy is available for maternal or congenital rubella infection. Women exposed to rubella early in pregnancy should be informed of the potential risks to the fetus. Some experts recommend giving nonspecific immune globulin (0.55 mL/kg IM) for exposure early in pregnancy, but this treatment does not prevent infection, and the use of immune globulin should be considered only in women who decline pregnancy termination.

Prevention

Rubella can easily be prevented by vaccination. In the US, infants should receive vaccination for rubella together with measles and mumps vaccinations at 12 to 15 mo of age and again at entry to grade school or junior high school (see p. 2469). Postpubertal nonpregnant females who are not immune to rubella should be vaccinated. (CAUTION: *Rubella vaccination is contraindicated in immunodeficient or pregnant women.*) After vaccination, women should be advised not to become pregnant for 28 days.

Efforts should also be made to screen and vaccinate high-risk groups, such as hospital and child care workers, military recruits, recent immigrants, and college students. Women who are found to be susceptible during prenatal screening should be vaccinated after delivery and before hospital discharge. Theoretically, vaccination of nonimmune people exposed to rubella might prevent infection if done within 3 days of exposure, but this treatment has not proved to be beneficial.

People with documented vaccination with at least one dose of live-attenuated rubella virus-containing vaccine after age 1 yr or who have serologic evidence of immunity can be considered immune to rubella.

KEY POINTS

- Maternal rubella infection, particularly during the 1st trimester, can cause intrauterine growth restriction and serious developmental abnormalities.
- Routine rubella vaccination has made congenital rubella rare in the US.
- Rubella vaccine is contraindicated in pregnancy, so pregnant women with rubella or exposed to it should be informed of the potential risk to the fetus.

CONGENITAL SYPHILIS

Congenital syphilis is a multisystem infection caused by *Treponema pallidum* and transmitted to the fetus via the placenta. Early signs are characteristic skin lesions, lymphadenopathy, hepatosplenomegaly, failure to thrive, blood-stained nasal discharge, perioral fissures, meningitis, choroiditis, hydrocephalus, seizures, intellectual disability, osteochondritis, and pseudoparalysis (Parrot atrophy of newborn). Later signs are gummatous ulcers, periosteal lesions, paresis, tabes, optic atrophy, interstitial keratitis,

sensorineural deafness, and dental deformities. Diagnosis is clinical, confirmed by microscopy or serology. Treatment is penicillin.

Overall risk of transplacental infection of the fetus is about 60 to 80%, and likelihood is increased during the 2nd half of the pregnancy. Untreated primary or secondary syphilis in the mother usually is transmitted, but latent or tertiary syphilis is transmitted in only about 20% of cases. Untreated syphilis in pregnancy is also associated with a significant risk of stillbirth and neonatal death. In infected neonates, manifestations of syphilis are classified as early congenital (ie, birth through age 2 yr) and late congenital (ie, after age 2 yr).

Symptoms and Signs

Many patients are asymptomatic, and the infection may remain clinically silent throughout their life.

Early congenital syphilis commonly manifests during the first 3 mo of life. Manifestations include characteristic vesiculobullous eruptions or a macular, copper-colored rash on the palms and soles and papular lesions around the nose and mouth and in the diaper area, as well as petechial lesions. Generalized lymphadenopathy and hepatosplenomegaly often occur. The infant may fail to thrive and have a characteristic mucopurulent or blood-stained nasal discharge causing snuffles. A few infants develop meningitis, choroiditis, hydrocephalus, or seizures, and others may be intellectually disabled. Within the first 8 mo of life, osteochondritis (chondroepiphysitis), especially of the long bones and ribs, may cause pseudoparalysis of the limbs with characteristic radiologic changes in the bones.

Late congenital syphilis typically manifests after 2 yr of life and causes gummatous ulcers that tend to involve the nose, septum, and hard palate and periosteal lesions that result in saber shins and bossing of the frontal and parietal bones. Neurosyphilis is usually asymptomatic, but juvenile paresis and tabes may develop. Optic atrophy, sometimes leading to blindness, may occur. Interstitial keratitis, the most common eye lesion, frequently recurs, often resulting in corneal scarring. Sensorineural deafness, which is often progressive, may appear at any age. Hutchinson incisors, mulberry molars, perioral fissures (rhagades), and maldevelopment of the maxilla resulting in "bulldog" facies are characteristic, if infrequent, sequelae.

Diagnosis

- **Early congenital syphilis:** Clinical evaluation; darkfield microscopy of lesions, placenta, or umbilical cord; serologic testing of mother and neonate; possibly CSF analysis
- **Late congenital syphilis:** Clinical evaluation, serologic testing of mother and child

Early congenital syphilis: Diagnosis of early congenital syphilis is usually suspected based on maternal serologic testing, which is routinely done early in pregnancy, and often repeated in the 3rd trimester and at delivery. Neonates of mothers with serologic evidence of syphilis should have a thorough examination, darkfield microscopy or immunofluorescent staining of any skin or mucosal lesions, and a quantitative nontreponemal serum test (eg, rapid plasma reagin [RPR], Venereal Disease Research Laboratory [VDRL]); cord blood is not used for serum testing because results are less sensitive and specific. The placenta or umbilical cord should be analyzed using darkfield microscopy or fluorescent antibody staining if available.

Infants and young children with clinical signs of illness or suggestive serologic test results also should have a lumbar puncture with CSF analysis for cell count, VDRL, and protein; CBC with platelet count; liver function tests; long-bone x-rays; and other tests as clinically indicated (ophthalmologic evaluation, chest x-rays, neuroimaging, and auditory brain stem response).

Syphilis can cause many different abnormalities on long-bone x-rays, including

- Periosteal reactions
- Diffuse or localized osteitis
- Metaphysitis

The osteitis is sometimes described as "diffuse moth-eaten changes of the shaft." Metaphysitis commonly appears as lucent or dense bands that can alternate to give a sandwich or celery stalk appearance. The Wimberger sign is symmetric erosions of the upper tibia but there can also be erosions in the metaphysis of other long bones. Excessive callus formation at the ends of long bones has been described. Many affected infants have more than one of these findings.

Diagnosis is confirmed by microscopic visualization of spirochetes in samples from the neonate or the placenta. Diagnosis based on neonatal serologic testing is complicated by the transplacental transfer of maternal IgG antibodies, which can cause a positive test in the absence of infection. However, a neonatal nontreponemal antibody titer > 4 times the maternal titer would not generally result from passive transfer, and diagnosis is considered confirmed or highly probable. Maternal disease acquired late in pregnancy may be transmitted before development of antibodies. Thus, in neonates with lower titers but typical clinical manifestations, syphilis is also considered highly probable. In neonates with no signs of illness and low or negative serologic titers, syphilis is considered possible; subsequent approach depends on various maternal and neonatal factors.

The utility of fluorescent assays for antitreponemal IgM, which is not transferred across the placenta, is controversial, but such assays have been used to detect neonatal infection. Any positive nontreponemal test should be confirmed with a specific treponemal test to exclude false-positive results, but confirmative testing should not delay treatment in a symptomatic infant or an infant at high risk of infection.

Late congenital syphilis: Diagnosis of late congenital syphilis is by clinical history, distinctive physical signs, and positive serologic tests (see p. 1710). The Hutchinson triad of interstitial keratitis, Hutchinson incisors, and 8th cranial nerve deafness is diagnostic. Sometimes the standard nontreponemal serologic tests for syphilis are negative, but the fluorescent treponemal antibody absorption test (FTA-ABS) is positive. The diagnosis should be considered in cases of unexplained deafness, progressive intellectual deterioration, or keratitis.

Follow up: All seropositive infants and those whose mothers were seropositive should have VDRL or RPR titers every 2 to 3 mo until the test is nonreactive or the titer has decreased 4-fold. In uninfected and successfully treated infants, nontreponemal antibody titers are usually nonreactive by 6 mo. Passively acquired treponemal antibodies may be present for longer, perhaps 15 mo. It is important to remember to use the same specific nontreponemal test to monitor titers in mothers, neonates, infants, and young children over time.

If VDRL or RPR remain reactive past 6 to 12 mo of age or titers increase, the infant should be reevaluated (including lumbar puncture for CSF analysis, and CBC with platelet count, long-bone x-rays, and other tests as clinically indicated).

Treatment

- Parenteral penicillin

Pregnant women: Pregnant women in the early stages of syphilis receive benzathine penicillin G (2.4 million units IM in a single dose). For later stages of syphilis or neurosyphilis, the appropriate regimen for nonpregnant patients should be followed (see p. 1711). Occasionally, a severe Jarisch-Herxheimer reaction occurs after such therapy, leading to spontaneous abortion. Patients allergic to penicillin may be desensitized and then treated with penicillin.

After adequate treatment, RPR and VDRL test results decrease 4-fold by 6 to 12 mo in most patients and revert to negative by 2 yr in nearly all patients. Erythromycin therapy is inadequate for both the mother and fetus and is not recommended. Tetracycline is *contraindicated*.

Early congenital syphilis: In confirmed or highly probable cases, 2015 Centers for Disease Control and Prevention (CDC) guidelines for congenital syphilis recommend aqueous crystalline penicillin G 50,000 units/kg IV q 12 h for the first 7 days of life and q 8 h thereafter for a total of 10 days or procaine penicillin G 50,000 units/kg IM once/day for 10 days (see Table 314–1). If ≥ 1 day of therapy is missed, the entire course must be repeated. This regimen is also recommended for infants with possible syphilis if the mother fits any of the following criteria:

- Untreated
- Treatment status unknown
- Treated ≤ 4 wk before delivery
- Inadequately treated (a nonpenicillin regimen)
- Maternal evidence of relapse or reinfection (≥ 4-fold increase in maternal titer)

In infants with possible syphilis whose mothers were not adequately treated but who are clinically well and have a completely negative full evaluation, a single dose of benzathine penicillin 50,000 units/kg IM is an alternative treatment choice in selected circumstances, but only if follow-up is assured.

Infants with possible syphilis whose mothers were adequately treated and who are clinically well can also be given a single dose of benzathine penicillin 50,000 units/kg IM. Alternatively, if close follow-up is assured, some clinicians defer penicillin and do nontreponemal serologic testing monthly for 3 mo and then at 6 mo; antibiotics are given if titers rise or are positive at 6 mo.

Older infants and children with newly diagnosed congenital syphilis: CSF should be examined before treatment starts. The CDC recommends that any child with late congenital syphilis be treated with aqueous crystalline penicillin G 50,000 units/kg IV q 4 to 6 h for 10 days. A single dose of benzathine penicillin G 50,000 units/kg IM may also be given at the completion of the IV therapy. Alternatively, if a full evaluation is completely negative and the child is asymptomatic, benzathine penicillin G 50,000 units/kg IM once/wk for 3 doses may be used.

Many patients do not revert to seronegativity but do have a 4-fold decrease in titer of reagin (eg, VDRL) antibody. Patients should be reevaluated at regular intervals to ensure the appropriate serologic response to therapy has occurred and that there is no indication of relapse.

Interstitial keratitis is usually treated with corticosteroid and atropine drops in consultation with an ophthalmologist. Patients with sensorineural hearing loss may benefit from penicillin plus a corticosteroid such as prednisone 0.5 mg/kg po once/day for 1 wk, followed by 0.3 mg/kg once/day for 4 wk, after which the dose is gradually reduced over 2 to 3 mo. Corticosteroids have not been critically evaluated in these conditions.

Prevention

Pregnant women should be routinely tested for syphilis in the 1st trimester and retested if they acquire other sexually transmitted diseases during pregnancy. In 99% of cases, adequate treatment during pregnancy cures both mother and fetus. However, in some cases, syphilis treatment late in pregnancy eliminates the infection but not some signs of syphilis that appear at birth. Treatment of the mother < 4 wk before delivery may not eradicate fetal infection.

When congenital syphilis is diagnosed, other family members should be examined for physical and serologic evidence of infection. Retreatment of the mother in subsequent pregnancies is necessary only if serologic titers suggest relapse or reinfection. Women who remain seropositive after adequate treatment may have been reinfected and should be reevaluated. A mother without lesions who is seronegative but who has had venereal exposure to a person known to have syphilis should be treated, because there is a 25 to 50% chance that she acquired syphilis.

KEY POINTS

- Manifestations of syphilis are classified as early congenital (birth through age 2 yr) and late congenital (after age 2 yr).
- Risk of transmission of maternal primary or secondary syphilis is 60 to 80%; risk of transmission of latent or tertiary syphilis is about 20%.
- Diagnose clinically and by serologic testing of mother and child; darkfield examination of skin lesions and sometimes of placenta and umbilical cord samples may help diagnose early congenital syphilis.
- Treat with parenteral penicillin.

CONGENITAL TOXOPLASMOSIS

Congenital toxoplasmosis is caused by transplacental acquisition of *Toxoplasma gondii*. Manifestations, if present, are prematurity, intrauterine growth restriction, jaundice, hepatosplenomegaly, myocarditis, pneumonitis, rash, chorioretinitis, hydrocephalus, intracranial calcifications, microcephaly, and seizures. Diagnosis is by serologic testing or PCR. Treatment is with pyrimethamine, sulfadiazine, and leucovorin.

Toxoplasma gondii, a parasite found worldwide, causes congenital infection in about 1/10,000 to 80/10,000 births.

Etiology

Congenital toxoplasmosis is almost exclusively due to a primary maternal infection during pregnancy; however, there are exceptions, including reinfection with a new serotype of *T. gondii* or reactivation of toxoplasmosis in mothers with severe cell-mediated immunodeficiencies. Infection with *T. gondii* occurs primarily from ingestion of inadequately cooked meat containing cysts or from ingestion of oocysts derived from food or water contaminated with cat feces.

The rate of transmission to the fetus is higher in women infected later during pregnancy. However, fetuses infected earlier in gestation generally have more severe disease. Overall, 30 to 40% of women infected during pregnancy will have a congenitally infected child.

Symptoms and Signs

Pregnant women infected with *T. gondii* generally do not have clinical manifestations, but some may have a mild mononucleosis-like syndrome, regional lymphadenopathy, or occasionally chorioretinitis. Similarly, infected neonates are usually asymptomatic at birth, but manifestations may include

- Prematurity
- Intrauterine growth restriction
- Jaundice
- Hepatosplenomegaly
- Myocarditis
- Pneumonitis
- Various rashes

Neurologic involvement, often prominent, includes chorioretinitis, hydrocephalus, intracranial calcifications, microcephaly, and seizures. The classic triad of findings consists of chorioretinitis, hydrocephalus, and intracranial calcifications. Neurologic and ophthalmologic sequelae may be delayed for years or decades.

Diagnosis

- Serial IgG measurement (for maternal infection)
- Amniotic fluid PCR (for fetal infection)
- Serologic testing, brain imaging, CSF analysis, ophthalmologic evaluation (for neonatal infection), and PCR testing of various body fluids or tissues

Serologic testing is important in diagnosing maternal and congenital infection. Maternal infection should be suspected if women have a mononucleosis-like syndrome and negative Epstein-Barr virus, HIV, and CMV (antibody or PCR) testing, isolated regional adenopathy not due to another cause (eg, HIV), or chorioretinitis. Acute maternal infection is suggested by seroconversion or a ≥ 4-fold rise between acute and convalescent IgG titers. However, maternal IgG antibodies may be detectable in the infant through the first year.

PCR analysis of amniotic fluid is emerging as the method of choice for diagnosing fetal infection. There are numerous other serologic tests, some of which are done only in reference laboratories. The most reliable are the Sabin-Feldman dye test, the indirect immunofluorescent antibody (IFA) test, and the direct agglutination assay. Tests to isolate the organism include inoculation into mice and tissue culture, but these tests are not usually done because they are expensive, not highly sensitive, and can take weeks before yielding results.

In suspected congenital toxoplasmosis, serologic tests, MRI or CT imaging of the brain, CSF analysis, and a thorough eye examination by an ophthalmologist should be done. CSF abnormalities include xanthochromia, pleocytosis, and increased protein concentration. The placenta is inspected for characteristic signs of *T. gondii* infection (eg, placentitis). Nonspecific laboratory findings include thrombocytopenia, lymphocytosis, monocytosis, eosinophilia, and elevated transaminases. PCR testing of body fluids, including CSF, and tissues (placenta) can also be done to confirm infection.

Prognosis

Some children have a fulminant course with early death, whereas others have long-term neurologic sequelae. Occasionally, neurologic manifestations (eg, chorioretinitis, intellectual disability, deafness, seizures) develop years later in children who appeared normal at birth. Consequently, children with congenital toxoplasmosis should be closely monitored beyond the neonatal period.

Treatment

- Sometimes spiramycin for pregnant women
- Pyrimethamine, sulfadiazine, and leucovorin

Limited data suggest that treatment of infected women during pregnancy may be beneficial to the fetus. Spiramycin (available in the US with special permission from the FDA) has been used to prevent maternofetal transmission but does not provide treatment to the fetus. Pyrimethamine and sulfonamides have been used later in gestation to treat the infected fetus.

Treatment of symptomatic and asymptomatic neonates may improve outcome. Therefore, treatment is begun with pyrimethamine (initial loading dose of 2 mg/kg po once/day for 2 days followed by 1 mg/kg po once/day, maximum 25 mg) and leucovorin (10 mg po 3 times/wk). Sulfadiazine (50 mg/kg po bid, maximum 4 g) is begun after neonatal jaundice has resolved. After the initial 6 mo of treatment, sulfadiazine and leucovorin are continued at the same dose, but pyrimethamine is given less frequently (only on Monday, Wednesday, and Friday). This regimen is continued for at least 6 more mo. All treatment should be overseen by an expert. The use of corticosteroids is controversial and should be determined case by case but may be considered for active chorioretinitis or if CSF protein is > 1 gm/dL.

Prevention

Pregnant women should be counseled to avoid contact with cat litter boxes and other areas contaminated with cat feces. Because oocysts require > 24 h after excretion to become infectious, conscientiously changing the entire litter box on a daily basis while wearing gloves followed by careful handwashing should reduce infection by this route.

Meat should be thoroughly cooked before consumption by pregnant women. Fruits and vegetables should be washed thoroughly or peeled, and all food preparation should be followed immediately by handwashing.

Women at risk of primary infection (eg, those frequently exposed to cat feces) should be screened during pregnancy. Women infected during the 1st or 2nd trimester should be counseled regarding available treatments.

KEY POINTS

- Congenital toxoplasmosis is usually due to a primary maternal infection acquired during pregnancy; reactivation of prior infection is of low risk except in immunocompromised women.
- Many organs may be affected, including heart, liver, lungs, and CNS; the classic triad of findings consists of chorioretinitis, hydrocephalus, and intracranial calcifications.
- Some children have a fulminant course with early death, whereas others have long-term neurologic and ophthalmologic sequelae (which may not develop for several years or even decades).
- Do PCR analysis of amniotic fluid (for fetal infection) or of body fluids (including CSF) and tissues for neonatal infection; serologic testing may also be used.
- Do MRI or CT of the brain.
- Pyrimethamine, sulfadiazine, and leucovorin may help.
- Pregnant women should avoid contact with cat litter boxes and other areas contaminated with cat feces.

NEONATAL CONJUNCTIVITIS

(Ophthalmia Neonatorum)

Neonatal conjunctivitis is watery or purulent ocular drainage due to a chemical irritant or a pathogenic organism. Prevention with antigonococcal topical treatment at birth

is routine. Diagnosis is clinical and usually confirmed by laboratory testing. Treatment is with organism-specific antimicrobials.

Etiology

The major causes (in decreasing order) are

- Bacterial infection
- Chemical inflammation
- Viral infection (see p. 939)

Infection is acquired from infected mothers during passage through the birth canal. Chlamydial ophthalmia (caused by *Chlamydia trachomatis*) is the most common bacterial cause; it accounts for up to 40% of conjunctivitis in neonates < 4 wk of age. The prevalence of maternal chlamydial infection ranges from 2 to 20%. About 30 to 50% of neonates born to acutely infected women acquire infection, and 25 to 50% of those develop conjunctivitis (and 5 to 20% develop pneumonia). Other bacteria, including *Streptococcus pneumoniae* and nontypeable *Haemophilus influenzae,* account for another 30 to 50% of cases, whereas gonococcal ophthalmia (conjunctivitis due to *Neisseria gonorrhoeae*) accounts for < 1% of cases.

Chemical conjunctivitis is usually secondary to the instillation of topical therapy for ocular prophylaxis.

The major viral cause is herpes simplex virus types 1 and 2 (herpetic keratoconjunctivitis), but this virus causes < 1% of cases.

Symptoms and Signs

Because they overlap in both manifestation and onset, causes of neonatal conjunctivitis are difficult to distinguish clinically. Conjunctivae are injected, and discharge (watery or purulent) is present.

Chemical conjunctivitis secondary to topical prophylaxis usually appears within 6 to 8 h after instillation and disappears spontaneously within 48 to 96 h.

Chlamydial ophthalmia usually occurs 5 to 14 days after birth. It may range from mild conjunctivitis with minimal mucopurulent discharge to severe eyelid edema with copious drainage and pseudomembrane formation. Follicles are not present in the conjunctiva, as they are in older children and adults.

Gonococcal ophthalmia causes an acute purulent conjunctivitis that appears 2 to 5 days after birth or earlier with premature rupture of membranes. The neonate has severe eyelid edema followed by chemosis and a profuse purulent exudate that may be under pressure. If untreated, corneal ulcerations and blindness may occur.

Conjunctivitis caused by other bacteria has a variable onset, ranging from 4 days to several weeks.

Herpetic keratoconjunctivitis can occur as an isolated infection or with disseminated or CNS infection. It can be mistaken for bacterial or chemical conjunctivitis, but the presence of dendritic keratitis is pathognomonic.

Diagnosis

- Testing of conjunctival material for pathogens including gonorrhea, chlamydia, and, sometimes, herpes

Conjunctival material is Gram stained, cultured for gonorrhea (eg, on modified Thayer-Martin medium) and other bacteria, and tested for chlamydia (eg, by culture, direct immunofluorescence, or enzyme-linked immunosorbent assay [samples must contain cells]). Conjunctival scrapings can also be examined with Giemsa stain; if blue intracytoplasmic inclusions are identified, chlamydial ophthalmia is confirmed. Nucleic acid amplification tests may provide equivalent or better sensitivity for the detection of chlamydia from conjunctival material compared to older methods. Viral culture is done only if viral infection is suspected because of skin lesions or maternal infection.

Treatment

- Systemic, topical, or combined antimicrobial therapy

Neonates with conjunctivitis and known maternal gonococcal infection or with gram-negative intracellular diplococci identified in conjunctival exudates should be treated with ceftriaxone or cefotaxime (see Table 314–1) before results of confirmatory tests are available.

In **chlamydial ophthalmia,** systemic therapy is the treatment of choice, because at least half of affected neonates also have nasopharyngeal infection and some develop chlamydial pneumonia. Erythromycin ethylsuccinate 12.5 mg/kg po q 6 h for 2 wk is recommended (see Table 314–3). Efficacy of this therapy is only 80%, so a 2nd treatment course may be needed. Because use of erythromycin in neonates is associated with the development of hypertrophic pyloric stenosis (HPS), all neonates treated with erythromycin should be monitored for symptoms and signs of HPS, and their parents should be counseled regarding the potential risks. Azithromycin 20 mg/kg po once/day for 3 days may also be effective but is not yet recommended by the American Academy of Pediatrics.

A neonate with **gonococcal ophthalmia** is hospitalized for evaluation of possible systemic gonococcal infection and given a single dose of ceftriaxone 25 to 50 mg/kg IM to a maximum dose of 125 mg. Infants with hyperbilirubinemia or those receiving Ca-containing fluids should not receive ceftriaxone and may be given a single dose of cefotaxime 100 mg/kg IV or IM. Frequent saline irrigation of the eye prevents secretions from adhering. Topical antimicrobial ointments alone are ineffective and not needed when systemic therapy is provided.

Conjunctivitis due to other bacteria usually responds to topical ointments containing polymyxin plus bacitracin, erythromycin, or tetracycline.

Herpetic keratoconjunctivitis should be treated (with an ophthalmologist's consultation) with systemic acyclovir 20 mg/kg q 8 h for 14 to 21 days and topical 1% trifluridine ophthalmic drops or ointment, vidarabine 3% ointment, or 0.1% iododeoxyuridine q 2 to 3 h, with a maximum of 9 doses/24 h. Systemic therapy is important, because dissemination to the CNS and other organs can occur.

Corticosteroid-containing ointments may seriously exacerbate eye infections due to *C. trachomatis* and herpes simplex virus and should be avoided.

Prevention

Routine use of 1% silver nitrate drops, 0.5% erythromycin, or 1% tetracycline ophthalmic ointments or drops instilled into each eye after delivery effectively prevents gonococcal ophthalmia. However, none of these agents prevents chlamydial ophthalmia; povidone iodine 2.5% drops may be effective against chlamydia and gonococci but is not available in the US. Silver nitrate and tetracycline ophthalmic ointments are also no longer available in the US.

Neonates of mothers with untreated gonorrhea should receive a single injection of ceftriaxone 25 to 50 mg/kg IM or IV, up to 125 mg (ceftriaxone should not be used in neonates with hyperbilirubinemia or those receiving Ca-containing fluids), and both mother and neonate should be screened for chlamydia infection, HIV, and syphilis.

KEY POINTS

- *C. trachomatis, S. pneumoniae,* and nontypeable *H. influenzae* cause most bacterial conjunctivitis; *N. gonorrhoeae* is a rare cause.
- Conjunctivae are injected, and discharge (watery or purulent) is present.
- Test conjunctival material for pathogens (including gonorrhea and chlamydia) using culture, and sometimes nucleic acid amplification tests.
- Give antibiotics active against the infecting organism; neonates with gonococcal infection should be hospitalized.
- Give systemic therapy for chlamydial ophthalmia.
- Chemical conjunctivitis can result from antimicrobial drops or silver nitrate given at birth to prevent bacterial conjunctivitis.

NEONATAL HEPATITIS B VIRUS INFECTION

Neonatal hepatitis B virus infection is usually acquired during delivery. It is usually asymptomatic but can cause chronic subclinical disease in later childhood or adulthood. Symptomatic infection causes jaundice, lethargy, failure to thrive, abdominal distention, and clay-colored stools. Diagnosis is by serology. Rarely, severe illness may cause acute liver failure requiring liver transplantation. Less severe illness is treated supportively. Active and passive immunization help prevent vertical transmission.

Of the recognized forms of primary viral hepatitis, only hepatitis B virus (HBV) is a cause of neonatal hepatitis. Infection with other viruses (eg, CMV, herpes simplex virus) may cause liver inflammation along with other manifestations.

Etiology

HBV infection occurs during delivery from an infected mother. The risk of transmission is 70 to 90% from women seropositive for hepatitis B surface antigen (HBsAg) and hepatitis B e antigen (HBeAg—see p. 225) at the time of delivery. Women without the e antigen or with anti-HBe transmit the infection only 5 to 20% of the time.

Mother–infant HBV transmission results primarily from maternofetal microtransfusions during labor or contact with infectious secretions in the birth canal. Transplacental transmission is identified in < 2% of infections. Postpartum transmission occurs rarely through exposure to infectious maternal blood, saliva, stool, urine, or breast milk. Up to 90% of infants infected perinatally will develop chronic infection, and perinatally acquired HBV infection may be an important viral reservoir in certain communities.

Symptoms and Signs

Most neonates with HBV infection are asymptomatic but develop chronic, subclinical infection characterized by persistent HBsAg antigenemia and variably elevated transaminase activity. Many neonates born to women with acute hepatitis B during pregnancy are of low birth weight, regardless of whether they are infected.

Infrequently, infected neonates develop acute hepatitis B, which is usually mild and self-limited. They develop jaundice, lethargy, failure to thrive, abdominal distention, and clay-colored stools. Occasionally, severe infection with hepatomegaly, ascites, and hyperbilirubinemia (primarily conjugated bilirubin) occurs. Rarely, the disease is fulminant and even fatal. Fulminant disease occurs more often in neonates whose mothers are chronic carriers of hepatitis B.

Diagnosis

- Serologic testing

Diagnosis of neonatal HBV infection is by serologic testing, including measurement of HBsAg, HBeAg, antibody to hepatitis B e antigen (anti-HBe), and quantitation of HBV DNA in blood. Other initial tests include CBC with platelets, ALT and α-fetoprotein levels, and liver ultrasonography. Family history of liver cancer or liver disease is noted because of the long-term risk of hepatocellular carcinoma. If testing suggests HBV infection, consultation with a pediatric hepatologist is recommended.

Prognosis

Long-term prognosis is not predictable, although chronic HBV infection early in life increases the risk of subsequent liver disease including chronic hepatitis, cirrhosis, end-stage liver disease, and hepatocellular carcinoma.

Treatment

- Supportive care

Symptomatic care and adequate nutrition are needed. Neither corticosteroids nor hepatitis B immune globulin (HBIG) is helpful for acute infection. No therapy prevents the development of chronic, subclinical hepatitis once infection is acquired.

All children with chronic HBV infection should be immunized with hepatitis A vaccine. Children with chronic HBV infection may benefit from antiviral drugs (eg, interferon alfa, lamivudine, adefovir) but these should be used only in consultation with a pediatric hepatologist.

Prevention

Pregnant women should be tested for HBsAg during an early prenatal visit. Failing that, they should be tested when admitted for delivery. Some women who are HBsAg-positive are treated with lamivudine or telbivudine during the 3rd trimester, which may prevent perinatal transmission of HBV.

Neonates whose mothers are HBsAg-positive should be given 1 dose of HBIG 0.5 mL IM within 12 h of birth. Recombinant HBV vaccine should be given IM in a series of 3 doses, as is recommended for all infants in the US. (NOTE: Doses vary among proprietary vaccines.) The first dose is given concurrently with HBIG but at a different site. The 2nd dose is given at 1 to 2 mo, and the 3rd dose is given 6 mo after the first. If the infant weighs < 2 kg, the first dose of vaccine may be less effective. Subsequent vaccine doses are given at age 30 days (or when discharged from the hospital), and then 2 other doses are given at 1 to 2 mo and 6 mo after the 30-day dose.

Neonates whose mothers have unknown HBsAg status at the time of delivery should also receive their first dose of vaccine within 12 h of birth. For infants < 2 kg, the first dose is given concurrently with HBIG (0.5 mL IM) at a different site. For infants ≥ 2 kg and whose mothers can be tested for HBsAg and in whom follow up is assured, HBIG (0.5 mL IM) can be delayed up to 7 days pending a positive maternal test for HBsAg. Testing for HBsAg and anti-HBs at 9 to 15 mo is recommended for all infants born to HBsAg-positive mothers.

Separating a neonate from its HBsAg-positive mother is not recommended, and breastfeeding does not seem to increase the risk of postpartum HBV transmission, particularly if HBIG and HBV vaccine have been given. However, if a mother has cracked nipples, abscesses, or other breast pathology, breastfeeding could potentially transmit HBV.

KEY POINTS

- Only HBV is a major cause of neonatal hepatitis; it is typically transmitted during delivery.
- Most neonates are asymptomatic but develop chronic, subclinical HBsAg antigenemia and elevated transaminase levels.
- Some infants develop mild hepatitis, and a few have fulminant liver disease.
- Do serologic testing of infant and mother.
- Neonates whose mothers are HBsAg-positive should be given 1 dose of HBIG 0.5 mL IM and HBV vaccine within 12 h of birth.
- HBV-infected children should be immunized with hepatitis A vaccine; anti-HBV drugs (eg, interferon alfa) may help but should be used only in consultation with a pediatric hepatologist.

NEONATAL HERPES SIMPLEX VIRUS INFECTION

Neonatal herpes simplex virus infection is usually transmitted during delivery. A typical sign is vesicular eruption, which may be accompanied by or progress to disseminated disease. Diagnosis is by viral culture, PCR, immunofluorescence, or electron microscopy. Treatment is with high-dose parenteral acyclovir and supportive care.

Neonatal herpes simplex virus (HSV) infection has high mortality and significant morbidity. Incidence estimates range from 1/3,000 to 1/20,000 births. HSV type 2 causes more cases than HSV type 1.

HSV is usually transmitted during delivery through an infected maternal genital tract. Transplacental transmission of virus and hospital-acquired spread from one neonate to another by hospital personnel or family may account for some cases. Mothers of neonates with HSV infection tend to have newly acquired genital infection, but many have not had symptoms at the time of delivery.

Symptoms and Signs

Manifestations generally occur between the 1st and 3rd wk of life but rarely may not appear until as late as the 4th wk. Neonates may present with local or disseminated disease. Skin vesicles are common with either type, occurring in about 70% overall. Neonates with no skin vesicles usually present with localized CNS disease. In neonates with isolated skin or mucosal disease, progressive or more serious forms of disease frequently follow within 7 to 10 days if left untreated.

Localized disease: Neonates with localized disease can be divided into 2 groups. One group has encephalitis manifested by neurologic findings, CSF pleocytosis, and elevated protein concentration, with or without concomitant involvement of the skin, eyes, and mouth. The other group has only skin, eye, and mouth involvement and no evidence of CNS or organ disease.

Disseminated disease: Neonates with disseminated disease and visceral organ involvement have hepatitis, pneumonitis, disseminated intravascular coagulation, or a combination, with or without encephalitis or skin disease.

Other signs, which can occur singly or in combination, include temperature instability, lethargy, hypotonia, respiratory distress, apnea, and seizures.

Diagnosis

- HSV culture or PCR
- Sometimes immunofluorescent testing of lesions or electron microscopy

Rapid diagnosis by viral culture or HSV PCR is essential. The most common site of retrieval is skin vesicles. The nasopharynx, eyes, rectum, blood, and CSF should also be tested. In some neonates with encephalitis, virus is present only in the CNS. Diagnosis of neonatal HSV also can be made by immunofluorescence of lesion scrapings, particularly with use of monoclonal antibodies; and electron microscopy.

If no diagnostic virology facilities are available, a Tzanck test of the lesion base may show characteristic multinucleated giant cells and intranuclear inclusions, but this test is less sensitive than culture, and false-positives can occur.

Prognosis

The mortality rate of untreated disseminated disease is 85%; among neonates with untreated encephalitis, it is about 50%. Without treatment, at least 65% of survivors of disseminated disease or encephalitis have severe neurologic sequelae. Appropriate treatment, including parenteral acyclovir, decreases the mortality rate in CNS and disseminated disease by 50% and increases the percentage of children who develop normally from about 35% to 50 to 80%.

Death is uncommon in neonates with local disease limited to the skin, eyes, or mouth. However, without treatment, many of these neonates will progress to disseminated disease or CNS disease that may be unrecognized.

Treatment

- Parenteral acyclovir
- Supportive therapy

Acyclovir should be started immediately and presumptively in suspected cases while awaiting confirmatory diagnostic tests. Infants with disseminated and/or CNS disease are given 20 mg/kg IV q 8 h for 21 days. After this regimen, infants with CNS disease are given oral acyclovir 300 mg/m^2 tid for 6 mo; this long-term regimen improves neurodevelopmental outcomes at 1 yr of age but may cause neutropenia.

Vigorous supportive therapy is required, including appropriate IV fluids, alimentation, respiratory support, correction of clotting abnormalities, and control of seizures.

For localized disease (skin, mouth, or conjunctivae), treatment is acyclovir 20 mg/kg IV q 8 h for 14 days. Herpetic keratoconjunctivitis requires concomitant topical therapy with a drug such as trifluridine, iododeoxyuridine, or vidarabine (see p. 2629).

Prevention

Efforts to prevent neonatal transmission have not been very effective. Universal screening has not been recommended or shown to be effective, and most maternal infections with risk of transmission are asymptomatic. However, women with genital lesions at term should have testing and serology to diagnose HSV and determine the risk of transmission as well as to direct the care of the exposed but asymptomatic neonate. Cesarean delivery for women known to have a high risk of transmission (eg, active genital lesions present at term) has been shown to decrease transmission and is recommended even if the membranes have ruptured. Also, fetal scalp monitors should not be used during labor on infants whose mothers have suspected active genital herpes. Asymptomatic neonates born to women with active genital lesions at the time of delivery should be evaluated and tested for HSV infection. Additional information is available from the American Academy of Pediatrics.[1]

Giving oral acyclovir or valacyclovir during in the last few weeks of pregnancy to women with a history of genital HSV may prevent recurrences at the time of delivery and decrease the need for cesarean delivery.

1. Kimberlin DW, Baley J, Committee on infectious diseases, Committee on fetus and newborn: Guidance on management of asymptomatic neonates born to women with active genital herpes lesions. *Pediatrics* 131(2):e635-646, 2013.

KEY POINTS

- Neonatal herpes may be localized to the skin, eyes, or mouth, the CNS, or may be disseminated.
- Encephalitis and disseminated disease have a high mortality rate, and neurologic sequelae are common among survivors.
- In suspected cases, presumptive therapy and rapid diagnosis by HSV PCR of CSF, blood, or lesions are essential to optimize outcomes.
- Give parenteral acyclovir for both localized and disseminated disease.
- Do cesarean delivery if the mother has active genital herpes lesions present at term.

NEONATAL HOSPITAL-ACQUIRED INFECTION

Some infections are acquired after admission to the nursery rather than from the mother in utero or intrapartum. For some infections (eg, group B streptococci, herpes simplex virus) it may not be clear whether the source is maternal or the hospital environment.

Hospital-acquired (nosocomial) infection is primarily a problem for premature infants and for term infants with medical disorders requiring prolonged hospitalization. Healthy, term neonates have infection rates < 1%. For neonates in special care nurseries, the incidence increases as birth weight decreases. The most common nosocomial infections are central line-associated bloodstream infections (CLABSI) and healthcare-associated pneumonia.

Etiology

In **term neonates,** skin infection due to *Staphylococcus aureus* (both methicillin-sensitive and methicillin-resistant) is the most frequent hospital-acquired infection. Although nursery personnel who are *S. aureus* nasal carriers are potential sources of infection, colonized neonates and mothers also may be reservoirs. The umbilical stump, nose, and groin are frequently colonized during the first few days of life. Often, infections do not manifest until the neonate is at home.

In **very-low-birth-weight** (VLBW; < 1500 g) infants, gram-positive organisms cause about 70% of infections, the majority being with coagulase-negative staphylococci. Gram-negative organisms, including *Escherichia coli, Klebsiella, Pseudomonas, Enterobacter,* and *Serratia,* cause about 20%. Fungi (*Candida albicans* and *C. parapsilosis*) cause about 10%. Patterns of infection (and antibiotic resistance) vary among institutions and units and change with time. Intermittent "epidemics" sometimes occur as a particularly virulent organism colonizes a unit.

Infection is facilitated by the multiple invasive procedures VLBW infants undergo (eg, long-term arterial and venous catheterization, endotracheal intubation, continuous positive airway pressure, NGTs or nasojejunal feeding tubes). The longer the stay in special care nurseries and the more procedures done, the higher is the likelihood of infection.

Prevention

- Measures to reduce *S. aureus* colonization
- Prevention of colonization and infection in special care nurseries and neonatal ICUs
- Hand hygiene
- Surveillance for infection
- Sometimes antibiotics
- Vaccination

Colonization reduction: Bathing neonates with 3% hexachlorophene decreases frequency of *S. aureus* colonization, but this product can cause neurotoxicity, particularly in low-birth-weight infants, and is not used. The American Academy of Pediatrics recommends dry umbilical cord care, but this practice may result in high rates of colonization with *S. aureus,* and epidemics have occurred in some hospitals. During disease outbreaks, application of triple dye to the cord area or bacitracin or mupirocin ointment to the cord, nares, and circumcision site reduces colonization. Routine cultures of personnel or of the environment are not recommended.

Special care nurseries and neonatal ICUs: Prevention of colonization and infection in special care nurseries requires provision of sufficient space and personnel. In intensive care, multipatient rooms should provide 120 sq ft (about 11.2 sq m)/infant and 8 ft (about 2.4 m) between incubators or warmers, edge-to-edge in each direction. A nurse:patient ratio of 1:1 to 1:2 is required. In intermediate care, multipatient rooms should provide 120 sq ft (about 11.2 sq m)/infant and 4 ft (about 1.2 m) between incubators or warmers, edge-to-edge in each direction. A nurse:patient ratio of 1:3 to 1:4 is required.

Proper techniques are required, particularly for placement and care of invasive devices and for meticulous cleaning and disinfection or sterilization of equipment. Active monitoring of adherence to techniques is essential. Formal evidence-based protocols for inserting and maintaining central catheters have significantly decreased the rate of central line-associated bloodstream infection.

Similarly, a group of procedures and protocols that reduce healthcare-associated pneumonia in the neonatal ICU have been identified; these include staff education and training, active surveillance for healthcare-associated pneumonia, raising the head of an intubated neonate's bed 30 to 45°, and providing comprehensive oral hygiene. Placing the neonate in a lateral position with the endotracheal tube horizontal with the ventilator circuit also may be helpful.

Hand hygiene: Other preventive measures include meticulous attention to hand hygiene. Cleansing with alcohol preparations is as effective as soap and water in decreasing bacterial colony counts on hands, but if hands are visibly soiled, they should be washed with soap and water. Incubators provide limited protective isolation; the exteriors and interiors of the units rapidly become heavily contaminated, and personnel are likely to contaminate their hands and forearms. Universal blood and body fluid precautions add further protection.

Infection surveillance: Active surveillance for infection is done. In an epidemic, establishing a cohort of diseased or colonized infants and assigning them a separate nursing staff are useful. Continuing surveillance for 1 mo after discharge is necessary to assess the adequacy of controls instituted to end an epidemic.

Antibiotics: Prophylactic antimicrobial therapy is generally not effective, hastens development of resistant bacteria, and alters the balance of normal flora in the neonate. However, during a confirmed nursery epidemic, antibiotics against specific pathogens may be considered—eg, penicillin G for prophylaxis against group A streptococcal infection (see Table 314–1).

Vaccination: Inactivated vaccines should be given according to the routine schedule (see Table 291–2 on p. 2462) to any infant who is in the hospital at that time. Live viral vaccines (eg, rotavirus vaccine) are not given until the time of discharge to prevent spread of vaccine virus in the hospital.

KEY POINTS

- Nosocomial infection is primarily a problem for premature infants and for term infants with disorders requiring prolonged hospitalization.
- The lower the birth weight, the higher the risk of infection, particularly in neonates with central catheters, endotracheal tubes, or both.
- Meticulous technique for inserting and maintaining catheters, tubes, and devices is essential for prevention; formal protocols improve adherence.
- Prophylactic antibiotics are not recommended except possibly during a confirmed nursery epidemic involving a specific pathogen.

NEONATAL LISTERIOSIS

Neonatal listeriosis is acquired transplacentally or during or after delivery. Symptoms are those of sepsis. Diagnosis is by culture of mother and infant. Treatment is antibiotics, initially ampicillin plus an aminoglycoside.

In utero infection with *Listeria monocytogenes* can result in fetal dissemination with granuloma formation (eg, in the skin, liver, adrenal glands, lymphatic tissue, lungs, and brain). If a rash is present, it is referred to as granulomatosis infantisepticum. Aspiration or swallowing of amniotic fluid or vaginal secretions can lead to in utero or perinatal infection of the lungs, manifesting in the first several days of life with respiratory distress, shock, and a fulminant course.

Symptoms and Signs

Infections in pregnant women may be asymptomatic or characterized by a primary bacteremia manifesting first as a nonspecific flu-like illness.

In the fetus and neonate, clinical presentation depends on the timing and route of infection. Abortion, premature delivery with amnionitis (with a characteristic brown, murky amniotic fluid), stillbirth, or neonatal sepsis (see p. 2637) is common. Infection may be apparent within hours or days of birth (early onset) or it may be delayed up to several weeks.

Neonates with early-onset disease frequently are of low birth weight, have associated obstetric complications, and show evidence of sepsis soon after birth with circulatory or respiratory insufficiency or both. Neonates with the delayed-onset form are usually full-term, previously healthy neonates presenting with meningitis or sepsis.

Diagnosis

- Culture of blood, cervix, and amniotic fluid (if available) of febrile pregnant woman
- Culture of blood, CSF, gastric aspirate, meconium, and infected tissues of sick neonate

Blood and cervix specimens should be obtained from any pregnant woman with an unexplained febrile disease and cultured for *L. monocytogenes*. A sick neonate whose mother has listeriosis should be evaluated for sepsis, including cultures of either umbilical cord or peripheral blood, CSF, gastric aspirate, meconium, any potentially infected tissue, the mother's lochia and exudates from cervix and vagina, grossly diseased parts of the placenta, and amniotic fluid (if available).

CSF examination may show a predominance of mononuclear cells, but usually polymorphonuclear cells predominate. Gram-stained smears frequently are negative but may show pleomorphic, gram-variable coccobacillary forms, which should not be disregarded as diphtheroid contaminants.

Laboratory confirmation of the organism involves biochemical testing and observation of motility using a slide test or showing motility in semisolid media. To do the slide test, colonies of the organism that have grown on solid media are mixed with saline and examined under a microscope. *L. monocytogenes* exhibits a distinctive end-over-end "tumbling" motility due to the presence of flagella at both ends. Serologic tests are not useful. Molecular detection via PCR appears to be sensitive and specific but remains a research tool at present.

Prognosis

Mortality, ranging from 10 to 50%, is higher in neonates with early-onset disease.

Treatment

- Ampicillin plus an aminoglycoside

Treatment of the newborn is with ampicillin plus an aminoglycoside (see Table 314–1). A 14-day course is usually satisfactory (21 days for meningitis), but the optimal duration is unknown. Other possible drugs include ampicillin or penicillin with rifampin or trimethoprim/sulfamethoxazole, trimethoprim/sulfamethoxazole alone, and meropenem, but they have not been well evaluated.

Neonates with sepsis require other measures (see p. 2638). In heavy infection, drainage/secretion precautions may be considered.

Prevention

Food products that may be contaminated by *L. monocytogenes* (eg, unpasteurized dairy products, soft cheeses, raw vegetables, prepared deli meats and salads, refrigerated meat spreads or smoked seafood) should be avoided by pregnant women. Proper food handling, in particular separating uncooked meats from other items during preparation and washing hands, utensils, and cutting boards after handling uncooked foods, is critical.

If infection during pregnancy is recognized, treatment may then be given before delivery or intrapartum to prevent vertical transmission, but the usefulness of such treatment is unproved.

KEY POINTS

- Infection may be acquired in utero or during delivery, and clinical manifestations may appear within hours or days of birth (early onset) or may be delayed up to several weeks (delayed onset).
- Early-onset listeriosis manifests soon after birth as sepsis with circulatory insufficiency, respiratory insufficiency, or both.
- In delayed-onset listeriosis, full-term, previously healthy neonates present with meningitis or sepsis.
- Do cultures for *L. monocytogenes* on pregnant women with unexplained febrile illness.

- Treat with ampicillin plus an aminoglycoside.
- Pregnant women should avoid food products that may be contaminated by *L. monocytogenes*.

NEONATAL BACTERIAL MENINGITIS

Neonatal bacterial meningitis is inflammation of the meninges due to bacterial invasion. Signs are those of sepsis, CNS irritation (eg, lethargy, seizures, vomiting, irritability [particularly paradoxical irritability], nuchal rigidity, a bulging or full fontanelle), and cranial nerve abnormalities. Diagnosis is by lumbar puncture. Treatment is with antibiotics.

Neonatal bacterial meningitis occurs in 2/10,000 full-term and 2/1,000 low-birth-weight (LBW) neonates, with a male predominance. It occurs in about 15% of neonates with sepsis and occasionally occurs in isolation.

Etiology

The predominant pathogens are

- Group B streptococcus (GBS—predominantly type III)
- *Escherichia coli* (particularly those strains containing the K1 polysaccharide)
- *Listeria monocytogenes*

Enterococci, nonenterococcal group D streptococci, α-hemolytic streptococci, *Staphylococcus aureus*, coagulase-negative staphylococci, and gram-negative enteric organisms (eg, *Klebsiella* sp, *Enterobacter* sp, *Citrobacter diversus*) also are pathogens. *Haemophilus influenzae, Neisseria meningitidis,* and *Streptococcus pneumoniae* have been reported as causes.

Neonatal bacterial meningitis most frequently results from the bacteremia that occurs with neonatal sepsis; the higher the colony count in the blood culture, the higher the risk of meningitis. Neonatal bacterial meningitis may also result from scalp lesions, particularly when developmental defects lead to communication between the skin surface and the subarachnoid space, which predisposes to thrombophlebitis of the diploic veins. Rarely, there is direct extension to the CNS from a contiguous otic focus (eg, otitis media).

Symptoms and Signs

Frequently, only those findings typical of neonatal sepsis (eg, temperature instability, respiratory distress, jaundice, apnea) are manifest. CNS signs (eg, lethargy, seizures [particularly focal], vomiting, irritability) more specifically suggest neonatal bacterial meningitis. So-called paradoxical irritability, in which cuddling and consoling by a parent irritates rather than comforts the neonate, is more specific for the diagnosis. A bulging or full fontanelle occurs in about 25% and nuchal rigidity in only 15%. The younger the patient, the less common are these findings. Cranial nerve abnormalities (particularly those involving the 3rd, 6th, and 7th nerves) may also be present.

Meningitis due to GBS (GBS meningitis) may occur in the first week of life, accompanying early-onset neonatal sepsis and frequently manifesting initially as a systemic illness with prominent respiratory signs. Often, however, GBS meningitis occurs after this period (most commonly in the first 3 mo of life) as an isolated illness characterized by absence of antecedent obstetric or perinatal complications and the presence of more specific signs of meningitis (eg, fever, lethargy, seizures).

Ventriculitis frequently accompanies neonatal bacterial meningitis, particularly when caused by gram-negative enteric bacilli. Organisms that cause meningitis together with severe vasculitis, particularly *C. diversus* and *Cronobacter (*formerly *Enterobacter) sakazakii,* are likely to cause cysts and abscesses. *Pseudomonas aeruginosa, E. coli* K1, and *Serratia* sp also may cause brain abscesses. An early clinical sign of brain abscess is increased intracranial pressure (ICP), commonly manifested by vomiting, a bulging fontanelle, and sometimes enlarging head size. Deterioration in an otherwise stable neonate with meningitis suggests progressive increased ICP caused by abscess or hydrocephalus, or rupture of an abscess into the ventricular system.

PEARLS & PITFALLS

- Classic signs of meningitis are uncommon; a bulging or full fontanelle occurs in only about 25% of neonates and nuchal rigidity occurs in only 15% of neonates.

Diagnosis

- CSF cell counts, glucose and protein levels, Gram stain, and culture
- Sometimes ultrasonography or CT or MRI of the brain

Definitive diagnosis of neonatal bacterial meningitis is made by CSF examination via lumbar puncture (LP), which should be done in any neonate suspected of having sepsis or meningitis. However, LP can be difficult to do in a neonate, and there is some risk of hypoxia. Poor clinical condition (eg, respiratory distress, shock, thrombocytopenia) makes LP risky. If LP is delayed, the neonate should be treated as though meningitis is present. Even when the clinical condition improves, the presence of inflammatory cells and abnormal glucose and protein levels in CSF days after illness onset can still suggest the diagnosis. A needle with a trocar should be used for LP to avoid introducing epithelial rests and subsequent development of epitheliomas.

The CSF, even if bloody or acellular, should be cultured. About 15 to 35% of neonates with negative blood cultures have positive CSF cultures depending on the population studied. LP should be repeated at 24 to 48 h if clinical response is questionable and at 72 h when gram-negative organisms are involved (to ensure sterilization).

Repeating the CSF analysis helps guide duration of therapy and predict prognosis. Some experts believe that a repeat LP at 24 to 48 h in neonates with GBS meningitis has prognostic value. LP should not be repeated at the end of therapy if the neonate is doing well.

Normal CSF values are controversial and in part age-related. In general, both term and preterm infants without meningitis have ≤ 20 WBCs/μL (one fifth of which may be polymorphonuclear leukocytes) in their CSF. CSF protein levels in the absence of meningitis are more variable; term infants have levels of < 100 mg/dL, whereas preterm infants have levels up to 150 mg/dL. CSF glucose levels in the absence of meningitis are > 75% of the serum value measured at the same time. These levels may be as low as 20 to 30 mg/dL (1.1 to 1.7 mmol/L). Bacterial meningitis has been identified by culture in neonates with normal CSF indices, showing that normal CSF values do not exclude a diagnosis of meningitis.

Ventriculitis is suspected in a neonate not responding appropriately to antimicrobial therapy. The diagnosis is made when a ventricular puncture yields a WBC count greater than that from the LP, by a positive Gram stain or culture of ventricular fluid, or by increased ventricular pressure. When ventriculitis or brain abscess is suspected, ultrasonography or MRI or CT with contrast may aid diagnosis; dilated ventricles also confirm ventriculitis.

Prognosis

Without treatment, the mortality rate for neonatal bacterial meningitis approaches 100%. With treatment, prognosis is determined by birth weight, organism, and clinical severity. Mortality rate for treated neonatal bacterial meningitis is 5 to 20%. For organisms that cause vasculitis or brain abscess (necrotizing meningitis), the mortality rate may approach 75%. Neurologic sequelae (eg, hydrocephalus, hearing loss, intellectual disability) develop in 20 to 50% of infants who survive, with a poorer prognosis when gram-negative enteric bacilli are the cause.

Prognosis also depends partly on the number of organisms present in CSF at diagnosis. The duration of positive CSF cultures correlates directly with the incidence of complications. In general, CSF cultures from neonates with GBS are usually sterilized within the first 24 h of antimicrobial therapy. Those from gram-negative bacillary meningitis remain positive longer, with a median of 2 days.

GBS meningitis has a mortality rate significantly lower than that of early-onset GBS sepsis.

Treatment

- Empiric ampicillin plus gentamicin, cefotaxime, or both, followed by culture-specific drugs

See Table 314–1.

Empiric antibiotic therapy: Initial empiric treatment depends on patient age and is still debated. For neonates, many experts recommend ampicillin plus an aminoglycoside. A 3rd-generation cephalosporin (eg, cefotaxime) is also added until culture and sensitivity results are available if meningitis due to a gram-negative organism is suspected. However, resistance may develop more rapidly when cefotaxime is used routinely for empiric therapy, and prolonged use of 3rd-generation cephalosporins is a risk factor for invasive candidiasis. Ampicillin is active against organisms such as GBS, enterococci, and *Listeria*. Gentamicin provides synergy against these organisms and also treats many gram-negative infections. Third-generation cephalosporins provide adequate coverage for most gram-negative pathogens.

Hospitalized neonates who previously received antibiotics (eg, for early-onset sepsis) may have resistant organisms; fungal disease may also be considered in a septic-appearing neonate after prolonged hospitalization. Ill neonates with hospital-acquired infection should initially receive vancomycin plus an aminoglycoside with or without a 3rd-generation cephalosporin or a carbapenem with activity against *Pseudomonas aeruginosa,* such as cefepime or meropenem, depending on the concern for meningitis.

Antibiotics are adjusted when results of CSF culture and sensitivities are known. The results of the Gram stain should not be used to narrow coverage before culture results are available.

Organism-specific antibiotic therapy: The recommended initial treatment for GBS meningitis in neonates < 1 wk of age is penicillin G 100,000 to 150,000 units/kg IV q 8 h or ampicillin 100 to 150 mg/kg IV q 8 h. Additionally, gentamicin 3 mg/kg IV once/day is given for synergy if neonates are < 35 wk gestational age or 4 mg/kg IV once/day is given if neonates are > 35 wk gestational age. If clinical improvement occurs or sterilization of CSF is documented, gentamicin can be stopped.

For enterococci or *L. monocytogenes,* treatment is generally ampicillin plus gentamicin for the entire course.

In gram-negative bacillary meningitis, treatment is difficult. The traditional regimen of ampicillin plus an aminoglycoside results in a 15 to 20% mortality rate, with a high rate of sequelae in survivors. Instead, a 3rd-generation cephalosporin (eg, cefotaxime) should be used in neonates with *proven* gram-negative meningitis. If antibiotic resistance is a concern, both an aminoglycoside and a 3rd-generation cephalosporin or extended-spectrum β-lactam (eg, meropenem) may be used until sensitivities are known.

Parenteral therapy for gram-positive meningitis is given for a minimum of 14 days, and for complicated gram-positive or gram-negative meningitis, a minimum of 21 days. Intraventricular instillation of antibiotics is not recommended.

Adjunctive measures: Because meningitis may be considered part of the continuum of neonatal sepsis, the adjunctive measures used in treating neonatal sepsis should also be used to treat neonatal meningitis. Corticosteroids are not used in treatment of neonatal meningitis. Patients should be closely monitored for neurologic complications during early childhood, including for sensorineural hearing loss.

KEY POINTS

- The most common causes are GBS, *E. coli,* and *L. monocytogenes*.
- Manifestations are often nonspecific (eg, temperature instability, respiratory distress, jaundice, apnea).
- Although CNS signs (eg, lethargy, seizures, vomiting, irritability) may be present, classic findings such as a bulging or full fontanelle and nuchal rigidity are not common.
- CSF culture is critical because some neonates with meningitis have normal CSF indices (eg, WBC count, protein and glucose levels).
- Begin empiric treatment with ampicillin, gentamicin, and cefotaxime followed by specific drugs based on the results of cultures and susceptibility testing.
- Corticosteroids are not used in neonatal meningitis.

NEONATAL PNEUMONIA

Neonatal pneumonia is lung infection in a neonate. Onset may be within hours of birth and part of a generalized sepsis syndrome or after 7 days and confined to the lungs. Signs may be limited to respiratory distress or progress to shock and death. Diagnosis is by clinical and laboratory evaluation for sepsis. Treatment is initial broad-spectrum antibiotics changed to organism-specific drugs as soon as possible.

Pneumonia is the most common invasive bacterial infection after primary sepsis. Early-onset pneumonia is part of generalized sepsis that first manifests at or within hours of birth (see p. 2636). Late-onset pneumonia usually occurs after 7 days of age, most commonly in neonatal ICUs among infants who require prolonged endotracheal intubation because of lung disease (called healthcare-associated pneumonia).

Etiology

Organisms are acquired from the maternal genital tract or the nursery. These organisms include gram-positive cocci (eg, groups A and B streptococci, both methicillin-sensitive and methicillin-resistant *Staphylococcus aureus*) and gram-negative bacilli (eg, *Escherichia coli, Klebsiella* sp, *Proteus* sp). In infants who have received broad-spectrum antibiotics, many other pathogens may be found, including *Pseudomonas, Citrobacter, Bacillus,* and *Serratia*. Viruses or fungi cause some cases.

Symptoms and Signs

Late-onset health-care associated pneumonia manifests with unexplained worsening of the patient's respiratory status and increased quantities and a change in the quality of the respiratory secretions (eg, thick and brown). Infants may be acutely ill, with temperature instability and neutropenia.

Diagnosis

- Chest x-ray

Evaluation includes chest x-ray, pulse oximetry, blood cultures, and Gram stain and culture of tracheal aspirate.

New, persistent infiltrates should be visible on chest x-ray but may be difficult to recognize if the infant has severe bronchopulmonary dysplasia.

If Gram stain shows a significant number of polymorphonuclear leukocytes and a single organism that is consistent with the one that grows from culture of the tracheal aspirate, the likelihood increases that this organism is the cause of the pneumonia. Because bacterial pneumonia in neonates may disseminate, a full evaluation for sepsis, including a lumbar puncture, should also be done. However, blood cultures are positive in only 2 to 5% of cases of healthcare-associated pneumonia.

Treatment

- Usually vancomycin and a broad-spectrum β-lactam drug

Antimicrobial therapy in early-onset disease is similar to that for neonatal sepsis. Vancomycin and a broad-spectrum β-lactam drug such as meropenem, piperacillin/tazobactam, or cefepime (see Table 314–1), are the initial treatment of choice for most late-onset healthcare-associated pneumonia. This regimen treats sepsis as well as pneumonia with typical hospital-acquired pathogens including *P. aeruginosa.* Local patterns of infection and bacterial resistance should always be used to help guide empiric choices of antimicrobials. More specific antibiotics are substituted after sensitivity results are available. General treatment is the same as that for neonatal sepsis.

Chlamydial Pneumonia

Exposure to chlamydial organisms during delivery may result in development of chlamydial pneumonia at 2 to 18 wk. Infants are tachypneic but usually not critically ill and may also have a history of conjunctivitis caused by the same organism. Eosinophilia may be present, and x-rays show bilateral interstitial infiltrates with hyperinflation.

Treatment

- Erythromycin

Treatment with erythromycin leads to rapid resolution (see Table 314–3). Because erythromycin in neonates may cause HPS, all neonates treated with erythromycin should be monitored for symptoms and signs of HPS and their parents counseled regarding potential risks. Azithromycin 20 mg/kg po once/day for 3 days may also be effective. The diagnosis of pneumonia secondary to *Chlamydia trachomatis* should prompt an evaluation of the mother and her partner because untreated maternal chlamydial infection may have complications such as pelvic inflammatory disease and sterility.

NEONATAL SEPSIS

(Sepsis Neonatorum)

Neonatal sepsis is invasive infection, usually bacterial, occurring during the neonatal period. Signs are multiple, nonspecific, and include diminished spontaneous activity, less vigorous sucking, apnea, bradycardia, temperature instability, respiratory distress, vomiting, diarrhea, abdominal distention, jitteriness, seizures, and jaundice. Diagnosis is clinical and based on culture results. Treatment is initially with ampicillin plus either gentamicin or cefotaxime, narrowed to organism-specific drugs as soon as possible.

Neonatal sepsis occurs in 0.5 to 8.0/1000 births. The highest rates occur in

- Low-birth-weight (LBW) infants
- Infants with depressed function at birth as manifested by a low Apgar score
- Infants with maternal perinatal risk factors (eg, low socioeconomic status, premature rupture of membranes)
- Minorities
- Males

Etiology

Onset of neonatal sepsis can be early (≤ 3 days of birth) or late (after 3 days).

Early onset: Early-onset neonatal sepsis usually results from organisms acquired intrapartum. Most infants have symptoms within 6 h of birth.

GBS and gram-negative enteric organisms (predominantly *Escherichia coli*) account for most cases of early-onset sepsis. Vaginal or rectal cultures of women at term may show GBS colonization rates of up to 35%. At least 35% of their infants also become colonized. The density of infant colonization determines the risk of early-onset invasive disease, which is 40 times higher with heavy colonization. Although only 1/100 of infants colonized develop invasive disease due to GBS, > 50% of those present within the first 6 h of life. Nontypeable *Haemophilus influenzae* sepsis has also been identified in neonates, especially premature neonates.

Other gram-negative enteric bacilli (eg, *Klebsiella* sp) and gram-positive organisms—*Listeria monocytogenes,* enterococci (eg, *Enterococcus faecalis, E. faecium*), group D streptococci (eg, *Streptococcus bovis*), α-hemolytic streptococci, and staphylococci—account for most other cases. *S. pneumoniae, H. influenzae* type b, and, less commonly, *Neisseria meningitidis* have been isolated. Asymptomatic gonorrhea occurs occasionally in pregnancy, so *N. gonorrhoeae* may rarely be a pathogen.

Late onset: Late-onset neonatal sepsis is usually acquired from the environment (see p. 2632). Staphylococci account for 30 to 60% of late-onset cases and are most frequently due to intravascular devices (particularly central vascular catheters). *E. coli* is also becoming increasingly recognized as a significant cause of late-onset sepsis, especially in extremely LBW infants. Isolation of *Enterobacter cloacae* or *Cronobacter* (formerly *Enterobacter) sakazakii* from blood or CSF may be due to contaminated feedings. Contaminated respiratory equipment is suspected in outbreaks of hospital-acquired *Pseudomonas aeruginosa* pneumonia or sepsis.

Although universal screening and intrapartum antibiotic prophylaxis for GBS have significantly decreased the rate of early-onset disease due to this organism, the rate of late-onset GBS sepsis has remained unchanged, which is consistent with the hypothesis that late-onset disease is usually acquired from the environment.

The role of anaerobes (particularly *Bacteroides fragilis*) in late-onset sepsis remains unclear, although deaths have been attributed to *Bacteroides* bacteremia.

Candida sp are increasingly important causes of late-onset sepsis, occurring in 12 to 18% of extremely LBW infants.

Early and late onset: Certain viral infections (eg, disseminated herpes simplex, enterovirus, adenovirus, respiratory syncytial virus) may manifest as early-onset or late-onset sepsis.

Pathophysiology

Early onset: Certain maternal perinatal and obstetric factors increase risk, particularly of early-onset neonatal sepsis, such as the following:

- Premature rupture of membranes (PROM) occurring ≥ 18 h before birth
- Maternal chorioamnionitis (most commonly manifesting as maternal fever shortly before or during delivery with maternal leukocytosis, tachycardia, uterine tenderness, and/or foul-smelling amniotic fluid)
- Colonization with GBS
- Preterm delivery

Hematogenous and transplacental dissemination of maternal infection occurs in the transmission of certain viral (eg, rubella, CMV), protozoal (eg, *Toxoplasma gondii*), and treponemal (eg, *Treponema pallidum*) pathogens. A few bacterial pathogens (eg, *L. monocytogenes, Mycobacterium tuberculosis*) may reach the fetus transplacentally, but most are acquired by the ascending route in utero or as the fetus passes through the colonized birth canal.

Though the intensity of maternal colonization is directly related to risk of invasive disease in the neonate, many mothers with low-density colonization give birth to infants with high-density colonization who are therefore at risk. Amniotic fluid contaminated with meconium or vernix caseosa promotes growth of GBS and *E. coli*. Hence, the few organisms in the vaginal vault are able to proliferate rapidly after PROM, possibly contributing to this paradox. Organisms usually reach the bloodstream by fetal aspiration or swallowing of contaminated amniotic fluid, leading to bacteremia.

The ascending route of infection helps to explain such phenomena as the high incidence of PROM in neonatal infections, the significance of adnexal inflammation (amnionitis is more commonly associated with neonatal sepsis than is central placentitis), the increased risk of infection in the twin closer to the birth canal, and the bacteriologic characteristics of early-onset neonatal sepsis, which reflect the flora of the maternal vaginal vault.

Late onset: The most important risk factor in late-onset sepsis is preterm delivery. Others include

- Prolonged use of intravascular catheters
- Associated illnesses (which may, however, be only a marker for the use of invasive procedures)
- Exposure to antibiotics (which selects resistant bacterial strains)
- Prolonged hospitalization
- Contaminated equipment or IV or enteral solutions

Gram-positive organisms (eg, coagulase-negative staphylococci and *Staphylococcus aureus*) may be introduced from the environment or the patient's skin. Gram-negative enteric bacteria are usually derived from the patient's endogenous flora, which may have been altered by antecedent antibiotic therapy or populated by resistant organisms transferred from the hands of personnel (the major means of spread) or contaminated equipment. Therefore, situations that increase exposure to these bacteria (eg, crowding, inadequate nurse staffing, or inconsistent provider hand washing) result in higher rates of hospital-acquired infection.

Risk factors for *Candida* sp sepsis include prolonged (> 10 days) use of central IV catheters, hyperalimentation, use of antecedent antibiotics (especially 3rd-generation cephalosporins), and abdominal pathology.

Initial foci of infection can be in the urinary tract, paranasal sinuses, middle ear, lungs, or GI tract, and may later disseminate to meninges, kidneys, bones, joints, peritoneum, and skin.

Symptoms and Signs

Early signs of neonatal sepsis are frequently nonspecific and subtle and do not distinguish among organisms (including viral). Particularly common early signs include

- Diminished spontaneous activity
- Less vigorous sucking
- Anorexia
- Apnea
- Bradycardia
- Temperature instability (hypothermia or hyperthermia)

Fever is present in only 10 to 15% but, when sustained (eg, > 1 h), generally indicates infection. Other symptoms and signs include respiratory distress, neurologic findings (eg, seizures, jitteriness), jaundice (especially occurring within the first 24 h of life without Rh or ABO blood group incompatibility and with a higher than expected direct bilirubin concentration), vomiting, diarrhea, and abdominal distention.

Specific signs of an infected organ may pinpoint the primary site or a metastatic site.

- Most neonates with early-onset GBS (and many with *L. monocytogenes*) infection present with respiratory distress that is difficult to distinguish from respiratory distress syndrome.
- Periumbilical erythema, discharge, or bleeding without a hemorrhagic diathesis suggests omphalitis (infection prevents obliteration of the umbilical vessels).
- Coma, seizures, opisthotonos, or a bulging fontanelle suggests meningitis, encephalitis, or brain abscess.
- Decreased spontaneous movement of an extremity and swelling, warmth, erythema, or tenderness over a joint indicates osteomyelitis or pyogenic arthritis.
- Unexplained abdominal distention may indicate peritonitis or necrotizing enterocolitis (particularly when accompanied by bloody diarrhea and fecal leukocytes).
- Cutaneous vesicles, mouth ulcers, and hepatosplenomegaly (particularly with disseminated intravascular coagulation [DIC]) can indicate disseminated herpes simplex.

Early-onset GBS infection may manifest as a fulminating pneumonia. Often, obstetric complications (particularly prematurity, PROM, or chorioamnionitis) have occurred. In > 50% of neonates, GBS infection manifests within 6 h of birth; 45% have an Apgar score of < 5. Meningitis may also be present but is not common. In late-onset GBS infection (at > 3 days to 12 wk), meningitis is often present. Late-onset GBS infection is generally not associated with perinatal risk factors or demonstrable maternal cervical colonization and may be acquired postpartum.

Diagnosis

- High index of suspicion
- Blood, CSF, and sometimes urine culture

Early diagnosis of neonatal sepsis is important and requires awareness of risk factors (particularly in LBW neonates) and a high index of suspicion when any neonate deviates from the norm in the first few weeks of life.

Neonates with clinical signs of sepsis should have a CBC, differential with smear, blood culture, urine culture (not necessary for evaluation of early-onset sepsis), and lumbar puncture (LP), if clinically feasible, as soon as possible. Neonates with respiratory symptoms require chest x-ray. Diagnosis is confirmed by isolation of a pathogen in culture. Other tests may have abnormal results but are not necessarily diagnostic. Infants should be given broad-spectrum empiric antimicrobial therapy.

Neonates who appear well are managed depending on several factors as discussed below under Prevention.

CBC, differential, and smear: The total WBC count and absolute band count in neonates are poor predictors of early-onset sepsis. However, an elevated ratio of immature:total polymorphonuclear leukocytes of > 0.16 is sensitive, and values below this cutoff have a high negative predictive value. However, specificity is poor; up to 50% of term neonates have an elevated ratio. Values obtained after 6 h of life are more likely to be abnormal and clinically useful than those obtained immediately after birth.

The platelet count may fall hours to days before the onset of clinical sepsis but more often remains elevated until a day or so after the neonate becomes ill. This fall is sometimes accompanied by other findings of DIC (eg, increased fibrin degradation products, decreased fibrinogen, prolonged INR). Given the timing of these changes, the platelet count is not typically helpful in evaluating a neonate for sepsis.

Because of large numbers of circulating bacteria, organisms can sometimes be seen in or associated with polymorphonuclear leukocytes by applying Gram stain, methylene blue, or acridine orange to the buffy coat.

Regardless of the results of CBC or LP, in all neonates with suspected sepsis (eg, those who look sick or are febrile or hypothermic), antibiotics should be started immediately after cultures (eg, blood and CSF [if possible]) are taken.

Lumbar puncture: There is a risk of increasing hypoxia during an LP in already hypoxemic neonates. However, LP should be done in neonates with suspected sepsis as soon as they are able to tolerate the procedure (see also p. 2634 under Neonatal Bacterial Meningitis). Supplemental O_2 is given before and during LP to prevent hypoxia. Because GBS pneumonia manifesting in the first day of life can be confused with respiratory distress syndrome, LP is often done routinely in neonates suspected of having these diseases.

Blood cultures: Umbilical vessels are frequently contaminated by organisms on the umbilical stump, especially after a number of hours, so blood cultures from umbilical venous lines may not be reliable. Therefore, blood for culture should be obtained by venipuncture, preferably at 2 peripheral sites. Although the optimal skin preparation to perform before obtaining blood cultures in neonates is not defined, clinicians can apply an iodine-containing liquid and allow the site to dry. Alternatively, blood obtained soon after placement of an umbilical arterial catheter may also be used for culture if necessary.

Blood should be cultured for both aerobic and anaerobic organisms. However, the minimum amount of blood per blood culture bottle is 1.0 mL; if < 2 mL is obtained, it should all be placed in a single aerobic blood culture bottle. If catheter-associated sepsis is suspected, a culture specimen should be obtained through the catheter as well as peripherally. In > 90% of positive bacterial blood cultures, growth occurs within 48 h of incubation. Data on capillary blood cultures are insufficient to recommend them.

Candida sp grow in blood cultures and on blood agar plates, but if other fungi are suspected, a fungal culture medium should be used. For species other than *Candida,* fungal blood cultures may require 4 to 5 days of incubation before becoming positive and may be negative even in obviously disseminated disease. Proof of colonization (in mouth or stool or on skin) may be helpful before culture results are available. Neonates with candidemia should undergo LP to identify candidal meningitis. Indirect ophthalmoscopy with dilation of the pupils is done to identify retinal candidal lesions. Renal ultrasonography is done to detect renal mycetoma.

Urinalysis and culture: Urine testing is needed only for evaluation of late-onset sepsis. Urine should be obtained by catheterization or suprapubic aspiration, not by urine collection bags. Although only culture is diagnostic, a finding of ≥ 5 WBCs/high-power field in the spun urine or any organisms in a fresh unspun gram-stained sample is presumptive evidence of a UTI. Absence of pyuria does not rule out UTI.

Other tests for infection and inflammation: Numerous tests are often abnormal in sepsis and have been evaluated as possible early markers. In general, however, sensitivities tend to be low until later in illness, and specificities are suboptimal.

Acute-phase reactants are proteins produced by the liver under the influence of IL-1 when inflammation is present. The most valuable of these is quantitative C-reactive protein. A concentration of ≥ 1 mg/dL (measured by nephelometry) is abnormal. Elevated levels occur within 6 to 8 h of developing sepsis and peak at 1 day. The sensitivity of C-reactive protein measurements is higher if measured after 6 to 8 h of life. Two normal values obtained between 8 h and 24 h after birth and then 24 h later have a negative predictive value of 99.7%.

Procalcitonin is being investigated as an acute-phase reactant marker for neonatal sepsis. Although procalcitonin appears more sensitive than C-reactive protein, it is less specific.

Prognosis

The fatality rate is 2 to 4 times higher in LBW infants than in full-term infants. The overall mortality rate of early-onset sepsis is 3 to 40% (that of early-onset GBS infection is 2 to 10%) and of late-onset sepsis is 2 to 20% (that of late-onset GBS is about 2%). Mortality in late-onset sepsis highly depends on the etiology of the infection; infections caused by gram-negative bacilli or *Candida* spp have rates of up to 32 to 36%. In addition to mortality, extremely LBW infants who develop bacterial or candidal sepsis have a significantly greater risk of poor neurodevelopmental outcome.

Treatment

- Antibiotic therapy
- Supportive therapy

Because sepsis may manifest with nonspecific clinical signs and its effects may be devastating, rapid empiric antibiotic therapy is recommended (see p. 1495); drugs are later adjusted according to sensitivities and the site of infection. Generally, if no source of infection is identified clinically, the infant appears well, and cultures are negative, antibiotics can be stopped after 48 h (up to 72 h in small preterm infants).

General supportive measures, including respiratory and hemodynamic management, are combined with antibiotic treatment.

Antimicrobials: In early-onset sepsis, initial therapy should include ampicillin plus an aminoglycoside. Cefotaxime may be added to or substituted for the aminoglycoside if meningitis caused by a gram-negative organism is suspected. Antibiotics may be changed as soon as an organism is identified.

Previously well infants admitted from the community with presumed late-onset sepsis should also receive therapy with ampicillin plus gentamicin or ampicillin plus cefotaxime. If gram-negative meningitis is suspected, ampicillin, cefotaxime, and an aminoglycoside may be used. In late-onset hospital-acquired sepsis, initial therapy should include vancomycin (active against methicillin-resistant *S. aureus*) plus an aminoglycoside. If *P. aeruginosa* is prevalent in the nursery, ceftazidime, cefepime, or piperacillin/tazobactam may be used in addition to or instead of an aminoglycoside depending on local susceptibilities.

For neonates previously treated with a full 7- to 14-day aminoglycoside course who need retreatment, a different aminoglycoside or a 3rd-generation cephalosporin should be considered.

If coagulase-negative staphylococci are suspected (eg, an indwelling catheter has been in place for > 72 h) or are isolated from blood or other normally sterile fluid and considered a pathogen, initial therapy for late-onset sepsis should include vancomycin. However, if the organism is sensitive to nafcillin, cefazolin or nafcillin should replace vancomycin. Removal of the presumptive source of the organism (usually an indwelling intravascular catheter) may be necessary to cure the infection because coagulase-negative staphylococci may be protected by a biofilm (a covering that encourages adherence of organisms to the catheter).

Because *Candida* may take 2 to 3 days to grow in blood culture, empiric initiation of amphotericin B deoxycholate therapy and removal of the infected catheter before cultures confirm yeast infection may be lifesaving.

Other treatment: Exchange transfusions have been used for severely ill (particularly hypotensive and metabolically acidotic) neonates. Their purported value is to increase levels of circulating immunoglobulins, decrease circulating endotoxin, increase Hb levels (with higher 2,3-diphosphoglycerate levels), and improve perfusion. However, no controlled prospective studies of their use have been conducted.

Fresh frozen plasma may help reverse the heat-stable and heat-labile opsonin deficiencies that occur in LBW neonates, but controlled studies of its use are unavailable, and transfusion-associated risks must be considered.

Granulocyte transfusions (see p. 1212) have been used in septic and granulocytopenic neonates but have not convincingly improved outcome.

Recombinant colony-stimulating factors (granulocyte colony-stimulating factor [G-CSF] and granulocyte-macrophage colony-stimulating factor [GM-CSF]) have increased neutrophil number and function in neonates with presumed sepsis but do not seem to be of routine benefit in neonates with severe neutropenia; further study is required.

Prevention

Neonates who appear well may be at risk of GBS infection. They are managed depending on several factors.[1,2] including

- Presence of chorioamnionitis
- Whether maternal GBS prophylaxis was indicated and given appropriately
- Gestational age and the duration of membrane rupture

If there is neither chorioamnionitis nor indication for GBS prophylaxis, no testing or treatment is indicated.

If **chorioamnionitis is present or strongly suspected,** preterm and term neonates should have a blood culture at birth and begin empiric broad-spectrum antibiotic therapy. Testing should also include WBC count and differential and C-reactive protein at 6 to 12 h of life. Further management depends on the clinical course and results of the laboratory tests.

If **maternal GBS prophylaxis was indicated and given appropriately** (ie, penicillin, ampicillin, or cefazolin given IV for ≥ 4 h), infants should be observed in the hospital for 48 h; testing and treatment are done only if symptoms develop. Selected patients ≥ 37 wk gestation who have reliable caretakers and ready access to follow-up may go home after 24 h.

If **adequate GBS prophylaxis was not given,** infants are observed in the hospital for 48 h without antimicrobial therapy. If membranes ruptured ≥ 18 h before birth or gestational age is < 37 wk, blood culture, CBC with differential, and perhaps a C-reactive protein level is recommended at birth and/or at 6 to 12 h of life. The clinical course and results of the laboratory evaluation guide management.

Giving IV immune globulin to augment the neonate's immune response has not been shown to help prevent or treat sepsis.

Maternal indications for GBS prophylaxis: All pregnant women should be screened for GBS colonization late in gestation.

Women with a positive GBS screen should be given intrapartum antibiotic prophylaxis unless they are undergoing cesarean delivery before labor starts and before membrane rupture.

Women with a negative GBS screen should receive intrapartum antibiotics if they previously gave birth to an infant with GBS disease.

Women whose GBS status is unknown (eg, because they were not tested or results are unavailable) should receive intrapartum antibiotics if ≥ 1 of the following factors are present:

- < 37 wk gestation
- Rupture of membranes for ≥ 18 h
- Temperature ≥ 38° C

Antibiotics typically used include penicillin, ampicillin, or cefazolin and should be given IV for ≥ 4 hr before delivery. Selection should take into account local GBS antimicrobial resistance patterns.

1. Brady MT, Polin RA: Prevention and management of infants with suspected or proven neonatal sepsis. *Pediatrics* 132:166–168, 2013.
2. Polin RA and the Committee on Fetus and Newborn: Management of neonates with suspected or proven early-onset bacterial sepsis. *Pediatrics* 129:1006–1015, 2012.

KEY POINTS

- Neonatal sepsis can be early onset (≤ 3 days of birth) or late onset (after 3 days).
- Early-onset sepsis usually results from organisms acquired intrapartum, and symptoms appear within 6 h of birth.
- Late-onset sepsis is usually acquired from the environment and is more likely in preterm infants, particularly those with prolonged hospitalization, use of IV catheters, or both.
- Early signs are frequently nonspecific and subtle, and fever is present in only 10 to 15% of neonates.
- Do blood and CSF cultures and, for late-onset sepsis, also do urine culture.
- Treat early-onset sepsis initially with ampicillin plus gentamicin (and/or cefotaxime if gram-negative meningitis is suspected), narrowed to organism-specific drugs as soon as possible.

PERINATAL TUBERCULOSIS

Tuberculosis can be acquired during the perinatal period. Symptoms and signs are nonspecific. Diagnosis is by culture and sometimes x-ray and biopsy. Treatment is with isoniazid and other antituberculous drugs.

Infants may acquire tuberculosis by the following means:

- Transplacental spread through the umbilical vein to the fetal liver
- Aspiration or ingestion of infected amniotic fluid
- Airborne inoculation from close contacts (family members or nursery personnel)

About 50% of children born to mothers with active pulmonary tuberculosis develop the disease during the first year of life if chemoprophylaxis or BCG vaccine is not given.

Symptoms and Signs

The clinical presentation of neonatal tuberculosis is nonspecific but is usually marked by multiple organ involvement. The neonate may look acutely or chronically ill and may have fever, lethargy, respiratory distress or non-responsive pneumonia, hepatosplenomegaly, or failure to thrive.

Diagnosis

- Culture of tracheal aspirate, gastric washings, urine, and CSF
- Chest x-ray
- Sometimes skin testing

All neonates with suspected congenital tuberculosis and infants born to mothers who have active TB should have a chest x-ray and culture of tracheal aspirates, gastric washings, and urine for acid-fast bacilli; a lumbar puncture should be done to measure cell counts, glucose, and protein as well as obtain CSF culture. The placenta should be examined and cultured as well. Skin testing is not extremely sensitive, particularly initially, but should be done. Biopsy of the liver, lymph nodes, lungs, or pleurae may be needed to confirm the diagnosis. HIV testing of the infant should be done.

Well-appearing neonates whose mothers have a positive skin test but a negative chest x-ray and no evidence of active disease should have close follow-up, and all household members should be evaluated. If there is no exposure to a case of active TB, the neonate does not need treatment or testing. If significant exposure to a case of active TB is found in the neonate's environment after birth, the neonate should be evaluated for suspected TB as described previously.

PEARLS & PITFALLS

- Skin testing is not extremely sensitive for perinatal TB, particularly initially, but should be done.

Treatment

- Isoniazid (INH) for positive skin test or high-risk exposure
- Addition of other drugs (eg, rifampin, ethambutol, ethionamide, pyrazinamide, an aminoglycoside) if TB is present

Management depends on the whether there is active TB disease or only a positive skin test (in mother, infant, or both) indicating infection without disease.

Pregnant women with a positive tuberculin test: Women are evaluated for active TB. If active disease is excluded, INH use may be deferred until after the postpartum period because the hepatotoxicity of INH is increased in pregnancy and because the risk of contracting TB from a mother with a positive tuberculin test is greater for the neonate than for the fetus. However, if the woman has had recent contact with a person with contagious TB (in which case the benefit outweighs the risk), treatment is given for 9 mo, along with supplemental pyridoxine. Treatment for a pregnant woman exposed to contagious TB should be deferred until the 1st trimester is complete.

Neonates with a positive tuberculin test: If there is no clinical, laboratory, or x-ray evidence of disease, neonates should receive INH 10 to 15 mg/kg po once/day for 9 mo and should be closely monitored. Exclusively breastfed neonates should receive pyridoxine 1 to 2 mg/kg once/day.

Pregnant women with active TB: INH, ethambutol, and rifampin use in recommended doses during pregnancy has not been shown to be teratogenic to the human fetus. The recommended initial treatment regimen in the US includes INH 300 mg po, ethambutol 15 to 25 mg/kg (maximum 2.5 g) po, and rifampin 600 mg po. All pregnant and breastfeeding women receiving INH should also receive pyridoxine 25 to 30 mg po. All these drugs can be given once daily. The recommended duration of therapy is at least 9 mo; if the organism is drug-resistant, an infectious disease consultation is recommended, and therapy may need to be extended to 18 mo.

Streptomycin is potentially ototoxic to the developing fetus and should not be used early in pregnancy unless rifampin is contraindicated. If possible, other antituberculous drugs should be avoided because of teratogenicity (eg, ethionamide) or lack of clinical experience during pregnancy.

Breastfeeding is not contraindicated for mothers receiving therapy who are not infective.

Patients with active TB should be reported to the local health department. Mothers with active TB should be tested for HIV.

Asymptomatic neonates whose mother or close contacts have active TB: The neonate is evaluated for congenital TB as above and is usually separated from the mother only until effective treatment of both mother and neonate is under way. If congenital TB is excluded and once the neonate is receiving INH, separation is no longer necessary unless the mother (or a household contact) has possible multidrug-resistant organisms or poorly adheres to treatment (including not wearing a mask if TB is active) and directly observed therapy is not possible. Family contacts should be investigated for undiagnosed TB before the infant goes home.

If adherence can be reasonably assured and the family is nontuberculous (ie, the mother is being treated and no other transmission risks are present), the neonate is started on a regimen of INH 10 to 15 mg/kg po once/day and sent home at the usual time. Exclusively breastfed infants should receive pyridoxine 1 to 2 mg/kg once/day.

Skin testing should be done at age 3 or 4 mo. If the neonate is tuberculin-negative and the initial infectious contact has adhered to treatment and has a positive response, INH is stopped. If the skin test is positive, chest x-ray and cultures for acid-fast bacilli are done as described previously and, if active disease is excluded, treatment with INH is continued for a total of 9 mo. If cultures become positive for TB at any time, the neonate should be treated for active TB disease.

If adherence in a nontuberculous environment cannot be ensured, BCG vaccine may be considered for the neonate, and INH therapy should be started as soon as possible. (Although INH inhibits the multiplication of BCG organisms, the combination of BCG vaccine and INH is supported by clinical trials and anecdotal reports.) BCG vaccination does not ensure against exposure to and development of TB, but offers significant protection against serious and widespread invasion (eg, tuberculous meningitis). BCG should only be given if skin and HIV test results of the neonate are negative. Neonates should be monitored for development of TB, particularly during the first year. (CAUTION: *BCG vaccine is contraindicated in immunosuppressed patients and those suspected of being infected with HIV. However, in high-risk populations, the WHO [unlike the American Academy of Pediatrics] recommends that asymptomatic HIV-infected neonates receive BCG vaccine at birth or shortly thereafter.)*

Neonates with active TB: For congenital TB, the American Academy of Pediatrics recommends treatment once/day with INH 10 to 15 mg/kg po, rifampin 10 to 20 mg/kg po, pyrazinamide 30 to 40 mg/kg po, and an aminoglycoside (eg, amikacin). This regimen should be modified as indicated based on results of testing for resistance. Pyridoxine is given if the neonate is exclusively breastfed. Ethambutol is usually avoided because it causes ocular toxicity, which is impossible to assess in neonates.

For TB acquired after birth, the suggested regimen is treatment once/day with INH 10 to 15 mg/kg po, rifampin 10 to 20 mg/kg po, and pyrazinamide 30 to 40 mg/kg. A fourth drug such as ethambutol 20 to 25 mg/kg po once/day, ethionamide 7.5 to 10 mg/kg po bid (or 5 to 6.67 mg/kg po tid), or an aminoglycoside should be added if drug resistance or tuberculous meningitis is suspected or the child lives in an area where HIV prevalence among TB patients is ≥ 5%. After the first 2 mo of treatment, INH and rifampin are continued to complete a 6- to 12-mo course (depending on disease category) and other drugs are stopped. Breastfed infants should also receive pyridoxine.

When the CNS is involved, initial therapy also includes corticosteroids (prednisone 2 mg/kg po once/day [maximum 60 mg/day] for 4 to 6 wk, then gradually tapered). Other therapy continues until all signs of meningitis have disappeared and cultures are negative on 2 successive lumbar punctures at least 1 wk apart. Therapy can then be continued with INH and rifampin once/day or twice/wk for another 10 mo. Corticosteroids may also be considered for infants and children with severe miliary disease, pleural or pericardial effusions, or endobronchial disease or those with abdominal TB.

TB in infants and children that is not congenitally acquired or disseminated, does not involve the CNS, bones, or joints, and results from drug-susceptible organisms can be treated effectively with a 6- to 9-mo (total) course of therapy. Organisms recovered from the child or mother should be tested for drug sensitivity. Hematologic, hepatic, and otologic symptoms should be monitored frequently to determine response to therapy and drug toxicity. Frequent laboratory analysis is not usually necessary.

Directly observed therapy is used whenever possible to improve adherence and the success of therapy. Many anti-TB drugs are not available in pediatric dosages. When possible, experienced personnel should give these drugs to children.

Prevention

Universal neonatal BCG vaccination is not routinely indicated in developed countries but may curb the incidence of childhood TB or decrease its severity in populations at increased risk of infection.

KEY POINTS

- TB may be acquired transplacentally, through aspiration of infected amniotic fluid, or by respiratory transmission after birth.
- Manifestations of neonatal TB are nonspecific, but multiple organs (including lungs, liver, and/or CNS) are usually involved.
- Do chest x-ray and TB culture of tracheal aspirate, gastric washings, urine, and CSF.
- Give INH for positive skin test or high-risk exposure.
- Add other drugs (eg, rifampin, ethambutol, pyrazinamide, ethionamide, an aminoglycoside) for active TB.

315 Inherited Disorders of Metabolism

Most inherited disorders of metabolism (also called inborn errors of metabolism) are caused by mutations in genes that code for enzymes; enzyme deficiency or inactivity leads to accumulation of substrate precursors or metabolites or to deficiencies of the enzyme's products. Hundreds of disorders exist, and although most inherited disorders of metabolism are extremely rare individually, collectively they are not rare. The disorders are typically grouped by the affected substrate (eg, carbohydrates, amino acids, fatty acids).

Most states routinely do neonatal screening of all newborns for specific inherited disorders of metabolism and other conditions, including phenylketonuria, tyrosinemia, biotinidase deficiency, homocystinuria, maple syrup urine disease, and galactosemia. Many states have an expanded screening program that covers many more inherited disorders of metabolism, including disorders of fatty acid oxidation and other organic acidemias. For a comprehensive review of each of these conditions, see also the American College of Medical Genetics and Genomics' (ACMG) newborn screening ACT sheets and algorithm table (available at www.acmg.net).

Metabolic defects that primarily cause disease in adults (eg, gout, porphyria), are organ-specific (eg, Wilson disease, congenital adrenal hypoplasia), or are common (eg, cystic fibrosis, X) are discussed elsewhere in THE MANUAL. For inherited disorders of lipoprotein metabolism, see Table 168–3 on p. 1304.

APPROACH TO THE PATIENT WITH A SUSPECTED INHERITED DISORDER OF METABOLISM

Most inherited disorders of metabolism are rare, and therefore their diagnosis requires a high index of suspicion. Timely diagnosis leads to early treatment and may help avoid acute and chronic complications, developmental compromise, and even death.

Evaluation

Symptoms and signs tend to be nonspecific and are more often caused by something other than an inherited disorder of metabolism (eg, infection); these more likely causes should also be investigated.

History and physical examination: Disorders manifesting in the neonatal period tend to be more serious; manifestations of many of the disorders typically include lethargy, poor feeding, vomiting, and seizures. Disorders that manifest later tend to affect growth and development, but vomiting, seizures, and weakness may also appear.

Growth delay suggests decreased anabolism or increased catabolism and may be due to decreased availability of energy-generating substrates (eg, in glycogen storage disease [GSD]) or inefficient energy or protein use (eg, in organic acidemias or urea cycle defects).

Developmental delay may reflect chronic energy deficit in the brain (eg, oxidative phosphorylation defects), decreased supply of needed carbohydrates that are non-energy substrates for the brain (eg, lack of uridine-5′-diphosphate-galactose [UDP-galactose] in untreated galactosemia), or chronic amino acid deficit in the brain (eg, tyrosine deficiency in phenylketonuria).

Neuromuscular symptoms, such as seizures, muscle weakness, hypotonia, myoclonus, muscle pain, strokes, or coma, may suggest acute energy deficit in the brain (eg, hypoglycemic seizures in GSD type I, strokes in mitochondrial oxidative phosphorylation defects) or muscle (eg, muscle weakness in muscle forms of GSD). Neuromuscular symptoms may also reflect accumulation of toxic compounds in the brain (eg, hyperammonemic coma in urea cycle defects) or tissue breakdown (eg, rhabdomyolysis and myoglobinuria in patients with long-chain hydroxyacyl dehydrogenase deficiency or muscle forms of GSD).

Congenital brain malformation may reflect decreased availability of energy (eg, decreased ATP output in pyruvate dehydrogenase deficiency) or critical precursors (eg, decreased cholesterol in 7-dehydrocholestrol reductase deficiency or Smith-Lemli-Opitz syndrome) during fetal development.

Autonomic symptoms can result from hypoglycemia caused by increased glucose consumption or decreased glucose production (eg, vomiting, diaphoresis, pallor, and tachycardia in GSD or hereditary fructose intolerance) or from metabolic acidosis (eg, vomiting and Kussmaul respirations in organic acidemias). Some conditions cause both (ie, in propionic acidemia, accumulation of acyl-CoAs causes metabolic acidosis and inhibits gluconeogenesis, thus causing hypoglycemia).

Nonphysiologic jaundice after the neonatal period usually reflects intrinsic hepatic disease, especially when accompanied by elevation of liver enzymes, but may be due to inherited disorders of metabolism (eg, untreated galactosemia, hereditary fructose intolerance, tyrosinemia type I).

Unusual odors in body fluids reflect accumulation of specific compounds (eg, sweaty feet odor in isovaleric acidemia, smoky-sweet odor in maple syrup urine disease, mousy or musty odor in phenylketonuria, boiled cabbage odor in tyrosinemia).

Change in urine color on exposure to air occurs in some disorders (eg, darkish brown in alkaptonuria, purplish brown in porphyria).

Organomegaly may reflect a failure in substrate degradation resulting in substrate accumulation within the organ cells (eg, hepatomegaly in hepatic forms of GSD and many lysosomal storage diseases, cardiomegaly in GSD type II).

Eye changes include cataracts in galactokinase deficiency or classic galactosemia, and ophthalmoplegia and retinal degeneration in oxidative phosphorylation defects.

Testing: When an inherited disorder of metabolism is suspected, evaluation begins with a review of neonatal screening test results and ordering of basic metabolic screening tests, which typically include the following:

- Glucose
- Electrolytes
- CBC and peripheral smear
- Liver function tests
- Ammonia levels
- Serum amino acid levels
- Urinalysis
- Urine organic acids

Glucose measurement detects hypoglycemia or hyperglycemia; measurement may have to be timed relative to meals (eg, fasting hypoglycemia in GSD).

Electrolyte measurement detects metabolic acidosis and presence or absence of an anion gap; metabolic acidosis may need to be corroborated by ABG measurement. Non-anion gap acidosis occurs in inherited disorders of metabolism that cause renal tubular damage (eg, galactosemia, tyrosinemia type I). Anion gap acidosis occurs in inherited disorders of metabolism in which accumulation of titratable acids is typical, such as methylmalonic and propionic acidemias; it can also be caused by lactic acidosis (eg, in pyruvate decarboxylase deficiency or mitochondrial oxidative phosphorylation defects). When the anion gap is elevated, lactate and pyruvate levels should be obtained. An increase in the lactate:pyruvate ratio distinguishes oxidative phosphorylation defects from disorders of pyruvate metabolism, in which the lactate:pyruvate ratio remains normal.

CBC and peripheral smear detect hemolysis caused by RBC energy deficits or WBC defects (eg, in some pentose phosphate pathway disorders and GSD type Ib) and cytopenia caused by metabolite accumulation (eg, neutropenia in propionic acidemia due to propionyl CoA accumulation).

Liver function tests detect hepatocellular damage, dysfunction, or both (eg, in untreated galactosemia, hereditary fructose intolerance, or tyrosinemia type I).

Ammonia levels are elevated in urea cycle defects, organic acidemias, and fatty acid oxidation defects.

Urinalysis detects ketonuria (present in some GSDs and many organic acidemias); absence of ketones in the presence of acidosis suggests a fatty acid oxidation defect.

More specific tests may be indicated when ≥ 1 of the previously described simple screening tests support an inherited disorder of metabolism. Carbohydrate metabolites, mucopolysaccharides, and amino and organic acids can be measured directly by chromatography and mass spectrometry. Quantitative plasma amino acid tests should include a plasma acylcarnitine profile. Urine organic acid tests should include a urine acylglycine profile.

Confirmatory tests may also include biopsy (eg, liver biopsy to distinguish hepatic forms of GSDs from other disorders associated with hepatomegaly, muscle biopsy to detect ragged red fibers in mitochondrial myopathy); enzyme studies (eg, using blood and skin cells to diagnose lysosomal storage diseases); and DNA studies, which identify gene mutations that cause disease. DNA testing can be done on almost all cells (except RBCs and platelets), thus avoiding the need for tissue biopsies; however, sensitivity for any given disease is often suboptimal because not all mutations that cause disease have been characterized.

Challenge testing is used judiciously to detect symptoms, signs, or measurable biochemical abnormalities not detectable in the normal state. The need for challenge testing has diminished with the availability of highly sensitive metabolite detection methods, but it is still occasionally used. Examples include fasting tests (eg, to provoke hypoglycemia in hepatic forms of GSD); provocative tests (eg, fructose challenge to trigger symptoms in hereditary fructose intolerance, glucagon challenge in hepatic forms of GSD [failure to observe hyperglycemia suggests disease]); and physiologic challenge (eg, exercise stress testing to elicit lactic acid production and other deformities in muscle forms of GSD). Challenge tests are often associated with an element of risk so they must be done under well-controlled conditions with a clear plan for reversing symptoms and signs.

MITOCHONDRIAL OXIDATIVE PHOSPHORYLATION DISORDERS

Impairment of oxidative phosphorylation often, but not always, causes lactic acidosis, particularly affecting the CNS, retina, and muscle.

Cellular respiration (oxidative phosphorylation) occurs in the mitochondria, where a series of enzymes catalyze the transfer of electrons to molecular oxygen and the generation of energy-storing ATP. Mitochondrial or nuclear genetic defects involving enzymes used in this process impair cellular respiration, decreasing the ATP:ADP ratio. Tissues with a high energy demand (eg, brain, nerves, retina, skeletal and cardiac muscle) are particularly vulnerable. The most common clinical manifestations are seizures, hypotonia, ophthalmoplegia, strokelike episodes, muscle weakness, severe constipation, and cardiomyopathy.

Biochemically, there is profound lactic acidosis because the NADH:NAD ratio increases, shifting the equilibrium of the lactate dehydrogenase reaction toward lactate. The increase in the lactate:pyruvate ratio distinguishes oxidative phosphorylation defects from other genetic causes of lactic acidosis, such as pyruvate carboxylase or pyruvate dehydrogenase deficiency, in which the lactate:pyruvate ratio remains normal. A large number of oxidative phosphorylation defects have been described; only the most common ones are outlined here, along with their distinguishing features.

Mitochondrial mutations and variants have also been implicated in a number of diseases of aging (eg, Parkinson disease, Alzheimer disease, diabetes, deafness, cancer).

The following disorders are conditions with a known phenotype/genotype correlation. Other less well-defined defects in mitochondrial function exist. Additionally, there are a number of conditions in which a genetic defect causes secondary mitochondrial dysfunction.

Leber hereditary optic neuropathy (LHON): This disease is characterized by acute or subacute bilateral central vision loss caused by retinal degeneration. Onset usually occurs in the patient's 20s or 30s but can occur from childhood to adulthood. Male:female ratio is 4:1. Many mutations have been defined, but 3 common ones account for 90% of those in European patients. LHON pedigrees usually show a pattern of maternal inheritance typical of mitochondrial disorders.

Mitochondrial encephalomyopathy, lactic acidosis, and strokelike episodes (MELAS): Mutations in the mitochondrial-$tRNA^{leu}$ gene cause this progressive neurodegenerative disease characterized by repeated episodes of "chemical strokes," myopathy, and lactic acidosis. In many cases, cells contain both wild-type and mutant mitochondrial DNA (heteroplasmy); thus, expression is variable.

Myoclonic epilepsy with ragged-red fibers (MERRF): This progressive disorder is characterized by uncontrolled muscle contractions (myoclonic seizures), dementia, ataxia, and myopathy, which shows ragged-red fibers (indicating mitochondrial proliferation) with specialized stains when biopsied. Mutations are in the mitochondrial $tRNA^{lys}$ gene. Heteroplasmy is common; thus, expression is variable.

Kearns-Sayre syndrome and chronic progressive external ophthalmoplegia (CPEO): These disorders are characterized by ophthalmoplegia, ptosis, atypical retinitis pigmentosa, ragged-red fiber myopathy, ataxia, deafness, and cardiomyopathy typically occurring before age 20 yr. Most mutations involve contiguous deletion/duplication of part of the mitochondrial transfer RNA and other protein-coding genes.

Neurogenic muscle atrophy and retinitis pigmentosa (NARP) and Leigh disease: Pigmentary retinopathy in the presence of neuromuscular degeneration and Leigh disease (subacute necrotizing encephalopathy characterized by ataxias and basal ganglia degeneration) is a genetically heterogeneous syndrome. Mutations can be seen in the *ATP6* gene of the mitochondrial genomes.

PEROXISOMAL DISORDERS

Peroxisomes are intracellular organelles that contain enzymes for β-oxidation. These enzymes overlap in function with those in mitochondria, with the exception that mitochondria lack enzymes to metabolize very long-chain fatty acids (VLCFA), those 20 to 26 carbons in length. Therefore, peroxisomal disorders generally manifest with elevated VLCFA levels (except rhizomelic chondrodysplasia). Although VLCFA levels may help screen for these disorders, other assays are also required (eg, plasma levels of phytanic, pristanic, and pipecolic acids; RBC plasmalogen levels). For information on other disorders affecting fatty acid metabolism, see Overview of Fatty Acid and Glycerol Metabolism Disorders (p. 2667). See also Approach to the Patient With a Suspected Inherited Disorder of Metabolism (p. 2641).

There are 2 types of peroxisomal disorders:

- Those with defective peroxisome formation
- Those with defects in single peroxisomal enzymes

X-linked adrenoleukodystrophy is the most common peroxisomal disorder (incidence 1/17,000 births); all others are autosomal recessive, with a combined incidence of about 1/50,000 births.

For more information, see Table 315–1.

Zellweger syndrome (ZS), neonatal adrenoleukodystrophy, and infantile Refsum disease (IRD): These disorders are 3 expressions of a disease continuum, from most (ZS) to least (IRD) severe. The responsible genetic defect occurs in 1 of at least 11 genes involved in peroxisomal formation or protein import (the *PEX* gene family).

Manifestations include facial dysmorphism, CNS malformations, demyelination, neonatal seizures, hypotonia, hepatomegaly, cystic kidneys, short limbs with stippled epiphyses (chondrodysplasia punctata), cataracts, retinopathy, hearing deficit, psychomotor delay, and peripheral neuropathy.

Diagnosis is by detecting elevated blood levels of VLCFA, phytanic acid, bile acid intermediates, and pipecolic acid.

Experimental treatment with docosahexaenoic acid (DHA—levels of which are reduced in patients with disorders of peroxisome formation) has shown some promise.

Rhizomelic chondrodysplasia punctata: This defect of peroxisomal biogenesis is caused by *PEX7* gene mutations and characterized by skeletal changes that include midface hypoplasia, strikingly short proximal limbs, frontal bossing, small nares, cataracts, ichthyosis, and profound psychomotor retardation. Vertebral clefts are also common.

Diagnosis of rhizomelic chondrodysplasia punctata is by x-ray findings, serum elevation of phytanic acid, and low RBC plasmalogen levels; VLCFA levels are normal.

There is no effective treatment for rhizomelic chondrodysplasia punctata.

X-linked adrenoleukodystrophy: This disorder is caused by deficiency of the peroxisomal membrane transporter ALDP, which is coded for by the gene *ABCD1*.

The cerebral form affects 40% of patients. Onset occurs between age 4 yr and 8 yr, and symptoms of attention deficit

Table 315–1. PEROXISOME BIOGENESIS AND VERY LONG-CHAIN FATTY ACID METABOLISM DISORDERS

DISEASE (OMIM NUMBER)	DEFECTIVE PROTEINS OR ENZYMES	DEFECTIVE GENE OR GENES (CHROMOSOMAL LOCATION)	COMMENTS
Cerebrohepatorenal syndrome (Zellweger syndrome; 214100)	Peroxin-1 Peroxin-2 Peroxin-3 Peroxin-5 Peroxin-6 Peroxin-12 Peroxin-14 Peroxin-26	PEX1 (7q21-q22)* PEX2 (8q21.1)* PEX3 (6q23-q24)* PEX5 (12p13.3)* PEX6 (6p21.1)* PEX12 (17)* PEX14 (1p36.2)* PEX26 (22q11.21)*	**Biochemical profile:** Decreased dihydroxyacetone phosphate acyltransferase and plasmalogen; elevated VLCFA, phytanic acid, pipecolate, iron, and total iron-binding capacity **Clinical features:** Growth failure, large fontanelles, macrocephaly, turribrachycephaly, dysmorphic facies, cataracts, nystagmus, congenital heart disease, hepatomegaly, biliary dysgenesis, hypospadias, renal cysts, hypotonia, brain malformation **Treatment:** No effective treatment Ether lipids, low phytanic acid diet, and docosahexaenoic acid possibly helpful
Neonatal adrenoleukodystrophy (202370)	Peroxin-1 Peroxin-5 Peroxin-10 Peroxin-13 Peroxin-26	PEX1 (7q21-q22)* PEX5 (12p13.3)* PEX10 (1)* PEX13 (2p15)* PEX26 (22q11.21)*	**Biochemical profile:** Elevated VLCFA **Clinical features:** Dolichocephaly, dysmorphic facies, cataracts, hyperpigmentation, seizures, developmental delay, adrenal insufficiency **Treatment:** Similar to that for Zellweger syndrome
Infantile Refsum disease (266510)	Peroxin-1 Peroxin-2 Peroxin-26	PEX1 (7q21-q22)* PEX2 (8q21.1)* PEX26 (22q11.21)*	**Biochemical profile:** Elevated plasma phytanic acid, cholesterol, VLCFA, dihydroxycholestanoic acid, trihydroxycholestanoic acid, and pipecolic acid **Clinical features:** Growth and developmental delay, peripheral neuropathy, hypotonia, deafness, facial dysmorphism, retinopathy, osteoporosis, steatorrhea, episodic bleeding, hepatomegaly **Treatment:** Similar to that for Zellweger syndrome
Rhizomelic chondrodysplasia punctata			**Biochemical profile:** In type 1, plasmalogen deficiency, elevated plasma phytanic acid and unprocessed 3-oxoacyl CoA thiolase, acyl-CoA dihydroxyacetonephosphate acyltransferase deficiency
Type 1 (215100)	Peroxin-7	PEX7 (6q22-q24)*	
Type 2 (222765)	Dihydroxyacetonephosphate acyltransferase	GNPAT (1)*	In type 2, normal plasmalogen, phytanic acid, alkyl dihydroxyacetonephosphate synthase, and peroxisomal thiolase; dihydroacetonephosphate acyltransferase deficiency
Type 3 (600121)	Alkyldihydroxyacetonephosphate synthase	AGPS (2q31)*	In type 3, abnormal peroxisomes, alkyl dihydroxyacetonephosphate synthase deficiency **Clinical features:** Dwarfism with rhizomelic limb shortening, punctuate epiphyseal calcification, and metaphyseal splaying; severe growth and developmental delay; microcephaly; midface hypoplasia; micrognathia; sensorineural deafness; cataracts; cleft palate; ichthyosis; respiratory difficulties; kyphoscoliosis; vertebral clefts; spasticity; cortical atrophy; seizures; death before 2 yr **Treatment:** Similar to that for Zellweger syndrome
Hyperpipecolicacidemia (239400)	Pipecolate oxidase		**Biochemical profile:** Elevated plasma pipecolate, mild generalized aminoaciduria **Clinical features:** Hepatomegaly, demyelination, CNS degeneration, severe intellectual disability and developmental delay, retinopathy **Treatment:** Reduced intake of VLCFA

Table 315–1. PEROXISOME BIOGENESIS AND VERY LONG-CHAIN FATTY ACID METABOLISM DISORDERS (*Continued*)

DISEASE (OMIM NUMBER)	DEFECTIVE PROTEINS OR ENZYMES	DEFECTIVE GENE OR GENES (CHROMOSOMAL LOCATION)	COMMENTS
X-linked adrenoleukodystrophy (300100)	ATP-binding cassette transporter 1	ABCD1 (Xq28)*	**Biochemical profile:** Elevated plasma VLCFA, peroxisomal lignoceroyl-CoA ligase deficiency **Clinical features:** Hyperpigmentation, blindness, cognitive hearing loss, spastic paraplegia, impotence, sphincter disturbance, ataxia, dysarthria, adrenal insufficiency, hypogonadism, pontine and cerebellar atrophy **Treatment:** Adrenal hormone replacement, bone marrow transplantation 4:1 mixture of glyceryl trioleate and glycerol trierucate (Lorenzo's oil) apparently of no clinical benefit
Acyl-CoA oxidase 1 deficiency (pseudoneonatal adrenoleukodystrophy; 264470)	Straight-chain peroxisomal acyl-CoA oxidase	ACOX (17q25)*	**Biochemical profile:** Elevated plasma VLCFA; normal peroxisomal phytanate, pipecolate, dihydroxycholestanoic acid, and trihydroxycholestanoic acid **Clinical features:** Neonatal hypotonia, developmental delay, sensorineural deafness, retinopathy, no dysmorphic features, leukodystrophy at age 2 to 3 yr **Treatment:** Not established
D-Bifunctional protein deficiency (261515)	D-bifunctional enzyme	HSD17B4 (5q2)*	**Biochemical profile:** Elevated serum VLCFA and pipecolate, elevated trihydroxycholestanoic acid in duodenal aspirate, peroxisomal 3-oxoacyl-CoA thiolase defect **Clinical features:** Hypotonia, exaggerated startle reflex, facial diplegia, seizures, high-pitched and weak cry, developmental delay, myopathic facies, high-arched palate, abducted limbs, ventricular heart disease **Treatment:** Not established
2-Methylacyl-CoA racemase deficiency	2-Methylacyl-CoA racemase	AMACR (5p13.2-q11.1)*	**Biochemical profile:** Elevated plasma pristanic acid **Clinical features:** Adult-onset sensorimotor neuropathy, retinopathy **Treatment:** Not established
Primary oxaluria			**Biochemical profile:** Elevated urinary oxalate excretion, glycolic aciduria **Clinical features:** Ca oxalate urolithiasis, nephrocalcinosis, renal failure, heart block, peripheral vascular insufficiency, arterial occlusion, intermittent claudication, optic neuropathy, fractures, death during childhood or early adulthood Type 2 milder than type 1 **Treatment:** Hepatorenal transplantation
Hyperoxaluria type 1 (259900)	Peroxisomal alanine-glyoxylate aminotransferase	AGXT (2q36-q37)*	
Hyperoxaluria type 2 (260000)	D-Glycerate dehydrogenase glyoxylate reductase	GRHPR (9cen)*	
Refsum disease (266500)	Phytanoyl-CoA hydroxylase	PAHX (10pter-p11.2)*	**Biochemical profile:** Elevated plasma and tissue phytanic acid **Clinical features:** Retinitis pigmentosa, ataxia, ptosis, miosis, peripheral neuropathy, anosmia, heart failure, deafness, ichthyosis, short 4th metacarpal **Treatment:** Low phytanic acid diet, plasmapheresis
	Peorxin-7	PEX7 (6q22-q24)*	
Glutaric aciduria type 3 (231690)	Peroxisomal glutaryl CoA oxidase		**Biochemical profile:** Glutaric aciduria exacerbated by lysine loading **Clinical features:** Failure to thrive, postprandial vomiting **Treatment:** Not established

Table continues on the following page.

Table 315–1. PEROXISOME BIOGENESIS AND VERY LONG-CHAIN FATTY ACID METABOLISM DISORDERS (*Continued*)

DISEASE (OMIM NUMBER)	DEFECTIVE PROTEINS OR ENZYMES	DEFECTIVE GENE OR GENES (CHROMOSOMAL LOCATION)	COMMENTS
Mevalonic aciduria	See Table 315–9 on p. 2652	—	—
Acatalasemia (115500)	Catalase	CAT (11p13)*	**Biochemical profile:** Failure of tissue to cause hydrogen peroxide frothing **Clinical features:** Ulcerating oral lesions in Japanese patients but not in Swiss patients **Treatment:** Symptomatic

*Gene has been identified, and molecular basis has been elucidated.
OMIM = online mendelian inheritance in man (see the OMIM database at www.ncbi.nlm.nih.gov/omim).

progress over time to severe behavioral problems, dementia, and vision, hearing, and motor deficits, causing total disability and death 2 to 3 yr after diagnosis. Milder adolescent and adult forms have also been described.

About 45% of patients have a milder form called adrenomyeloneuropathy (AMN); onset occurs in the 20s or 30s, with progressive paraparesis, and sphincter and sexual disturbance. About one third of these patients also develop cerebral symptoms.

Patients with any form may also develop adrenal insufficiency; about 15% have isolated Addison disease without neurologic involvement.

Diagnosis of X-linked adrenoleukodystrophy is confirmed by isolated elevation of VLCFA.

Bone marrow or stem cell transplantation may help stabilize symptoms in some cases. Adrenal steroid replacement is needed for patients with adrenal insufficiency. Dietary supplement with a 4:1 mixture of glyceryl trioleate and glyceryl trierucate (Lorenzo's oil) can normalize plasma VLCFA levels and may be beneficial in some cases but is under study.

Classic Refsum disease: Genetic deficiency of a single peroxisomal enzyme, phytanoyl-CoA hydroxylase, which catalyzes metabolism of phytanic acid (a common dietary plant component), causes phytanic acid accumulation.

Clinical manifestations include progressive peripheral neuropathy, impaired vision caused by retinitis pigmentosa, hearing deficit, anosmia, cardiomyopathy and conduction defects, and ichthyosis. Onset is usually in the 20s.

Diagnosis of Refsum disease is confirmed by elevation of serum phytanic acid and decreased levels of pristanic acid (phytanic acid elevation is accompanied by pristanic acid elevation in several other peroxisomal disorders).

Treatment of Refsum disease is dietary restriction of phytanic acid (< 10 mg/day), which can be effective in preventing or delaying symptoms when started before symptom onset.

OVERVIEW OF AMINO ACID AND ORGANIC ACID METABOLISM DISORDERS

Defects of amino acid transport in the renal tubule include cystinuria and Hartnup disease, which are discussed in Ch. 302. Amino acid and organic acid metabolism disorders include

- Branched-chain amino acid disorders
- Methionine metabolism disorders
- Phenylketonuria
- Tyrosine metabolism disorders
- Urea cycle disorders (UCD)

In addition, there are a number of other disorders of amino acid and organic acid metabolism, including those involving beta- and gamma-amino acids, the gamma-glutamyl cycle, glycine, histidine, lysine, proline and hydroxyproline, and miscellaneous other amino acid disorders (see Tables 315–2 through 315-8).

BRANCHED-CHAIN AMINO ACID METABOLISM DISORDERS

Valine, leucine, and isoleucine are branched-chain amino acids; deficiency of enzymes involved in their metabolism leads to accumulation of organic acids with severe metabolic acidosis.

There are numerous disorders of branched-chain amino acid metabolism (see Table 315–9 on p. 2652) as well as many other amino acid and organic acid metabolism disorders.

Maple syrup urine disease: This is a group of autosomal recessive disorders caused by deficiency of one or more subunits of a dehydrogenase active in the 2nd step of branched-chain amino acid catabolism. Although quite rare, incidence is significant (perhaps 1/200 births) in Amish and Mennonite populations.

Clinical manifestations include body fluid odor that smells like maple syrup (particularly strong in cerumen) and overwhelming illness in the first days of life, beginning with vomiting and lethargy, and progressing to seizures, coma, and death if untreated. Patients with milder forms of the disease may manifest symptoms only during stress (eg, infection, surgery).

Biochemical findings are profound ketonemia and acidemia. Diagnosis of maple syrup urine disease is by finding elevated plasma levels of branched-chain amino acids (particularly leucine). (Also see testing for suspected inherited disorders of metabolism—p. 2642.)

Acutely, treatment of maple syrup urine disease with peritoneal dialysis or hemodialysis may be required, along with IV hydration and nutrition (including protein restriction and high-dose dextrose). Patients should be closely monitored for cerebral edema and acute pancreatitis. Long-term management is restriction of dietary branched-chain amino acids; however, small amounts are required for normal metabolic function. Thiamin is a cofactor for the decarboxylation, and some patients respond favorably to high-dose thiamin (up to 200 mg po once/day). An emergency plan for how to manage

Table 315–2. BETA-AMINO ACID AND GAMMA-AMINO ACID DISORDERS

DISEASE (OMIM NUMBER)	DEFECTIVE PROTEINS OR ENZYMES	DEFECTIVE GENE OR GENES (CHROMOSOMAL LOCATION)	COMMENTS
Hyper-β-alaninemia (237400)	β-Alanine-α-ketoglutarate aminotransferase	Not determined	**Biochemical profile:** Elevated urinary β-alanine, taurine, γ-aminobutyrate (GABA), and β-aminoisobutyrate **Clinical features:** Seizures, somnolence, death **Treatment:** Pyridoxine
Methylmalonate/malonate semialdehyde dehydrogenase deficiency with 3-amino and 3-hydroxy aciduria (236795)	Methylmalonate/ malonate semialdehyde dehydrogenase	ALDH6A1 (14q24.3)*	**Biochemical profile:** Elevated 3-hydroxyisobutyrate 3-aminoisobutyrate, 3-hydroxypropionate β-alanine, and 2-ethyl-3-hydroxypropionate **Clinical features:** None to mild **Treatment:** Not determined
Methylmalonic semialdehyde dehydrogenase deficiency with mild methylmalonic acidemia	Methylmalonic semialdehyde dehydrogenase (see also Branched-chain amino acid metabolism, above)	ALDH6A1 (14q24.1)	**Biochemical profile:** Moderately elevated urine methylmalonate **Clinical features:** Developmental delay, seizures **Treatment:** No effective treatment
Hyper-β-aminoisobutyric aciduria (210100)	D(R)-3-Aminoisobutyrate: pyruvate aminotransferase	Not determined	**Biochemical profile:** Elevated β-aminoisobutyric acid **Clinical features:** Benign **Treatment:** None needed
Pyridoxine dependency with seizures (266100)	Not determined	Specific gene not determined (5q31.2-q31.3)	**Biochemical profile:** Elevated CSF glutamate **Clinical features:** Seizure disorder refractory to conventional anticonvulsants, high-pitched cry, hypothermia, jitteriness, dystonia, hepatomegaly, hypotonia, dyspraxia, developmental delay **Treatment:** Pyridoxine
GABA-transaminase deficiency (137150)	4-Aminobutyrate-α-ketoglutarate aminotransferase	ABAT (16p13.3)*	**Biochemical profile:** Elevated plasma and CSF GABA and β-alanine, elevated carnosine **Clinical features:** Accelerated linear growth, seizures, cerebellar hypoplasia, psychomotor delay, leukodystrophy, burst suppression EEG pattern **Treatment:** No known treatment
4-Hydroxybutyric aciduria (271980)	Succinic semialdehyde dehydrogenase	ALDH5A1 (6p22)*	**Biochemical profile:** Elevated urinary 4-hydroxybutyrate and glycine **Clinical features:** Psychomotor retardation, specch delay, hypotonia **Treatment:** Vigabatrin
Carnosinemia, homocarnosinosis, or both (236130, 212200)	Carnosinase	Specific gene not determined (18q21.3)	**Biochemical profile:** In carnosinemia phenotype, carnosinuria despite meat-free diet, elevated urine anserine after ingestion of food containing imidazole dipeptides, normal CSF In homocarnosinosis phenotype, elevated CSF homocarnosine, normal serum carnosine **Clinical features:** Usually benign; reported symptoms probably due to ascertainment bias **Treatment:** None needed

*Gene has been identified, and molecular basis has been elucidated.
OMIM = online mendelian inheritance in man (see the OMIM database).

Table 315–3. GAMMA-GLUTAMYL CYCLE DISORDERS

DISEASE (OMIM NUMBER)	DEFECTIVE PROTEINS OR ENZYMES	DEFECTIVE GENE OR GENES (CHROMOSOMAL LOCATION)	COMMENTS
γ-Glutamylcysteine synthetase deficiency (230450)	γ-Glutamylcysteine synthetase	GGLC (6p12)*	**Biochemical profile:** Aminoaciduria, glutathione deficiency **Clinical features:** Hemolysis, spinocerebellar degeneration, peripheral neuropathy, myopathy **Treatment:** No clear treatment; avoidance of drugs that trigger hemolytic crisis in G6PD deficiency
Pyroglutamic aciduria (5-oxoprolinuria; 266130, 231900)	Glutathione synthetase	GSS (20q11.2)*	**Biochemical profile:** Elevated urinary, plasma, and CSF 5-oxoproline; increased γ-glutamylcysteine; decreased glutathione level **Clinical features:** Hemolysis, ataxia, seizures, intellectual disability, spasticity, metabolic acidosis In mild form, no evidence of neurologic damage **Treatment:** Na bicarbonate or citrate, vitamins E and C, avoidance of drugs that trigger hemolytic crisis in G6PD deficiency
γ-Glutamyltranspeptidase deficiency (glutathionuria; 231950)	γ-Glutamyltranspeptidase	Specific gene not determined (22q11.1-q11.2)	**Biochemical profile:** Elevated plasma and urinary glutathione **Clinical features:** Intellectual disability **Treatment:** No specific treatment
5-Oxoprolinase deficiency (260005)	5-Oxoprolinase	Not determined	**Biochemical profile:** Elevated urinary 5-oxoproline **Clinical features:** Probably benign **Treatment:** None needed

*Gene has been identified, and molecular basis has been elucidated.
OMIM = online mendelian inheritance in man (see the OMIM database at www.ncbi.nlm.nih.gov/omim).

acute illness, which may provoke a metabolic crisis, should be in place. Liver transplantation is curative.

Isovaleric acidemia: The 3rd step of leucine metabolism is the conversion of isovaleryl CoA to 3-methylcrotonyl CoA, a dehydrogenation step. Deficiency of this dehydrogenase results in isovaleric acidemia, also known as "sweaty feet" syndrome, because accumulated isovaleric acid emits an odor that smells like sweat.

Clinical manifestations of the acute form occur in the first few days of life with poor feeding, vomiting, and respiratory distress as infants develop profound anion gap metabolic acidosis, hypoglycemia, and hyperammonemia. Bone marrow suppression often occurs. A chronic intermittent form may not manifest for several months or years.

Diagnosis of isovaleric acidemia is made by detecting elevated levels of isovaleric acid and its metabolites in blood or

Table 315–4. GLYCINE METABOLISM DISORDERS

DISEASE (OMIM NUMBER)	DEFECTIVE PROTEINS OR ENZYMES	DEFECTIVE GENE OR GENES (CHROMOSOMAL LOCATION)	COMMENTS
Nonketotic hyperglycinemia (605899)	Glycine cleavage enzyme system P protein H protein T protein L protein	 GLDC (9p22)* GCSH (16q23)* ATM (3p21)* Not determined	**Biochemical profile:** Elevated plasma and CSF glycine **Clinical features:** In neonatal form, hypotonia, seizures, myoclonus, apnea, death In infantile and episodic forms, seizures, intellectual disability, episodic delirium, chorea, vertical gaze palsy In late-onset form, progressive spastic diplegia, optic atrophy, but no cognitive impairment or seizures **Treatment:** No effective treatment; in some patients, temporary benefit from Na benzoate and dextromethorphan

*Gene has been identified, and molecular basis has been elucidated.
OMIM = online mendelian inheritance in man (see the OMIM database at www.ncbi.nlm.nih.gov/omim).

Table 315–5. HISTIDINE METABOLISM DISORDERS

DISEASE (OMIM NUMBER)	DEFECTIVE PROTEINS OR ENZYMES	DEFECTIVE GENE OR GENES (CHROMOSOMAL LOCATION)	COMMENTS
Histidinemia (235800)	Classic: l-Histidine ammonia-lyase (liver and skin) Variant: l-Histidine ammonia-lyase (liver only)	HAL (12q22-q23)*	**Biochemical profile:** Elevated plasma histidine **Clinical features:** Frequently benign; neurologic manifestations in some patients **Treatment:** Low-protein diet For symptomatic patients only, controlled histidine intake
Urocanic aciduria (276880)	Urocanase	Not determined	**Biochemical profile:** Elevated urine urocanic acid **Clinical features:** Probably benign **Treatment:** None needed

*Gene has been identified, and molecular basis has been elucidated.
OMIM = online mendelian inheritance in man (see the OMIM database at www.ncbi.nlm.nih.gov/omim).

urine. (Also see testing for suspected inherited disorders of metabolism—p. 2641.)

Acute treatment of isovaleric acidemia is with IV hydration and nutrition (including high-dose dextrose) and measures to increase renal isovaleric acid excretion by conjugation with glycine. If these measures are insufficient, exchange transfusion and peritoneal dialysis may be needed. Long-term treatment is with dietary leucine restriction and continuation of glycine and carnitine supplements. Prognosis is excellent with treatment.

Propionic acidemia: Deficiency of propionyl CoA carboxylase, the enzyme responsible for metabolizing propionic acid to methylmalonate, causes propionic acid accumulation.

Illness begins in the first days or weeks of life with poor feeding, vomiting, and respiratory distress due to profound anion gap metabolic acidosis, hypoglycemia, and hyperammonemia. Seizures may occur, and bone marrow suppression is common. Physiologic stresses may trigger recurrent attacks. Survivors may have tubular nephropathies, intellectual disability, and

Table 315–6. LYSINE METABOLISM DISORDERS

DISEASE (OMIM NUMBER)	DEFECTIVE PROTEINS OR ENZYMES	DEFECTIVE GENE OR GENES (CHROMOSOMAL LOCATION)	COMMENTS
Hyperlysinemia (238700)	Lysine:α-ketoglutarate reductase	AASS (7q31.3)*	**Biochemical profile:** Hyperlysinemia **Clinical features:** Muscle weakness, seizures, mild anemia, intellectual disability, joint and muscular laxity, ectopia lentis; sometimes benign **Treatment:** Limited lysine intake
2-Ketoadipic acidemia (245130)	2-Ketoadipic dehydrogenase	Not determined	**Biochemical profile:** Elevated urine 2-ketoadipate, 2-aminoadipate, and 2-hydroxyadipate **Clinical features:** Benign **Treatment:** None needed
Glutaric acidemia type I (231670)	Glutaryl CoA dehydrogenase	(19q13.2)*	**Biochemical profile:** Elevated urinary glutaric acid and 2-hydroxyglytaric acid **Clinical features:** Dystonia, dyskinesia, degeneration of the caudate and putamen, frontotemporal atrophy, arachnoid cysts **Treatment:** Aggressive treatment of intercurrent illness, carnitine, Protein, lysine, and tryptophan restriction possibly helpful
Saccharopinuria (268700)	α-Aminoadipic semialdehyde-glutamate reductase	AASS (7q31.3)*	**Biochemical profile:** Elevated urine lysine, citrulline, histidine, and saccharopine **Clinical features:** Intellectual disability, spastic diplegia, short stature, EEG abnormality **Treatment:** No clear treatment

*Gene has been identified, and molecular basis has been elucidated.
OMIM = online mendelian inheritance in man (see the OMIM database at www.ncbi.nlm.nih.gov/omim).

Table 315–7. PROLINE AND HYDROXYPROLINE METABOLISM DISORDERS

DISEASE (OMIM NUMBER)	DEFECTIVE PROTEINS OR ENZYMES	DEFECTIVE GENE OR GENES (CHROMOSOMAL LOCATION)	COMMENTS
Hyperprolinemia, type I (239500)	Proline oxidase (proline dehydrogenase)	PRODH (22q11.2)*	**Biochemical profile:** Elevated plasma proline and urinary proline, hydroxyproline, and glycine **Clinical features:** Usually benign; hereditary nephritis, nerve deafness **Treatment:** None needed
Hyperprolinemia, type II (239510)	Δ1-Pyrroline-5-carboxylate dehydrogenase	P5CDH (1p36)*	**Biochemical profile:** Elevated plasma proline and pyrroline-5-carboxylate (P5C); elevated urinary P5C, Δ1-pyrroline-5-carboxylate, proline, hydroxyproline, and glycine **Clinical features:** During childhood, seizures, intellectual disability During adulthood, benign **Treatment:** None needed
Δ1-Pyrroline-5-carboxylate synthetase deficiency (138250)	Δ1-Pyrroline-5-carboxylate synthetase	PYCS (10q24.3)*	**Biochemical profile:** Low plasma proline, citrulline, arginine, and ornithine **Clinical features:** Hyperammonemia, cataracts, intellectual disability, joint laxity **Treatment:** Avoidance of fasting
Hyperhydroxyprolinemia (237000)	4-Hydroxyproline oxidase	Not determined	**Biochemical profile:** Hydroxyprolinemia **Clinical features:** Disease association not proven **Treatment:** None needed
Prolidase deficiency (170100)	Prolidase	PEPD (19q12-q13.11)*	**Biochemical profile:** Amino acid profile normal in unhydrolyzed urine, but excessive proline and hydroxyproline in acid-hydrolyzed urine **Clinical features:** Skin ulcers, frequent infections, dysmorphic features, immunodeficiency, intellectual disability **Treatment:** Proline supplement, Mn++ and ascorbic acid, essential amino acids, blood transfusion (packed RBC), topical proline and glycine ointment

*Gene has been identified, and molecular basis has been elucidated.
OMIM = online mendelian inheritance in man (see the OMIM database at www.ncbi.nlm.nih.gov/omim).

neurologic abnormalities. Propionic acidemia can also be seen as part of multiple carboxylase deficiency, biotin deficiency, or biotinidase deficiency.

Diagnosis of propionic acidemia is suggested by elevated levels of propionic acid metabolites, including methylcitrate and tiglate and their glycine conjugates in blood and urine, and confirmed by measuring propionyl CoA carboxylase activity in WBCs or cultured fibroblasts. (Also see testing for suspected inherited disorders of metabolism—p. 2641.)

Acute treatment of propionic acidemia is with IV hydration (including high-dose dextrose), nutrition, and protein restriction; carnitine may be helpful. If these measures are insufficient, peritoneal dialysis or hemodialysis may be needed. Long-term propionic acidemia treatment is dietary restriction of precursor amino acids and odd-chain fatty acids and possibly continuation of carnitine supplementation. A few patients respond to high-dose biotin because it is a cofactor for propionyl CoA and other carboxylases. Intermittent courses of antibiotics should be considered for reducing a proprionic acid load resulting from intestinal bacteria. An emergency plan for how to manage acute illness, which may provoke a metabolic crisis, should be in place.

Methylmalonic acidemia: This disorder is caused by deficiency of methylmalonyl CoA mutase, which converts methylmalonyl CoA (a product of the propionyl CoA carboxylation) into succinyl CoA. Adenosylcobalamin, a metabolite of vitamin B_{12}, is a cofactor; its deficiency also may cause methylmalonic acidemia (and also homocystinuria and megaloblastic anemia). Methylmalonic acid accumulates. Age of onset, clinical manifestations, and treatment are similar to those of propionic acidemia except that cobalamin, instead of biotin, may be helpful for some patients.

METHIONINE METABOLISM DISORDERS

A number of defects in methionine metabolism lead to accumulation of homocysteine (and its dimer, homocystine) with adverse effects including thrombotic tendency, lens dislocation, and CNS and skeletal abnormalities.

There are numerous disorders of methionine and sulfur metabolism (see Table 315–10 on p. 2657) as well as many other amino acid and organic acid metabolism disorders.

Table 315–8. MISCELLANEOUS AMINO ACID AND ORGANIC ACID METABOLISM DISORDERS

DISEASE (OMIM NUMBER)	DEFECTIVE PROTEINS OR ENZYMES	DEFECTIVE GENE OR GENES (CHROMOSOMAL LOCATION)	COMMENTS
Sarcosinemia (268900)	Sarcosine dehydrogenase	Specific gene not determined (9q34)	**Biochemical profile:** Elevated plasma sarcosine **Clinical features:** Benign; intellectual disability reported **Treatment:** None needed
D-glyceric aciduria (220120)	D-glycerate kinase	Not determined	**Biochemical profile:** Elevated urinary D-glyceric acid **Clinical features:** Chronic acidosis, hypotonia, seizures, intellectual disability **Treatment:** Bicarbonate or citrate for acidosis
Hartnup disease (234500)	System B(0) neutral amino acid transporter	SLC6A19 (5p15)*	**Biochemical profile:** Neutral aminoaciduria **Clinical features:** Atrophic glossitis, photodermatitis, intermittent ataxia, hypertonia, seizures, psychosis **Treatment:** Nicotinamide
Cystinuria	Renal dibasic amino acid transporter	—	**Biochemical profile:** Elevated urinary cystine, lysine, arginine, and ornithine **Clinical features:** Nephrolithiasis, increased risk of impaired cerebral function **Treatment:** Maintenance of fluid intake, bicarbonate or citrate, penicillamine or mercaptopropionylglycine
Type I (220100)	Heavy subunit	SLC3A1 (2p16.3)*	
Types II and III (600918)	Light subunit	SLC7A9 (19q13.1)*	
Iminoglycinuria (242600)	Renal transporter of proline, hydroxyproline, and glycine	Not determined	**Biochemical profile:** Elevated urinary proline, hydroxyproline, and glycine but normal plasma levels **Clinical features:** Probably benign **Treatment:** None needed
Guanidinoacetate methyltransferase deficiency (601240)	Guanidinoacetate methyltransferase	GAMT (19p13.3)*	**Biochemical profile:** Elevated guanidinoacetate, decreased creatine and phosphocreatine **Clinical features:** Developmental delay, hypotonia, extrapyramidal movements, seizures, autistic behavior **Treatment:** Creatine supplementation
Cystinosis	See Table 315–23 on p. 2683		

*Gene has been identified, and molecular basis has been elucidated.
OMIM = online mendelian inheritance in man (see the OMIM database at http://www.ncbi.nlm.nih.gov/omim).

Homocysteine is an intermediate in methionine metabolism; it is either remethylated to regenerate methionine or combined with serine in a series of transsulfuration reactions to form cystathionine and then cysteine. Cysteine is then metabolized to sulfite, taurine, and glutathione. Various defects in remethylation or transsulfuration can cause homocysteine to accumulate, resulting in disease.

The first step in methionine metabolism is its conversion to adenosylmethionine; this conversion requires the enzyme methionine adenosyltransferase. Deficiency of this enzyme results in methionine elevation, which is not clinically significant except that it causes false-positive neonatal screening results for homocystinuria.

Classic homocystinuria: This disorder is caused by an autosomal recessive deficiency of cystathionine β-synthase, which catalyzes cystathionine formation from homocysteine and serine. Homocysteine accumulates and dimerizes to form the disulfide homocystine, which is excreted in the urine. Because remethylation is intact, some of the additional homocysteine is converted to methionine, which accumulates in the blood. Excess homocysteine predisposes to thrombosis and has adverse effects on connective tissue (perhaps involving fibrillin), particularly the eyes and skeleton; adverse neurologic effects may be due to thrombosis or a direct effect.

Arterial and venous thromboembolic phenomena can occur at any age. Many patients develop ectopia lentis (lens subluxation), intellectual disability, and osteoporosis. Patients can have a marfanoid habitus even though they are not usually tall.

Diagnosis of classic homocystinuria is by neonatal screening for elevated serum methionine; elevated total plasma homocysteine levels are confirmatory. Enzymatic assay in skin fibroblasts can also be done.

Table 315–9. BRANCHED-CHAIN AMINO ACID* METABOLISM DISORDERS

DISEASE (OMIM NUMBER)	DEFECTIVE PROTEINS OR ENZYMES	DEFECTIVE GENE OR GENES (CHROMOSOMAL LOCATION)	COMMENTS
Maple syrup urine disease, or branched-chain ketoaciduria (248600)	Branched-chain α-ketoacid dehydrogenase complex (BCKD)		**Biochemical profile:** Elevated plasma valine, leucine, isoleucine, and alloisoleucine **Clinical features** (molecular forms do not correlate with clinical forms except that a high percentage of type II mutations are associated with thiamin responsiveness): In classic form, hypertonia, seizures, coma, death In intermediate form, intellectual disability, neurologic symptoms, full-blown picture developing with stress In intermittent form, symptoms only with stress (eg, fever, infection) In thiamin-responsive form, features similar to mild intermediate form In E3 subunit deficient form, features similar to intermediate form but accompanied by severe lactic acidosis because E3 is needed for pyruvate dehydrogenase and α-ketoglutarate dehydrogenase **Acute treatment:** Peritoneal dialysis, hemodialysis, or both; aggressive nutrition management, including protein restriction, high-dose glucose, insulin, and special hyperalimentation; close monitoring for cerebral edema and acute pancreatitis **Chronic treatment:** Dietary branched-chain amino acid restriction, thiamin supplementation as needed Emergency plan for acute illness, which may provoke a metabolic crisis Liver transplantation
Type IA	BCKD E1α component	BCKDHA (19q13)†	
Type IB	BCKD E1β component	BCKDHB (6p22-p21)†	
Type II	BCKD E2 component	DBT (1p31)†	
Type III	BCKD E3 component	DLD (7q31-q32)†	
Propionic acidemia (606054)	Propionyl-CoA carboxylase		**Biochemical profile:** Elevated plasma glycine, urine methylcitrate, 3-hydroxypropionate, propionylglycine, and tiglylglycine **Clinical features:** Hypotonia, vomiting, lethargy, coma, ketoacidosis, hypoglycemia, hyperammonemia, bone marrow suppression, growth delay, intellectual disability, physical disability **Treatment:** During acute episodes, high-dose glucose and aggressive fluid resuscitation, protein restriction For extreme hyperammonemia, may need hemodialysis or peritoneal dialysis. For long-term management, controlled intake of threonine, valine, isoleucine, and methionine; carnitine supplementation; biotin for responsive patients (see also Multiple carboxylase deficiency and Biotinidase deficiency, below) Intermittent courses of antibiotics considered for reduction of propionic acid load from intestinal bacteria Emergency plan for acute illness, which may provoke a metabolic crisis
Type I	α-Subunit	PCCA (13q32)†	

Table 315–9. BRANCHED-CHAIN AMINO ACID* METABOLISM DISORDERS (*Continued*)

DISEASE (OMIM NUMBER)	DEFECTIVE PROTEINS OR ENZYMES	DEFECTIVE GENE OR GENES (CHROMOSOMAL LOCATION)	COMMENTS
Type II	β-Subunit	PCCB (3q21-q22)†	
Multiple carboxylase deficiency (253270)	Holocarboxylase synthetase	HLCS (21q22.1)†	**Biochemical profile:** Same as for propionic acidemia but also elevated lactate and 3-methylcrotonate **Clinical features:** Skin rash, alopecia, seizures, hypotonia, developmental delay, ketoacidosis, defective T- and B-cell immunity, hearing loss **Treatment:** Biotin, carnitine
Biotinidase deficiency (253260)	Biotinidase	BTD (3p25)†	Similar to multiple carboxylase deficiency
Methylmalonic acidemia (mut defects; 251000)	Methylmalonyl-CoA mutase Mut0 (no enzyme activity) Mut- (some residual enzyme activity)	MUT (6p21)†	**Biochemical profile:** Elevated plasma glycine; increased urine methylmalonate, 3-hydroxypropionate, methylcitrate, and tiglylglycine **Clinical features:** Hypotonia, vomiting, lethargy, coma, ketoacidosis, hypoglycemia, hyperammonemia, bone marrow suppression, growth delay, intellectual disability, and physical disability **Treatment:** During acute episodes, high-dose glucose, aggressive fluid resuscitation, and protein restriction Close monitoring for stroke, renal failure, and acute pancreatitis For extreme hyperammonemia, may need hemodialysis or peritoneal dialysis For long-term management, controlled intake of threonine, valine, isoleucine, and methionine; carnitine supplementation; vitamin B_{12} for patients with mut- type Intermittent courses of antibiotics considered for reduction of propionic acid load from intestinal bacteria Emergency plan for acute illness, which may provoke a metabolic crisis
Methylmalonic acidemia (cblA; 251100)	Mitochondrial cobalamin translocase	MMAA (4q31.1-q31.2)†	**Biochemical profile:** Similar to methylmalonic acidemia due to mutase deficiency **Clinical features:** Similar to methylmalonic acidemia due to mutase deficiency **Treatment:** Responsive to high-dose hydroxycobalamin
Methylmalonic acidemia (cblB; 251110)	ATP:cob(1)alamin adenosyl transferase	MMMB (12q24)†	**Biochemical profile:** Similar to methylmalonic acidemia due to mutase deficiency **Clinical features:** Similar to methylmalonic acidemia due to mutase deficiency **Treatment:** Responsive to high-dose hydroxycobalamin
Methylmalonic acidemia-homocystinuria-megaloblastic anemia (cblC; 277400)	Methylmalonyl-CoA mutase and methylene tetrahydrofolate:-homocysteine methyltransferase	Genetically heterogeneous	**Biochemical profile:** Similar to methylmalonic acidemia cblA and cblB but also homocystinemia, homocystinuria, low methionine, and high cystathionine; normal serum cobalamin **Clinical features:** Similar to cblA and cblB but also megaloblastic anemia **Treatment:** Protein restriction, high-dose hydroxycobalamin
Methylmalonic acidemia-homocystinuria-megaloblastic anemia (cblD; 277410)	Not determined	Genetically heterogeneous	Similar to methylmalonic acidemia cblC

Table continues on the following page.

Table 315–9. BRANCHED-CHAIN AMINO ACID* METABOLISM DISORDERS (*Continued*)

DISEASE (OMIM NUMBER)	DEFECTIVE PROTEINS OR ENZYMES	DEFECTIVE GENE OR GENES (CHROMOSOMAL LOCATION)	COMMENTS
Methylmalonic acidemia-homocystinuria-megaloblastic anemia (cblF; 277380)	Defective lysosomal release of cobalamin	Genetically heterogeneous	Similar to methylmalonic acidemia cblC
Methylmalonic acidemia-homocystinuria-megaloblastic anemia (intrinsic factor deficiency; 261000)	Intrinsic factor	GIF (11q13)†	Similar to methylmalonic acidemia cblC
Methylmalonic acidemia-homocystinuria-megaloblastic anemia (Imerslund-Graesbeck syndrome; 261100)	Cubilin (intrinsic factor receptor)	CUBN (10p12.1)†	Similar to methylmalonic acidemia cblC
Methylmalonic acidemia-homocystinuria-megaloblastic anemia (transcobalamin II deficiency; 275350)	Transcobalamin II	TC2 (22q11.2)†	Similar to methylmalonic acidemia cblC
Methylmalonic semialdehyde dehydrogenase deficiency with mild methylmalonic acidemia (603178)	Methylmalonic semialdehyde dehydrogenase (see also disorders of β- and γ-amino acids, below)	ALDH6A1 (14q24.1)	**Biochemical profile:** Moderate urine methylmalonate **Clinical features:** Developmental delay, seizures **Treatment:** No effective treatment
Methylmalonic acidemia-homocystinuria (cblH; 606169)	Not determined	Genetically heterogeneous	Similar to methylmalonic acidemia cblA
Isovaleric acidemia (243500)	Isovaleryl-CoA dehydrogenase	IVD(15q14-q15)†	**Biochemical profile:** Isovaleryl glycine, 3-hydroxyisovalerate **Clinical features:** Characteristic sweaty feet odor, vomiting, lethargy, acidosis, intellectual disability, bone marrow suppression, hypoglycemia; ketoacidosis, hyperammonemia, neonatal death **Treatment:** Controlled leucine intake, glycine, carnitine
3-Methylcrotonyl-CoA carboxylase deficiency	3-Methylcrotonyl CoA carboxylase		**Biochemical profile:** Elevated 3-hydroxyisovalerate, 3-methylcrontylglycine, and 3-hydroxyisovalerylcarnitine **Clinical features:** Episodic vomiting, acidosis, hypoglycemia, hypotonia, intellectual disability, coma; sometimes asymptomatic intellectual disability **Treatment:** Controlled leucine intake (see also Multiple carboxylase deficiency and Biotinidase deficiency, above)
Type I (210200)	α-Subunit	MCCC1 (3q25-q27)†	
Type II (210210)	β-Subunit	MCCC2 (5q12-q13)†	
3-Methylglutaconic aciduria type I (250950)	3-Methylglutaconyl-CoA hydratase	AUH (9)†	**Biochemical profile:** Elevated urine 3-methylglutaconate and 3-hydroxyisolvalerate **Clinical features:** Acidosis, hypotonia, hepatomegaly, speech delay **Treatment:** Carnitine; benefit of leucine restriction unclear

Table 315–9. BRANCHED-CHAIN AMINO ACID* METABOLISM DISORDERS (*Continued*)

DISEASE (OMIM NUMBER)	DEFECTIVE PROTEINS OR ENZYMES	DEFECTIVE GENE OR GENES (CHROMOSOMAL LOCATION)	COMMENTS
3-Methylglutaconic aciduria type II (Barth syndrome; 302060)	Tafazzin	TAZ (Xq28)†	**Biochemical profile:** Elevated urine 3-methylglutaconate and 3-methylglutarate **Clinical features:** Myopathy, dilated cardiomyopathy, mitochondrial abnormality, neutropenia, developmental delay **Treatment:** Pantothenic acid
3-Methylglutaconic aciduria type III (Costeff optic atrophy; 258501)	Not determined	OPA3 (19q13)†	**Biochemical profile:** Elevated urine 3-methylglutaconate and 3-methylglutarate **Clinical features:** Optic atrophy, ataxia, spasticity, choreiform movement **Treatment:** No effective treatment
3-Methylglutaconic aciduria type IV (250951)	Not determined	Not determined	**Biochemical profile:** Elevated urine 3-methylglutaconate and 3-methylglutarate **Clinical features:** Variable expression, growth and developmental delay, hypotonia, seizures, optic atrophy, deafness, cardiomyopathy, acidosis **Treatment:** No effective treatment
3-Hydroxy-3-methylglutaryl-CoA lyase deficiency (246450)	3-Hydroxy-3-methylglutaryl-CoA lyase	HMGCL (1pter-p33)†	**Biochemical profile:** Elevated urine 3-hydroxy-3-methylglutarate, 3-methylglutaconate, and 3-hydroxyisovalerate; elevated plasma 3-methylglutarylcarnitine **Clinical features:** Reye-like syndrome, vomiting, hypotonia, acidosis, hypoglycemia, lethargy, hyperammonemia without ketosis **Treatment:** Restricted leucine intake, control of hypoglycemia
Mevalonic aciduria (251170, 260920)	Mevalonate kinase	MVK (12q24)†	**Biochemical profile:** Elevated creatine kinase, transaminase, leukotriene, and urinary mevalonic acid; decreased cholesterol **Clinical features:** In classic form, short stature, hypotonia, developmental delay, dysmorphic features, cataracts, vomiting, diarrhea, hepatosplenomegaly, arthralgia, lymphadenopathy, cerebral and cerebellar atrophy, anemia, thrombocytopenia, early death In hyper IgD form, recurrent febrile episodes, vomiting, diarrhea, arthralgia, abdominal pain, rash, splenomegaly, elevated serum IgD and IgA levels **Treatment:** No effective treatment; corticosteroids during acute attacks possibly helpful
Mitochondrial acetoacetyl-CoA thiolase deficiency (607809)	Acetyl-CoA thiolase	ACAT1 (11q22.3-a23.1)†	**Biochemical profile:** Elevated urine 2-methyl-3-hydroxybutyrate and 2-methylacetoacetate, elevated plasma tiglylglycine **Clinical features:** Episodes of ketoacidosis, vomiting, diarrhea, coma, intellectual disability **Treatment:** Low-protein diet, controlled isoleucine intake
Isobutyryl-CoA dehydrogenase deficiency	Isobutyryl-CoA dehydrogenase	Not determined	**Biochemical profile:** Elevated C-4 carnitine, low free carnitine **Clinical features:** Anemia, cardiomyopathy **Treatment:** Carnitine
3-Hydroxyisobutyryl-CoA deacylase deficiency (methacrylic aciduria; 250620)	3-Hydroxyisobutyryl-CoA deacylase	Not determined	**Biochemical profile:** Elevated *S*-(2-carboxypropyl)-cysteine and *S*-(2-carboxypropyl)-cysteamine **Clinical features:** Growth and developmental delay, dysmorphic feature, vertebral anomaly, CNS malformations, death **Treatment:** No effective treatment

Table continues on the following page.

Table 315–9. BRANCHED-CHAIN AMINO ACID* METABOLISM DISORDERS (*Continued*)

DISEASE (OMIM NUMBER)	DEFECTIVE PROTEINS OR ENZYMES	DEFECTIVE GENE OR GENES (CHROMOSOMAL LOCATION)	COMMENTS
3-Hydroxyisobutyric aciduria (236795)	3-Hydroxyisobutyrate dehydrogenase	HIBADH (chromosomal location not determined)	**Biochemical profile:** Elevated urine 3-hydroxyisobutyrate; in 50% patients, elevated lactate **Clinical features:** Dysmorphic features, CNS malformations, hypotonia, ketoacidosis **Treatment:** Low-protein diet, carnitine
2-Methylbutyryl glycinuria (600301)	Short branched-chain acyl-CoA dehydrogenase	ACADSB (10q25-q26)†	**Biochemical profile:** Elevated urine 2-methylbutyrulglycine **Clinical features:** Hypotonia, muscular atrophy, lethargy, hypoglycemia, hypothermia **Treatment:** No effective treatment
Ethylmalonic encephalopathy (602473)	Mitochondrial protein of undetermined function	ETHE1 (19q13.32)†	**Biochemical profile:** Elevated urine ethylmalonic and methylsuccinic acids, elevated serum lactate **Clinical features:** Retinopathy, acrocyanosis, diarrhea, petechiae, developmental delay, intellectual disability, extrapyramidal symptoms, ataxia, seizures, hyperintense lesions in the basal ganglia **Treatment:** No effective treatment
Malonic aciduria (248360)	Malonyl-CoA decarboxylase	MLYCD (16q24)†	**Biochemical profile:** Elevated lactate, malonate, methylmalonate, and malonylcarnitine **Clinical features:** Hypotonia, developmental delay, hypoglycemia, acidosis **Treatment:** No effective treatment; low-fat, high-carbohydrate diet Carnitine possibly helpful in some patients
Hypervalinemia or hyperisoleucine-hyperleucinemia (277100)	Mitochondrial branched-chain aminotransferase 2	BCAT2 (19q13)	**Biochemical profile:** Elevated urine and serum valine **Clinical features:** Growth retardation **Treatment:** Controlled valine intake

*The branched-chain amino acids are valine, leucine, and isoleucine.
†Gene has been identified, and molecular basis has been elucidated.
OMIM = online mendelian inheritance in man (see the OMIM database at www.ncbi.nlm.nih.gov/omim).

Treatment of classic homocystinuria is a low-methionine diet, combined with high-dose pyridoxine (a cystathionine synthetase cofactor) 100 to 500 mg po once/day. Because about half of patients respond to high-dose pyridoxine alone, some clinicians do not restrict methionine intake in these patients. Betaine (trimethylglycine), which enhances remethylation, can also help lower homocysteine; dosage is 100 to 125 mg/kg po bid. Folate 500 to 1000 μg once/day is also given. With early treatment, intellectual outcome is normal or near normal.

Other forms of homocystinuria: Various defects in the remethylation process can result in homocystinuria. Defects include deficiencies of methionine synthase (MS) and MS reductase (MSR), delivery of methylcobalamin and adenosylcobalamin, and deficiency of methylenetetrahydrofolate reductase (MTHFR, which is required to generate the 5-methyltetrahydrofolate needed for the MS reaction). Because there is no methionine elevation in these forms of homocystinuria, they are not detected by neonatal screening.

Clinical manifestations are similar to other forms of homocystinuria. In addition, MS and MSR deficiencies are accompanied by neurologic deficits and megaloblastic anemia. Clinical manifestation of MTHFR deficiency is variable, including intellectual disability, psychosis, weakness, ataxia, and spasticity.

Diagnosis of MS and MSR deficiencies is suggested by homocystinuria and megaloblastic anemia and confirmed by DNA testing. Patients with cobalamin defects have megaloblastic anemia and methylmalonic acidemia. MTHFR deficiency is diagnosed by DNA testing.

Treatment is by replacement of hydroxycobalamin 1 mg IM once/day (for patients with MS, MSR, and cobalamin defects) and folate in supplementation similar to characteristic homocystinuria.

Cystathioninuria: This disorder is caused by deficiency of cystathionase, which converts cystathionine to cysteine. Cystathionine accumulation results in increased urinary excretion but no clinical symptoms.

Sulfite oxidase deficiency: Sulfite oxidase converts sulfite to sulfate in the last step of cysteine and methionine degradation; it requires a molybdenum cofactor. Deficiency of either the enzyme or the cofactor causes similar disease; inheritance for both is autosomal recessive.

In its most severe form, clinical manifestations appear in neonates and include seizures, hypotonia, and myoclonus, progressing to early death. Patients with milder forms may present similarly to cerebral palsy and may have choreiform movements.

Table 315–10. METHIONINE AND SULFUR METABOLISM DISORDERS

DISEASE (OMIM NUMBER)	DEFECTIVE PROTEINS OR ENZYMES	DEFECTIVE GENE OR GENES (CHROMOSOMAL LOCATION)	COMMENTS
Homocystinuria (236200)	Cystathionine β-synthase	CBS (21q22.3)*	**Biochemical profile:** Methioninuria, homocystinuria **Clinical features:** Osteoporosis, scoliosis, fair complexion, ectopia lentis, progressive intellectual disability, thromboembolism **Treatment:** Pyridoxine, folate, betaine for unresponsive patients, low methionine diet with some L-cysteine supplementation
Methylenetetrahydrofolate reductase deficiency (236250)	Methylenetetrahydrofolate reductase	MTHFR (1p36.3)*	**Biochemical profile:** Low to normal plasma methionine, homocystinemia, homocystinuria **Clinical features:** Varies from asymptomatic to microcephaly, hypotonia, seizures, gait abnormality, and intellectual disability to apnea, coma, and death **Treatment:** Pyridoxine, folate (folic acid), hydroxycobalamin, methionine, betaine
Methylmalonic acidemia-homocystinuria (cblE; 236270)	Methionine synthase reductase	MTRR (5p15)*	**Biochemical profile:** Homocystinuria, homocystinemia, low plasma methionine, no methylmalonic aciduria, normal B_{12} and folate **Clinical features:** Feeding difficulty, growth failure, intellectual disability, ataxia, cerebral atrophy **Treatment:** Hydroxycobalamin, folate, L-methionine
Methylmalonic acidemia-homocystinuria (cblG; 250940)	Methylene tetrahydrofolate homocysteine methyltransferase	MTR (1q43)*	Same as methylmalonic acidemia-homocystinuria cblE
Hypermethioninemia (250850)	Methionine adenosyltransferase I and III	MAT1A (10q22)*	**Biochemical profile:** Elevated plasma methionine **Clinical features:** Mainly asymptomatic, fetid breath **Treatment:** None needed
Cystathioninuria (219500)	γ-Cystathionase	CTH (16)*	**Biochemical profile:** Cystathioninuria **Clinical features:** Usually normal; intellectual disability reported **Treatment:** Pyridoxine
Sulfite oxidase deficiency (606887)	Sulfite oxidase	SUOX (12q13)*	**Biochemical profile:** Elevated urine sulfite, thiosulfate, and S-sulfocysteine; decreased sulfate **Clinical features:** Developmental delay, ectopia lentis, eczema, delayed dentition, fine hair, hemiplegia, infantile hypotonia, hypertonia, seizures, choreoathetosis, ataxia, dystonia, death **Treatment:** No effective treatment
Molybdenum cofactor defect (252150)	MOCS1A and MOCS1B proteins Molybdopterin synthase Gephyrin	MCOS1 (14q24)* MCOS2 (6p21.3)* GEPH (5q21)*	**Biochemical profile:** Elevated urinary sulfite, thiosulfate, S-sulfocysteine, taurine, hypoxanthine, and xanthine; decreased sulfate and urate **Clinical features:** Similar to sulfite oxidase deficiency but also urinary stones **Treatment:** No effective treatment Low sulfur diet possibly helpful in patients with milder symptoms

*Gene has been identified, and molecular basis has been elucidated.
OMIM = online mendelian inheritance in man (see the OMIM database at www.ncbi.nlm.nih.gov/omim).

Diagnosis of sulfite oxidase deficiency is suggested by elevated urinary sulfite and confirmed by measuring enzyme levels in fibroblasts and cofactor levels in liver biopsy specimens. Treatment is supportive.

PHENYLKETONURIA

Phenylketonuria (PKU) is a disorder of amino acid metabolism that causes a clinical syndrome of intellectual disability with cognitive and behavioral abnormalities caused by elevated serum phenylalanine. The primary cause is deficient phenylalanine hydroxylase activity. Diagnosis is by detecting high phenylalanine levels and normal or low tyrosine levels. Treatment is lifelong dietary phenylalanine restriction. Prognosis is excellent with treatment.

PKU is most common among all white populations and relatively less common among Ashkenazi Jews, Chinese, and blacks. Inheritance is autosomal recessive; incidence is about 1/10,000 births among whites.

For information on other related amino acid disorders, see Table 315–11.

Pathophysiology

Excess dietary phenylalanine (ie, that not used for protein synthesis) is normally converted to tyrosine by phenylalanine hydroxylase; tetrahydrobiopterin (BH4) is an essential cofactor for this reaction. When one of several gene mutations results in deficiency or absence of phenylalanine hydroxylase, dietary phenylalanine accumulates; the brain is the main organ affected, possibly due to disturbance of myelination.

Some of the excess phenylalanine is metabolized to phenylketones, which are excreted in the urine, giving rise to the term PKU. The degree of enzyme deficiency, and hence severity of hyperphenylalaninemia, varies among patients depending on the specific mutation.

Variant forms: Although nearly all cases (98 to 99%) of PKU result from phenylalanine hydroxylase deficiency, phenylalanine can also accumulate if BH4 is not synthesized because of deficiencies of dihydrobiopterin synthase or not regenerated because of deficiencies of dihydropteridine reductase. Additionally, because BH4 is also a cofactor for tyrosine hydroxylase, which is involved in the synthesis of dopamine and serotonin, BH4 deficiency alters synthesis of neurotransmitters, causing neurologic symptoms independently of phenylalanine accumulation.

Symptoms and Signs

Most children with PKU are normal at birth but develop symptoms and signs slowly over several months as phenylalanine accumulates. The hallmark of untreated PKU is severe intellectual disability. Children also manifest extreme hyperactivity, gait disturbance, and psychoses and often exhibit an unpleasant, mousy body odor caused by phenylacetic acid (a breakdown product of phenylalanine) in urine and sweat. Children also tend to have a lighter skin, hair, and eye color than unaffected family members, and some may develop a rash similar to infantile eczema.

Diagnosis

- Routine neonatal screening
- Phenylalanine levels

In the US and many developed countries, all neonates are screened for PKU 24 to 48 h after birth with one of several blood tests; abnormal results are confirmed by directly measuring phenylalanine levels. In classic PKU, neonates often have phenylalanine levels > 20 mg/dL (1.2 mM/L). Those with partial deficiencies typically have levels < 8 to 10 mg/dL while on a normal diet (levels > 6 mg/dL require treatment); distinction from classic PKU requires a liver phenylalanine hydroxylase activity assay showing activity between 5% and 15% of normal or a mutation analysis identifying mild mutations in the gene.

BH4 deficiency is distinguished from other forms of PKU by elevated concentrations of biopterin or neopterin in urine, blood, CSF, or all 3; recognition is important, and the urine biopterin profile should be determined routinely at initial diagnosis because standard PKU treatment does not prevent neurologic damage.

Children in families with a positive family history can be diagnosed prenatally by using direct mutation studies after chorionic villus sampling or amniocentesis.

Prognosis

Adequate treatment begun in the first days of life prevents all manifestations of disease. Treatment begun after 2 to 3 yr may be effective only in controlling the extreme hyperactivity and intractable seizures. Children born to mothers with poorly controlled PKU (ie, they have high phenylalanine levels) during pregnancy are at high risk of microcephaly and developmental deficit.

Treatment

- Dietary phenylalanine restriction

Treatment of PKU is lifelong dietary phenylalanine restriction. All natural protein contains about 4% phenylalanine. Therefore dietary staples include low-protein natural foods (eg, fruits, vegetables, certain cereals), protein hydrolysates treated to remove phenylalanine, and phenylalanine-free elemental amino acid mixtures. Examples of commercially available phenylalanine-free products include XPhe products (PKU Anamix® for infants, XP Maxamaid® for children 1 to 8 yr, XP Maxamum® for children > 8 yr); Phenex®-1 and Phenex®-2; Phenyl-Free® 1 and Phenyl-Free® 2; pku 1, pku 2, and pku 3; PhenylAde® (varieties); PKU Lophlex LQ®; and Phlexy-10® (multiple formulations). Some phenylalanine is required for growth and metabolism; this requirement is met by measured quantities of natural protein from milk or low-protein foods.

Frequent monitoring of plasma phenylalanine levels is required; recommended targets are between 2 mg/dL and 4 mg/dL (120 to 240μmol/L) for children < 12 yr and between 2 mg/dL and 10 mg/dL (120 to 600 μmol/L) for children > 12 yr. Dietary planning and management need to be initiated in women of childbearing age before pregnancy to ensure a good outcome for the child. Tyrosine supplementation is increasingly used because it is an essential amino acid in patients with PKU. In addition, sapropterin is increasingly being used.

For those with BH4 deficiency, treatment also includes tetrahydrobiopterin 1 to 5 mg/kg po tid; levodopa, carbidopa, and 5-OH tryptophan; and folinic acid 10 to 20 mg po once/day in cases of dihydropteridine reductase deficiency. However, treatment goals and approach are the same as those for PKU.

KEY POINTS

- PKU is caused by one of several gene mutations that result in deficiency or absence of phenylalanine hydroxylase so that dietary phenylalanine accumulates; the brain is the main organ affected, possibly because of disturbance of myelination.
- PKU causes a clinical syndrome of intellectual disability with cognitive and behavioral abnormalities; if untreated, the intellectual disability is severe.

- In the US and many developed countries, all neonates are screened for PKU 24 to 48 h after birth with one of several blood tests; abnormal results are confirmed by directly measuring phenylalanine levels.
- Treatment is lifelong dietary phenylalanine restriction; adequate treatment begun in the first days of life prevents all manifestations of disease.
- Although prognosis is excellent with treatment, frequent monitoring of plasma phenylalanine levels is required; recommended targets are between 2 mg/dL and 4 mg/dL (120 to 240 μmol/L) for children < 12 yr and between 2 mg/dL and 10 mg/dL (120 to 600 μmol/L) for children > 12 yr.

TYROSINE METABOLISM DISORDERS

Tyrosine is an amino acid that is a precursor of several neurotransmitters (eg, dopamine, norepinephrine, epinephrine), hormones (eg, thyroxine), and melanin; deficiencies of enzymes involved in its metabolism lead to a variety of syndromes.

There are numerous disorders of phenylalanine and tyrosine metabolism (see Table 315–11).

Transient tyrosinemia of the newborn: Transient immaturity of metabolic enzymes, particularly 4-hydroxyphenylpyruvic acid dioxygenase, sometimes leads to elevated plasma tyrosine levels (usually in premature infants, particularly those receiving high-protein diets); metabolites may show up on routine neonatal screening for PKU.

Most infants are asymptomatic, but some have lethargy and poor feeding.

Tyrosinemia is distinguished from PKU by elevated plasma tyrosine levels.

Most cases resolve spontaneously. Symptomatic patients should have dietary tyrosine restriction (2 g/kg/day) and be given vitamin C 200 to 400 mg po once/day.

Tyrosinemia type I: This disorder is an autosomal recessive trait caused by deficiency of fumarylacetoacetate hydroxylase, an enzyme important for tyrosine metabolism.

Disease may manifest as fulminant liver failure in the neonatal period or as indolent subclinical hepatitis, painful peripheral neuropathy, and renal tubular disorders (eg, normal anion gap metabolic acidosis, hypophosphatemia, vitamin D–resistant rickets) in older infants and children. Children who do not die of associated liver failure in infancy have a significant risk of developing liver cancer.

Diagnosis of tyrosinemia type I is suggested by elevated plasma levels of tyrosine; it is confirmed by a high level of succinylacetone in plasma or urine and by low fumarylacetoacetate hydroxylase activity in blood cells or liver biopsy specimens. Treatment with nitisinone is effective in acute episodes and slows progression.

A diet low in phenylalanine and tyrosine is recommended. Liver transplantation is effective.

Tyrosinemia type II: This rare autosomal recessive disorder is caused by tyrosine transaminase deficiency.

Accumulation of tyrosine causes cutaneous and corneal ulcers. Secondary elevation of phenylalanine, though mild, may cause neuropsychiatric abnormalities if not treated.

Diagnosis of tyrosinemia type II is by elevation of tyrosine in plasma, absence of succinylacetone in plasma or urine, and measurement of decreased enzyme activity in liver biopsy.

This disorder is easily treated with mild to moderate restriction of dietary phenylalanine and tyrosine.

Table 315–11. PHENYLALANINE AND TYROSINE METABOLISM DISORDERS

DISEASE (OMIM NUMBER)	DEFECTIVE PROTEINS OR ENZYMES	DEFECTIVE GENE OR GENES (CHROMOSOMAL LOCATION)	COMMENTS
Phenylketonuria (PKU), with classic and mild forms (261600)	Phenylalanine hydroxylase	PAH (12q24.1)*	**Biochemical profile:** Elevated plasma phenylalanine **Clinical features:** Intellectual disability, behavioral problems **Treatment:** Dietary phenylalanine restriction, tyrosine supplementation
Dihydropteridine reductase deficiency (261630)	Dihydropteridine reductase	QDPR (4p15.31)*	**Biochemical profile:** Elevated plasma phenylalanine, high urine biopterin, low plasma biopterin **Clinical features:** Similar to mild PKU, but if neurotransmitter deficiency is unrecognized, development of intellectual disability, seizures, and dystonia **Treatment:** Dietary phenylalanine restriction, tyrosine supplementation, folinic acid, neurotransmitter replacement
Pterin-4α-carbinolamine dehydratase deficiency (264070)	Pterin-4α-carbinolamine dehydratase	PCBD (10q22)*	**Biochemical profile:** Elevated plasma phenylalanine, high urine neopterin and primapterin, low plasma biopterin **Clinical features:** Similar to mild PKU, but if neurotransmitter deficiency is unrecognized, development of intellectual disability, seizures, and dystonia **Treatment:** Dietary phenylalanine restriction, tyrosine supplementation, neurotransmitter replacement

Table continues on the following page.

Table 315–11. PHENYLALANINE AND TYROSINE METABOLISM DISORDERS (*Continued*)

DISEASE (OMIM NUMBER)	DEFECTIVE PROTEINS OR ENZYMES	DEFECTIVE GENE OR GENES (CHROMOSOMAL LOCATION)	COMMENTS
Biopterin synthesis deficiency	GTP-cyclohydrolase (233910) 6-Pyruvoyl-tetrahydropterin synthase (261640) Sepiapterin reductase (182125)	GCH1 (14q22)* PTS (11q22-q23)* SPR (2p14-p12)*	**Biochemical profile:** Elevated plasma phenylalanine, low urine biopterin, low (GCH) or high (PTS and SPR) urine neopterin **Clinical features:** Similar to mild PKU, but if neurotransmitter deficiency is unrecognized, development of intellectual disability, seizures, and dystonia **Treatment:** Tetrahydrobiopterin and neurotransmitter supplementation
Tyrosinemia type I (hepatorenal; 276700)	Fumarylacetoacetate hydrolase	FAH (15q23-q25)*	**Biochemical profile:** Elevated plasma tyrosine, elevated plasma and urinary succinylacetone **Clinical features:** Cirrhosis, acute liver failure, peripheral neuropathy, Fanconi syndrome **Treatment:** Dietary phenylalanine, tyrosine, and methionine restriction; nitisinone; liver transplantation
Tyrosinemia type II (oculocutaneous; 276600)	Tyrosine aminotransferase	TAT (16q22.1-q22.3)*	**Biochemical profile:** Elevated plasma tyrosine and phenylalanine **Clinical features:** Intellectual disability, palmoplantar hyperkeratitis, corneal ulcers **Treatment:** Dietary phenylalanine and tyrosine restriction
Tyrosinemia type III (276710)	4-Hydroxyphenylpyruvate dioxygenase	HPD (12q24-qter)*	**Biochemical profile:** Elevated plasma tyrosine, elevated urinary 4-hydroxyphenyl derivatives **Clinical features:** Developmental delay, seizures, ataxia **Treatment:** Dietary phenylalanine and tyrosine restriction, ascorbate supplementation
Transient tyrosinemia of the newborn	4-Hydroxyphenylpyruvate dioxygenase	Not genetic	**Biochemical profile:** Elevated plasma phenylalanine and tyrosine **Clinical features:** Usually occurring in premature infants; mostly asymptomatic Occasionally poor feeding and lethargy **Treatment:** Tyrosine restriction and ascorbate supplementation for symptomatic patients only
Hawkinsinuria (140350)	4-Hydroxyphenylpyruvate dioxygenase complex	HPD (12q24-qter)*	**Biochemical profile:** Mild hypertyrosinemia, elevated urinary hawkinsin **Clinical features:** Failure to thrive, ketotic metabolic acidosis **Treatment:** Dietary phenylalanine and tyrosine restriction, ascorbate supplementation
Alkaptonuria (203500)	Homogentisate oxidase	HGD (3q21-q23)*	**Biochemical profile:** Elevated urine homogentisic acid **Clinical features:** Dark urine, ochronosis, arthritis **Treatment:** None; ascorbate supplementation to reduce pigmentation
Oculocutaneous albinism type I (A and B; 203100)	Tyrosinase	TYR (11q21)*	**Biochemical profile:** No abnormality in plasma and urine amino acids, absent (IA) or decreased (IB) tyrosinase **Clinical features:** Absent (IA) or decreased (IB) pigment in skin, hair, iris, and retina; nystagmus; blindness; skin cancer **Treatment:** Protection of skin and eyes from actinic radiation

*Gene has been identified, and molecular basis has been elucidated.
OMIM = online mendelian inheritance in man (see the OMIM database at www.ncbi.nlm.nih.gov/omim).

Alkaptonuria: This rare autosomal recessive disorder is caused by homogentisic acid oxidase deficiency; homogentisic acid oxidation products accumulate in and darken skin, and crystals precipitate in joints.

The condition is usually diagnosed in adults and causes dark skin pigmentation (ochronosis) and arthritis. Urine turns dark when exposed to air because of oxidation products of homogentisic acid. Diagnosis of alkaptonuria is by finding elevated urinary levels of homogentisic acid (> 4 to 8 g/24 h).

There is no effective treatment for alkaptonuria, but ascorbic acid 1 g po once/day may diminish pigment deposition by increasing renal excretion of homogentisic acid.

Oculocutaneous albinism: Tyrosinase deficiency results in absence of skin and retinal pigmentation, causing a much increased risk of skin cancer and considerable vision loss. Nystagmus is often present, and photophobia is common.

UREA CYCLE DISORDERS

Urea cycle disorders (UCD) are characterized by hyperammonemia under catabolic or protein-loading conditions.

There are many types of urea cycle and related disorders (see Table 315–12) as well as many other amino acid and organic acid metabolism disorders.

Primary UCDs include carbamoyl phosphate synthase (CPS) deficiency, ornithine transcarbamylase (OTC) deficiency, argininosuccinate synthetase deficiency (citrullinemia), argininosuccinate lyase deficiency (argininosuccinic aciduria), and arginase deficiency (argininemia). In addition, N-acetylglutamate synthetase (NAGS) deficiency has been reported. The more "proximal" the enzyme deficiency is, the more severe the hyperammonemia; thus, disease severity in descending order is NAGS deficiency, CPS deficiency, OTC deficiency, citrullinemia, argininosuccinic aciduria, and argininemia.

Inheritance for all UCDs is autosomal recessive, except for OTC deficiency, which is X-linked.

Symptoms and Signs

Clinical manifestations range from mild (eg, failure to thrive, intellectual disability, episodic hyperammonemia) to severe (eg, altered mental status, coma, death). Manifestations in females with OTC deficiency range from growth failure, developmental delay, psychiatric abnormalities, and episodic (especially postpartum) hyperammonemia to a phenotype similar to that of affected males (ie, recurrent vomiting, irritability, lethargy, hyperammonemic coma, cerebral edema, spasticity, intellectual disability, seizures, death).

Diagnosis

- Serum amino acid profiles

Diagnosis of UCD is based on amino acid profiles. For example, elevated ornithine indicates CPS deficiency or OTC deficiency, whereas elevated citrulline indicates citrullinemia. To distinguish between CPS deficiency and OTC deficiency, orotic acid measurement is helpful because accumulation of carbamoyl phosphate in OTC deficiency results in its alternative metabolism to orotic acid.

Treatment

- Dietary protein restriction
- Arginine or citrulline supplementation
- Sodium phenylbutyrate
- Possible liver transplantation

Treatment of urea cycle disorders is dietary protein restriction that still provides adequate amino acids for growth, development, and normal protein turnover.

Arginine has become a staple of treatment. It supplies adequate urea cycle intermediates to encourage the incorporation of more nitrogen moieties into urea cycle intermediates, each of which is readily excretable. Arginine is also a positive regulator of acetylglutamate synthesis. Recent studies suggest that oral citrulline is more effective than arginine in patients with OTC deficiency.

Additional treatment is with sodium benzoate, phenylbutyrate, or phenylacetate, which by conjugating glycine (sodium benzoate) and glutamine (phenylbutyrate and phenylacetate) provides a "nitrogen sink."

Despite these therapeutic advances, many UCDs remain difficult to treat, and liver transplantation is eventually required for many patients. Timing of liver transplantation is critical. Optimally, the infant should grow to an age when transplantation is less risky (> 1 yr), but it is important to not wait so long as to allow an intercurrent episode of hyperammonemia (often associated with illness) to cause irreparable harm to the CNS.

OVERVIEW OF CARBOHYDRATE METABOLISM DISORDERS

Carbohydrate metabolism disorders are errors of metabolism that affect the catabolism and anabolism of carbohydrates. The inability to effectively use metabolites of carbohydrates accounts for the majority of these disorders. These disorders include

- Fructose metabolism disorders
- Galactosemia
- GSDs
- Pyruvate metabolism disorders
- Other carbohydrate metabolism disorders

FRUCTOSE METABOLISM DISORDERS

Deficiency of enzymes that metabolize fructose may be asymptomatic or cause hypoglycemia.

Fructose is a monosaccharide that is present in high concentrations in fruit and honey and is a constituent of sucrose and sorbitol. Fructose metabolism disorders are one of the many carbohydrate metabolism disorders.

Fructose 1-phosphate aldolase (aldolase B) deficiency: This deficiency causes the clinical syndrome of hereditary fructose intolerance. Inheritance is autosomal recessive; incidence is estimated at 1/20,000 births. Infants are healthy until they ingest fructose; fructose 1-phosphate then accumulates, causing hypoglycemia, nausea and vomiting, abdominal pain, sweating, tremors, confusion, lethargy, seizures, and coma. Prolonged ingestion may cause cirrhosis, mental deterioration, and proximal renal tubular acidosis with urinary loss of phosphate and glucose.

Diagnosis of fructose 1-phosphate aldolase deficiency is suggested by symptoms in relation to recent fructose intake and is confirmed by enzyme analysis of liver biopsy tissue or by induction of hypoglycemia by fructose infusion 200 mg/kg IV.

Table 315–12. UREA CYCLE AND RELATED DISORDERS

DISEASE (OMIM NUMBER)	DEFECTIVE PROTEINS OR ENZYMES	DEFECTIVE GENE OR GENES (CHROMOSOMAL LOCATION)	COMMENTS
OTC deficiency (311250)	OTC	OTC (Xp21.1)*	**Biochemical profile:** Elevated ornithine and glutamine, decreased citrulline and arginine, markedly increased urine orotate **Clinical features:** In males, recurrent vomiting, irritability, lethargy, hyperammonemic coma, cerebral edema, spasticity, intellectual disability, seizures, death In female carriers, variable manifestations, ranging from growth delay, small stature, protein aversion, and postpartum hyperammonemia to symptoms as severe as those in males with the deficiency **Treatment:** Hemodialysis for emergent hyperammonemic crisis, Na benzoate, Na phenylacetate, Na phenylbutyrate, low-protein diet supplemented with essential amino acid mixture and arginine, citrulline, experimental attempts at gene therapy, liver transplantation (which is curative)
N-Acetylglutamate synthetase deficiency (237310)	*N*-Acetylglutamate synthetase	NAGS (17q21.31)	**Biochemical profile:** Similar to OTC deficiency except for normal to low urine orotate **Clinical features:** Similar to OTC deficiency except carriers are asymptomatic **Treatment:** Similar to OTC deficiency but also N-carbamylglutamate supplementation
CPS deficiency (237300)	Carbamoyl phosphate synthetase	CPS1 (2q35)*	**Biochemical profile:** Similar to OTC deficiency except for normal to low urine orotate **Clinical features:** Similar to OTC deficiency except carriers are asymptomatic **Treatment:** Na benzoate and arginine
Citrullinemia type I (215700)	Argininosuccinic acid synthetase	ASS (9q34)*	**Biochemical profile:** High plasma citrulline and glutamine, citrullinuria, orotic aciduria **Clinical features:** Episodic hyperammonemia, growth failure, protein aversion, lethargy, vomiting, coma, seizures, cerebral edema, developmental delay **Treatment:** Similar to that for OTC deficiency except citrulline supplementation is not recommended Liver transplantation
Citrullinemia type II (603814, 603471)	Citrin	SCL25A13 (7q21.3)*	**Biochemical profile:** Elevated plasma citrulline, methionine, galactose, and bilirubin **Clinical features:** With neonatal onset, cholestasis resolved by 3 mo With adult onset, enuresis, delayed menarche, sleep reversal, vomiting, delusions, hallucinations, psychosis, coma **Treatment:** Liver transplantation; otherwise no clear treatment
Argininosuccinic aciduria (207900)	Argininosuccinate lyase	ASL (7cen-q11.2)*	**Biochemical profile:** Elevated plasma citrulline and glutamine, elevated urine argininosuccinate **Clinical features:** Episodic hyperammonemia, hepatic fibrosis, elevated liver enzymes, hepatomegaly, protein aversion, vomiting, seizures, intellectual disability, ataxia, lethargy, coma, trichorrhexis nodosa **Treatment:** Arginine supplementation

Table 315–12. UREA CYCLE AND RELATED DISORDERS (*Continued*)

DISEASE (OMIM NUMBER)	DEFECTIVE PROTEINS OR ENZYMES	DEFECTIVE GENE OR GENES (CHROMOSOMAL LOCATION)	COMMENTS
Argininemia (107830)	Arginase I	ARG1 (6q23)*	**Biochemical profile:** Elevated plasma arginine, diaminoaciduria (argininuria, lysinuria, cystinuria, ornithinuria), orotic aciduria, pyrimidinuria **Clinical features:** Growth and developmental delay, anorexia, vomiting, seizures, spasticity, irritability, hyperactivity, protein intolerance, hyperammonemia **Treatment:** Low-protein diet, benzoate, phenylacetate
Lysinuric protein intolerance (dibasic aminoaciduria II; 222700)	Dibasic amino acid transporter	SLC7A7 (14q11.2)*	**Biochemical profile:** Elevated urine lysine, ornithine, and arginine **Clinical features:** Protein intolerance, episodic hyperammonemia, growth and developmental delay, diarrhea, vomiting, hepatomegaly, cirrhosis, leucopenia, osteopenia, skeletal fragility, coma **Treatment:** Low-protein diet, citrulline
Hyperornithinemia, hyperammonemia, and homocitrullinemia (238970)	Mitochondrial ornithine translocase	SLC25A15 (13q14)*	**Biochemical profile:** Elevated plasma ornithine, homocitrullinemia **Clinical features:** Intellectual disability, progressive spastic paraparesis, episodic confusion, hyperammonemia, dyspraxia, seizures, vomiting, retinopathy, abnormal nerve conduction and evoked potentials, leukodystrophy **Treatment:** Lysine, ornithine, or citrulline supplementation
Ornithinemia (258870)	Ornithine aminotransferase	OAT (10q26)*	**Biochemical profile:** Elevated plasma ornithine and urine ornithine, lysine, and arginine; low plasma lysine, glutamic acid, and glutamine **Clinical features:** Myopia, night blindness, blindness, progressive loss of peripheral vision, progressive gyrate atrophy of choroid and retina, mild proximal hypotonia, myopathy **Treatment:** Pyridoxine, low-arginine diet, lysine and α-aminoisobutyrate to increase renal loss of ornithine; proline or creatine supplementation
Hyperinsulinism-hyperammonemia syndrome (606762)	Hyperactivity of glutamate dehydrogenase	GLUD1 (10q23.3)*	**Biochemical profile:** Elevated urine α-ketoglutarate **Clinical features:** Seizures, recurrent hypoglycemia, hyperinsulinism, asymptomatic hyperammonemia **Treatment:** Prevention of hypoglycemia

*Gene has been identified, and molecular basis has been elucidated.
OMIM = online mendelian inheritance in man (see the OMIM database at www.ncbi.nlm.nih.gov/omim).

Diagnosis and identification of heterozygous carriers of the mutated gene can also be made by direct DNA analysis.

Short-term treatment of fructose 1-phosphate aldolase deficiency is glucose for hypoglycemia; long-term treatment is exclusion of dietary fructose, sucrose, and sorbitol. Many patients develop a natural aversion to fructose-containing food. Prognosis is excellent with treatment.

Fructokinase deficiency: This deficiency causes benign elevation of blood and urine fructose levels (benign fructosuria). Inheritance is autosomal recessive; incidence is about 1/130,000 births.

The condition is asymptomatic and diagnosed accidentally when a non-glucose reducing substance is detected in urine.

Deficiency of fructose-1,6-biphosphatase: This deficiency compromises gluconeogenesis and results in fasting hypoglycemia, ketosis, and acidosis. This deficiency can be fatal in neonates. Inheritance is autosomal recessive; incidence is unknown. Febrile illness can trigger episodes.

Acute treatment of fructose-1,6-biphosphatase deficiency is oral or IV glucose. Tolerance to fasting generally increases with age.

GALACTOSEMIA

Galactosemia is a carbohydrate metabolism disorder caused by inherited deficiencies in enzymes that convert galactose to glucose. Symptoms and signs include hepatic and renal dysfunction, cognitive deficits, cataracts, and premature ovarian failure. Diagnosis is by enzyme analysis of RBCs. Treatment is dietary elimination of galactose. Physical prognosis is good with treatment, but cognitive and performance parameters are often subnormal.

Galactose is found in dairy products, fruits, and vegetables. Autosomal recessive enzyme deficiencies cause 3 clinical syndromes.

Galactose-1-phosphate uridyl transferase deficiency: This deficiency causes classic galactosemia. Incidence is 1/62,000 births; carrier frequency is 1/125. Infants become anorectic and jaundiced within a few days or weeks of consuming breast milk or lactose-containing formula. Vomiting, hepatomegaly, poor growth, lethargy, diarrhea, and septicemia (usually *Escherichia coli*) develop, as does renal dysfunction (eg, proteinuria, aminoaciduria, Fanconi syndrome), leading to metabolic acidosis and edema. Hemolytic anemia may also occur.

Without treatment, children remain short and develop cognitive, speech, gait, and balance deficits in their teenage years; many also have cataracts, osteomalacia (caused by hypercalciuria), and premature ovarian failure. Patients with the Duarte variant have a much milder phenotype.

Galactokinase deficiency: Patients develop cataracts from production of galactitol, which osmotically damages lens fibers; idiopathic intracranial hypertension (pseudotumor cerebri) is rare. Incidence is 1/40,000 births.

Uridine diphosphate galactose 4-epimerase deficiency: There are benign and severe phenotypes. Incidence of the benign form is 1/23,000 births in Japan; no incidence data are available for the more severe form. The benign form is restricted to RBCs and WBCs and causes no clinical abnormalities. The severe form causes a syndrome indistinguishable from classic galactosemia, although sometimes with hearing loss.

Diagnosis

- Galactose levels
- Enzyme analysis

Diagnosis of galactosemia is suggested clinically and supported by elevated galactose levels and the presence of reducing substances other than glucose (eg, galactose, galactose 1-phosphate) in the urine; it is confirmed by enzyme analysis of RBCs, hepatic tissue, or both. Most states require routine neonatal screening for galactose-1-phosphate uridyl transferase deficiency.

Treatment

- Dietary galactose restriction

Treatment of galactosemia is elimination of all sources of galactose in the diet, most notably lactose, which is a source of galactose present in all dairy products, including milk-based infant formulas and a sweetener used in many foods. A lactose-free diet prevents acute toxicity and reverses some manifestations (eg, cataracts) but may not prevent neurocognitive deficits. Many patients require supplemental calcium and vitamins. For patients with epimerase deficiency, some galactose intake is critical to ensure a supply of uridine-5′-diphosphate-galactose (UDP-galactose) for various metabolic processes.

GLYCOGEN STORAGE DISEASES

Glycogen storage diseases (GSDs) are carbohydrate metabolism disorders and are caused by deficiencies of enzymes involved in glycogen synthesis or breakdown; the deficiencies may occur in the liver or muscles and cause hypoglycemia or deposition of abnormal amounts or types of glycogen (or its intermediate metabolites) in tissues.

Inheritance for GSDs is autosomal recessive except for GSD type VIII/IX, which is X-linked. Incidence is estimated at about 1/25,000 births, which may be an underestimate because milder subclinical forms may be undiagnosed. For a more complete listing of GSDs, see Table 315–13.

Age of onset, clinical manifestations, and severity vary by type, but symptoms and signs are most commonly those of hypoglycemia and myopathy.

Diagnosis of GSDs is suspected by history, examination, and detection of glycogen and intermediate metabolites in tissues by MRI or biopsy. Diagnosis is confirmed by significant decrease of enzyme activity in liver (types I, III, VI, and VIII/IX), muscle (types IIb, III, VII, and VIII/IX), skin fibroblasts (types IIa and IV), or RBCs (type VII) or by lack of an increase in venous lactate with forearm activity/ischemia (types V and VII).

Prognosis and treatment of GSDs vary by type, but treatment typically includes dietary supplementation with cornstarch to provide a sustained source of glucose for the hepatic forms of GSD and exercise avoidance for the muscle forms.

Defects in glycolysis (rare) may cause syndromes similar to GSDs. Deficiencies of phosphoglycerate kinase, phosphoglycerate mutase, and lactate dehydrogenase mimic the myopathies of GSD types V and VII; deficiencies of glucose transport protein 2 (Fanconi-Bickel syndrome) mimic the hepatopathy of other GSD types (eg, I, III, IV, VI).

PYRUVATE METABOLISM DISORDERS

Inability to metabolize pyruvate causes lactic acidosis and a variety of CNS abnormalities.

Pyruvate is an important substrate in carbohydrate metabolism. Pyruvate metabolism disorders are included among the carbohydrate metabolism disorders.

Pyruvate dehydrogenase deficiency: Pyruvate dehydrogenase is a multi-enzyme complex responsible for the generation of acetyl CoA from pyruvate for the Krebs cycle. Deficiency results in elevation of pyruvate and thus elevation of lactic acid levels. Inheritance is X-linked or autosomal recessive.

Clinical manifestations vary in severity but include lactic acidosis and CNS malformations and other postnatal changes, including cystic lesions of the cerebral cortex, brain stem, and basal ganglia; ataxia; and psychomotor retardation.

Diagnosis of pyruvate dehydrogenase deficiency is confirmed by enzyme analysis of skin fibroblasts, DNA testing, or both.

Table 315–13. GLYCOGEN STORAGE DISEASES AND DISORDERS OF GLUCONEOGENESIS

DISEASE (OMIM NUMBER)	DEFECTIVE PROTEINS OR ENZYMES	DEFECTIVE GENE OR GENES (CHROMOSOMAL LOCATION)	COMMENTS
GSD I (Von Gierke disease)			Most common type of GSD I: Ia (> 80%) **Onset:** Before 1 yr **Clinical features:** Before 1 yr, severe hypoglycemia, lactic acidosis, and hepatomegaly; later, hepatic adenomas, renomegaly with progressive renal insufficiency and hypertension, short stature, hypertriglyceridemia, hyperuricemia, platelet dysfunction with epistaxis, and anemia In type Ib, less severe but including neutropenia, neutrophil dysfunction with recurrent infections, and inflammatory bowel disease **Treatment:** Uncooked cornstarch 1.5–2.5 g/kg po q 4–6 h or lactose-free formula with maltodextrin to maintain normoglycemia; nocturnal feedings (important); fructose and galactose restriction; for lactic acidosis, bicarbonate 0.25 to 0.5 mmol/kg qid; allopurinol to keep uric acid to < 6.4 mg/dL; liver and kidney transplantation (may be successful) For type Ib patients with neutropenia, G-CSF
Type Ia (232200)	Glucose-6-phosphatase	G6PC (17q21)*	
Type Ib (232220)	Glucose-6-phosphate translocase	G6PT1 (11q23)*	
Type Ic (232240)	Microsomal phosphate or pyrophosphate transporter	G6PT1 (11q23)*	
Type Id	Microsomal glucose transporter	Probably same as Ic	
GSD II (Pompe disease, 232300)			**Onset:** Infancy, childhood, or adulthood; residual enzyme activity in child and adult forms **Clinical features:** In infantile form, cardiomyopathy with heart failure, severe hypotonia, macroglossia In juvenile and adult forms, skeletal myopathy with delayed motor development, progressive peripheral and respiratory muscle weakness In type IIb, intellectual disability **Treatment:** None known For cardiomyopathy, heart transplantation
Type IIa	Lysosomal acid α-glucosidase	GAA (17q25)*	
Type IIb (Danon)	Lysosomal membrane protein-2	LAMP2 (Xq24)*	
GSD III (Forbes disease, Cori disease, limit dextrinosis; 232400)			**Frequency:** IIIa, 85%; IIIb, 15%; IIIc and IIId, rare **Onset:** Infancy or childhood **Clinical features:** In type IIIa, liver and muscle involvement with features of type Ia and II In type IIIb, only liver involvement plus features of type Ia In types IIIc and IIId, various features depending on tissue affected **Treatment:** Uncooked cornstarch and continuous feeding to maintain normoglycemia, high-protein diet to stimulate gluconeogenesis
Types IIIa and IIIb	Debrancher enzyme (amyloglucosidase and oligoglucanotransferase)	AGL (1p21)*	
Type IIIc	Amyloglucosidase only		
Type IIId	Oligoglucanotransferase only		
GSD IV (Andersen disease; 232500)	Branching enzyme	GBE1 (3p12)*	**Onset:** Early infancy; rarely, the neonatal period, late childhood, or adulthood (manifesting as a variant nonprogressive or a neuromuscular form) **Clinical features:** Hepatomegaly with progressive cirrhosis and hypoglycemia, esophageal varices, and ascites; splenomegaly; failure to thrive In neuromuscular forms, hypotonia and muscle atrophy **Treatment:** None known For cirrhosis, liver transplantation, which treats the primary disease as well
GSD V (McArdle disease; 232600)	Muscle phosphorylase	PYGM (11q13)*	**Onset:** Adolescence or early adulthood **Clinical features:** Exercise intolerance due to muscle cramps, rhabdomyolysis **Treatment:** Carbohydrate administration before exercise, high-protein diet

Table continues on the following page.

Table 315–13. GSDS AND DISORDERS OF GLUCONEOGENESIS (*Continued*)

DISEASE (OMIM NUMBER)	DEFECTIVE PROTEINS OR ENZYMES	DEFECTIVE GENE OR GENES (CHROMOSOMAL LOCATION)	COMMENTS
GSD VI (Hers disease; 232700)	Liver phosphorylase	PYGL (14q21-q22)*	**Frequency:** Rare **Onset:** Early childhood **Clinical features:** Benign course with symptoms lessening with aging; growth retardation, hepatomegaly, hypoglycemia, hyperlipidemia, ketosis **Treatment:** None necessary
GSD VII (Tarui disease; 232800)	Phosphofructokinase	PFKM (12q13.3)*	**Onset:** Middle childhood **Clinical features:** Exercise intolerance due to muscle cramps, rhabdomyolysis, hemolysis **Treatment:** Nonspecific, avoidance of exercise
GSD VIII/IX (306000, 172490, 604549, 311870)	—	—	**Onset:** Heterogeneous **Clinical features:** Heterogeneous; hepatomegaly, growth retardation, muscle hypotonia, hypercholesterolemia **Treatment:** Nonspecific
Type VIII/IXa	X-linked phosphorylase kinase	PHKA2 (Xp22)*	
Type IXb	Liver and muscle phosphorylase kinase	PHKB (16q12-q13)*	
Type IXc	Liver phosphorylase kinase	PHKG2 (16p12.1-p11.2)*	
Type IXd	Muscle phosphorylase kinase	PHKA1 (Xq13)*	
GSD O (240600)	Glycogen synthase	GYS2 (12p12)*	**Onset:** Variable but often after cessation of nighttime feedings or intercurrent illness **Clinical features:** Fasting hypoglycemia and ketosis, postprandial lactic acidosis **Treatment:** Frequent protein-rich meals, uncooked cornstarch at bedtime
Fanconi-Bickel syndrome (227810)	Glucose transporter-2	GLUT2 (3q26)*	**Onset:** Infancy **Clinical features:** Failure to thrive, abdominal distention, hepatomegaly, renomegaly, mild fasting hypoglycemia and hyperlipidemia, glucose intolerance, renal Fanconi syndrome **Treatment:** Diet similar to that for diabetes, replacement of renally lost electrolytes, vitamin D
Fructose 1,6-biphosphatase deficiency (229700)	Fructose 1,6-biphosphatase	FBP1 (9q22)*	**Onset:** Infancy or early childhood **Clinical features:** Episodic hyperventilation, apnea, hypoglycemia, ketosis, or lactic acidosis; episodes provoked by fasting, febrile infection, or ingestion of fructose, sorbitol, or glycerol **Treatment:** Avoidance of fasting and fructose, sorbitol, and glycerol; uncooked cornstarch
Phosphoenolpyruvate carboxykinase deficiency (261680)	Phosphoenolpyruvate carboxykinase	PCK1 (20q13.31)*	**Onset:** Childhood **Clinical features:** Failure to thrive, hypotonia, hepatomegaly, lactic acidosis, hypoglycemia **Treatment:** Avoidance of fasting, uncooked cornstarch

*Gene has been identified, and molecular basis has been elucidated.

G-CSF = granulocyte colony-stimulating factor; GSD = glycogen storage disease; OMIM = online mendelian inheritance in man (see the OMIM database at www.ncbi.nlm.nih.gov/omim).

There is no clearly effective treatment for pyruvate dehydrogenase deficiency, although a low-carbohydrate or ketogenic diet and dietary thiamin supplementation have been beneficial for some patients.

Pyruvate carboxylase deficiency: Pyruvate carboxylase is an enzyme important for gluconeogenesis from pyruvate and alanine generated in muscle. Deficiency may be primary, or secondary to deficiency of holocarboxylase synthetase, biotin, or biotinidase; inheritance for both is autosomal recessive, and both result in lactic acidosis.

Primary deficiency incidence is < 1/250,000 births but may be higher in certain American Indian populations. Psychomotor retardation with seizures and spasticity are the major clinical manifestations. Laboratory abnormalities include hyperammonemia; lactic acidosis; ketoacidosis; elevated levels of plasma lysine, citrulline, alanine, and proline; and increased excretion of α-ketoglutarate.

Secondary deficiency is clinically similar, with failure to thrive, seizures, and other organic acidurias.

Diagnosis of pyruvate carboxylase deficiency is confirmed by enzyme analysis of cultured skin fibroblasts or DNA analysis.

There is no effective treatment for pyruvate carboxylase deficiency, but some patients with primary deficiency and all those with secondary deficiencies should be given biotin supplementation 5 to 20 mg po once/day.

OTHER CARBOHYDRATE METABOLISM DISORDERS

See also Table 315–13.

Phosphoenolpyruvate carboxykinase deficiency impairs gluconeogenesis and results in symptoms and signs similar to the hepatic forms of GSD but without hepatic glycogen accumulation.

Other deficiencies include those of glycolytic enzymes or enzymes in the pentose phosphate pathway. Common examples are pyruvate kinase deficiency (see p. 1106) and glucose-6-phosphate dehydrogenase (G6PD) deficiency, both of which may result in hemolytic anemia. Wernicke-Korsakoff syndrome is caused by a partial deficiency of transketolase, which is an enzyme for the pentose phosphate pathway that requires thiamin as a cofactor.

OVERVIEW OF FATTY ACID AND GLYCEROL METABOLISM DISORDERS

Fatty acids are the preferred energy source for the heart and an important energy source for skeletal muscle during prolonged exertion. Also, during fasting, the bulk of the body's energy needs must be supplied by fat metabolism. Using fat as an energy source requires catabolizing adipose tissue into free fatty acid and glycerol. The free fatty acid is metabolized in the liver and peripheral tissue via β-oxidation into acetyl CoA; the glycerol is used by the liver for triglyceride synthesis or for gluconeogenesis. Carnitine is required for long-chain fatty acid oxidation. Carnitine deficiencies can be primary or secondary. Secondary carnitine deficiency is a secondary biochemical feature of many organic acidemias and fatty acid oxidation defects.

There are a number of other disorders of fatty acid and glycerol metabolism, including those involving

- Fatty acid transport and mitochondrial oxidation
- Glycerol
- Ketones (see Table 315–14)
- Peroxisome biogenesis and VLCFA
- Other disorders of fat metabolism (see Table 315–15)

BETA-OXIDATION CYCLE DISORDERS

In these processes, there are numerous inherited defects, which typically manifest during fasting with hypoglycemia and acidosis; some cause cardiomyopathy and muscle weakness.

Table 315–14. KETONE METABOLISM DISORDERS

DISEASE (OMIM NUMBER)	DEFECTIVE PROTEINS OR ENZYMES	DEFECTIVE GENE OR GENES (CHROMOSOMAL LOCATION)	COMMENTS
3-Hydroxy-3-methylglutaryl-CoA synthase deficiency (605911)	3-Hydroxy-3-methylglutaryl-CoA synthase	HMGCS2 (600234)	**Biochemical profile:** See below **Clinical features:** Episodic nonketotic hypoglycemia **Treatment:** Avoidance of fasting
3-Hydroxy-3-methylglutaryl-CoA lyase deficiency	See Table 315–9 on p. 2652	—	—
Succinyl-CoA 3-oxoacid-CoA transferase deficiency (245050)	Succinyl-CoA 3-oxoacid-CoA transferase	OXCT (5p13)*	**Biochemical profile:** Ketonuria **Clinical features:** Severe episodic ketoacidosis, vomiting, hyperventilation **Treatment:** Glucose during acute episode plus judicious use of bicarbonate, high-carbohydrate diet with some restriction of protein and fat
Mitochondrial acetoacetyl-CoA thiolase deficiency (607809)	See Table 315–9 on p. 2652	—	—
Cytoplasmic aceto-acetyl-CoA thiolase deficiency (100678)	Cytoplasmic acetoacetyl-CoA thiolase	ACAT2 (6q25.3-q26)	**Biochemical profile:** Nonspecific **Clinical features:** Intellectual disability, hypotonia **Treatment:** Not established

*Gene has been identified, and molecular basis has been elucidated.
OMIM = online mendelian inheritance in man (see the OMIM database at www.ncbi.nlm.nih.gov/omim).

Table 315–15. OTHER FAT METABOLISM DISORDERS

DISEASE (OMIM NUMBER)	DEFECTIVE PROTEINS OR ENZYMES	DEFECTIVE GENE OR GENES (CHROMOSOMAL LOCATION)	COMMENTS
Sjögren-Larsson syndrome (270200)	Fatty aldehyde dehydrogenase	ALDH3A2 (17p11.2)*	**Biochemical profile:** No readily detectable plasma or urinary abnormality **Clinical features:** Ichthyosis, intellectual disability, spastic diplegia or tetraplegia, retinopathy, seizures **Treatment:** Symptomatic; topical keratolytics or systemic retinoids, reduced long-chain fat and increased medium-chain triglycerides in diet

*Gene has been identified, and molecular basis has been elucidated.
OMIM = online mendelian inheritance in man (see the OMIM database at www.ncbi.nlm.nih.gov/omim.).

Beta-oxidation cycle disorders are among the fatty acid and glycerol metabolism disorders.

Acetyl CoA is generated from fatty acids through repeated beta-oxidation cycles. Sets of 4 enzymes (an acyl dehydrogenase, a hydratase, a hydroxyacyl dehydrogenase, and a lyase) specific for different chain lengths (very long chain, long chain, medium chain, and short chain) are required to catabolize a long-chain fatty acid completely (see Table 315–16). Inheritance for all fatty acid oxidation defects is autosomal recessive.

Medium-chain acyl-CoA dehydrogenase deficiency (MCADD): This deficiency is the most common defect in the β-oxidation cycle and has been incorporated into expanded neonatal screening in many states.

Clinical manifestations typically begin after 2 to 3 mo of age and usually follow fasting (as little as 12 h). Patients have vomiting and lethargy that may progress rapidly to seizures, coma, and sometimes death (which can also appear as SIDS). During attacks, patients have hypoglycemia, hyperammonemia, and unexpectedly low urinary and serum ketones. Metabolic acidosis is often present but may be a late manifestation.

Diagnosis of MCADD is by detecting medium-chain fatty acid conjugates of carnitine in plasma or glycine in urine or by detecting enzyme deficiency in cultured fibroblasts; however, DNA testing can confirm most cases.

Treatment of acute attacks is with 10% dextrose IV at 1.5 times the fluid maintenance rate (see p. 2556); some clinicians also advocate carnitine supplementation during acute episodes. Prevention is a low-fat, high-carbohydrate diet and avoidance of prolonged fasting. Cornstarch therapy is often used to provide a margin of safety during overnight fasting.

Long-chain 3-hydroxyacyl-CoA dehydrogenase deficiency (LCHADD): This deficiency is the 2nd most common fatty acid oxidation defect. It shares many features of MCADD, but patients may also have cardiomyopathy; rhabdomyolysis, massive creatine kinase elevations, and myoglobinuria with muscle exertion; peripheral neuropathy; and abnormal liver function. Mothers with an LCHADD fetus often have HELLP syndrome (hemolysis, elevated liver function tests, and low platelet count) during pregnancy.

Diagnosis of LCHADD is based on the presence of excess long-chain hydroxy acids on organic acid analysis and on the presence of their carnitine conjugates in an acylcarnitine profile or glycine conjugates in an acylglycine profile. LCHADD can be confirmed by enzyme study in skin fibroblasts.

Treatment during acute exacerbations includes hydration, high-dose glucose, bed rest, urine alkalinization, and carnitine supplementation. Long-term treatment includes a high-carbohydrate diet, medium-chain triglyceride supplementation, and avoidance of fasting and strenuous exercise.

Very long-chain acyl-CoA dehydrogenase deficiency (VLCADD): This deficiency is similar to LCHADD but is commonly associated with significant cardiomyopathy.

Table 315–16. FATTY ACID TRANSPORT AND MITOCHONDRIAL OXIDATION DISORDERS

DISEASE (OMIM NUMBER)	DEFECTIVE PROTEINS OR ENZYMES	DEFECTIVE GENE OR GENES (CHROMOSOMAL LOCATION)	COMMENTS
Systemic primary carnitine deficiency (212140)	Plasma membrane carnitine transport OCTN2	SLC22A5 (5q31.1)*	**Biochemical profile:** High urinary carnitine excretion despite very low plasma carnitine, absence of significant dicarboxylic aciduria **Clinical features:** Hypoketotic hypoglycemia, fasting intolerance with hypotonia, depressed CNS, apnea, seizures, dilated cardiomyopathy, developmental delay **Treatment:** L-Carnitine
Long-chain fatty acid transport deficiency (603376)	—	—	**Biochemical profile:** Low to normal free carnitine; during acute episodes, elevated plasma C8–C18 acylcarnitine esters **Clinical features:** Episodic acute liver failure, hyperammonemia, encephalopathy **Treatment:** Liver transplantation

Table 315–16. FATTY ACID TRANSPORT AND MITOCHONDRIAL OXIDATION DISORDERS (*Continued*)

DISEASE (OMIM NUMBER)	DEFECTIVE PROTEINS OR ENZYMES	DEFECTIVE GENE OR GENES (CHROMOSOMAL LOCATION)	COMMENTS
Carnitine palmitoyl transferase I (CPT-I) deficiency (255120)	CPT-I	CPT1A (11q13)*	**Biochemical profile:** Normal to elevated total and free plasma carnitine, no dicarboxylic aciduria **Clinical features:** Fasting intolerance, hypoketotic hypoglycemia, hepatomegaly, seizures, coma, elevated creatine kinase **Treatment:** Avoidance of fasting; frequent feeding; during acute episodes, high-dose glucose; replacement of long-chain dietary fat with medium-chain fat
Carnitine/acylcarnitine translocase deficiency (212138)	Carnitine/ acylcarnitine translocase	SLC25A20 (3p21.31)*	**Biochemical profile:** Low total plasma carnitine, with most conjugated to long-chain fatty acids; elevated C16 carnitine ester **Clinical features:** In the neonatal form, fasting intolerance with hypoglycemic coma, vomiting, weakness, cardiomyopathy, arrhythmia, mild hyperammonemia In the mild form, recurrent hypoglycemia with no cardiac involvement **Treatment:** Avoidance of fasting; frequent feeding; if plasma level is low, carnitine; during acute episodes, high-dose glucose
Carnitine palmitoyl transferase II (CPT-II) deficiency (255100, 600649, 608836)	CPT-II	CPTII (1p32)*	**Biochemical profile:** Elevated C16 carnitine ester In the classical muscle form, carnitine usually normal In the severe form, low total plasma carnitine, with most conjugated to long-chain fatty acids **Clinical features:** In the classical muscle form, presentation in adulthood with episodic myoglobinuria and weakness after prolonged exercise, fasting, intercurrent illness, or stress In the severe form, presentation in neonatal period or infancy with hypoketotic hypoglycemia, cardiomyopathy, arrhythmia, hepatomegaly, coma, or seizures **Treatment:** Avoidance of fasting; frequent feeding; if plasma level is low, carnitine; during acute episodes, high-dose glucose
Very long-chain acyl-CoA dehydrogenase (VLCAD) deficiency (201475)	VLCAD	ACADVL (17p12-p11.1)*	**Biochemical profile:** Elevated saturated and unsaturated C14–C18 acylcarnitine esters, elevated urinary C6–C14 dicarboxylic acids **Clinical features:** In the VLCAD-C type, arrhythmia, hypertrophic cardiomyopathy, sudden death In the VLCAD-H type, recurrent hypoketotic hypoglycemia, encephalopathy, mild acidosis, mild hepatomegaly, hyperammonemia, elevated liver enzymes **Treatment:** Avoidance of fasting; high-carbohydrate diet; carnitine; medium-chain triglycerides; during acute episodes, high-dose glucose
Long-chain 3-hydroxyacyl-CoA dehydrogenase (LCHAD) deficiency (600890)	LCHAD	HADHA (2p23)*	**Biochemical profile:** Elevated saturated and unsaturated C16–C18 acylcarnitine esters, elevated urinary C6–C14 3-hydroxydicarboxylic acids **Clinical features:** Fasting-induced hypoketotic hypoglycemia, exercise-induced rhabdomyolysis, cardiomyopathy, cholestatic liver disease, retinopathy, maternal HELLP syndrome **Treatment:** Avoidance of fasting; high-carbohydrate diet; carnitine; medium-chain triglycerides; during acute episodes, high-dose glucose For retinopathy, docosahexanoic acid possibly useful

Table continues on the following page.

Table 315–16. FATTY ACID TRANSPORT AND MITOCHONDRIAL OXIDATION DISORDERS (*Continued*)

DISEASE (OMIM NUMBER)	DEFECTIVE PROTEINS OR ENZYMES	DEFECTIVE GENE OR GENES (CHROMOSOMAL LOCATION)	COMMENTS
Mitochondrial trifunctional protein (TFP) deficiency (609015)	Mitochondrial TFP α-Subunit β-Subunit	 HADHA (2p23)* HADHB (2p23)*	**Biochemical profile:** Similar to LCHAD deficiency **Clinical features:** Liver failure, cardiomyopathy, fasting hypoglycemia, myopathy, sudden death **Treatment:** Similar to that for LCHAD deficiency
Medium-chain acyl-CoA dehydrogenase (MCAD) deficiency (201450)	MCAD	ACADM (1p31)*	**Biochemical profile:** Elevated saturated and unsaturated C8–C10 acylcarnitine esters; elevated urinary C6–C10 dicarboxylic acids, suberylglycine, and hexanoylglycine; low free carnitine **Clinical features:** Episodic hypoketotic hypoglycemia after fasting, vomiting, hepatomegaly, lethargy, coma, acidosis, SIDS, Reye-like syndrome **Treatment:** Avoidance of fasting; frequent feeding, including bedtime snacks; high-carbohydrate diet; carnitine; during acute episodes, high-dose glucose
Short-chain acyl-CoA dehydrogenase (SCAD) deficiency (201470)	SCAD	ACADS (12q22-qter)*	**Biochemical profile:** In the neonatal form, intermittent ethylmalonic aciduria In the chronic form, low muscle carnitine **Clinical features:** In the neonatal form, neonatal acidosis, vomiting, growth and developmental delay In the chronic form, progressive myopathy **Treatment:** Avoidance of fasting
Glutaric aciduria type II (231680)	Electron transfer flavoprotein (ETF) α-Subunit β-Subunit ETF:ubiquinone oxidoreductase (ETF:QO)	— ETFA (15q23-q25)* ETFB (19q13.3)* ETFDH (4q32-qter)*	**Biochemical profile:** Elevated urinary ethylmalonic, glutaric, 2-hydroxyglutaric, 3-hydroxyisovaleric, and C6–C10 dicarboxylic acids and isovalerylglycine; elevated glutarylcarnitine, isovalerylcarnitine, and straight-chain acylcarnitine esters of C4, C8, C10, C10:1, and C12 fatty acids; low serum carnitine; increased serum sarcosine **Clinical features:** Fasting hypoketotic hypoglycemia, acidosis, sudden death, CNS anomalies, myopathy, possibly liver and cardiac involvement **Treatment:** Avoidance of fasting; frequent feeding; carnitine; riboflavin; during acute episodes, high-dose glucose
Short-chain 3-hydroxyacyl-CoA dehydrogenase (SCHAD) deficiency (601609)	SCHAD	HADHSC (4q22-q26)	**Biochemical profile:** Ketotic C8–C14 3-hydroxydicarboxylic aciduria **Clinical features:** Recurrent myoglobinuria, ketonuria, hypoglycemia, encephalopathy, cardiomyopathy **Treatment:** Avoidance of fasting
Short/medium-chain 3-hydroxyacyl-CoA dehydrogenase (S/MCHAD) deficiency	S/MCHAD	—	**Biochemical profile:** Marked elevation of MCHADs and acylcarnitines **Clinical features:** Liver failure, encephalopathy **Treatment:** Avoidance of fasting
Medium-chain 3-ketoacyl-CoA thiolase (MCKAT) deficiency (602199)	MCKAT		**Biochemical profile:** Lactic aciduria, ketosis, elevated urinary C4–C12 dicarboxylic aciduria (especially C10 and C12) **Clinical features:** Fasting intolerance, vomiting, dehydration, metabolic acidosis, liver dysfunction, rhabdomyolysis **Treatment:** Avoidance of fasting
2,4-Dienoyl-CoA reductase deficiency (222745)	2,4-Dienoyl-CoA reductase	DECR1 (8q21.3)*	**Biochemical profile:** Hyperlysinemia, low plasma carnitine, 2-trans,4-cis decadienoylcarnitine in plasma and urine **Clinical features:** Neonatal hypotonia, respiratory acidosis **Treatment:** Not established

*Gene has been identified, and molecular basis has been elucidated.
HELLP = hemolysis, elevated liver enzymes, and low platelet count; OMIM = online mendelian inheritance in man (see the OMIM database at www.ncbi.nlm.nih.gov/omim).

Glutaric acidemia type II: A defect in the transfer of electrons from the coenzyme of fatty acyl dehydrogenases to the electronic transport chain affects reactions involving fatty acids of all chain lengths (multiple acyl-coA dehydrogenase deficiency); oxidation of several amino acids is also affected.

Clinical manifestations thus include fasting hypoglycemia, severe metabolic acidosis, and hyperammonemia.

Diagnosis of glutaric acidemia type II is by increased ethylmalonic, glutaric, 2- and 3-hydroxyglutaric, and other dicarboxylic acids in organic acid analysis, and glutaryl and isovaleryl and other acylcarnitines in tandem mass spectrometry studies. Enzyme deficiencies in skin fibroblasts can be confirmatory.

Treatment of glutaric acidemia type II is similar to that for MCADD, except that riboflavin may be effective in some patients.

GLYCEROL METABOLISM DISORDERS

Glycerol is converted to glycerol-3-phosphate by the hepatic enzyme glycerol kinase; deficiency results in episodic vomiting, lethargy, and hypotonia.

Glycerol metabolism disorders (see Table 315–17) are among the fatty acid and glycerol metabolism disorders.

Glycerol kinase deficiency is X-linked; many patients with this deficiency also have a chromosomal deletion that extends beyond the glycerol kinase gene into the contiguous gene region, which contains the genes for congenital adrenal hypoplasia and Duchenne muscular dystrophy. Thus, patients with glycerol kinase deficiency may have one or more of these disease entities.

Symptoms of glycerol metabolism disorders begin at any age and are usually accompanied by acidosis, hypoglycemia, and elevated blood and urine levels of glycerol.

Diagnosis of glycerol metabolism disorders is by detecting an elevated level of glycerol in serum and urine and is confirmed by DNA analysis.

Glycerol metabolism disorder treatment is with a low-fat diet, but glucocorticoid replacement is critical for patients with adrenal hypoplasia.

OVERVIEW OF LYSOSOMAL STORAGE DISORDERS

Lysosomal enzymes break down macromolecules, either those from the cell itself (eg, when cellular structural components are being recycled) or those acquired outside the cell. Inherited defects or deficiencies of lysosomal enzymes (or other lysosomal components) can result in accumulation of undegraded metabolites. Because there are numerous specific deficiencies, storage diseases are usually grouped biochemically by the accumulated metabolite. Subgroups include

- Mucopolysaccharidoses
- Sphingolipidoses (lipidoses)
- Mucolipidoses

The most important are the mucopolysaccharidoses and sphingolipidoses. Type 2 glycogenosis is a lysosomal storage disorder, but most glycogenoses are not.

Because reticuloendothelial cells (eg, in the spleen) are rich in lysosomes, reticuloendothelial tissues are involved in a number of lysosomal storage disorders, but, generally, tissues richest in the substrate are most affected. Thus the brain, which is rich in gangliosides, is particularly affected by gangliosidoses, whereas mucopolysaccharidoses affect many tissues because mucopolysaccharides are present throughout the body.

Mucopolysaccharidoses (MPS): MPS are inherited deficiencies of enzymes involved in glycosaminoglycan breakdown. Glycosaminoglycans (previously termed mucopolysaccharides) are polysaccharides abundant on cell surfaces and in extracellular matrix and structures. Enzyme deficiencies that prevent glycosaminoglycan breakdown cause accumulation of glycosaminoglycan fragments in lysosomes and cause extensive bone, soft tissue, and CNS changes. Inheritance is usually autosomal recessive (except for MPS type II).

Table 315–17. GLYCEROL METABOLISM DISORDERS

DISEASE (OMIM NUMBER)	DEFECTIVE PROTEINS OR ENZYMES	DEFECTIVE GENE OR GENES (CHROMOSOMAL LOCATION)	COMMENTS
Glycerol kinase deficiency (307030)	Glycerol kinase	GK (xp21.3-p21.2)* (Complex form: Deletion of the *GK* gene and contiguous genes including congenital adrenal hypoplasia, Duchenne muscular dystrophy, or both Juvenile and adult forms: Isolated *GK* gene mutation)	**Biochemical profile:** Hyperglycerolemia **Clinical features:** In the complex form, symptoms of the juvenile form, in addition to those due to the specific gene or genes deleted In the juvenile form, episodic vomiting, acidosis, hypotonia, CNS depression, Reye-like syndrome In the adult form, pseudohypertriglyceridemia **Treatment:** Low-fat diet, avoidance of prolonged fasting
Glycerol intolerance syndrome	—	—	**Biochemical profile:** Hypoglycemia, ketonuria, reports of decreased activity of fructose-1,6-biphosphatase and increased sensitivity of this enzyme to the inhibition of glycerol-3-phosphate **Clinical features:** History of prematurity; after exposure to glycerol, hypoglycemia, lethargy, sweating, seizure, coma **Treatment:** Low-fat diet

*Gene has been identified, and molecular basis has been elucidated.
OMIM = online mendelian inheritance in man (see the OMIM database at www.ncbi.nlm.nih.gov/omim).

Age at presentation, clinical manifestations, and severity vary by type (see Table 315–18). Common manifestations include coarse facial features, neurodevelopmental delays and regression, joint contractures, organomegaly, stiff hair, progressive respiratory insufficiency (caused by airway obstruction and sleep apnea), cardiac valvular disease, skeletal changes, and cervical vertebral subluxation.

Diagnosis of MPS is suggested by history, physical examination, bone abnormalities (eg, dysostosis multiplex) found during skeletal survey, and elevated total and fractionated urinary glycosaminoglycans. Diagnosis is confirmed by enzyme analysis of cultured fibroblasts (prenatal) or peripheral WBCs (postnatal). Additional testing is required to monitor organ-specific changes (eg, echocardiography for valvular disease, audiometry for hearing changes).

Treatment of MPS type I (Hurler disease) is enzyme replacement with α-l-iduronidase, which effectively halts progression and reverses all non-CNS complications of the disease. Hematopoietic stem cell (HSC) transplantation has also been used. The combination of enzyme replacement and HSC transplantation is under study. For patients with MPS type IV-A (Morquio A syndrome), enzyme replacement with elosulfase alfa may improve functional status, including mobility.

Sphingolipidoses: Sphingolipids are normal lipid components of cell membranes; they accumulate in lysosomes and cause extensive neuronal, bone, and other changes when enzyme deficiencies prevent their breakdown. Although incidence is low, carrier rate of some forms is high.

There are many types of sphingolipidosis (see Table 315–19); the **most common sphingolipidosis** is

- Gaucher disease

Other sphingolipidoses include

- Cholesteryl ester storage disease
- Fabry disease
- Krabbe disease
- Metachromatic leukodystrophy
- Niemann-Pick disease
- Sandhoff disease
- Tay-Sachs disease
- Wolman disease

Mucolipidoses and other lysosomal disorders: In addition to mucolipidoses, there are many other lysosomal disorders including (see Table 315–20)

- Other lipidoses (see Table 315–21)
- Oligosaccharidosis and related disorders (see Table 315–22)
- Lysosomal transport defects (see Table 315–23)
- Other lysosomal disorders (see Table 315–24)

CHOLESTERYL ESTER STORAGE DISEASE AND WOLMAN DISEASE

Cholesteryl ester storage disease and Wolman disease are sphingolipidoses, an inherited disorder of metabolism, caused by lysosomal acid lipase deficiency resulting in hyperlipidemia and hepatomegaly.

For more information, see Tables 315–19 and 315–21.

These diseases are rare, autosomal recessive disorders that result in accumulation of cholesteryl esters and triglycerides, mainly in lysosomes of histiocytes, resulting in foam cells in the liver, spleen, lymph nodes, and other tissues. Serum low-density lipoprotein (LDL) is usually elevated.

Wolman disease is the more severe form, manifesting in the first weeks of life with poor feeding, vomiting, and abdominal distention secondary to hepatosplenomegaly; infants usually die within 6 mo.

Cholesteryl ester storage disease is less severe and may not manifest until later in life, even adulthood, at which time hepatomegaly may be detected; premature atherosclerosis, often severe, may develop.

Diagnosis is based on clinical features and detection of acid lipase deficiency in liver biopsy specimens or cultured skin fibroblasts, lymphocytes, or other tissues. Prenatal diagnosis is based on the absence of acid lipase activity in cultured chorionic villi.

There is no proven treatment, but statins reduce plasma LDL levels, and cholestyramine combined with a low-cholesterol diet has reportedly alleviated other signs.

Table 315–18. MUCOPOLYSACCHARIDOSIS (MPS)

DISEASE (OMIM NUMBER)	DEFECTIVE PROTEINS OR ENZYMES	DEFECTIVE GENE OR GENES (CHROMOSOMAL LOCATION)	COMMENTS
MPS I-H (Hurler syndrome; 607014) MPS I-S (Scheie syndrome; 607016) MPS I H/S (Hurler-Scheie syndrome; 607015)	α-l-Iduronidase	IDUA (4p16.3)*	**Onset:** In I-H, 1st yr In I-S, > 5 yr In I-H/S, 3–8 yr **Urine metabolites:** Dermatan sulfate, heparin sulfate **Clinical features:** Corneal clouding, stiff joints, contractures, dysostosis multiplex, coarse facies, coarse hair, macroglossia, organomegaly, intellectual disability with regression, valvular heart disease, hearing and vision impairment, inguinal and umbilical hernia, sleep apnea, hydrocephalus **Treatment:** Supportive care, enzyme replacement, stem cell or bone marrow transplantation

Table 315–18. MUCOPOLYSACCHARIDOSIS (MPS) (*Continued*)

DISEASE (OMIM NUMBER)	DEFECTIVE PROTEINS OR ENZYMES	DEFECTIVE GENE OR GENES (CHROMOSOMAL LOCATION)	COMMENTS
MPS II (Hunter syndrome; 309900)	Iduronate sulfate sulfatase	IDS (Xq28)*	**Onset:** 2–4 yr **Urine metabolites:** Dermatan sulfate, heparin sulfate **Clinical features:** Similar to Hurler syndrome but milder and no corneal clouding In mild form, normal intelligence In severe form, progressive intellectual and physical disability, death before age 15 **Treatment:** Supportive care, stem cell or bone marrow transplantation
MPS III (Sanfilippo syndrome)			**Onset:** 2–6 yr **Urine metabolites:** Heparin sulfate **Clinical features:** Similar to Hurler syndrome but with severe intellectual disability and mild somatic manifestations **Treatment:** Supportive care
Type III-A (252900)	Heparan-S-sulfate sulfamidase	SGSH (17q25.3)*	
Type III-B (252920)	*N*-acetyl-D-glucosaminidase	NAGLU (17q21)*	
Type III-C (252930)	Acetyl-CoA-glucosaminide *N*-acetyltransferase	(14)	
Type III-D (252940)	*N*-acetyl-glucosaminine-6-sulfate sulfatase	GNS (12q14)*	
MPS IV (Morquio syndrome			**Onset:** 1–4 yr **Urine metabolites:** Keratin sulfate; in IV-B, also chondroitin 6-sulfate **Clinical features:** Similar to Hurler syndrome but with severe bone changes including odontoid hypoplasia; possibly normal intelligence **Treatment:** Supportive care For type IV-A, enzyme replacement therapy with elosulfase alfa
Type IV-A (253000)	Galactosamine-6-sulfate sulfatase	GALNS (16q24.3)*	
Type IV-B (253010)	β-Galactosidase	GLB1 (3p21.33*—see also GM1 gangliosidosis in Table 315–19)	
MPS VI (Maroteaux-Lamy syndrome; 253200)	*N*-Acetyl galactosamine α-4-sulfate sulfatase (arylsulfatase B)	ARSB (5q11-q13)*	**Onset:** Variable but can be similar to Hurler syndrome **Urine metabolites:** Dermatan sulfate **Clinical features:** Similar to Hurler syndrome but normal intelligence **Treatment:** Supportive care
MPS VII (Sly syndrome; 253220)	β-Glucuronidase	GUSB (7q21.11)*	**Onset:** 1–4 yr **Urine metabolites:** Dermatan sulfate, heparin sulfate, chondroitin 4-, 6-sulfate **Clinical features:** Similar to Hurler syndrome but greater variation in severity **Treatment:** Supportive care, stem cell or bone marrow transplantation
MPS IX (hyaluronidase deficiency; 601492)	Hyaluronidase deficiency	HYAL1 (3p21.3-p21.2)*	**Onset:** 6 mo **Urine metabolites:** None **Clinical features:** Bilateral soft-tissue periarticular masses, dysmorphic features, short stature, normal intelligence **Treatment:** Not established

*Gene has been identified, and molecular basis has been elucidated.
OMIM = online mendelian inheritance in man (see the OMIM database at www.ncbi.nlm.nih.gov/omim).

Table 315–19. SPHINGOLIPIDOSIS

DISEASE (OMIM NUMBER)	DEFECTIVE PROTEINS OR ENZYMES	DEFECTIVE GENE OR GENES (CHROMOSOMAL LOCATION)	COMMENTS
GM1 gangliosidosis, generalized	Ganglioside β-galactosidase	GLB1 (3p21.33*; allelic to MPS IVB)	—
Type I (230500)			**Type I onset:** 0–6 mo **Urine metabolites:** None **Clinical features:** Coarse facies; clear cornea, cherry-red macular spot, gingival hyperplasia, organomegaly, dysostosis multiplex, hypertrichosis, angiokeratoma corporis diffusum, cerebral degeneration; death in infancy **Treatment:** Supportive care
Type II (juvenile type; 230600)			**Type II onset:** 6–12 mo **Urine metabolites:** None **Clinical features:** Gait disturbance, spasticity, dystonia, loss of psychomotor milestones, mild visceromegaly and bone abnormality **Treatment:** Supportive care
Type III (adult type; 230650)			**Type III onset:** 3–50 yr **Urine metabolites:** None **Clinical features:** Angiokeratoma corporis diffusum, spondyloepiphyseal dysplasia, dysarthria, cerebellar dysfunction; no macular red spots or visceromegaly **Treatment:** Supportive care
GM2 gangliosidosis			**Onset:** In types I and II, 5–6 mo In type III, 2–6 yr **Urine metabolites:** None **Clinical features:** Doll-like facies; cherry-red retina; early blindness; exaggerated startle reflex; initial hypotonia followed by hypertonia; psychomotor retardation followed by regression, seizures, and impaired sweating; death by age 5 yr In type I, increased frequency in Ashkenazi Jews **Treatment:** Supportive care
Type I (Tay-Sachs disease; 272800)	β-Hexosaminidase A	HEXA (15q23-q24)*	
Type II (Sandhoff disease; 268800)	β-Hexosaminidase B	HEXB (5q13)*	
Type III (juvenile type)	β-Hexosaminidase A	—	
GM2 activator protein deficiency (Tay-Sachs disease AB variant, GM2A; 272750)	GM2 activator protein	GM2A (5q31.3-q33.1)*	**Treatment:** Supportive care, stem cell or bone marrow transplantation Same as that for GM2 types I and II
Niemann-Pick disease (see also Niemann-Pick disease types C and D in Table 315–21)	Sphingomyelinase	SMPD1 (11p15.4-p15.1)*	
Type A (257200)			**Onset:** < 6 mo **Clinical features:** Growth delay, cherry-red retina, frequent respiratory infections, hepatosplenomegaly, vomiting, constipation, osteoporosis, lymphadenopathy, hypotonia followed by spasticity, sea-blue histiocytes on tissue biopsies, large vacuolated foam cells in bone marrow (NP cells), death by age 3 yr **Treatment:** Supportive care, stem cell or bone marrow transplantation
Type B (607616)			**Onset:** Variable **Clinical features:** Much milder symptoms, no neurologic involvement, survival to adulthood Increased frequency in Ashkenazi Jews **Treatment:** Supportive care, stem cell or bone marrow transplantation

Table 315–19. SPHINGOLIPIDOSIS (*Continued*)

DISEASE (OMIM NUMBER)	DEFECTIVE PROTEINS OR ENZYMES	DEFECTIVE GENE OR GENES (CHROMOSOMAL LOCATION)	COMMENTS
Gaucher disease	Glucosylceramide β-glucosidase	GBA (1q21)*	
Type I (adult or chronic form; 230800)			**Onset:** Childhood or adolescence **Urine metabolites:** None **Clinical features:** Hepatosplenomegaly, osteolytic lesions with bone pain, avascular necrosis of the femoral head, vertebral compression, thrombocytopenia, anemia Increased frequency in Ashkenazi Jews **Treatment:** Supportive care Splenectomy Enzyme replacement (eliglustat) Bone marrow or stem cell transplantation
Type II (infantile form; 230900)			**Onset:** Infancy **Urine metabolites:** None **Clinical features:** Infantile hydrops, hepatosplenomegaly, dysphagia, bone lesions, hypertonicity, pseudobulbar palsy, laryngeal spasm, ichthyosis, developmental delay, hypersplenism, death by age 2 yr **Treatment:** Supportive care
Type III (juvenile form, Norrbottnian type; 231000)			**Onset:** 4–8 yr **Urine metabolites:** None **Clinical features:** Similar to type II except milder, possible survival into adulthood **Treatment:** Supportive care
Farber disease (lipogranulomatosis; 228000)	Ceramidase	ASAII (8p22-p21.3)*	**Onset:** First weeks of life **Urine metabolites:** Ceramide **Clinical features:** Lipogranulomatosis, periarticular subcutaneous nodules, irritability, hoarse cry, psychomotor and growth delay, respiratory insufficiency, histiocytosis in multiple tissues, nephropathy, hepatosplenomegaly, cherry-red macular spot Milder variants sometimes divided into 7 subtypes according to severity **Treatment:** Supportive care
Fabry disease (301500)	Trihexosylceramide α-galactosidase	GLA (Xq22)*	**Onset:** Childhood or adolescence **Urine metabolites:** Globosylceramide **Clinical features:** Painful crisis involving extremities and abdomen precipitated by stress, fatigue, or exercise; angiokeratoma; growth and pubertal delay; corneal dystrophy; renal failure; cardiomyopathy; MI and heart failure, hypertension; lymphedema; obstructive lung disease; strokes; seizures; death Generally, only males affected but occasionally females **Treatment:** Supportive care, enzyme replacement
Metachromatic leukodystrophy (250100) • Late infantile form • Juvenile form • Adult form • Pseudodeficiency form	Arylsulfatase A	ARSA (22q13.31)*	**Onset:** For late infantile form, 1–2 yr For juvenile form, 4 yr to puberty For adult form, any age after puberty **Urine metabolites:** Sulfatides **Clinical features:** Optic atrophy, gall bladder dysfunction, urinary incontinence, hypotonia, gait disturbance, hyporeflexia followed by hyperreflexia, bulbar palsies, ataxia, chorea, demyelination and developmental regression, increased CSF protein In adult form, also schizophrenia-like symptoms pseudodeficiency characterized by mild decrease in enzyme activity without neurologic degeneration **Treatment:** Supportive care, consideration of bone marrow or stem cell transplantation

Table continues on the following page.

Table 315–19. SPHINGOLIPIDOSIS (*Continued*)

DISEASE (OMIM NUMBER)	DEFECTIVE PROTEINS OR ENZYMES	DEFECTIVE GENE OR GENES (CHROMOSOMAL LOCATION)	COMMENTS
Mucosulfatidosis (multiple sulfatase deficiency; 272200)	Sulfatase-modifying factor-1	SUMF1 (3p26)*	**Onset:** Infancy **Urine metabolites:** Sulfatides, mucopolysaccharides **Clinical features:** Similar to late infantile form of metachromatic leukodystrophy, plus ichthyosis and dysostosis multiplex **Treatment:** Supportive care
Krabbe disease (245200) • Infantile form • Late infantile form • Juvenile form • Adult form	Galactosylceramide β-galactosidase	GALC (14q31)*	**Onset:** In infantile form, 3–6 mo In late infantile and juvenile forms, 15 mo–17 yr In adult form, variable Urine metabolites: None **Clinical features:** Growth delay, developmental delay followed by regression, deafness, blindness, vomiting, hyperirritability, hypersensitivity to stimuli, increased deep-tendon reflex, and spasticity; seizures; diffuse cerebral atrophy and demyelination; elevated CSF protein; peripheral neuropathy; episodic fever In adult form, mentation generally preserved **Treatment:** Supportive care, bone marrow or stem cell transplantation
Sphingolipid activator protein deficiencies			**Onset:** Infancy to early childhood **Urine metabolites:** Sulfatides **Clinical features:** In saposin B deficiency, features similar to those of metachromatic leukodystrophy In saposin C deficiency, features similar to those of Gaucher disease type III In prosaposin deficiency, features of saposin B and C deficiencies **Treatment:** Supportive care; consideration of bone marrow or stem cell transplantation; for features of Gaucher disease, consideration of enzyme replacement
Prosaposin deficiency (176801)	Prosaposin	PSAP (10q22.1)*	
Saposin B deficiency (sulfatide activator deficiency)	Saposin B	PSAP (10q22.1)*	
Saposin C deficiency (Gaucher activator deficiency)	Saposin C	PSAP (10q22.1)*	

*Gene has been identified, and molecular basis has been elucidated.

MPS = mucopolysaccharidosis; OMIM = online mendelian inheritance in man (see the OMIM database at www.ncbi.nlm.nih.gov/omim).

FABRY DISEASE

(Angiokeratoma Corporis Diffusum)

Fabry disease is a sphingolipidosis, an inherited disorder of metabolism, caused by deficiency of α-galactosidase A, which causes angiokeratomas, acroparesthesias, corneal opacities, recurrent febrile episodes, and renal or heart failure.

For more information, see Table 315–19.

Fabry disease is an X-linked deficiency of the lysosomal enzyme α-galactosidase A, which is needed for normal trihexosylceramide catabolism. Glycolipid (globotriaosylceramide) accumulates in many tissues (eg, vascular endothelium, lymph vessels, heart, kidney).

Diagnosis in males is clinical, based on appearance of typical skin lesions (angiokeratomas) over the lower trunk and by characteristic features of peripheral neuropathy (causing recurrent burning pain in the extremities), corneal opacities, and recurrent febrile episodes. Death results from renal failure or cardiac or cerebral complications of hypertension or other vascular disease. Heterozygous females are usually asymptomatic but may have an attenuated form of disease often characterized by corneal opacities.

Diagnosis of Fabry disease is by assay of galactosidase activity—prenatally in amniocytes or chorionic villi and postnatally in serum or WBCs.

Treatment of Fabry disease is enzyme replacement with recombinant α-galactosidase A (agalsidase beta) combined with supportive measures for fever and pain. Kidney transplantation is effective for treating renal failure.

GAUCHER DISEASE

Gaucher disease is a sphingolipidosis, an inherited disorder of metabolism, resulting from glucocerebrosidase deficiency, causing deposition of glucocerebroside and related compounds. Symptoms and signs vary by type but are most commonly hepatosplenomegaly or CNS changes. Diagnosis is by enzyme analysis of WBCs.

For more information, see Table 315–19.

Glucocerebrosidase normally hydrolyzes glucocerebroside to glucose and ceramide. Genetic defects of the enzyme cause glucocerebroside accumulation in tissue macrophages through phagocytosis, forming Gaucher cells. Accumulation of Gaucher

Table 315–20. MUCOLIPIDOSIS (ML)

DISEASE (OMIM NUMBER)	DEFECTIVE PROTEINS OR ENZYMES	DEFECTIVE GENE OR GENES (CHROMOSOMAL LOCATION)	COMMENTS
ML I	See Sialidosis type I in Table 315–22		
ML II (I-cell disease; 252500)	*N*-Acetylglucosaminyl-1-phosphotransfeerase catalytic subunit	GNPTA (4q21-q23)	**Onset:** 1st yr **Urine metabolites:** No mucopolysaccharides **Clinical features:** Similar to Hurler syndrome but more severe; presence of phase-dense inclusion bodies in fibroblasts (I-cells) **Treatment:** Supportive care
ML III (pseudo-Hurler polydystrophy)	N-acetylglucosaminyl-1-phosphotransfeerase		**Onset:** 2–4 yr **Urine metabolites:** None **Clinical features:** Similar to ML II but later onset and possible survival to adulthood **Treatment:** Supportive care
Type III-A (252600)	Catalytic subunit	GNPTA (4q21-q23)*	
Type III-C (252605)	Substrate-recognition subunit	GNPTAG (16p)*	
ML IV	See Sialolipidosis in Table 315–22	—	—

*Gene has been identified, and molecular basis has been elucidated.
OMIM = online mendelian inheritance in man (see the OMIM database at www.ncbi.nlm.nih.gov/omim.).

cells in the perivascular spaces in the brain causes gliosis in the neuronopathic forms. There are 3 types, which vary in epidemiology, enzyme activity, and manifestations.

Type I (nonneuronopathic) is most common (90% of all patients). Residual enzyme activity is highest. Ashkenazi Jews are at greatest risk; 1/12 is a carrier. Onset ranges from age 2 yr to late adulthood. Symptoms and signs include splenohepatomegaly, bone disease (eg, osteopenia, pain crises, osteolytic lesions with fractures), growth failure, delayed puberty, ecchymoses, and pingueculae. Epistaxis and ecchymoses resulting from thrombocytopenia are common. X-rays show flaring of the ends of the long bones (Erlenmeyer flask deformity) and cortical thinning.

Type II (acute neuronopathic) is rarest, and residual enzyme activity in this type is lowest. Onset occurs during infancy. Symptoms and signs are progressive neurologic deterioration (eg, rigidity, seizures) and death by age 2 yr.

Type III (subacute neuronopathic) falls between types I and II in incidence, enzyme activity, and clinical severity. Onset occurs at any time during childhood. Clinical manifestations vary by subtype and include progressive dementia and ataxia (IIIa), bone and visceral involvement (IIIb), and supranuclear palsies with corneal opacities (IIIc). Patients who survive to adolescence may live for many years.

Diagnosis

- Enzyme analysis

Diagnosis of Gaucher disease is by enzyme analysis of WBCs. Carriers are detected, and types are distinguished by mutation analysis. Although biopsy is unnecessary, Gaucher cells—lipid-laden tissue macrophages in the liver, spleen, lymph nodes, bone marrow, or brain that have a wrinkled tissue-paper

Table 315–21. OTHER LIPIDOSES

DISEASE (OMIM NUMBER)	DEFECTIVE PROTEINS OR ENZYMES	DEFECTIVE GENE OR GENES (CHROMOSOMAL LOCATION)	COMMENTS
Niemann-Pick disease (see also Niemann-Pick disease, types A and B in Table 315–19)			**Onset:** Highly variable (early or late infancy, adolescence, adulthood) **Urine metabolites:** None **Clinical features:** Vertical gaze palsy, hepatosplenomegaly, neonatal jaundice, dysphagia, hypotonia followed by spasticity, seizures, cerebellar ataxia, dysarthria, psychomotor delay and degeneration, psychosis and behavioral problem, fetal ascites, foam cells and sea-blue histiocytes as in Niemann-Pick disease types A and B Earlier onset associated with faster progression and shorter lifespan **Treatment:** Supportive care
Type C1/Type D ((257220)	NPC1 protein	NPC1 (18q11-q12)*	
Type C2 (607625)	Epididymal secretory protein 1 (HE1; NPC2 protein)	NPC2 (14q24.3)*	

Table 315–21. OTHER LIPIDOSES (*Continued*)

DISEASE (OMIM NUMBER)	DEFECTIVE PROTEINS OR ENZYMES	DEFECTIVE GENE OR GENES (CHROMOSOMAL LOCATION)	COMMENTS
Lysosomal acid lipase deficiency (278000) • Wolman disease • Cholesteryl ester storage disease (CESD)	Lysosomal acid lipase	LIPA (10q24-q25)*	**Onset:** In Wolman disease, infancy In CESD, variable **Urine metabolites:** None **Clinical features:** Growth failure; vomiting; diarrhea; steatorrhea; hepatosplenomegaly; hepatic fibrosis; pulmonary hypertension; adrenal calcification; xanthomatous changes in liver, adrenal glands, lymph nodes, bone marrow, small intestine, lungs, and thymus; hypercholesterolemia and normal to elevated plasma lipids; foam cells in marrow In Wolman disease, death during infancy In CESD, premature atherosclerosis **Treatment:** Enzyme replacement with sebelipase, a new recombinant human lysosomal acid lipase For CESD, also statins plus a low-cholesterol diet helpful
Cerebrotendinous xanthomatosis (cholestanol lipidosis; 213700)	Sterol 27-hydroxylase	CYP27A (2q33-qter)*	**Onset:** Adolescence **Urine metabolites:** Elevated 7-α-hydroxylated bile alcohol **Clinical features:** Juvenile cataracts, tendon and skin xanthomas, xanthelasma, fractures, atherosclerosis, dementia, spinal cord paresis, cerebellar ataxia, developmental disability, pseudobulbar paralysis, leukodystrophy, peripheral neuropathy **Treatment:** Chenodeoxycholic acid, statins
Neuronal ceroid lipofuscinosis			**Onset:** In infantile form, 6–12 mo In late infantile form, 2–4 yr In juvenile forms (including CLN9), 4–10 yr In adult form, 20–39 yr In variant infantile forms, 4–7 yr In progressive epilepsy form, 5–10 yr **Urine metabolites:** None **Clinical features:** In infantile and late infantile forms, developmental delay, microcephaly, optic and cerebral atrophy, retinal degeneration, blindness, flexion contractures, hypotonia, ataxia, myoclonus, seizures, loss of speech, hyperexcitability, autofluorescence in neurons, granular osmiophilic deposits in cells, increased serum arachidonic acid, decreased linoleic acid In juvenile and adult forms, features of above forms plus extrapyramidal signs, progressive loss of walking ability, school and behavioral difficulties **Treatment:** Supportive care
Infantile form (CLN1, Santavuori-Haltia disease; 256730)	Palmitoyl-protein thioesterase-1	PPT1 (1p32)*	
Late infantile form (CLN2, Jansky-Bielschowsky disease; 204500)	Lysosomal pepstatin-insensitive peptidase	CLN2 (11p15.5)*	
Juvenile form (CLN3, Batten disease, Vogt-Spielmeyer disease; 204200)	Lysosomal transmembrane CLN3 protein	CLN3 (16p12.1)*	
Adult form (CLN4, Kufs disease; 204300)	Palmitoyl-protein thioesterase-1	PPT1 (1p32)*	
Variant late infantile form, Finnish type (CLN5; 256731)	Lysosomal transmembrane CLN5 protein	CLN5 (13q21-q32)*	
Variant late infantile form (CLN6; 601780)	Transmembrane CLN6 protein	CLN6 (15q21-q23)*	
Progressive epilepsy with intellectual disability (600143)	Transmembrane CLN8 protein	CLN8 (8pter-p22)*	
CLN9 (609055)	—	—	

*Gene has been identified, and molecular basis has been elucidated.
OMIM = online mendelian inheritance in man (see the OMIM database at www.ncbi.nlm.nih.gov/omim).

Table 315–22. OLIGOSACCHARIDOSIS AND RELATED DISORDERS

DISEASE (OMIM NUMBER)	DEFECTIVE PROTEINS OR ENZYMES	DEFECTIVE GENE OR GENES (CHROMOSOMAL LOCATION)	COMMENTS
Sialidosis (256550) Type I (cherry-red macular spot-myoclonus syndrome, mild form)	Neuraminidase 1 (sialidase)	NEU1 (6p21.3)*	**Onset:** 8–25 yr **Urine metabolites:** Increased sialyloligosaccharides **Clinical features:** Cherry-red macular spot, insidious vision loss, cataracts, progressive myoclonus and ataxia, normal intelligence, increased deep tendon reflex **Treatment:** Supportive care
Type II (congenital, infantile, juvenile, and childhood forms)			**Onset:** In congenital form, in utero In infantile form, birth to 12 mo In juvenile and childhood forms, 2–20 yr **Urine metabolites:** Increased sialyloligosaccharides **Clinical features:** All of features of type I plus coarse facies, hypotonia, hepatomegaly, ascites, inguinal hernia, growth delay, muscle wasting, laryngomalacia, dysostosis multiplex **Treatment:** Supportive care
Galactosialidosis (Goldberg syndrome, combined neuraminidase and β-galactosidase deficiency; 256540) • Neonatal form • Late infantile form • Juvenile/adult form	Protective protein/cathepsin A (PPCA)	PPGB (20q13.1)*	**Onset:** In neonatal form, birth to 3 mo In late infantile form, 1st mo In juvenile/adult form, adolescence but with wide variability **Urine metabolites:** Elevated sialyloligosaccharides but no free sialic acid **Clinical features:** Coarse facies, corneal clouding, cherry-red macular spot, intellectual disability, seizures, dysostosis multiplex, hearing loss, hemangiomas, valvular heart disease **Treatment:** Supportive care
Sialolipidosis (phospholipidosis; mucolipidosis IV, Berman disease; 252650)		MCOLN1 (19p13.3-p13.2)*	**Onset:** 1st yr **Urine metabolites:** No mucopolysaccharides **Clinical features:** Severe (Berman disease) and mild forms Developmental delay, corneal opacities, visual deficiency, strabismus, hypotonia, increased deep tendon reflexes; no radiographic skeletal abnormality, macrocephaly, or organomegaly **Treatment:** Supportive care
Mannosidosis α-Mannosidosis (248500), type I (severe) or II (mild)	α-D-Mannosidase	MAN2B1 (19cen-q12)*	**Onset:** In type I, 3–12 mo In type II, 1–4 yr **Urine metabolites:** Mannose-rich oligosaccharides **Clinical features:** Coarse facies, macrocephaly, macroglossia, cataracts, gingival hypertrophy, slight hepatosplenomegaly, dysostosis multiplex, hypotonia, hearing loss, bowed femur, pancytopenia, recurrent respiratory infections, immunodeficiency and autoimmunity, developmental disabilities **Treatment:** Supportive care, consideration of bone marrow or stem cell transplantation
β-Mannosidosis (248510)	β-D-Mannosidase	MANBA (4q22-q25)*	**Onset:** 1–6 yr **Urine metabolites:** Disaccharides, mannosyl-(1-4)-*N*-acetylglucosamine, heparin sulfate **Clinical features:** Coarse facies, deafness, delayed speech, hyperactivity, genital angiokeratoma, tortuous conjunctival vessels **Treatment:** Supportive care, consideration of bone marrow or stem cell transplantation

Table continues on the following page.

Table 315–22. OLIGOSACCHARIDOSIS AND RELATED DISORDERS (*Continued*)

DISEASE (OMIM NUMBER)	DEFECTIVE PROTEINS OR ENZYMES	DEFECTIVE GENE OR GENES (CHROMOSOMAL LOCATION)	COMMENTS
Fucosidosis (230000) • Type I (severe infantile form) • Type II (mild form)	α-L-Fucosidase	FUCA1 (1p34)*	**Onset:** In type I, 3–18 mo In type II, 1–2 yr **Urine metabolites:** Oligosaccharides **Clinical features:** Short stature, growth delay, coarse facies, macroglossia, cardiomegaly, recurrent respiratory infections, dysostosis multiplex, hernias, hepatosplenomegaly, angiokeratoma, anhidrosis and elevated sweat chloride, developmental disability, hypotonia changing to hypertonia, cerebral atrophy, seizures, spastic quadriplegia, vacuolated lymphocytes Most patients from Italy or southwestern US **Treatment:** Supportive care, consideration of bone marrow or stem cell transplantation
Aspartylglucosaminuria (208400)	*N*-Aspartylglucosaminidase	AGA (4q32-q33)*	**Onset:** 2–6 yr **Urine metabolites:** Aspartylglucosamine **Clinical features:** Growth delay, microcephaly, cataracts, coarse facies, macroglossia, mitral insufficiency, hepatomegaly, diarrhea, hernias, recurrent respiratory infections, macro-orchidism, mild dysostosis multiplex, angiokeratoma corporis diffusum, acne, developmental disabilities, hypotonia, spasticity, cerebral atrophy, seizures, speech delay, hoarse voice Increased frequency in Finnish populations **Treatment:** Supportive care, consideration of bone marrow or stem cell transplantation
Winchester syndrome (277950)	Metalloproteinase-2	MMP2 (16q13)*	**Onset:** Early infancy **Urine metabolites:** None **Clinical features:** Short stature, coarse facies, corneal opacities, gingival hyperplasia, joint contractures, osteoporosis, kyphoscoliosis, vertebral compression, carpotarsal osteolysis, ankylosis of small joints of feet, diffuse thickened skin, hyperpigmentation, hypertrichosis **Treatment:** Supportive care
Schindler disease Type I (infantile severe form; 609241)	*N*-Acetyl-galactosaminidase α-NAGA (22q13)*		**Onset:** 8–15 mo **Urine metabolites:** Oligosaccharides and O-linked sialopeptides **Clinical features:** Cortical blindness, optic atrophy, nystagmus, strabismus, osteopenia, joint contracture, muscular atrophy, developmental delay and regression, myoclonus, seizures, spasticity, hyperreflexia, decorticate posturing, neuraxonal dystrophy **Treatment:** Supportive care
Type II (Kanzaki disease, adult-onset form; 609242)			**Onset:** Adulthood **Urine metabolites:** Oligosaccharides and O-linked sialopeptides **Clinical features:** Coarse facies, deafness, conjunctival and retinal vascular tortuosity, angiokeratoma corporis diffusum, telangiectasia, lymphedema, mild intellectual impairment, peripheral axonal neuropathy **Treatment:** Supportive care

Table 315–22. OLIGOSACCHARIDOSIS AND RELATED DISORDERS (*Continued*)

DISEASE (OMIM NUMBER)	DEFECTIVE PROTEINS OR ENZYMES	DEFECTIVE GENE OR GENES (CHROMOSOMAL LOCATION)	COMMENTS
Type III (intermediate form; 609241)			**Onset:** Childhood **Urine metabolites:** Oligosaccharides and O-linked sialopeptides **Clinical features:** Intermediate between types I and II; variable and ranging from seizures and moderate psychomotor retardation to mild autistic features with speech and language delay **Treatment:** Supportive care
Congenital disorders of *N*-glycosylation, type I (pre-Golgi glycosylation defects)			**Onset:** Mostly infancy or childhood **Clinical features** (some or most of the following): Growth failure, prominent forehead with large ears, high-arched or cleft palate, strabismus, retinitis pigmentosa, pericardial effusion, cardiomyopathy, hepatomegaly, vomiting, diarrhea, liver fibrosis, primary ovarian failure, renal cysts, nephrosis, proximal tubulopathy, kyphosis, joint contractures, ectopic fat pads, orange-peel skin, muscle weakness, hypotonia, strokelike episodes, seizures, olivopontine hypoplasia, peripheral neuropathy, hypothyroidism, hyperinsulinism, factor XI deficiency, antithrombin III deficiency, thrombocytosis, decreased IgA and IgG, leukocyte adhesion defect (in type IIc), hypoalbuminemia, hypocholesterolemia, increased disialotransferrin and asialotransferrin bands when isoelectric focusing of serum transferrin is done **Treatment:** Supportive care
CDG Ia (solely neurologic and neurologic-multivisceral forms; 212065)	Phosphomannomutase-2	PMM2 (16p13.3-p13.2)*	
CDG Ib (602579)	Mannose (Man) phosphate (P) isomerase	MPI (15q22-qter)*	
CDG Ic (603147)	Dolicho-P-Glc:-Man9GlcNAc2-PP-dolichol glucosyltransferase	ALG6 (1p22.3)*	
CDG Id (601110)	Dolicho-P-Man:-Man5GlcNAc2-PP-dolichol mannosyltransferase	ALG3 (3q27)*	
CDG Ie (608799)	Dolichol-P-mannose synthase	DPM1 (20q13.31)*	
CDG If (609180)	Protein involved in mannose-P-dolichol utilization	MPUD1 (17p13.1-p12)*	
CDG Ig (607143)	Dolichyl-P-mannose:-Man-7-GlcNAc-2-PP-dolichyl-α-6-mannosyltransferase	ALG12 (22)*	
CDG Ih (608104)	Dolichyl-P-glucose: Glc-1-Man-9-GlcNAc-2-PP-dolichyl-α-3-glucosyltransferase	ALG8 (11pter-p15.5)*	
CDG Ii (607906)	α-1,3-Mannosyltransferase	ALG2 (9q22)*	
CDG Ij (608093)	UDP-GlcNAc: dolichyl-P NAcGlc phosphotransferase	DPAGT1 (11q23.3)*	
CDG Ik (608540)	β-1,4-Mannosyltransferase	ALG1 (16p13.3)*	
CDG Il (608776)	α-1,2-Mannosyltransferase	ALG9 (11q23)*	

Table continues on the following page.

Table 315–22. OLIGOSACCHARIDOSIS AND RELATED DISORDERS (*Continued*)

DISEASE (OMIM NUMBER)	DEFECTIVE PROTEINS OR ENZYMES	DEFECTIVE GENE OR GENES (CHROMOSOMAL LOCATION)	COMMENTS
Congenital disorders of *N*-glycosylation, type II (Golgi defects)			Same as for type I, except isoelectric focusing of serum transferrin shows increased monosialotransferrin, disialotransferrin, trisialotransferrin, and asialotransferrin bands For type IIb, normal pattern
CDG IIa (212066)	Mannosyl-α-1,6-glycoprotein-β-1,2-*N*-acetylglucosminyltransferase	MGAT2 (14q21)*	
CDG IIb (606056)	Glucosidase I	GCS1 (1p13-p12)*	
CDG IIc (Rambam-Hasharon syndrome; 266265	GDP-fucose transporter-1	FUCT1 (11p11.2)*	
CDG IId (607091)	β-1,4-Galactosyltransferase	B4GALT1 (9p13)*	
CDG IIe (608779)	Oligomeric Golgi complex-7	COG7 (16p)*	

*Gene has been identified, and molecular basis has been elucidated.
OMIM = online mendelian inheritance in man (see the OMIM database at www.ncbi.nlm.nih.gov/omim).

appearance—are diagnostic. DNA analysis is being done more and more frequently.

Treatment

- Types I and III: Enzyme replacement with glucocerebrosidase
- Sometimes miglustat, eliglustat, splenectomy, or stem cell or bone marrow transplantation

Enzyme replacement with IV glucocerebrosidase is effective in types I and III; there is no treatment for type II. The enzyme is modified for efficient delivery to lysosomes. Patients receiving enzyme replacement require routine Hb and platelet monitoring, routine assessment of spleen and liver volume by CT or MRI, and routine assessment of bone disease by skeletal survey, dual-energy x-ray absorptiometry scanning, or MRI.

Miglustat (100 mg po tid), a glucosylceramide synthase inhibitor, reduces glucocerebroside concentration (the substrate for glucocerebrosidase) and is an alternative for patients unable to receive enzyme replacement.

Eliglustat (84 mg po once/day or bid), another glucosylceramide synthase inhibitor, also reduces glucocerebroside concentration.

Splenectomy may be helpful for patients with anemia, leukopenia, or thrombocytopenia or when spleen size causes discomfort. Patients with anemia may also need blood transfusions.

Bone marrow transplantation or stem cell transplantation provides a definitive cure but is considered a last resort because of substantial morbidity and mortality.

KEY POINTS

- Gaucher disease is a sphingolipidosis resulting from glucocerebrosidase deficiency, causing deposition of glucocerebroside.
- There are 3 types, which vary in epidemiology, enzyme activity, and manifestations.
- Symptoms and signs vary by type but are most commonly hepatosplenomegaly or CNS changes.
- Diagnosis of Gaucher disease is by enzyme analysis of WBCs; carriers are detected, and types are distinguished by mutation analysis.
- Treatment for types I and III include enzyme replacement with glucocerebrosidase, and sometimes miglustat, eliglustat, splenectomy, or stem cell or bone marrow transplantation; there is no treatment for type II.

KRABBE DISEASE

(Galactosylceramide Lipidosis; Globoid Cell Leukodystrophy)

Krabbe disease is a sphingolipidosis, an inherited disorder of metabolism, that causes intellectual disability, paralysis, blindness, deafness, and pseudobulbar palsy, progressing to death.

For more information, see Table 315–19.

Krabbe disease is caused by an autosomal recessive galactocerebroside β-galactosidase deficiency.

It affects infants and is characterized by intellectual disability, paralysis, blindness, deafness, and pseudobulbar palsy, progressing to death.

Diagnosis of Krabbe disease is by detecting enzyme deficiency in WBCs or cultured skin fibroblasts.

Because bone marrow transplantation effectively delays onset of symptoms, prenatal testing or neonatal screening (routine in New York) is sometimes done.

METACHROMATIC LEUKODYSTROPHY

(Sulfatide Lipidosis)

Metachromatic leukodystrophy is a sphingolipidosis, an inherited disorder of metabolism, caused by arylsulfatase A deficiency, which causes progressive paralysis and dementia resulting in death by age 10 yr.

Table 315–23. LYSOSOMAL TRANSPORT DEFECTS

DISEASE (OMIM NUMBER)	DEFECTIVE PROTEINS OR ENZYMES	DEFECTIVE GENE OR GENES (CHROMOSOMAL LOCATION)	COMMENTS
Sialuria			
Infantile sialic acid storage disorder (269920)	Na phosphate cotransporter	SLC17A5 (6q14-q15)*	**Onset:** At birth **Urine metabolites:** Increased free sialic acid **Clinical features:** Growth failure, coarse facial features, dysostosis multiplex, nystagmus, ptosis, gingival hypertrophy, cardiomegaly, heart failure, hepatosplenomegaly, nephrosis, death at about age 1 yr **Treatment:** Supportive care
Finnish type (Salla disease; 604369)	Na phosphate cotransporter	SLC17A5 (6q14-q15)*	**Onset:** 6–9 mo **Urine metabolites:** Increased free sialic acid **Clinical features:** Growth failure, developmental disability, ataxia, hypotonia, hypotonia, spasticity, dyspraxia, dysarthria, seizures, gait problems, athetosis; increased frequency in Finland **Treatment:** Supportive care
French type (269921)	UDP-N-acetylglucosamine-2-epimerase/*N*-acetylmannosamine kinase	GNE (9p12-p11)*	**Onset:** Infancy to early childhood **Urine metabolites:** Increased free sialic acid **Clinical features:** Coarse facies with normal growth, developmental delay, sleep apnea, hypoplastic nipples, hepatosplenomegaly, inguinal hernias, generalized hirsutism, seizures **Treatment:** Supportive care
Neuronal ceroid lipofuscinosis (CLN3, CLN5, CLN6, CLN8)	see Table 315–21		
Cystinosis	Cystinosin (lysosomal cystine transporter)	CTNS (17p13)*	
Infantile nephropathic form (219800)			**Onset:** 1st yr **Urine metabolites:** Renal Fanconi syndrome **Clinical features:** Growth failure, frontal bossing, photophobia, peripheral retinopathy with decreased acuity, corneal crystals and erosion, rickets, hepatosplenomegaly, pancreatic insufficiency, renal calculi, renal failure, renal Fanconi syndrome, decreased sweating, myopathy, dysphagia, cerebral atrophy, normal intelligence but neurologic deterioration in long-term survivors Cystine accumulation throughout reticuloendothelial system, WBC, and cornea **Treatment:** Replacement therapy for Fanconi syndrome, renal transplant for failure, cysteamine orally or as eyedrops, growth hormone
Late-onset juvenile form (219900)			**Onset:** 12–15 yr **Urine metabolites:** Renal Fanconi syndrome **Clinical features:** Similar to infantile form but milder **Treatment:** Similar to that for infantile form
Adult non-nephropathic form (219750)			**Onset:** Early teens to adulthood **Urine metabolites:** Renal Fanconi syndrome **Clinical features:** Similar to infantile form but no renal disorders **Treatment:** Cysteamine orally or as eyedrops, growth hormone

*Gene has been identified, and molecular basis has been elucidated.
OMIM = online mendelian inheritance in man (see the OMIM database at www.ncbi.nlm.nih.gov/omim).

Table 315–24. OTHER LYSOSOMAL DISORDERS

DISEASE (OMIM NUMBER)	DEFECTIVE PROTEINS OR ENZYMES	DEFECTIVE GENE OR GENES (CHROMOSOMAL LOCATION)	COMMENTS
Pycnodysostosis (265800)	Cathepsin K	CTSK (1q21)*	**Onset:** Early childhood **Urine metabolites:** None **Clinical features:** Short stature, frontal and occipital prominence, delayed closure of anterior fontanel, micrognathia, narrow palate, delayed eruption and persistence of deciduous teeth, hypodontia, aplasia or hypoplasia of clavicles, osteosclerosis, susceptibility to fracture, scoliosis, spondylolysis, brachydactyly, grooved nails **Treatment:** Supportive care, growth hormone possibly helpful
Glutamyl ribose-5-phosphate storage disease (305920)	ADP-ribose protein hydrolase		**Onset:** 1st yr **Urine metabolites:** Proteinuria **Clinical features:** Coarse facies, hypotonia, muscle wasting and atrophy, loss of speech and vision, seizures, neurologic deterioration, optic atrophy, nephrosis, hypertension, renal failure, developmental disabilities **Treatment:** Supportive care
Glycogen storage disease type 2 (Pompe disease)	See Table 315–13 on p. 2665		

*Gene has been identified, and molecular basis has been elucidated.
OMIM = online mendelian inheritance in man (see the OMIM database at www.ncbi.nlm.nih.gov/omim).

For more information, see Table 315–19.

In metachromatic leukodystrophy, arylsulfatase A deficiency causes metachromatic lipids to accumulate in the white matter of the CNS, peripheral nerves, kidney, spleen, and other visceral organs; accumulation in the nervous system causes central and peripheral demyelination. Numerous mutations exist; patients vary in age at onset and speed of progression.

The **infantile form** is characterized by progressive paralysis and dementia usually beginning before age 4 yr and resulting in death about 5 yr after onset of symptoms.

The **juvenile form** manifests between 4 yr and 16 yr of age with gait disturbance, intellectual impairment, and findings of peripheral neuropathy. Contrary to the infantile form, deep tendon reflexes are usually brisk. There is also a milder adult form.

Diagnosis of metachromatic leukodystrophy is suggested clinically and by findings of decreased nerve conduction velocity; it is confirmed by detecting enzyme deficiency in WBCs or cultured skin fibroblasts.

There is no effective treatment for metachromatic leukodystrophy.

NIEMANN-PICK DISEASE

Niemann-Pick disease is a sphingolipidosis, an inherited disorder of metabolism, caused by deficient sphingomyelinase activity, resulting in accumulation of sphingomyelin (ceramide phosphorylcholine) in reticuloendothelial cells.

For more information, see Tables 315–19 and 315–21.

Niemann-Pick disease inheritance is autosomal recessive and appears most often in Ashkenazi Jews; 2 types, A and B, exist. Type C Niemann-Pick disease is an unrelated enzymatic defect involving abnormal cholesterol storage.

Children with **type A** have < 5% of normal sphingomyelinase activity. The disease is characterized by hepatosplenomegaly, failure to thrive, and rapidly progressive neurodegeneration. Death occurs by age 2 or 3 yr.

Patients with **type B** have sphingomyelinase activity within 5 to 10% of normal. Type B is more variable clinically than type A. Hepatosplenomegaly and lymphadenopathy may occur. Pancytopenia is common. Most patients with type B have little or no neurologic involvement and survive into adulthood; they may be clinically indistinguishable from those with type I Gaucher disease. In severe cases of type B, progressive pulmonary infiltrates cause major complications.

Diagnosis

- Prenatal screening
- WBC sphingomyelinase assay

Both types are usually suspected by history and examination, most notably hepatosplenomegaly. Diagnosis of Niemann-Pick disease can be confirmed by sphingomyelinase assay on WBCs and can be made prenatally by using amniocentesis or chorionic villus sampling. DNA tests can be done to diagnose carriers.

Treatment

- Possible bone marrow transplantation, stem cell transplantation, and enzyme replacement

Bone marrow transplantation, stem cell transplantation, and enzyme replacement are under investigation as potential treatment options.

TAY-SACHS DISEASE AND SANDHOFF DISEASE

Tay-Sachs disease and Sandhoff disease are sphingolipidoses, inherited disorders of metabolism, caused by hexosaminidase deficiency that causes severe neurologic symptoms and early death.

Gangliosides are complex sphingolipids present in the brain. There are 2 major forms, GM_1 and GM_2, both of which may be involved in lysosomal storage disorders; there are 2 main types of GM_2 gangliosidosis, each of which can be caused by numerous different mutations.

For more information, see Table 315–19.

Tay-Sachs disease: Deficiency of hexosaminidase A results in accumulation of GM_2 in the brain. Inheritance is autosomal recessive; the most common mutations are carried by 1/27 normal adults of Eastern European (Ashkenazi) Jewish origin, although other mutations cluster in some French-Canadian and Cajun populations.

Children with Tay-Sachs disease start missing developmental milestones after age 6 mo and develop progressive cognitive and motor deterioration resulting in seizures, intellectual disability, paralysis, and death by age 5 yr. A cherry-red macular spot is common.

Diagnosis of Tay-Sachs disease is clinical and can be confirmed by enzyme assay.

In the absence of effective treatment, management is focused on screening adults of childbearing age in high-risk populations to identify carriers (by way of enzyme activity and mutation testing) combined with genetic counseling.

Sandhoff disease: There is a combined hexosaminidase A and B deficiency. Clinical manifestations include progressive cerebral degeneration beginning at 6 mo, accompanied by blindness, cherry-red macular spot, and hyperacusis. It is almost indistinguishable from Tay-Sachs disease in course, diagnosis, and management, except that there is visceral involvement (hepatomegaly and bone change) and no ethnic association.

OVERVIEW OF PURINE AND PYRIMIDINE METABOLISM DISORDERS

Purines are key components of cellular energy systems (eg, ATP, NAD), signaling (eg, GTP, cAMP, cGMP), and, along with pyrimidines, RNA and DNA production. Purines and pyrimidines may be synthesized de novo or recycled by a salvage pathway from normal catabolism. The end product of complete catabolism of purines is uric acid; catabolism of pyrimidines produces citric acid cycle intermediates.

Purine and pyrimidine metabolism disorders include

- Purine catabolism disorders
- Purine nucleotide synthesis disorders
- Purine salvage disorders
- Pyrimidine metabolism disorders

PURINE CATABOLISM DISORDERS

Purines are key components of cellular energy systems (eg, ATP, NAD), signaling (eg, GTP, cAMP, cGMP), and, along with pyrimidines, RNA and DNA production. Purines and pyrimidines may be synthesized de novo or recycled by a salvage pathway from normal catabolism. The end product of complete catabolism of purines is uric acid.

Table 315–25. PURINE METABOLISM DISORDERS

DISEASE (OMIM NUMBER)	DEFECTIVE PROTEINS OR ENZYMES	DEFECTIVE GENE OR GENES (CHROMOSOMAL LOCATION)	COMMENTS
Ca pyrophosphate arthropathy (chondrocalcinosis-2; 118600)	Increased nucleoside triphosphate pyrophosphohydrolase	ANKH (5p15.2-p14.1)*	**Biochemical profile:** Ca pyrophosphate dihydrate crystals in joints **Clinical features:** Recurrent episodes of monoarticular or multiarticular arthritis **Treatment:** No clear treatment
Lesch-Nyhan syndrome (300322) • Classic form • Variant form	Hypoxanthine-guanine phosphoribosyltransferase	HPRT (Xq26-q27.2)*	**Biochemical profile:** Hyperuricemia, hyperuricosuria **Clinical features:** Orange sandy crystals in diapers, growth failure, uric acid nephropathy and arthropathy, motor delay, hypotonia, self-injurious behavior, spasticity, hyperreflexia, extrapyramidal signs with choreoathetosis, dysarthria, dysphagia, developmental disabilities, megaloblastic anemia In variant form, no self-injurious behavior **Treatment:** Supportive care, protective measures, allopurinol, benzodiazepines, certain experimental approaches
Increased activity of phosphoribosylpyrophosphate synthetase (311850)	Phosphoribosylpyrophosphate synthetase	PRPS1 (Xq22-q24)*	**Biochemical profile:** Hyperuricemia **Clinical features:** Megaloblastic bone marrow, ataxia, hypotonia, hypertonia, psychomotor delay, polyneuropathy, cardiomyopathy, heart failure, uric acid nephropathy and arthropathy, diabetes mellitus, intracerebral calcification **Treatment:** Allopurinol, anti-inflammatory drugs, colchicines, probenecid, sulfinpyrazone

Table 315–25. PURINE METABOLISM DISORDERS (*Continued*)

DISEASE (OMIM NUMBER)	DEFECTIVE PROTEINS OR ENZYMES	DEFECTIVE GENE OR GENES (CHROMOSOMAL LOCATION)	COMMENTS
Phosphoribosylpyrophosphate synthetase deficiency (311850)	Phosphoribosylpyrophosphate synthetase	PRPS1 (Xq22-q24) PRPS2 (Xp22.3-p22.2)	**Biochemical profile:** Increased urinary orotate, hypouricemia **Clinical features:** Developmental disabilities, seizures with hypsarrhythmia, megaloblastic bone marrow **Treatment:** ACTH
Hereditary xanthinuria			**Biochemical profile:** Xanthinuria, hypouricemia, hypouricosuria **Clinical features:** Xanthine stones, nephropathy, myopathy **Treatment:** High fluid intake; low-purine diet
Type I (278300)	Xanthine dehydrogenase	XDH (2p23-p22)*	
Type II (603592)	Xanthine dehydrogenase and aldehyde oxidase		
Adenine phosphoribosyltransferase deficiency (102600)	Adenine phosphoribosyltransferase	APRT (16q24.3)*	**Biochemical profile:** Urinary 2,8-dihydroxyadenine **Clinical features:** Urolithiasis, nephropathy, round yellow-brown urine crystals **Treatment:** High fluid intake, low-purine diet, avoidance of dietary alkalis, renal transplantation
Type I	No enzyme activity		
Type II	Residual enzyme activity		
Adenosine deaminase deficiency (102700)	Adenosine deaminase	ADA (20q13.11)*	**Biochemical profile:** Elevated serum adenosine and 2′-deoxyadenosine **Clinical features:** Growth failure, skeletal changes, recurrent infections, severe combined immunodeficiency, B-cell lymphoma, hemolytic anemia, idiopathic thrombocytopenia, hepatosplenomegaly, mesangial sclerosis **Treatment:** Supportive care, enzyme replacement, bone marrow or stem cell transplantation, experimental gene therapy
Increased adenosine deaminase (102730)	Adenosine deaminase	ADA	**Biochemical profile:** Mild hyperuricemia **Clinical features:** Hemolytic anemia with aniso-poikilocytosis and stomatocytosis **Treatment:** Deoxycoformycin
Purine nucleoside phosphorylase deficiency (164050)	Purine nucleoside phosphorylase	NP (14q13.1)*	**Biochemical profile:** Hypouricemia; hypouricosuria; high serum inosine and guanine; high urinary inosine, 2′-deoxyinosine, and 2′-deodyguanosine **Clinical features:** Growth failure, cellular immunodeficiency, recurrent infections, hepatosplenomegaly, cerebral vasculitis, spastic diplegia, tetraparesis, ataxia, tremors, hypotonia, hypertonia, developmental disabilities, autoimmune hemolytic anemia, idiopathic thrombocytopenia, lymphoma, lymphosarcoma **Treatment:** Supportive care, stem cell transplantation
Myoadenylate deaminase deficiency (adenosine monophosphate deaminase I; 102770)	Myoadenylate deaminase	AMPD1 (1p21-p13)*	**Biochemical profile:** No specific change **Clinical features:** Neonatal weakness and hypotonia; exercise-induced weakness or cramping; after exercise, decreased purine release and low increase in serum ammonia (relative to lactate) **Treatment:** Ribose or xylitol
Adenylate kinase deficiency (103000)	Adenylate kinase	AK1 (9q34.1)*	**Biochemical profile:** No specific change **Clinical features:** Hemolytic anemia **Treatment:** Supportive care
Adenylosuccinate lyase deficiency (103050) • Type I (severe form) • Type II (mild form)	Adenylosuccinate lyase	ADSL (22Q13.1)*	**Biochemical profile:** Elevated succinyladenosine and succinylaminoimidazole carboxamide ribotides in body fluids **Clinical features:** Autism, severe psychomotor delay, seizures, growth delay, muscle wasting **Treatment:** Supportive care, adenine, and ribose

*Gene has been identified, and molecular basis has been elucidated.
OMIM = online mendelian inheritance in man (see the OMIM database at www.ncbi.nlm.nih.gov/omim).

In addition to purine catabolism disorders, purine metabolism disorders (see Table 315–25) include

- Purine nucleotide synthesis disorders
- Purine salvage disorders

Myoadenylate deaminase deficiency (or muscle adenosine monophosphate deaminase deficiency): The enzyme myoadenylate deaminase converts AMP to inosine and ammonia. Deficiency may be asymptomatic or it may cause exercise-induced myalgias or cramping; expression seems to be variable because, despite the high frequency of the mutant allele (10 to 14%), the frequency of the muscle phenotype is quite low in patients homozygous for the mutant allele. When symptomatic patients exercise, they do not accumulate ammonia or inosine monophosphate as do unaffected people; this is how the disorder is diagnosed.

Treatment of myoadenylate deaminase deficiency is exercise modulation as appropriate.

Adenosine deaminase deficiency: Adenosine deaminase converts adenosine and deoxyadenosine to inosine and deoxyinosine, which are further broken down and excreted. Enzyme deficiency (from 1 of > 60 known mutations) results in accumulation of adenosine, which is converted to its ribonucleotide and deoxyribonucleotide (dATP) forms by cellular kinases. The dATP increase results in inhibition of ribonucleotide reductase and underproduction of other deoxyribonucleotides. DNA replication is compromised as a result. Immune cells are especially sensitive to this defect; adenosine deaminase deficiency causes one form of severe combined immunodeficiency.

Diagnosis of adenosine deaminase deficiency is by low RBC and WBC enzyme activity.

Treatment of adenosine deaminase deficiency is by bone marrow or stem cell transplantation and enzyme replacement therapy. Somatic cell gene therapy is being evaluated as well.

Purine nucleoside phosphorylase deficiency: This rare, autosomal recessive deficiency is characterized by immunodeficiency with severe T-cell dysfunction and often neurologic symptoms. Manifestations are lymphopenia, thymic deficiency, recurrent infections, and hypouricemia. Many patients have developmental delay, ataxia, or spasticity.

Diagnosis of purine nucleoside phosphorylase deficiency is by low enzyme activity in RBCs.

Treatment is with bone marrow or stem cell transplantation.

Xanthine oxidase deficiency: Xanthine oxidase is the enzyme that catalyzes uric acid production from xanthine and hypoxanthine. Deficiency causes buildup of xanthine, which may precipitate in the urine, causing symptomatic stones with hematuria, urinary colic, and UTIs.

Diagnosis of xanthine oxidase deficiency is by low serum uric acid and high urine and plasma hypoxanthine and xanthine. Enzyme determination requires liver or intestinal mucosal biopsy and is rarely indicated.

Treatment of xanthine oxidase deficiency is high fluid intake to minimize likelihood of stone formation and allopurinol in some patients.

PURINE NUCLEOTIDE SYNTHESIS DISORDERS

Purines are key components of cellular energy systems (eg, ATP, NAD), signaling (eg, GTP, cAMP, cGMP), and, along with pyrimidines, RNA and DNA production. Purines may be synthesized de novo or recycled by a salvage pathway from normal catabolism. The end product of complete catabolism of purines is uric acid.

In addition to purine nucleotide synthesis disorders, purine metabolism disorders (see Table 315–25) include

- Purine catabolism disorders
- Purine salvage disorders

Phosphoribosylpyrophosphate synthetase superactivity: This X-linked, recessive disorder causes purine overproduction. Excess purine is degraded, resulting in hyperuricemia and gout and neurologic and developmental abnormalities.

Diagnosis of phosphoribosylpyrophosphate synthetase superactivity is by enzyme studies on RBCs and cultured skin fibroblasts.

Phosphoribosylpyrophosphate synthetase superactivity treatment is with allopurinol and a low-purine diet.

Adenylosuccinase deficiency: This autosomal recessive disorder causes profound intellectual disability, autistic behavior, and seizures.

Diagnosis of adenylosuccinase deficiency is by identifying elevated levels of succinylaminoimidazole carboxamide riboside and succinyladenosine in CSF and urine.

There is no effective treatment for adenylosuccinase deficiency.

PURINE SALVAGE DISORDERS

Purines are key components of cellular energy systems (eg, ATP, NAD), signaling (eg, GTP, cAMP, cGMP), and, along with pyrimidines, RNA and DNA production. Purines may be synthesized de novo or recycled by a salvage pathway from normal catabolism. The end product of complete catabolism of purines is uric acid.

In addition to purine salvage disorders, purine metabolism disorders (see Table 315–25) include

- Purine catabolism disorders
- Purine nucleotide synthesis disorders

Lesch-Nyhan syndrome: This is a rare, X-linked, recessive disorder caused by deficiency of hypoxanthine-guanine phosphoribosyl transferase (HPRT); degree of deficiency (and hence manifestations) vary with the specific mutation. HPRT deficiency results in failure of the salvage pathway for hypoxanthine and guanine. These purines are instead degraded to uric acid. Additionally, a decrease in inositol monophosphate and guanosyl monophosphate leads to an increase in conversion of 5-phosphoribosyl-1-pyrophosphate (PRPP) to 5-phosphoribosylamine, which further exacerbates uric acid overproduction. Hyperuricemia predisposes to gout and its complications. Patients also have a number of cognitive and behavioral dysfunctions, etiology of which is unclear; they do not seem related to uric acid.

The disease usually manifests between 3 mo and 12 mo of age with the appearance of orange sandy precipitate (xanthine) in the urine; it progresses to CNS involvement with intellectual disability, spastic cerebral palsy, involuntary movements, and self-mutilating behavior (particularly biting). Later, chronic hyperuricemia causes symptoms of gout (eg, urolithiasis, nephropathy, gouty arthritis, tophi).

Diagnosis of Lesch-Nyhan syndrome is suggested by the combination of dystonia, intellectual disability, and self-mutilation. Serum uric acid levels are usually elevated, but confirmation by HPRT enzyme assay is usually done.

CNS dysfunction has no known treatment; management is supportive. Self-mutilation may require physical restraint, dental extraction, and sometimes drug therapy; a variety of drugs has been used. Hyperuricemia is treated with a low-purine diet (eg, avoiding organ meats, beans, sardines) and allopurinol, a xanthine oxidase inhibitor (the last enzyme in the purine catabolic pathway). Allopurinol prevents conversion of accumulated hypoxanthine to uric acid; because hypoxanthine is highly soluble, it is excreted.

Adenine phosphoribosyltransferase deficiency: This is a rare autosomal recessive disorder that results in the inability to salvage adenine for purine synthesis. Accumulated adenine is oxidized to 2,8-dihyroxyadenine, which precipitates in the urinary tract, causing problems similar to those of uric acid nephropathy (eg, renal colic, frequent infections, and, if diagnosed late, renal failure). Onset can occur at any age.

Diagnosis of adenine phosphoribosyltransferase deficiency is by detecting elevated levels of 2, 8-dihyroxyadenine, 8-hyroxyadenine, and adenine in urine and confirmed by enzyme assay; serum uric acid is normal.

Treatment of adenine phosphoribosyltransferase deficiency is with dietary purine restriction, high fluid intake, and avoidance of urine alkalinization. Allopurinol can prevent oxidation of adenine; renal transplantation may be needed for end-stage renal disease.

Table 315–26. PYRIMIDINE METABOLISM DISORDERS

DISEASE (OMIM NUMBER)	DEFECTIVE PROTEINS OR ENZYMES	DEFECTIVE GENE OR GENES (CHROMOSOMAL LOCATION)	COMMENTS
Hereditary orotic aciduria			**Biochemical profile:** Elevated urinary orotate **Clinical features:** Megaloblastic anemia, recurrent infections, cellular immunodeficiency, developmental disabilities **Treatment:** Uridine, uridylic and cytidylic acid
Type I (258900)	UMP synthase (orotidine-5′-pyrophosphorylase and decarboxylase)	UMPS (3q13)*	
Type II (258920)	Orotidine-5′-decarboxylase	—	
Dihydropyrimidine dehydrogenase deficiency (274270) • Inborn error form • Pharmacogenetic form	Dihydropyrimidine dehydrogenase	DPYD (1p22)*	**Biochemical profile:** Elevated urinary uracil, thymine, and 5-hydroxymethyluracil **Clinical features:** In inborn error form, growth and deve`lopmental delay, seizures, spasticity, microcephaly In pharmacogenetic form, adverse reactions to 5-flurouracil, including myelosuppression, neurotoxicity, GI and skin symptoms, death **Treatment:** No specific treatment except for withdrawal of offending drug
Dihydropyrimidinuria (222748)	Dihydropyrimidinase	DPYS (8q22)*	**Biochemical profile:** Elevated urinary dihydrouracil and dihydrothymine **Clinical features:** Variable; feeding problems, seizures, lethargy, somnolence, metabolic acidosis Sometimes benign **Treatment:** Not established
β-Ureido propionase deficiency (210100)	β-Ureido propionase (β-alanine synthase)	UPB1 (22q11.2)	**Biochemical profile:** Elevated urinary ureidopropionate and ureidobutyrate **Clinical features:** Microcephaly, developmental delay, dystonia, scoliosis **Treatment:** Not established
Pyrimidine 5′nucleotidase deficiency (266120)	5′-Monophosphate hydrolase	NT5C3 (7p15-p14)*	**Biochemical profile:** No specific profile **Clinical features:** Hemolytic anemia, basophilic stippling **Treatment:** Supportive care
Activation-induced cytidine deaminase deficiency (hyper IgM syndrome type II; 605257)	Activation-induced cytidine deaminase	AICDA (12p13)*	**Biochemical profile:** High IgM, low to absent IgG and IgA **Clinical features:** Recurrent bacterial infections, defective Ig class switching **Treatment:** Control of infections

*Gene has been identified, and molecular basis has been elucidated.
OMIM = online mendelian inheritance in man (see the OMIM database at www.ncbi.nlm.nih.gov/omim).

PYRIMIDINE METABOLISM DISORDERS

Pyrimidines may be synthesized de novo or recycled by a salvage pathway from normal catabolism. The catabolism of pyrimidines produces citric acid cycle intermediates. There are several disorders of pyrimidine metabolism (see Table 315–26).

Uridine monophosphate synthase deficiency (hereditary orotic aciduria): Uridine monophosphate is the enzyme that catalyzes orotate phosphoribosyltransferase and orotidine-5′-monophosphate decarboxylase reactions. With deficiency, orotic acid accumulates, causing clinical manifestations of megaloblastic anemia, orotic crystalluria and nephropathy, cardiac malformations, strabismus, and recurrent infections.

Diagnosis of uridine monophosphate synthase deficiency is by enzyme assay in a variety of tissues.

Treatment of uridine monophosphate synthase deficiency is with oral uridine supplementation.

316 Inherited Muscular Disorders

Muscular dystrophies are inherited, progressive muscle disorders resulting from defects in one or more genes needed for normal muscle structure and function. Facioscapulohumeral dystrophy is the most common form of muscular dystrophy, and Duchenne dystrophy is the second most common and most severe form. Becker dystrophy, although closely related to Duchenne, has a later onset and causes milder symptoms.

Other forms include Emery-Dreifuss dystrophy, myotonic dystrophy, limb-girdle dystrophy, oculopharyngeal muscular dystrophy, and congenital dystrophies.

Muscular dystrophies are distinguished by the selective distribution of weakness and the specific nature of the genetic abnormality involved.

Other inherited muscular disorders include congenital myopathies and familial periodic paralysis.

Inherited metabolic disorders affecting the muscles, such as mitochondrial oxidative phosphorylation disorders and glycogen storage diseases, are discussed elsewhere. Only those disorders that have all or most of their effects on muscle are discussed in this chapter.

DUCHENNE MUSCULAR DYSTROPHY AND BECKER MUSCULAR DYSTROPHY

Duchenne muscular dystrophy and Becker muscular dystrophy are X-linked recessive disorders characterized by progressive proximal muscle weakness caused by muscle fiber degeneration. Becker dystrophy has later onset and causes milder symptoms. Diagnosis is suggested clinically and is confirmed by analysis of the protein product (dystrophin) of the mutated gene. Treatment focuses on maintaining function through physical therapy and the use of braces and orthotics. Patients who have Duchenne dystrophy should be offered prednisone or deflazacort.

Duchenne dystrophy and Becker dystrophy are the second most prevalent muscular dystrophy. They are caused by mutations of the *dystrophin* gene, the largest known human gene, at the Xp21.2 locus. In Duchenne dystrophy, this mutation results in the severe absence (< 5%) of dystrophin, a protein in the muscle cell membrane. In Becker dystrophy, the mutation results in production of abnormal dystrophin or insufficient dystrophin.

Duchenne dystrophy and Becker dystrophy together affect 5/1000 people; the majority have Duchenne. Female carriers may have asymptomatic elevated CK levels and possibly calf hypertrophy.

Symptoms and Signs

Duchenne dystrophy: This disorder manifests typically between ages 2 yr and 3 yr. Weakness affects proximal muscles, typically in the lower limbs initially. Children frequently toe walk and have a waddling gait and lordosis. They have difficulty running, jumping, climbing stairs, and rising from the floor. Children fall frequently, often causing arm or leg fractures (in about 20% of patients). Progression of weakness is steady, and limb flexion contractures and scoliosis develop in nearly all children. Firm pseudohypertrophy (fatty and fibrous replacement of certain enlarged muscle groups, notably the calves) develops. Most children are confined to a wheelchair by age 12 and die of respiratory complications by age 20.

Consequences of cardiac muscle involvement include dilated cardiomyopathy, conduction abnormalities, and arrhythmias. Such complications occur in about one third of patients by age 14 and in all patients over age 18; however, because these patients are not able to exercise, cardiac involvement is usually asymptomatic until late in the disease. About one third have mild, nonprogressive intellectual impairment that affects verbal ability more than performance.

Becker dystrophy: This disorder typically becomes symptomatic much later and is milder. Ambulation is usually preserved until at least age 15, and many children remain ambulatory into adulthood. Most affected children survive into their 30s and 40s.

Diagnosis

- Muscle biopsy with immunostaining analysis of dystrophin
- DNA mutation analysis

Diagnosis is suspected by characteristic clinical findings, age at onset, and family history suggestive of X-linked recessive inheritance. Myopathic changes are noted on electromyography (rapidly recruited, short duration, low-amplitude motor unit potentials) and muscle biopsy (necrosis and marked variation in muscle fiber size not segregated by motor unit). CK levels are elevated up to 100 times normal.

Diagnosis is confirmed by analysis of dystrophin with immunostaining of biopsy samples. Dystrophin is undetectable in patients with Duchenne dystrophy. In patients with Becker dystrophy, dystrophin is typically abnormal (lower molecular weight) or present in low concentration. Mutation analysis of DNA from peripheral blood leukocytes can also confirm the diagnosis by identifying abnormalities in the *dystrophin* gene (deletions in about 70% of patients with Duchenne dystrophy and 85% of patients with Becker dystrophy; duplications in about 10% of both groups).

Patients with Duchenne dystrophy should have a baseline assessment of cardiac function with ECG and echocardiography at the time of diagnosis or by age 6 yr.

Carrier detection and prenatal diagnosis are possible by using conventional studies (eg, pedigree analysis, CK determinations, fetal sex determination) combined with recombinant DNA analysis and dystrophin immunostaining of muscle tissue.

Treatment

- Supportive measures
- Sometimes prednisone or deflazacort
- Sometimes, for cardiomyopathy, an ACE inhibitor and/or beta-blocker
- Sometimes corrective surgery

No specific treatment exists. Gentle (ie, submaximal) active exercise is encouraged for as long as possible to avoid disuse atrophy or complications of inactivity. Passive exercises may extend the period of ambulation. Orthopedic interventions should be aimed at maintaining function and preventing contractures. Ankle-foot orthoses worn during sleep may help prevent flexion contractures. Leg braces may temporarily help preserve ambulation or standing. Corrective surgery is sometimes needed, particularly for scoliosis. Obesity should be avoided; caloric requirements are likely to be less than normal because of decreased physical activity.

Respiratory insufficiency may be treated with noninvasive ventilatory support (eg, nasal mask—see p. 567). Elective tracheotomy is gaining acceptance, allowing children with Duchenne dystrophy to live into their 20s.

For children with dilated cardiomyopathy, an ACE inhibitor and/or a beta-blocker may help prevent or slow progression.

In Duchenne dystrophy, daily prednisone or deflazacort is considered for patients > age 5 yr who are no longer gaining or have declining motor skills. These drugs start working as early as 10 days after initiation of therapy; efficacy peaks at 3 mo and persists for 6 mo. Long-term use improves strength, delays the age at which ambulation is lost by 1.4 to 2.5 yr, improves timed function testing (a measurement of how fast a child completes a functional task, such as walking or getting up from the floor), improves pulmonary function, reduces orthopedic complications (eg, the need for scoliosis surgery), stabilizes cardiac function (eg, delays onset of cardiomyopathy until 18 yr of age), and increases survival by 5 to 15 yr.[1] Alternate-day prednisone is not effective. Weight gain and cushingoid facies are common adverse effects after 6 to 18 mo. Risk of vertebral compression and long bone fractures also is increased. Deflazacort may be associated with a greater risk of cataracts than prednisone.

Use of prednisone or deflazacort in Becker dystrophy has not been adequately studied.

Gene therapy is not yet available. Genetic counseling is indicated.

1. Gloss D, Moxley RT 3rd, Ashwal S, Oskoui M: Practice guideline update summary: Corticosteroid treatment of Duchenne muscular dystrophy: Report of the Guideline Development Subcommittee of the American Academy of Neurology. *Neurology* 86:465–472, 2016. doi: 10.1212/WNL.0000000000002337.

KEY POINTS

- Duchenne dystrophy and Becker dystrophy are X-linked recessive disorders that cause a decrease in dystrophin, a protein in muscle cell membranes.
- Patients have significant, progressive weakness that causes severe disability, including difficulty walking, frequent falls, dilated cardiomyopathy, and early death due to respiratory insufficiency.
- Active and passive exercise is helpful, along with leg braces and ankle-foot orthoses.
- In Duchenne dystrophy, daily prednisone or deflazacort can improve muscle strength and mass, improve pulmonary function, and help delay onset of cardiomyopathy, although adverse effects are common.
- An ACE inhibitor and/or a beta-blocker may help prevent or slow progression of cardiomyopathy.
- Ventilatory support (noninvasive and, later on, invasive) can help prolong life.

OTHER FORMS OF MUSCULAR DYSTROPHY

Congenital Muscular Dystrophy

Congenital muscular dystrophy is not a single disorder but instead refers to muscular dystrophy evident at birth, occurring from any of several rare forms of muscular dystrophy. All such dystrophies are genetically recessive and result from mutations in a variety of different genes including those that encode for structural proteins of the basal membrane or the extracellular matrix of skeletal muscle fibers.

The diagnosis of congenital muscular dystrophy is suspected in any floppy neonate but must be distinguished from a congenital myopathy by muscle biopsy.

Treatment of congenital muscular dystrophy consists of supportive care including physical therapy, which may help preserve function.

Emery-Dreifuss Dystrophy

This disorder can be inherited as an autosomal dominant, autosomal recessive (the rarest), or X-linked recessive disorder. The overall incidence is unknown. Females can be carriers, but only males are affected clinically by X-linked inheritance. Genes associated with Emery-Dreifuss dystrophy encode for the nuclear membrane proteins lamin A/C (autosomal) and emerin (X-linked).

Symptoms and Signs

Muscle weakness and wasting can begin any time before age 20 and commonly affect the biceps and triceps and, less often, distal leg muscles. Early contractures are characteristic. The heart is frequently involved, with atrial paralysis, conduction abnormalities (atrioventricular block), cardiomyopathy, and a high likelihood of sudden death.

Diagnosis

- Muscle biopsy
- DNA mutation analysis

Diagnosis of Emery-Dreifuss dystrophy is indicated by clinical findings, age at onset, and family history. The diagnosis is supported by mildly increased serum CK levels and myopathic features on electromyography and muscle biopsy and is confirmed by DNA testing.

Treatment

- Therapy to prevent contractures

Treatment of Emery-Dreifuss dystrophy involves therapy to prevent contractures. Cardiac pacemakers are sometimes lifesaving in patients with abnormal conduction.

Facioscapulohumeral Muscular Dystrophy

Facioscapulohumeral muscular dystrophy (FSHMD) is the most prevalent type of muscular dystrophy and occurs in 7/1000 people vs 5/1000 people with Duchenne or Becker muscular dystrophy. It is an autosomal dominant disorder. In about 98% of patients, FSHMD is caused by a deletion on the long arm of chromosome 4, at the 4q35 locus. In about 10 to 33% of patients, the mutation is de novo (sporadic) rather than inherited.[1]

1. Tawil R, Kissel JT, Heatwole C, et al: Evidence-based guideline summary: Evaluation, diagnosis, and management of FSHMD: Report of the Guideline Development, Dissemination, and Implementation Subcommittee of the American Academy of Neurology and the Practice Issues Review Panel of the American Association of Neuromuscular & Electrodiagnostic Medicine. *Neurology* 85:357–364, 2015. doi: 10.1212/WNL.0000000000001783.

Symptoms and Signs

FSHMD is characterized by weakness of the facial muscles and shoulder girdle. Symptoms may develop in early childhood and are usually noticeable in the teenage years; 95% of cases manifest by age 20. Initial symptoms are slowly progressive and may include difficulty whistling, closing the eyes, and raising the arms (due to weakness of the scapular stabilizer muscles). Patients eventually notice a change in facial expression.

The course is variable. Many patients do not become disabled and have a normal life expectancy. Other patients are confined to a wheelchair in adulthood. An infantile variety, characterized by facial, shoulder, and hip-girdle weakness, is rapidly progressive, and disability is always severe. Nonmuscular symptoms frequently associated with this disorder include sensorineural hearing loss and retinal vascular abnormalities.

Diagnosis

- DNA mutation analysis

Diagnosis of FSHMD is indicated by characteristic clinical findings, age at onset, and family history and is confirmed by DNA testing.

Treatment

- Physical therapy

There is no treatment for the weakness, but physical therapy may help maintain function. Monitoring for retinal vascular abnormalities is essential to prevent blindness.

Limb-Girdle Dystrophy

Limb-girdle dystrophy at last count has 31 known subtypes, 23 autosomal recessive and 8 autosomal dominant. The overall incidence is estimated to be around 20 to 40/1,000,000. Males and females are affected equally.

Insights from molecular biology have redefined the way these disorders are classified. Autosomal dominant forms are classified as LGMD 1A, -1B, -1C, and so on, and recessive forms are classified as LGMD 2A, -2B, -2C, and so on. Several chromosomal loci have been identified for autosomal dominant (5q [no known gene product]) and recessive (2q, 4q [beta-sarcoglycan], 13q [gamma-sarcoglycan], 15q [calpain, a calcium-activated protease], and 17q [alpha-sarcoglycan or adhalin]) forms. Structural (eg, dystrophin-associated glycoproteins) or nonstructural (eg, proteases) proteins can be affected.

Symptoms and Signs

Patients typically present with slowly progressive, symmetric, proximal muscle weakness with or without facial involvement and diminished or absent tendon reflexes. The pelvic or the shoulder girdle muscles can be affected first. Onset of symptoms for autosomal dominant types ranges from early childhood to adulthood. Onset of symptoms for autosomal recessive types tends to be during childhood, and these types primarily have a pelvic-girdle distribution.

Diagnosis

- Muscle biopsy
- DNA mutation analysis

Diagnosis of limb-girdle dystrophy is indicated by characteristic clinical findings, age at onset, and family history and requires muscle histology, immunocytochemistry, Western blot analysis, and genetic testing for specific proteins.

Treatment

- Maintenance of function and prevention of contractures

Treatment of limb-girdle dystrophy focuses on maintaining function and preventing contractures. Guidelines issued by the American Academy of Neurology recommend that newly diagnosed LGMD patients at high risk of cardiac complications be referred for cardiac evaluation, even in the absence of cardiac symptoms. Those at high risk of respiratory failure should undergo pulmonary function testing. All LGMD patients should ideally be referred to a multi-specialty clinic with expertise in neuromuscular disorders.

There is currently no role for gene therapy, myoblast transplantation, neutralizing antibody to myostatin, or growth hormone other than in a research study.[2]

2. Narayanaswami P, Weiss M, Selcen D, et al: Evidence-based guideline summary: Diagnosis and treatment of limb-girdle and distal dystrophies: Report of the Guideline Development Subcommittee of the American Academy of Neurology and the Practice Issues Review Panel of the American Association of Neuromuscular & Electrodiagnostic Medicine. *Neurology* 83:1453–1463, 2014. doi: 10.1212/WNL.0000000000000892.

Myotonic Dystrophy

Myotonic dystrophy affects about 1/8000 in the general population. Inheritance is autosomal dominant with variable penetrance. Two genetic loci—DM 1 and DM 2—cause the abnormality.

Congenital myotonic dystrophy: Affected mothers and, rarely, fathers with DM 1 mutations may have offspring with a severe form of myotonia referred to as congenital myotonic dystrophy. This form is characterized by severe hypotonia (floppy infant), feeding and respiratory difficulties, skeletal deformities, facial weakness, and delayed psychomotor development. Up to 40% of infants do not survive, usually because of respiratory failure and perhaps cardiomyopathy. Up to 60% of survivors have intellectual disability.

Symptoms and Signs

Symptoms and signs of myotonic dystrophy begin during adolescence or young adulthood and include myotonia (delayed relaxation after muscle contraction), weakness and wasting of distal limb muscles (especially in the hand) and facial muscles (ptosis is especially common), and cardiomyopathy. Intellectual disability, cataracts, and endocrine disorders can also occur.

Death is most commonly due to respiratory and cardiac disease, and patients who develop cardiac arrhythmias and severe muscle weakness at a younger age are at increased risk of premature death. Mean age at death is 54 yr.

Diagnosis

- DNA mutation analysis

Diagnosis of myotonic dystrophy is indicated by characteristic clinical findings, age at onset, and family history and is confirmed by DNA testing.

Treatment

- Membrane-stabilizing drugs

Myotonia may respond to membrane-stabilizing drugs (eg, mexiletine, procainamide, quinidine, phenytoin, carbamazepine). Of these, mexiletine has been shown to significantly reduce myotonia in nondystrophic myotonia and is thus the first-line drug for myotonic dystrophy patients who have functionally limiting myotonia. Because mexiletine can rarely precipitate arrhythmias in patients with underlying ventricular arrhythmias, the drug is contraindicated in patients with 2nd- or 3rd-degree atrioventricular block; consultation with a cardiologist is recommended before initiating mexiletine therapy, particularly in those with an abnormal ECG.

However, it is weakness, for which no treatment is available, and not myotonia that usually disables the patient; braces for footdrop are usually required as the disease progresses.

CONGENITAL MYOPATHIES

Congenital myopathy is a term sometimes applied to hundreds of distinct neuromuscular disorders that may be present at birth, but it is usually reserved for a group of rare, inherited, primary muscle disorders that cause hypotonia and weakness at birth or during the neonatal period and, in some cases, delayed motor development later in childhood.

The 3 most common types of congenital myopathy, in order, are

- Central core and multiminicore myopathies (core myopathies)
- Centronuclear myopathy
- Nemaline myopathy

The types are distinguished primarily by their histologic features, symptoms, and prognosis.

Diagnosis of congenital myopathy is indicated by characteristic clinical findings and is confirmed by muscle biopsy.

Treatment of congenital myopathy is supportive and includes physical therapy, which may help preserve function.

Central core myopathy and multiminicore myopathy (core myopathies): Central core myopathy and multiminicore myopathy (core myopathies) are the most common form of congenital myopathy and are most commonly associated with RYR1 mutations. Inheritance is usually autosomal dominant, but recessive and sporadic forms exist. Core myopathies are characterized by regions (cores) on muscle biopsy specimens in which oxidative enzyme staining is absent; regions may be peripheral or central, focal, multiple, or extensive. Central core myopathy was the first congenital myopathy to be identified.

Most affected patients develop hypotonia and mild proximal muscle weakness as neonates, but sometimes symptoms of core myopathy do not manifest until adulthood. Many also have facial weakness. Weakness is nonprogressive, and life expectancy is normal, but some patients are severely affected and require a wheelchair. The gene mutation associated with central core myopathy is also associated with increased susceptibility to malignant hyperthermia.

Centronuclear myopathy: Centronuclear myopathy is characterized by an abundance of central nuclei on muscle biopsy. This myopathy may be X-linked, autosomal dominant, or autosomal recessive, but most genes implicated encode membrane-trafficking proteins.

X-linked forms are the most common and most severe, and most affected children do not survive beyond the first year of life.

Autosomal dominant forms typically manifest in adolescence or adulthood with exercise-induced myalgia, bifacial weakness, ptosis, and external ophthalmoplegia.

Nemaline myopathy: This myopathy, one of the more common congenital myopathies, can be autosomal dominant or recessive. Causative mutations have been identified in 10 genes and all are related to the production of thin-filament proteins.

Nemaline myopathy may be severe, moderate, or mild. Severely affected patients may have weakness of respiratory muscles and respiratory failure. Moderate disease causes progressive weakness in muscles of the face, neck, trunk, and feet, but life expectancy may be nearly normal. Mild disease is nonprogressive, and life expectancy is normal.

FAMILIAL PERIODIC PARALYSIS

Familial periodic paralysis is a rare autosomal dominant condition with considerable variation in penetrance characterized by episodes of flaccid paralysis with loss of deep tendon reflexes and failure of muscle to respond to electrical stimulation. There are 4 forms: hypokalemic, hyperkalemic, thyrotoxic, and Andersen-Tawil syndrome. Diagnosis is indicated by history and is confirmed by provoking an episode (eg, by giving dextrose and insulin to

cause hypokalemia or potassium chloride to cause hyperkalemia). Treatment depends on the form.

Each form of familial periodic paralysis involves a different gene and electrolyte channel. In 70% of affected people, the hypokalemic form is due to a mutation in the alpha-subunit of the voltage-sensitive muscle calcium channel gene on chromosome 1q (HypoPP type I). In some families, the mutation is in the alpha-subunit of the sodium channel gene on chromosome 17 (HypoPP type II).

Although the hypokalemic form is the most common form of familial periodic paralysis, it is nonetheless quite rare, with a prevalence of 1/100,000.

The hyperkalemic form is due to mutations in the gene that encodes the alpha-subunit of the skeletal muscle sodium channel (SCN4A).

The mutations and affected electrolyte channels in the thyrotoxic form are unknown, but this form usually involves hypokalemia and is associated with symptoms of thyrotoxicosis. Incidence of the thyrotoxic form is highest in Asian men.

Andersen-Tawil syndrome is due to an autosomal dominant defect of the inward-rectifying potassium channel; patients can have a high, low, or normal serum potassium level.

Symptoms and Signs

Hypokalemic periodic paralysis: Episodes usually begin before age 16. The day after vigorous exercise, the patient often awakens with weakness, which may be mild and limited to certain muscle groups or may affect all four limbs. Episodes are also precipitated by carbohydrate-rich meals, emotional or physical stress, alcohol ingestion, and cold exposure. Ocular, bulbar, and respiratory muscles are spared. Consciousness is not altered. Serum and urine potassium are decreased. Weakness may last up to 24 h.

Hyperkalemic periodic paralysis: Episodes often begin at an earlier age and usually are shorter, more frequent, and less severe. Episodes are precipitated by rest after exercise, exercise after meals, or fasting. Myotonia (delayed relaxation after muscle contraction) is common. Eyelid myotonia may be the only symptom.

Thyrotoxic periodic paralysis: Episodes last hours to days and are usually precipitated by exercise, stress, or a carbohydrate load, similar to the hypokalemic form. Symptoms of thyrotoxicosis (eg, anxiety, emotional lability, weakness, tremor, palpitations, heat intolerance, increased perspiration, weight loss) are typically present. Clinical features of hyperthyroidism often precede the onset of periodic paralysis by months or years; however, features have been noted to occur at the same time as (in up to 60% of patients) or after the development of (in up to 17% of patients) periodic paralysis.

Andersen-Tawil syndrome: Episodes usually begin before age 20 with all or some of the clinical triad:

- Periodic paralysis
- Prolonged QT interval and ventricular arrhythmias
- Dysmorphic physical features

Dysmorphic physical features include short stature, high-arched palate, low-set ears, broad nose, micrognathia, hypertelorism, clinodactyly of the fingers, short index fingers, and syndactyly of the toes.

Episodes are precipitated by rest after exercise, may last for days, and occur monthly.

Diagnosis

- Clinical evaluation
- Serum potassium level during symptoms
- Sometimes provocative testing

The best diagnostic indicator is a history of typical episodes. If measured during an episode, serum potassium may be abnormal. Episodes can sometimes be provoked by giving dextrose and insulin (to cause the hypokalemic form) or potassium chloride (to cause the hyperkalemic form), but only experienced physicians should attempt provocative testing, because respiratory paralysis or cardiac conduction abnormalities may occur with provoked episodes.

Diagnosis of the hyperkalemic form is based on clinical findings and/or the identification of a heterozygous pathogenic variant in SNC4A.

Treatment

- Varies with type and severity

Hypokalemic periodic paralysis: Episodes of paralysis are managed by giving potassium chloride 2 to 10 g in an unsweetened oral solution or giving potassium chloride IV. Following a low-carbohydrate, low-sodium diet, avoiding strenuous activity, avoiding alcohol after periods of rest, and taking acetazolamide 250 mg po bid may help prevent hypokalemic episodes.

Hyperkalemic periodic paralysis: Episodes of paralysis, if mild, can be aborted at onset by light exercise and a 2-g/kg oral carbohydrate load. Established episodes require thiazides, acetazolamide, or inhaled beta-agonists. Severe episodes require calcium gluconate and insulin and dextrose IV (see also treatment of severe hyperkalemia). Regularly ingesting carbohydrate-rich, low-potassium meals and avoiding fasting, strenuous activity after meals, and cold exposure help prevent hyperkalemic episodes.

Thyrotoxic periodic paralysis: Acute episodes are treated with potassium chloride, and serum potassium levels are closely monitored. Episodes are prevented by maintaining a euthyroid state (see treatment of hyperthyroidism—p. 1347) and giving beta-blockers (eg, propranolol).

Andersen-Tawil syndrome: In addition to lifestyle changes including tightly controlled levels of exercise or activity, episodes may be prevented by giving a carbonic anhydrase inhibitor (eg, acetazolamide). The major complication of Andersen-Tawil syndrome is sudden death from cardiac arrhythmias, and a cardiac pacemaker or implantable cardioverter-defibrillator may be required to control cardiac symptoms.

KEY POINTS

- There are 4 types of familial periodic paralysis, which are caused by rare mutations of membrane electrolyte channels.
- Serum potassium is usually but not always abnormal but may be low or high.
- Patients have intermittent episodes of weakness, typically precipitated by exercise and sometimes meals (particularly containing carbohydrates) or alcohol.
- Diagnose by typical symptoms and measuring serum potassium during symptoms.
- Treat episodes by correcting serum potassium and prevent episodes by recommending lifestyle changes.

317 Juvenile Idiopathic Arthritis

Juvenile idiopathic arthritis (JIA) is a group of rheumatic diseases that begins by age 16. Arthritis, fever, rash, adenopathy, splenomegaly, and iridocyclitis are typical of some forms. Diagnosis is clinical. Treatment involves NSAIDs, intra-articular corticosteroids, and disease-modifying antirheumatic drugs.

JIA is uncommon. The cause is unknown, but there seems to be a genetic predisposition as well as autoimmune and autoinflammatory pathophysiology. JIA is distinct from adult rheumatoid arthritis, despite occasional similarities.

Classification

JIA is not a single disease; the term applies to a number of chronic arthritides that occur in children and share certain features. The current classification system, from the International League of Associations for Rheumatology, defines categories of disease based on clinical and laboratory findings. Some of the categories are subdivided into different forms. Categories include the following:

- Oligoarticular JIA (persistent or extended)
- Polyarticular JIA (rheumatoid factor [RF] negative or positive)
- Enthesitis-related arthritis
- Psoriatic JIA
- Undifferentiated JIA
- Systemic JIA

Many of these categories likely include more than one disease but are useful to help group children with a similar prognosis and response to treatment. Also, children sometimes move to different categories during the course of their illness.

Oligoarticular JIA is the most common form and usually affects young girls. It is characterized by involvement of ≤ 4 joints during the first 6 mo of disease. Oligoarticular JIA is further divided into 2 types: persistent (always ≤ 4 joints involved) and extended (≥ 5 joints involved after the first 6 mo of disease).

Polyarticular JIA is the second most common form. It affects ≥ 5 joints at onset and is divided into 2 types: RF negative and RF positive. Typically, young girls are RF negative and have a better prognosis. The RF-positive type typically occurs in adolescent girls and is often similar to adult RA. In both types, arthritis can be symmetric and frequently involves the small joints.

Enthesitis-related arthritis involves arthritis and enthesitis (painful inflammation at the insertion of tendons and ligaments). It is more common among older boys who may subsequently develop classic features of one of the spondyloarthritides such as ankylosing spondylitis or reactive arthritis. The arthritis tends to be in the lower extremities and asymmetric. The HLA-B27 allele is more common in this form of JIA.

Psoriatic JIA has a bimodal age distribution. One peak occurs in young girls, and the other peak occurs in older males and females (who are equally affected). It is associated with psoriasis, dactylitis (swollen digits), nail pits, or a family history of psoriasis in a 1st-degree relative. Arthritis is frequently oligoarticular.

Undifferentiated JIA is diagnosed when patients do not meet criteria for any one category or meet criteria for more than one.

Systemic JIA (Still disease) involves fever and systemic manifestations.

Symptoms and Signs

Manifestations involve the joints and sometimes the eyes and/or skin; systemic JIA may affect multiple organs.

Children typically have joint stiffness, swelling, effusion, pain, and tenderness, but some children have no pain. Joint manifestations may be symmetric or asymmetric, and involve large or small joints. Enthesitis typically causes tenderness of the iliac crest and spine, greater trochanter of the femur, patella, tibial tuberosity, or Achilles and plantar fascia insertions.

Sometimes, JIA interferes with growth and development. Micrognathia (receded chin) due to early closure of mandibular epiphyses or limb length inequality (usually the affected limb is longer) may occur.

The most common ocular abnormality is iridocyclitis (inflammation of the anterior chamber and anterior vitreous) that is typically asymptomatic but sometimes causes blurring of vision and miosis. Rarely, in enthesitis-related arthritis, there is conjunctival injection, pain, and photophobia. Iridocyclitis can result in scarring (synechia), cataracts, glaucoma, or band keratopathy. Iridocyclitis is most common in oligoarticular JIA, developing in nearly 20% of patients, especially if patients are positive for antinuclear antibodies (ANA). It may occur in the other forms but is rare in polyarticular RF-positive JIA and systemic JIA.

Skin abnormalities are present mainly in psoriatic JIA, in which psoriatic skin lesions, dactylitis, and/or nail pits may be present, and in systemic JIA, in which a typical transient rash often appears with fever. Rash in systemic JIA may be diffuse and migratory, with urticarial or macular lesions with central clearing.

Systemic abnormalities in systemic JIA include high fever, rash, splenomegaly, generalized adenopathy (especially of the axillary nodes), and serositis with pericarditis or pleuritis. These symptoms may precede the development of arthritis. Fever occurs daily (quotidian) and is often highest in the afternoon or evening and may recur for weeks.

Diagnosis

- Clinical criteria
- RF, antinuclear antibodies (ANA), anticyclic citrullinated peptide antibody (anti-CCP), and HLA-B27 tests

JIA should be suspected in children with symptoms of arthritis, signs of iridocyclitis, generalized adenopathy, splenomegaly, or unexplained rash or prolonged fever, especially if quotidian. Diagnosis of JIA is primarily clinical. Patients with JIA should be tested for RF, anti-CCP antibodies, ANA, and HLA-B27 because these tests may be helpful in distinguishing between forms. In systemic JIA, RF and ANA are usually absent. In oligoarticular JIA, ANA are present in up to 75% of patients and RF is usually absent. In polyarticular JIA, RF usually is negative, but in some patients, mostly adolescent girls, it can be positive. HLA-B27 is present more commonly in enthesitis-related arthritis.

To diagnose iridocyclitis, a slit-lamp examination should be done even in the absence of ocular symptoms. A recently diagnosed patient with oligoarticular or polyarticular JIA should have an eye examination every 3 month if ANA test results are positive and every 6 mo if ANA test results are negative.

Prognosis

Remissions occur in 50 to 70% of treated patients. Patients with RF-positive polyarticular JIA have a less favorable prognosis.

Treatment

- Drugs that slow disease progression (particularly methotrexate, etanercept, and anakinra)
- Intra-articular corticosteroid injections
- NSAIDs

Similar to the therapy of patients with adult rheumatoid arthritis, disease-modifying antirheumatic drugs (DMARDs), particularly methotrexate and the biologic agents (eg, etanercept, anakinra), have dramatically changed the therapeutic approach.[1]

Symptoms of JIA may be reduced with NSAIDs but they do not alter long-term joint disease or prevent complications. NSAIDs are most useful for enthesitis. Naproxen 5 to 10 mg/kg po bid, ibuprofen 5 to 10 mg/kg po qid, and indomethacin 0.5 to 1.0 mg/kg po tid are among the most useful.

Except for severe systemic disease, systemic corticosteroids can usually be avoided. When necessary, the lowest possible dose is used (eg, range for oral prednisone, 0.0125 to 0.5 mg/kg qid, or the same daily dose given once or twice daily). Growth retardation, osteoporosis, and osteonecrosis are the major hazards of prolonged corticosteroid use in children. Intra-articular corticosteroid injections can be given. The dosage for children is adjusted based on weight. A few children may need to be sedated for intra-articular injection, especially if multiple joints require injection.

Methotrexate is useful for oligoarticular, psoriatic, and polyarticular forms of JIA. Adverse effects are monitored as in adults. Bone marrow depression and hepatic toxicity are monitored with CBC, AST, ALT, and albumin. Occasionally, sulfasalazine is used, especially in cases of suspected spondyloarthropathy.

TNF-alpha blockade is used if methotrexate is not effective. Etanercept is used most commonly at doses of 0.4 mg/kg sc (up to a maximum of 25 mg) twice/wk or 0.8 mg/kg sc (up to 50 mg) once/wk. Adalimumab and infliximab are different TNF-alpha antagonists that have been shown to be effective. IL-1 blockade with anakinra or canakinumab is particularly effective for systemic JIA. Tocilizumab is an IL-6 receptor antagonist that is indicated for the treatment of systemic JIA.[2]

Physical therapy, exercises, splints, and other supportive measures may help prevent flexion contractures. Adaptive devices can improve function and minimize unnecessary stresses on inflamed joints. Iridocyclitis is treated with ophthalmic corticosteroid drops and mydriatics and may require systemic methotrexate and anti-TNF therapy.

1. Beukelman T, Patkar NM, Saag KG, et al: 2011 American College of Rheumatology recommendations for the treatment of JIA: Initiation and safety monitoring of therapeutic agents for the treatment of arthritis and systemic features. *Arthritis Care Res (Hoboken)* 63(4):465–482, 2011. doi: 10.1002/acr.20460.
2. De Benedetti F, Brunner H, Ruperto N, et al: Tocilizumab in patients with systemic JIA: Efficacy from the placebo-controlled 12-week part of the phase 3 TENDER trial. *Arthritis Rheum* 62 (supplement 10):1434, 2010. doi: 10.1002/art.29200.

KEY POINTS

- JIA encompasses a number of different arthritides in children that differ in clinical and laboratory manifestations.
- Suspect JIA in children with symptoms of arthritis, signs of iridocyclitis, generalized adenopathy, splenomegaly, or unexplained rash or prolonged fever.
- Diagnose JIA clinically; use laboratory testing (of RF, anti-CCP antibodies, ANA, and HLA-B27) mainly to distinguish between forms.
- Slow disease progression with methotrexate and/or biologic drugs (eg, etanercept, anakinra) and treat symptoms with intra-articular corticosteroid injections and/or NSAIDs.
- Treat iridocyclitis with ophthalmic corticosteroid drops and mydriatics, or systemic therapy if refractory.

318 Learning and Developmental Disorders

ATTENTION-DEFICIT/HYPERACTIVITY DISORDER

Attention-deficit/hyperactivity disorder (ADHD) is a syndrome of inattention, hyperactivity, and impulsivity. The 3 types of ADHD are predominantly inattentive, predominantly hyperactive/impulsive, and combined. Diagnosis is made by clinical criteria. Treatment usually includes drug therapy with stimulant drugs, behavioral therapy, and educational interventions.

Attention-deficit/hyperactivity disorder is considered a neurodevelopmental disorder. Neurodevelopmental disorders are neurologically based conditions that appear early in childhood, typically before school entry, and impair development of personal, social, academic, and/or occupational functioning. They typically involve difficulties with the acquisition, retention, or application of specific skills or sets of information. Neurodevelopmental disorders may involve dysfunction in attention, memory, perception, language, problem-solving, or social interaction. Other common neurodevelopmental disorders in-0clude autism spectrum disorders, learning disorders (eg, dyslexia), and intellectual disability.

Although some experts previously considered ADHD a behavior disorder, this was probably because comorbid behavior disorders, particularly oppositional-defiant disorder and conduct disorder, are common.

ADHD affects an estimated 5 to 11% of school-aged children. However, many experts think ADHD is overdiagnosed, largely because criteria are applied inaccurately. According to the *Diagnostic and Statistical Manual of Mental Disorders*, Fifth Edition (DSM-5), there are 3 types:

- Predominantly inattentive
- Predominantly hyperactive/impulsive
- Combined

Overall, ADHD is about twice as common in boys, although the ratios vary by type. The predominantly hyperactive/impulsive type occurs 2 to 9 times more frequently in boys; the predominantly inattentive type occurs with about equal frequency in both sexes. ADHD tends to run in families.

ADHD has no known single, specific cause. Potential causes include genetic, biochemical, sensorimotor, physiologic, and behavioral factors. Some risk factors include birth weight < 1500 g, head trauma, iron deficiency, obstructive sleep apnea, and lead exposure, as well as prenatal exposure to alcohol, tobacco, and cocaine. Fewer than 5% of children with ADHD have evidence of neurologic injury. Increasing evidence implicates abnormalities in dopaminergic and noradrenergic systems with decreased activity or stimulation in upper brain stem and frontal-midbrain tracts.

ADHD in adults: Although ADHD is considered a disorder of children and always starts during childhood, it persists into adulthood in about half of cases. Although the diagnosis occasionally may not be recognized until adolescence or adulthood, some manifestations should have been present before age 12.

In adults, symptoms include

- Difficulty concentrating
- Difficulty completing tasks
- Mood swings
- Impatience
- Difficulty in maintaining relationships

Hyperactivity in adults usually manifests as restlessness and fidgetiness rather than the overt motor hyperactivity that occurs in young children. Adults with ADHD tend to be at higher risk for unemployment, reduced educational achievement, and increased rates of substance abuse and criminality. Motor vehicle crashes and violations are more common.

ADHD can be more difficult to diagnose during adulthood. Symptoms may be similar to those of mood disorders, anxiety disorders, and substance use disorders. Because self-reporting of childhood symptoms may be unreliable, clinicians may need to review school records or interview family members to confirm existence of manifestations before age 12.

Adults with ADHD may benefit from the same types of stimulant drugs that children with ADHD take. They may also benefit from counseling to improve time management and other coping skills.

Symptoms and Signs

Onset often occurs before age 4 and invariably before age 12. The peak age for diagnosis is between ages 8 and 10; however, patients with the predominantly inattentive type may not be diagnosed until after adolescence.

Core symptoms and signs of ADHD involve

- Inattention
- Impulsivity
- Hyperactivity

Inattention tends to appear when a child is involved in tasks that require vigilance, rapid reaction time, visual and perceptual search, and systematic and sustained listening.

Impulsivity refers to hasty actions that have the potential for a negative outcome (eg, in children, running across a street without looking, in adolescents and adults, suddenly quitting school or a job without thought for the consequences).

Hyperactivity involves excessive motor activity. Children, particularly younger ones, may have trouble sitting quietly when expected to (eg, in school or church). Older patients may simply be fidgety, restless, or talkative—sometimes to the extent that others feel worn out watching them.

Inattention and impulsivity impede development of academic skills and thinking and reasoning strategies, motivation for school, and adjustment to social demands. Children who have predominantly inattentive ADHD tend to be hands-on learners who have difficulty in passive learning situations that require continuous performance and task completion.

Overall, about 20 to 60% of children with ADHD have learning disabilities, but some school dysfunction occurs in most children with ADHD due to inattention (resulting in missed details) and impulsivity (resulting in responding without thinking through the question).

Behavioral history can reveal low frustration tolerance, opposition, temper tantrums, aggressiveness, poor social skills and peer relationships, sleep disturbances, anxiety, dysphoria, depression, and mood swings.

Although there are no specific physical examination or laboratory findings associated with ADHD, signs can include

- Motor incoordination or clumsiness
- Nonlocalized, "soft" neurologic findings
- Perceptual-motor dysfunctions

Diagnosis

- Clinical criteria based on the DSM-5

Diagnosis is clinical and is based on comprehensive medical, developmental, educational, and psychologic evaluations (see also the American Academy of Pediatrics ADHD: Clinical Practice Guideline for the Diagnosis, Evaluation, and Treatment of Attention-Deficit/Hyperactivity Disorder in (ADHD) Children and Adolescents).

DSM-5 diagnostic criteria for ADHD: DSM-5 diagnostic criteria include 9 symptoms and signs of inattention and 9 of hyperactivity and impulsivity. Diagnosis using these criteria requires that ≥ 6 symptoms and signs from at least one group

- Be present often for ≥ 6 mo
- Be more pronounced than expected for the child's developmental level
- Occur in at least 2 situations (eg, home and school)
- Be present before age 12 (at least some symptoms)
- Interfere with functioning at home, school, or work

Inattention symptoms:

- Does not pay attention to details or makes careless mistakes in schoolwork or with other activities
- Has difficulty sustaining attention on tasks at school or during play
- Does not seem to listen when spoken to directly
- Does not follow through on instructions or finish tasks
- Has difficulty organizing tasks and activities
- Avoids, dislikes, or is reluctant to engage in tasks that require sustained mental effort over a long period of time
- Often loses things necessary for school tasks or activities
- Is easily distracted
- Is forgetful in daily activities

Hyperactivity and impulsivity symptoms:

- Often fidgets with hands or feet or squirms
- Often leaves seat in classroom or elsewhere
- Often runs about or climbs excessively where such activity is inappropriate
- Has difficulty playing quietly
- Often on the go, acting as if driven by a motor
- Often talks excessively
- Often blurts out answers before questions are completed
- Often has difficulty awaiting turn
- Often interrupts or intrudes on others

Diagnosis of the predominantly inattentive type requires ≥ 6 symptoms and signs of inattention. Diagnosis of the hyperactive/impulsive type requires ≥ 6 symptoms and signs of hyperactivity and impulsivity. Diagnosis of the combined type requires ≥ 6 symptoms and signs each of inattention and hyperactivity/impulsivity.

Other diagnostic considerations: Differentiating between ADHD and other conditions can be challenging. Overdiagnosis must be avoided, and other conditions must be accurately identified. Many ADHD signs expressed during the preschool years could also indicate communication problems that can occur in other neurodevelopmental disorders (eg, autism spectrum disorders) or in certain learning disorders, anxiety, depression, or behavioral disorders (eg, conduct disorder).

Clinicians should consider whether the child is distracted by external factors (ie, environmental input) or by internal factors (ie, thoughts, anxieties, worries). However, during later childhood, ADHD signs become more qualitatively distinct; children with the hyperactive/impulsive or combined types often exhibit continuous movement of the lower extremities, motor impersistence (eg, purposeless movement, fidgeting of hands), impulsive talking, and a seeming lack of awareness of their environment. Children with the predominantly inattentive type may have no physical signs.

Medical assessment focuses on identifying potentially treatable conditions that may contribute to or worsen symptoms and signs. Assessment should include seeking a history of prenatal exposures (eg, drugs, alcohol, tobacco), perinatal complications or infections, CNS infections, traumatic brain injury, cardiac disease, sleep-disordered breathing, poor appetite and/or picky eating, and a family history of ADHD.

Developmental assessment focuses on determining the onset and course of symptoms and signs. The assessment includes checking developmental milestones, particularly language milestones and the use of ADHD-specific rating scales (eg, the Vanderbilt Assessment Scale, the Conners Comprehensive Behavior Rating Scale, the ADHD Rating Scale IV).

Educational assessment focuses on documenting core symptoms and signs; it may involve reviewing educational records and using rating scales or checklists. However, rating scales and checklists alone often cannot distinguish ADHD from other developmental disorders or from behavioral disorders.

Prognosis

Traditional classrooms and academic activities often exacerbate symptoms and signs in children with untreated or inadequately treated ADHD. Social and emotional adjustment problems may be persistent. Poor acceptance by peers and loneliness tend to increase with age and with the obvious display of symptoms. Substance abuse may result if ADHD is not identified and adequately treated because many adolescents and adults with ADHD self-medicate with both legal (eg, caffeine) and illegal (eg, cocaine) substances.

Although hyperactivity symptoms and signs tend to diminish with age, adolescents and adults may display residual difficulties. Predictors of poor outcomes in adolescence and adulthood include

- Coexisting low intelligence
- Aggressiveness
- Social and interpersonal problems
- Parental psychopathology

Problems in adolescence and adulthood manifest predominantly as academic failure, low self-esteem, and difficulty learning appropriate social behavior. Adolescents and adults who have predominately impulsive ADHD may have an increased incidence of personality trait disorders and antisocial behavior; many continue to display impulsivity, restlessness, and poor social skills. People with ADHD seem to adjust better to work than to academic and home situations, particularly if they can find jobs that do not require intense attention to perform.

Treatment

- Behavioral therapy
- Drug therapy, typically with stimulants such as methylphenidate or dextroamphetamine (in short- and long-acting preparations)

Randomized, controlled studies show behavioral therapy alone is less effective than therapy with stimulant drugs alone for school-aged children, but behavioral or combination therapy is recommended for younger children. Although correction of the underlying neurophysiologic differences of patients with ADHD does not occur with drug therapy, drugs are effective in alleviating ADHD symptoms and they permit participation in activities previously inaccessible because of poor attention and impulsivity. Drugs often interrupt the cycle of inappropriate behavior, enhancing behavioral and academic interventions, motivation, and self-esteem.

Treatment of adults follows similar principles, but drug selection and dosing are determined on an individual basis, depending on other medical conditions.

Stimulant drugs: Stimulant preparations that include methylphenidate or amphetamine salts are most widely used. Response varies greatly, and dosage depends on the severity of the behavior and the child's ability to tolerate the drug. Dosing is adjusted in frequency and amount until the optimal response is achieved.

Methylphenidate is usually started at 0.3 mg/kg po once/day (immediate-release form) and increased in frequency weekly, usually to about 3 times per day or every 4 h. If response is inadequate but the drug is tolerated, dose can be increased. Most children find an optimal balance between benefits and adverse effects at individual doses between 0.3 and 0.6 mg/kg. The dextro isomer of methylphenidate is the active moiety and is available for prescription at one half the dose.

Dextroamphetamine is typically started (often in combination with racemic amphetamine) at 0.15 to 0.2 mg/kg po once/day, which can then be increased to 2 or 3 times per day or every 4 h. Individual doses in the range of 0.15 to 0.4 mg/kg are usually effective. Dose titration should balance effectiveness against adverse effects. In general, dextroamphetamine doses are about two thirds those of methylphenidate doses.

For methylphenidate or dextroamphetamine, once an optimal dosage is reached, an equivalent dosage of the same drug in a sustained-release form is often substituted to avoid the need for drug administration in school. Long-acting preparations include wax matrix slow-release tablets, biphasic capsules containing the equivalent of 2 doses, and osmotic release pills and transdermal patches that provide up to 12 h of coverage. Both short-acting and long-acting liquid preparations are now available. Pure dextro preparations (eg, dextromethylphenidate) are often used to minimize adverse effects such as anxiety; doses are typically half those of mixed preparations. Prodrug preparations are also sometimes used because of their smoother release, longer duration of action, fewer adverse effects, and lower abuse potential. Learning is often enhanced by low doses, but improvement in behavior often requires higher doses.

Dosing schedules of stimulant drugs can be adjusted to cover specific days and times (eg, during school hours, while doing homework). Drug holidays may be tried on weekends, on holidays, or during summer vacations. Placebo periods (for 5 to 10 school days to ensure reliability of observations) are recommended to determine whether the drugs are still needed.

Common adverse effects of stimulant drugs include

- Sleep disturbances (eg, insomnia)
- Depression
- Headache
- Stomachache
- Appetite suppression
- Elevated heart rate and blood pressure

Some studies have shown slowing of growth over 2 yr of stimulant drug use, but results have not been consistent, and whether slowing persists over longer periods of use remains unclear. Some patients who are sensitive to stimulant drug effects appear overfocused or dulled; decreasing the stimulant drug dosage or trying a different drug may be helpful.

Nonstimulant drugs: Atomoxetine, a selective norepinephrinereuptake inhibitor, is also used. The drug is effective, but data are mixed regarding its efficacy compared with stimulant drugs. Many children experience nausea, sedation, irritability, and temper tantrums; rarely, liver toxicity and suicidal ideation occur. A typical starting dose is 0.5 mg/kg po once/day, titrated weekly to 1.2 to 1.4 mg/kg once/day. The long half-life allows once/day dosing but requires continuous use to be effective. The maximum recommended daily dosage is 100 mg.

Antidepressants such as bupropion, alpha-2 agonists such as clonidine and guanfacine, and other psychoactive drugs are sometimes used in cases of stimulant drug ineffectiveness or unacceptable adverse effects, but they are less effective and are not recommended as first-line drugs. Sometimes these drugs are used in combination with stimulants for synergistic effects; close monitoring for adverse effects is essential.

Behavioral management: Counseling, including cognitive-behavioral therapy (eg, goal-setting, self-monitoring, modeling, role-playing), is often effective and helps children understand ADHD. Structure and routines are essential.

Classroom behavior is often improved by environmental control of noise and visual stimulation, appropriate task length, novelty, coaching, and teacher proximity.

When difficulties persist at home, parents should be encouraged to seek additional professional assistance and training in behavioral management techniques. Adding incentives and token rewards reinforces behavioral management and is often effective. Children with ADHD in whom hyperactivity and poor impulse control predominate are often helped at home when structure, consistent parenting techniques, and well-defined limits are established.

Elimination diets, megavitamin treatments, use of antioxidants or other compounds, and nutritional and biochemical interventions have had the least consistent effects. Biofeedback can be helpful in some cases but is not recommended for routine use because evidence of sustained benefit is lacking.

KEY POINTS

- ADHD involves inattention, hyperactivity/impulsivity, or a combination; it typically appears before age 12, including in preschoolers.
- Cause is unknown, but there are numerous suspected risk factors.
- Diagnose using clinical criteria, and be alert for other disorders that may initially manifest similarly (eg, autism spectrum disorders, certain learning or behavioral disorders, anxiety, or depression).
- Manifestations tend to diminish with age, but adolescents and adults may have residual difficulties.
- Treat with stimulant drugs and cognitive-behavioral therapy; behavioral therapy alone may be appropriate for preschool-aged children.

Further Reading

American Academy of Pediatrics: ADHD: Clinical Practice Guideline for the Diagnosis, Evaluation, and Treatment of Attention-Deficit/Hyperactivity Disorder in Children and Adolescents

National Institute for Children's Health Quality

AUTISM SPECTRUM DISORDERS

Autism spectrum disorders are neurodevelopmental disorders characterized by impaired social interaction and communication, repetitive and stereotyped patterns of behavior, and uneven intellectual development often with intellectual disability. Symptoms begin in early childhood. The cause in most children is unknown, although evidence supports a genetic component; in some patients, the disorders may be caused by a medical condition. Diagnosis is based on developmental history and observation. Treatment consists of behavioral management and sometimes drug therapy.

Autism spectrum disorders represent a range of neurodevelopmental differences that are considered neurodevelopmental disorders. Neurodevelopmental disorders are neurologically based conditions that appear early in childhood, typically before school entry and affect development of personal, social, academic, and/or occupational functioning. They typically involve difficulties with the acquisition, retention, or application of specific skills or sets of information. Neurodevelopmental disorders may involve dysfunction in attention, memory, perception, language, problem-solving, or social interaction. Other common neurodevelopmental disorders include attention-deficit/hyperactivity disorder, learning disorders (eg, dyslexia), and intellectual disability.

Current estimates of prevalence of autism spectrum disorders are in the range of 1/68 in the US, with similar ranges in other countries. Autism is about 4 times more common among boys. In recent years, there has been a rapid rise in the diagnosis of autism spectrum disorders, partially because of changes in diagnostic criteria.

Etiology

The specific cause in most cases of autism spectrum disorders remains elusive. However, some cases have occurred with congenital rubella syndrome, cytomegalic inclusion disease, phenylketonuria, or fragile X syndrome.

Strong evidence supports a genetic component. For parents of one child with an autism spectrum disorder, risk of having a subsequent child with an autism spectrum disorder is 50 to 100 times greater. The concordance rate of autism is high in monozygotic twins. Research on families has suggested several potential target gene areas, including those related to neurotransmitter receptors (serotonin and gamma-aminobutyric acid [GABA]) and CNS structural control (*HOX* genes). Environmental causes have been suspected but are unproved. There is **strong evidence** that vaccinations do not cause autism, and the primary study that suggested this association has been withdrawn because its author falsified data (see also MMR vaccine and autism—p. 2461).

Differences in brain structure and function probably underlie much of the etiology of autism spectrum disorders. Some children with autism spectrum disorders have enlarged ventricles, some have hypoplasia of the cerebellar vermis, and others have abnormalities of brain stem nuclei.

Symptoms and Signs

Autism spectrum disorders may manifest during the first year of life but, depending on severity of symptoms, diagnosis may not be clear until school age.

Two main features characterize autism spectrum disorders:

- Persistent deficits in social communication and interaction
- Restricted, repetitive patterns of behavior, interests, and/or activities

Both of these features must be present at a young age (although they may not be recognized at the time) and must be severe enough to significantly impair the child's ability to function at home, school, or other situations. Manifestations must be more pronounced than expected for the child's developmental level and adjusted for norms in different cultures.

Examples of **deficits in social communication and interaction** include

- Deficits in social and/or emotional reciprocity (eg, failure to initiate or respond to social interactions or conversation, no sharing of emotions)
- Deficits in nonverbal social communication (eg, difficulty interpreting others' body language, gestures, and expressions; diminished facial expressions and gestures and/or eye contact)
- Deficits in developing and maintaining relationships (eg, making friends, adjusting behavior to different situations)

The first manifestations noticed by parents may be delayed language development and lack of interest in parents or typical play.

Examples of **restricted, repetitive patterns of behavior, interests, and/or activities** include

- Stereotyped or repetitive movements or speech (eg, repeated hand flapping or finger flicking, repeating idiosyncratic phrases or echolalia, lining up toys)
- Inflexible adherence to routines and/or rituals (eg, having extreme distress with small changes in meals or clothing, having stereotyped greeting rituals)
- Highly restricted, abnormally intense fixated interests (eg, preoccupation with vacuum cleaners, older patients writing out airline schedules)
- Extreme over- or under-reaction to sensory input (eg, extreme aversion to specific smells, tastes, or textures; apparent indifference to pain or temperature)

Some affected children injure themselves. About 25% of affected children experience a documented loss of previously acquired skills.

All children with an autism spectrum disorder have at least some difficulty with interaction, behavior, and communication; however, the severity of the problems varies widely.

Current theory holds that a fundamental problem in autism spectrum disorders is "mind blindness," the inability to imagine what another person might be thinking. This difficulty is thought to result in interaction abnormalities that, in turn, lead to abnormal language development. One of the earliest and most sensitive markers for autism is a 1-yr-old child's inability to point communicatively at objects at a distance. It is theorized that the child cannot imagine that another person would understand what was being indicated; instead, the child indicates wants only by physically touching the desired object or using the adult's hand as a tool.

Comorbid conditions are common, particularly intellectual disability and learning disorders. Nonfocal neurologic findings include poorly coordinated gait and stereotyped motor movements. Seizures occur in 20 to 40% of these children (particularly those with an IQ < 50).

Diagnosis

- Clinical evaluation

Diagnosis is made clinically based on criteria in the *Diagnostic and Statistical Manual of Mental Disorders,* Fifth Edition (DSM-5), and requires evidence of impairment of social interaction and communication and presence of ≥ 2 restricted, repetitive, stereotyped behaviors or interests. Although the manifestations of autism spectrum disorders can vary significantly in scope and severity, previous categorizations such as Asperger syndrome, childhood disintegrative disorder, and pervasive developmental disorder are encompassed under autism spectrum disorders and are no longer distinguished.

Screening tests include the Social Communication Questionnaire and the Modified Checklist for Autism in Toddlers (M-CHAT-R). M-CHAT is available online. See also the American Academy of Neurology's Practice Parameter: Screening and Diagnosis of Autism and the American Academy of Pediatrics' Identification and Evaluation of Children with Autism Spectrum Disorders. Formal standard diagnostic tests such as the Autism Diagnostic Observation Schedule-2 (ADOS-2), based on criteria in the DSM-5, are usually given by psychologists or developmental-behavioral pediatricians. Children with autism spectrum disorders can be difficult to test; they often do better on performance items than verbal items in IQ tests and may show instances of age-appropriate performance despite cognitive limitation in most areas. Nonetheless, reliable diagnosis of autism spectrum disorders is becoming increasingly possible at younger ages. An IQ test given by an experienced examiner often can provide a useful predictor of outcome.

Treatment

- Behavioral therapy
- Speech and language therapy
- Sometimes physical and occupational therapy
- Drug therapy

Treatment is usually multidisciplinary, and recent studies show measurable benefits from intensive, behaviorally based approaches that encourage interaction and meaningful communication. Psychologists and educators typically focus on behavioral analysis and then match behavioral management strategies to specific behavioral problems at home and at school. See also the American Academy of Pediatrics' Management of Children with Autism Spectrum Disorders.

Speech and language therapy should begin early and use a range of media, including signing, picture exchange, and augmentative communication devices such as those that generate speech based on symbols children select on a tablet or other handheld device, as well as speech. Physical and occupational therapists plan and implement strategies to help affected children compensate for specific deficits in motor function, motor planning, and sensory processing.

Drug treatment may help relieve symptoms. There is evidence that atypical antipsychotic drugs (eg, risperidone, aripiprazole) help relieve behavioral problems, such as ritualistic, self-injurious, and aggressive behaviors. Other drugs are sometimes used for control of specific symptoms, including SSRIs for ritualistic behaviors, mood stabilizers (eg, valproate) for self-injury and outburst behaviors, and stimulants and other attention-deficit/hyperactivity disorder (ADHD) drugs for inattention, impulsivity, and hyperactivity.

Dietary interventions, including some vitamin supplements and a gluten-free and casein-free diet, are not helpful enough to be recommended; however, many families choose to use them, leading to needs to monitor for dietary insufficiencies and excesses. Other complementary and investigational approaches to therapy (eg, facilitated communication, chelation therapy, auditory integration training, and hyperbaric oxygen therapy) have not shown efficacy.

KEY POINTS

- Children have some combination of impaired social interaction and communication, repetitive and stereotyped patterns of behavior, and uneven intellectual development often with intellectual disability.
- Cause is usually unknown, but there appears to be a genetic component; vaccines are not causative.
- Screening tests include the Social Communication Questionnaire and the Modified Checklist for Autism in Toddlers (M-CHAT-R)
- Formal diagnostic testing is usually done by psychologists or developmental-behavioral pediatricians.
- Treatment is usually multidisciplinary, using intensive, behaviorally based approaches that encourage interaction and communication.
- Drugs (eg, atypical antipsychotics) may help severe behavioral disturbances (eg, self-injury, aggression).

INTELLECTUAL DISABILITY

Intellectual disability is characterized by significantly subaverage intellectual functioning (often expressed as an intelligence quotient < 70 to 75) combined with limitations of > 2 of the following: communication, self-direction, social skills, self-care, use of community resources, and maintenance of personal safety. Management consists of education, family counseling, and social support.

Intellectual disability is considered a neurodevelopmental disorder. Neurodevelopmental disorders are neurologically based conditions that appear early in childhood, typically before school entry and impair development of personal, social, academic, and/or occupational functioning. They typically involve difficulties with the acquisition, retention, or application of specific skills or sets of information. Neurodevelopmental disorders may involve dysfunction in attention, memory, perception, language, problem-solving, or social interaction. Other common neurodevelopmental disorders include attention-deficit/hyperactivity disorder, autism spectrum disorders, and learning disorders (eg, dyslexia).

Intellectual disability must involve early-childhood onset of deficits in both of the following:

- Intellectual functioning (eg, in reasoning, planning and problem solving, abstract thinking, learning at school or from experience)
- Adaptive functioning (ie, ability to meet age- and socioculturally appropriate standards for independent functioning in activities of daily life)

Basing severity on IQ alone (eg, mild, 52 to 70 or 75; moderate, 36 to 51; severe, 20 to 35; and profound, < 20) is inadequate. Classification must also account for the level of support needed, ranging from intermittent to ongoing high-level support for all activities. Such an approach focuses on a person's strengths and weaknesses, relating them to the demands of the person's environment and the expectations and attitudes of the family and community.

About 3% of the population functions at an IQ of < 70, which is at least 2 standard deviations below the mean IQ of the general population (IQ of 100); if the need for support is considered, only about 1% of the population has severe intellectual disability. Severe intellectual disability occurs in families from all socioeconomic groups and educational levels. Less severe ID (requiring intermittent or limited support) occurs most often in lower socioeconomic groups, paralleling with observations that IQ correlates best with success in school and socioeconomic status rather than specific organic factors. Nevertheless, recent studies suggest that genetic factors play roles even in milder cognitive disabilities.

Etiology

Intelligence is both genetically and environmentally determined. Children born to parents with intellectual disability are at increased risk of a range of developmental disabilities, but clear genetic transmission of intellectual disability is unusual. Although advances in genetics, such as chromosomal microarray analysis and whole genome sequencing of the coding regions (exome), have increased the likelihood of identifying the cause of an intellectual disability, a specific cause often cannot be identified. A cause is most likely to be identified in severe cases. Deficits in language and personal-social skills may be due to emotional problems, environmental deprivation, learning disorders, or deafness rather than intellectual disability.

Prenatal: A number of chromosomal anomalies and genetic metabolic and neurologic disorders can cause intellectual disability (see Table 318–1).

Congenital infections that can cause intellectual disability include rubella and those due to cytomegalovirus, *Toxoplasma gondii*, *Treponema pallidum*, herpes simplex virus, or HIV. Prenatal Zika virus infection has been associated recently with congenital microcephaly and associated intellectual disability.

Prenatal drug and toxin exposure can cause intellectual disability. Fetal alcohol syndrome is the most common of these conditions. Anticonvulsants such as phenytoin or valproate, chemotherapy drugs, radiation exposure, lead, and methylmercury are also causes.

Table 318–1. SOME CHROMOSOMAL AND GENETIC CAUSES OF INTELLECTUAL DISABILITY*

CAUSE	EXAMPLE
Chromosomal abnormalities	5p-deletion (Cri du chat syndrome) Down syndrome Fragile X syndrome Klinefelter syndrome Mosaicisms Trisomy 13 (Patau syndrome) Trisomy 18 (Edwards syndrome) Turner syndrome
Genetic metabolic disorders	Autosomal recessive disorders: • Aminoacidurias and acidemias • Galactosemia • Maple syrup urine disease • Phenylketonuria • Lysosomal defects • Gaucher disease • Hurler syndrome (mucopolysaccharidosis) • Niemann-Pick disease • Tay-Sachs disease • Peroxisomal disorders X-linked recessive disorders: • Hunter syndrome (a variant of mucopolysaccharidosis) • Lesch-Nyhan syndrome (hyperuricemia) • Oculocerebrorenal (Lowe) syndrome
Genetic neurologic disorders	Autosomal dominant disorders: • Myotonic dystrophy • Neurofibromatosis • Tuberous sclerosis Autosomal recessive disorders: • Primary microcephaly

*This is a partial list of disorders.

Severe undernutrition during pregnancy may affect fetal brain development, resulting in intellectual disability.

Perinatal: Complications related to prematurity, CNS bleeding, periventricular leukomalacia, breech or high forceps delivery, multiple births, placenta previa, preeclampsia, and perinatal asphyxia may increase the risk of intellectual disability. The risk is increased in small-for-gestational-age infants; intellectual impairment and decreased weight share similar causes. Very low- and extremely low-birth-weight infants have variably increased chances of having intellectual disability, depending on gestational age, perinatal events, and quality of care.

Postnatal: Undernutrition and environmental deprivation (lack of physical, emotional, and cognitive support required for growth, development, and social adaptation) during infancy and early childhood may be the most common causes of intellectual disability worldwide. Viral and bacterial encephalitides (including AIDS-associated neuroencephalopathy) and meningitides (eg, pneumococcal infections, *Haemophilus influenzae* infection), poisoning (eg, lead, mercury), and accidents that cause severe head injuries or asphyxia may result in intellectual disability.

Symptoms and Signs

The primary manifestations are

- Slowed acquisition of new knowledge and skills
- Immature behavior
- Limited self-care skills

Some children with mild intellectual disability may not develop recognizable symptoms until preschool age. However, early identification is common among children with moderate to severe intellectual disability and among children in whom intellectual disability is accompanied by physical abnormalities or signs of a condition (eg, cerebral palsy) that may be associated with a particular cause of intellectual disability (eg, perinatal asphyxia). Delayed development is usually apparent by preschool age. Among older children, hallmark features are a low IQ combined with limitations in adaptive behavior skills. Although developmental patterns may vary, it is much more common for children with intellectual disability to experience slow progress than developmental arrest.

Behavioral disorders are the reason for most psychiatric referrals and out-of-home placements for people with intellectual disability. Behavioral problems are often situational, and precipitating factors can usually be identified. Factors that predispose to unacceptable behavior include

- Lack of training in socially responsible behavior
- Inconsistent discipline
- Reinforcement of faulty behavior
- Impaired ability to communicate
- Discomfort due to coexisting physical problems and mental health disorders such as depression or anxiety

In institutional settings (now uncommon in the US), overcrowding, understaffing, and lack of activities contribute to both behavior challenges and to limited functional progress. Avoidance of long-term placement in large congregate care settings is extremely important in maximizing the individual's success.

Comorbid disorders: Comorbid disorders are common, particularly attention-deficit/hyperactivity disorder, mood disorders (depression, bipolar disorder), autism spectrum disorders, anxiety disorder, and others.

Some children may have cerebral palsy or other motor deficits, language delays, or hearing loss. Such motor or sensory impairments can mimic cognitive impairment but are not in themselves causes of it. As children mature, some develop anxiety or depression if they are socially rejected by other children or if they are disturbed by the realization that others see them as different and deficient. Well-managed, inclusive school programs can help maximize social integration, thereby minimizing such emotional responses.

Diagnosis

- Developmental and intelligence assessment
- Imaging of the CNS
- Genetic testing

For suspected cases, development and intelligence are assessed, typically by early intervention or school staff. Standardized intelligence tests can measure subaverage intellectual ability but are subject to error, and results should be questioned when they do not match clinical findings; illness, motor or sensory impairments, language barriers, or cultural differences may hamper a child's test performance. Such tests also have a middle-class bias but are generally reasonable in appraising intellectual ability in children, particularly in older ones.

Developmental screening tests such as the Ages and Stages Questionnaire (ASQ) or the Parents' Evaluation of Developmental Status (PEDS) provide gross assessments of development for young children and can be given by a physician or others. Such measures should be used only for screening and not as substitutes for standardized intelligence tests, which should be given by qualified psychologists. A neurodevelopmental assessment should be initiated as soon as developmental delays are suspected.

A developmental pediatrician or pediatric neurologist should investigate all cases of

- Moderate to severe developmental delays
- Progressive disability
- Neuromuscular deterioration
- Suspected seizure disorders

Establishing intellectual disability is followed by efforts to determine a cause. Accurate determination of the cause may provide a developmental prognosis, suggest plans for educational and training programs, help in genetic counseling, and relieve parental guilt.

Diagnosis of cause: History (including perinatal, developmental, neurologic, and familial) may identify causes. An algorithm for the diagnostic evaluation of the child with intellectual disability (global developmental delay) has been proposed by the Child Neurology Society.

Cranial imaging (eg, MRI) can show CNS malformations (as seen in neurodermatoses such as neurofibromatosis or tuberous sclerosis), treatable hydrocephalus, or more severe brain malformations such as schizencephaly.

Genetic tests may help identify disorders.

- Standard karyotyping shows Down syndrome (trisomy 21)
- Chromosome microarray identifies copy number variants such as might be found in 5p-deletion (cri du chat syndrome) or DiGeorge syndrome (chromosome 22q deletion)
- Direct DNA studies identify Fragile X syndrome

Chromosomal microarray analysis has become the preferred investigative tool; it can be used to identify specifically suspected syndromes and when no specific syndrome is suspected. It affords opportunities for identifying otherwise unrecognized chromosome disruptions but requires parental testing to interpret positive findings. Whole genome sequencing of the coding regions (whole exome sequencing) is a newer method that may uncover additional causes of intellectual disability.

Clinical manifestations (eg, failure to thrive, lethargy, vomiting, seizures, hypotonia, hepatosplenomegaly, coarse facial features, abnormal urinary odor, macroglossia) may suggest genetic metabolic disorders. Isolated delays in sitting or walking (gross motor skills) and in pincer grasp, drawing, or writing (fine motor skills) may indicate a neuromuscular disorder.

Specific laboratory tests are done depending on the suspected cause (see Table 318–2). Visual and auditory assessments should be done at an early age, and screening for lead poisoning is often appropriate.

Prognosis

Many people with mild to moderate intellectual disability can support themselves, live independently, and be successful at jobs that require basic intellectual skills. Life expectancy may

Table 318–2. TESTS FOR SOME CAUSES OF INTELLECTUAL DISABILITY

SUSPECTED CAUSE	INDICATED TESTS
Single major anomaly or multiple minor anomalies Family history of cognitive disability	Chromosome analysis Chromosomal microarray analysis Cranial MRI* Possibly exome sequencing
Failure to thrive Idiopathic hypotonia Genetic metabolic disorders	HIV screening in high-risk infants Nutritional and psychosocial history Urine and serum amino acid and organic acid analysis and enzyme studies for storage diseases or peroxisomal disorders Muscle enzymes SMA 12 (includes albumin, alkaline phosphatase, AST, total bilirubin, BUN, Ca, cholesterol, creatinine, glucose, P, total protein, and uric acid) Bone age, skeletal x-rays
Seizures	EEG Cranial MRI* Blood calcium, phosphorus, magnesium, amino acids, glucose, and lead levels
Cranial abnormalities (eg, premature closure of the sutures, microcephaly, macrocephaly, craniostenosis, hydrocephalus) Cerebral atrophy Cerebral malformations CNS hemorrhage Tumor Intracranial calcifications due to toxoplasmosis, cytomegalovirus infection, or tuberous sclerosis	Cranial MRI* TORCH screening Urine culture for virus Chromosome analysis Chromosomal microarray analysis

*After neurologic consultation.

SMA = sequential multiple analyzer; TORCH = toxoplasmosis, rubella, cytomegalovirus, herpes.

be shortened, depending on the etiology of the disability, but health care is improving long-term health outcomes for people with all types of developmental disabilities. People with severe intellectual disability are likely to require life-long support. The more severe the cognitive disability and the greater the immobility, the higher the mortality risk.

Treatment

- Early intervention program
- Multidisciplinary team support

Treatment and support needs depend on social competence and cognitive function. Referral to an early intervention program during infancy may prevent or decrease the severity of disability resulting from a perinatal insult. Realistic methods of caring for affected children must be established.

Family support and counseling are crucial. As soon as intellectual disability is confirmed or strongly suspected, the parents should be informed and given ample time to discuss causes, effects, prognosis, education and training of the child, and the importance of balancing known prognostic risks against negative self-fulfilling prophecies in which diminished expectations result in poor functional outcomes later in life. Sensitive ongoing counseling is essential for family adaptation. If the family's physician cannot provide coordination and counseling, the child and family should be referred to a center with a multidisciplinary team that evaluates and serves children with intellectual disability; however, the family's physician should provide continuing medical care and advice.

A comprehensive, individualized program is developed with the help of appropriate specialists, including educators.

A multidisciplinary team includes

- Neurologists or developmental-behavioral pediatricians
- Orthopedists
- Physical therapists and occupational therapists (who assist in managing comorbidities in children with motor deficits)
- Speech pathologists and audiologists (who help with language delays or with suspected hearing loss)
- Nutritionists (who help with treatment of undernutrition)
- Social workers (who help reduce environmental deprivation and identify key resources)

Affected children with concomitant mental health disorders such as depression may be given appropriate psychoactive drugs in dosages similar to those used in children without intellectual disability. Use of psychoactive drugs without behavioral therapy and environmental changes is rarely helpful.

Every effort should be made to have children live at home or in community-based residences. Although the presence of a child with intellectual disability in the home can be disruptive, it can also be extremely rewarding. The family may benefit from psychologic support and help with daily care provided by day care centers, homemakers, and respite services. The living environment must encourage independence and reinforce learning of skills needed to accomplish this goal.

Whenever possible, children with intellectual disability should attend an appropriately adapted day care center or school with peers without cognitive disability. The Individuals with Disabilities Education Act (IDEA), the primary US special education law, stipulates that all children with disabilities should receive appropriate educational opportunities and programming in the least restrictive and most inclusive environments.

As people with intellectual disability reach adulthood, an array of supportive living and work settings is available. Large residential institutions are being replaced by small group or individual residences matched to the affected person's functional abilities and needs.

Prevention

Genetic counseling may help high-risk couples understand possible risks. If a child has intellectual disability, evaluation of the etiology can provide the family with appropriate risk information for future pregnancies.

Prenatal testing may be done in high-risk couples who choose to have children. Prenatal testing enables couples to consider pregnancy termination and subsequent family planning. Testing includes

- Amniocentesis or chorionic villus sampling
- Ultrasonography
- Maternal serum alpha-fetoprotein

Amniocentesis or chorionic villus sampling may detect inherited metabolic and chromosomal disorders, carrier states, and CNS malformations (eg, neural tube defects, anencephaly). Amniocentesis may be considered for all pregnant women > 35 yr (because their risk of having an infant with Down syndrome is increased) and for women with family histories of inherited metabolic disorders.

Ultrasonography may also identify CNS defects.

Maternal serum alpha-fetoprotein is a helpful screen for neural tube defects, Down syndrome, and other abnormalities.

Vaccines have all but eliminated congenital rubella and pneumococcal and *H. influenzae* meningitis as causes of intellectual disability.

Continuing improvements in and increased availability of obstetric and neonatal care and the use of exchange transfusion and Rh_0(D) immune globulin to prevent hemolytic disease of the newborn have reduced the incidence of intellectual disability; the increase in survival of very low-birth-weight infants has kept the prevalence constant.

KEY POINTS

- Intellectual disability involves slow intellectual development with subaverage intellectual functioning, immature behavior, and limited self-care skills that in combination are severe enough to require some level of support.
- A number of prenatal, perinatal, and postnatal disorders can cause intellectual disability, but a specific cause often cannot be identified.
- Deficits in language and personal-social skills may be due to emotional problems, environmental deprivation, learning disorders, or deafness rather than intellectual disability.
- Screen using tests such as the Ages and Stages Questionnaire (ASQ) or the Parents' Evaluation of Developmental Status (PEDS) and refer suspected cases for standardized intelligence testing and neurodevelopmental assessment.
- Search for specific causes with cranial imaging, genetic tests (eg, chromosomal microarray analysis, exome sequencing), and other tests as clinically indicated.
- Provide a comprehensive, individualized program (including family support and counseling) using a multidisciplinary team.

OVERVIEW OF LEARNING DISORDERS

Learning disorders are conditions that cause a discrepancy between potential and actual levels of academic performance as predicted by the person's intellectual abilities.

Learning disorders involve impairments or difficulties in concentration or attention, language development, or visual and aural information processing. Diagnosis includes cognitive, educational, speech and language, medical, and psychologic evaluations. Treatment consists primarily of educational management and sometimes medical, behavioral, and psychologic therapy.

Learning disorders are considered a type of neurodevelopmental disorder. Neurodevelopmental disorders are neurologically based conditions that appear early in childhood, typically before school entry. These disorders impair development of personal, social, academic, and/or occupational functioning and typically involve difficulties with the acquisition, retention, or application of specific skills or sets of information. The disorders may involve dysfunction in attention, memory, perception, language, problem-solving, or social interaction. Other common neurodevelopmental disorders include attention-deficit/hyperactivity disorder, autism spectrum disorders, and intellectual disability.

Specific learning disorders affect the ability to

- Understand or use spoken language
- Understand or use written language
- Do mathematical calculations
- Coordinate movements
- Focus attention on a task

Thus, these disorders involve problems in reading, mathematics, spelling, written expression or handwriting, and understanding or using verbal and nonverbal language (see Table 318–3). Most learning disorders are complex or mixed, with deficits in more than one system.

Although the number of children with learning disorders is unknown, about 5% of the school-age population in the US receives special educational services for learning disorders. Among affected children, boys outnumber girls 5:1.

Learning disorders may be congenital or acquired. No single cause has been defined, but neurologic deficits are evident or presumed. Genetic influences are often implicated. Other possible causes include

- Maternal illness or use of toxic drugs during pregnancy
- Complications during pregnancy or delivery (eg, spotting, toxemia, prolonged labor, precipitous delivery)
- Neonatal problems (eg, prematurity, low birth weight, severe jaundice, perinatal asphyxia, postmaturity, respiratory distress)

Potential postnatal factors include exposure to environmental toxins (eg, lead), CNS infections, cancers and their treatments, trauma, undernutrition, and severe social isolation or deprivation.

Table 318–3. COMMON SPECIFIC LEARNING DISORDERS

DISORDER	MANIFESTATION
Dyslexia (impairment in reading)	Problems with reading
Phonologic dyslexia	Problems with sound analysis and memory
Surface dyslexia	Problems with visual recognition of forms and structures of words
Dysgraphia (impairment in written expression)	Problems with spelling, written expression, or handwriting
Dyscalculia (impairment in mathematics)	Problems with mathematics and difficulties with problem-solving
Ageometria (ageometresia)	Problems due to disturbances in mathematical reasoning
Anarithmia	Disturbances in basic concept formation and inability to acquire computational skills
Anomic aphasia (dysnomia)	Difficulty recalling words and information from memory on demand

Symptoms and Signs

Children with learning disorders typically have at least average intelligence, although such disorders can occur in children with lower cognitive function as well. Symptoms and signs of severe disorders may manifest at an early age, but most mild to moderate learning disorders are not recognized until school age, when the rigors of academic learning are encountered.

Academic impairments: Affected children may have trouble learning the alphabet and may be delayed in paired associative learning (eg, color naming, labeling, counting, letter naming). Speech perception may be limited, language may be learned at a slower rate, and vocabulary may be decreased. Affected children may not understand what is read, have very messy handwriting or hold a pencil awkwardly, have trouble organizing or beginning tasks or retelling a story in sequential order, or confuse math symbols and misread numbers.

Executive function impairments: Disturbances or delays in expressive language or listening comprehension are predictors of academic problems beyond the preschool years. Memory may be defective, including short-term and long-term memory, memory use (eg, rehearsal), and verbal recall or retrieval. Problems may occur in conceptualizing, abstracting, generalizing, reasoning, and organizing and planning information for problem solving.

Visual perception and auditory processing problems may occur; they include difficulties in spatial cognition and orientation (eg, object localization, spatial memory, awareness of position and place), visual attention and memory, and sound discrimination and analysis.

Behavior problems: Some children with learning disabilities have difficulty following social conventions (eg, taking turns, standing too close to the listener, not understanding jokes); these difficulties are often components of mild autism spectrum disorders as well.

Short attention span, motor restlessness, fine motor problems (eg, poor printing and copying), and variability in performance and behavior over time are other early signs.

Difficulties with impulse control, non–goal-directed behavior and overactivity, discipline problems, aggressiveness, withdrawal and avoidance behavior, excessive shyness, and excessive fear may occur. Learning disabilities and attention-deficit/hyperactivity disorder (ADHD) often occur together.

Diagnosis

- Cognitive, educational, medical, and psychologic evaluations
- Clinical criteria

Children with learning disorders are typically identified when a discrepancy is recognized between academic potential and academic performance. Speech and language, cognitive, educational, medical, and psychologic evaluations are necessary for determining deficiencies in skills and cognitive processes.

Social and emotional-behavioral evaluations are also necessary for planning treatment and monitoring progress.

Evaluation: Cognitive evaluation typically includes verbal and nonverbal intelligence testing and is usually done by school personnel. Psychoeducational testing may be helpful in describing the child's preferred manner of processing information (eg, holistically or analytically, visually or aurally). Neuropsychologic assessment is particularly useful in children with known CNS injury or illness to map the areas of the brain that correspond to specific functional strengths and weaknesses. Speech and language evaluations establish integrity of comprehension and language use, phonologic processing, and verbal memory.

Educational assessment and performance evaluation by teachers' observations of classroom behavior and determination of academic performance are essential. Reading evaluations measure abilities in word decoding and recognition, comprehension, and fluency. Writing samples should be obtained to evaluate spelling, syntax, and fluency of ideas. Mathematical ability should be assessed in terms of computation skills, knowledge of operations, understanding of concepts, and interpretation of "word problems."

Medical evaluation includes a detailed family history, the child's medical history, a physical examination, and a neurologic or neurodevelopmental examination to look for underlying disorders. Although infrequent, physical abnormalities and neurologic signs may indicate medically treatable causes of learning disabilities. Gross motor coordination problems may indicate neurologic deficits or neurodevelopmental delays. Developmental level is evaluated according to standardized criteria.

Psychologic evaluation helps identify ADHD, conduct disorder, anxiety disorders, depression, and poor self-esteem, which frequently accompany and must be differentiated from learning disabilities. Attitude toward school, motivation, peer relationships, and self-confidence are assessed.

Clinical criteria: Diagnosis is made clinically based on criteria in the *Diagnostic and Statistical Manual of Mental Disorders,* Fifth Edition (DSM-5), and requires evidence that at least one of the following has been present for ≥ 6 mo despite targeted intervention:

- Inaccurate, slow and/or effortful word reading
- Difficulty understanding the meaning of written material
- Difficulty spelling
- Difficulty writing (eg, multiple grammar and punctuation errors; ideas not expressed clearly)
- Difficulty mastering number sense (eg, understanding the relative magnitude and relationship of numbers; in older children, difficulty doing simple calculations)
- Difficulty with mathematical reasoning (eg, using mathematical concepts to solve problems)

Skills must be substantially below the level expected for the child's age and also significantly impair performance at school or in daily activities.

Treatment

- Educational management
- Medical, behavioral, and psychologic therapy
- Occasionally drug therapy

Treatment centers on educational management but may also involve medical, behavioral, and psychologic therapy. Effective teaching programs may take a remedial, compensatory, or strategic (ie, teaching the child how to learn) approach. A mismatch of instructional method and a child's learning disorder and learning preference aggravates the disability.

Some children require specialized instruction in only one area while they continue to attend regular classes. Other children need separate and intense educational programs. Optimally and as required by US law, affected children should participate as much as possible in inclusive classes with peers who do not have learning disabilities.

Drugs minimally affect academic achievement, intelligence, and general learning ability, although certain drugs (eg, psychostimulants, such as methylphenidate and several amphetamine preparations) may enhance attention and concentration, allowing children to respond more efficiently to instruction.

Many popular remedies and therapies (eg, eliminating food additives, using antioxidants or megadoses of vitamins, patterning by sensory stimulation and passive movement, sensory integrative therapy through postural exercises, auditory nerve training, optometric training to remedy visual-perceptual and sensorimotor coordination processes) are unproved.

DYSLEXIA

Dyslexia is a general term for primary reading disorder. Diagnosis is based on intellectual, educational, speech and language, medical, and psychologic evaluations. Treatment is primarily educational management, consisting of instruction in word recognition and component skills.

Dyslexia is a specific type of learning disorder. Learning disorders involve problems in reading, mathematics, spelling, written expression or handwriting, and understanding or using verbal and nonverbal language (see Table 318–3).

No definition of dyslexia is universally accepted; thus, incidence is undetermined. An estimated 15% of public school children receive special instruction for reading problems; about half of these children may have persistent reading disabilities. Dyslexia is identified more often in boys than girls, but sex is not a proven risk factor for developing dyslexia.

The inability to learn derivational rules of printed language is often considered part of dyslexia. Affected children may have difficulty determining root words or word stems and determining which letters in words follow others.

Reading problems other than dyslexia are usually caused by difficulties in language comprehension or low cognitive ability. Visual-perceptual problems and abnormal eye movements are not dyslexia. However, these problems can interfere further with word learning.

Etiology

Aural, rather than visual, problems are now thought to be the predominant causes of reading disabilities. Phonologic processing problems cause deficits in discrimination, blending, memory, and analysis of sounds. Dyslexia may affect both production and understanding of written language, which is often restricted further by problems with auditory memory, speech production, and naming or word finding. Underlying weaknesses in verbal language are often present.

Pathophysiology

Dyslexia tends to run in families. Children with a family history of reading or learning difficulties are at higher risk. Because changes have been identified in the brains of people with dyslexia, experts believe dyslexia results predominantly from cortical dysfunction stemming from congenital neurodevelopmental abnormalities. Lesions affecting the integration or interactions of specific brain functions are suspected. Most researchers concur that dyslexia is left hemisphere–related and linked to dysfunctions in brain areas responsible for language association (Wernicke motor speech area) and sound and speech production (Broca motor speech area) and in the interconnection of these areas via the fasciculus arcuatus. Dysfunctions or defects in the angular gyrus, the medial occipital area, and the right hemisphere cause word recognition problems. Research suggests some malleability of brain systems in response to training.

Symptoms and Signs

Dyslexia may manifest as

- Delayed language production
- Speech articulation difficulties
- Difficulties remembering the names of letters, numbers, and colors

Children with phonologic processing problems often have difficulty blending sounds, rhyming words, identifying the positions of sounds in words, and segmenting words into pronounceable components. They may reverse the order of sounds in words. Delay or hesitation in choosing words, substituting words, or naming letters and pictures is often an early sign. Short-term auditory memory and auditory sequencing difficulties are common.

Fewer than 20% of children with dyslexia have difficulties with the visual demands of reading. However, some children confuse letters and words with similar configurations or have difficulty visually selecting or identifying letter patterns and clusters (sound-symbol association) in words. Reversals or visual confusions can occur, most often because of retention or retrieval difficulties that cause affected children to forget or confuse the names of letters and words that have similar structures; subsequently, *d* becomes *b, m* becomes *w, h* becomes *n, was* becomes *saw, on* becomes *no*. However, such reversals are normal in children < 8 yr.

Although dyslexia is a lifelong problem, many children develop functional reading skills. However, other children never reach adequate literacy.

Diagnosis

- Reading evaluation
- Speech, language, and auditory evaluations
- Psychologic evaluations

Most children with dyslexia are not identified until kindergarten or 1st grade, when they encounter symbolic learning. Children with a history of delayed language acquisition or use, who are not accelerating in word learning by the end of 1st grade, or who are not reading at the level expected for their verbal or intellectual abilities at any grade level should be evaluated. Often, the best diagnostic indicator is the child's inability to respond to traditional or typical reading approaches during 1st grade, although wide variation in reading skills can still be seen at this level. Demonstration of phonologic processing problems is essential for diagnosis.

Children suspected of having dyslexia should undergo reading, speech and language, auditory, cognitive, and psychologic evaluations to identify their functional strengths and weaknesses and their preferred learning styles. Such evaluations can be requested of school staff by the child's teacher or family based on the Individuals with Disabilities Education Act (IDEA), the primary US special education law. Evaluation findings then guide the most effective instructional approach.

Comprehensive reading evaluations test word recognition and analysis, fluency, reading or listening comprehension, and level of understanding of vocabulary and the reading process.

Speech, language, and auditory evaluations assess spoken language and deficits in processing phonemes (sound elements) of spoken language. Receptive and expressive language functions are also assessed. Cognitive abilities (eg, attention, memory, reasoning) are tested.

Psychologic evaluations address emotional concerns that can exacerbate a reading disability. A complete family history of mental disorders and emotional problems is obtained.

Physicians should ensure that children have normal vision and hearing, either through office-based screening or referral for formal audiologic or vision testing. Neurologic evaluations may help detect secondary features (eg, neurodevelopmental immaturity or minor neurologic abnormalities) and rule out other disorders (eg, seizures).

Treatment

- Educational interventions

Treatment consists of educational interventions, including direct and indirect instruction in word recognition and component skills.

Direct instruction includes teaching specific phonics skills separate from other reading instruction. Indirect instruction includes integrating phonics skills into reading programs. Instruction may teach reading from a whole-word or whole-language approach or by following a hierarchy of skills from the sound unit to the word to the sentence. Multisensory approaches that include whole-word learning and the integration of visual, auditory, and tactual procedures to teach sounds, words, and sentences are then recommended.

Component skills instruction consists of teaching children to blend sounds to form words, segment words into word parts, and identify the positions of sounds in words. Component skills for reading comprehension include identifying the main idea, answering questions, isolating facts and details, and reading inferentially. Many children benefit from using a computer to help isolate words within text samples or for word processing of written work.

Compensatory strategies, such as using audiobooks and taking notes using a digital recorder, can help children in later elementary school grades master content while continuing to build reading skills.

Other treatments (eg, optometric training, perceptual training, auditory integration training) and drug therapies are unproved and not recommended.

KEY POINTS

- Dyslexia involves difficulty reading, and producing and understanding written language; there may also be problems with auditory memory, speech production, and naming or word finding.
- Dyslexia probably results from congenital neurodevelopmental abnormalities that affect left hemisphere brain areas responsible for language association, sound and speech production, the interconnections between these areas, or a combination.
- Children may have delayed language production, but sometimes the first indicator is inability to respond to typical reading instruction during early elementary grades.
- Rule out cognitive, psychologic, hearing, and vision disorders.
- Various educational interventions are used.

RETT SYNDROME

Rett syndrome is a neurodevelopmental disorder occurring almost exclusively in females that affects development after an initial 6-mo period of normal development. Diagnosis is based on clinical observation of signs and symptoms during the child's early growth and development, regular ongoing evaluations of the child's physical and neurologic status and genetic testing to search for the *MECP2* gene mutation on the child's X chromosome (Xq28). Treatment involves a multidisciplinary approach that focuses on the management of symptoms.

Rett syndrome is estimated to affect 1 in every 10,000 to 15,000 live female births in all racial and ethnic groups worldwide. Most cases are random, spontaneous mutations; < 1% of recorded cases are inherited or passed from one generation to the next. Girls with the typical clinical picture of Rett syndrome are usually born at term after an uneventful pregnancy and delivery. Boys are rarely affected.

Etiology

Usually Rett syndrome is caused by a mutation in the methyl CpG binding protein 2 (*MECP2*) gene. The *MECP2* gene is involved in the production of a protein called methyl-cystine binding protein 2 (MeCP2) which is needed for brain development and acts as a biochemical switch that can either increase gene expression or tell other genes when to turn off and stop producing their own unique proteins. The *MECP2* gene does not function normally in Rett syndrome so that structural abnormal forms or inadequate amounts of the protein are produced and can cause other genes to have abnormal gene expression.

Rett syndrome is not always caused by a *MECP2* mutation but may be caused by partial gene deletions, mutations in other genes (eg, *CDKL5* and *FOXG1* genes) that affect brain development in atypical Rett syndrome, mutations in other parts of the *MECP2* gene, and possibly other genes that have not yet been identified.

Now that a genetic cause of Rett syndrome has been identified, it has been separated from the autism spectrum disorders (inconsistently associated with genetic causes) based on criteria from the *Diagnostic and Statistical Manual of Mental Disorders*, Fifth Edition (DSM-5).

Symptoms and Signs

The course, age of onset, and severity of symptoms of Rett syndrome vary from child to child.

Rett syndrome is characterized by normal early growth and development followed by slowing of developmental milestones, and then regression of skills with loss of purposeful hand use with compulsive hand wringing and washing behavior, slowed head and brain growth, seizures, walking difficulty, and intellectual disability.

There are 4 stages used to describe the symptoms of Rett syndrome:

- **Stage 1** (early onset) usually begins when the child is between 6 and 18 mo old with subtle slowing of development. Symptoms may include less eye contact, decreased interest in toys, delays in sitting or crawling, decreased head growth, and hand-wringing.
- **Stage 2** (developmental regression or rapid destructive stage) usually begins between ages 1 and 4 yr. The onset may be rapid or gradual with loss of purposeful hand skills and spoken language. During this stage, characteristic hand movements begin such as wringing, clapping, washing, tapping and repeatedly bringing the hands to the mouth. The movements disappear during sleep. Breathing irregularities may occur, such as episodes of apnea and hyperventilation. Walking may be unsteady, and initiating motor movements may be difficult. Some girls may also have symptoms similar to those of autism spectrum disorders, such as impaired social interaction and impaired communication.
- **Stage 3** (pseudostationary stage) usually begins between ages 2 and 10 yr and can last for years. Seizures, motor deficits, and apraxia are common during this stage. Sometimes, symptoms such as crying, irritability, and autism-like symptoms decline during this stage. Alertness, communication skills, attention span, and interest in the surroundings may increase during this stage.
- **Stage 4** (late motor deterioration stage) can last for years or decades. Common characteristics include scoliosis, decreased mobility, muscle weakness, spasticity, or rigidity. Sometimes walking may stop. Eye gaze for communication purposes becomes prominent as spoken language is absent, and repetitive hand movements may decrease.

Children may develop scoliosis. Cardiac abnormalities (such as prolonged QT interval) are often present. Affected children may have slowed growth and tend to have difficulty maintaining weight.

Diagnosis

- Clinical
- Genetic testing

Diagnosis is made clinically by observing signs and symptoms during the child's early growth and development. Ongoing evaluation of the child's physical and neurologic status is needed.

Genetic testing for the *MECP2* mutation on the X chromosome (Xq28) is used to complement the clinical diagnosis.

The National Institute of Neurological Disorders and Stroke (NINDS) provides guidelines used to confirm the clinical diagnosis of Rett syndrome. These guidelines divide the clinical diagnostic criteria into main, supportive and exclusion.

The **main diagnostic criteria** include loss of all or part of purposeful hand skills, repetitive hand movements (such as wringing or squeezing, clapping or rubbing), loss of all or part of spoken language, and gait abnormalities including toe-walking, unsteady, wide-based or stiff-legged walk.

The **supportive criteria** are not required for a diagnosis of Rett syndrome but may occur in some children. A child with supportive criteria but none of the main criteria does not have Rett syndrome. Supportive criteria include scoliosis, teeth-grinding, abnormal sleep patterns, small hands and feet in relation to height, cold hands and feet, abnormal muscle tone, intense eye communication, inappropriate laughing or screaming, and decreased response to pain.

The **exclusion criteria** include the presence of other disorders that cause similar symptoms, including traumatic brain injury, grossly abnormal psychomotor development during the first 6 mo, and severe infection causing neurologic problems.

Prognosis

Rett syndrome is rare, so there is little information about long-term prognosis and life expectancy beyond about age 40. Sometimes cardiac abnormalities may predispose children with Rett syndrome to sudden death but usually children survive well into adulthood with comprehensive, multidisciplinary team support.

Treatment

- Management of symptoms
- Multidisciplinary team support

There is no cure for Rett syndrome. Treatment is optimal with a multidisciplinary approach to address symptoms and signs.

A program of occupational therapy, physical therapy, and communication therapy (with a speech and language therapist) should be provided to address self-help skills such as feeding and dressing, limited mobility, walking difficulty, and communication deficits.

Drugs may be needed to control seizures, for breathing dysfunction or motor difficulties

Regular re-evaluation is needed for scoliosis progression and to follow cardiac abnormalities.

Nutrition support may be needed to help affected children maintain weight. Special education programs and social and support services are needed.

319 Mental Disorders in Children and Adolescents

Although it is sometimes assumed that childhood and adolescence are times of carefree bliss, as many as 20% of children and adolescents have one or more diagnosable mental disorders. Most of these disorders may be viewed as exaggerations or distortions of normal behaviors and emotions.

Like adults, children and adolescents vary in temperament. Some are shy and reticent; others are socially exuberant. Some are methodical and cautious; others are impulsive and careless. Whether a child is behaving like a typical child or has a disorder is determined by the presence of impairment and the degree of distress related to the symptoms. For example, a 12-yr-old girl may be frightened by the prospect of delivering a book report in front of her class. This fear would be viewed as social anxiety disorder only if her fears were severe enough to cause significant distress and avoidance.

There is much overlap between the symptoms of many disorders and the challenging behaviors and emotions of normal children. Thus, many strategies useful for managing behavioral problems in children can also be used in children who have mental disorders. Furthermore, appropriate management of childhood behavioral problems may decrease the risk of temperamentally vulnerable children developing a full-blown disorder. Also, effective treatment of some disorders (eg, anxiety) during childhood may decrease the risk of mood disorders later in life.

The **most common mental disorders** of childhood and adolescence fall into the following categories:

- Anxiety disorders
- Stress-related disorders
- Mood disorders
- Obsessive-compulsive disorder
- Disruptive behavioral disorders (eg, attention-deficit/hyperactivity disorder [ADHD], conduct disorder, and oppositional defiant disorder)

Schizophrenia and related disorders are much less common.

However, more often than not, children and adolescents have symptoms and problems that cut across diagnostic boundaries. For example, > 25% of children with ADHD also have an anxiety disorder, and 25% meet the criteria for a mood disorder.

Evaluation

Evaluation of mental complaints or symptoms in children and adolescents differs from that in adults in 3 important ways:

- Developmental context is critically important in children. Behaviors that are normal at a young age may indicate a serious mental disorder at an older age.
- Children exist in the context of a family system, and that system has a profound effect on children's symptoms and behaviors; normal children living in a family troubled by domestic violence and substance abuse may superficially appear to have one or more mental disorders.
- Children often do not have the cognitive and linguistic sophistication needed to accurately describe their symptoms. Thus, the clinician must rely very heavily on direct observation, corroborated by observations of other people, such as parents and teachers.

In many cases, developmental and behavioral problems (eg, poor academic progress, delays in language acquisition, deficits in social skills) are difficult to distinguish from those due to a mental disorder. In such cases, formal developmental and neuropsychologic testing should be part of the evaluation process.

Because of these factors, evaluation of children with a mental disorder is typically more complex than that of adults. However, most cases are not severe and can be competently managed by an appropriately trained primary care practitioner. However, uncertain or severe cases are best managed in consultation with a child and adolescent psychiatrist.

OVERVIEW OF ANXIETY DISORDERS IN CHILDREN AND ADOLESCENTS

Anxiety disorders are characterized by fear, worry, or dread that greatly impairs the ability to function normally and that is disproportionate to the circumstances at hand. Anxiety may result in physical symptoms. Diagnosis is clinical. Treatment is with behavioral therapy and drugs, usually SSRIs.

Some anxiety is a normal aspect of development, as in the following:

- Most toddlers become fearful when separated from their mother, especially in unfamiliar surroundings.
- Fears of the dark, monsters, bugs, and spiders are common in 3- to 4-yr-olds.
- Shy children may initially react to new situations with fear or withdrawal.
- Fears of injury and death are more common among older children.
- Older children and adolescents often become anxious when giving a book report in front of their classmates.

Such difficulties should not be viewed as evidence of a disorder. However, if manifestations of anxiety become so exaggerated that they greatly impair function or cause severe distress and/or avoidance, an anxiety disorder should be considered.

Anxiety disorders often emerge during childhood and adolescence. At some point during childhood, about 10 to 15% of children experience an anxiety disorder. Children with an anxiety disorder have an increased risk of depressive and anxiety disorders later in life.

Anxiety disorders that can occur in children and adolescents include

- Agoraphobia
- Generalized anxiety disorder (GAD)
- Panic disorder
- Separation anxiety disorder
- Social anxiety disorder
- Specific phobias

Etiology

Evidence suggests that anxiety disorders involve dysfunction in the parts of the limbic system and hippocampus that regulate emotions and response to fear. Heritability studies indicate a role for genetic and environmental factors. No specific genes have been identified; many genetic variants are probably involved.

Anxious parents tend to have anxious children; having such parents may make children's problems worse than they otherwise might be. Even normal children have difficulty remaining calm and composed in the presence of an anxious parent, and children who are genetically predisposed to anxiety have even greater difficulty. In as many as 30% of cases, treating the parents' anxiety in conjunction with the child's anxiety is helpful (for anxiety disorders in adults, see p. 1741).

Symptoms and Signs

Perhaps the most common manifestation of an anxiety disorder in children and adolescents is school refusal. "School refusal" has largely supplanted the term "school phobia." Actual fear of school is exceedingly rare. Most children who refuse to go to school probably have separation anxiety, social anxiety disorder, panic disorder, or a combination. Some have a specific phobia. The possibility that the child is being bullied at school must also be considered.

Some children complain directly about their anxiety, describing it in terms of worries—eg, "I am worried that I will never see you again" (separation anxiety) or "I am worried the kids will laugh at me" (social anxiety disorder). However, most children couch their discomfort in terms of somatic complaints: "I cannot go to school because I have a stomachache." These children are often telling the truth because an upset stomach, nausea, and headaches often develop in children with anxiety. Several long-term follow-up studies confirm that many children with somatic complaints, especially abdominal pain, have an underlying anxiety disorder.

Diagnosis

- Clinical evaluation

Diagnosis of an anxiety disorder is clinical. A thorough psychosocial history can usually confirm it.

The physical symptoms that anxiety can cause in children can complicate the evaluation. In many children, considerable testing for physical disorders is done before clinicians consider an anxiety disorder.

Prognosis

Prognosis depends on severity, availability of competent treatment, and the child's resiliency. Many children struggle with anxiety symptoms into adulthood. However, with early treatment, many children learn how to control their anxiety.

Treatment

- Behavioral therapy (exposure-based cognitive-behavioral therapy)
- Parent-child and family interventions
- Drugs, usually SSRIs for long-term treatment and sometimes benzodiazepines to relieve acute symptoms

Anxiety disorders in children are treated with behavioral therapy (using principles of exposure and response prevention), sometimes in conjunction with drug therapy.

In exposure-based cognitive-behavioral therapy, children are systematically exposed to the anxiety-provoking situation in a graded fashion. By helping children remain in the anxiety-provoking situation (response prevention), therapists enable them to gradually become desensitized and feel less anxiety. Behavioral therapy is most effective when an experienced therapist knowledgeable in child development individualizes these principles.

In mild cases, behavioral therapy alone is usually sufficient, but drug therapy may be needed when cases are more severe or when access to an experienced child behavior therapist is limited. SSRIs are usually the first choice for long-term treatment (see Table 319–1). Benzodiazepines are better for acute anxiety (eg, due to a medical procedure) but are not preferred for long-term treatment. Benzodiazepines with a short-half life (eg, lorazepam 0.05 mg/kg to a maximum of 2 mg in a single dose) are the best choice.

Most children tolerate SSRIs without difficulty. Occasionally, upset stomach, diarrhea, insomnia, or weight gain may occur. Some children have behavioral adverse effects (eg, agitation, disinhibition); these effects are usually mild to moderate. Usually, decreasing the drug dose or changing to a different drug eliminates or reduces these effects. Rarely, behavioral adverse effects (eg, aggressiveness, increased suicidality) are severe. Behavioral adverse effects are idiosyncratic and may occur with any antidepressant and at any time during treatment. As a result, children and adolescents taking such drugs must be closely monitored.

KEY POINTS

- The most common manifestation of an anxiety disorder may be school refusal; most children couch their discomfort in terms of somatic complaints.
- Consider anxiety as a disorder in children only when anxiety becomes so exaggerated that it greatly impairs functioning or causes severe distress and/or avoidance.
- The physical symptoms that anxiety can cause in children can complicate the evaluation.
- Behavioral therapy (using principles of exposure and response prevention) is most effective when done by an experienced therapist who is knowledgeable about child development and who tailors these principles to the child.
- When cases are more severe or when access to an experienced child behavior therapist is limited, drugs may be needed.

Table 319–1. DRUGS FOR LONG-TERM TREATMENT OF ANXIETY AND RELATED DISORDERS

DRUG	USES	STARTING DOSE*	DOSE RANGE	COMMENTS/PRECAUTIONS†
Citalopram	OCD children ≥ 7 yr	10 mg	10–40 mg/day	—
Duloxetine	GAD in children 7–17 yr	30 mg	30–100 mg/day	—
Escitalopram	Major depression in children ≥ 7 yr	5 mg	5–20 mg/day	—
Fluoxetine‡	OCD, GAD, separation anxiety, social anxiety, major depression in children > 8 yr	10 mg	10–60 mg/day	Long-half life
Fluvoxamine	GAD, separation anxiety, social anxiety, OCD in children > 8 yr	25 mg (titrated up as needed)	50–200 mg/day	For doses > 50 mg/day, divided into 2 doses/day, with the larger dose given at bedtime)
Paroxetine‡	OCD in children > 6 yr	10 mg	10–60 mg/day	Increased weight
Sertraline	OCD, GAD, separation anxiety, social anxiety in children ≥ 6 yr	25 mg	25–200 mg/day	—
Venlafaxine, immediate-release	Depression in children ≥ 8 yr	12.5 mg	25–75 mg/day bid or tid	Limited data about dose and concerns about increased suicidal behavior; not as effective as other drugs, possibly because low doses have been used
Venlafaxine, extended-release	GAD in children > 7 yr	37.5 mg	37.5–225 mg/day	

*Unless otherwise stated, dose is given once/day. Starting dose is increased only if needed. Dose ranges are approximate. Interindividual variability in therapeutic response and adverse effects is considerable. This table is not a substitute for the full prescribing information.

†Behavioral adverse effects (eg, disinhibition, agitation) are common but are usually mild to moderate. Usually, decreasing the drug dose or changing to a different drug eliminates or reduces these effects. Rarely, such effects are severe (eg, aggressiveness, increased suicidality). Behavioral adverse effects are idiosyncratic and may occur with any antidepressant and at any time during treatment. As a result, children and adolescents taking such drugs must be closely monitored.

‡Fluoxetine and paroxetine are potent inhibitors of the liver enzymes that metabolize many other drugs (eg, beta-blockers, clonidine, lidocaine).

GAD = generalized anxiety disorder; OCD = obsessive compulsive disorder.

AGORAPHOBIA IN CHILDREN AND ADOLESCENTS

Agoraphobia is a persistent fear of being trapped in situations or places without a way to escape easily and without help. Diagnosis is by history. Treatment is with benzodiazepines or SSRIs and behavioral therapy.

During a typical agoraphobic situation (eg, standing in line, sitting in the middle of a long row in a classroom), some people have panic attacks; others simply feel uncomfortable. Agoraphobia is uncommon among children, but it may develop in adolescents, particularly those who also have panic attacks.

Agoraphobia often interferes with function and, if severe enough, can cause people to become housebound.

Diagnosis

- Clinical criteria

For agoraphobia to be diagnosed, patients must consistently have fear or anxiety about ≥ 2 of the following for ≥ 6 mo:

- Using public transportation
- Being in open spaces
- Being in enclosed spaces
- Standing in line or being in a crowd
- Being outside the home alone

Also, the fear must cause patients to avoid the distressing situation to the extent that they have difficulty functioning normally (eg, going to school, visiting the mall, doing other typical activities).

Agoraphobia must be distinguished from the following:

- Specific phobias (eg, to a certain situation)
- Social anxiety disorder
- Panic disorder
- Depression, which can cause patients to avoid leaving the house for reasons unrelated to anxiety

Treatment

- Behavioral therapy

Behavioral therapy is especially useful for agoraphobia symptoms. Drugs are rarely useful except to control any associated panic attacks.

GENERALIZED ANXIETY DISORDER IN CHILDREN AND ADOLESCENTS

Generalized anxiety disorder (GAD) is a persistent state of heightened anxiety and apprehension characterized by excessive worrying, fear, and dread. Physical symptoms can include tremor, sweating, multiple somatic complaints, and

exhaustion. Diagnosis is by history. Treatment is often with relaxation therapy, sometimes combined with drug therapy.

Symptoms and Signs

Children with GAD have multiple and diffuse worries, which are exacerbated by stress. These children often have difficulty paying attention and may be hyperactive and restless. They may sleep poorly, sweat excessively, feel exhausted, and complain of physical discomfort (eg, stomachache, muscle aches, headache).

Diagnosis

- Clinical criteria

GAD is diagnosed in children and adolescents who have prominent and impairing anxiety symptoms that are not focused enough to meet criteria for a specific disorder such as social anxiety disorder or panic disorder. GAD is also an appropriate diagnosis for children who have a specific anxiety disorder, such as separation anxiety, but also have other significant anxiety symptoms above and beyond those of the specific anxiety disorder.

Specific criteria include excessive anxiety and worry that patients have difficulty controlling and that is present on more days than not for ≥ 6 mo. The symptoms must cause significant distress or impair functioning socially or at school and must be accompanied by ≥ 1 of the following:

- Restlessness or a keyed-up or on-edge feeling
- Being easily fatigued
- Difficulty concentrating
- Irritability
- Muscle tension
- Sleep disturbance

Occasionally, GAD can be confused with attention-deficit/hyperactivity disorder (ADHD) because GAD can cause difficulty paying attention and can result in psychomotor agitation (ie, hyperactivity). However, in ADHD, children also have difficulty concentrating and feel restless when they are not anxious. Some children have both ADHD and an anxiety disorder.

Treatment

- Relaxation therapy
- Sometimes anxiolytic drugs, usually SSRIs

Because the focus of symptoms is diffuse, GAD is especially challenging to treat with behavioral therapy. Relaxation training is often more appropriate.

Patients who have severe GAD or who do not respond to psychotherapeutic interventions may need anxiolytic drugs. As with other anxiety disorders, SSRIs (see Table 319–1) are typically the drugs of choice. Buspirone is sometimes used for children who cannot tolerate SSRIs; however, it is much less effective. The starting dose for buspirone is 5 mg po bid; the dose may be gradually increased to 30 mg bid (or 20 mg tid) as tolerated. GI distress or headache may be limiting factors in dosage escalation.

KEY POINTS

- Children with GAD have multiple and diffuse worries, rather than a single, specific one.
- Diagnose GAD when symptoms cause significant distress to the child or impair social or academic functioning socially and the child has ≥ 1 of specific symptoms (eg, restlessness, a keyed-up or on-edge feeling).
- Relaxation therapy may help; if children have severe GAD or do not respond to psychotherapeutic interventions, consider anxiolytic drugs (preferably SSRIs).

PANIC DISORDER IN CHILDREN AND ADOLESCENTS

Panic disorder is characterized by recurrent, frequent (at least once/wk) panic attacks. Panic attacks are discrete spells lasting about 20 min; during attacks, children experience somatic symptoms, cognitive symptoms, or both. Diagnosis is by history. Treatment is with benzodiazepines or SSRIs and behavioral therapy.

Panic disorder is much less common among prepubertal children than among adolescents.

Panic attacks can occur alone or in other anxiety disorders (eg, agoraphobia, separation anxiety), other mental disorders (eg, OCD), or certain medical disorders (eg, asthma). Panic attacks can trigger an asthma attack and vice versa.

Symptoms and Signs

Symptoms of a panic attack involve a sudden surge of intense fear, accompanied by somatic symptoms (eg, palpitations, sweating, trembling, shortness of breath or choking, chest pain, nausea, dizziness). Compared with those in adults (see p. 1743), panic attacks in children and adolescents are often more dramatic in presentation (eg, with screaming, weeping, and hyperventilation). This display can be alarming to parents and others.

Panic attacks usually develop spontaneously, but over time, children begin to attribute them to certain situations and environments. Affected children then attempt to avoid those situations, which can lead to agoraphobia. Avoidance behaviors are considered agoraphobia if they greatly impair normal functioning, such as going to school, visiting the mall, or doing other typical activities.

Diagnosis

- Clinical evaluation
- Evaluation for other causes

Panic disorder is diagnosed based on a history of recurrent panic attacks, usually after a physical examination is done to rule out physical causes of somatic symptoms. Many children undergo considerable diagnostic testing before panic disorder is suspected. The presence of other disorders, especially asthma, can also complicate the diagnosis. Thorough screening for other disorders (eg, OCD, social anxiety disorder) is needed because any one of these disorders may be the primary problem causing panic attacks as a symptom.

In adults, important diagnostic criteria for panic disorder include concerns about future attacks, the implications of the attacks, and changes in behavior. However, children and younger adolescents usually lack the insight and forethought needed to develop these features, except they may change behavior to avoid situations they believe are related to the panic attack.

Prognosis

Prognosis is good with treatment. Without treatment, adolescents may drop out of school, withdraw from society, and become reclusive and suicidal.

Panic disorder often waxes and wanes in severity without any discernible reason. Some patients experience long periods of spontaneous symptom remission, only to experience a relapse years later.

Treatment

- Usually benzodiazepines or SSRIs plus behavioral therapy

Treatment of panic disorder is usually a combination of drug therapy and behavioral therapy. In children, it is difficult to even begin behavioral therapy until after the panic attacks have been controlled by drugs.

Benzodiazepines are the most effective drugs, but SSRIs are often preferred because benzodiazepines are sedating and may greatly impair learning and memory. However, SSRIs do not work quickly, and a short course of a benzodiazepine (eg, lorazepam 0.5 to 2.0 mg po tid) may be helpful until the SSRI is effective.

KEY POINTS

- Panic attacks are characterized by a sudden surge of intense fear, accompanied by somatic symptoms.
- Panic attacks in children and adolescents are often more dramatic (eg, with screaming, weeping, and hyperventilation) than those in adults.
- Panic disorder often waxes and wanes in severity without any discernible reason.
- Treat panic disorder with benzodiazepines or SSRIs to control symptoms, then with behavioral therapy.

SEPARATION ANXIETY DISORDER

Separation anxiety disorder is a persistent, intense, and developmentally inappropriate fear of separation from a major attachment figure (usually the mother). Affected children desperately attempt to avoid such separations. When separation is forced, these children are distressfully preoccupied with reunification. Diagnosis is by history. Treatment is with behavioral therapy for the child and family and, for severe cases, SSRIs.

Separation anxiety is a normal emotion in children between about age 8 mo and 24 mo; it typically resolves as children develop a sense of object permanence and realize their parents will return. In some children, separation anxiety persists beyond this time or returns later; it may be severe enough to be considered a disorder. Separation anxiety disorder commonly occurs in younger children and is rare after puberty.

Life stresses (eg, death of a relative, friend, or pet; a geographic move, a change in schools) may trigger separation anxiety disorder. Also, some people have a genetic predisposition to anxiety.

Symptoms and Signs

Like social anxiety disorder, separation anxiety disorder often manifests as school (or preschool) refusal.

Dramatic scenes typically occur at the time of separation. Separation scenes are typically painful for both the child and attachment figure (usually the mother but can be either parent or a caregiver). Children often wail and plead with such desperation that the parent cannot leave, resulting in protracted scenes that are difficult to interrupt. When separated, children fixate on reunification with the attachment figure and are often worried that this person has been harmed (eg, in a car accident, by a serious illness). Children may refuse to sleep alone and may even insist on always being in the same room as the attachment figure.

Children often develop somatic complaints (eg, headache, stomachache).

The child's demeanor is often normal when the attachment figure is present. This normal demeanor can sometimes give a false impression that the problem is minor. However, some children have persistent and excessive worry about losing the attachment figure (eg, to illness, kidnapping, or death).

Separation anxiety is often compounded by a parent's anxiety, which exacerbates the child's anxiety; the result is a vicious circle that can be interrupted only by sensitive and appropriate treatment of parent and child simultaneously.

Diagnosis

- Clinical evaluation

Diagnosis of separation anxiety disorder is by history and by observation of separation scenes. Manifestations must be present ≥ 4 wk and cause significant distress or impair functioning (eg, children are unable to participate in age-appropriate social or scholastic activities).

Treatment

- Behavioral therapy
- Rarely anxiolytics

Treatment of separation anxiety disorder is with behavioral therapy that systematically enforces regular separations. The goodbye scenes should be kept as brief as possible, and the attachment figure should be coached to react to protestations matter-of-factly. Assisting children in forming an attachment to one of the adults in the preschool or school may be helpful.

In extreme cases, children may benefit from an anxiolytic such as an SSRI (see Table 319–1). However, separation anxiety disorder often affects children as young as 3 yr, and experience with these drugs in the very young is limited.

Successfully treated children are prone to relapses after holidays and breaks from school. Because of these relapses, parents are often advised to plan regular separations during these periods to help the child remain accustomed to being away from the parents.

KEY POINTS

- Separation anxiety is a normal emotion in children between about age 8 mo and 24 mo; if it persists beyond this time or returns later, it may be severe enough to be considered a disorder.
- Dramatic, painful scenes, with desperate wailing and pleading, typically occur at the time of separation.
- A normal demeanor when the attachment figure is present does not mean that the problem is minor.
- Treatment involves planning regular separations (including during holidays) and coaching the attachment figure to react to the child's protestations matter-of-factly.

SOCIAL ANXIETY DISORDER IN CHILDREN AND ADOLESCENTS

(Social Phobia)

Social anxiety disorder is a persistent fear of embarrassment, ridicule, or humiliation in social settings. Typically, affected children avoid situations that might provoke social scrutiny (eg, school). Diagnosis is by history. Treatment is with behavioral therapy; in severe cases, SSRIs are used.

Symptoms and Signs

The first symptoms of social anxiety disorder in adolescents may be excessive worrying before attending a social event or excessive preparation for a class presentation. The first symptoms in children may be tantrums, crying, freezing, clinging, or withdrawing in social situations. Avoidant behaviors (eg, refusing to go to school, not going to parties, not eating in front of others) can follow. Complaints often have a somatic focus (eg, "My stomach hurts," "I have a headache"). Some children have a history of many medical appointments and evaluations in response to these somatic complaints.

Affected children are terrified that they will humiliate themselves in front of their peers by giving the wrong answer, saying something inappropriate, becoming embarrassed, or even vomiting. In some cases, social anxiety disorder emerges after an unfortunate and embarrassing incident. In severe cases, children may refuse to talk on the telephone or even refuse to leave the house.

Diagnosis

- Clinical evaluation

For social anxiety disorder to be diagnosed, the anxiety must persist for ≥ 6 mo and be consistently present in similar settings (eg, children are anxious about all classroom presentations rather than only occasional ones or ones for a specific class). The anxiety must occur in peer settings and not only during interactions with adults.

Treatment

- Behavioral therapy
- Sometimes an anxiolytic

Behavioral therapy is the cornerstone of treatment for social anxiety disorder. Children should not be allowed to miss school. Absence serves only to make them even more reluctant to attend school.

If children and adolescents are not sufficiently motivated to participate in behavioral therapy or do not respond adequately to it, an anxiolytic such as an SSRI may help (see Table 319–1). Treatment with an SSRI may reduce anxiety enough to facilitate children's participation in behavioral therapy.

ACUTE AND POSTTRAUMATIC STRESS DISORDERS IN CHILDREN AND ADOLESCENTS

Acute stress disorder (ASD) and posttraumatic stress disorder (PTSD) are reactions to traumatic events. The reactions involve intrusive thoughts or dreams, avoidance of reminders of the event, and negative effects on mood, cognition, arousal, and reactivity. ASD typically begins immediately after the trauma and lasts from 3 days to 1 mo. PTSD can be a continuation of ASD or may manifest up to 6 mo after the trauma and lasts for > 1 mo. Diagnosis is by clinical criteria. Treatment is with behavioral therapy and sometimes with SSRIs or antiadrenergic drugs.

ASD and PTSD are trauma- and stressor-related disorders. They used to be considered anxiety disorders but are now considered distinct because many patients do not have anxiety but have other symptoms instead.

Because vulnerability and temperament are different, not all children who are exposed to a severe traumatic event develop a stress disorder. Traumatic events commonly associated with these disorders include assaults, sexual assaults, car accidents, dog attacks, and injuries (especially burns). In young children, domestic violence is the most common cause of PTSD.

Children do not have to directly experience the traumatic event; they may develop a stress disorder if they witness a traumatic event happening to others or learn that one occurred to a close family member.

Symptoms and Signs

Symptoms of ASD and PTSD are similar and generally involve a combination of the following:

- **Intrusion symptoms:** Recurrent, involuntary, and distressing memories or dreams of the traumatic event (in children < 6 yr, it may not be clear whether their distressing dreams are related to the event); dissociative reactions (typically flashbacks in which patients reexperience the trauma, although young children may frequently reenact the event in play); and distress at internal or external cues that resemble some aspect of the trauma (eg, seeing a dog or someone who resembles a perpetrator)
- **Avoidance symptoms:** Persistent avoidance of memories, feelings, or external reminders of the trauma
- **Negative effects on cognition and/or mood:** Inability to remember important aspects of the traumatic event, distorted thinking about the causes and/or consequences of the trauma (eg, that they are to blame or could have avoided the event by certain actions), a decrease in positive emotions and an increase in negative emotions (fear, guilt, sadness, shame, confusion), general lack of interest, social withdrawal, a subjective sense of feeling numb, and a foreshortened expectation of the future (eg, thinking "I will not live to see 20")
- **Altered arousal and/or reactivity** (eg, hyperarousal): Jitteriness, exaggerated startle response, difficulty relaxing, difficulty concentrating, disrupted sleep (sometimes with frequent nightmares), and aggressive or reckless behavior
- **Dissociative symptoms:** Feeling detached from one's body as if in a dream and feeling that the world is unreal

Typically, children with ASD are in a daze and may seem dissociated from everyday surroundings.

Children with PTSD have intrusive recollections that cause them to reexperience the traumatic event. The most dramatic kind of recollection is a flashback. Flashbacks may be spontaneous but are most commonly triggered by something associated with the original trauma. For example, the sight of a dog may trigger a flashback in children who experienced a dog attack. During a flashback, children may be in a terrified state and unaware of their current surroundings while desperately searching for a way to hide or escape; they may temporarily lose touch with reality and believe they are in grave danger. Some children have nightmares. When children reexperience the event in other ways (eg, in thoughts, mental images, or recollections), they remain aware of current surroundings, although they may still be greatly distressed.

Diagnosis

- Clinical evaluation

Diagnosis of ASD and PTSD is based on a history of exposure to severely frightening and horrifying trauma followed by reexperiencing, emotional numbing, and hyperarousal. These symptoms must be severe enough to cause impairment or distress.

Symptoms lasting ≥ 3 days and < 1 mo are considered ASD. Symptoms lasting > 1 mo are considered PTSD, which can be a continuation of ASD or may manifest up to 6 mo after the trauma.

Patients must have a number of manifestations in different symptom areas; specific criteria for ASD and PTSD in the *Diagnostic and Statistical Manual of Mental Disorders*, Fifth Edition (DSM-5) differ slightly.

Prognosis

Prognosis is much better for children with ASD than for those with PTSD, but both benefit from early treatment.

Risk factors include

- Severity of the trauma
- Associated physical injuries
- The underlying resiliency and temperament of children and family members
- Socioeconomic status
- Adversity during childhood
- Family dysfunction
- Minority status
- Family psychiatric history

Family and social support before and after the trauma moderates the final outcome.

Treatment

- SSRIs and sometimes antiadrenergic drugs
- Sometimes psychotherapy
- Behavioral therapy

SSRIs often help reduce emotional numbing and reexperiencing of symptoms but are less effective for hyperarousal. Antiadrenergic drugs (eg, clonidine, guanfacine, prazosin) may help relieve hyperarousal symptoms, but supportive data are preliminary.

Supportive psychotherapy may help children who have adjustment issues associated with trauma, as may result from disfigurement due to burns. Behavioral therapy can be used to systematically desensitize children to situations that cause them to reexperience the event (exposure therapy). Behavioral therapy is clearly effective in reducing distress and impairment in children and adolescents with PTSD.

KEY POINTS

- ASD typically begins immediately after the trauma and lasts from 3 days to 1 mo; PTSD lasts for > 1 mo and can be a continuation of ASD or may manifest up to 6 mo after the trauma.
- Stress disorders may start after children directly experience a traumatic event, if they witness one or learn that one happened to a close family member.
- Symptoms of ASD and PTSD are similar and usually involve a combination of intrusion symptoms (eg, reexperiencing the event), avoidance symptoms, negative effects on cognition and/or mood (eg, emotional numbing), altered arousal and/or reactivity, and dissociative symptoms.
- Treat with SSRIs and sometimes antiadrenergic drugs and supportive psychotherapy and/or exposure therapy.

BIPOLAR DISORDER IN CHILDREN AND ADOLESCENTS

Bipolar disorder is characterized by alternating periods of mania, depression, and normal mood, each lasting for weeks to months at a time. Diagnosis is based on clinical criteria. Treatment is a combination of mood stabilizers (eg, lithium, certain anticonvulsants, antipsychotic drugs), psychotherapy, and antidepressants.

Bipolar disorder typically begins during mid-adolescence through the mid-20s (see also. p. 1766). In many children, the initial manifestation is one or more episodes of depression.

Bipolar disorder is rare in children. In the past, bipolar disorder was diagnosed in prepubertal children who were disabled by intense, unstable moods. However, because such children typically progress to a depressive rather than bipolar disorder, they are now classified as having disruptive mood dysregulation disorder.

Etiology

Etiology of bipolar disorder is unknown, but heredity is involved. Dysregulation of serotonin and norepinephrine may be involved, as may a stressful life event.

Certain drugs (eg, cocaine, amphetamines, phencyclidines, certain antidepressants) and environmental toxins (eg, lead) can exacerbate or mimic the disorder. Certain disorders (eg, thyroid disorders) can cause similar symptoms.

Symptoms and Signs

The hallmark of bipolar disorder is the manic episode. Manic episodes alternate with depressive episodes, which can be more frequent. During a manic episode in adolescents, mood may be very positive or hyperirritable and often alternates between the 2 moods depending on social circumstances. Speech is rapid and pressured, sleep is decreased, and self-esteem is inflated. Mania may reach psychotic proportions (eg, "I have become one with God"). Judgment may be severely impaired, and adolescents may engage in risky behaviors (eg, promiscuous sex, reckless driving).

Prepubertal children may experience dramatic moods, but the duration of these moods is much shorter (often lasting only a few moments) than that in adolescents.

Onset is characteristically insidious, and children typically have a history of always being very temperamental and difficult to manage.

Diagnosis

- Clinical evaluation
- Testing for toxicologic causes

Diagnosis of bipolar disorder is based on identification of symptoms of mania as described above, plus a history of remission and relapse.

A number of medical disorders (eg, thyroid disorders, brain infections or tumors) and drug intoxication must be ruled out with appropriate medical assessment, including a toxicology screen for drugs of abuse and environmental toxins. The interviewer should also search for precipitating events, such as severe psychologic stress, including sexual abuse or incest.

Prognosis

Prognosis for adolescents with bipolar disorder varies. Those who have mild to moderate symptoms, who have a good response to treatment, and who remain adherent and cooperative with treatment have an excellent prognosis. However, treatment response is often incomplete, and adolescents are notoriously nonadherent to drug regimens. For such adolescents, the long-term prognosis is not as good.

Little is known about the long-term prognosis of prepubertal children diagnosed with bipolar disorder based on highly unstable and intense moods.

Treatment

- Mood stabilizers and antidepressants
- Psychotherapy

For adolescents and prepubertal children, mood stabilizers are used to treat manic or agitated episodes, and psychotherapy and antidepressants are used to treat the depressive episodes.

Mood stabilizers (see Table 319–2) roughly fall into 3 categories:

- Mood-stabilizing anticonvulsants
- Mood-stabilizing antipsychotics
- Lithium

All mood stabilizers have a potential for troubling and even dangerous adverse effects. Thus, treatment must be

Table 319–2. SELECTED DRUGS FOR BIPOLAR DISORDER*

DRUG	INDICATION	STARTING DOSE†	MAINTENANCE DOSE†	COMMENTS
Lithium				
Lithium extended-release,‡,§ in adolescents ≥ 12 yr	Acute mania and maintenance	—	450–900 mg bid	Dose titrated to a blood level of 0.8–1.2 mEq/L
Lithium, immediate-release,‡,§ in adolescents	Acute mania and maintenance	200–300 mg tid	300–600 mg tid up to 2400 mg/day	
Antipsychotics				
Aripiprazole§ in children ≥ 10 yr	Acute mania Psychosis	2–5 mg once/day	Up to 30 mg once/day	Limited experience in children
Chlorpromazine in children > 5 yr‡,§	Acute mania Psychosis	0.6–1.5 mg/kg q 6 h up to 200 mg/day	—	Rarely used because newer drugs have a more favorable adverse effect profile
Olanzapine in children > 13 yr§	Acute mania Psychosis	2.5–5 mg once/day	Up to 10 mg bid	Causes weight gain, which may limit use in some patients
Olanzapine/fluoxetine fixed combination children > 10 yr‡,§	Bipolar depression	3 mg/25 mg once/day	Up to 12 mg/50 mg once/day	Limited experience in children
Paliperidone in children > 12 yr ‡,§	Acute mania Psychosis	3 mg once/day	Up to 3 mg bid	Closely related to risperidone Very limited experience in children
Quetiapine, immediate-release, in children > 10 yr§	Acute mania Psychosis	25 mg bid	Up to 200 mg bid	Causes sedation that may limit dose increases
Risperidone in children > 10 yr§	Acute mania Psychosis	0.5 mg once/day	Up to 2.5 mg/day in divided doses (eg, 0.5 mg tid) up to 6 mg/day	Maintenance dose highly variable In high doses, increased risk of neurologic adverse effects
Ziprasidone in children > 10 yr§	Acute mania Psychosis	20 mg bid	Up to 80 mg bid	Very limited experience in children
Anticonvulsants				
Carbamazepine	Acute mania and mixed episode	200 mg bid	Up to 600 mg bid	Metabolic enzyme induction, possibly requiring dose adjustments
Divalproex	Acute mania	5 mg/kg bid or tid	Up to 10–20 mg/kg tid	Dose titrated to a blood level of 50–125 μg/mL
Lamotrigine	Maintenance	25 mg once/day	Up to 100 mg bid	Requires that dosing guidelines in the package insert be followed closely

*These drugs pose a small but serious risk for a wide variety of major adverse effects. Therefore, benefits must be carefully weighed against potential risks.

†Dose ranges are approximate. Interindividual variability in therapeutic response and adverse effects is considerable. This table is not a substitute for the full prescribing information.

‡These drugs have not been studied in children. For dosing in children < 12 yr, see the prescribing information.

§These drugs increase the risk of weight gain, negative effects on the lipid profile, increases in glucose and prolactin levels, and QT prolongation.

individualized. Furthermore, drugs that are highly successful during initial stabilization may be unacceptable for maintenance because of adverse effects, most notably weight gain.

Antidepressants may trigger a switch from depression to mania; therefore, they are usually used with a mood stabilizer.

PEARLS & PITFALLS

- In patients with bipolar disorder, antidepressants may trigger a switch from depression to mania, so they are usually used with a mood stabilizer.

KEY POINTS

- Bipolar disorder is characterized by alternating periods of mania, depression, and normal mood, each lasting for weeks to months at a time.
- Bipolar disorder typically begins during mid-adolescence through the mid-20s; it is rare in children.
- Typically, onset is insidious; children have a history of being very temperamental and difficult to manage.
- In adolescents and prepubertal children, treat manic or agitated episodes with mood stabilizers and depressive episodes with psychotherapy and antidepressants (usually with a mood stabilizer).

CONDUCT DISORDER

Conduct disorder is a recurrent or persistent pattern of behavior that violates the rights of others or violates major age-appropriate societal norms or rules. Diagnosis is by history. Treatment of comorbid disorders and psychotherapy may help; however, many children require considerable supervision.

Prevalence of some level of conduct disorder (CD) is about 10%. Onset is usually during late childhood or early adolescence, and the disorder is much more common among boys than girls.

Etiology is likely a complex interplay of genetic and environmental factors. Parents of adolescents with conduct disorder often have engaged in substance abuse and antisocial behaviors and frequently have been diagnosed with ADHD, mood disorders, schizophrenia, or antisocial personality disorder. However, conduct disorder can occur in children from high-functioning, healthy families.

Symptoms and Signs

Children or adolescents with conduct disorder lack sensitivity to the feelings and well-being of others and sometimes misperceive the behavior of others as threatening. They may act aggressively, by bullying and making threats, brandishing or using a weapon, committing acts of physical cruelty, or forcing someone into sexual activity, and have few or no feelings of remorse. Sometimes their aggression and cruelty is directed at animals. These children or adolescents may destroy property, lie, and steal. They tolerate frustration poorly and are commonly reckless, violating rules and parental prohibitions (eg, by running away from home, being frequently truant from school).

Aberrant behaviors differ between the sexes: Boys tend to fight, steal, and vandalize; girls are likely to lie, run away, and engage in prostitution. Both sexes are likely to use and abuse illicit drugs and have difficulties in school. Suicidal ideation is common, and suicide attempts must be taken seriously.

Diagnosis

- Clinical criteria

Conduct disorder is diagnosed in children or adolescents who have demonstrated ≥ 3 of the following behaviors in the previous 12 mo plus at least 1 in the previous 6 mo:

- Aggression toward people and animals
- Destruction of property
- Deceitfulness, lying, or stealing
- Serious violations of parental rules

Symptoms or behaviors must be significant enough to impair functioning in relationships, at school, or at work.

Prognosis

Usually, disruptive behaviors stop during early adulthood, but in about one third of cases, they persist. Many of these cases meet the criteria for antisocial personality disorder. Early onset is associated with a poorer prognosis.

Some children and adolescents subsequently develop mood or anxiety disorders, somatic symptom or related disorders, substance-related disorders, or early adult–onset psychotic disorders. Children and adolescents with conduct disorder tend to have higher rates of physical and other mental disorders.

Treatment

- Drugs to treat comorbid disorders
- Psychotherapy
- Sometimes placement in a residential center

Treating comorbid disorders with drugs and psychotherapy may improve self-esteem and self-control and ultimately improve control of conduct disorder. Drugs may include stimulants, mood stabilizers, and atypical antipsychotics, especially short-term use of risperidone.

Moralization and dire admonitions are ineffective and should be avoided. Individual psychotherapy, including cognitive therapy and behavior modification, may help. Often, seriously disturbed children and adolescents must be placed in residential centers where their behavior can be managed appropriately, thus separating them from the environment that may contribute to their aberrant behavior.

KEY POINTS

- Children with conduct disorder repeatedly act aggressively, violating the rights of others and/or societal norms or rules; they have few or no feelings of remorse.
- Disruptive behaviors continue into adulthood in about one third of patients; many of these cases then meet the criteria for antisocial personality disorder.

DEPRESSIVE DISORDERS IN CHILDREN AND ADOLESCENTS

Depressive disorders are characterized by sadness or irritability that is severe or persistent enough to interfere with functioning or cause considerable distress. Diagnosis is by history and examination. Treatment is

with antidepressants, supportive and cognitive-behavioral therapy, or both.

Depressive disorders in children and adolescents include

- Disruptive mood dysregulation disorder
- Major depressive disorder
- Persistent depressive disorder (dysthymia)

The term depression is often loosely used to describe the low or discouraged mood that results from disappointment (eg, serious illness) or loss (eg, death of a loved one). However, such low moods, unlike depression, occur in waves that tend to be tied to thoughts or reminders of the triggering event, resolve when circumstances or events improve, may be interspersed with periods of positive emotion and humor, and are not accompanied by pervasive feelings of worthlessness and self-loathing. The low mood usually lasts days rather than weeks or months, and suicidal thoughts and prolonged loss of function are much less likely. Such low moods are more appropriately called demoralization or grief. However, events and stressors that cause demoralization and grief can also precipitate a major depressive episode.

The etiology of depression in children and adolescents is unknown but is similar to etiology in adults (see p. 1758); it is believed to result from interactions of genetically determined risk factors and environmental stress (particularly deprivation and loss early in life).

Symptoms and Signs

Basic manifestations of depressive disorders in children and adolescents are similar to those in adults but are related to typical concerns of children, such as schoolwork and play. Children may be unable to explain inner feelings or moods. Depression should be considered when previously well-performing children do poorly in school, withdraw from society, or commit delinquent acts.

In some children with a depressive disorder, the predominant mood is irritability rather than sadness (an important difference between childhood and adult forms). The irritability associated with childhood depression may manifest as overactivity and aggressive, antisocial behavior.

In children with intellectual disability, depressive or other mood disorders may manifest as somatic symptoms and behavioral disturbances.

Disruptive mood dysregulation disorder: Disruptive mood dysregulation disorder involves persistent irritability and frequent episodes of behavior that is very out of control, with onset at age 6 to 10 yr. Many children also have other disorders, particularly oppositional defiant disorder, attention-deficit/hyperactivity disorder (ADHD), or an anxiety disorder. The diagnosis is not made before age 6 yr or after age 18 yr. As adults, patients may develop unipolar (rather than bipolar) depression or an anxiety disorder.

Manifestations include the presence of the following for ≥ 12 mo (with no period of ≥ 3 mo without all of them):

- Severe recurrent temper outbursts (eg, verbal rage and/or physical aggression toward people or property) that are grossly out of proportion to the situation and that occur ≥ 3 times/wk on average
- Temper outbursts that are inconsistent with developmental level
- An irritable, angry mood present every day for most of the day and observed by others (eg, parents, teachers, peers)

The outbursts and angry mood must occur in 2 of 3 settings (at home or school, with peers).

Major depressive disorder: Major depressive disorder is a discrete depressive episode lasting ≥ 2 wk. It occurs in as many as 2% of children and 5% of adolescents. Major depressive disorder can first occur at any age but is more common after puberty. Untreated, major depression may remit in 6 to 12 mo. Risk of recurrence is higher in patients who have severe episodes, who are younger, or who have had multiple episodes. Persistence of even mild depressive symptoms during remission is a strong predictor of recurrence.

For diagnosis, ≥ 1 of the following must be present for most of the day nearly every day during the same 2-wk period:

- Feeling sad or being observed by others to be sad (eg, tearful) or irritable
- Loss of interest or pleasure in almost all activities (often expressed as profound boredom)

In addition, ≥ 4 of the following must be present:

- Decrease in weight (in children, failure to make the expected weight gain) or decrease or increase in appetite
- Insomnia or hypersomnia
- Psychomotor agitation or retardation observed by others (not self-reported)
- Fatigue or loss of energy
- Decreased ability to think, concentrate, and make choices
- Recurrent thoughts of death (not just fear of dying) and/or suicidal ideation or plans
- Feelings of worthlessness (ie, feeling rejected and unloved) or excessive or inappropriate guilt

Major depression in adolescents is a risk factor for academic failure, substance abuse, and suicidal behavior. While depressed, children and adolescents tend to fall far behind academically and lose important peer relationships.

Persistent depressive disorder (dysthymia): Dysthymia is a persistent depressed or irritable mood that lasts for most of the day for more days than not for ≥ 1 yr plus ≥ 2 of the following:

- Poor appetite or overeating
- Insomnia or hypersomnia
- Low energy or fatigue
- Low self-esteem
- Poor concentration
- Feelings of hopelessness

Symptoms may be more or less intense than those of a major depressive disorder.

A major depressive episode may occur before the onset or during the first year (ie, before the duration criterion is met for persistent depressive disorder).

Diagnosis

- Clinical evaluation

Diagnosis of depressive disorders is based on symptoms and signs, including the criteria listed above.

Sources of information include an interview with the child or adolescent and information from parents and teachers. Several brief questionnaires are available for screening. They help identify some depressive symptoms but cannot be used alone for diagnosis. Specific close-ended questions help determine whether patients have the symptoms required for diagnosis of major depression, based on *Diagnostic and Statistical Manual of Mental Disorders*, Fifth Edition (DSM-5) criteria.

History should include causative factors such as domestic violence, sexual abuse and exploitation, and drug adverse effects. Questions about suicidal behavior (eg, ideation, gestures, attempts) should be asked.

A careful review of the history and appropriate laboratory tests are needed to exclude other disorders (eg, infectious mononucleosis, thyroid disorders, drug abuse) that can cause similar symptoms.

Other mental disorders that can increase the risk and/or modify the course of depressive symptoms (eg, anxiety, bipolar disorders) must be considered. Some children who eventually develop a bipolar disorder or schizophrenia may present initially with major depression.

After depression is diagnosed, the family and social setting must be evaluated to identify stresses that may have precipitated depression.

Treatment

- Concurrent measures directed at the family and school
- For adolescents, usually antidepressants plus psychotherapy
- For preadolescents, psychotherapy followed, if needed, by antidepressants

Appropriate measures directed at the family and school must accompany direct treatment of the child to enhance continued functioning and provide appropriate educational accommodations. Brief hospitalization may be necessary in acute crises, especially when suicidal behavior is identified.

For adolescents (as for adults), a combination of psychotherapy and antidepressants usually greatly outperforms either modality used alone. For preadolescents, the situation is much less clear. Most clinicians opt for psychotherapy in younger children; however, drugs can be used in younger children (fluoxetine can be used in children ≥ 8 yr), especially when depression is severe or has not previously responded to psychotherapy.

Usually, an SSRI (see Table 319–3) is the first choice when an antidepressant is indicated. Children should be closely monitored for the emergence of behavioral side effects (eg, disinhibition, behavioral activation), which are common but are usually mild to moderate. Usually, decreasing the drug dose or changing to a different drug eliminates or reduces these effects. Rarely, such effects are severe (eg, aggressiveness, increased suicidality). Behavioral adverse effects are idiosyncratic and may occur with any antidepressant and at any time during treatment. As a result, children and adolescents taking such drugs must be closely monitored.

Adult-based research has suggested that antidepressants that act on both the serotonergic and adrenergic/dopaminergic systems may be modestly more effective; however, such drugs (eg, duloxetine, venlafaxine, mirtazapine; certain tricyclics, particularly clomipramine) also tend to have more adverse effects. Such drugs may be especially useful in treatment-resistant cases. Nonserotonergic antidepressants such as bupropion and desipramine may also be used with an SSRI to enhance efficacy.

As in adults, relapse and recurrence are common. Children and adolescents should remain in treatment for at least 1 yr after symptoms have remitted. Most experts recommend that children who have experienced ≥ 2 episodes of major depression be treated indefinitely.

Suicide risk and antidepressants: Suicide risk and treatment with antidepressants have been a topic of debate and

Table 319–3. DRUGS FOR LONG-TERM TREATMENT OF ANXIETY AND RELATED DISORDERS

DRUG	USES	STARTING DOSE*	DOSE RANGE	COMMENTS/PRECAUTIONS†
Citalopram	OCD children ≥ 7 yr	10 mg	10–40 mg/day	—
Duloxetine	GAD in children 7–17 yr	30 mg	30–100 mg/day	—
Escitalopram	Major depression in children ≥ 7 yr	5 mg	5–20 mg/day	—
Fluoxetine‡	OCD, GAD, separation anxiety, social anxiety, major depression in children > 8 yr	10 mg	10–60 mg/day	Long-half life
Fluvoxamine	GAD, separation anxiety, social anxiety, OCD in children > 8 yr	25 mg (titrated up as needed)	50–200 mg/day	For doses > 50 mg/day, divided into 2 doses/day, with the larger dose given at bedtime)
Paroxetine‡	OCD in children > 6 yr	10 mg	10–60 mg/day	Increased weight
Sertraline	OCD, GAD, separation anxiety, social anxiety in children ≥ 6 yr	25 mg	25–200 mg/day	—
Venlafaxine, immediate-release	Depression in children ≥ 8 yr	12.5 mg	25–75 mg/day bid or tid	Limited data about dose and concerns about increased suicidal behavior; not as effective as other drugs, possibly because low doses have been used
Venlafaxine, extended-release	GAD in children > 7 yr	37.5 mg	37.5–225 mg/day	

*Unless otherwise stated, dose is given once/day. Starting dose is increased only if needed. Dose ranges are approximate. Interindividual variability in therapeutic response and adverse effects is considerable. This table is not a substitute for the full prescribing information.

†Behavioral adverse effects (eg, disinhibition, agitation) are common but are usually mild to moderate. Usually, decreasing the drug dose or changing to a different drug eliminates or reduces these effects. Rarely, such effects are severe (eg, aggressiveness, increased suicidality). Behavioral adverse effects are idiosyncratic and may occur with any antidepressant and at any time during treatment. As a result, children and adolescents taking such drugs must be closely monitored.

‡Fluoxetine and paroxetine are potent inhibitors of the liver enzymes that metabolize many other drugs (eg, beta-blockers, clonidine, lidocaine).

GAD = generalized anxiety disorder; OCD = obsessive compulsive disorder.

research.[1] In 2004, the US FDA did a meta-analysis of 23 previously conducted trials of 9 different antidepressants.[2] Although no patients completed suicide in these trials, a small but statistically significant increase in suicidal ideation was noted in children and adolescents taking an antidepressant (about 4% vs about 2%), leading to a black box warning on all classes of antidepressants (eg, tricyclic antidepressants, SSRIs, serotonin-norepinephrine reuptake inhibitors such as venlafaxine, tetracyclic antidepressants such as mirtazapine).

In 2006, a meta-analysis (from the United Kingdom) of children and adolescents being treated for depression[3] found that compared with patients taking a placebo, those taking an antidepressant had a small increase in self-harm or suicide-related events (4.8% vs 3.0% of those treated with placebo). However, whether the difference was statistically significant or not varied depending on the type of analysis (fixed-effects analysis or random-effects analysis). There was a nonsignificant trend toward an increase in suicidal ideation (1.2% vs 0.8%), self-harm (3.3% vs 2.6%), and suicide attempts (1.9% vs 1.2%). There appear to have been some differences in risk between different drugs; however, no direct head-to-head studies have been done, and it is difficult to control for severity of depression and other confounding risk factors.

Observational and epidemiologic studies[4,5] have found no increase in the rate of suicide attempts or completed suicide in patients takings antidepressants. Also, despite a decrease in prescriptions for antidepressants, the suicide rate has increased.

In general, although antidepressants have limited efficacy in children and adolescents, the benefits appear to outweigh risks. The best approach seems to be combining drug treatment with psychotherapy and minimizing risk by closely monitoring treatment.

Whether or not drugs are used, suicide is always a concern in a child or adolescent with depression. The following should be done to reduce risk:

- Parents and mental health care practitioners should discuss the issues in depth.
- The child or adolescent should be supervised at an appropriate level.
- Psychotherapy with regularly scheduled appointments should be included in the treatment plan.

PEARLS & PITFALLS

- Suicide risk is always a concern in children or adolescents with depression whether they are taking antidepressants or not.

1. Hetrick SE, McKenzie JE, Merry SN: Newer generation antidepressants for depressive disorders in children and adolescents. *Cochrane Database Syst Rev* Nov 11 2012.
2. US FDA: Review and evaluation of clinical data: Relationship between psychotropic drugs and pediatric suicidality. 2004. Accessed 11/4/16.
3. Dubicka B, Hadley S, Roberts C: Suicidal behaviour in youths with depression treated with new-generation antidepressants: Meta-analysis. *Br J Psychiatry* Nov 189:393–398, 2006.
4. Adegbite-Adeniyi C, et al: An update on antidepressant use and suicidality in pediatric depression. *Expert Opin Pharmacother* 13(15):2119–2130, 2012.
5. Gibbons RD, Brown CH, Hur K, et al: Early evidence on the effects of regulators' suicidality warnings on SSRI prescriptions and suicide in children and adolescents. *Am J Psychiatry* 164(9):1356–1363, 2007.

KEY POINTS

- In children, depressive disorders may manifest as sadness or irritability.
- Major depressive disorder involves feeling sad or irritable or losing interest or pleasure in almost all activities for most of the day nearly every day during a 2-wk period plus other specific symptoms.
- Diagnose a depressive disorder based on specific clinical criteria, and do appropriate laboratory tests to exclude other disorders (eg, infectious mononucleosis, thyroid disorders, drug abuse).
- Involve the family and school while treating the child to enhance the child's continued functioning and provide appropriate educational accommodations.
- For adolescents (as for adults), a combination of psychotherapy and antidepressants usually greatly outperforms either modality used alone; in younger children, most clinicians opt for psychotherapy although if needed, drugs can be used (depending on the child's age).
- In 2004, the FDA did a meta-analysis that led to a black box warning of a increased risk of suicidal ideation and behavior in children, adolescents, and young adults with all classes of antidepressants; subsequent analyses have cast doubt on this conclusion.

OBSESSIVE-COMPULSIVE DISORDER AND RELATED DISORDERS IN CHILDREN AND ADOLESCENTS

Obsessive-compulsive disorder is characterized by obsessions, compulsions, or both. Obsessions are irresistible, persistent ideas, images, or impulses to do something. Compulsions are pathologic urges to act on an impulse, which, if resisted, result in excessive anxiety and distress. The obsessions and compulsions cause great distress and interfere with academic or social functioning. Diagnosis is by history. Treatment is with behavioral therapy and SSRIs.

Mean age of onset of obsessive-compulsive disorder (OCD) is 19 to 20 yr; about 25% of cases begin before age 14.

OCD encompasses several related disorders, including

- Body dysmorphic disorder
- Hoarding disorder
- Trichotillomania (hair pulling)
- Skin picking disorder

Some children, particularly boys, also have a tic disorder.

Etiology

Studies suggest that there is a familial component. However, no specific genes have been identified, although animal studies suggest an abnormality in the genes that affect the function of microglia.

Although some experts remain unconvinced, there is evidence that some cases with acute (overnight) onset have been associated with infection.[1,2] Those associated with group A beta-hemolytic streptococci are called PANDAS (pediatric autoimmune neuropsychiatric disorder associated with streptococcus). Those associated with other infections are called PANS (pediatric acute-onset neuropsychiatric syndrome).

Research in this area is ongoing, and if PANDAS or PANS is suspected, consultation with a specialist in these disorders is recommended.

1. Murphy TK, Roger Kurlan R, James Leckman J: The immunobiology of Tourette's disorder, pediatric autoimmune neuropsychiatric disorders associated with Streptococcus, and related disorders: A way forward. *J Child Adolesc Psychopharmacol* 20(4):317–331, 2010. doi: 10.1089/cap.2010.0043.
2. Esposito S, Bianchini S, Baggi E, Fattizzo M, Rigante D: Pediatric autoimmune neuropsychiatric disorders associated with streptococcal infections: An overview. *Eur J Clin Microbiol Infect Dis* 33(12):2105–2109, 2014.

Symptoms and Signs

Typically, OCD has a gradual, insidious onset. Most children initially hide their symptoms and report struggling with symptoms years before a definitive diagnosis is made.

Obsessions are typically experienced as worries or fears of harm (eg, contracting a deadly disease, sinning and going to hell, injuring themselves or others). Compulsions are deliberate volitional acts, usually done to neutralize or offset obsessional fears; they include checking behaviors; excessive washing, counting, or arranging; and many more. Obsessions and compulsions may have some logical connection (eg, handwashing to avoid disease) or may be illogical and idiosyncratic (eg, counting to 50 over and over to prevent grandpa from having a heart attack). If children are prevented from carrying out their compulsions, they become excessively anxious and concerned.

Most children have some awareness that their obsessions and compulsions are abnormal. Many affected children are embarrassed and secretive. Common symptoms include

- Having raw, chapped hands (the presenting symptom in children who compulsively wash)
- Spending excessively long periods of time in the bathroom
- Doing schoolwork very slowly (because of an obsession about mistakes)
- Making many corrections in schoolwork
- Engaging in repetitive or odd behaviors such as checking door locks, chewing food a certain number of times, or avoiding touching certain things
- Making frequent and tedious requests for reassurance, sometimes dozens or even hundreds of times per day—asking, eg, "Do you think I have a fever? Could we have a tornado? Do you think the car will start? What if we're late? What if the milk is sour? What if a burglar comes?"

Diagnosis

- Clinical evaluation

Diagnosis of OCD is by history. Once a comfortable relationship with a nonjudgmental therapist is established, the child with OCD usually discloses many obsessions and related compulsions. However, usually several appointments are needed to first establish trust.

For OCD to be diagnosed, the obsessions and compulsions must cause great distress and interfere with academic or social functioning.

Children with OCD often have symptoms of other anxiety disorders, including panic attacks, separation problems, and specific phobias. This symptom overlap sometimes confuses the diagnosis.

Diagnostic criteria for PANDAS and PANS have been developed.[1,2]

1. Chang K, Frankovich J, Cooperstock M, et al: Clinical evaluation of youth with pediatric acute-onset neuropsychiatric syndrome (PANS): Recommendations from the 2013 PANS Consensus Conference. *J Child Adolesc Psychopharmacol* 25(1):3–13, 2015. doi: 10.1089/cap.2014.0084.
2. Swedo S, Leckman J, Rose N: From research subgroup to clinical syndrome: Modifying the PANDAS criteria to describe PANS (pediatric acute-onset neuropsychiatric syndrome). *Pediatr Therapeutics* 2:1–8, 2012.

Prognosis

In about 5% of children, the disorder remits after a few years, and in about 40%, it remits by early adulthood. Treatment can then be stopped. In other children, the disorder tends to be chronic, but normal functioning can usually be maintained with ongoing treatment. About 5% of children do not respond to treatment and remain greatly impaired.

Treatment

- Cognitive-behavioral therapy
- Usually SSRIs

Cognitive-behavioral therapy is helpful if children are motivated and can carry out the tasks.

SSRIs are the most effective drugs and are generally well-tolerated (see Table 319–1); all are equally effective. However, about 50% of patients respond only partially to SSRIs and may require an SSRI plus other drugs that have serotonergic activity (eg, lithium) or glutamatergic activity (eg, riluzole). Another alternative is clomipramine, a tricyclic antidepressant, which may be more effective and have a better response rate than SSRIs, although it has a higher risk of cardiac effects and seizures.

If criteria for PANS/PANDAS are met, clinicians may try antibiotics (such as beta-lactams, which reduce glutamatergic activity). However, if symptoms persist, the typical treatments for OCD are helpful and should be implemented.

KEY POINTS

- Children typically experience obsessions as worries or fears of harm (eg, contracting a deadly disease, sinning and going to hell, injuring themselves).
- Compulsions (eg, excessive washing, counting, arranging) are done deliberately, usually to neutralize or offset obsessional fears.
- Not being able to carry out their compulsions makes children excessively anxious and concerned.
- Establish a comfortable relationship with the child and maintain a nonjudgmental attitude so that the child feels able to disclose obsessions and related compulsions.
- Try cognitive-behavioral therapy if children are motivated and can carry out the tasks, but drugs (usually SSRIs) may be needed.

OPPOSITIONAL DEFIANT DISORDER

Oppositional defiant disorder is a recurrent or persistent pattern of negative, defiant, or even hostile behavior directed at authority figures. Diagnosis is by history. Treatment is with individual psychotherapy combined with family or caregiver therapy. Occasionally, drugs may be used to reduce irritability.

Prevalence estimates of oppositional defiant disorder (ODD) vary widely because the diagnostic criteria are highly subjective; prevalence in children and adolescents may be as high as 15%. Before puberty, affected boys greatly outnumber girls; after puberty, the difference narrows.

Although oppositional defiant disorder is sometimes viewed as a mild version of conduct disorder, similarities between the 2 disorders are only superficial. The hallmark of this disorder is an interpersonal style characterized by irritability and defiance. However, children with a conduct disorder seemingly lack a conscience and repeatedly violate the rights of others (eg, bullying, threatening or causing harm, being cruel to animals), sometimes without any evidence of irritability.

Etiology of oppositional defiant disorder is unknown, but it is probably most common among children from families in which the adults engage in loud, argumentative, interpersonal conflicts. This diagnosis should not be viewed as a circumscribed disorder but rather as an indication of underlying problems that may require further investigation and treatment.

Symptoms and Signs

Typically, children with oppositional defiant disorder tend to frequently do the following:

- Lose their temper easily and repeatedly
- Argue with adults
- Defy adults
- Refuse to obey rules
- Deliberately annoy people
- Blame others for their own mistakes or misbehavior
- Be easily annoyed and angered
- Be spiteful or vindictive

Many affected children also lack social skills.

Diagnosis

- Clinical criteria

Oppositional defiant disorder is diagnosed if children have had ≥ 4 of the above symptoms for at least 6 mo. Symptoms must also be severe and disruptive.

Oppositional defiant disorder must be distinguished from the following, which may cause similar symptoms:

- Mild to moderate oppositional behaviors: Such behaviors occur periodically in nearly all children and adolescents.
- Untreated attention-deficit/hyperactivity disorder (ADHD): The symptoms that resemble those of oppositional defiant disorder often resolve when ADHD is adequately treated.
- Mood disorders: Irritability caused by depression can be distinguished from oppositional defiant disorder by the presence of anhedonia and neurovegetative symptoms (eg, sleep and appetite disruption); these symptoms are easily overlooked in children.
- Anxiety disorders and obsessive-compulsive disorder: In these disorders, the oppositional behaviors occur when children have overwhelming anxiety or when they are prevented from carrying out their rituals.

Treatment

- Behavior modification therapy
- Sometimes drugs

Underlying problems (eg, family dysfunction) and coexisting disorders (eg, ADHD) should be identified and corrected. However, even without corrective measures or treatment, most children with ODD gradually improve over time.

Initially, the treatment of choice for oppositional defiant disorder is a rewards-based behavior modification program designed to make the child's behaviors more socially appropriate. Many children can benefit from group-based therapy that builds social skills.

Sometimes drugs used to treat depressive or anxiety disorders (see Table 319–1) may be beneficial.

KEY POINTS

- In oppositional defiant disorder, children typically lose their temper frequently, defy adults, disregard rules, and deliberately annoy other people.
- Initially, use a rewards-based behavior modification program to make the child's behaviors more socially appropriate; sometimes drugs used to treat depressive and anxiety disorders can help.

SCHIZOPHRENIA IN CHILDREN AND ADOLESCENTS

Schizophrenia is the presence of hallucinations and delusions causing considerable psychosocial dysfunction and lasting ≥ 6 mo.

Onset of schizophrenia is typically from mid-adolescence to the mid-30s, with a peak age of onset in the 20s. Features in adolescents and young adults are similar (see p. 1789). Schizophrenia in prepubertal children (childhood-onset schizophrenia [COS]), in which symptoms similar to those of the adolescent/young adult-onset form develop before age 12, is extremely rare.

Although the first episode usually occurs in young adults, some contributory neurodevelopmental events and experiences occur earlier (eg, during the perinatal period).

These **perinatal risk factors** include the following:

- Genetic disorders (particularly those that increase risk of childhood onset)
- Exposure to certain drugs or substances (eg, cannabis) during a vulnerable period
- Prenatal undernutrition
- Labor complications, hypoxia, perinatal infection, placental abruption or insufficiency
- Childhood brain injury

Other risk factors, which occur later (eg, drug use later in adolescence), may then trigger the onset of schizophrenia.

Manifestations of childhood-onset schizophrenia are usually similar to those in adolescents and adults, but delusions and visual hallucinations (which may be more common among children) may be less elaborate. Additional characteristics also help distinguish childhood-onset schizophrenia from the adolescent/young adult form:

- More severe symptoms
- A strong family history
- Increased prevalence of genetic abnormalities, developmental abnormalities (eg, pervasive developmental disorder, intellectual disability), and motor abnormalities
- Increased prevalence of premorbid social difficulties
- Insidious onset
- Cognitive deterioration
- Neuroanatomic changes (progressive loss of cortical gray matter volume, increase in ventricular volume)

Sudden-onset psychosis in young children should always be treated as a medical emergency with a thorough medical assessment to search for a physiologic cause of the mental status change; these causes include

- Drugs (in younger children, stimulants and corticosteroids; in adolescents, drugs of abuse)
- CNS infection or injury
- Thyroid disorders
- Autoimmune encephalopathies (eg, anti-NMDA [*N*-methyl-D-aspartate] receptor encephalitis[1]
- SLE[2]
- Porphyria[3]
- Wilson disease[4]

Treatment of schizophrenia in children and adolescents is complex, with variable outcomes, and referral to a child and adolescent psychiatrist is strongly recommended.

1. Dalmau J, Lancaster E, Martinez-Hernandez E, et al: Clinical experience and laboratory investigations in patients with anti-NMDAR encephalitis. *Lancet Neurol* 10(1):63–74, 2011. doi: 10.1016/S1474-4422(10)70253.
2. Muscal E, Nadeem T, Li X, et al: Evaluation and treatment of acute psychosis in children with systemic lupus erythematosus (SLE): Consultation-liaison service experiences at a tertiary-care pediatric institution. *Psychosomatics* 51(6):508–514, 2010. doi: 10.1176/appi.psy.51.6.508.
3. Kumar B: Acute intermittent porphyria presenting solely with psychosis: A case report and discussion. *Psychosomatics* 53(5):494–498, 2012. doi: 10.1016/j.psym.2012.03.008.
4. Grover S, Sarkar S, Jhanda S, et al: Psychosis in an adolescent with Wilson's disease: A case report and review of the literature. *Indian J Psychiatry* 56(4): 395–398, 2014. doi: 10.4103/0019-5545.146530.

SOMATIC SYMPTOM AND RELATED DISORDERS IN CHILDREN

Somatic symptom disorder and related disorders are characterized by persistent physical symptoms that are associated with excessive or maladaptive thoughts, feelings, and behaviors in response to these symptoms and associated health concerns. These disorders are distressing and often impair functioning.

Somatic symptom and related disorders include the following:

- **Conversion disorder:** Typically, symptoms involve apparent deficits in voluntary motor or sensory function but sometimes include shaking movements and impaired consciousness (suggesting seizures) and abnormal limb posturing (suggesting another neurologic or general physical disorder). Children may present with impaired coordination or balance, weakness, paralysis of an arm or a leg, loss of sensation in a body part, seizures, unresponsiveness, blindness, double vision, deafness, aphonia, difficulty swallowing, sensation of a lump in the throat, or urinary retention.
- **Factitious disorder imposed on another:** Caregivers (typically a parent) intentionally falsify or produce physical symptoms in a child. For example, they may add blood or other substances to urine specimens to simulate a urine infection.
- **Illness anxiety disorder:** Children are extremely afraid that they have or will acquire a serious disorder. They are so preoccupied with the idea that they are or might become ill that their anxiety impairs daily functioning or causes significant distress. Children may or may not have physical symptoms, but if they do, their concern is more about the possible implications of the symptoms than the symptoms themselves.
- **Somatic symptom disorder:** Children may develop multiple somatic symptoms or only one severe symptom, typically pain. Symptoms may be specific (eg, pain in the abdomen) or vague (eg, fatigue). Any part of the body may be the focus of concern. The symptoms themselves or excessive worry about them is distressing or disrupts daily life.

Somatic symptom and related disorders are equally common among young boys and young girls but are more common among adolescent girls than adolescent boys.

Symptoms and treatment of somatic symptom and related disorders are very similar to those of anxiety disorders. The symptoms are not consciously fabricated, and children are actually experiencing the symptoms they describe.

Diagnosis

- Usually clinical criteria
- Sometimes tests to rule out other disorders

Diagnosis of somatic or related disorders is based on criteria from the *Diagnostic and Statistical Manual of Mental Disorders*, Fifth Edition (DSM-5). Generally, for one of these disorders to be diagnosed, symptoms must cause significant distress and/or interfere with daily functioning, and children must be excessively concerned about their health and/or symptoms in thoughts and actions.

At first presentation, physicians take an extensive history (sometimes conferring with family members) and do a thorough examination and often testing to determine whether a physical disorder is the cause. Because children with somatic symptom disorder may subsequently develop physical disorders, appropriate examinations and tests should be done whenever symptoms change significantly or when objective signs develop. However, extensive laboratory tests are generally avoided because they may further convince children that a physical problem exists and unnecessary diagnostic tests may themselves traumatize children.

If no physical problem can be identified, doctors may use standardized mental health tests to help determine whether symptoms are due to a somatic symptom or related disorder. Doctors also talk to the children and family members to try to identify underlying psychologic problems or troubled family relationships.

Treatment

- Psychotherapy
- Sometimes drugs to relieve symptoms

Children, even when there is a satisfactory relationship with a primary physician, are commonly referred to a psychotherapist. Children may balk at the idea of visiting a psychotherapist because they think their symptoms are purely physical. However, individual and family psychotherapy, often using cognitive-behavioral techniques, can help children and family members recognize patterns of thought and behavior that perpetuate the symptoms. Therapists may use hypnosis, biofeedback, and relaxation therapy.

Psychotherapy is usually combined with a rehabilitation program that aims to help children get back into a normal routine. It can include physical therapy, which has the following benefits:

- It may treat actual physical effects, such as reduced mobility or loss of muscle, caused by a somatic symptom or related disorder.
- It makes children feel as if something concrete is being done to treat them.
- It enables children to participate actively in their treatment.

Drugs to treat concurrent mental disorders (eg, depression, anxiety) may help; however, the primary intervention is psychotherapy.

Children also benefit from having a supportive relationship with a primary care physician, who coordinates all of their health care, offers symptomatic relief, sees them regularly, and protects them from unnecessary tests and procedures.

KEY POINTS

- Children are preoccupied with and excessively worried about their health, physical symptoms, or the possibility of having or acquiring a serious illness.
- Children may have multiple symptoms (eg, impaired coordination or balance, weakness, paralysis or loss of sensation, seizures, blindness, double vision, deafness) or one severe symptom, typically pain.
- Do appropriate examinations and tests initially to rule out a physical disorder as the cause of symptoms and, if symptoms change significantly or objective signs develop, to check for a new physical disorder.
- Treatment may involve psychotherapy, usually combined with a rehabilitation program that aims to help children get back into a normal routine.

SUICIDAL BEHAVIOR IN CHILDREN AND ADOLESCENTS

Suicidal behavior includes completed suicide, attempted suicide (with at least some intent to die), and suicide gestures; suicidal ideation is thoughts and plans about suicide. Psychiatric referral is usually required.

Youth suicide rates have declined in recent years after more than a decade of steady increase, only to have started climbing again. The exact reasons for these fluctuations are unclear. Many experts believe that the changing rates with which antidepressants are prescribed may be a factor (see p. 2718). Some experts hypothesize that antidepressants have paradoxical effects, making children and adolescents more vocal about suicidal feelings but less likely to commit suicide. Nonetheless, although rare in prepubertal children, suicide is the 2nd or 3rd leading cause of death in 15- to 19-yr-olds and remains a considerable public health concern.

Etiology

In children and adolescents, risk of suicidal behavior is influenced by the presence of other mental disorders and other disorders that affect the brain, family history, psychosocial factors, and environmental factors (see Table 319–4).

Other contributing factors may include

- A lack of structure and boundaries, leading to an overwhelming feeling of lack of direction
- Intense parental pressure to succeed accompanied by the feeling of falling short of expectations

A frequent motive for a suicide attempt is an effort to manipulate or punish others with the fantasy "You will be sorry after I am dead."

Table 319–4. RISK FACTORS FOR SUICIDAL BEHAVIOR IN CHILDREN AND ADOLESCENTS

TYPE	EXAMPLES
Mental disorders and physical disorders that affect the brain	Mood disorders* (eg, bipolar disorder, depressive disorders) Schizophrenia Alcohol and/or substance use in adolescents Aggressive, impulsive tendencies (conduct disorder) Previous suicide attempts Traumatic head injury Posttraumatic stress disorder (PTSD)
Family history	Family history of suicidal behavior Mother with a mood disorder Father with a history of trouble with the police Poor communication with parents
Psychosocial factors	Recent disciplinary action† (most commonly, school suspension) Interpersonal loss (loss of a girlfriend or boyfriend, especially in boys); separation from parents) Difficulties in school Social isolation (particularly not working or going to college) Minority in upwardly mobile home Victim of bullying Media reports of suicide (copycat suicide)
Environmental factors	Easy access to lethal methods (eg, guns) Barriers to and/or stigma associated with accessing mental health services

*Mood disorders are present in more than one-half of suicidal adolescents.
†Almost half of completed suicides occur after recent disciplinary action.

Protective factors include

- Effective clinical care for mental, physical, and substance use disorders
- Easy access to clinical interventions
- Family and community support (connectedness)
- Skills in conflict resolution
- Cultural and religious beliefs that discourage suicide

Treatment

- Crisis intervention, possibly including hospitalization
- Psychotherapy
- Possibly drugs to treat underlying disorders, usually combined with psychotherapy
- Psychiatric referral

Every suicide attempt is a serious matter that requires thoughtful and appropriate intervention. Once the immediate threat to life is removed, a decision regarding the need for hospitalization must be made. The decision involves balancing the degree of risk with the family's capacity to provide support. Hospitalization (even in an open medical or pediatric ward with special-duty nursing) is the surest form of short-term protection and is usually indicated if depression, psychosis, or both are suspected.

Lethality of suicidal intent can be assessed based on the following:

- Degree of forethought evidenced (eg, by writing a suicide note)
- Steps taken to prevent discovery
- Method used (eg, firearms are more lethal than pills)
- Degree of self-injury sustained
- Circumstances or immediate precipitating factors surrounding the attempt
- Mental state at the time of the episode (acute agitation is especially concerning)
- Recent discharge from inpatient care
- Recent discontinuation of psychoactive drugs

Drugs may be indicated for any underlying disorder (eg, depression, bipolar or conduct disorder, psychosis) but cannot prevent suicide. Antidepressant use may increase risk of suicide in some adolescents (see p. 2718). Use of drugs should be carefully monitored, and only sublethal amounts should be supplied.

Psychiatric referral is usually needed to provide appropriate drug treatment and psychotherapy. Cognitive-behavioral therapy for suicide prevention and dialectical behavioral therapy may be preferred. Treatment is most successful if the primary care practitioner continues to be involved.

Rebuilding morale and restoring emotional equilibrium within the family are essential. A negative or unsupportive parental response is a serious concern and may suggest a need for a more intensive intervention such as out-of-home placement. A positive outcome is most likely if the family shows love and concern.

Response to suicide: Family members of children and adolescents who committed suicide have complicated reactions to the suicide, including grief, guilt, and depression. Counseling can help them understand the psychiatric context of the suicide and reflect on and acknowledge the child's difficulties before the suicide.

After a suicide, the risk of suicide may increase in other people in the community, especially friends and classmates of the person who committed suicide. Resources (eg, a toolkit for schools) are available to help schools and communities after a suicide. School and community officials can arrange for mental health care practitioners to be available to provide information and consultation.

Prevention

Suicidal incidents are often preceded by behavioral changes (eg, despondent mood, low self-esteem, sleep and appetite disturbances, inability to concentrate, truancy from school, somatic complaints, and suicidal preoccupation), which often bring the child or adolescent to the physician's office. Statements such as "I wish I had never been born" or "I would like to go to sleep and never wake up" should be taken seriously as possible indications of suicidal intent. A suicidal threat or attempt represents an important communication about the intensity of experienced despair.

Early recognition of the risk factors mentioned above may help prevent a suicide attempt. In response to these early cues, to threatened or attempted suicide, or to severe risk-taking behavior, vigorous intervention is appropriate. Adolescents should be directly questioned about their unhappy or self-destructive feelings; such direct questioning may diminish suicide risk. A physician should not provide unfounded reassurance, which can undermine the physician's credibility and further lower the adolescent's self-esteem.

Physicians should help patients do the following, which may help reduce the risk of suicide:

- Get effective care for mental, physical, and substance use disorders
- Access mental health services
- Get support from the family and community
- Learn ways to peacefully resolve conflict

Suicide prevention programs can help. The most effective programs are those that strive to ensure that the child has the following:

- A supportive nurturing environment
- Ready access to mental health services
- A social setting that is characterized by respect for individual, racial, and cultural differences

In the US, the Suicide Prevention Resource Center lists some of these programs, and the National Suicide Prevention Lifeline (1-800-273-TALK) provides crisis intervention for people threatening suicide.

KEY POINTS

- Suicide is rare in prepubertal children but is the 2nd or 3rd leading cause of death in 15- to 19-yr-olds.
- Consider drug treatment for any underlying disorder (eg, mood disorders, psychosis); however, antidepressants may increase risk of suicide in some adolescents, so carefully monitor use of drugs, and supply only sublethal amounts.
- Look for early warning changes in behavior (eg, skipping school, sleeping or eating too much or too little, making statements suggesting suicidal intent, engaging in very risky behavior).

NONSUICIDAL SELF-INJURY IN CHILDREN AND ADOLESCENTS

Nonsuicidal self-injurious (NSSI) behaviors can include superficial scratching, cutting, or burning the skin (using cigarettes or curling irons), as well as stabbing, hitting, and repeated rubbing the skin with an eraser or salt.

In some communities, self-injurious behaviors suddenly sweep through a high school in fad-like fashion and then gradually diminish over time. Such behaviors are often associated with illicit substance abuse and suggest that an adolescent is in great distress.

In many adolescents, these behaviors do not indicate suicidality but instead are self-punishing actions that they may feel they deserve; these behaviors are used to gain the attention of parents and/or significant others, express anger, or identify with a peer group. However, these adolescents, especially those who have used multiple methods of self-harm, have an increased risk of suicide.[1]

All self-injurious behaviors should be evaluated by a clinician experienced in working with troubled adolescents to assess whether suicidality is an issue and to identify the underlying distress leading to the self-injurious behaviors.

1. Greydanus DE, Apple RW: The relationship between deliberate self-harm behavior, body dissatisfaction, and suicide in adolescents: Current concepts. *J Multidiscip Healthc* 4:183–189, 2011. doi: 10.2147/JMDH.S11569.

320 Metabolic, Electrolyte, and Toxic Disorders in Neonates

NEONATAL HYPERBILIRUBINEMIA

(Jaundice in Neonates)

Jaundice is a yellow discoloration of the skin and eyes caused by hyperbilirubinemia (elevated serum bilirubin concentration—see p. 186). The serum bilirubin level required to cause jaundice varies with skin tone and body region, but jaundice usually becomes visible on the sclera at a level of 2 to 3 mg/dL (34 to 51 μmol/L) and on the face at about 4 to 5 mg/dL (68 to 86 μmol/L). With increasing bilirubin levels, jaundice seems to advance in a head-to-foot direction, appearing at the umbilicus at about 15 mg/dL (258 μmol/L) and at the feet at about 20 mg/dL (340 μmol/L). Slightly more than half of all neonates become visibly jaundiced in the first week of life.

Consequences of hyperbilirubinemia: Hyperbilirubinemia may be harmless or harmful depending on its cause and the degree of elevation. Some causes of jaundice are intrinsically dangerous whatever the bilirubin level. But hyperbilirubinemia of any etiology is a concern once the level is high enough. The threshold for concern varies by

- Age
- Degree of prematurity
- Health status

Among healthy term infants, the threshold typically is considered to be a level > 18 mg/dL (> 308 μmol/L)—see Fig. 320–1. However, infants who are premature, small for gestational age, and/or ill (eg, with sepsis, hypothermia, or hypoxia) are at much greater risk. In such infants, although risk increases with increasing hyperbilirubinemia, there is no level of hyperbilirubinemia that is considered safe; treatment is given based on age and clinical factors. There are now suggested operational thresholds to initiate phototherapy based on gestational age.

Neurotoxicity is the major consequence of neonatal hyperbilirubinemia. An acute encephalopathy can be followed by a variety of neurologic impairments, including cerebral palsy and sensorimotor deficits; cognition is usually spared. Kernicterus is the most severe form of neurotoxicity. Although it is now rare, kernicterus still occurs and can nearly always be prevented. Kernicterus is brain damage caused by unconjugated bilirubin deposition in basal ganglia and brain stem nuclei, caused by either acute or chronic hyperbilirubinemia. Normally, bilirubin bound to serum albumin stays in the intravascular space. However, bilirubin can cross the blood-brain barrier and cause kernicterus in certain situations:

- When serum bilirubin concentration is markedly elevated
- When serum albumin concentration is markedly low (eg, in preterm infants)
- When bilirubin is displaced from albumin by competitive binders

Competitive binders include drugs (eg, sulfisoxazole, ceftriaxone, aspirin) and free fatty acids and hydrogen ions (eg, in fasting, septic, or acidotic infants).

Pathophysiology

The majority of bilirubin is produced from the breakdown of Hb into unconjugated bilirubin (and other substances). Unconjugated bilirubin binds to albumin in the blood for transport to the liver, where it is taken up by hepatocytes and conjugated with glucuronic acid by the enzyme uridine diphosphoglucon-urate glucuronosyltransferase (UGT) to make it water-soluble. The conjugated bilirubin is excreted in bile into the duodenum. In adults, conjugated bilirubin is reduced by gut bacteria to urobilin and excreted. Neonates, however, have less bacteria in their digestive tracts, so less bilirubin is reduced to urobilin and excreted. They also have the enzyme β-glucuronidase, which deconjugates bilirubin. The now unconjugated bilirubin can be reabsorbed and recycled into the circulation. This is called enterohepatic circulation of bilirubin (see also Bilirubin metabolism on p. 2789).

Mechanisms of hyperbilirubinemia: Hyperbilirubinemia can be caused by one or more of the following processes:

- Increased production
- Decreased hepatic uptake
- Decreased conjugation
- Impaired excretion
- Impaired bile flow (cholestasis)
- Increased enterohepatic circulation

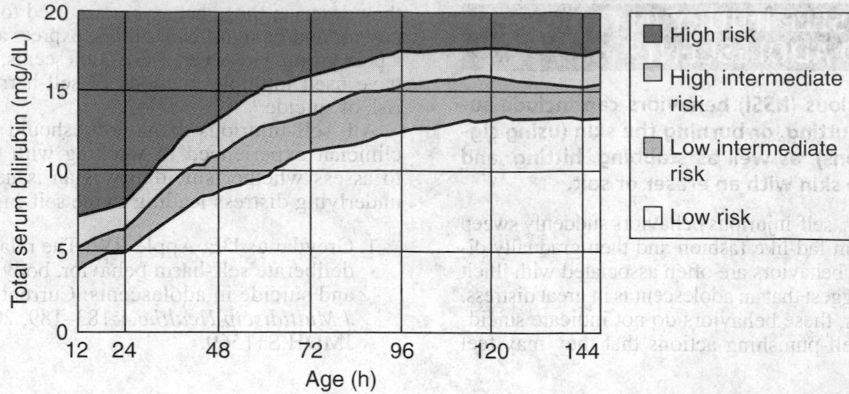

Fig. 320–1. Risk of hyperbilirubinemia in neonates ≥ 35 wk gestation. Risk is based on total serum bilirubin levels. (Adapted from Bhutani VK, Johnson L, Sivieri EM: Predictive ability of a predischarge hour-specific serum bilirubin for subsequent significant hyperbilirubinemia in healthy term and near-term newborns. *Pediatrics* 103(1):6–14, 1999.)

Etiology

Classification: There are several ways to classify and discuss causes of hyperbilirubinemia. Because transient jaundice is common among healthy neonates (unlike adults, in whom jaundice always signifies a disorder), hyperbilirubinemia can be classified as physiologic or pathologic. It can be classified by whether the hyperbilirubinemia is unconjugated, conjugated, or both. It also can be classified by mechanism (see Table 320–1).

Causes: Most cases involve unconjugated hyperbilirubinemia. Some of the most common causes of neonatal jaundice include

- Physiologic hyperbilirubinemia
- Breastfeeding jaundice
- Breast milk jaundice
- Pathologic hyperbilirubinemia due to hemolytic disease

Liver dysfunction (eg, caused by parenteral alimentation causing cholestasis, neonatal sepsis, neonatal hepatitis) may cause a conjugated or mixed hyperbilirubinemia.

Physiologic hyperbilirubinemia occurs in almost all neonates. Shorter neonatal RBC life span increases bilirubin production; deficient conjugation due to the deficiency of UGT decreases clearance; and low bacterial levels in the intestine combined with increased hydrolysis of conjugated bilirubin increase enterohepatic circulation. Bilirubin levels can rise up to 18 mg/dL by 3 to 4 days of life (7 days in Asian infants) and fall thereafter.

Breastfeeding jaundice develops in one sixth of breastfed infants during the first week of life. Breastfeeding increases enterohepatic circulation of bilirubin in some infants who have decreased milk intake and who also have dehydration or low caloric intake. The increased enterohepatic circulation also may result from reduced intestinal bacteria that convert bilirubin to nonresorbed metabolites.

Breast milk jaundice is different from breastfeeding jaundice. It develops after the first 5 to 7 days of life and peaks at about 2 wk. It is thought to be caused by an increased concentration of β-glucuronidase in breast milk, causing an increase in the deconjugation and reabsorption of bilirubin.

Pathologic hyperbilirubinemia in term infants is diagnosed if

- Jaundice appears in the first 24 h, after the first week of life, or lasts > 2 wk
- Total serum bilirubin (TSB) rises by > 5 mg/dL/day
- TSB is > 18 mg/dL
- Infant shows symptoms or signs of a serious illness

Some of the most common pathologic causes are

- Immune and nonimmune hemolytic anemia
- G6PD deficiency
- Hematoma resorption
- Sepsis
- Hypothyroidism

Evaluation

History: History of present illness should note age of onset and duration of jaundice. Important associated symptoms include lethargy and poor feeding (suggesting possible kernicterus), which may progress to stupor, hypotonia, or seizures and eventually to hypertonia. Patterns of feeding can be suggestive of possible breastfeeding failure or underfeeding. Therefore, history should include what the infant is being fed, how much and how frequently, urine and stool production (possible breastfeeding failure or underfeeding), how well the infant is latching on to the breast or taking the nipple of the bottle, whether the mother feels that her milk has come in, and whether the infant is swallowing during feedings and seems satiated after feedings.

Review of systems should seek symptoms of causes, including respiratory distress, fever, and irritability or lethargy (sepsis); hypotonia and poor feeding (hypothyroidism, metabolic disorder); and repeated episodes of vomiting (intestinal obstruction).

Past medical history should focus on maternal infections (toxoplasmosis, other pathogens, rubella, cytomegalovirus, and herpes simplex [TORCH] infections), disorders that can cause early hyperbilirubinemia (maternal diabetes), maternal Rh factor and blood group (maternofetal blood group incompatibility), and a history of a prolonged or difficult birth (hematoma or forceps trauma).

Table 320–1. CAUSES OF NEONATAL HYPERBILIRUBINEMIA

MECHANISM	CAUSES
Increased enterohepatic circulation	Breast milk (breast milk jaundice) Breastfeeding failure (breastfeeding jaundice) Drug-induced paralytic ileus (magnesium sulfate or morphine) Fasting or other cause for hypoperistalsis Hirschsprung disease Intestinal atresia or stenosis, including annular pancreas Meconium ileus or meconium plug syndrome Pyloric stenosis* Swallowed blood
Overproduction	Breakdown of extravascular blood (eg, hematomas; petechiae; pulmonary, cerebral, or occult hemorrhage) Polycythemia due to maternofetal or fetofetal transfusion or delayed umbilical cord clamping
Overproduction due to hemolytic anemia	Certain drugs and agents in neonates with G6PD deficiency (eg, acetaminophen, alcohol, antimalarials, aspirin, bupivacaine, corticosteroids, diazepam, nitrofurantoin, oxytocin, penicillin, phenothiazine, sulfonamides) Maternofetal blood group incompatibility (eg, Rh, ABO) RBC enzyme deficiencies (eg, of G6PD or pyruvate kinase) Spherocytosis Thalassemias (α, β–γ)
Undersecretion due to biliary obstruction	α_1-Antitrypsin deficiency* Biliary atresia* Choledochal cyst* Cystic fibrosis* (inspissated bile) Dubin-Johnson syndrome and Rotor syndrome* Parenteral nutrition Tumor or band* (extrinsic obstruction)
Undersecretion due to metabolic-endocrine conditions	Crigler-Najjar syndrome (familial nonhemolytic jaundice types 1 and 2) Drugs and hormones Gilbert syndrome Hypermethioninemia Hypopituitarism and anencephaly Hypothyroidism Lucey-Driscoll syndrome Maternal diabetes Prematurity Tyrosinosis
Mixed overproduction and undersecretion	Asphyxia Intrauterine infections Maternal diabetes Respiratory distress syndrome Sepsis Severe erythroblastosis fetalis Syphilis TORCH infections

*Jaundice may also occur outside the neonatal period.
TORCH = toxoplasmosis, other pathogens, rubella, cytomegalovirus, and herpes simplex.
Adapted from Poland RL, Ostrea EM Jr: Neonatal hyperbilirubinemia. In *Care of the High-Risk Neonate,* ed. 3, edited by MH Klaus and AA Fanaroff. Philadelphia, WB Saunders Company, 1986.

Family history should note known inherited disorders that can cause jaundice, including G6PD deficiency, thalassemias, and spherocytosis, and also any history of siblings who have had jaundice.

Drug history should specifically note drugs that may promote jaundice (eg, ceftriaxone, sulfonamides, antimalarials).

Physical examination: Overall clinical appearance and vital signs are reviewed (see Table 320–2).

The skin is inspected for extent of jaundice. Gentle pressure on the skin can help reveal the presence of jaundice. Also, ecchymoses or petechiae (suggestive of hemolytic anemia) are noted.

The physical examination should focus on signs of causative disorders.

The general appearance is inspected for plethora (maternofetal transfusion); macrosomia (maternal diabetes); lethargy or extreme irritability (sepsis or infection); and any dysmorphic features such as macroglossia (hypothyroidism) and flat nasal bridge or bilateral epicanthal folds (Down syndrome).

For the head and neck examination, any bruising and swelling of the scalp consistent with a cephalohematoma are noted. Lungs are examined for crackles (rales), rhonchi, and decreased breath sounds (pneumonia). The abdomen is examined for distention, mass (hepatosplenomegaly), or pain (intestinal obstruction). Neurologic examination should focus on signs of hypotonia or weakness (metabolic disorder, hypothyroidism, sepsis).

Red flags: The following findings are of particular concern:

- Jaundice in the first day of life
- TSB > 18 mg/dL
- Rate of rise of TSB > 0.2 mg/dL/h (> 3.4 μmol/L/h) or > 5 mg/dL/day
- Conjugated bilirubin concentration > 1 mg/dL (> 17 μmol/L) if TSB is < 5 mg/dL or > 20% of TSB (suggests neonatal cholestasis)
- Jaundice after 2 wk of age
- Lethargy, irritability, respiratory distress

Interpretation of findings: Evaluation should focus on distinguishing physiologic from pathologic jaundice. History, physical examination, and timing can help, but typically TSB and conjugated serum bilirubin levels are measured.

Timing: Jaundice that develops in the first 24 to 48 h, or that persists > 2 wk, is most likely pathologic. Jaundice that does not become evident until after 2 to 3 days is more consistent with physiologic, breastfeeding, or breast milk jaundice. An exception is undersecretion of bilirubin due to metabolic factors (eg, Crigler-Najjar syndrome, hypothyroidism, drugs), which may take 2 to 3 days to become evident. In such cases, bilirubin typically peaks in the first week, accumulates at a rate of < 5 mg/dL/day, and can remain evident for a prolonged period. Because most neonates are now discharged from the hospital or nursery within 48 h, many cases of hyperbilirubinemia are detected only after discharge.

Testing: Diagnosis is suspected by the infant's color and is confirmed by measurement of serum bilirubin. Noninvasive techniques for transcutaneous measurement of bilirubin levels in infants are being used increasingly, with good correlation with serum bilirubin measurements. Risk of hyperbilirubinemia is based on age-specific TSB levels.

A bilirubin concentration > 10 mg/dL (> 170 μmol/L) in preterm infants or > 18 mg/dL in term infants warrants additional testing, including Hct, blood smear, reticulocyte count, direct Coombs test, TSB and direct serum bilirubin concentrations, and blood type and Rh group of the infant and mother.

Other tests, such as blood, urine, and CSF cultures to detect sepsis and measurement of RBC enzyme levels to detect unusual causes of hemolysis, may be indicated by the history and physical examination. Such tests also may be indicated for any neonates with an initial bilirubin level > 25 mg/dL (> 428 μmol/L).

Treatment

Treatment of hyperbilirubinemia is directed at the underlying disorder. In addition, treatment for hyperbilirubinemia itself may be necessary.

Table 320–2. PHYSICAL FINDINGS IN NEONATAL JAUNDICE

FINDINGS	TIMING OF JAUNDICE	CAUSE
General examination		
Fever, tachycardia, respiratory distress	First 24 h Accumulates > 5 mg/dL/day (> 86 μmol/L/day)	Pneumonia, TORCH infection, sepsis
Lethargy, hypotonia	May appear in the first 24–48 h Can be prolonged (> 2 wk)	Hypothyroidism, metabolic disorder
Macrosomia	24–48 h Can accumulate > 5 mg/dL	Maternal diabetes
Petechiae	First 24 h Accumulates > 5 mg/dL	Hemolytic states (eg, maternofetal blood group incompatibility, RBC enzyme deficiencies, hereditary spherocytosis, thalassemias, sepsis)
Plethora	First 24 h Accumulates > 5 mg/dL	Maternofetal or fetofetal transfusion, delayed umbilical cord clamping
Head and neck examination		
Bilateral slanting palpebral fissures, flat nasal bridge, macroglossia, flattened occiput	First 2–3 days	Down syndrome (possible duodenal atresia, Hirschsprung disease, intestinal obstruction, wide spacing between 1st and 2nd toes)
Cephalohematoma	24–48 h Can accumulate > 5 mg/dL	Birth trauma
Macroglossia	24–48 h Can be prolonged (> 2 wk)	Hypothyroidism
Abdominal examination		
Abdominal distention, decreased bowel sounds	Possible delayed manifestation (2–3 days or later)	Intestinal obstruction (eg, cystic fibrosis, Hirschsprung disease, intestinal atresia or stenosis, pyloric stenosis, biliary atresia)

TORCH = toxoplasmosis, other pathogens, rubella, cytomegalovirus, and herpes simplex.

Physiologic jaundice usually is not clinically significant and resolves within 1 wk. Frequent formula feedings can reduce the incidence and severity of hyperbilirubinemia by increasing GI motility and frequency of stools, thereby minimizing the enterohepatic circulation of bilirubin. The type of formula does not seem important in increasing bilirubin excretion.

Breastfeeding jaundice may be prevented or reduced by increasing the frequency of feedings. If the bilirubin level continues to increase > 18 mg/dL in a term infant with early breastfeeding jaundice, a temporary change from breast milk to formula may be appropriate; phototherapy also may be indicated at higher levels. Stopping breastfeeding is necessary for only 1 or 2 days, and the mother should be encouraged to continue expressing breast milk regularly so she can resume nursing as soon as the infant's bilirubin level starts to decline. She also should be assured that the hyperbilirubinemia has not caused any harm and that she may safely resume breastfeeding. It is not advisable to supplement with water or dextrose because that may disrupt the mother's production of milk.

Definitive treatment of hyperbilirubinemia involves

- Phototherapy
- Exchange transfusion

Phototherapy: This treatment remains the standard of care, most commonly using fluorescent white light. (Blue light, wavelength 425 to 475 nm, is most effective for intensive phototherapy.) Phototherapy is the use of light to photoisomerize unconjugated bilirubin into forms that are more water-soluble and can be excreted rapidly by the liver and kidney without glucuronidation. It provides definitive treatment of neonatal hyperbilirubinemia and prevention of kernicterus.

For neonates born at ≥ 35 wk gestation, phototherapy is an option when unconjugated bilirubin is > 12 mg/dL (> 205.2 μmol/L) and may be indicated when unconjugated bilirubin is > 15 mg/dL at 25 to 48 h, 18 mg/dL at 49 to 72 h, and 20 mg/dL at > 72 h (see Fig. 320–1). Phototherapy is not indicated for conjugated hyperbilirubinemia.

For neonates born at < 35 wk gestation, threshold bilirubin levels for treatment are lower because premature infants are at a greater risk of neurotoxicity. The more preterm the infant, the lower the threshold (see Table 320–3).

Because visible jaundice may disappear during phototherapy even though serum bilirubin remains elevated, skin color cannot be used to evaluate jaundice severity. Blood taken for bilirubin determinations should be shielded from bright light, because bilirubin in the collection tubes may rapidly photo-oxidize.

Exchange transfusion: This treatment can rapidly remove bilirubin from circulation and is indicated for severe hyperbilirubinemia, which most often occurs with immune-mediated hemolysis. Small amounts of blood are withdrawn and replaced through an umbilical vein catheter to remove partially hemolyzed and antibody-coated RBCs as well as circulating Igs. The blood is replaced with uncoated donor RBCs that do not have the RBC membrane antigen that binds the circulating antibodies. That is, type O blood is used if the neonate is sensitized to AB antigens and Rh-negative blood is used if the neonate is sensitized to Rh antigen. Because adult donor RBCs have more ABO antigen sites than fetal cells, type-specific transfusion will intensify the hemolysis. Only unconjugated hyperbilirubinemia can cause kernicterus, so if conjugated bilirubin is elevated, the level of unconjugated rather than total bilirubin is used to determine the need for exchange transfusion.

For term infants, specific indications are serum bilirubin ≥ 20 mg/dL at 24 to 48 h or ≥ 25 mg/dL at > 48 h and failure of phototherapy to result in a 1- to 2-mg/dL (17- to 34-μmol/L) decrease within 4 to 6 h of initiation or at the first clinical signs of kernicterus regardless of bilirubin levels. If the serum bilirubin level is > 25 mg/dL when the neonate is initially examined, preparation for an exchange transfusion should be made in case intensive phototherapy fails to lower the bilirubin level.

Thresholds have been suggested for neonates born at < 35 wk gestation (see Table 320–3). Previously, some clinicians used criteria based solely on patient weight, but these criteria have been replaced by the more specific guidelines described above.

Most often, 160 mL/kg (twice the infant's total blood volume) of packed RBCs is exchanged over 2 to 4 h; an alternative is to give 2 successive exchanges of 80 mL/kg each over 1 to 2 h. To do an exchange, 20 mL of blood is withdrawn and then immediately replaced by 20 mL of transfused blood. This procedure is repeated until the total desired volume is exchanged. For critically ill or premature infants, aliquots of 5 to 10 mL are used to avoid sudden major changes in blood volume. The goal is to reduce bilirubin by nearly 50%, with the knowledge that hyperbilirubinemia may rebound to about 60% of pretransfusion level within 1 to 2 h. It is also customary to lower the target level by 1 to 2 mg/dL in conditions that increase the risk of kernicterus (eg, fasting, sepsis, acidosis). Exchange transfusions may need to be repeated if bilirubin levels remain high. Finally, there are risks and complications with the procedure, and the success of phototherapy has reduced the frequency of exchange transfusion.

Table 320–3. SUGGESTED THRESHOLDS* FOR STARTING PHOTOTHERAPY OR EXCHANGE TRANSFUSION IN INFANTS < 35 WK GESTATION

GESTATIONAL AGE (wk)	PHOTOTHERAPY (TSB, mg/dL)	EXCHANGE TRANSFUSION (TSB, mg/dL)
< 28	5–6	11–14
28 to < 30	6–8	12–14
30 to < 32	8–10	13–16
32 to < 34	10–12	15–18
34 to < 35	12–14	17–19

*Consensus-based recommendations adapted from Maisels MJ, Watchko JF, Bhutani VK, Stevenson DK: An approach to the management of hyperbilirubinemia in the preterm infant less than 35 weeks of gestation. *Journal of Perinatology* 32:660–664, 2012.

TSB = Total serum bilirubin.

KEY POINTS

- Neonatal jaundice is caused by increased bilirubin production, decreased bilirubin clearance, or increased enterohepatic circulation.
- Some jaundice is normal in neonates.
- Risk varies with postnatal age, TSB value, prematurity, and health of the neonate.
- Treatment depends on cause and degree of bilirubin elevation; the more preterm the infant, the lower the threshold level for treatment.
- Definitive treatments include phototherapy and exchange transfusion.

KERNICTERUS

(Bilirubin Encephalopathy)

Kernicterus is brain damage caused by unconjugated bilirubin deposition in basal ganglia and brain stem nuclei.

Normally, bilirubin bound to serum albumin stays in the intravascular space. However, bilirubin can cross the blood-brain barrier and cause kernicterus when serum bilirubin concentration is markedly elevated (hyperbilirubinemia); serum albumin concentration is markedly low (eg, in preterm infants); or bilirubin is displaced from albumin by competitive binders (eg, sulfisoxazole, ceftriaxone, and aspirin; free fatty acids and hydrogen ions in fasting, septic, or acidotic infants).

Symptoms and Signs

In preterm infants, kernicterus may not cause recognizable clinical symptoms or signs. Early symptoms of kernicterus in term infants are lethargy, poor feeding, and vomiting. Opisthotonos, oculogyric crisis, seizures, and death may follow. Kernicterus may result in intellectual disability, choreoathetoid cerebral palsy, sensorineural hearing loss, and paralysis of upward gaze later in childhood. It is unknown whether minor degrees of kernicterus can cause less severe neurologic impairment (eg, perceptual-motor problems, learning disorders).

Diagnosis

- Clinical evaluation

There is no reliable test to determine the risk of kernicterus, and the diagnosis is made presumptively. A definite diagnosis of kernicterus can be made only by autopsy.

Treatment

- Prevention of hyperbilirubinemia

There is no treatment once kernicterus develops; it must be prevented by treating hyperbilirubinemia.

NEONATAL HYPERCALCEMIA

Hypercalcemia is total serum calcium > 12 mg/dL (> 3 mmol/L) or ionized calcium > 6 mg/dL (> 1.5 mmol/L). The most common cause is iatrogenic. GI signs may occur (eg, anorexia, vomiting, constipation) and sometimes lethargy or seizures. Treatment is IV normal saline plus furosemide and sometimes corticosteroids, calcitonin, and bisphosphonates.

Etiology

The **most common cause** of neonatal hypercalcemia is

- Iatrogenic

Iatrogenic causes usually involve excess calcium or vitamin D, or phosphate deprivation, which can result from prolonged feeding with incorrectly prepared formula.

Other causes include maternal hypoparathyroidism, subcutaneous fat necrosis, parathyroid hyperplasia, abnormal renal function, Williams syndrome, and idiopathic. Williams syndrome includes supravalvular aortic stenosis, pulmonary valvular or peripheral pulmonary artery stenosis, atrial septal defect and/or ventricular septal defect, renal artery stenosis, aortic anomalies, elfin facies, and hypercalcemia of unknown pathophysiology; infants may also be small for gestational age, and hypercalcemia can be noted early in infancy, usually resolving by age 12 mo. Idiopathic neonatal hypercalcemia is a diagnosis of exclusion and is difficult to differentiate from Williams syndrome and often requires genetic testing. Neonatal hyperparathyroidism is very rare. Subcutaneous fat necrosis may occur after major trauma and causes hypercalcemia that usually resolves spontaneously. Maternal hypoparathyroidism or maternal hypocalcemia may cause secondary fetal hyperparathyroidism, with changes in fetal mineralization (eg, osteopenia).

Symptoms and Signs

Symptoms and signs of neonatal hypercalcemia may be noted when total serum calcium is > 12 mg/dL (> 3 mmol/L). These signs can include anorexia, GI reflux, nausea, vomiting, lethargy or seizures or generalized irritability, and hypertension. Other symptoms and signs include constipation, abdominal pain, dehydration, feeding intolerance, and failure to thrive. Some neonates have vague symptoms of muscle or joint aches and weakness. With subcutaneous fat necrosis, firm purple nodules may be observed on trunk, buttocks, or legs.

Diagnosis

- Total or ionized serum calcium level

Diagnosis of neonatal hypercalcemia is made by measuring total or ionized serum calcium level.

Treatment

- IV normal saline plus furosemide
- Sometimes corticosteroids, calcitonin, and bisphosphonates

Marked elevation of serum calcium may be treated with normal saline 20 mL/kg IV plus furosemide 2 mg/kg IV and, when persistent, with corticosteroids and calcitonin. Bisphosphonates are also increasingly used in this context (eg, etidronate by mouth or pamidronate IV). Treatment of subcutaneous fat necrosis is with a low-calcium formula; fluids, furosemide, calcitonin, and corticosteroids are used as indicated by the degree of hypercalcemia. Fetal hypercalcemia caused by maternal hypoparathyroidism can be treated expectantly, because it usually resolves spontaneously within a few weeks. Treatment of chronic conditions includes a low-calcium, low-vitamin D formula.

NEONATAL HYPOCALCEMIA

Hypocalcemia is a total serum calcium concentration < 8 mg/dL (< 2 mmol/L) in term infants or < 7 mg/dL (< 1.75 mmol/L) in preterm infants. It is also defined as an ionized calcium level < 3.0 to 4.4 mg/dL (< 0.75 to

1.10 mmol/L), depending on the method (type of electrode) used. Signs are primarily neurologic and include hypotonia, apnea, and tetany. Treatment is IV or oral calcium supplementation.

Etiology

Neonatal hypocalcemia occurs in 2 forms:

- Early onset (in the first 2 days of life)
- Late onset (> 3 days), which is rare

Some infants with congenital hypoparathyroidism (eg, caused by DiGeorge syndrome with agenesis or dysgenesis of the parathyroid glands) have both early and late (prolonged) hypocalcemia.

Early-onset hypocalcemia: Risk factors for early-onset hypocalcemia include prematurity, being small for gestational age, maternal diabetes, and perinatal asphyxia. Mechanisms vary. Normally, parathyroid hormone helps maintain normal calcium levels when the constant infusion of ionized calcium across the placenta is interrupted at birth. A transient, relative hypoparathyroidism may cause hypocalcemia in preterm neonates and some small-for-gestational-age neonates, who have parathyroid glands that do not yet function adequately, and in infants of mothers with diabetes or hyperparathyroidism, because these women have higher-than-normal ionized calcium levels during pregnancy. Perinatal asphyxia may also increase serum calcitonin, which inhibits calcium release from bone and results in hypocalcemia. In other neonates, the normal phosphaturic renal response to parathyroid hormone is absent; the elevated phosphate level leads to hypocalcemia.

Late-onset hypocalcemia: The cause of late-onset hypocalcemia is usually ingestion of cow's milk or formula with a too-high phosphate load; elevated serum phosphate leads to hypocalcemia.

Symptoms and Signs

Symptoms and signs of neonatal hypocalcemia rarely occur unless total serum calcium is < 7 mg/dL (< 1.75 mmol/L) or the ionized calcium is < 3.0 mg/dL (< 0.75 mmol/L). Signs include hypotonia, tachycardia, tachypnea, apnea, poor feeding, jitteriness, tetany, and seizures. Similar symptoms may occur with hypoglycemia and opioid withdrawal.

Diagnosis

- Total or ionized serum calcium level

Diagnosis of neonatal hypocalcemia is by measurement of total or ionized serum calcium; ionized calcium is the more physiologic measurement, because it does not require correction for protein concentration and pH. Prolongation of the corrected QT interval (QT_c) on ECG also suggests hypocalcemia.

Treatment

- Early onset: IV 10% calcium gluconate
- Late onset: Oral calcitriol or calcium

Early-onset hypocalcemia ordinarily resolves in a few days, and asymptomatic neonates with serum calcium levels > 7 mg/dL or ionized calcium > 3.5 mg/dL rarely require treatment. Those term infants with levels < 7 mg/dL and preterm infants with calcium < 6 mg/dL (< 1.5 mmol/L) should be treated with 2 mL/kg of 10% calcium gluconate (200 mg/kg) by slow IV infusion over 30 min. Too-rapid infusion can cause bradycardia, so heart rate should be monitored during the infusion. The IV site should also be watched closely because tissue infiltration by a calcium solution is irritating and may cause local tissue damage or necrosis. Manifestations of calcium infiltration include skin redness, calcification, and necrosis or slough; there can be radial nerve damage at the wrist.

After acute correction of hypocalcemia, calcium gluconate may be mixed in the maintenance IV infusion and given continuously. Starting with 400 mg/kg/day of calcium gluconate, the dose may be increased gradually to 800 mg/kg/day, if needed, to prevent a recurrence. When oral feedings are begun, the formula may be supplemented with the same daily dose of calcium gluconate, if needed, by adding the 10% calcium gluconate solution into the day's formula. Supplementation is usually required for only a few days.

Late-onset hypocalcemia treatment is addition of calcitriol or additional calcium to infant formula to provide a 4:1 molar ratio of calcium:phosphate until normal calcium levels are maintained. Oral calcium preparations have a high sucrose content, which may lead to diarrhea in preterm infants.

KEY POINTS

- Neonatal hypocalcemia usually occurs within the first 2 days of life and is most often caused by prematurity, being small for gestational age, maternal diabetes or hyperparathyroidism, and perinatal asphyxia.
- Neonates may have hypotonia, tachycardia, tachypnea, apnea, poor feeding, jitteriness, tetany, and/or seizures.
- Diagnose by measuring total or ionized serum calcium level; measure glucose level to rule out hypoglycemia.
- Treat early-onset hypocalcemia with IV 10% calcium gluconate, followed by several days of oral calcium supplementation.

NEONATAL HYPERGLYCEMIA

Hyperglycemia is a serum glucose concentration > 150 mg/dL (> 8.3 mmol/L).

The **most common cause** of neonatal hyperglycemia is

- Iatrogenic

Iatrogenic causes usually involve too-rapid IV infusions of dextrose during the first few days of life in very low-birth-weight infants (< 1.5 kg).

The other important cause is physiologic stress caused by surgery, hypoxia, respiratory distress syndrome, or sepsis; fungal sepsis poses a special risk. In premature infants, partially defective processing of proinsulin to insulin and relative insulin resistance may cause hyperglycemia. In addition, transient neonatal diabetes mellitus is a rare self-limited cause that usually occurs in small-for-gestational-age infants; corticosteroid therapy may also result in transient hyperglycemia. Hyperglycemia is less common than hypoglycemia, but it is important because it increases morbidity and mortality of the underlying causes.

Symptoms and Signs

Symptoms and signs of neonatal hyperglycemia are those of the underlying disorder.

Diagnosis

- Serum glucose testing

Diagnosis of neonatal hyperglycemia is by serum glucose testing. Additional laboratory findings may include glycosuria and marked serum hyperosmolarity.

Treatment

- Reduction of IV dextrose concentration, rate, or both
- Sometimes IV insulin

Treatment of iatrogenic hyperglycemia is reduction of the IV dextrose concentration (eg, from 10% to 5%) or of the infusion rate; hyperglycemia persisting at low dextrose infusion rates (eg, 4 mg/kg/min) may indicate relative insulin deficiency or insulin resistance.

Treatment of other causes is fast-acting insulin. One approach is to add fast-acting insulin to an IV infusion of 10% dextrose at a uniform rate of 0.01 to 0.1 unit/kg/h, then titrate the rate until the glucose level is normalized. Another approach is to add insulin to a separate IV of 10% D/W given simultaneously with the maintenance IV infusion so that the insulin can be adjusted without changing the total infusion rate. Responses to insulin are unpredictable, and it is extremely important to monitor serum glucose levels and to titrate the insulin infusion rate carefully.

In transient neonatal diabetes mellitus, glucose levels and hydration should be carefully maintained until hyperglycemia resolves spontaneously, usually within a few weeks.

Any fluid or electrolytes lost through osmotic diuresis should be replaced.

NEONATAL HYPOGLYCEMIA

Hypoglycemia is a serum glucose concentration < 40 mg/dL (< 2.2 mmol/L) in term neonates or < 30 mg/dL (< 1.7 mmol/L) in preterm neonates. Risk factors include prematurity, being small for gestational age, maternal diabetes, and perinatal asphyxia. The most common causes are deficient glycogen stores, delayed feeding, and hyperinsulinemia. Signs include tachycardia, cyanosis, seizures, and apnea. Diagnosis is suspected empirically and is confirmed by glucose testing. Prognosis depends on the underlying condition. Treatment is enteral feeding or IV dextrose.

Etiology

Neonatal hypoglycemia may be transient or persistent.

Causes of **transient hypoglycemia** are

- Inadequate substrate (eg, glycogen)
- Immature enzyme function leading to deficient glycogen stores

Deficiency of glycogen stores at birth is common in very low-birth-weight preterm infants, infants who are small for gestational age because of placental insufficiency, and infants who have perinatal asphyxia. Anaerobic glycolysis consumes glycogen stores in these infants, and hypoglycemia may develop at any time in the first few hours or days, especially if there is a prolonged interval between feedings or if nutritional intake is poor. A sustained input of exogenous glucose is therefore important to prevent hypoglycemia.

Causes of **persistent hypoglycemia** include

- Hyperinsulinism
- Defective counter-regulatory hormone release (growth hormone, corticosteroids, glucagon, catecholamines)
- Inherited disorders of metabolism (eg, glycogen storage diseases, disorders of gluconeogenesis, fatty acid oxidation disorders)

Hyperinsulinism most often occurs in infants of diabetic mothers and is inversely related to the degree of maternal diabetic control. When a mother has diabetes, her fetus is exposed to increased levels of glucose because of the elevated maternal blood glucose levels. The infant responds by producing increased levels of insulin. When the umbilical cord is cut, the infusion of glucose to the neonate ceases, and it may take hours or even days for the neonate to decrease its insulin production. Hyperinsulinism also commonly occurs in physiologically stressed infants who are small for gestational age. In both cases, the hyperinsulinism is transient. Less common and longer lasting causes include congenital hyperinsulinism (genetic conditions transmitted in both autosomal dominant and recessive fashion), severe erythroblastosis fetalis, and Beckwith-Wiedemann syndrome (in which islet cell hyperplasia accompanies features of macroglossia and umbilical hernia). Hyperinsulinemia characteristically results in a rapid fall in serum glucose in the first 1 to 2 h after birth when the continuous supply of glucose from the placenta is interrupted.

Blood glucose levels are dependent on multiple interacting factors. Although insulin is the primary factor, glucose levels are also dependent on growth hormone, cortisol, and thyroid hormone levels. Any condition that interferes with the appropriate secretion of these hormones can lead to hypoglycemia.

Hypoglycemia may also occur if an IV infusion of D/W is abruptly interrupted. Finally, hypoglycemia can be due to malposition of an umbilical catheter or sepsis.

Symptoms and Signs

Many infants remain asymptomatic. Prolonged or severe hypoglycemia causes both adrenergic and neuroglycopenic signs. Adrenergic signs include diaphoresis, tachycardia, lethargy or weakness, and shakiness. Neuroglycopenic signs include seizure, coma, cyanotic episodes, apnea, bradycardia or respiratory distress, and hypothermia. Listlessness, poor feeding, hypotonia, and tachypnea may occur.

Diagnosis

- Bedside glucose check

All signs are nonspecific and also occur in neonates who have asphyxia, sepsis or hypocalcemia, or opioid withdrawal. Therefore, at-risk neonates with or without these signs require an immediate bedside serum glucose check from a capillary sample. Abnormally low levels are confirmed by a venous sample.

Treatment

- IV dextrose (for prevention and treatment)
- Enteral feeding
- Sometimes IM glucagon

Most high-risk neonates are treated preventively. For example, infants of diabetic women who have been using insulin are often started at birth on a 10% D/W infusion IV or given oral glucose, as are those who are sick, are extremely premature, or have respiratory distress. Other at-risk neonates who are not sick should be started on early, frequent formula feedings to provide carbohydrates.

Any neonate whose glucose falls to ≤ 50 mg/dL (≤ 2.75 mmol/L) should begin prompt treatment with enteral feeding or with an IV infusion of up to 12.5% D/W, 2 mL/kg over 10 min; higher concentrations of dextrose can be infused if necessary through a central catheter. The infusion should then continue at a rate that provides 4 to 8 mg/kg/min of glucose (ie, 10% D/W at about 2.5 to 5 mL/kg/h). Serum glucose levels must be monitored to guide adjustments in the infusion rate.

Once the neonate's condition has improved, enteral feedings can gradually replace the IV infusion while the glucose concentration continues to be monitored. IV dextrose infusion should always be tapered, because sudden discontinuation can cause hypoglycemia.

If starting an IV infusion promptly in a hypoglycemic neonate is difficult, glucagon 100 to 300 mcg/kg IM (maximum, 1 mg) usually raises the serum glucose rapidly, an effect that lasts 2 to 3 h, except in neonates with depleted glycogen stores. Hypoglycemia refractory to high rates of glucose infusion may be treated with hydrocortisone 2.5 mg/kg IM bid. If hypoglycemia is refractory to treatment, other causes (eg, sepsis) and possibly an endocrine evaluation for persistent hyperinsulinism and disorders of defective gluconeogenesis or glycogenolysis should be considered.

KEY POINTS

- Small and/or premature infants often have low glycogen stores and become hypoglycemic unless they are fed early and often.
- Infants of diabetic mothers have hyperinsulinemia caused by high maternal glucose levels; they may develop transient hypoglycemia after birth, when maternal glucose is withdrawn.
- Signs include diaphoresis, tachycardia, lethargy, poor feeding, hypothermia, seizures, and coma.
- Give preventive treatment (using oral or IV glucose) to infants of diabetic mothers, extremely premature infants, and infants with respiratory distress.
- If glucose falls to ≤ 50 mg/dL (≤ 2.75 mmol/L), promptly give enteral feeding or an IV infusion of 10% to 12.5% D/W, 2 mL/kg over 10 min; follow this bolus with supplemental IV or enteral glucose and closely monitor glucose levels.

NEONATAL HYPERNATREMIA

Hypernatremia is a serum sodium concentration > 150 mEq/L, usually caused by dehydration. Signs include lethargy and seizures. Treatment is cautious hydration with IV saline solution.

Etiology

Hypernatremia develops when

- Water is lost in excess of sodium (hypernatremic dehydration)
- Sodium intake exceeds sodium losses (salt poisoning)
- Both

Water loss in excess of sodium intake is most commonly caused by diarrhea, vomiting, or high fever. It may also be caused by poor feeding in the early days of life (eg, when mother and infant are both learning to breastfeed) and may occur in very low-birth-weight (VLBW) infants born at 24 to 28 wk. In VLBW infants, insensible water losses through an immature, water-permeable stratum corneum combine with immature renal function and a reduced ability to produce concentrated urine to facilitate free water loss. Insensible water loss through the skin is also significantly increased by radiant warmers and phototherapy lights; exposed VLBW infants may require up to 250 mL/kg/day of water IV in the first few days, after which the stratum corneum develops and insensible water loss decreases. A rare cause is central or nephrogenic diabetes insipidus. Infants with hypernatremia and dehydration are often more dehydrated than is apparent by physical examination, because the increased osmolality helps maintain the extracellular fluid space (and hence circulating blood volume).

Solute overload most commonly results from adding too much salt when preparing homemade infant formula or from giving hyperosmolar solutions. Fresh frozen plasma and human albumin contain sodium and can contribute to hypernatremia when given repeatedly to very premature infants.

Symptoms and Signs

Symptoms and signs of hypernatremia include lethargy, restlessness, hyperreflexia, spasticity, hyperthermia, and seizures. Skin texture may be doughy rather than diminished. Intracranial hemorrhage, venous sinus thrombosis, and acute renal tubular necrosis are major complications.

Diagnosis

- Serum sodium concentration

Diagnosis of hypernatremia is suspected by symptoms and signs and is confirmed by measuring serum sodium concentration.

Additional laboratory findings may include an increase in BUN, a modest increase in serum glucose, and, if serum potassium is low, a depression in the level of serum calcium.

Treatment

- IV 0.9% saline, then hypotonic saline (0.3% or 0.45% saline)

Severely dehydrated infants must have their circulating blood volume restored first, usually with 0.9% saline in aliquots of 20 mL/kg IV. Treatment is then with 5% D/W/0.3% to 0.45% saline solution IV in volumes equal to the calculated fluid deficit (see also p. 2555), given over 2 to 3 days to avoid a rapid fall in serum osmolality, which would cause rapid movement of water into cells and potentially lead to cerebral edema. Maintenance fluids should be provided concurrently. The goal of treatment is to decrease serum sodium by about 10 mEq/L/day. Body weight, serum electrolytes, and urine volume and specific gravity must be monitored regularly so that fluid therapy can be adjusted appropriately. Once adequate urine output is shown, potassium is added to provide maintenance requirements or replace urinary losses.

Extreme hypernatremia (sodium > 200 mEq/L) caused by salt poisoning should be treated with peritoneal dialysis, especially if poisoning causes a rapid rise in serum sodium.

Prevention

Prevention of hypernatremia requires attention to the volume and composition of unusual fluid losses and of solutions used to maintain homeostasis. In neonates and young infants, who are unable to signal thirst effectively and to replace losses voluntarily, the risk of dehydration is greatest. The composition of feedings whenever mixing is involved (eg, some infant formulas and concentrated preparations for tube feeding) requires particular attention, especially when the potential for developing dehydration is high, such as during episodes of diarrhea, poor fluid intake, vomiting, or high fever.

KEY POINTS

- Hypernatremia is usually due to dehydration (eg, caused by diarrhea, vomiting, high fever); sodium overload is rare.
- Signs include lethargy, restlessness, hyperreflexia, spasticity, hyperthermia, and seizures.

- Intracranial hemorrhage, venous sinus thrombosis, and acute renal tubular necrosis may occur.
- Diagnose by finding serum sodium concentration > 150 mEq/L.
- If the cause is dehydration, restore circulating blood volume with 0.9% saline and then give 5% D/W/0.3% to 0.45% saline solution IV in volumes equal to the calculated fluid deficit.
- Rehydrate over 2 to 3 days to avoid a too-rapid fall in serum sodium.

NEONATAL HYPONATREMIA

Hyponatremia is a serum sodium concentration < 135 mEq/L. Significant hyponatremia may cause seizures or coma. Treatment is cautious sodium replacement with IV 0.9% saline solution; rarely, 3% saline solution is required, particularly if seizures are occurring.

Etiology

The most frequent cause of neonatal hyponatremia is hypovolemic dehydration caused by vomiting, diarrhea, or both when large GI losses are replaced with fluids that have little or no sodium (eg, some juices).

A less frequent cause is euvolemic hyponatremia caused by inappropriate ADH secretion and consequent water retention. Possible causes of inappropriate ADH secretion include CNS tumors and infection. Also, overdilution of infant formula can lead to water intoxication.

Finally, hypervolemic hyponatremia occurs in the setting of water retention and excess sodium retention, such as in heart failure or renal failure.

Symptoms and Signs

Symptoms and signs of neonatal hyponatremia include nausea and vomiting, apathy, headache, seizures, hypothermia, and coma; other symptoms include cramps and weakness. Infants with hyponatremic dehydration may appear quite ill, because hyponatremia causes disproportionate reductions in ECF volume. Symptoms and signs are related to duration and degree of hyponatremia.

Diagnosis

- Serum sodium concentration

Diagnosis of neonatal hyponatremia is suspected because of symptoms and signs and confirmed by measuring serum sodium concentration. In dehydration, an increase in BUN may be observed.

Treatment

- IV 5% D/W/0.45% to 0.9% saline solution
- Rarely IV hypertonic (3%) saline solution

Treatment of neonatal hyponatremia is with 5% D/W/0.45% to 0.9% saline solution IV in volumes equal to the calculated deficit, given over as many days as it takes to correct the sodium concentration by no more than 10 to 12 mEq/L/day to avoid rapid fluid shifts in the brain. Neonates with hypovolemic hyponatremia need volume expansion, using a solution containing salt to correct the sodium deficit (10 to 12 mEq/kg of body weight or even 15 mEq/kg in young infants with severe hyponatremia) and include sodium maintenance needs (3 mEq/kg/day in 5% D/W solution). Neonates with symptomatic hyponatremia (eg, lethargy, confusion) require emergency treatment with 3% saline solution IV to prevent seizure or coma.

PRENATAL DRUG EXPOSURE

Alcohol and illicit drugs are toxic to the placenta and developing fetus and can cause congenital syndromes and withdrawal symptoms. Prescription drugs also may have adverse effects on the fetus (see Table 283–1 on p. 2360). Fetal alcohol syndrome and the effects of cigarette smoking on the fetus are discussed elsewhere.

A fetus that has been exposed to drugs in utero (termed fetuses exposed to noxious substances [FENS]) can become dependent on the drug during gestation. Although some toxic substances used by the mother are not illegal, many are. In any case, the home situation should be evaluated to determine whether the infant will be safely cared for after discharge. With the supportive help of relatives, friends, and visiting nurses, the mother may be able to care for her infant. If not, foster home care or an alternative care plan may be best.

Amphetamines: Prenatal exposure to amphetamines has lasting subtle effects on neonatal brain structure and function. Some studies have shown decreased volume of the caudate, putamen, and globus pallidus (anatomic components of brain) in methamphetamine-exposed children, whereas other studies have not uniformly confirmed these findings. Other studies indicate that prenatal methamphetamine exposure may be associated with abnormal neurobehavioral patterns or fetal growth restriction, but these findings are not yet fully established.

Barbiturates: Prolonged maternal abuse of barbiturates may cause neonatal drug withdrawal with jitteriness, irritability, and fussiness that often do not develop until 7 to 10 days postpartum, after the neonate has been discharged home. Sedation with phenobarbital 0.75 to 1.5 mg/kg po or IM q 6 h may be required and then tapered over a few days or weeks, depending on the duration of symptoms.

Cocaine: Cocaine inhibits reuptake of the neurotransmitters norepinephrine and epinephrine; it crosses the placenta and causes vasoconstriction and hypertension in the fetus. Cocaine abuse in pregnancy is associated with a higher rate of placental abruption and spontaneous abortion, perhaps caused by reduced maternal blood flow to the placental vascular bed; abruption may also lead to intrauterine fetal death or to neurologic damage if the infant survives.

Neonates born to addicted mothers have low birth weight, reduced body length and head circumference, and lower Apgar scores. Cerebral infarcts may occur, and rare anomalies associated with prenatal cocaine use include limb amputations; GU malformations, including prune-belly syndrome; and intestinal atresia or necrosis. All are caused by vascular disruption, presumably secondary to local ischemia caused by the intense vasoconstriction of fetal arteries caused by cocaine. In addition, a pattern of mild neurobehavioral effects has also been observed, including decreases in attention and alertness, lower IQ, and impaired gross and fine motor skills.

Some neonates may show withdrawal symptoms if the mother used cocaine shortly before delivery, but symptoms are less common and less severe than for opioid withdrawal, and signs and treatment are the same.

Marijuana: Marijuana does not consistently seem to increase risk of congenital malformations, fetal growth restriction, or postnatal neurobehavioral abnormalities. However, women who use marijuana during pregnancy often also use alcohol, cigarettes, or both, which can cause fetal problems.

Opioids: Opioid exposure in utero can cause withdrawal on delivery. The neonate of a woman who used opioids chronically during pregnancy should be observed for withdrawal symptoms (narcotic abstinence syndrome [NAS]). NAS usually occurs within 72 h after delivery, although many neonatal units observe infants for 4 or 5 days to be sure there are no significant signs of withdrawal.

Characteristic signs of withdrawal include

- Irritability
- Jitteriness
- Hypertonicity
- Vomiting and/or diarrhea
- Sweating
- Seizures
- Hyperventilation that causes respiratory alkalosis

Prenatal benzodiazepine exposure may cause similar effects.

There are many scoring systems to help quantify the severity of withdrawal (The Opioid Exposed Newborn: Assessment and Pharmacologic Management). Mild withdrawal symptoms are treated by a few days of swaddling and soothing care to alleviate the physical overarousal and by giving frequent feedings to reduce restlessness. With patience, some problems resolve in no more than a week. However, up to 80% of infants with NAS require drug treatment, typically using an opioid, sometimes with the addition of clonidine. Phenobarbital (0.75 to 1.5 mg/kg po q 6 h) may help but is now considered 2nd-line treatment. Treatment is tapered and stopped over several days or weeks as symptoms subside; many infants require up to 5 wk of therapy.

There is no consensus on the best drug, but most experts use methadone, morphine, or sometimes tincture of opium. Dosing is based on the weight of the infant and the severity of the symptoms. Typically, a starting dose is given and increased until symptoms are controlled and then slowly tapered (see Table 320–4).

The addition of clonidine 1 mcg/kg po q 4 h may reduce the duration of drug treatment needed in full-term infants. However, clonidine should not be given to premature infants, because of the risk of bradycardia. If clonidine is used, BP should be monitored as the clonidine dose is tapered, because there can be rebound hypertension.

The incidence of SIDS is greater among infants born to women addicted to opioids but still is < 10/1000 infants, so routine use of home cardiorespiratory monitors is not recommended for these infants.

FETAL ALCOHOL SYNDROME

Alcohol exposure in utero increases the risk of spontaneous abortion, decreases birth weight, and can cause fetal alcohol syndrome, a constellation of variable physical and cognitive abnormalities.

At birth, infants with fetal alcohol syndrome (FAS) can be identified by small stature and a typical set of facial traits including microcephaly, microphthalmia, short palpebral fissures, epicanthal folds, a small or flat midface, a flat elongated philtrum, a thin upper lip, and a small chin. Abnormal palmar creases, cardiac defects, and joint contractures may also be evident.

After birth, cognitive deficits become apparent. The most serious manifestation is severe intellectual disability, which is thought to be a teratogenic effect of alcohol given the high number of intellectually disabled infants of alcoholic women; FAS may be the most common cause of noninherited intellectual disability.

Diagnosis

- Clinical evaluation

Diagnosis of FAS is given to infants with characteristic findings born to women who used alcohol excessively during pregnancy.

No single physical or cognitive finding is pathognomonic; lesser degrees of alcohol use cause less severe manifestations, and the diagnosis of mild cases can be difficult because partial expression occurs. It is often difficult to distinguish the effects of alcohol on the developing fetus from those of other exposures (eg, tobacco, other drugs) and factors (eg, poor nutrition, lack of health care, violence) that affect women who drink excessively.

Treatment

- Supportive care

There is no treatment for FAS. Supportive care should include an appropriate stimulating and nurturing environment. Good nutrition and growth are especially important. Many children with FAS will need learning support in school.

Because it is unknown when during pregnancy alcohol is most likely to harm the fetus and whether there is a lower limit of alcohol use that is completely safe, pregnant women should be advised to avoid all alcohol intake. Siblings of an infant diagnosed with FAS should be examined for subtle manifestations of the disorder.

Table 320–4. ONE DRUG REGIMEN FOR NEONATAL OPIOID WITHDRAWAL

DRUG	STARTING DOSE	INCREMENTAL INCREASE	TAPER
Morphine	0.04 mg/kg po q 3–4 h	0.04 mg/kg/dose	10–20% q 2–3 days
Methadone	0.05–0.1 mg/kg po q 6 h	0.05 mg/kg/dose	10–20% q wk

Adapted from Hudak ML, Tan RC, The Committee on Drugs, The Committee on Fetus and Newborn: Neonatal drug withdrawal. *Pediatrics* 129:E540–E560, 2012.

321 Miscellaneous Bacterial Infections in Infants and Children

BACTERIAL MENINGITIS IN INFANTS OVER 3 MONTHS OF AGE

Bacterial meningitis in infants is a serious infection of the meninges and subarachnoid space. Infants may present with nonspecific symptoms and signs (eg, lethargy, irritability, poor feeding, fever or hypothermia). Diagnosis is by CSF analysis. Treatment is with antimicrobials and, for selected infants, dexamethasone.

Etiology

The etiology and incidence of bacterial meningitis are closely related to age and whether the infants have received routine immunization with *Haemophilus influenzae* type b and *Streptococcus pneumoniae* conjugate vaccines.

In infants who have not received routine immunizations, common causes of bacterial meningitis include

- *Neisseria meningitidis* (especially serogroup B, but occasionally groups A, C, Y, or W135)
- *S. pneumoniae* (many serotypes; particularly in infants with no record of *S. pneumoniae* conjugate vaccination)
- *H. influenzae* type b (particularly in infants with no record of *H. influenzae* type b conjugate vaccination)

Symptoms and Signs

The younger the patient, the less specific are the symptoms and signs of meningitis.

The initial manifestations of bacterial meningitis may be an acute febrile illness with respiratory or GI symptoms followed only later by signs of serious illness. Young infants may have a bulging anterior fontanelle, but only rarely do they have nuchal rigidity or other classic meningeal signs (eg, Kernig sign or Brudzinski sign) typically present in older children. In children < 12 mo, the absence of nuchal rigidity must not be used to exclude meningitis.

PEARLS & PITFALLS

- In children < 12 mo, the absence of nuchal rigidity must not be used to exclude meningitis. However, if present, nuchal rigidity should not be ignored.

As bacterial meningitis progresses, children develop CNS manifestations, sometimes very rapidly. The degree of CNS derangement ranges from irritability to coma. As many as 15% of children who have bacterial meningitis are comatose or semicomatose at the time of hospitalization. Seizures sometimes occur with bacterial meningitis but in only about 20% of children—typically those who are already toxic, obtunded, or comatose. Infants who are alert and appear normal after a brief, non-focal seizure with fever are unlikely to have bacterial meningitis (see also p. 2772).

Papilledema is very uncommon in children of any age with bacterial meningitis. When papilledema is present, other causes of papilledema should be sought; bacterial meningitis progresses so quickly that there is usually insufficient time for papilledema to develop.

Diagnosis

- CSF analysis

In general, lumbar puncture should be done whenever the diagnosis of meningitis is known or suspected in an infant.

However, lumbar puncture may be delayed for the following reasons:

- Clinically important cardiorespiratory compromise (most often in young infants)
- Signs of significantly increased intracranial pressure, including retinal changes; altered pupillary responses; hypertension, bradycardia, and respiratory depression (Cushing triad); and focal neurologic signs
- Suspected intracranial injury, including presence of visible injuries, particularly to the head, or history suggestive of nonaccidental injury
- Infection at the site of lumbar puncture
- Suspicion or history of bleeding disorders (eg, hemophilia, severe thrombocytopenia)

In these circumstances, blood cultures should be done and antibiotics should be given empirically without doing the lumbar puncture. In cases of suspected increased intracranial pressure, arrangements should be made for a neuroimaging study (eg, cranial CT with and without contrast enhancement) during or immediately after antibiotics administration. If the results of the imaging study suggest it is safe, lumbar puncture may be done. However, it is not necessary to routinely do CT before lumbar puncture in young children with suspected meningitis; herniation of the brain is rare in bacterial meningitis of young children, even though all patients with meningitis have some degree of increased intracranial pressure.

CSF is sent for analysis, typically cell count, protein, glucose, Gram stain, culture, and, in selected infants, PCR tests for enteroviruses (eg, in infants with meningitis during the late summer and autumn months in the US) or herpes simplex virus (eg, infants < 3 mo of age). Simultaneously, a blood sample should be drawn and sent to have the CSF:blood glucose ratio determined.

Typical CSF findings in bacterial meningitis include

- High WBC count (> 500 WBC/μL [range, 10,000 to 20,000 WBC] with a predominance of polymorphonuclear leukocytes [> 80%])
- Elevated protein (> 100 mg/dL)
- Low glucose (< 40 mg/dL, often < 10 mg/dL, and CSF:blood glucose ratio typically < 0.33)

Gram stain often shows organisms in the CSF in bacterial meningitis. Although findings may vary somewhat, infants who have bacterial meningitis very rarely have completely normal CSF at examination.

Infants also should have 2 sets of blood cultures (if possible), serum electrolytes, CBC and differential, and a urinalysis and urine culture.

Differential diagnosis: Symptoms and signs of bacterial meningitis may also be caused by other CNS infections, including viral meningitis (typically enteroviral), HSV encephalitis (almost exclusively in the infant < 3 mo of age), and brain abscess. Other causes of CNS infections that affect older children and adults (eg, Lyme neuroborreliosis; fungal meningitis; tuberculous meningitis; *Bartonella* infection; chemical meningitis resulting from use of NSAIDs, trimethoprim/sulfamethoxazole, or IV immune globulin; cancer) rarely occur in children < 12 mo and should be distinguishable based on history, physical examination, and examination of the CSF.

In these other causes of meningitis, CSF findings most often include < 500 WBC/μL with < 50% polymorphonuclear leukocytes, protein < 100 mg/dL, normal glucose, and a negative Gram stain for organisms.

Prognosis

Among older infants and children, the mortality rate with bacterial meningitis is about 5 to 10%, and neurologic morbidity (eg, sensorineural hearing loss, intellectual disability, spasticity and paresis, seizure disorder) occurs in 15 to 25%. Sensorineural deafness is most common after pneumococcal meningitis.

Treatment

- Antimicrobial therapy

As soon as bacterial meningitis is diagnosed, IV access should be secured and appropriate antimicrobial drugs (and possibly corticosteroids) should be given.

Empiric antimicrobial therapy for infants > 3 mo is directed at the common pathogens: pneumococci, meningococci, and *H. influenzae* type b. A typical drug regimen includes

- Ceftriaxone or cefotaxime *plus*
- Vancomycin

Cefotaxime and ceftriaxone are extremely effective against the organisms that usually cause bacterial meningitis in infants > 3 mo. The major difference between these drugs is that ceftriaxone has a much longer serum half-life than cefotaxime. Vancomycin is given because some pneumococcal strains in certain areas are not susceptible to 3rd-generation cephalosporins. In areas (and institutions) where most pneumococci are susceptible to penicillin, vancomycin may not be necessary, particularly if no gram-positive cocci are seen on the CSF Gram stain; decision to withhold vancomycin should typically be made in consultation with an infectious disease specialist.

Once the infecting organism is identified, more specifically targeted drugs are used; for example, vancomycin may no longer be required.

Organism-specific antimicrobial therapy: After immediate empiric antimicrobial drugs have been started, results of CSF and/or blood cultures are used to select a more specifically targeted drug while waiting for microbial identification and susceptibility test results (see Tables 321–1 and 321–2).

If *S. pneumoniae* is suspected (eg, because gram-positive cocci in pairs are seen on a Gram stain of the CSF), the empiric vancomycin should be continued until susceptibility test results are available. Vancomycin is stopped if the isolate is susceptible to penicillin or the 3rd-generation cephalosporins; if the isolate is *not* susceptible, vancomycin is continued (and some clinicians add rifampin). Because dexamethasone can decrease the CSF penetrance (and thus effectiveness) of vancomycin, some experts advise that either dexamethasone should not be given, or if given, that rifampin be added concurrently.

If *H. influenzae type b* is suspected or proven, disease may be treated reliably with either ceftriaxone or cefotaxime; ampicillin may be used only if the isolate is proved susceptible. If ampicillin therapy is used, it is followed by a 4-day course of once-daily rifampin to clear the carrier state and prevent relapse (rifampin is not necessary if a 3rd-generation cephalosporin is used to complete therapy).

Disease caused by *N. meningitidis* is treated reliably with penicillin G or ampicillin at high doses, or alternatively by a 3rd-generation cephalosporin. If penicillin or ampicillin therapy is used, it is followed by a 2-day course of twice-daily rifampin to clear the carrier state and prevent relapse (rifampin is not necessary if a 3rd-generation cephalosporin is used to complete therapy).

Other etiologies of bacterial meningitis in infants and children > 3 mo of age have been reported but are very rare. *Listeria monocytogenes, S. agalactiae,* and *E. coli* cause disease in infants < 3 mo of age; they rarely are found in extremely premature infants who have survived to become > 3 mo of age. *S. aureus* meningitis may occur in infants who have had trauma or neurologic surgery. Specific antimicrobial therapy for these types of rare infections should be selected in consultation with an infectious disease specialist.

Corticosteroids for bacterial meningitis: The use of corticosteroids (eg, dexamethasone) as adjunctive therapy in bacterial meningitis has been studied for decades and continues to be controversial. The beneficial effects of corticosteroids in reducing neurologic morbidity appear to vary with the age of the patient, (child or adult), the specific bacterial etiology, and even

Table 321–1. SPECIFIC THERAPY FOR BACTERIAL MENINGITIS IN INFANTS OVER 3 MONTHS ONCE IDENTIFICATION AND SUSCEPTIBILITY RESULTS ARE KNOWN

PATHOGEN	THERAPY
Streptococcus pneumoniae	Penicillin MIC ≤ 0.06 μg/mL and ceftriaxone or cefotaxime MIC ≤ 0.5 μg/mL: Penicillin G or ampicillin for 10–14 days; ceftriaxone or cefotaxime also acceptable Penicillin MIC ≥ 0.12 μg/mL and ceftriaxone or cefotaxime MIC ≤ 0.5 μg/mL: Ceftriaxone or cefotaxime for 10–14 days Penicillin MIC ≥ 0.12 μg/mL and ceftriaxone or cefotaxime MIC ≥ 1.0 μg/mL: Ceftriaxone or cefotaxime) plus vancomycin with or without rifampin for 10–14 days
Neisseria meningitidis	Penicillin G or ampicillin for 7 days (must be followed by rifampin to eliminate carrier state) **Alternatives:** Ceftriaxone or cefotaxime
Haemophilus influenzae type b	Ceftriaxone or cefotaxime for 10 days **Alternative:** Ampicillin if isolate is susceptible (must be followed by rifampin to eliminate carrier state)

MIC = minimum inhibitory concentration.

Table 321–2. RECOMMENDED DOSAGES OF ANTIMICROBIAL DRUGS FOR INFANTS AND CHILDREN WITH BACTERIAL MENINGITIS

DRUG	INFANTS AND CHILDREN
Ampicillin	50–75 mg/kg q 6 h
Cefotaxime	50–75 mg/kg q 6 h
Ceftriaxone	40–50 mg/kg q 12 h *or* 80–100 mg/kg q 24 h
Penicillin G	50,000–66,667 units/kg q 4 h *or* 75,000–100,000 units/kg q 6 h
Rifampin	10 mg/kg q 12 h
Vancomycin	10–15 mg/kg q 6 h

whether the patient lives in an industrialized country or in the developing world.

At present, evidence suggests that dexamethasone reduces hearing impairment in infants and children living in industrialized countries who have bacterial meningitis caused by *H. influenzae* type b. The effectiveness of dexamethasone in meningitis caused by other organisms remains unproved, although some studies of adults in industrialized countries with meningitis caused by *S. pneumoniae* report improved neurologic outcomes and reduced mortality. Dexamethasone does not appear to benefit children or adults with bacterial meningitis who live in developing countries, nor does it seem to benefit neonates with meningitis.

Thus, dexamethasone 0.15 mg/kg IV should be given before, or within 1 h after, antimicrobial therapy in children > 6 wk of age with meningitis caused by *H. influenzae* type b. The drug is continued q 6 h for 4 days in confirmed *H. influenzae* type b meningitis. Some experts also recommend using this same dexamethasone regimen in children with pneumococcal meningitis who are > 6 wk of age.

For optimal efficacy, dexamethasone must be started at the time of diagnosis; this is not always possible, unless the Gram stain of the fluid or epidemiologic factors (eg, disease contact history) can yield an immediate etiologic diagnosis. In regions where children have been given routine *H. influenzae* type b and pneumococcal conjugate vaccines, bacterial meningitis caused by these organisms will be rare. For these reasons, along with the conflicting evidence regarding the benefits of dexamethasone therapy, many pediatric infectious disease experts no longer routinely give corticosteroids to infants with meningitis.

Prevention

Prevention of bacterial meningitis involves vaccination and sometimes chemoprophylaxis.

Vaccination: A conjugate pneumococcal vaccine effective against 13 serotypes, including > 90% of the pneumococcal serotypes that cause meningitis in infants, is recommended for all children beginning at 2 mo of age (see Table 291–2 on p. 2462).

Routine vaccination with an H. influenzae type b conjugate vaccine also is highly effective and begins at age 2 mo.

The Advisory Committee on Immunization Practices (ACIP) recommends that infants > 6 wk who are at high risk of meningococcal disease receive a meningococcal conjugate vaccine. For infants not at high risk, routine meningococcal conjugate vaccination is recommended at age 11 or 12 yr (see Table 291–3 on p. 2467). High-risk infants include those who

- Have functional or anatomic asplenia
- Have persistent complement component pathway deficiencies
- Are traveling to a high-risk area (eg, sub-Saharan Africa, Saudi Arabia during the Hajj)

Two serogroup B meningococcal vaccines have been approved by the ACIP for use in children ≥10 yr of age who are at high risk of meningococcal group B disease (same categories as above); routine meningococcal B vaccination is not yet currently given. For further information, see current ACIP meningococcal vaccine recommendations.

Chemoprophylaxis for meningitis: Antimicrobial chemoprophylaxis is necessary for

- *N. meningitidis* meningitis: All close contacts
- *H. influenzae* meningitis: Selected close contacts

Contacts of children who have meningitis caused by other bacteria do not require chemoprophylaxis.

For **meningococcal meningitis,** close contacts have a risk of infection that may be 25 to 500 times higher than that of the general population. Close contacts are defined as

- Household members, especially children < 2 yr of age
- Child care center contacts exposed in the 7 days before symptom onset
- Anyone directly exposed to the patient's oral secretions (eg, through kissing, sharing toothbrushes or utensils, mouth-to-mouth resuscitation, endotracheal intubation, endotracheal tube management) in the 7 days before symptom onset

Not every health care practitioner who has cared for an infant with meningitis is considered a close contact. Health care personnel should receive chemoprophylaxis only if they were managing the patient's airway or were directly exposed to the patient's respiratory secretions. Chemoprophylaxis should be given as soon as possible (ideally within 24 h of identification of the index patient); chemoprophylaxis given > 2 wk after exposure is likely of little to no value. Rifampin, ceftriaxone, and ciprofloxacin are appropriate drugs depending on the age of the contact (see Table 321–3). For young children, oral rifampin or injectable ceftriaxone is preferred.

For ***H. influenzae* type b meningitis,** the risk of infection in contacts is lower than with meningococcal disease but can be substantial in young, unvaccinated infant or toddler contacts residing in the household of an index patient. Also, household contacts may be asymptomatic carriers of *H. influenzae* type b. Close contacts are defined more explicitly than for meningococcal prophylaxis because caretakers who spend time in the household but do not live there may nevertheless have become colonized with *H. influenzae* type b. Thus for this organism, **household contacts** are defined as the following:

- People who live with the index patient
- People who have spent ≥ 4 h with the index patient for ≥ 5 of the 7 days preceding the index patient's hospital admission

Chemoprophylaxis is then recommended *for each member* of a household, as just defined, if that household *also* has

- At least 1 contact < 4 yr who is incompletely immunized or unimmunized
- A child < 12 mo who has not completed the primary Hib conjugate immunization series
- An immunocompromised child (regardless of previous immunization status)

Table 321–3. RECOMMENDED CHEMOPROPHYLAXIS FOR HIGH-RISK CONTACTS* OF CHILDREN WITH MENINGOCOCCAL OR *H. INFLUENZAE* TYPE B MENINGITIS

DRUG AND INDICATION	AGE	DOSE	DURATION
Rifampin† (for *N. meningitidis*)	< 1 mo	5 mg/kg IV or po q 12 h	2 days
	≥ 1 mo	10 mg/kg IV or po q 12 h (maximum 600 mg po q 12 h)	2 days
Rifampin† (for *H. influenzae*)	< 1 mo	10 mg/kg IV or po once/day	4 days
	≥ 1 mo	20 mg/kg IV or po once/day (maximum 600 mg po once/day)	4 days
Ceftriaxone (for either pathogen)	< 15 yr	125 mg IM	Single dose
	≥ 15 yr	250 mg IM	Single dose
Ciprofloxacin‡ (for either pathogen)	> 1 m	20 mg/kg po (maximum 500 mg)	Single dose

*See text for definitions of high-risk close contacts.
†Rifampin is not recommended for pregnant women.
‡Ciprofloxacin is not routinely recommended for children < 18 yr; however, it may be used for certain children > 1 mo if risks and benefits have been assessed. If fluoroquinolone-resistant strains of meningococci have been identified in a community, ciprofloxacin should not be used for chemoprophylaxis.

Complete immunization against *H. influenzae* type b is defined as having had at least 1 dose of Hib conjugate vaccine at age ≥ 15 mo, or 2 doses between 12 mo and 14 mo, or the 2- or 3-dose primary series for children < 12 mo with a booster dose at ≥ 12 mo.

In addition, if a preschool or child care center has had ≥ 2 cases of invasive Hib disease within 60 days among its members, many experts recommend chemoprophylaxis for all attendees and staff to eliminate asymptomatic nasal carriage regardless of immunization status.

Close contacts most at risk of secondary infection are children < 4 yr who are incompletely immunized against *H. influenzae* type b. Chemoprophylaxis should be given < 24 h after identification of the index patient; chemoprophylaxis given > 2 wk after exposure is likely of little to no value. Oral rifampin or injectable ceftriaxone is preferred, and ciprofloxacin is acceptable for older contacts (see Table 321–3).

KEY POINTS

- Infants with bacterial meningitis may first present with nonspecific symptoms and signs (eg, of upper respiratory or GI illness) but then decompensate rapidly.
- The most common bacterial causes of meningitis are *Neisseria meningitidis, Haemophilus influenzae* type b, and *Streptococcus pneumoniae*.
- If meningitis is suspected, do lumbar puncture and give empiric antimicrobial therapy (and possibly dexamethasone) as soon as possible.
- Empiric antimicrobial therapy in infants > 3 mo is with cefotaxime or ceftriaxone plus vancomycin.

OCCULT BACTEREMIA AND FEVER WITHOUT APPARENT SOURCE IN INFANTS AND YOUNG CHILDREN

Occult bacteremia is the presence of bacteria in the bloodstream of febrile young children who have no apparent foci of infection and look well. Diagnosis is by blood culture and exclusion of focal infection. Treatment is with antibiotics, either in the hospital or as outpatients; select children are treated pending blood culture results.

The causes, evaluation, and management of possible occult bacteremia vary by childrens' age and immunization status.

Children 3 to 36 mo of age: In the era before conjugate vaccines, about 3 to 5% of children aged 3 to 36 mo with a febrile illness (temperature ≥ 39° C) and no localizing abnormalities (ie, fever without a source) had occult bacteremia. In contrast, children > 36 mo with bacteremia almost always looked ill and had an identifiable (ie, non-occult) focus of infection. The majority (80%) of occult bacteremia prior to routine conjugate immunization was caused by *Streptococcus pneumoniae*. A smaller percentage (10%) was caused by *Haemophilus influenzae* type b, and an even smaller percentage (5%) by *Neisseria meningitidis*.

Occult bacteremia is a concern because about 5 to 10% of the children develop serious bacterial infections (SBIs)—typically defined as sepsis, meningitis, and urinary tract infection, but also including septic arthritis and osteomyelitis. Such infections could be minimized by early identification and treatment of the bacteremia. The likelihood of progression to serious focal illness depended on the cause: 7 to 25% for bacteremia caused by *H. influenzae* type b but 4 to 6% for bacteremia caused by *S. pneumoniae*.

Currently in the US, routine vaccination of infants with polysaccharide conjugate vaccines against *S. pneumoniae* and *H. influenzae* type b has eliminated (> 99%) *H. influenzae* type b infections and substantially reduced (≥ 70%) invasive *S. pneumoniae* infections. Thus, in this age group, occult bacteremia has become rare except in underimmunized or nonimmunized children, and in children with immunodeficiency.

Children < 3 mo of age: In contrast, febrile infants < 3 mo of age continue to have a greater risk of SBI than older infants, about 8 to 10%. In the past, SBIs in young infants < 3 mo of age were more commonly caused by group B β-hemolytic *Streptococcus, S. pneumoniae,* and *H. influenzae* type b. However, chemoprophylaxis during labor in pregnant women colonized with group B β-hemolytic *Streptococcus* has reduced early-onset (infection occurring at < 7 days of age) group B streptococcal disease by > 80%. In addition, routine conjugate immunization has decreased colonization among older siblings immunized against *S. pneumoniae* and *H. influenzae* type b such that the rate of SBI caused by those organisms has decreased as well (herd immunity).

Notably, late-onset (infection occurring at > 7 days of age) group B streptococcal infection is not affected by chemoprophylaxis during labor, and other serious bacterial illnesses such as urinary tract infection (UTI) (most commonly caused by *Escherichia coli*) and occasional cases of *Salmonella* bacteremia continue to be important causes of fever without apparent source on physical examination in infants < 3 mo.

Symptoms and Signs

The major symptom of occult bacteremia is fever—temperature ≥ 39° C (≥ 38° C for infants < 3 mo). By definition, children with apparent focal disease (eg, cough, dyspnea, and pulmonary crackles suggesting pneumonia; skin erythema suggesting cellulitis or septic arthritis) are excluded (ie, because their disease is not occult). A toxic appearance (eg, limpness and listlessness, lethargy, signs of poor perfusion, cyanosis, marked hypoventilation or hyperventilation) suggests sepsis or septic shock; bacteremia in such children is also not classified as occult or fever without a source. However, early sepsis can be difficult to distinguish from occult bacteremia.

Diagnosis

- Blood cultures
- Urine culture and urinalysis
- Complete blood count and differential
- Sometimes other tests depending on age and clinical circumstances

Diagnosis of bacteremia requires blood cultures; ideally, two samples are taken from separate sites, which helps minimize the problem of false positives due to skin contaminants, and results should be made available within 24 h.

Recommendations for testing and choice of tests vary with age, temperature, and clinical appearance; the goal is to minimize testing without missing an SBI. Children who have indications of focal infection on history or physical examination are evaluated based on those findings.

When available, rapid diagnostic tests for enteroviruses, respiratory syncytial virus, and influenza virus are useful in the evaluation of infants with fever without apparent source, because infants whose test results are positive for these viruses likely have fever resulting from that virus and require few or no further tests for SBI. There also are rapid tests for other viruses but these have not been studied sufficiently to justify using their results to alter testing for SBI.

In infants with SBI, the CBC usually shows an elevated WBC count; however, only about 10% of children with WBC counts of > 15,000/μL are bacteremic, so specificity is low. Acute-phase reactants (eg, ESR, C-reactive protein [CRP] with or without procalcitonin) are used by some clinicians but add little information; some clinicians believe that elevated procalcitonin levels may be more specific for serious illness. In children < 3 mo, band counts > 1500/μL and either low (< 5000/μL) or high (> 15,000/μL) WBC counts may indicate bacteremia.

Children 3 to 36 mo of age: It is important to note that any febrile infant, regardless of immunization history, who appears seriously ill or toxic requires complete clinical and laboratory evaluation (CBC with differential, blood cultures, urine cultures, lumbar puncture, and in most cases, admission to the hospital with empiric antimicrobial therapy). Unimmunized, underimmunized, and immunocompromised febrile infants in this age range are more susceptible to SBI than their peers and also typically require the same full clinical and laboratory evaluation for SBI and empiric antibiotics. Children with dyspnea or low O_2 saturation should also have chest x-ray.

In previously immunized febrile infants aged 3 to 36 mo who appear well (nontoxic), the risk of bacteremia is now as low or even lower than the rate of false-positive blood cultures due to skin contaminants, leading many experts to forego blood cultures in these children. However, a urinalysis with microscopic examination and urine culture is typically recommended but not additional laboratory examination (eg, CBC, chest x-ray). Although the vast majority of these children have a viral infection, a very small number of well-appearing children will have an early SBI so caretakers should be advised to monitor the child's symptoms, give antipyretics, and follow up with the clinician (by visit or telephone depending on the circumstances and the caretakers' reliability) in 24 to 48 h. Children who worsen or remain febrile should have testing done (eg, CBC with differential, blood cultures, possibly chest x-ray or lumbar puncture).

Children < 3 mo of age: Toxic-appearing or seriously ill-appearing infants require immediate clinical evaluation and collection of blood, urine, and spinal fluid cultures and hospitalization for empiric antibiotic therapy. Unlike in older infants, in those < 3 mo of age, a nontoxic clinical appearance does not routinely allow deferral of testing.

Algorithms have been developed to help guide evaluation of infants in this age group (for one example, see Fig. 321–1). In using the algorithm, many experts consider age < 30 days by itself to be a high-risk criterion (and thus routinely admit them and do additional testing), whereas others do not and manage all infants < 90 days of age using the same criteria. This algorithm is sensitive for SBI but relatively nonspecific. Thus, given the relatively low incidence of SBI even among the population of febrile young infants, the algorithm has a high negative predictive value but a low positive predictive value (see p. 3141), making it much more effective in identifying children at low risk of infection who can be treated expectantly (ie, SBI or bacteremia ruled out) rather than in identifying children with true SBI or bacteremia.

Treatment

- Antibiotics (empirically, for select patients pending culture results, as well as for those patients with positive cultures)
- Antipyretics for discomfort
- Adequate hydration (because of increased losses with fever and possible anorexia; oral hydration if possible, parenteral if not)

Children who receive antibiotics before bacteremia is confirmed by blood culture seem less likely to develop focal infections, but data are inconsistent. However, because of the low overall incidence of bacteremia, many children would receive unnecessary treatment if all who were tested were empirically treated. As above, management varies by age and other clinical factors.

Regardless of age, all children are reexamined in 24 to 48 h. Those with persistent fever or positive blood or urine cultures who have not been treated already have more cultures done and are hospitalized for evaluation of possible sepsis and parenteral antibiotic therapy. If new signs of focal infection are found on reexamination, evaluation and therapy are directed by the findings.

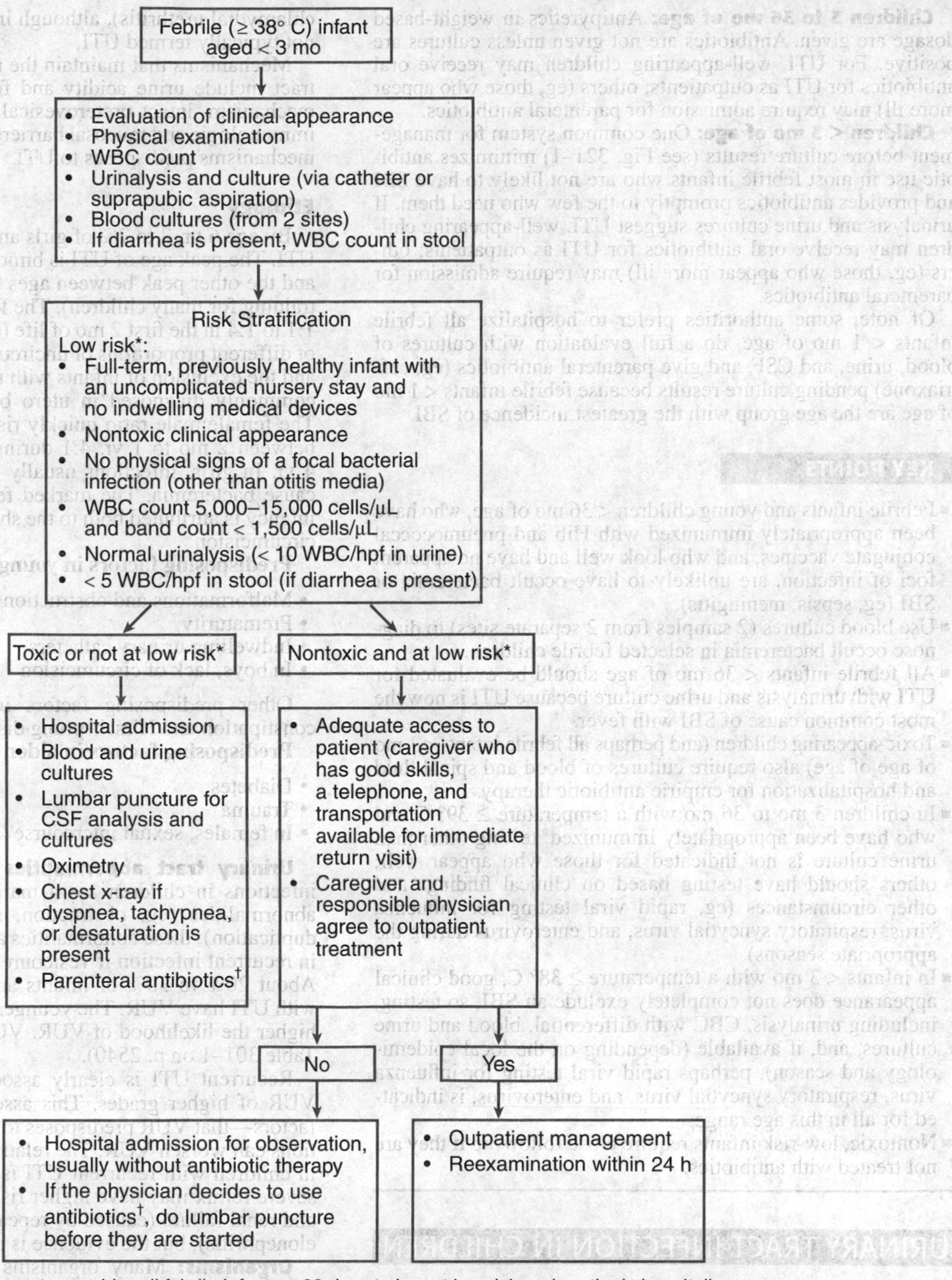

* Some experts consider all febrile infants < 28 days to be not low risk and routinely hospitalize, do lumbar puncture, and give parenteral antibiotics to all such infants.

† Typically, ceftriaxone 50 mg/kg IM or IV once/day (or for infants < 1 mo, ampicillin 50 mg/kg IM or IV qid plus gentamicin 5 mg/kg IM or IV once/day) is given, with adjustments made depending on culture results. Abnormal lumbar puncture or suspected meningitis may require higher doses.

Fig. 321–1. Evaluation and management of the febrile infant aged < 3 mo. hpf = high-power field.

Children 3 to 36 mo of age: Antipyretics in weight-based dosage are given. Antibiotics are not given unless cultures are positive. For UTI, well-appearing children may receive oral antibiotics for UTI as outpatients; others (eg, those who appear more ill) may require admission for parenteral antibiotics.

Children < 3 mo of age: One common system for management before culture results (see Fig. 321–1) minimizes antibiotic use in most febrile infants who are not likely to have SBI and provides antibiotics promptly to the few who need them. If urinalysis and urine cultures suggest UTI, well-appearing children may receive oral antibiotics for UTI as outpatients; others (eg, those who appear more ill) may require admission for parenteral antibiotics.

Of note, some authorities prefer to hospitalize all febrile infants < 1 mo of age, do a full evaluation with cultures of blood, urine, and CSF, and give parenteral antibiotics (eg, ceftriaxone) pending culture results because febrile infants < 1 mo of age are the age group with the greatest incidence of SBI.

KEY POINTS

- Febrile infants and young children < 36 mo of age, who have been appropriately immunized with Hib and pneumococcal conjugate vaccines, and who look well and have no apparent foci of infection, are unlikely to have occult bacteremia or SBI (eg, sepsis, meningitis).
- Use blood cultures (2 samples from 2 separate sites) to diagnose occult bacteremia in selected febrile children.
- All febrile infants < 36 mo of age should be evaluated for UTI with urinalysis and urine culture because UTI is now the most common cause of SBI with fever.
- Toxic-appearing children (and perhaps all febrile infants < 1 mo of age of age) also require cultures of blood and spinal fluid and hospitalization for empiric antibiotic therapy.
- In children 3 mo to 36 mo with a temperature ≥ 39° C and who have been appropriately immunized, testing other than urine culture is not indicated for those who appear well; others should have testing based on clinical findings and other circumstances (eg, rapid viral testing for influenza virus, respiratory syncytial virus, and enterovirus during the appropriate seasons).
- In infants < 3 mo with a temperature ≥ 38° C, good clinical appearance does not completely exclude an SBI, so testing, including urinalysis, CBC with differential, blood and urine cultures, and, if available (depending on the local epidemiology and season), perhaps rapid viral testing for influenza virus, respiratory syncytial virus, and enterovirus, is indicated for all in this age range.
- Nontoxic, low-risk infants require close follow-up if they are not treated with antibiotics.

URINARY TRACT INFECTION IN CHILDREN

UTI is defined by ≥ 5 × 10^4 colonies/mL in a catheterized urine specimen or, in older children, by repeated voided specimens with ≥ 10^5 colonies/mL. In younger children, UTIs are frequently associated with anatomic abnormalities. UTI may cause fever, failure to thrive, flank pain, and signs of sepsis, especially in young children. Treatment is with antibiotics. Follow-up imaging studies of the urinary tract are done.

UTI may involve the kidneys, bladder, or both. Sexually transmitted infections of the urethra (eg, gonococcal or chlamydial urethritis), although involving the urinary tract, are not typically termed UTI.

Mechanisms that maintain the normal sterility of the urinary tract include urine acidity and free flow, a normal emptying mechanism, intact ureterovesical and urethral sphincters, and immunologic and mucosal barriers. Abnormality of any of these mechanisms predisposes to UTI.

Etiology

By age 6 yr, 3 to 7% of girls and 1 to 2% of boys have had a UTI. The peak age of UTI is bimodal, with one peak in infancy and the other peak between ages 2 to 4 yr (at the time of toilet training for many children). The female:male ratio ranges from 1:1 to 1:4 in the first 2 mo of life (estimates vary, likely because of different proportions of uncircumcised males in study groups and the exclusion of infants with urologic anomalies now more commonly diagnosed in utero by prenatal ultrasonography). The female:male ratio quickly rises with age, being about 2:1 between 2 mo to 1 yr, 4:1 during the 2nd yr, and > 5:1 after 4 yr. In girls, infections usually are ascending and less often cause bacteremia. The marked female preponderance beyond infancy is attributed both to the shorter female urethra and male circumcision.

Predisposing factors in younger children include

- Malformations and obstructions of the urinary tract
- Prematurity
- Indwelling urinary catheters
- In boys, lack of circumcision

Other predisposing factors in younger children include constipation and Hirschsprung disease.

Predisposing factors in older children include

- Diabetes
- Trauma
- In females, sexual intercourse

Urinary tract abnormalities in children: Urinary tract infections in children are a marker of possible urinary tract abnormalities (eg, obstruction, neurogenic bladder, ureteral duplication); these abnormalities are particularly likely to result in recurrent infection if vesicoureteral reflux (VUR) is present. About 20% to 30% of infants and children age 12 to 36 mo with UTI have VUR. The younger the child at the first UTI, the higher the likelihood of VUR. VUR is classified by grade (see Table 301–1 on p. 2540).

Recurrent UTI is clearly associated with VUR, especially VUR of higher grades. This association is likely due to two factors—that VUR predisposes to infection and recurrent infections can worsen VUR. The relative contribution of each factor in children with recurrent UTI is unclear. Children with more severe reflux may have higher risk of developing hypertension and renal failure (caused by repeated infection and chronic pyelonephritis), but the evidence is not definitive (see p. 2744).

Organisms: Many organisms cause UTI in anatomically abnormal urinary tracts.

In relatively normal urinary tracts, the most common pathogens are

- Strains of *Escherichia coli* with specific attachment factors for transitional epithelium of the bladder and ureters

E. coli causes > 80 to 90% of UTIs in all pediatric age groups.

The remaining causes are other gram-negative enterobacteria, especially *Klebsiella, Proteus mirabilis,* and *Pseudomonas aeruginosa*. Enterococci (group D streptococci) and coagulase-negative staphylococci (eg, *Staphylococcus saprophyticus*) are the most frequently implicated gram-positive organisms.

Fungi and mycobacteria are rare causes, occurring in immunocompromised hosts.

Adenoviruses rarely cause UTIs, and when they do, the disorder is predominantly hemorrhagic cystitis, also predominantly among immunocompromised hosts.

Symptoms and Signs

In **neonates,** symptoms and signs of UTI are nonspecific and include poor feeding, diarrhea, failure to thrive, vomiting, mild jaundice (which is usually direct bilirubin elevation), lethargy, fever, and hypothermia. Neonatal sepsis may develop.

Infants and children < 2 yr with UTI may also present with poorly localizing signs, such as fever, GI symptoms (eg, vomiting, diarrhea, abdominal pain), or foul-smelling urine. About 4 to 10% of febrile infants without localizing signs have UTI.

In **children > 2 yr,** the more classic picture of cystitis or pyelonephritis can occur. Symptoms of cystitis include dysuria, frequency, hematuria, urinary retention, suprapubic pain, urgency, pruritus, incontinence, foul-smelling urine, and enuresis. Symptoms of pyelonephritis include high fever, chills, and costovertebral pain and tenderness.

Physical findings suggesting associated urinary tract abnormalities include abdominal masses, enlarged kidneys, abnormality of the urethral orifice, and signs of lower spinal malformations. Diminished force of the urinary stream may be the only clue to obstruction or neurogenic bladder.

Diagnosis

- Urine analysis and culture
- Often urinary tract imaging

Urine tests: A reliable diagnosis of UTI requires the presence of pyuria on urinalysis and positive bacterial culture in properly collected urine, before an antimicrobial is given. A diagnosis of probable UTI may be made by the presence of pyuria on urinalysis, while culture results are pending. Most clinicians obtain urine by transurethral catheterization in infants and young children, reserving suprapubic aspiration of the bladder for boys with moderate to severe phimosis. Both procedures require technical expertise, but catheterization is less invasive, slightly safer, and has sensitivity of 95% and specificity of 99% compared with suprapubic aspiration. Bagged specimens are unreliable and should not be used for diagnosis.

Urine culture results are interpreted based on colony counts. If urine is obtained by catheterization or suprapubic aspiration, $\geq 5 \times 10^4$ colonies/mL commonly defines UTI. Clean-catch, midstream-voided specimens are significant when colony counts of a single pathogen (ie, not the total count of mixed flora) are $\geq 10^5$ colonies/mL. However, at times symptomatic children may have UTI despite lower colony counts on urine cultures. Urine should be examined by urinalysis and cultured as soon as possible or stored at 4° C if a delay of > 10 min is expected. Occasionally, UTI may be present despite colony counts lower than the described guidelines, possibly because of prior antibiotic therapy, very dilute urine (specific gravity < 1.003), or obstruction to the flow of grossly infected urine. Sterile cultures generally rule out UTI unless the child is receiving antibiotics or the urine is contaminated with antibacterial skin-cleaning agents.

Microscopic examination of urine is very useful but not definitive. Pyuria (> 3 WBCs/high-power field in spun urine sediment) is about 96% sensitive for UTI and 91% specific. Raising the threshold of pyuria to > 10 WBCs/high-power field in spun urine sediment decreases the sensitivity to 81% but is more specific (97%). A WBC count (using a hemocytometer) > 10/μL in *unspun* urine has greater sensitivity (90%) but is not used by many laboratories. Presence of bacteria on urinalysis of spun or unspun fresh urine is about 80 to 90% sensitive but only 66% specific; Gram stain of the urine to detect the presence of bacteria is about 80% sensitive and 80% specific.

Dipstick tests on urine to detect gram-negative bacteria (nitrite test) or WBC (leukocyte esterase test) are typically done together; if both are positive, the diagnostic sensitivity for UTI is about 93 to 97% and the specificity is about 72 to 93%. Sensitivity is lower for each individual test, especially for the nitrite test (about 50% sensitivity), because it may take several hours for bacterial metabolism to produce nitrites, and frequent voiding by children may preclude nitrite detection. The specificity of the nitrite test is quite high (about 98%); a positive result on a freshly voided specimen is highly predictive of UTI. Sensitivity of the leukocyte esterase test is 83 to 96% and specificity is 78 to 90%.

Differentiating an upper UTI from a lower UTI can be difficult. High fever, costovertebral angle tenderness, and gross pyuria with casts indicate pyelonephritis; an elevated CRP level also tends to be associated with pyelonephritis. However, many children without these symptoms and signs have an upper UTI. Tests to distinguish upper infection from lower infection are not indicated in most clinical settings because treatment is not altered.

Blood tests: A CBC and tests for inflammation (eg, ESR, CRP) may help diagnose infection in children with borderline urine findings. Some authorities measure serum BUN and creatinine during a first UTI. Blood cultures are appropriate for infants with UTIs and for children > 1 to 2 yr who appear toxic.

Urinary tract imaging: Many major renal or urologic anomalies now are diagnosed in utero by routine prenatal ultrasonography, but a normal result does not completely exclude the possibility of anatomic anomalies. Thus, renal and bladder ultrasound imaging is typically done in children < 3 yr of age after their first febrile UTI. Some clinicians do imaging on children up to 7 yr of age or older.

Renal and bladder ultrasonography helps exclude obstruction and hydronephrosis in children with febrile UTIs and is typically done within a week of diagnosing UTI in infants. Ultrasonography is done within 48 h if infants do not respond quickly to antimicrobials or if their illness is unusually severe. Beyond infancy, ultrasonography may be done in the few weeks after the UTI diagnosis.

Voiding cystourethrography (VCUG) and **radionuclide cystography** (RNC) are better than ultrasonography for detecting VUR and anatomic abnormalities and previously were recommended for most children after a first UTI. However, VCUG and RNC both involve use of radiation and are more uncomfortable than ultrasonography. Also, the role VUR plays in the development of chronic renal disease is undergoing re-evaluation, making the immediate diagnosis of VUR less urgent. Thus, VCUG is no longer routinely recommended after the first UTI in children, especially if ultrasonography is normal and if children respond quickly to antibiotic therapy. VCUG is reserved for children with the following:

- Ultrasonographic abnormalities (eg, scarring, significant hydronephrosis, evidence of obstructive uropathy or suggestion of VUR)
- Complex UTI (ie, persistent high fever, organism other than *E. coli*)
- Recurrent febrile UTIs

If VCUG is to be done, it is done at the earliest convenient time after clinical response, typically toward the end of therapy, when bladder reactivity has resolved and urine sterility has been regained. If imaging is not scheduled until after therapy is due to be completed, children should continue antibiotics at prophylactic doses until VUR is excluded.

Radionuclide scanning is now used mainly to detect evidence of renal scarring. It is done using technetium-99m-labeled dimercaptosuccinic acid (DMSA), which images the renal parenchyma. DMSA scanning is not a routine test, but it may be done if children have risk factors such as abnormal ultrasound results, high fever, and organisms other than *E. coli*.

Prognosis

Properly managed children rarely progress to renal failure unless they have uncorrectable urinary tract abnormalities. However, repeated infection, particularly in the presence of VUR, is thought (but not proved) to cause renal scarring, which may lead to hypertension and end-stage renal disease. In children with high-grade VUR, long-term scarring is detected at a 4- to 6-fold greater rate than in children with low-grade VUR and at an 8- to 10-fold greater rate than in children without VUR.

Treatment

- Antibiotics
- For severe VUR, sometimes antibiotic prophylaxis and surgical repair

Treatment of UTI aims to eliminate the acute infection, prevent urosepsis, and preserve renal parenchymal function. Antibiotics are begun presumptively in all toxic-appearing children and in nontoxic children with a probable UTI (positive leukocyte esterase or nitrite test, or microscopy showing pyuria). Others can await the results of the urine culture, which are important for both confirming the diagnosis of UTI and yielding antimicrobial susceptibility results.

In infants 2 mo to 2 yr with toxicity, dehydration, or inability to retain oral intake, parenteral antibiotics are used, typically a 3rd-generation cephalosporin (eg, ceftriaxone 75 mg/kg IV/IM q 24 h, cefotaxime 50 mg/kg IV q 6 or 8 h). A 1st-generation cephalosporin (eg, cefazolin) may be used if typical local pathogens are known to be sensitive. Aminoglycosides (eg, gentamicin), although potentially nephrotoxic, may be useful in complex UTIs (eg, urinary tract abnormalities, presence of indwelling catheters, recurrent UTIs) to treat potentially resistant gram-negative bacilli such as *Pseudomonas*.

If blood cultures are negative and clinical response is good, an appropriate oral antibiotic (eg, cefixime, cephalexin, trimethoprim/sulfamethoxazole [TMP/SMX], amoxicillin/clavulanic acid, or, for selected children such as those > 1 yr with complicated UTI caused by multidrug-resistant *E. coli, P. aeruginosa,* or other gram-negative bacteria, a fluoroquinolone) selected on the basis of antimicrobial sensitivities can be used to complete a 7- to 14-day course. A poor clinical response suggests a resistant organism or an obstructive lesion and warrants urgent evaluation with ultrasonography and repeat urine culture.

In nontoxic, nondehydrated infants and children who are able to retain oral intake, oral antibiotics may be given initially. The drug of choice is TMP/SMX 5 to 6 mg/kg (of TMP component) bid. Alternatives include cephalosporins such as cefixime 8 mg/kg once/day, cephalexin 25 mg/kg qid, or amoxicillin/clavulanic acid 15 mg/kg/dose tid. Therapy is changed based on the results of cultures and antimicrobial sensitivities. Treatment is typically for 7 to 14 days. Urine culture is repeated 2 to 3 days after therapy starts only if efficacy is not clinically apparent.

Vesicoureteral reflux: It has long been thought that antibiotic prophylaxis reduces UTI recurrences and prevents kidney damage and should be started after a first or second febrile UTI in children with VUR. However, this conclusion was not based on long-term, placebo-controlled trials (important because it has been observed that much VUR abates with time as children mature). A recent large, controlled trial, the Randomized Intervention for Children with Vesicoureteral Reflux (RIVUR) trial,[1] did show that antibiotic prophylaxis using TMP/SMX reduced UTI recurrences by 50% (from about 25% to 13%) compared to placebo but did not show a difference in the rate of renal scarring at 2 yr (8% in each group). Also, the children in the trial who did develop UTI while taking prophylactic antibiotics were 3 times as likely to be infected with resistant organisms. However, because the 2-yr follow-up period is likely too short to draw firm conclusions regarding prevention of renal scarring, additional study may show that antibiotic prophylaxis does provide some renal protection but at the risk of more antibiotic-resistant infections. Thus, the optimal strategy remains somewhat uncertain.

Nonetheless, for children with grade IV or grade V VUR, open repair or endoscopic injection of polymeric bulking agents is usually recommended, often along with antibiotic prophylaxis until repair is completed. For children with lesser grades of VUR, further research is required. Because renal complications are probably unlikely after only one or two UTIs, pending further research one acceptable strategy may be to closely monitor children for UTIs, treat them as they occur, and then reconsider antimicrobial prophylaxis in those children with recurrent infections.

Drugs commonly used for prophylaxis, if prophylaxis is desired, include nitrofurantoin 2 mg/kg po once/day or TMP/SMX 3 mg/kg po (of TMP component) once/day, usually given at bedtime.

1. The RIVUR Trial Investigators: Antimicrobial prophylaxis for children with vesicoureteral reflux. *NEJM* 370:2367–2376, 2014.

KEY POINTS

- UTIs in children are frequently associated with urinary tract abnormalities such as obstruction, neurogenic bladder, and ureteral duplication.
- The peak age of UTI is bimodal, one peak in infancy and the other peak usually at the time of toilet training for many children.
- *E. coli* causes most UTIs in all pediatric age groups; the remaining causes are usually gram-negative enterobacteria (eg, *Klebsiella, P. mirabilis, P. aeruginosa*); frequently implicated gram-positive organisms are group D streptococci and coagulase-negative staphylococci (eg, *S. saprophyticus*).
- Neonates and children < 2 yr with nonspecific symptoms and signs (eg, poor feeding, diarrhea, failure to thrive, vomiting) may have a UTI; children > 2 yr usually present with the symptoms and signs of cystitis or pyelonephritis.
- Antibiotics are initiated presumptively in all toxic-appearing children and in nontoxic children with evidence of positive leukocyte esterase or nitrite test, or microscopy showing pyuria.
- For children with high-grade VUR, antibiotic prophylaxis is given until surgical correction is done; with lesser grades of VUR, the benefit of prophylactic antibiotics is unclear and close monitoring for recurrent UTI may be an acceptable management strategy for individual children.

RHEUMATIC FEVER

Rheumatic fever is a nonsuppurative, acute inflammatory complication of group A streptococcal (GAS) pharyngeal infection, causing combinations of arthritis, carditis, subcutaneous nodules, erythema marginatum, and chorea. Diagnosis is based on applying the modified Jones criteria to information gleaned from history, examination, and laboratory testing. Treatment includes aspirin or other NSAIDs, corticosteroids during severe carditis, and antimicrobials to eradicate residual streptococcal infection and prevent reinfection.

A first episode of acute rheumatic fever (ARF) can occur at any age but occurs most often between 5 yr and 15 yr, which are the peak years of age for streptococcal pharyngitis. ARF is uncommon before 3 yr and after 21 yr. However, preceding symptomatic pharyngitis is recognized in only about two thirds of patients with ARF.

Worldwide, incidence is 19/100,000 (range, 5 to 51/100,000), with lowest rates (< 10/100,000) in North America and Western Europe and highest rates (> 10/100,000) in Eastern Europe, the Middle East, Asia, Africa, Australia, and New Zealand. The attack rate (percentage of patients with untreated GAS pharyngitis who develop ARF) varies from < 1.0 to 3.0%. Higher attack rates occur with certain streptococcal M protein serotypes and a stronger host immune response (likely resulting from as-yet-uncharacterized genetic tendencies).

In patients with a prior episode of ARF, the rate of recurrence of ARF in untreated group A streptococcal (GAS) pharyngitis approaches 50%, underscoring the importance of long-term antistreptococcal prophylaxis. Incidence has declined in most developed countries but remains high in less developed parts of the world, especially parts with aboriginal or native populations, such as Alaskan Native, Canadian Inuit, Native American, Australian Aboriginal, and Maori New Zealander, where incidence is as high as 50 to 250/100,000. However, the continued occurrence in the US of local outbreaks of ARF suggest that more rheumatogenic strains of streptococci are still present in the US.

The prevalence of chronic rheumatic heart disease is uncertain because criteria are not standardized and autopsy is not done routinely, but it is estimated that worldwide there are ≥ 15 million patients with rheumatic heart disease, resulting in about 200,000 deaths annually.

PEARLS & PITFALLS

- Patients who have had rheumatic fever have about a 50% likelihood of having a recurrence if they have another episode of GAS pharyngitis that is untreated.

Pathophysiology

GAS pharyngitis is the etiologic precursor of ARF, but host and environmental factors are important. GAS M proteins share epitopes (antigenic-determinant sites that are recognized by antibodies) with proteins found in synovium, heart muscle, and heart valve, suggesting that molecular mimicry by GAS antigens from rheumatogenic strains contributes to the arthritis, carditis, and valvular damage. Genetic host risk factors include the D8/17 B-cell antigen and certain class II histocompatibility antigens. Undernutrition, overcrowding, and lower socioeconomic status predispose to streptococcal infections and subsequent episodes of rheumatic fever.

Remarkably, although GAS infections of both the pharynx and of other areas of the body (skin and soft-tissue structures, bones or joints, lungs, and bloodstream) may cause poststreptococcal glomerulonephritis, nonpharyngitis GAS infections do not lead to ARF. The reason for this distinct difference in complications resulting from infection by the same organism is not well understood.

The joints, heart, skin, and CNS are most often affected. Pathology varies by site.

Joints: Joint involvement manifests as nonspecific synovial inflammation, which if biopsied sometimes shows small foci resembling Aschoff bodies (granulomatous collections of leukocytes, myocytes, and interstitial collagen). Unlike the cardiac findings, however, the abnormalities of the joints are not chronic and do not leave scarring or residual abnormalities ("ARF licks the joints but bites the heart").

Heart: Cardiac involvement manifests as carditis, typically affecting the heart from the inside out, ie, valves and endocardium, then myocardium, and finally pericardium. It is sometimes followed years to decades later by chronic rheumatic heart disease, primarily manifested by valvular stenosis, but also sometimes by regurgitation, arrhythmias, and ventricular dysfunction.

In **ARF,** Aschoff bodies often develop in the myocardium and other parts of the heart. Fibrinous nonspecific pericarditis, sometimes with effusion, occurs only in patients with endocardial inflammation and usually subsides without permanent damage. Characteristic and potentially dangerous valve changes may occur. Acute interstitial valvulitis may cause valvular edema.

In **chronic rheumatic heart disease,** valve thickening, fusion, and retraction or other destruction of leaflets and cusps may occur, leading to stenosis or insufficiency. Similarly, chordae tendineae can shorten, thicken, or fuse, worsening regurgitation of damaged valves or causing regurgitation of an otherwise unaffected valve. Dilation of valve rings may also cause regurgitation.

Rheumatic valvular disease most commonly involves the mitral and aortic valves. The tricuspid and pulmonic valves are seldom if ever affected in isolation.

In **ARF,** the most common cardiac manifestations are

- Mitral regurgitation
- Pericarditis
- Sometimes aortic regurgitation

In **chronic rheumatic heart disease,** the most common cardiac manifestations are

- Mitral stenosis
- Aortic regurgitation (often with some degree of stenosis)
- Perhaps tricuspid regurgitation (often along with mitral stenosis)

Skin: Subcutaneous nodules appear indistinguishable from those of juvenile idiopathic arthritis (JIA), but biopsy shows features resembling Aschoff bodies. Erythema marginatum differs histologically from other skin lesions with similar macroscopic appearance, eg, the rash of systemic JIA, Henoch-Schönlein purpura, erythema chronicum migrans, and erythema multiforme. Perivascular neutrophilic and mononuclear infiltrates of the dermis occur.

CNS: Sydenham chorea, the form of chorea that occurs with ARF, manifests in the CNS as hyperperfusion and increased metabolism in the basal ganglia. Increased levels of antineuronal antibodies have also been shown.

Symptoms and Signs

An initial episode of symptoms of rheumatic fever occurs typically about 2 to 3 wk after the streptococcal infection. Manifestations typically involve some combination of the joints, heart, skin, and CNS.[1]

Joints: Migratory polyarthritis is the most common manifestation of ARF, occurring in about 35 to 66% of children; it is often accompanied by fever. Migratory means the arthritis appears in one or a few joints, resolves but then appears in others, thus seeming to move from one joint to another. Occasionally monarthritis occurs in high-risk indigenous populations (eg, in Australia, India, Fiji) but very rarely in the US. Joints become extremely painful and tender; these symptoms are often out of proportion to the modest warmth and swelling present on examination (this is in contrast to the arthritis of Lyme disease, in which the examination findings tend to be more severe than the symptoms).

Ankles, knees, elbows, and wrists are usually involved. Shoulders, hips, and small joints of the hands and feet also may be involved, but almost never alone. If vertebral joints are affected, another disorder should be suspected.

Arthralgia-like symptoms may be due to nonspecific myalgia or tenodynia in the periarticular zone; tenosynovitis may develop at the site of muscle insertions. Joint pain and fever usually subside within 2 wk and seldom last > 1 mo.

Heart: Carditis can occur alone or in combination with pericardial rub, murmurs, cardiac enlargement, or heart failure. In the first episode of ARF, carditis occurs in about 50 to 70%. Patients may have high fever, chest pain, or both; tachycardia is common, especially during sleep. In about 50% of cases, cardiac damage (ie, persistent valve dysfunction) occurs much later.

Although the carditis of ARF is considered to be a pancarditis (involving the endocardium, myocardium, and pericardium), valvulitis is the most consistent feature of ARF, and if it is not present, the diagnosis should be reconsidered. The diagnosis of valvulitis has classically been made by auscultation of murmurs, but subclinical cases (ie, valvular dysfunction not manifested by murmurs but recognized on echocardiography and Doppler studies) may occur in up to 18% of cases of ARF.

Heart murmurs are common and, although usually evident early, may not be heard at initial examination; in such cases, repeated clinical examinations as well as echocardiography are recommended to determine the presence of carditis. Mitral regurgitation is characterized by an apical pansystolic blowing murmur radiating to the axilla. The soft diastolic blow at the left sternal border of aortic regurgitation, and the presystolic murmur of mitral stenosis, may be difficult to detect. Murmurs often persist indefinitely. If no worsening occurs during the next 2 to 3 wk, new manifestations of carditis seldom follow. ARF typically does not cause chronic, smoldering carditis. Scars left by acute valvular damage may contract and change, and secondary hemodynamic difficulties may develop in the myocardium without persistence of acute inflammation.

Pericarditis may be manifested by chest pain and a pericardial rub.

Heart failure caused by the combination of carditis and valvular dysfunction may cause dyspnea without rales, nausea and vomiting, a right upper quadrant or epigastric ache, and a hacking, nonproductive cough. Marked lethargy and fatigue may be early manifestations of heart failure.

Skin: Cutaneous and subcutaneous features are uncommon and almost never occur alone, usually developing in a patient who already has carditis, arthritis, or chorea.

Subcutaneous nodules, which occur most frequently on the extensor surfaces of large joints (eg, knees, elbows, wrists), usually coexist with arthritis and carditis. Fewer than 10% of children with ARF have nodules. Ordinarily, the nodules are painless and transitory and respond to treatment of joint or heart inflammation.

Erythema marginatum is a serpiginous, flat or slightly raised, nonscarring, and painless rash. Fewer than 6% of children have this rash. The rash usually appears on the trunk and proximal extremities but not the face. It sometimes lasts < 1 day. Its appearance is often delayed after the inciting streptococcal infection; it may appear with or after the other manifestations of rheumatic inflammation.

CNS: Sydenham chorea occurs in about 10 to 30% of children. It may develop along with other manifestations but frequently arises after the other manifestations have subsided (often months after the acute streptococcal infection) and thus may be overlooked as an indicator of ARF. Onset of chorea is typically insidious and may be preceded by inappropriate laughing or crying. Chorea consists of rapid and irregular jerking movements that may begin in the hands but often becomes generalized, involving the feet and face.

Characteristic findings include fluctuating grip strength (milkmaid's grip), tongue fasciculations or tongue darting (the tongue cannot protrude without darting in and out), facial grimacing, and explosive speech with or without tongue clucking. Associated motor symptoms include loss of fine motor control, and weakness and hypotonia (that can be severe enough to be mistaken for paralysis).

Previously undiagnosed obsessive-compulsive behavior may be unmasked in many patients.

Other: Fever (≥ 38.5° C) and other systemic manifestations such as anorexia and malaise can be prominent but are not specific. ARF can occasionally manifest as FUO until a more identifiable sign develops. Abdominal pain and anorexia can occur because of the hepatic involvement in heart failure or because of concomitant mesenteric adenitis, and rarely the situation may resemble acute appendicitis.

Recurrence: Recurrent episodes of ARF often mimic the initial episode; carditis tends to recur in patients who have had moderate to severe carditis in the past, and chorea without carditis recurs in patients who had chorea without carditis initially.

1. Gewitz MH, Baltimore RS, Tani LY, et al: Revision of Jones criteria for the diagnosis of ARF in the era of Doppler echocardiography: A scientific statement from the American Heart Association. *Circulation* 131: 1806–18, 2015.

Diagnosis

- Modified Jones criteria (for initial diagnosis)
- Testing for GAS (culture, rapid strep test, or antistreptolysin O and anti-DNase B titers)
- ECG
- Echocardiography with Doppler
- ESR and CRP level

Diagnosis of a first episode of ARF is based on the modified Jones criteria (see Table 321–4);[1] 2 major criteria or 1 major and 2 minor criteria are required, each along with evidence of preceding GAS infection. Sydenham chorea alone (ie, without minor criteria) fulfills diagnostic criteria if other causes of movement disorder are ruled out.

The modified Jones criteria were designed for the evaluation of ARF rather than for a possible recurrence. However, if patients have a reliable past history of ARF or rheumatic heart disease and also have documented GAS infection, the criteria may be used to establish the presence of a recurrence.

Table 321–4. MODIFIED JONES CRITERIA FOR A FIRST EPISODE OF ACUTE RHEUMATIC FEVER*

MANIFESTATIONS	SPECIFIC FINDING
Major	Carditis[†] Chorea Erythema marginatum Polyarthritis Subcutaneous nodules
Minor	Polyarthralgia[‡] Elevated ESR (> 60 mm/h) or CRP (> 30 mg/L) Fever (≥ 38.5° C) Prolonged PR interval (on ECG)[§]

*Diagnosis of ARF requires 2 major or 1 major and 2 minor manifestations and evidence of group A streptococcal infection (elevated or rising antistreptococcal antibody titer [eg, antistreptolysin O, anti-DNase B], positive throat culture, or positive rapid antigen test in a child with clinical manifestations suggestive of streptococcal pharyngitis).

[†]Carditis can be clinical and/or subclinical. Subclinical carditis is defined by strict echocardiographic criteria.

[‡]Polyarthralgia is not used for diagnosis if polyarthritis is a major criterion for the patient.

[§]PR interval is adjusted for age and is not used for diagnosis if carditis is a major criterion for the patient.

Adapted from Gewitz MH, Baltimore RS, Tani LY, et al: Revision of Jones criteria for the diagnosis of acute rheumatic fever in the era of Doppler echocardiography: A scientific statement from the American Heart Association. *Circulation* 131:1806 1818, 2015.

A **preceding streptococcal infection** is suggested by a recent history of pharyngitis and is confirmed by one or more of the following:

- Positive throat culture
- Increased or preferably rising antistreptolysin O titer
- Positive rapid GAS antigen test in a child with clinical manifestations suggestive of streptococcal pharyngitis

Recent scarlet fever is highly suggestive. Throat cultures and rapid strep antigen tests are often negative by the time ARF manifests, whereas titers of antistreptolysin O and anti-DNase B typically peak 3 to 6 wk after GAS pharyngitis. About 80% of children with ARF have a significantly elevated antistreptolysin O titer; if an anti-DNase B antibody level is also done, the percentage with confirmed GAS infection is higher, especially if acute and convalescent samples are tested.

Joint aspiration may be needed to exclude other causes of arthritis (eg, infection). The joint fluid is usually cloudy and yellow, with an elevated WBC count composed primarily of neutrophils; culture is negative. Complement levels are usually normal or slightly decreased, compared with decreased levels in other inflammatory arthritides.

ECG is done during the initial evaluation. Serum cardiac marker levels are obtained; normal cardiac troponin I levels exclude prominent myocardial damage. ECG abnormalities such as PR prolongation do not correlate with other evidence of carditis. Only 35% of children with ARF have a prolonged PR interval; higher-degree heart block may occur but is uncommon. Other ECG abnormalities may be due to pericarditis, enlargement of ventricles or atria, or arrhythmias.

Echocardiography can detect evidence of carditis even in patients without apparent murmurs and is recommended for all patients with confirmed or suspected ARF. Echocardiography is also used to detect subclinical carditis in patients with apparently isolated Sydenham chorea and to monitor the status of patients with recurrences of carditis or chronic rheumatic heart disease. However, not all echocardiographic abnormalities represent rheumatic carditis; isolated trivial valvar regurgitation or trivial pericardial effusion may be a nonspecific finding. To maintain specificity, echocardiographic and Doppler results should meet the following criteria[1] for acute rheumatic carditis:

Doppler flow criteria:

- Pathologic mitral regurgitation: Must be seen in at least 2 views, and have a jet length ≥ 2 cm in at least 1 view, a peak velocity of > 3 m/sec, and a pansystolic jet in at least 1 envelope
- Pathologic aortic regurgitation: Must be seen in at least 2 views, and have a jet length ≥ 1 cm in at least 1 view, a peak velocity of > 3 m/sec, and a pandiastolic jet in at least 1 envelope

Echocardiographic morphologic criteria:

- Pathologic mitral valve morphologic changes include annular dilation, chordal elongation or rupture with flail leaflet, anterior (or less commonly posterior) leaflet tip prolapse, or beading/nodularity of leaflet tips.
- Pathologic aortic valve morphologic changes include irregular or focal leaflet thickening, coaptation defect, restricted leaflet motion, or leaflet prolapse.

Chest x-rays are not routinely done but can detect cardiomegaly, a common manifestation of carditis in ARF.

Biopsy of a subcutaneous nodule can aid in early diagnosis, especially when other major clinical manifestations are absent.

ESR and serum CRP are sensitive but not specific. The ESR is typically > 60 mm/h. CRP is typically > 30 mg/L and often > 70 mg/L; because it rises and falls faster than ESR, a normal CRP may confirm that inflammation is resolving in a patient with prolonged ESR elevation after acute symptoms have subsided. In the absence of carditis, ESR usually returns to normal within 3 mo. Evidence of acute inflammation, including ESR, usually subsides within 5 mo in uncomplicated carditis. The WBC count reaches 12,000 to 20,000/μL and may go higher with corticosteroid therapy.

The differential diagnosis includes JIA (especially systemic JIA and, less so, polyarticular JIA), Lyme disease, reactive arthritis, arthropathy of sickle cell disease, leukemia or other cancer, SLE, embolic bacterial endocarditis, serum sickness, Kawasaki disease, drug reactions, and gonococcal arthritis. These are frequently distinguished by history or specific laboratory tests. The absence of an antecedent GAS infection, the diurnal variation of the fever, evanescent rash, and prolonged symptomatic joint inflammation usually distinguish systemic JIA from ARF.

1. Gewitz MH, Baltimore RS, Tani LY, et al: Revision of Jones criteria for the diagnosis of ARF in the era of Doppler echocardiography: A scientific statement from the American Heart Association. *Circulation* 131: 1806–1818, 2015.

Prognosis

Prognosis following an initial episode of ARF depends mostly on how severely the heart is affected, and whether there is a recurrent episode of ARF. Murmurs eventually disappear in about half of patients whose acute episodes were manifested by mild carditis without major cardiac enlargement or decompensation. However, many others develop chronic valvular disease, including some who recovered from the acute episode without evidence of valvular disease.

Episodes of Sydenham chorea usually last several months and resolve completely in most patients, but about one third of patients have recurrences.

Joint inflammation may take 1 mo to subside if not treated but does not lead to residual damage.

In patients with chronic valvular disease, symptoms develop and progress slowly, typically over several decades. However, once significant symptoms develop, intervention is usually necessary. In developing countries, chronic rheumatic heart disease is the cause of 25 to 45% of all cardiovascular disease.

Treatment

- Antibiotics
- Aspirin
- Sometimes corticosteroids

The primary goals of rheumatic fever treatment are eradication of GAS infection, relief of acute symptoms, suppression of inflammation, and prophylaxis against future infection to prevent recurrent heart disease.

For general management, patients should limit their activities if they have symptoms of arthritis, chorea, or heart failure. In the absence of carditis, no physical restrictions are needed after the initial episode subsides. In asymptomatic patients with carditis, strict bed rest has no proven value, despite its traditional usage.

The management of chronic cardiac valvular disease and heart failure is discussed elsewhere in The Manual.

Antibiotic treatment: Although poststreptococcal inflammation is well developed by the time ARF is detected, a 10-day course of oral penicillin or amoxicillin, or a single injection of benzathine penicillin, is used to eradicate any lingering organisms and prevent reinfection. For specific regimens, see treatment of streptococcal pharyngitis. Antibiotic prophylaxis is continued as described below.

Aspirin and other anti-inflammatory drugs: Aspirin controls fever and pain and should be given to all patients with arthritis and/or mild carditis. Although aspirin has been used for many decades, there are surprisingly few data from controlled trials to define the optimal dosing schedule. Most experts would give children and adolescents 15 to 25 mg/kg po qid (to a maximum daily dose of 4 to 6 g) for 2 to 4 wk and then taper the dose over another 4 wk. Symptomatic ARF responds dramatically to aspirin. If no improvement is seen after 24 to 48 h of high-dose aspirin therapy, the diagnosis of ARF should be reconsidered. Salicylate toxicity is the limiting factor to aspirin therapy and is manifested by tinnitus, headache, or hyperpnea; it may not appear until after 1 wk of therapy. Salicylate levels are measured only to manage toxicity. Enteric-coated, buffered, or complex salicylate molecules provide no advantage.

For patients with minimal to mild carditis, there are no controlled data to suggest that adding prednisone to aspirin therapy speeds resolution of illness or prevents rheumatic heart disease.

Other NSAIDs have been reported in small trials to be effective; naproxen (7.5 to 10 mg/kg po bid) is the most studied. However, other NSAIDs have few advantages over aspirin, especially in the first week of therapy when salicylism is uncommon. Acetaminophen is not effective for symptoms of ARF.

Prednisone 1 mg/kg po bid (up to 60 mg/day) is recommended instead of aspirin for patients with moderate to severe carditis (as judged by a combination of clinical findings, presence of cardiac enlargement, and possibly by severely abnormal echocardiography results). If inflammation is not suppressed after 2 days or for severe heart failure, an IV corticosteroid pulse of methylprednisolone succinate (30 mg/kg IV once/day, maximum 1 g/day, for 3 successive days) may be given. Oral corticosteroids typically are given for 2 to 4 wk and then tapered over another 2 to 3 wk. Aspirin should be started during the corticosteroid taper and continued for 2 to 4 wk after the corticosteroid has been stopped. Aspirin dose is the same as above. Inflammatory markers such as ESR and CRP may be used to monitor disease activity and response to treatment.

Recurrences of mild cardiac inflammation (indicated by fever or chest pain) may subside spontaneously; aspirin or corticosteroids should be resumed if recurrent symptoms last longer than a few days or if heart failure is uncontrolled by standard management (eg, diuretics, ACE inhibitors, β-blockers, inotropic agents).

Antibiotic prophylaxis: Antistreptococcal prophylaxis should be maintained continuously after the initial episode of ARF to prevent recurrences (see Table 321–5). Antibiotics taken orally are slightly less effective as those given by injection. However, with the oral route, painful injections are avoided, and clinic visits and observation for postinjection reactions are not needed.

The optimal duration of antistreptococcal prophylaxis is uncertain. Children without carditis should receive prophylaxis for 5 yr or until age 21 (whichever is longer). The American Academy of Pediatrics recommends that patients with carditis without evidence of residual heart damage receive prophylaxis for 10 yr or until age 21 (whichever is longer). Children with carditis and evidence of residual heart damage should receive prophylaxis for > 10 yr; many experts recommend that such patients continue prophylaxis indefinitely or, alternatively, until age 40. Prophylaxis should be life long in all patients with severe valvular disease who have close contact with young children because young children have a high rate of GAS carriage.

The American Heart Association no longer recommends that patients with known or suspected rheumatic valvular disease

Table 321–5. RECOMMENDED PROPHYLAXIS AGAINST RECURRENT GROUP A STREPTOCOCCAL INFECTION

REGIMEN	DRUG	DOSE
Standard	Penicillin G benzathine	1.2 million units IM q 3–4 wk* ≤ 27 kg: 600,000 units IM q 3–4 wk*
Alternatives (eg, for patients unwilling to receive injections)	Penicillin V *or* Sulfadiazine *or* Sulfisoxazole	250 mg po bid ≤ 27 kg: 500 mg po once/day > 27 kg: 1 g po once/day
For patients allergic to penicillin and sulfa drugs	Erythromycin *or* Azithromycin	250 mg po bid 250 mg po once/day

*In less developed parts of the world with high ARF endemicity, IM prophylaxis q 3 wk is superior to q 4 wk.

(*who are not currently taking prophylactic antibiotics*) take short-term antibiotic prophylaxis against bacterial endocarditis for dental or oral surgical procedures (see p. 711).

KEY POINTS

- Rheumatic fever is a nonsuppurative, acute, inflammatory complication of GAS pharyngeal infection occurring most often initially between age 5 yr and 15 yr.
- Symptoms and signs may include migratory polyarthritis, carditis, subcutaneous nodules, erythema marginatum, and chorea.
- Chronic rheumatic heart disease, particularly involving the mitral and/or aortic valves, may progress over decades and is a major cause of heart disease in the developing world.
- Diagnosis of ARF requires 2 major or 1 major and 2 minor manifestations (modified Jones criteria for a first episode of ARF) and evidence of GAS infection.
- Give antibiotics to eliminate GAS infection, aspirin to control fever and pain caused by arthritis and mild carditis, and corticosteroids for patients with moderate to severe carditis.
- Give prophylactic antistreptococcal antibiotics after the initial episode of ARF to prevent recurrences.

Poststreptococcal Reactive Arthritis

Poststreptococcal reactive arthritis is development of arthritis after group A streptococcal infection in patients who do not meet the criteria for ARF.

Poststreptococcal reactive arthritis may or may not represent an attenuated variant of ARF. Patients do not have symptoms or signs of the carditis common in ARF.

Compared with the arthritis of ARF, poststreptococcal reactive arthritis typically involves only 1 or 2 joints, is less migratory but more protracted, and does not respond as well or as quickly to aspirin. Other, nonrheumatic disorders causing similar symptoms (eg, Lyme arthritis, JIA) should be excluded.

It can be treated with other NSAIDs (eg, ibuprofen, naproxen).

Although clinical practice for secondary prevention of cardiac involvement varies greatly, it is reasonable to give antistreptococcal prophylaxis for several months to 1 yr and then to reevaluate the patient. If cardiac lesions are detected by echocardiography, long-term prophylaxis is indicated.

322 Miscellaneous Disorders in Infants and Children

APPARENT LIFE-THREATENING EVENT AND BRIEF, RESOLVED, UNEXPLAINED EVENT

Apparent life-threatening event (ALTE) and brief, resolved, unexplained event (BRUE) are not specific disorders but terms for a group of alarming symptoms that can occur in infants. They involve the sudden appearance of respiratory symptoms (eg, apnea), change in color or muscle tone, and/or altered responsiveness. The caregiver may fear that the child is dead or that his or her life is in jeopardy. Events typically occur in children < 1 yr with peak incidence at 10 to 12 wk. Some of these events are unexplained (and designated BRUEs), but others result from numerous possible causes including digestive, neurologic, respiratory, infectious, cardiac, metabolic, or traumatic (eg, resulting from abuse) disorders. Treatment is aimed at specific causes when identified.

Some infants have transient events involving some combination of altered respiration, consciousness, muscle tone, and/or skin color that are alarming for caregivers—some of whom even begin doing cardiopulmonary resuscitation (CPR). Because of their concerning manifestations, these events have been referred to as an "apparent life-threatening event." However, although a small minority of these infants are found to have a significant underlying disorder, a large number have neither recurrences nor complications and go on to develop normally. Thus, a recent clinical practice guideline from the American Academy of Pediatrics recommended eliminating the term "life-threatening" so that parents are not unnecessarily alarmed and clinicians do not feel compelled to do extensive testing, which is unnecessary in many cases. The new term is "brief, resolved, unexplained event."

BRUE refers to events lasting < 1 min in an infant < 1 yr of age that are associated with ≥ 1 of the following:

- Absent, decreased, or irregular breathing
- Cyanosis or pallor
- Altered level of responsiveness
- Marked change in muscle tone (hypertonia or hypotonia)

In addition, infants must otherwise appear well and be back at their baseline state of health at the time of presentation. Thus, infants who are febrile, coughing, or showing any signs of distress or other abnormalities are not considered to have a possible BRUE.

It must be noted that the term BRUE applies only to events for which there is no underlying cause (hence "unexplained"), which can be determined only after a thorough history and physical examination and sometimes testing. Also, BRUE does not apply to infants with a similar presentation in whom a cause *was* identified; for these infants, some clinicians still consider the term ALTE useful.

Etiology

Although by definition BRUE is diagnosed only when there is no explanation for the event, a number of disorders can manifest with similar abnormalities of breathing, responsiveness, tone, and/or skin color. Thus, it is important to search for a cause.

The **most common causes** include

- Digestive: Gastroesophageal reflux disease or swallowing difficulty when associated with laryngospasm or aspiration
- Neurologic: Neurologic disorders (eg, seizures, brain tumors, breath holding or abnormal brain stem neuroregulation

of cardiorespiratory control, hydrocephalus, brain malformations)
- Respiratory: Infections (eg, respiratory syncytial virus, influenza, pertussis)
- Infectious: Sepsis, meningitis

Less common causes include

- Cardiac disorders
- Metabolic disorders
- Upper airway obstruction (eg, obstructive sleep apnea)
- Other (eg, drug-related, anaphylaxis, abuse)

Causes may be genetic or acquired. If an infant is under the care of one person and has repeated episodes with no clear etiology, child abuse should be considered.

Evaluation

Evaluation of infants with any other manifestations (eg, cough, fever, nausea and vomiting, seizures) besides those defined as BRUE is described elsewhere.

History: Evaluation of an event initially involves a thorough history, including

- Observations by the caregiver who witnessed the event, particularly a description of changes in breathing, color, muscle tone, and eyes; noises made; length of episode; and any preceding signs such as respiratory distress or hypotonia
- Interventions taken (eg, gentle stimulation, mouth-to-mouth breathing, CPR)
- Prenatal (maternal) and current family use of drugs, tobacco, and alcohol
- Information about the infant's birth (eg, gestational age, perinatal complications)
- Feeding habits (whether gagging, coughing, vomiting, or poor weight gain has occurred)
- Growth and development history (eg, length and weight percentiles, developmental milestones)
- Prior events, including recent illness or trauma
- Recent exposure to infectious illness
- Family history of similar events, early deaths, long QT syndrome or other arrhythmias, or possible causative disorders

Features in the history suggestive of child abuse should be sensitively assessed. Recurrent events that are concerning for abuse include those that begin only in the presence of a parent or caretaker.

Because disposition depends in part on family capabilities and resources, it is also important to assess the housing and family situation, the level of caregiver anxiety, and whether the infant has ready access to follow-up medical care.

Physical examination: Physical examination is done to check for abnormal vital signs, respiratory signs, obvious malformations and deformities, neurologic abnormalities (eg, posturing, inappropriate head lag), signs of infection or trauma (particularly including retinal hemorrhage on funduscopy), and indicators of possible physical abuse.

Risk classification: Possible BRUEs are classified as low or high risk based on history and physical examination.

Low-risk infants are those who meet the following criteria:

- Age > 60 days
- Gestational age > 32 wk and post-conceptual age > 45 wk
- One event only, no prior BRUE, no cluster of BRUEs
- No CPR required by trained medical provider
- No features of concern in history (eg, concern for child abuse, family history of sudden death)
- Normal physical examination (eg, afebrile, normotensive)

Low-risk infants are very unlikely to have a serious underlying disorder, and the new guidelines recommend few or no interventions other than caregiver education.

High-risk infants include all those who do not meet low-risk criteria. The new guidelines do not contain recommendations for their evaluation and management.

Testing: For **low-risk infants,** current guidelines recommend minimal testing. It is reasonable to observe the infant (including monitoring pulse oximetry) in the emergency department or office for a brief period and do 12-lead ECG and testing nasopharyngeal swab for pertussis (culture or PCR). Other tests, including imaging studies and blood tests, are not necessary. Routine hospital admission also is not necessary; however, infants may be hospitalized for cardiorespiratory monitoring if caregivers are extremely anxious or are unable to bring the infant for follow-up in 24 h.

For **high-risk infants,** laboratory and imaging tests are done to check for possible causes. Some tests are done routinely and others should be done based on clinical suspicion (see Table 322–1), including whether the infant is still symptomatic or has required medical intervention. Infants are often hospitalized for cardiorespiratory monitoring, particularly if they required resuscitation or if evaluation detected any abnormalities.

Prognosis

Most often, BRUE is harmless and not a sign of more serious health problems or death. BRUE is unlikely to be a risk factor for sudden infant death syndrome (SIDS). Most victims of SIDS do not have any types of events beforehand.

Prognosis of a high-risk event depends on the cause. For example, risk of death is higher if the cause is a serious neurologic disorder. When no cause is identified, the relationship of such events to SIDS is unclear. About 4 to 10% of infants who die of SIDS have a history of such events, and the risk of SIDS is higher if an infant has had 2 or more. Also, infants who have had an event share many of the same characteristics with infants who die of SIDS. However, incidence of ALTE, unlike that of SIDS, has not decreased in response to the Safe to Sleep® campaign.

There seem to be no long-term effects on development from the ALTE itself, but the causative disorder (eg, cardiac or neurologic) may have such effects.

Treatment

- Treatment of cause
- Sometimes home monitoring devices
- Close follow-up

Low-risk infants: Parents and caregivers should be educated about BRUEs and offered training in CPR for infants and in safe infant care. Home cardiorespiratory monitoring is not necessary. Infants should be reevaluated within 24 h.

High-risk infants: The cause, if identified, is treated.

If parents and caregivers are interested and seem capable of using them, they may be prescribed apnea monitoring devices to use at home for a specified period of time. Monitors should be equipped with event recorders. Parents should be taught how to use the monitor and be advised that false alarms are common and that home monitoring has not been shown to reduce the mortality rate. Also, exposure to tobacco smoke must be eliminated.

Infants who were not hospitalized should receive follow-up with their primary care physician within 24 h.

Table 322–1. DIAGNOSTIC TESTS FOR HIGH-RISK INFANTS

TESTS	POSSIBLE CAUSES
Typical initial testing	
Blood tests, typically including • CBC and differential • Electrolytes (magnesium, calcium, sodium, potassium), bicarbonate, and glucose • Liver function tests • Lactate	Acidosis Anemia Dehydration Infection Liver disorders Metabolic disorders
Chest x-ray	Cardiomegaly, pneumonia
Cultures (blood, stool, urine, CSF)	Infection
ECG Cardiac monitoring in hospital	Arrhythmias QT abnormalities
Echocardiography	Cardiomegaly
Lumbar puncture	Meningitis
Pertussis testing	Pertussis
Skeletal survey	Fractures
Toxicology screen	Drugs or toxins
Urinalysis	Infection
Additional tests based on clinical suspicion	
ABGs	Acidosis
Brain imaging (head CT, MRI)	Trauma, hemorrhage, tumor
EEG	Seizures
Esophageal pH monitoring*	Gastroesophageal reflux disease
Genetic testing	Possible genetic/metabolic disorder
Nasal swab	Respiratory syncytial virus infection
Sleep study	Breathing or other problems during sleep
Upper GI with radioisotope milk scanning*	Gastroesophageal reflux disease

*In infants with a history of spitting up, gagging, vomiting, coughing, or difficulty feeding.

KEY POINTS

- Some infants have transient, alarming events involving alterations of respiration, consciousness, muscle tone, and/or skin color.
- Events can be divided into low-risk and high-risk based on history and physical examination.
- Events meeting low-risk criteria are unlikely to have a dangerous cause and require minimal assessment.
- BRUE is present only when there is no explanation for the event after a thorough history and examination.
- High-risk events have many possible causes, but often no etiology is found.
- Respiratory, neurologic, infectious, cardiac, metabolic, and GI disorders as well as abuse should be considered, with testing done based on clinical findings.
- Prognosis depends on cause; risk of death is increased in children with a neurologic disorder, who have had 2 or more events, who have experienced nonaccidental trauma, or who are > 6 mo and have had an event of longer duration, especially if they have heart disease.
- Children with abnormal examination findings or laboratory results or who required intervention or had a worrisome history are hospitalized.
- Treatment is directed at the cause; home monitoring may be done but has not been shown to decrease mortality.

FAILURE TO THRIVE

Failure to thrive (FTT) is weight consistently below the 3rd to 5th percentile for age and sex, progressive decrease in weight to below the 3rd to 5th percentile, or a decrease in the percentile rank of 2 major growth parameters in a short period. The cause may be an identified medical condition or may be related to environmental factors. Both types relate to inadequate nutrition. Treatment aims to restore proper nutrition.

Etiology

The physiologic basis for FTT of any etiology is inadequate nutrition and is divided into

- Organic FTT
- Nonorganic FTT
- Mixed FTT

Most cases of FTT are multifactorial.

Organic FTT: Growth failure is due to an acute or chronic disorder that interferes with nutrient intake, absorption, metabolism, or excretion or that increases energy requirements (see Table 322–2). Illness of any organ system can be a cause.

Nonorganic FTT: Up to 80% of children with growth failure do not have an apparent growth-inhibiting (organic) disorder; growth failure occurs because of environmental neglect (eg, lack of food), stimulus deprivation, or both.

Lack of food may be due to

- Impoverishment
- Poor understanding of feeding techniques
- Improperly prepared formula (eg, overdiluting formula to stretch it because of financial difficulties)
- Inadequate supply of breast milk (eg, because the mother is under stress, exhausted, or poorly nourished)

Nonorganic FTT is often a complex of disordered interaction between a child and caregiver. In some cases, the psychologic basis of nonorganic FTT seems similar to that of hospitalism, a syndrome observed in infants who have depression secondary to stimulus deprivation. The unstimulated child becomes depressed, apathetic, and ultimately anorexic. Stimulation may be lacking because the caregiver

- Is depressed or apathetic
- Has poor parenting skills
- Is anxious about or unfulfilled by the caregiver role
- Feels hostile toward the child
- Is responding to real or perceived external stresses (eg, demands of other children in large or chaotic families, marital dysfunction, a significant loss, financial difficulties)

Table 322–2. SOME CAUSES OF ORGANIC FAILURE TO THRIVE

MECHANISM	DISORDER
Decreased nutrient intake	Cleft lip or palate CNS disorder (eg, cerebral palsy) Gastroesophageal reflux disease Parasites Pyloric stenosis Rumination
Malabsorption	Celiac disease Cystic fibrosis Disaccharidase (eg, lactase) deficiency Inflammatory bowel disease Short gut
Impaired metabolism	Chromosomal abnormality (eg, Down syndrome, Turner syndrome) Fructose intolerance Galactose-1-phosphate uridyl transferase deficiency (classic galactosemia) Inborn errors of metabolism
Increased excretion	Diabetes mellitus Proteinuria
Increased energy requirements	Bronchopulmonary dysplasia Cystic fibrosis Heart failure Hyperthyroidism Infection

Poor caregiving does not fully account for all cases of nonorganic FTT. The child's temperament, capacities, and responses help shape caregiver nurturance patterns. Common scenarios involve parent-child mismatches, in which the child's demands, although not pathologic, cannot be adequately met by the parents, who might, however, do well with a child who has different needs or even with the same child under different circumstances.

Mixed FTT: In mixed FTT, organic and nonorganic causes can overlap; children with organic disorders also have disturbed environments or dysfunctional parental interactions. Likewise, children with severe undernutrition caused by nonorganic FTT can develop organic medical problems.

Diagnosis

- Frequent weight monitoring
- Thorough medical, family, and social history
- Diet history
- Laboratory testing

Children with organic FTT may present at any age depending on the underlying disorder. Most children with nonorganic FTT manifest growth failure before age 1 yr and many by age 6 mo. Age should be plotted against weight, height, and head size on growth standards and growth charts, such as those recommended by the WHO and the CDC. (For children 0 to 2 yr, see WHO Growth Charts; for children 2 yr and older, see CDC Growth Charts.) Until premature infants reach 2 yr, age should be corrected for gestation.

Weight is the most sensitive indicator of nutritional status. When FTT is due to inadequate caloric intake, weight falls from the baseline percentile before length does. Reduced linear growth usually indicates severe, prolonged undernutrition. Simultaneous fall off of length and weight suggests a primary disorder of growth or a prolonged inflammatory state. Because the brain is preferentially spared in protein-energy undernutrition, reduced growth in head circumference occurs late and indicates very severe or long-standing undernutrition. Children who are underweight may be smaller and shorter than their peers and may present with fussiness or crying, lethargy or sleepiness, and constipation. FTT is associated with physical delays (eg, sitting, walking), social delays (eg, interacting, learning), and, if occurring in older children, delayed puberty.

Usually, when growth failure is noted, a history (including diet history—see Table 322–3) is obtained, diet counseling is provided, and the child's weight is monitored frequently. A child who does not gain weight satisfactorily in spite of outpatient assessment and intervention usually is admitted to the hospital so that all necessary observations can be made and diagnostic tests can be done quickly.

Without historic or physical evidence of a specific underlying etiology for growth failure, no single clinical feature or test can reliably distinguish organic from nonorganic FTT. Because children may have both organic and nonorganic FTT, the physician should search simultaneously for an underlying physical problem and for personal, family, and child-family characteristics that support a psychosocial etiology. Optimally, evaluation is multidisciplinary, involving a physician, a nurse, a social worker, a nutritionist, an expert in child development, and often a psychiatrist or psychologist. The child's feeding behaviors with health care practitioners and with the parents must be observed, whether the setting is inpatient or outpatient.

Engaging the parents as co-investigators is essential. It helps foster their self-esteem and avoids blaming parents who may already feel frustrated or guilty because of a perceived inability to nurture their child. The family should be encouraged to visit as often and as long as possible. Staff members should make them feel welcome, support their attempts to feed the child, and provide toys and ideas that promote parent-child play and other interactions.

Parental adequacy and sense of responsibility should be evaluated. Suspected neglect or abuse must be reported to social services, but in many instances, referral for preventive services that are targeted to meet the family's needs for support and education (eg, additional food stamps, more accessible child care, parenting classes) is more appropriate.

During hospitalization, the child's interaction with people in the environment is closely observed, and evidence of self-stimulatory behaviors (eg, rocking, head banging) is noted. Some children with nonorganic FTT have been described as hypervigilant and wary of close contact with people, preferring interactions with inanimate objects if they interact at all. Although nonorganic FTT is more consistent with neglectful than abusive parenting, the child should be examined closely for evidence of abuse. A screening test of developmental level should be done and, if indicated, followed with more sophisticated assessment. Hospitalized children who begin gaining weight well with proper feeding techniques, formula preparation, and amount of calories are more likely to have nonorganic FTT.

Testing: Extensive laboratory testing is usually nonproductive. If a thorough history or physical examination does not indicate a particular cause, most experts recommend limiting screening tests to

- CBC with differential
- ESR
- BUN and serum creatinine and electrolyte levels
- Urinalysis (including ability to concentrate and acidify) and culture
- Stool for pH, reducing substances, odor, color, consistency, and fat content

Table 322–3. ESSENTIALS OF THE HISTORY FOR FAILURE TO THRIVE

ITEM	COMMENTS
Growth chart	Measurements, including those taken at birth if possible, should be examined to determine the trend in growth rate. Because of wide normal variations, diagnosis of FTT should not be based on a single measurement, except when undernutrition is obvious.
Diet history (3 days)	Diet history should be detailed, including feeding schedule and techniques for the preparation and feeding of formula or adequacy of breast milk supply. As soon as possible, parents should be observed feeding the infant to evaluate their technique and the infant's vigor of sucking. An infant who tires easily during feeding may have underlying cardiac or pulmonary disease. Enthusiastic burping or rapid rocking of the infant during feeding may result in excessive regurgitation or even vomiting. A disinterested parent may be depressed or apathetic, suggesting a psychosocial environment that is lacking stimulation for and interaction with the infant.
Assessment of the child's elimination pattern	Abnormalities of urine or stool and frequent emesis should trigger an investigation to detect underlying renal disease, malabsorption syndrome, pyloric stenosis, or gastroesophageal reflux.
Medical history and birth history	Of concern is any evidence of intrauterine growth restriction or prematurity with growth delay that has not been compensated; developmental delay; unusual, prolonged, or chronic infections (eg, TB, parasitic, HIV); neurologic, cardiac, pulmonary, or renal disease; illness or hospitalization; and possible food intolerance.
Family history	Included is information about familial growth patterns, especially in parents and siblings; the occurrence of diseases known to affect growth (eg, cystic fibrosis); and a parent's recent physical or psychiatric illness resulting in inability to provide consistent stimulation and nurturance.
Social history	Attention is focused on family composition, socioeconomic status, desire for pregnancy with and acceptance of the child, and stresses (eg, job changes, family moves, separation, divorce, deaths, other losses).

Depending on prevalence of specific disorders in the community, blood lead level, HIV, or TB testing may be warranted.

Other tests that are sometimes appropriate include a thyroxine (T_4) level if growth in height is more severely affected than growth in weight or when height and weight fall off simultaneously (in which case growth hormone deficiency should also be suspected) and a sweat test for cystic fibrosis if the child has a history of recurrent upper or lower respiratory tract disease, a salty taste when kissed, a ravenous appetite, foul-smelling bulky stools, hepatomegaly, or a family history of cystic fibrosis. Newborn screening test results should be reviewed for indications of genetic diseases.

Investigation for infectious diseases should be reserved for children with evidence of infection (eg, fever, vomiting, cough, diarrhea); however, a urine culture may be helpful because some children with FTT due to UTI lack other symptoms and signs.

Radiologic investigation should be reserved for children with evidence of anatomic or functional pathology (eg, pyloric stenosis, gastroesophageal reflux). However, if an endocrine cause is suspected, bone age is sometimes determined.

Prognosis

Prognosis with organic FTT depends on the cause.

With nonorganic FTT, the majority of children age > 1 yr achieve a stable weight above the 3rd percentile. Children who develop FTT before age 1 yr are at high risk of cognitive delay, especially verbal and math skills. Children diagnosed at age < 6 mo, when the rate of postnatal brain growth is maximal, are at highest risk. General behavioral problems, identified by teachers or mental health practitioners, occur in about 50% of children. Problems specifically related to eating (eg, pickiness, slowness) or elimination tend to occur in a similar proportion of children, usually those with other behavioral or personality disturbances.

Treatment

- Sufficient nutrition
- Treatment of underlying disorder
- Long-term social support

Treatment of FTT is aimed at providing sufficient health and environmental resources to promote satisfactory growth. A nutritious diet containing adequate calories for catch-up growth (about 150% of normal caloric requirement) and individualized medical and social supports are usually necessary. Ability to gain weight in the hospital does not always differentiate infants with nonorganic FTT from those with organic FTT; all children grow when given sufficient nutrition. However, some children with nonorganic FTT lose weight in the hospital, highlighting the complexity of this condition.

For children with organic or mixed FTT, the underlying disorder should be treated quickly. For children with apparent nonorganic FTT or mixed FTT, management includes provision of education and emotional support to correct problems interfering with the parent-child relationship. Because long-term social support or psychiatric treatment is often required, the evaluation team may be able only to define the family's needs, provide initial instruction and support, and institute appropriate referrals to community agencies. The parents should understand why the referrals are being made and, if options exist, should participate in decisions concerning which agencies will be involved. If the child is hospitalized in a tertiary care center, the referring physician should be consulted regarding local agencies and the level of expertise available in the community.

A predischarge planning conference involving hospital-based personnel, representatives from the community agencies that will provide follow-up services, and the child's primary physician is ideal. Areas of responsibility and lines of accountability must be clearly defined, preferably in writing, and distributed to everyone involved. The parents should be invited to a summary session after the conference so that they can meet the community workers, ask questions, and arrange follow-up appointments.

In some cases, the child must be placed in foster care. If the child is expected to eventually return to the biologic parents, parenting skill training and psychologic counseling must be provided for them. Their child's progress must be monitored scrupulously. Return to the biologic parents should be based on the parents' demonstrated ability to care for the child adequately, not only on the passage of time.

KEY POINTS

- FTT should be suspected in children with a significant drop in percentile rank on growth parameters or a consistently low rank (eg, below 3rd to 5th percentile).
- Organic FTT is due to a medical disorder (eg, malabsorption, inborn error of metabolism).
- Nonorganic FTT is due to psychosocial problems (eg, neglect, poverty).
- In addition to a taking a thorough medical, social, and dietary history, health care providers should observe parents/caregivers feeding the child.
- Hospitalization may be necessary to evaluate the child, to observe the child's response to appropriate feeding, and to involve a feeding team if needed.

KAWASAKI DISEASE

Kawasaki disease (KD) is a vasculitis, sometimes involving the coronary arteries, that tends to occur in infants and children between ages 1 yr and 8 yr. It is characterized by prolonged fever, exanthem, conjunctivitis, mucous membrane inflammation, and lymphadenopathy. Coronary artery aneurysms may develop and rupture or cause myocardial infarction. Diagnosis is by clinical criteria; once the disease is diagnosed, echocardiography is done. Treatment is aspirin and IV immune globulin. Coronary thrombosis may require fibrinolysis or percutaneous interventions.

KD is a vasculitis of medium-sized arteries, most significantly the coronary arteries, which are involved in about 20% of untreated patients. Early manifestations include acute myocarditis with heart failure, arrhythmias, endocarditis, and pericarditis. Coronary artery aneurysms may subsequently form. Giant coronary artery aneurysms (> 8 mm internal diameter on echocardiography), though rare, have the greatest risk of causing cardiac tamponade, thrombosis, or infarction. KD is the leading cause of acquired heart disease in children. Extravascular tissue also may become inflamed, including the upper respiratory tract, pancreas, biliary tract, kidneys, mucous membranes, and lymph nodes.

Etiology

The etiology of KD is unknown, but the epidemiology and clinical presentation suggest an infection or an abnormal immunologic response to an infection in genetically predisposed children. Autoimmune disease is also a possibility. Children of Japanese descent have a particularly high incidence, but KD occurs worldwide. In the US, 3000 to 5000 cases occur annually. The male:female ratio is about 1.5:1. Eighty percent of patients are < 5 yr (peak, 18 to 24 mo). Cases in adolescents, adults, and infants < 4 mo are rare.

Cases occur year-round but most often in spring or winter. Clusters have been reported in communities without clear evidence of person-to-person spread. About 2% of patients have recurrences, typically months to years later. There is no known prevention.

Symptoms and Signs

The illness tends to progress in stages, beginning with fever lasting at least 5 days, usually unremittent (however, unless treated with antipyretics, temperature does not return to normal) and > 39° C (about 102° F), and is associated with irritability, occasional lethargy, or intermittent colicky abdominal pain. Usually within a day or two of fever onset, bilateral bulbar conjunctival injection appears without exudate.

Within 5 days, a polymorphous, erythematous macular rash appears, primarily over the trunk, often with accentuation in the perineal region. The rash may be urticarial, morbilliform, erythema multiforme, or scarlatiniform. It is accompanied by injected pharynx; reddened, dry, fissured lips; and a red strawberry tongue (see Plate 94).

During the first week, pallor of the proximal portion of the fingernails or toenails (leukonychia partialis) may occur. Erythema or a purple-red discoloration and variable edema of the palms and soles usually appear on about the 3rd to 5th day. Although edema may be slight, it is often tense, hard, and nonpitting. Periungual, palmar, plantar, and perineal desquamation begins on about the 10th day. The superficial layer of the skin sometimes comes off in large casts, revealing new normal skin.

Tender, nonsuppurative cervical lymphadenopathy (≥ 1 node ≥ 1.5 cm in diameter) is present throughout the course in about 50% of patients. The illness may last from 2 to 12 wk or longer. Incomplete or atypical cases can occur, especially in younger infants, who have higher risk of developing coronary artery disease. These findings manifest in about 90% of patients.

Other less specific findings indicate involvement of many systems. Arthritis or arthralgias (mainly involving large joints) occur in about 33% of patients. Other clinical features include urethritis, aseptic meningitis, hepatitis, otitis, vomiting, diarrhea, hydrops of the gallbladder, upper respiratory symptoms, and anterior uveitis.

Cardiac manifestations usually begin in the subacute phase of the syndrome about 1 to 4 wk after onset as the rash, fever, and other early acute clinical symptoms begin to subside.

Diagnosis

- Clinical criteria
- Serial ECG and echocardiography
- Testing to rule out other disorders: CBC, ESR, C-reactive protein, antinuclear antibody (ANA), rheumatoid factor (RF), albumin, liver enzymes, throat and blood cultures, urinalysis, chest x-ray

Diagnosis of KD is by clinical criteria (see Table 322–4). Similar symptoms can result from scarlet fever, staphylococcal exfoliative syndromes, measles, drug reactions, and juvenile idiopathic arthritis. Less common mimics are leptospirosis and Rocky Mountain spotted fever.

Some febrile children who have fewer than 4 of the 5 diagnostic criteria nonetheless develop vasculitic complications, including coronary artery aneurysms. Such children are considered to have atypical (or incomplete) KD. Atypical KD should be considered, and testing should be initiated if the child has had ≥ 5 days of fever > 39° C (about 102° F) plus ≥ 2 of the 5 criteria for KD.

Laboratory tests are not diagnostic but may be done to exclude other disorders. Patients generally undergo CBC, ANA, RF, ESR, and throat and blood cultures. Leukocytosis, often with a marked increase in immature cells, is common acutely.

Table 322–4. CRITERIA FOR DIAGNOSIS OF KAWASAKI DISEASE

Diagnosis is made if fever of ≥ 5 days has occurred and 4 of the following 5 criteria are noted:

1. Bilateral nonexudative conjunctival injection
2. Changes in the lips, tongue, or oral mucosa (injection, drying, fissuring, red strawberry tongue)
3. Changes in the peripheral extremities (edema, erythema, desquamation)
4. Polymorphous truncal exanthem
5. Cervical lymphadenopathy (at least 1 node ≥ 1.5 cm in diameter)

Other hematologic findings include a mild normocytic anemia, thrombocytosis (≥ 450,000/μL) in the 2nd or 3rd wk of illness, and elevated ESR or C-reactive protein. ANA, RF, and cultures are negative. Other abnormalities, depending on the organ systems involved, include sterile pyuria, elevated liver enzymes, proteinuria, reduced serum albumin, and CSF pleocytosis.

Consultation with a pediatric cardiologist is important. At diagnosis, ECG and echocardiography are done. Because abnormalities may not appear until later, these tests are repeated 2 to 3 wk, 6 to 8 wk, and perhaps 6 to 12 mo after onset. ECG may show arrhythmias, decreased voltage, or left ventricular hypertrophy. Echocardiography should detect coronary artery aneurysms, valvular regurgitation, pericarditis, or myocarditis. Coronary arteriography occasionally is useful in patients with aneurysms and abnormal stress test results.

Prognosis

Without therapy, mortality may approach 1%, usually occurring within 6 wk of onset. With adequate therapy, the mortality rate in the US is 0.17%. Long duration of fever increases cardiac risk. Deaths most commonly result from cardiac complications and can be sudden and unpredictable: > 50% occur within 1 mo of onset, 75% within 2 mo, and 95% within 6 mo but may occur as long as 10 yr later. Effective therapy reduces acute symptoms and, more importantly, lowers the incidence of coronary artery aneurysms from 20% to < 5%.

In the absence of coronary artery disease, the prognosis for complete recovery is excellent. About two thirds of coronary aneurysms regress within 1 yr, although it is unknown whether residual coronary stenosis remains. Giant coronary aneurysms are less likely to regress and require more intensive follow-up and therapy.

Treatment

- High-dose IV immune globulin (IVIG)
- High-dose aspirin

Children should be treated by or in close consultation with an experienced pediatric cardiologist, pediatric infectious disease specialist, or pediatric rheumatologist. Because infants with atypical KD are at high risk of coronary artery aneurysms, treatment should not be delayed. Therapy is started as soon as possible, optimally within the first 10 days of illness, with a combination of high-dose IVIG (single dose of 2 g/kg given over 10 to 12 h) and oral high-dose aspirin 20 to 25 mg/kg po qid. The aspirin dose is reduced to 3 to 5 mg/kg once/day after the child has been afebrile for 4 to 5 days; some authorities prefer to continue high-dose aspirin until the 14th day of illness. Aspirin metabolism is erratic during acute KD, which partially explains the high dose requirements. Some authorities monitor serum aspirin levels during high-dose therapy, especially if therapy is given for 14 days and/or fever persists despite IVIG treatment.

Most patients have a brisk response over the first 24 h of therapy. A small fraction continues to be ill with fever for several days and requires repeated dosing with IVIG. An alternative regimen, which may lead to slightly slower resolution of symptoms but may benefit patients with cardiac dysfunction who could not tolerate the volume of a 2 g/kg IGIV infusion, is IVIG 400 mg/kg once/day for 4 days (again in combination with high-dose aspirin). The efficacy of IVIG/aspirin therapy when begun > 10 days after onset of illness is unknown, but therapy should still be considered.

After the child's symptoms have abated for 4 to 5 days, aspirin 3 to 5 mg/kg once/day is continued for at least 8 wk after onset until repeated echocardiographic testing is completed. If there are no coronary artery aneurysms and signs of inflammation are absent (shown by normalization of ESR and platelets), aspirin may be stopped. Because of its antithrombotic effect, aspirin is continued indefinitely for children with coronary artery abnormalities. Children with giant coronary aneurysms may require additional anticoagulant therapy (eg, warfarin, antiplatelet drugs).

Children who receive IVIG therapy may have a lower response rate to live viral vaccines. Thus, measles-mumps-rubella vaccine should generally be delayed for 11 mo after IVIG therapy, and varicella vaccine should be delayed for ≥ 11 mo. If the risk of measles exposure is high, vaccination should proceed, but revaccination (or serologic testing) should be done 11 mo later.

A small risk of Reye syndrome exists in children receiving long-term aspirin therapy during outbreaks of influenza or varicella; thus, annual influenza vaccination is especially important for children (≥ 6 mo of age) receiving long-term aspirin therapy. Further, parents of children receiving aspirin should be instructed to contact their child's physician promptly if the child is exposed to or develops symptoms of influenza or varicella. Temporary interruption of aspirin may be considered (with substitution of dipyridamole for children with documented aneurysms).

KEY POINTS

- KD is a childhood systemic vasculitis of unknown etiology.
- The most serious complications involve the heart and include acute myocarditis with heart failure, arrhythmias, and coronary artery aneurysms.
- Children have fever, cutaneous rash (which later desquamates), oral and conjunctival inflammation, and lymphadenopathy; atypical cases with fewer of these classic criteria can occur.
- Diagnosis is made by clinical criteria; children meeting criteria should have a serial ECG and echocardiography and consult with a specialist.
- Early use of high-dose aspirin and IV immune globulin relieves symptoms and helps prevent cardiac complications.

PROGERIA

(Hutchinson-Gilford Syndrome)

Progeria is a rare syndrome of accelerated aging that manifests early in childhood and causes premature death.

Progeria is caused by a sporadic mutation in the *LMNA* gene that codes for a protein (lamin A) that provides the molecular scaffolding of cell nuclei. The defective protein leads to nuclear instability from cell division and early death of every body cell.

Symptoms and signs of progeria develop within 2 yr and include

- Growth failure (eg, short stature, delayed tooth eruption)
- Craniofacial abnormalities (eg, craniofacial disproportion, micrognathia, beaked nose, macrocephaly, large fontanelle)
- Physical changes of aging (eg, wrinkled skin, balding, decreased range of motion of joints, tough skin that resembles scleroderma)

Diagnosis of progeria is usually obvious by appearance but must be distinguished from segmental progerias (eg, acrogeria, metageria) and other causes of growth failure. Median age at death is 12 yr; cause is coronary artery and cerebrovascular disease. Insulin resistance and atherosclerosis may develop. Of note is that other problems associated with normal aging (eg, increased cancer risk, degenerative arthritis) are not present.

There is no known progeria treatment. Support groups are available.

Other progeroid syndromes: Premature aging is a feature of other rare progeroid syndromes.

Werner syndrome is premature aging after puberty with hair thinning and development of conditions of old age (eg, cataracts, diabetes, osteoporosis, atherosclerosis). **Rothmund-Thomson syndrome** is premature aging with increased susceptibility to cancer. Both are caused by gene mutations leading to defective RecQ DNA helicases, which normally repair DNA.

Cockayne syndrome is an autosomal recessive disease caused by mutation in the *ERCC8* gene, which is important in DNA excision repair. Clinical features include severe growth failure, cachectic appearance, retinopathy, hypertension, renal failure, skin photosensitivity, and intellectual disability.

Neonatal progeroid syndrome (Wiedemann-Rautenstrauch syndrome) is a recessively inherited syndrome of aging causing death by 2 yr.

Other syndromes (eg, Down, Ehlers-Danlos) occasionally have progeroid features.

REYE SYNDROME

Reye syndrome is a rare form of acute encephalopathy and fatty infiltration of the liver that tends to occur after some acute viral infections, particularly when salicylates are used. Diagnosis is clinical. Treatment is supportive.

The cause of Reye syndrome is unknown, but many cases seem to follow infection with influenza A or B or varicella. Using salicylates (generally aspirin) during such illness increases the risk by as much as 35-fold. This finding has led to a marked decrease in salicylate use in the US since the mid-1980s (except when specifically indicated, such as in juvenile idiopathic arthritis and KD) and a corresponding decrease in the incidence of Reye syndrome from several hundred annual cases to about 2. The syndrome occurs almost exclusively in children < 18 yr. In the US, most cases occur in late fall and winter.

The disease affects mitochondrial function, causing disturbance in fatty acid and carnitine metabolism. Pathophysiology and clinical manifestations are similar to a number of inherited metabolic disorders of fatty acid transport and mitochondrial oxidation (see p. 2641).

Symptoms and Signs

The disease varies greatly in severity but is characteristically biphasic. Initial viral symptoms (URI or sometimes chickenpox) are followed in 5 to 7 days by pernicious nausea and vomiting and a sudden change in mental status. The changes in mental status may vary from a mild amnesia, weakness, vision and hearing changes, and lethargy to intermittent episodes of disorientation and agitation, which can progress rapidly to deepening stages of coma manifested by

- Progressive unresponsiveness
- Decorticate and decerebrate posturing
- Seizures
- Flaccidity
- Fixed dilated pupils
- Respiratory arrest

Focal neurologic findings usually are not present. Hepatomegaly occurs in about 40% of cases, but jaundice is absent.

Complications of Reye syndrome: Complications include

- Electrolyte and fluid disturbances
- Increased intracranial pressure (ICP)
- Diabetes insipidus
- Syndrome of inappropriate ADH secretion
- Hypotension
- Arrhythmias
- Bleeding diatheses (especially GI)
- Pancreatitis
- Respiratory insufficiency
- Hyperammonemia
- Aspiration pneumonia
- Poor temperature regulation
- Uncal herniation and death

Diagnosis

- Clinical findings in association with laboratory testing
- Liver biopsy

Reye syndrome should be suspected in any child exhibiting the acute onset of an encephalopathy (without known heavy metal or toxin exposure) and pernicious vomiting associated with hepatic dysfunction. Liver biopsy provides the definitive diagnosis, showing microvesicular, fatty changes, and is especially useful in sporadic cases and in children < 2 yr. The diagnosis may also be made when the typical clinical findings and history are associated with the following laboratory findings: increased liver transaminases (AST, ALT > 3 times normal), normal bilirubin, increased blood ammonia level, and prolonged PT.

Head CT or MRI is done as for any child with encephalopathy. If head CT or MRI is normal, a lumbar puncture can be done. CSF examination usually shows increased pressure, < 8 to 10 WBCs/μL, and normal protein levels; the CSF glutamine level may be elevated. Hypoglycemia and hypoglycorrhachia (a very low concentration of CSF glucose) occur in 15% of cases, especially in children < 4 yr; they should be screened for metabolic disease. The condition is staged from I to V according to severity.

Signs of metabolic derangement include elevated serum amino acid levels, acid-base disturbances (usually with hyperventilation, mixed respiratory alkalosis–metabolic acidosis), osmolar changes, hypernatremia, hypokalemia, and hypophosphatemia.

Differential diagnosis: The differential diagnosis of coma and liver dysfunction includes

- Sepsis or hyperthermia (especially in infants)
- Potentially treatable inborn abnormalities of urea synthesis (eg, ornithine transcarbamylase deficiency) or fatty acid oxidation (eg, systemic carnitine deficiency, medium chain acyl-CoA dehydrogenase deficiency)

- Phosphorus or carbon tetrachloride intoxication
- Acute encephalopathy caused by salicylism, other drugs (eg, valproate), or poisons; viral encephalitis or meningoencephalitis
- Acute hepatitis

Illnesses such as idiopathic steatosis of pregnancy and tetracycline liver toxicity may show similar light microscopic findings.

Prognosis

Outcome is related to the duration of cerebral dysfunction, severity and rate of progression of coma, severity of increased ICP, and degree of blood ammonia elevation. Progression from stage I to higher stages is likely when the initial blood ammonia level is > 100 μg/dL (> 60 μmol/L) and the PT is ≥ 3 sec longer than that of the control. In fatal cases, the mean time from hospitalization to death is 4 days. Fatality rates average 21% but range from < 2% among patients in stage I to > 80% among patients in stage IV or V.

Prognosis for survivors usually is good, and recurrences are rare. However, the incidence of neurologic sequelae (eg, intellectual disability, seizure disorders, cranial nerve palsies, motor dysfunction) is as high as 30% among survivors who developed seizures or decerebrate posturing during illness.

Treatment

- Support measures

Treatment of Reye syndrome is supportive, with particular attention paid to control of ICP and blood glucose because glycogen depletion is common.

Treatment of elevated ICP includes intubation, hyperventilation, fluid restriction of 1500 mL/m²/day, elevating the head of the bed, osmotic diuretics, direct ICP monitoring, and decompressing craniotomy. Infusion of 10 or 15% dextrose is common to maintain euglycemia. Coagulopathy may require fresh frozen plasma or vitamin K. Other treatments (eg, exchange transfusion, hemodialysis, barbiturate-induced deep coma) have not been proved effective but are sometimes used.

KEY POINTS

- Reye syndrome of acute encephalopathy and hepatic dysfunction, typically occurring after viral infection (particularly with salicylate use), has become rare since routine use of aspirin in children has been reduced.
- Diagnosis is by exclusion of similarly manifesting infectious, toxic, and metabolic disorders; liver biopsy may help confirm it.
- Treatment is supportive, particularly with measures to lower ICP.

SUDDEN INFANT DEATH SYNDROME

Sudden infant death syndrome (SIDS) is the sudden and unexpected death of an infant or young child between 2 wk and 1 yr of age in which an examination of the death scene, thorough postmortem examination, and clinical history fail to show cause.

SIDS is the most common cause of death of infants between 2 wk and 1 yr of age, accounting for 35 to 55% of all deaths in this age group. The rate of SIDS occurrence is 0.5/1000 births in the US; there are racial and ethnic disparities (African American and Native American children have twice the average risk of SIDS). Peak incidence is between the 2nd and 4th mo of life. Almost all SIDS deaths occur when the infant is thought to be sleeping.

Etiology

The cause of SIDS is unknown, although it is most likely due to dysfunction of neural cardiorespiratory control mechanisms. The dysfunction may be intermittent or transient, and multiple mechanisms are probably involved. Factors that may be involved are the infant having a poor sleep arousal mechanism, an inability to detect elevated CO_2 levels in the blood, or a cardiac channelopathy that affects heart rhythm.

Fewer than 5% of infants with SIDS have episodes of prolonged apnea before their death, so the overlap between the SIDS population and infants with recurrent prolonged apnea is very small.

Risk factors for SIDS: The association between a prone (on stomach) sleeping position and an increased risk of SIDS has been documented strongly.

Other risk factors (see Table 322–5) include old or unsafe cribs, soft bedding (eg, lamb's wool), waterbed mattresses, bed-sharing with a parent/caregiver, smoking in the home, and an overheated environment. Siblings of infants who die of SIDS are 5 times more likely to die of SIDS; it is not clear whether

Table 322–5. RISK FACTORS FOR SUDDEN INFANT DEATH SYNDROME

African American or Native American ethnicity
Bed-sharing with parent/caregiver
Cold temperatures/winter months
Episodes of apnea requiring resuscitation
Growth failure
Increased parity
Low birth weight
Lower socioeconomic group
Male sex
Maternal age < 20 yr
Maternal drug use during pregnancy
Maternal smoking during pregnancy
No pacifier
Old or unsafe cribs
Overheating (eg, blankets, hot room)
Poor prenatal care
Prematurity
Prone sleeping position*
Recent illness
Short interval between pregnancies
Sibling of a SIDS victim
Smoking in the home
Soft bedding
Waterbed mattress

*Most important.

this is related to genetics or environment (including possible abuse by the affected infant's family).

Many risk factors for SIDS apply to non-SIDS infant deaths as well.

Diagnosis

- Exclusion of other causes by autopsy

The diagnosis of SIDS, while largely one of exclusion, cannot be made without an adequate autopsy to rule out other causes of sudden, unexpected death (eg, intracranial hemorrhage, meningitis, myocarditis). An autopsy may be required in many states. Also, the care team (including social workers) should sensitively assess the likelihood of infant suffocation or nonaccidental trauma; concern for this etiology should increase when the affected infant was outside the highest-risk age group (1 to 5 mo) or another infant in the family had SIDS or frequent ALTEs.

Management

Parents who have lost a child to SIDS are grief-stricken and unprepared for the tragedy. Because no definitive cause can be found for their child's death, they usually have excessive guilt feelings, which may be aggravated by investigations conducted by police, social workers, or others. Family members require support not only during the days immediately after the infant's death but for at least several months to help them with their grief and dispel guilt feelings. Such support includes, whenever possible, an immediate home visit to observe the circumstances in which SIDS occurred and to inform and counsel the parents concerning the cause of death.

Autopsy should be done quickly. As soon as the preliminary results are known (usually within 12 h), they should be communicated to the parents. Some clinicians advise a series of home or office visits over the first month to continue the earlier discussions, answer questions, and give the family the final (microscopic) autopsy results. At the last meeting, it is appropriate to discuss the parents' adjustment to their loss, especially their attitude toward having other children. Much of the counseling and support can be complemented by specially trained nurses or by lay people who have themselves experienced the tragedy of and adjustment to SIDS (visit www.sids.org for more information and resources).

Prevention

The American Academy of Pediatrics recommends that infants be placed supine (on their back—the Safe to Sleep® campaign) for sleep unless other medical conditions prevent this. Side sleeping or propping is too unstable. The incidence of SIDS increases with overheating (eg, clothing, blankets, hot room) and in cold weather. Thus, every effort should be made to avoid an overly hot or an overly cold environment, to avoid overwrapping the infant, and to remove soft bedding, such as sheepskin, pillows, stuffed toys/animals, and comforters, from the crib. Pacifiers may be helpful, because they help open the airway. Parents/caregivers should not have the infant sleep in their bed.

Mothers should avoid smoking during pregnancy, and infants should not be exposed to smoke. Breastfeeding is encouraged to help prevent infections. There is no evidence that home apnea monitors reduce the incidence of SIDS and therefore are not suggested for prevention.

KEY POINTS

- Specific causes, including child abuse, must be ruled out by clinical evaluation and autopsy.
- Etiology is unclear, although a number of risk factors have been identified.
- The most important modifiable risk factors involve the sleep setting, particularly prone sleeping, along with bed-sharing and sleeping on very soft surfaces or with loose bedding.
- Apneic episodes and ALTEs do not appear to be risk factors.

TEETHING

Teething is the process of tooth eruption through the gums.

A child's first tooth usually erupts by 6 mo of age, and a complete set of 20 deciduous teeth usually develops by 2½ yr.

Before a tooth erupts, the child may cry, be fussy, and sleep and eat poorly. During tooth eruption (see Table 310–1 on p. 2590), the child may drool, have red and tender gums, and chew constantly on objects such as toys and crib rails. Teething does not cause fever.

Children who have fever and who are especially fussy should be evaluated for a viral or bacterial infection, because these symptoms are not caused by teething.

Teething infants get some relief from chewing on hard (eg, teething biscuits) or cold objects (eg, firm rubber or gel-containing teething rings). Massaging the child's gums with or without ice also may help. Children may be treated with weight-based doses of acetaminophen or ibuprofen.

Teething gels are not recommended because they are not any more effective than other measures, and some contain benzocaine. Benzocaine can rarely cause methemoglobinemia.

323 Miscellaneous Viral Infections in Infants and Children

Many viruses cause human disease. Most viruses can infect adults and children and are discussed elsewhere in THE MANUAL. Viruses with specific effects on neonates are discussed in Ch. 314. This chapter covers viral infections that are typically acquired during childhood (although many may also affect adults).

ERYTHEMA INFECTIOSUM

(Fifth Disease; Parvovirus B19 Infection)

Erythema infectiosum, acute infection with parvovirus B19, causes mild constitutional symptoms and a blotchy or

maculopapular rash beginning on the cheeks and spreading primarily to exposed extremities. Diagnosis is clinical, and treatment is generally not needed.

The disease is caused by human parvovirus B19. It occurs mostly during the spring, commonly causing localized outbreaks every few years among children (particularly children aged 5 to 7 yr). Spread seems to be by respiratory droplets and by percutaneous exposure to blood or blood products, with high rates of secondary infection among household contacts; infection can occur without symptoms or signs.

Pathophysiology

Parvovirus B19 causes transient suppression of erythropoiesis that is mild and asymptomatic except in children with underlying hemoglobinopathies (eg, sickle cell disease) or other RBC disorders (eg, hereditary spherocytosis), who may develop transient aplastic crisis. Also, immunocompromised children can develop protracted viremia (lasting weeks to months), leading to severe anemia (pure RBC aplasia).

Erythema infectiosum can be transmitted transplacentally, sometimes resulting in stillbirth or severe fetal anemia with widespread edema (hydrops fetalis). However, about half of pregnant women are immune because of previous infection. The risk of fetal death is 2 to 6% after maternal infection, with risk greatest during the first half of pregnancy.

Symptoms and Signs

The incubation period is 4 to 14 days. Typical initial manifestations are nonspecific flu-like symptoms (eg, low-grade fever, slight malaise). Several days later, an indurated, confluent erythema appears over the cheeks ("slapped-cheek" appearance) and a symmetric rash appears that is most prominent on the arms, legs (often extensor surfaces), and trunk, usually sparing the palms and soles. The rash is maculopapular, tending toward confluence; it forms reticular or lacy patterns of slightly raised, blotchy areas with central clearing, usually most prominent on exposed areas. The rash, and the entire illness, typically lasts 5 to 10 days. However, the rash may recur for several weeks, exacerbated by sunlight, exercise, heat, fever, or emotional stress.

Mild joint pain and swelling (nonerosive arthritis) that may persist or recur for weeks to months sometimes occurs in adults. A few patients (more commonly children) develop papular-purpuric gloves-and-socks syndrome (PPGSS), which causes papular, purpuric, or petechial lesions limited to the hands and feet and is often accompanied by fever and oral and/or genital lesions.

Diagnosis

- Clinical evaluation

The appearance and pattern of spread of the rash are the only diagnostic features; however, some enteroviruses may cause similar rashes. Rubella can be ruled out by serologic testing; an exposure history is also helpful. Serologic testing is not required in otherwise healthy children; however, children with a known hemoglobinopathy or immunocompromised state should have CBC and reticulocyte count to detect hematopoietic suppression as well as viral testing. In children with transient aplastic crisis or adults with arthropathy, the presence of IgM-specific antibody to parvovirus B19 in the late acute or early convalescent phase strongly supports the diagnosis. Parvovirus B19 viremia also can be detected by quantitative PCR techniques, which are generally used for patients with transient aplastic crisis, immunocompromised patients with pure RBC aplasia, and infants with hydrops fetalis or congenital infection.

Treatment

- Supportive care

Only symptomatic treatment is needed. IV immune globulin has been used to curtail viremia and increase erythropoiesis in immunocompromised patients with pure RBC aplasia.

KEY POINTS

- Children develop low-grade fever and slight malaise followed several days later by an indurated, confluent erythema on the cheeks ("slapped-cheek" appearance) and a symmetric rash that is most prominent on the arms, legs, and trunk.
- There is mild, transient suppression of erythropoiesis that is asymptomatic except sometimes in children with hemoglobinopathies (eg, sickle cell disease) or other RBC disorders (eg, hereditary spherocytosis), or immunosuppression.
- Risk of fetal death is 2 to 6% after maternal infection.
- Testing is done mainly in children with transient aplastic crisis or adults with arthropathy.
- Treatment is symptomatic, but immunocompromised children may benefit from IV immune globulin.

MEASLES

(Rubeola; Morbilli; 9-Day Measles)

Measles is a highly contagious viral infection that is most common among children. It is characterized by fever, cough, coryza, conjunctivitis, an enanthem (Koplik spots) on the oral mucosa, and a maculopapular rash that spreads cephalocaudally. Diagnosis is usually clinical. Treatment is supportive. Vaccination is highly effective.

Worldwide, measles infects about 20 million people and causes about 200,000 deaths annually, primarily in children. These numbers can vary dramatically over a short period of time depending on the vaccination status of the population. Measles is rare in the US because of routine childhood vaccination; an average of 63 cases/yr were reported to the Centers for Disease Control and Prevention (CDC) from 2000 to 2007. However, since 2013, cases in the US have been increasing in record numbers, primarily because of imported cases with subsequent spread among unvaccinated groups.

Pathophysiology

Measles is caused by a paramyxovirus and is a human disease with no known animal reservoir or asymptomatic carrier state. It is extremely communicable; the secondary attack rate is > 90% among susceptible people who are exposed.

Measles is spread mainly by secretions from the nose, throat, and mouth during the prodromal or early eruptive stage. Communicability begins several days before and continues until several days after the rash appears. Measles is not communicable once the rash begins to desquamate.

Transmission is typically by large respiratory droplets that are discharged by cough and briefly remain airborne for a short distance. Transmission may also occur by small aerosolized droplets that can remain airborne (and thus can be inhaled) for up to 2 h in closed areas (eg, in an office examination room). Transmission by fomites seems less likely than airborne transmission because the measles virus is thought to survive only for a short time on dry surfaces.

An infant whose mother has immunity to measles (eg, because of previous illness or vaccination) receives antibodies transplacentally; these antibodies are protective for most of the first 6 to 12 mo of life. Lifelong immunity is conferred by infection. In the US, almost all measles cases are imported by travelers or immigrants, with subsequent indigenous transmission occurring primarily among unvaccinated people.

Symptoms and Signs

After a 7- to 14-day incubation period, measles begins with a prodrome of fever, coryza, hacking cough, and tarsal conjunctivitis. Pathognomonic Koplik spots appear during the prodrome, before the onset of rash, usually on the oral mucosa opposite the 1st and 2nd upper molars. The spots resemble grains of white sand surrounded by red areolae. They may be extensive, producing diffuse mottled erythema of the oral mucosa. Sore throat develops.

The rash appears 3 to 5 days after symptom onset, usually 1 to 2 days after Koplik spots appear. It begins on the face in front of and below the ears and on the side of the neck as irregular macules, soon mixed with papules. Within 24 to 48 h, lesions spread to the trunk and extremities (including the palms and soles) as they begin to fade on the face. Petechiae or ecchymoses may occur with severe rashes.

During peak disease severity, a patient's temperature may exceed 40° C, with periorbital edema, conjunctivitis, photophobia, a hacking cough, extensive rash, prostration, and mild itching. Constitutional symptoms and signs parallel the severity of the eruption and the epidemic. In 3 to 5 days, the fever falls, the patient feels more comfortable, and the rash fades rapidly, leaving a coppery brown discoloration followed by desquamation.

Immunocompromised patients may not have a rash and can develop severe, progressive giant cell pneumonia.

Complications: Complications include

- Atypical measles syndrome
- Pneumonia
- Bacterial superinfection
- Acute thrombocytopenic purpura
- Encephalitis
- Transient hepatitis
- Subacute sclerosing panencephalitis

Atypical measles syndrome usually occurs in people previously immunized with the original killed-virus measles vaccines, which have been unavailable since 1968. The older vaccines can alter disease expression after infection with wild-type measles. Atypical measles syndrome may begin abruptly, with high fever, prostration, headache, abdominal pain, and cough. The rash may appear 1 to 2 days later, often beginning on the extremities, and may be maculopapular, vesicular, urticarial, or purpuric. Edema of the hands and feet may occur. Pneumonia, pleural effusion, and hilar adenopathy may develop; chest x-ray abnormalities may persist for weeks to months. Symptomatic hypoxemia may occur.

Pneumonia (see p. 478) due to measles virus infection of the lungs occurs in about 5% of patients, even during apparently uncomplicated infection; in infants, it is a common cause of death.

Bacterial superinfections include pneumonia, laryngotracheobronchitis, and otitis media. Measles transiently suppresses delayed hypersensitivity, which can worsen active TB and temporarily prevent reaction to tuberculin and histoplasmin antigens in skin tests. Bacterial superinfection is suggested by pertinent focal signs or a relapse of fever, leukocytosis, or prostration.

Acute thrombocytopenic purpura may occur after infection resolves and cause a mild, self-limited bleeding tendency; occasionally, bleeding is severe.

Encephalitis (see p. 1851) occurs in 1/1000 to 2000 cases, usually 2 days to 2 wk after onset of the rash, often beginning with recrudescence of high fever, headache, seizures, and coma. CSF usually has a lymphocyte count of 50 to 500/μL and a mildly elevated protein level but may be normal initially. Encephalitis may resolve in about 1 wk or may persist longer, causing morbidity or death.

Transient hepatitis and diarrhea may occur during an acute infection.

Subacute sclerosing panencephalitis (see p. 2766) is a rare, progressive, ultimately fatal, late complication of measles.

Diagnosis

- Clinical evaluation
- Serologic testing
- Viral detection via culture or reverse transcription–PCR

Typical measles may be suspected in an exposed patient who has coryza, conjunctivitis, photophobia, and cough but is usually suspected only after the rash appears. Diagnosis is usually clinical, by identifying Koplik spots or the rash. CBC is unnecessary but, if obtained, may show leukopenia with a relative lymphocytosis. Laboratory identification is necessary for public health and outbreak control purposes. It is most easily done by demonstration of the presence of measles IgM antibody in an acute serum specimen or by viral culture or reverse transcription–PCR of throat swabs, blood, nasopharyngeal swabs, or urine samples. A rise in IgG antibody levels between acute and convalescent sera is highly accurate, but obtaining this information delays diagnosis. All cases of suspected measles should be reported to the local health department even before laboratory confirmation.

Differential diagnosis includes rubella (see p. 2764), scarlet fever (see p. 1605), drug rashes (eg, resulting from phenobarbital or sulfonamides), serum sickness (see Table 119–3 on p. 981), roseola infantum (see p. 2764), infectious mononucleosis (see p. 1625), erythema infectiosum (see p. 2758), and echovirus and coxsackievirus infections (see Table 205–1 on p. 1727). Manifestations can also resemble Kawasaki disease (see p. 2754) and cause diagnostic confusion in areas where measles is very rare. Atypical measles, because of its greater variability, can simulate even more conditions than typical measles, including Rocky Mountain spotted fever, toxic shock syndromes, and meningococcemia.

Some of these conditions can be distinguished from typical measles as follows:

- Rubella: A recognizable prodrome is absent, fever and other constitutional symptoms are absent or less severe, postauricular and suboccipital lymph nodes are enlarged (and usually tender), and duration is short.
- Drug rashes: A drug rash often resembles the measles rash, but a prodrome is absent, there is no cephalocaudal progression or cough, and there is usually a history of recent drug exposure.
- Roseola infantum: The rash resembles that of measles, but it seldom occurs in children > 3 yr. Initial temperature is usually high, Koplik spots and malaise are absent, and defervescence and rash occur simultaneously.

Prognosis

Mortality is about 2/1000 in the US but is much higher in the developing world. Undernutrition and vitamin A deficiency may predispose to mortality.

Treatment

- Supportive care
- For children, vitamin A

Treatment is supportive, including for encephalitis.

Hospitalized patients with measles should be managed with standard contact and airborne precautions. Single-patient airborne infection isolation rooms and N-95 respirators or similar personal protective equipment are recommended. Otherwise healthy outpatients with measles are most contagious for 4 days after the development of the rash and should severely limit contact with others during their illness.

Vitamin A supplementation has been shown to reduce morbidity and mortality due to measles in children in the developing world. Because low serum levels of vitamin A are associated with severe disease due to measles, vitamin A treatment is recommended for all children with measles. The dose is given orally once/day for 2 days and depends on the child's age:

- > 1 yr: 200,000 IU
- 6 to 11 mo: 100,000 IU
- < 6 mo: 50,000 IU

In children with clinical signs of vitamin A deficiency (see p. 44), an additional single, age-specific dose of vitamin A is repeated 2 to 4 wk later.

Prevention

A live-attenuated virus vaccine containing measles, mumps, and rubella is routinely given to children in most developed countries (see also p. 1456 and see Table 291–2 on p. 2462). Two doses are recommended:

- The first dose is recommended at age 12 to 15 mo but can be given as young as age 6 mo during a measles outbreak or before international travel.
- The second is given at age 4 to 6 yr.

Infants immunized at < 1 yr of age still require 2 further doses given after the first birthday. Vaccine provides long-lasting immunity and has decreased measles incidence in the US by 99%. The vaccine causes mild or inapparent, noncommunicable infection. Fever > 38° C occurs 5 to 12 days after inoculation in 5 to 15% of vaccinees and can be followed by a rash. CNS reactions are exceedingly rare; the vaccine does not cause autism.

Contraindications to the vaccine include generalized cancers (eg, leukemia, lymphoma), immunodeficiency, and therapy with immunosuppressants (eg, corticosteroids, irradiation, alkylating agents, antimetabolites). HIV infection is a contraindication only if immunosuppression is severe (CDC immunologic category 3 with CD4 < 15%); if not, the risks of wild measles outweigh the risk of acquiring measles from the live vaccine. Reasons to defer vaccination include pregnancy, serious febrile illness, active untreated TB, or recent administration of antibody (as whole blood, plasma, or any immune globulin). Duration of deferral depends on the type and dose of immune globulin preparation given but may be as long as 11 mo.

Postexposure prophylaxis: Prevention in susceptible contacts is possible by giving the vaccine within 3 days of exposure. If vaccine should be deferred, immune globulin 0.25 mL/kg IM (maximum dose, 15 mL) is given immediately (within 6 days), with vaccination given 5 to 6 mo later if medically appropriate (eg, if the patient is no longer pregnant). An exposed immunodeficient patient with a contraindication to vaccination is given immune globulin 0.5 mL/kg IM (maximum, 15 mL). Immune globulin should not be given simultaneously with vaccine.

In an institutional outbreak (eg, schools), susceptible contacts who refuse or cannot receive vaccination and who also do not receive immune globulin should be excluded from the affected institution until 21 days after onset of rash in the last case. Exposed, susceptible healthcare workers should be excluded from duty from 5 days after their first exposure to 21 days after their last exposure, even if they receive postexposure prophylaxis.

KEY POINTS

- Incidence of measles is highly variable depending on the vaccination rate in the population.
- Measles is highly transmissible, developing in > 90% of susceptible contacts.
- Measles causes about 200,000 deaths annually, primarily in children in the developing world; pneumonia is a common cause, whereas encephalitis is less common.
- Treatment is mainly supportive, but children should also receive vitamin A supplementation.
- Universal childhood vaccination is imperative unless contraindicated (eg, by active cancer, use of immunosuppressants, or HIV infection with severe immunosuppression).
- Give postexposure prophylaxis to susceptible contacts within 3 days of exposure; use vaccine unless contraindicated, in which case give immune globulin.

MUMPS

(Epidemic Parotitis)

Mumps is an acute, contagious, systemic viral disease, usually causing painful enlargement of the salivary glands, most commonly the parotids. Complications may include orchitis, meningoencephalitis, and pancreatitis. Diagnosis is usually clinical; all cases are reported promptly to public health authorities. Treatment is supportive. Vaccination is effective for prevention.

The causative agent, a paramyxovirus, is spread by droplets or saliva. The virus probably enters through the nose or mouth. It is in saliva up to 7 days before salivary gland swelling appears with maximal transmissibility just before the development of parotitis. It is also in blood and urine and, if the CNS is involved, in CSF. One attack usually confers permanent immunity.

Mumps is less communicable than measles. It occurs mainly in unimmunized populations, but outbreaks among largely immunized populations have occurred. A combination of primary vaccine failure (failure to develop immunity after vaccination) and waning immunity may have played a part in these outbreaks. In 2006, there was a resurgence of mumps in the US with 6584 cases, which occurred primarily in young adults with prior vaccination. Two smaller outbreaks occurred in 2009 to 2010, one with 3000 cases, mainly among high school–age people in a religious community in New York City. In the first half of 2014, 871 cases have occurred, many in outbreaks at 4 US universities.

As with measles, mumps cases may be imported, leading to indigenous transmission, especially in congregate settings (eg, college campuses) or closed communities (eg, tradition-observant Jewish communities). Peak incidence of mumps is during late winter and early spring. Disease occurs at any age but is unusual in children < 2 yr, particularly those < 1 yr. About 25 to 30% of cases are clinically inapparent.

Symptoms and Signs

After a 12- to 24-day incubation period, most people develop headache, anorexia, malaise, and a low- to moderate-grade fever. The salivary glands become involved 12 to 24 h later, with fever up to 39.5 to 40° C. Fever persists 24 to 72 h. Glandular swelling peaks on about the 2nd day and lasts 5 to 7 days. Involved glands are extremely tender during the febrile period.

Parotitis is usually bilateral but may be unilateral, especially at the onset. Pain while chewing or swallowing, especially while swallowing acidic liquids such as vinegar or citrus juice, is its earliest symptom. It later causes swelling beyond the parotid in front of and below the ear. Occasionally, the submandibular and sublingual glands also swell and, more rarely, are the only glands affected. Submandibular gland involvement causes neck swelling beneath the jaw, and suprasternal edema may develop, perhaps because of lymphatic obstruction by enlarged salivary glands. When sublingual glands are involved, the tongue may swell. The oral duct openings of the affected glands are edematous and slightly inflamed. The skin over the glands may become tense and shiny.

Complications: Mumps may involve organs other than the salivary glands, particularly in postpubertal patients. Such complications include

- Orchitis or oophoritis
- Meningitis or encephalitis
- Pancreatitis

About 20% of postpubertal male patients develop orchitis (testicular inflammation), usually unilateral, with pain, tenderness, edema, erythema, and warmth of the scrotum. Some testicular atrophy may ensue, but testosterone production and fertility are usually preserved. In females, oophoritis (gonadal involvement) is less commonly recognized, is less painful, and does not impair fertility.

Meningitis, typically with headache, vomiting, stiff neck, and CSF pleocytosis, occurs in 1 to 10% of patients with parotitis (see p. 1917). Encephalitis, with drowsiness, seizures, or coma, occurs in about 1/1000 to 5000 cases (see p. 1851). About 50% of CNS mumps infections occur without parotitis.

Pancreatitis, typically with sudden severe nausea, vomiting, and epigastric pain, may occur toward the end of the first week (see p. 154). These symptoms disappear in about 1 wk, leading to complete recovery.

Prostatitis, nephritis, myocarditis, hepatitis, mastitis, polyarthritis, deafness, and lacrimal gland involvement occur extremely rarely. Inflammation of the thyroid and thymus glands may cause edema and swelling over the sternum, but sternal swelling more often results from submandibular gland involvement with obstruction of lymphatic drainage.

Diagnosis

- Clinical evaluation
- Viral detection via reverse transcription–PCR (RT-PCR)
- Serologic testing

Mumps is suspected in patients with salivary gland inflammation and typical systemic symptoms, particularly if there is parotitis or a known mumps outbreak. Laboratory testing is not needed to make a diagnosis but is strongly recommended for public health purposes. Other conditions can cause similar glandular involvement (see Table 323–1). Mumps is also suspected in patients with unexplained aseptic meningitis or encephalitis during mumps outbreaks. Lumbar puncture is necessary for patients with meningeal signs.

Table 323–1. CAUSES OF PAROTID AND OTHER SALIVARY GLAND ENLARGEMENT

Suppurative bacterial parotitis
HIV parotitis
Other viral parotitis
Metabolic disorders (eg, uremia, diabetes mellitus)
Mikulicz syndrome (a chronic, usually painless parotid and lacrimal gland swelling of unknown etiology that occurs with TB, sarcoidosis, SLE, leukemia, and lymphosarcoma)
Malignant and benign salivary gland tumors
Drug-related parotid enlargement (eg, due to iodides, phenylbutazone, or propylthiouracil)

Laboratory diagnosis is necessary if disease is

- Unilateral
- Recurrent
- Occurs in previously immunized patients
- Causes prominent involvement of tissues other than the salivary glands

Testing is also recommended for all patients with parotitis lasting ≥ 2 days without an identified cause. RT-PCR is the preferred method of diagnosis; however, serologic testing of acute and convalescent sera by complement fixation or enzyme-linked immunosorbent assays (ELISA) and viral culture of the throat, CSF, and occasionally the urine can be done. In previously immunized populations, IgM testing may be falsely negative; therefore, RT-PCR assays should be done on samples of saliva or throat washings as early in the course of the disease as possible.

Other laboratory tests are generally unnecessary. In undifferentiated aseptic meningitis, an elevated serum amylase level can be a helpful clue in the diagnosis of mumps despite the absence of parotitis. WBC count is nonspecific; it may be normal but usually shows slight leukopenia and neutropenia. In meningitis, CSF glucose is usually normal but is occasionally between 20 and 40 mg/dL (1.1 and 2.2 mmol/L), as in bacterial meningitis. CSF protein is only mildly elevated.

Prognosis

Uncomplicated mumps usually resolves, although a relapse occurs rarely after about 2 wk. Prognosis of patients with meningitis is usually good, although permanent sequelae, such as unilateral (or rarely bilateral) nerve deafness or facial paralysis, may result. Postinfectious encephalitis, acute cerebellar ataxia, transverse myelitis, and polyneuritis occur rarely.

Treatment

- Supportive care

Treatment of mumps and its complications is supportive. The patient is isolated until glandular swelling subsides. A soft diet reduces pain caused by chewing. Acidic substances (eg, citrus fruit juices) that cause discomfort should be avoided.

Repeated vomiting due to pancreatitis may necessitate IV hydration. For orchitis, bed rest and support of the scrotum in cotton on an adhesive-tape bridge between the thighs to minimize tension or use of ice packs often relieves pain. Corticosteroids have not been shown to hasten resolution of orchitis.

Prevention

Vaccination with live mumps virus vaccine (see p. 1456 and see Table 291–2 on p. 2462) provides effective prevention and causes no significant local or systemic reactions. Two doses, given as a combined measles, mumps, and rubella vaccine, are recommended for children:

- The first dose at age 12 to 15 mo
- The second dose at age 4 to 6 yr

Adults born during or after 1957 should have 1 dose, unless they have had mumps diagnosed by a health care practitioner. Pregnant women and people with an impaired immune system should not be given such live-attenuated vaccines.

Postexposure vaccination does not protect against mumps from that exposure. Mumps immune globulin is no longer available, and serum immune globulin is not helpful. The Centers for Disease Control and Prevention now recommend isolation of infected patients with standard and respiratory droplet precautions for 5 days after the onset of parotitis. Susceptible contacts should be vaccinated, but this intervention is unlikely to abort an outbreak in progress. Nonimmune asymptomatic healthcare providers should be excused from work from 11 days after the initial exposure until 25 days after the last exposure.

KEY POINTS

- Mumps causes painful enlargement of the salivary glands, most commonly the parotids.
- Cases may occur in vaccinated people because of primary vaccination failure or waning immunity.
- About 20% of infected postpubertal males develop orchitis, usually unilateral; some testicular atrophy may occur, but testosterone production and fertility are usually preserved.
- Other complications include meningoencephalitis and pancreatitis.
- Laboratory diagnosis is done mainly for public health purposes and when disease manifestations are atypical, such as absence of parotitis, unilateral or recurrent parotitis, parotitis in previously immunized patients, or prominent involvement of tissues other than the salivary glands.
- Universal vaccination is imperative unless contraindicated (eg, by pregnancy or severe immunosuppression).

PROGRESSIVE RUBELLA PANENCEPHALITIS

Progressive rubella panencephalitis is a neurologic disorder occurring in children with congenital rubella. It is presumably due to persistence or reactivation of rubella virus infection.

Some children with congenital rubella syndrome (eg, with deafness, cataracts, microcephaly, and intellectual disability) develop neurologic deficits in early adolescence (see p. 2624).

Diagnosis

- CSF examination and serologic testing
- CT
- Sometimes brain biopsy

The diagnosis is considered when a child with congenital rubella develops progressive spasticity, ataxia, mental deterioration, and seizures. Testing involves at least CSF examination and serologic testing. CSF total protein and globulin and rubella antibody titers in CSF and serum are elevated. CT may show ventricular enlargement due to cerebellar atrophy and white matter disease. Brain biopsy may be necessary to exclude other causes of encephalitis or encephalopathy. Rubella virus usually cannot be recovered by viral culture or immunohistologic testing.

Treatment

No specific treatment exists.

RESPIRATORY SYNCYTIAL VIRUS AND HUMAN METAPNEUMOVIRUS INFECTIONS

Respiratory syncytial virus (RSV) and human metapneumovirus (hMPV) infections cause seasonal lower respiratory tract disease, particularly in infants and young children. Disease may be asymptomatic, mild, or severe, including bronchiolitis and pneumonia. Although diagnosis is usually clinical, laboratory diagnosis is available. Treatment is supportive.

RSV is an RNA virus, classified as a pneumovirus. Subgroups A and B have been identified. RSV is ubiquitous; almost all children are infected by age 4 yr. Outbreaks occur annually in winter or early spring in temperate climates. Because the immune response to RSV does not protect against reinfection, the attack rate is about 40% for all exposed people. However, antibody to RSV decreases illness severity. RSV is the most common cause of lower respiratory tract illness in young infants and is responsible for > 50,000 hospitalizations annually in the US in children under the age of 5 yr.

hMPV is a similar but separate virus. The seasonal epidemiology of hMPV appears to be similar to that of RSV, but the incidence of infection and illness appears to be substantially lower.

Symptoms and Signs

RSV and hMPV illness manifest similarly. The most recognizable clinical syndromes are bronchiolitis (see p. 2825) and pneumonia (see p. 478). These illnesses typically begin with upper respiratory symptoms and fever, then progress over several days to dyspnea, cough, wheezing, and/or crackles on chest auscultation. Apnea may be the initial symptom of RSV in infants < 6 mo. In healthy adults and older children, illness is usually mild and may be inapparent or manifested only as an afebrile common cold. However, severe disease may develop in the following:

- Patients who are < 6 mo, elderly, or immunocompromised
- Patients who have underlying cardiopulmonary disorders

Diagnosis

- Clinical evaluation
- Sometimes rapid antigen tests of nasal washings or swabs, reverse-transcription–PCR (RT-PCR), or viral culture

RSV (and possibly hMPV) infection is suspected in infants and young children with bronchiolitis or pneumonia during RSV season. Because antiviral treatment is not typically recommended, a specific laboratory diagnosis is unnecessary for patient management. However, a laboratory diagnosis may facilitate hospital infection control by allowing segregation of children infected with the same virus. Rapid antigen tests with high sensitivities for RSV and other respiratory viruses are available for use in children; nasal washings or swabs are used. These tests are less sensitive in adults. Molecular diagnostic assays such as RT-PCR have improved sensitivity and are generally available as single or multiplex assays.

Treatment

- Supportive care

Treatment of RSV and hMPV infections is supportive and includes supplemental O_2 and hydration as needed (see Bronchiolitis on p. 2825).

Corticosteroids and bronchodilators are generally not helpful and are currently not recommended.

Antibiotics are reserved for patients with fever, evidence of pneumonia on chest x-ray, and clinical suspicion of a bacterial coinfection.

Palivizumab (monoclonal antibody to RSV) is not effective for treatment.

Inhaled ribavirin, an antiviral drug with activity against RSV, has marginal efficacy, is potentially toxic to health care practitioners, and is no longer recommended except for infection in severely immunocompromised patients.

Prevention

Contact precautions (eg, hand washing, gloves, isolation) are important, particularly in hospitals.

Passive prophylaxis with palivizumab decreases the frequency of hospitalization for RSV in high-risk infants. It is cost-effective only for infants at high risk of hospitalization, including those who

- Are < 1 yr with hemodynamically significant congenital heart disease
- Are < 1 yr with chronic lung disease of prematurity (gestational age < 32 wk and 0 days with the need for O_2 therapy for at least 28 days after birth)
- Are born at < 29 wk gestation and are < 1 yr old at the start of RSV season
- Have chronic lung disease of prematurity in the 2nd yr of life and have received treatment (chronic corticosteroid or diuretic treatment or continued need for O_2 therapy) within 6 mo of RSV season

Prophylaxis may also be considered for

- Infants in the 1st yr of life who have anatomic pulmonary abnormalities that impair the ability to effectively clear the upper airways
- Infants who have neuromuscular disorders
- Children < 24 mo who have profound immunocompromise

The dose of palivizumab is 15 mg/kg IM. The first dose is given just before the usual onset of the RSV season (early November in North America). Subsequent doses are given at 1-mo intervals for the duration of the RSV season (usually a total of 5 doses).

KEY POINTS

- RSV and hMPV usually cause a syndrome of bronchiolitis, but pneumonia may occur.
- Diagnosis is usually clinical, but testing, including rapid antigen tests and molecular assays (eg, PCR), is available.
- Give supportive treatment; corticosteroids, bronchodilators, and palivizumab are not recommended.
- Inhaled ribavirin may be useful for RSV but only in severely immunocompromised patients.
- Passive prophylaxis with palivizumab just before and during RSV season decreases the frequency of hospitalization in high-risk infants.

ROSEOLA INFANTUM

(Exanthem Subitum; Pseudorubella)

Roseola infantum is an infection of infants or very young children caused by human herpesvirus 6B (HHV-6B) or, less commonly, HHV-7. The infection causes high fever and a rubelliform eruption that occurs during or after defervescence, but localizing symptoms or signs are absent. Diagnosis is clinical, and treatment is symptomatic.

Roseola infantum is the most well-described illness to result from HHV-6. HHV-6B may also cause CNS disease in immunocompromised patients (eg, hematopoietic stem cell transplant recipients). Roseola infantum occurs most often in the spring and fall. Minor local epidemics have been reported.

Symptoms and Signs

The incubation period is about 5 to 15 days. Fever of 39.5 to 40.5° C begins abruptly and persists 3 to 5 days without any localizing symptoms or signs. Despite the high fever, the child is usually alert and active, although febrile seizures may occur (see p. 2772). Cervical and posterior auricular lymphadenopathy often develops. Encephalitis or hepatitis occurs rarely.

The fever usually falls rapidly on the 4th day, and when the fall occurs, a macular or maculopapular exanthem usually appears prominently on the chest and abdomen and, to a lesser extent, on the face and extremities; it lasts for a few hours to 2 days and may be unnoticed in mild cases. In 70% of HHV-6 infections, the classic exanthem does not occur.

PEARLS & PITFALLS

- In roseola infantum, the characteristic rash occurs with defervescence.

Diagnosis

- Clinical evaluation

It may be suspected when a child aged 6 mo to 3 yr develops typical symptoms and signs. Testing is rarely needed, but diagnosis can be confirmed by culture or serologic tests.

Treatment

- Supportive care

Treatment is generally symptomatic. Foscarnet or ganciclovir has been used to treat some immunosuppressed patients with severe disease, but controlled trials are lacking.

RUBELLA

(German Measles; 3-Day Measles)

(See also Congenital Rubella on p. 2624.)

Rubella is a contagious viral infection that may cause adenopathy, rash, and sometimes constitutional symptoms, which are usually mild and brief. Infection during early pregnancy can cause spontaneous abortion, stillbirth, or congenital defects. Diagnosis is usually clinical. Cases are reported to public health authorities. Treatment is usually unnecessary. Vaccination is effective for prevention.

Rubella is caused by an RNA virus, rubella virus, which is spread by respiratory droplets through close contact or through the air. Patients can transmit rubella during asymptomatic infection or from 7 days before the rash appears until 15 days after onset of the rash; the period of greatest risk is from a few days before the rash appears to 7 days after onset of the rash. Congenitally infected infants (see p. 2624) may transmit rubella for many months after birth.

Rubella is less contagious than measles. Immunity appears to be lifelong after natural infection. However, in unvaccinated populations, 10 to 15% of young adults have not had childhood infection and are susceptible. At present, incidence in the US is at a historic low because of routine childhood vaccination; all cases since 2004 have been linked to importation.

Symptoms and Signs

Many cases are mild. After a 14- to 21-day incubation period, a 1- to 5-day prodrome, usually consisting of low-grade fever, malaise, conjunctivitis, and lymphadenopathy, occurs in adults but may be minimal or absent in children. Tender swelling of the suboccipital, postauricular, and posterior cervical nodes is characteristic. There is pharyngeal injection at the onset.

The rash is similar to that of measles but is less extensive and more evanescent; it is often the first sign in children. It begins on the face and neck and quickly spreads to the trunk and extremities. At onset, a blanching, macular erythema may appear, particularly on the face. On the 2nd day, the rash often becomes more scarlatiniform (pinpoint) with a reddish flush. Petechiae form on the soft palate (Forschheimer spots), later coalescing into a red blush. The rash lasts 3 to 5 days.

Constitutional symptoms in children are absent or mild and may include malaise and occasional arthralgias. Adults usually have few or no constitutional symptoms but occasionally have fever, malaise, headache, stiff joints, transient arthritis, and mild rhinitis. Fever typically resolves by the 2nd day of the rash.

Encephalitis has occurred rarely during large military outbreaks. Complete resolution is typical, but encephalitis is occasionally fatal. Thrombocytopenic purpura and otitis media occur rarely.

Diagnosis

- Clinical evaluation
- Serologic testing

Rubella is suspected in patients with characteristic adenopathy and rash. Laboratory diagnosis is necessary for pregnant women, patients with encephalitis, and neonates. Also, laboratory evaluation is strongly encouraged for all suspected cases of rubella for public health purposes. A ≥ 4-fold rise between acute and convalescent (4 to 8 wk) antibody titers confirms the diagnosis, as can serum rubella IgM antibody testing. Detection of viral RNA by reverse transcription–PCR of throat, nasal, or urine specimens may also be done to confirm the diagnosis; genotype analysis is useful in epidemiologic investigations.

Differential diagnosis includes measles (see p. 2759), scarlet fever (see p. 1605), secondary syphilis (see p. 1708), drug rashes, erythema infectiosum (see p. 2758), and infectious mononucleosis (see p. 1625) as well as echovirus and coxsackievirus infections (see Table 205–1 on p. 1727). Infections with enteroviruses and parvovirus B19 (erythema infectiosum) may be clinically indistinguishable.

Some of these conditions can be distinguished from rubella as follows:

- Measles: Rubella is differentiated from measles by the milder, more evanescent rash, milder and briefer constitutional symptoms, and absence of Koplik spots, photophobia, and cough.
- Scarlet fever: Within a day of onset, scarlet fever usually causes more severe constitutional symptoms and pharyngitis than does rubella.
- Secondary syphilis: In secondary syphilis, adenopathy is not tender, and the rash is usually prominent on the palms and soles. Also, laboratory diagnosis of syphilis is usually readily available.
- Infectious mononucleosis: Infectious mononucleosis can be differentiated by its more severe pharyngitis, more prolonged malaise, and atypical lymphocytosis and with Epstein-Barr virus antibody testing (see p. 1625).

Treatment

- Supportive care

Treatment is symptomatic. No specific therapy for encephalitis is available.

Prevention

Live-virus vaccine is given routinely (see Tables 291–2 on p. 2462 and 291–3 on p. 2467). It produces immunity for ≥ 15 yr in > 95% of recipients and does not appear to transmit the infection. Because certain other infections are clinically indistinguishable from rubella, a reported history of rubella does not guarantee immunity.

Vaccination is given to children as a combined measles, mumps, and rubella vaccine in 2 doses:

- The first dose at age 12 to 15 mo
- The second dose at age 4 to 6 yr

One dose is recommended for all susceptible postpubertal people, especially college students, military recruits, health care practitioners, recent immigrants, and people working with young children. Routine vaccination is recommended for all susceptible mothers immediately after delivery. Screening women of childbearing age for rubella antibodies and immunizing those susceptible are also suggested. However, women receiving the vaccine should prevent conception for at least 28 days afterward. The vaccine virus may be capable of infecting a fetus during early pregnancy. The vaccine does not cause congenital rubella syndrome, but risk of fetal damage is estimated at ≤ 3%. *Vaccine use is contraindicated throughout pregnancy.*

Fever, rash, lymphadenopathy, polyneuropathy, arthralgia, and arthritis occur rarely after vaccination in children; painful joint swelling occasionally follows vaccination in adults, usually in nonimmune women.

KEY POINTS

- Rubella causes a scarlatiniform rash and often low-grade fever, malaise, conjunctivitis, and lymphadenopathy (characteristically involving the suboccipital, postauricular, and posterior cervical nodes).
- Most cases are mild and complications are few except for rare cases of encephalitis and the risk during early pregnancy that infection can cause spontaneous abortion, stillbirth, or congenital defects.
- Laboratory diagnosis is strongly encouraged for all suspected cases for public health purposes; serologic or PCR testing can be done.
- Screen women of childbearing age for rubella antibodies and immunize those susceptible, providing conception is prevented for ≥ 28 days afterwards.
- Vaccination is contraindicated during pregnancy.

SUBACUTE SCLEROSING PANENCEPHALITIS

Subacute sclerosing panencephalitis (SSPE) is a progressive, usually fatal brain disorder occurring months to usually years after an attack of measles. It causes mental deterioration, myoclonic jerks, and seizures. Diagnosis involves EEG, CT or MRI, CSF examination, and measles serologic testing. Treatment is supportive.

SSPE is probably a persistent measles virus infection (see p. 2759). The measles virus is present in brain tissue.

SSPE occurs in about 7 to 300 cases per million people who had wild measles and in about 1 case per million people who received measles vaccine; all cases are probably due to unrecognized measles before vaccination. Males are more often affected. Onset is usually before age 20. SSPE is exceedingly rare in the US and Western Europe.

Symptoms and Signs

Often, the first signs are subtle—diminished performance in schoolwork, forgetfulness, temper tantrums, distractibility, and sleeplessness. However, hallucinations and myoclonic jerks may then occur, followed by generalized seizures. There is further intellectual decline and speech deterioration. Dystonic movements and transient opisthotonos occur. Later, muscular rigidity, dysphagia, cortical blindness, and optic atrophy may occur. Focal chorioretinitis and other funduscopic abnormalities are common. In the final phases, hypothalamic involvement may cause intermittent hyperthermia, diaphoresis, and pulse and BP disturbances.

Diagnosis

- Serologic testing
- EEG
- Neuroimaging

SSPE is suspected in young patients with dementia and neuromuscular irritability. EEG, CT or MRI, CSF examination, and measles serologic testing are done. EEG shows periodic complexes with high-voltage diphasic waves occurring synchronously throughout the recording. CT or MRI may show cortical atrophy or white matter lesions. CSF examination usually reveals normal pressure, cell count, and total protein content; however, CSF globulin is almost always elevated, constituting up to 20 to 60% of CSF protein. Serum and CSF contain elevated levels of measles virus antibodies. Anti-measles IgG appears to increase as the disease progresses.

If test results are inconclusive, brain biopsy may be needed.

Prognosis

The disease is almost invariably fatal within 1 to 3 yr (often pneumonia is the terminal event), although some patients have a more protracted course. A few patients have remissions and exacerbations.

Treatment

- Supportive care

Anticonvulsants and other supportive measures are the only accepted treatments. Isoprinosine, interferon alfa, and lamivudine are controversial, and antiviral drugs have generally not proved helpful.

324 Neurocutaneous Syndromes

NEUROFIBROMATOSIS

Neurofibromatosis refers to several related disorders that have overlapping clinical manifestations but that are now understood to have distinct genetic causes. It causes various types of benign or malignant tumors that involve central or peripheral nerves and often causes pigmented skin macules and sometimes other manifestations. Diagnosis is clinical. There is no specific treatment, but benign tumors can be removed surgically, and malignant tumors (which are less common) can be treated with radiation therapy or chemotherapy.

Neurofibromatosis is a neurocutaneous syndrome (a syndrome with neurologic and cutaneous manifestations).

Types

There are several types of neurofibromatosis.

Neurofibromatosis type 1 (NF1, or von Recklinghausen disease) is most prevalent, occurring in 1 of 2500 to 3000 people. It causes neurologic, cutaneous, and sometimes soft-tissue or bone manifestations. The gene for NF1 is located on band 17q11.2 and encodes synthesis of neurofibromin; > 1000 mutations have been identified. Although it is an autosomal dominant disorder, 20 to 50% of cases are caused by a de novo germ cell mutation.

Neurofibromatosis type 2 (NF2) accounts for 10% of cases, occurring in about 1 of 35,000 people. It manifests primarily as congenital bilateral acoustic neuromas (vestibular schwannomas). The gene for NF2 is located on band 22q11 and encodes synthesis of merlin, a tumor suppressor; 200 mutations have been identified. Most people with NF2 inherited it from one of their parents.

Schwannomatosis, a rare disorder, is classified as a 3rd type of neurofibromatosis. In 15% of cases, this type is familial and related to a germline mutation in the *SMARCB1* gene, a tumor suppressor gene located at 22q11.23, very close to the *NF2* gene. In the remaining cases, the genetic basis is not well-understood, but in tissue from some patients, other mutations in the same gene are involved. Two or more schwannomas develop in peripheral nerves and are sometimes quite painful; however, acoustic neuromas do not develop. Schwannomatosis used to be considered a form of NF2 because multiple schwannomas are seen in both conditions; however, the clinical picture is different, and the genes involved are distinct.

Peripheral and central neurofibromas: Tumors may be peripheral or central.

Peripheral tumors are common in NF1 and can develop anywhere along the course of peripheral nerves. The tumors are neurofibromas, which develop from nerve sheaths and consist of mixtures of Schwann cells, fibroblasts, neural cells, and mast cells. Most appear during adolescence. Occasionally, they transform to malignant peripheral nerve sheath tumors. There are multiple forms:

- **Cutaneous neurofibromas** are soft and fleshy.
- **Subcutaneous neurofibromas** are firm and nodular.
- **Nodular plexiform neurofibromas** may involve spinal nerve roots, typically growing through an intervertebral foramen to cause intraspinal and extraspinal masses (dumbbell tumor). The intraspinal part may compress the spinal cord.
- **Diffuse plexiform neurofibromas** (subcutaneous nodules or amorphous overgrowth of underlying bone or Schwann cells) can be disfiguring and may cause deficits distal to the neurofibroma. These neurofibromas can become malignant.
- **Schwannomas** are derived from Schwann cells, rarely undergo malignant transformation, and can occur in peripheral nerves anywhere in the body.

Central tumors have several forms:

- **Optic gliomas:** These tumors are low-grade pilocytic astrocytomas, which may be asymptomatic or may progress enough to compress the optic nerve and cause blindness. They occur in younger children; these tumors can usually be identified by age 5 and rarely develop after age 10. They occur in NF1.
- **Acoustic neuromas (vestibular schwannomas):** These tumors may cause dizziness, ataxia, deafness, and tinnitus due to compression of the 8th cranial nerve; they sometimes cause facial weakness due to compression of the adjacent 7th nerve. They are the distinguishing feature of NF2.
- **Meningiomas:** These tumors develop in some people, particularly those with NF2.

Symptoms and Signs

Type 1: Most patients with type 1 neurofibromatosis are asymptomatic. Some present with neurologic symptoms or bone deformities. In > 90%, characteristic skin lesions are apparent at birth or develop during infancy.

Lesions are medium-brown (café-au-lait—see Plate 91), freckle-like macules, distributed most commonly over the trunk, pelvis, and flexor creases of elbows and knees. During late childhood, flesh-colored cutaneous tumors of various sizes and shapes appear, ranging in number from several to thousands. Rarely, plexiform neurofibromas develop, causing an irregularly thickened, distorted structure with grotesque deformities.

Although unaffected children may have 2 or 3 café-au-lait macules, children with NF1 have ≥ 6 such macules and often many more.

Neurologic symptoms vary, depending on location and number of neurofibromas.

Bone abnormalities include

- Fibrous dysplasia
- Subperiosteal bone cysts
- Vertebral scalloping
- Scoliosis
- Thinning of the long-bone cortex
- Pseudarthrosis
- Absence of the greater wing of the sphenoid bone (posterior orbital wall), with consequent pulsating exophthalmos

An optic glioma and Lisch nodules (iris hamartomas) occur in some patients. Changes in arterial walls may lead to Moyamoya disease or intracranial artery aneurysms. Some children have learning problems and slightly larger heads.

Children and adolescents with NF1 may have childhood chronic myelomonocytic leukemia (juvenile myelomonocytic leukemia) and rhabdomyosarcoma. Pheochromocytomas may occur at any age.

Malignant tumors are much less common but still more common than in the general population; they include supratentorial or brain stem gliomas and transformation of plexiform neurofibromas to malignant peripheral nerve sheath tumors. These tumors may develop at any age.

Type 2: In type 2 neurofibromatosis, bilateral acoustic neuromas develop and become symptomatic during childhood or early adulthood. They cause hearing loss, unsteadiness, and sometimes headache or facial weakness. Bilateral 8th cranial (vestibulocochlear) nerve masses may be present. Family members may have gliomas, meningiomas, or schwannomas.

Schwannomatosis: In schwannomatosis, multiple schwannomas develop on cranial, spinal, and peripheral nerves. Acoustic neuromas do not develop, and patients do not become deaf. Also, the other types of tumors that sometimes occur in neurocutaneous disorders do not develop.

The first symptom of schwannomatosis is usually pain, which may become chronic and severe. Other symptoms may develop, depending on the location of the schwannomas.

Diagnosis

- Clinical evaluation
- CT or MRI

Most patients with NF1 are identified during routine examination, examination for cosmetic complaints, or evaluation of a positive family history.

Diagnosis of all 3 types is clinical (see Table 324–1). For the few children who have 3 to 5 café-au-lait macules of > 5 mm diameter, the absence of Lisch nodules on ophthalmologic examination suggests NF1 is not present.

MRI is done in patients with neurologic symptoms or signs and, when detailed visual testing is not possible, in younger children who meet the clinical criteria for NF1 and who may have an optic glioma. T2-weighted MRI may show optic nerve swelling and parenchymal hyperintense lesions that change over time and correlate with small cystic structures in NF1; MRI may help identify acoustic neuromas or meningiomas in NF2. If acoustic neuroma is suspected, CT of the petrous ridge can be done; it typically shows widening of the auditory canal.

Genetic testing is not typically done in these disorders because not all mutations are known and the clinical criteria are clear.

Treatment

- Possibly surgery or irradiation

No general treatment for neurofibromatosis is available. Neurofibromas that cause severe symptoms may require surgical removal or irradiation, although surgery may obliterate function of the involved nerve. Optic gliomas or CNS lesions that have become malignant may be treated with radiation therapy or chemotherapy.

Genetic counseling is advisable. If either parent has neurofibromatosis, risk to subsequent offspring is 50%; if neither has it, risk for subsequent children is unclear because new mutations are common, particularly in NF1.

Table 324–1. DIAGNOSING NEUROFIBROMATOSIS

TYPE	CRITERIA
NF1	≥ 2 of the following must be present: • ≥ 6 café-au-lait macules with a diameter at the widest point of > 5 mm in prepubertal patients and > 15 mm in postpubertal patients • ≥ 2 neurofibromas of any type or 1 plexiform neurofibroma • Freckling in the axillary or inguinal region • Optic glioma • ≥ 2 Lisch nodules (iris hamartomas) • A distinctive osseous lesion (eg, sphenoid dysplasia, thinning of long-bone cortex), with or without pseudarthrosis • A parent or sibling with diagnosed type 1 neurofibromatosis
NF2	1 of the following must be present: • Bilateral 8th nerve masses seen with CT or MRI • A parent or sibling with type 2 neurofibromatosis and either a unilateral 8th nerve mass or any 2 of the following: Neurofibroma, meningioma, glioma, schwannoma, or juvenile posterior subcapsular lenticular opacity
Schwannomatosis	• ≥ 2 nonintradermal schwannomas (at least one pathologically determined) • No evidence of vestibular neuroma on high-resolution MRI • No known *NF1* gene mutation • A pathologically confirmed nonvestibular schwannoma and a 1st-degree relative who meets the criteria above

Adapted from Martuza RL, Eldredge R: Neurofibromatosis 2 (bilateral acoustic neurofibromatosis). Reprinted by permission of *The New England Journal of Medicine* 318:684–688, 1988; additional data from Plotkin SR, Blakeley JO, Evans DG, et al: Update from the 2011 International Schwannomatosis Workshop: From genetics to diagnostic criteria. *American Journal of Medical Genetics* (part A) 161(3):405–416, 2013 and Chen SL, Liu C, Liu B, et al: Schwannomatosis: a new member of neurofibromatosis family. *Chinese Medical Journal* (English) 126(14):2656–2660, 2013.

KEY POINTS

- There are 3 types of neurofibromatosis: NF1, NF2, and schwannomatosis, caused by gene mutations.
- NF1 causes cutaneous, neurologic, and bone abnormalities.
- NF2 causes bilateral acoustic neuromas.
- Schwannomatosis causes multiple nonintradermal schwannomas; it does not cause acoustic neuromas.
- Diagnosis is made using clinical criteria; neuroimaging is done if patients have neurologic abnormalities.
- There is no specific treatment, but neurofibromas that cause severe symptoms may be removed surgically or treated with radiation therapy.

STURGE-WEBER SYNDROME

Sturge-Weber syndrome is a congenital vascular disorder characterized by a facial port-wine nevus, a leptomeningeal angioma, and neurologic complications (eg, seizures, focal neurologic deficits, intellectual disability).

Sturge-Weber syndrome is a neurocutaneous syndrome that occurs in 1 in 50,000 people. Sturge-Weber syndrome is not inherited. It is caused by a somatic mutation (a change in DNA that occurs after conception in the precursors of the affected area) in the *GNAQ* gene on chromosome 9q21.

Sturge-Weber syndrome causes a capillary malformation called a port-wine nevus (or sometimes a stain or birth mark) typically on the forehead and upper eyelid in the distribution of the 1st and/or 2nd division of the trigeminal nerve. A similar vascular lesion—leptomeningeal angioma—occurs in 90% of patients when the port-wine nevus involves upper and lower eyelids on one side but in only 10 to 20% when only one eyelid is affected. Usually, the nevi and leptomeningeal angiomas are unilateral, but rarely, patients have bilateral port-wine nevi in the distribution of the 1st division of the trigeminal nerve and bilateral leptomeningeal angiomas.

A port-wine nevus may occur without a leptomeningeal angioma and its accompanying neurologic signs; in such cases, the eyes and eyelids may or may not be involved. Rarely, a leptomeningeal angioma occurs without the port-wine nevus and ocular involvement.

Neurologic complications include seizures, focal neurologic deficits (eg, hemiparesis), and intellectual disability.

Sturge-Weber syndrome can also cause glaucoma and vascular narrowing, which may increase risk of vascular events (eg, stroke, thrombosis, venous occlusion, infarction).

Often, the involved cerebral hemisphere progressively atrophies.

Symptoms and Signs

The port-wine nevus can vary in size and color, ranging from light pink to deep purple.

Seizures occur in about 75 to 90% of patients and typically start by age 1 yr. Seizures are usually focal but can become generalized. Hemiparesis of the side opposite the port-wine nevus occurs in 25 to 50% of patients. Sometimes the hemiparesis worsens, especially in patients whose seizures cannot be controlled.

About 50% of patients have intellectual disability, and more have some kind of learning difficulty. Development may be delayed.

Glaucoma may be present at birth or develop later. The eyeball may enlarge and bulge out of its socket (buphthalmos).

Diagnosis

- MRI or CT

Diagnosis of Sturge-Weber syndrome is suggested by a characteristic port-wine nevus.

MRI with contrast is used to check for a leptomeningeal angioma, but the angioma may not yet show up in very young children. If MRI is not available, CT may be done; it may show calcifications in the cortex under the leptomeningeal angioma. The parallel curvilinear railroad-track calcifications seen on skull x-rays as mentioned in older literature develop during adulthood.

A neurologic examination is done to check for neurologic complications, and an ophthalmologic examination is done to check for eye complications.

Treatment

- Symptomatic treatment

Treatment of Sturge-Weber syndrome focuses on symptoms. Anticonvulsants and drugs to treat glaucoma are used. Sometimes hemispherectomy is done if patients have intractable seizures.

Low-dose aspirin is usually given, starting at the time of diagnosis, to help prevent strokes or lessen the progressive hemispheric atrophy presumably by preventing sludging in the abnormal capillaries.

Selective photothermolysis can lighten the port-wine nevus.

TUBEROUS SCLEROSIS

Tuberous sclerosis (TS) is a dominantly inherited genetic disorder in which tumors (usually hamartomas) develop in multiple organs. Diagnosis requires imaging of the affected organ. Treatment is symptomatic or, if CNS tumors are growing, everolimus. Patients must be monitored regularly to check for complications.

TS is a neurocutaneous syndrome that occurs in 1 of 6000 children; 85% of cases involve mutations in the *TSC1* gene (9q34), which controls the production of hamartin, or the *TSC2* gene (16p13.3), which controls the production of tuberin. These proteins act as growth suppressors. If either parent has the disorder, children have a 50% risk of having it. However, new mutations account for two-thirds of cases.

Patients with TS (sometimes called tuberous sclerosis complex) have tumors or abnormalities that manifest at different ages and in multiple organs, including the

- Brain
- Heart
- Eyes
- Kidneys
- Lungs
- Skin

CNS tubers interrupt neural circuits, causing developmental delay and cognitive impairment and may cause seizures, including infantile spasms. Sometimes the tubers grow and obstruct CSF flow from the lateral ventricles, causing unilateral hydrocephalus. Sometimes tubers undergo malignant degeneration into gliomas, particularly subependymal giant cell astrocytomas.

Cardiac myomas may develop prenatally, sometimes causing heart failure in neonates. These myomas tend to disappear over time and usually do not cause symptoms later in childhood or in adulthood.

Kidney tumors (angiolipomas) may develop in adults, and polycystic kidney disease may develop at any age. Kidney disease may cause hypertension.

Pulmonary lesions, such as lymphangioleiomyomatosis, may develop, particularly in adolescent girls.

Symptoms and Signs

Manifestations vary greatly in severity. Skin lesions are typically present.

Infants with CNS lesions may present with a type of seizure called infantile spasms. Affected children may also have other types of seizures, intellectual disability, autism, learning disorders, or behavioral problems.

Retinal patches are common and may be visible with funduscopy.

Pitting of enamel in permanent teeth is common.

Skin findings include

- Initially pale, ash leaf–shaped macules, which develop during infancy or early childhood
- Angiofibromas of the face (adenoma sebaceum), which develop during later childhood
- Congenital shagreen patches (raised lesions resembling an orange peel), usually on the back
- Subcutaneous nodules
- Café-au-lait spots
- Subungual fibromas, which can develop any time during childhood or early adulthood

Diagnosis

- Identification of the skin lesions
- Imaging of affected organs
- Genetic testing

TS may be suspected when fetal ultrasonography detects cardiac myomas or when infantile spasms occur.

Physical examination is done to check for typical skin lesions. Funduscopy should be done to check for retinal patches.

Cardiac or cranial manifestations may be visible on routine prenatal ultrasonography. MRI or ultrasonography of the affected organs is necessary for confirmation.

Specific genetic testing is available.

Prognosis

Prognosis depends on symptom severity. Infants with mild symptoms generally do well and live long, productive lives; infants with severe symptoms may have serious disabilities.

Regardless of severity, most children show continued developmental progress.

Treatment

- Symptomatic treatment
- Everolimus

Treatment is both symptomatic and specific:

- For seizures: Anticonvulsants (especially vigabatrin for infantile spasms) or sometimes epilepsy surgery
- For skin lesions: Dermabrasion or laser techniques
- For neurobehavioral problems: Behavior management techniques or drugs
- For hypertension caused by renal problems: Antihypertensives or surgery to remove growing tumors
- For developmental delays: Special schooling or occupational therapy
- For malignant tumors and some of the benign tumors: Everolimus

Genetic counseling is indicated for adolescents and adults of childbearing age.

Screening for complications: All patients should be screened regularly to detect complications early.

Typically, the following is done:

- MRI of the head to check for intracranial complications at least every 3 yr
- Renal ultrasonography to check for kidney tumors every 3 yr in school-aged children and every 1 to 2 yr in adults

- Chest x-ray in girls in their late teens
- Neuropsychologic testing periodically in children to help plan for support at school

Use of sirolimus and its derivative, everolimus, to prevent and treat most of the complications of TS is under study.

Clinical monitoring is also important and sometimes prompts more frequent testing. Development of headaches, loss of skills, or new kinds of seizures may be caused by malignant degeneration or growth of CNS tubers and are indications for neuroimaging.

VON HIPPEL–LINDAU DISEASE

Von Hippel–Lindau (VHL) disease is a rare hereditary neurocutaneous disorder characterized by benign and malignant tumors in multiple organs. Diagnosis is with ophthalmoscopy or imaging to check for tumors. Treatment is with surgery or sometimes radiation therapy or, for retinal angiomas, laser coagulation or cryotherapy.

VHL is a neurocutaneous syndrome that occurs in 1 of 36,000 people and is inherited as an autosomal dominant trait with variable penetrance. The *VHL* gene is located on the short arm of chromosome 3 (3p25.3). Over 1500 different mutations in this gene have been identified in patients with VHL. In 20% of affected people, the abnormal gene appears to be a new mutation.

VHL most commonly causes cerebellar hemangioblastomas and retinal angiomas. Tumors, including pheochromocytomas and cysts (renal, hepatic, pancreatic, or genital tract), can occur in other organs. About 10% of people with VHL develop an endolymphatic tumor in the inner ear, threatening hearing. Risk of developing renal cell carcinoma increases with age and by age 60 may be as high as 70%.

Manifestations typically appear between ages 10 and 30 but can appear earlier.

Symptoms and Signs

Symptoms of VHL depend on the size and location of the tumors. Symptoms may include headaches, dizziness, weakness, ataxia, impaired vision, and high BP.

Retinal angiomas, detected by direct ophthalmoscopy, appear as a dilated artery leading from the disk to a peripheral tumor with an engorged vein. These angiomas are usually asymptomatic, but if they are centrally located and enlarge, they can result in substantial loss of vision. These tumors increase risk of retinal detachment, macular edema, and glaucoma.

Untreated, VHL can result in blindness, brain damage, or death. Death usually results from complications of cerebellar hemangioblastomas or renal cell carcinoma.

Diagnosis

- Direct ophthalmoscopy
- CNS imaging, typically MRI
- Genetic testing

VHL disease is diagnosed when typical tumors are detected and one of the following criteria is met:

- More than one tumor in the brain or eye
- Single tumor in the brain or eye and one elsewhere in the body
- Family history of VHL and presence of a tumor

Children who have a parent or sibling with the disorder should be evaluated before age 5 yr; evaluation should include ophthalmoscopy and brain MRI to determine whether the diagnostic criteria are met. If a specific mutation for VHL gene is identified in a patient, genetic testing should be done to determine whether at-risk family members also have that mutation.

Treatment

- Surgery or sometimes radiation therapy
- For retinal angiomas, laser coagulation or cryotherapy
- Regular monitoring

Treatment often involves surgical removal of the tumor before it becomes harmful. Some tumors can be treated with focused high-dose radiation. Typically, retinal angiomas are treated with laser coagulation or cryotherapy to preserve vision.

Use of propranolol to reduce the size of the hemangiomas is being studied.

Screening to check for complications and early treatment can improve prognosis.

Screening for complications: If the diagnostic criteria for VHL are met, patients should be regularly screened to check for complications of VHL because early detection is key to preventing serious complications.

Annual screening should include neurologic examination, BP monitoring, hearing screening, ophthalmoscopy, and measurement of urine or plasma fractionated metanephrines (to screen for pheochromocytoma). Formal audiologic evaluation should be done at least every 3 yr. After age 16, abdominal ultrasonography should be done annually to screen for renal tumors; every 2 yr, MRI of the brain and spinal cord should be done to screen for new CNS tumors or changes in existing tumors.

325 Neurologic Disorders in Children

CEREBRAL PALSY SYNDROMES

Cerebral palsy (CP) refers to nonprogressive syndromes characterized by impaired voluntary movement or posture and resulting from prenatal developmental malformations or perinatal or postnatal CNS damage. Syndromes manifest before age 2 yr. Diagnosis is clinical. Treatment may include physical and occupational therapy, braces, drug therapy or botulinum toxin injections, orthopedic surgery, intrathecal baclofen, or, in certain cases, dorsal rhizotomy.

CP is a group of syndromes that causes nonprogressive spasticity, ataxia, or involuntary movements; it is not a specific disorder or single syndrome. CP syndromes occur in 0.1 to 0.2% of children and affect up to 15% of premature infants.

Etiology

Etiology is multifactorial, and a specific cause is sometimes hard to establish. Prematurity, in utero disorders, neonatal encephalopathy, and kernicterus often contribute. Perinatal factors (eg, perinatal asphyxia, stroke, CNS infections) probably cause 15 to 20% of cases.

Examples of types of CP are

- Spastic diplegia after premature birth
- Spastic quadriparesis after perinatal asphyxia
- Athetoid and dystonic forms after perinatal asphyxia or kernicterus

CNS trauma or a severe systemic disorder (eg, stroke, meningitis, sepsis, dehydration) during early childhood (before age 2 yr) may also cause a CP syndrome.

Symptoms and Signs

Before a specific syndrome develops, symptoms include lagging motor development and often persistent infantile reflex patterns, hyperreflexia, and altered muscle tone.

Categories of CP syndromes: Syndromes are categorized mainly as one of the following, depending on which parts of the CNS are malformed or damaged:

- **Spastic syndromes** occur in > 70% of cases. Spasticity is a state of resistance to passive range of motion; resistance increases with increasing speed of that motion. It is due to upper motor neuron involvement and may mildly or severely affect motor function. These syndromes may cause hemiplegia, quadriplegia, diplegia, or paraplegia. Usually, deep tendon reflexes in affected limbs are increased, muscles are hypertonic, and voluntary movements are weak and poorly coordinated. Joint contractures develop, and joints may become misaligned. A scissors gait and toe walking are typical. In mild cases, impairment may occur only during certain activities (eg, running). Corticobulbar impairment of oral, lingual, and palatal movement, with consequent dysarthria or dysphagia, commonly occurs with quadriplegia.
- **Athetoid or dyskinetic syndromes** occur in about 20% of cases and result from basal ganglia involvement. The syndromes are defined by slow, writhing, involuntary movements of the proximal extremities and trunk (athetoid movements), often activated by attempts at voluntary movement or by excitement. Abrupt, jerky, distal (choreic) movements may also occur. Movements increase with emotional tension and disappear during sleep. Dysarthria occurs and is often severe.
- **Ataxic syndromes** occur in < 5% of cases and result from involvement of the cerebellum or its pathways. Weakness, incoordination, and intention tremor cause unsteadiness, a wide-based gait, and difficulty with rapid or fine movements.
- **Mixed syndromes** are common—most often with spasticity and athetosis.

Findings associated with CP: About 25% of patients, most often those with spasticity, have other manifestations. Strabismus and other visual defects may occur. Children with athetosis due to kernicterus commonly have nerve deafness and upward gaze paralysis.

Many children with spastic hemiplegia or paraplegia have normal intelligence; children with spastic quadriplegia or a mixed syndrome may have severe intellectual disability.

Diagnosis

- Cranial MRI
- Sometimes testing to exclude hereditary metabolic or neurologic disorders

If CP is suspected, identifying the underlying disorder is important. History may suggest a cause. A cranial MRI is done; it can detect abnormalities in most cases.

CP can rarely be confirmed during early infancy, and the specific syndrome often cannot be characterized until age 2 yr. High-risk children (eg, those with evidence of asphyxia, stroke, periventricular abnormalities seen on cranial ultrasonography in premature infants, jaundice, meningitis, neonatal seizures, hypertonia, hypotonia, or reflex suppression) should be followed closely.

Differential diagnosis: CP should be differentiated from progressive hereditary neurologic disorders and disorders requiring surgical or other specific neurologic treatments.

Ataxic forms are particularly hard to distinguish, and in many children with persistent ataxia, a progressive cerebellar degenerative disorder is ultimately identified as the cause.

Athetosis, self-mutilation, and hyperuricemia in boys indicate Lesch-Nyhan syndrome.

Cutaneous or ocular abnormalities may indicate tuberous sclerosis, neurofibromatosis, ataxia-telangiectasia, von Hippel–Lindau disease, or Sturge-Weber syndrome.

Infantile spinal muscular atrophy, muscular dystrophies, and neuromuscular junction disorders associated with hypotonia and hyporeflexia usually lack signs of cerebral disease.

Adrenoleukodystrophy begins later in childhood, but other leukodystrophies begin earlier and may be mistaken for CP at first.

Identification of a cause: When history and/or cranial MRI does not clearly identify a cause, laboratory tests should be done to exclude certain progressive storage disorders that involve the motor system (eg, Tay-Sachs disease, metachromatic leukodystrophy, mucopolysaccharidoses) and metabolic disorders (eg, organic or amino acid metabolism disorders).

Other progressive disorders (eg, infantile neuroaxonal dystrophy) may be suggested by nerve conduction studies and electromyography. These and many other brain disorders that cause CP (and other manifestations) are being increasingly identified with genetic testing, which may be done to check for a specific disorder or to screen for many disorders (microarray and whole genome testing).

Prognosis

Most children survive to adulthood. Severe limitations in sucking and swallowing, which may require feeding by gastrostomy tube, decrease life expectancy.

The goal is for children to develop maximal independence within the limits of their motor and associated deficits. With appropriate management, many children, especially those with spastic paraplegia or hemiplegia, can lead near-normal lives.

Treatment

- Physical and occupational therapy
- Braces, constraint therapy, drugs, or surgery to treat spasticity
- Botulinum toxin injections
- Intrathecal baclofen
- Assistive devices

Physical therapy and occupational therapy for stretching, strengthening, and facilitating good movement patterns are usually used first and are continued. Bracing, constraint therapy, and drugs may be added.

Botulinum toxin may be injected into muscles to decrease their uneven pull at joints and to prevent fixed contractures.

Baclofen, benzodiazepines (eg, diazepam), tizanidine, and sometimes dantrolene may diminish spasticity. Intrathecal baclofen (via subcutaneous pump and catheter) is the most effective treatment for severe spasticity.

Orthopedic surgery (eg, muscle-tendon release or transfer) may help reduce restricted joint motion or misalignment.

Selective dorsal rhizotomy, done by neurosurgeons, may help a few children if spasticity affects primarily the legs and if cognitive abilities are good.

When intellectual limitations are not severe, children may attend mainstream classes and take part in adapted exercise programs and even competition. Speech training or other forms of facilitated communication may be needed to enhance interactions.

Some severely affected children can benefit from training in activities of daily living (eg, washing, dressing, feeding), which increases their independence and self-esteem and greatly reduces the burden for family members or other caregivers. Assistive devices may increase mobility and communication, help maintain range of motion, and help with activities of daily living. Some children require varying degrees of lifelong supervision and assistance.

Many children's facilities are establishing transition programs for patients as they become adults and have fewer supports to help with special needs.

Parents of a child with chronic limitations need assistance and guidance in understanding the child's status and potential and in dealing with their own feelings of guilt, anger, denial, and sadness (see p. 2481). These children reach their maximal potential only with stable, sensible parental care and the assistance of public and private agencies (eg, community health agencies, vocational rehabilitation organizations, lay health organizations such as the United Cerebral Palsy Association.

KEY POINTS

- CP is a syndrome (not a specific disorder) that involves nonprogressive spasticity, ataxia, and/or involuntary movements.
- Etiology is often multifactorial and sometimes unclear but involves prenatal and perinatal factors that are associated with CNS malformation or damage (eg, genetic and in utero disorders, prematurity, kernicterus, perinatal asphyxia, stroke, CNS infections).
- Intellectual disability and other neurologic manifestations (eg, strabismus, deafness) are not part of the syndrome but may be present depending on the cause.
- Syndromes manifest before age 2 yr; later onset of similar symptoms suggests another neurologic disorder.
- Do cranial MRI and, if needed, testing for hereditary metabolic and neurologic disorders.
- Treatment depends on the nature and degree of disability, but physical therapy and occupational therapy are typically used; some children benefit from bracing, botulinum toxin, benzodiazepines, other muscle relaxants, intrathecal baclofen, and/or surgery (eg, muscle-tendon release or transfer, rarely dorsal rhizotomy).

FEBRILE SEIZURES

Febrile seizures are diagnosed in children < 6 yr with body temperature > 38° C and no previous afebrile seizures when no cause can be identified and no underlying developmental or neurologic problem exists. Diagnosis is clinical after exclusion of other causes. Treatment of seizures lasting < 15 min is supportive. Seizures lasting ≥ 15 min are treated with IV lorazepam, rectal diazepam, or intranasal midazolam and, if persistent, IV fosphenytoin, phenobarbital, valproate, or levetiracetam. Maintenance drug therapy is usually not indicated.

Febrile seizures occur in about 2 to 5% of children < 6 yr; most occur at age 6 to 36 mo. Febrile seizures may be simple or complex:

- **Simple febrile seizures** last < 15 min and have no focal features.
- **Complex febrile seizures** last ≥ 15 min continuously or with pauses, have focal features, or recur within 24 h.

Most (> 90%) febrile seizures are simple.

Febrile seizures occur during bacterial or viral infections. They sometimes occur after certain vaccinations such as measles, mumps, and rubella. Genetic and familial factors appear to increase susceptibility to febrile seizures. Monozygotic twins have a much higher concordance rate than dizygotic twins. Several genes associated with febrile seizures have been identified.

Symptoms and Signs

Often, febrile seizures occur during the initial rapid rise in body temperature, and most develop within 24 h of fever onset. Typically, seizures are generalized; most are clonic, but some manifest as periods of atonic or tonic posturing.

A postictal period of a few minutes is common but may last as long as a few hours. If the postictal period is longer than an hour or if children have focal features (eg, diminished movement on one side) during this period, it is important to immediately evaluate for an underlying acute CNS disorder.

Febrile status epilepticus is continuous or intermittent seizures that last ≥ 20 min without neurologic recovery between them.

Diagnosis

- Exclusion of other causes clinically or sometimes by testing

Seizures are diagnosed as febrile after exclusion of other causes. A fever may trigger seizures in children with previous afebrile seizures; such events are not termed febrile seizures because these children have already shown a tendency to have seizures.

Routine testing is not required for simple febrile seizures other than to look for the source of the fever, but if children have complex seizures, neurologic deficits, or signs of a serious underlying disorder (eg, meningitis, metabolic disorders), testing should be done.

Tests to exclude other disorders are determined clinically:

- CSF analysis to rule out meningitis and encephalitis if children are < 6 mo, have meningeal signs or signs of CNS depression, or have seizures after several days of febrile illness and consideration of CSF analysis if children are not fully immunized or are taking antibiotics
- Serum glucose, sodium, calcium, magnesium, and phosphorus and liver and kidney function tests to rule out metabolic disorders if the history includes recent vomiting, diarrhea, or impaired fluid intake; if there are signs of dehydration or edema; or if a complex febrile seizure occurs
- Cranial MRI if neurologic examination detects focal abnormalities or if focal features occur during the seizure or postictal period
- EEG if febrile seizures have focal features or are recurrent
- A diagnostic evaluation based on the underlying disorder if children have an already identified developmental or neurologic disorder (usually, the term febrile seizure is not used in such cases)

EEG typically does not identify specific abnormalities or help predict recurrent seizures; it is not recommended after an initial simple febrile seizure in children with a normal neurologic examination.

Prognosis

Recurrence and subsequent epilepsy: Overall recurrence rate of febrile seizures is about 35%. Risk of recurrence is higher if children are < 1 yr when the initial seizure occurs or have 1st-degree relatives who have had febrile seizures. Risk of developing an afebrile seizure disorder after having ≥ 1 simple febrile seizures is about 2 to 5%—slightly higher than the baseline risk of developing epilepsy (about 2%).

Most of the increased risk occurs in children who have additional risk factors (eg, complex febrile seizures, family history of seizures, developmental delay); in these children, risk is increased up to 10%. It is unclear whether having a febrile seizure can itself permanently lower the seizure threshold or whether some underlying factors predispose children to both febrile and nonfebrile seizures.

Neurologic sequelae: Simple febrile seizures themselves are not thought to cause neurologic abnormalities. However, in some children with an unrecognized neurologic disorder, a febrile seizure may be the first manifestation; signs of the disorder may be identified retrospectively or not appear until later. In either case, the febrile seizure is not thought to be causal.

Prolonged febrile status epilepticus may be associated with damage to vulnerable parts of the brain such as the hippocampus.

Treatment

- Antipyretic therapy
- Supportive therapy if seizures last < 15 min
- Anticonvulsants and sometimes intubation if seizures last ≥ 15 min

All children require antipyretic therapy; lowering temperature can help prevent another febrile seizure during the immediate illness and makes it easier to stop febrile status epilepticus.

Treatment is supportive if seizures last < 15 min.

Seizures lasting > 15 min may require drugs to end them, with careful monitoring of circulatory and respiratory status. Intubation may be necessary if response is not immediate and the seizure persists.

Drug therapy is usually IV, with a short-acting benzodiazepine (eg, lorazepam 0.05 to 0.1 mg/kg IV over 2 to 5 min repeated q 5 to 10 min for up to 3 doses). Fosphenytoin 15 to 20 mg PE (phenytoin equivalents)/kg IV may be given over 15 to 30 min if the seizure persists. In children up to 5 yr, diazepam rectal gel 0.5 mg/kg may be given once and repeated in 4 to 12 h if lorazepam cannot be given IV. Phenobarbital, valproate, or levetiracetam can also be used to treat a persistent seizure.

Prevention: Parents of a child who has had a febrile seizure should be advised to carefully monitor their child's temperature during illnesses and to give antipyretics if temperature is elevated (even though controlled studies have not shown that this treatment prevents febrile seizures from recurring).

Maintenance anticonvulsant drug therapy to prevent recurrent febrile seizures or development of afebrile seizures is usually not indicated unless multiple or prolonged episodes have occurred. Some clinicians prescribe rectal diazepam to be given by the parents at home for a prolonged febrile seizure.

KEY POINTS

- Febrile seizures are seizures that occur in neurologically normal children < 6 yr with a temperature of > 38° C and no previous afebrile seizures and that have no identifiable cause.
- Simple febrile seizures last < 15 min and have no focal features.
- Complex febrile seizures last > 15 min continuously or with pauses, have focal features, or recur within 24 h.
- Routine testing is not required, but if children have complex seizures, neurologic deficits, or signs of a serious underlying disorder (eg, meningitis, metabolic disorders), testing should be done.
- Seizures lasting ≥15 min require drug treatment (eg, lorazepam 0.05 to 0.1 mg/kg IV over 2 to 5 min repeated q 5 to 10 min for up to 3 doses).
- Risk of developing an afebrile seizure disorder after having a simple febrile seizure is about 2 to 5%.
- Giving an antipyretic at the beginning of a febrile illness has not been shown to prevent a febrile seizure.

INFANTILE SPASMS

(Salaam Seizures)

Infantile spasms are seizures characterized by sudden flexion of the arms, forward flexion of the trunk, extension of the legs, and hypsarrhythmia on EEG.

Infantile spasms last a few seconds and can recur many times a day. They usually manifest in children < 1 yr. Seizures may resolve spontaneously by about age 5 yr but are often replaced by other types of seizures.

Pathophysiology is unknown; however, infantile spasms may reflect abnormal interactions between the cortex and brain stem.

Causes

Usually, infantile spasms occur in infants with serious brain disorders and developmental abnormalities that often have already been recognized. These disorders may include

- Injuries to the brain during the perinatal period
- Metabolic disorders
- Brain malformations

Tuberous sclerosis is a common cause; prognosis is sometimes better when seizures are caused by this disorder than when seizures have other identifiable causes.

Sometimes the cause cannot be identified.

Symptoms and Signs

Spasms begin with a sudden, rapid, tonic contraction of the trunk and limbs, sometimes for several seconds. Spasms range from subtle head nodding to contraction of the whole body. They involve flexion, extension, or, more often, both (mixed). The spasms usually occur in clusters, often several dozens, in close succession; they occur typically after children wake up and occasionally during sleep. Sometimes at first, they are mistaken for startles.

Developmental defects are usually present. In the first stages of the disorder, developmental regression can occur (eg, children may stop smiling or lose the ability to sit up or roll over).

Rate of premature death ranges from 5 to 31% and is related to the etiology of the infantile spasms.

Diagnosis

- Waking and sleep EEG
- Neuroimaging, preferably MRI
- Testing to identify the cause unless an underlying significant neurologic disorder has already been identified

Previous history (eg, neonatal hypoxic-ischemic encephalopathy) and/or symptoms and signs suggest the diagnosis in some children. Physical and neurologic examinations are done, but often no pathognomonic findings are identified except in tuberous sclerosis.

Waking and sleep EEG is done to confirm the diagnosis and check for specific abnormalities. Typically, the interictal pattern is hypsarrhythmia (chaotic, high-voltage polymorphic delta and theta waves with superimposed multifocal spike discharges). Multiple variations (eg, focal or asymmetric hypsarrhythmia) are possible. The ictal pattern is usually a sudden, marked and diffuse attenuation of electrical activity.

Neuroimaging, preferably MRI, is done if it has not already recently been done.

Tests to determine the cause: If it is not clear from neuroimaging or the previous history, tests to determine the cause may include

- Laboratory tests (eg, CBC with differential; measurement of serum glucose, electrolytes, BUN, creatinine, sodium, calcium, magnesium, phosphorus, serum amino acids, and urine organic acids; liver function tests) if a metabolic disorder is suspected
- Genetic testing
- CSF analysis to check for metabolic disorders

Treatment

- Parenteral ACTH
- Vigabatrin (especially for tuberous sclerosis)
- Sometimes oral corticosteroids

Infantile spasms are not responsive to typical anticonvulsants.

ACTH is the most effective treatment. Both high-dose (150 units/m^2) ACTH and low-dose (20 units/m^2) ACTH, given daily IM, have been used, and evidence that the higher doses work better is not conclusive; however, generally, if low-dose therapy has not stopped spasms within 2 wk, higher doses are used. ACTH therapy is typically continued at the effective dose for 2 to 3 wk and then tapered off over 6 to 9 wk.

Vigabatrin is the only anticonvulsant with proven efficacy; it is the drug of choice when the spasms are caused by tuberous sclerosis and is often used in children with an established preexisting serious brain injury or malformation and in those who do not tolerate or respond to ACTH. Dosage of vigabatrin is 25 mg/kg twice/day, increased gradually up to 75 mg/kg twice/day if needed. There is insufficient evidence that any other anticonvulsants or the ketogenic diet is effective.

Corticosteroids (eg, prednisone 2 mg/kg/day po) are sometimes given for 4 to 7 wk as an alternative to ACTH.

In some patients with resistant spasms, focal cortical resection can eliminate seizures.

There is evidence that the more quickly effective therapy is initiated, the better the neurodevelopmental outcome, particularly when no cause is identified.

KEY POINTS

- Infantile spasms last a few seconds and can recur many times a day; they may resolve spontaneously by about age 5 yr but are often replaced by other types of seizures.
- Usually, infantile spasms occur in infants with serious brain disorders and developmental abnormalities that often have already been recognized; tuberous sclerosis is a common cause.
- Do waking and sleep EEG to confirm the diagnosis and to check for specific abnormalities; neuroimaging (preferably MRI), if not recently done, should be done.
- ACTH is the most effective treatment, but vigabatrin is the drug of choice for spasms caused by tuberous sclerosis and is often used in children who have an established preexisting serious brain injury or malformation or who do not tolerate or respond to ACTH.

NEONATAL SEIZURE DISORDERS

Neonatal seizures are abnormal electrical discharges in the CNS of neonates and usually manifest as stereotyped muscular activity or autonomic changes. Diagnosis is confirmed by EEG; testing for causes is indicated. Treatment depends on the cause.

Seizures occur in up to 1.4% of term infants and 20% of premature infants. Seizures may be related to a serious neonatal problem and require immediate evaluation. Most neonatal seizures are focal, probably because generalization of electrical activity is impeded in neonates by lack of myelination and incomplete formation of dendrites and synapses in the brain.

Some neonates undergoing EEG to assess seizures or other symptoms of encephalopathy (eg, hypoactivity, decreased responsiveness) are found to have clinically silent seizures (≥ 20 sec of rhythmic epileptiform electrical activity during an EEG but without any clinically visible seizure activity). Occasionally, clinically silent electrical activity is continuous and persists for > 20 min; at that point, it is defined as electrical status epilepticus.

Etiology

The abnormal CNS electrical discharge may be caused by a

- Primary intracranial process (eg, meningitis, ischemic stroke, encephalitis, intracranial hemorrhage, tumor, malformation)
- Systemic problem (eg, hypoxia-ischemia, hypoglycemia, hypocalcemia, hyponatremia, other disorders of metabolism)

Seizures resulting from an intracranial process usually cannot be differentiated from seizures resulting from a systemic problem by their clinical features (eg, focal vs generalized).

Hypoxia-ischemia, the most common cause of neonatal seizures, may occur before, during, or after delivery (see Overview of Perinatal Respiratory Disorders on p. 2807). Such seizures may be severe and difficult to treat, but they tend to abate after about 3 to 4 days. When neonatal hypoxia is treated with therapeutic hypothermia (usually whole-body cooling), seizures may be less severe but may recur during rewarming.

Ischemic stroke is more likely to occur in neonates with polycythemia, thrombophilia due to a genetic disorder, or severe hypotension but may occur in neonates without any risk factors. Stroke occurs typically in the middle cerebral artery distribution or, if associated with hypotension, in watershed zones. Seizures resulting from stroke tend to be focal and may cause apnea.

Neonatal infections such as meningitis and sepsis may cause seizures; in such cases, seizures are usually accompanied by other symptoms and signs. Group B streptococci and gram-negative bacteria are common causes of such infections in neonates. Encephalitis due to cytomegalovirus, herpes simplex virus, rubella virus, *Treponema pallidum*, or *Toxoplasma gondii* can also cause seizures.

Hypoglycemia is common among neonates whose mothers have diabetes, who are small for gestational age, or who have hypoxia-ischemia or other stresses. Seizures due to hypoglycemia tend to be focal and variable. Prolonged or recurrent hypoglycemia may permanently affect the CNS.

Intracranial hemorrhage, including subarachnoid, intracerebral, and intraventricular hemorrhage, may cause seizures. Intraventricular hemorrhage, which occurs more commonly in premature infants, results from bleeding in the germinal matrix (an area that is adjacent to the ventricles and that gives rise to neurons and glial cells during development).

Hypernatremia or **hyponatremia** may cause seizures. Hypernatremia can result from accidental oral or IV sodium chloride overload. Hyponatremia can result from dilution (when too much water is given po or IV) or may follow sodium loss in stool or urine.

Hypocalcemia (serum calcium level < 7.5 mg/dL [< 1.87 mmol/L]) is usually accompanied by a serum phosphorus level of > 3 mg/dL (> 0.95 mmol/L) and can be asymptomatic. Risk factors for hypocalcemia include prematurity and a difficult birth.

Hypomagnesemia is a rare cause of seizures, which may occur when the serum magnesium level is < 1.4 mEq/L (< 0.7 mmol/L). Hypomagnesemia often occurs with hypocalcemia and should be considered in neonates with hypocalcemia if seizures continue after adequate calcium therapy.

Inborn errors of metabolism (eg, amino or organic aciduria) can cause neonatal seizures. Rarely, pyridoxine deficiency or dependency causes seizures; it is readily treated.

CNS malformations can also cause seizures.

Maternal substance abuse (eg, cocaine, heroin, diazepam) is an increasingly common problem; seizures can accompany acute withdrawal after birth.

Neonatal seizures may be familial; some have genetic causes. Benign familial neonatal convulsions is a potassium channelopathy inherited in an autosomal dominant pattern. Early infantile epileptic encephalopathy (Ohtahara syndrome) is a rare disorder associated with a variety of mutations.

Symptoms and Signs

Neonatal seizures are usually focal and may be difficult to recognize. Common manifestations include migratory clonic jerks of extremities, alternating hemiseizures, and primitive subcortical seizures (which cause respiratory arrest, chewing movements, persistent eye deviations or nystagmoid movements, and episodic changes in muscle tone). Generalized tonic-clonic seizures are uncommon.

Clinically silent electrical seizure activity is often present after a hypoxic-ischemic insult (including perinatal asphyxia or stroke) and in neonates with CNS infections, especially after initial anticonvulsant treatment, which is more likely to stop clinical manifestations than electrical seizure activity.

Diagnosis

- EEG
- Laboratory testing (eg, serum glucose, electrolytes, CSF analysis, urine and blood cultures)
- Usually cranial imaging

Evaluation begins with a detailed family history and a physical examination.

Jitteriness (alternating contraction and relaxation of opposing muscles in the extremities) must be distinguished from true seizure activity. Jitteriness is usually stimulus-induced and can be stopped by holding the extremity still; in contrast, seizures occur spontaneously, and motor activity is felt even when the extremity is held still.

EEG: EEG (waking and sleep) is essential, especially when it is difficult to determine whether the neonate is having seizures. EEG is also helpful for monitoring response to treatment.

EEG should capture periods of active and quiet sleep and thus may require ≥ 2 h of recording. A normal EEG with expected variation during sleep stages is a good prognostic sign; an EEG with diffuse severe abnormalities (eg, suppressed voltage or burst suppression pattern) is a poor one.

Bedside EEG with video monitoring for ≥ 24 h may detect ongoing clinically silent electrical seizures, particularly in the first few days after a CNS insult.

Laboratory tests: Laboratory tests to look for underlying treatable disorders should be done immediately; tests include pulse oximetry; measurement of serum glucose, sodium, potassium, chloride, bicarbonate, calcium, and magnesium; and lumbar puncture for CSF analysis (cell count and differential, glucose, protein) and culture. Urine and blood cultures are obtained.

The need for other metabolic tests (eg, arterial pH, blood gases, serum bilirubin, urine amino or organic acids) or tests for commonly abused drugs (passed to the neonate transplacentally or by breastfeeding) depends on the clinical situation.

Imaging tests: Imaging tests are typically done unless the cause is immediately obvious (eg, glucose or electrolyte abnormality). MRI is preferred but may not be readily available; in such cases, cranial CT is done.

For very sick infants who cannot be moved to radiology, bedside cranial ultrasonography can be done; it may detect intraventricular but not subarachnoid hemorrhage. MRI or CT is done when infants are stable.

Cranial CT can detect intracranial bleeding and some brain malformations. MRI shows malformations more clearly and can detect ischemic tissue within a few hours of onset.

Magnetic resonance spectroscopy may help determine the extent of an ischemic injury or identify buildup of certain neurotransmitters associated with an underlying metabolic disorder.

Prognosis

Prognosis depends on the etiology:

- About 50% of neonates with seizures due to hypoxia-ischemia develop normally.
- Most neonates with seizures due to subarachnoid hemorrhage, hypocalcemia, or hyponatremia do well.
- Those with severe intraventricular hemorrhage have a high morbidity rate.
- For idiopathic seizures or seizures due to malformations, earlier onset is associated with worse neurodevelopmental outcomes.

Whether neonatal seizures cause damage beyond that caused by the underlying disorder is unknown, although there is concern that the metabolic stress of prolonged nerve cell firing during lengthy seizures may cause additional brain damage. When caused by acute injuries to the brain such as hypoxia-ischemia, stroke, or infection, neonates may have a series of seizures, but seizures typically abate after about 3 to 4 days; they may recur months to years later if brain damage has occurred. Seizures due to other conditions may be more persistent during the neonatal period.

Treatment

- Treatment of cause
- Anticonvulsants

Treatment focuses primarily on the underlying disorder and secondarily on seizures.

Treatment of the cause: For **low serum glucose,** 10% dextrose 2 mL/kg IV is given, and the serum glucose level is monitored; additional infusions are given as needed but cautiously, to avoid hyperglycemia.

For **hypocalcemia,** 10% calcium gluconate 1 mL/kg IV (9 mg/kg of elemental calcium) is given; this dosage can be repeated for persistent hypocalcemic seizures. Rate of calcium gluconate infusion should not exceed 0.5 mL/min (50 mg/min); continuous cardiac monitoring is necessary during the infusion. Extravasation should be avoided because skin may slough.

For **hypomagnesemia,** 0.2 mL/kg (100 mg/kg) of a 50% magnesium sulfate solution is given IM.

Bacterial infections are treated with antibiotics.

Herpes encephalitis is treated with acyclovir.

Anticonvulsants: Anticonvulsants are used unless seizures stop quickly after correction of reversible disorders such as hypoglycemia, hypocalcemia, hypomagnesemia, hyponatremia, or hypernatremia.

Phenobarbital is still the most commonly used drug; a loading dose of 15 to 20 mg/kg IV is given. If seizures continue, 5 to 10 mg/kg IV can be given q 15 to 30 min until seizures cease or until a maximum of 40 mg/kg is given. If seizures are persistent, maintenance therapy may be started about 24 h later at 1.5 to 2 mg/kg q 12 h and increased to 2.5 mg/kg q 12 h based on clinical or EEG response or serum drug levels. Phenobarbital is continued IV, especially if seizures are frequent or prolonged. When the infant is stable, phenobarbital can be given orally at 3 to 4 mg/kg once/day. Therapeutic serum levels of phenobarbital are 20 to 40 μg/mL (85 to 170 μmol/L).

Levetiracetam is being increasingly used to treat neonatal seizures because it is less sedating than phenobarbital. It is given IV as a 20- to 50-mg/kg IV loading dose, and therapy may be continued as 10 to 30 mg/kg IV q 12 h. Therapeutic levels are not well-established in the neonate.

Fosphenytoin can be used if seizures continue despite phenobarbital and levetiracetam. The loading dose is 20 mg PE (phenytoin equivalents)/kg IV. It is given over 30 min to avoid hypotension or arrhythmias. A maintenance dose may be started at 2 to 3 mg PE/kg q 12 h and adjusted based on clinical response or serum levels. Therapeutic serum levels for phenytoin in neonates are 8 to 15 μg/mL (32 to 60 μmol/L).

Lorazepam 0.1 mg/kg IV may be used initially for a prolonged seizure or for resistant seizures and repeated at 5- to 10-min intervals, up to 3 doses in any 8-h period.

Neonates given IV anticonvulsants are closely observed; large doses and combinations of drugs, particularly lorazepam plus phenobarbital, may result in respiratory depression.

The appropriate duration of therapy is not known for any of the anticonvulsants, but if seizures come under control, anticonvulsants may be stopped before discharge from the nursery.

KEY POINTS

- Neonatal seizures usually occur in reaction to a systemic or CNS event (eg, hypoxia/ischemia, stroke, hemorrhage, infection, metabolic disorder, structural brain abnormality).
- Neonatal seizures are usually focal and may be difficult to recognize; common manifestations include migratory clonic jerks of extremities, chewing movements, persistent eye deviations or nystagmoid movements, and episodic changes in muscle tone.
- EEG is essential for diagnosis; laboratory testing and usually neuroimaging are done to identify the cause.
- Treatment is directed at the cause.
- Give phenobarbital or levetiracetam if seizures do not stop when the cause is corrected; fosphenytoin and lorazepam may be added for persistent seizures.

TIC DISORDERS AND TOURETTE SYNDROME IN CHILDREN AND ADOLESCENTS

Tics are defined as repeated, sudden, rapid, nonrhythmic muscle movements including sounds or vocalizations. Tourette syndrome is diagnosed when people have had both motor and vocal tics for > 1 yr. Diagnosis is clinical. Tics are treated only if they interfere with a child's activities or self-image; treatment may include cognitive-behavioral therapy and clonidine or an antipsychotic.

Tics vary widely in severity; they occur in about 20% of children, many of whom are not evaluated or diagnosed. Tourette syndrome, the most severe type, occurs in 3 to 8/1000 children. Male to female ratio is 3:1.

Tics begin before age 18 years (typically between ages 4 and 6 yr); they increase in severity to a peak at about age 10 to 12 yr and decrease during adolescence. Eventually, most tics disappear spontaneously. However, in about 1% of children, tics persist into adulthood.

Etiology is not known, but tic disorders tend to be familial. In some families, they appear in a dominant pattern with incomplete penetrance.

Comorbidities

Comorbidities are common.

Children with tics may have one or more of the following:

- Attention-deficit/hyperactivity disorder (ADHD)
- Obsessive-compulsive disorder (OCD)
- Separation anxiety disorder
- Learning disorders

These disorders often interfere more with children's development and well-being than the tics. ADHD is the most common comorbidity, and sometimes tics first appear when children with ADHD are treated with a stimulant; these children probably have an underlying tendency to tics.

Adolescents (and adults) may have

- Depression
- Bipolar disorder
- Substance abuse

Classification

Tic disorders are divided into 3 categories by the *Diagnostic and Statistical Manual of Mental Disorders*, 5th edition (DSM-5):

- Tourette syndrome (Gilles de la Tourette syndrome): Both motor and vocal tics have been present for > 1 year.
- Persistent (chronic) tic disorder: Single or multiple motor or vocal tics (but not both motor and vocal) have been present for > 1 yr.
- Provisional tic disorder: Single or multiple motor and/or vocal tics have been present < 1 yr.

In all categories, age at onset must be < 18 yr, and the disturbance cannot be due to physiologic effects of a substance (eg, cocaine) or another disorder (eg, Huntington disease, postviral encephalitis).

Symptoms and Signs

Patients tend to manifest the same set of tics at any given time, although tics tend to vary in type (see Table 325–1), intensity, and frequency over a period of time. They may occur multiple times in an hour, then remit or barely be present for ≥ 3 mo. Typically, tics do not occur during sleep.

Tics can be

- Motor or vocal
- Simple or complex

Simple tics are a very brief movement or vocalization, typically without social meaning.

Complex tics last longer and may involve a combination of simple tics. Complex tics may appear to have social meaning (ie, be recognizable gestures or words) and thus seem intentional. However, although some patients can voluntarily suppress their tics for a short time (seconds to minutes) and some notice a premonitory urge to perform the tic, tics are not voluntary and do not represent misbehavior.

Stress and fatigue can make tics worse, but tics are often most prominent when the body is relaxed, as while watching TV. Tics may lessen when patients are engaged in tasks (eg, school or work activities). Tics rarely interfere with motor coordination. Mild tics often cause few problems, but severe tics, particularly coprolalia (which is rare), are physically and/or socially disabling.

Sometimes tics are explosive in onset, appearing and becoming constant within a day. Sometimes children with explosive-onset tics and/or related obsessive compulsiveness have a streptococcal infection—a phenomenon sometimes called pediatric autoimmune neuropsychiatric disorders associated with streptococcal infections (PANDAS). Many investigators do not believe that PANDAS is distinct from the spectrum of tic disorders.

Diagnosis

- Clinical evaluation

Diagnosis is clinical. To differentiate Tourette syndrome from transient tics, physicians may have to monitor patients over time. Tourette syndrome is diagnosed when people have had both motor and vocal tics for ≥ 1 yr.

Table 325–1. TYPES OF TICS

CLASSIFICATION	MOTOR	VOCAL
Simple	Blinking Grimacing Head jerking Shoulder shrugging	Grunting or barking Sniffing or snorting Throat clearing
Complex	Combinations of simple tics (eg, head turning plus shoulder shrugging) Copropraxia: Using sexual or obscene gestures Echopraxia: Imitating someone's movements	Coprolalia: Uttering socially inappropriate words (eg, obscenities, ethnic slurs) Echolalia: Repeating one's own or another's sounds or words

Treatment

- Cognitive-behavioral therapy
- Sometimes clonidine or antipsychotics
- Treatment of comorbidities

Treatment to suppress tics is recommended only if they are significantly interfering with children's activities or self-image; treatment does not alter the natural history of the disorder. Often, treatment may be avoided if clinicians help children and their families understand the natural history of tics and if school personnel can help classmates understand the disorder.

Sometimes the natural waxing and waning of tics makes it appear that the tics have responded to a particular treatment.

A type of behavioral therapy called comprehensive behavioral intervention for tics (CIBT) may help some older children control or reduce the number or severity of their tics. It includes cognitive-behavioral therapy such as habit reversal (learning a new behavior to replace the tic), education about tics, and relaxation techniques.

Drugs: Clonidine 0.05 to 0.1 mg po once/day to 4 times/day is effective in some patients. Adverse effects of fatigue may limit daytime dosage; hypotension is uncommon.

Antipsychotics may be required—for example,

- Risperidone 0.25 to 1.5 mg po bid
- Haloperidol 0.5 to 2 mg po bid or tid
- Pimozide 1 to 2 mg po bid
- Olanzapine 2.5 to 5 mg po once/day

Fluphenazine is also effective in suppressing tics.

With any drug, the lowest dose required to make tics tolerable is used; doses are tapered as tics wane. Adverse effects of dysphoria, parkinsonism, akathisia, and tardive dyskinesia are rare but may limit use of antipsychotics; using lower daytime doses and higher bedtime doses may decrease adverse effects.

Treatment of comorbidities: Treating comorbidities is important.

ADHD can sometimes be successfully treated with low doses of stimulants without exacerbating tics, but an alternative treatment (eg, atomoxetine) may be preferable.

If obsessive or compulsive traits are bothersome, an SSRI may be useful.

Children who have tics and who are struggling in school should be evaluated for learning disorders and provided with support as needed.

KEY POINTS

- Tics are repeated, sudden, rapid, nonrhythmic muscle movements or vocalizations that develop in children < 18 yr old.
- Tics are common, but the most severe manifestation of tics, coprolalia, is rare.
- Simple tics are a very brief movement or vocalization (eg, head jerk, grunt), typically without social meaning.
- Complex tics may appear to have social meaning (ie, be recognizable gestures or words) and thus seem intentional, but they are not.
- Use of cognitive-behavioral therapy, clonidine, or an antipsychotic may lessen severe or troublesome tics, which also tend to lessen with time although a few persist into adulthood.
- Comorbidities (eg, ADHD, OCD) are common and must also be diagnosed and treated.

326 Pediatric Cancers

Overall, childhood cancer is relatively rare, with fewer than 13,500 cases and about 1,500 deaths annually among children aged 0 to 14 yr. In comparison, there are 1.4 million cases and 575,000 deaths annually among adults. However, cancer is the 2nd leading cause of death among children, following only injuries.

Childhood cancers include many that also occur in adults. Leukemia is by far the most common (see p. 1141), representing about 33% of childhood cancers, brain tumors represent about 25%, lymphomas represent about 8% (see p. 1156), and certain bone cancers (osteosarcoma and Ewing sarcoma—see p. 340) represent about 4%.

Cancers that are exclusive to children include

- Neuroblastoma (7% of cases)
- Wilms tumor (5% of cases)
- Rhabdomyosarcoma (3 to 4% of cases)
- Retinoblastoma (3% of cases)

Currently, it is estimated that there are 350,000 adult survivors of childhood cancer in the United States. Children who survive cancer have more years than adults to develop long-term consequences of chemotherapy and radiation therapy, which include

- Infertility
- Poor growth
- Cardiac damage
- Development of second cancers (in 3 to 12% of survivors)

Consensus guidelines on screening for and management of long-term consequences are available from the Children's Oncology Group.

Because of the severe consequences and complexity of treatment, children with cancer are best treated in centers with expertise in childhood cancers.

The impact of being diagnosed with cancer and the intensity of the treatment are overwhelming to the child and family. Maintaining a sense of normalcy for the child is difficult, especially given the need for frequent hospitalizations and outpatient visits and potentially painful procedures. Overwhelming stress is typical, as parents struggle to continue to work, be attentive to siblings, and still attend to the many needs of the child with cancer. The situation is even more difficult when the child is being treated at a specialty center far from home.

OVERVIEW OF BRAIN TUMORS IN CHILDREN

Brain tumors are the most common solid cancer in children < 15 yr and are the 2nd leading cause of death due to cancer. Diagnosis is typically by imaging (usually MRI) and biopsy. Treatment may include surgical resection, chemotherapy, and radiation therapy.

The cause of most childhood CNS tumors is unknown, but two established risk factors are ionizing radiation (eg, high-dose cranial irradiation) and specific genetic syndromes (eg, neurofibromatosis).

The **most common CNS tumors** in children are (in order)

- Astrocytomas
- Medulloblastomas
- Ependymomas

Symptoms and Signs

Increased intracranial pressure is the cause of the most common manifestations, which include

- Headache
- Nausea and vomiting
- Irritability
- Lethargy
- Changes in behavior
- Gait and balance disorders

Diagnosis

- MRI
- Biopsy

MRI is the test of choice because it provides more detailed images of parenchymal tumors and can detect tumors within the posterior fossa, subarachnoid spaces, and the arachnoid and pia mater. CT may be done but is less sensitive and less specific.

Biopsy may be done to confirm the diagnosis and to determine tumor type and grade.

Once the diagnosis is made, staging, grading, and risk assessment are determined. Staging includes an MRI of the entire spine, a lumbar puncture for CSF cytology, and a postoperative MRI to assess for any residual tumor. The WHO has created a commonly used grading system. Risk assessment is based on age, degree of residual tumor, and evidence of spread of disease.

Treatment

- Surgical resection
- Radiation therapy, chemotherapy, or a combination

After tumor removal, radiation therapy, chemotherapy, or both are usually required.

Entry into a clinical trial should be considered for all children with a brain tumor. Optimal treatment requires a multidisciplinary team of pediatric oncologists, pediatric neuro-oncologists, pediatric neurosurgeons, neuropathologists, neuroradiologists, and radiation oncologists who have experience treating brain tumors in children. Because radiation therapy for brain tumors is technically demanding, children should be sent to centers that have experience in this area if possible.

ASTROCYTOMAS

Astrocytomas are childhood CNS tumors that develop from astrocytes. Diagnosis is based on MRI. Treatment is a combination of surgical resection, radiation therapy, and chemotherapy.

Astrocytomas range from low-grade indolent tumors (the most prevalent) to malignant high-grade tumors. As a group, astrocytomas are the most common brain tumor in children, representing about 40% of tumors. Most cases occur between ages 5 yr and 9 yr. These tumors can occur anywhere in the brain or spinal cord, but are most common in the cerebellum.

Symptoms and Signs

Most patients have symptoms consistent with increased intracranial pressure (eg, morning headaches, vomiting, lethargy). Location of the tumor determines other symptoms and signs, for example

- Cerebellum: Weakness, tremor, and ataxia
- Visual pathway: Visual loss, proptosis, or nystagmus
- Spinal cord: Pain, weakness, and gait disturbance

Diagnosis

- Contrast-enhanced MRI
- Biopsy

Contrast-enhanced MRI is the imaging test of choice for diagnosing the tumor, determining extent of disease, and detecting recurrence. Contrast-enhanced CT can also be used, although it is less specific and less sensitive.

Biopsy is needed for determining tumor type and grade. These tumors are typically classified as low grade (eg, juvenile pilocytic astrocytoma) or high grade (eg, glioblastoma—see Table 326–1). Many pathologists designate grades I and II tumors as low grade and grades III and IV tumors as high grade. However, because grade II tumors have a higher risk of relapse, some pathologists think these tumors should not be considered low grade.

Treatment

- Surgical resection
- Sometimes radiation therapy and/or chemotherapy

Treatment of astrocytoma depends on location and grade of tumor. As a general rule, the lower the grade of the tumor, the less intensive the therapy and the better the outcome.

- **Low grade:** Surgical resection is the primary treatment, and total resection is the goal. Even after local recurrence, a second surgical resection can be beneficial depending on the location of the tumor. Radiation therapy is usually reserved for children who are > 10 yr and whose tumors are unresectable, cannot be completely excised, or progress/recur after surgery. For children < 10 yr whose tumors are unresectable or progress/recur after surgery, chemotherapy is used instead because radiation therapy may cause long-term cognitive impairment. Most children with low-grade astrocytomas are cured.
- **High grade:** These tumors are treated with a combination of surgery (unless location precludes it), radiation therapy, and chemotherapy. Prognosis is poor; overall survival at 3 yr is only 20 to 30%.

MEDULLOBLASTOMA

Medulloblastomas are invasive and rapidly growing childhood CNS tumors that develop in the posterior fossa (containing the brain stem and cerebellum). Diagnosis is based on MRI and biopsy/tumor resection. Treatment is a combination of surgery, radiation therapy, and chemotherapy.

Medulloblastoma is the most common malignant posterior fossa tumor in children and represents about 20% of all pediatric CNS cancers. It has a bimodal peak at age 3 to 4 yr and at age 8 to 10 yr but can occur throughout childhood. Medulloblastoma is a type of primitive neuroectodermal tumor (PNET).

Etiology of medulloblastoma is unknown in most patients, but medulloblastoma may occur with certain syndromes (eg, Gorlin syndrome, Turcot syndrome).

Symptoms and Signs

Patients present most commonly with vomiting, headache, nausea, visual changes (eg, double vision), and unsteady walking or clumsiness.

Diagnosis

- MRI
- Histologic evaluation of biopsy specimen or entire resected tumor

MRI with gadolinium contrast is the test of choice for initial evaluation of possible medulloblastoma. Definitive diagnosis is made using tumor tissue obtained by biopsy or ideally by gross total resection of the tumor at initial presentation.

Once the initial diagnosis is established, staging and risk group determination are critical in medulloblastoma.

Table 326–1. WHO GRADING OF ASTROCYTIC TUMORS

TUMOR	TUMOR GRADE I	II	III	IV
Subependymal giant cell astrocytoma	X			
Pilocytic astrocytoma	X			
Pilomyxoid astrocytoma		X		
Diffuse astrocytoma		X		
Pleomorphic xanthoastrocytoma		X		
Anaplastic astrocytoma			X	
Glioblastoma				X
Giant cell glioblastoma				X
Gliosarcoma				X

Adapted from Louis DN, Ohgaki H, Wiestler OD, et al: WHO classification of tumors of the central nervous system. *Acta Neuropathologica* 114: 97–109, 2007.

Staging tests include

- MRI of the entire spine
- Lumbar puncture for CSF cytology
- Postoperative MRI to assess for any residual tumor

Risk assessment is based on amount of residual tumor and evidence of spread of disease:

- High risk: Postoperative residual disease is > 1.5 cm^2 or there is disseminated microscopic or gross disease.
- Average risk: Postoperative residual disease is < 1.5 cm^2 and there is no dissemination.

Prognosis

Prognosis depends on the stage, histology, and biologic (eg, histologic, cytogenetic, molecular) parameters of the tumor and patient age, but generally

- Age > 3 yr: Likelihood of 5-yr disease-free survival is 50 to 60% if the tumor is high risk and 80% if the tumor is average risk.
- Age ≤ 3 yr: Prognosis is more problematic, in part because up to 40% of children have disseminated disease at diagnosis. Children who survive are at risk of severe long-term neurocognitive deficits (eg, in memory, verbal learning, and executive function).

Treatment

- Surgery, radiation, and chemotherapy

Treatment of medulloblastoma includes surgery, radiation, and chemotherapy. Cure with chemotherapy alone has been shown in some children < 3 yr of age. Combination therapy typically provides the best long-term survival.

EPENDYMOMAS

Ependymomas are slow-growing CNS tumors that involve the ventricular system. Diagnosis is based on MRI and biopsy. Treatment is a combination of surgery, radiation therapy, and chemotherapy.

Ependymomas are the 3rd most common CNS tumor in children (after astrocytomas and medulloblastomas), representing 10% of pediatric brain tumors. Mean age at diagnosis is 6 yr; however, about 30% of ependymomas occur in children < 3 yr.

Ependymomas are derived from the ependymal lining of the ventricular system. Up to 70% of ependymomas occur in the posterior fossa; both high-grade and low-grade tumors in the posterior fossae tend to spread locally to the brain stem.

Symptoms and Signs

Initial symptoms are typically related to increased intracranial pressure. Infants may present with developmental delay and irritability.

Changes in mood, personality, or concentration may occur. Seizures, balance and gait disturbances, or symptoms of spinal cord compression (eg, back pain, loss of bladder and bowel control) may occur.

Diagnosis

- MRI
- Histologic evaluation of biopsy specimen or entire resected tumor

Diagnosis of ependymoma is based on MRI. Definitive diagnosis is made using tumor tissue obtained by biopsy or ideally by gross total resection of the tumor at initial presentation.

Prognosis

Survival rate depends on age and on how much of the tumor can be removed:

- Total or near-total removal: 51 to 80% survival
- Less than 90% removal: 0 to 26% survival

Children who survive are at risk of neurologic deficits.

Treatment

- Surgical resection, usually followed by radiation therapy
- Sometimes chemotherapy

Surgical resection is critical, and the degree of resection is one of the most important prognostic factors.

Radiation therapy has been shown to increase survival and should be given after surgery; however, a small subset of ependymomas can potentially can be cured by surgery alone.

Chemotherapy has not been clearly shown to improve survival but, in some children, may be used to shrink the tumor before gross total resection or a second-look surgery.

NEUROBLASTOMA

Neuroblastoma is a cancer arising in the adrenal gland or less often from the extra-adrenal sympathetic chain, including the retroperitoneum, chest, and neck. Diagnosis is confirmed by biopsy. Treatment may include surgical resection, chemotherapy, radiation therapy, high-dose chemotherapy with stem cell transplantation, *cis*-retinoic acid, and immunotherapy.

Neuroblastoma is the most common cancer among infants. Almost 90% of neuroblastomas occur in children < 5 yr. Most neuroblastomas occur spontaneously, but 1 to 2% appear to be inherited. Some markers (eg, *MYCN* oncogene amplification, hyperdiploidy, histopathology) correlate with progression and prognosis. Although *MYCN* amplification is associated with advanced disease and unfavorable biology, it is also predictive of survival even in the absence of high-risk features. *MYCN* amplification occurs in about 20% of cases.

PEARLS & PITFALLS

- Neuroblastoma is the most common cancer among infants.

Neuroblastomas may begin in the abdomen (about 65%), thorax (15 to 20%), neck, pelvis, or other sites. Neuroblastoma occurs very rarely as a primary CNS cancer.

Most neuroblastomas produce catecholamines, which can be detected as elevated levels of urinary catecholamine breakdown products. Neuroblastomas do not typically cause severe hypertension because these tumors do not usually secrete epinephrine. Ganglioneuroma is a fully differentiated, benign variant of neuroblastoma.

About 40 to 50% of children have localized or regional disease at diagnosis; 50 to 60% have metastases at diagnosis. Neuroblastoma may metastasize to bone marrow, bone, liver, lymph nodes, or, less commonly, skin or brain. Bone marrow metastases may cause anemia and/or thrombocytopenia. Anemia also occasionally occurs when bleeding into these highly vascular tumors causes a rapid drop in Hb.

Symptoms and Signs

Symptoms and signs of neuroblastoma depend on the site of the primary cancer and pattern of disease spread. The most common symptoms are abdominal pain, discomfort, and a sense of fullness due to an abdominal mass.

Certain symptoms may result from metastases. These include bone pain due to widespread bone metastases, periorbital ecchymosis and proptosis due to retrobulbar metastasis, and abdominal distention and respiratory problems due to liver metastases, especially in infants. Children with anemia may have pallor, and those with thrombocytopenia may have petechiae.

Children occasionally present with focal neurologic deficits or paralysis due to direct extension of the cancer into the spinal canal. They may also present with paraneoplastic syndromes, such as cerebellar ataxia, opsoclonus-myoclonus, watery diarrhea, or hypertension.

ROHHADNET (rapid-onset obesity with hypothalamic dysfunction, hypoventilation, autonomic dysregulation, and neuroendocrine tumors) is a very rare disease that can be associated with ganglioneuroblastomas and ganglioneuromas in the abdomen and lungs.

Diagnosis

- CT/MRI
- Biopsy
- Sometimes bone marrow aspirate or core biopsy plus measurement of urinary catecholamine intermediates

Routine prenatal ultrasonography occasionally detects neuroblastoma. Patients presenting with abdominal symptoms or a mass require CT or MRI. Diagnosis of neuroblastoma is then confirmed by biopsy of any identified mass.

Alternatively, diagnosis can be established without biopsy or surgery of the primary tumor by finding characteristic cancer cells in a bone marrow aspirate or core biopsy plus elevated urinary catecholamine intermediates. These methods of diagnosis are not commonly done but can be useful in situations where biopsy and/or surgery is considered high risk because of patient or tumor characteristics.

Urinary vanillylmandelic acid (VMA), homovanillic acid (HVA), or both are elevated in ≥ 90% of patients. A 24-h urine collection can be used, but a spot urine test is usually sufficient. If the primary site of the neuroblastoma is adrenal, it must be differentiated from Wilms tumor and other renal masses. It may also need to be differentiated from rhabdomyosarcoma, hepatoblastoma, lymphoma, and tumors of genital origin.

Staging of neuroblastoma: The following should be done to evaluate for metastases:

- Bone marrow aspirates and core biopsies from multiple sites (typically, both posterior iliac crests)
- Skeletal survey
- Bone scan or ^{131}I-metaiodobenzylguanidine (MIBG) scan
- Abdominal, pelvis, and chest CT or MRI

Cranial imaging with CT or MRI is indicated if symptoms or signs suggest brain metastases.

Results of these tests determine stage (extent of spread) of disease. The International Neuroblastoma Staging System (INSS) requires the results of surgery to determine stage. The International Neuroblastoma Risk Group Staging System (INRGSS) uses imaging-defined risk factors rather than surgery to stage neuroblastoma.

Neuroblastoma also has a unique stage called 4S (per INSS) or MS (per INGRSS) that often regresses spontaneously without treatment. This stage includes children < age 12 mo (4S) or 18 mo (MS) who have a localized primary tumor that has dissemination limited to skin, liver, and/or bone marrow. Marrow involvement should be minimal and limited to < 10% of the total nucleated cells and cannot involve the cortex of the bone.

Risk stratification of neuroblastoma: At diagnosis, attempts should be made to obtain adequate tumor tissue to analyze for DNA index (the ratio of the amount of DNA in a tumor cell to the amount in a normal cell; the DNA index is thus a quantitative measure of chromosome content) and amplification of the *MYCN* oncogene. These factors help determine prognosis and guide intensity of therapy.

Risk categorization is complex, and two major risk group stratification systems exist: one developed by the Children's Oncology Group (COG) and the other by INRGSS. These systems are based on patient age, stage, histology, *MYCN* amplification, and DNA index. In addition, the INRG considers chromosome 11q aberrations in the evaluation. In both systems, these factors are used to stratify patients into low-, intermediate-, and high-risk categories that help determine prognosis and guide the intensity of treatment.

Prognosis

Prognosis of neuroblastoma depends on age at diagnosis, stage, and biologic factors (eg, histopathology, tumor cell ploidy in younger patients, *MYCN* amplification). Younger children with localized disease have the best outcome.

Survival rates for low-risk and intermediate-risk disease are about 90%. Historically, the survival rate for high-risk disease was about 15%. This rate has improved to > 50% with use of more intensified therapy. And a recent randomized study showed intensive therapy combined with immunotherapy resulted in a 2-yr event-free survival rate of 66%.

Treatment

- Surgical resection
- Usually chemotherapy
- Sometimes high-dose chemotherapy followed by stem cell transplantation
- Sometimes radiation therapy
- *Cis*-retinoic acid for maintenance therapy in high-risk disease
- Immunotherapy

Treatment of neuroblastoma is based on the risk category (see also National Cancer Institute's Overview of Neuroblastoma Treatment at www.cancer.gov).

Surgical resection is important for low-risk and intermediate-risk disease. It is often delayed until adjuvant chemotherapy is given to improve the chance of adequate surgical resection.

Chemotherapy (typical drugs include vincristine, cyclophosphamide, doxorubicin, cisplatin, carboplatin, ifosfamide, and etoposide) is usually necessary for children with intermediate-risk disease. High-dose chemotherapy with stem cell transplantation and *cis*-retinoic acid are frequently used for children with high-risk disease.

Radiation therapy is sometimes needed for children with intermediate-risk or high-risk disease or for inoperable tumors.

Immunotherapy using monoclonal antibodies against neuroblastoma antigens combined with cytokines is the latest approach to treating high-risk disease.

RETINOBLASTOMA

Retinoblastoma is a cancer arising from the immature retina. Symptoms and signs commonly include leukocoria (a white reflex in the pupil), strabismus, and, less often, inflammation and impaired vision. Diagnosis is based on ophthalmoscopic examination and ultrasonography, CT, or MRI. Treatment of small cancers and bilateral disease may include photocoagulation, cryotherapy, and radiation therapy. Treatment of advanced and some larger cancers is enucleation. Chemotherapy is sometimes used to reduce cancer volume and to treat cancers that have spread beyond the eye.

Retinoblastoma occurs in 1/15,000 to 1/30,000 live births and represents about 3% of childhood cancers. It is usually diagnosed in children < 2 yr; < 5% of cases are diagnosed in those > 5 yr. The cancer may be hereditary; inheritance is mainly autosomal dominant but with incomplete penetrance (clinical symptoms are not always present in individuals who have the disease-causing mutation). About 25% of patients have bilateral disease, which is always heritable. Another 15% of patients have heritable unilateral disease, and the remaining 60% have nonhereditary unilateral disease.

The pathogenesis of inheritance appears to involve mutational deactivation of both alleles of a retinoblastoma suppressor gene (*RB1*) located on chromosome 13q14. In the hereditary form, a germline mutation alters one allele in all cells, and a later somatic mutation alters the other allele in the retinal cells (the 2nd hit in this 2-hit model), resulting in the cancer. The nonhereditary form probably involves somatic mutation of both alleles in a retinal cell.

Symptoms and Signs

Patients typically present with leukocoria (a white reflex in the pupil, sometimes referred to as cat's-eye pupil—see Plate 93) or strabismus. Much less often, patients present with inflammation of the eye or impaired vision.

Rarely, the cancer has already spread, via the optic nerve or the choroid or hematogenously, resulting in an orbital or soft-tissue mass, local bone pain, headache, anorexia, or vomiting.

When the diagnosis is suspected, both fundi must be closely examined by indirect ophthalmoscopy with the pupils widely dilated and the child under general anesthesia. The cancers appear as single or multiple gray-white elevations in the retina; cancer seeds may be visible in the vitreous.

Diagnosis

- Orbital ultrasonography, CT, or MRI
- Sometimes bone scan, bone marrow aspirate and biopsy, and lumbar puncture

Diagnosis of retinoblastoma is usually confirmed by orbital ultrasonography, MRI, or CT. In almost all cancers, calcification can be detected by CT. However, if the optic nerve appears abnormal during ophthalmoscopy, MRI is better for finding cancer extension into the optic nerve or choroid.

If optic nerve extension is suspected or extensive choroidal invasion is present, a lumbar puncture and brain MRI should be done to assess for metastasis. Because distant metastasis is rare, bone marrow evaluation and bone scan can be reserved for patients with bony symptoms.

Children who have a parent or sibling with a history of retinoblastoma should be evaluated by an ophthalmologist shortly after birth and then every 4 mo until age 4 yr. Patients with retinoblastoma require molecular genetic testing, and if a germline mutation is identified, parents should also be tested for the same mutation. If subsequent offspring of parents have the germline mutation, the same genetic testing and regular ophthalmologic examination are required. Recombinant DNA probes may be useful for detecting asymptomatic carriers.

Prognosis

If the cancer is treated when it is intraocular, > 90% of patients can be cured. Prognosis for patients with metastatic disease is poor.

In patients with hereditary retinoblastoma, incidence of 2nd cancers is increased; about 50% arise within the irradiated area. These cancers can include sarcomas and malignant melanoma. About 70% of patients who will develop a 2nd cancer develop it within 30 yr of the primary retinoblastoma.

Treatment

- Enucleation
- Photocoagulation, cryotherapy, and radiation therapy
- Sometimes chemotherapy

The goal of retinoblastoma treatment should be cure, but attempts to preserve as much vision as possible are appropriate. The treatment team should include a pediatric ophthalmologist with expertise in retinoblastoma, a pediatric oncologist, and a radiation oncologist.

Advanced unilateral retinoblastoma is managed by enucleation with removal of as much of the optic nerve as possible.

For patients with bilateral cancer, vision can usually be preserved. Options include bilateral photocoagulation or unilateral enucleation and photocoagulation, cryotherapy, and irradiation of the other eye. Radiation therapy is by external beam or, for very small cancers, brachytherapy (attachment of a radioactive plaque to the eye wall near the cancer).

Systemic chemotherapy, such as carboplatin plus etoposide, or cyclophosphamide plus vincristine, may be helpful to reduce the size of large cancers to allow for the use of other additional therapies (eg, cryotherapy, laser hyperthermia) or to treat cancer that has disseminated beyond the eye. However, chemotherapy alone can seldom cure this cancer.

Ophthalmologic re-examination of both eyes and retreatment, if necessary, are required at 2-mo to 4-mo intervals.

RHABDOMYOSARCOMA

Rhabdomyosarcoma is a childhood cancer arising from embryonal mesenchymal cells that have potential to differentiate into skeletal muscle cells. It can arise from almost any type of muscle tissue in any location, resulting in highly variable clinical manifestations. Cancers are typically detected by CT or MRI, and diagnosis is confirmed by biopsy. Treatment involves surgery, radiation therapy, and chemotherapy.

Rhabdomyosarcoma is the 3rd most common extra-CNS solid cancer in children (after Wilms tumor and neuroblastoma). Nonetheless, it accounts for only 3 to 4% of all childhood cancers. Rhabdomyosarcoma belongs to a group of tumors known as soft-tissue sarcomas and is the most common cancer in this group.

Incidence of rhabdomyosarcoma in children is 4.3/million/yr. Two-thirds of cancers are diagnosed in children < 7 yr. The disease is more common among whites than blacks (largely because frequency is lower in black girls) and is slightly more common among boys than girls.

Histology: There are 2 major histologic subtypes:

- Embryonal: Characterized by loss of heterozygosity on chromosome 11p15.5
- Alveolar: Associated with translocation t(2;13), which fuses the *PAX3* gene with the *FOXO1* (*FKHR*) gene, and t(1;13), which fuses the *PAX7* gene with the *FOXO1* (*FKHR*) gene

Location: Although rhabdomyosarcoma can occur almost anywhere in the body, the cancer has a predilection for several sites:

- Head and neck region (about 35%), usually in the orbit or nasopharyngeal passages: Most common among school-aged children
- GU system (about 25%), usually in the bladder, prostate, or vagina: Usually occurring in infants and toddlers
- Extremities (about 20%): Most common among adolescents
- Trunk/miscellaneous sites (20%)

About 15 to 25% of children present with metastatic disease. The lung is the most common site of metastasis; bone, bone marrow, and lymph nodes are other possible sites.

Symptoms and Signs

Children do not typically have systemic symptoms such as fever, night sweats, or weight loss. Usually, children present with a firm, palpable mass or with organ dysfunction due to impingement on the organ by the cancer.

Orbital and nasopharyngeal cancers may cause tearing, eye pain, or proptosis. Nasopharyngeal cavity cancers may cause nasal congestion, a change in voice, or mucopurulent discharge.

GU cancers cause abdominal pain, a palpable abdominal mass, difficulty urinating, and hematuria.

Extremity cancers appear as firm, indiscrete masses anywhere on the arms or legs. Regional lymph node spread occurs frequently, and metastases in the lungs, bone marrow, and lymph nodes can occur and usually do not cause symptoms.

Diagnosis

- CT or MRI
- Biopsy or excision

Masses are evaluated by CT, although head and neck lesions are often better defined by MRI. Diagnosis of rhabdomyosarcoma is confirmed by biopsy or excision of the mass.

The standard metastatic evaluation includes chest CT, a bone scan, and bilateral bone marrow aspiration and biopsy.

Prognosis

Prognosis is based on

- Cancer location (eg, prognosis is better with nonparameningeal head/neck and nonbladder/nonprostate GU cancers)
- Completeness of resection
- Presence of metastasis
- Age (prognosis is worse for children < 1 yr of age or > 10 yr
- Histology (embryonal histology is associated with a better outcome than alveolar histology)

Combinations of these prognostic factors place children in a low-risk, intermediate-risk, or high-risk category. A complex risk stratification system exists based on two staging systems (see the National Cancer Institute's stage information for rhabdomyosarcoma at www.cancer.gov). Treatment intensifies with each risk category, and overall survival ranges from > 90% in children with low-risk disease to < 50% in children with high-risk disease.

Treatment

- Surgery and chemotherapy
- Radiation therapy for residual bulk or microscopic disease

Treatment of rhabdomyosarcoma consists of surgery, chemotherapy, and sometimes radiation therapy.

Complete excision of the primary cancer is recommended when it can be done safely. Because the cancer is responsive to chemotherapy and radiation therapy, aggressive resection is discouraged if it may result in organ damage or dysfunction.

Children in all risk categories are treated with chemotherapy; the most commonly used drugs are vincristine, actinomycin D, cyclophosphamide, doxorubicin, ifosfamide, and etoposide. Topotecan and irinotecan are newer drugs that have activity against this cancer.

Radiation therapy is generally reserved for children with residual bulk disease or microscopic residual tumor after surgery and for children with intermediate-risk or high-risk disease.

WILMS TUMOR

(Nephroblastoma)

Wilms tumor is an embryonal cancer of the kidney composed of blastemal, stromal, and epithelial elements. Genetic abnormalities have been implicated in the pathogenesis, but familial inheritance accounts for only 1 to 2% of cases. Diagnosis is by ultrasonography, abdominal CT, or MRI. Treatment may include surgical resection, chemotherapy, and radiation therapy.

Wilms tumor usually manifests in children < 5 yr but occasionally in older children and rarely in adults. Wilms tumor accounts for about 6% of cancers in children < 15 yr. Bilateral synchronous tumors occur in about 5% of patients.

A chromosomal deletion of *WT1* a Wilms tumor suppressor gene, has been identified in some cases. Other associated genetic abnormalities include deletion of *WT2* (a 2nd Wilms tumor suppressor gene), loss of heterozygosity of 16q and 1p, and inactivation of the *WTX* gene.

About 10% of cases manifest with other congenital abnormalities, especially GU abnormalities, but also hemihypertrophy (asymmetry of the body). WAGR syndrome is the combination of Wilms tumor (with *WT1* deletion), aniridia, GU malformations (eg, renal hypoplasia, cystic disease, hypospadias, cryptorchidism), and intellectual disablity.

Symptoms and Signs

The most frequent finding is a painless, palpable abdominal mass. Less frequent findings include abdominal pain, hematuria, fever, anorexia, nausea, and vomiting. Hematuria can be microscopic or gross. Hypertension may occur and is of variable severity.

Diagnosis

- Abdominal ultrasonography, CT, or MRI

Abdominal ultrasonography determines whether the mass is cystic or solid and whether the renal vein or vena cava is involved. Abdominal CT or MRI is needed to determine the extent of the tumor and check for spread to regional lymph nodes, the contralateral kidney, or liver. Chest CT is recommended to detect metastatic pulmonary involvement at initial diagnosis.

Diagnosis of Wilms tumor is typically made presumptively based on the results of the imaging studies, so nephrectomy rather than biopsy is done in most patients at the time of diagnosis. Biopsy is not done because of the risk of peritoneal contamination by tumor cells, which would spread the cancer and thus change the stage from a lower to a higher one requiring more intensive therapy.

During surgery, locoregional lymph nodes are sampled for pathologic and surgical staging (see also National Cancer Institute's Stages of Wilms Tumor at www.cancer.gov).

Prognosis

Prognosis for Wilms tumor depends on

- Histology (favorable or unfavorable)
- Stage at diagnosis
- Patient's age (older age is associated with a worse prognosis)

The outcome for children with Wilms tumor is excellent. Cure rates for lower-stage disease (localized to the kidney) range from 85% to 95%. Even children with more advanced disease fare well; cure rates range from 60% (unfavorable histology) to 90% (favorable histology).

The cancer may recur, typically within 2 yr of diagnosis. Cure is possible in children with recurrent cancer. Outcome after recurrence is better for children who present initially with lower-stage disease, whose tumors recur at a site that has not been irradiated, who relapse > 1 yr after presentation, and who receive less intensive treatment initially.

Treatment

- Surgery and chemotherapy
- Radiation therapy for patients with higher stage/risk disease

Initial treatment of unilateral Wilms tumor is primary surgical resection followed by adjuvant chemotherapy. A select group of younger patients with small tumors can be cured by surgery alone. The type of chemotherapy drug and the length of therapy depends on tumor histology and stage. The chemotherapy regimen depends on the risk group but usually consists of actinomycin D and vincristine with or without doxorubicin. For more aggressive tumors, intensive multiagent chemotherapy regimens are used.

Children with very large nonresectable tumors or bilateral tumors are candidates for chemotherapy followed by reevaluation and delayed resection.

Children who have higher-stage disease or tumors involving the regional lymph nodes are given radiation therapy.

327 Perinatal Hematologic Disorders

PERINATAL ANEMIA

Anemia is a reduction in red cell mass or Hb and is usually defined as Hb or Hct > 2 standard deviations below the mean for age. Some authorities also consider a relative anemia to exist when a Hb or Hct above that cutoff point is insufficient to meet tissue oxygen demand. Anemia and polycythemia are the most common hematologic disorders diagnosed at birth.

Both Hb and Hct change rapidly as a neonate matures, so lower limits of normal also change (see Table 327–1). Variables such as gestational age, sampling site (capillary vs vein), and position of the neonate relative to the placenta before cord clamping (lower position causes blood to transfer in to the neonate; higher position causes blood to transfer out of the neonate) also affect test results.

Table 327–1. AGE-SPECIFIC VALUES FOR HEMOGLOBIN AND HEMATOCRIT

AGE	HB (g/dL)	HCT (%)
28 wk gestation	14.5	45
32 wk gestation	15	47
Term	16.5	51
1–3 days	18.5	56
2 wk	16.6	53

Etiology

Causes of anemia in neonates include

- Physiologic processes
- Blood loss
- Decreased RBC production
- Increased RBC destruction (hemolysis)

Physiologic anemia: Physiologic anemia is the most common cause of anemia in the neonatal period. Normal physiologic processes often cause normocytic-normochromic anemia in term and preterm infants. Physiologic anemias do not generally require extensive evaluation or treatment.

In term infants, the increase in oxygenation that occurs with normal breathing after birth causes an abrupt rise in tissue oxygen level, resulting in negative feedback on erythropoietin production and erythropoiesis. This reduction in erythropoiesis, as well as the shorter life span of neonatal RBCs (90 days vs 120 days in adults), causes Hb concentration to fall over the first 2 to 3 mo of life (typical Hb nadir 9 to 11 g/dL). Hb remains stable over the next several weeks and then slowly rises in the 4th to 6th mo secondary to renewed erythropoietin stimulation.

Physiologic anemia is more pronounced in preterm infants, occurring earlier and with a lower nadir compared to term infants. This condition is also referred to as anemia of prematurity. A mechanism similar to the one that causes anemia in term infants causes anemia in preterm infants during the first 4 to 12 wk. Lower erythropoietin production, shorter RBC life span (35 to 50 days), rapid growth, and more frequent phlebotomy contribute to a faster and lower Hb nadir (8 to 10 g/dL) in preterm infants. Anemia of prematurity most commonly affects infants < 32 wk gestation. Almost all acutely ill and extremely preterm infants (< 28 wk gestation) will develop anemia that is severe enough to require RBC transfusion during their initial hospitalization.

Blood loss: Anemia may develop because of prenatal, perinatal (at delivery), or postpartum hemorrhage. In neonates, absolute blood volume is low (eg, preterm, 90 to 105 mL/kg; term, 78 to 86 mL/kg); therefore, acute loss of as little as 15 to 20 mL of blood may result in anemia. An infant with chronic blood loss can compensate physiologically and is typically more clinically stable than an infant with acute blood loss.

Prenatal hemorrhage may be caused by

- Fetal-to-maternal hemorrhage
- Twin-to-twin transfusion
- Cord malformations
- Placental abnormalities
- Diagnostic procedures

Fetal-to-maternal hemorrhage usually occurs spontaneously or may result from maternal trauma, amniocentesis, external cephalic version, or placental tumor. It affects about 50% of pregnancies, although in most cases the volume of blood lost is extremely small (about 2 mL); "massive" blood loss, defined as > 30 mL, occurs in 3/1000 pregnancies.

Twin-to-twin transfusion is the unequal sharing of blood supply between twins that affects 13 to 33% of monozygotic, monochorionic twin pregnancies. When significant blood transfer occurs, the donor twin may become very anemic and develop heart failure, while the recipient may become polycythemic and develop hyperviscosity syndrome.

Cord malformations include velamentous insertion of the umbilical cord, vasa previa, or abdominal or placental insertion; the mechanism of hemorrhage, which is often massive, rapid, and life threatening, is by cord vessel shearing or rupture.

The 2 important placental abnormalities causing hemorrhage are placenta previa and abruptio placentae.

Diagnostic procedures causing hemorrhage include amniocentesis, chorionic villus sampling, and umbilical cord blood sampling.

Perinatal hemorrhage may be caused by

- Precipitous delivery (ie, rapid and spontaneous delivery, which causes hemorrhage due to umbilical cord tearing)
- Obstetric accidents (eg, incision of the placenta during cesarean delivery, birth trauma)
- Coagulopathies

Cephalhematomas resulting from procedures such as vacuum or forceps delivery are usually relatively harmless, but subgaleal bleeds can rapidly extend into soft tissue, sequestering sufficient blood volume to result in anemia, hypotension, shock, and death. Neonates with intracranial hemorrhage can lose sufficient blood into their intracranial vault to cause anemia and sometimes hemodynamic compromise (unlike older children who have a lower head-to-body ratio and in whom intracranial hemorrhage is limited in volume because the fused cranial sutures do not allow the skull to expand; instead, intracranial pressure increases and stops the bleeding). Far less often, rupture of the liver, spleen, or adrenal gland during delivery may lead to internal bleeding. Intraventricular hemorrhage, most common among preterm infants (see p. 2797), as well as subarachnoid and subdural bleeding also can result in a significantly lowered Hct.

Hemorrhagic disease of the newborn (see p. 53) is hemorrhage within a few days of a normal delivery caused by transient physiologic deficiency in vitamin K–dependent coagulation factors (factors II, VII, IX, and X). These factors are poorly transferred across the placenta, and, because vitamin K is synthesized by intestinal bacteria, very little is produced in the initially sterile intestine of the newborn. Vitamin K–deficient bleeding has three forms:

- Early (1st 24 h)
- Classic (1st wk of life)
- Late (2 to 12 wk of age)

The early form is caused by maternal use of a drug that inhibits vitamin K (eg, certain anticonvulsants; isoniazid; rifampin; warfarin; prolonged maternal use of broad-spectrum antibiotics, which suppresses bowel bacterial colonization). The classic form occurs in neonates who do not receive vitamin K supplementation after birth. The late form occurs in exclusively breastfed neonates who do not receive vitamin K supplementation after birth. Giving vitamin K 0.5 to 1 mg IM after birth rapidly activates clotting factors and prevents hemorrhagic disease of the newborn.

Other possible causes of hemorrhage in the first few days of life are other coagulopathies (eg, hemophilia), disseminated intravascular coagulation caused by sepsis, or vascular malformations.

Decreased RBC production: Defects in RBC production may be

- Congenital
- Acquired

Congenital defects are extremely rare, but Diamond-Blackfan anemia and Fanconi anemia are the most common.

Diamond-Blackfan anemia is characterized by lack of RBC precursors in bone marrow, macrocytic RBCs, lack of reticulocytes in peripheral blood, and lack of involvement of other blood cell lineages. It is often (though no always) part of a syndrome of congenital anomalies including microcephaly, cleft palate, eye anomalies, thumb deformities, and webbed neck. Up to 25% of affected infants are anemic at birth, and low birth weight occurs in about 10%. It is thought to be caused by defective stem cell differentiation.

Fanconi anemia is an autosomal recessive disorder of bone marrow progenitor cells that causes macrocytosis and reticulocytopenia with progressive failure of all hematopoietic cell lines. It is usually diagnosed after the neonatal period. The cause is a genetic defect that prevents cells from repairing damaged DNA or removing toxic free radicals that damage cells.

Other congenital anemias include Pearson syndrome, a rare, multisystem disease involving mitochondrial defects that cause refractory sideroblastic anemia, pancytopenia, and variable hepatic, renal, and pancreatic insufficiency or failure; and congenital dyserythropoietic anemia, in which chronic anemia (typically macrocytic) results from ineffective or abnormal RBC production, and hemolysis caused by RBC abnormalities.

Acquired defects are those that occur after birth. The most common causes are

- Infections
- Nutritional deficiencies

Infections (eg, malaria, rubella, syphilis, HIV, cytomegalovirus, adenovirus, bacterial sepsis) may impair RBC production in the bone marrow. Congenital parvovirus B19 and human herpesvirus 6 infections may result in the absence of RBC production.

Nutritional deficiencies of iron, copper, folate (folic acid), and vitamins E and B_{12} may cause anemia in the early months of life but not usually at birth. The incidence of iron deficiency, the most common nutritional deficiency, is higher in less developed countries where it results from dietary insufficiency and exclusive and prolonged breastfeeding. Iron deficiency is common among neonates whose mothers have an iron deficit and among premature infants who have not been transfused and whose formula is not supplemented with iron; premature infants deplete iron stores by 10 to 14 wk if not supplemented.

Hemolysis: Hemolysis may be caused by

- Immune-mediated disorders
- RBC membrane disorders
- Enzyme deficiencies
- Hemoglobinopathies
- Infections

All also cause hyperbilirubinemia, which may cause jaundice and kernicterus.

Immune-mediated hemolysis may occur when fetal RBCs with surface antigens (most commonly Rh and ABO blood antigens but also Kell, Duffy, and other minor group antigens) that differ from maternal RBC antigens enter the maternal circulation and stimulate production of IgG antibody directed against fetal RBCs. The most common severe scenario is that an Rh (D antigen)-negative mother becomes sensitized to the D antigen during a previous pregnancy with an Rh-positive fetus; a 2nd Rh-positive pregnancy may then prompt an IgG response that may result in fetal and neonatal hemolysis (see p. 2347). Intrauterine hemolysis may be severe enough to cause hydrops or death; postpartum, there may be significant anemia and hyperbilirubinemia with ongoing hemolysis secondary to persistent maternal IgG (half-life about 28 days). With widespread prophylactic use of anti-Rh D to prevent sensitization, < 0.11% of pregnancies in Rh-negative women are affected.

ABO incompatibility may cause hemolysis by a similar mechanism. ABO incompatibility usually occurs in type O mothers. Mothers with type A, B, or AB blood make anti-A or anti-B antibodies that are predominantly IgM and are incapable of crossing the placenta. Hemolysis caused by ABO incompatibility is typically less severe than that caused by Rh sensitization, although some infants do develop more significant hemolysis and hyperbilirubinemia. Hemolysis caused by ABO incompatibility can occur in a first pregnancy. Mothers are often sensitized by antigens in foods or bacteria, causing an initial IgM response. Although the IgM does not cross the placenta, this sensitization causes an amnestic response that leads to IgG production when there is exposure to fetal blood during pregnancy.

RBC membrane disorders alter RBC shape and deformability, resulting in premature removal of RBCs from the circulation. The most common disorders are hereditary spherocytosis and hereditary elliptocytosis.

Enzyme deficiencies of G6PD and pyruvate kinase are the most common enzyme disorders causing hemolysis. G6PD deficiency is a sex-linked disorder common among people of Mediterranean, Middle Eastern, African, and Asian ancestry and affects > 400 million people worldwide. It is thought to help protect against malaria and has an estimated allele frequency of 8% in malarious regions. Pyruvate kinase deficiency is an autosomal dominant disorder that occurs in all ethnic groups. Pyruvate kinase deficiency is rare and occurs in about 51 of a million whites.

Hemoglobinopathies are caused by deficiencies and structural abnormalities of globin chains. At birth, 55 to 90% of the neonate's Hb is composed of 2 alpha and 2 gamma globin chains (fetal Hb or Hb F [alpha^2 gamma^2]). After birth, gamma-chain production decreases (to < 2% by 2 to 4 yr of age) and beta-chain production increases until adult Hb (Hb A [alpha^2 beta^2]) becomes predominant. Alpha-thalassemia is a genetically inherited disorder of depressed alpha globin chain production and is the most common hemoglobinopathy causing anemia in the neonatal period. Beta-thalassemia is an inherited decrease in beta-chain production. Because beta globin is naturally low at birth, beta-thalassemia and structural abnormalities of the beta globin chain (eg, Hb S [sickle cell disease], Hb C) are not clinically apparent at birth and symptoms do not appear until fetal Hb levels have fallen to sufficiently low levels at 3 to 4 mo of age.

Intrauterine infections by certain bacteria, viruses, fungi, and protozoa (most notably malaria) also may trigger hemolytic anemia. In malaria, the *Plasmodium* parasite invades and ultimately ruptures the RBC. Immune-mediated destruction of parasitized RBCs and excess removal of nonparasitized cells occur. Associated bone marrow dyserythropoiesis results in inadequate compensatory erythropoiesis. Intravascular hemolysis, extravascular phagocytosis, and dyserythropoiesis can lead to anemia.

Symptoms and Signs

Symptoms and signs are similar regardless of the cause but vary with severity and rate of onset of the anemia. Neonates are generally pale and, if anemia is severe, have tachypnea, tachycardia, and sometimes a flow murmur; hypotension is present with acute blood loss. Jaundice may be present with hemolysis.

Evaluation

History: History should focus on maternal factors (eg, bleeding diatheses, hereditary RBC disorders, nutritional deficiencies, drugs), family history of hereditary disorders that may cause neonatal anemia (eg, alpha-thalassemia, enzyme deficiencies, red cell membrane disorders, RBC aplasias), and obstetric factors (eg, infections, vaginal bleeding, obstetric interventions, mode of delivery, blood loss, treatment and appearance of the cord, placental pathology, fetal distress, number of fetuses).

Nonspecific maternal factors may provide additional clues. Splenectomy would indicate a possible history of hemolysis, red cell membrane disorder, or autoimmune anemia; cholecystectomy might indicate a history of hemolysis-induced gallstones. Important neonatal factors include gestational age at delivery, age at presentation, sex, race, and ethnicity.

Physical examination: Tachycardia and hypotension suggest acute, significant blood loss. Jaundice suggests hemolysis, either systemic (caused by ABO incompatibility or G6PD deficiency) or localized (caused by breakdown of sequestered blood in cephalhematomas). Hepatosplenomegaly suggests hemolysis, congenital infection, or heart failure. Hematomas, ecchymoses, or petechiae suggest bleeding diathesis. Congenital anomalies may suggest a bone marrow failure syndrome.

Testing: Anemia may be suspected prenatally if ultrasonography shows increased middle cerebral artery peak systolic velocity or hydrops fetalis, which, by definition, is abnormal, excessive fluid in ≥ 2 body compartments (eg, pleura, peritoneum, pericardium); cardiac, hepatic, and splenic enlargement may be present.

After birth, if anemia is suspected, Hb and Hct levels are done. If they are low, initial testing consists of

- Reticulocyte count
- Peripheral smear examination

If the **reticulocyte count is low** (it is normally elevated when Hb and Hct are low), anemia is caused by acquired or congenital bone marrow dysfunction, and the infant should be evaluated for causes of bone marrow suppression with

- Titers or PCR studies for congenital infection (rubella, syphilis, HIV, cytomegalovirus, adenovirus, parvovirus, human herpesvirus 6)
- Folate and vitamin B_{12} levels
- Iron and copper levels

If these studies do not identify a cause of anemia, a bone marrow biopsy, genetic testing for congenital disorders of RBC production, or both may be necessary.

If the **reticulocyte count is elevated or normal** (reflecting an appropriate bone marrow response), anemia is caused by blood loss or hemolysis. If there is no apparent blood loss or if signs of hemolysis are noted on the peripheral smear or the serum bilirubin level is elevated (which may occur with hemolysis), a direct antiglobulin test (DAT [Coombs test]) should be done.

If the **DAT is positive,** anemia is likely secondary to Rh, ABO, or other blood group incompatibility. The DAT is always positive with Rh incompatibility but sometimes negative with ABO incompatibility. Infants may have active hemolysis caused by ABO incompatibility and have a negative DAT; however, in such infants, the peripheral blood smear should reveal microspherocytes, and the indirect antiglobulin (Coombs) test is usually positive when done.

If the **DAT is negative,** the RBC mean corpuscular volume (MCV) may prove helpful. A significantly low MCV suggests α-thalassemia or, less commonly, iron deficiency due to chronic intrauterine blood loss; these can be distinguished by red cell distribution width (RDW), which is often normal with thalassemia but elevated with iron deficiency. With a normal or high MCV, peripheral blood smear may show abnormal RBC morphology compatible with a membrane disorder, microangiopathy, disseminated intravascular coagulation, vitamin E deficiency, or hemoglobinopathy. Infants with hereditary spherocytosis often have an elevated mean corpuscular hemoglobin concentration (MCHC). If the smear is normal, blood loss, enzyme deficiency, or infection should be considered and an appropriate assessment, including testing for fetal-to-maternal hemorrhage, should ensue.

Fetal-to-maternal hemorrhage can be diagnosed by testing for fetal RBCs in maternal blood. The Kleihauer-Betke acid elution technique is the most frequently used test, but other tests include fluorescent antibody techniques and differential or mixed agglutination testing. In the Kleihauer-Betke technique, citric acid-phosphate buffer of pH 3.5 elutes Hb from adult but not fetal RBCs; thus, fetal RBCs stain with eosin and are visible on microscopy, whereas adult RBCs appear as red cell ghosts. The Kleihauer-Betke technique is not useful when the mother has a hemoglobinopathy.

Treatment

Need for treatment of perinatal anemia varies with degree of anemia and associated medical conditions. Mild anemia in otherwise healthy term and preterm infants generally does not require specific treatment; treatment is directed at the underlying diagnosis. Some patients require transfusion or exchange transfusion of packed RBCs.

Transfusion: Transfusion is indicated to treat severe anemia. Infants should be considered for transfusion if symptomatic due to anemia or if a decrease in tissue oxygen delivery is suspected. The decision to transfuse should be based on symptoms, patient age, and degree of illness. Hct alone should not be the deciding factor regarding transfusion because some infants may be asymptomatic with lower levels and others may be symptomatic with higher levels.

Guidelines for when to transfuse vary, but one accepted set is described in Table 327–2.

Before the first transfusion, if not already done, maternal and fetal blood should be screened for ABO and Rh types and the presence of atypical RBC antibodies, and a DAT should be done on the infant's RBCs.

Blood for transfusion should be the same as or compatible with the neonate's ABO and Rh group and with any ABO or RBC antibody present in maternal or neonatal serum. Neonates produce RBC antibodies only rarely, so in cases where the need for transfusion persists, repeat antibody screening is usually not necessary until 4 mo of age.

Packed RBCs used for transfusion should be filtered (leukocyte depleted), irradiated, and given in aliquots of 10 to 20 mL/kg derived from a single donation; sequential transfusions from the same unit of blood minimize recipient exposure and transfusion complications. Blood from cytomegalovirus-negative donors should be considered for extremely premature infants.

Exchange transfusion: Exchange transfusion, in which blood from the neonate is removed in aliquots in sequence with packed RBC transfusion, is indicated for some cases of hemolytic anemia with elevation of serum bilirubin, some cases of severe anemia with heart failure, and cases when infants with chronic blood loss are euvolemic. This procedure decreases plasma antibody titers and bilirubin levels and minimizes fluid overload.

Serious adverse effects (eg, thrombocytopenia; necrotizing enterocolitis; hypoglycemia; hypocalcemia; shock, pulmonary edema, or both [caused by shifts in fluid balance]) are common, so the procedure should be done by experienced staff. Guidelines for when to begin exchange transfusion differ and are not evidence based.

Other treatments: Recombinant human erythropoietin is not routinely recommended, in part because it has not been shown to reduce transfusion requirements in the first 2 wk of life.

Iron therapy is restricted to cases of repetitive blood loss (eg, hemorrhagic diathesis, GI bleeding, frequent phlebotomy).

Table 327–2. TRANSFUSION GUIDELINES FOR INFANTS < 4 MO

HCT	CRITERIA* FOR TRANSFUSION OF RBCs
< 45%	Congenital cyanotic heart disease Use of ECMO
< 35%	Use of O_2 by hood at > 35% FIO_2 Use of CPAP or mechanical ventilation with mean airway pressure > 6–8 cm H_2O
< 30%	Use of any supplemental O_2 Use of any CPAP or mechanical ventilation Significant abnormalities of heart rate or respiratory rate†
< 20%	Low reticulocyte count and symptoms of anemia (eg, tachycardia, tachypnea, poor feeding)

*At least 1 of these criteria must also be present.

†Abnormalities include > 6 episodes of apnea in 12 h, 2 episodes of apnea in 24 h requiring bag-and-mask ventilation (while receiving therapeutic doses of methylxanthines), heart rate > 180/min for 24 h, clinically significant bradycardia, and respiratory rate > 80/min for 24 h.

CPAP = continuous positive airway pressure; ECMO = extracorporeal membrane oxygenation; FIO_2 = fractional inspired O_2.

Adapted from Roseff SD, Luban NLC, Manno CS: Guidelines for assessing appropriateness of pediatric transfusion. *Transfusion* 42(11):1398–1413, 2002.

Oral iron supplements are preferred; parenteral iron sometimes causes anaphylaxis, so therapy should be guided by a hematologist.

Treatment of more unusual causes of anemia is disorder specific (eg, corticosteroids in Diamond-Blackfan anemia, and vitamin B_{12} for B_{12} deficiency).

KEY POINTS

- Anemia is a reduction in red cell mass or Hb, and in neonates is usually defined as Hb or Hct > 2 standard deviations below the mean for age.
- Causes of anemia in newborns include physiologic processes, blood loss, decreased RBC production, and increased RBC destruction.
- Physiologic anemia is the most common cause of anemia in the neonatal period and does not generally require extensive evaluation or treatment.
- Neonates with anemia are generally pale and, if anemia is severe, have tachypnea, tachycardia, and sometimes a flow murmur.
- Need for treatment varies with degree of anemia and associated medical conditions.
- Mild anemia in otherwise healthy term and preterm infants generally does not require specific treatment; treatment is directed at the underlying diagnosis.

PERINATAL POLYCYTHEMIA AND HYPERVISCOSITY SYNDROME

Polycythemia is an abnormal increase in RBC mass, defined in neonates as a venous Hct ≥ 65%; this increase can lead to hyperviscosity with sludging of blood within vessels and sometimes thrombosis. The main symptoms and signs of neonatal polycythemia are nonspecific and include ruddy complexion, feeding difficulties, lethargy, hypoglycemia, hyperbilirubinemia, cyanosis, respiratory distress, and seizures. Diagnosis is made clinically and with an arterial or venous Hct measurement. Treatment is with partial exchange transfusion.

The terms polycythemia and hyperviscosity are often used interchangeably but are not equivalent. Polycythemia is significant only because it increases risk of hyperviscosity syndrome. Hyperviscosity is a clinical syndrome caused by sludging of blood within vessels. Sludging occurs because increased RBC mass causes a relative decrease in plasma volume and a relative increase in proteins and platelets.

Incidence of polycythemia is about 3 to 4% (range 0.4 to 12%), and about half of infants with polycythemia have hyperviscosity.

Etiology

Dehydration causing relative hemoconcentration and an elevated Hct mimics polycythemia, but RBC mass is not increased.

Causes of true polycythemia include intrauterine hypoxia, perinatal asphyxia, placental transfusion (including twin-to-twin transfusion), some congenital abnormalities (eg, cyanotic congenital heart disease, renovascular malformations, congenital adrenal hyperplasia), certain delivery procedures (eg, delayed cord clamping, holding neonate below the level of the mother before cord clamping, stripping the cord toward the neonate at delivery), maternal insulin-dependent diabetes, Down syndrome or other trisomies, Beckwith-Wiedemann syndrome, and intrauterine growth restriction. Polycythemia is also more common when the mother resides at a high altitude.

Premature infants rarely develop hyperviscosity syndrome.

Symptoms and Signs

Symptoms and signs of hyperviscosity syndrome are those of heart failure, thrombosis (cerebral and renal vessels), and CNS dysfunction, including tachypnea, respiratory distress, cyanosis, plethora, apnea, lethargy, irritability, hypotonia, tremulousness, seizures, and feeding problems. Renal vein thrombosis may also cause renal tubular damage, proteinuria, or both.

Diagnosis

- Hct
- Clinical evaluation

Diagnosis of polycythemia is by arterial or venous (not capillary) Hct. Diagnosis of hyperviscosity syndrome is clinical. Capillary samples often overestimate Hct, so a venous or arterial Hct should be obtained before the diagnosis is made; most published studies of polycythemia use spun Hcts, which are no longer routinely done and are generally higher than those done on automated counters. Laboratory measure of viscosity is not readily available.

Other laboratory abnormalities may include low blood glucose and Ca^{++} levels, maternal diabetes, or both; RBC lysis; thrombocytopenia (secondary to consumption with thrombosis); hyperbilirubinemia (caused by turnover of a higher number of RBCs); and reticulocytosis and increased peripheral nucleated RBCs (caused by increased erythropoiesis secondary to fetal hypoxia).

Treatment

- IV hydration
- Sometimes phlebotomy plus saline replacement (partial exchange transfusion)

Asymptomatic infants should be treated with IV hydration (see p. 2555). Symptomatic infants with Hct > 65 to 70% should undergo an isovolemic hemodilution (sometimes called partial exchange transfusion, although no blood products are given) to reduce the Hct to ≤ 55% and thereby decrease blood viscosity. Partial exchange is done by removing blood in aliquots of 5 mL/kg and immediately replacing it with an equal volume of 0.9% saline. Asymptomatic infants whose Hct remains persistently > 70% despite hydration may also benefit from this procedure.

Although many studies show immediate measurable effects of partial exchange, the long-term benefits remain in question. Most studies have failed to document differences in long-term growth or neurodevelopment between children who have received a partial exchange transfusion in the neonatal period and those who have not.

KEY POINTS

- Polycythemia in neonates is a venous Hct ≥ 65%.
- Hyperviscosity is a clinical syndrome involving sludging of blood within vessels and sometimes thrombosis.
- Manifestations are varied and can be severe (heart failure, thrombosis [cerebral and renal vessels], CNS dysfunction) or mild (tremulousness, lethargy, or hyperbilirubinemia).
- Treat with IV hydration and sometimes partial exchange transfusion.

328 Perinatal Physiology

The transition from life in utero to life outside the womb involves multiple changes in physiology and function.

Bilirubin metabolism: Aged or damaged fetal RBCs are removed from the circulation by reticuloendothelial cells, which convert heme to bilirubin (1 g of Hb yields 35 mg of bilirubin). This bilirubin is transported to the liver, where it is transferred into hepatocytes. Glucuronyl transferase then conjugates the bilirubin with uridine diphosphoglucuronic acid (UDPGA) to form bilirubin diglucuronide (conjugated bilirubin), which is secreted actively into the bile ducts. Bilirubin diglucuronide makes its way into meconium in the GI tract but cannot be eliminated from the body, because the fetus does not normally pass stool. The enzyme β-glucuronidase, present in the fetus' small-bowel luminal brush border, is released into the intestinal lumen, where it deconjugates bilirubin glucuronide; free (unconjugated) bilirubin is then reabsorbed from the intestinal tract and reenters the fetal circulation. Fetal bilirubin is cleared from the circulation by placental transfer into the mother's plasma following a concentration gradient. The maternal liver then conjugates and excretes the fetal bilirubin.

At birth, the placental connection is terminated, and although the neonatal liver continues to take up, conjugate, and excrete bilirubin into bile so it can be eliminated in the stool, neonates lack proper intestinal bacteria for oxidizing bilirubin to urobilinogen in the gut; consequently, unaltered bilirubin remains in the stool, imparting a typical bright-yellow color. Additionally, the neonatal GI tract (like that of the fetus) contains β-glucuronidase, which deconjugates some of the bilirubin. Feedings invoke the gastrocolic reflex, and bilirubin is excreted in stool before most of it can be deconjugated and reabsorbed. However in many neonates, the unconjugated bilirubin is reabsorbed and returned to the circulation from the intestinal lumen (enterohepatic circulation of bilirubin), contributing to physiologic hyperbilirubinemia and jaundice (see p. 2725).

Cardiovascular function: Fetal circulation is marked by right-to-left shunting of blood around the unventilated lungs through a patent ductus arteriosus (connecting the pulmonary artery to the aorta) and foramen ovale (connecting the right and left atria). Shunting is encouraged by high pulmonary arteriolar resistance and relatively low resistance to blood flow in the systemic (including placental) circulation. About 90 to 95% of the right heart output bypasses the lungs and goes directly to the systemic circulation. The fetal ductus arteriosus is kept open by low fetal systemic Pa_{O_2} (about 25 mm Hg) along with locally produced prostaglandins. The foramen ovale is kept open by differences in atrial pressures: left atrial pressure is relatively low because little blood is returned from the lungs, but right atrial pressure is relatively high because large volumes of blood return from the placenta.

Profound changes to this system occur after the first few breaths, resulting in increased pulmonary blood flow and functional closure of the foramen ovale. Pulmonary arteriolar resistance drops acutely as a result of vasodilation caused by lung expansion, increased Pa_{O_2}, and reduced Pa_{CO_2}. The elastic forces of the ribs and chest wall decrease pulmonary interstitial pressure, further enhancing blood flow through pulmonary capillaries. Increased venous return from the lungs raises left atrial pressure, thus reducing the pressure differential between left and right atria; this effect contributes to the functional closure of the foramen ovale.

As pulmonary blood flow is established, venous return from the lungs increases, raising left atrial pressure. Air breathing increases the Pa_{O_2}, which constricts the umbilical arteries. Placental blood flow is reduced or stops, reducing blood return to the right atrium. Thus, right atrial pressure decreases while left atrial pressure increases; as a result, the two fetal components of the interatrial septum (septum primum and septum secundum) are pushed together, stopping flow through the foramen ovale. In most people, the two septa eventually fuse and the foramen ovale ceases to exist.

Soon after birth, systemic resistance becomes higher than pulmonary resistance, a reversal from the fetal state. Therefore, the direction of blood flow through the patent ductus arteriosus reverses, creating left-to-right shunting of blood (called transitional circulation). This state lasts from moments after birth (when the pulmonary blood flow increases and functional closure of the foramen ovale occurs) until about 24 to 72 h of age, when the ductus arteriosus constricts. Blood entering the ductus and its vasa vasorum from the aorta has a high P_{O_2}, which, along with alterations in prostaglandin metabolism, leads to constriction and closure of the ductus arteriosus. Once the ductus arteriosus closes, an adult-type circulation exists. The 2 ventricles now pump in series, and there are no major shunts between the pulmonary and systemic circulations.

During the days immediately after birth, a stressed neonate may revert to a fetal-type circulation. Asphyxia with hypoxia and hypercarbia causes the pulmonary arterioles to constrict and the ductus arteriosus to dilate, reversing the processes described previously and resulting in right-to-left shunting through the now-patent ductus arteriosus, the reopened foramen ovale, or both. Consequently, the neonate becomes severely hypoxemic, a condition called persistent pulmonary hypertension (see p. 2815) or persistent fetal circulation (although there is no umbilical circulation). The goal of treatment is to reverse the conditions that caused pulmonary vasoconstriction.

Endocrine function: The fetus depends completely on the maternal supply of glucose via the placenta and does not contribute to glucose production. The fetus begins to build a hepatic glycogen supply early in gestation, accumulating most glycogen stores during the 2nd half of the 3rd trimester. The neonate's glucose supply terminates when the umbilical cord is cut; concurrently, levels of circulating epinephrine, norepinephrine, and glucagon surge, while insulin levels decline. These changes stimulate gluconeogenesis and mobilization of hepatic glycogen stores. In healthy, term neonates, glucose levels reach a nadir 30 to 90 min after birth, after which neonates are typically able to maintain normal glucose homeostasis. Infants at highest risk of neonatal hypoglycemia include those with reduced glycogen stores (small-for-gestational-age and premature infants), critically ill infants with increased glucose catabolism, and infants of diabetic mothers (secondary to temporary fetal hyperinsulinemia).

Hematopoietic function: In utero, RBC production is controlled exclusively by fetal erythropoietin produced in the liver; maternal erythropoietin does not cross the placenta. About 55 to 90% of fetal RBCs contain fetal Hb, which has high O_2 affinity. As a result, a high O_2 concentration gradient is maintained across the placenta, resulting in abundant O_2 transfer from the maternal to the fetal circulation. This increased O_2 affinity is less useful after birth, because fetal Hb gives up O_2 to tissues less readily, and it may be deleterious if severe pulmonary or cardiac disease with hypoxemia exists. The transition from fetal to adult Hb begins before birth; at delivery, the site of erythropoietin production changes from the liver to the more sensitive peritubular cells of the kidney by an unknown mechanism. The abrupt increase in Pa_{O_2} from about 25 to 30 mm Hg in the fetus to 90 to 95 mm Hg in the neonate just after delivery causes serum erythropoietin to fall, and RBC production shuts down between birth and about 6 to 8 wk, causing physiologic anemia and contributing to anemia of prematurity (see p. 2784).

Immunologic function: At term, most immune mechanisms are not fully functional, more so with increasing prematurity. Thus, all neonates and young infants are immunodeficient relative to adults and are at increased risk of overwhelming infection. This risk is enhanced by prematurity, maternal illness, neonatal stress, and drugs (eg, immunosuppressants, anticonvulsants). Neonates' decreased immune response may explain the absence of fever or localized clinical signs (eg, meningismus) with infection.

In the fetus, phagocytic cells, present at the yolk sac stage of development, are critical for the inflammatory response that combats bacterial and fungal infection. Granulocytes can be identified in the 2nd mo of gestation and monocytes can be identified in the 4th mo of gestation. Their level of function increases with gestational age but is still low at term.

At birth, the ultrastructure of neutrophils is normal, but in most neonates, chemotaxis of neutrophils and monocytes is decreased because of an intrinsic abnormality of cellular locomotion and adherence to surfaces. These functional deficits are more pronounced in premature infants.

By about the 14th wk of gestation, the thymus is functioning, and hematopoietic stem cell–produced lymphocytes accumulate in the thymus for development. Also by 14 wk, T cells are present in the fetal liver and spleen, indicating that mature T cells are established in the secondary peripheral lymphoid organs by this age. The thymus is most active during fetal development and in early postnatal life. It grows rapidly in utero and is readily noted on chest x-ray in a healthy neonate, reaching a peak size at age 10 yr then involuting gradually over many years.

The number of T cells in the fetal circulation gradually increases during the 2nd trimester and reaches nearly normal levels by 30 to 32 wk gestation. At birth, neonates have a relative T lymphocytosis compared to adults. However, neonatal T cells do not function as effectively as adult T cells. For example, neonatal T cells may not respond adequately to antigens and may not produce cytokines.

B cells are present in fetal bone marrow, blood, liver, and spleen by the 12th wk of gestation. Trace amounts of IgM and IgG can be detected by the 20th wk and trace amounts of IgA can be detected by the 30th wk; because the fetus is normally in an antigen-free environment, only small amounts of immunoglobulin (predominantly IgM) are produced in utero. Elevated levels of cord serum IgM indicate in utero antigen challenge, usually caused by congenital infection. Almost all IgG is acquired maternally from the placenta. After 22 wk gestation, placental transfer of IgG increases to reach maternal levels or greater at term. IgG levels at birth in premature infants are decreased relative to gestational age.

The passive transfer of maternal immunity from transplacental IgG and secretory IgA and antimicrobial factors in breast milk (eg, IgG, secretory IgA, WBCs, complement proteins, lysozyme, lactoferrin) compensate for the neonate's immature immune system and confer immunity to many bacteria and viruses. Protective immune factors in breast milk coat the GI and upper respiratory tracts via mucosa-associated lymphoid tissue and decrease the likelihood of invasion of mucous membranes by respiratory and enteric pathogens.

Over time, passive immunity begins to wane, reaching a nadir when the infant is 3 to 6 mo old. Premature infants, in particular, may become profoundly hypogammaglobulinemic during the first 6 mo of life. By 1 yr, the IgG level rises to about 60% of average adult levels. IgA, IgM, IgD, and IgE, which do not cross the placenta and therefore are detectable only in trace amounts at birth, increase slowly during childhood. IgG, IgM, and IgA reach adult levels by about age 10 yr.

Pulmonary function: Fetal lung development progresses through phases of organogenesis and differentiation. Fairly well-developed alveoli and type II surfactant–producing pneumocytes are present around the 25th wk and continue to mature throughout gestation. The lungs continually produce fluid—a transudate from pulmonary capillaries plus surfactant secreted by type II pneumocytes. For normal gas exchange to occur at birth, pulmonary alveolar fluid and interstitial fluid must be cleared promptly by compression of the fetal thorax during delivery and by absorption of fluid into cells in the lung via epithelial sodium channel activation. Transient tachypnea of the newborn (see p. 2807) is probably caused by delay in this clearance process.

On delivery, when elastic recoil of ribs and strong inspiratory efforts draw air into the pulmonary tree, air-fluid interfaces are formed in alveoli. At the first breath, surfactant is released into the air-fluid interfaces. Surfactant, a mixture of phospholipids (phosphatidylcholine, phosphatidyl glycerol, phosphatidylinositol), neutral lipids, and 4 surface-active proteins all stored in lamellar inclusions in type II pneumocytes, reduces high surface tension, which would otherwise cause atelectasis and increase the work of breathing. Surfactant works more effectively in small alveoli than in large alveoli, thus opposing the normal tendency of small alveoli to collapse into large alveoli (per Laplace's law, which states that in an elastic cavity, pressure *decreases* as volume increases).

In some neonates, surfactant may not be produced in sufficient quantities to prevent diffuse atelectasis, and respiratory distress syndrome develops (see p. 2808). Neonatal surfactant production in the preterm infant can be increased by giving corticosteroids to the mother before delivery. The production and function of surfactant may be decreased by maternal diabetes, neonatal meconium aspiration, and neonatal sepsis.

Renal function: At birth, renal function is generally reduced, particularly in premature infants. GFR increases progressively during gestation, particularly during the 3rd trimester. GFR rapidly increases in the first months of life; however, GFR, urea clearance, and maximum tubular clearances do not reach adult levels until age 1 to 2 yr.

329 Perinatal Problems

Extensive physiologic changes accompany the birth process, sometimes unmasking conditions that posed no problem during intrauterine life. For that reason, a person with neonatal resuscitation skills must attend each birth.

Gestational age and growth parameters help identify the risk of neonatal pathology.

GESTATIONAL AGE

Gestational age and growth parameters help identify the risk of neonatal pathology. Gestational age (menstrual age, postmenstrual age) is the time elapsed since the beginning of the woman's last menstrual period; it is usually counted in weeks. Because it is not based on the moment of fertilization, which is difficult to specify (except when in vitro fertilization is done), gestational age is not the actual age of the fetus. Gestational age is the primary determinant of organ maturity.

The best way to assess gestational age is with antenatal ultrasonography and menstrual history. Clinicians also estimate gestational age during the newborn physical examination (see p. 2411) using the new Ballard score (see Fig. 288–1 on p. 2412). The Ballard score is based on the neonate's physical and neuromuscular maturity and can be used up to 4 days after birth (in practice, the Ballard score is usually used in the first 24 h). The neuromuscular components are more consistent over time because the physical components mature quickly after birth. However, the neuromuscular components can be affected by illness and drugs (eg, Mg sulfate given during labor).

Based on gestational age, each neonate is classified as

- Premature: < 34 wk gestation
- Late pre-term: 34 to < 37 wk
- Early term: 37 0/7 wk through 38 6/7 wk
- Full term: 39 0/7 wk through 40 6/7 wk
- Late term: 41 0/7 wk through 41 6/7 wk
- Postterm: 42 0/7 wk and beyond
- Postmature: > 42 wk

GROWTH PARAMETERS IN NEONATES

(Length, Weight, and Head Circumference)

Growth parameters and gestational age help identify the risk of neonatal pathology. Growth is influenced by genetic and nutritional factors as well as intrauterine conditions. Growth parameters assessed at birth help predict subsequent growth and development and risk of disease. The parameters are length, weight, and head circumference.

By plotting weight vs gestational age, each infant is classified at birth as

- Small for gestational age: < 10th percentile (see p. 2806)
- Appropriate for gestational age: 10th to 90th percentile
- Large for gestational age (LGA): > 90th percentile (see p. 2799)

The Fenton growth charts (see Figs. 329–1 and 329–2) provide a more precise assessment of growth vs gestational age for all three parameters.

NEONATAL RESUSCITATION

About 10% of neonates require some respiratory assistance at birth. Less than 1% need extensive resuscitation. Causes are numerous (see Table 329–1), but most involve asphyxia or respiratory depression. Incidence rises significantly if birth weight is < 1500 g.

Assessment: The **Apgar score** is used at birth to evaluate a newborn's condition and possible need for resuscitation; it was not initially intended to determine long-term neurologic prognosis. The Apgar score assigns 0 to 2 points for each of 5 measures of neonatal health (Appearance, Pulse, Grimace, Activity, Respiration—see Table 288–1 on p. 2411). Scores depend on physiologic maturity, maternal perinatal therapy, and fetal cardiorespiratory and neurologic conditions. A score of 7 to 10 at 5 min is considered normal; 4 to 6, intermediate; and 0 to 3, low. A low Apgar score is not *by itself* diagnostic of perinatal asphyxia but is associated with a risk of long-term neurologic dysfunction. A persistently low Apgar score (0 to 3 at 5 min) is associated with increased neonatal mortality.

The earliest sign of asphyxia is cyanosis, followed by decreases in respiration, muscle tone, reflex response, and heart rate. Effective resuscitation leads initially to increased heart rate, followed by improved reflex response, color, respiration, and muscle tone. Evidence of intrapartum fetal distress, persistence of an Apgar score of 0 to 3 for > 5 min; an umbilical arterial blood pH < 7; and a sustained neonatal neurologic syndrome that includes hypotonia, coma, seizures, and evidence of multiorgan dysfunction are manifestations of hypoxic ischemic encephalopathy. The severity and prognosis of posthypoxic encephalopathy can be estimated with the Sarnat classification (see Table 329–2) in conjunction with EEG, neuroradiologic imaging, and brain stem auditory and cortical evoked responses.

Resuscitation: Initial measures for all neonates include providing warmth, drying, and stimulating breathing (eg, flicking the soles of the feet, rubbing the back). If there is obvious obstruction to spontaneous breathing, the airway is cleared using bulb suction or a suction catheter. Suctioning has not proved beneficial in infants without obvious obstruction, even if amniotic fluid was stained with meconium (suctioning was previously recommended in such infants). If deep suctioning is required, appropriately sized catheters and pressure limits of 100 mm Hg (136 cm H_2O) must be used. Infants not responding with appropriate respirations and heart rate may require positive pressure ventilation (PPV), O_2 therapy, and, less commonly, chest compressions.

The infant is quickly dried and placed supine under a preheated overhead warmer in the delivery room. The neck is supported in the neutral position (sniffing position) to maintain an open airway.

If spontaneous respirations are absent, the infant is gasping, or heart rate is < 100 beats/min, respirations are assisted with PPV via mask, or sometimes laryngeal mask airway or endotracheal tube. Note that infants with a sunken, convex (scaphoid) abdomen may have a congenital diaphragmatic hernia, in which case ventilation using a mask can be dangerous; if such infants require ventilatory assistance, they should undergo endotracheal intubation. O_2 saturation is monitored using a pulse oximeter placed to measure preductal saturation (typically on the right hand or wrist). Resuscitation should be started with room air or a blend of O_2 and air and titrated to achieve O_2 saturations within the target range, which increases over the first

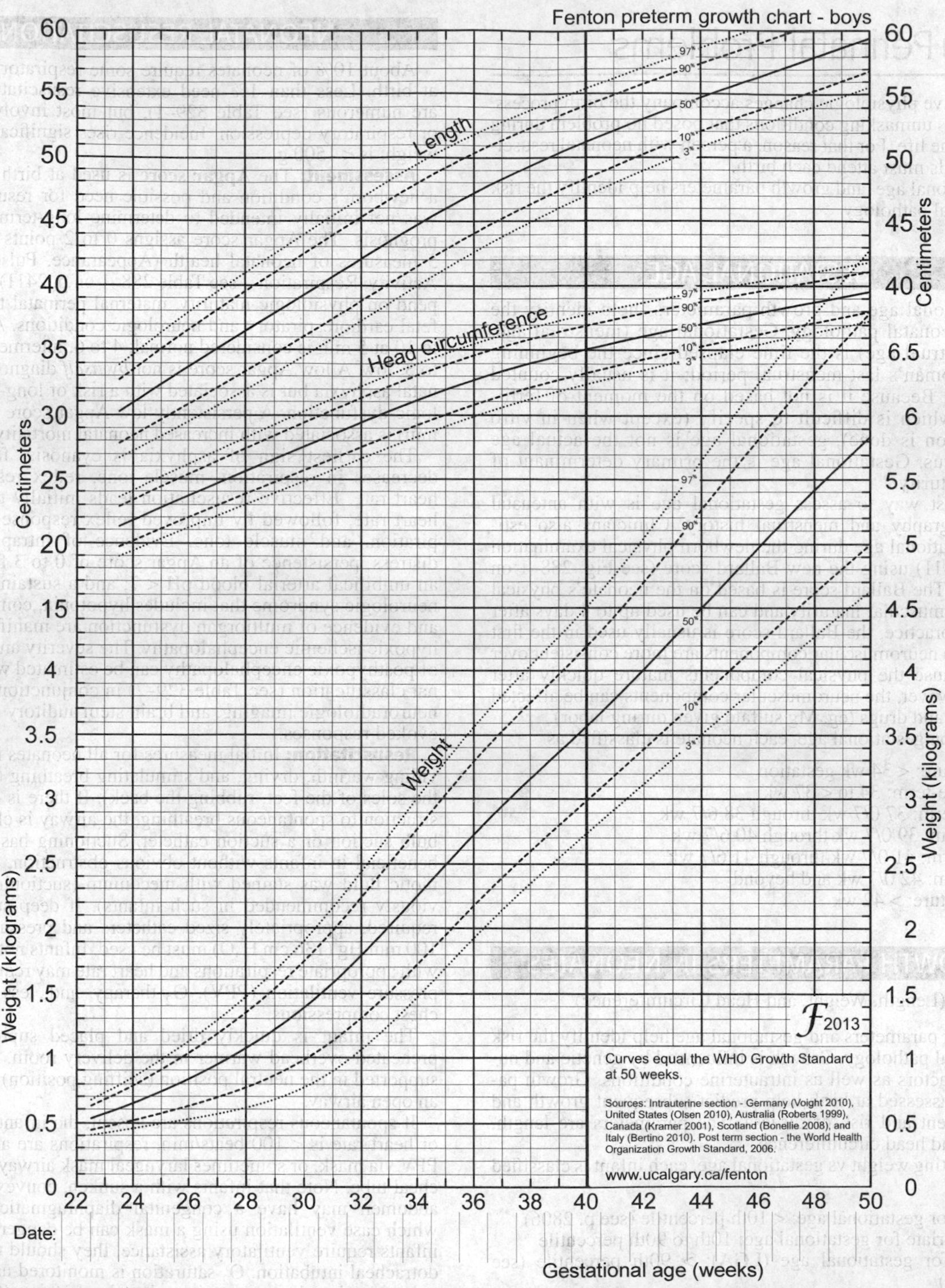

Fig. 329–1. Fenton Growth Chart for Preterm Boys. Fenton T, Kim J: A systematic review and meta-analysis to revise the Fenton growth chart for preterm infants. BMC Pediatrics 13:59, 2013; used with permission.

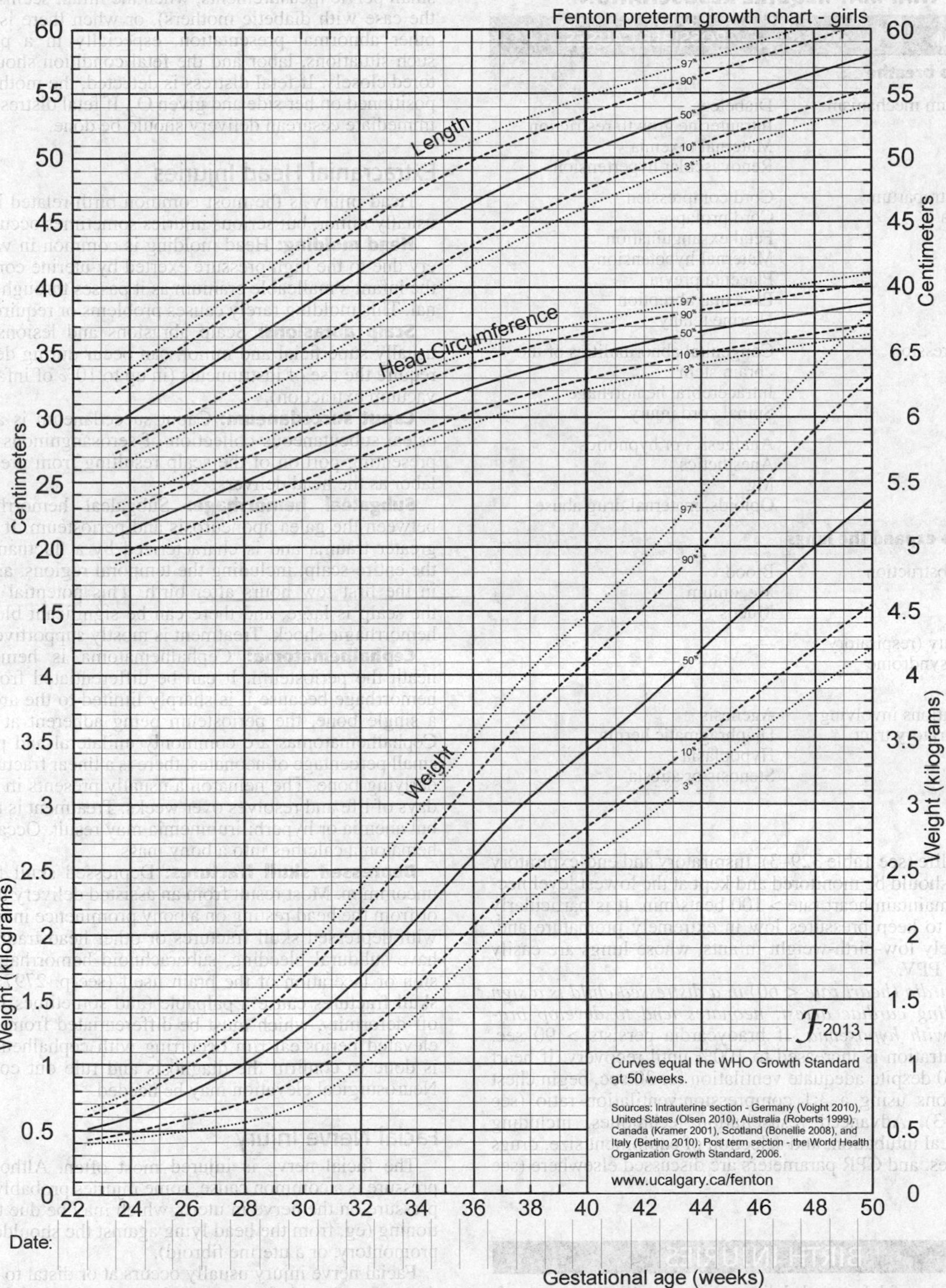

Fig. 329–2. Fenton Growth Chart for Preterm Girls. Fenton T, Kim J: A systematic review and meta-analysis to revise the Fenton growth chart for preterm infants. BMC Pediatrics 13:59, 2013; used with permission.

Table 329–1. PROBLEMS IN THE NEONATE THAT MAY REQUIRE RESUSCITATION

PROBLEM	POSSIBLE CAUSES
Failure to breathe	
Antepartum mechanism	Diabetes Intrauterine growth restriction Maternal toxemia Renovascular hypertension
Recent intrapartum asphyxia	Cord compression Cord prolapse Fetal exsanguination Maternal hypotension Placenta previa Placental abruption Uterine tetany
CNS depression	Congenital abnormalities of the brain stem Intracerebral hemorrhage Spinal cord injury
Drugs	Analgesics or hypnotics Anesthetics Mg Opioids, maternal drug abuse
Failure to expand the lungs	
Airway obstruction	Blood Meconium Mucus
Prematurity (respiratory distress syndrome [RDS])	—
Malformations involving the respiratory tract	Agenesis Diaphragmatic hernia Hypoplasia Stenosis or atresia

10 min of life (see Table 329–3). Inspiratory and end-expiratory pressures should be monitored and kept at the lowest level necessary to maintain heart rate > 100 beats/min. It is particularly important to keep pressures low in extremely premature and/or extremely low-birth-weight infants, whose lungs are easily injured by PPV.

Bradycardia (heart rate < 60) in a distressed child is a sign of impending cardiac arrest; neonates tend to develop bradycardia with hypoxemia. If bradycardia persists > 90 sec, O_2 concentration is increased to 100% until recovery. If heart rate is < 60 despite adequate ventilation for 30 sec, begin chest compressions using a 3:1 compression:ventilation ratio (see Fig. 329–3). Advanced resuscitation techniques, including endotracheal intubation, and selection of equipment size, drugs and dosages, and CPR parameters are discussed elsewhere (see p. 545).

BIRTH INJURIES

The forces of labor and delivery occasionally cause physical injury to the infant. The incidence of neonatal injury from difficult or traumatic deliveries is decreasing due to increasing use of cesarean delivery in place of difficult versions, vacuum extractions, or mid- or high-forceps deliveries.

A traumatic delivery is more likely when the mother has small pelvic measurements, when the infant seems LGA (often the case with diabetic mothers), or when there is a breech or other abnormal presentation, especially in a primipara. In such situations, labor and the fetal condition should be monitored closely. If fetal distress is detected, the mother should be positioned on her side and given O_2. If fetal distress persists, an immediate cesarean delivery should be done.

Extracranial Head Injuries

Head injury is the most common birth-related injury and is usually minor, but serious injuries sometimes occur.

Head molding: Head molding is common in vaginal delivery due to the high pressure exerted by uterine contractions on the infant's malleable cranium as it passes through the birth canal. This molding rarely causes problems or requires treatment.

Scalp abrasions: Scalp abrasions and lesions, which are usually superficial and minor, can occur during deliveries that require the use of instruments (in up to 10% of infants who had vacuum extraction).

Caput succedaneum: Caput succedaneum is an extraperiosteal subcutaneous collection of serosanguinous fluid on the presenting portion of the scalp resulting from pressure during labor as the head delivers.

Subgaleal hemorrhage: Subgaleal hemorrhage occurs between the galea aponeurosis and periosteum. It results from greater trauma and is characterized by a fluctuant mass over the entire scalp, including the temporal regions, and manifests in the first few hours after birth. This potential space under the scalp is large, and there can be significant blood loss and hemorrhagic shock. Treatment is mostly supportive.

Cephalhematoma: Cephalhematoma is hemorrhage beneath the periosteum. It can be differentiated from subgaleal hemorrhage because it is sharply limited to the area overlying a single bone, the periosteum being adherent at the sutures. Cephalhematomas are commonly unilateral and parietal. In a small percentage of neonates, there is a linear fracture of the underlying bone. The hematoma usually presents in the first few days of life and resolves over weeks. Treatment is not required, but anemia or hyperbilirubinemia may result. Occasionally, the hematoma calcifies into a bony mass.

Depressed skull fractures: Depressed skull fractures are uncommon. Most result from an assisted delivery using forceps or from the head resting on a bony prominence in utero. Infants with depressed skull fractures or other head trauma may also have subdural bleeding, subarachnoid hemorrhage, or contusion or laceration of the brain itself (see p. 2797). Depressed skull fractures cause a palpable (and sometimes visible) step-off deformity, which must be differentiated from the palpable elevated periosteal rim occurring with cephalhematomas. CT is done to confirm the diagnosis and rule out complications. Neurosurgical elevation may be needed.

Facial Nerve Injury

The facial nerve is injured most often. Although forceps pressure is a common cause, some injuries probably result from pressure on the nerve in utero, which may be due to fetal positioning (eg, from the head lying against the shoulder, the sacral promontory, or a uterine fibroid).

Facial nerve injury usually occurs at or distal to its exit from the stylomastoid foramen and results in facial asymmetry, especially during crying. Identifying which side of the face is affected can be confusing, but the facial muscles on the side of the nerve injury cannot move. Injury can also occur to individual branches of the nerve, most often the mandibular.

Table 329–2. CLINICAL STAGING OF POSTHYPOXIC ENCEPHALOPATHY

FACTOR	STAGE I (MILD)	STAGE II (MODERATE)	STAGE III (SEVERE)
Duration	< 24 h	2–14 days	Hours to weeks
Level of consciousness	Hyperalertness and irritability	Lethargy	Deep stupor or coma
Muscle tone	Normal	Hypotonia or proximal limb weakness	Flaccidity
Tendon reflexes	Increased	Increased	Depressed or absent
Myoclonus	Present	Present	Absent
Complex reflexes			
Sucking	Active	Weak	Absent
Moro response	Exaggerated	Incomplete	Absent
Grasping	Normal to exaggerated	Exaggerated	Absent
Oculocephalic (doll's eye)	Normal	Overreactive	Reduced or absent
Autonomic function			
Pupils	Dilated	Constricted	Variable or fixed
Respiration	Regular	Variable in rate and depth, periodic	Irregular apnea
Heart rate	Normal or tachycardic	Low resting < 120 beats/min	Bradycardia
Seizures	None	Common (70%)	Uncommon
EEG	Normal	Low voltage, periodic or paroxysmal, epileptiform activity	Periodic or isoelectric
Risk of death	< 1%	5%	> 60%
Risk of severe handicap	< 1%	20%	> 70%

Adapted from Sarnat HB, Sarnat MS: Neonatal encephalopathy following fetal distress. *Archives of Neurology* 33:696–705, 1975.

Another cause of facial asymmetry is mandibular asymmetry resulting from intrauterine pressure; in this case, muscle innervation is intact and both sides of the face can move. In mandibular asymmetry, the maxillary and the mandibular occlusal surfaces are not parallel, which differentiates it from a facial nerve injury. A congenital anomaly that can cause an asymmetric smile is unilateral absence of the depressor anguli oris muscle; this anomaly is clinically insignificant but must be differentiated from facial nerve injury.

Testing or treatment is not needed for peripheral facial nerve injuries or mandibular asymmetry. They usually resolve by age 2 to 3 mo.

Brachial Plexus Injuries

Brachial plexus injuries frequently follow lateral stretching of the neck during delivery caused by shoulder dystocia, breech extraction, or hyperabduction of the neck in cephalic presentations. Injuries can be due to simple stretching of the nerve, hemorrhage within a nerve, tearing of the nerve or root, or avulsion of the roots with accompanying cervical cord injury. Associated injuries (eg, fractures of the clavicle or humerus or subluxations of the shoulder or cervical spine) may occur. Intrauterine compression may also cause some cases.

Injuries may involve the

- Upper brachial plexus (C5 to C7): Affects muscles around the shoulder and elbow
- Lower plexus (C8 to T1): Primarily affects muscles of the forearm and hand
- Entire brachial plexus: Affects entire upper extremity and often sympathetic fibers of T1

The site and type of nerve root injury determine the prognosis.

Erb palsy is the most common brachial plexus injury. It is an upper brachial plexus (C5 to C7) injury causing adduction and internal rotation of the shoulder with pronation of the forearm (see Plate 92). Sometimes the biceps reflex is absent and the Moro reflex is asymmetric. Ipsilateral paralysis of the diaphragm due to phrenic nerve injury also is common. Treatment is usually supportive with physical therapy and protective positioning, which includes protecting the shoulder from excessive motion by immobilizing the arm across the upper abdomen and preventing contractures by gently doing passive range-of-motion exercises to involved joints every day starting at 1 wk of age.

Table 329–3. NEONATAL OXYGEN SATURATION TARGETS

TIME AFTER DELIVERY	PREDUCTAL* SPO_2
1 min	60–65%
2 min	65–70%
3 min	70–75%
4 min	75–80%
5 min	80–85%
≥ 10 min	85–95%

*The right upper extremity receives preductal blood.
SpO_2 = O_2 saturation.

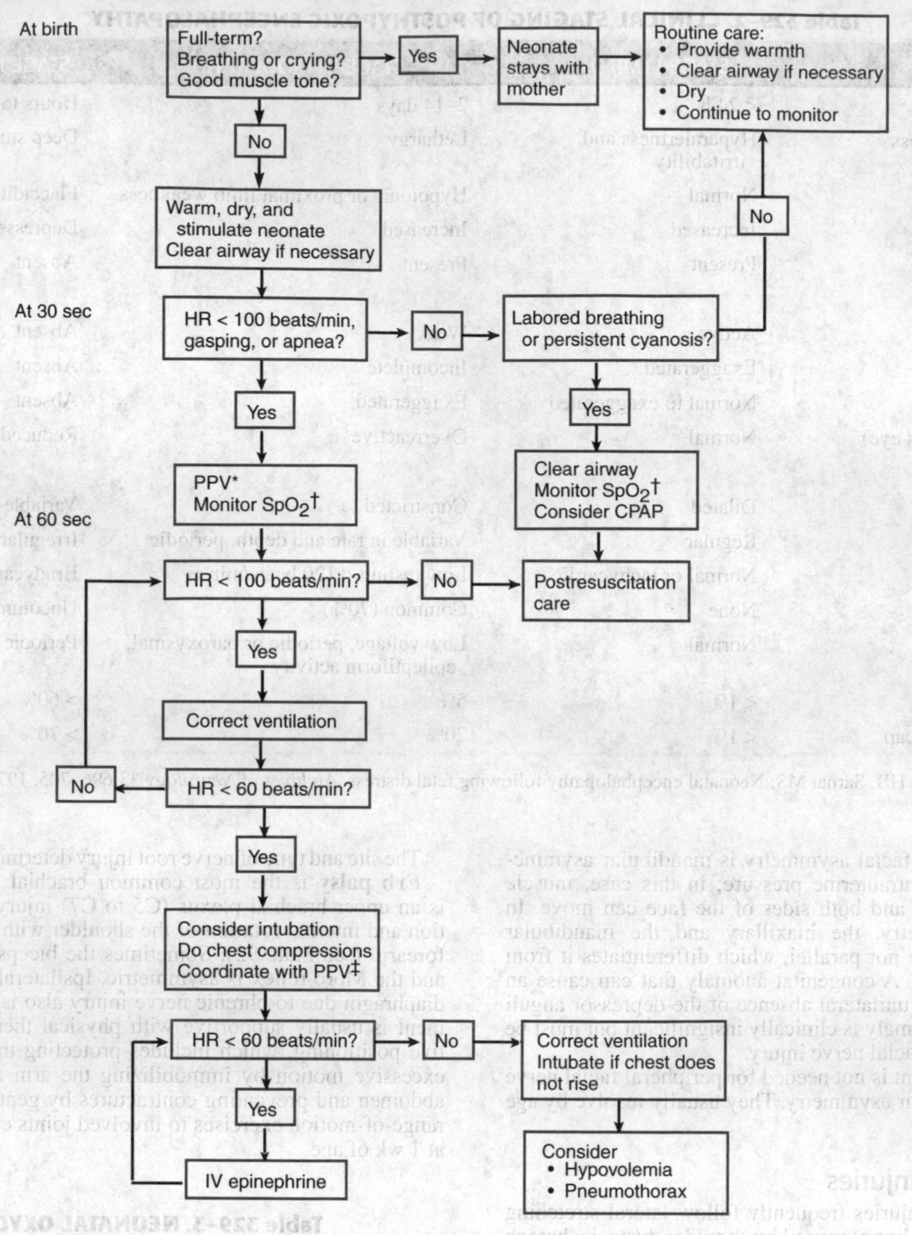

Fig. 329–3. Algorithm for resuscitation of neonates.

*PPV: Initiate resuscitation with room air. If SpO_2 targets are not achieved, titrate inhaled O_2 concentration upward. If HR is < 60 beats/min after 90 sec of resuscitation with a lower O_2 concentration, increase O_2 concentration to 100% until normal HR is recovered.

†For SpO_2 monitoring targets.

‡3:1 compression:ventilation ratio with a total of 90 compressions and 30 breaths/min. Compressions and ventilations are delivered sequentially, not simultaneously. Thus, give 3 compressions at a rate of 120/min, followed by 1 ventilation over 1/2 sec.

HR = heart rate; PPV = positive pressure ventilation; SpO_2 = O_2 saturation.

Adapted from Perlman JM, Wyllie J, Kattwinkel J, et al: American Heart Association guidelines for cardiopulmonary resuscitation and emergency cardiovascular care science, part 15: neonatal resuscitation. *Circulation* 122(supplement 2):S516–38, 2010.

Klumpke palsy is rare and is a lower plexus injury that causes weakness or paralysis of the hand and wrist. The grasp reflex is usually absent, but the biceps reflex is present. Often, the sympathetic fibers of T1 are involved causing an ipsilateral Horner syndrome (miosis, ptosis, facial anhidrosis—see p. 1848). Passive range-of-motion exercises are usually the only treatment needed.

Neither Erb palsy nor Klumpke palsy commonly causes demonstrable sensory loss, which suggests a tear or avulsion. These conditions usually improve rapidly, but deficits can persist. If a significant deficit persists > 3 mo, MRI is done to determine the extent of injury to the plexus, roots, and cervical cord. Surgical exploration and microsurgical repair of brachial plexus with nerve grafts have sometimes been helpful.

Involvement of the entire plexus is less common and results in a flaccid upper extremity with little or no movement, absent reflexes, and usually sensory loss. Ipsilateral Horner syndrome is present in the most severe cases. Ipsilateral pyramidal signs (eg, decreased movement, Babinski sign) indicate spinal cord trauma; an MRI should be done. The involved extremity's subsequent growth may be impaired. The prognosis for recovery is poor. Management may include neurosurgical exploration. Passive range-of-motion exercises can prevent contractures.

Phrenic Nerve Injuries

Most phrenic nerve injuries (about 75%) are associated with brachial plexus injury. Injury is usually unilateral and caused by a traction injury of the head and neck.

Infants have respiratory distress and decreased breath sounds on the affected side. Treatment is supportive and typically requires CPAP or mechanical ventilation. About one-third of infants recover spontaneously within the first month. Infants who do not recover may require surgical diaphragmatic plication.

Other Peripheral Nerve Injuries

Injuries to other peripheral nerves (eg, the radial, sciatic, obturator) are rare in neonates and are usually not related to labor and delivery. They are usually secondary to a local traumatic event (eg, an injection in or near the sciatic nerve). Treatment includes placing the muscles antagonistic to those paralyzed at rest until recovery. Neurosurgical exploration of the nerve is seldom indicated. In most peripheral nerve injuries, recovery is complete.

Spinal Cord Injury

Spinal cord injury (see also p. 3101) is rare and involves variable degrees of cord disruption, often with hemorrhage. Complete disruption of the cord is very rare. Trauma usually occurs in breech deliveries after excess longitudinal traction to the spine. It can also be caused by cord compression due to epidural hemorrhage or hyperextension of the fetal neck in utero (the "flying fetus"). Injury usually affects the lower cervical region (C5 to C7). When the injury is higher, lesions are usually fatal because respiration is completely compromised. Sometimes a click or snap is heard at delivery.

Spinal shock with flaccidity below the level of injury occurs initially. Usually, there is patchy retention of sensation or movement below the lesion. Spasticity develops within days or weeks. Breathing is diaphragmatic because the phrenic nerve remains intact because its origin is higher (at C3 to C5) than the typical cord lesion. When the spinal cord lesion is complete, the intercostal and abdominal muscles become paralyzed and rectal and bladder sphincters cannot develop voluntary control. Sensation and sweating are lost below the involved level, which can cause fluctuations of body temperature with environmental changes.

An MRI of the cervical cord may show the lesion and excludes surgically treatable lesions, such as congenital tumors or hematomas pressing on the cord. The CSF is usually bloody.

With appropriate care, most infants survive for many years. The usual causes of death are recurring pneumonia and progressive loss of renal function. Treatment includes nursing care to prevent skin ulcerations, prompt treatment of urinary and respiratory infections, and regular evaluations to identify obstructive uropathy early.

Intracranial Hemorrhage

Hemorrhage in or around the brain can occur in any neonate but is particularly common among those born prematurely; about 15 to 25% of premature infants < 1500 g have intracranial hemorrhage. Hypoxia-ischemia, variations in BP, hypoperfusion with reperfusion, and pressures exerted on the head during labor are major causes. The presence of the germinal matrix (a mass of embryonic cells lying over the caudate nucleus on the lateral wall of the lateral ventricles that is vulnerable to hemorrhage) makes hemorrhage more likely. Risk also is increased by hematologic disorders (eg, vitamin K deficiency, hemophilia, disseminated intravascular coagulation).

Hemorrhage can occur in several CNS spaces. Small hemorrhages in the subarachnoid space, falx, and tentorium are frequent incidental findings at autopsy of neonates that have died from non-CNS causes. Larger hemorrhages in the subarachnoid or subdural space, brain parenchyma, or ventricles are less common but more serious.

Intracranial hemorrhage is suspected in neonates with apnea, seizures, lethargy, or an abnormal neurologic examination. Such infants should have a cranial imaging study as part of the initial evaluation. Cranial ultrasonography is risk free, requires no sedation, and can readily identify blood within the ventricles or brain substance. CT is more sensitive than ultrasonography for thin layers of blood in the subarachnoid or subdural spaces and for bony injury. MRI is more sensitive and specific than CT or ultrasonography for intracranial blood and for brain injury. CT is done to rapidly identify intracranial hemorrhage.

Treatment depends on the location and severity of the hemorrhage but usually is only supportive, including giving vitamin K if not previously given and managing any underlying coagulation abnormality. In cases of significant hemorrhage (eg, subdural hemorrhage), neurosurgical consultation should be obtained to help identify infants requiring intervention.

Epidural hematoma: Epidural hematoma is a collection of blood between the skull and the dura mater. It is rare in neonates but can occur in association with a skull fracture or cephalhematoma. Infants may present with apnea, seizures, or focal neurologic abnormalities. The fontanelles may be bulging if intracranial pressure is increased. Most epidural hematomas are self-limiting and do not require treatment. If an intervention is required, surgical and nonsurgical options exist. Nonsurgical options are percutaneous epidural tapping or ultrasound-guided needle aspiration. Surgical options include craniotomy, which is reserved for cases that are rapidly progressing or not responsive to other interventions. If identified and treated promptly, neurologic outcomes are good.

Intraventricular and/or intraparenchymal hemorrhage: Intraventricular and/or intraparenchymal hemorrhage usually occurs during the first 3 days of life and is the most serious type of intracranial bleeding. Hemorrhages occur most often in premature infants, are often bilateral, and usually arise in the germinal matrix. Cases in term infants are rare. Most bleeding episodes are subependymal or intraventricular and involve a small amount of blood. In severe hemorrhage, there may be bleeding into the parenchyma or a cast of the ventricular system with large amounts of blood in the cisterna magna and basal cisterns. Hypoxia-ischemia often precedes intraventricular and subarachnoid bleeding. Hypoxia-ischemia damages the capillary endothelium, impairs cerebral vascular autoregulation, and can increase cerebral blood flow and venous pressure, all of which make hemorrhage more likely. Most intraventricular hemorrhages are asymptomatic, but larger hemorrhages may cause apnea, cyanosis, or sudden collapse.

Prognosis for infants with small intraventricular hemorrhages is good. However, infants with large intraventricular hemorrhages have a poor prognosis, especially if the hemorrhage extends into the parenchyma. Many infants who survive have residual neurologic deficits. Preterm infants with a history of severe intraventricular hemorrhage are at risk of developing posthemorrhagic hydrocephalus and must be monitored closely with serial cranial ultrasound examinations and frequent head circumference measurements.

Treatment for most hemorrhages is only supportive. However, infants with progressive hydrocephalus require CSF drainage by placement of a subcutaneous ventricular reservoir or one of the various types of ventricular shunts (eg, ventriculoperitoneal). Because many infants will have neurologic deficits, careful follow-up and referral for early intervention services are important.

Subarachnoid hemorrhage: Subarachnoid hemorrhage probably is the most common type of intracranial hemorrhage. It involves bleeding between the arachnoid membrane and the pia mater. Neonates typically present in the 2nd or 3rd day of life with apnea, seizures, lethargy, or an abnormal neurologic examination.

The prognosis is usually good, with no significant long-term sequelae. However, with large hemorrhages, the associated meningeal inflammation may lead to a communicating hydrocephalus as the infant grows.

Treatment is supportive.

Subdural hemorrhage: Subdural hemorrhage involves bleeding between the dura and the pia mater. It results from tears in the falx, tentorium, or bridging veins. Such tears tend to occur in neonates of primiparas, in large neonates, or after difficult deliveries—conditions that can produce unusual pressures on intracranial vessels. Some subdural hemorrhages are nontraumatic. Infants may present with apnea, seizures, a rapidly enlarging head, an abnormal neurologic examination with hypotonia, a poor Moro reflex, or extensive retinal hemorrhages.

The prognosis for subdural hemorrhage is guarded, but some infants do well.

Treatment is supportive, but neurosurgical drainage of the hematoma is usually needed for rapidly progressing bleeding with compression of vital intracranial structures and worsening clinical signs.

Fractures

Midclavicular fracture. the most common fracture during birth, occurs with shoulder dystocia and with normal, nontraumatic deliveries. Initially, the neonate is sometimes irritable and may not move the arm on the involved side either spontaneously or when the Moro reflex is elicited. Most clavicular fractures are greenstick and heal rapidly and uneventfully. A large callus forms at the fracture site within a week, and remodeling is completed within a month. Treatment consists of immobilizing the arm for 14 days by pinning the shirt sleeve of the involved side to the opposite side of the infant's shirt.

The **humerus and femur** may be fractured in difficult deliveries. Most of these are greenstick, mid-shaft fractures, and excellent remodeling of the bone usually follows, even if moderate angulation occurs initially. A long bone may be fractured through its epiphysis, but prognosis is excellent.

Soft-Tissue Injuries

All soft tissues are susceptible to injury during birth if they have been the presenting part or the fulcrum for the forces of uterine contraction. Edema and ecchymosis often follow injury, particularly of the periorbital and facial tissues in face presentations and of the scrotum or labia during breech deliveries. Breakdown of blood within the tissues and conversion of heme to bilirubin result whenever a hematoma develops. This added burden of bilirubin may cause sufficient neonatal hyperbilirubinemia to require phototherapy, and rarely, exchange transfusion. No other treatment is needed.

HYPOTHERMIA IN NEONATES

Hypothermia is a core temperature < 35 to 35.5° C. The condition may be purely environmental or represent intercurrent illness. Treatment is rewarming and correction of the cause.

Normal rectal temperature in term and preterm infants is 36.5 to 37.5° C. Although hypothermia is a core temperature < 35 to 35.5° C, there is cold stress at higher temperatures whenever heat loss requires an increase in metabolic heat production.

Pathophysiology

Thermal equilibrium is affected by relative humidity, air flow, proximity of cold surfaces, and ambient air temperature. Neonates are prone to rapid heat loss and consequent hypothermia because of a high surface area to volume ratio, which is even higher in low-birth-weight neonates. Radiant heat loss occurs when bare skin is exposed to an environment containing objects of cooler temperature. Evaporative heat loss occurs when neonates are wet with amniotic fluid. Conductive heat loss occurs when neonates are placed in contact with a cool surface or object. Convective heat loss occurs when a flow of cooler ambient air carries heat away from the neonate.

Prolonged, unrecognized cold stress may divert calories to produce heat, impairing growth. Neonates have a metabolic response to cooling that involves chemical (nonshivering) thermogenesis by sympathetic nerve discharge of norepinephrine in the brown fat. This specialized tissue of the neonate, located in the nape of the neck, between the scapulae, and around the kidneys and adrenals, responds by lipolysis followed by oxidation or re-esterification of the fatty acids that are released. These reactions produce heat locally, and a rich blood supply to the brown fat helps transfer this heat to the rest of the neonate's body. This reaction increases the metabolic rate and O_2 consumption 2- to 3-fold. Thus, in neonates with respiratory insufficiency (eg, the preterm infant with RDS), cold stress may also result in tissue hypoxia and neurologic damage. Activation of glycogen stores can cause transient hyperglycemia. Persistent hypothermia can result in hypoglycemia and metabolic acidosis and increases the risk of late-onset sepsis and mortality.

Despite their compensatory mechanisms, neonates, particularly low-birth-weight infants, have limited capacity to thermoregulate and are prone to decreased core temperature. Even before temperature decreases, cold stress occurs when heat loss requires an increase in metabolic heat production. The neutral thermal environment (thermoneutrality) is the optimal temperature zone for neonates; it is defined as the environmental temperature at which metabolic demands (and thus calorie expenditure) to maintain body temperature in the normal range (36.5 to 37.5° C rectal) are lowest. The neutral thermal environment has a narrow range from 36.7° to 37.3° C.

Etiology

Hypothermia may be caused by environmental factors, disorders that impair thermoregulation (eg, sepsis, intracranial hemorrhage, drug withdrawal), or a combination. Risk factors for hypothermia include maternal hypertension, cesarean delivery, and low Apgar scores.

Treatment

- Rewarming in an incubator or under a radiant warmer

Hypothermia is treated by rewarming in an incubator or under a radiant warmer. The neonate should be monitored and treated as needed for hypoglycemia, hypoxemia, and apnea. Underlying conditions such as sepsis, drug withdrawal, or intracranial hemorrhage require specific treatment.

Prevention

Hypothermia can be prevented by immediately drying and then swaddling the neonate (including the head) in a warm blanket to prevent evaporative, conductive, and convective losses. Preterm very-low-birth-weight infants also benefit from a polyethylene occlusive wrapping at the time of delivery. A neonate exposed for resuscitation or observation should be placed under a radiant warmer to prevent radiant losses. Sick neonates should be maintained in a neutral thermal environment to minimize the metabolic rate. The proper incubator temperature varies depending on the neonate's birth weight and postnatal age, and humidity in the incubator. Alternatively, heating can be adjusted with a servomechanism set to maintain skin temperature at 36.5° C.

KEY POINTS

- Neonates, particularly very low-birth-weight infants, are susceptible to environmental hypothermia; illness (eg, intracranial hemorrhage, sepsis) increases risk.
- The optimal ambient temperature for neonates is that at which calorie expenditure needed to maintain normal body temperature is lowest, typically between 36.7 and 37.3° C.
- Rewarm neonates in an incubator or under a radiant warmer and treat any underlying conditions.
- Prevent hypothermia by immediately drying and then swaddling the neonate.

LARGE-FOR-GESTATIONAL-AGE INFANT

Infants whose weight is > the 90th percentile for gestational age are classified as LGA. Macrosomia is birth weight > 4000 g in a term infant. The predominant cause is maternal diabetes. Complications include birth trauma, hypoglycemia, hyperviscosity, and hyperbilirubinemia.

The Fenton growth charts provide a more precise assessment of growth vs gestational age (see Figs. 329–1 and 329–2).

Etiology

Other than genetically determined size, maternal diabetes mellitus is the major cause of large-for-gestational-age (LGA) infants. The macrosomia results from the anabolic effects of high fetal insulin levels produced in response to excessive maternal blood glucose during gestation. The less well controlled the mother's diabetes during pregnancy, the more severe is the fetal macrosomia. Rare causes of macrosomia are Beckwith-Wiedemann syndrome (characterized by macrosomia, omphalocele, macroglossia, and hypoglycemia) and Sotos, Marshall, and Weaver syndromes.

Symptoms, Signs, and Treatment

LGA infants are large, obese, and plethoric. The 5-min Apgar score may be low. These infants may be listless and limp and feed poorly. Delivery complications can occur in any LGA infant. Congenital anomalies and some metabolic and cardiac complications are specific to LGA infants of diabetic mothers (IDMs).

Delivery complications: Because of the infant's large size, vaginal delivery may be difficult and occasionally results in birth injury (see p. 2794), particularly including

- Shoulder dystocia
- Fracture of the clavicle or limbs
- Perinatal asphyxia

Therefore, operative delivery (cesarean delivery) should be considered when the fetus is thought to be too large for the pelvis (true cephalopelvic disproportion).

Other complications occur when weight is > 4000 g. There is a proportional increase in morbidity and mortality due to the following:

- Respiratory distress (and need for ventilatory assistance)
- Meconium aspiration
- Hypoglycemia
- Polycythemia

Infants of diabetic mothers (IDMs): IDMs are at risk of

- Hypoglycemia
- Hypocalcemia and hypomagnesemia
- Polycythemia
- Hyperbilirubinemia
- Respiratory distress syndrome
- Certain congenital anomalies

Hypoglycemia is very likely in the first few hours after delivery because of the state of hyperinsulinism and the sudden termination of maternal glucose when the umbilical cord is cut. Neonatal hypoglycemia can be decreased by close prenatal control of the mother's diabetes and early frequent feedings. Blood glucose levels should be closely monitored by bedside testing from birth through the first 24 h. If there is persistent hypoglycemia, parenteral IV glucose is given.

Hypocalcemia and hypomagnesemia may occur but are usually transient and asymptomatic; serum levels should be checked within the first 72 h after birth. Good prenatal glycemic control decreases the risk of neonatal hypocalcemia. Hypocalcemia typically does not require treatment unless there are clinical signs of hypocalcemia or levels < 7 mg/dL in term infants. Treatment is usually given with IV supplementation of

Ca gluconate. Hypomagnesemia can interfere with the secretion of parathyroid hormone, so hypocalcemia may not respond to treatment until the Mg level is corrected.

Polycythemia is slightly more common among IDMs. Elevated insulin levels increase fetal metabolism and thus O_2 consumption. If the placenta is unable to meet the increased O_2 demand, fetal hypoxemia occurs, triggering an increase in erythropoietin and thus Hct.

Hyperbilirubinemia occurs for several reasons. IDMs have decreased tolerance for oral feedings (particularly when they are preterm) in the earliest days of life, which increases the enterohepatic circulation of bilirubin. Also, if polycythemia is present, the bilirubin load increases.

Respiratory distress syndrome (RDS) may occur because elevated insulin levels decrease surfactant production; pulmonary maturation may thus be delayed until late in gestation. RDS may develop even if the infant is delivered late preterm or term. The lecithin/sphingomyelin ratio, and especially the presence of phosphatidyl glycerol, in amniotic fluid obtained by amniocentesis can evaluate fetal lung maturity and help determine the optimal time for safe delivery. Lung maturity can be assumed only if phosphatidyl glycerol is present. Good prenatal glycemic control decreases the risk of RDS. Treatment is discussed elsewhere (see p. 2808). Transient tachypnea of the newborn (see p. 2807) is 2 to 3 times more likely in IDMs because of the delay in fetal lung fluid clearance.

Congenital anomalies are more likely in IDMs because maternal hyperglycemia at the time of organogenesis is detrimental. Specific anomalies include

- Congenital heart disease (hypertrophic cardiomyopathy, ventricular septal defect, transposition of the great arteries, and aortic stenosis)
- Caudal regression syndrome
- Spina bifida
- Small left colon syndrome

Persistently elevated insulin levels can also lead to increased deposition of glycogen and fat into cardiomyocytes. This deposition can cause transient hypertrophic cardiomyopathy, predominantly of the septum.

KEY POINTS

- Maternal diabetes mellitus is the major cause of LGA infants.
- Large size itself increases risk of birth injury (eg, clavicle or extremity long bone fracture) and perinatal asphyxia.
- IDMs also may have metabolic complications immediately after delivery, including hypoglycemia, hypocalcemia, and polycythemia.
- IDMs are also at risk of respiratory distress syndrome and congenital anomalies.
- Good control of maternal glucose levels minimizes risk of complications.

POSTMATURE INFANT

A postmature infant is an infant born after 42 wk gestation.

The cause of postmaturity is generally unknown, but previous postterm delivery increases the risk 2- to 3-fold. Postmaturity may be caused by abnormalities that affect the fetal pituitary-adrenal axis (eg, anencephaly, adrenal gland hypoplasia, congenital adrenal hyperplasia) and by x-linked ichthyosis associated with placental sulfatase deficiency.

Pathophysiology

In most cases, continued fetal growth between 39 and 43 wk gestation results in a macrosomic infant. However, sometimes the placenta involutes, and multiple infarcts and villous degeneration cause placental insufficiency syndrome. In this syndrome, the fetus receives inadequate nutrients and O_2 from the mother, resulting in a thin (due to soft-tissue wasting), small-for-gestational-age (SGA), undernourished infant with depleted glycogen stores. Post term, the amniotic fluid volume eventually decreases (oligohydramnios).

Complications: Postmature infants have higher morbidity and mortality than term infants. During labor, postmature infants are prone to develop

- Asphyxia
- Meconium aspiration syndrome
- Hypoglycemia

Asphyxia may result from cord compression secondary to oligohydramnios. Meconium aspiration syndrome may be unusually severe because amniotic fluid volume is decreased and thus the aspirated meconium is less dilute. Neonatal hypoglycemia is caused by insufficient glycogen stores at birth. Because anaerobic metabolism rapidly uses the remaining glycogen stores, hypoglycemia is exaggerated if perinatal asphyxia has occurred.

Symptoms and Signs

Postmature infants are alert and appear mature but have a decreased amount of soft-tissue mass, particularly subcutaneous fat. The skin may hang loosely on the extremities and is often dry and peeling. The fingernails and toenails are long. The nails and umbilical cord may be stained with meconium passed in utero.

Diagnosis

- Clinical evaluation

Diagnosis is by clinical appearance (see Fig. 288–1 on p. 2412) and estimated date of delivery.

Treatment

- Treatment of complications

Prognosis and treatment depend on complications. Neonates with meconium aspiration may have chronic respiratory insufficiency and secondary pulmonary hypertension if untreated; surfactant replacement therapy is frequently helpful.

LATE PRETERM INFANT

A late preterm infant is an infant born ≥ 34 wk and < 37 wk gestation.

Full-term gestation is 40 wk (range 37 to 42 wk). Late preterm infants often appear to be the size of full-term infants but have increased morbidity due to their prematurity. Late preterm births represent nearly three quarters of all preterm births. The rate of late preterm birth has increased in the past 2 decades from 7.2% in 1990 to 8.3% in 2011; many late preterm deliveries are medically indicated.

Etiology

Late preterm delivery is sometimes medically indicated (eg, because of preeclampsia, placenta previa/placenta accreta, or premature rupture of membranes) and is often done using cesarean delivery.

In a given patient, the cause of spontaneous late preterm labor and delivery is usually unknown. However, risk factors are similar to those of preterm birth in general (see below), and chronic chorioamnionitis may be associated with spontaneous late preterm deliveries.

Complications

Although clinicians tend to focus on the more dramatic and obvious complications of premature infants born < 34 wk gestation, late preterm infants are at risk of many of the same disorders. They have longer hospital stays and higher incidence of readmission and diagnosed medical disorders than term infants. Most complications relate to dysfunction of immature organ systems and are similar to, but typically less severe than, those of infants born more prematurely (see p. 2802). However, some complications of prematurity (eg, necrotizing enterocolitis, retinopathy of prematurity, bronchopulmonary dysplasia (BPD), intraventricular hemorrhage) are rare in late preterm infants. In most cases, complications resolve completely.

Complications include the following:

- CNS: Apneic episodes
- GI tract: Poor feeding due to delayed maturation of the suck and swallow mechanism (primary reason for prolonged hospital stay and/or readmission)
- Hyperbilirubinemia: Caused by immature mechanisms for hepatic bilirubin metabolism and/or increased intestinal reabsorption of bilirubin (eg, if feeding difficulties cause decreased intestinal motility)
- Hypoglycemia: Caused by low glycogen stores
- Lungs: Respiratory distress syndrome (caused by inadequate surfactant production); transient tachypnea of the newborn
- Temperature instability: Some degree of hypothermia in half of infants (caused by increased surface area to volume ratio, decreased adipose tissue, and ineffective thermogenesis from brown fat)

Diagnosis

- Gestational age estimated by new Ballard score
- Routine screening for metabolic complications

Findings on physical examination correlate with gestational age (see Fig. 288–1 on p. 2412).

Glucose monitoring is necessary for at least 24 h, particularly if regular feedings have not been well established. Routine evaluations include pulse oximetry, serum Ca and electrolytes, CBC, and bilirubin level.

Infants must be monitored for apnea and bradycardia until they are 34.5 to 35 wk adjusted age or until event free. Glucose levels are monitored for at least 24 h, particularly if regular feedings have not been well established. Bilirubin levels are monitored clinically in the first week of life.

Prognosis

Prognosis varies with presence and severity of complications, but usually mortality and likelihood of complications decrease greatly with increasing gestational age and birth weight.

Most CNS problems resolve. Breathing control is usually mature by 37 to 38 wk gestation, and apneic events cease by 43 wk. However, some children have mild delays in development and school-related problems, so all should have neurodevelopmental follow-up and appropriate early referral to intervention programs as needed.

Lung problems usually resolve, but some infants develop pulmonary hypertension.

Treatment

- Supportive care

Identified disorders are treated. For infants without specific conditions, support focuses on body temperature and feeding.

Preterm infants can be stressed by the metabolic demands of maintaining core body temperature (see p. 2798). Thus, they should be kept in a neutral thermal environment, which is the environmental temperature at which metabolic demands (and thus calorie expenditure) to maintain body temperature in the normal range are lowest. The neutral thermal environment has a narrow range from 36.7 to 37.3° C.

Breastfeeding is strongly encouraged. Most late preterm infants tolerate breast milk, which provides immunologic and nutritional factors that are absent in cow's milk formulas. If infants do not suck and/or swallow adequately, feedings should be given by NGT beginning with small amounts and gradually increasing over time.

KEY POINTS

- Although late preterm infants (≥ 34 wk and < 37 wk gestation) may appear to be similar in size and appearance to term infants, they are at increased risk of complications.
- Complications include hypothermia, hypoglycemia, respiratory distress syndrome, hyperbilirubinemia, and poor feeding.
- Treat disorders and support body temperature and feeding.
- Provide neurodevelopmental follow up to identify and address any disabilities.

PREMATURE INFANT

A premature infant is an infant born before 34 wk gestation.

Full-term gestation is 40 wk (range 37 to 42 wk). Infants born before 37 wk are preterm and have an increased incidence of complications and mortality roughly proportional to the degree of prematurity. Infants born < 34 wk are considered moderate premature and those born ≥ 34 wk and < 37 wk gestation are considered late preterm (see p. 2800). Infants born < 32 wk are considered very premature, and those < 28 wk are considered extremely premature.

The rate of preterm birth was 11.7% in 2011; 8.3% were late preterm and 3.4% were [premature], including 2% who were very premature.

Previously, any infant weighing < 2.5 kg was termed premature. This definition is inappropriate because many infants weighing < 2.5 kg are mature or postmature but small for gestational age; they have a different appearance and different problems. Infants < 2.5 kg at birth are considered low-birth-weight infants, and those < 1500 g are considered very low-birth-weight infants (VLBW).

Etiology

In a given patient, the specific cause of premature labor and delivery, whether preceded by premature rupture of the membranes (see p. 2340) or not, is usually unknown. There are many known maternal risk factors, which may involve

Socioeconomic factors

- Low socioeconomic status
- Mothers with less formal education
- Unwed mothers
- Cigarette smoking

Past obstetric history

- Prior premature births
- Prior multiple pregnancies
- Prior multiple therapeutic abortions and/or spontaneous miscarriages

Current pregnancy-related factors

- Pregnancy achieved by in vitro fertilization
- Little or no prenatal care
- Poor nutrition during gestation (and perhaps before)
- Untreated infections (eg, bacterial vaginosis, intra-amniotic infection [formerly chorioamnionitis])
- Multiple gestation (eg, twins, triplets)
- Cervical insufficiency (formerly cervical incompetence)
- Preeclampsia
- Placental abruption

However, most women who give birth preterm have no known risk factors.

Symptoms and Signs

The premature infant is small, usually weighing < 2.5 kg, and tends to have thin, shiny, pink skin through which the underlying veins are easily seen. Little subcutaneous fat, hair, or external ear cartilage exists. Spontaneous activity and tone are reduced, and extremities are not held in the flexed position typical of term infants. In males, the scrotum may have few rugae, and the testes may be undescended. In females, the labia majora do not yet cover the labia minora. Reflexes develop at different times during gestation. The Moro reflex begins by 28 to 32 wk gestation and is well established by 37 wk. The palmar reflex starts at 28 wk and is well established by 32 wk. The tonic neck reflex starts at 35 wk and is most prominent at 1 mo postterm.

Complications

Most complications relate to dysfunction of immature organ systems. In some cases, complications resolve completely; in others, there is residual organ dysfunction.

Cardiac: The most common cardiac complication is

- Patent ductus arteriosus (PDA)

The ductus arteriosus is more likely to fail to close after birth in premature infants. The incidence of PDA (see p. 2506) increases with increasing prematurity; PDA occurs in almost half of infants < 1750 g birth weight and in about 80% of those < 1000 g. About one third to one half of infants with PDA have some degree of heart failure. Premature infants ≤ 29 wk gestation at birth who have RDS have a 65 to 88% risk of a symptomatic PDA. If infants are ≥ 30 wk gestation at birth, the ductus closes spontaneously in 98% by the time of hospital discharge.

CNS: CNS complications include

- Poor sucking and swallowing reflexes
- Apneic episodes
- Intraventricular hemorrhage
- Developmental and/or cognitive delays

Infants born before 34 wk gestation have inadequate coordination of sucking and swallowing reflexes and need to be fed intravenously or by gavage. Immaturity of the respiratory center in the brain stem results in apneic spells (central apnea—see p. 2811). Apnea may also result from hypopharyngeal obstruction alone (obstructive apnea). Both may be present (mixed apnea).

The periventricular germinal matrix (a highly cellular mass of embryonic cells that lies over the caudate nucleus on the lateral wall of the lateral ventricles of a fetus) is prone to hemorrhage, which may extend into the cerebral ventricles (intraventricular hemorrhage—see p. 2797). Infarction of the periventricular white matter (periventricular leukomalacia) may also occur for reasons that are incompletely understood. Hypotension, inadequate or unstable brain perfusion, and BP peaks (as when fluid or colloid is given rapidly IV) may contribute to cerebral infarction or hemorrhage. Periventricular white matter injury is a major risk factor for cerebral palsy and neurodevelopmental delays.

Premature infants, particularly those with a history of sepsis, necrotizing enterocolitis, hypoxia, and intraventricular or periventricular hemorrhages, are at risk of developmental and cognitive delays. These infants require careful follow-up during the first year of life to identify auditory, visual, and neurodevelopmental delays. Careful attention must be paid to developmental milestones, muscle tone, language skills, and growth (weight, length, and head circumference). Infants with identified delays in visual skills should be referred to a pediatric ophthalmologist. Infants with auditory and neurodevelopmental delays (including increased muscle tone and abnormal protective reflexes) should be referred to early intervention programs that provide physical, occupational, and speech therapy. Infants with severe neurodevelopmental problems may need to be referred to a pediatric neurologist.

Eyes: Ocular complications include

- Retinopathy of prematurity (ROP)
- Myopia and/or strabismus

Retinal vascularization is not complete until near term. Preterm delivery may interfere with the normal vascularization process, resulting in abnormal vessel development and sometimes defects in vision including blindness (ROP—see p. 2805). Incidence of ROP is inversely proportional to gestational age. Disease usually manifests between 32 wk and 34 wk gestational age.

Incidence of myopia and strabismus (see p. 2580) increases independently of ROP.

GI tract: GI complications include

- Feeding intolerance, with increased risk of aspiration
- Necrotizing enterocolitis

Feeding intolerance is extremely common because premature infants have a small stomach, immature sucking and swallowing reflexes, and inadequate gastric and intestinal motility. These factors hinder the ability to tolerate both oral and NGT feedings and create a risk of aspiration. Feeding tolerance increases over time, particularly when infants are able to be given some enteral feedings.

Necrotizing enterocolitis (see p. 2586) usually manifests with bloody stool, feeding intolerance, and a distended, tender abdomen. Necrotizing enterocolitis is the most common surgical emergency in the premature infant. Complications of neonatal necrotizing enterocolitis include bowel perforation with pneumoperitoneum, intra-abdominal abscess formation, stricture formation, short bowel syndrome, septicemia, and death.

Infection: Infectious complications include

- Sepsis
- Meningitis

Sepsis (see p. 2636) or meningitis (see p. 2634) is about 4 times more likely in the premature infant, occurring in almost 25% of VLBW infants. The increased likelihood results from indwelling intravascular catheters and endotracheal tubes, areas of skin breakdown, and markedly reduced serum immunoglobulin levels.

Kidneys: Renal complications include

- Metabolic acidosis
- Growth failure

Renal function is limited, so the concentrating and diluting limits of urine are decreased. Late metabolic acidosis and growth failure may result from the immature kidneys' inability to excrete fixed acids, which accumulate with high-protein formula feedings and as a result of bone growth. Na and HCO_3 are lost in the urine.

Lungs: Pulmonary complications include

- Respiratory distress syndrome (RDS)
- Bronchopulmonary dysplasia (BPD)

Surfactant production is often inadequate to prevent alveolar collapse and atelectasis, which result in RDS (see p. 2808). Surfactant replacement therapy is used to both prevent and treat RDS. In spite of this therapy, many premature infants develop a chronic form of lung disease known as BPD (see p. 2812) with a prolonged need for ventilator therapy and supplemental O_2 therapy beyond 36 wk.

Palivizumab prophylaxis for respiratory syncytial virus is important for infants with chronic lung disease (see p. 2764).

Metabolic problems: Metabolic complications include

- Hypoglycemia
- Hyperbilirubinemia

Hypoglycemia (see p. 2732) and hyperglycemia (see p. 2731) are discussed elsewhere.

Hyperbilirubinemia (see also p. 2725) occurs more commonly in the premature as compared to the term infant, and kernicterus may occur at serum bilirubin levels as low as 10 mg/dL (170 μmol/L) in small, sick, premature infants. The higher bilirubin levels may be partially due to inadequately developed hepatic excretion mechanisms, including deficiencies in the uptake of bilirubin from the serum, its hepatic conjugation to bilirubin diglucuronide, and its excretion into the biliary tree. Decreased intestinal motility enables more bilirubin diglucuronide to be deconjugated within the intestinal lumen by the luminal enzyme β-glucuronidase, thus permitting increased reabsorption of unconjugated bilirubin (enterohepatic circulation of bilirubin). Conversely, early feedings increase intestinal motility and reduce bilirubin reabsorption and can thereby significantly decrease the incidence and severity of physiologic jaundice. Uncommonly, delayed clamping of the umbilical cord increases the risk of significant hyperbilirubinemia by allowing the transfusion of a large RBC mass, thus increasing RBC breakdown and bilirubin production.

Temperature regulation: The most common temperature regulation complication is

- Hypothermia

Premature infants have an exceptionally large body surface area to volume ratio. Therefore, when exposed to temperatures below the neutral thermal environment (see p. 2798), they rapidly lose heat and have difficulty maintaining body temperature.

Diagnosis

- Gestational age estimated by new Ballard score
- Routine screening for metabolic, CNS, and ocular complications

Findings on physical examination correlate with gestational age (see Fig. 288–1 on p. 2412). Estimated date of delivery and prenatal ultrasonography, if done, also determine gestational age.

Initial testing: Along with appropriate testing for any identified problems or disorders, routine evaluations include pulse oximetry, serum Ca and electrolytes, CBC, bilirubin level, blood culture, serum alkaline phosphatase and phosphorus levels (to screen for osteopenia of prematurity), hearing evaluation, cranial ultrasonography to screen for intraventricular hemorrhage and periventricular leukomalacia, and screening by an ophthalmologist for retinopathy of prematurity. Weight, length, and head circumference should be plotted on an appropriate growth chart at weekly intervals.

Subsequent screening: If initial laboratory testing was done before the infant was taking full enteral feedings, some of the tests for metabolic disorders may be false-positive and should be repeated. In particular, positive screening tests for thyroid function and congenital adrenal hyperplasia (eg, 17-hydroxyprogesterone) should be confirmed.

Preterm infants must be monitored for apnea and bradycardia until they are 34.5 to 35 wk adjusted age. Before discharge from the hospital, premature infants should undergo a car seat monitoring evaluation using pulse oximetry to make sure that they can maintain a patent airway and good O_2 saturation while positioned in the car seat. After discharge, premature infants should receive careful neurodevelopmental follow-up and appropriate early referral to intervention programs as needed for physical, occupational, and language therapy.

Prognosis

Prognosis varies with presence and severity of complications, but usually mortality and likelihood of complications decrease greatly with increasing gestational age and birth weight (see Fig. 329–4).

Treatment

- Supportive care

Specific disorders are treated as discussed elsewhere in THE MANUAL. General supportive care of the premature infant is best provided in a neonatal ICU or special care nursery and involves careful attention to the thermal environment, using servo-controlled incubators. Scrupulous adherence is paid to handwashing before and after all patient contact. Infants are continually monitored for apnea, bradycardia, and hypoxemia until 34.5 or 35 wk gestation.

Parents should be encouraged to visit and interact with the infant as much as possible within the constraints of the infant's medical condition. Skin-to-skin contact between the infant and mother (kangaroo care) is beneficial for infant health and facilitates maternal bonding. It is feasible and safe even when infants are supported by ventilators and infusions.

Preterm infants should be transitioned to the supine sleeping position before hospital discharge. Parents should be instructed to keep cribs free of fluffy materials including blankets, quilts, pillows, and stuffed toys, which have been associated with an increased risk of SIDS (see p. 2757).

Feeding: Feeding should be by NGT until coordination of sucking, swallowing, and breathing is established at about 34 wk gestation, at which time breastfeeding is strongly encouraged. Most premature infants tolerate breast milk, which provides immunologic and nutritional factors that are absent in cow's milk formulas. However, breast milk does not provide sufficient Ca, phosphorus, and protein for very low-birth-weight infants (ie, < 1500 g), for whom it should be mixed with a breast milk fortifier. Alternatively, specific premature infant formulas that contain 20 to 24 kcal/oz (2.8 to 3.3 joules/mL) can be used.

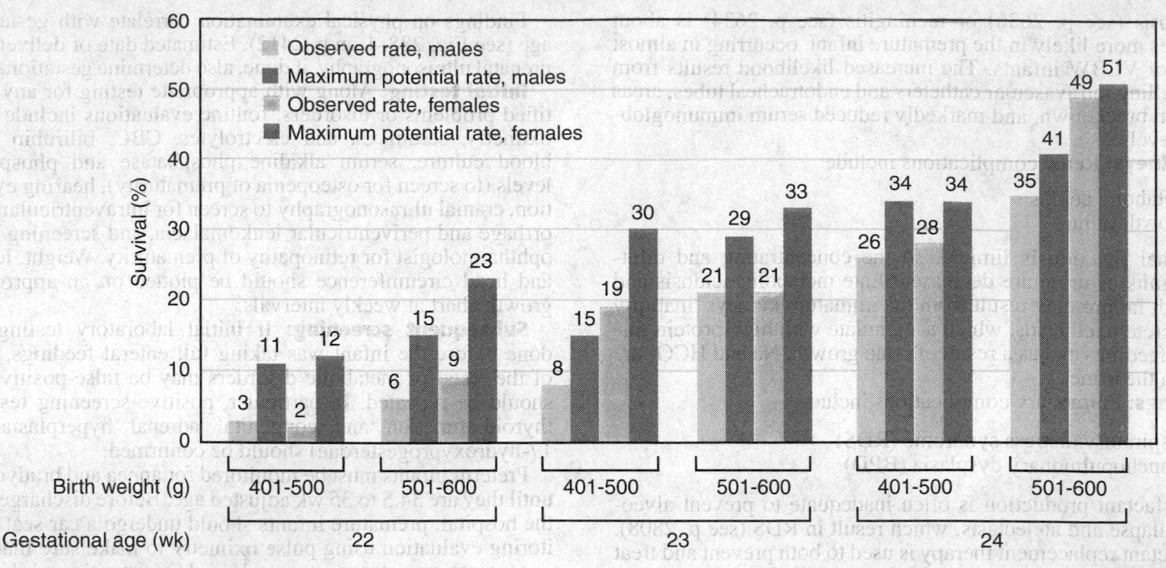

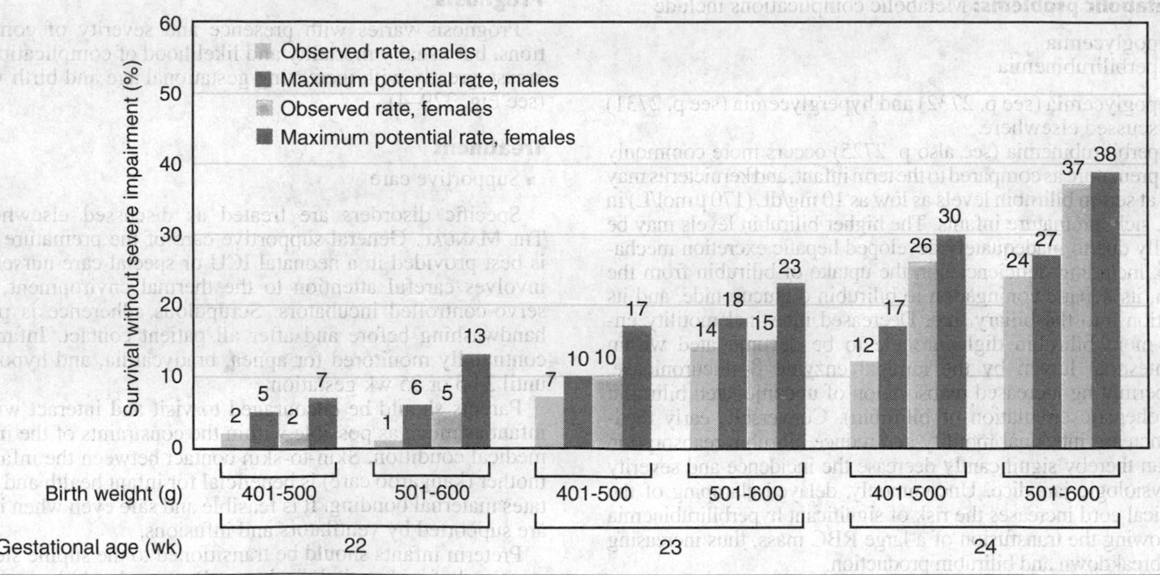

Fig. 329–4. Survival and survival without severe impairment in extremely low-birth-weight infants. Observed and maximal potential rates of survival (top) and survival without severe impairment (bottom) in extremely low-birth-weight infants. (Adapted from Tyson JE, Parikh NA, Langer J, et al: Intensive care for extreme prematurity—moving beyond gestational age. *The New England Journal of Medicine* 358:1672–1681, 2008.)

In the initial 1 or 2 days, if adequate fluids and calories cannot be given by mouth or NGT because of the infant's condition, IV parenteral nutrition with protein, glucose, and fats is given to prevent dehydration and undernutrition. Breast milk or preterm formula feeding via NGT can satisfactorily maintain caloric intake in small, sick, premature infants, especially those with respiratory distress or recurrent apneic spells. Feedings are begun with small amounts (eg, 1 to 2 mL q 3 to 6 h) to stimulate the GI tract. When tolerated, the volume and concentration of feedings are slowly increased over 7 to 10 days. In very small or critically sick infants, total parenteral hyperalimentation via a peripheral IV or a percutaneously or surgically placed central catheter may be required for a prolonged period of time until full enteral feedings can be tolerated.

Prevention

Although early and appropriate prenatal care is important overall, there is no good evidence that such care or any other interventions decrease the incidence of premature birth.

The use of tocolytics to arrest premature labor and provide time for prenatal administration of corticosteroids to hasten lung maturation is discussed elsewhere (see p. 2341).

KEY POINTS

- There are many risk factors for premature birth but they are not present in most cases.
- Complications include hypothermia, hypoglycemia, RDS, apneic episodes, intraventricular hemorrhage, developmental delay, sepsis, retinopathy of prematurity, hyperbilirubinemia, necrotizing enterocolitis, and poor feeding.
- Mortality and likelihood of complications decrease greatly with increasing gestational age and birth weight.
- Treat disorders and support body temperature and feeding.
- There is no evidence that improved prenatal care or other interventions decrease the incidence of premature birth.

RETINOPATHY OF PREMATURITY

(Retrolental Fibroplasia)

Retinopathy of prematurity (ROP) is a bilateral disorder of abnormal retinal vascularization in premature infants, especially those of lowest birth weight. Outcomes range from normal vision to blindness. Diagnosis is by ophthalmoscopy. Treatment of severe disease may include cryotherapy, laser photocoagulation, or bevacizumab; other treatment is directed at complications (eg, retinal detachment).

The inner retinal blood vessels start growing about midpregnancy, but the retina is not fully vascularized until term. ROP results if these vessels continue their growth in an abnormal pattern, forming a ridge of tissue between the vascularized central retina and the nonvascularized peripheral retina. In severe ROP, these new vessels invade the vitreous. Sometimes the entire vasculature of the eye becomes engorged (plus disease).

Susceptibility to ROP correlates with the proportion of retina that remains avascular at birth. In neonates weighing < 1 kg at birth, ROP occurs in 47 to 80%, and severe ROP occurs in 21 to 43%. The percentage is higher when many medical complications exist (eg, infection, intraventricular hemorrhage, bronchopulmonary dysplasia). Excessive (especially prolonged) O_2 therapy increases the risk. However, supplemental O_2 is often needed to adequately oxygenate the infant even though a safe level and duration of O_2 therapy have not been determined.

Diagnosis

- Ophthalmoscopy

Diagnosis is made by ophthalmoscopic examination, done by an ophthalmologist, which shows a line of demarcation and a ridge in mild cases and proliferation of retinal vessels in more severe cases.

Screening ophthalmoscopy is done in all infants weighing < 1500 g or < 30 wk gestation at birth. Because disease onset is usually at 32 to 34 wk gestational age, screening begins at 31 wk. Ophthalmologic examinations continue every 1 to 3 wk (depending on the severity of the eye disease) until infants have growth of vessels into the periphery (equivalent to term). Because significant ROP is rare in appropriately managed infants weighing > 1500 g at birth, alternative diagnoses should be considered in these infants (eg, familial exudative retinopathy, Norrie disease).

Prognosis

Abnormal vessel growth often subsides spontaneously but, in about 4% of survivors weighing < 1 kg at birth, progresses to produce retinal detachments and vision loss within 2 to 12 mo postpartum. Children with healed ROP have a higher incidence of myopia, strabismus, and amblyopia. A few children with moderate, healed ROP are left with cicatricial scars (eg, dragged retina or retinal folds) and are at risk of retinal detachments later in life; rarely, glaucoma and cataracts can also occur.

Treatment

- Laser photocoagulation
- Bevacizumab

In severe ROP, laser photocoagulation to ablate the peripheral avascular retina reduces the incidence of retinal fold and detachment. Retinal vascularization must be followed at 1- to 2-wk intervals until the vessels have matured sufficiently. If retinal detachments occur in infancy, scleral buckling surgery or vitrectomy with lensectomy may be considered, but these procedures are late rescue efforts with low benefit.

Patients with residual scarring should be followed at least annually for life. Treatment of amblyopia and refractive errors in the first year optimizes vision. Infants with total retinal detachments should be monitored for secondary glaucoma and poor eye growth and referred to intervention programs for the visually impaired.

Bevacizumab is a new antivascular endothelial growth factor monoclonal antibody that can stop the progression of ROP. Compared to laser therapy, bevacizumab has a lower rate of recurrence and fewer structural abnormalities. When disease did recur, it recurred months later; long-term ophthalmology follow-up is required. Concerns regarding systemic absorption and possible infection coupled with the need for optimal dose and timing of follow-up are reasons why this drug has remained a 2nd-line therapy that can be used to treat severe disease or in conjunction with laser therapy.

Prevention

After a preterm birth, O_2 should be supplemented only as needed to avoid swings in O_2 as both hyperoxia and hypoxia increase ROP risk. Vitamin E and restricted light are not effective.

KEY POINTS

- ROP typically develops in infants weighing < 1500 g and < 30 wk gestation at birth, particularly those who had serious medical complications or who received excessive and/or prolonged O_2 therapy.
- Risk increases with increasing prematurity.
- Most cases subside spontaneously, but a small number develop retinal detachment and vision loss 2 to 12 mo postpartum.
- Screen at-risk infants by ophthalmoscopic examination (done by an ophthalmologist) beginning at 31 wk gestation.
- Minimize use of supplemental O_2 after premature birth.
- Treat severe ROP using laser photocoagulation or bevacizumab.

SMALL-FOR-GESTATIONAL-AGE INFANT

(Dysmaturity; Intrauterine Growth Restriction)

Infants whose weight is < the 10th percentile for gestational age are classified as small for gestational age (SGA). Complications include perinatal asphyxia, meconium aspiration, and hypoglycemia.

The Fenton growth charts provide a more precise assessment of growth vs gestational age (see Figs. 329–1 and 329–2 on pp. 2792 and 2793).

Etiology

Causes may be divided into those in which the growth restriction is

- Symmetric: Height, weight, and head circumference are about equally affected.
- Asymmetric: Weight is most affected, with a relative sparing of growth of the brain, cranium, and long bones.

Symmetric growth restriction usually results from a fetal problem that begins early in gestation, often during the 1st trimester. When the cause begins relatively early in gestation, all of the body is affected, resulting in fewer cells of all types. Common causes include

- Many genetic disorders
- First-trimester congenital infections (eg, with cytomegalovirus, rubella virus, or *Toxoplasma gondii*)

Asymmetric growth restriction usually results from placental or maternal problems that typically manifest in the late 2nd or the 3rd trimester. When the cause begins relatively late in gestation, organs and tissues are not equally affected, resulting in asymmetric growth restriction. Common causes include

- Placental insufficiency resulting from maternal disease involving the small blood vessels (eg, preeclampsia, hypertension, renal disease, antiphospholipid antibody syndrome, long-standing diabetes)
- Relative placental insufficiency caused by multiple gestation
- Placental involution accompanying postmaturity
- Chronic maternal hypoxemia caused by pulmonary or cardiac disease
- Maternal malnutrition
- Conception using assisted reproductive technology

An infant may also have asymmetric growth restriction and be small for gestational age (SGA) if the mother is a heavy user of opioids, cocaine, alcohol, and/or tobacco during pregnancy.

Symptoms and Signs

Despite their size, SGA infants have physical characteristics (eg, skin appearance, ear cartilage, sole creases) and behavior (eg, alertness, spontaneous activity, zest for feeding) similar to those of normal-sized infants of like gestational age. However, they may appear thin with decreased muscle mass and subcutaneous fat tissue. Facial features may appear sunken, resembling those of an elderly person ("wizened facies"). The umbilical cord can appear thin and small.

Complications: Full-term SGA infants do not have the complications related to organ system immaturity that premature infants of similar size have. They are, however, at risk of

- Perinatal asphyxia
- Meconium aspiration
- Hypoglycemia
- Hypothermia

Perinatal asphyxia during labor is the most serious potential complication. It is a risk if intrauterine growth restriction is caused by placental insufficiency (with marginally adequate placental perfusion) because each uterine contraction slows or stops maternal placental perfusion by compressing the spiral arteries. Therefore, when placental insufficiency is suspected, the fetus should be assessed before labor and the fetal heart rate should be monitored during labor. If fetal compromise is detected, rapid delivery, often by cesarean delivery, is indicated.

Meconium aspiration may occur during perinatal asphyxia. SGA infants, especially those who are postmature, may pass meconium into the amniotic sac and begin deep gasping movements. The consequent aspiration is likely to result in meconium aspiration syndrome (often most severe in growth-restricted or postmature infants, because the meconium is contained in a smaller volume of amniotic fluid and thus more concentrated—see also p. 2814).

Hypoglycemia often occurs in the early hours and days of life because of a lack of adequate glycogen synthesis and thus decreased glycogen stores and must be treated quickly with IV glucose (see p. 2732).

Polycythemia (see p. 2788) may occur when SGA fetuses experience chronic mild hypoxia caused by placental insufficiency. Erythropoietin release is increased, leading to an increased rate of erythrocyte production. The neonate with polycythemia at birth appears ruddy and may be tachypneic or lethargic.

Hypothermia (see p. 2798) may occur because of impaired thermoregulation, which involves multiple factors including increased heat loss due to the decrease in subcutaneous fat, decreased heat production due to intrauterine stress and depletion of nutrient stores, and increased surface to volume ratio due to small size. SGA infants should be in a thermoneutral environment to minimize O_2 consumption.

Prognosis

If asphyxia can be avoided, neurologic prognosis for term SGA infants is quite good. However, later in life there is probably increased risk of ischemic heart disease, hypertension, and stroke, which are thought to be caused by abnormal vascular development.

Infants who are SGA because of genetic factors, congenital infection, or maternal drug use often have a worse prognosis, depending on the specific diagnosis. If intrauterine growth restriction is caused by chronic placental insufficiency, adequate nutrition may allow SGA infants to demonstrate remarkable "catch-up" growth after delivery.

Treatment

- Supportive care

Underlying conditions and complications are treated. There is no specific intervention for the SGA state, but prevention is aided by prenatal advice on the importance of avoiding alcohol, tobacco, and illicit drugs.

KEY POINTS

- Infants whose weight is < the 10th percentile for gestational age are small for gestational age (SGA).
- Disorders early in gestation cause symmetric growth restriction, in which height, weight, and head circumference are about equally affected.

- Disorders late in gestation cause asymmetric growth restriction, in which weight is most affected, with relatively normal growth of the brain, cranium, and long bones.
- Although small, SGA infants do not have the complications related to organ system immaturity that premature infants of similar size have.
- Complications are mainly those of the underlying cause but generally also include perinatal asphyxia, meconium aspiration, hypoglycemia, polycythemia, and hypothermia.

TRANSIENT TACHYPNEA OF THE NEWBORN

(Neonatal Wet Lung Syndrome)

Transient tachypnea of the newborn is transient respiratory distress caused by delayed resorption of fetal lung fluid.

Transient tachypnea of the newborn affects premature infants, term infants delivered by elective cesarean delivery without labor, and infants born with respiratory depression, all of whom have delayed clearance of fetal lung fluid. Part of the cause is immaturity of the Na channels in lung epithelial cells; these channels are responsible for absorbing Na (and thus water) from the alveoli. (Mechanisms for normal resorption of fetal lung fluid are on p. 2790.) Other risk factors include macrosomia, maternal diabetes and/or asthma, lower gestational age, and male sex.

Transient tachypnea of the newborn is suspected when the infant develops respiratory distress shortly after birth. Symptoms include tachypnea, intracostal and subcostal retractions, grunting, nasal flaring, and possible cyanosis.

Pneumonia, RDS, and sepsis may have similar manifestations, so chest x-ray, CBC, and blood cultures usually are done. Chest x-ray shows hyperinflated lungs with streaky perihilar markings, giving the appearance of a shaggy heart border while the periphery of the lungs is clear. Fluid is often seen in the lung fissures. If initial findings are indeterminate or suggest infection, antibiotics (eg, ampicillin, gentamicin) are given while awaiting culture results.

Recovery usually occurs within 2 to 3 days. Treatment is supportive and involves giving O_2 by hood and monitoring ABGs or pulse oximetry. Rarely, extremely premature infants, those with neurologic depression at birth, or both require CPAP and occasionally even mechanical ventilation.

OVERVIEW OF PERINATAL RESPIRATORY DISORDERS

Symptoms and signs of respiratory distress vary and include nasal flaring; intercostal, subcostal, and suprasternal retractions; weak breathing, irregular breathing, or a combination; tachypnea and apneic spells; cyanosis, pallor, mottling, delayed capillary refill, or a combination; and hypotension. In neonates, symptoms and signs may be apparent immediately on delivery or develop minutes or hours afterward.

Etiology

Respiratory distress in neonates and infants has multiple causes (see Table 329–4).

Physiology

There are several significant differences in the physiology of the respiratory system in neonates and infants compared with that of older children and adults. These differences include

- A more compliant collapsible chest wall
- More reliance on diaphragmatic excursions over intercostal muscles
- Collapsible extrathoracic airways

Also, infants' smaller airway caliber gives increased airway resistance, and absence of collateral ventilation increases tendency toward atelectasis. Yet, other principles of respiration are similar in adults and children.

Evaluation

Evaluation starts with a thorough history and physical examination.

History in the neonate focuses on maternal and prenatal history, particularly gestational age, maternal infection or bleeding, meconium staining of amniotic fluid, and oligohydramnios or polyhydramnios.

Table 329–4. CAUSES OF RESPIRATORY DISTRESS IN NEONATES AND INFANTS

CATEGORY	CAUSES
Cardiac	**Right-to-left shunting with normal or increased pulmonary flow:** Transposition of the great vessels, total anomalous venous return, truncus arteriosus, hypoplastic left heart syndrome **Right-to-left shunting with decreased pulmonary flow:** Pulmonary atresia, tetralogy of Fallot, critical pulmonic stenosis, tricuspid atresia, single ventricle with pulmonic stenosis, Ebstein anomaly, persistent fetal circulation/persistent pulmonary hypertension
Respiratory	**Upper tract:** Choanal atresia or stenosis, tracheobronch

olaryngeal stenosis, compressive obstruction (eg, vascular ring), tracheoesophageal anomalies (eg, cleft, fistula)
Lower tract: RDS, transient tachypnea of the newborn, meconium aspiration, pneumonia, sepsis, pneumothorax, congenital diaphragmatic hernia, pulmonary hypoplasia, cystic malformation of the lung, congenital deficiency of surfactant proteins B or C |
Neurologic	Intracranial hemorrhage or hypertension, oversedation (infant or maternal), diaphragmatic paralysis, neuromuscular disease, seizure disorder
Hematologic	Methemoglobinemia, polycythemia, severe anemia
Miscellaneous	Hypoglycemia, blood loss, metabolic disorders (eg, acid-base disorders, hyperammonemia), hypovolemic shock

Physical examination focuses on the heart and lungs. Chest wall asymmetry or sunken abdomen suggests diaphragmatic hernia. Asymmetric breath sounds suggest pneumothorax, pneumonia, or asthma. A displaced left apical impulse, heart murmur, or both suggest a congenital heart defect. Assessment of BP and femoral pulses may identify circulatory collapse with or without congenital defects. Poor capillary refill reflects circulatory compromise.

In both neonates and infants, it is important to assess oxygenation and response to O_2 therapy by pulse oximetry or blood gases. Chest x-ray also is recommended.

RESPIRATORY DISTRESS SYNDROME IN NEONATES

(Hyaline Membrane Disease)

Respiratory distress syndrome (RDS) is caused by pulmonary surfactant deficiency in the lungs of neonates, most commonly in those born at < 37 wk gestation. Risk increases with degree of prematurity. Symptoms and signs include grunting respirations, use of accessory muscles, and nasal flaring appearing soon after birth. Diagnosis is clinical; prenatal risk can be assessed with tests of fetal lung maturity. Treatment is surfactant therapy and supportive care.

Etiology

Surfactant is not produced in adequate amounts until relatively late in gestation (34 to 36 wk); thus, risk of RDS increases with greater prematurity. Other risk factors include multifetal pregnancies, maternal diabetes, and being male and white.

Risk decreases with fetal growth restriction, preeclampsia or eclampsia, maternal hypertension, prolonged rupture of membranes, and maternal corticosteroid use.

Rare cases are hereditary, caused by mutations in surfactant protein (SP-B and SP-C) and ATP-binding cassette transporter *A3* (*ABCA3*) genes.

Pathophysiology

Pulmonary surfactant is a mixture of phospholipids and lipoproteins secreted by type II pneumocytes (see p. 2790). It diminishes the surface tension of the water film that lines alveoli, thereby decreasing the tendency of alveoli to collapse and the work required to inflate them.

With surfactant deficiency, a greater pressure is needed to open the alveoli. Without adequate airway pressure, the lungs become diffusely atelectatic, triggering inflammation and pulmonary edema. Because blood passing through the atelectatic portions of lung is not oxygenated (forming a right-to-left intrapulmonary shunt), the infant becomes hypoxemic. Lung compliance is decreased, thereby increasing the work of breathing. In severe cases, the diaphragm and intercostal muscles fatigue, and CO_2 retention and respiratory acidosis develop.

Complications: Complications of RDS include intraventricular hemorrhage, periventricular white matter injury, tension pneumothorax, bronchopulmonary dysplasia (BPD), sepsis, and neonatal death. Intracranial complications have been linked to hypoxemia, hypercarbia, hypotension, swings in arterial BP, and low cerebral perfusion.

Symptoms and Signs

Symptoms and signs include rapid, labored, grunting respirations appearing immediately or within a few hours after delivery, with suprasternal and substernal retractions and flaring of the nasal alae. As atelectasis and respiratory failure progress, symptoms worsen, with cyanosis, lethargy, irregular breathing, and apnea.

Neonates weighing < 1000 g may have lungs so stiff that they are unable to initiate or sustain respirations in the delivery room.

On examination, breath sounds are decreased. Peripheral pulses may be decreased with peripheral extremity edema and decreased urine output.

Diagnosis

- Clinical evaluation
- ABG (hypoxemia and hypercapnia)
- Chest x-ray
- Blood, CSF, and tracheal aspirate cultures

Diagnosis is by clinical presentation, including recognition of risk factors; ABGs showing hypoxemia and hypercapnia; and chest x-ray. Chest x-ray shows diffuse atelectasis classically described as having a ground-glass appearance with visible air bronchograms; appearance correlates loosely with clinical severity.

Differential diagnosis includes group B streptococcal pneumonia and sepsis, transient tachypnea of the newborn (see p. 2807), persistent pulmonary hypertension, aspiration, pulmonary edema, and congenital cardiopulmonary anomalies. Neonates typically require cultures of blood, CSF, and possibly tracheal aspirate. Clinically, group B streptococcal pneumonia is extremely difficult to differentiate from RDS; thus, antibiotics should be started pending culture results.

Screening: RDS can be anticipated prenatally using tests of fetal lung maturity, which are done on amniotic fluid obtained by amniocentesis or collected from the vagina (if membranes have ruptured) and which can help determine the optimal timing of delivery. These are indicated for elective deliveries before 39 wk when fetal heart tones, human chorionic gonadotropin levels, and ultrasound measurements cannot confirm gestational age and for nonelective deliveries between 34 wk and 36 wk.

Amniotic fluid tests include the

- Lecithin/sphingomyelin ratio
- Foam stability index test (the more surfactant in amniotic fluid, the greater the stability of the foam that forms when the fluid is combined with ethanol and shaken)
- Surfactant/albumin ratio

Risk of RDS is low when lecithin/sphingomyelin ratio is > 2, phosphatidyl glycerol is present, foam stability index = 47, or surfactant/albumin ratio is > 55 mg/g.

Treatment

- Surfactant
- Supplementary O_2 as needed
- Mechanical ventilation as needed

Prognosis with treatment is excellent; mortality is < 10%. With adequate ventilatory support alone, surfactant production eventually begins, and once production begins, RDS resolves within 4 or 5 days. However, in the meantime, severe hypoxemia can result in multiple organ failure and death.

Specific treatment is intratracheal surfactant therapy. This therapy requires endotracheal intubation, which also may be necessary to achieve adequate ventilation and oxygenation. Less premature infants (those > 1 kg) and those with lower O_2 requirements (fraction of inspired O_2 [FIO_2] < 40 to 50%) may respond well to supplemental O_2 alone or to treatment with nasal CPAP (continuous positive airway pressure). A treatment strategy of early (within 20 to 30 min after birth) surfactant therapy is associated with significant decrease in duration of mechanical ventilation, lesser incidence of air leak syndromes, and lower incidence of BPD.

Surfactant hastens recovery and decreases risk of pneumothorax, interstitial emphysema, intraventricular hemorrhage, BPD, and neonatal mortality in the hospital and at 1 yr. However, neonates who receive surfactant for established RDS have an increased risk of apnea of prematurity (see p. 2811). Options for surfactant replacement include

- Beractant
- Poractant alfa
- Calfactant
- Lucinactant

Beractant is a lipid bovine lung extract supplemented with proteins B and C, colfosceril palmitate, palmitic acid, and tripalmitin); dose is 100 mg/kg q 6 h prn up to 4 doses.

Poractant alfa is a modified porcine-derived minced lung extract containing phospholipids, neutral lipids, fatty acids, and surfactant-associated proteins B and C; dose is 200 mg/kg followed by up to 2 doses of 100 mg/kg 12 h apart prn.

Calfactant is a calf lung extract containing phospholipids, neutral lipids, fatty acids, and surfactant-associated proteins B and C; dose is 105 mg/kg q 12 h up to 3 doses prn.

Lucinactant is a synthetic surfactant with a pulmonary surfactant protein B analog, sinapultide (KL4) peptide, phospholipids, and fatty acids; dose is 175 mg/kg q 6 h up to 4 doses.

Lung compliance can improve rapidly after therapy. The ventilator peak inspiratory pressure may need to be lowered rapidly to reduce risk of a pulmonary air leak. Other ventilator parameters (eg, FIO_2, rate) also may need to be reduced.

Prevention

When a fetus must be delivered between 24 wk and 34 wk, giving the mother 2 doses of betamethasone 12 mg IM 24 h apart or 4 doses of dexamethasone 6 mg IV or IM q 12 h at least 48 h before delivery induces fetal surfactant production and reduces the risk of RDS or decreases its severity.

Prophylactic intratracheal surfactant therapy given to neonates that are at high risk of developing RDS (infants < 30 wk completed gestation especially in absence of antenatal corticosteroid exposure) has been shown to decrease risk of neonatal death and certain forms of pulmonary morbidity (eg, pneumothorax).

KEY POINTS

- RDS is caused by pulmonary surfactant deficiency, which typically occurs only in neonates born at < 37 wk gestation; deficiency is worse with increasing prematurity.
- With surfactant deficiency, alveoli close or fail to open, and the lungs become diffusely atelectatic, triggering inflammation and pulmonary edema.
- In addition to causing respiratory insufficiency, RDS increases risk of intraventricular hemorrhage, tension pneumothorax, BPD, sepsis, and death.
- Diagnose clinically and with chest x-ray; exclude pneumonia and sepsis by appropriate cultures.
- If premature delivery is anticipated, assess lung maturity by testing amniotic fluid for lecithin/sphingomyelin ratio, foam stability, or the surfactant/albumin ratio.
- Treat with intratracheal surfactant and give respiratory support as needed.
- Give the mother several doses of a parenteral corticosteroid (betamethasone, dexamethasone) if she must deliver between 24 wk and 34 wk gestation; corticosteroids induce fetal surfactant production and reduce the risk and/or severity of RDS.

RESPIRATORY SUPPORT IN NEONATES AND INFANTS

Initial stabilization maneuvers include mild tactile stimulation, head positioning, and suctioning of the mouth and nose followed as needed by

- Supplemental O_2
- Continuous positive airway pressure (CPAP)
- Noninvasive positive pressure ventilation (NIPPV)
- Bag-and-mask ventilation or mechanical ventilation

Neonates who cannot be oxygenated by any of these means may require a full cardiac evaluation to exclude congenital heart disease and treatment with high-frequency oscillatory ventilation, nitric oxide, extracorporeal membrane oxygenation (ECMO), or a combination.

Oxygen: O_2 may be given using a nasal cannula, face mask, or O_2 hood, with O_2 concentration set to achieve a PaO_2 of 50 to 70 mm Hg in preterm infants and 50 to 80 mm Hg in term infants or an O_2 saturation of 90 to 94% in preterm infants and 92 to 96% in term infants. Lower PaO_2 in preterm infants provides almost full saturation of Hb, because fetal Hb has a higher affinity for O_2; maintaining higher PaO_2 increases the risk of retinopathy of prematurity. No matter how O_2 is delivered, it should be warmed (36 to 37° C) and humidified to prevent secretions from cooling and drying and to prevent bronchospasm.

An umbilical artery catheter (UAC) is usually placed for sampling ABGs in neonates who require fraction of inspired O_2 (FIO_2) ≥ 40%. If a UAC cannot be placed, a percutaneous radial artery catheter can be used for continuous BP monitoring and blood sampling.

Neonates who are unresponsive to these maneuvers may require fluids to improve cardiac output and are candidates for CPAP ventilation or bag-and-mask ventilation (40 to 60 breaths/min). If the infant does not oxygenate with or requires prolonged bag-and-mask ventilation, endotracheal intubation with mechanical ventilation is indicated, although very immature neonates (eg, < 28 wk gestation or < 1000 g) are typically begun on ventilatory support immediately after delivery so that they can receive preventive surfactant therapy. Because bacterial sepsis is a common cause of respiratory distress in neonates, it is common practice to draw blood cultures and give antibiotics to neonates with high O_2 requirements pending culture results.

CPAP: CPAP delivers O_2 at a positive pressure, usually 5 to 7 cm H_2O, which keeps alveoli open and improves oxygenation by reducing the amount of blood shunted through atelectatic areas while the infant breathes spontaneously. CPAP can be provided using nasal prongs and various apparatuses to provide the positive pressure; it also can be given using an endotracheal tube connected to a conventional ventilator with the rate set to zero. CPAP is indicated when FIO_2 ≥ 40% is required to maintain acceptable PaO_2 (50 to 70 mm Hg) in infants with respiratory disorders that are of limited duration (eg, diffuse atelectasis, mild RDS, lung edema). In these infants, CPAP may preempt the need for positive pressure ventilation.

NIPPV: NIPPV (see also p. 561) delivers positive pressure ventilation using nasal prongs or nasal masks. It can be synchronized (ie, triggered by the infant's inspiratory effort) or nonsynchronized. NIPPV can provide a back-up rate and can augment an infant's spontaneous breaths. Peak pressure can be set to desired limits. It is particularly useful in patients with apnea to facilitate extubation and to help prevent atelectasis.

Mechanical ventilation: Endotracheal tubes are required for mechanical ventilation (see also p. 554):

- Endotracheal tubes 2.5 mm in diameter (the smallest) typically used for infants < 1250 g
- 3 mm for infants 1250 to 2500 g
- 3.5 mm for infants > 2500 g

Intubation is safer if O_2 is insufflated into the infant's airway during the procedure. Orotracheal intubation is preferred. The tube should be inserted such that the

- 7-cm mark is at the lip for infants who weigh 1 kg
- 8-cm mark for 2 kg
- 9-cm mark for 3 kg

The endotracheal tube is properly placed when its tip can be palpated through the anterior tracheal wall at the suprasternal notch. It should be positioned about halfway between the clavicles and the carina on chest x-ray, coinciding roughly with vertebral level T2. If position or patency is in doubt, the tube should be removed and the infant should be supported by bag-and-mask ventilation until a new tube is inserted. Acute deterioration of the infant's condition (sudden changes in oxygenation, ABGs, BP, or perfusion) should trigger suspicion of changes in the position of the tube, patency of the tube, or both.

Ventilators can be set to deliver fixed pressures or volumes; can provide assist control (AC, in which the ventilator is triggered to deliver a full breath with each patient inspiration) or intermittent mandatory ventilation (IMV, in which the ventilator delivers a set number of breaths within a time period, and patients can take spontaneous breaths in between without triggering the ventilator); and can be normal or high frequency (delivering 400 to 900 breaths/min). Optimal mode or type of ventilation depends on the infant's response. Volume ventilators are considered useful for larger infants with varying pulmonary compliance or resistance (eg, in BPD), because delivering a set volume of gas with each breath ensures adequate ventilation. AC mode is often used for treating less severe pulmonary disease and for decreasing ventilator dependence while providing a small increase in airway pressure or a small volume of gas with each spontaneous breath. High-frequency jet, oscillatory, and flow-interrupter ventilators are used in extremely premature infants (< 28 wk) and in some infants with air leaks, widespread atelectasis, or pulmonary edema.

Initial ventilator settings are estimated by judging the severity of respiratory impairment. Typical settings for an infant in moderate respiratory distress are FIO_2 = 40%; inspiratory time (IT) = 0.4 sec; expiratory time = 1.1 sec; IMV or AC rate = 40 breaths/min; peak inspiratory pressure (PIP) = 15 cm H_2O for very low-birth-weight infants and up to 25 cm H_2O for near-term infants; and positive end-expiratory pressure (PEEP) = 5 cm H_2O. These settings are adjusted based on the infant's oxygenation, chest wall movement, breath sounds, and respiratory efforts along with arterial or capillary blood gases.

- **$PaCO_2$** is lowered by increasing the minute ventilation through an increase in tidal volume (increasing PIP or decreasing PEEP) or an increase in rate.
- **PaO_2** is increased by increasing the FIO_2 or increasing the mean airway pressure (increasing PIP, PEEP, or rate or prolonging IT).

Patient-triggered ventilation often is used to synchronize the positive pressure ventilator breaths with the onset of the patient's own spontaneous respirations. This seems to shorten the time on a ventilator and may reduce barotrauma. A pressure-sensitive air-filled balloon attached to a pressure transducer (Graseby capsule) taped to the infant's abdomen just below the xiphoid process can detect the onset of diaphragmatic contraction, or a flow or temperature sensor placed at the endotracheal tube adapter can detect the onset of a spontaneous inhalation.

Ventilator pressures or volumes should be as low as possible to prevent barotrauma and BPD; an elevated $Paco_2$ is acceptable as long as pH remains ≥ 7.25 (permissive hypercapnia). Likewise, a PaO_2 as low as 40 mm Hg is acceptable if BP is normal and metabolic acidosis is not present.

Adjunctive treatments used with mechanical ventilation in some patients include

- Paralytics
- Sedation
- Nitric oxide

Paralytics (eg, vecuronium or pancuronium bromide 0.03 to 0.1 mg/kg IV q 1 to 2 h prn [with pancuronium, a test dose of 0.02 mg/kg is recommended in neonates]) and sedatives (eg, fentanyl 1 to 4 mcg/kg IV push q 2 to 4 h or midazolam 0.05 to 0.15 mg/kg IV over 5 min q 2 to 4 h) may facilitate endotracheal intubation and can help stabilize infants whose movements and spontaneous breathing prevent optimal ventilation. These drugs should be used selectively, however, because paralyzed infants may need greater ventilator support, which can increase barotrauma. Inhaled nitric oxide 5 to 20 ppm may be used for refractory hypoxemia when pulmonary vasoconstriction is a contributor to hypoxia (eg, in idiopathic pulmonary hypertension, pneumonia, or congenital diaphragmatic hernia) and may prevent the need for extracorporeal membrane oxygenation.

Weaning from the ventilator can occur as respiratory status improves. The infant can be weaned by lowering

- FIO_2
- Inspiratory pressure
- Rate

Continuous-flow positive pressure ventilators permit the infant to breathe spontaneously against PEEP while the ventilator rate is progressively slowed. As the rate is reduced, the infant takes on more of the work of breathing. Infants who can maintain adequate oxygenation and ventilation on lower settings typically tolerate extubation. The final steps in ventilator weaning involve extubation, possibly support with nasal (or nasopharyngeal) CPAP or NIPPV, and, finally, use of a hood or nasal cannula to provide humidified O_2 or air.

Very low-birth-weight infants may benefit from the addition of a methylxanthine (eg, aminophylline, theophylline, caffeine) during the weaning process. Methylxanthines are CNS-mediated respiratory stimulants that increase ventilatory effort and may reduce apneic and bradycardic episodes that may interfere with successful weaning. Caffeine is the preferred agent because it is better tolerated, easier to give, safer, and requires less monitoring. Corticosteroids, once used routinely for weaning and treatment of chronic lung disease, are no longer recommended in premature infants because risks (eg, impaired growth and neurodevelopmental delay) outweigh benefits. A possible exception is as a last resort in near-terminal illness, in which case parents should be fully informed of risks.

Complications: Mechanical ventilation complications more common among neonates include

- Pneumothorax
- Asphyxia from endotracheal tube obstruction
- Ulceration, erosion, or narrowing of airway structures due to adjacent pressure
- Bronchopulmonary dysplasia

Extracorporeal membrane oxygenation (ECMO): ECMO is a form of cardiopulmonary bypass used for infants who cannot be oxygenated adequately or ventilated with conventional ventilators. Eligibility criteria vary by center, but in general, infants should have reversible disease (eg, persistent pulmonary hypertension of the newborn, congenital diaphragmatic hernia, overwhelming pneumonia) and should have been on mechanical ventilation < 7 days.

After systemic heparinization, blood is circulated through large-diameter catheters from the internal jugular vein into a membrane oxygenator, which serves as an artificial lung to remove CO_2 and add O_2. Oxygenated blood is then circulated back to the internal jugular vein (venovenous ECMO) or to the carotid artery (venoarterial ECMO). Venoarterial ECMO is used when both circulatory support and ventilatory support are needed (eg, in overwhelming sepsis). Flow rates can be adjusted to obtain desired O_2 saturation and BP.

ECMO is contraindicated in infants < 34 wk, < 2 kg, or both because of the risk of intraventricular hemorrhage with systemic heparinization. Complications include thromboembolism, air embolization, neurologic (eg, stroke, seizures) and hematologic (eg, hemolysis, neutropenia, thrombocytopenia) problems, and cholestatic jaundice.

APNEA OF PREMATURITY

Apnea of prematurity is defined as respiratory pauses > 20 sec or pauses < 20 sec that are associated with bradycardia (< 80 beats/min), central cyanosis, and/or O_2 saturation < 85% in neonates born at < 37 wk gestation and with no underlying disorders causing apnea. Cause may be CNS immaturity (central) or airway obstruction. Diagnosis is by multichannel respiratory monitoring. Treatment is with respiratory stimulants for central apnea and head positioning for obstructive apnea. Prognosis is excellent; apnea resolves in most neonates by 37 wk.

About 25% of preterm infants have apnea of prematurity, which usually begins 2 to 3 days after birth and only rarely on the first day. Apnea that develops > 14 days after birth in an otherwise healthy infant signifies a serious illness other than apnea of prematurity (eg, sepsis). Risk increases with earlier gestational age.

Pathophysiology

Apnea of prematurity is a developmental disorder caused by immaturity of neurologic and/or mechanical function of the respiratory system. Apnea may be characterized as

- Central
- Obstructive
- A mixed pattern (most common)

Central apnea is caused by immature medullary respiratory control centers. The specific pathophysiology is not understood completely but appears to involve a number of factors, including abnormal responses to hypoxia and hypercapnia.

Obstructive apnea is caused by obstructed airflow, neck flexion causing opposition of hypopharyngeal soft tissues, nasal occlusion, or reflex laryngospasm.

Mixed apnea is a combination of central and obstructive apnea.

All types of apnea can cause hypoxemia, cyanosis, and bradycardia if the apnea is prolonged. Among infants dying of sudden infant death syndrome (SIDS), 18% have a history of prematurity, but apnea of prematurity is not a precursor to SIDS.

Periodic breathing is repeated cycles of 5 to 20 sec of normal breathing alternating with brief (< 20 sec) periods of apnea. This phenomenon is common among premature infants and has little or no clinical significance.

Diagnosis

- Clinical evaluation
- Cardiorespiratory monitoring, physiologic parameter recordings
- Other causes (eg, hypoglycemia, sepsis, intracranial hemorrhage) ruled out

Although frequently attributable to immature respiratory control mechanisms, apnea in premature infants can be sign of infectious, metabolic, thermoregulatory, respiratory, cardiac, or CNS dysfunction. Thorough history, physical assessment, and, when necessary, testing should be done before accepting prematurity as the cause of apnea. Gastroesophageal reflux disease (GERD) is no longer thought to cause apnea in preterm infants, so the presence of GERD should not be considered an explanation for apneic episodes.

Diagnosis of apnea usually is made by visual observation or by use of impedance-type cardiorespiratory monitors used continuously during assessment and ongoing care of preterm infants. Multichannel recordings of multiple physiologic parameters (eg, chest wall movement, airflow, O_2 saturation, heart rate, brain electric activity) taken for up to 24 h can be used as adjuncts for diagnosis and planning and monitoring treatment. However, these more advanced tests are not necessary for discharge planning.

Prognosis

Most preterm infants stop having apneic spells by the time they reach about 37 wk gestation. Apnea may continue for weeks in infants born at extremely early gestational ages (eg, 23 to 27 wk). Death is rare.

Treatment

- Stimulation
- Treatment of underlying disorder
- Respiratory stimulants (eg, caffeine)

When apnea is noted, either by observation or monitor alarm, infants are stimulated, which may be all that is required; if breathing does not resume, bag-valve-mask or mouth-to-mouth-and-nose ventilation is provided (see p. 552). For infants at home, the physician is contacted if apnea occurs but ceases after stimulation; if intervention beyond stimulation is required, the infant should be rehospitalized and evaluated.

Frequent or severe episodes should be quickly and thoroughly evaluated, and identifiable causes should be treated. If no infectious or other treatable underlying disorder is found, respiratory stimulants are indicated for treatment of frequent or severe episodes, characterized by hypoxemia, cyanosis, bradycardia, or a combination. Caffeine is the safest and most commonly used respiratory stimulant drug. It can be given as caffeine base (loading dose 10 mg/kg followed by a maintenance dose of 2.5 mg/kg po q 24 h) or caffeine citrate, a caffeine salt that is 50% caffeine (loading dose 20 mg/kg followed by a maintenance dose of 5 to 10 mg/kg q 24 h). Caffeine is preferred because of ease of administration, fewer adverse effects, larger therapeutic window, and less need to monitor drug levels. Treatment continues until the infant is 34 to 35 wk gestation and free from apnea requiring physical intervention for at least 5 to 7 days. Monitoring continues until the infant is free of apnea requiring intervention for 5 to 10 days.

If apnea continues despite respiratory stimulants, the infant may be given CPAP (see p. 2809) starting at 5 to 8 cm H_2O pressure. Intractable apneic spells require ventilator support. Discharge practices vary; some practitioners observe infants for 7 days after treatment has ended to ensure that apnea or bradycardia does not recur, whereas others discharge with caffeine if treatment seems effective.

Prevention

Home monitoring: Hospitalized high-risk infants who have not had clinically significant cardiopulmonary events (eg, apnea > 20 sec, apnea accompanied by central cyanosis, apnea associated with heart rate < 80 for > 5 sec) during 3 to 10 days of continuous cardiorespiratory monitoring can be discharged home safely without a monitor. Sometimes a home cardiorespiratory monitor and/or oral caffeine may be prescribed to shorten the hospital stay for infants who are otherwise ready for discharge but are still having cardiopulmonary events that reverse without intervention. However, infants who have events that require intervention, including stimulation, are not discharged from the hospital.

Parents should be taught how to properly use equipment, assess alarm situations, intervene (eg, CPR—see p. 545), and keep a log of events. Round-the-clock telephone support and triage as well as outpatient follow-up regarding the decision to stop using the monitor should be provided. Monitors that store event information are preferred. Parents should be informed that home cardiorespiratory monitors have not been shown to reduce the incidence of SIDS (see p. 2757) or apparent life-threatening events (ALTE—see p. 2749).

PEARLS & PITFALLS

- Home cardiorespiratory monitors have not been shown to reduce the incidence of SIDS or ALTEs.

Positioning: Infants should always be placed on their back to sleep. The infant's head should be kept in the midline, and the neck should be kept in the neutral position or slightly extended to prevent upper airway obstruction. All premature infants, especially those with apnea of prematurity, are at risk of apnea, bradycardia, and O_2 desaturation while in a car seat and should undergo a car seat challenge test before discharge.

KEY POINTS

- Apnea of prematurity is caused by immaturity of neurologic and/or mechanical function of the respiratory system.
- Infants have respiratory pauses > 20 sec or pauses < 20 sec combined with bradycardia (< 80 beats/min) and/or O_2 saturation < 85%.
- Diagnose by observation and exclude other, more serious causes of apnea (eg, infectious, metabolic, thermoregulatory, respiratory, cardiac, or CNS disorders).
- Monitor respiration and give physical stimulation for apnea; if breathing does not resume, give bag-valve-mask or mouth-to-mouth-and-nose ventilation.
- Give oral caffeine to neonates who have recurrent episodes.

BRONCHOPULMONARY DYSPLASIA

Bronchopulmonary dysplasia (BPD) is chronic lung disease of the neonate that typically is caused by prolonged ventilation and is further defined by age of prematurity and extent of O_2 requirement.

BPD is considered present when there is need for supplemental O_2 in premature infants who do not have other conditions requiring O_2 (eg, pneumonia, congenital heart disease).

Etiology

BPD has a multifactorial etiology

Significant risk factors include

- Prolonged mechanical ventilation
- High concentrations of inspired O_2
- Infection (eg, chorioamnionitis or sepsis)
- Degree of prematurity

Additional risk factors include

- Pulmonary interstitial emphysema
- High peak inspiratory pressures
- Large end-tidal volumes
- Repeated alveolar collapse
- Increased airway resistance
- Increased pulmonary artery pressures
- Male sex

The lungs of premature infants are more vulnerable to the inflammatory changes that result from mechanical ventilation. The development of normal lung architecture is interrupted; fewer and larger alveoli develop, and the interstitium is thickened. Also, the pulmonary vasculature develops abnormally, with fewer and/or abnormally distributed alveolar capillaries; pulmonary resistance may be increased and pulmonary hypertension (see p. 2815) can develop.

Diagnosis

- National Institute of Child Health and Human Development (NICHD) criteria
- Characteristic x-ray findings

BPD typically is suspected when a ventilated infant is unable to wean from O_2 therapy, mechanical ventilation, or both. Infants typically develop worsening hypoxemia, hypercapnia, and increasing O_2 requirements. Additionally, when an infant cannot be weaned within the expected time, possible underlying disorders, including patent ductus arteriosus and nursery-acquired pneumonia, should be sought.

For diagnosis, the patient has to have required at least 28 days of > 21% O_2. Specific additional diagnostic criteria (see Table 329–5) have been developed by the NICHD.

Chest x-ray initially shows diffuse haziness due to accumulation of exudative fluid; appearance then becomes multicystic or spongelike, with alternating areas of emphysema, pulmonary scarring, and atelectasis. Alveolar epithelium may slough, and macrophages, neutrophils, and inflammatory mediators may be found in the tracheal aspirate.

Prognosis

Prognosis varies with severity. Most infants gradually transition from mechanical ventilation to CPAP to low-flow O_2 over 2 to 4 mo. Infants who still depend on mechanical ventilation at 36 wk gestation have a 20 to 30% mortality rate in infancy. Infants who develop pulmonary arterial hypertension also are at higher risk of mortality during the first year of life.

Infants with BPD have a 3- to 4-fold increased rate of growth failure and neurodevelopmental problems. For several years, infants are at increased risk of lower respiratory tract infections (particularly viral pneumonia or bronchiolitis) and may quickly develop respiratory decompensation if pulmonary infection occurs. The threshold for hospitalization should be

Table 329–5. NATIONAL INSTITUTE OF CHILD HEALTH AND HUMAN DEVELOPMENT CRITERIA FOR DIAGNOSIS OF BRONCHOPULMONARY DYSPLASIA*

< 32 WK GESTATIONAL AGE†	≥ 32 WK GESTATIONAL AGE‡	DIAGNOSIS
Breathing room air at 36 wk PMA or discharge, whichever comes first	Breathing room air by 56 days postnatal age or discharge, whichever comes first	Mild BPD
Need for < 30% O_2 at 36 wk PMA or discharge, whichever comes first	Need for < 30% O_2 at 56 days postnatal age or discharge, whichever comes first	Moderate BPD
Need for ≥ 30% O_2, positive pressure, or both at 35 wk PMA or discharge, whichever comes first	Need for ≥ 30% O_2, positive pressure, or both at 56 days postnatal age or discharge, whichever comes first	Severe BPD

*These criteria are in addition to the baseline requirement of > 21% O_2 for at least 28 days.
†Assessed at 36 wk PMA.
‡Assessed at age 29 to 55 days.
BPD = bronchopulmonary dysplasia; PMA = postmenstrual age.

low if signs of a respiratory infection or respiratory distress develop.

Treatment

- Nutrition supplementation
- Fluid restriction
- Diuretics
- O_2 supplementation as needed
- Respiratory syncytial virus (RSV) monoclonal antibody

Treatment is supportive and includes nutritional supplementation, fluid restriction, diuretics, and perhaps inhaled bronchodilators. Respiratory infections must be diagnosed early and treated aggressively. Weaning from mechanical ventilation and supplemental O_2 should be accomplished as early as possible.

Feedings should achieve an intake of 150 calories/kg/day including protein 3.5 to 4 g/kg/day; caloric requirements are increased because of the increased work of breathing and to aid lung healing and growth.

Because pulmonary congestion and edema may develop, daily fluid intake is often restricted to about 120 to 140 mL/kg/day. Diuretic therapy transiently improves pulmonary mechanics but not long-term clinical outcome. Thiazide or loop diuretics can be used for short-term benefit in patients who do not respond adequately to or cannot tolerate fluid restriction. Chlorothiazide 10 to 20 mg/kg po bid with or without spironolactone 1 to 3 mg/kg po once/day or split into twice-daily doses is often tried first. Furosemide (1 to 2 mg/kg IV or IM or 1 to 4 mg/kg po q 12 to 24 h for neonates and q 8 h for older infants) may be used for short periods, but prolonged use causes hypercalciuria with resultant osteoporosis, fractures, and renal calculi. If long-term diuretic use is required, chlorothiazide is preferred because it has fewer adverse effects. Hydration and serum electrolytes should be monitored closely during diuretic therapy.

Inhaled bronchodilators (eg, albuterol) do not appear to improve long-term outcome and are not used routinely. However, they may be helpful for acute episodes of bronchoconstriction.

Weeks or months of additional ventilator support, supplemental O_2, or both may be required for advanced BPD. Ventilator pressures or volumes and fraction of inspired O_2 (FIO_2) should be reduced as rapidly as tolerated, but the infant should not be allowed to become hypoxemic. Arterial oxygenation should be continuously monitored with a pulse oximeter and maintained at ≥ 89% saturation. Respiratory acidosis may occur during ventilator weaning and treatment and is acceptable as long as the pH remains > 7.25 and the infant does not develop severe respiratory distress.

Passive immunoprophylaxis with palivizumab, a monoclonal antibody to RSV, decreases RSV-related hospitalizations and ICU stays but is costly and is indicated primarily in high-risk infants (see p. 2764 for indications). During RSV season (November through April), children are given 15 mg/kg IM q 30 days until 6 mo after treatment of the acute illness. Infants > 6 mo also should be vaccinated against influenza.

Systemic or inhaled corticosteroids are discouraged except as a last-resort therapy for established BPD with rapidly worsening pulmonary status and impending death. Informed parental consent is required.

Prevention

Practices for prevention of BPD include

- Use of antenatal corticosteroids
- Prophylactic use of exogenous surfactant in selected high-risk infants (eg, weighing < 1000 g and requiring ventilator support)
- Early therapeutic continuous positive airway pressure
- Early use of surfactant for treatment of RDS
- Prophylactic use of methylxanthines (eg, caffeine 5 to 10 mg/kg po once/day), particularly when birth weight is < 1250 g
- Permissive hypercarbia and hypoxemia to achieve low ventilator pressures, volumes, or both
- Prophylactic use of vitamin A (5000 units IM 3 times/wk for a total of 12 doses) for infants with birth weight < 1000 g
- Avoidance of large volumes of fluid

Inhaled nitric oxide has been studied and may help prevent of BPD. However, optimal dosage, duration, and timing are unclear, so nitric oxide is not yet recommended outside of research protocols.

KEY POINTS

- BPD is chronic lung disease of premature infants.
- BPD develops in neonates who required prolonged mechanical ventilation and/or O_2 supplementation, which can disrupt normal lung development.
- Diagnosis is based on prolonged (≥ 28 days) need for O_2 supplementation and sometimes ventilatory support.
- Wean from respiratory support as soon as possible and use nutritional supplementation, fluid restriction, and sometimes diuretics.
- Prevent by using antenatal corticosteroids, surfactant, caffeine, and vitamin A and use lowest FIO_2 and airway pressure as possible.

MECONIUM ASPIRATION SYNDROME

Intrapartum meconium aspiration can cause inflammatory pneumonitis and mechanical bronchial obstruction, causing a syndrome of respiratory distress. Findings include tachypnea, rales and rhonchi, and cyanosis or desaturation. Diagnosis is suspected when there is respiratory distress after delivery through meconium-tinged amniotic fluid and is confirmed by chest x-ray. Treatment is vigorous suction immediately on delivery before neonates take their first breath, followed by respiratory support as needed. Prognosis depends on the underlying physiologic stressors.

Etiology

Physiologic stress at the time of labor and delivery (eg, due to hypoxia caused by umbilical cord compression or placental insufficiency or caused by infection) may cause the fetus to pass meconium into the amniotic fluid before delivery; meconium passage is noted in about 10 to 15% of births. During delivery, perhaps 5% of neonates with meconium passage aspirate the meconium, triggering lung injury and respiratory distress, termed meconium aspiration syndrome. Postterm infants delivered through reduced amniotic fluid volume are at risk of more severe disease because the less dilute meconium is more likely to cause airway obstruction.

Pathophysiology

The mechanisms by which aspiration induces the clinical syndrome probably include

- Nonspecific cytokine release
- Airway obstruction
- Surfactant inactivation
- Chemical pneumonitis

Underlying physiologic stressors also may contribute. If complete bronchial obstruction occurs, atelectasis results; partial blockage leads to air trapping on expiration, resulting in hyperexpansion of the lungs and possibly pulmonary air leak (see p. 2816) with pneumomediastinum or pneumothorax. Persistent pulmonary hypertension can be associated with meconium aspiration as a comorbid condition or because of continuing hypoxia.

Neonates also may aspirate vernix caseosa, amniotic fluid, or blood of maternal or fetal origin during delivery, which can cause respiratory distress and signs of aspiration pneumonia on chest x-ray.

Symptoms and Signs

Signs include tachypnea, nasal flaring, retractions, cyanosis or desaturation, rales, rhonchi, and greenish yellow staining of the umbilical cord, nail beds, or skin. Meconium staining may be visible in the oropharynx and (on intubation) in the larynx and trachea. Neonates with air trapping may have a barrel-shaped chest and also symptoms and signs of pneumothorax, pulmonary interstitial emphysema, and pneumomediastinum.

Diagnosis

- Meconium passage
- Respiratory distress
- Characteristic x-ray findings

Diagnosis is suspected when a neonate shows respiratory distress in the setting of meconium-tinged amniotic fluid. Diagnosis is confirmed by chest x-ray showing hyperinflation with variable areas of atelectasis and flattening of the diaphragm. Initial x-ray findings can be confused with the findings of transient tachypnea of the newborn. Fluid may be seen in the lung fissures or pleural spaces, and air may be seen in the soft tissues or mediastinum. Because meconium may enhance bacterial growth and meconium aspiration syndrome is difficult to distinguish from bacterial pneumonia, cultures of blood and tracheal aspirate also should be taken.

Prognosis

Prognosis is generally good, although it varies with the underlying physiologic stressors; overall mortality is slightly increased. Infants with meconium aspiration syndrome may be at greater risk of asthma in later life.

Treatment

- Suctioning at birth before the first breath
- Endotracheal intubation as needed
- Mechanical ventilation as needed
- Supplemental O_2 as needed
- IV antibiotics

Routine suctioning of neonates delivered with meconium-stained fluid has not been shown to improve outcome. However, if the neonate's breathing appears obstructed, suctioning is done. If the neonate is nonvigorous at delivery (ie, with poor muscle tone or absent or depressed respiratory effort) or is bradycardic (< 100 beats/min), the trachea should be intubated and suctioned with a meconium aspirator. Suction is maintained while the endotracheal tube is removed. Reintubation and CPAP (see p. 2809) are indicated for continued respiratory distress, followed by mechanical ventilation (see p. 2810) and admission to the neonatal ICU as needed. Because positive pressure ventilation enhances risk of pulmonary air-leak syndrome, regular evaluation (including physical examination and chest x-ray) is important to detect this complication, which should be sought immediately in any intubated neonate whose BP, perfusion, or O_2 saturation suddenly worsens. See p. 2816 for treatment of air-leak syndromes.

Additional treatments may include surfactant for mechanically ventilated neonates with high O_2 requirements, which can decrease the need for extracorporeal membrane oxygenation (ECMO), and antibiotics (usually ampicillin and an aminoglycoside). Inhaled nitric oxide at 20 ppm and high-frequency ventilation are other therapies that are used if refractory hypoxemia develops; they also may decrease need for ECMO.

KEY POINTS

- About 5% of neonates with meconium passage aspirate the meconium, triggering lung injury and respiratory distress.
- Suspect the diagnosis when respiratory distress occurs in neonates who had meconium-tinged amniotic fluid.
- Neonates may have tachypnea, nasal flaring, retractions, cyanosis or desaturation, rales, rhonchi, and visible meconium staining in the oropharynx.
- Do cultures of blood and tracheal aspirates to exclude pneumonia.
- After delivery, suction infants who have signs of obstructed breathing; if there is weak respiratory effort or bradycardia, insert an endotracheal tube and suction using a meconium aspirator.
- Severe cases require mechanical ventilation and sometimes antibiotics, inhaled nitric oxide, or ECMO.

PERSISTENT PULMONARY HYPERTENSION OF THE NEWBORN

Persistent pulmonary hypertension of the newborn is the persistence of or reversion to pulmonary arteriolar constriction, causing a severe reduction in pulmonary blood flow and right-to-left shunting. Symptoms and signs include tachypnea, retractions, and severe cyanosis or desaturation unresponsive to O_2. Diagnosis is by history, examination, chest x-ray, and response to O_2. Treatment includes O_2, high-frequency ventilation, nitric oxide, and pressors and/or inotropes; extracorporeal membrane oxygenation (ECMO) is done if other therapies fail.

Persistent pulmonary hypertension of the newborn is a disorder of pulmonary vasculature that affects term or postterm infants.

Etiology

The **most common causes** involve

- Perinatal asphyxia or hypoxia

A history of meconium staining of amniotic fluid or meconium in the trachea is common. Hypoxia triggers reversion to or persistence of intense pulmonary arteriolar constriction, a normal state in the fetus.

Additional causes include

- Respiratory distress syndrome (RDS)
- Premature ductus arteriosus or foramen ovale closure, which increases fetal pulmonary blood flow and may be triggered by maternal NSAID use
- Pulmonary hypoplasia
- Congenital diaphragmatic hernia, in which one lung is severely hypoplastic, forcing most of the pulmonary blood flow through the other lung
- Neonatal sepsis or pneumonia presumably because vasoconstrictive prostaglandins are produced by activation of the cyclooxygenase pathway by bacterial phospholipids

Pathophysiology

Whatever the cause, elevated pressure in the pulmonary arteries causes abnormal smooth muscle development and hypertrophy in the walls of the small pulmonary arteries and arterioles and right-to-left shunting via the ductus arteriosus or a foramen ovale, resulting in intractable systemic hypoxemia. Both pulmonary and systemic resistances are high, which leads to an increased load on the heart. This load increase may result in right heart dilation, tricuspid insufficiency, and right heart failure.

Symptoms and Signs

Symptoms and signs include tachypnea, retractions, and severe cyanosis or desaturation unresponsive to supplemental O_2. In infants with a right-to-left shunt via a patent ductus arteriosus, oxygenation is higher in the right brachial artery than in the descending aorta; thus cyanosis may be differential (ie, O_2 saturation in the lower extremities is $\geq 5\%$ lower than in the right upper extremity).

Diagnosis

- Cyanosis unresponsive to O_2 therapy
- Echocardiogram
- X-ray to identify underlying disorders

Diagnosis should be suspected in any near-term infant with arterial hypoxemia, cyanosis, or both, especially one with a suggestive history whose O_2 saturation does not improve with administration of 100% O_2. Diagnosis is confirmed by echocardiogram, which can confirm the presence of elevated pressures in the pulmonary artery and simultaneously can exclude congenital heart disease. On x-ray, lung fields may be normal or may show changes due to the underlying disorder (eg, meconium aspiration syndrome, neonatal pneumonia, congenital diaphragmatic hernia).

Prognosis

The oxygenation index (mean airway pressure [cm H_2O] × fraction of inspired O_2[F_{IO_2}] × 100/Pa_{O_2}) is used to assess disease severity and determine timing of interventions (in particular for inhaled nitric oxide [oxygenation index 15 to 25] and ECMO [oxygenation index > 40]). Overall mortality ranges from 10 to 60% and is related to the underlying disorder. However, 25% of survivors exhibit developmental delay, hearing deficits, functional disabilities, or a combination. This rate of disability may be no different from that of other infants with severe illness.

Treatment

- O_2 to dilate pulmonary vasculature and improve oxygenation
- Mechanical ventilation support
- Inhaled nitric oxide
- ECMO as needed
- Circulatory support

Treatment with O_2, which is a potent pulmonary vasodilator, is begun immediately to prevent disease progression. O_2 is delivered via bag-and-mask or mechanical ventilation (see p. 2810); mechanical distention of alveoli aids vasodilation. F_{IO_2} should initially be 1 but can be titrated downward to maintain PaO_2 between 50 and 90 mm Hg to minimize lung injury. Once PaO_2 is stabilized, weaning can be attempted by reducing F_{IO_2} in decrements of 2 to 3%, then reducing ventilator pressures; changes should be gradual, because a large drop in PaO_2 can cause recurrent pulmonary artery vasoconstriction. High-frequency oscillatory ventilation expands and ventilates the lungs while minimizing barotrauma and should be considered for infants with underlying lung disease in whom atelectasis and ventilation/perfusion (V/Q) mismatch may exacerbate the hypoxemia of persistent pulmonary hypertension of the newborn.

Inhaled nitric oxide relaxes endothelial smooth muscle, dilating pulmonary arterioles, which increases pulmonary blood flow and rapidly improves oxygenation in as many as half of patients. Initial dose is 20 ppm, titrated downward by effect.

ECMO (see p. 2811) may be used in newborns with severe hypoxic respiratory failure defined by an oxygenation index > 35 to 40 despite maximum respiratory support.

Normal fluid, electrolyte, glucose, and Ca levels must be maintained. Infants should be kept in a neutral thermal environment and treated with antibiotics for possible sepsis until culture results are known. Inotropes and pressors may be required as part of circulatory support.

KEY POINTS

- Prolonged hypoxia or disorders that increase pulmonary blood flow cause smooth muscle hypertrophy in small pulmonary arteries, resulting in persistent pulmonary hypertension.

- Persistent pulmonary hypertension causes right-to-left shunting via the ductus arteriosus or a foramen ovale, resulting in intractable systemic hypoxemia; right-sided heart failure may develop.
- Confirm diagnosis by echocardiography.
- Give O_2 to dilate pulmonary vasculature, mechanical ventilation, inhaled nitric oxide, and, for severe cases, ECMO.

PULMONARY AIR-LEAK SYNDROMES

Pulmonary air-leak syndromes involve dissection of air out of the normal pulmonary airspaces.

Air-leak syndromes include

- Pulmonary interstitial emphysema
- Pneumomediastinum
- Pneumothorax
- Pneumopericardium
- Pneumoperitoneum or subcutaneous emphysema (rare)

Pneumothorax and pneumomediastinum occur in 1 to 2% of normal neonates, probably because large negative intrathoracic forces created when the neonate starts breathing occasionally disrupt alveolar epithelium, which allows air to move from the alveoli into extra-alveolar soft tissues or spaces.

Air leak is more common and severe among neonates with lung disease, who are at risk because of poor lung compliance and the need for high airway pressures (eg, in respiratory distress) or because of air trapping (eg, meconium aspiration syndrome), which leads to alveolar overdistention.

Many affected neonates are asymptomatic; diagnosis is suspected clinically or because of deterioration in O_2 status and is confirmed by x-ray. Treatment varies by type of air leak but in ventilated infants always involves lowering inspiratory pressures to lowest tolerated settings. High-frequency ventilators may be helpful but are of unproven benefit.

Pulmonary interstitial emphysema: Pulmonary interstitial emphysema is leakage of air from alveoli into the pulmonary interstitium, lymphatics, or subpleural space. It usually occurs in infants with poor lung compliance, such as those with respiratory distress syndrome (see p. 2808) who are being treated with mechanical ventilation, but it may occur spontaneously. One or both lungs may be involved, and pathology may be focal or generalized within each lung. If dissection of air is widespread, respiratory status may acutely worsen because lung compliance suddenly is reduced.

Chest x-ray shows a variable number of cystic or linear lucencies in the lung fields. Some lucencies are elongated; others appear as enlarged subpleural cysts ranging from a few millimeters to several centimeters in diameter.

Pulmonary interstitial emphysema may resolve dramatically over 1 or 2 days or persist on x-ray for weeks. Some infants with severe respiratory disease and pulmonary interstitial emphysema develop bronchopulmonary dysplasia (see p. 2812), and the cystic changes of long-standing pulmonary interstitial emphysema then merge into the x-ray picture of bronchopulmonary dysplasia.

Treatment is mainly supportive. For mechanically ventilated infants, lowering tidal volume and airway pressure by switching to a high-frequency oscillatory ventilator or high-frequency jet ventilator may help. If one lung is significantly more involved than the other, the infant may be laid down on the side of the lung with the more severe pulmonary interstitial emphysema; this will help to compress the lung with pulmonary interstitial emphysema, thereby decreasing air leakage and perhaps improving ventilation of the normal (elevated) lung. If one lung is very severely affected and the other is mildly affected or uninvolved, differential bronchial intubation and ventilation of the less-involved lung also may be attempted; total atelectasis of the nonintubated lung soon results. Because only one lung is now being ventilated, ventilator settings and fraction of inspired O_2 may need to be altered. After 24 to 48 h, the endotracheal tube is pulled back into the trachea, at which time the air leak may have stopped.

Pneumomediastinum: Pneumomediastinum is dissection of air into connective tissue of the mediastinum (see p. 475); the air may further dissect into the subcutaneous tissues of the neck and scalp. Pneumomediastinum usually causes no symptoms or signs, but subcutaneous air causes crepitus. Diagnosis is by x-ray; in an anteroposterior view, air may form a lucency around the heart, whereas on a lateral view, air lifts the lobes of the thymus away from the cardiac silhouette (spinnaker sail sign). No treatment is usually needed, and the condition resolves spontaneously.

Pneumopericardium: Pneumopericardium is dissection of air into the pericardial sac. It affects mechanically ventilated infants almost exclusively. Most cases are asymptomatic, but if sufficient air accumulates, it can cause cardiac tamponade (see p. 744). Diagnosis is suspected if infants experience acute circulatory collapse and is confirmed by lucency around the heart on x-ray or by return of air on pericardiocentesis using an angiocatheter and syringe. Treatment is pericardiocentesis followed by surgical insertion of a pericardial tube.

Pneumoperitoneum: Pneumoperitoneum is dissection of air into the peritoneum. It is generally not clinically significant but must be distinguished from pneumoperitoneum due to a ruptured abdominal viscus, which is a surgical emergency. Diagnosis is made by abdominal x-ray and physical examination. Clinical symptoms that include abdominal rigidity, absent bowel sounds, and signs of sepsis suggest abdominal viscus injury.

Pneumothorax: Pneumothorax is dissection of air into the pleural space; sufficient accumulation of air causes tension pneumothorax (see p. 475). Although sometimes asymptomatic, pneumothorax typically causes worsening of tachypnea, grunting, and cyanosis. Breath sounds decrease, and the chest enlarges on the affected side. Tension pneumothorax causes cardiovascular collapse.

Diagnosis is suspected by deterioration of respiratory status, by transillumination of the chest with a fiberoptic probe, or both. Diagnosis is confirmed by chest x-ray or, in the case of tension pneumothorax, return of air during thoracentesis.

Most small pneumothoraces resolve spontaneously, but larger and tension pneumothoraces require evacuation of the air in the pleural cavity. In tension pneumothorax, a small (23- or 25-gauge) needle or an angiocatheter (18- or 20-gauge) and syringe can be used to temporarily evacuate free air from the pleural space. Definitive treatment is insertion of an 8 or 10 French chest tube attached to continuous suction. Follow-up auscultation, transillumination, and x-ray confirm that the tube is functioning properly.

330 Principles of Drug Treatment in Children

Drug treatment in children differs from that in adults, most obviously because it is usually based on weight or surface area. Doses (and dosing intervals) differ because of age-related variations in drug absorption, distribution, metabolism, and elimination. A child cannot safely receive an adult drug dose, nor can it be assumed that a child's dose is proportional to an adult's dose (ie, that a 7-kg child requires 1/10 the dose of a 70-kg adult). Most drugs have not been adequately studied in children, although federal legislation (the Best Pharmaceuticals for Children Act of 2001 and the Pediatric Research Equity Act of 2003 [both renewed in 2012]) provides the statutory and regulatory authority to begin those studies.

Adverse effects and toxicity: Children are generally subject to the same adverse effects as adults (see p. 2903), but they have increased risk with certain drugs because of differences in pharmacokinetics or because of drug effects on growth and development. Common drugs with unique or higher risk of adverse effects in children are listed in Table 330–1.

Younger children are at especially high risk of accidental poisoning when they discover and take caregivers' vitamins or drugs. Infants are at risk of toxicity from drugs used by adults; toxicity can occur prenatally when they are exposed via placental transfer or postnatally when exposed through breast milk (numerous agents—see p. 2416 and Table 288–4 on p. 2417) or skin contact with caregivers who have recently applied certain topical drugs (eg, scopolamine for motion sickness, malathion for lice, diphenhydramine for poison ivy).

Adverse effects, including death, have occurred in children receiving OTC cough and cold preparations containing some combination of an antihistamine, sympathomimetic decongestant, and the antitussive dextromethorphan. Current recommendations are that such products should not be given to children < 4 yr.

PHARMACOKINETICS IN CHILDREN

Pharmacokinetics refers to the processes of drug absorption, distribution, metabolism, and elimination (see p. 2914).

Absorption: Absorption from the GI tract is affected by

- Gastric acid secretion
- Bile salt formation
- Gastric emptying time
- Intestinal motility
- Bowel length and effective absorptive surface
- Microbial flora

All these factors are reduced in neonates (full-term and premature) and all may be reduced or increased in an ill child of any age. Reduced gastric acid secretion increases bioavailability of acid-labile drugs (eg, penicillin) and decreases bioavailability of weakly acidic drugs (eg, phenobarbital). Reduced bile salt formation decreases bioavailability of lipophilic drugs (eg, diazepam). Reduced gastric emptying and intestinal motility increase the time it takes to reach therapeutic concentrations when enteral drugs are given to infants < 3 mo. Drug-metabolizing

Table 330–1. DRUGS MANIFESTING UNUSUAL TOXICITY IN CHILDREN

DRUG	CLINICAL SYNDROME	MECHANISM	COMMENTS
Anesthetics, topical (eg, benzocaine, mixture of lidocaine and prilocaine)	Cyanosis	Formation of methemoglobin (ferrous iron oxidized to ferric iron)	Incidence rare
Ceftriaxone	Jaundice Kernicterus	Bilirubin displaced from albumin	Affects only neonates
Codeine	Respiratory depression Death	Ultrarapid metabolization of codeine to morphine	Genetic variant Deaths have occurred after surgery and in a breastfed infant whose mother took codeine
Diphenoxylate	Respiratory depression Death	CNS depression (in immature CNS)	Overdose syndrome, usually in children < 2 yr
Fluoroquinolones	Cartilage toxicity	Unknown	Suspected based on animal studies, but adverse effects in humans unproved—short-term use may be safe
Lindane (topical)	Seizures CNS toxicity	Probably enhanced absorption in children	Should not be used in children < 50 kg (alternative should be used)
Prochlorperazine	Altered CNS function Extrapyramidal effects Opisthotonus Bulging fontanelles	Actions via multiple CNS receptors	Febrile and dehydrated infants especially at risk
SSRIs	Suicidal ideation	Unknown	Increased incidence of suicidal ideation in children and adolescents
Tetracycline	Discoloration and pitting of tooth enamel	Chelation with Ca in growing teeth	Not given to children < 8 yr

enzymes present in the intestines of young infants are another cause of reduced drug absorption. Infants with congenital atretic bowel or surgically removed bowel or who have jejunal feeding tubes may have specific absorptive defects depending on the length of bowel lost or bypassed and the location of the lost segment.

Injected drugs are often erratically absorbed because of

- Variability in their chemical characteristics
- Differences in absorption by site of injection (IM or sc)
- Variability in muscle mass among children
- Illness (eg, compromised circulatory status)
- Variability in depth of injection (too deep or too shallow)

IM injections are generally avoided in children because of pain and the possibility of tissue damage, but, when needed, water-soluble drugs are best because they do not precipitate at the injection site.

Transdermal absorption may be enhanced in neonates and young infants because the stratum corneum is thin and because the ratio of surface area to weight is much greater than for older children and adults. Skin disruptions (eg, abrasions, eczema, burns) increase absorption in children of any age.

Transrectal drug therapy is generally appropriate only for emergencies when an IV route is not available (eg, use of rectal diazepam for status epilepticus). Site of placement of the drug within the rectal cavity may influence absorption because of the difference in venous drainage systems. Young infants may also expel the drug before significant absorption has occurred.

Absorption of drugs from the lungs (eg, β-agonists for asthma, pulmonary surfactant for respiratory distress syndrome) varies less by physiologic parameters and more by reliability of the delivery device and patient or caregiver technique.

Distribution: The volume of distribution of drugs changes in children with aging. These age-related changes are due to changes in body composition (especially the extracellular and total body water spaces) and plasma protein binding.

Higher doses (per kg of body weight) of water-soluble drugs are required in younger children because a higher percentage of their body weight is water (see Fig. 330–1). Conversely, lower doses are required to avoid toxicity as children grow older because of the decline in water as a percentage of body weight.

Many drugs bind to proteins (primarily albumin, α_1-acid glycoprotein, and lipoproteins); protein binding limits distribution of free drug throughout the body. Albumin and total protein concentrations are lower in neonates but approach adult levels by 10 to 12 mo. Decreased protein binding in neonates is also due to qualitative differences in binding proteins and to competitive binding by molecules such as bilirubin and free fatty acids, which circulate in higher concentrations in neonates and infants. The net result may be increased free drug concentrations, greater drug availability at receptor sites, and both pharmacologic effects and higher frequency of adverse effects at lower drug concentrations.

Metabolism and elimination: Drug metabolism and elimination vary with age and depend on the substrate or drug, but most drugs, and most notably phenytoin, barbiturates, analgesics, and cardiac glycosides, have plasma half-lives 2 to 3 times longer in neonates than in adults.

The cytochrome P-450 (CYP450) enzyme system in the small bowel and liver is the most important known system for drug metabolism. CYP450 enzymes inactivate drugs via

- Oxidation, reduction, and hydrolysis (phase I metabolism)
- Hydroxylation and conjugation (phase II metabolism)

Phase I activity is reduced in neonates, increases progressively during the first 6 mo of life, exceeds adult rates by the first few years for some drugs, slows during adolescence, and usually attains adult rates by late puberty. However, adult rates of metabolism may be achieved for some drugs (eg, barbiturates, phenytoin) 2 to 4 wk postnatally. CYP450 activity can also be induced (reducing drug concentrations and effect) or inhibited (augmenting concentrations and effect) by coadministered drugs. These drug interactions may lead to drug toxicity when CYP450 activity is inhibited or an inadequate drug level when CYP450 activity is induced. Kidneys, lungs, and skin also play a role in the metabolism of some drugs, as do intestinal drug-metabolizing enzymes in neonates. Phase II metabolism varies considerably by substrate. Maturation of enzymes responsible for bilirubin and acetaminophen conjugation is delayed; enzymes responsible for morphine conjugation are fully mature even in preterm infants.

Drug metabolites are eliminated primarily through bile or the kidneys. Renal elimination depends on

- Plasma protein binding
- Renal blood flow
- GFR
- Tubular secretion

All of these factors are altered in the first 2 yr of life. Renal plasma flow is low at birth (12 mL/min) and reaches adult levels of 140 mL/min by age 1 yr. Similarly, GFR is 2 to 4 mL/min at birth, increases to 8 to 20 mL/min by 2 to 3 days, and reaches adult levels of 120 mL/min by 3 to 5 mo.

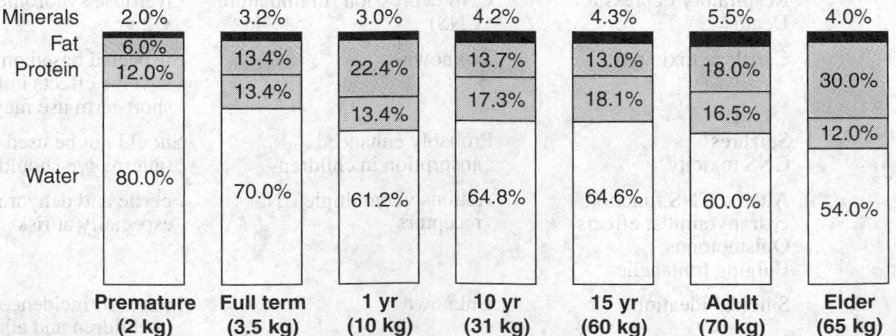

Fig. 330–1. Changes in body composition with growth and aging. Adapted from Puig M: Body composition and growth. In *Nutrition in Pediatrics*, ed. 2, edited by WA Walker and JB Watkins. Hamilton, Ontario, BC Decker, 1996.

Drug dosing: Because of the above factors, drug dosing in children < 12 yr is always a function of age, body weight, or both. This approach is practical but not ideal. Even within a population of similar age and weight, drug requirements may differ because of maturational differences in absorption, metabolism, and elimination. Thus, when practical, dose adjustments should be based on plasma drug concentration (however, plasma drug concentration may not reflect the drug concentration in the target organ). Unfortunately, these adjustments are not feasible for most drugs. Studies done as a result of federal legislation (the Best Pharmaceuticals for Children Act of 2001 and the Pediatric Research Equity Act of 2003 [both renewed in 2012]) have provided dosing for > 450 drugs that previously did not have pediatric dosing information.

NONADHERENCE IN CHILDREN

Nonadherence with drug recommendations (see p. 2908) may occur at any age because of cost; painful or inconvenient administration; or the need for frequent doses, complex regimens, or both. But many unique factors contribute to nonadherence in children. Children < 6 yr may have difficulty swallowing pills and may resist taking forms of drugs that taste bad. Older children often resist drugs or regimens (eg, insulin, metered-dose inhalers) that require them to leave their classes or activities or that make them appear different from their peers. Adolescents may express rebellion and assert independence from parents by not taking their drugs. Parents or caregivers of younger children may only partially remember or understand the rationale and instructions for taking a drug, and their work schedules may preclude their being available to give children their scheduled doses. Some parents may wish to try folk or herbal remedies initially. Some caregivers have limited incomes and are forced to spend their money on other priorities, such as food; others have beliefs and attitudes that prevent them from giving children drugs.

To minimize nonadherence, a prescribing provider can do the following:

- Ascertain whether the patient or caregiver agrees with the diagnosis, perceives it as serious, and believes the treatment will work.
- Correct misunderstandings and guide the patient or caregiver toward reliable sources of information.
- Give written as well as oral instructions in a language the patient or caregiver can review and understand.
- Make early follow-up telephone calls to families to answer residual questions.
- Assess progress and remind the patient or caregiver of follow-up visits.
- Review drug bottles at follow-up office visits for pill counts.
- Educate the patient or caregiver about how to keep a daily symptom or drug diary.

Adolescents in particular need to feel in control of their illness and treatment and should be encouraged to communicate freely and to take as much responsibility as is possible for their own treatment. Regimens should be simplified (eg, synchronizing multiple drugs and minimizing the number of daily doses while maintaining efficacy) and matched to the patient's and caregivers' schedules. Critical aspects of the treatment should be emphasized (eg, taking the full course of an antibiotic). If lifestyle changes (eg, in diet or exercise) are also needed, such changes should be introduced incrementally over several visits, and realistic goals should be set (eg, to lose 1 of 14 kg [2 of 30 lb] by a 2-wk follow-up visit). Success in achieving a goal should be reinforced with praise, and only then should the next goal be added. For patients who require expensive long-term regimens, a list of pharmaceutical patient-assistance programs is available at www.needymeds.org.

331 Problems in Adolescents

Fortunately, most adolescents enjoy good physical and mental health. However, the incidence and prevalence of chronic diseases in adolescence are on the rise and likely are due to an earlier onset of obesity-associated disorders, longer survival after serious childhood disorders, and other unknown factors.

The **most common problems** among adolescents relate to growth and development, school, childhood illnesses that continue into adolescence, mental health disorders, and the consequences of risky or illegal behaviors, including injury, legal consequences, pregnancy, infectious diseases, and addiction. Unintentional injuries resulting from motor vehicle crashes and injuries resulting from interpersonal violence are leading causes of death and disability among adolescents.

Psychosocial adjustment is a hallmark of this phase of development because even normal individuals struggle with issues of identity, autonomy, sexuality, and relationships. "Who am I, where am I going, and how do I relate to all of these people in my life?" are frequent preoccupations for most adolescents. Psychosocial disorders are more common during adolescence than during childhood, and many unhealthy behaviors begin during adolescence. Having an eating disorder, poor diet, obesity, smoking, using drugs, and violent behavior can lead to acute health problems, chronic disorders, or morbidity later in life.

BEHAVIOR PROBLEMS IN ADOLESCENTS

Adolescence is a time for developing independence. Typically, adolescents exercise their independence by questioning their parents' rules, which at times leads to rule breaking. Parents and health care practitioners must distinguish occasional errors of judgment from a degree of misbehavior that requires professional intervention. The severity and frequency of infractions are guides. For example, recurrent binge drinking and engaging in recurrent truancy or theft are much more significant than isolated episodes of the same activities. Warning signs that suggest disruptive behaviors are impairing functioning include deterioration of performance at school and running away from home. Of particular concern are adolescents who cause serious injury or use a weapon in a fight.

Because adolescents are much more independent and mobile than they were as children, they are often out of the direct physical control of adults. In these circumstances, adolescents' behavior is determined by their own moral and behavioral code. Parents guide rather than directly control their children's actions. Adolescents who feel warmth and support from their parents are less likely to engage in risky behaviors, as are those whose parents convey clear expectations regarding their children's behavior and show consistent limit setting and monitoring.

Authoritative parenting is a parenting style in which children participate in establishing family expectations and rules. This parenting style, as opposed to harsh or permissive parenting, is most likely to promote mature behaviors.

Authoritative parents typically use a system of graduated privileges, in which adolescents initially are given small bits of responsibility and freedom (eg, caring for a pet, doing household chores, purchasing clothing, decorating their room, managing an allowance, going to social events with friends, driving). If adolescents handle this responsibility well over a period of time, more privileges are granted. By contrast, poor judgment or lack of responsibility leads to loss of privileges. Each new privilege requires close monitoring by parents to make sure adolescents comply with the agreed-upon rules.

Some parents and their adolescents clash over almost everything. In these situations, the core issue is really control. Adolescents want to feel in control of their lives, but parents are not ready to give up that control. In these situations, everyone may benefit from the parents picking their battles and focusing their efforts on the adolescent's actions (eg, attending school and complying with household responsibilities) rather than on expressions (eg, dress, hairstyle, and preferred entertainment).

Adolescents whose behavior is dangerous or otherwise unacceptable despite their parents' best efforts may need professional intervention. Substance use disorders are a common trigger of behavioral problems, and substance use disorders require specific treatment. Behavioral problems also may be a symptom of learning disabilities, depression, or other mental health disorders. Such disorders typically require treatment with drugs as well as counseling. If parents are not able to limit their child's dangerous behavior, they may request help from the court system and be assigned to a probation officer who can help enforce reasonable household rules.

Specific Behavioral Disorders

Disruptive behavioral disorders are common during adolescence.

Attention-deficit/hyperactivity disorder (ADHD) is the most common mental health disorder of childhood and often persists into adolescence and adulthood. Once thought of as a "nuisance" disorder of childhood, research has shown poor long-term functional outcomes in children diagnosed with ADHD as compared to their peers. Behavioral and drug therapy can improve outcomes. Clinicians should continue to treat and monitor adolescent patients diagnosed with ADHD in childhood. Although substance use disorders are more common among people with ADHD, treating with stimulants does not appear to increase the risk of developing a substance use disorder and may even decrease the risk.

Clinicians are cautioned to make the diagnosis of ADHD carefully before initiating treatment because other conditions, such as depression or learning disabilities, may manifest primarily with symptoms of inattention and can mimic ADHD. In some cases, an adolescent may complain of symptoms of inattention in an attempt to obtain a prescription for stimulants, either to be used as a study aid or recreationally. Because of the high potential for misuse and dependence, stimulants should be prescribed only after a diagnosis of ADHD has been confirmed.

Other common disruptive behaviors of childhood include oppositional defiant disorder and conduct disorder. These conditions are typically treated with psychotherapy for the child and advice and support for parents.

Violence

Children occasionally engage in physical confrontation and bullying. During adolescence, the frequency and severity of violent interactions may increase. Although episodes of violence at school are highly publicized, adolescents are much more likely to be involved in violent episodes (or more often the threat of violence) at home and outside of school. Many factors contribute to an increased risk of violence for adolescents, including

- Developmental issues
- Gang membership
- Access to firearms
- Substance use
- Poverty

There is little evidence to suggest a relationship between violence and genetic defects or chromosomal abnormalities.

Gang membership has been linked with violent behavior. Youth gangs are self-formed associations made up of 3 or more members, typically ranging in age from 13 to 24. Gangs usually adopt a name and identifying symbols, such as a particular style of clothing, the use of certain hand signs, or graffiti. Some gangs require prospective members to perform random acts of violence before membership is granted.

Increasing youth gang violence has been blamed at least in part on gang involvement in drug distribution and drug use, particularly methamphetamines and heroin. Firearms and other weapons are frequent features of gang violence.

Violence prevention begins in early childhood with violence-free discipline. Limiting exposure to violence through media and video games may also help because exposure to these violent images has been shown to desensitize children to violence and cause children to accept violence as part of their life. School-age children should have access to a safe school environment. Older children and adolescents should not have unsupervised access to weapons and should be taught to avoid high-risk situations (such as places or settings where others have weapons or are using alcohol or drugs) and to use strategies to defuse tense situations.

All victims of gang violence should be encouraged to talk to parents, teachers, and even their doctor about problems they are experiencing.

CONTRACEPTION AND ADOLESCENT PREGNANCY

Many adolescents engage in sexual activity but may not be fully informed about contraception, pregnancy, and sexually transmitted diseases, including HIV infection. Impulsivity, lack of planning, and concurrent drug and alcohol use decrease the likelihood that adolescents will use birth control and barrier protection.

Any of the adult contraceptive methods may be used by adolescents. The most common problem is adherence (eg, forgetting to take daily oral contraceptives or stopping them entirely—often without substituting another form of birth control). Although male condoms are the most frequently used form of contraception, there are still perceptions that may inhibit consistent use (eg, that condom use decreases pleasure and interferes with "romantic love"). Some female adolescents also are shy about asking male partners to use condoms during sex.

Pregnancy can be a source of significant emotional stress for adolescents. Pregnant adolescents and their partners tend to drop out of school or job training, thus worsening their economic status, lowering their self-esteem, and straining personal relationships. Adolescents (who account for 13% of all pregnancies in the US) are less likely than adults to get prenatal care, resulting in poorer pregnancy outcomes (eg, higher rates of prematurity). Adolescents, particularly the very young and those who are not receiving prenatal care, are more likely than women in their 20s to have medical problems during pregnancy, such as anemia and preeclampsia. Infants of young mothers (especially mothers < 15 yr) are more likely to be born prematurely and to have a low birth weight. However, with proper prenatal care, older adolescents have no higher risk of pregnancy problems than adults from similar backgrounds.

Having an abortion does not remove the psychologic problems of an unwanted pregnancy—either for the adolescent girl or her partner. Emotional crises may occur when pregnancy is diagnosed, when the decision to have an abortion is made, immediately after the abortion is done, when the infant would have been born, and when the anniversaries of that date occur. Family counseling and education about contraceptive methods, for both the girl and her partner, can be very helpful.

Parents may have different reactions when their daughter says she is pregnant or their son says he has impregnated someone. Emotions may range from apathy to disappointment and anger. It is important for parents to express their support and willingness to help the adolescent sort through his or her choices. Parents and adolescents need to communicate openly about abortion, adoption, and parenthood—all tough options for the adolescent to struggle with alone. However, before revealing a pregnancy to parents, practitioners should screen for domestic violence because revealing the pregnancy may put vulnerable adolescents at greater risk.

DRUG AND SUBSTANCE USE IN ADOLESCENTS

Substance use among adolescents ranges from sporadic use to severe substance use disorders. The consequences range from none to minor to life threatening, depending on the substance, the circumstances, and the frequency of use. However, even occasional use can put adolescents at increased risk of significant harm, including overdose, motor vehicle crashes, violent behaviors, and consequences of sexual contact (eg, pregnancy, sexually transmitted infection).

Adolescents use substances for a variety of reasons:

- To share a social experience or feel part of a social group
- To relieve stress
- To seek new experiences and take risks
- To relieve symptoms of mental health disorders (eg, depression, anxiety)

Additional risk factors include poor self-control, lack of parental monitoring, and various mental disorders (eg, ADHD and depression). Parental attitudes and the examples that parents set regarding their own use of alcohol, tobacco, prescription drugs, and other substances are a powerful influence.

According to national surveys, the proportion of high school seniors who report lifetime abstinence from all substances has been steadily increasing over the past 40 yr. However, at the same time, a broad range of more potent and dangerous products (eg, inhalable alcohol, pure tetrahydrocannabinol [THC], synthetic cannabinoids, prescription opioids) have become available. These products put adolescents who do initiate substance use at higher risk of developing both acute and long-term consequences.

Specific Substances

Alcohol: Alcohol use is common and is the substance most often used by adolescents. By 12th grade, > 70% of adolescents have tried alcohol, and nearly half are considered current drinkers (having consumed alcohol within the past month). Heavy alcohol use is also common, and adolescent drinkers may have significant alcohol toxicity. Nearly 90% of all alcohol consumed by adolescents occurs during a binge, putting them at risk of accidents, injuries, unwanted sexual activity and other bad outcomes.

Society and the media portray drinking as acceptable or even fashionable. Despite these influences, parents can make a difference by conveying clear expectations to their adolescent regarding drinking, setting limits consistently, and monitoring. On the other hand, adolescents whose family members drink excessively may think this behavior is acceptable. Some adolescents who try alcohol go on to develop an alcohol use disorder. Known risk factors for developing a disorder include starting drinking at a young age and genetics. Adolescents who have a family member with an alcohol use disorder should be made aware of their increased risk.

Tobacco: Rates of tobacco use among adolescents fell dramatically in the 1990s and 2000s but have now plateaued. The CDC reports that in 2015, about 11% of high school students reported current cigarette use (smoked in the previous 30 days), down from 27.5% in 1991; only about 2% report smoking every day. However, the majority of adults who smoke cigarettes begin smoking during adolescence. If adolescents do not try cigarettes before age 19, they are very unlikely to become smokers as adults. Children as young as age 10 may experiment with cigarettes. About 7 to 8% of 9th graders report smoking regularly.[1]

The strongest risk factors for adolescent smoking are having parents who smoke (the single most predictive factor) or having peers and role models (eg, celebrities) who smoke. Other risk factors include

- Poor school performance
- High-risk behavior (eg, excessive dieting, particularly among girls; physical fighting and drunk driving, particularly among boys; use of alcohol or other drugs)
- Poor problem-solving abilities
- Availability of cigarettes
- Poor self-esteem

Adolescents may also use tobacco in other forms. About 3.3% of people 18 and older and about 7.3% of high school students use smokeless tobacco; this rate has remained relatively constant since 1999. Smokeless tobacco can be chewed (chewing tobacco), placed between the lower lip and gum (dipping tobacco), or inhaled into the nose (snuff). Pipe smoking is relatively rare in the US, but use has increased among middle and high school students since 1999. The percentage of people > 12 yr who smoke cigars has declined.

Electronic cigarettes (e-cigarettes, e-cigs, vapes) have become increasingly popular among adolescents over the past several years, especially among adolescents of middle and upper socioeconomic status. Current e-cigarette use among middle and high school students has increased markedly from 4.5% in 2013 to 13.4% in 2014, and 24.1% in 2015 according to the CDC. About 45% of high school students have tried e-cigarettes. Electronic cigarettes do not contain tobacco but rather heat liquified nicotine into vapor that can be inhaled.

Because there are no combustion products of tobacco, these products do not cause most of the adverse health consequences of smoking. However, nicotine is highly addictive, and nicotine toxicity is possible. E-cigarettes are increasingly the initial form of exposure for adolescents to nicotine, but their effect on the rate of adult smoking is unclear. There are a number of other ingredients in e-cigarettes, some of which may be toxic. The long-term risks of e-cigarettes are unknown.[1]

Parents can help prevent their adolescent from smoking and using smokeless tobacco products by being positive role models (that is, by not smoking or chewing), openly discussing the hazards of tobacco, and encouraging adolescents who already smoke or chew to quit, including supporting them in seeking medical assistance if necessary (see p. 3264).

Other substances: Use of other substances among adolescents remains a serious problem. The Youth Risk Behavior Surveillance nationwide survey of high school students done annually by the CDC reported that in 2015 the prevalence of current marijuana use among high school students was 21.7% (which is below the peak rate of 25.3% in 1995) and about 39% reported having used marijuana one or more times in their life. In 2010, the rate of current marijuana use surpassed the rate of current tobacco use for the first time.

In the same survey, the following percentages of high school students reported using illicit substances one or more times in their life:

- Prescription drugs (without a prescription): 16.8%
- Inhalants (eg, glue, aerosols): 7.0%
- Hallucinogens (eg, LSD, PCP, mescaline, mushrooms): 6.4%
- Cocaine: 5.2%
- Anabolic steroids (oral or injectable): 3.5%
- Methamphetamines (nonprescription): 3.0%
- Heroin: 2.1%

Prescription drugs particularly abused include opioid analgesics (eg, oxycodone), stimulants (eg, ADHD drugs such as methylphenidate or dextroamphetamine), and sedatives (eg, benzodiazepines).

Nationwide, 1.8% of students had used a needle to inject any illegal drug into their body one or more times during their life.[1]

1. Kann L, McManus T, Harris WA, et al: Youth Risk Behavior Surveillance—United States, 2015. *MMWR Surveill Summ* 65(No. SS-6):1–174, 2016. doi: http://dx.doi.org/10.15585/mmwr.ss6506a. Clarification and additional information. *MMWR Morb Mortal Wkly Rep* 65:610, 2016. doi: http://dx.doi.org/10.15585/mmwr.mm6523a7.

Diagnosis

- Clinical evaluation, including routine screening

Behaviors that should prompt parental concern for possible substance abuse include

- Finding drugs or drug paraphernalia
- Erratic behavior
- Depression or mood swings
- A change in friends
- Declining school performance
- Loss of interest in hobbies

Screening adolescents for substance use: Clinicians should screen for use of tobacco, alcohol, and other drugs at every health maintenance visit and also should advise both adolescents and parents about safely using and monitoring OTC and prescription drugs.

There are a number of different screening tools. Some are brief and can be administered verbally; these may be helpful for identifying at-risk adolescents who might benefit from more detailed investigation. Other tools are more comprehensive paper or digital questionnaires that provide more information but require more time when administered by clinicians. Patient literacy may be an issue with a self-administered screening tool (eg, paper or digital questionnaire in office).

Alcohol screening: For **alcohol screening**, the National Institute on Alcohol Abuse and Alcoholism (NIAAA) has developed a guide that suggests beginning with two screening questions. The questions and interpretation of answers vary by age (see Table 331–1).

For moderate- and highest-risk patients, ask about

- Drinking patterns: Usual and maximal consumption
- Problems caused by or risks taken due to drinking: Missing school, fights, injuries, car crashes
- Use of other substances: Any other things taken to get high

The NIAA guide also provides useful strategies to address problems that are discovered.

The CRAFFT questionnaire is another validated screening tool that has been widely used. Adolescents with ≥ 2 positive answers require further evaluation. Clinicians ask adolescents whether they do or have done the following:

- C: Ride in a *C*ar driven by someone (including themselves) who is "high" or has been drinking alcohol or using drugs
- R: Drink alcohol or use drugs to *R*elax, feel better about themselves, or fit in
- A: Drink alcohol or use drugs while they are *A*lone
- F: *F*orget things they did while drinking or using drugs
- F: Are ever told by family members or *F*riends that they should drink less or use drugs less
- T: Get into *T*rouble while drinking or using drugs

General substance screening: Because the CRAFFT questionnaire does not screen for tobacco use, provide information on frequency of use, or discriminate between drug and alcohol use, other screening tools have been developed.

The Brief Screener for Tobacco, Alcohol, and other Drugs (BSTAD) and the Screening to Brief Intervention (S2BI) tools cover a broad range of substances and provide brief clinical guidance on how to respond to screening results. These tools will soon be available online.

Drug testing: Drug testing may be useful but has significant limitations. When parents demand a drug test, they may create an atmosphere of confrontation that makes it difficult to obtain an accurate substance use history and form a therapeutic alliance with the adolescent. Screening tests are typically rapid qualitative urine immunoassays that are associated with a number of false-positive and false-negative results. Furthermore, testing cannot determine frequency and intensity of substance use and thus cannot distinguish casual users from those with more serious problems. Clinicians must use other measures (eg, thorough history, questionnaires) to identify the degree to which substance use has affected each adolescent's life.

Given these concerns and limitations, it is often useful to consult with an expert in substance abuse to help determine whether drug testing is warranted in a given situation. However, the decision not to drug test should not prematurely terminate assessment for a possible substance use disorder or a mental health disorder. Adolescents with nonspecific signs of a substance use disorder or a mental health disorder should be referred to a specialist for a complete evaluation.

Table 331–1. NIAA ALCOHOL SCREENING QUESTIONS FOR CHILDREN AND ADOLESCENTS

AGE GROUP*	1ST QUESTION	2ND QUESTION	INTERPRETATION	RISK LEVELS BY AGE
Elementary school (typically 9–11 yr)	Do you have any friends who drank any drink containing alcohol in the past year?	In the past year, have you ever had more than a few sips of any drink containing alcohol?	Friends: Any drinking heightens concern Patient: Any drinking highest risk	≤ 11 yr: Any drinking highest risk
Middle school (typically 11–14 yr)	Do you have any friends who drank any drink containing alcohol in the past year?	In the past year, on how many days have you had more than a few sips of any drink containing alcohol?	Friends: Any drinking heightens concern Patient: Any drinking moderate to highest risk depending on age and number of days	≤ 11 yr: Any drinking highest risk 12–14 yr: Moderate risk 1–5 days; highest risk > 5 days
High school (typically 14–18 yr)	In the past year, on how many days have you had more than a few sips of any drink containing alcohol?	If your friends drink, how many drinks do they usually drink on an occasion?	Patient: Low, moderate or highest risk depending on age and number of days Friends: Binge drinking (3–5+ drinks) heightens concern	14–15 yr: Moderate risk 1–5 days; highest risk > 5 days 16 yr: Moderate risk 6–11 days; highest risk > 11 days 17 yr: Moderate risk 6–24 days; highest risk > 24 days 18 yr: Moderate risk 12–52 days; highest risk > 52 days

*School level is used because risk increases on transition to a higher level.
NIAA = National Institute on Alcohol Abuse and Alcoholism.

Treatment

- Behavioral therapy tailored for adolescents

Typically, adolescents with a moderate or severe substance use disorder are referred for further assessment and treatment. In general, the same behavioral therapies used for adults with substance use disorders can also be used for adolescents. However, these therapies should be adapted. Adolescents should not be treated in the same programs as adults; they should receive services from adolescent programs and therapists with expertise in treating adolescents with substance use disorders.

OBESITY IN ADOLESCENTS

Obesity is now twice as common among adolescents than it was 30 years ago and is one of the most common reasons for visits to adolescent clinics. Although fewer than one third of obese adults were obese as adolescents, most obese adolescents remain obese in adulthood.

Although most of the complications of obesity occur in adulthood, obese adolescents are more likely than their peers to have high blood pressure. Type 2 diabetes mellitus is occurring with increasing frequency in adolescents due to insulin resistance related to obesity. Because of society's stigma against obesity, many obese adolescents have a poor self-image and become increasingly sedentary and socially isolated.

Etiology

The factors that influence obesity among adolescents are the same as those among adults. Most cases are external (eg, consuming too many calories and/or a low-quality diet), often in conjunction with a sedentary lifestyle. Genetic influences are common, and responsible genes are now being identified (see p. 19).

Parents often are concerned that obesity is the result of some type of endocrine disease, such as hypothyroidism or hyperadrenocorticism, but such disorders are rarely the cause. Adolescents with weight gain caused by endocrine disorders are usually of small stature and have other signs of the underlying disorder.

Diagnosis

- Body mass index (BMI)

Determination of the BMI is an important aspect of physical assessment. Adolescents whose BMI is ≥ the 95th percentile for their age and sex are obese.

Primary endocrine (eg, hyperadrenocorticism, hypothyroidism) or metabolic causes are uncommon but should be ruled out if height growth slows significantly. If the child is short and has hypertension, Cushing syndrome should be considered.

Treatment

- Healthy eating and exercise habits

Despite many therapeutic approaches, obesity is one of the most difficult problems to treat, and long-term success rates remain low. Intervention for obese adolescents should be focused on developing healthy eating and exercise habits rather than on losing a specific amount of weight. Caloric intake is reduced by

- Establishing a well-balanced diet of ordinary foods
- Making permanent changes in eating habits

Calorie burning is increased by

- Increasing physical activity

Summer camps for obese adolescents may help them lose a significant amount of weight, but without continuing effort, the weight usually is regained. Counseling to help adolescents cope with their problems, including poor self-esteem, may be helpful.

Drugs that help reduce weight are generally not used during adolescence because of concerns about safety and possible abuse. One exception is for obese adolescents with a strong family history of type 2 diabetes. They are at high risk of developing diabetes. The drug metformin, which is used to treat diabetes, may help them lose weight and also lower their risk of becoming diabetic.

OVERVIEW OF PSYCHOSOCIAL PROBLEMS IN ADOLESCENTS

Clinicians must be aware of the high frequency of psychosocial disorders that occur during this stage of life. Screening for mental health disorders is considered a routine part of adolescent health care. Depression is common and should be screened for actively. Although suicide is a rare occurrence (5/100,000), suicidal ideation is common, with as many as 10% of adolescents reporting thoughts about suicide in their lifetime according to some studies. Anxiety often manifests during adolescence, as do mood disorders and disruptive behavioral disorders (eg, oppositional defiant disorder, conduct disorder). Individuals with thought disorders (psychosis) will often present with a "psychotic break" during adolescence. Eating disorders, especially in girls, are common. Some patients go to extraordinary lengths to hide symptoms of an eating disorder.

The clinician who has developed an open, trusting relationship with an adolescent often can identify these problems, develop a therapeutic relationship, offer practical advice and, when appropriate, encourage the adolescent to accept a referral to specialized care.

PHYSICAL PROBLEMS IN ADOLESCENTS

Although adolescents are susceptible to the same kinds of illness that afflict younger children, generally they are a healthy group. Adolescents should continue to receive vaccinations according to the recommended schedule (see Table 291–3 on p. 2467).

Acne is extremely common and needs to be addressed because of its impact on self-esteem.

Trauma is very common among adolescents, with sports and motor vehicle injuries most frequent. Motor vehicle crashes and other unintentional injuries, homicide, and suicide are the 4 leading causes of mortality in the adolescent age group.

Disorders that are common among all adolescents include

- Infectious mononucleosis
- Sexually transmitted diseases
- Endocrine disorders (particularly thyroid disorders)

Disorders that are common among adolescent girls include

- UTIs
- Menstrual abnormalities
- Iron deficiency

Pregnancy also is not a rare occurrence and must be kept in mind when treating adolescent girls.

Although not common, neoplastic diseases such as leukemia, lymphoma, bone cancers, and brain tumors also occur.

SCHOOL PROBLEMS IN ADOLESCENTS

School constitutes a large part of an adolescent's existence. Difficulties in almost any area of life often manifest as school problems.

Learning disorders may manifest for the first time as school becomes more demanding, particularly among bright children who previously had been able to accommodate for their areas of weakness.

Sometimes, mild intellectual disability that was not recognized earlier in life causes school problems. Behavior problems that developed earlier in childhood, such as attention-deficit/hyperactivity disorder, may continue to cause school problems for adolescents.

Particular school problems include

- Fear of going to school
- Absenteeism without permission (truancy)
- Dropping out
- Academic underachievement (particularly a change in grades or a drop in performance)

Between 1% and 5% of adolescents develop fear of going to school. This fear may be generalized or related to a particular person (a teacher or another student—see also Bullying on p. 2476) or event at school (such as physical education class). The adolescent may develop physical symptoms, such as abdominal pain, or may simply refuse to go to school. School personnel and family members should identify the reason, if any, for the fear and encourage the adolescent to attend school.

Adolescents who are repeatedly truant or drop out of school have made a conscious decision to miss school. These adolescents generally have poor academic achievement and have had little success with or felt little satisfaction resulting from participation in school-related activities. They often have engaged in high-risk behaviors, such as having unprotected sex, taking drugs, and engaging in violence. Adolescents at risk of dropping out should be made aware of other educational options, such as vocational training and alternative programs.

School problems during the adolescent years may be the result of

- Rebellion and a need for independence (most common)
- Mental health disorders, such as anxiety or depression
- Substance use
- Family conflict
- Learning disorders
- Behavior disorders

As adolescents begin to seek more freedom, their desire to do so may clash with their parents' desire to keep them safe. Adolescents rebel in various ways, such as refusing to attend school or drinking alcohol. Adolescents who are anxious or depressed may refuse therapy or stop taking their prescribed drugs. All of these challenging behaviors can cause problems within the family and at school.

Diagnosis

- Learning and mental health evaluations

In general, adolescents with significant school problems should undergo complete learning and mental health evaluations.

Treatment

- Treatment of cause

School problems, especially when related to learning or attention difficulties, should be addressed by clinicians, working together with school personnel and parents. If a learning disorder or intellectual disability is present, appropriate services should be provided through an individualized educational plan (IEP). Environmental changes and sometimes drug therapy can be of great help to struggling students.

332 Respiratory Disorders in Young Children

BACTERIAL TRACHEITIS

Bacterial tracheitis is bacterial infection of the trachea.

Bacterial tracheitis is uncommon and can affect children of any age. *Staphylococcus aureus* and group A β-hemolytic streptococci are involved most frequently.

Most children have symptoms of viral respiratory infection for 1 to 3 days before the onset of severe symptoms of stridor and dyspnea. In a few children, onset is acute and is characterized by respiratory stridor, high fever, and often copious purulent secretions. Rarely, bacterial tracheitis develops as a complication of viral croup or endotracheal intubation. As in patients with epiglottitis, the child may have marked toxicity and respiratory distress that may progress rapidly and may require intubation.

Complications of bacterial tracheitis include hypotension, cardiorespiratory arrest, bronchopneumonia, and sepsis. Subglottic stenosis secondary to prolonged intubation is uncommon. Most children treated appropriately recover without sequelae.

Diagnosis

- Clinical evaluation
- Direct laryngoscopy
- Characteristic x-ray findings

Diagnosis of bacterial tracheitis is suspected clinically and can be confirmed by direct laryngoscopy, which reveals purulent secretions and inflammation in the subglottic area with a shaggy, purulent membrane, or by lateral neck x-ray, which reveals subglottic narrowing that may be irregular as opposed to the symmetric tapering typical of croup. Direct laryngoscopy should be done in controlled circumstances where an artificial airway can be rapidly established if necessary.

Treatment

- Adequate airway ensured
- Antibiotics effective against *S. aureus* and streptococcal species

Treatment of bacterial tracheitis in severe cases is the same as that for epiglottitis; whenever possible, endotracheal intubation should be done in controlled circumstances by a clinician skilled in managing a pediatric airway.

Initial antibiotics should cover *S. aureus* and streptococcal species; cefuroxime or an equivalent IV preparation may be appropriate empirically unless methicillin-resistant staphylococcus is prevalent in the community, in which case vancomycin should be used. Therapy for critically ill children should be guided by a consultant knowledgeable in local susceptibility patterns. Once definitive microbial diagnosis is made, coverage is narrowed and continued for ≥ 10 days.

BRONCHIOLITIS

Bronchiolitis is an acute viral infection of the lower respiratory tract affecting infants < 24 mo and is characterized by respiratory distress, wheezing, and crackles. Diagnosis is suspected by history, including presentation during a known epidemic; the primary cause, respiratory syncytial virus, can be identified with a rapid assay. Treatment is supportive with oxygen and hydration. Prognosis is generally excellent, but some patients develop apnea or respiratory failure.

Bronchiolitis often occurs in epidemics and mostly in children < 24 mo, with a peak incidence between 2 mo and 6 mo of age. The annual incidence in the first year of life is about 11 cases/100 children. In the temperate northern hemisphere, most cases occur between November and April, with a peak incidence during January and February.

Etiology

Most cases of bronchiolitis are caused by

- Respiratory syncytial virus (RSV)
- Rhinovirus
- Parainfluenza virus type 3

Less frequent causes are influenza viruses A and B, parainfluenza viruses types 1 and 2, metapneumovirus, adenoviruses, and Mycoplasma pneumoniae.

Pathophysiology

The virus spreads from the upper respiratory tract to the medium and small bronchi and bronchioles, causing epithelial necrosis and initiating an inflammatory response. The developing edema and exudate result in partial obstruction, which is most pronounced on expiration and leads to alveolar air trapping. Complete obstruction and absorption of the trapped air may lead to multiple areas of atelectasis, which can be exacerbated by breathing high inspired oxygen concentrations.

Symptoms and Signs

Typically, an affected infant has URI symptoms with progressively increasing respiratory distress characterized by tachypnea, retractions, and a wheezy or hacking cough. Young infants (< 2 mo) and infants born prematurely may present with recurrent apneic spells followed by more typical symptoms and signs of bronchiolitis over 24 to 48 h. Signs of distress may include circumoral cyanosis, deepening retractions, and audible wheezing. Fever is usually but not always present. Infants initially appear nontoxic and in no distress, despite tachypnea and retractions, but may become increasingly lethargic as the infection progresses. Hypoxemia is the rule in more severely affected infants.

Dehydration may develop from vomiting and decreased oral intake. With fatigue, respirations may become more shallow and ineffective, leading to respiratory acidosis. Auscultation reveals wheezing, prolonged expiration, and, often, fine crackles. Many children have accompanying acute otitis media.

Diagnosis

- Clinical presentation
- Pulse oximetry
- Chest x-ray for more severe cases
- RSV antigen test on nasal washings or nasal aspirates for seriously ill children

Diagnosis of bronchiolitis is suspected by history, examination, and occurrence of the illness as part of an epidemic. Symptoms similar to bronchiolitis can result from an asthma exacerbation, which is often precipitated by a respiratory viral infection and is more likely in a child > 18 mo of age, especially if previous episodes of wheezing and a family history of asthma have been documented. Gastric reflux with aspiration of gastric contents also may cause the clinical picture of bronchiolitis; multiple episodes in an infant may be clues to this diagnosis. Foreign body aspiration occasionally causes wheezing and should be considered if the onset is sudden and not associated with manifestations of URI. Heart failure associated with a left-to-right shunt manifesting at age 2 to 3 mo also can be confused with bronchiolitis.

Patients suspected of having bronchiolitis should undergo pulse oximetry to evaluate oxygenation. No further testing is required for mild cases with normal oxygen levels, but in cases of hypoxemia and severe respiratory distress, a chest x-ray supports the diagnosis and typically shows hyperinflated lungs, depressed diaphragm, and prominent hilar markings. Infiltrates may be present resulting from atelectasis and/or RSV pneumonia; RSV pneumonia is relatively common among infants with RSV bronchiolitis.

RSV rapid antigen testing done on nasal washings or nasal aspirates is diagnostic but not generally necessary; it may be reserved for patients with illness severe enough to require hospitalization. Other laboratory testing is nonspecific and is not routinely indicated; about two thirds of the children have WBC counts of 10,000 to 15,000/μL. Most have 50 to 75% lymphocytes.

Prognosis

Prognosis is excellent. Most children recover in 3 to 5 days without sequelae, although wheezing and cough may continue for 2 to 4 wk. Mortality is < 0.1% when medical care is adequate. An increased incidence of asthma is suspected in children who have had bronchiolitis in early childhood, but the association is controversial and the incidence seems to decrease as children age.

Treatment

- Supportive therapy
- Oxygen supplementation as needed
- IV hydration as needed

Treatment of bronchiolitis is supportive, and most children can be managed at home with hydration and comfort measures.

Indications for hospitalization include accelerating respiratory distress, ill appearance (eg, cyanosis, lethargy, fatigue), apnea by history, hypoxemia, and inadequate oral intake. Children with underlying disorders such as cardiac disease, immunodeficiency, or bronchopulmonary dysplasia, which put them at high risk of severe or complicated disease, also should be considered candidates for hospitalization.

In hospitalized children, 30 to 40% oxygen delivered by nasal cannula, tent, or face mask is usually sufficient to maintain oxygen saturation > 90%. Endotracheal intubation is indicated for severe recurrent apnea, hypoxemia unresponsive to oxygen therapy, or CO_2 retention or if the child cannot clear bronchial secretions. High-flow nasal cannula therapy, continuous positive airway pressure (CPAP) therapy, or both are often used to avoid intubation in patients who are at risk of respiratory failure.

Hydration may be maintained with frequent small feedings of clear liquids. For sicker children, fluids should be given IV initially, and the level of hydration should be monitored by urine output and specific gravity and by serum electrolyte determinations.

There is some evidence that systemic corticosteroids are beneficial when given very early in the course of the illness in children with underlying corticosteroid-responsive conditions (eg, bronchopulmonary dysplasia, asthma), but there is no benefit in previously well infants.

Antibiotics should be withheld unless a secondary bacterial infection (a rare sequela) occurs.

Bronchodilators are not uniformly effective, but a substantial subset of children may respond with short-term improvement. This is particularly true of infants who have wheezed previously. Hospital stays probably are not shortened.

Ribavirin, an antiviral drug active in vitro against RSV, influenza, and measles, is probably not effective clinically and is no longer recommended except for immunosuppressed children with severe RSV infection; it also is potentially toxic to hospital staff. RSV immune globulin has been tried but is ineffective.

Prevention of RSV infection by passive immunoprophylaxis with monoclonal antibody to RSV (palivizumab) decreases the frequency of hospitalization but is costly and is indicated primarily in high-risk infants (see p. 2764 for indications and dosage).

KEY POINTS

- Bronchiolitis is an acute, viral, lower respiratory tract infection affecting infants < 24 mo and is typically caused by RSV or rhinovirus.
- Edema and exudate in medium and small bronchi and bronchioles cause partial obstruction and air trapping; atelectasis and/or pneumonia cause hypoxemia in more severe cases.
- Typical manifestations include fever, tachypnea, retractions, wheezing, and cough.
- Clinical evaluation is usually adequate for diagnosis, but more severely ill children should have pulse oximetry, chest x-ray, and rapid antigen testing for RSV.
- Indications for hospitalization include accelerating respiratory distress, ill appearance (eg, cyanosis, lethargy, fatigue), apnea by history, hypoxemia, and inadequate oral intake.
- Treatment is supportive; bronchodilators sometimes relieve symptoms but probably do not shorten hospitalization, and systemic corticosteroids are not indicated in previously well infants with bronchiolitis.
- There is no vaccine; monoclonal antibody to RSV (palivizumab) may be given to certain high-risk infants to decrease the frequency of hospitalization.

CROUP

(Laryngotracheobronchitis)

Croup is acute inflammation of the upper and lower respiratory tracts most commonly caused by parainfluenza virus type 1 infection. It is characterized by a brassy, barking cough and inspiratory stridor. Diagnosis is usually obvious clinically but can be made by anteroposterior neck x-ray. Treatment is antipyretics, hydration, nebulized racemic epinephrine, and corticosteroids. Prognosis is excellent.

Croup affects mainly children aged 6 mo to 3 yr.

Etiology

The **most common pathogens** are

- Parainfluenza viruses, especially type 1

Less common causes are respiratory syncytial virus (RSV) and adenovirus followed by influenza viruses A and B, enterovirus, rhinovirus, measles virus, and Mycoplasma pneumoniae. Croup caused by influenza may be particularly severe and may occur in a broader age range of children.

Seasonal outbreaks are common. Cases caused by parainfluenza viruses tend to occur in the fall; those caused by RSV and influenza viruses tend to occur in the winter and spring. Spread is usually through the air or by contact with infected secretions.

Pathophysiology

The infection causes inflammation of the larynx, trachea, bronchi, bronchioles, and lung parenchyma. Obstruction caused by swelling and inflammatory exudates develops and becomes pronounced in the subglottic region. Obstruction increases the work of breathing; rarely, tiring results in hypercapnia. Atelectasis may occur concurrently if the bronchioles become obstructed.

Symptoms and Signs

Croup is usually preceded by URI symptoms. A barking, often spasmodic, cough and hoarseness then occur, commonly at night; inspiratory stridor may be present as well. The child may awaken at night with respiratory distress, tachypnea, and retractions. In severe cases, cyanosis with increasingly shallow respirations may develop as the child tires.

The obvious respiratory distress and harsh inspiratory stridor are the most dramatic physical findings. Auscultation reveals prolonged inspiration and stridor. Crackles also may be present, indicating lower airway involvement. Breath sounds may be diminished with atelectasis. Fever is present in about half of children. The child's condition may seem to have improved in the morning but worsens again at night.

Recurrent episodes are often called spasmodic croup. Allergy or airway reactivity may play a role in spasmodic croup, but the clinical manifestations cannot be differentiated from those of viral croup. Also, spasmodic croup usually is initiated by a viral infection; however, fever is typically absent.

Diagnosis

- Clinical presentation (eg, barking cough, inspiratory stridor)
- Anteroposterior (AP) and lateral neck x-rays as needed

Diagnosis of croup is usually obvious by the barking nature of the cough. Similar inspiratory stridor can result from epiglottitis, bacterial tracheitis, airway foreign body, diphtheria, and retropharyngeal abscess. Epiglottitis, retropharyngeal abscess, and bacterial tracheitis have a more rapid onset and cause a more toxic appearance, odynophagia, and fewer upper respiratory tract symptoms. A foreign body may cause respiratory distress and a typical croupy cough, but fever and a preceding URI are absent. Diphtheria is excluded by a history of adequate immunization and is confirmed by identification of the organism in viral cultures of scrapings from a typical grayish diphtheritic membrane.

If the diagnosis is unclear, patients should have AP and lateral x-rays of the neck and chest; subepiglottic narrowing (steeple sign) seen on AP neck x-ray supports the diagnosis. Seriously ill patients, in whom epiglottitis is a concern, should be examined in the operating room by appropriate specialists able to establish an airway (see p. 841). Patients should have pulse oximetry, and those with respiratory distress should have ABG measurement.

PEARLS & PITFALLS

- Epiglottitis, retropharyngeal abscess, and bacterial tracheitis cause a more toxic appearance than croup and are not associated with a brassy, barking cough.

Treatment

- For outpatients, cool humidified air and possibly a single dose of corticosteroids
- For inpatients, humidified oxygen, racemic epinephrine, and corticosteroids

The illness usually lasts 3 to 4 days and resolves spontaneously. A mildly ill child may be cared for at home with hydration and antipyretics. Keeping the child comfortable is important because fatigue and crying can aggravate the condition. Humidification devices (eg, cold-steam vaporizers or humidifiers) may ameliorate upper airway drying and are frequently used at home by families but have not been shown to alter the course of the illness. The vast majority of children with croup recover completely.

Increasing or persistent respiratory distress, tachycardia, fatigue, cyanosis or hypoxemia, or dehydration indicates need for hospitalization. Pulse oximetry is helpful for assessing and monitoring severe cases. If oxygen saturation falls below 92%, humidified oxygen should be given and ABGs should be measured to assess CO_2 retention. A 30 to 40% inspired oxygen concentration is usually adequate. CO_2 retention ($PaCO_2$ > 45 mm Hg) generally indicates fatigue and the need for endotracheal intubation, as does inability to maintain oxygenation.

Nebulized racemic epinephrine 5 to 10 mg in 3 mL of saline q 2 h offers symptomatic relief and relieves fatigue. However, the effects are transient; the course of the illness, the underlying viral infection, and the Pao_2 are not altered by its use. Tachycardia and other adverse effects may occur. This drug is recommended mainly for patients with moderate to severe croup.

High-dose dexamethasone 0.6 mg/kg IM or po once (maximum dose 10 mg) may benefit children early in the first 24 h of the disease. It can help prevent hospitalization or help the child who is hospitalized with moderate to severe croup; hospitalized children who do not respond quickly may require several doses. The viruses that most commonly cause croup do not usually predispose to secondary bacterial infection, and antibiotics are rarely indicated.

KEY POINTS

- Croup is an acute, viral, respiratory tract infection affecting infants age 6 to 36 mo and is typically caused by parainfluenza viruses (mainly type 1).
- A barking, often spasmodic cough and sometimes inspiratory stridor (caused by subglottic edema) are the most prominent symptoms; symptoms are often worse at night.
- Diagnosis is usually clinical, but an anteroposterior x-ray of the neck and chest showing classic subepiglottic narrowing (steeple sign) supports the diagnosis.
- Give cool, humidified air or oxygen, and sometimes corticosteroids and nebulized racemic epinephrine.

WHEEZING AND ASTHMA IN INFANTS AND YOUNG CHILDREN

Wheezing is a relatively high-pitched whistling noise produced by movement of air through narrowed or

compressed small airways. It is common in the first few years of life and is typically caused by viral respiratory tract infection or asthma, but other possible causes include inhaled irritants or allergens, esophageal reflux, and heart failure.

Recurrent episodes of wheezing are common in the first few years of life; 1 in 3 children have at least one acute wheezing episode before 3 yr of age.[1] Because such wheezing typically responds to bronchodilators, this problem has historically been considered asthma. However, recent evidence that many children who have had recurrent wheezing in early childhood do not have asthma later in childhood or adolescence suggests that alternative diagnoses should be considered in young children with recurrent wheezing.

PEARLS & PITFALLS

- Not all wheezing in infants and young children is asthma.

1. Taussig LM, Wright AL, Holberg CJ, et al: Tucson Children's Respiratory Study: 1980 to present. *J Allergy Clin Immunol* 111:661–675, 2003.

Etiology

In some young children, recurrent wheezing episodes are the initial manifestations of asthma, and these children will continue to wheeze later in childhood or adolescence. In other children, wheezing episodes stop by age 6 to 10 yr and are not thought to represent asthma. In infants and young children, wheezing with viral illnesses, particularly those caused by respiratory syncytial virus and human rhinovirus, is associated with an increased risk of developing childhood asthma.[1] An eventual diagnosis of asthma is more likely in children who have atopic symptoms, more severe wheezing episodes, and/or a family history of atopy or asthma.

Wheezing usually results from bronchospasm that may be worsened by inflammation of the small and medium airways that causes edema and further airway narrowing. An acute wheezing episode in infants and young children is usually caused by respiratory viral infections, but airway inflammation may also be caused (or worsened) by allergies or inhaled irritants (eg, tobacco smoke). Recurrent wheezing may be caused by frequent viral respiratory infections, allergies, or asthma. Less common causes of recurrent wheezing include chronic dysphagia that causes recurrent aspiration, gastroesophageal reflux, airway malacia, a retained aspirated foreign body, or heart failure. Often, the cause of recurrent wheezing is unclear.

1. Sigurs N, Bjarnason R, Sigurbergsson F, et al: Respiratory syncytial virus bronchiolitis in infancy is an important risk factor for asthma and allergy at age 7. *Am J Respir Crit Care Med* 161:1501–1507, 2000. doi: 10.1164/ajrccm.161.5.9906076.

Symptoms and Signs

Wheezing is often accompanied by recurrent dry or productive cough. Other symptoms depend on the etiology and may include fever, runny nose (viral infection), and feeding difficulties (eg, due to heart failure or dysphagia).

On examination, wheezing manifests mainly on expiration, unless airway narrowing is severe, in which case wheezing can be heard on inspiration. Other findings present with more severe illness may include tachypnea, nasal flaring, intercostal and/or subxiphoid retractions, and cyanosis. Children with respiratory infection may have fever.

Diagnosis

- Chest x-ray for severe initial episode and sometimes for atypical or recurrent episodes

For a first episode of severe wheezing, most clinicians do a chest x-ray to detect signs of an aspirated foreign body, pneumonia, or heart failure and pulse oximetry to assess the need for oxygen therapy. The presence of generalized hyperinflation on plain x-rays suggests diffuse air trapping as seen in asthma, whereas localized findings suggest structural abnormalities or foreign body aspiration. Chest x-ray may also indicate the presence of a vascular ring as the cause of wheezing (eg, right aortic arch).

For children with recurrent episodes, exacerbations typically do not require testing unless there are signs of respiratory distress. Tests such as swallowing studies, contrast esophagram, CT, or bronchoscopy may be helpful for the few children with frequent or severe exacerbations or symptoms who do not respond to bronchodilators or other asthma drugs.

Prognosis

Many children with recurrent wheezing in early childhood will not have clinically important wheezing later in life. However, many older children and adults with difficult chronic asthma first developed symptoms in early childhood.

Treatment

- For acute wheezing episodes, inhaled bronchodilators and, if warranted, systemic corticosteroids
- For children with frequent severe wheezing episodes, a trial of maintenance therapy (eg, inhaled corticosteroids) as used for asthma

Infants and young children with acute wheezing are given inhaled bronchodilators and, if the wheezing is severe, systemic corticosteroids (see Treatment of acute exacerbation on p. 405).

Children who are unlikely to develop persistent asthma, such as children who do not have atopy or a family history of atopy or asthma, and whose wheezing episodes are relatively mild and infrequent can usually be managed with only intermittent inhaled bronchodilators used as needed. Most young children with more frequent and/or severe wheezing episodes benefit from maintenance therapy with bronchodilators and anti-inflammatory drugs (eg, inhaled corticosteroids) as used for asthma (see p. 404). However, although chronic use of a leukotriene modifier or low-dose inhaled corticosteroid decreases the severity and frequency of wheezing episodes, it does not alter the natural history of the disorder.

Geriatrics

333 Approach to the Geriatric Patient

Geriatrics refers to medical care for the elderly, an age group that is not easy to define precisely. "Older people" is sometimes preferred but is equally imprecise; > 65 is the age often used, but most people do not need geriatrics expertise in their care until age 70 or 75. Gerontology is the study of aging, including biologic, sociologic, and psychologic changes.

Around the year 1900 in the US, people > 65 accounted for 4% of the population; now they account for > 14% (nearly 50 million with a net gain of 10,000/day). In 2026, when post–World War II baby boomers begin to reach age 80, estimates suggest that > 20% (almost 80 million) will be > 65. Mean age of those > 65 is now a little more than 75, and the proportion of those > 85 is predicted to increase most rapidly.

Life expectancy is an additional 17 yr at age 65 and 10 yr at age 75 for men and an additional 20 yr at age 65 and 13 yr at age 75 for women. Overall, women live about 5 yr longer than men, probably because of genetic, biologic, and environmental factors. These differences in survival have changed little despite changes in women's lifestyle (eg, increased smoking, increased stress) over the late 20th century.

Aging

Aging (ie, pure aging) refers to the inevitable, irreversible decline in organ function that occurs over time even in the absence of injury, illness, environmental risks, or poor lifestyle choices (eg, unhealthy diet, lack of exercise, substance abuse). Initially, the changes in organ function (see Table 333–1) do not affect baseline function; the first manifestations are a reduced capacity of each organ to maintain homeostasis under stress (eg, illness, injury). The cardiovascular, renal, and central nervous systems are usually the most vulnerable (the weakest links).

Diseases interact with pure aging effects to cause geriatric-specific complications (now referred to as geriatric syndromes), particularly in the weak-link systems—even when those organs are not the primary ones affected by a disease. Typical examples are delirium complicating pneumonia or UTIs and the falls, dizziness, syncope, urinary incontinence, and weight loss that often accompany many minor illnesses in the elderly. Aging organs are also more susceptible to injury; eg, intracranial hemorrhage is more common and is triggered by less clinically important injury in the elderly.

The effects of aging must be taken into account during diagnosis and treatment of the elderly. Clinicians should not

- Mistake pure aging for disease (eg, slow information retrieval is not dementia)
- Mistake disease for pure aging (eg, ascribe debilitating arthritis, tremor, or dementia to old age)
- Ignore the increased risk of adverse drug effects on weak-link systems stressed by illness
- Forget that the elderly often have multiple underlying disorders (eg, hypertension, diabetes, atherosclerosis) that accelerate the potential for harm

In addition, clinicians should be alert for diseases and problems that are much more common among the elderly (eg, diastolic heart failure, Alzheimer disease, incontinence, atrial fibrillation). This approach enables clinicians to better understand and manage the complexity of the diseases that often coexist in older patients.

PHYSICAL CHANGES WITH AGING

Most age-related biologic functions peak before age 30 and gradually decline linearly thereafter (see Table 333–1);

Table 333–1. SELECTED PHYSIOLOGIC AGE-RELATED CHANGES

AFFECTED ORGAN OR SYSTEM	PHYSIOLOGIC CHANGE	CLINICAL MANIFESTATIONS
Body composition	↓ Lean body mass ↓ Muscle mass ↓ Creatinine production ↓ Skeletal mass ↓ Total body water ↑ Percentage adipose tissue (until age 60, then ↓ until death)	Changes in drug levels (usually ↑) ↓ Strength Tendency toward dehydration
Cells	↑ DNA damage and ↓ DNA repair capacity ↓ Oxidative capacity Accelerated cell senescence ↑ Fibrosis Lipofuscin accumulation	↑ Cancer risk
CNS	↓ Number of dopamine receptors ↑ Alpha-adrenergic responses ↑ Muscarinic parasympathetic responses	Tendency toward parkinsonian symptoms (eg, ↑ muscle tone, ↓ arm swing)
Ears	Loss of high-frequency hearing	↓ Ability to recognize speech
Endocrine system	↑ Insulin resistance and glucose intolerance	↑ Incidence of diabetes
	Menopause, ↓ estrogen and progesterone secretion ↓ Testosterone secretion ↓ Growth hormone secretion ↓ Vitamin D absorption and activation ↑ Incidence of thyroid abnormalities ↑ Bone mineral loss ↑ Secretion of ADH in response to osmolar stimuli	Vaginal dryness, dyspareunia ↓ Muscle mass ↓ Bone mass ↑ Fracture risk Changes in skin Tendency toward water intoxication
Eyes	↓ Lens flexibility ↑ Time for pupillary reflexes (constriction, dilation) ↑ Incidence of cataracts	Presbyopia ↑ Glare and difficulty adjusting to changes in lighting ↓ Visual acuity
GI tract	↓ Splanchnic blood flow ↑ Transit time	Tendency toward constipation and diarrhea
Heart	↓ Intrinsic heart rate and maximal heart rate Blunted baroreflex (less increase in heart rate in response to decrease in BP) ↓ Diastolic relaxation ↑ Atrioventricular conduction time ↑ Atrial and ventricular ectopy	Tendency toward syncope ↓ Ejection fraction ↑ Rates of atrial fibrillation ↑ Rates of diastolic dysfunction and diastolic heart failure
Immune system	↓ T-cell function ↓ B-cell function	↑ Susceptibility to infections and possibly cancer ↓ Antibody response to immunization or infection but ↑ autoantibodies
Joints	Degeneration of cartilaginous tissues Fibrosis ↑ Glycosylation and cross-linking of collagen Loss of tissue elasticity	Tightening of joints Tendency toward osteoarthritis
Kidneys	↓ Renal blood flow ↓ Renal mass ↓ Glomerular filtration ↓ Renal tubular secretion and reabsorption ↓ Ability to excrete a free-water load	Changes in drug levels with ↑ risk of adverse drug effects Tendency toward dehydration
Liver	↓ Hepatic mass ↓ Hepatic blood flow ↓ Activity of CYP 450 enzyme system	Changes in drug levels
Nose	↓ Smell	↓ Taste and consequent ↓ appetite ↑ Likelihood (slightly) of nosebleeds

Table continues on the following page.

Table 333–1. SELECTED PHYSIOLOGIC AGE-RELATED CHANGES (*Continued*)

AFFECTED ORGAN OR SYSTEM	PHYSIOLOGIC CHANGE	CLINICAL MANIFESTATIONS
Peripheral nervous system	↓ Baroreflex responses ↓ Beta-adrenergic responsiveness and number of receptors ↓ Signal transduction ↓ Muscarinic parasympathetic responses Preserved alpha-adrenergic responses	Tendency toward syncope ↓ Response to beta-blockers Exaggerated response to anticholinergic drugs
Pulmonary system	↓ Vital capacity ↓ Lung elasticity (compliance) ↑ Residual volume ↓ FEV_1 ↑ V/Q mismatch	↑ Likelihood of shortness of breath during vigorous exercise if people are normally sedentary or if exercise is done at high altitudes ↑ Risk of death due to pneumonia ↑ Risk of serious complications (eg, respiratory failure) for patients with a pulmonary disorder
Vasculature	↓ Endothelin-dependent vasodilation ↑ Peripheral resistance	Tendency toward hypertension

↓ = decreased; ↑ = increased; FEV_1 = forced expiratory volume in 1 sec; V/Q = ventilation/perfusion.
Adapted from the Institute of Medicine: *Pharmacokinetics and Drug Interactions in the Elderly Workshop*. Washington DC, National Academy Press, 1997, pp. 8–9.

the decline may be critical during stress, but it usually has little or no effect on daily activities. Therefore, disorders, rather than normal aging, are the primary cause of functional loss during old age.

In many cases, the declines that occur with aging may be due at least partly to lifestyle, behavior, diet, and environment and thus can be modified. For example, aerobic exercise can prevent or partially reverse a decline in maximal exercise capacity (O_2 consumption per unit time, or Vo_2 max), muscle strength, and glucose tolerance in healthy but sedentary older people (see Sidebar 333–1).

Only about 10% of the elderly participate in regular physical activity for > 30 min 5 times/wk (a common recommendation). About 35 to 45% participate in minimal activity. The elderly tend to be less active than other age groups for many reasons, most commonly because disorders limit their physical activity.

The benefits of physical activity for the elderly are many and far exceed its risks (eg, falls, torn ligaments, pulled muscles). Benefits include

- Reduced mortality rates, even for smokers and the obese
- Preservation of skeletal muscle strength, aerobic capacity, and bone density, contributing to greater mobility and independence
- Reduced risk of obesity
- Prevention and treatment of cardiovascular disorders (including rehabilitation after MI), diabetes, osteoporosis, colon cancer, and psychiatric disorders (especially mood disorders)
- Prevention of falls and fall-related injuries by improving muscle strength, balance, coordination, joint function, and endurance
- Improved functional ability
- Opportunities for social interaction
- Enhanced sense of well-being
- Possibly improved sleep quality

Physical activity is one of the few interventions that can restore physiologic capacity after it has been lost.

The unmodifiable effects of aging may be less dramatic than thought, and healthier, more vigorous aging may be possible for many people. Today, people > 65 are in better health than their ancestors and remain healthier longer.

EVALUATION OF THE ELDERLY PATIENT

Evaluation of the elderly usually differs from a standard medical evaluation. For elderly patients, especially those who are very old or frail, history-taking and physical examination may have to be done at different times, and physical examination may require 2 sessions because patients become fatigued.

The elderly also have different, often more complicated health care problems, such as multiple disorders, which may require use of many drugs (sometimes called polypharmacy) and thus greater likelihood of a high-risk drug being prescribed (see Table 335–5 on p. 2842). Diagnosis may be complicated, resulting in delayed, missed, or erroneous diagnoses leading to inappropriate use of drugs.

Early detection of problems results in early intervention, which can prevent deterioration and improve quality of life, often through relatively minor, inexpensive interventions (eg, lifestyle changes). Thus, some elderly patients, particularly the frail or chronically ill, are best evaluated using a comprehensive geriatric assessment, which includes evaluation of function and quality of life, best administered by an interdisciplinary team.

Multiple disorders: On average, elderly patients have 6 diagnosable disorders, and the primary care physician is often unaware of some of them. A disorder in one organ system can weaken another system, exacerbating the deterioration of both and leading to disability, dependence, and, without intervention, death. Multiple disorders complicate diagnosis and treatment, and effects of the disorders are magnified by social disadvantage (eg, isolation) and poverty (as patients outlive their resources and supportive peers) and by functional and financial problems.

Clinicians should also pay particular attention to certain common geriatric symptoms (eg, delirium, dizziness, syncope, falling, mobility problems, weight or appetite loss, urinary incontinence) because they may result from disorders of multiple organ systems.

If patients have multiple disorders, treatments (eg, bed rest, surgery, drugs) must be well-integrated; treating one disorder without treating associated disorders may accelerate decline. Also, careful monitoring is needed to avoid iatrogenic consequences. For example, with complete bed rest, elderly patients can lose 1 to 3% of muscle mass and strength each day (causing sarcopenia), and effects of bed rest alone can ultimately result in death.

Sidebar 333–1. Exercise

Exercise is usually used to mean movement that generates aerobic debt and increased heart rate and for many people is an important behavior with many positive outcomes. However, simple physical activity (eg, walking, gardening) has many of the same benefits for older people, especially those > 70; thus, physical activity, without aerobic debt or cardioacceleration, is recommended, even for those with mobility limitations.

All elderly patients starting an exercise program should be screened (by interview or questionnaire) to identify those with chronic disorders and to determine appropriate activities; however, virtually anyone can begin brief periods of walking, increased to 30 min 5 times/wk. Physical activity is inappropriate for only a few elderly people (eg, those with unstable medical conditions). Whether those with chronic disorders need a complete medical examination before starting an activity depends on the results of tests that have already been done and on clinical judgment. Some experts recommend such an examination, possibly with an exercise stress test, for patients who have ≥ 2 cardiac risk factors (eg, hypertension, obesity) and who plan on starting an activity more strenuous than walking.

Exercise programs that are more strenuous than walking may include any combination of 4 types of exercise: endurance, muscle strengthening, balance training (eg, tai chi), and flexibility. The combination of exercises recommended depends on the patient's medical condition and fitness level. For example, a seated exercise program that uses cuff weights for strength training and repeated movements for endurance training may be useful for patients who have difficulty standing and walking. An aquatics exercise program may be suggested for patients with arthritis. Patients should be able to select activities they enjoy but should be encouraged to include all 4 types of exercise. Of all types of exercise, endurance exercises (eg, walking, cycling, dancing, swimming, low-impact aerobics) have the most well-documented health benefits for the elderly.

Some patients, particularly those with a heart disorder (eg, angina, ≥ 2 MIs), require medical supervision during exercise.

High-intensity muscle-strengthening programs are particularly appropriate for frail elderly patients with sarcopenia. For these patients, machines that use air pressure rather than weights are useful because the resistance can be set lower and changed in smaller increments. High-intensity programs are safe even for nursing home residents > 80 in whom strength and mobility can be substantially improved. However, these programs are time-consuming because participants usually require close supervision.

Drugs and exercise: Doses of insulin and oral hypoglycemics in diabetics may need to be adjusted according to the amount of anticipated exercise to prevent hypoglycemia during exercise.

Doses of drugs that can cause orthostatic hypotension (eg, antidepressants, antihypertensives, hypnotics, anxiolytics, diuretics) may need to be lowered to avoid exacerbation of orthostasis by fluid loss during exercise. For patients taking such drugs, adequate fluid intake is essential during exercise.

Some sedative-hypnotics may reduce physical performance by reducing activity levels or by inhibiting muscles and nerves. These and other psychoactive drugs increase the risk of falls. Stopping such drugs or reducing their dose may be necessary to make exercise safe and to help patients adhere to their exercise regimen.

Missed or delayed diagnosis: Disorders that are common among the elderly are frequently missed, or the diagnosis is delayed. Clinicians should use the history, physical examination, and simple laboratory tests to actively screen elderly patients for disorders that occur only or commonly in the elderly (see Table 333–2); when diagnosed early, these disorders can often be more easily treated. Early diagnosis frequently depends on the clinician's familiarity with the patient's behavior and history, including mental status. Commonly, the first signs of a physical disorder are behavioral, mental, or emotional. If clinicians are unaware of this possibility and attribute these signs to dementia, diagnosis and treatment can be delayed.

Polypharmacy: Prescription and OTC drug use should be reviewed frequently, particularly for drug interactions and use of drugs considered inappropriate for the elderly (see p. 2856). When multiple drugs are used, electronic health record–based management is more efficient.

Caregiver problems: Occasionally, problems of elderly patients are related to neglect or abuse by their caregiver (see p. 2858). Clinicians should consider the possibility of patient abuse and drug abuse by the caregiver if circumstances and findings suggest it. Certain injury patterns or patient behaviors are particularly suggestive, including

- Frequent bruising, especially in difficult-to-reach areas (eg, middle of the back)
- Grip bruises of the upper arms
- Bruises of the genitals
- Peculiar burns
- Unexplained fearfulness of a caregiver in the patient

History

Often, more time is needed to interview and evaluate elderly patients, partly because they may have characteristics that interfere with the evaluation. The following should be considered:

- **Sensory deficits:** Dentures, eyeglasses, or hearing aids, if normally worn, should be worn to facilitate communication during the interview. Adequate lighting and elimination of visual or auditory distraction also help.
- **Underreporting of symptoms:** Elderly patients may not report symptoms that they consider part of normal aging (eg, dyspnea, hearing or vision deficits, memory problems, incontinence, gait disturbance, constipation, dizziness, falls). However, no symptom should be attributed to normal aging unless a thorough evaluation is done and other possible causes have been eliminated.
- **Unusual manifestations of a disorder:** In the elderly, typical manifestations of a disorder may be absent (see p. 2844). Instead, the elderly may present with nonspecific symptoms (eg, fatigue, confusion, weight loss).
- **Functional decline as the only manifestation:** Disorders may manifest solely as functional decline. In such cases, standard questions may not apply. For example, when asked about joint symptoms, patients with severe arthritis may not report pain, swelling, or stiffness, but if asked about changes in activities, they may, for example, report that they no longer take walks or volunteer at the hospital. Questions about duration of functional decline (eg, "How long have you been unable to do your own shopping?") can elicit useful information. Identifying people when they have just started to have difficulty doing basic activities of daily living (BADLs) or

Table 333–2. DISORDERS COMMON AMONG THE ELDERLY

FREQUENCY	DISORDERS
Almost exclusive in the elderly	Accidental hypothermia
	Normal-pressure hydrocephalus
	Urinary incontinence
	Diastolic heart failure
	Alzheimer disease
More common among the elderly than among other age groups	Atrial fibrillation
	Basal cell carcinoma
	Chronic lymphocytic leukemia
	Degenerative osteoarthritis
	Dementia
	Diabetic hyperosmolar nonketotic coma
	Falls
	Herpes zoster
	Hip fracture
	Monoclonal gammopathies
	Osteoporosis
	Parkinsonism
	Polymyalgia rheumatica
	Pressure ulcers
	Prostate cancer
	Stroke
	Temporal arteritis (giant cell arteritis)
Common among the elderly and treatable	Depression
	Diabetes mellitus
	Foot disorders interfering with mobility
	GI bleeding
	Hearing and vision abnormalities
	Heart failure
	Hypothyroidism
	Iron deficiency anemia
	Oral disorders interfering with eating
	Vitamin B_{12} deficiency

instrumental activities of daily living (IADLs) may provide more opportunities for interventions to restore function or to prevent further decline and thus maintain independence.

- **Difficulty recalling:** Patients may not accurately remember past illnesses, hospitalizations, operations, and drug use; clinicians may have to obtain these data elsewhere (eg, from family members, a home health aide, or medical records).
- **Fear:** The elderly may be reluctant to report symptoms because they fear hospitalization, which they may associate with dying.
- **Age-related disorders and problems:** Depression (common among elderly who are vulnerable and sick), the cumulative losses of old age, and discomfort due to a disorder may make the elderly less apt to provide health-related information to clinicians. Patients with impaired cognition may have difficulty describing problems, impeding the physician's evaluation.

Interview: A clinician's knowledge of an elderly patient's everyday concerns, social circumstances, mental function, emotional state, and sense of well-being helps orient and guide the interview. Asking patients to describe a typical day elicits information about their quality of life and mental and physical function. This approach is especially useful during the first meeting. Patients should be given time to speak about things of personal importance. Clinicians should also ask whether patients have specific concerns, such as fear of falling. The resulting rapport can help the clinician communicate better with patients and their family members.

A mental status examination may be necessary early in the interview to determine the patient's reliability; this examination should be conducted tactfully so that the patient does not become embarrassed, offended, or defensive. Routine screening for physical and psychologic disorders (see Table 341–1 on p. 2883) should be done annually, beginning at age 70.

Often, verbal and nonverbal clues (eg, the way the story is told, tempo of speech, tone of voice, eye contact) can provide information, as for the following:

- **Depression:** Elderly patients may omit or deny symptoms of anxiety or depression but betray them by a lowered voice, subdued enthusiasm, or even tears.
- **Physical and mental health:** What patients say about sleep and appetite may be revealing.
- **Weight gain or loss:** Clinicians should note any change in the fit of clothing or dentures.

Unless mental status is impaired, a patient should be interviewed alone to encourage the discussion of personal matters. Clinicians may also need to speak with a relative or caregiver, who often gives a different perspective on function, mental status, and emotional state. These interviews may be done with the patient absent or present.

The clinician should ask the patient's permission before inviting a relative or caregiver to be present and should explain that such interviews are routine. If the caregiver is interviewed alone, the patient should be kept usefully occupied (eg, filling out a standardized assessment questionnaire, being interviewed by another member of the interdisciplinary team).

If indicated, clinicians should consider the possibility of drug abuse by the patient and patient abuse by the caregiver.

Medical history: When asking patients about their past medical history, a clinician should ask about disorders that used to be more common (eg, rheumatic fever, poliomyelitis) and about outdated treatments (eg, pneumothorax therapy for TB, mercury for syphilis). A history of immunizations (eg, tetanus, influenza, pneumococcus), adverse reactions to immunizations, and skin test results for TB is needed. If patients recall having surgery but do not remember the procedure or its purpose, surgical records should be obtained if possible.

Clinicians should ask questions designed to systematically review each body area or system (review of systems) to check for other disorders and common problems that patients may have forgotten to mention (see Table 333–3).

Drug history: The drug history should be recorded, and a copy should be given to patients or their caregiver. It should contain

- Drugs used
- Dose
- Dosing schedule
- Prescriber
- Reason for prescribing the drugs
- Precise nature of any drug allergies

All drugs used should be recorded, including

- Topical drugs (which may be absorbed systemically)
- OTC drugs (which can have serious consequences if overused and may interact with prescription drugs)
- Dietary supplements
- Medicinal herb preparations (because many can interact adversely with prescription and OTC drugs)

Table 333–3. CLUES TO DISORDERS IN ELDERLY PATIENTS

REGION OR SYSTEM	SYMPTOM	POSSIBLE CAUSES
Skin	Itching	Allergic reaction, cancer, dry skin, hyperthyroidism, jaundice, lice, scabies, uremia
Head	Headaches	Anxiety, cervical osteoarthritis, depression, giant cell arteritis, subdural hematoma, tumors
Eyes	Glare from lights at night	Cataracts, glaucoma
	Loss of central vision	Macular degeneration
	Loss of near vision (presbyopia)	Decreased accommodation of the lens
	Loss of peripheral vision	Glaucoma, retinal detachment, stroke
	Pain	Giant cell arteritis, glaucoma
Ears	Hearing loss	Acoustic neuroma, cerumen, foreign body in the external canal, ototoxicity due to use of drugs (eg, aminoglycosides, aspirin, furosemide), Paget disease, presbycusis, trauma due to noise, tumor of the cerebellopontine angle, viral infection
	Loss of high-frequency range	Presbycusis (usually caused by age-related changes in the cochlea)
Mouth	Burning mouth	Pernicious anemia, stomatitis
	Denture pain	Dentures that fit poorly, oral cancer
	Dry mouth (xerostomia)	Autoimmune disorders (eg, RA, Sjögren syndrome, SLE), dehydration, drugs (eg, antidepressants including tricyclic antidepressants, antihistamines, antihypertensives, diuretics, psychoactive drugs), salivary gland damage due to infection or to radiation therapy for head and neck tumors
	Limited tongue motion	Oral cancer, stroke
	Loss of taste	Adrenal insufficiency, drugs (eg, antihistamines, antidepressants), infection of the mouth or nose, nasopharyngeal tumor, radiation therapy, smoking, xerostomia
Throat	Dysphagia	Anxiety, cancer, esophageal stricture, foreign body, Schatzki ring, stroke, Zenker diverticulum
	Voice changes	Hypothyroidism, recurrent laryngeal nerve dysfunction, vocal cord tumor
Neck	Pain	Cervical arthritis, carotid or vertebral artery dissection, polymyalgia rheumatica
Chest	Dyspnea during exertion	Cancer, COPD, functional decline, heart failure, infection
	Paroxysmal nocturnal dyspnea	Gastroesophageal reflux, heart failure
	Pain	Angina pectoris, anxiety, aortic dissection, costochondritis, esophageal motility disorders, gastroesophageal reflux, herpes zoster, MI, myocarditis, pericarditis, pleural effusion, pleuritis, pneumonia, pneumothorax
GI	Constipation with no other symptoms	Colorectal cancer, dehydration, drugs (eg, aluminum-containing antacids, anticholinergic drugs, iron supplements, opioids, tricyclic antidepressants), hypercalcemia (eg, due to hyperparathyroidism), hypokalemia, hypothyroidism, inadequate exercise, laxative abuse, low-fiber diet
	Constipation with pain, vomiting, and intermittent diarrhea	Fecal impaction, bowel obstruction
	Fecal incontinence	Cerebral dysfunction, fecal impaction, rectal cancer, spinal cord lesions
	Lower abdominal pain (crampy, sudden onset)	Diverticulitis, gastroenteritis, ischemic colitis, obstruction
	Postprandial abdominal pain (2–3 h after eating, lasting 1–3 h)	Chronic intestinal ischemia
	Rectal bleeding	Colon angiodysplasia, colon cancer, diverticulosis, hemorrhoids, ischemic colitis

Table continues on the following page.

Table 333–3. CLUES TO DISORDERS IN ELDERLY PATIENTS (*Continued*)

REGION OR SYSTEM	SYMPTOM	POSSIBLE CAUSES
GU	Frequency, dribbling, hesitancy, weak stream	Benign prostatic hyperplasia, constipation, drugs (eg, antihistamines, opioids), prostate cancer, urinary retention, UTI
	Dysuria with or without fever	Prostatitis, UTI
	Polyuria	Diabetes insipidus (decrease in ADH action), diabetes mellitus, diuretics
	Incontinence	Cystitis, functional decline, normal-pressure hydrocephalus, spinal cord dysfunction, stroke, urinary retention or overflow, UTI
Musculoskeletal	Back pain	Abdominal aortic aneurysm, compression fractures, infection, metastatic cancer, multiple myeloma, osteoarthritis, Paget disease, pyelonephritis, spinal stenosis
	Proximal muscle pain	Myopathies, polymyalgia rheumatica, use of statins
Extremities	Leg pain	Intermittent claudication, night cramps, osteoarthritis, radiculopathy (eg, disk herniation, lumbar stenosis), restless legs syndrome
	Swollen ankles	Heart failure (if swelling is bilateral), hypoalbuminemia, renal insufficiency, venous insufficiency
Neurologic	Change in mental status with fever	Delirium, encephalitis, meningitis, sepsis
	Change in mental status without fever	Acute illness, cognitive dysfunction, fecal impaction, delirium, depression, drugs, paranoia, urinary retention
	Clumsiness in tasks requiring fine motor coordination (eg, buttoning shirt)	Arthritis, parkinsonism, spondylotic cervical myelopathy, intention tremor
	Excessive sweating during meals	Autonomic neuropathy
	Fall without loss of consciousness	Bradycardia, drop attack, neuropathy, orthostatic hypotension, postural instability, tachycardia, transient ischemic attack, vision impairment
	Hesitant gait with intention tremor	Parkinson disease
	Numbness with tingling in fingers	Carpal tunnel syndrome, peripheral neuropathy, spondylotic cervical myelopathy
	Sleep disturbances	Anxiety, circadian rhythm disturbances, depression, drugs, pain, parkinsonism, periodic limb movement disorder, sleep apnea, urinary frequency
	Syncope	Aortic stenosis, cardiac arrhythmia, hypoglycemia, orthostatic hypotension (especially drug-related), seizure
	Transient interference with speech, muscle strength, sensation, or vision	Transient ischemic attack
	Tremor	Alcohol abuse, CNS disorder (eg, cerebellar disorders, poststroke), essential tremor, hyperthyroidism, parkinsonism

Patients or family members should be asked to bring in all of the above drugs and supplements at the initial visit and periodically thereafter. Clinicians can make sure patients have the prescribed drugs, but possession of these drugs does not guarantee adherence. Counting the number of tablets in each vial during the first and subsequent visits may be necessary. If someone other than a patient administers the drugs, that person is interviewed.

Patients should be asked to demonstrate their ability to read labels (often printed in small type), open containers (especially the child-resistant type), and recognize drugs. Patients should be advised not to put their drugs into one container.

Alcohol, tobacco, and recreational drug use history: Patients who smoke should be counseled to stop and, if they continue, not to smoke in bed because the elderly are more likely to fall asleep while doing so.

Patients should be checked for signs of alcohol use disorders, which are underdiagnosed in the elderly. Such signs include confusion, anger, hostility, alcohol odor on the breath, impaired balance and gait, tremors, peripheral neuropathy, and nutritional deficiencies. Screening questionnaires (eg, AUDIT—see Tables 341–3 on p. 2883 and 387–1 on p. 3234) and questions about quantity and frequency of alcohol consumption can help. The 4 CAGE questions are quick and straightforward; the clinician asks if the patient has ever felt

- Need to *C*ut down drinking
- *A*nnoyed by criticism about drinking
- *G*uilty about drinking
- Need for a morning "*E*ye-opener"

Two or more positive responses to the CAGE questions suggest the possibility of alcohol abuse. Questions about use of other recreational drugs or substances of abuse also are appropriate.

Nutrition history: Type, quantity, and frequency of food eaten are determined. Patients who eat ≤ 2 meals a day are at risk of undernutrition. Clinicians should ask about the following:

- Any special diets (eg, low-salt, low-carbohydrate) or self-prescribed fad diets
- Intake of dietary fiber and prescribed or OTC vitamins
- Weight loss and change of fit in clothing
- Amount of money patients have to spend on food
- Accessibility of food stores and suitable kitchen facilities
- Variety and freshness of foods

The ability to eat (eg, to chew and swallow) is evaluated. It may be impaired by xerostomia and/or dental problems, which are common among the elderly. Decreased taste or smell may reduce the pleasure of eating, so patients may eat less. Patients with decreased vision, arthritis, immobility, or tremors may have difficulty preparing meals and may injure or burn themselves when cooking. Patients who are worried about urinary incontinence may reduce their fluid intake; as a result, they may eat less food.

Mental health history: Mental health problems may not be detected easily in elderly patients. Symptoms that may indicate a mental health disorder in younger patients (eg, insomnia, changes in sleep patterns, constipation, cognitive dysfunction, anorexia, weight loss, fatigue, preoccupation with bodily functions, increased alcohol consumption) may have another cause in the elderly. Sadness, hopelessness, and crying episodes may indicate depression. Irritability may be the primary affective symptom of depression, or patients may present with cognitive dysfunction. Generalized anxiety is the most common mental disorder encountered in elderly patients and often is accompanied by depression.

Patients should be asked about delusions and hallucinations, past mental health care (including psychotherapy, institutionalization, and electroconvulsive therapy), use of psychoactive drugs, and recent changes in circumstances. Many circum stances (eg, recent loss of a loved one, hearing loss, a change in residence or living situation, loss of independence) may contribute to depression.

Patients' spiritual and religious preferences, including their personal interpretation of aging, declining health, and death, should be clarified.

Functional status: Whether patients can function independently, need some help with BADLs or IADLs, or need total assistance is determined as part of comprehensive geriatric assessment. Patients may be asked open-ended questions about their ability to do activities, or they may be asked to fill out a standardized assessment instrument with questions about specific ADLs and IADLs (eg, see Tables 333–4 and 388–3 on p. 3252).

Social history: Clinicians should obtain information about patients' living arrangements, particularly where and with whom they live (eg, alone in an isolated house, in a busy apartment building), accessibility of their residence (eg, up stairs or a hill), and what modes of transportation are available to them. Such factors affect the ability of the elderly to obtain food, health care, and other important resources. A home visit, although difficult to arrange, can provide critical information. For example, clinicians can gain insight about nutrition from the refrigerator's contents and about multiple ADLs from the bathroom's condition.

The number of rooms, number and type of phones, presence of smoke and carbon monoxide detectors, and condition of plumbing and heating system are determined, as is the availability of elevators, stairs, and air conditioning. Home safety evaluations can identify home features that can lead to falls (eg, poor lighting, slippery bathtubs, unanchored rugs), and solutions can be suggested.

Having patients describe a typical day, including activities such as reading, television viewing, work, exercise, hobbies, and interactions with other people, provides valuable information.

Clinicians should ask about the following:

- Frequency and nature of social contacts (eg, friends, senior citizens' groups), family visits, and religious or spiritual participation
- Driving and availability of other forms of transportation
- Caregivers and support systems (eg, church, senior citizens' groups, friends, neighbors) that are available to the patient
- The ability of family members to help the patient (eg, their employment status, their health, traveling time to the patient's home)
- The patient's attitude toward family members and their attitude toward the patient (including their level of interest in helping and willingness to help)

Marital status of patients is noted. Questions about sexual practices and satisfaction must be sensitive and tactful but thorough. The number and sex of sex partners are determined, and risk of sexually transmitted diseases (STDs) is evaluated. Many sexually active elderly people are not aware of the increasing incidence of STDs in the elderly and do not follow or even know about safe sex practices.

Patients should be asked about educational level, jobs held, known exposures to radioactivity or asbestos, and current and past hobbies. Economic difficulties due to retirement, a fixed income, or death of a spouse or partner are discussed. Financial or health problems may result in loss of a home, social status, or independence. Patients should be asked about past relationships with physicians; a long-time relationship with a physician may have been lost because the physician retired or died or because the patient relocated.

Advance directives: Patient wishes regarding measures for prolonging life must be documented. Patients are asked what provisions for surrogate decision making (advance directives) have been made in case they become incapacitated, and if none have been made, patients are encouraged to make them. Getting patients and their surrogates accustomed to discussing goals of care is important; then when circumstances require medical decisions and prior documentation is unavailable or not relevant to the circumstance (which is very common), appropriate decisions can be made.

KEY POINTS

- Unless corrected, sensory deficits, especially hearing deficits, may interfere with history-taking.
- Many disorders in the elderly manifest only as functional decline.
- As part of the drug history, the patient or a family member should be asked to bring in all the patient's drugs, including OTC drugs, at the initial visit and periodically thereafter.
- Health care practitioners must often interview caregivers to obtain the history of functionally dependent elderly patients.

Physical Examination

Observing patients and their movements (eg, walking into the examination room, sitting in or rising from a chair, getting on and off an examination table, taking off or putting on socks and shoes) can provide valuable information about their function.

Table 333–4. LAWTON INSTRUMENTAL ACTIVITIES OF DAILY LIVING SCALE

ACTIVITY	DESCRIPTION	SCORE*
Using the telephone	Uses a telephone, including looking up and dialing numbers	1
	Dials a few familiar numbers	1
	Answers the telephone but does not dial	1
	Does not use the telephone	0
Shopping	Does all the shopping without help	1
	Shops for small items without help	0
	Needs to be accompanied whenever shopping	0
	Cannot do any shopping	0
Preparing food	Plans, prepares, and serves adequate meals without help	1
	If given the ingredients, prepares adequate meals	0
	Heat and serves prepared meals or prepares meals but ones that are nutritionally inadequate	0
	Needs someone to prepare and serve meals	0
Doing household tasks	Does household tasks without help or occasionally with help for physically demanding tasks (eg, washing windows)	1
	Does light housework (eg, dish washing, dusting)	1
	Does light housework but does not keep the house adequately clean	1
	Needs help with all household tasks	1
	Does not do any household tasks	0
Doing laundry	Does laundry without help	1
	Washes small items (eg, stockings)	1
	Needs someone to do all laundry	0
Traveling other than by walking	Uses public transportation without help or drives a car	1
	Calls for taxis but does not use other public transportation	1
	Uses public transportation if accompanied by someone to help	1
	Travels only by taxi or car and only if helped by someone	0
	Does not travel	0
Taking prescription drugs as directed	Takes the correct doses of prescribed drugs at the correct time without help	1
	Takes prescribed drugs if they are prepared in advance in separate dosage	0
	Cannot dispense the prescribed drugs	0
Managing money	Manages finances (eg, making a budget, writing checks, paying rent, keeping track of income) without help	1
	Buys small items needed on a daily basis but requires help with banking and major purchases	1
	Cannot manage money	0

*People are asked to choose the description that most closely matches their highest functional level. Tasks are scored as either 1 (if they can do a task) or 0 (if they cannot).

Total scores range from 0 (unable to do all tasks and being dependent on help) to 8 (able to do all tasks and to function independently).

Adapted from Lawton MP, Brody EM: Assessment of older people: Self-maintaining and instrumental activities of daily living. *The Gerontologist* 9:179–186, 1969.

Their personal hygiene (eg, state of dress, cleanliness, odor) may provide information about mental status and the ability to care for themselves.

If patients become fatigued, the physical examination may need to be stopped and continued at another visit. Elderly patients may require additional time to undress and transfer to the examining table; they should not be rushed. The examining table should be adjusted to a height that patients can easily access; a footstool facilitates mounting. Frail patients must not be left alone on the table. Portions of the examination may be more comfortable if patients sit in a chair.

Clinicians should describe the general appearance of patients (eg, comfortable, restless, undernourished, inattentive, pale, dyspneic, cyanotic). If they are examined at bedside, use of protective padding or a protective mattress, bedside rails (partial or full), restraints, a urinary catheter, or an adult diaper should be noted.

Vital Signs

Weight should be recorded at each visit. During measurement, patients with balance problems may need to grasp grab bars placed near or on the scale. Height is recorded annually to check for height loss due to osteoporosis.

Temperature is recorded. Hypothermia can be missed if the thermometer cannot measure temperatures more than a few degrees lower than normal. Absence of fever does not exclude infection.

Pulses and BP are checked in both arms. Pulse is taken for 30 sec, and any irregularity is noted. Because many factors can alter BP, BP is measured several times after patients have rested > 5 min.

BP may be overestimated in elderly patients because their arteries are stiff. This rare condition, called pseudohypertension, should be suspected if dizziness develops after antihypertensives are begun or doses are increased to treat persistently elevated systolic BP.

All elderly patients are checked for orthostatic hypotension because it is common. BP is measured with patients in the supine position, then after they have been standing for 3 to 5 min. If systolic BP falls ≥ 20 mm Hg after patients stand, or any symptoms of hypotension are detected, orthostatic hypotension is diagnosed. Caution is required when testing hypovolemic patients.

A normal respiratory rate in elderly patients may be as high as 25 breaths/min. A rate of > 25 breaths/min may be the first sign of a lower respiratory tract infection, heart failure, or another disorder.

Skin

Initial observation includes color (normal rubor, pale, cyanotic). Examination includes a search for premalignant and malignant lesions, tissue ischemia, and pressure ulcers. In the elderly, the following should be considered:

- Ecchymoses may occur readily when skin is traumatized, often on the forearm, because the dermis thins with aging.
- Uneven tanning may be normal because melanocytes are progressively lost with aging.
- Longitudinal ridges on the nails and absence of the crescent-shaped lunula are normal age-related findings.
- Nail plate fractures may occur because with aging, the nail plate thins.
- Black splinter hemorrhages in the middle or distal third of the fingernail are more likely to be due to trauma than to bacteremia.
- A thickened, yellow toenail indicates onychomycosis, a fungal infection.
- Toenail borders that curve in and down indicate ingrown toenail (onychocryptosis).
- Whitish nails that scale easily, sometimes with a pitted surface, indicate psoriasis.
- Unexplained bruises may indicate abuse.

Head and Neck

Face: Normal age-related findings may include the following:

- Eyebrows that drop below the superior orbital rim
- Descent of the chin
- Loss of the angle between the submandibular line and neck
- Wrinkles
- Dry skin
- Thick terminal hairs on the ears, nose, upper lip, and chin

The temporal arteries should be palpated for tenderness and thickening, which may indicate giant cell arteritis, suspicion of which requires immediate evaluation and treatment.

Nose: Progressive descent of the nasal tip is a normal age-related finding. It may cause the upper and lower lateral cartilage to separate, enlarging and lengthening the nose.

Eyes: Normal age-related findings include the following:

- Loss of orbital fat: It may cause gradual sinking of the eye backward into the orbit (enophthalmos). Thus, enophthalmos is not necessarily a sign of dehydration in the elderly. Enophthalmos is accompanied by deepening of the upper eyelid fold and slight obstruction of peripheral vision.
- Pseudoptosis (decreased size of the palpebral aperture)
- Entropion (inversion of lower eyelid margins)
- Ectropion (eversion of lower eyelid margins)
- Arcus senilis (a white ring at the limbus)

With aging, presbyopia develops; the lens becomes less elastic and less able to change shape when focusing on close objects.

The eye examination should focus on testing visual acuity (eg, using a Snellen chart). Visual fields can be tested at the bedside by confrontation—ie, patients are asked to stare at the examiner so that the examiner can determine differences between their and the examiner's visual field. However, such testing has low sensitivity for most visual disorders. Tonometry is occasionally done in primary care; however, it is usually done by ophthalmologists or optometrists as part of routine eye examinations or by ophthalmologists when a patient is referred to them because glaucoma is clinically suspected.

Ophthalmoscopy is done to check for cataracts, optic nerve or macular degeneration, and evidence of glaucoma, hypertension, or diabetes. Findings may be unremarkable unless a disorder is present because the retina's appearance usually does not change much with aging. In elderly patients, mild to moderate elevated intracranial pressure may not result in papilledema because cortical atrophy occurs with aging; papilledema is more likely when pressure is markedly increased. Areas of black pigment or hemorrhages in and around the macula indicate macular degeneration.

For all elderly patients, an eye examination by an ophthalmologist or optometrist is recommended every 1 to 2 yr because such an examination may be much more sensitive for certain common eye disorders (eg, glaucoma, cataracts, retinal disorders).

Ears: Tophi, a normal age-related finding, may be noted during inspection of the pinna. The external auditory canal is examined for cerumen, especially if a hearing problem is noted during the interview. If a patient wears a hearing aid, it is removed and examined. The ear mold and plastic tubing can become plugged with wax, or the battery may be dead, indicated by absence of a whistle (feedback) when the volume of the hearing aid is turned up.

To evaluate hearing, examiners, with their face out of the patient's view, whisper 3 to 6 random words or letters into each of the patient's ears. If a patient correctly repeats at least half of these words for each ear, hearing is considered functional for one-on-one conversations. Patients with presbycusis (age-related, gradual, bilateral, symmetric, and predominantly high-frequency hearing deficits) are more likely to report difficulty in understanding speech than in hearing sounds. Evaluation with a portable audioscope, if available, is also recommended because the testing sounds are standardized; thus, this evaluation can be useful when multiple providers are caring for a patient.

Patients are asked whether hearing loss interferes with social, work, or family functioning, or they may be given the Hearing Handicap Inventory for the Elderly (HHIE), a self-assessment tool designed to determine the effects of hearing loss on the emotional and social adjustment of the elderly. If hearing loss interferes with functioning or if the HHIE score is positive, they are referred for formal audiologic testing.

Mouth: The mouth is examined for bleeding or swollen gums, loose or broken teeth, fungal infections, and signs of cancer (eg, leukoplakia, erythroplakia, ulceration, mass). Findings may include

- Darkened teeth: Due to extrinsic stains and less translucent enamel, which occur with aging
- Fissures in the mouth and tongue and a tongue that sticks to the buccal mucosa: Due to xerostomia
- Erythematous, edematous gingiva that bleeds easily: Usually indicating a gingival or periodontal disorder
- Bad breath: Possibly indicating caries, periodontitis, another oral disorder, or sometimes a pulmonary disorder

The dorsal and ventral surfaces of the tongue are examined. Common age-related changes include varicose veins on the ventral surface, benign migratory glossitis (geographic tongue), and atrophied papillae on the sides of the tongue. In edentulous patients, the tongue may enlarge to facilitate chewing; however, enlargement may also indicate amyloidosis or hypothyroidism. A smooth, painful tongue may indicate vitamin B_{12} deficiency.

Dentures should be removed before the mouth is examined. Dentures increase risk of oral candidiasis and resorption of the alveolar ridges. Inflammation of the palatal mucosa and ulcers of the alveolar ridges may result from poorly fitting dentures.

The interior of the mouth is palpated. A swollen, firm, and tender parotid gland may indicate parotitis, particularly in dehydrated patients; pus may be expressed from Stensen duct when bacterial parotitis is present. The infecting organisms are often staphylococci.

Painful, inflamed, fissured lesions at the lip commissures (angular cheilitis) may be noted in edentulous patients who do not wear dentures; these lesions are usually accompanied by a fungal infection.

Temporomandibular joint: This joint should be evaluated for degeneration (osteoarthrosis), a common age-related change. The joint can degenerate as teeth are lost and compressive forces in the joint become excessive. Degeneration may be indicated by joint crepitus felt at the head of the condyle as patients lower and raise their jaw, by painful jaw movements, or by both.

Neck: The thyroid gland, which is located low in the neck of elderly people, often beneath the sternum, is examined for enlargement and nodules.

Carotid bruits due to transmitted heart murmurs can be differentiated from those due to carotid artery stenosis by moving the stethoscope up the neck: A transmitted heart murmur becomes softer; the bruit of carotid artery stenosis becomes louder. Bruits due to carotid artery stenosis suggest systemic atherosclerosis. Whether asymptomatic patients with carotid bruits require evaluation or treatment for cerebrovascular disease is unclear.

The neck is checked for flexibility. Resistance to passive flexion, extension, and lateral rotation may indicate a cervical spine disorder. Resistance to flexion and extension can also occur in patients with meningitis, but unless meningitis is accompanied by a cervical spine disorder, the neck can be rotated passively from side to side without resistance.

Chest and Back

All areas of the lungs are examined by percussion and auscultation. Basilar rales may be heard in the lungs of healthy patients but should disappear after patients take a few deep breaths. The extent of respiratory excursions (movement of the diaphragm and ability to expand the chest) should be noted.

The back is examined for scoliosis and tenderness. Severe low back, hip, and leg pain with marked sacral tenderness may indicate spontaneous osteoporotic fractures of the sacrum, which can occur in elderly patients.

Breasts: In men and women, the breasts should be examined annually for irregularities and nodules. For women, self-examinations are sometimes recommended. Screening mammography is also recommended, especially for women who have a family history of breast cancer. If nipples are retracted, pressure should be applied around the nipples; pressure everts the nipples when retraction is due to aging but not when it is due to an underlying lesion.

Heart: Heart size can usually be assessed by palpating the apex. However, displacement caused by kyphoscoliosis may make assessment difficult.

Auscultation should be done systematically (rate, regularity, murmurs, clicks, and rubs). Unexplained and asymptomatic sinus bradycardia in apparently healthy elderly people may not be clinically important. An irregularly irregular rhythm suggests atrial fibrillation.

In elderly patients, a systolic murmur most commonly indicates

- **Aortic valve sclerosis:** Typically, this murmur is not hemodynamically significant, although risk of stroke may be increased. It peaks early during systole and is rarely heard in the carotid arteries. Rarely, sclerosis of the aortic valve progresses to hemodynamic significance and calcification; although infrequent, aortic valve sclerosis is now the most common lesion leading to symptomatic aortic stenosis and need for treatment.

However, systolic murmurs may be due to other disorders, which should be identified:

- **Aortic valve stenosis:** This murmur, in contrast to that of usual aortic valve sclerosis, typically peaks later during systole, is transmitted to the carotid arteries, and is loud (greater than grade 2); the 2nd heart sound is dampened, pulse pressure is narrow, and the carotid upstroke is slowed. However, in elderly patients, the murmur of aortic valve stenosis may be difficult to identify because it may be softer, a 2nd heart sound is rarely audible, and narrow pulse pressures are uncommon. Also, in many elderly patients with aortic valve stenosis, the carotid upstroke does not slow because vascular compliance is diminished.

- **Mitral regurgitation:** This murmur is usually loudest at the apex and radiates to the axilla.
- **Hypertrophic obstructive cardiomyopathy:** This murmur intensifies when patients do a Valsalva maneuver.

Diastolic murmurs are abnormal in people of any age.

Fourth heart sounds are common among elderly people without evidence of a cardiovascular disorder and are commonly absent among elderly people with evidence of a cardiovascular disorder.

If new neurologic or cardiovascular symptoms develop in patients with a pacemaker, evaluation for variable heart sounds, murmurs, and pulses and for hypotension and heart failure is required. These symptoms and signs may be due to loss of atrioventricular synchrony.

GI System

The abdomen is palpated to check for weak abdominal muscles, which are common among elderly people and which may predispose to hernias. Most abdominal aortic aneurysms are palpable as a pulsatile mass; however, only their lateral width can be assessed during physical examination. In some patients (particularly thin ones), a normal aorta is palpable, but the vessel and pulsations do not extend laterally. Screening ultrasonography of the aorta is recommended for all older men who have ever smoked. The liver and spleen are palpated for enlargement. Frequency and quality of bowel sounds are checked, and the suprapubic area is percussed for tenderness, discomfort, and evidence of urinary retention.

The anorectal area is examined externally for fissures, hemorrhoids, and other lesions. Sensation and the anal wink reflex are tested. A digital rectal examination (DRE) to detect a mass, stricture, tenderness, or fecal impaction is done in men and women. Fecal occult blood testing is also done.

Male GU System

The prostate gland is palpated for nodules, tenderness, and consistency. Estimating prostate size by DRE is inaccurate, and size does not correlate with urethral obstruction; however, DRE provides a qualitative evaluation.

Female Reproductive System

Regular pelvic examinations, with a Papanicolaou (Pap) test every 2 to 3 yr until age 65, are recommended. At age 65, testing can be stopped if results of the previous 2 consecutive tests were normal. If women ≥ 65 have not had regular Pap tests, they should have at least 2 negative tests, 1 yr apart, before testing is stopped. Once Pap testing has been stopped, it is restarted only if new symptoms or signs of a possible disorder develop. If women have had a hysterectomy, Pap tests are required only if cervical tissue remains.

For bimanual pelvic examination, patients who lack hip mobility may lie on their left side. Postmenopausal reduction of estrogen leads to atrophy of the vaginal and urethral mucosa; the vaginal mucosa appears dry and lacks rugal folds. The ovaries should not be palpable 10 yr after menopause; palpable ovaries suggest cancer. Patients should be examined for evidence of prolapse of the urethra, vagina, cervix, and uterus. They are asked to cough to check for urine leakage and intermittent prolapse.

Musculoskeletal System

Joints are examined for tenderness, swelling, subluxation, crepitus, warmth, redness, and other abnormalities, which may suggest a disorder:

- Heberden nodes (bony overgrowths at the distal interphalangeal joints) or Bouchard nodes (bony overgrowths at the proximal interphalangeal joints): Osteoarthritis
- Subluxation of the metacarpophalangeal joints with ulnar deviation of the fingers: Chronic RA
- Swan-neck deformity (hyperextension of the proximal interphalangeal joint with flexion of the distal interphalangeal joint) and boutonnière deformity (hyperextension of the distal interphalangeal joint with flexion of the proximal interphalangeal joint): RA

These deformities may interfere with functioning or usual activities.

Active and passive range of joint motion should be determined. The presence of contractures should be noted. Variable resistance to passive manipulation of the extremities (gegenhalten) sometimes occurs with aging.

Feet

Diagnosis and treatment of foot problems, which become common with aging, help elderly people maintain their independence. Common age-related findings include hallux valgus, medial prominence of the 1st metatarsal head with lateral deviation and rotation of the big toe, and lateral deviation of the 5th metatarsal head. Hammer toe (hyperflexion of the proximal interphalangeal joint) and claw toe (hyperflexion of the proximal and distal interphalangeal toe joints) may interfere with functioning and daily activities. Toe deformities may result from years of wearing poorly fitting shoes or from RA, diabetes, or neurologic disorders (eg, Charcot-Marie-Tooth disease). Occasionally, foot problems indicate other systemic disorders (see Table 36–1 on p. 278).

Patients with foot problems should be referred to a podiatrist for regular evaluation and treatment.

Neurologic System

Neurologic examination for elderly patients is similar to that for any adult (see Ch. 220). However, nonneurologic disorders that are common among elderly peo.ple may complicate this examination. For example, visual and hearing deficits may impede evaluation of cranial nerves, and periarthritis (inflammation of tissues around a joint) in certain joints, especially shoulders and hips, may interfere with evaluation of motor function.

Signs detected during the examination must be considered in light of the patient's age, history, and other findings. Symmetric findings unaccompanied by functional loss and other neurologic symptoms and signs may be noted in elderly patients. Clinicians must decide whether these findings justify a detailed evaluation to check for a neurologic lesion. Patients should be reevaluated periodically for functional changes, asymmetry, and new symptoms.

Cranial nerves: Evaluation may be complex (see also p. 1835). Elderly people often have small pupils; their pupillary light reflex may be sluggish, and their pupillary mitotic response to near vision may be diminished. Upward gaze and, to a lesser extent, downward gaze can be slightly limited. Eye movements, when tracking an examiner's finger during evaluation of visual fields, may appear jerky and irregular. Bell phenomenon (reflex upward movement of the eyes during closure) is sometimes absent. These changes occur normally with aging.

In many elderly people, sense of smell is diminished because they have fewer olfactory neurons, have had numerous upper respiratory infections, or have chronic rhinitis. However, asymmetric loss (loss of smell in one nostril) is abnormal. Taste may be altered because the sense of smell is diminished or because patients take drugs that decrease salivation.

Visual and hearing deficits may result from abnormalities in the eyes and ears rather than in nerve pathways.

Motor function: Patients can be evaluated for tremor during handshaking and other simple activities. If tremor is detected, amplitude, rhythm, distribution, frequency, and time of occurrence (at rest, with action, or with intention) are noted.

Muscle strength: Elderly people, particularly those who do not do resistance training regularly, may appear weak during routine testing. For example, during the physical examination, the clinician may easily straighten a patient's elbow despite the patient's effort to sustain a contraction. If weakness is symmetric, does not bother the patient, and has not changed the patient's function or activity level, it is likely to be due to disuse rather than neurologic disease. Such weakness is treatable with resistance training; for the legs especially, it can improve mobility and reduce fall risk. Strengthening the upper extremities is also beneficial for overall function. Increased muscle tone, measured by flexing and extending the elbow or knee, is a normal finding in elderly people; however, jerky movements during examination and cogwheel rigidity are abnormal.

Sarcopenia (a decrease in muscle mass) is a common age-related finding. It is insignificant unless accompanied by a decline or change in function (eg, patients can no longer rise from a chair without using chair arms). Sarcopenia affects the hand muscles (eg, interosseous and thenar muscles) in particular. Weak extensor muscles of the wrist, fingers, and thumb are common among patients who use wheelchairs because compression of the upper arm against the armrest injures the radial nerve. Arm function can be tested by having patients pick up an eating utensil or touch the back of their head with both hands.

Coordination: Motor coordination is tested. Coordination decreases because of changes in central mechanisms and can be measured in the neuro exam; this decrease is usually subtle and does not impair function.

Gait and posture: All components of gait should be assessed; they include initiation of walking; step length, height, symmetry, continuity, and cadence (rhythm); velocity (speed of walking); stride width; and walking posture. Sensation, musculoskeletal and motor control, and attention, which are necessary for independent, coordinated walking, must also be considered.

Normal age-related findings may include the following:

- Shorter steps, possibly because calf muscles are weak or because balance is poor
- Reduced gait velocity in patients > 70 because steps are shorter
- Increased time in double stance (when both feet are on the ground), which may be due to impaired balance or fear of falling
- Reduced motion in some joints (eg, ankle plantar flexion just before the back foot lifts off, pelvic motion in the frontal and transverse planes)
- Slight changes in walking posture (eg, greater downward pelvic rotation, possibly due to a combination of increased abdominal fat, abdominal muscle weakness, and tight hip flexor muscles; a slightly greater turn-out of the toes, possibly due to loss of hip internal rotation or to an attempt to increase lateral stability)

In people with a gait velocity of < 1 m/sec, mortality risk is significantly increased.

Aging has little effect on walking cadence or posture; typically, the elderly walk upright unless a disorder is present (see Table 333–5).

Overall postural control is evaluated using the Romberg test (patients stand with feet together and eyes closed). Safety is paramount, and a clinician doing the Romberg test must be in position to prevent the patient from falling. With aging, postural control is often impaired, and postural sway (movement in the anteroposterior plane when patients remain stationary and upright) may increase.

Table 333–5. SOME CAUSES OF GAIT DYSFUNCTION

PROBLEM	POSSIBLE CAUSES
Neurogenic claudication (pain, weakness, and numbness that occurs during walking and lessens during sitting)	Lumbar spinal stenosis
Difficulty initiating walking	Frontal or subcortical disorders Isolated gait initiation failure Parkinson disease
Truncal instability (eg, sway)	Arthritis in the hips or knees Cerebellar, subcortical, or basal ganglia dysfunction
Leaning forward during walking	Osteoporosis with kyphosis
Step asymmetry	Focal neurologic deficit Pain or weakness in one leg Unilateral musculoskeletal deficit
Step discontinuity	Fear of falling Frontal lobe disorder
Step length or height abnormalities	Arthritis Foot problem Stroke
Stride width abnormalities	Cerebellar disorders Hip disorders Normal-pressure hydrocephalus

Reflexes: The deep tendon reflexes are checked. Aging usually has little effect on them. However, eliciting the Achilles tendon reflex may require special techniques (eg, testing while patients kneel with their feet over the edge of a bed and with their hands clasped). A diminished or absent reflex, present in nearly half of elderly patients, may not indicate pathology, especially if symmetric. It occurs because tendon elasticity decreases and nerve conduction in the tendon's long reflex arc slows. Asymmetric Achilles tendon reflexes usually indicate a disorder (eg, sciatica).

Cortical release reflexes (known as pathologic reflexes), which include snout, sucking, and palmomental reflexes, commonly occur in elderly patients without detectable brain disorders (eg, dementia). A Babinski reflex (extensor plantar response) in elderly patients is abnormal; it indicates an upper motor neuron lesion, often cervical spondylosis with partial cord compression.

Sensation: Evaluation of sensation includes touch (using a skin prick test), cortical sensory function, temperature sense, proprioception (joint position sense), and vibration sense testing. Aging has limited effects on sensation. Many elderly patients report numbness, especially in the feet. It may result from a decrease in size of fibers in the peripheral nerves, particularly the large fibers. Nonetheless, patients with numbness should be checked for peripheral neuropathies. In many patients, no cause of numbness can be identified.

Many elderly people lose vibratory sensation below the knees. It is lost because small vessels in the posterior column of the spinal cord sclerose. However, proprioception, which is thought to use a similar pathway, is unaffected.

Mental status: A mental status examination is important. Patients who are disturbed by such a test should be reassured that it is routine. The examiner must make sure that patients can hear; hearing deficits that prevent patients from hearing and understanding questions may be mistaken for cognitive dysfunction. Evaluating the mental status of patients who have a speech or language disorder (eg, mutism, dysarthria, speech apraxia, aphasia) can be difficult.

Orientation may be normal in many patients with dementia or other cognitive disorders. Thus, evaluation may require questions that identify abnormalities in consciousness, judgment, calculations, speech, language, praxis, executive function, or memory, as well as orientation. Abnormalities in these areas cannot be attributed solely to age, and if abnormalities are noted, further evaluation, including a formal test of mental status, is needed.

With aging, information processing and memory retrieval slow but are essentially unimpaired. With extra time and encouragement, patients do such tasks satisfactorily (unless a neurologic abnormality is present).

Nutritional Status

Aging changes the interpretation of many measurements that reflect nutritional status in younger people. For example, aging can alter height. Weight changes can reflect alterations in nutrition, fluid balance, or both. The proportion of lean body mass and body fat content changes. Despite these age-related changes, body mass index (BMI) is still useful in elderly patients, although it underestimates obesity. Waist circumference and waist-to-hip ratio have been used instead. Risks due to obesity are increased if the waist circumference is > 102 cm (> 40 in) in men and > 88 cm (> 35 in) in women or if the waist-to-hip ratio is > 0.9 in men and > 0.85 in women.

If abnormalities in the nutrition history (eg, weight loss, suspected deficiencies in essential nutrients) or BMI are identified, thorough nutritional evaluation, including laboratory measurements, is indicated.

KEY POINTS

- Valuable information about a patient's function can be gained by observing the patient.
- Physical examination should include all systems, particularly mental status, and may require 2 sessions.

Comprehensive Geriatric Assessment

Comprehensive geriatric assessment is a multidimensional process designed to assess the functional ability, health (physical, cognitive, and mental), and socioenvironmental situation of elderly people.

The comprehensive geriatric assessment specifically and thoroughly evaluates functional and cognitive abilities, social support, financial status, and environmental factors, as well as physical and mental health. Ideally, a regular examination of elderly patients incorporates many aspects of the comprehensive geriatric assessment, making the 2 approaches very similar. Assessment results are coupled with sustained individually tailored interventions (eg, rehabilitation, education, counseling, supportive services).

The cost of geriatric assessment limits its use. Thus, this assessment may be used best mainly in high-risk elderly patients, such as the frail or chronically ill (eg, identified via mailed health questionnaires or interviews in the home or meeting places). Family members may also request a referral for geriatric assessment.

Assessment can have the following benefits:

- Improved care and clinical outcomes
- Greater diagnostic accuracy
- Improved functional and mental status
- Reduced mortality
- Decreased use of nursing homes and acute care hospitals
- Greater satisfaction with care

If elderly patients are relatively healthy, a standard medical evaluation may be appropriate.

Comprehensive geriatric assessment is most successful when done by a geriatric interdisciplinary team (typically, a geriatrician, nurse, social worker, and pharmacist). Usually, assessments are done in an outpatient setting. However, patients with physical or mental impairments and chronically ill patients may require inpatient assessment.

Assessment Domains

The principal domains (see Table 333–6) assessed are

- **Functional ability:** Ability to do activities of daily living (ADLs) and instrumental ADLs (IADLs) are assessed. ADLs include eating, dressing, bathing, transferring between the bed and a chair, using the toilet, and controlling bladder and bowel. IADLs enable people to live independently and include preparing meals, doing housework, taking drugs, going on errands, managing finances, and using a telephone (see also Tables 333–4 and 388–3 on p. 3252).
- **Physical health:** History and physical examination should include problems common among the elderly (eg, problems with vision, hearing, continence, gait, and balance).
- **Cognition and mental health:** Several validated screening tests for cognitive dysfunction (eg, mental status examination—see Sidebar 220–1 on p. 1836) and for depression (eg, Geriatric Depression Scale [see Table 333–7], Hamilton Depression Scale) can be used.

Table 333–6. A GERIATRIC ASSESSMENT INSTRUMENT

DOMAIN	ITEM
Daily functional ability	Degree of difficulty eating, dressing, bathing, transferring between bed and chair, using the toilet, and controlling bladder and bowel Degree of difficulty preparing meals, doing housework, taking drugs, going on errands (eg, shopping), managing finances, and using the telephone
Assistive devices	Use of personal devices (eg, cane, walker, wheelchair, oxygen) Use of environmental devices (eg, grab bars, shower bench, hospital bed)
Caregivers	Use of paid caregivers (eg, nurses, aides) Use of unpaid caregivers (eg, family members, friends, volunteers)
Drugs	Name of prescription drugs used Name of nonprescription drugs used
Nutrition	Height, weight Stability of weight (eg, Has the patient lost 4.54 kg [10 lb] in the past 6 mo without trying?)
Preventive measures	Regularity of BP measurements, guaiac test for occult blood in stool, sigmoidoscopy or colonoscopy, immunizations (influenza, pneumococcal, tetanus), thyroid-stimulating hormone assessment, and dental care Intake of calcium and vitamin D Regularity of exercise Use of smoke detectors
Cognition	Ability to remember 3 objects after 1 min and draw a clock face (mini-cog)
Affect	Feelings of sadness, depression, or hopelessness Lack of interest or pleasure in doing things
Advance directives	Possession of a living will Establishment of durable power of attorney for health care
Substance abuse/misuse	Use of alcohol Use of cigarettes Overuse of prescribed or unprescribed drugs
Gait and balance	Number of falls in the past 6 mo Time required to rise from a chair, walk 3.05 m (10 ft), turn around, return, and sit down Extent of maximal forward reach while standing
Sensory ability	Ability to report 3 numbers whispered 0.61 m (2 ft) behind the head Ability to read Snellen chart at 20/40 or better (with corrective lenses, if needed)
Upper extremities	Ability to clasp hands behind the head and back

- **Socioenvironmental situation:** The patient's social interaction network, available social support resources, special needs, and the safety and convenience of the patient's environment are determined, often by a nurse or social worker. Such factors influence the treatment approach used. A checklist can be used to assess home safety.

Standardized instruments make evaluation of these domains more reliable and efficient (see Table 333–6). They also facilitate communication of clinical information among health care practitioners and monitoring of changes in the patient's condition over time.

UNUSUAL PRESENTATIONS OF ILLNESS IN THE ELDERLY

In the elderly, many common conditions can exist without their characteristic features. Instead, the elderly may have ≥ 1 nonspecific geriatric syndromes (eg, delirium, dizziness, syncope, falling, weight loss, incontinence). These syndromes result from multiple disorders and impairments; nonetheless, patients may improve when only some of the precipitating factors are corrected. An even better strategy is to identify risk factors for these syndromes and correct as many as possible, thus reducing the likelihood of the syndrome's developing at all.

Although virtually any illness or drug intoxication can cause geriatric syndromes, the following disorders are especially likely to trigger one or more of them, sometimes instead of causing the typical symptoms and signs.

Acute bowel infarction may be indicated by acute confusion. Abdominal pain and tenderness may be minimal or absent.

Appendicitis pain tends to begin in the right lower quadrant rather than periumbilically. Eventually, pain may be diffuse in the abdomen rather than localized to the right lower quadrant. However, tenderness in this quadrant is a significant early sign.

Bacteremia causes a low-grade (at least) fever in most elderly patients, although fever may be absent. The source of bacteremia may be difficult to identify. Elderly patients may have nonspecific manifestations (eg, general malaise, anorexia, night sweats, unexplained change in mental status).

Biliary disorders may result in nonspecific mental and physical deterioration (eg, malaise, confusion, loss of mobility) without jaundice, fever, or abdominal pain. Abnormal liver function test results may be the only indication.

Table 333–7. GERIATRIC DEPRESSION SCALE (SHORT FORM)

QUESTION	RESPONSE	
1. Are you basically satisfied with your life?	Yes	No
2. Have you dropped many of your activities and interests?	Yes	No
3. Do you feel that life is empty?	Yes	No
4. Do you often get bored?	Yes	No
5. Are you in good spirits most of the time?	Yes	No
6. Are you afraid that something bad is going to happen to you?	Yes	No
7. Do you feel happy most of the time?	Yes	No
8. Do you often feel helpless?	Yes	No
9. Do you prefer to stay at home rather than go out and do new things?	Yes	No
10. Do you feel you have more problems with memory than most?	Yes	No
11. Do you think it is wonderful to be alive now?	Yes	No
12. Do you feel pretty worthless the way you are now?	Yes	No
13. Do you feel full of energy?	Yes	No
14. Do you feel that your situation is hopeless?	Yes	No
15. Do you think that most people are better off than you are?	Yes	No

Score: One point for "No" to questions 1, 5, 7, 11, 13.
One point for "Yes" to other questions.

- Normal = 3 ± 2
- Mildly depressed = 7 ± 3
- Very depressed = 12 ± 2

> 5 points suggests depression and warrants a follow-up evaluation.
≥ 10 points almost always indicates depression.

Adapted from Sheikh JI, Yesavage JA: Geriatric depression scale (GDS): Recent evidence and development of a shorter version. In *Clinical Gerontology: A Guide to Assessment and Intervention,* edited by TL Brink. Binghamton, NY, Haworth Press, 1986, pp. 165–173.

Heart failure may cause confusion, agitation, anorexia, weakness, insomnia, fatigue, weight loss, or lethargy; patients may not report dyspnea. Orthopnea may cause nocturnal agitation in patients who also have dementia. Peripheral edema is less specific as a sign of heart failure in elderly than in younger patients. In bedbound patients, edema may occur in the sacral area rather than in the lower extremities.

Hyperparathyroidism may cause nonspecific symptoms: fatigue, cognitive dysfunction, emotional instability, anorexia, constipation, and hypertension. Characteristic symptoms are often absent.

Hyperthyroidism may not cause the characteristic signs (eg, eye signs, enlarged thyroid gland). Instead, symptoms and signs may be subtle and may include tachycardia, weight loss, fatigue, weakness, palpitations, tremor, atrial fibrillation, and heart failure. Patients may appear apathetic rather than hyperkinetic.

Hypothyroidism may manifest subtly in elderly patients. The most common symptoms are nonspecific (eg, fatigue, weakness, falling). Anorexia, weight loss, and arthralgias may occur. Cold intolerance, weight gain, depression, paresthesias, hair loss, and muscle cramps are less common than among younger patients; cognitive dysfunction is more common. The most specific sign—delayed tendon reflex relaxation—may not be detectable in elderly patients because of decreased amplitude or absent reflexes.

Meningitis may cause fever and a change in mental status without symptoms of meningeal irritation (eg, headache, nuchal rigidity).

MI may manifest as diaphoresis, dyspnea, epigastric discomfort, syncope, weakness, vomiting, or confusion rather than as chest pain. After the onset of chest pain or other presenting symptoms of MI, elderly patients tend to delay longer than younger patients in seeking medical assistance.

Peptic ulcer disease may not cause characteristic ulcer symptoms; pain may be absent or nonspecific. Dyspepsia (usually epigastric discomfort with bloating, nausea, or early satiety) is more common among elderly than among younger patients. Elderly patients have more frequent, more severe GI bleeding, which may be painless. Slow, unrecognized blood loss may occur, resulting in severe anemia.

Pneumonia may be indicated by malaise, anorexia, or confusion. Tachycardia and tachypnea are common, but fever may be absent. Coughing may be mild and without copious, purulent sputum, especially in dehydrated patients.

TB may manifest differently in elderly patients with coexisting disorders. Symptoms may be nonspecific (eg, fever, weakness, confusion, anorexia). Pulmonary TB may manifest with fewer respiratory symptoms (eg, cough, excessive sputum production, hemoptysis) than in younger patients.

UTIs may be present in afebrile elderly patients. These patients may not report dysuria, frequency, or urgency but may experience dizziness, confusion, anorexia, fatigue, or weakness.

Other problems that manifest differently in the elderly include alcohol abuse, adverse drug effects, depression, pulmonary embolism, systemic infections, and unstable angina.

334 Aging and Quality of Life

Quality of life often depends on health and health care. However, health care practitioners, especially when establishing therapeutic objectives, may underemphasize its importance to patients.

Health-Related Quality of Life

How health affects quality of life is variable and subjective. Health-related quality of life has multiple dimensions, including the following:

- Absence of distressing physical symptoms (eg, pain, dyspnea, nausea, constipation)
- Emotional well-being (eg, happiness, absence of anxiety)
- Functional status (eg, capacity to do activities of daily living and higher-order functions, such as pleasurable activities)
- Quality of close interpersonal relationships (eg, with family members, friends)
- Participation in and enjoyment of social activities
- Satisfaction with medical and financial aspects of treatments
- Sexuality, body image, and intimacy

Influences: Some of the factors that influence health-related quality of life (eg, institutionalization, reduced life expectancy, cognitive impairment, disability, chronic pain, social isolation, functional status) may be obvious to health care practitioners. Practitioners may need to ask about others, especially social determinants of health (ie, the social, economic, and political conditions that people experience from birth to death and the systems put in place to prevent illness and treat it when it occurs). Other important factors include the nature and quality of close relationships, cultural influences, religion, personal values, and previous experiences with health care. However, how factors affect quality of life cannot necessarily be predicted, and some factors that cannot be anticipated may have effects.

Also, perspectives on quality of life can change. For example, after a stroke that caused severe disability, patients may choose treatment (eg, life-saving surgery) to sustain a quality of life that they would have considered poor or even unacceptable before the stroke.

Assessment

Barriers to assessment: Assessing patients' perspectives on quality of life may be difficult for the following reasons:

- Such an assessment is not always taught or emphasized sufficiently in traditional medical education.
- Quality of life is subjective, so decision models cannot be applied to individual patients.
- Assessing the patient's perspectives on quality of life takes time because it requires thoughtful conversation between patient and health care practitioner.

Method: Quality of life is best assessed by a direct interview with patients. During assessment, practitioners should be careful not to reveal their own biases. Determining a patient's preferences is usually possible; even patients with mild dementia or cognitive impairment can make their preferences known when practitioners use simple explanations and questions. Having family members present when discussing preferences of a patient with cognitive impairment is recommended.

Instruments that measure health-related quality of life can be useful in research studies for assessing group trends but tend not to be useful clinically for assessing individual patients.

THERAPEUTIC OBJECTIVES IN THE ELDERLY

Before a treatment or major diagnostic test is used, potential adverse effects should be weighed against potential benefits in the context of the patient's individual desires and goals.

Potential adverse effects include the following:

- Complications, including prolonged fatigue and disability
- Discomfort
- Inconvenience
- Cost
- Need for additional tests or treatments

Potential benefits include the following:

- Cure
- Prolongation of life
- Slowing of disease progression
- Functional improvement
- Symptom relief
- Prevention of complications

When treatments are very likely to achieve benefits and very unlikely to have adverse effects, decisions are relatively easy. However, assessing the relative importance of these quality of life factors to each patient is important when treatments may have discordant effects. For example, aggressive cancer therapy may prolong life but have severe adverse effects (eg, chronic nausea and vomiting, mouth ulcers) that greatly reduce quality of life. In this case, the patient's preference for quality vs duration of life and tolerance for risk and uncertainty help guide the decision whether to attempt cure, prolongation of life, or palliation.

The patient's perspective on quality of life may also affect treatment decisions when different treatments (eg, surgical vs drug treatment of severe angina or osteoarthritis) may have different efficacies, toxicities, or both. Practitioners can help patients understand the expected consequences of various treatments, enabling patients to make more informed decisions.

When predicting toxicities and benefits of various treatments, practitioners should use the patient's individual clinical characteristics, rather than chronologic age alone. In general, the patient's chronologic age is irrelevant when deciding among different treatments or therapeutic goals. However, life expectancy may affect treatment choice. For example, patients with a limited life expectancy may not live long enough to benefit from aggressive treatment of a slowly progressive disorder (eg, radical prostatectomy for a localized, slow-growing prostate cancer). Nevertheless, quality of life is important regardless of life expectancy. Thus, invasive treatments that may improve quality of life (eg, joint replacement, coronary artery bypass surgery) should not be automatically rejected for patients with a limited life expectancy.

Regardless of the overall therapeutic goal, symptom relief should always be offered.

335 Drug Therapy in the Elderly

Prevalence of prescription drug use among older adults increases substantially with age. Among people ≥ 65, 90% use at least 1 drug per week, > 40% use at least 5 different drugs per week, and 12% use ≥ 10 different drugs per week. Women take more drugs, particularly psychoactive and arthritis drugs. Drug use is greatest among the frail elderly, hospitalized patients, and nursing home residents; typically, a nursing home resident is given 7 to 8 different drugs on a regular basis.

Providing safe, effective drug therapy for the elderly is challenging for many reasons:

- They use more drugs than any other age group, increasing risk of adverse effects and drug interactions, and making adherence more difficult.
- They are more likely to have chronic disorders that may be worsened by the drug or affect drug response.
- Their physiologic reserves are generally reduced and can be further reduced by acute and chronic disorders.
- Aging can alter pharmacodynamics and pharmacokinetics.
- They may be less able to obtain or afford drugs.

There are 2 main approaches to optimizing drug therapy in the elderly:

- Using appropriate drugs as indicated to maximize cost-effectiveness
- Avoiding adverse drug effects

Because the risk of adverse drug effects is higher, overprescribing (polypharmacy) has been targeted as a major problem for the elderly. However, underprescribing appropriate drugs must also be avoided.

PHARMACOKINETICS IN THE ELDERLY

Pharmacokinetics (see also p. 2914) is best defined as what the body does to the drug; it includes

- Absorption
- Distribution across body compartments
- Metabolism
- Excretion

With aging, there are changes in all these areas; some changes are more clinically relevant. The metabolism and excretion of many drugs decrease, requiring that doses of some drugs be adjusted. Toxicity may develop slowly because levels of chronically used drugs increase for 5 to 6 half-lives, until a steady state is achieved. For example, certain benzodiazepines (diazepam, flurazepam, chlordiazepoxide) have half-lives of up to 96 h in elderly patients; signs of toxicity may not appear until days or weeks after therapy is started.

Absorption: Despite an age-related decrease in small-bowel surface area, slowed gastric emptying, and an increase in gastric pH, changes in drug absorption tend to be clinically inconsequential for most drugs. One exception is Ca carbonate, which requires an acidic environment for optimal absorption. Age-related increases in gastric pH decrease Ca absorption and increase the risk of constipation. Thus, elderly patients should use a Ca salt (eg, Ca citrate) that dissolves more easily in a less acidic environment. Another example of altered absorption is early release of enteric-coated dosage forms with increased gastric pH.

Distribution: With age, body fat generally increases and total body water decreases. Increased fat increases the volume of distribution for highly lipophilic drugs (eg, diazepam, chlordiazepoxide) and may increase their elimination half-lives.

Serum albumin decreases and α1-acid glycoprotein increases with age, but the clinical effect of these changes on serum drug binding is unclear. In patients with an acute disorder or malnutrition, rapid reductions in serum albumin may enhance drug effects because serum levels of unbound (free) drug may increase (only unbound drug has a pharmacologic effect). Phenytoin and warfarin are drugs with a high risk of toxic effects when serum albumin level decreases.

Hepatic metabolism: Overall hepatic metabolism of many drugs through the cytochrome P-450 enzyme system decreases with age. For drugs with decreased hepatic metabolism (see Table 335–1), clearance typically decreases 30 to 40%. Theoretically, maintenance drug doses should be decreased by this percentage; however, rate of drug metabolism varies greatly from person to person, and individual dose adjustment is required.

Hepatic clearance of drugs metabolized by phase I reactions (oxidation, reduction, hydrolysis—see Table 348–2 on p. 2919) is more likely to be prolonged in the elderly. Usually, age does not greatly affect clearance of drugs that are metabolized by conjugation (phase II reactions).

First-pass metabolism (metabolism, typically hepatic, that occurs before a drug reaches systemic circulation) is also affected by aging, decreasing by about 1%/yr after age 40. Thus, for a given oral dose, the elderly may have higher circulating drug levels. Important examples of drugs with a high risk of toxic effects include nitrates, propranolol, phenobarbital, and nifedipine.

Renal elimination: One of the most important pharmacokinetic changes associated with aging is decreased renal elimination of drugs. After age 30, creatinine clearance decreases an average of 8 mL/min/1.73 m^2/decade; however, the age-related decrease varies substantially from person to person. Serum creatinine levels often remain within normal limits despite a decrease in GFR because the elderly generally have less muscle mass and are generally less physically active than younger adults and thus produce less creatinine. Maintenance of normal serum creatinine levels can mislead clinicians who assume those levels reflect normal kidney function. Decreases in tubular function with age parallel those in glomerular function.

These changes decrease renal elimination of many drugs (see Table 335–1). Clinical implications depend on the extent that renal elimination contributes to total systemic elimination and on the drug's therapeutic index (ratio of maximum tolerated dose to minimum effective dose). Creatinine clearance (measured or estimated using computer programs or a formula, such as Cockcroft-Gault—see p. 2055) is used to guide drug dosing. The daily dose of drugs that rely heavily on renal elimination should be lower and/or the frequency of dosing should be decreased. Because renal function is dynamic, maintenance doses of drugs may need adjustment when patients become ill or dehydrated or have recently recovered from dehydration.

Table 335–1. EFFECT OF AGING ON METABOLISM* AND ELIMINATION OF SOME DRUGS

CLASS OR CATEGORY	DECREASED HEPATIC METABOLISM	DECREASED RENAL ELIMINATION
Analgesics and anti-inflammatory drugs	Ibuprofen Meperidine Morphine Naproxen	Meperidine Morphine Oxycodone
Antibiotics	—	Amikacin Ciprofloxacin Gentamicin Levofloxacin Nitrofurantoin Streptomycin Tobramycin
Cardiovascular drugs	Amlodipine Diltiazem Lidocaine† Nifedipine Propranolol Quinidine Theophylline Verapamil Warfarin	*N*-Acetylprocainamide Apixaban Captopril Dabigatran Digoxin Enalapril Enoxaparin Heparin Lisinopril Procainamide Quinapril Rivaroxaban
Diuretics	—	Amiloride Furosemide Hydrochlorothiazide Triamterene
Psychoactive drugs	Alprazolam† Chlordiazepoxide Desipramine† Diazepam Imipramine Nortriptyline Trazodone Triazolam†	Risperidone
Others	Levodopa	Amantadine Chlorpropamide Cimetidine Exenatide Gabapentin Glyburide Lithium Metoclopramide Ranitidine Sitagliptin

*When aging's effect on hepatic metabolism of a drug is controversial, effects reported in the majority of studies are listed.

†The effect occurs in men but not in women.

PHARMACODYNAMICS IN THE ELDERLY

Pharmacodynamics is defined as what the drug does to the body or the response of the body to the drug; it is affected by receptor binding, postreceptor effects, and chemical interactions (see p. 2914). In the elderly, the effects of similar drug concentrations at the site of action (sensitivity) may be greater or smaller than those in younger people (see Table 335–2). Differences may be due to changes in drug-receptor interaction, in postreceptor events, or in adaptive homeostatic responses and, among frail patients, are often due to pathologic changes in organs.

Elderly patients are particularly sensitive to anticholinergic drug effects. Many drugs (eg, tricyclic antidepressants, sedating antihistamines, urinary antimuscarinic agents, some antipsychotic drugs, antiparkinsonian drugs with atropine-like activity, many OTC hypnotics and cold preparations) have anticholinergic effects. The elderly, most notably those with cognitive impairment, are particularly prone to CNS adverse effects of such drugs and may become more confused and drowsy. Anticholinergic drugs also commonly cause constipation, urinary retention (especially in elderly men with benign prostatic hyperplasia), blurred vision, orthostatic hypotension, and dry mouth. Even in low doses, these drugs can increase risk of heatstroke by inhibiting diaphoresis. In general, older adults should avoid drugs with anticholinergic effects when possible.

DRUG-RELATED PROBLEMS IN THE ELDERLY

Drug-related problems are common in the elderly and include drug ineffectiveness, adverse drug effects, overdosage, underdosage, and drug interactions.

Drugs may be ineffective in the elderly because clinicians underprescribe (eg, because of increased concern about adverse effects) or because adherence is poor (eg, because of financial or cognitive limitations).

Adverse drug effects are effects that are unwanted, uncomfortable, or dangerous. Common examples are oversedation, confusion, hallucinations, falls, and bleeding. Among ambulatory people ≥ 65, adverse drug effects occur at a rate of about 50 events per 1000 person-years. Hospitalization rates due to adverse drug effects are 4 times higher in elderly patients (about 17%) than in younger patients (4%).

Reasons for Drug-Related Problems

Adverse drug effects can occur in any patient, but certain characteristics of the elderly make them more susceptible. For example, the elderly often take many drugs (polypharmacy) and have age-related changes in pharmacodynamics and pharmacokinetics; both increase the risk of adverse effects.

At any age, adverse drug effects may occur when drugs are prescribed and taken appropriately; eg, new-onset allergic reactions are not predictable or preventable. However, adverse effects are thought to be preventable in almost 90% of cases in the elderly (compared with only 24% in younger patients). Certain drug classes are commonly involved: antipsychotics, warfarin, antiplatelet agents, hypoglycemic drugs, antidepressants, and sedative-hypnotics.

In the elderly, a number of common reasons for adverse drug effects, ineffectiveness, or both are preventable (see Table 335–3). Several of these reasons involve inadequate communication with patients or between health care practitioners (particularly during health care transitions).

Drug-disease interactions: A drug given to treat one disease can exacerbate another disease regardless of patient age, but such interactions are of special concern in the elderly. Distinguishing often subtle adverse drug effects from the effects of disease is difficult (see Table 335–4) and may lead to a prescribing cascade.

A **prescribing cascade** occurs when the adverse effect of a drug is misinterpreted as a symptom or sign of a new disorder and a new drug is prescribed to treat it. The new, unnecessary

Table 335–2. EFFECT OF AGING ON DRUG RESPONSE

CLASS	DRUG	ACTION	EFFECT OF AGING
Analgesics	Morphine	Acute analgesic effect	↑
	Pentazocine	Analgesic effect	↑
Anticoagulants	Heparin	PTT	↔
	Warfarin	PT/INR	↑
Bronchodilators	Albuterol	Bronchodilation	↓
	Ipratropium	Bronchodilation	↔
Cardiovascular drugs	Angiotensin II receptor blockers	Decreased BP	↑
	Diltiazem	Acute antihypertensive effect	↑
	Dopamine	Increased creatinine clearance	↓
	Enalapril	Acute antihypertensive effect	↑
	Felodipine	Antihypertensive effect	↑
	Isoproterenol	Increased heart rate	↓
		Increased ejection fraction	↓
		Venodilation	↓
	Nitroglycerin	Venodilation	↔
	Norepinephrine	Acute vasoconstriction	↔
	Phenylephrine	Acute venoconstriction	↔
		Acute hypertensive effect	↔
	Prazosin	Acute antihypertensive effect	↔
	Propranolol (and other β-blockers)	Decreased heart rate	↓
	Verapamil	Acute antihypertensive effect, cardiac conduction effects	↑
Diuretics	Bumetanide	Increased urine flow and Na excretion	↓
	Furosemide	Latency and size of peak diuretic response	↓
Oral hypoglycemics	Glyburide	Chronic hypoglycemic effect	↔
	Tolbutamide	Acute hypoglycemic effect	↓
Psychoactive drugs	Diazepam	Sedation	↑
	Diphenhydramine	Psychomotor dysfunction	↑
	Haloperidol	Acute sedation	↑
	Midazolam	EEG activity	↑
		Sedation	↑
	Temazepam	Postural sway	↑
		Psychomotor effect	↑
		Sedation	↑
	Thiopental	Anesthesia	↔
	Triazolam	Sedation	↑
Others	Atropine	Impaired gastric emptying	↓
	Levodopa	Adverse effects	↑
	Metoclopramide	Sedation	↔

↔ = unchanged; ↑ = increased; ↓ = decreased.

Adapted and updated from Cusack BJ, Vestal RE: Clinical pharmacology: Special considerations in the elderly. In *Practice of Geriatric Medicine*, edited by E Calkins, PJ Davis, and AB Ford. Philadelphia, WB Saunders Company, 1986, pp. 115–136; used with permission.

Table 335–3. PREVENTABLE CAUSES OF DRUG-RELATED PROBLEMS

CATEGORY	DEFINITION
Drug interactions	Use of a drug results in a drug-drug, drug-food, drug-supplement, or drug-disease interaction, leading to adverse effects or decreased efficacy.
Inadequate monitoring	A medical problem is being treated with the correct drug, but the patient is not adequately monitored for complications, effectiveness, or both.
Inappropriate drug selection	A medical problem that requires drug therapy is being treated with a less-than-optimal drug.
Inappropriate treatment	A patient is taking a drug for no medically valid reason.
Lack of patient adherence	The correct drug for a medical problem is prescribed, but the patient is not taking it.
Overdosage	A medical problem is being treated with too much of the correct drug.
Poor communication	Drugs are inappropriately continued or stopped when care is transitioned between providers and/or facilities.
Underprescribing	A medical problem is being treated with too little of the correct drug.
Untreated medical problem	A medical problem requires drug therapy, but no drug is being used to treat that problem.

drug may cause additional adverse effects, which may then be misinterpreted as yet another disorder and treated unnecessarily, and so on.

Many drugs have adverse effects that resemble symptoms of disorders common among the elderly or changes due to aging. The following are examples:

- **Antipsychotics** may cause symptoms that resemble Parkinson disease. In elderly patients, these symptoms may be diagnosed as Parkinson disease and treated, possibly leading to adverse effects from the antiparkinson drugs (eg, orthostatic hypotension, delirium, nausea).
- **Cholinesterase inhibitors** (eg, donepezil) may be prescribed for patients with dementia. These drugs may cause diarrhea or urinary incontinence. Patients may then be prescribed an anticholinergic drug (eg, oxybutynin) to treat the new symptoms. Thus, an unnecessary drug is added, increasing the risk of adverse drug effects and drug-drug interactions. A better strategy is to reduce the dose of the cholinesterase inhibitor or consider a different treatment for dementia (eg, memantine) with a different mechanism of action.

In elderly patients, prescribers should always consider the possibility that a new symptom or sign is due to drug therapy.

Drug-drug interactions: Because the elderly often take many drugs, they are particularly vulnerable to drug-drug interactions. The elderly also frequently use medicinal herbs and other dietary supplements (see p. 3159) and may not tell their health care providers. Medicinal herbs can interact with prescribed drugs and lead to adverse effects. For example, ginkgo biloba extract taken with warfarin can increase risk of bleeding, and St. John's wort taken with an SSRI can increase risk of serotonin syndrome. Therefore, physicians should ask patients specifically about dietary supplements, including medicinal herbs and vitamin supplements.

Drug-drug interactions in the elderly differ little from those in the general population. However, induction of cytochrome P-450 (CYP450) drug metabolism (see p. 2918) by certain drugs (eg, phenytoin, carbamazepine, rifampin) may be decreased in the elderly; therefore, the change (increase) in drug metabolism may be less pronounced in the elderly. Many other drugs inhibit CYP450 metabolism and thus increase the risk of toxicity of drugs that depend on that pathway for elimination. Because the elderly typically use a larger number of drugs, they are at greater risk of multiple, difficult-to-predict CYP450 interactions. Also, concurrent use of ≥ 1 drug with similar adverse effects can increase risk or severity of adverse effects.

Inadequate monitoring: Monitoring drug use involves

- Documenting the indication for a new drug
- Keeping a current list of drugs used by the patient in medical records
- Monitoring for achievement of therapeutic goals and other responses to new drugs
- Monitoring necessary laboratory tests for efficacy or adverse effects
- Periodically reviewing drugs for continued need

Such measures are especially important for elderly patients. Lack of close monitoring, especially after new drugs are prescribed, increases risk of adverse effects and ineffectiveness. Criteria to facilitate monitoring have been developed by the Health Care Financing Administration expert consensus panel as part of drug utilization review criteria. The criteria focus on inappropriate dosage or duration of therapy, duplication of therapy, and possible drug-drug interactions.

Inappropriate drug selection: A drug is inappropriate if its potential for harm is greater than its potential for benefit. Inappropriate use of a drug may involve

- Choice of an unsuitable drug, dose, frequency of dosing, or duration of therapy
- Duplication of therapy
- Failure to consider drug interactions and correct indications for a drug
- Appropriate drugs that are mistakenly continued once an acute condition resolves (as may happen when patients move from one health care setting to another)

Adverse effects of inappropriate drugs account for about 7% of emergency hospitalizations for patients ≥ 65 yr, and 67% of these hospitalizations are due to 4 drugs or drug classes—warfarin, insulin, oral antiplatelet drugs, and oral hypoglycemic drugs. Some classes of drugs are of special concern in the elderly (see p. 2856). Some drugs are so problematic that they should be avoided altogether in the elderly, some should be avoided only in certain situations, and others can be used but with increased caution. The Beers Criteria (see Table 335–5) lists potentially inappropriate drugs for the elderly by drug class; other similar lists are available. However, currently, there are no similar lists of drugs that *should* be used in the elderly; clinicians must weigh benefits and risks of therapy in each patient.

Table 335–4. DRUG-DISEASE INTERACTIONS IN THE ELDERLY (BASED ON THE AMERICAN GERIATRICS SOCIETY 2012 BEERS CRITERIA UPDATE)

DISEASE	DRUGS	POSSIBLE ADVERSE EFFECTS
Cardiovascular		
Heart failure	Cilostazol, COX-2 inhibitors, dronedarone, nondihydropyridine Ca channel blockers* (diltiazem, verapamil), NSAIDs, pioglitazone, rosiglitazone	May promote fluid retention and exacerbate heart failure
Syncope	Acetylcholinesterase inhibitors, chlorpromazine, peripheral α-blockers (doxazosin, prazosin, terazosin), tertiary TCAs, thioridazine, olanzapine	Increased risk of orthostatic hypotension or bradycardia
CNS		
Chronic seizures or epilepsy	Bupropion, chlorpromazine, clozapine, maprotiline, olanzapine, thioridazine, thiothixene, tramadol	Lowered seizure threshold Possibly acceptable in patients with well-controlled seizures in whom alternative agents have not been effective
Delirium	All TCAs, benzodiazepines, drugs that have anticholinergic effects, chlorpromazine, corticosteroids, H_2 receptor blockers, meperidine, sedative hypnotics, thioridazine	Worsened delirium in older adults with or at high risk of delirium If discontinuing drugs used chronically, taper to avoid withdrawal symptoms
Dementia and cognitive impairment	Antipsychotics (chronic and as-needed use), benzodiazepines, drugs that have anticholinergic effects, H_2 receptor blockers, zolpidem	Adverse CNS effects For antipsychotics, increased risk of stroke and mortality in patients with dementia
History of falls or fractures	Anticonvulsants, antipsychotics, benzodiazepines, nonbenzodiazepine hypnotics (eszopiclone, zaleplon, zolpidem), TCAs, SSRIs	Ataxia, impaired psychomotor function, syncope, and additional falls; shorter-acting benzodiazepines are not safer than long-acting ones Can be used if safer alternatives are not available Avoid anticonvulsants except for seizure disorders
Insomnia	Oral decongestants (pseudoephedrine, phenylephrine), stimulants (amphetamine, methylphenidate, pemoline), theobromines (theophylline, caffeine)	CNS stimulant effects
Parkinson disease	Antiemetics (metoclopramide, prochlorperazine, promethazine), antipsychotics (except for quetiapine and clozapine)	Dopamine receptor antagonists with potential to worsen parkinsonian symptoms (less likely with quetiapine and clozapine)
GI		
Chronic constipation	Drugs that have antispasmodic and anticholinergic effects (antipsychotics, belladonna alkaloids, clidinium-chlordiazepoxide, dicyclomine, hyoscyamine, propantheline, scopolamine, tertiary TCAs [amitriptyline, clomipramine, doxepin, imipramine, and trimipramine]), first-generation antihistamines (brompheniramine carbinoxamine, chlorpheniramine, clemastine, cyproheptadine, dexbrompheniramine, dexchlorpheniramine, diphenhydramine, doxylamine, hydroxyzine, promethazine, triprolidine), nondihydropyridine Ca channel blockers (diltiazem, verapamil), oral antimuscarinics for urinary incontinence (darifenacin, fesoterodine, oxybutynin, solifenacin, tolterodine, trospium)	Can worsen constipation; agents for urinary incontinence: antimuscarinics overall differ in incidence of constipation; response variable; consider alternative agent if constipation develops
History of gastric or duodenal ulcers	Aspirin (> 325 mg/day), non–COX-2 selective NSAIDs	Exacerbate existing ulcers or cause new ulcers Avoid unless other alternatives are not effective and patients can take a gastroprotective drug (eg, a proton pump inhibitor or misoprostol)

Table continues on the following page.

Table 335–4. DRUG-DISEASE INTERACTIONS IN THE ELDERLY (BASED ON THE AMERICAN GERIATRICS SOCIETY 2012 BEERS CRITERIA UPDATE) (*Continued*)

DISEASE	DRUGS	POSSIBLE ADVERSE EFFECTS
Kidney and Urinary Tract		
Chronic kidney disease (stages IV and V)	NSAIDs, triamterene	Increased risk of kidney injury
Urinary incontinence (all types) in women	Estrogen, oral and transdermal (excludes intravaginal estrogen)	Worsened incontinence
Lower urinary tract symptoms, benign prostatic hyperplasia	Drugs that have strong anticholinergic effects (except antimuscarinics for urinary incontinence), inhaled agents that have anticholinergic effects	May decrease urinary flow and cause urinary retention in men
Stress or mixed urinary incontinence	α-Blockers (doxazosin, prazosin, terazosin)	Worsened incontinence in women

*Avoid only in patients who have systolic heart failure.
COX-2 = cyclooxygenase-2, TCAs = tricyclic antidepressants.
Adapted from The American Geriatrics Society 2012 Beers Criteria Update Expert Panel: American Geriatrics Society updated Beers criteria for potentially inappropriate medication use in older adults. *Journal of the American Geriatrics Society* 60: 616–631, 2012.

Despite the Beers and other criteria, inappropriate drugs are still being prescribed for the elderly; typically, about 20% of community-dwelling elderly received at least one inappropriate drug. In such patients, risk of adverse effects is increased. In nursing home patients, inappropriate use also increases risk of hospitalization and death. In one study of hospitalized patients, 27.5% received an inappropriate drug.

Some inappropriate drugs are available OTC; thus, clinicians should specifically question patients about use of OTC drugs and tell patients about the potential problems such drugs can cause.

The elderly are often given drugs (typically, analgesics, H_2 blockers, hypnotics, or laxatives) for minor symptoms (including adverse effects of other drugs) that may be better treated nonpharmacologically or by lowering the dose of the drug causing adverse effects. Initiating additional drugs is often inappropriate; benefit may be low, costs are increased, and the new drug may lead to additional toxicity.

Solving the problem of inappropriate use in the elderly requires more than avoiding a short list of drugs and noting drug categories of concern. A patient's entire drug regimen should also be assessed regularly to determine potential benefit vs harm.

Lack of patient adherence: Drug effectiveness is often compromised by lack of patient adherence among the ambulatory elderly. Adherence is affected by many factors but not by age per se. Up to half of elderly patients do not take drugs as directed, usually taking less than prescribed (underadherence). Causes are similar to those for younger adults (see p. 2908). In addition, the following contribute:

- Financial and physical constraints, which may make purchasing drugs difficult
- Cognitive problems, which may make taking drugs as instructed difficult
- Use of multiple drugs
- Use of drugs that must be taken several times a day or in a specific manner
- Lack of understanding about what a drug is intended to do (benefits) or how to recognize and manage adverse effects (harms)

A regimen using too frequent or too infrequent dosing, multiple drugs, or both may be too complicated for patients to follow. Clinicians should assess patients' health literacy and abilities to adhere to a drug regimen (eg, dexterity, hand strength, cognition, vision) and try to accommodate their limitations—eg, by arranging for or recommending easy-access containers, drug labels and instructions in large type, containers equipped with reminder alarms, containers filled based on daily drug needs, reminder telephone calls, or medication assistance. Pharmacists and nurses can help by providing education and reviewing prescription instructions with elderly patients at each encounter. Pharmacists may be able to identify a problem by noting whether patients obtain refills on schedule or whether a prescription seems illogical or incorrect.

Overdosage: An excessive dose of an appropriate drug may be prescribed for elderly patients if the prescriber does not consider age-related changes that affect pharmacokinetics (see p. 2914) and pharmacodynamics (see p. 2912). For example, doses of renally cleared drugs should be adjusted in patients with renal impairment.

Generally, although dose requirements vary considerably from person to person, drugs should be started at the lowest dose in the elderly. Typically, starting doses of about one third to one half the usual adult dose are indicated when a drug has a narrow therapeutic index or when another condition may be exacerbated by a drug. The dose is then titrated upward as tolerated to the desired effect. When the dose is increased, patients should be evaluated for adverse effects, and drug levels should be monitored when possible.

Overdosage can also occur when drug interactions (see p. 2850) increase the amount of drug available or when different practitioners prescribe a drug and are unaware that another practitioner prescribed the same or a similar drug (therapeutic duplication).

Poor communication: Poor communication of medical information at transition points (from one health care setting to another) causes up to 50% of all drug errors and up to 20% of adverse drug effects in the hospital. When patients are discharged from the hospital, drug regimens that were started and needed only in the hospital (eg, sedative hypnotics, laxatives, proton pump inhibitors) may be unnecessarily continued by another prescriber, who is reluctant to communicate with the previous prescriber. Conversely, at admission to a health care facility, lack of communication may result in unintentional omission of a necessary maintenance drug.

Table 335–5. POTENTIALLY INAPPROPRIATE DRUGS IN THE ELDERLY (BASED ON THE AMERICAN GERIATRICS SOCIETY 2012 BEERS CRITERIA UPDATE)

DRUG	PRESCRIBING CONCERN/RECOMMENDATIONS
Anticholinergics*	
First-generation antihistamines, as single agents or in combination products (brompheniramine, carbinoxamine, chlorpheniramine, clemastine, cyproheptadine, dexbrompheniramine, dexchlorpheniramine, diphenhydramine [oral], doxylamine, hydroxyzine, promethazine, triprolidine)	Highly anticholinergic; greater risk of confusion, dry mouth, constipation, and other anticholinergic effects and toxicity Clearance reduced with advanced age; tolerance develops when used as hypnotics Avoid, except use of diphenhydramine in special situations (eg, severe allergic reaction) may be appropriate
Antiparkinson drugs (benztropine [oral], trihexyphenidyl)	Not recommended for prevention of extrapyramidal symptoms with antipsychotics; more effective agents available for treatment of Parkinson disease
Antispasmodics (belladonna alkaloids, clidinium-chlordiazepoxide, dicyclomine, hyoscyamine, propantheline, scopolamine)	Highly anticholinergic, uncertain effectiveness Avoid except short-term use in palliative care to decrease oral secretions
Anti-infectives	
Nitrofurantoin	May cause pulmonary toxicity; safer alternatives available; lack of efficacy in patients with creatinine clearance < 60 mL/min due to inadequate drug concentration in the urine; do not use for long-term suppression or in patients with creatinine clearance < 60 mL/min
Antithrombotics	
Dipyridamole, oral short-acting[†] (does not apply to extended-release combination with aspirin)	Possible orthostatic hypotension; more effective alternatives available; avoid, except IV form acceptable for cardiac stress testing
Ticlopidine[†]	Safer effective alternatives available; avoid
Cardiovascular drugs	
Alpha-1 blockers (doxazosin, prazosin, terazosin)	High risk of orthostatic hypotension; alternative drugs have better risk/benefit ratio; avoid use as an antihypertensive
Alpha agonists, central (clonidine, guanabenz[†], guanfacine[†], methyldopa[†], reserpine [> 0.1 mg/day][†])	High risk of adverse CNS effects; may cause bradycardia and orthostatic hypotension; avoid clonidine as first-line hypertensive; others not recommended
Antiarrhythmic drugs, classes Ia, Ic, and III (amiodarone, dofetilide, dronedarone, flecainide, ibutilide, procainamide, propafenone, quinidine, sotalol)	Rate control preferred over rhythm control; avoid as first-line treatment for atrial fibrillation For amiodarone, increased risk of thyroid disease, pulmonary disorders, and QT interval prolongation
Disopyramide[†]	Potent negative inotrope (may induce heart failure); strongly anticholinergic; avoid, other antiarrhythmic drugs preferred
Dronedarone	Worse outcomes in patients who have permanent atrial fibrillation or heart failure; avoid Rate control preferred over rhythm control for atrial fibrillation
Digoxin (> 0.125 mg/day)	In patients with heart failure and/or low creatinine clearance, higher dosages associated with no additional benefit and increased risk of toxicity; avoid
Nifedipine, immediate release[†]	Risk of hypotension and myocardial ischemia; avoid
Spironolactone (> 25 mg/day)	In patients with heart failure, risk of hyperkalemia especially if also taking an NSAID, ACE inhibitor, angiotensin receptor blocker, or K supplement; avoid in heart failure or if creatinine clearance < 30 mL/min
CNS	
Tertiary TCAs, alone or in combination (amitriptyline, chlordiazepoxide-amitriptyline, clomipramine, doxepin [> 6 mg/day], imipramine, perphenazine-amitriptyline, trimipramine)	Highly anticholinergic and sedating and cause orthostatic hypotension; avoid
Antipsychotics, 1st (conventional) and 2nd (atypical) generations	Increased risk of stroke and mortality in patients with dementia Avoid in patients with dementia-related behavior problems unless nonpharmacologic options have failed and patients are a threat to themselves or others

Table continues on the following page.

Table 335–5. POTENTIALLY INAPPROPRIATE DRUGS IN THE ELDERLY (BASED ON THE AMERICAN GERIATRICS SOCIETY 2012 BEERS CRITERIA UPDATE) (*Continued*)

DRUG	PRESCRIBING CONCERN/RECOMMENDATIONS
Thioridazine Mesoridazine	Highly anticholinergic; risk of QT interval prolongation; avoid
Barbiturates (amobarbital†, butabarbital†, butalbital, mephobarbital†, pentobarbital†, phenobarbital, secobarbital†)	High rate of physical dependence and tolerance; risk of overdose at low dosages; avoid
Benzodiazepines, short- and intermediate-acting (alprazolam, estazolam, lorazepam, oxazepam, temazepam, triazolam) Benzodiazepines, long-acting (clorazepate, chlordiazepoxide, chlordiazepoxide-amitriptyline, clidinium-chlordiazepoxide, clonazepam, diazepam, flurazepam, quazepam)	Increased risk of cognitive impairment, delirium, falls, fractures, and motor vehicle crashes May be appropriate for seizure disorders, rapid eye movement sleep disorders, benzodiazepine withdrawal, ethanol withdrawal, severe generalized anxiety disorder, periprocedural anesthesia, end-of-life care Avoid use for insomnia, agitation, or delirium
Chloral hydrate†	Can overdose at only 3 times recommended dose; tolerance occurs within 10 days; risks outweigh benefits; avoid
Meprobamate	High rate of physical dependence; very sedating; avoid
Nonbenzodiazepine hypnotics (eszopiclone, zolpidem, zaleplon)	Similar to benzodiazepines (eg, delirium, falls, fractures); minimal improvement in sleep latency and duration Not to be used for > 90 days
Ergot mesylates† Isoxsuprine†	Lack of efficacy; avoid
Endocrine therapy	
Androgens (methyltestosterone†, testosterone)	Potential for cardiac problems; exacerbation of prostate cancer Avoid except for moderate to severe hypogonadism
Desiccated thyroid	Possible cardiac effects; safer alternatives available; avoid
Estrogens with or without progestins	Possible carcinogenic potential (breast and endometrium); lack of cardioprotective effect and cognitive protection in older women Topical vaginal cream low dose can be used for dyspareunia, lower UTIs, and other vaginal symptoms; evidence that low doses (estradiol < 25 mcg twice/wk) may be safe in women with breast cancer Avoid topical patch and oral
Growth hormone	Little effect on body composition; associated with edema, arthralgia, carpal tunnel syndrome, gynecomastia, impaired fasting glucose Avoid except for hormone replacement after pituitary gland removal
Insulin, sliding scale	Higher risk of hypoglycemia without improvement in glucose control regardless of care setting; avoid
Megestrol	Minimal effect on weight; increases risk of thrombotic events and possibly death; avoid
Sulfonylureas, long duration (chlorpropamide, glyburide)	Chlorpropamide: Prolonged half-life; can cause prolonged hypoglycemia, syndrome of inappropriate antidiuretic hormone secretion; avoid Glyburide: Greater risk of severe prolonged hypoglycemia; avoid
GI therapy	
Metoclopramide	Can cause extrapyramidal effects including tardive dyskinesia; risk may be greater in frail older adults; avoid except for gastroparesis
Mineral oil, oral	Potential for aspiration; safer alternatives available; avoid
Trimethobenzamide	One of the least effective antiemetics; can cause extrapyramidal effects; avoid
Pain management	
Meperidine	Not an effective oral analgesic in common dosages; may cause neurotoxicity; safer alternatives available; avoid

Table 335–5. POTENTIALLY INAPPROPRIATE DRUGS IN THE ELDERLY (BASED ON THE AMERICAN GERIATRICS SOCIETY 2012 BEERS CRITERIA UPDATE) (*Continued*)

DRUG	PRESCRIBING CONCERN/RECOMMENDATIONS
Non–COX-selective NSAIDs, oral (aspirin [> 325 mg/day], diclofenac, diflunisal, etodolac, fenoprofen, ibuprofen, ketoprofen, meclofenamate, mefenamic acid, meloxicam, nabumetone, naproxen, oxaprozin, piroxicam, sulindac, tolmetin)	Increased risk of GI bleeding and peptic ulcer disease in high-risk groups, including those aged > 75 or taking oral or parenteral corticosteroids, anticoagulants, or antiplatelet agents Upper GI ulcers, gross bleeding, or perforation occur in about 1% of patients treated for 3–6 mo and in about 2–4% of patients treated for 1 yr; these trends continue with longer duration of use Avoid chronic use unless other alternatives are ineffective and patients are able to take a proton pump inhibitor or misoprostol (which reduce but do not eliminate risk)
Indomethacin Ketorolac, includes parenteral	Increases risk of GI bleeding and peptic ulcer disease in high-risk groups (see above Non-COX selective NSAIDs) Of all the NSAIDs, indomethacin has most adverse effects; avoid
Pentazocine†	CNS adverse effects, including confusion and hallucinations, more common than with other opioids; is also a mixed agonist and antagonist; safer alternatives available; avoid
Skeletal muscle relaxants (carisoprodol, chlorzoxazone, cyclobenzaprine, metaxalone, methocarbamol, orphenadrine)	Poorly tolerated because of anticholinergic effects; sedation; risk of fracture; effectiveness at dosages tolerated by older adults is questionable; avoid

*TCAs are excluded.
†These drugs are used infrequently.
TCAs = tricyclic antidepressants.
Adapted from The American Geriatrics Society 2012 Beers Criteria Update Expert Panel: American Geriatrics Society updated Beers criteria for potentially inappropriate medication use in older adults. *Journal of the American Geriatrics Society* 60: 616–631, 2012.

Underprescribing: Appropriate drugs may be underprescribed—ie, not used for maximum effectiveness. Underprescribing may increase morbidity and mortality and reduce quality of life. Clinicians should use adequate drug doses and, when indicated, multidrug regimens.

Drugs that are often underprescribed in the elderly include those used to treat depression, Alzheimer disease, pain (eg, opioids), heart failure, post-MI (β-blockers), atrial fibrillation (warfarin), hypertension, glaucoma, and incontinence. Also, immunizations are not always given as recommended.

- **Opioids:** Clinicians are often reluctant to prescribe opioids for elderly patients with cancer or other types of chronic pain, typically because of concerns about adverse drug effects (eg, sedation, constipation, delirium) and development of dependence. When opioids are prescribed, the doses are often inadequate. Underprescribing opioids may mean that some elderly patients have needless pain and discomfort; elderly patients are more likely to report inadequate pain management than younger adults.
- **β-Blockers:** In patients with a history of MI and/or heart failure, even in elderly patients at high risk of complications (eg, those with pulmonary disorders or diabetes), these drugs reduce mortality rates and hospitalizations.
- **Antihypertensives:** Guidelines for treating hypertension in the elderly are available, and treatment appears to be beneficial (reducing risk of stroke and major cardiovascular events). Nonetheless, studies indicate that hypertension is often not controlled in elderly patients.
- **Drugs for Alzheimer disease:** Acetylcholinesterase inhibitors and NMDA (*N*-methyl-D-aspartate) antagonists have been shown to benefit patients with Alzheimer disease. The amount of benefit is unclear, but patients and family members should be given the opportunity to make an informed decision about their use.
- **Anticoagulants:** Anticoagulants reduce risk of stroke in patients with atrial fibrillation. Although there is an increased risk of bleeding with anticoagulation, some older adults who might nonetheless benefit from anticoagulation are not receiving it.
- **Immunizations:** Older adults are at greater risk of morbidity and mortality resulting from influenza, pneumococcal infection, and herpes zoster. Vaccination rates among older adults can still be improved.

In elderly patients with a chronic disorder, acute or unrelated disorders may be undertreated (eg, hypercholesterolemia may be untreated in patients with emphysema). Clinicians may withhold these treatments because they are concerned about increasing the risk of adverse effects or the time required to benefit from treatment. Clinicians may think that treatment of the primary problem is all patients can or want to handle or that patients cannot afford the additional drugs. Patients should participate in decision making about drug treatment so that clinicians can understand patients' priorities and concerns.

Prevention

Before starting a new drug: To reduce the risk of adverse drug effects in the elderly, clinicians should do the following before starting a new drug:

- Consider nondrug treatment
- Discuss goals of care with the patient
- Document the indication for each new drug (to avoid using unnecessary drugs)
- Consider age-related changes in pharmacokinetics or pharmacodynamics and their effect on dosing requirements

- Choose the safest possible alternative (eg, for noninflammatory arthritis, acetaminophen instead of an NSAID)
- Check for potential drug-disease and drug-drug interactions
- Start with a low dose
- Use the fewest drugs necessary
- Note coexisting disorders and their likelihood of contributing to adverse drug effects
- Explain the uses and adverse effects of each drug
- Provide clear instructions to patients about how to take their drugs (including generic and brand names, spelling of each drug name, indication for each drug, and explanation of formulations that contain more than one drug) and for how long the drug will likely be necessary
- Anticipate confusion due to sound-alike drug names and pointing out any names that could be confused (eg, Glucophage® and Glucovance®)

After starting a drug: The following should be done after starting a drug:

- Assume a new symptom may be drug-related until proved otherwise (to prevent a prescribing cascade).
- Monitor patients for signs of adverse drug effects, including measuring drug levels and doing other laboratory tests as necessary.
- Document the response to therapy and increase doses as necessary to achieve the desired effect.
- Regularly reevaluate the need to continue drug therapy and stop drugs that are no longer necessary.

Ongoing: The following should be ongoing:

Medication reconciliation is a process that helps ensure transfer of information about drug regimens at any transition point in the health care system. The process includes identifying and listing all drugs patients are taking (name, dose, frequency, route) and comparing the resulting list with the physician's orders at a transition point. Medication reconciliation should occur at each move (admission, transfer, and discharge).

Computerized physician ordering programs can alert clinicians to potential problems (eg, allergy, need for reduced dosage in patients with impaired renal function, drug-drug interactions). These programs can also cue clinicians to monitor certain patients closely for adverse drug effects.

DRUG CATEGORIES OF CONCERN IN THE ELDERLY

Some drug categories (eg, analgesics, anticoagulants, antihypertensives, antiparkinsonian drugs, diuretics, hypoglycemic drugs, psychoactive drugs) pose special risks for elderly patients. Some drugs, although reasonable for use in younger adults, are so risky they should be considered inappropriate for the elderly. The Beers Criteria are most commonly used to identify such inappropriate drugs (see Table 335–5). The 2012 American Geriatrics Society updates to the Beers criteria further categorize potentially inappropriate drugs into 3 groups:

- Inappropriate: Always to be avoided
- Potentially inappropriate: To be avoided in certain diseases or syndromes
- To be used with caution: Benefit may offset risk in some patients (see Table 335–6)

Analgesics: NSAIDs are used by > 30% of people aged 65 to 89, and half of all NSAID prescriptions are for people > 60. Several NSAIDs are available without prescription.

The elderly may be prone to adverse effects of these drugs, and adverse effects may be more severe because of the following:

- NSAIDs are highly lipid-soluble, and because adipose tissue increases with age, distribution of the drugs is extensive.
- Plasma protein is often decreased, resulting in higher levels of unbound drug and exaggerated pharmacologic effects.
- Renal function is reduced in many of the elderly, resulting in decreased renal clearance and higher drug levels.

Serious adverse effects include peptic ulceration and upper GI bleeding; risk is increased when an NSAID is begun and when dose is increased. Risk of upper GI bleeding increases when NSAIDs are given with warfarin, aspirin, or other antiplatelet drugs (eg, clopidogrel). NSAIDs may increase risk of cardiovascular events and can cause fluid retention and, rarely, nephropathy.

NSAIDs can also increase BP; this effect may be unrecognized and lead to intensification of antihypertensive treatment (a prescribing cascade—see p. 2848). Thus, clinicians should keep this effect in mind when BP increases in elderly patients and ask them about their use of NSAIDs, particularly OTC NSAIDs.

Selective COX-2 (cyclooxygenase-2) inhibitors (coxibs) cause less GI irritation and platelet inhibition than other NSAIDs. Nonetheless, coxibs still have a risk of GI bleeding, especially for patients taking warfarin or aspirin (even at a low dose) and for those who have had GI events. Coxibs, as a class, appear to increase risk of cardiovascular events, but risk may vary by drug; they should be used cautiously. Coxibs have renal effects comparable to those of other NSAIDs.

Lower-risk alternatives (eg, acetaminophen) should be used when possible. If NSAIDs are used in the elderly, the lowest effective dose should be used, and continued need should be reviewed frequently. If NSAIDs are used long-term, serum creatinine and BP should be monitored closely, especially in patients with other risk factors (eg, heart failure, renal impairment, cirrhosis with ascites, volume depletion, diuretic use).

Anticoagulants: Age may increase sensitivity to the anticoagulant effect of warfarin. Careful dosing and routine monitoring can largely overcome the increased risk of bleeding in elderly patients taking warfarin. Also, because drug interactions with warfarin are common, closer monitoring is necessary when new drugs are added or old ones are stopped; computerized drug interaction programs should be consulted if patients take multiple drugs. Patients should also be monitored for warfarin interactions with food, alcohol, and OTC drugs and supplements. The newer anticoagulants (dabigatran, rivaroxaban, apixaban) may be easier to dose and have fewer drug-drug interactions and food-drug interactions than warfarin, but still increase the risk of bleeding in elderly patients, particularly those with impaired renal function.

Antidepressants: Tricyclic antidepressants are effective but should rarely be used in the elderly. SSRIs and mixed reuptake inhibitors, such as serotonin-norepinephrine reuptake inhibitors (SNRIs), are as effective as tricyclic antidepressants and cause less toxicity; however, there are some concerns about some of these drugs:

- Paroxetine: This drug is more sedating than other SSRIs, has anticholinergic effects, and, like some other SSRIs, can inhibit hepatic cytochrome P-450 2D6 enzyme activity, possibly impairing the metabolism of several drugs, including tamoxifen, some antipsychotics, antiarrhythmics, and tricyclic antidepressants.

Table 335–6. DRUGS TO BE USED WITH CAUTION IN THE ELDERLY (BASED ON THE AMERICAN GERIATRICS SOCIETY 2012 BEERS CRITERIA UPDATE)

DRUG	REASON FOR CAUTION
Aspirin for primary prevention of cardiac events	Use with caution in patients ≥ 80 yr Lack of evidence regarding benefit vs risk in patients > 80 yr
Dabigatran	Use with caution in patients ≥ 75 yr or with creatinine clearance < 30 mL/min Greater risk of bleeding than warfarin in patients ≥ 75 yr Lack of evidence regarding efficacy and safety in patients with creatinine clearance < 30 mL/min
Prasugrel	Use with caution in patients ≥ 75 yr. Increased risk of bleeding; benefit may offset risk in highest-risk elderly (eg, those with previous MI or diabetes mellitus)
Antipsychotics Carbamazepine Carboplatin Cisplatin Mirtazapine Serotonin–norepinephrine reuptake inhibitors SSRIs Tricyclic antidepressants Vincristine	May worsen or cause syndrome of inappropriate antidiuretic hormone secretion or hyponatremia Monitor Na level closely when starting or changing dosages
Vasodilators	May increase episodes of syncope in patients with history of syncope

Adapted from The American Geriatrics Society 2012 Beers Criteria Update Expert Panel: American Geriatrics Society updated Beers criteria for potentially inappropriate medication use in older adults. *Journal of the American Geriatrics Society* 60: 616–631, 2012.

- Citalopram: Doses in the elderly should be limited to a maximum of 20 mg/day because QT prolongation is a concern.
- Venlafaxine: This drug may increase BP.
- Mirtazapine: This drug can be sedating and may stimulate appetite/weight gain.

Antihyperglycemics: Doses of antihyperglycemics should be titrated carefully in patients with diabetes mellitus. Risk of hypoglycemia due to sulfonylureas may increase with age. As described in Table 335–5, chlorpropamide is not recommended in elderly patients because of the increased risk of hypoglycemia and of hyponatremia due to the syndrome of inappropriate antidiuretic hormone secretion (SIADH). Risk of hypoglycemia is also greater with glyburide than with other oral antihyperglycemics because its renal clearance is reduced in the elderly.

Metformin, a biguanide excreted by the kidneys, increases peripheral tissue sensitivity to insulin and can be effective given alone or with sulfonylureas. Risk of lactic acidosis, a rare but serious complication, increases with degree of renal impairment and with patient age. Heart failure is a contraindication.

Antihypertensives: In many elderly patients, lower starting doses of antihypertensives may be necessary to reduce risk of adverse effects; however, for most elderly patients with hypertension, achieving BP goals requires standard doses and multidrug therapy. Initial treatment of hypertension in the elderly typically involves a thiazide-type diuretic, ACE inhibitor, angiotensin II receptor blocker, or dihydropyridine Ca channel blocker, depending on comorbidities. β-blockers should be reserved for 2nd-line therapy. Short-acting dihydropyridines (eg, nifedipine) may increase mortality risk and should not be used. Sitting and standing BP can be monitored, particularly when multiple antihypertensives are used, to check for orthostatic hypotension, which may increase risk of falls and fractures.

Antiparkinsonian drugs: Levodopa clearance is reduced in elderly patients, who are also more susceptible to the drug's adverse effects, particularly orthostatic hypotension and confusion. Therefore, elderly patients should be given a lower starting dose of levodopa and carefully monitored for adverse effects (see p. 1938). Patients who become confused while taking levodopa may also not tolerate dopamine agonists ß(eg, pramipexole, ropinirole). Because elderly patients with parkinsonism may be cognitively impaired, drugs with anticholinergic effects should be avoided.

Antipsychotics: Antipsychotics should be used only for psychosis. In nonpsychotic, agitated patients, antipsychotics control symptoms only marginally better than placebo and can have severe adverse effects. In people with dementia, studies showed antipsychotics increased mortality and risk of stroke, leading the FDA to issue a black box warning on their use in such patients. Generally, dementia-related behavior problems (eg, wandering, yelling, uncooperativeness) do not respond to antipsychotics.

When an antipsychotic is used, the starting dose should be about one quarter the usual starting adult dose and should be increased gradually with frequent monitoring for response and adverse effects. Once the patient responds, the dose should be titrated down, if possible, to the lowest effective dose. The drug needs to be stopped if it is ineffective. Clinical trial data relating to dosing, efficacy, and safety of these drugs in the elderly are limited.

Antipsychotics can reduce paranoia but may worsen confusion (see also p. 1791). Elderly patients, especially women, are at increased risk of tardive dyskinesia, which is often irreversible. Sedation, orthostatic hypotension, anticholinergic effects, and akathisia (subjective motor restlessness) can occur in up to 20% of elderly patients taking an antipsychotic, and drug-induced parkinsonism can persist for up to 6 to 9 mo after the drug is stopped.

Extrapyramidal dysfunction can develop even when 2nd-generation antipsychotics (eg, olanzapine, quetiapine, risperidone) are used, especially at higher doses. Risks and benefits of using an antipsychotic should be discussed with the patient or the person responsible for the patient's care. Antipsychotics should be considered for behavior problems only when nonpharmacologic options have failed and patients are a threat to themselves or others.

Anxiolytics and hypnotics: Treatable causes of insomnia should be sought and managed before using hypnotics (see also p. 2016). Nonpharmacologic measures, such as cognitive-behavioral therapy, and sleep hygiene (eg, avoiding caffeinated beverages, limiting daytime napping, modifying bedtime) should be tried first. If they are ineffective, nonbenzodiazepine hypnotics (eg, zolpidem, eszopiclone, zaleplon) are options for short-term use. These drugs bind mainly to a benzodiazepine receptor subtype and disturb the sleep pattern less than benzodiazepines. They have a more rapid onset, fewer rebound effects, fewer next-day effects, and less potential for dependence. As described in Table 335–5, short-, intermediate-, and long-acting benzodiazepines are associated with increased risk of cognitive impairment, delirium, falls, fractures, and motor vehicle crashes in the elderly and should be avoided for the treatment of insomnia. Benzodiazepines may be appropriate for treatment of anxiety or panic attacks in the elderly.

Duration of anxiolytic or hypnotic therapy should be limited if possible because tolerance and dependence may develop; withdrawal may lead to rebound anxiety or insomnia.

Antihistamines (eg, diphenhydramine, hydroxyzine) are not recommended as anxiolytics or hypnotics because they have anticholinergic effects, and tolerance to the sedative effects develops quickly.

Buspirone, a partial serotonin agonist, can be effective for general anxiety disorder; elderly patients tolerate doses up to 30 mg/day well. The slow onset of anxiolytic action (up to 2 to 3 wk) can be a disadvantage in urgent cases.

Digoxin: Digoxin, a cardiac glycoside, is used to increase the force of myocardial contractions and to treat supraventricular arrhythmias. However, it must be used with caution in elderly patients. In men with heart failure and a left ventricular ejection fraction of ≤ 45%, serum digoxin levels > 0.8 ng/mL are associated with increased mortality risk. Adverse effects are typically related to its narrow therapeutic index. One study found digoxin to be beneficial in women when serum levels were 0.5 to 0.9 ng/mL but possibly harmful when levels were ≥ 1.2 ng/mL. A number of factors increase the likelihood of digoxin toxicity in the elderly. Renal impairment, temporary dehydration, and NSAID use (all common among the elderly) can reduce renal clearance of digoxin. Furthermore, digoxin clearance decreases an average of 50% in elderly patients with normal serum creatinine levels. Also, if lean body mass is reduced, as may occur with aging, volume of distribution for digoxin is reduced. Therefore, starting doses should be low (0.125 mg/day) and adjusted according to response and serum digoxin levels (normal range 0.8 to 2.0 ng/mL). However, serum digoxin level does not always correlate with likelihood of toxicity.

Diuretics: Lower doses of thiazide diuretics (eg, hydrochlorothiazide or chlorthalidone 12.5 to 25 mg) can effectively control hypertension in many elderly patients and have less risk of hypokalemia and hyperglycemia than other diuretics (see also p. 732). Thus, K supplements may be required less often.

K-sparing diuretics should be used with caution in the elderly; the K level must be carefully monitored, particularly when these diuretics are given with ACE inhibitors or angiotensin II receptor blockers or when the patient has impaired kidney function.

336 Elder Abuse

Elder abuse is physical or psychologic mistreatment, neglect, or financial exploitation of the elderly.

Common types of elder abuse include physical abuse, psychologic abuse, neglect, and financial abuse. Each type may be intentional or unintentional. The perpetrators are usually adult children but may be other family members or paid or informal caregivers. Abuse usually becomes more frequent and severe over time. Fewer than 20% of abuse cases are reported; thus, physicians must remain vigilant in identifying elderly patients at risk of mistreatment.

Physical abuse is use of force resulting in physical or psychologic injury or discomfort. It includes striking, shoving, shaking, beating, restraining, forceful feeding, and unwarranted administration of drugs. It may include sexual assault (any form of sexual intimacy without consent or by force or threat of force).

Psychologic abuse is use of words, acts, or other means to cause emotional stress or anguish. It includes issuing threats (eg, of institutionalization), insults, and harsh commands, as well as remaining silent and ignoring the person. It also includes infantilization (a patronizing form of ageism in which the perpetrator treats the elderly person as a child), which encourages the elderly person to become dependent on the perpetrator.

Neglect is the failure or refusal to provide food, medicine, personal care, or other necessities; it also includes abandonment. Neglect that results in physical or psychologic harm is considered abuse.

Financial abuse is exploitation of or inattention to a person's possessions or funds. It includes swindling, pressuring a person to distribute assets, and managing a person's money irresponsibly.

Although the true incidence is unclear, elder abuse appears to be a growing public health problem in the US. The National Center on Elder Abuse cites studies reporting as many as 1 in 10 older adults are victims of physical abuse, psychologic abuse, or neglect. Because certain forms of abuse (eg, financial exploitation) were not included, the actual incidence of mistreatment was probably higher. In Canadian and western European studies, incidence of abuse was comparable to that in the US.

Risk Factors

For the victim, risk factors for elder abuse include impairment (chronic disorders, functional impairment, cognitive impairment) and social isolation. For the perpetrator, risk factors include substance abuse, psychiatric disorders, a history of violence, stress, and dependence on the victim (including shared living arrangements—see Table 336–1).

Diagnosis

Elder abuse is difficult to detect because many of the signs are subtle, and the victim is often unwilling or unable to discuss the abuse. Victims may hide abuse because of shame, fear

Table 336–1. RISK FACTORS FOR ELDER ABUSE

FACTOR	COMMENTS
For the victim	
Social isolation	Abuse of isolated people is less likely to be detected and stopped. Social isolation can intensify stress.
A chronic disorder, functional impairment, or both	The ability to escape, seek help, and defend self is reduced. Such elderly people may require more care, increasing stress for the caregiver.
Cognitive impairment	Risk of financial abuse and neglect is particularly high. People with dementia may be difficult to care for, frustrating caregivers, and may be aggressive and disruptive, precipitating abuse by overwhelmed caregivers.
For the perpetrator	
Substance abuse	Alcohol or drug abuse, intoxication, or substance withdrawal may lead to abusive behavior. Substance-dependent caregivers may attempt to use or sell drugs prescribed to the elderly person, depriving the person of treatment.
Psychiatric disorders	Psychiatric disorders (eg, schizophrenia, other psychoses) may lead to abusive behavior. Patients discharged from an inpatient psychiatric institution may return to their elderly parents' home for care. These patients, even if not violent in the institution, may become abusive at home.
History of violence	A history of violence in a relationship (particularly between spouses) and outside the family may predict elder abuse. One theory is that violence is a learned response to difficult life experiences and a learned method of expressing anger and frustration. Because reliable information about past family violence is difficult to obtain, this theory is unsubstantiated.
Dependence of the perpetrator on the elderly person	Dependence on the elderly person for financial support, housing, emotional support, and other needs can cause resentment, contributing to abuse. If the elderly person refuses to provide resources to a family member (especially an adult child), abuse is more likely.
Stress	Stressful life events (eg, chronic financial problems, death in the family) and the responsibilities of caregiving increase the likelihood of abuse.
For both victim and perpetrator	
Shared living arrangements	Elderly people living alone are much less likely to be abused. When living arrangements are shared, opportunities for the tension and conflict that usually precede abuse are greater.

Adapted from Lachs MS, Pillemer K: Current concepts: Abuse and neglect of elderly persons. *New England Journal of Medicine* 332: 437–443, 1995.

of retaliation, or a desire to protect the perpetrator. Sometimes when abuse victims seek help, they encounter ageist responses from health care practitioners, who may, for example, dismiss complaints of abuse as confusion, paranoia, or dementia.

Social isolation of the elderly victim often makes detecting elder abuse difficult. Abuse tends to increase the isolation because the perpetrator often limits the victim's access to the outside world (eg, denies the victim visitors and telephone calls).

Symptoms and signs of elder abuse may erroneously be attributed to a chronic disorder (eg, a hip fracture attributed to osteoporosis). However, the following clinical situations are particularly suggestive of abuse:

- Delay between an injury or illness and the seeking of medical attention
- Disparities in the patient's and caregiver's accounts
- Injury severity that is incompatible with the caregiver's explanation
- Implausible or vague explanation of the injury by the patient or caregiver
- Frequent visits to the emergency department for exacerbations of a chronic disorder despite an appropriate care plan and adequate resources
- Absence of the caregiver when a functionally impaired patient presents to the physician
- Laboratory findings that are inconsistent with the history
- Reluctance of the caregiver to accept home health care (eg, a visiting nurse) or leave the elderly patient alone with a health care practitioner

History: If elder abuse is suspected, the patient should be interviewed alone, at least for part of the time. Other involved people may also be interviewed separately. The patient interview may start with general questions about feelings of safety but should also include direct questions about possible mistreatment (eg, physical violence, restraints, neglect). If abuse is confirmed, the nature, frequency, and severity of events should be elicited. The circumstances precipitating the abuse (eg, alcohol intoxication) should also be sought.

Social and financial resources of the patient should be assessed because they affect management decisions (eg, living arrangements, hiring of a professional caregiver). The examiner should inquire whether the patient has family members or friends able and willing to nurture, listen, and assist. If financial resources are adequate but basic needs are not being met, the examiner should determine why. Assessing these resources can also help identify risk factors for abuse (eg, financial stress, financial exploitation of the patient).

In the interview with the family caregiver, confrontation should be avoided. The interviewer should explore whether caregiving responsibilities are burdensome for the family member and, if appropriate, acknowledge the caregiver's difficult role. The caregiver is asked about recent stressful events (eg, bereavement, financial stresses), the patient's illness (eg, care needs, prognosis), and the reported cause of any recent injuries.

Physical examination: The patient should be thoroughly examined, preferably at the first visit, for signs of elder abuse (see Table 336–2). The physician may need help from a trusted family member or friend of the patient, state adult protective services, or, occasionally, law enforcement agencies to encourage the caregiver or patient to permit the evaluation. If abuse is identified or suspected, a referral to Adult Protective Services is mandatory in most states.

Table 336–2. SIGNS OF ELDER ABUSE

ITEM	SIGN
Behavior	Withdrawal by the patient Infantilization of the patient by the caregiver Caregiver's insistence on providing the history
General appearance	Poor hygiene (eg, unkempt appearance, uncleanliness) Inappropriate dress
Skin and mucous membranes	Poor skin turgor or other signs of dehydration Bruises, particularly multiple bruises in various stages of evolution Pressure ulcers Deficient care of established skin lesions
Head and neck	Traumatic alopecia (distinguished from male- or female-pattern alopecia by distribution)
Trunk	Bruises Welts (shape may suggest implement—eg, utensil, stick, belt)
GU region	Rectal bleeding Vaginal bleeding Pressure ulcers Infestations
Extremities	Wrist or ankle lesions suggesting use of restraints or immersion burns (ie, in a stocking-glove distribution)
Musculoskeletal system	Previously undiagnosed fracture Unexplained pain Unexplained gait disturbance
Mental and emotional health	Depressive symptoms Anxiety

Cognitive status should be assessed, eg, using the Mini-Mental State Examination (see Sidebar 220–1 on p. 1836). Cognitive impairment is a risk factor for elder abuse and may affect the reliability of the history and the patient's ability to make management decisions.

Mood and emotional status should be assessed. If the patient feels depressed, ashamed, guilty, anxious, fearful, or angry, the beliefs underlying the emotion should be explored. If the patient minimizes or rationalizes family tension or conflict or is reluctant to discuss abuse, the examiner should determine whether these attitudes are interfering with recognition or admission of abuse.

Functional status, including the ability to do activities of daily living (ADLs), should be assessed and any physical limitations that impair self-protection noted. If help with ADLs is needed, the examiner should determine whether the current caregiver has sufficient emotional, financial, and intellectual ability for the task. Otherwise, a new caregiver needs to be identified.

Coexisting disorders caused or exacerbated by the abuse should be sought.

Laboratory tests: Imaging and laboratory tests (eg, electrolytes to determine hydration, albumin to determine nutritional status, drug levels to document compliance with prescribed regimens) are done as necessary to identify and document the abuse.

Documentation: The medical record should contain a complete report of the actual or suspected abuse, preferably in the patient's own words. A detailed description of any injuries should be included, supported by photographs, drawings, x-rays, and other objective documentation (eg, laboratory test results) when possible. Specific examples of how needs are not being met, despite an agreed-on care plan and adequate resources, should be documented.

Prognosis

Abused elderly people are at high risk of death. In a large 13-yr longitudinal study, the survival rate was 9% for abuse victims compared with 40% for nonabused controls. Multivariate analysis to determine the independent effect of abuse indicated that risk of mortality for abused patients over a 3-yr period after abuse was 3 times higher than that for controls over a similar period.

Treatment

An interdisciplinary team approach (involving physicians, nurses, social workers, lawyers, law enforcement officials, psychiatrists, and other practitioners) is essential. Any previous intervention (eg, court orders of protection) and the reason for its failure should be investigated to avoid repeating any mistakes.

Intervention: If the patient is in immediate danger, the physician, in consultation with the patient, should consider hospital admission, law enforcement intervention, or relocation to a safe home. The patient should be informed of the risks and consequences of each option.

If the patient is not in immediate danger, steps to reduce risk should be taken but are less urgent. The choice of intervention depends on the perpetrator's intent to harm. For example, if a family member administers too much of a drug because the physician's directions are misunderstood, the only intervention needed may be to give clearer instructions. A deliberate overdose requires more intensive intervention.

In general, interventions need to be tailored to each situation. Interventions may include

- Medical assistance
- Education (eg, teaching victims about abuse and available options, helping them devise safety plans)
- Psychologic support (eg, psychotherapy, support groups)
- Law enforcement and legal intervention (eg, arrest of the perpetrator, orders of protection, legal advocacy including asset protection)
- Alternative housing (eg, sheltered senior housing, nursing home placement)
- Counseling the victim, which usually requires many sessions (progress may be slow)

If victims have decision-making capacity, they should help determine their own intervention. If they do not, the interdisciplinary team, ideally with a guardian or objective conservator, should make most decisions. Decisions are based on the severity of the violence, the victim's previous lifestyle choices, and legal ramifications. Often, there is no single correct decision; each case must be carefully monitored.

Nursing and social work issues: As members of the interdisciplinary team, nurses and social workers can help prevent elder abuse and monitor the results of interventions. A nurse, social worker, or both can be appointed as coordinator to ensure that pertinent information is accurately recorded, that relevant parties are contacted and kept informed, and that necessary care is available 24 h/day.

In-service education about elder abuse should be offered to all nurses and social workers annually. In some states, education about child abuse is mandatory for physician, nursing, and social work licensure. However, mandated professional education on elder abuse is established in just a few states.

Reporting: All states require that suspected or confirmed abuse in an institution be reported, and most states require that abuse in the home also be reported. All US states have laws protecting and providing services for vulnerable, incapacitated, or disabled adults.

In > 75% of US states, the agency designated to receive abuse reports is the state social service department (Adult Protective Services). In the remaining states, the designated agency is the state unit on aging. For abuse within an institution, the local long-term care ombudsman office should be contacted. Telephone numbers for these agencies and offices in any part of the US can be found by contacting the Eldercare Locator (800-677-1116 or www.eldercare.gov) or the National Center on Elder Abuse (855-500-3537 or www.ncea.acl.gov) and giving the patient's county and city of residence or zip code. Health care practitioners should know reporting laws and procedures for their own states.

Caregiver issues: Caregivers of a physically or cognitively impaired elderly person may not be able to provide adequate care or may not realize that their behavior sometimes borders on abuse. These caregivers may be so immersed in their caregiving roles that they become socially isolated and lack an objective frame of reference for what constitutes normal caregiving. The deleterious effects of caregiver burden, including depression, an increase in stress-related disorders, and a shrinking social network, are well-documented. Physicians need to point out these effects to caregivers. Services to help caregivers include adult day care, respite programs, and home health care. Families should be referred for such services by using the Eldercare Locator (800-677-1116 or www.eldercare.gov) or the National Association of Area Agencies on Aging (202-872-0888 or www.n4a.org).

Prevention

A physician or other health care practitioner may be the only person an abuse victim has contact with other than the perpetrator and should therefore be vigilant for risk factors and signs of abuse. Recognizing high-risk situations can prevent elder abuse—eg, when a frail or cognitively impaired elderly person is being cared for by someone with a history of substance abuse, violence, a psychiatric disorder, or caregiver burden. Physicians should pay particular attention when a frail elderly person (eg, a person with a recent history of stroke or a newly diagnosed condition) is discharged into a precarious home environment. Physicians should also remember that perpetrators and victims may not fit stereotypes.

Elderly people often agree to share their homes with family members who have drug or alcohol problems or serious psychiatric disorders. A family member may have been discharged from a mental or other institution to an elderly person's home without having been screened for risk of causing abuse. Physicians should therefore counsel elderly patients considering such living arrangements, especially if the relationship was fraught with tension in the past.

Additional considerations should be made for the screening and hiring of in-home helpers, both from formal service agencies and informal private arrangements. A small, but meaningful, proportion of patients who utilize in-home helpers report concerns of theft, neglect, or mistreatment. Screening and training for such workers may help in preventing mistreatment. The National Center on Elder Abuse (www.ncea.acl.gov) offers a comprehensive review titled Preventing Elder Abuse by In-Home Helpers, and elderly patients and their families should be directed to this resource if considering such forms of assistance.

Patients can also actively decrease their risk of abuse (eg, by maintaining social relationships, by increasing social and community contacts). They should seek legal advice before signing any documents related to where they live or who makes financial decisions for them.

337 Falls in the Elderly

A fall is defined as a person coming to rest on the ground or another lower level; sometimes a body part strikes against an object that breaks the fall. Typically, events caused by acute disorders (eg, stroke, seizure) or overwhelming environmental hazards (eg, being struck by a moving object) are not considered falls.

Annually, 30 to 40% of elderly people living in the community fall; 50% of nursing home residents fall. In the US, falls are the leading cause of accidental death and the 7th leading cause of death in people ≥ 65; 75% of deaths caused by falls occur in the 13% of the population who are ≥ 65. Medical costs to Medicare alone for fall injuries were $31 billion in 2015 and will undoubtedly increase.

Falls threaten the independence of elderly people and cause a cascade of individual and socioeconomic consequences. However, physicians are often unaware of falls in patients who do not present with an injury because a routine history and physical examination typically do not include a specific evaluation for falls. Many elderly people are reluctant to report a fall because they attribute falling to the aging process or because they fear being subsequently restricted in their activities or institutionalized.

Etiology

The best predictor of falling is a previous fall. However, falls in elderly people rarely have a single cause or risk factor. A fall is usually caused by a complex interaction among the following:

- Intrinsic factors (age-related decline in function, disorders, and adverse drug effects)
- Extrinsic factors (environmental hazards)
- Situational factors (related to the activity being done, eg, rushing to the bathroom)

Intrinsic factors: Age-related changes can impair systems involved in maintaining balance and stability (eg, while standing, walking, or sitting) and increase the risk of falls. Visual acuity, contrast sensitivity, depth perception, and dark adaptation decline. Changes in muscle activation patterns and ability to generate sufficient muscle power and velocity may impair the ability to maintain or recover balance in response to perturbations (eg, stepping onto an uneven surface, being bumped). In fact, muscle weakness of any type is a major predictor of falls.

Chronic and acute disorders (see Table 337–1) and use of drugs (see Table 337–2) are major risk factors for falls. The risk of falls increases with the number of drugs taken. Psychoactive drugs are the drugs most commonly reported as increasing the risk of falls and fall-related injuries.

Extrinsic factors: Environmental factors can increase the risk of falls independently or, more importantly, by interacting with intrinsic factors. Risk is highest when the environment requires greater postural control and mobility (eg, when walking on a slippery surface) and when the environment is unfamiliar (eg, when relocated to a new home).

Situational factors: Certain activities or decisions may increase the risk of falls and fall-related injuries. Examples are walking while talking or being distracted by multitasking and then failing to notice an environmental hazard (eg, a curb or step), rushing to the bathroom (especially at night when not fully awake or when lighting may be inadequate), and rushing to answer the telephone.

Complications: Falling, particularly falling repeatedly, increases risk of injury, hospitalization, and death, particularly in elderly people who are frail and have preexisting disease comorbidities (eg, osteoporosis) and deficits in activities of daily living (eg, incontinence). Longer-term complications can include decreased physical function, fear of falling, and institutionalization. Falls reportedly contribute to > 40% of nursing home admissions.

Over 50% of falls among elderly people result in an injury. Although most injuries are not serious (eg, contusions, abrasions), fall-related injuries account for about 5% of hospitalizations in patients ≥ 65. About 5% of falls result in fractures of the humerus, wrist, or pelvis. About 2% of falls result in a hip fracture. Other serious injuries (eg, head and internal injuries, lacerations) occur in about 10% of falls. Some fall-related injuries are fatal. About 5% of elderly people with hip fractures die while hospitalized. Overall mortality in the 12 mo after a hip fracture ranges from 18 to 33%.

About half of elderly people who fall cannot get up without help. Remaining on the floor for > 2 h after a fall increases risk of dehydration, pressure ulcers, rhabdomyolysis, hypothermia, and pneumonia.

Function and quality of life may deteriorate drastically after a fall; at least 50% of elderly people who were ambulatory before fracturing a hip do not recover their previous level of mobility. After falling, elderly people may fear falling again, so mobility is sometimes reduced because confidence is lost. Some people may even avoid certain activities (eg, shopping, cleaning) because of this fear. Decreased activity can increase joint stiffness and weakness, further reducing mobility.

Table 337–1. SOME DISORDERS THAT CONTRIBUTE TO RISK OF FALLS

FUNCTIONAL IMPAIRMENT	DISORDER
BP regulation	Anemia Arrhythmias Cardioinhibitory carotid sinus hypersensitivity COPD Dehydration Infections (eg, pneumonia, sepsis) Metabolic disorders (eg, diabetes, thyroid disorders, hypoglycemia, hyperosmolar states) Neurocardiogenic inhibition after micturition Postural hypotension Postprandial hypotension Valvular heart disorders
Central processing	Delirium Dementia Stroke
Gait	Arthritis Foot deformities Muscle weakness
Postural and neuromotor function	Cerebellar degeneration Myelopathy (eg, due to cervical or lumbar spondylosis) Parkinson disease Peripheral neuropathy Stroke Vertebrobasilar insufficiency
Proprioception	Peripheral neuropathy (eg, due to diabetes mellitus) Vitamin B_{12} deficiency
Otolaryngologic function	Acute labyrinthitis Benign paroxysmal positional vertigo Hearing loss Meniere disease
Vision	Cataract Glaucoma Macular degeneration (age-related)

Evaluation

- Clinical evaluation
- Performance testing
- Sometimes laboratory testing

After treatment of acute injuries, assessment aims to identify risk factors and appropriate interventions, thus decreasing the risk of future falls and fall-related injuries.[1,2]

Table 337–2. SOME DRUGS THAT CONTRIBUTE TO RISK OF FALLS

DRUGS	MECHANISM
Aminoglycosides	Direct vestibular damage
Analgesics (especially opioids)	Reduced alertness or slow central processing
Antiarrhythmics	Impaired cerebral perfusion
Anticholinergics	Confusion/delirium
Antihypertensives (especially vasodilators)	Impaired cerebral perfusion
Antipsychotics	Extrapyramidal syndromes, other antiadrenergic effects, reduced alertness, or slow central processing
Diuretics (especially when patients are dehydrated)	Impaired cerebral perfusion
Loop diuretics (high-dose)	Direct vestibular damage
Psychoactive drugs (especially antidepressants, antipsychotics, and benzodiazepines)	Reduced alertness or slow central processing

Some falls are promptly recognized because of an obvious fall-related injury or concern about a possible injury. However, because elderly people often do not report falls, they should be asked about falls or mobility problems at least once per year.

Patients who report a single fall should be evaluated for a balance or gait problem using the basic Get-Up-and-Go Test. For the test, patients are observed as they rise from a standard armchair, walk 3 m (about 10 ft) in a straight line, turn, walk back to the chair, and sit back down. Observation may detect lower-extremity weakness, imbalance while standing or sitting, or an unsteady gait. Sometimes the test is timed. A time of > 12 sec indicates a significantly increased risk of falls.

Patients who require a more complete assessment of risk factors for falls include

- Those who have difficulty during the Get-Up-and-Go Test
- Those who report multiple falls during screening
- Those who are being evaluated after a recent fall (after acute injuries are identified and treated)

History and physical examination: When a more complete assessment of risk factors is needed, the focus is on identifying intrinsic, extrinsic, and situational factors that can be reduced by interventions targeted at them.

Patients are asked open-ended questions about the most recent fall or falls, followed by more specific questions about when and where a fall occurred and what they were doing. Witnesses are asked the same questions. Patients should be asked whether they had premonitory or associated symptoms (eg, palpitations, shortness of breath, chest pain, vertigo, light-headedness) and whether consciousness was lost. Patients should also be asked whether any obvious extrinsic or situational factors may have been involved. The history should include questions about past and present medical problems, use of prescription and OTC drugs, and use of alcohol. Because eliminating all risk of future falls may be impossible, patients should be asked whether they were able to get back up without help after falling and whether any injuries occurred; the goal is reducing the risk of complications due to future falls.

The physical examination should be comprehensive enough to exclude obvious intrinsic causes of falls. If the fall occurred recently, temperature should be measured to determine whether fever was a factor. Heart rate and rhythm should be assessed to identify obvious bradycardia, resting tachycardia, or irregular rhythms. BP should be measured with patients supine and after patients stand for 1 and 3 min to rule out orthostatic hypotension. Auscultation can detect many types of valvular heart disorders. Visual acuity should be evaluated with patients wearing their usual corrective lenses if needed. Abnormalities in visual acuity should trigger a more detailed visual examination by an optometrist or ophthalmologist. The neck, spine, and extremities (especially the legs and feet) should be evaluated for weakness, deformities, pain, and limitation in range of motion.

A neurologic examination should be done; it includes testing muscle strength and tone, sensation (including proprioception), coordination (including cerebellar function), stationary balance, and gait. Basic postural control and the proprioceptive and vestibular systems are evaluated using the Romberg test (in which patients stand with feet together and eyes both open and closed). Tests to establish high-level balance function include the one-legged stance and tandem gait. If patients can stand on one leg for 10 sec with their eyes open and have an accurate 3-m (10-ft) tandem gait, any intrinsic postural control deficit is likely to be minimal. Physicians should evaluate positional vestibular function (eg, with the Dix-Hallpike maneuver—see Sidebar 91–1 on p. 785) and mental status (see Sidebar 220–1 on p. 1836).

Performance tests: The Performance-Oriented Assessment of Mobility or the Timed Up-and-Go test can identify problems with balance and stability during walking and other movements that may indicate increased risk of falls. These tests are especially helpful if the patient had difficulty doing the basic Get-Up-and-Go test.

Laboratory tests: There is no standard diagnostic evaluation. Testing should be based on the history and examination and helps rule out various causes:

- A CBC for anemia or leukocytosis
- Blood glucose measurement for hypoglycemia or hyperglycemia
- Electrolyte measurement for dehydration

Tests such as ECG, ambulatory cardiac monitoring, and echocardiography are recommended only when a cardiac cause is suspected. Carotid massage under controlled conditions (IV access and cardiac monitoring) has been proposed to determine carotid hypersensitivity and ultimately who might respond to pacemaker treatment. Spinal x-rays and cranial CT or MRI are indicated only when the history and physical examination detect new neurologic abnormalities.

1. National Institute for Health and Care Excellence: Falls in older people: Assessing risk and prevention (Clinical Guideline [CG] 161), 2013.
2. U.S. Preventive Services Task Force (USPSTF): Final Evidence Summary: Falls prevention in older adults: Counseling and preventive medication. *Ann Intern Med*, 2012.

Prevention

The focus should be on preventing or reducing the number of future falls and fall-related injuries and complications while maintaining as much of the patient's function and independence

Table 337–3. HOME ASSESSMENT CHECKLIST FOR HAZARDS THAT INCREASE RISK OF FALLING

LOCATION	HAZARD	CORRECTION	RATIONALE
General household			
Lighting	Too dim	Provide ample lighting in all areas	Improves visual acuity and contrast sensitivity
	Too direct, creating glare	Reduce glare with evenly distributed light, indirect lighting, or translucent shades	Improves visual acuity and contrast sensitivity
	Inaccessible light switches	Provide night-lights or touch-activated lights Install switches that are immediately accessible when entering a room or motion sensors that activate lights	Reduces risk of tripping over or bumping into unseen obstacles in a dark room
Carpets, rugs, linoleum	Torn	Repair or replace torn carpet	Reduces risk of tripping and slipping, especially for people who have difficulty stepping
	Slippery	Provide rugs with nonskid backs	Reduces risk of slipping
	Curled edges	Tack or tape down rugs or linoleum to prevent curling Replace rugs or linoleum	Reduces risk of tripping
Chairs, tables, other furnishings	Unstable	Provide furniture stable enough to support the weight of a person leaning on table edges or chair arms and backs Do not use chairs that have wheels or that swivel Repair legs that are loose	Increases support for people with impaired balance and helps with transferring
	Chairs without armrests	Provide chairs with armrests that extend forward enough to provide leverage when getting up or sitting down	Helps people with proximal muscle weakness and helps with transferring
	Obstructed pathways	Arrange furnishings so that pathways are not obstructed Remove clutter from hallways	Reduces risk of tripping over or bumping into obstacles, making movement in the home easier and safer, especially for people with impaired peripheral vision
Wires and cords	Exposed in pathways	Tack cords above the floor or run beneath floor coverings	Reduces risk of tripping
Kitchen			
Cabinets, shelves	Too high	Keep frequently used items at waist level Install shelves and cupboards at an accessible height	Reduces risk of falls due to frequent reaching or climbing on ladders or chairs
Floors	Wet or waxed	Place a rubber mat on the floor in the sink area Wear rubber-soled shoes in the kitchen Use nonslip wax	Reduces risk of slipping, especially for people with a gait disorder
Bathroom			
Bathtub or shower	Slippery tub or shower floor	Install skid-resistant strips or rubber mat Use shower shoes or a bath seat (a bath seat enables people with impaired balance to sit while showering)	Reduces risk of sliding on a wet tub or shower floor
	Need to use the side of the bathtub for support or transfer	Install grab bars in shower Install a portable grab bar on the side of the tub Take grab bar on trips	Helps with transferring

Table 337–3. HOME ASSESSMENT CHECKLIST FOR HAZARDS THAT INCREASE RISK OF FALLING (*Continued*)

LOCATION	HAZARD	CORRECTION	RATIONALE
Towel racks, sink tops	Unstable for use as support while transferring from the toilet, tub, or shower	Fasten grab rails to wall studs	Helps with transferring
Toilet seat	Too low	Use elevated toilet seat	Helps with transferring to and from the toilet
Doors	Locks	Remove locks from bathroom doors or use locks that can be opened from both sides of the door	Enables other people to enter if a person falls
Stairways			
Height	Height of steps too high	Correct step height to < 15 cm	Reduces risk of tripping, especially for people who have difficulty stepping
Handrails	Missing	Install and anchor rails well on both sides of the stairway Use cylindrical rails placed 2.5–5 cm from the wall	Provides support and enables people to grasp the rail with either hand
	Too short and end of rail unclear	Extend beyond the top and bottom step and turn ends inward	Signals that the top or bottom step has been reached
Configuration	Too steep or too long	Install landings on stairways when feasible or select a residence with a stairway landing	Provides a rest stop, especially for people with heart or pulmonary disorders
Condition	Slippery	Place nonskid treads securely on all steps	Prevents slipping
Lighting	Inadequate	Install adequate lighting at both the top and bottom of stairway Provide night-lights or bright-colored adhesive strips to clearly mark steps	Outlines location of steps, especially for people with impaired vision or perception

as possible. In the periodic physical or wellness examination, patients should be asked about falls in the past year and difficulty with balance or ambulation.[1,2]

Patients who report a single fall and who do not have problems with balance or gait on the Get-Up-and-Go Test or a similar test should be given general information about reducing risk of falls. It should include how to use drugs safely and reduce environmental hazards (see Table 337–3).

Patients who report more than one fall or a problem with balance or gait should receive a fall evaluation to identify risk factors and opportunities to lower risk.

For more information regarding preventing falls in the elderly, see the Cochrane review abstract interventions for preventing falls in older people living in the community (www.cochrane.org), the American Geriatrics Society/British Geriatrics Society guideline for the prevention of falls in older persons (www.onlinelibrary.wiley.com), and the British Medical Journal interventions for the prevention of falls in older adults (www.ncbi.nlm.nih.gov).

Physical therapy and exercise: Patients who have fallen more than once or who have problems during initial balance and gait testing should be referred to physical therapy or an exercise program. Physical therapy and exercise programs can be done in the home if patients have limited mobility.

Physical therapists customize exercise programs to improve balance and gait and to correct specific problems contributing to fall risk.

More general exercise programs in health care or community settings can also improve balance and gait. For example, tai chi may be effective and can be done alone or in groups. The most effective exercise programs to reduce fall risk are those that

- Are tailored to the patient's deficit
- Are provided by a trained professional
- Have a sufficient balance challenge component
- Are provided over the long term (eg, ≥ 4 mo)

Many senior citizen centers, YMCAs, or other health clubs offer free or low-cost group exercise classes tailored to senior citizens, and these classes can help with accessibility and adherence. The savings from decreased fall-related expenses exceed the costs of these programs.[3]

Assistive devices: Some patients benefit from use of an assistive device (eg, cane, walker). Canes may be adequate for patients with minimal unilateral muscle or joint impairment, but walkers, especially wheeled walkers, are more appropriate for patients with increased risk of falls attributable to bilateral leg weakness or impaired coordination (wheeled walkers can be dangerous for patients who cannot control them properly). Physical therapists can help fit or size the devices and teach patients how to use them (see p. 3253).

Medical management: Drugs that can increase the risk of falls should be stopped, or the dosage should be adjusted to the lowest effective dose (see Table 337–2). Patients should be evaluated for osteoporosis and, if osteoporosis is diagnosed, treated to reduce risk of fractures from any future falls.

If any other specific disorder is identified as a risk factor, targeted interventions are required. For example, drugs and physical therapy may reduce risk for patients with Parkinson disease. Vitamin D, particularly taken with calcium, can reduce fall risk, especially in patients with reduced blood vitamin D levels. Pain management, physical therapy, and sometimes joint replacement surgery may reduce risk for patients with arthritis. A change to appropriate lenses (single lenses rather than bifocals or trifocals) or surgery, particularly for removal of cataracts, may help patients with visual impairment.

Environmental management: Correcting environmental hazards in the home may reduce the risk of falls (see Table 337–3). Patients should also be advised on how to reduce risk due to situational factors. For example, footwear should have flat heels, some ankle support, and firm, nonskid midsoles. Many patients with chronic limited mobility (eg, caused by severe arthritis or paresis) benefit from combined medical, rehabilitative, and environmental strategies. Wheelchair adaptations (eg, removable foot plates to reduce tripping during transfers, antitip bars to prevent backward tipping), removable belts, and wedge seating may prevent falls in patients with poor sitting balance or severe weakness when they are sitting or transferring.

Restraints may lead to more falls and other complications and should generally not be used. Surveillance by a caregiver is more effective and safer. Motion detectors may be used, but a caregiver must be present to respond promptly to the triggered alarm.

Hip protectors (padding sewn into special undergarments) have been shown to reduce hip fractures in high-risk patients, but many patients are reluctant to wear protectors indefinitely. Compliant flooring (eg, firm rubber) can help dissipate the impact force, but a floor that is too compliant (eg, soft foam) may destabilize patients.

Patients should also be taught what to do if they fall and cannot get up. Useful techniques include turning from the supine position to the prone position, getting on all fours, crawling to a strong support surface, and pulling up. Having frequent contact with family members or friends, a phone that can be reached from the floor, a remote alarm, or a wearable emergency response system device can decrease the likelihood of lying on the floor for a long time after a fall.

1. National Institute for Health and Care Excellence: Falls in older people: assessing risk and prevention (CG161), 2013.
2. U.S. Preventive Services Task Force (USPSTF): Falls Prevention in Older Adults: Counseling and Preventive Medication. *Ann Intern Med*, 2012.
3. Carande-Kulis V, Stevens JA, Florence CS, et al: A cost-benefit analysis of three older adult fall prevention interventions. *J Safety Res* 52: 65-70, 2015. doi: 10.1016/j.jsr.2014.12.007.

KEY POINTS

- Each year, 30 to 40% of elderly people living in the community and 50% of nursing home residents fall.
- Falls contribute to > 40% of nursing home admissions and are the 7th leading cause of death in people ≥ 65.
- Causes are multifactorial and include age- and illness-related decline in function, environmental hazards, and adverse drug effects.
- Assess the patient for predisposing factors and assess the home for hazards.
- To the extent possible, treat causative disorders, change or stop causative drugs, and correct environmental hazards.
- Patients who have fallen more than once or who have problems during balance and gait testing may benefit from physical therapy or an exercise program.
- Teach techniques for getting off the floor and consider use of a wearable emergency response device.

338 Funding Health Care for the Elderly

In the US, health care services for the elderly are funded mainly by Medicare, Medicaid, the Veterans Health Administration, private insurance, and out-of-pocket payments. In addition, many states offer health-related benefits and programs, such as subsidies for transportation, housing, utilities, telephone, and food expenses, as well as help at home and nutrition services. Health care workers should help elderly patients learn about health benefits and programs they are entitled to.

MEDICARE

Medicare, administered by the Center for Medicare and Medicaid Services (CMS), is primarily a health insurance program for the elderly. (Medicare funds are also used to support certain components of postgraduate medical training and programs that regulate and monitor quality of care.) The following groups are eligible for Medicare:

- US citizens who are ≥ 65 and are eligible for benefits under Social Security, Civil Service Retirement, or Railroad Retirement
- People of all ages with end-stage renal disease requiring dialysis or transplantation or with amyotrophic lateral sclerosis
- Some people who are < 65 and have certain disabilities

The type and range of services that Medicare covers change regularly with new statutory and regulatory amendments (current information is available at www.medicare.gov). Each state has a State Health Insurance Assistance Program, which patients can call for assistance in understanding and choosing Medicare plans, understanding bills, and dealing with payment denials or appeals.

Physicians should understand basic Medicare rules, supply documentation used to determine whether patients are eligible for benefits, and make referrals to legal and social services for counseling and support.

If a patient's claim is denied, a Medicare Summary Notice is issued to the patient to provide information about services or supplies that Medicare does not cover. The denial of coverage may be reversed by a challenge made within 120 days of the notice. The challenge must be supported by an appeal in a fair hearing administrative forum, in which the insurance company handling Medicare claims reviews the case. If unsatisfied with the outcome of that review, the patient has the right to a hearing before a judge.

The original Medicare Plan (sometimes referred to as the fee-for-service plan) has 2 parts:

- Part A (hospital insurance)
- Part B (medical insurance)

The original Medicare Plan is available nationwide. A complete description of Part A and B services and other provisions (called *Medicare & You*) is available at www.medicare.gov or by calling 800-633-4227.

Medicare also provides reimbursement for health care services (including prescription drugs) in models other than traditional fee-for-service, such as

- Medicare Advantage Plans (Part C), which includes managed care plans, preferred provider organization plans, and private fee-for-service plans
- Part D (for prescription drugs)

Each part covers specific health care services (see Table 338–1). Medicare does not cover intermediate or long-term nursing care (except for the Part A services noted below), nor does it cover routine eye, foot, or dental examinations.

Part A

More than 95% of people ≥ 65 are enrolled in Part A. Part A is supported by a payroll tax collected from people who are working; it represents prepaid hospital insurance for Medicare-qualified retirees. Generally, only people who receive monthly Social Security payments are eligible, and most of those who are eligible do not pay premiums. However, people may be required to pay premiums if they or their spouses have worked < 40 quarters at a job that is considered Medicare eligible (ie, if they or their employer paid the payroll tax required by the Federal Insurance Contributions Act [FICA]). Premiums vary depending on how long people have been employed; in 2017, they were $227/mo for people with 30 to 39 quarters of eligible employment and $413/mo for those with 0 to 29 quarters of eligible employment. People whose income and assets are below certain thresholds are eligible for financial assistance from the Medicare Savings Programs (see p. 2871).

Part A covers the following under the circumstances outlined below:

- Inpatient hospital care
- Posthospital care in a skilled nursing facility or a rehabilitation facility

Table 338–1. FUNDING SOURCES BY TYPE OF CARE

TYPE OF CARE	SERVICES	POSSIBLE FUNDING SOURCE
Hospital care	Inpatient care, including mental health care General nursing and other hospital services and supplies Drugs used during hospitalization A semiprivate room (a private room only if medically necessary) Meals	Medicare Part A Medicare Advantage (Part C) Medicaid VA*
Short-term care in a certified skilled nursing facility (nursing home)	Skilled nursing care Social services Drugs used in the facility Medical supplies and equipment used in the facility Dietary counseling Physical, occupational, and speech therapy (if needed) to meet the patient's health goals Transportation by ambulance (when other transportation endangers health) to the nearest facility providing needed services unavailable at the skilled nursing facility A semiprivate room Meals	Medicare Part A if patients need short-term care temporarily after a hospital stay Medicare Advantage if patients need short-term care temporarily after a hospital stay Medicaid VA*
Outpatient care	Physician's, nurse practitioner's, and physician assistant's fees Emergency department visits Transportation by ambulance (when other transportation endangers health) Outpatient surgery (with no overnight stay in the hospital) Rehabilitation (physical, occupational, and speech therapy) Diagnostic tests (eg, x-rays, laboratory tests) Outpatient mental health care Outpatient dialysis A second opinion if surgery is recommended and a third opinion if opinions differ For patients with diabetes, diabetes supplies, self-management training, eye examinations, and nutritional counseling Smoking cessation Durable medical equipment (eg, wheelchairs, hospital beds, oxygen, walkers)	Medicare Part B Medicare Advantage Medicaid VA*

Table continues on the following page.

Table 338–1. FUNDING SOURCES BY TYPE OF CARE (*Continued*)

TYPE OF CARE	SERVICES	POSSIBLE FUNDING SOURCE
Home health care	Personal care, including help with eating, bathing, going to the bathroom, and dressing Part-time skilled nursing care Physical, occupational, and speech therapy Home health aide services Social services Medical supplies (eg, wound dressings), but not prescription drugs	Medicare Part A if patients are homebound and need part-time skilled nursing care or rehabilitation on a daily basis Medicare Part B Medicare Advantage Medicaid VA*
Preventive care	Screening tests for prostate and colorectal cancer Mammography Papanicolaou (Pap) test Bone density measurements Glaucoma tests Influenza, pneumococcal, and hepatitis B vaccination Diabetes screening Cholesterol screening	Medicare Part B Medicare Advantage Medicaid VA*
Extra benefits	Prescription drugs Eyeglasses Hearing aids	Medicare Advantage Medicare Part D (prescription drug plans) Medicaid in some states VA*
Long-term care in an assisted living community	Varies greatly from community to community Meals Help with daily activities Some social and recreational activities Some health care	Medicaid in a few states (partial coverage) VA* in some situations
Long-term care in a skilled-nursing facility (nursing home)	Varies from state to state	Medicaid VA*
Hospice care	Physical care and counseling Room and meals only during inpatient respite care and short-term hospital stays	Medicare Part A Medicare Advantage

*For the Veterans Administration, rules of eligibility vary for different services and change frequently.
VA = Department of Veterans Affairs.

- Hospice care
- Limited custodial care
- Limited home health care

Care in a hospital or a skilled nursing facility is paid for based on benefit periods. A benefit period begins when a person is admitted to a facility and ends when the person has been out of the facility for 60 consecutive days. If a person is readmitted after the 60 days, a new benefit period begins, and another deductible must be paid. If a person is readmitted in < 60 days, an additional deductible is not paid, but the hospital or facility may not receive full payment for the 2nd admission. There is no limit to the number of benefit periods.

Medicare Prospective Payment Systems determine what Medicare will pay for each aspect of care it covers (eg, for hospital inpatient care, skilled nursing facility care, or home health care).

Inpatient hospital care: Under Part A, the beneficiary pays only a deductible for the first 60 full coverage days of the benefit period; the deductible is established annually ($1316 in 2017). If the hospital stay exceeds 60 days, the beneficiary pays a daily co-payment equal to one fourth of the deductible (in 2017, $329 per day for days 61 to 90). If the hospital stay exceeds 90 days, the beneficiary pays a daily co-payment equal to half of the deductible (in 2017, $658 per day for days 91 and beyond). Days 91 to 150 during a hospital stay are designated as reserve days. Part A benefits include 60 lifetime reserve days for use after a 90-day benefit period has exhausted. The 90-day benefit period renews each year, but the 60 reserve days are not renewable and can be used only once during a beneficiary's lifetime. Payment is automatically made for such additional days of hospital care after the 90 days of benefits have been exhausted unless the beneficiary chooses not to have such payment made (thus saving the reserve days for a later time). Even if all reserve days are available, the beneficiary is responsible for all charges beyond 150 days.

Part A covers virtually all medically necessary hospital services, except it provides only limited coverage for inpatient mental health care services. Part A pays for a semi-private room or, if medically necessary, a private room, but not for amenities. Other covered services include discharge planning and medical social services, such as identification of eligibility for public programs and referrals to community agencies.

The prospective payment system determines payment for inpatient hospital care based on the diagnosis-related group (DRG). The DRG is determined by the beneficiary's principal diagnosis with some adjustment for age, severity, sex, comorbidities, and complications. Hospitals are reimbursed a set amount for a given DRG regardless of their actual expenses in providing care. Thus, a hospital's financial profit or loss depends partly on length of stay and costs of diagnosis and therapy for each patient. Under the prospective payment system, the financial pressure for early discharge and limited intervention may conflict with medical judgment. When a patient cannot be discharged home safely or to a nursing home because no bed is available, Medicare typically pays a relatively low per diem cost for an alternative level of care.

Inpatient care in a skilled nursing facility: Coverage of skilled nursing care and skilled rehabilitation services is complex and can change every year. These services are covered only if initiated immediately or shortly after discharge from a hospital. The period of coverage is usually < 1 mo (specific duration of coverage depends on documented improvement in the patient's condition or level of function). In 2017, the first 20 days were covered completely; the next 80 days were covered but required a co-payment of $164.50/day. Benefits are limited to 100 days per benefit period.

Medicare's prospective payment system assigns patients in skilled nursing facilities to a resource utilization group system (RUGS III) based on 7 categories:

- Special care
- Rehabilitation
- Clinically complex problems
- Severe behavioral problems
- Impaired cognition
- Reduced physical functioning
- Need for extensive services

These categories reflect the types and amounts of resources a patient's care is expected to cost. They are subdivided based primarily on the patient's functional dependence. This system is updated annually. The goal is to increase efficiency and avoid excessive payment for patients who require little care. Prospective per diem rates cover routine, ancillary, and capital costs of care for a patient in a skilled nursing facility.

RUGS III uses data from the Minimum Data Set (MDS), the mandated uniform assessment instrument for patients in skilled nursing facilities. The MDS requires ongoing review of patients, making it possible to link patient outcomes with RUGS categories.

Home health care: Generally, part A covers certain medical services provided in the home (eg, part-time or intermittent skilled nursing care; home health aide services incidental to skilled care; physical, speech, and occupational therapy) if they are part of a physician-approved care plan for a homebound patient. However, amount and duration of coverage is limited. The recent implementation of a prospective payment system now limits the amount of coverage. Medical supplies are covered when billed by a home health agency.

Hospice services: Medical and support services for a terminal illness are generally covered if a physician certifies that the patient is terminally ill (estimated life expectancy of 6 mo). However, the patient must choose to receive hospice care instead of standard Medicare benefits.

Custodial care: Assistance with activities of daily living (ADLs), such as eating, dressing, toileting, and bathing, is covered in the home only when skilled care (services of a professional nurse or therapist under a physician-authorized plan of home care) is also required. Such custodial care in a skilled nursing facility is covered when it is part of posthospital acute or rehabilitation care.

Part B

The federal government pays an average of about 75% of Part B costs, and beneficiaries pay 25%. Part B is optional; although Social Security beneficiaries are automatically enrolled in Part B at age 65, they may decline coverage (95% elect to keep Part B coverage). All beneficiaries pay a monthly premium, which varies by income—$134 in 2017 for new beneficiaries whose income in 2015 was ≤ $85,000 (≤ $170,000 if they were married and filing a joint return). Premiums are higher for people with a higher income. Premiums are automatically deducted from monthly Social Security checks. People who decline coverage but later change their minds must pay a surcharge based on how long they delayed enrollment. Premiums generally increase by 10% for each year's delay in enrollment, except for people who delay because they are covered by group insurance through their, their spouse's, or a family member's employer; such people do not pay the surcharge if they enroll when employment or health care coverage ends (whichever comes first). Most states have Medicare Savings Programs (see p. 2871) that pay Part B premiums for people who meet certain financial qualifications.

Participants may stop coverage at any time but must pay a surcharge on the premium if they reenroll.

Covered services: Part B covers a percentage of the following: cost of physician services; outpatient hospital care (eg, emergency department care, outpatient surgery, dialysis), with certain restrictions; outpatient physical, speech, and occupational therapy; diagnostic tests, including portable x-ray services in the home; prosthetics and orthotics; and durable medical equipment for home use. If surgery is recommended, Part B covers part of the cost of an optional 2nd opinion and, if these opinions differ, a 3rd opinion.

Part B also covers medically necessary ambulance services, certain services and supplies not covered by Part A (eg, colostomy bags, prostheses), spinal manipulation by a licensed chiropractor for subluxation shown on x-ray, drugs and dental services if deemed necessary for medical treatment, optometry services related to lenses for cataracts, smoking cessation counseling, and the services of physician assistants, nurse practitioners, clinical psychologists, and clinical social workers. Outpatient mental health care, with certain limitations, is covered.

Drugs and biologicals that cannot be administered by the patient (eg, drugs given IV), some oral anticancer drugs, and certain drugs for hospice patients are covered by Part B. However, unless the patient is enrolled in a managed care program, Part B generally does not cover outpatient drugs.

Part B covers several preventive services, including bone mass measurement, serum cholesterol screening, abdominal aortic aneurysm screening, diabetes services (screening, supplies, self-care training, and eye and foot examinations), colorectal cancer screening, prostate cancer screening and prostate-specific antigen tests, an initial physical examination (the "Welcome to Medicare" examination), glaucoma screening, vaccinations (influenza, pneumococcal, hepatitis B), mammograms, and Papanicolaou (Pap) tests. Part B does not cover routine eye, hearing, foot, or dental examinations and does not cover hearing aids.

Physician reimbursement: Under Part B, physicians may elect to be paid directly by Medicare (assignment), receiving 80% of the allowable charge directly from the program, once the deductible has been met. If physicians accept assignment, their patients are responsible for paying only the deductible. Physicians who do not accept assignment of Medicare payments (or do so selectively) may bill patients up to 115% of the allowable charge; the patient receives reimbursement (80% of the allowable charge) from Medicare. Physicians are subject to fines if their charges exceed the maximum allowable Medicare fees. Physicians who do not accept assignment from Medicare must give patients a written estimate for elective surgery if it is > $500. Otherwise, patients can later claim a refund from physicians for any amount paid over the allowable charge.

Medicare payments to physicians have been criticized as inadequate for the time involved in giving physical and mental status examinations and obtaining the patient history from family members. A Medicare fee schedule based on a resource-based relative value scale for physician services became effective in January 1992 in an attempt to correct this problem.

Part C (Medicare Advantage Plans)

This program (formerly called Medicare + Choice) offers several alternatives to the traditional fee-for-service programs. The alternatives are provided by private insurance companies; Medicare pays these companies a fixed amount for each beneficiary. Several different types of plans are available; they include managed care, preferred provider organizations, private fee-for-service, medical savings accounts, and special needs plans.

Medicare Advantage plans must cover at least the same level and types of benefits covered by Medicare A and B. However, Medicare Advantage plans may include additional benefits (eg, coverage for dentures, prescription drugs, or routine eyeglasses), although participants may pay an additional monthly premium for the additional benefits. Plans differ on whether participants are free to choose any physician and hospital they want, whether they can keep coverage from an employer or union, and what costs are paid out-of-pocket, including how much (if at all) they charge for a premium, whether they pay any of the Part B premium, and how much their deductible and co-payments are.

Part D

Medicare Part D helps cover costs of prescription drugs. It is optional. Plans are provided by insurance or other private companies working with Medicare. There are over 1000 plans available nationwide. Premiums generally increase by an additional 1% for each month that people delay enrolling after they first become eligible for Medicare.

Covered drugs: Plans vary in the drugs they cover (formulary) as well as in pharmacies that can be used. However, formularies must include ≥ 2 effective drugs in the categories and classes of drugs most commonly prescribed for people who use Medicare. Formularies must also cover all available drugs for the following 6 classes: anticonvulsants, antidepressants, antiretroviral drugs, antineoplastics, antipsychotics, and immunosuppressants. Formularies may change over time (often annually). Formularies must also have an appeals process by which nonformulary drugs can be approved if necessary.

Benefits and costs: Costs in 2017 are as follows for the basic benefits (see also Costs for Medicare drug coverage at www.medicare.gov):

- **Premiums:** Premiums vary by plan and income but average about $40/mo for people earning ≤ $85,000/yr (≤ $170,000 if married and filing jointly); those earning more pay an additional $13.30 to $76.20/mo above the plan premium.
- **Annual deductible:** Patients pay the first $400 of drug costs (some plans do not have a deductible).
- **Co-payments:** For the next $3300 of drug costs (after the $400 deductible), patients pay 25% of drug costs (co-payment). Thus, the amount patients pay for the first $3700 of drug costs is $1225 ($400 deductible + $825 co-pay).
- **Coverage gap (doughnut hole):** After the first $3700 of drug costs, people must pay a higher percentage of drug costs (40% for brand-name drugs, 51% for generic) until total out-of-pocket drug costs equal $4950.
- **Reduced co-payments:** Once the out-of-pocket threshold is reached, Medicare pays most of additional drug costs until the end of the year.

The costs during the doughnut hole will decline each year at least until 2020.

Many companies also offer enhanced plans that provide more coverage (eg, lower deductibles or co-payments), although these plans have higher monthly premiums. Specific drug costs may vary depending on whether the drug is on the plan's formulary and whether the prescription is filled by a pharmacy in the plan's network (if the plan has any).

People with low income and minimal assets (eg, those who have full Medicaid coverage, who belong to a Medicare Savings Program, or who get Supplemental Security Income) may be eligible for financial assistance with premiums, deductibles, and co-payments. In addition to providing insurance assistance, many states have state pharmacy assistance programs that help pay for prescription drugs, based on some combination of the person's need, age, and medical disorders; information about these programs is available from the State Health Insurance Assistance Program.

MEDICAID

Funded by a federal-state partnership, Medicaid pays for health services for certain categories of the poor (including the aged poor, the blind or disabled, and low-income families with dependent children). The federal government contributes between 50% and about 76% of the payments made under each state's program; the state pays the remainder. Federal reimbursement is higher for states where incomes are lower. About 10% of the elderly receive services under Medicaid, accounting for about 40% of all Medicaid expenditures. Medicaid is the major public payer for long-term care.

Covered services: Services covered under federal guidelines include inpatient and outpatient hospital care, laboratory and x-ray services, physician services, skilled nursing care, nursing home care not covered by Medicare, and many home health services for people > 21 yr.

States may cover certain other services and items, including prescription drugs (or the premiums for Medicare Part D if patients are eligible for Part D), dental services, eyeglasses, physical therapy, rehabilitation services, and intermediate-level nursing care. Each state determines eligibility requirements, which therefore vary, but people receiving funds from cash-assistance programs (eg, the Supplemental Security Income program) must be included. Several states offer enriched packages of Medicaid services under waiver programs, which are intended to delay or prevent nursing home admission by providing additional home and community-based services (eg, day care, personal care, respite care).

Eligibility: Eligibility depends on income, assets, and personal characteristics. The Affordable Care Act will expand Medicaid coverage to all people < 65 with an income < 133% of the federal poverty level if they reside in a state that elects to expand Medicaid.

Most states have other criteria that allow people to qualify for Medicaid.

Assets, excluding equity in a home and certain other assets, are also considered. If the remaining assets exceed the limit, people are not eligible for Medicaid, even if their income is low. Thus, the elderly may have to spend down (ie, pay for care from personal savings and sale of assets until stringent state eligibility requirements are met) to qualify for Medicaid. How much of monthly income and of the couple's assets that the spouse of a nursing home resident may keep varies by state. Divestment of assets at below fair-market value during the 3 yr before entrance into a nursing home may delay eligibility for Medicaid benefits. Medicaid denies coverage for a period of time that is determined by the amount of inappropriately divested funds divided by the average monthly cost of nursing home care in the state. For example, if a person gives away $10,000 in a state where the average monthly cost of care is $3500, Medicaid coverage is delayed by about 3 mo.

Medicaid estate recovery: Under certain circumstances, Medicaid is entitled (and sometimes required) to recover expenditures from the estates of deceased Medicaid recipients. Typically, recovery may be made only from estates of recipients who were ≥ 55 yr when they received Medicaid benefits or were permanently institutionalized regardless of age. The definition of estate varies by state. Some states include only property that passes through probate; others include assets that pass directly (eg, through joint tenancy with right of survivorship, living trusts, or life insurance payouts). Some states protect the family home from Medicaid claims. The vigor with which claims are pursued varies by state and by case.

Medicare Savings Programs: People who are currently eligible for Medicare and whose income and assets are below certain thresholds are eligible for Medicare Savings Programs. These programs are run by individual state Medicaid programs and cover certain out-of-pocket expenses not covered by Medicare. There are several programs. The Qualified Medicare Beneficiary Program covers Part A and Part B premiums, deductibles, and co-insurance; the Specified Low-Income Medicare Beneficiary Program and the Qualified Disabled Working Individual Program pay part B premiums.

The federal government has set eligibility requirements based on income and asset value. States are free to adopt less restrictive requirements (eg, permitting enrollment at a higher income level). People enroll through state Medicaid offices.

OTHER FEDERAL PROGRAMS AFFECTING THE ELDERLY

Veterans Health Administration: This Department of Veterans Affairs (VA) program provides health care to eligible veterans. Determining eligibility for VA benefits can be complex, and care is not always free. The VA operates > 160 hospitals, 43 domiciliary facilities, and > 130 nursing homes. It also contracts to provide care in community hospitals and nursing homes. Several innovative geriatric programs (including geriatric assessment units; Geriatric Research, Education, and Clinical Centers; and hospital-based home health care programs) have been developed within the VA system.

Tricare: This healthcare program is for active-duty service members, retired service members, and their families.

Older Americans Act (OAA): Enacted in 1965, the OAA has evolved from a program of small grants and research projects into a network of 57 state, territorial, and Indian tribal units on aging; 670 area agencies on aging; and thousands of community agencies. The primary purpose of the OAA is to develop, coordinate, and deliver a comprehensive system of services for elderly people at the community level; services include information and referral, outreach, transportation, senior centers, nutritional programs, advocacy, protective services, senior employment, ombudsman programs, and supportive services. The OAA also funds research and training. People > 60 are eligible regardless of income level.

Social Security: Although not usually considered a health program, Social Security provides basic pension payments that the elderly use for health care services. The elderly receive 2 types of payments:

- Old Age and Survivors Insurance, which is financed by Social Security trust funds and provides payments to retirees, surviving spouses, or qualified dependents
- Supplementary Security Income, which is financed from general revenues and provides a guaranteed minimum income to aged, blind, and disabled people

Title XX of the Social Security Act: This program authorizes reimbursements to states for social services, including various home health services and homemaker services (eg, meal preparation, laundry, light housekeeping, grocery shopping) for the frail elderly. These funds have shifted to the Social Services Block Grant Program, which was designed to prevent or reduce inappropriate institutional care by providing for community-based care and other assistance that enables the elderly to maintain autonomy in the community. The program is defined, administered, and implemented by states; it does not support institutional care or any service covered by Medicare or Medicaid. The program covers health services only when they are an "integral but subordinate" component of an overall social service program.

PRIVATE INSURANCE FOR THE ELDERLY

Medigap: About 87% of beneficiaries enrolled in fee-for-service Medicare programs have Medicare supplemental insurance policies (most are a form of Medigap insurance), which pay for some or all of Medicare deductibles and co-payments, typically in Parts A and B. People must be enrolled in Parts A and B to be eligible to purchase Medigap insurance. People enrolled in the Medicare Advantage plan (Part C—see p. 2870) cannot purchase a Medigap policy unless they leave the Medicare Advantage plan and return to original Medicare. Most Medigap insurance is purchased individually from private insurers, although employers may provide it to retirees.

There are 14 different types of Medigap insurance available, labeled A through N. Benefits are the same for all plans with the same letter, regardless of insurance carrier. No plan may duplicate Medicare benefits. The basic plan (Plan A) covers

- Hospital co-payments
- 100% of expenses eligible for coverage by Medicare Part A after Medicare hospital benefits are exhausted
- Part B co-payments

The other plans, which have higher premiums than Plan A, may provide additional coverage in a skilled nursing facility and may cover Part A and Part B deductibles, preventive medical services, and short-term home-based help with activities of daily living (ADLs) during recovery from an illness, injury, or surgery. Some of these plans, if purchased before Medicare Part D took effect, covered a percentage of the cost of outpatient prescribed drugs.

The Medigap open enrollment period begins the month people turn 65 and lasts 6 mo. During this period, people who have preexisting conditions cannot be denied coverage or charged more; however, they may be made to wait up to 6 mo before preexisting conditions are covered.

Long-term care insurance: Very few private medical insurance policies cover services such as long-term home health care or long-term nursing home care. However, some private insurers offer long-term care insurance. Such plans are useful for people who want to preserve their assets and who can afford to pay the premiums until care is needed, possibly for an extended period of time. This insurance is not recommended for people with few assets and may not be worthwhile for people who can easily pay for long-term care.

Benefits usually begin when a person can no longer do a certain number of ADLs.

Some plans, called tax-qualified plans, offer tax advantages (eg, deduction of premiums from taxable income as medical expenses).

For all long-term care services, private insurance pays for only 9%, and people pay for 22% out-of-pocket. A large proportion of out-of-pocket spending occurs as the elderly spend down to qualify for Medicaid.

MODELS FOR COMPREHENSIVE HEALTH CARE COVERAGE FOR THE ELDERLY

Individually, Medicare, Medicaid, Medigap, and private long-term care insurance have shortcomings in providing comprehensive geriatric care:

- Medicare excludes long-term custodial care, some preventive services, and large amounts of prescription drug costs.
- Medicaid belatedly intervenes after the patient is impoverished.
- Medigap, like Medicare, excludes long-term care.
- Private insurance is too expensive for most of the elderly, leaves them vulnerable to financial catastrophe, and supports only fragments of long-term care.

Collectively, these programs rarely promote integration of acute and long-term care or coordination of health and social services. However, several model projects have demonstrated that with organized delivery of services using combinations of public funding and private insurance, comprehensive geriatric care, including some long-term care, can be adequately financed.

Social health maintenance organizations (SHMOs): SHMOs are demonstration programs financed by Medicare. They use Medicare, Medicaid, and private patient payments to cover a wide range of care benefits managed by nurses, social workers, and physicians. Patients not eligible for Medicaid benefits use private payments to cover a limited amount of long-term care, principally in the home. Like an HMO, an SHMO is at financial risk for the cost of services and therefore has an incentive to manage resources carefully.

Program of All-Inclusive Care for the Elderly (PACE): PACE is designed to keep patients in the community as long as medically, socially, and financially possible. A PACE interdisciplinary team assesses patient needs and develops and implements a care plan.

PACE includes medical and dental care, adult day care (including transportation to and from the facility), health and personal care at home, prescription drugs, social services, rehabilitation, meals, nutritional counseling, and hospital and long-term care when needed. PACE programs provide social and medical services primarily in an adult day health center, supplemented by in-home and referral services. The PACE service package must include all Medicare and Medicaid covered services, and other services determined necessary by the interdisciplinary team for the care of the PACE participant. PACE may require a monthly fee.

Extended care communities: A life-care community or continuing care retirement community provides housing, health care, and other services under packaged financing and management. These communities may have a clinic, an infirmary, or even a nursing home on the site, and housing is designed to accommodate disabled people. Many of these communities serve wealthy retirees willing to sign long-term contracts for their housing and care.

Some life-care communities fail because inflation and an aging population cause costs for services to exceed income. Some communities keep costs down by providing housing and minimal services with options to purchase additional services.

339 Gait Disorders in the Elderly

Gait disorders encompass a number of issues, including slowing of gait speed and loss of smoothness, symmetry, or synchrony of body movement.

For the elderly, walking, standing up from a chair, turning, and leaning are necessary for independent mobility. Gait speed, chair rise time, and the ability to do tandem stance (standing with one foot in front of the other—a measure of balance) are independent predictors of the ability to do instrumental activities of daily living (eg, shopping, traveling, cooking) and of the risk of nursing home admission and death.

Walking without assistance requires adequate attention and muscle strength plus effective motor control to coordinate sensory input and muscle contraction.

PEARLS & PITFALLS

- Gait speed, chair rise time, and the ability to do tandem stance are independent predictors of the ability to do instrumental activities of daily living and of the risk of nursing home admission and death.

Normal Age-Related Changes in Gait

Some elements of gait normally change with aging; others do not.

Gait velocity (speed of walking) remains stable until about age 70; it then declines about 15%/decade for usual gait and 20%/decade for fast walking. Gait velocity is a powerful predictor of mortality—as powerful as an elderly person's number of chronic medical conditions and hospitalizations. At age 75, slow walkers die ≥ 6 yr earlier than normal velocity walkers and ≥ 10 yr earlier than fast velocity walkers. Gait velocity slows because elderly people take shorter steps at the same rate (cadence). The most likely reason for shortened step length (the distance from one heel strike to the next) is weakness of the calf muscles, which propel the body forward; calf muscle strength is substantially decreased in elderly people. However, elderly people seem to compensate for decreased lower calf power by using their hip flexor and extensor muscles more than young adults.

Cadence (reported as steps/min) does not change with aging. Each person has a preferred cadence, which is related to leg length and usually represents the most energy-efficient rhythm. Tall people take longer steps at a slower cadence; short people take shorter steps at a faster cadence.

Double stance time (ie, time with both feet on the ground during ambulation—a more stable position for moving the center of mass forward) increases with age. The percentage of time in double stance goes from 18% in young adults to ≥ 26% in healthy elderly people. Increased time in double stance reduces the time the swing leg has to advance and shortens step length. Elderly people may increase their double stance time even more when they walk on uneven or slippery surfaces, when they have impaired balance, or when they are afraid of falling. They may appear as if they are walking on slippery ice.

Walking posture changes only slightly with aging. Elderly people walk upright, with no forward lean. However, elderly people walk with greater anterior (downward) pelvic rotation and increased lumbar lordosis. This posture change is usually due to a combination of weak abdominal muscles, tight hip flexor muscles, and increased abdominal fat. Elderly people also walk with their legs rotated laterally (toes out) about 5°, possibly because of a loss of hip internal rotation or in order to increase lateral stability. Foot clearance in swing is unchanged with advancing age.

Joint motion changes slightly with aging. Ankle plantar flexion is reduced during the late stage of stance (just before the back foot lifts off). The overall motion of the knee is unchanged. Hip flexion and extension are unchanged, but the hips have increased adduction. Pelvic motion is reduced in all planes.

Abnormal Changes in Gait

Causes: A number of disorders can contribute to dysfunctional or unsafe gait. They particularly include

- Neurologic disorders
- Musculoskeletal disorders (eg, spinal stenosis—see p. 319)

Causative neurologic disorders include dementias (see p. 1874), movement and cerebellar disorders (see p. 1928), and sensory or motor neuropathies (see p. 1984).

Manifestations: There are many manifestations of gait abnormality. Some help suggest certain causes.

Loss of symmetry of motion and timing between left and right sides usually indicates a disorder. When healthy, the body moves symmetrically; step length, cadence, torso movement, and ankle, knee, hip, and pelvis motion are equal on the right and left sides. A *regular* asymmetry occurs with unilateral neurologic or musculoskeletal disorders (eg, a limp caused by a painful ankle). Unpredictable or highly variable gait cadence, step length, or stride width indicates breakdown of motor control of gait due to a cerebellar or frontal lobe syndrome or use of multiple psychoactive drugs.

Difficulty initiating or maintaining gait may occur. When patients first start walking, their feet may appear stuck to the floor, typically because patients do not shift their weight to one foot to allow the other foot to move forward. This problem may represent isolated gait initiation failure, Parkinson disease, or frontal or subcortical disease. Once gait is initiated, steps should be continuous, with little variability in the timing of the steps. Freezing, stopping, or almost stopping usually suggests a cautious gait, a fear of falling, or a frontal gait disorder. Scuffing the feet is not normal (and is a risk factor for tripping).

Retropulsion is walking backwards when initiating gait or falling backwards while walking. It may occur with frontal gait disorders, parkinsonism, CNS syphilis, and progressive supranuclear palsy.

Footdrop causes toe dragging or a stepping gait (ie, exaggerated lift of the leg to avoid catching the toe). It may be secondary to anterior tibialis weakness (eg, caused by trauma to the peroneal nerve at the lateral aspect of the knee or a peroneal mononeuropathy usually associated with diabetes), spasticity of calf muscles (gastrocnemius and soleus), or lowering of the pelvis due to muscle weakness of the proximal muscles on the stance side (particularly the gluteus medius). Low foot swing (eg, due to reduced knee flexion) may resemble footdrop.

Short step length is nonspecific and may represent a fear of falling or a neurologic or musculoskeletal problem. The side with short step length is usually the healthy side, and the short step is usually due to a problem during the stance phase of the opposite (problem) leg. For example, a patient with a weak or painful left leg spends less time in single stance on the left leg and develops less power to move the body forward, resulting in shorter swing time for the right leg and a shorter right step. The normal right leg has a normal single stance duration, resulting in a normal swing time for the abnormal left leg and a longer step length for the left leg than for the right leg.

Wide-based gait (increased step width) is determined by observing the patient's gait on a floor with 12-in (30-cm) tiles. The gait is considered wide based if the outside of the patient's feet do not stay within the width of the tile. As gait speed decreases, step width increases slightly. Wide-based gait can be caused by cerebellar disease or bilateral knee or hip disease. Variable step width (lurching to one side or the other) suggests poor motor control, which may be due to frontal or subcortical gait disorders.

Circumduction (moving the foot in an arc rather than a straight line when stepping forward) occurs in patients with pelvic muscle weakness or difficulty bending the knee. Spasticity of the knee extensor muscles is a common cause.

Forward lean can occur with kyphosis and with Parkinson disease or disorders with parkinsonian features associated with dementia (particularly vascular dementia and Lewy body dementia).

Festination is a progressive quickening of steps (usually with forward lean), whereby patients may break into a run to prevent falling forward. Festination can occur with Parkinson disease and rarely as an adverse effect of dopamine-blocking drugs (typical and atypical antipsychotics).

Sideward trunk lean that is consistent or predictable to the side of the stance leg may be a strategy to reduce joint pain due to hip arthritis or, less commonly, knee arthritis (antalgic gait). In a hemiparetic gait, the trunk may lean to the strong side. In this pattern, the patient leans to lift the pelvis on the opposite side to permit the limb with spasticity (inability to flex the knee) to clear the floor during the swing phase.

Irregular and unpredictable trunk instability can be caused by cerebellar, subcortical, or basal ganglia dysfunction.

Deviations from path are strong indicators of motor control deficits.

Arm swing may be reduced or absent in Parkinson disease and vascular dementias. Arm swing disorders may also be adverse effects of dopamine-blocking drugs (typical and atypical antipsychotics).

Evaluation

The goal is to determine as many potential contributing factors to gait disorders as possible. A performance-oriented mobility assessment tool may be helpful (Table 339–1), as may other clinical tests (eg, a screening cognitive examination for patients with gait problems possibly due to frontal lobe syndromes).

Evaluation is best approached in 4 parts:

- Discussing the patient's complaints, fears, and goals related to mobility
- Observing gait with and without an assistive device (if safe)
- Assessing all components of gait (Table 339–1)
- Observing gait again with a knowledge of the patient's gait components

Table 339–1. PERFORMANCE-ORIENTED ASSESSMENT OF MOBILITY

COMPONENT	FINDINGS	SCORE*	CLINICAL MEANING
Initiation of gait (immediately after being told to go)	Any hesitancy or multiple attempts to start	0	Parkinson disease Isolated gait initiation failure (stroke or dementia) Frontal gait disorder
	No hesitancy	1	
Right step length and height (right swing foot)	Does not pass left stance foot with step or does not clear floor completely with step	0	Arthritis Foot problem Stroke
	Passes left stance foot	1	
	Completely clears floor	1	
Left step length and height (left swing foot)	Does not pass right stance foot with step or does not clear floor completely with step	0	Arthritis Foot problem Stroke
	Passes right stance foot	1	
	Completely clears floor	1	
Step symmetry	Right and left step length not equal (estimated)	0	Unilateral Musculoskeletal or focal neurologic deficit
	Right and left step length equal (estimated)	1	
Step continuity	Stopping or discontinuity between steps	0	Frontal gait disorder Fear of falling
	Steps appear continuous	1	
Path (estimated in relation to floor tiles that are 12 in [30 cm] wide; observed excursion of one foot over about 10 ft of the course)	Marked deviation	0	Frontal gait disorder
	Mild to moderate deviation or use of a walking aid	1	
	Straight without a walking aid	2	
Trunk	Marked sway or use of a walking aid	0	Cerebellar, subcortical, and basal ganglia dysfunction Antalgic gait (hip or knee arthritis)
	No sway but flexion of knees, back pain, or arms spread out while walking	1	Fear of falling
	No sway, no flexion, no use of arms, and no use of a walking aid	2	
Stride width (step width)	Heels wide apart while walking	0	Hip disease Cerebellar disease Normal-pressure hydrocephalus
	Heels almost touching while walking	1	

*A perfect score is 12. A score of < 10 is usually associated with limitations in mobility-related function.

Adapted from Tinetti M: Performance-oriented assessment of mobility problems in elderly patients. *Journal of the American Geriatrics Society* 34:119–126, 1986; used with permission.

History: In addition to the standard medical history, elderly patients should be asked about gait-related issues. First, they are asked open-ended questions regarding any difficulty with walking, balance, or both, including whether they have fallen (or fear they might fall). Then specific capabilities are assessed; they include whether patients can go up and down stairs; get in and out of a chair, shower, or tub; and walk as needed to buy and prepare food and do household chores. If they report any difficulties, details of the onset, duration, and progression are sought. History of neurologic and musculoskeletal symptoms and known disorders is important.

Physical examination: A thorough physical examination is done with emphasis on the musculoskeletal examination (see p. 251) and the neurologic examination (see p. 1835).

Lower-extremity strength is assessed. Proximal muscle strength is tested by having patients get out of a chair without using their arms. Calf strength is measured by having patients face a wall, put their palms on the wall, and rise onto their toes first using both feet and then using one foot at a time. Strength of hip internal rotation is assessed.

Gait assessment: Routine gait assessment can be done by a primary care practitioner; an expert may be needed for complex gait disorders. Assessment requires a straight hallway without distractions or obstructions and a stopwatch.

Patients should be prepared for the examination. They should be asked to wear pants or shorts that reveal the knees and be informed that several observations may be needed but that they will be allowed to rest if fatigued.

Assistive devices provide stability but also affect gait. Use of walkers often results in a flexed posture and discontinuous gait, particularly if the walker has no wheels. If safe to do so, the practitioner should have the patient walk without an assistive device, while remaining close to or walking with the patient with a gait belt for safety. If patients use a cane, the practitioner can walk with them on the cane side or take their arm and walk with them. Patients with a suspected peripheral neuropathy should walk touching the practitioner's forearm. If gait improves with this intervention, proprioception from the arm is being used to supplement the missing proprioception from the leg; such patients usually benefit from using a cane, which transmits information about the type of surface or floor to the cane-holding hand.

Balance is assessed by measuring the time patients can stand on both feet in tandem stance (heel to toe) and on one foot (single stance); normal is ≥ 5 sec.

Gait velocity is measured using a stopwatch. Patients are timed while walking a fixed distance (preferably 6 or 8 m) at their preferred speed. The test may need to be repeated with patients walking as quickly as possible. Normal gait speed in healthy elderly people ranges from 1.1 to 1.5 m/sec.

Cadence is measured as steps/min. Cadence varies with leg length—about 90 steps/min for tall adults (1.83 m [72 in]) to about 125 steps/min for short adults (1.5 m [60 in]).

Step length can be determined by measuring the distance covered in 10 steps and dividing that number by 10. Because shorter people take shorter steps and foot size is directly related to height, normal step length is 3 foot lengths, and abnormal step length is < 2 foot lengths. A rule of thumb is that if at least 1 foot length is visible between the patient's steps, step length is normal.

Step height can be assessed by observing the swing foot; if it touches the floor, particularly in the middle of the swing phase, patients may trip. Some patients with fear of falling or a cautious gait syndrome purposefully slide their feet over the floor surface. This gait pattern may be safe on a smooth surface but is a risky strategy when walking on rugs because patients may trip.

Asymmetry or variability of gait rhythm can be detected when practitioners whisper "dum . . . dum . . . dum" to themselves with each of the patient's steps. Some practitioners have a better ear than an eye for gait rhythm.

Testing: Testing is sometimes required.

CT or MRI of the brain is often done, particularly when there is poor gait initiation, chaotic cadence, or the appearance of a very stiff gait. These tests help identify lacunar infarcts, white matter disease, and focal atrophy and can help determine whether normal-pressure hydrocephalus should be considered.

Treatment

- Strength training
- Balance training
- Assistive devices

Although determining why gait is abnormal is important, interventions to alter gait are not always indicated. A slowed, aesthetically abnormal gait may enable the elderly person to walk safely and without assistance. However, some treatment interventions can lead to improvement; they include exercise, balance training, and assistive devices (Table 339–2).

Strength training: Frail elderly people with mobility problems achieve modest improvements with exercise programs. In elderly people with arthritis, walking or resistance training reduces knee pain, and gait may improve.

Resistance exercises can improve strength and gait velocity, especially in frail patients with slowed gait. Two or three training sessions a week are usually needed; resistance exercises consist of 3 sets of 8 to 14 repetitions during each session. The load is increased every week or two until a plateau of strength is reached.

Leg press machines train all the large muscle groups of the leg and provide back and pelvic support during lifting. However, these machines are not always accessible to elderly patients. Chair rises with weight vests or weights attached to the waist (waist belts) are an alternative. Instructions are required to reduce the risk of back injury due to excess lumbar lordosis. Step-ups and stair climbing with the same weights are also useful. Ankle plantar flexion can be done with the same weights.

Knee extension machines are effective to strengthen quadriceps. Attaching weights to the ankle strengthens the quadriceps in very frail elderly patients. The usual starting weight for frail people is 3 kg (7 lb). Resistance for all exercises should be increased every week or after the patient can complete 10 or 12 repetitions until the patient reaches a plateau of strength. Then, exercise is continued at the maximum tolerable weight for maintenance.

Balance training: Many patients with balance deficits benefit from balance training. Good standing posture and static balance are taught first. Patients are then taught to be aware of the location of pressure on their feet and how the location of pressure moves with slow leaning or turning the torso to look to the left or right. Leaning forward (using a wall or counter for support), backward (with a wall directly behind), and to each side is then practiced. The goal is for the patient to be able stand on one leg for 10 sec.

Dynamic balance training can involve slow movements in single stance, simple tai chi movements, tandem walking, turns while walking, walking backwards, walking over a virtual object (eg, a 15-cm stripe on the floor), slow forward lunges, and slow dance movements. Multicomponent balance training is probably most effective in improving balance.

Assistive devices: Assistive devices can help maintain mobility and quality of life (see p. 3253). New motor strategies must be learned. Physical therapists should be involved in choice of and training with assistive devices.

Canes are particularly helpful for patients with pain caused by knee or hip arthritis or with peripheral neuropathy

Table 339–2. TREATMENT OF GAIT DISORDERS

COMMON PROBLEM	TREATMENT	COMMENTS
Bone structure		
Kyphotic posture due to compression fractures of the thoracic spine or poor posture	Thoracic extension, shoulder rotation, chin tuck exercises Osteoporosis treatment to prevent new fractures	Compression fracture can be diagnosed by x-ray, and osteoporosis can be identified by bone mineral density testing.
Leg length differences	Heel lift	Usually, heel lift correction is not 100%.
Severe genu varus or valgus	Orthotics, bracing, strengthening of quadriceps	Knee replacement criteria should be reviewed.
Foot abnormality or pain Hallux valgus (bunion) Loss of longitudinal arch	Orthotics, podiatry care, custom shoes	Testing for plantar neuropathy with monofilament nylon is always done to detect risk of plantar ulceration.
Joint range of motion		
Decreased hip internal rotation	Stretching of adductors, strengthening of abductors	Attempting to increase internal rotation by stretching is not usually effective but may prevent further loss of range of motion.
Decreased hip extension	Stretching of hip flexors, strengthening of hip extensors	Lying prone and doing thoracic extension is often recommended.
Decreased ankle dorsiflexion	Stretching of calf muscles	Height of high-heel shoes is reduced.
Hallux rigidus (loss of dorsiflexion of the great toe)	Podiatry or orthopedic referral	An orthotic should be considered.
Muscle power		
Weak hip extension	Chair rise exercises	Chair rise test may be helpful in diagnosis.
Weak knee extension	Chair rise exercises, knee extension with ankle sandbags, squats	Chair rise test may be helpful in diagnosis.
Weak ankle plantar flexion	Heel raises (using body weight)	To increase resistance during heel raises, patients can wear a weighted vest, backpack, or waist belt; they may need to stabilize themselves against a wall.
Weak ankle dorsiflexion	Muscle strengthening (eg, toe rises), ankle foot orthotic for footdrop	Patients place sandbag weights over their metatarsals. With their back to the wall for safety, patients rise on their heels (ie, lift toes off the floor).
Weak hip abduction	Hip abduction with ankle weights, side-lying position on the floor	—
Sensory systems		
Decreased or impaired position sense or balance when eyes are closed during a Romberg test	Appropriate footwear	Vitamin B_{12} level should be checked.
Decreased or impaired plantar touch sensation as measured by Semmes-Weinstein monofilaments	Appropriate footwear	The patient should be assessed for diabetes and alcohol abuse.
Dizziness or vertigo	See p. 795	—
Motor control/balance		
Tandem stance or single-leg stance < 5 sec or turning 360° (both to right and left) requires > 10 steps or patient is unsteady during turning	Balance training involving static and dynamic balance, tai chi, or the equivalent	Vitamin D supplementation (1000–2000 IU once/day) for frail elderly patients with limited sun exposure reduces risk of falls and injury.
Forward lean Bradykinesia Leg hypertonia Parkinsonian signs	Physical therapy training to maintain or improve motor control/balance	CT or MRI can detect lacunar infarcts or white matter disease. Vitamin B_{12} level should be checked.

Table 339–2. TREATMENT OF GAIT DISORDERS (*Continued*)

COMMON PROBLEM	TREATMENT	COMMENTS
Physical and cardiovascular fitness		
Dizziness due to postural hypotension	Review of drugs for possible cause, compression stockings	See pp. 597 and 792
Fatigue, shortness of breath, inability to walk < 400 m at usual pace	Regular walking program	Patients should be assessed for angina, heart failure, pulmonary disease, and claudication. A 6-min walking distance is measured.

of the feet because a cane transmits information about the type of surface or floor to the cane-holding hand. A quad cane can stabilize the patient but usually slows gait. Canes are usually used on the side opposite the painful or weak leg. Many store-bought canes are too long but can be adjusted to the correct height (see Fig. 388–2 on p. 3253) by cutting (a wooden cane) or moving the pin settings (an adjustable cane). For maximal support, cane length should be such that patients have their elbow flexed 20 to 30° when holding the cane.

Walkers can reduce the force and pain at arthritic joints more than a cane, assuming adequate arm and shoulder strength. Walkers provide good lateral stability and moderate protection from forward falls but do little or nothing to help prevent backward falls for patients with balance problems. When prescribing a walker, the physical therapist should consider the sometimes competing needs of providing stability and maximizing efficiency (energy efficiency) of walking. Four-wheeled walkers with larger wheels and brakes maximize gait efficiency but provide less lateral stability. These walkers have the added advantage of a small seat to sit on if patients become fatigued.

Prevention

Primary prevention: High levels of physical activity have been shown to help maintain mobility, even in patients with disease.

Secondary prevention: Exercise has improved gait and measures of mobility in short and long term trials.

Regular walking or maintaining a physically active lifestyle is the most important recommendation. The adverse effects of deconditioning and of inactivity cannot be overstated. A regular walking program of 30 min/day is the best single activity for maintaining mobility; however, an active lifestyle that includes multiple shorter walking episodes is probably equivalent to a single 30-min walk. A safe walking course should be recommended. The patient should be instructed to increase gait speed and duration over several months.

Prevention also includes resistance and balance training. The effects of an active lifestyle on mood and confidence are probably as important as their effect on physiology.

340 The Older Driver

For adults, driving is the most important method of independent transportation. In 2015, there were 40 million licensed drivers ≥ 65 yr in the US, including many ≥ 80 yr (see Table 340–1). Progressive disease that impairs driving in older adults may have two serious adverse outcomes: injury or death resulting from a motor vehicle crash (MVC) or driving cessation. In 2015, over 6,000 older adults (> 65 yr) died in MVCs, and 240,000 were injured. Drivers > age 65 accounted for 18% of all traffic fatalities in 2015.

Table 340–1. PERCENTAGE OF DRIVERS BY AGE AND SEX

AGE	MEN	WOMEN
60–69	95.1%	88.2%
70–79	90.8%	77.1%
≥ 80	77.4%	52.4%

Adapted from the U.S. Department of Transportation 2009 National Household Travel Survey.

Older drivers on average have a lower number of MVCs than drivers of all other ages. However, because the number of miles driven per year also declines with age (see Table 340–2), the crash rate per mile for drivers ≥ 70 yr is higher than that for drivers of all other ages except those < 20 yr (see Fig. 340–1). The overall motor vehicle fatality rate has dropped for older adults—as it has for people of all ages (see Fig. 340–2)—probably because of improved vehicle crashworthiness, improved trauma systems, and roadway improvements. Older drivers also

Table 340–2. ANNUAL MILES PER LICENSED DRIVER BY AGE, 2009

AGE OF DRIVER	ANNUAL MILES
16–19	6,244
20–34	13,709
35–54	15,117
55–64	12,528
≥ 65	8,250

Adapted from the U.S. Department of Transportation 2009 National Household Travel Survey.

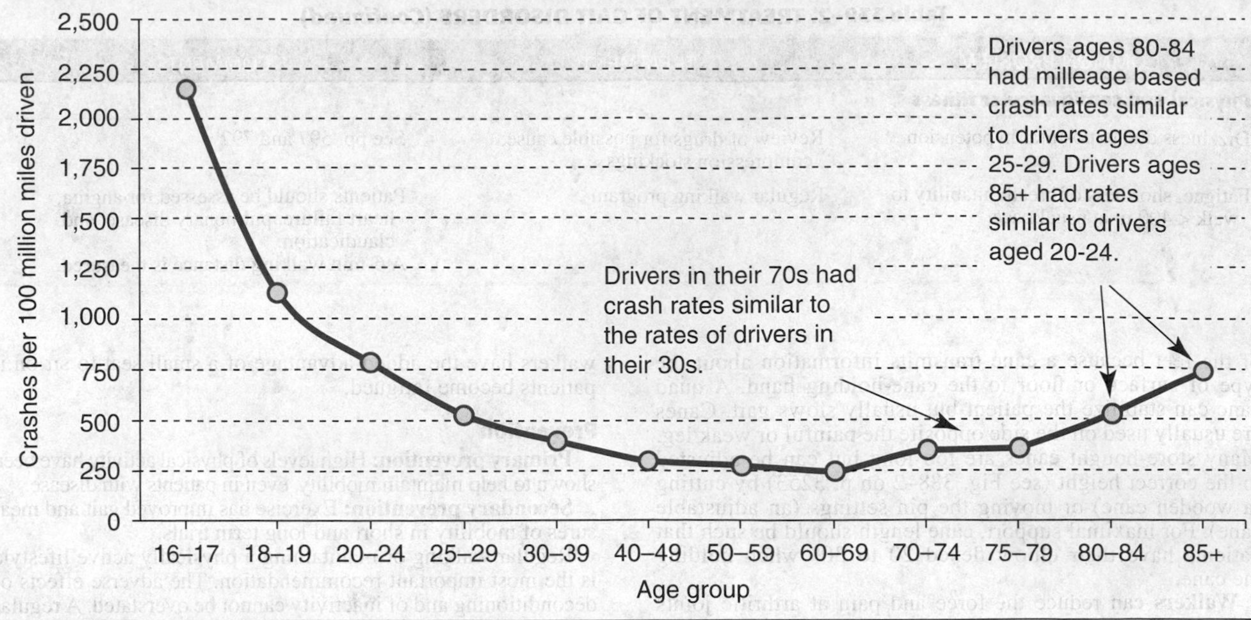

Fig. 340–1. Motor vehicle crashes per 100 million miles driven by age group (2008–2009).

Figure from Online Auto Insurance News; used with permission. Available at http://news.onlineautoinsurance.com/consumer/aaa-study-older-drivers-98576. Data adapted from the AAA Foundation for Traffic Safety.

have the lowest absolute crash rate per year. However, the oldest old (> 80 yr) have the highest traffic death rates per 100,000 population among all age groups, which, given their lower absolute number of MVCs, indicates a higher degree of vulnerability for a given MVC.

Safe driving requires the integration of complex visual, physical, and cognitive processes, and some older drivers may have mild to moderate deficits in one or more of these domains. Many older drivers successfully self-regulate their behavior and compensate for deficits by avoiding rush hour, driving fewer miles per year, limiting trips to shorter distances, and avoiding driving during twilight, nighttime, or inclement weather. Also, older drivers tend to be more cautious, drive more slowly, and take fewer risks. However, some older adults, because they deny or lack insight regarding limitations (eg, vision impairment, dementia, slower reaction time) or have a strong desire to maintain independence, continue to drive despite significant impairment of skills that relate to safe driving ability.

Most MVCs involving older drivers occur during the daytime and on weekdays. These MVCs often result from failing to yield the right-of-way, not heeding stop signs or red lights, or not maintaining proper lane positioning and tend to occur in more complex driving situations (eg, while going through intersections, making left turns, or merging into traffic). MVCs are more likely to involve multiple vehicles and to result in serious injuries and fatalities. Unlike in younger drivers, alcohol, texting, cell phone use, and speeding rarely play a role in MVCs involving older drivers; however, this situation may change in future aging cohorts.

When MVCs do occur, older adults seem to be more vulnerable to injury because

- They have less capacity to withstand trauma.
- They often have more comorbidities.
- Many MVCs are driver-side impact (eg, occur while making left turns), making the driver more vulnerable and likely to be injured.
- They may be more likely than younger drivers to drive very old cars without air bags or other improvements in crash protection.

Assessment: Health care practitioners become involved in driving decisions when deficits are identified during routine examination, a serious medical condition or illness manifests, patients solicit advice, family members express concern, or law enforcement cites unsafe driving behaviors. The role of practitioners is to do detailed functional (see p. 2879) and medical (see p. 2880) assessments related to driving safety. Another useful resource is the American Geriatric Association's Physician's Guide to Assessing and Counseling Older Drivers at www.geriatricscareonline.org.

Driving history should be reviewed; details of driving habits and past violations, MVCs, close calls, or getting lost may point to general or specific impairments. The Alzheimer's Association's warning signs of unsafe driving include the following:

- Forgetting how to locate familiar destinations
- Not obeying traffic signs
- Making slow or poor decisions while driving
- Driving at an inappropriate speed
- Becoming angry or confused while driving
- Hitting curbs
- Not keeping within lanes
- Making errors at intersections
- Confusing the gas and brake pedals
- Returning late from a routine drive
- Forgetting the destination during a drive

Some impairments may obligate practitioners to refer a patient to the state Department of Motor Vehicles for additional testing or driving restrictions. (See the National Highway Traffic Safety

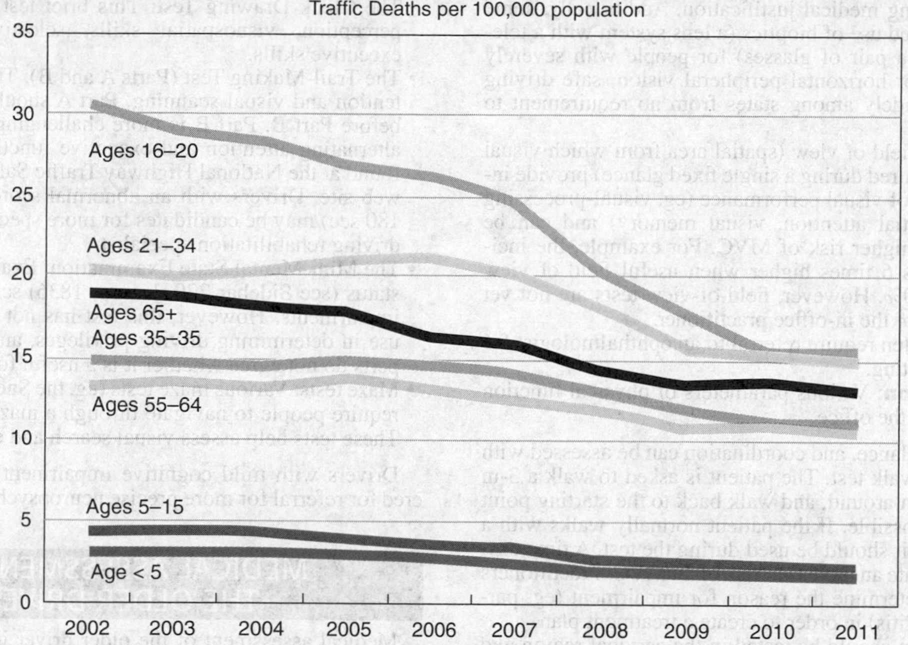

Fig. 340-2. Motor vehicle traffic fatality rates by age group (2002–2011).
Adapted from the National Highway Traffic Safety Administration's (NHTSA) Safety Facts 2011. Available at http://www-nrd.nhtsa.dot.gov/Pubs/811745.pdf.

Administration's [NHTSA] Physician's Guide to Assessing and Counseling Older Drivers for state licensing requirements and reporting regulations at www.nhtsa.gov/people/injury/olddrive/OlderDriversBook.)

KEY POINTS

- The number of older adults is growing rapidly.
- Driving cessation is inevitable for many older adults and can have negative outcomes (eg, social isolation, depression, fewer driving destinations).
- Age-related and disease-related changes in physical, motor, sensory, and cognitive function can impair driving ability and account for some of the increase in MVC rates per miles driven.
- Many older drivers self-regulate their behavior.
- Older adults are more vulnerable to injury in an MVC than younger adults.
- The role of practitioners is to do functional and medical assessments, which may help determine overall driving safety, and to communicate recommendations effectively to older drivers and their family members.
- State licensing requirements and reporting regulations that pertain to older drivers are available from the National Highway Traffic Safety Administration.

FUNCTIONAL ASSESSMENT OF THE OLDER DRIVER

Functional assessment involves assessment of a patient's visual, physical, and cognitive abilities. Adequate function in these areas is needed to drive safely. Most of a functional assessment can be done by primary health care practitioners, but specialists (eg, ophthalmologists, neuropsychologists, subspecialists, occupational and physical therapists, driving rehabilitation specialists) may need to be consulted. Identified deficits may require interventions (see p. 2881), including driving rehabilitation, assistive devices, reporting to the state Department of Motor Vehicles, driving restrictions or cessation, or a combination. Some complicated cases may be referred to state medical advisory boards.

Visual function: Visual function is vital to safe driving. Age-related and pathologic changes in vision are common and can contribute to driving impairment.

Changes with aging include

- Decreased retinal illuminance (amount of light reaching the retina), visual acuity, and peripheral vision
- Presbyopia (decreased ability to accommodate), which impairs depth perception
- Decreased ability to adapt to changes in light and heightened sensitivity to glare, which impair night driving

Ocular diseases common with aging include

- Age-related macular degeneration
- Cataracts
- Glaucoma
- Diabetic retinopathy

In many states, central visual acuity and peripheral vision are routinely tested by the Department of Motor Vehicles when a license is renewed. Most states require 20/40 visual acuity in at least one eye for unrestricted licensing (glasses or contacts are allowed). However, in some states, practitioners can extend the requirement pending medical justification. Additionally, some states have approved use of bioptics (a lens system with a telescope attached to a pair of glasses) for people with severely reduced vision. For horizontal peripheral vision, safe driving thresholds vary widely among states from no requirement to about 140°.

Tests of useful field of view (spatial area from which visual stimuli can be acquired during a single fixed glance) provide integrated measures of visual performance (eg, visual-processing speeds, visual-spatial attention, visual memory) and can be used to predict a higher risk of MVC. For example, the incidence of MVCs is 6 times higher when useful field of view is reduced by > 40%. However, field-of-view tests are not yet widely available for the in-office practitioner.

Older drivers often require referral to an ophthalmologist for comprehensive testing.

Physical function: Various parameters of physical function can be assessed in the office.

- Motor speed, balance, and coordination can be assessed with the rapid-pace walk test. The patient is asked to walk a 3-m (10-ft) path, turn around, and walk back to the starting point as quickly as possible. If the patient normally walks with a walker or cane, it should be used during the test. A time of > 9 sec may indicate an increased risk of an MVC. Practitioners should try to determine the reason for impairment (eg, parkinsonism, arthritis) in order to create a treatment plan.
- Range of motion should be tested in the cervical region and in all joints of the upper and lower extremities. Decreased cervical range of motion impairs ability to turn the head and scan for traffic (particularly in the blind spot). Older adults should have ≥ 30° of lateral rotation to each side; if range of motion is less, they can be referred to a physical therapist to improve range of motion or to a driving rehabilitation specialist for installation of larger, wide-angle mirrors in the vehicle. Decreased range of motion in the extremities impairs ability to operate vehicle controls.
- Strength in upper and lower extremities should be assessed qualitatively (in terms of meeting the needs of driving a vehicle). Grip strength can be measured with a dynamometer. A grip strength of < 16 kg for men or < 14 kg for women may reflect decreased ability to manipulate the steering wheel.
- Lower extremity proprioception and peripheral sensory function should be tested. Decreased sensation can impair ability to modulate pressure on foot controls.

Physical and occupational therapists who specialize in driving rehabilitation can provide comprehensive testing of motor function related to driving ability. A rehabilitation driving assessment sometimes also involves the specialist going out in a vehicle with the patient to evaluate actual driving skills. The vehicle used during the evaluation should be equipped with features that allow the specialist to maintain safe control (eg, passenger-side brake). Driving rehabilitation specialists can be located by contacting local rehabilitation facilities or going to www.driver-ed.org. However, in most states, the cost of a rehabilitation driving assessment is not covered by insurance (Medicare or private) and may be an out-of-pocket cost.

Cognitive function: The incidence of cognitive impairment increases in people ≥ 65. People with cognitive impairment often do not recognize their limitations and are at higher risk of MVCs; risk increases with severity of impairment. Although no one test has been found to completely and accurately predict driving safety, some tests are able to provide some level of predictability regarding impaired driving performance in older adults. These tests include the following:

- The Clock Drawing Test: This brief test screens for visual perception, visuospatial skills, selective attention, and executive skills.
- The Trail-Making Test (Parts A and B): This test assesses attention and visual scanning. Part A should always be given before Part B. Part B is more challenging and also assesses alternating attention and executive function. Part B can be found at the National Highway Traffic Safety Administration web site. Drivers with an abnormal score on Part B (eg, > 180 sec) may be candidates for more specialized testing by a driving rehabilitation specialist.
- The Mini-Mental State Examination: Examination of mental status (see Sidebar 220–1 on p. 1836) screens for cognitive impairments. However, this test has not been validated for use in determining driving privileges, and traffic safety experts do not agree whether it is a useful for this purpose.
- Maze tests: Various maze tests (eg, the Snellgrove Maze Test) require people to navigate through a maze printed on paper. These tests help assess visual search and executive skills.

Drivers with mild cognitive impairment should be considered for referral for more precise neuropsychologic assessment.

MEDICAL ASSESSMENT OF THE OLDER DRIVER

Medical assessment of the older driver includes a thorough review of medical conditions and/or drugs that can impair driving ability. Such medical conditions can be chronic disorders that impair important functional abilities needed for driving (eg, macular degeneration that decreases vision) or acute events that impair consciousness (eg, seizure, syncope). The following are a few of the more common medical illnesses or syndromes that are associated with increased driving risk (eg, MVCs, poor performance on road tests).

Falls: Falls and MVCs share common causative factors (eg, impaired vision, muscle strength, cognition). A history of falls in the past 1 to 2 yr indicates increased risk of MVCs and should prompt further evaluation of physical functioning (see above).

Cardiac disorders: Cardiac disorders may increase driving risk. General guidelines include refraining from driving for

- At least 1 mo after MI, coronary artery bypass surgery, or stabilization of unstable angina symptoms
- 3 mo after arrhythmia with syncope
- 6 mo after internal cardioverter-defibrillator placement or after resuscitation required because of sustained ventricular tachycardia or ventricular fibrillation

However, patients should discuss these specific recommendations with their cardiologist or primary care physician.

Patients with severe heart failure (eg, class IV heart failure, dyspnea at rest or while driving) should refrain from driving until they can be evaluated with on-road testing.

Neurologic disorders: Neurologic disorders also increase driving risk. Specific disorders include

- Stroke or transient ischemic attack (TIA): Drivers with a single TIA should wait 1 mo before resuming driving; those with recurrent TIAs or stroke should be event-free for at least 3 mo before resuming driving. Physical examination should be done to assess how residual disability due to stroke may affect driving ability.
- Seizures: Regulations for drivers who have seizures are state-specific, but most states require a seizure-free interval (often 6 mo) before they reinstate driving privileges. Anticonvulsants can adequately control seizures in about 70% of

patients, although relapses may occur when these drugs are withdrawn.

Alzheimer disease or progressive dementing disorders will eventually impair all functional abilities, including those required for driving. Monitoring patients for new driving errors that can be attributed to changes in cognition or identifying significant impairments in psychometric tests (see p. 2880) may be useful in determining referrals for on-road evaluation or possibly driving cessation.

Many other neurologic disorders (eg, Parkinson disease) cause disability and should be monitored by functional assessment and possibly an on-road test.

Diabetes mellitus: Diabetes mellitus poses a risk because patients may become hypoglycemic while driving. Patients who have had a recent hypoglycemic episode with unawareness should not drive for 3 mo or until factors contributing to the episode (eg, diet, activity, timing and dose of insulin or antihyperglycemic drug) have been assessed and managed. Sensory changes in the extremities, retinopathy, or both caused by diabetes can also impair driving ability.

Sleep disorders: Sleep disorders, most notably obstructive sleep apnea syndrome, can cause drowsiness leading to MVCs, and patients should refrain from driving until they are adequately treated.

Drugs: When starting a new drug that could affect visual, physical, or cognitive function, patients should refrain from driving for several days (depending on the time required to reach a steady state) to be sure no adverse effects occur.

A large number of drugs potentially can impair driving, typically those with CNS adverse effects (eg, confusion, sedation). Many of these drugs have been shown to impair actual driving in road tests and/or driving simulators and to increase MVC risk. These drugs can also increase fall risk. Despite these risks, many of these drugs should not be stopped abruptly because they may need to be tapered.

Drugs that increase driving risk include

- Antihistamines, benzodiazepines, opioids, anticholinergics, hypnotics, antihypertensives, or tricyclic antidepressants: These drugs increase driving risk because they can cause drowsiness; some can also cause hypotension or arrhythmias.
- Antiparkinsonian dopamine agonists (eg, pergolide, pramipexole, ropinirole): These drugs occasionally cause acute sleep attacks, which may pose an increased risk of an MVC.
- Antiemetics (eg, prochlorperazine) and muscle relaxants (eg, cyclobenzaprine): These drugs are cause for concern because of their potential for altering sensory perception.

Instructing patients to bring all drug containers to the office can help identify drugs that increase risk.

Older adults are involved in fewer alcohol-related fatal MVCs. Fewer older adults consume alcohol, but limiting alcohol consumption is still important because blood alcohol level per amount of alcohol consumed is higher in older adults. Also, concurrent use of alcohol and other drugs, particularly multiple drugs, further impairs cognition, increasing the risk of MVCs.

INTERVENTIONS WITH THE OLDER DRIVER

If older drivers with significant functional deficits decide to limit or stop driving, the role of health care practitioners is largely supportive. If the medical evaluation identifies potentially correctable deficits and older drivers acknowledge these deficits but still wish to continue driving, practitioners can offer treatment to help correct the deficits or impairments. However, aside from treating medical conditions that impair driving ability, most practitioners are ill-equipped to formulate or execute a driving rehabilitation plan; referral to specialists is often helpful.

Driving rehabilitation programs: Although some older drivers can benefit from driving refresher courses (eg, American Association of Retired Persons Driver Safety Program available at www.aarp.org), most should be referred to occupational therapists that specialize in driving rehabilitation (called driving rehabilitation specialists—to find one of these specialists, contact local rehabilitation facilities). Driving rehabilitation specialists usually do comprehensive driving assessments that include clinical tests of vision, motor, and cognitive skills as well as on-road evaluations. During on-road evaluations, the specialist goes in a vehicle with the older driver to evaluate actual driving skills in varied traffic conditions. The vehicle used during the evaluation should be equipped with features that allow the specialist to maintain safe control (eg, passenger-side brake). These specialists can also assist by

- Instituting a tailored rehabilitation plan to increase motor skills or cognition and perception in the driver's daily life
- Providing adaptive equipment, such as a spinner knob, to help with one-handed steering or more complicated devices such as hand controls
- Evaluating the response to the rehabilitation plan and providing feedback to the driver, involved relatives, and the physician as to whether the driver's driving abilities are adequate to continue driving or whether driving restrictions are indicated
- Providing mobility counseling or advice on alternate modes of transportation

In most states, the cost of a rehabilitation driving assessment is not covered by insurance (Medicare or private) and may be an out-of-pocket cost.

Driving cessation: If older drivers deny or are unaware of their limitations or if deficits do not respond to treatment, practitioners may need to be more proactive. In these situations, practitioners should discuss issues relevant to driving safety, potential driving cessation, patient transportation needs, and alternative transportation resources with the patient and family members.

The practitioner should balance the benefits of safety to the patient, pedestrians, and other drivers against the costs of social isolation, worsening functional status, impaired quality of life, and clinical depression. For some patients (eg, those with severe dementia), the benefits of driving cessation clearly outweigh the costs.

Alternative transportation options should be discussed; they vary from community to community, and contact with local resources such as the Alzheimer's Association (www.alz.org) or American Automobile Association Foundation for Traffic Safety (seniordriving.aaa.com) may provide updated information on options. Family members can find publications and online information about having conversations with older drivers.

The loss of driving privileges can be relatively devastating in terms of maintaining independence. If alternative transportation cannot be arranged and the ability to maintain activities of daily living is adversely affected, loss of driving privileges sometimes prompts the need to move in with a family member or transition to an assisted-living facility or retirement community.

Reporting: If the driver's functional limitations or medical status seems to warrant driving cessation, practitioners should follow the reporting requirements of their state Department of Motor Vehicles. States vary in their reporting laws. All states have voluntary reporting laws, but some states have mandatory reporting laws. (See the National Highway Traffic Safety

Administration's [NHTSA] Physician's Guide to Assessing and Counseling Older Drivers for state licensing requirements and reporting regulations at www.nhtsa.gov/people/injury/olddrive/OlderDriversBook). In most states, statutes protect the practitioner's anonymity or provide immunity to the practitioner. Legal consultation may be beneficial when an office or institution is developing a reporting policy and procedure.

Before making a report, practitioners should discuss recommendations for driving cessation directly with the patient and family rather than simply filing a report. Practitioners should make every attempt to persuade the patient to cooperate with driving restrictions. Such discussion should include why the patient's limitations make driving unsafe and why the practitioner is obligated to report.

In some situations, practitioners must report functional limitations or medical status to state agencies against the wishes of their patients; this action often has a negative impact on the practitioner-patient relationship. Regardless, medical information can be legally disclosed if a patient's driving impairment might jeopardize public safety; practitioners who do not notify appropriate authorities may be legally liable for subsequent injuries.

341 Prevention of Disease and Disability in the Elderly

For the elderly, prevention focuses mainly on disease, frailty, accidents (ie, unintentional injury), iatrogenic complications, and psychosocial problems. Not all elderly patients benefit from every preventive measure. Choice of preventive measures is guided by the patient's general condition:

- Healthy: These elderly people have minimal or no chronic disease and are functionally independent. Primary and secondary prevention of disease and prevention of frailty are the most beneficial measures for this group.
- Chronically ill: These people typically have several noncurable but treatable diseases, are usually functionally independent or minimally dependent, often take several prescription drugs, and occasionally are hospitalized for exacerbations of their chronic diseases. Secondary and tertiary prevention of disease and prevention of frailty are priorities, as are primary prevention of disease and prevention of iatrogenic complications and accidents.
- Frail/complex: These people typically have many severe chronic diseases, are functionally dependent, and have lost their physiologic reserve. They are frequently hospitalized and institutionalized. For them, prevention of accidents and iatrogenic complications is most important.

Some preventive measures apply to all elderly people. For example, exercise can help prevent frailty in healthy or chronically ill elderly people. In frail elderly people, exercise can help preserve functional ability and reduce the incidence of accidents. Influenza vaccination (yearly) and pneumococcal vaccination (needed only once, except for patients at high risk) are effective, inexpensive, and associated with minimal morbidity.

Patient and caregiver issues: Healthy elderly people should visit their primary care physician at least annually to ensure timely completion of primary and secondary disease prevention measures, including screening (see Tables 341–1 and 341–2) and chemoprevention (eg, vaccination, aspirin—see Table 341–3). For more information, see recommendations for clinical preventive services from the U.S. Preventive Services Task Force (USPSTF).

Medicare covers a comprehensive "Welcome to Medicare" preventive physical examination, which must occur within 12 mo of Part B enrollment, and an annual wellness visit every 12 mo thereafter.

Regular exercise (see p. 3182) and a healthy diet (see Table 341–4) help prevent or postpone frailty and many diseases, as can other disease prevention measures (see Table 341–5). Chronically ill patients should learn about their diseases and treatment plans, as should their caregivers. Regular physician visits and prompt reporting of a change in symptoms can help reduce severe disease exacerbations, which can lead to hospitalization and functional decline.

Caregivers of the frail elderly must work assiduously to prevent accidents by completing a home safety checklist and correcting any potential problems that are identified. Caregivers should watch for even subtle functional changes in elderly patients and promptly report any changes to a health care practitioner. If a patient has multiple unmet needs, especially when coupled with functional decline, a caregiver should consider seeking the care of a geriatric interdisciplinary team.

PREVENTION OF DISEASE IN THE ELDERLY

Primary and Secondary Prevention

Primary prevention aims to stop disease before it starts, often by reducing or eliminating risk factors. Primary prevention may include immunoprophylaxis (vaccinations), chemoprophylaxis (see Table 341–3), and lifestyle changes (see Table 341–5). In secondary prevention, disease is detected and treated at an early stage, before symptoms or functional losses occur, thereby minimizing morbidity and mortality.

Screening can be a primary or secondary preventive measure (see Tables 341–1 and 341–2). Screening can be used to detect risk factors, which may be altered to prevent disease, or to detect disease in asymptomatic people, who can then be treated early.

Tertiary Prevention

In tertiary prevention, an existing symptomatic, usually chronic disease is appropriately managed to prevent further functional loss. Disease management is enhanced by using disease-specific practice guidelines and protocols. Several disease management programs have been developed:

- Disease-specific care management: A specially trained nurse, working with a primary care physician or geriatrician, coordinates protocol-driven care, arranges support services, and teaches patients.
- Chronic care clinics: Patients with the same chronic disease are taught in groups and are visited by a health care practitioner; this approach can help patients with diabetes achieve better glucose control.

Table 341–1. SCREENING RECOMMENDATIONS FOR ELDERLY PATIENTS

DISEASE TO BE DETECTED	TEST	FREQUENCY	COMMENTS*, †
Abdominal aortic aneurysm	Abdominal ultrasonography	Once between age 65–75	For men who have ever smoked: B recommendation by USPSTF For men who have never smoked: C recommendation For women: D recommendation
Abuse or neglect	Inquire about mistreatment (eg, "Are there any problems with family or household members that you would like to tell me about?")	At least once	For all elderly patients: I recommendation by USPSTF
Alcohol misuse	Alcoholism screening questionnaire (eg, AUDIT, AUDIT-C)	Yearly	For all adults, including those ≥ 65: B recommendation by USPSTF For patients who are ≥ 65 and have a positive screening test: B recommendation by USPSTF for brief behavioral counseling interventions For patients who meet the criteria for alcoholism: Abstinence recommended
Cognitive impairment (eg, dementia, delirium)	Cognitive impairment screening instrument (eg, Mini-Cog)	NA	I recommendation by USPSTF
Depression (major depressive disorder)	Depression screening questionnaire (eg, PHQ-2)	Yearly	For all adults, including those ≥ 65: B recommendation by USPSTF‡
Diabetes mellitus, type 2	Plasma glucose level	Yearly	For everyone with BP ≥ 130/85: B recommendation by USPSTF For general population ≥ 65: I recommendation For adults with cholesterol levels near the threshold for treatment: Screening for diabetes as part of assessment of cardiovascular risk Medicare coverage: Screening every 6 mo for people with hypertension, dyslipidemia, or a history of high plasma glucose levels
Dyslipidemia	Fasting serum total, LDL, and HDL cholesterol levels; triglyceride levels optional	At least every 5 yr More frequently for people who have coronary artery disease, diabetes, or peripheral arterial disease or who have had a stroke	For women ≥ 45 who have risk factors for coronary artery disease and for all men ≥ 35: A recommendation by USPSTF Medicare coverage: Screening every 5 yr
Fall risk	Inquiry about falls during the previous year and about difficulty with walking or balance, Get-Up-and-Go test	Yearly	Recommendation by the AGS and BGS For community-dwelling patients ≥ 65 who are at increased risk of falls: B recommendation by USPSTF for exercise and vitamin D supplementation
Glaucoma	Intraocular pressure measurement	Yearly	I recommendation by USPSTF Medicare coverage: Yearly screening for high-risk patients (anyone with diabetes or a family history of glaucoma, blacks ≥ 50, and Hispanics ≥ 65)
Hearing deficits	Bedside hearing test	Yearly	For everyone ≥ 65: I recommendation by USPSTF
HIV	HIV test of serum, blood, or oral fluid	At least once	For everyone 15–65 and for patients > 65 with HIV risk factors: A recommendation by USPSTF

Table continues on the following page.

Table 341–1. SCREENING RECOMMENDATIONS FOR ELDERLY PATIENTS (*Continued*)

DISEASE TO BE DETECTED	TEST	FREQUENCY	COMMENTS*, †
Hypertension	BP measurement	At least every 2 yr for people with BP < 120/80 mm Hg More frequently for people with higher BP	For everyone ≥ 18: A recommendation by USPSTF
Obesity or undernutrition	Height and weight measurement BMI (kg/m²) calculation§	At least yearly	For all adults: B recommendation by USPSTF
Osteoporosis	Dual-energy x-ray absorptiometry	At most, every 2 yr	For all women ≥ 65 and for women < 65 with a ≥ 9.3% risk of osteoporotic fracture over 10 yr as calculated by the FRAX (Fracture Risk Assessment) tool: B recommendation by USPSTF Medicare coverage: Screening every 2 yr after age 50 or, if medically necessary, more often
Thyroid dysfunction (hypothyroidism or hyperthyroidism)	Thyroid-stimulating hormone level	NA	I recommendation by USPSTF
Tobacco use	Inquiry about tobacco use	At least once	A recommendation by USPSTF For all patients who report tobacco use: Cessation counseling and appropriate drug therapy
Visual deficits	Snellen visual acuity test	Yearly	For everyone ≥ 65: I recommendation by USPSTF

*USPSTF recommendations based on strength of evidence and net benefit (benefit minus harm):

- A = Strong evidence in support
- B = Good evidence in support
- C = Balance of benefit and harm too close to justify recommendation
- D = Evidence against
- I = Insufficient evidence to recommend for or against

†Medicare coverage, if provided, is listed. Patients may have to pay co-payments and deductibles, depending on the test.
‡USPSTF recommends screening only in practices with systems to ensure accurate diagnosis, effective treatment, and follow-up.
§BMI ≥ 25 = overweight; BMI ≥ 30 = obesity.
AAOS = American Academy of Orthopedic Surgeons; AGS = American Geriatrics Society; AUDIT = Alcohol Use Disorder Identification Test; AUDIT-C = abbreviated AUDIT Consumption Test; BGS = British Geriatrics Society; BMI = body mass index; NA = not applicable; PHQ-2 = Patient Health Questionnaire-2; USPSTF = U.S. Preventive Services Task Force.

- Specialists: Patients with a chronic disease that is difficult to stabilize can be referred to a specialist. This approach works best when the specialist and primary care physician work collaboratively.

Patients with the following chronic disorders, which are common among the elderly, can potentially benefit from tertiary prevention.

Arthritis: Arthritis (primarily osteoarthritis; much less commonly, RA) affects about half of people ≥ 65. It leads to impaired mobility and increases risk of osteoporosis, aerobic and muscular deconditioning, falls, and pressure ulcers.

Osteoporosis: Tests to measure bone density can detect osteoporosis before it leads to a fracture. Ca and vitamin D supplementation, exercise, and, if needed, cessation of cigarette smoking can help prevent osteoporosis from progressing, and treatment can prevent new fractures.

Diabetes: Hyperglycemia, especially when the glycosylated hemoglobin (Hb A_{1c}) concentration is > 7.9% for at least 7 yr, increases the risk of retinopathy, neuropathy, nephropathy, and coronary artery disease. Glycemic treatment goals should be adjusted based on patient preferences, comorbid conditions, and life expectancy. For example, appropriate HbA_{1c} goals might be

- < 7.5% for otherwise healthy diabetic older patients with a life expectancy of > 10 yr
- < 8.0% for patients with comorbidities and a life expectancy of < 10 yr
- < 9.0% for frail patients with a limited life expectancy

Control of hypertension and dyslipidemia in diabetic patients is particularly important.

Patient education and foot examinations at each visit can help prevent foot ulcers.

Vascular disorders: Elderly patients with a history of coronary artery disease, cerebrovascular disease, or peripheral vascular disease are at high risk of disabling events. Risk can be reduced by aggressive management of vascular risk factors (eg, hypertension, smoking, diabetes, obesity, atrial fibrillation, dyslipidemia).

Heart failure: Morbidity due to heart failure is significant among the elderly, and the mortality rate is higher than that of many cancers. Appropriate, aggressive treatment, especially of systolic dysfunction, reduces functional decline, hospitalization, and mortality rate.

Table 341–2. CANCER SCREENING RECOMMENDATIONS FOR ELDERLY PATIENTS

CANCER TO BE DETECTED	TEST	FREQUENCY	COMMENTS*, †
Breast cancer	Mammography	Every 2 yr	For women 50–74: B recommendation by USPSTF For women ≥ 75: I recommendation by USPSTF; suggestion by AGS to continue screening unless life expectancy is < 10 yr Medicare coverage: Yearly screening
Cervical or uterine cancer	Papanicolaou (Pap) test (evidence for newer methods is insufficient)	At least every 3 yr	For women > 65: D recommendation by USPSTF against screening if results of adequate recent screening have been normal and women are not at high risk For women who have had a total hysterectomy for a benign disorder: D recommendation by USPSTF against having Pap tests Suggestion by AGS and ACS to stop screening in women > 70 if the last 2 results were normal (if women > 70 have never been screened, screening should be done, and if results of 2 tests done 1 yr apart are normal, screening may be stopped) Medicare coverage: Screening every 1 yr for women at high risk; otherwise, every 2 yr
Colon cancer	Screening test (FOBT, flexible sigmoidoscopy, colonoscopy)	—	For everyone 50–75: A recommendation by USPSTF For patients 76–85, C recommendation by USPSTF against routine screening (citing a very small net benefit) For patients > 85: D recommendation by USPSTF against screening
	FOBT	Yearly	Medicare coverage: Yearly FOBT
	Flexible sigmoidoscopy	Every 5 yr	Sometimes used with FOBT Medicare coverage: Flexible sigmoidoscopy every 4 yr or 10 yr after colonoscopy
	Colonoscopy	Every 10 yr	Medicare coverage: Colonoscopy every 2 yr for high-risk patients or otherwise every 10 yr (but not within 4 yr of previous sigmoidoscopy)
Prostate cancer	PSA measurement DRE	PSA commonly measured every 1–4 yr	D recommendation by USPSTF against screening Medicare coverage: Yearly PSA measurement and DRE

*USPSTF recommendations based on strength of evidence and net benefit (benefit minus harm):

- A = Strong evidence in support
- B = Good evidence in support
- C = Balance of benefit and harm too close to justify recommendation
- D = Evidence against
- I = Insufficient evidence to recommend for or against

†Medicare coverage, if provided, is listed. Patients may have to pay co-payments and deductibles, depending on the test.

ACS = American Cancer Society; AGS = American Geriatrics Society; DRE = digital rectal examination; FOBT = fecal occult blood test; PSA = prostate-specific antigen; USPSTF = U.S. Preventive Services Task Force.

Chronic obstructive pulmonary disease (COPD): Smoking cessation, appropriate use of inhalers and other drugs, and patient education regarding energy-conserving behavioral techniques can decrease the number and severity of exacerbations of COPD leading to hospitalization.

PREVENTION OF FRAILTY

Frailty is loss of physiologic reserve, which makes people susceptible to disability due to minor stresses. Common features of frailty include weakness, slowed motor function, weight loss, muscle wasting (sarcopenia), exercise intolerance, frequent falls, immobility, incontinence, and frequent exacerbations of chronic diseases.

Exercise (see p. 3182) and a healthy diet (see Table 341–4) are recommended for preventing or reducing frailty. Elderly people who engage in regular aerobic exercise (eg, walking, swimming, running) increase their life expectancy and have less functional decline than those who are sedentary. Mood and possibly cognitive function may also be improved. Weight training can help increase bone mass and reduce risk of falls and fractures. A healthy diet may prevent or reduce risk of many diseases that contribute to frailty, including breast and colon

Table 341–3. CHEMOPREVENTION AND IMMUNIZATION FOR ELDERLY PATIENTS

DISEASE TO BE PREVENTED	MEASURE	FREQUENCY	COMMENTS*, †
Atherosclerotic cardiovascular disease (coronary artery disease, stroke)	Aspirin chemoprevention	Daily	For men 45–79 if risk of MI exceeds risk of GI bleeding and for women 55–79 if risk of ischemic stroke exceeds risk of GI bleeding: A recommendation by USPSTF For patients > 80: I recommendation by USPSTF Optimal dose unknown (but 75 mg po once/day may be as effective as higher doses and may have a lower risk of GI bleeding)
Influenza	Vaccination	Yearly	For everyone: Recommendation by CDC‡ Medicare coverage: Vaccination once during an influenza season
Pneumococcal infection	Vaccination	Once at age 65	For everyone ≥ 65: Recommendation by CDC (which also recommends one-time revaccination for people ≥ 65 if they were vaccinated ≥ 5 yr previously and were < 65 at the time of primary vaccination) Medicare coverage: Vaccination once in a lifetime (revaccination coverage depends on patient's status)
Tetanus	Vaccination	Every 10 yr	For everyone ≥ 65: Recommendation by CDC to maintain booster schedule or, if people were never vaccinated, to be given the primary vaccine series
Zoster	Vaccination	Once at age 60	For everyone ≥ 60: Recommendation by CDC for vaccination once, regardless of history of zoster or varicella

*USPSTF recommendations based on strength of evidence and net benefit (benefit minus harm):

- A = Strong evidence in support
- B = Good evidence in support
- C = Balance of benefit and harm too close to justify recommendation
- D = Evidence against
- I = Insufficient evidence to recommend for or against

†Medicare coverage, if provided, is listed. Patients may have to pay co-payments and deductibles, depending on the test.

‡For people at high risk of influenza A (eg, during institutional outbreaks), oseltamivir or zanamivir may be started at the time of vaccination and continued for 2 wk.

CDC = Centers for Disease Control and Prevention; USPSTF = U.S. Preventive Services Task Force.

cancers, osteoporosis, obesity, and undernutrition; morbidity and mortality may also be reduced.

PREVENTION OF INJURIES IN THE ELDERLY

Falls: The elderly are vulnerable to injury due to falls (see p. 2861). A falls prevention program, including exercise (with or without physical therapy) and vitamin D supplementation, should be implemented for people who are at high risk of falls or who have already fallen.

Driving hazards: All elderly people should be reminded to use lap and shoulder belts and to refrain from driving when they are under the influence of alcohol or psychoactive drugs.

For the elderly, risk of injuring themselves and others while driving is higher than that for younger adults because of age-associated changes and conditions common among the elderly (see also Ch. 340). Driving ability should be investigated with further questions and, if indicated, with formal assessment for any of the following:

- Poor visual acuity
- Dementia
- Functionally significant impairment of neck or trunk movement
- Poor motor coordination
- Bradykinesia

Also, a family member's or friend's concern about the patient's driving ability should prompt further inquiry and assessment.

Formal assessment of driving ability can be done by an occupational therapist (see p. 2880). Many states have laws that mandate physician reporting of suspected impaired drivers. Sensitivity is required when a health care practitioner must recommend cessation of driving because such a recommendation threatens autonomy.

Home hazards: The home may have many hazards. For example, people with peripheral neuropathy are at increased risk of burns from excessively hot water; burns can be prevented by setting the hot water heater temperature at < 49° C. For people with dementia, using electrical and gas appliances is particularly dangerous; use of alarms and automatic shut-off

Table 341–4. NUTRITIONAL RECOMMENDATIONS FOR PREVENTION OF FRAILTY

MEASURE	DESCRIPTION	RATIONALE
Low-fat diet	Fats limited to less than about 20 g/day, with 6–10 g polyunsaturated (with ω-3s and ω-6s in equal proportions), ≤ 2 g saturated fats, and the rest as monounsaturated fats Some sources of healthful oils: Oily fish (eg, tuna, salmon, mackerel, herring), certain vegetable oils (flaxseed, canola, soybean), flax seed, and walnuts	Decreases risk of cardiovascular disease
Reduced Na diet	Optimal level of intake unknown but some evidence to support reducing intake to 2.3 g/day	Lowers BP in some people
High Ca diet and Ca supplements	For the elderly, 1200 mg/day (most American diets contain only 500–700 mg/day)	Helps maintain bone density and reduce risk of fractures
Adequate intake of vitamins and minerals	Largely by eating fruits and vegetables Supplementation with vitamin D (at least 600 IU/day for patients ≤ 70, 800 IU/day for patients > 70) for people with average or low dietary Ca	For vitamin D, prevents bone loss, falls, and fractures May prevent various chronic diseases
High-fiber diet	Best obtained by eating fruits, vegetables, and grains	May prevent colon cancer Has a beneficial effect on serum lipids
Moderate alcohol intake	About 1 oz of alcohol/day (more can be harmful)	May decrease risk of cardiovascular disease

features on appliances can help. Smoke and carbon monoxide detectors should be installed and maintained. Firearms should be safely stored or removed from the home.

All patients or their caregivers can complete a home safety checklist to identify hazards. Physical and occupational therapists may visit a patient's home to assess its safety.

PREVENTION OF IATROGENIC COMPLICATIONS IN THE ELDERLY

Iatrogenic complications are more common and often more severe among the elderly than among younger patients. These complications include adverse drug effects (eg,

Table 341–5. LIFESTYLE MEASURES THAT HELP PREVENT COMMON CHRONIC DISEASES

MEASURE	EXAMPLES OF DISEASES
Smoking cessation	Atherosclerotic cardiovascular disease (coronary artery disease, stroke), cancer, COPD, diabetes mellitus type 2, hypertension, osteoporosis
Achievement of and maintenance of a desirable body weight	Atherosclerotic cardiovascular disease (coronary artery disease, stroke), diabetes mellitus type 2, hypertension, osteoarthritis
Reduction of dietary saturated fat and avoidance of trans fats	Atherosclerotic cardiovascular disease (coronary artery disease, stroke), cancer, diabetes mellitus type 2, hypertension
Increased intake of fruits, vegetables, and fiber	Atherosclerotic cardiovascular disease (coronary artery disease, stroke), cancer (possibly), hypertension
Increased aerobic exercise	Atherosclerotic cardiovascular disease (coronary artery disease, stroke), cancer
Reduction of dietary Na	Atherosclerotic cardiovascular disease (coronary artery disease, stroke), hypertension
Reduced intake of salt- or smoke-cured food	Cancer
Minimized radiation and sun exposure	Cancer
Muscle strengthening and stretching	Osteoarthritis
Moderate physical activity	Osteoarthritis
Adequate Ca and vitamin D intake and sun exposure	Osteoporosis
Regular weight-bearing exercise	Osteoporosis
Limited caffeine intake	Osteoporosis
Limited alcohol intake (to 1 drink/day)*	Osteoporosis

*1 drink = one 12-oz can of beer, one 5-oz glass of wine, 1.5 oz of distilled liquor.

interactions), falls, nosocomial infections, pressure ulcers, delirium, and complications related to surgery. Prevention is often possible.

Risk Factors

The first step in prevention is to identify patients at high risk. Risk factors include the following.

Multiple chronic diseases: The greater the number of chronic diseases, the greater the risk that treatment of one disease will exacerbate others. For example, treatment of arthritis with an NSAID may exacerbate heart failure, coronary artery disease, or chronic gastritis.

Multiple physicians: Having multiple physicians can result in uncoordinated care and polypharmacy. Consultation among multiple physicians every time one of them sees a common patient is difficult. As a result, a patient's therapeutic regimen is frequently changed without the input of the patient's other physicians, thereby increasing risk of iatrogenic complications.

Multiple drugs (polypharmacy) and inappropriate drugs: Taking multiple drugs concurrently and having multiple chronic diseases markedly increase risk of adverse drug-drug or drug-disease interactions (see p. 2848). Risk of such interactions is particularly high among patients who are undernourished or who have renal failure. Also, certain drugs have an especially high risk of adverse effects in the elderly (see p. 2856).

Hospitalization: Risks due to hospitalization include hospital-acquired infection, polypharmacy, and transfusion reactions. Hospitalized patients who have dementia or who are immobilized (eg, after surgery) are at high risk of iatrogenic complications.

Medical technology may contribute to iatrogenic complications, including sudden death or MI after valvular replacement surgery, stroke after carotid endarterectomy, fluid overload after transfusions and infusions, unwanted prolongation of life via artificial life support, and hypoxic encephalopathy after potentially life-prolonging CPR.

Prevention

Interventions that can prevent iatrogenic complications include the following.

Care management: Care managers facilitate communication among health care practitioners, ensure that needed services are provided, and prevent duplication of services. Care managers may be employed by physician groups, health plans, or community or governmental organizations. The frail elderly benefit the most from case management.

Geriatric interdisciplinary team: A geriatric interdisciplinary team (see p. 2889) evaluates all of the patient's needs, develops a coordinated care plan, and manages (or, along with the primary care physician, co-manages) care. Because this intervention is resource-intensive, it is best reserved for very complex cases.

Pharmacist consultation: A pharmacist can help prevent potential complications caused by polypharmacy and inappropriate drug use.

Acute Care for the Elderly (ACE) units: These units are hospital wards with protocols to ensure that elderly patients are thoroughly evaluated for potential iatrogenic problems before problems occur and that such problems are identified and appropriately managed.

Advance directives: Patients are encouraged to prepare advance directives, including designation of a proxy to make medical decisions (see p. 3212). These documents can help prevent unwanted treatment for critically ill patients who cannot speak for themselves.

PREVENTION OF PSYCHOSOCIAL PROBLEMS IN THE ELDERLY

Depression screening is recommended because depression is common among the elderly. Screening is relatively easy; several instruments do not require a physician for administration. For patients who feel lonely or isolated, social worker assistance to increase social contacts may prevent morbidity and postpone death. For those who are depressed, appropriate intervention with counseling or drugs is warranted.

A sense of self-worth may contribute to better health. Patients should be encouraged to remain productive, engage in leisure activities, and remain or become involved with other people. These actions can enhance self-worth. Suggesting activities that confirm a sense of social connectedness, such as obtaining a pet, contributing to household chores, or doing volunteer work, may help prevent psychosocial problems (and physical disability).

342 Provision of Care to the Elderly

Because older adults tend to have multiple disorders and may have social or functional problems, they use a disproportionately large amount of health care resources. In the US, people ≥ 65 account for

- > 40% of acute hospital bed days
- > 30% of prescription and OTC drug purchases
- $329 billion or almost 44% of the national health budget
- > 75% of the federal health budget

The elderly are likely to see several health care practitioners and to move from one health care setting to another. Providing consistent, integrated care across specific care settings, sometimes called continuity of care, is thus particularly important for elderly patients. Communication among primary care physicians, specialists, other health care practitioners, and patients and their family members, particularly when patients are transferred between settings, is critical to ensuring that patients receive appropriate care in all settings. Electronic health records may help facilitate communication.

Health care settings: Care may be delivered in the following settings:

- **Physician's office:** The most common reasons for visits are routine diagnosis and management of acute and chronic problems, health promotion and disease prevention, and presurgical or postsurgical evaluation.
- **Patient's home:** Home care (see p. 2889) is most commonly used after hospital discharge, but hospitalization is not a

prerequisite. Also, a small but growing number of health care practitioners deliver care for acute and chronic problems and sometimes end-of-life care in a patient's home.

- **Long-term care facilities:** These facilities include assisted-living facilities (see p. 2897), board-and-care facilities (see p. 2897), nursing homes (see p. 2894), and life-care communities (see p. 2897). Whether patients require care in a long-term care facility depends partly on the patient's wishes and needs and on the family's ability to meet the patient's needs.
- **Day care facilities:** These facilities provide medical, rehabilitative, cognitive, and social services several hours a day for several days a week.
- **Hospitals:** Only seriously ill elderly patients should be hospitalized (see p. 2891). Hospitalization itself poses risks to elderly patients because of confinement, immobility, diagnostic testing, and treatments.
- **Hospice:** Hospices provide care for the dying (see p. 3175). The goal is to alleviate symptoms and keep people comfortable rather than to cure a disorder. Hospice care can be provided in the home, a nursing home, or an inpatient facility.

In general, the lowest, least restrictive level of care suitable to a patient's needs should be used. This approach conserves financial resources and helps preserve the patient's independence and functioning.

Geriatric Interdisciplinary Teams

Geriatric interdisciplinary teams consist of practitioners from different disciplines who provide coordinated, integrated care with collectively set goals and shared resources and responsibilities.

Not all elderly patients need a formal geriatric interdisciplinary team. However, if patients have complex medical, psychologic, and social needs, such teams are more effective in assessing patient needs and creating an effective care plan than are practitioners working alone. If interdisciplinary care is not available, an alternative is management by a geriatrician or a primary care physician with experience and interest in geriatric medicine.

Interdisciplinary teams aim to ensure the following:

- That patients move safely and easily from one care setting to another and from one practitioner to another
- That the most qualified practitioner provides care for each problem
- That care is not duplicated

To create, monitor, or revise the care plan, interdisciplinary teams must communicate openly, freely, and regularly. Core team members must collaborate, with trust and respect for the contributions of others, and coordinate the care plan (eg, by delegating, sharing accountability, jointly implementing it). Team members may work together at the same site, making communication informal and expeditious.

A team typically includes physicians, nurses, pharmacists, social workers, and sometimes a dietitian, physical and occupational therapists, an ethicist, or a hospice physician. Team members should have knowledge of geriatric medicine, familiarity with the patient, dedication to the team process, and good communication skills.

To function effectively, teams need a formal structure. Teams should set deadlines for reaching their goals, have regular meetings (to discuss team structure, process, and communication), and continuously monitor their progress (using quality improvement measures). In general, team leadership should rotate, depending on the needs of the patient; the key provider of care reports on the patient's progress. For example, if the main concern is the patient's medical condition, a physician leads the meeting and introduces the team to the patient and family members. The physician determines what medical conditions a patient has, informs the team (including differential diagnoses), and explains how these conditions affect care. The team's input is incorporated into medical orders. The physician must write medical orders agreed on through the team process and discusses team decisions with the patient, family members, and caregivers.

If a formally structured interdisciplinary team is not available or practical, a virtual team can be used. Such teams are usually led by the primary care physician but can be organized and managed by an advanced practice nurse, a care coordinator, or a case manager. The virtual team uses information technologies (eg, handheld devices, email, video conferencing, teleconferencing) to communicate and collaborate with team members in the community or within a health care system.

Patient and caregiver participation: Practitioner team members must treat patients and caregivers as active members of the team—eg, in the following ways:

- Patients and caregivers should be included in team meetings when appropriate.
- Patients should be asked to help the team set goals (eg, advance directives, end-of-life care).
- Patients and caregivers should be included in discussions of drug treatment, rehabilitation, dietary plans, and other therapies.
- Patients should be asked what their ideas and preferences are; thus, if patients will not take a particular drug or change certain dietary habits, care can be modified accordingly.

Patients and practitioners must communicate honestly to prevent patients from suppressing an opinion and agreeing to every suggestion. Cognitively impaired patients should be included in decision making provided that practitioners adjust their communication to a level that patients can understand. Capacity to make health care decisions (see p. 3209) is specific to each particular decision; patients who are not capable of making complex decisions may still be able to decide less complicated issues.

Caregivers, including family members, can help by identifying realistic and unrealistic expectations based on the patient's habits and lifestyle. Caregivers should also indicate what kind of support they can provide.

HOME HEALTH CARE

Usually, home health care is indicated when patients need monitoring, adjustment of drugs, dressing changes, and limited physical therapy. Home health care is commonly used

- After hospital discharge (postacute care), although hospitalization is not a prerequisite, particularly for the elderly

Home health care can also be used for

- Patients with conditions that require many days of hospitalization each year (medically complex care)
- Medically stable patients with severe functional impairment (long-term care)
- Sometimes patients with acute or chronic problems
- Sometimes patients who are dying (end-of-life care)

Home health care is being increasingly used to meet the demand for long-term care. Home health care, which can reduce nursing home placement of patients by 23%, is less expensive than institutional care when home health aide and skilled care visits are scheduled appropriately.

Home health care is provided by agencies, which vary in ownership, size, location, and services. Some are certified. To be certified, an agency must meet state licensing requirements and federal conditions for participation in Medicare. Such agencies provide skilled nursing care under the direction of referring physicians. Nurses provide services under the supervision of a physician, who consults with them as changes in care are needed. Caring for patients at home requires communication among health care practitioners to ensure that patients are maintaining function and are progressing as expected. The patients or caregivers need to promptly report changes in the patient's condition to nurses or physicians to ensure that patients are monitored appropriately.

Home health care may provide medical and nonmedical services (see Table 342–1).

Reimbursement: Few patients with a serious, chronic disorder can afford full home care even though most would prefer to remain at home. Medicare covers some home care services for patients who are homebound, but it has certain requirements, which depend on the Medicare option chosen (see p. 2866). Some private insurance companies cover some home health care services (eg, infusion services) for patients who are not homebound.

For patients' care to be reimbursed by a third party, physicians must certify that home care is required and, for Medicare, that patients meet Medicare requirements for home care. Medicare requires that home health care agencies tell patients which services are reimbursable. Home care services that are delivered are based on a detailed assessment (Outcome and Assessment Information Set [OASIS]) that is completed by a registered nurse or therapist when the patient is admitted to Medicare. Third-party payers are increasingly limiting personal services to control costs. Home health care agencies are directly reimbursed by Medicare, Medicaid, or private insurers.

Table 342–1. SERVICES THAT MAY BE PROVIDED IN HOME HEALTH CARE

TYPE	SPECIFIC SERVICES
Medical	Nursing Skilled professional and paraprofessional care Hospice and respite services Durable medical equipment (eg, commodes, wheelchairs, walkers) IV therapy Dialysis Parenteral and enteral nutrition Ventilator support Diagnostic procedures (eg, x-rays, ECG, blood tests)
Nonmedical	Personal care (eg, help with bathing, washing hair, using the toilet, and dressing) Housekeeping services Personal emergency response systems Alarm devices Security surveillance Food programs (eg, meals-on-wheels)

DAY CARE FOR THE ELDERLY

Day care provides medical, rehabilitative, and cognitive support services several hours a day for several days a week. All day care facilities provide certain core services: transportation, nutrition, and recreational and social activity programs. In the US, there are only about 2,900 day care programs compared with > 16,000 nursing homes. Most day care programs are small, averaging 20 clients.

There are several models.

- **Day hospital:** This model emphasizes rehabilitation or intensive skilled care. It is designed for patients recovering from an acute condition (eg, stroke, amputation, fracture). Programs are usually limited in duration (6 wk to 6 mo) and are costly because the ratio of staff members to patients is high.
- **Maintenance:** This model combines limited skilled care (screening for and monitoring of chronic disorders) with physical exercise. Goals are to prevent deterioration, to maintain or improve the patient's functional level for as long as possible, to improve self-image, to eliminate the monotony of daily life, to prevent exacerbation of chronic disorders, and to prevent loneliness, isolation, and withdrawal. Maintenance programs provide long-term care and are less costly than day hospital programs.
- **Social:** This model provides counseling, group therapy, and cognitive retraining. It may resemble a typical senior citizens' center, which provides care to elderly people with various psychosocial needs, or a mental health center, which provides care to elderly people with dementia or psychiatric disorders.

Programs are increasingly accepting patients who are in wheelchairs and those who are incontinent; however, patients cannot be socially disruptive. Care may be long-term or limited in duration.

In addition to providing needed medical care, these facilities also provide respite care. By doing so, they may help delay or avoid placement in a nursing home.

Reimbursement: Medicare does not reimburse for day care services. Funds generally come from the Older Americans Act, Medicaid waiver programs, long-term care insurance, and private funds. Some centers use donated funds to subsidize transportation and a sliding-fee scale to match aid with the patient's financial need.

RESPITE CARE

Respite care is provision of temporary care by a substitute caregiver to provide relief to the regular caregiver. Over 50% of US states have respite programs. Programs may be provided in different settings:

- In the home by respite care agencies or by home health care agencies
- In the community by adult day care centers, respite care cooperatives, or freestanding respite facilities
- In a long-term care facility (eg, by board-and-care facilities or nursing homes)
- In a hospital

Duration of care may vary (eg, limited to 28 days in a calendar year).

Support comes from Medicaid (almost 50%), grants (25%), and private funds (25%).

HOSPITAL CARE AND THE ELDERLY

A hospital may provide emergency medical care, diagnostic testing, intensive treatment, or surgery, which may or may not require admission. The elderly use hospitals more than younger patients; they have more admissions to the hospital from the emergency department and more and longer hospital stays, and they use more resources while in the hospital.

Emergency Department Care

In 2011, about 20% of people aged 65 to 74 and 27% of those ≥ 75 had at least one emergency department (ED) visit. Elderly patients tend to be sicker. More than 40% of elderly patients seen in an ED are admitted to the hospital; 6% go to ICUs. More than 50% are prescribed new drugs. The elderly may use the ED as a substitute for primary care or may come because they are not receiving adequate attention from their primary care physician. ED visits are often caused by a breakdown in the social structure of a frail elderly patient—eg, absence or illness of their caregiver may result in people calling an ambulance rather than going to their physician's office. However, in many cases, the reasons for coming are true emergencies.

A visit to an ED may create more stress for the elderly because there are typically no special accommodations for them (eg, quiet rooms, lower beds, extra pillows, indirect lighting).

Evaluation of the elderly usually takes longer and requires more diagnostic tests because many elderly patients do not present with clear-cut or typical symptoms and signs of a disorder (see p. 2844). For example, MI manifests as chest pain in < 50% of patients > 80 yr. Instead, elderly patients may complain of feeling generally weak or just not feeling themselves.

Factors that are not apparent (eg, polypharmacy, adverse drug effects) may affect an elderly patient's presentation. For example, a fall may result from elder abuse, an adverse drug effect (eg, oversedation), hazards in the home, physical problems (eg, poor vision), depression, or chronic alcoholism. Adverse drug effects account for at least 5% of hospital admissions for the elderly.

About 30 to 40% of elderly patients who come to the ED are cognitively impaired but do not have a diagnosis of dementia; in 10%, cognitive impairment consistent with delirium is unrecognized. When indicated (eg, if an elderly patient is having difficulty with orientation to person, place, or time), a standardized cognitive assessment (see p. 1835) should be done in the ED. However, a standardized cognitive assessment is appropriate for any elderly patient coming to the ED. Cognitive impairment affects the reliability of the patient history as well as the diagnosis, increases the risk of delirium during a hospital stay, and must be considered when planning the patient's disposition. Knowing whether onset of cognitive impairment is recent helps determine whether the impairment should be fully assessed in the ED. Cognitive impairment of recent onset may indicate sepsis, occult subdural hemorrhage, or an adverse drug effect.

Suicide risk, fall risk, incontinence, and nutritional and immunization status should be assessed in the ED so that follow-up care can be arranged.

Communication among practitioners: Good communication among ED physicians and patients, caregivers, primary care physicians, and staff members of long-term care facilities greatly enhances the outcome of elderly patients with complicated problems. Advance directives should be promptly and clearly communicated to emergency medicine practitioners. Baseline information from the patient's personal physician facilitates assessment and management planning in the ED. Reports to the patient's primary care physician should describe even simple injuries (eg, ankle sprain, Colles wrist fracture) because such injuries can dramatically affect functional ability and independence.

Disposition: Discharge planning may be complex because acute illness or injury may impair functional ability more in elderly patients (eg, a simple ankle sprain may be incapacitating unless patients have good support at home). Discharge planning may be improved when nurses, social workers, and primary care physicians are involved. It should include the following:

- Functional status assessment (see p. 2837)
- Strategies to manage problems (eg, depression, alcoholism, impaired functional status) identified during the ED assessment
- Determination of whether patients can obtain and take drugs as directed and can obtain the necessary follow-up care
- Assessment of caregiver capabilities (eg, whether respite services are needed)

Many elderly patients are hospitalized after they are evaluated in the ED.

Occasionally, elderly patients are brought to the ED by a caregiver who refuses to take them home or who leaves, abandoning them in the hospital.

Hospitalization

Almost half of adults who occupy hospital beds are ≥ 65 yr; this proportion is expected to increase as the population ages. Hospital care costs Medicare > $100 billion/yr, representing 30% of health care expenditures for hospital care in the US.

Hospitalization can magnify age-related physiologic changes and increase morbidity.

Only seriously ill elderly patients who cannot be appropriately cared for elsewhere should be hospitalized. Hospitalization itself poses risks to elderly patients because it involves confinement, immobility, diagnostic testing, and treatments (particularly changes in drug regimens). When patients are transferred to or from a hospital, drugs are likely to be added or changed, leading to a higher risk of adverse effects (see p. 2848). Treatment in hospitals can be dehumanizing and impersonal. Acute hospital care should last only long enough to allow successful transition to home care, a skilled nursing facility, or an outpatient rehabilitation program.

The outcome of hospitalization appears to be poorer with increasing age, although physiologic age is a more important predictor of outcome than is chronologic age. Outcome is better for patients hospitalized because of elective procedures (eg, joint replacement) than for those hospitalized because of serious disorders (eg, multisystem organ failure).

About 75% of patients who are ≥ 75 and functionally independent at admission are not functionally independent when they are discharged; 15% of patients ≥ 75 are discharged to skilled nursing facilities (SNFs). The trend toward abbreviated acute hospital stays followed by subacute care and rehabilitation in a skilled nursing facility may explain why these percentages are high. However, even when a disorder is treatable or appears uncomplicated, patients may not return to prehospital functional status.

Improving outcomes: The following strategies can help reduce functional decline and improve care of elderly patients:

- **Geriatric interdisciplinary team:** To identify and meet the complex needs of elderly patients and to watch for and prevent problems that are common among the elderly and that may develop or worsen during hospitalization (see also p. 2889)

- **Primary care nurse** (one nurse with around-the-clock responsibility for a particular patient): To administer the team's care plan, to monitor response to nursing and medical care, and to teach and counsel patients, staff members, and family members
- **Changes in the hospital environment, often made by nurses:** Eg, to move disruptive patients into the hall near the nursing station or to change roommates for a patient
- **Rooming-in programs for a family member:** To provide better one-on-one care, to relieve staff members of some caregiving tasks, to allay patient anxiety (particularly if patients have delirium or dementia), and to enable a family member to participate actively in the patient's recovery
- **Good communication among practitioners:** To prevent errors in and duplication of diagnostic procedures and treatments (particularly drugs)
- **Documentation of drug regimen:** To state the indication for each new drug, to maintain a daily list of drugs prescribed and received, and thus to avoid using unnecessary drugs and help prevent drug interactions
- **Advance directives:** To document the patient's choice of health care proxy and health care decisions (see p. 3212)
- **Early mobilization and participation in functional activity:** To prevent physical deterioration due to decreased activity during illness and hospitalization
- **Discharge planning:** To ensure that appropriate care is continued
- **Acute care of the elderly (ACE) units:** To provide effective care for the hospitalized elderly by using most of the strategies listed above

Advance directives, if already prepared, should be brought to the hospital as soon as possible. Practitioners should reaffirm these choices during acute hospitalization. If directives were not documented, practitioners should make every effort to determine the patient's wishes.

Problems common among the elderly require specific consideration during hospitalization, particularly after surgery (see p. 3182); many of them can be remembered using the acronym ELDERSS (Table 342–2). In the hospital, elderly patients frequently experience nighttime confusion (sundowning), fracture a bone with no identifiable trauma, fall, or become unable to walk. Hospitalization may precipitate or worsen undernutrition, pressure ulcers, urinary incontinence, fecal impaction, and urinary retention. Such problems can prolong convalescence.

Table 342–2. ELDERSS: SOME IMPORTANT ISSUES FOR THE HOSPITALIZED ELDERLY

ACRONYM	ISSUE
E	Eating (nutritional status)
L	Lucidity (mental status)
D	Directives for limiting care (eg, do not resuscitate)
E	Elimination (incontinence)
R	Rehabilitation (needed because of bed rest effects)
S	Skin care (to prevent and treat pressure ulcers)
S	Social services (discharge planning)

Adverse Drug Effects

Hospitalization rates due to adverse drug effects are 4 times higher for elderly patients (≈ 17%) than for younger patients (4%). Reasons for these effects include

- Polypharmacy
- Age-related changes in pharmacokinetics and pharmacodynamics
- Changes in drugs (intentional and unintentional) during hospitalization and at discharge (see p. 2848)

Prevention: Maintaining a daily list of drugs prescribed and received can help prevent adverse drug effects and drug interactions.

Because drug distribution, metabolism, and elimination vary widely among elderly patients, the following should be done:

- Drug doses should be carefully titrated.
- Creatinine clearance for renally excreted drugs should be calculated when doses are adjusted.
- Serum drug levels should be measured.
- Patient responses should be observed.

Certain drugs or drug categories should be avoided in the elderly (see Table 335–5 on p. 2853). Use of hypnotic drugs should be minimized because tachyphylaxis may occur and risk of falls and delirium is increased; measures to improve sleep hygiene should be tried before drugs (see Table 239–5 on p. 2017). If drugs are necessary, short-acting benzodiazepines are usually the best choice. Antihistamines have anticholinergic effects and should not be used for sedation.

Bed Rest Effects

Prolonged bed rest, as can occur during hospitalization, causes deconditioning and is seldom warranted. The resulting inactivity has the following effects:

- With complete inactivity, muscle strength decreases by 5% per day, increasing risk of falls.
- Muscles shorten and periarticular and cartilaginous joint structure changes (most rapidly in the legs), limiting motion and contributing to development of contractures.
- Aerobic capacity decreases markedly, substantially reducing maximum O_2 uptake.
- Bone loss (demineralization) is accelerated.
- Risk of deep venous thrombosis is increased.

After even a few days of bed rest, elderly patients who have reduced physiologic reserves but can still function independently may lose that ability. Even if the loss is reversible, rehabilitation requires extensive, expensive, and relatively lengthy intervention.

In elderly patients, bed rest can cause vertebral bone loss 50 times faster than in younger patients. The loss incurred from 10 days of bed rest takes 4 mo to restore.

Prevention: Unless prohibited for a specific reason, activity (particularly walking) should be encouraged. If assistance with walking is needed, therapists may provide it at scheduled times. However, physicians, nurses, and family members should also assist patients with walking throughout the day. Hospital orders should emphasize the need for activity.

If immobilization is necessary or results from prolonged illness, procedures to prevent deep venous thrombosis are recommended unless contraindicated.

Rehabilitation is often needed. Realistic goals for rehabilitation at home can be based on the patient's prehospitalization activity level and current needs.

Falls

Age-related changes (eg, baroreceptor insensitivity, decreased body water and plasma volume) result in a tendency to develop orthostatic hypotension. These changes plus effects of bed rest and use of sedatives and certain antihypertensives increase risk of falls (and syncope).

Among hospitalized elderly patients, > 60% of falls occur in the bathroom; often, patients hit hard objects. Some patients fall while getting out of hospital beds. Patients are in a strange bed and in a strange environment, and they may easily become confused. Although bed rails may help remind elderly patients to call for assistance before attempting to get up, bed rails may also tempt patients to climb over or around them and thus may contribute to patient falls.

Prevention: Usually, bed rails should be removed or kept down. The best alternatives to the use of physical or chemical restraints are to identify, carefully analyze, and modify or correct risk factors for falling (including agitation) and to closely observe patients at risk. Using low beds and keeping pathways in rooms and hallways clear may also help reduce the risk of falls.

Incontinence

Urinary or fecal incontinence develops in > 40% of hospitalized patients ≥ 65, often within a day of admission. Reasons include

- An unfamiliar environment
- A cluttered path to the toilet
- Disorders that impair ambulation
- A bed that is too high
- Bed rails
- Hampering equipment such as IV lines, nasal oxygen lines, cardiac monitors, and catheters
- Psychoactive drugs that may reduce the perception of the need to void, inhibit bladder or bowel function, or impair ambulation
- Drugs that may result in urinary incontinence (eg, anticholinergic drugs and opioids, causing overflow urinary incontinence; diuretics, causing urge incontinence)

Bedpans may be uncomfortable, especially for postsurgical patients or patients with chronic arthritis. Patients with dementia or a neurologic disorder may be unable to use the call bell to request toileting assistance.

Fecal impaction, GI tract infection (eg, *Clostridium difficile*–induced colitis), adverse effects of drugs, and liquid nutritional supplements may cause uncontrollable diarrhea.

With appropriate diagnosis and treatment, continence can be reestablished.

Mental Status Changes

Elderly patients may appear confused because they have dementia, delirium, depression, or a combination. However, health care practitioners must always remember that confusion may have other causes, and its presence requires thorough evaluation.

Confusion may be due to a specific disorder (see Table 226–2 on p. 1872). However, it may develop or be exacerbated because the hospital setting exacerbates the effects of acute illness and age-related changes in cognition. For example, elderly patients who do not have their eyeglasses and hearing aids may become disoriented in a quiet, dimly lit hospital room. Patients may also become confused by hospital procedures, schedules (eg, frequent awakenings in strange settings and rooms), the effects of psychoactive drugs, and the stress of surgery or illness. In an ICU, the constant light and noise can result in agitation, paranoid ideation, and mental and physical exhaustion.

Prevention: Family members can be asked to bring missing eyeglasses and hearing aids. Placing a wall clock, a calendar, and family photographs in the room can help keep patients oriented. The room should be lit well enough to enable patients to recognize what and who is in their room and where they are. When appropriate, staff and family members should periodically remind patients of the time and place. Procedures should be explained before and as they are done.

Use of physical restraints is discouraged. For agitated patients, restraints invariably increase the level of agitation. Identifying and modifying risk factors for agitation and closely observing patients can help prevent or minimize it. Invasive and noninvasive devices attached to patients (eg, pulse oximeters, urinary catheters, IV lines) can also cause agitation; the risk:benefit ratio of these interventions should considered.

Pressure Ulcers

Pressure ulcers often develop in elderly hospitalized patients because of age-related changes in the skin. Direct pressure may cause skin necrosis in as few as 2 h if the pressure is greater than the capillary perfusion pressure of 32 mm Hg. During a typical ED visit, pressure ulcers can start developing while elderly patients are lying on a hard stretcher waiting to be examined. After short periods of immobilization, sacral pressures reach 70 mm Hg, and pressure under an unsupported heel averages 45 mm Hg. Shearing forces result when patients sitting in wheelchairs or propped up in beds slide downward. Incontinence, poor nutrition, and chronic disorders may contribute to pressure ulcer development.

Prevention: A protocol to prevent and treat pressure ulcers should be started immediately, at admission (see p. 1069). It should be followed daily by the patient's care providers and reviewed regularly by an interdisciplinary team. Pressure ulcers may be the only reason patients are discharged to a nursing home rather than to the community.

Undernutrition

In the hospital, elderly patients can become undernourished quickly, or they may be undernourished when admitted. Prolonged hospitalization exacerbates preexisting problems and often results in significant nutritional loss. Undernutrition is particularly serious for hospitalized patients because it makes them less able to fight off infection, maintain skin integrity, and participate in rehabilitation; surgical wounds may not heal as well.

Hospitalization contributes to undernutritioin several ways:

- Rigidly scheduled meals, use of drugs, and changes in environment can affect appetite and nutritional intake.
- Hospital food and therapeutic diets (eg, low-salt diets) are unfamiliar and often unappetizing.
- Eating in a hospital bed with a tray is difficult, particularly when bed rails and restraints limit movement.
- Elderly patients may need help with eating; help may be slow to come, resulting in cold, even less appetizing food.
- The elderly may not drink enough water because their thirst perception is decreased, water is difficult to reach, or both; severe dehydration may develop (sometimes leading to stupor and confusion).
- Dentures may be left at home or misplaced, making chewing difficult; labeling dentures helps prevent them from being lost or discarded with the food tray.

Prevention: Patients with preexisting nutritional abnormalities should be identified when admitted and be treated appropriately. Physicians and staff members should anticipate nutritional deficiencies in elderly patients.

The following measures can help:

- Rescinding restrictive dietary orders as soon as possible
- Monitoring nutritional intake daily
- Conferring with patients and family members about food preferences and attempting to tailor a reasonable diet specific to each patient
- Encouraging family members to join the patient at mealtimes because people eat more when they eat with others
- Making sure patients are fed adequately at all times (eg, ensuring that meals are saved if patients are out of their unit for tests or treatment during mealtime)
- Considering use of temporary parenteral nutrition or GI tube feedings for patients too sick to swallow
- Giving explicit oral fluid orders (eg, providing a fresh and readily accessible bedside water pitcher or other fluids unless fluids are restricted; advising family members, friends, and staff members to regularly offer patients a drink)

Discharge Planning and Transfers

Early, effective discharge planning has many benefits:

- Shortening the hospital stay
- Reducing the likelihood of readmission
- Identifying less expensive care alternatives
- Facilitating placement of equipment (eg, hospital bed, O_2) in the patient's home
- Helping increase patient satisfaction
- Possibly preventing placement in a nursing home

As soon as a patient is admitted, all members of the interdisciplinary team begin discharge planning. A social worker or discharge planning coordinator evaluates the patient's needs within 24 h of admission. Nurses help physicians determine when discharge is safe and which setting is most appropriate.

To home: Patients being discharged to their home need detailed instructions about follow-up care, and family members or other caregivers may need training to provide care. If patients and family members are not taught how to give drugs, implement treatment, and monitor recovery, adverse outcomes and readmission are more likely. Writing down follow-up appointments and drug schedules may help patients and family members. At discharge, a copy of a brief discharge summary plan should be given to patients or family members in case they have questions about care before the primary care physician receives the official summary plan.

To another health care facility: When a patient is discharged to a nursing home or to another facility, a written summary should be sent with the patient, and a full copy should be sent electronically to the receiving institution. The summary must include complete, accurate information about the following:

- The patient's mental and functional status
- Times the patient last received drugs
- List of drugs being currently taken and the dosage
- Known drug allergies
- Advance directives, including resuscitation status
- Family contacts and support status
- Follow-up appointments and tests
- Names and phone numbers of a nurse and physician who can provide additional information

A written copy of the patient's medical and social history should accompany the patient during transfer and may be sent electronically to the receiving facility to ensure that there are no information gaps.

Effective communication between staff members of institutions helps ensure continuity of care. For example, the patient's nurse can call the receiving institution to review the information shortly before the patient is transferred and can call the nurse who will care for the patient after discharge.

SKILLED NURSING FACILITIES

(Nursing Homes)

Skilled nursing facilities (SNFs) are licensed and certified by each state according to federal Medicare criteria. SNFs typically provide a broad range of health-related services for people ≥ 65 yr (and for younger disabled people—Table 342–3). Services include

- Skilled nursing care (ie, care that is ordered by a physician and can be given only by a registered nurse)
- Rehabilitation services (eg, physical, speech, and occupational therapy)
- Custodial care (ie, meals, assistance with personal care activities)
- Medically related social services
- Pharmaceutical services
- Dietary services appropriate to each person's needs

Many nursing homes also provide additional community-based services (eg, day care, respite care). Many provide short-term postacute care (including intensive physical, occupational, respiratory, and speech therapy) after an injury or illness (eg, hip fracture, MI, stroke). Hospitals (including rural hospitals with swing-beds) or freestanding facilities that may or may not be affiliated with a hospital may act as nursing homes.

Placement in a nursing home may be unnecessary if community-based long-term care services (eg, independent housing for the elderly, board-and-care facilities, assisted living, life-care communities) are available, accessible, and affordable.

The percentage of people in nursing homes has declined, partly because assisted-living facilities and home health care, which depend substantially on informal caregiving, are being used more.

About 45% of people ≥ 65 spend some time in a nursing home; of these, ≥ 50% stay ≥ 1 yr, and a minority of these die there. The probability of nursing home placement within a person's lifetime is closely related to age; for people aged 65 to 74, the probability is 17%, but for those > 85, it is 60%.

However, twice as many functionally dependent elderly live in the community as in nursing homes. About 25% of all community-dwelling elderly have no family members to help with their care. Special attention to health and health care needs of the community-dwelling elderly could add quality and years to their life and limit costs by preventing institutionalization.

Supervision of care: Physicians must complete the initial admission of residents to a nursing home. Then they may delegate routine follow-up of residents to a nurse practitioner or physician's assistant, who alternate with the physician in visiting residents. Visits must be done as often as medically necessary but not less than every 30 days for the first 90 days and at least once every 60 days thereafter.

During routine visits, patients should be examined, drug status assessed, and laboratory tests ordered as needed. Findings must be documented in the patient's chart to keep other staff members informed. Some physicians limit their practice

Table 342–3. NURSING HOMES AT A GLANCE

FACTOR	DETAILS
Statistics	
Number of certified homes	About 16,000
Number of beds	About 1.7 million
Occupancy rate	81.6%
Number of residents	1.39 million
Average monthly charge (varies significantly by state)	$6752
Resident	
Requirements for Medicare coverage	Must need daily skilled nursing care or daily rehabilitation therapy Must be admitted to the nursing home or rehabilitation service within 30 days after a minimum 3-day hospital stay
Risk factors for nursing home placement	Older age Living alone Inability to care for self Immobility Impaired mental status (eg, dementia) Incontinence Lack of social or informal support Poverty Female sex
Potential benefits for residents	Increased structure Opportunities for socialization Nutritional encouragement Exercise and activities Access to nursing care Help with adherence to the drug regimen
Potential problems for residents	Inability to leave the facility Infrequent visitors Complaints that may not be believed or taken seriously because residents are ill or old Abuse, which may be subtle (eg, using drugs and physical restraints inappropriately to manage disruptive behavior) or not subtle (eg, pinching, slapping, yanking) Decline in functional ability* Undernutrition and weight loss* Pressure ulcers* Incontinence* Constipation* Infections* Depression* Polypharmacy*
Facility	
Requirements for Medicare reimbursement	A licensed charge nurse on site 24 h/day Certified nurse assistants A full-time social worker if the facility has > 120 beds A medical director and licensed nursing home administrator A qualified recreational therapist to provide recreational programs A rehabilitative therapist A dietitian Physicians, pharmacists, dentists, and pastoral services to be available as needed, but not required on site

Table continues on the following page.

Table 342–3. NURSING HOMES AT A GLANCE (*Continued*)

FACTOR	DETAILS
Possible additional services	Medical specialty services (eg, ophthalmologic, otolaryngologic, neurologic, psychiatric, psychologic), which may require transport of patients to other facilities IV therapy Enteral nutrition through feeding tubes Long-term O_2 treatment or ventilator support Special care units (eg, for patients with Alzheimer disease or cancer)[†] Scheduled recreational events for groups Choices of leisure-time activities for patients, especially those who are cognitively impaired or bedbound Personal services (eg, hairdressing, makeup), usually paid for by the patient's personal funds

*These problems, which commonly develop or worsen among nursing home residents, can sometimes be prevented with attentive care.

[†]Special care units must specify programs and admissions criteria, train staff specifically for the unit, meet regulations and reimbursement requirements, and have an identifiable area or discrete physical space.

to nursing homes. They are available to participate in team activities and to consult with other staff members, thus promoting better care than that given in hurried visits every other month. Some nurse practitioners and physicians collaborate to manage patients' disorders. By administering antibiotics and monitoring IV lines, suctioning equipment, and sometimes ventilators, nurse practitioners may help prevent patients from being hospitalized.

Detecting and preventing abuse is also a function of physicians, nurses, and other health care practitioners. All practitioners involved in care of the elderly should be familiar with signs of abuse or neglect and be ready to intervene if elder abuse is suspected. A public advocacy system exists, and nursing homes can be cited by regulatory agencies.

The federal and state governments are legally responsible for ensuring that a facility is providing good care; surveyors attempt to assess a facility's performance and to detect deficiencies by monitoring outcome measures, observing care, interviewing patients and staff members, and reviewing clinical records.

Hospitalization: If hospitalization becomes necessary and if possible, the physician who cares for a patient in the nursing home should coordinate with the treating physician for that patient in the hospital. However, hospitalization is avoided whenever possible because of its risks (see p. 2891).

When patients are transferred to a hospital, their medical records, as well as their advance directives and Medical (or Physician) Orders for Life-Sustaining Treatment (MOLST or POLST) forms), should accompany them. A phone call from a nursing home nurse to a hospital nurse is useful to explain the diagnosis and reason for transfer and to describe the patient's baseline functional and mental status, drugs, and advance directives. Similarly, when patients are returned to the nursing home from the hospital, a hospital nurse should call a nursing home nurse.

Costs: Nursing home care is expensive, averaging over $80,000 per year in the US. Costs widely vary from person to person, both because of geographical difference in rates and because lengths of stay differ. Medicare covers up to 100 days of convalescent care in a Medicare-certified skilled nursing facility immediately following discharge from a 3-day hospital stay for medically necessary care (www.medicare.gov). If a patient does not have enough savings to cover the cost of a nursing home–or if the cost of a lengthy stay exhausts the patient's assets–the patient can become eligible for assistance from Medicaid (www.medicaid.gov). Patient's private insurance and funds are also often used to pay for nursing home care.

Problems related to reimbursement: Critics suggest the following:

- The rate of reimbursement may be too low, limiting patient access to rehabilitation and services that enhance quality of life, especially for patients with dementia.
- Financial incentives to provide restorative care and rehabilitation for patients with limited functioning may be insufficient.
- Nursing homes may be motivated to foster dependence or to maintain the need for high-level care so that reimbursement is maximized.

Nursing home placement: A patient's preferences and needs can be determined most effectively through comprehensive geriatric assessment, including identification and evaluation of all disorders and evaluation of the patient's functional ability (see p. 2843). Disabling or burdensome disorders—most commonly dementia, incontinence, and immobility—may trigger consideration of nursing home placement. However, even modest amelioration of a disorder may forestall the need for a nursing home (see Table 342–4).

Selection: Nursing homes vary in the types of medical, nursing, and social services provided. Some states set minimum nurse-to-patient ratios that are more stringent than federal requirements; the ratio of other staff members to patients varies considerably.

Physicians should help families select a nursing home that matches the needs of the patient with the services of a nursing home. Physicians should consider the following:

- Which clinical care practice model the nursing home uses (eg, private single-physician practices, large networks of primary care practitioners who routinely visit a certain set of nursing homes)
- Which hospitals have transfer agreements with the nursing home
- Which special therapeutic services, palliative care, hospice, and other services are available
- Whether staff members are employed full-time or part-time
- What the patient's medical coverage is, particularly if it is a Medicare capitated program, which covers certain aspects of ongoing medical care but does not cover long-term custodial care

Table 342–4. STRATEGIES FOR AVOIDING NURSING HOME PLACEMENT

PROBLEM	POSSIBLE SOLUTIONS
Urinary incontinence	Treating the cause may enable patients to remain at home.
Dementia	Family members or other caregivers can be taught strategies for managing frustrating or disruptive behavior. For example, using purchased or rented monitoring devices can help with behaviors such as nocturnal wandering.
Functional impairments	Physical and occupational therapists and home health nurses can • Assess patients in their homes • Help determine whether placement in a nursing home or in an assisted-living facility is necessary • Suggest ways to help patients function better • Teach patients to use adaptive devices • Encourage exercise Durable medical equipment, if needed, can be provided.
Need for elaborate and detailed care	Support and respite services can help prevent family members or other caregivers from becoming resentful or worn out. Physicians can help by listening when caregivers discuss their burdens and by providing them with information about community caregiving support groups and about options for paid respite care.

BOARD-AND-CARE FACILITIES

Board-and-care facilities provide care for elderly people who cannot live independently but who do not need the constant supervision provided in nursing homes. Board-and-care facilities (also called rest homes) typically provide the following:

- A room
- Meals in a communal dining room
- Housekeeping services (eg, laundry, cleaning)
- Minimal assistance with personal care
- Sometimes supervision of drug administration

The number of board-and-care facilities is increasing because they offer an economic, federally funded means of accommodating the increasing number of elderly people who would otherwise require nursing home care paid for with state Medicaid funds.

Minimally regulated and sometimes unlicensed, these facilities principally serve 2 groups, often cared for together—the elderly and the deinstitutionalized mentally ill. Although excellent homes exist, some facilities tend to warehouse the disabled in substandard buildings and to employ few skilled staff members.

Physicians should try to ensure that their patients in board-and-care facilities are safe and are receiving appropriate care. Physicians may need to visit the facility or send a nurse or social worker to evaluate it.

ASSISTED-LIVING PROGRAMS

Assisted-living programs enable residents who have problems doing activities of daily living to maintain their independence in personalized settings by providing or arranging for the provision of daily meals, personal and other supportive services, health care, and 24-h oversight as needed.

Assisted-living programs typically provide the following:

- Meals
- Personal care
- Housekeeping services
- Transportation
- 24-h oversight if needed

The average annual cost of assisted living programs is over $42,000. These programs are paid for by private funds, long-term care insurance, community-based charity organizations, or church groups. Some states provide some waivers to help cover services in these settings.

LIFE-CARE COMMUNITIES

Life-care communities offer a contract intended to remain in effect for the resident's lifetime and, at a minimum, to guarantee shelter and access to various health care services.

Life-care communities (continuing care retirement communities) offer different levels of care:

- For people who can live independently
- For those who need assistance
- For those who need skilled nursing care

Generally, people pay a substantial entrance fee ($50,000 to $500,000) when moving to the community and monthly fees thereafter. In some communities, residents pay only a monthly fee for rent plus service or health packages. In others, residents can purchase a condominium, cooperative, or membership; service or health packages are purchased separately.

There are 3 main types of communities:

- Those covered by an all-inclusive contract
- Those covered by a modified contract limiting the amount of long-term care provided before the monthly fee is increased
- Those covered by a fee-for-service contract with billing for health services as they are used

If well-financed and well-managed, life-care communities provide a broad range of housing, social, supportive, and health services that enable their residents to live comfortably. However, some communities are not well-regulated; in some, residents' assets have been wiped out because of unscrupulous real estate dealers or well-intentioned but inept management.

Communities may occupy a single building or be spread across multiacre campuses with housing options ranging from efficiency apartments to cottages with several rooms. Many have community buildings for organized social events, dining rooms, clubs, sports facilities, planned outings, and vacation options. Access to physicians is usually provided, and most programs are affiliated with local acute care facilities.

Medicare and Medicaid usually do not pay for residence in a life-care community but may help pay for skilled nursing care when it is needed. Long-term care insurance may reimburse residents for monthly fees as well as personal care services.

PROGRAM OF ALL-INCLUSIVE CARE FOR THE ELDERLY

Program of All-Inclusive Care for the Elderly (PACE) is designed for elderly people who meet criteria for nursing home admission but wish to live at home as long as possible. The program involves an interdisciplinary team that includes physicians, nurses, physical and occupational therapists, social workers, dieticians, and drivers. The services are typically provided in an adult day health center and are available every day. The program provides transportation to the center. However, some services may be provided in the home.

PACE is available only in certain areas of the country. It combines funds from Medicare and Medicaid. The Department of Health and Human Services web site explains the PACE program and provides an up-to-date list of participating health care practitioners.

PHARMACISTS AND THE ELDERLY

For elderly patients, developing a relationship with a pharmacist and using one pharmacy can help ensure consistency in care. A pharmacist can help prevent drug-related problems, which are a particular risk for the elderly (see also Ch. 335).

For elderly patients, pharmacists are sometimes the most accessible health care practitioner. In addition to dispensing drugs, pharmacists provide drug information to patients and providers, monitor drug use (including adherence), and liaise between physicians or other health care practitioners and patients to ensure optimal pharmaceutical care. Pharmacists also provide information about interactions between drugs and other substances, including OTC drugs, dietary supplements (eg, medicinal herbs), and foods.

Patient adherence: Pharmacists can help improve patient adherence by doing the following:

- Assessing the patient's ability to adhere to a drug regimen by noticing certain impairments (eg, poor dexterity, lack of hand strength, cognitive impairment, loss of vision)
- Teaching patients how to take certain drugs (eg, inhalers, transdermal patches, injectable drugs, eye or ear drops) or how to measure doses of liquid drugs
- Supplying drugs in ways that are accessible to patients (eg, easy-open bottles, pills without wrappers)
- Making sure that drug labels and take-home printed materials are in large type and in the patient's native language

Table 342–5. VARIOUS DUTIES OF PHARMACISTS

SETTING	DUTIES
Hospital	Help obtain a detailed drug history from the patient or caregiver Accompany physicians and other practitioners on patient rounds Make drug recommendations Provide drug information when appropriate When discharge is imminent, provide oral and written drug-related information to the patient or caregiver
Long-term facilities*	May accompany physicians and other practitioners on rounds Participate in facility quality-improvement committees Assess and interview patients Assess drug effectiveness and monitor patients for drug interactions, adverse drug effects, and therapeutic failures If pharmacists identify a problem or a high risk of drug-related problems, contact the patient's nurse or physician directly As required by federal law, conduct a monthly drug regimen review for all patients
Mail service and online pharmacies	Provide consultation by telephone to patients and health care practitioners Review and validate prescription orders Participate in drug utilization review and formulary management Help ensure quality control Develop education materials for patients and health care practitioners
Organized health care systems	May develop, implement, and manage formularies, computer-based adverse event tracking systems, and performance measurement indicators (to improve quality) May help design therapeutic guidelines and manage drug utilization programs
Hospice	Make recommendations for appropriate drugs to control symptoms Ensure the timeliness of drug delivery Minimize duplicative and interacting drugs Help improve cost-effective use of drugs Teach patients about the best way to use the prescribed drugs Monitor therapeutic responses and recognize drug-related problems Advise hospice team members about appropriate drugs and potential drug interactions with other substances (eg, medicinal herbs) Compound drugs or dosage forms extemporaneously as needed

*Pharmacists who work in long-term care facilities are called consultant pharmacists.

- Teaching patients how to use drug calendar reminders, commercially available drug boxes, electronic drug-dispensing devices, and pill splitters or crushers
- Eliminating unnecessary complexity and duplication from the overall drug regimen

Settings: Many pharmacists work in a community pharmacy. But they may also work in any health care setting, including hospitals, long-term care facilities, the home (with a home health care agency), mail service and online pharmacies, organized health care systems, and hospice settings (see Table 342–5).

343 Social Issues in the Elderly

Social issues influence an elderly person's risk and experience of illness as well as a health care practitioner's ability to deliver timely and appropriate care.

A social history helps members of the interdisciplinary team evaluate care needs and social supports. It should include questions about the following:

- Family and marital or companion status
- Living arrangements
- Financial status
- Work history
- Education
- Typical daily activities (eg, how meals are prepared, what activities add meaning to life, where problems may be occurring)
- Need for and availability of caregivers (to help plan care)
- History of trauma, losses, and coping strengths
- History of substance use and legal issues
- Patients' own caregiving responsibilities (which may make patients reluctant to report their own symptoms lest their symptoms or any resulting interventions interfere with caregiving)

FAMILY CAREGIVING FOR THE ELDERLY

Family caregivers play a key role in delaying and possibly preventing institutionalization of chronically ill elderly patients. Although neighbors and friends may help, about 80% of help in the home (physical, emotional, social, economic) is provided by family caregivers. When the patient is mildly or moderately impaired, a spouse or adult children often provide care, but when the patient is severely disabled, a spouse (usually a wife) is more likely to be the caregiver. Approximately 34 million Americans, more than 10% of the US population, were estimated to have served as an unpaid caregiver for someone age 50 or older in the year 2015.

The amount and type of care provided by family members depend on economic resources, family structure, quality of relationships, and other demands on the family members' time and energy. Family caregiving ranges from minimal assistance (eg, periodically checking in) to elaborate full-time care. On average, family caregiving for older adults consumes about 24 hours per week, and about 20% of the time more than 40 hours per week. Caregivers of the elderly report that 63% of their care recipients have long-term physical conditions and 29% have cognitive impairment.

Although society tends to view family members as having a responsibility to care for one another, the limits of filial and spousal obligations vary among cultures, families, and individual family members. The willingness of family members to provide care may be bolstered by supportive services (eg, technical assistance in learning new skills, counseling services, family mental health services) and supplemental services (eg, personal care [assistance with grooming, feeding, and dressing], home health care, adult day care, meals programs). Supplemental services may be provided on a regular schedule or as respite care for a few hours or days.

Changes in demographics and social values have reduced the number of family members available to care for impaired elderly relatives because of the following:

- Increased life span: As a result, the population of the very old has been increasing. Thus, their children, who are potential caregivers, are likely to be old also.
- Delayed procreation: Combined with increased longevity, this delay has created a sandwich generation of caregivers who care simultaneously for their children and their parents.
- Increasing mobility of US society and the increased divorce rate: As a result, families are more likely to be geographically separated, and family ties are more complex. Nonetheless, 80% of people ≥ 65 live within 20 min of one child.
- An increasing number of women in the workforce: Previously, women may have provided care for elderly parents, but the demands of a job may diminish or eliminate their ability to do so.
- The number of dependent and very sick elderly people is increasing.

These factors predict an increasing demand for home health care services provided by someone other than family members, friends, and neighbors.

Effects: Although caregiving can be very rewarding, it can also have negative effects. Family caregivers may experience considerable stress (called caregiver burden) and subsequent health problems, isolation, fatigue, and frustration, sometimes leading to a sense of helplessness and exhaustion (caregiver burnout) or elder abuse.

Caregiving may also become a financial burden. Couples in which one partner cares for the other tend to be disproportionately poor.

Caregivers can often obtain reassurance or learn helpful information or strategies for caregiving from physicians, nurses, social workers, or case managers. Caregivers can also take the following measures to prepare themselves for caregiving and to avoid caregiver burnout:

- Attending to their own physical, emotional, recreational, spiritual, and financial needs
- When appropriate, asking for help with caregiving or support from other family members and friends
- Investigating outside groups that can offer psychologic support (eg, support groups) or help with caregiving (eg, counseling, home health care, adult day care, meals programs, respite care)
- If their loved one is hostile or difficult, not taking it personally

THE ELDERLY LIVING ALONE

In the US, nearly 29% of the 46 million community-dwelling elderly live alone. About half of the community-dwelling oldest old (≥ 85 yr) live alone. About 70% of elderly people living alone are women, and 46% of all women age ≥ 75 yr live alone. Men are more likely to die before their wives, and widowed or divorced men are more likely to remarry than are widowed or divorced women.

The elderly who live alone are more likely to be poor, especially with advancing age. Many report feelings of loneliness (in 60% of those > 75) and social isolation. In those with health problems or sensory deficits, new or worsening symptoms may be unnoticed. Many have difficulty complying with prescribed treatment regimens. Because they have physical limitations and because eating is a social activity, some elderly people who live alone do not prepare full, balanced meals, making undernutrition a concern.

Despite these problems, almost 90% of elderly people living alone express a keen desire to maintain their independence. Many fear being too dependent on others and, despite the loneliness, want to continue to live alone. To help them maintain their independence, physicians should encourage them to engage in regular physical activity and social interactions and should provide social work referrals to help them do so.

Coordination and delivery of services during convalescence are difficult for patients living alone. Physicians should ensure that home care is available and recommend additional services as appropriate. A passive or individually activated emergency response device may reassure patients that help can be obtained if needed.

SELF-NEGLECT IN THE ELDERLY

Self-neglect implies not caring for self. It can include ignoring personal hygiene, not paying bills, not maintaining the integrity or cleanliness of the home, not obtaining or preparing food (leading to undernutrition), not seeking medical care for potentially serious symptoms, not filling prescriptions or taking drugs, and skipping follow-up visits.

Risk factors for self-neglect include

- Social isolation
- Disorders that impair memory or judgment (eg, dementia)
- The presence of multiple chronic disorders
- Substance abuse
- Severe depression

Differentiating between self-neglect and simply choosing to live in a way that others find undesirable can be difficult. Social workers are often in the best position to make this determination.

Adult Protective Services or the state unit on aging (whose numbers are available through the Eldercare Locator at 800-677-1116) can help by coordinating in-home safety assessments and helping the elderly obtain counseling services, emergency response systems, referrals to additional support services, and, if necessary, hospitalization.

ALTERNATIVE LIVING ARRANGEMENTS FOR THE ELDERLY

Living arrangements and relationships that do not involve living with a spouse, with an adult child, or alone are fairly common among the elderly. For example, a substantial proportion of elderly people who never married, are divorced, or are widowed have long-standing and close relationships with siblings, friends, and partners. Understanding the nature of these relationships helps practitioners plan care that is in keeping with a patient's wishes.

Consideration of the Homosexual Elderly

About 6 to 10% of the US population are estimated to be homosexual adults, including as many as 4 million of the elderly. Elderly people in a homosexual relationship face special challenges. The health care system may not be aware of their sexual preference, may not recognize their partner as having a role in caregiving decisions or as being part of the patient's family, and may not provide services that are appropriate for their circumstances. For example, an unmarried partner may not have legal standing in decision making for a cognitively impaired patient and may not be able to share a room in a nursing home or other congregate living setting. Health care practitioners should ask questions about partners and marital status or living arrangements, and try to accommodate patient preferences.

EFFECTS OF LIFE TRANSITIONS ON THE ELDERLY

Late life is commonly a period of transitions (eg, retirement, relocation) and adjustment to losses.

Retirement is often the first major transition faced by the elderly. Its effects on physical and mental health differ from person to person, depending on attitude toward and reason for retiring. About one third of retirees have difficulty adjusting to certain aspects of retirement, such as reduced income and altered social role and entitlements. Some people choose to retire, having looked forward to quitting work; others are forced to retire (eg, because of health problems or job loss). Appropriate preparation for retirement and counseling for retirees and families who experience difficulties may help.

Relocation may occur several times during old age—eg, to retirement housing with desirable amenities, to smaller quarters to reduce the burden of upkeep, to the homes of siblings or adult children, or to a residential care facility. Physical and mental status are significant predictors of relocation adjustment, as is thoughtful and adequate preparation. People who respond poorly to relocation are more likely to be living alone, socially isolated, poor, and depressed. Men respond less well than women.

The less control people perceive they have over the move and the less predictable the new environment seems, the greater the stress of relocation. People should become acquainted with the new setting well in advance. For the cognitively impaired, a move away from familiar surroundings may exacerbate functional dependence and disruptive behavior. Because of financial, social, and other complications, some older adults feel they must remain in problematic homes or neighborhoods despite their desire to relocate. Social workers can help such people assess their options for relocation or home modification.

Bereavement affects many aspects of an elderly person's life. For example, social interaction and companionship decrease, and social status may change. The death of a spouse affects men and women differently. In the 2 yr after death of a wife, the mortality rate in men tends to increase, especially if the wife's death was unexpected. For women who lose a husband, data are less clear but generally do not indicate an increased mortality rate.

With bereavement, some sleep disturbance and anxiety are normal; these effects usually resolve in months without drug treatment. In contrast, prolonged, pathologic grief is characterized by the following:

- Symptoms that are typical of a major depressive episode and that last > 2 mo
- Feelings of guilt about things not directly related to the loss
- Thoughts of death unrelated to survivorship
- Morbid preoccupation with worthlessness
- Hallucinations other than hearing and seeing the decedent

Caregivers and health care practitioners should look for such symptoms and be aware that bereaved patients are at high risk of suicide and declining health status.

Timely screening for depression and suicidal ideation is essential. Counseling and supportive services (eg, support groups for widows) may facilitate difficult transitions. Short-term use of anxiolytic drugs can help patients with excessive anxiety. However, excessive or prolonged use should be avoided because it may interfere with the process of grieving and adjustment. Prolonged, pathologic grief usually requires psychiatric evaluation and treatment.

INTIMACY AND THE ELDERLY

Intimacy refers to a close feeling shared between 2 people, based on knowledge of and familiarity with the other person. It includes emotional, social (based on shared experiences), and physical intimacy (eg, touching, cuddling, sexual intercourse).

The desire for intimacy does not decrease with age, and there is no age at which intimacy, including physical intimacy, is inappropriate. However, the disorders and emotional changes that often occur with aging can interfere with developing and maintaining an intimate relationship. Aging can also change the way intimacy is expressed.

Intimacy, particularly physical intimacy, may be lost because of the following:

- **Loss of a partner:** Loss or absence of a partner is probably the most common age-related barrier to intimacy.
- **Disorders:** Various disorders that become more common with aging can interfere with physical intimacy. Vascular disorders and diabetes can cause erectile dysfunction; arthritis can limit movements and make them painful. The pain, discomfort, drugs, and worry associated with a disorder can dampen the desire for intimacy. Moderate to severe cognitive impairment complicates issues of consent to and comfort during intercourse. For the partner, the stress and demands of caregiving may interfere with intimacy.
- **Use of drugs:** The elderly are more likely to take drugs (eg, antihypertensives, psychoactive drugs) that can cause problems affecting intimacy (eg, erectile dysfunction, reduced libido).
- **Age-related changes:** Levels of sex hormones decrease, causing changes (eg, vaginal atrophy, reduced vaginal lubrication) that make sexual intercourse uncomfortable or difficult. Libido may decrease.
- **Reluctance to discuss effects of aging:** If elderly people develop problems that interfere with physical intimacy or if they feel embarrassed about changes in their body (eg, wrinkles, sagging flesh), they may not want to discuss these changes with their partner or with a health care practitioner, who may be able to suggest solutions.
- **Discrepancy in expectations of partners:** One partner may want certain physical expressions of intimacy, but the other does not.
- **Lack of privacy:** Elderly people who live with family members or in a long-term care facility have fewer opportunities for privacy, which are necessary for physical intimacy.
- **Shift to other forms of intimacy:** Some couples grow to prefer other forms of intimacy (eg, touching, massaging, kissing, verbal expressions of affection) that express familiarity, caring, or engagement with their partner.

Nonetheless, many elderly people continue to have a healthy sexual relationship. Intimacy, particularly physical intimacy, can help prevent depression and improve self-esteem and physical health. If elderly people have a new sex partner, they should practice safe sex. Acquiring sexually transmitted diseases, including AIDS, is a risk, regardless of age, and physicians should discuss safe sex measures with elderly patients.

Many elderly people, especially those that live alone, find satisfaction and a sense of companionship in interactions with a pet. Caring for a pet can give people a sense of purpose and connectedness.

RELIGION AND SPIRITUALITY IN THE ELDERLY

Religion and spirituality are similar but not identical concepts. Religion is often viewed as more institutionally based, more structured, and involving more traditional activities, rituals and practices. Spirituality refers to the intangible and immaterial and thus may be considered a more general term, not associated with a particular group or organization. It can refer to feelings, thoughts, experiences, and behaviors related to the soul or to a search for the sacred.

Traditional religion involves accountability and responsibility; spirituality has fewer requirements. People may reject traditional religion but consider themselves spiritual. In the US, > 90% of elderly people consider themselves religious or spiritual; about 6 to 10% are atheists and do not seek meaning through religion or a spiritual life. Most research assesses religion, not spirituality, using measures such as attendance at religious services, frequency of private religious practices, use of religious coping mechanisms (eg, praying, trusting in God, turning problems over to God, receiving support from the clergy), and intrinsic religiosity (internalized religious commitment).

For most of the elderly in the US, religion has a major role in their life, with about half attending religious services at least weekly.

The elderly's level of religious participation is greater than that in any other age group. For the elderly, the religious community is the largest source of social support outside of the family, and involvement in religious organizations is the most common type of voluntary social activity—more common than all other forms of voluntary social activity combined.

Benefits

Religion correlates with improved physical and mental health, and religious people may propose that God's intervention facilitates these benefits. However, experts cannot determine whether participation in organized religion contributes to health or whether psychologically or physically healthier people are attracted to religious groups. If religion is helpful, the reason—whether it is the religious beliefs themselves or other factors—is not clear. Many such factors (eg, psychologic benefits, encouragement of healthful practices, social support) have been proposed.

Psychologic benefits: Religion may provide the following psychologic benefits:

- A positive and hopeful attitude about life and illness, which predicts improved health outcomes and lower mortality rates
- A sense of meaning and purpose in life, which affects health behaviors and social and family relationships
- A greater ability to cope with illness and disability

Many elderly people report that religion is the most important factor enabling them to cope with physical health problems and life stresses (eg, declining financial resources, loss of a spouse or partner). In one study, > 90% of elderly patients relied on religion, at least to a moderate degree, when coping with health problems and difficult social circumstances. For example, having a hopeful, positive attitude about the future helps people with physical problems remain motivated to recover.

People who use religious coping mechanisms are less likely to develop depression and anxiety than those who do not; this inverse association is strongest among people with greater physical disability. Even the perception of disability appears to be altered by the degree of religiousness. Of elderly women with hip fractures, the most religious had the lowest rates of depression and were able to walk significantly further when discharged from the hospital than those who were less religious. Religious people also tend to recover from depression more quickly.

Health-promoting practices: In the elderly, active involvement in a religious community correlates with better maintained physical functioning and health. Some religious groups (eg, Mormons, Seventh-Day Adventists) advocate behaviors that enhance health, such as avoidance of tobacco and heavy alcohol use. Members of these groups are less likely to develop substance-related disorders, and they live longer than the general population.

Social benefits: Religious beliefs and practices often foster the development of community and broad social support networks. Increased social contact for the elderly increases the likelihood that disease will be detected early and that elderly people will comply with treatment regimens because members of their community interact with them and ask them questions about their health and medical care. Elderly people who have such community networks are less likely to neglect themselves.

Caregivers: Religious faith also benefits caregivers. In a study of caregivers of patients with Alzheimer disease or terminal cancer, caregivers with a strong personal religious faith and many social contacts were better able to cope with the stresses of caregiving during a 2-yr period.

Harmful Effects

Religion is not always beneficial to the elderly. Religious devotion may promote excessive guilt, inflexibility, and anxiety. Religious preoccupations and delusions may develop in patients with obsessive-compulsive disorder, bipolar disorder, schizophrenia, or psychoses.

Certain religious groups discourage mental and physical health care, including potentially lifesaving therapies (eg, blood transfusions, treatment of life-threatening infections, insulin therapy), and may substitute religious rituals (eg, praying, chanting, lighting candles). Some more rigid religious groups may isolate and alienate elderly people from nonparticipating family members and the broader social community.

Role of the Health Care Practitioner

Talking to elderly patients about their religious beliefs and practices helps health care practitioners provide care because these beliefs can affect the patients' mental and physical health. Inquiring about religious issues during a medical visit is appropriate under certain circumstances, including the following:

- When patients are severely ill, under substantial stress, or near death and ask or suggest that a practitioner talk about religious issues
- When patients tell a practitioner that they are religious and that religion helps them cope with illness
- When religious needs are evident and may be affecting patients' health or health behaviors

The elderly often have distinct spiritual needs that may overlap with but are not the same as psychologic needs. Ascertaining a patient's spiritual needs can help mobilize the necessary resources (eg, spiritual counseling or support groups, participation in religious activities, social contacts from members of a religious community).

Spiritual history: Taking a spiritual history shows elderly patients that the health care practitioner is willing to discuss spiritual topics. Practitioners may ask patients whether their spiritual beliefs are an important part of their life, how these beliefs influence the way they take care of themselves, whether they are a part of a religious or spiritual community, and how they would like the health care practitioner to handle their spiritual needs.

Alternatively, a practitioner may ask patients to describe their most important coping mechanism. If the response is not a religious one, patients may be asked whether religious or spiritual resources are of any help. If the response is no, patients may be sensitively asked about barriers to those activities (eg, transportation problems, hearing difficulties, lack of financial resources, depression, lack of motivation, unresolved conflicts) to determine whether the reason is circumstances or their choice. However, practitioners should not force religious beliefs or opinions on patients or intrude if patients do not want help.

Referral to clergy: Many clergy members provide counseling services to the elderly at home and in the hospital, often free of charge. Many elderly patients prefer such counseling to that from a mental health care practitioner because they are more satisfied with the results and because they believe such counseling does not have the stigma that mental health care does. However, many clergy members in the community do not have extensive training in mental health counseling and may not recognize when elderly patients need professional mental health care. In contrast, many hospital clergy have extensive training in the mental, social, and spiritual needs of the elderly. Thus, including hospital clergy as part of the health care team can be helpful. They can often bridge the gap between hospital care and care in the community by communicating with clergy in the community. For example, when a patient is discharged from the hospital, the hospital clergy may call the patient's clergy, so that support teams in the patient's religious community can be mobilized to help during the patient's convalescence (eg, by providing housekeeping services, meals, or transportation, by visiting the patient or caregiver).

Support of patients' religious beliefs and practices: Patients seek medical care for health-related reasons, not religious ones. However, health care practitioners should not discourage a patient's religious involvement as long as it does not interfere with necessary medical care, because such involvement may contribute to good health. People who are actively involved in religious groups, particularly those in major religious traditions, tend to be healthier.

If patients are not already involved in religious activities, suggesting such activities requires sensitivity. However, health care practitioners may suggest that patients consider religious activities if patients seem receptive and may benefit from such activities, which can provide social contact, reduce alienation and isolation, and increase a sense of belonging, of meaning, and of life purpose. These activities may also help the elderly focus on positive activities rather than on their own problems. However, some activities are appropriate only for more religious patients.

SECTION 22

Clinical Pharmacology

344 Adverse Drug Reactions

(Adverse Drug Effects)

Adverse drug reaction (ADR, or adverse drug effect) is a broad term referring to unwanted, uncomfortable, or dangerous effects that a drug may have.

ADRs can be considered a form of toxicity; however, toxicity is most commonly applied to effects of overingestion (accidental or intentional) or to elevated blood levels or enhanced drug effects that occur during appropriate use (eg, when drug metabolism is temporarily inhibited by a disorder or another drug). For information on toxicity of specific drugs see Table 366–8 on p. 3069. *Side effect* is an imprecise term often used to refer to a drug's unintended effects that occur within the therapeutic range.

Because all drugs have the potential for ADRs, risk-benefit analysis (analyzing the likelihood of benefit vs risk of ADRs) is necessary whenever a drug is prescribed.

In the US, 3 to 7% of all hospitalizations are due to ADRs. ADRs occur during 10 to 20% of hospitalizations; about 10 to 20% of these ADRs are severe. Incidence of death due to ADRs is unknown; suggested rates of 0.5 to 0.9% may be falsely high because many of the patients included had serious and complex disorders.

Incidence and severity of ADRs vary by patient characteristics (eg, age, sex, ethnicity, coexisting disorders, genetic or geographic factors) and by drug factors (eg, type of drug, administration route, treatment duration, dosage, bioavailability). Incidence is higher with advanced age and polypharmacy. ADRs are more severe among the elderly (see p. 2848), although age per se may not be the primary cause. The contribution of prescribing and adherence errors to the incidence of ADRs is unclear.

PEARLS & PITFALLS

- ADRs occur in 10 to 20% of hospitalizations.
- About 10 to 20% of these reactions are severe.

Etiology

Most ADRs are dose-related; others are allergic or idiosyncratic. Dose-related ADRs are usually predictable; ADRs unrelated to dose are usually unpredictable.

Dose-related ADRs are particularly a concern when drugs have a narrow therapeutic index (eg, hemorrhage with oral anticoagulants). ADRs may result from decreased drug clearance in patients with impaired renal or hepatic function or from drug-drug interactions.

Allergic ADRs are not dose-related and require prior exposure. Allergies develop when a drug acts as an antigen or allergen. After a patient is sensitized, subsequent exposure to the drug produces one of several different types of allergic reaction. Clinical history and appropriate skin tests can sometimes help predict allergic ADRs.

Idiosyncratic ADRs are unexpected ADRs that are not dose-related or allergic. They occur in a small percentage of patients given a drug. Idiosyncrasy is an imprecise term that has been defined as a genetically determined abnormal response to a drug, but not all idiosyncratic reactions have a pharmacogenetic cause. The term may become obsolete as specific mechanisms of ADRs become known.

Symptoms and Signs

ADRs are usually classified as mild, moderate, severe, or lethal (see Table 344–1). Severe or lethal ADRs may be specifically mentioned in black box warnings in the physician prescribing information provided by the manufacturer.

Symptoms and signs may manifest soon after the first dose or only after chronic use. They may obviously result from drug use or be too subtle to identify as drug-related. In the elderly, subtle ADRs can cause functional deterioration, changes in mental status, failure to thrive, loss of appetite, confusion, and depression.

Allergic ADRs typically occur soon after a drug is taken but generally do not occur after the first dose; typically, they occur when the drug is given after an initial exposure. Symptoms include itching, rash, fixed-drug eruption, upper or lower airway edema with difficulty breathing, and hypotension.

Idiosyncratic ADRs can produce almost any symptom or sign and usually cannot be predicted.

Diagnosis

- Consideration of rechallenge
- Reporting of suspected ADRs to MedWatch

Symptoms that occur soon after a drug is taken are often easily connected with use of a drug. However, diagnosing symptoms due to chronic drug use requires a significant level of suspicion and is often complicated. Stopping a drug is sometimes necessary but is difficult if the drug is essential and does not have an acceptable substitute. When proof of the relationship between drug and symptoms is important, rechallenge should be considered, except in the case of serious allergic reactions.

Table 344–1. CLASSIFICATION OF ADVERSE DRUG REACTIONS

SEVERITY	DESCRIPTION	EXAMPLE
Mild	No antidote or treatment is required; hospitalization is not prolonged.	Antihistamines (some): Drowsiness Opioids: Constipation
Moderate	A change in treatment (eg, modified dosage, addition of a drug), but not necessarily discontinuation of the drug, is required; hospitalization may be prolonged, or specific treatment may be required.	Hormonal contraceptives: Venous thrombosis NSAIDs: Hypertension and edema
Severe	An ADR is potentially life threatening and requires discontinuation of the drug and specific treatment of the ADR.	ACE inhibitors: Angioedema Phenothiazines: Abnormal heart rhythm
Lethal	An ADR directly or indirectly contributes to a patient's death.	Acetaminophen overdosage: Liver failure Anticoagulants: Hemorrhage

Physicians should report most suspected ADRs to MedWatch (the Food and Drug Administration's [FDA's] ADR monitoring program), which is an early alert system. Only through such reporting can unexpected ADRs be identified and investigated. MedWatch also monitors changes in the nature and frequency of ADRs. Forms for and information about reporting ADRs are available in the Physicians' Desk Reference and the FDA News Daily Drug Bulletin, as well as at www.fda.gov/Safety/MedWatch/default.htm; forms may also be obtained by calling 800-FDA-1088. Nurses, pharmacists, and other health care practitioners should also report ADRs.

The incidence of severe or fatal ADRs is very low (typically < 1 in 1000) and may not be apparent during clinical trials, which are typically not powered to detect low-incidence ADRs. Thus, these ADRs may not be detected until after a drug is released to the general public and is in widespread use. Clinicians should not assume that because a drug is on the market that all ADRs are known. Postmarketing surveillance is extremely important for tracking low-incidence ADRs.

Treatment

- Modification of dosage
- Discontinuation of drug if necessary
- Switching to a different drug

For dose-related ADRs, modifying the dose or eliminating or reducing precipitating factors may suffice. Increasing the rate of drug elimination is rarely necessary. For allergic and idiosyncratic ADRs, the drug usually should be discontinued and not tried again. Switching to a different drug class is often required for allergic ADRs and sometimes required for dose-related ADRs.

Prevention

Prevention of ADRs requires familiarity with the drug and potential reactions to it. Computer-based analysis should be used to check for potential drug interactions; analysis should be repeated whenever drugs are changed or added. Drugs and initial dosage must be carefully selected for the elderly (see p. 2848). If patients develop nonspecific symptoms, ADRs should always be considered before beginning symptomatic treatment.

345 Concepts in Pharmacotherapy

Drugs are selected based on characteristics of the drug (eg, efficacy, safety profile, route of administration, route of elimination, dosing frequency, cost) and of the patient (eg, age, sex, other medical problems, likelihood of pregnancy, ethnicity, other genetic determinants). Risks and benefits of the drug are also assessed; every drug poses some risk.

Response to a drug depends partly on the patient's characteristics and behaviors (eg, consumption of foods or supplements; adherence to a dosing regimen; differences in metabolism due to age, sex, race, genetic polymorphisms, or hepatic or renal insufficiency), coexistence of other disorders, and use of other drugs.

Drug errors (eg, prescribing an inappropriate drug, misreading a prescription, administering a drug incorrectly) can also affect response.

DRUG DEVELOPMENT

Promising compounds can be identified by mass screening of hundreds or thousands of molecules for biologic activity. In other cases, knowledge of the specific molecular pathophysiology of various diseases allows for rational drug design via computer modeling or modification of existing pharmaceutical agents.

During **early development,** potentially useful compounds are studied in animals to evaluate desired effects and toxicity. Compounds that seem effective and safe are candidates for human studies. A protocol describing the clinical study must be approved by an appropriate institutional review board (IRB) and the FDA, which then issues an investigational new drug (IND) exemption permit. At this point, the patent time period for the compound begins, which usually provides the owner with exclusive rights for the next 20 yr; however, the drug cannot be sold until it is approved by the FDA.

Phase 1 evaluates safety and toxicity in humans. Different amounts of the compound are given to a small number (often 20 to 80) of healthy, young, usually male volunteers to determine the dose at which toxicity first appears.

Phase 2 determines whether the compound is active against the target disorder. The compound is given to up to about 100 patients for treatment or prevention of the target disorder. An additional goal is to determine an optimal dose-response range.

Phase 3 evaluates the drug's effect in larger (often hundreds to thousands of people), more heterogeneous populations in an attempt to duplicate the drug's proposed clinical use. This phase also compares the drug with existing treatments, a placebo, or both. Studies may involve many practicing physicians and multiple research sites. The purpose is to verify efficacy and detect effects—good and bad—that may not have been observed during phases 1 and 2.

When sufficient data have been collected to justify and request approval of the drug, a new drug application (NDA) is submitted to the FDA. The process from early development to approval of a drug may sometimes take up to 10 yr.

Phase 4 (postmarketing surveillance, pharmacovigilance) occurs after the drug is approved and marketed and can include formal research studies along with ongoing reporting of adverse effects. Phase 4 typically involves larger populations and longer time periods than phases 1 to 3, which helps detect uncommon or slowly developing adverse effects that are unlikely to be recognized in shorter, smaller studies. Also, real-world use of drugs is not limited to patients fulfilling the strict eligibility criteria used in clinical trials; drugs tend to be used in patients at higher risk of adverse effects. Often, special subpopulations (eg, pregnant women, children, the elderly) are studied. Some drugs approved by the FDA after phase 3 have been withdrawn from the market after newly recognized and serious adverse effects have occurred in phase 4.

DRUG EFFICACY AND SAFETY

Obviously, a drug (or any medical treatment) should be used only when it will benefit a patient. Benefit takes into account both the drug's ability to produce the desired result (efficacy) and the type and likelihood of adverse effects (safety). Cost is commonly also balanced with benefit (see p. 3146).

Efficacy and Effectiveness

Efficacy is the capacity to produce an effect (eg, lower BP). Efficacy can be assessed accurately only in ideal conditions (ie, when patients are selected by proper criteria and strictly adhere to the dosing schedule). Thus, efficacy is measured under expert supervision in a group of patients most likely to have a response to a drug, such as in a controlled clinical trial.

Effectiveness differs from efficacy in that it takes into account how well a drug works in real-world use; often, a drug that is efficacious in clinical trials is not very effective in actual use. For example, a drug may have high efficacy in lowering BP but may have low effectiveness because it causes so many adverse effects that patients stop taking it. Effectiveness also may be lower than efficacy if clinicians inadvertently prescribe the drug inappropriately (eg, giving a fibrinolytic drug to a patient thought to have an ischemic stroke, but who had an unrecognized cerebral hemorrhage on CT scan). Thus, effectiveness tends to be lower than efficacy.

Patient-oriented outcomes, rather than surrogate or intermediate outcomes, should be used to judge efficacy and effectiveness.

Patient-oriented outcomes: Patient-oriented outcomes are those that affect patients' well being. They involve the following:

- Prolongation of life
- Improved function (eg, prevention of disability)
- Relief of symptoms

Surrogate outcomes: Surrogate, or intermediate, outcomes involve things that do not directly involve patients' well-being.

They are often such things as physiologic parameters (eg, BP) or test results (eg, concentrations of glucose or cholesterol, tumor size on CT scan) that are thought to *predict* actual patient-oriented outcomes. For example, clinicians typically presume that lowering BP will prevent the patient-oriented outcome of uncontrolled hypertension (eg, death resulting from MI or stroke). However, it is conceivable that a drug could lower BP but not decrease mortality, perhaps because it has fatal adverse effects. Also, if the surrogate is merely a marker of disease (eg, HbA_{1c}) rather than a cause of disease (eg, elevated BP), an intervention might lower the marker by means that do not affect the underlying disorder. Thus, surrogate outcomes are less desirable measures of efficacy than patient-oriented outcomes.

On the other hand, surrogate outcomes can be much more feasible to use, for example, when patient-oriented outcomes take a long time to appear (eg, kidney failure resulting from uncontrolled hypertension) or are rare. In such cases, clinical trials would need to be very large and run for a long time unless a surrogate outcome (eg, lowered BP) is used. In addition, the main patient-oriented outcomes, death and disability, are dichotomous (ie, yes/no), whereas surrogate outcomes are often continuous, numerical variables (eg, BP, blood glucose). Numerical variables, unlike dichotomous outcomes, may indicate the magnitude of an effect. Thus, use of surrogate outcomes can often provide much more data for analysis than can patient-oriented outcomes, allowing clinical trials to be done using many fewer patients.

However, surrogate outcomes should ideally be proved to correlate with patient-oriented outcomes. There are many studies in which such correlation appeared reasonable but was not actually present. For example, treatment of certain postmenopausal women with estrogen and progesterone resulted in a more favorable lipid profile but failed to achieve the hypothesized corresponding reduction in MI or cardiac death. Similarly, lowering blood glucose to near-normal concentrations in patients with diabetes in the ICU resulted in higher mortality and morbidity (possibly by triggering episodes of hypoglycemia) than did lowering blood glucose to a slightly higher level. Some oral antihyperglycemic drugs lower blood glucose, including HbA_{1c} concentrations, but do not decrease risk of cardiac events. Some antihypertensive drugs decrease BP but do not decrease risk of stroke.

Adverse Effects

Similarly, clinically relevant adverse effects are patient-oriented outcomes; examples include the following:

- Death
- Disability
- Discomfort

Surrogate adverse effects (eg, alteration of concentrations of serum markers) are often used but, as with surrogate efficacy outcomes, should ideally correlate with patient-oriented adverse effects. Clinical trials that are carefully designed to prove efficacy can still have difficulty identifying adverse effects if the time needed to develop an adverse effect is longer than the time needed for benefit to occur or if the adverse effect is rare. For example, cyclooxygenase-2 (COX-2) inhibitors relieve pain quickly, and thus their efficacy can be shown in a comparatively brief study. However, the increased incidence of MI caused by some COX-2 inhibitors occurred over a longer period of time and was not apparent in shorter, smaller trials. For this reason, and because clinical trials may exclude certain subgroups and high-risk patients, adverse effects may not be fully known until a drug has been in widespread clinical use for years. Many drug adverse effects are dose-related.

Balancing Drug Benefits and Adverse Effects

Whether a drug is indicated depends on the balance of its benefits and harms. In making such judgments, clinicians often consider factors that are somewhat subjective, such as personal experience, anecdotes, peer practices, and expert opinions.

The **number needed to treat (NNT)** is a less subjective accounting of the likely benefits of a drug (or any other intervention). NNT is the number of patients who need to be treated for one patient to benefit. For example, consider a drug that decreases mortality of a certain disease from 10% to 5%, an absolute risk reduction of 5% (1 in 20). That means that of 100 patients, 90 would live even without treatment, and thus would not benefit from the drug. Also, 5 of the 100 patients will die even though they take the drug and thus also do not benefit. Only 5 of the 100 patients (1 in 20) benefit from taking the drug; thus, 20 need to be treated for 1 to benefit, and the NNT is 20. NNT can be simply calculated as the inverse of the absolute risk reduction; if the absolute risk reduction is 5% (0.05), the NNT = 1/0.05 = 20. NNT can be calculated for adverse effects also, in which case it is sometimes called the number needed to harm (NNH).

Importantly, NNT is based on changes in *absolute* risk; it cannot be calculated from changes in *relative* risk. Relative risk is the proportional difference between two risk levels. For example, a drug that decreases mortality from 10% to 5% decreases absolute mortality by 5% but decreases relative mortality by 50% (ie, a 5% death rate indicates 50% fewer deaths than a 10% death rate). Most often, benefits are reported in the literature as relative risk reductions because these make a drug look more effective than the absolute risk reductions (in the previous example, a 50% reduction in mortality sounds much better than a 5% reduction). In contrast, adverse effects are usually reported as absolute risk increases because they make a drug appear safer. For example, if a drug increases the incidence of bleeding from 0.1% to 1%, the increase is more likely to be reported as 0.9% than 1000%.

PEARLS & PITFALLS

- Calculate the NNT based on absolute, rather than relative, changes in risks.

When balancing NNT against NNH, it is important to weigh the magnitude of specific benefits and harms. For example, a drug that causes many more harms than benefits may be worth prescribing if those harms are minor (eg, reversible, mild) and the benefits are major (eg, preventing mortality or morbidity). In all cases, patient-oriented outcomes are best used.

Genetic profiling is increasingly being used to identify subgroups of patients that are more susceptible to the benefits and adverse effects of some drugs. For example, breast cancers can be analyzed for the HER2 genetic marker that predicts response to particular chemotherapy drugs. Patients with HIV/AIDS can be tested for the allele HLA-B*57:01, which predicts hypersensitivity to abacavir, reducing the incidence of hypersensitivity reactions and thus increasing NNH. Genetic variations in various drug-metabolizing enzymes help predict how patients respond to drugs (see p. 2910) and also often affect the probability of benefit, harm, or both.

Therapeutic index: One goal in drug development is to have a large difference between the dose that is efficacious and the dose that causes adverse effects. A large difference is called a wide therapeutic index, therapeutic ratio, or therapeutic window. If the therapeutic index is narrow (eg, < 2), factors that are usually clinically inconsequential (eg, food-drug interactions, drug-drug interactions, small errors in dosing) can have harmful clinical effects. For example, warfarin has a narrow therapeutic index and interacts with many drugs and foods. Insufficient anticoagulation increases the risk of complications resulting from the disorder being treated by anticoagulation (eg, increased risk of stroke in atrial fibrillation), whereas excessive anticoagulation increases risk of bleeding.

DRUG ERRORS

Drug errors contribute to morbidity and mortality. They are estimated to cost the US health care system up to $177 billion (depending on definitions) annually. Drug errors may involve

- The wrong choice of a drug or a prescription for the wrong dose, frequency, or duration
- An error in reading the prescription by the pharmacist so that the wrong drug or dose is dispensed
- An error in reading the label of the drug container by the caregiver so that the wrong drug or dose is given
- Incorrect instructions to the patient
- Incorrect administration by a clinician, caregiver, or patient
- Incorrect storage of a drug by the pharmacist or patient, altering the drug's potency
- Use of an outdated drug, altering the drug's potency
- Confusion of the patient so that the drug is taken incorrectly
- Inaccurate transmission of prescription information between different providers

Special subpopulations: Errors in prescribing are common, especially for certain populations. The elderly, women of childbearing age, and children are particularly at risk. Drug interactions particularly affect people taking many drugs. To minimize risk, clinicians should know all drugs being taken—including those prescribed by others and OTC drugs—and keep a complete problem list. Patients should be encouraged to write and update a list of their current drugs and dosages and bring the list to every health care appointment or emergency department visit. If there is any doubt as to which drugs are being used, patients should be instructed to bring all their drugs to their health care appointments for review.

Unclear prescriptions: Prescriptions must be written as clearly as possible. The names of some drugs are similar and, if not written clearly, cause confusion. Changing some traditional but easily confused notations may also help reduce errors. For example, "qd" (once/day) may be confused with "qid" (4 times/day). Writing "once/day" or "once a day" is preferred. Electronically transmitted or computer-printed prescriptions can avoid problems with illegible handwriting or inappropriate abbreviations. However, electronic prescribing systems that use check boxes or pull-down lists may increase the risk of inadvertently selecting the wrong drug or dose.

Inappropriate use of drugs: Drugs may be given incorrectly, especially in institutions. A drug may be given to the wrong patient, at the wrong time, or by the wrong route. Certain drugs must be given slowly when given IV, and some drugs cannot be given simultaneously. When an error is recognized, it should be reported immediately to a clinician, and a pharmacist should be consulted. Bar codes and computerized pharmacy systems may help decrease the incidence of drug errors.

Improper storage of drugs: A pharmacist should store drugs in a manner that ensures their potency. Mail-order pharmacies should follow procedures to ensure proper transportation. Storage by patients is often suboptimal. The bathroom medicine cabinet is not an ideal storage place for drugs because of the heat and humidity. If stored incorrectly, drugs are likely to decrease in potency long before the stated expiration date. Labeling should clearly state whether a drug needs to be stored in the refrigerator or kept cool, needs to be kept out of excessive heat or sun, or otherwise requires special storage. On the other hand, unnecessary precautions decrease adherence and waste the patient's time. For example, unopened insulin should be refrigerated, but a bottle in use can be stored safely outside the refrigerator for a relatively long time if not exposed to excessive heat and sun.

Drug expiration date exceeded: Use of outdated drugs is common. Outdated drugs may be ineffective, and some (eg, aspirin, tetracycline) can be harmful if used when outdated.

Patient error: Drug error often results from a patient's confusion about how to take drugs. Patients may take the wrong drug or dose. Dosing instructions for each drug, including why the drug has been prescribed, should be completely explained to patients and given in writing when possible. They should be advised to ask their pharmacist for additional advice about taking their drugs. Packaging should be convenient but safe. If children will not have access to the drug and patients may have difficulty opening the container, drugs do not need to be provided in childproof containers.

Miscommunication among health care providers: Another common source of error is inaccurate transmission of prescription information when a patient's care is transferred from one facility or provider to another (eg, from hospital to rehabilitation facility, from nursing home to hospital, or between a specialist and primary care provider). Communication between different busy providers usually requires active effort, and changes to a drug regimen are common when care is transitioned. Increased attention to communication can help decrease the risk of such errors. Risk has been decreased by various formal drug reconciliation programs, such as preparing a full list of current drugs each time a patient transfers from one facility to another.

PLACEBOS

Placebos are inactive substances or interventions, most often used in controlled studies for comparison with potentially active drugs.

The term placebo (Latin for "I will please") initially referred to an inactive, harmless substance given to patients to make them feel better by the power of suggestion. More recently, sham interventions (eg, mock electrical stimulation or simulated surgical procedures in clinical trials) have also been considered placebos. The term is sometimes used for an active drug that is given solely for its placebo effect on a disorder in which the drug is inactive (eg, an antibiotic for patients with viral illness).

Placebo effects: Placebos, although physiologically inactive, may have substantial effects—good and bad. These effects seem to be related to anticipation that the product will work; anticipation of *adverse* effects is sometimes called the nocebo effect. The placebo effect typically occurs with subjective responses (eg, pain, nausea) rather than objective ones (eg, rate of healing of leg ulcers, infection rate of burn wounds).

The magnitude of the response varies with many factors, including the

- Expressed confidence of the clinician ("this is going to make you feel a lot better" vs "there is a chance this might help")
- Certainty of the patient's beliefs (effect is larger when patients are sure they are receiving an active drug than when they know there is a chance they are getting a placebo)
- Type of placebo (eg, injectable drugs have a larger placebo effect than oral ones)

Not everyone responds to placebos, and it is not possible to predict who will respond; correlations between personality characteristics and response to placebos have been theorized but not well established. However, people who have a dependent personality and who want to please their clinicians may be more likely to report beneficial effects; those with a histrionic personality may be more likely to report any effect, good or bad.

Use of placebos in clinical trials: Many clinical trials compare an active treatment with a placebo. The apparent effects of the placebo are then subtracted from the apparent effects of the active treatment to identify the true treatment effect; to be meaningful, a clinically and statistically significant difference is required. In some studies, the placebo relieves the disorder in a high percentage of patients, making it more difficult to show the active treatment's efficacy.

Use of placebos in clinical practice: Rarely today, when a clinician determines that a patient has a mild, self-limited disorder for which an active drug does not exist or is not indicated (eg, for nonspecific malaise or tiredness), a placebo may be prescribed. The reasoning is that the placebo satisfies patients' demands for treatment without exposing them to potential adverse effects and often makes them feel better—due to the placebo effect or spontaneous improvement.

Ethical considerations: In clinical studies, the ethical consideration is whether a placebo should be given at all. When effective treatment exists (eg, opioid analgesics for severe pain), it is typically considered unethical to deprive study participants of treatment by giving a placebo; in such cases, control groups are given an active treatment. Because participants acknowledge in advance that they may be given a placebo, there is no concern about deception.

However, when a placebo is given in medical practice, patients are not told they are receiving an inactive treatment. This deception is controversial. Some clinicians argue that it is prima facie (Latin for "at first view") unethical and, if discovered, may damage the clinician-patient relationship. Others suggest that it is more unethical to not give something that may make patients feel better. Giving an active treatment solely for placebo effect may be further considered unethical because it exposes patients to actual adverse effects (as opposed to nocebo adverse effects).

346 Factors Affecting Response to Drugs

ADHERENCE TO A DRUG REGIMEN

Adherence (compliance) is the degree to which a patient follows a treatment regimen. For drugs, adherence requires that the prescription be obtained promptly and the drug be taken as prescribed in terms of dose, dosing interval, duration of treatment, and any additional special instructions (eg, taking the drug without food). Patients should be told to alert their physician if they stop or alter the way they take a drug but they rarely do so.

Only about half of patients who leave a physician's office with a prescription take the drug as directed. The most common reasons for nonadherence are

- Frequent dosing
- Denial of illness
- Poor comprehension of the benefits of taking the drug
- Cost

Many other reasons contribute to nonadherence (see Table 346–1).

Children are less likely than adults to adhere to a treatment regimen. Adherence is worse with chronic disorders requiring complex, long-term treatment (eg, juvenile diabetes, asthma). Parents may not clearly understand prescription instructions and, within 15 min, forget about half the information given by the physician.

The elderly adhere to treatment regimens as well as other adults. However, factors that decrease adherence (eg, inadequate finances, use of multiple drugs or drugs that must be taken several times a day) are more common among the elderly (see p. 2848). Cognitive impairment may further decrease adherence. Sometimes a prescriber must be creative by picking a drug that is easier to use even though it may not be the first choice. For example, a clonidine patch applied weekly by a visiting nurse or family member may be tried for hypertension in patients who cannot adhere to a more preferable daily regimen of oral drugs.

The most obvious result of nonadherence is that the disorder may not be relieved or cured. Nonadherence is estimated to result in 125,000 deaths due to cardiovascular disorders each year in the US. If patients took their drugs as directed, up to 23% of nursing home admissions, 10% of hospital admissions, many physician visits, many diagnostic tests, and many unnecessary treatments could be avoided. In some cases, nonadherence can actually lead to worsening of disease. For example, missed doses or early cessation of antibiotic or antiviral therapy may lead to resistant organisms.

Table 346–1. CAUSES OF NONADHERENCE

SOURCE	CAUSE
Patient	Apathy
	Concern about taking drugs (eg, adverse effects, addiction)
	Denial of the disorder or its significance
	Financial concerns
	Forgetfulness
	Misunderstanding of prescribing instructions
	No faith in the drug's efficacy
	Physical difficulties (eg, with swallowing tablets or capsules, opening bottles, or obtaining prescriptions)
	Reduction, fluctuation, or disappearance of symptoms
Drug	Adverse effects (real or imagined)
	Complex regimen (eg, frequent dosing, many drugs)
	Inconvenient or restrictive precautions (eg, no alcohol or cheese)
	Similar appearance of drugs
	Unpleasant taste or smell

Pharmacists and nurses may detect and help solve adherence problems. For example, a pharmacist may note that a patient does not obtain refills or that a prescription is being refilled too soon. In reviewing prescription directions with the patient, a pharmacist or nurse may uncover a patient's misunderstandings or fears and alleviate them. Physicians can alter complicated or frequent dosing or substitute safe, effective, but less expensive drugs. Communication among all health care practitioners that provide care for a patient is important.

DRUG INTERACTIONS

Drug interactions are changes in a drug's effects due to recent or concurrent use of another drug or drugs (drug-drug interactions), ingestion of food (drug-nutrient interactions), or ingestion of dietary supplements (dietary supplement-drug interactions).

A drug-drug interaction may increase or decrease the effects of one or both drugs. Clinically significant interactions are often predictable and usually undesired (see Table 346–2). Adverse effects or therapeutic failure may result. Rarely, clinicians can use predictable drug-drug interactions to produce a desired therapeutic effect. For example, coadministration of lopinavir and ritonavir to patients with HIV infection results in altered metabolism of lopinavir and increases serum lopinavir concentrations and effectiveness.

In therapeutic duplication, 2 drugs with similar properties are taken at the same time and have additive effects. For example, taking a benzodiazepine for anxiety and another benzodiazepine at bedtime for insomnia may have a cumulative effect, leading to toxicity.

Drug interactions involve

- Pharmacodynamics
- Pharmacokinetics

In **pharmacodynamic interactions,** one drug alters the sensitivity or responsiveness of tissues to another drug by having the same (agonistic) or a blocking (antagonistic) effect. These effects usually occur at the receptor level but may occur intracellularly.

In **pharmacokinetic interactions,** a drug usually alters absorption, distribution, protein binding, metabolism, or excretion of another drug. Thus, the amount and persistence

Table 346–2. SOME DRUGS WITH POTENTIALLY SERIOUS DRUG-DRUG INTERACTIONS*

MECHANISM	EXAMPLES
Narrow margin of safety[†]	Antiarrhythmic drugs (eg, quinidine) Antineoplastic drugs (eg, methotrexate) Digoxin Lithium Theophylline Warfarin
Extensive metabolism by certain hepatic enzymes	Alprazolam Amitriptyline Atorvastatin Carbamazepine Clozapine Corticosteroids Cyclosporine Diazepam HIV protease inhibitors Imipramine Lovastatin Midazolam Olanzapine Phenytoin Sildenafil Simvastatin Tacrolimus Tadalafil Theophylline Triazolam Vardenafil Warfarin
Inhibition of certain hepatic enzymes[‡]	Aprepitant Boceprevir Cimetidine Ciprofloxacin Clarithromycin Cobicistat Conivaptan Diltiazem Erythromycin Fluconazole Fluoxetine Fluvoxamine Itraconazole Ketoconazole Paroxetine Posaconazole Ritonavir Telaprevir Telithromycin Verapamil Voriconazole
Induction of certain hepatic enzymes	Barbiturates (eg, phenobarbital) Bosentan Carbamazepine Efavirenz Phenytoin Rifabutin Rifampin St. John's wort

*Any drug to be used concurrently with one of these drugs should be thoroughly evaluated for possible interactions.

[†]Even when used alone, these drugs may have serious adverse effects. Concurrent use of another drug that increases the action of these drugs further increases risk of adverse effects. For additional research on potential drug-drug interactions, consult a reliable source, such as Drug.com's Drugs Interaction Checker.

[‡]Inhibition also can occur after ingestion of grapefruit products.

of available drug at receptor sites change. Pharmacokinetic interactions alter magnitude and duration, not type, of effect. They are often predicted based on knowledge of the individual drugs or detected by monitoring drug concentrations or clinical signs.

Minimizing drug interactions: Clinicians should know all of their patients' current drugs, including drugs prescribed by other clinicians and all OTC drugs, herbal products, and nutritional supplements. Asking patients relevant questions about diet and alcohol consumption is recommended. The fewest drugs in the lowest doses for the shortest possible time should be prescribed. The effects, desired and undesired, of all drugs taken should be determined because these effects usually include the spectrum of drug interactions. If possible, drugs with a wide safety margin should be used so that any unforeseen interactions do not cause toxicity.

Patients should be observed and monitored for adverse effects, particularly after a change in treatment; some interactions (eg, effects that are influenced by enzyme induction) may take ≥ 1 wk to appear. Drug interactions should be considered as a possible cause of any unexpected problems. When unexpected clinical responses occur, prescribers should determine serum concentrations of selected drugs being taken, consult the literature or an expert in drug interactions, and adjust the dosage until the desired effect is produced. If dosage adjustment is ineffective, the drug should be replaced by one that does not interact with other drugs being taken.

PHARMACOGENETICS

Pharmacogenetics involves variations in drug response due to genetic makeup.

The activity of drug-metabolizing enzymes often varies widely among healthy people, making metabolism highly variable. Drug elimination rates vary up to 40-fold. Genetic factors and aging seem to account for most of these variations.

Pharmacogenetic variation (eg, in acetylation, hydrolysis, oxidation, or drug-metabolizing enzymes) can have clinical consequences (see Table 346–3). For example, if patients metabolize certain drugs rapidly, they may require higher, more frequent doses to achieve therapeutic concentrations; if patients metabolize certain drugs slowly, they may need lower, less frequent doses to avoid toxicity, particularly of drugs with a narrow margin of safety. For example, patients with inflammatory bowel disease who require azathioprine therapy are now routinely tested for thiopurine methyltransferase (TPMT) genotype to determine the most appropriate starting dose for drug therapy. Most genetic differences cannot be predicted before drug therapy, but for an increasing number of drugs (eg, carbamazepine, clopidogrel, warfarin), changes in effectiveness and risk of toxicity have been specifically associated with certain genetic variations. Also, many environmental and developmental factors can interact with each other and with genetic factors to affect drug response (see Fig. 346–1).

Table 346–3. EXAMPLES OF PHARMACOGENETIC VARIATIONS

VARIATION	INCIDENCE	EFFECTS
Acetylation, fast	—	Need for higher or more frequent doses of drugs that are acetylated (eg, isoniazid) to produce the desired therapeutic response
Acetylation, slow (drug inactivation by hepatic *N*-acetyltransferase)	About 50% of the US population	Increased susceptibility to adverse effects of drugs that are acetylated (eg, with isoniazid, peripheral neuritis; with hydralazine or procainamide, lupus)
Aldehyde dehydrogenase-2 deficiency	About 50% of Japanese, Chinese, and other Asian populations	With alcohol ingestion, marked elevations of blood acetaldehyde, causing facial flushing, increased heart rate, diaphoresis, muscle weakness, and sometimes catecholamine-mediated vasodilation with euphoria
CYP2C9 genetic polymorphisms	30% in one study More common among East Asians	Reduced enzymatic activation of clopidogrel, resulting in reduced antiplatelet effect and increased risk of thrombosis in high-risk patients
G6PD deficiency	10% of black males Higher prevalence in people of Mediterranean descent	With use of oxidant drugs, such as certain antimalarials (eg, chloroquine, primaquine), increased risk of hemolytic anemia
Genetic polymorphisms of *CYP2C9* and vitamin K epoxide reductase complex subunit 1 (*VKORC1*)	—	Increased action of warfarin,* increasing risk of bleeding events
HLA-B*1502	1 to 6/10,000 in countries with mainly white populations In some Asian countries, about 10 times higher	Increased risk of adverse reactions to carbamazepine, including serious dermatologic reactions (eg, Stevens-Johnson syndrome)
Plasma pseudocholinesterase deficiency	About 1/1500 people	Decreased succinylcholine inactivation With conventional succinylcholine doses, prolonged paralysis of respiratory muscles and sometimes persistent apnea requiring mechanical ventilation until the drug can be eliminated by alternate pathways

*In one study, variations in *CYP2C9* or *VKORC1* genes accounted for about 40% of variance in warfarin dosage.

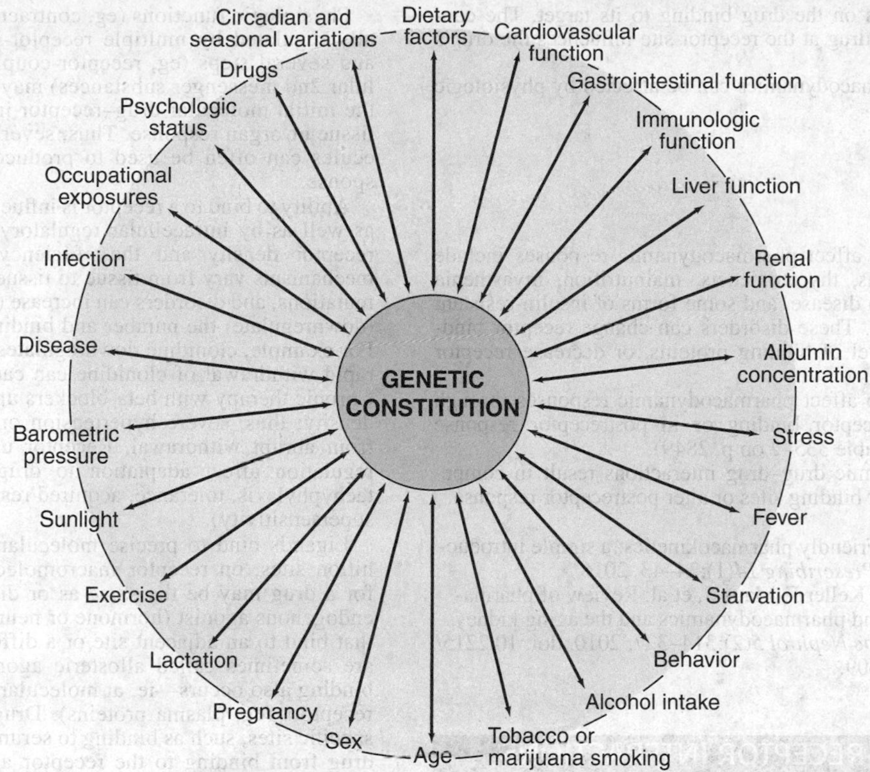

Fig. 346–1. Genetic, environmental, and developmental factors that can interact, causing variations in drug response among patients.

TOLERANCE AND RESISTANCE

Tolerance is a decrease in response to a drug that is used repeatedly. Resistance is development of the ability to withstand the previously destructive effect of a drug by microorganisms or tumor cells.

Examples of drugs that result in tolerance include alcohol and opioids. One mechanism responsible for tolerance is accelerated metabolism, for example, by induction of hepatic enzymes such as the cytochrome P-450 system enzymes. Generally, tolerance leads to increasing doses of a drug being required to produce the same effect. Other possible mechanisms are a decrease in binding affinity between a drug and receptor and a decrease in the number of receptors. The mechanisms responsible for drug tolerance are not always known.

Examples of resistance include the following:

- Strains of microorganisms are resistant when they are no longer killed or inhibited by previously effective antimicrobial drugs. The mechanism begins with a genetic change resulting from a mutation or gene acquisition. Because the previously effective antimicrobial drug preferentially eliminates nonresistant organisms, the resistant organisms become the predominant species (see p. 1506).
- Tumors can become resistant if a mutation develops that confers resistance to an anticancer drug and that anticancer drug is used repeatedly, preferentially eliminating nonresistant tumor cells. For example, many patients with chronic myeloid leukemia have become resistant to the tyrosine kinase inhibitor imatinib because of the presence of the *T315I* mutation.
- Corticosteroid resistance can affect the treatment of a number of disorders such as asthma or inflammatory bowel disease. The mechanism of this type of resistance is not fully understood but may involve a number of different factors (eg, infection, oxidative stress, allergen exposure, inflammation, deficient vitamin D_3, genetic mutations or variations).

347 Pharmacodynamics

Pharmacodynamics (sometimes described as what a drug does to the body) is the study of the biochemical, physiologic, and molecular effects of drugs on the body and involves receptor binding (including receptor sensitivity), postreceptor effects, and chemical interactions. Pharmacodynamics, with pharmacokinetics (what the body does to a drug, or the fate of a drug within the body[1-2]), helps explain the relationship between the dose and response, ie, the drug's effects. The pharmacologic response depends on the drug binding to its target. The concentration of the drug at the receptor site influences the drug's effect.

A drug's pharmacodynamics can be affected by physiologic changes due to

- A disorder
- Aging
- Other drugs

Disorders that affect pharmacodynamic responses include genetic mutations, thyrotoxicosis, malnutrition, myasthenia gravis, Parkinson disease, and some forms of insulin-resistant diabetes mellitus. These disorders can change receptor binding, alter the level of binding proteins, or decrease receptor sensitivity.

Aging tends to affect pharmacodynamic responses through alterations in receptor binding or in postreceptor response sensitivity (see Table 335–2 on p. 2849).

Pharmacodynamic drug–drug interactions result in competition for receptor binding sites or alter postreceptor response.

1. Hughes G: Friendly pharmacokinetics: a simple introduction. *Nurse Prescribing 14*(1):34–43, 2016.
2. Aymanns C, Keller F, Maus S, et al: Review of pharmacokinetics and pharmacodynamics and the aging kidney. *Clin J Am Soc Nephrol 5*(2):314–327, 2010. doi: 10.2215/CJN.03960609.

DRUG–RECEPTOR INTERACTIONS

Receptors are macromolecules involved in chemical signaling between and within cells; they may be located on the cell surface membrane or within the cytoplasm (see Table 347–1). Activated receptors directly or indirectly regulate cellular biochemical processes (eg, ion conductance, protein phosphorylation, DNA transcription, enzymatic activity).

Molecules (eg, drugs, hormones, neurotransmitters) that bind to a receptor are called ligands. The binding can be specific and reversible. A ligand may activate or inactivate a receptor; activation may increase or decrease a particular cell function. Each ligand may interact with multiple receptor subtypes. Few if any drugs are absolutely specific for one receptor or subtype, but most have relative selectivity. Selectivity is the degree to which a drug acts on a given site relative to other sites; selectivity relates largely to physicochemical binding of the drug to cellular receptors.

A drug's ability to affect a given receptor is related to the drug's affinity (probability of the drug occupying a receptor at any given instant) and intrinsic efficacy (intrinsic activity—degree to which a ligand activates receptors and leads to cellular response). A drug's affinity and activity are determined by its chemical structure.

The pharmacologic effect is also determined by the duration of time that the drug-receptor complex persists (residence time). The lifetime of the drug-receptor complex is affected by dynamic processes (conformation changes) that control the rate of drug association and dissociation from the target. A longer residence time explains a prolonged pharmacologic effect. Drugs with long residence times include finasteride and darunavir. A longer residence time can be a potential disadvantage when it prolongs a drug's toxicity. For some receptors, transient drug occupancy produces the desired pharmacologic effect, whereas prolonged occupancy causes toxicity.

Physiologic functions (eg, contraction, secretion) are usually regulated by multiple receptor-mediated mechanisms, and several steps (eg, receptor-coupling, multiple intracellular 2nd messenger substances) may be interposed between the initial molecular drug–receptor interaction and ultimate tissue or organ response. Thus, several dissimilar drug molecules can often be used to produce the same desired response.

Ability to bind to a receptor is influenced by external factors as well as by intracellular regulatory mechanisms. Baseline receptor density and the efficiency of stimulus-response mechanisms vary from tissue to tissue. Drugs, aging, genetic mutations, and disorders can increase (upregulate) or decrease (downregulate) the number and binding affinity of receptors. For example, clonidine downregulates alpha$_2$-receptors; thus, rapid withdrawal of clonidine can cause hypertensive crisis. Chronic therapy with beta-blockers upregulates beta-receptor density; thus, severe hypertension or tachycardia can result from abrupt withdrawal. Receptor upregulation and downregulation affect adaptation to drugs (eg, desensitization, tachyphylaxis, tolerance, acquired resistance, postwithdrawal supersensitivity).

Ligands bind to precise molecular regions, called recognition sites, on receptor macromolecules. The binding site for a drug may be the same as or different from that of an endogenous agonist (hormone or neurotransmitter). Agonists that bind to an adjacent site or a different site on a receptor are sometimes called allosteric agonists. Nonspecific drug binding also occurs—ie, at molecular sites not designated as receptors (eg, plasma proteins). Drug binding to such nonspecific sites, such as binding to serum proteins, prohibits the drug from binding to the receptor and thus inactivates the drug. Unbound drug is available to bind to receptors and thus have an effect.

Agonists and antagonists: Agonists activate receptors to produce the desired response. Conventional agonists increase the proportion of activated receptors. Inverse agonists stabilize the receptor in its inactive conformation and act similarly to competitive antagonists. Many hormones, neurotransmitters (eg, acetylcholine, histamine, norepinephrine), and drugs (eg, morphine, phenylephrine, isoproterenol, benzodiazepines, barbiturates) act as agonists.

Antagonists prevent receptor activation. Preventing activation has many effects. Antagonists increase cellular function if they block the action of a substance that normally decreases cellular function. Antagonists decrease cellular function if they block the action of a substance that normally increases cellular function.

Receptor antagonists can be classified as reversible or irreversible. Reversible antagonists readily dissociate from their receptor; irreversible antagonists form a stable, permanent or nearly permanent chemical bond with their receptor (eg, by alkylation). Pseudo-irreversible antagonists slowly dissociate from their receptor.

In **competitive antagonism,** binding of the antagonist to the receptor prevents binding of the agonist to the receptor.

In **noncompetitive antagonism,** agonist and antagonist can be bound simultaneously, but antagonist binding reduces or prevents the action of the agonist.

In **reversible competitive antagonism,** agonist and antagonist form short-lasting bonds with the receptor, and a steady state among agonist, antagonist, and receptor is reached. Such antagonism can be overcome by increasing the concentration of the agonist. For example, naloxone (an opioid receptor antagonist that is structurally similar to morphine), when given shortly

Table 347–1. SOME TYPES OF PHYSIOLOGIC AND DRUG-RECEPTOR PROTEINS

TYPE	STRUCTURE	CELLULAR LOCATION	EXAMPLES
Multisubunit ion channels	Out; Cell membrane; In; Ion flux	Cell surface transmembrane	Acetylcholine (nicotinic) $GABA_A$ Glutamate Glycine
G-protein-coupled receptors	Out; Cell membrane; In; G protein; GTP; GDP	Cell surface transmembrane	Acetylcholine (muscarinic) α- and β-adrenergic receptor proteins Eicosanoids
Protein kinases	Binding Site; Out; Cell membrane; In; Catalysis	Cell surface transmembrane	Growth factors Insulin Peptide hormones
Transcription factors	Nucleus; Ligand; Cytosol; Receptor; Activation/suppression of DNA transcription	Cytoplasm	Steroid hormones Thyroid hormone Vitamin D

GABA = γ-aminobutyric acid; GDP = guanosine diphosphate; GTP = guanosine triphosphate.

before or after morphine, blocks morphine's effects. However, competitive antagonism by naloxone can be overcome by giving more morphine.

Structural analogs of agonist molecules frequently have agonist and antagonist properties; such drugs are called partial (low-efficacy) agonists, or agonist-antagonists. For example, pentazocine activates opioid receptors but blocks their activation by other opioids. Thus, pentazocine provides opioid effects but blunts the effects of another opioid if the opioid is given while pentazocine is still bound. A drug that acts as a partial agonist in one tissue may act as a full agonist in another.

CHEMICAL INTERACTIONS

Some drugs produce effects without altering cellular function and without binding to a receptor. For example, most antacids decrease gastric acidity through simple chemical reactions; antacids are bases that chemically interact with acids to produce neutral salts. The primary action of cholestyramine, a bile acid sequestrant, is to bind bile acids in the GI tract.

DOSE-RESPONSE RELATIONSHIPS

Regardless of how a drug effect occurs—through binding or chemical interaction—the concentration of the drug at the site of action controls the effect. However, response to concentration may be complex and is often nonlinear. The relationship between the drug dose, regardless of route used, and the drug concentration at the cellular level is even more complex (see p. 2914).

Dose-response data are typically graphed with the dose or dose function (eg, $\log_{10}$ dose) on the x-axis and the measured effect (response) on the y-axis. Because a drug effect is a function of dose and time, such a graph depicts the dose-response relationship independent of time. Measured effects are frequently recorded as maxima at time of peak effect or under steady-state conditions (eg, during continuous IV infusion). Drug effects may be quantified at the level of molecule, cell, tissue, organ, organ system, or organism.

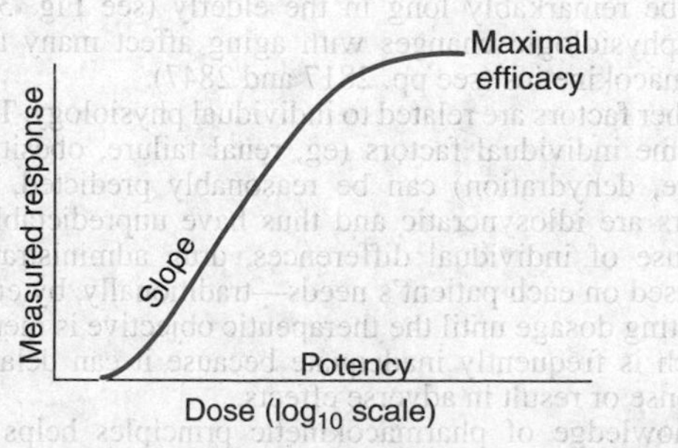

Fig. 347–1. Hypothetical dose-response curve.

A hypothetical dose-response curve has features that vary (see Fig. 347–1):

- Potency (location of curve along the dose axis)
- Maximal efficacy or ceiling effect (greatest attainable response)
- Slope (change in response per unit dose)

Biologic variation (variation in magnitude of response among test subjects in the same population given the same dose of drug) also occurs. Graphing dose-response curves of drugs studied under identical conditions can help compare the pharmacologic profiles of the drugs (see Fig. 347–2). This information helps determine the dose necessary to achieve the desired effect.

Dose-response, which involves the principles of pharmacokinetics and pharmacodynamics, determines the required dose and frequency as well as the therapeutic index for a drug in a population. The therapeutic index (ratio of the minimum toxic concentration to the median effective concentration) helps determine the efficacy and safety of a drug. Increasing the dose of a drug with a small therapeutic index increases the probability of toxicity or ineffectiveness of the drug. However, these features differ by population and are affected by patient-related factors, such as pregnancy, age, and organ function (eg, estimated GFR).

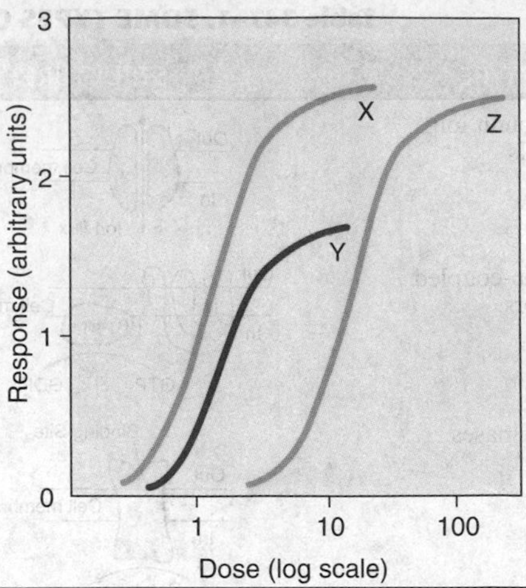

Fig. 347–2. Comparison of dose-response curves. Drug X has greater biologic activity per dosing equivalent and is thus more potent than drugs Y or Z. Drugs X and Z have equal efficacy, indicated by their maximal attainable response (ceiling effect). Drug Y is more potent than drug Z, but its maximal efficacy is lower.

348 Pharmacokinetics

Pharmacokinetics, sometimes described as what the body does to a drug, refers to the movement of drug into, through, and out of the body—the time course of its absorption, bioavailability, distribution, metabolism, and excretion.

Pharmacodynamics, described as what a drug does to the body, involves receptor binding, postreceptor effects, and chemical interactions. Drug pharmacokinetics determines the onset, duration, and intensity of a drug's effect. Formulas relating these processes summarize the pharmacokinetic behavior of most drugs (see Table 348–1).

Pharmacokinetics of a drug depends on patient-related factors as well as on the drug's chemical properties. Some patient-related factors (eg, renal function, genetic makeup, sex, age) can be used to predict the pharmacokinetic parameters in populations. For example, the half-life of some drugs, especially those that require both metabolism and excretion, may be remarkably long in the elderly (see Fig. 348–1). In fact, physiologic changes with aging affect many aspects of pharmacokinetics (see pp. 2817 and 2847).

Other factors are related to individual physiology. The effects of some individual factors (eg, renal failure, obesity, hepatic failure, dehydration) can be reasonably predicted, but other factors are idiosyncratic and thus have unpredictable effects. Because of individual differences, drug administration must be based on each patient's needs—traditionally, by empirically adjusting dosage until the therapeutic objective is met. This approach is frequently inadequate because it can delay optimal response or result in adverse effects.

Knowledge of pharmacokinetic principles helps prescribers adjust dosage more accurately and rapidly. Application of pharmacokinetic principles to individualize pharmacotherapy is termed therapeutic drug monitoring.

DRUG ABSORPTION

Drug absorption is determined by the drug's physicochemical properties, formulation, and route of administration. Dosage forms (eg, tablets, capsules, solutions), consisting of the drug plus other ingredients, are formulated to be given by various routes (eg, oral, buccal, sublingual, rectal, parenteral, topical, inhalational). Regardless of the route of administration, drugs must be in solution to be absorbed. Thus, solid forms (eg, tablets) must be able to disintegrate and deaggregate.

Unless given IV, a drug must cross several semipermeable cell membranes before it reaches the systemic circulation. Cell membranes are biologic barriers that selectively inhibit passage of drug molecules. The membranes are composed primarily of a bimolecular lipid matrix, which determines membrane permeability characteristics. Drugs may cross cell membranes by

- Passive diffusion
- Facilitated passive diffusion
- Active transport
- Pinocytosis

Sometimes various globular proteins embedded in the matrix function as receptors and help transport molecules across the membrane.

Passive diffusion: Drugs diffuse across a cell membrane from a region of high concentration (eg, GI fluids) to one of low concentration (eg, blood). Diffusion rate is directly proportional to the gradient but also depends on the molecule's lipid solubility, size, degree of ionization, and the area of absorptive surface. Because the cell membrane is lipoid, lipid-soluble

Table 348–1. FORMULAS DEFINING BASIC PHARMACOKINETIC PARAMETERS

CATEGORY	PARAMETER	FORMULA
Absorption	Absorption rate constant	Rate of drug absorption ÷ amount of drug remaining to be absorbed
	Bioavailability	Amount of drug absorbed ÷ drug dose
Distribution	Apparent volume of distribution	Amount of drug in body ÷ plasma drug concentration
	Unbound fraction	Plasma concentration of unbound drug ÷ total plasma drug concentration
Elimination (metabolism and excretion)	Rate of elimination	Renal excretion + extrarenal (usually metabolic) elimination
	Clearance	Rate of drug elimination ÷ plasma drug concentration, or elimination rate constant × apparent volume of distribution
	Renal clearance	Rate of renal excretion of drug ÷ plasma drug concentration
	Metabolic clearance	Rate of drug metabolism ÷ plasma drug concentration
	Fraction excreted unchanged	Rate of renal excretion of drug ÷ rate of drug elimination
	Elimination rate constant	Rate of drug elimination ÷ amount of drug in body
		Clearance ÷ volume of distribution
	Biologic half-life	0.693 ÷ elimination rate constant (for first-order elimination only—see p. 2918)

drugs diffuse most rapidly. Small molecules tend to penetrate membranes more rapidly than larger ones.

Most drugs are weak organic acids or bases, existing in un-ionized and ionized forms in an aqueous environment. The un-ionized form is usually lipid soluble (lipophilic) and diffuses readily across cell membranes. The ionized form has low lipid solubility (but high water solubility—ie, hydrophilic) and high electrical resistance and thus cannot penetrate cell membranes easily.

The proportion of the un-ionized form present (and thus the drug's ability to cross a membrane) is determined by the environmental pH and the drug's pK_a (acid dissociation constant). The pK_a is the pH at which concentrations of ionized and un-ionized forms are equal. When the pH is lower than the pK_a, the un-ionized form of a weak acid predominates, but the ionized form of a weak base predominates. Thus, in plasma (pH 7.4), the ratio of un-ionized to ionized forms for a weak acid (eg, with a pK_a of 4.4) is 1:1000; in gastric fluid (pH 1.4), the ratio is reversed (1000:1). Therefore, when a weak acid is given orally, most of the drug in the stomach is un-ionized, favoring diffusion through the gastric mucosa. For a weak base with a pK_a of 4.4, the outcome is reversed; most of the drug in the stomach is ionized.

Theoretically, weakly acidic drugs (eg, aspirin) are more readily absorbed from an acid medium (stomach) than are weakly basic drugs (eg, quinidine). However, whether a drug is acidic or basic, most absorption occurs in the small intestine because the surface area is larger and membranes are more permeable (see p. 2916).

Facilitated passive diffusion: Certain molecules with low lipid solubility (eg, glucose) penetrate membranes more rapidly than expected. One theory is facilitated passive diffusion: A carrier molecule in the membrane combines reversibly with the substrate molecule outside the cell membrane, and the carrier-substrate complex diffuses rapidly across the membrane, releasing the substrate at the interior surface. In such cases, the membrane transports only substrates with a relatively specific

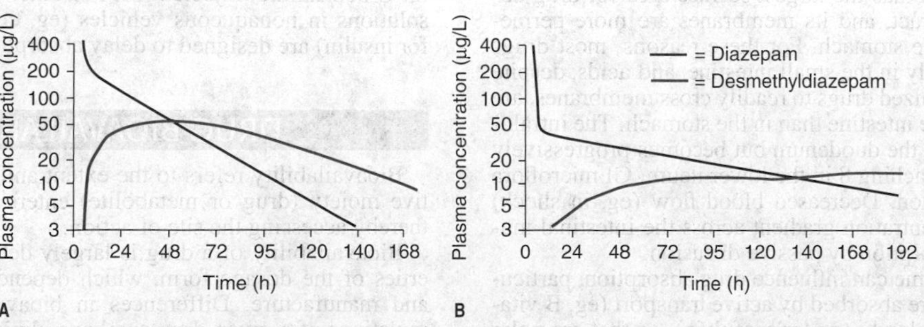

Fig. 348–1. Comparison of pharmacokinetic outcomes for diazepam in a younger man (A) and an older man (B). Diazepam is metabolized in the liver to desmethyldiazepam through P-450 enzymes. Desmethyldiazepam is an active sedative, which is excreted by the kidneys. Elimination half-life is inversely proportional to the terminal slopes of the curves; flat slopes correspond to long half-lives. 0 = time of dosing. (Adapted from Greenblatt DJ, Allen MD, Harmatz JS, Shader RI: Diazepam disposition determinants. *Clinical Pharmacology and Therapeutics.* 27:301–312, 1980.)

molecular configuration, and the availability of carriers limits the process. The process does not require energy expenditure, and transport against a concentration gradient cannot occur.

Active transport: Active transport is selective, requires energy expenditure, and may involve transport against a concentration gradient. Active transport seems to be limited to drugs structurally similar to endogenous substances (eg, ions, vitamins, sugars, amino acids). These drugs are usually absorbed from specific sites in the small intestine.

Pinocytosis: In pinocytosis, fluid or particles are engulfed by a cell. The cell membrane invaginates, encloses the fluid or particles, then fuses again, forming a vesicle that later detaches and moves to the cell interior. Energy expenditure is required. Pinocytosis probably plays a small role in drug transport, except for protein drugs.

Oral Administration

To be absorbed, a drug given orally must survive encounters with low pH and numerous GI secretions, including potentially degrading enzymes. Peptide drugs (eg, insulin) are particularly susceptible to degradation and are not given orally. Absorption of oral drugs involves transport across membranes of the epithelial cells in the GI tract. Absorption is affected by

- Differences in luminal pH along the GI tract
- Surface area per luminal volume
- Blood perfusion
- Presence of bile and mucus
- The nature of epithelial membranes

The oral mucosa has a thin epithelium and rich vascularity, which favor absorption; however, contact is usually too brief for substantial absorption. A drug placed between the gums and cheek (buccal administration) or under the tongue (sublingual administration) is retained longer, enhancing absorption.

The stomach has a relatively large epithelial surface, but its thick mucous layer and short transit time limit absorption. Because most absorption occurs in the small intestine, gastric emptying is often the rate-limiting step. Food, especially fatty food, slows gastric emptying (and rate of drug absorption), explaining why taking some drugs on an empty stomach speeds absorption. Drugs that affect gastric emptying (eg, parasympatholytic drugs) affect the absorption rate of other drugs. Food may enhance the extent of absorption for poorly soluble drugs (eg, griseofulvin), reduce it for drugs degraded in the stomach (eg, penicillin G), or have little or no effect.

The small intestine has the largest surface area for drug absorption in the GI tract, and its membranes are more permeable than those in the stomach. For these reasons, most drugs are absorbed primarily in the small intestine, and acids, despite their ability as un-ionized drugs to readily cross membranes, are absorbed faster in the intestine than in the stomach. The intraluminal pH is 4 to 5 in the duodenum but becomes progressively more alkaline, approaching 8 in the lower ileum. GI microflora may reduce absorption. Decreased blood flow (eg, in shock) may lower the concentration gradient across the intestinal mucosa and reduce absorption by passive diffusion.

Intestinal transit time can influence drug absorption, particularly for drugs that are absorbed by active transport (eg, B vitamins), that dissolve slowly (eg, griseofulvin), or that are polar (ie, with low lipid solubility; eg, many antibiotics).

To maximize adherence, clinicians should prescribe oral suspensions and chewable tablets for children < 8 yr. In adolescents and adults, most drugs are given orally as tablets or capsules primarily for convenience, economy, stability, and patient acceptance. Because solid drug forms must dissolve before absorption can occur, dissolution rate determines availability of the drug for absorption. Dissolution, if slower than absorption, becomes the rate-limiting step. Manipulating the formulation (ie, the drug's form as salt, crystal, or hydrate) can change the dissolution rate and thus control overall absorption.

Parenteral Administration

Drugs given IV enter the systemic circulation directly. However, drugs injected IM or sc must cross one or more biologic membranes to reach the systemic circulation. If protein drugs with a molecular mass > 20,000 g/mol are injected IM or sc, movement across capillary membranes is so slow that most absorption occurs via the lymphatic system. In such cases, drug delivery to systemic circulation is slow and often incomplete because of first-pass metabolism (metabolism of a drug before it reaches systemic circulation) by proteolytic enzymes in the lymphatics.

Perfusion (blood flow/gram of tissue) greatly affects capillary absorption of small molecules injected IM or sc. Thus, injection site can affect absorption rate. Absorption after IM or sc injection may be delayed or erratic for salts of poorly soluble bases and acids (eg, parenteral form of phenytoin) and in patients with poor peripheral perfusion (eg, during hypotension or shock).

Controlled-Release Forms

Controlled-release forms are designed to reduce dosing frequency for drugs with a short elimination half-life and duration of effect. These forms also limit fluctuation in plasma drug concentration, providing a more uniform therapeutic effect while minimizing adverse effects. Absorption rate is slowed by coating drug particles with wax or other water-insoluble material, by embedding the drug in a matrix that releases it slowly during transit through the GI tract, or by complexing the drug with ion-exchange resins. Most absorption of these forms occurs in the large intestine. Crushing or otherwise disturbing a controlled-release tablet or capsule can often be dangerous.

Transdermal controlled-release forms are designed to release the drug for extended periods, sometimes for several days. Drugs for transdermal delivery must have suitable skin penetration characteristics and high potency because the penetration rate and area of application are limited.

Many non-IV parenteral forms are designed to sustain plasma drug concentrations. Absorption of antimicrobials can be extended by using their relatively insoluble salt form (eg, penicillin G benzathine) injected IM. For other drugs, suspensions or solutions in nonaqueous vehicles (eg, crystalline suspensions for insulin) are designed to delay absorption.

DRUG BIOAVAILABILITY

Bioavailability refers to the extent and rate at which the active moiety (drug or metabolite) enters systemic circulation, thereby accessing the site of action.

Bioavailability of a drug is largely determined by the properties of the dosage form, which depend partly on its design and manufacture. Differences in bioavailability among formulations of a given drug can have clinical significance; thus, knowing whether drug formulations are equivalent is essential.

Chemical equivalence indicates that drug products contain the same active compound in the same amount and meet current official standards; however, inactive ingredients in drug products may differ. **Bioequivalence** indicates that the drug products, when given to the same patient in the same dosage regimen, result in equivalent concentrations of drug in plasma and tissues. **Therapeutic equivalence** indicates that drug products, when given to the same patient in the same dosage regimen, have the same therapeutic and adverse effects.

Bioequivalent products are expected to be therapeutically equivalent. Therapeutic nonequivalence (eg, more adverse effects, less efficacy) is usually discovered during long-term treatment when patients who are stabilized on one formulation are given a nonequivalent substitute.

Sometimes therapeutic equivalence is possible despite differences in bioavailability. For example, the therapeutic index (ratio of the minimum toxic concentration to the median effective concentration) of penicillin is so wide that efficacy and safety are usually not affected by the moderate differences in plasma concentration due to bioavailability differences in penicillin products. In contrast, for drugs with a relatively narrow therapeutic index, bioavailability differences may cause substantial therapeutic nonequivalence.

Causes of low bioavailability: Orally administered drugs must pass through the intestinal wall and then the portal circulation to the liver; both are common sites of first-pass metabolism (metabolism that occurs before a drug reaches systemic circulation). Thus, many drugs may be metabolized before adequate plasma concentrations are reached. Low bioavailability is most common with oral dosage forms of poorly water-soluble, slowly absorbed drugs.

Insufficient time for absorption in the GI tract is a common cause of low bioavailability. If the drug does not dissolve readily or cannot penetrate the epithelial membrane (eg, if it is highly ionized and polar), time at the absorption site may be insufficient. In such cases, bioavailability tends to be highly variable as well as low.

Age, sex, physical activity, genetic phenotype, stress, disorders (eg, achlorhydria, malabsorption syndromes), or previous GI surgery (eg, bariatric surgery) can also affect drug bioavailability.

Chemical reactions that reduce absorption can decrease bioavailability. They include formation of a complex (eg, between tetracycline and polyvalent metal ions), hydrolysis by gastric acid or digestive enzymes (eg, penicillin and chloramphenicol palmitate hydrolysis), conjugation in the intestinal wall (eg, sulfoconjugation of isoproterenol), adsorption to other drugs (eg, digoxin to cholestyramine), and metabolism by luminal microflora.

Assessing bioavailability: Bioavailability is usually assessed by determining the area under the plasma concentration–time curve (AUC—see Fig. 348–2). The most reliable measure of a drug's bioavailability is AUC. AUC is directly proportional to the total amount of unchanged drug that reaches systemic circulation. Drug products may be considered bioequivalent in extent and rate of absorption if their plasma concentration curves are essentially superimposable.

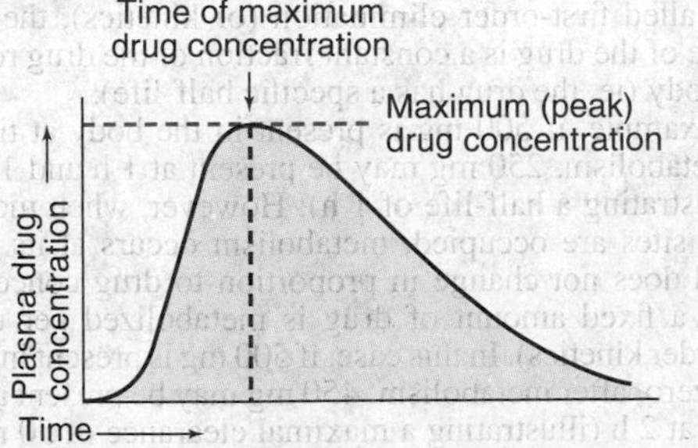

Fig. 348–2. Representative plasma concentration–time relationship after a single oral dose of a hypothetical drug.

Plasma drug concentration increases with extent of absorption; the maximum (peak) plasma concentration is reached when drug elimination rate equals absorption rate. Bioavailability determinations based on the peak plasma concentration can be misleading because drug elimination begins as soon as the drug enters the bloodstream. Peak time (when maximum plasma drug concentration occurs) is the most widely used general index of absorption rate; the slower the absorption, the later the peak time.

For drugs excreted primarily unchanged in urine, bioavailability can be estimated by measuring the total amount of drug excreted after a single dose. Ideally, urine is collected over a period of 7 to 10 elimination half-lives for complete urinary recovery of the absorbed drug. After multiple dosing, bioavailability may be estimated by measuring unchanged drug recovered from urine over a 24-h period under steady-state conditions.

DRUG DISTRIBUTION TO TISSUES

After a drug enters the systemic circulation, it is distributed to the body's tissues. Distribution is generally uneven because of differences in blood perfusion, tissue binding (eg, because of lipid content), regional pH, and permeability of cell membranes.

The entry rate of a drug into a tissue depends on the rate of blood flow to the tissue, tissue mass, and partition characteristics between blood and tissue. Distribution equilibrium (when entry and exit rates are the same) between blood and tissue is reached more rapidly in richly vascularized areas, unless diffusion across cell membranes is the rate-limiting step. After equilibrium, drug concentrations in tissues and in extracellular fluids are reflected by the plasma concentration. Metabolism and excretion occur simultaneously with distribution, making the process dynamic and complex.

After a drug has entered tissues, drug distribution to the interstitial fluid is determined primarily by perfusion. For poorly perfused tissues (eg, muscle, fat), distribution is very slow, especially if the tissue has a high affinity for the drug.

Volume of distribution: The apparent volume of distribution is the theoretical volume of fluid into which the total drug administered would have to be diluted to produce the concentration in plasma. For example, if 1000 mg of a drug is given and the subsequent plasma concentration is 10 mg/L, that 1000 mg seems to be distributed in 100 L (dose/volume = concentration; 1000 mg/x L = 10 mg/L; therefore, x = 1000 mg/10 mg/L = 100 L).

Volume of distribution has nothing to do with the actual volume of the body or its fluid compartments but rather involves the distribution of the drug within the body. For a drug that is highly tissue-bound, very little drug remains in the circulation; thus, plasma concentration is low and volume of distribution is high. Drugs that remain in the circulation tend to have a low volume of distribution.

Volume of distribution provides a reference for the plasma concentration expected for a given dose but provides little information about the specific pattern of distribution. Each drug is uniquely distributed in the body. Some drugs distribute mostly into fat, others remain in extracellular fluid, and others are bound extensively to specific tissues.

Many acidic drugs (eg, warfarin, aspirin) are highly protein-bound and thus have a small apparent volume of distribution. Many basic drugs (eg, amphetamine, meperidine) are extensively taken up by tissues and thus have an apparent volume of distribution larger than the volume of the entire body.

Binding: The extent of drug distribution into tissues depends on the degree of plasma protein and tissue binding. In the bloodstream, drugs are transported partly in solution as free (unbound) drug and partly reversibly bound to blood components (eg, plasma proteins, blood cells). Of the many plasma proteins that can interact with drugs, the most important are albumin, alpha-1 acid glycoprotein, and lipoproteins. Acidic drugs are usually bound more extensively to albumin; basic drugs are usually bound more extensively to alpha-1 acid glycoprotein, lipoproteins, or both.

Only unbound drug is available for passive diffusion to extravascular or tissue sites where the pharmacologic effects of the drug occur. Therefore, the unbound drug concentration in systemic circulation typically determines drug concentration at the active site and thus efficacy.

At high drug concentrations, the amount of bound drug approaches an upper limit determined by the number of available binding sites. Saturation of binding sites is the basis of displacement interactions among drugs (see Drug–Receptor Interactions on p. 2912).

Drugs bind to many substances other than proteins. Binding usually occurs when a drug associates with a macromolecule in an aqueous environment but may occur when a drug is partitioned into body fat. Because fat is poorly perfused, equilibration time is long, especially if the drug is highly lipophilic.

Accumulation of drugs in tissues or body compartments can prolong drug action because the tissues release the accumulated drug as plasma drug concentration decreases. For example, thiopental is highly lipid soluble, rapidly enters the brain after a single IV injection, and has a marked and rapid anesthetic effect; the effect ends within a few minutes as the drug is redistributed to more slowly perfused fatty tissues. Thiopental is then slowly released from fat storage, maintaining subanesthetic plasma levels. These levels may become significant if doses of thiopental are repeated, causing large amounts to be stored in fat. Thus, storage in fat initially shortens the drug's effect but then prolongs it.

Some drugs accumulate within cells because they bind with proteins, phospholipids, or nucleic acids. For example, chloroquine concentrations in WBCs and liver cells can be thousands of times higher than those in plasma. Drug in cells is in equilibrium with drug in plasma and moves into plasma as the drug is eliminated from the body.

Blood-brain barrier: Drugs reach the CNS via brain capillaries and CSF. Although the brain receives about one sixth of cardiac output, drug penetration is restricted because of the brain's permeability characteristics. Although some lipid-soluble drugs (eg, thiopental) enter the brain readily, polar compounds do not. The reason is the blood-brain barrier, which consists of the endothelium of brain capillaries and the astrocytic sheath. The endothelial cells of brain capillaries, which appear to be more tightly joined to one another than those of most capillaries, slow the diffusion of water-soluble drugs. The astrocytic sheath consists of a layer of glial connective tissue cells (astrocytes) close to the basement membrane of the capillary endothelium. With aging, the blood-brain barrier may become less effective, allowing increased passage of compounds into the brain.

Drugs may enter ventricular CSF directly via the choroid plexus, then passively diffuse into brain tissue from CSF. Also in the choroid plexus, organic acids (eg, penicillin) are actively transported from CSF to blood.

The drug penetration rate into CSF, similar to other tissue cells, is determined mainly by the extent of protein binding, degree of ionization, and lipid-water partition coefficient of the drug. The penetration rate into the brain is slow for highly protein-bound drugs and nearly nonexistent for the ionized form of weak acids and bases. Because the CNS is so well perfused, the drug distribution rate is determined primarily by permeability.

DRUG METABOLISM

The liver is the principal site of drug metabolism. Although metabolism typically inactivates drugs, some drug metabolites are pharmacologically active—sometimes even more so than the parent compound. An inactive or weakly active substance that has an active metabolite is called a prodrug, especially if designed to deliver the active moiety more effectively.

Drugs can be metabolized by oxidation, reduction, hydrolysis, hydration, conjugation, condensation, or isomerization; whatever the process, the goal is to make the drug easier to excrete. The enzymes involved in metabolism are present in many tissues but generally are more concentrated in the liver. Drug metabolism rates vary among patients. Some patients metabolize a drug so rapidly that therapeutically effective blood and tissue concentrations are not reached; in others, metabolism may be so slow that usual doses have toxic effects. Individual drug metabolism rates are influenced by genetic factors, coexisting disorders (particularly chronic liver disorders and advanced heart failure), and drug interactions (especially those involving induction or inhibition of metabolism).

For many drugs, metabolism occurs in 2 phases. Phase I reactions involve formation of a new or modified functional group or cleavage (oxidation, reduction, hydrolysis); these reactions are nonsynthetic. Phase II reactions involve conjugation with an endogenous substance (eg, glucuronic acid, sulfate, glycine); these reactions are synthetic. Metabolites formed in synthetic reactions are more polar and thus more readily excreted by the kidneys (in urine) and the liver (in bile) than those formed in nonsynthetic reactions. Some drugs undergo only phase I or phase II reactions; thus, phase numbers reflect functional rather than sequential classification.

Rate: For almost all drugs, the metabolism rate in any given pathway has an upper limit (capacity limitation). However, at therapeutic concentrations of most drugs, usually only a small fraction of the metabolizing enzyme's sites are occupied, and the metabolism rate increases with drug concentration. In such cases, called first-order elimination (or kinetics), the metabolism rate of the drug is a constant fraction of the drug remaining in the body (ie, the drug has a specific half-life).

For example, if 500 mg is present in the body at time zero, after metabolism, 250 mg may be present at 1 h and 125 mg at 2 h (illustrating a half-life of 1 h). However, when most of the enzyme sites are occupied, metabolism occurs at its maximal rate and does not change in proportion to drug concentration; instead, a fixed amount of drug is metabolized per unit time (zero-order kinetics). In this case, if 500 mg is present in the body at time zero, after metabolism, 450 mg may be present at 1 h and 400 mg at 2 h (illustrating a maximal clearance of 50 mg/h and no specific half-life). As drug concentration increases, metabolism shifts from first-order to zero-order kinetics.

Cytochrome P-450: The most important enzyme system of phase I metabolism is cytochrome P-450 (CYP450), a microsomal superfamily of isoenzymes that catalyzes the oxidation of many drugs. The electrons are supplied by NADPH–CYP450 reductase, a flavoprotein that transfers electrons from NADPH (the reduced form of nicotinamide adenine dinucleotide phosphate) to CYP450.

CYP450 enzymes can be induced or inhibited by many drugs and substances resulting in drug interactions in which one drug enhances the toxicity or reduces the therapeutic effect of another drug. For examples of drugs that interact with specific enzymes, see Tables 346–2 on p. 2909 and 348–2.

With aging, the liver's capacity for metabolism through the CYP450 enzyme system is reduced by ≥ 30% because hepatic volume and blood flow are decreased. Thus, drugs that are metabolized through this system reach higher levels and have prolonged half-lives in the elderly (see Fig. 348–1). Because neonates have partially developed hepatic microsomal enzyme systems, they also have difficulty metabolizing many drugs.

Conjugation: Glucuronidation, the most common phase II reaction, is the only one that occurs in the liver microsomal enzyme system. Glucuronides are secreted in bile and eliminated in urine. Thus, conjugation makes most drugs more soluble and easily excreted by the kidneys. Amino acid conjugation with glutamine or glycine produces conjugates that are readily excreted in urine but not extensively secreted in bile. Aging does not affect glucuronidation. However, in neonates, conversion to glucuronide is slow, potentially resulting in serious effects (eg, as with chloramphenicol).

Conjugation may also occur through acetylation or sulfoconjugation. Sulfate esters are polar and readily excreted in urine. Aging does not affect these processes.

DRUG EXCRETION

The kidneys are the principal organs for excreting water-soluble substances. The biliary system contributes to excretion to the degree that drug is not reabsorbed from the GI tract. Generally, the contribution of intestine, saliva, sweat, breast milk, and lungs to excretion is small, except for exhalation of volatile anesthetics. Excretion via breast milk may affect the breastfeeding infant (see Table 288–4 on p. 2417).

Hepatic metabolism often increases drug polarity and water solubility. The resulting metabolites are then more readily excreted.

Renal excretion: Renal filtration accounts for most drug excretion. About one fifth of the plasma reaching the glomerulus is filtered through pores in the glomerular endothelium; nearly all water and most electrolytes are passively and actively reabsorbed from the renal tubules back into the circulation. However, polar compounds, which account for most drug metabolites, cannot diffuse back into the circulation and are excreted unless a specific transport mechanism exists for their reabsorption (eg, as for glucose, ascorbic acid, and B vitamins). With aging, renal drug excretion decreases (see Table 335–1 on p. 2848); at age 80, clearance is typically reduced to half of what it was at age 30.

Table 348–2. COMMON SUBSTANCES THAT INTERACT WITH CYTOCHROME P-450 ENZYMES

ENZYME	SUBSTRATES	INHIBITORS	INDUCERS
CYP1A2	Acetaminophen Caffeine Clarithromycin Estradiol Haloperidol Lidocaine Methadone Olanzapine Propranolol Ritonavir Tacrine Theophylline Tricyclic antidepressants Verapamil *(R)*-Warfarin	Amiodarone Cimetidine Ciprofloxacin Erythromycin Fluvoxamine Ticlopidine	Charcoal-broiled beef Cigarette smoke Omeprazole Phenobarbital Phenytoin Rifampin
CYP2C9	Celecoxib Diclofenac Fluoxetine Glipizide Glyburide Indomethacin Nifedipine Phenytoin Piroxicam Progesterone Testosterone Tricyclic antidepressants Valproate Voriconazole *(S)*-Warfarin	Amiodarone Cimetidine Fluconazole Lovastatin Ritonavir Sertraline Sulfamethoxazole Topiramate Trimethoprim Voriconazole Zafirlukast	Dexamethasone Phenobarbital Other barbiturates Phenytoin Rifampin

Table continues on the following page.

Table 348–2. COMMON SUBSTANCES THAT INTERACT WITH CYTOCHROME P-450 ENZYMES (*Continued*)

ENZYME	SUBSTRATES	INHIBITORS	INDUCERS
CYP2C19	Diazepam *(S)*-Mephenytoin Omeprazole Pentamidine Propranolol Voriconazole *(R)*-Warfarin	Cimetidine Fluoxetine Fluvoxamine Ketoconazole Lansoprazole Omeprazole Paroxetine Ticlopidine	Carbamazepine Phenobarbital Prednisone Rifampin
CYP2D6	Beta blockers Codeine Dextromethorphan Flecainide Haloperidol Lidocaine Mexiletine Morphine Omeprazole Phenothiazines Quinidine Risperidone SSRIs Tamoxifen Testosterone Tramadol Trazodone Tricyclic antidepressants Venlafaxine	Amiodarone Bupropion Celecoxib Cimetidine Fluoxetine Fluvoxamine Metoclopramide Methadone Paroxetine Quinidine Ritonavir Sertraline	Carbamazepine Dexamethasone Phenobarbital Phenytoin Rifampin
CYP2E1	Acetaminophen Alcohol	Disulfiram	Alcohol Isoniazid Tobacco use
CYP3A4	Amiodarone Aprepitant Azole antifungals Benzodiazepines Ca channel blockers Caffeine Carbamazepine Clarithromycin Cyclosporine Delavirdine Enalapril Estradiol Estrogen Erythromycin Fentanyl Finasteride Indinavir Lidocaine Lopinavir Loratidine Methadone Nelfinavir Omeprazole Opioid analgesics Prednisone Progesterone Ritonavir Saquinavir Sildenafil Sirolimus Statins Tacrolimus Tamoxifen Tricyclic antidepressants *(R)*-Warfarin	Amiodarone Amprenavir Atazanavir Azole antifungals Cimetidine Ciprofloxacin Clarithromycin Delavirdine Diltiazem Erythromycin Fluoxetine Fluvoxamine Grapefruit juice Indinavir Metronidazole Nefazodone Nelfinavir Nifedipine Omeprazole Paroxetine Posaconazole Propoxyphene Ritonavir Saquinavir Sertraline Verapamil Voriconazole	Carbamazepine Dexamethasone Isoniazid Phenobarbital Phenytoin Prednisone Rifampin

The principles of transmembrane passage govern renal handling of drugs. Drugs bound to plasma proteins remain in the circulation; only unbound drug is contained in the glomerular filtrate. Un-ionized forms of drugs and their metabolites tend to be reabsorbed readily from tubular fluids.

Urine pH, which varies from 4.5 to 8.0, may markedly affect drug reabsorption and excretion because urine pH determines the ionization state of a weak acid or base (see p. 2914). Acidification of urine increases reabsorption and decreases excretion of weak acids, and, in contrast, decreases reabsorption of weak bases. Alkalinization of urine has the opposite effect. In some cases of overdose, these principles are used to enhance the excretion of weak bases or acids; eg, urine is alkalinized to enhance excretion of acetylsalicylic acid. The extent to which changes in urinary pH alter the rate of drug elimination depends on the contribution of the renal route to total elimination, the polarity of the un-ionized form, and the molecule's degree of ionization.

Active tubular secretion in the proximal tubule is important in the elimination of many drugs. This energy-dependent process may be blocked by metabolic inhibitors. When drug concentration is high, secretory transport can reach an upper limit (transport maximum); each substance has a characteristic transport maximum.

Anions and cations are handled by separate transport mechanisms. Normally, the anion secretory system eliminates metabolites conjugated with glycine, sulfate, or glucuronic acid. Anions compete with each other for secretion. This competition can be used therapeutically; eg, probenecid blocks the normally rapid tubular secretion of penicillin, resulting in higher plasma penicillin concentrations for a longer time. In the cation transport system, cations or organic bases (eg, pramipexole, dofetilide) are secreted by the renal tubules; this process can be inhibited by cimetidine, trimethoprim, prochlorperazine, megestrol, or ketoconazole.

Biliary excretion: Some drugs and their metabolites are extensively excreted in bile. Because they are transported across the biliary epithelium against a concentration gradient, active secretory transport is required. When plasma drug concentrations are high, secretory transport may approach an upper limit (transport maximum). Substances with similar physicochemical properties may compete for excretion.

Drugs with a molecular weight of > 300 g/mol and with both polar and lipophilic groups are more likely to be excreted in bile; smaller molecules are generally excreted only in negligible amounts. Conjugation, particularly with glucuronic acid, facilitates biliary excretion.

In the enterohepatic cycle, a drug secreted in bile is reabsorbed into the circulation from the intestine. Biliary excretion eliminates substances from the body only to the extent that enterohepatic cycling is incomplete—when some of the secreted drug is not reabsorbed from the intestine.

SECTION 23

Injuries; Poisoning

349 Approach to the Trauma Patient

Injury is the number one cause of death for people aged 1 to 44. In the US, there were 199,756 trauma deaths in 2014, about two-thirds being accidental. Of intentional injury deaths, more than 70% were due to self-harm. In addition to deaths, injury results in about 41 million emergency department visits and 2.3 million hospital admissions annually.

Patients whose injuries are serious but not immediately fatal benefit the most from treatment in designated trauma centers, hospitals that have special staffing and protocols to provide immediate care to critically injured patients. Criteria for such designation (and for the necessity of transport to them) vary by state but usually follow the guidelines of the American College of Surgeons' Committee on Trauma.

Many traumatic injuries are discussed elsewhere in THE MANUAL:

- Bone and joint injuries (see Ch. 359)
- Spinal cord injuries (see Ch. 368)
- Head injuries (see Ch. 371)
- Facial injuries (see Ch. 358)
- Eye injuries (see Ch. 357)
- Genitourinary injuries (see Ch. 360)
- Lacerations (see Ch. 363)

Etiology

Of the myriad ways people are injured, most can be categorized as blunt or penetrating. Blunt injury involves a forceful impact (eg, blow, kick, strike with an object, fall, motor vehicle crash, blast). Penetrating injury involves breach of the skin by an object (eg, knife, broken glass) or projectile (eg, bullet, shrapnel from an explosion).

Other injury types include thermal and chemical burns, toxic inhalations or ingestions, and radiation injury.

Pathophysiology

All injuries, by definition, cause *direct* tissue damage, the nature and extent depending on the anatomic site, mechanism, and intensity of trauma. Severe direct tissue damage to critical organs (eg, to the heart, brain, spinal cord) is responsible for most immediate trauma deaths.

Additionally, patients surviving the initial insult may develop *indirect* injury effects. Disruption of blood vessels causes hemorrhage, which may be external (and hence visible) or internal, either confined within an organ as a contusion or hematoma, or as free hemorrhage into a body compartment (eg, peritoneal cavity, thorax). Small amounts of hemorrhage (ie, < 10% of blood volume) are tolerated well by most patients. Larger amounts cause progressive declines in BP and organ perfusion (shock—see p. 572), leading to cellular dysfunction, organ failure, and eventually death. Hemorrhagic shock causes most short-term (ie, within hours) deaths, and multiple organ failure due to prolonged shock causes many of the near-term (ie, first 14 days) deaths. Additional near-term deaths result from infection because of disruption of normal anatomic barriers and immune system dysfunction.

Evaluation and Treatment

- Primary survey: A, B, C, D, E evaluation and stabilization of *A*irway, *B*reathing, *C*irculation, *D*isability (neurologic status), and *E*xposure/*e*nvironmental control
- Secondary survey: Head-to-toe examination after initial stabilization
- Selective use of CT and other imaging studies

Care in the emergency department rather than emergency care delivered at the accident site is discussed here. Evaluation and treatment are done simultaneously, beginning with systems that pose the most immediate threat to life if damaged. *Attending to dramatic but not deadly injuries (eg, open lower-extremity fracture, finger amputations) before evaluating immediate life threats can be a fatal mistake.* A helpful mnemonic is A, B, C, D, E. Systems are rapidly examined for serious abnormalities (primary survey); a more detailed examination (secondary survey) is done after the patient is stable.

PEARLS & PITFALLS

- Attending to dramatic but not deadly injuries (eg, open lower-extremity fracture, finger amputations) before evaluating immediate life threats can be a fatal mistake.

Airway: Airway patency is threatened by blood clots, teeth, or foreign bodies in the oropharynx; soft-tissue laxity and posterior retraction of the tongue caused by obtundation (eg, due to head injury, shock, intoxication); and edema or hematoma due to direct neck trauma. These obstructions are readily visible on direct inspection of the mouth or neck; having the patient speak can rapidly confirm that the airway is not likely in immediate danger.

Blood and foreign material are removed by suction or manually. Obtunded patients whose airway patency, airway protective mechanisms, oxygenation, or ventilation is in doubt and patients with significant oropharyngeal injury require endotracheal intubation (see p. 554); usually drugs are given for paralysis and sedation before intubation is done. Multiple tools are available to assist with airway management including extraglottic devices, gum elastic bougie, and video laryngoscopy. A CO_2 colorimetric device or, preferably, capnography can help confirm proper endotracheal tube placement.

If patients require an artificial airway and endotracheal intubation is not possible (eg, due to edema of the airway caused by a thermal burn) or contraindicated (eg, due to severe maxillofacial injury), surgical or percutaneous cricothyrotomy is indicated. NOTE: When evaluating or manipulating a patient's airway, cervical spine immobilization should be maintained (eg, by rigid collar, inline immobilization techniques) until cervical spine injury has been excluded by examination, imaging, or both.

Breathing: Adequate ventilation is threatened by decreased central respiratory drive (usually due to head injury, intoxication, or nearly fatal shock) or by chest injury (eg, hemothorax or pneumothorax, multiple rib fractures, pulmonary contusion—see p. 3109).

The chest wall is fully exposed to look for ample chest wall expansion, external signs of trauma, and paradoxical wall motion (ie, retraction of the chest wall on inspiration), which indicates a flail chest. The chest wall is palpated for rib fractures and the presence of subcutaneous air (sometimes the only finding in pneumothorax).

Adequacy of air exchange is usually apparent on auscultation. Tension pneumothorax, simple pneumothorax, or hemothorax (see p. 476) may cause decreased breath sounds on the affected side. Tension pneumothorax may also cause distended neck veins; hypotension and deviation of the trachea to the side opposite the injury are later findings.

Pneumothorax is decompressed by chest tube (see p. 390). In patients with findings consistent with a pneumothorax, a chest x-ray or bedside ultrasonography should be done before initiating positive-pressure ventilation. Positive-pressure ventilation may enlarge a simple pneumothorax or convert it to a tension pneumothorax. Suspected tension pneumothorax can be decompressed with needle thoracostomy (eg, a 14-gauge needle inserted in the midclavicular line, 2nd intercostal space or the midaxillary line, 5th intercostal space) to stabilize the patient if a chest tube cannot be inserted immediately. Inadequate ventilation is treated with endotracheal intubation and mechanical ventilation. A flail chest is stabilized by applying gentle pressure over the flail segment. An open pneumothorax is covered with an occlusive dressing attached on 3 sides; the 4th side is left untaped to release pressure that might build up and cause a tension pneumothorax.

Circulation: Significant external hemorrhage can occur from any major vessel but is always apparent. Life-threatening internal hemorrhage is often less obvious. However, this volume of hemorrhage can occur in only a few body compartments: the chest, abdomen, and soft tissues of the pelvis or thigh (eg, from a pelvic or femoral fracture).

Pulse and BP are assessed, and signs of shock are noted (eg, tachypnea, dusky color, diaphoresis, altered mental status, poor capillary refill). Abdominal distention and tenderness, pelvis instability, and thigh deformity and instability are often present when internal hemorrhage in those areas is large enough to be life-threatening.

External hemorrhage is controlled by direct pressure. Two large-bore (eg, 14- or 16-gauge) IVs are started with 0.9% saline or lactated Ringer's solution; rapid infusion of 1 to 2 L (20 mL/kg for children) is given for signs of shock and hypovolemia (see p. 575). Subsequently, additional fluids and, if necessary, blood component therapy is given as indicated. Protocols have been developed for patients requiring large volumes of blood products (massive transfusion protocols). When there is strong clinical suspicion of serious intra-abdominal hemorrhage, patients may require immediate laparotomy. Patients with massive intrathoracic hemorrhage may require immediate thoracotomy and possibly autotransfusion of blood recovered via tube thoracostomy.

PEARLS & PITFALLS

- Signs of hypovolemic shock in patients with apparently isolated head injury should prompt reevaluation for internal bleeding, because isolated head injury does not cause shock.

Disability (neurologic dysfunction): Neurologic function is evaluated for serious deficits involving the brain and spinal cord. The Glasgow Coma Scale (GCS—see Tables 224–4 on p. 1862 and 349–1) and pupillary response to light are used to screen for serious intracranial injury.

Gross motor movement and sensation in each extremity are used to screen for serious spinal cord injury. The cervical spine is palpated for tenderness and deformity and stabilized in a rigid collar until cervical spine injury is excluded. With careful manual stabilization of the head and neck, the patient is logrolled onto a side to allow palpation of the thoracic and lumbar spine, inspection of the back, and rectal examination if indicated to check tone (decreased tone indicates possible spinal cord injury), the prostate (a high-riding prostate suggests urethral or pelvic injury), and presence of blood.

In the US, most patients arriving by ambulance are immobilized on a long, rigid board for ease of transport and to stabilize possible spinal fractures. Patients should be taken off the board as soon as possible because it is quite uncomfortable and pressure ulcers may occur within a few hours.

Patients with severe traumatic brain injury (GCS < 9) require endotracheal intubation for airway protection, brain imaging, neurosurgical evaluation, and therapy to prevent secondary brain injury (eg, optimization of BP and oxygenation, seizure prophylaxis, osmotic diuresis for elevated intracranial pressure, sometimes hyperventilation for patients with signs of impending brain herniation—see Fig. 224–1 on p. 1858).

Exposure/environmental control: To ensure injuries are not missed, patients are completely undressed (by cutting off garments) and the entire body surface is examined for signs of occult trauma. The patient is kept warm (eg, with heated blankets and by using only warmed IV fluids) to prevent hypothermia.

Secondary survey: After immediate life threats are assessed and the patient is stable, a more thorough evaluation is done, and a focused history is obtained. If only limited conversation is possible, an "AMPLE" history covers essential information:

- *A*llergies
- *M*edications
- *P*ast medical history
- *L*ast meal
- *E*vents of the injury

After the patient is completely undressed, the examination generally proceeds from head to toe; it typically includes all orifices and a more detailed look at areas examined in the initial survey. All soft tissues are inspected for lesions and swelling, all bones are palpated for tenderness, and range of motion is assessed in joints (unless there is obvious fracture or deformity).

A urinary catheter is usually placed in seriously injured and obtunded patients provided there is no evidence of urethral injury (eg, blood at the meatus, ecchymosis of the perineum, high-riding prostate). Intubated, seriously injured patients often also have an orogastric tube placed.

Open wounds are covered with sterile dressings, but cleansing and repair are deferred until completion of evaluation and treatment of more serious injuries. Serious clinically apparent dislocations with marked deformity or neurovascular compromise are imaged and reduced as soon as immediate life threats have been addressed.

Obvious or suspected fractures are splinted pending full assessment of serious injuries and appropriate imaging studies. A clinically apparent unstable pelvic fracture is stabilized with a sheet or commercial stabilizing device to help close the pelvic space and decrease bleeding; severe bleeding may require urgent angiographic embolization, surgical fixation, or direct surgical control.

In **pregnant trauma patients,** initial priority is stabilization of the woman, which is the best way to ensure fetal stability. Near term, immobilization in the supine position may cause the uterofetoplacental unit to compress the inferior vena cava, obstructing blood return and causing hypotension. If so, the uterus can be manually pushed to the patient's left or the entire backboard can be tilted to the left to relieve the compression. Fetal monitoring is done if the fetus is > 20 wk gestation and continued for at least 4 to 6 h. An obstetrician should be consulted early for patients with serious trauma or signs of pregnancy complications (eg, abnormal fetal heart rate, vaginal bleeding, contractions). Rh_0 (D) immune globulin is given to all Rh-negative women following even minor trauma. If the woman has cardiac

Table 349–1. MODIFIED GLASGOW COMA SCALE FOR INFANTS AND CHILDREN

AREA ASSESSED	INFANTS	CHILDREN	SCORE*
Eye opening	Open spontaneously	Open spontaneously	4
	Open in response to verbal stimuli	Open in response to verbal stimuli	3
	Open in response to pain only	Open in response to pain only	2
	No response	No response	1
Verbal response	Coos and babbles	Oriented, appropriate	5
	Irritable cries	Confused	4
	Cries in response to pain	Inappropriate words	3
	Moans in response to pain	Incomprehensible words or nonspecific sounds	2
	No response	No response	1
Motor response†	Moves spontaneously and purposefully	Obeys commands	6
	Withdraws to touch	Localizes painful stimulus	5
	Withdraws in response to pain	Withdraws in response to pain	4
	Responds to pain with decorticate posturing (abnormal flexion)	Responds to pain with decorticate posturing (abnormal flexion)	3
	Responds to pain with decerebrate posturing (abnormal extension)	Responds to pain with decerebrate posturing (abnormal extension)	2
	No response	No response	1

*Score ≤ 12 suggests a severe head injury. Score < 8 suggests need for intubation and ventilation. Score ≤ 6 suggests need for intracranial pressure monitoring.

†If the patient is intubated, unconscious, or preverbal, the most important part of this scale is motor response. This section should be carefully evaluated.

Adapted from Davis RJ, et al: Head and spinal cord injury. In *Textbook of Pediatric Intensive Care*, edited by MC Rogers. Baltimore, Williams & Wilkins, 1987; James H, Anas N, Perkin RM: *Brain Insults in Infants and Children*. New York, Grune & Stratton, 1985; and Morray JP, et al: Coma scale for use in brain-injured children. *Critical Care Medicine* 12:1018, 1984.

arrest and cannot be resuscitated, a perimortem cesarean delivery can be done if the fetus is > 24 wk gestation (corresponding to a uterine fundal height of about 4 cm above the umbilicus).

Testing: Imaging tests are the cornerstone; laboratory tests are generally ancillary, except for possibly serial point-of-care hemoglobin testing for ongoing blood loss. Patients with penetrating trauma typically have focal injuries that can limit imaging to the obviously involved region or regions. Blunt trauma, particularly when significant deceleration is involved (eg, serious fall, motor vehicle crash), can affect any part of the body, and imaging is used more liberally. Previously, x-rays or CT of the neck, chest, and pelvis were routinely done on most patients with blunt trauma. However, most trauma centers are now doing only imaging studies that are indicated by the mechanism of injury and findings on examination.

Cervical spine imaging can be deferred in patients who are not intoxicated, do not have focal neurologic findings, have no midline cervical spine tenderness or distracting injuries (eg, femur fracture), and are awake and alert. All others should have cervical spine imaging, preferably using CT.

Chest x-ray can identify airway disruption, lung injury, hemothorax, and pneumothorax; it can also suggest thoracic aorta tears (eg, by mediastinal widening). However, chest CT is more sensitive for most intrathoracic injuries and is often preferred. Chest imaging is now commonly done at the bedside using ultrasonography E-FAST (extended focused assessment with sonography in trauma), particularly if patients are unstable. Pneumothoraces, hemothoraces, and hemopericardium can be identified.

CT of the chest, abdomen, pelvis, spine, or head or, particularly, combinations of these studies are frequently used for patients who require imaging after severe multiple blunt trauma.

Identification of intra-abdominal injury is essential. Historically, diagnostic peritoneal lavage (DPL) was used to assess for intraperitoneal blood. In DPL, a peritoneal dialysis catheter is inserted through the abdominal wall into the peritoneal cavity. If > 10 mL of blood is aspirated, immediate laparotomy is indicated. If blood is not aspirated, 1 L of 0.9% saline is infused through the catheter and drained out; analysis of the returned fluid is used to guide management. However, in all but low-resource areas, DPL has largely been replaced by bedside ultrasonography (E-FAST examination), particularly for unstable patients; it is sensitive for significant volumes of intraperitoneal blood and thus the need for immediate laparotomy. If patients are stable, CT is the preferred study; it is very accurate, allows imaging of the retroperitoneal structures and bones, and shows the volume and sometimes the origin of hemorrhage.

If pelvic fracture is suspected, CT of the pelvis is done; it is more accurate than plain x-rays.

Head CT is typically done in patients with altered mental status or focal neurologic abnormalities and in patients who sustained loss of consciousness. Some evidence suggests that CT is not necessary in patients with brief loss of consciousness (ie, < 5 sec) or transient amnesia or disorientation but who are alert with a GCS of 15 during examination. Imaging is done more liberally in patients with persistent headache, vomiting, amnesia, seizures, age > 60 yr, and drug or alcohol intoxication and in patients taking anticoagulant or antiplatelet drugs. Clinical decision rules have been developed to help determine which patients should have a head CT.[1] These decision rules should be used to aid, but not replace, clinical judgment.

For children with head injury, the Pediatric Emergency Care Applied Research Network (PECARN) has developed an algorithm that may help limit radiation exposure from head CT (see Figs. 349–1 and 349–2); clinical observation is used in children who may otherwise have received CT.

Aortic injury should be considered in patients with severe deceleration chest injury or suggestive signs (eg, pulse deficits or asymmetric BP measurements, end-organ ischemia, suggestive findings on chest x-ray); these patients may require CT angiography or other aortic imaging (see p. 3111).

All patients suspected of having significant blunt chest injury should be placed on a cardiac monitor and have an ECG to detect myocardial injury and arrhythmias. Patients with abnormalities on ECG usually have blood levels of cardiac markers measured and sometimes echocardiography to evaluate the patient for possible cardiac contusion.

Vascular injury to the carotid and vertebral vessels should be considered in patients with trauma to the head and neck, particularly those with unilateral neurologic findings, a neck

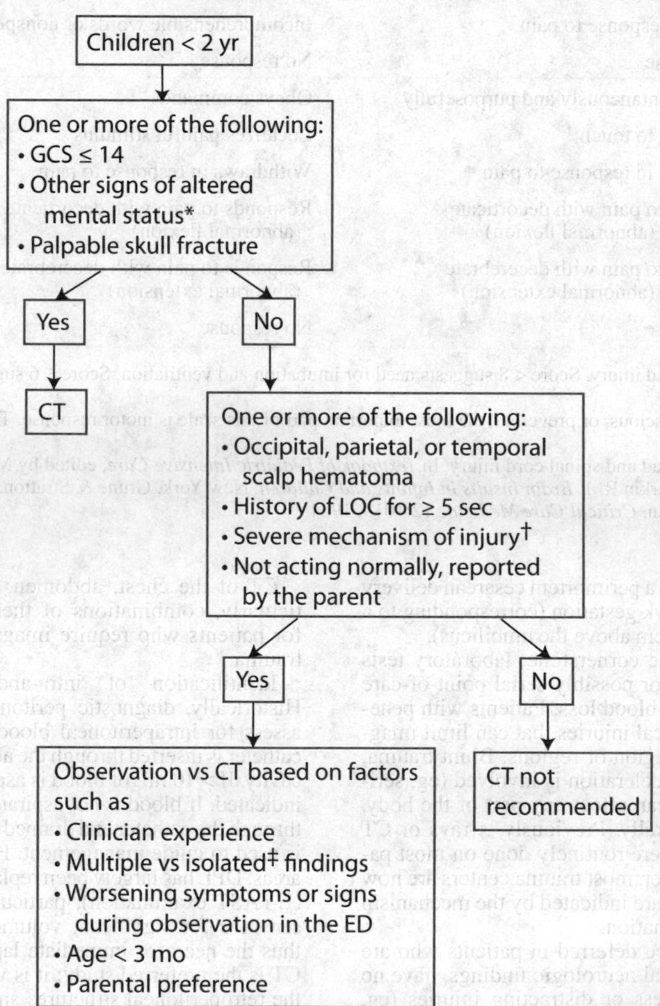

Fig. 349–1. Evaluation of children < 2 yr with a head injury.

*Include agitation, somnolence, repetitive questioning, and slow response to verbal communication.

†Include motor vehicle crash involving ejection of patient, death of another passenger, or rollover; collision of a motor vehicle with a pedestrian or bicyclist not wearing a helmet; and a fall of > 0.9 m for children < 2 yr; and a blow to the head by a high-impact object.

‡No other findings suggesting traumatic brain injury, such as only LOC, headache, vomiting, and certain scalp hematomas in children > 3 mo.

ED = emergency department; GCS = Glasgow Coma Scale; LOC = loss of consciousness.

Adapted from Kupperman N, Holmes JF, Dayton PS, et al for the Pediatric Emergency Care Applied Research Network: Identification of children at very low risk of clinically-important brain injuries after head trauma: a prospective cohort study. *Lancet* 374:1160–1170, 2009.

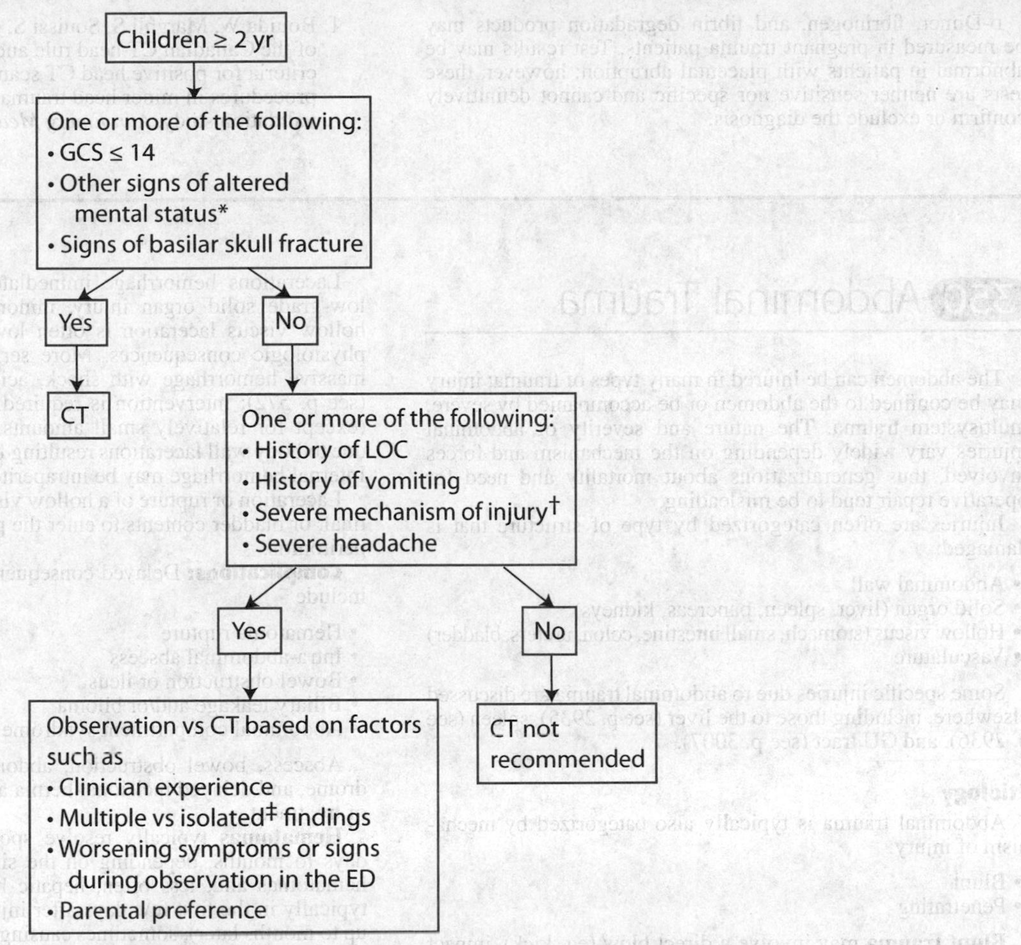

Fig. 349–2. Evaluation of children ≥ 2 yr with a head injury.

*Include agitation, somnolence, repetitive questioning, and slow response to verbal communication.

†Include motor vehicle crash involving ejection of patient, death of another passenger, or rollover; collision of a motor vehicle with a pedestrian or bicyclist not wearing a helmet; and a fall of > 1.5 m for children ≥ 2 yr; and a blow to the head by a high-impact object.

‡No other findings suggesting traumatic brain injury, such as only LOC, headache, vomiting, and certain scalp hematomas in children > 3 mo.

ED = emergency department; GCS = Glasgow Coma Scale; LOC = loss of consciousness.

Adapted from Kupperman N, Holmes JF, Dayton PS, et al for the Pediatric Emergency Care Applied Research Network: Identification of children at very low risk of clinically-important brain injuries after head trauma: a prospective cohort study. *Lancet* 374:1160–1170, 2009.

seat belt sign (linear ecchymosis due to the shoulder strap), or a predisposing injury (eg, fracture of C1, C2, or C3; other C-spine fracture with subluxation; hanging mechanism). Such patients typically should have CT angiography.

Plain x-rays are obtained of any suspected fractures and dislocations. Other imaging tests are obtained for specific indications (eg, angiography to diagnose and sometimes embolize vascular injury; CT to better delineate spinal, pelvic, or complex joint fractures).

Laboratory tests that may be useful include

- Serial Hb levels to assess for bleeding
- ABGs for Po_2, Pco_2, and base deficit
- Urine examination for blood
- CBC to establish a baseline to monitor ongoing hemorrhage
- Glucose to evaluate for hypoglycemia
- Type and crossmatch for possible blood transfusion

Measures of perfusion (serum lactate, base deficit on ABG measurement, and, in patients with a catheterized central vein, central venous O_2 saturation) are indicated to help identify early or partially treated shock. Other reflexively obtained tests (eg, electrolytes and other chemistries, coagulation studies) are unlikely to be helpful unless suggested by relevant medical history (eg, renal insufficiency, diuretic use).

Toxicology screening (eg, blood alcohol, urine drug screen) is often done; results of this testing rarely change immediate management but can help identify substance abuse causative of injury, allowing intervention to prevent subsequent trauma.

D-Dimer, fibrinogen, and fibrin degradation products may be measured in pregnant trauma patients. Test results may be abnormal in patients with placental abruption; however, these tests are neither sensitive nor specific and cannot definitively confirm or exclude the diagnosis.

1. Bouida W, Marghli S, Souissi S, et al: Prediction value of the Canadian CT head rule and the New Orleans criteria for positive head CT scan and acute neurosurgical procedures in minor head trauma: a multicenter external validation study. *Ann Emerg Med* 61(5):521–527, 2013.

350 Abdominal Trauma

The abdomen can be injured in many types of trauma; injury may be confined to the abdomen or be accompanied by severe, multisystem trauma. The nature and severity of abdominal injuries vary widely depending on the mechanism and forces involved, thus generalizations about mortality and need for operative repair tend to be misleading.

Injuries are often categorized by type of structure that is damaged:

- Abdominal wall
- Solid organ (liver, spleen, pancreas, kidneys)
- Hollow viscus (stomach, small intestine, colon, ureters, bladder)
- Vasculature

Some specific injuries due to abdominal trauma are discussed elsewhere, including those to the liver (see p. 2935), spleen (see p. 2936), and GU tract (see p. 3007).

Etiology

Abdominal trauma is typically also categorized by mechanism of injury:

- Blunt
- Penetrating

Blunt trauma may involve a direct blow (eg, kick), impact with an object (eg, fall on bicycle handlebars), or sudden deceleration (eg, fall from a height, vehicle crash). The spleen is the organ damaged most commonly, followed by the liver and a hollow viscus (typically the small intestine).

Penetrating injuries may or may not penetrate peritoneum and if they do, may not cause organ injury. Stab wounds are less likely than gunshot wounds to damage intra-abdominal structures; in both, any structure can be affected. Penetrating wounds to the lower chest may cross the diaphragm and damage abdominal structures.

Classification: Injury scales have been devised that classify organ injury severity from grade 1 (minimal) to grades 5 or 6 (massive); mortality and need for operative repair increase as grade increases. Scales exist for the liver (see Table 350–1), spleen (see Table 350–2), and kidneys (see Fig. 360–2 on p. 3009).

Associated injuries: Blunt or penetrating injury that affects intra-abdominal structures may also damage the spine, ribs, and/or pelvis. Patients who experience significant deceleration often have injuries to other parts of the body, including the thoracic aorta.

Pathophysiology

Blunt or penetrating trauma may lacerate or rupture intra-abdominal structures. Blunt injury may alternatively cause only a hematoma in a solid organ or the wall of a hollow viscus.

Lacerations hemorrhage immediately. Hemorrhage due to low-grade solid organ injury, minor vascular laceration, or hollow viscus laceration is often low-volume, with minimal physiologic consequences. More serious injuries may cause massive hemorrhage with shock, acidosis, and coagulopathy (see p. 572); intervention is required. Hemorrhage is internal (except for relatively small amounts of external hemorrhage due to body wall lacerations resulting from penetrating trauma). Internal hemorrhage may be intraperitoneal or retroperitoneal.

Laceration or rupture of a hollow viscus allows gastric, intestinal, or bladder contents to enter the peritoneal cavity, causing peritonitis.

Complications: Delayed consequences of abdominal injury include

- Hematoma rupture
- Intra-abdominal abscess
- Bowel obstruction or ileus
- Biliary leakage and/or biloma
- Abdominal compartment syndrome

Abscess, bowel obstruction, abdominal compartment syndrome, and delayed incisional hernia also can be complications of treatment.

Hematomas typically resolve spontaneously over several days to months, depending on the size and location. Splenic hematomas and, less often, hepatic hematomas may rupture, typically in the first few days after injury (although sometimes up to months later), sometimes causing significant delayed hemorrhage. Intestinal wall hematomas sometimes perforate, typically within 48 to 72 h after injury, releasing intestinal contents and causing peritonitis, but without causing significant hemorrhage. Intestinal wall hematomas rarely can cause intestinal stricture, typically months to years later, although there are case reports of bowel obstruction as early as 2 wk after blunt trauma.

Intra-abdominal abscess typically is the result of undetected hollow viscus perforation but may be a complication of laparotomy. Rate of abscess formation ranges from 0% after nontherapeutic laparotomies to about 10% after therapeutic laparotomies, although the rate may be as high as 50% after surgery to repair severe liver lacerations.

Bowel obstruction rarely develops in weeks to years after injury due to intestinal wall hematoma or adhesions caused by intestinal serosal or mesenteric tears. More commonly bowel obstruction is a complication of exploratory laparotomy. Even nontherapeutic laparotomies occasionally cause adhesions, which develop in 0 to 2% of such cases.

Biliary leakage and/or biloma is a rare complication of liver injury and, even less commonly, of bile duct injury. Bile can be excreted from the raw surface of a liver injury or from an injured bile duct. It may be disseminated throughout the peritoneal cavity or become walled off into a distinct fluid collection, or biloma. Biliary leakage can result in pain, a systemic inflammatory response, and/or hyperbilirubinemia.

Abdominal compartment syndrome is analogous to extremity compartment syndrome after orthopedic injury. In abdominal compartment syndrome, mesenteric and intestinal capillary leakage (eg, due to shock, prolonged abdominal surgical procedures, systemic ischemia-reperfusion injury, and the systemic inflammatory response syndrome [SIRS]) causes tissue edema within the abdomen. Although there is more room for expansion in the peritoneal cavity than in an extremity, unchecked edema, and occasionally ascites, ultimately elevates intra-abdominal pressure (defined as > 20 mm Hg), causing pain and organ ischemia and dysfunction. Intestinal ischemia further worsens vascular leakage, causing a vicious circle. Other affected organs include the

- Kidneys (causing renal insufficiency)
- Lungs (elevated abdominal pressure can interfere with respiration, causing hypoxemia and hypercarbia)
- Cardiovascular system (elevated abdominal pressure decreases venous return from the lower extremities, causing hypotension)
- CNS (intracranial pressure increases, possibly due to rise in central venous pressure preventing adequate venous drainage from brain, decreasing cerebral perfusion, which can worsen intracranial injuries)

Abdominal compartment syndrome typically occurs in conditions in which there is both vascular leak and high-volume fluid resuscitation (usually > 10 L). Thus, it often develops after laparotomy for severe abdominal injury accompanied by shock but may occur in conditions not primarily affecting the abdomen, such as severe burns, sepsis, and pancreatitis. Once multiorgan dysfunction develops, the only way to prevent mortality is to decompress the abdominal contents, typically with a laparotomy. Large-volume paracentesis may be effective when there is significant ascites.

Symptoms and Signs

Abdominal pain typically is present; however, pain is often mild and thus easily obscured by other, more painful injuries (eg, fractures) and by altered sensorium (eg, due to head injury, substance abuse, shock). Pain from splenic injury sometimes radiates to the left shoulder. Pain from a small intestinal perforation typically is minimal initially but steadily worsens over the first few hours. Patients with renal injury may notice hematuria.

On examination, vital signs may show evidence of hypovolemia (tachycardia) or shock (eg, dusky color, diaphoresis, altered sensorium, hypotension).

Inspection: Penetrating injuries by definition cause a break in the skin, but clinicians must be sure to inspect the back, buttocks, flank, and lower chest in addition to the abdomen, particularly when firearms or explosive devices are involved. Cutaneous lesions are often small, with minimal bleeding, although occasionally wounds are large, sometimes accompanied by evisceration.

PEARLS & PITFALLS

- Not all penetrating abdominal injuries originate from wounds on the abdominal wall; be suspicious of entrance wounds on the back, buttocks, flank, perineum, and lower chest.

Blunt trauma may cause ecchymosis (eg, the transverse, linear ecchymosis termed seat belt sign), but this finding has poor sensitivity and specificity. Abdominal distention after trauma typically indicates severe hemorrhage (2 to 3 L), but distention may not be apparent even in patients who have lost several units of blood.

Palpation: Abdominal tenderness is often present. This sign is very unreliable because abdominal wall contusions can be tender and many patients with intra-abdominal injury have equivocal examinations if they are distracted by other injuries or have altered sensorium or if their injuries are mainly retroperitoneal. Although not very sensitive, when detected, peritoneal signs (eg, guarding, rebound) strongly suggest the presence of intraperitoneal blood and/or intestinal contents.

Rectal examination may show gross blood due to a penetrating colonic lesion, and there may be blood at the urethral meatus or perineal hematoma due to GU tract injury. Although these findings are quite specific, they are not very sensitive.

Diagnosis

- Clinical evaluation
- Often CT or ultrasonography

As in all patients experiencing significant trauma, clinicians do a thorough, organized trauma evaluation simultaneous with resuscitation (see p. 2927). Because many intra-abdominal injuries heal without specific treatment, the clinician's primary goal is to identify injuries requiring intervention.

Following clinical evaluation, a few patients clearly require exploratory laparotomy rather than testing, including those with

- Peritonitis
- Hemodynamic instability due to penetrating abdominal trauma
- Gunshot wounds (most)
- Evisceration

Conversely, a few patients are at very low risk and may be discharged or observed briefly without any testing other than visual inspection of the urine for gross blood. These patients typically have isolated blunt abdominal trauma and a minor mechanism of injury, normal sensorium, and no tenderness or peritoneal signs; they should be instructed to return immediately if pain worsens. Patients with isolated anterior abdominal stab wounds that have not penetrated the fascia can also be observed briefly and discharged.[1]

However, most patients do not have such clear-cut positive or negative manifestations and thus require testing to evaluate for intra-abdominal injury. Testing options include

- Imaging studies (ultrasonography, CT)
- Procedures (wound exploration, diagnostic peritoneal lavage)

In addition, patients usually should have a chest x-ray to look for free air under the diaphragm (indicating perforation of a hollow viscus) and an elevated hemidiaphragm (suggesting diaphragmatic rupture). Pelvis x-ray is done in patients with pelvic tenderness or significant deceleration and an unreliable clinical examination.

Laboratory testing is secondary. Urinalysis to detect hematuria (gross or microscopic) is helpful, and for patients with apparently serious injuries, CBC is valuable to establish baseline Hct. Pancreatic and liver enzyme levels are not sufficiently sensitive or specific for significant organ injury to be recommended. The blood bank should do a type and screen in case blood transfusions are necessary; type and cross-match is done if transfusion is very likely. Serum lactate level or base deficit calculation (from arterial blood gas testing) may help identify occult shock.

The method chosen to detect intra-abdominal injury varies by mechanism of injury and the clinical examination.

Penetrating abdominal trauma: Blindly probing wounds with a blunt instrument (eg, cotton swab, fingertip) should not be done. If the peritoneum *has* been violated, probing may introduce infection or cause further damage.

Stab wounds (including impalements) to the anterior abdomen (between the 2 anterior axillary lines) in hemodynamically stable patients without peritoneal signs can be explored locally. Typically, local anesthesia is given and the wound is opened enough to allow complete visualization of the entire tract. If the anterior fascia is penetrated, patients are admitted for serial clinical examinations; exploratory laparotomy is done if peritoneal signs or hemodynamic instability develop. If the fascia is not violated, the wound is cleansed and repaired and the patient discharged. Alternatively, some centers do CT, or less commonly, DPL, to evaluate patients with fascial penetration. CT is recommended for stab wounds to the flank (between the anterior and posterior axillary lines) or back (between the 2 posterior axillary lines) because injuries to the retroperitoneal structures underlying these areas can be missed when serial abdominal examinations are done.

For **gunshot wounds,** most clinicians do exploratory laparotomy unless the wound is clearly grazing or tangential and peritonitis and hypotension are absent. However, some centers that use nonoperative management of select patients with only solid organ (typically liver) injury do CT of stable patients with gunshot wounds. Local wound exploration is typically not done for gunshot wounds.

Blunt abdominal trauma: Most patients with multiple trauma and distracting injuries and/or altered sensorium should have testing of the abdomen as should patients with findings on examination. Typically, clinicians use ultrasonography or CT, or sometimes both.

Ultrasonography (sometimes termed focused assessment with sonography in trauma [FAST]) can be done during the initial assessment without moving the patient to the radiology suite. The FAST images the pericardium, right and left upper quadrants, and pelvis; its primary aim is to find abnormal pericardial fluid or intraperitoneal free fluid. An extended FAST (E-FAST) adds images of the chest aimed at detecting pneumothorax. Ultrasonography gives no radiation exposure and is sensitive for detecting larger amounts of abdominal fluid but does not identify specific solid organ injuries well, is poor at detecting viscus perforation, and is limited in obese patients and in patients with subcutaneous air (eg, due to pneumothorax).

CT is typically done with IV but not an oral contrast agent; this test is very sensitive for free fluid and solid organ injury but less so for small viscus perforations (albeit better than ultrasonography), and it can simultaneously detect injury to the spine or pelvis. However, CT exposes patients to radiation, which is a particular concern in children and in patients who may require repeat studies (eg, stable patients with small amounts of free fluid), and requires patient transport away from the resuscitation area.

Choice between ultrasonography and CT is based on patient status. If the patient needs CT to assess another body region (eg, cervical spine, pelvis), CT is probably the reasonable choice to evaluate the abdomen. Some clinicians do a FAST scan during the resuscitation phase and proceed to laparotomy if a large amount of free fluid is seen (in hypotensive patients). If FAST results are negative or weakly positive, clinicians do CT if there is still concern about the abdomen after the patient is stabilized. Reasons for such concern include increasing abdominal pain or anticipated inability to monitor the patient clinically (eg, patients who require heavy sedation or who will be undergoing lengthy surgical procedures).

In **diagnostic peritoneal lavage (DPL),** a peritoneal dialysis catheter is placed through the abdominal wall near the umbilicus into the pelvic/peritoneal cavity. Aspiration of blood is considered positive for abdominal injury. If no blood is aspirated, 1 L of crystalloid is run in and allowed to drain back out. Finding > 100,000 RBCs/mL of effluent is very sensitive for abdominal injury. However, DPL has largely been replaced by the FAST examination and CT. DPL has low specificity, identifying many lesions that do not require operative repair and thus resulting in a high negative laparotomy rate. DPL also misses retroperitoneal injuries. DPL may be useful in limited clinical situations such as when there is free pelvic fluid in the absence of a solid organ injury or a hypotensive patient with an unclear FAST examination result.

Recognizing complications of abdominal trauma: Patients with sudden worsening of abdominal pain in the days following injury should be suspected of having a ruptured solid organ hematoma or a delayed hollow viscus perforation, particularly if they have tachycardia and/or hypotension. Steadily worsening pain within the first day suggests hollow viscus perforation or, if after several days, abscess formation, particularly if accompanied by fever and leukocytosis. In both cases, imaging with ultrasonography or CT is usually done in stable patients, followed by operative repair.

Following severe abdominal trauma, abdominal compartment syndrome should be suspected in patients with decreased urine output, ventilatory insufficiency, and/or hypotension, particularly if the abdomen is tense or distended (however, physical findings are not very sensitive). Because such manifestations can also be signs of decompensation due to the underlying injuries, a high degree of suspicion is required in at-risk patients. Diagnosis requires measuring intra-abdominal pressure, typically with a pressure transducer connected to the bladder catheter; values > 20 mm Hg are diagnostic of intra-abdominal hypertension and are concerning. When patients with such a reading also have signs of organ dysfunction (eg, hypotension, hypoxia/hypercarbia, decreased urine output, increased intracranial pressure), surgical decompression is done. Typically the abdomen is left open with the wound covered by a vacuum pack dressing or other temporary device.

1. Como JJ, Bokhari F, Chiu WC, et al. Practice management guidelines for selective nonoperative management of penetrating abdominal trauma. *J Trauma* 68(3): 721–733, 2010.

Treatment

- Sometimes laparotomy for hemorrhage control, organ repair, or both
- Rarely arterial embolization

Patients are given intravenous fluid resuscitation as needed, typically with crystalloid fluids, either 0.9% saline or lactated Ringer solution. However, patients who appear to be in hemorrhagic shock should receive damage control resuscitation until hemorrhage can be controlled. Damage control resuscitation uses blood products in an approximately 1:1:1 ratio of plasma to platelets to red blood cells to minimize the use of crystalloid solutions.[1] Some hemodynamically unstable patients are taken for immediate exploratory laparotomy as described above. For the majority of patients who do not require immediate surgery but who have intra-abdominal injuries identified during imaging, management options include observation, angiographic embolization, and less frequently operative intervention. Prophylactic antibiotics are not indicated when patients are managed without surgery. However, antibiotics are often given before surgical exploration when patients develop an indication for surgery.

Observation: Observation (beginning in an ICU) is often appropriate for hemodynamically stable patients with solid organ injury, many of which heal spontaneously. Patients with free fluid seen during CT but no specific organ injury identified may also be observed provided they have no peritoneal signs. However, free fluid without evidence of solid organ injury is also the most frequent radiographic finding in hollow viscus injury, although this finding has low specificity. Because observation is not appropriate for hollow viscus perforation (patients typically develop sepsis due to peritonitis), clinicians should have a lower threshold for operative exploration when patients with isolated free fluid worsen or fail to improve during a period of observation.

During observation, patients are examined several times per day (preferably by the same examiner), and CBC is done, typically every 4 to 6 h. Assessment seeks to identify ongoing hemorrhage and peritonitis.

Ongoing hemorrhage is suggested by

- Worsening hemodynamic status
- Significant ongoing transfusion needs (eg, more than 2 to 4 units over a 12-h period)
- A significant decrease in Hct (eg, by > 10 to 12%)

The significance of transfusion requirements and change in Hct depend somewhat on the organ injured and other associated injuries (ie, that may also have caused blood loss) as well as the patient's physiologic reserves. However, patients suspected of significant ongoing hemorrhage should be considered for angiography with embolization or immediate laparotomy.

Peritonitis requires further investigation by DPL, CT, or in some cases, exploratory laparotomy.

Patients who remain stable are typically transferred to a regular floor after 12 to 48 h, depending on the severity of their abdominal and other injuries. Their activity and diet are advanced as tolerated. Typically, patients may be discharged home after 2 to 3 days. They are instructed to restrict activity for a minimum of 6 to 8 wk.

It is not clear which asymptomatic patients require an imaging study before resuming full activity, especially when heavy lifting, contact sports, or torso trauma are likely to occur. Patients with high grade (ie, grade 4 and 5) injuries are at the highest risk for postinjury complications and should have the lowest threshold for repeat imaging.

Laparotomy: Laparotomy is elected either because of the initial nature of the injury and clinical status (eg, hemodynamic instability) or because of subsequent clinical decompensation. Most patients can have a single procedure during which hemorrhage is controlled and injuries repaired.

However, patients with extensive intra-abdominal injuries who undergo a prolonged initial surgical procedure tend to fare poorly, particularly when they have other serious injuries, have been in shock for a prolonged period, or both. The more extensive and lengthy the initial surgical procedure, the more likely such patients are to develop the highly lethal combination of acidosis, coagulopathy, and hypothermia with subsequent multiple organ dysfunction. In such cases, mortality can be lessened if the surgeon initially does a much briefer procedure (termed damage control surgery) in which the hemorrhage and enteric spillage is controlled (eg, by packing, ligation, shunting, oversewing or stapling bowel) without definitive repair and the abdomen temporarily closed.

Temporary closure can be achieved using a closed suction vacuum system constructed from towels, drains, and large bio-occlusive dressings or through use of a commercially available negative-pressure abdominal dressing. Patients are then stabilized in the ICU and taken for packing removal and definitive repair once normal physiology has been restored (particularly correction of pH and temperature), typically within 24 h—or sooner if they deteriorate clinically despite resuscitation. Because patients requiring damage control procedures are the most seriously injured, mortality is still significant and subsequent intra-abdominal complications are common.

Angiographic embolization: Ongoing bleeding can sometimes be stopped without surgery by embolizing the bleeding vessel using a percutaneous angiographic procedure (angiographic embolization). Hemostasis is obtained by injecting a thrombogenic substance (eg, powdered gelatin) or metallic coils into the bleeding vessel. Although there is not complete consensus, generally accepted indications for angiographic embolization include

- Pseudoaneurysm
- Arteriovenous fistula
- Solid organ injury (particularly of the liver) or pelvic fracture with bleeding severe enough to require postresuscitation transfusion

Angiographic embolization is not recommended for unstable patients because the radiology suite is a suboptimal area for providing critical care. Additionally, prolonged attempts at embolization should be discouraged in patients whose bleeding requires continued transfusion; operative management is more appropriate. However, with increasing availability of hybrid operating suites (operating room with angiographic intervention capabilities), some unstable patients may be able to undergo angiography and surgical management in rapid succession if needed.

1. Holcomb JB, Tilley BC, Baraniuk S, et al: Transfusion of plasma, platelets, and red blood cells in a 1:1:1 vs a 1:1:2 ratio and mortality in patients with severe trauma. *JAMA* 313(5):471–482, 2015.

KEY POINTS

- Complications of abdominal injuries can be acute (eg, bleeding) or delayed (eg, abscess, obstruction or ileus, delayed hematoma rupture).
- The abdominal examination does not reliably indicate the severity of abdominal injury.
- If patients have evisceration, shock due to penetrating abdominal trauma, or peritonitis, do exploratory laparotomy without delay for diagnostic testing.
- Unless there is clear evidence that laparotomy is indicated or the mechanism of injury is minor, imaging (typically ultrasonography or CT) is typically required after blunt or penetrating trauma.
- If pain gradually increases or clinical signs suggest deterioration, suspect a delayed complication.

HEPATIC INJURY

Hepatic injury can result from blunt or penetrating trauma. Patients have abdominal pain, sometimes radiating to the shoulder, and tenderness. Diagnosis is made by CT or ultrasonography. Treatment is with observation and sometimes surgical repair; rarely, partial hepatectomy is necessary.

Etiology

Significant impact (eg, motor vehicle crash) can damage the liver, as can penetrating trauma (eg, knife wound, gunshot

Table 350–1. GRADES OF HEPATIC INJURY

GRADE	INJURY
1	Subcapsular hematoma < 10% of surface area Laceration < 1 cm deep
2	Subcapsular hematoma 10–50% of surface area, intraparenchymal hematoma < 10 cm Laceration 1–3 cm deep and < 10 cm long
3	Subcapsular hematoma > 50% of surface area, intraparenchymal hematoma > 10 cm or any expanding or ruptured hematoma Laceration > 3 cm deep
4	Parenchymal disruption involving 25–75% of a hepatic lobe or 1–3 Couinaud segments within a single lobe
5	Parenchymal disruption involving > 75% of a hepatic lobe or > 3 Couinaud segments Juxtahepatic venous injuries (ie, retrohepatic vena cava or central major hepatic veins)
6	Hepatic avulsion

wound). Hepatic injuries range from subcapsular hematomas and small capsular lacerations to deep parenchymal lacerations, major crush injury, and vascular avulsion.

Classification: Hepatic injuries are classified according to severity into 6 grades (see Table 350–1).

Pathophysiology

The main immediate consequence is hemorrhage. The amount of hemorrhage may be small or large, depending on the nature and degree of injury. Many small lacerations, particularly in children, cease bleeding spontaneously. Larger injuries hemorrhage extensively, often causing hemorrhagic shock. Mortality is significant in high-grade liver injuries.

Complications: The overall incidence of complications is < 7% but can be as high as 15 to 20% in high-grade injuries. Deep parenchymal lacerations can lead to a biliary fistula or biloma formation. In biliary fistula, bile leaks freely into the abdominal or thoracic cavity. A biloma is a contained collection of bile similar to an abscess. Bilomas are typically treated with percutaneous drainage. For biliary fistulas, biliary decompression through endoscopic retrograde cholangiopancreatography (ERCP) is highly successful.

Abscesses develop in about 3 to 5% of injuries, often because of devitalized tissue being exposed to biliary contents. Diagnosis is suspected in patients in whom pain, temperature, and WBC count increase in the days after injury; confirmation is by CT. Abscesses are usually treated with percutaneous drainage, but laparotomy may be necessary when percutaneous management fails.

Symptoms and Signs

The manifestations of severe abdominal hemorrhage, including hemorrhagic shock, and abdominal pain, tenderness, and distention, are usually clinically obvious. Lesser hemorrhage or hematomas cause right upper quadrant abdominal pain and tenderness.

Diagnosis

- Imaging (CT or ultrasonography)

The diagnosis is confirmed with CT in stable patients and with bedside ultrasonography or exploratory laparotomy in unstable patients.

Treatment

- Observation
- Sometimes embolization or surgical repair

Hemodynamically stable patients who have no other indications for laparotomy (eg, hollow viscus perforation) can be observed with monitoring of vital signs and serial Hct levels. Patients with significant ongoing hemorrhage (ie, those with hypotension and shock, significant ongoing transfusion requirements, or declining Hct) require intervention. Patients whose vital signs are stable but who require ongoing transfusion may be candidates for angiography with selective embolization of bleeding vessels. Unstable patients should undergo laparotomy.

Success rates for nonoperative management are about 92% for grade 1 and 2 injuries, 80% for grade 3 injuries, 72% for grade 4 injuries, and 62% for grade 5 injuries. Following nonoperative management, there is no consensus in the literature regarding length of ICU stay, hospital stay, resumption of diet, duration of bedrest, or limitation of activity once discharged.[1]

When surgery is done, small lacerations can typically be sutured or treated with hemostatic agents (eg, oxidized cellulose, fibrin glue, mixtures of thrombin and powdered gelatin). Surgical management of deeper and more complex injuries can be complicated.

1. Stassen NA, Bhullar I, Cheng JD: Nonoperative management of blunt hepatic injury: an Eastern Association for the Surgery of Trauma practice management guideline. *J Trauma Acute Care Surg* 73:S288-S293, 2012.

KEY POINTS

- The main immediate consequence is bleeding, which often stops spontaneously, particularly if injuries are grade 1 or 2, but may require embolization or surgical repair; mortality and morbidity can be significant in high-grade injuries.
- Complications include formation of biliary fistulas, bilomas, and abscesses.
- Confirm the diagnosis by CT in stable patients.
- Treat patients using laparotomy (if unstable), observation (if stable), or sometimes selective angiographic embolization (eg, if stable but requiring ongoing transfusion).

SPLENIC INJURY

Splenic injury usually results from blunt abdominal trauma. Patients often have abdominal pain, sometimes radiating to the shoulder, and tenderness. Diagnosis is made by CT or ultrasonography. Treatment is with observation and sometimes surgical repair; rarely, splenectomy is necessary.

Etiology

Significant impact (eg, motor vehicle crash) can damage the spleen as can penetrating trauma (eg, knife wound, gunshot wound). Splenic enlargement as a result of fulminant Epstein-Barr viral disease (infectious mononucleosis or

Table 350–2. GRADES OF SPLENIC INJURY

GRADE	INJURY
1	Subcapsular hematoma < 10% of surface area Laceration < 1 cm deep
2	Subcapsular hematoma 10–50% of surface area, intraparenchymal hematoma < 5 cm Laceration 1–3 cm deep and not involving a trabecular vessel
3	Subcapsular hematoma > 50% of surface area, intraparenchymal hematoma ≥ 5 cm, any expanding or ruptured hematoma Laceration > 3 cm deep or involving a trabecular vessel
4	Laceration involving segmental or hilar vessels and that devascularizes > 25% of spleen
5	Completely shattered spleen Hilar vascular injury that devascularizes spleen

posttransplant Epstein-Barr virus–mediated pseudolymphoma) predisposes to rupture with minimal trauma or even spontaneously. Splenic injuries range from subcapsular hematomas and small capsular lacerations to deep parenchymal lacerations, crush injury, and avulsion from the pedicle.

Classification: Splenic injuries are classified according to severity into 5 grades (see Table 350–2).

Pathophysiology

The main immediate consequence is hemorrhage into the peritoneal cavity. The amount of hemorrhage ranges from small to massive, depending on the nature and degree of injury. Many small lacerations, particularly in children, cease bleeding spontaneously. Larger injuries hemorrhage extensively, often causing hemorrhagic shock. A splenic hematoma sometimes ruptures, usually in the first few days, although rupture can occur from hours to even months after injury.

Symptoms and Signs

The manifestations of major hemorrhage, including hemorrhagic shock, abdominal pain, and distention, are usually clinically obvious. Lesser hemorrhage causes left upper quadrant abdominal pain, which sometimes radiates to the left shoulder. Patients with unexplained left upper quadrant pain, particularly if there is evidence of hypovolemia or shock, should be asked about recent trauma. Maintain a high index of suspicion for splenic injury in patients who have left rib fractures.

PEARLS & PITFALLS

- Ask patients with unexplained left upper quadrant abdominal pain about recent trauma (including contact sports), particularly if there is hypovolemia or shock.

Diagnosis

- Imaging (CT or ultrasonography)

The diagnosis is confirmed with CT in stable patients and with bedside (point of care) ultrasonography or exploratory laparotomy in unstable patients.

Treatment

- Observation
- Angioembolization
- Sometimes surgical repair or splenectomy

In the past, treatment for any splenic injury was splenectomy. However, splenectomy should be avoided if possible, particularly in children, the elderly, and patients with hematologic malignancy, to avoid the resulting permanent susceptibility to bacterial infections, increasing the risk of overwhelming postsplenectomy sepsis. The most common pathogen is *Streptococcus pneumoniae*, but other encapsulated bacteria such as *Neisseria* sp and *Haemophilus* sp may also be involved.

Currently, most low-grade and many high-grade splenic injuries can be managed nonoperatively, even in older patients (ie, > 55 yr). Hemodynamically stable patients who have no other indications for laparotomy (eg, hollow viscus perforation) can be observed with monitoring of vital signs and serial abdominal examinations and Hct levels. Need for transfusion is compatible with nonoperative management, particularly when there are other associated injuries (eg, long-bone fractures). However, there should be a predetermined transfusion threshold (typically 2 units for isolated splenic injuries) beyond which surgery should be done to prevent morbidity and mortality. In one high-volume trauma center, of those who fail nonoperative management, 75% fail within two days, 88% within five days, and 93% within seven days of injury.[1]

Similar to hepatic injuries, there is no consensus in the literature regarding duration of restricted activity, optimum length of stay in the ICU or hospital, timing of resumption of diet, or need for repeat imaging for splenic injuries managed nonoperatively.

Patients with significant ongoing hemorrhage (ie, significant ongoing transfusion requirements and/or declining Hct) require laparotomy. Sometimes when patients are hemodynamically stable, angiography with selective embolization of bleeding vessels is done.

When surgery is needed, hemorrhage can sometimes be controlled by suturing, topical hemostatic agents (eg, oxidized cellulose, thrombin compounds, fibrin glue), or partial splenectomy, but splenectomy is still sometimes necessary. Splenectomized patients should receive the pneumococcal vaccine; many clinicians also vaccinate against *Neisseria* and *Haemophilus* spp.

1. Stassen NA, Bhullar I, Cheng JD: Nonoperative management of blunt hepatic injury: an Eastern Association for the Surgery of Trauma practice management guideline. *J Trauma Acute Care Surg* 73:S288–S293, 2012.

KEY POINTS

- Splenic injury is common and can occur with minimal trauma if the spleen is enlarged.
- The main complications are immediate bleeding and delayed hematoma rupture.
- Confirm the diagnosis with CT in stable patients and with exploratory laparotomy in unstable patients.
- To avoid permanently increasing the patient's susceptibility to bacterial infections (caused by splenectomy), manage splenic injuries nonoperatively when possible.
- Do laparotomy or angiography with embolization in patients who have significant ongoing transfusion requirements and/or declining Hct.

351 Altitude Diseases

Altitude diseases (AD) are caused by the decreased availability of O_2 at high altitudes. Acute mountain sickness (AMS), the mildest form of AD, is characterized by headache plus one or more systemic manifestations; it may occur in recreational hikers and skiers and others traveling to high altitude. High-altitude cerebral edema (HACE) is encephalopathy in people with AMS. High-altitude pulmonary edema (HAPE) is a form of noncardiogenic pulmonary edema causing severe dyspnea and hypoxemia. Diagnosis is clinical. Treatment of mild AMS is with analgesics and acetazolamide. Severe AMS may require descent and supplemental O_2 if available. Both HACE and HAPE are potentially life-threatening and require immediate descent. In addition, dexamethasone may be useful for HACE, and nifedipine or phosphodiesterase inhibitors may be useful for HAPE. Prevention of AMS is by gradual ascent and use of acetazolamide.

As altitude increases, atmospheric pressure decreases while the percentage of O_2 in air remains constant; thus, the partial pressure of O_2 decreases with altitude and, at 5800 m (19,000 ft), is about one half-that at sea level.

Most people can ascend to 1500 to 2000 m (5000 to 6500 ft) in one day without problems, but about 20% of those who ascend to 2500 m (8000 ft) and 40% of those who ascend to 3000 m (10,000 ft) develop AMS. Rate of ascent, maximum altitude reached, and sleeping altitude influence the likelihood of developing the disorder.

Risk factors: Effects of high altitude vary greatly among individuals. But generally, risk is increased by the following:

- History of previous AD
- Living near sea level
- Going too high too fast
- Overexertion
- Sleeping at too high an altitude

Young children and young adults are probably more susceptible. Disorders such as asthma, hypertension, diabetes, coronary artery disease, and mild COPD are not risk factors for AD, but hypoxia may adversely affect these disorders. Physical fitness is not protective.

PEARLS & PITFALLS

- Physical fitness is not protective against AD.

Pathophysiology

Acute hypoxia (eg, as occurs during rapid ascent to high altitude in an unpressurized aircraft) alters CNS function within minutes. However, AD results from the body's neurohumoral and hemodynamic responses to hypoxia and develops over hours to days. The primary manifestations involve the CNS and the lungs.

The pathogenesis of AMS and HACE is thought to be similar, with HACE representing the extreme of the spectrum. Although it is not certain, pathogenesis may involve mild cerebral edema, possibly related to the increased cerebral blood flow caused by hypoxia.

HAPE is caused by hypoxia-induced elevation of pulmonary artery pressure which causes interstitial and alveolar pulmonary edema, resulting in impaired oxygenation. Small-vessel hypoxic vasoconstriction is patchy, causing elevated pressure, capillary wall damage, and capillary leakage in less constricted areas. Other factors, such as sympathetic overactivity, may also be involved.

Long-time high-altitude residents can develop HAPE when they return after a brief stay at low altitude, a phenomenon referred to as reentry pulmonary edema.

Acclimatization: Acclimatization is an integrated series of responses that gradually restores tissue oxygenation toward normal in people exposed to altitude. However, in spite of acclimatization, all people at high altitude have tissue hypoxia. Most people acclimatize reasonably well to altitudes of up to 3000 m (10,000 ft) within a few days. The higher the altitude, the longer acclimatization takes. However, no one can fully acclimatize to long-term residence at altitudes > 5100 m (> 17,000 ft).

Features of acclimatization include sustained hyperventilation, which increases tissue oxygenation but also causes respiratory alkalosis. Blood pH tends to normalize within days as HCO_3 is excreted in urine; as pH normalizes, ventilation can increase further. Cardiac output increases initially; RBC mass and tolerance for aerobic work also increase.

Symptoms and Signs

AMS is by far the most common form of AD.

Acute mountain sickness (AMS): This disease is unlikely unless altitude is above 2440 m (8000 ft), but it can develop at lower elevations in some highly susceptible people. It may be due to mild cerebral edema and is characterized by headache plus at least one of the following: fatigue, GI symptoms (anorexia, nausea, vomiting), persistent dizziness, and sleep disturbance. Exertion aggravates the symptoms. Symptoms typically develop 6 to 10 h after ascent and subside in 24 to 48 h. AMS is common at ski resorts, and some people affected by it mistakenly attribute it to excessive alcohol intake (hangover) or a viral illness.

High-altitude cerebral edema (HACE): Marked cerebral edema manifests as headache and diffuse encephalopathy with confusion, drowsiness, stupor, and coma. Gait ataxia is a reliable early warning sign. Seizures, focal deficits (eg, cranial nerve palsy, hemiplegia), fever, and meningeal signs are uncommon and should prompt concern for other diagnoses. Papilledema and retinal hemorrhage may be present but are not necessary for diagnosis. Coma and death may occur within a few hours.

High-altitude pulmonary edema (HAPE): HAPE typically develops 24 to 96 h after rapid ascent to > 2500 m (> 8000 ft) and is responsible for most deaths due to AD.

Initially, patients have dyspnea on exertion, decreased exertion tolerance, and dry cough. Later, dyspnea is present at rest. Pink or bloody sputum and respiratory distress are late findings. On examination, cyanosis, tachycardia, tachypnea, and low-grade fever (< 38.5° C) are common. Focal or diffuse crackles (sometimes audible without a stethoscope) are usually present. HAPE may worsen rapidly; coma and death may occur within hours.

Other manifestations: Peripheral and facial edema is common at high altitude.

Headache, without other symptoms of AMS, is also common.

Retinal hemorrhages may develop at altitudes as low as 2700 m (9000 ft) and are common at > 5000 m (> 16,000 ft). They are usually asymptomatic unless they occur in the macular region; they resolve over weeks without sequelae, but if they develop, descent is indicated and further ascent is contraindicated until hemorrhages have resolved.

People who have had radial keratotomy may have significant visual disturbances at altitudes > 5000 m (> 16,000 ft). These symptoms disappear rapidly after descent.

Chronic mountain sickness (Monge disease) is a disease that affects long-time high-altitude residents; it is characterized by excessive polycythemia, fatigue, dyspnea, aches and pains, and cyanosis. The disorder often involves alveolar hypoventilation. Patients should descend to low altitude and remain there permanently if possible, but economic factors often prevent them from doing so. Repeated phlebotomy can help by reducing polycythemia. In some patients, long-term treatment with acetazolamide results in improvement.

Diagnosis

- Clinical evaluation

Diagnosis of most forms of AD is clinical; laboratory tests are usually unnecessary. In HAPE, hypoxemia is often severe, with pulse oximetry showing 40 to 70% saturation, depending on the elevation at which the individual becomes ill. If obtained, chest x-ray shows a normal-sized heart and patchy lung edema. HACE can usually be differentiated from other causes of headache and coma (eg, infection, brain hemorrhage, uncontrolled diabetes) by history and clinical findings; CT imaging of the head is not usually done.

Treatment

- For mild or moderate AMS, halting ascent and treatment with fluids, nonopioid analgesics, and sometimes acetazolamide
- For severe AMS, descent
- For HACE and HAPE, immediate descent and treatment with O_2, drugs, and pressurization

AMS: Patients should halt ascent and reduce exertion until symptoms resolve.[1,2] Other treatment includes fluids and nonopioid analgesics for headache. For severe symptoms, descent of 500 to 1000 m (1650 to 3200 ft) is often rapidly effective. Acetazolamide 250 mg po bid may relieve symptoms and improve sleep. Dexamethasone 2 to 4 mg po, IM, or IV q 6 h is also highly effective for treating symptoms of AMS.

HACE and HAPE: Patients should descend to low altitude immediately. Helicopter evacuation may be life-saving.[1] If descent is delayed, patients should rest and be given O_2. If descent is impossible, O_2 (to raise the O_2 saturation to > 90%), drugs, and pressurization in a portable hyperbaric bag help buy time but are not substitutes for descent.

For **HACE** (and severe AMS)

- Dexamethasone

Dexamethasone 8 mg initially, followed by 4 mg q 6 h, may help. It should be given po but if this is impossible, dexamethasone may be given IM or IV. Acetazolamide 250 mg po bid may be added.

For **HAPE**

- Nifedipine or a phosphodiesterase inhibitor

Nifedipine 30 mg slow-release po q 12 h lowers pulmonary artery pressure and is beneficial, although systemic hypotension is a possible complication. A phosphodiesterase inhibitor, such as sildenafil (50 mg po q 12 h) or tadalafil (10 mg po q 12 h), may be used instead of nifedipine. Diuretics (eg, furosemide) are contraindicated; they have no efficacy and many patients have concomitant volume depletion. The heart is normal in HAPE, and digoxin and afterload reduction with ACE inhibitors are of no value. When promptly treated by descent, patients usually recover from HAPE within 24 to 48 h. Exertion should be avoided during descent. People who have had one episode of HAPE are likely to have another and should be so warned.

PEARLS & PITFALLS

- Diuretics are contraindicated in high altitude pulmonary edema.

1. Luks AM, McIntosh SE, Grissom CK, et al: Wilderness Medical Society consensus guidelines for the prevention and treatment of acute altitude illness: 2014 update. *Wilderness Environ Med* 25(4S):S4–S14, 2014.
2. Bartsch P, Swenson ER: Acute high-altitude illnesses. *N Engl J Med* 368:2294–2302, 2013. doi: 10.1056/NEJMcp1214870.

Prevention

- Slow ascent
- Sometimes acetazolamide or dexamethasone

Although physical fitness enables greater exertion at altitude, it does not protect against any form of AD. Maintaining adequate fluid intake does not prevent AMS but does protect against dehydration, the symptoms of which closely resemble AMS. Opioids and heavy alcohol consumption, particularly shortly before sleep, should be avoided.

Ascent: The most important measure is a slow ascent.[1,2] Graded ascent is essential for activity at > 2500 m (> 8000 ft). Above 3000 m (10,000 ft), climbers should not increase their sleeping altitude by more than 500 m per day and should include a rest day (ie, sleep at the same altitude) every 3 to 4 days. During rest days, climbers can engage in physical activity and ascend to higher altitudes but should return to the lower level for sleep. Climbers vary in ability to ascend without developing symptoms; a climbing party should be paced for its slowest member.

Acclimatization is gradually lost after a few days at low altitude, and climbers returning to high altitude after this duration should once more follow a graded ascent.

Drugs: Acetazolamide 125 to 250 mg po q 12 h reduces the incidence of altitude illness. Sustained-release capsules (500 mg once/day) are also available. Acetazolamide can be started on the day of the ascent; it acts by inhibiting carbonic anhydrase and thus increasing ventilation. Acetazolamide 125 mg po at bedtime reduces the amount of periodic breathing (almost universal during sleep at high altitude), thus limiting sharp falls in blood O_2. Acetazolamide should not be given to patients allergic to sulfa drugs. Analogs of acetazolamide offer no advantage. Acetazolamide may cause numbness and paresthesias of the fingers; these symptoms are benign but can be annoying. Carbonated drinks taste flat to people taking acetazolamide.

Dexamethasone 2 mg po q 6 h (or 4 mg po q 12 h) is an alternative to acetazolamide.

Low-flow O_2 during sleep at altitude is effective but inconvenient and may pose logistic difficulties.

Patients who have had a previous episode of HAPE should in addition consider prophylaxis with sustained-release nifedipine 30 mg po bid or tadalafil 10 mg po bid.[3] Salmeterol,

125 micrograms inhaled q 12 h, can be added as an adjunct to a pulmonary vasodilator but should not be used as monotherapy for prevention.

Analgesics (eg, acetaminophen, ibuprofen) may prevent high-altitude headache.

1. Luks AM, McIntosh SE, Grissom CK, et al: Wilderness Medical Society consensus guidelines for the prevention and treatment of acute altitude illness: 2014 update. *Wilderness Environ Med* 25(4S):S4–S14, 2014.
2. Bartsch P, Swenson ER: Acute high-altitude illnesses. *N Engl J Med* 368:2294–2302, 2013. doi: 10.1056/NEJMcp1214870.
3. Maggiorini M, Brunner-La Rocca HP, Peth S, et al: Both tadalafil and dexamethasone may reduce the incidence of high-altitude pulmonary edema: a randomized trial. *Ann Intern Med* 3;145(7):497–506, 2006.

KEY POINTS

- About 20% of people who ascend to 2500 m (8000 ft) and 40% of those who ascend to 3000 m (10,000 ft) in one day develop AMS.
- AMS causes headache plus fatigue, GI symptoms (anorexia, nausea, vomiting), dizziness, and/or sleep disturbance.
- HACE causes ataxia and encephalopathy.
- HAPE causes dyspnea, decreased exertion tolerance, and dry cough initially which may become productive.
- Diagnose AD based on clinical findings.
- Treat mild AMS with fluids, analgesics, sometimes acetazolamide, and by stopping further ascent.
- Arrange immediate descent for patients with HACE, HAPE, or very severe AMS.
- Prevent AD by gradual ascent and use of acetazolamide.

352 Bites and Stings

CENTIPEDE AND MILLIPEDE BITES

Some larger centipedes can inflict a painful bite, causing swelling and redness. Symptoms rarely persist for more than 48 h. Millipedes do not bite but may secrete a toxin that is irritating, particularly when accidentally rubbed into the eye.

An ice cube wrapped in a cloth and placed on a centipede bite usually relieves the pain. Toxic secretions of millipedes should be washed from the skin with large amounts of soap and water. If a skin reaction develops, a corticosteroid cream should be applied. Eye injuries should be irrigated immediately.

Tetanus prophylaxis (see Table 181–2 on p. 1472) should be given.

HUMAN AND MAMMAL BITES

Human and other mammal (mostly dog and cat, but also squirrel, gerbil, rabbit, guinea pig, and monkey) bites are common and occasionally cause significant morbidity and disability. The hands, extremities, and face are most frequently affected, although human bites can occasionally involve breasts and genitals.

Bites by large animals sometimes cause significant tissue trauma; about 10 to 20 people, mostly children, die from dog bites each year. However, most bites cause relatively minor wounds.

Infection: In addition to tissue trauma, infection due to the biting organism's oral flora is a major concern. Human bites can theoretically transmit viral hepatitis and HIV. However, HIV transmission is unlikely because the concentration of HIV in saliva is much lower than in blood and salivary inhibitors render the virus ineffective.

Rabies is a risk with certain mammal bites (see p. 1853). Monkey bites, usually restricted in the US to animal laboratory workers, carry a small risk of herpes simian B virus (*Herpesvirus simiae*) infection, which causes vesicular skin lesions at the inoculation site and can progress to encephalitis, which is often fatal.

Bites to the hand (see p. 291) carry a higher risk of infection than bites to other sites. Specific infections include

- Cellulitis
- Tenosynovitis
- Infectious arthritis
- Osteomyelitis

A **fight bite** is the most common human bite wound. It results from a clenched-fist strike to the mouth and is a particular risk for infection. In fight bites, the skin wound moves away from the underlying damaged structures when the hand is opened, trapping bacteria inside. Patients often delay seeking treatment, allowing bacteria to multiply.

Cat bites to the hand also have a high risk of infection because cats' long, slender teeth often penetrate deep structures, such as joints and tendons, and the small punctures are then sealed off.

Human bites to sites other than the hand have not been proved to carry a greater risk of infection than bites from other mammals.

Diagnosis

- Evaluation of hand bites while the hand is in the same position as when the bite was inflicted
- Assessment for damage to underlying nerve, tendon, bone, and vasculature and for presence of foreign bodies

Human bites sustained in an altercation are often attributed to other or vague causes to avoid involvement of the authorities or to ensure insurance coverage. Domestic violence is often denied.

PEARLS & PITFALLS

- For any dorsal hand wound near the metacarpophalangeal joint, consider a human bite, particularly if the history is vague.

Wounds are evaluated (see p. 3030) for damage to underlying structures (eg, nerves, vasculature, tendons, bone) and for foreign bodies. Evaluation should focus on careful assessment of function and the extent of the bite. Wounds over or near joints should be examined while the injured area is held in the same position as when the bite was inflicted (eg, with fist clenched). Wounds are explored under sterile conditions to assess tendon, bone, and joint involvement and to detect retained foreign bodies. Wounds inflicted by chomping may appear to be minor abrasions but should be examined to rule out deep injury.

Culturing fresh wounds is not valuable for targeting antimicrobial therapy, but infected wounds should be cultured. For patients with human bites, screening for hepatitis or HIV is recommended only if the attacker is known or suspected to be seropositive.

Treatment

- Meticulous wound care
- Selective wound closure
- Selective use of prophylactic antibiotics

Hospitalization is indicated if complications mandate very close monitoring, particularly when patient characteristics predict a high risk of nonadherence with outpatient follow-up. Hospitalization should be considered in the following circumstances:

- When a human bite is infected (including clenched-fist injuries)
- When a nonhuman bite is moderately or severely infected
- When loss of function is evident
- When the wound threatens or has damaged deep structures
- When a wound is disabling or difficult to care for at home (eg, significant wounds to both hands or both feet, hand wounds that require continuous elevation)

Priorities of treatment include wound cleaning, debridement, closure, and infection prophylaxis, including for tetanus (see Table 181–2 on p. 1472).

Wound care: Wounds should first be cleaned with a mild antibacterial soap and water (tap water is sufficient), then pressure irrigated with copious volumes of saline solution using a syringe and IV catheter. A local anesthetic should be used as needed. Dead and devitalized tissue should be debrided, taking particular care in wounds involving the face or the hand.

Wound closure is done only for select wounds (ie, that have minimal damage and can be cleansed effectively). Many wounds should initially be left open, including the following:

- Puncture wounds
- Wounds to the hands, feet, perineum, or genitals
- Wounds more than several hours old
- Wounds that are heavily contaminated
- Wounds that are markedly edematous
- Wounds that show signs of inflammation
- Wounds that involve deeper structures (eg, tendon, cartilage, bone)
- Wounds due to human bites
- Wounds sustained in a contaminated environment (eg, marine, field, sewers)

In addition, in immunocompromised patients, wound healing may be better with delayed closure. Other wounds (ie, fresh, cutaneous lacerations) can usually be closed after appropriate wound hygiene. Results with delayed primary closure are comparable to those with primary closure, so little is lost by leaving the wound open initially if there is any question.

Hand bites should be wrapped in sterile gauze, splinted in position of function (slight wrist extension, metacarpophalangeal and both interphalangeal joints in flexion). If wounds are moderate or severe, the hand should be continuously elevated (eg, hanging from an IV pole).

Facial bites may require reconstructive surgery given the cosmetic sensitivity of the area and the potential for scarring. Primary closure of dog bites of the face in children has shown good results, but consultation with a plastic surgeon may be indicated.

Infected wounds may require debridement, suture removal, soaking, splinting, elevation, and IV antibiotics, depending on the specific infection and clinical scenario. Joint infections and osteomyelitis require prolonged IV antibiotic therapy and orthopedic consultation.

Antimicrobials: Thorough wound cleansing is the most effective and essential way to prevent infection and often suffices. There is no consensus on indications for prophylactic antibiotics. Studies have not confirmed a definite benefit, and widespread use of prophylactic antibiotics has the potential to select resistant organisms. Drugs do not prevent infection in heavily contaminated or inadequately cleaned wounds. However, many practitioners prescribe prophylactic antibiotics for bites to the hand and some other bites (eg, cat bites, monkey bites).

Infections are treated with antimicrobials initially chosen based on animal species (see Table 352–1). Culture results, when available, guide subsequent therapy.

Patients with human bites that cause bleeding or exposure to the biter's blood should receive postexposure prophylaxis for viral hepatitis (see p. 222) and HIV (see p. 1627) as indicated by patient and attacker serostatus. If status is unknown, prophylaxis is not indicated.

KEY POINTS

- Infectious risk is high for hand wounds, particularly clenched-fist injuries.
- Evaluate hand wounds with the hand in the position it was when the wound was inflicted.
- Evaluate wounds for damage to nerve, tendon, bone, and vasculature and for the presence of foreign bodies.
- Close only wounds that have minimal damage and can be cleansed effectively.
- Decrease risk of infection by thorough mechanical cleaning, debridement, and sometimes antimicrobial prophylaxis.

INSECT STINGS

Stinging insects are members of the order Hymenoptera of the class Insecta. Hymenoptera venoms cause local toxic reactions in all people and allergic reactions only in those previously sensitized. Severity depends on the dose of venom and degree of previous sensitization. Patients exposed to swarm attacks and patients with high venom-specific IgE levels are most at risk of anaphylaxis; many children never outgrow the risk. The average unsensitized person can safely tolerate 22 stings/kg body weight; thus, the average adult can withstand > 1000 stings, whereas 500 stings can kill a child.

Unexpectedly large numbers of people seek medical attention for stings and their complications after hurricanes and possibly other environmental disasters.

Major Hymenoptera subgroups are

- Apids (eg, honeybees, bumblebees)
- Vespids (eg, wasps, yellow jackets, hornets)
- Formicids (eg, nonwinged fire ants)

Apids usually do not sting unless provoked; however, Africanized honeybees (killer bees), migrants from South America that reside in some southern and southwestern US states,

Table 352–1. ANTIMICROBIALS FOR BITE WOUNDS

DRUG	DOSE	COMMENTS
Human and dog bites		
Amoxicillin/clavulanate	500–875 mg po bid	For outpatients Prophylaxis: Give for 3 days Treatment: Give for 5–7 days
Ampicillin/sulbactam	1.5–3.0 g IV q 6 h	For inpatients Effective against alpha-hemolytic streptococci, *Staphylococcus aureus*, and *Eikenella corrodens*
Trimethoprim/sulfamethoxazole *plus*	160/800 mg IV q 12 h	For penicillin-allergic patients (use weight-appropriate doses for children)
Clindamycin	150–300 mg IV q 6 h	
Doxycycline	100 mg po or IV q 12 h	Alternative for dog bites in penicillin-allergic patients, except children < 8 yr and pregnant women
Clindamycin *plus*	150–300 mg po or IV q 6 h	Alternative for dog bites in adults
A fluoroquinolone (eg, ciprofloxacin)	500 mg po q 12 h (ciprofloxacin)	
Cat bites*		
A fluoroquinolone (eg, ciprofloxacin)	500 mg po bid for 5–7 days	For prophylaxis and treatment in adults Effective against *P. multocida*†
Clarithromycin	500 mg po bid for 7–10 days	Alternative for children
Clindamycin	150–300 mg po qid for 7–10 days	Alternative for children
Monkey bites‡		
Acyclovir	800 mg IV 5 times/day for 14 days	For prophylaxis

*Squirrel, gerbil, rabbit, and guinea pig bites rarely become infected, but when they do, they can be treated with the same drugs used to treat infected cat bites.

†*Bartonella henselae*—see p. 1578—is also transmitted by cat bites.

‡For treatment of infected monkey bites, use antibacterial drugs similar to those used for infected human and dog bites.

are especially aggressive when agitated. Apids typically sting once and dislodge their barbed stinger into the wound, introducing venom and killing the insect. Melittin is thought to be the main pain-inducing component of the venom. The venom of Africanized honeybees is no more potent than that of other honeybees but causes more severe consequences because these insects attack in swarms and inflict multiple stings, increasing the dose of venom. In the US, bee stings cause 3 to 4 times more deaths than do venomous snakebites.

Vespid stingers have few barbs and do not stay in the skin, so these insects can inflict multiple stings. The venom contains phospholipase, hyaluronidases, and the antigen 5 protein, which is the most allergenic. Although vespids also avoid stinging unless provoked, they nest close to humans, so provocative encounters are more frequent. Yellow jackets are the major cause of allergic reactions to insect stings in the US.

Fire ants are present in the southern US, particularly in the Gulf region, where in urban areas, they may sting as many as 40% of the population, causing at least 30 deaths/yr. There are several species, but *Solenopsis invicta* predominates and is responsible for an increasing number of allergic reactions. The ant bites to anchor itself to the person and stings repeatedly as it rotates its body in an arc around the bite, producing a characteristic central bite partially encircled by a reddened sting line. The venom has hemolytic, cytolytic, antimicrobial, and insecticidal properties; 3 or 4 small aqueous protein fractions are probably responsible for allergic reactions.

Symptoms and Signs

Local apid and vespid reactions are immediate burning, transient pain, and itching, with an area of erythema, swelling, and induration up to a few centimeters across. Swelling and erythema usually peak at 48 h, can persist for a week, and can involve an entire extremity. This local chemical cellulitis is often confused with secondary bacterial cellulitis, which is more painful and uncommon after envenomation. Allergic reactions may manifest with urticaria, angioedema, bronchospasm, refractory hypotension, or a combination; swelling alone is not a manifestation of allergic reaction.

Symptoms and signs of a fire ant sting are immediate pain followed by a wheal and flare lesion, which often resolves within 45 min and gives rise to a sterile pustule, which breaks down within 30 to 70 h. The lesion sometimes becomes infected and can lead to sepsis. In some cases, an edematous, erythematous, and pruritic lesion, rather than a pustule, develops. Anaphylaxis due to fire ant stings probably occurs in < 1% of patients. Mononeuritis and seizures have been reported.

Diagnosis

- Clinical evaluation

Diagnosis is clinical. Apid stings are checked for the stinger. Upper and lower airways are assessed for signs of allergic reaction. Secondary bacterial cellulitis is rare but is considered when erythema and swelling begin a day or two after the sting (rather than immediately), there are systemic signs of infection (eg, fever, chills), and pain is significant.

Treatment

- Parenteral epinephrine and antihistamines for systemic allergic reactions
- Removal of any apid stingers
- Analgesics and antihistamines for local reactions

Stingers, if present, should be removed as quickly as possible. Suggested methods include scraping with a thin dull edge (eg, edge of a credit card, dull side of a scalpel, thin table knife).

Pain, burning, and itching can be reduced by placing an ice cube wrapped in a cloth over the sting as soon as possible and giving oral H_1 blockers, NSAIDs, or both. Other possibly effective local measures include antihistamine lotion (eg, with diphenhydramine or tripelennamine), lidocaine patches, eutectic mixture of local anesthetic cream, intradermal injection of 1% lidocaine (with or without 1:100,000 epinephrine), and mid-potency corticosteroid creams or ointments (eg, triamcinolone 0.1%). Most folk remedies (eg, application of meat tenderizer) are of limited effectiveness.

Allergic reactions are treated with IV antihistamines; anaphylaxis is treated with parenteral epinephrine and IV fluids and vasopressors if necessary (see p. 1378).

People with known hypersensitivity to stings should carry a kit containing a prefilled syringe of epinephrine. They should use it as soon as possible after a sting and seek medical care immediately. People who have a history of anaphylaxis or a known allergy to insect bites should wear identification such as an alert bracelet.

Prevention

People who have had anaphylaxis are at risk from subsequent stings. Desensitization immunotherapy can be considered. Venom immunotherapy (see p. 1374) is highly effective, reducing the chance of recurrent anaphylaxis from 50% to about 10% after 2 yr of therapy and to about 2% after 3 to 5 yr of therapy. Children who receive venom immunotherapy have a significantly lower risk of systemic reaction to stings 10 to 20 yr after treatment. Venom immunotherapy seems to be safe for use during pregnancy. Single-venom therapy is adequate. After initial immunotherapy, maintenance doses may be needed for up to 5 yr.

KEY POINTS

- Apid and vespid stings cause immediate pain, burning, itching, erythema, and swelling.
- Fire ant stings cause immediate pain, wheal, and flare, often followed by a pustule within an hour and sometimes infection within hours or days.
- Suspect secondary infection when significant pain, a delay of a day or 2 in erythema and swelling, or systemic findings occur.
- Suspect an allergic reaction when urticaria, angioedema, bronchospasm, and/or refractory hypotension occurs, but not with swelling alone.
- Remove apid stingers and treat local reactions with ice, oral H_1 blockers, and/or NSAIDs.
- Treat allergic reactions and infections.
- Consider desensitization immunotherapy for patients with anaphylactic reactions.

PUSS MOTH CATERPILLAR STINGS

(Asp Stings)

Puss moth caterpillars (*Megalopyge opercularis*), of the order Lepidoptera, are also known as asps. They are one of the most toxic caterpillars in North America. Puss moth caterpillars are endemic to the southern US and live in shade trees and shrubbery around homes and schools and in parks. The asp caterpillar produces 2 generations a year, leading to a bimodal peak in late spring and late fall. They are teardrop shaped and, because they have long silky hair, resemble a tuft of cotton or fur. Their color varies from yellow or gray to reddish brown. When a puss moth caterpillar rubs or is pressed against skin, venomous hairs become embedded.

Envenomation causes intense throbbing pain, burning, and a rash with erythematous spots. More susceptible patients can experience swelling, nausea, abdominal pain, headache, lymphadenopathy, lymphadenitis, shock, and respiratory distress. Wound pain usually subsides within an hour, and the erythematous spots disappear in a day.

Treatment

- Local cooling measures

Treatment for local reactions includes washing the skin with soap and water (using noncontact drying such as a hair dryer), local cooling measures such as an ice pack, or topical isopropyl alcohol, and putting tape on the site and pulling it off to remove embedded hairs. Applying a baking soda slurry or calamine lotion can be soothing. Treatment of systemic reactions is symptomatic. Treatment of severe reactions is like that for insect stings.

OVERVIEW OF MARINE BITES AND STINGS

Some marine bites and stings are toxic (see below and p. 2944). All create wounds at risk of infection with marine organisms, most notably *Vibrio* sp, *Aeromonas* sp, and *Mycobacterium marinum*.

Shark bites result in jagged lacerations with near-total or total amputations and should be treated in the same way as other major trauma (see p. 2927).

CNIDARIA STINGS

Cnidaria (coelenterates) include the following:

- Corals
- Sea anemones
- Jellyfish (including sea nettles)
- Hydroids (eg, Portuguese man-of-war)

Cnidaria are responsible for more envenomations than any other marine animal. However, of the 9000 species, only about 100 are toxic to humans. The multiple, highly developed stinging units (nematocysts) on cnidaria tentacles can penetrate human skin; one tentacle may fire thousands of nematocysts into the skin on contact.

Symptoms and Signs

Lesions vary with the type of cnidaria. Usually, lesions initially appear as small, linear, papular eruptions that develop rapidly in one or several discontinuous lines, at times surrounded by a raised erythematous zone. Pain is immediate and may be severe; itching is common. The papules may vesiculate and proceed to pustulation, hemorrhage, and desquamation.

Systemic manifestations include weakness, nausea, headache, muscle pain and spasms, lacrimation and nasal discharge, increased perspiration, changes in pulse rate, and pleuritic chest pain. Uncommonly, fatal injuries have been inflicted by the Portuguese man-of-war in North American waters and by members of the Cubomedusae order, particularly the box jellyfish (sea wasp, *Chironex fleckeri*), in Indo-Pacific waters.

Treatment

- Removal of tentacles
- Symptomatic treatment
- Various rinses to treat pain and deactivate nematocysts, depending on the specific animal

Cnidaria sting treatment includes removal of adherent tentacles with a forceps (preferably) or fingers (double-gloved if possible) and liberal rinsing to remove invisible stinging cells. The type of rinse varies by the stinging organism:

- For jellyfish stings sustained in nontropical waters and for coral stings, seawater rinse can be used.
- For jellyfish stings sustained in tropical waters, vinegar rinse followed by seawater rinse can be used. Fresh water should not be used because it can activate undischarged nematocysts.
- For box jellyfish stings, vinegar inhibits nematocyst firing and is used as the initial rinse if available, followed by seawater rinse. Fresh water should not be used because it can activate undischarged nematocysts.
- For Portuguese man-of-war stings, saltwater rinse can be used. Vinegar should not be used because it can activate undischarged nematocysts.

Any difficulty breathing or alteration in level of consciousness, no matter how mild, is a medical emergency, requiring transport to a medical center and possibly injection of epinephrine.

Symptoms are treated supportively. Pain caused by sea nettle stings, usually short-lived, can be relieved with baking soda in a 50:50 slurry applied to the skin. For other stings, hot water or cold packs, whichever feels better, can help relieve pain, as can an NSAID or other analgesic. For severe pain, opioids are preferred. Painful muscle spasms may be treated with benzodiazepines. IV fluids and epinephrine can be given if shock develops. Antivenom is available for the stings of the box jellyfish *C. fleckeri* but not for the stings of North American species.

Tetanus prophylaxis (see Table 181–2 on p. 1472) should be given.

Seabather's eruption: This stinging, pruritic, maculopapular rash affects swimmers in some Atlantic locales (eg, Florida, Caribbean, Long Island). It is caused by hypersensitivity to stings from the larvae of the sea anemone (eg, *Edwardsiella lineate*) or the thimble jellyfish (*Linuche unguiculata*). The rash appears where the bathing suit contacts the skin. People exposed to these larvae should shower after taking off their bathing suit. Cutaneous manifestations can be treated with hydrocortisone lotion and, if needed, an oral antihistamine. More severe reactions may require the addition of oral or IV prednisone.

MOLLUSK STINGS

Mollusks include cones (including cone snails), cephalopods (including octopi and squids), and bivalves.

Conus californicus: This type is the only known dangerous cone in North American waters. Its sting causes localized pain, swelling, redness, and numbness that rarely progresses to paralysis or shock.

Treatment is largely supportive. Local measures seem to be of little value, and reports that local injection of epinephrine and neostigmine are helpful are unproved. Severe *Conus* stings may require mechanical ventilation and measures to reverse shock.

Cone snails: These snails are a rare cause of marine envenomation among divers and shell collectors in the Indian and Pacific Oceans. When the snail is aggressively handled (eg, during shell cleaning, when placed in a pocket), it injects its venom through a harpoon-like tooth. Multiple neurotoxins in the venom block ion channels and neurotransmitter receptors, resulting in paralysis, which is usually reversible but has resulted in some deaths.

Treatment is supportive and may include local pressure immobilization (eg, by wrapping wide crepe or other fabric bandages around the limb), immersion in hot water, and tetanus prophylaxis (see Table 181–2 on p. 1472). Severe cases may require respiratory support.

Octopi: The bites of North American octopi are rarely serious. Bites from the blue-ringed octopus, most common in Australian waters, cause tetrodotoxin envenomation, with local anesthesia, neuromuscular paralysis, and respiratory failure; treatment is supportive.

Squid: The large (up to 1.5 m), aggressive Humboldt squid is present off the west coast of the Americas; it has reportedly bitten fishermen and divers. Other squid species are of less concern.

SEA URCHIN STINGS

Sea urchins are present worldwide. Most sea urchin injuries result when spines break off in the skin and cause local tissue reactions. Without treatment, the spines may migrate into deeper tissues, causing a granulomatous nodular lesion, or they may wedge against bone or nerve. Joint and muscle pain and dermatitis may also occur. A few sea urchins (eg, *Globiferous pedicellariae*) have calcareous jaws with venom organs, enabling them to inject venom, but injuries are rare.

Diagnosis is usually obvious by history. A bluish discoloration at the entry site may help locate the spine. X-rays can help when the location is not obvious during examination.

Treatment

- Spine removal

Treatment is immediate removal. Vinegar dissolves most superficial spines; soaking the wound in vinegar several times a day or applying a wet vinegar compress may be sufficient. Hot soaks may help relieve pain. Rarely, a small incision must be made to extract the spine; care must be taken because the spine is very fragile. A spine that has migrated into deeper tissues may require surgical removal. Once spines are removed, pain may continue for days; pain beyond 5 to 7 days should trigger suspicion of infection or a retained foreign body.

G. pedicellariae stings are treated by washing the area and applying a mentholated balm.

Tetanus prophylaxis (see Table 181–2 on p. 1472) should be given.

STINGRAY STINGS

Stingrays once caused about 750 stings/yr along North American coasts; the present incidence is unknown, and most cases are not reported. Venom is contained in the one or more spines on the dorsum of the animal's tail. Injuries usually occur when an unwary swimmer wading in ocean surf, bay, or backwater steps on a stingray buried in the sand and provokes it to thrust its tail upward and forward, driving the dorsal spine (or spines) into the patient's foot or leg. The integumentary sheath surrounding the spine ruptures, and the venom escapes into the patient's tissues.

Symptoms and Signs

The main symptom is immediate severe pain. Although often limited to the injured area, the pain may spread rapidly, reaching its greatest intensity in < 90 min; in most cases, pain gradually diminishes over 6 to 48 h but occasionally lasts days or weeks. Syncope, weakness, nausea, and anxiety are common and may be due, in part, to peripheral vasodilation. Lymphangitis, vomiting, diarrhea, sweating, generalized cramps, inguinal or axillary pain, respiratory distress, and death have been reported.

The wound is usually jagged, bleeds freely, and is often contaminated with parts of the integumentary sheath. The edges of the wound are often discolored, and some localized tissue destruction may occur. Generally, some swelling is present. Open wounds are subject to infection.

Treatment

- Irrigation and debridement

Injuries to an extremity should be gently irrigated with salt water in an attempt to remove fragments of spine, glandular tissue, and integument. The spine should be removed in the field only if it is superficially embedded and is not penetrating the neck, thorax, or abdomen or creating a through-and-through injury of a limb. Significant bleeding should be staunched with local pressure. Warm water immersion, although recommended by some experts, has not been verified as an effective early treatment for stingray injuries.

In the emergency department, the wound should be reexamined for remnants of the sheath and debrided; a local anesthetic may be given as needed. Embedded spines are treated similarly to other foreign bodies. Patients stung on the trunk should be evaluated closely for puncture of viscera. Treatment of systemic manifestations is supportive. Tetanus prophylaxis (see Table 181–2 on p. 1472) should be given, and an injured extremity should be elevated for several days. Use of antibiotics and surgical wound closure may be necessary.

MITE BITES

There are multiple kinds of biting mites. Chiggers are probably the most common. Chiggers are mite larvae that are ubiquitous outdoors except in arid regions; they bite, feed in the skin, then fall off. Outside the US, chiggers may carry *Orientia tsutsugamushi* (see p. 1698). They do not burrow into the skin, but because they are small, they are not readily seen on the skin surface.

Common mite species that bite and burrow into the skin include *Sarcoptes scabiei*, which causes scabies (see p. 1058), and *Demodex* mites, which cause a scabies-like dermatitis (sometimes referred to as mange).

Dermatitis is caused by mites that occasionally bite humans but are ordinarily ectoparasites of birds, rodents, or pets and by mites associated with plant materials or stored food or feed.

- Bird mites may bite people who handle live poultry or pet birds or who have birds' nests on their homes.
- Rodent mites from cats, dogs (especially puppies), and rabbits may bite people.
- Swine mange mites (*S. scabiei var suis*) from pig farms or pet pigs may also bite humans.
- The straw itch mite (*Pyemotes tritici*) is often associated with seeds, straw, hay, and other plant material; it is a parasite of soft-bodied insects that are or have been present in such materials. These mites often bite people who handle the infested items. Granary workers, people who handle grass seeds or grass hay, and people who make dried plant arrangements are most at risk.

Allergic dermatitis or grocer's itch is caused by several species of mites associated with stored grain products, cheese, and other foods. These mites do not bite but cause allergic dermatitis because people become sensitized to allergens on the mites or their waste products.

House dust mites do not bite but feed on sloughed skin cells in pillows and mattresses and on floors (especially on carpets). They are significant because many people develop pulmonary hypersensitivity to allergens in the exoskeletons and feces of house dust mites.

Symptoms and Signs

Most bites cause some version of pruritic dermatitis; pruritus due to chigger bites is especially intense.

Diagnosis

- Clinical evaluation

Diagnosis of nonburrowing mite bites is presumptive based on the patient's history (eg, living, working, and recreational environments) and physical examination. The mites themselves are rarely found because they fall off after biting, the skin reaction is usually delayed, and most patients seek a physician's assistance only after several days. Lesions caused by different mites are usually indistinguishable and may superficially resemble other skin conditions (eg, other insect bites, contact dermatitis, folliculitis).

Diagnosis of burrowing mites can often be made presumptively based on history and a scabies-like pattern of skin lesions. If the diagnosis is unclear or if treatment is ineffective, the diagnosis can be confirmed by skin biopsy.

Treatment

- Topical corticosteroids or oral antihistamines
- Antimicrobial therapy for burrowing mites
- See treatment of scabies

Treatment of nonburrowing mite bites is symptomatic. Topical corticosteroids or oral antihistamines are used as needed to control pruritus until the hypersensitivity reaction resolves. Through discussion of possible sources, the physician can help patients avoid repeated exposure to mites. For *Demodex* bites, veterinary consultation is needed.

KEY POINTS

- Mites that bite include chiggers (too small to see) and occasionally mites that are ectoparasites of birds, rodents, or pets and mites associated with plant materials or stored food or feed.
- Mites that bite and burrow include *Sarcoptes scabiei*, which causes scabies, and *Demodex* mites, which cause a scabies-like dermatitis.
- Mites that bite usually cause pruritic dermatitis.
- Diagnose patients by history and, for burrowing mites, scabies-like pattern of skin lesions.
- Treat symptoms (eg, topical corticosteroids or oral antihistamines for itching) and treat burrowing mite bites with antimicrobial therapy.

SCORPION STINGS

Although all scorpions in North America sting, most are relatively harmless. The stings usually cause only localized pain with minimal swelling, some lymphangitis with regional lymphadenopathy, increased skin temperature, and tenderness around the wound.

A significant exception in North America is the bark scorpion (*Centruroides sculpturatus*, also known as *C. exilicauda*), present in Arizona, in New Mexico, and on the California side of the Colorado River. This species is venomous and can cause more serious injury and illness.

Initial symptoms are immediate pain and sometimes numbness or tingling over the involved part. Swelling is usually absent, and there are few skin changes. Serious symptoms, most common among children, include

- Restlessness
- Muscle spasms
- Abnormal and random head, neck, and eye movements
- Anxiety and agitation
- Sialorrhea and diaphoresis

In adults, tachycardia, hypertension, increased respirations, weakness, muscle spasms, and fasciculations may predominate. Respiratory difficulties are rare in both age groups.

C. sculpturatus stings have resulted in death in children < 6 yr and in hypersensitive people.

Diagnosis

- Clinical evaluation

Diagnosis is obvious from the history. Determining the scorpion species is usually not. Several species of scorpions kept as exotic pets in the US (known by names that falsely suggest toxicity, such as yellow death stalker and black death scorpion) are similar in appearance to foreign species with dangerously toxic venom. However, the actual species of pet scorpion is seldom known by the patient or, if provided, may be unreliable. Stings should be treated as potentially dangerous until signs or lack of signs indicates otherwise.

Treatment

- Supportive care
- Antivenom for severe cases in North America

Treatment of nonvenomous scorpion stings is based on symptoms. An ice pack over the wound and oral NSAIDs reduce pain. Treatment of venomous *Centruroides* stings consists of bed rest, benzodiazepines for muscle spasms, and IV drugs as needed to control hypertension, agitation, and pain. Patients should be kept npo for 8 to 12 h after the bite. For serious stings by scorpions not native to North America, prazosin may help prevent pulmonary edema due to extreme hypertension, and opioids may be indicated for pain control.

An antivenom that is specific for *Centruroides* is available in the US and should be given to all patients with severe symptoms and to patients who are unresponsive to supportive care, particularly children. Information about availability and dosing may be obtained by contacting a regional poison center (1-800-222-1222).

Tetanus prophylaxis (see Table 181–2 on p. 1472) should be given.

SNAKEBITES

Of about 3000 snake species throughout the world, only about 15% worldwide and 20% in the US are dangerous to humans because of venom or toxic salivary secretions (see Table 352–2). At least one species of venomous snake is native to every state in the US except Alaska, Maine, and Hawaii. Almost all are crotalines (also called pit vipers because of pitlike depressions on either side of the head, which are heat-sensing organs):

- Rattlesnakes
- Copperheads
- Cottonmouths (water moccasins)

More than 60,000 bites and stings are reported to poison centers and result in about 100 deaths each year in the US. About 45,000 are snakebites (of which 7000 to 8000 are venomous

Table 352–2. SIGNIFICANT VENOMOUS SNAKES BY REGION

GEOGRAPHIC REGION	SNAKES
Africa	Bird snake Boomslang Burrowing asp Gaboon viper Mamba Mole viper Natal black snake Puff adder
Asia	Asiatic pit vipers King cobra Krait Malaysian pit viper Red-necked keelback Russell's viper
Australia	Death adder King brown snake Red-bellied black snake Taipan Tiger snake
Central and South America	Bushmaster Cantil pit viper Coral snake Fer-de-lance Palm pit viper Rattlesnake
Europe	Adder Asp viper Blunt nose viper Nose-horned viper Ottoman viper
Indo-Pacific	Sea kraits Sea snakes
Middle East	Burrowing asp Egyptian cobra Horned or desert vipers Mole vipers Natal black snake Palestinian viper Saw-scaled viper Sinai desert snake
North America	Copperhead Coral snakes Cottonmouth (water moccasin) Rattlesnake (eg, diamondback, sidewinder, timber, prairie, Mojave)

and cause about 5 deaths). Rattlesnakes account for the majority of snakebites and almost all deaths. Copperheads and, to a lesser extent, cottonmouths account for most other venomous bites. Coral snakes (elapids) and imported species (in zoos, schools, snake farms, and amateur and professional collections) account for < 1% of all bites.

Most patients are males between 17 and 27 yr; 50% of them are intoxicated and deliberately handled or molested the snake. Most bites occur on the upper extremities. Five or 6 deaths occur annually in the US. Risk factors for death include age extremes, handling of captive snakes (rather than wild encounters), delay in treatment, and undertreatment.

Outside the US, fatal snakebites are much more common, accounting for > 100,000 deaths yearly.

Pathophysiology

Snake venoms are complex substances, chiefly proteins, with enzymatic activity. Although enzymes play an important role, the lethal properties of venom are caused by certain smaller polypeptides. Most venom components appear to bind to multiple physiologic receptors, and attempts to classify venom as toxic to a specific system (eg, neurotoxin, hemotoxin, cardiotoxin, myotoxin) are misleading and can lead to errors in clinical judgment.

Pit vipers: The complex venom of most North American pit vipers has local effects as well as systemic effects such as coagulopathy. Effects may include

- Local tissue damage, causing edema and ecchymosis
- Vascular endothelial damage
- Hemolysis
- A disseminated intravascular coagulation (DIC) like (defibrination) syndrome
- Pulmonary, cardiac, renal, and neurologic defects

Venom alters capillary membrane permeability, causing extravasation of electrolytes, albumin, and RBCs through vessel walls into the envenomated site. This process may occur in the lungs, myocardium, kidneys, peritoneum, and, rarely, the CNS. Common clinical syndromes secondary to severe pit viper envenomation include the following:

- **Edema:** Initially, edema, hypoalbuminemia, and hemoconcentration occur.
- **Hypovolemia:** Later, blood and fluids pool in the microcirculation, causing hypotension, lactic acidemia, shock, and, in severe cases, multisystem organ failure. Effective circulating blood volume falls and may contribute to cardiac and renal failure.
- **Bleeding:** Clinically significant thrombocytopenia (platelet count < 20,000/μL) is common in severe rattlesnake bites and may occur alone or with other coagulopathies. Venom-induced intravascular clotting may trigger DIC-like syndrome, resulting in bleeding.
- **Renal failure:** Renal failure may result from severe hypotension, hemolysis, rhabdomyolysis, nephrotoxic venom effects, or a DIC-like syndrome. Proteinuria, hemoglobinuria, and myoglobinuria may occur in reaction to severe rattlesnake bites.

The venom of most North American pit vipers causes very minor changes in neuromuscular conduction, except for Mojave and eastern diamondback rattlesnake venom, which may cause serious neurologic deficits.

Coral snakes: Venom of these snakes contains primarily neurotoxic components, which cause a presynaptic neuromuscular blockade, potentially causing respiratory paralysis. The lack of significant proteolytic enzyme activity accounts for the paucity of symptoms and signs at the bite site.

Symptoms and Signs

A snakebite, whether from a venomous or nonvenomous snake, usually causes terror, often with autonomic manifestations (eg, nausea, vomiting, tachycardia, diarrhea, diaphoresis), which may be difficult to distinguish from systemic manifestations of envenomation.

Nonvenomous snakebites cause only local injury, usually pain and 2 to 4 rows of scratches from the snake's upper jaw at the bite site.

Symptoms and signs of envenomation may be local, systemic, or a combination, depending on degree of envenomation and species of snake. Anaphylaxis can occur, particularly in snake handlers who have been previously sensitized.

Pit vipers: About 25% of pit viper bites are dry (venom is not deposited), and no systemic symptoms or signs develop.

Local signs include ≥ 1 fang marks and scratches. If envenomation has occurred, edema and erythema at the bite site and in adjacent tissues occur, usually within 30 to 60 min. Oozing from the wound suggests envenomation. Edema can progress rapidly and may involve the entire extremity within hours. Lymphangitis and enlarged, tender regional lymph nodes may develop; temperature increases over the bite area. In moderate or severe envenomations (see p. 2949), ecchymosis is common and may appear at and around the bite site within 3 to 6 h. Ecchymosis is most severe after bites by

- Eastern and western diamondbacks
- Cottonmouths
- Prairie, Pacific, and timber rattlesnakes

The skin around the bite may appear tense and discolored. Bullae—serous, hemorrhagic, or both—usually appear at the bite site within 8 h. Edema resulting from North American rattlesnake envenomations may be severe but is usually limited to dermal and subcutaneous tissues, although severe envenomation rarely causes edema in subfascial tissue, causing compartment syndrome (defined as compartment pressures ≥ 30 mm Hg for > 1 h, or as < 30 mm Hg below the diastolic pressure). Necrosis around the bite site is common after rattlesnake envenomations. Most venom effects on soft tissues peak within 2 to 4 days.

Ecchymosis is less common after copperhead and Mojave rattlesnake bites.

Systemic manifestations of envenomation can include nausea, vomiting, diarrhea, diaphoresis, anxiety, confusion, spontaneous bleeding, fever, chest pain, difficulty breathing, paresthesias, hypotension, and shock. Some patients with rattlesnake bites experience a rubbery, minty, or metallic taste in their mouth. The venom of most North American pit vipers causes minor neuromuscular conduction changes, including generalized weakness and paresthesias and muscle fasciculations. Some patients have alterations in mental status. Venom of Mojave and eastern diamondback rattlesnakes may cause serious neurologic deficits, including respiratory depression.

Anaphylaxis can cause systemic symptoms immediately.

Rattlesnake envenomations may induce various coagulation abnormalities, including thrombocytopenia, prolongation of PT (measured by the INR) or activated PTT, hypofibrinogenemia, elevated fibrin degradation products, or a combination of these disorders, resembling a DIC-like syndrome. Thrombocytopenia is usually the first manifestation and may be asymptomatic or, in the presence of a multicomponent coagulopathy, cause spontaneous bleeding. Patients with coagulopathy typically hemorrhage from the bite site or from venipuncture sites or mucous membranes, with epistaxis, gingival bleeding, hematemesis, hematochezia, hematuria, or a combination. A rise in Hct is an early finding secondary to edema and hemoconcentration. Later, Hct may fall as a result of fluid replacement and blood loss due to DIC-like syndrome. In severe cases, hemolysis may cause a rapid fall in Hct.

Coral snakes: Pain and swelling may be minimal or absent and are often transitory. The absence of local symptoms and signs may erroneously suggest a dry bite, producing a false sense of security for both patient and clinician.

PEARLS & PITFALLS

- Suspect envenomation with all bites caused by venomous snakes, even if there are no signs of envenomation soon after the bite.

Weakness of the bitten extremity may become evident within several hours. Systemic neuromuscular manifestations may be delayed for 12 h and include weakness and lethargy; altered sensorium (eg, euphoria, drowsiness); cranial nerve palsies causing ptosis, diplopia, blurred vision, dysarthria, and dysphagia; increased salivation; muscle flaccidity; and respiratory distress or failure. Once the neurotoxic venom effects manifest, they are difficult to reverse and may last 3 to 6 days. Untreated, respiratory muscle paralysis may be fatal.

Diagnosis

- Identification of the snake
- Grading severity of envenomation

Definitive diagnosis is aided by positive identification of the snake and clinical manifestations of envenomation. History should include the time of bite, description of the snake, type of field therapy, underlying medical conditions, allergy to horse or sheep products, and history of previous venomous snakebites and therapy. A complete physical examination should be done. A marker should be used to indicate the leading edge of edema on the affected limb or area, and the time the mark was made should be recorded.

Snakebites should be assumed to be venomous until proved otherwise by clear identification of the species or by a period of observation.

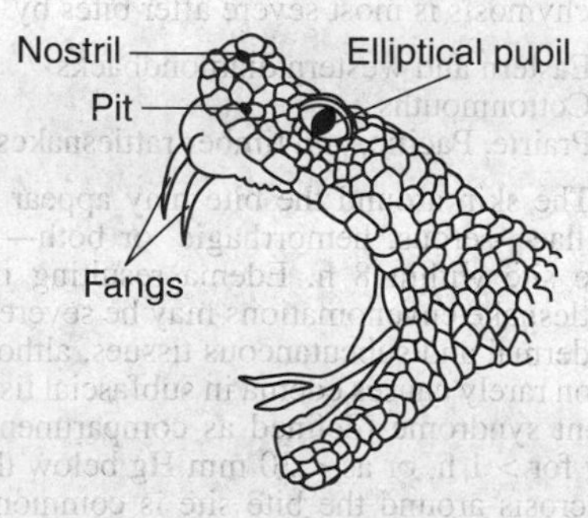

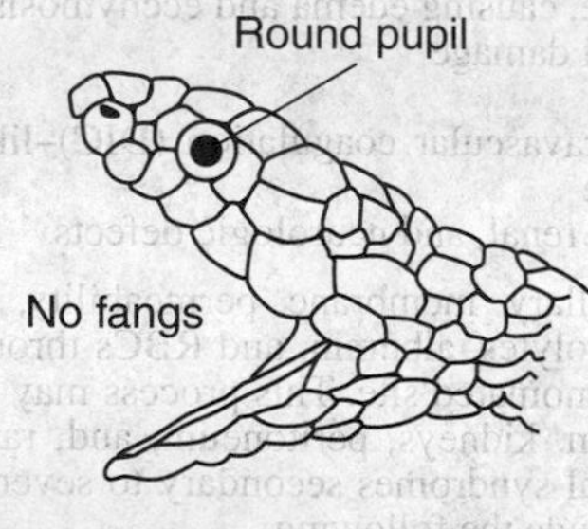

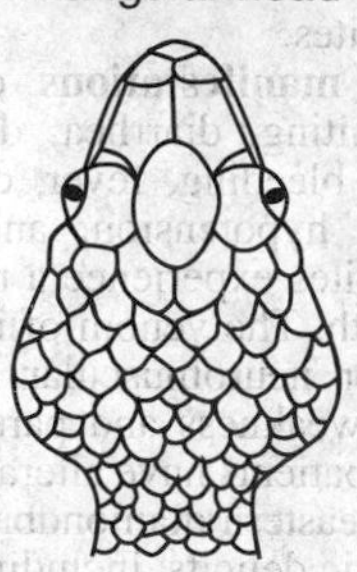

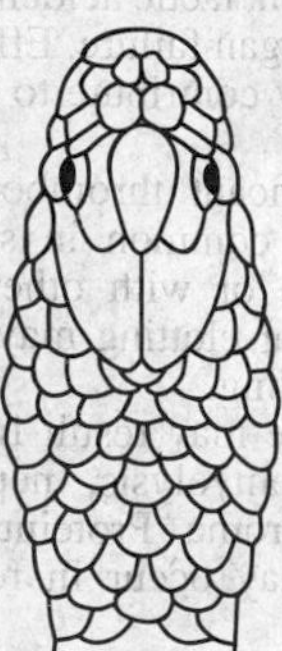

Fig. 352–1. Identifying pit vipers. Pit vipers have the following features, which help differentiate them from nonvenomous snakes:

- Arrowhead-shaped (triangular) heads
- Elliptical pupils
- Heat-sensing pits between the eyes and nose
- Retractable fangs
- A single row of subcaudal plates extending from the anal plate on the underside of the tail

Snake identification: Patients often cannot recall details of the snake's appearance. Pit vipers and nonvenomous snakes can be distinguished by some physical features (see Fig. 352–1). Consultation with a zoo, an aquarium, or a poison center (1-800-222-1222) can help in the identification of snake species.

Coral snakes in the US have round pupils and black snouts but lack facial pits. They have blunt or cigar-shaped heads and alternating bands of red, yellow (cream), and black, often causing them to be mistaken for the common nonvenomous scarlet king snake, which has alternating bands of red, black, and yellow. The distinguishing feature in the coral snake is that the red bands are adjacent to only yellow bands, not black bands ("red on yellow, kill a fellow; red on black, venom lack"). Coral snakes have short, fixed fangs and inject venom through successive chewing movements.

Fang marks are suggestive but not conclusive; rattlesnakes may leave single or double fang marks or other teeth marks, whereas bites by nonvenomous snakes usually leave multiple superficial teeth marks. However, the number of teeth marks and bite sites may vary because snakes may strike and bite multiple times.

A dry pit viper bite is diagnosed when no symptoms or signs of envenomation appear within 8 h after the bite.

Severity of envenomation: Severity of envenomation depends on the following:

- Size and species of the snake (rattlesnakes > cottonmouths > copperheads)
- Amount of venom injected per bite (cannot be determined by history)
- Number of bites
- Location and depth of the bite (eg, envenomation in bites to the head and trunk tends to be more severe than in bites to the extremities)
- Age, size, and health of the patient
- Time elapsed before treatment
- Patient's susceptibility (response) to the venom

Severity of envenomation can be graded as minimal, moderate, or severe based on local findings, systemic symptoms and signs, coagulation parameters, and laboratory results (see Table 352–3). Grading should be determined by the most severe symptom, sign, or laboratory finding.

Envenomation may progress rapidly from minimal to severe and must be reassessed continually.

If systemic symptoms begin immediately, anaphylaxis should be assumed.

Table 352–3. SEVERITY OF PIT VIPER ENVENOMATION

GRADE	DESCRIPTION
Minimal	Changes at bite site only No systemic symptoms or signs or abnormal laboratory findings
Moderate	Changes extending beyond the bite site Non-life-threatening systemic symptoms and signs (eg, nausea, vomiting, paresthesias) Mildly abnormal coagulation or laboratory changes without clinically significant bleeding
Severe	Changes involving the entire extremity Severe systemic symptoms and signs (eg, hypotension, dyspnea, shock) Markedly abnormal coagulation and laboratory changes with or without clinically significant bleeding

Treatment

- First aid
- Supportive care
- Antivenom
- Wound care

General approach: Treatment begins immediately, before patients are moved to a medical facility.

In the field, patients should move or be moved beyond the snake's striking distance. They should avoid exertion and be reassured, kept warm, and transported rapidly to the nearest medical facility. A bitten extremity should be wrapped loosely and immobilized in a functional position at about heart level, and all rings, watches, and constrictive clothing should be removed. Pressure immobilization to delay systemic absorption of venom (eg, by wrapping wide crepe or other fabric bandages around the limb) may be appropriate for coral snake bites but is not recommended in the US, where most bites are from pit vipers; pressure immobilization may cause arterial insufficiency and necrosis.

First responders should support airway and breathing, administer O_2, and establish IV access in an unaffected extremity while transporting patients. All other out-of-hospital interventions (eg, tourniquets, topical preparations, any form of wound suction with or without incision, cryotherapy, electrical shock) are of no proven benefit, may be harmful, and may delay appropriate treatment. However, tourniquets that are already placed, unless causing limb-threatening ischemia, should remain in place until patients are transported to the hospital and envenomation is excluded or definitive treatment is initiated.

PEARLS & PITFALLS

- Do not incise or apply tourniquets to snakebite wounds.

Serial assessment and testing begin in the emergency department. Outlining the leading margin of local edema with an indelible marker every 15 to 30 min can help clinicians assess progression of local envenomation. Extremity circumference should also be measured on arrival and at regular intervals until local progression subsides. All but trivial pit viper bites require

- A baseline CBC (including platelets)
- Coagulation profile (eg, PT, PTT, fibrinogen)
- Measurement of fibrin degradation products
- Urinalysis
- Measurement of serum electrolytes, BUN, and creatinine

For moderate and severe envenomations, patients require blood typing and cross-matching, ECG, chest x-ray, and CK tests, as governed by the patient's status, often as frequently as every 4 h for the first 12 h and then daily. In the management of patients with coral snake bites, neurotoxic venom effects necessitate monitoring of oxygen saturation and baseline and serial pulmonary function tests (ie, peak flow, vital capacity).

Duration of close observation for all patients with pit viper bites should be at least 8 h. Patients without evidence of envenomation after 8 h may be sent home after adequate wound care (see p. 2950). Patients with coral snake bites should be monitored closely for at least 12 h in case respiratory paralysis develops. Envenomation initially assessed as mild may progress to severe within several hours.

Supportive care may include respiratory support, benzodiazepines for anxiety and sedation, opioids for pain, and fluid replacement and vasopressor support for shock. Transfusions (eg, packed RBCs, fresh frozen plasma, cryoprecipitate, platelets) may be required but should not be given before patients have received adequate quantities of neutralizing antivenom because most coagulopathies respond to sufficient quantities of neutralizing antivenom. Suspected anaphylaxis (eg, with immediate onset of systemic symptoms) is treated with standard measures, including epinephrine. Tracheostomy may be needed if trismus, laryngeal spasm, or excessive salivation is present.

Antivenom: Along with aggressive supportive care, antivenom is the mainstay of treatment for patients with anything more than the mildest envenomation grade.

For pit viper envenomation, the mainstay of treatment in the US is an ovine-derived Crotalidae polyvalent immune FAb antivenom (purified FAb fragments of IgG harvested from pit viper venom–immunized sheep). The effectiveness of this antivenom is time and dose related; it is most effective in preventing venom-induced tissue damage when given early. It is less effective if delayed but can reverse coagulopathies and be effective even when started 24 h after envenomation. Crotalidae polyvalent immune FAb is very safe, although it can still cause acute (cutaneous or anaphylactic) reactions and delayed hypersensitivity reactions (serum sickness). Serum sickness develops in up to 16% of patients 1 to 3 wk after administration of the FAb product.

A loading dose of 4 to 6 vials of reconstituted Crotalidae polyvalent immune FAb diluted in 250 mL of normal saline should be infused slowly at 20 to 50 mL/h for the first 10 min; then, if no adverse reactions occur, the remainder is infused over the next hour. The same dose can be repeated 2 times as needed to achieve initial control of symptoms, reverse coagulopathies, and correct physiologic parameters. In children, the dose is not decreased (eg, based on weight or size). Measuring the circumference of the involved extremity at 3 points proximal to the bite and measuring the advancing border of edema every 15 to 30 min can guide decisions about the need for additional doses. Once control is achieved, a 2-vial dose in 250 mL saline is given at 6, 12, and 18 h to prevent recurrence of limb swelling and other venom effects.

PEARLS & PITFALLS

- Give children envenomated by a pit viper bite full adult doses of antivenom.

Pit viper species may affect dose. Cottonmouth, copperhead, and pygmy rattlesnake envenomations may require smaller doses of antivenom. However, antivenom should not be withheld based on the species of snake and should be given based on envenomation grading regardless of the species. Special attention is warranted for children, the elderly, and patients with medical conditions (eg, diabetes mellitus, coronary artery disease), who may be more susceptible to venom effects.

For **coral snake envenomation,** equine-derived polyvalent coral snake antivenom is given at a dose of 5 vials for suspected envenomation and an additional 10 to 15 vials if symptoms develop. Dose is similar for adults and children. This dosing recommendation may be reduced during national shortages of coral snake antivenom.

Antivenom pretreatment precautions should be considered for patients with known hypersensitivity to Crotalidae polyvalent immune FAb or sheep serum and those with a history of asthma or multiple allergies. In such patients, if the envenomation is considered life or limb threatening, H_1 and H_2 blockers should be given before antivenom in a critical care setting equipped to treat anaphylaxis. Early anaphylactoid reactions to antivenom have been noted and usually result from too-rapid infusion; treatment is to temporarily stop the infusion and give epinephrine, H_1 and H_2 blockers, and IV fluid, depending on severity. Usually, antivenom can be resumed after diluting the antivenom further and infusing it at a slower rate.

Serum sickness may develop, manifesting 7 to 21 days after treatment as fever, rash, malaise, urticaria, arthralgia, and lymphadenopathy (see p. 2947). Treatment is H_1 blockers and a tapering course of oral corticosteroids.

Adjunctive measures: Patients should receive tetanus prophylaxis (toxoid and sometimes Ig) as indicated by their history (see Table 181–2 on p. 1472). Snakebites rarely become infected, and antibiotics are indicated only for patients with clinical evidence of infection. If necessary, options include a 1st-generation cephalosporin (eg, oral cephalexin, IV cefazolin) or a broad-spectrum penicillin (eg, oral amoxicillin/clavulanate, IV ampicillin/sulbactam). Subsequent antibiotic choices should be based on culture and sensitivity results from wound cultures.

Wound care for bites is similar to that for other puncture wounds. The area is cleaned and dressed. For limb bites, the extremity is splinted in a functional position and elevated. Wounds should be examined and cleaned daily and covered with a sterile dressing. Blebs, bloody vesicles, or superficial necrosis should be surgically debrided between days 3 and 10, in stages if needed. Sterile whirlpool sessions may be indicated for wound debridement and physical therapy. Fasciotomy (ie, for compartment syndrome) is rarely indicated and should be considered only when compartment pressure is ≥ 30 mm Hg for > 1 h or < 30 mm Hg below the diastolic pressure, causes severe vascular compromise, is unresponsive to limb elevation and mannitol 1 to 2 g/kg IV, and appropriate doses of antivenom have failed. Massive edema alone is *not* an indication for fasciotomy. Joint motion, muscle strength, sensation, and limb girth should be evaluated within 2 days after the bite. Contractures can be prevented by interrupting immobilization with frequent periods of gentle exercise, progressing from passive to active.

Regional poison centers and zoos are excellent resources when dealing with snakebites, including those by nonnative snakes. These facilities maintain a list of physicians trained in snake identification and snakebite care as well as the Antivenom Index, published and periodically updated by the American Zoo and Aquarium Association and the American Association of Poison Control Centers. This index catalogs the location and number of vials of antivenom available for all native venomous snakes and most exotic species. A national help line is available at 1-800-222-1222.

KEY POINTS

- In the US, common venomous snakes include rattlesnakes, copperheads, and cottonmouths (all pit vipers), but rattlesnakes account for most bites and almost all deaths.
- Pit viper envenomation can cause local effects (eg, pain, progressive swelling, ecchymosis) and systemic effects (eg, vomiting, diaphoresis, confusion, bleeding, fever, chest pain, dyspnea, paresthesias, hypotension).
- Features that can help differentiate pit vipers from nonvenomous snakes include an elliptical pupil, a triangular head, retractable fangs, heat-sensing pits between the eyes and nose, and a single row of subcaudal plates extending from the anal plate on the underside of the tail.
- In the field, remove the patient out of striking distance from the snake, arrange rapid transport, wrap a bitten limb loosely,

immobilize it in a position at about heart level, and remove constricting devices such as rings and watches; do not incise bite wounds or apply tourniquets.

- Monitor patients with pit viper bites serially for at least 8 h, longer if any findings suggest envenomation.
- Treat wounds and symptoms, and consult a poison center.
- Give antivenom early and at adequate doses, including full adult doses for children.

ALLIGATOR, CROCODILE, IGUANA, AND VENOMOUS LIZARD BITES

Venomous lizards, alligators and crocodiles, and iguanas are other reptiles that can cause clinically significant bites. Tetanus prophylaxis (see Table 181–2 on p. 1472) should be given.

Venomous lizards: These lizards include the following:

- Gila monster (*Heloderma suspectum*), present in the southwestern US and Mexico
- Beaded lizard (*H. horridum*) of Mexico

The complex venom of these lizards contains serotonin, arginine esterase, hyaluronidase, phospholipase A_2, and ≥ 1 salivary kallikreins but lacks neurotoxic components or coagulopathic enzymes. Bites are rarely fatal. Varanids (eg, Komodo dragon [*Varanus komodoensis*], crocodile monitor lizard [*Varanus salvadorii*]) are also venomous and pose little risk to humans. When venomous lizards bite, they clamp on firmly and chew the venom into the person.

Symptoms and signs include intense pain, swelling, ecchymosis, lymphangitis, and lymphadenopathy. Systemic manifestations, including weakness, sweating, thirst, headache, and tinnitus, may develop in moderate or severe cases. Cardiovascular collapse occurs rarely. The clinical course is similar to that of a minimal to moderate envenomation by a larger species of rattlesnake (see p. 2947).

Treatment in the field involves removing the lizard's jaws by using pliers, applying a flame to the lizard's chin, or immersing the animal entirely underwater. In a hospital, treatment is supportive and similar to that for pit viper envenomation; no antivenom is available. The wound should be probed with a small needle for broken or shed teeth and then cleaned. If the wound is deep, an x-ray can be done to rule out a retained foreign body or bone fracture. Prophylactic antibiotics are usually not recommended.

Iguanas: Bites and claw injuries are becoming more frequent as more iguanas are kept as pets. Wounds are superficial, and treatment is local. Soft-tissue infection is uncommon, but when infection occurs, *Salmonella* is a common cause; infection can be treated with a fluoroquinolone. A secondary but growing concern is infection with *Serratia marcescens*, which is usually sensitive to trimethoprim/sulfamethoxazole.

Alligators and crocodiles: Bites usually result from handling; however, rarely, native encounters occur. Bites are not venomous, are notable for a high frequency of soft-tissue infections by *Aeromonas* sp (usually *Aeromonas hydrophila*), and are generally treated as major trauma.

Wounds should be irrigated and debrided; then delayed primary closure can be done or the wounds allowed to heal by secondary intention. Optimal antibiotic coverage may include trimethoprim/sulfamethoxazole, a fluoroquinolone, a 3rd-generation cephalosporin, an aminoglycoside, or a combination. Additionally, patients can be treated preventively with clindamycin and trimethoprim/sulfamethoxazole (first choice) or tetracycline.

SPIDER BITES

Almost all of the 40,000 species of spiders are venomous. However, the fangs of most species are too short or too fragile to penetrate the skin. Serious systemic reactions most frequently occur with bites from

- Brown spiders: Violin, fiddleback, brown recluse (*Loxosceles* sp)
- Widow spiders: Black widow (*Latrodectus* sp), brown widow (*L. geometricus*)

Brown spiders are present in the Midwest and south central US, not in the coastal and Canadian border states, except when imported through clothing or luggage. Black widow spiders are present throughout the US. Distribution of the brown widow recently spread from Florida to all of the Gulf Coast states. Several other venomous spider species (eg, *Pamphobeteus*, *Cupiennius*, *Phoneutria*) are not native to the US but may be imported on produce or other materials or through commercial trade in spiders as novelty pets. Spider bites cause < 3 deaths/yr in the US, usually in children.

Only a few spider venoms have been studied in detail. Of greatest significance are those having

- Necrotizing venom components (in brown and some house spiders)
- Neurotoxic venom components (in widow spiders)

Sphingomyelinase D is the protein component that seems to be responsible for most of the tissue destruction and hemolysis caused by brown spider envenomations. The most toxic component of widow spider venom seems to be a peptide, alpha-latrotoxin, that affects neuromuscular transmission.

Symptoms and Signs

Brown spider bites are most common in the US. Some bites are painless initially, but pain, which can be severe and involve the entire extremity, develops within 30 to 60 min in all cases. The bite area becomes erythematous and ecchymotic and may be pruritic. Generalized pruritus may also be present. A central bleb forms at the bite site, often surrounded by an irregular ecchymotic area (bull's eye lesion). The lesion may mimic pyoderma gangrenosum. The central bleb becomes larger, fills with blood, ruptures, and leaves an ulcer. A black eschar forms over the ulcer and eventually sloughs (see Plate 95).

Most bites leave minimal residual scarring but some can leave a large tissue defect, which may involve muscle. Loxoscelism, a venom-induced systemic syndrome, may not be detected until 24 to 72 h after the bite and is uncommon but more prevalent in children and adolescents. Systemic effects (eg, fever, chills, nausea, vomiting, arthralgias, myalgias, generalized rash, seizures, hypotension, disseminated intravascular coagulation, thrombocytopenia, hemolysis, renal failure) are responsible for all reported fatalities.

Widow spider bites usually cause an immediate, sharp, stinging sensation. The pain may be described as dull and numbing and may be disproportionate to the clinical signs. Within 1 h after envenomation, there may be progression to persistent local pain, diaphoresis, erythema, and piloerection at the bite site. Sometimes remote and/or systemic symptoms develop.

Widow spider envenomations are graded as mild, moderate, or severe.

- Mild: Pain restricted to the bite site, normal vital signs
- Moderate: Diaphoresis and piloerection in the area of the bite, cramping pain in large muscle groups of the trunk, normal vital signs

- Severe (also called latrodectism): Diaphoresis at a remote site; intense generalized cramping pain in large muscle groups of the trunk; hypertension and tachycardia; often headache, nausea, and vomiting.

Latrodectism, a systemic syndrome caused by neurotoxic venom components of widow spider bites, manifests as restlessness, anxiety, sweating, headache, dizziness, nausea, vomiting, hypertension, salivation, weakness, diffuse erythematous rash, pruritus, ptosis, eyelid and extremity edema, respiratory distress, increased skin temperature over the affected area, and cramping pain and muscular rigidity in the abdomen, shoulders, chest, and back. Abdominal pain may be severe and mimic acute surgical abdomen, rabies, or tetanus. Symptoms tend to resolve over 1 to 3 days, but residual spasms, paresthesias, agitation, and weakness can last weeks to months.

Tarantula bites are extremely rare and nonvenomous with North or South American ("new world") tarantulas. However, agitation of the spider may cause it to throw needle-like hairs. The hairs act as foreign bodies in skin or eyes and can trigger mast cell degranulation and an anaphylactoid reaction (eg, urticaria, angioedema, bronchospasm, hypotension) in sensitized people, usually pet owners who handle the spider daily. Tarantula species native to non-American continents ("old-world" tarantulas) are occasionally kept as pets. They are more aggressive than new world tarantulas, lack needle-like hairs, and can be venomous.

Diagnosis

- Clinical evaluation
- Careful consideration of alternative diagnoses

Spider bites are often falsely suspected by patients. Diagnosis is typically suspected based on history and physical signs, but confirmation is rare because it requires witnessed biting, identification of the spider (the spider is rarely recovered intact), and exclusion of other causes.

In nonendemic areas, a brown spider bite should not be diagnosed without identifying the spider. Many patients incorrectly attribute much more common methicillin-resistant *Staphylococcus aureus* (MRSA) skin infections to brown recluse spider bites. Such infections should be excluded, as should other conditions that mimic spider bites (see Table 352–4). Severe cases of latrodectism should be distinguished from acute abdomen, rabies, or tetanus.

Spiders are identified by location and markings. Widow spiders live outdoors in protected spaces (eg, rock piles, firewood cords, hay bales, outhouses) and have a red or orange hourglass marking on the ventral abdomen. Brown spiders live indoors or in protected spaces (eg, in barns, attics, and wood piles; behind furniture; under baseboards) and have a fiddle- or violin-like marking on the dorsal cephalothorax, ranging from the eyes to the abdomen. This marking may be difficult to recognize even in the intact spider.

Treatment

- Routine wound care
- Delayed excision for necrotic brown spider bites
- Parenteral opioids, benzodiazepines, and antivenom for severe and sometimes moderate widow spider bites

Treatment common to all spider bites includes wound cleaning, ice to reduce pain, extremity elevation, tetanus prophylaxis (see Table 181–2 on p. 1472), and observation. Most local reactions respond to these measures alone.

Table 352–4. DISORDERS THAT MIMIC SPIDER BITES

CATEGORY	EXAMPLES
Insect bites	Ant bites Bedbug bites Flea bites Fly bites Reduviid (eg, assassin, wheel, kissing) bug bites
Other arachnid bites	Mite bites Tick bites
Skin disorders	Erythema chronicum migrans Erythema nodosum Leukocytoclastic vasculitis Sporotrichosis Toxic epidermal necrolysis
Infections	Chronic herpes simplex Cutaneous anthrax Disseminated gonococcal infection Methicillin-resistant *Staphylococcus aureus* Septic emboli in endocarditis or IV drug use
Trauma	Self-inflicted injuries Subcutaneous drug injection

For **brown spider bites,** limiting intervention to standard wound care and measures that minimize infection risk is usually most prudent:

- Ulcerating lesions should be cleaned daily and debrided as needed; topical antibiotic ointment (eg, polymyxin/bacitracin/neomycin) may be used.
- Urticarial lesions can be treated with antihistamines, topical corticosteroids, or both.
- Necrotic lesions caused by brown recluse spider bites should be cleaned and bandaged. Surgical excision, if necessary, should be delayed until the area of necrosis is fully demarcated, a process that may take weeks.

No intervention has been proved to reduce morbidity or improve outcome after a brown spider bite. Commonly touted or poorly studied treatment options are controversial or potentially harmful. Dapsone (eg, 100 mg po once/day until inflammation subsides) is often considered for ulcers > 2 cm, but its benefit is unproved and dose-related hemolysis almost always develops; agranulocytosis, aplastic anemia, and methemoglobinemia have been documented. Tetracycline has been suggested to prevent the dermonecrosis caused by brown spider envenomation but efficacy is unproven. Corticosteroids, colchicine, nitroglycerin, electric shock therapy, and surgical excision are of no value.

For **widow spider bites,** medical attention is necessary if symptoms are moderate or severe; initial treatment is parenteral opioids and benzodiazepines. Myalgias and muscle spasms resulting from widow spider bites respond poorly to muscle relaxants and calcium salts.

Symptomatic envenomation is initially treated supportively. Equine-derived antivenom is available, and a new F(ab)2 antivenom is currently being studied. Because death from widow spider envenomation is rare, antivenom treatment has historically been reserved for patients at extremes of age and those with comorbid medical conditions. But because symptoms may persist for weeks or months, antivenom is being used more broadly (eg, if envenomation is severe or sometimes moderate). Antivenom is most effective when used early, but can be effective up to 36 h after the bite. Clinical response is usually dramatic. The dose for children and adults is 1 vial (6000 units) IV in 50 mL of normal saline, usually over 15 min. Although the manufacturer recommends skin testing before administering the antivenom, testing does not always predict adverse reactions such as acute anaphylaxis and is not often done.

All **tarantula bites** are treated supportively.

KEY POINTS

- Brown spiders (eg, violin, fiddleback, brown recluse—*Loxosceles* sp) are present in the Midwest and south central US, not in the coastal and Canadian border states.
- Widow spiders (eg, black widow—*Latrodectus* sp) are present throughout the US.
- Brown spider bites tend to cause pain (sometimes delayed for 30 to 60 min), erythema, ecchymosis, and bleb formation, sometimes with surrounding ulceration.
- Widow spider bites cause immediate pain and sometimes regional or generalized manifestations such as muscle cramping, diaphoresis, hypertension and tachycardia, and weakness.
- Diagnose spider bites (often falsely suspected by patients) clinically.
- For brown spider bites, use wound care, local symptomatic measures, and sometimes delayed excision.
- For widow spider bites, use wound care, local symptomatic measures, and sometimes parenteral opioids, benzodiazepines, and antivenom.

TICK BITES

Most tick bites in the US are from various species of Ixodidae, which attach and feed for several days if not removed. Disease transmission is the main concern and becomes more likely if ticks are attached for a longer duration.

Tick bites most often occur in spring and summer and are painless. The vast majority are uncomplicated and do not transmit disease. However, they often cause a red papule at the bite site and may induce hypersensitivity or granulomatous foreign body reactions. The bites of *Ornithodoros coriaceus* ticks (pajaroello) cause local vesiculation, pustulation with rupture, ulceration, and eschar, with varying degrees of local swelling and pain. Similar reactions have resulted from bites of other ticks.

Diagnosis

Diagnosis is by clinical evaluation and identification of the attached tick.

Treatment

- Tick removal with blunt, curved forceps
- Sometimes prophylactic doxycycline

Tick removal should occur as soon as possible to reduce the cutaneous immune response and the likelihood of disease transmission. If the patient presents with the tick still attached, the best method of extracting the tick and all of its mouth parts from the skin is by using a blunt forceps with medium-sized, curved tips. The forceps should be placed parallel to the skin to grasp the tick's mouth parts firmly as close to the skin as possible. Care should be taken to avoid puncturing the patient's skin and the tick's body. The forceps should be pulled slowly and steadily, directly away from the skin without twisting. Curved-tip forceps are best because the outer curve can be laid against the skin while the handle remains far enough from the skin to grasp easily.

Tick mouth parts that remain in the skin and are readily visible should be removed carefully. However, if the presence of mouth parts is questionable, attempts at surgical removal may cause more tissue trauma than would occur if the parts are left in the skin; leaving mouth parts in the skin does not affect disease transmission and, at most, prolongs irritation. Other methods of tick removal, such as burning it with a match (which can damage the patient's tissues) or covering it with petroleum jelly (which is ineffective), are not recommended.

After tick removal, an antiseptic should be applied. If local swelling and discoloration are present, an oral antihistamine may be helpful. Although rarely practical, the tick may be saved for laboratory analysis to check for etiologic agents of tick-borne disease in the geographic area where the patient acquired the tick.

Pajaroello tick lesions should be cleaned, soaked in 1:20 Burow's solution, and debrided when necessary. Corticosteroids are helpful in severe cases. Infections are common during the ulcer stage but rarely require more than local antiseptic measures.

Lyme disease prophylaxis: A single dose of doxycycline (200 mg for adults and 4 mg/kg to a maximum of 200 mg for children ≥ 8 yr) should be considered when all of the following criteria are met:

- The tick is an adult or nymphal *Ixodes scapularis*.
- The tick is estimated to have been attached for ≥ 36 h based on degree of engorgement or certainty about time of exposure.
- Prophylaxis can be started within 72 h after the tick was removed.
- The local rate of infection of ticks with *Borrelia burgdorferi* is ≥ 20%.
- Doxycycline is not contraindicated.

Some experts recommend a longer course of doxycycline (100 mg po bid for 10 to 20 days) to ensure eradication (see also p. 1715).

TICK PARALYSIS

Tick paralysis is a rare, ascending, flaccid paralysis that occurs when toxin-secreting Ixodidae ticks bite and remain attached for several days.

In North America, some species of *Dermacentor* and *Amblyomma* cause tick paralysis due to a neurotoxin secreted in tick saliva. The toxin is not present in tick saliva during early stages of feeding, so paralysis occurs only when a tick has fed for several days or more. A single tick can cause paralysis, especially if it is attached to the back of the skull or near the spine.

Symptoms and signs include anorexia, lethargy, muscle weakness, impaired coordination, nystagmus, and ascending flaccid paralysis. Bulbar or respiratory paralysis may develop.

Diagnosis is based on clinical findings. Tick paralysis should be considered in North American patients with acute ascending flaccid paralysis or bulbar paralysis; ticks should be sought over the entire body surface and be removed. Differential diagnosis includes Guillain-Barré syndrome, botulism, myasthenia gravis, hypokalemia, and spinal cord tumor.

Treatment

- Removal of ticks
- Supportive care

Tick paralysis can be fatal, but the paralysis is reversible with rapid removal of the tick or ticks. Paralysis usually begins to resolve in a few hours after tick removal, but paralysis may progress for 24 to 48 h after tick removal. If breathing is impaired, O_2 therapy or respiratory assistance may be needed.

OTHER ARTHROPOD BITES

The more common biting non-tick arthropods in the US include

- Sand flies
- Horseflies
- Deerflies
- Blackflies
- Stable flies
- Mosquitoes
- Fleas
- Kissing bugs
- Lice
- Bedbugs
- Wheel bugs
- Certain water bugs

All of these arthropods, except wheel bugs and water bugs, also suck blood, but none is venomous.

Disease transmission is the main concern related to mosquito bites. Mosquitoes may transmit

- Chikungunya virus, dengue
- Some types of encephalitis
- Malaria
- Yellow fever
- Zika virus

Arthropod saliva composition varies considerably, and the lesions caused by bites vary from small papules to large ulcers with swelling and acute pain. Dermatitis may also occur. Most serious consequences result from secondary infection or hypersensitivity reactions, which can be fatal in sensitized people. Flea allergens may trigger respiratory allergy even without a bite in some people.

The location and pattern of wheals and lesions are sometimes diagnostic of the bite source. For example, blackfly bites are usually on the neck, ears, and face; flea bites may be numerous, mostly on the feet and legs; and bedbug bites often occur in linear patterns, most commonly on the torso.

Treatment

- Routine wound care
- For itching, a topical antihistamine or corticosteroid

The bite should be cleaned, and an antihistamine or corticosteroid cream or ointment should be applied for itching. Severe hypersensitivity reactions should be treated.

353 Burns

Burns are injuries of skin or other tissue caused by thermal, radiation, chemical, or electrical contact. Burns are classified by depth (superficial and deep partial-thickness, and full-thickness) and percentage of total body surface area (TBSA) involved. Complications and associated problems include hypovolemic shock, inhalation injury, infection, scarring, and contractures. Patients with large burns (> 20% TBSA) require fluid resuscitation. Treatments for burn wounds includes topical antibacterials, regular cleaning, elevation, and sometimes skin grafting. Intensive rehabilitation, consisting of range-of-motion exercises and splinting, is often necessary.

Burns cause about 3000 deaths/yr in the US and about 2 million physician visits.

Etiology

Thermal burns may result from any external heat source (flame, hot liquids, hot solid objects, or, occasionally, steam). Fires may also result in toxic smoke inhalation.

PEARLS & PITFALLS

- Assess the airway and prepare for intubation if patients have respiratory symptoms, carbonaceous sputum, perioral burns, singed nasal hairs, or were confined in a burning environment.

Radiation burns most commonly result from prolonged exposure to solar ultraviolet radiation (sunburn—see p. 1079) but may result from prolonged or intense exposure to other sources of ultraviolet radiation (eg, tanning beds) or from exposure to sources of x-ray or other nonsolar radiation (see p. 3090).

Chemical burns may result from strong acids, strong alkalis (eg, lye, cement), phenols, cresols, mustard gas, phosphorus, and certain petroleum products (eg, gasoline, paint thinner). Skin and deeper tissue necrosis caused by these agents may progress over several hours.

Electrical burns (see p. 2965) result from heat generation and electroporation of cell membranes associated with massive current of electrons. Electrical burns often cause extensive deep tissue damage to electrically conductive tissues, such as muscles, nerves, and blood vessels, despite minimal apparent cutaneous injury.

Events associated with a burn (eg, jumping from a burning building, being struck by debris, motor vehicle crash) may cause other injuries. Abuse should be considered in young children and elderly patients with burns.

Smoke inhalation: Burns and smoke inhalation often occur together but may occur separately. When smoke is inhaled, toxic products of combustion injure airway tissues. Hot smoke usually burns only the pharynx because the incoming gas cools quickly. An exception is steam, which carries much more heat energy than smoke and thus can also burn the lower airways (below the glottis). Many toxic chemicals produced in routine house fires (eg, hydrogen chloride, phosgene, sulfur dioxide, toxic aldehydes, ammonia) cause chemical burns. Some toxic products of combustion, such as carbon monoxide (p. 3060) or cyanide, impair cellular respiration systemically.

Upper airway injury usually causes symptoms within minutes but occasionally over several hours; upper airway edema may cause stridor. Lower airway injury may also occur with upper airway injury and usually causes symptoms (eg, oxygenation problems highlighted by increasing oxygen requirements or decreases in lung compliance) 24 h or later.

Smoke inhalation is suspected in patients with respiratory symptoms, a history of confinement in a burning environment, or carbonaceous sputum. Perioral burns and singed nasal hair may also be clues.

Diagnosis of upper airway injury is by endoscopy (laryngoscopy or bronchoscopy) that is adequate to see the upper airways and trachea and shows edema, tissue damage, or soot in the airways; however, injury occasionally develops after an initial normal study. Endoscopy is done as soon as possible, usually with a flexible fiberoptic scope, typically after or simultaneously with endotracheal intubation in patients with significant findings. Diagnosis of lower airway injury is by chest x-ray and oximetry or ABGs; abnormalities may develop early or only days later. Cyanide and carbon monoxide toxicity should be considered; carboxyhemoglobin levels are measured in patients with significant smoke inhalation.

All patients at risk of smoke inhalation injury are given 100% oxygen by face mask initially. Patients with airway obstruction or respiratory distress require endotracheal intubation or another artificial airway and mechanical ventilation (see p. 561). Patients with edema or significant soot in the upper airways require intubation as soon as possible because the airway becomes more difficult to intubate as edema increases. Bronchoscopy is usually done at the same time as intubation. Patients with lower airway injury may require supplemental oxygen, bronchodilators, and other supportive measures.

Pathophysiology

Burns cause protein denaturation and thus coagulative necrosis. Around the coagulated tissue, platelets aggregate, vessels constrict, and marginally perfused tissue (known as the zone of stasis) can extend around the injury. In the zone of stasis, tissue is hyperemic and inflamed.

Damage to the normal epidermal barrier allows bacterial invasion and external fluid loss; damaged tissues often become edematous, further enhancing volume loss. Heat loss can be significant because thermoregulation of the damaged dermis is absent, particularly in wounds that are exposed.

Burn depth: First-degree burns are limited to the epidermis.

Partial-thickness (also called 2nd-degree) burns involve part of the dermis and can be superficial or deep.

Superficial partial-thickness burns involve the papillary (more superficial) dermis (see Plate 100). These burns heal within 1 to 2 wk, and scarring is usually minimal. Healing occurs from epidermal cells lining sweat gland ducts and hair follicles; these cells grow to the surface, then migrate across the surface to meet cells from neighboring glands and follicles.

Deep partial-thickness burns involve the deeper dermis and take ≥ 2 wk to heal. Healing occurs only from hair follicles, and scarring is common and may be severe.

Full-thickness (3rd-degree) burns extend through the entire dermis and into the underlying fat (see Plate 98). Healing occurs only from the periphery; these burns, unless small, require excision and skin grafting.

Complications

Burns cause both systemic and local complications. The major factors contributing to systemic complications are breakdown of skin integrity and fluid loss. Local complications include eschars and contractures and scarring.

Systemic: The greater the percentage of TBSA involved, the greater the risk of developing systemic complications. Risk factors for severe systemic complications and mortality include all of the following:

- Second- and third-degree burns of > 40% of TBSA
- Age > 60 yr or < 2 yr
- Presence of simultaneous major trauma or smoke inhalation

The most common systemic complications are hypovolemia and infection.

Hypovolemia, causing hypoperfusion of burned tissue and sometimes shock, can result from fluid losses due to burns that are deep or that involve large parts of the body surface; whole-body edema from escape of intravascular volume into the interstitium and cells also develops. Hypoperfusion of burned tissue also may result from direct damage to blood vessels or from vasoconstriction secondary to hypovolemia.

Infection, even in small burns, is a common cause of sepsis and mortality, as well as local complications. Impaired host defenses and devitalized tissue enhance bacterial invasion and growth. The most common pathogens are streptococci and staphylococci during the first few days and gram-negative bacteria after 5 to 7 days; however, flora are almost always mixed.

Metabolic abnormalities may include hypoalbuminemia that is partly due to hemodilution (secondary to replacement fluids) and partly due to protein loss into the extravascular space through damaged capillaries. Dilutional electrolyte deficiencies can develop; they include hypomagnesemia, hypophosphatemia, and hypokalemia. Metabolic acidosis may result from shock. Rhabdomyolysis or hemolysis can result from deep thermal or electrical burns of muscle or from muscle ischemia due to constricting eschars. Rhabdomyolysis causing myoglobinuria or hemolysis causing hemoglobinuria can lead to acute tubular necrosis and acute kidney injury.

Hypothermia may result from large volumes of cool IV fluids and extensive exposure of body surfaces to a cool emergency department environment, particularly in patients with extensive burns.

Ileus is common after extensive burns.

Local: Eschar is stiff, dead tissue caused by deep burns. A circumferential eschar, which completely encircles a limb (or sometimes the neck or torso), is potentially constricting. A constricting eschar limits tissue expansion in response to edema; instead, tissue pressure increases, eventually causing local ischemia. The ischemia threatens viability of limbs and digits distal to the eschar, and an eschar around the neck or thorax can compromise ventilation.

Scarring and contractures result from healing of deep burns. Depending on the extent of the scar, contracture deformities can appear at the joints. If the burn is located near joints (particularly in the hands), in the feet, or in the perineum, function can be severely impaired. Infection can increase scarring. Keloids form in some patients with burns, especially in patients with darker skin.

Symptoms and Signs

Wound symptoms and signs depend on burn depth:

- **First-degree burns:** These burns are red, blanch markedly and widely with light pressure, and are painful and tender. Vesicles or bullae do not develop.
- **Superficial partial-thickness burns:** These burns blanch with pressure and are painful and tender. Vesicles or bullae develop within 24 h. The bases of vesicles and bullae are pink and subsequently develop a fibrinous exudate.
- **Deep partial-thickness burns:** These burns may be white, red, or mottled red and white. They do not blanch and are less

painful and tender than more superficial burns. A pinprick is often interpreted as pressure rather than sharp. Vesicles or bullae may develop; these burns are usually dry.

- **Full-thickness burns:** These burns may be white and pliable, black and charred, brown and leathery, or bright red because of fixed Hb in the subdermal region. Pale full-thickness burns may simulate normal skin except the skin does not blanch to pressure. Full-thickness burns are usually anesthetic or hypoesthetic. Hairs can be pulled easily from their follicles. Vesicles and bullae usually do not develop. Sometimes features that differentiate full thickness from deep partial thickness burns take 24 to 48 hours to develop.

Diagnosis

- Clinical assessment of burn extent and depth
- Laboratory testing and chest x-ray in admitted patients

Location and depth of burned areas are recorded on a burn diagram. Burns with an appearance compatible with both deep partial-thickness and full-thickness are presumed to be full-thickness.

The percentage of TBSA involved is calculated; only partial-thickness and full-thickness burns are included in this calculation.[1] For adults, the percentage TBSA for parts of the body is estimated by the rule of nines (see Fig. 353–1); for smaller scattered burns, estimates can be based on the size of the patient's entire opened hand (not the palm only), which is about 1% of TBSA. Children have proportionally larger heads and smaller lower extremities, so the percentage TBSA is more accurately estimated using the Lund-Browder chart (see Fig. 353–1).

In hospitalized patients, Hb and Hct, serum electrolytes, BUN, creatinine, albumin, protein, phosphate, and ionized calcium should be measured. ECG, urinalysis for myoglobin, and a chest x-ray are also required. Myoglobinuria (suggesting hemolysis or rhabdomyolysis) is suggested by urine that is grossly dark or that tests positive for blood on dipstick in the absence of microscopic RBCs. These tests are repeated as needed. Muscle compartments are evaluated in patients with myoglobinuria.

Infection is suggested by wound exudate, impaired wound healing, or systemic evidence of infection (eg, feeding intolerance, decrease in platelet count, increase in serum glucose level). Fever and WBC count elevation are common in burns without infection and therefore are unreliable signs of developing sepsis. If the diagnosis is unclear, infection can be confirmed by biopsy; cultures from the wound surface or exudate are unreliable.

1. Kamolz LP, Parvizi D, Giretzlehner M, et al: Burn surface area calculation: what do we need in future. *Burns* 40(1):171–172, 2014. doi: 10.1016/j.burns.2013.07.021.

Treatment

- IV fluids for burns > 10% TBSA
- Wound cleaning, dressing, and serial assessment
- Supportive measures
- Transfer or referral of selected patients to burn centers
- Surgery and physical therapy for deep partial-thickness and full-thickness burns

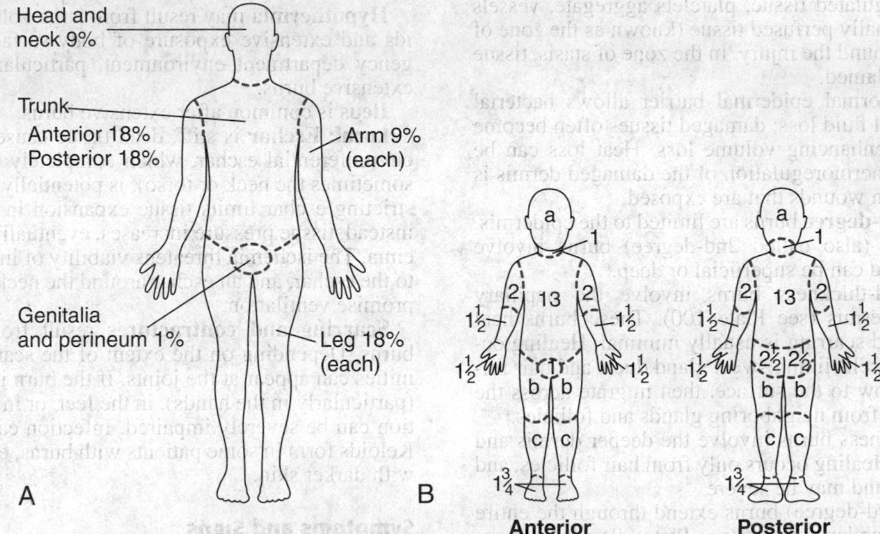

Relative percentage of body surface area (% BSA) affected by growth

Body Part	Age 0 yr	1 yr	5 yr	10 yr	15 yr
a = 1/2 of head	9 1/2	8 1/2	6 1/2	5 1/2	4 1/2
b = 1/2 of 1 thigh	2 3/4	3 1/4	4	4 1/4	4 1/2
c = 1/2 of 1 lower leg	2 1/2	2 1/2	2 3/4	3	3 1/4

Fig. 353–1. (A) Rule of nines (for adults) and (B) Lund-Browder chart (for children) for estimating extent of burns. (Redrawn from Artz CP, JA Moncrief: *The Treatment of Burns*, ed. 2. Philadelphia, WB Saunders Company, 1969; used with permission.)

Initial treatment: Treatment begins in the prehospital setting. The first priorities are the same as for any injured patient: ABC (airway, breathing, and circulation). An airway is provided, ventilation is supported, and possible associated smoke inhalation (see p. 2954) is treated with 100% oxygen. Ongoing burning is extinguished, and smoldering and hot material is removed. All clothing is removed. Chemicals, except powders, are flushed with water; powders should be brushed off before wetting. Burns caused by acids, alkalis, or organic compounds (eg, phenols, cresols, petrochemicals) are flushed with copious amounts of water continuing for at least 20 min after nothing of the original solution seems to remain.

Intravenous fluids: IV fluids are given to patients in shock or with burns > 10% TBSA. A 14- to 16-gauge venous cannula is placed in 1 or 2 peripheral veins through unburned skin if possible. Venous cutdown, which has a high risk of infection, is avoided.

Initial fluid volume is guided by treatment of clinically evident shock (see p. 572).[1] If shock is absent, fluid administration aims to replace the predicted deficit and supply maintenance fluids. The Parkland formula (4 mL/kg) × % TBSA burned (second-degree and third-degree burns) is used to estimate fluid volume needs in the first 24 h after the burn (not after presentation to the hospital) and determines the rate of IV fluid administration. Half the calculated amount is given over the first 8 h; the remainder is given over the next 16 h. Fluid is given as lactated Ringer's solution because large amounts of normal saline could result in hyperchloremic acidosis.

For example, in a 100-kg man with a 50% TBSA burn, fluid volume by the Parkland formula would be $4 \times 100 \times 50 = 20{,}000$ mL. Half of the volume, 10 L, is given in the first 8 h after injury as a constant infusion, and the remaining 10 L is given over the following 16 h. In practice, this formula is only a starting point, and infusion rates are adjusted based on clinical response. Urine output, typically measured with an indwelling catheter, is the usual indicator of clinical response; the goal is to maintain output between 30 and 50 mL/h in adults and between 0.5 and 1.0 mL/kg/h in children. When giving typical large volumes of fluid, it is also important to avoid fluid overload and consequent heart failure and compartment syndrome. Clinical parameters, including urine output and signs of shock or heart failure, are recorded at least hourly on a flow chart.

Some clinicians give colloid, usually albumin, after 12 h to patients who have larger burns, are very young or very old, or have heart disease and require large fluid volumes.

If urine output is inadequate despite administration of a large volume of crystalloid, consultation with a burn center is necessary. Such patients may respond to an infusion of colloid or other measures. Patients with inadequate urine output despite administration of a large volume of crystalloid are at risk of resuscitation complications including compartment syndromes of the abdomen and extremities.

For patients of any age with rhabdomyolysis, fluid should be given to maintain urine output between 0.5 and 1 mL/kg/h. Some authorities recommend alkalinizing the urine by adding 50 mEq $NaHCO_3$ (one 50-mL ampule of 8.4% solution) to a liter of IV fluid.

Initial wound care: After adequate analgesia, the wound is cleaned with soap and water, and all loose debris is removed. Water should be room temperature or warmer to avoid inducing hypothermia. Ruptured blisters, except for small ones on palms, fingers, and soles, are debrided. Unruptured blisters can sometimes be left intact, but should be treated by application of a topical antimicrobial. In patients who are to be transferred to a burn center, clean dry dressings can be applied (burn creams may interfere with burn wound assessment at the receiving facility), and patients are kept warm and relatively comfortable with IV opioids.

After the wound is cleaned and is assessed by the final treatment provider, burns can be treated topically. For shallow partial-thickness burns, topical treatment alone is usually adequate. All deep partial-thickness burns and full-thickness burns should ultimately be treated with excision and grafting, but in the interim, topical treatments are appropriate.

Topical treatment may be with antimicrobial salves (eg, 1% silver sulfadiazine), commercial dressings incorporating silver (eg, sustained-release nanocrystalline silver dressings), or biosynthetic wound dressings (also called artificial skin products). Topical salves must be changed daily, and silver sulfadiazine may induce transient leukopenia. Some (but not all) silver-impregnated dressings must be kept moist but can be changed as infrequently as every 7 days (to minimize pain associated with repeated wound care). Artificial skin products are not changed routinely but can result in underlying purulence necessitating removal, particularly when wounds are deep. Burned extremities should be elevated.

A tetanus toxoid booster (0.5 mL sc or IM) is given to patients with all but minor burns who have been previously fully vaccinated and who have not received a booster within the past 5 yr. Patients whose booster was more remote or who had not received a full vaccine series are given tetanus immune globulin 250 units IM and concomitant active vaccination (see p. 1472).

Escharotomy (incision of the eschar) of constricting eschars may be necessary to allow adequate expansion of the thorax or perfusion of an extremity. However, constricting eschars rarely threaten extremity viability during the first few hours, so if transfer to a burn center can occur within that time, escharotomy can typically be deferred until then.

Supportive measures: Hypothermia is treated (see p. 2961), and pain is relieved. Opioids (eg, morphine) should always be given IV, and large doses may be needed for adequate pain control. Treatment of electrolyte deficits may require supplemental calcium (Ca), magnesium (Mg), potassium (K), or phosphate (PO_4).

Nutritional support is indicated for patients with burns > 20% TBSA or preexisting undernutrition. Support with a feeding tube begins as soon as possible. Parenteral support is rarely necessary.

Hospitalization and referral: After initial treatment and stabilization, the need for hospitalization is assessed. Inpatient treatment, optimally at a burn center, is strongly suggested for

- Full-thickness burns > 1% TBSA
- Partial-thickness burns > 5% TBSA
- Burns of the hands, face, feet, or perineum (partial-thickness or deeper)

In addition, hospitalization may be necessary if

- Patients are < 2 yr or > 60 yr.
- Adherence to home care measures is likely to be poor or difficult (eg, if continuous elevation of the hands or feet, usually difficult at home, is required).

Many experts recommend that all burns, except for 1st-degree burns < 1% TBSA, be treated by experienced physicians and that brief inpatient care be strongly considered for all burns > 2% TBSA. Maintaining adequate analgesia and exercise can be difficult for many patients and caregivers.

Infection: Prophylactic systemic antibiotics are not given.

Initial empiric antibiotic treatment for apparent infection during the first 5 days should target staphylococci and streptococci (eg, with vancomycin for inpatients). Infections that develop after 5 days are treated with broad-spectrum antibiotics that are effective against gram-positive and gram-negative bacteria. Antibiotic selection is subsequently adjusted based on culture and sensitivity results.

Surgery: Surgery is indicated for burns that are not expected to heal within 2 wk, including most deep partial-thickness burns and all full-thickness burns. Eschars are removed as soon as possible, ideally within 3 days to prevent sepsis and facilitate early wound grafting, which shortens hospitalization and improves the functional result. If burns are extensive and life-threatening, the largest eschars are removed first to close as much burn area as early as possible.

After excision, grafting proceeds ideally using partial-thickness autografts (the patient's skin), which are permanent.[2] Autografts can be transplanted as sheets (solid pieces of skin) or meshed grafts (sheets of donor skin that are stretched to cover a larger area by making multiple, regularly spaced, small incisions). Meshed grafts are used in areas where appearance is less of a concern when burns are > 20% TBSA and donor skin is scarce. Meshed grafts heal with an uneven gridlike appearance, sometimes with excessive hypertrophic scarring.

When burns are > 40% TBSA and the supply of autograft material appears insufficient, an artificial dermal regeneration template can be used as temporary coverage.[2] Allografts (viable skin usually from cadaver donors) or xenografts (eg, pig skin) can also be used temporarily; they are rejected, sometimes within 10 to 14 days. Both types of temporary coverage must ultimately be replaced with autografts.

Fasciotomy is done when edema within a muscle compartment elevates compartment pressure > 30 mm Hg.

Physical and occupational therapy: Physical and occupational therapy are begun at admission to help minimize scarring and contractures, particularly for body surfaces with high skin tension and frequent movement (eg, face, hands), and to optimize function. Active and passive range-of-motion exercises become easier as the initial edema subsides; they are done once or twice daily. After grafting, exercises are usually suspended for 3 days, then resumed. Extremities affected by deep partial-thickness burns or full-thickness burns are splinted in functional positions as soon as possible and kept splinted continuously (except during exercise) until the graft has been placed, healing has occurred, or both.

Outpatient treatment: Outpatient treatment includes keeping burns clean and, to the extent possible, keeping the affected body part elevated. Dressings should be changed daily for burns treated with topical salves. The salve is applied and then covered with a dry nonadherent gauze dressing and compression wraps. Silver dressings should be changed every 3 to 7 days. Dressing change simply involves removing the older dressing and replacing it with new one. Biosynthetic wound dressings should not be changed in the absence of purulence. Biosynthetic dressings should simply be covered with dry gauze, which is changed daily.

Outpatient follow-up visits are scheduled as needed depending on burn severity (eg, for very minor burns, initial visit within 24 h, then subsequent visits every 5 to 7 days). Visits include debridement if indicated, reassessment of burn depth, and evaluation of the need for physical therapy and grafting. Patients should return earlier if they note signs of infection, such as increasing redness extending from the wound edges, increasing purulence and pain, or a change in the appearance of the wound with development of black or red spots. Should these signs occur, medical evaluation should ensue urgently. Outpatient treatment is acceptable for minor burn-wound cellulitis in healthy patients aged 2 to 60 yr; hospitalization is indicated for other infections.

1. Pham TN, Cancio CL, Gibran NS: American Burn Association practice guidelines burn shock resuscitation. *J Burn Care Res* J 29(1):257–266, 2008. doi: 10.1097/BCR.0b013e31815f3876.
2. Kagan RJ, Peck MD, Ahrenholz DH, et al: Surgical management of the burn wound and use of skin substitutes: an expert panel white paper. *J Burn Care Res* 34:e60–79. doi: 10.1097/BCR.0b013e31827039a6.

KEY POINTS

- Clues to burn depth include presence of vesicles or bullae (suggesting a partial-thickness burn); and decreased sensation, dry leathery eschar, hypoesthesia, and ability to easily pull hairs (suggesting a full-thickness burn).
- If burns are > 10% TBSA, give IV lactated Ringer's solution at an initial rate guided by the Parkland formula (4 mL × wgt (kg) × %TBSA burned during the 1st 24 h after the burn) and adjusted based on hourly urine output.
- For eschars that are circumferential or constricting, consider escharotomy.
- Supportive measures include adequate analgesia and, if burns are > 20% TBSA, early nutritional support.
- Strongly consider hospitalization if burns involve the hands, feet, or perineum (partial-thickness or deeper); are > 5% TBSA (partial-thickness or deeper); are > 1% TBSA (full-thickness); or if patients are > 60 or < 2 yr or are unlikely to fully adhere to home care measures.
- Treat surgically if an eschar is present, compartmental pressure is > 30 mm Hg, or, usually, if burns are full or deep partial-thickness.
- For infections, apply topical antimicrobials (for prevention); routinely inspect burns (for early diagnosis); and use systemic antibiotics, change topical treatment as needed, and occasionally excise the infected area (for treatment).
- Begin physical and occupational therapy early to minimize scarring and contractures.

354 Cold Injury

Exposure to cold may cause decreased body temperature (hypothermia) and focal soft-tissue injury.

- Tissue injury without freezing includes frostnip, immersion foot, and chilblains.
- Tissue injury with freezing is frostbite.

Treatment is rewarming and selective, usually delayed, surgical treatment for injured tissues.

Susceptibility to all cold injury is increased by exhaustion, undernutrition, dehydration, hypoxia, impaired cardiovascular function, and contact with moisture or metal.

Prevention

Prevention is crucial. Several layers of warm clothing and protection against moisture and wind are important even when the weather does not seem to threaten cold injury. Clothing that remains insulating when wet (eg, made of wool or polypropylene) should be worn. Gloves and socks should be kept as dry as possible; insulated boots that do not impede circulation should be worn in very cold weather. A warm head covering is also important.

Consuming ample fluids and food helps sustain metabolic heat production.

Paying attention to when body parts become cold or numb and immediately warming them may prevent cold injury.

FROSTBITE

Frostbite is injury due to freezing of tissue. Initial manifestations may be deceptively benign. Skin may appear white or blistered and is numb; rewarming causes substantial pain. Gangrene may develop. Severely damaged tissue may autoamputate. Treatment is rewarming in warm (40 to 42° C) water and local care. Surgical amputation is occasionally necessary, but a decision, often guided by imaging results, should usually be delayed until after definitive demarcation of necrotic tissue.

Frostbite usually occurs in extreme cold, especially at high altitude, and is aggravated by hypothermia. Distal extremities and exposed skin are affected most often (see Plate 97).

Ice crystals form within or between tissue cells, essentially freezing the tissue and causing cell death. Adjacent unfrozen areas are at risk because local vasoconstriction and thrombosis can cause endothelial and ischemic damage. With reperfusion during rewarming, inflammatory cytokines (eg, thromboxanes, prostaglandins) are released, exacerbating tissue injury. Depth of tissue loss depends on duration and depth of freezing.

Symptoms and Signs

The affected area is cold, hard, white, and numb. When warmed, the area becomes blotchy red, swollen, and painful. Blisters form within 4 to 6 h, but the full extent of injury may not be apparent for several days.

- Blisters filled with clear serum indicate superficial damage; superficial damage heals without residual tissue loss.
- Blood-filled, proximal blisters indicate deep damage and likely tissue loss.

Freezing of deep tissue causes dry gangrene with a hard black carapace over healthy tissue. Wet gangrene, which is gray, edematous, and soft, is less common. Wet gangrene is characterized by infection, but dry gangrene is less likely to become infected.

Severely damaged tissue may autoamputate. Compartment syndrome may develop. All degrees of frostbite may cause long-term neuropathic symptoms: sensitivity to cold, excessive sweating, faulty nail growth, and numbness (symptoms resembling those of complex regional pain syndrome), although any relationship is speculative.

Diagnosis

- Clinical evaluation

Diagnosis is based on clinical findings. However, because many of the early characteristics of frostbite (eg, coldness, numbness, white or red color, blisters) are also characteristic of nonfreezing cold injuries, differentiation of frostbite may require repeated observation until more specific characteristics (eg, black carapace, gangrene) develop.

Treatment

- Rewarming in warm (40 to 42° C) water
- Supportive measures
- Local wound care
- Sometimes delayed surgery

Prehospital care: In the field, frostbitten extremities should be rewarmed rapidly by totally immersing the affected area in water that is tolerably warm to the touch (40 to 42° C, ideally about 40.5° C). Because the area is numb, rewarming with an uncontrolled dry heat source (eg, fire, heating pad) risks burns. Rubbing may further damage tissue and is avoided.

The longer an area remains frozen, the greater the ultimate damage may be. However, thawing the feet is inadvisable if a patient must walk any distance to receive care because thawed tissue is particularly sensitive to the trauma of walking and, if refrozen, will be more severely damaged than if left frozen. If thawing must be delayed, the frozen area is gently cleaned, dried, and protected in sterile compresses. Patients are given analgesics, if available, and the whole body is kept warm.

Acute care: Once the patient is in the hospital, core temperature is stabilized and extremities are rapidly rewarmed in large containers of circulating water kept at about 40.5° C; 15 to 30 min is usually adequate. Thawing is often mistakenly ended prematurely because pain may be severe during rewarming. Parenteral analgesics, including opioids, may be used. Patients are encouraged to move the affected part gently during thawing. Large, clear blisters are left intact or aspirated using sterile technique. Hemorrhagic blisters are left intact to avoid secondary desiccation of deep dermal layers. Broken vesicles are debrided. If there is no perfusion after thawing, the administration of papaverine (a vasodilator) followed by intra-arterial thrombolytic (fibrinolytic) therapy may be considered.

Anti-inflammatory measures (eg, topical aloe vera q 6 h, ibuprofen 400 mg po q 8 h, ketorolac 30 to 60 mg IV) probably help. Affected areas are left open to warm air, and extremities are elevated to decrease edema. Anticoagulants, IV low molecular weight dextran, and intra-arterial vasodilators (eg, reserpine, tolazoline) have no proven clinical benefit. Phenoxybenzamine, a long-acting alpha-blocker, at a dosage of 10 to 60 mg po once/day may theoretically decrease vasospasm and improve blood flow.

Preventing infection is fundamental; streptococcal prophylaxis (eg, with penicillin) is sometimes provided. If wet gangrene is present, broad-spectrum antibiotics are used. Tetanus toxoid is given if vaccination is not up to date. If tissue damage is severe, tissue pressure is monitored.

Ongoing care: Adequate nutrition is important to sustain metabolic heat production.

Imaging tests (eg, radionuclide scanning, MRI, microwave thermography, laser-Doppler flowmetry) can help assess circulation, determine tissue viability, and thus guide treatment. MRI and particularly magnetic resonance angiography may establish the line of demarcation before clinical demarcation and thus make earlier surgical debridement or amputation possible. However, whether earlier surgery improves long-term outcome is unclear. Usually, surgery is delayed as long as possible because the black carapace is often shed, leaving viable tissue. Patients with severe frostbite are warned that many weeks of observation may be required before demarcation and the extent of tissue loss become apparent.

Whirlpool baths at 37° C 3 times/day followed by gentle drying, rest, and time are the best long-term management. No totally effective treatment for the long-lasting symptoms of frostbite (eg, numbness, hypersensitivity to cold) is known, although chemical or surgical sympathectomy may be useful for late neuropathic symptoms.

KEY POINTS

- Depth of injury is difficult to recognize initially, although blood-filled blisters indicate deeper damage.
- Thaw frostbitten tissue as soon as possible using water that is tolerably warm to the touch (40 to 42° C); analgesia is usually required.
- Avoid thawing and refreezing.
- Keep affected areas uncovered, clean, dry, and elevated.
- Black tissue may represent a black carapace that will be shed or gangrene that will require amputation; surgery may be delayed until the distinction is clear.
- Neuropathic symptoms (eg, sensitivity to cold, numbness) may persist indefinitely.

HYPOTHERMIA

Hypothermia is a core body temperature < 35° C. Symptoms progress from shivering and lethargy to confusion, coma, and death. Mild hypothermia requires a warm environment and insulating blankets (passive rewarming). Severe hypothermia requires active rewarming of the body surface (eg, with forced-air warming systems, radiant sources) and core (eg, inhalation, heated infusion and lavage, extracorporeal blood rewarming).

Primary hypothermia causes about 600 deaths each year in the US. Hypothermia also has a significant and underrecognized effect on mortality risk in cardiovascular and neurologic disorders.

Etiology

Hypothermia results when body heat loss exceeds body heat production. Hypothermia is most common during cold weather or immersion in cold water, but it may occur in warm climates when people lie immobile on a cool surface (eg, when they are intoxicated) or after very prolonged immersion in swimming-temperature water (eg, 20 to 24° C). Wet clothing and wind increase risk of hypothermia.

Conditions that cause loss of consciousness, immobility, or both (eg, trauma, hypoglycemia, seizure disorders, stroke, drug or alcohol intoxication) are common predisposing factors. The elderly and the very young also are at high risk:

- The elderly often have diminished temperature sensation and impaired mobility and communication, resulting in a tendency to remain in an overly cool environment. These impairments, combined with diminished subcutaneous fat, contribute to hypothermia in the elderly—sometimes even indoors in cool rooms.
- The very young have similarly diminished mobility and communication and have an increased surface area/mass ratio, which enhances heat loss. Intoxicated people who lose consciousness in a cold environment are likely to become hypothermic.

Pathophysiology

Hypothermia slows all physiologic functions, including cardiovascular and respiratory systems, nerve conduction, mental acuity, neuromuscular reaction time, and metabolic rate. Thermoregulation ceases below about 30° C; the body must then depend on an external heat source for rewarming.

Renal cell dysfunction and decreased levels of vasopressin (ADH) lead to production of a large volume of dilute urine (cold diuresis). Diuresis plus fluid leakage into the interstitial tissues causes hypovolemia. Vasoconstriction, which occurs with hypothermia, may mask hypovolemia, which then manifests as sudden shock or cardiac arrest during rewarming (rewarming collapse) when peripheral vasculature dilates.

PEARLS & PITFALLS

- With moderate to severe hypothermia, core temperature must be stabilized before rewarming the extremities, to prevent sudden cardiovascular collapse (rewarming collapse) when peripheral vasculature dilates.

Immersion in cold water can trigger the diving reflex, which involves reflex vasoconstriction in visceral muscles; blood is shunted to essential organs (eg, heart, brain). The reflex is most pronounced in small children and may help protect them. Also, hypothermia due to total immersion in near-freezing water may protect the brain from hypoxia by decreasing metabolic demands. The decreased demand probably accounts for the occasional survival after prolonged cardiac arrest due to extreme hypothermia.

Symptoms and Signs

Intense shivering occurs initially, but it ceases below about 31° C, allowing body temperature to drop more precipitously. CNS dysfunction progresses as body temperature decreases; people do not sense the cold. Lethargy and clumsiness are followed by confusion, irritability, sometimes hallucinations, and eventually coma. Pupils may become unreactive. Respirations and heartbeat slow and ultimately cease. Initially, sinus bradycardia is followed by slow atrial fibrillation; the terminal rhythm is ventricular fibrillation or asystole.

Diagnosis

- Core temperature measurement
- Consideration of intoxication, myxedema, sepsis, hypoglycemia, and trauma

Diagnosis is by core temperature, not oral temperature. Electronic thermometers are preferred; many standard mercury thermometers have a lower limit of 34° C. Rectal and esophageal probes are most accurate.

Laboratory tests include CBC, glucose (including bedside measurement), electrolytes, BUN, creatinine, and ABGs. ABGs are not corrected for low temperature. ECG may show J (Osborn) waves (see Fig. 354–1) and interval prolongation (PR, QRS, QT). Causes are sought. If the cause is unclear, alcohol level is measured, and drug screening and thyroid function tests are done. Sepsis and occult head or skeletal trauma must be considered.

Prognosis

Patients who have been immersed in icy water for 1 h or (rarely) longer have sometimes been successfully rewarmed without permanent brain damage (see p. 2963), even when core temperatures were very low or when pupils were unreactive. Outcome is difficult to predict and cannot be based on the Glasgow Coma Scale. Grave prognostic markers include

- Evidence of cell lysis (hyperkalemia > 10 mEq/L)
- Intravascular thrombosis (fibrinogen < 50 mg/dL)
- A nonperfusing cardiac rhythm (ventricular fibrillation or asystole)

For a given degree and duration of hypothermia, children are more likely to recover than adults.

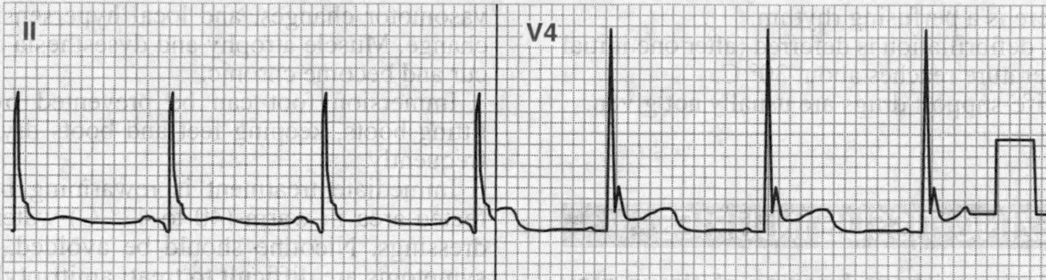

Fig. 354–1. Abnormal ECG showing J (Osborn) waves (V4).

Treatment

- Drying and insulation
- Fluid resuscitation
- Active rewarming unless hypothermia is mild, accidental, and uncomplicated

The first priority is to prevent further heat loss by removing wet clothing and insulating the patient. Subsequent measures depend on how severe hypothermia is and whether cardiovascular instability or cardiac arrest is present. Returning patients to a normal temperature is less urgent in hypothermia than in severe hyperthermia. For stable patients, elevation of core temperature by 1° C/h is acceptable.

Fluid resuscitation is essential for hypovolemia. Patients are given 1 to 2 L of 0.9% saline solution (20 mL/kg for children) IV; if possible, the solution is heated to 40 to 42° C. More fluid is given as needed to maintain perfusion.

Passive rewarming: In **mild hypothermia** (temperature 32.2 to 35° C) with intact thermoregulation (indicated by shivering), insulation with heated blankets and warm fluids to drink are adequate.

Active rewarming: Active rewarming is required if patients have temperature < 32.2° C, cardiovascular instability, hormone insufficiency (such as hypoadrenalism or hypothyroidism), or hypothermia secondary to trauma, toxins, or predisposing disorders.

In **moderate hypothermia**, body temperature is at the warmer end of the range (28 to 32.2° C), and external rewarming with forced hot air enclosures may be used. External heat is best applied to the thorax because warming the extremities may increase metabolic demands on a depressed cardiovascular system.

In **severe hypothermia**, patients with lower temperatures (< 28° C), particularly those with low BP or cardiac arrest, require core rewarming.

Core rewarming options include

- Inhalation
- IV infusion
- Lavage
- Extracorporeal core rewarming (ECR)

Inhalation of heated (40 to 45° C), humidified O_2 via mask or endotracheal tube eliminates respiratory heat loss and can add 1 to 2° C/h to the rewarming rate.

IV crystalloids or blood should be heated to 40 to 42° C, especially with massive volume resuscitations.

Closed thoracic lavage through 2 thoracostomy tubes (see p. 390) is very efficient in severe cases. Peritoneal lavage with dialysate heated to 40 to 45° C requires 2 catheters with outflow suction and is especially useful for severely hypothermic patients who have rhabdomyolysis, toxin ingestions, or electrolyte abnormalities. Heated lavage of the bladder or GI tract transfers minimal heat.

There are 5 types of ECR: hemodialysis, venovenous, continuous arteriovenous, cardiopulmonary bypass, and extracorporeal membrane oxygenation. ECR measures require a prearranged protocol with appropriate specialists. Although they are intuitively attractive and heroic, these measures are not routinely available, and they are not commonly used in most hospitals.

CPR: Hypotension and bradycardia are expected when core temperature is low and, if due solely to hypothermia, need not be aggressively treated.

When needed, endotracheal intubation after oxygenation must be done gently to avoid converting the unstable heart to a nonperfusing rhythm.

CPR should be withheld if patients have a perfusing rhythm unless true cardiac arrest is confirmed by absence of cardiac motion on bedside cardiac ultrasonography. Treat with fluids and active rewarming. Chest compressions are not done, because

- Pulses may quickly return with rewarming
- Chest compressions may convert the perfusing rhythm to a nonperfusing one.

Patients with a nonperfusing rhythm (ventricular fibrillation or asystole) require CPR. Chest compressions and endotracheal intubation are done. Defibrillation is difficult if body temperature is low; one attempt with a 2 watt sec/Kg charge may be made, but if ineffective, further attempts are generally deferred until temperature reaches > 30° C.

Advanced life support should be continued until temperature reaches 32° C unless obviously lethal injuries or disorders are present. However, advanced cardiac life-support drugs (eg, antiarrhythmics, vasopressors, inotropes) are usually not given. Low-dose dopamine (1 to 5 mcg/kg/min) or other catecholamine infusions are typically reserved for patients who have disproportionately severe hypotension and who do not respond to fluid resuscitation and rewarming. Severe hyperkalemia (> 10 mEq/L) during resuscitation typically indicates a fatal outcome and can guide resuscitation efforts.

KEY POINTS

- Measure core temperature using an electronic thermometer or probe.
- Above about 32° C, heated or forced-air blankets and warm drinks are adequate treatment.
- Below about 32° C, active rewarming should be done, typically using forced-air hot air enclosures, heated, humidified oxygen, warm IV fluid, and sometimes heated lavage or extracorporeal methods (eg, cardiopulmonary bypass, hemodialysis).
- At lower temperatures, patients are hypovolemic and require fluid resuscitation.

- CPR not done if there is a perfusing rhythm.
- When CPR is done, defibrillation is deferred (after one initial attempt) until temperature reaches about 30° C.
- Advanced cardiac life-support drugs are usually not given.

NONFREEZING TISSUE INJURIES

Acute or chronic injuries without freezing of tissue may result from cold exposure.

Frostnip: The mildest cold injury is frostnip. Affected areas are numb, swollen, and red. Treatment is rewarming, which causes pain and itching. Rarely, mild hypersensitivity to cold persists for months to years.

Immersion (trench) foot: Prolonged exposure to wet cold can cause immersion foot. Peripheral nerves and the vasculature are usually injured; muscle and skin tissue may be injured in severe cases.

Initially, the foot is pale, edematous, clammy, cold, and numb. Tissue maceration may occur if patients walk extensively. Rewarming causes hyperemia, pain, and often hypersensitivity to light touch, which can persist for 6 to 10 wk. Skin may ulcerate, or a black eschar may develop. Autonomic dysfunction is common, with increased or decreased sweating, vasomotor changes, and local hypersensitivity to temperature change. Muscle atrophy and dysesthesia or anesthesia may occur and become chronic.

Immersion foot can be prevented by not wearing tight-fitting boots, keeping feet and boots dry, and changing socks frequently.

Immediate treatment is rewarming by immersing the affected area in warm (40 to 42° C) water, followed by sterile dressings. Nicotine should be avoided. Chronic neuropathic symptoms are difficult to treat; amitriptyline may be tried (see p. 1975).

Chilblains (pernio): Localized areas of erythema, swelling, pain, and pruritus result from repeated exposure to damp nonfreezing cold; the mechanism is unclear. Blistering or ulceration may occur. Chilblains most commonly affects the fingers and pretibial area and is self-limited. Occasionally, symptoms recur.

Pernio is often used to refer to a vasculitic disorder most common among young females with a history of Raynaud syndrome. Endothelial and neuronal damage results in vasospasm and exaggerated sympathetic response when exposed to cold. Nifedipine 20 mg po tid, limaprost 20 mcg po tid (not available in the USA), or corticosteroids (oral, eg, prednisolone 0.25 mg/kg bid, plus topical corticosteroids) may be effective for refractory pernio. Sympatholytic drugs and avoidance of nicotine may also help.

355 Drowning

(Fatal Drowning; Nonfatal Drowning)

Drowning is respiratory impairment resulting from submersion in a liquid medium. It can be nonfatal (previously called near drowning) or fatal. Drowning results in hypoxia, which can damage multiple organs, including the lungs and brain. Treatment is supportive, including reversal of respiratory arrest and cardiac arrest, hypoxia, hypoventilation, and hypothermia.

Drowning is among the top 10 causes of mortality for children and young people worldwide. In the US, drowning is the 10th most common cause of unintentional death. In 2013 in the US, drowning was the leading cause of injury mortality in children ages 1 to 4 yr and was second only to motor vehicle crashes for children ages 5 to 14 yr. Other groups at higher risk of drowning death include the following:

- Children from African American, immigrant, or impoverished families
- Males
- People who have used alcohol or sedatives
- People with conditions that cause temporary incapacitation (eg, seizure, hypoglycemia, stroke, MI, cardiac arrhythmia)
- People with a long QT syndrome (swimming can trigger arrhythmias that cause unexplained drowning in people with a long QT syndrome, particularly LQT1)
- People who engage in dangerous underwater breath-holding behaviors (DUBBs)

Drowning is common in pools, hot tubs, and natural water settings, and, among infants and toddlers, in toilets, bathtubs, and buckets of water or cleaning fluids. About 4 times as many people are hospitalized for nonfatal drowning as die as a result of drowning.

Pathophysiology

Hypoxia: Hypoxia is the major insult in drowning, affecting the brain, heart, and other tissues; respiratory arrest followed by cardiac arrest may occur. Brain hypoxia may cause cerebral edema and, occasionally, permanent neurologic sequelae. Generalized tissue hypoxia may cause metabolic acidosis. Immediate hypoxia results from aspiration of fluid or gastric contents, acute reflex laryngospasm (previously called dry drowning), or both. Lung injury due to aspiration or hypoxia itself may cause delayed hypoxia (previously called secondary drowning). Aspiration, especially with particulate matter or chemicals, may cause chemical pneumonitis or secondary bacterial pneumonia and may impair alveolar secretion of surfactant, resulting in patchy atelectasis. Extensive atelectasis may make the affected areas of the lungs stiff, noncompliant, and poorly ventilated, potentially causing respiratory failure (see p. 559) with hypercapnia and respiratory acidosis. Perfusion of poorly ventilated areas of the lungs (V/Q mismatch) worsens hypoxia. Alveolar hypoxia may cause noncardiogenic pulmonary edema.

Hypothermia: Exposure to cold water induces systemic hypothermia (see p. 2960), which can be a significant problem. However, hypothermia can be protective by stimulating the mammalian diving reflex, slowing the heart rate, and constricting the peripheral arteries, shunting oxygenated blood away from the extremities and the gut to the heart and brain. Also, hypothermia decreases the O_2 needs of tissues, possibly prolonging survival and delaying the onset of hypoxic tissue damage. The diving reflex and overall clinically protective effects of cold water are usually greatest in young children.

Fluid aspiration: Laryngospasm often limits the volume of fluid aspirated; however, large volumes of water are occasionally aspirated, on rare fatal drownings enough to change electrolyte concentrations and blood volume. Seawater may increase Na and Cl slightly. In contrast, large quantities of freshwater can decrease electrolyte concentration significantly, increase blood volume, and cause hemolysis. Aspiration can lead to pneumonia, sometimes with anaerobic pathogens.

Dangerous underwater breath-holding behaviors (DUBBs): DUBBs are practiced mostly by healthy young men (often good swimmers) trying to prolong their capacity to remain submerged. There are 3 described types of DUBBs:

- Intentional hyperventilation—blowing off CO_2 before submerged swimming, thereby delaying central hypercarbic ventilatory responses
- Hypoxic training—extending capacity for underwater distance swimming or breath-holding
- Static apnea—breath-holding for as long as possible while submerged and motionless, including as a game

In DUBB, while submerged, hypoxia occurs first, followed by loss of consciousness (hypoxic blackout, breath-hold blackout) and then drowning.

Associated injuries: Skeletal, soft-tissue, head, and internal injuries may occur, particularly among surfers, water skiers, boaters, flood victims, and occupants of submerged vehicles. People who dive into shallow water may sustain cervical and other spine injuries (which may be the cause of drowning).

Rarely, drowning occurs when people develop carbon monoxide poisoning when they are swimming near an exhaust port of a boat. Only a few breaths may cause unconsciousness.

Symptoms and Signs

During drowning, panic and air hunger occur. Children who are unable to swim may become submerged in < 1 min, more rapidly than adults. After rescue, anxiety, vomiting, wheezing, and altered consciousness are common. Patients may have respiratory failure with tachypnea, intercostal retractions, or cyanosis. Sometimes respiratory symptoms are delayed until several hours after submersion. Patients may have symptoms due to injuries or exacerbations of underlying disorders.

PEARLS & PITFALLS

- Sometimes respiratory symptoms and hypoxia are delayed until several hours after submersion.

Diagnosis

- Clinical evaluation
- For concomitant injuries, imaging studies as indicated
- Pulse oximetry and, if results are abnormal or if respiratory symptoms and signs are present, ABG and chest x-ray
- Core temperature measurement to rule out hypothermia
- Evaluation for causative or contributing disorders (eg, hypoglycemia, MI, intoxication, injury)
- Ongoing monitoring as indicated for delayed respiratory complications

Most people are found in or near water, making the diagnosis obvious clinically. Resuscitation, if indicated, should precede completion of the diagnostic assessment. Cervical spine injury is considered, and the spine is immobilized in patients who have altered consciousness or whose mechanism of injury involves diving or trauma. Secondary head injury and conditions that may have contributed to drowning (eg, hypoglycemia, MI, stroke, intoxication, arrhythmia) are considered.

All patients undergo assessment of oxygenation by oximetry or, if results are abnormal or if there are respiratory symptoms or signs, ABG and chest x-ray. Because respiratory symptoms may be delayed, even asymptomatic patients are transported to the hospital and observed for several hours.

In patients with symptoms or a history of prolonged submersion, core body temperature is measured, ECG and serum electrolytes are obtained, and continuous oximetry and cardiac monitoring are done. Patients with possible cervical spine injury undergo cervical spine imaging.

Patients with altered consciousness undergo head CT. Any other suspected predisposing or secondary conditions are evaluated with appropriate testing (eg, fingerstick glucose for hypoglycemia, ECG for MI, cardiac monitoring for arrhythmia, evaluation for intoxication). Patients who drown without apparent risk factors are evaluated for long QT syndrome and torsades de points ventricular tachycardia. In patients with pulmonary infiltrates, bacterial pneumonia is differentiated from chemical pneumonitis using blood cultures and sputum Gram stain and culture. If indicated (eg, bacterial pneumonia is suspected but the pathogen cannot be otherwise identified), bronchial washings are obtained for testing, including culture. Anaerobic pathogens should be considered.

Prognosis

Factors that increase the chance of surviving submersion without permanent injury include the following:

- Brief duration of submersion
- Cold water temperature
- Young age
- Absence of underlying medical conditions, secondary trauma, and aspiration of particulate matter or chemicals
- Rapid institution of resuscitation (most important)

Survival may be possible in cold water submersion that lasts > 1 h, especially among children; thus, even patients with prolonged submersion are vigorously resuscitated.

Treatment

- Resuscitation
- Correction of O_2 and CO_2 levels and other physiologic abnormalities
- Intensive respiratory support

Treatment aims to correct cardiac arrest, hypoxia, hypoventilation, hypothermia, and other physiologic insults.

Resuscitation after drowning: In apneic patients, rescue breathing is started immediately—in the water, if necessary. If spinal immobilization is necessary, it is done in a neutral position, and rescue breathing is done using a jaw thrust without head tilt or chin lift. Emergency medical services are called. If the patient does not respond to rescue breathing, cardiac compression is started, followed by advanced cardiac life support (see p. 539). Although the 2015 American Heart Association Guidelines for CPR recommend chest compressions as the first step in resuscitation of patients in cardiac arrest, drowning is an exception to this recommendation. Attempts to remove water from the lungs are avoided because they delay ventilation and increase the risk of vomiting. Oxygenation, endotracheal intubation, or both should proceed as soon as possible. Hypothermic patients are warmed as soon as possible (see p. 2961). Immediate treatment measures may include removing clothing, drying, and insulation.

PEARLS & PITFALLS

- Avoid attempts to remove water from the lungs; this only delays ventilation and increases risk of vomiting.

Hospital care for drowning patients: All hypoxic or moderately symptomatic patients are hospitalized. In the hospital, supportive treatment continues, aimed primarily at achieving acceptable arterial O_2 and CO_2 levels. Mechanical ventilation may be necessary. Patients are initially given 100% O_2; the concentration is titrated lower based on ABG results. Positive end-expiratory pressure ventilation (see p. 561) is usually necessary to help expand or maintain patency of alveoli to maintain adequate oxygenation. Pulmonary support may be necessary for hours or days. If adequate oxygenation is impossible despite maximizing ventilator settings, extracorporeal membrane oxygenation may be considered. Nebulized β_2-agonists may help reduce bronchospasm and wheezing. Patients with bacterial pneumonia are treated with antibiotics targeting organisms identified or suspected based on results of sputum testing and/or blood cultures. Corticosteroids are not used. Core body temperature is monitored, and hypothermia is treated.

Fluids or electrolytes are rarely required to correct significant electrolyte imbalances. Fluid restriction is rarely indicated, unless pulmonary or cerebral edema occurs. Concomitant injuries and disorders (eg, head or cervical injury, carbon monoxide poisoning) may also require treatment.

Discharge of drowning patients: Patients with mild symptoms, clear lungs, and normal oxygenation can be observed in the emergency department for several hours. If symptoms resolve and the examination and oxygenation remain normal, patients can be discharged with instructions to return if symptoms recur.

Prevention

Drugs, alcohol, and drowning: Use of alcohol or drugs, a major risk factor, should be avoided before and during swimming and boating and when supervising children around water.

Swimming safety: Swimmers should use common sense and be aware of weather and water conditions. Swimmers should be accompanied by an experienced swimmer or swim only in guarded areas. Swimming should stop if the swimmer looks or feels very cold, because hypothermia may impair judgment. Ocean swimmers should learn to escape rip currents by swimming parallel to the beach rather than toward the beach. Swimmers should be discouraged from DUBBs. If they practice them, they should be supervised and should know their dangers. Swimmers should avoid swimming near a boat exhaust port, which can cause carbon monoxide poisoning.

Public swimming areas should be supervised by lifeguards trained in water safety and resuscitation as well as rescue techniques. Life preservers, life jackets, and a shepherd's crook should be available close to poolside. Emergency airway equipment, automated external defibrillators (AEDs), and immediate telephone access to emergency medical services should be available. Comprehensive community prevention programs should target high-risk groups, teach children to swim as early as possible, and teach CPR to as many adolescents and adults as possible. Owners of private pools should also have immediate telephone access to emergency medical services and know about resuscitation after drowning.

Water safety for children: Children should wear Coast Guard–approved flotation devices when in or around water. Air-filled swimming aids and foam toys (water wings, noodles, etc) are not designed to keep swimmers from drowning and should not be used as a substitute for US Coast Guard–approved equipment. Children must be constantly supervised by an adult when around water, including beaches, pools, and ponds. Infants and toddlers should also be supervised, ideally within arm's length, when near toilets, bathtubs, or any collection of water. Studies in the US and China have shown that formal swimming lessons reduce the risk of fatal drowning among children ages 1 to 4; however, even children who have been taught how to swim require constant supervision when in or around water. Adults should remove water from containers such as pails and buckets immediately after use. Swimming pools should be surrounded with a locked fence ≥ 1.5 m in height.

Boating safety: Before embarking, boaters should wear Coast Guard–approved life jackets and should check weather and water conditions. Nonswimmers and small children in a boat should wear Coast Guard–approved life jackets at all times. Because consuming any quantity of alcohol increases the risk of drowning, operators and passengers on recreational boats should generally avoid consuming alcohol.

Special populations at risk for drowning: People who are debilitated or elderly or have seizure disorders or other medical conditions that can alter consciousness require constant supervision when they are boating or swimming and when in bathtubs.

People with a personal or family history of unexplained drowning not attributable to alcohol use, drug use, or a seizure disorder merit evaluation for long QT syndrome.

KEY POINTS

- Evaluate patients for suspected or feasible causes of drowning (eg, cervical spine injury, head injury, carbon monoxide toxicity, arrhythmias, hypoglycemia) as well as injuries or consequences of drowning (eg, head or cervical spine injury, aspiration).
- Vigorously resuscitate cold water drowning victims even if submersion was prolonged; survival is possible even after 1 h of submersion.
- Resuscitation begins with rescue breathing, not chest compressions.
- Preventive measures (eg, swimming lessons, child supervision, use of Coast Guard–approved floatation devices or life jackets, avoiding alcohol, access to trained lifeguards and emergency medical services) can have significant public health benefits.

356 Electrical and Lightning Injuries

ELECTRICAL INJURIES

Electrical injury is damage caused by generated electrical current passing through the body. Symptoms range from skin burns, damage to internal organs and other soft tissues to cardiac arrhythmias and respiratory arrest. Diagnosis is based on history, clinical criteria, and selective laboratory testing. Treatment is supportive, with aggressive care for severe injuries.

Although accidental electrical injuries encountered in the home (eg, touching an electrical outlet or getting shocked by a small appliance) rarely result in significant injury or sequelae, accidental exposure to high voltage results in about 400 deaths annually in the US. There are > 30,000 nonfatal shock incidents/yr in the US and electrical burns account for about 5% of admissions to burn units in the US.

Pathophysiology

Traditional teaching is that the severity of electrical injury depends on Kouwenhoven's factors:

- Type of current (direct [DC] or alternating [AC])
- Voltage and amperage (measures of current strength)
- Duration of exposure (longer exposure increases injury severity)
- Body resistance
- Pathway of current (which determines the specific tissue damaged)

However, electrical field strength, a newer concept, seems to predict injury severity more accurately.

Kouwenhoven's factors: AC changes direction frequently; it is the current usually supplied by household electrical outlets in the US and Europe. DC flows in the same direction constantly; it is the current supplied by batteries. Defibrillators and cardioverters usually deliver DC current. How AC affects the body depends largely on frequency. Low-frequency (50- to 60-Hz) AC is used in US (60 Hz) and European (50 Hz) households. Because low-frequency AC causes extended muscle contraction (tetany), which may freeze the hand to the current's source and prolong exposure, it can be more dangerous than high-frequency AC and is 3 to 5 times more dangerous than DC of the same voltage and amperage. DC exposure is likely to cause a single convulsive contraction, which often throws the person away from the current's source.

For both AC and DC, the higher the voltage (V) and amperage, the greater the ensuing electrical injury (for the same duration of exposure). Household current in the US is 110 V (standard electrical outlet) to 220 V (used for large appliances, eg, refrigerator, dryer). High-voltage (> 500 V) currents tend to cause deep burns, and low-voltage (110 to 220 V) currents tend to cause muscle tetany and freezing contact to the current's source. The maximum amperage that can cause flexors of the arm to contract but that allows release of the hand from the current's source is called the let-go current. Let-go current varies with weight and muscle mass. For an average 70-kg man, let-go current is about 75 mA for DC and about 15 mA for AC.

Low-voltage 60-Hz AC traveling through the chest for even a fraction of a second can cause ventricular fibrillation at amperage as low as 60 to 100 mA; for DC, about 300 to 500 mA are required. If current has a direct pathway to the heart (eg, via a cardiac catheter or pacemaker electrodes), < 1 mA (AC or DC) can cause ventricular fibrillation.

Tissue damage due to electrical exposure is caused primarily by the conversion of electric energy to heat, resulting in thermal injury. Amount of dissipated heat energy equals amperage^2 × resistance × time; thus, for any given current and duration, tissue with the highest resistance tends to suffer the most damage. Body resistance (measured in ohms/cm^2) is provided primarily by the skin, because all internal tissue (except bone) has negligible resistance. Skin thickness and dryness increase resistance; dry, well-keratinized, intact skin averages 20,000 to 30,000 ohms/cm^2. For a thickly calloused palm or sole, resistance may be 2 to 3 million ohms/cm^2; in contrast, moist, thin skin has a resistance of about 500 ohms/cm^2. Resistance for punctured skin (eg, cut, abrasion, needle puncture) or moist mucous membranes (eg, mouth, rectum, vagina) may be as low as 200 to 300 ohms/cm^2.

If skin resistance is high, more electrical energy may be dissipated at the skin, resulting in large skin burns but less internal damage. If skin resistance is low, skin burns are less extensive or absent, and more electrical energy is transmitted to internal structures. Thus, the absence of external burns does not predict the absence of electrical injury, and the severity of external burns does not predict the severity of electrical injury.

PEARLS & PITFALLS

- The absence of external burns does not predict the absence of electrical injury, and the severity of external burns does not predict the severity of electrical injury.

Damage to internal tissues depends on their resistance as well as on current density (current per unit area; energy is concentrated when the same current flows through a smaller area). For example, as electrical energy flows in an arm (primarily through lower-resistance tissues, eg, muscle, vessels, nerves), current density increases at joints because a significant proportion of the joint's cross-sectional area consists of higher-resistance tissues (eg, bone, tendon), which decreases the area of lower-resistance tissue; thus, damage to the lower-resistance tissues tends to be most severe at joints.

The current's pathway through the body determines which structures are injured. Because AC current continually reverses direction, the commonly used terms "entry" and "exit" are inappropriate; "source" and "ground" are more precise. The hand is the most common source point, followed by the head. The foot is the most common ground point. Current traveling between arm and arm or between arm and foot is likely to traverse the heart, possibly causing arrhythmia. This current tends to be more dangerous than current traveling from one foot to the other. Current to the head may damage the CNS.

Electrical field strength: In addition to Kouwenhoven's factors, electrical field strength also determines the degree of tissue injury. For instance, 20,000 volts (20 kV) distributed across the body of a man who is about 2 m (6 ft) tall result in a field strength of about 10 kV/m. Similarly, 110 volts, if applied only to 1 cm (eg, across a young child's lip), result in a similar field strength of 11 kV/m; this relationship is why such a low-voltage injury can cause the same severity of tissue injury as some high-voltage injuries applied to a larger area. Conversely, when considering voltage rather than electrical field strength, minor or trivial electrical injuries technically could be classified as high voltage. For example, the shock received from shuffling across a carpet in the winter involves thousands of volts but causes inconsequential injury.

The electrical field effect can cause cell membrane damage (electroporation) even when the energy is insufficient to cause any thermal damage.

Pathology: Application of low electrical field strength causes an immediate, unpleasant feeling (being "shocked") but seldom results in serious or permanent injury. Application of high electrical field strength causes thermal or electrochemical damage to internal tissues. Damage may include

- Hemolysis
- Protein coagulation
- Coagulation necrosis of muscle and other tissues
- Thrombosis
- Dehydration
- Muscle and tendon avulsion

High electrical field strength injuries may result in massive edema, which, as blood in veins coagulates and muscles swell, results in compartment syndrome. Massive edema may also cause hypovolemia and hypotension. Muscle destruction can result in rhabdomyolysis and myoglobinuria, and electrolyte disturbances. Myoglobinuria, hypovolemia, and hypotension increase risk of acute kidney injury. The consequences of organ dysfunction do not always correlate with the amount of tissue destroyed (eg, ventricular fibrillation may occur with relatively little tissue destruction).

Symptoms and Signs

Burns may be sharply demarcated on the skin even when current penetrates irregularly into deeper tissues. Severe involuntary muscular contractions, seizures, ventricular fibrillation, or respiratory arrest due to CNS damage or muscle paralysis may occur. Brain, spinal cord, and peripheral nerve damage may result in various neurologic deficits. Cardiac arrest may occur in the absence of burns as in bathtub accidents (when a wet [grounded] person contacts a 110-V circuit—eg, from a hair dryer or radio).

Young children who bite or suck on extension cords can burn their mouth and lips. Such burns may cause cosmetic deformities and impair growth of the teeth, mandible, and maxilla. Labial artery hemorrhage, which results when the eschar separates 5 to 10 days after injury, occurs in up to 10% of these young children.

An electrical shock can cause powerful muscle contractions or falls (eg, from a ladder or roof), resulting in dislocations (electrical shock is one of the few causes of posterior shoulder dislocation), vertebral or other fractures, injuries to internal organs, and other blunt force injuries.

Subtle or vaguely defined neurologic, psychologic, and physical sequelae can develop 1 to 5 yr after the injury and result in significant morbidity.

Diagnosis

- Head to toe examination
- Sometimes ECG, cardiac enzyme measurement, and urinalysis

The patient, once away from current, is assessed for cardiac arrest (see p. 538) and respiratory arrest (see p. 550). Necessary resuscitation is done. After initial resuscitation, patients are examined from head to toe for traumatic injuries, particularly if the patient fell or was thrown.

Asymptomatic patients who are not pregnant, have no known heart disorders, and who have had only brief exposure to household current usually have no significant acute internal or external injuries and do not require testing or monitoring. For other patients, ECG, CBC, measurement of cardiac enzymes, and urinalysis (to check for myoglobin) should be considered. Patients with impaired consciousness may require CT or MRI.

Treatment

- Shutting off current
- Resuscitation
- Analgesia
- Sometimes cardiac monitoring for 6 to 12 h
- Wound care

Prehospital care: The first priority is to break contact between the patient and the current source by shutting off the current (eg, by throwing a circuit breaker or switch, by disconnecting the device from its electrical outlet). High- and low-voltage power lines are not always easily differentiated, particularly outdoors. CAUTION: *If power lines could be high voltage, no attempts to disengage the patient should be made until the power is shut off.*

Resuscitation: Patients are resuscitated while being assessed. Shock, which may result from trauma or massive burns, is treated (see p. 575). Standard burn fluid resuscitation formulas, which are based on the extent of skin burns, may underestimate the fluid requirement in electrical burns; thus, such formulas are not used. Instead, fluids are titrated to maintain adequate urine output (about 100 mL/h in adults and 1.5 mL/kg/h in children). For myoglobinuria, maintaining adequate urine output is particularly important, while alkalinizing the urine may help decrease the risk of renal failure. Surgical debridement of large amounts of muscle tissue may also help to decrease myoglobinuric renal failure.

Severe pain due to an electrical burn is treated by the judicious titration of IV opioids.

Other measures: Asymptomatic patients who are not pregnant, have no known heart disorders, and who have had only brief exposure to household current usually have no significant acute internal or external injuries that would necessitate admission and can be discharged.

Cardiac monitoring for 6 to 12 h is indicated for patients with the following conditions:

- Arrhythmias
- Chest pain
- Any suggestion of cardiac damage
- Pregnancy (possibly)
- Known heart disorders (possibly)

Appropriate tetanus prophylaxis (see p. 1472) and topical burn wound care (see p. 2957) are required. Pain is treated with NSAIDs or other analgesics.

All patients with significant electrical burns should be referred to a specialized burn unit. Young children with lip burns should be referred to a pediatric orthodontist or oral surgeon familiar with such injuries.

Prevention

Electrical devices that touch or may be touched by the body should be properly insulated, grounded, and incorporated into circuits containing protective circuit-breaking equipment. Ground-fault circuit breakers, which trip when as little as 5 mA of current leaks to ground, are effective and readily available. Outlet guards reduce risk in homes with infants or young children.

KEY POINTS

- In addition to burn injuries, AC can freeze the patient's hand to the current source, while DC can throw the patient, causing injury.
- Although skin burn severity does not predict the degree of internal damage, internal damage is more severe if the skin has low resistance.
- Examine patients completely, including for traumatic injuries.
- Consider ECG, CBC, cardiac enzymes, urinalysis, and monitoring unless patients are asymptomatic, are not pregnant, have no known heart disorders, and have had only brief exposure to household current.
- Refer patients with significant electrical burns to a specialized burn unit and, if significant internal damage is suspected, begin fluid resuscitation.

LIGHTNING INJURIES

Lightning injuries include cardiac arrest, loss of consciousness, and temporary or permanent neurologic deficits; serious burns and internal tissue injury are rare. Diagnosis is clinical; evaluation requires ECG and cardiac monitoring. Treatment is supportive.

Although injury and deaths due to lightning strikes have decreased significantly over the last 50 yr, lightning strikes still cause about 30 deaths and several hundred injuries annually in the US. Lightning tends to strike tall or isolated objects, including trees, towers, shelters, flagpoles, bleachers, and fences. A person may be the tallest object in an open field. Metal objects and water do not attract lightning but easily transmit electricity once they are hit. Lightning can strike a person directly, or the current can be transferred to the person through the ground or a nearby object. Lightning can also travel from outdoor power or electrical lines to indoor electrical equipment or telephone lines. The force of a lightning strike can throw the person up to several meters.

Because the physics of lightning injury is different from that of generated electrical energy, knowledge of the effects of exposure to household current or high voltage cannot be extrapolated to lightning injuries. For example, damage from lightning injury is not determined by voltage or amperage. Although lightning current contains a large amount of energy, it flows for an extremely brief period (1/10,000 to 1/1000 sec). It rarely, if ever, causes serious skin wounds and seldom causes rhabdomyolysis or serious internal tissue damage, unlike high-voltage and high-current electrical injury from generated sources. Patients may have intracranial hemorrhage resulting from secondary injury or, rarely, from lightning itself.

Lightning can affect the heart but primarily affects the nervous system, damaging the brain, autonomic nervous system, and peripheral nerves.

PEARLS & PITFALLS

- Unlike high-voltage and high-current electrical injury from generated sources, lightning rarely, if ever, causes serious skin wounds and seldom causes rhabdomyolysis or serious internal tissue damage.

Symptoms and Signs

The electrical charge can cause asystole or other arrhythmias or cause symptoms of brain dysfunction, such as loss of consciousness, confusion, or amnesia.

Keraunoparalysis is paralysis and mottling, coldness, and pulselessness of the lower and sometimes upper extremities plus sensory deficits; the cause is likely injury to the sympathetic nervous system. Keraunoparalysis is common and usually resolves within several hours, although some degree of permanent paresis occasionally results. Other manifestations of lightning injury may include

- Minor skin burns in a punctate or feathered, branched pattern
- Tympanic membrane perforation
- Cataracts (within days)

Neurologic problems may include confusion, cognitive deficits, and peripheral neuropathy. Neuropsychologic problems (eg, sleep disturbances, attention deficit, memory problems) may occur. Cardiopulmonary arrest at the time of the strike is the most common cause of death. Cognitive deficits, pain syndromes, and sympathetic nervous system damage are the most common long-term sequelae.

Diagnosis

- Recognition of cardiac and brain complications

Lightning injuries may be witnessed or unwitnessed. Unwitnessed injuries should be suspected when people found outside during or after storms have amnesia or are unconscious. All patients struck by lightning should be evaluated for traumatic injuries.

ECG may be done if injury is severe. Cardiac enzymes are measured for patients with the following:

- Chest pain
- Abnormal ECG
- Altered mental status

Patients with initially abnormal or deteriorating mental status or focal neurologic deficits compatible with a brain lesion require a head CT or MRI.

Treatment

- Supportive care

CPR is initiated for cardiac or respiratory arrest or both. If an automated external defibrillator is available, it should be used. Patients who are in cardiac arrest following a lightning strike, unlike patients in cardiac arrest from other types of trauma, often have an excellent prognosis if resuscitated. Thus, unlike in a typical mass casualty event, in which patients in cardiac arrest are given low triage priority, such patients are given high priority when multiple casualties are caused by lightning strike.

Supportive care is provided. Fluids are usually restricted to minimize potential brain edema. Most patients who have been injured by lightning can be safely discharged unless cardiac effects or brain lesions are suspected.

Prevention

Most lightning injuries can be prevented by following lightning safety guidelines. People should know the weather forecast and have an escape plan involving evacuation to a safer area (ideally a large, habitable building). They should pay attention to the weather while outdoors so they can implement the escape plan if a storm comes up. By the time thunder is heard, people are already in danger and should seek shelter (eg, in a building or fully enclosed metal vehicle). Small, open structures, such as gazebos, are not safe. People should not go outdoors until 30 min after the last lightning is seen or thunder is heard.

When indoors during an electrical storm, people should avoid plumbing and electrical appliances, stay away from windows and doors, and not use hard-wired telephones, video game consoles, or computers. Cellular phones and other handheld devices and laptop computers are safe when used with battery power only because they do not attract lightning.

KEY POINTS

- Lightning injuries tend to cause arrhythmias and brain dysfunction, unlike electrical injuries from generated sources, which tend to cause skin burns and internal tissue injury.
- Suspect lightning injury if patients are found unconscious or amnestic outside after a storm.
- When evaluating patients, consider traumatic injuries, arrhythmias, and brain and heart damage.
- Treat patients supportively.
- Most lightning injuries can be prevented by following lightning safety guidelines.

357 Eye Trauma

Common causes of eye injury include domestic accidents (eg, during hammering or exposure to household chemicals or cleaners), assault, car battery explosions, sporting injuries (including air- or paint pellet-gun injuries), and motor vehicle crashes (including airbag injuries). Injury may be to the eyeball (globe), surrounding soft tissues (including muscles, nerves, and tendons), or bones of the orbit.

General evaluation should include the following:

- Tests of visual acuity
- Range of extraocular motion
- Visual fields to confrontation
- Pupillary appearance and responses
- Location and depth of lid and conjunctival lacerations and of foreign bodies
- Depth of anterior chamber
- Presence of anterior chamber or vitreous hemorrhage, cataract, or red reflex
- Retinal examination
- Intraocular pressure determination

Detailed examination of the sclera, anterior segment (cornea, anterior chamber, ciliary body, iris), lens, and anterior vitreous is best done with a slit lamp. Although direct ophthalmoscopy can be used to examine the lens and posterior structures of the eye, indirect ophthalmoscopy, usually done by an ophthalmologist, provides a more detailed view of these structures. Indications for indirect ophthalmoscopy include clinical suspicion of traumatic cataracts, vitreous abnormalities (eg, hemorrhage, foreign body), and retinal abnormalities; clinical suspicion may be based on injury mechanism, absence of the red reflex, or retinal abnormalities (visible with direct ophthalmoscopy). Because direct and indirect ophthalmoscopy are best done through a dilated pupil, about 15 to 30 min before this examination, mydriatics (such as 1 drop of cyclopentolate 1% and 1 drop of phenylephrine 2.5%) can be instilled. If an intraocular or orbital foreign body or an orbital fracture is suspected, CT is done.

Use of eye guards, goggles, or special eyeglasses, such as those constructed of polycarbonate lenses in a wrap-around polyamide frame, is a simple precaution that greatly reduces the risk of injury.

When eye drops are prescribed, each dose includes only one drop.

OCULAR BURNS

Thermal burns: The blink reflex usually causes the eye to close in response to a thermal stimulus. Thus, thermal burns tend to affect the eyelid rather than the conjunctiva or cornea. Eyelid burns should be cleansed thoroughly with sterile isotonic saline solution followed by application of an antimicrobial ointment (eg, bacitracin bid). Most thermal burns affecting the conjunctiva or cornea are mild and heal without significant sequellae. They are treated with oral analgesics (acetaminophen with or without oxycodone), cycloplegic mydriatics (eg, homatropine 5% qid), and topical ophthalmic antibiotics (eg, bacitracin/polymyxin B ointment or ciprofloxacin 0.3% ointment qid for 3 to 5 days).

Chemical burns: Burns of the cornea and conjunctiva can be serious, particularly when strong acid or alkali is involved. Alkali burns tend to be more serious than acid burns.

PEARLS & PITFALLS

- Chemical burns to the cornea and conjunctiva are a true emergency; treatment must begin immediately.

Burns should be irrigated with copious amounts of water or with 0.9% saline if available. The eye may be anesthetized with one drop of proparacaine 0.5%, but irrigation should not be delayed and should last for at least 30 min. Irrigation may be facilitated by using an irrigating lens placed under the lids. In acid and alkali burns, some experts suggest 1 to 2 h of irrigation; others recommend that the pH of the conjunctiva be measured with expanded pH paper (a type that measures pH over a limited range for more accurate assessment) and irrigation continued until pH is normal.

After irrigation, the conjunctival fornices should be examined for chemical embedded in the tissue and swept with a swab to remove trapped particles. The superior fornices are exposed by using double eyelid eversion (ie, first everting the eyelid and then inserting a swab under the everted eyelid and lifting it up until the fornix is visible).

Chemical iritis is suspected in patients with photophobia (deep eye pain with exposure to light) that develops hours or days after a chemical burn and is diagnosed by finding flare and WBCs in the anterior chamber during slit-lamp examination. Chemical iritis is treated by instilling a long-acting cycloplegic (eg, a single dose of homatropine 2% or 5% or scopolamine 0.25% solution). Because topical corticosteroids can cause corneal perforation after chemical burns, they should be given only by an ophthalmologist. Corneal epithelial defects are treated by applying an antibiotic ointment (eg, erythromycin 0.5%) 4 times a day until they are healed (eg, about 3 to 5 days in mild burns). Topical anesthetics should be avoided after initial irrigation; significant pain may be treated with acetaminophen with or without oxycodone.

Severe chemical burns require treatment by an ophthalmologist to save vision and prevent complications such as uveitis, perforation of the globe, and lid deformities. Patients with severe conjunctival hyperemia, ciliary flush (prominent conjunctival injection around the limbus), true photophobia (ie, not just sensitivity to light), avascular areas of conjunctiva, or loss of conjunctival or corneal epithelium as demonstrated by fluorescein staining should be examined by an ophthalmologist as soon as possible and no longer than 24 h after the exposure.

CORNEAL ABRASIONS AND FOREIGN BODIES

Corneal abrasions are self-limited, superficial epithelial defects.

The most common conjunctival and corneal injuries are foreign bodies and abrasions. Improper use of contact lenses can damage the cornea. Although superficial foreign bodies often spontaneously exit the cornea in the tear film, occasionally leaving a residual abrasion, other foreign bodies remain on or within the cornea. Sometimes, a foreign body trapped under the upper lid causes one or more vertical corneal abrasions that worsen as a result of blinking. Intraocular penetration can occur with seemingly minor trauma, particularly when foreign bodies result from high-speed machines (eg, drills, saws, anything with a metal-on-metal mechanism), hammering, or explosions. Infection generally does not develop from a corneal injury. However, if intraocular penetration is not recognized, infection within the eye (endophthalmitis), although somewhat rare, may develop.

Symptoms and Signs

Symptoms and signs of abrasion or foreign body include foreign body sensation, tearing, redness, and occasionally discharge. Vision is rarely affected (other than by tearing).

Diagnosis

- Slit-lamp examination, usually with fluorescein staining

After an anesthetic (eg, 2 drops of proparacaine 0.5%) is instilled into the inferior fornix, each lid is everted, and the entire conjunctiva and cornea are inspected with a binocular lens (loupe) or a slit lamp. Fluorescein staining (see p. 894) with cobalt light illumination renders abrasions and nonmetallic foreign bodies more apparent. Seidel sign is streaming of fluorescein away from a corneal defect, visible during slit-lamp examination. A positive Seidel sign suggests leakage of aqueous fluid through a corneal perforation. Patients with multiple vertical linear abrasions should have their eyelids everted to search for a foreign body under the upper lid. Patients with a high-risk intraocular injury or (more rarely) visible globe perforation or a teardrop-shaped pupil should undergo CT to rule out intraocular foreign body and be seen by an ophthalmologist as soon as possible.

Treatment

- For surface foreign bodies, irrigation or removal with a damp, cotton-tipped swab or a small needle
- For corneal abrasions, antibiotic ointment and pupillary dilation
- For intraocular foreign bodies, surgical removal

After an anesthetic is instilled into the conjunctiva, clinicians can remove conjunctival foreign bodies by irrigation or lift them out with a moist sterile cotton applicator. A corneal foreign body that cannot be dislodged by irrigation may be lifted out carefully on the point of a sterile spud (an instrument designed to remove ocular foreign bodies) or of a 25- or 27-gauge hypodermic needle under loupe or, preferably, slit-lamp magnification; the patient must be able to stare without moving the eye during removal.

Steel or iron foreign bodies remaining on the cornea for more than a few hours may leave a rust ring on the cornea that also requires removal under slit-lamp magnification by scraping or using a low-speed rotary burr; removal is usually done by an ophthalmologist.

Abrasions: An antibiotic ointment (eg, bacitracin/polymyxin B or ciprofloxacin 0.3% qid for 3 to 5 days) is used for most abrasions until the epithelial defect is healed. Contact lens wearers with corneal abrasions require an antibiotic with optimal antipseudomonal coverage (eg, ciprofloxacin 0.3% ointment qid). For symptomatic relief of larger abrasions (eg, area > 10 mm^2), the pupil is also dilated once with a short-acting cycloplegic (eg, one drop cyclopentolate 1% or homatropine 5%).

Eye patches may increase risk of infection and are usually not used, particularly for an abrasion caused by a contact lens or an object that may be contaminated with soil or vegetation. Ophthalmic corticosteroids tend to promote the growth of fungi and reactivation of herpes simplex virus and are contraindicated. Continued use of topical anesthetics can impair healing and is thus contraindicated. Pain can be managed with oral analgesics.

The corneal epithelium regenerates rapidly; even large abrasions heal within 1 to 3 days. A contact lens should not be worn for 5 to 7 days. Follow-up examination by an ophthalmologist 1 or 2 days after injury is wise, especially if a foreign body was removed with a needle or spud.

Intraocular foreign bodies: Intraocular foreign bodies require immediate surgical removal by an ophthalmologist. Systemic and topical antimicrobials (effective against *Bacillus cereus* if the injury involved contamination with soil or vegetation) are indicated; they include ceftazidime 1 g IV q 12 h, in combination with vancomycin 15 mg/kg IV q 12 h and moxifloxacin 0.5% ophthalmic solution q 1 to 2 h. Ointment should be avoided if the globe is lacerated. A protective shield (such as a Fox shield or the bottom third of a paper cup) is placed and taped over the eye to avoid inadvertent pressure that could extrude ocular contents through the penetration site. Tetanus prophylaxis is indicated after open globe injuries. As with any laceration of the globe, vomiting, which can increase intraocular pressure, should be prevented. If nausea occurs, an antiemetic is given.

KEY POINTS

- Symptoms of corneal abrasion or foreign body include foreign body sensation, tearing, and redness; visual acuity is typically unchanged.
- Diagnosis is usually by slit-lamp examination with fluorescein staining.
- Suspect an intraocular foreign body if fluorescein streams away from a corneal defect, if the pupil is teardrop shaped,

or if the mechanism of injury involves a high-speed machine (eg, drill, saw, anything with a metal-on-metal mechanism), hammering, or explosion.

- Treat corneal abrasions and foreign bodies by removing foreign material, prescribing a topical antibiotic, and sometimes instilling a cycloplegic.
- For intraocular foreign bodies, give systemic and topical antibiotics, apply a shield, and consult an ophthalmologict for surgical removal.

EYE CONTUSIONS AND LACERATIONS

Consequences of blunt trauma to the eye range from eyelid to orbital injury.

Eyelids: Eyelid **contusions** (which result in black eyes) are more cosmetically than clinically significant, although more serious injuries may sometimes accompany them and should not be overlooked. Uncomplicated contusions are treated with ice packs to inhibit swelling during the first 24 to 48 h, followed by hot compresses to aid absorption of the hematoma.

Minor lid **laceration** s not involving the lid margin or tarsal plate may be repaired with nylon (or, in children, plain gut) 6-0 or 7-0 sutures. Lacerations of the lid margin are best repaired by an ophthalmic surgeon to ensure accurate apposition and to avoid a notch in the contour. Complicated lid lacerations, which include those of the medial portion of the lower or upper eyelid (possibly involving the lacrimal canaliculus), through-and-through lacerations, those in which the patient has ptosis, and those that expose orbital fat or involve the tarsal plate, should also be repaired by an ophthalmic surgeon.

Globe: Trauma may cause the following:

- Conjunctival, anterior chamber, and vitreous hemorrhage
- Retinal hemorrhage, edema, or detachment (see p. 963)
- Laceration of the iris
- Cataract
- Dislocated lens
- Glaucoma
- Globe rupture (laceration)

Evaluation can be difficult when massive lid edema or laceration is present. Even so, unless the need for immediate eye surgery is obvious (necessitating evaluation by an ophthalmologist as soon as possible), the lid is opened, taking care not to exert pressure on the globe, and as complete an examination as possible is conducted. At a minimum, the following are noted:

- Visual acuity (see Sidebar 357–1)
- Pupil shape and pupillary responses
- Extraocular movements
- Anterior chamber depth or hemorrhage
- Presence of red reflex

Sidebar 357–1. Assessing Visual Acuity

In descending order of acuity, vision is assessed as

- Reading a Snellen chart
- Counting fingers
- Detecting motion (eg, seeing hand motion)
- Perceiving light
- Lacking light perception

An analgesic or, after obtaining any surgical consent, an anxiolytic may be given to facilitate examination. Gentle and careful use of eyelid retractors or an eyelid speculum makes it possible to open the lids. If a commercial instrument is not available, the eyelids can be separated with makeshift retractors fashioned by opening a paperclip to an S shape, then bending the U-shaped ends to 180°. Globe laceration should be suspected with any of the following:

- A corneal or scleral laceration is visible.
- Aqueous humor is leaking (positive Seidel sign).
- The anterior chamber is very shallow (eg, making the cornea appear to have folds) or very deep (due to rupture posterior to the lens).
- The pupil is irregular.

If globe laceration is suspected, measures that can be taken before an ophthalmologist is available consist of applying a protective shield (see p. 2969) and combating possible infection with systemic antimicrobials as for intraocular foreign bodies (see p. 2969). Topical antibiotics are avoided. Vomiting, which can increase intraocular pressure (IOP) and contribute to extravasation of ocular contents, is suppressed using antiemetics as needed. Because fungal contamination of open wounds is dangerous, corticosteroids are contraindicated until after wounds are closed surgically. Tetanus prophylaxis is indicated after open globe injuries. Very rarely, after laceration of the globe, the uninjured, contralateral eye becomes inflamed (sympathetic ophthalmia—see p. 969) and may lose vision to the point of blindness unless treated. The mechanism is an autoimmune reaction; corticosteroid drops can prevent the process and may be prescribed by an ophthalmologist.

Hyphema (anterior chamber hemorrhage—see Plate 99): Hyphema may be followed by recurrent bleeding, glaucoma, and blood staining of the cornea, any of which may result in permanent vision loss. Symptoms are of associated injuries unless the hyphema is large enough to obstruct vision. Direct inspection typically reveals layering of blood or the presence of clot or both in the anterior chamber. Layering is seen as a meniscus-like blood level in the dependent (usually inferior) part of the anterior chamber. Microhyphema, a less severe form, may be detectable by direct inspection as haziness in the anterior chamber or by slit-lamp examination as suspended RBCs.

An ophthalmologist should attend to the patient as soon as possible. The patient is placed on bed rest with the head elevated 30 to 45° and is given an eye shield to protect the eye from further trauma (see p. 2969). Patients who are at high risk of recurrent bleeding (eg, those with large hyphemas, bleeding diatheses, anticoagulant use, or sickle cell disease), who have IOP that is difficult to control, or who are likely to be nonadherent to recommended treatment may be hospitalized. Oral and topical NSAIDs are contraindicated because they may contribute to recurrent bleeding.

IOP can rise acutely (within hours, usually in patients with sickle cell disease or trait) or months to years later. Thus, IOP is monitored daily for several days and then regularly over subsequent weeks and months and if symptoms develop (eg, eye ache, decreased vision, nausea—similar to symptoms of acute angle-closure glaucoma). If pressure rises, timolol 0.5% bid, brimonidine 0.2% or 0.15% bid, or both are given. Response to treatment is determined by pressure, often checked every 1 or 2 h until controlled or until a significant rate of reduction is demonstrated; thereafter, it is usually checked once or twice daily. Mydriatic drops (eg, scopolamine 0.25% tid or atropine 1% tid for 5 days) and topical corticosteroids (eg, prednisolone acetate 1% 4 to 8 times/day for 2 to 3 wk) are often given.

If bleeding is recurrent, an ophthalmologist should be consulted for management. Administration of aminocaproic acid 50 to 100 mg/kg po q 4 h (not exceeding 30 g/day) for 5 days may reduce recurrent bleeding, and miotic or mydriatic drugs must also be given. Rarely, recurrent bleeding with secondary glaucoma requires surgical evacuation of the blood.

Blowout fracture: Blowout fracture occurs when blunt trauma forces the orbital contents through one of the most fragile portions of the orbital wall, typically the floor. Medial and roof fractures also can occur. Symptoms include diplopia, enophthalmos, inferiorly displaced globe, hypesthesia of the cheek and upper lip (due to infraorbital nerve injury), and subcutaneous emphysema. Epistaxis, lid edema, and ecchymosis may occur. Diagnosis is best made using CT with thin cuts through the facial bones. If diplopia or cosmetically unacceptable enophthalmos persists beyond 2 wk, surgical repair is indicated. Patients should be told to avoid blowing the nose to prevent subcutaneous dissection of air. Using a topical vasoconstrictor for 2 to 3 days may alleviate epistaxis.

KEY POINTS

- Consult an ophthalmologist if an eyelid laceration is complicated (eg, through the margin, tarsal plate, or canaliculus, causing ptosis, or exposing orbital fat).
- Globe trauma may cause iris laceration, cataract, lens dislocation, glaucoma, vitreous hemorrhage, or retinal damage (hemorrhage, detachment, or edema).
- Suspect globe rupture if trauma results in a visible corneal or scleral laceration, leaking aqueous humor, an unusually shallow or deep anterior chamber, or an irregular pupil.
- Hyphema, best diagnosed by slit-lamp examination, requires bed rest with head elevation at 30 to 45° and close monitoring of intraocular pressure.
- Refer patients for surgical repair of blowout fractures that cause > 2 wk of diplopia or unacceptable enophthalmos.

POSTTRAUMATIC IRIDOCYCLITIS

(Traumatic Anterior Uveitis; Traumatic Iritis)

Posttraumatic iridocyclitis is an inflammatory reaction of the uvea and iris, typically developing within 3 days of blunt eye trauma.

Symptoms of posttraumatic iridocyclitis include tearing, throbbing ache and redness of the eye, photophobia, and blurred vision. The pupil may be dilated. Diagnosis is by history, symptoms, and slit-lamp examination, which typically reveals flare (due to an increase in protein content of the aqueous humor from the inflammatory exudate) and WBCs in the anterior chamber. Treatment involves a cycloplegic (usually scopolamine 0.25% tid or homatropine 5% tid). Topical corticosteroids (eg, prednisolone acetate 1% 4 to 8 times/day) are often used to shorten symptom duration.

358 Facial Trauma

EXTERNAL EAR TRAUMA

Trauma to the external ear may result in hematoma, laceration, avulsion, or fracture.

Subperichondrial hematoma (cauliflower ear): The perichondrium supplies blood to the auricular cartilage. Blunt trauma to the pinna may cause a subperichondrial hematoma; the accumulation of large amounts of blood between the perichondrium and cartilage can interrupt the blood supply to the cartilage and render all or part of the pinna a shapeless, reddish purple mass. Avascular necrosis of the cartilage may follow. The resultant destruction causes the cauliflower ear characteristic of wrestlers and boxers.

Treatment consists of promptly evacuating the clot through an incision and preventing reaccumulation of the hematoma with through-and-through ear sutures over dental gauze rolls or insertion of a Penrose drain plus a pressure dressing. Because these injuries are prone to infection and abscess formation, an oral antibiotic effective against staphylococci (eg, cephalexin 500 mg tid) is given for 5 days.

PEARLS & PITFALLS

- Failure to drain a subperichondrial hematoma may lead to permanent external ear deformity.

Lacerations: In lacerations of the pinna, the skin margins are sutured whenever possible. If the cartilage is penetrated, it is repaired unless there is not enough skin to cover it. Damaged cartilage, whether repaired or not, is splinted externally with benzoin-impregnated cotton, and a protective dressing is applied. Oral antibiotics are given as for a hematoma.

Human bite wounds are at high risk of infection, including infection of the cartilage, a potentially severe complication. Treatment includes meticulous debridement of devitalized tissue, prophylactic antibiotics (eg, amoxicillin/clavulanate 500 to 875 mg po bid for 3 days) and possibly antivirals (see Table 352–1 on p. 2942). Wounds < 12 h old can be closed but older wounds should be allowed to heal secondarily, with cosmetic deformities treated later.

Avulsions: Complete or partial avulsions are repaired by an otolaryngologist, facial plastic surgeon, or plastic surgeon.

Trauma secondary to mandibular fractures: Forceful blows to the mandible may be transmitted to the anterior wall of the ear canal (posterior wall of the glenoid fossa). Displaced fragments from a fractured anterior wall may cause stenosis of the canal and must be reduced or removed surgically after a general anesthetic is given.

FRACTURES OF THE MANDIBLE AND MIDFACE

Blunt facial trauma can fracture the jaw and other bones of the midface. Symptoms depend on the location of the fracture. A dental x-ray or CT is diagnostic. Treatment may include surgery and/or external fixation.

Fractures of the lower jaw (mandible) are suspected in patients with post-traumatic malocclusion or focal swelling and tenderness over a segment of the mandible. Other clues include defects (stepoff) of the dental occlusal surface, alveolar ridge disruptions, and anesthesia in the distribution of the inferior alveolar or mental nerve. Some fractures result in palpable instability. Fractures of the mandibular condyle usually cause preauricular pain, swelling, and limited opening of the mouth (trismus). With a unilateral condylar fracture, the jaw deviates to the affected side when the mouth is opened.

Fractures of the midface, which includes the area from the superior orbital rim to the maxillary teeth, can cause irregularity in the smooth contour of the cheeks, malar eminences, zygomatic arch, or orbital rims. The Le Fort classification (see Fig. 358–1) can be used to describe midface fractures. Traumatic malocclusion and upper alveolar ridge fractures may suggest a maxillary fracture that involves the occlusal surface.

Orbital floor fracture (see p. 2971) is suggested by infraorbital nerve anesthesia, enophthalmos, or diplopia. An injury near the orbit requires an eye examination, including, at least, assessment of visual acuity, pupils, and extraocular movements.

Zygomatic arch fracture is suggested by trismus and a defect on palpation of the zygomatic arch.

Brain injury and fractured cervical vertebrae are possible when trauma has been severe enough to fracture facial bones. In major impact injuries, hemorrhage and edema due to a facial fracture may compromise the airway.

Diagnosis

- X-ray and/or CT

A panoramic dental x-ray is preferred for an isolated mandibular fracture. Fine-cut CT (1-mm slices) is done in axial and coronal planes to diagnose facial fractures.

Treatment

- Fracture management
- Sometimes endotracheal intubation, antibiotics

An oral endotracheal airway may be required to maintain airway patency in patients with hemorrhage, edema, or significant tissue disruption. Definitive facial fracture management is complex and may include internal fixation.

Tooth socket fractures: Fractures through a tooth socket are open fractures. They require antibiotic prophylaxis (typically with a broad-spectrum antibiotic that is particularly effective against anaerobes, such as penicillin) given orally as a liquid or parenterally.

Mandible fractures: For a fractured mandible, treatment ranges from soft diet alone to maxillomandibular fixation (wiring the jaw shut), rigid open fixation, or both. If fixation is available within the first few hours after injury, closure of any lip or oral lacerations should be delayed until the fracture has been reduced. For maxillomandibular fixation, metal bars (arch bars) are attached to the buccal surface of the upper and lower teeth and then wired to each other after correct occlusion has been established. Patients with maxillomandibular fixation should always carry wire cutters in case of vomiting. Fixation may need to last several weeks. Eating is restricted to liquids, pureed foods, and supplements.

Because only part of the teeth surfaces can be brushed, control of plaque formation, infection, and halitosis is accomplished using a 60-sec rinse with 30 mL of chlorhexidine 0.12% every morning and evening. Jaw-opening exercises usually help restore function after fixation is discontinued.

PEARLS & PITFALLS

- Ensure that patients with maxillomandibular fixation always carry wire cutters.

Condylar fractures may require only 2 to 3 wk of maxillomandibular fixation, followed by a soft diet. However, severely displaced, bilaterally fractured condyles may require open reduction and fixation. Condylar fractures in children should not be rigidly immobilized because ankylosis and abnormal facial development may result. Flexible (elastic) fixation for 5 to 10 days is usually sufficient.

Midface fractures: Fractures of the midface are treated surgically if they cause malocclusion, enophthalmos, diplopia, infraorbital nerve anesthesia, or unacceptable cosmetic deformity. Surgical treatment usually consists of internal stabilization using fine screws and plates. Surgery can often be delayed until swelling subsides, particularly if the indication for surgery is not clear. However, if surgery is required, it is best done within 14 days of injury because after this time, bone callus can make reduction difficult.

FRACTURES OF THE NOSE

Fractures of the nasal bones or cartilaginous injury may result in swelling, point tenderness, hypermobility, crepitus, epistaxis, and periorbital bruising. Diagnosis is

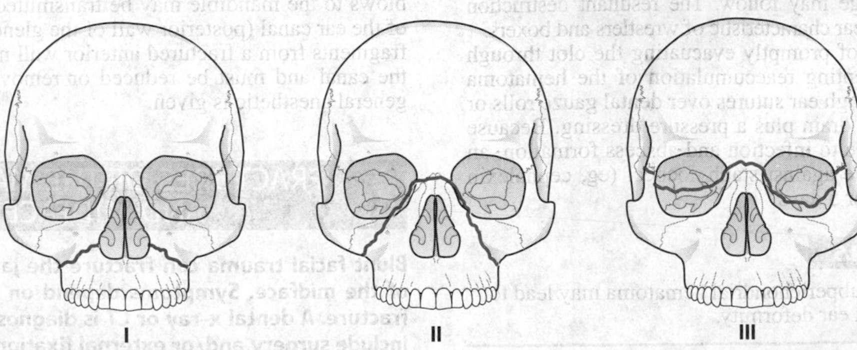

Fig. 358–1. Le Fort classification of midface fractures. I: only the lower maxilla; II: the infraorbital rim; III: complete detachment of the midface from the skull (craniofacial dissociation).

usually clinical. Treatment may include reduction, stabilization through internal packing, and splinting. A septal hematoma is drained without delay.

The nasal bones are the most frequently fractured facial bones because of their central location and protrusion. Depending on the mechanism of injury, fractures of the maxilla, orbit, or cribriform plate and injury to the nasolacrimal ducts may also occur.

Complications include cosmetic deformity and functional obstruction. Septal hematomas are subperichondrial blood collections that may lead to avascular or septic necrosis of the cartilage with resultant deformity (saddle nose). Cribriform plate fracture may cause a CSF leak, with increased risk of meningitis or brain abscess. Fortunately, this complication is rare.

Symptoms and Signs

Facial trauma resulting in epistaxis may indicate a nasal fracture. Other symptoms and signs include obvious or subtle nasal deformity, swelling, point tenderness, crepitus, and instability. Lacerations, ecchymosis (nasal and periorbital), septal deviation, and nasal obstruction may be present. Septal hematoma appears as a purplish bulge on the septum. CSF rhinorrhea appears as clear drainage but may be mixed with blood, making it difficult to identify.

Diagnosis

- Physical examination

Diagnosis is based on physical examination. Plain x-rays of an uncomplicated nasal fracture are not helpful because their sensitivity and specificity are poor. If other facial fractures or complications are suspected, CT of facial bones is done.

Treatment

- Symptomatic care
- For septal hematomas, immediate drainage
- For deformities, delayed reduction

Immediate treatment includes symptomatic control with ice and analgesics. Septal hematomas must be immediately incised and drained to prevent infection and cartilage necrosis.

Reduction is needed only for fractures causing clinically visible deformity or nasal airway obstruction. The end-point of reduction is determined by clinical appearance or improved airway. Reduction is usually deferred for 3 to 5 days after injury to allow swelling to subside but should take place within 2 to 3 wk of the injury, before bony callus formation. Nasal fractures in adults may be reduced after a local anesthetic is given; children require general anesthesia.

A blunt elevator is passed through the nares and placed under the depressed nasal bone, which is lifted anteriorly and laterally while pressure is applied to the other side of the nose to bring the nasal dorsum to the midline. The nose may be stabilized with internal packing (consisting of antibiotic-impregnated strip gauze) placed high within the nasal vestibule, as well as with external splinting. Internal packing is left in place for 4 to 7 days; external splinting is left for 7 to 14 days. Antibiotic prophylaxis effective against staphylococci is required for the duration of nasal packing, to decrease the risk of toxic shock syndrome.

Cartilaginous injuries often do not require reduction. In the rare circumstance that a deformity persists after swelling subsides, a reduction and splinting after a local anesthetic is given are usually sufficient.

Septal fractures are difficult to hold in position and often require septal surgery later.

Cribriform plate fractures with CSF leak require hospital admission with bed rest, head elevation, and placement of a lumbar drain. Drain management and need for antibiotics vary by institution. If the CSF leak does not resolve, surgical repair of the skull base may be required.

KEY POINTS

- The main concerns with nasal fractures are septal hematoma, epistaxis, nasal obstruction, cosmetic problems, and rare cribriform plate fractures.
- Nasal x-rays are unnecessary.
- Immediately drain septal hematomas.
- Delay reduction and some other treatments for 3 to 5 days to allow edema to resolve.

TEMPORAL BONE FRACTURES

Temporal bone fractures can occur after severe blunt trauma to the head and sometimes involve structures of the ear, causing hearing loss, vertigo, balance disturbance, or facial paralysis.

Temporal bone fractures are suggested by

- Battle sign (postauricular ecchymosis)
- Bleeding from the ear

Bleeding may come from the middle ear (hemotympanum) through a ruptured tympanic membrane (see p. 834) or from a fracture line in the ear canal. A hemotympanum makes the tympanic membrane appear blue-black. CSF otorrhea indicates a communication between the middle ear and the subarachnoid space.

Temporal bone fractures have been classified by orientation with respect to the long axis of the petrous portion of the temporal bone. Longitudinal fractures make up 70 to 90% of temporal bone fractures, and transverse fractures make up 10 to 30%. Some fractures may have characteristics of both patterns.

Longitudinal fractures can extend through the middle ear and rupture the tympanic membrane; they cause facial paralysis in 20% of cases and may cause hearing loss (usually conductive).

Transverse fractures cross the fallopian canal and otic capsule, causing facial paralysis in about 40% of patients and sometimes hearing loss (usually sensorineural) and vestibular dysfunction (eg, vertigo, balance disturbance).

Rarely, fluctuating sensorineural hearing loss and vestibular dysfunction occur with temporal bone fracture and may be due to a perilymph fistula. Immediate complete facial paralysis may indicate a severed or crushed facial nerve, whereas delayed-onset complete facial paralysis usually indicates edema within an intact nerve.

Diagnosis

- CT
- Assessment of hearing and facial nerve function

If a temporal bone fracture is suspected, immediate CT of the head with special attention to the temporal bone is recommended. The Weber and Rinne tuning fork tests can be done during the initial physical examination in conscious patients to help differentiate between conductive and sensorineural hearing loss. However, formal audiometric examination is required for all patients with temporal bone fractures. If facial paralysis is present, electrical testing of the facial nerve is warranted.

Treatment

- Management of facial nerve injury, hearing loss, vestibular dysfunction, and CSF leakage

Treatment is based on managing facial nerve injury, hearing loss, vestibular dysfunction, and CSF leakage. If immediate facial nerve paralysis occurs with loss of electrical response, surgical exploration may be warranted. Delayed-onset or incomplete facial paralysis almost always resolves with conservative management, including use of corticosteroids, which are gradually tapered.

Conductive hearing loss requires ossicular chain reconstruction several weeks to months after the injury. Good results can be expected. When sensorineural hearing loss occurs, it is typically permanent, and there are no medical or surgical therapies available to improve hearing. However, in the rare case of fluctuating sensorineural hearing loss, an exploratory tympanotomy to search for a perilymph fistula may be indicated.

When vestibular dysfunction results from perilymph fistula, repair may reduce severity and frequency of vertiginous episodes. When dysfunction results from injury to the vestibular nerve or vestibular labyrinth, few interventions can improve outcome. Symptoms may subside when benzodiazepines are used. More lasting improvement may occur with vestibular rehabilitation.

Patients who have a temporal bone fracture and CSF otorrhea should be hospitalized because meningitis is a risk. The leak usually stops spontaneously within a few days, although a lumbar drain or surgical closure of the defect is occasionally required. The ear canal is not irrigated or manipulated. Prophylactic antibiotics are used in some institutions.

KEY POINTS

- Temporal bone fracture can cause blood coming from the ear, blood behind the tympanic membrane, hearing loss, vestibular dysfunction, and/or facial nerve paralysis.
- Do CT with attention to the temporal bone, refer patients for audiometry, and, if facial nerve paralysis is suspected, arrange electrical testing of the facial nerve.
- Direct treatment toward management of facial nerve injury, hearing loss, vestibular dysfunction, and CSF leakage.

359 Fractures, Dislocations, and Sprains

Musculoskeletal injuries include

- Fractures
- Joint dislocations
- Ligament sprains
- Muscle strains
- Tendon injuries

These injuries are common and vary greatly in mechanism, severity, and treatment. The extremities, spine and pelvis can all be affected.

Some injuries are discussed elsewhere in THE MANUAL: spinal trauma (see p. 3098); fractures of the temporal bone, jaw and contiguous structures, and nose (see p. 2971); metatarsal stress fractures (see p. 3108); orbital fractures (see p. 2972); rib fractures (see p. 3116); fractures that occur during birth (see p. 2974); spinal subluxation (see p. 319); and mandibular dislocation (see p. 880). For dental fractures, see p. 879.

Musculoskeletal injuries may occur in isolation or as part of multisystem trauma (see p. 2927). Most musculoskeletal injuries result from blunt trauma, but penetrating trauma can also damage musculoskeletal structures.

Fractures and dislocations may be open (in communication with the environment via a skin wound) or closed.

Pathophysiology

Fractures: A fracture is a break in a bone. Most involve a single, significant force applied to normal bone.

In a closed fracture, the overlying skin is intact. In an open fracture, the overlying skin is disrupted and the broken bone is in communication with the environment.

Pathologic fractures occur when mild or minimal force fractures an area of bone weakened by a disorder (eg, osteoporosis, cancer, infection, bone cyst). When the disorder is osteoporosis, they are often called insufficiency or fragility fractures.

Stress fractures (see p. 3108) result from repetitive application of moderate force, as may occur in long-distance runners or in soldiers marching while carrying a heavy load. Normally, bone damaged by microtrauma from moderate force self-repairs during periods of rest, but repeated application of force to the same location predisposes to further injury and causes the microtrauma to propagate.

Dislocations: A dislocation is a complete separation of the 2 bones that form a joint. Subluxation is partial separation. Often, a dislocated joint remains dislocated until reduced (realigned) by a clinician, but sometimes it reduces spontaneously.

Sprains and strains: Ligaments connect one bone to another. Tears may occur in ligaments (sprains) or in muscles (strains).

Tears may be graded as

- 1st degree: Minimal (fibers are stretched but intact, or only a few fibers are torn)
- 2nd degree: Partial (some to almost all fibers are torn)
- 3rd degree: Complete (all fibers are torn)

Tendon injuries: Tendons connect muscles to bones. Tendon tears can also be partial or complete.

With **complete tears,** the motion produced by the detached muscle is usually lost.

Partial tears can result from a single traumatic event (eg, penetrating trauma) or repeated stress (chronically, causing tendinopathy). Motion is often intact, but partial tears may progress to complete tears, particularly when significant or repetitive force is applied.

Healing: Bone heals at various rates, depending on the patient's age and coexisting disorders. For example, children heal much faster than adults; disorders that impair peripheral circulation (eg, diabetes, peripheral vascular disease) slow healing.

Fractures heal in 3 overlapping stages:

- Inflammatory
- Reparative
- Remodeling

The **inflammatory phase** occurs first. A hematoma forms at the fracture site, and a small amount of bone in the distal fracture fragments is resorbed. If a fracture line is not evident initially (eg, in some nondisplaced fractures), one typically becomes evident about 1 wk after the injury as this small amount of bone is resorbed.

During the **reparative phase,** a callus is formed. New blood vessels develop, enabling cartilage to form across the fracture line. Immobilization (eg, casting) is needed during the first 2 stages to allow new blood vessels to grow. The reparative phase ends with clinical union of the fracture (ie, when there is no pain at fracture site, the injured extremity can be used without pain, and clinical examination detects no bone movement).

In the **remodeling stage,** the callus, which was originally cartilaginous, becomes ossified, and the bone is broken down and rebuilt (remodeled). During this stage, patients should be instructed to gradually resume moving the injured part normally, including putting load-bearing stress on it.

Most **joint dislocations** can be reduced (returned to the normal anatomic position) without surgery. Occasionally, dislocations cannot be reduced using closed manipulative techniques, and open surgery is required. Once a joint is reduced, additional surgery is often not necessary, However, surgery is sometimes required to manage associated fractures, debris in the joint, or residual instability.

Many **partial tears** to ligaments, tendons, or muscles heal spontaneously. Complete tears often require surgery to restore anatomy and function. Prognosis and treatment vary greatly depending on the location and severity of the injury.

Complications: Serious complications are unusual but may threaten life or limb viability or cause permanent limb dysfunction. Risk of complications is high with open injuries (which predispose to infection) and with injuries that disrupt blood vessels, tissue perfusion, and/or nerves. Dislocations, particularly if not rapidly reduced, tend to have a higher risk of vascular and nerve injuries than do fractures. Closed injuries that do not involve blood vessels or nerves, particularly those that are quickly reduced, are least likely to result in serious complications.

Acute complications (associated injuries) include the following:

- **Bleeding:** Bleeding accompanies all fractures and soft-tissue injuries. Rarely, internal or external bleeding is severe enough to cause hemorrhagic shock (eg, in pelvic, femoral, and some open fractures).
- **Vascular injuries:** Some open fractures disrupt blood vessels. Some closed injuries, particularly knee or hip dislocations and posteriorly displaced supracondylar humeral fractures, disrupt the vascular supply sufficiently to cause distal limb ischemia; this vascular disruption may be clinically occult for hours after the injury.
- **Nerve injuries:** Nerves may be injured when stretched by displaced pieces of a fractured bone or by a dislocated joint, when bruised by a blunt blow, when crushed in a severe crush injury, or when torn by sharp bone fragments. When nerves are bruised (called neurapraxia), nerve conduction is blocked, but the nerve is not torn. Neurapraxia causes temporary motor and/or sensory deficits; neurologic function returns completely in about 6 to 8 wk. When nerves are crushed (called axonotmesis), the axon is injured, but the myelin sheath is not. This injury is more severe than neurapraxia. Depending on the extent of the damage, the nerve can regenerate over weeks to years. Usually, nerves are torn (called neurotmesis) in open injuries. Torn nerves do not heal spontaneously and may have to be repaired surgically.
- **Fat embolism:** Fractures of long bones may release fat (and other marrow contents) that embolizes to the lungs and causes respiratory complications.
- **Compartment syndrome:** Tissue pressure increases in a closed fascial space, disrupting the vascular supply and reducing tissue perfusion. Crush injuries or markedly comminuted fractures are a common cause, increasing tissue pressure as edema develops. Risk is high with forearm fractures that involve both the radius and ulna, tibial plateau fractures (proximal tibial fractures that extend into the joint space), or tibial shaft fractures. Untreated compartment syndrome can lead to rhabdomyolysis, hyperkalemia, and infection. It can also cause contractures, sensory deficits, and paralysis. Compartment syndrome threatens limb viability (possibly requiring amputation) and survival.
- **Infection:** Any injury can become infected, but risk is highest with those that are open or surgically treated. Acute infection can lead to osteomyelitis (see p. 298), which can be difficult to cure.

Long-term complications include the following:

- **Instability:** Various fractures, dislocations, and ligament injuries, particularly 3rd-degree sprains, can lead to joint instability. Instability can be disabling and increases the risk of osteoarthritis.
- **Stiffness and impaired range of motion:** Fractures that extend into joints usually disrupt articular cartilage; misaligned articular cartilage tends to scar, causing osteoarthritis and impairing joint motion. Stiffness is more likely if a joint needs prolonged immobilization. The knee, elbow, and shoulder are particularly prone to posttraumatic stiffness, especially in the elderly.
- **Nonunion or delayed union:** Occasionally, fractures do not heal (called nonunion), or union is delayed. Major contributing factors include incomplete immobilization, partial disruption of the vascular supply, and patient factors that impair healing (eg, use of corticosteroids or thyroid hormone).
- **Malunion:** Malunion is healing with residual deformity. It is more likely if a fracture is not adequately reduced and stabilized.
- **Osteonecrosis:** Part of a fracture fragment can become necrotic, primarily when the vascular supply is damaged. Closed injuries prone to osteonecrosis include scaphoid fractures, displaced femoral neck fractures, dislocations of a native (not prosthetic) hip, and displaced talar neck fractures.
- **Osteoarthritis:** Injuries that disrupt the weight-bearing surfaces of joints or that result in joint malalignment and instability predispose to joint cartilage degeneration and osteoarthritis.

Evaluation

- Evaluation for serious injuries
- History and physical examination
- X-rays to identify fractures
- Sometimes MRI or CT

In the emergency department, if the mechanism suggests potentially severe or multiple injuries (as in a high-speed motor vehicle crash or fall from a height), patients are first evaluated from head to toe for serious injuries to all organ systems and, if needed, are resuscitated (see p. 2927). Patients, especially those with pelvic or femoral fractures, are evaluated for hemorrhagic shock due to occult blood loss. If a limb is injured, it is immediately evaluated for open wounds and symptoms or signs of neurovascular injury (numbness, paresis, poor perfusion) and compartment syndrome (eg, pain out of proportion to injuries, pallor, paresthesias, coolness, pulselessness).

Patients should be checked for ligament, tendon, and muscle injuries as well as fractures; sometimes parts of this evaluation are deferred until fracture is excluded. The joint above and below the injured joint should also be examined.

History: The mechanism (eg, the direction and magnitude of force) may suggest the type of injury. However, many patients do not remember or cannot describe the exact mechanism.

If a patient reports a deformity that has resolved before the patient is medically evaluated, the deformity should be assumed to be a true deformity that spontaneously reduced. A perceived snap or pop at the time of injury may signal a fracture or a ligament or tendon injury. Fractures and serious ligamentous injuries usually cause immediate pain; pain that begins hours to days after the injury suggests minor injury. Pain that is out of proportion to the apparent severity of the injury or that steadily worsens in the first hours to days immediately after injury suggests compartment syndrome (see p. 2997) or ischemia.

Physical examination: Examination includes

- Vascular and neurologic assessment
- Inspection for deformity, swelling, ecchymoses, open wounds, and decreased or abnormal motion
- Palpation for tenderness, crepitation, and gross defects in bone or tendon
- Examination of the joints above and below the injured area
- After fracture and dislocation are excluded (clinically or by imaging), stress testing of the affected joints for pain and instability

If muscle spasm and pain limit physical examination (particularly stress testing), examination is sometimes easier after the patient is given a systemic analgesic or local anesthetic. Or the injury can be immobilized until muscle spasm subsides, usually for a few days, and then the patient can be reexamined.

Deformity suggests dislocation, subluxation (partial separation of bones in a joint), or fracture.

If a **wound** is near a dislocation or fracture, the injury is assumed to be open. Open fractures can be classified using the Gustilo-Anderson system:

- **Grade I:** Wound < 1 cm, with minimal contamination, comminution, and soft-tissue damage
- **Grade II:** Wound > 1 cm, with moderate soft-tissue damage and minimal periosteal stripping
- **Grade IIIA:** Severe soft-tissue damage and substantial contamination, with adequate soft-tissue coverage
- **Grade IIIB:** Severe soft-tissue damage and substantial contamination, with inadequate soft-tissue coverage
- **Grade IIIC:** Open fracture with arterial injury requiring repair

Higher grades indicate a higher risk of osteomyelitis; however, interobserver reliability using this system is not high (often about 60%), and certain aspects can be best assessed intraoperatively.

Swelling commonly indicates a significant musculoskeletal injury but may require several hours to develop. If no swelling occurs within this time, fracture or severe ligament disruption is unlikely. With some fractures (eg, buckle fractures, small fractures without displacement), swelling may be subtle but is rarely absent.

Tenderness accompanies nearly all injuries, and for many patients, palpation anywhere around the injured area causes discomfort. However, a noticeable increase in tenderness in one localized area (point tenderness) suggests a fracture or sprain. Localized ligamentous tenderness and pain when the joint is stressed are consistent with sprain. With some fractures and complete muscle or tendon tears, a defect may be palpable in the affected structure.

Crepitus (a characteristic palpable and/or audible grinding produced when the joint is moved) may be a sign of fracture.

Gross joint instability suggests dislocation or severe ligamentous disruption.

Stress testing is done to evaluate the stability of an injured joint (see p. 3006); however, if a fracture is suspected, stress testing is deferred until x-rays exclude fracture. Bedside stress testing involves passively opening the joint in a direction usually perpendicular to the normal range of motion (stressing). Because muscle spasm during acutely painful injuries may mask joint instability, the surrounding muscles are relaxed as much as possible, and examinations are begun gently, then repeated, with slightly more force each time. Findings are compared with those for the opposite, normal side but can be limited by their subjective nature.

Findings can help differentiate between 2nd- and 3rd-degree sprains:

- **2nd-degree sprains:** Stress is painful, and joint opening is limited.
- **3rd-degree sprains:** Stress is less painful because the ligament is completely torn and is not being stretched, and joint opening is significant.

If muscle spasm is severe despite use of analgesia or anesthetic injection, the examination should be repeated a few days later, when the spasm has subsided.

PEARLS & PITFALLS

- Stress testing may be less painful with 3rd-degree sprains than with 2nd-degree sprains.

Some **partial tendon tears** escape initial clinical detection because function appears intact. Any of the following suggests partial tendon tears:

- Tendon tenderness
- Pain when the joint is moved through its range of motion
- Dysfunction
- Weakness
- Palpable defects

Partial tendon tears may progress to complete tears if patients continue to use the injured part. If the mechanism of injury or examination suggests a partial tendon injury or if the examination is inconclusive, a splint should be applied to limit motion and thus the potential for further injury. Subsequent examination, occasionally supplemented with MRI, may further delineate the extent of injury.

Attention to certain areas during examination can help detect commonly missed injuries (see Table 359–1).

If physical examination is normal in a joint that patients identify as painful, the cause may be referred pain. For example, patients with a slipped capital femoral epiphysis (or less often hip fracture) may feel pain in their knee.

Imaging: Not all limb injuries require imaging. Some fractures are minor and are treated similarly to soft-tissue injuries. For example, most injuries of toes 2 through 5 and many fingertip injuries are treated symptomatically whether a fracture is present or not; thus, x-rays are not needed. Many ankle sprains do not require x-rays during the initial evaluation because the probability of finding a fracture that would require a change in treatment is acceptably low; for ankle sprains, explicit, generally accepted criteria for obtaining x-rays (Ottawa ankle rules—see p. 3005) can help limit x-rays to patients that are more likely to have a fracture requiring specific treatment.

Table 359–1. EXAMINATION FOR SOME COMMONLY MISSED INJURIES

SYMPTOM	CHARACTERISTIC HISTORY	FINDING	INJURY
Shoulder pain	Seizure Electric shock	Restriction of passive external rotation with the elbow flexed	Posterior shoulder (glenohumeral) dislocation, possibly bilateral
	History of shoulder dislocation in patients > 40	Inability to maintain a position at 90° of abduction when slight downward pressure is applied (drop-arm test)	Acute complete rotator cuff tear
	Various mechanisms (eg, pile-on injury in football, direct blow to joint)	Tenderness over the sternoclavicular joint	Sternoclavicular joint injury
	Most often, fall on the point of the shoulder	Tenderness over the acromioclavicular area	Acromioclavicular strain or disruption (shoulder separation)
Wrist pain or swelling	Fall on an outstretched hand	Tenderness over the anatomic snuffbox (located just distal to the radius, between the extensor pollicis longus, extensor pollicis brevis, and abductor pollicis longus tendons)	Scaphoid fracture
	Various mechanisms	Tenderness over the lunate fossa (in the wrist at the base of the 3rd metacarpal) and pain with axial compression of the 3rd metacarpal	Lunate fracture Lunate or perilunate dislocation
Hip pain	Fall	Pain during passive hip rotation when the knee is flexed Inability to flex the hip Leg externally rotated and shortened Inability to bear weight even though plain x-rays are normal (particularly in patients with osteoporosis)	Hip fracture
Knee pain in a child or an adolescent	Various mechanisms	Pain during passive hip rotation when the knee is flexed	Hip injury (eg, slipped capital femoral epiphysis [see p. 2480], Legg-Calvé-Perthes disease [see p. 2477])
Knee pain or swelling	Various mechanisms	Weak or absent active knee extension and normal knee x-rays	Quadriceps tendon rupture Patellar tendon rupture

Plain x-rays are done first; they show primarily bone (and joint effusion secondary to bleeding or occult fracture) and thus are useful for diagnosing dislocations and fractures rather than sprains. They should include at least 2 views taken in different planes (usually anteroposterior and lateral views).

Additional views (eg, oblique) may be done when

- The evaluation suggests fracture and 2 projections are negative.
- They are routine for certain joints (eg, a mortise view for evaluating an ankle, an oblique view for evaluating a foot).
- Certain abnormalities are suspected (eg, Y view of the shoulder when posterior dislocation is suspected).

For lateral views of digits, the digit of interest should be separated from the others.

MRI or **CT** can be used if a fracture is not visible on plain x-rays but is strongly suspected clinically (common with scaphoid fractures and impacted femoral neck (subcapital) hip fractures) or if more detail is needed to guide treatment (eg, for scapular fractures, pelvic fractures, or intraarticular fractures). For example, if findings after a fall suggest hip fracture but x-rays are normal, MRI should be done to check for an occult hip fracture. MRI can also be done to identify soft-tissue injuries, including ligament, tendon, cartilage, and muscle injuries.

Arteriography or **CT angiography** may be indicated for suspected arterial injuries.

Nerve conduction studies may be indicated if nerve symptoms persist weeks to months after injuries. These tests help identify focal peripheral nervous system dysfunction as occurs in entrapment neuropathies (eg, carpal tunnel syndrome). These studies are usually done weeks to months after the initial injury.

Fracture description: A fracture's appearance on x-rays can be described relatively precisely using the following terms:

- Type of fracture line (see Fig. 359–1)
- Location of fracture line
- Displacement (see Fig. 359–2)
- Open or closed

Terms for location include

- Dorsal or volar
- Epiphysis (sometimes involving the articular surface), which can refer to the proximal end of the bone [the head] or the distal end
- Metaphysis (neck—the part of a long bone between the epiphysis and diaphysis)
- Diaphysis (shaft, divided into the proximal, middle, or distal third)

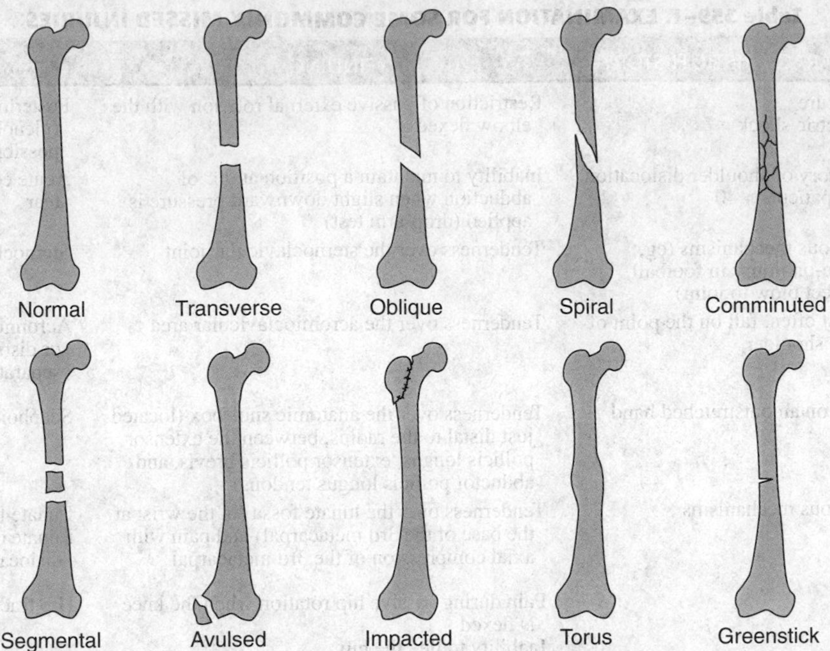

Fig. 359–1. Common types of fracture lines. Transverse fractures are perpendicular to the long axis of a bone. **Oblique** fractures occur at an angle. **Spiral** fractures result from a rotatory mechanism; on x-rays, they are differentiated from oblique fractures by a component parallel to the long axis of bone in at least 1 view. **Comminuted** fractures have > 2 bone fragments. Comminuted fractures include segmental fractures (2 separate breaks in a bone). **Avulsion** fractures are caused by a tendon dislodging a bone fragment. In **impacted** fractures, bone fragments are driven into each other, shortening the bone; these fractures may be visible as a focal abnormal density in trabeculae or irregularities in bone cortex. **Torus** fractures (buckling of the bone cortex) and **greenstick** fractures (cracks in only 1 side of the cortex) are childhood fractures.

Treatment

- Treatment of associated injuries
- Reduction as indicated, splinting, and analgesia
- RICE (rest, ice, compression, and elevation) or PRICE (including protection) as indicated
- Usually immobilization
- Sometimes surgery

Initial treatment: Hemorrhagic shock is treated immediately (see p. 573). Injuries to arteries are surgically repaired unless they affect only small arteries with good collateral circulation. Compartment syndrome is treated (see p. 2997). Severed nerves are surgically repaired; for neuropraxia and axonotmesis, initial treatment is usually observation, supportive measures, and sometimes physical therapy. Suspected open fractures or dislocations require sterile wound dressings, tetanus prophylaxis, broad-spectrum antibiotics (eg, a 2nd-generation cephalosporin plus an aminoglycoside), and surgery to irrigate and debride them (and thus prevent infection).

Most moderate and severe injuries, particularly grossly unstable ones, are immobilized immediately by splinting (immobilization with a nonrigid or noncircumferential device) to decrease pain and to prevent further injury to soft tissues by unstable injuries. In patients with long-bone fractures, splinting may prevent fat embolism.

Pain is treated as soon as possible, typically with opioids (see p. 1969).

After initial treatment, injuries are reduced, immobilized, and treated symptomatically as indicated.

Many 3rd-degree sprains and tendon tears and some dislocations in which structures supporting the joint are damaged require surgical repair.

Reduction: Rotational malalignment or significant angulation or displacement of fractures is typically treated with reduction (realignment of bones or bone fragments by manipulation), which usually requires analgesia and/or sedation. Exceptions include some fractures in children in which remodeling over time can correct significant deformities.

Dislocations are reduced.

Closed reduction (by manipulation, without skin incision) is done when possible; if not, open reduction (with skin incision) is done.

Closed reduction of fractures is usually maintained by casting; some dislocations require only a splint or sling.

Open reduction of fractures is usually maintained by various surgical hardware, external and/or internal. In open reduction with internal fixation (ORIF), fracture fragments are aligned and held in place using a combination of pins, screws, and plates. ORIF is usually indicated when

- Intra-articular fractures are displaced (to precisely align the joint surface).
- ORIF has better results than nonsurgical treatment for a particular type of fracture.
- Closed reduction was ineffective.

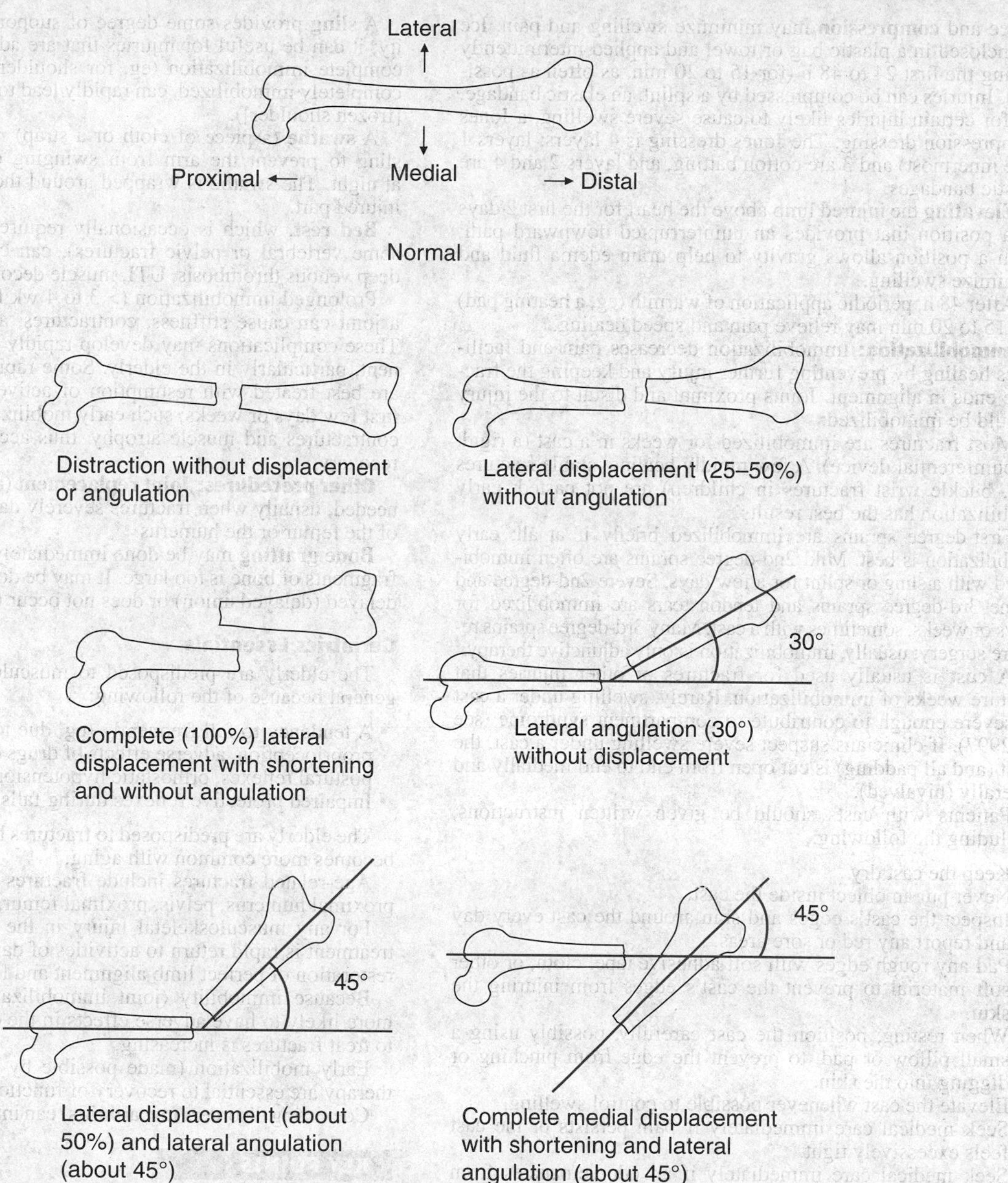

Fig. 359–2. Spatial relationship between fracture fragments. Distraction, displacement, angulation, or shortening (overriding) may occur. **Distraction** is separation in the longitudinal axis. **Displacement** is the degree to which the fractured ends are out of alignment with each other; it is described in millimeters or bone width percentage. **Angulation** is the angle of the distal fragment measured from the proximal fragment. Displacement and angulation may occur in the ventral-dorsal plane, lateral-medial plane, or both.

- Pathologic fractures occur in a bone weakened by cancer; such bone does not heal normally, and ORIF reduces pain more quickly than other treatments and makes early ambulation possible.
- Prolonged immobility (required for fracture healing) is undesirable (eg, for hip or femoral shaft fractures); ORIF provides early structural stability, minimizes pain, and facilitates mobilization.

PRICE: Patients who have soft-tissue injuries, with or without other musculoskeletal injuries, may benefit from PRICE (protection, rest, ice, compression, elevation), although this practice is not supported by strong evidence.

Protection helps prevent further injury. It may involve limiting the use of an injured part, applying a splint or cast, or using crutches.

Rest may prevent further injury and speed healing.

Ice and **compression** may minimize swelling and pain. Ice is enclosed in a plastic bag or towel and applied intermittently during the first 24 to 48 h (for 15 to 20 min, as often as possible). Injuries can be compressed by a splint, an elastic bandage, or, for certain injuries likely to cause severe swelling, a Jones compression dressing. The Jones dressing is 4 layers; layers 1 (the innermost) and 3 are cotton batting, and layers 2 and 4 are elastic bandages.

Elevating the injured limb above the heart for the first 2 days in a position that provides an uninterrupted downward path; such a position allows gravity to help drain edema fluid and minimize swelling.

After 48 h, periodic application of warmth (eg, a heating pad) for 15 to 20 min may relieve pain and speed healing.

Immobilization: Immobilization decreases pain and facilitates healing by preventing further injury and keeping the fracture ends in alignment. Joints proximal and distal to the injury should be immobilized.

Most fractures are immobilized for weeks in a cast (a rigid, circumferential device). A few rapidly healing, stable fractures (eg, buckle wrist fractures in children) are not casted; early mobilization has the best results.

First-degree sprains are immobilized briefly if at all; early mobilization is best. Mild 2nd-degree sprains are often immobilized with a sling or splint for a few days. Severe 2nd-degree and some 3rd-degree sprains and tendon tears are immobilized for days or weeks, sometimes with a cast. Many 3rd-degree sprains require surgery; usually, immobilization is only adjunctive therapy.

A **cast** is usually used for fractures or other injuries that require weeks of immobilization. Rarely, swelling under a cast is severe enough to contribute to compartment syndrome (see p. 2997). If clinicians suspect severe swelling under a cast, the cast (and all padding) is cut open from end to end medially and laterally (bivalved).

Patients with casts should be given written instructions, including the following:

- Keep the cast dry.
- Never put an object inside the cast.
- Inspect the cast's edges and skin around the cast every day and report any red or sore areas.
- Pad any rough edges with soft adhesive tape, cloth, or other soft material to prevent the cast's edges from injuring the skin.
- When resting, position the cast carefully, possibly using a small pillow or pad, to prevent the edge from pinching or digging into the skin.
- Elevate the cast whenever possible to control swelling.
- Seek medical care immediately if pain persists or the cast feels excessively tight.
- Seek medical care immediately if an odor emanates from within the cast or if a fever, which may indicate infection, develops.
- Seek care immediately for progressively worsening pain or any new numbness or weakness (see p. 2997).

Good hygiene is important.

A **splint** (see Fig. 359–3) can be used to immobilize some stable injuries, including some suspected but unproven fractures, rapidly healing fractures, sprains, and other injuries that require immobilization for several days or less. A splint is noncircumferential; thus, it enables patients to apply ice and to move more than a cast does. Also, it allows for some swelling, so it does not contribute to compartment syndrome. Some injuries that ultimately require casting are immobilized initially with a splint until most of the swelling resolves.

A **sling** provides some degree of support and limits mobility; it can be useful for injuries that are adversely affected by complete immobilization (eg, for shoulder injuries, which, if completely immobilized, can rapidly lead to adhesive capsulitis [frozen shoulder]).

A **swathe** (a piece of cloth or a strap) may be used with a sling to prevent the arm from swinging outward, especially at night. The swathe is wrapped around the back and over the injured part.

Bed rest, which is occasionally required for fractures (eg, some vertebral or pelvic fractures), can cause problems (eg, deep venous thrombosis, UTI, muscle deconditioning).

Prolonged immobilization (> 3 to 4 wk for young adults) of a joint can cause stiffness, contractures, and muscle atrophy. These complications may develop rapidly and may be permanent, particularly in the elderly. Some rapidly healing injuries are best treated with resumption of active motion within the first few days or weeks; such early mobilization may minimize contractures and muscle atrophy, thus accelerating functional recovery.

Other procedures: Joint replacement (arthroplasty) may be needed, usually when fractures severely damage the upper end of the femur or the humerus.

Bone grafting may be done immediately if the gap between fragments of bone is too large. It may be done later if healing is delayed (delayed union) or does not occur (nonunion).

Geriatrics Essentials

The elderly are predisposed to musculoskeletal injuries in general because of the following:

- A tendency to fall frequently (eg, due to age-related loss of proprioception, adverse effects of drugs on proprioception or postural reflexes, orthostatic hypotension)
- Impaired protective reflexes during falls

The elderly are predisposed to fractures because osteoporosis becomes more common with aging.

Age-related fractures include fractures of the distal radius, proximal humerus, pelvis, proximal femur, and vertebrae.

For any musculoskeletal injury in the elderly, the goal of treatment is rapid return to activities of daily living rather than restoration of perfect limb alignment and length.

Because immobility (joint immobilization or bed rest) is more likely to have adverse effects in the elderly, use of ORIF to treat fractures is increasing.

Early mobilization (made possible by ORIF) and physical therapy are essential to recovery of function.

Coexisting disorders (eg, arthritis) can interfere with recovery.

KEY POINTS

- Injuries that disrupt arterial supply and compartment syndrome threaten limb viability and may ultimately threaten life.
- Check for ligament, tendon, and muscle injuries as well as fractures (sometimes part of this evaluation is deferred until fracture is excluded).
- Examine the joints above and below the injured area.
- Consider referred pain, particularly if physical findings are normal in a joint that patients identify as painful (eg, knee pain in patients with a slipped capital femoral epiphysis).
- X-rays are not necessary for many distal extremity injuries (eg, most injuries of toes 2 through 5, many fingertip injuries and ankle sprains).
- Consider MRI (sometimes CT) when x-rays are normal but a fracture is strongly suspected clinically (eg, in an elderly

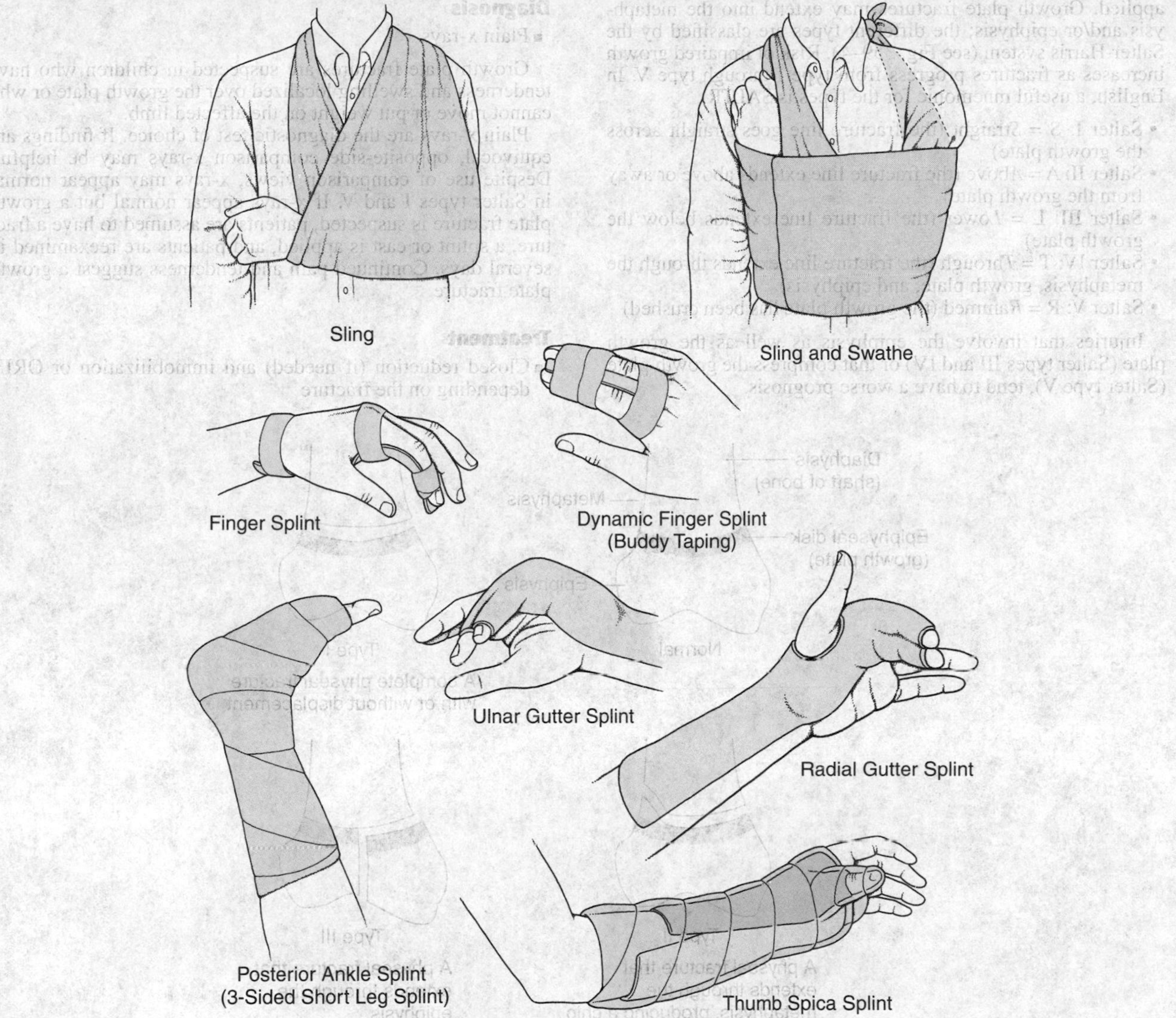

Fig. 359–3. Joint immobilization as acute treatment: Some commonly used techniques.

person who has hip pain and cannot walk after a fall); MRI can also be done to diagnose soft-tissue injuries.

- Immediately treat serious associated injuries, splint unstable injuries, and, as soon as possible, treat pain and reduce dislocations.
- Immobilize unstable injuries immediately; immobilize all injuries that require reduction as soon as they are reduced using a cast or splint
- Treat most minor injuries with PRICE (protection, rest, ice, compression, elevation).
- Provide patients with explicit, written instructions about cast care.
- When treating the elderly, usually choose the method that results in the earliest mobilization.

PEDIATRIC PHYSEAL FRACTURES

(Growth Plate Fractures)

Open growth plates in children are often involved in fractures. Diagnosis is by plain x-ray. Treatment is with closed reduction and immobilization or ORIF.

Bone grows as tissue is added at the physeal disk (growth plate), which is bordered by the metaphysis proximally and the epiphysis distally (see Fig. 359–4). The age at which the growth plate closes and bone growth stops varies by bone, but the growth plate is closed in all bones by age 20 (see Fig. 359–5).

Before closure, the growth plate is the most fragile part of the bone and is therefore frequently disrupted when force is applied. Growth plate fractures may extend into the metaphysis and/or epiphysis; the different types are classified by the Salter-Harris system (see Fig. 359–4). Risk of impaired growth increases as fractures progress from type I through type V. In English, a useful mnemonic for the types is SALTR:

- Salter I: S = *S*traight (the fracture line goes straight across the growth plate)
- Salter II: A = *A*bove (the fracture line extends above or away from the growth plate)
- Salter III: L = *L*ower (the fracture line extends below the growth plate)
- Salter IV: T = *T*hrough (the fracture line extends through the metaphysis, growth plate, and epiphysis)
- Salter V: R = *R*ammed (the growth plate has been crushed)

Injuries that involve the epiphysis as well as the growth plate (Salter types III and IV) or that compress the growth plate (Salter type V), tend to have a worse prognosis.

Diagnosis

- Plain x-rays

Growth plate fractures are suspected in children who have tenderness and swelling localized over the growth plate or who cannot move or put weight on the affected limb.

Plain x-rays are the diagnostic test of choice. If findings are equivocal, opposite-side comparison x-rays may be helpful. Despite use of comparison views, x-rays may appear normal in Salter types I and V. If x-rays appear normal but a growth plate fracture is suspected, patients are assumed to have a fracture, a splint or cast is applied, and patients are reexamined in several days. Continued pain and tenderness suggest a growth plate fracture.

Treatment

- Closed reduction (if needed) and immobilization or ORIF, depending on the fracture

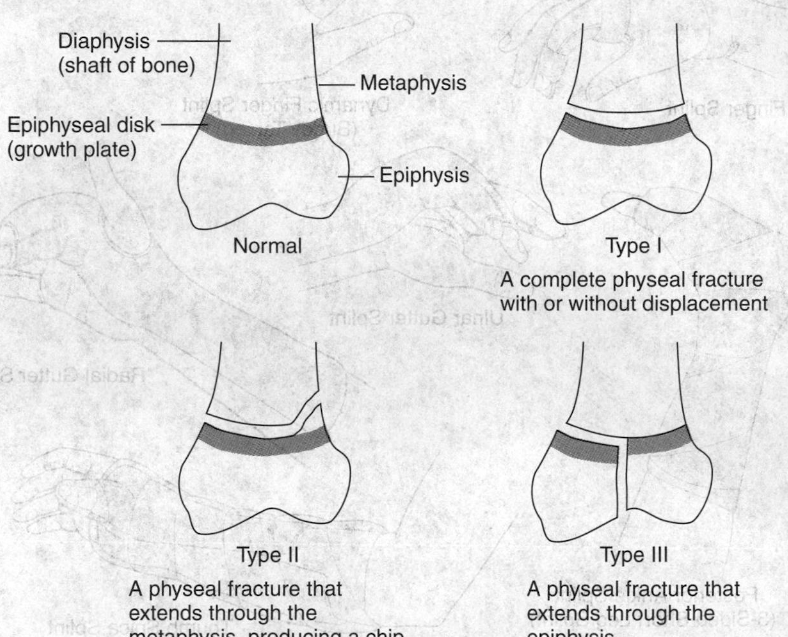

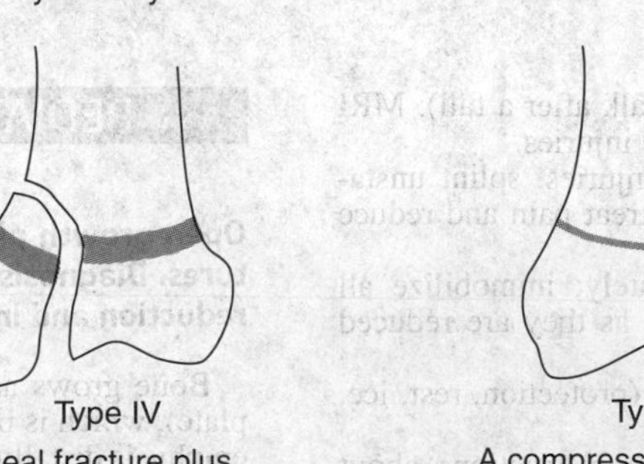

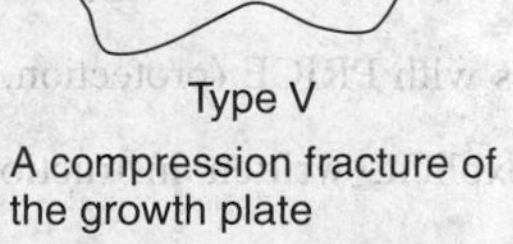

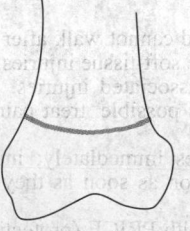

Fig. 359–4. Salter-Harris classification of physeal disk (growth plate) fractures. Types I through IV are physeal separations; the growth plate is separated from the metaphysis. Type II is the most common, and type V is the least common.

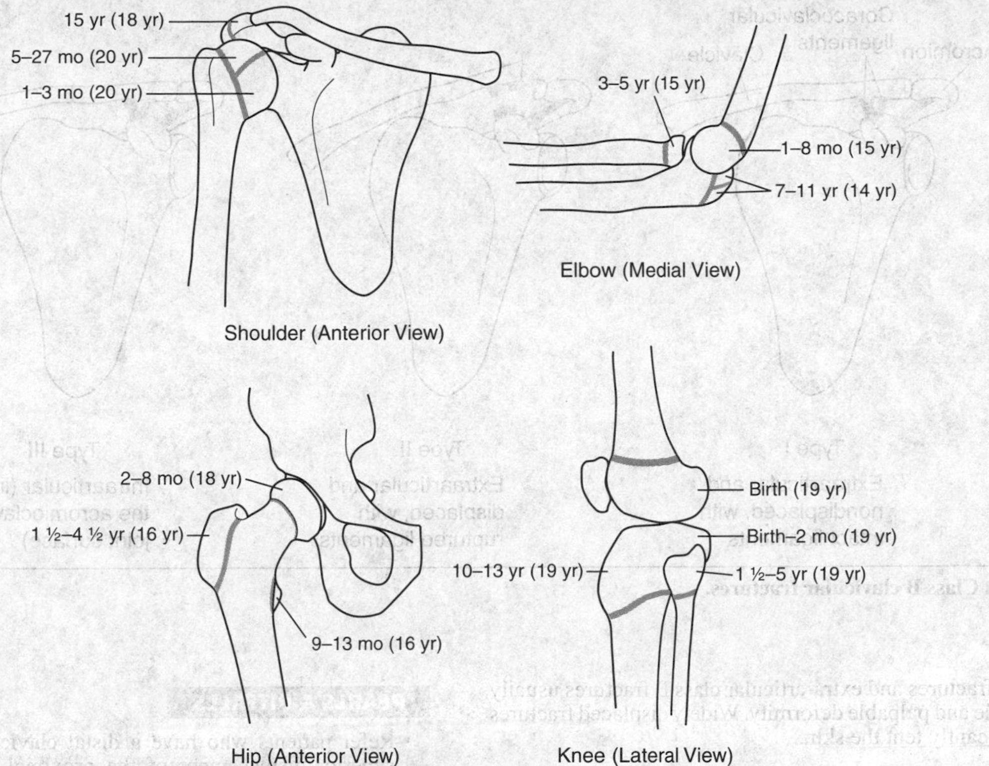

Fig. 359–5. Epiphyseal disks (growth plates). The first numbers are the age at which ossification first appears on x-ray; the numbers in parentheses are the age at which union occurs.

Depending on the particular fracture, closed treatment is usually sufficient for types I and II; ORIF is often required for types III and IV.

Patients with type V injuries should be referred to a pediatric orthopedist because such injuries almost always lead to growth abnormalities.

KEY POINTS

- Because the growth plate is more fragile in children, it is often disrupted before other stabilizing structures (eg, major ligaments).
- The prognosis tends to be worse for children with Salter types III, IV, and V than for those with types I and II.
- Consider comparison x-rays of the uninjured side if fracture is suspected but is not visible on x-rays of the injured side.
- ORIF is often required for types III and IV.

CLAVICLE FRACTURES

Clavicle fractures are among the most common fractures, particularly among children. Diagnosis is by plain x-ray. Most types are treated with a sling.

Etiology

Clavicle fractures usually result from a fall on the lateral shoulder or, less often, a direct blow.

Classification: Traditionally, treatment has been based on the following classification.

Class A fractures involve the middle third of the bone and account for about 80% of clavicle fractures. The proximal fragment is often displaced upward because it is pulled by the sternocleidomastoid muscle. Subclavian vessels are rarely damaged.

Class B fractures involve the distal third of the bone and account for about 15% of clavicle fractures. They usually result from a direct blow. There are 3 subtypes:

- **Type I:** Extra-articular and nondisplaced, generally indicating a functionally intact coracoclavicular ligament (a strong and structurally important ligament)
- **Type II:** Extra-articular and displaced, generally indicating rupture of the coracoclavicular ligament, with the proximal fragment typically displaced upward because it is pulled by the sternocleidomastoid muscle
- **Type III:** Involving the intra-articular surface of the acromioclavicular joint, thus increasing the risk of osteoarthritis (see Fig. 359–6)

Class C fractures involve the proximal third of the bone and account for about 5% of clavicle fractures. These fractures usually result from great force and thus may be accompanied by intrathoracic injuries or sternoclavicular joint damage.

Symptoms and Signs

The area over the fracture is painful, and patients may sense movement of the fracture fragments and instability. Some patients report pain in the shoulder. Arm abduction is painful.

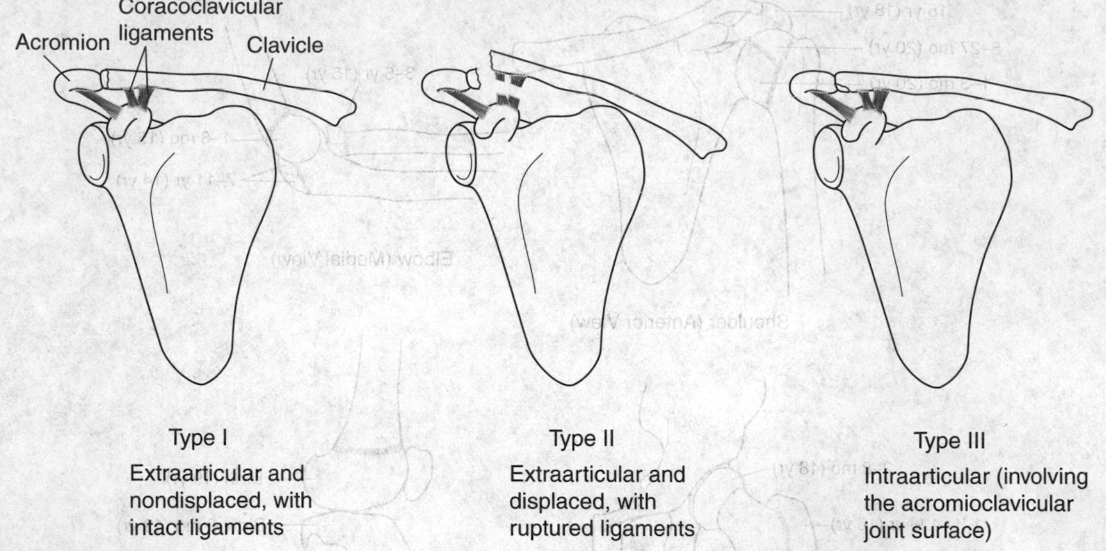

Fig. 359–6. Class B clavicular fractures.

Class A fractures and extra-articular class B fractures usually cause visible and palpable deformity. Widely displaced fractures may significantly tent the skin.

Diagnosis

- Plain x-rays

Clinical evaluation is often diagnostic, but anteroposterior plain x-rays are usually taken, and sometimes an apical lordotic view or an x-ray at a 45° angle upward is included. However, some class C and intra-articular class B fractures require other imaging studies (eg, CT).

Treatment

- Sling
- If the coracoclavicular ligament is ruptured, usually surgical repair

Many fractures are minimally displaced and can be treated with a sling for comfort for 4 to 6 weeks. Figure-of-eight braces are not recommended anymore because a simple sling is just as effective and often more comfortable.

Usually, reduction is not necessary, even for greatly angulated fractures.

However, if the skin is significantly tented (usually in class A fractures), immediate consultation with an orthopedic specialist may be needed. Usually, such fractures are still successfully managed with a sling, but if they are not treated promptly, the bone may pierce the skin, causing an open fracture.

In class B type II fractures, the ruptured coracoclavicular ligament usually requires surgical repair by an orthopedic surgeon. For example, if patients have a distal clavicle fracture with superior displacement of the proximal fragment, they should be referred to an orthopedic surgeon for consideration of surgical repair of the coracoclavicular ligament.

For class B type III fractures, early mobilization may help decrease the risk of osteoarthritis.

PEARLS & PITFALLS

- Refer patients who have a distal clavicle fracture with superior displacement of the proximal fragment to an orthopedic surgeon for consideration of surgical repair of the coracoclavicular ligament.

Displaced class C fractures require reduction by an orthopedic surgeon.

KEY POINTS

- Most clavicle fractures are evident based on clinical findings.
- Treat most clavicle fractures with a sling.
- An orthopedic surgeon is needed to reduce displaced class C fractures and usually to surgically repair class B type II fractures.

PROXIMAL HUMERAL FRACTURES

(Shoulder Fracture)

Proximal humeral fractures are proximal to the surgical neck (see Fig. 359–7). Most are minimally displaced and angulated. Diagnosis is by plain x-ray or sometimes CT. Most of these fractures can be treated with a sling, a swathe, and early mobilization.

Proximal humeral fractures are especially common among the elderly. A few patients have axillary nerve damage (reducing sensation over the middle deltoid) or axillary artery damage. Contractures may develop after only a few days of immobilization, particularly in the elderly.

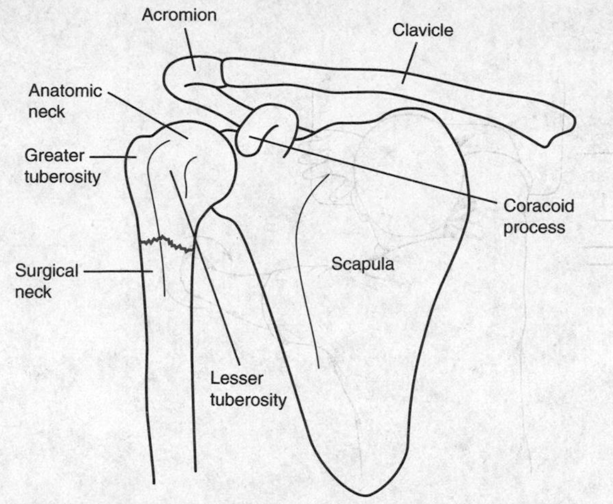

Fig. 359–7. Key anatomic landmarks in the proximal humerus. The surgical neck of the humerus is fractured.

Etiology

Most of these fractures result from a fall on an outstretched arm; less often, a direct blow is involved.

Classification: Fractures are classified by the number of parts that result; a part is defined as a key anatomic structure that is displaced (> 1 cm) or angulated (> 45°) in relation to its normal anatomic position. The 4 key anatomic structures of the proximal humerus are the

- Anatomic neck
- Surgical neck
- Greater tuberosity
- Lesser tuberosity

For example, if no structures are displaced or angulated, the fracture has one part. If one structure is angulated or displaced, the fracture has 2 parts (see Fig. 359–8). Almost 80% of proximal humeral fractures have only one part; they are usually stable, held together by the joint capsule, rotator cuff, and/or periosteum. Fractures with ≥ 3 parts are uncommon.

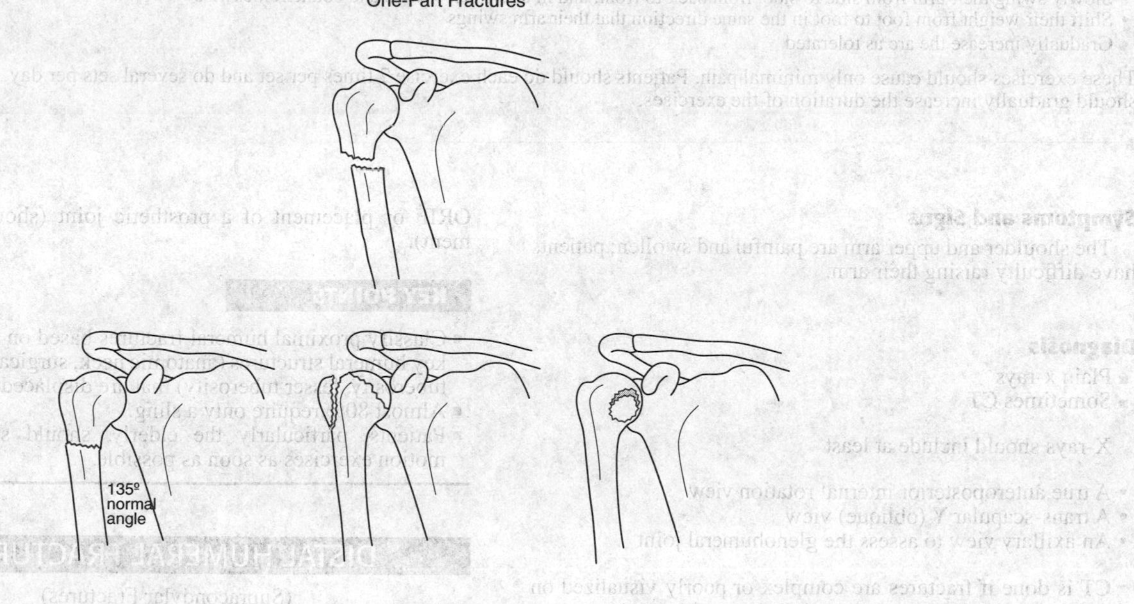

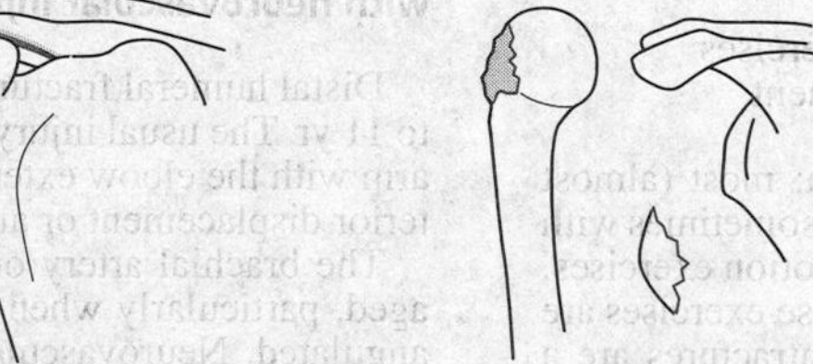

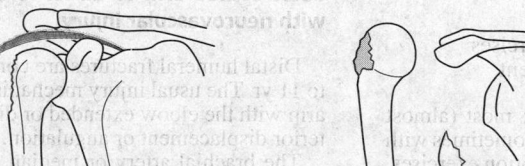

Fig. 359–8. One- and 2-part fractures of the proximal humerus. If no structures are displaced or angulated, the fracture has one part. If one structure is angulated or displaced, the fracture has 2 parts.

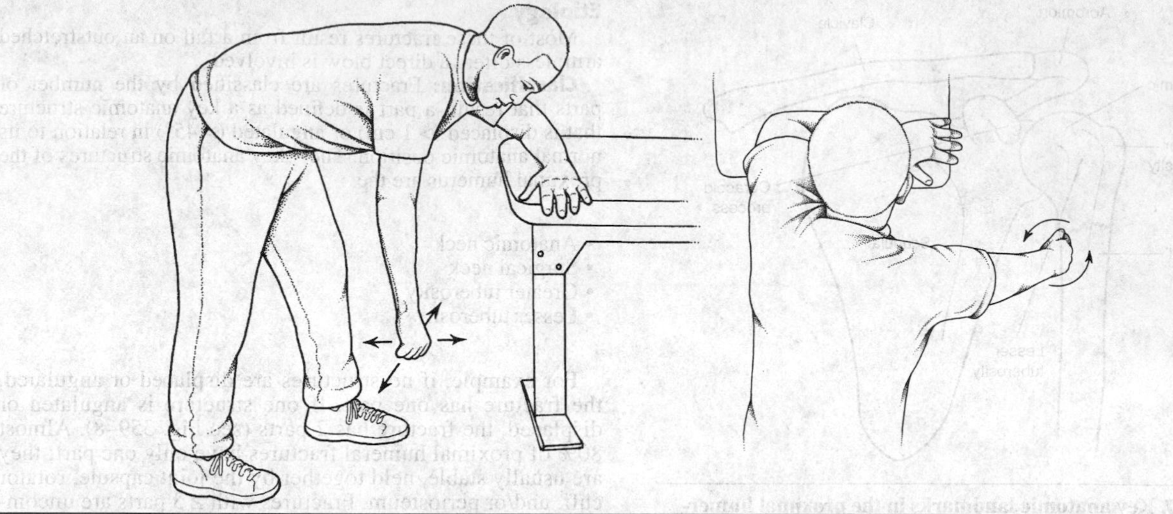

Fig. 359–9. Codman exercises. The patient bends at the waist with the affected arm hanging down perpendicular to the floor. The arm and shoulder should be relaxed, and knees bent. Patients should

- Slowly swing their arm from side to side, from back to front, and in circles clockwise and counterclockwise
- Shift their weight from foot to foot in the same direction that their arm swings
- Gradually increase the arc as tolerated

These exercises should cause only minimal pain. Patients should do each exercise 2 times per set and do several sets per day. Patients should gradually increase the duration of the exercises.

Symptoms and Signs

The shoulder and upper arm are painful and swollen; patients have difficulty raising their arm.

Diagnosis

- Plain x-rays
- Sometimes CT

X-rays should include at least

- A true anteroposterior internal rotation view
- A trans-scapular Y (oblique) view
- An axillary view to assess the glenohumeral joint

CT is done if fractures are complex or poorly visualized on plain x-rays.

Treatment

- Usually a sling and early range-of-motion exercises
- Sometimes ORIF or prosthetic joint replacement

One-part fractures rarely require reduction; most (almost 80%) are treated with immobilization in a sling, sometimes with a swathe (see Fig. 359–3), and early range-of-motion exercises, such as Codman exercises (see Fig. 359–9). These exercises are particularly useful for the elderly. Because contractures are a risk, early mobilization is desirable, even if alignment is anatomically imperfect.

Fractures with ≥ 2 parts are immobilized, and patients are referred to an orthopedic surgeon. These fractures may require ORIF or placement of a prosthetic joint (shoulder replacement).

KEY POINTS

- Classify proximal humeral fractures based on the number of key humeral structures (anatomic neck, surgical neck, greater tuberosity, lesser tuberosity) that are displaced or angulated.
- Almost 80% require only a sling.
- Patients, particularly the elderly, should start range-of-motion exercises as soon as possible.

DISTAL HUMERAL FRACTURES

(Supracondylar Fractures)

Distal humeral fractures usually result from a fall on an outstretched arm or direct force; they may be associated with neurovascular injury.

Distal humeral fractures are common among children aged 3 to 11 yr. The usual injury mechanism is a fall on an outstretched arm with the elbow extended or direct force, often causing posterior displacement or angulation.

The brachial artery or median or radial nerve may be damaged, particularly when the fracture is posteriorly displaced or angulated. Neurovascular injury sometimes leads to compartment syndrome of the forearm, which can cause Volkmann ischemic contracture (a flexion contracture at the wrist resulting in a clawlike hand deformity). Fractures are usually intra-articular, causing hemarthrosis.

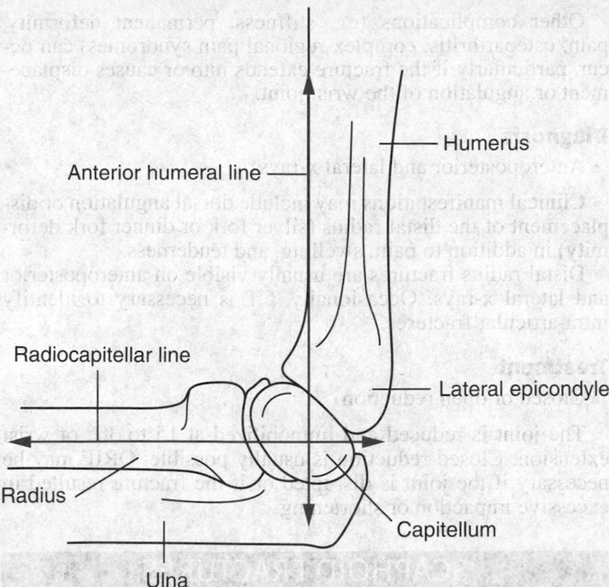

Fig. 359–10. Anterior humeral line and radiocapitellar line. Normally, the anterior humeral line, which is drawn along the anterior border of the humerus on a lateral x-ray, transects the middle of the capitellum. If the line transects none or only the anterior part of the capitellum, a distal humeral fracture with posterior displacement may be present. The radiocapitellar line, which is drawn through the midshaft of the radius, normally bisects the capitellum. If it does not, an occult fracture should be suspected.

Diagnosis

- Anteroposterior and lateral x-rays

A fracture line may not be visible, but other x-ray findings may suggest fracture. They include

- Posterior fat pad
- Anterior fat pad (sail sign)
- Abnormal anterior humeral line
- Abnormal radiocapitellar line

A **posterior fat pad** on a true lateral x-ray of the elbow is always abnormal; this finding is specific for joint effusion but not highly sensitive.

A **displaced anterior fat pad** may indicate joint effusion but is not specific.

However, if a posterior fat pad is seen or if a large anterior fat pad (sail sign) is present, an occult fracture should be assumed and should be treated as such.

The **anterior humeral line** is a line drawn along the anterior border of the humerus on a true lateral x-ray. Normally, this line transects the middle of the capitellum (see Fig. 359–10). If the line transects none or only the anterior part of the capitellum, a posteriorly displaced distal humeral fracture is possible; then oblique views are taken, and other imaging may be done.

The **radiocapitellar line** is a line drawn through the midshaft of the radius on a true lateral x-ray of the elbow; normally, it bisects the capitellum. If it does not, an occult fracture should be suspected.

If findings in children are compatible with a distal humeral fracture, x-rays should be reviewed closely for evidence of occult fracture (eg, a posterior fat pad, abnormalities in the anterior humeral or radiocapitellar line.

PEARLS & PITFALLS

- If findings in children are compatible with a distal humeral fracture, review x-rays closely for evidence of occult fracture (eg, a posterior fat pad, abnormalities in the anterior humeral or radiocapitellar line.

A complete neurovascular examination is done if a fracture is suspected.

Treatment

- Early orthopedic consultation
- For nondisplaced fractures or occult fractures, splinting
- For displaced fractures, often ORIF

Most fractures are managed by an orthopedic surgeon because long-term complications are a risk. Most patients are admitted for neurovascular observation, although some clinicians splint and discharge patients who have nondisplaced fractures if patients can be trusted to return for follow-up the next day.

Posteriorly displaced or angulated distal humeral fractures, in particular, should be reduced by a specialist because nerves and/or the radial artery can be injured during reduction. Casting with closed reduction may be tried but is typically not recommended because ORIF is usually necessary.

KEY POINTS

- Distal humeral fractures are more common among children.
- These fractures can injure the radial artery or median nerve.
- Check x-rays for posterior and anterior fat pads, and use the anterior humeral line and radiocapitellar line to determine whether an occult fracture is likely.
- For treatment, consult an orthopedic surgeon.

RADIAL HEAD FRACTURES

Radial head fractures frequently result from a fall on an outstretched arm and may be difficult to see on x-rays.

The radial head is palpated on the lateral elbow as a structure that rotates during pronation and supination and that articulates with the lateral epicondyle. The lateral epicondyle and radial head typically form an isosceles triangle with the olecranon. Joint effusions (common with radial head fractures) may be palpable over this triangle.

Symptoms and Signs

When the radial head is fractured, pain at the radial head is worse during supination, and the radial head is tender. Swelling due to hemarthrosis is usually present. Passive motion of the elbow may be limited. Capitellum fracture may occur simultaneously.

Diagnosis

- X-rays

Anteroposterior, lateral, and oblique views are taken. But because x-rays may show only indirect evidence of fracture, diagnosis relies heavily on physical examination.

Routine anteroposterior and lateral x-rays often do not show the fracture but usually show a joint effusion, which is indicated by the presence of abnormal fat pads on x-rays. Displacement of the anterior fat pad may indicate joint effusion but is not specific; visibility of the posterior fat pad on a true lateral view is specific for joint effusion but not highly sensitive. Patients with localized radial head tenderness and effusion require oblique views (which are more sensitive for fracture) or presumptive treatment of a fracture.

The **radiocapitellar line** is a line through the midshaft of the radius on a lateral x-ray of the elbow. Normally, this line transects the middle of the capitellum (see Fig. 359–10). Sometimes in children, the only sign of fracture on x-rays is displacement of this line.

PEARLS & PITFALLS

- If the radial head is tender and there is clinical or radiographic evidence of an elbow effusion, treat presumptively for radial head fracture even if the x-ray shows no fracture.

Arthrocentesis (see p. 253) may be done to remove blood from the joint to help differentiate mechanical blockage of passive joint motion from restriction due to pain and muscle spasm. Then, a local anesthetic is injected to relieve pain.

Stability is tested by applying stress to the elbow medially and laterally and checking for laxity or increased motion. If the joint does not move when stress is applied, the fracture is stable and associated ligaments are probably uninjured.

Treatment

- Usually a sling and range-of-motion exercises
- Rarely surgical repair

Fractures with minimal displacement and no restriction of passive elbow motion or instability can be treated with a sling, which can be applied for comfort with the elbow flexed 90°. Elbow range of motion exercises should be started as soon as patients can tolerate them.

If the elbow is unstable or motion is mechanically blocked, fractures are treated surgically.

DISTAL RADIUS FRACTURES

(Colles Fractures; Smith Fractures; Wrist Fractures)

Distal radius fractures usually result from a fall on an outstretched hand.

Most distal radius fractures are dorsally displaced or angulated (sometimes called Colles fractures); they are common, particularly among the elderly. Often, the ulnar styloid process is also fractured. Less often, volar displacement (called Smith fracture) occurs because the wrist was flexed during the injury.

Symptoms and Signs

A wrist fracture (Colles or Smith) can cause deformity or swelling, which can injure the median nerve; when the median nerve is injured, the tip of the index finger is numb and the pinch of the thumb to the little finger is weak.

Other complications (eg, stiffness, permanent deformity, pain, osteoarthritis, complex regional pain syndromes) can occur, particularly if the fracture extends into or causes displacement or angulation of the wrist joint.

Diagnosis

- Anteroposterior and lateral x-rays

Clinical manifestations may include dorsal angulation or displacement of the distal radius (silver fork or dinner fork deformity) in addition to pain, swelling, and tenderness.

Distal radius fractures are usually visible on anteroposterior and lateral x-rays. Occasionally, CT is necessary to identify intra-articular fractures.

Treatment

- Closed or open reduction

The joint is reduced and immobilized at 15 to 30° of wrist extension. Closed reduction is usually possible. ORIF may be necessary if the joint is disrupted or if the fracture resulted in excessive impaction or shortening.

SCAPHOID FRACTURES

(Navicular Fractures)

Scaphoid fractures usually result from wrist hyperextension. They may not be visible on initial x-rays. Complications can be severe.

The scaphoid is the most commonly injured carpal bone. Scaphoid fractures usually result from wrist hyperextension, typically during a fall on an outstretched hand. They can disrupt the blood supply to the proximal scaphoid. Osteonecrosis is thus a common complication, even when initial care is optimal, and can cause disabling, degenerative arthritis of the wrist.

Symptoms and Signs

The radial wrist is swollen and tender. If patients have these symptoms, scaphoid fracture should be considered. More specific signs include

- Pain during axial compression of the thumb
- Pain during wrist supination against resistance
- Particularly tenderness in the anatomic snuffbox during ulnar wrist deviation

The anatomic snuffbox is palpated just distal to the radius between the extensor pollicis longus, extensor pollicis brevis, and abductor pollicis longus tendons.

Diagnosis

- Plain x-rays
- Sometimes MRI or presumptive treatment

Initially, plain x-rays (anteroposterior, lateral, and oblique views) are taken, but up to 20% of these x-rays are normal. If x-rays are normal but a fracture is still suspected, MRI can be done. Or a fracture is presumed and is treated with a thumb spica splint. Then, if the patient is still in pain or if the wrist is tender when examined after 1 to 2 wk, a follow-up plain x-ray is taken.

PEARLS & PITFALLS

- If clinical findings suggest a scaphoid fracture, do MRI or immobilize with thumb spica splint, even if no fracture is evident on x-ray.

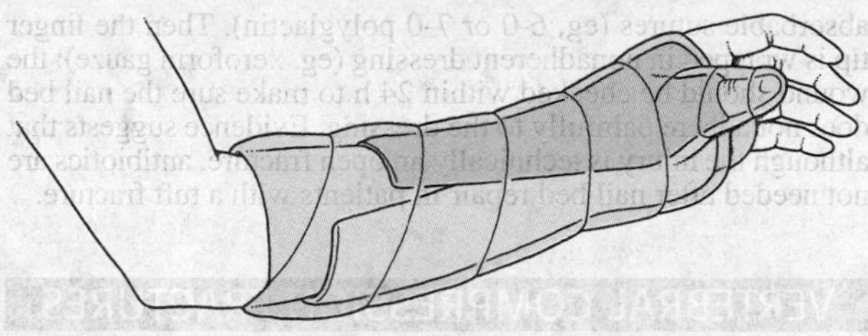

Fig. 359–11. Thumb spica splint.

Treatment

- Thumb spica cast

Many nondisplaced fractures can be treated definitively with a thumb spica cast (see Fig. 359–11), which is worn for up to 8 wk.

Sometimes open reduction and internal fixation (ORIF) is required.

METACARPAL NECK FRACTURES (EXCEPT THUMB)

Metacarpal neck fractures usually result from an axial load (eg, from punching with a clenched fist).

Metacarpal neck fractures are common. They cause pain, swelling, tenderness, and sometimes deformity. Rotational deformity (see Fig. 359–12) may occur. The 5th metacarpal is most commonly injured by punching (boxer's fracture).

Diagnosis

- X-rays

Typically, anteroposterior, lateral, and oblique views are diagnostic.

Treatment

- Splinting
- For certain fractures, reduction

If patients have any wounds, particularly linear punctures, near the metacarpophalangeal joint, they should be specifically questioned about whether they punched someone in the mouth. If they did, contamination with human oral flora is possible, and measures to prevent infection (eg, wound exploration and cleaning, prophylactic antibiotics) are often required (see p. 2941).

Reduction is not necessary for dorsal or volar angulation of

- < 35° for the 4th metacarpal
- < 45° for the 5th metacarpal

Reduction is necessary for

- Rotational deformity of any metacarpal
- Fractures of the 2nd and 3rd metacarpals with angulation

Usually, closed reduction is possible.

Treatment is a splint (eg, an ulnar gutter splint for fractures of the 4th or 5th metacarpal—see Fig. 359–13), usually for at least a few weeks. Then patients can gradually begin range-of-motion exercises.

FINGERTIP FRACTURES

Fingertip (tuft) fractures occur in the distal phalanx. The usual mechanism is a crush injury (eg, in a door jamb).

Fingertip fractures are common. They range from simple transverse fractures to complex comminution of the tuft (the flat, wide area at the tip of the distal phalanges). They are often associated with a nail bed laceration, although the nail itself is frequently intact.

Symptoms and Signs

The fingertip is swollen and tender. A fracture with significant soft-tissue injury may cause hyperesthesia, which frequently

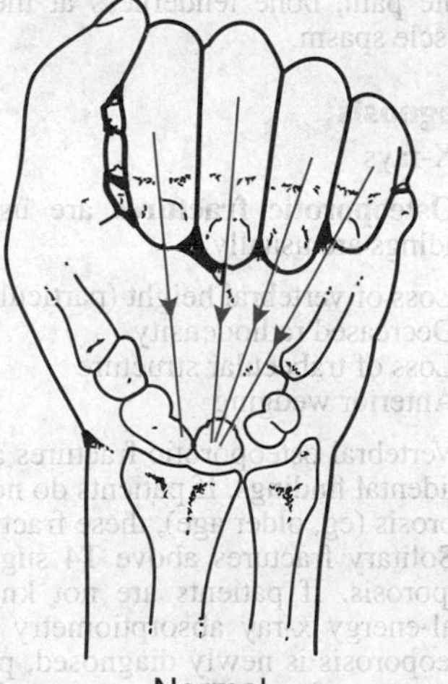

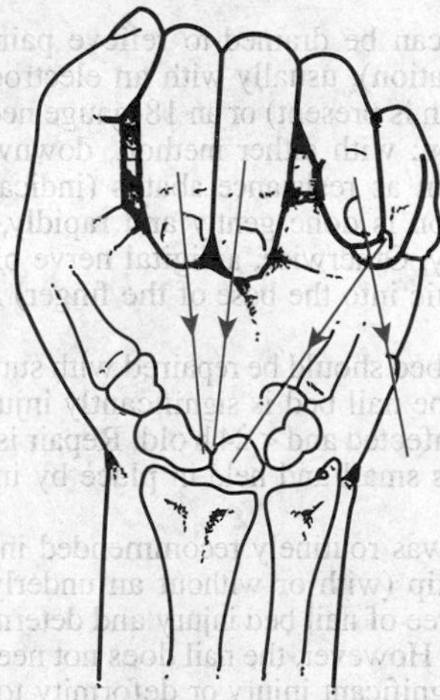

Fig. 359–12. Rotational deformity due to a fracture in the hand. Normally, when the proximal interphalangeal joints are flexed to 90°, lines from the distal phalanges converge at a point on the proximal carpal bones. Deviation of one of these lines suggests a metacarpal fracture.

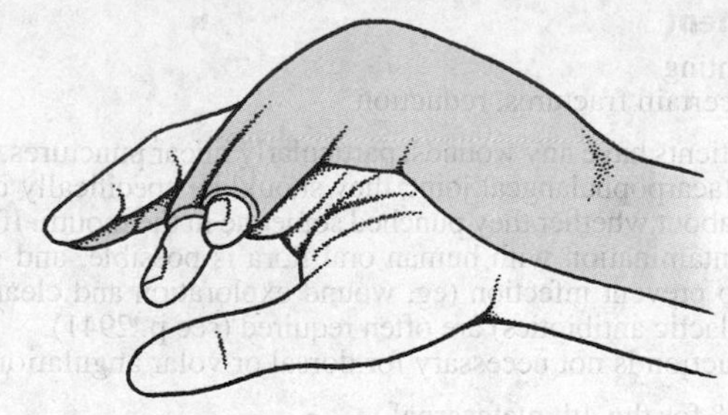

Fig. 359–13. Ulnar gutter splint.

persists long after the fracture heals. Usually, blood becomes trapped between the nail plate and nail bed (subungual hematoma), causing a bluish black discoloration under all or part of the nail, which may be elevated. Subungual hematoma commonly occurs when the nail bed is lacerated.

Marked disruption of the nail bed can result in a permanently deformed nail.

Diagnosis

- X-rays

Diagnosis is based on x-rays, which include anteroposterior, oblique, and lateral views. For the lateral view, the affected digit is separated from the others.

Treatment

- Protective covering or a finger splint for 2 wk
- For a large or painful subungual hematoma, nail trephination

Most fingertip fractures are treated symptomatically with a protective covering (eg, commercially available aluminum and foam splint material) wrapped around the fingertip, often for 2 wk. Rarely, fractures are displaced enough to require surgical repair.

Persistent hyperesthesia may resolve when treated with desensitization therapy.

Subungual hematomas can be drained to relieve pain by puncturing the nail (trephination), usually with an electrocautery device (unless nail polish is present) or an 18-gauge needle in a rotatory, drilling motion; with either method, downward pressure should stop as soon as resistance abates (indicating nail puncture). If trephination is done gently and rapidly, anesthesia is often unnecessary. Otherwise, a digital nerve block (injection of a local anesthetic into the base of the finger) may be used.

Nail bed injury: The nail bed should be repaired with sutures (requiring nail removal) if the nail bed is significantly injured, as long as the wound is not infected and < 24 h old. Repair is not necessary if the laceration is small and held in place by intact nail folds.

Previously, nail removal was routinely recommended in patients with a crushed fingertip (with or without an underlying fracture) to evaluate the degree of nail bed injury and determine whether repair was required. However, the nail does not need to be removed if there is no significant injury or deformity to the nail itself. In such cases, nail bed laceration, if present, is likely to heal well on its own when a splint is applied; trephination is done as needed to relieve pain caused by a subungual hematoma.

If the nail appears severely injured or deformed, the nail should be removed, and the nail bed repaired with thin, absorbable sutures (eg, 6-0 or 7-0 polyglactin). Then the finger tip is wrapped in nonadherent dressing (eg, xeroform gauze); the wound should be checked within 24 h to make sure the nail bed does not adhere painfully to the dressing. Evidence suggests that although the injury is technically an open fracture, antibiotics are not needed after nail bed repair in patients with a tuft fracture.

VERTEBRAL COMPRESSION FRACTURES

Most vertebral compression fractures are a consequence of osteoporosis, are asymptomatic or minimally symptomatic, and occur with no or minimal trauma.

Vertebral osteoporotic compression fractures (see p. 323) are common in the thoracic spine (usually below T6) and lumbar spine, particularly near the T12-L1 junction. There may be no preceding trauma or only minimal trauma (eg, a minor fall, sudden bending, lifting, coughing). Patients who have had an osteoporotic vertebral fracture are at higher risk of other vertebral and nonvertebral fractures.

Occasionally, compression or other vertebral fractures result from significant force (eg, a motor vehicle crash, a fall from a height, a gunshot wound). In such cases, the spinal cord is often also injured (see p. 3098), and the spine may be fractured in > 1 place. If the cause was a fall or jump from a height, one or both heels may also be fractured (see Calcaneal Fractures on p. 2995); 10% of all patients with a calcaneal fracture also have a thoracolumbar fracture (because of the axial load to the skeleton when landing on the heels).

Symptoms and Signs

Osteoporotic vertebral fractures are asymptomatic or cause only loss of height or kyphosis in about two-thirds of patients. In other patients, pain may develop immediately or later. The pain may radiate into the abdomen. Radicular pain, weakness, and reflex or sphincter abnormalities are uncommon. The pain typically decreases after about 4 wk and resolves after about 12 wk.

Nonosteoporotic vertebral compression fractures cause acute pain, bone tenderness at the fracture site, and usually muscle spasm.

Diagnosis

- X-rays

Osteoporotic fractures are usually diagnosed by x-ray. Findings are usually

- Loss of vertebral height (particularly > 6 cm)
- Decreased radiodensity
- Loss of trabecular structure
- Anterior wedging

Vertebral osteoporotic fractures are commonly diagnosed as incidental findings. If patients do not have risk factors for osteoporosis (eg, older age), these fractures are unlikely.

Solitary fractures above T4 suggest cancer rather than osteoporosis. If patients are not known to have osteoporosis, dual-energy x-ray absorptiometry (DXA) should be done. If osteoporosis is newly diagnosed, patients should be evaluated for causes of secondary osteoporosis (see p. 325).

If **significant trauma** has occurred, CT is done to evaluate the entire spinal column, and if neurologic deficits or symptoms are present, MRI of the appropriate section of the spinal cord is done (see p. 3099).

If the cause was a fall or jump from a height from a height, clinicians should check for calcaneus fractures and for additional vertebral fractures.

Treatment

- Analgesics
- Early mobilization and physical therapy

Treatment focuses on pain relief and early mobilization. Analgesics are given. Early resumption of normal activity helps limit further bone loss and disability.

Physical therapists can help by teaching correct lifting techniques and prescribing exercises to strengthen paravertebral muscles, but therapy may need to be delayed until pain is controlled.

Osteoporosis, if present, should be treated (eg, with a bisphosphonate—see p. 326). Calcitonin may also be used and can help relieve pain and increase bone density.

Bracing is commonly prescribed, but its efficacy is unclear.

In some cases, vertebroplasty, sometimes preceded by kyphoplasty, can relieve severe pain. In vertebroplasty, methyl methacrylate is injected into the vertebral body. In kyphoplasty, the vertebral body is expanded with a balloon.

These procedures may reduce deformity in the injected vertebrae but do not reduce and may even increase the risk of fractures in adjacent vertebrae. Other risks may include rib fractures, cement leakage, and pulmonary edema or MI.

If fractures result from significant trauma, the spine is immobilized immediately, and CT or MRI is done to evaluate the stability of the fractures. Spinal cord injuries, if present, are treated promptly (see p. 3098), and supportive care (eg, analgesics, early mobilization) is provided.

KEY POINTS

- Most vertebral fractures result from osteoporosis.
- About two-thirds of vertebral osteoporotic fractures are asymptomatic or cause only loss of height or kyphosis.
- Suspect cancer if patients have a solitary fracture above T4.
- If patients are not known to have osteoporosis, schedule dual-energy x-ray absorptiometry.
- Encourage early mobilization.

PELVIC FRACTURES

Pelvic fractures can involve the pubic symphysis, innominate bones, acetabulum, sacroiliac joint or sacrum. They range from minimally displaced stable injuries caused by low energy falls to dramatically displaced and unstable injures that can cause massive hemorrhage. GU, intestinal, and neurologic injuries may also occur. Diagnosis is by plain x-rays and usually CT. Minor stable fractures require only symptomatic treatment. Unstable fractures and fractures with significant hemorrhage usually require external fixation or open reduction with internal fixation.

Pathophysiology

The pelvic bones, with the anterior and posterior sacroiliac ligaments and fibrous joints between bones (syndesmoses), form a ring. Pelvic fractures may or may not disrupt the ring; ring disruption results from fractures in ≥ 2 places and results in instability.

Complications: Many significant anatomic structures traverse the pelvis and are often damaged. Vascular injuries (eg, iliac vein injuries) may occur and cause significant hemorrhage, especially with posterior pelvic fractures. Hemorrhage may be external (indicating open fracture) or only internal; either can cause hemorrhagic shock.

Concomitant GU injuries (eg, urethral or bladder tears) are common, particularly in anterior fractures. Intestinal injuries may occur, particularly in patients with posterior fractures. Nerve roots and plexuses near the sacral foramina may be damaged in posterior fractures.

Etiology

Most pelvic fractures result from high-energy injuries, most commonly caused by motor vehicle crashes (including motor vehicle–pedestrian collisions) or a fall from a height. Some (eg, symphyseal or pubic ramus fractures) result from minor or low-energy injuries (eg, falls at home), especially in patients with osteoporosis.

Some pelvic fractures, typically in adolescents with open growth plates, are small avulsion fractures of the anterior or inferior iliac spine or of the ischial tuberosity.

There are complex classification systems based on the mechanism, location, and/or stability of the injury.

Symptoms and Signs

Most patients with a pelvic fracture have groin and/or lower back pain. Compression of the pubic symphysis or simultaneous compression of both anterior superior iliac spines is usually painful, particularly in severe fractures, and may indicate instability.

Depending on the severity of the fracture, patients may or may not be able to walk.

Signs of GU and/or gynecologic (usually vaginal) injuries include

- Blood at the urethral meatus
- Scrotal or perineal hematoma
- Hematuria
- Anuria
- A high-riding prostate
- Vaginal bleeding

Intestinal or rectal injuries can cause

- Abdominal or pelvic pain
- Rectal bleeding
- Later development of peritonitis

Neurologic injuries can cause

- Weakness or loss of sensation and reflexes in the lower extremities, rectum, or perineum
- Incontinence
- Urinary retention

Mortality rate is high when fractures are unstable or posterior or when they cause hemorrhagic shock.

Diagnosis

- Plain x-rays
- Usually CT

Pelvic fractures should be considered if patients have pain in the pelvic region or hip or have had major trauma. An anteroposterior pelvis x-ray shows most fractures.

A displaced fracture indicates that the pelvic ring is disrupted, suggesting another fracture or syndesmotic or ligamentous disruption. Specialized x-ray views (eg, Judet views to visualize the acetabulum) may be necessary.

CT is more sensitive than x-rays and is usually done to identify all fracture fragments and certain associated injuries when the fracture is due to a high-energy injury. CT is often unnecessary when patients have an isolated pubic ramus fracture due to a low-energy injury or a small avulsion fracture.

Diagnosis and treatment of associated injuries takes precedence over full definition of the pelvic fracture. Bladder and urethral injuries should be considered and evaluated (see p. 3007). Tests include

- Urinalysis to check for hematuria
- Neurologic examination
- Pelvic examination in women to check for vaginal injury

Traditionally, digital rectal examination is done in men to check for a high-riding prostate, which suggests increased risk of posterior urethral injury. However, the usefulness of this examination is not clear.

Treatment

- For stable fractures, usually only symptomatic treatment
- For unstable fractures, external fixation, or open reduction and internal fixation (ORIF)
- For significant hemorrhage, external fixation or sometimes angiographic embolization or pelvic packing

Typically, an orthopedic surgeon is consulted.

Stable fractures often require only symptomatic treatment, particularly when patients can walk unaided. Acetabular fractures result from a high-energy injury (eg, a fall from height or a motor vehicle crash). Acetabular fractures are treated surgically if the fractures are displaced or instability persists after closed reduction. Acetabular fractures with posterior wall injuries are managed nonsurgically. Orthopedic consultation is recommended for these injuries.

Unstable fractures should be wrapped (eg, in sheets) or stabilized with a commercially available pelvic binder as soon as possible in the emergency department; such stabilization can often decrease or stop bleeding. Orthopedic consultation is needed when pelvic fractures are unstable to determine whether ORIF or external screw fixation should be done. External screw fixation can be done in the emergency department by orthopedic surgeons.

Indications for external screw fixation include

- Ongoing hemorrhage or hemodynamic instability, particularly in patients with large pelvic disruption
- Multisystem trauma
- Need for stabilization before transfer for definitive care

Percutaneous screw fixation reduces morbidity and the length of stay in a hospital.

PEARLS & PITFALLS

- Wrap the pelvis or apply an external fixator as soon as possible to stabilize an unstable pelvic fracture.

If bleeding persists, angiographic embolization or surgery for pelvic packing and/or internal pelvic fixation is required.

Unstable fractures without significant hemorrhage require a pelvic binder, applied in the emergency department; ORIF is the definitive treatment.

Other associated injuries are treated.

KEY POINTS

- Serious pelvic fractures due to high-energy injuries are often associated with GU and vascular injuries.
- Some (eg, symphyseal or pubic ramus fractures), particularly in patients with osteoporosis, result from minor injuries (eg, falls at home).
- Do CT for high-energy injuries.
- Stabilize fractures, control bleeding, and treat associated injuries and symptoms.

HIP FRACTURES

Hip fractures may occur in the head, neck, or area between or below the trochanters (prominences) of the femur. These fractures are most common among the elderly, particularly those with osteoporosis, and usually result from ground level falls. Diagnosis is by x-rays or, if needed, MRI. Treatment is usually with open reduction and internal fixation (ORIF) or sometimes hemiarthroplasty or total hip arthroplasty.

Most hip fractures result from falls, but in the elderly, seemingly minimal force (eg, rolling over in bed, getting up from a chair, walking) can result in fracture, usually because osteoporosis has weakened the bone. Fracture locations include

- Femoral head
- Femoral neck (subcapital)
- Intertrochanteric
- Subtrochanteric

Subcapital and intertrochanteric fractures are the most common types.

Complications include

- Osteonecrosis of the femoral head
- Fracture nonunion
- Osteoarthritis

Complications are more common among elderly patients with a displaced femoral neck fracture.

Symptoms and Signs

Hip fractures most often result in groin pain and inability to ambulate. Sometimes pain is referred to the knee and is thus misinterpreted as a knee abnormality. Similarly, pubic ramus fractures can cause groin pain.

Patients with displaced fractures cannot walk and have significant pain; the affected leg may appear shortened and externally rotated. In contrast, patients with impacted fractures may be able to walk and have only mild pain and no visible deformity. However, such patients are usually unable to flex the entire lower limb against resistance with the knee extended.

Passive hip rotation with the knee flexed aggravates the pain, helping to distinguish hip fracture from extra-articular disorders such as trochanteric bursitis.

Diagnosis

- Plain x-rays
- Rarely MRI or CT

Diagnosis begins with an anteroposterior pelvis x-ray and a cross-table lateral view. If a fracture is identified, x-rays of the entire femur should be done. Subtle evidence of fracture (eg, as when fractures are minimally displaced or impacted) can include irregularities in femoral neck trabecular density or bone cortex. However, x-rays are occasionally normal, particularly in patients with subcapital fractures or severe osteoporosis.

If a fracture is not seen on x-rays but is still suspected clinically, MRI is done because it has almost 100% sensitivity and specificity for occult fractures. CT is a less sensitive alternative.

PEARLS & PITFALLS

- If x-rays do not show a fracture but fracture is suspected clinically, do MRI.

Treatment

- Usually ORIF
- Sometimes femoral head replacement or total hip replacement

The vast majority of hip fractures are treated surgically to minimize the duration of pain and because the prolonged bed rest (see p. 2892), which is required after nonsurgical treatment, increases the risk of serious complications (eg, deep venous thrombosis, pressure ulcers, deconditioning, pneumonia, death), particularly in the elderly. Rehabilitation is started as soon as possible (see p. 3259).

Prophylactic anticoagulation may reduce the incidence of venous thrombosis after hip fracture.

Femoral neck fractures: Nondisplaced and impacted femoral neck fractures in the elderly and all femoral neck fractures in younger patients are typically treated with ORIF.

Displaced femoral neck fractures in the elderly are usually treated with hip arthroplasty (replacement) to allow early unrestricted weight-bearing and to minimize the likelihood that additional surgery will be required. Elderly patients who walk very little and thus put little stress on the hip joint are usually treated with hemiarthroplasty (only the proximal femur is replaced); more active elderly patients are increasingly being treated with total hip arthroplasty (the proximal femur is replaced, and the acetabulum is resurfaced). Total hip arthroplasty surgery is more extensive and poses greater risk but results in better function.

Intertrochanteric fractures: Intertrochanteric fractures are usually treated with ORIF (see Fig. 359–14).

KEY POINTS

- Hip (particularly subcapital and intertrochanteric) fractures are common among older patients with osteoporosis.
- Osteonecrosis of the femoral head, fracture nonunion, and osteoarthritis are common complications.
- For all patients with unexplained hip or knee pain and difficulty walking due to pain, rotate their hip with their knee flexed; if this maneuver aggravates the pain, hip fracture is possible.
- If a fracture is suspected based on clinical findings but is not seen on x-rays, do MRI.
- Treat most fractures surgically (ORIF or hip arthroplasty) so that patients can walk as soon as possible.

FEMORAL SHAFT FRACTURES

Femoral shaft fractures usually result from severe force and are clinically obvious. Treatment is with immediate splinting with traction followed by open reduction and internal fixation (ORIF).

The usual injury mechanism is severe direct force or an axial load to the flexed knee (typically in a motor vehicle crash or automobile-pedestrian collision). Thus, other serious injuries are often present.

Fracture causes obvious swelling, deformity (often with shortening), and instability. Up to 1.5 L of blood for each fracture may be lost. Hemorrhagic shock is possible, particularly when the cause is blunt trauma and there are other injuries.

Diagnosis

- X rays

Anteroposterior and lateral x-rays are diagnostic. If the fracture resulted from great force, hip x-rays should always be done to look for an ipsilateral femoral neck fracture. The knee also needs to be carefully evaluated.

Treatment

- Immediate splinting with traction
- ORIF

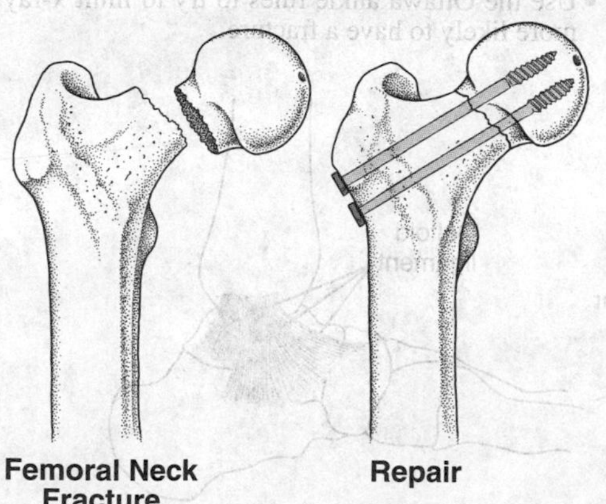

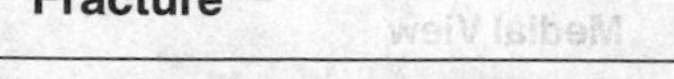

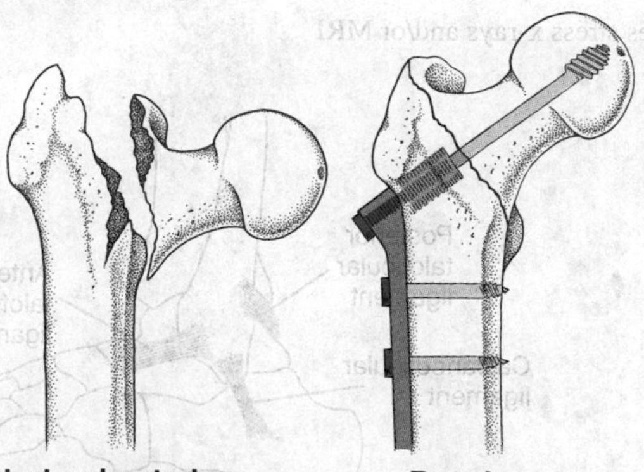

Fig. 359–14. Open reduction and internal fixation.

Immediate treatment is splinting, usually with distraction force (such as with a Hare traction or Sager traction splint), followed by ORIF. Because traction splints apply traction to the lower leg, they should not be used if patients also have a tibial fracture.

ANKLE FRACTURES

Ankle fractures occur in the medial or posterior malleolus of the tibia and/or lateral malleolus of the fibula. These fractures may be stable or unstable. Diagnosis is with x-rays and sometimes MRI. Treatment is usually casting or a walking boot for stable fractures and often open reduction and internal fixation for unstable fractures.

Ankle fractures are common and can result from multiple injury mechanisms, but inversion injury while running or jumping is most common.

The ankle bones and ligaments form a ring that connects the tibia and fibula to the talus and calcaneus. Within the ring, stability is provided by

- 2 bones: Medial malleolus of the tibia and lateral malleolus of the fibula
- 2 ligament complexes: Medially, the deltoid ligament; laterally, mainly the anterior and posterior talofibular ligaments and calcaneofibular ligament—see Fig. 359–15)

Fractures that disrupt the ring in one place often disrupt it in another (eg, if only one bone is fractured, a ligament is often simultaneously and severely torn). If fractures disrupt ≥ 2 of the structures that stabilize the ankle ring, the ankle is unstable. Disruption of the medial deltoid ligament also causes instability.

The proximal fibula may also be fractured (called a Maisonneuve fracture) when the medial malleolus is fractured, the ankle mortise (the joint between the tibia and the talus) is open, and the distal fibula is not fractured; without a fracture of the distal fibula, the joint can be disrupted only if the interosseous ligament between the tibia and fibula tears, as sometimes occurs when the proximal fibula is fractured.

Pain and swelling occur first at the injury site, then often extend diffusely around the ankle.

Diagnosis

- X-rays
- Sometimes stress x-rays and/or MRI

Ankle x-rays are taken in anteroposterior, lateral, and oblique (mortise) views. Specific criteria (eg, Ottawa ankle rules—see p. 3005) are often used to avoid x-rays in patients unlikely to have a fracture.

Fractures are usually evident on x-rays.

Determining stability helps guide treatment. Instability may be obvious when the ankle is inspected or gently palpated. The knee, particularly the proximal fibula, should also be examined.

If both the medial and lateral malleoli are fractured, the injury is probably unstable.

If only the fibula is fractured and the tibiotalar joint appears normal, an external rotation stress x-ray can be done; it may detect tibiotalar subluxation, which suggests deltoid ligament and thus ankle joint instability.

PEARLS & PITFALLS

- If the medial malleolus is fractured, particularly if it is displaced and the mortise is open on the medial side, take knee x-rays to look for fracture of the proximal fibula.

If a proximal fibula fracture seems possible, x-rays of the knee should also be taken.

Treatment

- Walking boot or casting
- Sometimes open reduction and internal fixation (ORIF)

Most stable ankle fractures can be treated nonsurgically with a walking boot or cast.

For unstable injuries, ORIF is often done to align the bone fragments correctly and to better maintain alignment during fracture healing.

The prognosis is usually good if the ankle is stable and if treatment results in correct alignment. If bone fragments do not remain correctly aligned, arthritis may develop and fractures may recur.

KEY POINTS

- If an ankle fracture disrupts the ankle ring (formed by the ankle bones and ligaments) in one place, it often disrupts it in another; if ≥ 2 of the structures that stabilize the ankle ring are disrupted, the ankle is unstable.
- Use the Ottawa ankle rules to try to limit x-rays to patients more likely to have a fracture.

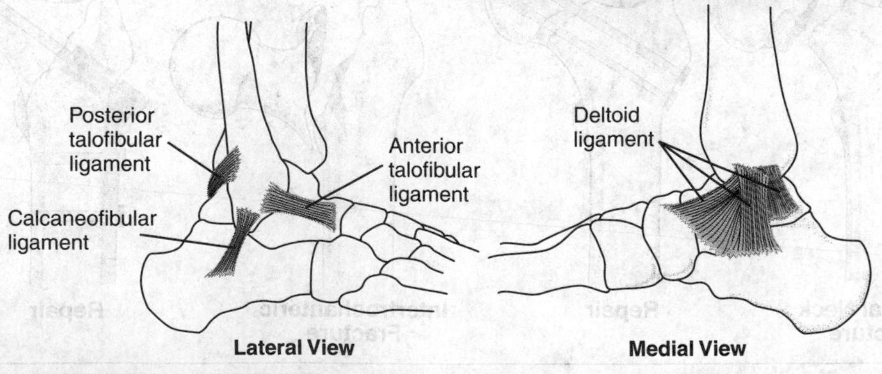

Fig. 359–15. Ligaments of the ankle.

- Evaluate ankle stability (which determines treatment) by physical examination and, if needed, x-rays.
- Treat most stable ankle fractures with a walking boot or cast and many unstable fractures with ORIF.

CALCANEAL FRACTURES

Calcaneal fractures occur in the calcaneus (heel bone), often resulting from great force. Diagnosis is by x-rays and, if needed, CT. Treatment requires orthopedic consultation and includes casting and sometimes surgery.

Calcaneal fractures are serious but uncommon injuries; they account for only 1 to 2% of all fractures. However, if not diagnosed and treated promptly, they can result in long-term disability. Up to 10% of these fractures are missed at initial presentation in an emergency department.

Typically, these fractures result from a high-energy axial load to the foot (eg, a fall from a height onto the heels). Because these fractures require great force, they are often accompanied by other serious injuries; 10% of patients with a calcaneal fracture have a thoracolumbar compression fracture.

Stress fractures may also occur in the calcaneus, particularly in athletes, such as long-distance runners.

Calcaneal fractures may be intra-articular.

Symptoms and Signs

Usually, the area around the heel and the hindfoot is tender and very swollen.

Acute compartment syndrome (see p. 2997) occurs in up to 10% of patients.

Diagnosis

- X-rays
- Sometimes CT

X-rays include axial and lateral views.

CT is done if

- X-rays are negative but clinical findings suggest a calcaneal fracture.
- The Bohler angle is < 20°.
- More detail about the fracture is needed.

The Bohler angle is determined on the lateral x-ray. This angle is formed by the intersection of a line drawn from the superior aspect of the posterior calcaneal tuberosity to the superior subtalar articular surface and a line drawn from the superior subtalar articular surface to the superior aspect of the anterior calcaneal process. Normally, the angle is 20 to 40°. An angle < 20° suggests a fracture.

PEARLS & PITFALLS

- If patients have calcaneal swelling and tenderness after a high-energy axial load to the calcaneus, check the Bohler angle on x-ray, and check for thoracolumbar compression fracture and compartment syndrome.

Clinicians should also check for other injuries, such as thoracolumbar fractures.

Treatment

- Orthopedic consultation
- Casting or possibly surgery, depending on the type of fracture

Orthopedic consultation is necessary.

Whether **intra-articular calcaneal fractures** should be treated surgically or nonsurgically is much debated.

Extra-articular calcaneal fractures are treated symptomatically with rest (avoiding weight bearing), a compression dressing (which also provides protection), ice, and elevation (PRICE). When the swelling resolves, a cast is applied.

KEY POINTS

- If calcaneal fractures are not diagnosed and treated promptly, they can result in long-term disability.
- Because these fractures usually result from a high-energy axial load to the foot, other injuries (eg, thoracolumbar compression fracture) are often also present; other complications include compartment syndrome (in up to 10%).
- Diagnose based on x-rays and, if needed, CT.
- Whether intra-articular calcaneal fractures should be treated surgically or nonsurgically is controversial.
- Treat extra-articular calcaneal fractures symptomatically with PRICE, followed by casting.

FRACTURE-DISLOCATION OF THE MIDFOOT

(Lisfranc Fracture-Dislocation; Lisfranc Injury)

A Lisfranc injury is a fracture and/or dislocation of the midfoot that disrupts one or more tarsometatarsal joints. Diagnosis is by x-rays and often CT. Treatment requires referral to an orthopedic surgeon and usually open reduction and internal fixation or sometimes fusion of the midfoot.

These injuries are common. The usual mechanism is a direct blow or an indirect twisting force applied to a foot in plantar flexion (eg, fall on a foot in plantar flexion).

The Lisfranc joint complex consists of the 5 tarsometatarsal joints that connect the forefoot and midfoot. There are multiple ligaments in this complex. The Lisfranc ligament itself is the ligament that attaches the base of the 2nd metatarsal to the 1st cuneiform (see Fig. 359–16). Lisfranc complex injuries vary widely in severity from strains to dislocation of one or more tarsometatarsal joints with or without fracture. When fracture occurs, it often involves the 2nd metatarsal. Lisfranc injuries often cause instability of the midfoot.

Severity varies widely. Some injuries cause only mild swelling and pain in the midfoot; others cause severe soft-tissue pain and swelling, deformity, a hematoma on the sole of the midfoot, and sometimes paresthesias. The foot may appear shortened.

Complications (eg, osteoarthritis, compartment syndrome) can be serious and chronic disability is common.

Diagnosis

- X-rays
- Sometimes CT

Anteroposterior, lateral, and oblique x-rays of the foot are taken, but findings may be subtle, leading to misdiagnosis. Up to 20% of these fractures are missed at the initial presentation.

X-rays can show a fracture at the base of the 2nd metatarsal or chip fractures of the cuneiform but may not show disruption of the tarsometatarsal joint, which should be suspected even if it is not visible on plain x-rays. Normally in this joint, the medial aspect of the 2nd cuneiform aligns directly with the medial aspect of the 2nd metatarsal. Comparison views or CT may be necessary to identify disruption of the joint.

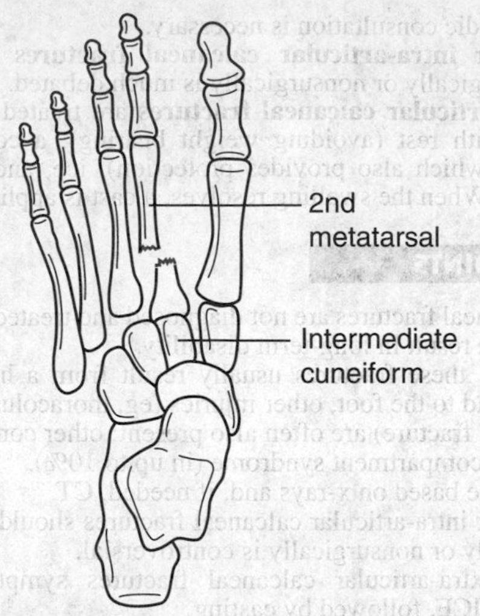

Fig. 359–16. Fracture of the 2nd metatarsal base with tarsometatarsal joint dislocation. Fracture of the 2nd metatarsal base may disrupt one or more of the tarsometatarsal joints. In this figure, the 2nd metatarsal fracture displaces the 3rd through 5th metatarsals laterally.

PEARLS & PITFALLS

- If the midfoot is extremely swollen and tender, closely examine the x-ray to determine whether the medial aspect of the 2nd cuneiform directly aligns with the medial aspect of the 2nd metatarsal.

If CT is not readily available, stress x-rays can be used. X-rays are taken while the foot is under stress (eg, the patient is standing on the foot). The patient's body weight can cause the space between the 1st and 2nd metatarsals to widen, making the diagnosis much easier. However, CT is more sensitive than stress x-rays and so is preferred in equivocal cases.

Treatment

- Orthopedic consultation
- Usually, open reduction and internal fixation (ORIF) or sometimes fusion of the midfoot

Dislocations often spontaneously reduce. Nonetheless, because these injuries usually compromise foot function and cause residual pain and arthritis, patients should be immediately referred to an orthopedic specialist, usually for surgery. Typically, definitive treatment is ORIF or fusion of the midfoot.

After ORIF, CT is usually done to confirm correct alignment.

If surgery is not considered necessary, patients are immobilized, with no weight-bearing for ≥ 6 wk.

KEY POINTS

- Lisfranc injuries involve disruption of ≥ 1 ligaments that stabilize the midfoot, sometimes disrupting ≥ 1 tarsometatarsal joints.
- Complications (eg, compartment syndrome, chronic pain, disability) may be serious.
- Because x-ray findings may be subtle, stress x-rays or CT may be needed.
- Refer patients to an orthopedic surgeon; usually, ORIF or fusion of the midfoot is required.

FRACTURES OF THE 5TH METATARSAL BONE

Fractures of the 5th metatarsal may occur in the base or shaft (diaphysis). Fractures of the diaphysis can be acute or stress fractures. Because these fractures have very different treatments and prognoses, accurate diagnosis is important. Diagnosis is with x-rays. Treatment depends on the location of the fracture.

Pain, swelling, and tenderness are usually well-localized to the fracture site.

Diagnosis is based on anteroposterior, lateral, and oblique foot x-rays.

Fractures of the 5th Metatarsal Diaphysis

Fractures of the 5th metatarsal diaphysis can be acute or stress fractures (see p. 3108). Acute diaphyseal fractures tend to occur near the metaphysis and are sometimes called Jones fractures.

Because the blood supply may be disrupted, nonunion and delayed union can result.

Treatment

- Casting
- Orthopedic consultation

Treatment involves a short leg cast with no weight bearing for 6 wk; patients are referred to an orthopedic surgeon to determine whether ORIF should be done.

Fractures of the 5th Metatarsal Base

Fractures of the base are sometimes called dancer's or pseudo-Jones fractures. The mechanism is usually a crush injury or an inversion force that causes avulsion by the peroneus brevis tendon. These fractures are more common than acute diaphyseal fractures (Jones fractures).

Because the base, unlike the diaphysis, has abundant collateral circulation, delayed union and nonunion are rare.

Treatment

- Symptomatic

Treatment is symptomatic and may include a hard-soled shoe or walking boot and weight bearing as tolerated.

TOE FRACTURES

Most toe fractures are minimally displaced and require only taping to an adjacent toe (buddy taping).

Pain, swelling, and tenderness are common. Subungual hematoma (between the nail plate and nail bed) is also common, particularly when the mechanism is a crush injury.

Diagnosis

- If certain injuries are suspected, x-rays

Unless rotational deformity or joint involvement is suspected or the proximal phalanx of the great toe is injured, x-rays are usually unnecessary because treatment is the same whether fracture is present or not. When x-rays are indicated, anteroposterior, lateral, and oblique views of each toe are taken.

Treatment

- Buddy taping
- For certain injuries, reduction and fixation

Treatment involves taping the injured toe to an adjacent toe (dynamic splinting, or buddy taping). If the toe is displaced or deformed, reduction may be needed beforc buddy taping. Fixation is sometimes indicated (eg, for fractures with marked displacement or rotational deformity of the great toe).

COMPARTMENT SYNDROME

Compartment syndrome is increased tissue pressure within a closed fascial space, resulting in tissue ischemia. The earliest symptom is pain out of proportion to the severity of injury. Diagnosis is usually by measuring compartment pressure. Treatment is fasciotomy.

Compartment syndrome is a self-perpetuating cascade of events. It begins with the tissue edema that normally occurs after injury (eg, because of soft-tissue swelling or a hematoma). If edema develops within a closed fascial compartment, typically in the anterior or posterior compartments of the leg, therc is little room for tissue expansion, so interstitial (compartment pressure) increases. As compartmental pressure exceeds the normal capillary pressure of about 8 mm Hg, cellular perfusion slows and may ultimately stop. (NOTE: Because 8 mm Hg is much lower than arterial pressure, cellular perfusion can stop long before pulses disappear.) Resultant tissue ischemia further worsens edema in a vicious circle.

As ischemia progresses, muscles necrose, sometimes leading to rhabdomyolysis, infections, and hyperkalemia; these complications can cause loss of limb and, if untreated, death. Hypotension or arterial insufficiency can compromise tissue perfusion with even mildly elevated compartment pressures, causing or worsening compartment syndrome. Contractures may develop after necrotic tissue heals.

Compartment syndrome is mainly a disorder of the extremities and is most common in the lower leg and the forearm. However, compartment syndrome can also occur in other locations (eg, upper arm, abdomen, buttock).

Etiology

Common causes include

- Fractures
- Severe contusions or crush injuries
- Reperfusion injury after vascular injury and repair

Rare causes include snakebites, burns, severe exertion, drug overdose (of heroin or cocaine), casts, tight bandages, and other rigid circumferential devices that limit swelling and thus increase compartment pressure. Prolonged pressure on a muscle during coma may cause rhabdomyolysis.

Symptoms and Signs

The **earliest symptom** is

- Worsening pain

It is typically out of proportion to the severity of the apparent injury and is exacerbated by passive stretching of the muscles within the compartment (eg, for the anterior leg compartment, by passive ankle plantar flexion and toe flexion, which stretches the anterior compartment muscles). Pain, one of the 5 Ps of tissue ischemia, is followed by the other 4: paresthesias, paralysis, pallor, and pulselessness. Compartments may feel tense when palpated.

PEARLS & PITFALLS

- If pain is more than expected for the severity of the apparent injury, consider compartment syndrome; check for exacerbation of pain with passive muscle stretching, and if compartments are palpable, check for tenseness.

Diagnosis

- Measurement of compartmental pressure

Diagnosis must be made and treatment started before pallor or pulselessness develops, indicating necrosis. Clinical evaluation is difficult for several reasons:

- Typical symptoms and signs may be absent.
- Findings are not specific because similar findings are sometimes caused by the fracture itself.
- Many trauma patients have altered mental status due to other injuries and/or sedation.

Thus, in patients with at-risk injuries, clinicians must have a low threshold for measuring compartment pressure (normal ≤ 8 mm Hg), usually with a commercially available pressure monitor. Compartment syndrome is confirmed if compartmental pressure is more than about 30 mm Hg or within about 30 mm Hg of diastolic BP.

Treatment

- Fasciotomy

Initial treatment is removal of any constricting structure (eg, cast, splint) around the limb, correction of hypotension, analgesia, and supplemental oxygen as needed.

Usually, unless compartment pressure decreases rapidly and symptoms abate, urgent fasciotomy is required. Fasciotomy should be done through large skin incisions to open all fascial compartments in the limb and thus relieve the pressure. All muscle should be carefully inspected for viability, and any nonviable tissue should be debrided.

Amputation is indicated if necrosis is extensive.

KEY POINTS

- Once the process triggering compartment syndrome begins, compartment syndrome tends to increase in severity.
- Consider compartment syndrome if pain appears to be out of proportion to the severity of injury and is increased by passive stretch of muscles within the compartment or if the compartment is tense.
- Measure compartment pressure to confirm the diagnosis; a finding of more than about 30 mm Hg or within about 30 mm Hg of diastolic BP confirms it.
- Unless the disorder resolves rapidly after initial treatment, fasciotomy must be done as soon as possible.

SHOULDER DISLOCATIONS

In shoulder (glenohumeral) dislocations, the humeral head separates from the glenoid fossa; displacement is almost always anterior.

Shoulder dislocations account for about half of major joint dislocations.

Shoulder dislocations may be

- Anterior
- Posterior
- Inferior

Anterior dislocations: Shoulder dislocations are anterior in ≥ 95% of patients; the mechanism is abduction and external rotation. Associated injuries can include brachial plexus injuries, rotator cuff tears (particularly in elderly patients), fracture of the greater tuberosity, and axillary nerve injury. Shoulder instability and thus recurrent dislocation are common in patients < 30 yr.

The acromion is prominent, and the elbow is held slightly out from the side; the humeral head is displaced anteriorly and inferiorly and cannot be palpated in its usual position. Patients are unwilling to move the arm. They may have motor and sensory deficits (eg, if the axillary nerve is injured, decreased sensation over the deltoid).

True anteroposterior (AP) and axillary x-rays are diagnostic for anterior dislocations, showing the humeral head outside the glenoid fossa.

Treatment is usually closed reduction using local anesthesia (intra-articular block) or conscious sedation. Commonly used methods of reduction include

- Traction-countertraction (see Fig. 359–17)
- External rotation (eg, Hennepin technique—see Fig. 359–18)
- Scapular manipulation
- Cunningham (massage) technique

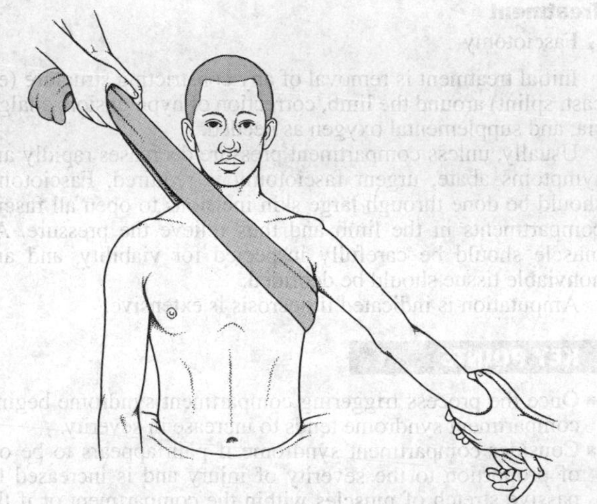

Fig. 359–17. Traction-countertraction technique for reducing anterior shoulder dislocations. The patient lies on a stretcher, and its wheels are locked. One practitioner pulls on a folded sheet wrapped around the patient's chest. Another practitioner pulls the affected limb down and laterally 45°. After the humerus is free, slight lateral traction on the upper humerus may be needed.

Many techniques (eg, Hennepin, scapular manipulation, Cunningham) can be done without sedation, but they require time for muscles affected by spasm to adequately relax; patients must be able to focus their attention on relaxation.

After reduction, the joint is immobilized immediately with a sling and swathe (see Fig. 359–3 on p. 2981).

Hennepin technique (external rotation) can be done with the patient supine or seated. The dislocated arm is adducted with the elbow held at 90°. The arm is then externally rotated slowly (eg, over 5 to 10 min) to allow time for muscle spasms to resolve. Reduction commonly occurs at 70 to 110° of external rotation. This technique is effective in about 80 to 90% of cases.

Scapular manipulation can be done with the patient upright or prone. The practitioner flexes the patient's elbow 90° and slowly externally rotates the arm. An assistant applies gentle traction on the arm. The practitioner then rotates the scapula so that the inferior tip moves medially, toward the spine. Scapular manipulation can be used with other techniques (eg, Stimson technique).

The **Cunningham technique** involves massage of the muscles around the glenohumeral joint while the patient is sitting. The practitioner does the following:

- Sits facing and just to the side of the patient
- Puts the patient's hand on the practitioner's shoulder, keeping the patient's elbow flexed
- Puts the practitioner's hand in the depression in the bend of the patient's elbow (antecubital fossa) and holds the dislocated arm in place
- Massages the biceps, mid-deltoid, and trapezius to relax muscle spasms
- Instructs the patient to try to relax rather than tense up if the shoulder feels as if it is moving (relaxation is crucial to reduction using this technique)
- Instructs the patient to sit up straight (no slouching forward or to the side) and to shrug the shoulders back, trying to make the upper ends of the right and left scapula touch each other

The shoulder slips back into place within minutes.

The **Stimson technique** (also called the dangling weights technique) is done less commonly. It is done with the patient prone and the affected extremity hanging over the side of a bed. Weights are attached to the wrist. After about 30 min, the muscle spasm usually relaxes enough to allow the humeral head to reduce. Because the patient is prone, conscious sedation is not recommended. This position may be too uncomfortable for pregnant patients and extremely obese patients. This technique can also be used with scapular manipulation; the practitioner applies scapular manipulation while the patient is prone. This approach shortens the time needed for shoulder to relocate.

Posterior dislocations: Occasionally, dislocations are posterior—a commonly missed injury (see Table 359–1 on p. 2977). It is classically caused by seizures, electric shock, or electroconvulsive therapy done without muscle relaxants.

Deformity may not be obvious. The arm is held adducted and internally rotated. Typically, when the elbow is flexed, passive external rotation is impossible. If such rotation is impossible, an AP shoulder x-ray should be taken. If it shows no obvious fracture or dislocation, posterior shoulder dislocation should be considered. A clue to the diagnosis on the AP view is the light bulb or ice cream cone sign; the humeral head is internally rotated, and the tuberosities do not project laterally, making the humeral head appear circular.

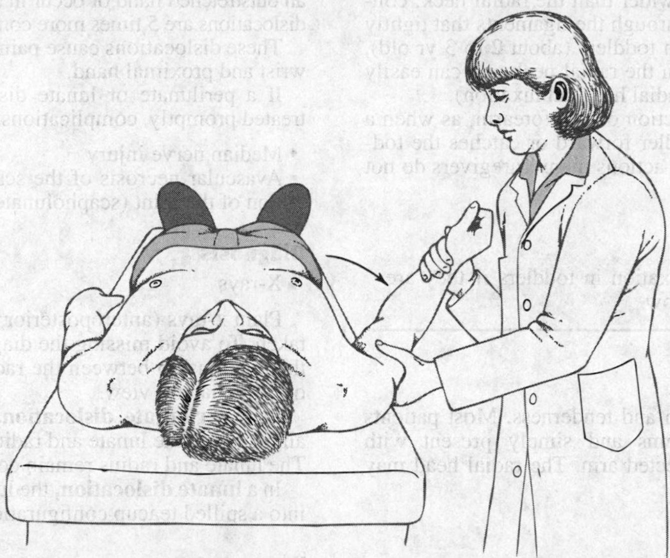

Fig. 359–18. Hennepin technique for reducing anterior shoulder dislocations. The practitioner adducts the dislocated arm with the elbow held at 90°. The arm is then externally rotated slowly (eg, over 5 to 10 min) to allow time for muscle spasms to resolve. Reduction commonly occurs at 70 to 110° of external rotation.

PEARLS & PITFALLS

- Suspect posterior shoulder location if patients have shoulder pain, keep their arm adducted, and cannot externally rotate their arm and x-rays show no obvious abnormality.

The axillary view or trans-scapular Y view is diagnostic.

Reduction is often possible using longitudinal traction (as with the traction-countertraction technique).

Inferior dislocations: Inferior dislocations (luxatio erecta) are rare and usually clinically obvious; patients hold their arm over their head (ie, abducted to almost 180°), usually with the forearm resting on the head. The arm is shortened; the humeral head is often palpable in the axilla. The joint capsule is disrupted, and the rotator cuff may be torn. The brachial artery is injured in < 5% of cases. The axillary nerve or another nerve is usually damaged, but deficits often resolve after reduction.

X-rays are diagnostic.

Reduction is done using traction-countertraction of the abducted arm. Closed reduction is usually successful unless there is a buttonhole deformity (humeral head is trapped in a tear of the inferior capsule); in such cases, open reduction is required.

ELBOW DISLOCATIONS

Most elbow dislocations are posterior and usually result from a fall on an extended arm.

Posterior elbow dislocations are common. Associated injuries may include fractures, injuries to the ulnar or median nerve, and possibly injury to the brachial artery. The joint is usually flexed about 45°, and the olecranon is prominent and posterior to the humeral epicondyles; however, these anatomic relationships may be difficult to determine because of swelling.

X-rays are diagnostic.

Treatment

- Traction to reduce the joint

Reduction is usually with sustained, gentle traction and correction of deformity after patients are sedated and given analgesics. The following technique is commonly used:

- With the patient supine, the practitioner flexes the elbow to about 90° and supinates the forearm.
- An assistant stabilizes the upper arm against the stretcher.
- The practitioner grasps the wrist and applies slow, steady axial traction to the forearm while keeping the elbow flexed and the forearm supinated.
- Traction is maintained until the dislocation is reduced.

After reduction, the practitioner checks the elbow for stability by fully flexing and extending the elbow while pronating and supinating the forearm. These movements should be easy after reduction.

The joint is usually immobilized (eg, in a splint) for up to 1 wk until pain and swelling resolve; then active range-of-motion exercises are started, and a sling is worn for 2 to 3 wk.

RADIAL HEAD SUBLUXATIONS

(Nursemaid's Elbow)

Radial head subluxation, common among toddlers, is caused by traction on the forearm and usually manifests as refusal to move the elbow (pseudoparalysis).

In adults, the radial head is wider than the radial neck; consequently, the head cannot fit through the ligaments that tightly surround the neck. However, in toddlers (about 2 to 3 yr old), the radial head is no wider than the radial neck and can easily slip through these ligaments (radial head subluxation).

Subluxation results from traction on the forearm, as when a caregiver pulls a reluctant toddler forward or catches the toddler by the wrist during a fall—actions many caregivers do not remember.

PEARLS & PITFALLS

- Consider radial head subluxation in toddlers if they are unwilling to move their elbow.

Symptoms

Symptoms may include pain and tenderness. Most patients cannot describe their symptoms and simply present with unwillingness to move the affected arm. The radial head may be only mildly tender.

Diagnosis

- Usually history

Plain x-rays are normal and considered unnecessary by some experts when patients have a clear history of a traction injury, unless an alternate diagnosis is clinically suspected.

Using a reduction maneuver may be diagnostic and therapeutic.

Treatment

- Reduction

Reduction may be done using

- Supination-flexion
- Hyperpronation

Neither technique requires sedation or analgesia; the child experiences pain only for a few seconds.

In **supination-flexion,** the elbow is completely extended and supinated, then flexed. A subtle palpable pop or click is often detected when the radial head resumes its normal position.

In **hyperpronation,** the practitioner supports the child's arm at the elbow and places moderate pressure with a finger on the radial head. The practitioner then grips the distal forearm with the other hand and hyperpronates the forearm. A pop can be felt at the radial head when it is reduced.

Children usually start to move the elbow after about 10 to 20 min. If they do not move it, x-rays of the elbow should be taken. If they do move it, x-rays and immobilization are unnecessary.

If pain or dysfunction lasts > 24 h, incomplete reduction or an occult fracture should be suspected. Radial head subluxation recurs in 20 to 40% of children.

PERILUNATE AND LUNATE DISLOCATIONS

A perilunate dislocation is disruption of the normal relationship between the lunate and capitate. A lunate dislocation is separation of the lunate from both the capitate and the radius.

Perilunate and lunate dislocations result when great force is applied to a hyperextended wrist. They usually result from a fall on an outstretched hand or occur in a motor vehicle crash. Perilunate dislocations are 5 times more common than lunate dislocations.

These dislocations cause pain, swelling, and deformity in the wrist and proximal hand.

If a perilunate or lunate dislocation is not diagnosed and treated promptly, complications can develop. They include

- Median nerve injury
- Avascular necrosis of the scaphoid or lunate and deterioration of the joint (scapholunate advanced collapse).

Diagnosis

- X-rays

Plain x-rays (anteroposterior, lateral, and oblique views) are taken. To avoid missing the diagnosis, clinicians should assess the relationship between the radius, lunate, and capitate bones on a true lateral view.

In a **perilunate dislocation,** the capitate is not vertically aligned with the lunate and radius on a lateral view of the wrist. The lunate and radius remain correctly aligned.

In a **lunate dislocation,** the lunate is rotated out of alignment into a spilled teacup configuration.

Treatment

- Closed reduction and splinting
- Usually surgical repair

Treatment of both perilunate and lunate dislocations is closed reduction and splinting in the emergency department. Both the wrist and elbow should be immobilized in the neutral position (eg, with a sugar-tong splint).

Patients should be immediately referred to an orthopedic surgeon; most dislocations must be surgically repaired because function is better after surgical repair.

FINGER DISLOCATIONS

Most finger dislocations occur at the proximal interphalangeal (PIP) joint; they are usually caused by hyperextension and thus are usually dorsal.

Finger dislocations can be dorsal, lateral, or volar. They may rupture various combinations of supporting ligaments. Most cause obvious deformities, as well as pain and swelling.

Anteroposterior, lateral, and oblique x-rays are taken. Lateral views should be taken with the affected digit visibly separated from the others.

For most dislocations, closed reduction is done after a digital nerve block is used. For all PIP dislocations, stability of the lateral ligaments is assessed by stress testing after the dislocation is reduced.

Dorsal dislocations: Dorsal dislocations result from hyperextension. They occasionally displace the volar joint structures intra-articularly (volar plate injury).

In volar plate injuries, x-rays occasionally show a small bone fragment avulsed from the middle phalanx.

Dorsal dislocations are reduced using axial traction and volar force. If volar plate injury is suspected or if closed reduction is difficult (suggesting volar plate injury), open reduction may be necessary.

Dorsal dislocations are usually splinted in 15° of flexion for 3 wk.

Lateral dislocations: Lateral dislocations may occur when abduction or adduction forces are applied to an extended finger joint.

The joint is tender and unstable when lateral stress is applied. The joint is reduced, then splinted in 35° of flexion.

Volar dislocations: Volar dislocations are uncommon and occur when volar forces are applied to a rotated finger joint.

Usually, the central slip of the extensor tendon ruptures, causing boutonnière deformity (see p. 288).

Volar dislocations are reduced using axial traction and dorsal force, then splinted in extension for 1 to 2 wk. Subsequently, patients should be evaluated to determine whether surgery is needed to repair a ruptured central slip of the extensor tendon.

HIP DISLOCATIONS

Most hip dislocations are posterior and result from severe posteriorly directed force to the knee while the knee and hip are flexed (eg, against a car dashboard).

Complications may include

- Sciatic nerve injury
- Delayed osteonecrosis of the femoral head

Associated injuries include

- Patella fractures
- Posterior cruciate ligament injuries
- Acetabular and femoral head fractures

In patients with posterior dislocations, the leg is shortened, adducted, and internally rotated. Anterior dislocations are rare and result in the leg being abducted and externally rotated.

Diagnosis

- X-rays

Routine hip x-rays are diagnostic.

Treatment

- Closed reduction

Treatment is closed reduction as soon as possible, preferably in ≤ 6 h; delay increases the risk of osteonecrosis.

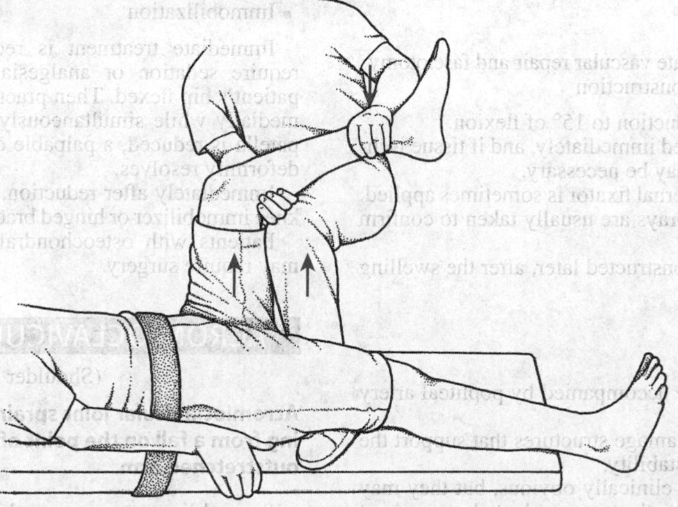

Fig. 359–19. Captain Morgan technique.

The hip can be reduced using one of the following techniques:

- Allis technique
- Captain Morgan technique

When either technique is done, the patient requires sedation and muscle relaxation and is in the supine position.

For the **Allis technique,** the hip is gently flexed to 90°, and vertical traction is applied to the femur; this maneuver may be easiest and safest when the patient is temporarily placed on a rigid backboard that is put on the floor.

For the **Captain Morgan technique,** the patient's hips are held down by a sheet or belt, and the dislocated hip is flexed. Practitioners then place their knee under the patient's knee and lift up while applying vertical traction to the femur (see Fig. 359–19).

After reduction, CT is usually done to identify fractures and intra-articular debris.

Dislocated Prosthetic Hip

After total hip replacement, the prosthetic hip dislocates in up to 2% of patients. Posterior dislocations are more common.

Closed reduction is often successful, particularly for first-time dislocations, but hip revision surgery is sometimes required.

KNEE DISLOCATIONS

(Tibiofemoral Dislocations)

Knee dislocations are commonly accompanied by arterial or nerve injuries. These dislocations may spontaneously reduce before medical evaluation. Diagnosis is by x-ray. Vascular and neurologic evaluation is required. Immediate treatment is closed reduction and treatment of vascular injuries.

Most anterior dislocations result from hyperextension; most posterior dislocations result from a posteriorly directed force to the proximal tibia while the knee is slightly flexed. Most knee dislocations result from severe trauma (eg, in high-speed motor vehicle crashes), but seemingly slight trauma, such as stepping in a hole and twisting the knee) can sometimes dislocate the knee, particularly in morbidly obese patients.

Dislocation always damages

- Structures that support the knee joint, causing joint instability

Joint instability due to extensive ligament injury is a common long-term complication of knee injury.

Other structures that are commonly injured include the

- Popliteal artery (particularly in anterior dislocations)
- Peroneal and tibial nerves

Popliteal artery injury may initially affect only the intima and thus does not cause distal limb ischemia until the artery later becomes occluded. Undiagnosed arterial injury has a high risk of ischemic complications, which may lead to amputation.

Symptoms and Signs

Dislocation causes deformity that is clinically obvious. However, some dislocations spontaneously reduce before medical evaluation; in such cases, the knee remains very swollen and grossly unstable.

Fullness in the popliteal fossa suggests hematoma or popliteal artery injury.

Diagnosis

- X-rays
- Vascular evaluation

Dislocation should be suspected if an injured knee is grossly unstable. Anteroposterior and lateral x-rays are diagnostic for dislocations that have not spontaneously reduced.

Vascular and neurologic evaluations are particularly important.

Popliteal artery injury should be suspected regardless of whether ischemia is evident. Some experts believe that serial clinical evaluations of the distal pulse can rule out a popliteal artery injury if the pulse is normal over a period of time. The ankle-brachial BP index (ABI) should always be measured (see p. 751); values ≤ 0.9 are very sensitive for vascular injury. Some experts also recommend duplex ultrasonography even if the ABI is > 0.9 and no findings suggest ischemia. If the ABI is ≤ 0.9 or if any findings suggest ischemia, immediate vascular surgical consultation and/or diagnostic testing is required. Tests may include CT angiography (which should be done liberally), conventional angiography, and ultrasonography.

Treatment

- Immediate reduction
- For vascular injury, immediate vascular repair and fasciotomy
- Later elective ligament reconstruction

Treatment is immediate reduction to 15° of flexion.

Vascular injuries are repaired immediately, and if tissue ischemia is present, fasciotomy may be necessary.

For gross instability, an external fixator is sometimes applied. Anteroposterior and lateral x-rays are usually taken to confirm reduction.

Knee ligaments can be reconstructed later, after the swelling resolves.

KEY POINTS

- Many knee dislocations are accompanied by popliteal artery or nerve injuries.
- Knee dislocations always damage structures that support the knee joint, causing joint instability.
- Most knee dislocations are clinically obvious, but they may spontaneously reduce before they are evaluated; so suspect dislocation if an injured knee is grossly unstable.
- Always measure the ankle-brachial index because the popliteal artery is commonly injured by knee dislocation.
- Immediately reduce the dislocated knee and repair vascular injuries.

PATELLAR DISLOCATIONS

Patellar dislocations are common and almost always lateral. Diagnosis is clinical; x-rays are taken to exclude fracture. Treatment is reduction, immobilization, and sometimes surgery.

Patellar dislocation is distinct from knee dislocation (see p. 3001), which is a much more serious injury.

Most patients are adolescent females and have an underlying chronic patellofemoral abnormality. Many dislocations spontaneously reduce before medical evaluation.

Associated injuries include

- Osteochondral fracture of the patella or lateral femoral condyle

Complications can include

- Osteoarthritis
- In patients with patellofemoral abnormalities, recurrent dislocation or subluxation

Diagnosis

- Clinical evaluation
- X-rays to exclude fracture

Dislocation, unless spontaneously reduced, is clinically obvious; ie, the patella is visibly and palpably displaced laterally, and the patient holds the knee in a slightly flexed position and is unwilling to straighten it. If the dislocation has spontaneously reduced, hemarthrosis is often present, and the peripatellar area is usually tender.

Anteroposterior and lateral knee x-rays and patellar views are taken to exclude fracture, even if the dislocation has obviously reduced.

Treatment

- Reduction
- Immobilization

Immediate treatment is reduction; most patients do not require sedation or analgesia. Reduction is done with the patient's hip flexed. Then practitioners gently move the patella medially while simultaneously extending the knee. When the patella is reduced, a palpable clunk is usually evident and the deformity resolves.

Immediately after reduction, the knee is immobilized with a knee immobilizer or hinged brace with the knee in 20° of flexion.

Patients with osteochondral injury or recurrent instability may require surgery.

ACROMIOCLAVICULAR JOINT SPRAINS

(Shoulder Separation)

Acromioclavicular joint sprains are common, usually resulting from a fall on the point of the shoulder or, less often, an outstretched arm.

Several ligaments surround this joint, and depending on the severity of the injury, one or all of the ligaments may be torn.

Severe sprains tear the acromioclavicular and coracoclavicular ligaments.

The acromioclavicular joint is commonly injured when the clavicle is fractured.

Patients have pain and tenderness at the acromioclavicular joint.

Diagnosis

- X-rays

Anteroposterior x-rays of both sides of the clavicle are taken. Sprains are classified based on x-ray findings:

- **Type I:** No joint disruption
- **Type II:** Subluxation with some overlap of the clavicle and acromion
- **Type III:** Complete joint dislocation, usually because the coracoclavicular ligament is torn
- **Type IV:** Posterior displacement of the distal clavicle
- **Type V:** Superior displacement of the distal clavicle
- **Type VI:** Inferior displacement of the distal clavicle

Types IV, V, and VI are variants of type III.

Treatment

- Immobilization
- Early range-of-motion exercises

Treatment is usually immobilization (eg, with a sling) and early range-of-motion exercises. Some severe sprains (usually type III) are surgically repaired.

ULNAR COLLATERAL LIGAMENT SPRAINS

(Gamekeeper's Thumb; Skier's Thumb)

Ulnar collateral ligament sprains of the thumb are common and sometimes disabling.

The ulnar collateral ligament connects the base of the thumb's proximal phalanx to the thumb's metacarpal bone on the ulnar aspect of the joint. The usual injury mechanism is radial deviation of the thumb, commonly caused by falling on the hand while holding a ski pole.

Sometimes when the ligament tears, it avulses part of the proximal phalanx at the ligament attachment.

Initially, patients have pain and point tenderness on the ulnar aspect of the thumb metacarpal joint. Long-term complications can include weakness and instability of the joint.

Diagnosis

- Stress testing
- X-rays

Stress testing is done to check for radial deviation of the thumb; before testing, some patients require anesthesia (infiltration of a local anesthetic). The examiner stabilizes the radial side of the metacarpophalangeal joint of the thumb and pulls on the distal thumb in a radial direction. Both thumbs are tested, and the degree of laxity is compared.

Anteroposterior and lateral x-rays are taken to check for an avulsion fracture of the proximal phalanx. Sometimes stress x-rays are taken.

Treatment

- Thumb spica splint
- Sometimes surgery

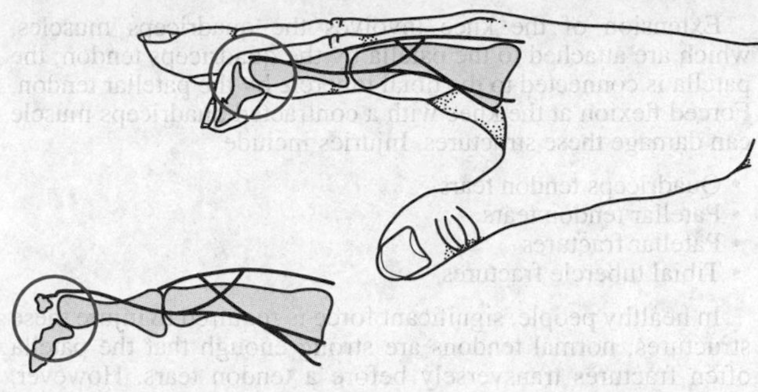

Fig. 359–20. Mallet finger. The extensor tendon is avulsed from the proximal end of the distal phalanx (top); sometimes the tendon avulses a piece of the distal phalangeal bone (bottom).

Initial treatment is immobilization with a thumb spica splint (see Fig. 359–11 on p. 2989) for several weeks.

Surgical repair is sometimes necessary (eg, if instability persists). After surgery, a thumb spica cast is worn for 6 to 8 wk.

MALLET FINGER

Mallet finger is a flexion deformity of the fingertip caused by avulsion of the extensor tendon, with or without fracture, from the proximal end of the distal phalanx.

The usual mechanism is forced flexion of the distal phalanx, typically when hit with a ball. The extensor tendon may avulse part of the proximal aspect of the distal phalangeal bone (see Fig. 359–20). The avulsed part involves the articular surface.

The affected dorsal interphalangeal (DIP) joint rests in a more flexed position than the other DIP joints and cannot be actively straightened but can easily be passively straightened, usually with minimal pain.

Diagnosis

- Clinical evaluation
- X-rays

Mallet finger can usually be diagnosed by examining the finger. Anteroposterior, lateral, and usually oblique x-rays are taken. A fracture, if present, is usually visible on the lateral view.

Treatment

- Splinting

Treatment is with a dorsal splint that holds the DIP joint in extension for 6 to 8 wk; during this time, the tip cannot be allowed to flex (eg, when cleaning the finger).

Fractures that involve > 25% of the joint surface or that cause joint subluxation may require surgical fixation.

KNEE EXTENSOR MECHANISM INJURIES

(Quadriceps Tendon Tear; Patellar Fracture; Patellar Tendon Tear; Tibial Tubercle Fracture)

Knee extensor mechanism injuries can involve the quadriceps tendon, patellar tendon, patella, or tibial tubercle. Surgical repair is usually required.

Extension of the knee involves the quadriceps muscles, which are attached to the patella by the quadriceps tendon; the patella is connected to the tibial tubercle by the patellar tendon. Forced flexion at the knee with a contracted quadriceps muscle can damage these structures. Injuries include

- Quadriceps tendon tears
- Patellar tendon tears
- Patellar fractures
- Tibial tubercle fractures

In healthy people, significant force is required to injure these structures; normal tendons are strong enough that the patella often fractures transversely before a tendon tears. However, certain people are at risk of tendon tears. They include the elderly and people who take certain drugs (eg, fluoroquinolones, corticosteroids). In these people, the injury can result from minor trauma (eg, when descending stairs). The quadriceps tendon is injured more often than the patellar tendon, particularly in the elderly.

The affected area is painful and swollen.

Patients with complete tendon tears cannot stand, do a straight leg raise while lying on their back, or extend their knee while seated. Long-term complications (eg, loss of motion, weakness) are common.

Diagnosis

- Clinical evaluation
- X-rays
- MRI

Examination of the knee can suggest which structure is injured:

- Quadriceps tendon tear: The patella is palpably displaced inferiorly.
- Patella tendon tear: The patella is displaced superiorly.
- Transverse patellar fracture: There is often a palpable gap between the 2 bone fragments.

However, swelling in the area can be significant and mask these findings so that the injury may be misinterpreted as a ligamentous knee joint injury with hemarthrosis.

PEARLS & PITFALLS

- Always test active knee extension if patients have knee swelling and pain after an injury.

Routine knee x-rays are taken. X-rays often show displacement or fracture of the patella but may appear normal. MRI confirms the diagnosis.

Treatment

- Surgical repair

Treatment is surgical repair as soon as possible.

ANKLE SPRAINS

Ankle sprains are very common, most often resulting from turning the foot inward (inversion). Common findings are pain, swelling, and tenderness, which are maximal at the anterolateral ankle. Diagnosis is by stress testing and sometimes x-rays. Treatment is protection, rest, ice, compression, and elevation (PRICE) and early weight bearing for mild sprains and immobilization followed by physical therapy for moderate and severe sprains; some very severe sprains require surgical repair.

The most important ankle ligaments are the deltoid (the strong, medial ligament), the anterior and posterior talofibular (lateral ligaments), and the calcaneofibular (lateral ligaments—see Fig. 359–15 on p. 2994).

Inversion (turning the foot inward) tears the lateral ligaments, usually beginning with the anterior talofibular ligament. Severe 2nd- and 3rd-degree sprains sometimes cause chronic joint instability and predispose to additional sprains. Inversion can also cause talar dome fractures, with or without an ankle sprain.

Eversion (turning the foot outward) stresses the joint medially. This stress often causes an avulsion fracture of the medial malleolus rather than a ligament sprain because the deltoid ligament is so strong. However, eversion can also cause a sprain. Eversion also compresses the joint laterally; this compression, often combined with dorsiflexion, may fracture the distal fibula or tear the syndesmotic ligaments between the tibia and fibula just proximal to the ankle (called a high ankle sprain). Sometimes eversion forces are transmitted up the fibula, fracturing the fibular head just below the knee (called a Maisonneuve fracture).

Recurrent ankle sprains can damage ankle proprioception and thus predispose to future ankle sprains. Most ankle sprains are mild (1st- or 2nd-degree).

Symptoms and Signs

Ankle sprains cause pain and swelling, The location of pain and swelling varies with the type of injury:

- Inversion sprains: Usually maximal at the anterolateral ankle
- Eversion injuries: Maximal over the deltoid ligament
- Maisonneuve fracture: Over the proximal fibula as well as the medial and sometimes lateral ankle
- Third-degree sprains (complete tears, often involving both medial and lateral ligaments): Often diffuse (sometimes the ankle appears egg-shaped)

Generally, tenderness is maximal over the damaged ligaments rather than over the bone; tenderness that is greater over bone than over ligaments suggests fracture.

Diagnosis

- Stress testing
- Sometimes x-rays to exclude fractures
- Occasionally MRI

Diagnosis is primarily clinical; not every patient requires x-rays.

Stress testing to evaluate ligament integrity is important. However, if patients have marked pain and swelling or spasm, the examination is typically delayed until x-rays exclude fractures. Also, swelling and spasm may make joint stability difficult to evaluate; thus, reexamination after several days is helpful. The ankle may be immobilized until examination is possible.

The ankle anterior drawer test is done to evaluate the stability of the anterior talofibular ligament and thus help differentiate between 2nd- and 3rd-degree lateral ligament sprains. For this test, patients sit or lie supine with the knee at least slightly flexed; one of the practitioner's hands prevents forward movement of the anterior distal tibia while the other hand cups the heel, pulling it anteriorly.

High ankle sprains should be considered when eversion is the mechanism and when eversion reproduces pain; the distal tibiofibular joint, just proximal to the talar dome, may be tender.

If findings suggest a deltoid ligament or high ankle sprain, practitioners should check for evidence of a proximal fibular fracture.

Ankle sprains should be differentiated from avulsion fractures of the base of the 5th metatarsal, Achilles tendon injuries, and talar dome fractures, which may cause similar symptoms.

Imaging: Anteroposterior, lateral, and oblique (mortise) ankle x-rays are taken to exclude clinically significant fractures. Clinical criteria (Ottawa ankle rules) are used to determine whether x-rays are needed; these criteria are used to help limit x-rays to patients more likely to have a fracture that requires specific treatment. Ankle x-ray is required only if patients have ankle pain and one of the following:

- Age > 55
- Inability to bear weight without assistance immediately after the injury and in the emergency department (for 4 steps), with or without limping
- Bone tenderness within 6 cm of the posterior edge or tip of either malleolus

Sprains that are painful after 6 wk may require additional testing (eg, MRI) to identify overlooked and subtle injuries, such as talar dome fractures, high ankle sprains, or other complex ankle sprains.

Treatment

- RICE and early mobilization for mild sprains
- Immobilization and/or surgical repair for moderate or severe sprains

Most ankle sprains heal well with minimal intervention and early mobilization. Splinting alleviates pain but does not appear to affect final outcome. Crutches are used for all sprains until gait is normal.

Other treatment depends on severity of the sprain:

- Mild (eg, 1st-degree) sprains: RICE and weight bearing and mobilization as soon as it can be tolerated (usually within a few days)
- Moderate (eg, 2nd-degree) sprains: PRICE, including immobilization of the ankle in a neutral position with a posterior splint or a commercially available boot, followed by mobilization and physical therapy
- Severe (eg, 3rd-degree) sprains: Immobilization (possibly with a cast), possibly surgical repair, and physical therapy

High ankle sprains usually require a cast for several weeks.

If evaluation of the injury is impossible (eg, because of muscle spasm or pain), the ankle may be immobilized for a few days and then reexamined after pain and spasm subside.

KEY POINTS

- Before diagnosing an ankle sprain, consider an avulsion fracture of the base of the 5th metatarsal, an Achilles tendon injury, and a talar dome fracture.
- Use the Ottawa ankle rules to help decide whether x-rays are necessary.
- Evaluate joint stability by stress testing (eg, anterior drawer test), but if needed, delay this testing until swelling and pain subside.
- Encourage early mobilization if the sprain is mild.

ACHILLES TENDON TEARS

Achilles tendon tears (ruptures) most often result from ankle dorsiflexion, particularly when the tendon is taut. Diagnosis is by examination and sometimes ultrasonography or, if unavailable, MRI. Treatment is splinting and immediate referral to an orthopedic surgeon; sometimes surgical repair is necessary.

Achilles tendon tears are common. They typically occur during running or jumping and are most common among middle-aged men and athletes. Very rarely, spontaneous Achilles tendon tears have occurred in people who take fluoroquinolone antibiotics.

Pain in the distal calf makes walking difficult, particularly when the tear is complete. The calf may be swollen and bruised. Complete tears may result in a palpable defect and usually occur 2 to 6 cm proximal to the tendon's insertion.

Diagnosis

- Clinical evaluation
- Sometimes ultrasonography or, if unavailable, MRI

Diagnosis is by examination. The patient's ability to flex the ankle does not rule out a tear.

For the Thompson test (calf squeeze test), the calf is squeezed to elicit plantar flexion while the patient is prone; results may include

- For complete tears: Absent or decreased ankle plantar flexion
- For partial tears: Sometimes normal results, so these tears are often missed

If the Thompson test is normal but a partial Achilles tendon tear is suspected, ultrasonography is the test of choice. However, if ultrasonography is not available, MRI can be done.

Treatment

- Splinting
- Immediate orthopedic referral
- Sometimes surgical repair

Initial treatment consists of splinting with the ankle in plantar flexion and immediate referral to an orthopedic surgeon.

Whether tendon tears should be treated surgically is controversial.

Treatment may involve a posterior ankle splint with the ankle in plantar flexion for 4 wk and avoidance of weight bearing.

Some complete tears are surgically repaired immediately.

KNEE SPRAINS AND MENISCAL INJURIES

Sprains of the external (medial and lateral collateral) or internal (anterior and posterior cruciate) ligaments or injuries of the menisci may result from knee trauma. Symptoms include pain, joint effusion, instability (with severe sprains), and locking (with some meniscal injuries). Diagnosis is by physical examination and sometimes MRI. Treatment is PRICE (protection, rest, ice, compression, elevation) and, for severe injuries, casting or surgical repair.

Many structures that help stabilize the knee are located mainly outside the joint; they include muscles (eg, quadriceps, hamstrings), their insertions (eg, pes anserinus), and extracapsular ligaments. The lateral collateral ligament is extracapsular; the medial (tibial) collateral ligament has a superficial extracapsular portion and a deep portion that is part of the joint capsule.

Inside the knee, the joint capsule and the posterior and highly vascular anterior cruciate ligaments help stabilize the joint. The medial and lateral menisci are intra-articular cartilaginous structures that act mainly as shock absorbers but provide some stabilization (see Fig. 359–21).

The most commonly injured knee structures are the

- Medial collateral and anterior cruciate ligaments

Mechanism predicts the type of injury:

- Inward (valgus) force: Usually, the medial collateral ligament, followed by the anterior cruciate ligament, then the medial meniscus (this mechanism is the most common and is usually accompanied by some external rotation and flexion, as when being tackled in football)
- Outward (varus) force: Often, the lateral collateral ligament, anterior cruciate ligament, or both (this mechanism is the 2nd most common)
- Anterior or posterior forces and hyperextension: Typically, the cruciate ligaments
- Weight bearing and rotation at the time of injury: Usually, menisci

Symptoms and Signs

Swelling and muscle spasm progress over the first few hours. With 2nd-degree sprains, pain is typically moderate or severe. With 3rd-degree sprains, pain may be mild, and surprisingly, some patients can walk unaided.

Some patients hear or feel a pop when the injury occurs. This finding suggests an anterior cruciate ligament tear but is not a reliable indicator.

Location of the tenderness and pain depends on the injury:

- Sprained medial or lateral ligaments: Tenderness over the damaged ligament
- Medial meniscal injuries: Tenderness in the joint plane (joint line tenderness) medially

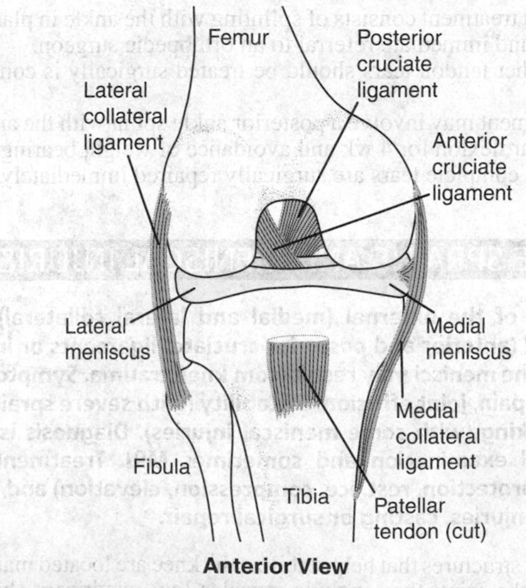

Fig. 359–21. Ligaments of the knee.

- Lateral meniscal injuries: Tenderness in the joint plane laterally
- Medial and lateral meniscal injuries: Pain made worse by extreme flexion or extension and restricted passive knee motion (locking)

Injuries of any of the knee ligaments or menisci cause a visible and palpable joint effusion.

Diagnosis

- Stress testing
- X-rays to exclude fractures
- Sometimes MRI

Diagnosis is primarily clinical.

A spontaneously reduced knee dislocation should be suspected in patients with a large hemarthrosis, gross instability, or both; detailed vascular evaluation, including ankle-brachial BP index, should be done immediately (see p. 582). Next, the knee is fully examined. Active knee extension is assessed in all patients with knee pain and effusion to check for disruption of the extensor mechanism (eg, tears of the quadriceps or patellar tendon, fracture of the patella or tibial tubercle—see p. 3003).

PEARLS & PITFALLS

- Immediately check for vascular injuries if patients have a large knee hemarthrosis, gross knee instability, or both.

Stress testing: Stress testing to evaluate ligament integrity helps distinguish partial from complete tears. However, if patients have significant pain and swelling or muscle spasm, testing is typically delayed until x-rays exclude fractures. Also, significant swelling and spasm may make joint stability difficult to evaluate. Such patients should be examined after injection of a local anesthetic, after use of systemic analgesia and sedation, or at a follow-up examination 2 to 3 days later (after swelling and spasm have subsided).

Bedside stress testing is done to check for specific injuries, although most of these tests are not highly accurate or reliable. For bedside stress testing, practitioners move the joint in a direction in which the ligament being tested normally prevents excessive joint movement.

For the **Apley test,** the patient is prone, and the examiner stabilizes the patient's thigh. The examiner flexes the patient's knee 90° and rotates the lower leg while pressing the lower leg downward toward the knee (compression), then rotates the lower leg while pulling it away from the knee (distraction). Pain during compression and rotation suggests a meniscal injury; pain during distraction and rotation suggests a ligamentous or joint capsule injury.

For **evaluation of the medial and lateral collateral ligaments,** the patient is supine, with the knee flexed about 20° and the hamstring muscles relaxed. The examiner puts one hand over the side of the knee opposite the ligament being tested. With the other hand, the examiner cups the heel and pulls the lower leg outward to test the medial collateral ligament or inward to test the lateral collateral ligament. Moderate instability after acute injury suggests that a meniscus or cruciate ligament is torn as well as the collateral ligament.

The **Lachman test** is the most sensitive physical test for acute anterior cruciate ligament tears. With the patient supine, the examiner supports the patient's thigh and calf, and the patient's knee is flexed 20°. The lower leg is moved anteriorly. Excessive passive anterior motion of the lower leg from the femur suggests a significant tear.

Imaging: Not every patient requires x-rays. However, anteroposterior, lateral, and oblique x-rays are often taken to exclude fractures. The Ottawa knee rules are used to limit x-rays to patients more likely to have a fracture that requires specific treatments. X-rays should be taken only if one of the following is present:

- Age > 55
- Isolated tenderness of the patella (with no other bone tenderness of the knee)
- Tenderness of fibular head
- Inability to flex the knee 90°
- Inability to bear weight both immediately and in the emergency department for 4 steps (with or without limping)

Use of MRI at the initial evaluation is much debated. A reasonable approach is to do MRI if symptoms do not resolve after a few weeks of conservative management. However, MRI is often done when severe injury or significant intra-articular injury is suspected or cannot be otherwise excluded.

Treatment

- Mild sprains: Protection, rest, ice, compression, and elevation (PRICE) and early immobilization
- Severe injuries: Splinting or a knee immobilizer and referral to an orthopedic surgeon for surgical repair

Draining large effusions (see Fig. 32–3 on p. 254) may decrease pain and spasm.

Most 1st-degree and moderate 2nd-degree injuries can be treated initially with PRICE, including immobilization of the knee at 20° of flexion with a commercially available knee immobilizer or splint. Early range of motion exercises are usually encouraged. Severe 2nd-degree and most 3rd-degree sprains require casting for ≥ 6 wk. Some 3rd-degree injuries of the medial collateral ligament and anterior cruciate ligament require arthroscopic surgical repair. Patients with severe injuries are referred to an orthopedic surgeon for surgical repair.

Meniscal injuries vary widely in their characteristics and treatments. Large, complex, or vertical tears and injuries that result in persistent effusions or disabling symptoms are more likely to require surgery. Patient preference can influence choice of treatment.

Physical therapy may be helpful, depending on the patient and the type of injury.

KEY POINTS

- Stress testing (sometimes done days after the injury) is necessary for differentiation of partial from complete ligamentous tears.
- Consider injury to the anterior cruciate ligament and other intra-articular structures if patients have an effusion after an injury.
- Consider knee dislocation and popliteal artery injury if patients have a large hemarthrosis, gross instability, or both.
- If patients have knee pain and effusion, test active knee extension to check for disruption of the extensor mechanism (eg, tears of the quadriceps or patellar tendon, fracture of the patella or tibial tubercle).
- Do MRI if symptoms do not resolve after a few weeks of conservative management or possibly when severe injury or significant intra-articular injury is suspected or cannot be otherwise excluded.

360 Genitourinary Tract Trauma

BLADDER TRAUMA

External bladder injuries are caused by either blunt or penetrating trauma to the lower abdomen, pelvis, or perineum. Blunt trauma is the more common mechanism, usually by a sudden deceleration, such as in a high-speed motor vehicle crash or fall, or from an external blow to the lower abdomen. The most frequently accompanying injury is a pelvic fracture, occurring in > 95% of bladder ruptures caused by blunt trauma. Other concomitant injuries include long bone fractures and CNS and chest injuries. Penetrating injuries, most often gunshot wounds, account for < 10% of bladder injuries.

The bladder is the most frequently injured organ during pelvic surgery. Such injuries can occur during transurethral surgery, gynecologic procedures (most commonly abdominal hysterectomy, cesarean section, pelvic mass excision), or colon resection. Predisposing factors include scarring from prior surgery or radiation therapy, inflammation, and extensive tumor burden.

Bladder injuries are classified as contusions or ruptures based on the extent of injury seen radiographically. They can be extraperitoneal, intraperitoneal, or both.

Complications of bladder injuries include uroascites (free urine in the peritoneal cavity) due to intraperitoneal rupture, infection (including sepsis), persistent hematuria, incontinence, bladder instability and fistula. Mortality with bladder rupture approaches 20%; this is due to concomitant organ injuries rather than the bladder injury.

Symptoms and Signs

Symptoms may include suprapubic pain and inability to void; signs may include hematuria, suprapubic tenderness, distention, hypovolemic shock (due to hemorrhage), and, in the case of intraperitoneal rupture, peritoneal signs. Blunt bladder ruptures almost always present with a pelvic fracture *and* gross hematuria.

Bladder injuries occurring during surgery are usually identified intraoperatively. Findings can include urinary extravasation, a sudden increase in bleeding, appearance of the bladder catheter in the wound, and, during laparoscopy, distention of the urinary drainage bag with gas.

Diagnosis

- Retrograde cystography, usually with CT

Symptoms and signs are often subtle or nonspecific; therefore, diagnosis requires a high level of suspicion. Diagnosis is suspected on the basis of history and physical examination findings and hematuria (predominantly gross). Confirmation is by retrograde cystography using 350 mL of diluted contrast to directly fill the bladder. Plain film x-rays or CT can be used, but CT provides the additional advantage of evaluating concomitant intra-abdominal injuries and pelvic fractures. Drainage films should be obtained only when plain film x-rays are used. If urethral disruption is suspected in a male, retrograde catheter placement is avoided, pending results of urethrography.

A rectal examination should be done in all patients with a blunt or penetrating mechanism of injury to assess for blood which is highly suggestive of a concomitant bowel injury. Similarly, female patients should be examined for genital lacerations.

Treatment

- Catheter drainage
- Sometimes surgical repair

All penetrating trauma and intraperitoneal ruptures due to blunt trauma require surgical exploration and repair. Contusions require only catheter drainage until gross hematuria resolves. Most extraperitoneal ruptures require only catheter drainage if urine is draining freely and the bladder neck is spared. If the bladder neck is involved, surgical exploration and repair are required to limit the likelihood of incontinence. Most bladder injuries during surgery are identified and repaired intraoperatively.

KEY POINTS

- Most bladder injuries are caused by blunt mechanisms, which are accompanied by pelvic fractures and gross hematuria.
- Consider the diagnosis when there is a compatible mechanism of injury and suprapubic pain and tenderness, inability to void, hematuria, bladder distention, and/or unexplained shock or peritoneal signs.
- Confirm the diagnosis using retrograde cystography.
- Contusions and most extraperitoneal ruptures can be managed with catheter drainage alone. Intraperitoneal ruptures should be surgically explored.
- Most bladder injuries during surgery are identified and repaired intraoperatively.

GENITAL TRAUMA

Most genital trauma occurs in men and includes injury to the testes, scrotum, and penis. Genital mutilation of women by removing the clitoris, which is done in some cultures, is a form of genital trauma and child abuse (see p. 2486).

Most **testicular injuries** result from blunt trauma (eg, assaults, motor vehicle crashes, sports injuries); penetrating testicular injuries are far less common. Testicular injuries are classified as contusions or, if the tunica albuginea is disrupted, as ruptures.

Scrotal injury may be caused by penetrating trauma, burns, avulsions, and bites.

Penile injuries have diverse mechanisms. Zipper injuries are common. Penile fractures, which are ruptures of the corpus cavernosum, occur most often when the penis is forcibly bent during sexual activity; urethral injury may also be present. Amputations (usually self-inflicted or due to clothing trapped by heavy machinery) and strangulations (usually due to constricting penile rings used to enhance erections) are additional mechanisms. Penetrating injuries, including animal and human bites and gunshot wounds, are less common; gunshot wounds often involve the urethra.

Complications of genital injuries include infection, tissue loss, erectile dysfunction, male hypogonadism, and urethral scarring.

Symptoms and Signs

Symptoms after a direct scrotal blow are usually scrotal pain and swelling. Signs may include scrotal discoloration and a tender, firm scrotal mass that fails to transilluminate, suggesting a hematocele. Scrotal penetration suggests the possibility of testicular involvement. Often the examination is limited by patient discomfort. Penile fracture typically occurs during intercourse and results in a cracking sound, immediate pain, marked penile swelling and ecchymosis, and usually a visible deformity. The presence of hematuria suggests the possibility of a concomitant urethral injury; in such cases a retrograde urethrography should be performed.

Diagnosis

- Clinical evaluation
- Ultrasonography (for testicular injury)
- Retrograde urethrography (for some penile injuries with possible urethral injuries)

Diagnosis of external scrotal and penile injury is made clinically. Clinical diagnosis of testicular contusion and rupture can be difficult because the degree of injury may be out of proportion to the physical findings, so patients with blunt testicular injury typically require scrotal ultrasonography. Most penile injuries are evident on physical examination. An x-ray with urethral contrast (retrograde urethrography) should be done for any patient with penile fracture or penetrating penile injury in which urethral injury is suspected (eg, with hematuria or inability to void).

Treatment

- Sometimes surgical repair

Patients with penetrating testicular injuries or clinical or sonographic characteristics that suggest testicular rupture require surgical exploration and repair. Similarly, all penile fractures and penetrating injuries should be surgically explored and the defects repaired. Penile amputations should be repaired by microsurgical reimplantation if the amputated segment is viable. Strangulation injuries can usually be managed simply by removing the constricting agent, which may require the use of metal cutters. Animal and human bites involving the genitalia should be managed with copious irrigation, appropriate debridement and antibiotic prophylaxis; primary wound closure is contraindicated. Zippers should be removed (see Fig. 360–1).

To remove a zipper, local anesthetic is injected into the area. Mineral oil is used to lubricate the zipper, and then one attempt is made to unzip the zipper. If this attempt is unsuccessful, a sturdy wire cutter (diagonal cutter) is used to cut the median bar on the top of the zipper slider, which connects its front and back plates. Then the slider falls off in 2 pieces, and the zipper teeth come apart readily.

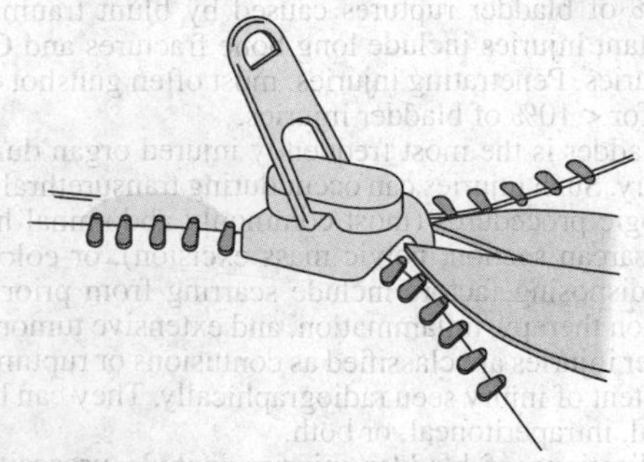

Fig. 360–1. Zipper removal from penile skin.

KEY POINTS

- Diagnose external scrotal and penile injuries clinically.
- Diagnose most blunt testicular injuries with ultrasonography.
- Do retrograde urethrography to diagnose concomitant urethral injury if patients have either a penile fracture or a penetrating penile injury with hematuria or inability to void.
- Surgically repair certain injuries (eg, testicular rupture or penetrating trauma; penile fractures, amputations, and penetrating injuries).

RENAL TRAUMA

The kidney is injured in up to 10% of patients who sustain significant abdominal trauma. Overall about 65% of GU injuries involve the kidney. It is the most commonly injured GU organ.

Most renal injuries (85 to 90% of cases) result from blunt trauma, typically due to motor vehicle crashes, falls, or assaults. Most injuries are low grade. The most common accompanying injuries are to the head, CNS, chest, spleen, and liver. Penetrating injuries usually result from gunshot wounds and are usually associated with multiple intra-abdominal injuries, most commonly to the chest, liver, intestine, and spleen.

Renal injuries are classified according to severity into 5 grades (see Fig. 360–2).

Diagnosis

- Hct and urinalysis
- Clinical evaluation, including repeated vital sign determinations
- If moderate or severe injury is suspected, contrast-enhanced CT

Diagnosis should be suspected in any patient with the following situations:

- Penetrating injury between the mid chest and lower abdomen
- Significant deceleration injury
- Direct blow to the flank

In such patients, hematuria strongly suggests renal injury; other indicators include the following:

- Seat belt marks
- Diffuse abdominal tenderness
- Flank contusions
- Lower rib fractures

Patients who develop gross hematuria after relatively minor trauma may have a previously undiagnosed congenital renal anomaly.

Laboratory testing should include Hct and urinalysis. When imaging is indicated, contrast-enhanced CT should be used to determine the grade of renal injury and identify accompanying intra-abdominal trauma and complications, including retroperitoneal hemorrhage and urinary extravasation. Patients with

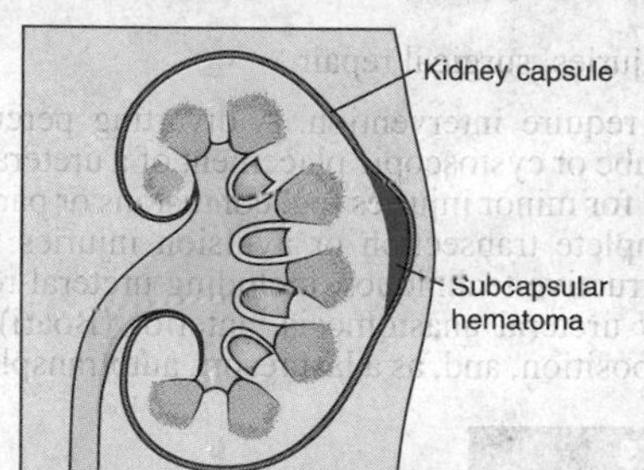

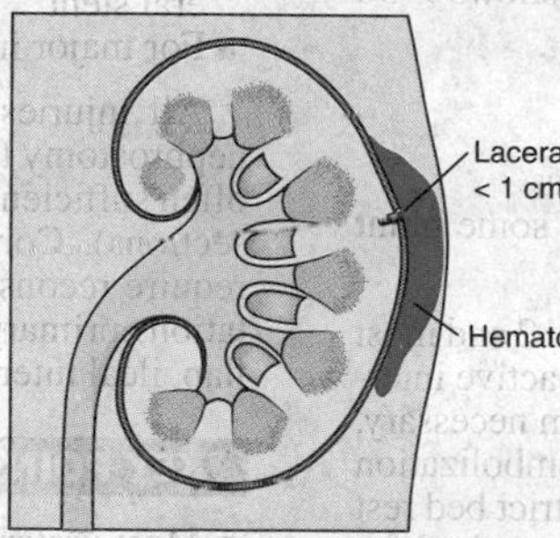

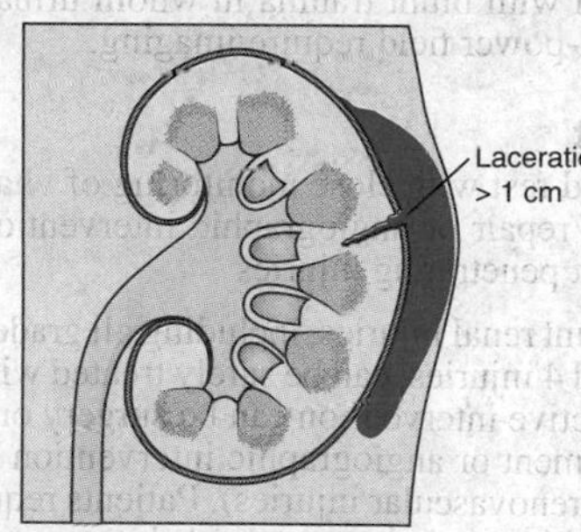

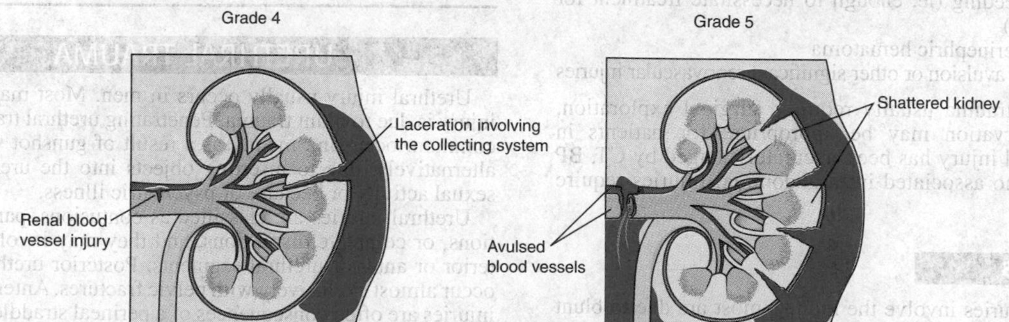

Fig. 360–2. Grades of renal injury. Renal injuries are classified by severity as follows:

- Grade 1: Renal contusion and/or nonexpanding subcapsular hematoma
- Grade 2: Laceration < 1 cm in depth sparing the renal medulla and collecting system and/or nonexpanding retroperitoneal hematoma
- Grade 3: Laceration > 1 cm sparing the collecting system
- Grade 4: Laceration > 1 cm involving the collecting system and/or renal vessel injury with hemorrhage
- Grade 5: Shattered kidney and/or avulsed renal vessels

blunt trauma and microscopic hematuria usually have minor renal injuries that almost never require surgical repair; thus, CT is usually unnecessary. CT is indicated in blunt trauma in any of the following:

- The mechanism involves a fall from a significant height or a high-speed motor vehicle crash
- Gross hematuria
- Microscopic hematuria with hypotension (systolic pressure < 90 mm Hg)
- Clinical signs potentially suggesting severe renal injury (eg, flank contusion, seat belt marks, lower rib or vertebral transverse process fractures)

PEARLS & PITFALLS

- Most patients with only microscopic hematuria after blunt trauma do not require imaging for diagnosis of renal injury.
- The degree of hematuria may not correlate with the extent of injury.

For **penetrating trauma,** CT is indicated for all patients with microscopic or gross hematuria. Angiography may be indicated to assess persistent or delayed bleeding and can be combined with selective arterial embolization.

Pediatric renal injuries are evaluated similarly, except that all children with blunt trauma in whom urinalysis shows > 50 RBCs/high-power field require imaging.

Treatment

- Strict bed rest with close monitoring of vital signs
- Surgical repair or angiographic intervention for some blunt and most penetrating injuries

Most blunt renal injuries, including all grade 1 and 2 and most grade 3 and 4 injuries, can be safely treated without active intervention. Active intervention can be surgery or, when necessary, stent placement or angiographic intervention (eg, embolization for certain renovascular injuries). Patients require strict bed rest until gross hematuria has resolved. Intervention is required for patients with the following:

- Persistent bleeding (ie, enough to necessitate treatment for hypovolemia)
- Expanding perinephric hematoma
- Renal pedicle avulsion or other significant renovascular injuries

Penetrating trauma usually requires surgical exploration, although observation may be appropriate for patients in whom the renal injury has been accurately staged by CT, BP is stable, and no associated intra-abdominal injuries require surgery.

KEY POINTS

- Most GU injuries involve the kidney, most are due to blunt mechanisms, and most are low grade.
- Begin urologic testing with urinalysis and Hct.
- Obtain contrast-enhanced CT for suspected moderate or severe injury (eg, mechanism or findings suggesting severe injury, gross hematuria, hypotension).
- Consider surgery or angiographic intervention for persistent bleeding, expanding perinephric hematoma, renal pedicle avulsions, and significant renovascular injuries.

URETERAL TRAUMA

Most ureteral injuries occur during surgery. Procedures that most often injure a ureter include ureteroscopy, hysterectomy, low anterior colon resection, and abdominal aneurysm repair; mechanisms include ligation, transection, avulsion, crush, devascularization, kinking, and electrocoagulation.

Noniatrogenic ureteral injury accounts for only about 1 to 3% of all GU trauma. It usually results from gunshot wounds and rarely from stab wounds. In children, avulsion injuries are more common. Complications include peritoneal or retroperitoneal urinary leakage; perinephric abscess; fistula (eg, ureterovaginal, ureterocutaneous) formation; and ureteral stricture, obstruction, or both.

Diagnosis

- Imaging, exploratory surgery, or both

Diagnosis is suspected on the basis of history and requires a high index of suspicion, because symptoms are nonspecific and hematuria is absent in > 30% of patients. Diagnosis is confirmed by imaging (eg, CT with contrast that includes delayed images, retrograde pyelography), exploratory surgery, or both. Fever, flank tenderness, prolonged ileus, urinary leakage, obstruction, and sepsis are the most common delayed signs of otherwise occult injuries.

Treatment

- For minor injuries, percutaneous nephrostomy tube or ureteral stent
- For major injuries, surgical repair

All injuries require intervention. A diverting percutaneous nephrostomy tube or cystoscopic placement of a ureteral stent is often sufficient for minor injuries (eg, contusions or partial transections). Complete transection or avulsion injuries typically require reconstructive techniques, including ureteral reimplantation, primary ureteral anastomosis, anterior (Boari) bladder flap, ileal interposition, and, as a last resort, autotransplantation.

KEY POINTS

- Most ureteral injuries occur during surgery.
- Have a high index of suspicion because findings are nonspecific and hematuria is commonly absent.

URETHRAL TRAUMA

Urethral injury usually occurs in men. Most major urethral injury is due to blunt trauma. Penetrating urethral trauma is less common, occurring mainly as a result of gunshot wounds, or, alternatively, due to inserting objects into the urethra during sexual activity or because of psychiatric illness.

Urethral injuries are classified as contusions, partial disruptions, or complete disruptions, and they may involve the posterior or anterior urethral segments. Posterior urethral injuries occur almost exclusively with pelvic fractures. Anterior urethral injuries are often consequences of a perineal straddle injury due to a fall, perineal blow, or motor vehicle crash.

Complications include infection, incontinence, erectile dysfunction, and stricture formation.

Symptoms and Signs

Symptoms include pain with voiding or inability to void. Blood at the urethral meatus is the most important sign of a urethral injury. Additional signs include perineal, scrotal, penile, and labial ecchymosis, edema, or both. Abnormal location of the prostate on rectal examination (so-called high-riding prostate) is an inaccurate indicator of a urethral injury. Blood on digital, rectal, or vaginal examination requires thorough evaluation.

Diagnosis

- Retrograde urethrography

In any male patient with suggestive symptoms or signs, the diagnosis is confirmed by retrograde urethrography. This procedure should always precede catheterization. Urethral catheterization in a male with an undetected significant urethral injury may potentiate urethral disruption (eg, convert a partial disruption to a complete disruption). Female patients require prompt cystoscopy and a thorough vaginal examination

PEARLS & PITFALLS

- If male urethral injury is suspected, do not insert a urethral catheter until after urethrography.

Treatment

- Usually urethral catheterization (for contusions) or suprapubic cystostomy
- Sometimes endoscopic realignment or surgical repair (for select injuries)
- Delayed definitive surgery

Contusions can be safely treated with an indwelling transurethral catheter for 7 days. Partial disruptions are best treated with bladder drainage via suprapubic cystostomy. In selected cases of posterior partial disruptions, primary endoscopic urethral realignment may be attempted; if successful, this approach may limit subsequent urethral strictures.

Complete disruptions usually are treated with bladder drainage via suprapubic cystostomy. This option is simplest and can be used safely in all patients. Definitive surgery is deferred for about 8 to 12 wk until the urethral scar tissue has stabilized and the patient has recovered from any accompanying injuries.

Open repair of urethral injuries is limited to those associated with penile fractures, certain penetrating transections, and injuries in females.

KEY POINTS

- Consider urethral injuries particularly in patients who have pelvic fractures or straddle injuries and who have difficulty voiding or blood at the urethral meatus.
- In males, do retrograde urethrography before urethral catheterization.
- In females, perform cystoscopy and vaginal examination.
- Treat contusions with urethral catheterization and complete and many partial disruptions initially with suprapubic cystostomy.
- Surgical reconstruction should be delayed except in select injuries (ie, penile fractures, certain penetrating injuries, and female urethral injuries).

361 Heat Illness

Heat illness encompasses a number of disorders ranging in severity from muscle cramps and heat exhaustion to heatstroke (which is a life-threatening emergency). Heat illness, although preventable, affects thousands of people each year in the US and can be fatal; it is the second leading cause of death in young athletes. When heatstroke is not treated promptly and effectively, mortality approaches 80%.

Patients with heat exhaustion maintain the ability to dissipate heat and have normal CNS function. In heatstroke, compensatory mechanisms for heat dissipation fail (although sweating may still be present) and CNS function is impaired. Heatstroke should be considered in patients with hyperthermia and an altered mental status or other CNS dysfunction, regardless of sweating.

Pathophysiology

Heat input comes from

- The environment
- Metabolism

Heat output occurs through the skin via the following:

- Radiation: Transfer of body heat directly into a cooler environment by infrared radiation, a process that does not require air motion or direct contact
- Evaporation: Cooling by water vaporization (eg, sweat)
- Convection: Transfer of heat to cooler air (or liquid) that passes over exposed skin
- Conduction: Transfer of heat from a warmer surface to a cooler surface that is in direct contact

The contribution of each of these mechanisms varies with environmental temperature and humidity. When environmental temperature is lower than body temperature, radiation provides 65% of cooling. Evaporation normally provides 30% of cooling, and exhalation of water vapor and production of urine and feces provide about 5%.

When environmental temperature is > 35° C, evaporation accounts for virtually all dissipation of heat because the other mechanisms function only when environmental temperature is lower than body temperature. However, effectiveness of sweating is limited. Sweat that drips from the skin is not evaporated and does not contribute to cooling. Effectiveness of sweating is also limited by body surface area and humidity. When humidity is > 75%, evaporative heat loss markedly decreases. Thus, if both environmental temperature and humidity are high, all mechanisms for heat dissipation are lost, markedly increasing risk of heat illness.

The body can compensate for large variations in heat load, but significant or prolonged exposure to heat that exceeds capacity for heat dissipation increases core temperature. Modest, transient core temperature elevations are tolerable, but severe elevations (typically > 41° C) lead to protein denaturation and, especially during hard work in the heat, release of inflammatory cytokines (eg, tumor necrosis factor-α, IL-1b). As a result, cellular dysfunction occurs and the inflammatory cascade is activated, leading to dysfunction of most organs and activation of the coagulation cascade. These pathophysiologic processes are similar to those of multiple organ dysfunction syndrome (see p. 573), which follows prolonged shock.

Compensatory mechanisms include an acute-phase response by other cytokines that moderate the inflammatory response (eg, by stimulating production of proteins that decrease production of free radicals and inhibit release of proteolytic enzymes). Also, increased core temperature triggers expression of heat-shock proteins. These proteins transiently enhance heat tolerance by poorly understood mechanisms (eg, possibly by preventing protein denaturation) and by regulation of cardiovascular responses. With prolonged or extreme temperature elevation, compensatory mechanisms are overwhelmed or malfunction, allowing inflammation and multiple organ dysfunction syndrome to occur.

Heat output is modulated by changes in cutaneous blood flow and sweat production. Cutaneous blood flow is 200 to 250 mL/min at normal temperatures but increases to 7 to 8 L/min with heat stress (and facilitates heat loss by convective, conductive, radiant and evaporative mechanisms), requiring a marked increase in cardiac output. Also, heat stress increases sweat production from negligible to > 2 L/h; however, although sweat that is dripped from the skin does not contribute to cooling, it still contributes to dehydration. Significant sweating can occur less perceptibly in very hot, very dry air, in which sweat evaporates very quickly. With sweat production of > 2L/h, dehydration can develop very rapidly. Because sweat contains electrolytes, electrolyte loss may be substantial. However, prolonged exposure triggers physiologic changes to accommodate heat load (acclimatization); eg, sweat Na levels are 40 to 100 mEq/L in people who are not acclimatized but decrease to 10 to 70 mEq/L in acclimatized people.

Etiology

Heat disorders are caused by some combination of increased heat input and decreased output (see Table 361–1).

Excess heat input typically results from strenuous exertion, high environmental temperatures, or both. Medical disorders and use of stimulant drugs can increase heat production.

Impaired cooling can result from obesity, high humidity, high environmental temperatures, wearing heavy clothing, and anything that impairs sweating or evaporation of sweat.

Clinical effects of heat illnesses are exacerbated by the following:

- Inability to tolerate increased cardiovascular demands (eg, due to aging, heart failure, chronic kidney disease, respiratory disorders, liver failure)
- Dehydration
- Electrolyte disturbance
- Use of certain drugs (see Table 361–1)

The elderly and very young are at increased risk. The elderly are at high risk because they more often use drugs that can increase risk, have higher rates of dehydration and heart failure, and have age-related loss of heat-shock proteins. Children are at high risk due to their greater surface area to body mass ratio (resulting in greater heat gain from the environment on a hot day), and slower rates of sweat production. Children are slower to acclimatize and have less of a thirst response. Both the elderly and young children may be relatively immobile and thus have difficulty leaving a hot environment.

Prevention

Common sense is the best prevention. Physicians should recommend the following measures:

- During excessively hot weather, the elderly and the young should not remain in unventilated residences without air-conditioning.

Table 361–1. COMMON FACTORS CONTRIBUTING TO HEAT DISORDERS

CONDITION	EXAMPLES
Excess heat input	
Certain disorders	Hyperthyroidism Infections Malignant hyperthermia Neuroleptic malignant syndrome Salicylate poisoning, severe Seizures Serotonin syndrome
High environmental temperatures	—
Strenuous exertion	Exercise Physical labor
Stimulant drugs	Amphetamines Cocaine Methylenedioxymethamphetamine (MDMA, or Ecstasy) Monoamine oxidase inhibitors Phencyclidine (PCP)
Withdrawal from certain drugs	Alcohol Opioids
Impaired cooling	
Heavy clothing	Protective gear for workers and athletes (eg, football pads)
High humidity	—
Obesity and/or poor cardiovascular fitness	—
High environmental temperatures	—
Impaired sweating*	
Skin disorders	Burn scars, extensive Eczema, extensive Heat rash Psoriasis, extensive Systemic sclerosis
Anticholinergic drugs	Antihistamines Antiparkinsonian drugs Atropine Phenothiazines Scopolamine
Cystic fibrosis	—

*Impaired sweating is a cause of impaired cooling.

- Children should not be left in automobiles in the hot sun.
  - If possible, strenuous exertion in a very hot environment or an inadequately ventilated space should be avoided, and heavy, insulating clothing should not be worn.
  - Weight loss after exercise or work can be used to monitor dehydration; people who lose 2 to 3% of their body weight should be reminded to drink extra fluids and should be within 1 kg of starting weight before the next day's exposure. If people lose > 4%, activity should be limited for 1 day.
  - If exertion in the heat is unavoidable, fluid should be replaced by drinking frequently, and evaporation should be facilitated by wearing open-mesh clothing or by using fans.

Temperature (°C)

Relative humidity (%)	20	21	22	23	24	25	26	27	28	29	30	31	32	33	34	35	36	37	38	39	40	41	42	43	44	45	46	47	48	49	50
0	15	16	16	17	18	18	19	19	20	20	21	22	22	23	23	24	24	25	25	26	27	27	28	28	29	29	30	31	31	32	32
5	16	16	17	18	18	19	19	20	21	21	22	22	23	24	24	25	26	26	27	27	28	29	29	30	31	31	32	33	33	34	35
10	16	17	17	18	19	19	20	21	21	22	23	23	24	25	25	26	27	27	28	29	30	30	31	32	32	33	34	35	36	36	37
15	17	17	18	19	19	20	21	21	22	23	23	24	25	26	26	27	28	29	29	30	31	32	33	33	34	35	36	37	38	39	
20	17	18	18	19	20	21	21	22	23	24	24	25	26	27	27	28	29	30	31	32	32	33	34	35	36	37	38	39			
25	18	18	19	20	20	21	22	23	24	24	25	26	27	28	28	29	30	31	32	33	34	35	36	37	38	39					
30	18	19	20	20	21	22	23	23	24	25	26	27	28	29	29	30	31	32	33	34	35	36	37	39							
35	18	19	20	21	22	22	23	24	25	26	27	28	29	30	31	32	33	34	35	36	37	38	39								
40	19	20	21	21	22	23	24	25	26	27	28	29	30	31	32	33	34	35	36	37	38	39									
45	19	20	21	22	23	24	25	26	27	27	28	29	30	32	33	34	35	36	37	38											
50	20	21	22	23	23	24	25	26	27	28	29	30	31	33	34	35	36	37	39												
55	20	21	22	23	24	25	26	27	28	29	30	31	32	34	35	36	37	38													
60	21	22	23	24	25	26	27	28	29	30	31	32	33	35	36	37	38														
65	21	22	23	24	25	26	27	28	29	31	32	33	34	36	37	38															
70	22	23	24	25	26	27	28	29	30	31	33	34	35	36	38	39															
75	22	23	24	25	26	27	29	30	31	32	33	35	36	37	39																
80	23	24	25	26	27	28	29	30	32	33	34	36	37	38																	
85	23	24	25	26	28	29	30	31	32	34	35	37	38	39																	
90	24	25	26	27	28	29	31	32	33	35	36	37	39																		
95	24	25	26	27	29	30	31	33	34	35	37	38																			
100	24	26	27	28	29	31	32	33	35	36	38	39																			

Fig. 361–1. Wet bulb globe temperature based on temperature and relative humidity. Values are derived from an approximate formula that depends on temperature and humidity and that is valid for full sunshine and a light wind. Heat stress may be overestimated in other conditions.

Hydration: Maintaining adequate levels of fluid and Na helps prevent heat illnesses. Thirst is a poor indicator of dehydration and the need for fluid replacement during exertion because thirst is not stimulated until plasma osmolality rises 1 to 2% above normal. Thus, fluids should be drunk every few hours regardless of thirst. Because maximum net water absorption in the gut is about 20 mL/min (1200 mL/h—lower than the maximum sweating rate of 2000 mL/h), prolonged exertion that causes very high sweat loss requires rest periods that reduce sweating rate and allow time for rehydration.

The best hydrating fluid to use depends on the expected loss of water and electrolytes, which depends on the duration and degree of exertion along with environmental factors and whether the person is acclimatized. For maximum fluid absorption, a carbohydrate-containing beverage can be absorbed by the body up to 30% faster than plain water. A beverage containing 6 or 7% carbohydrate concentration is absorbed most rapidly. Higher carbohydrate concentrations should be avoided because they can cause stomach cramps and delay absorption. However, for most situations and activities, plain water is adequate for hydration as long as overhydration is avoided. Significant hyponatremia (see p. 1272) has occurred in endurance athletes who drink free water very frequently before, during, and after exercise without replacing Na losses. Special hydrating solutions (eg, sports drinks) are not required, but their flavoring enhances consumption, and their modest salt content is helpful if fluid requirements are high.

Laborers, soldiers, endurance athletes, or others who sweat heavily can lose ≥ 20 g of Na/day, making heat cramps more likely; such people need to replace the Na loss with drink and food. In most situations, consuming generously salted foods is adequate; people on low-salt diets should increase salt intake. For more extreme circumstances (eg, prolonged exertion by unacclimatized people) an oral salt solution can be used. The ideal concentration is 0.1% NaCl, which can be prepared by dissolving a 1-g salt tablet or one quarter of a teaspoon of table salt in a liter (or quart) of water. People should drink this solution under moderate to extreme circumstances. Undissolved salt tablets should not be ingested. They irritate the stomach, can cause vomiting, and do not treat the underlying dehydration.

PEARLS & PITFALLS

- Salt tablets should not be swallowed because they can cause gastric irritation. Instead, they are dissolved in water to be drunk.

Acclimatization: Successively and incrementally increasing the level and amount of work done in the heat eventually results in acclimatization, which enables people to work safely at temperatures that were previously intolerable or life-threatening. To reach maximum benefit, acclimatization usually requires spending 8 to 11 days in the hot environment with some daily exercise (eg, 1 to 2 h/day with intensity increased from day to day). Acclimatization markedly increases the amount of sweat (and hence cooling) produced at a given level of exertion and markedly decreases the electrolyte content of sweat. Acclimatization significantly decreases risk of a heat illness.

Moderation of activity level: When possible, people should adjust their activity level based on the environment and any heat loss-impairing gear (eg, firefighting or chemical protective outfits) that must be worn. Work periods should shorten and rest periods increase when

- Temperature increases
- Humidity increases

Table 361–2. WET BULB GLOBE TEMPERATURE AND RECOMMENDED ACTIVITY LEVELS

TEMPERATURE ° C (° F)	RECOMMENDATIONS
≤ 15.6 (≤ 60)	No precautions
> 15.6–21.1 (> 60–70)	No precautions if adequate hydration maintained
> 21.1–23.9 (> 70–75)	Unacclimatized: Stop or restrict exercise Acclimatized: Exercise with caution; rest periods and water breaks every 20 to 30 min
> 23.9–26.7 (> 75–80)	Unacclimatized: Avoid hiking, sports, and sun exposure Acclimatized: Heavy to moderate activity permissible with caution
> 26.7–31.1 (> 80–88)	Unacclimatized: Avoid activity Acclimatized: Limited brief activity permissible, only if fit
≥ 31.1 (> 88)	Avoid activity and sun exposure

- Workload is heavier
- Sun gets stronger
- There is no air movement
- When protective clothing or gear is worn

The best indicator of environmental heat stress is the wet bulb globe temperature (WBGT), which is widely used by the military, industry, and sports. In addition to temperature, the WBGT reflects the effects of humidity, wind, and solar radiation. The WBGT can be used as a guide for recommended activity (see Table 361–2).

Although the WBGT is complex and may not be available, it can be estimated based on only temperature and relative humidity in sunny conditions and when the wind is light (see Fig. 361–1).

KEY POINTS

- When environmental temperature is > 35° C, cooling relies largely on evaporation, but when humidity is > 75%, evaporation markedly decreases, so when temperature and humidity are both high, risk of heat illness is high.
- Among the many risk factors for heat illness are certain drugs and disorders (including those that disturb electrolyte balance or decrease cardiovascular reserve) and extremes of age.
- Prevention includes common sense measures and maintaining and replacing fluids and sodium.
- Acclimatization, requiring daily exercise for 8 to 11 days, decreases risk of heat illness.
- Activity levels should be restricted as temperature, humidity, sunlight, and amount of clothing or gear increases and when air movement decreases.

HEAT CRAMPS

Heat cramps are painful spasmodic muscle cramps that usually occur in heavily exercised muscles in hot and humid environments.

Although exertion may induce cramps during cool weather, such cramps are not heat related and probably reflect lack of fitness. In contrast, heat cramps can occur in physically fit people who sweat profusely and replace lost water but not salt, thereby causing hyponatremia. Heat cramps are common among the following:

- Manual laborers (eg, engine room personnel, steel workers, roofers, miners)
- Military trainees
- Athletes

Cramping is abrupt, usually occurring in muscles of the extremities. Cramping can begin during or after exercise. Severe pain and carpopedal spasm may incapacitate the hands and feet. Temperature is normal, and other findings are unremarkable. The cramp usually lasts minutes to hours. Diagnosis is by history and clinical evaluation.

Treatment

Cramps may be relieved immediately by firm passive stretching of the involved muscle (eg, ankle dorsiflexion for a calf cramp). The patient should rest in a cool environment. Fluids and electrolytes should be replenished orally (1 to 2 L water containing 10 g [2 level tsp] salt or sufficient amounts of a commercial sports drink) or, for more rapid relief or when oral repletion is not possible, IV (1 to 2 L 0.9% saline solution). Adequate conditioning, acclimatization, and appropriate management of salt balance help prevent cramps.

HEAT EXHAUSTION

Heat exhaustion is a non-life-threatening clinical syndrome of weakness, malaise, nausea, syncope, and other nonspecific symptoms caused by heat exposure. Thermoregulation and CNS function are not impaired, but patients are usually dehydrated and may have mild elevations of body temperature (< 40° C). Treatment involves rest in a cool environment and replacing fluids and electrolytes.

Rarely, severe heat exhaustion after hard work may be complicated by rhabdomyolysis, myoglobinuria, and acute kidney injury. It is distinguished from heat stroke by the absence of brain dysfunction (eg, confusion, ataxia).

Symptoms and Signs

Symptoms are often vague, and patients may not realize that heat is the cause. Symptoms may include malaise, weakness, dizziness, headache, nausea, and sometimes vomiting. Syncope due to standing for long periods in the heat (heat syncope) may occur. On examination, patients appear tired, are usually sweaty and tachycardic, and may have orthostatic hypotension. Mental status is intact, unlike in heatstroke. Temperature is usually normal and, when elevated, usually does not exceed 40° C.

Diagnosis

- Clinical evaluation

Diagnosis is clinical and requires exclusion of other possible causes (eg, hypoglycemia, acute coronary syndrome, various infections). Laboratory testing is required only if needed to rule out such disorders. Electrolyte levels should be measured to exclude severe hyponatremia in patients who have had excessive free water intake, particularly if they develop findings of brain dysfunction.

Treatment

- Oral or IV fluid and electrolyte replacement

Treatment involves stopping all exertion and removing patients to a cool environment, having them lie flat, and attempting oral rehydration with a solution of 0.1% NaCl. Patients should drink about 1L/h. If vomiting or nausea prevents oral rehydration, IV fluid and electrolyte replacement therapy, typically using 0.9% saline solution, is indicated. Also, if symptoms do not resolve after 30 to 60 min, patients should be transported to an emergency department, where rehydration is usually done IV. Rate and volume of IV rehydration are guided by age, underlying disorders, and clinical response. Replacement of 1 to 2 L at 500 mL/h is often adequate. Elderly patients and patients with heart disorders may require lower rates. External cooling measures (see p. 3016) are usually not required. However, if patients with heat exhaustion have a core temperature of ≥ 40° C, measures may be taken to reduce it.

KEY POINTS

- In heat exhaustion, symptoms tend to be nonspecific, temperature is usually < 40° C, and CNS function is not impaired.
- Diagnose heat exhaustion clinically, testing as indicated to exclude other clinically suspected disorders.
- Have patients rest in a cool environment and try oral rehydration, transporting patients to an emergency department if these measures are unsuccessful.

HEATSTROKE

Heatstroke is hyperthermia accompanied by a systemic inflammatory response causing multiple organ dysfunction and often death. Symptoms include temperature > 40° C and altered mental status; sweating may be absent or present. Diagnosis is clinical. Treatment includes rapid external cooling, IV fluid resuscitation, and support as needed for organ dysfunction.

Heatstroke occurs when compensatory mechanisms for dissipating heat fail and core temperature increase substantially. Inflammatory cytokines are activated, and multiple organ dysfunction may develop. Endotoxin from GI flora may also play a role. Organ dysfunction may occur in the CNS, skeletal muscle (rhabdomyolysis), liver, kidneys, lungs (acute respiratory distress syndrome), and heart. The coagulation cascade is activated, sometimes causing disseminated intravascular coagulation. Hyperkalemia and hypoglycemia may occur.

Heatstroke is sometimes divided into 2 variants, although the usefulness of this classification is controversial (see Table 361–3):

- Classic
- Exertional

Classic heatstroke takes 2 to 3 days of exposure to develop. It occurs during summer heat waves, typically in elderly, sedentary people with no air-conditioning and often with limited access to fluids.

Exertional heatstroke occurs more abruptly and affects healthy active people (eg, athletes, military recruits, factory workers). It is the 2nd most common cause of death in young athletes. Intense exertion in a hot environment causes a sudden massive heat load that the body cannot modulate. Rhabdomyolysis is common; acute kidney injury and coagulopathy are somewhat more likely and severe. Heat exhaustion can transition to heatstroke as heat illness progresses and is characterized by impairment of mental status and neurologic function.

Heatstroke may occur after using certain drugs (eg, cocaine, phencyclidine [PCP], amphetamines, monoamine oxidase inhibitors) that cause a hypermetabolic state. Usually, an overdose is required, but exertion and environmental conditions can be additive.

Malignant hyperthermia (see p. 3017) can result from exposure to some anesthetics in genetically predisposed patients. Neuroleptic malignant syndrome (see p. 3018) can develop in patients taking antipsychotics. These disorders are life-threatening.

Symptoms and Signs

CNS dysfunction, ranging from confusion or bizarre behavior to delirium, seizures, and coma, is the hallmark. Ataxia may be an early manifestation. Tachycardia, even when the patient is supine, and tachypnea are common. Sweating may be present or absent. Temperature is > 40° C.

Diagnosis

- Clinical evaluation, including core temperature measurement
- Laboratory testing for organ dysfunction

Diagnosis is usually clear from a history of exertion and environmental heat. Heatstroke is differentiated from heat exhaustion by presence of the following:

- CNS dysfunction
- Temperature > 40° C

When the diagnosis of heatstroke is not obvious, other disorders that can cause CNS dysfunction and hyperthermia should be considered. These disorders include the following:

- Acute infection (eg, sepsis, malaria, meningitis, toxic shock syndrome)
- Drugs
- Neuroleptic malignant syndrome
- Serotonin syndrome
- Status epilepticus (interictal)
- Stroke
- Thyroid storm

Laboratory testing includes CBC, PT, PTT, electrolytes, BUN, creatinine, Ca, CK, and hepatic profile to evaluate organ function. A urethral catheter is placed to obtain urine, which is checked for occult blood by dipstick, and to monitor output. Tests to detect myoglobin are unnecessary. If a urine sample contains no RBCs but has a positive reaction for blood and if serum CK is elevated, myoglobinuria is likely. A urine drug screen may be helpful. Continual monitoring of core temperature, usually by rectal, esophageal, or bladder probe, is desired.

Prognosis

Mortality rate and morbidity are significant but vary markedly with age, underlying disorders, maximum temperature, and, most importantly, duration of hyperthermia and promptness of cooling. Without prompt and effective treatment, mortality approaches 80%. About 20% of survivors have residual brain damage, regardless of intervention. In some patients, renal insufficiency persists. Temperature may be labile for weeks.

Treatment

- Aggressive cooling
- Aggressive supportive care

Classic and exertional heatstroke are treated similarly. The importance of rapid recognition and effective, aggressive cooling cannot be overemphasized.

Cooling techniques: The main cooling techniques are

- Cold water immersion
- Evaporative cooling

Cold water immersion results in the lowest morbidity and mortality rates and is the treatment of choice when available. Large cooling tanks are often used at outdoor activities such as football practices and endurance races. In more remote areas, patients may be immersed in a cool pond or stream. Immersion can be used in an emergency department if suitable equipment is available and the patient is stable enough (eg, no need for endotracheal intubation, absence of seizures). The rate of heat loss during cooling may be decreased by vasoconstriction and shivering; shivering can be decreased by giving a benzodiazepine (eg, diazepam 5 mg or lorazepam 2 to 4 mg IV, with additional doses as needed) or chlorpromazine 25 to 50 mg IV.

Evaporative cooling can also be effective but works best if the environment is dry and the patient has adequate peripheral circulation (requiring adequate cardiac output). When humidity is high or profound shock is present, cold water immersion should be used. Evaporative cooling can be accomplished by splashing or spraying tepid water over the patient while fanning. Evaporative cooling is more effective when using warm rather than cold water. Warm water maximizes skin-to-air vapor pressure gradient and minimizes vasoconstriction and shivering. Some specially designed body cooling units suspend patients naked on a net over a drainage table while finely misted water at 15° C is sprayed over the entire body from above and below. Fans are used to circulate air warmed to 45 to 48° C around the body. With this technique, most patients who have heatstroke can be cooled in < 60 min. In addition, ice or chemical cold packs can be applied to the neck, axillae, and groin or to hairless skin surfaces (ie, palms of hands, soles of feet, cheeks) that contain densely packed subcutaneous vessels to augment cooling, but are not adequate as the sole cooling method.

Table 361–3. SOME DIFFERENCES BETWEEN CLASSIC AND EXERTIONAL HEATSTROKE

CHARACTERISTIC	CLASSIC HEATSTROKE	EXERTIONAL HEATSTROKE
Onset	2–3 days	Hours
Patients usually affected	Elderly, sedentary people	Healthy active people (eg, athletes, military recruits, factory workers)
Risk factors	No air-conditioning during summer heat waves	Intense exertion, particularly without acclimatization
Skin	Usually hot and dry but sometimes moist with sweat	Often moist with sweat

Other measures: Necessary resuscitation should proceed while cooling is done. Endotracheal intubation and mechanical ventilation (sometimes with paralysis) may be needed to prevent aspiration in obtunded patients, who commonly develop vomiting and seizures. Supplemental O_2 is given because heatstroke increases metabolic demand. The patient is admitted to an ICU, and IV hydration with 0.9% saline solution is begun as in heat exhaustion (see p. 3015). Theoretically, giving 1 to 2 L of IV 0.9% saline cooled to 4° C, as used in protocols to induce hypothermia after cardiac arrest, may also help decrease core temperature. Fluid deficits range from minimal (eg, 1 to 2 L) to severe dehydration. IV fluids should be given as boluses, assessing responses and the need for additional boluses by monitoring BP, urine output, and central venous pressures. Excessive amounts of IV fluids, particularly if patients develop heatstroke-induced acute kidney injury, can cause acute pulmonary edema.

Organ dysfunction and rhabdomyolysis are treated (see elsewhere in THE MANUAL). An injectable benzodiazepine (eg, lorazepam, diazepam) may be used aggressively to prevent agitation and to treat seizures (which increase heat production).

Platelets and fresh frozen plasma may be required for severe disseminated intravascular coagulation. If myoglobinuria is present, giving enough fluids to maintain urine output of ≥ 0.5 mL/kg/h and giving IV $NaHCO_3$ to alkalinize the urine can help prevent or minimize nephrotoxicity. IV Ca salts may be necessary to treat hyperkalemic cardiotoxicity. Vasoconstrictors used to treat hypotension may reduce cutaneous blood flow and decrease heat loss. When vasoconstrictors are used in an ICU, a pulmonary artery catheter may be used to monitor filling pressures. Catecholamines (epinephrine, norepinephrine, and dopamine) may increase heat production. Hemodialysis may be required. Antipyretics (eg, acetaminophen) are of no value and may contribute to liver or kidney damage. Dantrolene is used to treat anesthetic-induced malignant hyperthermia but has no proven benefit for other causes of severe hyperthermia. Activated protein C shows promising results in animal models, but is unproven in humans.

KEY POINTS

- Heatstroke differs from heat exhaustion by the failure of mechanisms to dissipate body heat, the presence of CNS dysfunction, and temperature > 40° C.
- If the diagnosis of heatstroke is not obvious in febrile, obtunded patients, consider a wide variety of other disorders, such as infection, intoxication, thyroid storm, stroke, seizures (interictal), neuroleptic malignant syndrome, and serotonin syndrome.
- Rapid recognition and effective, aggressive cooling is extremely important.
- Use cool water immersion if feasible.
- Evaporative cooling can also be effective, but requires a dry environment and adequate peripheral circulation; use tepid (not cold) water, and fanning.
- Monitor patients closely (including their fluid status), and provide aggressive supportive treatment.

MALIGNANT HYPERTHERMIA

Malignant hyperthermia is a life-threatening elevation in body temperature usually resulting from a hypermetabolic response to concurrent use of a depolarizing muscle relaxant and a potent, volatile inhalational general anesthetic. Manifestations can include muscle rigidity, hyperthermia, tachycardia, tachypnea, rhabdomyolysis, and respiratory and metabolic acidosis. Diagnosis is clinical; patients at risk can be tested for their susceptibility. The highest priority treatments are rapid cooling and aggressive supportive measures.

The muscle relaxant involved is usually succinylcholine; the inhalational anesthetic is most often halothane, but other anesthetics (eg, isoflurane, sevoflurane, desflurane) may also be involved. This drug combination causes a similar reaction in some patients with muscular dystrophy and myotonia. Although malignant hyperthermia may develop after the first exposure to these drugs, on average, patients require 3 exposures.

Pathophysiology

Malignant hyperthermia affects about 1/20,000 people. Susceptibility is inherited, with autosomal dominant inheritance and variable penetrance. Most often, the causative mutation affects the ryanodine receptor of skeletal muscle; however, > 22 other causative mutations have been identified.

The mechanism may involve anesthetic-induced potentiation of Ca exit from the sarcoplasmic reticulum of skeletal muscle in susceptible patients. As a result, Ca-induced biochemical reactions are accelerated, causing severe muscle contractions and elevation of the metabolic rate, resulting in respiratory and metabolic acidosis. In response to the acidosis, patients breathing spontaneously develop tachypnea that only partially compensates.

Complications: Hyperkalemia, respiratory and metabolic acidosis, hypocalcemia, and rhabdomyolysis with CK elevation and myoglobinemia may occur, as may coagulation abnormalities (particularly disseminated intravascular coagulation [DIC]). In older patients and patients with comorbidities, DIC may increase the risk of death.

Symptoms and Signs

Malignant hyperthermia may develop during anesthesia or the early postoperative period. Clinical presentation varies depending on the drugs used and the patient's susceptibility. Muscular rigidity, especially in the jaw, is often the first sign, followed by tachycardia, other arrhythmias, tachypnea, acidosis, shock, and hyperthermia. Hypercapnia (detected by increased end-tidal CO_2) may be an early sign. Temperature is usually ≥ 40° C and may be extremely high (ie, > 43° C). Urine may appear brown or bloody if rhabdomyolysis and myoglobinuria have occurred.

Diagnosis

- Clinical evaluation
- Testing for complications
- Susceptibility testing for people at risk

The diagnosis is suspected by the appearance of typical symptoms and signs within 10 min to, occasionally, several hours after inhalational anesthesia is begun. Early diagnosis can be facilitated by prompt recognition of jaw rigidity, tachypnea, tachycardia, and increased end-tidal CO_2.

There are no immediately confirmatory tests, but patients should have testing for complications, including ECG, blood tests (CBC with platelets, electrolytes, BUN, creatinine, CK, Ca, PT, PTT, fibrinogen, D-dimer), and urine testing for myoglobinuria.

Other diagnoses must be excluded. Perioperative sepsis may cause hyperthermia but rarely as soon after anesthetic induction. Inadequate anesthesia can cause increased muscle tone and tachycardia but not elevated temperature. Thyroid storm and pheochromocytoma rarely manifest immediately after anesthetic induction.

Susceptibility testing: Testing for susceptibility to malignant hyperthermia is recommended for people at risk based on a family history of the disorder or a personal history of a severe or incompletely characterized previous adverse reaction to general anesthesia. The caffeine halothane contracture test (CHCT) is the most accurate. It measures the response of a muscle tissue sample to caffeine and halothane. This test can be done only at certain referral centers and requires excision of about 2 g of muscle tissue. Because multiple mutations may be involved, genetic testing has limited sensitivity (about 30%) but is quite specific; patients in whom a mutation is identified do not require the CHCT.

Treatment

- Rapid cooling and supportive measures
- Dantrolene

It is critical to cool patients as quickly and effectively as possible (see p. 3016) to prevent damage to the CNS and also to give patients supportive treatment to correct metabolic abnormalities. Outcome is best when treatment begins before muscular rigidity becomes generalized and before development of rhabdomyolysis, severe hyperthermia, and DIC. Dantrolene 2.5 mg/kg IV q 5 min as needed, up to a total dose of 10 mg/kg should be given in addition to the usual physical cooling measures. The dose of dantrolene is titrated based on heart rate and end-tidal CO_2. In some patients, tracheal intubation (see p. 554), paralysis, and induced coma are required to control symptoms and provide support. Benzodiazepines given IV, often in high doses, can be used to control agitation. Malignant hyperthermia has a high mortality and may not respond to even early and aggressive therapy.

Prevention

Local or regional anesthesia is preferred to general anesthesia when possible. Potent inhalational anesthetics and depolarizing muscular relaxants should be avoided in patients who are susceptible and those with a strong family history. Nondepolarizing muscular blockers are the preferred preanesthetic drugs. Preferred anesthetics include barbiturates (eg, thiopental), etomidate, and propofol. Dantrolene should be available at the bedside.

KEY POINTS

- Malignant hyperthermia develops in genetically susceptible patients who have been exposed (usually more than once) simultaneously to a depolarizing muscle relaxant (most often succinylcholine) and a potent, volatile inhalational general anesthetic (most often halothane).
- Complications can include hyperkalemia, respiratory and metabolic acidosis, hypocalcemia, rhabdomyolysis, and DIC.
- Suspect the diagnosis if patients develop jaw rigidity, tachypnea, tachycardia, or increased end-tidal CO_2 within minutes or sometimes hours after inhalational anesthesia is begun.
- Test people at risk by the caffeine halothane contracture test or genetic testing if those tests are available.
- Treat with aggressive, early cooling and IV dantrolene.

NEUROLEPTIC MALIGNANT SYNDROME

Neuroleptic malignant syndrome is characterized by altered mental status, muscle rigidity, hyperthermia, and autonomic hyperactivity that occur when certain neuroleptic drugs are used. Clinically, neuroleptic malignant syndrome resembles malignant hyperthermia. Diagnosis is clinical. Treatment is aggressive supportive care.

Among patients taking neuroleptic drugs, about 0.02 to 3% develop neuroleptic malignant syndrome. Patients of all ages can be affected.

Etiology

Many antipsychotics and antiemetics can be causative (see Table 361–4). The factor common to all drug causes is a decrease in dopaminergic transmission; however, the reaction is not allergic but rather idiosyncratic. Etiology and mechanism are unknown. Risk factors appear to include high drug doses, rapid dose increases, parenteral administration, and switching from one potentially causative drug to another.

Neuroleptic malignant syndrome can also occur in patients withdrawing from levodopa or dopamine agonists.

Symptoms and Signs

Symptoms begin most often during the first 2 wk of treatment but may occur earlier or after many years.

The 4 characteristic symptoms usually develop over a few days and often in the following order:

- Altered mental status: Usually the earliest manifestation is a change in mental status, often an agitated delirium, and may progress to lethargy or unresponsiveness (reflecting encephalopathy).
- Motor abnormalities: Patients may have generalized, severe muscle rigidity (sometimes with simultaneous tremor, leading to cogwheel rigidity), or, less often, dystonias, chorea, or other abnormalities. Reflex responses tend to be decreased.
- Hyperthermia: Temperature is usually > 38° C and often > 40° C.
- Autonomic hyperactivity: Autonomic activity is increased, tending to cause tachycardia, arrhythmias, tachypnea, and labile hypertension.

Table 361–4. DRUGS THAT CAN CAUSE NEUROLEPTIC MALIGNANT SYNDROME

CLASS	DRUGS
Antipsychotics, traditional	Chlorpromazine Fluphenazine Haloperidol Loxapine Mesoridazine Molindone Perphenazine Pimozide Thioridazine Thiothixene Trifluoperazine
Antipsychotics, newer	Aripiprazole Clozapine Olanzapine Paliperidone Quetiapine Risperidone Ziprasidone
Antiemetics	Domperidone Droperidol Metoclopramide Prochlorperazine Promethazine

Diagnosis

- Clinical evaluation
- Exclusion of other disorders and complications

The diagnosis should be suspected based on clinical findings. Early manifestations can be missed because mental status changes may be overlooked or dismissed in patients with psychosis.

Other disorders can cause similar findings. For example:

- Serotonin syndrome tends to cause rigidity, hyperthermia, and autonomic hyperactivity, but it is usually caused by SSRIs or other serotonergic drugs, and patients typically have hyperreflexia. Also, temperature elevations and muscle rigidity are usually less severe than in neuroleptic malignant syndrome, onset may be rapid (eg, < 24 h), and nausea and diarrhea may precede serotonin syndrome.
- Malignant hyperthermia (see p. 3017) and withdrawal of intrathecal baclofen can cause findings similar to those of neuroleptic malignant syndrome, but they are usually easily differentiated by history.
- Systemic infections, including sepsis (see p. 569), pneumonia, and CNS infection, can cause altered mental status, hyperthermia, and tachypnea and tachycardia, but generalized motor abnormalities are not expected. Also, in neuroleptic malignant syndrome, unlike most infections, altered mental status and motor abnormalities tend to precede hyperthermia.

There are no confirmatory tests, but patients should have testing for complications, including serum electrolytes, BUN, creatinine, glucose, Ca, Mg, and CK, urine myoglobin, and usually neuroimaging and CSF analysis. EEG may be done to exclude nonconvulsive status epilepticus.

Treatment

- Rapid cooling, control of agitation, and other aggressive supportive measures

The causative drug is stopped and complications are treated supportively, usually in an ICU. Severe hyperthermia is treated very aggressively, mainly with physical cooling (see p. 3016). Some patients may require tracheal intubation (see p. 554) and induced coma. Benzodiazepines, given IV in high doses, can be used to control agitation. Adjunctive drug therapy can be used, although efficacy has not been shown in clinical trials. Dantrolene 0.25 to 2 mg/kg IV q 6 to 12 h to a maximum of 10 mg/kg/24 h can be given for hyperthermia. Bromocriptine 2.5 mg q 6 to 8 h or, alternatively, amantadine 100 to 200 mg q 12 h can be given po or via NGT to help restore some dopaminergic activity. This condition may not respond to even rapid and aggressive therapy, and mortality in treated cases is about 10 to 20%.

KEY POINTS

- Neuroleptic malignant syndrome develops infrequently in patients taking neuroleptic or other drugs that decrease dopaminergic transmission.
- Suspect the disorder if patients develop altered mental status, muscle rigidity or involuntary movements, hyperthermia, and autonomic hyperactivity.
- Serotonin syndrome can often be differentiated from neuroleptic malignant syndrome by use of an SSRI or other serotonergic drug (and often developing within 24 h of administration of its drug trigger) and hyperreflexia.
- Stop the causative drug, initiate rapid cooling, and begin aggressive supportive care, usually in an ICU.

SEROTONIN SYNDROME

Serotonin syndrome is a potentially life-threatening condition resulting from increased CNS serotonergic activity that is usually drug related. Symptoms may include mental status changes, hyperthermia, and autonomic and neuromuscular hyperactivity. Diagnosis is clinical. Treatment is supportive.

Serotonin syndrome can occur with therapeutic drug use, self-poisoning, or, most commonly, unintended drug interactions when 2 serotonergic drugs are used (see Table 361–5). It can occur in all age groups.

Complications in severe serotonin syndrome can include metabolic acidosis, rhabdomyolysis, seizures, acute kidney injury, and disseminated intravascular coagulation (DIC). Causes probably include severe hyperthermia and excessive muscle activity.

Symptoms and Signs

In most cases, serotonin syndrome manifests within 24 h, and most occur within 6 h, of a change in dose or initiation of a drug. Manifestations can range widely in severity. They can be grouped into the following categories:

- Mental status alterations: Anxiety, agitation and restlessness, easy startling, delirium
- Autonomic hyperactivity: Tachycardia, hypertension, hyperthermia, diaphoresis, shivering, vomiting, diarrhea
- Neuromuscular hyperactivity: Tremor, muscle hypertonia or rigidity, myoclonus, hyperreflexia, clonus (including ocular clonus), extensor plantar responses

Neuromuscular hyperactivity may be more pronounced in the lower than the upper extremities.

Symptoms usually resolve in 24 h, but symptoms may last longer after use of drugs that have a long half-life or active metabolites (eg, monoamine oxidase inhibitors, SSRIs).

Diagnosis

- Clinical criteria

Diagnosis is clinical. Various explicit criteria have been proposed.

The **Hunter criteria** are currently preferred because of ease of use and high accuracy (almost 85% sensitivity and > 95% specificity compared with diagnosis by a toxicologist). These criteria require that patients have taken a serotonergic drug and have one of the following:

- Muscle hypertonia
- Spontaneous clonus
- Tremor plus hyperreflexia
- Ocular or inducible clonus, plus either agitation, diaphoresis, or temperature > 38° C

Systemic infections, drug or alcohol withdrawal syndromes, and toxicity caused by sympathomimetic or anticholinergic drugs should also be considered in the differential diagnosis. Differentiation of serotonin syndrome from neuroleptic malignant syndrome (see p. 3018) may be difficult because symptoms (eg, muscle rigidity, hyperthermia, autonomic hyperactivity, altered mental status) overlap. Clues to serotonin syndrome include use of serotonergic drugs, rapid onset (eg, within 24 h), and hyperreflexia, in contrast to the often decreased reflex responses in neuroleptic malignant syndrome.

Table 361–5. DRUGS THAT CAN CAUSE SEROTONIN SYNDROME

CLASS	DRUGS	CLASS	DRUGS
Antidepressants: Monoamine oxidase inhibitors	Isocarboxazid Linezolid Phenelzine Selegiline Tranylcypromine	Hallucinogens	Lysergic acid diethylamide (LSD) 5-Methoxy-diisopropyltryptamine
Antidepressants: Serotonin-norepinephrine reuptake inhibitors	Bupropion Nefazodone Trazodone Venlafaxine	Herbs	Nutmeg Panax (Asian or American) ginseng St John's wort Syrian rue
Antidepressants: SSRIs	Citalopram Escitalopram Fluoxetine Fluvoxamine Paroxetine Sertraline	5-Hydroxytryptamine (5-HT$_1$) agonists (triptans)	Almotriptan Eletriptan Frovatriptan Naratriptan Rizatriptan Sumatriptan Zolmitriptan
Antidepressants: Tricyclic antidepressants	Amitriptyline Amoxapine Desipramine Doxepin Imipramine Maprotiline Nortriptyline Protriptyline Trimipramine	Opioids	Buprenorphine Fentanyl Hydrocodone Meperidine Oxycodone Pentazocine Pethidine Tramadol
CNS stimulants	Amphetamine Cocaine Diethylpropion Methamphetamine 3,4-Methylenedioxyamphetamine (MDA) 3,4-Methylenedioxymethamphetamine (MDMA, or Ecstasy) Methylphenidate Phentermine Sibutramine	Others	Buspirone Chlorpheniramine Dextromethorphan Granisetron 5-Hydroxytryptophan Levodopa Lithium Metoclopramide Olanzapine Ondansetron Risperidone Ritonavir Tryptophan Valproate

There are no confirmatory tests, but patients should have testing to exclude other disorders (eg, CSF analysis for possible CNS infection, urine testing for drugs of abuse). Also, some tests (eg, serum electrolytes, platelet count, renal function tests, CK, PT, testing for urine myoglobin) may be necessary to identify complications in severe serotonin syndrome.

Treatment

- Supportive measures
- Sometimes cyproheptadine

When serotonin syndrome is recognized and treated promptly, the prognosis is usually good.

All serotonergic drugs should be stopped. Mild symptoms are often relieved with sedation using a benzodiazepine, with resolution occurring in 24 to 72 hours. If symptoms resolve more rapidly, patients should be observed for at least several hours. However, most patients require hospitalization for further testing, treatment, and monitoring.

In severe cases, admission to an ICU is required. Hyperthermia is treated by cooling (see p. 3016). Neuromuscular blockade with appropriate sedation, muscle paralysis, and other supportive measures may be necessary. Drug treatment of autonomic abnormalities (eg, hypertension, tachycardia) should be with shorter-acting drugs (eg, nitroprusside, esmolol) because autonomic effects can change rapidly.

If symptoms persist despite supportive measures, the serotonin antagonist cyproheptadine can be given orally or, after crushing, via NGT (12 mg, then 2 mg q 2 h until response occurs). Chlorpromazine and olanzapine may be effective, but are not routinely used because of the potential for adverse effects. Unlike in malignant hyperthermia or neuroleptic malignant syndrome, dantrolene should not be used.

Consultation with a toxicologist is encouraged and can be accomplished by calling the United States Poison Control Network (1-800-222-1222) or accessing the WHO's list of international poison centers (http://www.who.int/gho/phe/chemical_safety/poisons_centres/en/index.html).

KEY POINTS

- Drugs that increase serotonergic activity can lead to hyperthermia and neuromuscular hyperactivity, with complications of metabolic acidosis, rhabdomyolysis, seizures, acute kidney injury, and DIC.
- The diagnosis is likely if patients have taken a serotonergic drug and have muscle hypertonia, spontaneous clonus, tremor plus hyperreflexia, or the combination of ocular or inducible clonus, plus either agitation, diaphoresis, or temperature > 38° C.
- Serotonin syndrome can often be differentiated from neuroleptic malignant syndrome by use of serotonergic drugs, rapid onset (eg, within 24 h of its drug trigger), and hyperreflexia.
- Stop all serotonergic drugs and give a benzodiazepine.
- Treat complications aggressively and consider cyproheptadine.

362 Injury During Diving or Work in Compressed Air

More than 1000 diving-related injuries occur annually in the US; > 10% are fatal. Similar injuries can befall workers in tunnels or caissons (watertight retaining structures used for construction), in which pressurized air is used to exclude water from work sites.

Many injuries are related to high pressure, which, at depth or in a caisson, results from the water weight above plus the atmospheric pressure at the surface. At a depth of 10 m (33 ft), seawater exerts a pressure equivalent to standard sea level atmospheric pressure, which is 1.03 kg/cm^2 (14.7 lb/sq in), 760 mm Hg, or 1 atmosphere absolute (atm abs); thus, the total pressure at that depth is 2 atm abs. Every additional 10 m of descent adds 1 atm.

The volume of gases in body compartments is inversely related to external pressure; an increase or a decrease in gas volume due to pressure change exerts direct physical forces that can disrupt various body tissues (barotrauma). The amount of gas dissolved in the bloodstream increases as ambient pressure increases. Increased gas content can cause injury directly (eg, nitrogen narcosis, oxygen toxicity) or indirectly during ascent when decompression of the supersaturated blood or tissues releases N_2 bubbles (decompression sickness). Arterial gas embolism can result from barotrauma or decompression.

Some medical disorders, if they cause symptoms at depth, may be disabling or disorienting and thus lead to drowning.

Other diving-related injuries are discussed elsewhere (eg, drowning—see p. 2962; hypothermia—see p. 2960; trauma—see p. 3117).

BAROTRAUMA

Barotrauma is tissue injury caused by a pressure-related change in body compartment gas volume; it affects air-containing areas, including lungs, ears, sinuses, GI tract, air spaces in tooth fillings, and space contained by the diving face mask. Manifestations depend on the affected area. Diagnosis is clinical but sometimes requires imaging tests. Treatment generally is supportive but may include O_2 and chest tube placement for pneumothorax.

Risk of barotrauma (often called squeeze by divers) is greatest from the surface to 10 m (33 ft). Risk is increased by any condition that can interfere with equilibration of pressure (eg, sinus congestion, eustachian tube blockage, structural anomaly, infection) in the air-containing spaces of the body.

Ear barotrauma constitutes about two thirds of all diving injuries.

In divers who inspire even a single breath of air or other gas at depth and do not let it escape freely during ascent, or when ascent is rapid, the expanding gas may overinflate the lungs, causing pulmonary barotrauma. Lung overinflation occurs mostly in divers breathing compressed air but can occur even in swimming pools when compressed air is inspired at the bottom of the pool (eg, when scuba gear is used there) and, rarely, from an inverted bucket.

Barotrauma can also affect the GI tract (gastrointestinal barotrauma), teeth (dental barotrauma), eyes (eye barotrauma), and face (mask barotrauma).

Symptoms

Manifestations depend on the affected area; all occur almost immediately when pressure changes. Symptoms may include ear pain, vertigo, hearing loss, sinus pain, epistaxis, and abdominal pain. Dyspnea and loss of consciousness can be life-threatening and may result from alveolar rupture and pneumothorax.

Some medical disorders, if they cause symptoms at depth, may be disabling or disorienting and thus lead to drowning. Secondary infection is sometimes a late complication.

Diagnosis

- Clinical evaluation
- Imaging tests

Diagnosis is primarily clinical; imaging tests can sometimes confirm barotrauma. Sometimes patients are evaluated for other problems or organ dysfunction.

Treatment

- Symptomatic treatment
- Other treatment dependent on specific injury

Most barotrauma injuries require only symptomatic treatment and outpatient follow-up; however, some injuries are life-threatening. Potentially life-threatening barotrauma emergencies are those involving alveolar or GI rupture, particularly in patients who present with any of the following:

- Neurologic symptoms
- Pneumothorax
- Peritoneal signs
- Abnormal vital signs

Initial stabilizing treatment includes high-flow 100% O_2 and, if respiratory failure appears imminent, endotracheal intubation. Positive pressure ventilation may cause or exacerbate pneumothorax.

Patients with suspected pneumothorax who are hemodynamically unstable or have signs of tension pneumothorax require immediate chest decompression (see p. 476) with a large-bore (eg, 14-gauge) needle placed into the 2nd intercostal space in the midclavicular line, followed by tube thoracostomy. Patients with neurologic symptoms or other evidence of arterial gas embolism are transported to a recompression chamber (see p. 3027) for treatment as soon as transportation can be arranged.

When stable, patients are treated for the specific type of barotrauma sustained.

Patients treated for severe or recurrent diving-related injuries should not return to diving until they have consulted with a diving medicine specialist.

Prevention of other diving injuries is discussed elsewhere (see p. 3028).

KEY POINTS

- Most barotrauma is ear barotrauma.
- Symptomatic treatment is sufficient for barotrauma unless patients have manifestation of potential life-threats (neurologic symptoms, pneumothorax, peritoneal signs, abnormal vital signs).
- Treat patients who have potentially life-threatening injuries with 100% O_2 and other stabilizing measures as necessary.
- When patients are stable, treat the specific type of barotrauma sustained.

EAR AND SINUS BAROTRAUMA

Barotrauma is tissue injury caused by a pressure-related change in body compartment gas volume. It can affect the ear (causing ear pain, hearing loss, and/or vestibular symptoms) or the sinuses (causing pain and congestion). Diagnosis sometimes requires audiometry and vestibular testing. Treatment, when required, may involve decongestants, analgesics, and sometimes oral corticosteroids or surgical repair of serious inner or middle ear or sinus injuries.

Diving can affect the external, middle, and inner ear. Typically, divers experience ear fullness and pain during descent; if pressure is not quickly equilibrated, middle ear hemorrhage or tympanic membrane rupture may occur. Inflow of cold water to the middle ear may result in vertigo, nausea, and disorientation while submerged. On examination of the ear canal, the tympanic membrane may show congestion, hemotympanum, perforation, or lack of mobility during air insufflation with a pneumatic otoscope; conductive hearing loss is usually present.

Inner ear barotrauma often involves rupture of the round or oval window, which causes tinnitus, sensorineural hearing loss, vertigo, nausea, and vomiting. The resulting labyrinthine fistula and perilymph leakage can permanently damage the inner ear.

Sinus barotrauma most often affects the frontal sinuses, followed by the ethmoid and maxillary sinuses. Divers experience mild pressure to severe pain, with a feeling of congestion in the involved sinus compartments during ascent or descent and sometimes epistaxis. Pain can be severe, sometimes accompanied by facial tenderness on palpation.

Rarely, the sinus may rupture and cause pneumocephalus with facial or oral pain, nausea, vertigo, or headache. Rupture of a maxillary sinus can cause retro-orbital air with diplopia due to oculomotor dysfunction. Compression of the trigeminal nerve in the maxillary sinus can cause facial paresthesias. Physical examination may detect tenderness in the sinuses or nasal hemorrhage.

Diagnosis

- Audiometry and vestibular testing

Patients with symptoms of inner ear trauma should be examined for signs of vestibular dysfunction and referred for formal audiometry and vestibular testing (see pp. 795 and 813).

Imaging (eg, plain x-rays, CT) is not necessary for diagnosis of uncomplicated sinus barotrauma, but CT is useful if sinus rupture is suspected.

Treatment

- Decongestants and analgesics
- Sometimes oral corticosteroids, surgical repair, or both

Most ear and sinus barotrauma injuries resolve spontaneously and require only symptomatic treatment and outpatient follow-up.

Drug treatment for sinus and middle ear barotrauma is identical. Decongestants (usually oxymetazoline 0.05%, 2 sprays each nostril bid for 3 to 5 days or pseudoephedrine 60 to 120 mg po bid to qid up to a maximum of 240 mg/day for 3 to 5 days) can help open occluded chambers. Severe cases can be treated with nasal corticosteroids. Doing the Valsalva maneuver immediately after nasal spray therapy may help distribute the decongestant into the occluded chamber. Pain can be controlled with NSAIDs or opioids.

If bleeding or evidence of effusion is present, antibiotics are given (eg, amoxicillin 500 mg po q 12 h for 10 days, trimethoprim/sulfamethoxazole 1 double-strength tablet po bid for 10 days).

For middle ear barotrauma, some physicians also advocate a short course of oral corticosteroids (eg, prednisone 60 mg po once/day for 6 days, then tapered over 7 to 10 days).

Referral to an otorhinolaryngologist is indicated for severe or persistent symptoms. Surgery (eg, tympanotomy for direct repair of a ruptured round or oval window, myringotomy to drain fluid from the middle ear, sinus decompression) may be necessary for serious inner or middle ear or sinus injuries.

Prevention

Ear barotrauma may be avoided by frequently swallowing or exhaling against pinched nostrils to open the eustachian tubes and equalize pressure between the middle ear and the environment. Pressure behind ear plugs cannot be equalized, so they should not be used for diving.

Prophylaxis with pseudoephedrine 60 to 120 mg po bid or qid up to a maximum of 240 mg/day, beginning 12 to 24 h before a dive, can reduce the incidence of ear and sinus barotrauma. Diving should not be done if congestion does not resolve or if a URI or uncontrolled allergic rhinitis is present.

KEY POINTS

- If patients have tinnitus, hearing loss, or vertigo, arrange audiometry and vestibular testing.
- Consider CT if sinus rupture is suspected.
- If symptoms are severe, prescribe an analgesic and a decongestant.
- Decrease risk of ear and sinus barotrauma by counseling against diving when the nose is congested and sometimes by prescribing prophylactic pseudoephedrine.

PULMONARY BAROTRAUMA

Barotrauma is tissue injury caused by a pressure-related change in body compartment gas volume. Factors increasing risk of pulmonary barotrauma include certain behaviors (eg, rapid ascent, breath-holding, breathing compressed air) and lung disorders (eg, COPD). Pneumothorax and pneumomediastinum are common manifestations. Patients require neurologic examination and chest imaging. Pneumothorax is treated. Prevention involves decreasing risky behaviors and counseling high-risk divers.

Overexpansion and alveolar rupture can occur when breath-holding occurs (usually while breathing compressed air) during ascent, particularly rapid ascent. The result can be pneumothorax (causing dyspnea, chest pain, and unilateral decrease in breath sounds) or pneumomediastinum (causing sensation of fullness in the chest, neck pain, pleuritic chest pain that may radiate to the shoulders, dyspnea, coughing, hoarseness, and dysphagia). Pneumomediastinum may cause crepitation in the neck, due to associated subcutaneous emphysema, and a crackling sound may rarely be heard over the heart during systole (Hamman sign). Tension pneumothorax, although rare with barotrauma, can cause hypotension, distended neck veins, hyperresonance to percussion, and, as a late finding, tracheal deviation. Alveolar rupture can allow air into the pulmonary venous circulation with subsequent arterial gas embolism (see p. 3024).

During very deep breath-hold diving, compression of the lungs during descent may rarely lead to a decrease in volume below residual volume, causing mucosal edema, vascular engorgement, and hemorrhage, which manifest clinically as dyspnea and hemoptysis on ascent.

Diagnosis

- Clinical evaluation
- Chest imaging

Patients require a neurologic examination for signs of brain dysfunction due to arterial gas embolism.

Chest x-ray is done to look for signs of pneumothorax or pneumomediastinum (radiolucent band along the cardiac border). If chest x-ray is negative but there is strong clinical suspicion, then chest CT, which may be more sensitive than plain film x-rays, may be diagnostic. Ultrasound may also be useful for rapid bedside diagnosis of pneumothorax.

Treatment

- 100% O_2
- Sometimes tube thoracostomy

Suspected tension pneumothorax is treated with needle decompression followed by tube thoracostomy (see p. 390). If a smaller (eg, 10 to 20%) pneumothorax is present and there is no sign of hemodynamic or respiratory instability, the pneumothorax may resolve when high-flow 100% O_2 is given for 24 to 48 h. If this treatment is ineffective or if a larger pneumothorax is present, tube thoracostomy (using a pigtail catheter or small chest tube) is done.

No specific treatment is required for pneumomediastinum; symptoms usually resolve spontaneously within hours to days. After a few hours of observation, most patients can be treated as outpatients; high-flow 100% O_2 is recommended to hasten resorption of extra-alveolar gas in these patients. Rarely, mediastinotomy is required to relieve tension pneumomediastinum.

Prevention

Prevention of pulmonary barotrauma is usually the top priority. Proper ascent timing and techniques are essential. Patients with pulmonary blebs, Marfan syndrome, or COPD are at very high risk of pneumothorax and should not dive or work in areas of compressed air. Patients with asthma may be at risk of pulmonary barotrauma, although many people with asthma can dive safely after they are evaluated and treated appropriately.

KEY POINTS

- Although rare, pulmonary barotrauma can result in tension pneumothorax, which must be immediately decompressed.
- Examine all patients who have pulmonary barotrauma for signs of brain dysfunction, which suggests arterial gas embolism.
- Treat all patients with suspected pulmonary barotrauma with 100% O_2 pending diagnostic testing.

GASTROINTESTINAL BAROTRAUMA

Small amounts of air swallowed when diving may expand during ascent (gastrointestinal barotrauma), usually causing self-limited symptoms.

Breathing improperly from a regulator or using ear and sinus pressure-equalization techniques may cause divers to swallow small amounts of air during a dive. This air expands during ascent, causing abdominal fullness, cramps, pain, belching, and flatulence; these symptoms are self-limited. GI rupture rarely occurs, manifesting with severe abdominal pain and tenderness with rebound and guarding.

If signs of GI rupture are present, immediate upright chest x-ray or CT is done to detect free air. Milder symptoms require no testing.

Patients with GI rupture require aggressive fluid resuscitation, broad-spectrum antibiotic therapy, and immediate surgical consultation for possible exploratory laparotomy.

DENTAL, MASK, AND EYE BAROTRAUMA

Barotrauma is tissue injury caused by a pressure-related change in body compartment gas volume. It can affect the spaces around teeth, behind a face mask, or underneath hard contact lenses.

Dental barotrauma can occur during descent or ascent, when pressure in the air spaces at the roots of infected teeth or adjacent to fillings changes rapidly and causes pain or tooth damage. The affected tooth may be tender when percussed with a tongue blade.

Mask barotrauma occurs when the pressure in the space behind the face mask is not equalized during descent. The resulting relative vacuum can lead to local pain, conjunctival hemorrhage, and ecchymosis of the skin enclosed by the mask. Retro-orbital hemorrhage is possible but rare.

If retro-orbital hemorrhage is suspected, complete eye examination (including visual acuity, extraocular movements, and intraocular pressure measurement) and head CT are done. Mask barotrauma may be avoided when pressures are equalized within the face mask by exhaling from the nose into the mask.

Eye barotrauma occurs when small air bubbles are trapped behind hard contact lenses. The air bubbles can damage the eye and cause soreness, decreased visual acuity, and halos around lights. A screening ophthalmic examination should be done to rule out other causes. Pressure behind goggles cannot be equalized, so they should not be used for diving.

Treatment

- Symptomatic

Usually symptomatic treatment suffices.

ARTERIAL GAS EMBOLISM

(Air Embolism)

Arterial gas embolism is a potentially catastrophic event that occurs when gas bubbles enter or form in the arterial vasculature and occlude blood flow, causing organ ischemia. Arterial gas embolism can cause CNS ischemia with rapid loss of consciousness, other CNS manifestations, or both; it also may affect other organs. Diagnosis is clinical and may be corroborated by imaging tests. Treatment is 100% O_2 and immediate recompression.

Gas emboli may enter the arterial circulation in any of the following ways:

- From ruptured alveoli after lung barotrauma
- From within the arterial circulation itself in severe decompression sickness
- Via migration from the venous circulation (venous gas embolism) either via a right-to-left shunt (patent foramen ovale, atrial septal defect) or by overwhelming the filtering capacity of the lungs

Even an otherwise asymptomatic venous gas embolism can cause serious manifestations (eg, stroke) in the presence of a right-to-left shunt. Venous gas embolism that does not enter the arterial circulation is less serious.

Although cerebral embolism is considered the most serious manifestation, arterial gas embolism can cause significant ischemia in other organs (eg, spinal cord, heart, skin, kidneys, spleen, GI tract).

Symptoms and Signs

Symptoms occur within a few minutes of surfacing and may include altered mental status, hemiparesis, focal motor or sensory deficits, seizures, loss of consciousness, apnea, and shock; death may follow. Signs of pulmonary barotrauma (see p. 3023) or type II decompression sickness (see p. 3026) may also be present.

Other symptoms may result from arterial gas embolism in any of the following:

- Coronary arteries (eg, arrhythmias, MI, cardiac arrest)
- Skin (eg, cyanotic marbling of the skin, focal pallor of the tongue)
- Kidneys (eg, hematuria, proteinuria, renal failure)

PEARLS & PITFALLS

- Any unconscious diver should be assumed to have arterial gas embolism and should be recompressed promptly.

Diagnosis

- Clinical evaluation
- Sometimes confirmation by imaging

Diagnosis is primarily clinical. A high level of suspicion is necessary when divers lose consciousness during or immediately after ascent. Confirming the diagnosis is difficult because air may be reabsorbed from the affected artery before testing. However, imaging techniques that may support the diagnosis (each with limited sensitivity) include the following:

- Echocardiography (showing air in the cardiac chambers)
- Ventilation-perfusion scan (showing results consistent with pulmonary emboli)
- Chest CT (showing local lung injury or hemorrhage)
- Head CT (showing intravascular gas and diffuse edema)

Sometimes decompression sickness can cause similar symptoms and signs (for a comparison of features, see Table 362–1).

Treatment

- Immediate 100% O_2
- Recompression therapy

Divers thought to have arterial gas embolism should be recompressed promptly. Transport to a recompression chamber (see p. 3027) takes precedence over nonessential procedures. Transport by air may be justified if it saves significant time, but exposure to reduced pressure at altitude must be minimized.

Before transport, high-flow 100% O_2 enhances N_2 washout by widening the N_2 pressure gradient between the lungs and the circulation, thus accelerating reabsorption of embolic bubbles. Patients should remain in a supine position to decrease the risk of brain embolism. Mechanical ventilation, vasopressors, and volume resuscitation are used as needed. Placing patients in the left lateral decubitus position (Durant's maneuver) or Trendelenburg position is no longer recommended.

KEY POINTS

- Strongly consider arterial gas embolism if patients have neurologic symptoms within minutes after surfacing or manifestations of ischemia in another organ.
- Do not exclude arterial gas embolism based on negative test results.
- Start high-flow 100% O_2 and initiate transport to a recompression chamber if gas embolism is suspected.

IMMERSION PULMONARY EDEMA

Immersion pulmonary edema is sudden-onset pulmonary edema that typically occurs early during a dive while at depth.

Immersion pulmonary edema has become more common over the past 2 decades. This disorder is similar to negative pressure pulmonary edema encountered during induction of anesthesia or after extubation, when a patient with laryngospasm attempts to take deep breaths against a closed larynx, thereby causing negative intra-alveolar pressure. Abnormal left ventricular systolic or diastolic function may contribute. Immersion pulmonary edema is not related to pulmonary barotrauma or decompression sickness. Cold water and a history of hypertension are risk factors. This syndrome occurs in competitive open water swimmers.

Table 362–1. COMPARISON OF GAS EMBOLISM AND DECOMPRESSION SICKNESS

FEATURE	GAS EMBOLISM	DECOMPRESSION SICKNESS
Symptoms and signs	**Common:** Unconsciousness, often with seizures (*any unconscious diver should be assumed to have gas embolism and should be recompressed promptly*) **Less common:** Milder cerebral manifestations, signs of pulmonary barotrauma (eg, mediastinal or subcutaneous emphysema, pneumothorax)	Extremely variable—the bends (pain, most often in or near a joint), neurologic manifestations of almost any type or degree, and the chokes (respiratory distress followed by circulatory collapse—*an extreme emergency*), occurring alone or with other symptoms
Onset	Sudden, usually during or within a few minutes after surfacing	Gradual or sudden, with symptoms developing ≥ 1 h after surfacing in about 50%; onset up to 24 h after dives* of > 10 m (> 33 ft) or hyperbaric exposures of > 2 atm abs
Proximate cause	**Usual:** Breath holding or airway obstruction during ascent (even from a few feet of depth, particularly when ascent is rapid); air trapped in the lungs expands during ascent and causes lung tissue injury **Occasional:** Severe decompression sickness	**Usual:** Diving or hyperbaric exposure beyond no-stop limits and without appropriate decompression stops **Occasional:** Diving or hyperbaric exposure within no-stop limits or with appropriate decompression stops; low-pressure exposure (eg, flying after diving)
Mechanism	**Usual:** Overinflation of lungs causing entry of free gas into pulmonary vessels followed by embolization of cerebral vessels **Occasional:** Coronary, renal, or cutaneous circulatory obstruction by free gas from any source	Formation of bubbles from excess dissolved gas in blood or tissue when external pressure decreases
Emergency treatment	Essential emergency care as needed (eg, airway patency, hemostasis, CPR or mechanical ventilation) Prompt transport to nearest recompression chamber Horizontal position 100% O_2 by close-fitting mask Fluids orally if patient is conscious; otherwise, IV	Essential emergency care as needed (eg, airway patency, CPR or mechanical ventilation) Prompt transport to nearest recompression chamber 100% O_2 by close-fitting mask Fluids orally if patient is conscious; otherwise, IV

*Repeat dives are frequently involved.
atm abs = atmospheres absolute.

Severe dyspnea develops. Divers usually ascend rapidly and have cough, frothy sputum, scattered crackles throughout both lung fields, and sometimes cyanosis. Hypoxia is present.

Chest x-ray shows typical pulmonary edema. Cardiac evaluation usually shows normal right and left ventricular function and normal coronary arteries. Diastolic dysfunction can be documented by echocardiography.

Diuretic therapy and O_2 by positive pressure mask are usually sufficient therapy. Mechanical ventilation may be necessary. Recompression therapy is not indicated.

DECOMPRESSION SICKNESS

(Caisson Disease; The Bends)

Decompression sickness occurs when rapid pressure reduction (eg, during ascent from a dive, exit from a caisson or hyperbaric chamber, or ascent to altitude) causes gas previously dissolved in blood or tissues to form bubbles in blood vessels. Symptoms typically include pain, neurologic symptoms, or both. Severe cases can be fatal. Diagnosis is clinical. Definitive treatment is recompression therapy. Proper diving techniques are essential for prevention.

Henry's law states that the solubility of a gas in a liquid is directly proportional to the pressure exerted on the gas and liquid. Thus, the amount of inert gases (eg, N_2, helium) dissolved in the blood and tissues increases at higher pressure.

During ascent, when the surrounding pressure decreases, bubbles (mainly N_2) may form. The liberated gas bubbles can arise in any tissue and cause local symptoms, or they can travel via the blood to distant organs (arterial gas embolism). Bubbles cause symptoms by blocking vessels, rupturing or compressing tissue, or activating clotting and inflammatory cascades. Because N_2 dissolves readily in fat, tissues with a high lipid content (eg, in the CNS) are particularly susceptible.

Risk factors of decompression sickness: Decompression sickness occurs in about 2 to 4/10,000 dives among recreational divers. The incidence is higher among commercial divers, who often have minor musculoskeletal injuries. Risk factors include all of the following:

- Cold-temperature dives
- Dehydration
- Exercise after diving
- Fatigue
- Flying after diving
- Obesity
- Older age
- Prolonged or deep dives
- Rapid ascents
- Right-to-left cardiac shunts

Because excess N_2 remains dissolved in body tissues for at least 12 h after each dive, repeated dives within 1 day are more likely to cause decompression sickness. Decompression sickness can also develop if pressure decreases below atmospheric pressure (eg, by exposure to altitude).

Classification of decompression sickness: Generally, there are 2 types of decompression sickness:

- **Type I,** which involves joints, skin, and lymphatics, is milder and not typically life-threatening.
- **Type II** is serious, is sometimes life-threatening, and affects various organ systems.

The spinal cord is especially vulnerable; other vulnerable areas include the brain, respiratory system (eg, pulmonary emboli), and circulatory system (eg, heart failure, cardiogenic shock).

The bends refers to local joint or muscle pain due to decompression sickness but is often used as a synonym for any component of the disorder.

Symptoms and Signs

Severe symptoms may manifest within minutes of surfacing, but in most patients, symptoms begin gradually, sometimes with a prodrome of malaise, fatigue, anorexia, and headache. Symptoms occur within 1 h of surfacing in about 50% of patients and by 6 h in 90%. Rarely, symptoms can manifest 24 to 48 h after surfacing, particularly by exposure to altitude after diving (such as air travel).

Type I decompression sickness typically causes progressively worsening pain in the joints (typically elbows and shoulders), back, and muscles; the pain intensifies during movement and is described as "deep" and "boring." Other manifestations include lymphadenopathy, skin mottling, itching, and rash.

Type II decompression sickness tends to cause neurologic and sometimes respiratory symptoms. It typically manifests with paresis, numbness and tingling, difficulty urinating, and loss of bowel or bladder control. Headache and fatigue may be present but are nonspecific. Dizziness, tinnitus, and hearing loss may result if the inner ear is affected. Severe symptoms include seizures, slurred speech, vision loss, confusion, and coma. Death can occur.

The chokes (respiratory decompression sickness) is a rare but grave manifestation; symptoms include shortness of breath, chest pain, and cough. Massive bubble embolization of the pulmonary vascular tree can result in rapid circulatory collapse and death.

Dysbaric osteonecrosis is a late manifestation of decompression sickness. It is an insidious form of osteonecrosis caused by prolonged or closely repeated exposures to increased pressure (typically in people working in compressed air and in deep commercial rather than recreational divers). Deterioration of shoulder and hip articular surfaces can cause chronic pain and severe disability.

Diagnosis

- Clinical evaluation

Diagnosis is clinical. CT and MRI may be helpful to rule out other disorders that cause similar symptoms (eg, herniated intervertebral disk, ischemic stroke, CNS hemorrhage). Although these studies may show brain or spinal cord abnormalities, they are not sensitive for decompression sickness, and treatment should usually begin based on clinical suspicion.

Arterial gas embolism can have similar manifestations (for a comparison of features, see Table 362–1).

For dysbaric osteonecrosis, skeletal x-rays may show joint degeneration, which cannot be distinguished from that caused by other joint disorders; MRI is usually diagnostic.

PEARLS & PITFALLS

- If decompression sickness is suspected, begin recompression immediately, without delays for diagnostic studies.

Treatment

- 100% O_2
- Recompression therapy

About 80% of patients recover completely.

Initially, high-flow 100% O_2 enhances N_2 washout by widening the N_2 pressure gradient between the lungs and the circulation, thus accelerating reabsorption of embolic bubbles.

Recompression therapy is indicated for all patients except perhaps those whose symptoms are limited to itching, skin mottling, and fatigue; they should be observed for deterioration. Other patients are transported to a suitable recompression facility. Because time to treatment and severity of the injury are important determinants of outcome, transport should not be delayed for performance of nonessential procedures.

If air evacuation is required, an aircraft capable of 1 atmosphere internal pressure is preferred. In unpressurized aircraft, low altitude (< 609 m [< 2000 ft]) must be maintained. Commercial aircraft, although pressurized, typically have a cabin pressure equivalent to 2438 m (8000 ft) at normal cruise altitude, which may exacerbate symptoms. Flying in commercial aircraft shortly after a dive can precipitate symptoms.

Prevention

Significant bubble formation can usually be avoided by limiting the depth and duration of dives to a range that does not need decompression stops during ascent (called no-stop limits) or by ascending with decompression stops as specified in published guidelines (eg, the decompression table in the chapter *Diagnosis and Treatment of Decompression Sickness* in the US Navy Diving Manual). Many divers wear a portable dive computer that continually tracks depth and time at depth and calculates a decompression schedule.

In addition to following published and computer-generated guidelines, many divers make a safety stop for a few minutes at about 4.6 m (15 ft) below the surface. However, a few cases develop after appropriately identified no-stop dives, and the incidence of decompression sickness has not decreased despite widespread use of dive computers. The reason may be that published tables and computer programs do not completely account for the variation in risk factors among divers or that people do not follow the recommendations precisely.

Dives < 24 h apart (repetitive dives) require special techniques to determine proper decompression procedures.

KEY POINTS

- Symptoms of decompression sickness develop within 1 h of surfacing in 50% of affected patients and within 6 h in 90%.
- Severe decompression sickness with brain dysfunction within minutes of surfacing may be difficult to differentiate from arterial gas embolism.
- If the disorder is suspected, start high-flow 100% O_2 and arrange the most expeditious transport to a recompression facility possible, using ground transportation or an aircraft capable of 1 atmosphere of internal pressure.
- Counsel divers to follow established recommendations (eg, diving depth and duration, use of decompression stops during ascent) that decrease the risk of decompression sickness.

GAS TOXICITY DURING DIVING

Various physiologic (eg, O_2, N_2, CO_2) and nonphysiologic (eg, carbon monoxide) gases can cause symptoms during diving.

Oxygen toxicity: O_2 toxicity typically occurs when the partial pressure of O_2 exceeds 1.4 atmospheres (atm), equivalent to about 57 m (187 ft) depth when air is breathed. Symptoms include paresthesias, focal seizures, vertigo, nausea, vomiting, and constricted (tunnel) vision. About 10% of patients have generalized seizures or syncope, which typically results in drowning. Risk is increased when divers breathe mixtures of O_2 and N_2 (nitrox) that have an increased percentage of O_2.

Nitrogen narcosis: When compressed air is breathed at depths of > 30 m (> 100 ft), the elevated partial pressure of N_2 can exert an anesthetic-like effect similar to that of nitrous oxide. Nitrogen narcosis (rapture of the deep) causes symptoms and signs similar to those of alcohol intoxication (eg, impaired intellectual and neuromuscular performance, changes in behavior and personality). Impairment of judgment can lead to drowning. Hallucinations and loss of consciousness can occur at depths of > 91 m (> 300 ft).

Because divers recover rapidly during ascent, diagnosis is often based on history. Treatment entails immediate but controlled ascent. Nitrogen narcosis can be prevented by using helium to dilute O_2 for deep diving because helium lacks the narcotic properties of N_2. However, using pure helium/O_2 mixtures in very deep dives (> 180 m [> 600 ft]) increases the risk of developing high-pressure neurologic syndrome.

Carbon dioxide poisoning: CO_2 poisoning may be caused by any of the following:

- Inadequate respiratory effort (hypoventilation)
- A tight wetsuit
- Overexertion
- Regulator malfunction
- Deep diving
- Air supply contamination by exhaled gases (as occurs with a CO_2 scrubber failure in a rebreather air supply)

Hypoventilation can increase blood CO_2 levels and cause shortness of breath and sedation. Severe CO_2 poisoning can cause nausea, vomiting, dizziness, headache, rapid breathing, flushing, confusion, seizures, and loss of consciousness.

Mild CO_2 poisoning is suspected if divers frequently have dive-related headaches or low air-use rates.

CO_2 intoxication usually resolves during ascent; thus, ABG testing after a dive typically does not detect any increase in CO_2 levels. Treatment is gradual ascent and termination of the diving exercise or correction of the precipitating cause.

Carbon monoxide poisoning: Carbon monoxide can enter a diver's air supply if the air compressor intake valve is placed too close to engine exhaust or if the lubricating oil in a malfunctioning compressor becomes hot enough to partially combust (flashing), producing carbon monoxide.

Symptoms include nausea, headache, weakness, clumsiness, and mental changes. Severe carbon monoxide poisoning can cause seizures, syncope, or coma (see also p. 3060).

Diagnosis is by detecting an elevated carboxyhemoglobin (COHb) level in blood; pulse oximetry readings are nondiagnostic and usually normal because pulse oximeters cannot distinguish between oxyhemoglobin and COHb. The diver's air supply can be tested for carbon monoxide.

Treatment is with high-flow 100% O_2, best given via a nonrebreather mask, which decreases the half-life of COHb from 4 to 8 h in room air to 40 to 80 min. For severe cases, hyperbaric oxygen therapy may be considered if readily available. COHb levels will drop quickly in the hyperbaric chamber (half-life 15 to 30 min); however, the benefit of hyperbaric O_2 therapy is controversial. Some studies indicate that hyperbaric O_2 therapy lessens neurologic sequelae, but others do not support this finding.

High-pressure neurologic syndrome: A poorly understood syndrome of neuromuscular and cerebral abnormalities can develop at ≥ 180 m (≥ 600 ft), particularly when divers are compressed rapidly while breathing helium/O_2 mixtures. Symptoms include nausea, vomiting, fine tremors, incoordination, dizziness, fatigue, somnolence, myoclonic jerking, stomach cramps, and decrements in intellectual and psychomotor performance.

Diagnosis is clinical. Prevention is usually accomplished by slowing the rate of compression.

RECOMPRESSION THERAPY

(Hyperbaric O_2 Therapy)

Recompression therapy is administration of 100% O_2 for several hours in a sealed chamber pressurized to > 1 atmosphere, gradually lowered to atmospheric pressure. In divers, this therapy is used primarily for decompression sickness and arterial gas embolism. A shorter time to start of therapy is associated with a better patient outcome, but therapy should be started anytime within 48 hours of surfacing. Despite therapy, severe injury predicts a poor outcome. Untreated pneumothorax requires chest tube placement before or at the start of recompression therapy.

The goals of recompression therapy in diving injuries include all of the following:

- Increasing O_2 solubility and delivery
- Increasing N_2 washout
- Decreasing CO concentration
- Decreasing gas bubble size
- Reducing tissue ischemia

For carbon monoxide poisoning, mechanisms include decreasing the half-life of carboxyhemoglobin, reducing ischemia, and possibly improving mitochondrial function.

Hyperbaric O_2 therapy is also used for several disorders unrelated to diving (see Table 362–2).

Because recompression is relatively well tolerated, it should be started if there is any likelihood that it would promote recovery; recompression may help even if started up to 48 h after surfacing. However, success is usually low if started > 48 h after symptom onset, except for exposure to altitude (eg, flying) after diving, in which case therapy could be successful even a few days after altitude exposure.

Recompression chambers are either multiplace, with space for one or more patients on a gurney and for a medical attendant, or monoplace, with space for only one patient. Although monoplace chambers are less expensive, because patients cannot be accessed during recompression, their use for critically ill patients, who may require intervention, can be risky.

Information regarding the location of the nearest recompression chamber, the most rapid means of reaching it, and the most appropriate source to consult by telephone should be known by most divers, medical staff members, and rescue and police personnel in popular diving areas.

Table 362–2. HYPERBARIC O_2 THERAPY*

SUPPORTING EVIDENCE	DISORDERS
Good	Arterial gas embolism Clostridial infection Decompression sickness Osteoradionecrosis Poorly healing skin grafts
Some	Anemia (severe) with hemorrhagic shock Burns Carbon monoxide poisoning (severe) Intracranial abscess with actinomycosis Necrotizing fasciitis Radiation soft-tissue injury Refractory osteomyelitis Traumatic crush injury and compartment syndrome Wound healing in ischemic limbs Acute retinal artery or vein occlusion

*Hyperbaric O_2 therapy (HBO) is the mainstay of treatment for diving-related decompression injury and arterial gas embolism. It is also tried for other disorders, but its efficacy is more strongly established for some conditions than others. Relative contraindications include chronic lung disorders, sinus problems, seizure disorders, and claustrophobia. Pregnancy is not a contraindication. In the US, HBO chambers can be located by contacting the Divers Alert Network at 919-684-9111 for emergencies and 919-684-2948 for other information; see also www.diversalertnetwork.org.

Recompression protocols: Pressure and duration of treatment are usually decided by a hyperbaric medicine specialist at the recompression facility. Treatments are given once or twice/day for 45 to 300 min until symptoms abate; 5- to 10-min air breaks are added to reduce risk of O_2 toxicity. Chamber pressure is usually maintained between 2.5 and 3.0 atmospheres (atm), but patients with life-threatening neurologic symptoms due to gas embolism may begin with an excursion to 6 atm to rapidly compress cerebral gas bubbles.

Although recompression therapy is usually done with 100% O_2 or compressed air, special gas mixtures (eg, helium/O_2 or N_2/O_2 in nonatmospheric proportions) may be indicated if the diver used an unusual gas mixture or if depth or duration of the dive was extraordinary. Specific protocol tables for treatment are included in the US Navy Diving Manual.

Patients with residual neurologic deficits should be given repetitive, intermittent hyperbaric treatments and may require several days to reach maximum improvement.

Complications of recompression therapy: Recompression therapy can cause problems similar to those that occur with barotrauma, including ear and sinus barotrauma. O_2 toxicity can cause reversible myopia. Rarely, pulmonary barotrauma, pulmonary O_2 toxicity, hypoglycemia, or seizures result. Sedatives and opioids may obscure symptoms and cause respiratory insufficiency; they should be avoided or used only in the lowest effective doses.

Contraindications to recompression therapy: Patients with pneumothorax require tube thoracostomy before recompression therapy.

Relative contraindications include

- Obstructive lung disorders
- Upper respiratory or sinus infections
- Severe heart failure
- Recent ear surgery or injury
- Fever
- Claustrophobia
- Seizure disorder
- Chest surgery

KEY POINTS

- Arrange for indicated recompression therapy to be done as soon as possible.
- Do not exclude recompression therapy based on the amount of time elapsed since surfacing; however, except for altitude exposure after diving, success rate for recompression therapy is low when started > 48 h after symptom onset.
- If an unstable patient needs recompression therapy, use a multiplace chamber if possible.
- Patients with pneumothorax require tube thoracostomy before recompression therapy.

DIVING PRECAUTIONS AND PREVENTION OF DIVING INJURIES

Diving is a relatively safe recreational activity for healthy people who have been appropriately trained and educated. Diving safety courses offered by national diving organizations are widely available.

Safety precautions: Incidence of barotrauma can be decreased through active equalization of various air spaces, including the face mask (by blowing out air from the nose into the mask) and the middle ear (by yawning, swallowing, or performing a Valsalva maneuver). Divers should avoid holding their breath and breathe normally during ascent, which should be no faster than 0.15 to 0.3 m/sec (0.5 to 1 ft/sec), a rate that allows for gradual offloading of N_2 and emptying of air-filled spaces (eg, lungs, sinuses). Divers should ascend with decompression stops as specified in published guidelines (eg, the decompression table in *Diagnosis and Treatment of Decompression Sickness and Arterial Gas Embolism*, a chapter in the US Navy Diving Manual at www.navsea.navy.mil). Current recommendations also include a 3- to 5-min safety stop at 4.6 m (15 ft) for further equilibration. Also, divers should not fly for 15 to 18 h after diving.

Divers should be aware of and avoid certain diving conditions, eg,

- Poor visibility
- Currents requiring excessive effort
- Cold temperatures
- Diving alone
- Recreational or sedative drugs and alcohol

Cold temperatures are a particular hazard because hypothermia can develop rapidly and affect judgment and dexterity or induce fatal cardiac arrhythmias in susceptible people. Diving alone is not recommended.

Recreational or sedative drugs and alcohol in any amount may have unpredictable or unanticipated effects at depth and should be strictly avoided. Otherwise, prescription drugs rarely interfere with recreational diving, but if the disorder being treated is a contraindication to diving, the dive should not be pursued.

Contraindications to diving: Because diving can involve heavy exertion, divers should not have a functionally significant cardiovascular or pulmonary disorder and should have above-average aerobic capacity. Disorders that can impair consciousness, alertness, or judgment generally prohibit diving. If there is any doubt as to whether diving is contraindicated by a specific disorder, a recognized expert should be consulted. For specific diving contraindications, see Table 362–3.

Table 362–3. SPECIFIC MEDICAL CONTRAINDICATIONS TO DIVING

CONTRAINDICATION	SPECIFIC EXAMPLES OR ADVERSE EFFECTS
Lung disorders	Active asthma Bronchiectasis COPD Cystic fibrosis History of spontaneous pneumothorax Interstitial lung disease Lung cysts Marfan syndrome
Cardiovascular disorders	Heart failure History of significant ventricular arrhythmias Hemodynamically significant intracardiac shunt Significant coronary artery disease
Psychologic disorders	Panic or phobia
Structural disorder	Unrepaired inguinal hernia
Neurologic disorders	Seizure disorder Syncope
Metabolic disorders	Extreme obesity Type 1 or type 2 diabetes mellitus treated with insulin (a relative contraindication)
Ear, nose, and throat disorders	Allergic rhinitis Perforated tympanic membrane Upper respiratory infection
Pregnancy	Possible risk of birth defects and fetal injury due to decompression sickness
Habitual air-swallowing	GI overinflation during ascent due to swallowing pressurized air at depth
Poor exercise tolerance	Inadequate physiologic response to adverse diving conditions
Severe gastroesophageal reflux	Aggravated by loss of gravity effect on the abdomen during submersion
Children < 10 yr	Incomplete understanding of the physics and physiology needed for safe diving

363 Lacerations

Care of lacerations

- Enables prompt healing
- Minimizes risk of infection
- Optimizes cosmetic results

Physiology

Healing begins immediately after injury with coagulation and introduction of WBCs; neutrophils and macrophages remove debris (including devitalized tissue) and bacteria. Macrophages also encourage fibroblast replication and neovascularization. Fibroblasts deposit collagen, typically beginning within 48 h and reaching a maximum in about 7 days. Collagen deposition is essentially complete in 1 mo, but collagen fiber strength builds more slowly as fibers undergo crosslinking. Wound tensile strength is only about 20% of ultimate by 3 wk, 60% by 4 mo, and maximum at 1 yr; strength never becomes equivalent to the undamaged state.

Epithelial cells from the wound edge migrate across the wound shortly after injury. In a surgically repaired wound (healing by primary intention), they form an effective protective barrier to water and bacteria in 12 to 24 h and resemble normal epidermis within 5 days. In a wound that is not repaired (ie, heals by secondary intention), epithelialization is prolonged proportionally to the defect size.

There are static forces on the skin because of its natural elasticity and the underlying muscles (see Fig. 363–1). Because scar tissue is not as strong as adjacent undamaged skin, these forces tend to widen scars, sometimes resulting in a cosmetically unacceptable appearance after apparently adequate wound closure. Scar widening is particularly likely when the forces are perpendicular to the wound edge. This tendency (and resultant wound stress) is readily observed in the fresh wound; gaping edges indicate perpendicular tension, and relatively well approximated edges indicate parallel forces.

Scars tend to be red and prominent for about 8 wk. As collagen remodeling occurs, the scar becomes thinner and loses its erythema. In some patients, however, the scar hypertrophies, becoming unsightly and raised. Keloids are exuberant scars that extend beyond the limits of the original wound (see p. 1003).

The most common factors that interfere with wound healing involve tissue ischemia, infection, or both (see Table 363–1); tissue ischemia predisposes to infection.

Lower extremities are usually at greatest risk of poor healing due to impaired circulation. The scalp and face are at lowest risk. Certain drugs and disorders can also interfere with wound healing.

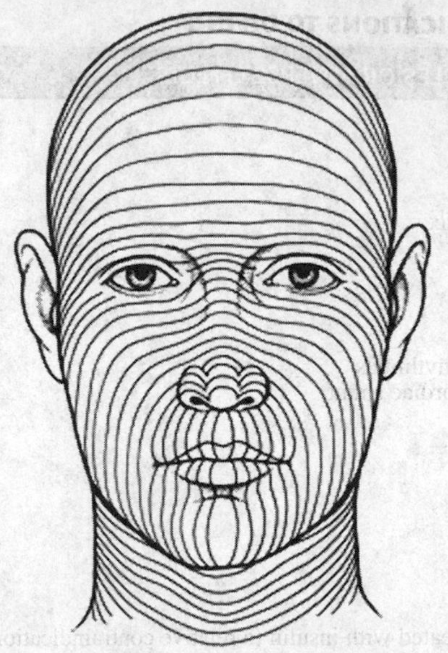

Fig. 363–1. Representative minimal skin tension lines. Direction of force is along each line. Cuts perpendicular to these lines are thus under greatest tension and most likely to widen.

Bite wounds are usually heavily contaminated.

Evaluation

Sequential steps in evaluation include the following:

- Finding and treating serious injuries
- Obtaining hemostasis
- Looking for damage to underlying structures

Clinicians must find and treat serious injuries (see p. 2927) before focusing on skin lacerations, however dramatic.

Actively bleeding wounds require hemostasis before evaluation. Hemostasis is best obtained by direct pressure and, when possible, elevation; clamping bleeding vessels with instruments is generally avoided because of the possibility of damaging adjacent nerves. Use of topical anesthetics containing epinephrine may also help reduce bleeding. Careful and temporary placement of a proximal tourniquet may enhance visualization of hand and finger wounds.

Wound evaluation also requires good lighting. Magnification (eg, with magnifying glasses) can help, particularly for examiners with imperfect near-vision. Full wound evaluation may require probing or manipulation, and thus local anesthesia, but sensory examination should precede administration of a local anesthetic.

Associated injuries: The wound is evaluated for damage to underlying structures, including nerves, tendons, vessels, joints, and bones, as well as the presence of foreign bodies or body cavity penetration (eg, peritoneum, thorax). Failure to recognize these complications is one of the most significant errors in wound management.

Nerve injury is suggested by sensory or motor abnormality distal to the wound; suspicion is increased for lacerations near the course of significant nerves. Examination should test light touch and motor function. Two-point discrimination is useful for hand and finger injuries; the clinician touches the skin with 2 ends of a bent paper clip simultaneously to determine the minimum separation that allows perception of 2 points (usually 2 to 3 mm). Normal varies among patients and by location on the hand; the identical site on the uninjured side is the best control.

Tendon injury is suspected in any laceration over the course of a tendon. Complete tendon laceration usually causes a resting deformity (eg, foot drop due to Achilles tendon laceration, loss of normal resting finger flexion due to digital flexor laceration) because forces from antagonist muscles are unopposed. Resting deformity does not occur with partial tendon laceration, which may manifest with only pain or relative weakness on strength testing or be discovered only on exploration of the wound. The injured area should be examined through the full range of motion; the injured tendon may sometimes retract and not be visible on inspection or wound exploration when the injured area is in the resting position.

Vascular injury is suggested by signs of ischemia, such as pallor, decreased pulses, or perhaps delayed capillary refill distal to the laceration (all compared with the uninjured side). Vascular injury is occasionally suspected in the absence of ischemia when a laceration traverses the territory of a major artery and is deep or complex or results from penetrating trauma. Other signs of vascular injury can include a rapidly expanding or pulsatile mass or a bruit.

Bone injury is possible, particularly after blunt trauma or when injury occurs over a bony prominence. If the mechanism or location of injury is concerning, plain x-rays are taken to rule out fracture.

Foreign bodies are sometimes present in wounds, depending on the mechanism. Wounds involving glass are likely to have foreign bodies, lacerations due to sharp metal rarely do, and wounds involving other substances are of intermediate risk. Although not very sensitive, a patient's complaint of feeling a foreign body is fairly specific and should not be ignored. Localized pain or

Table 363–1. FACTORS THAT INTERFERE WITH WOUND HEALING

FACTOR	EXAMPLES
Tissue ischemia (due to features of the wound or locally poor circulation)	Disorders affecting peripheral vasculature (eg, diabetes, arterial insufficiency) Type of injury (eg, a crush-type injury, which damages the microvasculature) Repair techniques (eg, overly tight sutures) Use of cautery
Bacterial proliferation	Wound hematoma Foreign material (including deep dermal suture material) Delayed treatment (eg, > 6 h for lower-extremity injuries; > 12 to 24 h for face and scalp injuries) Significant wound contamination (as typically occurs in bite wounds)
Drugs	Antiplatelet drugs and anticoagulants Drugs that suppress inflammation (eg, corticosteroids, immunosuppressants)
Certain disorders	Disorders that suppress the immune system or impair healing (eg, chronic kidney disease) Undernutrition (eg, protein-calorie undernutrition, deficiencies of specific nutrients such as vitamin C) Disorders of collagen synthesis (eg, Marfan syndrome, Ehlers-Danlos syndrome)

tenderness in a high-risk wound also is suggestive, particularly if pain worsens with active or passive motion. Wound examination and exploration are not sensitive for small foreign bodies unless the wound is superficial and its full depth is visible.

PEARLS & PITFALLS

- Do not ignore a patient's complaint of feeling a foreign body; although not very sensitive, this complaint is fairly specific.

Joint penetration should be suspected when wounds near a joint are deep or involve penetrating trauma.

Penetration of the abdominal or thoracic cavity should be considered in any wound over those locations in which the bottom of the laceration is not clearly visible. Wounds should not be blindly probed; blind probing is unreliable and may cause further injury. Patients with suspected thoracic lacerations require a chest x-ray initially, with a repeat film after 4 to 6 h of observation; any slowly developing pneumothorax should be visible by that time. In patients with abdominal lacerations, local anesthesia facilitates exploration (lacerations can be extended horizontally if necessary). Patients with wounds penetrating the fascia should be observed in the hospital; sometimes abdominal CT is used to identify hemoperitoneum. Bedside ultrasonography may also help identify injuries such as a pneumothorax, hemothorax, or hemoperitoneum, especially in unstable patients who cannot be transported to CT.

Imaging of lacerations: Imaging studies are recommended for all wounds involving glass and for other wounds if a foreign body is suspected because of the mechanism, the symptoms, or an inability to examine the wound's full depth. If glass or inorganic material (eg, stones, metal fragments) is involved, plain x-rays are taken; glass bits as small as 1 mm are usually visible. Organic materials (eg, wood splinters, plastic) are rarely detected with plain x-rays (although the outline of larger objects may be visible because of their displacement of normal tissue); various other modalities have been used, including ultrasonography, CT, and MRI. None of these is 100% sensitive, but CT may offer the best balance between accuracy and practicality. A high index of suspicion and careful exploration of all wounds are always appropriate.

Treatment

Treatment involves

- Cleansing and local anesthesia (sequence can vary)
- Exploration
- Debridement
- Closure

Tissue should be handled as gently as possible.

Cleansing lacerations: Both the wound and the surrounding skin are cleaned. Subepidermal tissue in the wound is relatively delicate and should not be exposed to harsh substances (eg, full-strength povidone iodine, chlorhexidine, hydrogen peroxide) and vigorous scrubbing.

Removing hair from laceration edges is not necessary for wound hygiene but can make markedly hairy areas (eg, scalp) easier to work on. If necessary, hair is removed with electric clippers or scissors, not shaving; razors create microtrauma, allowing skin pathogens to enter and increasing risk of infection. Hair is clipped before wound irrigation so that any clipped hair entering the wound is removed. Eyebrows are never trimmed because the hair-skin border is needed for proper alignment of wound edges. Furthermore, eyebrows may grow back abnormally or not at all.

Although wound cleansing is not particularly painful, local anesthesia is usually administered first, except for heavily contaminated wounds; these wounds are best initially cleansed with running tap water and mild soap before a local anesthetic is administered. Tap water is clean and free of typical wound pathogens, and, used in this manner, does not seem to increase risk of infection. Wounds are then cleansed by a high-velocity stream of liquid and sometimes scrubbed with a fine-pore sponge; brushes and rough materials are avoided. An appropriate irrigation stream can be created using a 20-, 35-, or 50-mL syringe with a 20-gauge needle or IV catheter; commercially available devices incorporating a splash guard help limit splatter. Sterile 0.9% saline is an effective irrigant; specialized surfactant irrigants are costly and of doubtful additional benefit. If bacterial contamination is of particular concern (eg, bites, old wounds, organic debris), povidone iodine solution diluted 1:10 in 0.9% saline may be beneficial and is not harmful to tissues at this concentration. The volume necessary varies. Irrigation continues until visible contamination is removed and at least 100 to 300 mL has been applied (more for large wounds).

Painting the skin with a mixture of chlorhexidine and alcohol before suturing may reduce skin flora, but the substance should not be introduced into the wound.

Local anesthesia for laceration treatment: Generally, injectable local anesthetics are used. Topical anesthetics are beneficial in certain cases, especially for wounds of the face and scalp and when topical skin adhesives are used to close wounds.

Common injectable agents are lidocaine 0.5%, 1%, and 2%, and bupivacaine 0.25% and 0.5%, both from the amide group of local anesthetics; the ester group includes procaine, tetracaine, and benzocaine. Lidocaine is most commonly used. Bupivacaine has a slightly slower onset (several minutes vs almost immediate) and a significantly longer duration (2 to 4 h vs 30 to 60 min). Duration of action of both can be prolonged by adding epinephrine 1:100,000, a vasoconstrictor. Because vasoconstriction may impair wound vascularity (and thus defenses), epinephrine is mostly used for wounds in highly vascular areas (eg, face, scalp). Although traditional teaching has been to avoid using epinephrine in distal parts (eg, nose, ears, fingers, penis) to prevent tissue ischemia, complications from use on distal parts are rare, and such use is now considered safe. Epinephrine can be particularly helpful in achieving hemostasis in wounds that are bleeding heavily.

The maximum dose of lidocaine is 3 to 5 mg/kg (1% solution = 1 g/100 mL = 10 mg/mL), and that of bupivacaine is 2.5 mg/kg. Addition of epinephrine increases the allowable dose of lidocaine to 7 mg/kg, and of bupivacaine to 3.5 mg/kg.

Adverse reactions to local anesthetics include allergic reactions (hives and, occasionally, anaphylaxis) and sympathomimetic effects from epinephrine (eg, palpitations, tachycardia). True allergic reaction is rare, particularly to amide anesthetics; many patient-reported events represent anxiety or vagal reactions. Furthermore, allergic reactions are often due to methylparaben, the preservative used in multidose vials of anesthetic. If the offending agent can be identified, a drug from another class (eg, ester instead of amide) can be used. Otherwise, a test dose of 0.1 mL preservative-free (single-dose vial) lidocaine can be given intradermally; if there is no reaction within 30 min, that anesthetic can be used.

Techniques recommended to minimize the pain of injection include the following:

- Using a small needle (a 27-gauge needle is best, and a 25-gauge is acceptable; a 30-gauge may be too flimsy)
- Giving the injection slowly
- Giving the injection into the subcutaneous plane instead of intradermally

- Buffering lidocaine with 1 mL of $NaHCO_3$ (concentration from 4.2 to 7.4%) for every 9 to 10 mL of lidocaine solution (Note: Buffering decreases the shelf life of multidose lidocaine vials, and buffering is less effective for bupivacaine.)
- Warming the anesthetic solution to body temperature

Regional nerve blocks are sometimes preferred to wound injection. Nerve blocks cause less distortion of wound edges by injected anesthetic; this decreased distortion is important when alignment of wound edges must be particularly precise (eg, infraorbital nerve block for lacerations through the vermilion border of the lip) or when wound injection would be difficult because the space for injection is small (eg, digital nerve block for finger lacerations). Also, large areas can be anesthetized without using toxic doses of anesthetic. Slight disadvantages of nerve blocks are slower onset of anesthesia and sometimes ≤ 100% effectiveness with the first injection.

Use of **topical anesthesia** makes injection unnecessary and is completely painless—factors particularly desirable in children and fearful adults. The most common solution is LET, which consists of lidocaine 2 to 4%, epinephrine 1:1000 or 1:2000, and tetracaine 0.5 to 2%. A cotton dental pledget (or cotton ball) the length of the wound soaked in several milliliters of the solution and placed within the wound for 30 min usually provides adequate anesthesia. If anesthesia is incomplete after application of a topical anesthetic, supplementary local anesthetic can be injected, usually with minimal pain.

Exploration of lacerations: The full extent of the wound is explored to look for foreign material and possible tendon injury. Foreign material may also often be discerned by palpating gently with the tip of a blunt forceps, feeling for a discrete object and listening for a click characteristic of glass or metal foreign bodies. Occasionally, contaminated puncture wounds (eg, human bite wounds near the metacarpophalangeal joint) must be extended so that they can be adequately explored and cleansed. Deep wounds near a major artery should be explored in the operating room by a surgeon.

Debridement of lacerations: Laceration debridement uses a scalpel, scissors, or both to remove dead tissue, devitalized tissue (eg, tissue with a narrow base and no viable blood supply), and sometimes firmly adherent wound contaminants (eg, grease, paint). Macerated or ragged wound edges are excised; usually 1 to 2 mm is sufficient. Otherwise, debridement is not used to convert irregular wounds into straight lines. Sharply beveled wound edges are sometimes trimmed so that they are perpendicular.

Closure of lacerations: Decision to close a wound depends on the wound's location, age, cause, and degree of contamination and on patient risk factors.

Most wounds can be closed immediately (primary closure). Primary closure is usually appropriate for uninfected and relatively uncontaminated wounds < 6 to 8 h old (< 12 to 24 h for face and scalp wounds).

Many other wounds can be closed after several days (delayed primary closure). Delayed primary closure is appropriate for wounds too old for primary closure, particularly if signs of infection have begun to appear, and for wounds of any age with significant contamination, particularly if organic debris is involved. The threshold for using delayed primary closure is lowered for patients with risk factors for poor healing.

At initial presentation, anesthesia, exploration, and debridement are done at least as thoroughly as for other wounds, but the wound is loosely packed with moist gauze. The dressing is changed at least daily and evaluated for closure after 3 to 5 days. If there are no signs of infection, the laceration is closed by standard techniques. Loosely closing such wounds initially may be ineffective and inappropriate because the wound edges nonetheless typically seal shut within 12 to 24 h.

Some wounds should not be closed. These wounds include the following:

- Small bites to hands or feet (p. 2941)
- Puncture wounds
- High-velocity missile wounds

Materials and methods for laceration repair: Traditionally, sutures have been used for laceration repair, but metal staples, adhesive strips, and liquid topical skin adhesives are now used for certain wounds, mainly linear lacerations subject to only small amounts of tension. Whatever the material used, preliminary wound care is the same; a common error is to do cursory exploration and no debridement because a noninvasive closure not requiring local anesthesia is planned.

Staples are quick and easy to apply and, because there is minimal foreign material in the skin, are less likely to cause infection than sutures. However, they are suited mainly for straight, smooth cuts with perpendicular edges in areas of low skin tension. Improper wound edge apposition (sometimes causing wound edges to overlap) is the most common error.

Topical skin adhesives usually contain octyl cyanoacrylate, butyl cyanoacrylate, or both. They harden within a minute; are strong, nontoxic, and waterproof; form a microbial barrier; and have some antibacterial properties. However, adhesive should not be allowed into the wound. Infections are very unlikely, and cosmetic results are generally good.

Adhesive is best for simple, regular lacerations; it should not be used for wounds under tension unless tension is relieved with deep dermal sutures, immobilization, or both. In wounds requiring debridement, deep dermal suturing, or exploration under local anesthesia, the advantages of decreased pain and time are minimized. However, patients do not require follow up for suture or staple removal. With long lacerations, skin edges can be held together by a 2nd person or with skin tapes while the adhesive is applied. One or 2 layers are applied as recommended by the manufacturer. The adhesive sloughs spontaneously in about a week. Excess or inadvertently applied adhesive can be removed with any petrolatum-based ointment or, in areas away from the eyes or open wounds, acetone.

Adhesive strips are probably the quickest repair method and have a very low infection rate. They are useful for wounds not subject to tension. Use on lax tissue (eg, dorsum of hand) is difficult because edges tend to invert. Adhesive strips cannot be used on hairy areas. Adhesive strips are particularly advantageous for lacerations in an extremity that is to be casted (thus blocking appropriate suture removal). Adhesive strips can also be used to reinforce wounds after suture or staple removal. Skin must be dry before application. Many clinicians apply tincture of benzoin to boost adhesion. Improper application may result in blister formation. Adhesive strips may be removed by the patient or eventually will fall off on their own.

Sutures are the best choice for

- Irregular, heavily bleeding, or complex lacerations
- Areas of loose skin
- Areas under tension
- Wounds requiring deep dermal closure

Because sutures can serve as an entry site for bacteria and there is a significant amount of foreign material under the skin, they have the highest rate of infection. Suture materials can be monofilament or braided and absorbable or nonabsorbable. Characteristics and uses vary (see Table 363–2); generally, absorbable material is used for deep dermal sutures, and nonabsorbable material is used for percutaneous ones. Outcomes using rapidly absorbing absorbable

Table 363–2. SUTURE MATERIALS

CATEGORY	MATERIAL	COMMENTS
Nonabsorbable (preferred for cutaneous repair)		
Monofilament	Nylon	Strong Stiff Moderately hard to work with
	Polypropylene	Poorest knot security Soft, more pliable Most difficult to work with
	Polybutester	Somewhat elastic, so lengthens with wound edema and contracts as edema resolves
Braided	Polyester	Low reactivity Not preferred to monofilament for cutaneous use
	Silk	Soft, easy to work with Good knot security High tissue reactivity Typically limited to use on the mouth, lips, eyelids, and intraorally, where patient comfort is significantly better (because removal of intraoral sutures can be difficult, most clinicians use absorbable sutures in that area)
Absorbable (preferred for deep dermal sutures)		
Monofilament	Poliglecaprone 25	Handles like nonabsorbable sutures Easily passes through tissues Low tissue reactivity Rapid absorption (1–2 wk)
	Polydioxanone	Very strong and long lasting (absorption, 180 days) Stiffer, more difficult to handle than other absorbable sutures Lowest tissue reactivity among absorbable sutures May extrude over time
Natural	Gut, chromic gut	From sheep intima Weak, rapidly absorbed (1 wk) Poor knot security High tissue reactivity Not preferred
Braided	Polyglycolic acid	Easy handling Good knot security Mild reactivity Most strength gone in 1 wk First absorbable suture
	Polyglactic acid	Easy handling Good knot security Mild reactivity Most strength gone in 3 wk Probably current preference

sutures are comparable to those using nonabsorbable sutures. Rapidly absorbing absorbable sutures should be considered when suture removal is undesirable, such as in children and non-adherent patients. Braided material generally has higher tissue reactivity and thus poses a slightly higher risk of infection than does monofilament but is soft and easy to handle and has good knot security. Absorbable sutures containing antiseptic agents such as triclosan are available and may help reduce infection.

Suture technique for laceration repair: General goals include the following:

- Closely approximating skin margins
- Everting wound edges
- Eliminating dead space
- Minimizing tension in the wound and of individual sutures
- Minimizing the amount of subcutaneous material

The relative importance of minimizing wound tension and minimizing the amount of material buried under the skin (eg, deep dermal sutures) vary by wound location. For example, in facial wounds, cosmetic result is very important and, because of the excellent vascular supply, infection risk is low. Thus, for gaping wounds, deep dermal sutures, which decrease wound tension and improve cosmetic result, are desired; infection risk is low even if they are used. In areas where vascular supply or cosmetic result is less important, deep dermal sutures are less desirable.

Sutures may be placed and tied individually (interrupted sutures) or be continuous (running suture). They may be completely buried under the skin (subcuticular or deep dermal sutures) or enter and exit the skin to be tied externally (percutaneous sutures).

If the wound is gaping, deep dermal suturing tends to be used initially (see Fig. 363–2); the resultant narrow epidermal gap is

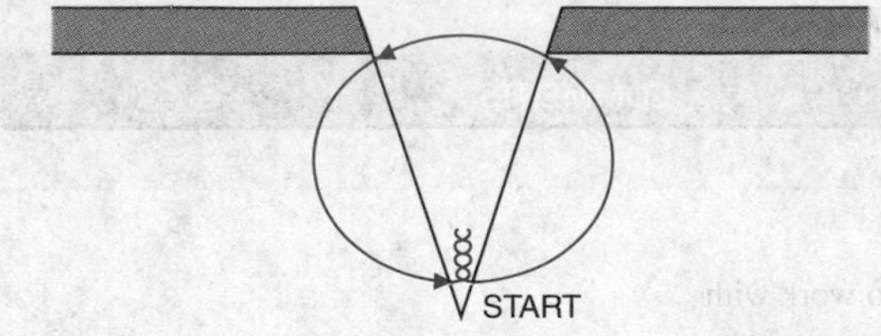

Fig. 363–2. Simple deep dermal suture. The suture begins and ends at the bottom of the wound so that the knot is deeply buried.

then closed by percutaneous sutures. For wounds on the face, any gaping > 5 to 10 mm may benefit from deep dermal suturing (not used on nose and eyelids); in other body areas, a wider gap is acceptable. Interrupted sutures using size 4-0 or 5-0 (smaller numbers indicate thicker material with greater tensile strength) absorbable material (eg, polyglactic acid, poliglecaprone 25) are most common. They are placed with the knot at the bottom of the wound to avoid a palpable lump and must not be too tight. A running subcuticular suture is sometimes used, especially for cosmetic repairs.

Epidermal closure is typically with simple, interrupted sutures (see Fig. 363–3) of nonabsorbable monofilament (eg, nylon, polypropylene). Suture size depends on where the wound is located.

- In areas over large joints and the scalp, size 3-0 or 4-0 sutures are used
- For facial wounds, size 5-0 or 6-0 sutures are used
- For wounds in the hand, size 5-0 sutures are used
- In most other areas, size 4-0 or 5-0 sutures are used

Suture size can vary slightly depending on how much static and dynamic tension is predicted (eg, for facial lacerations subject to frequent movement or high tension, size 5-0 sutures may be used).

Sutures are placed about as deep as they are wide and are spaced as far apart as the distance from the needle entry point to wound edge (see Fig. 363–4). Small bites (suture typically inserted 1 to 3 mm from the wound edge) are used for repairs in areas where cosmetic results are of particular concern and when tissues are thin. For other repairs, wider bites are used, varying with the tissue thickness. Wound edges can be everted by making the width of the bite greater at the deepest part of the wound than at the surface. Eversion is more easily obtained when the skin is entered with the needle at a 90° angle and angled slightly away from the skin edge.

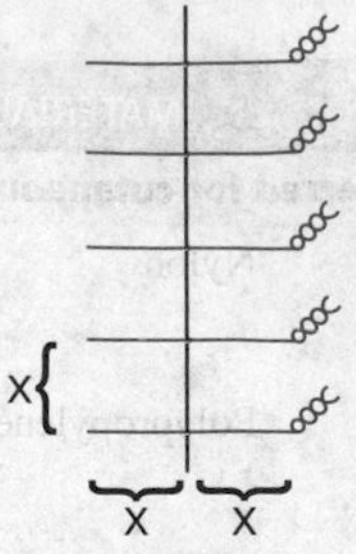

Fig. 363–4. Suture spacing. Spacing between sutures is typically equal to the distance from needle entry to wound margin. Sutures should enter and exit at an equal distance from the wound margin.

A vertical mattress suture (see Fig. 363–5) is sometimes used instead of a layered closure, provided skin tension is not marked; it also helps ensure proper edge eversion in loose tissue. A running suture (see Fig. 363–6) is quicker to place than interrupted sutures and can be used when wound edges are well aligned.

In all cases, epidermal closure must precisely realign edges horizontally using natural skin landmarks (eg, folds, creases, lip margins) when available. Vertical alignment is equally important to avoid a step-off deformity. Excess tension after closure is evidenced by indenting of the skin or a sausage link appearance. Such a repair should be redone, adding deep dermal sutures, additional percutaneous sutures, or both as needed. Adjustments to suture technique are needed to achieve optimal alignment when wound edges are beveled. For example, edges may be debrided or suture bite size may differ from one side of the wound to the other.

Aftercare: Tetanus immunization is given if necessary (see Table 181–2 on p. 1472).

Topical antibiotic ointment is applied daily; it can reduce risk of infection and help maintain a moist wound environment that optimizes healing. However, ointment is not used over tissue adhesives or adhesive strips.

Prophylactic systemic antibiotics are not indicated except for the following cases:

- Bite wounds on the extremities
- Human bites
- Wounds involving tendons, bones, or joints
- Possibly intraoral lacerations
- Some heavily contaminated wounds

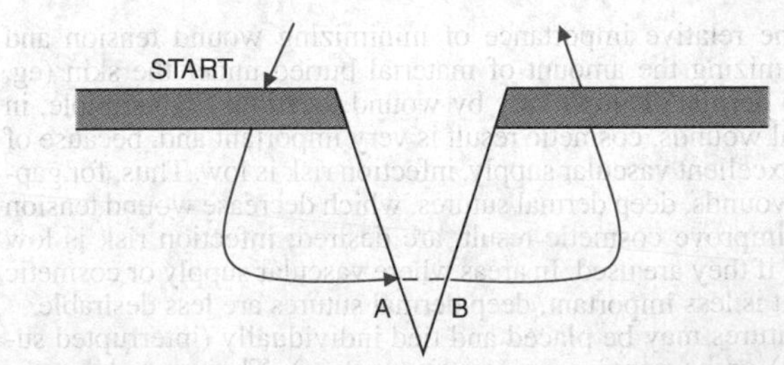

Fig. 363–3. Simple cutaneous suture. The suture begins and ends equidistant from the wound margins. Points A and B are at the same depth. The suture is farther from the wound edge at the depth of the wound. The skin edges should be everted by making the width of the bite greater at the deepest part of the wound than at the surface.

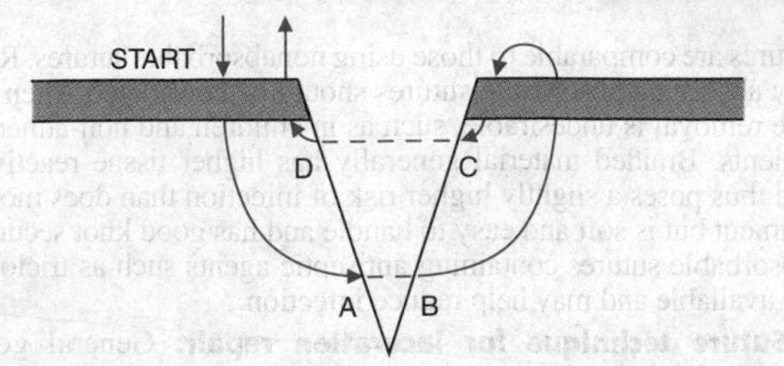

Fig. 363–5. Vertical mattress suture. The first pass of the needle is the same as a large simple suture, but instead of tying off, another smaller bite is taken back across the wound to end on the starting side. Both ends are pulled up to closely align (approximate) the wound edges. Points A and B must be at the same depth, as must points C and D; this placement results in correct vertical alignment.

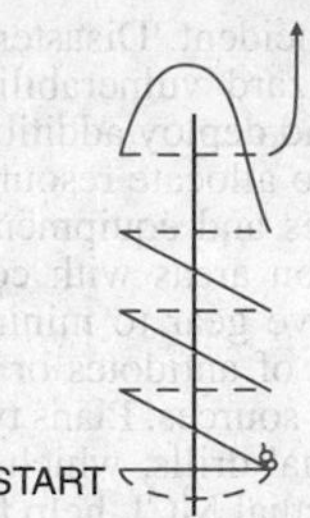

Fig. 363–6. Running suture. This suture begins with a simple suture at one end of the wound. The non-needle end is cut, and then suturing continues; the bite under the skin is perpendicular to the wound, and the crossover is at about a 65° angle. Sutures should be evenly spaced and are snugged up as they are done, except for the last one, which is left as a loop; this loop is tied to the needle end.

If deemed necessary, antibiotics are given as early as possible; the first dose may be given parenterally.

Wounds are immobilized because excess movement of the affected area may interfere with healing. Wounds near joints should be immobilized with splints. Bulky dressings are used to immobilize fingers and hands. Wounds should be elevated, above heart level when feasible, for the first 48 h after suturing. A sling may help maintain some degree of elevation of an upper extremity wound. Patients with distal lower extremity lacerations (other than minor) should probably stay off their feet for several days (eg, by using crutches); restrictions on walking probably result in better healing.

Wound care is meticulous. The wound is kept clean and dry; dressings that are nonadherent and impermeable to bacteria are usually applied. Antibiotic ointment is applied daily until the wound closure device is removed. A reliable patient may inspect minor, clean lacerations, but early physician examination is preferable for higher risk wounds and wounds in unreliable patients. After 12 h, well-healing wounds can be cleansed gently of residual secretions with water, half-strength hydrogen peroxide, or soap and water. Brief wetting in the shower is safe, but prolonged soaking should be avoided.

Wound infection occurs in 2 to 5% of lacerations; steadily increasing pain ≥ 12 h after closure is often the earliest manifestation, and initial signs are redness more than about 0.5 cm from the wound edge, swelling, tenderness, and warmth. Later signs may include fever, purulent drainage, and ascending lymphangitis. Systemic antibiotics effective against skin flora are begun; a 1st-generation cephalosporin (eg, cephalexin 500 mg po qid) or, for intraoral infection, penicillin 500 mg po qid, is typically used. Infection beginning > 5 to 7 days after injury suggests a retained foreign body.

Closure material (except for tissue adhesive) is removed after various intervals depending on location. For facial lacerations, sutures are removed in 3 to 5 days to prevent cross-hatching and visible needle entrance marks; some clinicians apply adhesive strips to bolster the wound for a few more days. Sutures and staples on the torso and upper extremities are removed in 7 to 10 days. Sutures and staples on the extensor surface of the elbow, knee, and anywhere below the knee should remain for 10 to 12 days.

ABRASIONS

Abrasions are skin scrapes that may involve epidermis or part or all of the dermis.

Abrasions are evaluated, cleansed, and debrided similarly to lacerations. They are harder to anesthetize, however, which is particularly problematic when large amounts of dirt, stones, or glass are embedded as is frequently the case, particularly with deep, scraping wounds; a regional nerve block or IV sedation may be needed.

Treatment

- Cleansing
- Antibiotics

After thoroughly removing all debris (vigorous scrubbing may be needed), antibiotic ointment (eg, bacitracin, bacitracin/neomycin/polymyxin) and a nonadherent gauze dressing that is impermeable to bacteria can be applied.

Other commercial wound dressings may be used; the goals are to keep the wound from drying out, because drying interferes with re-epithelialization, and to keep the dressing from adhering. Close observation and follow-up are necessary if defects are large, to check for purulent discharge (indicating infection) or lack of wound healing.

364 Mass Casualty Weapons

OVERVIEW OF INCIDENTS INVOLVING MASS CASUALTY WEAPONS

Mass casualty incidents (MCIs) are events that generate sufficiently high numbers of casualties to overwhelm available medical resources. They include natural disasters (eg, hurricanes) and several types of intentional and unintentional man-made events, including transportation disasters, releases of dangerous substances, explosions, and mass shootings.

Mass casualty weapons (MCWs) are weapons capable of producing MCIs. They include a variety of

- Chemicals
- Toxins
- Biological (infectious) agents
- Radiation sources
- Explosives

The weapon types are sometimes referred to as CBRNE (chemical, biological, radiological, nuclear, explosive) or NBC (nuclear, biological, chemical). The effects of an MCW agent can be local (at or near the site of exposure) or systemic (because of absorption and distribution in the circulation).

MCWs are sometimes termed weapons of mass destruction (WMD), but this term is less appropriate because it implies significant physical destruction of infrastructure, which occurs only with explosive MCWs. Also, although "weapon" signifies intentional use (eg, by warring states or terrorists), most MCWs have unintentional equivalents (eg, an industrial or transportation leak of a toxic or radioactive substance, an infectious disease outbreak, or an industrial explosion) for which the basic principles and response are the same.

Exposure: Exposure is contact with an epithelial surface, and absorption means penetration of an epithelial barrier to result in an internal dose. For radiation events, exposure also means the passage of electromagnetic radiation through the body (termed irradiation), which may occur without physical contact with the radiation source (see p. 3090). For all types of MCWs, contamination refers to agent present on an epithelial surface (external contamination) or in depots within the body (internal contamination). Internal contamination most commonly refers only to radioactive particles in the body rather than other MCW agents.

Exposure to an MCW may be readily apparent, as occurs with an explosion or visible leak or spill, and may even be announced in advance by a perpetrator. However, NBC exposure may be hidden, even if the NBC agent is dispersed as a result of an explosion. Because most NBC agents do not have a readily identifiable odor or appearance and because there is usually an appreciable time between exposure and development of symptoms or signs, an explosion may not be recognized as an NBC exposure event until some time later. Covert exposure can be particularly difficult to identify or distinguish from an outbreak of natural illness. An exception occurs with exposures to high doses of certain chemicals (eg, cyanides, nerve agents), which may cause obvious effects after only a few seconds or minutes, especially when they are inhaled.

Once disseminated into the environment, MCWs may exist as a combination of solid, liquid, gas, or vapor (the gaseous form of a substance that is liquid at room temperature). Fine dust particles or small liquid droplets may be suspended in the air as aerosols (eg, smokes, fogs, mists, fumes). The state of the agent affects its persistence in the environment and the potential routes of exposure. Persistent agents, typically solids and low-volatility liquids, remain in the environment for more than a day under usual conditions; some may persist for weeks. Nonpersistent agents, typically gases and high-volatility liquids, disperse in < 24 h. Particulate aerosols may settle to the ground in minutes to days depending upon particle size and weather conditions but then may still act as surface contaminants.

Besides dose and substance, the route of exposure is a major factor in the clinical manifestations of an MCW event. Gases, vapors, and particulates can be inhaled. Solids and liquids can contaminate the skin, from which they may be absorbed or transferred to the mouth and ingested. Contaminated objects (eg, debris from an explosion) can penetrate the skin and thus introduce NBC agents parenterally. Decontamination usually refers to external decontamination, the removal of chemicals, toxins, or infectious agents from epithelial surfaces. The removal of radioactive substances from within the body is termed internal decontamination.

Initial Approach

The approach to an MCW incident includes

- Preparedness
- Recognition
- Primary assessment and triage
- Secondary assessment
- Treatment

These steps often overlap. Recognition, assessment, and treatment may take place simultaneously depending on the nature, number, and severity of the casualties.

Preparedness: Prevention, which typically is handled by civil rather than medical agencies, eliminates the need for a medical response. But if prevention fails, preparedness efforts are crucial. Hospitals and prehospital services must have a disaster plan along with appropriate supplies and equipment to respond to an MCW incident. Disaster preparedness activities typically include a hazard vulnerability analysis (HVA) and protocols to activate and deploy additional staff to specified locations and roles and to allocate resources (eg, beds, operating rooms, blood). Supplies and equipment typically include designated decontamination areas with contained drainage, floor coverings and protective gear to minimize spread of contamination, and stockpiles of antidotes or formal arrangements to obtain them from other sources. Plans typically include requirements for regular formal drills, which although only a distant approximation of an actual MCI, help familiarize staff with the process, including the location of written procedures, supplies, and equipment (particularly those for decontamination).

Recognition: Recognizing MCIs involving explosives, firearms, and transportation crashes is straightforward. However, recognizing covert MCW events requires a high degree of clinical suspicion by first responders and physicians. Health care providers must first recognize that an event or cluster of illness may represent the of use of an MCW. They must then determine the type of MCW and class of agent.

Recognition of an MCW incident may come via intelligence or announcement by the perpetrators, environmental clues (eg, dead or dying animals, unusual odors), or environmental monitors (chemical, biological, or radiation), which may not be available at every hospital. The only clue may be observations of a large number of people presenting with unusual symptoms. However, initial reports of the identity of the agent or agents used in an MCW incident are often incomplete or in error, and a high index of clinical suspicion is invaluable. As casualties are evaluated, characteristic symptoms and signs may be recognized. Toxidromes (constellations of symptoms and signs that are typical of exposure to a class of agents) exist for several classes of chemical agents and toxins (see Table 366–2 on p. 3052) and are crucial to clinical recognition. Ultimately, laboratory analysis of clinical or environmental specimens may be required. However, diagnosis and initial treatment may need to occur without laboratory confirmation, especially for those chemical agents with short latent periods.

Primary assessment and triage: Primary assessment and triage of casualties from an MCI differs from normal trauma assessment and triage (see Table 364–1). The large number of casualties in an MCI requires initial encounters and decision making to be brief, particularly when casualties involve agents with short latent periods. Triage can be particularly challenging because many patients affected by MCWs have no visible injuries and because many people at or near an MCI who were not exposed to the agent may have stress reactions (eg, hyperventilation, shaking, nausea, weakness) that mimic effects of MCW agents. In some incidents, up to 80% of patients presenting to hospitals had only a stress reaction. Differentiating purely psychologic effects from toxic, infectious, or radiological effects may be difficult. A good first step is to separate patients who are able to walk from those unable to walk; this differentiation

Table 364–1. TRIAGE CLASSIFICATION

CLASSIFICATION	EXPLANATION
Morgue	No pulse Not breathing
Immediate	Life-threatening injury or poisoning
Delayed	Serious injury or poisoning but not life-threatening
Minimal	Minor or resolving injury or poisoning

will identify the most seriously affected. However, frequent re-triage of ambulatory patients is needed to detect those beginning to deteriorate after a latent period.

The **hot zone** is the area immediately surrounding the release of the MCW agent. Risk of contamination of medical providers is greatest in the hot zone, and normally, only emergency response personnel with appropriate personal protective equipment are allowed into this zone. Such equipment typically includes toxicologic agent protective (TAP) level A gear, which affords full encapsulation with self-contained breathing apparatus.

The **warm zone** (decontamination corridor) borders the hot zone. Comprehensive, whole-body decontamination (thorough decontamination) should occur in this zone. Medical personnel may need to don protective gear for primary assessment, triage, and initial treatment of casualties, especially patients exposed to chemicals. This gear typically is TAP B gear, which includes air-purifying respirators.

The **cold zone** (clean zone) includes hospital emergency departments. Because decontamination should have taken place in the warm zone, medical staff in the cold zone should normally be safe with standard precautions. However, hospitals still need decontamination capability because many patients who bypassed site triage and decontamination (ie, left the scene on their own and self-transported) may arrive. Inadvertent entry of contaminated patients into a hospital emergency department will change its classification to a warm or even a hot zone.

Secondary assessment: Because definitive information is often lacking early in an MCI, initial assessment of the agent involved may be wrong or incomplete. Thus, it is essential to systematically reassess individual patients and the overall situation using a fast, reproducible method. Such a method should use a logical progression that addresses each of the 3 components—agent, environment, and host (patient)—of the epidemiologic triad and that considers (or reconsiders)

- Possible agent(s)
- State(s) of the agent(s) in the environment
- Transition of the agent to the patient (routes of entry or routes of exposure and absorption)
- Clinical effects of the agent, including whether the effects are local (at or near the entry site), systemic (due to distribution in the bloodstream), or both
- Temporal progression (duration of exposure, time of exposure, latent period, current trend of symptoms, and prognosis)
- Differential diagnosis and concurrent exposures or conditions
- Possible interactions among concurrent exposures or conditions

A useful acronym to facilitate rapid secondary assessment is ASBESTOS (see Table 364–2).

Treatment

Initial management of MCW casualties aims to

- Protect health care providers
- Stop exposure to the agent (remove patient from contaminated area, remove contamination from patient)
- Stabilize patients medically

Table 364–2. ASBESTOS: SECONDARY ASSESSMENT OF MASS CASUALTIES DUE TO CHEMICAL OR RADIOLOGICAL WEAPONS

INITIAL	IN EVALUATING CHEMICAL WEAPON INJURIES	IN EVALUATING RADIOLOGICAL WEAPON INJURIES
*A*gents	Type (Is a toxidrome present?) Estimated dose	Type (α, β, γ, neutron) Estimated dose
*S*tate(s)	Is the agent a • Solid • Liquid* • Gas • Vapor* • Aerosol • Combination	The same as for chemical weapons
*B*ody site(s)	Routes of entry (exposure and absorption)	Exposure (passage through whole body)? Where? External contamination? Where? Internal contamination? Where? Combinations?
*E*ffect(s)	Distribution • Local • Systemic • Both	The same as for chemical weapons
*S*everity	Of effects Of exposure	The same as for chemical weapons
*T*ime course	Past (onset, latent period) Present (Getting better or worse? Stable?) Future (expected prognosis)	The same as for chemical weapons
*O*ther diagnoses?	Instead of (differential diagnosis) In addition to (coexisting diagnoses)	The same as for chemical weapons
*S*ynergism	Combined effects of multiple exposures	The same as for chemical weapons

*Most common states.

A useful aid to memory uses the ABCDDs: *A*irway, *B*reathing, *C*irculation, Immediate *D*econtamination, and *D*rugs. However, these steps are done as nearly simultaneously as possible rather than following a strict order. For example, bronchospasm in patients exposed to nerve agents may be so severe that patients cannot be ventilated (B) until atropine is given (D), and drugs may be ineffective as long as chemical agents remain in contact with the patient. As these steps are taken, responders to NBC emergencies, particularly chemical ones, must be careful to protect themselves from exposure (from the environment and directly from casualties) before administering care.

Airway, Breathing, and **Circulation** (ABCs) are addressed in standard fashion, as discussed elsewhere in THE MANUAL. These steps are typically done first, whether the cause is physical or NBC trauma. An exception is with certain patients with chemical exposure (eg, nerve agents) for whom immediate decontamination and administration of antidotes may be lifesaving (and prevent development of or allow effective treatment of airway or breathing problems). Medical stabilization of the ABCs sometimes needs to be done in the warm zone.

Decontamination priority varies by the type of MCW agent and the medical condition of the patient. Patients exposed to dispersed aerosols of biological or radiological agents (see p. 3096) typically have skin and/or clothing contamination. Because most such agents cannot quickly penetrate intact skin, disrobing and showering usually suffice for decontamination; such decontamination should not be unduly delayed but is not as urgent as when certain chemical agents are involved. Because certain chemical agents (eg, sulfur mustard, liquid nerve agents) begin penetrating skin upon contact and may also start damaging tissue immediately, patients exposed to such agents need immediate decontamination to stop ongoing absorption and prevent the spread of contamination to other areas on the patient and to medical personnel and facilities. Immediate decontamination is most effective with a specially formulated commercial topical skin decontamination product (Reactive Skin Decontamination Lotion, or RSDL®), which inactivates nerve agents and sulfur mustard on the skin (it should not be used in eyes or in wounds). However, soap and water are also effective. Water alone is less effective for oily chemicals but should still be used when soap is unavailable. A 0.5% solution of sodium hypochlorite (made by diluting standard 5% household bleach in a 1:9 ratio of bleach to water) is also effective but should not be used in eyes or in wounds. In an emergency, any available adsorbent (eg, paper towels, tissue, talc, clay-rich soil, bread) can be applied to the affected area for a few seconds and then removed by copious flushing. Wounds must be inspected and all debris removed; wounds must then be flushed with water or saline.

Drugs for initial stabilization should be given as needed as for any unstable patient. Most definitive drug treatment for MCW casualties can wait until admission to a hospital. The exceptions are management of shock and management of acute effects of chemical agents such as cyanides and nerve agents. Appropriate antidotes for these agents should be available for prompt administration in a prehospital setting.

CHEMICAL WARFARE AGENTS

Chemical warfare (CW) agents are chemical MCWs developed by governments for wartime use and include

- Toxic agents (intended to cause serious injury or death)
- Incapacitating agents (intended to cause only temporary, non–life-threatening effects)

Although incapacitating agents are sometimes referred to as nonlethal, in high doses, these agents can cause serious injury or death.

Toxic industrial chemicals (TICs) are chemicals produced for industrial uses that are capable of causing mass casualties. Some chemicals (eg, chlorine, phosgene, cyanide compounds) have both industrial and CW uses and are called dual-use agents.

Classification

Toxic CW agents are divided into four major classes:

- Pulmonary agents
- Systemic asphyxiants (blood agents)
- Vesicants (blistering agents)
- Nerve agents

Because **pulmonary agents** include substances that also affect primarily the upper respiratory tract rather than lung parenchyma, some experts prefer to call this class "agents with acute local effects on the respiratory tract." Because most TICs capable of generating mass casualties affect the respiratory tract, they are discussed with pulmonary CW agents.

Systemic asphyxiants, specifically cyanide compounds and hydrogen sulfide, interfere with mitochondrial energy transport, blocking cellular respiration. They are distributed in the blood (and are thus termed blood agents in military references) and thus affect most tissues.

Vesicants damage the dermoepidermal junction, causing pain and typically blistering. Many can affect the lungs if inhaled.

Nerve agents inhibit the enzyme acetylcholinesterase, causing excess cholinergic stimulation and cholinergic crisis (eg, diarrhea, urination, miosis, bronchorrhea, bronchoconstriction, emesis, lacrimation, salivation).

Incapacitating agents can be divided into

- Anticholinergic agents
- Riot-control agents (often incorrectly called tear gas) are dispersed as solid aerosols or as solutions (Note: The US military does not consider riot-control agents to be CW agents.)

In addition to their chemical designations, most CW agents also have a one- to three-letter North Atlantic Treaty Organization (NATO) code.

Incendiary agents, designed to create light and flame, may also cause thermal burns in large numbers of casualties. Hydrogen fluoride (HF) may likewise cause chemical burns. Some of these burns require specific management apart from the typical management of thermal burns.

Pulmonary CW Agents

Pulmonary agents include traditional CW "choking" agents such as chlorine, phosgene, diphosgene, and chloropicrin and some vesicants such as sulfur mustard, lewisite, and phosgene oxime (which also affect the skin) as well as military smokes, products of combustion, and many toxic industrial chemicals. Most of these compounds are gases or highly volatile liquids.

Pathophysiology

Toxic CW agents that affect the respiratory tract are divided into 2 types depending on which part of the tract is predominantly affected (see Table 364–3):

- Type 1 agents: Affect large airways
- Type 2 agents: Affect terminal and respiratory bronchioles, alveolar sacs, and alveoli
- Mixed-effect agents: Affect large airways and small airways and alveoli

Table 364–3. REPRESENTATIVE TYPE 1, TYPE 2, AND MIXED-EFFECT CHEMICALS WITH ACUTE LOCAL EFFECTS ON THE RESPIRATORY TRACT

TYPE	EXAMPLE
Type 1	Acetaldehyde Acetic acid Acrolein Ammonia Formaldehyde Hydrogen chloride Hydrogen fluoride Ozone Riot-control agents Smoke products Sulfur dioxide Sulfur mustard (H, HD)
Type 2	Carbon tetrachloride Chloropicrin (PS) Diphosgene (DP) Methyl isocyanate Oxides of nitrogen Perfluoroisobutylene (PFIB) Phosgene (CG) Phosgene oxime (CX)
Mixed effect	Chloramines Chlorine (CL) HC (hexachloroethane plus zinc oxide) smoke Lewisite (L)

Type 1 agents usually are those with inhaled particles (eg, smoke), which tend to settle out before reaching the alveoli, or highly water-soluble and/or highly reactive chemicals, which dissolve into respiratory mucosa before reaching the alveoli. Type 1 agents cause necrosis and sloughing of the respiratory epithelium in the large airways, which may cause partial or total airway obstruction. Chemical pneumonitis and secondary bacterial pneumonitis may occur as a consequence of type 1 local damage. High doses of type 2 agents also can cause type 1 (large-airway) effects, although the type 1 effects are more likely to be transient.

Type 2 agents usually are lower-solubility and/or less-reactive chemicals, which travel to the alveoli before dissolving. These agents damage pulmonary capillary endothelium, causing fluid leakage into interstitial spaces and alveoli; pulmonary edema may result. With some type 2 agents (eg, oxides of nitrogen and HC smoke [hexachloroethane plus zinc oxide]), acute pulmonary edema may be followed days to weeks later by progressive and potentially irreversible pulmonary fibrosis. The mechanism is presumed to be immunologic. High doses of type 1 agents can also cause pulmonary edema.

Mixed-effect agents act in both large airways and alveoli in low to moderate doses.

Symptoms and Signs

Initial exposure to type 1 agents causes sneezing, coughing, and laryngospasm (eye irritation can also occur). Patients with airway obstruction have hoarseness, wheezing, and inspiratory stridor. With a high dose of a type 1 agent, chest tightness or shortness of breath may subsequently develop as a result of incipient pulmonary edema.

With type 2 agents, symptoms and signs are usually delayed several hours following exposure. Patients initially complain of chest tightness or shortness of breath. Physical findings may be minimal except for rare expiratory crackles and dullness to percussion. Time of onset is shorter with higher doses; development of dyspnea within 4 h of exposure suggests a potentially lethal dose.

Diagnosis

- Clinical evaluation
- Frequent re-evaluation for deterioration
- Sometimes bronchoscopy, chest x-ray

Clinical diagnosis is used to recognize exposure and distinguish type of damage (not necessarily the type of agent, because both types can cause similar effects depending upon the dose). Patients with an initially noisy chest and prominent symptoms are presumed to have type 1 involvement (large airways). Delayed onset of shortness of breath with a relatively quiet chest suggests type 2 damage. Although a high dose of type 2 agent may initially cause coughing, sneezing, and wheezing, these signs typically decrease over time; the patient then appears well until developing progressive shortness of breath.

Chest x-ray may be normal initially. Scattered opacities due to chemical or secondary pneumonitis may develop with type 1 damage. Eventually, as pulmonary edema becomes radiographically evident, Kerley B lines and fluffy interstitial infiltrates due to type 2 damage will be visible.

Bronchoscopy can confirm type 1 damage but may miss early type 2 damage.

Laboratory testing is not helpful in initial diagnosis, but pulse oximetry and/or ABG measurements can help monitor for clinical deterioration.

Triage: Severe signs of type 1 damage (eg, severe wheezing, inspiratory stridor, soot around the nose or mouth due to smoke inhalation) should lower the threshold for early intubation. With a type 2 agent, it is important to re-triage patients frequently. Initially asymptomatic patients also require monitoring for deterioration; even mild symptoms are grounds for prompt transport to a medical facility because such patients often deteriorate further. Most patients with shortness of breath due to early pulmonary edema can be triaged as delayed for medical treatment; they can usually tolerate a short delay if more immediate casualties require treatment. However, such patients should have highest priority (urgent) for evacuation because they may require definitive, life-saving treatment in a pulmonary intensive care unit.

Treatment

- Supportive care
- For type 1: Early intubation and bronchodilators, sometimes inhaled corticosteroids, and antibiotics for documented secondary bacterial infection
- For type 2: O_2 and positive-pressure ventilation (continuous positive airway pressure in conscious patients; positive end-expiratory pressure in ventilated patients), bronchodilators, and rarely corticosteroids

It is important to treat the damage rather than the agent because some agents cause both type 1 and type 2 effects even at low doses and since at high doses both types of damage will occur. Decontamination of vapor or gas exposure is not indicated, and there are no specific antidotes for these agents.

For type 1 effects, give warm, humidified 100% O_2 by face mask. Bronchoscopy may be both diagnostic and therapeutic, via the removal of necrotic debris from the large airways. Early intubation and assisted ventilation may be needed. Bronchodilators may help by increasing the caliber of airways. Inhaled corticosteroids may decrease the inflammation that often accompanies large-airway damage. For management of smoke inhalation, see p. 2954.

For type 2 effects, patients should be admitted to an ICU. O_2 should be given via continuous positive airway pressure (CPAP) in conscious patients or via positive end-expiratory pressure (PEEP) in intubated patients. Positive-pressure ventilation may help force fluid from the alveolar spaces back into the pulmonary capillaries. A central line may help monitor pulmonary pressures so that they can be controlled without inducing hypovolemic shock. For guidelines for the hospital treatment of pulmonary edema, see p. 724. Although bronchodilators are indicated mainly to dilate large airways in cases of type 1 damage, recent evidence suggests that they act via independent pathways to alleviate type 2 damage as well. Corticosteroids do not relieve pulmonary edema but oral corticosteroids may be indicated early for patients exposed to HC smoke or to oxides of nitrogen in an effort to prevent late-onset pulmonary fibrosis.

Prophylactic antibiotics do not help either type of injury. Antibiotics should be given only after diagnosis of bacterial infection is made, including isolating an organism and determining antibiotic sensitivities.

Systemic Asphyxiants

Systemic asphyxiants include

- Cyanide compounds
- Hydrogen sulfide

Systemic asphyxiants have also been called blood agents because they are systemically distributed via the blood. However, their site of action is not the blood but rather at the cellular level throughout the body.

Although cyanide salts have been used to murder via ingestion, mass casualties would more likely result from inhalation of hydrogen cyanide or cyanogen chloride, which are highly volatile liquids or gases at ambient temperatures. Cyanides are also products of combustion of numerous household and industrial contents, and patients with smoke inhalation may also have cyanide poisoning. Cyanide has a characteristic bitter-almonds odor, but ability to detect this odor is conferred by a single gene that is absent in half the population.

Hydrogen sulfide is always a gas at ambient temperatures. Exposure is thus usually by inhalation. Hydrogen sulfide can be produced by mixing sulfur-containing household chemicals with acids; this combination has been used for suicide (termed detergent suicide), and residual gas can affect rescuers, causing multiple casualties. Hydrogen sulfide is also produced when manure decomposes. Large farm manure pits often contain lethal quantities of the gas, which may cause multiple casualties as would-be rescuers without proper protective gear succumb. Hydrogen sulfide has a characteristic rotten egg odor, but high concentrations damage olfactory fibers so that this odor will not be perceived in the most lethal environments.

Pathophysiology

Cyanides and hydrogen sulfides both enter mitochondria, where they inactivate cytochrome oxidase, an enzyme needed for oxidative phosphorylation (cellular respiration). Suppression of oxidative phosphorylation leads to cellular anoxia, with ATP depletion, inability to extract oxygen from blood delivered to tissues, and lactic acidosis resulting from the body's attempts to generate energy nonoxidatively. All organs and tissues are affected, but neurons are more sensitive than muscle; central apnea is the usual mechanism of death.

Symptoms and Signs

Cyanide initially causes gasping, tachycardia, and hypertension. Loss of consciousness and convulsions may occur in as little as 30 sec. Tetanus-like signs, including trismus (lockjaw), risus sardonicus (grimacing), and opisthotonus (neck arching), may occur. The skin may be flushed, but about half of casualties are cyanotic. Apnea usually precedes bradycardia and hypotension, and decorticate posturing may be noted prior to death.

Hydrogen sulfide in high doses also causes abrupt loss of consciousness with convulsions. Direct damage to myocardium may be prominent. Continued exposure to initially sublethal concentrations may induce eye irritation with conjunctivitis and corneal abrasions and ulcerations (gas eye), irritation of nasal and pharyngeal mucous membranes, headache, weakness, ataxia, nausea, vomiting, chest tightness, and hyperventilation. Some of these manifestations appear to be a reaction to the offensive odor of the compound. A green discoloration or darkening of coins carried by the patient should lead to a heightened suspicion of hydrogen-sulfide poisoning.

Diagnosis

- Clinical evaluation

Severely affected patients must be treated before testing is available, so diagnosis is mainly clinical. Laboratory findings include a decreased arteriovenous O_2 difference (due to higher-than-usual venous O_2 content) and high-anion-gap acidemia with increased lactate.

Triage: All unconscious patients with a pulse are potentially salvageable and should be triaged for immediate medical treatment. Because patients with inhalational exposure usually do not get worse after removal from the contaminated environment, conscious patients who are reporting decreasing symptoms may be triaged as delayed (ie, able to tolerate a short delay while immediate casualties are being treated).

Treatment

- Airway support and 100% O_2
- For cyanide, specific antidotes

Attention should be given to airway, breathing, and circulation. Water with or without soap suffices for skin decontamination; patients exposed only to vapor or gas usually do not require decontamination.

Cyanide casualties require prompt antidotal therapy with inhaled amyl nitrite 0.2 mL (1 ampule) for 30 sec of each min; 3% Na nitrite 10 mL at 2.5 to 5 mL/min IV (in children, 10 mg/kg), then 25% Na thiosulfate 25 to 50 mL at 2.5 to 5 mL/min IV. Where available, hydroxocobalamin 5 to 10 g IV may be given instead. Antidotes may be effective even in apneic patients. In the absence of antidotes, ventilation and administration of 100% O_2 may be life-saving. However, unprotected mouth-to-mouth resuscitation may expose the rescuer to cyanide in the patient's breath. Cyanide casualties resulting from smoke inhalation may also have carbon monoxide poisoning; previous concerns about administering nitrites in this situation are probably overstated. Hyperbaric O_2 has not been proven to improve outcomes in patients poisoned with cyanide.

Hydrogen-sulfide casualties are managed with supportive care, including administration of 100% O_2. Amyl nitrite and especially Na nitrite may be of use, but there is no indication for Na thiosulfate or hydroxocobalamin. Hyperbaric O_2 has not proven to be of benefit.

Vesicants

Vesicants are blistering agents and include

- Mustards, including sulfur mustard and nitrogen mustards
- Lewisite
- Phosgene oxime (technically an urticant and a corrosive agent rather than a vesicant, although it is classified as a vesicant)

These agents also affect the respiratory tract: mustards are predominantly type 1 agents, phosgene oxime is a type 2 agent, and lewisite is a mixed agent (see p. 3039).

Sulfur mustard has been variously described as smelling like mustard, garlic, horseradish, or asphalt. Lewisite may have a geranium-like odor, and phosgene oxime has been described simply as irritating. The perceptions of these odors are so subjective that they are not reliable indicators of the presence of these compounds.

Pathophysiology

Sulfur mustard and nitrogen mustard alkylate many cellular components, including DNA, and also release inflammatory cytokines. They have similar acute local effects on the skin, eyes, and airways; at lethal concentrations, they suppress bone marrow. Damage to cells in the basal layer of the epidermis results in separation of the epidermis from the dermis or, at high doses, in direct necrosis and sloughing of the epidermis. Blister fluid does not contain active sulfur mustard. Type 1 damage to the large airways involves sloughing of airway mucosa as pseudomembranes. Pulmonary edema (type 2 damage) may occur at high doses. Mustards may also induce nausea, presumably via a cholinergic mechanism. Bone marrow suppression may lead to sepsis a week or two after exposure. Long-term effects can include eye changes (eg, chronic keratitis) and cancer of the skin and respiratory tract.

Lewisite causes skin damage similar to that caused by sulfur mustard, although the mechanism of damage is different and involves effects on glutathione and sulfhydryl groups in enzymes as well as inhibition of pyruvate dehydrogenase. In the respiratory tract, the arsenic moiety of lewisite leads to leakage of pulmonary capillaries and pulmonary edema; with high doses, systemic hypotension—so-called lewisite shock—may occur. Unlike the mustards, lewisite does not cause immunosuppression.

Phosgene oxime causes urticaria and then tissue necrosis by mechanisms that are currently unclear.

Symptoms and Signs

Mustard compounds cause intense and increasing skin pain, erythema, and blister formation after a latent period. The latent period is inversely correlated with dose but is usually at least a few hours (and up to 36 h). Blisters caused by sulfur mustard sometimes resemble a string of pearls around a centrally unaffected area; blisters caused by nitrogen mustard are less likely to show this pattern. Blisters may become large and pendulous. Painful chemical conjunctivitis causing reflex lid closure occurs earlier than skin symptoms but still after a delay often of hours. The cornea may become cloudy. Respiratory manifestations include cough, laryngospasm, hoarseness, wheezing, and inspiratory stridor. Chest tightness and dyspnea may occur with severe exposure. Nausea may occur after moderate to high doses.

Lewisite causes pain within a minute or so of skin exposure. Erythema is often noticeable in 15 to 30 min, and blisters develop after several hours. The blisters usually form at the center of the erythematous area and spread peripherally. Pain is usually not so severe as that caused by mustard and begins to subside after blisters form. Irritation of mucosal membranes and large airways occurs soon after inhalation and leads to coughing, sneezing, and wheezing. Later, after a few hours, type 2 symptoms (chest tightness and shortness of breath) occur.

Skin contact with phosgene oxime causes intense, “nettling” pain and blanching within 5 to 20 sec. The affected skin then turns gray with an erythematous border. Between 5 and 30 min after exposure, edema leads to wheal formation (urticaria). During the next 7 days, the skin becomes dark brown and then black as necrosis of skin and underlying subcutis and muscle occurs. If not surgically excised, the lesion may persist for more than 6 mo. In the respiratory tract, phosgene oxime causes pulmonary edema even at low doses.

Diagnosis

- Clinical evaluation

Pain occurring at or shortly after exposure suggests that lewisite or phosgene oxime is the agent; the early onset of skin changes distinguishes phosgene oxime. Delayed onset of pain (sometimes until a day after exposure) suggests sulfur mustard. Clinical diagnosis can be confirmed by laboratory tests, but these tests are available only from specialized laboratories.

Patients exposed to mustard should have regular CBC with differential for the first 2 wk to monitor for lymphopenia and neutropenia.

Triage: All casualties with potential skin or eye exposure to vesicants should be prioritized for immediate decontamination. Skin decontamination within 2 min is ideal, but decontamination up to 15 or 20 min after exposure can potentially decrease the size of the eventual blisters. However, even patients arriving after this time should still be decontaminated as soon as possible to stop continuing absorption and thus accumulation of a lethal dose, which for mustard and lewisite is about 3 to 7 g. However, except for patients with impending airway compromise, most patients exposed to vesicants can tolerate a short delay in treatment while more immediate casualties are being stabilized.

Treatment

- Decontamination
- Treat skin lesions similar to thermal burns
- Airway support as needed

Eye and skin decontamination should occur as soon as possible, preferably using Reactive Skin Decontamination Lotion (RSDL®). A 0.5% solution of sodium hypochlorite is less effective but still useful if RSDL® is unavailable. Physical or mechanical decontamination can be tried, but soap and water are minimally effective.

Skin lesions are managed as thermal burns (see p. 2957). However, because fluid loss in patients exposed to vesicants is lower than in patients with thermal burns, less fluid should be used than is called for in the Brooke or Parkland fluid-replacement formulas. Scrupulous hygiene is important to prevent secondary infection. Antibiotic ointment should be applied to the edges of the eyelids to prevent lid adhesion.

Supportive respiratory care, including attention to airway and breathing, is indicated for patients with respiratory manifestations (see p. 3039). Because nausea is cholinergic in origin, it can be treated with atropine (eg, 0.1 to 1.3 mg IV q 1 to 2 h prn).

Bone-marrow suppression requires reverse isolation and treatment with colony-stimulating factors.

Nerve Agents

There are 2 types of nerve agents:

- G-series agents
- V-series agents

G-series agents, or G agents, include GA (tabun), GB (sarin), GD (soman), and GF (cyclosarin), which were developed by Nazi Germany before and during World War II. V-series agents include VX; these compounds were synthesized after World War II. All nerve agents are organophosphorus esters, as are organophosphate (OP) pesticides (see p. 3065). However, nerve agents are far more potent; the LD_{50} (the amount required to cause death in half of people receiving that dose) of VX is approximately 3 mg.

At room temperature, G agents are watery liquids with high volatilities and pose both skin-contact and inhalational hazards. VX is a liquid with the consistency of motor oil and that evaporates relatively slowly. None of these agents has a pronounced odor or causes local skin irritation.

Pathophysiology

Nerve agents inhibit the enzyme acetylcholinesterase (AChE), which hydrolyzes the neurotransmitter acetylcholine (ACh) once ACh has finished activating receptors in neurons, muscles, and glands. ACh receptors are present in the CNS, autonomic ganglia, skeletal-muscle fibers, smooth-muscle fibers, and exocrine glands.

The binding of nerve agent to AChE is essentially irreversible without treatment; treatment with an oxime can regenerate the enzyme as long as the bond has not been further stabilized (a process termed aging) over time. Most nerve agents, like OP insecticides, take hours to age fully, but GD (soman) can age essentially completely within 10 min of binding. Inhibition of AChE leads to an excess of ACh at all of its receptors (cholinergic crisis) first causing increased activity of the affected tissue, followed eventually in the CNS and in skeletal muscle by fatigue and failure of the tissue.

Symptoms and Signs

The clinical manifestations depend on the state of the agent, route of exposure, and dose. Vapor exposure to the face causes local effects such as miosis, rhinorrhea, and bronchoconstriction within seconds, progressing to the full range of systemic manifestations of cholinergic excess. However, if vapor is inhaled, collapse will occur within seconds. Liquid exposure to the skin first causes local effects (local twitching, fasciculations, sweating). Systemic effects occur after a latent period that can be as long as 18 h after exposure to a very small droplet; even fatal doses usually take up to 20 to 30 min to cause symptoms and signs, which may include sudden collapse and convulsions without warning.

Patients exhibit parts or all of the cholinergic toxidrome (see Tables 366–2 on p. 3052 and 366–8 on p. 3069). Overstimulation and eventual fatigue of the CNS lead to agitation, confusion, unconsciousness, and seizures, progressing to failure of the respiratory center in the medulla. Overstimulation and eventual fatigue of skeletal muscles cause twitching and fasciculations that progress to weakness and paralysis. Overstimulation of cholinergically activated smooth muscle leads to miosis, bronchospasm, and hyperperistalsis (with nausea, vomiting, and cramping), and overstimulation of exocrine glands causes excessive tearing, nasal secretions, salivation, bronchial secretions, digestive secretions, and sweating. Death is usually due to central apnea, but direct paralysis of the diaphragm, bronchospasm, and bronchorrhea can also contribute.

Diagnosis

- Clinical evaluation

Diagnosis is made clinically, although laboratory analysis of erythrocyte cholinesterase or plasma cholinesterase levels as well as more specialized laboratory tests can confirm nerve-agent exposure.

Triage: All people with suspicious liquid on their skin need to be prioritized for immediate decontamination of the affected area. Patients can then be triaged for medical treatment based on their symptoms and signs. All patients exposed to nerve agents who have significant difficulty breathing or systemic effects should be triaged as immediate for medical treatment.

Treatment

- Anticholinergics (atropine, 2-PAM)
- Benzodiazepines
- Respiratory support as needed

Attention to *A*irway, *B*reathing, *C*irculation, Immediate *D*econtamination, and *D*rugs (the ABCDDs) is paramount. Bronchoconstriction may be so severe that ventilation may be impossible until atropine is given (see Table 366–8 on p. 3069).

Two drugs are given, atropine and 2-pyridine aldoxime methyl chloride (2-PAM—also called pralidoxime). Atropine blocks the action of ACh. 2-PAM reactivates AChE that has been phosphorylated by nerve agents (or OP insecticides) but that has not yet undergone aging. 2-PAM reverses the peripheral effects of nerve agents, most importantly the paralysis of respiratory muscles, but has less pronounced effects in the CNS (eg, to reverse respiratory depression) and on smooth muscles and so is always given with atropine.

For prehospital care, 2 autoinjectors for intramuscular use are typically used, one containing 2.0 or 2.1 mg of atropine and another containing 600 mg of 2-PAM. Newer autoinjectors combine both drugs in one autoinjector. The drugs are given into the belly of a large muscle (eg, thigh) before establishing IV access. Once IV access is obtained, subsequent doses are given IV.

Adult patients with significant difficulty breathing or with systemic effects should promptly receive three 2.0-mg or 2.1-mg doses of atropine and three 600-mg doses of 2-PAM followed immediately by 2 to 4 mg of diazepam (also available as 2-mg autoinjectors) or 1 to 2 mg of midazolam (which is better absorbed intramuscularly than diazepam). Patients with less severe signs and symptoms can be given one autoinjector repeated in 3 to 5 min if symptoms have not resolved; a benzodiazepine is not automatically given unless 3 autoinjectors are required to be given all at once. Additional 2-mg doses of atropine are given every 2 to 3 min until muscarinic effects (airway resistance, secretions) resolve. Additional 600-mg doses of 2-PAM may be given hourly as needed for the control of skeletal-muscle effects (twitching, fasciculations, weakness, paralysis). Additional doses of benzodiazepines are given as needed for seizures. Note that paralyzed patients may have seizures in the absence of visible convulsions. Transition to IV administration should be done at the first opportunity. Dosages are adjusted downward for children.

Decontaminate all suspicious liquid on skin as soon as possible using Reactive Skin Decontamination Lotion (RSDL®); a 0.5% hypochlorite solution may also be used, as may soap and water. Possibly contaminated wounds require inspection, removal of all debris, and copious flushing with water or saline. Severe symptoms and death may occur after skin decontamination because decontamination may not completely remove nerve agents that are passing through the skin.

Anticholinergic Compounds

Anticholinergic drugs have been used as incapacitating agents, designed not to cause serious injury or death but rather to cause sufficient disorientation to prevent military personnel from carrying out their missions. One anticholinergic CW agent is 3-quinuclidinyl benzilate, NATO code BZ.

BZ is a solid that can be disseminated by heat-generating artillery rounds without being inactivated. It can persist in the environment for 3 to 4 wk. Mass casualties due to BZ exposure would likely result from inhalation of aerosolized BZ, although the compound can also be dissolved in a solvent and placed on an environmental surface from which it can be absorbed through the skin following contact.

Pathophysiology

BZ binds to muscarinic cholinergic receptors in the CNS, smooth muscle, and exocrine glands and blocks acetylcholine (ACh) at these sites. The decrease in cholinergic stimulation produces the anticholinergic toxidrome (see Table 366–2 on p. 3052).

Symptoms and Signs

Patients have dry mouth and skin and dilated pupils (causing blurring of vision) and may develop hyperthermia. Cholinergic blockade in the CNS causes first lethargy and then characteristic anticholinergic illusions and hallucinations; hallucinations may be visual or auditory and are typically concrete and easily describable (eg, voices of known contacts, imaginary television programs, sharing of imaginary cigarettes, odd shapes) in contrast to the abstract, geometric, and ineffable nature of psychedelic hallucinations. Anticholinergic visual hallucinations may also be lilliputian (ie, items hallucinated decrease in size over time—eg, a cow transforms into a dog and then into a mouse or a butterfly). Speech may be slurred, and patients exhibit stereotypical picking or plucking motions (woolgathering) and may confabulate. Stupor and coma may last hours to days, with gradual recovery.

Diagnosis

- Clinical evaluation
- Sometimes diagnostic challenge with physostigmine

Diagnosis is made by recognizing the typical anticholinergic toxidrome. No common laboratory tests detect BZ exposure. Although many drugs and plants have anticholinergic effects (see Table 366–2 on p. 3052), the simultaneous appearance of an anticholinergic toxidrome in many individuals who did not all ingest an anticholinergic drug or plant suggests an intentional or CW exposure. Physostigmine, a cholinergic drug, can be used as a diagnostic challenge; reduction of anticholinergic manifestations after physostigmine is given strongly suggests an anticholinergic compound.

Triage: Most patients exposed to BZ can be triaged as delayed.

Treatment

- Supportive care, including cooling as needed
- Rarely physostigmine

Patients are usually quiet but may become disruptive and may need to be reassured and in some cases restrained. Patients with elevated body temperature require cooling (see p. 3016). Most patients do not require drug treatment, but those who are disruptive or who are markedly distressed as a result of hallucinations may benefit from being given physostigmine slowly; dose is 0.5 to 20 mg IV in adults and 0.02 mg/kg IV in children (see Table 366–8 on p. 3069.) Exceeding recommended doses may cause cholinergic effects, including seizures.

Incendiary Agents and Hydrogen Fluoride (HF)

Military incendiary agents are designed to illuminate the battlefield, to start fires, to create smoke to obscure terrain and personnel, or for combinations of these effects. Agents include thickened gasoline (napalm), thermite (TH), white phosphorus (WP), and magnesium.

Hydrofluoric acid, used in industry and in other applications, is often confused with hydrochloric acid; for this reason, it is recommended that it be referred to as HF. Any of these compounds can create mass casualties.

Napalm has a jelly-like consistency; the other incendiary agents are usually weaponized as powdered solids. HF can exist at ambient temperatures as a liquid or a vapor. The most common routes of exposure are percutaneous, ocular, and inhalational.

Pathophysiology

Incendiary agents cause thermal burns. Some of them may be used in exploding projectiles which cause shrapnel that may lodge in tissue. White phosphorus may continue to burn on skin or clothing as long as it has access to air, and because magnesium will burn under water, it will continue to burn within tissue. White phosphorus is toxic and may also cause systemic effects, due to uncoupling of oxidative phosphorylation in hepatocytes, hyperphosphatemia, hypocalcemia (from binding of calcium to phosphorus), renal injury, and hyperkalemia (from hypocalcemia or from renal damage).

HF penetrates deeply and quickly into exposed tissue but generates hydronium ions relatively slowly. The fluoride released from the dissociation of hydrogen fluoride binds avidly to calcium and magnesium and may produce systemic effects due to hypocalcemia, hypomagnesemia, and hyperkalemia; coagulopathy and fatal cardiac dysrhythmias may occur.

Symptoms and Signs

Thermal burns due to incendiary agents have manifestations similar to those of other thermal burns.

The onset of pain after HF exposure depends on the concentration of HF; pain may appear within an hour but typically occurs after 2 or 3 h. However, once pain occurs, it is often deep and intense. Affected skin is erythematous but does not seem as severely affected as the intense pain would suggest.

Diagnosis

- Clinical evaluation

Most incendiary burns are readily apparent. However, burns due to low concentrations of HF may appear deceptively innocuous, and a high index of suspicion must be maintained for deep tissue injury and systemic toxicity. WP burns may glow or smoke when exposed to air.

Triage: Triage of incendiary burns should occur as for thermal burns.

HF burns should be triaged more urgently than their appearance would otherwise indicate; patients with large areas of exposure should be triaged immediate because of the danger of systemic toxicity.

Treatment

- Treat as thermal burns
- For HF, topical and sometimes systemic Ca

See p. 2956 for the general management of thermal burns.

For WP burns, the affected areas are flooded with water or smothered to avoid exposure to air. WP particles are removed mechanically (they often adhere tightly to skin) and placed in water. Smoking trails may be good indicators of the location of small particles. A bicarbonate solution may be used to flood the burns and to wet the burn dressings, but cupric sulfate ($CuSO_4$) is no longer recommended for these burns.

Mg reacts with water to generate highly flammable gas and with carbon dioxide to produce magnesium oxide and carbon. Burning or smoking Mg particles in the skin or subcutis should be removed as promptly as possible. If not all particles can be removed at once (eg, because of the number of wounds), oil can be used to cover wounds until removal can be accomplished.

Patients exposed to HF require prompt decontamination by copious flushing with water; a topical skin decontamination product (RSDL®) has not been tested in patients with skin exposures to HF. However, because HF penetrates quickly, significant local and systemic effects may occur even after thorough decontamination. Ca gluconate or Ca carbonate paste is applied to local burns. Sometimes local injection of 10% Ca gluconate is also given; some clinicians give Ca gluconate intra-arterially. Patients with significant exposure are hospitalized to undergo cardiac monitoring and treatment with CaCl or Ca gluconate (see Table 366–8 on p. 3069).

Riot-Control Agents

Riot-control agents are compounds that were initially developed for crowd control but that have also been used in military conflicts. They are also referred to as harassing agents, tear agents, or lacrimators and are often incorrectly called tear gas, but in fact they do not exist as gases or vapors. Instead, they are solids that can be dispersed as liquids (by dissolving the solid agent to form a solution and then spraying the solution) or as aerosols (small particles released explosively or as smoke). Like anticholinergic agents, they are intended to cause incapacitation rather than serious injury or death, although deaths due to pulmonary edema (acute lung injury) have occurred. Military versions of these agents include chloroacetophenone (CN, also marketed as Mace®), chlorobenzylidenemalononitrile (CS), dibenzoxazepine (CR), and diphenylaminoarsine (adamsite, or DM, a so-called vomiting agent). Oleoresin capsicum (OC, pepper spray) is a more recently developed riot-control agent used primarily for law enforcement and personal protection. Chloropicrin (PS) is a compound used during World War I that is occasionally regarded as a riot-control agent, although it is more properly classified as a pulmonary agent.

Pathophysiology

CN and CS alkylate enzymes such as lactic dehydrogenase; this mechanism may be responsible for transient tissue injury that resolves with rapid replacement of the inactivated enzymes. Release of cytokines such as bradykinin contributes to the pain caused by these compounds, as does generation of hydrochloric acid at high doses. CR appears to have a similar mechanism of action. DM is thought to exert its effects partly via the oxidation of its arsenic moiety from As(III) to As(V) and the subsequent release of chlorine. OC causes pain by binding to transient receptor potential vanilloid (TRPV1) receptors in neurons that are then stimulated to release neurokinin A, calcitonin-gene-related peptide, and substance P. These compounds induce neurogenic inflammation associated with pain, capillary leakage, edema, mucous production, and bronchoconstriction.

Symptoms and Signs

Although there are minor differences between compounds, most riot-control agents cause nearly immediate irritation and pain involving the eyes, mucous membranes, and skin, which may also become briefly erythematous. Respiratory effects resulting from inhalation are typically obviously audible (eg, coughing, sneezing, and wheezing) due to type 1 damage, although type 2 damage (delayed-onset shortness of breath due to incipient acute lung injury) can occur with high doses. Deaths are usually due to pulmonary edema resulting from high doses delivered in confined spaces. The largely obsolete agent DM may cause either immediate or delayed-onset irritation along with vomiting.

Effects of all of the riot-control agents typically resolve within a half an hour, although agent left on the skin may cause blisters. Reactive airways dysfunction syndrome (RADS) can occur long after exposure and persist indefinitely, although it is impossible to predict which patients will develop this complication.

Diagnosis

- Clinical evaluation

Diagnosis is made by history, signs (lacrimation, blepharospasm, erythema, type 1 respiratory signs), and symptoms (transient irritation and pain with, at high doses, delayed-onset shortness of breath or chest tightness). Chest x-rays are usually clear and not needed unless patients develop dyspnea, which suggests pulmonary edema. Laboratory studies do not contribute to diagnosis.

Triage: Casualties typically need prompt removal from exposure but are then usually triaged as delayed or minimal, since except at high doses effects are self-limiting. Evidence of incipient pulmonary edema should prompt urgent evacuation to a pulmonary intensive care unit.

Treatment

- Termination of exposure
- Skin decontamination
- If eye pain does not resolve spontaneously, eye decontamination
- Cold compresses and analgesics if necessary for pain

At the first sign of exposure or potential exposure, masks are applied when available. People are removed from the affected area when possible.

Decontamination is by physical or mechanical removal (brushing, washing, rinsing) of solid or liquid agents. Water may transiently exacerbate the pain caused by CS and OC but is still effective, although fat-containing oils or soaps may be more effective against OC. Eyes are decontaminated by copious flushing with sterile water or saline or (with OC) open-eye exposure to wind from a fan. Referral to an ophthalmologist is needed if slit-lamp examination shows impaction of solid particles of agent.

Most effects resulting from riot-control agents are transient and do not require treatment beyond decontamination, and most patients do not need observation beyond 4 h. However, patients should be instructed to return if they develop effects such as vesication or delayed-onset shortness of breath.

TOXINS AS MASS-CASUALTY WEAPONS

"Toxin" is often loosely used to refer to any poison, but technically refers only to a poisonous chemical produced by an organism (although some toxins can now also be produced synthetically). Because toxins used as MCWs do not include the infectious agents from which they are derived, they do not replicate in the body and are not transmissible from person to person. Thus, toxins are more like chemical agents than biological agents; they cause poisoning rather than infection.

Hundreds of toxins are known. However, because of difficulties in isolating sufficient quantities, and problems with dissemination or environmental fragility, most toxins are more suited to assassination than to production of mass casualties. Only four toxins are considered high-threat agents by the US Centers for Disease Control and Prevention (CDC):

- Botulinum toxin
- Epsilon toxin from *Clostridium perfringens*
- Ricin toxin
- Staphylococcal enterotoxin B

Of these, only botulinum toxin is classified among the highest priority agents. Epsilon toxin from *C. perfringens* is mainly of historical interest as an agent reportedly developed by Iraq in the 1980s; its main action is to increase capillary permeability, especially in the intestine.

Botulinum Toxin

Botulinum toxin, or botulinum neurotoxin (BoNT), refers to any of 7 known types of neurotoxins produced by *Clostridium botulinum*. Botulism is the poisoning produced by exposure to botulinum toxin; infection with *C. botulinum* is not required. Food-borne, wound, and infant botulism are described elsewhere (see p. 1464). Mass casualties from BoNT could occur from widespread contamination of food or water, but the most likely scenario would be inhalation of aerosolized BoNT.

BoNT blocks the action of acetylcholine (ACh) at muscarinic receptors in smooth muscle and exocrine glands but does not penetrate the blood-brain barrier to gain entry to the CNS. As with wound botulism, neurologic symptoms (typically bilaterally symmetrical descending paralysis with mydriasis) without nausea, vomiting, cramping, or diarrhea would be expected 12 to 36 h (range 2 h to 8 days) after exposure. Sensation and mentation are intact.

Clinical diagnosis is sufficient to make the decision to administer antitoxin, which becomes progressively less effective as symptoms and signs develop. One vial of equine heptavalent botulism immune globulin diluted 1:10 in 0.9% saline solution is given slowly IV.

Ricin and Abrin

Ricin (from beans of the castor plant) and abrin (from jequirity, or rosary pea) both inactivate ribosomes catalytically; one molecule of either toxin is capable of poisoning all of the ribosomes in a cell. Although ricin has been injected in assassination attempts, mass casualties would probably involve inhalation of aerosolized toxin.

The clinical manifestations of ricin intoxication vary by route of exposure. Following inhalation, there is a latent period of 4 to 8 h followed by cough, respiratory distress, and fever. Multiple organ systems are progressively affected over the next 12 to 24 h, culminating in respiratory failure. Diagnosis is by clinical suspicion, no specific antidote or antitoxin is available, and treatment is supportive.

Staphylococcal Enterotoxin B

Staphylococcal enterotoxin B (SEB) is one of 7 enterotoxins (toxins acting in the intestine) produced by *Staphylococcus aureus*. SEB is responsible for staphylococcal food poisoning when ingested (see p. 1603). Mass casualties could result from food adulteration but also from inhalation of aerosolized toxin; SEB was developed for use as an aerosol to cause incapacitation in military personnel.

The latent period is typically 1 to 12 h after ingestion and 2 to 12 h (with a range of 1.5 to 24 h) after inhalation. After initial influenza-like symptoms of fever, chills, headache, and myalgias, subsequent symptoms and signs depend on the route of exposure. Ingestion causes nausea, vomiting, and diarrhea for 1 to 2 days. Inhalation causes nonproductive cough, retrosternal chest pain, and often nasal irritation and congestion. Conjunctivitis can result from contact of aerosol with the eyes. Although SEB was intended to be an incapacitating agent, inhalation can cause death due to pulmonary edema and circulatory collapse. In survivors, fever may persist up to 5 days and cough for 4 wk. Specialized toxin assays may help confirm the diagnosis. Treatment is supportive.

BIOLOGICAL AGENTS AS WEAPONS

Biological warfare (BW) is the use of microbiological agents for hostile purposes. Such use is contrary to international law and has rarely taken place during formal warfare in modern history, despite the extensive preparations and stockpiling of biological agents carried out during the 20th century by most major powers (including development of strains resistant to multiple drugs). The area of most concern is the use of BW agents by terrorist groups. BW agents are thought by some to be an ideal weapon for terrorists. These agents may be delivered clandestinely, and they have delayed effects, allowing the user to remain undetected.

The US Centers for Disease Control and Prevention (CDC) has created a priority list of biological agents and toxins (see Table 364–4). The highest priority is Category A.

The deliberate use of BW agents to cause mass casualties would probably entail dissemination of aerosols to create disease via inhalation, and thus inhalational anthrax and pneumonic plague are the 2 diseases most likely to occur under these circumstances.

Recognition

It can be difficult to distinguish use of a BW from a natural outbreak of disease. Clues to the deliberate rather than a natural origin of a disease outbreak include the following:

- Cases of diseases not usually seen in the geographic area
- Unusual distribution of cases among segments of the population
- Significantly different attack rates between those inside and those outside buildings
- Separate outbreaks in geographically noncontiguous areas
- Multiple simultaneous or serial outbreaks of different diseases in the same population
- Unusual routes of exposure (eg, inhalation)
- Zoonotic disease occurring in humans rather than in animals
- Zoonotic disease occurring first in humans and then in its typical vector
- Zoonotic disease arising in an area with a low prevalence of the typical vector for the disease
- Unusual severity of disease
- Unusual strains of infectious agents
- Failure to respond to standard therapy

Epidemiologic investigation of cases and cooperation with law-enforcement resources are crucial, as is risk communication to the general public.

The clinical presentation, diagnosis, and treatment of patients with disease caused by high-risk BW agents are discussed elsewhere in The Manual: Anthrax (see p. 1609), plague (see p. 1590), smallpox (see p. 1682), tularemia (see p. 1597), and

Table 364–4. CDC HIGH-PRIORITY BIOLOGICAL AGENTS AND TOXINS

CATEGORY	AGENT
A: Highest priority	*Bacillus anthracis*, causing anthrax Botulinum toxin from *Clostridium botulinum*, causing botulism *Yersinia pestis*, causing plague Variola virus, causing variola major (classic smallpox) *Francisella tularensis*, causing tularemia Viral-hemorrhagic-fever (VHF) viruses • Arenaviruses, causing Lassa fever and New World VHFs (Machupo, Junin, Guanarito, and Sabia hemorrhagic fevers) • Bunyaviridae, causing Crimean Congo hemorrhagic fever and Rift Valley fever • Filoviridae, causing Ebola virus disease and Marburg virus disease • Flaviviridae, causing yellow fever, Omsk hemorrhagic fever, and Kyasanur Forest disease
B: 2nd-highest priority	*Brucella* species, causing brucellosis Epsilon toxin of *Clostridium perfringens* *Salmonella* sp, *Escherichia coli* 0157:H7, and *Shigella*, causing food poisoning *Burkholderia mallei*, causing glanders *Burkholderia pseudomallei*, causing melioidosis *Chlamydia psittaci*, causing psittacosis *Coxiella burnetii*, causing Q fever Ricin toxin from *Ricinus communis* Staphylococcal enterotoxin B *Rickettsia prowazekii*, causing typhus fever Alphaviruses causing viral encephalitides (eg, Venezuelan, eastern, and western equine encephalitides) *Vibrio cholerae*, *Cryptosporidium parvum*, and other agents, causing waterborne diseases
C: 3rd-highest priority	Nipah virus, hantavirus, SARS coronavirus, and influenza viruses capable of causing pandemic influenza Other agents associated with emerging infectious diseases

CDC = US Centers for Disease Control and Prevention; SARS = severe acute respiratory syndrome.

viral hemorrhagic fevers (see p. 1480). Management of outbreaks due to BW does not differ from that of natural outbreaks except that clinicians must be alert for unusual antibiotic resistance patterns.

Isolation (of patients) and quarantine (of contacts) may be necessary. The most communicable deliberately disseminated diseases are smallpox (for which airborne precautions are necessary) and pneumonic plague (necessitating droplet precautions).

Response

Because of the relatively long incubation periods of diseases caused by BW agents, most lives will be saved or lost in a hospital setting. Adequate supplies of vaccines, antibiotics, and antivirals for hospitalized patients and for contacts are needed, and systems for distributing such medical countermeasures to members of the general public at high risk of exposure are crucial.

RADIOLOGICAL WEAPONS

Ionizing radiation is discussed in detail elsewhere (see p. 3090). Mass casualties due to ionizing radiation can result from the detonation of a nuclear (fission) or a thermonuclear (fusion) device, from the contamination of conventional explosives with radioactive material (such a weapon is called a radiation dispersal device [RDD], or a dirty bomb), or from placement (eg, under a subway seat) of a concealed point source of radiation. In cases of the deliberate use of radiation as a weapon, it must be determined whether patients have been exposed (irradiated), contaminated, or both. If contamination has occurred, determination of whether it is external, internal, or both is needed. Use of the ASBESTOS acronym (see Table 364–2) is helpful in making these determinations. Another useful clinical resource is the online and downloadable module, Radiation Emergency Medical Management (REMM), available at www.remm.nlm.gov.

EXPLOSIVES AND BLAST INJURIES

High-energy events in which a solid or liquid is converted rapidly to a gas can occur at 3 rates:

- Deflagration: Rapid burning but minimal blast
- Explosion: Subsonic ignition and blast wind (low-grade explosive)
- Detonation: Supersonic ignition and blast wave (high-grade explosive)

An example of deflagration would be the rapid flash (without a bang) that results when an open pile of black powder is ignited. The same black powder confined tightly in a container would cause a low-grade explosion. In high-grade explosives, the ignition wave travels through the material at supersonic speed and causes a supersonic blast (detonation) wave; common examples include nitroglycerin and trinitrotoluene (TNT—see Table 364–5).

In MCIs involving explosions, 3 concentric zones are identified:

- Blast epicenter
- Secondary perimeter
- Blast periphery

In the blast epicenter (kill zone), any survivors are probably mortally injured, technical rescue capabilities and extrication are likely to be required, and advanced life support and high victim-to-care-provider ratios are required for any survivors. In the secondary perimeter (critical casualty zone), survivors

Table 364–5. EXAMPLES OF LOW-GRADE AND HIGH-GRADE EXPLOSIVES

Low-grade explosives
Nitrocellulose
"Smokeless" gunpowder
Black powder
Most solid rocket fuels
Pipe bombs
Fireworks
High-grade explosives
Ammonium nitrate (NH_4NO_3)
Amatol 80/20 (NH_4NO_3 + TNT)
Ammonal (NH_4NO_3 + TNT + aluminum)
ANFO (NH_4NO_3 + fuel oil)
RDX (cyclotrimethylenetrinitramine)
TNT (trinitrotoluene)
Nitroglycerin (the explosive component in dynamite)
PETN (pentaerythritol tetranitrate)
Composition B (TNT + RDX)
Composition C-4 (RDX + plasticizer)
Picric acid

will have multiple injuries, and standard rescue capabilities and moderate victim-to-care-provider ratios are required. In the blast periphery (walking-wounded zone), most casualties will have non–life-threatening injuries and psychologic trauma, no rescue is required, and basic life support and self help are needed.

Pathophysiology

Blast injuries include both physical and psychologic trauma. Physical trauma includes fractures, respiratory compromise, injuries to soft tissue and internal organs, internal and external blood loss with shock, burns, and sensory impairment, especially of hearing and sight. Five mechanisms of blast injury have been described (see Table 364–6).

The supersonic blast wave in primary blast injury (PBI) compresses gas-filled spaces, which then rapidly reexpand, causing shearing and tearing forces that can damage tissue and perforate organs. Blood is forced from the vasculature into air spaces and surrounding tissue. Pulmonary involvement (blast lung injury) may cause pulmonary contusion, systemic air embolism (especially in the brain and spinal cord), and free-radical-associated injuries (thrombosis, lipo-oxygenation, and disseminated intravascular coagulation); it is a common cause of delayed mortality. PBI also includes intestinal barotrauma (particularly with underwater explosions), acoustic barotrauma (including tympanic-membrane rupture, hemotympanum without rupture, and fracture or dislocation of ossicles in the middle ear), and traumatic brain injury.

Symptoms and Signs

Most injuries (eg, fractures, lacerations, brain injuries) manifest the same as in other types of trauma. Blast lung injury may cause dyspnea, hemoptysis, cough, chest pain, tachypnea, wheezing, decreased breath sounds, apnea, hypoxia, cyanosis, and hemodynamic instability. Air embolism may manifest as stroke, MI, acute abdomen, blindness, deafness, spinal cord injury, or claudication. Damage to the tympanic membrane and the inner ear may impair hearing, which should always be assessed. Patients with abdominal blast injury may have abdominal pain, nausea, vomiting, hematemesis, rectal pain, tenesmus, testicular pain, and unexplained hypovolemia.

Diagnosis

- Clinical evaluation
- Imaging studies as indicated by findings

Patients are evaluated as for most multiple trauma casualties (see p. 2927), except that special effort is directed at identifying blast injury, particularly blast lung (and consequent air embolism), ear trauma, occult penetrating injury, and crush injury. Apnea, bradycardia, and hypotension are the clinical triad classically associated with blast lung injury. Tympanic membrane rupture has been considered to predict blast lung injury, but

Table 364–6. MECHANISMS OF BLAST INJURY

TYPE	MECHANISM	TYPICAL INJURIES
Primary	Impact of supersonic blast wave on body Preferentially affects hollow or gas-filled structures	Pulmonary barotrauma (blast lung) Tympanic membrane rupture and middle ear damage Abdominal hemorrhage and intestinal perforation Eyeball rupture Mild traumatic brain injury (concussion)
Secondary	Impact of debris from blast onto body	Penetrating or blunt injuries Eye penetration (evident or occult)
Tertiary	Impact of body thrown by blast onto environmental surfaces or debris	Fractures and traumatic amputations Closed and open brain injury
Quaternary	Processes independent of primary, secondary, or tertiary blast injury (eg, burns, toxic inhalation, crush injury from entrapment under debris, aggravation of medical disorders)	Burns Crush injuries with rhabdomyolysis and compartment syndrome Respiratory tract injury from inhaled toxicants Asthma, angina, or MI triggered by the event
Quinary	Thought to result from toxic materials absorbed by the body from the blast Affects the immune system and perhaps the autonomic nervous system, leading to an immediate hyperinflammatory state	Fever Diaphoresis Low central venous pressure Tissue edema

pharyngeal petechiae may be a better predictor. Chest radiography is done, and x-rays may show a characteristic butterfly pattern. Cardiac monitoring is done in all patients. Patients with possible crush injury are tested for myoglobinuria, hyperkalemia, and ECG changes.

Triage: In blast injuries, less seriously injured patients often bypass prehospital triage and go directly to hospitals, possibly overwhelming medical resources in advance of the later arrival of more seriously injured patients. On-scene triage differs from standard trauma triage mainly in that blast injuries may be more difficult to recognize initially, so initial triage should be geared toward identifying blast lung, blast abdomen, and acute crush syndrome in addition to more obvious injuries.

Treatment

Attention should be given to airway, breathing, circulation, disability (neurologic status), and exposure of the patient (see p. 2927). High-flow O_2 and fluid administration are priorities, and early chest tube placement should be considered. Most injuries (eg, lacerations, fractures, burns, internal injuries, head injuries) are managed as discussed elsewhere in THE MANUAL.

Because air embolism may worsen after initiation of positive-pressure ventilation, positive-pressure ventilation should be avoided unless absolutely necessary. If it is used, slower rates and lower inspiratory pressure settings should be chosen. Patients suspected of having air-gas embolism should be placed in the coma position, halfway between left lateral decubitus and prone, with the head at or below the level of the heart. Hyperbaric O_2 (HBO) therapy may be useful (see p. 3027).

If acute crush syndrome is diagnosed or suspected, urinary catheterization is done to allow continual monitoring of urine output. Forced diuresis using an alkaline mannitol solution to maintain urine output up to 8 L/day and a urinary pH of ≥ 5 may help. ABGs, electrolytes, and muscle enzymes should be monitored. Control hyperkalemia with calcium, insulin, and glucose (see p. 1283). Hyperbaric oxygen therapy may be particularly useful in patients with deep tissue infections. Monitoring for compartment syndrome is done clinically and by measuring compartment pressure. Patients may need fasciotomy if the difference between diastolic BP and compartment pressure is < 30 mm Hg. Hypovolemia and hypotension may not be apparent initially but may suddenly occur after tissue release and reperfusion, so large volumes of intravenous fluid (eg, 1 to 2 L normal saline) are given both before and after reperfusion. Fluids are continued at a rate sufficient to maintain a urine output of 300 to 500 mL/h.

The views expressed in this chapter are those of the author and do not reflect the official policy of the Department of Army, Department of Defense, or the US Government.

365 Motion Sickness

(Mal de Mer; Seasickness)

Motion sickness is a symptom complex that usually includes nausea, often accompanied by vague abdominal discomfort, vomiting, dizziness, pallor, diaphoresis, and related symptoms. It is induced by specific forms of motion, particularly repetitive angular and linear acceleration and deceleration, or as a result of conflicting vestibular, visual, and proprioceptive inputs. Behavioral change and drug therapy can help prevent or control symptoms.

Motion sickness is a normal physiologic response to a provocative stimulus. Individual susceptibility to motion sickness varies greatly; however, it occurs more frequently in women and in children between the ages of 2 and 12 yr. Motion sickness is uncommon after the age of 50 and in infants < 2 yr. The incidence ranges from < 1% on airplanes to nearly 100% on ships in rough seas and upon becoming weightless during space travel.

Etiology

Excessive stimulation of the vestibular apparatus by motion is the primary cause. Vestibular stimulation can result from angular motion (sensed by the semicircular canals) or linear acceleration or gravity (sensed by the otolithic organs [utricle and saccule]). CNS components that mediate motion sickness include the vestibular system and brain stem nuclei, the hypothalamus, the nodulus and uvula of the cerebellum, and emetic pathways (eg, medullary chemoreceptor trigger zone, vomiting center, and emetic efferents).

The exact pathophysiology is undefined, but motion sickness occurs only when the 8th cranial nerve and cerebellar vestibular tracts are intact; those lacking a functional vestibulo-cochlear system are immune to motion sickness. Movement via any form of transportation, including ship, motor vehicle, train, plane, spacecraft, and playground or amusement park rides can cause excessive vestibular stimulation.

The trigger may involve conflicting vestibular, visual, and proprioceptive inputs. For example, visual input that indicates being stationary may conflict with the sensation of movement (eg, looking at an apparently unmoving ship cabin wall while sensing the ship rolling). Alternatively, moving visual input may conflict with lack of perception of movement, eg, viewing a rapidly moving slide with a microscope or watching a virtual reality game while sitting still (also termed pseudomotion sickness or pseudokinetosis, given the lack of actual acceleration). When watching waves from a boat, a person may experience conflicting visual input (the movement of the waves in one direction) and vestibular input (the vertical motion of the boat itself).

Another possible trigger is a conflict in inputs between angular motion and linear acceleration or gravity, as can occur in a zero gravity environment when turning (angular acceleration). Also, a pattern of motion that differs from the expected pattern (eg, in a zero gravity environment, floating instead of falling) can be a trigger.

Risk factors: Factors that may increase the risk of developing motion sickness or increase the severity of symptoms include the following:

- Poor ventilation (eg, with exposure to fumes, smoke, or carbon monoxide)
- Emotional factors (eg, fear, anxiety)
- Migraine headaches
- Labyrinthitis
- Hormonal factors (eg, pregnancy, use of hormonal contraceptives)

In **space adaptation syndrome** (motion sickness during space travel), weightlessness (zero gravity) is an etiologic factor. This syndrome reduces the efficiency of astronauts during the first few days of space flight, but adaptation occurs over several days.

Symptoms and Signs

Characteristic manifestations are nausea, vomiting, pallor, diaphoresis, and vague abdominal discomfort. Other symptoms, which may precede the characteristic manifestations, include yawning, hyperventilation, salivation, and somnolence. Aerophagia, dizziness, headache, fatigue, weakness, and inability to concentrate may also occur. Pain, shortness of breath, focal weakness or neurologic deficits, and visual and speech disturbances are absent. With continuous exposure to motion, patients often adapt within several days. However, symptoms may recur if motion increases or if motion resumes after a short respite from the inciting trigger.

Prolonged vomiting due to motion sickness may rarely lead to dehydration with hypotension, inanition, and depression.

Diagnosis

- Clinical evaluation

The diagnosis is suspected in patients with compatible symptoms who have been exposed to typical triggers. Diagnosis is clinical and usually straightforward. However, the possibility of another diagnosis (eg, CNS hemorrhage or infarction) should be considered in some people, particularly the elderly, patients with no prior history of motion sickness, or those with risk factors for CNS hemorrhage or infarction who develop acute dizziness and vomiting during travel. Patients with focal neurologic symptoms or signs, significant headache, or other findings atypical of motion sickness should be further evaluated.

Treatment

- Prophylactic drugs (eg, scopolamine, antihistamines, antidopaminergic drugs)
- Nondrug prophylaxis and treatment measures
- Antiemetic drugs (eg, serotonin antagonists)
- Sometimes IV fluid and electrolyte replacement

People prone to motion sickness should take prophylactic drugs and use other preventive measures before symptoms start; interventions are less effective after symptoms develop. If vomiting occurs, an antiemetic, given rectally or parenterally, can be effective. If vomiting is prolonged, IV fluids and electrolytes may be required for replacement and maintenance.

Scopolamine: Scopolamine, an anticholinergic prescription drug, is effective for prevention, but efficacy in treatment is uncertain. Scopolamine is available as a 1.5-mg transdermal patch or in oral form. The patch is a good choice for longer trips because it is effective for up to 72 h. It is applied behind the ear 4 h before its effect is required. If treatment is needed after 72 h, the patch is removed and a fresh one is placed behind the other ear. The oral form of scopolamine is effective within 30 min and is given as 0.4 mg to 0.8 mg 1 h before travel and then every 8 h as needed.

Anticholinergic adverse effects, which include drowsiness, blurred vision, dry mouth, and bradycardia, occur less commonly with patches. Inadvertent contamination of the eye with patch residue may cause a fixed and widely dilated pupil. Additional adverse effects of scopolamine in the elderly can include confusion, hallucinations, and urinary retention. Scopolamine is contraindicated in people who are at risk of angle-closure glaucoma.

PEARLS & PITFALLS

- If an elderly person becomes confused and develops a fixed, dilated pupil while traveling, consider scopolamine toxicity (as well as intracranial hematoma with brain herniation).

Scopolamine can be used by children > 12 yr in the same dosages as for adults. Use in children ≤ 12 yr may be safe but is not recommended due to the higher risk of adverse effects.

Antihistamines: The mechanism of action for antihistamines is probably anticholinergic. All effective ones are sedating; nonsedating antihistamines do not appear to be effective. These drugs can be effective for prevention and possibly treatment. Anticholinergic adverse effects may be troublesome, particularly in the elderly. Beginning 1 h before departure, susceptible people may be given nonprescription dimenhydrinate, diphenhydramine, meclizine, or cyclizine in the following doses:

- Diphenhydramine: Adults, 25 to 50 mg po q 4 to 8 h; children ≥ 12 yr, 25 to 50 mg po q 4 to 6 h; children 6 to 11 yr 12.5 to 25 mg po q 4 to 6 h; children 2 to 5 yr, 6.25 mg po q 4 to 6 h
- Dimenhydrinate: Adults and children > 12 yr, 50 to 100 mg po q 4 to 6 h (not to exceed 400 mg/day); children 6 to 12 yr, 25 to 50 mg po q 6 to 8 h (not to exceed 150 mg/day); children 2 to 5 yr, 12.5 to 25 mg po q 6 to 8 h (not to exceed 75 mg/day)
- Meclizine: Adults and children ≥ 12 yr, 25 to 50 mg po q 24 h
- Cyclizine: Adults, 50 mg po q 4 to 6 h; children 6 to 12 yr, 25 mg tid or qid

Cyclizine and dimenhydrinate can minimize vagally mediated GI symptoms.

Antidopaminergic drugs: Promethazine 25 to 50 mg po 1 h before departure and then bid appears to be effective for prevention and treatment. The dosage in children 2 yr to 12 yr is 0.5 mg/kg po 1 h before departure and then bid; it should not be used in children < 2 yr because of the risk of respiratory depression. Adding caffeine may increase efficacy. Metoclopramide may also be effective, but evidence suggests it is less so than promethazine. Adverse effects include extrapyramidal symptoms and sedation.

Benzodiazepines: Benzodiazepines may also have some benefit in the treatment of motion sickness but do have sedative effects.

Serotonin antagonists: Serotonin (5-HT_3) antagonists, such as ondansetron and granisetron, are highly effective antiemetics.

Nondrug measures: Susceptible people should minimize exposure by positioning themselves where motion is the least (eg, in the middle of a ship close to water level, over the wings in an airplane). Also, they should try to minimize the discrepancy between visual and vestibular stimuli. If traveling in a motor vehicle, then driving or riding in the front passenger seat, where vehicle motion is most evident, is best. When traveling on a ship, viewing the horizon or land masses is usually better than viewing a cabin wall. Whatever the form of transportation, reading and rear-facing seats should be avoided. A supine or semirecumbent position with the head supported is best. Sleeping can also help by reducing vestibular sensory input. In space adaptation syndrome, movement, which aggravates the symptoms, should be avoided.

Adequate ventilation helps prevent symptoms. Consuming alcoholic beverages and overeating before or during travel increase the likelihood of motion sickness. Small amounts of fluids and bland food consumed frequently are preferred to large meals during extended travel; some people find that dry crackers and carbonated beverages, especially ginger ale, are best. If travel time is short, food and fluids should be avoided.

Adaptation is one of the most effective prophylactic therapies for motion sickness and is accomplished by repeated exposure to the same stimulus. However, adaptation is specific to the stimulus (eg, sailors who adapt to motion on large boats may still develop motion sickness when on smaller boats).

Alternative therapies: Some alternative therapies are unproven but may be helpful. These alternative therapies include wristbands that apply acupressure and wristbands that apply electrical stimulation. Both can be safely used by people of all ages. Ginger 0.5 to 1 g, which can be repeated but should be limited to 4 g/day, has been used but has not been shown to be more effective than placebo.

KEY POINTS

- Motion sickness is triggered by excessive stimulation of the vestibular system or conflicts among proprioceptive, visual, and vestibular sensory inputs.
- The diagnosis, based on clinical findings, is usually straightforward.
- Drug therapy is more effective prophylactically and usually involves scopolamine or an antihistamine.
- Once vomiting is established, serotonin antagonist antiemetics are preferred.
- To minimize motion sickness, it is recommended that people seek the position in the vehicle least subject to motion, sleep when possible, obtain adequate ventilation, and avoid alcohol and unnecessary food and drink.

366 Poisoning

GENERAL PRINCIPLES OF POISONING

Poisoning is contact with a substance that results in toxicity. Symptoms vary, but certain common syndromes may suggest particular classes of poisons. Diagnosis is primarily clinical, but for some poisonings, blood and urine tests can help. Treatment is supportive for most poisonings; specific antidotes are necessary for a few. Prevention includes labeling drug containers clearly and keeping poisons out of the reach of children.

Most poisonings are dose-related. Dose is determined by concentration over time. Toxicity may result from exposure to excess amounts of normally nontoxic substances. Some poisonings result from exposure to substances that are poisonous at all doses. Poisoning is distinguished from hypersensitivity and idiosyncratic reactions, which are unpredictable and not dose-related, and from intolerance, which is a toxic reaction to a usually nontoxic dose of a substance.

Poisoning is commonly due to ingestion but can result from injection, inhalation, or exposure of body surfaces (eg, skin, eye, mucous membranes). Many commonly ingested nonfood substances are generally nontoxic (see Table 366–1); however, almost any substance can be toxic if ingested in excessive amounts.

Accidental poisoning is common among young children, who are curious and ingest items indiscriminately despite noxious tastes and odors; usually, only a single substance is involved. Poisoning is also common among older children, adolescents, and adults attempting suicide; multiple drugs, including alcohol, acetaminophen, and other OTC drugs, may be involved. Accidental poisoning may occur in the elderly because of confusion, poor eyesight, mental impairment, or multiple prescriptions of the same drug by different physicians.

Occasionally, people are poisoned by someone who intends to kill or disable them (eg, to rape or rob them). Drugs used to disable (eg, scopolamine, benzodiazepines, γ-hydroxybutyrate) tend to have sedative or amnestic properties or both. Rarely, parents, who may have some medical knowledge, poison their children because of unclear psychiatric reasons or a desire to cause illness and thus gain medical attention (a disorder called factitious disorder imposed on another—see p. 1804 [formerly called Munchausen syndrome by proxy]).

After exposure or ingestion and absorption, most poisons are metabolized, pass through the GI tract, or are excreted. Occasionally, tablets (eg, aspirin, iron, enteric-coated drugs) form large concretions (bezoars) in the GI tract, where they tend to remain, continuing to be absorbed and causing toxicity.

Symptoms and Signs

Symptoms and signs of poisoning vary depending on the substance (see Table 366–8 on p. 3069). Also, different patients poisoned with the same substance may present with very different symptoms. However, 6 clusters of symptoms (toxic syndromes, or toxidromes) occur commonly and may suggest particular classes of substances (see Table 366–2). Patients who ingest multiple substances are less likely to have symptoms characteristic of a single substance.

Symptoms typically begin soon after contact but, with certain poisons, are delayed. The delay may occur because only a metabolite is toxic rather than the parent substance (eg, methanol, ethylene glycol, hepatotoxins). Ingestion of hepatotoxins (eg, acetaminophen, iron, *Amanita phalloides* mushrooms) may cause acute liver failure that occurs one to a few days later. With metals or hydrocarbon solvents, symptoms typically occur only after chronic exposure to the toxin.

Ingested and absorbed toxins generally cause systemic symptoms. Caustics and corrosive liquids damage mainly the mucous membranes of the GI tract, causing stomatitis, enteritis, or perforation. Some toxins (eg, alcohol, hydrocarbons) cause characteristic breath odors. Skin contact with toxins can cause various acute cutaneous symptoms (eg, rashes, pain, blistering); chronic exposure may cause dermatitis.

Inhaled toxins are likely to cause symptoms of upper airway injury if they are water-soluble (eg, chlorine, ammonia) and symptoms of lower airway injury and noncardiogenic pulmonary edema if they are less water-soluble (eg, phosgene). Inhalation of carbon monoxide, cyanide, or hydrogen sulfide gas can cause organ ischemia or cardiac or respiratory arrest. Eye contact with toxins (solid, liquid, or vapor) may damage the cornea, sclera, and lens, causing eye pain, redness, and loss of vision.

Table 366–1. SUBSTANCES USUALLY NOT DANGEROUS WHEN INGESTED*

Adhesives
Antibiotics, topical
Antifungals, topical
Barium sulfate
Bathtub toys (floating)
Blackboard chalk (Ca carbonate)
Bleach, hypochlorite (Na hypochlorite concentration < 6% and Na hydroxide concentration < 0.5%)
Candles (insect-repellent type may be toxic)
Carbowax (polyethylene glycol)
Carboxymethylcellulose (dehydrating material packed with drugs, film, and other products)
Castor oil
Cetyl alcohol
Cigarettes (small amounts ingested by a child)
Clay, art and craft
Contraceptives
Corticosteroids, topical
Crayons (children's; marked A.P., C.P., or C.S. 130–46)
Detergent, dishwashing, liquid
Dichloral (herbicide)
Diaper rash cream and ointment
Dry cell battery (alkaline)
Fabric softeners, solid sheets
Glow products (eg, glow sticks, glow necklaces)
Glycerol
Glyceryl monostearate
Graphite
Gums (eg, acacia, agar, ghatti)
Ink (amount in one ballpoint pen)
Iodide salts
Kaolin
Lanolin
Linoleic acid
Linseed oil (not boiled)
Lipstick
Lotion, calamine (excluding products with antihistamines or local anesthetics)
Lozenges, throat (without local anesthetics)
Magnesium silicate (antacid)
Make-up
Matches
Methylcellulose
Mineral oil (if not aspirated)
Newspaper
Paint, water-color or water-based
Paraffin, chlorinated
Pencil lead (graphite)
Petrolatum jelly
Plant food (household)
Polyethylene glycols
Polyethylene glycol stearate
Polysorbate
Putty
Shaving cream
Silica (silicon dioxide)
Soap (bath or dishwashing)
Spermaceti
Starch and sizing
Stearic acid
Talc (except when inhaled)
Titanium dioxide
Toothpaste (with or without fluoride)
Triacetin (glyceryl triacetate)
Vitamins, children's multiple with or without iron
Vitamins, multiple without iron
Zinc oxide
Zirconium oxide

*This table is intended only as a guide. Substances may be combined with phenol, petroleum distillate vehicles, or other toxic chemicals. A poison control center should be consulted for up-to-date information. Almost any substance can be toxic if ingested in sufficient amounts.

Some substances (eg, cocaine, phencyclidine, amphetamine) can cause severe agitation, which can result in hyperthermia, acidosis, and rhabdomyolysis.

Diagnosis

- Consideration of poisoning in patients with altered consciousness or unexplained symptoms
- History from all available sources
- Selective, directed testing

The first step of diagnosis of poisoning is to assess the overall status of the patient. Severe poisoning may require rapid intervention to treat airway compromise or cardiopulmonary collapse.

Poisoning may be known at presentation. It should be suspected if patients have unexplained symptoms, especially altered consciousness (which can range from agitation to somnolence to coma). If purposeful self-poisoning occurs in adults, multiple substances should be suspected.

History is often the most valuable tool. Because many patients (eg, preverbal children, suicidal or psychotic adults, patients with altered consciousness) cannot provide reliable information, friends, relatives, and rescue personnel should be questioned. Even seemingly reliable patients may incorrectly report the amount or time of ingestion. When possible, the patient's living quarters should be inspected for clues (eg, partially empty pill containers, a suicide note, evidence of recreational drug use). Pharmacy and medical records may provide useful information. In potential workplace poisonings, coworkers and supervisors should be questioned. All industrial chemicals must have a material safety data sheet (MSDS) readily available at the workplace; the MSDS provides detailed information about toxicity and any specific treatment.

In many parts of the world, information about household and industrial chemicals can be obtained from poison control centers. Consultation with the centers is encouraged because ingredients, first-aid measures, and antidotes printed on product containers are occasionally inaccurate or outdated. Also, the container may have been replaced, or the package may have been tampered with. Poison control centers may be able to help identify unknown pills based on their appearance. The centers have ready access to toxicologists. The telephone number of the nearest center is often listed with other emergency numbers in the front of the local telephone book; the number is also available from the telephone operator or, in the US, by dialing 1-800-222-1222. More information is available at the American Association of Poison Control Centers (www.aapcc.org).

Physical examination sometimes detects signs suggesting particular types of substances (eg, toxidromes [see Table 366–2], breath odor, presence of topical drugs, needle marks or tracks suggesting injected drug use, stigmata of chronic alcohol use).

Even if a patient is known to be poisoned, altered consciousness may be due to other causes (eg, CNS infection, head trauma, hypoglycemia, stroke, hepatic encephalopathy, Wernicke

Table 366–2. COMMON TOXIC SYNDROMES (TOXIDROMES)

SYNDROME	SYMPTOMS	COMMON CAUSES
Anticholinergic	Tachycardia, hyperthermia, mydriasis, warm and dry skin, urinary retention, ileus, delirium ("mad as a hatter, blind as a bat, red as a beet, hot as a hare, and dry as a bone"*)	Antihistamines Atropine Belladonna alkaloids Datura (angel's trumpet) Jimson weed Mushrooms (some) Psychoactive drugs (many) Scopolamine Tricyclic antidepressants
Cholinergic, muscarinic	*S*alivation, *l*acrimation, *u*rination, *d*efecation, *G*I cramps, *e*mesis (mnemonic device: SLUDGE) *or* *D*iarrhea; *u*rination; *m*iosis; *b*ronchorrhea, *b*radycardia, and *b*ronchoconstriction; *e*mesis; *l*acrimation; and *s*alivation (mnemonic device: DUMBELS) Wheezing	Carbamates Mushrooms (some) Organophosphates Physostigmine Pilocarpine Pyridostigmine
Cholinergic, nicotinic	*M*ydriasis, *t*achycardia, *w*eakness, *h*ypertension and *h*yperglycemia, *f*asciculations, *s*weating (mnemonic device: MTWT[h]FS) Abdominal pain, paresis	Black widow spider bites Carbamates Nicotine Organophosphates (some)
Opioid	Hypoventilation, hypotension, miosis, sedation, possibly hypothermia	Opioids (eg, diphenoxylate, fentanyl, heroin, methadone, morphine, pentazocine, propoxyphene)
Sympathomimetic	Tachycardia, hypertension, mydriasis, agitation, seizures, diaphoresis, hyperthermia, psychosis (after chronic use)	Amphetamines Caffeine Cocaine Ephedrine Herbal and synthetic marijuana and common substitutes MDMA (Ecstasy) Phenylpropanolamine Theophylline
Withdrawal	Tachycardia, mild hypertension, mydriasis, diaphoresis, agitation, restlessness, anxiety, hyperreflexia, piloerection, yawning, abdominal cramps, lacrimation, flu-like symptoms, insomnia, vomiting and diarrhea	Withdrawal from the following sedating or recreational drugs: • Barbiturates • Marijuana • Opioids
	Agitation, hallucinations, confusion, disorientation, seizures, hyperreflexia, hypertension, tachycardia, arrhythmias, dehydration, autonomic instability, death Baclofen: Severe muscle spasm	Withdrawal from the following drugs with sedative-hypnotic effects: • Alcohol • Baclofen • Benzodiazepines • GHB
	Decreased mental alertness, lethargy, coma, decreased blood pressure, decreased heart rate	Withdrawal from the following drugs with sympathomimetic effects: • Amphetamine • Cocaine • Phencyclidine • Synthetic cathinones (bath salts)
	Mild flu-like symptoms, insomnia, restlessness and anxiety	Withdrawal from the following drugs with antidepressant effects: • MAOIs • SSRIs • Tricyclic antidepressants

*From Carroll L: *Alice's Adventures in Wonderland*. London, MacMillan & Co., 1865.
GHB = gamma-hydroxybutyrate; MDMA = methylenedioxymethamphetamine.

encephalopathy), which should also be considered. Attempted suicide must always be considered in older children, adolescents, and adults who have ingested a drug. After such patients are stabilized, psychiatric intervention should be considered.

Testing: In most cases, laboratory testing provides limited help. Standard, readily available tests to identify common drugs of abuse (often called toxic screens) are qualitative, not quantitative. These tests may provide false-positive or false-negative results, and they check for only a limited number of substances. Also, the presence of a drug of abuse does not necessarily indicate that the drug caused the patient's symptoms or signs. Urine drug screening is used most often but has limited value and usually detects classes of drugs or metabolites rather than specific drugs. For example, an opioid urine immunoassay test does not detect fentanyl or methadone but does react with very small amounts of morphine or codeine analogues. The test used to identify cocaine detects a metabolite rather than cocaine itself.

For most substances, blood levels cannot be easily determined or do not help guide treatment. For a few substances (eg, acetaminophen, aspirin, carbon monoxide, digoxin, ethylene glycol, iron, lithium, methanol, phenobarbital, phenytoin, theophylline), blood levels may help guide treatment. Many authorities recommend measuring acetaminophen levels in all patients with mixed ingestions because acetaminophen ingestion is common, is often asymptomatic during the early stages, and can cause serious delayed toxicity that can be prevented by an antidote. For some substances, other blood tests (eg, PT for warfarin overdose, methemoglobin levels for certain substances) help guide treatment. For patients who have altered consciousness or abnormal vital signs or who have ingested certain substances, tests should include serum electrolytes, BUN, creatinine, serum osmolality, glucose, coagulation studies, and ABGs. Other tests (eg, methemoglobin level, carbon monoxide level, brain CT) may be indicated for certain suspected poisons or in certain clinical situations.

For certain poisonings (eg, due to iron, lead, arsenic, other metals, or to packets of cocaine or other illicit drugs ingested by so-called body packers), plain abdominal x-rays may show the presence and location of ingested substances.

For poisonings with drugs that have cardiovascular effects or with an unknown substance, ECG and cardiac monitoring are indicated.

If blood levels of a substance or symptoms of toxicity increase after initially decreasing or persist for an unusually long time, a bezoar, a sustained-release preparation, or reexposure (ie, repeated covert exposure to a recreationally used drug) should be suspected.

Treatment

- Supportive care
- Activated charcoal for serious oral poisonings
- Occasional use of specific antidotes or dialysis
- Only rare use of gastric emptying

Seriously poisoned patients may require assisted ventilation or treatment of cardiovascular collapse. Patients with impaired consciousness may require continuous monitoring or restraints. The discussion of treatment for specific poisonings, below and in Tables 366–3, 366–4, and 366–8 on p. 3069, is general and does not include specific complexities and details. Consultation with a poison control center is recommended for any poisonings except the mildest and most routine.

Initial stabilization:

- Maintain airway, breathing, and circulation
- IV naloxone
- IV dextrose and thiamine
- IV fluids, sometimes vasopressors

Table 366–3. COMMON SPECIFIC ANTIDOTES

TOXIN	ANTIDOTE
Acetaminophen	*N*-Acetylcysteine
Anticholinergics	Physostigmine*
Benzodiazepines	Flumazenil*
Black widow spider bite	Lactrodectus antivenom
Botulism	Botulinum antitoxin
β-Blockers	Glucagon IV lipid emulsion
Ca channel blockers	Ca IV insulin in high doses with IV glucose IV lipid emulsion
Carbamates	Atropine Pralidoxime chloride
Crotaline snake bites (US)	Crotalinae polyvalent immune Fab (ovine)
Cyanide	Hydroxocobalamin Cyanide antidote kit (includes amyl nitrate, Na nitrite, and Na thiosulfate)
Digitalis glycosides (eg, digoxin, digitoxin, oleander, foxglove)	Digoxin-specific Fab fragments
Ethylene glycol	Fomepizole Ethanol
Heavy metals	Chelating drugs (see Table 366–4)
Ionizing radiation	Potassium iodide
Iron	Deferoxamine
Isoniazid	Pyridoxine (vitamin B_6)
Methanol	Fomepizole Ethanol
Methemoglobin-forming agents (eg, aniline dyes, some local anesthetics, nitrates, nitrites, phenacetin, sulfonamides)	Methylene blue
Methotrexate	Leucovorin (folinic acid) Glucarpidase (carboxypeptidase-G2)
Opioids	Naloxone
Organophosphates	Atropine Pralidoxime
Scorpion envenomation (*Centruroides* sp)	Centruroides immune F(ab')2
Sulfonylurea	Octreotide
Thallium	Prussian blue
Tricyclic antidepressants	$NaHCO_3$
Unfractionated heparin	Protamine
Valproic acid	L-Carnitine
Warfarin	Vitamin K Fresh frozen plasma Prothrombin complex concentrate (PCC)

*Use is controversial.
Fab = fractionated antibodies.

Table 366–4. GUIDELINES FOR CHELATION THERAPY

CHELATING DRUG*	METAL	DOSAGE†
Deferoxamine	Iron	See Treatment of Iron Poisoning—p. 3067
Dimercaprol, 10% in oil	Antimony Arsenic Bismuth Copper salts Gold Lead Mercury Thallium*	3–4 mg/kg via deep IM injection q 4 h on day 1, 2 mg/kg IM q 4 h on day 2, 3 mg/kg IM q 6 h on day 3, then 3 mg/kg IM q 12 h for 7–10 days until recovery
Edetate Ca disodium (Ca disodium edathamil) diluted to ≤ 3%	Cobalt Lead Zinc Zinc salts	25–35 mg/kg via deep IM injection or IV slowly (over 1 h) q 12 h for 5–7 days, followed by 7 days without the drug; then repeated
Penicillamine	Arsenic Copper salts Gold Lead	5–7.5 mg/kg po qid (usual starting dose is 250 mg qid) to a maximum adult dose of 2 g/day
Succimer	Arsenic (occupational exposure in adults) Cadmium salts Lead if children have blood lead levels > 45 μg/dL (> 2.15 μmol/L) Lead (occupational exposure in adults) Mercury (occupational exposure in adults)	10 mg/kg po q 8 h for 5 days, then 10 mg/kg po q 12 h for 14 days

*Thallium salts are chelated with varying success by this drug (see thallium salts in Table 366–8).
†Dosages depend on type and severity of poisoning.

Airway, breathing, and circulation must be maintained in patients suspected of a systemic poisoning. Patients without a pulse or BP require emergency cardiopulmonary resuscitation.

If patients have apnea or compromised airways (eg, foreign material in the oropharynx, decreased gag reflex), an endotracheal tube should be inserted (see p. 554). If patients have respiratory depression or hypoxia, supplemental O_2 or mechanical ventilation should be provided as needed.

IV naloxone (2 mg in adults; 0.1 mg/kg in children) should be tried in patients with apnea or severe respiratory depression while maintaining airway support. In opioid addicts, naloxone may precipitate withdrawal, but withdrawal is preferable to severe respiratory depression. If respiratory depression persists despite use of naloxone, endotracheal intubation and continuous mechanical ventilation are required. If naloxone relieves respiratory depression, patients are monitored; if respiratory depression recurs, patients should be treated with another bolus of IV naloxone or endotracheal intubation and mechanical ventilation. Using a low-dose continuous naloxone infusion to maintain respiratory drive without precipitating withdrawal has been suggested but in reality can be very difficult to accomplish.

IV dextrose (50 mL of a 50% solution for adults; 2 to 4 mL/kg of a 25% solution for children) should be given to patients with altered consciousness or CNS depression, unless hypoglycemia has been ruled out by immediate bedside determination of blood glucose.

Thiamine (100 mg IV) is given with or before glucose to adults with suspected thiamine deficiency (eg, alcoholics, undernourished patients).

IV fluids are given for hypotension. If fluids are ineffective, invasive hemodynamic monitoring may be necessary to guide fluid and vasopressor therapy. The first-choice vasopressor for most poison-induced hypotension is norepinephrine 0.5 to 1 mg/min IV infusion, but treatment should not be delayed if another vasopressor is more immediately available.

Topical decontamination: Any body surface (including the eyes) exposed to a toxin is flushed with large amounts of water or saline. Contaminated clothing, including shoes and socks, and jewelry should be removed. Topical patches and transdermal delivery systems are removed.

Activated charcoal: Charcoal is usually given, particularly when multiple or unknown substances have been ingested. Use of charcoal adds little risk (unless patients are at risk of vomiting and aspiration) but has not been proved to reduce overall morbidity or mortality. When used, charcoal is given as soon as possible. Activated charcoal adsorbs most toxins because of its molecular configuration and large surface area. Multiple doses of activated charcoal may be effective for substances that undergo enterohepatic recirculation (eg, phenobarbital, theophylline) and for sustained-release preparations. Charcoal may be given at 4- to 6-h intervals for serious poisoning with such substances unless bowel sounds are hypoactive. Charcoal is ineffective for caustics, alcohols, and simple ions (eg, cyanide, iron, other metals, lithium).

The recommended dose is 5 to 10 times that of the suspected toxin ingested. However, because the amount of toxin ingested is usually unknown, the usual dose is 1 to 2 g/kg, which is about 10 to 25 g for children < 5 yr and 50 to 100 g for older children and adults. Charcoal is given as a slurry in water or soft drinks. It may be unpalatable and results in vomiting in 30% of patients. Administration via a gastric tube may be considered, but caution should be used to prevent trauma caused by tube insertion or aspiration of charcoal; potential benefits must outweigh risks. Activated charcoal should probably be used without sorbitol or other cathartics, which have no clear benefit and can cause dehydration and electrolyte abnormalities.

Gastric emptying: Gastric emptying, which used to be well-accepted and seems intuitively beneficial, should not be routinely done. It does not clearly reduce overall morbidity or mortality and has risks. Gastric emptying is considered if it can be done within 1 h of a life-threatening ingestion. However, many poisonings manifest too late, and whether a poisoning is life-threatening is not always clear. Thus, gastric emptying is seldom indicated and, if a caustic substance has been ingested, is contraindicated (see p. 3061).

If gastric emptying is used, gastric lavage is the preferred method. Gastric lavage may cause complications such as epistaxis, aspiration, or, rarely, oropharyngeal or esophageal injury. Syrup of ipecac has unpredictable effects, often causes prolonged vomiting, and may not remove substantial amounts of poison from the stomach. Syrup of ipecac may be warranted if the ingested agent is highly toxic and transport time to the emergency department is unusually long, but this is uncommon in the US.

For gastric lavage, tap water is instilled and withdrawn from the stomach via a tube. The largest tube possible (usually > 36 French for adults or 24 French for children) is used so that tablet fragments can be retrieved. If patients have altered consciousness or a weak gag reflex, endotracheal intubation should be done before lavage to prevent aspiration. Patients are placed in the left lateral decubitus position to prevent aspiration, and the tube is inserted orally. Because lavage sometimes forces substances farther into the GI tract, stomach contents should be aspirated and a 25-g dose of charcoal should be instilled through the tube immediately after insertion. Then aliquots (about 3 mL/kg) of tap water are instilled, and the gastric contents are withdrawn by gravity or syringe. Lavage continues until the withdrawn fluids appear free of the substance; usually, 500 to 3000 mL of fluid must be instilled. After lavage, a 2nd 25-g dose of charcoal is instilled.

Whole-bowel irrigation: This procedure flushes the GI tract and theoretically decreases GI transit time for pills and tablets. Irrigation has not been proved to reduce morbidity or mortality. Irrigation is indicated for any of the following:

- Some serious poisonings due to sustained-release preparations or substances that are not adsorbed by charcoal (eg, heavy metals)
- Drug packets (eg, latex-coated packets of heroin or cocaine ingested by body packers)
- A suspected bezoar

A commercially prepared solution of polyethylene glycol (which is nonabsorbable) and electrolytes is given at a rate of 1 to 2 L/h for adults or at 25 to 40 mL/kg/h for children until the rectal effluent is clear; this process may require many hours or even days. The solution is usually given via a gastric tube, although some motivated patients can drink these large volumes.

Alkaline diuresis: Alkaline diuresis enhances elimination of weak acids (eg, salicylates, phenobarbital). A solution made by combining 1 L of 5% D/W with 3 50-mEq ampules of $NaHCO_3$ and 20 to 40 mEq of K can be given at a rate of 250 mL/h in adults and 2 to 3 mL/kg/h in children. Urine pH is kept at > 8, and K must be repleted. Hypernatremia, alkalemia, and fluid overload may occur but are usually not serious. However, alkaline diuresis is contraindicated in patients with renal insufficiency.

Dialysis: Common toxins that may require dialysis or hemoperfusion include

- Ethylene glycol
- Lithium
- Methanol
- Salicylates
- Theophylline

These therapies are less useful if the poison is a large or charged (polar) molecule, has a large volume of distribution (ie, if it is stored in fatty tissue), or is extensively bound to tissue protein (as with digoxin, phencyclidine, phenothiazines, or tricyclic antidepressants). The need for dialysis is usually determined by both laboratory values and clinical status. Methods of dialysis include hemodialysis, peritoneal dialysis, and lipid dialysis (which removes lipid-soluble substances from the blood), as well as hemoperfusion (which more rapidly and efficiently clears specific poisons—see p. 2145).

Specific antidotes: For the most commonly used antidotes, see Table 366–3. Chelating drugs are used for poisoning with heavy metals and occasionally with other drugs (see Table 366–4). IV fat emulsions in 10% and 20% concentrations and high-dose insulin therapy have been used to successfully treat several different cardiac toxins (eg, bupivacaine, verapamil).

Ongoing supportive measures: Most symptoms (eg, agitation, sedation, coma, cerebral edema, hypertension, arrhythmias, renal failure, hypoglycemia) are treated with the usual supportive measures (see elsewhere in THE MANUAL).

Drug-induced hypotension and arrhythmias may not respond to the usual drug treatments. For refractory hypotension, dopamine, epinephrine, other vasopressors, an intra-aortic balloon pump, or even extracorporeal circulatory support may be considered.

For refractory arrhythmias, cardiac pacing may be necessary. Often, torsades de pointes can be treated with Mg sulfate 2 to 4 g IV, overdrive pacing, or a titrated isoproterenol infusion.

Seizures are first treated with benzodiazepines. Phenobarbital or phenytoin can also be used. Severe agitation must be controlled; benzodiazepines in large doses, other potent sedatives (eg, propofol), or, in extreme cases, induction of paralysis and mechanical ventilation may be required.

Hyperthermia is treated with aggressive sedation and physical cooling measures rather than with antipyretics. Organ failure may ultimately require kidney or liver transplantation.

Hospital admission: General indications for hospital admission include altered consciousness, persistently abnormal vital signs, and predicted delayed toxicity. For example, admission is considered if patients have ingested sustained-release preparations, particularly of drugs with potentially serious effects (eg, cardiovascular drugs). If there are no other reasons for admission, if indicated laboratory test results are normal, and if symptoms are gone after patients have been observed for 4 to 6 h, most patients can be discharged. However, if ingestion was intentional, patients require a psychiatric evaluation.

Prevention

In the US, widespread use of child-resistant containers with safety caps has greatly reduced the number of poisoning deaths in children < 5 yr. Limiting the amount of OTC analgesics in a single container and eliminating confusing and redundant formulations reduces the severity of poisonings, particularly with acetaminophen, aspirin, or ibuprofen.

Other preventive measures include

- Clearly labeling household products and prescription drugs
- Storing drugs and toxic substances in cabinets that are locked and inaccessible to children
- Promptly disposing of expired drugs by mixing them in cat litter or some other nontempting substance and putting them in a trash container that is inaccessible to children
- Using carbon monoxide detectors

Public education measures to encourage storage of substances in their original containers (eg, not placing insecticides in drink bottles) are important. Use of imprint identifications on solid drugs helps prevent confusion and errors by patients, pharmacists, and health care practitioners.

KEY POINTS

- Poisoning is distinguished from hypersensitivity and idiosyncratic reactions, which are unpredictable and not dose-related, and from intolerance, which is a toxic reaction to a usually nontoxic dose of a substance.
- Recognizing a toxidrome (eg, anticholinergic, muscarinic cholinergic, nicotinic cholinergic, opioid, sympathomimetic, withdrawal) can help narrow the differential diagnosis.
- Toxicity may be immediate, delayed (eg, acetaminophen, iron, *Amanita phalloides* mushrooms causing delayed hepatotoxicity), or occur only after repeated exposure.
- Maximize recognition of poisoning and identification of the specific poison by considering poisoning in all patients with unexplained alterations in consciousness and by searching thoroughly for clues from the history.
- Consider other causes (eg, CNS infection, head trauma, hypoglycemia, stroke, hepatic encephalopathy, Wernicke encephalopathy) if consciousness is altered, even if poisoning is suspected.
- Use toxicology testing (eg, drug immunoassays) selectively because it can provide incomplete or incorrect information.
- Treat all poisoning supportively and use activated charcoal for serious oral poisoning and other methods selectively.

ACETAMINOPHEN POISONING

Acetaminophen poisoning can cause gastroenteritis within hours and hepatotoxicity 1 to 3 days after ingestion. Severity of hepatotoxicity after a single acute overdose is predicted by serum acetaminophen levels. Treatment is with *N*-acetylcysteine to prevent or minimize hepatotoxicity.

Acetaminophen is contained in > 100 products sold OTC. Products include many children's preparations in liquid, tablet, and capsule form and many cough and cold preparations. Many prescription drugs also contain acetaminophen. Consequently, acetaminophen overdose is common.

Pathophysiology

The principal toxic metabolite of acetaminophen, *N*-acetyl-*p*-benzoquinone imine (NAPQI), is produced by the hepatic cytochrome P-450 enzyme system; glutathione stores in the liver detoxify this metabolite. An acute overdose depletes glutathione stores in the liver. As a result, NAPQI accumulates, causing hepatocellular necrosis and possibly damage to other organs (eg, kidneys, pancreas). Theoretically, alcoholic liver disease or undernutrition could increase risk of toxicity because hepatic enzyme preconditioning may increase formation of NAPQI and because undernutrition (also common among alcoholics) reduces hepatic glutathione stores. However, therapeutic doses of acetaminophen in alcoholic patients are not associated with hepatic injury.

Acute Acetaminophen Poisoning

To cause toxicity, an acute oral overdose must total ≥ 150 mg/kg (about 7.5 g in adults) within 24 h.

IV acetaminophen: An IV formulation of acetaminophen that is designed for use in hospitals and in patients > 2 yr of age has been associated with several hundred reports of overdoses, including several dozen fatalities, 3 in children. Most of these adverse events were the result of dosing errors because the drug is dosed in milligrams but dispensed in milliliters. Because these overdoses are iatrogenic, reliable information regarding time and total dose is available. The Rumack-Matthew nomogram (see Fig. 366–1) has thus been used with success to predict toxicity. Overdoses < 150 mg/kg are unlikely to result in toxicity. However, definitive treatment of IV acetaminophen overdose has not been determined, and consultation with a toxicologist or a poison control center is recommended.

Symptoms and Signs

Mild poisoning may not cause symptoms, and when present, symptoms of acute acetaminophen poisoning are usually minor until ≥ 48 h after ingestion. Symptoms, which occur in 4 stages (see Table 366–5), include anorexia, nausea, vomiting, and right upper quadrant abdominal pain. Renal failure and pancreatitis may occur, occasionally without liver failure. After > 5 days, hepatotoxicity resolves or progresses to multiple organ failure, which can be fatal.

Diagnosis

- Serum acetaminophen levels
- Rumack-Matthew nomogram

Acetaminophen overdose should be considered in all patients with nonaccidental ingestions that may be suicide attempts and in children with ingestions because formulations containing acetaminophen are frequently ingested in such overdoses and are not reported. Also, because acetaminophen often causes minimal symptoms during the early stages and is potentially lethal but treatable, ingestion should be considered in all patients with accidental ingestions as well.

Table 366–5. STAGES OF ACUTE ACETAMINOPHEN POISONING

STAGE	TIME POSTINGESTION	DESCRIPTION
I	0–24 h	Anorexia, nausea, vomiting
II	24–72 h	Right upper quadrant abdominal pain (common) AST, ALT, and, if poisoning is severe, bilirubin and PT (usually reported as the INR) sometimes elevated
III	72–96 h	Vomiting and symptoms of liver failure Peaking of AST, ALT, bilirubin, and INR Sometimes renal failure and pancreatitis
IV	> 5 days	Resolution of hepatotoxicity or progression to multiple organ failure (sometimes fatal)

PEARLS & PITFALLS

- Consider occult acetaminophen toxicity in all patients who have ingestions.

Likelihood and severity of hepatotoxicity caused by an acute ingestion can be predicted by the amount ingested or, more accurately, by the serum acetaminophen level. If the time of acute ingestion is known, the Rumack-Matthew nomogram (see Fig. 366–1) is used to estimate likelihood of hepatotoxicity; if the time of acute ingestion is unknown, the nomogram cannot be used. For a single acute overdose of traditional acetaminophen or rapid-relief acetaminophen (which is absorbed 7 to 8 min faster), levels are measured ≥ 4 h after ingestion and plotted on the nomogram. A level ≤ 150 μg/mL (≤ 990 μmol/L) and absence of toxic symptoms indicate that hepatotoxicity is very unlikely. Higher levels indicate possible hepatotoxicity. For a single acute overdose with extended-relief acetaminophen(which has 2 peak serum levels about 4 h apart), acetaminophen levels are measured ≥ 4 h after ingestion and 4 h later; if either level is above the Rumack-Matthew line of toxicity, treatment is required.

If poisoning is confirmed or strongly suspected or if the time of ingestion is unclear or unknown, additional testing is indicated. Liver function tests are done and, in suspected severe poisoning, PT is measured. AST and ALT results correlate with the stage of poisoning (see Table 366–5). AST levels > 1000 IU/L are more likely to result from acetaminophen poisoning than from chronic hepatitis or alcoholic liver disease. If poisoning is severe, bilirubin and INR may be elevated.

Low-level transaminase elevations (eg, up to 2 or 3 times the upper limit of normal) may occur in adults taking therapeutic doses of acetaminophen for days or weeks. These elevations appear to be transient, usually resolve or decrease (even with continued acetaminophen use), are usually clinically asymptomatic, and are probably insignificant.

Acetaminophen/cysteine protein adducts are new biomarkers developed and marketed as indicators of acetaminophen-induced hepatotoxicity. Although the biomarkers may indicate

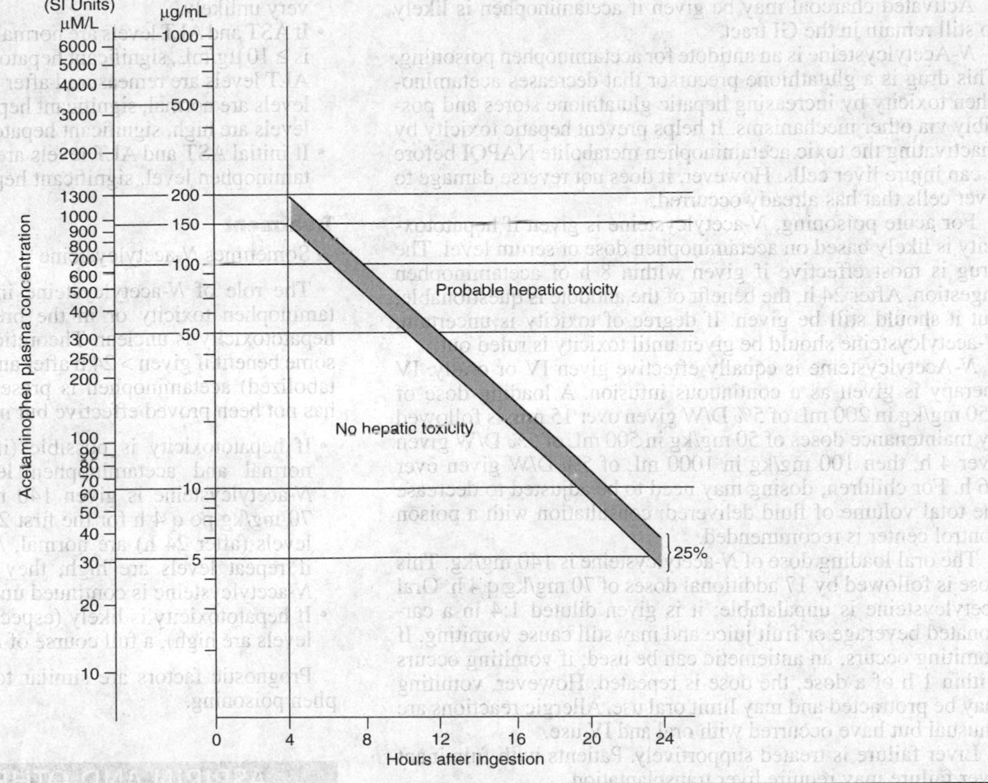

Fig. 366–1. Rumack-Matthew nomogram for single acute acetaminophen ingestions. Semilogarithmic plot of plasma acetaminophen levels vs time. *Cautions for use of this nomogram:*

- The time coordinates refer to time of ingestion.
- Serum levels drawn before 4 h may not represent peak levels.
- The graph should be used only in relation to a single acute ingestion.
- The lower solid line 25% below the standard nomogram is included to allow for possible errors in acetaminophenplasma assays and estimated time from
- ingestion of an overdose.

Adapted from Rumack BH, Matthew H: Acetaminophen poisoning and toxicity. *Pediatrics* 55(6):871–876, 1975; reproduced by permission of *Pediatrics*.

exposure to acetaminophen, they do not conclusively indicate acetaminophen-induced hepatotoxicity.

Prognosis

With appropriate treatment, mortality is uncommon.

Poor prognostic indicators at 24 to 48 h postingestion include all of the following:

- pH < 7.3 after adequate resuscitation
- INR > 3
- Serum creatinine > 2.6
- Hepatic encephalopathy grade III (confusion and somnolence) or grade IV (stupor and coma)
- Hypoglycemia
- Thrombocytopenia

Acute acetaminophen toxicity does not predispose patients to cirrhosis.

Treatment

- Oral or IV *N*-acetylcysteine
- Possibly activated charcoal

Activated charcoal may be given if acetaminophen is likely to still remain in the GI tract.

N-Acetylcysteine is an antidote for acetaminophen poisoning. This drug is a glutathione precursor that decreases acetaminophen toxicity by increasing hepatic glutathione stores and possibly via other mechanisms. It helps prevent hepatic toxicity by inactivating the toxic acetaminophen metabolite NAPQI before it can injure liver cells. However, it does not reverse damage to liver cells that has already occurred.

For acute poisoning, *N*-acetylcysteine is given if hepatotoxicity is likely based on acetaminophen dose or serum level. The drug is most effective if given within 8 h of acetaminophen ingestion. After 24 h, the benefit of the antidote is questionable, but it should still be given. If degree of toxicity is uncertain, *N*-acetylcysteine should be given until toxicity is ruled out.

N-Acetylcysteine is equally effective given IV or orally. IV therapy is given as a continuous infusion. A loading dose of 150 mg/kg in 200 mL of 5% D/W given over 15 min is followed by maintenance doses of 50 mg/kg in 500 mL of 5% D/W given over 4 h, then 100 mg/kg in 1000 mL of 5% D/W given over 16 h. For children, dosing may need to be adjusted to decrease the total volume of fluid delivered; consultation with a poison control center is recommended.

The oral loading dose of *N*-acetylcysteine is 140 mg/kg. This dose is followed by 17 additional doses of 70 mg/kg q 4 h. Oral acetylcysteine is unpalatable; it is given diluted 1:4 in a carbonated beverage or fruit juice and may still cause vomiting. If vomiting occurs, an antiemetic can be used; if vomiting occurs within 1 h of a dose, the dose is repeated. However, vomiting may be protracted and may limit oral use. Allergic reactions are unusual but have occurred with oral and IV use.

Liver failure is treated supportively. Patients with fulminant liver failure may require liver transplantation.

KEY POINTS

- Because acetaminophen is ubiquitous and initially asymptomatic and treatable in overdose, consider toxicity in all possibly poisoned patients.
- Use the Rumack-Matthew nomogram when time of ingestion is known to predict risk of hepatotoxicity based on serum acetaminophen levels.
- If hepatotoxicity is likely, give oral or IV *N*-acetylcysteine.
- If acetaminophen is still probably in the GI tract, give activated charcoal.
- If degree of toxicity is uncertain, begin IV or oral *N*-acetylcysteine until more conclusive definitive information is available.

Chronic Acetaminophen Poisoning

Chronic excessive use or repeated overdoses cause hepatotoxicity in a few patients. Usually, chronic overdose is not an attempt at self-injury but instead results from taking inappropriately high doses to treat pain. Symptoms may be absent or may include any of those that occur with acute overdose.

Diagnosis

- AST, ALT, and serum acetaminophen levels

The Rumack-Matthew nomogram cannot be used, but likelihood of clinically significant hepatotoxicity can be estimated based on AST, ALT, and serum acetaminophen levels.

- If AST and ALT levels are normal (< 50 IU/L) and the acetaminophen level is < 10 μg/mL, significant hepatotoxicity is very unlikely.
- If AST and ALT levels are normal but the acetaminophen level is ≥ 10 μg/mL, significant hepatotoxicity is possible; AST and ALT levels are remeasured after 24 h. If repeat AST and ALT levels are normal, significant hepatotoxicity is unlikely; if the levels are high, significant hepatotoxicity is assumed.
- If initial AST and ALT levels are high, regardless of the acetaminophen level, significant hepatotoxicity is assumed.

Treatment

- Sometimes *N*-acetylcysteine

The role of *N*-acetylcysteine in treatment of chronic acetaminophen toxicity or in the presence of established acute hepatotoxicity is unclear. Theoretically, the antidote may have some benefit if given > 24 h after an ingestion if residual (unmetabolized) acetaminophen is present. The following approach has not been proved effective but may be used:

- If hepatotoxicity is possible (if AST and ALT levels are normal and acetaminophen level is initially elevated), *N*-acetylcysteine is given 140 mg/kg po loading dose and 70 mg/kg po q 4 h for the first 24 h. If repeat AST and ALT levels (after 24 h) are normal, *N*-acetylcysteine is stopped; if repeat levels are high, they are remeasured daily, and *N*-acetylcysteine is continued until levels are normal.
- If hepatotoxicity is likely (especially if initial AST and ALT levels are high), a full course of *N*-acetylcysteine is given.

Prognostic factors are similar to those in acute acetaminophen poisoning.

ASPIRIN AND OTHER SALICYLATE POISONING

(Salicylism)

Salicylate poisoning can cause vomiting, tinnitus, confusion, hyperthermia, respiratory alkalosis, metabolic acidosis, and multiple organ failure. Diagnosis is clinical, supplemented by measurement of the anion gap, ABGs, and serum salicylate levels. Treatment is with activated charcoal and alkaline diuresis or hemodialysis.

Acute ingestion of > 150 mg/kg can cause severe toxicity. Salicylate tablets may form bezoars, prolonging absorption and toxicity. Chronic toxicity can occur after several days or more of high therapeutic doses; it is common, often undiagnosed, and often more serious than acute toxicity. Chronic toxicity tends to occur in elderly patients.

The most concentrated and toxic form of salicylate is oil of wintergreen (methyl salicylate, a component of some liniments and solutions used in hot vaporizers); ingestion of < 5 mL can kill a young child. Any exposure should be considered serious. Bismuth subsalicylate (8.7 mg salicylate/mL) is another potentially unexpected source of large amounts of salicylate.

PEARLS & PITFALLS

- Ingestion of < 5 mL of oil of wintergreen (methyl salicylate, a component of some liniments and solutions used in hot vaporizers) can kill a young child.

Pathophysiology

Salicylates impair cellular respiration by uncoupling oxidative phosphorylation. They stimulate respiratory centers in the medulla, causing primary respiratory alkalosis, which is often unrecognized in young children. Salicylates simultaneously and independently cause primary metabolic acidosis. Eventually, as salicylates disappear from the blood, enter the cells, and poison mitochondria, metabolic acidosis becomes the primary acid-base abnormality.

Salicylate poisoning also causes ketosis, fever, and, even when systemic hypoglycemia is absent, low brain glucose levels. Renal Na, K, and water loss and increased but imperceptible respiratory water loss due to hyperventilation lead to dehydration.

Salicylates are weak acids that cross cell membranes relatively easily; thus, they are more toxic when blood pH is low. Dehydration, hyperthermia, and chronic ingestion increase salicylate toxicity because they result in greater distribution of salicylate to tissues. Excretion of salicylates increases when urine pH increases.

Symptoms and Signs

With **acute overdose,** early symptoms include nausea, vomiting, tinnitus, and hyperventilation. Later symptoms include hyperactivity, fever, confusion, and seizures. Rhabdomyolysis, acute renal failure, and respiratory failure may eventually develop. Hyperactivity may quickly turn to lethargy; hyperventilation (with respiratory alkalosis) progresses to hypoventilation (with mixed respiratory and metabolic acidosis) and respiratory failure.

With **chronic overdose,** symptoms and signs tend to be nonspecific, vary greatly, and may suggest sepsis. They include subtle confusion, changes in mental status, fever, hypoxia, noncardiogenic pulmonary edema, dehydration, lactic acidosis, and hypotension.

PEARLS & PITFALLS

- Consider occult salicylate poisoning in elderly patients with findings that are nonspecific and/or compatible with sepsis (eg, subtle confusion, changes in mental status, fever, hypoxia, noncardiogenic pulmonary edema, dehydration, lactic acidosis, hypotension).

Diagnosis

- Serum salicylate level
- ABGs

Salicylate poisoning is suspected in patients with any of the following:

- History of a single acute overdose
- Repeated ingestions of therapeutic doses
- Unexplained metabolic acidosis
- Unexplained confusion and fever (in elderly patients)
- Other findings compatible with sepsis (eg, fever, hypoxia, noncardiogenic pulmonary edema, dehydration, hypotension)

If poisoning is suspected, serum salicylate level (drawn at least a few hours after ingestion), urine pH, ABGs, serum electrolytes, serum creatinine, plasma glucose, and BUN are measured. If rhabdomyolysis is suspected, serum CK and urine myoglobin are measured.

Significant salicylate toxicity is suggested by serum levels much higher than therapeutic (therapeutic range, 10 to 20 mg/dL), particularly 6 h after ingestion (when absorption is usually almost complete), and by acidemia plus ABG results compatible with salicylate poisoning. Serum levels are helpful in confirming the diagnosis and may help guide therapy, but levels may be misleading and should be clinically correlated.

Usually, ABGs show primary respiratory alkalosis during the first few hours after ingestion; later, they show compensated metabolic acidosis or mixed metabolic acidosis/respiratory alkalosis. Eventually, usually as salicylate levels decrease, poorly compensated or uncompensated metabolic acidosis is the primary finding. If respiratory failure occurs, ABGs suggest combined metabolic and respiratory acidosis, and chest x-ray shows diffuse pulmonary infiltrates. Plasma glucose levels may be normal, low, or high. Serial salicylate levels help determine whether absorption is continuing; ABGs and serum electrolytes should always be determined simultaneously. Increased serum CK and urine myoglobin levels suggest rhabdomyolysis.

Treatment

- Activated charcoal
- Alkaline diuresis with extra KCl

Unless contraindicated (eg, by altered mental status), activated charcoal is given as soon as possible and, if bowel sounds are present, may be repeated every 4 h until charcoal appears in the stool.

After volume and electrolyte abnormalities are corrected, alkaline diuresis can be used to increase urine pH, ideally to ≥ 8. Alkaline diuresis is indicated for patients with any symptoms of poisoning and should not be delayed until salicylate levels are determined. This intervention is usually safe and exponentially increases salicylate excretion. Because hypokalemia may interfere with alkaline diuresis, patients are given a solution consisting of 1 L of 5% D/W, 3 50-mEq ampules of $NaHCO_3$, and 40 mEq of KCl at 1.5 to 2 times the maintenance IV fluid rate. Serum K is monitored. Because fluid overload can result in pulmonary edema, patients are monitored for respiratory findings.

Drugs that increase urinary HCO_3 (eg, acetazolamide) should be avoided because they worsen metabolic acidosis and decrease blood pH. Drugs that decrease respiratory drive should be avoided if possible because they may impair hyperventilation and respiratory alkalosis, decreasing blood pH.

Fever can be treated with physical measures such as external cooling. Seizures are treated with benzodiazepines. In patients with rhabdomyolysis, adequate hydration and urine output are crucial; alkaline diuresis may also help prevent renal failure.

Hemodialysis may be required to enhance salicylate elimination in patients with severe neurologic impairment, renal or respiratory insufficiency, acidemia despite other measures, or very high serum salicylate levels (> 100 mg/dL [> 7.25 mmol/L] with acute overdose or > 60 mg/dL [> 4.35 mmol/L] with chronic overdose).

Treating acid-base alterations in salicylate-poisoned patients who require endotracheal intubation and mechanical ventilation for airway protection or oxygenation can be extremely challenging. In general, intubated patients should probably be dialyzed and closely monitored by a critical care specialist.

KEY POINTS

- Salicylate poisoning causes respiratory alkalosis and, by an independent mechanism, metabolic acidosis.
- Consider salicylate toxicity in patients with nonspecific findings (eg, alteration in mental status, metabolic acidosis, noncardiogenic pulmonary edema, fever), even when a history of ingestion is lacking.
- Estimate the severity of toxicity by the salicylate level and ABGs.
- Treat with activated charcoal and alkaline diuresis with extra KCl.
- Consider hemodialysis if poisoning is severe.

CARBON MONOXIDE POISONING

Carbon monoxide (CO) poisoning causes acute symptoms such as headache, nausea, weakness, angina, dyspnea, loss of consciousness, seizures, and coma. Neuropsychiatric symptoms may develop weeks later. Diagnosis is by carboxyhemoglobin levels and ABGs, including measured O_2 saturation. Treatment is with supplemental O_2. Prevention is often possible with household CO detectors.

CO poisoning, one of the most common fatal poisonings, occurs by inhalation. CO is a colorless, odorless gas that results from incomplete combustion of hydrocarbons. Common sources of CO in poisonings include house fires and improperly vented automobiles, gas heaters, furnaces, hot water heaters, wood- or charcoal-burning stoves, and kerosene heaters. CO is produced when natural gas (methane or propane) burns. Inhaling tobacco smoke results in CO in the blood but not enough to cause poisoning.

Pathophysiology

The elimination half-life of CO is about 4.5 h with inhalation of room air, 1.5 h with 100% O_2, and 20 min with 3 atmospheres (pressure) of O_2 (as in a hyperbaric chamber—see p. 3027).

Mechanisms of CO toxicity are not completely understood. They appear to involve

- Displacement of O_2 from Hb (because CO has greater affinity for Hb than does O_2)
- Shifting of the O_2-Hb dissociation curve to the left (decreasing release of O_2 from Hb to tissues—see Fig. 50–4 on p. 397)
- Inhibition of mitochondrial respiration
- Possibly direct toxic effects on brain tissue

Symptoms and Signs

CO poisoning symptoms tend to correlate well with the patient's peak blood carboxyhemoglobin levels. Many symptoms are nonspecific.

- Headache and nausea can begin when levels are 10 to 20%.
- Levels > 20% commonly cause vague dizziness, generalized weakness, difficulty concentrating, and impaired judgment.
- Levels > 30% commonly cause dyspnea during exertion, chest pain (in patients with coronary artery disease), and confusion.
- Higher levels can cause syncope, seizures, and obtundation.

Hypotension, coma, respiratory failure, and death may occur, usually when levels are > 60%.

Patients may also have many other symptoms, including visual deficits, abdominal pain, and focal neurologic deficits. If poisoning is severe, neuropsychiatric symptoms and signs (eg, dementia, psychosis, parkinsonism, chorea, amnestic syndromes) can develop days to weeks after exposure and become permanent. Because CO poisoning often results from house fires, patients may have concomitant airway injuries (see p. 2954), which may increase risk of respiratory failure.

Diagnosis

- Diagnosis considered when patients at risk have nonspecific symptoms or metabolic acidosis
- Venous carboxyhemoglobin level

Because symptoms can be vague, nonspecific, and variable, the diagnosis of CO poisoning is easily missed. Many cases of mild poisoning with nonspecific symptoms are mistaken for viral syndromes. Physicians must maintain a high level of suspicion. If people from the same dwelling, particularly a heated dwelling, experience nonspecific flu-like symptoms, CO exposure should be considered.

If CO poisoning is suspected, the carboxyhemoglobin level is measured with a CO-oximeter; venous samples can be used because arteriovenous differences are trivial. ABGs are not measured routinely. ABGs and pulse oximetry, alone or combined, are inadequate for diagnosis of CO poisoning because O_2 saturation reported in ABGs represents dissolved O_2 and is thus unaffected by carboxyhemoglobin concentration; furthermore, the pulse oximeter cannot differentiate normal Hb from carboxyhemoglobin and thus provides a falsely elevated oxyhemoglobin reading. Noninvasive CO detectors have not been shown to be accurate or useful in the diagnosis of CO exposure or toxicity.

Although elevated carboxyhemoglobin levels are clear evidence of poisoning, levels may be falsely low because they decrease rapidly after CO exposure ends, particularly in patients treated with supplemental O_2 (eg, in an ambulance). Metabolic acidosis can be a clue to the diagnosis. Other tests may help evaluate specific symptoms (eg, ECG for chest pain, CT for neurologic symptoms).

Treatment

- 100% O_2
- Possibly hyperbaric O_2

Patients should be removed from the source of CO and stabilized as necessary. They are given 100% O_2 (by nonrebreather mask) and treated supportively. Although its use is becoming increasingly controversial, hyperbaric O_2 therapy (in a chamber at 2 to 3 atmospheres of 100% O_2) typically should be considered for patients who have any of the following:

- Life-threatening cardiopulmonary complications
- Ongoing chest pain
- Altered consciousness
- Loss of consciousness (no matter how brief)
- A carboxyhemoglobin level > 25%

Hyperbaric O_2 therapy should also be considered for pregnant patients, possibly at lower serum CO levels than in nonpregnant patients.

Hyperbaric O_2 therapy may decrease the incidence of delayed neuropsychiatric symptoms. However, this therapy may cause barotrauma and, because therapy is not available at most hospitals, may require transfer of patients, who may not be stable; also, a chamber may not be available locally. Evidence for the efficacy of hyperbaric O_2 therapy is becoming more controversial, with some studies suggesting harm. In cases where hyperbaric O_2 therapy is considered, consultation with a poison control center or hyperbaric expert is strongly recommended.

Prevention

Prevention involves checking sources of indoor combustion to make sure they are correctly installed and vented to the outdoors. Exhaust pipes should be inspected periodically for leaks. Cars should never be left running in an enclosed garage. CO detectors should be installed because they provide early warning that CO is free in a dwelling's atmosphere. If CO is suspected in a dwelling, windows should be opened, and the dwelling should be evacuated and evaluated for the source of CO.

KEY POINTS

- CO poisoning (eg, caused by house fires, improperly vented automobiles, gas heaters, furnaces, hot water heaters, wood- or charcoal-burning stoves, or kerosene heaters) is one of the most common fatal poisonings.
- Consider toxicity is patients with nonspecific symptoms (eg, flu-like symptoms in winter) or unexplained metabolic acidosis.
- Measure CO level with a CO-oximeter.
- Do not rule out toxicity based on a normal CO level because levels can decrease rapidly, particularly after treatment with supplemental O_2.
- Treat with 100% O_2.
- For severe poisoning, consult an expert or poison control center to discuss treatment with hyperbaric O_2.

CAUSTIC INGESTION

Caustics (strong acids and alkalis), when ingested, burn upper GI tract tissues, sometimes resulting in esophageal or gastric perforation. Symptoms may include drooling, dysphagia, and pain in the mouth, chest, or stomach; strictures may develop later. Diagnostic endoscopy may be required. Treatment is supportive. Gastric emptying and activated charcoal are contraindicated. Perforation is treated surgically.

Worldwide, 80% of caustic ingestions occur in young children; these are usually accidental ingestions of small amounts and are often benign. In adults, caustic ingestions are frequently intentional ingestions of large amounts by suicidal people and are life-threatening. Common sources of caustics include solid and liquid drain and toilet bowl cleaners. Industrial products are usually more concentrated than household products and thus tend to be more damaging.

Pathophysiology

Acids cause coagulation necrosis; an eschar forms, limiting further damage. Acids tend to affect the stomach more than the esophagus. Alkalis cause rapid liquefaction necrosis; no eschar forms, and damage continues until the alkali is neutralized or diluted. Alkalis tend to affect the esophagus more than the stomach, but ingestion of large quantities severely affects both.

Solid products tend to leave particles that stick to and burn tissues, discouraging further ingestion and causing localized damage. Because liquid preparations do not stick, larger quantities are easily ingested, and damage may be widespread. Liquids may also be aspirated, leading to upper airway injury.

Symptoms and Signs

Initial symptoms of caustic ingestion include drooling and dysphagia. In severe cases, pain, vomiting, and sometimes bleeding develop immediately in the mouth, throat, chest, or abdomen. Airway burns may cause coughing, tachypnea, or stridor.

Swollen, erythematous tissue may be visible intraorally; however, caustic liquids may cause no intraoral burns despite serious injury farther down the GI tract.

Esophageal perforation may result in mediastinitis, with severe chest pain, tachycardia, fever, tachypnea, and shock. Gastric perforation may result in peritonitis. Esophageal or gastric perforation may occur within hours, after weeks, or any time in between.

Esophageal strictures can develop over weeks, even if initial symptoms had been mild and treatment had been adequate.

Diagnosis

- Endoscopy

Because the presence or absence of intraoral burns does not reliably indicate whether the esophagus and stomach are burned, meticulous endoscopy is indicated to check for the presence and severity of esophageal and gastric burns when symptoms or history suggests more than trivial ingestion.

Treatment

- Avoidance of gastric emptying
- Sometimes dilution with oral fluids

Treatment of caustic ingestion is supportive. (CAUTION: *Gastric emptying by emesis or lavage is contraindicated because it can reexpose the upper GI tract to the caustic. Attempts to neutralize a caustic acid by correcting pH with an alkaline substance [and vice versa] are contraindicated because severe exothermic reactions may result. Activated charcoal is contraindicated because it may infiltrate burned tissue and interfere with endoscopic evaluation and insertion of an NGT is contraindicated because it can damage already compromised mucosal surfaces.*)

PEARLS & PITFALLS

- Do not do gastric emptying by emesis or lavage with a caustic ingestion because it reexposes the upper GI tract to the caustic.
- Do not attempt to neutralize a caustic acid with an alkaline substance (and vice versa) because it will produce heat that may worsen tissue damage.

Dilution with milk or water is only useful in the first few minutes after ingesting a liquid caustic, but delayed dilution may be useful after ingesting a solid caustic. Dilution should be avoided if patients have nausea, drooling, stridor, or abdominal distention.

Esophageal or gastric perforation is treated with antibiotics and surgery (see p. 87). IV corticosteroids and prophylactic antibiotics are not recommended. Strictures are treated with bougienage or, if they are severe or unresponsive, with esophageal bypass by colonic interposition.

KEY POINTS

- Suspect severe consequences if a large volume of a caustic or an industrial-strength caustic product is ingested.
- Alkalis, by causing liquefaction, can cause damage until they are sufficiently diluted.
- Do not do gastric emptying or give activated charcoal, or neutralize an acid or alkali.
- Consider esophageal and stomach burns and do endoscopy, even if intraoral burns are absent.
- Treat perforation with antibiotics and surgery.

MUSHROOM POISONING

Numerous mushroom species cause toxicity when ingested. Symptoms vary by species. Identification of specific species is difficult, so treatment usually is guided by symptoms.

Differentiating toxic and nontoxic species in the wild is difficult, even for highly knowledgeable people. Folklore rules are unreliable, and the same species may have varying degrees of toxicity depending on where and when they are harvested. If patients have eaten an unidentified mushroom, identifying the species can help determine specific treatment. However, because an experienced mycologist is seldom available for immediate consultation, treatment of patients who become ill after mushroom ingestion is usually guided by symptoms. If a sample of the mushroom, uningested or from the patient's emesis, is available, it can be sent to a mycologist for analysis.

All toxic mushrooms cause vomiting and abdominal pain; other manifestations vary significantly by mushroom type. Generally, mushrooms that cause symptoms early (within 2 h) are less dangerous than those that cause symptoms later (usually after 6 h).

Treatment for most mushroom poisonings is symptomatic and supportive. Activated charcoal may be useful to limit absorption. Numerous antidotal therapies have been tried, especially for *Amanita* species, but none have shown consistently positive results.

Early GI symptoms: Mushrooms that cause early GI symptoms (eg, *Chlorophyllum molybdites* and the little brown mushrooms that often grow in lawns) cause gastroenteritis, sometimes with headaches or myalgias. Diarrhea is occasionally bloody.

Symptoms usually resolve within 24 h.

Treatment is supportive.

Early neurologic symptoms: Mushrooms that cause early neurologic symptoms include hallucinogenic mushrooms, which are usually ingested recreationally because they contain psilocybin, a hallucinogen. The most common are members of the *Psilocybe* genus, but some other genera contain psilocybin.

Symptoms begin within 15 to 30 min and include euphoria, enhanced imagination, and hallucinations. Tachycardia and hypertension are common, and hyperpyrexia occurs in some children; however, serious consequences are rare.

Treatment occasionally involves sedation (eg, with benzodiazepines).

Early muscarinic symptoms: Mushrooms that cause early muscarinic symptoms include members of the *Inocybe* and *Clitocybe* genera.

Symptoms may include the SLUDGE syndrome (see Table 366–2), including miosis, bronchorrhea, bradycardia, diaphoresis, wheezing, and fasciculations. Symptoms are usually mild, begin within 30 min, and resolve within 12 h.

Atropine may be given to treat severe muscarinic symptoms (eg, wheezing, bradycardia).

Delayed GI symptoms: Mushrooms that cause delayed GI symptoms include members of the *Amanita, Gyromitra,* and *Cortinarius* genera.

The most toxic *Amanita* mushroom is *Amanita phalloides,* which causes 95% of mushroom poisoning deaths. Initial gastroenteritis, which may occur 6 to 12 h after ingestion, can be severe; hypoglycemia can occur. Initial symptoms abate for a few days; then liver failure and sometimes renal failure develop. Initial care involves close monitoring for hypoglycemia and possibly repeated doses of activated charcoal. Treatment of liver failure may require liver transplantation; other specific treatments (eg, *N*-acetylcysteine, high-dose penicillin, silibinin, IV fat emulsion) are unproved.

Amanita smithiana mushrooms cause delayed gastroenteritis, usually 6 to 12 h after ingestion, and acute renal failure (usually within 1 to 2 wk after ingestion) that often requires dialysis.

Gyromitra mushrooms can cause hypoglycemia simultaneously with or shortly after gastroenteritis. Other manifestations may include CNS toxicity (eg, seizures) and, after a few days, hepatorenal syndrome. Initial care involves close monitoring for hypoglycemia and possibly repeated doses of activated charcoal. Neurologic symptoms are treated with pyridoxine 70 mg/kg slow IV infusion over 4 to 6 h (maximum daily dose of 5 g); liver failure is treated supportively.

Most *Cortinarius* mushrooms are indigenous to Europe. Gastroenteritis may last for 3 days. Renal failure, with symptoms of flank pain and decreased urine output, may occur 3 to 20 days after ingestion. Renal failure often resolves spontaneously.

PLANT POISONING

A few commonly grown plants are highly poisonous, and many plants are moderately poisonous (see Table 366–6). Few plant poisonings have specific antidotes. Most plant ingestions, including the plants listed in Table 366–6, result in minimal symptoms unless the leaves and other components are concentrated into a paste or brewed into a tea.

Highly toxic and potentially fatal plants include the following:

- Castor beans and jequirity beans
- Oleander and foxglove
- Hemlock

Castor beans and jequirity beans: Castor beans contain ricin, an extremely concentrated cellular poison. Jequirity beans contain abrin, a related and even more potent toxin. In both, the beans have a relatively impervious shell; thus, the bean must be chewed to release the toxin. However, the seed coating of the jequirity bean is often not intact, and simple bacterial digestion can release the abrin toxin.

Symptoms of either poisoning may include delayed gastroenteritis, sometimes severe and hemorrhagic, followed by delirium, seizures, coma, and death. Whole-bowel irrigation should be considered because it aims to remove all beans ingested.

Oleander and foxglove: These plants and lily of the valley (which is similar but less toxic) contain digitalis glycosides.

Table 366–6. MODERATELY POISONOUS PLANTS

PLANT	SYMPTOMS	TREATMENT
Aconitine (eg, derived from monkshood)	Bradycardia, dysrhythmias, paresthesia, weakness	Supportive care Sodium bicarbonate
Aloe spp	Gastroenteritis, nephritis, skin irritation	Supportive care and irrigation with soap and water
Aristolochia spp (birthworts, pipevines)	Tubulointerstitial nephropathy	Supportive care
Azalea	Cholinergic symptoms	Supportive care and atropine
Caladium spp (elephant ear, angel's wings)	Oral mucosal damage due to Ca oxalate crystals in leaves	Supportive care and demulsification (eg, with milk or ice cream)
Capsicum spp (peppers)	Mucous membrane irritation and swelling	Supportive care, irrigation
Colchicine (autumn crocus, meadow saffron, glory lily)	Delayed gastroenteritis, multiple organ failure Bone marrow suppression	Supportive care and possibly, as a last resort, experimental colchicine-specific Fab fragments*
Cyanogenic glycosides (eg, in *Prunus* spp [eg, peach, apricot, and wild cherry pits], *Malus* spp [eg, apple seeds], and other seeds)	Symptoms of cyanide poisoning	Hydroxocobalamin Cyanide antidote kit (includes amyl nitrate, Na nitrite, and Na thiosulfate)
Deadly nightshade	Anticholinergic symptoms, hyperthermia, seizures, hallucinations	Supportive care For severe hyperthermia or seizures, possibly physostigmine
Dieffenbachia (dumbcane)	Oral mucosal damage due to Ca oxalate crystals in leaves	Supportive care and demulsification (eg, with milk or ice cream)
Fava beans	In patients with G6PD deficiency, gastroenteritis, fever, headache, hemolytic anemia	Supportive care For severe anemia and poisoning, consideration of exchange transfusion
Green potato and potato sprout	Gastroenteritis, hallucinations, delirium	Supportive care
Holly berries	Gastroenteritis	Supportive care
Jimsonweed	Anticholinergic symptoms, hyperthermia, seizures, hallucinations	Supportive care For severe hyperthermia or seizures, possibly physostigmine
Licorice (not the artificially flavored licorice candy)	Hypokalemia, hypertension, and retention of water and Na (pseudohyperaldosteronism)	Supportive
Lily of the valley	Hyperkalemia, gastroenteritis, confusion, arrhythmias	See Digitalis preparations on p. 723
Mistletoe	Gastroenteritis	Supportive care
Nettle	Local stinging and burning	Supportive care
Nightshade, common or woody	Gastroenteritis, hallucinations, delirium	Supportive care
Pennyroyal	Hepatotoxicity	*N*-Acetylcysteine
Philodendron spp	Oral mucosal damage due to Ca oxalate crystals in leaves	Supportive care and demulsification (eg, with milk or ice cream)
Poinsettia	Minor mucous membrane irritation	Unnecessary
Poison ivy	Dermatitis	See Contact Dermatitis on p. 1024
Pokeweed	Mucous membrane irritation, gastroenteritis	Supportive care
Pothos	Oral mucosal damage due to Ca oxalate crystals in leaves	Supportive care and demulsification (eg, with milk or ice cream)
Yew	Gastroenteritis Rarely, seizures, arrhythmias, coma	Supportive care

*Available only in France.
Fab = fractionated antibodies.

Toxicity includes gastroenteritis, confusion, hyperkalemia, and arrhythmias. The serum digoxin level can confirm ingestion but is not useful as quantitative information.

K levels are closely monitored. Hyperkalemia may respond only to hemodialysis. Ca is not recommended for arrhythmias. Digoxin-specific fractionated antibody (Fab) fragments have been used to treat ventricular arrhythmias.

Hemlock: Hemlock poisoning (poison hemlock and water hemlock) can cause symptoms within 15 min.

Poison hemlock has nicotinic effects, beginning with dry mouth and progressing to tachycardia, tremors, diaphoresis, mydriasis, seizures, and muscle paresis. Rhabdomyolysis and bradycardia may occur.

Water hemlock seems to enhance γ-aminobutyric acid (GABA) activity. Symptoms may include gastroenteritis, delirium, refractory seizures, and coma.

FISH POISONING AND SHELLFISH POISONING

Fish poisoning and shellfish poisoning commonly cause GI, neurologic, or histamine-mediated manifestations.

Ciguatera poisoning: Ciguatera poisoning may result from eating any of > 400 species of fish from the tropical reefs of Florida, the West Indies, or the Pacific, where a dinoflagellate produces a toxin that accumulates in the flesh of the fish. Older fish and large fish (eg, grouper, snapper, kingfish) contain more toxin. No known processing procedures, including cooking, are protective, and flavor is unaffected. A commercial product is available to test for ciguatoxin in fish.

Symptoms may begin 2 to 8 h after eating. Abdominal cramps, nausea, vomiting, and diarrhea last 6 to 17 h; then, pruritus, paresthesias, headache, myalgia, reversal of hot and cold sensation, and face pain may occur. For months afterward, unusual sensory phenomena and nervousness may cause debilitation.

IV mannitol has been suggested as a treatment, but no clear benefit has been shown.

Scombroid poisoning: Scombroid poisoning is caused by high histamine levels in fish flesh due to bacterial decomposition after the fish is caught. Commonly affected species include

- Tuna
- Mackerel
- Bonito
- Skipjack
- Mahi mahi

The fish may taste peppery or bitter. Facial flushing and possibly nausea, vomiting, epigastric pain, and urticaria occur within a few minutes of eating and resolve within 24 h. Symptoms are often mistaken for those of a seafood allergy. Unlike other fish poisonings, this poisoning can be prevented by properly storing the fish after it is caught.

Treatment may include H_1 and H_2 blockers.

Tetrodotoxin poisoning: Tetrodotoxin poisoning is most commonly due to eating the puffer fish (fugu), a sushi delicacy, but > 100 fresh and salt water species contain tetrodotoxin. Symptoms are similar to those of ciguatera poisoning; potentially fatal respiratory paralysis can also occur. Treatment is supportive care with attention to ventilatory assistance until the toxin is metabolized, which may take days.

The toxin cannot be destroyed by cooking or freezing.

Shellfish poisoning: Paralytic shellfish poisoning can occur from June to October, especially on the Pacific and New England coasts, when mussels, clams, oysters, and scallops are contaminated by the poisonous dinoflagellate responsible for red tide. This dinoflagellate produces the neurotoxin saxitoxin, which is resistant to cooking. Circumoral paresthesias occur 5 to 30 min after eating. Nausea, vomiting, and abdominal cramps then develop, followed by muscle weakness. Untreated respiratory paralysis may be fatal; for survivors, recovery is usually complete.

HYDROCARBON POISONING

Hydrocarbon poisoning may result from ingestion or inhalation. Ingestion, most common among children < 5 yr, can result in aspiration pneumonitis. Inhalation, most common among adolescents, can result in ventricular fibrillation, usually without warning symptoms. Diagnosis of pneumonitis is by clinical evaluation, chest x-ray, and oximetry. Gastric emptying is contraindicated because aspiration is a risk. Treatment is supportive.

Ingestion of hydrocarbons, such as petroleum distillates (eg, gasoline, kerosene, mineral oil, lamp oil, paint thinners), results in minimal systemic effects but can cause severe aspiration pneumonitis. Toxic potential mainly depends on viscosity, measured in Saybolt seconds universal (SSU). Hydrocarbon liquids with low viscosity (SSU < 60), such as gasoline and mineral oil, can spread rapidly over large surface areas and are more likely to cause aspiration pneumonitis than are hydrocarbons with SSU > 60, such as tar. Hydrocarbons, if ingested in large amounts, may be absorbed systemically and cause CNS or hepatic toxicity, which is more likely with halogenated hydrocarbons (eg, carbon tetrachloride, trichloroethylene).

Recreational inhalation of halogenated hydrocarbons (eg, glues, paint, solvents, cleaning sprays, gasoline, fluorocarbons used as refrigerants or propellants in aerosols—see p. 3247), called huffing or bagging, is common among adolescents. It can cause euphoria and mental status changes and can sensitize the heart to endogenous catecholamines. Fatal ventricular arrhythmias may result; they usually occur without premonitory palpitations or other warning, often when patients are startled or chased.

Chronic toluene ingestion can cause long-term CNS toxicity, characterized by .periventricular, occipital, and thalamic destruction.

Symptoms and Signs

After ingestion of even a very small amount of liquid hydrocarbon, patients initially cough, choke, and may vomit. Young children may have cyanosis, hold their breath, and cough persistently. Older children and adults may report burning in the stomach.

Aspiration pneumonitis causes hypoxia and respiratory distress. Symptoms and signs of pneumonitis may develop a few hours before infiltrates are visible on x-ray. Substantial systemic absorption, particularly of a halogenated hydrocarbon, may cause lethargy, coma, and seizures. Nonfatal pneumonitis usually resolves in about 1 wk; mineral or lamp oil ingestion usually resolves in 5 to 6 wk.

Arrhythmias usually occur before presentation and are unlikely to recur after presentation unless patients have excessive agitation.

Diagnosis

- Chest x-ray and oximetry done about 6 h after ingestion

If patients are too obtunded to provide a history, hydrocarbon exposure may be suspected if their breath or clothing has an odor or if a container is found near them. Paint residue on the hands or around the mouth may suggest recent paint sniffing.

Diagnosis of aspiration pneumonitis is by symptoms and signs as well as by chest x-ray and oximetry, which are done about 6 h after ingestion or sooner if symptoms are severe. If respiratory failure is suspected, ABGs are measured.

CNS toxicity is diagnosed by neurologic examination and MRI.

Treatment

- Supportive care
- Avoidance of gastric emptying

Any contaminated clothing is removed, and the skin is washed. (CAUTION: *Gastric emptying, which increases risk of aspiration, is contraindicated.*) Charcoal is not recommended. Patients who do not have aspiration pneumonitis or other symptoms after 4 to 6 h are discharged. Patients who have symptoms are admitted and treated supportively; antibiotics and corticosteroids are not indicated.

PEARLS & PITFALLS

- Avoid gastric emptying if hydrocarbon ingestion is suspected (sometimes suspected based on odor of breath or clothing).

ORGANOPHOSPHATE POISONING AND CARBAMATE POISONING

Organophosphates and carbamates are common insecticides that inhibit cholinesterase activity, causing acute muscarinic manifestations (eg, salivation, lacrimation, urination, diarrhea, emesis, bronchorrhea, bronchospasm, bradycardia, miosis) and some nicotinic symptoms, including muscle fasciculations and weakness. Neuropathy can develop days to weeks after exposure. Diagnosis is clinical and sometimes with a trial of atropine, measurement of RBC acetylcholinesterase level, or both. Bronchorrhea and bronchospasm are treated with titrated high-dose atropine. Neuromuscular toxicity is treated with IV pralidoxime.

Organophosphates and carbamates, although different structurally, both inhibit cholinesterase activity. Some are used medically to reverse neuromuscular blockade (eg, neostigmine, pyridostigmine, edrophonium) or to treat glaucoma, myasthenia gravis, and Alzheimer disease (eg, echothiophate, pyridostigmine, tacrine, donepezil).

Some organophosphates were developed as nerve gases. One, sarin, has been used by terrorists. Organophosphates and carbamates are commonly used as insecticides (see Table 366–8). Those most often implicated in human poisoning include

- Carbamates: Aldicarb and methomyl
- Organophosphates: Chlorpyrifos, diazinon, dursban, fenthion, malathion, and parathion

Organophosphates and carbamates are common causes of poisoning and poison-related deaths worldwide.

Pathophysiology

Organophosphates and carbamates are absorbed through the GI tract, lungs, and skin. They inhibit plasma and RBC cholinesterase, preventing breakdown of acetylcholine, which then accumulates in synapses. Carbamates are cleared spontaneously within about 48 h after exposure. Organophosphates, however, can irreversibly bind to cholinesterase.

Symptoms and Signs

Acute: Organophosphates and carbamates cause similar initial findings characterized by acute muscarinic and nicotinic cholinergic toxidromes (see Table 366–2). Muscle fasciculations and weakness are typical. Respiratory findings include rhonchi, wheezing, and hypoxia, which may be severe. Most patients have bradycardia and, if poisoning is severe, hypotension. CNS toxicity is common, sometimes with seizures and excitability and often with lethargy and coma. Pancreatitis is possible, and organophosphates may cause arrhythmias such as heart block and QTc interval prolongation.

Delayed: Weakness, particularly of proximal, cranial, and respiratory muscles, may develop 1 to 3 days after exposure to organophosphates or rarely carbamates despite treatment (the intermediate syndrome); these symptoms resolve in 2 to 3 wk. A few organophosphates (eg, chlorpyrifos, triorthocresyl phosphate) may cause an axonal neuropathy that begins 1 to 3 wk after exposure. The mechanism may be independent of RBC cholinesterase, and the risk is independent of the severity of poisoning. Long-term, persistent sequelae of organophosphate poisoning may include cognitive deficits or parkinsonism.

Diagnosis

- Muscarinic toxidrome with prominent respiratory findings, pinpoint pupils, muscle fasciculations, and weakness
- Sometimes RBC cholinesterase levels

The diagnosis is usually based on the characteristic muscarinic toxidrome in patients with neuromuscular and respiratory findings, particularly in patients at risk. If findings are equivocal, reversal or abatement of muscarinic symptoms after 1 mg of atropine (0.01 to 0.02 mg/kg in children) supports the diagnosis. The specific toxin should be identified if possible. Many organophosphates have characteristic garliclike or petroleum odors.

RBC cholinesterase activity, which can be measured by some laboratories, indicates the severity of poisoning. If it can be measured rapidly, values can be used to monitor the effectiveness of treatment; however, patient response is the primary marker of effectiveness.

Treatment

- Supportive therapy
- Atropine for respiratory manifestations
- Decontamination
- Pralidoxime for neuromuscular manifestations

In-hospital treatment: Supportive therapy is key. Patients should be closely monitored for respiratory failure due to weakness of respiratory muscles.

Atropine is given in amounts sufficient to relieve bronchospasm and bronchorrhea rather than to normalize pupil size or heart rate. Initial dosage is 2 to 5 mg IV (0.05 mg/kg in children); the dose can be doubled every 3 to 5 min prn. Grams of atropine may be necessary for severely poisoned patients.

Decontamination is pursued as soon as possible after stabilization. Caregivers should avoid self-contamination while providing care. For topical exposure, clothes are removed, and the body surface is flushed thoroughly. For ingestion within 1 h of presentation, activated charcoal can be used. Gastric emptying is usually avoided. If done, the trachea is intubated beforehand to prevent aspiration.

Pralidoxime (2-PAM) is given after atropine to relieve neuromuscular symptoms. 2-PAM (1 to 2 g in adults; 20 to 40 mg/kg in children) is given over 15 to 30 min IV after exposure to an organophosphate or carbamate because, frequently, whether the poison is an organophosphate or carbamate is unknown at the time of treatment. An infusion can be used after the bolus (8 mg/kg/h in adults; 10 to 20 mg/kg/h in children).

Benzodiazepines are used for seizures. Prophylactic diazepam may help prevent neurocognitive sequelae after moderate to severe organophosphate poisoning.

Out-of-hospital exposure: People exposed to these toxins away from a hospital can give themselves low doses of atropine using commercially prepared autoinjectors (2 mg for adults and for children > 41 kg; 1 mg for children 19 to 41 kg; 0.5 mg for children < 19 kg). Autoinjection of 10 mg diazepam has been recommended for people exposed to a chemical attack.

KEY POINTS

- Organophosphates have been used in insecticides, medical treatments, and biologic weapons.
- Suspect toxicity if patients have a muscarinic cholinergic toxidrome with prominent respiratory and neuromuscular findings.
- Confirm the diagnosis by the response to atropine and sometimes RBC cholinesterase levels.
- Treat supportively by giving atropine to relieve bronchospasm and bronchorrhea and by giving 2-PAM to relieve neuromuscular symptoms.

IRON POISONING

Iron poisoning is a leading cause of poisoning deaths in children. Symptoms begin with acute gastroenteritis, followed by a quiescent period, then shock and liver failure. Diagnosis is by measuring serum iron, detecting radiopaque iron tablets in the GI tract, or detecting unexplained metabolic acidosis in patients with other findings suggesting iron poisoning. Treatment of a substantial ingestion is usually whole-bowel irrigation and chelation therapy with IV deferoxamine.

Many commonly used OTC preparations contain iron. Of the many iron compounds used in OTC and prescription preparations, the most common are

- Ferrous sulfate (20% elemental iron)
- Ferrous gluconate (12% elemental iron)
- Ferrous fumarate (33% elemental iron)

To children, iron tablets may look like candy. Prenatal multivitamins are the source of iron in most lethal ingestions among children. Children's chewable multivitamins with iron usually have such small amounts that toxicity rarely occurs.

Pathophysiology

Iron is toxic to the GI system, cardiovascular system, and CNS. Specific mechanisms are unclear, but excess free iron is inserted into enzymatic processes and interferes with oxidative phosphorylation, causing metabolic acidosis. Iron also catalyzes free radical formation, acts as an oxidizer, and, when plasma protein binding is saturated, combines with water to form iron hydroxide and free H^+ ions, compounding the metabolic acidosis. Coagulopathy may appear early because of interference with the coagulation cascade and later because of liver injury.

Toxicity depends on the amount of elemental iron that has been ingested. Up to 20 mg/kg of elemental iron is not toxic, 20 to 60 mg/kg is mildly to moderately toxic, and > 60 mg/kg can cause severe symptoms and morbidity.

Symptoms and Signs

Symptoms of iron poisoning occur in 5 stages (see Table 366–7); however, symptoms and their progression vary significantly. The severity of stage 1 symptoms usually reflects the overall severity of poisoning; late-stage symptoms develop only if stage 1 symptoms are moderate or severe. If no symptoms develop within the first 6 h after ingestion, risk of serious toxicity is minimal. If shock and coma develop within the first 6 h, the mortality rate is about 10%.

Diagnosis

- Abdominal x-ray
- Determination of serum iron, electrolytes, and pH 3 to 4 h after ingestion

Iron poisoning should be considered in mixed ingestions (because iron is ubiquitous) and in small children with access to iron and unexplained metabolic acidosis or severe or hemorrhagic gastroenteritis. Because children often share, siblings and playmates of small children who have ingested iron should be evaluated.

Abdominal x-ray is usually recommended to confirm ingestion; it detects intact iron tablets or iron concretions but misses chewed and dissolved tablets, liquid iron preparations, and iron in multivitamin preparations. Serum iron, electrolytes, and pH are determined 3 to 4 h after ingestion. Toxicity is assumed if suspected ingestion is accompanied by any of the following:

- Vomiting and abdominal pain
- Serum iron levels > 350 μg/dL (63 μmol/L)
- Iron visible on x-ray
- Unexplained metabolic acidosis

These iron levels may indicate toxicity; however, iron levels alone do not predict toxicity accurately. Total iron binding capacity is often inaccurate and not helpful in diagnosing

Table 366–7. STAGES OF IRON POISONING

STAGE	TIME POSTINGESTION	DESCRIPTION
1	Within 6 h	Vomiting, hematemesis, explosive diarrhea, irritability, abdominal pain, lethargy If toxicity is severe, tachypnea, tachycardia, hypotension, coma, metabolic acidosis
2	Within 6–48 h	Up to 24 h of apparent improvement (latent period)
3	12–48 h	Shock, seizures, fever, coagulopathy, metabolic acidosis
4	2–5 days	Liver failure, jaundice, coagulopathy, hypoglycemia
5	2–5 wk	Gastric outlet or duodenal obstruction secondary to scarring

serious poisoning and is not recommended. The most accurate approach is to serially measure levels of serum iron, HCO_3, and pH (with calculation of the anion gap); these findings are then evaluated together, and results are correlated with the patient's clinical status. For example, toxicity is suggested by increasing iron levels, metabolic acidosis, worsening symptoms, or, more typically, some combination of these findings.

Treatment

- Whole-bowel irrigation
- For severe toxicity, IV deferoxamine

If radiopaque tablets are visible on abdominal x-ray, whole-bowel irrigation with polyethylene glycol 1 to 2 L/h for adults or 25 to 40 mL/kg/h for children is done until no iron is visible on repeat abdominal x-ray. Administration via NGT may be necessary to deliver these large volumes and care must be taken to protect the airway; intubation may be necessary (see p. 554). Gastric lavage is usually not helpful because vomiting tends to empty the stomach more efficiently. Activated charcoal does not adsorb iron and should be used only if other toxins also were ingested.

All patients with more than mild gastroenteritis are hospitalized. Patients with severe toxicity (metabolic acidosis, shock, severe gastroenteritis, or serum iron level > 500 μg/dL) are treated with IV deferoxamine to chelate free serum iron. Deferoxamine is infused at rates up to 15 mg/kg/h IV, titrated until hypotension occurs. Because both deferoxamine and iron poisoning can decrease BP, patients receiving deferoxamine require IV hydration.

KEY POINTS

- Iron toxicity, like some other hepatotoxins, can cause gastroenteritis followed by a quiescent phase, then shock and liver failure.
- Suspect iron poisoning in mixed ingestions (because iron is ubiquitous) and in small children with access to iron and unexplained metabolic acidosis or severe or hemorrhagic gastroenteritis.
- Suspect that toxicity is severe with increasing iron levels, metabolic acidosis, worsening symptoms, or a combination.
- Do whole-bowel irrigation until an abdominal x-ray shows absence of radiopaque iron products.
- Give IV deferoxamine to treat severe poisoning (eg, metabolic acidosis, shock, severe gastroenteritis, serum iron level > 500 μg/dL).

LEAD POISONING

(Plumbism)

Lead poisoning often causes minimal symptoms at first but can cause acute encephalopathy or irreversible organ damage, commonly resulting in cognitive deficits in children. Diagnosis is by whole blood lead level. Treatment involves stopping lead exposure and sometimes using chelation therapy with succimer or edetate Ca disodium, with or without dimercaprol.

There is no blood lead level that does not have deleterious effects. The Centers for Disease Control and Prevention (CDC) recommend that children with blood lead levels > 5 μg/dL must have remediation, retesting, and serial monitoring as well as assessment for vitamin deficiency and general nutritional status.

Etiology

Leaded paint was commonly used until 1960, used to some degree until the early 1970s, and mostly eliminated in 1978. Thus, for a significant number of older housing units, leaded paint still poses some hazard. Lead poisoning is usually caused by direct ingestion of leaded paint chips (from cracked, peeling paint). During home remodeling, patients may be exposed to significant amounts of aerosolized lead in the form of particles scraped or sanded off during surface preparation for repainting.

Some ceramic glazes contain lead; ceramic ware (eg, pitchers, cups, plates) that is made with these glazes (common outside the US) can leach lead, particularly when in contact with acidic substances (eg, fruits, cola drinks, tomatoes, wine, cider). Lead-contaminated moonshine whiskey and folk remedies are possible sources, as are occasional lead foreign objects in the stomach or tissues (eg, bullets, curtain or fishing weights). Bullets lodged in soft tissues near synovial fluid or CSF may increase blood lead levels, but that process takes years.

Occupational exposure can occur during battery manufacture and recycling, bronzing, brass making, glass making, pipe cutting, soldering and welding, smelting, or working with pottery or pigments. Certain ethnic cosmetic products and imported herbal products and medicinal herbs contain lead and have caused cluster outbreaks of lead poisoning in immigrant communities. Fumes of leaded gasoline (in countries other than the US) recreationally inhaled for CNS effects may cause lead poisoning.

Symptoms and Signs

Lead poisoning is most often a chronic disorder and may not cause acute symptoms. With or without acute symptoms, poisoning eventually has irreversible effects (eg, cognitive deficits, peripheral neuropathy, progressive renal dysfunction).

Symptoms of lead poisoning are roughly proportional to lead levels, but there are no safe levels of lead. Risk of cognitive deficits increases when the whole blood lead level (PbB) is ≥ 10 μg/dL (≥ 0.48 mmol/L) for an extended period, although the cutoff may be even lower. Other symptoms (eg, abdominal cramping, constipation, tremors, mood changes) may occur if PbB is > 50 μg/dL (> 2.4 mmol/L). Encephalopathy is likely if PbB is > 100 μg/dL (> 4.8 mmol/L).

In children: Acute lead poisoning may cause irritability, decreased attentiveness, and acute encephalopathy. Cerebral edema develops over 1 to 5 days, causing persistent and forceful vomiting, ataxic gait, seizures, altered consciousness, and, finally, intractable seizures and coma. Encephalopathy may be preceded by several weeks of irritability and decreased play activity.

Chronic lead poisoning in children may cause intellectual disability, seizure disorders, aggressive behavior disorders, developmental regression, chronic abdominal pain, and anemia.

In adults: Adults with occupational exposure characteristically develop symptoms (eg, personality changes, headache, abdominal pain, neuropathy) over several weeks or longer. Encephalopathy is unusual. Adults may develop loss of sex drive, infertility, and, in men, erectile dysfunction.

In children and adults: Anemia may develop because lead interferes with the normal formation of Hb. Children and adults who inhale tetra-ethyl or tetra-methyl lead (in leaded gasoline) may develop toxic psychosis in addition to more characteristic symptoms of lead poisoning.

Diagnosis

- Lead levels in capillary or whole blood

Lead poisoning is suspected in patients with characteristic symptoms. However, because symptoms are often nonspecific, diagnosis of lead poisoning is often delayed. Evaluation includes CBC and measurement of serum electrolytes, BUN, serum creatinine, plasma glucose, and PbBs. An abdominal x-ray should be taken to look for lead particles, which are radiopaque. X-rays of long bones are taken in children. Horizontal, metaphyseal lead bands representing lack of RBC remodeling and increased Ca deposition in the zones of provisional calcification in children's long bones are somewhat specific for poisoning with lead or other heavy metals but are insensitive. Normocytic or microcytic anemia suggests lead toxicity, particularly when the reticulocyte count is elevated or RBC basophilic stippling occurs; however, sensitivity and specificity are limited. Diagnosis is definitive if PbB is ≥ 5 μg/dL.

Because measuring PbB is not always possible and can be expensive, other preliminary or screening tests for lead poisoning can be used. Capillary blood testing for lead is accurate, inexpensive, and quick. All positive tests should be confirmed with PbB. The erythrocyte protoporphyrin (also called zinc protoporphyrin or free erythrocyte protoporphyrin) test is often inaccurate and now is seldom used.

Children with PbB > 5 μg/dL should be assessed clinically and, if necessary, with testing for nutritional and vitamin deficiencies (eg, iron, Ca, vitamin C deficiencies).

Provocative testing: Provocative urine metal testing for lead and other metals in which chelation agents (eg, dimercaptosuccinic acid, dimercaptopropane sulfonic acid, calcium disodium edetate) are given to the patient and then urinary levels of excreted metals are measured has not been scientifically validated, has no shown benefit, and may be harmful in the assessment and treatment of patients in whom there is concern for metal poisoning.

Treatment

- Source of lead eliminated (eg, whole-bowel irrigation if lead in GI tract)
- Chelation for adults with symptoms of poisoning plus PbB > 70 μg/dL
- Chelation for children with encephalopathy or PbB > 45 μg/dL (> 2.15 mmol/L)

For all patients, the source of lead is eliminated. If lead chips are visible on abdominal x-ray, whole-bowel irrigation with a polyethylene glycol electrolyte solution at 1 to 2 L/h for adults or 25 to 40 mL/kg/h for children is done until repeat x-ray shows no lead. Administration via NGT may be necessary to deliver these large volumes and care must be taken to protect the airway; intubation may be necessary. If the cause is bullets, surgical removal should be considered. Children with PbB > 70 μg/dL (> 3.40 μmol/L) and all patients with neurologic symptoms should be hospitalized. Patients with acute encephalopathy are admitted to an ICU.

Chelating drugs (eg, succimer [meso-2,3-dimercaptosuccinic acid], $CaNa_2$ EDTA, dimercaprol [British antilewisite, or BAL]) can be given to bind lead into forms that can be excreted. Chelation should be supervised by an experienced toxicologist. Chelation is indicated for adults with symptoms of poisoning plus PbB > 70 μg/dL and for children with encephalopathy or PbB > 45 μg/dL (> 2.15 μmol/L). Liver and kidney disorders are relative contraindications for chelating drugs. Chelating drugs should not be given to any patient with ongoing exposure to lead because chelation can increase GI absorption of lead. Chelation removes only relatively small amounts of metal. If total body burden of lead is very large, multiple chelations over many years may be required.

Regimens: Patients with encephalopathy are treated with dimercaprol 75 mg/m^2 (or 4 mg/kg) IM q 4 h and $CaNa_2$ EDTA 1000 to 1500 mg/m^2 IV (infusion) once/day. The first dose of dimercaprol should precede the first dose of $CaNa_2$ EDTA by at least 4 h to prevent redistribution of lead into the brain. Dimercaprol may be stopped after the first few doses depending on lead levels and symptom severity. Dimercaprol-$CaNa_2$ EDTA combination therapy is given for 5 days, followed by a 3-day washout period; then the need for continued chelation is reassessed.

Patients without encephalopathy are usually treated with succimer 10 mg/kg po q 8 h for 5 days, followed by 10 mg/kg po q 12 h for 14 days. If these patients have symptoms, they can alternatively be treated for 5 days with dimercaprol 50 mg/m^2 via deep IM injection q 4 h plus $CaNa_2$ EDTA 1000 mg/m^2 IV once/day.

Drugs: Dimercaprol, which can cause vomiting, is given with parenteral or oral fluids. Dimercaprol can also cause pain at the injection site, numerous systemic symptoms, and, in patients with G6PD deficiency, moderate to severe acute intravascular hemolysis. This drug should not be given concurrently with iron supplements. Dimercaprol is formulated with peanut derivatives and thus is contraindicated in patients with known or suspected peanut allergy.

$CaNa_2$ EDTA can cause thrombophlebitis, which can be prevented by giving the drug IM, not IV, and by using an IV concentration of < 0.5%. Before beginning treatment with $CaNa_2$ EDTA, adequate urine flow must be confirmed. Serious reactions to $CaNa_2$ EDTA include renal insufficiency, proteinuria, microscopic hematuria, fever, and diarrhea. Renal toxicity, which is dose-related, is usually reversible. Adverse effects of $CaNa_2$ EDTA are probably due to zinc depletion.

Succimer may cause rash, GI symptoms (eg, anorexia, nausea, vomiting, diarrhea, metallic taste), and transient elevations of liver enzymes.

Lower lead levels: Patients with PbB > 5 μg/dL should be monitored closely with retesting as needed, and they or their parents should be taught how to reduce their exposure to lead.

Prevention

Patients at risk should be screened by measuring PbB. Measures that reduce risk of household poisoning include regular hand washing, regular washing of children's toys and pacifiers, and regular cleaning of household surfaces; drinking water, household paint (except in houses built after 1978), and ceramic ware made outside the US should be tested for lead. Adults exposed to lead dust at work should use appropriate personal protective equipment, change their clothing and shoes before going home, and shower before going to bed.

KEY POINTS

- Houses painted before 1978 (particularly when remodeled or repainted), certain ceramic ware (eg, pitchers, cups, plates) that has a leaded glaze, and certain occupational exposures increase the risk of lead poisoning.
- Test patients by measuring capillary levels or PbB.
- Remove the source of lead (eg, by whole-bowel irrigation for lead in the GI tract).
- Arrange chelation therapy for adults with PbB > 70 μg/dL and for children with encephalopathy or PbB > 45 μg/dL.
- Use succimer or $CaNa_2$ EDTA, with or without dimercaprol, for chelation therapy.

SPECIFIC POISONS

Symptoms and treatment of specific poisons vary (see Table 366–8); including all the specific complexities and details is impossible. Consultation with a poison control center is recommended for any poisonings except the mildest and most routine.

Table 366–8. SYMPTOMS AND TREATMENT OF SPECIFIC POISONS

POISON*	SYMPTOMS	TREATMENT
ACE inhibitors	Angioedema, hypotension	Charcoal, supportive care, a bradykinin inhibitor (ecallantide or icatibant) For angioedema, epinephrine, antihistamines, or corticosteroids unlikely to be effective For hypotension, consideration of naloxone
Acephate	See Organophosphates	—
Acetaminophen	See Acetaminophen Poisoning on p. 3056	See Acetaminophen Poisoning on p. 3056
Acetanilide Aniline dyes and oil Chloroaniline Phenacetin (acetophenetidin, phenylacetamide)	Cyanosis due to formation of methemoglobin and sulfhemoglobin, dyspnea, weakness, vertigo, angina, rashes and urticaria, vomiting, delirium, depression, respiratory and circulatory failure	**Ingestion:** Charcoal; then as for inhalation **Skin contact:** Clothing removed and area washed with copious soap and water; then as for inhalation **Inhalation:** O_2, respiratory support, blood transfusion For severe cyanosis, methylene blue 1–2 mg/kg IV
Acetic acid	**Low concentration:** Mild mucosal irritation **High concentration:** See Caustic Ingestion on p. 3061	Supportive care with irrigation and dilution
Acetone Ketones • Model airplane glues or cements • Nail polish remover	**Ingestion:** As for inhalation, except for direct pulmonary effect **Inhalation:** Bronchial irritation, pneumonia (pulmonary congestion and edema, decreased respiration, dyspnea), drunkenness, stupor, ketosis, cardiac arrhythmias	Removal from source Respiratory support, O_2 and fluids, correction of metabolic acidosis
Acetonitrile Cosmetic nail adhesive	Converted to cyanide, with usual symptoms and signs	See Cyanides
Acetophenetidin	See Acetanilide	—
Acetylsalicylic acid	See Aspirin and Other Salicylate Poisoning on p. 3058	—
Acids and alkalis	See specific acids and alkalis (eg, Boric acid, Fluorides); see Caustic Ingestion on p. 3061 **Eye contact:** See p. 2968 **Skin contact:** See p. 2954	—
Airplane glues or cements (model-building)	See Acetone, Benzene (toluene), and Petroleum distillates	—
Alcohol, ethyl (ethanol) • Brandy • Whiskey • Other liquors	Emotional lability, impaired coordination, flushing, nausea, vomiting, stupor to coma, respiratory depression	Supportive care, IV glucose to prevent hypoglycemia
Alcohol, isopropyl • Rubbing alcohol	Dizziness, incoordination, stupor to coma, gastroenteritis, hemorrhagic gastritis, hypotension Ketosis without acidosis No retinal injury or acidosis	Supportive care, IV glucose, correction of dehydration and electrolyte abnormalities For gastritis, IV H_2 blockers or proton pump inhibitors
Alcohol, methyl (methanol, wood alcohol) • Antifreeze • Paint solvent • Solid canned fuel • Varnish	Severe toxicity with 60–250 mL (2–8 oz) in adults or 8–10 mL (2 tsp) in children Latency period 12–18 h Headache, weakness, leg cramps, vertigo, seizures, retinal injury, dimmed vision, metabolic acidosis, decreased respiration	Fomepizole (15 mg/kg, then 10 mg/kg q 12 h); alternatively, 10% ethanol/5% D/W IV with an initial loading dose of 10 mL/kg over 1 h, then 1–2 mL/kg/h to maintain a blood ethanol level of 100 mg/dL (22 mmol/L) Hemodialysis (which is definitive treatment)
Aldrin	See Chlorinated and other halogenated hydrocarbons	—
Alkalis	See Acids and alkalis	—
Alphaprodine	See Opioids	—

Table continues on the following page.

Table 366–8. SYMPTOMS AND TREATMENT OF SPECIFIC POISONS (*Continued*)

POISON*	SYMPTOMS	TREATMENT
Aminophylline Caffeine Guarana Theophylline	Wakefulness, restlessness, anorexia, vomiting, dehydration, seizures, tachycardia In adults, greater toxicity after acute overdose added to chronic intake	Charcoal (for ingestion), discontinuation of drug, measurement of blood theophylline level, phenobarbital or diazepam for seizures, parenteral fluids, maintenance of BP For theophylline, serum level > 50–100 mg/L (> 278–555 μmol/L), acidosis, seizures, or coma, possibly dialysis For patients without asthma, possibly a β-blocker (eg, esmolol)
Amitriptyline	See Tricyclic antidepressants	—
Ammonia gas (anhydrous ammonia [NH_3])	Irritation of eyes and respiratory tract, cough, choking, abdominal pain	Flushing of eyes for 15 min with tap water or saline If severe toxicity, positive pressure O_2 to manage pulmonary edema, respiratory support
Ammonia water (ammonium hydroxide [NH_4OH])	See Caustic Ingestion on p. 3061	—
Ammoniated mercury (NH_2HgCl)	See Mercury	
Ammonium carbonate ($[NH_4]_2CO_3$)	See Caustic Ingestion on p. 3061	—
Ammonium fluoride (NH_4F)	See Fluorides	
Amobarbital	See Barbiturates	—
Amphetamines • Amphetamine sulfate or phosphate • Dextroamphetamine • Methamphetamine • Phenmetrazine • Synthetic cathinones (bath salts)	Increased activity, exhilaration, talkativeness, insomnia, irritability, exaggerated reflexes, anorexia, diaphoresis, tachyarrhythmia, anginal chest pain, psychotic-like states, inability to concentrate or sit still, paranoia	Charcoal possibly effective long after ingestion because of recycling via enterohepatic circulation, benzodiazepines for sedation and seizures, reduction of external stimuli, external cooling, prevention of cerebral edema For patients without asthma, β-blockers possibly helpful but rarely necessary
Amyl nitrite	See Nitrites	—
Aniline	See Acetanilide	—
Anticoagulants, direct thrombin inhibitors • Argatroban • Bivalirudin • Dabigatran etexilate • Desirudin	Bleeding secondary to thrombin inhibition	Supportive care (eg, whole blood transfusion, consideration of prothrombin complex concentrates or hemodialysis)
Anticoagulants, factor Xa inhibitors • Fondaparinux • Apixaban • Rivaroxaban	Bleeding secondary to factor Xa inhibition	For control of bleeding complications, supportive care (eg, whole blood transfusion) and/or prothrombin complex concentrate Oral activated charcoal and supportive care
Anticoagulants, heparin and low mol wt heparins • Heparin (unfractionated) • Dalteparin • Enoxaparin • Tinzaparin	Bleeding secondary to decreased thrombin and fibrin clot formation	Supportive care (eg, whole blood transfusion) Protamine sulfate (to reverse unfractionated heparin, but only partially neutralizes low mol wt heparins)
Anticoagulants, warfarins • Dicumarol • Superwarfarins • Warfarin	See Warfarin	—
Antidepressants	See Bupropion, Mirtazapine, SSRIs, Trazodone, Tricyclic antidepressants, and Venlafaxine	—

Table 366–8. SYMPTOMS AND TREATMENT OF SPECIFIC POISONS (*Continued*)

POISON*	SYMPTOMS	TREATMENT
Antifreeze	See Alcohol, methyl and Ethylene glycol	—
Antihistamines	Anticholinergic symptoms (eg, tachycardia, hyperthermia, mydriasis, warm and dry skin, urinary retention, ileus, delirium)	For diagnostic or therapeutic trial or for treatment of severe symptoms refractory to sedation (CAUTION: *Seizures—see Physostigmine*), consideration of physostigmine 0.5–2.0 mg in adults or 0.02 mg/kg in children IV (slowly)
Antihyperglycemic drugs, oral	See Hypoglycemic drugs, oral	—
Antimony • Stibophen • Tartar emetic	Throat constriction, dysphagia, burning GI pain, vomiting, diarrhea, GI hemorrhage, dehydration, pulmonary edema, renal failure, lactic acidosis, liver failure, shock	Chelation with penicillamine, dimercaprol for patients who cannot take oral drugs, hydration, treatment of shock and pain
Antineoplastic drugs • Mercaptopurine • Methotrexate • Vincristine • > 50 others	Effects on hematopoiesis, nausea, vomiting, specific acute vs chronic effects depending on drug	Supportive care, leucovorin rescue, observation for postacute problems (> 24–48 h)
Antipsychotic drugs (conventional) • Chlorpromazine • Fluphenazine • Haloperidol • Loxapine • Mesoridazine • Molindone • Perphenazine • Pimozide • Prochlorperazine • Thioridazine • Thiothixene • Trifluoperazine • Triflupromazine	A wide range of effects (eg, sedation, seizures, excitement, coma, dystonia, hypotension, tachycardia, ventricular arrhythmias or torsades de pointes, anticholinergic effects, hyperthermia, agranulocytosis, or hypothermia)	For dystonia, diphenhydramine or benztropine For hypotension refractory to fluids, norepinephrine For ventricular arrhythmias, consideration of alkalinization
Antipsychotic drugs (2nd-generation) • Clozapine • Olanzapine • Quetiapine • Risperidone • Ziprasidone	CNS depression (particularly with olanzapine), miosis, anticholinergic effects, hypotension, dystonia, QT prolongation (occasionally), fatal bone marrow suppression (rare)	For dystonia, diphenhydramine or benztropine For hypotension refractory to fluids, norepinephrine For ventricular arrhythmias, consideration of alkalinization
Ant poison	See Arsenic (sodium arsenate) and Boric acid	—
Arsenic • Donovan solution • Fowler solution • Herbicides • Paris green • Pesticides • Selenium • Sodium arsenate	Same as for Antimony —	Same as for Antimony
Arsine gas	Acute hemolytic anemia	Transfusions, diuresis
Artificial bitter almond oil	See Cyanides	—
Asphalt	See Petroleum distillates	
Aspirin	See Aspirin and Other Salicylate Poisoning on p. 3058	—
Atropine	See Belladonna	
Automobile exhaust	See Carbon monoxide	—

Table continues on the following page.

Table 366–8. SYMPTOMS AND TREATMENT OF SPECIFIC POISONS (*Continued*)

POISON*	SYMPTOMS	TREATMENT
Barbiturates • Amobarbital • Meprobamate • Pentobarbital • Phenobarbital • Secobarbital	Bradycardia, hypothermia, confusion, delirium, loss of corneal reflex, respiratory failure, drowsiness, ataxia, coma	Charcoal up to 24 h after ingestion, supportive care, forced alkaline diuresis for phenobarbital (to aid in elimination) For severe cases, hemodialysis
Barium compounds (soluble) • Barium acetate • Barium carbonate • Barium chloride • Barium hydroxide • Barium nitrate • Barium sulfide • Depilatories • Explosives • Fireworks • Rat poisons	Vomiting, abdominal pain, diarrhea, tremors, seizures, colic, hypertension, cardiac arrest, dyspnea and cyanosis, ventricular fibrillation, severe hypokalemia, skeletal muscle weakness	KCl 10–15 mEq/h IV, Na or Mg sulfate 60 g po to precipitate barium in stomach, then possibly gastric lavage Diazepam to control seizures For dyspnea and cyanosis, O_2
Belladonna • Atropine • Hyoscyamine • Hyoscyamus • Scopolamine (hyoscine) • Stramonium	Anticholinergic symptoms (eg, tachycardia, hyperthermia, mydriasis, warm and dry skin, urinary retention, ileus, delirium)	For diagnostic or therapeutic trial or for treatment of severe symptoms refractory to sedation, which is rarely needed (CAUTION: *Seizures—see Physostigmine*), consideration of physostigmine 0.5–2.0 mg in adults or 0.02 mg/kg in children IV (slowly)
Benzene • Benzol • Hydrocarbons • Model airplane glue • Toluene • Toluol • Xylene	Dizziness, weakness, headache, euphoria, nausea, vomiting, ventricular arrhythmia, paralysis, seizures With chronic poisoning, aplastic anemia, hypokalemia, leukemia, CNS depression	Decontamination with water, avoidance of vomiting and aspiration, O_2, respiratory support, ECG monitoring (ventricular fibrillation can occur early) Diazepam to control seizures For severe anemia, blood transfusions Replacement of K as necessary *Epinephrine contraindicated*
γ-Benzene hexachloride Benzene hexachloride Hexachlorocyclohexane Lindane	Irritability, CNS excitation, muscle spasms, atonia, tonic-clonic seizures, respiratory failure, pulmonary edema, nausea, vomiting, obtundation, coma	Supportive care, activated charcoal after airway control Diazepam to control seizures
Benzine (benzin)	See Petroleum distillates	—
Benzodiazepines • Alprazolam • Chlordiazepoxide • Diazepam • Flurazepam	Sedation to coma, particularly if drugs are accompanied by alcohol Hypotension	Airway control For hypotension, IV fluids and vasopressors Avoidance of flumazenil (CAUTION: *If tricyclic antidepressants are involved, flumazenil may precipitate seizures; in patients who depend on benzodiazepines, flumazenil may precipitate withdrawal.*)
Benzol	See Benzene	—
Beta-blockers	Hypotension, bradycardia, seizures, cardiac arrhythmias, hypoglycemia, altered mental status	Close monitoring and attention to airway maintenance For symptomatic patients, consideration of dopamine, epinephrine, other vasopressors, glucagon 3–5 mg IV followed by infusion, $CaCl_2$, IV insulin and glucose, cardiac pacing, intra-aortic balloon pump, and IV lipid emulsion
Bichloride of mercury	See Mercury	—
Bichromates	See Chromic acid	—
Bidrin (dicrotophos)	See Organophosphates	—
Bifenthrin	See Pyrethroids	—

Table 366–8. SYMPTOMS AND TREATMENT OF SPECIFIC POISONS (*Continued*)

POISON*	SYMPTOMS	TREATMENT
Bishydroxycoumarin	See Warfarin	—
Bismuth compounds	**Acute:** Abdominal pain, oliguria, acute renal failure **Chronic:** Poor absorption, ulcerative stomatitis, anorexia, progressive encephalopathy	Respiratory support, consideration of chelation with dimercaprol and succimer (Table 366–4 on p. 3054)
Bitter almond oil	See Cyanides	—
Bleach, chlorine	See Hypochlorites	—
β-Blockers	See Beta-blockers	—
Bluing	See Selenium	—
Boric acid	Nausea, vomiting, diarrhea, hemorrhagic gastroenteritis, weakness, lethargy, CNS depression, seizures, "boiled lobster" rash, shock	Removal from skin, prevention or treatment of electrolyte abnormalities and shock, control of seizures For severe poisoning (rare), dialysis
Brandy	See Alcohol, ethyl	—
Bromates	Vomiting, diarrhea, epigastric pain, acidosis, deafness	Supportive care, thiosulfate to reduce bromate to less toxic bromide For renal failure, hemodialysis
Bromides	Nausea, vomiting, rash (may be acneiform), slurred speech, ataxia, confusion, psychotic behavior, coma, paralysis, negative anion gap	Discontinuation of drug, hydration and NaCl IV to promote diuresis, furosemide 10 mg IV q 6 h For severe poisoning, hemodialysis
Bromine	Highly corrosive With exposure to liquid or vapor, skin and mucous membrane burns	Aggressive decontamination, supportive care
Bupropion HCl	Respiratory depression, ataxia, seizures	Charcoal, benzodiazepines, supportive care
Butyl nitrate	See Nitrites	—
Cadmium • Cadmium oxide fumes (eg, from welding)	**Ingestion:** Severe gastric cramps, vomiting, diarrhea, dry throat, cough, dyspnea, headache, shock, coma, brown urine, renal failure **Inhalation:** Pneumonitis with dyspnea and bilateral pulmonary infiltrates, hypoxia, death	Dilution with milk or albumin, respiratory support, hydration, possibly chelation with succimer or dimercaptopropane sulfonate *Dimercaprol contraindicated* For inhalation, O_2, sometimes bronchodilators and corticosteroids
Caffeine	See Aminophylline	—
Ca channel blockers • Diltiazem • Nifedipine • Verapamil • Others	Nausea, vomiting, confusion, bradycardia, hypotension, total cardiovascular collapse Toxicity sometimes occurring after hyperglycemia	For sustained-release preparations, consideration of whole-bowel irrigation Glucagon 5–10 mg IV For hypotension or severe arrhythmias, consideration of $CaCl_2$ (eg, 1 g–10 mL of a 10% solution) or 3 times as much Ca gluconate IV with additional amounts as needed, pacemaker, or intra-aortic balloon pump Consideration of regular insulin 10–100 units IV and 50–100 mL 50% dextrose plus 50–100 mL/h 10% dextrose IV infusion Consideration of IV lipid emulsion
Calomel	See Mercury	—
Camphor • Camphorated oils	Camphor odor on breath, headache, confusion, delirium, hallucinations, seizures, coma	Diazepam to prevent and treat seizures, respiratory support
Cannabinoid research chemicals • Cannabicyclohexanol • CP-47 • JWH-018 • JWH-073 • JWH-200	Hypertension, tachycardia, MI, nausea, vomiting, agitation, hallucinations, psychoses, seizures, convulsions, stroke	Supportive care with IV fluids, benzodiazepines for agitation and seizures, phenobarbital for seizures Beta-blockers may help relieve cardiac symptoms, but are rarely necessary

Table continues on the following page.

Table 366–8. SYMPTOMS AND TREATMENT OF SPECIFIC POISONS (*Continued*)

POISON*	SYMPTOMS	TREATMENT
Canned fuel, solid	See Alcohol, methyl	—
Cantharides • Cantharidin • Spanish fly	Irritated skin and mucous membranes, skin vesicles, nausea, vomiting, bloody diarrhea, burning pain in back and urethra, respiratory depression, seizures, coma, abortion, menorrhagia	Avoidance of all oils, respiratory support, treatment of seizures, maintenance of fluid balance No specific antidote
Carbamates • Aldicarb • Bendiocarb • Benomyl • Carbaryl • Carbofuran • Fenothiocarb • Methiocarb • Methomyl • Oxamyl • Propoxur	Slightly to highly toxic effects; similar to those of organophosphates except cholinesterase inhibition is not permanent	See Organophosphates
Carbamazepine	Progressive CNS depression, seizures (occasional), cardiac arrhythmia (rare)	Supportive care after decontamination, heart rate monitoring For arrhythmias, consideration of IV Na bicarbonate
Carbolic acid	See Phenols	—
Carbonates (ammonium, potassium, sodium)	See Caustic Ingestion on p. 3061	—
Carbon bisulfide	See Carbon disulfide	—
Carbon dioxide	Dyspnea, weakness, tinnitus, palpitations, asphyxia	Respiratory support, O_2
Carbon disulfide • Carbon bisulfide	Garlic odor on breath, irritability, weakness, mania, narcosis, delirium, mydriasis, blindness, parkinsonism, seizures, coma, paralysis, respiratory failure	Washing of skin, O_2, diazepam sedation, respiratory and circulatory support
Carbon monoxide • Acetylene gas • Automobile exhaust • Coal gas • Furnace gas • Illuminating gas • Marsh gas	Variable toxicity depending on length of exposure, concentration inhaled, and respiratory and circulatory rates Various symptoms depending on % carboxyhemoglobin in blood Headache, vertigo, vomiting, dyspnea, confusion, dilated pupils, seizures, coma	100% O_2 by mask, respiratory support if needed, immediate measurement of carboxyhemoglobin level; if carboxyhemoglobin is more than about 25%, consideration of hyperbaric O_2 in consultation with poison control center (see Carbon Monoxide Poisoning on p. 3060)
Carbon tetrachloride (sometimes used in chemical manufacturing) • Cleaning fluids (nonflammable)	Nausea, vomiting, abdominal pain, headache, confusion, visual disturbances, CNS depression, ventricular fibrillation, kidney injury, liver injury, cirrhosis	Washing of skin, O_2, respiratory support, monitoring of kidney and liver function and appropriate treatment
Carbonyl iron	See Iron	—
Caustic soda (sodium hydroxide)	See Caustic Ingestion on p. 3061	—
Chloral hydrate Chloral amide	Drowsiness, confusion, shock, coma, respiratory depression, kidney injury, liver injury	For ventricular arrhythmias, respiratory support, assessment of concomitant ingestions, β-blockers
Chlorates and nitrates • Herbicides • Manufacture of explosives and matches	Vomiting, nausea, diarrhea, cyanosis (methemoglobin), toxic nephritis, shock, seizures, CNS depression, coma, jaundice	Methylene blue for methemoglobinemia, 10% thiosulfate to reduce chlorate to the less toxic chloride, transfusion for severe cyanosis, ascorbic acid, treatment of shock, O_2 For complex cases, possibly dialysis
Chlordane	See Chlorinated and other halogenated hydrocarbons	—
Chlorethoxyfos	See Organophosphates	—

Table 366–8. SYMPTOMS AND TREATMENT OF SPECIFIC POISONS (*Continued*)

POISON*	SYMPTOMS	TREATMENT
Chlorinated and other halogenated hydrocarbons • Aldrin • Benzene hexachloride • Chlordane • Chlorothalonil • DDD (2-dichlorethane) • DDT (chlorophenothane) • Dicofol • Dieldrin • Dienochlor • Dilan • Endosulfan • Endrin • Heptachlor • Lindane • Methoxychlor • Perchlordecone • Prolan • Toxaphene • Other chlorinated organic insecticides and industrial compounds	Slightly toxic effects (eg, with methoxychlor) to highly toxic effects (eg, with dieldrin) Vomiting (early or delayed), paresthesias, malaise, coarse tremors, seizures, pulmonary edema, ventricular fibrillation, respiratory failure	Diazepam or phenobarbital to prevent and control tremors and seizures, cautious use of epinephrine, avoidance of sudden stimuli, parenteral fluids For renal and liver failure, monitoring
Chlorinated lime	See Chlorine	—
Chlorine (see also Hypochlorites) • Chlorinated lime • Chlorine water • Tear gas	**Ingestion:** Irritation, corrosion of mouth and GI tract, possible ulceration or perforation, abdominal pain, tachycardia, prostration, circulatory collapse **Inhalation:** Severe respiratory and ocular irritation, glottal spasm, cough, choking, vomiting, pulmonary edema, cyanosis	**Ingestion:** Dilution with water or milk, treatment of shock **Inhalation:** O_2, respiratory support, observation for and treatment of pulmonary edema, nebulized $NaHCO_3$ (4 mL of 4.2% $NaHCO_3$)
Chloroaniline	See Acetanilide	—
Chloroform	Asphyxiation Drowsiness, coma Possible acute liver injury	**Ingestion:** Observation for kidney and liver damage; respiratory, cardiac, and circulatory support **Inhalation:** Respiratory, cardiac, and circulatory support
Chlorothalonil	See Chlorinated and other halogenated hydrocarbons	—
Chlorothion	See Organophosphates	—
Chlorpromazine	See Phenothiazines	—
Chlorpyrifos	See Organophosphates	—
Chromates	See Chromic acid	—
Chromic acid • Bichromates • Chromates • Chromium trioxide	Corrosive effects due to oxidation, ulcerated and perforated nasal septum, severe gastroenteritis, shock, vertigo, coma, nephritis	Dilution with milk or water, cautious use of fluids and electrolytes to support kidney function, consideration of *N*-acetylcysteine and ascorbic acid to convert hexavalent to the less toxic trivalent compound
Chromium	Irritation of skin and mucous membranes	Thorough washing with water and 10% ascorbic acid solution for 15 min
Chromium trioxide	See Chromic acid	—
Cimetidine Ranitidine	Slight dryness and drowsiness, possible altered metabolism of concomitant drugs	No specific antidote available Monitoring for effect on metabolism of other drugs being taken

Table continues on the following page.

Table 366–8. SYMPTOMS AND TREATMENT OF SPECIFIC POISONS (*Continued*)

POISON*	SYMPTOMS	TREATMENT
Clonidine	Bradycardia, sedation, periodic apnea, hypotension, hypothermia	Supportive care; vasopressors; naloxone 5 mcg/kg up to 2–20 mg, repeated prn, to possibly reduce sedation
Coal gas	See Carbon monoxide	—
Cobalt	Tachycardia, tachypnea and hypoxia after inhalation, skin and mucous membrane irritation, glomerulonephritis, hypothyroidism (rare)	Supportive care, decontamination with water and soap
Cobaltous chloride	See Nitrogen oxides	—
Cocaine[†]	Stimulation then depression, nausea, vomiting, loss of self-control, anxiety, hallucinations, sweating, hyperthermia, seizures, MI (rare)	Diazepam for excitation (primary treatment), O_2, respiratory and circulatory support if needed, IV $NaHCO_3$ For arrhythmias, extremely cautious use of IV esmolol Observation for myocardial or pulmonary disorder (usually before emergency department arrival) For hyperthermia, external cooling
Codeine	See Opioids	—
Colchicine	Nausea, hemorrhagic gastritis, multiorgan failure, sepsis	Multiple-dose activated charcoal, IV fluids, supportive care, granulocyte colony-stimulating factor
Copper	See Copper salts	—
Copper salts • Cupric sulfate, acetate, or subacetate • Cuprous chloride or oxide • Zinc salts	Vomiting, burning sensation, metallic taste, diarrhea, pain, shock, jaundice, anuria, seizures	Penicillamine or dimercaprol (see Table 366–4 on p. 3054), electrolyte and fluid balance, respiratory support, monitoring of GI tract, treatment of shock, control of seizures, monitoring for liver and renal failure
Corrosive sublimate (mercuric chloride)	See Mercury	—
Coumaphos	See Organophosphates	—
Creosote, cresols	See Phenols	—
Cyanides • Bitter almond oil • Hydrocyanic acid • Nitroprusside • Potassium cyanide • Prussic acid • Sodium cyanide • Wild cherry syrup	Tachycardia, headache, drowsiness, hypotension, coma, rapid severe acidosis, seizures, death, possibly bitter almond odor on breath, bright red venous blood *Very rapidly lethal* (in 1–15 min)	*Speed essential* **Inhalation:** Removal from source **Inhalation or ingestion:** 100% O_2, respiratory support Inhalation of amyl nitrite 0.2 mL (1 ampule) for 30 sec of each min; 3% Na nitrite 10 mL at 2.5–5 mL/min IV (in children, 10 mg/kg), then 25% Na thiosulfate 25–50 mL at 2.5–5 mL/min IV (Lilly cyanide kit); treatment repeated if symptoms recur Hydroxocobalamin 5 g IV (becoming the preferred treatment)
Cyfluthrin	See Pyrethroids	—
Cypermethrin	See Pyrethroids	—
DDD (2-dichlorethane)	See Chlorinated and other halogenated hydrocarbons	—
DDT (chlorophenothane)	See Chlorinated and other halogenated hydrocarbons	—
Demeton	See Organophosphates	—
Deodorizers, household	See Naphthalene and Paradichlorobenzene	—
Depilatories	See Barium compounds	—

Table 366–8. SYMPTOMS AND TREATMENT OF SPECIFIC POISONS (*Continued*)

POISON*	SYMPTOMS	TREATMENT
Desipramine	See Tricyclic antidepressants	—
Detergent powders	See Caustic Ingestion on p. 3061	—
Dextroamphetamine	Amphetamines	—
Diazinon	Organophosphates	—
Dichlorvos	Organophosphates	—
Dicofol	See Chlorinated and other halogenated hydrocarbons	—
Dicumarol	See Warfarin	—
Dieldrin	See Chlorinated and other halogenated hydrocarbons	—
Dienochlor	See Chlorinated and other halogenated hydrocarbons	—
Diethylene glycol	See Ethylene glycol	—
Digitalis Digitoxin Digoxin	See Digoxin on p. 723	—
Dilan	See Chlorinated and other halogenated hydrocarbons	—
Dimethoate	See Organophosphates	—
Dinitrobenzene	See Nitrobenzene	—
Dinitro-*o*-cresol • Herbicides • Pesticides	Fatigue, thirst, flushing, nausea, vomiting, abdominal pain, hyperpyrexia, tachycardia, loss of consciousness, dyspnea, respiratory arrest, skin absorption	Fluid therapy, O_2, anticipation of kidney and liver toxicity, no specific antidote, detergents to rinse skin
Diphenoxylate with atropine	Lethargy, nystagmus, pinpoint pupils, tachycardia, coma, respiratory depression (NOTE: Toxicity may be delayed up to 12 h.)	Activated charcoal, naloxone, careful monitoring of all children for 12–18 h if ingestion is verified, supportive care
Diquat	See Paraquat	—
Dishwasher detergents	See Caustic Ingestion on p. 3061	—
Disulfoton	See Organophosphates	—
Diuretics, mercurial	See Mercury	—
Donovan solution	See Arsenic	—
Doxepin	See Tricyclic antidepressants	—
Drain cleaners	See Caustic Ingestion on p. 3061	—
Endosulfan	See Chlorinated and other halogenated hydrocarbons	—
Endrin	See Chlorinated and other halogenated hydrocarbons	—
Ergot derivatives	Thirst, diarrhea, vomiting, light-headedness, burning feet, increased heart rate and BP, cardiovascular collapse, seizures, hypotension, coma, abortion, gangrene of feet, cataracts	Benzodiazepine or a short-acting barbiturate for seizures For peripheral ischemia, heparin plus phentolamine 5–10 mg in 10 mL normal saline IV or intra-arterially or nitroprusside 1–2 mcg/kg/min IV For coronary vasospasm, IV nitroglycerin and nifedipine
Eserine	See Physostigmine	—
Esfenvalerate	See Pyrethroids	—

Table continues on the following page.

Table 366–8. SYMPTOMS AND TREATMENT OF SPECIFIC POISONS (*Continued*)

POISON*	SYMPTOMS	TREATMENT
Ethanol	See Alcohol, ethyl	—
Ether	See Chloroform	—
Ethion	See Organophosphates	—
Ethyl alcohol	See Alcohol, ethyl	—
Ethyl biscoumacetate	See Warfarin	—
Ethylene glycol Diethylene glycol • Most automotive antifreeze	**Ingestion:** Inebriation but no alcohol odor on breath, nausea, vomiting Later, carpopedal spasm, lumbar pain, oxalate crystalluria, oliguria progressing to anuria and acute renal failure, respiratory distress, seizures, coma **Eye contact:** Iridocyclitis	**Ingestion:** Respiratory support, correction of electrolyte imbalance (anion gap), consideration of correcting acidemia, ethanol (see treatment of methyl alcohol) or fomepizole 15 mg/kg IV (loading dose) followed by 10 mg/kg IV q 12 h Hemodialysis, which is definitive treatment **Eye contact:** Flushing of eyes
Explosives	See Barium compounds (fireworks) and Nitrogen oxides	—
Famphur	See Organophosphates	—
Fava bean (favism)	Symptoms of hemolysis (see p. 1107)	—
Fenthion	See Organophosphates	—
Ferric salts	See Iron	—
Ferrous salts (eg, gluconate, sulfate)	See Iron	—
Fireworks	See Barium compounds	—
Fluorides • Ammonium fluoride • Fluorine • Hydrofluoric acid • Rat poisons • Roach poisons • Sodium fluoride • Soluble fluorides generally	**Ingestion:** Salty or soapy taste **With large doses:** Tremors, seizures, CNS depression, shock, renal failure **Skin and mucosal contact:** Painful superficial or deep burns **Inhalation:** Intense eye and nasal irritation, headache, dyspnea, sense of suffocation, glottal edema, pulmonary edema, bronchitis, pneumonia, mediastinal and subcutaneous emphysema due to bleb rupture	**Ingestion:** Dilution with milk or water, IV glucose and saline, 10% Ca gluconate 30 mL IV (in children, 0.6 mL/kg) or 10% $CaCl_2$ 10 mL IV (in children, 0.1–0.2 mL/kg), monitoring for cardiac irritability, treatment of shock and dehydration **Skin and mucosal contact:** Copious flushing with water, debridement of white tissue, sometimes injection of 10% Ca gluconate locally but may be given intra-arterially, application of Ca gluconate or Ca carbonate paste or gel **Inhalation:** O_2, respiratory support, prednisone for chemical pneumonitis (in adults, 15–40 mg po bid), management of pulmonary edema
Fluvalinate	See Pyrethroids	—
Formaldehyde • Formalin (may contain methyl alcohol)	**Ingestion:** Oral and gastric pain, nausea, vomiting, hematemesis, shock, hematuria, anuria, coma, respiratory failure **Skin contact:** Irritation, coagulation necrosis (with high concentrations), dermatitis, hypersensitivity **Inhalation:** Eye, nose, and respiratory tract irritation; laryngeal spasm and edema; dysphagia; bronchitis; pneumonia	**Ingestion:** Dilution with water or milk; treatment of shock, $NaHCO_3$ to correct acidosis, respiratory support, observation for perforations **Skin contact:** Washing with copious soap and water **Inhalation:** Flushing of eyes with saline, O_2, respiratory support
Fowler solution	See Arsenic	—
Fuel, canned	See Alcohol, methyl	—
Fuel oil	See Petroleum distillates	—
Furnace gas	See Carbon monoxide	—

Table 366–8. SYMPTOMS AND TREATMENT OF SPECIFIC POISONS (*Continued*)

POISON*	SYMPTOMS	TREATMENT
Gas	See Ammonia gas, Carbon monoxide (acetylene gas, automobile exhaust, coal gas, furnace gas, illuminating gas, marsh gas), Chlorine (tear gas), Hydrogen sulfide (sewer gas, volatile hydrides), and Organophosphates (nerve gas)	—
Gasoline	See Petroleum distillates	—
Glues, model airplane	See Acetone, Benzene (toluene), and Petroleum distillates	—
Glutethimide	Drowsiness, areflexia, mydriasis, hypotension, respiratory depression, coma	Activated charcoal, respiratory support, maintenance of fluid and electrolyte balance, hemodialysis possibly helpful, treatment of shock
Gold salts	Gold chloride: Liver and kidney toxicity Cyanide gold salts: Cyanide toxicity	See Cynanide See Table 366–4 on p. 3054
Guaiacol	See Phenols	—
H_2 blockers (eg, cimetidine, ranitidine)	Minor GI problems, possibly altered levels of other drugs	Nonspecific supportive measures
Heptachlor	See Chlorinated and other halogenated hydrocarbons	—
Herbicides	See specific ingredient (eg, Arsenic, Dinitro-*o*-cresol, Chlorates and nitrates)	—
Heroin	See Opioids	—
Hexachlorocyclohexane	See γ-Benzene hexachloride	—
Hexaethyltetraphosphate	See Organophosphates	—
Histamine-2 blockers	See H_2 blockers	—
Hydrides, volatile	See Hydrogen sulfide	—
Hydrocarbons	See Benzene	—
Hydrocarbons, chlorinated	See Chlorinated and other halogenated hydrocarbons	—
Hydrocarbons, halogenated	See Chlorinated and other halogenated hydrocarbons	—
Hydrochloric acid	See Caustic Ingestion on p. 3061	—
Hydrocodone	See Opioids	—
Hydrocyanic acid	See Cyanides	—
Hydrofluoric acid	See Fluorides	—
Hydrogen chloride or fluoride	See Nitrogen oxides	—
Hydrogen sulfide • Alkali sulfides • Phosphine • Sewer or manure gas • Volatile hydrides	Gas eye (subacute keratoconjunctivitis), lacrimation and burning, cough, dyspnea, pulmonary edema, caustic skin burns, erythema, pain, profuse salivation, nausea, vomiting, diarrhea, confusion, vertigo, sudden collapse, unconsciousness	O_2, respiratory support
Hyoscine (scopolamine) Hyoscyamine Hyoscyamus	See Belladonna	—
Hypochlorites • Bleach, chlorine • Javelle water	Usually mild pain and inflammation of oral and GI mucosa Cough, dyspnea, vomiting, skin vesicles	If usual 6% household preparations have been ingested, dilution with milk (little else required); treatment of shock If concentrated forms have been ingested, esophagoscopy

Table continues on the following page.

Table 366–8. SYMPTOMS AND TREATMENT OF SPECIFIC POISONS (*Continued*)

POISON*	SYMPTOMS	TREATMENT
Hypoglycemic drugs, oral Sulfonylureas • Chlorpropamide • Glipizide • Glyburide	Hypoglycemia, diaphoresis, lethargy, confusion	Admission to the hospital, IV dextrose as needed, frequent feeding (not just sugar) plus careful observation of behavior and periodic measurement of blood glucose For persistent hypoglycemia, consideration of octreotide 50–100 mcg IV or sc bid or tid For lactic acidosis, supportive care and hemodialysis
Illuminating gas	See Carbon monoxide	—
Imipramine	See Tricyclic antidepressants	—
Inhalational anesthetics • Chloroform • Ether • Nitrous oxide • Trichloromethane	Asphyxiation Drowsiness, coma With nitrous oxide, delirium With chloroform, possible acute liver injury	**Ingestion:** Observation for kidney and liver damage; respiratory, cardiac, and circulatory support **Inhalation:** Respiratory, cardiac, and circulatory support
Insecticides	See Chlorinated and other halogenated hydrocarbons, Organophosphates, Paradichlorobenzene, and Pyrethroids	
Iodine	Burning pain in mouth and esophagus, brown-stained mucous membranes, laryngeal edema, vomiting, abdominal pain, diarrhea, shock, nephritis, circulatory collapse	Milk, starch, or flour po; early airway support; fluid and electrolytes; treatment of shock; early, aggressive airway management
Iodoform (triiodomethane)	Dermatitis, vomiting, cerebral depression, excitation, coma, respiratory difficulty	**Ingestion:** Dilution with milk or water, respiratory support **Skin contact:** Washing with $NaHCO_3$ or alcohol
Iron • Carbonyl iron (see Carbon monoxide) • Ferric salts • Ferrous salts • Ferrous gluconate • Ferrous sulfate • Vitamins with iron (NOTE: Children's chewables with iron are remarkably safe.)	Vomiting, upper abdominal pain, pallor, cyanosis, diarrhea, drowsiness, shock; possible toxicity if > 20 mg/kg of elemental iron is ingested	For serum iron > 400–500 µg/dL (> 72–90 µmol/L) at 3–6 h plus GI symptoms, deferoxamine IV infusion starting at 15 mg/kg/h and titrated to BP
Isofenphos	See Organophosphates	—
Isoniazid	CNS stimulation, seizures, obtundation, coma, hepatotoxicity	For seizures, pyridoxine given IV mg for mg ingested or, if amount ingested is unknown, 5 mg IV For acidosis, $NaHCO_3$
Isopropyl alcohol	See Alcohol, isopropyl	—
Javelle water	See Hypochlorites	—
Kerosene	See Petroleum distillates	—
Ketones	See Acetone	—
Lambda-cyhalothrin	See Pyrethroids	—
Lead • Lead salts • Solder • Some paints and painted surfaces	**Acute ingestion:** Thirst, burning abdominal pain, vomiting, diarrhea; CNS symptoms (eg, irritability, inattentiveness, decreased level of consciousness, seizures) **Acute inhalation:** Insomnia, headache, ataxia, mania, seizures **Chronic exposure:** Anemia, peripheral neuropathy, confusion, lead encephalopathy, acceleration of atherosclerosis	See Lead Poisoning on p. 3067

Table 366–8. SYMPTOMS AND TREATMENT OF SPECIFIC POISONS (*Continued*)

POISON*	SYMPTOMS	TREATMENT
Lead, tetraethyl	**Vapor inhalation, skin absorption, or ingestion:** CNS symptoms (eg, insomnia, restlessness, ataxia, delusions, mania, seizures)	Supportive care, diazepam to control seizures, fluid and electrolytes, elimination of source
Lime, chlorinated	See Chlorine	—
Lindane	See γ-Benzene hexachloride and Chlorinated and other halogenated hydrocarbons	—
Liquor	See Alcohol, ethyl	—
Lithium salts	Nausea, vomiting, diarrhea, tremors, fasciculations, drowsiness, diabetes insipidus, ataxia, seizures, hypothyroidism	**Acute:** Hydration, diazepam, possibly dialysis for end-organ damage or serum lithium level > 4 mEq/L **Chronic:** If symptoms are severe, dialysis
Lye (sodium hydroxide [NaOH])	See Caustic Ingestion on p. 3061	—
Lysergic acid diethylamide (LSD)	Confusion, hallucinations, hyperexcitability, coma, flashbacks	Supportive care, benzodiazepines For severe agitation, haloperidol 2–10 mg IV or IM in adults (repeated as necessary)
Malathion	See Organophosphates	—
Manganese	See Potassium permanganate	—
Marsh gas	See Carbon monoxide	—
Meperidine	See Opioids	—
Meprobamate	See Barbiturates	—
Mercury, compounds of • Ammoniated mercury • Bichloride of mercury • Calomel • Corrosive sublimate • Diuretics, mercurial • Mercuric chloride • Merthiolate	**Acute:** Severe gastroenteritis, burning mouth pain, salivation, abdominal pain, vomiting, colitis, nephrosis, anuria, uremia With alkyl and phenyl mercurials, skin burns **Chronic:** Gingivitis, mental disturbance, neurologic deficits	Consideration of gastric lavage, activated charcoal, penicillamine (or succimer—see Table 366–4 on p. 3054) Maintenance of fluid and electrolyte balance, hemodialysis for renal failure, observation for GI perforation **Skin contact:** Soap and water for scrubbing
Mercury, elemental • Liquid (skin contact, ingestion) • Vapor	**Liquid:** If ingested, no symptoms If injected IV, pulmonary emboli **Mercury vapor:** Severe pneumonitis	**Liquid:** If ingested, no treatment needed If injected IV, supportive care **Mercury vapor:** Supportive care
Merthiolate (thimerosal)	See Mercury—usually nontoxic	
Metaldehyde • Slug bait	Nausea, vomiting, retching, abdominal pain, muscular rigidity, hyperventilation, seizures, coma	Supportive care, diazepam
Metals	See specific metals	See Table 366–4 on p. 3054
Metformin	Lactic acidosis	For lactic acidosis, supportive care and hemodialysis
Methadone	See Opioids	—
Methamphetamine	See Amphetamines	—
Methanol	See Alcohol, methyl	—
Methidathion	See Organophosphates	—
Methotrexate	Nausea, vomiting, diarrhea, stomatitis, bone marrow suppression, thrombocytopenia, cirrhosis	IV fluids, urinary alkalinization, folinic acid (leucovorin rescue), glucarpidase to deactivate methotrexate
Methoxychlor	See Chlorinated and other halogenated hydrocarbons	—

Table continues on the following page.

Table 366–8. SYMPTOMS AND TREATMENT OF SPECIFIC POISONS (*Continued*)

POISON*	SYMPTOMS	TREATMENT
Methyl alcohol	See Alcohol, methyl	—
Methyl parathion	See Organophosphates	—
Methyl salicylate	See Aspirin and Other Salicylate Poisoning on p. 3058	—
Methylene chloride	See Carbon monoxide	See Carbon monoxide
Mineral spirits	See Petroleum distillates	—
Mirtazapine	Usually benign Most commonly, sedation, confusion, tachycardia	Observation for ≥ 8 h
Model airplane glues, solvents	See Acetone, Benzene, Petroleum distillates, and Toluene	—
Monoamine oxidase (MAO) inhibitors • Isocarboxazid • Phenelzine • Selegiline • Tranylcypromine	Nonspecific and highly variable symptoms, which are often delayed 6–24 h Sympathomimetic toxidromes, headache, nausea, dystonia, hallucinations, nystagmus, fasciculations, diarrhea, seizures, agitation, muscle rigidity Hypotension and bradycardia (which may be ominous)	Consideration of gastric decontamination, supportive care
Monosodium glutamate	Burning sensations throughout the body, facial pressure, anxiety, chest pain (Chinese restaurant syndrome)	Supportive care
Morphine	See Opioids	—
Moth balls, crystals, or repellent cakes	See Naphthalene, Camphor, and Paradichlorobenzene	—
Mushrooms, poisonous	See Mushroom Poisoning on p. 3062	—
Nail polish remover	See Acetone	—
Naled	See Organophosphates	—
Naphtha	See Petroleum distillates	—
Naphthalene • Deodorizer cakes • Moth balls, crystals, or repellent cakes (see also Paradichlorobenzene)	**Ingestion:** Abdominal cramps, nausea, vomiting, headache, confusion, dysuria, intravascular hemolysis, seizures, hemolytic anemia in people with G6PD deficiency **Skin contact:** Dermatitis, corneal ulceration **Inhalation:** Headache, confusion, vomiting, dyspnea	**Ingestion:** Blood transfusion for severe hemolysis, urine alkalinization for hemoglobinuria, benzodiazepines to control seizures **Skin contact:** Clothing removed if formerly stored with naphthalene moth balls, flushing of skin and eyes
Naphthols	See Phenols	—
Narcotics	See Opioids	—
Nefazodone	See Trazodone	—
Neostigmine	See Physostigmine	—
Nerve gas agents	See Organophosphates	—
Nickel	Hypersensitivity dermatitis **Chronic inhalation:** Pulmonary inflammation	Removal from the source, irrigation with water
Nickel carbonyl	Pneumonitis, cyanosis, delirium, seizures (see also Nickel)	Removal from source, decontamination, consideration of Na diethyldithiocarbamate po (mild exposure) or IV (severe exposure) or disulfiram if Na diethyldithiocarbamate is unavailable

Table 366–8. SYMPTOMS AND TREATMENT OF SPECIFIC POISONS (*Continued*)

POISON*	SYMPTOMS	TREATMENT
Nicotine	See Tobacco	—
Nitrates	See Chlorates and nitrates	—
Nitric acid	See Caustic Ingestion on p. 3061	—
Nitrites • Amyl nitrite • Butyl nitrite • Nitroglycerin • Potassium nitrite • Sodium nitrite	Methemoglobinemia, cyanosis, anoxia, GI disturbance, vomiting, headache, dizziness, hypotension, respiratory failure, coma	O_2 For methemoglobinemia, 1% methylene blue 1–2 mg/kg IV slowly
Nitrobenzene • Artificial bitter almond oil • Dinitrobenzene	Bitter almond odor (suggests cyanides), drowsiness, headache, vomiting, ataxia, nystagmus, brown urine, convulsive movements, delirium, cyanosis, coma, respiratory arrest	See Acetanilide
Nitrogen oxides (see also Chlorine, Fluorides, Hydrogen sulfide, Sulfur dioxide, and see p. 438) • Air contaminants that form atmospheric oxidants and that have been liberated from missile fuels, explosives, or agricultural wastes • Cobaltous chloride • Hydrogen chloride • Hydrogen fluoride	Delayed onset of symptoms with nitrogen oxides unless heavy concentration Fatigue, cough, dyspnea, pulmonary edema Later, bronchitis, pneumonia	Bed rest, O_2 as soon as symptoms develop For excessive pulmonary edema, suction, postural drainage, mechanical ventilation, prednisone 30–80 mg/day in adults and dexamethasone 1 mg/m^2 BSA in children to possibly prevent pulmonary fibrosis
Nitroglycerin	See Nitrites	—
Nitroprusside	See Cyanides	—
Nitrous oxide	See Chloroform	—
NSAIDs • Ibuprofen • Naproxen	Nausea, vomiting, CNS toxicity (eg, seizures with massive overdoses)	Clinical observation, supportive care
Nortriptyline	See Tricyclic antidepressants	—
Octamethyl pyrophosphoramide	See Organophosphates	—
Oil of wintergreen	See Aspirin and Other Salicylate Poisoning on p. 3058	—
Oils	See Acetanilide (aniline oil) and Petroleum distillates (fuel oil, lubricating oils)	—
Opioids (see also p. 3244) • Alphaprodine • Codeine • Fentanyl • Heroin • Hydrocodone • Meperidine • Methadone • Morphine • Opium • Oxycodone • Propoxyphene	Pinpoint pupils, drowsiness, shallow respirations, spasticity, respiratory failure Meperidine: Seizures	Charcoal, respiratory support, naloxone IV as required to awaken patients and improve respiration, IV fluids to support circulation
Opium	See Opioids	—

Table continues on the following page.

Table 366–8. SYMPTOMS AND TREATMENT OF SPECIFIC POISONS (*Continued*)

POISON*	SYMPTOMS	TREATMENT
Organophosphates • Acephate • Bidrin • Chlorethoxyfos • Chlorothion • Chlorpyrifos • Coumaphos • Demeton • Diazinon • Dichlorvos • Dimethoate • Disulfoton • Ethion • Famphur • Fenthion • Hexaethyltetraphosphate • Isofenphos • Leptophos • Malathion • Merphos • Methidathion • Methyl parathion • Mipafox • Naled • Nerve gas agents • Octamethyl pyrophosphoramide • Oxydemeton-methyl • Parathion • Phorate • Phosdrin • Phosmet • Pirimiphos-methyl • Temefos • Terbufos • Tetrachlorvinphos • Trichlorfon • Triorthocresyl phosphate	**Absorption via skin, inhalation, or ingestion:** Nausea, vomiting, abdominal cramping, excessive salivation, increased pulmonary secretion, headache, rhinorrhea, blurred vision, miosis, slurred speech, mental confusion, difficulty breathing, frothing at the mouth, coma	Removal of clothing, flushing and washing of skin For increased secretions, atropine 2–5 mg in adults or 0.05 mg/kg in children IV or IM q 15–60 min, repeated and increased prn (massive amounts may be necessary) as often as q 3–5 min; pralidoxime chloride 1–2 g in adults or 20–40 mg/kg in children IV over 15–30 min, repeated in 1 h if needed; O_2; respiratory support; correction of dehydration For attendants, avoidance of self-contamination
Oxalic acid Oxalates	Burning pain in throat, vomiting, intense pain, hypotension, tetany, shock, glottal and kidney damage, oxaluria	Milk or Ca lactate, 10% Ca gluconate 10–20 mL IV, pain control, saline IV for shock, observation for glottal edema and stricture
Oxycodone	See Opioids	—
Oxydemeton-methyl	See Organophosphates	—
Paints	See Lead	—
Paint solvents	See Alcohol, methyl; Petroleum distillates (mineral spirits); and Turpentine	—
Paradichlorobenzene • Insecticides • Moth repellents • Pesticides • Toilet bowl deodorizers	Abdominal pain, nausea, vomiting, diarrhea, seizures, tetany (rare)	Fluid replacement, diazepam to control seizures
Paraldehyde	Acetic acid odor on breath, incoherence, miosis, depressed respiration, coma	O_2, respiratory support
Paraquat (a strong corrosive) Diquat	**Immediate:** GI pain and vomiting **Within 24 h:** Respiratory failure (but no pulmonary problems with diquat)	Activated charcoal, fuller's earth, limited O_2, consultation with poison control center or manufacturer
Parathion	See Organophosphates	—
Paris green	See Arsenic	—

Table 366–8. SYMPTOMS AND TREATMENT OF SPECIFIC POISONS (*Continued*)

POISON*	SYMPTOMS	TREATMENT
Pentobarbital	See Barbiturates	—
Perchlordecone	See Chlorinated and other halogenated hydrocarbons	—
Permanent wave neutralizers	See Bromates	—
Permethrin	See Pyrethroids	—
Pesticides	See specific compounds	—
Petroleum distillates (see also Hydrocarbon Poisoning on p. 3064) • Asphalt • Benzine (benzin) • Fuel oil • Gasoline • Kerosene • Lubricating oils • Mineral spirits • Model airplane glue • Naphtha • Petroleum ether • Tar	**Ingestion:** Burning throat and stomach, vomiting, diarrhea, pneumonia only if aspiration has occurred **Vapor inhalation:** Euphoria, burning in chest, headache, nausea, weakness, CNS depression, confusion, dyspnea, tachypnea, rales, possibly myocardial sensitization to catecholamines (which can result in cardiac arrhythmias) **Aspiration:** Early acute pulmonary changes	Because major problems result from aspiration and not GI absorption, gastric evacuation usually not warranted Supportive care for pulmonary edema, O_2, respiratory support
Phenacetin	See Acetanilide	—
Phencyclidine (PCP)	Inattentiveness with eyes open, agitation, violent behavior, unconsciousness, tachycardia, hypertension	Quiet environment Benzodiazepines if needed to provide sedation
Phenmetrazine	See Amphetamines	—
Phenobarbital	See Barbiturates	—
Phenols • Carbolic acid • Creosote • Cresols • Guaiacol • Naphthols	Corrosive effects, mucous membrane burns, pallor, weakness, shock, seizures in children, pulmonary edema, smoky urine, esophageal stricture (rare) Respiratory, cardiac, and circulatory failure	Removal of clothing, washing of external burns with water, activated charcoal, pain relief, O_2, respiratory support, correction of fluid imbalance, observation for esophageal stricture
Phenothiazines • Chlorpromazine • Prochlorperazine • Promazine • Trifluoperazine	Extrapyramidal symptoms (eg, ataxia, muscular and carpopedal spasms, torticollis), usually idiosyncratic With overdose, dry mouth, drowsiness, seizures, coma, respiratory depression	Diphenhydramine 2–3 mg/kg IV or IM for extrapyramidal symptoms, diazepam to control seizures
Phenylpropanolamine	Nervousness, irritability, bradycardia, hypertension plus other sympathomimetic effects	Supportive care, diazepam For hypertension, phentolamine 5 mg IV over about 1 min or nitroprusside IV
Phorate	See Organophosphates	—
Phosdrin	See Organophosphates	—
Phosmet	See Organophosphates	—
Phosphine	See Hydrogen sulfide	—
Phosphodiesterase (PDE) 5 inhibitors • Avanafil • Sildenafil • Tadalafil • Vardenafil	Hypotension, tachycardia, chest pain, arrhythmias, vision loss, priapism	Supportive care, IV fluids and vasopressors, urologic consultation to treat priapism, avoidance of nitrates
Phosphoric acid	See Caustic Ingestion on p. 3061	—

Table continues on the following page.

Table 366–8. SYMPTOMS AND TREATMENT OF SPECIFIC POISONS (*Continued*)

POISON*	SYMPTOMS	TREATMENT
Phosphorus (yellow or white) • Rat poisons • Roach powders (NOTE: Red phosphorus is unabsorbable and nontoxic.)	**Stage 1:** Garlicky taste, garlic odor on the breath, local irritation, nausea, vomiting, diarrhea, corrosive burns of skin, throat, and mucous membranes (due to explosiveness and flammability of phosphorus) **Stage 2:** Symptom-free 8 h to several days **Stage 3:** Nausea, vomiting, diarrhea, liver enlargement, jaundice, hemorrhages, kidney damage, seizures, coma Toxicity enhanced by alcohol, fats, or digestible oils	Protection of patient and attendant from vomitus and feces GI lavage with dilute K permanganate (1:5000) or hydrogen peroxide (eg, 1–2%), which may change phosphorus to nontoxic oxides **For phosphorus embedded in skin:** • Submersion of the patient's body in water • Irrigation with dilute K permanganate or cupric sulfate (250 mg in 250 mL of water), recommended by some experts • Mineral oil 100 mL (applied topically to prevent absorption), repeated in 2 h • Prevention of shock • Meticulous surgical debridement • 5% $NaHCO_3$ plus 3% cupric sulfate plus 1% hydroxyethyl cellulose as a paste, which is applied to exposed skin and is thoroughly washed off after 30 min (prolonged contact with cupric sulfate may result in copper poisoning)
Physostigmine • Eserine • Neostigmine • Pilocarpine • *Pilocarpus* genus	Dizziness, weakness, vomiting, cramping pain, bradycardia, possibly seizures, agitation	Atropine sulfate 0.6–1 mg in adults or 0.01 mg/kg in children sc or IV, repeated prn Benzodiazepine prn to provide sedation
Pilocarpine	See Physostigmine	—
Pilocarpus genus	See Physostigmine	—
Pirimiphos-methyl	See Organophosphates	—
Potash (potassium hydroxide or potassium carbonate)	See Acids and alkalis	—
Potassium cyanide	See Cyanides	—
Potassium nitrite	See Nitrites	—
Potassium permanganate	Brown discoloration and burns of oral mucosa, glottal edema, hypotension, kidney involvement	Dilution with water or milk, consideration of early endoscopy, maintenance of fluid balance
Pregabalin	Agitation, sinus tachycardia, seizures, coma Withdrawal syndrome similar to withdrawal symptoms after stopping gamma-hydroxybutyrate (GHB)	Supportive care, benzodiazepines for seizures and agitation
Prochlorperazine	See Phenothiazines	—
Prolan	See Chlorinated and other halogenated hydrocarbons	—
Promazine	See Phenothiazines	—
Propoxyphene	See Opioids	—
Protriptyline	See Tricyclic antidepressants	—
Prussic acid	See Cyanides	—
Pyrethrin	See Pyrethroids	—
Pyrethroids • Bifenthrin • Cyfluthrin • Cypermethrin • Esfenvalerate • Fluvalinate • Lambda-cyhalothrin • Permethrin • Pyrethrin • Resmethrin • Sumithrin • Tefluthrin • Tetramethrin	Allergic response (including anaphylactic reactions and skin sensitivity) in sensitive people; otherwise, low toxicity unless vehicle is a petroleum distillate	Thorough washing of skin, symptomatic and supportive care

Table 366–8. SYMPTOMS AND TREATMENT OF SPECIFIC POISONS (*Continued*)

POISON*	SYMPTOMS	TREATMENT
Ranitidine	See Cimetidine	—
Rat poisons	See specific components (eg, Barium compounds, Fluorides, Phosphorus, Thallium salts, Warfarin)	—
Resmethrin	See Pyrethroids	—
Resorcinol (resorcin)	Vomiting, dizziness, tinnitus, chills, tremor, delirium, seizures, respiratory depression, coma, methemoglobinemia	Respiratory support, methylene blue for methemoglobinemia
Roach poisons	See Fluorides, Phosphorus, and Thallium salts	—
Rubbing alcohol	See Alcohol, isopropyl	—
Salicylates	See Aspirin and Other Salicylate Poisoning on p. 3058	—
Salicylic acid	See Aspirin and Other Salicylate Poisoning on p. 3058	—
Scopolamine (hyoscine)	See Belladonna	—
Secobarbital	See Barbiturates	—
Selenium	See Arsenic and Thallium salts	—
Sewer gas	See Hydrogen sulfide	—
Silver salts Silver nitrate	Stained lips (white, brown, then black), argyria (slate gray or blue skin discoloration), gastroenteritis, shock, vertigo, seizures	Control of pain, diazepam to control seizures
Smog	See Sulfur dioxide	—
Soda, caustic (Na hydroxide)	See Caustic Ingestion on p. 3061	—
Sodium carbonate	See Acids and alkalis	—
Sodium cyanide	See Cyanides	—
Sodium fluoride	See Fluorides	—
Sodium hydroxide	See Caustic Ingestion on p. 3061	—
Sodium nitrite	See Nitrites	—
Sodium salicylate	See Aspirin and Other Salicylate Poisoning on p. 3058	—
Solder	See Cadmium and Lead	—
SSRIs • Citalopram • Escitalopram • Fluoxetine • Fluvoxamine • Paroxetine • Sertraline	Commonly, sedation, vomiting, tremor, tachycardia Possibly, seizures, hallucinations, hypotension, serotonin syndrome Rarely, death With citalopram, QRS prolongation possible	Airway protection, consideration of alkalinization for QRS widening, admission of patients who have symptoms > 6 h after ingestion For severe symptoms, consideration of IV lipid emulsion
Stibophen	See Arsenic	—
Stramonium	See Belladonna	—
Strychnine	Restlessness; hyperacuity of hearing, vision, and tactile sensation Violent myoclonus that simulates generalized seizures but with intact mental status, caused by minor stimuli; complete muscle relaxation between apparent seizures; perspiration; respiratory arrest	Isolation and restricted stimulation to prevent seizures, activated charcoal po, IV diazepam, respiratory support For severe seizures, neuromuscular blockade and mechanical ventilatory support

Table continues on the following page.

Table 366–8. SYMPTOMS AND TREATMENT OF SPECIFIC POISONS (*Continued*)

POISON*	SYMPTOMS	TREATMENT
Sulfur dioxide • Smog	Respiratory tract irritation, sneezing, cough, dyspnea, pulmonary edema	Removal from contaminated area, O_2, positive pressure breathing, respiratory support
Sulfuric acid	See Caustic Ingestion on p. 3061	—
Sumithrin	See Pyrethroids	—
Syrup of wild cherry	See Cyanides	—
Tar	See Petroleum distillates	—
Tartar emetic	See Arsenic	—
Tear gas	See Chlorine	—
Tefluthrin	See Pyrethroids	—
Temefos	See Organophosphates	—
Terbufos	See Organophosphates	—
Tetrachlorvinphos	See Organophosphates	—
Tetraethyl lead	See Lead, tetraethyl	—
Tetramethrin	See Pyrethroids	—
Thallium salts (formerly used in ant, rat, and roach poisons)	Abdominal pain (colic), vomiting (may be bloody), diarrhea (may be bloody), stomatitis, excessive salivation, tremors, leg pains, paresthesias, polyneuritis, ocular and facial palsy, delirium, seizures, respiratory failure, loss of hair about 3 wk after poisoning	Treatment of shock, supportive care, diazepam to control seizures, activated charcoal (which effectively binds thallium and interrupts enterohepatic circulation), Prussian blue 60 mg/kg qid via NGT (same purpose as charcoal), chelation therapy with dimercaprol (used with varying success) Avoidance of penicillamine and diethyldithiocarbamate (which may redistribute thallium into the CNS) Consultation with poison control center for latest information advisable
Theophylline	See Aminophylline	—
Thyroxine	Usually asymptomatic Rarely, increasing irritability progressing to thyroid storm in 5–7 days	Emesis, observation at home, diazepam, possibly antithyroid preparations and propranolol but only if symptoms occur
Tobacco • Nicotine	Excitement, confusion, muscular twitching, weakness, abdominal cramps, generalized myoclonus, CNS depression, rapid respirations, palpitations, cardiovascular collapse, coma, respiratory failure	Activated charcoal, respiratory support, O_2, diazepam for seizures, thorough washing of skin if contaminated
Toilet bowl cleaners, deodorizers	See Caustic Ingestion on p. 3061 and see Paradichlorobenzene	—
Toluene, toluol	See Benzene	—
Toxaphene	See Chlorinated and other halogenated hydrocarbons	—
Trazodone	CNS depression, orthostatic hypotension, seizures, QRS prolongation (but torsades de pointes is rare), hypotension (rare)	Airway protection For hypotension refractory to fluids, norepinephrine
Trichlorfon	See Organophosphates	—
Trichloromethane	See Chloroform	—

Table 366–8. SYMPTOMS AND TREATMENT OF SPECIFIC POISONS (*Continued*)

POISON*	SYMPTOMS	TREATMENT
Tricyclic antidepressants • Amitriptyline • Desipramine • Doxepin • Imipramine • Nortriptyline • Protriptyline	Anticholinergic effects (eg, blurred vision, urinary hesitation), CNS effects (eg, drowsiness, stupor, coma, ataxia, restlessness, agitation, hyperactive reflexes, muscle rigidity, seizures), cardiovascular effects (eg, tachycardia, other arrhythmias, bundle branch block, QRS widening, impaired conduction, heart failure), respiratory depression, hypotension, shock, vomiting, hyperpyrexia, mydriasis, diaphoresis	Symptomatic treatment and supportive care, charcoal, monitoring of vital signs and ECG, maintenance of airway $NaHCO_3$ as a rapid IV injection (0.5–2 mEq/kg), repeated periodically to narrow the QRS, prevent arrhythmias, and maintain blood pH > 7.45 (constant infusion may be needed) Diazepam to control seizures Vasopressors (eg, norepinephrine) to maintain BP For severe poisoning, consideration of IV lipid emulsion
Trifluoperazine	See Phenothiazines	
Triiodomethane	See Iodoform	—
Tungsten	See p. 449	
Turpentine • Some paint solvents • Some varnishes	Turpentine odor, burning oral and abdominal pain, coughing, choking, respiratory failure, nephritis	Respiratory support, O_2, control of pain, monitoring of kidney function
Valproate	Progressive CNS and respiratory depression Hyperammonemia with or without hepatic toxicity	Respiratory and cardiovascular supportive measures, monitoring of liver function Symptomatic hyperammonemia: L-Carnitine 100 mg/kg (6 g maximum) IV over 30 min with maintenance dose of 15 mg/kg q 4 h Asymptomatic hyperammonemia: L-Carnitine 100 mg/kg po q 6 h (3 g/day maximum)
Varnish	See Alcohol, methyl and Turpentine	—
Venlafaxine	Possibly sedation, seizures, QRS prolongation, sympathomimetic symptoms (eg, tremor, mydriasis, tachycardia, hypertension, diaphoresis), hypotension Rarely death	Observation for ≥ 6 h For QRS prolongation, consideration of alkalinization
Vitamins with iron	See Iron	—
Warfarin (sometimes used in pesticides) • Bishydroxycoumarin • Dicumarol • Ethyl biscoumacetate • Superwarfarins (sometimes used in pesticides)	Single ingestion not serious With multiple ingestions, coagulopathy with increased PT/INR	For single ingestion, observation For hemorrhagic manifestations, vitamin K_1 (phytonadione) until INR is normal, transfusion with fresh frozen plasma if necessary To achieve rapid reversal, prothrombin complex concentrate
Wild cherry syrup (natural, not artificially flavored)	See Cyanides	—
Wintergreen oil	See Aspirin and Other Salicylate Poisoning on p. 3058	—
Wood alcohol	See Alcohol, methyl	—
Xylene	See Benzene	—
Zinc	—	See Table 366-4 on p. 3054
Zinc salts	See Copper salts	—

*Inclusion of one poison with another (eg, toluene with benzene) in a single row indicates that the terms are synonymous, that the poisons are chemically related, or that one poison is an ingredient or impurity of the other. Lists of substances containing the poison are examples and are not all-inclusive.

†Physicians should be aware of people who smuggle plastic bags of cocaine in the GI tract (inserted through the mouth or rectum) or the vagina (so-called packers) and people who hurriedly ingest poorly wrapped packs of drugs to avoid criminal consequences when being pursued by police (so-called stuffers).

367 Radiation Exposure and Contamination

Ionizing radiation injures tissues variably, depending on factors such as radiation dose, rate of exposure, type of radiation, and part of the body exposed. Symptoms may be local (eg, burns) or systemic (eg, acute radiation sickness). Diagnosis is by history of exposure, symptoms and signs, and sometimes use of radiation detection equipment to localize and identify radionuclide contamination. Management focuses on associated traumatic injuries, decontamination, supportive measures, and minimizing exposure of health care workers. Patients with severe acute radiation sickness receive reverse isolation and bone marrow support. Patients internally contaminated with certain specific radionuclides may receive uptake inhibitors or chelating agents. Prognosis is initially estimated by the time between exposure and symptom onset, the severity of those symptoms, and by the lymphocyte count during the initial 24 to 72 h.

Ionizing radiation is emitted by radioactive elements and by equipment such as x-ray and radiation therapy machines.

Types of radiation: Radiation includes

- High-energy electromagnetic waves (x-rays, gamma rays)
- Particles (alpha particles, beta particles, neutrons)

Alpha particles are energetic helium nuclei emitted by some radionuclides with high atomic numbers (eg, plutonium, radium, uranium); they cannot penetrate skin beyond a shallow depth (< 0.1 mm).

Beta particles are high-energy electrons that are emitted from the nuclei of unstable atoms (eg, cesium-137, iodine-131). These particles can penetrate more deeply into skin (1 to 2 cm) and cause both epithelial and subepithelial damage.

Neutrons are electrically neutral particles emitted by a few radionuclides (eg, californium-252) and produced in nuclear fission reactions (eg, in nuclear reactors); their depth of tissue penetration varies from a few millimeters to several tens of centimeters, depending on their energy. They collide with the nuclei of stable atoms, resulting in emission of energetic protons, alpha and beta particles, and gamma radiation.

Gamma radiation and x-rays are electromagnetic radiation (ie, photons) of very short wavelength that can penetrate deeply into tissue (many centimeters). While some photons deposit all their energy in the body, other photons of the same energy may only deposit a fraction of their energy and others may pass completely through the body without interacting.

Because of these characteristics, alpha and beta particles cause the most damage when the radioactive atoms that emit them are *within* the body (internal contamination) or, in the case of beta-emitters, directly *on* the body; only tissue in close proximity to the radionuclide is affected. Gamma rays and x-rays can cause damage distant from their source and are typically responsible for acute radiation syndromes (ARS—see p. 3093).

Measurement of radiation: Conventional units of measurement include the roentgen, rad, and rem. The roentgen (R) is a unit of exposure measuring the ionizing ability of x-rays or gamma radiation in air. The radiation absorbed dose (rad) is the amount of that radiation energy absorbed per unit of mass. Because biologic damage per rad varies with radiation type (eg, it is higher for neutrons than for x-rays or gamma radiation), the dose in rad is corrected by a quality factor; the resulting equivalent dose unit is the roentgen equivalent in man (rem). Outside the US and in the scientific literature, SI (International System) units are used, in which the rad is replaced by the gray (Gy) and the rem by the sievert (Sv); 1 Gy = 100 rad and 1 Sv = 100 rem. The rad and rem (and hence Gy and Sv) are essentially equal (ie, the quality factor equals 1) when describing x-rays or gamma or beta radiation.

The amount (quantity) of radioactivity is expressed in terms of the number of nuclear disintegrations (transformations) per second. The becquerel (Bq) is the SI unit of radioactivity; one Bq is 1 disintegration per second (dps). In the US system, one curie is 37 billion Bq.

Types of exposure: Radiation exposure may involve

- Contamination
- Irradiation

Radioactive contamination is the unintended contact with and retention of radioactive material, usually as a dust or liquid. Contamination may be

- External
- Internal

External contamination is that on skin or clothing, from which some can fall or be rubbed off, contaminating other people and objects. Internal contamination is unintended radioactive material within the body, which it may enter by ingestion, inhalation, or through breaks in the skin. Once in the body, radioactive material may be transported to various sites (eg, bone marrow), where it continues to emit radiation until it is removed or decays. Internal contamination is more difficult to remove. Although internal contamination with any radionuclide is possible, historically, most cases in which contamination posed a significant risk to the patient involved a relatively small number of radionuclides, such as phosphorus-32, cobalt-60, strontium-90, cesium-137, iodine-131, iodine-125, radium-226, uranium-235, uranium-238, plutonium-238, plutonium-239, polonium-210, and americium-241.

Irradiation is exposure to radiation but not radioactive material (ie, no contamination is involved). Radiation exposure can occur without the source of radiation (eg, radioactive material, x-ray machine) being in contact with the person. When the source of the radiation is removed or turned off, exposure ends. Irradiation can involve the whole body, which, if the dose is high enough, can result in systemic symptoms and radiation syndromes (see p. 3093), or a small part of the body (eg, from radiation therapy), which can result in local effects. People do not emit radiation (ie, become radioactive) following irradiation.

Sources of exposure: Sources may be naturally occurring or artificial (see Table 367–1).

People are constantly exposed to low levels of naturally occurring radiation called background radiation. Background radiation comes from cosmic radiation and from radioactive elements in the air, water, and ground. Cosmic radiation is concentrated at the poles by the earth's magnetic field and is attenuated by the atmosphere. Thus, exposure is greater for people living at high latitudes, at high altitudes, or both and during airplane flights. Terrestrial sources of external radiation exposure are primarily due to the presence of radioactive elements with half-lives comparable to the age of the earth (~ 4.5 billion

Table 367–1. AVERAGE ANNUAL RADIATION EXPOSURE IN THE US*

SOURCE	EFFECTIVE DOSE (MILLISIEVERTS)
Naturally occurring sources	
Radon gas	2.3
Other terrestrial sources	0.2
Solar and cosmic radiation	0.3
Natural internal radioactive elements	0.3
Subtotal	**3.1**
Man-made sources (average person's exposure)	
Diagnostic x-rays and nuclear medicine	3.0
Consumer products	0.1
Fallout from weapons testing	< 0.01
Nuclear industry	< 0.01
Subtotal	**3.1**
Total annual exposure	**6.2**
Other sources of exposure (average per exposure or procedure)	
Airline travel	0.001–0.014/h of flight
Dental x-rays	0.005
Chest x-ray (posteroanterior view)	0.02
Chest x-ray (2 views: posteroanterior and lateral)	0.1
Mammography	0.4
CT, head	2
CT, body (chest, abdomen, pelvis)	6–8
Barium enema	8
Nuclear medicine (eg, bone scan)	4.2

*National Council on Radiation Protection and Measurements. Ionizing radiation exposure of the population of the United States. NCRP Report No. 160 National Council on Radiation Protection and Measurements, Bethesda, MD, 2009.

years). In particular, uranium (^{238}U) and thorium (^{232}Th) along with several dozen of their radioactive progeny and a radioactive isotope of potassium (^{40}K) are present in many rocks and minerals. Small quantities of these radionuclides are in the food, water, and air and thus contribute to internal exposure as these radionuclides are invariably incorporated into the body. The majority of the dose from internally incorporated radionuclides is from radioisotopes of carbon (^{14}C) and potassium (^{40}K), and because these and other elements (stable and radioactive forms) are constantly replenished in the body by ingestion and inhalation, there are approximately 7,000 atoms undergoing radioactive decay each second.

Internal exposure from the inhalation of radioactive isotopes of the noble gas radon (^{222}Rn and ^{220}Rn), which are also formed from the Uranium (^{238}U) decay series, accounts for the largest portion (73%) of the US population's average per capita naturally occurring radiation dose. Cosmic radiation accounts for 11%, radioactive elements in the body for 9%, and external terrestrial radiation for 7%. In the US, people receive an average effective dose of about 3 millisieverts (mSv)/yr from natural sources (range ~ 0.5 to 20 mSv/yr). However, in some parts of the world, people receive > 50 mSv/yr. The doses from natural background radiation are far too low to cause radiation injuries; they may result in a small increase in the risk of cancer, although some experts think there is no increased risk.

In the US, people receive on the average about 3 mSv/yr from man-made sources, the vast majority of which involve medical imaging. On a per capita basis, the contribution of exposure from medical imaging is highest for CT and nuclear cardiology procedures. However, medical diagnostic procedures rarely impart doses sufficient to cause radiation injury, although there is a small theoretical increase in the risk of cancer. Exceptions may include certain prolonged fluoroscopically guided interventional procedures (eg, endovascular reconstruction, vascular embolization, cardiac and tumor radiofrequency ablation); these procedures have caused injuries to skin and underlying tissues. Radiation therapy can also cause injury to normal tissues near the target tissue.

A very small portion of average public exposure results from radiation accidents and fallout from nuclear weapons testing. Accidents may involve industrial irradiators, industrial radiography sources, and nuclear reactors. These accidents commonly result from failure to follow safety procedures (eg, interlocks being bypassed). Radiation injuries have also been caused by lost or stolen medical or industrial sources containing large quantities of the radionuclide. People seeking medical care for these injuries may be unaware that they were exposed to radiation.

Unintended releases of radioactive material have occurred, including from the Three Mile Island plant in Pennsylvania in 1979, the Chernobyl reactor in Ukraine in 1986, and the Fukushima Daiichi nuclear power facility in Japan in 2011. Exposure from Three Mile Island was minimal because there was no breach of the containment vessel as occurred at Chernobyl and no hydrogen explosion as occurred at Fukushima. People living within 1.6 km of Three Mile Island received at most only about 0.08 mSv (a fraction of what is received from natural sources in a month). However, the 115,000 people who were eventually evacuated from the area around the Chernobyl plant received an average effective dose of about 30 mSv and an average thyroid dose of about 490 mGy. People working at the Chernobyl plant at the time of the accident received significantly higher doses. More than 30 workers and emergency responders died within a few months of the accident, and many more experienced acute radiation sickness. Low-level contamination from that accident was detected as far away as Europe, Asia, and even (to a lesser extent) North America. The average cumulative exposure for the general population in various affected regions of Belarus, Russia, and Ukraine over a 20-yr period after the accident was estimated to be about 9 mSv. The earthquake and tsunami in Japan in 2011 led to releases of radioactive material into the environment from several reactors at the Fukushima Daiichi nuclear power plant. There were no serious radiation-induced injuries to on-site workers. Among nearly 400,000 residents in Fukushima prefecture, the estimated effective dose (based on interviews and dose reconstruction modeling) was < 2 mSv for 95% of the people and < 5 mSv for 99.8%. WHO estimates were somewhat higher because of intentionally more conservative assumptions regarding exposure. The effective dose in prefectures not immediately adjacent to Fukushima was estimated to be between 0.1 to 1 mSv, and the dose to populations outside of Japan was negligible (< 0.01 mSv).

Another significant radiation event was the detonation of 2 atomic bombs over Japan in August 1945, which caused about 110,000 deaths from the immediate trauma of the blast and heat. A much smaller number (< 600) of excess deaths due to radiation-induced cancer have occurred over the ensuing 60 yr. Ongoing health surveillance of the survivors remains among the most important sources of estimates of radiation-induced cancer risk.

While several criminal cases of intentional contamination of individuals have been reported, radiation exposure to a population as a result of terrorist activities has not occurred but remains a concern. A possible scenario involves the use of a device to contaminate an area by dispersing radioactive material (eg, from a discarded radiotherapy source of cesium-137). A radiation dispersal device (RDD) that uses conventional explosives is referred to as a dirty bomb. Other terrorist scenarios include using a hidden radiation source to expose unsuspecting people to large doses of radiation, attacking a nuclear reactor or radioactive material storage facility, and detonating a nuclear weapon (eg, an improvised nuclear device [IND], a stolen weapon).

Pathophysiology

Ionizing radiation can damage DNA, RNA, and proteins directly, but more often the damage to these molecules is indirect, caused by highly reactive free radicals generated by radiation's interaction with intracellular water molecules. Large doses of radiation can cause cell death, and lower doses may interfere with cellular proliferation. Damage to other cellular components can result in progressive tissue hypoplasia, atrophy, and eventually fibrosis.

Factors affecting response: Biologic response to radiation varies with

- Tissue radiosensitivity
- Dose
- Duration of exposure
- The age of the patient

Cells and tissues differ in their radiosensitivity. In general, cells that are undifferentiated and those that have high mitotic rates (eg, stem cells, cancer cells) are particularly vulnerable to radiation. Because radiation preferentially depletes rapidly dividing stem cells over the more resistant mature cells, there is typically a latent period between radiation exposure and overt radiation injury. Injury does not manifest until a significant fraction of the mature cells die of natural senescence and, due to loss of stem cells, are not replaced.

Cellular sensitivities in approximate descending order from most to least sensitive are

- Lymphoid cells
- Germ cells
- Proliferating bone marrow cells
- Intestinal epithelial cells
- Epidermal stem cells
- Hepatic cells
- Epithelium of lung alveoli and biliary passages
- Kidney epithelial cells
- Endothelial cells (pleura and peritoneum)
- Connective tissue cells
- Bone cells
- Muscle, brain, and spinal cord cells

The severity of radiation injury depends on the dose and the length of time over which it is delivered. A single rapid dose is more damaging than the same dose given over weeks or months. Dose response also depends on the fraction of the body exposed. Significant illness is certain, and death is possible, after a whole-body dose > 4.5 Gy delivered over a short time interval; however, 10s of Gy can be well tolerated when delivered over a long period to a small area of tissue (eg, for cancer therapy).

Other factors can increase the sensitivity to radiation injury. Children are more susceptible to radiation injury because they have a higher rate of cellular proliferation. People who are homozygous for the ataxia-telangiectasia gene exhibit greatly increased sensitivity to radiation injury. Disorders, such as connective tissue disorders and diabetes, may increase sensitivity to radiation injury. Chemotherapeutic agents may also increase sensitivity to radiation injury.

Cancer and teratogenicity: Genetic damage to somatic cells may result in malignant transformation, and damage to germ cells raises the theoretical possibility of transmissible genetic defects.

Protracted whole-body exposure to 0.5 Gy is estimated to increase an average adult's lifetime risk of cancer mortality from approximately 22% to about 24.5%, an 11% relative risk increase but only a 2.5% absolute risk increase. The chance of developing cancer due to commonly encountered doses (ie, from background radiation and typical imaging tests (see p. 3221) is much less and may be zero. Estimates of increased risk of radiation-induced cancer as a result of the typically low doses experienced by people in the vicinity of reactor incidents such as Fukushima have been made by extrapolating downward from known effects of much higher doses. The very small resultant theoretical effect is multiplied by a large population to give what may appear to be a concerning number of additional cancer deaths. The validity of such extrapolations cannot be confirmed because the hypothesized increase in risk is too small to be detected in epidemiologic studies, and the possibility that there is no increased cancer risk due to this exposure cannot be excluded.

Children are more susceptible because they have a higher number of future cell divisions and a longer life span during which cancer may manifest. CT of the abdomen done in a 1-yr-old child is estimated to increase the child's estimated lifetime absolute risk of developing cancer by about 0.1%. Radionuclides that are incorporated into specific tissues are potentially carcinogenic at those sites (eg, the Chernobyl reactor accident resulted in substantial radioactive iodine uptake due to consumption of contaminated milk, and subsequent excess thyroid cancers occurred among exposed children).

The fetus is exceptionally susceptible to high-dose radiation injury. However, at doses < 100 mGy, teratogenic effects are unlikely. The fetal risk from radiation at doses typical of imaging tests that pregnant women are likely to undergo is very small compared with the overall risk of birth defects (2 to 6 % observable at birth) and the potential diagnostic benefit of the examination. The increased risk of developing cancer as a result of in-utero radiation exposure is about the same as that from radiation exposure of children which is about 2 to 3 times the adult risk of 5%/Sv.

The potential risks from radiation exposure mandate giving careful consideration to the need for (or alternatives to) imaging tests involving radiation, optimizing the radiation exposure for body habitus and clinical question, and attention to the use of proper radiation protection procedures, especially in children and pregnant women.

Damage to reproductive cells has been shown to cause birth anomalies in progeny of severely irradiated animals.

However, hereditary effects have not been found in children of radiation-exposed humans, including the children of Japanese atomic bomb survivors or the children of cancer survivors treated with radiotherapy. The average dose to the ovaries was ~ 0.5 Gy and to the testes 1.2 Gy.

Symptoms and Signs

Clinical manifestations depend on whether radiation exposure involves the whole body (acute radiation syndrome) or is limited to a small portion of the body (focal radiation injury).

Acute radiation syndromes: After the whole body, or a large portion of the body, receives a high dose of penetrating radiation, several distinct syndromes may occur:

- Cerebrovascular syndrome
- Gastrointestinal (GI) syndrome
- Hematopoietic syndrome

These syndromes have 3 different phases:

- Prodromal phase (minutes to 2 days after exposure): Lethargy and GI symptoms (nausea, anorexia, vomiting, diarrhea) are possible.
- Latent asymptomatic phase (hours to 21 days after exposure)
- Overt systemic illness phase (hours to > 60 days after exposure): Illness is classified by the main organ system affected

Which syndrome develops, how severe it is, and how quickly it progresses depend on radiation dose (see Table 367–2). The symptoms and time course are fairly consistent for a given dose of radiation and thus can help estimate radiation exposure.

The **cerebrovascular syndrome,** the dominant manifestation of extremely high whole-body doses of radiation (> 30 Gy), is always fatal. The prodrome develops within minutes to 1 h after exposure. There is little or no latent phase. Patients develop tremors, seizures, ataxia, and cerebral edema and die within hours to 1 or 2 days.

The **GI syndrome** is the dominant manifestation after whole-body doses of about 6 to 30 Gy. Prodromal symptoms, often marked, develop within about 1 h and resolve within 2 days. During the latent period of 4 to 5 days, GI mucosal cells die. Cell death is followed by intractable nausea, vomiting, and diarrhea, which lead to severe dehydration and electrolyte imbalances, diminished plasma volume, and vascular collapse. Necrosis of intestine may also occur, predisposing to intestinal perforation, bacteremia, and sepsis. Death is common. Patients receiving > 10 Gy may have cerebrovascular symptoms (suggesting a lethal dose). Survivors also have the hematopoietic syndrome.

The **hematopoietic syndrome** is the dominant manifestation after whole-body doses of about 1 to 6 Gy and consists of a generalized pancytopenia. A mild prodrome may begin after 1 to 6 h, lasting 24 to 48 h. Bone marrow stem cells are significantly depleted, but mature blood cells in circulation are largely unaffected. Circulating lymphocytes are an exception, and lymphopenia may be evident within hours to days after exposure. As the cells in circulation die by senescence, they are not replaced in sufficient numbers, resulting in pancytopenia. Thus, patients remain asymptomatic during a latent period of up to 4.5 wk after a 1-Gy dose as the impediment of hematopoiesis progresses. Risk of various infections is increased as a result of the neutropenia (most prominent at 2 to 4 wk) and decreased antibody production. Petechiae and mucosal bleeding result from thrombocytopenia, which develops within 3 to 4 wk and may persist for months. Anemia develops slowly, because preexisting RBCs have a longer life span than WBCs and platelets. Survivors have an increased incidence of radiation-induced cancer, including leukemia.

Cutaneous radiation injury (CRI) is injury to the skin and underlying tissues due to acute radiation doses as low as 3 Gy (see Table 367–3). CRI can occur with ARS or with focal radiation exposure and ranges from mild transient erythema to necrosis. Delayed effects (> 6 mo after exposure) include hyperpigmentation and hypopigmentation, progressive fibrosis, and diffuse telangiectasia. Thin atrophic skin can be easily damaged by mild mechanical trauma. Exposed skin is at increased risk of squamous cell carcinoma. In particular, the possibility of radiation exposure should be considered when patients present with a painful nonhealing skin burn without a history of thermal injury.

Focal injury: Radiation to almost any organ can have both acute and chronic adverse effects (see Table 367–3). In most patients, these adverse effects result from radiation therapy (see p. 1185). Other common sources of exposure include inadvertent contact with unsecured food irradiators, radiation therapy equipment, x-ray diffraction equipment, and other industrial or medical radiation sources capable of producing high dose rates. Also, prolonged exposure to x-rays during certain interventional procedures done under fluoroscopic guidance can result in CRI. Radiation-induced sores or ulcers may take months or years to fully develop. Patients with severe CRI have severe pain and often require surgical intervention.

Diagnosis

- Symptoms, severity, and symptom latency
- Serial absolute lymphocyte counts and serum amylase levels

Diagnosis is by history of exposure, symptoms and signs, and laboratory testing. The onset, time course, and severity of symptoms can help determine radiation dose and thus also help triage patients relative to their likely consequences. However, some prodromal symptoms (eg, nausea, vomiting, diarrhea, tremors) are nonspecific, and causes other than radiation should be considered. Many patients *without* sufficient exposure to cause acute radiation syndromes may present with similar, nonspecific symptoms, particularly after a terrorist attack or reactor accident, when anxiety is high.

After acute radiation exposure, CBC with differential and calculation of absolute lymphocyte count is done and repeated 24, 48, and 72 h after exposure to estimate the initial radiation dose and prognosis (see Table 367–4). The relationship between dose and lymphocyte counts can be altered by physical trauma, which can shift lymphocytes from the interstitial spaces into the vasculature, raising the lymphocyte count. This stress-related increase is transient and typically resolves within 24 to 48 h after the physical insult. The CBC is repeated weekly to monitor bone marrow activity and as needed based on the clinical course. Serum amylase level rises in a dose-dependent fashion beginning 24 h after significant radiation exposure, so levels are measured at baseline and daily thereafter. Other laboratory tests are done if feasible:

- C-reactive protein (CRP) level: CRP increases with radiation dose; levels show promise to discriminate between minimally and heavily exposed patients.
- Blood citrulline level: Decreasing citrulline levels indicate GI damage.
- Blood fms-related tyrosine kinase-3 (FLT-3) ligand levels: FLT-3 is a marker for hematopoietic damage.
- IL-6: Marker is increased at higher radiation doses.
- Quantitative granulocyte colony-stimulating factor (G-CSF) test: Levels are increased at higher radiation doses.
- Cytogenetic studies with over dispersion index: These studies are used to evaluate for partial body exposure.

Table 367–2. EFFECTS OF WHOLE-BODY IRRADIATION FROM EXTERNAL RADIATION OR INTERNAL ABSORPTION

PHASE OF SYNDROME	FEATURE	DOSE RANGE (GY)*,†				
		1–2	2–6	6–8	8–30	> 30
Prodrome	Incidence of nausea and vomiting	5–50%	50–100%	75–100%	90–100%	100%
	Time of onset of nausea and vomiting after exposure‡	2–6 h	1–2 h	10–60 min	< 10 min	Minutes
	Duration of nausea and vomiting	< 24 h	24–48 h	< 48 h	< 48 h	N/A (patients die in < 48 h)
	Severity and incidence of diarrhea	None	None to mild (< 10%)	Heavy (> 10%)	Heavy (> 95%)	Heavy (100%)
	Time of onset of diarrhea after exposure	—	3–8 h	1–3 h	< 1 h	< 1 h
	Severity and incidence of headache	Slight	Mild to moderate (50%)	Moderate (80%)	Severe (80–90%)	Severe (100%)
	Time of onset of headache after exposure	—	4–24 h	3–4 h	1–2 h	< 1 h
	Severity of fever	Afebrile	Moderate increase	Moderate to severe	Severe	Severe
	Incidence of fever	—	10–100%	100%	100%	100%
	Time of onset of fever after exposure	—	1–3 h	< 1 h	< 1 h	< 1 h
	CNS function	No impairment	Cognitive impairment for 6–20 h	Cognitive impairment for > 24 h	At higher doses, rapid incapacitation May have a lucid interval of several hours	Ataxia Seizures Tremor Lethargy
Latent period	No symptoms	28–31 days	7–28 days	< 7 days	None	None
Overt illness	Clinical manifestations	Mild to moderate leukopenia Fatigue Weakness	Moderate to severe leukopenia Purpura Hemorrhage Infections Epilation after 3 Gy	Severe leukopenia High fever Diarrhea Vomiting Dizziness and disorientation Hypotension Electrolyte disturbance	Nausea Vomiting Severe diarrhea High fever Electrolyte disturbance Shock	N/A (patients die in < 48 h)
	Dominant organ system syndrome	Hematopoietic	Hematopoietic	GI (mucosal cells)	GI (mucosal cells)	CNS
	Hospitalization	Outpatient observation	Recommended to necessary	Urgent	Palliative treatment (symptomatic only)	Palliative treatment (symptomatic only)
	Acute mortality without medical care	0–5%	5–100%	95–100%	100%	100%
	Acute mortality with medical care	0–5%	5–50%	50–100%	100%	100%
	Death	6–8 wk	4–6 wk	2–4 wk	2 days–2 wk	1–2 days

*1 rad = 1 cGy; 100 rad = 1 Gy.

†Whole-body irradiation of up to ~ 1 Gy is unlikely to cause any symptoms.

‡Although time to emesis is a rapid and inexpensive method for estimating radiation dose, it should be used with caution because it is imprecise and has a high false-positive rate. Additional information, such as lymphocyte counts and details of the potential for exposure, improve accuracy.

Adapted from Military Medical Operations Armed Forces Radiobiology Research Institute: *Medical Management of Radiological Casualties*, edition 2. April 2003. Available at the Armed Forces Radiobiology Research Institute web site.

Table 367–3. FOCAL RADIATION INJURY*

TISSUE EXPOSED	ADVERSE EFFECTS
Brain	See p. 1912
Heart and blood vessels	Chest pain, radiation pericarditis, radiation myocarditis
Skin	Dose 2–4 Gy: Transient erythema Dose 4–5 Gy: Transient erythema, temporary epilation (within 2–3 wk of exposure to > ~ 4 Gy) Dose 5–10 Gy: Prolonged erythema, possibly permanent epilation, dry desquamation (with exposures at the high end of the range) Dose 10–15 Gy: Dry desquamation (within 2–8 wk of exposure) Dose 15–20 Gy: Moist desquamation (within 2–4 wk of exposure) Dose 15–25 Gy: Blister formation (within 2–3 wk of exposure) Dose > 20 Gy: Ulceration (within 2–3 wk of exposure) Dose > 25 Gy: Necrosis (> 3 wk after exposure)
Gonads	Depressed spermatogenesis, amenorrhea, decreased libido Threshold dose (~ 1% incidence) for sterility: • Testes: > 6 Gy, onset ~ 3 wk • Ovaries: > 3 Gy, onset < 1 wk
Head and neck	Mucositis, odynophagia, thyroid carcinoma
Muscle and bone	Myopathy, neoplastic changes, osteosarcoma
Eyes	Dose > ~ 0.5 Gy: Cataracts (after ~ 20 yr latent period; the higher the dose and the younger the age at exposure, the shorter the latent period)
Lungs	Acute pneumonitis Fractionated exposure > 30 Gy: Sometimes fatal (LD_{50} ~ >10 Gy single high-dose exposure) Pulmonary fibrosis
Kidneys	Decreased GFR, decreased renal tubular function High doses (after 6 mo–1 yr latent period): Proteinuria, renal insufficiency, anemia, hypertension Cumulative dose > 20 Gy in < 5 wk: Radiation fibrosis, oliguric renal failure
Spinal cord	Dose > 50 Gy: Myelopathy
Fetus	Growth restriction, congenital malformations, in-born errors of metabolism, fetal death Dose < 0.1 Gy: No significant effect Future cancer risk about the same as exposure of a child: ~ 10–15% per Gy

*Typically due to radiation therapy.
LD_{50} = dose expected to be fatal to 50% of patients.

Contamination: When contamination is suspected, the entire body should be surveyed with a thin window Geiger-Muller probe attached to a survey meter (Geiger counter) to identify the location and extent of external contamination. Additionally, to detect possible internal contamination, the nares, ears, mouth, and wounds are wiped with moistened swabs that are then tested with the counter. Urine, feces, and emesis should also be tested for radioactivity if internal contamination is suspected.

Prognosis

Without medical care, the $LD_{50/60}$ (dose expected to be fatal to 50% of patients within 60 days) for whole-body radiation is about 3 Gy; 6 Gy exposure is nearly always fatal. When exposure is < 6 Gy, survival is possible and is inversely related to total dose. Time to death decreases as the dose increases. Death may occur within hours to a few days in patients with the cerebrovascular syndrome and usually within 2 days to several weeks in patients with the GI syndrome. In patients with the hematopoietic syndrome, death may occur within 4 to 8 wk because of a supervening infection or massive hemorrhage. Patients exposed to whole-body doses < 2 Gy should fully recover within 1 mo, although long-term sequelae (eg, cancer) may occur.

With medical care, the $LD_{50/60}$ is 6 Gy. Occasional patients have survived exposures of up to 10 Gy. Significant comorbidities, injuries, and burns worsen prognosis.

Treatment

- Treatment of severe traumatic injuries or life-threatening medical conditions first
- Minimization of health care worker radiation exposure and contamination
- Treatment of external and internal contamination
- Sometimes specific measures for particular radionuclides
- Supportive care

Radiation exposure may be accompanied by physical injuries (eg, from burn, blast, fall). *Associated trauma is more immediately life-threatening than radiation exposure and must be treated expeditiously* (see p. 2927). Trauma resuscitation of the

Table 367–4. RELATIONSHIP BETWEEN ABSOLUTE LYMPHOCYTE COUNT IN THE ADULT AT 48 H, RADIATION DOSE,* AND PROGNOSIS

LOWEST ABSOLUTE LYMPHOCYTE COUNT (cells/mL)	RADIATION DOSE (Gy)	PROGNOSIS
> 1500 (normal adults)†	0.4	Excellent
1000–1499	0.5–1.9	Good
500–999	2.0–3.9	Fair
100–499	4.0–7.9	Poor
< 100	8.0	Almost always fatal

*Whole-body irradiation (approximate dose).
†Children normally have higher counts that decrease with age from a median of 4600/mL at 0–2 yr to 3100/mL at 2–6 yr, and 2300/mL at 7–17 yr.

Adapted from Mettler FA Jr, Voelz GL: Major radiation exposure—what to expect and how to respond. *New England Journal of Medicine* 346:1554–1561, 2002.

seriously injured takes priority over decontamination efforts and must not be delayed awaiting special radiation management equipment and personnel. Standard universal precautions, as routinely used in trauma care, adequately protect the critical care team.

Extensive, reliable information about principles of radiation injuries, including management, is available at the US Department of Health and Human Services Radiation Event Medical Management web site (www.remm.nlm.gov). This information can be downloaded to a personal computer or personal digital assistant (PDA) in case Internet connectivity is lost during a radiation incident.

Preparation: The Joint Commission mandates that all hospitals have protocols and that personnel have training to deal with patients contaminated with hazardous material, including radioactive material. Identification of radioactive contamination on patients should prompt their isolation in a designated area (if practical), decontamination, and notification of the hospital radiation safety officer, public health officials, hazardous material teams, and law enforcement agencies as appropriate to investigate the source of radioactivity.

Treatment area surfaces may be covered with plastic sheeting to aid in facility decontamination. This preparation should never take precedence over provision of medical stabilization procedures. Waste receptacles (labeled "Caution, Radioactive Material"), sample containers, and Geiger counters should be readily available. All equipment that has come into contact with the room or with the patient (including ambulance equipment) should remain isolated until lack of contamination has been verified. An exception is a mass casualty situation, during which lightly contaminated critical equipment such as helicopters, ambulances, trauma rooms, and x-ray, CT, and surgical facilities, should be quickly decontaminated to the extent possible and returned to service.

Personnel involved in treating or transporting the patient should follow standard precautions, wearing caps, masks, gowns, gloves, and shoe covers. Used gear should be placed in specially marked bags or containers. Dosimeter badges should be worn to monitor radiation exposure. Personnel may be rotated to minimize exposure, and pregnant personnel should be excluded from the treatment area.

Due to the low exposure rates anticipated from most contaminated patients, medical staff members caring for typical patients are unlikely to receive doses in excess of the occupational limit of 0.05 Sv/yr. Even in the extreme case of radiation casualties from the Chernobyl nuclear reactor accident, medical personnel who treated patients in the hospital received < 0.01 Sv. Several authoritative sources suggest that a dose of up to at least 0.5 Gy may be considered an acceptable risk for lifesaving activity.

External decontamination: Typical sequence and priorities are

- Removing clothing and external debris
- Decontaminating wounds before intact skin
- Cleaning the most contaminated areas first
- Using a radiation survey meter to monitor progress of decontamination
- Continuing decontamination until areas are below 2 to 3 times background radiation or there is no significant reduction between decontamination efforts

Clothes are removed carefully to minimize the spread of contamination and placed in labeled containers. Clothing removal eliminates about 90% of external contamination. Foreign objects should be considered contaminated until checked with a radiation survey meter.

Contaminated wounds are decontaminated before intact skin; they are irrigated with saline and gently scrubbed with a surgical sponge. Minimal debridement of wound edges may be done if there is residual contamination after multiple attempts at cleaning. Debridement beyond the wound margin is not required, although embedded radioactive shrapnel should be removed and placed in a lead container.

If necessary, consultation is available 24 h/day from the Department of Energy Radiation Emergency Assistance Center/Training Site (REAC/TS) at (865) 576–1005.

Contaminated skin and hair are washed with lukewarm water and mild detergent until radiation survey meter measurements indicate levels below 2 to 3 times normal background radiation or until successive washings do not significantly reduce contamination levels. All wounds are covered during washing to prevent the introduction of radioactive material. Scrubbing may be firm but should not abrade the skin. Special attention is usually required for fingernails and skinfolds. Hair that remains contaminated is removed with scissors or electric clippers; shaving is avoided. Inducing sweating (eg, placing a rubber glove over a contaminated hand) may help remove residual skin contamination.

Burns are rinsed gently because scrubbing may increase injury severity. Subsequent dressing changes help remove residual contamination.

Decontamination is not necessary for patients who have been irradiated by an external source and are not contaminated.

Internal decontamination: Ingested radioactive material should be removed promptly by induced vomiting or lavage if exposure is recent. Frequent mouth rinsing with saline or dilute hydrogen peroxide is indicated for oral contamination. Exposed eyes should be decontaminated by directing a stream of water or saline laterally to avoid contaminating the nasolacrimal duct.

The urgency and importance of using more specific treatment measures depend on the type and amount of the radionuclide, its chemical form and metabolic characteristics (eg, solubility, affinity for specific target organs), the route of contamination (eg, inhalation, ingestion, contaminated wounds), and the efficacy of the therapeutic method. The decision to treat internal contamination requires knowledge of the potential risks; consultation with a specialist (eg, CDC or REAC/TS) is recommended.

Current methods to remove radioactive contaminants from the body (decorporation) include

- Saturation of the target organ (eg, potassium iodide [KI] for iodine isotopes)
- Chelation at the site of entry or in body fluids followed by rapid excretion (eg, calcium or zinc diethylenetriamine penta-acetate [DTPA] for americium, californium, plutonium, and yttrium)
- Acceleration of the metabolic cycle of the radionuclide by isotope dilution, (eg, water for hydrogen-3)
- Precipitation of the radionuclide in the intestinal lumen followed by fecal excretion (eg, oral calcium or aluminum phosphate solutions for strontium-90)
- Ion exchange in the GI tract (eg, Prussian blue for cesium-137, rubidium-82, thallium-201)

Because a serious nuclear power reactor accident that releases fission products into the environment could expose large groups of people to radioiodine, decorporation using oral potassium iodide (KI) has been studied in great detail. KI is > 95% effective when given at the optimal time (1 h before exposure). However, effectiveness of KI diminishes significantly over time

(~ 80% effective at 2 h after exposure). KI can be given either in tablet form or as a supersaturated solution (dosage: adults and children > 68 kg, 130 mg; age 3 to 18 yr [< 68 kg], 65 mg; age 1 to 36 mo, 32 mg; age < 1 mo, 16 mg). KI is effective only for internal contamination with radioactive iodides and has no benefit in internal contamination with any other radioactive elements. Most other drugs used for decorporation are much less effective than KI and reduce the dose to the patient only by 25 to 75%. Contraindications to KI include iodine allergies and certain skin disorders associated with iodine sensitivity (eg, dermatitis herpetiformis, urticaria vasculitis).

Specific management: Symptomatic treatment is given as needed and includes managing shock and hypoxia, relieving pain and anxiety, and giving sedatives (lorazepam 1 to 2 mg IV prn) to control seizures, antiemetics (metoclopramide 10 to 20 mg IV q 4 to 6 h, prochlorperazine 5 to 10 mg IV q 4 to 6 h, or ondansetron 4 to 8 mg IV q 8 to 12 h) to control vomiting, and antidiarrheal agents (kaolin/pectin 30 to 60 mL po with each loose stool or loperamide 4 mg po initially, then 2 mg po with each loose stool) for diarrhea.

There is no specific treatment for the cerebrovascular syndrome. It is universally fatal; care should address patient comfort.

The GI syndrome is treated with aggressive fluid resuscitation and electrolyte replacement. Parenteral nutrition should be initiated to promote bowel rest. In febrile patients, broad-spectrum antibiotics (eg, imipenem 500 mg IV q 6 h) should be initiated immediately. Septic shock from overwhelming infection remains the most likely cause of death.

Management of the hematopoietic syndrome is similar to that of bone marrow hypoplasia and pancytopenia of any cause. Blood products should be transfused to treat anemia and thrombocytopenia, and hematopoietic growth factors (granulocyte colony-stimulating factor and granulocyte macrophage colony-stimulating factor) and broad-spectrum antibiotics should be given to treat neutropenia and neutropenic fever, respectively (see p. 1155). Patients with neutropenia should also be placed in reverse isolation. With a whole-body radiation dose > 4 Gy, the probability of bone marrow recovery is poor, and hematopoietic growth factors should be given as soon as possible. Stem cell transplantation has had limited success but should be considered for exposure > 7 to 10 Gy (see p. 1413).

Cytokines may be helpful. Recommended drugs and dosages are

- Filgrastim (G-CSF) 2.5 to 5 mcg/kg sc once/day or the equivalent (100 to 200 mcg/m^2 sc once/day)
- Sargramostim (granulocyte macrophage colony-stimulating factor [GM-CSF]) 5 to 10 mcg/kg sc once/day or 200 to 400 mcg/m^2 sc once/day
- Pegfilgrastim (pegylated G-CSF) 6 mg sc once

Radiation-induced sores or ulcers that fail to heal satisfactorily may be repaired by skin grafting or other surgical procedures.

Aside from regular monitoring for signs of certain disorders (eg, ophthalmic examination for cataracts, thyroid function studies for thyroid disorders), there is no specific monitoring, screening, or treatment for specific organ injury or cancer.

Prevention

Protection from radiation exposure is accomplished by avoiding contamination with radioactive material and by minimizing the duration of exposure, maximizing the distance from the source of radiation, and shielding the source. During imaging procedures that involve ionizing radiation and especially during radiation therapy for cancer, the most susceptible parts of the body (eg, gonads, thyroid, female breasts) that are not being treated or imaged are shielded by lead aprons or blocks.

Although shielding of personnel with lead aprons or commercially available transparent shields effectively reduces exposure to low-energy scattered x-rays from diagnostic and interventional imaging studies, these aprons and shields are almost useless in reducing exposure to the high-energy gamma rays produced by radionuclides that would likely be used in a terrorist incident or be released in a nuclear power plant accident. In such cases, measures that can minimize exposure include using standard precautions, undergoing decontamination efforts, and maintaining distance from contaminated patients when not actively providing care. All personnel working around radiation sources should wear dosimeter badges if they are at risk for exposures > 10% of the maximum permissible occupational dose (0.05 Sv). Self-reading electronic dosimeters are helpful for monitoring the cumulative dose received during an incident.

Public response: After widespread high-level environmental contamination from a nuclear power plant accident or intentional release of radioactive material, exposure can be reduced either by

- Sheltering in place
- Evacuating the contaminated area

The better approach depends on many event-specific variables, including the elapsed time since initial release, whether release has stopped or is ongoing, weather conditions, availability and type of shelter, and evacuation conditions (eg, traffic, transportation availability). The public should follow the advice of local public health officials as broadcast on television or radio as to which response option is best. If in doubt, shelter in place is the best option until additional information becomes available. If sheltering is recommended, the center of a concrete or metal structure above or below grade (eg, in a basement) is best.

Consistent and concise messages from public health officials can help reduce unnecessary panic and reduce the number of emergency department visits from people at low risk, thus keeping the emergency department from being overwhelmed. Such a communication plan should be developed prior to any event. A plan to decrease the demand on emergency department resources by providing an alternative location for first aid, decontamination, and counseling of people without emergent medical problems is also recommended.

People living within 16 km (10 miles) of a nuclear power plant should have ready access to KI tablets. These tablets can be obtained from local pharmacies and some public health agencies.

Preventive drugs: Radioprotective drugs, such as thiol compounds with radical scavenging properties, have been shown to reduce mortality when given before or at the time of irradiation. Amifostine is a powerful injectable radioprotective agent in this category. It prevents xerostomia in patients undergoing radiation therapy. Although thiol compounds have good efficacy in radioprotection, these compounds cause adverse effects, such as hypotension, nausea, vomiting, and allergic reactions. Other experimental drugs and chemicals have also been shown to increase survival rates in animals if given before or during irradiation. However, these drugs can be very toxic at doses necessary to provide substantial protection, and none currently are recommended.

368 Spinal Trauma

Trauma to the spine may cause injuries involving the spinal cord, vertebrae, or both. Occasionally, the spinal nerves are affected. The anatomy of the spinal column is reviewed elsewhere (see p. 2027).

Spinal cord injury may be

- Complete
- Incomplete

Etiology

Spinal cord injury: During a typical year, there are about 11,000 spinal cord injuries in the US.

The **most common** causes of spinal cord injuries are

- Motor vehicle crashes (48%)
- Falls (23%)

The remainder of spinal cord injuries are attributed to assault (14%), sports (9%), and work-related accidents. About 80% of patients are male.

In the elderly, falls are the most common cause. Osteoporotic bones and degenerative joint disease may increase the risk of cord injury at lower impact velocities due to angulations formed by the degenerated joints, osteophytes impinging on the cord, and brittle bone allowing for easy fracture through critical structures.

Spinal cord injuries occur when blunt physical force damages the vertebrae, ligaments, or disks of the spinal column, causing bruising, crushing, or tearing of spinal cord tissue, and when the spinal cord is penetrated (eg, by a gunshot or a knife wound). Such injuries can also cause vascular injury with resultant ischemia or hematoma (typically extradural), leading to further damage. All forms of injury can cause spinal cord edema, further decreasing blood flow and oxygenation. Damage may be mediated by excessive release of neurotransmitters from damaged cells, an inflammatory immune response with release of cytokines, accumulation of free radicals, and apoptosis.

Vertebral injury: Vertebral injuries may be

- Fractures, which may involve the vertebral body, lamina, and pedicles as well as the spinous, articular, and transverse processes
- Dislocations, which typically involve the facets
- Subluxations, which may involve ligament rupture without bony injury

In the neck, fractures of the posterior elements and dislocations can damage the vertebral arteries, causing a syndrome resembling a brain stem stroke.

Unstable vertebral injuries are those in which bony and ligamentous integrity is disrupted sufficiently that free movement can occur, potentially compressing the spinal cord or its vascular supply and resulting in marked pain and potential worsening of neurologic function. Such vertebral movement may occur even with a shift in patient position (eg, for ambulance transport, during initial evaluation). **Stable fractures** are able to resist such movement.

Specific injuries typically vary with mechanism of trauma. Flexion injuries can cause wedge fractures of the vertebral body or spinous process fractures. Greater flexion force may cause bilateral facet dislocation, or if the force occurs at the level of C1 or C2, odontoid fracture, atlanto-occipital or atlantoaxial subluxation, or both fracture and subluxation. Rotational injury can cause unilateral facet dislocation. Extension injury most often causes posterior neural arch fracture. Compression injuries can cause burst fractures of vertebral bodies.

Cauda equina injury: The lower tip of the spinal cord (conus medullaris) is usually at the level of the L1 vertebra. Spinal nerves below this level comprise the cauda equina. Findings in spinal injuries below this level may mimic those of spinal cord injury, particularly conus medullaris syndrome.

Symptoms and Signs

The cardinal sign of spinal cord injury is a discrete injury level in which neurologic function above the injury is intact, and function below the injury is absent or markedly diminished. Muscle strength is assessed using the standard 0 to 5 scale. Specific manifestations depend on the exact level (see Table 368–1) and whether cord injury is complete or incomplete. Priapism may occur in the acute phase of spinal cord injury.

In addition to motor and sensory function, upper motor neuron signs are an important finding in cord injury. These signs include increased deep tendon reflexes and muscle tone, a plantar extensor response (upgoing toe), clonus (most commonly found at the ankle by rapidly flexing the foot upward), and a Hoffman reflex (a positive response is flexion of the terminal phalanx of the thumb after flicking the nail of the middle finger).

Vertebral injury, as with other fractures and dislocations, typically is painful, but patients who are distracted by other painful injuries (eg, long bone fractures) or whose level of consciousness is altered by intoxicants or head injury may not complain of pain.

Complete cord injury: Complete cord injury leads to immediate, complete, flaccid paralysis (including loss of anal sphincter tone), loss of all sensation and reflex activity, and autonomic dysfunction below the level of the injury.

High cervical injury (at or above C5) affects the muscles controlling respiration, causing respiratory insufficiency; ventilator dependence may occur, especially in patients with injuries at or above C3. Autonomic dysfunction from cervical cord injury can result in bradycardia and hypotension, termed neurogenic shock; unlike in other forms of shock, the skin remains warm and dry. Arrhythmias and blood pressure instability may develop. Pneumonia is a frequent cause of death in people with a high spinal cord injury, especially in those who are ventilator dependent.

Flaccid paralysis gradually changes over hours or days to spastic paralysis with increased deep tendon reflexes due to loss of descending inhibition. Later, if the lumbosacral cord is intact, flexor muscle spasms appear and autonomic reflexes return.

Incomplete cord injury: Incomplete motor and sensory loss occurs, and deep tendon reflexes may be hyperactive. Motor and sensory loss may be permanent or temporary depending on the etiology; function may be lost briefly due to concussion or more lastingly due to a contusion or laceration. Sometimes, however, rapid swelling of the cord results in total neurologic dysfunction resembling complete cord injury, which is termed spinal shock (not to be confused with neurogenic shock). Symptoms resolve over one to several days; residual disability often remains.

Manifestations depend on which portion of the cord is involved; several discrete syndromes are recognized.

Brown-Séquard syndrome results from unilateral hemisection of the cord. Patients have ipsilateral spastic paralysis and loss of position sense below the lesion, and contralateral loss of pain and temperature sensation.

Table 368–1. EFFECTS OF SPINAL CORD INJURY BY LOCATION

LOCATION OF INJURY*	POSSIBLE EFFECTS†
At or above C5	Respiratory paralysis and quadriplegia
Between C5 and C6	Paralysis of legs, wrists, and hands; weakened shoulder abduction and elbow flexion; loss of brachioradialis reflex
Between C6 and C7	Paralysis of legs, wrists, and hands, but shoulder movement and elbow flexion usually possible; loss of biceps jerk reflex
Between C7 and C8	Paralysis of legs and hands
At C8 to T1	With transverse lesions, Horner syndrome (ptosis, miotic pupils, facial anhidrosis), paralysis of legs
Between T11 and T12	Paralysis of leg muscles above and below the knee
At T12 to L1	Paralysis below the knee
Cauda equina	Hyporeflexic or areflexic paresis of the lower extremities, usually pain and hyperesthesia in the distribution of the affected nerve roots, and usually loss of bowel and bladder control
At S3 to S5 or conus medullaris at L1	Complete loss of bowel and bladder control

*Abbreviations refer to vertebrae; the cord is shorter than the spine, so that moving down the spine, the cord segments and vertebral levels are increasingly out of alignment.

†Priapism, reduced rectal tone, and changes in caudal reflexes may occur with injury at any level.

Anterior cord syndrome results from direct injury to the anterior spinal cord or to the anterior spinal artery. Patients lose motor and pain sensation bilaterally below the lesion. Posterior cord function (vibration, proprioception) is intact.

Central cord syndrome usually occurs in patients with a narrowed spinal canal (congenital or degenerative) after a hyperextension injury. Motor function in the arms is impaired to a greater extent than that in the legs. If the posterior columns are affected, posture, vibration, and light touch are lost. If the spinothalamic tracts are affected, pain, temperature, and, often, light or deep touch are lost. Hemorrhage in the spinal cord resulting from trauma (hematomyelia) is usually confined to the cervical central gray matter, resulting in signs of lower motor neuron damage (muscle weakness and wasting, fasciculations, and diminished tendon reflexes in the arms), which is usually permanent. Motor weakness is often proximal and accompanied by selective impairment of pain and temperature sensation.

Cauda equina lesions: Motor or sensory loss, or both, usually partial, occurs in the distal legs. Sensation is usually diminished in the perineal region (saddle anesthesia). Bowel and bladder dysfunction, either incontinence or retention, may occur. Men may have erectile dysfunction, and women diminished sexual response. Anal sphincter tone is lax, and bulbocavernosus and anal wink reflexes are abnormal. These findings may be similar to those of conus medullaris syndrome, a spinal cord injury.

Complications of spinal cord injury: Sequelae depend on the severity and level of the injury. Breathing may be impaired if the injury is at or above the C5 segment. Reduced mobility increases the risk of blood clots, UTIs, contractures, atelectasis and pneumonia, and pressure ulcers. Disabling spasticity may develop. Autonomic dysreflexia may occur in response to triggering events such as pain or pressure on the body. Chronic neurogenic pain may manifest as burning or stinging.

Diagnosis

- Consideration of injury in high-risk patients, even those without symptoms
- CT

Spinal injuries resulting from trauma are not always obvious. Injury to the spine and spinal cord must be considered in patients with

- Injuries that involve the head
- Pelvic fractures
- Penetrating injuries in the area of the spine
- Injuries sustained in motor vehicle crashes
- Severe blunt injuries
- Injuries related to falling from heights or diving into water

In elderly patients, spinal cord injury must also be considered after minor falls.

Injury should also be considered in patients with altered sensorium, localized spinal tenderness, painful distracting injuries, or compatible neurologic deficits.

Motor function is tested in all extremities. Sensation testing should involve both light touch (posterior column function), pinprick (anterior spinothalamic tract), and position sense. Identification of the sensory level is best done by testing from distal to proximal and by testing thoracic roots on the back to avoid being misled by the cervical cape. Priapism indicates spinal cord damage. Rectal tone may be decreased, and deep tendon reflexes may be exuberant or absent.

Traditionally, plain x-rays are taken of any possibly injured areas. CT is done of areas that appear abnormal on x-rays and areas at risk of injury based on clinical findings. However, CT is being used increasingly as the primary imaging study for spinal trauma because it has better diagnostic accuracy and, at many trauma centers, can be obtained rapidly.

MRI helps identify the type and location of cord injury; it is the most accurate study for imaging the spinal cord and other soft tissues but may not be immediately available. Manifestations of injury may be characterized using the ASIA (American Spinal Injury Association) Impairment Scale or a similar instrument (see Table 368–2).

If a fracture passes through the transverse foramen of a cervical vertebrae, a vascular study is usually warranted (typically, CT angiography) to rule out a dissection.

Table 368–2. SPINAL INJURY IMPAIRMENT SCALE*

LEVEL	IMPAIRMENT
A	Complete: There is no motor or sensory function, including in the sacral segments S4–S5.
B	Incomplete: Sensory but not motor function is preserved below the spinal cord level, including in the sacral segments S4–S5.
C	Incomplete: Motor function is preserved below the neurologic level, and more than half of key muscles below the spinal cord level have a muscle strength grade of < 3.
D	Incomplete: Motor function is preserved below the neurologic level, and at least half of key muscles below the spinal cord level have a muscle grade of ≥ 3.
E	Normal: Motor and sensory function are normal.

*According to the American Spinal Injury Association.

Prognosis

Transected or degenerated nerves in the cord usually do not recover, and functional damage is often permanent. Compressed nerve tissue can recover its function. Return of a movement or sensation during the first week after injury heralds a favorable recovery. Dysfunction remaining after 6 mo is likely to be permanent; however, ASIA grade may improve by one grade for up to one year after injury. Some new research demonstrates return of some function in previous complete spinal cord injuries with spinal cord stimulation.

Treatment

- Immobilization
- Maintenance of oxygenation and spinal cord perfusion
- Supportive care
- Surgical stabilization when appropriate
- Long-term symptomatic care and rehabilitation

Immediate care: An important goal is to prevent secondary injury to the spine or spinal cord.

In unstable injuries, flexion or extension of the spine can contuse or transect the cord. Thus, when injured people are moved, inappropriate handling can precipitate paraplegia, quadriplegia, or even death due to spinal injury.

Patients who may have a spinal injury should have the spine immobilized immediately; the neck is held straight manually (in line stabilization) during endotracheal intubation. As soon as possible, the spine is fully immobilized on a firm, flat, padded backboard or similar surface to stabilize the position without excessive pressure. A rigid collar should be used to immobilize the cervical spine. Patients with thoracic or lumbar spine injuries can be carried prone or supine. Those with cervical cord damage that could induce respiratory difficulties should be carried supine, with attention to maintaining a patent airway and avoiding chest constriction. Transfer to a trauma center is desirable.

Medical care should be directed at avoiding hypoxia and hypotension, both of which can further stress the injured cord. In cervical injuries higher than C5, intubation and respiratory support are usually needed.

Large doses of corticosteroids, started within 8 h after spinal cord injury, have long been used in attempt to improve the outcome in blunt injuries, but this finding has not been firmly established and is no longer standard treatment.

Injuries are treated with rest, analgesics, and muscle-relaxing drugs with or without surgery until swelling and local pain have subsided. Additional general treatment for trauma patients is provided as necessary (see p. 2927).

Unstable injuries are immobilized until bone and soft tissues have healed in proper alignment; surgery with fusion and internal fixation is sometimes needed. Patients with incomplete cord injuries can have significant neurologic improvement after decompression. In contrast, in complete injury, return of useful neurologic function below the level of the injury is unlikely. Thus, surgery aims to stabilize the spine to allow early mobilization.

Early surgery allows for earlier mobilization and rehabilitation. Recent studies suggest that the optimal timing of decompression surgery for incomplete cord injuries is within 24 h of injury. For complete injuries, surgery is sometimes done in the first few days, but it is not clear that this timing affects outcome.

Nursing care includes preventing urinary and pulmonary infections and pressure ulcers—eg, by turning the immobile patient every 2 h (on a Stryker frame when necessary). Deep venous thrombosis prophylaxis is required. An inferior vena cava filter could be considered in immobile patients.

Long-term care after spinal cord injury: Drugs effectively control spasticity in some patients. Drugs such as baclofen 5 mg po tid (maximum, 80 mg during a 24-h period) and tizanidine 4 mg po tid (maximum, 36 mg during a 24-h period) are typically used for spasticity occurring after spinal cord injury. Intrathecal baclofen 50 to 100 mcg once/day may be considered in patients in whom oral drugs are ineffective.

Rehabilitation is needed to help people recover as fully as possible (see p. 3260). Rehabilitation, best provided through a team approach, combines physical therapies, skill-building activities, and counseling to meet social and emotional needs. The rehabilitation team is best directed by a physician with training and expertise in rehabilitation (physiatrist); it usually includes nurses, social workers, nutritionists, psychologists, physical and occupational therapists, recreational therapists, and vocational counselors.

Physical therapy focuses on exercises for muscle strengthening, passive stretch exercises to prevent contractures, and appropriate use of assistive devices such as braces, a walker, or a wheelchair that may be needed to improve mobility. Strategies for controlling spasticity, autonomic dysreflexia, and neurogenic pain are taught.

Occupational therapy focuses on redeveloping fine motor skills. Bladder and bowel management programs teach toileting techniques, which may require intermittent catheterization. A bowel regimen, involving timed stimulation with laxatives, is often needed.

Vocational rehabilitation involves assessing both fine and gross motor skills, as well as cognitive capabilities, to determine the likelihood for meaningful employment. The vocational specialist then helps identify possible work sites and determines need for assistive equipment and workplace modifications. Recreation therapists use a similar approach in identifying and facilitating participation in hobbies, athletics, and other activities.

Emotional care aims to combat the depersonalization and the almost unavoidable depression that occur after losing control of the body. Emotional care is fundamental to the success of all other components of rehabilitation and must be accompanied by efforts to educate the patient and encourage active involvement of family and friends.

Investigational treatments: Treatments to promote nerve regeneration and minimize scar tissue formation in the injured cord are under study. Such treatments include injections of autologous, incubated macrophages; human-derived embryonic stem cell oligodendrocytes; neural stem cells; and trophic factors. Stem cell research is under study; many animal studies have shown promising results and there have been several phase I and II human clinical trials.

Implantation of an epidural stimulator is another treatment modality under investigation to improve voluntary movement after spinal cord injury. During epidural stimulation, electrical pulses are delivered to the surface of the spinal cord below the injury.

KEY POINTS

- Suspect spinal cord injuries in patients who have a high-risk injury mechanism (including minor falls in the elderly), an altered sensorium, neurologic deficits suggesting cord injury, or localized spinal tenderness.
- To ensure recognition of incomplete spinal cord injuries, test motor function and sensory function (including light touch, pinprick, and position sensation) and check for disproportionate weakness in the upper extremities.
- Immediately immobilize the spine in patients at risk.
- Arrange for immediate CT or, if available, MRI.
- Arrange for surgery within 24 h of injury if patients have incomplete cord injuries.
- Treat irreversible spinal cord injury with multimodal rehabilitation and drugs that control spasticity.

SPINAL CORD INJURY IN CHILDREN

Although children < 10 yr have the lowest rate of spinal cord injuries (SCI), such injuries are not rare. In children < 8 yr, **cervical** spine injuries occur most commonly above C4 and are most commonly caused by motor vehicle crashes, falls, and child abuse. In children > 8 yr, injuries at C5 to C8 are more common and due to motor vehicle crashes and sports injuries, particularly gymnastics, diving, horseback riding, American football, and wrestling. Compared with adults, children have distinct anatomic features (eg, larger head size-to-body, elasticity of spinal ligaments capsules) that predispose them to hypermobility of the spinal column without apparent bony injury.

Of increasing importance has been the recognition of spinal cord injury without evidence of radiologic abnormality (SCIWORA), which often occurs in the cervical spine. SCIWORA occurs in children with neurologic findings suggestive of spinal cord injury (eg, paresthesias, weakness) with normal anatomic alignment and no bony abnormalities seen on imaging studies (plain x-rays, CT, and/or MRI). This type of injury occurs almost exclusively in children and is related to direct spinal cord traction, spinal cord impingement, spinal cord concussion, and vascular injury.

Diagnosis

- X-rays (cross-table lateral view, anteroposterior view, and open-mouth odontoid view)
- Usually CT, particularly for bony or ligamentous injury
- MRI to confirm injury to the spinal cord

Spinal cord injury should be suspected in any child that has been in a motor vehicle crash, has fallen from a height ≥ 3 m, or has had a submersion injury.

SCIWORA is suspected in children who have even transient symptoms of neurologic dysfunction or lancinating pains down the spine or extremities and a mechanism of injury compatible with spinal cord injury. In about 25% of children, onset of neurologic signs (such as partial neurologic deficits, complete paralysis) is delayed, from 30 min to 4 days after injury, making immediate diagnosis difficult.

Imaging usually begins with x-rays, including cross-table lateral, anteroposterior, and open-mouth odontoid views. If fracture, dislocation, or subluxation is suspected based on x-ray findings or a very high-risk mechanism of injury, CT is usually done. MRI is usually done with any of the following:

- Spinal cord injury is suspected or confirmed by x-ray or CT
- Spinal cord injury is suggested by neurologic deficits on examination
- Spinal cord injury is suggested by a history of even transient neurologic deficits

Treatment

- Immobilization
- Maintenance of oxygenation and spinal cord perfusion
- Supportive care
- Surgical stabilization when appropriate
- Long-term symptomatic care and rehabilitation

Children with a spinal injury should be transferred to a pediatric trauma center.

Treatment acutely is similar to that in adults, with immobilization and attention to the adequacy of oxygenation, ventilation, and circulation. Treatment may also include high-dose corticosteroids (same weight-based dose as for adults).

369 Sports Injury

Regular exercise enhances health and a sense of well-being. However, injury, particularly overuse injury, is a risk for people who exercise regularly. (For musculoskeletal injuries not specifically associated with sports, see p. 2974.)

SCREENING FOR SPORTS PARTICIPATION

Cardiovascular screening: Screening for all children and adults should include a thorough cardiovascular history, with questions about

- Known hypertension or heart murmur
- Chest pain
- Exercise-induced or unexplained syncope (including convulsive syncope), near-syncope, chest pain, or palpitations
- Family history of sudden cardiac death at age < 50 yr, arrhythmias, dilated or hypertrophic cardiomyopathy, long QT syndrome, or Marfan syndrome
- Risk factors for coronary artery disease in adults (see p. 666)

Physical examination should routinely include BP in both arms, supine and standing cardiac auscultation, and inspection for features of Marfan syndrome. These measures aim to identify adults as well as rare, apparently healthy young people at high risk of life-threatening cardiac events (eg, people with arrhythmias, hypertrophic cardiomyopathy, or other structural heart disorders).

Testing is directed at clinically suspected disorders (eg, exercise stress testing for coronary artery disease, echocardiography for structural heart disease, ECG for arrhythmia or long QT syndrome). Routine stress testing in the absence of symptoms, signs, or risk factors is not recommended.

Other screening measures: Noncardiovascular risk factors are more common than cardiovascular risk factors. Adults are asked about the following:

- Previous or current musculoskeletal injuries (including easily triggered dislocations)
- Arthritic disorders, particularly those involving major weight-bearing joints (eg, hips, knees, ankles)
- Concussions
- Asthma
- Symptoms suggesting systemic infection
- Heat-related illness
- Seizure

Two populations at risk for injuries are commonly overlooked:

- Boys who physically mature late are assumed to be at greater risk of injury in contact sports if competing against larger and stronger children.
- Overweight or obese people are at increased risk of musculoskeletal problems because of excess body weight and associated forces on the joints and tissues. One risk is overuse injury and soft-tissue inflammation, particularly if people increase intensity and duration of exercise too rapidly. A long-term risk is osteoarthritis affecting weight-bearing joints. Another risk may be injury due to sudden stops and starts if they participate in activities that require jumping or high levels of agility.

Adolescents and young adults should be asked about use of illicit and performance-enhancing drugs.

In girls and young women, screening should detect delayed onset of menarche. Girls and young women should be screened for the presence of the female athlete triad (eating disorders, amenorrhea or other menstrual dysfunction, and diminished bone mineral density). Two questions are validated screening measures for eating disorders:

- Have you ever had an eating disorder?
- Are you happy with your weight?

Contraindications: There are almost no absolute contraindications to sports participation.

Exceptions in children include

- Myocarditis, which increases the risk of sudden cardiac death
- Hypertrophic cardiomyopathy, in which increases in heart rate can increase risk of sudden cardiac death
- Acute splenic enlargement or recent infectious mononucleosis (Epstein-Barr virus infection) because splenic rupture is a risk
- Fever, which decreases exercise tolerance, increases risk of heat-related disorders, and may be a sign of serious illness
- Possibly significant diarrhea and/or recent significant vomiting because dehydration is a risk

Exceptions in adults include

- Angina pectoris
- Recent MI (within 6 wk)
- Known aneurysms in the brain or large vessels

Relative contraindications are more common and lead to recommendations for precautions or for participation in some sports rather than others, for example:

- People with a history of frequent and easily triggered dislocations or multiple concussions (see p. 3123) should participate in noncollision sports.
- Males with a single testis should wear a protective cup for most contact sports.
- People at risk of heat intolerance and dehydration (eg, those with diabetes, cystic fibrosis, or previous heat-related illness) should hydrate frequently during activity.
- People with suboptimal seizure control should avoid swimming, weight lifting, and, to prevent injury to others, sports such as archery and riflery.
- People who have asthma need to monitor their symptoms closely.

APPROACH TO SPORTS INJURIES

Sports participation always has a risk of injury.

Generally, sports injury can be divided into

- Overuse injuries
- Blunt trauma
- Fractures and dislocations (see p. 2974)
- Acute soft-tissue sprains and strains

Many injuries (eg, fractures, dislocations, soft-tissue contusions, blunt trauma, sprains, strains) are not unique to sports participation and can result from activities that are not athletic or from accidents. Such injuries are described elsewhere in THE MANUAL (see also p. 2974). However, athletes may need to learn how to modify faulty techniques that predispose to injuries or may resist taking an adequate period of rest to recover from a sports injury (working through the pain).

Overuse: Overuse is one of the most common causes of athletic injury and is the cumulative effect of excessive, repetitive stress on anatomic structures. It results in trauma to muscles, tendons, cartilage, ligaments, bursae, fascia, and bone in any combination. Risk of overuse injury depends on complex interactions between individual and extrinsic factors.

Individual factors include

- Muscle weakness and inflexibility
- Joint laxity
- Previous injury
- Bone malalignment
- Limb asymmetries

Extrinsic factors include

- Training errors (eg, exercise without sufficient recovery time, excess load, building one group of muscles without training the opposing group, and extensive use of the same movement patterns)
- Environmental conditions (eg, excessive running on banked tracks or crowned roads—which stresses the limbs asymmetrically)
- Training equipment characteristics (eg, unusual or unaccustomed motions, such as those made while on an elliptical trainer)

Runners most often sustain injury after too rapidly increasing their intensity or length of workouts. Swimmers may be least prone to overuse injuries because buoyancy has protective effects, although they still are at risk, particularly in the shoulders, from which most movement occurs.

Blunt trauma: Blunt athletic trauma can result in injuries such as soft-tissue contusions, concussions, and fractures. The mechanism of injury usually involves high-impact collisions with other athletes or objects (eg, being tackled in football or checked into the sideboards in hockey), falls, and direct blows (eg, in boxing or the martial arts).

Sprains and strains: Sprains are injuries to ligaments, and strains are injuries to muscles. They typically occur with sudden, forceful exertion, most commonly during running, particularly with sudden changes of direction (eg, dodging and avoiding competitors in football). Such injuries also are common in strength training, when a person quickly drops or yanks at the load rather than moving slowly and smoothly with constant controlled tension.

Symptoms and Signs

Injury always results in pain, which ranges from mild to severe. Physical signs may be absent or may include any combination of soft-tissue edema, erythema, warmth, point tenderness, ecchymosis, instability, and loss of mobility.

Diagnosis

Diagnosis should include a thorough history and physical examination. History should focus on the mechanism of injury, physical stresses of the activity, past injuries, timing of pain onset, and extent and duration of pain before, during, and after activity. Patients should be asked about exposure to quinolone antibiotics, which can predispose to tendon rupture. Diagnostic testing (eg, x-rays, ultrasonography, CT, MRI, bone scans, electromyography) and referral to a specialist may be required.

Treatment

- Rest, ice, compression, elevation (RICE)
- Analgesics
- Cross training
- Gradual return to activity

RICE: Immediate treatment of most acute sports injuries is RICE.

Rest prevents further injury and helps to reduce swelling.

Ice (or a commercial cold pack) causes vasoconstriction and reduces soft-tissue swelling, inflammation, and pain. Ice and cold packs should not be applied directly to the skin. They should be enclosed in plastic or a towel. They should be left in place for no more than 20 min at a time. An elastic bandage can be wrapped around a tightly closed plastic bag containing ice to keep it in place.

Wrapping an injured extremity with an elastic bandage for compression reduces edema and pain. The bandage should not be wrapped too firmly because doing so may cause swelling in the distal extremity.

The injured area should be elevated above heart level so that gravity can facilitate drainage of fluid, which reduces swelling and thus pain. Ideally, fluid should drain on an entirely downhill path from the injured area to the heart (eg, for a hand injury, the elbow, as well as the hand, should be elevated). Ice and elevation should be used periodically throughout the initial 24 h after an acute injury.

Pain control: Pain control usually involves use of analgesics, typically acetaminophen or NSAIDs. NSAIDs should be avoided in patients with renal insufficiency or a history of gastritis or peptic ulcer disease. However, if pain persists for > 72 h after a seemingly minor injury, referral to a specialist is recommended. For persistent pain, evaluation for additional or more severe injuries is indicated. These injuries are treated as appropriate (eg, with immobilization, sometimes with oral or injectable corticosteroids). Corticosteroids should be given only by a specialist and when necessary because corticosteroids can delay soft-tissue healing and sometimes weaken injured tendons and muscles. The frequency of corticosteroid injections should be monitored by a specialist because too-frequent injections may increase the risk of tissue degeneration and ligament or tendon rupture.

Activity: In general, injured athletes should avoid the specific activity that caused the injury until after healing occurs. To minimize deconditioning, athletes can cross-train (ie, do different or related exercises that do not cause reinjury or pain). Injury may also necessitate reducing exercise range-of-motion if there is intolerable pain at certain points of movement. Initially, exercise of previously injured areas should be low in intensity to gradually strengthen weak muscles, tendons, and ligaments without risking reinjury. It is more important to maintain a good range-of-motion, which helps direct blood to the injured area to accelerate healing, than to rapidly resume full intensity training for fear of losing conditioning. Resumption of full activity should be gradual once pain subsides. Competitive athletes should consider consultation with a professional (eg, physical therapist, athletic trainer).

Athletes should be placed in a graduated program of exercises and physical therapy to restore flexibility, strength, and endurance. They also need to feel psychologically ready before re-engaging in an activity at full capacity. Competitive athletes may benefit from motivational counseling.

Prevention

Exercise itself helps prevent injuries because tissues become more resilient and tolerant of the forces they experience during vigorous activities. In general, flexibility and generalized conditioning are important for all athletes as a means to avoid injury.

General warming up raises muscle temperature and makes muscles more pliable, stronger, and more resistant to injury; it also improves workout performance by enhancing mental and physical preparedness. However, stretching before exercise has not been shown to prevent injury. Cooling down (ie, a brief period of lower-level exertion immediately after a workout) is sometimes thought to prevent dizziness and syncope after aerobic exercise and help remove metabolic byproducts of exercise, such as lactic acid, from muscles and the bloodstream. However, studies fail to show that cooling down decreases postexercise stiffness and soreness. Removing lactic acid may help decrease muscle soreness. Cooling down also helps decrease heart rate slowly and gradually to near-resting levels.

ROTATOR CUFF INJURY/SUBACROMIAL BURSITIS

Rotator cuff injury includes tendinitis and partial or complete tears; subacromial bursitis may result from tendinitis. Symptoms are shoulder area pain and, with severe tears, weakness. Diagnosis is by examination and, sometimes, diagnostic testing. Treatment includes NSAIDs, maintenance of range of motion, and rotator cuff strengthening exercises.

The rotator cuff, consisting of the supraspinatus, infraspinatus, teres minor, and subscapularis (SITS) muscles, together with the triceps and biceps, helps stabilize the humeral head in the glenoid fossa of the scapula during overhead arm motions (eg, pitching, swimming, weightlifting, serving in racket sports).

Etiology

Rotator cuff injury can be an acute or chronic sports injury, but it commonly occurs for reasons unrelated to sports activities and in people with no history of overuse.

A strain of the rotator cuff is a single acute, traumatic injury to the muscles. Tendinitis typically results from chronic impingement of the supraspinatus tendon between the humeral head and coracoacromial arch (the acromion, acromioclavicular joint, coracoid process, and coracoacromial ligament). Activities that require the arm to be moved over the head repeatedly, such as pitching in baseball, lifting heavy weights over the shoulder, serving the ball in racket sports, and swimming freestyle, butterfly, or backstroke, increase the risk.

The supraspinatus tendon is thought to be particularly susceptible because it has an under-vascularized region near its insertion on the greater tuberosity. The resultant inflammatory reaction and edema further narrow the subacromial space, accelerating tendon irritation or damage. If the process is not interrupted, the resulting inflammation can lead to partial or complete tear of the rotator cuff. Degenerative rotator cuff tendinitis is common among older (> 40 yr) people who are not athletes for the same reason. Subacromial bursitis (inflammation, swelling, and fibrosis of the bursal area above the rotator cuff) commonly results from tendinitis of the cuff.

Symptoms and Signs

Subacromial bursitis, rotator cuff tendinitis, and partial rotator cuff tears cause shoulder pain, especially when the arm is moved overhead. The pain usually is worse between 60° and 120° (painful arc of motion) of shoulder abduction or flexion and is usually minimal or absent at < 60° or > 120°. The pain may be described as a dull ache that is poorly localized. Complete rotator cuff tears result in acute pain and weakness of the shoulder. In larger tears of the rotator cuff, weakness of external rotation is particularly apparent.

Diagnosis

- Physical examination
- Sometimes MRI or arthroscopy

Diagnosis is by history and physical examination, including provocative maneuvers. The rotator cuff cannot be palpated directly, but it can be assessed indirectly by provocative maneuvers that test its individual muscular components; significant pain or weakness is considered a positive result.

The **supraspinatus** is assessed by having the patient resist downward pressure on the arms held in forward flexion with the thumbs pointing downward (empty can, or Jobe test).

The **infraspinatus** and **teres minor** are assessed by having the patient resist external rotation pressure with the arms held at the sides with elbows flexed to 90°; this position isolates rotator cuff muscle function from that of other muscles such as the deltoid. Weakness during this test suggests significant rotator cuff dysfunction (eg, a complete tear).

The **subscapularis** is assessed by having the patient place the hand behind the back with the back of the hand resting on the lower back. The examiner lifts the hand off the lower back. The patient should be able to keep the hand off the skin of the back (Gerber lift-off test).

The **Neer test** checks for impingement of the rotator cuff tendons under the coracoacromial arch. It is done by placing the arm in forced forward flexion (arm lifted overhead) with the arm fully pronated.

The **Hawkins test** also checks for impingement. It is done by elevating the arm to 90°, flexing the elbow 90°, and then forcibly rotating the shoulder internally.

The **Apley scratch test** assesses combined shoulder range of motion by having the patient attempt to touch the opposite scapula: Reaching overhead, behind the neck, and to the opposite scapula with the tips of the fingers tests abduction and external rotation; reaching under, behind the back, and across to the opposite scapula with the back of the hand tests adduction and internal rotation.

Other areas that may be the source of shoulder pain include the acromioclavicular and sternoclavicular joints, cervical spine, biceps tendon, and scapula. These areas should be assessed for any tenderness or deformity indicating a problem in those areas.

The **neck** is examined as part of any shoulder evaluation because pain can be referred to the shoulder from the cervical spine (particularly with C5 radiculopathy).

Suspected rotator cuff injury can be further evaluated with MRI should a brief course of conservative treatment not result in resolution of symptoms.

Treatment

- NSAIDs
- Exercises
- Sometimes surgery

In most cases of tendinitis and bursitis, rest, NSAIDs, and rotator cuff strengthening exercises are sufficient. Injections of corticosteroids into the subacromial space are occasionally indicated (eg, when symptoms are acute and severe or when prior treatment has been ineffective). Surgery may be necessary in chronic bursitis that is resistant to conservative management to remove excess bone and decrease impingement. Surgical repair may be recommended if a rotator cuff injury is severe (eg, a complete tear).

KEY POINTS

- The rotator cuff consists of the supraspinatus, infraspinatus, teres minor, and subscapularis muscles; these muscles help stabilize the humeral head during overhead arm motions (eg, pitching, swimming, weightlifting, serving in racket sports) and assist in elevation and rotation of the shoulder.
- Rotator cuff muscles may be torn acutely; shoulder instability, rotator cuff weakness, or mechanical impingement in the subacromial space may cause tendinitis (particularly of the supraspinatus tendon) and result in subacromial bursitis.
- Diagnosis is usually made by examination, but some patients require MRI and/or arthroscopy.
- Treat with NSAIDs, rest, and rotator cuff exercises.
- Surgical repair may be recommended if injury is severe (eg, a complete tear).

GLENOID LABRAL TEAR

The glenoid labrum usually tears as a result of a specific trauma, such as a fall onto an outstretched arm. Tears can also result from chronic overhead movement, as occurs in pitching. A glenoid labral tear causes pain during motion. Treatment is with physical therapy and sometimes surgery.

The shoulder (unlike the hip or elbow) is an inherently unstable joint; it has been likened to a golf ball sitting on a tee. To enhance structural stability, the glenoid (anatomically, a very shallow socket) is deepened by the labrum, which is a rubbery, fibrocartilaginous material attached around the lip of the glenoid. This structure can tear during athletics, especially during throwing sports, or as a result of blunt trauma when falling and landing on an outstretched upper extremity.

Symptoms and Signs

A glenoid labral tear results in deep shoulder pain during motion, especially when pitching a baseball. This discomfort may be accompanied by a painful clicking or clunking sensation and a feeling of catching in the shoulder.

Diagnosis

- Usually contrast-enhanced MRI

A thorough shoulder and neck physical examination should be done initially, but referral to a specialist is frequently needed because more sophisticated diagnostic tests (eg, contrast-enhanced MRI) are often the only way to definitively identify the pathology.

Treatment

- Physical therapy
- Sometimes surgery

Physical therapy is the initial treatment. If symptoms do not subside with physical therapy, and the diagnosis has been confirmed by MRI, surgical debridement or repair is the treatment of choice. Surgery is usually done arthroscopically.

LATERAL EPICONDYLITIS

(Tennis Elbow)

Lateral epicondylitis results from inflammation and microtearing of fibers in the extensor tendons of the forearm. Symptoms include pain at the lateral epicondyle of the elbow, which can radiate into the forearm. Diagnosis is by examination and provocative testing. Treatment is with rest, NSAIDs, and physical therapy.

Theories about the pathophysiology of lateral epicondylitis include nonathletic and occupational activities that require repetitive and forceful forearm supination and pronation, as well as overuse or weakness (or both) of the extensor carpi radialis brevis and longus muscles of the forearm, which originate from the lateral epicondyle of the elbow. For example, during a backhand return in racket sports such as tennis, the elbow and wrist are extended, and the extensor tendons, particularly the extensor carpi radialis brevis, can be damaged when they roll over the lateral epicondyle and radial head. Contributing factors include weak shoulder and wrist muscles, a racket strung too tightly, an undersized grip, hitting heavy wet balls, and hitting off-center on the racket.

In resistance trainees, injuries often are caused by overuse (too much activity or doing the same movements too often) or by muscle imbalance between the forearm extensors and flexors. Nonathletic activities that can cause or contribute to lateral epicondylitis include those involving repetitive grasping and twisting the elbow (eg, turning a screwdriver, perhaps typing).

With time, subperiosteal hemorrhage, calcification, spur formation on the lateral epicondyle, and, most importantly, tendon degeneration can occur.

Symptoms and Signs

Pain initially occurs in the extensor tendons of the forearm and around the lateral elbow when the wrist is extended against resistance (eg, as in using a manual screw driver or hitting a backhand shot with a racket). In resistance trainees, lateral epicondylitis is most noticeable during various rowing and chin-up exercises for the back muscles, particularly when the hands are pronated. Pain can extend from the lateral epicondyle to the mid forearm.

Diagnosis

- Provocative testing

Pain along the common extensor tendon when the long finger is extended against resistance and the elbow is held straight is diagnostic. Alternatively, the diagnosis is confirmed if the same pain occurs during the following maneuver: The patient sits on a chair with the forearm on the examination table and the elbow held flexed (bent) and the hand held palm downward; the examiner places a hand firmly on top of that of the patient, who tries to raise the hand by extending the wrist.

Treatment

- Rest, ice, NSAIDs, extensor muscle stretches
- Modification of activity
- Later, resistive exercises

Treatment involves a 2-phased approach. Initially, rest, ice, NSAIDs, and stretching of the extensor muscles are used. Occasionally a corticosteroid injection into the painful area around the tendon is needed. When the pain subsides, gentle resistive exercises of the extensor and flexor muscles in the forearm are done followed by eccentric and concentric resistive exercises. Activity that hurts when the wrist is extended or supinated should be avoided. Use of a tennis elbow (counter force) brace is often advised. Adjusting the fit and type of racket used can also help prevent further injury.

Although surgery is not usually needed, surgical techniques to treat lateral epicondylitis involve removing scar and degenerative tissue from the involved extensor tendons at the elbow. Surgery is usually considered only after at least 9 to 12 mo of unsuccessful conservative treatment; patients should be advised that surgery may not provide satisfactory relief of symptoms.

KEY POINTS

- Lateral epicondylitis can result from repetitive and forceful forearm supination and pronation, and/or extension of the forearm and wrist; such motions involve the extensor carpi radialis brevis and longus muscles of the forearm, which originate from the lateral epicondyle of the elbow.
- Typical activities that involve such motions include a backhand return in racket sports (eg, tennis) and using a screwdriver.
- Pain along the common extensor tendon when the long finger is extended against resistance and the elbow is held straight is diagnostic.
- Treat initially with rest, ice, NSAIDs, and stretching of the extensor muscles, followed by exercises to strengthen wrist extensors and flexors.
- Sometimes corticosteroid injections and rarely surgery may help.

MEDIAL EPICONDYLITIS

(Golfer's Elbow)

Medial epicondylitis is inflammation of the flexor pronator muscle mass originating at the medial epicondyle of the elbow. Diagnosis is with provocative testing. Treatment is rest and ice and then exercises and gradual return to activity.

Medial epicondylitis is caused by any activity that places a valgus force on the elbow or that involves forcefully flexing the volar forearm muscles, as occurs during pitching, golfing with improper technique, serving a tennis ball (particularly with top spin, with a racket that is too heavy or too tightly strung or has an undersized grip, or with heavy balls), and throwing a javelin. Nonathletic activities that may cause medial epicondylitis include bricklaying, hammering, and typing.

Symptoms and Signs

Pain occurs in the flexor pronator tendons (attached to the medial epicondyle) and in the medial epicondyle when the wrist is flexed or pronated against resistance.

Diagnosis

- Provocative testing

To confirm the diagnosis, the examiner has the patient sit in a chair with the forearm resting on a table and the hand supinated. The patient tries to raise the fist by bending the wrist while the examiner holds it down. Pain around the medial epicondyle and in the flexor tendon origin confirms the diagnosis.

Treatment

- Rest, ice, and muscle stretches
- Modification of activity
- Later, resistive exercises

Treatment is symptomatic and similar to that of lateral epicondylitis (see p. 3105). Patients should avoid any activity that causes pain. Initially, rest, ice, NSAIDs, and stretching are used, occasionally with a corticosteroid injection into the painful area around the tendon. When pain subsides, gentle resistive exercises of the extensor and flexor muscles of the forearm are done, followed by eccentric and concentric resistive exercises. In general, surgery is considered only after at least 9 to 12 mo of failed conservative management. Surgical techniques to treat medial epicondylitis involve removing scar tissue and reattaching damaged tissues.

PIRIFORMIS SYNDROME

Piriformis syndrome is compression of the sciatic nerve by the piriformis muscle in the posterior pelvis, causing pain in the buttocks and occasionally sciatica. Diagnosis is by examination. Treatment is symptomatic.

The piriformis muscle extends from the pelvic surface of the sacrum to the upper border of the greater trochanter of the femur. During running or sitting, this muscle can compress the sciatic nerve at the site where it emerges from under the piriformis to pass over the hip rotator muscles. Piriformis syndrome is uncommon.

Symptoms and Signs

A chronic nagging ache, pain, tingling, or numbness starts in the buttocks and can extend along the course of the sciatic nerve, down the entire back of the thigh and calf, and sometimes into the foot. Pain worsens when the piriformis is pressed against the sciatic nerve (eg, while sitting on a toilet, a car seat, or a narrow bicycle seat or while running).

Diagnosis

- Physical examination and provocative testing

Diagnosis is by physical examination. Pain with forceful internal rotation of the flexed thigh (Freiberg maneuver), abduction of the affected leg while sitting (Pace maneuver), raising of the knee several centimeters off the table while lying on a table on the side of the unaffected leg (Beatty maneuver), or pressure into the buttocks where the sciatic nerve crosses the piriformis muscle while the patient slowly bends to the floor (Mirkin test) is diagnostic. Imaging is not useful except to rule out other causes of sciatic compression. Unlike piriformis pain, lumbar disk compression of the sciatic nerve (sciatica—see p. 319) can result in radiation of pain down the lower extremity below the knee and often is associated with back pain. However, differentiation from a lumbar disk disorder can be difficult, and referral to a specialist may be needed.

Treatment

- Modification of activity
- Stretches

Patients should temporarily stop running, bicycling, or doing any activity that elicits pain. Patients whose pain is aggravated by sitting should stand or, if unable to do so, change positions to remove the source of pressure around the buttock. Specific stretching exercises for the posterior hip and piriformis can be beneficial. Surgery is rarely warranted. A carefully directed corticosteroid injection near the site where the piriformis muscle crosses the sciatic nerve often helps temporarily. NSAIDs can also provide temporary pain relief.

KNEE PAIN

Etiology

There are many causes of pain in or around the knee in athletes, particularly runners, including

- Subluxation of the patella when bending the knee
- Chondromalacia of the undersurface of the patella (runner's knee, which is softening of the knee cap cartilage—see p. 2544)
- Intra-articular pathology, such as meniscal tears and plicae (infolding of the normal synovial lining of the knee)
- Fat pad inflammation
- Stress fractures of the tibia
- Malalignment of the lower extremities
- Patellar (or infrapatellar) tendinitis (jumper's knee, which is an overuse injury to the patellar tendon at the attachment to the lower pole of the patella—see p. 2545)

Knee pain may be referred from the lumbar spine or hip or result from foot problems (eg, excessive pronation or rolling inward of the foot during walking or running).

Diagnosis

Diagnosis requires a thorough review of the injured athlete's training program, including a history of symptom onset and aggravating factors, and a complete lower-extremity examination (for knee examination, see pp. 252 and 3005).

Mechanical symptoms, such as locking or catching, suggest an internal derangement of the knee such as a meniscal tear. Instability symptoms, such as giving way and loss of confidence in the extremity when twisting or turning on the knee, suggest ligamentous injury or subluxation of the patella.

Chondromalacia is suggested by anterior knee pain after running, especially on hills, as well as pain and stiffness after sitting for any length of time (positive movie sign). On examination, pain is typically reproduced by compression of the patella against the femur.

Pain that becomes worse with weight-bearing suggests a stress fracture.

Treatment

Treatment is tailored to the specific cause of the pain.

Treatment of chondromalacia includes quadriceps strengthening exercises with balanced strengthening exercises for the hamstrings, use of arch supports if excessive pronation is a possible contributor, and use of NSAIDs.

For patellar subluxation, use of patella-stabilizing pads or braces may be necessary, especially in sports that require rapid, agile movements in various planes (eg, basketball, tennis).

If there is excessive pronation of the foot, and all other possible causes of knee pain have been excluded, use of an orthotic insert is sometimes useful.

Stress fractures require rest and cessation of weight-bearing activity.

Intra-articular pathology often requires surgery.

SHIN SPLINTS

The term shin splints refers to nonspecific pain that occurs in the lower legs during running sports.

Repetitive impact forces during jogging, running, or vigorous walking (eg, hiking) can overload the musculotendinous unit and cause shin pain. Such pain sometimes results from a specific injury (eg, tibial stress fracture, exercise-induced compartment syndrome, tibial periostitis, excessive foot pronation), but often an exact cause cannot be identified. In such cases, the term shin splints is used.

Symptoms and Signs

Shin pain can occur in the anterior or posterior aspect of the leg and typically begins at the start of activity but then lessens as activity continues. Pain that persists during rest suggests another cause, such as stress fracture of the tibia.

Diagnosis

- Usually clinical

On examination, severe localized tenderness is usually present over the anterior compartment muscles, and sometimes there is palpable bone pain.

X-ray findings are usually unremarkable, regardless of the cause. If a stress fracture is suspected, a bone scan may be necessary.

Exercise-induced compartment syndrome is diagnosed by using a specialized manometer to document increased intra-compartmental pressure during exercise.

Treatment

- Modification of activity
- Stretches, NSAIDs

Running must be stopped until it causes no pain. Early treatment is ice, NSAIDs, and stretching of the anterior and posterior calf muscles. During the rest phase of treatment, deconditioning can be minimized by encouraging cross-training techniques that do not require repetitive weight-bearing activity, such as swimming.

Once symptoms have resolved, it is advised that a return to running be gradual. Wearing supportive shoes with rigid heel counters and arch supports helps support the foot and ankle during running and can aid recovery and prevent further symptoms. Avoiding running on hard surfaces (eg, cement roads) can also help. Exercising the front of the calves by dorsiflexing the ankle against resistance (eg, rubber bands or a dorsiflexion machine) increases leg muscle strength and can help prevent shin pain.

ACHILLES TENDINITIS

Achilles tendon injuries include inflammation of the paratenon and partial or complete tears.

Achilles tendinitis is very common among running athletes. The calf muscles attach to the calcaneus via the Achilles tendon. During running, the calf muscles help with the lift-off phase of gait. Repetitive forces from running combined with insufficient recovery time can initially cause inflammation in the tendon paratenon (fatty areolar tissue that surrounds the tendon). A complete tear of the Achilles tendon is a serious injury, usually resulting from sudden, forceful stress (see p. 3005). Tendon tears can occur with minimal exertion in people who have taken fluoroquinolone antibiotics.

Symptoms and Signs

The primary symptom of Achilles tendon inflammation is pain in the back of the heel, which initially increases when exercise is begun and often lessens as exercise continues. A complete tear of the Achilles tendon typically occurs with a sudden forceful change in direction when running or playing tennis and is often accompanied by a sensation of having been struck in the back of the ankle and calf with an object such as a baseball bat.

Diagnosis

- Clinical evaluation

On examination, an inflamed or partially torn Achilles tendon is tender when squeezed between the fingers. Complete tears are differentiated by

- Sudden, severe pain and inability to walk on the extremity
- A palpable defect along the course of the tendon
- A positive Thompson test (while the patient lies prone on the examination table, the examiner squeezes the calf muscle; this maneuver by the examiner does not cause the normally expected plantar flexion of the foot)

Treatment

- Ice, NSAIDs, and stretches
- Modification of activities

Tendon inflammation should initially be treated with ice, gentle calf muscle stretching, and use of NSAIDs. A heel lift can be placed in the shoes to take tension off the tendon. Athletes should be instructed to avoid uphill and downhill running until the tendon is not painful and to engage in cross-training aerobic conditioning. Complete tears of the Achilles tendon usually require surgical repair.

STRESS FRACTURES

Stress fractures are small incomplete fractures that often involve the metatarsal shafts. They are caused by repetitive weight-bearing stress.

Stress fractures do not usually result from a discrete injury (eg, fall, blow) but occur instead following repeated stress and overuse that exceeds the ability of the supporting muscles to absorb the stress. Stress fractures can involve the proximal femur, pelvis, or lower extremity. Over 50% involve the lower leg and, in particular, the metatarsal shafts of the foot. Metatarsal stress fractures (march fractures) usually occur in

- Runners who too quickly change intensity of workouts, time of workouts, or both
- Poorly conditioned people who walk long distances carrying a load (eg, newly recruited soldiers)

They most commonly occur in the 2nd metatarsal. Other risk factors include the following:

- Cavus foot (a foot with a high arch)
- Shoes with inadequate shock-absorbing qualities
- Osteoporosis

Stress fractures also may be a sign of the female athlete triad (amenorrhea, eating disorder, and osteoporosis).

Symptoms and Signs

Forefoot pain that occurs after a long or intense workout, then disappears shortly after stopping exercise is the typical initial manifestation of a metatarsal stress fracture. With subsequent exercise, onset of pain is progressively earlier, and pain may become so severe that it prohibits exercise and persists even when patients are not bearing weight.

Patients who have groin pain with weight bearing must be evaluated for a proximal femur stress fracture. Patients with such fractures should be referred to a specialist.

Diagnosis

- X-ray or bone scan

Standard x-rays are recommended but may be normal until a callus forms 2 to 3 wk after the injury. Often, technetium diphosphonate bone scanning is necessary for early diagnosis. Women with stress fractures may have osteoporosis and should undergo dual-energy x-ray absorptiometry (see p. 324).

Treatment

- Restriction of weight-bearing activity

Treatment includes cessation of weight bearing on the involved foot (in case patients have a metatarsal stress fracture) and use of crutches. Although casting is sometimes used, a wooden shoe or other commercially available supportive shoe or boot is preferable to casting to avoid muscle atrophy. Healing can take anywhere from 6 to 12 wk.

POPLITEUS TENDINITIS

Popliteus tendinitis is inflammation in the popliteus tendon, which extends from the outer surface of the bottom of the femur diagonally across the posterior knee to the medial superior tibia.

Popliteus tendinitis is very uncommon.

The popliteus tendon prevents the lower leg from twisting outward during running as well as helping to prevent forward movement of the femur on the tibia. Excessive running downhill tends to put excessive stress on this tendon.

Pain and soreness, particularly when running downhill, develop along the posterolateral knee. Diagnosis is by physical examination. The patient sits with the involved extremity in a cross-legged position (ie, the hip flexed, abducted, and externally rotated and the knee flexed with the leg crossed over the opposite extremity). The examiner then palpates the posterior lateral corner for tenderness. The differential diagnosis of reported posterior knee pain should always include intra-articular pathology, such as a posterior horn tear of the meniscus.

Treatment includes rest, NSAIDs, ice, and occasionally physical therapy. Patients should not run until the area is free of pain and then should limit their workouts and downhill running for at least 6 wk. Bicycling is a good alternative exercise during healing.

HAMSTRING STRAIN

A hamstring strain is a partial tear of the hamstring muscles most commonly at the musculotendinous junction.

Hamstring strains are common among runners. Athletes at risk include those with poor flexibility of the hamstring muscles, inadequate pre-participation warm-up, and previous injury. Older athletes are also at higher risk. As with any muscle strain, the amount of force that caused the muscle to tear determines the degree of injury.

Symptoms and Signs

Strains of the hamstring muscles can manifest as an acute painful area in the posterior thigh when sprinting or running or develop more slowly, usually because of inadequate flexibility training.

Diagnosis

- Clinical evaluation

The diagnosis is confirmed by finding hamstring pain with knee flexion against resistance as well as on palpation of the posterior thigh. In mild strains, tenderness and mild swelling are present. In more severe strains, ecchymosis, moderate to severe swelling, and poor muscle function caused by pain and weakness are present.

Treatment

- Rest, ice, and compression
- Stretching, then strengthening exercises

Ice and compression with use of a thigh sleeve should begin as soon as possible. NSAIDs and analgesics are prescribed as necessary, and crutches may be required initially if walking is painful.

Once pain begins to resolve, patients should begin gentle hamstring stretching. When the pain has completely resolved, gradual strengthening of the quadriceps and hamstrings is begun.

Only when satisfactory strength has been achieved should patients resume running. Athletes must be made aware that recovery from hamstring injury can often take up to several months, depending on the severity.

370 Thoracic Trauma

Thoracic trauma causes about 25% of traumatic deaths in the US. Many chest injuries cause death during the first minutes or hours after trauma; they can frequently be treated at the bedside with definitive or temporizing measures that do not require advanced surgical training.

Etiology

Chest injuries can result from blunt or penetrating trauma. The most important chest injuries include the following:

- Aortic disruption
- Blunt cardiac injury
- Cardiac tamponade
- Flail chest
- Hemothorax
- Pneumothorax (traumatic pneumothorax, open pneumothorax, and tension pneumothorax)
- Pulmonary contusion

Many patients have simultaneous hemothorax and pneumothorax (hemopneumothorax).

Bone injuries are common, typically involving the ribs and clavicle, but fractures of the sternum and scapula may occur. The esophagus and diaphragm (see p. 2932) also can be damaged by chest trauma. Because the diaphragm can be as high as the nipple line during exhalation, penetrating trauma to the chest at or below nipple level can also cause intra-abdominal injuries.

Pathophysiology

Most morbidity and mortality due to chest trauma occurs because injuries interfere with respiration, circulation, or both.

Respiration can be compromised by

- Direct damage to the lungs or airways
- Altered mechanics of breathing

Injuries that directly damage the lung or airways include pulmonary contusion and tracheobronchial disruption. Injuries that alter the mechanics of breathing include hemothorax, pneumothorax, and flail chest. Injury to the lung, tracheobronchial tree, or rarely esophagus may allow air to enter the soft tissues of the chest and/or neck (subcutaneous emphysema) or mediastinum (pneumomediastinum). This air itself rarely has significant physiologic consequence; the underlying injury is the problem. Tension pneumothorax impairs respiration as well as circulation.

Circulation can be impaired by

- Bleeding
- Decreased venous return
- Direct cardiac injury

Bleeding, as occurs in hemothorax, can be massive, causing shock (respiration is also impaired if hemothorax is large). Decreased venous return impairs cardiac filling, causing hypotension. Decreased venous return can occur due to increased intrathoracic pressure in tension pneumothorax or to increased intrapericardial pressure in cardiac tamponade. Heart failure and/or conduction abnormalities can result from blunt cardiac injury that damages the myocardium or the heart valves.

Complications: Because chest wall injuries typically make breathing very painful, patients often limit inspiration (splinting). A common complication of splinting is atelectasis, which can lead to hypoxemia, pneumonia, or both.

Patients treated with tube thoracostomy, particularly if a hemothorax is incompletely drained, may develop purulent intrathoracic infection (empyema).

Symptoms and Signs

Symptoms include pain, which usually worsens with breathing if the chest wall is injured, and sometimes shortness of breath.

Common findings include chest tenderness, ecchymoses, and respiratory distress; hypotension or shock may be present.

Neck vein distention can occur in tension pneumothorax or cardiac tamponade if patients have sufficient intravascular volume.

Decreased breath sounds can result from pneumothorax or hemothorax; percussion over the affected areas is dull with hemothorax and hyperresonant with pneumothorax.

The trachea can deviate away from the side of a tension pneumothorax.

In flail chest, a segment of the chest wall moves paradoxically—that is, in the opposite direction of the rest of the chest wall (outward during expiration and inward during inspiration); the flail segment is often palpable.

Subcutaneous emphysema causes a crackling or crunch when palpated. Findings may be localized to a small area or involve a large portion of the chest wall and/or extend to the neck. Most often, pneumothorax is the cause; when extensive, injury to the tracheobronchial tree or upper airway should be considered. Air in the mediastinum may produce a characteristic crunching sound synchronous with the heartbeat (Hamman sign or Hamman crunch). Hamman sign suggests pneumomediastinum and often tracheobronchial tree injury or, rarely, esophageal injury.

Diagnosis

- Clinical evaluation
- Chest x-ray
- Sometimes other imaging studies (eg, CT, ultrasonography, aortic imaging studies)

Clinical evaluation: Five conditions are immediately life-threatening and rapidly correctable:

- Massive hemothorax
- Tension pneumothorax
- Open pneumothorax
- Flail chest
- Pericardial tamponade

Diagnosis and treatment begin during the primary survey (see p. 2927) and are based first on clinical findings. Depth and symmetry of chest wall excursion are assessed, the lungs are auscultated, and the entire chest wall and neck are inspected and palpated. Patients in respiratory distress should be monitored with serial assessments of clinical status and of oxygenation plus ventilation (eg, with pulse oximetry, ABGs, capnometry if intubated).

Penetrating chest wounds should not be probed. However, their location helps predict risk of injury. High-risk wounds are those medial to the nipples or scapulae and those that traverse the chest from side to side (ie, entering one hemithorax and exiting the other). Such wounds may injure the hilar or great vessels, heart, tracheobronchial tree, or rarely the esophagus.

Patients with symptoms of partial or complete **airway** obstruction following blunt trauma should be immediately intubated to control the airway.

In patients with difficulty **breathing,** severe injuries to consider during the primary survey include the following:

- Tension pneumothorax
- Open pneumothorax
- Massive hemothorax
- Flail chest

There is a simplified, rapid approach to help differentiate these injuries (see Fig. 370–1).

In patients with thoracic trauma and impaired **circulation** (signs of shock), severe injuries to consider during the primary survey include the following:

- Massive hemothorax
- Tension pneumothorax
- Cardiac tamponade

Other chest injuries (eg, blunt cardiac injury, aortic disruption) may cause shock but are not treated during the primary survey. Simplified, rapid approaches can help differentiate among rapidly correctable causes of shock due to chest injuries (see Fig. 370–2). However, hemorrhage should be excluded in all patients who have shock after major trauma, regardless of whether a chest injury that could cause shock is identified.

Treatment of injuries affecting the airway, breathing, or circulation begins during the primary survey. After the primary survey, patients are clinically assessed in more detail for other severe chest injuries as well as less severe manifestations of the injuries considered during the primary survey.

Imaging: Imaging studies are typically required in patients with significant chest trauma. Chest x-ray is virtually always done. Results are usually diagnostic of certain injuries (eg, pneumothorax, hemothorax, moderate or severe pulmonary contusion, clavicle fracture, some rib fractures) and suggestive for others (eg, aortic disruption, diaphragmatic rupture). However, findings may evolve over hours (eg, in pulmonary contusion and diaphragmatic injury). Plain x-rays of the scapula or sternum are sometimes done when there is tenderness over those structures.

In trauma centers, ultrasonography of the heart is typically done during the resuscitation phase to look for pericardial tamponade; some pneumothoraces can also be seen.

CT of the chest is often done when aortic injury is suspected and to diagnose small pneumothoraces, sternal fractures, or mediastinal (eg, heart, esophageal, bronchial) injuries; thoracic spine injuries also will be identified.

Other tests for aortic injury include aortography and transesophageal echocardiography.

Laboratory and other testing: CBC is often done but is mainly valuable as a baseline for detecting ongoing hemorrhage. ABG results help monitor patients with hypoxia or respiratory distress. Cardiac markers (eg, troponin, CPK-MB) can help exclude blunt cardiac injury.

ECG is typically done for chest trauma that is severe or compatible with cardiac injury. Cardiac injury may cause

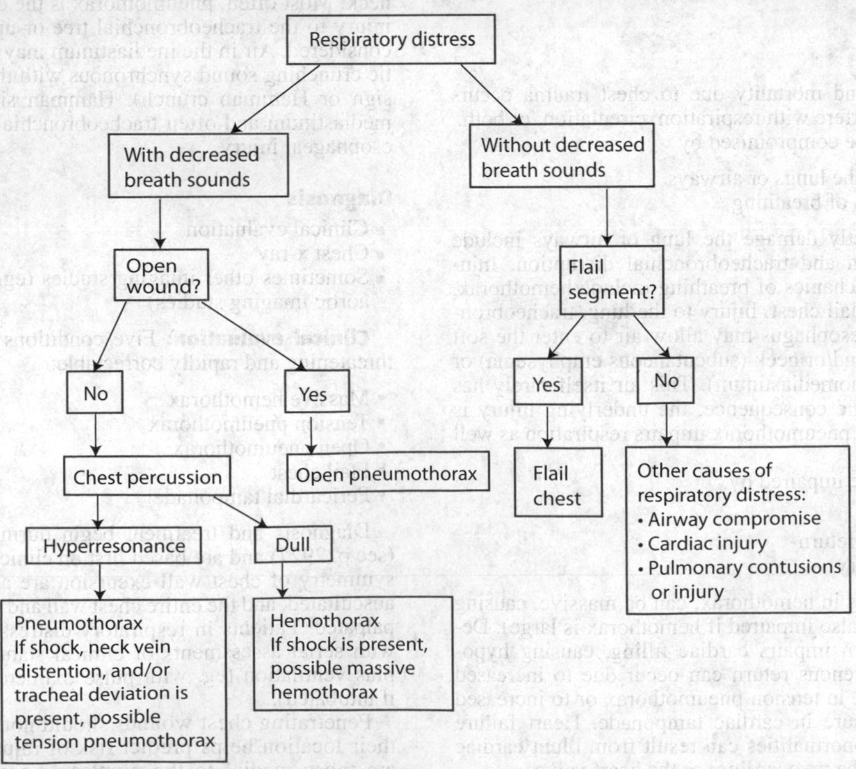

Fig. 370–1. A simple, rapid assessment of patients with thoracic trauma and respiratory distress during the primary survey.

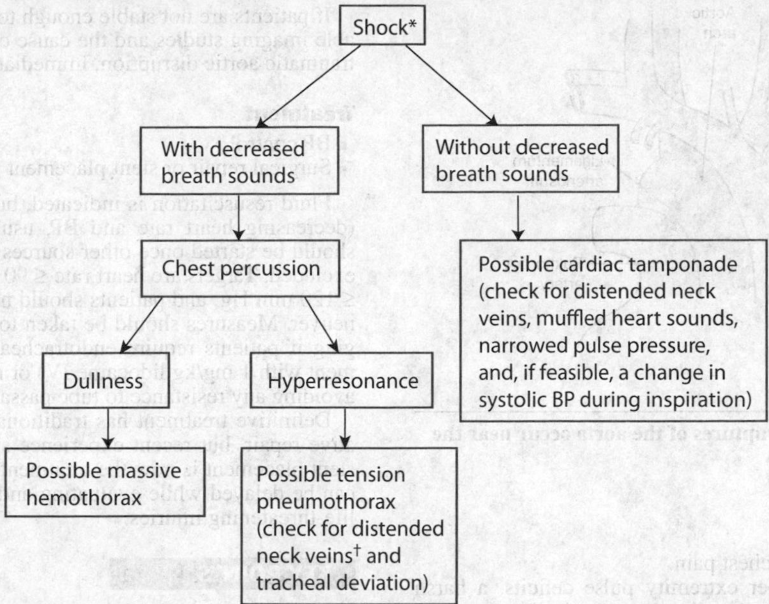
Shock*
With decreased breath sounds
Without decreased breath sounds
Chest percussion
Possible cardiac tamponade (check for distended neck veins, muffled heart sounds, narrowed pulse pressure, and, if feasible, a change in systolic BP during inspiration)
Dullness
Hyperresonance
Possible massive hemothorax
Possible tension pneumothorax (check for distended neck veins† and tracheal deviation)

Fig. 370–2. A simple, rapid assessment for chest injuries in patients with shock during the primary survey.

*Hemorrhage should be excluded in all patients who are in shock after major trauma, regardless of whether a chest injury that could cause shock is identified

†Neck vein distention may be absent in patients with hypovolemic shock.

dysrhythmia, conduction abnormalities, ST segment abnormalities, or a combination.

Treatment

- Supportive care
- Treatment of specific injuries

Immediately life-threatening injuries are treated at the bedside at the time of diagnosis:

- Suspected tension pneumothorax: Needle decompression
- Respiratory distress or shock and decreased breath sounds: Tube thoracostomy
- Shock with suspected cardiac tamponade: Pericardiocentesis
- Suspected hypovolemic shock: Fluid resuscitation

Immediate resuscitative thoracotomy can be considered for trauma victims if the clinician is proficient in the procedure and the patient has one of the following indications:

- Penetrating thoracic injury with a need for CPR of < 15 min
- Penetrating nonthoracic trauma with a need for CPR of < 5 min
- Blunt trauma with a need for CPR of < 10 min
- Persistent systolic BP of < 60 mm Hg due to suspected cardiac tamponade, hemorrhage, or air embolism

PEARLS & PITFALLS

- In trauma patients with respiratory distress or shock and decreased breath sounds, tube thoracostomy can be done before imaging studies are obtained.

In the absence of any of these criteria, resuscitative thoracotomy is contraindicated because the procedure has significant risks (eg, transmission of blood-borne diseases, injury to clinician) and costs.

Specific treatment is directed at the injury. Supportive therapy typically includes analgesics, supplemental oxygen, and sometimes mechanical ventilation.

AORTIC DISRUPTION (TRAUMATIC)

The aorta can rupture completely or incompletely after blunt or penetrating chest trauma. Signs may include asymmetric pulses or BP, decreased blood flow to the lower extremities, and precordial systolic murmur. Diagnosis is often suspected because of the mechanism of injury and/or chest x-ray findings and confirmed by CT, ultrasonography, or aortography. Treatment is open repair or stent placement.

Etiology

With **blunt trauma,** the usual mechanism is a severe deceleration injury; patients often have multiple rib fractures, 1st and/or 2nd rib fractures, or other manifestations of severe chest trauma.

With **penetrating trauma,** the usual wound traverses the mediastinum (eg, entering between the nipples or the scapulae).

Pathophysiology

Complete rupture causes rapid death by exsanguination. Partial disruption with contained rupture tends to occur near the ligamentum arteriosum (see Fig. 370–3) and to have blood flow maintained, usually by an intact adventitial layer. However, partial ruptures may also cause limited mediastinal hematomas.

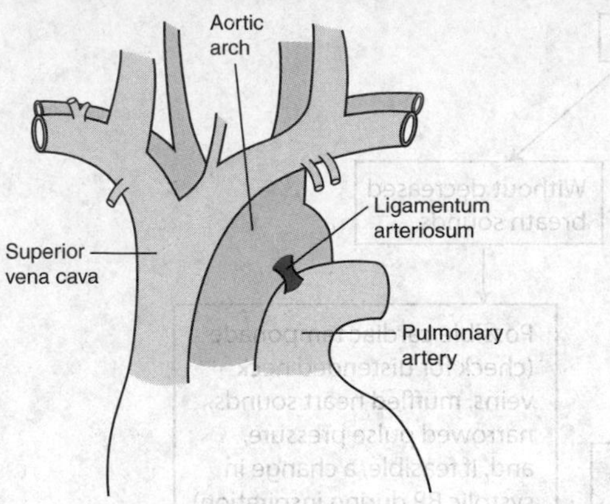

Fig. 370–3. Most partial ruptures of the aorta occur near the ligamentum arteriosum.

Symptoms and Signs

Patients typically have chest pain.

Signs can include upper extremity pulse deficits, a harsh systolic murmur over the precordium or posterior interscapular space, hoarseness, and evidence of impaired blood flow to the lower extremities, including decreased pulse strength or BP in the lower extremities compared to the upper extremities.

Diagnosis

- Aortic imaging

The diagnosis should be suspected in patients with a suggestive mechanism or suggestive findings. Chest x-ray is done.

Suggestive chest x-ray findings include the following:

- Widened mediastinum (high sensitivity except among elderly patients)
- 1st or 2nd rib fracture
- Obliteration of the aortic knob
- Deviation of the trachea or esophagus (and thus also any nasogastric tube) to the right
- Depression of the left mainstem bronchus
- Pleural or apical cap
- Hemothorax, pneumothorax, or pulmonary contusion

However, some of these suggestive chest x-ray findings may not be present immediately. Also, no finding or combination of findings is sufficiently sensitive or specific; thus, many authorities recommend aortic imaging for all patients who have had a severe deceleration injury, even in the absence of suggestive findings on examination or chest x-ray.

The **aortic imaging study of choice** varies by institution. Studies that are reasonably accurate include the following:

- CT angiography: Immediately available (in most trauma centers) and rapid.
- Aortography: Considered the most accurate but is invasive (resulting in a higher complication rate) and takes longer to complete (usually 1 to 2 h).
- Transesophageal echocardiography: Rapid (usually < 30 min), has low complication rate, can detect certain associated injuries (eg, to the innominate vessels) that can be missed on CT, and, because it is a bedside test, can be used in unstable patients. However, accuracy is operator-dependent, and it is not always available.

If patients are not stable enough to undergo any of the available imaging studies and the cause of shock is suspected to be traumatic aortic disruption, immediate surgery is indicated.

Treatment

- BP control
- Surgical repair or stent placement

Fluid resuscitation is indicated, but impulse control therapy (decreasing heart rate and BP, usually with a beta-blocker) should be started once other sources of hemorrhage have been excluded. Targets are heart rate ≤ 90 beats/min and systolic BP ≤ 120 mm Hg; and patients should not perform a Valsalva maneuver. Measures should be taken to avoid coughing and gagging if patients require endotracheal intubation (eg, pretreatment with 1 mg/kg lidocaine IV) or nasogastric intubation (eg, avoiding any resistance to tube passage).

Definitive treatment has traditionally been immediate operative repair, but recent experience suggests that endovascular stent placement is now the treatment of choice. Surgical repair can be delayed while evaluating and treating other potentially life-threatening injuries.

KEY POINTS

- Partial disruption of the aorta should be considered in patients with a chest injury caused by severe deceleration.
- Chest x-ray abnormalities are common but may be absent and are often nonspecific; better aortic imaging studies include CT angiography, aortography, and transesophageal echocardiography.
- Control heart rate and BP (usually with a beta-blocker) and place an endovascular stent or do operative repair.

BLUNT CARDIAC INJURY

(Cardiac Contusion)

Blunt cardiac injury is blunt chest trauma that causes contusion of myocardial muscle, rupture of a cardiac chamber, or disruption of a heart valve. Sometimes a blow to the anterior chest wall causes cardiac arrest without any structural lesion (commotio cordis).

Manifestations vary with the injury.

Myocardial contusion may be minor and asymptomatic, although tachycardia may be present. Some patients develop conduction abnormalities and/or dysrhythmias.

Ventricular rupture is usually rapidly fatal, but patients with smaller, particularly right-sided, lesions may survive to present with cardiac tamponade. Tamponade due to atrial rupture may manifest more gradually.

Valve disruption may occur, causing a heart murmur and sometimes manifestations of heart failure (eg, dyspnea, pulmonary crackles, sometimes hypotension), which may develop rapidly.

Septal rupture may not cause symptoms initially, but patients may present later with heart failure.

Commotio cordis is sudden cardiac arrest that follows a blow to the anterior chest wall in patients who do not have pre-existing or traumatic structural heart disease. Typically this blow involves a fast, hard projectile (eg, baseball, hockey puck) with relatively low kinetic energy. Pathophysiology is unclear, but the timing of the blow in relation to the cardiac cycle may be important. Initial rhythm is usually ventricular fibrillation.

Diagnosis

- ECG
- Echocardiography
- Cardiac enzymes

Cardiac injury should be suspected in patients with significant chest or multiple blunt trauma and any palpitations, dysrhythmia, new cardiac murmur, or unexplained tachycardia or hypotension.

Most patients with significant blunt chest trauma should have 12-lead ECG. With myocardial contusion, ECG may reveal ST segment changes that mimic cardiac ischemia or infarction. The most common conduction abnormalities include atrial fibrillation, bundle branch block (usually right), unexplained sinus tachycardia, and single or multiple premature ventricular contractions. Echocardiography is sometimes done during the initial resuscitation and may show wall motion abnormalities, pericardial fluid, or chamber or valvular rupture. Patients suspected of having blunt cardiac injury because of clinical or ECG findings should have formal echocardiography to evaluate function and anatomic abnormalities.

Cardiac markers (eg, troponin, CPK-MB) are most useful to screen for and thus help exclude blunt cardiac injury. If cardiac markers and ECG are normal and there are no arrhythmias, blunt cardiac injury can be safely excluded.

Treatment

- Supportive care

Patients with myocardial contusion causing conduction abnormalities require cardiac monitoring for 24 h because they are at risk for sudden dysrhythmias during this time. Treatment is mainly supportive (eg, treatment of symptomatic dysrhythmias or heart failure) and is seldom needed. Surgical repair is indicated for rare cases of myocardial or valvular rupture.

Patients with commotio cordis are treated for their dysrhythmia (eg, resuscitation with CPR and defibrillation followed by in-hospital observation).

KEY POINTS

- Blunt cardiac injury should be suspected in patients with significant chest or multiple blunt trauma and any palpitations, dysrhythmia, new cardiac murmur, or unexplained tachycardia or hypotension.
- ECG and cardiac markers are useful to screen for injury, and echocardiography is helpful to evaluate function and anatomic abnormalities.
- Patients with conduction abnormalities or dysrhythmias require cardiac monitoring.

CARDIAC TAMPONADE

Cardiac tamponade is accumulation of blood in the pericardial sac of sufficient volume and pressure to impair cardiac filling. Patients typically have hypotension, muffled heart tones, and distended neck veins. Diagnosis is made clinically and often with bedside echocardiography. Treatment is immediate pericardiocentesis or pericardiotomy.

Fluid in the pericardial sac can impair cardiac filling, leading to low cardiac output and sometimes shock and death. If fluid accumulates slowly (eg, due to chronic inflammation), the pericardium can stretch to accommodate up to 1 to 1.5 L of fluid before cardiac output is compromised. However, with rapid fluid accumulation, as occurs with traumatic hemorrhage, as little as 150 mL may cause tamponade.

In trauma, the cause is more often penetrating than blunt trauma. The wound is often medial to the nipples (for anterior wounds) or the scapulae (for posterior wounds). Tamponade due to blunt trauma involves cardiac chamber rupture, which is typically fatal before patients can be brought for treatment.

Symptoms and Signs

Classically, patients have Beck's triad, which consists of the following:

- Hypotension
- Muffled heart tones
- Venous pressure increase (eg, neck vein distention)

However, hypotension has multiple potential causes in trauma patients, muffled heart tones can be difficult to assess during a noisy trauma resuscitation, and neck vein distention can be absent due to hypovolemia. Pulsus paradoxus, a decrease in systolic BP during inspiration of > 10 mm Hg, is also suggestive, but again not easy to assess in a noisy setting.

Diagnosis

- Clinical evaluation
- Often bedside echocardiography

Diagnosis can be difficult. Beck's triad is considered diagnostic but may not be present or easy to recognize. In addition, tension pneumothorax also should be considered in patients with hypotension and neck vein distention, although this disorder typically causes markedly decreased breath sounds and hyperresonance on the affected hemithorax. Bedside transthoracic echocardiography can be diagnostic and can be done during the initial evaluation and resuscitation but may be falsely negative. The diagnosis sometimes is suggested by unexplained failure to respond to volume resuscitation.

Treatment

- Pericardiocentesis
- Sometimes pericardiotomy or creation of a pericardial window

Subxiphoidal pericardiocentesis is done in unstable patients when cardiac tamponade is suspected. Electrocardiographic monitoring during the insertion needle for ST segment elevation (indicating contact with the epicardium and the need to withdraw the needle) is done if possible. Pericardiocentesis is a temporizing measure. Removal of as little as 10 mL of blood may normalize BP. However, failure to aspirate blood does not exclude the diagnosis; fresh blood in the pericardium is often clotted.

Thoracotomy with pericardiotomy or establishment of a subxiphoidal pericardial window are more definitive treatments, which are indicated in patients in whom the diagnosis is confirmed or strongly suspected. If adequately trained personnel are available and the patient is unstable and fails to respond to other resuscitative measures, one of these procedures can be done at the bedside in the emergency setting. Otherwise, the procedure is done in the operating room as soon as feasible.

KEY POINTS

- Cardiac tamponade is most often caused by a penetrating wound medial to the nipples (for anterior wounds) or the scapulae (for posterior wounds).

- The triad of muffled heart tones, hypotension, and neck vein distention is diagnostic but not always present; in their absence, bedside echocardiography should be done if the diagnosis is suspected.
- Subxiphoidal pericardiocentesis is a temporizing measure and may be falsely negative; a pericardial window or pericardiotomy are more definitive.

FLAIL CHEST

Flail chest is multiple adjacent rib fractures that result in a segment of the chest wall separating from the rest of the thoracic cage; it is a marker for injury to the underlying lung.

A single rib may fracture in more than one place. If multiple adjacent ribs fracture in ≥ 2 places, the breaks in each rib result in a segment of chest wall that is not mechanically connected to the rest of the thoracic cage (flail segment). This flail segment moves paradoxically (ie, outward during expiration and inward during inspiration—see Fig. 370–4).

Patients are at high risk for respiratory complications, mainly because the large amount of force required to cause a flail chest typically causes a significant underlying pulmonary contusion. In addition, the paradoxical motion of flail chest increases the work of breathing, and chest wall pain tends to limit deep inspiration and thus maximal ventilation.

Diagnosis

- Clinical evaluation

Diagnosis is clinical, ideally by observing the paradoxical motion of the flail segment during breathing. However, this motion may be difficult to see if inspiratory depth is limited by pain or obtundation due to other injuries. The paradoxical motion does not occur if the patient is mechanically ventilated, but the flail segment may be identified by its more extreme outward movement during lung inflation. Palpation can often detect crepitus of the flail segment and confirm abnormal chest wall motion.

Chest x-ray can help confirm bone fractures and usually shows underlying pulmonary contusion; x-ray does not show cartilaginous disruption.

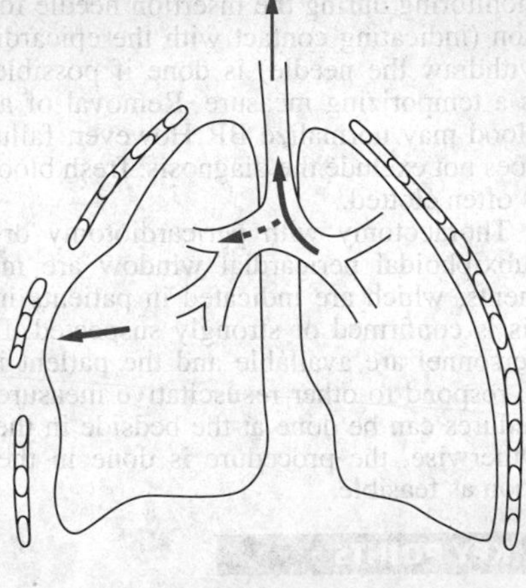

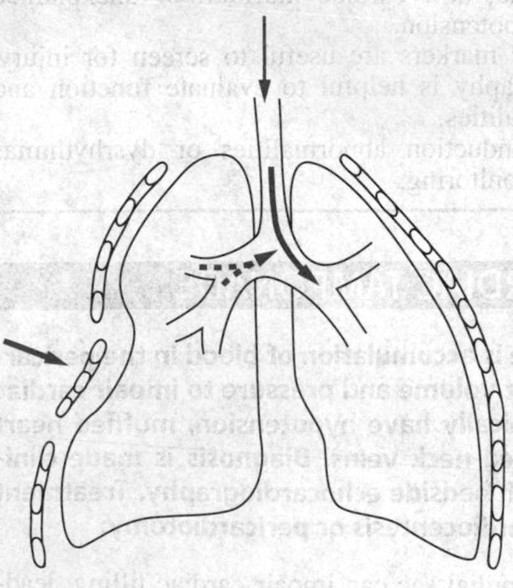

Fig. 370–4. Flail chest.

Treatment

- Supportive care
- Sometimes mechanical ventilation

Humidified oxygen is given. Analgesics may help improve ventilation by decreasing pain during breathing, but ventilation may need to be supported mechanically. Volume status should be closely monitored because harm can result from either hypovolemia (due to lung hypoperfusion) or hypervolemia (due to pulmonary edema).

HEMOTHORAX

Hemothorax is accumulation of blood in the pleural space.

The usual cause of hemothorax is laceration of the lung, intercostal vessel, or an internal mammary artery. It can result from penetrating or blunt trauma. Hemothorax is often accompanied by pneumothorax (hemopneumothorax).

Hemorrhage volume ranges from minimal to massive. Massive hemothorax is most often defined as rapid accumulation of ≥ 1000 mL of blood. Shock is common.

Patients with large hemorrhage volume are often dyspneic and have decreased breath sounds and dullness to percussion (often difficult to appreciate during initial evaluation of patients with multiple injuries). Findings may be unremarkable in patients with smaller hemothoraces.

Diagnosis

- Chest x-ray

Hemothorax is suspected based on symptoms and physical findings. Diagnosis is typically confirmed by chest x-ray.

Treatment

- Fluid resuscitation as needed
- Usually tube thoracostomy
- Sometimes thoracotomy

Patients with signs of hypovolemia (eg, tachycardia, hypotension) are given IV crystalloid and sometimes blood transfusion (see p. 576).

If blood volume is sufficient to be visible on chest x-ray (usually requiring about 500 mL), or if pneumothorax is present, a large-caliber (eg, 32 to 38 Fr) chest tube is inserted in the 5th or 6th intercostal space in the midaxillary line. Tube drainage improves ventilation, decreases risk of clotted hemothorax (which can lead to empyema or fibrothorax), and facilitates assessment of ongoing blood loss and diaphragmatic integrity. Blood collected via tube thoracostomy can be transfused, decreasing the requirement for crystalloid and exogenous blood.

Urgent thoracotomy is indicated in either of the following situations:

- Initial bleeding is > 1500 mL
- Bleeding is > 200 mL/h for > 2 to 4 h and causes respiratory or hemodynamic compromise or the need for repeated blood transfusions.

OPEN PNEUMOTHORAX

(Sucking Chest Wound)

Open pneumothorax is a pneumothorax involving an unsealed opening in the chest wall; when the opening is sufficiently large, respiratory mechanics are impaired.

Some patients with traumatic pneumothorax have an unsealed opening in the chest wall. When patients with an open pneumothorax inhale, the negative intrathoracic pressure generated by inspiration causes air to flow into the lungs through the trachea and simultaneously into the intrapleural space through the chest wall defect. There is little airflow through small chest wall defects and hence few adverse effects. However, when the opening in the chest wall is sufficiently large (when the defect is about two-thirds the diameter of the trachea or larger), more air passes through the chest wall defect than through the trachea into the lung. Larger defects can eliminate ventilation on the affected side. Inability to ventilate the lungs causes respiratory distress and respiratory failure.

In awake patients, the chest wound is painful and patients have respiratory distress and other manifestations of pneumothorax (see p. 3116). The air entering the wound typically makes a characteristic sucking sound.

Diagnosis

- Clinical evaluation

The diagnosis is made clinically and requires inspecting the entire chest wall surface.

Treatment

- Partially occlusive dressing followed by tube thoracostomy

Immediate management is to cover the wound with a rectangular sterile occlusive dressing that is closed securely with tape on only 3 sides. Thus, the dressing prevents atmospheric air from entering the chest wall during inspiration but allows any intrapleural air out during expiration. Tube thoracostomy should be done when the patient is stabilized. The wound may require later surgical repair.

TENSION PNEUMOTHORAX

Tension pneumothorax is accumulation of air in the pleural space under pressure, compressing the lungs and decreasing venous return to the heart.

Tension pneumothorax develops when a lung or chest wall injury is such that it allows air into the pleural space but not out of it (a one-way valve). As a result, air accumulates and compresses the lung, eventually shifting the mediastinum, compressing the contralateral lung, and increasing intrathoracic pressure enough to decrease venous return to the heart, causing shock. These effects can develop rapidly, particularly in patients undergoing positive pressure ventilation.

Causes include mechanical ventilation (most commonly) and simple (uncomplicated) pneumothorax with lung injury that fails to seal following penetrating or blunt chest trauma or failed central venous cannulation.

Symptoms and Signs

Symptoms and signs initially are those of simple pneumothorax (see p. 475). As intrathoracic pressure increases, patients develop hypotension, tracheal deviation, and neck vein distention. The affected hemithorax is hyperresonant to percussion and often feels somewhat distended, tense, and poorly compressible to palpation.

Diagnosis

- Clinical evaluation

Tension pneumothorax should be diagnosed by clinical findings. Treatment should not be delayed pending radiographic confirmation. Although cardiac tamponade also can cause hypotension, neck vein distention, and sometimes respiratory distress, tension pneumothorax can be differentiated clinically by its unilateral absence of breath sounds and hyperresonance to percussion.

PEARLS & PITFALLS

- Tension pneumothorax should be diagnosed at the bedside based on clinical findings and treated immediately with needle decompression and/or tube thoracostomy.

Treatment

- Needle decompression followed by tube thoracostomy

Treatment is immediate needle decompression by inserting a large-bore (eg, 14 or 16 gauge) needle into the 2nd intercostal space in the midclavicular line. Air will usually gush out. Because needle decompression causes a simple pneumothorax, tube thoracostomy should be done immediately thereafter.

TRAUMATIC PNEUMOTHORAX

Traumatic pneumothorax is air in the pleural space resulting from trauma and causing partial or complete lung collapse. Symptoms include chest pain from the causative injury and sometimes dyspnea. Diagnosis is made by chest x-ray. Treatment is usually with tube thoracostomy.

Pneumothorax can be caused by penetrating or blunt trauma; many patients also have a hemothorax (hemopneumothorax). In patients with penetrating wounds that traverse the mediastinum (eg, wounds medial to the nipples or to the scapulae), or with severe blunt trauma, pneumothorax may be caused by disruption of the tracheobronchial tree. Air from the pneumothorax may enter the soft tissues of the chest and/or neck (subcutaneous emphysema), or mediastinum (pneumomediastinum).

A simple unilateral pneumothorax, even when large, is well tolerated by most patients unless they have significant underlying pulmonary disease. However, tension pneumothorax can cause severe hypotension, and open pneumothorax can compromise ventilation.

Symptoms and Signs

Patients commonly have pleuritic chest pain, dyspnea, tachypnea, and tachycardia.

Breath sounds may be diminished and the affected hemithorax hyperresonant to percussion—mainly with larger pneumothoraces. However, these findings are not always present and may be hard to detect in a noisy resuscitation setting. Subcutaneous emphysema causes a crackle or crunch when palpated; findings may be localized to a small area or involve a large portion of the chest wall and/or extend to the neck; extensive involvement suggests disruption of the tracheobronchial tree.

Air in the mediastinum may produce a characteristic crunching sound synchronous with the heartbeat (Hamman sign or Hamman crunch), but this finding is not always present and also is occasionally caused by injury to the esophagus.

Diagnosis

- Chest x-ray

Diagnosis is usually made by chest x-ray. Ultrasonography (done at the bedside during initial resuscitation) and CT are more sensitive for small pneumothoraces than chest x-ray.

The size of the pneumothorax, stated as percent of the hemithorax that is vacant, can be estimated by x-ray findings (see p. 476). The numerical size is valuable mainly for quantifying progression and resolution rather than for determining prognosis.

Treatment

- Usually tube thoracostomy

Treatment of most pneumothoraces is with insertion of a thoracostomy tube (eg, 28 Fr) into the 5th or 6th intercostal space anterior to the midaxillary line.

Patients with small pneumothoraces and no respiratory symptoms may simply be observed with serial chest x-rays until the lung re-expands. Alternatively, a small pigtail catheter drain can be placed. However, tube thoracostomy should be done in patients who will undergo general anesthesia, positive pressure ventilation, and/or air transport because these interventions can convert a small, simple (uncomplicated) pneumothorax to a tension pneumothorax.

If a large air leak persists after tube thoracostomy, tracheobronchial tree injury should be suspected and bronchoscopy or immediate surgical consultation should be arranged.

KEY POINTS

- Physical findings can be subtle or normal, particularly if pneumothorax is small.
- Although CT and ultrasonography are more sensitive, chest x-ray is usually considered sufficient for diagnosis.
- Tube thoracostomy is indicated if pneumothorax causes respiratory symptoms or is moderate or large or if air transport, positive pressure ventilation, or general anesthesia is necessary.

PULMONARY CONTUSION

Pulmonary contusion is trauma-induced lung hemorrhage and edema without laceration.

Pulmonary contusion is a common and potentially lethal chest injury that results from significant blunt or penetrating chest trauma. Patients may have associated rib fracture, pneumothorax, or other chest injuries. Larger contusions can impair oxygenation. Late complications include pneumonia and sometimes acute respiratory distress syndrome (ARDS).

Symptoms include pain (mainly due to injury to the overlying chest wall) and sometimes dyspnea. The chest wall is tender; other physical findings are those of any associated injuries.

Diagnosis

- Imaging, typically chest x-ray

The diagnosis should be suspected when respiratory distress develops after chest trauma, particularly when symptoms worsen gradually. Chest x-ray is typically done, along with pulse oximetry. Contusions cause opacification of affected lung tissue on imaging, but opacification may not be apparent for 24 to 48 h because opacification increases with time. CT is highly sensitive but is usually done only when other injuries are also under consideration.

Patients should be monitored for respiratory failure with serial clinical assessments and pulse oximetry. If hypoxemia or dyspnea is noted, capnometry or ABG measurement is indicated.

Treatment

- Supportive care with analgesics and oxygen
- Sometimes mechanical ventilation

Analgesics are given as needed to facilitate deep respirations. Supplemental oxygen (O_2) is given for mild hypoxemia (SaO_2 91 to 94%). Usual indications for mechanical ventilation are moderate or severe hypoxemia (usually $PaO_2 < 65$ or $SaO_2 < 90\%$ while breathing room air) and hypercarbia. Patients with COPD or chronic kidney disease are at increased risk of the need for mechanical ventilation.

RIB FRACTURE

One or more ribs can be fractured due to blunt chest injury.

Typically, rib fractures result from blunt injury to the chest wall, usually involving a strong force (eg, due to high-speed deceleration, a baseball bat, a major fall); however, sometimes in the elderly, only mild or moderate force (eg, in a minor fall) is required. If ≥ 2 adjacent ribs fracture in 2 separate places, the breaks in each rib result in a flail chest.

PEARLS & PITFALLS

- Minor trauma (eg, due to a fall) in the elderly can cause rib fractures that may have fatal consequences.

Concomitant chest injuries may occur, including

- Aortic, subclavian, or cardiac injuries (uncommon but can occur with high-speed deceleration, particularly if rib 1 or 2 is fractured)
- Splenic or abdominal injuries (with fractures of any of ribs 7 through 12)
- Pulmonary laceration or pulmonary contusion
- Pneumothorax (see p. 3115)
- Hemothorax
- Tracheobronchial injuries (uncommon)

Complications: Most complications result from concomitant injuries. Isolated rib fractures are painful but rarely cause complications. However, inspiratory splinting (incomplete inspiration due to pain) can cause atelectasis and pneumonia, especially in the elderly or patients with multiple fractures. As a result, elderly patients have high mortality rates (up to 20%) due to rib fractures. Young healthy patients and those with 1 or 2 rib fractures rarely develop these complications.

Symptoms and Signs

Pain is severe, is aggravated by movement of the trunk (including coughing or deep breathing), and lasts for several weeks. The affected ribs are quite tender; sometimes the clinician can detect crepitance over the affected rib as the fracture segment moves during palpation.

Diagnosis

- Usually chest x-ray

Palpation of the chest wall may identify some fractures. Some clinicians feel clinical evaluation is adequate in healthy patients with minor trauma. However, in patients with significant blunt trauma, a chest x-ray is typically done to check for concomitant injuries (eg, pneumothorax, pulmonary contusion). Many rib fractures are not visible on a chest x-ray; specific rib views can be done, but identifying all rib fractures by x-ray is usually unnecessary. Other tests are done to check for concomitant injuries that are clinically suspected.

Treatment

- Analgesia
- Pulmonary toilet

Treatment usually requires opioid analgesics, although opioids can also depress respiration and worsen atelectasis. Some clinicians prescribe NSAIDs simultaneously.

To minimize pulmonary complications, patients should consciously and frequently (eg, hourly while awake) breathe deeply or cough. Holding (essentially splinting) the affected area with the flat palm of the hand or a pillow can minimize the pain during deep breathing or coughing. Patients are hospitalized if they have ≥ 3 fractures or underlying cardiopulmonary insufficiency. Immobilization (eg, by strapping or taping) should usually be avoided; it constricts respiration and may predispose to atelectasis and pneumonia. If patients cannot cough or breathe deeply despite oral or IV analgesics, epidural drug administration or intercostal nerve blocks can be considered.

KEY POINTS

- Morbidity results from underlying lung, splenic, or vascular injury or development of pneumonia due to splinting, rather than rib fractures themselves.
- X-ray identification of all rib fractures is usually unnecessary.
- Pain can be severe and last for weeks, usually requiring opioid analgesics.
- Strapping or taping should usually be avoided because it constricts respiration and may predispose to atelectasis and pneumonia.

371 Traumatic Brain Injury

Traumatic brain injury (TBI) is physical injury to brain tissue that temporarily or permanently impairs brain function. Diagnosis is suspected clinically and confirmed by imaging (primarily CT). Initial treatment consists of ensuring a reliable airway and maintaining adequate ventilation, oxygenation, and blood pressure. Surgery is often needed in patients with more severe injury to place monitors to track and treat intracranial pressure elevation, decompress the brain if intracranial pressure is increased, or remove intracranial hematomas. In the first few days after the injury, maintaining adequate brain perfusion and oxygenation and preventing complications of altered sensorium are important. Subsequently, many patients require rehabilitation.

In the US, as in much of the world, TBI is a common cause of death and disability. Causes include motor vehicle crashes and other transportation-related causes (eg, bicycle crashes, collisions with pedestrians), falls (especially in older adults and young children), assaults, and sports activities (see p. 3123).

Pathology

Structural changes from head injury may be gross or microscopic, depending on the mechanism and forces involved. Patients with less severe injuries may have no gross structural damage. Clinical manifestations vary markedly in severity and consequences. Injuries are commonly categorized as open or closed.

Open injuries involve penetration of the scalp and skull (and usually the meninges and underlying brain tissue). They typically involve bullets or sharp objects, but a skull fracture with overlying laceration due to severe blunt force is also considered an open injury.

Closed injuries typically occur when the head is struck, strikes an object, or is shaken violently, causing rapid brain acceleration and deceleration. Acceleration or deceleration can injure tissue at the point of impact (coup), at its opposite pole (contrecoup), or diffusely; the frontal and temporal lobes are particularly vulnerable. Axons, blood vessels, or both can be sheared or torn. Disrupted blood vessels leak, causing contusions, intracerebral or subarachnoid hemorrhage, and epidural or subdural hematomas (see Table 371–1).

Concussion: Concussion (see p. 3123) is defined as a transient and reversible posttraumatic alteration in mental status (eg, loss of consciousness or memory, confusion) lasting from seconds to minutes and, by arbitrary definition, < 6 h. Gross structural brain lesions and serious neurologic residua are not part of concussion, although temporary disability can occur due to symptoms, such as nausea, headache, dizziness, memory disturbance, and difficulty concentrating (postconcussion syndrome) that usually resolve within weeks.

Brain contusions: Contusions (bruises of the brain) can occur with open or closed injuries and can impair a wide range of brain functions, depending on contusion size and location. Larger

Table 371–1. COMMON TYPES OF TRAUMATIC BRAIN INJURY

DISORDER	CLINICAL FINDINGS	DIAGNOSIS
Acute subdural hematoma	Typically, acute neurologic dysfunction, which may be focal, nonfocal, or both With small hematomas, normal function possible	CT: Hyperdensity in subdural space, classically crescent-shaped Degree of midline shift important
Basilar skull fracture	Leakage of CSF from the nose or ear Blood behind the tympanic membrane (hemotympanum) or in the external ear Ecchymosis behind the ear (Battle sign) or around the eye (raccoon eyes)	CT: Usually visible
Brain contusion	Widely variable degrees of neurologic dysfunction or normal function	CT: Hyperdensities resulting from punctate hemorrhages of varied sizes
Concussion	Transient mental status alteration (eg, loss of consciousness or memory) lasting < 6 h	Based on clinical findings CT: Rarely abnormal
Chronic subdural hematoma	Gradual headache, somnolence, confusion, sometimes with focal deficits or seizures	CT: Hypodensity in subdural space (abnormality is isodense during subacute transition from hyperdense to hypodense)
Diffuse axonal injury	Loss of consciousness lasting > 6 h but no focal deficits or motor posturing	Based on clinical findings CT: At first, may be normal or show small hyperdensities (microhemorrhages) in corpus callosum, centrum semiovale, basal ganglia, or brain stem MRI: Often abnormal
Epidural hematoma	Headache, impaired consciousness within hours, sometimes with a lucid interval Herniation typically causing contralateral hemiparesis and ipsilateral pupillary dilation	CT: Hyperdensity in epidural space, classically lenticular-shaped and located over the middle meningeal artery (temporal fossa) due to a temporal bone fracture
Subarachnoid hemorrhage	Typically, normal function Occasionally, acute neurologic dysfunction	CT: Hyperdensity within subarachnoid space on the surface of the brain; often lining sulci

contusions may cause brain edema and increased intracranial pressure (ICP). Contusions may enlarge in the hours and days following the initial injury and cause neurologic deterioration.

Diffuse axonal injury: Diffuse axonal injury (DAI) occurs when rotational deceleration causes shear-type forces that result in generalized, widespread disruption of axonal fibers and myelin sheaths. A few DAI lesions may also result from minor head injury. Gross structural lesions are not part of DAI, but small petechial hemorrhages in the white matter are often observed on CT and on histopathologic examination. DAI is sometimes defined clinically as a loss of consciousness lasting > 6 h in the absence of a specific focal lesion. Edema from the injury often increases ICP, leading to various manifestations (see p. 3119). DAI is typically the underlying injury in shaken baby syndrome.

Hematomas: Hematomas (collections of blood in or around the brain) can occur with open or closed injuries and may be epidural, subdural, or intracerebral. Subarachnoid hemorrhage (SAH—bleeding into the subarachnoid space; see p. 2045) is common in TBI, although the appearance on CT is not usually the same as aneurysmal SAH.

Subdural hematomas are collections of blood between the dura mater and the pia-arachnoid mater. Acute subdural hematomas arise from laceration of cortical veins or avulsion of bridging veins between the cortex and dural sinuses. They often occur with head trauma from falls and motor vehicle crashes. Compression of the brain by the hematoma and swelling of the brain due to edema or hyperemia (increased blood flow due to engorged blood vessels) can increase ICP. When these processes both occur, mortality and morbidity can be high. A chronic subdural hematoma may appear and cause symptoms gradually over several weeks after trauma. These hematomas occur more often in alcoholics and elderly patients (especially in those taking antiplatelet or anticoagulant drugs, or in those with brain atrophy). Elderly patients may consider the head injury relatively trivial or may have even forgotten it. In contrast to acute subdural hematomas, edema and increased ICP are unusual.

Epidural hematomas are collections of blood between the skull and dura mater and are less common than subdural hematomas. Epidural hematomas that are large or rapidly expanding are usually caused by arterial bleeding, classically due to damage to the middle meningeal artery by a temporal bone fracture. Without intervention, patients with arterial epidural hematomas may rapidly deteriorate and die. Small, venous epidural hematomas are rarely lethal.

Intracerebral hematomas are collections of blood within the brain itself. In the traumatic setting, they result from coalescence of contusions. Exactly when one or more contusions become a hematoma is not well defined. Increased ICP, herniation, and brain stem failure can subsequently develop, particularly with lesions in the temporal lobes.

Skull fractures: Penetrating injuries by definition involve fractures. Closed injuries may also cause skull fractures, which may be linear, depressed, or comminuted. The presence of a fracture suggests that significant force was involved in the injury. Although most patients with simple linear fractures and no neurologic impairment are not at high risk of brain injuries, patients with any fracture associated with neurologic impairment are at increased risk of intracranial hematomas. Fractures that involve special risks include

- Depressed fractures: These fractures have the highest risk of tearing the dura, damaging the underlying brain, or both.

- Temporal bone fractures that cross the area of the middle meningeal artery: In these fractures, an epidural hematoma is a risk.
- Fractures that cross one of the major dural sinuses: These fractures may cause significant hemorrhage and venous epidural or venous subdural hematoma. Injured venous sinuses can later thrombose and cause cerebral infarction.
- Fractures that involve the carotid canal: These fractures can result in carotid artery dissection.
- Fractures of the occipital bone and base of the skull (basilar bones): These bones are thick and strong, so fractures in these areas indicate a high-intensity impact and meaningfully increase risk of brain injury. Basilar skull fractures that extend into the petrous part of the temporal bone often damage middle and inner ear structures and can impair facial, acoustic, and vestibular nerve function.
- Fractures in infants: The meninges may become trapped in a linear skull fracture with subsequent development of a leptomeningeal cyst and expansion of the original fracture (growing fracture).

Pathophysiology

Brain function may be immediately impaired by direct damage (eg, crush, laceration) of brain tissue. Further damage may occur shortly thereafter from the cascade of events triggered by the initial injury.

TBI of any sort can cause cerebral edema and decrease brain blood flow. The cranial vault is fixed in size (constrained by the skull) and filled by noncompressible CSF and minimally compressible brain tissue; consequently, any swelling from edema or an intracranial hematoma has nowhere to expand and thus increases ICP. Cerebral blood flow is proportional to the cerebral perfusion pressure (CPP), which is the difference between mean arterial pressure (MAP) and mean ICP. Thus, as ICP increases (or MAP decreases), CPP decreases. When CPP falls below 50 mm Hg, the brain may become ischemic. Ischemia and edema may trigger various secondary mechanisms of injury (eg, release of excitatory neurotransmitters, intracellular Ca, free radicals, and cytokines), causing further cell damage, further edema, and further increases in ICP. Systemic complications from trauma (eg, hypotension, hypoxia) can also contribute to cerebral ischemia and are often called secondary brain insults.

Excessive ICP initially causes global cerebral dysfunction. If excessive ICP is unrelieved, it can push brain tissue across the tentorium or through the foramen magnum, causing herniation (see Fig. 224–1 on p. 1858) and increased morbidity and mortality. If ICP increases to equal MAP, CPP becomes zero, resulting in complete brain ischemia and brain death; absent cranial blood flow is objective evidence of brain death (see p. 1868).

Hyperemia and increased brain blood flow may result from concussive injury in adolescents or children. Second impact syndrome is a rare and debated entity defined by sudden increased ICP and sometimes death after a second traumatic insult that is sustained before complete recovery from a previous minor head injury. It is attributed to loss of autoregulation of cerebral blood flow that leads to vascular engorgement, increased ICP, and herniation.

Symptoms and Signs

Initially, most patients with moderate or severe TBI lose consciousness (usually for seconds or minutes), although some patients with minor injuries have only confusion or amnesia (amnesia is usually retrograde and results in memory loss of a period of seconds to a few hours before the injury). Young children may simply become irritable. Some patients have seizures, often within the first hour or day. After these initial symptoms, patients may be fully awake and alert, or consciousness and function may be altered to some degree, from mild confusion to stupor to coma. Duration of unconsciousness and severity of obtundation are roughly proportional to injury severity but are not specific.

The **Glasgow Coma Scale** (GCS—see Table 224–4 on p. 1862) is a quick, reproducible scoring system to be used during the initial examination to estimate severity of TBI. It is based on eye opening, verbal response, and the best motor response. The lowest total score (3) indicates likely fatal damage, especially if both pupils fail to respond to light and oculovestibular responses are absent. Higher initial scores tend to predict better recovery. By convention, the severity of head injury is initially defined by the GCS:

- 14 or 15 is mild TBI
- 9 to 13 is moderate TBI
- 3 to 8 is severe TBI

Prediction of the severity of TBI and prognosis can be refined by also considering CT findings and other factors. Some patients with initially moderate TBI and a few patients with initially mild TBI deteriorate. For infants and young children, the Modified GCS for Infants and Children is used (see Table 349–1 on p. 2929). Because hypoxia and hypotension can decrease the GCS, GCS values after resuscitation from cardiopulmonary insults are more specific for brain dysfunction than values determined before resuscitation. Similarly, sedatives and paralytics can decrease GCS values and should be avoided before full neurologic examination is done.

PEARLS & PITFALLS

- Delay use of sedative and paralytic drugs until after full neurologic examination whenever possible.

Symptoms of specific types of TBI: Symptoms of various types of TBI may overlap considerably.

Epidural hematoma symptoms usually develop within minutes to several hours after the injury (the period without symptoms is the so-called lucid interval) and consist of increasing headache, decreased level of consciousness, and focal neurologic deficits (eg, hemiparesis). Pupillary dilation with loss of light reactivity usually indicates herniation. Some patients lose consciousness, then have a transient lucid interval, and then gradual neurologic deterioration. Most patients with subdural hematomas have immediate loss of consciousness. Intracerebral hematoma and subdural hematoma can cause focal neurologic deficits such as hemiparesis, progressive decrease in consciousness, or both. Progressive decrease in consciousness may result from anything that increases ICP (eg, hematoma, edema, hyperemia).

Increased ICP sometimes causes vomiting but vomiting is nonspecific. Markedly increased ICP classically manifests as a combination of hypertension (usually with increased pulse pressure), bradycardia, and respiratory depression (Cushing triad); respirations are usually slow and irregular. Severe diffuse brain injury or markedly increased ICP may cause decorticate or decerebrate posturing. Both are poor prognostic signs.

Transtentorial herniation (see Fig. 224–1 on p. 1858) may result in coma, unilaterally or bilaterally dilated and unreactive pupils, hemiplegia (usually on the side opposite a unilaterally dilated pupil), and Cushing triad.

Basilar skull fracture may result in leakage of CSF from the nose (CSF rhinorrhea) or ear (CSF otorrhea), blood behind the tympanic membrane (hemotympanum) or in the external ear canal if the tympanic membrane has ruptured, and ecchymosis behind the ear (Battle sign—see Plate 96) or in the periorbital area (raccoon eyes). Loss of smell and hearing is usually immediate, although these losses may not be noticed until the patient regains consciousness. Facial nerve function may be impaired immediately or after a delay. Other fractures of the cranial vault are sometimes palpable, particularly through a scalp laceration, as a depression or step-off deformity. However, blood under the galea aponeurotica may mimic such a step-off deformity.

Chronic subdural hematoma may manifest with increasing daily headache, fluctuating drowsiness or confusion (which may mimic early dementia), and mild-to-moderate hemiparesis or other focal neurologic deficits.

Long-term symptoms: Amnesia may persist and be both retrograde and anterograde (ie, for events following the injury). Postconcussion syndrome, which commonly follows a moderate or severe concussion, includes headache, dizziness, fatigue, difficulty concentrating, variable amnesia, depression, apathy, and anxiety. Commonly smell (and thus taste), sometimes hearing, or rarely vision is altered or lost. Symptoms usually resolve spontaneously over weeks to months.

A range of cognitive and neuropsychiatric deficits can persist after severe, moderate, and even mild TBI, particularly if structural damage was significant. Common problems include amnesia, behavioral changes (eg, agitation, impulsivity, disinhibition, lack of motivation), emotional lability, sleep disturbances, and decreased intellectual function.

Late seizures (> 7 days after the injury) develop in a small percentage of patients, often weeks, months, or even years later. Spastic motor impairment, gait and balance disturbances, ataxia, and sensory losses may occur.

A persistent vegetative state (see p. 1866) can result from a TBI that destroys forebrain cognitive functions but spares the brain stem. The capacity for self-awareness and other mental activity is absent; however, autonomic and motor reflexes are preserved, and sleep-wake cycles are normal. Few patients recover normal neurologic function when a persistent vegetative state lasts for 3 mo after injury, and almost none recover after 6 mo.

Neurologic function may continue to improve for a few years after TBI, most rapidly during the initial 6 mo.

Diagnosis

- Initial rapid trauma assessment
- Glasgow coma scale (GCS) and neurologic examination
- CT

(For an example of how to triage, diagnose, and treat head injuries in a system in which CT and specialty trauma care are used more selectively than in the US, see also the practice guideline of the National Institute for Clinical Excellence of the United Kingdom Head injury: assessment and early management.)

Initial measures: An initial overall assessment of injuries should be done (see p. 2927). Diagnosis and treatment occur simultaneously in seriously injured patients.

A rapid, focused neurologic evaluation is part of the initial assessment, including assessment of the components of the GCS, adequacy of the airway and breathing, and pupillary light response. Patients are ideally assessed before paralytics and sedatives are given. Patients are reassessed at frequent intervals (eg, every 15 to 30 min initially, then every 1 h after stabilization). Subsequent improvement or deterioration helps estimate injury severity and prognosis.

Complete clinical evaluation: Complete neurologic examination is done as soon as the patient is sufficiently stable. Infants and children should be examined carefully for retinal hemorrhages, which may indicate shaken baby syndrome. Funduscopic examination in adults may disclose traumatic retinal detachment and absence of retinal venous pulsations due to elevated ICP, but examination may be normal despite brain injury. Concussion is diagnosed when loss of consciousness or memory lasts < 6 h and symptoms are not explained by brain injury seen on neuroimaging. DAI is suspected when loss of consciousness exceeds 6 h and microhemorrhages are seen on CT. Diagnosis of other types of TBI is made by CT or MRI.

Neuroimaging: Imaging should always be done in patients with more than transiently impaired consciousness, GCS score < 15, focal neurologic findings, persistent vomiting, seizures, a history of loss of consciousness, or clinically suspected fractures. A case can be made for obtaining a CT scan of the head in all patients with more than a trivial head injury, because the clinical and medicolegal consequences of missing a hematoma are severe, but clinicians should balance this against the possible risk for radiation-related adverse effects from CT in younger patients.

Although plain x-rays can detect some skull fractures, they cannot help assess the brain and they delay more definitive brain imaging; thus, plain x-rays are usually not done. CT is the best choice for initial imaging, because it can detect hematomas, contusions, skull fractures (thin cuts are obtained to reveal clinically suspected basilar skull fractures, which may otherwise not be visible), and sometimes DAI. On CT, contusions and acute bleeding appear opaque (dense) compared with brain tissue. Arterial epidural hematomas classically appear as lenticular-shaped opacities over brain tissue, often in the territory of the middle meningeal artery. Subdural hematomas classically appear as crescent-shaped opacities overlying brain tissue. A chronic subdural hematoma appears hypodense compared with brain tissue, whereas a subacute subdural hematoma may have a similar radiopacity as brain tissue (isodense). Isodense subdural hematoma, particularly if bilateral and symmetric, may appear only subtly abnormal. In patients with severe anemia, an acute subdural hematoma may appear isodense with brain tissue. Among individual patients, findings may differ from these classic appearances. Signs of mass effect include sulcal effacement, ventricular and cisternal compression, and midline shift. Absence of these findings does not exclude increased ICP, and mass effect may be present with normal ICP. A shift of > 5 mm from the midline is generally considered to be an indication for surgical evacuation of the hematoma.

PEARLS & PITFALLS

- Consider chronic subdural hematoma in patients who have unexplained mental status changes and risk factors, including elderly patients taking antiplatelet or anticoagulant drugs or who have brain atrophy and alcoholics, even if there is no history of trauma and even if brain imaging at first shows no obvious abnormalities.

MRI may be useful later in the clinical course to detect more subtle contusions, DAI, and brain stem injury. It is usually more sensitive than CT for the diagnosis of very small acute or isodense subacute and isodense chronic subdural hematomas. Preliminary, unconfirmed evidence suggests that certain MRI findings predict prognosis. Angiography, CT angiography, and magnetic resonance angiography are all useful for the evaluation of vascular injury. For example, vascular injury is suspected when CT findings are inconsistent with the physical examination findings (eg, hemiparesis with a normal or nondiagnostic CT due to suspected evolving ischemia secondary to vascular thrombosis or embolism due to a carotid artery dissection).

Prognosis

In the US, adults with severe TBI who are treated have a mortality rate of about 25 to 33%. Mortality is lower with higher GCS scores. Mortality rates are lower in children ≥ 5 yr (≤ 10% with a GCS score of 5 to 7). Children overall do better than adults with a comparable injury.

The vast majority of patients with mild TBI retain good neurologic function. With moderate or severe TBI, the prognosis is not as good but is much better than is generally believed. The most commonly used scale to assess outcome in TBI patients is the Glasgow Outcome Scale. On this scale the possible outcomes are

- Good recovery (return to previous level of function)
- Moderate disability (capable of self-care)
- Severe disability (incapable of self-care)
- Vegetative (no cognitive function)
- Death

Over 50% of adults with severe TBI have a good recovery or only moderate disability. Occurrence and duration of coma after a TBI are strong predictors of disability. Of patients whose coma exceeds 24 h, 50% have severe persistent neurologic sequelae, and 2 to 6% remain in a persistent vegetative state at 6 mo. In adults with severe TBI, recovery occurs most rapidly within the initial 6 mo. Smaller improvements continue for perhaps as long as several years. Children have a better immediate recovery from TBI regardless of severity and continue to improve for a longer period of time.

Cognitive deficits, with impaired concentration, attention, and memory, and various personality changes are a more common cause of disability in social relations and employment than are focal motor or sensory impairments. Posttraumatic anosmia and acute traumatic blindness seldom resolve after 3 to 4 mo. Hemiparesis and aphasia usually resolve at least partially, except in the elderly.

Treatment

- For mild injuries, discharge and home observation
- For moderate and severe injuries, optimization of ventilation, oxygenation, and brain perfusion; treatment of complications (eg, increased ICP, seizures, hematomas); and rehabilitation

Multiple noncranial injuries, which are likely with motor vehicle crashes and falls, often require simultaneous treatment. Initial resuscitation of trauma patients is discussed elsewhere (see p. 2927).

At the injury scene, a clear airway is secured and external bleeding is controlled before the patient is moved. Particular care is taken to avoid displacement of the spine or other bones to protect the spinal cord and blood vessels. Proper immobilization should be maintained with a cervical collar and long spine board until stability of the entire spine has been established by appropriate examination and imaging (see p. 3099). After the initial rapid neurologic assessment, pain should be relieved with a short-acting opioid (eg, fentanyl).

In the hospital, after quick initial evaluation, neurologic findings (GCS and pupillary reaction), BP, pulse, and temperature should be recorded frequently for several hours because any deterioration demands prompt attention. Serial GCS and CT results stratify injury severity, which helps guide treatment (see Table 371–2).

The cornerstone of management for all patients is maintenance of adequate ventilation, oxygenation, and brain perfusion to avoid secondary brain insult. Aggressive early management of hypoxia, hypercapnia, hypotension, and increased ICP helps avoid secondary complications. Bleeding from injuries (external and internal) is rapidly controlled, and intravascular volume is promptly replaced with crystalloid (eg, 0.9% saline) or sometimes blood transfusion to maintain cerebral perfusion. Hypotonic fluids (especially 5% D/W) are contraindicated because they contain excess free water, which can increase brain edema and ICP.

Table 371–2. MANAGEMENT OF TRAUMATIC BRAIN INJURY BASED ON SEVERITY OF INJURY

SEVERITY	GCS SCORE	MANAGEMENT
Mild	14–15	Observation at home
Moderate	9–13	Observation in hospital
Severe	3–8	Rapid sequence intubation Intensive supportive care Monitoring and treatment of increased intracranial pressure as indicated

GCS = Glasgow Coma Scale.

Other complications to check for and to prevent include hyperthermia, hyponatremia, hyperglycemia, and fluid imbalance.

Mild injury: Injury is mild (by GCS score) in 80% of patients who have TBI and present to an emergency department. If there is brief or no loss of consciousness and if patients have stable vital signs, a normal head CT scan, and normal mental and neurologic function (including resolution of any intoxication), they may be discharged home provided family members or friends can observe them closely for an additional 24 h. These observers are instructed to return patients to the hospital if any of the following develop:

- Decreased level of consciousness
- Focal neurologic deficits
- Worsening headache
- Vomiting
- Deterioration of mental function (eg, seems confused, cannot recognize people, behaves abnormally)
- Seizures

Patients who have had loss of consciousness or have any abnormalities in mental or neurologic function and cannot be observed closely after discharge are generally observed in the emergency department or overnight in the hospital, and follow-up CT may be done in 8 to 12 h if symptoms persist. Patients who have no neurologic changes but minor abnormalities on head CT (eg, small contusions, small subdural hematomas with no mass effect, or punctuate or small traumatic subarachnoid hemorrhage) may need only a follow-up CT within 24 h. With a stable CT and normal neurologic examination results, these patients may be discharged home.

Moderate and severe injury: (See also the practice guideline of the Brain Trauma Foundation of the American Association of Neurological Surgeons Guidelines for the acute medical management of severe traumatic brain injury in infants, children, and adolescents at www.guideline.gov.) Injury is moderate in 10% of patients who have TBI and present to an emergency department. They often do not require intubation and mechanical ventilation (unless other injuries are present) or ICP monitoring. However, because deterioration is possible, these patients should be admitted and observed even if head CT is normal.

Injury is severe in 10% of patients who have TBI and present to an emergency department. They are admitted to a critical care unit. Because airway protective reflexes are usually impaired and ICP may be increased, patients are intubated endotracheally while measures are taken to avoid increasing ICP. Close monitoring using the GCS and pupillary response should continue, and CT is repeated, particularly if there is an unexplained ICP rise.

Increased intracranial pressure: Treatment principles for patients with increased ICP include

- Rapid sequence orotracheal intubation
- Mechanical ventilation
- Monitoring of ICP and CPP
- Ongoing sedation as needed
- Maintaining euvolemia and serum osmolality of 295 to 320 mOsm/kg
- For intractable increased ICP, possibly CSF drainage, temporary hyperventilation, decompressive craniotomy, or pentobarbital coma

Patients with TBI who require airway support or mechanical ventilation undergo rapid sequence oral intubation (using paralysis) rather than awake nasotracheal intubation (see p. 559), which can cause coughing and gagging and thereby raise the ICP. Drugs are used to minimize the ICP increase when the airway is manipulated—eg, lidocaine 1.5 mg/kg IV 1 to 2 min before giving the paralytic. Etomidate is an excellent induction agent because it has minimal effects on BP; IV dose in adults is 0.3 mg/kg (or 20 mg for an average-sized adult) and in children is 0.2 to 0.3 mg/kg. An alternative, if hypotension is absent and unlikely, is propofol 0.2 to 1.5 mg/kg IV. Succinylcholine 1.5 mg/kg IV is typically used as a paralytic.

Pulse oximetry and ABGs (if possible, end-tidal CO_2) should be used to assess adequacy of oxygenation and ventilation. The goal is a normal $Paco_2$ level (38 to 42 mm Hg). Prophylactic hyperventilation ($Paco_2$ 25 to 35 mm Hg) is no longer recommended. The lower $Paco_2$ reduces ICP by causing cerebral vasoconstriction, but this vasoconstriction also decreases cerebral perfusion, thus potentiating ischemia. Therefore, hyperventilation (target $Paco_2$ of 30 to 35 mm Hg) is used only during the first several hours and if ICP is unresponsive to other measures.

In patients with severe TBI who cannot follow simple commands, especially those with an abnormal head CT, ICP and CPP monitoring (see p. 530) and control are recommended. The goal is to maintain ICP at < 20 mm Hg and CPP as close as possible to 60 mm Hg. Cerebral venous drainage can be enhanced (thus lowering ICP) by elevating the head of the bed to 30° and by keeping the patient's head in a midline position. If needed, a ventricular catheter can be inserted for CSF drainage to lower the ICP. A recent multicenter study found no difference in TBI recovery with ICP treatment directed by an ICP monitor versus care directed by clinical and CT findings. However, interpretation of these findings is controversial, in part because care was provided in settings that differ from those in the US, limiting extrapolation of results.

Preventing agitation, excessive muscular activity (eg, due to delirium), and pain can also help prevent increases in ICP. For sedation, propofol is often used in adults (contraindicated in children) because it has quick onset and very brief duration of action; dose is 0.3 mg/kg/h continuous IV infusion, titrated gradually upward as needed (up to 3 mg/kg/h). An initial bolus is not used. The most common adverse effect is hypotension. Prolonged use at high doses can cause pancreatitis. Benzodiazepines (eg, midazolam, lorazepam) can also be used for sedation, but they are not as rapidly acting as propofol and individual dose-response can be hard to predict. Antipsychotics can delay recovery and should be avoided if possible. Rarely, paralytics may be needed; if so, adequate sedation must be ensured. Opioids are often needed for adequate pain control.

Patients should be kept euvolemic and iso-osmolar or slightly hyperosmolar (target serum osmolality 295 to 320 mOsm kg). To control ICP, recent studies have found that hypertonic saline solution (usually 2% to 3%) is a more effective osmotic agent than mannitol. It is given as a bolus of 2 to 3 mL/kg IV as needed or as a continuous infusion of 1 mL/kg/h. Serum Na level is monitored and kept ≤ 155 mEq/L. Osmotic diuretics (eg, mannitol) given IV are an alternative to lower ICP and maintain serum osmolality. However, they should be reserved for patients whose condition is deteriorating or used preoperatively for patients with hematomas. Mannitol 20% solution is given 0.5 to 1 g/kg IV (2.5 to 5 mL/kg) over 15 to 30 min and repeated in a dose ranging from 0.25 to 0.5 g/kg (1.25 to 2.5 mL/kg) given as often as needed (usually q 6 to 8 h); it lowers ICP for a few hours. Mannitol must be used cautiously in patients with severe coronary artery disease, heart failure, renal insufficiency, or pulmonary vascular congestion because mannitol rapidly expands intravascular volume. Because osmotic diuretics increase renal excretion of water relative to Na, prolonged use of mannitol may also result in water depletion and hypernatremia. Furosemide 1 mg/kg IV is also helpful to decrease total body water, particularly when the transient hypervolemia associated with mannitol is to be avoided. Fluid and electrolyte balance should be monitored closely while osmotic diuretics are used.

When increased ICP is refractory to other interventions, decompressive craniotomy can be considered. For this procedure, a bone flap is removed (to be replaced later), and duraplasty is done to allow outward brain swelling.

A more involved and currently less popular option for intractable increased ICP is pentobarbital coma. Coma is induced by giving pentobarbital 10 mg/kg IV over 30 min, 5 mg/kg/h for 3 h, then 1 mg/kg/h maintenance infusion. The dose may be adjusted to suppress bursts of EEG activity, which is continuously monitored. Hypotension is common and managed by giving fluids and, if necessary, vasopressors.

Therapeutic systemic hypothermia has not proved helpful. Corticosteroids are not useful to control ICP and are not recommended; they were associated with a worse outcome in a previous multinational study. A variety of neuroprotective agents are being studied, but thus far, none has demonstrated efficacy in clinical trials.

Seizures: Seizures can worsen brain damage and increase ICP and therefore should be treated promptly. In patients with significant structural injury (eg, larger contusions or hematomas, brain laceration, depressed skull fracture) or a GCS score < 10, a prophylactic anticonvulsant should be considered. If phenytoin is used, a loading dose of 20 mg/kg IV is given (at a maximum rate of 50 mg/min to prevent cardiovascular adverse effects such as hypotension and bradycardia). The starting maintenance IV dose for adults is 2 to 2.7 mg/kg tid; children require higher doses (up to 5 mg/kg bid for children < 4 yr). Serum levels should be measured to adjust the dose. Duration of treatment depends on the type of injury and EEG results. If no seizures develop within 1 wk, anticonvulsants should be stopped because their value in preventing future seizures is not established. Newer anticonvulsants are under study. Fosphenytoin, a form of phenytoin that has better water solubility, is being used in some patients without central venous access because it decreases the risk of thrombophlebitis when given through a peripheral IV. Dosing is the same as for phenytoin. Levetiracetam is used increasingly, particularly in patients with liver disorders.

Skull fractures: Aligned closed fractures require no specific treatment. Depressed fractures sometimes require surgery to elevate fragments, manage lacerated cortical vessels, repair dura mater, and debride injured brain. Open fractures may require surgical debridement unless there is no CSF leak and the fracture is not depressed by greater than the thickness of the skull. Use of antibiotic prophylaxis is controversial because of limited data on its efficacy and the concern that it promotes drug-resistant strains.

Surgery: Intracranial hematomas may require urgent surgical evacuation to prevent or treat brain shift, compression, and herniation; hence, early neurosurgical consultation is mandatory. However, not all hematomas require surgical removal. Small intracerebral hematomas rarely require surgery. Patients with small subdural hematomas can often be treated without surgery. Factors that suggest a need for surgery include a midline brain shift of > 5 mm, compression of the basal cisterns, and worsening neurologic examination findings. Chronic subdural hematomas may require surgical drainage but much less urgently than acute subdural hematomas. Large or arterial epidural hematomas are treated surgically, but small epidural hematomas that are thought to be venous in origin can be followed with serial CT.

Rehabilitation: When neurologic deficits persist, rehabilitation is needed. Rehabilitation is best provided through a team approach that combines physical, occupational, and speech therapy, skill-building activities, and counseling to meet the patient's social and emotional needs (see also p. 3260). Brain injury support groups may provide assistance to the families of brain-injured patients.

For patients whose coma exceeds 24 h, 50% of whom have severe persistent neurologic sequelae, a prolonged period of rehabilitation, particularly in cognitive and emotional areas, is often required. Rehabilitation services should be planned early.

KEY POINTS

- TBI can cause a wide variety of neurologic symptoms, sometimes even in the absence of detectable structural brain damage on imaging studies.
- Follow assessment (trauma assessment and stabilization, GCS scoring, rapid and focussed neurologic examination) with a more detailed neurologic examination when the patient is stable.
- Obtain neuroimaging (usually CT) acutely if patients have more than transiently impaired consciousness, GCS score < 15, focal neurologic findings, persistent vomiting, seizures, a history of loss of consciousness, clinically suspected fractures, and possibly other findings.
- Most patients can be discharged home if TBI is mild; they can be observed at home if neuroimaging (if indicated) is normal and neurologic examination is normal.
- Admit patients with severe TBI to a critical care unit and, to avoid secondary brain insult, treat them aggressively to maintain adequate ventilation, oxygenation, and brain perfusion.
- Treat increased ICP usually with rapid sequence intubation, ICP monitoring, sedation, maintenance of euvolemia and normal serum osmolality, and sometimes surgical interventions (eg, CSF drainage, decompressive craniotomy).
- Treat some lesions surgically (eg, large or arterial epidural hematomas, intracranial hematomas with midline brain shift of > 5 mm, compression of the basal cisterns, worsening neurologic examination findings).

SPORTS-RELATED CONCUSSION

Sports activities are a common cause of concussion, a form of mild traumatic brain injury (TBI). Symptoms include loss of consciousness, confusion, memory difficulties, and other signs of brain dysfunction. Diagnosis is clinical with neuroimaging done as needed, as there is rarely any evidence of structural brain injury. Early return to competition can be harmful; once symptoms are resolved, athletes can gradually resume athletic activity.

Concussion is a transient disturbance in brain function caused by head injury, usually a blow. By definition, there are no structural brain abnormalities visible directly or on imaging studies (for more serious brain injuries, see p. 3117). Pathophysiology is still being clarified, but brain dysfunction is thought to involve excitotoxicity, which is neuronal damage caused by excessive release of excitatory neurotransmitters, particularly glutamate.

Estimates of the incidence of sports-related concussion in the US vary from 200,000/yr up to 3.8 million/yr; the highest numbers include rough estimates of injuries that are not evaluated in a hospital or otherwise reported. The awareness and thus reporting of concussions has risen significantly in the past decade—the incidence of serious and fatal sports-related TBI has not increased similarly. Sports that routinely involve high-speed collision (eg, football, rugby, ice hockey, lacrosse) have the highest rates of concussion, but no sport is free of risk, including cheerleading. An estimated 19% of participants in contact sports have a concussive injury over the course of a season.

Repeat injury: Unlike with other causes of concussion (eg, vehicular crashes, falls), which are usually isolated events, sports participants are continually exposed to risk of concussion. Thus, repeat injury is common. Athletes are particularly vulnerable if the repeat injury occurs before they have fully recovered from a previous concussion, but even after recovery, athletes who have suffered one concussion are 2 to 4 times more likely to suffer another concussion at some point. Also, repeat concussions may occur following a less severe impact.

Furthermore, although most athletes eventually recover fully from a single concussion, about 3% of those who had multiple (even apparently minor) concussions develop chronic traumatic encephalopathy (CTE, initially described in boxers and termed dementia pugilistica). In CTE, patients have structural neurodegenerative changes, including cortical atrophy, somewhat similar to changes present in patients with Alzheimer disease. Symptoms can include memory problems, impaired judgment and decision making, personality change (eg, irascibility, volatility), and parkinsonism. Several prominent retired athletes who had sustained recurrent TBI have committed suicide.

Symptoms and Signs

The most obvious disturbance of brain function with a concussion is

- Loss of consciousness

However, many patients do not lose consciousness but instead manifest symptoms and signs such as

- Confusion: Appears dazed or stunned, unsure of opponent or score, answers slowly
- Memory loss: Does not know plays or assignment, does not recall events before the injury (retrograde amnesia) or afterward (anterograde amnesia)
- Vision disturbance: Double vision, light sensitivity
- Dizziness, clumsy movements, impaired balance
- Headache

Postconcussive symptoms are cognitive and/or behavioral manifestations that may be present for a few days to weeks following concussion, including

- Chronic headaches
- Short-term memory difficulties
- Fatigue

- Difficulty sleeping
- Personality changes (irritability, mood swings)
- Sensitivity to light and noise

Postconcussive symptoms typically resolve in a few days to several weeks.

PEARLS & PITFALLS

- Patients may have concussion without loss of consciousness.

Diagnosis

- Clinical evaluation
- Sometimes neuroimaging to exclude more serious injuries

Athletes with possible concussion should be evaluated by a clinician with experience in evaluation and management of concussions. Sometimes such clinicians are on site at high-level athletic events; otherwise, sideline staff should have training in recognizing concussive symptoms and protocols for referring patients for evaluation. Diagnostic tools, such as the Standardized Assessment of Concussion (SAC), Sports Concussion Assessment Tool 2 (SCAT2), or SCAT3 can help coaching staff, trainers, and inexperienced clinicians screen athletes on site. SCAT2 and SCAT3 are available free online and can also be downloaded to handheld devices. The CDC has tools and training information for nonclinicians (CDC "Heads Up" programs).

Neuroimaging is not helpful to diagnose concussion itself but is done if there is suspicion of more serious brain injury (eg, hematoma, contusion). Typically, patients should have CT scan if they had loss of consciousness, have a Glasgow Coma Scale (GCS) score < 15 (see Table 224–4 on p. 1862), have focal neurologic deficit, have persistently altered mental status, or appear to be deteriorating (see p. 3120).

Formal neurocognitive testing would likely show abnormalities on symptomatic patients but is not typically done unless postconcussive symptoms last longer than expected or the individual is manifesting profound cognitive issues. However, some athletic programs do baseline neurocognitive tests on all participants and repeat them following concussion so that more subtle abnormalities can be identified and further participation deferred until the person returns to baseline. One of the more commonly used tests is a commercial computer-based tool called ImPACT.

Prognosis

Patients recover fully, although postconcussive symptoms can persist for up to several weeks.

CTE causes progressive brain dysfunction typically leading to death within 10 to15 yr of initial presentation.

Treatment

- Removal from contest or activity
- Rest, acetaminophen for headache
- Graduated increase to full athletic activity

Patients who had any concussive symptoms or signs should not return to play that day and are advised to rest. School and work activities, driving, and alcohol and excessive brain stimulation (eg, using computers, television, video games) should be avoided. No drugs have been shown to improve recovery from concussion, but specific symptoms can be treated with appropriate drugs (eg, acetaminophen or NSAIDs for headache). Family members are advised to watch for signs of deterioration (see p. 3121) and take the person to the hospital should they occur.

Return to play: Typically, a graduated approach is recommended. Athletes should refrain from athletic activities until they are completely asymptomatic and require no medication. Then they may begin light aerobic exercise and advance through sport-specific training, non-contact drills, full-contact drills, and finally competitive play. Patients who remain asymptomatic at one level can be advanced to the next. But however quickly they improve, patients are typically not advised to return to full play until they have been asymptomatic for 1 wk. Those who had severe symptoms (eg, unconsciousness for > 5 min, > 24 h of amnesia) should wait at least 1 mo. Athletes who have had multiple concussions in one season need to be fully advised of the risks versus benefits of continued participation. Parents of school-aged children should be involved in these discussions as well.

KEY POINTS

- Concussion involves transient, traumatic brain dysfunction; consciousness may be lost but sometimes patients manifest only confusion, memory loss, and gait or balance difficulties.
- Symptoms may resolve quickly or persist for up to several weeks.
- Athletes with possible concussion should be removed from play and evaluated; screening tools such as SCAT2 may be helpful.
- Neuroimaging is done if there is loss of consciousness, GCS < 15, focal neurologic deficit, persistently altered mental status, or clinical deterioration.
- After concussion, patients are more susceptible to repeat concussion for a period of time and must refrain from sports activities until they have been asymptomatic for 1 wk or more (depending on severity of injury).
- Athletic activities are resumed gradually.

Special Subjects

372 Care of the Surgical Patient

Before elective surgical procedures, a thorough preoperative medical evaluation by nonsurgical consultants (eg, internists, cardiologists, pulmonologists) may be necessary to help assess surgical risk. Such consultants may also help manage preexisting disease (eg, diabetes) and help prevent and treat perioperative and postoperative complications (eg, cardiac, pulmonary, infectious). Psychiatric consultation is occasionally needed to assess capacity or help deal with underlying psychiatric problems that can interfere with recovery.

Elderly patients may benefit from involvement of an interdisciplinary geriatric team, which may need to involve social workers, therapists, ethicists, and other practitioners.

PREOPERATIVE EVALUATION

If an **emergency procedure** is required (eg, for intra-abdominal hemorrhage, perforated viscus, necrotizing fasciitis), there is usually no time for a full preoperative evaluation. However, the patient's history should be reviewed as expeditiously as possible, particularly for allergies and to help identify factors that increase risk of emergency surgery (eg, history of bleeding problems or adverse anesthetic reactions).

Before **elective surgery,** the surgical team may consult an internist for a formal preoperative evaluation to minimize risk by identifying correctable abnormalities and by determining whether additional perioperative monitoring and treatment are needed. Additionally, elective procedures should be delayed when possible so that certain underlying disorders (eg, hypertension, diabetes, hematologic abnormalities) can be optimally controlled.

Routine preoperative evaluation varies substantially from patient to patient because surgical risk varies depending on the patient's risk factors, and risks of the procedure.

History: A relevant preoperative history includes information about all of the following:

- Current symptoms suggesting an active cardiopulmonary disorder (eg, cough, chest pain, dyspnea during exertion, ankle swelling) or infection (eg, fever, dysuria)
- Risk factors for excessive bleeding (eg, known bleeding disorder, history of bleeding excessively with dental procedures, elective surgeries, or childbirth)
- Risk factors for thromboembolism (see p. 757)
- Risk factors for infection
- Risk factors for cardiac disease
- Known disorders that increase risk of complications, particularly hypertension, heart disease, kidney disease, liver disease, diabetes, asthma, and COPD

- Previous surgery, anesthesia, or both, particularly their complications
- Allergies
- Tobacco and alcohol use
- Current prescription and nonprescription drug and supplement use
- History of obstructive sleep apnea or excessive snoring

If an indwelling bladder catheter may be needed, patients should be asked about prior urinary retention and prostate surgery.

Physical examination: Physical examination should address not only areas affected by the surgical procedure but also the cardiopulmonary system as well as a search for any signs of ongoing infection (eg, upper respiratory tract, skin). When spinal anesthesia is likely to be used, patients should be evaluated for scoliosis and other anatomic abnormalities that may complicate lumbar puncture. Any cognitive dysfunction, especially in elderly patients who will be given a general anesthetic, should be noted. Preexisting dysfunction may become more apparent postoperatively and, if undetected beforehand, may be misinterpreted as a surgical complication.

Testing: No preoperative tests are required in healthy patients undergoing operations with very low risk of bleeding or other complications; abnormal results are more likely to be false positives than in patients with symptoms or risk factors.

In symptomatic patients or in patients undergoing operations with a higher risk of significant bleeding or other complications, laboratory evaluation may include the following tests:

- CBC and urinalysis (glucose, protein, and cells) usually are done.
- Serum electrolytes and creatinine and plasma glucose are measured unless patients are extremely healthy and < 50 yr of age, the procedure is considered very low risk, and use of nephrotoxic drugs is not expected.
- Liver enzymes are measured if abnormalities are suspected based on the patient's history or examination.
- Coagulation studies and bleeding time are needed only if patients have a history of bleeding diathesis or a disorder associated with bleeding.
- ECG is done for patients at risk of coronary artery disease (CAD), including all men > 45 and women > 50.
- If a general anesthetic is to be used, a chest x-ray typically is done (or a recent x-ray is reviewed), but its usefulness is limited, particularly in younger patients and in patients without suspicion of heart or lung disease.
- Pulmonary function testing may be done if patients have a known chronic pulmonary disorder or symptoms or signs of pulmonary disease.

Patients with symptomatic CAD need additional tests (eg, stress testing, coronary angiography) before surgery.

Procedural Risk Factors

Procedural risk is highest with the following:

- Heart or lung surgery
- Hepatic resection
- Intra-abdominal surgeries that are estimated to require a prolonged operative time or that have a risk of large-volume hemorrhage (eg, Whipple procedure, aortic surgery, retroperitoneal surgery)
- Prostatectomy
- Major orthopedic procedures (eg, hip replacement)

Patients undergoing elective surgery that has a significant risk of hemorrhage should consider autologous transfusion. Autologous transfusion decreases the risks of infection and transfusion reactions.

Emergency surgery has a higher risk of morbidity and mortality than the same surgery done electively.

Patient Risk Factors

Patient risk factors are stratified by some clinicians using published criteria. Older age is associated with decreased physiologic reserve and greater morbidity if a complication occurs. However, chronic disorders are more closely associated with increased postoperative morbidity and mortality than is age alone. Older age is not an absolute contraindication to surgery.

Cardiac risk factors: Cardiac risk factors dramatically increase surgical risk. Perioperative cardiac risk is typically assessed using the American College of Cardiology/American Heart Association's Revised Cardiac Risk Index (see Fig. 372–1). It considers the following independent predictors of cardiac risk:

- History of CAD
- History of heart failure
- History of cerebrovascular disease
- Diabetes requiring treatment with insulin
- Serum creatinine (2.0 mg/dL)

Risk of cardiac complications increases with increasing risk factors:

- No risk factors: 0.4% (95% confidence interval 0.1 to 0.8%)
- 1 risk factor: 1.0% (95% confidence interval 0.5 to 1.4%)
- 2 risk factors: 2.4% (95% confidence interval 1.3 to 3.5%)
- ≥ 3 risk factors: 5.4% (95% confidence interval 2.8 to 7.9%)

A high-risk surgical procedure (eg, vascular surgery, open intrathoracic or intraperitoneal procedure) also independently predicts a high cardiac perioperative risk.

Patients with active cardiac symptoms (eg, of heart failure or unstable angina) have a particularly high perioperative risk. Patients with unstable angina have about a 28% risk of perioperative MI. In patients with stable angina, risk is proportional to their degree of exercise tolerance. Patients with active cardiac symptoms thus require thorough evaluation. For example, the cause of heart failure should be determined so that perioperative cardiac monitoring and treatment can be optimized before elective surgery. Other cardiac testing, such as stress echocardiography or even angiography, should be considered if there is evidence of reversible cardiac ischemia on preoperative evaluation.

Preoperative care should aim to control active disorders (eg, heart failure, diabetes) using standard treatments. Also, measures should be taken to minimize perioperative tachycardia, which can worsen heart failure and increase risk of MI; for example, pain control should be optimized and β-blocker therapy should be considered, especially if patients are already taking β-blockers. Coronary revascularization should be considered for patients with unstable angina. If a heart disorder cannot be corrected before surgery or if a patient is at high risk of cardiac complications, intraoperative and sometimes preoperative monitoring with pulmonary artery catheterization (see p. 528) may be advised. Sometimes the cardiac risk outweighs the benefit of surgery.

Infections: Incidental bacterial infections discovered preoperatively should be treated with antibiotics. However, infections should not delay surgery unless prosthetic material is being implanted; in such cases, surgery should be postponed until the infection is controlled or eliminated.

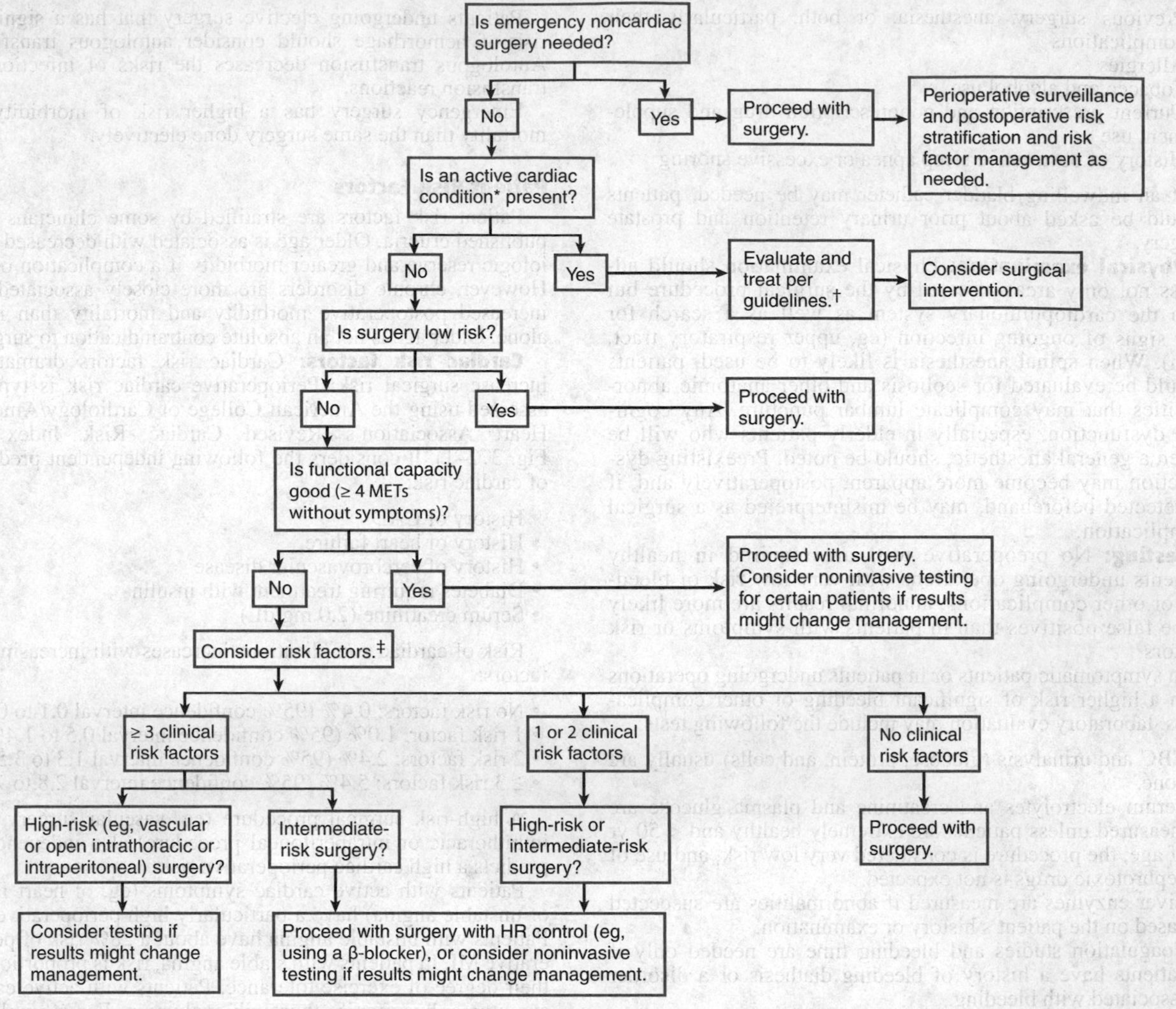

Fig. 372–1. Algorithm for risk stratification for noncardiac surgery.

*Active clinical conditions include unstable coronary syndromes, decompensated heart failure, significant arrhythmias, and severe valvular disorders.
†See the ACC/AHA guidelines.
‡Clinical risk factors include coronary artery disease, history of heart failure, history of cerebrovascular disease, diabetes mellitus, and preoperative creatinine > 2.0 mg/dL.

ACC = American College of Cardiology; AHA = American Heart Association; HR = heart rate; MET = metabolic equivalent.

Adapted from Fleisher LA, Beckman JA, Brown KA, et al: ACC/AHA 2007 guidelines on perioperative cardiovascular evaluation and care for noncardiac surgery; a report of the American College of Cardiology/American Heart Association Task Force on Practice Guidelines. *Circulation* 116: e418–e500, 2007.

Patients with respiratory infections should be treated and have evidence that the infection has resolved before receiving inhalational anesthesia.

Viral infections with or without fever should be resolved before elective surgery is done, especially if a general anesthetic is going to be used.

Fluid and electrolyte imbalances: Fluid and electrolyte imbalances should be corrected before surgery. Hypokalemia and hyperkalemia must be corrected before general anesthesia to decrease risk of potentially lethal arrhythmias. Dehydration and hypovolemia should be treated with IV fluids before general anesthesia to prevent severe hypotension on induction—BP tends to fall when general anesthesia is induced.

Nutritional disorders: **Undernutrition** increases risk of postoperative complications in adults. Nutritional status is assessed preoperatively using history, physical examination, and laboratory tests. Indicators of undernutrition include the following:

- A history of weight loss > 10% of body weight over 6 mo or 5% over 1 mo
- Suggestive physical examination findings (eg, muscle wasting, signs of specific nutritional deficiencies)
- Low serum albumin levels

Serum albumin is an inexpensive, widely available, and reliable indicator of undernutrition; it should be measured preoperatively in patients who may be undernourished. Values < 2.8 g/dL predict increased morbidity and mortality. Because the half-life of serum albumin is 14 to 18 days, levels may not reflect acute undernutrition. If more acute undernutrition is suspected, a protein with a shorter half-life can be measured; for example transferrin (half-life 7 days) or transthyretin (half-life 3 to 5 days). Preoperative and perioperative nutritional support is most likely to improve outcomes in patients whose histories of weight loss and protein levels indicate severe undernutrition. In some cases, surgery can be delayed so patients can receive nutritional support, sometimes for several weeks.

Significant obesity (BMI > 40 kg/m^2) increases perioperative mortality risk because such patients have increased risk of cardiac and pulmonary disorders (eg, hypertension, pulmonary hypertension, left ventricular hypertrophy, heart failure, CAD). Obesity is an independent risk factor for deep venous thrombosis and pulmonary embolism; preoperative venous thromboembolism prophylaxis is indicated in most obese patients. Obesity also increases risk of postoperative wound complications (eg, fat necrosis, infection, dehiscence).

PERIOPERATIVE MANAGEMENT

The American College of Surgeons (ACS) National Surgical Quality Improvement Program (NSQIP) has published guidelines and recommendations to standardize and improve surgical care. The guidelines include a set of measures created by the Surgical Care Improvement Project (SCIP) referred to as the SCIP guidelines. The SCIP guidelines are published as part of a continually evolving manual that is intended to provide standard quality measures to unify documentation and track standards of care. The SCIP guidelines target complications that account for a significant portion of preventable morbidity as well as cost. Seven SCIP initiatives pertain to perioperative care. Among the general recommendations are the following:

- Maintain a near-normal blood glucose level (eg, < 180 mg/dL) during the first 2 postoperative days, particularly in cardiac surgery patients.
- Use clippers or depilatory methods, not a blade, to remove hair from the surgical site immediately before surgery.
- Remove urinary catheters within the first 2 postoperative days except when required by specific clinical circumstances.
- Standardize antibiotic choices based on type of surgery and patient factors (see p. 3132).

Perioperative care is based on individual as well as general recommendations. Many drugs can interact with anesthetic drugs or have adverse effects during or after surgery. Thus, usually before surgery the patient's drugs are reviewed and which should be taken on the day of surgery is decided.

Anticoagulants and antiplatelets: Antiplatelet drugs (eg, aspirin) are usually stopped 5 to 7 days before surgery. Warfarin is stopped for 5 days before surgery; INR at the time of surgery should be ≤ 1.5. Patients who are at significant risk of an embolic event (eg, patients who have history of pulmonary embolism or atrial fibrillation with history of stroke) are given a short-acting anticoagulant such as low molecular weight heparin after stopping warfarin (called bridging anticoagulation—see p. 757). Because it takes up to 5 days for warfarin to achieve therapeutic anticoagulation, it can be started the day of or after surgery unless the risk of postoperative bleeding is high. Patients should receive bridging anticoagulation until the INR has reached the therapeutic target.

Corticosteroids: Patients may require supplemental corticosteroids to help prevent inadequate responses to perioperative stress if they have taken > 5 mg of prednisone daily (or an equivalent dose of another corticosteroid) for > 3 wk within the past year. Corticosteroids are unnecessary for minor procedures.

Diabetes: On the day of surgery, patients with insulin-dependent diabetes are typically given one third of their usual insulin dose in the morning. Patients who take oral drugs are given half of their usual dose. If possible, surgery is done early in the day. The anesthesiologist monitors glucose levels during surgery and gives additional insulin or dextrose as needed. Close monitoring with fingerstick testing continues throughout the perioperative period. In the immediate postoperative period, insulin is given on a sliding scale. The usual at-home insulin regimen is not restarted until patients resume their regular diet.

Drug dependence: Patients who are dependent on drugs or alcohol may experience withdrawal during the perioperative period. Alcoholics should be given prophylactic benzodiazepines (eg, chlordiazepoxide, diazepam, lorazepam) starting at admission. Opioid addicts may be given opioid analgesics to prevent withdrawal; for pain relief, they may require larger doses than patients who are not addicted. Rarely, opioid addicts require methadone to prevent withdrawal during the perioperative period.

Heart disease: Patients with known coronary artery disease or heart failure should undergo preoperative evaluation and risk stratification by their cardiologist. If patients are not medically optimized, they should undergo additional testing before elective surgery.

Other drugs that control chronic disorders: Most drugs taken to control chronic disorders, especially cardiovascular drugs (including antihypertensives), should be continued throughout the perioperative period. Most oral drugs can be given with a small sip of water on the day of surgery. Other drugs may have to be given parenterally or delayed until after surgery. Anticonvulsant levels should be measured preoperatively in patients with a seizure disorder.

Preprocedural checklist: In the operating room, before the procedure begins, a time out is held during which the team confirms several important factors:

- Patient identity
- Correct procedure and operative site (if applicable)
- Availability of all needed equipment
- Completion of indicated prophylaxis (eg, antibiotics, anticoagulants)

Smoking: Smokers are advised to stop smoking as early as possible before any procedure involving the chest or abdomen. Several weeks of smoking cessation are required for ciliary mechanisms to recover. An incentive inspirometer should be used before and after surgery.

Upper airway: Before intubation, dentures must be removed. Ideally, before patients are moved from the preanesthetic holding area, they should give dentures to a family member. Patients with a deviated septum or another airway abnormality should be evaluated by an anesthesiologist before surgery requiring intubation.

OUTPATIENT PROCEDURES

Many surgical procedures are done in outpatient settings. Patients are evaluated (eg, with laboratory tests—see p. 3128) one to several days before the procedure.

Preparation: The general rule is for patients to have no oral intake after midnight the night before surgery. For certain GI procedures, cleansing enemas or oral solutions must be started 1 to 2 days before surgery. When prophylactic antibiotics are needed before a procedure, the initial dose must be given within 1 h before the surgical incision.

Discharge precautions: Before discharge, patients should be free of severe pain and should be able to think clearly, breathe normally, drink, walk, and urinate.

If sedatives (eg, opioids, benzodiazepines) were used during an outpatient procedure, patients should not leave the hospital unaccompanied. Even after anesthetic effects have apparently worn off and patients feel fine, they are likely to be weak and have subtle residual effects that make driving inadvisable; many patients require opioids for pain. Elderly patients may be temporarily disoriented because of the combined effects of anesthesia and surgical stress and may develop urinary retention caused by immobility and anticholinergic drug effects.

ANTIBIOTIC PROPHYLAXIS FOR SURGICAL PROCEDURES

Most surgical procedures do not require prophylactic or postoperative antibiotics. However, certain patient-related and procedure-related factors alter the risk/benefit ratio in favor of prophylactic use.

Patient-related risk factors suggesting need for antibiotics include

- Certain valvular heart disorders
- Immunosuppression

Procedures with higher risk involve areas where bacterial seeding is likely:

- Mouth
- GI tract
- Respiratory tract
- GU tract

In so-called clean (likely to be sterile) procedures, prophylaxis generally is beneficial only when prosthetic material or devices are being inserted or when the consequence of infection is known to be serious (eg, mediastinitis after coronary artery bypass grafting).

Choice of antibiotics is based on the Surgical Care Improvement Project (SCIP) guidelines (see p. 3131). There is strong evidence that standardizing antibiotic choices and adhering to SCIP protocols or another standardized and validated protocol reduce the risk of surgical infection. Some regions of the US that followed SCIP guidelines were able to decrease surgical site infections by 25% from 2006 to 2010. Drug choice is based on the drug's activity against the bacteria most likely to contaminate the wound during the specific procedure (see Table 372–1). The antibiotic is given within 1 h before the surgical incision (2 h for vancomycin and fluoroquinolones). Antibiotics may be given orally or IV, depending on the procedure. For most cephalosporins, another dose is given if the procedure lasts > 4 h. For clean procedures, no additional doses are needed, but, for other cases, it is unclear whether additional doses are beneficial. Antibiotics are continued > 24 h postoperatively only when an active infection is detected during surgery; antibiotics are then considered treatment, not prophylaxis.

POSTOPERATIVE CARE

Postoperative care begins at the end of the operation and continues in the recovery room and throughout the hospitalization and outpatient period. Critical immediate concerns are airway protection, pain control, mental status, and wound healing. Other important concerns are preventing urinary retention, constipation, deep venous thrombosis (DVT), and BP variability (high or low). For patients with diabetes, blood glucose levels are monitored closely by fingerstick testing every 1 to 4 h until patients are awake and eating because better glycemic control improves outcome.

Airway: Most patients are extubated before leaving the operating room and soon become able to clear secretions from their airway. Patients should not leave the recovery room until they can clear and protect their airway (unless they are going to an ICU). After intubation, patients with normal lungs and trachea may have a mild cough for 24 h after extubation; for smokers and patients with a history of bronchitis, postextubation coughing lasts longer. Most patients who have been intubated, especially smokers and patients with a lung disorder, benefit from an incentive inspirometer.

Table 372–1. ANTIBIOTIC REGIMENS FOR CERTAIN SURGICAL PROCEDURES

SURGICAL PROCEDURE	APPROVED ANTIBIOTICS
Cardiac or vascular	Cefazolin, cefuroxime, or vancomycin If β-lactam allergy: Vancomycin or clindamycin
Hip/knee arthroplasty	Cefazolin, cefuroxime, or vancomycin If β-lactam allergy: Vancomycin or clindamycin
Colon	Cefotetan, cefoxitin, ampicillin/sulbactam, or ertapenem *or* cefazolin plus Metronidazole *or* cefuroxime plus metronidazole *or* ceftriaxone plus metronidazole If β-lactam allergy: Clindamycin plus gentamicin *or* clindamycin plus ciprofloxacin *or* clindamycin plus aztreonam *or* metronidazole plus gentamicin *or* metronidazole plus ciprofloxacin
Hysterectomy	Cefotetan, cefazolin, cefoxitin, cefuroxime, or ampicillin/sulbactam If β-lactam allergy: Clindamycin plus gentamicin *or* clindamycin plus ciprofloxacin *or* clindamycin plus aztreonam *or* metronidazole plus gentamicin *or* metronidazole plus ciprofloxacin *or* vancomycin plus aminoglycoside *or* vancomycin plus aztreonam *or* vancomycin plus quinolone

Adapted from the Specifications Manual for National Hospital Inpatient Quality Measures, Section 2.4 Surgical Care Improvement Project (SCIP), version 4.3:38–39, 2014. Available at www.qualitynet.org.

Postoperative dyspnea may be caused by pain secondary to chest or abdominal incisions (nonhypoxic dyspnea) or by hypoxemia (hypoxic dyspnea—see also p. 533). Hypoxemia secondary to pulmonary dysfunction is usually accompanied by dyspnea, tachypnea, or both; however, oversedation may cause hypoxemia but blunt dyspnea, tachypnea, or both. Thus, sedated patients should be monitored with pulse oximetry or capnometry. Hypoxic dyspnea may result from atelectasis or, especially in patients with a history of heart failure or chronic kidney disease, fluid overload. Whether dyspnea is hypoxic or nonhypoxic must be determined by pulse oximetry and sometimes ABGs; chest x-ray can help differentiate fluid overload from atelectasis.

Hypoxic dyspnea is treated with O_2. Nonhypoxic dyspnea may be treated with anxiolytics or analgesics.

Pain: Pain control may be necessary as soon as patients are conscious (see p. 1968). Opioids are typically the first-line choice and can be given orally or parenterally. Often, oxycodone/acetaminophen 1 or 2 tablets (each tablet can contain 2.5 to 10 mg oxycodone and 325 to 650 mg acetaminophen) po q 4 to 6 h or morphine 2 to 4 mg IV q 3 h is given as a starting dose, which is subsequently adjusted as needed; individual needs and tolerances can vary several-fold. With less frequent dosing, breakthrough pain, which should be avoided, is possible. For more severe pain, IV patient-controlled, on-demand dosing is best (see Dosing and titration). If patients do not have a renal disorder or a history of GI bleeding, giving NSAIDs at regular intervals may reduce breakthrough pain, allowing the opioid dosage to be reduced.

Mental status: All patients are briefly confused when they come out of anesthesia. The elderly, especially those with dementia, are at risk of postoperative delirium, which can delay discharge and increase risk of death. Risk of delirium is high when anticholinergics are used. These drugs are sometimes used before or during surgery to decrease upper airway secretions, but they should be avoided whenever possible. Opioids, given postoperatively, may also cause delirium, as can high doses of H_2 blockers. The mental status of elderly patients should be assessed frequently during the postoperative period. If delirium occurs, oxygenation should be assessed, and all nonessential drugs should be stopped. Patients should be mobilized as they are able, and any electrolyte or fluid imbalances should be corrected.

Wound care: The surgeon must individualize care of each wound, but the sterile dressing placed in the operating room is generally left intact for 24 to 48 h unless signs of infection (eg, increasing pain, erythema, drainage) develop. After the operative dressing is removed, the site should be checked twice daily for signs of infection. If they occur, wound exploration and drainage of abscesses, systemic antibiotics, or both may be required. Topical antibiotics are usually not helpful. A drain tube, if present, must be monitored for quantity and quality of the fluid collected. Sutures, skin staples, and other closures are usually left in place 7 days or longer depending on the site and the patient. Face and neck wounds may be superficially healed in 3 days; wounds on the lower extremities may take weeks to heal to a similar degree.

Deep venous thrombosis (DVT) prophylaxis: Risk of DVT after surgery is small, but because consequences can be severe and risk is still higher than that in the general population, prophylaxis is often warranted. Surgery itself increases coagulability and often requires prolonged immobility, which is another risk factor for DVT (see pp. 490 and 755). Prophylaxis for DVT usually begins in the operating room (see Table 88–4 on p. 763). Alternatively, heparin may be started shortly after surgery, when risk of bleeding has decreased. Patients should begin moving their limbs as soon as it is safe for them to do so.

Fever: A common cause of postoperative fever is an inflammatory or hypermetabolic response to an operation. Other causes include pneumonia, UTIs, wound infections, and DVTs. Additional possibilities are drug-induced fever and infections affecting implantable devices and drains. Common causes of fever during the days or weeks after surgery include the so-called "six Ws":

- *W*ound infections
- *W*ater (eg, UTIs)
- *W*ind (eg, atelectasis, pneumonia)
- *W*alking (eg, DVTs)
- *W*onder drugs (eg, drug-induced fever)
- *W*idgets (eg, implantable devices, drains)

Optimal postoperative care (eg, early ambulation and removal of bladder catheters, meticulous wound care) can decrease risk of DVTs, UTIs, and wound infections. Incentive spirometry and periodic coughing can help decrease risk of pneumonia.

Urinary retention and constipation: Urinary retention and constipation are common after surgery. Causes include

- Anticholinergics
- Opioids
- Immobility
- Decreased oral intake

Urine output must be monitored. Straight catheterization is typically necessary for patients who have a distended bladder and are uncomfortable or who have not urinated for 6 to 8 h after surgery; the Credé maneuver sometimes helps and may make catheterization unnecessary. Chronic retention is best treated by avoiding causative drugs and by having patients sit up as often as possible. Bethanechol 5 to 10 mg po can be tried in patients unlikely to have any bladder obstruction and who have not had a laparotomy; doses can be repeated every hour up to a maximum of 50 mg/day. Sometimes an indwelling bladder catheter is needed, especially if patients have a history of retention or a large initial output after straight catheterization.

Constipation is common and typically secondary to anesthetic drugs, bowel surgery, postoperative immobility, and opioids. Constipation is treated by minimizing use of opioids and other constipating drugs, by beginning postoperative ambulation early, and, if patients have not had GI surgery, by giving stimulant laxatives (eg, bisacodyl, senna, cascara). Stool softeners (eg, docusate) do not alleviate postoperative constipation.

Loss of muscle mass (sarcopenia): Loss of muscle mass (sarcopenia) and strength occur in all patients who require prolonged bed rest. With complete bed rest, young adults lose about 1% of muscle mass/day, but the elderly lose up to 5%/day because growth hormone levels decrease with age. Avoiding sarcopenia is essential to recovery. Thus, patients should sit up in bed, transfer to a chair, stand, and exercise as much as and as soon as is safe for their surgical and medical condition. Nutritional deficiencies may also contribute to sarcopenia. Thus, nutritional intake of patients on complete bed rest should be optimized. Oral intake should be encouraged, and tube feeding or, rarely, parenteral feeding may be necessary.

Other issues: Certain types of surgery require additional precautions. For example, hip surgery requires that patients be moved and positioned so that the hip does not dislocate. Any physician moving such patients for any reason, including auscultating the lungs, must know the positioning protocol to avoid doing harm; often, a nurse is the best instructor.

373 Chronic Fatigue Syndrome

(SEID; Systemic Exertion Intolerance Disease)

Chronic fatigue syndrome (CFS) is a syndrome of life-altering fatigue lasting > 6 mo that is unexplained and is accompanied by a number of associated symptoms. Management includes validating the patient's disability, treating specific symptoms, cognitive-behavioral therapy, and a graded exercise program.

Although as many as 25% of people report being chronically fatigued (see p. 3214), only about 0.5% of people meet criteria for having CFS. Although the term CFS was first used in 1988, the disorder has been well described since at least the mid 1700s but has had different names (eg, febricula, neurasthenia, chronic brucellosis, effort syndrome). CFS is most common among young and middle-aged women but has been described in all ages, including children, and in both sexes.

CFS is not malingering (intentional feigning of symptoms). CFS does share many features with fibromyalgia, such as sleep disorders, mental cloudiness, fatigue, pain, and exacerbation of symptoms with activity.

Etiology

Etiology is unknown. No infectious, hormonal, immunologic, or psychiatric cause has been established. Among the many proposed infectious causes, Epstein-Barr virus, Lyme disease, candidiasis, and cytomegalovirus have been proven not to cause CFS. Similarly, there are no allergic markers and no immunosuppression.

Various minor immunologic abnormalities have been reported. These abnormalities include low levels of IgG, abnormal IgG, decreased lymphocytic proliferation, low interferon-gamma levels in response to mitogens, poor cytotoxicity of natural killer cells, circulating autoantibodies and immune complexes, and many other immunologic findings. However, there is no consistent or reliably reproducible pattern of immunologic abnormalities, and none provide adequate sensitivity and specificity for defining CFS.

Relatives of patients with CFS have an increased risk of developing the syndrome, suggesting a genetic component or common environmental exposure. Recent studies have identified some genetic markers that might predispose to CFS. Some researchers believe the etiology will eventually be shown to be multifactorial, including a genetic predisposition, and exposure to microbes, toxins, and other physical and/or emotional trauma.

Symptoms and Signs

Before onset of CFS, most patients are highly functioning and successful.

Onset is usually abrupt, and many patients report an initial viral-like illness with swollen lymph nodes, extreme fatigue, fever, and upper respiratory symptoms. The initial syndrome resolves but seems to trigger protracted severe fatigue, which interferes with daily activities, and many of the other features of the syndrome. In February 2015, the Institute of Medicine (now the Health and Medicine Division of The National Academies of Science, Engineering, and Medicine) published an extensive review of this disease called Beyond Myalgic Encephalomyelitis/Chronic Fatigue Syndrome: Redefining an Illness. In this review they proposed a new name, systemic exertion intolerance disease (SEID), and new diagnostic criteria that simplified the diagnosis and emphasized the most consistent features (see Table 373–1). In addition, the review clearly emphasized the validity of this debilitating disease.

The physical examination is normal, with no objective signs of muscle weakness, arthritis, neuropathy, or organomegaly. However, some patients have low-grade fever, nonexudative pharyngitis, and/or palpable or tender (but not enlarged) lymph nodes. Any abnormal physical findings must be evaluated and alternative diagnoses that cause chronic fatigue excluded before the diagnosis of CFS can be made.

Diagnosis

- Clinical criteria
- Laboratory evaluation to exclude non-CFS disorders

The diagnosis is made by the characteristic history combined with a normal physical examination and normal laboratory test results. The case definition is sometimes useful but is mainly an epidemiologic and research tool and should not be strictly applied to individual patients.

Testing is directed at any non-CFS causes suspected based on objective clinical findings. If no cause is evident or suspected, a reasonable laboratory assessment includes CBC and measurement of electrolytes, BUN, creatinine, ESR, and TSH. If indicated by clinical findings, further testing may include chest x-ray, sleep studies, and testing for adrenal insufficiency in selected patients. Serologic testing for infections, antinuclear antibodies, and neuroimaging are not indicated without objective evidence of disease on examination (ie, not

Table 373–1. DIAGNOSTIC CRITERIA FOR CHRONIC FATIGUE SYNDROME*

Diagnosis requires that the patient have the following 3 symptoms:

1. A substantial reduction or impairment in the ability to engage in pre-illness levels of occupational, educational, social, or personal activities that persists for more than 6 mo and is accompanied by fatigue, which is often profound, is of new or definite onset (not lifelong), is not the result of ongoing excessive exertion, and is not substantially alleviated by rest
2. Post-exertional malaise†
3. Unrefreshing sleep†

At least one of the following manifestations is also required:

1. Cognitive impairment†
2. Orthostatic intolerance

*Diagnostic criteria proposed by the Institute of Medicine (now the Health and Medicine Division of The National Academies of Science, Engineering, and Medicine) in February 2015.

†Frequency and severity of symptoms should be assessed. The diagnosis of ME/CFS should be questioned if patients do not have these symptoms at least half of the time with moderate, substantial, or severe intensity.

just subjective complaints) or on basic testing; in such cases, pretest probability is low and so the risk of false-positive results (and thus unnecessary treatment and/or confirmatory testing) is high.

Prognosis

Most patients improve over time though not necessarily back to their pre-illness state. However, that time is typically years and improvement is often only partial. Some evidence indicates that earlier diagnosis and intervention improve the prognosis.

Treatment

- Acknowledgment of patient's symptoms
- Cognitive-behavioral therapy
- Graded exercise
- Drugs for depression, sleep, or pain if indicated

To provide effective care, physicians must acknowledge and accept the validity of patients' symptoms. Whatever the underlying cause, these patients are suffering and strongly desire a return to their previous state of health. However, patients need to reframe expectations. They need to accept and accommodate their disability, focusing on what they can still do instead of lamenting what they cannot do.

Cognitive-behavioral therapy and a graded exercise program are the only interventions proven helpful. Depression should be treated with antidepressants and/or psychiatric referral. Sleep disturbances should be aggressively managed with relaxation techniques and improved sleep hygiene (see Table 239–5 on p. 2017).

If these measures are ineffective, hypnotic drugs and/or referral to a sleep specialist may be necessary. Patients with pain (usually due to a component of fibromyalgia) can be treated using a number of drugs such as pregabalin, duloxetine, amitriptyline, or gabapentin. Physical therapy is also often helpful.

Unproven or disproven treatments, such as antivirals, immunosuppressants, elimination diets, and amalgam extractions, should be avoided.

KEY POINTS

- CFS is life-altering fatigue lasting > 6 mo that typically affects previously healthy and active people; it is not malingering.
- Etiology is unclear but probably involves multiple factors, including genetic susceptibility, microbial exposure, and environmental and psychologic factors.
- Diagnose CFS based on characteristic symptoms in patients with a normal examination and normal basic laboratory test results; Institute of Medicine (now the Health and Medicine Division of The National Academies of Science, Engineering, and Medicine) criteria may be helpful but are not strictly applied to individual patients.
- Validate patients' symptoms, encourage them to accept and accommodate to their disabilities, and treat using cognitive-behavioral therapy and graded exercise.
- Use drugs as needed to treat specific symptoms (eg, pain, depression, insomnia).

374 Clinical Decision Making

Clinicians must integrate a huge variety of clinical data while facing conflicting pressures to decrease diagnostic uncertainty, risks to patients, and costs. Deciding what information to gather, which tests to order, how to interpret and integrate this information to draw diagnostic conclusions, and which treatments to give is known as clinical decision making.

When presented with a patient, clinicians usually must answer the following questions:

- What disease does this patient have?
- Should this patient be treated?
- Should testing be done?

In straightforward or common situations, clinicians often make such decisions informally; diagnoses are made by recognizing disease patterns, and testing and treatment are initiated based on customary practice. For example, during a flu epidemic, a healthy adult who has had fever, aches, and harsh cough for 2 days is likely to be recognized as another case of influenza and provided only appropriate symptomatic relief. Such pattern recognition is efficient and easy to use but may be subject to error because other diagnostic and therapeutic possibilities are not seriously or systematically considered. For example, a patient with that flu pattern and decreased O_2 saturation might instead have bacterial pneumonia and require antibiotics.

In more complex cases, a structured, quantitative, analytical methodology may be a better approach to decision making. Even when pattern recognition provides the most likely diagnostic possibility, analytic decision making is often used to confirm the diagnosis. Analytic methods may include application of the principles of evidence-based medicine (EBM), use of clinical guidelines, and use of various specific quantitative techniques (eg, Bayes theorem).

EVIDENCE-BASED MEDICINE AND CLINICAL GUIDELINES

Physicians have always felt that their decisions were based on evidence; thus, the current term "evidence-based medicine" is somewhat of a misnomer. However, for many clinicians, the "evidence" is often a vague combination of recollected strategies effective in previous patients, advice given by mentors and colleagues, and a general impression of "what is being done" based on random journal articles, abstracts, symposia, and advertisements. This kind of practice results in wide variations in strategies for diagnosing and managing similar conditions, even when strong evidence exists for favoring one particular strategy over another. Variations exist among different countries, different regions, different hospitals, and even within individual group practices. These variations have led to a call for a more systematic approach to identifying the most appropriate strategy for an individual patient; this approach is called EBM. EBM is built on reviews of relevant medical literature and follows a discrete series of steps.

Evidence-Based Medicine

EBM is not the blind application of advice gleaned from recently published literature to individual patient problems. Rather, EBM requires the use of a series of steps to gather sufficiently useful information to answer a carefully crafted question for an individual patient. Fully integrating the principles of EBM also incorporates the patient's value system, which includes such things as costs incurred, the patient's religious or moral beliefs, and patient autonomy. Applying the principles of EBM typically involves the following steps:

- Formulating a clinical question
- Gathering evidence to answer the question
- Evaluating the quality and validity of the evidence
- Deciding how to apply the evidence to the care of a given patient

Formulating a clinical question: Questions must be specific. Specific questions are most likely to be addressed in the medical literature. A well-designed question specifies the population, intervention (diagnostic test, treatment), comparison (treatment A vs treatment B), and outcome. "What is the best way to evaluate someone with abdominal pain?" is not a good question. A better, more specific question may be "Is CT or ultrasonography preferable for diagnosing acute appendicitis in a 30-yr-old male with acute lower abdominal pain?"

Gathering evidence to answer the question: A broad selection of relevant studies is obtained from a review of the literature. Standard resources are consulted (eg, MEDLINE, the Cochrane Collaboration [treatment options], the National Guideline Clearinghouse, ACP Journal Club).

Evaluating the quality and validity of the evidence: Not all scientific studies are of equal value. Different types of studies have different scientific strengths and legitimacy, and for any given type of study, individual examples often vary in quality of the methodology, internal validity, and generalizability of results (external validity).

Levels of evidence are graded 1 through 5 in decreasing order of quality. Types of studies at each level vary somewhat with the clinical question (eg, of diagnosis, treatment, or economic analysis), but typically level 1 evidence (the highest quality) consists of systematic reviews or meta-analyses of randomized controlled trials and high-quality, single, randomized controlled trials. Level 2 evidence is well-designed cohort studies. Level 3 evidence is systematically reviewed case-control studies. Level 4 evidence is case series and poor-quality cohort and case-control studies. Level 5 evidence is expert opinion not based on critical appraisal but is based on reasoning from physiology, bench research, or underlying principles.

For EBM analysis, the highest level of evidence available is selected. Ideally, a significant number of large, well-conducted level 1 studies are available. However, because the number of high-quality, randomized, controlled trials is vanishingly small compared with the number of possible clinical questions, less reliable level 4 or 5 evidence is very often all that is available. Lower-quality evidence does not mean that the EBM process cannot be followed, just that the strength of the conclusion is weaker.

Deciding how to apply the evidence to the care of a given patient: Because the best available evidence may have come from patient populations with different characteristics from those of the patient in question, some judgment is required. Additionally, patients' wishes regarding aggressive or invasive tests and treatment must be taken into account as well as their tolerance for discomfort, risk, and uncertainty. For example, even though an EBM review may definitively show a 3-mo survival advantage from an aggressive chemotherapy regimen in a certain form of cancer, patients may differ on whether they prefer to gain the extra time or avoid the extra discomfort. The cost of tests and treatments may also influence physician and patient decision making, especially when some of the alternatives are significantly costlier for the patient.

Limitations: Dozens of clinical questions are faced during the course of even one day in a busy practice. Although some of them may be the subject of an existing EBM review available for reference, most are not, and preparing an EBM analysis is too time-consuming to be useful in answering an immediate clinical question. Even when time is not a consideration, many clinical questions do not have any relevant studies in the literature.

Clinical Guidelines

Clinical guidelines have become common in the practice of medicine; many specialty societies have published such guidelines. Most well-conceived clinical guidelines are developed using a specified method that incorporates principles of EBM and consensus recommendations made by a panel of experts. Although clinical guidelines may describe standard practice, clinical guidelines alone do not establish the standard of care for an individual patient.

Some clinical guidelines follow "if, then" rules (eg, if a patient is febrile and neutropenic, then institute broad-spectrum antibiotics). More complex, multistep rules may be formalized as algorithms. Guidelines and algorithms are generally straightforward and easy to use but should be applied only to patients whose clinical characteristics (eg, demographics, comorbidities, clinical features) are similar to those of the patient group used to create the guideline. Furthermore, guidelines do not take into account the degree of uncertainty inherent in test results, the likelihood of treatment success, and the relative risks and benefits of each course of action. To incorporate uncertainty and the value of outcomes into clinical decision making, clinicians must often apply the principles of quantitative or analytical medical decision making.

CLINICAL DECISION-MAKING STRATEGIES

One of the most commonly used strategies for medical decision making mirrors the scientific method of hypothesis generation followed by hypothesis testing. Diagnostic hypotheses are accepted or rejected based on testing.

Hypothesis Generation

Hypothesis generation involves the identification of the main diagnostic possibilities (differential diagnosis) that might account for the patient's clinical problem. The patient's chief complaint (eg, chest pain) and basic demographic data (age, sex, race) are the starting points for the differential diagnosis, which is usually generated by pattern recognition. Each element on the list of possibilities is ideally assigned an estimated probability, or likelihood, of its being the correct diagnosis (pre-test probability—see Table 374–1).

Clinicians often use vague terms such as "highly likely," "improbable," and "cannot rule out" to describe the likelihood of disease. Both clinicians and patients often misinterpret such semiquantitative terms; explicit statistical terminology should be used instead when available. Mathematical computations assist clinical decision making and, even when exact numbers are unavailable, can better define clinical probabilities and narrow the list of hypothetical diseases further.

Table 374–1. HYPOTHETICAL DIFFERENTIAL DIAGNOSIS AND PRE-TEST AND POST-TEST PROBABILITIES FOR A 50-YR-OLD HYPERTENSIVE, DIABETIC CIGARETTE SMOKER WITH CHEST PAIN

DIAGNOSIS	PRE-TEST PROBABILITY	POST-TEST PROBABILITY I (ADDITIONAL FINDINGS OF LEG PAIN, SWELLING, AND NORMAL ECG AND CHEST X-RAY)	POST-TEST PROBABILITY II (ADDITIONAL FINDINGS OF SEGMENTAL DEFECT ON CHEST CT ANGIOGRAPHY AND NORMAL SERUM TROPONIN I LEVEL)
Acute coronary syndrome	40%	28%	1%
ST-segment elevation MI	20%	< 1%	< 1%
Chest wall pain	30%	20%	< 1%
Pulmonary embolism	5%	50%	98%
Dissecting thoracic aortic aneurysm	< 3%	< 1%	< 1%
Spontaneous pneumothorax	< 2%	< 1%	< 1%

Probability and odds: The **probability** of a disease (or event) occurring in a patient whose clinical information is unknown is the frequency with which that disease or event occurs in a population. Probabilities range from 0.0 (impossible) to 1.0 (certain) and are often expressed as percentages (from 0 to 100). A disease that occurs in 2 of 10 patients has a probability of 2/10 (0.2 or 20%). Rounding very small probabilities to 0, thus excluding all possibility of disease (sometimes done in implicit clinical reasoning), can lead to erroneous conclusions when quantitative methods are used.

Odds represent the ratio of affected to unaffected patients (ie, the ratio of disease to no disease). Thus, a disease that occurs in 2 of 10 patients (probability of 2/10) has odds of 2/8 (0.25, often expressed as 1 to 4). Odds (Ω) and probabilities (p) can be converted one to the other, as in $\Omega = p/(1 - p)$ or $p = \Omega/(1 + \Omega)$.

Hypothesis Testing

The initial differential diagnosis based on chief complaint and demographics is usually very large, so the clinician first tests the hypothetical possibilities during the history and physical examination, asking questions or doing specific examinations that support or refute a suspected diagnosis. For instance, in a patient with chest pain, a history of leg pain and a swollen, tender leg detected during examination increases the probability of pulmonary embolism.

When the history and physical examination form a clear-cut pattern, a presumptive diagnosis is made. Diagnostic testing is used when uncertainties persist after the history and physical examination, particularly when the diseases remaining under consideration are serious or have dangerous or costly treatment. Test results further modify the probabilities of different diagnoses (post-test probability). For example, Table 374–1 shows how the additional findings that the hypothetical patient had leg pain and swelling and a normal ECG and chest x-ray modify diagnostic probabilities—the probability of acute coronary syndrome (ACS), dissecting aneurysm, and pneumothorax decreases, and the probability of pulmonary embolism increases. These changes in probability may lead to additional testing (in this example, probably chest CT angiography) that further modifies post-test probability (see Table 374–1) and, in some cases, confirms or refutes a diagnosis.

It may seem intuitive that the sum of probabilities of all diagnostic possibilities should equal nearly 100% and that a single diagnosis can be derived from a complex array of symptoms and signs. However, applying this principle that the best explanation for a complex situation involves a single cause (often referred to as Occam's razor) can lead clinicians astray. Rigid application of this principle discounts the possibility that a patient may have more than one active disease. For example, a dyspneic patient with known COPD may be presumed to be having an exacerbation of COPD but actually is also suffering from a pulmonary embolism.

Probability Estimations and the Testing Threshold

Even when diagnosis is uncertain, testing is not always useful. A test should be done only if its results will affect management. When disease pre test probability is above a certain threshold, treatment is warranted (treatment threshold) and testing is not indicated.

Below the treatment threshold, testing is indicated only when a positive test result would raise the post-test probability *above* the treatment threshold. The lowest pre-test probability at which this can occur depends on test characteristics and is termed the testing threshold. The testing threshold is discussed in greater detail elsewhere.

Probability Estimations and the Treatment Threshold

The disease probability at and above which treatment is given and no further testing is warranted is termed the treatment threshold (TT).

The above hypothetical example of a patient with chest pain converged on a near-certain diagnosis (98% probability). When diagnosis of a disease is certain, the decision to treat is a straightforward determination that there is a benefit of treatment (compared with no treatment, and taking into account adverse effects of treatment). When the diagnosis has some degree of uncertainty, as is almost always the case, the decision to treat also must balance the benefit of treating a sick person against the risk of erroneously treating a well person or a person with a different disorder; benefit and risk encompass both financial and medical consequences. This balance must take into account both the likelihood of disease and the magnitude of the benefit and risk. This balance determines where the clinician sets the TT.

PEARLS & PITFALLS

- When there is some uncertainty about the diagnosis, the decision to treat must balance the benefit of treating a sick person against the risk of erroneously treating a well person or a person with a different disorder.

Conceptually, if the benefit of treatment is very high and the risk is very low (as when giving a safe antibiotic to a patient with diabetes who possibly has a life-threatening infection), clinicians tend to accept high diagnostic uncertainty and might initiate treatment even if probability of infection is fairly low (eg, 30%—see Fig. 374–1). However, when the risk of treatment is very high (as when doing a pneumonectomy for possible lung cancer), clinicians want to be extremely sure of the diagnosis and might recommend treatment only when the probability of cancer is very high, perhaps > 95% (see Fig. 374–1). Note that the TT does not necessarily correspond to the probability at which a disease might be considered confirmed or ruled in. It is simply the point at which the risk of not treating is greater than the risk of treating.

Quantitatively, the TT can be described as the point at which probability of disease (p) times benefit of treating a person with disease (B) equals probability of no disease (1 – p) times risk of treating a person without disease (R). Thus, at the TT

$$p \times B = (1 - p) \times R$$

Solving for p, this equation reduces to

$$p = R/(B + R)$$

From this equation, it is apparent that if B (benefit) and R (risk) are the same, the TT becomes 1/(1 + 1) = 0.5, which means that when the probability of disease is > 50%, clinicians would treat, and when probability is < 50%, clinicians would not treat.

For a clinical example, a patient with chest pain can be considered. How high should the clinical likelihood of acute MI be before thrombolytic therapy should be given, assuming the only risk considered is short-term mortality? If it is postulated (for illustration) that mortality due to intracranial hemorrhage with thrombolytic therapy is 1%, then 1% is R, the fatality rate of mistakenly treating a patient who does not have an MI. If net mortality in patients with MI is decreased by 3% with thrombolytic therapy, then 3% is B. Then, TT is 1/(3 + 1), or 25%; thus, treatment should be given if the probability of acute MI is > 25%.

Alternatively, the TT equation can be rearranged to show that the TT is the point at which the odds of disease p/(1 – p) equal the risk:benefit ratio (R/B). The same numerical result is obtained as in the previously described example, with the TT occurring at the odds of the risk:benefit ratio (1/3); 1/3 odds corresponds to the previously obtained probability of 25% (see probability and odds—p. 3137).

Limitations of quantitative decision methods: Quantitative clinical decision making seems precise, but because many elements in the calculations are often imprecisely known (if they are known at all), this methodology is difficult to use in all but the most well-defined and studied clinical situations.

COGNITIVE ERRORS IN CLINICAL DECISION MAKING

Although quantitative mathematical models can guide clinical decision making, clinicians rarely use formal computations to make patient care decisions in day-to-day practice. Rather, an intuitive understanding of probabilities is combined with cognitive processes called heuristics to guide clinical judgment. Heuristics are often referred to as rules of thumb, educated guesses, or mental shortcuts. Heuristics usually involve pattern recognition and rely on a subconscious integration of somewhat haphazardly gathered patient data with prior experience rather than on a conscious generation of a rigorous differential diagnosis that is formally evaluated using specific data from the literature.

Such informal reasoning is often fallible because heuristics may cause several types of unconscious errors (cognitive errors). Studies suggest that more medical errors involve cognitive error than lack of knowledge or information.

Types of cognitive error: There are many types of cognitive errors, and although it is obviously more important to avoid errors than to properly classify them once made, being aware of common types of cognitive errors can help clinicians recognize and avoid them.

Cognitive errors may roughly be classified as those involving

- Faulty assessment of pre-test probability (overestimating or underestimating disease likelihood)
- Failure to seriously consider all relevant possibilities

Both types of error can easily lead to improper testing (too much or too little) and missed diagnoses.

Availability error occurs when clinicians misestimate the prior probability of disease because of recent experience. Experience often leads to overestimation of probability when there is memory of a case that was dramatic, involved a patient who fared poorly, or a lawsuit. For example, a clinician who recently missed the diagnosis of pulmonary embolism in a healthy young woman who had vague chest discomfort but no other findings or apparent risk factors might then overestimate the risk of pulmonary embolism in similar patients and become more likely to order chest CT angiography for similar patients despite the very small probability of disease. Experience can also lead to underestimation. For example, a junior resident who has seen only a few patients with chest pain, all of whom turned out to have benign causes, may begin to do cursory evaluations of that complaint even among populations in which disease prevalence is high.

Representation error occurs when clinicians judge the probability of disease based on how closely the patient's findings fit classic manifestations of a disease without taking into account disease prevalence. For example, although several hours of vague chest discomfort in a thin, athletic, healthy-appearing

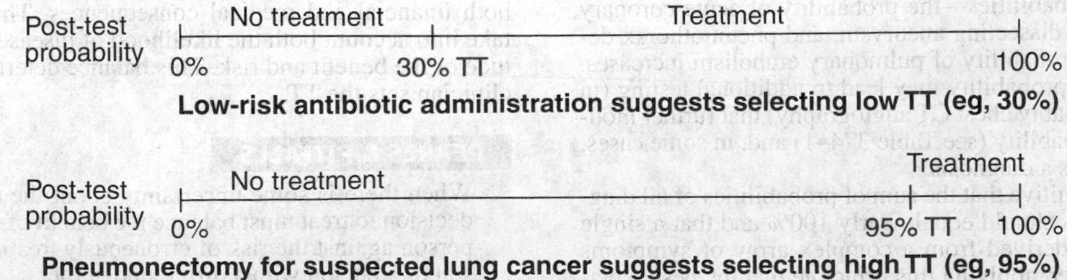

Fig. 374–1. Variation of treatment threshold (TT) with risk of treatment. Horizontal lines represent post-test probability.

60-yr-old man who has no known medical problems and who now looks and feels well does not match the typical profile of an MI, it would be unwise to dismiss that possibility because MI is common among men of that age and has highly variable manifestations. Conversely, a 20-yr-old healthy man with sudden onset of severe, sharp chest pain and back pain may be suspected of having a dissecting thoracic aortic aneurysm because those clinical features are common in aortic dissection. The cognitive error is not taking into account the fact that aortic dissections are exceptionally rare in a 20-yr-old, otherwise healthy patient; that disorder can be dismissed and other, more likely causes (eg, pneumothorax, pleuritis) should be considered. Representation error also occurs when clinicians fail to recognize that positive test results in a population where the tested disease is rare are more likely to be false positive than true positive.

Premature closure is one of the most common errors; clinicians make a quick diagnosis (often based on pattern recognition), fail to consider other possible diagnoses, and stop collecting data (jump to conclusions). The suspected diagnosis is often not even confirmed by appropriate testing. Premature closure errors may occur in any case but are particularly common when patients seem to be having an exacerbation of a known disorder—eg, if a woman with a long history of migraine presents with a severe headache (and actually has a new subarachnoid hemorrhage), the headache may be mistakenly assumed to be another attack of migraine. A variation of premature closure occurs when subsequent clinicians (eg, consultants on a complicated case) unquestioningly accept a previous working diagnosis without independently collecting and reviewing relevant data. Electronic medical records may exacerbate premature closure errors because incorrect diagnoses may be propagated until they are removed.

Anchoring errors occur when clinicians steadfastly cling to an initial impression even as conflicting and contradictory data accumulate. For example, a working diagnosis of acute pancreatitis is quite reasonable in a 60-yr-old man who has epigastric pain and nausea, who is sitting forward clutching his abdomen, and who has a history of several bouts of alcoholic pancreatitis that he states have felt similar to what he is currently feeling. However, if the patient states that he has had no alcohol in many years and has normal blood levels of pancreatic enzymes, clinicians who simply dismiss or excuse (eg, the patient is lying, his pancreas is burned out, the laboratory made a mistake) these conflicting data are committing an anchoring error. Clinicians should regard conflicting data as evidence of the need to continue to seek the true diagnosis (acute MI) rather than as anomalies to be disregarded. There may be no supporting evidence (ie, for the misdiagnosis) in some cases in which anchoring errors are committed.

Confirmation bias occurs when clinicians selectively accept clinical data that support a desired hypothesis and ignore data that do not (cherry-picking). Confirmation bias often compounds an anchoring error when the clinician uses confirmatory data to support the anchored hypothesis even when clearly contradictory evidence is also available. For example, a clinician may steadfastly cling to patient history elements suggesting ACS to confirm the original suspicion of ACS even when serial ECGs and cardiac enzymes are normal.

Attribution errors involve negative stereotypes that lead clinicians to ignore or minimize the possibility of serious disease. For example, clinicians might assume that an unconscious patient with an odor of alcohol is "just another drunk" and miss hypoglycemia or intracranial injury, or they might assume that a known drug abuser with back pain is simply seeking drugs and miss an epidural abscess caused by use of dirty needles. Psychiatric patients who develop a physical disorder are particularly likely to be subject to attribution errors because not only may they be subject to negative stereotyping but they often describe their symptoms in unclear, inconsistent, or confusing ways, leading unwary clinicians to assume their complaints are of mental origin.

Affective error involves avoiding unpleasant but necessary tests or examinations because of fondness or sympathy for the patient (eg, avoiding a pelvic examination on a modest patient or blood cultures on a seriously ill patient who has poor veins).

Minimizing cognitive errors: Some specific strategies can help minimize cognitive errors. Typically, after history and physical examination are done, clinicians often form a working diagnosis based on heuristics. At this point, it is relatively easy to insert a formal pause for reflection, asking several questions:

- If it is *not* the working diagnosis, what else could it be?
- What are the most dangerous things it could be?
- Is there any evidence that is at odds with the working diagnosis?

These questions can help expand the differential diagnosis to include things that may have been left out because of cognitive errors and thus trigger clinicians to obtain further necessary information.

UNDERSTANDING MEDICAL TESTS AND TEST RESULTS

Test results may help make a diagnosis in symptomatic patients (diagnostic testing) or identify occult disease in asymptomatic patients (screening). However, test results may interfere with clinical decision making if the test poorly discriminates between patients with and without disease, if the result is inconsistent with the clinical picture, or if the test result is improperly integrated into the clinical context.

Laboratory tests are imperfect and may mistakenly identify some healthy people as diseased (a false-positive result) or may mistakenly identify some affected people as disease-free (a false-negative result). A test's ability to correctly identify patients with disease depends on how likely a person is to have a disease (prior probability) and on the test's intrinsic operating characteristics.

Although diagnostic testing is often a critical contributor to clinical decision making, testing can have undesired or unintended consequences. Testing must be done with deliberation and purpose and with the expectation that the test result will reduce ambiguity surrounding patient problems and contribute to their health. In addition to the risk of providing incorrect information (thereby delaying initiation of treatment or inducing unnecessary treatment), laboratory tests consume limited resources and may themselves have adverse effects (eg, pneumothorax caused by lung biopsy) or may prompt additional unnecessary testing.

Defining a Positive Test Result

Among the most common tests are those that provide results along a continuous, quantitative scale (eg, blood glucose, WBC count). Such tests may provide useful clinical information throughout their ranges, but clinicians often use them to diagnose a condition by requiring that the result be classified as positive or negative (ie, disease present or absent) based on comparison to some established criterion or cutoff point. Such cutoff points are usually selected based on statistical and conceptual analysis that attempts to balance the rate of false-positive results (prompting unnecessary, expensive, and possibly dangerous tests or treatments) and false-negative results (failing to diagnose a treatable disease). Identifying a

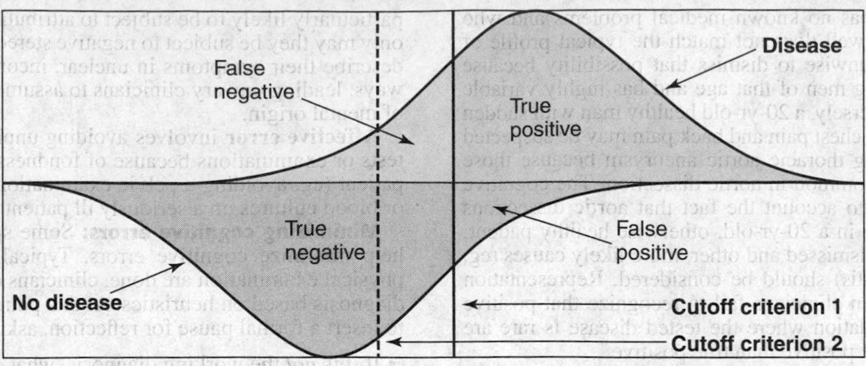

Fig. 374–2. Distributions of test results. Patients with disease are shown in the upper distribution; patients without disease are shown in the lower distribution. For patients with disease, the region beneath the distribution of results that lies to the right of (above) the cutoff criterion corresponds to the test's true-positive rate (ie, its sensitivity); the region that lies to the left of (below) the criterion corresponds to the false-negative rate. For patients without disease, the region to the right of the cut-off criterion corresponds to the false-positive rate, and the region to the left corresponds to the true-negative rate (ie, its specificity). For 2 overlapping distributions (eg, patients with and without disease), moving the cutoff criterion line affects sensitivity and specificity, but in opposite directions; changing the cutoff criterion from 1 to 2 decreases the number of false negatives (increases sensitivity) but also increases the number of false positives (decreases specificity).

cutoff point also depends on having a gold standard to identify the disease in question.

Typically, such quantitative test results (eg, WBC count in cases of suspected appendicitis) follow some type of distribution curve (not necessarily a normal curve, although commonly depicted as such). The distribution of test results for patients with disease is centered on a different point than that for patients without disease. Some patients with disease will have a very high or very low result, but most have a result centered on a mean. Conversely, some disease-free patients have a very high or very low result, but most have a result centered on a different mean from that for patients with disease. For most tests, the distributions overlap such that many of the possible test results occur in patients with and without disease; such results are more clearly illustrated when the curves are depicted on the same graph (see Fig. 374–2). Some patients above and below the selected cutoff point will be incorrectly characterized. Adjusting a cutoff point to identify more patients with disease (increase test sensitivity) also increases the number of false positives (poor specificity), and moving the cutoff point the other way to avoid falsely diagnosing patients as having disease increases the number of false negatives. Each cutoff point is associated with a specific probability of true-positive and false-positive results.

Receiver operating characteristic (ROC) curves: Graphing the fraction of true-positive results (number of true positives/number with disease) against the fraction of false-positive results (number of false positives/number without disease) for a series of cutoff points generates what is known as an ROC curve. The ROC curve graphically depicts the tradeoff between the sensitivity and specificity when the cutoff point is adjusted (see Fig. 374–3). By convention, the true-positive fraction is

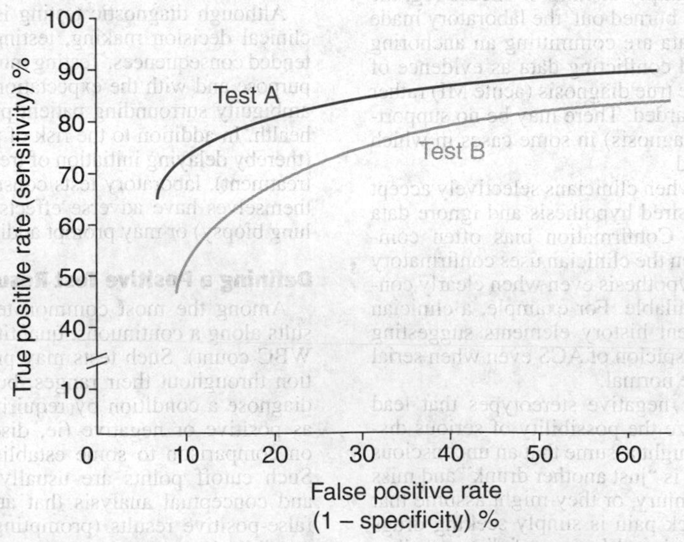

Fig. 374–3. Typical receiver operating characteristic (ROC) curve.

placed on the y-axis, and the false-positive fraction is placed on the x-axis. The greater the area under the ROC curve, the better the test discriminates between patients with or without disease.

ROC curves allow tests to be compared over a variety of cutoff points. In the example, Test A performs better than Test B over all ranges. ROC curves also assist in the selection of the cutoff point designed to maximize a test's utility. If a test is designed to confirm a disease, a cutoff point with greater specificity and lower sensitivity is selected. If a test is designed to screen for occult disease, a cutoff point with greater sensitivity and lower specificity is selected.

Test Characteristics

Some clinical variables have only 2 possible results (eg, alive/dead, pregnant/not pregnant); such variables are termed categorical and dichotomous. Other categorical results may have many discrete values (eg, blood type, Glasgow Coma Scale) and are termed nominal or ordinal. Nominal variables such as blood type have no particular order. Ordinal variables such as the Glasgow Coma Scale have discrete values that are arranged in a particular order. Other clinical variables, including many typical diagnostic tests, are continuous and have an infinite number of possible results (eg, WBC count, blood glucose level). Many clinicians select a cutoff point that can cause a continuous variable to be treated as a dichotomous variable (eg, patients with a fasting blood glucose level > 126 mg/dL are considered to have diabetes). Other continuous diagnostic tests have diagnostic utility when they have multiple cutoff points or when ranges of results have different diagnostic value.

When test results can be defined as positive or negative, all possible outcomes can be recorded in a simple 2×2 table (see Table 374–2) from which important discriminatory test characteristics, including sensitivity, specificity, positive and negative predictive value, and likelihood ratio (LR), can be calculated (see Table 374–3).

Sensitivity, specificity, and predictive values: Sensitivity, specificity, and predictive values are typically considered characteristics of the test itself, independent of the patient population.

Sensitivity is the likelihood of a positive test result in patients with disease (true-positive rate); a test that is positive in 8 of 10 patients with a disease has a sensitivity of 0.8 (also expressed as 80%). Sensitivity represents how well a test detects the disease; a test with low sensitivity does not identify many patients with disease, and a test with high sensitivity is useful to exclude a diagnosis when results are negative. Sensitivity is

Table 374–2. DISTRIBUTION OF HYPOTHETICAL TEST RESULTS

RESULTS	DISEASE PRESENT	DISEASE ABSENT
Test positive	True positive	False positive
Test negative	False negative	True negative
Total patients	All patients with disease	All patients without disease

the complement of the false-negative rate (ie, the false-negative rate plus the sensitivity = 100%).

Specificity is the likelihood of a negative test result in patients without disease (true-negative rate); a test that is negative in 9 of 10 patients without disease has a specificity of 0.9 (or 90%). Specificity represents how well a test correctly identifies patients with disease because tests with high specificity have a low false-positive rate. A test with low specificity diagnoses many patients without disease as having disease. It is the complement of the false-positive rate.

Positive predictive value (PPV) is the proportion of patients with a positive test that actually have disease; if 9 of 10 positive test results are correct (true positive), the PPV is 90%. Because all positive test results have some number of true positives and some false positives, the PPV describes how likely it is that a positive test result in a given patient population represents a true positive.

Negative predictive value (NPV) is the proportion of patients with a negative test result that are actually disease free; if 8 of 10 negative test results are correct (true negative), the NPV is 80%. Because not all negative test results are true negatives, some patients with a negative test result actually have disease. The NPV describes how likely it is that a negative test result in a given patient population represents a true negative.

Likelihood ratios (LRs): Unlike sensitivity and specificity, which do not apply to specific patient probabilities, the LR allows clinicians to interpret test results in a specific patient provided there is a known (albeit often estimated) pre-test probability of disease.

The LR describes the change in pre-test probability of disease when the test result is known and answers the question, "How much has the post-test probability changed now that the test result is known?" Many clinical tests are dichotomous; they are either above the cutoff point (positive) or below the cutoff point (negative) and there are only 2 possible results.

Table 374–3. DISTRIBUTION OF TEST RESULTS OF A HYPOTHETICAL LEUKOCYTE ESTERASE TEST IN A COHORT OF 1000 WOMEN WITH AN ASSUMED 30% PREVALENCE OF UTI

RESULTS	DISEASE PRESENT	DISEASE ABSENT	TOTAL PATIENTS
Test positive	True positive (TP) 213 patients (71% of 300)	False positive (FP) 105 patients (700–595)	318 patients with a positive test
Test negative	False negative (FN) 87 patients (300–213)	True negative (TN) 595 patients (85% of 700)	682 patients with a negative test
Total patients	300 patients with UTI (assumed)	700 patients without UTI (assumed)	1000 patients

Positive predictive value (PPV) = TP/(all patients with a positive test) = TP/(TP + FP) = 213/(213 + 105) = 67%.
Negative predictive value (NPV) = TN/(all patients with a negative test) = TN/(TN + FN) = 595/(595 + 87) = 87%.
Positive likelihood ratio (LR+) = sensitivity/(1 − specificity) = 0.71/(1 − 0.85) = 4.73.
Negative likelihood ratio (LR−) = (1 − sensitivity)/specificity = (1 − 0.71)/0.85 = 0.34.

Other tests give results that are continuous or occur over a range where multiple cutoff points are selected. The actual post-test probability depends on the magnitude of the LR (which depends on test operating characteristics) and the pre-test probability estimation of disease. When the test being done is dichotomous and the result is either positive or negative, the sensitivity and specificity can be used to calculate positive LR (LR+) or negative LR (LR–).

- **LR+:** The ratio of the likelihood of a positive test result occurring in patients with disease (true positive) to the likelihood of a positive test result in patients without disease (false positive)
- **LR–:** The ratio of the likelihood of a negative test result in patients with disease (false negative) to the likelihood of a negative test result in patients without disease (true negative)

When the result is continuous or has multiple cutoff points, the ROC curve, not sensitivity and specificity, is used to calculate an LR that is no longer described as LR+ or LR–.

Because the LR is a ratio of mutually exclusive events rather than a proportion of a total, it represents odds rather than probability. For a given test, the LR is different for positive and negative results.

For example, given a positive test result, an LR of 2.0 indicates the odds are 2:1 (true positives:false positives) that a positive test result represents a patient with disease. Of 3 positive tests, 2 would occur in patients with disease (true positive) and 1 would occur in a patient without disease (false positive). Because true positives and false positives are components of sensitivity and specificity calculations, the LR+ can also be calculated as sensitivity/(1 – specificity). The greater the LR+, the more information a positive test result provides; a positive result on a test with an LR+ > 10 is considered strong evidence in favor of a diagnosis. In other words, the pre-test probability estimation moves strongly toward 100% when a positive test has a high LR+.

For a negative test result, an LR– of 0.25 indicates that the odds are 1:4 (false negatives:true negatives) that a negative test result represents a patient with disease. Of 5 negative test results, 1 would occur in a patient with disease (false negative) and 4 would occur in patients without disease (true negative). The LR– can also be calculated as (1 – sensitivity)/specificity. The smaller the LR–, the more information a negative test result provides; a negative result on a test with an LR < 0.1 is considered strong evidence against a diagnosis. In other words, the pre-test probability estimation moves strongly toward 0% probability when a negative test has a low LR–.

Test results with LRs of 1.0 carry no information and do not affect the post-test probability of disease.

LRs are convenient for comparing tests and are also used in Bayesian analysis to interpret test results. Just as sensitivity and specificity change as cutoff points change, so do LRs. As a hypothetical example, a high cutoff for WBC count (eg, 20,000/μL) in a possible case of acute appendicitis is more specific and would have a high LR+ but also a high (and thus not very informative) LR–; choosing a much lower and very sensitive cutoff (eg, 10,000/μL) would have a low LR– but also a low LR+.

Dichotomous Tests

An ideal dichotomous test would have no false positives or false negatives; all patients with a positive test result would have disease (100% PPV), and all patients with a negative test result would not have disease (100% NPV).

In reality, all tests have false positives and false negatives, some tests more than others. To illustrate the consequences of imperfect sensitivity and specificity on test results, consider hypothetical results (see Table 374–3) of urine dipstick leukocyte esterase testing in a group of 1000 women, 300 (30%) of whom have a UTI (as determined by a gold-standard test such as urine culture). This scenario assumes for illustrative purposes that the dipstick test has sensitivity of 71% and specificity of 85%.

Sensitivity of 71% means that only 213 (71% of 300) women *with* UTI would have a positive test result. The remaining 87 would have a negative test result. Specificity of 85% means that 595 (85% of 700) women *without* UTI would have a negative test result. The remaining 105 would have a positive test result. Thus, of 318 positive test results, only 213 would be correct (213/318 = 67% PPV); a positive test result makes the diagnosis of UTI more likely than not but not certain. There would also be 682 negative tests, of which 595 are correct (595/682 = 87% NPV), making the diagnosis of UTI much less likely but still possible; 13% of patients with a negative test result would actually have a UTI.

However, the PPVs and NPVs derived in this patient cohort cannot be used to interpret results of the same test when the underlying incidence of disease (pre-test or prior probability) is different. Note the effects of changing disease incidence to 5% (see Table 374–4). Now most positive test results are false, and the PPV is only 20%; a patient with a positive test result is actually more likely to *not* have a UTI. However, the NPV is now very high (98%); a negative result essentially rules out UTI.

Note that in both patient cohorts, even though the PPV and NPV are very different, the LRs do not change because the LRs are determined only by test sensitivity and specificity.

Table 374–4. DISTRIBUTION OF TEST RESULTS OF A HYPOTHETICAL LEUKOCYTE ESTERASE TEST IN A COHORT OF 1000 WOMEN WITH AN ASSUMED 5% PREVALENCE OF UTI

RESULTS	DISEASE PRESENT	DISEASE ABSENT	TOTAL PATIENTS
Test positive	True positive (TP) 36 patients (71% of 50)	False positive (FP) 144 patients (950 – 806)	180 patients with a positive test
Test negative	False negative (FN) 14 patients (50 – 36)	True negative (TN) 806 patients (85% of 950)	820 patients with a negative test
Total patients	50 patients with UTI (assumed)	950 patients without UTI (assumed)	1000 patients

Positive predictive value (PPV) = TP/(all with a positive test) = TP/(TP + FP) = 36/(36 + 144) = 20%.
Negative predictive value (NPV) = TN/(all with a negative test) = TN/(TN + FN) = 806/(806 + 14) = 98%.
Positive likelihood ratio (LR+) = sensitivity/(1 – specificity) = 0.71/(1 – 0.85) = 4.73.
Negative likelihood ratio (LR–) = (1 – sensitivity)/specificity = (1 – 0.71)/0.85 = 0.34.

Clearly, a test result does not provide a definitive diagnosis but only estimates the probability of a disease being present or absent, and this post-test probability (likelihood of disease given a specific test result) varies greatly based on the pre-test probability of disease as well as the test's sensitivity and specificity (and thus its LR).

Pre-test probability is not a precise measurement; it is based on clinical judgment of how strongly the symptoms and signs suggest the disease is present, what factors in the patient's history support the diagnosis, and how common the disease is in a representative population. Many clinical scoring systems are designed to estimate pre-test probability; adding points for various clinical features facilitates the calculation of a score. These examples illustrate the importance of accurate pre-test prevalence estimation because the prevalence of disease in the considered population dramatically influences the test's utility. Validated, published prevalence-estimating tools should be used when they are available. For example, there are criteria for predicting pre-test probability of pulmonary embolism (see p. 492). Higher calculated scores yield higher estimated probabilities.

Continuous Tests

Many test results are continuous and may provide useful clinical information over a wide range of results. Clinicians often select a certain cutoff point to maximize the test's utility. For example, a WBC count > 15,000 may be characterized as positive; values < 15,000 as negative. When a test yields continuous results but a certain cutoff point is selected, the test operates like a dichotomous test. Multiple cutoff points can also be selected. Sensitivity, specificity, PPV, NPV, LR+, and LR− can be calculated for single or multiple cutoff points. Table 374–5 illustrates the effect of changing the cutoff point of the WBC count in patients suspected of having appendicitis.

Alternatively, it can be useful to group continuous test results into levels. In this case, results are not characterized as positive or negative because there are multiple possible results, so although an LR can be determined for each level of results, there is no longer a distinct LR+ or LR−. For example, Table 374–6 illustrates the relationship between WBC count and bacteremia in febrile children. Because the LR is the probability of a given result in patients with disease divided by the probability of that result in patients without the disease, the LR for each grouping of WBC count is the probability of bacteremia in that group divided by the probability of no bacteremia.

Grouping continuous variables allows for much greater use of the test result than when a single cutoff point is established. Using Bayesian analyses, the LRs in Table 374–6 can be used to calculate the post-test probability.

For continuous test results, if an ROC curve is known, calculations as shown in Table 374–6 do not have to be done; LRs can be found for various points over the range of results using the slope of the ROC curve at the desired point.

Bayes Theorem

The process of using the pre-test probability of disease and the test characteristics to calculate the post-test probability is referred to as Bayes theorem or Bayesian revision. For routine clinical use, Bayesian methodology typically takes several forms:

- Odds-likelihood formulation (calculation or nomogram)
- Tabular approach

Odds-likelihood calculation: If the pre-test probability of disease is expressed as its odds and because a test's LR represents odds, the product of the 2 represents the post-test odds of disease (analogous to multiplying 2 probabilities together to calculate the probability of simultaneous occurrence of 2 events):

$$\text{Pre-test odds} \times \text{LR} = \text{post-test odds}$$

Because clinicians typically think in terms of probabilities rather than odds, probability can be converted to odds (and vice versa) with these formulas:

$$\text{Odds} = \text{probability}/1 - \text{probability}$$

$$\text{Probability} = \text{odds}/\text{odds} + 1$$

Consider the example of UTI as given in Table 374–3, in which the pre-test probability of UTI is 0.3, and the test being used has an LR+ of 4.73 and an LR− of 0.34. A pre-test probability of 0.3 corresponds to odds of $0.3/(1 - 0.3) = 0.43$. Thus, the post-test odds that a UTI is present in a patient with a positive test result equals the product of the pre-test odds and the LR+; $4.73 \times 0.43 = 2.03$, which represents a post-test probability of $2.03/(1 + 2.03) = 0.67$. Thus, Bayesian calculations show that a positive test result increases the pre-test probability from 30% to 67%, the same result obtained in the PPV calculation in Table 374–3.

A similar calculation is done for a negative test; post-test odds $= 0.34 \times 0.43 = 0.15$, corresponding to a probability of $0.15/(1 + 0.15) = 0.13$. Thus, a negative test result decreases the pre-test probability from 30% to 13%, again the same result obtained in the NPV calculation in Table 374–3.

Many medical calculator programs that run on handheld devices are available to calculate post-test probability from pre-test probability and LRs.

Table 374–5. EFFECT OF CHANGING THE CUTOFF POINT OF THE WBC COUNT IN PATIENTS SUSPECTED OF HAVING APPENDICITIS

WBC CUTOFF*	SENSITIVITY	SPECIFICITY	LR+	LR–
> 10,500	84%	53.13%	1.79	0.3
> 11,500	78%	62.5%	2.13	0.32
> 12,850	68%	75%	2.72	0.43
> 13,400	61.33%	78.12%	2.86	0.45
> 14,300	56.67%	81.25%	3.2	0.49

*Various cutoff points are selected for a continuous variable such as WBC count; results above the cutoff point are considered positive and those below the cutoff point are considered negative.

LR = likelihood ratio.

Adapted from Keskek M, Tez M, Yoldas O, et al: Receiver operating characteristic analysis of leukocyte counts in operations for suspected appendicitis. *American Journal of Emergency Medicine* 26:769–772, 2008.

Table 374–6. USING WBC COUNT GROUPS TO DETERMINE LIKELIHOOD RATIO OF BACTEREMIA IN FEBRILE CHILDREN*

WBC COUNT	NUMBER OF CHILDREN WITH BACTEREMIA, N = 127 (%)	NUMBER OF CHILDREN WITHOUT BACTEREMIA, N = 8629 (%)	LR (% WITH BACTEREMIA/ % WITHOUT BACTEREMIA)
0–5000	0 (0.0%)	543 (6.3%)	0.00
5,001–10,000	3 (2.4%)	3291 (38.1%)	0.06
10,001–15,000	15 (11.8%)	2767 (32.1%)	0.37
15,001–20,000	48 (37.8%)	1337 (15.5%)	2.4
20,001–25,000	34 (26.8%)	469 (5.4%)	4.9
25,001–30,000	12 (9.4%)	155 (1.8%)	5.3
> 30,001	15 (11.8%)	67 (0.8%)	15.2

*Incidence of bacteremia in 8756 febrile children grouped by WBC count. LR for each group is calculated by dividing the probability of bacteremia by the probability of no bacteremia.

LR = likelihood ratio.

Adapted from Lee GM, Harper MB: Risk of bacteremia for febrile young children in the post-*Haemophilus influenzae* type b era. *Archives of Pediatric and Adolescent Medicine* 152:624–628, 1998.

Odds-likelihood nomogram: Using a nomogram is particularly convenient because it avoids the need to convert between odds and probabilities or create 2 × 2 tables.

The Fagan nomogram is depicted in Fig. 374–4. To use the nomogram, a line is drawn from the pre-test probability through the LR. The post-test probability is the point at which this line intersects the post-test probability line. Sample lines in the figure are drawn using data from the UTI test in Table 374–3. Line A represents a positive test result; it is drawn from pre-test probability of 0.3 through the LR+ of 4.73 and gives a post-test value of slightly < 0.7, similar to the calculated probability of 0.67. Line B represents a negative test result; it is drawn from pre-test probability of 0.3 through the LR– value of 0.34 and gives a post-test value slightly > 0.1, similar to the calculated probability of 13%.

Although the nomogram appears less precise than calculations, typical values for pre-test probability are often estimates, so the apparent precision of calculations is usually misleading.

Tabular approach: Often, LRs of a test are not known, but sensitivity and specificity are known, and pre-test probability can be estimated. In this case, Bayesian methodology can be done using a 2 × 2 table illustrated in Table 374–7 using the example from Table 374–3. Note that this method shows that a positive test result increases the probability of a UTI to 67%, and a negative result decreases it to 13%, the same results obtained by calculation using LRs.

Sequential Testing

Clinicians often do tests in sequence during many diagnostic evaluations. If the pre-test odds before sequential testing are known and the LR for each of the tests in sequence is known, post-test odds can be calculated using the following formula:

Pre-test odds × LR1 × LR2 × LR3 = post-test odds

This method is limited by the important assumption that each of the tests is conditionally independent of each other.

Screening Tests

Patients often must consider whether to be screened for occult disease. The premises of a screening program are that early detection improves outcome in patients with occult disease and that the false-positive results that often occur in screening do not create a burden (eg, costs and adverse effects of confirmatory testing, unwarranted treatment) that exceeds such benefit. To minimize these possible burdens, clinicians must choose the proper screening test. Screening is not appropriate when treatments are ineffective or the disease is very uncommon (unless a subpopulation can be identified in which prevalence is higher).

Theoretically, the best test for both screening and diagnosis is the one with the highest sensitivity *and* specificity. However, such highly accurate tests are often complex, expensive, and invasive (eg, coronary angiography) and are thus not practical for screening large numbers of asymptomatic people. Typically, some tradeoff in sensitivity, specificity, or both must be made when selecting a screening test.

Whether a clinician chooses a test that optimizes sensitivity or specificity depends on the consequences of a false-positive or false-negative test result as well as the pre-test probability of disease. An ideal screening test is one that is always positive in nearly every patient with disease so that a negative result confidently excludes disease in healthy patients. For example, in testing for a serious disease for which an effective treatment is available (eg, coronary artery disease), clinicians would be willing to tolerate more false positives than false negatives (lower specificity and high sensitivity). Although high sensitivity is a very important attribute for screening tests, specificity also is important in certain screening strategies. Among populations with a higher prevalence of disease, the PPV of a screening test increases; as prevalence decreases, the post-test or posterior probability of a positive result decreases. Therefore, when screening for disease in high-risk populations, tests with a higher sensitivity are preferred over those with a higher specificity because they are better at ruling out disease (fewer false negatives). On the other hand, in low-risk populations or for uncommon diseases for which therapy has lower benefit or higher risk, tests with a higher specificity are preferred.

Multiple screening tests: With the expanding array of available screening tests, clinicians must consider the implications of a panel of such tests. For example, test panels containing 8, 12, or sometimes 20 blood tests are often done when a patient is admitted to the hospital or is first examined by a new clinician. Although this type of testing may be helpful in screening patients for certain diseases, using the large panel of tests has potentially negative consequences. By definition,

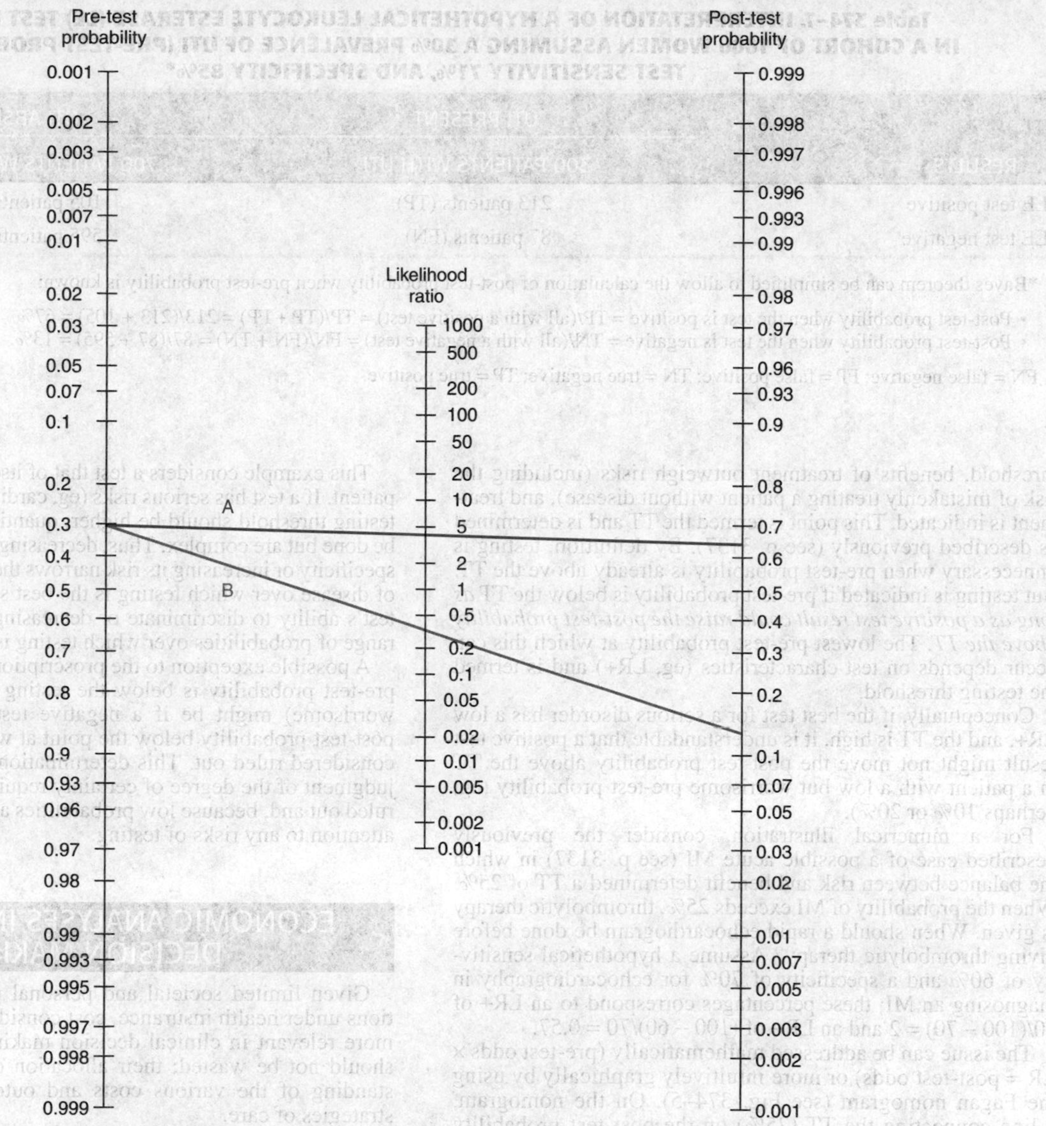

Fig. 374–4. Fagan nomogram. Illustrative lines are drawn using data from the UTI test in Table 374–3. Line A represents a positive test result, drawn from a pre-test probability of 0.3 through an LR+ of 4.73 to a post-test value of slightly < 0.7, similar to the calculated probability of 0.67. Line B represents a negative test result drawn from pre-test probability of 0.3 through an LR– of 0.34 to a post-test value slightly > 0.1, similar to the calculated probability of 13%.LR+ = likelihood ratio for a positive result; LR– = LR for a negative result.Adapted from Fagan TJ. Letter: Nomogram for Bayes theorem. *New England Journal of Medicine* 293:257, 1975.

a test with a specificity of 95% gives false-positive results in 5% of healthy, normal patients. If 2 different tests with such characteristics are done, each for a different occult disease, in a patient who actually does not have either disease, the chance that both tests will be negative is 95% × 95%, or about 90%; thus, there is a 10% chance of at least one false-positive result. For 3 such tests, the chance that all 3 would be negative is 95% × 95% × 95%, or 86%, corresponding to a 14% chance of at least one false-positive result. If 12 different tests for 12 different diseases are done, the chance of obtaining at least one false-positive result is 46%. This high probability underscores the need for caution when deciding to do a screening test panel and when interpreting its results.

Testing Thresholds

A laboratory test should be done only if its results will affect management; otherwise the expense and risk to the patient are for naught. Clinicians can sometimes make the determination of when to test by comparing pre-test and post-test probability estimations with certain thresholds. Above a certain probability

Table 374–7. INTERPRETATION OF A HYPOTHETICAL LEUKOCYTE ESTERASE (LE) TEST RESULT IN A COHORT OF 1000 WOMEN ASSUMING A 30% PREVALENCE OF UTI (PRE-TEST PROBABILITY), TEST SENSITIVITY 71%, AND SPECIFICITY 85%*

	UTI PRESENT	UTI ABSENT
RESULTS	300 PATIENTS WITH UTI	700 PATIENTS WITHOUT UTI
LE test positive	213 patients (TP)	105 patients (FP)
LE test negative	87 patients (FN)	595 patients (TN)

*Bayes theorem can be simplified to allow the calculation of post-test probability when pre-test probability is known:

- Post-test probability when the test is positive = TP/(all with a positive test) = TP/(TP + FP) = 213/(213 + 105) = 67%.
- Post-test probability when the test is negative = TN/(all with a negative test) = FN/(FN + TN) = 87/(87 + 595) = 13%.

FN = false negative; FP = false positive; TN = true negative; TP = true positive.

threshold, benefits of treatment outweigh risks (including the risk of mistakenly treating a patient without disease), and treatment is indicated. This point is termed the TT and is determined as described previously (see p. 3137). By definition, testing is unnecessary when pre-test probability is already above the TT. But testing is indicated if pre-test probability is below the TT *as long as a positive test result could raise the post-test probability above the TT*. The lowest pre-test probability at which this can occur depends on test characteristics (eg, LR+) and is termed the testing threshold.

Conceptually, if the best test for a serious disorder has a low LR+, and the TT is high, it is understandable that a positive test result might not move the post-test probability above the TT in a patient with a low but worrisome pre-test probability (eg, perhaps 10% or 20%).

For a numerical illustration, consider the previously described case of a possible acute MI (see p. 3137) in which the balance between risk and benefit determined a TT of 25%. When the probability of MI exceeds 25%, thrombolytic therapy is given. When should a rapid echocardiogram be done before giving thrombolytic therapy? Assume a hypothetical sensitivity of 60% and a specificity of 70% for echocardiography in diagnosing an MI; these percentages correspond to an LR+ of 60/(100 – 70) = 2 and an LR– of (100 – 60)/70 = 0.57.

The issue can be addressed mathematically (pre-test odds × LR = post-test odds) or more intuitively graphically by using the Fagan nomogram (see Fig. 374–5). On the nomogram, a line connecting the TT (25%) on the post-test probability line through the LR+ (2.0) on the middle LR line intersects a pre-test probability of about 0.14. Clearly, a positive test in a patient with any pre-test probability < 14% would still result in a post-test probability less than the TT. In this case, echocardiography would be useless because even a positive result would not lead to a decision to treat; thus, 14% pre-test probability is the testing threshold *for this particular test* (see Fig. 374–6). Another test with a different LR+ would have a different testing threshold.

Because 14% still represents a significant risk of MI, it is clear that a disease probability below the testing threshold (eg, a 10% pre-test probability) does not necessarily mean disease is ruled out, just that a positive test result on the particular test in question would not change management and thus *that* test is not indicated. In this situation, the clinician would observe the patient for further findings that might elevate the pre-test probability above the testing threshold. In practice, because multiple tests are often available for a given disease, sequential testing might be used.

This example considers a test that of itself poses no risk to the patient. If a test has serious risks (eg, cardiac catheterization), the testing threshold should be higher; quantitative calculations can be done but are complex. Thus, decreasing a test's sensitivity and specificity or increasing its risk narrows the range of probabilities of disease over which testing is the best strategy. Improving the test's ability to discriminate or decreasing its risk broadens the range of probabilities over which testing is the best strategy.

A possible exception to the proscription against testing when pre-test probability is below the testing threshold (but is still worrisome) might be if a negative test result could *reduce* post-test probability below the point at which disease could be considered ruled out. This determination requires a subjective judgment of the degree of certainty required to say a disease is ruled out and, because low probabilities are involved, particular attention to any risks of testing.

ECONOMIC ANALYSES IN CLINICAL DECISION MAKING

Given limited societal and personal resources and restrictions under health insurance, cost considerations have become more relevant in clinical decision making. Limited resources should not be wasted; their allocation depends on an understanding of the various costs and outcomes resulting from strategies of care.

Cost

The elements included in cost analysis are determined by the perspective of the analysis. Different perspectives often result in different conclusions based on which costs and outcomes are considered.

- **Providers** (eg, health care practitioners, institutions) typically consider only costs within the organization (eg, personnel, supplies, overhead).
- **Payors** (eg, insurance companies) consider only the reimbursements they have to make.
- **Patients** consider out-of-pocket expenses (eg, cost of insurance, deductibles, transportation, parking) and lost income (for themselves and their family).

From a societal perspective, all such costs are taken into account along with the costs of lost productivity and costs of treating other diseases (iatrogenic and naturally occurring) that may develop in patients who recover from the disease

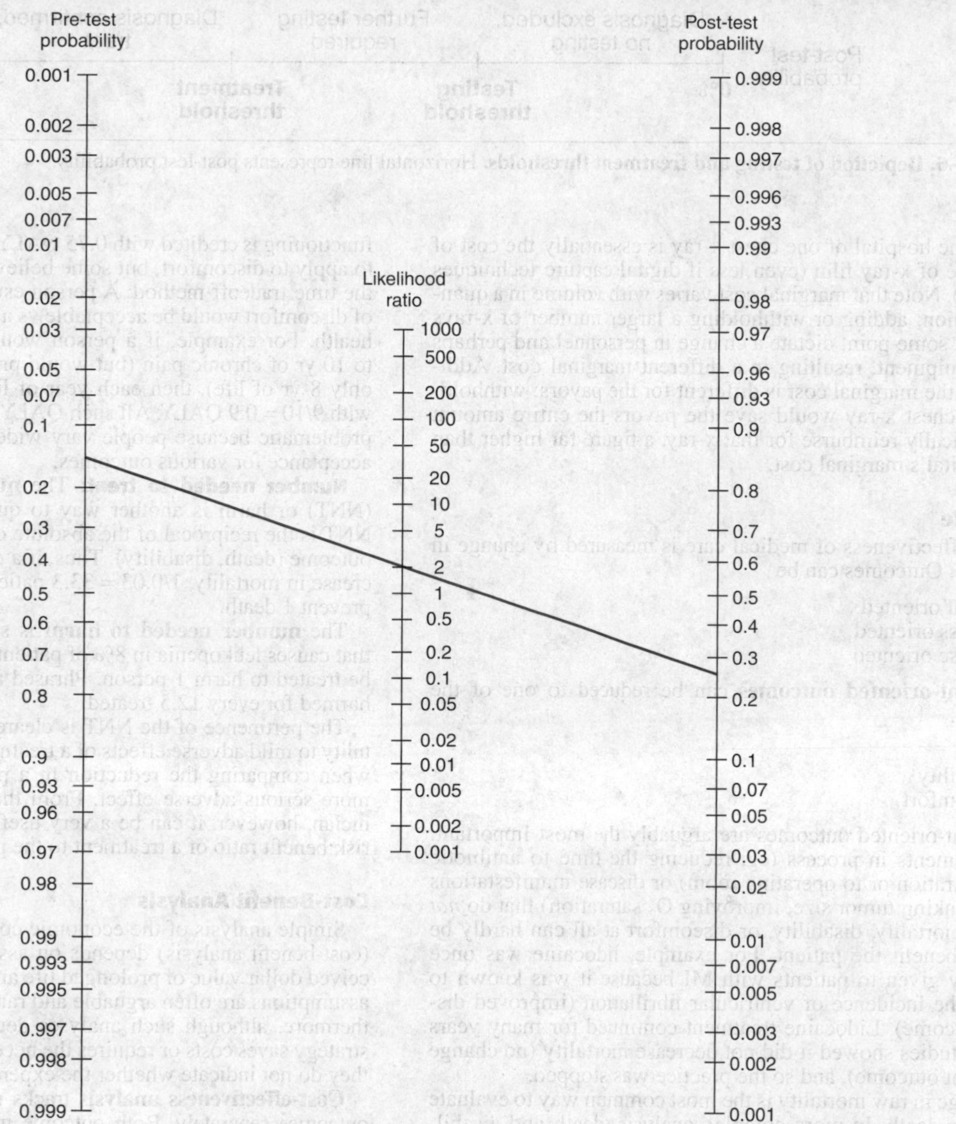

Fig. 374–5. Fagan nomogram used to determine need to test. In this example, a patient is assumed to have a TT of 25% for acute MI. When the probability of MI exceeds 25%, thrombolytic therapy is given. Clinicians can use the Fagan nomogram to determine when rapid echocardiography should be done before giving thrombolytic therapy. Assuming that echocardiography has a hypothetical sensitivity of 60% and a specificity of 70% for a new MI, these percentages correspond to a likelihood ratio (LR) of a positive test result (LR+) of 60/(100 – 70) = 2. A line connecting a 25% TT on the post-test probability line with LR+ (2.0) on the middle LR line intersects a pre-test probability of about 0.14. A positive test result in a patient with a pre-test probability of < 14% still results in a post-test probability of less than the TT.Adapted from Fagan TJ. Letter: Nomogram for Bayes theorem. *New England Journal of Medicine* 293:257, 1975.

being treated. For example, a young man cured of lymphoma may develop leukemia or coronary artery disease years later. Cost analysis of a screening program needs to include the costs of pursuing false-positive results, which in a screening test for a disease with a low prevalence often exceed the costs of evaluating and treating patients who actually have the disease.

Marginal cost: The marginal cost is the cost of providing (or withholding) an additional unit of service. This cost is often one of the most relevant for an individual clinician's medical decision making and is typically quite different from the overall cost allocated to that service. For example, a hospital may have determined that $50 is the cost of providing a chest x-ray. However, a clinical protocol to better identify patients requiring x-rays that resulted in one fewer chest x-ray a day (with no change in outcome) would not "save" the hospital $50 because personnel and overhead expenses would be unchanged; only the expense of x-ray film would be eliminated. Hence the marginal

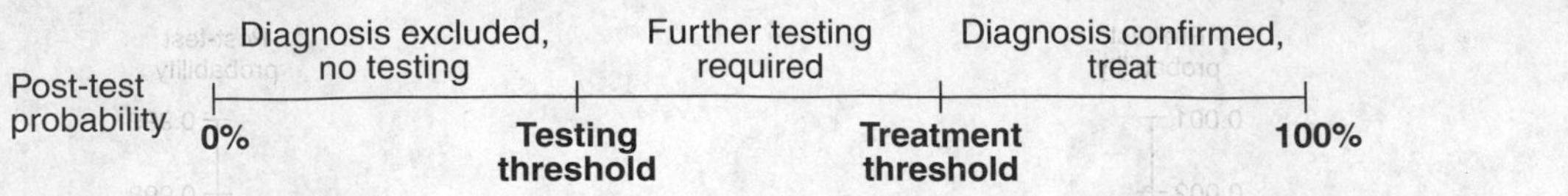

Fig. 374–6. Depiction of testing and treatment thresholds. Horizontal line represents post-test probability.

cost to the hospital of one chest x-ray is essentially the cost of one piece of x-ray film (even less if digital capture techniques are used). Note that marginal cost varies with volume in a quantum fashion; adding or withholding a larger number of x-rays would at some point dictate a change in personnel and perhaps x-ray equipment, resulting in a different marginal cost. Additionally, the marginal cost is different for the payors; withholding one chest x-ray would save the payors the entire amount they typically reimburse for that x-ray, a figure far higher than the hospital's marginal cost.

Outcome

The effectiveness of medical care is measured by change in outcome. Outcomes can be

- Patient oriented
- Process oriented
- Disease oriented

Patient-oriented outcomes can be reduced to one of the three Ds:

- Death
- Disability
- Discomfort

Patient-oriented outcomes are arguably the most important. Improvements in process (eg, reducing the time to antibiotic administration or to operating room) or disease manifestations (eg, shrinking tumor size, improving O_2 saturation) that do *not* reduce mortality, disability, or discomfort at all can hardly be said to benefit the patient. For example, lidocaine was once routinely given to patients with MI because it was known to reduce the incidence of ventricular fibrillation (improved disease outcome). Lidocaine treatment continued for many years before studies showed it did not decrease mortality (no change in patient outcome), and so the practice was stopped.

Change in raw mortality is the most common way to evaluate effect on death. In more complex analysis, death and disability are often evaluated in combination as the quality-adjusted life year (QALY); treatment that results in an additional year of life at 100% of normal functioning is credited with 1 QALY; treatment that results in an additional year of life at only 75% functioning is credited with 0.75 QALY. QALY is more difficult to apply to discomfort, but some believe it can be estimated by the time tradeoff method: A person estimates how many years of discomfort would be acceptable vs a shorter period of perfect health. For example, if a person would prefer 9 yr of health to 10 yr of chronic pain (but would prefer the 10 yr of pain to only 8 yr of life), then each year of life with pain is credited with 9/10 = 0.9 QALY. All such QALY estimates are somewhat problematic because people vary widely in risk tolerance and acceptance for various outcomes.

Number needed to treat: The **number needed to treat** (NNT) or harm is another way to quantify patient outcome; NNT is the reciprocal of the absolute change in a dichotomous outcome (death, disability). Thus, if a drug causes a 3% net decrease in mortality, 1/0.03 = 33.3 patients need to be treated to prevent 1 death.

The **number needed to harm** is similar. Thus, for a drug that causes leukopenia in 8% of patients, 1/0.08 or 12.5 need to be treated to harm 1 person. Phrased another way, 1 person is harmed for every 12.5 treated.

The pertinence of the NNT is clearer when comparing mortality to mild adverse effects of a treatment. It becomes cloudier when comparing the reduction in a particular morbidity to a more serious adverse effect. From the perspective of the clinician, however, it can be a very useful tool in explaining the risk:benefit ratio of a treatment to the patient.

Cost-Benefit Analysis

Simple analysis of the economic consequences of outcomes (cost-benefit analysis) depends on assumptions about the perceived dollar value of prolonged life and improved health. Such assumptions are often arguable and rarely straightforward. Furthermore, although such analyses determine whether a given strategy saves costs or requires the net expenditure of resources, they do not indicate whether the expenditures are worthwhile.

Cost-effectiveness analysis tracks medical costs and health outcomes separately. Both outcome measures can be strongly affected by the perspective and duration of the analysis and by the underlying assumptions. Comparison of the costs and health outcomes of 2 management strategies results in 1 of 9 pairings (see Table 374–8). When health outcomes are equivalent (center

Table 374–8. COST-EFFECTIVENESS COMPARISON OF MANAGEMENT STRATEGIES A AND B

	HEALTH OUTCOME		
COST	A > B	A = B	A < B
A > B	Calculate marginal cost-effectiveness ratio*.	B is less expensive: Choose B.	B dominates A: Choose B.
A = B	A has a better outcome: Choose A.	It makes no difference.	B has a better outcome: Choose B.
A < B	A dominates B: Choose A.	A is less expensive: Choose A.	Calculate marginal cost-effectiveness ratio*.

*See Table 374–9.

Table 374–9. CALCULATING A MARGINAL COST-EFFECTIVENESS RATIO

STRATEGY	COST* ($)	EFFECTIVENESS (QALY)	MARGINAL COST ($)	MARGINAL EFFECTIVENESS (QALY)	MARGINAL COST- EFFECTIVENESS RATIO ($/QALY)
Analysis 1 (2 strategies)					
No antiarrhythmic therapy	78,300	7.42	—	—	—
ICD	131,400	7.87	53,100	0.45	118,000
Analysis 2 (3 strategies)					
No antiarrhythmic therapy	78,300	7.42	—	—	—
Amiodarone	96,800	7.69	18,500	0.27	68,519
ICD	131,400	7.87	34,600	0.18	192,222

*For illustrative purposes only.
ICD = implantable cardioverter defibrillator; QALY = quality-adjusted life year.

column), the choice should be based on cost; when costs are equivalent (center row), the choice should be based on outcome. When one strategy has better outcomes *and* lower costs (upper right and lower left cells), the choice is clear. The decision is difficult only when the strategy that is more expensive also produces better outcomes (upper left and lower right cells); in such cases, the marginal cost-effectiveness ratio should be determined.

Marginal cost-effectiveness ratio: The marginal cost-effectiveness ratio is the additional cost of a strategy divided by the additional health outcome it achieves and thus pertains to the situation in which there is a choice between ≥ 2 effective management strategies. Greater health improvement for a given resource expenditure is derived when the ratio is lower.

For policy analysis, the most common measure of effectiveness is the QALY, making the units of the corresponding marginal cost-effectiveness ratio "additional dollars spent per QALY gained." However, the marginal cost-effectiveness ratio has been criticized because elderly patients or patients with life-limiting comorbidities have a smaller potential gain in survival from a treatment and therefore have a higher (less advantageous) cost-effectiveness ratio.

For example (see Table 374–9), consider no antiarrhythmic therapy vs prophylactic use of an implantable cardioverter-defibrillator (ICD) for patients who have survived several months after an acute anterior MI and who have a mildly depressed ejection fraction (between 0.3 and 0.4). (All figures and costs in this example are hypothetical.) Both strategies assume similar baseline costs for routine care ($78,300), but the ICD has an additional (marginal) cost of $53,100, based on the cost of the device and professional fees, initial hospitalization, and ongoing therapy (including extra physician visits, laboratory tests, drugs, rehospitalizations for ICD-related complications, and replacement of ICD generator or leads). If patients with an ICD have a slightly increased life expectancy (7.87 vs 7.42 QALY), the marginal effectiveness of ICD therapy is 7.87 − 7.42 = 0.45 QALY. Thus, prophylactic ICD enhances survival compared to no antiarrhythmic therapy at a cost of $53,100/0.45 QALY, or $118,000/QALY.

Now assume that a third strategy, prophylactic amiodarone therapy, is available. This therapy is less expensive but also less effective than ICD. The effect of adding this third intermediate strategy is noteworthy because marginal cost-effectiveness ratios are calculated sequentially when there are multiple strategies (see Table 374–9, Analysis 2). The marginal cost-effectiveness ratio of amiodarone is lower ($68,519/QALY gained) than that for an ICD calculated in the previous example, and furthermore, because the effectiveness of an ICD is now compared to amiodarone rather than to no therapy, the addition of this intermediate cost strategy with partial effectiveness increases the ICD's marginal cost-effectiveness ratio from $118,000 to $192,222/QALY gained. This analysis suggests that for an expensive therapy such as an ICD, an attempt should be made to identify subpopulations expected to reap the greatest benefit.

375 Complementary and Alternative Medicine

(See also Ch. 376.)

Complementary and alternative medicine (CAM) refers to an eclectic mixture of healing approaches and therapies that historically have not been included in conventional, mainstream Western medicine.

CAM is often thought of as medicine that is not based on the principles of mainstream Western medicine. However, this characterization is not strictly accurate.

Probably the key differences between CAM and mainstream medicine (see Table 375–1) are the following:

- Scientific validation (if scientifically validated, practices are considered mainstream)
- The basis for their practices (a related issue)

Most CAM therapies have not been scientifically validated, and this standard has been used to distinguish the 2 types of medicine. However, use of some nutritional supplements, which are often included in CAM, has been scientifically validated and can be considered mainstream. Some CAM therapies are now offered in hospitals and are sometimes reimbursed by

Table 375–1. DIFFERENCES BETWEEN CONVENTIONAL AND ALTERNATIVE MEDICINE

FACTOR	CONVENTIONAL MEDICINE	ALTERNATIVE MEDICINE
Definition of health	A condition of physical, mental, and social well-being and the absence of disease and other abnormalities	Optimal balance, resilience, and integrity of the body, mind, and spirit and their interrelationships
Definition of illness	Organ dysfunction, disordered biochemical processes, or undesirable symptoms	Symptom and individual based: Imbalance of body, mind, and spirit
Concept of life force	Life processes that are based on known physical laws and that involve physical and biochemical events	A nonphysical, scientifically inaccessible life force that unites mind and body, interconnects all living beings, and is the underpinning of health (often called vitalism)
Understanding of consciousness	Results only from physical processes in the brain	Not localized to the brain; can exert healing effects on the body
Method of treatment	Any evidence-based intervention, including drugs, surgery, radiation therapy, electrical treatments, medical devices, physical therapy, exercise, and nutritional and lifestyle interventions	Support and strengthening of patients' inherent capacity for self-healing
Reliance on scientific evidence	Strict reliance on established principles of scientific evidence	Flexible use of scientific evidence; treatments often based on tradition and/or anecdotal support instead

insurance companies, further blurring the boundaries. Some traditional medical schools, including 45 North American medical schools in the Consortium of Academic Health Centers for Integrative Medicine, provide education about CAM and integrative medicine.

Mainstream medicine intends to base its practices only on the best scientific evidence available. In contrast, CAM tends to base its practices on philosophy—sometimes conflicting and even mutually exclusive philosophies—and does not rely on strict evidence-based standards.

As many as 38% of adults and 12% of children have used CAM at some point, depending on how broadly CAM is defined. A National Health Interview survey (2012) indicates that commonly used CAM therapies include

- Deep breathing exercises (11%)
- Yoga, tai chi, and qi gong (10%)
- Manipulative therapy (8%)
- Meditation (8%)

Use of other CAM therapies and approaches remains low: homeopathy (2.2%), naturopathy (0.4%), and energy healing (0.5%). A 2012 survey reported that in the US, 17.7% of adults used at least one dietary supplement.

Because patients worry about being criticized, they do not always volunteer information about their use of CAM to physicians. Therefore, it is very important for physicians to specifically ask their patients about CAM use (including use of medicinal herbs and nutritional supplements) in an open, nonjudgmental way. Learning about patients' use of CAM can do the following:

- Strengthen rapport and build trust
- Provide an opportunity to discuss evidence for CAM and its plausibility and risks
- Sometimes help physicians identify and avoid potentially harmful interactions between drugs and CAM therapies or nutritional supplements
- Monitor patient progress
- Help patients determine whether they should use specific certified or licensed CAM practitioners
- Learn from patients' experiences with CAM

Sidebar 375–1. CAM Terms

Several different terms are used for CAM practices:

- **Complementary medicine** refers to unconventional practices used with mainstream medicine.
- **Alternative medicine** refers to unconventional practices used instead of mainstream medicine.
- **Integrative medicine** is health care that uses all appropriate therapeutic approaches—conventional and alternative—within a framework that focuses on the therapeutic relationship and the whole person.

CAM = complementary and alternative medicine.

Efficacy

In 1992, the Office of Alternative Medicine in the National Institutes of Health (NIH) was formed to study the efficacy and safety of alternative therapies. In 1998, this office became the National Center for Complementary and Alternative Medicine (NCCAM), and in 2015, it became the National Center for Complementary and Integrative Health (NCCIH). Other NIH offices (eg, National Cancer Institute) also fund some CAM research. A 2009 review of research funded by the NCCAM found that in their first 10 yr, NCCAM spent 2.5 billion dollars on studies of CAM therapies without providing clear evidence of efficacy for any CAM therapy.

There are 3 types of support for CAM therapies:

- Efficacy on clinical outcomes as shown in controlled clinical trials (considered the strongest evidence for clinical uses)
- Evidence of established physiologic mechanisms of action (eg, modification of γ-aminobutyric acid [GABA] activity in the brain by valerian), although evidence of a validated physiologic mechanism of action does not necessarily indicate efficacy on clinical outcomes
- Use over periods of time ranging from decades to centuries (considered an anecdotal and unreliable form of evidence)

A substantial amount of information about CAM is available in peer-reviewed publications, evidence-based reviews, expert panel consensus documents, and authoritative textbooks; much of it has been published in languages other than English (eg, German, Chinese). Many CAM therapies have been studied and found to be ineffective, or at best, the studies had conflicting and inconsistent results. Some CAM therapies have not been tested in definitive clinical trials. Factors that limit such research include the following:

- Industry has no financial incentive to fund research.
- Often, CAM is not practiced in a culture of evidence-based medicine.
- Manufacturers of CAM products do not have to prove disease-specific efficacy.

The FDA, under the Dietary Supplement Health and Education Act of 1994, allows marketing of dietary supplements and use of CAM devices but significantly restricts efficacy claims. Generally, manufacturers of dietary supplements can claim, without having to provide evidence for safety or efficacy to the FDA, benefit to the body's structure or function (eg, improves cardiovascular health) but cannot claim benefit for treating disease (eg, treats hypertension).

Research: Designing studies of CAM therapies poses challenges beyond those faced by researchers of conventional therapies:

- Therapies may not be standardized. For example, there are different systems of acupuncture, and the contents and biologic activity of extracts made from the same plant species vary widely (chemical identification and standardization of active ingredients is not considered part of CAM).
- Diagnoses may not be standardized; use of many CAM therapies (eg, traditional herbal medicine, homeopathy, acupuncture) is based on the patient's unique characteristics rather than on a specific disease or disorder.
- Double- or single-blinding is often difficult or impossible. For example, patients cannot be blinded as to whether they are practicing meditation. Reiki practitioners cannot be blinded as to whether or not they are using energy healing.
- Outcomes are difficult to standardize because they are often specific to the individual rather than objective and uniform (as mean arterial pressure, Hb A_{1c} level, and mortality are).
- Placebos may be difficult to devise because identifying the effective component of a CAM therapy may be difficult. For example, in massage, the effective component could be touching, the specific area of the body massaged, the particular massage technique used, or time spent with the patient.

From a conventional research perspective, use of a placebo control is particularly important when subjective outcomes (eg, pain, nausea, indigestion) are used and when disorders that are intermittent, self-limited, or both (eg, headaches) are being studied; such end points and disorders are often the targets of CAM therapies. However, CAM systems interpret placebo effects as nonspecific healing effects that arise out of the therapeutic interaction and are inseparable from specific treatments. In practice, alternative therapies are intended to enhance the quality of the healing environment and therapeutic relationship and thus optimize the patient's capacity for self-healing (placebo response) as well as treatment-specific effects, making it hard to separate the effects of the specific treatment from those of a placebo. Thus, studying the effective components of a CAM therapy without undermining the integrity of that therapy in a research setting remains a methodologic challenge.

This interpretation of placebo is controversial. Many studies suggest that placebo effects (eg, regression to the mean) are mostly subjective and statistical and do not represent any meaningful self-healing. Researchers can reasonably isolate specific variables of individual treatments and determine whether those variables add to overall efficacy.

Despite these challenges, many high-quality studies of CAM therapies (eg, acupuncture, homeopathy) have been designed and done. For example, one study determined that double-blinding was possible for acupuncture when an opaque sheath that contained a penetrating or nonpenetrating needle was used.[1] Another studycompared the effects of acupuncture (individualized or standardized) with those of simulated acupuncture using a toothpick in a needle guide tube (and usual care).[2] Thus, by using carefully designed placebos, researchers can isolate the effects of some CAM therapies on the overall clinical response. For CAM therapies to be considered efficacious, evidence must show that they are more efficacious than placebo.

1. Takakura N, Yajima H: A placebo acupuncture needle with potential for double blinding—a validation study. *Acupunct Med* 26(4):224–230, 2008.
2. Cherkin DC, Sherman KJ, Avins AL, et al: A randomized trial comparing acupuncture, simulated acupuncture, and usual care for chronic low back pain. *Arch Intern Med* 169(9):858–866, 2009.

Safety

Although the safety of most CAM therapies has not been studied in clinical trials, many of these therapies have a good safety record. Many CAM therapies (eg, nontoxic botanicals, mind-body techniques such as meditation and yoga, body-based practices such as massage) have been used for thousands of years with no evidence of harm, and many seem to have no potential for harm. However, there are some safety considerations, including the following:

- Use of an alternative approach to treat a life-threatening disorder that can be effectively treated conventionally (eg, meningitis, diabetic ketoacidosis, acute leukemia)—perhaps the greatest risk of CAM, rather than the risk of direct harm from a CAM therapy
- Toxicity from certain herbal preparations (eg, hepatotoxicity from pyrrolizidine alkaloids, *Atractylis gummifera*, chaparral, germander, greater celandine, Jin Bu Huan, kava, pennyroyal, or others; nephrotoxicity from *Aristolochia*; adrenergic stimulation from ephedra)
- Contamination (eg, heavy metal contamination of some Chinese and Ayurvedic herbal preparations; contamination of other products, such as PC-SPES and some Chinese herbs, with other drugs)
- Interactions between CAM therapies (eg, botanicals, micronutrients, other dietary supplements) and other drugs (eg, induction of cytochrome P-450 [CYP3A4] enzymes by St. John's wort, resulting in reduced activity of antiretrovirals, immunosuppressants, and other drugs), particularly when the drug has a narrow therapeutic index
- As with any physical manipulation of the body (including mainstream techniques such as physical therapy), injury (eg, nerve or cord damage due to spinal manipulation in patients at risk, bruising in patients with bleeding disorders)

Current alerts about harmful dietary supplements are available at the FDA web site (Safety Alerts and Advisories). Historically, the FDA did not tightly regulate the production of dietary supplements. However, new FDA regulations now require compliance with manufacturing practices that guarantee quality and safety of supplements.

To help prevent injuries due to physical manipulations, patients should look for CAM practitioners who graduated from accredited schools and are professionally licensed. Rates of complications are very low when chiropractic or acupuncture is provided by practitioners with full credentials.

TYPES OF ALTERNATIVE MEDICINE

Five categories of alternative medicine are generally recognized:

- Alternative whole medical systems
- Mind-body medicine
- Biologically based practices
- Manipulative and body-based practices
- Energy medicine

The name of many therapies only partially describes their components.

ALTERNATIVE WHOLE MEDICAL SYSTEMS

Alternative medical systems are complete systems with explanation of disease, diagnosis, and therapy. They include the following:

- Ayurveda
- Homeopathy
- Naturopathy
- Traditional Chinese medicine

MIND-BODY MEDICINE

Mind-body medicine is based on the theory that mental and emotional factors regulate physical health through a system of interdependent neuronal, hormonal, and immunologic connections throughout the body. Behavioral, psychologic, social, and spiritual techniques are used to enhance the mind's capacity to affect the body and thus to preserve health and to prevent or cure disease.

Because scientific evidence supporting the benefits of mind-body medicine is abundant, many of these approaches are now considered mainstream. For example, the following techniques are used in the treatment of chronic pain, coronary artery disease, headaches, insomnia, and incontinence and as aids during childbirth:

- Biofeedback
- Guided imagery
- Hypnotherapy
- Meditation
- Relaxation

These techniques are also used to help patients cope with disease-related and treatment-related symptoms of cancer and to prepare patients for surgery.

Efficacy of mind-body techniques in patients with asthma, hypertension, or tinnitus is not as clear.

The benefits of relaxation are well-established and science-based; generally, the other mind-body techniques have no well-established specific benefit other than promoting relaxation.

BIOLOGICALLY BASED PRACTICES

Biologically based practices use naturally occurring substances to affect health. These practices include the following:

- Chelation therapy
- Diet therapies
- Herbalism
- Orthomolecular medicine
- Biologic therapies

Biologic Therapies

Biologic therapies use substances that occur naturally in animals to treat disease. These substances include the following:

- Shark cartilage to treat cancer
- S-adenosyl-L-methionine (SAMe) to treat depression or osteoarthritis
- Glucosamine to treat osteoarthritis

MANIPULATIVE AND BODY-BASED PRACTICES

Manipulative and body-based practices focus primarily on the body's structures and systems (eg, bones, joints, soft tissues). These practices are based on the belief that the body can regulate and heal itself and that its parts are interdependent. They include

- Chiropractic
- Massage therapy
- Postural reeducation
- Reflexology
- Structural integration

Several lesser known therapies are used in various cultures. They include the following:

- Cupping
- Scraping (eg, coining, spooning)
- Moxibustion

Some of these therapies result in lesions that may be mistaken for signs of child abuse. These therapies are thought to stimulate the body's energy and to enable toxins to leave the body. However, no research has verified their efficacy.

Cupping

Cupping is used in traditional Chinese medicine and in Middle Eastern, Asian, Latin American, and Eastern European cultures. The practice derives from older traditions of bloodletting, which is still done in some cultures.

The air inside a cup is heated, often using a cotton ball soaked in alcohol, then ignited. The heated cup is immediately inverted and placed on the skin. The resulting vacuum sucks the skin partway into the cup, which may be left in place for several minutes.

Cupping has been used to treat bronchitis, asthma, digestive disorders, and certain types of pain.

Cupping may redden or burn the skin.

Scraping

Scraping involves rubbing an implement across lubricated (oiled or wet) skin, usually on the back, neck, and shoulders. Coining uses a coin; spooning uses a spoon.

These therapies are used to treat the common cold, influenza, muscle pain and stiffness, and other disorders.

Coining results in linear red marks; spooning results in ecchymosis.

Moxibustion

Dried moxa herb (a mugwort) is burned usually just above but sometimes directly on the skin over acupuncture points. The herb may be in the form of incense sticks.

Moxibustion is used to treat fever, digestive problems, and pain due to injury or arthritis.

Moxibustion can result in circular burns (which resemble burns from cigarette tips) and vesicobullous lesions.

ENERGY MEDICINE

Energy medicine intends to manipulate subtle energy fields (also called biofields) thought to exist in and around the body and thus affect health. All energy therapies are based on the belief that a universal life force (qi) or subtle energy resides in and around the body (vitalism). Historically, a vitalistic force was posited to explain biologic processes that were not yet understood. As science advanced, a vitalistic force was discarded as an unnecessary notion. No scientific evidence supports the existence of a universal (vitalistic) life force.

Energy therapies include the following:

- Acupuncture
- Magnets
- Therapeutic touch (eg, Reiki)
- External qi gong

In external qi gong, master healers use the energy of their own biofield to bring the patient's energy into balance. Qi gong is used in traditional Chinese medicine.

AYURVEDA

Ayurveda, the traditional medical system of India, originated > 4000 yr ago. It is based on the theory that disease results from an imbalance of the body's life force (prana). It aims to restore balance within the body. The balance of prana is determined by equilibrium of the 3 bodily qualities (doshas): vata, pitta, and kapha. Most people have a dominant dosha; the specific balance is unique to each person.

Evidence for Ayurveda

Few well-designed studies of Ayurvedic practices have been done. Use of Ayurvedic herbal combinations to relieve symptoms in patients with RA has been studied. A 2005 systematic review identified randomized controlled trials that studied the efficacy of Ayurvedic herbal combinations for treatment of RA.[1] Only a few high-quality studies were identified, but existing evidence did not demonstrate efficacy for treatment of RA. Use of Ayurvedic practices to treat diabetes is being studied.

1. Park J, Ernst E: Ayurvedic medicine for rheumatoid arthritis: a systematic review. *Semin Arthritis Rheum* 34(5):705–713, 2005.

Uses for Ayurveda

After determining the balance of doshas, practitioners design a treatment specifically tailored to each patient. Ayurveda uses diet, herbs, massage, meditation, yoga, and therapeutic detoxification (panchakarma)—typically with enemas, oil massages, or nasal lavage—to restore balance within the body and with nature.

Possible Adverse Effects

In some of the herbal combinations used, heavy metals (mainly lead, mercury, and arsenic) are included because they are thought to have therapeutic effects. Several studies found that about 20% of Ayurvedic herbal supplements were contaminated with heavy metals in doses that, if taken as directed, could cause toxicity;[1,2] cases of heavy metal toxicity have been reported.[3]

1. Saper RB, et al: Heavy metal content of Ayurvedic herbal medicine products. *JAMA* 292(23):2868–2873, 2004.
2. Martena MJ, Van Der Wielen JC, Rietjens IM, et al: Monitoring of mercury, arsenic, and lead in traditional Asian herbal preparations on the Dutch market and estimation of associated risks. *Food Addit Contam Part A Chem Anal Control Expo Risk Assess* 27(2): 190–205, 2010.
3. Gair R: Heavy metal poisoning from Ayurvedic medicines. *BCMJ* 50(2):105, 2008.

HOMEOPATHY

Developed in Germany in the late 1700s, homeopathy is a medical system based on the principle that like cures like (the law of similars). A substance that, when given in large doses, causes a certain set of symptoms is believed to cure the same symptoms when it is given in minute to nonexistent doses. The minute dose is thought to stimulate the body's healing mechanisms.

Treatments are based on the patient's unique characteristics, including personality and lifestyle, as well as symptoms and general health. Homeopathy aims to restore the flow of the body's innate life force (vitalism); it is not based on principles of chemistry or physiology.

Remedies used in homeopathy are derived from naturally occurring substances, such as plant extracts and minerals. Extremely low concentrations are prepared in a specific way. The more dilute the homeopathic remedy, the stronger it is considered to be. Many solutions are so dilute that they contain no molecules of the active ingredient. For example, 30C dilution is diluted 1 to 100 in 30 serial dilutions, resulting in a final dilution of 1×10^{60}.

Homeopathic products are available over the counter or by prescription.

Regulation of Homeopathy

Unlike herbal and nutritional supplements, homeopathic remedies are regulated by the FDA. Only homeopathic remedies that are approved by the FDA can be manufactured. Because so little active ingredient is left after dilution, active ingredients are tested before dilution.

The FDA exempts homeopathic remedies from several requirements that exist for other drugs:

- The identity and strength of each active ingredient do not have to be confirmed by a laboratory before the remedy is distributed.
- Manufacturers of homeopathic products are not required to provide evidence of efficacy.
- Homeopathic remedies have been temporarily exempted from limits on the amount of alcohol (the usual diluent) that they can contain.

However, the label is required to list the following:

- Manufacturer
- The label "homeopathic"
- At least one indication
- Instructions for safe use
- Unless specifically exempted, the active ingredient and degree of dilution

Evidence for Homeopathy

The principles of homeopathy—like cures like and diluting makes preparations stronger—have no scientific basis. Expecting a preparation diluted so much that it has no active ingredient to have physiologic effects other than those of a placebo is biologically and chemically implausible. However, some homeopathic preparations do contain active ingredients in concentration sufficient to have physiologic effects (eg, Zicam®, which contains a measurable amount of zinc).

Efficacy of homeopathic remedies for various disorders has been extensively studied. A 2010 analysis of systematic reviews found that homeopathy is no more efficacious than placebo for any indication,[1] as did the United Kingdom's House of Commons Science and Technology Committee after an exhaustive review of systematic reviews and meta-analyses of homeopathy (2010).[2] The Australian government's exhaustive review of the clinical evidence for homeopathy (2013) found that for 61 indications,[3] there was evidence of lack of efficacy for homeopathy, and for another 7 indications, there was no good-quality evidence.

Proponents often cite the preliminary evidence in 3 studies published in 2003 supporting the efficacy of homeopathy for diarrhea in children.[4] However, an independent review of that evidence found it unconvincing, and a larger, more rigorous follow-up study in 2006 concluded that homeopathy did not effectively treat diarrhea in children.[5] Critics also point out that because all 3 studies were done by the same researcher, there has been no independent replication.

1. Ernst E: Homeopathy: what does the "best" evidence tell us? *Med J Aust* 192(8):458–460, 2010.
2. United Kingdom's House of Commons Science and Technology Committee: Homeopathy, 2010. Accessed 9/17/14.
3. National Health and Medical Research Council: Effectiveness of homeopathy for clinical conditions: evaluation of the evidence. Accessed 7/13/15.
4. Jacobs J, Jonas WB, Jiménez-Pérez M, et al: Homeopathy for childhood diarrhea: combined results and metaanalysis from three randomized, controlled clinical trials. *Pediatr Infect Dis J* 22(3):229–234, 2003.
5. Jacobs J, Guthrie BL, Montes GA, et al: Homeopathic combination remedy in the treatment of acute childhood diarrhea in Honduras. *J Altern Complement Med* 12(8):723–732, 2006.

Uses of Homeopathy

Homeopathy is commonly used in Europe and India, largely because of a long history of use; as a result, the practice has become part of the culture.

Homeopathy has been used to treat various disorders, such as allergies, rhinitis, digestive problems, musculoskeletal pain, and vertigo.

Possible Adverse Effects

Homeopathy is well-tolerated and has few risks; rarely, an allergic or toxic reaction occurs.

A 2012 review of reported cases of adverse effects identified 38 reports involving 1159 patients.[1] Adverse effects included

- Direct reactions to homeopathic treatments, presumably due to active ingredients
- Indirect harm caused by substituting homeopathy for effective conventional treatment

Conventional clinicians should not assume that a homeopathic remedy taken by a patient is biologically inactive and thus could not have adverse effects. Also, some homeopathic remedies contain other active ingredients that can have physiologic effects. Whether patients are taking homeopathic remedies may be unclear because patients often use the term homeopathic erroneously in reference to a dietary supplement they are taking. Also, the FDA allows many medicinal herbs to be registered and labeled as homeopathic if they undergo a particular pharmaceutical process.

PEARLS & PITFALLS

- Do not assume homeopathic remedies are biologically inactive; although the ingredients in homeopathic remedies are usually so dilute that they have no potential for harm, some remedies do contain ingredients in amounts that can have physiologic effects.

1. Posadzki P, Alotaibi A, Ernst E: Adverse effects of homeopathy: a systematic review of published case reports and case series. *Int J Clin Pract* 66(12):1178–1188, 2012.

NATUROPATHY

Naturopathy began as a formal health care system in the US during the early 1900s. Founded on the healing power of nature, naturopathy emphasizes

- Prevention and treatment of disease through a healthy lifestyle
- Treatment of the whole patient
- Use of the body's natural healing abilities

Some of this system's principles are not that different from those of traditional healing systems such as Ayurveda and traditional Chinese medicine.

Naturopathy uses a combination of therapies, including acupuncture, counseling, exercise therapy, medicinal herbs, homeopathy, hydrotherapy, natural childbirth, nutrition, physical therapies (eg, heat or cold therapy, ultrasound, massage), guided imagery, and stress management.

The American Association of Naturopathic Physicians tends to discourage childhood vaccinations.

Evidence for Naturopathy

Many naturopathic diagnostic and treatment methods are unproved or even disproved. An example is hydrotherapy (application of cold or hot water compresses), which is used to treat many conditions; this therapy is specific to naturopathy. Despite a wide range of claims made for hydrotherapy, no published studies demonstrate its efficacy.[1]

1. Kamioka H, Tsutani K, Okuizumi H, et al: Effectiveness of aquatic exercise and balneotherapy: a summary of systematic reviews based on randomized controlled trials of water immersion therapies. *J Epidemiol* 20(1):2–12, 2010. [Epub 2009 Oct 31.]

TRADITIONAL CHINESE MEDICINE

Originating > 2000 yr ago, traditional Chinese medicine (TCM) is a medical system based on the philosophy that illness results from improper flow of the life force (qi). The movement of qi is restored by balancing the opposing forces of yin and yang, which manifest in the body as cold and heat, internal and external, and deficiency and excess.

Various practices are used to preserve and restore qi and thus health. Most commonly used are

- Medicinal herbs
- Acupuncture

Other practices include diet, massage, and meditative exercise called qi gong.

TCM often uses diagnostic categories that do not correspond to current scientific understanding of biology and illness (eg, general deficiency, excess of yin or yang).

Evidence for Traditional Chinese Medicine

Obtaining high-quality evidence is difficult, mainly because the active ingredients in TCM herbs are not purified, are often unidentified, and may be numerous. Thus, determining the dose is difficult or impossible, and the dose may vary from one source of herbs to another. Information about bioavailability, pharmacokinetics, and pharmacodynamics is usually unavailable. Also, active ingredients may interact with each other in complex and variable ways.

Chinese herbal medicine traditionally uses formulas containing mixtures of herbs to treat various disorders. Traditional formulas can be studied as a whole, or each herb in the formula can be studied separately. One herb, used by itself, may not be as effective and may have adverse effects. Nevertheless, current conventional research favors study of single herbs to better control for variables. Another problem is the large number of herbal mixtures that could be studied.

Studies of TCM herbs and herbal mixtures for irritable bowel syndrome have had mixed results, and reviews of these studies conclude that more rigorous studies are required.

Preliminary studies of *Tripterygium wilfordii* (thunder god vine) has demonstrated anti-inflammatory properties and suggested clinical efficacy in treating RA, but reviews have found that existing evidence is insufficient to prove efficacy and concluded that more research is needed.[1]

Preliminary studies show that *Astragalus* may improve quality of life for patients being treated with chemotherapy for lung cancer, but it does not prolong survival or slow progression of cancer, as assessed by biomarkers.[2]

1. Liu Y, Tu S, Gao W, et al: Extracts of *Tripterygium wilfordii* Hook F in the treatment of rheumatoid arthritis: a systemic review and meta-analysis of randomised controlled trials. *Evid Based Complement Alternat Med* 410793, 2013. [Epub 2013 Dec 4.]
2. McCulloch M, See C, Shu XJ, et al: Astragalus-based Chinese herbs and platinum-based chemotherapy for advanced non-small-cell lung cancer: meta-analysis of randomized trials. *J Clin Oncol* 20;24(3):419–430, 2006.

Possible Adverse Effects

One problem is the standardization and quality control of Chinese herbs. Many are unregulated in Asia; they may be contaminated with heavy metals from polluted ground water or may be adulterated with drugs such as antibiotics or corticosteroids. Ingredients are often substituted, partly because the names of the herbs are translated incorrectly. A 2013 study found that 32% of herbal supplements did not contain the main active ingredient on the label,[1] 20% contained contaminants (physiologically active compounds other than the ingredients desired or on the label), and another 21% contained fillers not listed on the label. However, high-quality products are available through certain manufacturers that comply with FDA Good Manufacturing Practices.

In herbal mixtures, adverse effects may also result from interactions between active ingredients.

1. Newmaster SG, Grguric M, Shanmughanandhan D, et al: DNA barcoding detects contamination and substitution in North American herbal products. *BMC Med* 11; 11–222, 2013.

BIOFEEDBACK

For biofeedback, a type of mind-body medicine, electronic devices are used to provide information to patients about biologic functions (eg, heart rate, BP, muscle activity, skin temperature, skin resistance, brain surface electrical activity) and to teach patients to control these functions.

Uses for Biofeedback

With the help of a therapist or with training, patients can then use information from biofeedback to modify the function or to relax, thereby lessening the effects of conditions such as pain, stress, insomnia, and headaches.

Biofeedback is also used in patients with fecal or urinary incontinence, chronic abdominal pain, tinnitus, Raynaud syndrome, or attention or memory disorders (eg, attention-deficit/hyperactivity disorder, traumatic brain injury).

Generally, biofeedback does not seem to be useful in asthma; a possible exception is heart rate variability biofeedback, which may help reduce asthma symptoms and drug use and improve pulmonary function.

GUIDED IMAGERY

Guided imagery, a type of mind-body medicine, involves using mental images, self-directed or guided by a practitioner, to help patients relax (eg, before a procedure) and to promote wellness and healing (to try to effect physical changes—eg, by mobilizing the immune system). The images can involve any of the senses.

Uses for Guided Imagery

Imagery used with relaxation techniques (muscle relaxation and deep breathing) may help reduce pain and improve quality of life in patients with cancer. Imagery has also been used in patients with psychologic trauma.

HYPNOTHERAPY

Hypnotherapy, a type of mind-body medicine, is derived from western psychotherapeutic practice. Patients are put into an advanced state of relaxation and focused concentration to help them change their behavior and thus improve their health. They become absorbed in the images presented by the hypnotherapist and are relatively distracted from but not unconscious of their surroundings and the experiences they are undergoing. Some patients learn to hypnotize themselves.

Uses for Hypnotherapy

Hypnotherapy is used to treat pain syndromes, phobias, and conversion disorders and has been used with some success to manage smoking cessation and weight loss. It can reduce pain and anxiety during medical procedures in adults and children. It may be useful in irritable bowel syndrome, headaches, asthma, and some skin disorders (eg, warts, psoriasis). It may help lower BP.

Hypnotherapy helps control nausea and vomiting (particularly anticipatory) related to chemotherapy and is useful in palliative cancer care. Some evidence suggests that hypnotherapy helps lessen anxiety and improve quality of life in patients with cancer.

MEDITATION

In meditation, a type of mind-body medicine, patients regulate their attention or systematically focus on particular aspects of inner or outer experience. The most highly studied forms of meditation are transcendental meditation (TM) and mindfulness meditation. Although research is incomplete, results to date suggest that meditation could work via at least 2 mechanisms:

- Producing a relaxed state that counters excessive activation of neurohormonal pathways resulting from repeated stress
- Developing the capacity for metacognitive awareness (the ability to stand back from and witness the contents of consciousness), thus theoretically helping patients not react to stress automatically (with highly conditioned, learned patterns of behavior) and helping them tolerate and regulate emotional distress better

Most meditation practices were developed in a religious or spiritual context; their ultimate goal was some type of spiritual growth, personal transformation, or transcendental experience. However, studies suggest that as a health care intervention, meditation can often be beneficial regardless of a person's cultural or religious background.

Uses for Meditation

Meditation has been used to relieve anxiety, pain, depression, stress, insomnia, and symptoms of chronic disorders such as cancer or cardiovascular disorders. It is also used to promote wellness.

RELAXATION TECHNIQUES

Relaxation techniques, a type of mind-body medicine, are practices specifically designed to relieve tension and strain. The specific technique may be aimed at

- Reducing activity of the sympathetic nervous system
- Lowering BP
- Easing muscle tension
- Slowing metabolic processes
- Altering brain wave activity

Relaxation techniques may be used with other techniques, such as meditation, guided imagery, or hypnotherapy.

CHELATION THERAPY

In chelation therapy, a biologically based practice, a drug is used to bind with and remove hypothesized excess or toxic amounts of a metal or mineral (eg, lead, copper, iron, calcium) from the bloodstream. In conventional medicine, chelation therapy is a widely accepted way to treat lead and other heavy metal poisoning (see Table 366–4 on p. 3054).

Chelation therapy with EDTA (ethylene diamine tetraacetic acid) has also been suggested as a way to remove calcium and thus treat atherosclerosis. However, despite > 50 yr of study, researchers have not identified any theoretical mechanism to explain how chelation therapy could treat atherosclerosis or prevent heart attacks or strokes.

Also, until recently, clinical trials showed no significant benefit from chelation therapy, and systematic reviews have all concluded that EDTA chelation therapy is ineffective.[1] In 2012, a large randomized, placebo-controlled trial of alternative medicine (the Trial to Assess Chelation Therapy [TACT])[2] found a barely significant benefit for chelation over placebo for aggregated outcomes (26.5% vs 30% for placebo), but not for individual outcomes (eg, death, cardiovascular events, stroke, hospitalizations). However, this study had a high drop-out rate, and there were questions about blinding and the heterogeneity of treatment centers; thus, this study did not end the controversy over chelation therapy.

Risks of chelation therapy include hypocalcemia (which is potentially serious) and delay of more effective treatment.

- Hypocalcemia (which is potentially serious)
- Delay of more effective treatment

1. Villarruz MV, Dans A, Tan F:Chelation therapy for atherosclerotic cardiovascular disease. *Cochrane Database Syst Rev* (4):CD002785, 2002.
2. Lamas GA, Goertz C, Boineau R, et al: Effect of disodium EDTA chelation regimen on cardiovascular events in patients with previous myocardial infarction: the TACT randomized trial. *JAMA*. 309(12):1241–1250, 2013.

DIET THERAPY

Diet therapy, a biologically based practice, uses specialized dietary regimens (eg, Gerson therapy, macrobiotic diets, Pritikin diet) to

- Treat or prevent a specific disorder (eg, cancer, cardiovascular disorders)
- Generally promote wellness
- Detoxify the body (ie, neutralize or eliminate toxins from the body)

Some diets (eg, Mediterranean diet) are widely accepted and encouraged in traditional western medicine.

Diet therapy usually takes months or years for its maximal effects to occur and is more likely to have effects if started at a young age.

Ornish Diet

This very low-fat vegetarian diet aims to help reverse arterial blockages that cause coronary artery disease and may help prevent or slow the progression of prostate and other cancers. However, its efficacy is not yet clear because definitive clinical trials have not been done.

Gerson Diet

This diet involves consuming the equivalent of 15 to 20 lb of fruits and vegetables (in solid food and juices) each day, plus taking supplements and using coffee enemas. Proponents claim that this protocol is effective for treating cancer, heart disease, arthritis, autoimmune disorders, and diabetes; however, there are no rigorous clinical trials to support any of these claims. Also, claims of detoxification are not based on identification and measurement of any specific toxin.

One **risk** with this therapy is that its unsubstantiated claims for efficacy (eg, against cancer) can delay treatment with efficacious conventional therapies and worsen outcome.

Macrobiotic Diet

This diet consists mainly of vegetables, whole grains, fruits, and cereals. Some proponents claim that this diet can prevent and treat cancer and other chronic disorders; however, no evidence supports efficacy of a macrobiotic diet for treatment of cancer.

Risks include inadequate nutrition if the diet is not followed carefully.

Paleo Diet

This diet consists of types of food allegedly consumed during the Paleolithic era, when food was hunted or gathered (ie, animals and wild plants). Thus, the diet includes

- Increased protein intake
- Decreased carbohydrate intake (with intake consisting mainly of nonstarchy fresh fruits and vegetables)
- Increased fiber intake
- A moderate to higher fat intake (with intake mainly of monounsaturated and polyunsaturated fats)

Foods thought not to be available during the Paleolithic era (eg, dairy products, grains, legumes, processed oils, refined sugar, salt, coffee) are avoided. Proponents claim that human metabolism has not adapted to handle many of these foods.

Proponents of the Paleo diet claim that it reduces the risk of coronary artery disease, type 2 diabetes, and many chronic degenerative disorders. They also claim it promotes weight loss in overweight people, improves athletic performance, enhances sleep, and improves mental function. However, there is no good-quality evidence concerning the efficacy of this diet.

Risks include inadequate nutrition (due to decreased intake of whole grains and dairy) and possibly an increased risk of coronary artery disease (due to increased intake of fat and protein).

Knowledge of what was eaten in the Paleolithic era is limited; however, some evidence suggests that the diet of the Paleolithic era was not as limited as the modern Paleo diet.

ORTHOMOLECULAR MEDICINE

Orthomolecular medicine, also called nutritional medicine, is a biologically based practice. It aims to provide the body with optimal amounts of substances that naturally occur in the body (eg, hormones, vitamins) as a way to treat disease and promote wellness. Nutrition is the focus in diagnosis and treatment.

This therapy differs from diet therapy because it uses supradietary doses of individual micronutrients. High doses of vitamins, minerals, enzymes, hormones (eg, melatonin), amino acids, or various combinations may be used. Practitioners believe that people's nutritional needs far exceed the recommended daily allowances and that nutritional therapy must be individualized based on each patient's medical profile. High doses of micronutrients are also used as biologic response modifiers in an attempt to modulate inflammation and other disease processes. Doses may be administered orally or, far less often, intravenously.

Evidence and Uses

Treatment claims include benefit for a wide range of disorders (eg, cancer, cardiovascular disease, chronic fatigue, chronic pain, autism, psychiatric disorders). These treatments are widely used, and many patients report clinical improvement. However, no clinical study data support the usefulness of most of these practices. Exceptions include use of high-dose fish oil to treat hypertriglyceridemia (and possibly inflammatory and mood disorders); however, high doses of fish oil have been linked to increased risk of prostate cancer.

Preliminary evidence supported use of high-dose antioxidants to prevent macular degeneration, but later studies found no benefit. In addition, high doses of antioxidants may increase cardiovascular risk.

Preliminary studies of high-dose melatonin for the prevention or treatment cancer have had mixed results; further study is necessary.

If sufficient evidence of usefulness is shown, treatments (eg, high-dose fish oils to treat hypertriglyceridemia) become part of conventional medicine.

Possible Adverse Effects

Clinicians should be aware that high-dose micronutrients may cause harm; eg, some micronutrients may increase the risk of developing prostate cancer or blunt the effects of certain cancer treatments.

CHIROPRACTIC

In chiropractic (a manipulative and body-based practice), the relationship between the structure of the spine and function of the nervous system is thought to be the key to maintaining or restoring health. The main method for restoring this relationship is spinal manipulation. Other joints and soft tissues may also be manipulated. Chiropractors may provide physical therapies (eg, heat and cold, electrical stimulation, rehabilitation strategies), massage, or acupressure and may recommend exercises, ergonomic measures, or lifestyle changes.

Some chiropractors, called straight chiropractors, practice a form of vitalistic medicine. They use manipulation to correct hypothesized misalignments in the vertebrae in an attempt to restore the flow of a life energy (called innate). They believe that this method can heal most disorders. Other chiropractors reject this notion to various degrees; some of them restrict themselves to evidence-based musculoskeletal treatments.

Uses for Chiropractic

Evidence for chiropractic manipulation is sufficient only for

- Short-term relief of acute uncomplicated low back strain

After the acute stage, continuing adjustments may not provide additional benefit. Thus, the usefulness of chiropractic for chronic back pain is unclear. Chiropractic is sometimes useful in treating headache disorders (although data are inconsistent) and nerve impingement syndromes; it has also been used to treat neck pain.

Some chiropractors treat other disorders (eg, asthma in adults and children; enuresis, colic, torticollis, and otitis media in children), although only a few studies of chiropractic as treatment for these disorders have been done, and they do not support efficacy.

The usefulness of manipulation for conditions not directly related to the musculoskeletal system has not been established.

Possible Adverse Effects

Serious complications resulting from spinal manipulation (eg, low back pain, damage to cervical nerves, damage to arteries in the neck) are rare. Spinal manipulation is not recommended for patients with osteoporosis or symptoms of neuropathy (eg, paresthesias, loss of strength in a limb). Whether it is safe for patients who have had spinal surgery or stroke or who have a vascular disorder is unclear.

MASSAGE THERAPY

In massage therapy (a manipulative and body-based practice), body tissues are manipulated to promote wellness and reduce pain and stress. The therapeutic value of massage for many musculoskeletal symptoms and stress is widely accepted. Massage has been shown to help relieve the following:

- Muscle soreness
- Pain due to back injuries
- Fibromyalgia
- Anxiety, fatigue, pain, nausea, and vomiting in cancer patients

Massage therapy is reported to be effective in treating low-birth-weight infants, preventing injury to the mother's genitals during childbirth, relieving chronic constipation, and controlling asthma. A 2004 Cochrane review of massage therapy for low-birth-weight infants concluded that the evidence for efficacy was weak and wider use is not warranted.[1] Evidence for the other reported uses is preliminary only; further study is required.

Massage can cause bruising and bleeding in patients with thrombocytopenia or bleeding disorders. Therapists must avoid putting pressure on bones affected by osteoporosis or metastatic cancer.

1. Vickers A, Ohlsson A, Lacy JB, et al: Massage for promoting growth and development of preterm and/or low birth-weight infants. *Cochrane Database Syst Rev* (2):CD000390, 2004.

REFLEXOLOGY

Reflexology (a manipulative and body-based practice) is a variant of massage therapy that relies on manual pressure applied to specific areas of the foot; these areas are believed to correspond to different organs or body systems via meridians. Stimulation of these areas is believed to eliminate the blockage of energy responsible for pain or disease in the corresponding body part.

Reflexology is considered a homunculus-based therapy because it presumes that the entire body is represented on the bottom of the feet. No homunculus-based therapy, including reflexology, has any basis in science. In most clinical studies of reflexology, methodology has been poor, and findings tend to be nonspecific effects on subjective symptoms (eg, causing relaxation, indistinguishable from that caused by massage). A systematic review of randomized clinical trials concluded that the best available clinical evidence does not support the efficacy of reflexology as treatment for any indication; the review also noted that methodology in studies of reflexology is often poor.[1]

1. Ernst E, Posadzki P, Lee MS:Reflexology: an update of a systematic review of randomised clinical trials. *Maturitas* 68(2):116–120, 2011.

STRUCTURAL INTEGRATION

Structural integration (a manipulative and body-based practice) is based on the theory that good health depends on correct body alignment. It is a form of deep tissue manipulation that is typically done over a series of sessions. Practitioners believe that they can correct the alignment of bone and muscle and thus restore good health by manipulating and stretching muscles and fascia. However, neither the basic principles nor efficacy of this therapy has been proved[1].

1. Jacobson E: Structural integration, an alternative method of manual therapy and sensorimotor education. *J Altern Complement Med* 17(10):891–899, 2011.

POSTURAL REEDUCATION

Postural reeducation (a manipulative and body-based practice) uses movement and touch to help people relearn healthy posture, move more easily, and become more aware of their body. The therapies involved seek to release habitual, harmful ways of holding the body by focusing on awareness through movement.

The effectiveness of postural reeducation is not clear.

ACUPUNCTURE

Acupuncture, a therapy within traditional Chinese medicine, is one of the most widely accepted alternative therapies in the western world. Specific points on the body are stimulated, usually by inserting thin needles into the skin and underlying tissues. Stimulating these specific points is believed to unblock the flow of qi along energy pathways (meridians) and thus restore balance. In classic acupuncture, there were 365 defined points that corresponded to the 365 days of the year and reflected the historical connection between acupuncture and astrology. Over time, the number of points has increased to > 2000.

The procedure is generally not painful but may cause a tingling sensation. Sometimes stimulation is increased by twisting or warming the needle.

Acupuncture points may also be stimulated by

- Pressure (called acupressure)
- Lasers
- Ultrasound
- A very low voltage electrical current (called electroacupuncture) applied to the needle

Evidence and Uses

Despite extensive study, no high-quality evidence supports clinically meaningful efficacy of acupuncture for any indication. High-quality studies compare true (verum) acupuncture with sham acupuncture (needle insertion at points not used in acupuncture) or placebo acupuncture (use of opaque sheaths containing a blunt needle or toothpick that is pressed against the skin but not inserted). Because placebo acupuncture studies also use opaque sheaths for true acupuncture, neither patient nor acupuncturist know which treatment is being used (double-blinding). Such high-quality studies generally show no differences in efficacy. Therefore, the best evidence indicates that neither where the needle is inserted nor whether it is inserted affect outcome and that acupuncture has only nonspecific placebo effects.

In some cultures, publication bias tends to favor efficacy for acupuncture; for example, 99% of studies published in China supported efficacy, despite a worldwide average of about 75%. Thus, positive results of existing studies should be interpreted carefully.

Systematic reviews of acupuncture for pain, the most commonly promoted indication, show either no differences between verum, sham, and placebo acupuncture or a small statistical difference that is clinically insignificant or imperceptible. Proponents also claim efficacy of acupuncture for specific disorders (eg, carpal tunnel syndrome, addiction, asthma, stroke, RA); however, in all cases, systematic reviews conclude that the evidence is negative or that methodology is too poor to produce conclusive results.

Possible Adverse Effects and Contraindications

Reliable data are uncommon and often nonexistent, and adverse effects of acupuncture are probably underreported. A 2012 review of adverse effects that were reported after acupuncture noted the following:[1]

- Retained needles (31%)
- Dizziness (30%)
- Loss of consciousness or unresponsiveness (19%)
- Falls (4%)
- Bruising or soreness at the needle site (2%)
- Pneumothorax (1%)
- Other adverse effects (12%)

Most (95%) were classified as causing little or no harm.

When correctly done, acupuncture is fairly safe, but skill and care vary among practitioners; also, some do not follow antiseptic standards.

1. Wheway J, Agbabiaka TB, Ernst E: Patient safety incidents from acupuncture treatments: a review of reports to the National Patient Safety Agency. *Int J Risk Saf Med* 24(3):163–169, 2012.

MAGNETS

Energy therapy may rely on static magnetic fields (constant fields produced by permanent magnets) or pulsed electromagnetic fields (intermittent magnetic fields produced by an electromagnet). Practitioners place magnets on the body or place injured body parts in an induced electrical field to reduce pain or enhance healing.

Evidence and Uses

Magnets, in particular, are a popular treatment for various musculoskeletal disorders, although multiple studies have shown no effectiveness, especially for pain relief, one of their most common applications.

For static magnetic therapy, systematic reviews found no benefit for chronic pain, and high-quality studies found no benefit for osteoarthritis and RA.[1]

The biologic effect of pulsed electromagnetic therapy is significantly different from that of static magnetic. Preliminary evidence suggests that pulsed electromagnetic therapy may relieve pain. Using pulsed electromagnetic fields to speed healing of nonunion fractures is well-established.

1. Pittler MH, Brown EM, Ernst E: Static magnets for reducing pain: systematic review and meta-analysis of randomized trials. *CMAJ* 177(7):736–742, 2007.

Possible Contraindications

Possible contraindications for magnets include pregnancy (effects on the fetus are unknown) and use of implanted cardiac devices, an insulin pump, or a drug given by patch.

THERAPEUTIC TOUCH

Therapeutic touch, sometimes referred to as laying on of hands, is a type of energy medicine. It claims to use the therapist's healing energy to identify and repair imbalances in a patient's biofield. Usually, practitioners do not touch the patient; instead, they move their hands back and forth over the patient. Therapeutic touch has been used to lessen anxiety and improve the sense of well-being in patients with cancer, but these effects have not been rigorously studied. In the US, nurses have introduced therapeutic touch into ICUs and other hospital settings.

Existing evidence does not support the claim that therapeutic touch practitioners can detect a human biofield nor that a human biofield even exists. For example, a 1998 study[1] found that therapeutic touch practitioners could not detect the presence of a biofield. High-quality clinical studies are lacking, but systematic reviews[2] of existing studies have not found sufficient evidence to support therapeutic touch's effectiveness for treating for any disorder.

1. Rosa L, Rosa E, Sarner L, Barrett S: A close look at therapeutic touch. *JAMA* 279(13):1005–1010, 1998.
2. Hammerschlag R, Marx BL, Aickin M: Nontouch biofield therapy: a systematic review of human randomized controlled trials reporting use of only nonphysical contact treatment. *J Altern Complement Med* 2014.

Reiki

Reiki, which originated in Japan, is similar to therapeutic touch; in Reiki, practitioners channel energy through their hands and transfer it into the patient's body to promote healing. Practitioners are thought to have special healing powers, which are required for these treatments.

High-quality clinical trials of Reiki are lacking. Preliminary evidence is mixed. A blinded controlled trial[1] of Reiki for fibromyalgia found no benefit.

1. Assefi N, Bogart A, Goldberg J, et al: Reiki for the treatment of fibromyalgia: a randomized controlled trial. *J Altern Complement Med* 14(9):1115–1122, 2008.

376 Dietary Supplements

Dietary supplements are the most commonly used of all complementary and alternative therapies (see Ch. 375), primarily because they are widely available, relatively inexpensive, and can be bought without consulting a health care practitioner.

The Food and Drug Administration (FDA) regulates dietary supplements differently from drugs. The FDA regulates only quality control and good manufacturing processes but does not ensure standardization of the active ingredients or efficacy.

Definition: The Dietary Supplement Health Education Act (DSHEA) of 1994 defines a dietary supplement as

- Any product (except tobacco)—in pill, capsule, tablet, or liquid form—containing a vitamin, mineral, herb or other plant product, amino acid, or other known dietary substance that is intended as a supplement to the normal diet

In addition, certain hormones, such as dehydroepiandrosterone (DHEA, a precursor to androgens and estrogens) and melatonin, are regulated as dietary supplements and not as prescription drugs.

Labeling: The DSHEA requires that the product label identify the product as a dietary supplement and notify the consumer that the claims for the supplement have not been evaluated by the FDA. The label must also list each ingredient by name, quantity, and total weight and identify plant parts from which ingredients are derived. Manufacturers are permitted to make claims about the product's structure and function (eg, good for urinary tract health) but cannot make or imply claims for the product as a drug or therapy (eg, treats UTIs). Expiration dates should also be included on the standardized product labels.

Safety and efficacy: Most people who use dietary supplements assume that they are good for health generally, are safe and effective for treating and/or preventing specific conditions, or both because dietary supplements are natural (ie, derived from plants or animals) and because some are supported by centuries of use in traditional systems of medicine. However, the FDA does not require manufacturers of dietary supplements to prove safety or efficacy (although supplements must have a history of safety). Most supplements have not been rigorously studied. For most, evidence suggesting safety or efficacy comes from

- Traditional use
- In vitro studies
- Certain case reports
- Animal studies

However, manufacturers and distributors of supplements now must report serious adverse events to the FDA through the MedWatch system. There are a few supplements (eg, fish oil, chondroitin/glucosamine, St. John's wort) now proved to be safe and useful complements to standard drugs.

Evidence concerning the safety and efficacy of dietary supplements is increasing rapidly as more and more clinically based studies are being done. Information about such studies is available at the National Institutes of Health's National Center for Complementary and Alternative Medicine (NCCAM) web site (www.nccam.nih.gov/research/clinicaltrials).

Purity and standardization: Lack of regulation and government monitoring also means that supplements are not monitored to ensure that they contain the ingredients or amount of active ingredient the manufacturer claims they contain. The supplement may have unlisted ingredients, which may be inert or harmful (eg, natural toxins, bacteria, pesticides, lead or other heavy metals, unapproved dyes), or it may contain variable amounts of active ingredients, especially when whole herbs are ground or made into extracts. Consumers are at risk of getting less, more, or, in some cases, none of the active ingredient, if the active ingredient(s) is even known. Most herbal products are mixtures of several substances, and which ingredient is the most active is not always known.

The lack of standardization means not only that products from different manufacturers may vary, but also that separate batches produced by the same manufacturer may differ. This product variability is a particular source of difficulty in conducting rigorous clinical trials and comparing the results among different trials. However, some supplements have been standardized and may include a designation of standardization on the label.

New regulations governing supplement production in the US include rules for Good Manufacturing Practices (GMPs). These rules strengthen standards for keeping manufacturing facilities and equipment clean and raw materials pure and uncontaminated. GMPs also ensure proper labeling, packaging, and storage of the finished product.

Other concerns: Additional areas of concern include

- Use of dietary supplements instead of conventional drugs
- Stability of supplements (especially herbal products) once manufactured
- Toxicity
- Interactions between supplements and drugs
- Contribution to incorrect diagnosis

Most information about these concerns comes from sporadic individual reports (see Table 376–1) and some references.

Despite these concerns, many patients strongly believe in the benefits of supplements and continue to use them with or without a physician's involvement. Patients may not think to disclose or may wish to conceal their use of dietary supplements. For this reason, the outpatient history should periodically include explicit questions about past and new use of complementary and alternative therapies, including dietary supplements. Many physicians incorporate some supplement use into their practice; their reasons include proven benefit of the supplement, a desire to ensure that supplements are used safely by patients who will use supplements anyway, and the physician's belief that the supplements are safe and effective.

Common concerns about the use of supplements include the following:

- Placebo effects can simulate true efficacy, particularly if the patient and/or physician strongly believes in the supplement.
- Therapeutic responses to supplements, placebo-mediated or otherwise, could be mistaken as evidence that confirms a particular, possibly incorrect, diagnosis.

There are few data to guide patient counseling regarding supplement safety. But some experts believe that the overall number of problems due to dietary supplements is rare compared with the overall number of doses taken and that the supplement, if correctly manufactured, is likely to be safe. As a result, these experts advise purchase of supplements from a well-known manufacturer, and many recommend buying supplements made in Germany because there they are regulated as drugs and thus oversight is stricter than in the US.

The following supplements are ones that are most popular, are effective, or have some questions about their safety. More complete information is available through the NCCAM web site (www.nccam.nih.gov).

BLACK COHOSH

Black cohosh is the underground stem of a plant that can be ingested directly in powdered form or extracted into tablet or liquid form. It should be standardized to contain certain triterpenes. Black cohosh contains no phytoestrogens that can account for its purported estrogen-like effects, but it contains small amounts of anti-inflammatory compounds, including salicylic acid.

Claims: Black cohosh is said to be useful for menopausal symptoms (eg, hot flushes, mood lability, tachycardia, vaginal dryness), for menstrual symptoms, and for arthralgias in rheumatoid arthritis or osteoarthritis.

Evidence: Evidence regarding benefit in relieving menstrual symptoms is conflicting.[1] There are few reliable data on its effectiveness for other disorders and symptoms.

A recent review included 16 randomized controlled trials of women (n = 2027) using oral preparations of black cohosh (average dose 40 mg). There was no significant difference between black cohosh and placebo in the frequency of

Table 376–1. SOME POSSIBLE DIETARY SUPPLEMENT–DRUG INTERACTIONS*

DIETARY SUPPLEMENT	AFFECTED DRUGS	INTERACTION
Chamomile	Barbiturates and other sedatives	May intensify or prolong effects of sedatives because its volatile oils have additive effects
	Iron supplements	May reduce iron absorption via tannins in the plant
	Warfarin	May increase risk of bleeding because chamomile contains phytocoumarins, which may have additive effects
Echinacea	Potentially hepatotoxic drugs metabolized by cytochrome P-450 enzymes (eg, amiodarone, anabolic steroids, ketoconazole, methotrexate)	May slow metabolism of these drugs and increase risk of hepatotoxicity if taken for > 8 wk
	Immunosuppressants (eg, corticosteroids, cyclosporine)	May lessen immunosuppressive effects via T-cell stimulation
Ephedra[†]	Stimulant drugs (eg, caffeine, epinephrine, phenylpropanolamine, pseudoephedrine)	Increases the stimulant effects of other drugs, increasing risk of irregular or rapid heartbeat and hypertension
	MAOIs	May intensify effects of these drugs and increase risk of side effects (eg, headache, tremors, irregular or rapid heartbeat, hypertension)
Feverfew	Antimigraine drugs (eg, ergotamine—see Table 229–2 on p. 1902)	May increase heart rate and BP because it has additive vasoconstrictive effects
	Antiplatelet drugs	May increase risk of bleeding because feverfew inhibits platelet aggregation (has additive effects)
	Iron supplements	May reduce iron absorption via tannins in the plant
	NSAIDs	Feverfew's efficacy in preventing and managing migraine headaches reduced by NSAIDs
	Warfarin	May increase risk of bleeding because warfarin may have additive effects
Garlic	Antihypertensives	May augment antihypertensive effect
	Antiplatelet drugs	May increase risk of bleeding because these drugs enhance garlic's inhibition of platelet aggregation and fibrinolytic effects
	Protease inhibitors (eg, saquinavir)	Blood level of protease inhibitors reduced by garlic
	Warfarin	May increase risk of bleeding by augmenting warfarin's anticoagulant effects
Ginger	Antiplatelet drugs	May increase risk of bleeding by augmenting inhibition of platelet aggregation
	Warfarin	May increase risk of bleeding by augmenting warfarin's anticoagulant effects
Ginkgo	Anticonvulsants (eg, phenytoin)	May reduce efficacy of anticonvulsants because contaminants in ginkgo preparations may reduce anticonvulsant effects
	MAOIs (eg, tranylcypromine)	May intensify effects of these drugs and increase risk of side effects (eg, headache, tremors, manic episodes)
	NSAIDs	May increase risk of bleeding by augmenting inhibition of antiplatelet aggregation
	Warfarin	May increase risk of bleeding by augmenting warfarin's anticoagulant effects
Ginseng	Antihyperglycemic drugs (eg, glipizide)	May intensify effects of these drugs, causing hypoglycemia
	Aspirin and other NSAIDs	May increase risk of bleeding by augmenting inhibition of antiplatelet aggregation
	Corticosteroids	May intensify adverse effects of corticosteroids because ginseng has anti-inflammatory effects
	Digoxin	May increase digoxin levels
	Estrogens	May intensify adverse effects of estrogen
	MAOIs	Can cause headache, tremors, and manic episodes
	Opioids	May reduce the effectiveness of opioids
	Warfarin	May increase risk of bleeding by augmenting warfarin's anticoagulant effects

Table continues on the following page.

Table 376–1. SOME POSSIBLE DIETARY SUPPLEMENT–DRUG INTERACTIONS* (*Continued*)

DIETARY SUPPLEMENT	AFFECTED DRUGS	INTERACTION
Goldenseal	Warfarin and heparin	May oppose effects of warfarin and heparin, increasing risk of thromboembolism
Green tea	Warfarin	May reduce efficacy of warfarin, increasing risk of thromboembolism
Kava	Sedatives (eg, barbiturates, benzodiazepines)	May intensify or prolong the effects of sedatives
Licorice (glycyrriza glabra)‡	Antiarrhythmics	May increase risk of an abnormal heart rhythm, making antiarrhythmic therapy less effective
	Antihypertensives	May increase salt and water retention and increase BP, making antihypertensives less effective
	Digoxin	May decrease levels of K, which increases risk of digoxin toxicity
	Diuretics	May intensify the K-wasting effects of most diuretics and interfere with the effectiveness of K-sparing diuretics (eg, spironolactone)
	MAOIs	May intensify effects of these drugs and increase risk of adverse effects (eg, headache, tremors, manic episodes)
Milk thistle	Antihyperglycemic drugs	May intensify effects of these drugs, causing hypoglycemia
	Protease inhibitors (eg, indinavir, saquinavir)	May interfere with metabolizing enzymes, lowering blood levels of indinavir
Saw palmetto	Estrogens (eg, oral contraceptives)	May augment effects of these drugs
St. John's wort	Cyclosporine	May reduce blood level of cyclosporine, increasing risk of organ transplant rejection
	Digoxin	May reduce blood level of digoxin, making it less effective, with potentially dangerous results
	Iron supplements	May reduce iron absorption
	MAOIs	May augment effects of MAOIs, possibly causing very high BP requiring emergency treatment
	Nonnucleoside reverse transcriptase inhibitors	Increases metabolism of these drugs, reducing their efficacy
	Oral contraceptives	Increases metabolism of these drugs, reducing their efficacy
	Photosensitizing drugs (eg, lansoprazole, omeprazole, piroxicam, sulfonamide antibiotics)	May increase sun sensitivity
	Protease inhibitors	May reduce blood level of protease inhibitors, reducing their efficacy
	SSRIs (eg, fluoxetine, paroxetine, sertraline)	May augment effects of these drugs
	Tricyclic antidepressants	May augment effects of these drugs
	Warfarin	May reduce blood level of warfarin, increasing risk of thromboembolism
Valerian	Sedatives (eg, barbiturates, benzodiazepines)	May intensify effects of sedatives

*Caution is required when dietary supplements are used because these products are not standardized and thus vary considerably and because information about their use is continually changing. The theoretical status of many published interactions does not obviate the need for cautious use. Before prescribing any drug, health care practitioners should ask patients whether they are taking dietary supplements and, if so, which ones. Practitioners must identify any potential adverse interactions of drugs and supplements taken by a patient and then determine appropriate drugs and dosages.

†Sale of supplements containing ephedra is banned in the US.

‡This substance is true, natural licorice, not the more common, artificially flavored licorice candy.

MAOIs = monoamine oxidase inhibitors; NSAIDs = nonsteroidal anti-inflammatory drugs; SSRIs = selective serotonin reuptake inhibitors.

hot flushes (3 trials; 393 women) or in menopausal symptom scores (4 trials; 357 women).[1] A lack of standardization of the supplement product used between studies indicates that more research is necessary to reach definitive conclusions.

Adverse effects: Adverse effects are uncommon. The most likely are headache and GI distress. Dizziness, diaphoresis, and hypotension (if high doses are taken) may occur.

Theoretically, black cohosh is contraindicated in patients with aspirin sensitivity, liver disease, hormone-sensitive cancers (eg, certain kinds of breast cancer), stroke, or high blood pressure. The US Pharmacopeia (USP), based on a few case reports,[2] has recommended that black cohosh products be labeled with a warning declaring that they may be hepatotoxic.

Drug interactions: There is little clinical evidence that black cohosh interferes with drugs. However, a recent in vitro study suggests that black cohosh may inhibit the biotransformation or effectiveness of tamoxifen and irinotecan, both chemotherapy drugs.[3]

1. Leach MJ, Moore V. Black cohosh (Cimicifuga spp.) for menopausal symptoms. *Cochrane Database Syst Rev* 9:CD007244, 2012.
2. Lim TY, Considine A, Quaglia A, et al. Subacute liver failure secondary to black cohosh leading to liver transplantation. *BMJ Case Rep*, Published online: 5 July 2013. doi:10.1136/bcr-2013-009325.
3. Gorman GS, Coward L, Darby A, et al. Effects of herbal supplements on the bioactivation of chemotherapeutic agents. *J Pharm Pharmacol* 65(7):1014-1025, 2013.

CHAMOMILE

The flower of chamomile is dried and drunk as a tea, consumed as a capsule, or used topically as an extract.

Claims: Chamomile tea is said to reduce inflammation and fever, to act as a mild sedative, to provide antidepressant activity, to relieve stomach cramps and indigestion, and to promote healing of gastric ulcers. Chamomile extract applied topically in a compress is said to soothe irritated skin. Mechanism is due to essential oil containing bisabolol constituents and the flavonoids apigenin and luteolin.

Evidence: Limited clinical trial evidence supports any use of chamomile. However, randomized, double-blind, placebo-controlled trials using oral capsules of chamomile extract (standardized to 1.2% apigenin) in patients with mild-to-moderate anxiety[1] showed possible modest anxiolytic activity and antidepressant activity.[2]

Adverse effects: Chamomile is generally safe; however, hypersensitivity reactions have been reported, especially in people allergic to members of the Asteraceae (eg, sunflower, ragweed) plant family and pollen of all flowering plants. Typical symptoms include lacrimation, sneezing, GI upset, dermatitis, and anaphylaxis.

Drug interactions: Chamomile may reduce the absorption of oral drugs. Chamomile may also increase the effects of anticoagulants and sedatives (including barbiturates and alcohol) and decrease the absorption of iron supplements.

1. Amsterdam JD, Li Y, Soeller I, et al: A randomized, double-blind, placebo-controlled trial of oral *Matricaria recutita* (chamomile) extract therapy for generalized anxiety disorder. *J Clin Psychopharmacol* 29(4):378–382, 2009.
2. Amsterdam JD, Shults J, Soeller I, et al. Chamomile (*Matricaria recutita*) may provide antidepressant activity in anxious, depressed humans: an exploratory study. *Altern Ther Health Med* 18(5):44-49, 2012.

CHONDROITIN SULFATE

Chondroitin sulfate is a glycosaminoglycan, a natural component of cartilage. It is extracted from shark or cow cartilage or manufactured synthetically. Its composition can vary. It is frequently combined with glucosamine.

Claims: Chondroitin sulfate is used to treat osteoarthritis. Scientific evidence shows no benefit when chondroitin sulfate is taken by itself. However, evidence suggests that in combination with glucosamine, it may reduce joint pain, improve joint mobility, and allow reduction of the doses of conventional anti-inflammatory drugs when it is taken for 6 to 24 mo. Effects over longer periods are unclear. Mechanism is unknown. Dose is 600 mg po once/day to 400 mg po tid.

Evidence: Evidence on efficacy of chondroitin sulfate is conflicting. Until recently, only small trials had studied chondroitin sulfate alone or in combination with glucosamine to treat osteoarthritis. The Glucosamine/Chondroitin Arthritis Intervention Trial (GAIT), a large, randomized, double-blinded, placebo-controlled, multicenter clinical trial studied use of glucosamine (500 mg po tid), chondroitin sulfate (400 mg po tid), and use of both drugs to treat osteoarthritis of the knee; in the group as a whole, pain was not reduced. However, exploratory subanalyses suggested efficacy in a subgroup of patients with moderate-to-severe knee pain.[1]

A meta-analysis has also suggested that the benefit of chondroitin, if any, is limited.[2] It has been suggested the reason for conflicting symptomatic benefit is due to the poor quality of several food-grade chondroitin sulfate supplements and that pharmaceutical-grade chondroitin sulfate with defined percent purity and sequences of oligosaccharides is efficacious and be used for treatment.[3] Heterogeneity of osteoarthritic symptoms and causes also contribute to the difficulty of use in clinical practice.

Adverse effects: No serious adverse effects have been reported. Among the most common adverse effects are stomach pain, nausea, and other GI symptoms.

Drug interactions: Chondroitin sulfate may increase the anticoagulant action of warfarin.[4]

1. Clegg DO, Reda DJ, Harris CL, et al: Glucosamine, chondroitin sulfate, and the two in combination for painful knee osteoarthritis. *N Engl J Med* 354(8):795–808, 2006.
2. Reichenbach S, Sterchi R, Scherer M, et al: Meta-analysis: chondroitin for osteoarthritis of the knee or hip. *Ann Intern Med* 146(8):580–590, 2007.
3. Hochberg M, Chevalier X, Henrotin Y, et al: Symptom and structure modification in osteoarthritis with pharmaceutical-grade chondroitin sulfate: what's the evidence? *Curr Med Res Opin* 29(3): 259–267, 2013.
4. Knudsen JF, Sokol GH: Potential glucosamine-warfarin interaction resulting in increased international normalized ratio: case report and review of the literature and MedWatch database. *Pharmacotherapy* 28(4): 540–548, 2008.

CHROMIUM

Chromium, a trace mineral, potentiates the action of insulin. Nutritional sources that contain sufficient amounts include carrots, potatoes, broccoli, whole grains, and molasses. Picolinate, a by-product of tryptophan that is paired with chromium in supplements, is said to help the body absorb chromium more efficiently. Chromium dinicocysteinate is a newer supplement complex of trivalent chromium with L-cysteine and niacin.

Claims: Chromium picolinate is said to promote weight loss, build muscle, reduce body fat, lower cholesterol and triglyceride (TG) levels, and enhance insulin function. Although chromium deficiency impairs insulin function, there is little evidence that supplementation helps patients with diabetes, nor is there evidence that it benefits body composition or lipid levels.

Evidence: The role of supplemental chromium is controversial, and the clinical data conflict. A 2002 meta-analysis evaluated 20 randomized clinical trials and concluded that the data indicated no effect of chromium on glucose or insulin levels in nondiabetic patients; results were inconclusive in diabetic patients.[1] However, a 2013 meta-analysis of data from a separate group of 20 randomized clinical trials indicated that supplementation in overweight or obese people resulted in statistically significant reductions in body weight.[2] The authors speculate that the effect is small and they are unsure of the clinical relevance, suggesting further long-term studies are warranted.

Randomized, controlled, clinical trials are needed to determine whether chromium can influence diabetes, lipid metabolism, or weight loss. These studies should control or adjust for baseline chromium status and the form of chromium used and be done in well-defined at-risk populations in whom food intake is monitored.

Adverse effects: Several studies have demonstrated that daily doses up to 1000 mcg of chromium are safe. Some in vitro evidence suggests that chromium picolinate damages chromosomes and may cause cancer. However, no clinical studies have shown an association. Some forms of chromium may contribute to GI irritation and ulcers. Isolated cases of impaired kidney and liver function have been reported; thus, people with preexisting kidney or liver disorders should avoid supplementation. Chromium supplements interfere with iron absorption.

Drug interactions: None are well documented.

1. Althuis MD, Jordan NE, Ludington EA, et al: Glucose and insulin responses to dietary chromium supplements: a meta-analysis. *Am J Clin Nutr* 76(1):148–155, 2002.
2. Onakpoya I, Posadzki P, Ernst E: Chromium supplementation in overweight and obesity: a systematic review and meta-analysis of randomized clinical trials. *Obes Rev* 14(6):496–507, 2013.

COENZYME Q10

Coenzyme Q10 (CoQ10, ubiquinone) is an antioxidant, produced naturally in humans, that is also a cofactor for mitochondrial ATP generation. The levels of CoQ10 seem to be lower in older people and in people with chronic diseases, such as cardiac problems, cancer, Parkinson disease, diabetes, HIV/AIDS, and muscular dystrophies. However, it is not known whether these low levels contribute to these disorders. Rich dietary sources are meat, fish, and vegetable oils. Most trials recommended that the supplement dose range between 100 and 300 mg/day (eg, 100 mg tid).

Claims: CoQ10 is said to be useful because of its antioxidant effect and role in energy metabolism. Specific claims include an anticancer effect mediated by immune stimulation, decreased insulin requirements in patients with diabetes, slowed progression of Parkinson disease, efficacy in treatment of heart failure, and protection against anthracycline cardiotoxicity. The most prominent claim may be ameliorating endothelial cell dysfunction that contributes to cardiovascular disease. Although some preliminary studies suggest CoQ10 may be useful in treating these disorders, results are unclear and more testing is needed.

Evidence: A 2012 meta-analysis evaluated 5 randomized, controlled trials with a total of 194 patients and found a significant improvement in endothelial function, as measured by flow-mediated peripheral arterial dilation.[1] A 2013 meta-analysis of randomized controlled trials suggested that CoQ10 may improve functional status in patients with heart failure.[2] However, this meta-analysis consisted of trials mainly of small size and short duration of treatment.

A 2014 randomized, controlled, multicenter study of 420 patients with heart failure showed that CoQ10, 100 mg po tid, when added to standard therapy, was safe, relieved symptoms, and reduced major cardiovascular events.[3] In these meta-analyses, the doses and target blood levels of CoQ10 were not standardized, a further limitation.

Adverse effects: There are relatively few case reports of GI symptoms (eg, loss of appetite, abdominal pain, nausea, vomiting) and CNS symptoms (eg, dizziness, photophobia, irritability, headache). Other adverse effects include itching, rash, fatigue, and flu-like symptoms.

Drug interactions: CoQ10 may decrease response to warfarin.

1. Gao L, Mao Q, Cao J, et al: Effects of coenzyme Q10 on vascular endothelial function in humans: a meta-analysis of randomized controlled trials. *Atherosclerosis* 221(2):311–316, 2012.
2. Fotino AD, Thompson-Paul AM, Bazzano LA: Effect of coenzyme Q10 supplementation on heart failure: a meta-analysis. *Am J Clin Nutr* 97(2):268–275, 2013.
3. Mortensen SA, Rosenfeldt F, Kumar A, et al: The effect of coenzyme Q10 on morbidity and mortality in chronic heart failure results from Q-SYMBIO: a randomized double-blind trial. *JACC Heart Fail* 2(6):641–649, 2014. doi:10.1016/j.jchf.2014.06.008

CRANBERRY

Cranberries are fruit that can be consumed whole or made into food products such as jellies and juices.

Claims: People most often take cranberries to help prevent and relieve the symptoms of UTIs. The effectiveness of cranberries in preventing UTIs has not been confirmed. Natural unprocessed cranberry juice contains anthocyanidins, which prevent *Escherichia coli* from attaching to the urinary tract wall.

Some people take cranberry juice to reduce fever and treat certain cancers; however, there is no scientific proof that it is effective for these uses.

Evidence: In 1966 the first clinical trial, uncontrolled, evaluating the positive effects of cranberry juice in preventing UTIs was published.[1] Since that time numerous trials have been performed evaluating different populations, severity of medical conditions, dosages, time, and form of supplement in juice or extract capsule/tablet.

The majority of evidence suggests that cranberry juice or extract can have a small, yet significant effect on preventing the recurrence of UTIs over 12 mo, but that supplementation cannot treat UTIs.[2,3] However, a 2012 Cochrane review of

24 studies (4473 participants) has placed some doubt on the effectiveness of the supplement, indicating a small trend toward fewer UTIs with supplementation, but that the finding was not statistically significant.[4] Standardization of cranberry products may help to clarify results and resolve the discrepancy. Physiologic differences in the urinary tract and proper hygiene of female individuals studied also could contribute to the variability in response.

Adverse effects: No adverse effects are known. However, because most cranberry juice is highly sweetened to offset its tart taste, people with diabetes should not consume cranberry juice unless it is artificially sweetened. Because cranberry increases urinary acidity, it may promote stone formation in patients with uric acid kidney stones.

Drug interactions: Cranberry products may increase the effects of warfarin.

1. Papas PN, Brusch CA, Ceresia GC: Cranberry juice in the treatment of urinary tract infections. *Southwest Med* 47(1):17–20, 1966.
2. Jepson RG, Craig JC: A systematic review of the evidence for cranberries and blueberries in UTI prevention. *Mol Nutr Food Res* 51(6):738–745, 2007.
3. Stothers L: A randomized trial to evaluate effectiveness and cost effectiveness of naturopathic cranberry products as prophylaxis against urinary tract infection in women. *Can J Urol* 9(3):1558–1562, 2002.
4. Jepson RG, Williams G, Craig JC: Cranberries for preventing urinary tract infections. *Cochrane Database Syst Rev* 10:CD001321, 2012.

CREATINE

Phosphocreatine is a compound stored in muscle; it donates phosphate to ADP and thereby rapidly replenishes ATP during anaerobic muscle contraction. It is synthesized endogenously in the liver from arginine, glycine, and methionine. Dietary sources are milk, steak, and some fish.

Claims: Creatine is said to improve physical and athletic performance and to reduce muscle fatigue.

Evidence: Some evidence suggests creatine is effective at increasing work done in a short maximal effort (eg, sprinting, weightlifting). It has proven therapeutic use in muscle phosphorylase deficiency (glycogen storage disease type V [McArdle disease]) and gyrate atrophy of the choroid and retina; early data also suggest possible effects in Parkinson disease and amyotrophic lateral sclerosis.

Numerous clinical trials have demonstrated that creatine supplementation is well tolerated and may increase muscle mass. The effects can be seen in normal healthy people as well as a means of aiding in the treatment of muscle disorders and improving physical function and quality of life in patients with osteoarthritis.[1-3]

Adverse effects: Creatine may cause weight gain (possibly because of an increase in muscle mass) and spurious increases in serum creatinine levels. Minor GI symptoms, dehydration, electrolyte imbalance, and muscle cramps have been reported anecdotally.

Drug interactions: None are well documented.

1. Kley RA, Vorgerd M, Tarnopolsky MA: Creatine for treating muscle disorders. *Cochrane Database Syst Rev* (1): CD004760, 2007.
2. Branch JD: Effect of creatine supplementation on body composition and performance: a meta-analysis. *Int J Sport Nutr Exerc Metab* 13(2):198–226, 2003.
3. Neves M Jr, Gualano B, Roschel H, et al: Beneficial effect of creatine supplementation in knee osteoarthritis. *Med Sci Sports Exerc* 43(8):1538–1543, 2011.

DEHYDROEPIANDROSTERONE

Dehydroepiandrosterone (DHEA) is a steroid produced by the adrenal gland and is a precursor of estrogens and androgens. Effects on the body are similar to those of testosterone. DHEA can also be synthesized from precursors in the wild Mexican yam; this form is the most commonly available. However, consumption of wild yam is not recommended as a supplement as the body is unable to convert the precursors to DHEA.

Claims: DHEA supplements are said to improve mood, energy, sense of well-being, and the ability to function well under stress. They are also said to improve athletic performance, stimulate the immune system, deepen nightly sleep, lower cholesterol levels, decrease body fat, build muscles, reverse aging, improve brain function in patients with Alzheimer disease, increase libido, and decrease symptoms of systemic lupus erythematosus.

Evidence: The medicinal claims of DHEA have not been fully supported by the evidence. In addition, DHEA is banned by numerous professional sports organizations as it is classified as a "prohormone."

DHEA levels are known to naturally decrease with age and therefore people in search of the unattainable fountain of youth have turned to DHEA supplementation as a possible solution to ailments associated with age. Studies have been reported showing both positive and negative results. More thorough studies are warranted not only with aging but with all clinical health conditions.

A 2013 meta-analysis of data collected from studying 1353 elderly men in a number of trials indicated that DHEA supplementation was associated with a reduction of fat mass; however, no effect was observed for numerous other clinical parameters, including lipid and glycemic metabolism, bone health, sexual function, or quality of life.[1] A similar analysis was performed in women with adrenal insufficiency and indicated that DHEA supplementation may improve the quality of life and symptoms of depression, while having no effect on anxiety and sexual well-being.[2]

Adverse effects: Adverse effects are unclear. There are theoretical risks of gynecomastia in men, hirsutism in women, acne, and stimulation of prostate and breast cancer. There is a case report of mania and one of seizure.

Drug interactions: None are well documented.

1. Corona G, Rastrelli G, Giagulli V, et al: Dehydroepiandrosterone supplementation in elderly men: a meta-analysis study of placebo controlled trials. *J Clin Endocrinol Metab* 98(9):3615–3626, 2013.
2. Alkatib AA, Cosma M, Elamin MB, et al: A systematic review and meta-analysis of randomized placebo-controlled trials of DHEA treatment effects on quality of life in women with adrenal insufficiency. *J Clin Endocrinol Metab* 94(10):3676–3781, 2009.

ECHINACEA

Echinacea, a North American wildflower, contains a variety of biologically active substances.

Claims: Echinacea is said to stimulate the immune system. When taken at the start of a cold, it is said to shorten the duration of cold symptoms. Well-designed studies have not supported this effect.

Topical preparations are used to promote wound healing.

Evidence: Studies of echinacea's role in preventing and/or treating the common cold are inconsistent. The largest factor contributing to inconsistency is the variability of plant preparations (including different plant parts and species) and ultimately composition of the supplement. According to a 2006 Cochrane review, the aerial parts of the plant might be effective for the early treatment of colds; also, the other preparations of echinacea, might have a role in prevention of colds.[1] However, more meticulous randomized, controlled trials are necessary.

Adverse effects: Most adverse effects are mild and transitory; they include dizziness, fatigue, headache, and GI symptoms. No other adverse effects are known. Theoretically, echinacea is contraindicated in patients with autoimmune disorders, multiple sclerosis, AIDS, tuberculosis, and organ transplants because it may stimulate T cells. Echinacea inhibits some cytochrome P-450 enzymes and stimulates others; it can therefore potentially interact with drugs metabolized by the same enzymes (eg, anabolic steroids, azole antifungals, methotrexate). Allergic reactions are possible in patients with allergies to ragweed, chrysanthemum, marigold, daisies, or related allergens.

Drug interactions: Echinacea inhibits some cytochrome P-450 enzymes and stimulates others; it can therefore potentially interact with drugs metabolized by the same enzymes (eg, anabolic steroids, azole antifungals, methotrexate, etoposide, and other chemotherapeutic drugs).

1. Linde K, Barrett B, Wölkart K, et al: Echinacea for preventing and treating the common cold. *Cochrane Database Syst Rev* (1):CD000530, 2006.

FEVERFEW

Feverfew is a bushy perennial herb. The dried leaves are used in capsules, tablets, and liquid extracts. Parthenolides and glycosides are thought to be the components responsible for its purported anti-inflammatory effects and relaxant effects on smooth muscle.

Claims: Feverfew is said to be effective in the prevention of migraine headaches and useful for relieving menstrual pain, asthma, and arthritis. In vitro, feverfew inhibits platelet aggregation.[1]

Evidence: Three of 5 relatively small but well-designed studies of feverfew's effect on migraine headaches support its efficacy in prevention,[2-4] but 2 larger and better-designed studies do not.[5,6] Differences among study findings may result from differences in formulations of feverfew used and dosage. Evaluations of feverfew on rheumatoid arthritis are few. One study showed no apparent benefit from oral feverfew in rheumatoid arthritis.[7]

Adverse effects: Mouth ulcers, contact dermatitis, dysgeusia, and mild GI symptoms may occur. Abrupt discontinuation may worsen migraines and cause nervousness and insomnia. Feverfew is contraindicated in pregnant women as it may cause the uterus to contract.

Drug interactions: Theoretically, feverfew is contraindicated in patients taking other antimigraine drugs, iron supplements, NSAIDs, antiplatelet drugs, or warfarin.

1. Groenewegen WA, Heptinstall S: A comparison of the effects of an extract of feverfew and parthenolide, a component of feverfew, on human platelet activity in-vitro. *J Pharm Pharmacol* 42:553–557, 1990.
2. Johnson ES, Kadam NP, Hylands DM, et al: Efficacy of feverfew as prophylactic treatment of migraine. *Br Med J (Clin Res Ed)* 291:569–573, 1985.
3. Murphy JJ, Heptinstall S, Mitchell JR: Randomised, double-blind, placebo-controlled trial of feverfew in migraine prevention. *Lancet* 2:189–192, 1988.
4. Palevitch D, Earon G, Carasso R: Feverfew (*Tanacetum parthenium*) as a prophylactic treatment for migraine—a double-blind, placebo-controlled study. *Phytotherapy Res* 11:508–511, 1997.
5. Pfaffenrath V, Diener HC, Fischer M, et al: The efficacy and safety of *Tanacetum parthenium* (feverfew) in migraine prophylaxis—a double-blind, multicentre, randomized placebo-controlled dose-response study. *Cephalalgia* 22:523–532, 2002.
6. de Weerdt GJ, Bootsman HPR, Hendriks H: Herbal medicines in migraine prevention. Randomized double-blind, placebo-controlled, crossover trial of a feverfew preparation. *Phytomedicine* 3:225–230, 1996.
7. Pattrick M, Heptinstall S, Doherty M: Feverfew in rheumatoid arthritis: a double-blind, placebo-controlled study. *Ann Rheum Dis* 48:547–549, 1989.

FISH OIL

Fish oil may be consumed by eating fish, extracted directly, or concentrated and put in capsule form. Active ingredients are omega-3 fatty acids (eicosapentaenoic acid [EPA] and docosahexaenoic acid [DHA]). Recently, genetically engineered yeast strains that can naturally produce substantial amounts of these oils have been engineered and are providing another source.[1] Western diets typically are low in omega-3 fatty acids. (Other non-fish dietary sources of omega-3 fatty acids are walnuts and flaxseed oil.)

Claims: Fish oil is used for prevention and treatment of atherosclerotic cardiovascular disease, specifically by lowering TG levels. Mechanisms are probably multiple but unknown. Benefits are suspected, but not yet supported, for primary prevention of atherosclerotic cardiovascular disease, lowering of cholesterol levels, treatment of rheumatoid arthritis, lowering blood pressure, and prevention of cyclosporine nephrotoxicity.

Evidence: Strong evidence indicates that EPA/DHA (EPA plus DHA in various combinations) 800 to 1500 mg/day reduces risk of myocardial infarction and death due to arrhythmia in patients who have preexisting coronary artery disease and are taking conventional drugs.[2] EPA/DHA also reduces TGs in a dose-dependent way (eg, 25 to 40% with EPA/DHA 4 g/day) and slightly lowers blood pressure (2 to 4 mm Hg with EPA/DHA > 3 g/day).

Adverse effects: Fishy eructation, nausea, and diarrhea may occur. Risk of bleeding increases with EPA/DHA > 3 g/day. Concerns about mercury contamination are not substantiated in laboratory testing. Even so, pregnant or breastfeeding women should not take omega-3 fatty acid supplements extracted from fish and should limit consumption of certain types and amounts of fish because of the potential risk of mercury contamination.

Drug interactions: Fish oil is contraindicated in patients on antihypertensives as it may lower blood pressure more than physiologically desired. Fish oil ingestion may increase the anticoagulant effect of warfarin, therefore patients taking warfarin should avoid fish oil.[3]

1. Xue Z, Sharpe PL, Hong SP, et al.: Production of omega-3 eicosapentaenoic acid by metabolic engineering of *Yarrowia lipolytica*. *Nat Biotechnol* 31(8):734–740, 2013.
2. Agency for Healthcare Research and Quality: Effects of omega-3 fatty acids on lipids and glycemic control in type II diabetes and the metabolic syndrome and on inflammatory bowel disease, rheumatoid arthritis, renal disease, systemic lupus erythematosus, and osteoporosis. AHRQ Publication No. 04-E012-1; 2004.
3. Buckley MS, Goff AD, Knapp WE: Fish oil interaction with warfarin. *Ann Pharmacother* 38(1):50–52, 2004.

GARLIC

Garlic (*Allium sativum*) bulbs are extracted and made into tablet, powder, and oil forms; the major active ingredient is allicin or S-allylcysteine, an amino acid by-product. Garlic can also be eaten raw or cooked. Because the active ingredients are volatile and destroyed by the act of crushing, the amount of active ingredient in the various forms of garlic varies greatly. Supplements are best standardized by the amount of active compound. Aged garlic extract (AGE), made from garlic allowed to age for at least 20 mo, has more stable active compounds than most forms. Consuming garlic supplements in this form appears to confer the greatest health benefits and freedom from adverse effects.

Claims: Garlic is said to have favorable effects on several cardiac risk factors, including reduction of BP and serum lipid and glucose levels; garlic inhibits platelets in vitro. Garlic is also said to protect against laryngeal, gastric, colorectal, and endometrial cancer and adenomatous colorectal polyps.

Evidence: The strongest evidence available for garlic supplementation, specifically AGE, is lowering blood pressure. A double-blind, randomized, placebo-controlled, dose-response trial of 79 general practice patients with uncontrolled systolic hypertension evaluated the effect of AGE supplementation for 12 wk. The study indicated that daily supplementation of 240, 480, and 960 mg AGE containing 0.6, 1.2, and 2.4 mg of S-allylcysteine, respectively, significantly reduced mean systolic blood pressure compared to placebo.[1]

Results of the lipid-lowering effects of garlic supplementation have been quite inconsistent. A 2012 meta-analysis of 26 randomized, double-blind, placebo-controlled trials indicated that garlic supplementation was superior to placebo in reducing serum total cholesterol (TC) and TG levels. The authors suggested that garlic supplementation could reduce serum TC and TG levels and that garlic therapy could benefit patients with risk of cardiovascular diseases.[2]

Scientific evidence of either garlic intake or garlic supplement use shows limited or no protection against cancer or regulation of glucose. A prospective cohort study evaluating garlic intake in relation to colorectal cancer incidence did not find any protective effect.[3] Evaluation of garlic supplement and glucose regulation is limited with little to no human placebo-controlled trials.

Garlic consumed in high doses has general antimicrobial effects in vitro.[4]

Most of these studies lack the specific details with regard to the supplement and/or concentration of active ingredients in the supplement, which may account for the variable results.

Adverse effects: Breath and body smell and nausea may occur; high doses may cause burning in the mouth, esophagus, and stomach.

Drug interactions: Theoretically, garlic is contraindicated in patients who have bleeding diatheses or who take antihypertensives, antiplatelet drugs, or warfarin. Garlic can reduce serum saquinavir levels.

1. Ried K, Frank OR, Stocks NP: Aged garlic extract reduces blood pressure in hypertensives: a dose-response trial. *Eur J Clin Nutr* 67(1):64–70, 2013.
2. Zeng T, Guo FF, Zhang CL, et al: A meta-analysis of randomized, double-blind, placebo-controlled trials for the effects of garlic on serum lipid profiles. *J Sci Food Agric* 92(9):1892–1902, 2012.
3. Meng S, Zhang X, Giovannucci EL, et al: No association between garlic intake and risk of colorectal cancer. *Cancer Epidemiol* 37(2):152–155, 2013.
4. Filocamo A, Nueno-Palop C, Bisignano C, et al: Effect of garlic powder on the growth of commensal bacteria from the gastrointestinal tract. *Phytomedicine.* 19(8-9):707–711, 2012.

GINGER

Ginger root (*Zingiber officinale*) is extracted and made into tablet form or can be used fresh, dried, or as a juice or oil. Active ingredients include gingerols (which give ginger its flavor and odor) and shogaols.

Claims: Ginger is said to be an effective antiemetic and antinauseant, especially for nausea caused by motion sickness or pregnancy, and to relieve intestinal cramps. Ginger is also used as an anti-inflammatory and analgesic.

Evidence: Ginger may have antibacterial properties and antiplatelet effects in vitro, but data are inconsistent.

Meta-analyses have suggested possible benefits of ginger in the control of postoperative[1] and pregnancy-related nausea and vomiting,[2] but no benefit for chemotherapy-induced nausea and vomiting.[3]

Ginger's anti-inflammatory and analgesic properties are less well supported. However, a review of 8 trials (481 participants) indicates a potential anti-inflammatory effect, which may reduce pain in some conditions, such as osteoarthritis.[4]

Adverse effects: Ginger is usually not harmful, although some people have a burning sensation when they eat it. Nausea, dyspepsia, and dysgeusia are possible.

Drug interactions: Theoretically, ginger is contraindicated in patients who have bleeding diatheses or who take antiplatelet drugs or warfarin.

1. Chaiyakunapruk N, Kitikannakorn N, Nathisuwan S, et al: The efficacy of ginger for the prevention of postoperative nausea and vomiting: a meta-analysis. *Am J Obstet Gynecol* 194(1):95–99, 2006.
2. Matthews A, Dowswell T, Haas DM, et al: Interventions for nausea and vomiting in early pregnancy. *Cochrane Database Syst Rev* (9):CD007575, 2010.
3. Lee J, Oh H: Ginger as an antiemetic modality for chemotherapy-induced nausea and vomiting: a systematic review and meta-analysis. *Oncol Nurs Forum* 40(2):163–170, 2013.
4. Terry R, Posadzki P, Watson LK, et al: The use of ginger (*Zingiber officinale*) for the treatment of pain: a systematic review of clinical trials. *Pain Med* 12(12):1808–1818, 2011.

GINKGO

Ginkgo (*Ginkgo biloba*) is prepared from leaves of the ginkgo tree (commonly planted in the US for ornamental purposes and botanically unique as it is the only surviving member of its family). Active ingredients are believed to be terpene ginkgolides and flavonoids.

The fruit of the gingko tree, which is quite malodorous, is not used in ginkgo products. Contact with the fruit pulp, which may be present under female ginkgo trees, can cause severe skin inflammation (dermatitis). The raw seeds of the fruit are toxic and can cause seizures and, in large amounts, death. Cooked ginkgo seeds are eaten in Asia and are available in Asian food shops in the US; because the seeds do not contain ginkgolides and flavonoids, they do not have known therapeutic effects.

Claims: Ginkgo leaf products are used for minor symptomatic relief of claudication, although exercise and cilostazol may be more effective. Gingko increases the distance that affected people can walk without pain.

Ginkgo has long been used in people with dementia. Gingko has also been used to alleviate memory loss, tinnitus, age-related macular degeneration, and altitude sickness. Gingko may prevent damage to the kidneys caused by the immunosuppressant cyclosporine.

Evidence: Ginkgo is thought to be a vasoactive agent. Although patients with intermittent claudication may be able to walk longer than placebo-treated patients, this benefit is quite minor according to a 2013 Cochrane review. This review looked at 14 trials with a total of 739 participants, of which 11 trials (477 participants) compared *Ginkgo biloba* to placebo.[1]

Early studies indicated that ginkgo temporarily stabilized mental and social function in people with mild-to-moderate dementia. However, recent large clinical trials showed that ginkgo supplementation (EGb 761) did not delay the development and progression of dementia and Alzheimer disease in older people.[2-4] It is obvious that further studies are warranted with regard to the clinical use of this supplement for dementia.

A 2013 Cochrane review of 2 studies suggested a potential role for ginkgo in slowing the progression of age-related macular degeneration.[5] A standard ginkgo extract compared to placebo was used in both studies, in which 119 people took the supplement for 6 mo. Future large-scale trials for longer periods of time are warranted before claims are supported.

A few small clinical trials suggest ginkgo may help relieve tinnitus[6] and prevent altitude sickness in some patients;[7,8] however, the effects are somewhat inconsistent and the source and composition of ginkgo extract may determine efficacy.

Adverse effects: Nausea, dyspepsia, headache, dizziness, and heart palpitations may occur.

Drug interactions: Ginkgo may interact with aspirin, other NSAIDs, and warfarin; it also may reduce the efficacy of anticonvulsants.

1. Nicolaï SP, Kruidenier LM, Bendermacher BL, et al: *Ginkgo biloba* for intermittent claudication. *Cochrane Database Syst Rev* 6: CD006888, 2013.
2. Vellas B, Coley N, Ousset PJ, et al: GuidAge Study Group. Long-term use of standardised *Ginkgo biloba* extract for the prevention of Alzheimer's disease (GuidAge): a randomised placebo-controlled trial. *Lancet Neurol* 11(10):851–859, 2012.
3. Snitz BE, O'Meara ES, Carlson MC, et al: Ginkgo Evaluation of Memory (GEM) Study Investigators. *Ginkgo biloba* for preventing cognitive decline in older adults: a randomized trial. *JAMA* 302(24): 2663–2670, 2009.
4. DeKosky ST, Williamson JD, Fitzpatrick AL, et al: Ginkgo Evaluation of Memory (GEM) Study Investigators. *Ginkgo biloba* for prevention of dementia: a randomized controlled trial. *JAMA* 300(19): 2253–2262, 2008.
5. Evans JR: *Ginkgo biloba* extract for age-related macular degeneration. *Cochrane Database Syst Rev* 31; 1:CD001775, 2013.
6. von Boetticher A: *Ginkgo biloba* extract in the treatment of tinnitus: a systematic review. *Neuropsychiatr Dis Treat* 7:441–447, 2011.
7. Moraga FA, Flores A, Serra J, et al: *Ginkgo biloba* decreases acute mountain sickness in people ascending to high altitude at Ollagüe (3696 m) in northern Chile. *Wilderness Environ Med* 18(4):251–257, 2007.
8. Leadbetter G, Keyes LE, Maakestad KM, et al: *Ginkgo biloba* does—and does not—prevent acute mountain sickness. *Wilderness Environ Med* 20(1):66–71, 2009.

GINSENG

Ginseng is a family of plants. Dietary supplements are derived from American ginseng (*Panax quinquefolius*) or Asian ginseng (*Panax ginseng*). Siberian ginseng (*Eleutherococcus senticosus*) is a different genus and does not contain the ingredients believed to be active in the 2 forms used in supplements.

Ginseng can be taken as fresh or dried roots, extracts, solutions, capsules, tablets, sodas, and teas or used as cosmetics. Active ingredients in American ginseng are panaxosides (saponin glycosides). Active ingredients in Asian ginseng are ginsenosides (triterpenoid glycosides).

Many ginseng products contain little or no detectable active ingredient. In very few cases, some ginseng products from Asia have been purposefully mixed with mandrake root, which has been used to induce vomiting, or with the drugs phenylbutazone or aminopyrine. These drugs have been removed from the US market because of significant adverse effects.

Claims: Ginseng is said to enhance physical (including sexual) and mental performance and to have adaptogenic effects (ie, to increase energy and resistance to the harmful effects of stress and aging). Other claims include reduction in plasma glucose levels; increases in high-density lipoprotein (HDL), Hb, and protein levels; stimulation of the immune system; and anticancer, cardiotonic, endocrine, CNS, and estrogenic effects. Another claim is possible beneficial effects on immune function.

Evidence: Studies of ginseng have all been limited, for example, by small size and number. Such studies have shown

- Enhancement of immune function[1]
- Anticarcinogenic effects[2]
- Decreases in blood glucose[3]
- Improvement of cognitive function[3-5]

A Canadian study showed that a polysaccharide extract of *P. quinquefolius* helped prevent colds.[6] A 2010 Cochrane review of 9 randomized, double-blind, placebo-controlled trials evaluated the efficacy and adverse effects of ginseng supplementation taken to improve cognitive function in healthy participants (8 trials) and those with age-associated memory impairment.[5] The analysis found no serious adverse events with ginseng supplementation, but there was no convincing evidence for enhanced cognitive function in healthy participants or people with diagnosed dementia.

Larger trials are needed to evaluate the effectiveness of ginseng. Also, further evaluation of the compounds found in the supplements is necessary to determine the components responsible for the observed beneficial effects. There is no evidence supporting other health claims for ginseng.

Adverse effects: Nervousness and excitability may occur but decrease after the first few days. Ability to concentrate may decrease, and plasma glucose may become abnormally low (causing hypoglycemia). Because ginseng has an estrogen-like effect, women who are pregnant or breastfeeding should not take it, nor should children. Occasionally, there are reports of more serious effects, such as asthma attacks, increased blood pressure, palpitations, and, in postmenopausal women, uterine bleeding. To many people, ginseng tastes unpleasant.

Drug interactions: Ginseng can interact with antihyperglycemic drugs, aspirin, other NSAIDs, corticosteroids, digoxin, estrogens, monoamine oxidase inhibitors and warfarin.

1. Assinewe VA, Amason JT, Aubry A, et al: Extractable polysaccharides of *Panax quinquefolius L.* (North American ginseng) root stimulate TNF-alpha production by alveolar macrophages. *Phytomedicine* 9(5):398–404, 2002.
2. Yun TK: Experimental and epidemiological evidence on non-organ specific cancer preventive effect of Korean ginseng and identification of active compounds. *Mutat Res* 523-524:63–74, 2003.
3. Reay JL, Kennedy DO, Scholey AB. Single doses of *Panax ginseng* (G115) reduce blood glucose levels and improve cognitive performance during sustained mental activity. *J Psychopharmacol* 19(4):357–365, 2005.
4. Kim J, Chung SY, Park S, et al: Enhancing effect of HT008-1 on cognitive function and quality of life in cognitively declined healthy adults: a randomized, double-blind, placebo-controlled, trial. *Pharmacol Biochem Behav* 90(4):517–524, 2008.
5. Geng J, Dong J, Ni H, et al: Ginseng for cognition. *Cochrane Database Syst Rev* (12):CD007769, 2010.
6. Predy GN, Goel V, Lovlin R, et al: Efficacy of an extract of North American ginseng containing poly-furanosyl-pyranosyl-saccharides for preventing upper respiratory tract infections: a randomized controlled trial. *CMAJ* 173(9):1043–1048, 2005.

GLUCOSAMINE

Glucosamine is a precursor of multiple cartilage constituents. It is extracted from chitin (in shells of crabs, oysters, and shrimp) and is taken in tablet or capsule form, usually as glucosamine sulfate, but sometimes as glucosamine hydrochloride. Efforts are being made to find alternative biorenewable sources including metabolically engineered fungi and *E. coli*.[1] Glucosamine is often taken with chondroitin sulfate.

Claims: Glucosamine is claimed to relieve pain due to osteoarthritis, possibly with both analgesic and disease-modifying effects. Mechanism is unknown. Mechanism for glucosamine sulfate may be related to improved glycosaminoglycan synthesis as a result of the sulfate moiety. Dosage of glucosamine in all its forms is 500 mg po tid.

Evidence: Evidence supports use of glucosamine sulfate from Rotta Research Laboratorium for treatment of mild-to-moderate osteoarthritis of the knee when given for at least 6 mo.[2,3] Other formulations still need to be rigorously evaluated. The role of glucosamine sulfate in the treatment of more severe knee osteoarthritis and osteoarthritis in other locations is less well-defined. The Glucosamine/Chondroitin Arthritis Intervention Trial (GAIT), a randomized, double-blinded, placebo-controlled, multicenter clinical trial of 1583 patients with symptomatic osteoarthritis of the knee reported that, alone and in combination with chondroitin sulfate (400 mg tid), glucosamine hydrochloride (500 mg tid) did not reduce pain effectively in the all-patient group. However, an exploratory analysis found pain relief with combination therapy in a subgroup of patients with moderate-to-severe knee pain.[4]

A recent review of randomized control trials evaluating the effect of glucosamine on chronic low back pain concluded that data were insufficient to demonstrate or exclude benefits of glucosamine.[5]

Adverse effects: Allergy (in patients who have shellfish allergy and take forms extracted from shellfish), dyspepsia, fatigue, insomnia, headache, photosensitivity, and nail changes may occur. Patients with chronic liver disease should also avoid glucosamine if possible, because of potential hepatotoxicity when taking glucosamine with or without chondroitin.[6]

Drug interactions: No definitive interactions are known.

1. Liu L, Liu Y, Shin HD, et al: Microbial production of glucosamine and N-acetylglucosamine: advances and perspectives. *Appl Microbiol Biotechnol* 97(14):6149–6158, 2013.
2. Wu D, Huang Y, Gu Y, et al: Efficacies of different preparations of glucosamine for the treatment of osteoarthritis: a meta-analysis of randomised, double-blind, placebo-controlled trials. *Int J Clin Pract* 67(6):585–594, 2013.
3. Towheed TE, Maxwell L, Anastassiades TP, et al: Glucosamine therapy for treating osteoarthritis. *Cochrane Database Syst Rev* (2):CD002946, 2005.
4. Clegg DO, Reda DJ, Harris CL, et al: Glucosamine, chondroitin sulfate, and the two in combination for painful knee osteoarthritis. *N Engl J Med* 354(8):795–808, 2006.
5. Sodha R, Sivanadarajah N, Alam M: The use of glucosamine for chronic low back pain: a systematic review of randomised control trials. *BMJ Open* 3(6). pii, 2013.
6. Cerda C, Bruguera M, Parés A: Hepatotoxicity associated with glucosamine and chondroitin sulfate in patients with chronic liver disease. *World J Gastroenterol* 19(32):5381–5384, 2013.

GOLDENSEAL

Goldenseal, an endangered US plant, is related to the buttercup (*Hydrastis canadensis*). Its active components are hydrastine and berberine, which have antiseptic activity. Goldenseal is available in liquid, tablet, and capsule forms standardized to the active components.

Claims: Various preparations of goldenseal are used as an antiseptic wash for mouth sores, inflamed and sore eyes, and irritated skin and as a douche for vaginal infections. It has been combined with echinacea as a cold remedy. Goldenseal is also used as a remedy for indigestion and diarrhea.

Evidence: Efficacy of goldenseal alone as a cold remedy has not been supported.[1] In 2 relatively well-designed but small studies, berberine isolated from goldenseal reduced diarrhea.[2,3] However, there are few, if any, recent, large, randomized, blinded clinical trials of goldenseal extract.

Adverse effects: Goldenseal can have many adverse effects, including nausea, anxiety, dyspepsia, uterine contractions, jaundice in neonates, and worsening of hypertension. If taken in large amounts, goldenseal can cause seizures and respiratory failure and may affect contraction of the heart. Women who are pregnant or breastfeeding, neonates, and people who have seizure disorders or problems with blood clotting should not take goldenseal. A recent in vitro study of the active ingredients of goldenseal, specifically berberine, indicates an increased risk of DNA damage leading to tumorigenic effects.[4]

Drug interactions: Goldenseal may interact with warfarin, and berberine may reduce the anticoagulant effect of heparin. In addition, a recent review of herbal extracts indicates that goldenseal, particularly berberine, is a weak inhibitor of CYP3A4 and CYP2D6 enzymes, which are important in the metabolism and elimination of many drugs.[5]

1. Rehman J, Dillow JM, Carter SM, et al: Increased production of antigen-specific immunoglobulins G and M following in vivo treatment with the medicinal plants *Echinacea angustifolia* and *Hydrastis canadensis*. *Immunol Lett* 68(2-3):391–395, 1999.
2. Khin-Maung-U, Myo-Khin, Nyunt-Nyunt-Wai, et al: Clinical trial of berberine in acute watery diarrhoea. *Br Med J (Clin Res Ed)* 291(6509):1601–1605, 1995.
3. Rabbani GH, Butler T, Knight J, et al: Randomized controlled trial of berberine sulfate therapy for diarrhea due to enterotoxigenic *Escherichia coli* and *Vibrio cholerae*. *J Infect Dis* 155(5):979–984, 1987.
4. Chen S, Wan L, Couch L, et al: Mechanism study of goldenseal-associated DNA damage. *Toxicol Lett* 221(1):64–72, 2013.
5. Hermann R, von Richter O: Clinical evidence of herbal drugs as perpetrators of pharmacokinetic drug interactions. *Planta Med* 78(13):1458–1477, 2012.

GREEN TEA

Green tea is made from the dried leaves of the same plant (*Camellia sinensis*) as traditional tea, an evergreen shrub native to Asia. However, traditional tea leaves are fermented, and green tea leaves are steamed but unfermented. Green tea may be brewed and drunk or ingested in extracted tablet or capsule form. It has multiple components that are thought to have antioxidant and anticancer effects. Green tea contains polyphenols and catechins as well as caffeine, but green tea is known to have lower amounts of caffeine than coffee, and many extracts have been decaffeinated.

Claims: Green tea is said to have multiple health benefits, few of which are supported by strong scientific evidence. It has been used to treat genital warts, increase mental alertness (because of its caffeine), prevent cancer, help in weight loss, reduce serum lipids, prevent coronary artery disease, enhance memory, relieve osteoarthritis pain, treat menopausal symptoms, and contribute to longevity.

Evidence: Green tea, the drink and the extract, is one of the most highly studied supplements on the market; however, the beneficial clinical evidence for the drink is limited. Recently, certain active ingredients found in green tea (sinecatechins, trade names Veregen and Polyphenon E) have been approved for the treatment of genital warts due to human papillomavirus infection. A randomized controlled study indicated that the defined extract (55% epigallocatechin gallate) is efficacious and safe for genital and perianal warts.[1] Another study indicated that the treatment with the green tea–derived extract yielded a lower cost of treatment compared to traditional pharmaceutical treatments.[2]

Numerous meta-analyses of the clinical trials available indicate that green tea is safe for moderate and regular consumption. In addition, small, most often nonsignificant, benefits are seen for weight loss and cardiovascular disease prevention, while there is insufficient and often conflicting evidence for any benefit from consumption of green tea for cancer prevention.[3-6] Further, more rigorously designed large scale clinical trials are needed before claims can be confirmed. Possibly confounding evidence from population studies is that in nations in which green tea is regularly consumed, other cultural, behavioral, or genetic factors may contribute to good health.

Adverse effects: Adverse effects are related to effects of caffeine. They include insomnia, anxiety, tachycardia, and mild tremor. Pregnant women should avoid excessive caffeine.

Drug interactions: Vitamin K in green tea may antagonize the anticoagulant effect of warfarin.

1. Stockfleth E, Beti H, Orasan R, et al: Topical Polyphenon E in the treatment of external genital and perianal warts: a randomized controlled trial. *Br J Dermatol* 158(6):1329–1338, 2008.
2. Langley PC: A cost-effectiveness analysis of sinecatechins in the treatment of external genital warts. *J Med Econ* 13(1):1–7, 2010.
3. Boehm K, Borrelli F, Ernst E, et al: Green tea (*Camellia sinensis*) for the prevention of cancer. *Cochrane Database Syst Rev* 8(3):CD005004, 2009.
4. Sturgeon JL, Williams M, van Servellen G: Efficacy of green tea in the prevention of cancers. *Nurs Health Sci* 11(4):436–446, 2009.
5. Jurgens TM, Whelan AM, Killian L, et al: Green tea for weight loss and weight maintenance in overweight or obese adults. *Cochrane Database Syst Rev*. 12: CD008650, 2012.
6. Hartley L, Flowers N, Holmes J, et al: Green and black tea for the primary prevention of cardiovascular disease. *Cochrane Database Syst Rev* 6:CD009934, 2013.

KAVA

Kava comes from the root of a shrub (*Piper methysticum*) that grows in the South Pacific. It is ingested as a tea or in capsule form. Active ingredients are thought to be kavalactones.

Claims: Strong scientific evidence supports use of kava as an anxiolytic and sleep aid. Mechanism is unknown. Some people use kava for asthma, menopausal symptoms, and UTIs. Dose is 100 mg of standardized extract tid.

Evidence: A 2003 Cochrane review evaluated 11 trials (total of 645 participants) to assess the effectiveness and safety of kava extract in clinical trials for treating anxiety. The meta-analysis concluded that kava extract appears to be an effective option for relieving anxiety compared to placebo.[1] This study also concluded that consumption of kava supplements for 1 to 24 wk appeared safe but suggested a need to study long-term safety. It is unclear how the supplements used in the meta-analysis above was standardized. Standardization of kava supplements to the active ingredient kavalactones (3 to 20%) should be included in future clinical trials.

Adverse effects: Since 1999 several cases of liver toxicity (including liver failure) in both Europe and the US after taking kava have prompted the FDA to mandate a warning label on kava products.[2] Safety is under continuing surveillance.

When kava is prepared traditionally (as tea) and used in high doses (> 6 to 12 g/day of dried root) or over long periods (up to 6 wk), there have been reports of scaly skin rash (kava dermopathy), blood changes (eg, macrocytosis, leukopenia), and neurologic changes (eg, torticollis, oculogyric crisis, worsening of Parkinson disease, movement disorders).

Drug interactions: Kava may prolong the effect of other sedatives (eg, barbiturates), which could affect driving or other activities requiring alertness.

1. Pittler MH, Ernst E: Kava extract for treating anxiety. *Cochrane Database Syst Rev* (1):CD003383, 2003.
2. Center for Food Safety and Applied Nutrition: Kava-containing dietary supplements may be associated with severe liver injury. United States Food and Drug Administration, 2002.

LICORICE

Natural licorice, which has a very sweet taste, is extracted from the root of a shrub (*Glycyrrhiza glabra*) and used medicinally as a capsule, tablet, or liquid extract. Most licorice candy made in the US is flavored artificially and does not contain natural licorice. Glycyrrhizin is the active ingredient in natural licorice. For people who are particularly sensitive to the effects of glycyrrhizin, specially treated licorice products that contain a much lower amount of glycyrrhizin (about one tenth) are available. These products are called deglycyrrhizinated licorice.

Claims: People most often take licorice to suppress coughs, to soothe a sore throat, and to relieve stomach upset. Applied externally, it is said to soothe skin irritation (eg, eczema). Licorice has also been claimed to help treat stomach ulcers and complications caused by hepatitis C.

Evidence: Evidence indicates that licorice in combination with other herbs provides relief from the symptoms of functional dyspepsia and irritable bowel syndrome.[1] However, clinical trials of both licorice alone and in combination are limited, and further evaluation is required. There are not enough data to determine whether licorice is effective for stomach ulcers or complications caused by hepatitis C.

Adverse effects: At lower dosages or normal consumption levels, few adverse reactions are evident. However, high doses of real licorice (> 1 oz/day) and glycyrrhizin cause renal sodium and water retention, possibly leading to high blood pressure, and potassium excretion, possibly causing low potassium levels (pseudoaldosteronism). Increased potassium excretion can be a particular problem for people who have heart disease and for those who take digoxin or diuretics that also increase potassium excretion. Such people and those who have high blood pressure should avoid taking licorice.

Licorice may increase the risk of premature delivery; thus, pregnant women should avoid licorice.

Drug interactions: Licorice may interact with warfarin and decrease its effectiveness, increasing the risk of blood clotting. As mentioned above, licorice may interact with digoxin by affecting potassium levels.

1. Ottillinger B, Storr M, Malfertheiner P, et al: STW 5 (Iberogast®)—a safe and effective standard in the treatment of functional gastrointestinal disorders. *Wien Med Wochenschr* 163(3-4): 65–72, 2013.

MELATONIN

Melatonin, a hormone produced by the pineal gland, regulates circadian rhythms. It can be derived from animals, but most melatonin is manufactured synthetically. In some countries, melatonin is considered a drug and is regulated as such.

Claims: Melatonin is used for the short-term regulation of sleep patterns, including jet lag and insomnia. Research into the use of melatonin supplementation for people affected by seasonal affective disorder, regulation of sleep patterns in people who work late shifts, and the resynchronization of the sleep/wake cycle in people with early Alzheimer disease is currently being evaluated.

Evidence: Some scientific evidence supports use of melatonin to minimize the effects of jet lag, especially in people traveling eastward over 2 to 5 time zones.[1,2] However, in one well-designed study, melatonin supplements did not relieve symptoms of jet lag,[3] and only a few small studies suggest that these supplements can relieve jet lag symptoms,[4,5] indicating that clinical trial results are inconsistent.

Standard dosage is not established and ranges from 0.5 to 5 mg po taken 1 h before usual bedtime on the day of travel and 2 to 4 nights after arrival. Evidence supporting use of melatonin as a sleep aid in adults and children with neuropsychiatric disorders (eg, pervasive developmental disorders) is less strong.

Adverse effects: Hangover drowsiness, headache, and transient depression may occur. Melatonin may worsen depression. Theoretically, prion infection caused by products derived from neurologic tissues of animals is a risk.

Drug interactions: Evidence suggests that melatonin may increase the effects of warfarin, increasing the risk of bleeding.

1. Herxheimer A, Petrie KJ: Melatonin for the prevention and treatment of jet lag. *Cochrane Database Syst Rev* (2):CD001520, 2002.
2. Buscemi N, Vandermeer B, Pandya R, et al: Melatonin for Treatment of Sleep Disorders. AHRQ Publication No. 05-E002-2, 2004.
3. Edwards BJ, Atkinson G, Waterhouse J, et al: Use of melatonin in recovery from jet-lag following an eastward flight across 10 time-zones. *Ergonomics* 43(10):1501–1513, 2000.
4. Claustrat B, Brun J, David M, et al: Melatonin and jet lag: confirmatory result using a simplified protocol. *Biol Psychiatry* 3(8):705–711, 1992.
5. Petrie K, Dawson AG, Thompson L, et al: A double-blind trial of melatonin as a treatment for jet lag in international cabin crew. *Biol Psychiatry* 33(7):526–530, 1993.

MILK THISTLE

(Silymarin)

Milk thistle (*Silybum marianum*) is a purple-flowered plant. Its sap and seeds contain the active ingredient silymarin, a potent antioxidant and a term often used interchangeably with milk thistle. Silymarin can be further divided into 3 primary flavonoids: silybin, silydianin, and silychristin. Extracts of milk thistle should be standardized to 80 percent silymarin.

Claims: Milk thistle is said to treat cirrhosis and to protect the liver from viral hepatitis, the damaging effects of alcohol, and hepatotoxic drugs.[1] Milk thistle may also improve glycemic control in type 2 diabetes[2] and individual case reports claim fatality reduction in mushroom poisoning.[3]

Evidence: A 2007 Cochrane review of 13 randomized clinical trials assessed milk thistle in 915 patients with alcoholic and/or hepatitis B or C virus liver diseases.[4] Data from this analysis determined that intervention had no significant effect on all-cause mortality, complications of liver disease, or liver histology. When all trials were included in the analysis, liver-related mortality was significantly reduced; however, in an analysis limited to high-quality studies, this reduction was not significant. Milk thistle was not associated with a significant increase in adverse effects. The design of these clinical trials did come into question, and the authors questioned the benefits of milk thistle and suggested the need for more well-designed placebo-controlled studies. In vitro, silymarin increases levels of intrahepatic glutathione, an antioxidant important for detoxification.[5]

Another recent analysis of 9 randomized, placebo-controlled trials (487 patients)[2] indicates that milk thistle may improve glycemic control in type 2 diabetes; however, the studies were small and therefore further high-quality, large controlled trials using standardized preparation are needed before beneficial claims are justified.

Recently, 2 cases of Amanita mushroom ingestion poisoning[3] showed favorable results after treatment with silybin.

Adverse effects: No serious adverse effects have been reported. Women who have hormone-sensitive conditions (eg, breast, uterine, and ovarian cancer; endometriosis; uterine fibroids) should avoid the above-ground parts of milk thistle.

Drug interactions: Milk thistle may intensify the effects of antihyperglycemic drugs[6] and may interfere with indinavir therapy.[7] Silybin inhibits phase 1 and 2 enzymes and inactivates cytochromes P450 3A4 and 2C9.

1. Loguercio C and Festi D: Silybin and the liver: from basic research to clinical practice. *World J Gastroenterol* 17(18):2288–2301, 2011.
2. Suksomboon N, Poolsup N, Boonkaew S, et al: Meta-analysis of the effect of herbal supplement on glycemic control in type 2 diabetes. *J Ethnopharmacol* 137(3):1328–1333, 2011.
3. Ward J, Kapadia K, Brush E, et al: Amatoxin poisoning: case reports and review of current therapies. *J Emerg Med* 44(1):116–121, 2013.
4. Rambaldi A, Jacobs BP, Gluud C: Milk thistle for alcoholic and/or hepatitis B or C virus liver diseases. *Cochrane Database Syst Rev* (4)CD003620, 2007.
5. Valenzuela A, Aspillaga M, Vial S, et al: Selectivity of silymarin on the increase of the glutathione content in different tissues of the rat. *Planta Med* 55(5):420–422, 1989.
6. Wu JW, Lin LC, Tsai TH: Drug-drug interactions of silymarin on the perspective of pharmacokinetics. *J Ethnopharmacol* 121(2):185–193, 2009.
7. van den Bout-van den Beukel CJ, Koopmans PP, van der Ven AJ, et al: Possible drug-metabolism interactions of medicinal herbs with antiretroviral agents. *Drug Metab Rev* 38(3):477–514, 2006.

S-ADENOSYL-L-METHIONINE

(SAMe)

S-Adenosyl-L-methionine (SAMe) is a derivative of methionine and a cofactor for multiple synthetic pathways, particularly as a methyl group donor. It is produced naturally in the body, mainly by the liver, and is manufactured synthetically in supplement form.

Claims: SAMe is said to be effective for treatment of depression,[1,2] osteoarthritis,[3-5] cholestasis,[6] and liver disorders.[7] In addition, mechanistically SAMe has been shown to be a platelet inhibitor.[8]

Evidence: The clinical studies evaluating the health benefits of SAMe either are very small, lacking in proper methodology, or yield conflicting results among different trials. However, a 2002 meta-analysis of osteoarthritis patients indicated that SAMe was more effective than placebo in reducing functional limitations associated with osteoarthritis.[5] More importantly, in 2 studies evaluated in this analysis, SAMe (1200 mg/day, eg, at 600 mg po bid) was as efficacious as nonsteroidal anti-inflammatory drugs (NSAIDs), but without the adverse effects common with NSAID use. More high-quality studies are needed with standardized supplements before recommendations can be made for the supplementation of SAMe for the treatment of depression, liver disorders, and osteoarthritis.

Adverse effects: No serious adverse effects have been reported with dosages between 200 and 1200 mg/day. SAMe is contraindicated in patients with bipolar disorder because SAMe can precipitate manic episodes.

Drug interactions: Some care should be taken with antidepressant drugs taken in combination with SAMe as both will increase serotonin levels, potentially resulting in adverse effects such as rapid heart rate and anxiety.

1. Papakostas GI: Evidence for S-adenosyl-L-methionine (SAM-e) for the treatment of major depressive disorder. *J Clin Psychiatry* 70(Suppl 5):18–22, 2009.
2. Turner P, Kantaria R, Young AH: A systematic review and meta-analysis of the evidence base for add-on treatment for patients with major depressive disorder who have not responded to antidepressant treatment: A European perspective. *J Psychopharmacol* 28(2):85–98, 2014.
3. Rutjes AW, Nüesch E, Reichenbach S, et al: S-Adenosylmethionine for osteoarthritis of the knee or hip. *Cochrane Database Syst Rev* (4) CD007321, 2009.
4. De Silva V, El-Metwally A, Ernst E, et al: Arthritis Research UK Working Group on Complementary and Alternative Medicines. Evidence for the efficacy of complementary and alternative medicines in the management of osteoarthritis: a systematic review. *Rheumatology (Oxford)* 50(5):911–920, 2011.
5. Soeken KL, Lee WL, Bausell RB, et al: Safety and efficacy of S-adenosylmethionine (SAMe) for osteoarthritis. *J Fam Pract* 51(5):425–430, 2002.
6. Gurung V, Middleton P, Milan SJ, et al: Interventions for treating cholestasis in pregnancy. *Cochrane Database Syst Rev* 6:CD000493, 2013.
7. Rambaldi A, Gluud C: S-adenosyl-L-methionine for alcoholic liver diseases. *Cochrane Database Syst Rev* (2):CD002235, 2006.
8. De la Cruz JP, Mérida M, González-Correa JA, et al: Effects of S-adenosyl-L-methionine on blood platelet activation. *Gen Pharmacol* 29(4):651–655, 1997.

SAW PALMETTO

Saw palmetto (*Serenoa repens, Serenoa serrulata*) berries contain the plant's active ingredients. The active ingredients, thought to be fatty acids, seem to inhibit 5-alpha-reductase, thus opposing the conversion of testosterone to dihydrotestosterone. The berries can be used to make a tea, or they can be extracted into tablets, capsules, or a liquid preparation. Most formulations evaluated in clinical studies are hexane extracts of saw palmetto berries, which are 80 to 90% essential fatty acids and phytosterols.

Claims: Many men report use of saw palmetto to treat symptoms (eg, frequent urination) of benign prostatic hyperplasia (BPH). Additional claims are that saw palmetto increases sperm production, breast size, and sexual vigor. Dose is 320 mg once/day or 160 mg bid.

Evidence: There is no scientific evidence to suggest that saw palmetto reverses BPH. A double-blind, multicenter, placebo-controlled randomized trial of 369 men found that increasing doses of a saw palmetto fruit extract did not reduce lower urinary tract symptoms more than placebo.[1] In addition, a 2012 Cochrane review of 32 randomized, controlled trials, determined that saw palmetto, at double and triple doses, did not improve urinary flow measures or prostate size in men with lower urinary tract symptoms consistent with BPH.[2] Claims that saw palmetto increases sperm production, breast size, or sexual vigor are unsupported.

Adverse effects: Headache and diarrhea may occur, but few serious adverse effects have been reported. One case report of a 58-yr-old white man taking 900 mg of dried extract and 660 mg of berry powder to ease the symptoms of BPH reported acute liver damage due to saw palmetto.[3] Another report of a 65-yr-old male indicated that supplementation with saw palmetto may have been responsible for acute pancreatitis.[4]

Saw palmetto may interact with estrogens; thus, women who are pregnant or who may become pregnant should not take it.

Drug interactions: No interactions have been reported for saw palmetto;[5] however, although strong evidence is not available, patients on warfarin should be careful when considering or taking saw palmetto because of a possible risk of hepatotoxicity.

1. Barry MJ, Meleth S, Lee JY, et al: Complementary and Alternative Medicine for Urological Symptoms (CAMUS) Study Group. Effect of increasing doses of saw palmetto extract on lower urinary tract symptoms: a randomized trial. *JAMA* 306(12):1344–1351, 2011.
2. Tacklind J, Macdonald R, Rutks I, et al: *Serenoa repens* for benign prostatic hyperplasia. *Cochrane Database Syst Rev* 12:CD001423, 2012.
3. Lapi F, Gallo E, Giocaliere E, et al: Acute liver damage due to *Serenoa repens*: a case report. *Br J Clin Pharmacol* 69(5):558–560, 2010.
4. Wargo KA, Allman E, Ibrahim F: A possible case of saw palmetto-induced pancreatitis. *South Med J* 103(7):683–685, 2010.
5. Izzo AA, Ernst E: Interactions between herbal medicines and prescribed drugs: an updated systematic review. *Drugs* 69(13):1777–1798, 2009.

ST. JOHN'S WORT

The flowers of St. John's wort (*Hypericum perforatum*) (SJW) contain its biologically active ingredients, hypericin and hyperforin. SJW may increase CNS serotonin and, in very high doses, acts like a monoamine oxidase inhibitor (MAOI).

Claims: Study findings are variable, but SJW may benefit patients with mild-to-moderate depression who have no suicidal ideation. Well-designed studies have been done on SJW treating major depression.

Recommended doses are 300 to 900 mg po once/day of a preparation standardized to 0.2 to 0.3% hypericin, to 1 to 4% hyperforin, or to both (usually). St. John's wort is also said to be useful for treating HIV infection because hypericin inhibits a variety of encapsulated viruses, including HIV, but has proven adverse interactions with protease inhibitors and non-nucleoside reverse transcriptase inhibitors (NNRTIs) and should therefore be avoided.[1,2] SJW has also been claimed to treat skin disorders, including psoriasis, and attention-deficit/hyperactivity disorder (ADHD) in children.

Evidence: Numerous randomized, placebo-controlled studies have evaluated safety and efficacy of SJW in treating mild-to-moderate depression and, recently, major depressive disorders.[3-8] SJW has also been compared with tricyclic antidepressants (amitryptilline, imipramine) and more recently with the SSRIs fluoxetine and sertraline.[(4-7)] Most placebo-controlled studies have shown that standardized extracts of SJW in the dose range of 300 mg to 900 mg once daily are moderately effective in the treatment of mild-to-moderate depressive symptoms. Some studies have shown equivalence of 900 mg of SJW to low-dose imipramine and low-dose fluoxetine. A study of patients with major depression failed to show significant improvement over either placebo or standard doses of sertraline over a short period of time.[7] However, the authors state that both SJW and sertraline were equally effective over long periods of time, indicating the potential alternative economic value of SJW as a therapeutic treatment of depression when taken at low doses and when drug interactions are not of concern.[7]

Overall, some studies show efficacy of SJW in treating mild depression, whereas in major depression most studies do not show efficacy. Differences in study design (lack of active control and placebo), study populations (major vs mild/moderate depression), length of time, and dosing of SJW or comparator agents are likely responsible for some variance in results.

Two very small pilot studies show potential topical application relief from skin disorders, including psoriasis.[9,10] A small trial showed SJW (standardized to hypericin but not hyperforin) did not relieve symptoms of ADHD in children.[11]

Adverse effects: Photosensitivity, dry mouth, constipation, dizziness, confusion, and mania (in patients with bipolar disorder) may occur. SJW is contraindicated in pregnant women.

Drug interactions: Potential adverse interactions occur with cyclosporine, digoxin, iron supplements, MAOIs, NNRTIs, oral contraceptives, protease inhibitors, SSRIs, tricyclic antidepressants, and warfarin.[12-14]

1. Maury W, Price JP, Brindley MA, et al: Identification of light-independent inhibition of human immunodeficiency virus-1 infection through bioguided fractionation of *Hypericum perforatum*. *Virol J* 6:101–113, 2009.
2. Kakuda TN, Schöller-Gyüre M, Hoetelmans RM: Pharmacokinetic interactions between etravirine and non-antiretroviral drugs. *Clin Pharmacokinet* 50(1):25–39, 2011.
3. Solomon D, Adams J, Graves N: Economic evaluation of St. John's wort (*Hypericum perforatum*) for the treatment of mild to moderate depression. *J Affect Disord* 148(2-3):228–234, 2013.
4. van Gurp G, Meterissian GB, Haiek LN, et al: St John's wort or sertraline? Randomized controlled trial in primary care. *Can Fam Physician* 48:905–912, 2002.
5. Woelk H: Comparison of St John's wort and imipramine for treating depression: randomised controlled trial. *BMJ* 321(7260):536–539, 2000.
6. Fava M, Alpert J, Nierenberg AA, et al: A double-blind, randomized trial of St John's wort, fluoxetine, and placebo in major depressive disorder. *J Clin Psychopharmacol* 25(5):441–447, 2005.
7. Sarris J, Fava M, Schweitzer I, et al: St John's wort (*Hypericum perforatum*) versus sertraline and placebo in major depressive disorder: continuation data from a 26-week RCT. *Pharmacopsychiatry* 45(7):275–278, 2012.
8. Shelton RC, Keller MB, Gelenberg A, et al: Effectiveness of St John's wort in major depression: a randomized controlled trial. *JAMA* 285(15):1978–86, 2001.
9. Najafizadeh P, Hashemian F, Mansouri P, et al: The evaluation of the clinical effect of topical St Johns wort

(*Hypericum perforatum L.*) in plaque type psoriasis vulgaris: a pilot study. *Australas J Dermatol* 53(2):131–135, 2012.
10. Rook AH, Wood GS, Duvic M, et al: A phase II placebo-controlled study of photodynamic therapy with topical hypericin and visible light irradiation in the treatment of cutaneous T-cell lymphoma and psoriasis. *J Am Acad Dermatol* 63(6):984–990, 2010.
11. Weber W, Vander Stoep A, McCarty RL, et al: *Hypericum perforatum* (St John's wort) for attention-deficit/hyperactivity disorder in children and adolescents: a randomized controlled trial. *JAMA* 299(22):633-2641, 2008.
12. Borrelli F, Izzo AA: Herb-drug interactions with St John's wort (*Hypericum perforatum*): an update on clinical observations. *AAPS J* 11(4):710-727, 2009.
13. Nadkarni A, Oldham MA, Howard M, et al: Drug-drug interactions between warfarin and psychotropics: updated review of the literature. *Pharmacotherapy* 32(10): 932–942, 2012.
14. Tsai HH, Lin HW, Simon Pickard A, et al: Evaluation of documented drug interactions and contraindications associated with herbs and dietary supplements: a systematic literature review. *Int J Clin Pract* 66(11):1056–1078, 2012.

VALERIAN

Valerian's (*Valeriana officinalis*) root and rhizomes (underground stems) contain its active ingredients, including valepotriates and pungent odiferous oils.

Claims: Valerian is used as a sedative and sleep aid and is especially popular in Europe.

Some people take valerian for headaches, depression, irregular heartbeat, and trembling. It is usually used for short periods of time (eg, 2 to 6 wk), at dosages of 400 to 600 mg of dried root once/day 1 hour before bedtime.

Evidence: In a 2006 meta-analysis of 16 randomized, placebo-controlled trials of valerian, the evidence suggested that valerian might improve sleep quality and shorten the time needed to fall asleep without producing adverse effects.[1] However, there are still insufficient clinical data to confirm whether valerian is effective for insomnia.[2,3] There is not enough scientific evidence to determine whether valerian works for headaches, depression, irregular heartbeat, and trembling.

Adverse effects: Studies suggest that it is generally safe to give valerian at the usual doses. Valerian may prolong the effect of other sedatives (eg, barbiturates) and affect driving or other activities requiring alertness.

Drug interactions: In vitro studies have suggested valerian to inhibit both CYP3A4 metabolism and p-glycoprotein activity,[4] but no clinical studies have shown any drug metabolism interactions.

1. Bent S, Padula A, Moore D, et al: Valerian for sleep: a systematic review and meta-analysis. *Am J Med* 119(12):1005–1012, 2006.
2. Fernández-San-Martín MI, Masa-Font R, Palacios-Soler L, et al: Effectiveness of valerian on insomnia: a meta-analysis of randomized placebo-controlled trials. *Sleep Med*11 (6):505–511, 2010.
3. Taibi D, Landis C, Petry H, et al: A systematic review of valerian as a sleep aid: safe but not effective. *Sleep Med Rev* 11(3):209–223, 2007.
4. Hellum BH, Nilsen OG: In vitro inhibition of CYP3A4 metabolism and P-glycoprotein-mediated transport by trade herbal products. *Basic Clin Pharmacol Toxicol* 102(5):466–475, 2008.

ZINC

Zinc, a mineral, is required in small quantities (adult RDA of 8 to 11 mg/day) for multiple metabolic processes. Dietary sources include oysters, beef, and fortified cereals.

Claims: Zinc has been claimed to reduce cold symptoms, help infants recover from infectious diseases, and slow progression of age-related macular degeneration.

Evidence: Some experts believe that when taken soon after cold symptoms develop, zinc taken as zinc gluconate or acetate lozenges can shorten the course of the common cold.[1] A 2013 Cochrane review of 16 therapeutic trials (1387 participants) and 2 preventive trials (394 participants) demonstrated that zinc reduced the duration (in days) but not the severity of common cold symptoms.[1] Although the proportion of participants with symptoms after 7 days of treatment was significantly smaller than those in the control groups, adverse effects, such as bad taste and nausea, were higher in the zinc group and should be taken into consideration.[1]

There is strong evidence that in developing countries, supplements containing zinc 20 mg and 20 mg iron taken once/wk, when given for the first 12 mo of life, reduce infant mortality due to diarrhea and respiratory infections.[2] There is also strong evidence that supplements containing zinc 40 to 80 mg and antioxidants (vitamin C and E and lutein/zeaxanthin) taken once/day slow progression of moderate to severe atrophic (dry form) age-related macular degeneration.[3,4]

Adverse effects: Zinc is generally safe, but toxicity can develop if high doses are used (see p. 14). The common adverse effects of zinc lozenges include nausea, vomiting, diarrhea, mouth irritation, mouth sores, and bad taste. Because zinc is a trace metal and can remove other necessary metals from the body, zinc lozenge dose should not exceed 75 mg day (total dose, regardless of dosing frequency) for 14 days. Zinc sprays may cause nose and throat irritation.

1. Singh M, Das RR: Zinc for the common cold. *Cochrane Database Syst Rev* 6:CD001364, 2013.
2. Baqui AH, Zaman K, Persson LA, et al: Simultaneous weekly supplementation of iron and zinc is associated with lower morbidity due to diarrhea and acute lower respiratory infection in Bangladeshi infants. *J Nutr* 133(12):4150–4157, 2003.
3. Age-Related Eye Disease Study Research Group: A randomized, placebo-controlled, clinical trial of high-dose supplementation with vitamins C and E, beta carotene, and zinc for age-related macular degeneration and vision loss: AREDS report no. 8. *Arch Ophthalmol* 119(10):1417–1436, 2001.
4. The Age-Related Eye Disease Study 2 (AREDS2) Research Group, Chew EY, Clemons TE, et al: Secondary analyses of the effects of lutein/zeaxanthin on age-related macular degeneration progression: AREDS2 report No. 3. *JAMA Ophthalmol* 132(2):142–149, 2014.

377 The Dying Patient

Dying patients can have needs that differ from those of other patients. So that their needs can be met, dying patients must first be identified. Before death, patients tend to follow 1 of 3 general trajectories of functional decline:

- A limited period of steadily progressive functional decline (eg, typical of progressive cancer)
- A prolonged indefinite period of severe dysfunction that may not be steadily progressive (eg, typical of severe dementia, disabling stroke, and severe frailty)
- Function that decreases irregularly, caused by periodic and sometimes unpredictable acute exacerbations of the underlying disorder (eg, typical of heart failure or COPD)

With the first trajectory (eg, in progressive cancer), the course of disease and time of death tend to be more predictable than with the other trajectories. For example, with prolonged dysfunction (eg, severe dementia), death may occur suddenly because of an infection such as pneumonia. With irregularly progressive dysfunction (eg, heart failure), people who do not appear near death may die suddenly during an acute exacerbation. As a result, although knowing the trajectory of functional decline can help, it is still often difficult to estimate with any precision when death will occur. Thus, clinicians are advised to consider patients that fulfill both of the following criteria as potentially dying patients, recognizing that these criteria may be overly inclusive:

- Presence of illness that is serious and expected to worsen
- Death within 1 yr would not surprise the clinician

If a patient is recognized as potentially dying, the clinician should

- Communicate the likely course of disease, including an estimation of the length of survival, to the patient, and, if the patient chooses, to family, friends, or both
- Discuss and clarify the goals of care (eg, palliation, cure)
- Arrange for desired palliative and hospice care
- Plan what to do when death is imminent
- Treat symptoms
- Help address financial, legal, and ethical concerns
- Help patients and caregivers deal with stress

Patients should be involved in decision making as much as they can. If patients lack capacity to make health care decisions (see p. 3209) and have a durable power of attorney for health care, the person appointed by that document makes health care decisions. If patients have no authorized surrogate, health care practitioners usually rely on the next of kin or even a close friend to gain insight into what the patient's wishes would be. However, the exact scope of authority and the priority of permissible surrogates vary by state. In states where default surrogate decision makers are authorized, the typical order of priority is the patient's

- Spouse (or domestic partner in jurisdictions that recognize this status)
- Adult child
- Parent
- Sibling
- Other relatives or a close friend (possibly)

If more than one person has the same priority (eg, several adult children), consensus is preferred, but some states allow health care practitioners to rely on a majority decision.

Communication and Clarification of Goals

A common mistake is to assume that patients and caregivers understand the course of disease or recognize when death is imminent; they need to be told specifically. When possible, a range of likely survival durations should be given, perhaps advising people to "hope for the best but plan for the worst." Educating patients early provides them time to address spiritual and psychosocial concerns and to deliberate and make reasoned decisions about priorities for their care. Priorities can differ when facing death. For example, some people value prolongation of life, even if it causes discomfort, costs money, or burdens family. Other people identify specific goals, such as maintaining function and independence, or relieving symptoms, such as pain. Some people are most concerned with seeking forgiveness, reconciling, or providing for a loved one.

Advance care plans should be documented and readily accessible to other health care providers (eg, emergency department) to offer the best chance of achieving the patient's desired care. State-authorized Portable Orders and Physician Orders for Life-Sustaining Treatment (POLST) are widely used and should be easily accessible in the home and in the medical record to direct emergency medical personnel regarding what medical care to give and to forgo. Decisions about specific treatments can be helpful. For example, CPR and transport to a hospital are usually not desirable if death is imminent; in contrast, certain aggressive treatments (eg, blood transfusions, chemotherapy) may be desired to relieve symptoms even if death is inevitable.

Palliative Care and Hospice

Palliative care: Palliative care aims to improve quality of life by helping relieve bothersome physical symptoms and psychosocial and spiritual distress. Palliative care is not incompatible with many curative treatments and can, in fact, be provided at the same time. For example, the palliative aspect of care emphasizes treatment of pain or delirium for a patient with liver failure who may be on a liver transplant list. However, to say that a patient's care has changed from curative to supportive or from treatment to palliation is an oversimplification of a complex decision process. Most patients need a customized mix of treatment to correct, prevent, and mitigate the effects of various illnesses and disabilities.

Clinicians should initiate palliative care as soon as patients are identified as seriously ill and especially when they are sick enough to die. Palliative care can be provided by individual practitioners, interdisciplinary teams, and hospice programs. Individual palliative care providers specialize in the recognition and treatment of pain and other bothersome symptoms. Interdisciplinary palliative care teams are made up of various professionals (eg, physicians, nurses, social workers, chaplains) who work together with patients' primary and specialty clinicians to relieve physical, psychosocial, and spiritual stress.

PEARLS & PITFALLS

- Consider palliative care for all potentially dying patients, even those pursuing aggressive or curative therapies.

Hospice: Hospice is a program of care and support for people who are very likely to die within a few months. Hospice care focuses on comfort and meaningfulness, not on cure. Services may include providing physical care, counseling, drugs, durable medical equipment, and supplies. In some countries, such as the US, hospice mostly provides services in the home; in others, such as England, hospice services are mainly in inpatient facilities.

In typical hospice care, family members serve as the primary caregivers, often with additional help from home health aides and volunteers. The hospice staff is available 24 hours a day every day. Hospice personnel are specially trained. The hospice team usually consists of the patient's personal physician, hospice physician, or medical director; nurses; home health aides; social workers; chaplains or other counselors; trained volunteers; and speech, physical, and occupational therapists as needed.

Physicians may be reluctant to use hospice because a treatable condition could develop. However, this reluctance is not justified because many treatable conditions are within the scope of hospice care. Medicare covers all medical care related to the hospice diagnosis, and patients are still eligible for medical coverage unrelated to the hospice diagnosis. Also, patients can leave hospice at any time and re-enroll later.

Advance Planning for Imminent Death

Planning for symptom relief as well as receiving patient and family support can help people deal with the most difficult parts of dying. When death is expected to occur at home, a hospice team typically provides drugs (a comfort kit) with instructions for how to use them to quickly suppress symptoms, such as pain or dyspnea. Family members should be told about changes that are likely during the dying process, including confusion, somnolence, irregular or noisy breathing, cool extremities, and purplish skin color. Planning can also help avert unnecessary, distressing hospital visits at the end of life. Family members should rehearse whom to call (eg, physician, hospice nurse, clergy) and know who not to call (eg, ambulance service).

Witnessing the last moments of a person's life can have a lasting effect on family, friends, and caregivers. The patient should be in an area that is peaceful, quiet, and physically comfortable. Clinicians should encourage family to maintain physical contact with the patient, such as holding hands. Hospice providers should inquire about and make accommodation for spiritual, cultural, ethnic, or personal rites of passage desired by the patient and family members. Families also often need help with burial or cremation services and arranging payment for them; social workers can provide information and advice. Regardless of setting (eg, home, hospital, nursing home, inpatient or home hospice), religious practices may affect care of the body after death and should be discussed in advance with the patient family, or both. Decisions about organ donation and autopsy are usually best made before death because that is usually a less stressful time than immediately after death.

Financial Concerns and Disability

One US study has shown that one third of families deplete most of their savings when caring for a dying relative. Families should be advised to investigate the cost of care for a family member's serious illness. Information about coverage and regulations can take substantial and diligent work to obtain. In addition to consulting the clinical care team, checking available services with the eldercare locator is a good place to start.

Progressive disability often accompanies fatal illnesses. Patients may gradually become unable to tend to a house or an apartment, prepare food, handle financial matters, walk, or care for themselves. Most dying patients need help during their last weeks. The clinical care team should anticipate disability and make appropriate preparations (eg, choosing housing that is wheelchair-accessible and close to family caregivers). Services such as occupational or physical therapy and hospice care may help a patient remain at home, even when the disability progresses. The clinical care team should know the financial effects of choices and discuss these issues with patients or family members. Some attorneys specialize in elder care and can help patients and their family members deal with these issues.

Legal and Ethical Concerns

Health care practitioners should know local laws and institutional policy governing living wills, durable powers of attorney, physician-assisted suicide, and procedures for forgoing resuscitation and hospitalization. This knowledge helps them ensure that the patient's wishes guide care, even when the patient can no longer make decisions (see p. 3212).

Many health care practitioners worry that medical treatments intended to relieve pain or other serious symptoms (eg, opioids for pain, dyspnea, or both) might hasten death, but this effect is actually quite uncommon. With skillful medical care and drug titration, health care practitioners avoid the most worrisome adverse drug effects, such as respiratory depression caused by opioids. Death is not hastened by common treatments for common symptoms in advanced illness. Even if intractable pain or dyspnea requires high doses of opioids that may also hasten death, the resulting death is not considered wrongful because the drugs had been given to relieve symptoms and had been appropriately titrated and dosed. Physicians who manage symptoms vigorously and forego life-sustaining treatment need to discuss these issues openly and sensitively and document decision making carefully.

A physician should usually not provide an intervention that is conventionally considered a means of homicide (eg, lethal injection) even if the intention is to relieve suffering. Assisting with suicide (eg, by directly providing a dying patient with lethal drugs and instructions for using them) is authorized under specific conditions in Oregon, Washington, Vermont, California, Colorado, and Montana but could be grounds for prosecution in all other parts of the United States. In states where physician-assisted suicide is legal, health care practitioners and patients must adhere to state-specific requirements, including patient residency, age, decision-making capacity, terminal illness, prognosis, and the timing of the request for assistance. In all other states and the District of Columbia, state or common laws specifically prohibit physician-assisted suicide or are unclear. In these locations, charges of homicide are plausible if the patient's interests are not carefully advocated, if the patient lacks capacity or is severely functionally impaired when decisions are made, or if decisions and their rationales are not documented.

Supporting Caregivers after Death

A physician, nurse, or other authorized person should pronounce the patient dead in a timely way to reduce the family's anxiety and uncertainty. The physician should complete the death certificate as soon as possible because funeral directors need a completed death certificate to make final arrangements. Even when death is expected, physicians may need to report the death to the coroner or police; knowledge of local law is important.

Telling family members about death, particularly unexpected death, requires planning and composure. The physician should use clear language when informing the family that death has occurred (eg, using the word "died"). Euphemisms (eg, "passed on") should not be used because they are easily misinterpreted. If the family was not present near death, clinicians should describe what happened, including resuscitative efforts and the patient's absence of pain and distress (if true). (If resuscitation is done, family or caregivers may prefer to witness it; no evidence indicates that their presence worsens resuscitative outcomes.) Prudence calls for trying to ensure that close kin do not hear the news alone. When told about death, especially unexpected death, family members may be overwhelmed and unable to process information given to them or to formulate questions.

Physicians, nurses, and other health care practitioners should respond to the psychologic needs of family members and provide appropriate counseling, a comfortable environment where family members can grieve together, and adequate time for them to be with the body. Before family members see the body, stains and tubes should be removed and odors should be masked whenever possible. When feasible, it may help for a clinician to be with the family members as they enter the room with the newly dead body because the situation is so unfamiliar to most people. Sometimes it is best to leave family members alone for a while, then return and offer explanations of treatments provided and give the family a chance to ask questions. Friends, neighbors, and clergy may be able to help provide support.

Clinicians should be sensitive to cultural differences in behavior at the time of death. The patient can decide about organ and tissue donation, if appropriate, before death, or family members and the clinical care team can discuss organ and tissue donation before or immediately after death; such discussions are ordinarily mandated by law. The attending physician should know how to arrange for organ donation and autopsy, even for patients who die at home or in a nursing home. Autopsy should be readily available regardless of where the death occurred, and decisions about autopsies can be made before death or just after death. A substantial minority of families welcome an autopsy to clear up uncertainties, and clinicians should appreciate the role of autopsy in quality assessment and improvement.

SYMPTOM RELIEF FOR THE DYING PATIENT

Physical, psychologic, emotional, and spiritual distress is common among patients living with fatal illness, and patients commonly fear protracted and unrelieved suffering. Health care providers can reassure patients that distressing symptoms can often be anticipated and prevented and, when present, can be treated.

Symptom treatment should be based on etiology when possible. For example, vomiting due to hypercalcemia requires different treatment from that due to elevated intracranial pressure. However, diagnosing the cause of a symptom may be inappropriate if testing is burdensome or risky or if specific treatment (eg, major surgery) has already been ruled out. For dying patients, comfort measures, including nonspecific treatment or a short sequential trial of empiric treatments, often serve patients better than an exhaustive diagnostic evaluation.

Because one symptom can have many causes and may respond differently to treatment as the patient's condition deteriorates, the clinical team must monitor and reevaluate the situation frequently. Drug overdosage or underdosage is harmful, and both become more likely as worsening physiology causes changes in drug metabolism and clearance.

When survival is likely to be brief, symptom severity frequently dictates initial treatment.

Pain

About half of patients dying of cancer have severe pain. Yet, only half of these patients receive reliable pain relief. Many patients dying of organ system failure and dementia also have severe pain. Sometimes pain can be controlled but persists because patients, family members, and physicians have misconceptions about pain and the drugs (especially opioids) that can relieve it, resulting in serious and persistent underdosing.

Patients perceive pain differently, depending partly on whether other factors (eg, fatigue, insomnia, anxiety, depression, nausea) are present. Analgesic choice depends largely on pain intensity and cause, which can be determined only by talking with and observing patients. Patients and physicians must recognize that all pain can be relieved by an appropriately potent drug at sufficient dosage, although aggressive treatment may also cause sedation or confusion. Commonly used drugs are aspirin, acetaminophen, or NSAIDs for mild pain; oxycodone for moderate pain; and hydromorphone, morphine, or fentanyl for severe pain (see p. 1968).

In dying patients, oral opioid therapy is convenient and cost-effective. Sublingual administration is also convenient particularly because it does not require patients to swallow. Long-acting opioids are best for long-lasting pain. Physicians should prescribe opioids in adequate dosages and on a continuous basis and make additional, short-acting opioids available for breakthrough pain. Unreasonable concerns by the public and by health care practitioners about addiction often limit appropriate use of opioids. Pharmacologic dependence may result from regular use but causes no problems in dying patients except the need to avoid inadvertent withdrawal. Addictive behaviors are rare and usually easy to control. In the unusual case where opioids cannot be given orally or sublingually, they can be given rectally, IM, IV, or sc.

Adverse effects of opioids include nausea, sedation, confusion, constipation, and respiratory depression. Opioid-induced constipation should be treated prophylactically (see p. 3178). Patients usually develop substantial tolerance to the respiratory depressant and sedative effects of morphine but develop much less tolerance for the analgesic and constipating effects. Opioids may also cause myoclonus, agitated delirium, hyperalgesia, and seizures. These neurotoxic effects may result from accumulation of toxic metabolites and usually resolve when another opioid is substituted. Patients with these adverse effects and serious pain often warrant consultation with a palliative care or pain specialist.

When a stable opioid dose becomes inadequate, increasing the dose by 1½ to 2 times the previous dose (eg, calculated based on daily dose) is reasonable. Usually, serious respiratory depression does not occur unless the new dose is much more than twice the previously tolerated dose.

Use of adjunctive drugs for pain relief often increases comfort and reduces the opioid dosage and consequent adverse effects. Corticosteroids can reduce the pain of inflammation and swelling. Tricyclic antidepressants (eg, nortriptyline, doxepin) help manage neuropathic pain; doxepin can provide bedtime sedation as well. Gabapentin 300 to 1200 mg po tid can relieve neuropathic pain. Methadone is effective for refractory or neuropathic pain; however, its kinetics vary, and it requires close monitoring. Benzodiazepines are useful for patients whose pain is worsened by anxiety.

For severe localized pain, regional nerve blocks given by an anesthesiologist experienced in pain management may provide relief with few adverse effects. Various nerve-blocking techniques may be used. Indwelling epidural or intrathecal catheters can provide continuous infusion of analgesics, often mixed with anesthetic drugs.

Pain-modification techniques (eg, guided mental imagery, hypnosis, acupuncture, relaxation, biofeedback) help some patients. Counseling for stress and anxiety may be very helpful, as may spiritual support from a chaplain.

Dyspnea

Dyspnea is one of the most feared symptoms and is extremely frightening to dying patients. The main causes of dyspnea are heart and lung disorders. Other factors include severe anemia and chest wall or abdominal disorders that cause painful respiration (eg, rib fracture) or that impede respiration (eg, massive ascites). Metabolic acidosis causes tachypnea but does not cause a sensation of dyspnea. Anxiety (sometimes due to delirium or pain) can cause tachypnea with or without a feeling of dyspnea.

Reversible causes should be treated specifically. For example, placing a chest tube for tension pneumothorax or draining a pleural effusion provides quick and definitive relief. Supplemental oxygen can sometimes correct hypoxemia. Nebulized albuterol and oral or injectable corticosteroids may relieve bronchospasm and bronchial inflammation. However, if death is imminent or a definitive treatment for the cause of dyspnea is not available, proper symptomatic treatment assures patients they will be comfortable, regardless of the cause. If death is expected and the goals of care focus on comfort, then pulse oximetry, ABGs, ECG, and imaging are not indicated. Clinicians should use general comfort-oriented treatments including positioning (eg, sitting up), increasing air movement with a fan or open window, and bedside relaxation techniques.

Opioids are the drugs of choice for dyspnea near the end of life. Low doses of morphine 2 to 10 mg sublingually or 2 to 4 mg sc q 2 h prn helps reduce breathlessness in an opioid-naive patient. Morphine may blunt the medullary response to CO_2 retention or O_2 decline, reducing dyspnea and decreasing anxiety without causing harmful respiratory depression. If patients are already taking opioids for pain, dosages that relieve dyspnea must often be more than double the patient's usual dosages. Benzodiazepines often help relieve anxiety associated with dyspnea and with fear of a return of dyspnea.

Oxygen may also give psychologic comfort to patients and family members even if it does not correct hypoxemia. Patients usually prefer oxygen via nasal cannula. An oxygen face mask may increase agitation of a dying patient. Nebulized saline may help patients with viscous secretions.

The death rattle is noisy breathing that results from air moving across pooled secretions in the oropharynx and bronchi and often portends death in hours or days. The death rattle is not a sign of discomfort in the dying patient but can disturb family members and caregivers. To minimize the death rattle, caregivers should limit patients' fluid intake (eg, oral, IV, enteral) and position patients on their side or semi-prone. Oropharyngeal suctioning is generally ineffective in reaching the pooled secretions and may cause discomfort. Airway congestion is best managed with an anticholinergic drug such as scopolamine, glycopyrrolate, or atropine (eg, glycopyrrolate beginning with 0.2 mg sc q 4 to 6 h or 0.2 to 0.4 mg po q 8 h, with dose increases prn). Adverse effects mostly occur with repeated doses and include blurred vision, sedation, delirium, palpitations, hallucinations, constipation, and urinary retention. Glycopyrrolate does not cross the blood-brain barrier and results in fewer neurotoxic adverse effects than other anticholinergics.

Anorexia

Anorexia and marked weight loss are common among dying patients. For family members, accepting the patient's poor oral intake is often difficult because it means accepting that the patient is dying. Patients should be offered their favorite foods whenever possible. Conditions that may cause poor intake and that can be easily treated—gastritis, constipation, toothache, oral candidiasis, pain, and nausea—should be treated. Some patients benefit from appetite stimulants such as oral corticosteroids (dexamethasone 2 to 8 mg bid or prednisone 10 to 30 mg once/day) or megestrol 160 to 480 mg po once/day. However, if a patient is close to death, family members should understand that neither food nor hydration is necessary to maintain the patient's comfort.

IV fluids, TPN, and tube feedings do not prolong the life of dying patients, may increase discomfort, and even hasten death. Adverse effects of artificial nutrition in dying patients can include pulmonary congestion, pneumonia, edema, and pain associated with inflammation. Conversely, dehydration and ketosis due to caloric restriction correlate with analgesic effects and absence of discomfort. The only reported discomfort due to dehydration near death is xerostomia, which can be prevented and relieved with oral swabs or ice chips.

Even debilitated and cachectic patients may live for several weeks with no food and minimal hydration. Family members should understand that stopping fluids does not result in the patient's immediate death and ordinarily does not hasten death. Supportive care, including good oral hygiene, is imperative for patient comfort during this time.

Nausea and Vomiting

Many seriously ill patients experience nausea, frequently without vomiting. Nausea may arise with GI problems (eg, constipation, gastritis), metabolic abnormalities (eg, hypercalcemia, uremia), drug adverse effects, increased intracranial pressure secondary to cerebral cancer, and psychosocial stress. When possible, treatment should match the likely cause—eg, stopping NSAIDs, treating gastritis with H_2 blockers, and trying corticosteroids for patients with known or suspected brain metastases. If nausea is due to gastric distention and reflux, metoclopramide (eg, 10 to 20 mg po or sc qid prn or given on a scheduled basis) is useful because it increases gastric tone and contractions while relaxing the pyloric sphincter.

Patients with no specific cause of nausea may benefit from treatment with a phenothiazine (eg, promethazine 25 mg po qid; prochlorperazine 10 mg po before meals or, for patients who cannot take oral drugs, 25 mg rectally bid). Anticholinergic drugs such as scopolamine and the antihistamines meclizine and diphenhydramine prevent recurrent nausea in many patients. Combining lower doses of the previously mentioned drugs often improves efficacy. Second-line drugs for intractable nausea include haloperidol (started at 1 mg po or sc q 6 to 8 h, then titrated to as much as 15 mg/day). The 5-hydroxytryptamine $(5\text{-HT})_3$ antagonists ondansetron and granisetron often dramatically relieve chemotherapy-induced nausea.

Nausea and pain due to intestinal obstruction are common among patients with widespread abdominal cancer. Generally, IV fluids and nasogastric suction are more burdensome than useful. Symptoms of nausea, pain, and intestinal spasm respond to hyoscyamine (0.125 to 0.25 mg q 4 h sublingually or sc), scopolamine (1.5 mg topically), morphine (given sc or rectally), or any of the other previously mentioned antiemetics. Octreotide 150 mcg sc or IV q 12 h inhibits GI secretions and dramatically reduces nausea and painful distention. Given with antiemetics, octreotide usually eliminates the need for nasogastric suctioning. Corticosteroids (eg, dexamethasone 4 to 6 mg IV, IM, or rectally tid) may decrease obstructive inflammation at the tumor site and temporarily relieve the obstruction. IV fluids may exacerbate obstructive edema.

Constipation

Constipation is common among dying patients because of inactivity, use of opioids and drugs with anticholinergic effects, and decreased intake of fluids and dietary fiber. Regular bowel movements are essential to the comfort of dying patients, at least until the last day or two of life. Laxatives help prevent fecal impaction, especially in patients receiving opioids. Monitoring bowel function regularly is essential. Most patients do well on a twice daily regimen of a mild stimulant laxative (eg, casanthranol, senna). If stimulant laxatives cause cramping discomfort, patients may respond to an osmotic laxative, such as lactulose or sorbitol started at 15 to 30 mL po bid and titrated to effect. However, there are a wide variety of appropriate laxatives with none that has proven superior in this clinical situation.

Soft fecal impaction may be treated with a bisacodyl suppository or saline enema. For a hard fecal impaction, a mineral oil enema may be given, possibly with an oral benzodiazepine (eg, lorazepam) or an analgesic, followed by digital disimpaction. After disimpaction, patients should be placed on a more aggressive bowel regimen to avoid recurrence.

Pressure Ulcers

Many dying patients are immobile, poorly nourished, incontinent, and cachectic and thus are at risk of pressure ulcers. Prevention requires relieving pressure by rotating the patient or shifting the patient's weight every 2 h; a specialized mattress or continuously inflated air-suspension bed may also help. Incontinent patients should be kept as dry as possible. Generally, use of an indwelling catheter, with its inconvenience and risk of infection, is justified only when bedding changes cause pain or when patients or family members strongly prefer it.

Delirium and Confusion

Mental changes that can accompany the terminal stage of a disorder may distress patients and family members; however, patients are often unaware of them. Delirium is common. Causes include drugs, hypoxia, metabolic disturbances, and intrinsic CNS disorders. If the cause can be determined, simple treatment may enable patients to communicate more meaningfully with family members and friends. Patients who are comfortable and less aware of their surroundings may do better with no treatment. When possible, the physician should ascertain the preferences of patients and family members and use them to guide treatment.

Simple causes of delirium should be sought. Agitation and restlessness often result from urinary retention, which resolves promptly with urinary catheterization. Confusion in debilitated patients is worsened by sleep deprivation. Agitated patients may benefit from benzodiazepines; however, benzodiazepines may also cause confusion. Poorly controlled pain may cause insomnia or agitation. If pain has been appropriately controlled, a nighttime sedative may help.

Family members and visitors may help lessen confusion by frequently holding the patient's hand and repeating where the patient is and what is happening. Patients with severe terminal agitation resistant to other measures may respond best to barbiturates. However, family members should be told that after these drugs are used, patients may not regain the capacity for coherent interaction. Pentobarbital, a rapid-onset, short-acting barbiturate, may be given as 100 to 200 mg IM q 4 h prn. Phenobarbital, which is longer-acting, may be given po, sc, or rectally.

Depression and Suicide

Most dying patients experience some depressive symptoms. Providing psychologic support and allowing patients to express concerns and feelings are usually the best approach. A skilled social worker, physician, nurse, or chaplain can help with these concerns.

A trial of antidepressants is often appropriate for patients who have persistent, clinically significant depression. SSRIs are useful for patients likely to live beyond the 4 wk usually needed for onset of the antidepressant effect. Depressed patients with anxiety and insomnia may benefit from a sedating tricyclic antidepressant given at bedtime. For patients who are withdrawn or who have vegetative signs, methylphenidate may be started at 2.5 mg po once/day and increased to 2.5 to 5 mg bid (given at breakfast and lunch) as necessary. Methylphenidate (same dosage) can provide a few days or weeks of increased energy for patients who are fatigued or somnolent because of analgesics. Methylphenidate has a rapid effect but may precipitate agitation. Although its duration of action is short, adverse effects are also short-lived.

Suicide: Serious medical illness is a significant risk factor for suicidality. Other risk factors for suicide are common among those sick enough to die; they include advanced age, male sex, psychiatric comorbidity, an AIDS diagnosis, and uncontrolled pain. Cancer patients have nearly twice the incidence of suicide than the general population, and patients with lung, stomach, and head and neck cancers have the highest suicide rates among all patients with cancer. Clinicians should routinely screen seriously ill patients for depression and suicidal thoughts. Psychiatrists should urgently evaluate all patients who seriously threaten self-harm or have serious suicidal thoughts.

Stress and Grief

Some people approach death peacefully, but more people and family members have stressful periods. Death is particularly stressful when interpersonal conflicts keep patients and family members from sharing their last moments together in peace. Such conflicts can lead to excessive guilt or inability to grieve in survivors and can cause anguish in patients. A family member who is caring for a dying relative at home may experience physical and emotional stress. Usually, stress in patients and family members responds to compassion, information, counseling, and sometimes brief psychotherapy. Community services may be available to help relieve caregiver burden. Sedatives should be used sparingly and briefly.

When a partner dies, the survivor may be overwhelmed by having to make decisions about legal or financial matters or household management. For an elderly couple, the death of one may reveal the survivor's cognitive impairment, for which the deceased partner had compensated. The clinical team should identify such high-risk situations so that they can mobilize the resources needed to prevent undue suffering and dysfunction.

Grief: Grieving is a normal process that usually begins before an anticipated death. For patients, grief often starts with denial caused by fears about loss of control, separation, suffering, an uncertain future, and loss of self. Traditionally, the stages after grief were thought to occur in the following order: denial, anger, bargaining, depression, and acceptance. However, the stages that patients go through and their order of occurrence vary. Members of the clinical team can help patients accept their prognosis by listening to their concerns, helping them understand that they can control important elements of their life, explaining how the disorder will worsen and how death will come, and assuring them that their physical symptoms will be controlled. If grief is still very severe or causes psychosis or suicidal ideation or if the patient has a previous severe mental disorder, referral for professional evaluation and grief counseling may help the person cope.

Family members may need support in expressing grief. Any clinical team member who has come to know the patient and family members can help them through this process and direct them to professional services if needed. Physicians and other clinical team members need to develop regular procedures that ensure follow-up of grieving family members.

378 Exercise

Exercise stimulates tissue change and adaptation (eg, increase in muscle mass and strength, cardiovascular endurance), whereas rest and recovery allow such change and adaptation to occur.[1,2] Recovery from exercise is as important as the exercise stimulus. Regular physical activity reduces the likelihood of medical illness, decreases the incidence of the major causes of death, and improves the overall health and quality of life for patients with most medical conditions.

By increasing muscle mass and strength and fostering cardiovascular endurance, exercise improves functional status for sports and activities of daily living and protects against injury. Specific exercise programs are also commonly prescribed to rehabilitate patients after MI, major surgery, and musculoskeletal injury. Preoperative exercise regimens are prescribed before many elective surgical procedures to enhance postoperative recovery.[2] Regardless of indication, recommendations for exercise should be based on 2 main principles:

- Goals for activity should be specific to the patient, accounting for motivation, needs, physical ability, and psychology, to maximize the likelihood of patient participation and desired outcome.
- Activity should be prescribed in a proper dose to achieve a desired effect. An exercise stimulus should be sufficient for the body to adapt to a higher state of function but not so great that it causes injury or nonadherence. More exercise or higher-intensity activity is not always better; too little or too much activity may prevent achievement of desired outcomes.

A prescription for exercise should specify intensity (level of exertion), volume (amount of activity in a session), frequency (number of exercise sessions), and progressive overload (either the amount of increase in one or more of these elements per workout or the actual load). The balance of these elements depends on individual tolerance and physiologic principles (ie, as intensity increases, volume and frequency may need to decrease, whereas as volume increases, intensity may need to decrease). Intensity, volume, and frequency can be increased concurrently, but increases are limited because human tolerance to strain is finite. The objective is to discover the appropriate amount of exercise for optimal benefit in the context of the patient's goals, health status, and current fitness level. Fixed and traditional generic recommendations (eg, 3 sets of 10 to 12 repetitions, running 30 min 3 times/wk) may be suboptimal because they do not address a person's specific requirements or capability (ie, people with marked deconditioning require a different program than people with the ability to train at higher intensity levels). Variation in the regimen helps avoid overadaptation (staleness) to the same stimulus as well as minor injuries due to repetitive actions.

Achieving long-term adherence is important and challenging. People differ greatly in their motivation and ability to sustain what they may perceive as arduous activity. To improve adherence, training programs typically start at low intensity levels and gradually increase to the target level. Some people require individually supervised exercise (eg, by a personal trainer), others benefit from the support of organized group activity (eg, an exercise class, group bike ride), and some are able to engage in solitary exercise long-term. For people to sustain motivation over the long term, exercise prescriptions should take into account their needs (eg, leg strengthening exercises for someone wheelchair dependent), what is actually required for them to achieve a particular goal (ie, how realistic the goal is), and preferences (the type of fitness program).

Exercise programs should encompass multiple dimensions of fitness, including

- Stretching and flexibility
- Aerobic capacity (cardiovascular endurance)
- Strength (including muscular endurance and muscle size or structure)
- Balance

1. Selye H: *The Stress of Life*, revised ed. New York, McGraw-Hill Companies, Inc., 1984.
2. Fletcher GF, Ades PA, Kligfield P, et al: Exercise standards for testing and training: a scientific statement from the American Heart Association. *Circulation* 128(8):873–934, 2013.

Pre-exercise medical evaluation: Before beginning a sports or vigorous exercise program, children and adults should undergo screening (ie, a history and physical examination), with emphasis on detecting cardiovascular risks. Testing is done only if disorders are clinically suspected.

Stretching and flexibility: Flexibility is important for safe, comfortable performance of physical activities. Stretching may be beneficial in strength training to improve range of motion and help relax muscles. These exercises can be done before or after other forms of training or as a regimen itself, as occurs in yoga and Pilates sessions. Although stretching before exercise enhances mental preparedness, there is no evidence that stretching decreases risk of injury. However, there is no need to discourage preactivity stretching if people enjoy it. General warming-up (eg, with low-intensity simulation of the exercise to be done, jogging on the spot, calisthenics, or other light activities that increase core temperature) seems to be more effective than stretching for facilitating safe exercise. Stretching after exercise is generally preferred because tissues stretch more effectively when warmed.

Specific flexibility exercises involve slowly and steadily stretching muscle groups without jerking or bouncing. To improve flexibility, a stretch should be held for at least 10 to 30 sec and not for more than 60 sec (there are no adverse effects from holding a stretch > 60 sec but there is no added benefit). Each stretch is repeated 2 to 3 times, and each time the stretch is held progressively further. Some mild discomfort is to be expected, but high pain levels should be avoided as pain can be a signal of unintended minor tissue tearing. For many muscles, flexibility increases sufficiently with a properly designed strength training program because muscles both stretch and work through the complete range of motion.

Aerobic exercise: Aerobic (cardiovascular) exercise is continuous, rhythmic physical activity. Exertion occurs at a level that can be supported by aerobic metabolism (although brief periods of more intense exertion triggering anaerobic metabolism may be interspersed) continuously for at least 5 min as a starting point and is increased slowly over time. Aerobic conditioning increases maximal oxygen uptake and cardiac output (mainly an increase in stroke volume), decreases resting heart rate, and reduces cardiac and all-cause mortality; however, too much activity causes excessive wear on the body and increases cellular oxidation. Examples of aerobic exercise include running, jogging, fast walking, swimming, bicycling, rowing, kayaking, skating, cross-country skiing, and using aerobic exercise machines (eg, treadmill, stair-climbing, or elliptical machines). Certain team sports such as basketball and soccer can also provide vigorous aerobic exercise but may stress knees and other joints. Recommendations should be based on patient preferences and abilities.

Aerobic metabolism starts within 2 min of beginning activity, but more sustained effort is needed to achieve health benefits. The usual recommendation is to exercise ≥ 30 min/day at least 3 times/wk with a 5-min warm-up and a 5-min cool-down period, but this recommendation is based as much on convenience as it is on evidence. Optimal aerobic conditioning can occur with as little as 10 to 15 min of activity per session 2 to 3 times/wk if interval cycling is implemented. In interval cycling, short periods of moderate activity are alternated with intense exertion. In one regimen, about 90 sec of moderate activity (60 to 80% maximum heart rate [HR_{max}]) is alternated with about 20 to 30 sec of intense sprint-type activity (85 to 95% HR_{max} or as hard as the person can exert for that time while maintaining proper body mechanics). This regimen, known as high-intensity interval training (HIIT), is more stressful on joints and tissues and so should be done infrequently or alternated with more conventional low- to moderate-intensity training.

Resistance training machines or free weights can be used for aerobic exercise provided that a sufficient number of repetitions are done per set, rest between sets is minimal (near zero to 60 sec), and intensity of effort is relatively high. In circuit training, the large muscles (of the legs, hips, back, and chest) are exercised followed by the smaller muscles (of the shoulders, arms, abdomen, and neck). Circuit training for only 15 to 20 min can benefit the cardiovascular system more than jogging or using aerobic exercise machines for the same amount of time because the more intense workout results in a greater increase in heart rate and oxygen uptake. This combined aerobic and resistance training enhances muscular endurance of all the involved muscles (ie, not just the heart).

Volume of aerobic exercise is graded simply by duration. Intensity is guided by heart rate. Target heart rate for appropriate intensity is 60 to 85% of a person's HR_{max} (the heart rate at peak O_2 consumption [VO_{2peak}], or the rate beyond which aerobic metabolism can no longer be sustained because O_2 is lacking and anaerobic metabolism begins). HR_{max} can be approximated by direct measurement,[1,2] or calculated using the following formula:

$$HR_{Max} = 205.8 - (0.685 \times Age)$$

Alternatively, the Karvonen formula can be used to calculate target heart rate:[2]

$$\text{Target Heart Rate} = [(0.50 \text{ to } 0.85) \times (HR_{Max} - HR_{Resting})] + HR_{Resting}$$

These formulas are based on the general population and may not provide accurate targets for people at the extremes of physical fitness (ie, highly trained athletes or physically deconditioned patients). In such people, metabolic or VO_2 testing may provide more accurate information.

Chronologic age should be distinguished from biologic age. People of any age who are less accustomed to aerobic exercise (less conditioned) will reach their target heart rate much sooner and with less effort, necessitating briefer exercise periods, at least initially. Obese people may be deconditioned and must move a larger body weight, thus causing the heart rate to increase much faster and to a greater extent with less vigorous activity than it does in thinner people. Patients with medical disorders or who are taking certain drugs (eg, beta-blockers) may also have a modified relationship between age and heart rate. A safe starting point for these patients may be 50 to 60% of the age-based target heart rate. These targets can be increased based on patient tolerance and progress.

1. Robergs RA, Landwehr R: The surprising history of the "HRmax=220-age" equation. *Am J Soc Exercise Physiol* 5(2), 2002.
2. Karvonen J, Vuorimaa T: Heart rate and exercise intensity during sports activities. Practical application. *Sports Med* 5(5):303–311, 1988.

Strength training: Strength (resistance) training involves forceful muscular contraction against a load—typically provided by free or machine weights, cable weights, or sometimes body weight (eg, push-ups, abdominal crunches, chin-ups). Such training increases muscle strength, muscle endurance, and muscle size. Strength training also improves functional ability and, depending on the pace of the program, aerobic performance. Cardiovascular endurance and flexibility increase concurrently.

Volume typically is categorized in terms of amount of weight lifted, the number of sets, and the number of repetitions per set. However, an equally important parameter is tension time, which is the total duration of lifting and lowering the weight during one set. To achieve moderate conditioning (developing both muscle mass and strength), appropriate tension time may be about 60 sec. A tension time of 90 to 120 sec is appropriate for injury rehabilitation and improving muscular endurance. When the goal is increasing strength, tension time is more important than number of repetitions, because the number of repetitions can vary within tension time due to differences in technique, set duration and how slowly each repetition is performed. When a person can achieve at least a 60-sec tension time with good technique, resistance (weight) can be increased so that a tension time of at least 60 sec is tolerable at the next weight level. Number of sets is determined by intensity of the training; more intense training necessitates fewer sets.

Intensity is essentially a subjective measure of perceived effort and how close a person comes to muscular fatigue in a given set (or exhaustion in a workout). Intensity may also be characterized objectively by the amount of weight lifted expressed as a percentage of the person's maximum for one repetition (1 RM) of a given exercise; ie, for a person who can deadlift at most 100 kg one time, 75 kg is 75% RM. A general guideline is to exercise with a load at 70 to 85% RM. Heavier loads increase risk of injury and are usually appropriate only for competitive strength athletes. Lifting < 30 to 40% RM provides minimal strength gain, although aerobic conditioning and muscular endurance may occur with sufficient tension time and effort. During strength training, the stimulus of tissue change is governed primarily by the quality and effort of training. For example, a person lifting 85% RM once (where 6 repetitions could be done with maximal effort) would have less stimulus for tissue change than if lifting 75% to 80% RM multiple times (close to or at muscular fatigue).

Intensity is limited by motivation and tolerance. For many patients undergoing rehabilitation, discomfort, pain, exercise inexperience, and/or limitation in range-of-motion (due to discomfort or pain) result in less effort than may be possible or tolerated. As a result, more sets are required to derive desired benefit (although the extent of adding more sets must take into consideration that doing too much activity can increase irritation and soreness to an injury). People should vary the intensity of workouts regularly to provide both a mental and a physical break. Exercise should be done at the highest intensity level during no more than half of the sets in a given workout. People should incorporate breaks from high-intensity training (eg, 1 wk every 3 mo, perhaps coordinated with holidays or vacations) into their fitness planning to allow for sufficient recovery. Continual high-intensity training is counterproductive, even for trained athletes. Symptoms such as fatigue or muscle heaviness when not exercising, lack of motivation to exercise, reduced exercise performance, joint and tendon pain (caused by inflammation), and increased resting heart rate suggest that exercise has been too intense.

Variation helps by providing different stimuli; use of the same stimulus repeatedly eventually fails to elicit the desired effects because muscles adapt to the stimulus. Variation also helps prevent minor injuries caused by repetitive actions.

Proper body mechanics are important for personal safety and effective strength training. People should strive for smooth body mechanics and avoid jerking or dropping weights, which can cause minor tissue injury due to sudden force. It is equally important to encourage controlled breathing, which prevents dizziness (and in extreme cases, fainting) that can occur with the Valsalva maneuver. People should exhale while lifting a weight and inhale while lowering a weight. If a movement is slow, such as lowering a weight for ≥ 5 sec, people may need to breathe in and out more than once, but breathing should still be coordinated so that a final breath is taken in just before the lifting phase and released during lifting. BP increases during resistance training (unrelated to atherosclerosis) and tends to be highest when gripping excessively (common during the leg press exercise when working the large lower body muscles and clenching the machine's hand grips very tightly). However, BP returns to normal quickly after exercise; the increase is minimal when breathing technique is correct, regardless of exertion.

Balance training: Balance training involves challenging the center of gravity by undertaking exercises in unstable environments, such as standing on one leg or using balance or wobble boards. Basic strength training improves balance because it increases muscle size and strength around the joints, thus improving stability indirectly. Balance training can help some people with impaired proprioception and is often used in an attempt to prevent falls in the elderly (see below).

Hydration: Proper hydration is important, particularly when exertion is prolonged or occurs in a hot environment. People should be well hydrated before activity, drink fluids regularly during extended exertion, and replace any deficit remaining after activity. During exertion, about 120 to 240 mL (½ to 1 cup) of fluid every 15 to 20 min is reasonable depending on heat and exertion level; however, *overhydration, which can cause hyponatremia and consequent seizures, is to be avoided.*

PEARLS & PITFALLS

- Avoid overhydration during exercise because it can cause hyponatremia sometimes severe enough to cause seizures.

Fluid deficit after exertion is calculated by comparing preexercise and postexercise body weight. Fluid deficit is replaced on a one-for-one basis (ie, 1 L for each kg lost, or 2 cups/lb). In most cases, plain water is acceptable. Electrolyte-containing sports drinks may be preferred. However, fluids with a carbohydrate content of > 8% (8 g/100 mL, or 20 g in a typical 250-mL serving) decrease gastric emptying and slow fluid absorption. Mixing plain water with sports drinks at a 50:50 ratio allows faster absorption of the glucose and electrolytes. Patients with findings suggesting heat illness or volume depletion may require oral or IV fluid and electrolyte replacement immediately.

EXERCISE IN THE ELDERLY

At least 75% of people age > 65 yr do not exercise at recommended levels despite the known health benefits of exercise:

- Longer survival
- Improved quality of life (eg, endurance, strength, mood, sleep, flexibility, insulin sensitivity, possibly cognitive function, bone density [with weight-bearing exercise])

Furthermore, many elderly people are not aware of how hard to exercise and also do not appreciate how much exercise they are capable of.

Exercise is one of the safest ways to improve health. Because of the decline in physical capability due to aging and age-related disorders, the elderly may benefit from exercise more than younger people. Exercise has proven benefits even when begun in later years. Basic, modest strength training helps elderly patients carry out activities of daily living. Many elderly patients need guidance regarding a safe and appropriate regular exercise regimen.

The largest health benefits occur, particularly with aerobic exercise, when sedentary patients begin exercising.

Strength decreases with age, and decreased strength can compromise function. For example, almost half of women > 65 and more than half of women > 75 cannot lift 4.5 kg. Strength training can increase muscle mass by 25 to 100% or more, meaningfully improving function. The same degree of muscle work demands less cardiovascular exertion; increasing leg muscle strength improves walking speed and stair climbing. Also, institutionalized elderly with more muscle mass have better nitrogen balance, less deconditioning, and a better prognosis during critical illness.

Contraindications: Absolute contraindications include[1]

- Acute myocardial infarction (MI), within 2 days
- Ongoing unstable angina
- Uncontrolled cardiac arrhythmia with hemodynamic compromise
- Active endocarditis
- Symptomatic severe aortic stenosis
- Decompensated heart failure
- Acute pulmonary embolism, pulmonary infarction, or deep vein thrombosis
- Acute myocarditis or pericarditis
- Acute aortic dissection
- Physical disability that precludes safe and adequate exercise

Relative contraindications include[1]

- Known obstructive left main coronary artery stenosis
- Moderate to severe aortic stenosis with uncertain relation to symptoms
- Tachyarrhythmias with uncontrolled ventricular rates
- Acquired advanced or complete heart block
- Hypertrophic obstructive cardiomyopathy with severe resting gradient
- Recent stroke or transient ischemic attack
- Mental impairment with limited ability to safely cooperate
- Resting hypertension with systolic or diastolic blood pressures > 200/110 mmHg
- Uncorrected medical conditions, such as significant anemia, important electrolyte imbalance, and hyperthyroidism

Most patients with relative contraindications can exercise in some form, although typically at lower levels of intensity and in more structured circumstances than other patients (see p. 3256). At times, shorter bursts of higher intensity exercise with rests between attempts can be more accommodating than sustained moderate-intensity exercise. The exercise program may be modified for patients with other disorders (eg, arthritic disorders, particularly those involving major weight-bearing joints, such as the knees, ankles, and hips).

Patients should be clearly told to stop exercising and seek medical attention if they develop chest pain, light-headedness, or palpitations.

Screening: Before beginning an exercise program, elderly people should undergo clinical evaluation aimed at detecting cardiac disorders and physical limitations to exercise. Routine ECG is not required unless history and physical examination indicate otherwise. Exercise stress testing is usually unnecessary for elderly people who plan to begin exercising slowly and increase intensity only gradually. For sedentary people who plan to begin intense exercise, stress testing should be considered if they have any of the following:[1]

- Known coronary artery disease
- Symptoms of coronary artery disease
- ≥ 2 cardiac risk factors (eg, hypercholesterolemia, hypertension, obesity, sedentary lifestyle, smoking, family history of early coronary artery disease)
- Lung disease, known or suspected
- Diabetes, known or suspected

1. Fletcher GF, Ades PA, Kligfield P, et al: Exercise standards for testing and training: a scientific statement from the American Heart Association. *Circulation* 128(8): 873–934, 2013.

Exercise program: A comprehensive exercise program should include

- Aerobic activity
- Strength training
- Flexibility and balance training
- Variation (regular change in exercise to avoid overadaptation to the same stimulus, but also to avoid minor injuries due to repetitive actions)

Often a single program can be designed to achieve all exercise goals. Strength training improves muscular mass, muscular endurance, and strength. If strength training is done through a full range of motion, many exercises improve flexibility, and the enhanced muscle strength improves joint stability and, consequently, balance. Moreover, if rests between sets are minimal, cardiovascular function also improves.

Duration of **aerobic activity** for elderly people is similar to that for younger adults, but exercise should be less intense. Usually during exercise, the person should be able to comfortably converse, and intensity should be ≤ 6/10 on a perceived scale of exertion. Elderly people who have no contraindications can gradually increase their target heart rate (HR_{max}) to the one calculated by use of age-based formulas.

Some deconditioned elderly people need to improve their functional abilities (eg, by strength training) before they will be capable of aerobic exercise.

Strength training is done according to the same principles and techniques as in younger adults. Lighter forces (loads/resistance) should be used initially (eg, using bands or weights as light as 1 kg or arising from a chair) and increased as tolerated. More aggressive training (the use of higher resistance initially) should be under the supervision of a qualified fitness professional.

To help increase **flexibility,** major muscle groups should be stretched once daily, ideally after exercise when muscles are most compliant.

Balance training traditionally involves challenging the center of gravity by undertaking exercises in unstable environments, such as standing on one leg or using balance or wobble boards. Balance training can help some people with impaired proprioception and is often used in an attempt to prevent falls in the elderly. However, it is often ineffective because any balance activity is skill specific (eg, good balance while standing on a balance board does not improve balance in dissimilar activities). For most elderly people, flexibility and strength training exercises prevent falls more effectively. Such a program develops strength around the joints and helps people hold body positions more effectively while standing and walking. In people who have difficulty standing and walking because of poor balance, more challenging balance tasks (eg, standing on a wobble board) are simply likely to facilitate injury and are contraindicated.

379 Financial Issues in Health Care

Health care in the US is technologically advanced but expensive, costing about $3.2 trillion dollars in 2015, which was 17.8% of gross domestic product (GDP). For decades, health care spending in the US has increased more than the rate of growth for the overall economy. The percentage of GDP spent on health care in the US is significantly higher than that in any other nation. According to the Organization for Economic Cooperation and Development (OECD), in 2013 the US spent 16.4% of GDP on health care compared to around 11% for the next highest countries, including the Netherlands, Switzerland, Sweden, Germany, and France.

Also, the amount of money spent per capita on health care is higher in the US than that in other countries. In 2013, the US spent more than $8700 per capita, which was 2 1/2 times more than the OECD average health expenditure per person and twice as much as that of relatively wealthy countries such as France and Canada. The absolute amount and the rate of increase in the US are widely regarded as unsustainable. Consequently, US health care is currently in flux, as the government attempts to find ways to provide universal health care and reduce its costs.

Consequences of increased US spending on health care include the following:

- Increased government spending (resulting in higher national debt, decreased funding for other programs, or both)
- Slowed growth or a real decline in workers' earnings due to higher payments for health insurance premiums
- Increased costs to employers (resulting in increased product cost and movement of jobs to countries with lower health care costs)

Even though US health care spending per capita is the highest in the world, many people in the US do not have health insurance, whereas other developed countries, despite lower per capita expenditures, ensure universal access to health care. Furthermore, the high spending may not lead to correspondingly superior outcomes; according to the OECD report, in 2013 the US ranked below the OECD average on many health care outcome measures, such as infant mortality and life expectancy at birth.

Funding

Health care providers in the US are paid by the following:

- Private insurance
- Government insurance programs
- Individual out-of-pocket funds

In addition, the government directly provides some health care in government hospitals and clinics staffed by government employees. Examples are the Veteran's Health Administration and the Indian Health Service.

Private insurance: Private insurance is purchased from for-profit and not-for-profit insurance companies, which are accredited separately in each state. Although there are many health insurance companies in the US, a given state tends to have a limited number.

Most private insurance is purchased by corporations as a benefit for employees. Premiums are typically shared by employers and employees. But because the cost of employer-provided health insurance is not considered taxable income for the employee, the government in effect provides some subsidization. People may also purchase private health insurance themselves.

The Patient Protection and Affordable Care Act (PPACA, or Affordable Care Act [ACA]) is US health care reform legislation intended, among other things, to increase the availability, affordability, and use of health insurance (www.hhs.gov/healthcare/rights). Many of the ACA's provisions involve an expansion of the private insurance market; it creates incentives for employers to provide health insurance and mandates that nearly all individuals not covered by their employer or a government insurance program (eg, Medicare, Medicaid) purchase private health insurance (individual mandate).

To enable risk pooling and minimize overhead, the ACA requires creation of health insurance exchanges within each state. These exchanges are government-regulated, standardized health plans that are administered and sold by private insurance companies. States may join together to run multistate exchanges. The federal government may establish exchanges in states that do not do so themselves. There will be separate exchanges for individuals and small businesses. To qualify for listing on an exchange, a plan must provide a defined minimum level of coverage (as well as higher levels of coverage). Subsidies may be available to individuals on a sliding scale depending on income.

The ACA requires that private insurance plans, including those available on the exchanges, do the following:

- Put no annual or lifetime limits on coverage
- Have no exclusions for preexisting conditions (guaranteed issue)
- Allow children to remain on their parent's health insurance up to age 26
- Provide limited variations in price (premiums can vary based only on age, geographic area, tobacco use, and number of family members)
- Allow for limited out-of-pocket expenses (in 2017, $7,150 for individuals and $14,300 for families)
- Not discontinue coverage (called rescission) except in cases of fraud
- Cover certain defined preventive services with no cost-sharing
- Spend at least 80% to 85% of premiums on medical costs

Government insurance programs: The main government insurance programs include

- Medicare, which funds the elderly, the disabled, and people receiving long-term dialysis therapy (www.medicare.gov)
- Medicaid, which funds certain people who are living near or below the poverty level and/or who have disabilities (www.medicaid.gov)

Other government programs include

- State Children's Health Insurance Program, which provides matching federal funds to states for health insurance for families with children and which was designed to help ensure coverage for uninsured children when family income was below average but too high to qualify for Medicaid
- Tricare, which covers about 9 million active duty and retired military personnel and their families (almost 9.5 million Tricare subscribers use government-provided care)
- Veterans Health Administration (VHA), which is a government-operated health care system that provides comprehensive health services to eligible military veterans (about 9 million veterans are enrolled)
- Indian Health Service, which is a system of government hospitals and clinics providing health services to about 2 million American Indians and Alaskan natives living on or near a reservation

Overall, about 30% of the population is covered by government insurance or government-provided care. The ACA expands the eligibility criteria for Medicaid and provides federal funding assistance to state Medicaid programs. However, it is still not yet clear how widely available states will make Medicaid and, thus, how many additional people will be enrolled.

Out of pocket: People pay for care not covered by other sources out of their own funds, often using their savings for small expenditures and borrowing (including using credit cards) for large expenditures.

Flexible spending accounts (FSAs) are offered by some employers. Through these accounts, employees can choose to have a limited amount of money deducted from their paychecks to pay for out-of-pocket health care expenses. The money deducted is not subject to federal income taxes. However, the account does not earn interest, and any unused money is forfeited at the end of the year.

Health savings accounts (HSAs) can also be used to pay out-of-pocket expenses; these accounts earn interest, and unused balances need not be forfeited. Most people who are eligible for these accounts are eligible because their health insurance plans limit their reimbursements enough to be classified as high-deductible health plans.

About 17% of health care costs in the US are funded out-of-pocket. Charges for health care services tend to be much larger for individuals than for large payors such as insurance companies that can negotiate discounts. Thus, individuals paying out-of-pocket charges that are not covered by insurance can have particularly large bills; these bills may be so large that expecting an individual to pay them is unrealistic. Out-of-pocket expenditures for health care contribute significantly to a large number of bankruptcies in the US.

The ACA requires that nearly all individuals have some type of health insurance coverage. However, the penalties for no doing so are only financial and are less costly than purchasing health insurance, so a significant number of individuals are likely to remain uncovered and to continue to pay out of pocket for health care.

KEY POINTS

- Costs of health care are much higher in the US than in other countries, but the US still ranks low on important outcome measures such as infant mortality and life expectancy.
- Health care is paid for by government programs (eg, Medicare, Medicaid), private health insurance plans (usually through employers), and personal funds (out-of-pocket).
- By not taxing employer-paid health insurance or money in flexible spending or health savings accounts, the government subsidizes private health insurance to some extent.

CAUSES OF HIGH HEALTH CARE COSTS

Health care costs in the US are disproportionately high for many reasons.

Use of costly new technologies and drugs: Such use may be the largest single factor increasing health care costs. Use may be appropriate or inappropriate, but in either case, cost is increased. An example of appropriate but costly treatment is the use of fibrinolysis or angioplasty to treat an MI; before the 1980s, when these treatments began to be used commonly, treating an MI was much less costly (but also less effective). On the other hand, many new and costly treatments, including some in popular use, are ineffective, offer only marginal advantages, or are used inappropriately for patients unlikely to benefit. An example is use of lower lumbar spinal fusion to treat chronic low back pain; many experts think this treatment is ineffective and/or grossly overused.

Use of many such costly treatments tends to vary considerably among geographic areas and among physician practices within a geographic area (termed practice variation). For some specific disorders (eg, coronary artery disease), health outcomes are no better in areas where adjusted health spending is high than in areas where it is low.

Corporate and governmental subsidization removes some economic disincentives to health care use and has been postulated to contribute to increased health care use (and thus costs).

Increased costs of health care goods and services: Drug costs have increased. One reason is the increasing cost of developing a new drug, often in the vicinity of $1 billion. The cost of drug development decreases the economic incentive to develop drugs with lower profit potentials, even those that could substantially benefit particular groups (eg, drugs to treat rare diseases) or public health in general (eg, vaccines, antibiotics).

Marketing of new drugs and devices: Intensive marketing to physicians and consumers (with direct-to-consumer advertising) has been suggested as a cause of overuse of costly new technologies and drugs. Some of these new measures may be no more effective than older, less costly ones.

Overuse of specialty care: Specialists are increasingly providing more care; reasons may include a decreasing number of primary care physicians and an increased desire by patients to see a specialist.

Specialty care is often more expensive than primary care; specialists have higher fees and may do more testing (often pursuing less common diagnoses) than primary care physicians. Also, evaluation and treatment of a patient who could have been managed by a single primary care physician may require more than one specialist.

High administrative costs: The percentage of health care dollars spent on administration is estimated to be 20 to > 30%. Most administrative costs are generated by private insurance, and most of those costs are generated by marketing and underwriting, processes that do not improve medical care; however, the Affordable Care Act limits the amount that private insurance can spend on administrative costs. Also, the existence of numerous private insurance plans in the same geographic area typically increases health care providers' costs by making processing (eg, claim submission, coding) complicated and time-consuming.

Physician fees: Physicians in the US are more highly compensated than other professionals in the US and more than physicians in many other countries. This disparity occurs partly because physicians in other countries typically spend far less on their medical education and malpractice insurance than those in the US and have lower office overhead. Because physician fees account for only about 20% of total health care costs, even a significant reduction in physician fees would have only a modest effect on overall costs.

Malpractice costs: The issue of malpractice adds to the cost of medicine directly and indirectly (by triggering defensive medicine).

The direct cost is the malpractice insurance premiums paid by physicians, other providers, health care institutions, and medical drug and device manufacturers. These premiums, which cover claim settlements and malpractice insurance company overhead and profits, must ultimately be paid from health care revenues.

As onerous as premiums and the threat of lawsuits can be for individual physicians (particularly in certain high-risk specialties and geographic areas), the total annual malpractice premium amount paid in 2008 by physicians and institutions was about $12 billion, representing only about 0.6% of total annual health care costs. Actual malpractice settlements paid out in 2014 were $3.9 billion (< 0.2% of health care costs). Thus, even a major reduction in malpractice settlements would not lower total health care costs significantly, although it could greatly affect certain physicians' practices.

Defensive medicine: Defensive medicine refers to diagnostic tests or treatments that providers do to guard against the possibility of malpractice litigation, even though such tests and treatments may not be warranted clinically. For example, a physician may hospitalize a patient who is likely to do well with outpatient treatment to avoid a lawsuit in the unlikely event of an adverse outcome.

The actual costs attributable to defensive medicine are difficult to measure. Few rigorous studies have assessed this cost, and estimates from these studies vary greatly, ranging from negligible to substantial (some experts believe that these costs are larger than direct malpractice costs). Some of the uncertainty lies in the fact that defensive medicine is defined subjectively (ie, it is the clinician's reason for doing a test, not how unlikely or uncommon the disorder being tested for is). A clinician's motivation is hard to determine, and different clinicians can reasonably vary in their assessment of the need for testing in a given case (except for a relatively few situations that have clear, sensitive, and specific guidelines for testing). In some survey studies of defensive medicine, physicians were asked whether and when they practice defensive medicine. However, such self-reporting may be unreliable, and such surveys often have a low response rate. Thus, the extent of defensive medicine is unknown.

Furthermore, even when defensive testing can be identified, calculating potential cost savings is not straightforward. Decreasing the amount of defensive testing involves a change in marginal costs (the cost of providing or withholding an additional unit of service), which are different from actual charges or reimbursements. In addition, studies of states that have enacted tort reforms to limit compensation to patients for iatrogenic injuries have had conflicting results about whether such reforms lower health care expenditures.

Aging of the population: Although often cited as a factor, population aging is probably not responsible for recent increased costs because the generation now in old age has not yet increased disproportionately; also, more effective health care has tended to delay serious illness in this generation. However, the aging of baby boomers may affect costs more as the proportion of the population > 65 increases from about 13% currently to almost 20% after 2030.

KEY POINTS

- Use of costly new technologies and drugs may be the largest single factor among the many that increase US health care costs.
- Use of such technologies sometimes varies widely between geographic areas, and increased use does not always result in better clinical outcomes.
- The percentage of US health care dollars spent on administration is 20 to > 30%.
- Reducing physician fees is not likely to decrease health care costs very much.
- Direct malpractice costs have a small effect on overall health care costs, but the costs of defensive medicine, done to guard against malpractice suits, are difficult to measure and largely unknown.
- Aging of the US population probably has not contributed greatly to the disproportionate increases in US health care costs but may do so as baby boomers age.

CONTAINING HEALTH CARE COSTS

Conceptually, total health care costs can be contained or decreased only by some combination of the following:

- Decreasing use of health care services
- Decreasing reimbursement for services that are used
- Decreasing overhead (payor, provider, or both)

Some strategies adversely affect access to care or outcomes; others may improve care. Evaluating different strategies is difficult, partly because accurately measuring patient-centered health outcomes (eg, morbidity and mortality, quality-adjusted life years [QALY]) tends to be expensive and to require large numbers of patients and long follow-up periods. As a result, most measures used to assess health care quality reflect processes (how care was delivered) rather than outcome. How well these process measures predict ultimate health outcomes is not always clear.

Decreasing Use of Health Care Services

Many strategies can decrease the use of health care services. Many involve limiting access to care (aimed at unnecessary care but sometimes affecting necessary care), but some limit need by improving health.

Limiting access to health care: Traditionally, limiting access has been the strategy used to limit health care costs.

Insurance companies have limited access to care by denying coverage to people likely to need care (eg, those with preexisting conditions) and by dropping coverage of heavy users (rescission). In the US, the Affordable Care Act, which became effective in 2014, has prohibited these practices.

Government may tighten eligibility criteria for medical assistance programs.

Payors may increase out-of-pocket costs, providing an economic incentive for patients to limit their own health care use. For example, payors may

- Limit the type and number of visits that are reimbursed (eg, mental health care, physical therapy)
- Increase deductibles and co-payments
- Decrease allowable amounts for covered procedures

These strategies probably adversely affect outcomes because evidence indicates that many patients avoid necessary as well as unnecessary care. For example, women may avoid screening (eg, Papanicolaou testing, mammography) and subsequently present with late-stage cancer; at-risk patients may avoid influenza vaccination.

By erecting administrative hurdles to care (eg, requiring approval for tests, referrals, and procedures; having complex enrollment procedures and regulations), payors, although not technically denying care, decrease use by a small amount.

State agencies may limit issuance of construction permits for new facilities and laboratories (called certificates of need).

Limiting access to health care can cause problems. For example, when people denied access become seriously ill (which is more likely when routine care is lacking), they are often treated in a hospital when a disorder is advanced. This care is largely uncompensated (not paid for by patient, insurance, or other source), increasing the burden on people who pay into the health care system, and may be more expensive than if routine care had been provided.

Eliminating unnecessary care: Unnecessary care is easy to define (care that does not improve patient outcome) but often difficult to recognize and still more difficult to eliminate. First steps include conducting more and better studies of comparative effectiveness and cost-effectiveness, so that best practices can be identified. Comparative effectiveness studies can evaluate areas other than drugs, such as effects of exercise, of physical therapy, and of different providers, systems, settings of medical care, and reimbursement systems. Education and monitoring of providers may decrease practice variation and increase cost-effectiveness. Eliminating the economic incentive for providing more intensive care (fee-for-service model) by using prospective payment systems (see below) and pay-for-performance models may encourage providers to eliminate cost-ineffective care processes.

Better coordination of services among providers (eg, by closer communication and use of universally readable electronic medical records) may make evaluation and treatment more efficient (eg, by eliminating duplication of tests).

Encouraging palliative hospice care, when appropriate, may help decrease use of costly, often technology-intensive, cure-directed care.

Improving health: Increased use of relatively inexpensive preventive services (eg, screening, diagnosis, and treatment of diabetes, hypertension, and hyperlipidemia; screening for breast and colon cancer) may decrease the subsequent need for expensive treatments (eg, for MI, stroke, or late-stage cancer). However, preventive measures may not decrease costs for a given private insurance company because savings are often not realized for many years; by that time, many patients have switched insurance plans. In the US, people stay with a given insurance company for an average of about 6 yr (usually determined by how often they change jobs)—too short to realize a savings via preventive care.

Strategies to increase preventive care include

- Incentives to increase the number of primary care physicians (who can often provide appropriate screening measures and help prevent complications)
- Pay-for-performance measures that financially reward adherence to preventive care guidelines
- Elimination of co-payments for preventive services
- Free preventive services, particularly for needy people

Whether care management programs that attempt to improve patient adherence to treatment plans and clinician adherence to guidelines can improve outcomes or reduce costs (eg, of potentially avoidable hospitalization or complications) is unclear; some studies do not show a benefit.

Decreasing Reimbursement for Care Used

Even when health care is provided, strategies can be used to limit payments.

Lower fees: Payors (government and private) may negotiate lower fees with institutions and providers or simply dictate such fees. In the US, reimbursement rates established by Medicare and Medicaid tend to influence rates paid by other plans, sometimes decreasing reimbursement.

Increased use of primary care: Measures may help increase the use of less costly primary care vs specialty care. For example, in the patient-centered medical home model, primary care practitioners coordinate and integrate all aspects of medical care, including specialty and interdisciplinary care, in various settings (eg, home, hospital, long-term care facility). Many authorities think that this model can decrease unnecessary specialty care, duplicative care, and care that may be inappropriate for the individual's health goals (eg, palliation rather than diagnosis).

Measures to increase the supply of primary care physicians have been proposed. They include increasing reimbursement for primary care, shifting more government funding of residency programs to primary care training, and making primary care more attractive to medical students, although how the last strategy could be implemented is unclear.

Prospective payment systems: In these systems, providers are paid a fixed amount regardless of how much care is provided. The amount may be based on a specified episode of care or be a fixed annual reimbursement per patient. For example, some Medicare reimbursement is based on diagnosis-related groups (DRGs); in such cases, Medicare pays a fixed amount based on the diagnosis. In capitated systems, providers are paid a fixed annual amount to provide health care for patients regardless of the services used.

Prospective payment systems reward less expensive care (and thus usually use of fewer services), in contrast to fee-for-service systems, which reward use of more services. However, prospective payment creates an economic disincentive to care for complex patients (eg, those who have multiple disorders or who are seriously ill) and may inhibit provision of necessary care. Because a decrease in the amount of care provided has the potential to decrease quality of care, quality control systems (eg, professional review organizations) are often also established.

Accountable Care Organizations: Accountable Care Organizations (ACOs) are integrated organizations of health care providers that agree to be accountable for the costs and quality of care for a defined group of beneficiaries assigned to them. Their reimbursement is based on measures of health care quality and reductions in the cost of care for their assigned beneficiaries rather than the volume of services provided. The amount of reimbursement to the ACO is based on the cost of care provided to similar patients not in ACOs. The ACOs share the differences in such costs (gains and losses) with the insurer. The ACO can use various payment models for its own providers, including capitation and sometimes fee for service.

Denial of claims: In the US, unlike in most of the developed world, insurance carriers routinely deny a significant percentage of claims for services delivered to patients. In one study in California, the denial rate averaged about 30% in 2009; some of the claims were paid after appeal, but appealing a claim is quite costly in time and effort for patients, providers, and payors alike.

Competition: Competition among providers for patients and among insurance companies for subscribers is thought to encourage lowering of charges (eg, by those who charge more than their competitors for a similar service). However, the ultimate consumers (ie, patients) usually do not know providers' charges in advance, and if they know, they often cannot act on this knowledge (eg, because patients are often limited to certain providers and limited in their ability to judge quality of care). Also, because the cost of medical care is subsidized for most consumers (eg, through employer-paid health insurance, tax deductions, and flexible spending accounts or medical savings accounts), consumers have less incentive to price shop than for most other purchases. Thus, competition is most effective in lowering costs and maintaining quality when it is among large organizations. For example, insurance companies can compete for contracts from employers such as corporations or the government; providers such as practitioner organizations and hospitals can compete for contracts with insurance companies.

Competition has some disadvantages. It results in multiple systems of claim submission and evaluation, which require more time from providers, their clerical staff, or both. Also, processes such as eligibility determination, referrals, co-payments, and coding must be coordinated between a large number of incompatible insurance company systems. Thus, competition increases the clerical (administrative) burden of the overall health care system.

Decreased drug costs: Using generic drugs or, when appropriate, more cost-effective brand-name drugs can help decrease drug costs. Strategies include

- Educating providers about cost-effective drug use
- Restricting drug marketing
- Establishing formularies and using pharmacy benefit managers
- Allowing the government to negotiate drug prices for patients covered by government insurance
- Allowing importation of drugs purchased from other countries to the US

Negative effects on medical research: In many academic medical centers, income from clinical practice has enabled physicians and institutions to participate in medical research. Similarly, income from drug sales supports pharmaceutical research. Thus, decreased reimbursement for care and drug sales may cause a decline in medical research. If other sources (eg, government or private grants) are used to fund research, these funds must be considered as health care costs and thus may offset savings realized from decreasing reimbursement.

Decreasing Overhead

Overhead is health care payments that do not go to health care providers (eg, administrative costs, malpractice insurance, corporate profits in for-profit hospitals and insurance companies).

Decreasing payor overhead: Government health care plans in developed countries (including the US) and private health plans outside the US have overhead costs that usually represent 3 to 5% of total costs (ie, ≥ 95% of all health care funds go to the delivery of health care). However, in the US, private insurers have had overhead costs of about 20 to 30%, partly because these insurers need staff to do extensive underwriting (identifying and rejecting applicants likely to require costly care, including those with preexisting conditions or a high likelihood of developing disorders), to evaluate claims for denial, and to adjudicate appeals by providers; they also typically need to show a profit. No evidence indicates that these activities and their higher administrative costs improve clinical care or outcomes. The Affordable Care Act now mandates that insurers spend 80% (for individual or small-group insurers) or 85% (for large-group insurers) of premium dollars on health costs and claims, leaving only 20% or 15%, respectively, for administrative costs and profits.

Strategies that may help minimize overhead costs include

- Increased use of standardized electronic health records
- Increased use of government plans and possibly not-for-profit plans, which have lower overhead than for-profit plans

Competition among payors is thought to encourage increased administrative efficiency, but it also increases the incentives to deny claims and coverage (which itself requires an extensive bureaucracy).

Decreasing provider overhead: Any payor reform that eliminates the need for the many billing and claims personnel who manage the billing of multiple payors and negotiate appeals and justify claims will decrease provider overhead. For example, some countries that have multiple insurance companies vying for business (eg, Germany, Japan) require the following:

- The payment amounts and rules are the same for all insurance companies.
- In many cases, payors are required to pay all provider bills.
- The cost of the same service is the same throughout the country.

Although malpractice costs are a small fraction of overall costs, malpractice costs for certain physicians can consume a considerable part of their annual income. Reforms that significantly decrease the number of suits and settlements should eventually lower premiums and greatly benefit these physicians; such reforms may also decrease the use of unnecessary, defensive medicine.

KEY POINTS

- Because of health care reform, limiting access to health care, which payors have traditionally done to contain costs, will probably decrease in the US.
- Unnecessary medical care is easier to define than eliminate and even to recognize.
- Whether improving health can reduce health care costs is unknown.
- Many strategies used to decrease reimbursement for health care (eg, decreasing provider fees, using prospective payment systems, denying claims, encouraging competition, decreasing drug costs) have significant disadvantages.
- Theoretically, decreasing overhead costs of payors and providers and reforming malpractice laws could substantially reduce costs.

380 General Principles of Medical Genetics

A gene, the basic unit of heredity, is a segment of DNA containing all the information necessary to synthesize a polypeptide (protein). Protein synthesis, folding, and tertiary and quaternary structure ultimately determine much of the body's structure and function.

Structure

Humans have about 20,000 to 23,000 genes. Genes are contained in chromosomes in the cell nucleus and mitochondria. In humans, somatic (nongerm) cell nuclei normally have 46 chromosomes in 23 pairs. Each pair consists of one chromosome from the mother and one from the father. Twenty-two of the pairs, the autosomes, are normally homologous (identical in size, shape, and position and number of genes). The 23rd pair, the sex chromosomes (X and Y), determines a person's sex as well as containing other functional genes. Women have 2 X chromosomes (which are homologous) in somatic cell nuclei; men have one X and one Y chromosome (which are heterologous). The X chromosome carries genes responsible for many hereditary traits; the smaller Y chromosome carries genes that initiate male sex differentiation, as well as a few other genes. Because the X chromosome has many more genes than the Y chromosome, many X chromosome genes in males are not paired; in order to maintain a balance of genetic material between men and women, one of the X chromosomes in women is randomly inactivated. A karyotype is the full set of chromosomes in a person's cells.

Germ cells (egg and sperm) undergo meiosis, which reduces the number of chromosomes to 23—half the number in somatic cells. In meiosis, the genetic information inherited from a person's mother and father is recombined through crossing over (exchange between homologous chromosomes). When an egg is fertilized by a sperm at conception, the normal number of 46 chromosomes is reconstituted.

Genes are arranged linearly along the DNA of chromosomes. Each gene has a specific location (locus), which is typically the same on each of the 2 homologous chromosomes. The genes that occupy the same locus on each chromosome of a pair (one inherited from the mother and one from the father) are called alleles. Each gene consists of a specific DNA sequence; 2 alleles may have slightly different or the same DNA sequences. Having a pair of identical alleles for a particular gene is homozygosity; having a pair of nonidentical alleles is heterozygosity. Some genes occur in multiple copies that may be next to each other or in different locations in the same or different chromosomes.

Gene Function

Genes consist of DNA. The length of the gene determines the length of the protein the gene codes for. DNA is a double helix in which nucleotides (bases) are paired; adenine (A) is paired with thymine (T) and guanine (G) is paired with cytosine (C). DNA is transcribed during protein synthesis, in which one strand of DNA is used as a template against which messenger RNA (mRNA) is made. RNA has the same base pairs as DNA, except that uracil (U) replaces T. Parts of mRNA travel from the nucleus to the cytoplasm and then to the ribosome, where protein synthesis occurs. Transfer RNA (tRNA) brings each amino acid back to the ribosome where it is added to the growing polypeptide chain in a sequence determined by the mRNA. As a chain of amino acids is assembled, it folds upon itself to create a complex 3-dimensional structure under the influence of nearby chaperone molecules.

The code in DNA is written in triplets containing 3 of the 4 possible nucleotides. Specific amino acids are coded by specific triplets. Because there are 4 nucleotides, the number of possible triplets is 4^3 (64). Because there are only 20 amino acids, there are redundant (extra) triplet combinations. Some triplets code for the same amino acids as other triplets. Other triplets may code for elements such as instructions to start or stop protein synthesis and the order in which to combine and assemble amino acids.

Genes consist of exons and introns. Exons code for amino acid components of the final protein. Introns contain other information that affects control and speed of protein production. Exons and introns together are transcribed onto mRNA, but the segments transcribed from introns are later spliced out. Many factors regulate transcription, including antisense RNA, which is synthesized from the DNA strand that is not transcribed into mRNA. In addition to DNA, chromosomes contain histones and other proteins that affect gene expression (which proteins and how many proteins are synthesized from a given gene).

Genotype refers to a specific genetic composition and sequence; it determines which proteins are coded for production. In contrast, genome refers to the entire composition of a set of haploid chromosomes, including the genes they contain.

Phenotype refers to the entire physical, biochemical, and physiologic makeup of a person—ie, how the cell (and thus the body) functions. Phenotype is determined by the types and amounts of proteins actually synthesized, ie, how the genes are actually expressed.

Expression refers to the process in which the information encoded in a gene is used to control the assembly of a molecule (usually protein or RNA). Gene expression depends on multiple factors such as whether a trait is dominant or recessive, the penetrance and expressivity of the gene (see p. 3191), degree of tissue differentiation (determined by tissue type and age), environmental factors, whether expression is sex-limited or subject to chromosomal inactivation or genomic imprinting, and other unknown factors.

Epigenetic factors: Factors that affect gene expression without changing the genome sequence are epigenetic factors.

Knowledge of the many biochemical mechanisms that mediate gene expression is growing rapidly. One mechanism is variability in intron splicing (also called alternative splicing). Because introns are spliced out, the exons may also be spliced out, and then the exons can be assembled in many combinations, resulting in many different mRNAs capable of coding for similar but different proteins. The number of proteins that can be synthesized by humans is > 100,000 even though the human genome has only about 20,000 genes. Other mechanisms mediating gene expression include DNA methylation and histone reactions such as methylation and acetylation. DNA methylation tends to silence a gene. Histones resemble spools around which DNA winds. Histone modifications such as methylation can increase or decrease the quantity of proteins synthesized from a particular gene. Histone acetylation is associated with decreased gene expression. The strand of DNA that is not transcribed to form mRNA may also be used as a template for synthesis of RNA that controls transcription of the opposite strand. Another important mechanism involves microRNAs (miRNAs). MiRNAs are short, hairpin-derived (hairpin refers to the shape the RNA sequences assume as they bind together) RNAs that repress target gene expression after transcription. They may be involved in regulation of as many as 60% of transcribed proteins.

Traits and Inheritance Patterns

A trait may be as simple as the color of the eyes or as complex as susceptibility to diabetes. Expression of a trait may involve one gene or many genes. Some single-gene defects cause abnormalities in multiple tissues, an effect called pleiotropy. For example, osteogenesis imperfecta (a connective tissue disorder that often results from abnormalities in a single collagen gene) may cause fragile bones, deafness, blue-colored sclerae, dysplastic teeth, hypermobile joints, and heart valve abnormalities.

Construction of a family pedigree: The family pedigree (family tree) can be used to diagram inheritance patterns. It is also commonly used in genetic counseling. The pedigree uses conventional symbols to represent family members and pertinent health information about them (see Fig. 380–1). Some familial disorders with identical phenotypes have multiple patterns of inheritance.

KEY POINTS

- Phenotype is determined by gene expression as well as the genotype.
- Mechanisms regulating gene expression are being elucidated and include intron splicing, DNA methylation, histone reactions, and microRNAs.

SINGLE-GENE DEFECTS

Genetic disorders determined by a single gene (Mendelian disorders) are easiest to analyze and the most well understood. If expression of a trait requires only one copy of a gene (one allele), that trait is considered dominant. If expression of a trait requires 2 copies of a gene (2 alleles), that trait is considered recessive. One exception is X-linked disorders. Because males usually have no paired allele to offset the effects of most alleles on the X chromosome, the X chromosome allele is expressed in males even if the trait is recessive. Other exceptions, such as mitochondrial disorders, exist as well. Mitochondrial genes are typically inherited only from the maternal oocyte.

Many specific disorders have been described (see Table 380–1).

Autosomal Dominant

Only one abnormal allele of a gene is needed to express an autosomal dominant trait; ie, heterozygotes and homozygotes

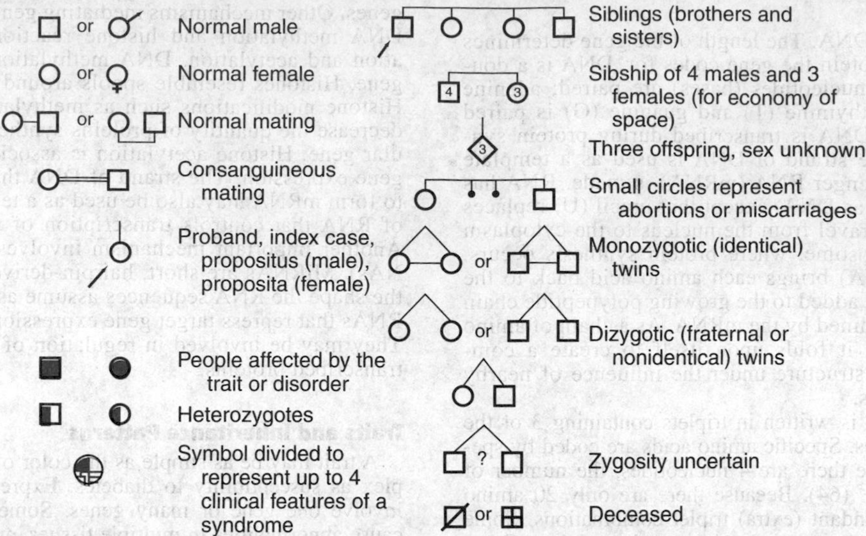

Fig. 380–1. Symbols for constructing a family pedigree. In the pedigree, symbols for each generation in the family are placed in a row and numbered with Roman numerals, starting with the older generation at the top and ending with the most recent at the bottom (see Figs. 380–2, 380–3, 380–4, and 380–5). Within each generation, people are numbered from left to right with Arabic numerals. Siblings are usually listed by age, with the oldest on the left. Thus, each member of the pedigree can be identified by 2 numbers (eg, II, 4). A spouse is also assigned an identifying number.

for the abnormal gene are affected. A typical pedigree of an autosomal dominant trait is shown in Fig. 380–2.

In general, the following rules apply:

- An affected person has an affected parent.
- A heterozygous affected parent and an unaffected parent have, on average, an equal number of affected and unaffected children; ie, risk of occurrence for each child of an affected parent is 50%.
- Unaffected children of an affected parent do not transmit the trait to their descendants.
- Males and females are equally likely to be affected.

Autosomal Recessive

Two copies of an abnormal allele are needed to express an autosomal recessive trait. An example of a pedigree is shown in Fig. 380–3.

Table 380–1. EXAMPLES OF GENETIC DISORDERS WITH MENDELIAN INHERITANCE

GENE	DOMINANT	RECESSIVE
Non–X-linked	Marfan syndrome Huntington disease	Cystic fibrosis
X-linked	Familial rickets Hereditary nephritis	Red–green color blindness Hemophilia

In general, the following rules of inheritance apply:

- If normal parents have an affected child, both parents are heterozygotes. On average, one fourth of their children are affected, half are heterozygotes, and one fourth are normal. Therefore, among the children, the chance of not developing the disorder (ie, being normal or a carrier) is three fourths, and among the unaffected children, the chance of being a carrier is two-thirds.
- All children of an affected parent and a genotypically normal parent are phenotypically normal heterozygotes.
- On average, half the children of an affected parent and a heterozygote are affected, and half are heterozygotes.
- All children of 2 affected parents are affected.
- Males and females are equally likely to be affected.
- Heterozygotes are phenotypically normal but carry the abnormal gene.

Relatives are more likely to carry the same mutant allele, so mating between close relatives (consanguinity) increases

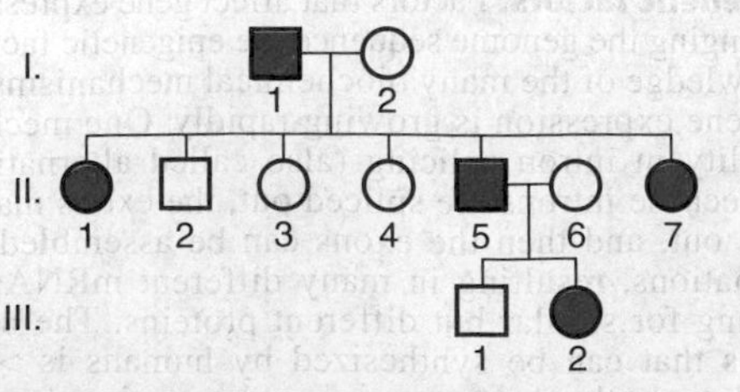

Fig. 380–2. Autosomal dominant inheritance.

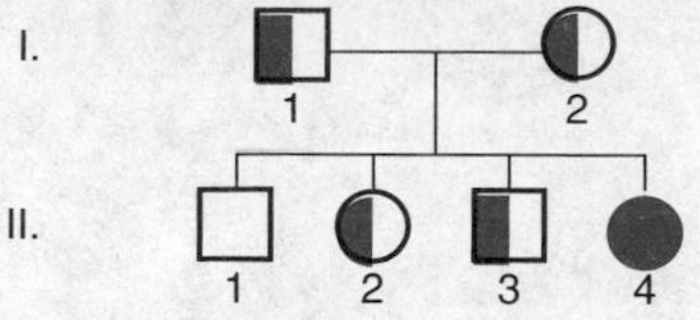

Fig. 380–3. Autosomal recessive inheritance.

the likelihood of having affected children. In parent-child or brother-sister unions (incest), the risk of having abnormal children is increased because so much of their genetic material is the same. In certain populations, the percentage of heterozygotes (carriers) is high because of a founder effect (ie, the group started with few members, one of whom was a carrier) or because carriers have a selective advantage (eg, heterozygosity for sickle cell anemia protects against malaria).

If the trait results in a defect of a specific protein (eg, an enzyme), heterozygotes usually have a reduced amount of that protein. If the mutation is known, molecular genetic techniques can identify heterozygous phenotypically normal people (eg, most of the time, people with cystic fibrosis).

X-Linked Dominant

X-linked dominant traits are carried on the X chromosome. Most are rare. Usually, males are more severely affected; some X-linked dominant disorders are often lethal in males. Females who carry only one abnormal allele are affected but less severely. A typical pedigree is shown in Fig. 380–4.

In general, the following rules of inheritance apply:

- Affected males transmit the trait to all of their daughters but to none of their sons.
- Affected heterozygous females transmit the trait to half of their children, regardless of sex.
- Affected homozygous females transmit the trait to all of their children.
- Because females can be heterozygous or homozygous, more females have the trait than males. The difference between the sexes is even larger if the disorder is lethal in males.

X-linked dominant inheritance may be difficult to differentiate from autosomal dominant inheritance by studying only inheritance patterns. Large pedigrees are required, with particular attention to children of affected males because male-to-male transmission rules out X-linkage (males pass only their Y chromosomes to their sons).

X-Linked Recessive

X-linked recessive traits are carried on the X chromosome. Thus, nearly all affected people are male because most females

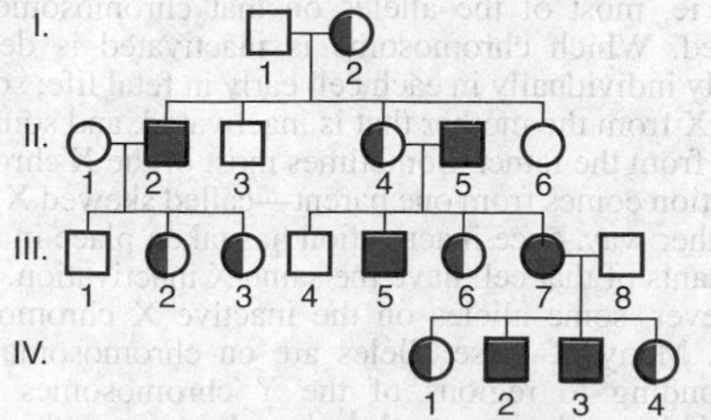

Fig. 380–4. X-linked dominant inheritance.

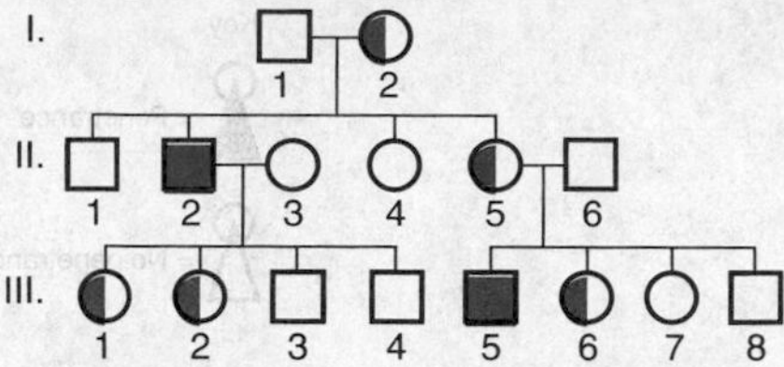

Fig. 380–5. X-linked recessive inheritance.

have one normal copy of the involved gene (ie, they are heterozygous). A typical pedigree is shown in Fig. 380–5.

In general, the following rules of inheritance apply:

- Nearly all affected people are male.
- Heterozygous females are usually phenotypically normal but, as carriers, transmit the abnormal gene to half of their children.
- Half the sons of a carrier female are affected, and half the daughters are carriers.
- An affected male never transmits the trait to his sons.
- All daughters of an affected male are carriers.
- No daughters of a carrier female and a normal father are affected, but half are carriers.

Occasionally, females who are heterozygous for X-linked mutations show some expression, but they are rarely affected as severely as affected males.

FACTORS AFFECTING GENE EXPRESSION

Many factors can affect gene expression. Some cause the expression of traits to deviate from the patterns predicted by Mendelian inheritance.

Penetrance and expressivity: Penetrance is how often a gene is expressed. It is defined as the percentage of people who have the gene and who develop the corresponding phenotype (see Fig. 380–6). A gene with incomplete (low) penetrance may not be expressed even when the trait is dominant or when it is recessive and the gene responsible for that trait is present on both chromosomes. Penetrance of the same gene may vary from person to person and may depend on a person's age. Even when an abnormal allele is not expressed (nonpenetrance), the unaffected carrier of the abnormal allele can pass it to children, who may have the clinical abnormality. In such cases, the pedigree appears to skip a generation. However, some cases of apparent nonpenetrance are due to the examiner's unfamiliarity with or inability to recognize minor manifestations of the disorder. Patients with minimal expression are sometimes considered to have a forme fruste of the disorder.

Expressivity is the extent to which a gene is expressed in one person. It can be graded as a percentage; eg, when a gene has 50% expressivity, only half the features are present or the severity is only half of what can occur with full expression. Expressivity may be influenced by the environment and by other genes, so people with the same gene may vary in phenotype. Expressivity can vary even among members of the same family.

Sex-limited inheritance: A trait that appears in only one sex is called sex-limited. Sex-limited inheritance is distinct from X-linked inheritance, which refers to traits carried on the X chromosome. Sex-limited inheritance, perhaps more correctly called sex-influenced inheritance, refers to special cases in which sex hormones and other physiologic differences between

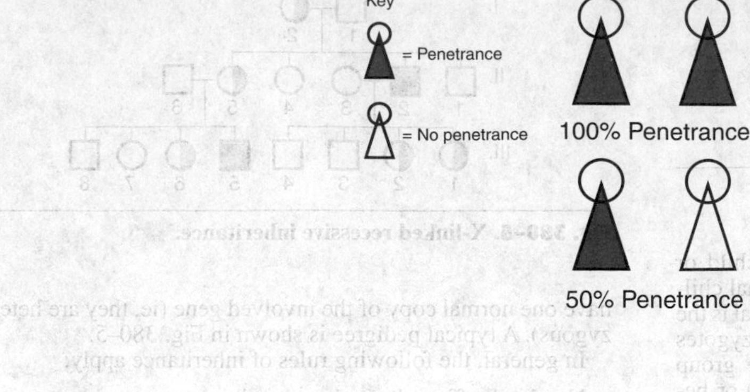

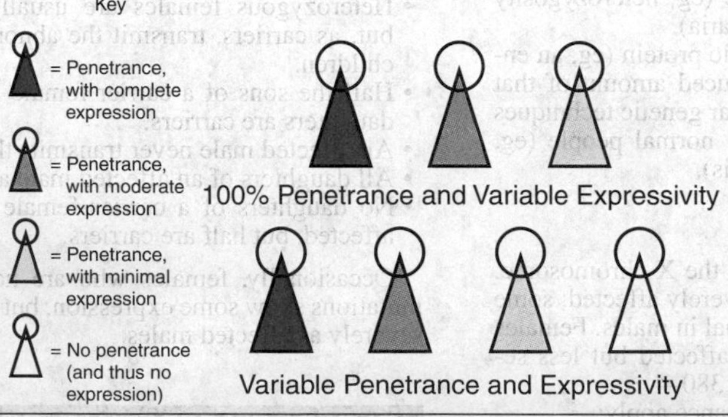

Fig. 380–6. Penetrance and expressivity.

How genotype is translated into phenotype depends on penetrance and expressivity.

Penetrance refers to whether the gene is expressed or not. That is, it refers to how many people with the gene have the trait associated with the gene. Penetrance may be complete (100%) or incomplete (eg, 50% when only half the people have the trait).

Expressivity determines how much the trait affects or how many features of the trait appear in the person. Expression, which can be stated as a percentage, ranges from complete to minimal, or it may not be present. Various factors, including genetic makeup, exposure to harmful substances, other environmental influences, and age, can affect expressivity.

Both penetrance and expressivity can vary: People with the gene may or may not have the trait and, in people with the trait, how the trait is expressed can vary.

males and females alter the expressivity and penetrance of a gene. For example, premature baldness (known as male-pattern baldness) is an autosomal dominant trait, but such baldness is rarely expressed in females and then usually only after menopause.

Genomic imprinting: Genomic imprinting is the differential expression of genetic material depending on whether it has been inherited from the father or mother. For most autosomes, both the parental and maternal alleles are expressed. However, in < 1% of alleles, expression is possible only from the paternal or maternal allele. For example, expression of the gene for insulin-like growth factor 2 is normally expressed only from the paternal allele. Genomic imprinting is usually determined by effects that occur normally in the development of gametes. Changes such as methylation of DNA may cause certain maternal or paternal alleles to be expressed to different degrees. A disorder may appear to skip a generation if genomic imprinting prevents the causative allele from being expressed. Defective imprinting, such as abnormal activation or silencing of alleles, can result in disorders (eg, Prader-Willi syndrome, Angelman syndrome).

Codominance: Codominant alleles are both observed. Thus, the phenotype of heterozygotes is distinct from that of either homozygote. For example, if a person has one allele coding for blood type A and one allele coding for blood type B, the person has both blood types (blood type AB).

Chromosomal inactivation: In females, who have 2 (or, with sex chromosomal abnormalities, > 2) X chromosomes (except in eggs), all but one of the X chromosomes is inactivated; ie, most of the alleles on that chromosome are not expressed. Which chromosome is inactivated is determined randomly individually in each cell early in fetal life; sometimes it is the X from the mother that is inactivated, and sometimes it is the X from the father. Sometimes most of the X chromosome inactivation comes from one parent—called skewed X inactivation. Either way, once inactivation has taken place in a cell, all descendants of that cell have the same X inactivation.

However, some alleles on the inactive X chromosome do express. Many of these alleles are on chromosomal regions corresponding to regions of the Y chromosomes (and are thus called pseudoautosomal regions because both males and females receive 2 copies of these regions).

KEY POINTS

- If a pedigree appears to skip a generation, consider incomplete penetrance, incomplete expression, and (less likely) genomic imprinting.
- Gene expression can also be modified by sex-limited inheritance, genomic imprinting, codominance of alleles, and X chromosome inactivation.

MULTIFACTORIAL (COMPLEX) INHERITANCE

Expression of many traits may involve multiple genes. Many such traits (eg, height) are distributed along a bell-shaped curve (normal distribution). Normally, each gene adds to or subtracts from the trait independently of other genes. In this distribution, few people are at the extremes and many are in the middle because people are unlikely to inherit multiple factors acting in the same direction. Environmental factors also add to or subtract from the final result.

Many relatively common congenital anomalies and familial disorders result from multifactorial inheritance. In an affected person, the disorder represents the sum of genetic and environmental influences. Risk of the occurrence of such a trait is much higher in 1st-degree relatives (siblings, parents, or children who share, on average, 50% of the affected person's genes) than in more distant relatives, who are likely to have inherited only a few high-liability genes.

Common disorders with multifactorial inheritance include hypertension, coronary artery disease, type II diabetes mellitus, cancer, cleft palate, and arthritis. Many specific genes contributing to these traits are being identified by using the most sensitive genetic tests available (called next-generation sequencing—see p. 3195) to test people with and without the traits for mutations. Genetically determined predisposing factors, including a family history and specific biochemical pathways often identified by molecular markers (eg, high cholesterol), can sometimes identify people who are at risk and are likely to benefit from preventive measures.

Multigenic, multifactorial traits seldom produce clear patterns of inheritance; however, these traits tend to occur more often among certain ethnic and geographic groups or among one sex or the other.

UNUSUAL ASPECTS OF INHERITANCE

Certain situations represent aberrant inheritance, often because genes or chromosomes are altered. However, some of these alterations, such as mosaicism, are very common; others, such as polymorphisms, are so common that they may be considered normal variants.

Mutations and polymorphisms: Variations in DNA can occur spontaneously or in response to cellular insults (eg, radiation, mutagenic drugs, viruses). Some variations are repaired by the cell's DNA error correction mechanisms. Other variations are not and can be passed on to subsequently replicated cells; in such cases, the variation is termed a mutation. However, offspring can inherit the mutation only if germ cells are affected. Mutations may be unique to an individual or family. Most mutations are rare. Polymorphisms begin as mutations. They are variations in DNA that have become common in a population (prevalence of ≥ 1%) through sufficient propagation or other mechanisms. Most polymorphisms are stable and do not noticeably change phenotype. A common example is human blood groups (A, B, AB, and O).

Mutations (including polymorphisms) involve random changes in DNA. Many mutations have little effect on cell function. Some mutations change cell function, often in a detrimental way, and some are lethal to the cell. Examples of detrimental changes in cell function are mutations that cause cancer by creating or activating oncogenes or altering tumor suppressor genes (see p. 1170). Rarely, a change in cell function confers a survival advantage. These mutations are more likely to be propagated. The mutation causing sickle cell anemia confers resistance to malaria. This resistance conferred a survival advantage in areas where malaria was endemic and often fatal. However, by causing symptoms and complications of sickle cell anemia, the mutation also has harmful effects usually when present in the homozygous state.

When and in what cell type mutations occur can explain certain abnormalities in inheritance patterns. Typically, an autosomal dominant disorder is expected to be present in one or both parents of an affected person. However, some disorders with autosomal dominant inheritance can appear de novo (in people whose parents have a normal phenotype). For example, about 80% of people with achondroplastic dwarfism have no family history of dwarfism and thus represent new (de novo) mutations. In many of these people, the mechanism is a spontaneous mutation occurring early in their embryonic life. Thus, other offspring have no increased risk of the disorder. However, in some of them, the disorder develops because of a germ cell mutation in their parents (eg, an autosomal dominant gene in a phenotypically normal parent). If so, other offspring have an increased risk of inheriting the mutation.

Mosaicism: Mosaicism occurs when a person starting from a single fertilized egg develops ≥ 2 cell lines differing in genotype. Mosaicism is a normal consequence of X inactivation in females; in most females, some cells have an inactive maternal X, and other cells have an inactive paternal X. Mosaicism can also result from mutations. Mutations are likely to occur during cell division in any large multicellular organism; each time a cell divides, 4 or 5 changes are estimated to occur in the DNA. Because these changes can be passed on to subsequently produced cells, large multicellular organisms have subclones of cells that have slightly different genotypes.

Mosaicism may be recognized as the cause of disorders in which patchy changes occur. For example, McCune-Albright syndrome is associated with patchy dysplastic changes in the bone, endocrine gland abnormalities, patchy pigmentary changes, and occasionally heart or liver abnormalities. Occurrence of the McCune-Albright mutation in all cells would cause early death; however, people with mosaicism survive because normal tissue supports the abnormal tissue. Occasionally, a parent with a single-gene disorder seems to have a mild form but actually represents a mosaic; the parent's offspring is more severely affected if they receive a germ cell with the mutant allele and thus have the abnormality in every cell.

Chromosomal abnormalities are most often fatal to the fetus. However, chromosomal mosaicism occurs in some embryos, resulting in some chromosomally normal cells, which can allow offspring to be born alive. Chromosomal mosaicism can be detected with prenatal genetic testing, particularly chorionic villus sampling.

Extra or missing chromosomes: Abnormal numbers of autosomes usually result in severe abnormalities. For example, extra autosomes typically cause abnormalities such as Down syndrome and other severe syndromes or can be fatal to the fetus. Absence of an autosome is generally fatal to the fetus.

Chromosomal abnormalities (see p. 2487) can usually be diagnosed before birth.

Because of X chromosomal inactivation, having an abnormal number of X chromosomes is usually much less severe than having an abnormal number of autosomes. For example, the abnormalities resulting from the absence of one X chromosome are usually relatively minor (eg, in Turner syndrome—see p. 2492). Also, females with 3 X chromosomes (trisomy X—see p. 2494) are often physically and mentally normal; only one X chromosome of genetic material is fully active even if a female has > 2 X chromosomes (the extra X chromosomes are also partly inactivated).

Uniparental disomy: Uniparental disomy occurs when both chromosomes have been inherited from only one parent. It is very rare and is thought to involve trisomy rescue; ie, the zygote started off as a trisomy (having 3 instead of 2 of a particular chromosome) and one of the 3 was lost, a process that leads to uniparental disomy when the 2 chromosomes that remain are from the same parent (in about one third of cases). Uniparental disomy may cause abnormal phenotypes and inheritance patterns. For example, if duplicates of the same chromosome (isodisomy) are present and carry an abnormal allele for an autosomal recessive disorder, affected people can have an autosomal recessive disorder even though only one parent is a carrier. Uniparental disomy can result in an imprinting disorder when the disomic chromosome results in the loss of appropriate expression of a critically imprinted region (eg, Prader-Willi syndrome may result from maternal isodisomy of chromosome 15).

Chromosomal translocation: Chromosomal translocation is exchange of chromosomal parts between nonpaired (nonhomologous) chromosomes. If chromosomes exchange equal parts of genetic material, the translocation is described as balanced. Unbalanced translocations result in loss of chromosomal material, usually the short arms of 2 fused chromosomes, leaving only 45 chromosomes remaining. Most people with translocations are phenotypically normal. However, translocations may cause or contribute to leukemia (acute myelocytic leukemia [AML] or chronic myelogenous leukemia [CML]) or Down syndrome. Translocations may increase risk of chromosomal abnormalities in offspring, particularly unbalanced translocations. Because chromosomal abnormalities are often fatal to an embryo or a fetus, a parental translocation may result in unexplained recurrent spontaneous abortions or infertility.

Triplet (trinucleotide) repeat disorders: A triplet repeat disorder results when a triplet of nucleotides is repeated an abnormal number of times within a gene (sometimes up to several hundred times). The number of triplets may increase when the gene is transmitted from one generation to the next or as cells divide within the body. When triplets increase enough, genes stop functioning normally. Triplet repeat disorders are infrequent but cause several neurologic disorders (eg, myotonic dystrophy, Fragile X syndrome), particularly those involving the CNS (eg, Huntington disease). Triplet repeat disorders can be detected by techniques that analyze DNA.

Anticipation: Anticipation occurs when a disorder has an earlier age of onset and is expressed more severely in each successive generation. Anticipation may occur when a parent is a mosaic and the child has the full mutation in all cells. It may also occur in triplet repeat disorders when the number of repeats and thus the severity of gene dysfunction increase with each generation.

KEY POINTS

- An apparently autosomal dominant mutation can arise spontaneously and thus may not indicate increased risk in siblings.
- Patchy changes in disorders may reflect mosaicism.
- Chromosomal translocations may have no phenotypic effects but can result in leukemias, Down syndrome, spontaneous abortions, or chromosomal abnormalities in offspring.
- Inherited disorders may become more severe and begin earlier in life with successive generations, sometimes because of triplet repeat disorders.

MITOCHONDRIAL DNA ABNORMALITIES

Each cell has several hundred mitochondria in its cytoplasm. Mitochondria contain DNA in a single circular chromosome that codes for 13 proteins, various RNAs, and several regulating enzymes. However, > 90% of mitochondrial proteins are coded by nuclear genes. For practical purposes, all mitochondria are inherited from the cytoplasm of the egg; thus, mitochondrial DNA comes only from the mother.

Mitochondrial disorders can be due to mitochondrial or nuclear DNA abnormalities (eg, deletions, duplications, mutations). High-energy tissues (eg, muscle, heart, brain) are particularly at risk of malfunction due to mitochondrial abnormalities. Particular mitochondrial DNA abnormalities result in characteristic manifestations (see Table 380–2). Mitochondrial disorders are equally common among males and females.

Mitochondrial abnormalities may occur in many common disorders such as some types of Parkinson disease (which may involve large mitochondrial deletions in the cells of the basal ganglia) and many types of muscle disorders.

Maternal inheritance patterns characterize abnormalities of mitochondrial DNA. Thus, all offspring of an affected female are at risk of inheriting the abnormality, but no offspring of

Table 380–2. SOME MITOCHONDRIAL DISORDERS

DISORDER	DESCRIPTION
Chronic progressive external ophthalmoplegia	Progressive paralysis of the extraocular muscles usually preceded by bilateral, symmetric, progressive ptosis that begins months to years earlier
Kearns-Sayre syndrome	A multisystem variant of chronic progressive external ophthalmoplegia that also includes heart block, retinitis pigmentosa, and CNS degeneration
Leber hereditary optic neuropathy	Variable but often devastating bilateral visual loss that often occurs in adolescents and that is due to a point mutation in mitochondrial DNA
MERRF syndrome	Myoclonic epilepsy with ragged red fibers, dementia, ataxia, and myopathy
MELAS syndrome	Mitochondrial encephalomyopathy with lactic acidosis, and strokelike episodes
Pearson syndrome	Sideroblastic anemia, pancreatic insufficiency, and progressive liver disease that begins in the first few months of life and is frequently fatal in infants

an affected male are at risk. Variability in clinical manifestations is the rule, and these abnormalities mimic a broad range of disorders, which often makes diagnosis extremely difficult. Variability may be due in part to variable mixtures of inherited mutant and normal mitochondrial genomes within cells and tissues.

KEY POINTS

- Mitochondrial disorders have maternal inheritance patterns.
- Because clinical manifestations can be subtle and variable, diagnosis can be very difficult.

GENETIC DIAGNOSTIC TECHNOLOGIES

Genetic diagnostic technology is rapidly improving. DNA or RNA can be amplified, producing many copies of a gene or gene segment, using PCR.

Gene probes can be used to locate specific segments of normal or mutated DNA. Different types of probes may investigate a broad range of sizes of DNA sequence. A known DNA segment may be cloned and then fluorescently tagged (using fluorescent in situ hybridization [FISH]); this segment is then combined with a test specimen. The tagged DNA binds to its complementary DNA segment and can be detected by measuring the amount and type of fluorescence. Gene probes can detect a number of disorders before and after birth.

Oligonucleotide arrays (probes) are another type of probe now routinely utilized to identify deleted or duplicated regions of DNA sequence in specific chromosomes on a genomewide basis. DNA from a patient is compared to a reference genome using many oligonucleotide probes. Using such probes, the entire genome can be tested (queried).

Microchips are powerful new tools that can be used to identify DNA mutations, pieces of RNA, or proteins. A single chip can test for millions of different DNA changes using only one sample. Microchips provide finer resolution for genome queries than oligonucleotide arrays.

Next-generation sequencing technologies have dramatically changed the approach to genetic diagnosis. This technology involves breaking the entire genome into small segments, sequencing the segments, and then reassembling the sequences using intensive computational techniques to provide the base-by-base sequence of the entire genome or more limited regions, such as the expressed portion of the genome known as the exome. This process helps identify single or multiple nucleotide variations as well as areas of insertion or deletion. The costs of this technology have dramatically fallen and continue to fall, and the equipment and computational methods continue to improve. Thus, this technology may become the mainstay of genetic diagnosis. However, the sheer volume of information generated results in a variety of interpretive problems that complicate understanding of the results.

CLINICAL USES OF GENETICS

Disease Understanding

Genetics has advanced understanding of many disorders, sometimes allowing them to be reclassified. For example, classification of many spinocerebellar ataxias has been changed from one based on clinical criteria to one based on genetic criteria. The Online Mendelian Inheritance in Man (OMIM) database is a searchable catalog of human genes and genetic disorders (available at www.ncbi.nlm.nih.gov/omim).

Diagnosis

Genetic testing is used to diagnose many disorders (eg, Turner syndrome, Klinefelter syndrome, hemochromatosis). Diagnosis of a genetic disorder often indicates that relatives of the affected person should be screened for the genetic defect or for carrier status. A catalog of genetic tests and reviews of many genetic diseases with diagnostic strategies and recommendations for risk counseling are available from the Genetic Testing Registry at www.ncbi.nlm.nih.gov/gtr.

Genetic Screening

Genetic screening may be indicated in populations at risk of a particular genetic disorder. The usual criteria for genetic screening are

- Genetic inheritance patterns are known.
- Effective therapy is available.
- Screening tests are sufficiently valid, reliable, sensitive and specific, noninvasive, and safe.

Prevalence in a defined population must be high enough to justify the cost of screening.

One aim of prenatal genetic screening (see p. 2298) is to identify asymptomatic parental heterozygotes carrying a gene for a recessive disorder. For example, Ashkenazi Jews are screened for Tay-Sachs disease, blacks are screened for sickle cell anemia, and several ethnic groups are screened for thalassemia (see Table 275–1 on p. 2298). If a heterozygote's mate is also a heterozygote, the couple is at risk of having an affected child. If the risk is high enough, prenatal diagnosis can be pursued (eg, with amniocentesis, chorionic villus sampling, umbilical cord blood sampling, maternal blood sampling, or fetal imaging). In some cases, genetic disorders diagnosed prenatally can be treated, preventing complications. For instance, special diet or replacement therapy can minimize or eliminate the effects of phenylketonuria, galactosemia, and hypothyroidism. Corticosteroids given to the mother before birth may decrease the severity of congenital virilizing adrenal hypoplasia.

Screening may be appropriate for people with a family history of a dominantly inherited disorder that manifests later in life, such as Huntington disease or cancers associated with abnormalities of the *BRCA1* and *BRCA2* genes. Screening clarifies the risk of developing the condition for that person, who can then make appropriate plans, such as for more frequent screening or preventive therapy.

Screening may also be indicated when a family member is diagnosed with a genetic disorder. A person who is identified as a carrier can make informed decisions about reproduction.

Treatment

Understanding the genetic and molecular basis of disorders may help guide therapy. For example, dietary restriction can eliminate compounds toxic to patients with certain genetic defects, such as phenylketonuria or homocystinuria. Vitamins or other agents can modify a biochemical pathway and thus reduce toxic levels of a compound; eg, folate (folic acid) reduces homocysteine levels in people with 5,10-methylene tetrahydrofolate reductase polymorphism. Therapy may involve replacing a deficient compound or blocking an overactive pathway.

Pharmacogenomics: Pharmacogenomics is the science of how genetic characteristics affect the response to drugs. One aspect of pharmacogenomics is how genes affect pharmacokinetics. Genetic characteristics of a person may help predict response to treatments. For example, metabolism of warfarin is determined partly by variants in genes for the CYP2C9 enzyme and for the vitamin K epoxide reductase complex protein 1. Genetic variations (eg, in production of UDP [uridine diphosphate]-glucoronosyltransferase 1A1) also help predict whether the anticancer drug irinotecan will have intolerable adverse effects.

Another aspect of pharmacogenomics is pharmacodynamics (how drugs interact with cell receptors—see p. 2911). Genetic and thus receptor characteristics of disordered tissue can help provide more precise targets when developing drugs (eg, anticancer drugs). For example, trastuzumab can target specific cancer cell receptors in metastatic breast cancers that amplify the *HER2/neu* gene. Presence of the Philadelphia chromosome in patients with CML helps guide chemotherapy.

Gene therapy: Gene therapy can broadly be considered any treatment that changes gene function. However, gene therapy is often considered specifically the insertion of normal genes into the cells of a person who lacks such normal genes because of a specific genetic disorder. The normal genes can be manufactured, using PCR, from normal DNA donated by another person. Because most genetic disorders are recessive, usually a dominant normal gene is inserted. Currently, such insertion gene therapy is most likely to be effective in the prevention or cure of single-gene defects, such as cystic fibrosis.

One way to transfer DNA into host cells is by viral transfection. The normal DNA is inserted into a virus, which then transfects the host cells, thereby transmitting the DNA into the cell nucleus. Some important concerns about insertion using a virus include reactions to the virus, rapid loss of (failure to propagate) the new normal DNA, and damage to the virus by antibodies developed against the transfected protein, which the immune system recognizes as foreign. Another way to transfer DNA uses liposomes, which are absorbed by the host cells and thereby deliver their DNA to the cell nucleus. Potential problems with liposome insertion methods include failure to absorb the liposomes into the cells, rapid degradation of the new normal DNA, and rapid loss of integration of the DNA.

With antisense technology, rather than inserting normal genes, gene expression can be altered; eg, drugs can combine with specific parts of the DNA, preventing or decreasing gene expression. Antisense technology is currently being tried for cancer therapy but is still very experimental. However, it seems to hold more promise than gene insertion therapy because the success rates may be higher and complications may be fewer.

Another approach to gene therapy is to modify gene expression chemically (eg, by modifying DNA methylation). Such methods have been tried experimentally in treating cancer. Chemical modification may also affect genomic imprinting, although this effect is not clear.

Gene therapy is also being studied experimentally in transplantation surgery. Altering the genes of the transplanted organs to make them more compatible with the recipient's genes makes rejection (and thus the need for immunosuppressive drugs) less likely. However, this process works only rarely.

KEY POINTS

- Genetic screening is justified only if disease prevalence is high enough, treatment is feasible, and tests are accurate enough.

ETHICAL CONTROVERSIES IN GENETICS

With new genetic diagnostic and therapeutic capabilities come many controversies about how they should be used. For example, there are concerns that genetic information might be used improperly to discriminate (eg, by denying health insurance coverage or employment) against people with genetic risk factors for particular disorders. Issues include the privacy of a person's own genetic information and the question of whether testing should be compulsory.

Prenatal screening for genetic abnormalities that cause serious disorders is widely supported; however, there is concern that screening could also be used to select for traits that are aesthetically desirable (eg, physical appearance, intelligence).

Cloning is highly controversial. Animal studies suggest cloning is much more likely than natural methods to result in defects that are lethal or cause serious health problems. Creating a human by cloning is widely seen as unethical, is usually illegal, and is technically difficult.

381 Idiopathic Environmental Intolerance

(Environmental Illness; Multiple Chemical Sensitivity)

Idiopathic environmental intolerance is characterized by recurrent, nonspecific symptoms attributed to low-level exposure to chemically unrelated substances commonly occurring in the environment. Symptoms are numerous, often involving multiple organ systems, but physical findings are unremarkable. Diagnosis is by exclusion. Treatment is psychologic support and avoidance of perceived triggers, although triggers rarely can be defined.

No universally accepted definition exists, but idiopathic environmental intolerance is generally defined as the development of multiple symptoms attributed to exposure to any number of identifiable or unidentifiable chemical substances (inhaled, touched, or ingested) in the absence of clinically detectable organ dysfunction or related physical signs.

Etiology

Triggers: Reported triggers for idiopathic environmental intolerance include

- Alcohol and drugs
- Caffeine and food additives
- Carpet and furniture odors
- Fuel odors and engine exhaust

- Painting materials
- Perfume and other scented products
- Pesticides and herbicides

Mechanism: Immunologic and nonimmunologic theories have been proposed. They are hampered by lack of a consistent dose response to proposed causative substances; ie, symptoms may not be replicated after exposure to high levels of a substance that previously, at much lower levels, seemed to provoke a reaction. Similarly, consistent objective evidence of systemic inflammation, cytokine excess, or immune system activation in relation to symptoms is lacking. Many physicians consider the etiology to be psychologic, probably a form of somatic symptom disorder. Others suggest that the syndrome is a type of panic attack or agoraphobia.

Idiopathic environmental intolerance occurs in 40% of people with chronic fatigue syndrome (also called systemic exertion intolerance disease) and in 16% of people with fibromyalgia. Idiopathic environmental intolerance is more prevalent in women.

Although measurable biologic abnormalities (eg, decreased levels of B cells, elevated levels of IgE) are rare, some patients have such abnormalities. However, these abnormalities appear without a consistent pattern, their significance is uncertain, and testing for these abnormalities to establish an immunologic basis for the disorder should be discouraged.

Symptoms and Signs

Symptoms (eg, palpitations, chest pain, sweating, shortness of breath, fatigue, flushing, dizziness, nausea, choking, trembling, numbness, coughing, hoarseness, difficulty concentrating) are numerous and usually involve more than one organ system. Most patients present with a long list of suspected agents, self-identified or identified by a physician during previous testing. Such patients often go to great lengths to avoid these agents by changing residence and employment, avoiding foods containing "chemicals," sometimes wearing masks in public, or avoiding public settings altogether. Physical examination is characteristically unremarkable.

Diagnosis

- Exclusion of other causes

Diagnosis initially involves exclusion of known disorders with similar manifestations:

- Allergies (eg, allergic rhinitis, food allergies)
- Atopic disorders (eg, asthma, angioedema)
- Building-related illnesses
- Connective tissue disorders (eg, systemic lupus erythematosus [SLE])
- Endocrine disorders (eg, carcinoid syndrome, pheochromocytoma, mastocytosis)

Atopic disorders are excluded based on a typical clinical history, skin-prick testing, serum assays of specific IgE, or all 3. Consultation with an allergy specialist may be helpful. Building-related illnesses, including sick building syndrome, in which many people who spend time in the same building develop symptoms should be considered.

If symptoms and signs are not strongly suggestive of a connective tissue or autoimmune rheumatologic disorder (eg, joint, skin and/or mucous membrane manifestations), testing for a wide range of autoantibodies (eg, antinuclear antibodies [ANA], rheumatoid factor, extractable nuclear antigens [ENA]) should be avoided. In such cases, pretest probability is low and false-positive results are far more likely than true-positive results; a weakly positive ANA is present in about 20% of the population.

Treatment

- Sometimes avoiding suspected triggers
- Psychologic treatments

Despite an uncertain cause-and-effect relationship, treatment is sometimes aimed at avoiding the suspected precipitating agents, which may be difficult because many are ubiquitous. However, social isolation and costly and highly disruptive avoidance behaviors should be discouraged. A supportive relationship with a primary care physician who offers reassurance and protects patients from unnecessary tests and procedures is helpful.

Psychologic evaluation and intervention may help, but characteristically many patients resist this approach. However, the point of this approach is not to convince patients that the cause is psychologic but rather to help them cope with their symptoms and improve quality of life.[1] Useful techniques include psychologic desensitization (often as part of cognitive-behavioral therapy) and graded exposure (see p. 1745).[1] Psychoactive drugs can be helpful if targeted toward coexisting psychiatric disorders (eg, major depression, panic disorder).

1. Hauge CR, Rasmussen A, Piet J, et al: Mindfulness-based cognitive therapy (MBCT) for multiple chemical sensitivity (MCS): results from a randomized controlled trial with 1 year follow-up. *J Psychosom Res* 79(6):628–634, 2015. doi: 10.1016/jpsychores.2015.06.010.

KEY POINTS

- Based on current evidence, idiopathic environmental intolerance cannot be explained by nonpsychologic factors.
- For diagnosis, exclude disorders that can have similar manifestations (eg, allergic disorders) and consider sick building syndrome.
- Test for immunologic abnormalities only if indicated by clinical findings.
- Encourage psychologic therapies such as graded exposure, and drug treatment of coexisting psychiatric disorders.

382 Limb Prosthetics

A prosthesis is an artificial device that replaces a missing body part.

A limb may be amputated or missing because of a blood vessel disorder (eg, atherosclerosis, damage due to diabetes), cancer, an injury (eg, in a motor vehicle accident, during combat), or a birth defect. In the US, slightly < 0.5% of people have an amputation. However, the percentage is likely to increase because of the rising rate of obesity, which increases the risk of atherosclerosis and diabetes.

An entire limb or part of one may be amputated. A lower-limb amputation may involve a toe, a foot, part of the leg below or above the knee, or an entire leg (at the hip). An amputation may even extend above the hip. An upper-limb amputation may involve ≥ 1 fingers, a hand, part of the arm below or above the elbow, or an entire arm (at the shoulder).

If a body part is missing, a prosthesis is often recommended to replace that part. At a minimum, a prosthesis should enable the user to perform daily activities (eg, walking, eating, dressing) independently and comfortably. However, a prosthesis may also enable the user to function as well or nearly as well as before the amputation. Because of recent advances in technology and prosthetic socket design, more functional and comfortable prostheses are available. Highly motivated, otherwise healthy people with a prosthesis can accomplish many extraordinary feats (eg, go skydiving, climb mountains, run marathons, complete triathlons, fully participate in sports, or return to demanding jobs or to active duty in the military). They can live life without limitations. Whether a prosthesis is used only for activities at home or for more demanding activities, it can provide profound psychologic benefits.

How well a prosthesis enables the user to function depends on the patient's anatomy and several other factors:

- Fit, stability, and comfort of the prosthesis
- Socket type and components selected
- User's goals, overall health, age, and frame of mind

Success is most likely when a clinical team (physician, prosthetist, therapist, rehabilitation counselor) works with the patient to determine the most appropriate type of prosthesis. (Prosthetists design, fit, build, and adjust prostheses and provide advice about how to use them.) A user who is motivated increases the likelihood of long-term success.

PROSTHETIC PARTS

A limb prosthesis (see Fig. 382–1) has 3 main parts:

- Interface
- Components
- Cover

Interface between the residual limb and prosthesis: The prosthesis attaches to the body at the interface, which consists of a socket and a rigid frame. At the socket (which is made of plastic or laminated material), the components attach to the user. The frame, which is made of graphite or similar materials, provides structural support for the socket.

A liner is worn between the residual limb (stump) and the socket to provide cushioning and to make the fit tight. The liner is made of soft polyurethane or silicone, which clings to the skin without causing friction. Ideally, users should have 2 liners for each prosthesis. Alternating the liners from day to day helps maintain their elasticity and shape and makes them last longer.

A prosthetic sock may be worn instead of or with a liner. Socks are made of wool, nylon, or synthetic fabrics, sometimes with gel sandwiched between the layers of fabric. Socks are available in different thicknesses (plies). By putting on several socks or socks of different thicknesses or by taking socks off, users can make the prosthesis fit better as the residual limb varies in size, as it does normally throughout the day when activities, weather, and other factors change.

The interface may include a suspension system, which helps hold the prosthesis on securely. The following suspension systems are commonly used:

- **Suction valve:** When the residual limb is put in the socket, air is forced out through an opening at the bottom of the socket. A one-way suction valve on the socket closes the opening and forms a seal that holds the prosthesis in place.

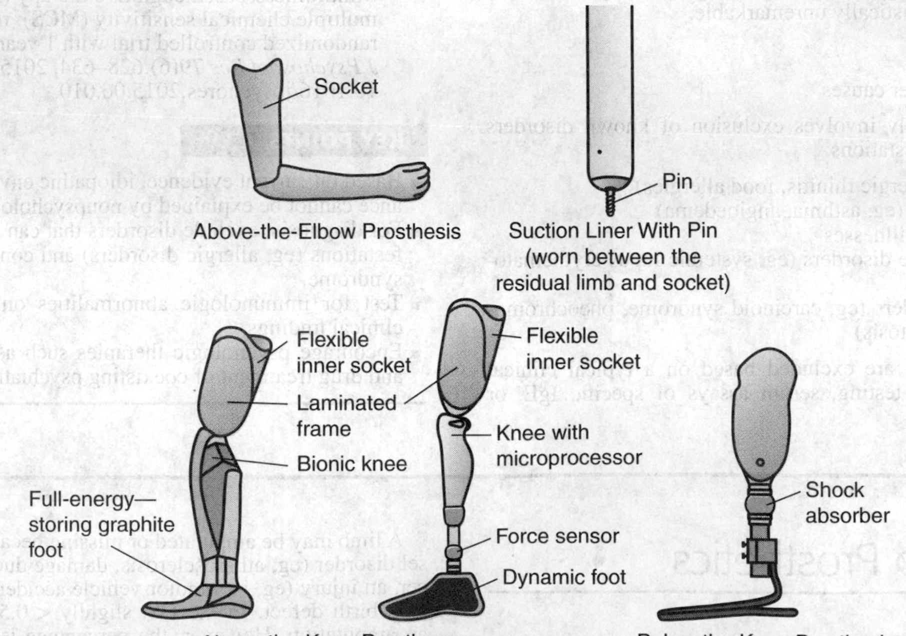

Fig. 382–1. Types of prostheses.

- **Liners with a locking pin:** Most liners are locked into the bottom of the socket by a notched pin. Because the pin is pressed tightly against the residual limb, the parts of the limb near it can become irritated and inflamed, fluid may accumulate, and sores may develop.
- **Belts and harnesses:** Sometimes the prosthesis is attached by a belt or harness. These devices may be used if keeping the prosthesis on with a suction valve or locking pin is difficult or the pin cannot be tolerated. However, the harness is relatively rigid and thus can be uncomfortable and cumbersome. It may also restrict movement.

Components of a limb prosthesis: Components include terminal devices (artificial fingers, hands, feet, and toes), and joints (wrists, elbows, hips, and knees). Metal shafts and customized carbon fiber structures, which function as bones, are used when extra strength, flexibility, and energy return are needed. For more advanced prostheses, there are control elements available that allow the user to move the prosthesis mechanically or electrically.

Components for upper extremity prostheses, which are controlled by microprocessors and powered myoelectrically, are replacing the older body-powered models. Myoelectric prostheses create movement using the electrical charges naturally produced when a muscle contracts. These electrical charges are picked up by surface electrodes and sent to an electric motor, which moves the limb. Components for microprocessor-controlled lower extremity prostheses utilize velocity, torque, and positioning sensors to help define function. These newer components are more efficient and require less effort to control the prosthesis.

Neural-integrated prosthetics, which are now in research and testing stages with upper-limb prosthetics, may enable people to function even better. The nerves that went to the amputated limb are rerouted to connect with healthy muscle (eg, to chest muscle for an amputated arm). These nerves direct impulses once sent to the amputated limb through electrodes on the skin's surface to microprocessors in the prosthetic limb; thus, the user can move the limb, as if by thinking, as with natural limbs.

Prosthesis cover: Some users choose to have the components enclosed by a cover. Covers consist of foam shaped by the prosthetist to look like the missing limb. The foam is often enclosed by a lifelike protective covering. How lifelike covers look depends on whether they are off-the-shelf or highly customized, designed by artisans to exactly match the user's skin pattern. Some users—especially athletes during competition—omit the cover, leaving the components exposed.

OPTIONS FOR LIMB PROSTHESES

The prosthetist explains the available options and helps users choose the type of prosthesis and options they need to accomplish their goals. For example, women who want to wear shoes with different heel heights may prefer a prosthetic ankle that can adjust to different heights. Swimmers can get a 2nd prosthetic leg that is designed for swimming and can withstand water, salt, and sand. Runners can get prosthetic feet specifically designed for running.

Hand Prostheses

Options for hand prostheses include

- Precision (pincher) grip
- Tripod (palmar) grip
- Lateral (key pinch)
- Hook
- Spherical
- Sport-specific
- Myoelectric

Hand prostheses with precision (pincher) and tripod (palmar) grips: These grips enable the user to pick up or pinch a small object. A hand prosthesis with a precision grip has a thumb that opposes the pad of the index finger; a hand prosthesis with a tripod grip has a thumb that opposes the pads of the index and middle fingers.

Lateral hand prosthesis: A lateral hand prosthesis enables the user to manipulate a small object (eg, turning a key in a lock) because it has a thumb that opposes the side of the index finger.

Hook prosthesis: A hook prosthesis enables the user to carry objects with a handle. It allows for thumb and finger flexion. A myoelectric hook improves the line of sight for functional grasp.

Spherical hand prosthesis: A spherical prosthesis allows thumb and fingertip flexion. A user with this type of prosthesis can grasp a round object (eg, door knob, electric bulb).

Sport-specific hand prosthesis: Sport-specific prostheses can include a hand with a gripping device (eg, for golf, archery, or weight-lifting) or a hand with a mesh pocket for catching a baseball.

Myoelectric functional hand prosthesis: New developments in small, wireless electronic devices that control movement and sensation in a patient's prosthetic hand introduce features that can help provide a more natural grip.

Elbow Prostheses

Options for elbow prostheses include

- Body-operated
- Friction-operated
- Myoelectric

Body-operated elbow prosthesis: A body-operated prosthesis consists of a cable and harness that uses shoulder and back movement to move the arm. Although body-operated elbow prostheses are lightweight, they are less attractive than other options and are sometimes bothersome to the user.

Friction-operated elbow prosthesis: A friction-operated prosthesis is raised or lowered by using the hand of the other arm. It is lightweight.

Myoelectric elbow prosthesis: Myoelectric prostheses require no cables and provide more function. However, they are heavy.

Foot Prostheses

Options for foot prostheses include

- Solid ankle, cushioned heel
- Single-axis design
- Multiple-axis (multiaxial) design
- Stored-energy (dynamic response) design
- Sport-specific

Solid ankle, cushioned heel (SACH) foot prosthesis: This type of prosthesis consists of a basic immovable foot made of rubber and wood. Stability is provided for the knee when the heel touches the ground because its soft heel allows the whole foot to contact the ground. However, less stability is provided when the user raises the heel and the opposite leg swings forward, resulting in uneven walking. A SACH prosthesis requires more energy to use than other types of prosthetic feet. It is appropriate for people who are limited in their activities and is not a good choice for active people.

Foot prosthesis with single-axis design: A prosthesis with single-axis design has an ankle joint that allows dorsiflexion and plantarflexion of the foot. This design allows the whole foot to quickly contact the ground after the heel touches the ground and for the knee to straighten quickly. Because of these features, the prosthesis provides good stability for the knee, which is particularly important for people with above-the-knee amputation. Single-axis design prostheses are not appropriate for active people.

Foot prosthesis with multiple-axis (multiaxial) design: A foot prosthesis with multiaxial design has an ankle joint that allows dorsiflexion and plantarflexion of the foot and inversion, eversion, and rotation of the ankle. This design enables users to walk on uneven terrain more easily and is thus appropriate for active people. With newer, lightweight models, minimal maintenance is required. The prosthesis can be made to look lifelike.

Foot prosthesis with stored-energy (dynamic response) design: A foot prosthesis with stored-energy design is made of carbon graphite, which is lightweight and strong. It requires less energy to use because the foot stores energy from when the heel touches the ground to when the toes push off, propelling the user forward. The design may include a shock absorber to reduce the force of contact with the ground during walking. Users are able to walk smoothly and relatively naturally. This type of foot prosthetic is appropriate for active people.

Sport-specific foot prosthesis: Foot prostheses can be customized for a specific sport. For example, for runners (long-distance and sprinting), the prosthesis is designed with the foot bent downward toward the sole and with the capacity to store energy needed to propel the user forward. For swimmers, the prosthesis is designed with an ankle that allows full range of motion in water.

Knee Prostheses

Options for knee prostheses include

- Single-axis, constant friction design
- Polycentric design
- Weight-activated stance control feature
- Manual lock feature
- Fluid control system
- Microprocessor feature

Knee prosthesis with single-axis, constant friction design: A prosthetic knee with single-axis, constant friction design has only one pivot point (the knee bends like a hinge). The design is simple, and the prosthesis is durable, lightweight, and inexpensive. The prosthesis uses friction that does not vary to control the leg when it swings forward. Users can walk normally at only one speed. The prosthesis relies on correct alignment by the prosthetist and muscle control by the user to provide stability.

Knee prosthesis with polycentric design: This type of knee prosthesis has several hinges with several pivot points that change as the knee moves, providing increased stability. The prosthesis shortens slightly when the knee is bent, so that the toe clears the ground more easily when the leg swings forward. The polycentric design of this type of prosthesis provides stability for people with a short residual limb and is appropriate for people whose leg has been amputated at the knee joint, enabling users to sit more comfortably without the knee protruding.

Knee prosthesis with weight-activated stance control feature: A prosthesis with weight-activated stance control feature locks the knee in a slightly bent position (to provide braking) when weight is put on the foot. Constant friction is used to control the leg when it swings forward, but the prosthesis has a knee extension aid, which helps swing the leg. Users can walk at only one speed. The prosthesis is appropriate for people with weak muscles.

Knee prosthesis with manual lock feature: A knee prosthesis with manual lock feature can be locked or unlocked by users as needed but requires a cable to do so. Although this type of prosthesis provides the most stability, it requires more energy to use than other types of prosthetic knees. Because the prosthesis does not provide swing-phase flexion, walking is stiff and awkward and is the least desirable choice.

Knee prosthesis with fluid control system: Knee prostheses with fluid control system may use compressed air (pneumatic system) or fluid (hydraulic system) to produce, store, and release energy as the knee bends and straightens. This type of prosthetic knee enables users to walk at different speeds and is the best choice for most people. It may be equipped with a microprocessor.

Knee prosthesis with microprocessor feature: Knee prostheses with microprocessor feature have sensors that detect movement and can adjust the hydraulic fluid or the magnetorheological fluid control system accordingly. The prosthetic knee provides good control when the foot is on the ground and when the leg swings forward. It can be programmed to compensate for stumbling and to enable users to descend stairs and ramps. Less energy is needed to use the prosthesis, and allow the user to achieve a more natural gait than would otherwise be possible.

PREPARING TO USE A LIMB PROSTHESIS

When amputation is elective, certain preoperative measures can help optimize recovery. After surgery, other steps to prepare for use of a limb prosthesis are helpful for all patients.

Preoperative Preparation for Amputation

Before surgery, the surgeon, prosthetist, and physical therapist should discuss plans and goals with the patient. Also before surgery, patients should, if possible, discuss what happens after surgery with a peer counselor who has had an amputation.

Exercises to increase muscle strength and flexibility are taught by a physical therapist before and after amputation. The stronger and more flexible patients are, the more they can do with or without their prosthesis. Some exercises depend on the type of amputation. All patients need to do exercises to help reduce edema in the residual limb and prevent contracture of tissues in the residual limb, which stiffens tissues, limits the joint's range of motion, and thus makes using a prosthesis more difficult.

Postoperative Preparation for Prosthetic Use

After surgery, the residual limb must heal before a prosthesis can be worn, and edema in the limb must be reduced before a prosthesis can be fitted for long-term use. To help reduce edema, patients are taught to apply an elastic sock (called a shrinker) or an elastic bandage over the residual limb. Wearing a shrinker or bandage also helps shape the residual limb and prevent irregularities that can make fitting the interface difficult. It increases circulation and makes phantom pain (pain seeming to come from the amputated limb) less likely. For a while after surgery, a shrinker, bandage, or both are worn whenever the prosthesis is off. The use of shrinkers can help control postsurgical edema and reduce phantom sensation (a feeling that the amputated limb is still there). How long it is worn varies from patient to patient.

Temporary limb prosthesis: Until edema resolves, a temporary (preparatory) prosthesis may be used. Because this prosthesis is lightweight and easy-to-use, some experts think it helps patients learn to use a prosthesis more quickly. Later, this prosthesis is replaced with a permanent prosthesis, which has higher-quality components. However, with this approach, patients must learn how to use 2 different prostheses. An alternative approach is to use a prosthesis with permanent components (eg, knee, foot, hand) but with a temporary socket and frame. Because some parts remain the same, this approach may enable patients to adjust to the new parts more quickly. In either case, the first socket and frame almost always need to be replaced within 4 to 6 mo of amputation because the residual limb changes in shape and size.

Learning to use a limb prosthesis: When the prosthesis is delivered, patients are taught the basics of using it:

- How to put the prosthesis on
- How to take it off
- How to walk with it
- How to care for the skin of the residual limb and the prosthesis

Training is usually continued, preferably by a team of specialists. A physical therapist provides a program of gait training as well as exercises to improve strength, flexibility, and cardiovascular fitness. An occupational therapist teaches the skills needed to do daily activities. Patients with lower-limb amputations also learn advanced gait training skills (eg, using stairs, walking up and down hills, walking on uneven surfaces). Rehabilitation for upper-limb amputations is coordinated by an occupational or physical therapist with the prosthetist. Rehabilitation consists of specific exercises designed to strengthen muscles and maintain flexibility in the residual limb, as well as teaching patients how to use the prosthesis for daily activities.

Counseling or psychotherapy may help when patients have prolonged difficulty adjusting to the loss of their limb and to prosthetic use.

FITTING THE PROSTHESIS

A prosthetist custom designs the interface (socket and frame), then constructs it by hand. The fit of the interface, particularly the socket, is crucial to success—much more so than the type of prosthesis, including the components. If the interface fits well and is comfortable, patients can function well even if the components are less than ideal. If the interface fits poorly or is uncomfortable, success is unlikely regardless of the patient's motivation or the components' sophistication.

The socket should be designed to distribute pressure and weight bearing over specific areas (see Figs. 382–2 and 382–3). This design increases comfort, provides the most control over the prosthesis, and helps prevent the residual limb (skin, bones, and nerves) from being damaged. The fit should be snug, producing the appropriate amount of suction to help hold the prosthesis firmly in the socket. Movement of the residual limb against the socket can produce friction and damage the skin.

Traditionally, prostheses were fitted by taking a plaster mold of the residual limb. Now, laser scanning, using computer-assisted design and manufacturing tools, can be used. This method is more comfortable and convenient. However, whether one method produces a better prosthesis than the other is unclear. The method used may depend on the preference and training of the prosthetist.

Once the socket is fitted, the prosthetist attaches the appropriate components to the interface, to each other, or to both and aligns them so that the patient can use them safely and efficiently.

SKIN CARE OF THE RESIDUAL LIMB

Skin that comes in contact with the prosthesis must be cared for meticulously to prevent skin damage such as irritation, skin breakdown (which may result in sores), and infection.

Usually, the disorders that put patients at risk of amputation such as blood vessel disorders and diabetes, which decrease circulation to the lower extremities, also increase the risk of skin breakdown and infection after amputation. Some of these disorders (eg, diabetes) and others (eg, neurologic disorders) impair sensation, so that patients may not feel discomfort or pain when skin breaks down or infection develops and thus do not notice these problems. These patients should remove their prosthesis several times a day to check the skin for redness and other signs of breakdown or infection. Other patients should check for these signs at least once daily.

Skin problems can be serious and should be evaluated and treated as necessary by the patient's health care practitioner in consultation with a prosthetist. As patients become familiar with recurrent problems, they may be able to identify which problems are minor and manage them on their own. However, anything unusual, persistent, painful, or worrisome should be evaluated by the practitioner.

Preventing skin breakdown: The skin next to the prosthesis tends to break down because the prosthesis puts pressure on and rubs against it and because moisture collects in the space between the residual limb and prosthetic socket. The first sign of skin breakdown is erythema, which may be followed by cuts, blisters, and ulcers. When skin breaks down, the prosthesis is often painful or impossible to wear for long periods of time, and infection can develop. Unrecognized or unchecked infection can lead to the need for a second operation (revision surgery).

Several measures can help prevent or delay skin breakdown:

- Having an interface that fits well is important. But even with a good fit, problems can occur. The residual limb changes in shape and size throughout the day, depending on activity level, diet, and the weather. Thus, there are times when the interface fits well and times when it fits less well. In response, patients can improve the fit by changing to a thicker or thinner liner or sock, by using a liner and a sock, or by adding or removing thin-ply socks. But even so, the change in the residual limb's size may vary too much and too often, making skin breakdown inevitable. Then, patients should see a prosthetist to have the interface adjusted without delay. Skin breakdown is often the first sign that the prosthesis needs adjustment.
- Maintaining a stable body weight is the best way to make sure the prosthesis continues to fit. Even small changes in weight can affect the fit.
- Eating a healthy diet and drinking lots of water help control body weight and maintain healthy skin.
- For patients with diabetes, monitoring and controlling blood sugar is important.
- For patients with a lower-limb prosthesis, avoiding changes in body alignment (the way they hold their body) can help. Such changes can cause skin breakdown because pressure is placed in different areas. Wearing different shoes can change

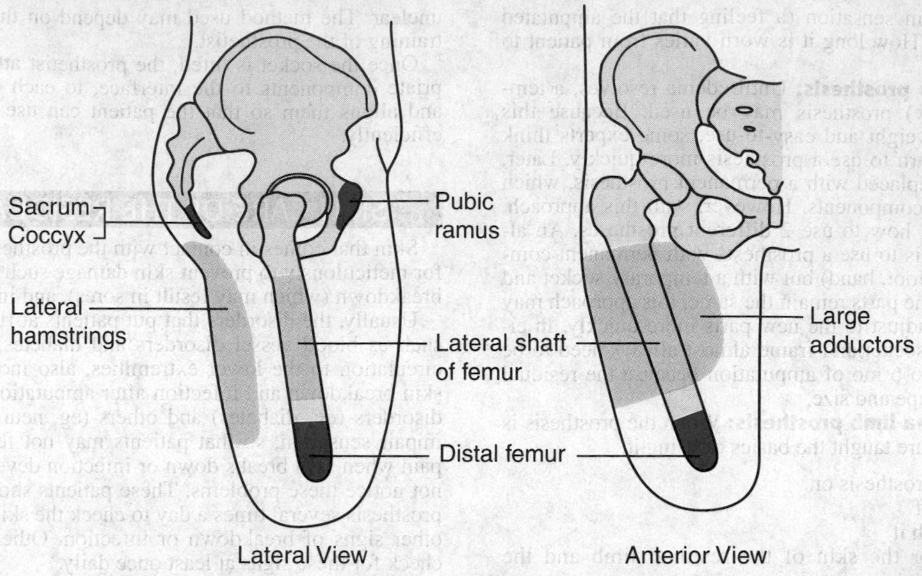

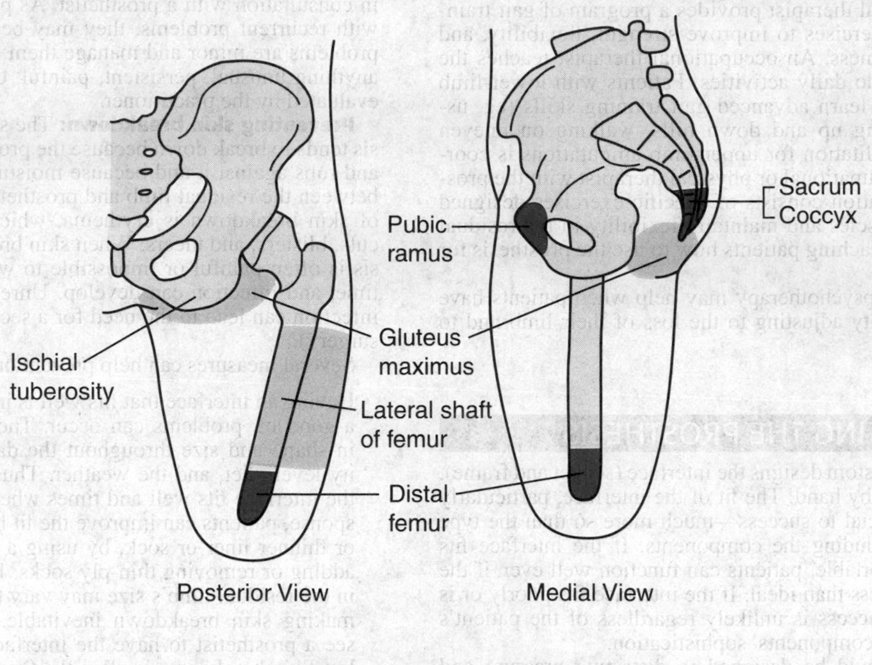

Fig. 382–2. Pressure-tolerant and pressure-sensitive areas after transfemoral amputation.

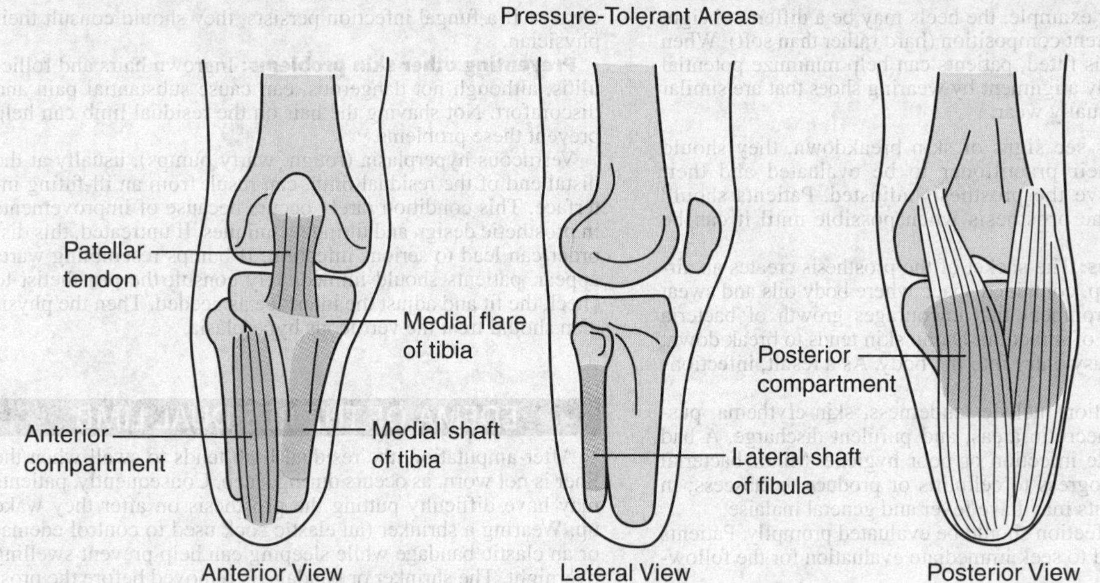

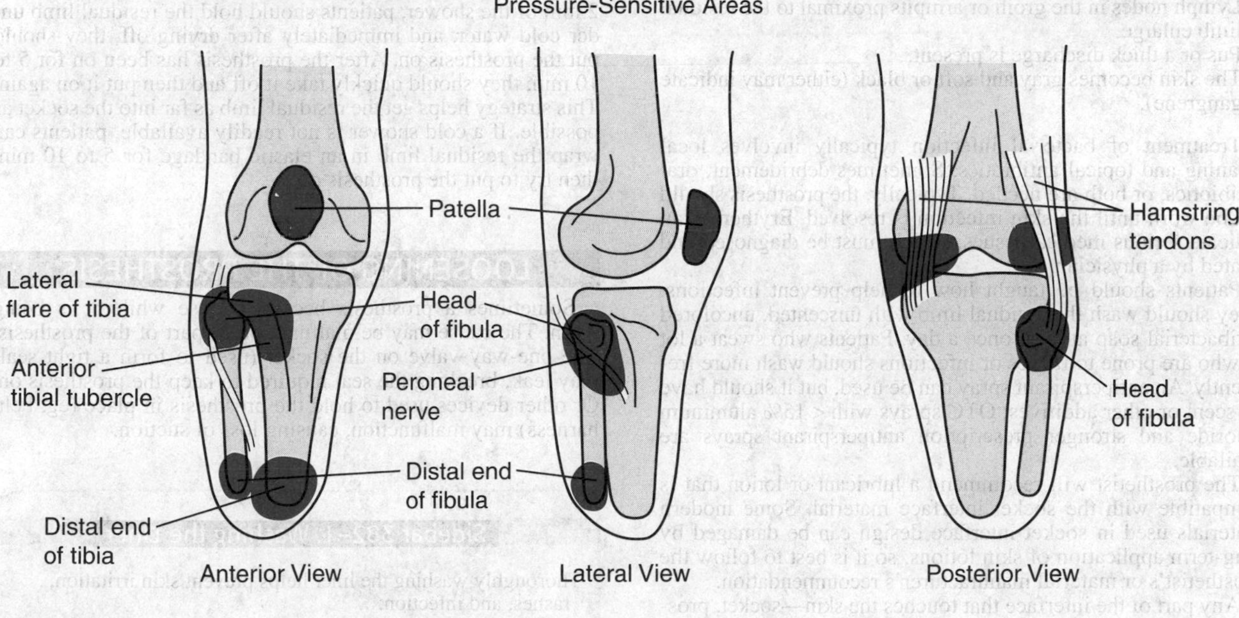

Fig. 382–3. Pressure-tolerant and pressure-sensitive areas after transtibial amputation.

alignment. For example, the heels may be a different height or have a different composition (hard rather than soft). When the prosthesis is fitted, patients can help minimize potential changes in body alignment by wearing shoes that are similar to ones they usually wear.

When patients see signs of skin breakdown, they should promptly see their practitioner to be evaluated and their prosthetist to have the prosthesis adjusted. Patients should avoid wearing the prosthesis when possible until it can be adjusted.

Skin infections: The socket of the prosthesis creates an airtight, warm, damp, contained space where body oils and sweat collect—an environment that encourages growth of bacteria and development of infection. Damp skin tends to break down, giving bacteria easy entry into the body. As a result, infections may spread.

Signs of infection include tenderness, skin erythema, pustules, ulcers or necrotic areas, and purulent discharge. A bad odor may indicate infection or poor hygiene. Minor bacterial infection may progress to cellulitis or produce an abscess; in such cases, patients may have fever and general malaise.

Any sign of infection should be evaluated promptly. Patients should be advised to seek immediate evaluation for the following symptoms:

- The residual limb feels cold (indicating decreased circulation).
- The affected area is red and tender.
- The affected area gives off a bad odor.
- Lymph nodes in the groin or armpits proximal to the residual limb enlarge.
- Pus or a thick discharge is present.
- The skin becomes gray and soft or black (either may indicate gangrene).

Treatment of bacterial infection typically involves local cleaning and topical antibiotics. Sometimes debridement, oral antibiotics, or both are needed. Typically, the prosthesis should not be worn until the skin infection is resolved. Erythema can indicate serious medical issues, which must be diagnosed and treated by a physician.

Patients should be taught how to help prevent infections. They should wash the residual limb with unscented, uncolored antibacterial soap at least once a day. Patients who sweat a lot or who are prone to rashes or infections should wash more frequently. An antiperspirant spray can be used, but it should have no scent or other additives; OTC sprays with < 15% aluminum chloride and stronger prescription antiperspirant sprays are available.

The prosthetist will recommend a lubricant or lotion that is compatible with the socket interface material. Some modern materials used in socket interface design can be damaged by long-term application of skin lotions, so it is best to follow the prosthetist's or material manufacturer's recommendation.

Any part of the interface that touches the skin—socket, prosthetic sock, or liner (see Sidebar 382–1)—should be washed thoroughly every day with hot water and antibacterial soap.

Liners and prosthetic socks should be dried thoroughly before wearing. Soap left in the socket or liner can cause rashes, so patients should make sure that the socket and liners are completely free of soap after washing. An itchy rash usually indicates irritation or an allergic reaction, not infection. A physician can prescribe a cream or ointment to treat rashes.

If patients can identify a fungal infection, they should apply an OTC antifungal cream. However, if the diagnosis is not clear or if a fungal infection persists, they should consult their physician.

Preventing other skin problems: Ingrown hairs and folliculitis, although not dangerous, can cause substantial pain and discomfort. Not shaving the hair on the residual limb can help prevent these problems.

Verrucous hyperplasia (rough, warty bumps), usually at the distal end of the residual limb, can result from an ill-fitting interface. This condition rarely occurs because of improvements in prosthetic design and fitting techniques. If untreated, this disorder can lead to serious infection. If bumps resembling warts appear, patients should immediately consult the prosthetist to check the fit and adjust the interface as needed. Then the physician should treat the verrucous hyperplasia.

EDEMA OF THE RESIDUAL LIMB

After amputation, the residual limb tends to swell when the liner is not worn, as occurs during sleep. Consequently, patients may have difficulty putting the prosthesis on after they wake up. Wearing a shrinker (an elastic sock used to control edema) or an elastic bandage while sleeping can help prevent swelling overnight. The shrinker or bandage is removed before the prosthesis is put on.

In hot and humid weather, the residual limb may swell and sweat, making the prosthesis hard to put on. Showering immediately before putting the prosthesis on may help. For the last 2 min of the shower, patients should hold the residual limb under cold water, and immediately after drying off, they should put the prosthesis on. After the prosthesis has been on for 5 to 10 min, they should quickly take it off and then put it on again. This strategy helps get the residual limb as far into the socket as possible. If a cold shower is not readily available, patients can wrap the residual limb in an elastic bandage for 5 to 10 min, then try to put the prosthesis on.

LOOSENING OF THE PROSTHESIS

Sometimes a prosthesis becomes loose while it is being worn. The cause may be malfunction of part of the prosthesis. The one-way valve on the socket (used to form a tight seal) may leak, breaking the seal required to keep the prosthesis on. Or other devices used to hold the prosthesis in place (eg, belt, harness) may malfunction, causing loss of suction.

Sidebar 382–1. Washing the Liner

Thoroughly washing the liner helps prevent skin irritation, rashes, and infection.

- Wash the liner with the outside surface turned out (right side out), not turned inside out.
- Fill the liner with hot water and antibacterial soap, and slosh the mixture inside the liner for 30 sec, then pour it out.
- Rinse the liner with hot water repeatedly until no soap remains, then pour the hot water out.
- Make sure the liner is completely dry before putting it on.
- Once a week, after washing the liner with soap, apply isopropyl rubbing alcohol to the inside surface of the liner, then rinse the liner with hot water.

Suction may also be lost because the residual limb shrinks, the person loses weight, or the sock worn between the residual limb and socket is not thick enough.

If suction is lost, patients should take the prosthesis off, put it back on, and verify that it is on correctly. If the problem persists, they should contact their prosthetist to assess the problem.

PAIN IN THE RESIDUAL LIMB

After amputation, the residual limb may be painful. Causes include

- Skin infection
- Deep tissue infection (eg, osteomyelitis, vascular graft infection)
- Pressure points with or without skin breakdown
- Neuroma
- Limb ischemia
- Phantom pain

Skin infection and breakdown have clear, visible manifestations and should be dealt with. Deep infection may be more difficult to diagnose because focal swelling and erythema may not become apparent until pain has been present for some time; systemic manifestations such as fever or tachycardia may appear first and should not be ignored. Painful neuroma can occur in any severed nerve (from surgery or trauma) and may cause focal pain that can be temporarily blocked (as a diagnostic maneuver) by local anesthetic injection. Patients whose amputation was necessitated by ischemic vascular disease are at risk for further ischemia, which can be difficult to diagnose but may be suggested by a very low transcutaneous O_2 tension (< 20 mmHg) on the skin of the distal limb. Phantom limb pain should be considered when more medically urgent causes have been excluded.

If there is no medical disorder causing the pain, massaging the residual limb sometimes relieves the pain. If massaging is ineffective, analgesics can be used. Typically, NSAIDs or acetaminophen is used, but sometimes opioid analgesics are required. If these measures do not relieve the pain or patients require prolonged opioid therapy, consultation with a pain management specialist may be required to supervise treatment, which may include using mechanical devices (eg, a vibrator), ultrasound, and drugs such as antidepressants (eg, nortriptyline, desipramine) and anticonvulsants (eg, gabapentin).

Sometimes pain is felt in other limbs or in the hips, spine, shoulders, or neck. This pain may occur because wearing a prosthesis makes patients change their gait or body alignment or causes them to repeat movements. Regularly doing specific stretching and strengthening exercises may help prevent or relieve this type of pain. A physical therapist can help design an appropriate exercise program.

Phantom pain: Many patients experience phantom pain at some time. The phantom aspect is not the pain, which is real, but the location of the pain—in a limb that has been amputated. Phantom pain is more likely if the pain before amputation was severe or lasted a long time. In some cases, the pain can be severe depending on the mechanism of amputation (eg, traumatic amputation vs elective surgical removal).

Phantom pain is often more severe soon after the amputation, then decreases over time. Postsurgical desensitizing therapies are available and recommended to reduce pain during initial weight-bearing in the prosthesis. For many patients, phantom pain is more common when the prosthesis is not being worn (because the limb and interface have no contact), for example, at night. The risk of having this pain is reduced if a spinal anesthetic and a general anesthetic are used during surgery.

There are a number of other, nonpharmacologic therapies that may be added to the treatment plan, among them transcutaneous electrical nerve stimulation (TENS), acupuncture, and spinal cord stimulation.

Phantom sensation: Most patients experience phantom sensation, which feels as though the amputated limb is still there. Phantom sensation can be painful during the immediate postoperative period. However, the pain tends to disappear for most amputees. Phantom sensation with new amputees can be a problem, especially at night when they have to go to the bathroom, and believing their limb is still there, do not remember to don their prosthesis. Many prosthetists recommend that a protective device be worn while sleeping, to protect the amputee from injury.

383 Medical Aspects of Travel

Planning and preparation reduce medical risks of travel, particularly risks involved with air travel and foreign travel. Travelers should carry their drugs, extra eyeglasses or other corrective lenses (as well as a current written prescription for either), and hearing-aid batteries in a carry-on bag in case their checked baggage is delayed, lost, or stolen. Drugs should be kept in their original labeled containers. Travelers who need to carry opioids, syringes, or large amounts of drugs should have a prescription or verifying letter from a physician to avoid possible security or customs complications. A medical record summary (including ECG for those with significant cardiac history) is invaluable if a traveler becomes ill. Travelers subject to disabling illness (eg, epilepsy) or those with chronic disease should wear a medical identification bracelet or necklace.

AIR TRAVEL

Air travel can cause or worsen certain medical problems; some are considered a contraindication to flight (see Table 383–1), and others may cause discomfort. Serious complications are rare.

During a flight, any health care practitioner among the passengers may be asked to help fellow passengers who become ill. Additionally, most commercial aircraft carry first-aid equipment, including an automatic external cardioverter defibrillator and limited medical supplies. Airline personnel are receiving more first-aid training now than in the past. Although physicians aiding ill or injured passengers are usually protected from litigation by the Good Samaritan concept, they should avoid practicing beyond their training or expertise.

Further information about air travel may be obtained from the medical department of major airlines, the Federal Aviation Administration (www.faa.gov), online travel information sources, or local travel clinics.

Table 383–1. CONTRAINDICATIONS TO FLYING

CONDITION	RISK
Bowel obstruction	Gas expansion* causing pain, tissue damage, or both
Chest or abdominal surgery if recent (< 10 days)	Gas expansion* causing pain, tissue damage, or both
Heart disease if severe	O_2 desaturation*,†
Immunodeficiency if severe	Acquisition or transmission of infection
Infections if highly contagious	Acquisition or transmission of infection
Intraocular gas injection if recent	Gas expansion* causing pain, tissue damage, or both
Jaw immobilization (unless the appliance is fitted with a quick-release device)	Aspiration (eg, if vomiting due to air sickness occurs)
MI, low-risk: • Age < 65 • LVEF > 45% • No complications No flight within 3 days	O_2 desaturation*,†
MI, medium-risk: • Not low risk • Ejection fraction > 40%, No flight within 10 days	O_2 desaturation*,†
MI, high-risk: • Any complications • Ejection fraction < 40% Defer travel until stable	O_2 desaturation*,†
Pneumothorax	Gas expansion* causing pain, tissue damage, or both
Pulmonary blebs or cavities if large	Gas expansion* causing pain, tissue damage, or both
Pulmonary dysfunction if severe	O_2 desaturation*,†
Unstable angina	O_2 desaturation*,†

*Risk mainly at high cabin altitude. Low-altitude flights (< 5000 ft [1524 m]; eg, MedEvac helicopters) are less likely to cause problems.

†If flying is essential, supplemental O_2 should be available.

Barometric pressure changes: Commercial airplanes and jet aircraft are pressurized only to the equivalent of an altitude of 6000 to 8000 ft (1830 to 2440 m), not to sea level pressure. Thus, air in body cavities or other closed spaces expands by about 25%; this expansion may aggravate certain medical conditions.

Untreated dental problems or recent dental procedures may become painful when air pressure changes. People with upper respiratory inflammation or allergic rhinitis may develop obstructed eustachian tubes (which may cause barotitis media) or obstructed sinus ostia (which may cause barosinusitis). Frequent yawning or closed-nose swallowing during descent, use of decongestant nasal sprays, or use of antihistamines before or during flight often prevents or relieves these conditions. Some people suck on hard candies during descent.

Air travel is contraindicated for patients who have or are likely to develop pneumothorax (eg, those who have large pulmonary blebs or cavities) and for those in whom air or gas is trapped (eg, those who have an incarcerated bowel, those traveling < 10 days after chest or abdominal surgery, those who have intraocular gas injection) because even modest expansion may cause pain or tissue damage.

Water should be substituted for air in devices secured by air-filled cuffs or balloons (eg, feeding tubes, urinary catheters). Patients with a colostomy should wear a large bag and expect frequent filling due to expansion of intestinal gas.

Children: Children are particularly susceptible to barotitis media and should be given fluids or food during descent to encourage swallowing, which can equalize pressures. Infants can be breastfed or given a bottle or pacifier. Precautions for children with chronic disease (eg, congenital heart disease, chronic lung disease, anemia) are the same as those for adults.

Circadian dysrhythmia (jet lag): Rapid travel across multiple time zones disrupts the normal circadian rhythm. Bright sunlight resets the internal clock. Exposure to bright late-afternoon or evening light delays the onset of normal sleep time, and exposure to early-morning light advances the biologic clock, so that sleep time is earlier than usual. Thus, managing exposure to light can help adaptation, particularly on the days after arrival in a new time zone. For example, people traveling westward could maximize exposure to bright afternoon light to help delay sleep time. People traveling eastward could maximize exposure to bright light in the early morning to help awakening and promote earlier sleep.

Short-acting hypnotics (see Table 239–7 on p. 2018) may help people fall asleep at the appropriate local time after eastward travel. However, hypnotics may have adverse effects, such as daytime drowsiness, amnesia, and nighttime insomnia. Long-acting hypnotics increase the likelihood of confusion and falls among the elderly and should be avoided.

Melatonin, a hormone secreted by the pineal gland, may provide a time-of-night cue; however, large placebo-controlled trials showing melatonin's safety and efficacy are lacking. Taking melatonin (0.5 to 5 mg po before the desired sleep time) may help those who need to go to sleep earlier because they have traveled east across several time zones.

Some therapeutic regimens must be altered to compensate for circadian dysrhythmia. For example, insulin dosage and timing may require modification depending on the number of time zones traversed, time spent at destination, available food, and activity; glucose must be monitored frequently. Target plasma glucose levels should be increased; because so many changes affect levels, tight control is more difficult, and the risk of hypoglycemia is increased. Regimens may require modification based on elapsed rather than local time.

Decreased O_2 tension: In passenger jets at cruising altitude, with a typical 8000-ft (2440-m) cabin altitude, the partial pressure of O_2 is about 25% less than at sea level, which, because of the O_2-Hb dissociation curve, represents a drop in arterial O_2 saturation of only about 4.4%. This decrease may be significant for people with severe heart or lung disease (see Table 383–1) but is harmless to most people; however, after 3 to 9 h at that altitude equivalent, some people report discomfort (eg, headache, malaise).

In general, anyone who can walk 50 m or climb one flight of stairs and whose disease is stable can tolerate normal passenger jet cabin conditions without additional O_2. However, problems may arise for travelers with moderate or severe pulmonary disease (eg, asthma, COPD, cystic fibrosis), heart failure, anemia with Hb < 8.5 g/dL, severe angina pectoris, sickle cell disease (but not trait), and some congenital heart diseases. When flying is essential, such patients can usually fly safely with specially designed continuous O_2 equipment, which must be provided by the airline. Mild ankle edema due to venous stasis commonly develops during long flights and should not be confused with heart failure.

Smoking can aggravate mild hypoxia and should be avoided before flying. Hypoxia and fatigue may increase the effects of alcohol.

Low cabin humidity: Dehydration may develop because of very low cabin humidity. It can be avoided with adequate fluid intake and alcohol avoidance. Contact lens wearers and people with dry eyes should instill artificial tears frequently to avoid corneal irritation resulting from low cabin humidity.

Motion sickness: Motion sickness is often triggered by turbulence and vibration and is made worse by warmth, anxiety, hunger, or overeating. Symptoms may include nausea, vomiting, sweating, and vertigo.

Motion sickness can be minimized before and during travel by moderating intake of food, fluids, and alcohol. Fixing the eyes on a stationary object or on the horizon can help, as can lying down and keeping the eyes closed. Other measures include choosing a seat where motion is felt least (eg, in the center of an airplane, over the wing), refraining from reading, and using an air vent. A scopolamine patch or an OTC or prescription antihistamine is often useful, especially if taken before travel. However, these drugs can cause drowsiness, dry mouth, confusion, falls, and other problems in the elderly.

Pregnancy: Uncomplicated pregnancy through 36 wk is not a contraindication to air travel; high-risk pregnancies must be individually evaluated. Flight during the 9th mo usually requires a physician's written approval dated within 72 h of departure and indicating expected delivery date. However, policies may vary by airline. Seat belts should be worn below the abdomen, across the hips.

To prevent effects on development of the fetal thyroid, pregnant women should avoid prolonged use of water purification tablets that contain iodine. Pregnant women should consider delaying travel to areas where malaria is endemic because malaria can be more virulent in pregnant women. Mefloquine is thought to be safe for use during all 3 trimesters of pregnancy (see also Malaria Prevention on p. 1559). When traveling, pregnant women should be particularly careful about following safe food guidelines and hand washing.

Psychologic stress: Hypnosis and behavior modification benefit some people with fear of flying or claustrophobia. Fearful passengers may also benefit from a short-acting anxiolytic (eg, zolpidem, alprazolam) taken before and, depending on duration, during flight. Hyperventilation commonly simulates heart disease and may cause tetany-like symptoms; anxiety and hyperventilation can cause panic, paranoia, and a sense of impending death. Psychotic tendencies may become more acute and troublesome during flight. Patients with violent or unpredictable tendencies must be accompanied by an attendant and appropriately sedated.

Restricted mobility: Deep venous thrombosis may develop in anyone sitting for long periods and may result in a pulmonary embolus. Risk factors include those for non–altitude-related deep venous thrombosis (eg, prior deep venous thrombosis, pregnancy, use of oral contraceptives—see Table 88–2 on p. 758). Frequent (every 1 to 2 h) ambulation, short-movement exercises while seated, and adequate hydration are recommended; however, studies showing benefit from these measures are lacking.

Turbulence: Turbulence may cause motion sickness or injury. While seated, passengers should keep their seat belts fastened at all times.

Other issues: Most implanted cardiac devices, including pacemakers and cardioverter defibrillators, are effectively shielded from interference from security devices. However, the metal content of some of these devices, as well as certain orthopedic prostheses and braces, may trigger a security alarm. A physician's letter should be carried to avoid security difficulties.

People with specific dietary and medical needs should plan carefully and carry their own food and supplies. With several days' notice, all airlines departing from or arriving in the US (and most others) can make reasonable efforts to accommodate passengers with physical handicaps and special needs, including those who require O_2 therapy. Wheelchairs can be accommodated on all US airlines and most foreign ones, but advance notice is advisable.

Some airlines accept passengers requiring more highly specialized equipment (eg, IV fluids, respirators) provided that appropriate personnel accompany the passenger and arrangements have been made in advance. If travelers cannot be accommodated on a commercial aircraft because of severe illness, air ambulance service is necessary.

FOREIGN TRAVEL

About 1 in 30 people traveling abroad requires emergency care. Illness in a foreign country may involve significant difficulties. Many US insurance plans, including Medicare, are not valid in foreign countries; overseas hospitals often require a substantial cash deposit for nonresidents, regardless of insurance. Travel insurance plans, including some that arrange for emergency evacuation, are available through commercial agents, travel agencies, and some major credit card companies.

Directories listing English-speaking physicians in foreign countries, US consulates who may assist in obtaining emergency medical services, and information about foreign travel risks are available (see Table 383–2). Patients with serious disorders should consider pretravel contact or arrangements with an organization that offers medically supervised evacuation from foreign countries. Certain infections are common when traveling to certain areas.

Vaccinations: Some countries require specific vaccinations (see Table 383–3). General travel and up-to-date immunization information is available from the Centers for Disease Control and Prevention (CDC) and malaria chemoprophylaxis requirements are available from the CDC's malaria hotline (855-856-4713) and web site (www.cdc.gov).

Injury and death: Road traffic accidents are the most frequent cause of death of nonelderly international travelers. Travelers should use seat belts in vehicles and a helmet when cycling. Travelers should avoid motorcycles and mopeds and avoid riding on bus roofs or in open truck beds. To prevent drowning (another common cause of death while abroad), travelers should avoid beaches with turbulent surf and avoid swimming after drinking alcoholic beverages.

Traveler's diarrhea: Traveler's diarrhea (TD) is the most common health problem among international travelers. TD is usually self-limited, typically resolving in 5 days; however, 3 to 10% of travelers with TD may have symptoms lasting > 2 wk, and up to 3% of travelers have TD lasting > 30 days. TD lasting < 1 wk requires no testing. For persistent TD, laboratory testing is done.

Self-initiated treatment is indicated for moderate to severe symptoms (≥ 3 unformed stools over 8 h), especially if vomiting,

Table 383–2. USEFUL CONTACTS FOR PEOPLE TRAVELING ABROAD

ORGANIZATION	PHONE NUMBERS	WEB SITE
International Association for Medical Assistance to Travellers (IAMAT)	US: (716) 754-4883 (Niagara Falls, NY) Canada: (519) 836-0102 (Guelph, Ontario); (416) 652-0137 (Toronto, Ontario)	www.iamat.org
Centers for Disease Control and Prevention (CDC)	US: Toll-free (800) CDC-INFO (800-232-4636) TTY: (888) 232-6348 (Atlanta, GA)	www.cdc.gov/travel
CDC Malaria Hotline	US: (770) 488-7788 or (855) 856-4713; after hours, (770) 488-7100 (Atlanta, GA)	www.cdc.gov/malaria
CDC Zika Pregnancy Hotline	US: (770) 488-7100 (Atlanta, GA)	www.cdc.gov/zika
US Department of State, Overseas Citizens Services	From US & Canada: (888) 407-4747 From Overseas: (202) 501-4444 (Washington, DC)	www.travel.state.gov
World Health Organization (WHO)	International: (+41 22) 791-2111 (Geneva, Switzerland) Americas: (202) 974-3000 (Washington, DC)	www.who.int/en

fever, abdominal cramps, or blood in the stool are present. Treatment is with an appropriate antibiotic (eg, a fluoroquinolone for most destinations, a macrolide such as azithromycin for Southeast Asia). Additional measures include loperamide (except in patients with fever, bloody stools, or abdominal pain and in children < 2 yr); replacement of fluids; and, in the elderly and small children, electrolytes (eg, oral rehydration solution).

Measures that may decrease the risk of TD include

- Drinking and brushing teeth with bottled, filtered, boiled, or chlorinated water
- Avoiding ice
- Eating freshly prepared foods only if they have been heated to steaming temperatures
- Eating only fruits and vegetables that travelers peel or shell themselves
- Avoiding food from street vendors
- Washing hands frequently
- Avoiding all foods likely to have been exposed to flies

Prophylactic antibiotics (eg, fluoroquinolones) are effective in preventing diarrhea, but because of concerns about adverse effects and development of resistance, they should probably be reserved for immunocompromised patients.

Schistosomiasis: Schistosomiasis is common and is caused by exposure to fresh water in Africa, Southeast Asia, China, and eastern South America. Risk of schistosomiasis can be reduced by avoiding freshwater activities in areas where schistosomiasis is common.

Table 383–3. VACCINES FOR INTERNATIONAL TRAVEL*,†,‡

INFECTION	REGIONS WHERE THE VACCINE IS RECOMMENDED	COMMENTS
Hepatitis A	All low-income countries	2 doses ≥ 6 mo apart; complete protection for 6–12 mo after the 1st dose and for life after the 2nd dose
Hepatitis B	All low-income countries, particularly China	Recommended for extended-stay travelers and all health care workers
Influenza	Year-round in the tropics April through September in the Southern Hemisphere; October through April in the Northern Hemisphere	Recommended for all travelers > 6 mo of age
Japanese encephalitis	Rural areas in most of Asia and South Asia, particularly in areas with rice and pig farming	2 doses at least 28 days apart Not recommended for pregnant women
Meningococcal infections	Northern sub-Saharan Africa from Mali to Ethiopia (the meningitis belt) Required for entry into Saudi Arabia during Hajj or Umrah Throughout the world, especially in crowded living situations (eg, dormitories)	Risk higher in Africa during the dry season (December through June)

Table 383–3. VACCINES FOR INTERNATIONAL TRAVEL*,†,‡ (*Continued*)

INFECTION	REGIONS WHERE THE VACCINE IS RECOMMENDED	COMMENTS
Rabies	All countries, including US	Recommended for travelers at risk of animal bites (eg, rural campers, veterinarians, field workers, people living in remote areas) Does not eliminate need for additional vaccinations after animal bite for added protection Recommended during pregnancy only if risk of infection is high
Typhoid fever	All low-income countries, especially in South Asia (including India)	Pill form: 1 pill taken every other day for a total of 4 pills; protects for 5 yr • Not safe for pregnant women Single injection form: Protects for 2 yr and is thought to be safer for pregnant women than the pill form of the vaccine.
Yellow fever	Tropical South America Tropical Africa	Although this infection is rare, proof of vaccination required for entry into many countries[§] Not safe for pregnant women Increased risk of adverse effects in the elderly[§] One dose provides protection for life

*In addition to the listed vaccinations, vaccinations for measles, mumps, rubella, tetanus, diphtheria, polio, pneumococcal disease, and varicella should be up to date.

†All recommendations are subject to change. For the latest recommendations, see the Centers for Disease Control and Prevention (www.cdc.gov or 800-CDC-INFO [800-232-4636]).

‡See also p. 1448.

§WHO no longer recommends a booster dose of yellow fever vaccine every 10 yr; however, this recommendation has not yet reached all international points of entry. For patients vaccinated > 10 yr previously who are traveling to countries that may require proof of vaccination *within* 10 yr, providers should consider completing the waiver section of the International Certificate of Vaccination or Prophylaxis (the "Yellow Card") to excuse elderly travelers from yellow fever vaccination (unless risk of exposure is high) rather than vaccinating, although there is theoretical risk of the waiver not being accepted at the border.

Problems after returning home: The **most common** medical problem after travel is

- Persistent traveler's diarrhea

The **most common potentially serious diseases** are

- Malaria
- Hepatitis A and B
- Typhoid fever
- Sexually transmitted diseases, including HIV infection
- Amebiasis
- Meningitis

People can also acquire lice and scabies after being in crowded living conditions or places where hygienic measures are poor.

Some diseases become evident months after a traveler has returned home; a travel history with exposure risks is a useful diagnostic clue when patients present with a puzzling illness. The International Society of Travel Medicine (www.istm.org) and the American Society of Tropical Medicine and Hygiene (www.astmh.org) have lists of travel clinics on their web sites. Many of these clinics specialize in assisting travelers who are ill after their return home.

384 Medicolegal Issues

CAPACITY (COMPETENCE) AND INCAPACITY

Historically, "incapacity" was considered primarily a clinical finding, and "incompetency" was considered a legal finding. That distinction, at least in terminology, is no longer firmly recognized; most state laws now use "incapacity" rather than "incompetency," although the terms are frequently used interchangeably. The more useful distinction in terminology now is between clinical incapacity and legal incapacity to make a health care decision.

People who have clinical and legal capacity with respect to health care have the right to make health care decisions, including refusal of medically necessary care, even if death may result from refusal. People who lack both capacities cannot make health care decisions. However, if a patient deemed by a physician to lack clinical capacity expresses a preference regarding a health care decision, the physician is not entitled to override that preference unless a court also deems the person lacks legal capacity to make that decision.

Clinical capacity: Clinical capacity to make health care decisions is the ability to understand the benefits and risks of the proposed health care, to understand possible alternatives, and to make and communicate a health care decision. Assessment of this capacity requires evaluation of the following:

- Medical factors (eg, the patient's medical condition, sensory deficits, drug side effects, emotional and psychiatric issues)
- Functional abilities (physical, cognitive, and psychologic)
- Environmental factors (eg, risks, supports, impediments to capacity)

Appropriate health care practitioners determine this type of capacity when needed and document the determination process. Qualified health care practitioners, as defined by state laws, are legally empowered to make these determinations in almost every state under state advance directive laws. The courts become involved only when the determination itself or another aspect of the process is challenged by the patient or someone else.

Clinical capacity is specific to a particular health care decision and thus is limited to that decision. The level of clinical capacity needed to make a health care decision depends on the complexity of that decision. A patient with some decrease in capacity, even one with fairly severe cognitive deficits, may still have enough capacity to make simple health care decisions, such as whether to allow a rectal examination or placement of an IV. However, the same patient may lack the capacity to decide whether to participate in a clinical trial.

All feasible attempts should be made to involve the patient in decision making. Ignoring the decision of patients with capacity or accepting the decision of patients without capacity is unethical and risks civil liability. A patient's ability to carry out a decision is also important for physicians to assess. For example, a patient with a broken leg may be able to make the decision to return home but be incapable of self-care during convalescence. Providing the necessary support to carry out a decision becomes an important goal of care.

Capacity may be intermittent, variable, and affected by the environment. Patients who lack capacity due to intoxication, delirium, coma, severe depression, agitation, or other impairment may regain capacity when their impairment resolves. To obtain consent to treat a patient who lacks clinical capacity, health care practitioners must contact an agent or proxy designated in the patient's durable power of attorney for health care or another legally authorized surrogate (see p. 3211). If urgent or emergency care is needed (eg, for an unconscious patient after an acute event) and there is no designated surrogate or the surrogate is unavailable, the doctrine of presumed consent applies: Patients are presumed to consent to any necessary emergency treatment. The process of making emergency health care decisions for people who cannot make decisions for themselves is rarely litigated in court.

Legal capacity: Legal capacity (also called competency) is a legal status; it cannot be determined by health care practitioners. However, health care practitioners play an important role in the assessment process. In the US, people aged 18 or older are presumptively considered legally capable of making health care decisions for themselves. Emancipated minors are people below the age of majority (usually 18) who are also considered legally capable. The definition of this group varies by state but generally includes minors who are married, who are in the armed forces, or who have obtained a court decree of emancipation.

People remain legally capable until a judge with appropriate jurisdiction declares them legally incapacitated with respect to some or all areas of functioning. This declaration usually occurs through a guardianship or conservatorship procedure in the courts. The legal requirements for declaring legal incapacity vary by state. However, substantiation of some combination of the following is typically required:

- A disabling condition (eg, intellectual disability, a mental disorder, dementia, altered consciousness, chronic use of drugs)
- A lack of cognitive ability to receive and evaluate information or to make or communicate decisions
- An inability to meet essential requirements of physical health, safety, or self-care without protective intervention
- A finding that guardianship or conservatorship is the least restrictive alternative for protecting the person

If physicians question a person's legal capacity, they may seek a court's determination. Physicians may be asked to testify at or provide documentation for a hearing to determine legal capacity.

When the court declares a person legally incapacitated, it appoints a guardian or conservator to make legally binding decisions for the person, either in all matters or in a limited range of matters specified by the court. Courts can also make decisions about specific issues in dispute (eg, a particular treatment decision or the meaning of a particular instruction in the person's living will).

INFORMED CONSENT

Consent of the patient is a prerequisite for any medical intervention. However, that consent often does not need to be explicit. For emergency care, consent is normally presumed, referred to as the doctrine of presumed consent. For interventions considered routine and unlikely to cause harm (eg, routine phlebotomy, placement of an IV line), circumstances are typically considered to imply consent. For example, by holding out their arm, patients are presumed to indicate consent to receive certain routine interventions. For more invasive or risky interventions, express informed consent is always required.

To give informed consent, patients must have legal and clinical capacity. Health care practitioners obtaining informed consent must be qualified to explain the risks and benefits of the intervention and to answer appropriate questions. The law requires that health care practitioners take reasonable steps to communicate adequately with patients who do not speak English or who have other communication barriers.

Ethical and legal authorities generally agree that health care practitioners are obligated to ensure, at a minimum, that patients understand

- Their current medical status, including its likely course if no treatment is pursued
- Potentially helpful treatments, including a description and explanation of potential risks and benefits
- Usually, the practitioner's professional opinion as to the best alternative
- Uncertainties associated with each of these elements

Practitioners should be clear about the prospects of recovery with treatment and, if treatment is successful, what life will be like afterward. Generally, these discussions are noted in the medical record, and a document describing the discussion is signed by the patient.

Although practitioners are ethically bound to provide sufficient information and to encourage decisions judged to be in the patient's best interest, patients have the right to refuse treatment. A patient's refusal of treatment is not considered to be attempted suicide or evidence by itself of diminished capacity, nor is the health care practitioner's compliance with the patient's refusal legally considered physician-assisted suicide. Rather, the subsequent death is considered legally to be a natural consequence of the disease process itself.

A refusal of care, if puzzling, should prompt the health care practitioner to initiate further discussion. If the patient's legal capacity seems questionable, such capacity should be assessed, but assessment should not be sought solely because the patient is refusing treatment. If refusal of treatment will hurt other people, such as a minor child or other dependent, ethical and legal consultation should be sought.

CONSENT AND SURROGATE DECISION MAKING

When immediate decisions are medically required, the doctrine of presumed consent applies. In other circumstances, consent must be obtained.

Children: For most nonemergency medical decisions affecting minors, medical care cannot proceed without a parent's or guardian's consent. The parent's or guardian's decision can be overridden only if a court determines that the decision constitutes neglect or abuse of the minor. In some states, minors can consent to certain medical treatments (eg, treatment of sexually transmitted diseases, prescriptions for birth control, abortion) without parental permission. Individual state law must be consulted.

Adults: When adult patients lack capacity to consent to or refuse medical treatment, health care practitioners must rely on an authorized surrogate for consent and decision making. All surrogates—whether appointed by the patient, by default pursuant to state law, or by the court—have an obligation to follow the expressed wishes of the patient and to act in the patient's best interests, taking into account the patient's personal values and wishes to the extent known.

If adult patients already have a court-appointed guardian with authority to make health care decisions, the guardian is the authorized surrogate. The guardianship order should be consulted to determine the extent of the guardian's health care decision-making authority. If patients who lack capacity have a durable power of attorney for health care, the agent or proxy appointed by that document is authorized to make health care decisions within the scope of authority granted by the document. Generally, specific instructions that are given in a living will, health care declaration, or other advance directive executed by patients while capacitated can be relied on to the extent that the document clarifies or explains the patient's wishes.

If the decision of an authorized agent or proxy seems to conflict directly with instructions in a living will or other clear instructions given by the patient, the outcome depends on the scope of discretion given to the agent or proxy. Normally, the durable power of attorney for health care confers broad decision-making discretion on the agent so that instructions serve as guidance, not mandates. Nevertheless, the health care practitioner should determine whether the document gives the agent broad discretion beyond the written instructions or limits the agent to the written instructions. Legal advice may be needed.

If patients have no authorized surrogate, health care practitioners usually rely on the next of kin or even a close friend. However, the exact scope of authority and the priority of permissible surrogates vary by state. In states where default surrogate decision makers are authorized, the typical order of priority is a spouse (or domestic partner in jurisdictions that recognize this status), an adult child, a parent, a sibling, and then possibly other relatives or a close friend. If more than one person has the same priority (eg, several adult children), consensus is preferred, but some states allow health care practitioners to rely on a majority decision.

If a patient's decision-making capacity, a surrogate's authority, or the ethical or legal appropriateness of a particular treatment decision is disputed, consultation with an institutional ethics committee or similar body is advisable. If agreement on an ethically and legally sound resolution cannot be reached, health care practitioners or their institution may need to request court review. Many institutions make the ethics committee available on short notice; judicial review is typically more time-consuming.

Scope: Patient choice is not limitless. For example, health care practitioners are not required to provide treatments that are medically or ethically inappropriate, such as those that are against generally accepted health care standards. However, sometimes there are legitimate differences of opinion regarding what is inappropriate. Labeling a treatment as "futile" does not generally help if said treatment may affect outcomes other than mortality or morbidity that are important to the patient. Physicians do not have to act against their conscience but if they cannot comply with a requested course of action, consultation with an ethics committee is advisable. They may also have a responsibility under state law to try to transfer a patient to another physician or institution of the patient's choice.

CONFIDENTIALITY AND HIPAA

Traditionally, ethical health care has always included the need to keep patients' medical information confidential. However, the Health Insurance Portability and Accountability Act (HIPAA—see www.hhs.gov/ocr/privacy) has codified the responsibility of health care providers, health plans, health care clearinghouses, and their business associates who electronically transmit health and related information (eg, health records, enrollment, billing, eligibility verification). Collectively, these are covered entities under HIPAA. Key provisions of HIPAA are embodied in three rules: the Privacy, Security, and Breach Notification rules, all of which are intended to protect the privacy and security of protected health information (PHI).

The Privacy Rule sets standards for the protection of PHI and gives patients important rights with respect to their health information. The Security Rule establishes safeguards that covered entities and their business associates must implement to protect the privacy, integrity, and security of electronic PHI. The Breach Notification Rule requires covered entities to notify affected individuals, the federal government, and in some cases, the media of a breach of unsecured PHI. The U.S. Department of Health and Human Services, Office for Civil Rights, enforces these three rules and provides guidance on complying with the rules (see www.hhs.gov/ocr/privacy).

Key aspects of the Privacy Rule are elaborated below.

Access to medical records: Typically, patients or their authorized representatives should be able to see and obtain copies of their medical records and request corrections if they identify errors.

Notice of privacy practices: Health care providers must provide a notice about their possible uses of personal medical information and about patient rights under HIPAA regulations.

Limits on use of personal medical information: HIPAA limits how health care providers may use individually identifiable (protected) health information. The act does not restrict physicians, nurses, and other practitioners from sharing information needed to treat their patients. However, practitioners may use or share only the minimum amount of protected information needed for a particular purpose. In most situations, personal health information may not be used for purposes unrelated to health care. For example, a patient must sign a specific authorization before a health care provider can release medical information to a life insurer, a bank, a marketing firm, or another outside business for purposes unrelated to the patient's current health care needs.

Marketing: Marketing is communication designed to encourage people to purchase a particular product or service. HIPAA requires that the patient's specific authorization must be obtained before disclosing information for marketing. Health care providers must disclose any payments that will be received as a result of marketing. However, health care providers can freely communicate with patients about treatment options, products, and other health-related services, including disease-management programs.

Confidential communications: Practitioners should take reasonable steps to ensure that their communications with the patient are confidential and in accord with patient preferences. For example, physician-patient medical discussions generally should be in private, or a patient might prefer that the physician call their office rather than home. Nonetheless, unless the patient objects, practitioners can share medical information with a patient's immediate family members or someone known to be a close personal friend if the information relates directly to that family member's or friend's involvement with the patient's care or payment for care. Practitioners are expected to exercise professional judgment.

For purposes of the privacy rule, an authorized personal representative of the patient (eg, a proxy appointed in a power of attorney for health care, a state-authorized health surrogate or someone given HIPAA-compliant written authorization to have access to confidential information) should be treated the same as the patient. Thus, the representative has the same access to information and may exercise the same rights regarding confidentiality of information, except that an express HIPAA authorization can specify limits on the representative's authority. Nevertheless, practitioners may restrict information or access if there are reasonable concerns about domestic violence, abuse, or neglect by the representative.

Some communication cannot remain confidential. Health care practitioners are sometimes required by law to disclose certain information, usually because the condition may present a danger to other people. For example, certain infectious diseases (eg, HIV, syphilis, TB) must be reported to state or local public health agencies. Signs of child and, in many states, adult or elder abuse or neglect, typically must be reported to protective services. Conditions that might seriously impair a patient's ability to drive, such as dementia or recent seizures, must be reported to the Department of Motor Vehicles in some states.

Complaints: Patients may file complaints about compliance with these privacy practices. Complaints can be made directly to the health care practitioner or to the Office for Civil Rights in the US Department of Health and Human Services. Patients do not have a right to file a private lawsuit under HIPAA. There are civil and criminal penalties for improper disclosure of personal health information. The soundest course for health care practitioners is to be well informed of HIPAA, to act in good faith, and make reasonable attempts to comply.

ADVANCE DIRECTIVES

Advance directives are legal documents that extend a person's control over health care decisions in the event that the person becomes incapacitated. They are called advance directives because they communicate preferences before incapacitation occurs. There are 2 primary types:

- Living will: Expresses preferences for end-of-life care
- Durable power of attorney for health care: Designates a surrogate decision maker

Every state in the US recognizes these documents and encourages their use as a simple legal tool by which people can express their wishes and have them honored. However, formal advance directives are not the only means of expressing such wishes. Both common law and constitutional principles direct that any authentic, clear expression of patients' wishes should be honored if within the scope of generally accepted medical standards.

An advance directive cannot be completed after a patient becomes too incapacitated to understand the nature and effect of an advance directive; and, in most states, the directive does not become effective until after incapacity to make health care decisions has been determined. If no advance directive has been prepared, an authorized surrogate must be identified or appointed to make health care decisions.

Living will: A living will is a limited document that expresses a person's preferences for end-of-life health care (it is called a "living" will because it is in effect while the person is still alive). In many states, the document is more formally called a medical directive to doctors or a declaration. State laws vary greatly regarding scope and applicability of living wills.

A living will allows people to express preferences for the amount and nature of their health care, from no interventions to maximum treatment. Detailed treatment preferences can be helpful because they provide more specific guidance to practitioners. However, living wills completed long before a person experiences a life-limiting disorder have not usually been very helpful because, among other reasons, many people change their preferences as their circumstances change. A living will cannot compel health care practitioners to provide health care that is medically or ethically unwarranted.

To be legally valid, a living will must comply with state law. Some states require that living wills be written in a fairly standardized way. Others are more flexible, permitting any language as long as the document is appropriately signed and witnessed. In most states, a health care practitioner involved in the patient's care cannot be a witness. A document that does not comply with state law requirements for statutory living wills may still serve as reliable evidence of a patient's wishes if it appears to be an authentic expression of the patient's wishes.

Living wills go into effect when people are no longer able to make their own health care decisions or a medical condition specified in the directive—typically a terminal condition, permanent vegetative state, or the end-stage of a chronic condition—is diagnosed. Often, state law provides a process for confirming and documenting the loss of decisional capacity and the medical condition.

Durable power of attorney for health care: In this document, one person (the principal) names another person (the agent, proxy, or health care representative) to make decisions about health care and *only* health care. In most states, these documents become legally effective when the principal loses clinical capacity to make health care decisions. Some states recognize *immediately* effective durable powers of attorney for health care, which in theory means that the agent can make health care decisions immediately; but as a practical matter, the principal can direct and override anything the agent does as long as the principal retains the capacity to make health care decisions. So, the difference is negligible. Like the living will, the durable power of attorney for health care may be referred to by different terms in different states.

People who have both a living will and a durable power of attorney for health care should stipulate which should be followed if the documents seem to conflict. The better option is to combine the two documents into the power of attorney. The strongest virtue of the power of attorney for health care is that it enables a designated decision maker to respond to here-and-now circumstances and options, rather than merely providing directions about hypothetical future medical circumstances such as those not addressed in a living will. The agent generally has the same authority the principal would have had if not incapacitated to know the medical facts and prognosis, discuss medical alternatives, and make decisions about any injury or illness. In most states, a health care practitioner providing care for the patient cannot serve as agent for health care matters. The durable power of attorney for health care can include a living will provision or any other specific instructions but, preferably, should do so only as guidance for the agent, rather than as a binding instruction.

The durable power of attorney for health care typically names an alternate or successor in case the first-named person is unable or unwilling to serve as agent. Two or more people may be named to serve together (jointly) or alone (severally), although reliance on multiple concurrent agents can be problematic. A **jointly held power** requires that all agents agree and act together. In this arrangement, any disagreement can result in a stalemate until it is resolved by the agents or the courts. A **severally held power** may be more functional because it allows any named agent to act alone. However, agents in this arrangement can also disagree, and, if irreconcilable, the courts may have to become involved.

The use of the durable power of attorney for health care is valuable for adults of all ages. It is especially critical for unmarried couples, same-sex partners, friends, or other individuals who are considered legally unrelated and who wish to grant each other the legal authority to make health care decisions and to ensure rights of visitation and access to medical information.

Ideally, physicians should obtain a copy of a patient's living will and durable power of attorney for health care, periodically review the contents with the patient while the patient is still capable, and make it part of the medical record. A copy of the durable power of attorney for health care should also be given to the patient's appointed agent and another copy placed with important papers. The patient's attorney should hold a copy of all documents. An increasing number of states offer optional electronic registries for recording advance directives.

DO-NOT-RESUSCITATE ORDERS AND PHYSICIAN ORDERS FOR LIFE-SUSTAINING TREATMENT

The do-not-resuscitate (DNR) order placed in a patient's medical record by a physician informs the medical staff that CPR should not be done in the event of cardiac arrest. This order has been useful in preventing unnecessary and unwanted invasive treatment at the end of life.

Physicians discuss with patients the possibility of cardiopulmonary arrest, describe CPR procedures and likely outcomes, and ask patients about treatment preferences. If the patient is incapable of making a decision about CPR, a surrogate may make the decision based on the patient's previously expressed preferences or, if such preferences are unknown, in accordance with the patient's best interests.

Living wills and durable powers of attorney for health care are not typically available in emergency situations and thus may be ineffective. Almost all states have specialized DNR protocols for patients who are living at home or in any non-hospital setting. These protocols typically require the signing of an out-of-hospital DNR order by both the physician and patient (or the patient's surrogate) and the use of a special identifier (eg, a bracelet or brightly colored form) that is worn by or kept near the patient. If emergency medical personnel are called in case of emergency and see an intact identifier, they will provide comfort care only and not attempt resuscitation. These protocols are important to know because, normally, emergency medical technicians are not expected to read or rely on a living will or durable power of attorney for health care.

Many patients with advanced illness face heightened challenges in having their wishes respected not only with respect to CPR but with respect to any critical care decision. To provide better care planning for patients with advanced illness, most states have adopted, or are in the process of adopting, some version of a program commonly called Physician Orders for Life-Sustaining Treatment (POLST). Other names for the program have included Medical Orders for Life-Sustaining Treatment (MOLST), Physician Orders for Scope of Treatment (POST), and Medical Orders for Scope of Treatment (MOST). The programs follow a common paradigm but typically have somewhat different forms and policies. The most common criterion for qualifying as advanced illness in these programs is if the clinician would not be surprised if the patient were to die within the next year.

The POLST process is initiated by health care providers and results in a set of medical orders that is portable across all health care settings and addresses CPR, along with overall goals of treatment (comfort care only, full curative treatments, or limited treatments in between) and other critical care decisions, such as the use of artificial nutrition and hydration. These programs can help physicians best honor their patients' wishes regarding goals of treatment and help ensure continuity across care settings.

POLST and similar programs do not exist in every state or community, but their development is spreading rapidly. A national POLST task force provides a clearinghouse at www.polst.org.

MEDICAL MALPRACTICE

Patients can sue health care practitioners if they feel they have been injured. However, successful medical malpractice lawsuits require proof of the following:

- The care provided was below the ordinary standard of care that would be provided by similar health care practitioners under similar circumstances.
- A professional relationship existed between the health care practitioner and the injured party.
- The patient was harmed because of the deviation from the standard of care.

Concern about lawsuits sometimes puts pressure on physicians to act in ways that are not necessarily in the best interest of their patients. For example, physicians may order tests that are not clearly medically necessary to avoid even a remote possibility of missing something and thus leaving themselves open to a lawsuit. This approach exposes patients to risks (eg, ionizing radiation, need for invasive and/or uncomfortable tests to confirm false-positive results) and expenses that are not justified by the medical benefit. However, such an approach is not required by law, may not protect against lawsuits, and is generally considered excessive and inappropriate. Explaining to patients the reasons why a particular test or treatment is not recommended and engaging patients in shared decision making about their care usually satisfies patients more. The best defense against malpractice lawsuits is providing excellent health care and building close, trusting, collaborative relationships with patients.

385 Nonspecific Symptoms

FATIGUE

Fatigue occurs most often as part of a symptom complex, but even when it is the sole or main presenting symptom, fatigue is one of the most common symptoms.

Fatigue is difficulty initiating and sustaining activity due to a lack of energy and accompanied by a desire to rest. Fatigue is normal after physical exertion, prolonged stress, and sleep deprivation.

Patients may refer to certain other symptoms as fatigue; differentiating between them and fatigue is usually, but not always, possible with detailed questioning.

- Weakness (see p. 1828), a symptom of nervous system or muscle disorders, is insufficient force of muscular contraction at maximum effort. Disorders such as myasthenia gravis and Eaton-Lambert syndrome can cause weakness that worsens with activity, simulating fatigue.
- Dyspnea on exertion, an early symptom of cardiac and pulmonary disorders, can decrease exercise tolerance, simulating fatigue. Respiratory symptoms usually can be elicited upon careful questioning or develop subsequently.
- Somnolence, a symptom of disorders causing sleep deprivation (eg, allergic rhinitis, esophageal reflux, painful musculoskeletal disorders, sleep apnea, severe chronic disorders), is an unusually strong desire to sleep. Yawning and lapsing into sleep during daytime hours are common. Patients can usually tell the difference between somnolence and fatigue. However, deprivation of deep nonrapid eye movement sleep can cause muscle aches and fatigue, and many patients with fatigue have disturbed sleep, so differentiating between fatigue and somnolence may be difficult.

Fatigue can be classified in various temporal categories, such as the following:

- Recent fatigue: < 1 mo duration
- Prolonged fatigue: 1 to 6 mo duration
- Chronic fatigue: > 6 mo duration

Chronic fatigue syndrome (see p. 3134) is one cause of chronic fatigue.

Etiology

Most serious (and many minor) acute and chronic illnesses produce fatigue. However, many of these have other more prominent manifestations (eg, pain, cough, fever, jaundice) as the presenting complaint. This discussion focuses on disorders that can manifest primarily as fatigue.

The most common disorders manifesting predominantly as recent fatigue (lasting < 1 mo) are

- Drug adverse effects
- Anemia
- Stress and/or depression

The most common causes manifesting predominantly as prolonged fatigue (lasting 1 to 6 mo) are

- Diabetes
- Hypothyroidism
- Sleep disturbances (eg, sleep apnea)
- Cancer

The most common causes manifesting predominantly as chronic fatigue (lasting > 6 mo) are

- Chronic fatigue syndrome
- Psychologic causes (eg, depression)
- Drugs

Table 385–1. SOME FACTORS COMMONLY CONTRIBUTING TO PROLONGED OR CHRONIC FATIGUE

CATEGORY	EXAMPLES
Chronic disorders	Chronic kidney disease, rheumatologic disorders (eg, giant cell arteritis, RA, SLE)
Drugs	Antidepressants, antihistamines (1st generation), antihypertensives, cocaine cessation (usually recent fatigue), diuretics that cause hypokalemia, muscle relaxants, recreational drugs, sedatives
Endocrine disorders	Adrenal insufficiency*, diabetes, hyperthyroidism* (usually apathetic), hypothyroidism, pituitary insufficiency
Infections	Cytomegalovirus infection, endocarditis, fungal pneumonias, hepatitis, HIV/AIDS, mononucleosis, parasitic infections*, TB
Psychologic disorders	Anxiety, depression, domestic violence, drug addiction, panic disorder, somatization disorder
Disorders of unknown cause	Chronic fatigue syndrome, fibromyalgia, idiopathic fatigue
Other causes	Anemias, cancers, deconditioning, pregnancy*, undernutrition, hypercalcemia*, multiple sclerosis

*Usually does not cause chronic fatigue.

Several factors commonly cause or contribute to a chief complaint of fatigue, usually prolonged or chronic fatigue (see Table 385–1).

Evaluation

Fatigue can be highly subjective. Patients vary in what they consider to be fatigue and how they describe it. There are also few ways to objectively confirm fatigue or tell how severe it is. History and physical examination focus on identifying subtle manifestations of underlying illness (particularly infections, endocrine and rheumatologic disorders, anemia, and depression) that can be used to guide testing.

History: History of present illness includes open-ended questions about what "fatigue" is, listening for descriptions that could suggest dyspnea on exertion, somnolence, or muscle weakness. The relationships between fatigue, activity, rest, and sleep should be elicited, as should the onset, time course and pattern, and factors that increase or decrease fatigue.

Review of systems should be thorough because potential causes of fatigue are so numerous and diverse. Among important nonspecific symptoms are fever, weight loss, and night sweats (possibly suggesting cancer, a rheumatologic disorder, or an infection). Menstrual history is obtained in women of child-bearing age. Unless a cause is evident, patients should be asked questions from screening questionnaires for psychologic disorders (eg, depression, anxiety, drug abuse, somatoform disorders, domestic violence).

Past medical history should address known disorders. Complete drug use history should include prescription, OTC, and recreational drugs.

Social history should elicit descriptions of diet, drug abuse, and the effect of fatigue on quality of life, employment, and social and family relationships.

Physical examination: Vital signs are checked for fever, tachycardia, tachypnea, and hypotension. General examination should be particularly comprehensive, including general appearance and examination of the heart, lungs, abdomen, head and neck, breasts, rectum (including prostate exam and testing for occult blood), genitals, liver, spleen, lymph nodes, joints, and skin. Neurologic examination should include testing of, at a minimum, mental status, cranial nerves, mood, affect, strength, muscle bulk and tone, reflexes, and gait. Usually if fatigue is of recent onset, a more focused examination will reveal the cause. If fatigue is chronic, examination is unlikely to reveal a cause; however, thorough physical examination is an important way to build rapport with the patient and occasionally is diagnostically helpful.

Red flags:

- Chronic weight loss
- Chronic fever or night sweats
- Generalized lymphadenopathy
- Muscle weakness or pain
- Serious non-fatigue symptoms (eg, hemoptysis, hematemesis, severe dyspnea, ascites, confusion, suicidal ideation)
- Involvement of > 1 organ system (eg, rash plus arthritis)
- New or different headache or loss of vision, particularly with muscle pains, in an older adult
- Older age (eg, > 65 yr)

Interpretation of findings: In general, a cause is more likely to be found when fatigue is one of many symptoms than when fatigue is the sole symptom. Fatigue that worsens with activity and lessens with rest suggests a physical disorder. Fatigue that is present constantly and does not lessen with rest, particularly with occasional bursts of energy, may indicate a psychologic disorder.

In the absence of red flag findings, a thorough history, physical examination, and routine laboratory testing (plus tests directed at specific findings—see Table 385–2) should suffice for an initial evaluation. If test results are negative, watchful waiting is usually appropriate; if fatigue worsens or other symptoms and signs develop, the patient is reevaluated.

Several causes can be considered for patients with prolonged or chronic fatigue and selected other common or specific clinical findings (see Table 385–2).

Testing: Testing is directed at causes suspected based on clinical findings. If no cause is evident or suspected based on clinical findings, laboratory testing is unlikely to reveal a cause. Still, many clinicians recommend testing with the following:

- CBC
- ESR
- TSH
- Chemistries, including electrolytes, glucose, Ca, and renal and liver function tests

CK is recommended if muscle pain or weakness is present. HIV testing and PPD placement are recommended if the patient has risk factors. Chest x-ray is recommended if cough or dyspnea are present. Other testing, such as for infections or immunologic deficiencies, is not recommended unless there are suggestive clinical findings. Diagnosis of chronic fatigue syndrome requires both of the following:

- Chronic fatigue that affects daily function, is not relieved by rest, and is not explained by clinical findings or abnormal findings on the laboratory tests mentioned above
- Presence of ≥ 4 of the following: sore throat, unrefreshing sleep, difficulty with concentration or short-term memory, myalgias, multiple joint pains without joint swelling, new or different headaches, and tender cervical or axillary nodes

Treatment

Treatment is directed at the cause. Patients with chronic fatigue syndrome (see p. 3134) and idiopathic chronic fatigue are treated similarly. They should be told clearly that there is no physical cause evident. Treatment is more often successful if the practitioner is patient and nonjudgmental and acknowledges the real effects of fatigue. Effective treatments include physical therapy (eg, graded exercise therapy) and psychologic support (eg, cognitive-behavioral therapy). Goals include returning to work and maintaining normal activity levels.

Geriatrics Essentials

Fatigue is more often the first symptom of a disorder in older patients. For example, the first symptom of a UTI in an older woman may be fatigue rather than urinary symptoms. Older patients with pneumonia may have fatigue before they have a cough or fever. The first symptom of other disorders, such as giant cell arteritis, may also be fatigue in an older patient. Because serious illness may become apparent soon after sudden fatigue in older patients, the cause should be determined as quickly as possible. Fatigue is also somewhat more likely to be caused by giant cell arteritis or another serious physical disorder in the elderly.

KEY POINTS

- Fatigue is a common symptom.
- Fatigue caused primarily by a physical disorder increases with activity and lessens with rest.
- Laboratory testing is low yield in the absence of suggestive clinical findings.
- Successful treatment is more likely if the practitioner is patient and understanding.

Table 385–2. INTERPRETATION OF SELECTED FINDINGS IN EVALUATING FATIGUE

SYMPTOMS	POSSIBLE CAUSES	TESTS TO CONSIDER*
Anorexia, abdominal pain, weight loss, or steatorrhea	Undernutrition secondary to GI tract disorder, cancer	Endoscopy, MRI of abdomen, MRCP
Anorexia, abdominal pain, weight loss, orthostatic hypotension, skin hyperpigmentation	Adrenal insufficiency	Blood electrolyte and cortisol levels
Fever, night sweats, or weight loss	Infection, rheumatologic disorder (including vasculitis)	CBC, ESR, blood or other cultures, rheumatoid factor and ANA
Dyspnea with cough or hemoptysis	HIV/AIDS (with *Pneumocystis jirovecii* pneumonia), fungal pneumonia, TB	Chest x-ray, chest CT or PET-CT, HIV test, sputum cytology and/or culture, pulmonary function tests, PPD
Dyspnea, orthopnea, and/or edema	Chronic kidney disease, heart failure	Chest x-ray, renal function tests, echocardiography (if orthopnea)
Dyspnea, Roth spots, Janeway lesions, new or changing heart murmurs, IV drug use	Endocarditis	Multiple blood cultures, echocardiography
Decreased exercise tolerance with dyspnea on exertion, pallor	Anemia	CBC
Generalized lymphadenopathy	HIV/AIDS, leukemia, lymphoma, mononucleosis	HIV test, CBC, EBV serologic tests
Combined arthritis, rash, and/or other organ involvement	Rheumatologic disorder (including vasculitis)	CBC, ESR, rheumatoid factor, ANA
Jaundice, ascites, confusion	Hepatitis	Liver function tests, viral hepatitis serologies
Polydipsia, polyuria, increased appetite, weight gain or loss	Diabetes	Fasting plasma glucose level, glucose tolerance testing
Cold intolerance, weight gain, constipation, coarse skin	Hypothyroidism, pituitary insufficiency	TSH
Weight loss or atrial fibrillation in elderly patient	Hyperthyroidism (apathetic)	Thyroid function tests
Fatigue worse with exposure to heat, past neurologic symptoms (eg, numbness, ataxia, weakness), particularly > 1 episode	Multiple sclerosis	Brain and/or spinal cord MRI with contrast
Headache, jaw claudication, temporal artery tenderness or thickening, and/or muscle pains in an older adult	Giant cell arteritis	ESR, brain MRI or CT, temporal artery biopsy
Anxiety, sadness, anorexia, unexplained sleep disturbance	Anxiety, depression, domestic violence, somatization disorder	Clinical evaluation
Recent sore throat, lymphadenopathy, splenomegaly	Mononucleosis, chronic fatigue syndrome	EBV serologic tests; CBC, ESR, TSH, chemistries (as for suspected chronic fatigue syndrome)
Lymphadenopathy, splenomegaly	CMV infection	EBV serologic tests, sometimes CMV antibody testing
Frequent or opportunistic infections, candidiasis, lymphadenopathy, splenomegaly	HIV/AIDS	HIV testing
Chronic, widespread musculoskeletal extra-articular pain, trigger points, irritable bowel symptoms, migraines, anxiety	Fibromyalgia	ESR or C-reactive protein, CK, TSH, hepatitis C serology
Weight loss, steatorrhea, inadequate oral intake	Undernutrition	Plasma albumin, total lymphocyte and CD4 counts, serum transferrin
Constipation, lethargy, bone pain (eg, at night)	Hypercalcemia	Serum chemistries, including Ca
Sore throat, unrefreshing sleep, difficulty with concentration or short-term memory, myalgias, multiple arthralgias, headaches, tender cervical or axillary nodes.	Chronic fatigue syndrome	CBC, ESR, TSH, serum electrolytes, glucose, Ca, and renal and liver function tests

*Choice of specific tests is dictated by which causes are clinically suspected.
ANA = antinuclear antibodies; CMV = cytomegalovirus; EBV = Epstein-Barr virus; MRCP = magnetic resonance cholangiopancreatography.

INVOLUNTARY WEIGHT LOSS

Involuntary weight loss generally develops over weeks or months. It can be a sign of a significant physical or mental disorder and is associated with an increased risk for mortality. The causative disorder may be obvious (eg, chronic diarrhea due to a malabsorption syndrome) or occult (eg, an undiagnosed cancer). This discussion focuses on patients who present for weight loss rather than those who lose weight as a more-or-less expected consequence of a known chronic disorder (eg, metastatic cancer, end-stage COPD).

Weight loss is typically considered clinically important if it exceeds 5% of body weight or 5 kg over 6 months. However, this traditional definition does not distinguish between loss of lean and fat body mass, which can lead to different outcomes. Also, accumulation of edema (eg, in heart failure or chronic kidney disease) can mask clinically important loss of lean body mass.

In addition to weight loss, patients may have other symptoms, such as anorexia, fever, or night sweats, due to the underlying disorder. Depending on the cause and its severity, symptoms and signs of nutritional deficiency (see p. 37) may also be present.

The overall incidence of significant involuntary weight loss is about 5% per year in the US. However, incidence increases with aging, often reaching 50% among nursing home patients.

Pathophysiology

Weight loss results when more calories are expended than taken in (ingested and absorbed). Disorders that increase expenditure or decrease absorption tend to *increase* appetite. More commonly, inadequate caloric intake is the mechanism for weight loss and such patients tend to have *decreased* appetite. Sometimes, several mechanisms are involved. For example, cancer tends to decrease appetite but also increases basal caloric expenditure by cytokine-mediated mechanisms.

Etiology

Many disorders cause involuntary weight loss, including almost any chronic illness of sufficient severity. However, many of these are clinically obvious and have typically been diagnosed by the time weight loss occurs. Other disorders are more likely to manifest as involuntary weight loss (see Table 385–3).

With **increased appetite,** the most common occult causes of involuntary weight loss are

- Hyperthyroidism
- Uncontrolled diabetes
- Disorders that cause malabsorption

With **decreased appetite,** the most common occult causes of involuntary weight loss are

- Mental disorders (eg, depression)
- Cancer
- Drug adverse effects
- Drug abuse

In some disorders that cause involuntary weight loss, other symptoms tend to be more prominent, so that weight loss is usually not the chief complaint. Examples include the following:

- Some malabsorptive disorders: GI tract surgery and cystic fibrosis
- Chronic inflammatory disorders: Severe RA

Table 385–3. SOME CAUSES OF A PRESENTING SYMPTOM OF INVOLUNTARY WEIGHT LOSS

CAUSE	SUGGESTIVE FINDINGS	DIAGNOSTIC APPROACH
Endocrine disorders		
Hyperthyroidism	Increased appetite Heat intolerance, sweating, tremor, anxiety, tachycardia, diarrhea	Thyroid function tests
Diabetes mellitus, type 1 (new onset or poorly controlled)	Increased appetite Polydipsia, polyuria	Plasma glucose measurement
Chronic primary adrenal insufficiency	Abdominal pain, fatigue, hyperpigmentation, orthostatic light-headedness	Serum electrolytes, cortisol, and ACTH levels
Drugs		
Alcohol	History of excess consumption Vascular spiders, Dupuytren's contractures, testicular atrophy, peripheral neuropathy Sometimes ascites, asterixis	Clinical evaluation Sometimes liver function tests and/or liver biopsy
Drugs (see Table 385–4) • Of abuse • Herbal and OTC products • Prescription	History of use	Clinical evaluation When possible, trial of stopping drug
Mental disorders		
Anorexia nervosa	Inappropriate fear of weight gain in an emaciated young woman or adolescent female, amenorrhea	Clinical evaluation
Depression	Sadness, fatigue, loss of sexual desire and/or pleasure, sleep disturbance, psychomotor retardation	Clinical evaluation

Table 385–3. SOME CAUSES OF A PRESENTING SYMPTOM OF INVOLUNTARY WEIGHT LOSS (*Continued*)

CAUSE	SUGGESTIVE FINDINGS	DIAGNOSTIC APPROACH
Renal disorders*		
Chronic kidney disease	Edema, nausea, vomiting, stomatitis, dysgeusia, nocturia, fatigue, pruritus, decreased mental acuity, muscle twitches and cramps, peripheral neuropathy, seizures	Serum BUN and creatinine measurement
Nephrotic syndrome	Edema, hypertension, proteinuria, fatigue, frothy urine	24-h Urinary protein measurement Alternatively, spot urinary/serum protein ratio
Infections		
Fungal infections (usually primary fungal infections)	Fever, night sweats, fatigue, cough, dyspnea Often risk of exposure based on geography Sometimes other organ-specific manifestations	Usually cultures and stains Sometimes serologic tests Sometimes biopsy
Helminthic (worm) infections	Fever, abdominal pain, bloating, flatulence, diarrhea, eosinophilia Usually residence or travel in developing countries	Disorder-specific tests (eg, microscopic examination of stool, culture, serology)
HIV/AIDS	Fever, dyspnea, cough, lymphadenopathy, diarrhea, candidiasis	Blood antibody or antigen testing
Subacute bacterial endocarditis	Fever, night sweats, arthralgias, dyspnea, fatigue, Roth spots, Janeway lesions, Osler nodes, splinter hemorrhages, retinal artery emboli, stroke Often in patients with valvular heart disease or IV drug use	Blood cultures Echocardiography
TB	Fever, night sweats, cough, hemoptysis Sometimes risk factors (eg, exposure, poor living conditions)	Sputum culture and smear
Other systemic disorders		
Cancer	Often night sweats, fatigue, fever Sometimes bone pain at night or other organ-specific symptoms	Organ-specific evaluation
Giant cell arteritis	Headache, muscle pains, jaw claudication, fever, and/or visual disturbances in an older adult	ESR and, if elevated, temporal artery biopsy
Sarcoidosis	Cough, dyspnea, crackles Fever, fatigue, lymphadenopathy Sometimes symptoms of other organ involvement (eg, ocular, hepatic, GI, bone)	Chest x-ray Sometimes chest CT Biopsy
Dental and taste disorders		
Dysgeusia (loss of taste)	Usually risk factors (eg, cranial nerve dysfunction, use of certain drugs, aging)	Clinical evaluation
Poor dentition	Tooth or gum pain Halitosis, periodontitis, missing and/or decayed teeth	Clinical evaluation

*Accumulation of edema may mask loss of lean body weight.

Table 385–4. DRUGS AND HERBAL PRODUCTS THAT CAN CAUSE WEIGHT LOSS

CATEGORY	EXAMPLES
Prescription drugs	Antiretroviral drugs, cancer chemotherapy drugs, digoxin, exenatide, levodopa. liraglutide, metformin, NSAIDs, SSRIs, topiramate, zonisamide Withdrawal after chronic high-dose psychotropic drugs
Herbal products and OTC drugs	Aloe, caffeine, cascara, chitosan, chromium, dandelion, ephedra, 5-hydroxytryptophan, garcinia, guarana, guar gum, glucomannan, herbal diuretics, ma huang, pyruvate, St. John's wort, yerba mate
Drugs of abuse	Alcohol, amphetamines, cocaine, opioids

- Gastrointestinal disorders: Achalasia, Crohn disease, chronic pancreatitis, esophageal obstructive disorders, ischemic colitis, diabetic enteropathy, peptic ulcer disease, progressive systemic sclerosis, ulcerative colitis (late)
- Severe, chronic heart and lung disorders: COPD, heart failure (stage III or IV), restrictive lung disease
- Mental disorders (known and poorly controlled): Anxiety, bipolar disorder, depression, schizophrenia
- Neurologic disorders: Amyotrophic lateral sclerosis, dementia, multiple sclerosis, myasthenia gravis, Parkinson disease, stroke
- Social problems: Poverty, social isolation

With chronic kidney disease and heart failure, accumulation of edema may mask loss of lean body weight.

Evaluation

Evaluation focuses on detection of otherwise occult causes. Because these are numerous, evaluation must be comprehensive.

History: History of present illness includes questions about the amount and time course of weight loss. A report of weight loss may be inaccurate; thus, corroborating evidence should be sought, such as weight measurement in old medical records, changes in size of clothes, or confirmation by family members. Appetite, food intake, swallowing, and bowel patterns should be described. For repeat evaluations, patients should keep a food diary because recollections of food intake are often inaccurate. Nonspecific symptoms of potential causes are noted, such as fatigue, malaise, fevers, and night sweats.

Review of systems must be complete, seeking symptoms in all major organ systems.

Past medical history may reveal a disorder capable of causing weight loss. Also addressed should be use of prescription drugs, OTC drugs, recreational drugs, and herbal products. Social history may reveal changes in living situations that could explain why food intake is decreased (eg, loss of loved one, loss of independence or job, loss of communal eating routine).

Physical examination: Vital signs are checked for fever, tachycardia, tachypnea, and hypotension. Weight is measured and body mass index (BMI) is calculated (see p. 20). Triceps skinfold thickness and mid upper arm circumference can be measured to estimate lean body mass (see p. 31). BMI and lean body mass estimates are helpful mainly for detecting a trend in follow-up visits.

General examination should be particularly comprehensive, including examination of the heart, lungs, abdomen, head and neck, breasts, neurologic system, rectum (including prostate examination and testing for occult blood), genitals, liver, spleen, lymph nodes, joints, skin, mood, and affect.

Red flags:

- Fever, night sweats, generalized lymphadenopathy
- Bone pain
- Dyspnea, cough, hemoptysis
- Inappropriate fear of weight gain in an adolescent or young woman
- Polydipsia and polyuria
- Headache, jaw claudication, and/or visual disturbances in an older adult
- Roth spots, Janeway lesions, Osler nodes, splinter hemorrhages, retinal artery emboli

Interpretation of findings: Interpretations of some findings are listed in Table 385–5. Abnormal findings suggest the cause of weight loss in about half or more patients, including patients eventually diagnosed with cancer.

Although many chronic disorders can cause weight loss, the clinician must not be too quick to assume that an existing disorder is the cause. Although the existing disorder is the likely cause in patients whose condition has remained poorly controlled or is deteriorating, stable patients who suddenly begin losing weight without a worsening of that disorder may have developed a new condition (eg, patients with stable ulcerative colitis may begin losing weight because they developed a colon cancer).

PEARLS & PITFALLS

- When a chronic disease has been stable, do not assume that it is the cause of acute weight loss.

Testing: Age-appropriate cancer screening (eg, colonoscopy, mammography) is indicated if not previously done. Other testing is done for disorders suspected based on abnormal findings in the history or examination. There are no widely accepted guidelines on other testing for patients without such focal abnormal findings. One suggested approach is to do the following tests:

- Chest x-ray
- Urinalysis
- CBC with differential count
- ESR or C-reactive protein
- HIV testing
- Serum chemistries (serum electrolytes, calcium, hepatic and renal function tests)
- TSH level

Abnormal results on these tests are followed with additional testing as indicated. If all test results are normal and clinical findings are otherwise normal, extensive further testing (eg, CT, MRI) is not recommended. Such testing is very low yield and can be misleading and harmful by revealing incidental, unrelated findings. Such patients should be taught how to ensure adequate caloric intake and have a follow-up evaluation in about 1 mo that includes a weight measurement. If patients

Table 385–5. INTERPRETATION OF SELECTED FINDINGS IN INVOLUNTARY WEIGHT LOSS

FINDING	SOME CAUSES TO CONSIDER
Fatigue	Adrenal insufficiency, cancer, chronic kidney disease, depression, infections, giant cell arteritis, nephrotic syndrome, sarcoidosis
Fever, night sweats	Cancer, infections, giant cell arteritis
Lymphadenopathy	Infections, cancer, sarcoidosis
Rectal bleeding, abdominal pain	Colorectal cancer
Cough, dyspnea, hemoptysis	Lung cancer, TB, sarcoidosis, fungal pneumonias, HIV/AIDS
Hematuria	Renal or prostate cancer
Heat intolerance, tremor, anxiety, sweating	Hyperthyroidism
Polydipsia, polyuria	Diabetes
Bone pain (eg, unrelated to activity, prominent at night)	Cancer (eg, multiple myeloma, bone metastases from breast, prostate, or lung cancer)
Headache or visual symptoms and muscle pains in an older adult	Giant cell arteritis
Arthralgias	Endocarditis, giant cell arteritis
Abdominal pain, fatigue, orthostatic light-headedness	Adrenal insufficiency
Abdominal pain	Adrenal insufficiency, diabetes, helminthic infections
Ascites	Alcoholism, nephrotic syndrome
Edema	Chronic kidney disease, nephrotic syndrome
Fever	Cancer, infections, inflammatory disorders
Sleep disturbance, loss of libido, sadness	Depression

have continued to lose weight, the entire history and physical examination should be repeated because patients may share important, previously undisclosed, information, and new, subtle physical abnormalities may then be detected. If weight loss continues and all other findings remain normal, further testing (eg, CT, MRI) should be considered.

Treatment

The underlying disorder is treated. If an underlying disorder causes undernutrition and is difficult to treat, nutritional support should be considered (see p. 14). Helpful general behavioral measures include encouraging patients to eat, assisting them with feeding, offering snacks between meals and before bedtime, providing favorite or strongly flavored foods, and offering only small portions. If behavioral measures are ineffective and weight loss is extreme, enteral tube feeding can be tried if patients have a functioning GI tract. Measures of lean body mass are followed serially. Appetite stimulants have not been shown to prolong life.

Geriatrics Essentials

Normal age-related changes that can contribute to weight loss include the following:

- Decreased sensitivity to certain appetite-stimulating mediators (eg, orexins, ghrelin, neuropeptide Y) and increased sensitivity to certain inhibitory mediators (eg, cholecystokinin, serotonin, corticotropin-releasing factor)
- A decreased rate of gastric-emptying (prolonging satiety)
- Decreased sensitivities of taste and smell
- Loss of muscle mass (sarcopenia)

In the elderly, multiple chronic disorders often contribute to weight loss. Social isolation tends to decrease food intake. Particularly in nursing home patients, depression is a very common contributing factor. It is difficult to sort out the exact contribution of specific factors because of the interactions between factors such as depression, loss of function, drugs, dysphagia, dementia, and social isolation.

When evaluating elderly patients with weight loss, a useful checklist is of potential contributing factors beginning with the letter D:

- Dentition
- Dementia
- Depression
- Diarrhea
- Disorders (eg, severe renal, cardiac, or pulmonary disorders)
- Drugs
- Dysfunction
- Dysgeusia
- Dysphagia

Elderly patients who have lost weight should be evaluated for deficiencies of vitamins D (see p. 50) and B_{12} (see p. 47).

Enteral feeding is rarely beneficial in elderly patients, except for specific patients in whom such feeding may possibly be a short-term bridge to eating normally.

KEY POINTS

- Particularly among nursing home patients, multiple factors commonly contribute to weight loss.
- Involuntary weight loss > 5% of body weight or 5 kg warrants investigation.
- The highest yield aspects of the evaluation are a thorough history and physical examination.
- Advanced imaging or other extensive testing is not usually recommended unless suggested by clinical findings.
- Emphasize behavioral measures that encourage eating and try to avoid enteral feeding, particularly in the elderly.

386 Principles of Radiologic Imaging

Imaging helps with initial diagnosis, staging, and monitoring. Primary care physicians and specialists work with radiologists who specialize in diagnostic imaging to choose the best imaging test; choice is based on the type of lesion suspected and its anatomic location.

Many imaging tests (eg, x-rays, CT, radionuclide scanning) use ionizing radiation and radiographic contrast agents; the associated risks to patients are usually small but should be considered.

RISKS OF MEDICAL RADIATION

Ionizing radiation (see also p. 3090) includes

- High-energy electromagnetic waves (x-rays, gamma rays)
- Particles (alpha particles, beta particles, neutrons)

Ionizing radiation is emitted by radioactive elements and by equipment such as x-ray and radiation therapy machines.

Most diagnostic tests that use ionizing radiation (eg, x-rays, CT, radionuclide scanning) expose patients to relatively low doses of radiation that are generally considered safe. However, all ionizing radiation is potentially harmful, and there is no threshold below which no harmful effect occurs, so every effort is made to minimize radiation exposure.

There are various ways to measure radiation exposure:

- The **absorbed dose** is the amount of radiation absorbed per unit mass. It is expressed in special units of gray (Gy) and milligray (mGy). It was previously expressed as radiation-absorbed dose (rad); 1 mGy = 0.1 rad.
- The **equivalent dose** is the absorbed dose multiplied by a radiation weighting factor that adjusts for tissue effects based on the type of radiation delivered (eg, x-rays, gamma rays, electrons). It is expressed in sieverts (Sv) and millisieverts (mSv). It was previously expressed in roentgen equivalents in man (rem; 1 mSv = 0.1 rem). For x-rays, including CT, the radiation weighting factor is 1.
- The **effective dose** is a measure of cancer risk; it adjusts the equivalent dose based on the susceptibility of the tissue exposed to radiation (eg, gonads are most susceptible). It is expressed in Sv and mSv. The effective dose is higher in young people.

Medical imaging is only one source of exposure to ionizing radiation (see Table 386–1). Another source is environmental background exposure (from cosmic radiation and natural isotopes), which can be significant, particularly at high altitudes; airplane flights result in increased exposure to environmental radiation as follows:

- From a single coast-to-coast airplane flight: 0.01 to .03 mSv
- From average yearly background radiation exposure in the US: About 3 mSv
- From yearly exposure at high altitudes (eg, Denver, Colorado): Possibly > 10 mSv

Radiation may be harmful if the total accumulated dose for a person is high, as when multiple CT scans are done, because CT scans require a higher doses than most other imaging studies.

Radiation exposure is also a concern in certain high-risk situations, as during the following:

- Pregnancy
- Infancy
- Early childhood
- Young adulthood for women who require mammography

In the US, CT accounts for about 15% of all imaging tests but for up to 70% of total radiation delivered during diagnostic imaging. Multidetector CT scanners, which are the type most commonly used in the US, deliver about 40 to 70% more radiation per scan than do older single detector CT scanners. However, recent advances (eg, automated exposure control, iterative reconstruction algorithms, 3rd-generation CT detectors), are likely to significantly lower radiation doses used for CT scans. The American College of Radiology has initiated programs—Image Gently (for children) and Image Wisely (for adults)—to respond to concerns about the surge in exposure to ionizing radiation used in medical imaging. These programs provide resources and information about minimizing radiation exposure

Table 386–1. TYPICAL RADIATION DOSES*

IMAGING TEST	AVERAGE EFFECTIVE RADIATION DOSE (mSv)
X-ray, chest (posteroanterior view)	0.02
X-ray, chest (2 views: posteroanterior and lateral)	0.1
X-ray, lumbar spine series	1.5
X-ray, extremity	0.001–0.01
X-ray, abdomen	0.7
Barium enema	8
Mammogram	0.4
CT, head	2
CT, body (chest, abdomen, or pelvis)	6–8
Coronary angiogram	7
Coronary angiogram with interventions	15
Lung perfusion scan	2.0
PET scan (without whole-body CT)	7
Bone scan	6.3
Hepatobiliary scan	2.1–3.1
Technetium sestimibi heart scan	9.4–12.8

*Doses may vary.

Data from Mettler FA, Huda W, Yoshizumi TT, Mahesh M: Effective doses in radiology and diagnostic nuclear medicine: A catalog. *Radiology* 248:254-263, 2008.

to radiologists, medical physicists, other imaging practitioners, and patients.

Radiation and cancer: Estimated risk of cancer due to radiation exposure in diagnostic imaging has been extrapolated from studies of people exposed to very high radiation doses (eg, survivors of the atomic bomb explosions at Hiroshima and Nagasaki). This analysis suggests a small but real risk of cancer if radiation doses are in the tens of mGy (as used in CT). A CT pulmonary angiogram, routinely done to detect pulmonary embolism, delivers about as much radiation to the breasts as about 10 to 25 two-view mammograms.

Risk is higher in young patients because

- They live longer, giving cancers more time to develop.
- More cellular growth (and thus susceptibility to DNA damage) occurs in the young.

For a 1-yr-old who has a CT scan of the abdomen, estimated lifetime risk of developing cancer is increased by 0.18%. If an elderly patient has this test, risk is lower.

Risk also depends on the tissue being irradiated. Lymphoid tissue, bone marrow, blood, and the testes, ovaries, and intestines are considered very radiosensitve; in adults the CNS and musculoskeletal system are relatively radioresistant.

Radiation during pregnancy: Risks of radiation depend on

- Dose
- Type of test
- Area being examined

The fetus may be exposed to much less radiation than the mother; exposure to the fetus is negligible during x-rays of the following:

- Head
- Cervical spine
- Extremities
- Breasts (mammography) when the uterus is shielded

The extent of uterine exposure depends on gestational age and thus uterine size. The effects of radiation depend on the age of the conceptus (the time from conception).

Recommendations: Diagnostic imaging using ionizing radiation, especially CT, should be done only when clearly required. Alternatives should be considered. For example, in young children, minor head injury can often be diagnosed and treated based on clinical findings, and appendicitis can often be diagnosed by ultrasonography. However, necessary tests should not be withheld, even if the radiation dose is high (eg, as with CT scans), as long as the benefit outweighs the potential risk.

PEARLS & PITFALLS

- During imaging tests that use radiation, shield the uterus in all women of child-bearing age when possible because radiation risks are highest during early (often unrecognized) pregnancy.

Before diagnostic tests are done in women of child-bearing age, pregnancy should be considered, particularly because risks of radiation exposure are highest during early, often unrecognized pregnancy during the 1st trimester. The uterus should be shielded in such women when possible.

RADIOGRAPHIC CONTRAST AGENTS AND CONTRAST REACTIONS

Radiopaque contrast agents are often used in radiography and fluoroscopy to help delineate borders between tissues with similar radiodensity. Most contrast agents are iodine-based.

Iodinated contrast agents may be

- Ionic
- Nonionic

Ionic contrast agents, which are salts, are hyperosmolar to blood. These agents should not be used for myelography or in injections that may enter the spinal canal (because neurotoxicity is a risk) or the bronchial tree (because pulmonary edema is a risk).

Nonionic contrast agents are low-osmolar (but still hyperosmolar relative to blood) or iso-osmolar (with the same osmolarity as blood). Newer nonionic contrast agents are now routinely used at nearly all institutions because they have fewer adverse effects.

The most serious contrast reactions are

- Allergic-type reactions
- Contrast nephropathy (renal damage after intravascular injection of a contrast agent)

Allergic-type contrast reactions: Reactions vary in severity:

- Mild (eg, cough, itching, nasal congestion)
- Moderate (eg, dyspnea, wheezing, slight changes in pulse or BP)
- Severe (eg, respiratory distress, arrhythmias such as bradycardia, seizures, shock, cardiopulmonary arrest)

The mechanism is anaphylactoid (see p. 1378); risk factors include the following:

- A previous reaction to injected contrast agents
- Asthma
- Allergies

Treatment begins by stopping contrast infusion.

For **mild or moderate reactions,** diphenhydramine 25 to 50 mg IV is usually effective.

For **severe reactions,** treatment depends on the type of reaction and may include oxygen, epinephrine, IV fluids, and possibly atropine (for bradycardia).

In patients at high risk of contrast reactions, imaging tests that do not require iodinated contrast should be used. If contrast is necessary, a nonionic agent should be used, and patients should be premedicated with prednisone (50 mg po 13 h, 7 h, and 1 h before injection of contrast) and diphenhydramine (50 mg po or IM 1 h before the injection). If patients require imaging immediately, they can be given diphenhydramine 50 mg po or IM 1 h before injection of contrast and hydrocortisone 200 mg IV q 4 h until imaging is completed.

Contrast nephropathy: In contrast-induced nephropathy, serum creatinine typically begins to increase within 24 h after administration of IV contrast; it peaks between days 3 and 5 and returns to baseline within 7 to 10 days.

Common risk factors include the following:

- Preexisting renal insufficiency (elevated creatinine)
- Diabetes mellitus, especially in patients with associated chronic kidney disease
- Hypertension
- Heart failure
- Multiple myeloma
- Age > 70
- Use of other nephrotoxic drugs
- Dehydration

In patients at risk of acute kidney injury after receiving iodinated intravascular contrast, the following measures should be considered:

- A reduced dose of contrast
- Use of an iso-osmolar agent
- Hydration

Many hydration regimens exist; one example is IV administration of 0.9% normal saline at 1 mL/kg for 24 h beginning a few hours before the procedure.

Acetylcysteine may be given as premedication for patients at risk of developing nephrotoxicity, but its efficacy is uncertain. Oral antihyperglycemic drugs, such as metformin, should be withheld for 48 h after IV contrast administration to avoid drug accumulation if contrast-induced nephrotoxicity occurs.

Because many protocols dealing with contrast agents and reactions are specific and continually updated, it is important to discuss such details with the imaging department.

ANGIOGRAPHY

Angiography is sometimes called conventional angiography to distinguish it from CT angiography (CTA—see p. 3224) and magnetic resonance angiography (MRA—see p. 3225). Angiography provides detailed images of blood vessels, commonly those in the heart, lungs, brain, and legs. Angiography can provide still images or motion pictures (called cineangiography).

IV contrast is injected through a catheter inserted into a blood vessel that connects with the vessel to be imaged. A local anesthetic or a sedative may be used. If the catheter is inserted into an artery, the insertion site must be steadily compressed for 10 to 20 min after all instruments are removed to reduce the risk of bleeding at the puncture site. Patients may also need to lie flat for several hours or be hospitalized to reduce this risk.

Angiography, although invasive, is relatively safe.

Uses of Angiography

CTA and MRA are often done instead of conventional angiography. However, conventional angiography is the traditional gold standard for evaluating vascular lesions (eg, stenosis, obstruction, arteriovenous or other vascular malformations, aneurysms, dissections, vasculitis).

Common uses of conventional angiography include the following:

- **Coronary angiography** is usually done before percutaneous or surgical interventions involving the coronary arteries or heart valves. It is usually done with cardiac catheterization (see p. 606).
- **Cerebral angiography** may be indicated after stroke or transient ischemic attack (TIA)—eg, if stenting or carotid endarterectomy is being considered.
- **Iliac and femoral angiography** may be indicated before interventions to treat peripheral arterial disease.
- **Aortography** is sometimes done to diagnose and provide anatomic detail about aortic aneurysms, aortic dissection, and aortic regurgitation.
- **Angiography of the eye arteries** can be done using fluorescein dye.

Conventional pulmonary angiography used to be the gold standard for diagnosis of pulmonary embolism; now, it has largely been replaced by CT pulmonary angiography [CTPA], which is less invasive.

Conventional angiography is usually done before therapeutic angiographic procedures such as angioplasty, vascular stenting, and embolization of tumors and vascular malformations.

Variations of Angiography

Digital subtraction angiography: Images of blood vessels are taken before and after contrast injection; then a computer subtracts the precontrast image from the postcontrast image. Images of extraneous structures are thus eliminated, isolating images of the blood vessel lumens opacified by contrast.

Disadvantages of Angiography

Contrast reactions occasionally occur (see p. 3222).

The injection site may bleed if the injected blood vessel ruptures; a painful hematoma can form. Rarely, the site becomes infected; it becomes red and swollen and exudes a purulent discharge within a few days after the injection.

Rarely, an artery is injured by the catheter, or an atherosclerotic plaque dislodges, causing an embolism distally. Very rarely, shock, seizures, renal failure, and cardiac arrest occur.

Risk of complications is higher in the elderly, although it is still low.

The radiation dose used in angiography can vary and be significant (eg, coronary angiography is associated with an effective radiation dose of 4.6 to 15.8 mSv).

Angiography must be done by highly skilled physicians, usually specially trained interventional radiologists or cardiologists.

COMPUTED TOMOGRAPHY

In CT, an x-ray source and x-ray detector housed in a doughnut-shaped assembly move circularly around a patient who lies on a motorized table that is moved through the machine. Usually, multidetector scanners with 4 to 64 or more rows of detectors are used because more detectors allow quicker scanning and higher-resolution images, which are particularly important for imaging the heart and abdominal organs.

Data from the detectors essentially represent a series of x-ray images taken from multiple angles all around the patient. The images are not viewed directly but are sent to a computer, which quickly reconstructs them into 2-dimensional images (tomograms) representing a slice of the body in any plane desired. Data can also be used to construct detailed 3-dimensional images.

For some CT scans, the table moves incrementally and stops when each scan (slice) is taken. For other CT scans, the table moves continuously during scanning; because the patient is moving in a straight line and the detectors are moving in a circle, the series of images appear to be taken in a spiral fashion around the patient—hence the term helical (spiral) CT.

These same principles of tomographic imaging can also be applied to radionuclide scanning, in which the sensors for emitted radiation encircle the patient and computer techniques convert the sensor data into tomographic images; examples include single-photon emission CT (SPECT—see p. 3227) and positron-emission tomography (PET—see p. 3228).

Uses of CT

CT provides better differentiation between various soft-tissue densities than do x-rays. Because CT provides so much more information, it is preferred to conventional x-rays for imaging most intracranial, head and neck, spinal, intrathoracic, and intra-abdominal structures. Three-dimensional images of lesions can help surgeons plan surgery.

CT is the most accurate study for detecting and localizing urinary calculi.

CT may be done with or without IV contrast.

Noncontrast CT is used

- To detect acute hemorrhage in the brain, urinary calculi, and lung nodules
- To characterize bone fractures and other skeletal abnormalities

IV contrast is used

- To improve imaging of tumors, infection, inflammation, and trauma in soft tissues
- To assess the vascular system, as when pulmonary embolism, aortic aneurysm, or aortic dissection is suspected

Oral or occasionally rectal contrast is used for abdominal imaging; sometimes gas is used to distend the lower GI tract and make it visible. Contrast in the GI tract helps distinguish the GI tract from surrounding structures. Standard oral contrast is barium-based, but low-osmolar iodinated contrast should be used when intestinal perforation is suspected.

Variations of CT

Virtual colonoscopy and CT enterography: For **virtual (CT) colonoscopy** (CT colonography), oral contrast is given, and air is introduced into the rectum via a flexible, thin-diameter rubber catheter; then thin-section CT of the entire colon is done. CT colonoscopy produces high-resolution 3-dimensional images of the colon that closely simulate the detail and appearance of optical colonoscopy. This technique can show colon polyps and colon mucosal lesions as small as 5 mm. It is an alternative to conventional colonoscopy. Virtual colonoscopy is more comfortable than conventional colonoscopy and does not require conscious sedation. It provides clearer, more detailed images than a conventional lower GI series and can show extrinsic soft-tissue masses. The entire colon is visualized during virtual colonoscopy; in contrast, in about 1 in 10 patients, conventional colonoscopy does not allow the right colon to be evaluated completely.

The main disadvantages of virtual colonoscopy include

- The inability to biopsy the polyps at the time of examination
- Radiation exposure

CT enterography is similar, but it provides images of the stomach and entire small intestine. A large volume of low-density oral contrast agent (eg, 1300 to 2100 mL of 0.1% barium sulfate) is given to distend the entire small intestine; use of neutral or low-density contrast helps show detail of intestinal mucosa that might be obscured by use of contrast that is more radiopaque.

Thus, the unique advantage of CT enterography is in

- Identifying inflammatory bowel disease

CT enterography often involves using IV contrast. Thin-slice high-resolution CT images of the entire abdomen and pelvis are obtained. These images are reconstructed in multiple anatomic planes, forming 3-dimensional reconstructions.

CT enterography can also be used to detect and evaluate disorders other than inflammatory bowel disease, including the following:

- Lesions obstructing the small intestine
- Tumors
- Abscesses
- Fistulas
- Bleeding sources

CT IV pyelography (CT IVP) or urography: IV contrast is injected to produce detailed images of the kidneys, ureters, and bladder. IV contrast concentrates in the kidneys and is excreted into the renal-collecting structures, ureters, and bladder. Multiple CT images are obtained, producing high-resolution images of the urinary tract during maximal contrast opacification.

CT urography has replaced conventional IV urography in most institutions.

CT angiography: After a rapid bolus injection of IV contrast, thin-slice images are rapidly taken as the contrast opacifies arteries and veins. Advanced computer graphics techniques are used to remove images of surrounding soft tissues and to provide highly detailed images of blood vessels similar to those of conventional angiography.

CTA is a safer, less invasive alternative to conventional angiography.

Disadvantages of CT

CT accounts for most diagnostic radiation exposure to patients collectively. If multiple scans are done, the total radiation dose may be relatively high, placing the patient at potential risk (see p. 3221). Patients who have recurrent urinary tract stones or who have had major trauma are most likely to have multiple CT scans. The risk of radiation exposure vs benefit of the examination must always be considered because the effective radiation dose of one abdomen CT is equal to 500 chest x-rays.

Current practice dictates that CT scanning use the lowest radiation dose possible. Modern CT scanners and revised imaging protocols have dramatically lowered radiation exposure from CT. The American College of Radiology has initiated effective programs to limit radiation dose from CT: Image Wisely for adults and Image Gently initiative for children. Also, newer, investigational methods are evaluating the use of even much lower radiation doses for certain CT scans and certain indications; in some cases, these doses would be comparable to the radiation delivered by x-rays.

Some CT scans use IV contrast, which has certain risks (see p. 3222). However, oral and rectal contrast also has risks, such as the following:

- If barium, given orally or rectally, extravasates outside the GI tract lumen, it can induce severe inflammation in the peritoneal cavity. Iodinated oral contrast agents are used if there is a risk of intestinal perforation.
- Aspiration of iodinated contrast agents can induce severe chemical pneumonitis.
- Barium retained in the intestinal tract can become hard and inspissated, potentially causing intestinal obstruction.

MAGNETIC RESONANCE IMAGING

MRI uses magnetic fields and radio waves to produce images of thin slices of tissues (tomographic images). Normally, protons within tissues spin to produce tiny magnetic fields that are randomly aligned. When surrounded by the strong magnetic field of an MRI device, the magnetic axes align along that field. A radiofrequency pulse is then applied, causing the axes of many protons to momentarily align against the field in a high-energy state. After the pulse, protons relax and resume their baseline alignment within the magnetic field of the MRI device. The magnitude and rate of energy release that occurs as the protons resume this alignment (T1 relaxation) and as they wobble (precess) during the process (T2 relaxation) are recorded as spatially localized signal intensities by a coil (antenna) built within the MRI device. Computer algorithms analyze these signals and produce detailed anatomic images.

The relative signal intensity (brightness) of tissues in an MRI image is determined by factors such as

- The radiofrequency pulse and gradient waveforms used to obtain the image
- Intrinsic T1 and T2 characteristics of different tissues
- The proton density of different tissues

By controlling the radiofrequency pulse and gradient waveforms, computer programs produce specific pulse sequences that determine how an image is obtained (weighted) and how various tissues appear. Images can be

- T1-weighted
- T2-weighted
- Proton density–weighted

For example, fat appears bright (high signal intensity) on T1-weighted images and relatively dark (low signal intensity) on T2-weighted images; water and fluids appear relatively dark on T1-weighted images and bright on T2-weighted images. T1-weighted images optimally show normal soft-tissue anatomy and fat (eg, to confirm a fat-containing mass). T2-weighted images optimally show fluid and abnormalities (eg, tumors, inflammation, trauma). In practice, T1- and T2-weighted images provide complementary information, so both are important for characterizing abnormalities.

Recently introduced high-resolution MRI scanners increase image quality and diagnostic accuracy.

Uses of MRI

MRI is preferred to CT when soft-tissue contrast resolution must be highly detailed (eg, to evaluate intracranial or spinal cord abnormalities, inflammation, trauma, suspected musculoskeletal tumors, or internal joint derangement). MRI is also useful for the following:

- **Vascular imaging:** Magnetic resonance angiography (MRA) is used to image arteries with good diagnostic accuracy and is less invasive than conventional angiography. Gadolinium contrast is sometimes used. MRA can be used to image the thoracic and abdominal aorta and arteries of the brain, neck, abdominal organs, kidneys, and lower extremities. Venous imaging (magnetic resonance venography, or MRV) provides the best images of venous abnormalities, including thrombosis and anomalies.
- **Hepatic and biliary tract abnormalities:** Magnetic resonance cholangiopancreatography (MRCP) is particularly valuable as a noninvasive, highly accurate method of imaging the biliary and pancreatic duct systems.
- **Masses in the female reproductive organs:** MRI supplements ultrasonography to further characterize adnexal masses and to stage uterine tumors.
- **Certain fractures:** For example, MRI can provide accurate images of hip fractures in patients with osteopenia.
- **Bone marrow infiltration and bone metastases**

MRI can also be substituted for CT with contrast in patients with a high risk of reactions to iodinated contrast agents.

Contrast: With MRI, contrast agents are often used to highlight vascular structures and to help characterize inflammation and tumors.

The most commonly used agents are gadolinium derivatives, which have magnetic properties that affect proton relaxation times. MRI of intra-articular structures may include injection of a diluted gadolinium derivative into a joint.

Variations of MRI

Diffusion (diffusion-weighted) MRI: Signal intensities are related to diffusion of water molecules in tissue. This type of MRI can be used

- To detect early cerebral ischemia and infarction
- To detect white matter disease of the brain
- To stage various tumors such as non–small cell lung cancer

Echo planar imaging: This ultrafast technique (images obtained in > 1 sec) is used for diffusion, perfusion, and functional imaging of the brain and heart. Its potential advantages include showing brain and heart activity and reducing motion artifacts. However, its use is limited because it requires special technical hardware and is more sensitive to various artifacts than conventional MRI.

Functional MRI: Functional MRI is used to assess brain activity by location.

In the most common type, the brain is scanned at low resolution very frequently (eg, every 2 to 3 sec). The change in oxygenated Hb can be discerned and used to estimate metabolic activity of different parts of the brain.

Researchers sometimes do functional MRI while subjects do different cognitive tasks (eg, solve a math equation); the metabolically active parts of the brain are presumed to be the structures most involved in that particular task. Correlating brain function and anatomy this way is called brain mapping.

Functional MRI is used primarily in research but is being increasingly used clinically.

Gradient echo imaging: Gradient echo is a pulse sequence that can be used for fast imaging of moving blood and CSF (eg, in MRA). Because this technique is fast, it can reduce motion artifacts (eg, blurring) during imaging that requires patients to hold their breath (eg, during imaging of cardiac. pulmonary, and abdominal structures).

Magnetic resonance spectroscopy (MRS): MRS combines the information obtained by MRI (mainly based on water and fat content of tissues) with that of nuclear magnetic resonance (NMR). NMR provides information about tissue metabolites and biochemical abnormalities; this information can help differentiate certain types of tumors and other abnormalities.

Magnetic resonance enterography: Magnetic resonance enterography has become popular, especially for follow-up imaging of children with known inflammatory conditions of the small bowel.

Because magnetic resonance enterography does not require ionizing radiation, it has an advantage over CT enterography.

Perfusion MRI: Perfusion MRI is a method of assessing relative cerebral blood flow. It can be used to detect

- Areas of ischemia during imaging for stroke
- Areas of increased vascularity that can indicate tumors

This information can help direct biopsy.

PET MRI: PET MRI combines functional PET (see p. 3228) with whole-body MRI. T1-weighted and short T1 inversion recovery (STIR) sequences are frequently used. This method is new and is available in only a few major medical centers.

Disadvantages of MRI

MRI is relatively expensive, requires longer imaging times than CT and may not be immediately available in all areas.

Other disadvantages include problems related to

- The magnetic field
- Patient claustrophobia
- Contrast reactions

Magnetic field: MRI is relatively contraindicated in patients with implanted materials that can be affected by powerful magnetic fields. These materials include

- Ferromagnetic metal (ie, containing iron)
- Magnetically activated or electronically controlled medical devices (eg, pacemakers, implantable cardioverter defibrillators, cochlear implants)
- Nonferromagnetic electrical wires or materials (eg, pacemaker wires, certain pulmonary artery catheters)

Ferromagnetic material may be displaced by the strong magnetic field, injuring a nearby organ; for example, displacement of vascular clips can result in hemorrhage. Displacement is more likely if the material has been in place < 6 wk (before scar tissue forms). Ferromagnetic material can also cause imaging artifacts.

Magnetically activated medical devices may malfunction when exposed to magnetic fields.

Magnetic fields may induce current in any conductive materials strong enough to produce enough heat to burn tissues.

Whether a specific device is compatible with MRI depends on the type of device, its components, and its manufacturer (see the MRI safety web site). Patients with an implantable device should not be placed in the MRI magnetic field until practitioners are sure that MRI is safe with such a device in place. Also, MRI machines with different magnetic field strengths have different effects on materials, so safety in one machine does not ensure safety in another.

The MRI magnetic field is very strong and may always be on. Thus, a ferromagnetic object (eg, an O_2 tank, a metal pole) at the entrance of the scanning room may be pulled into the magnet bore at high velocity and injure anyone in its path. The only way to separate the object from the magnet may be to turn off (quench) the magnetic field.

Claustrophobia: The imaging tube of an MRI machine is a tight, enclosed space that can trigger claustrophobia even in patients without preexisting phobias or anxiety. Also, some obese patients do not fit on the table or within the machine. Premedication with an anxiolytic (eg, alprazolam or lorazepam 1 to 2 mg po) 15 to 30 min before scanning is effective for most anxious patients.

MRI scanners with an open side can be used for patients with claustrophobia (or those who are very obese). Images obtained during open MRI may be inferior to those of enclosed scanners depending on the field strength of the magnet, but they are usually sufficient for making a diagnosis.

Patients should be warned that the MRI machine makes loud, banging noises during scanning.

Contrast reactions: Gadolinium-based contrast agents injected IV can cause headache, nausea, pain, and distortion of taste, as well as sensation of cold at the injection site.

Serious contrast reactions are rare and much less common than with iodinated contrast agents.

However, **nephrogenic systemic fibrosis** is a risk in patients with impaired renal function. Nephrogenic systemic fibrosis is a rare but life-threatening disorder that involves fibrosis of the skin, blood vessels, and internal organs, resulting in severe disability or death. For patients with impaired renal function, the risks and benefits of contrast MRI should be weighed; in addition the following is recommended:

- Use gadolinium only when necessary and at the lowest dose possible.
- Check renal function if diabetes, dehydration, or heart failure is clinically suspected, if patients are taking certain drugs that can cause renal insufficiency, or if patients are elderly. (Patients who have a GFR of < 30 mL/min/1.73 m^2 should not be given gadolinium contrast agents. If GFR is between 30 and 60 mL/min/1.73m^2, patients can be hydrated IV before contrast administration.
- Consider alternative imaging methods.

CONVENTIONAL RADIOGRAPHY

Conventional radiography involves the use of x-rays; the term "plain x-rays" is sometimes used to distinguish x-rays used alone from x-rays combined with other techniques (eg, CT).

For conventional radiography, an x-ray beam is generated and passed through a patient to a piece of film or a radiation detector, producing an image. Different soft tissues attenuate x-ray photons differently, depending on tissue density; the denser the tissue, the whiter (more radiopaque) the image. The range of densities, from most to least dense, is represented by metal (white, or radiopaque), bone cortex (less white), muscle and fluid (gray), fat (darker gray), and air or gas (black, or radiolucent).

Uses of Conventional Radiography

Radiography is the most readily available imaging method. Typically, it is the first imaging method indicated to evaluate the extremities, chest, and sometimes the spine and abdomen. These areas contain important structures with densities that differ from those of adjacent tissues. For example, radiography is a first-line test for detecting the following:

- **Fractures:** White bone is well seen because it is adjacent to gray soft tissues.
- **Pneumonia:** Inflammatory exudate that fills the lungs is well seen because it contrasts with adjacent, more radiolucent air spaces.
- **Intestinal obstruction:** Dilated, air-filled loops of intestine are well seen amidst the surrounding soft tissue.

Variations of Conventional Radiography

Contrast studies: When the density of adjacent tissues is similar, a radiopaque contrast agent (see p. 3222) is often added to one tissue or structure to differentiate it from its surroundings. Structures typically requiring a contrast agent include blood vessels (for angiography) and the lumina of the GI, biliary, and GU tracts. Gas may be used to distend the lower GI tract and make it visible.

Other imaging tests (eg, CT, MRI) have largely replaced contrast studies because their tomographic images provide better anatomic localization of an abnormality. Endoscopic procedures have largely replaced barium contrast studies of the esophagus, stomach, and upper intestinal tract.

Fluoroscopy: A continuous x-ray beam is used to produce real-time images of moving structures or objects. Fluoroscopy is most often used

- With contrast agents (eg, in swallowing studies or coronary artery catheterization)
- During medical procedures to guide placement of a lead, catheter, or needle (eg, in electrophysiologic testing or percutaneous coronary interventions)

Fluoroscopy can also be used in real time to detect motion of the diaphragm and of bones and joints (eg, to assess the stability of musculoskeletal injuries).

Disadvantages of Conventional Radiography

Diagnostic accuracy is limited in many situations. Other imaging tests may have advantages, such as providing better detail or being safer or faster.

Contrast agents such as barium and gastrografin, if used, have disadvantages (see p. 3224), and IV contrast agents have risks (see p. 3222).

Fluoroscopy may involve high doses of radiation (see p. 3221).

MAMMOGRAPHY

Mammograms are breast x-rays, which usually include ≥ 2 views of each breast taken at different angles. The breasts are compressed with plastic paddles to optimize visualization of breast tissue and abnormalities.

Screening mammograms are used to check for breast cancer in asymptomatic women (see also p. 2219).

Diagnostic mammograms are used to diagnose breast disorders in women who have

- Breast symptoms
- Palpable breast masses
- Abnormal results on screening mammograms that require further investigation

Diagnostic mammograms can include standard and specialized views.

Typically, mammography exposes the breasts to about 0.4 mSv of radiation. This dose is relatively low compared with other imaging tests that use radiation (see Table 386–1). However, radiation exposure is a concern with mammography because breast tissue is sensitive to radiation (see p. 3221). Mammography is sometimes recommended only for women > 40 partly because breast tissue in older women is less sensitive to the adverse effects of radiation. Specialized mammography units and digital imaging techniques are used to minimize radiation exposure.

Variations of mammography: Tomosynthesis, a 3-dimensional technique, can be used in mammography. In tomosynthesis, an x-ray source moves over an arc of excursion, providing thin, tomographic slices, which are reconstructed into 3-dimensional images. This technique minimizes the effect of overlapping structures in the breast. Thus, abnormalities can be better separated from the background. As a result, the need for repeat mammograms may be reduced, and clinicians may be able to detect cancers more accurately, especially in patients with dense breasts.

The total radiation dose used in 3-dimensional mammography (1.0 mSv) is higher than that used in conventional mammography (0.5 mSv). although it is relatively low, compared with some other imaging tests.

RADIONUCLIDE SCANNING

Radionuclide scanning uses the radiation released by radionuclides (called nuclear decay) to produce images. A radionuclide is an unstable isotope that becomes more stable by releasing energy as radiation. This radiation can include gamma-ray photons or particulate emission (such as positrons, used in PET).

Radiation produced by radionuclides may be used for imaging or for treatment of certain disorders (eg, thyroid disorders).

A radionuclide, usually technetium-99m, is combined with different stable, metabolically active compounds to form a radiopharmaceutical that localizes to a particular anatomic or diseased structure (target tissue). The radiopharmaceutical is given by mouth or by injection. After the radionuclide has had time to reach the target tissue, images are taken with a gamma camera. Gamma rays emitted by the radionuclide interact with scintillation crystals in the camera, creating light photons that are converted into electrical signals by photomultiplier tubes. A computer summarizes and analyzes the signals and integrates them into 2-dimensional images. However, only signals near the camera's face can be accurately analyzed; thus, imaging is limited by the thickness of the tissue and the range of the camera.

Portable gamma cameras can provide radionuclide imaging at bedside.

Generally, radionuclide scanning is considered safe; it uses a relatively low dose of radiation and provides valuable information (eg, it enables clinicians to image the entire skeleton when they suspect cancer has metastasized to bone.

Uses of Radionuclide Scanning

The compound labeled with the radionuclide depends on the target tissue or indication:

- For imaging the skeleton, technetium-99m is combined with diphosphonate and used to check for bone metastasis or infection.
- For identifying inflammation, WBCs are labeled and used to identify focal inflammation.
- For localizing GI bleeding, RBCs are labeled to determine whether they have been extravasated from blood vessels.
- For imaging the liver, spleen, or bone marrow, sulfur colloid is labeled.
- For imaging the biliary tract, iminodiacetic acid derivatives are labeled and used to check for biliary obstruction, bile leaks, and gallbladder disorders.

Radionuclide scanning is also used to image the thyroid gland and the cerebrovascular, cardiovascular, respiratory, and GU systems. For example, in myocardial perfusion imaging, heart tissue takes up radionuclides (eg, thallium) in proportion to perfusion. This technique can be combined with stress testing.

Radionuclide scanning is also used to evaluate tumors.

Variations of Radionuclide Scanning

Single-photon emission CT (SPECT): SPECT uses a gamma camera that rotates around the patient. The resultant series of images are reconstructed by computer into 2-dimensional tomographic slices in a similar manner to that done in conventional CT. The 2-dimensional images can be used for tomographic reconstruction to yield 3-dimensional images.

Disadvantages of Radionuclide Scanning

Radiation exposure depends on the radionuclide and dose used. Effective doses tend to range from 1.5 to 17 mSv, as in the following:

- For lung scans: About 1.5 mSv
- For bone and hepatobiliary scans: About 3.5 to 4.5 mSv
- For technetium sestimibi heart scans: About 17 mSv

Reactions to radionuclides are rare.

The area that can be imaged accurately is limited because only signals near the gamma camera's face can be accurately localized. Image detail may also be limited.

Often, imaging must be delayed for up to several hours to give the radionuclide time to reach the target tissue.

POSITRON EMISSION TOMOGRAPHY

Positron emission tomography (PET), a type of radionuclide scanning, uses compounds containing radionuclides that decay by releasing a positron (the positively charged antimatter equivalent of an electron). The released positron combines with an electron and produces 2 photons whose paths are 180° apart. Ring detector systems encircling the positron-emitting source simultaneously detect the 2 photons to localize the source and to produce color tomographic images of the area. Because PET incorporates positron-emitting radionuclides into metabolically active compounds, it can provide information about tissue function. Standard uptake value (SUV) indicates metabolic activity of a lesion; typically intensity of color is increased with higher SUVs.

The most commonly used compound in clinical PET is

- Fluorine-18 [^{18}F]–labeled deoxyglucose (FDG)

FDG is an analog of glucose, and its uptake is proportional to glucose metabolic rates. A patient's relative glucose metabolic rate (SUV) is calculated: The amount of FDG taken up from the injected dose is divided by the patient's body weight.

Uses of PET

PET has several clinical indications, such as

- Cancer (eg, staging and evaluating specific types of cancer and evaluating response to treatment), which accounts for about 80% of PET usage
- Cardiac function (eg, evaluating myocardial viability, detecting hibernating myocardium)
- Neurologic function (eg, evaluation of dementia and seizures)

PET applications continue to be investigated. Not all applications are reimbursable in the US.

Variations

PET-CT: Functional information provided by PET is superimposed on anatomic information provided by CT.

Disadvantages of PET

The typical effective radiation dose during PET is about 7 mSv. The effective radiation dose with PET-CT is 5 to 18 mSv.

Production of FDG requires a cyclotron. FDG has a short half-life (110 min); thus, shipment from the manufacturer and completion of the scan must occur very rapidly. The resulting expense, inconvenience, and impracticality greatly limit the availability of PET.

ULTRASONOGRAPHY

In ultrasonography, a signal generator is combined with a transducer. Piezoelectric crystals in the signal generator convert electricity into high-frequency sound waves, which are sent into tissues. The tissues scatter, reflect, and absorb the sound waves to various degrees. The sound waves that are reflected back (echoes) are converted into electric signals. A computer analyzes the signals and displays an anatomic image on a screen.

Ultrasonography is portable, widely available, relatively inexpensive, and safe. No radiation is used.

Uses of Ultrasonography

Ultrasonography can identify superficial growths and foreign bodies (eg, in the thyroid gland, breasts, testes, limbs, and some lymph nodes). With deeper structures, other tissues and densities (eg, bone, gas) can interfere with images.

Ultrasonography is commonly used to evaluate the following:

- **Heart (echocardiography):** For example, to detect valvular and chamber size abnormalities and to estimate ejection fraction and myocardial strain (see p. 610)
- **Gallbladder and biliary tract:** For example, to detect gallstones and biliary tract obstruction (see p. 199)
- **Urinary tract:** For example, to distinguish cysts (usually benign) from solid masses (often malignant) in the kidneys or to detect obstruction such as calculi or other structural abnormalities in the kidneys, ureters, or bladder (see p. 2074)
- **Female reproductive organs:** For example, to detect tumors and inflammation in the ovaries, fallopian tubes, or uterus (see p. 2201)
- **Pregnancy:** For example, to evaluate the growth and development of the fetus and to detect abnormalities of the placenta (eg, placenta previa—see p. 2322).
- **Musculoskeletal:** To evaluate muscles, tendons, and nerves.

Ultrasonography can also be used to guide biopsy sampling.

Ultrasonography is sometimes done internally, using a small transducer on the tip of an endoscope or vascular catheter.

Variations of Ultrasonography

Ultrasound information can be displayed in several ways.

A-mode: This display mode is the simplest; signals are recorded as spikes on a graph. The vertical (Y) axis of the display shows the echo amplitude, and the horizontal (X) axis shows depth or distance into the patient.

This type of ultrasonography is used for ophthalmologic scanning.

B-mode (gray-scale): This mode is most often used in diagnostic imaging; signals are displayed as a 2-dimensional anatomic image.

B-mode is commonly used to evaluate the developing fetus and to evaluate organs, including the liver, spleen, kidneys, thyroid gland, testes, breasts, uterus, ovaries, and prostate gland.

B-mode ultrasonography is fast enough to show real-time motion, such as the motion of the beating heart or pulsating blood vessels. Real-time imaging provides anatomic and functional information.

M-mode: This mode is used to image moving structures; signals reflected by the moving structures are converted into waves that are displayed continuously across a vertical axis.

M-mode is used primarily for assessment of fetal heartbeat and, in cardiac imaging, most notably to evaluate valvular disorders.

Doppler: This type of ultrasonography is used to assess blood flow. Doppler ultrasonography uses the Doppler effect (alteration of sound frequency by reflection off a moving object). The moving objects are RBCs in blood.

Direction and velocity of blood flow can be determined by analyzing changes in the frequency of sound waves:

- If a reflected sound wave is lower in frequency than the transmitted sound wave, blood flow is away from the transducer.

- If a reflected sound wave is higher in frequency than the transmitted sound wave, blood flow is toward the transducer.
- The magnitude of the change in frequency is proportional to blood flow velocity.

Changes in frequency of the reflected sound waves are converted into images showing blood flow direction and velocity.

Doppler ultrasonography is also used

- To evaluate vascularity of tumors and organs
- To evaluate heart function (eg, as for echocardiography)
- To detect occlusion and stenosis of blood vessels
- To detect blood clots in blood vessels (eg, in deep venous thrombosis)

Spectral Doppler ultrasonography displays blood flow information as a graph with velocity on the vertical axis and time on the horizontal axis. Specific velocities can be measured if the Doppler angle (the angle between the direction of the ultrasound beam and the direction of blood flow) can be determined. Velocity measurements and the appearance of the spectral Doppler tracing can indicate the severity of vascular stenoses.

Duplex Doppler ultrasonography combines the graphic display of spectral ultrasonography with the images of B-mode.

Color Doppler ultrasonography converts the Doppler blood flow information into a color image with blood flow in color; it is displayed on a gray-scale anatomic ultrasound image. Direction of blood flow is indicated by the shade of color (eg, red for blood flow toward the transducer, blue for blood flow away from the transducer). Average blood flow velocity is indicated by the brightness of the color (eg, bright red indicates high-velocity flow toward the transducer; dark blue indicates low-velocity flow away from the transducer).

Disadvantages of Ultrasonography

Quality of images depends on the skills of the operator.

Obtaining clear images of the target structures can be technically difficult in overweight patients.

Ultrasonography cannot be used to image through bone or gas, so certain images may be difficult to obtain.

387 Recreational Drugs and Intoxicants

BODY PACKING AND BODY STUFFING

Body packing and body stuffing involve swallowing drug-filled packets or placing them in body cavities to evade detection by law enforcement. The risks and consequences vary depending on the amount and type of drug and the way it is packaged.

Body packing: Body packing often involves drugs with a high street value (primarily heroin or cocaine) and is done to smuggle drugs across borders or other security checkpoints. The drugs may be placed in condoms or in packets enclosed by several layers of polyethylene or latex and sometimes covered with an outer layer of wax. After body packers ("mules") swallow multiple packets, they typically take antimotility drugs to decrease intestinal motility until the packets can be retrieved. The total amount of drug involved represents a supra-lethal dose. Rupture of one or more packets is a risk, resulting in abrupt toxicity and overdose.

Specific symptoms depend on the drug, but intractable seizures, tachycardia, hypertension, and hyperthermia are common with cocaine. Coma and respiratory depression are common with heroin. Intestinal obstruction or rupture and peritonitis are also risks.

Body stuffing: Body stuffing is similar to body packing; it occurs when people about to be apprehended by law enforcement swallow drug packets to avoid detection. Sometimes packets are placed in the rectum or vagina. Body stuffing usually involves much smaller amounts of drugs than does body packing, but the drugs are usually less securely wrapped, so overdose is still a concern.

Diagnosis

- Known history and clinical suspicion
- Pelvic and/or digital rectal examination
- Sometimes plain x-ray

Suspected body packers and stuffers are usually brought to medical attention by law enforcement officials, but clinicians should consider body packing if recent travelers and newly incarcerated people present with coma or seizures of unknown etiology. Pelvic examination and digital rectal examination should be done to check those areas for drug packets. Plain x-rays can often confirm the presence of packets in the GI tract.

Treatment

- Supportive treatment for complications
- Sometimes measures to remove drug packets

Treatment of patients with symptoms of overdose (and presumed packet rupture) is supportive and includes airway protection, respiratory and circulatory support, and anticonvulsants, depending on patient symptoms. Sometimes, specific antidotes are indicated (see under specific drugs).

Usually, unruptured packets in the GI tract can be removed by whole-bowel irrigation. However, once packets rupture, immediate surgical or endoscopic removal (depending on location in the GI tract) of all packets is indicated but can rarely be done in time; death commonly occurs because the quantity of drug released is large. Patients with intestinal obstruction or perforation also need immediate surgery. Activated charcoal may be helpful but is contraindicated in patients with obstruction or perforation.

Vaginal and rectal packets should be removed manually.

Asymptomatic body packers (and stuffers who have swallowed drug packets) should be observed for development of symptoms until the packets are passed and followed by several packet-free stools. Some clinicians use whole-bowel irrigation with a polyethylene glycol solution with or without metoclopramide as a promotility agent. Emergency endoscopy is not indicated for asymptomatic patients.

DRUG TESTING

Drug testing is done primarily to screen people systematically or randomly for evidence of use of one or more substances with potential for abuse. Testing is done in the following:

- Certain groups of people, commonly including students, athletes, and prisoners
- People who are applying for or who already hold certain types of jobs (eg, pilots, commercial truck drivers)
- People who have been involved in motor vehicle or boating accidents or accidents at work
- People who have attempted suicide by unclear means
- People in a court-ordered treatment program or with terms of probation or parole requiring abstinence (to monitor adherence)
- People in a substance abuse treatment program (as a standard feature, to obtain objective evidence about substance abuse and thus optimize treatment)
- People required to participate in a drug testing program as part of custody or parental rights
- Members of the military

Notification or consent may be a requirement before testing, depending on jurisdiction and circumstances. Mere documentation of use may be sufficient for legal purposes; however, testing cannot determine frequency and intensity of substance use and thus cannot distinguish casual users from those with more serious problems. Also, drug testing targets only a limited number of substances and thus does not identify many others. The clinician must use other measures (eg, history, questionnaires) to identify the degree to which substance use has affected each patient's life.

The substances most commonly tested for are

- Alcohol
- Amphetamines
- Cocaine
- Marijuana
- Natural and semisynthetic opioids
- Phencyclidine

Testing for benzodiazepines and barbiturates may also be done. Urine, blood, breath, saliva, sweat, or hair samples may be used. Urine testing is most common because it is noninvasive, quick, and able to qualitatively detect a wide range of drugs. The window of detection depends on the frequency and amount of drug intake but is about 1 to 4 days for most drugs. Because cannabinoid metabolites persist, urine tests for marijuana can remain positive longer after use is stopped. Blood testing can be used to quantify levels of certain drugs but is less commonly done because it is invasive and the window of detection for many drugs is much shorter, often only hours. Hair analysis is not as widely available but provides the longest window of detection, ≥ 100 days for some drugs.

Validity of testing depends on the type of test done. Screening tests are typically rapid qualitative urine immunoassays. Such screening tests are associated with a number of false-positive and false-negative results, and they do not detect the opioids meperidine and fentanyl. Also, lysergic acid diethylamide (LSD), gamma hydroxybutyrate (GHB), mescaline, and inhaled hydrocarbons are not detected on readily available screens. Confirmatory tests, which may require several hours, typically use gas chromatography or mass spectroscopy.

False results: Several factors can produce false-negative results, particularly in urine testing. Patients may submit samples provided by others (presumably drug-free). This possibility can be eliminated by directly observing sample collection and by sealing samples immediately with tamper-evident seals. Some people attempt to defeat urine drug testing by drinking large quantities of fluids or by taking diuretics before the test; however, samples that appear too clear can be rejected if specific gravity of the sample is very low.

False positives can result from ingesting prescription and nonprescription therapeutic drugs and from consuming certain foods. Poppy seeds may produce false-positive results for opioids. Pseudoephedrine, tricyclic antidepressants, and quetiapine may produce false-positive results for amphetamines, and ibuprofen may produce false-positive results for marijuana. With cocaine testing, which detects benzoylecgonine, the primary metabolite, other substances do not cause false-positive results.

INJECTION DRUG USE

A number of drugs of abuse are given by injection to achieve a more rapid or potent effect or both. Drugs are typically injected IV but may be injected sc, IM, or even sublingually. Users typically access peripheral veins, but when these have sclerosed due to chronic use, some learn to inject into large central veins (eg, internal jugular, femoral, axillary).

Complications

People who inject illicit drugs risk not only the adverse pharmacodynamic effects of the drugs but also complications related to contaminants, adulterants, and infectious agents that may be injected with the drug.

Adulterants: Some drug users crush tablets of prescription drugs, dissolve them, and inject the solution IV, thus injecting themselves with an array of filler agents commonly present in tablets, including cellulose, talc, and cornstarch. Filler agents can become trapped by the pulmonary capillary bed and result in chronic inflammation and foreign body granulomatosis. Filler agents can also damage the endothelium of heart valves, thus increasing the risk of endocarditis.

Street drugs such as heroin and cocaine are often "cut" with various adulterants (eg, amphetamines, clenbuterol, dextromethorphan, fentanyl, ketamine, levamisole, lidocaine, lysergic acid diethylamide [LSD], pseudoephedrine, quinine, scopolamine, xylazine). Adulterants may be added to enhance mind-altering properties or to substitute for pure drug; their presence can make diagnostic and therapeutic decisions difficult.

Infectious agents: Needle sharing and use of nonsterile techniques can lead to many infectious complications. Injection site complications include cutaneous abscesses, cellulitis, lymphangitis, lymphadenitis, and thrombophlebitis. Distant focal infectious complications due to septic emboli and bacteremia include bacterial endocarditis and abscesses in various organs and sites. Septic lung emboli and osteomyelitis (particularly lumbar vertebral) are particularly common. Infectious spondylitis and sacroiliitis may occur.

Systemic infectious diseases are primarily hepatitis B and C and HIV infection. IV drug users are at high risk of pneumonia, resulting from aspiration or hematogenous spread of bacteria. Other infections that are not directly caused by drug injection but are common among IV drug users include TB, syphilis, and other sexually transmitted diseases. Even botulism and tetanus can result from IV drug abuse.

Diagnosis

- History, physical examination, or both

Some patients readily admit to injection drug use, but for others, a thorough physical examination is needed to detect evidence of injection.

Chronic IV drug use can be confirmed by observing track marks due to repeated injections into subcutaneous veins. Track marks are a linear area of tiny, dark punctate lesions (needle punctures) surrounded by an area of darkened or discolored skin due to chronic inflammation. Track marks are often found in easily accessible sites (eg, antecubital fossa, forearms), but some drug users try to hide evidence of their injections by choosing less obvious sites (eg, axillae).

Subcutaneous injection (skin popping) can cause characteristic circular scars or ulcers; there may be signs of previous abscesses. Addicts may deny stigmata of drug use by attributing track marks to frequent blood donations, bug bites, or previous trauma.

Treatment

- Prevention and treatment of infectious complications

Drug users, especially those with a history of injection drug use, should be thoroughly evaluated for viral hepatitis, HIV infection, and the wide range of other infectious diseases common among these patients (eg, TB, syphilis, other sexually transmitted diseases). Also, vaccination to prevent hepatitis, influenza, pneumococcal infections, tetanus infection, and other infections should be offered to all appropriate patients (see p. 1448 as well as specific vaccine topics).

The AIDS epidemic has triggered a harm-reduction movement, which aims to reduce the harm of drug use without necessarily requiring cessation. For example, providing clean needles and syringes for users who cannot stop injecting drugs reduces the spread of HIV and hepatitis.

Treatment of infectious complications is the same as that for similar infections resulting from other conditions; it includes use of antibiotics and incision and drainage of abscesses. Treatment may be complicated by difficulty obtaining venous access (and keeping the patient from using it to inject more drugs) and by poor adherence to treatment regimens.

ALCOHOL TOXICITY AND WITHDRAWAL

Alcohol (ethanol) is a CNS depressant. Large amounts consumed rapidly can cause respiratory depression, coma, and death. Large amounts chronically consumed damage the liver and many other organs. Alcohol withdrawal manifests as a continuum, ranging from tremor to seizures, hallucinations, and life-threatening autonomic instability in severe withdrawal (delirium tremens). Diagnosis is clinical.

About half of adults in the US are current drinkers, 20% are former drinkers, and 30 to 35% are lifetime abstainers. Alcohol use is also becoming an increasing problem in preteens and teenagers. For most drinkers, the frequency and amount of alcohol consumption does not impair physical or mental health or the ability to safely carry out daily activities. However, acute alcohol intoxication is a significant factor in injuries, particularly those due to interpersonal violence, suicide, and motor vehicle crashes.

Chronic alcohol abuse interferes with the ability to socialize and work. About 7 to 10% of adults meet criteria for an alcohol use disorder (abuse or dependence) in any given year. Binge drinking, defined as consuming ≥ 5 drinks per occasion for men and ≥ 4 drinks per occasion for women, is a particular problem among younger people.

Pathophysiology

One serving of alcohol (one 12-oz can of beer, one 6-oz glass of wine, or 1.5 oz of distilled liquor) contains 10 to 15 g of ethanol. Alcohol is absorbed into the blood mainly from the small bowel, although some is absorbed from the stomach. Alcohol accumulates in blood because absorption is more rapid than oxidation and elimination. The concentration peaks about 30 to 90 min after ingestion if the stomach was previously empty.

About 5 to 10% of ingested alcohol is excreted unchanged in urine, sweat, and expired air; the remainder is metabolized mainly by the liver, where alcohol dehydrogenase converts ethanol to acetaldehyde. Acetaldehyde is ultimately oxidized to CO_2 and water at a rate of 5 to 10 mL/h (of absolute alcohol); each milliliter yields about 7 kcal. Alcohol dehydrogenase in the gastric mucosa accounts for some metabolism; much less gastric metabolism occurs in women.

Alcohol exerts its effects by several mechanisms. Alcohol binds directly to gamma-aminobutyric acid (GABA) receptors in the CNS, causing sedation. Alcohol also directly affects cardiac, hepatic, and thyroid tissue.

Chronic effects: Tolerance to alcohol develops rapidly; similar amounts cause less intoxication. Tolerance is caused by adaptational changes of CNS cells (cellular, or pharmacodynamic, tolerance) and by induction of metabolic enzymes. People who develop tolerance may reach an incredibly high blood alcohol content (BAC). However, ethanol tolerance is incomplete, and considerable intoxication and impairment occur with a large enough amount. But even these drinkers may die of respiratory depression secondary to alcohol overdose.

Alcohol-tolerant people are susceptible to alcoholic ketoacidosis, especially during binge drinking. Alcohol-tolerant people are cross-tolerant to many other CNS depressants (eg, barbiturates, nonbarbiturate sedatives, benzodiazepines).

The physical dependence accompanying tolerance is profound, and alcohol withdrawal has potentially fatal adverse effects.

Chronic heavy alcohol intake typically leads to liver disorders (eg, fatty liver, alcoholic hepatitis, cirrhosis); the amount and duration required vary (see p. 201). Patients with a severe liver disorder often have coagulopathy due to decreased hepatic synthesis of coagulation factors, increasing the risk of significant bleeding due to trauma (eg, from falls or vehicle crashes) and of GI bleeding (eg, due to gastritis, from esophageal varices due to portal hypertension); alcohol abusers are at particular risk of GI bleeding.

Chronic heavy intake also commonly causes the following:

- Gastritis
- Pancreatitis
- Cardiomyopathy, often accompanied by arrhythmias and hypertension
- Peripheral neuropathy
- Brain damage, including Wernicke encephalopathy, Korsakoff psychosis, Marchiafava-Bignami disease, and alcoholic dementia
- Certain cancers (eg, head and neck, esophageal), especially when drinking is combined with smoking

Indirect long-term effects include undernutrition, particularly vitamin deficiencies.

On the other hand, low to moderate levels of alcohol consumption (≤ 1 to 2 drinks/day) may decrease the risk of death due to cardiovascular disorders. Numerous explanations, including increased high density lipoprotein (HDL) levels and a direct antithrombotic effect, have been suggested. Nonetheless, alcohol should not be recommended for this purpose, especially when there are several safer, more effective approaches to reduce cardiovascular risk.

Special populations: Young children who drink alcohol are at significant risk of hypoglycemia because alcohol impairs gluconeogenesis and their smaller stores of glycogen are rapidly depleted. Women may be more sensitive than men, even on a per-weight basis, because their gastric (first-pass) metabolism of alcohol is less. Drinking during pregnancy increases the risk of fetal alcohol syndrome.

Symptoms and Signs

Acute effects: Symptoms progress proportionately to the BAC. Actual levels required to cause given symptoms vary with tolerance, but in typical users

- 20 to 50 mg/dL: Tranquility, mild sedation, and some decrease in fine motor coordination
- 50 to 100 mg/dL: Impaired judgment and a further decrease in coordination
- 100 to 150 mg/dL: Unsteady gait, nystagmus, slurred speech, loss of behavioral inhibitions, and memory impairment
- 150 to 300 mg/dL: Delirium and lethargy (likely)

Emesis is common with moderate to severe intoxication; because emesis usually occurs with obtundation, aspiration is a significant risk.

In most US states, the legal definition of intoxication is a BAC of ≥ 0.08 to 0.10% (≥ 80 to 100 mg/dL); 0.08% is used most commonly.

Toxicity or overdose: In alcohol-naive people, a BAC of 300 to 400 mg/dL often causes unconsciousness, and a BAC ≥ 400 mg/dL may be fatal. Sudden death due to respiratory depression or arrhythmias may occur, especially when large quantities are drunk rapidly. This problem is emerging in US colleges but has been known in other countries where it is more common. Other common effects include hypotension and hypoglycemia.

The effect of a particular BAC varies widely; some chronic drinkers seem unaffected and appear to function normally with a BAC in the 300 to 400 mg/dL range, whereas nondrinkers and social drinkers are impaired at a BAC that is inconsequential in chronic drinkers.

Chronic effects: Stigmata of chronic use include Dupuytren contracture of the palmar fascia, vascular spiders, and, in men, signs of hypogonadism and feminization (eg, smooth skin, lack of male-pattern baldness, gynecomastia, testicular atrophy). Undernutrition may lead to enlarged parotid glands.

Withdrawal: A continuum of symptoms and signs of CNS (including autonomic) hyperactivity may accompany cessation of alcohol intake.

A mild alcohol withdrawal syndrome includes tremor, weakness, headache, sweating, hyperreflexia, and GI symptoms. Symptoms usually begin within about 6 h of cessation. Some patients have generalized tonic-clonic seizures (called alcoholic epilepsy, or rum fits) but usually not > 2 in short succession.

Alcoholic hallucinosis (hallucinations without other impairment of consciousness) follows abrupt cessation from prolonged, excessive alcohol use, usually within 12 to 24 h. Hallucinations are typically visual. Symptoms may also include auditory illusions and hallucinations that frequently are accusatory and threatening; patients are usually apprehensive and may be terrified by the hallucinations and by vivid, frightening dreams.

Alcoholic hallucinosis may resemble schizophrenia, although thought is usually not disordered and the history is not typical of schizophrenia. Symptoms do not resemble the delirious state of an acute organic brain syndrome as much as does delirium tremens (DT) or other pathologic reactions associated with withdrawal. Consciousness remains clear, and the signs of autonomic lability that occur in DT are usually absent. When hallucinosis occurs, it usually precedes DT and is transient.

Delirium tremens usually begins 48 to 72 h after alcohol withdrawal; anxiety attacks, increasing confusion, poor sleep (with frightening dreams or nocturnal illusions), profuse sweating, and severe depression also occur. Fleeting hallucinations that arouse restlessness, fear, and even terror are common. Typical of the initial delirious, confused, and disoriented state is a return to a habitual activity; eg, patients frequently imagine that they are back at work and attempt to do some related activity.

Autonomic lability, evidenced by diaphoresis and increased pulse rate and temperature, accompanies the delirium and progresses with it. Mild delirium is usually accompanied by marked diaphoresis, a pulse rate of 100 to 120 beats/min, and a temperature of 37.2 to 37.8° C. Marked delirium, with gross disorientation and cognitive disruption, is accompanied by significant restlessness, a pulse of > 120 beats/min, and a temperature of > 37.8° C; risk of death is high.

During DT, patients are suggestible to many sensory stimuli, particularly to objects seen in dim light. Vestibular disturbances may cause them to believe that the floor is moving, the walls are falling, or the room is rotating. As the delirium progresses, resting tremor of the hand develops, sometimes extending to the head and trunk. Ataxia is marked; care must be taken to prevent self-injury. Symptoms vary among patients but are usually the same for a particular patient with each recurrence.

Diagnosis

- Usually clinical
- Acute: BAC, evaluation to rule out hypoglycemia and occult trauma and possible co-ingestion
- Chronic: CBC, magnesium, liver function tests, and PT/PTT
- Withdrawal: Evaluation to rule out CNS injury and infection

In acute intoxication, laboratory tests, except for fingerstick glucose to rule out hypoglycemia and tests to determine BAC, are generally not helpful; diagnosis is usually made clinically. Confirmation by breath or blood alcohol levels is useful for legal purposes (eg, to document intoxication in drivers or employees who appear impaired). However, finding a low BAC in patients who have altered mental status and smell of alcohol is helpful because it expedites the search for an alternate cause.

Clinicians should not assume that a high BAC in patients with apparently minor trauma accounts for their obtundation, which may be due to intracranial injury or other abnormalities. Such patients should also have toxicology tests to search for evidence of toxicity due to other substances.

Chronic alcohol abuse and dependence are clinical diagnoses; experimental markers of long-term use have not proved sufficiently sensitive or specific for general use. Screening tests such as AUDIT (Alcohol Use Disorders Identification Test) or the CAGE questionnaire can be used. However, heavy alcohol users may have a number of metabolic derangements that are worth screening for, so CBC, electrolytes (including magnesium), liver function tests (including coagulation profile [PT/PTT]), and serum albumin are often recommended.

In severe withdrawal and toxicity, symptoms may resemble those of CNS injury or infection, so medical evaluation with CT and lumbar puncture may be needed. Patients with mild symptoms do not require routine testing unless improvement is not marked within 2 to 3 days. A clinical assessment tool for severity of alcohol withdrawal is available.

Treatment

- Supportive measures
- For withdrawal, benzodiazepines and sometimes also phenobarbital or propofol

Toxicity or overdose: Treatment of alcohol toxicity may include the following:

- Airway protection
- Sometimes IV fluids with thiamin, Mg, and vitamins

The first priority is ensuring an adequate airway; endotracheal intubation and mechanical ventilation are required for apnea or inadequate respirations. IV hydration is needed for hypotension or evidence of volume depletion but does not significantly enhance ethanol clearance. When IV fluids are used, a single dose of thiamin 100 mg IV is given to treat or prevent Wernicke encephalopathy. Many clinicians also add multivitamins and Mg to the IV fluids.

Disposition of the acutely intoxicated patient depends on clinical response, not a specific BAC.

Withdrawal: Patients with severe alcohol withdrawal or DT should be managed in an ICU until these symptoms abate. Treatment may include the following to prevent Wernicke-Korsakoff syndrome and other complications:

- IV thiamin
- Benzodiazepines

Thiamin 100 mg IV is given to prevent Wernicke-Korsakoff syndrome.

Alcohol-tolerant people are cross-tolerant to some drugs commonly used to treat withdrawal (eg, benzodiazepines).

Benzodiazepines are the mainstay of therapy. Dosage and route depend on degree of agitation, vital signs, and mental status. Diazepam, given 5 to 10 mg IV or po hourly until sedation occurs, is a common initial intervention; lorazepam 1 to 2 mg IV or po is an alternative. Chlordiazepoxide 50 to 100 mg po q 4 to 6 h, then tapered, is an older acceptable alternative for less severe cases of withdrawal. Phenobarbital may help if benzodiazepines are ineffective, but respiratory depression is a risk with concomitant use.

Phenothiazines and haloperidol are not recommended initially because they may lower the seizure threshold. For patients with a significant liver disorder, a short-acting benzodiazepine (lorazepam) or one metabolized by glucuronidation (oxazepam) is preferred. (Note: Benzodiazepines may cause intoxication, physical dependence, and withdrawal in alcoholics and therefore should not be continued after the detoxification period. Carbamazepine 200 mg po qid may be used as an alternative and then tapered.) For severe hyperadrenergic activity or to reduce benzodiazepine requirements, short-term therapy (12 to 48 h) with titrated beta-blockers (eg, metoprolol 25 to 50 mg po or 5 mg IV q 4 to 6 h) and clonidine 0.1 to 0.2 mg IV q 2 to 4 h can be used.

A **seizure,** if brief and isolated, needs no specific therapy; however, some clinicians routinely give a single dose of lorazepam 1 to 2 mg IV as prophylaxis against another seizure. Repeated or longer-lasting (ie, > 2 to 3 min) seizures should be treated and often respond to lorazepam 1 to 3 mg IV. Routine use of phenytoin is unnecessary and unlikely to be effective. Outpatient therapy with phenytoin is rarely indicated for patients with simple alcohol withdrawal seizures when no other source of seizure activity has been identified because seizures occur only under the stress of alcohol withdrawal, and patients who are withdrawing or heavily drinking may not take the anticonvulsant.

Delirium tremens may be fatal and thus must be treated promptly with high-dose IV benzodiazepines, preferably in an ICU. Dosing is higher and more frequent than in mild withdrawal. Very high doses of benzodiazepines may be required, and there is no maximum dose or specific treatment regimen. Diazepam 5 to 10 mg IV or lorazepam 1 to 2 mg IV q 10 min is given as needed to control delirium; some patients require several hundred milligrams over the first few hours. Patients refractory to high-dose benzodiazepines may respond to phenobarbital 120 to 240 mg IV q 20 min as needed.

Severe drug-resistant DT can be treated with a continuous infusion of lorazepam, diazepam, midazolam, or propofol, usually with concomitant mechanical ventilation. Physical restraints should be avoided if possible to minimize additional agitation, but patients must not be allowed to elope, remove IVs, or otherwise endanger themselves. Intravascular volume must be maintained with IV fluids, and large doses of vitamins B and C, particularly thiamin, must be given promptly. Appreciably elevated temperature with DT is a poor prognostic sign.

ALCOHOL USE DISORDERS AND REHABILITATION

Alcohol use disorder involves a pattern of alcohol use that typically includes craving and manifestations of tolerance and/ or withdrawal along with adverse psychosocial consequences. Alcoholism and alcohol abuse are common but less rigorously defined terms applied to people with problems related to alcohol.

Alcohol use disorder is quite common. It is estimated to be present in 8.5% of adults in the US in any 12-mo period. Among people age 18 to 29 yr, estimated 12-mo prevalence is 16.2%.

At-risk drinking is defined solely by quantity and frequency of drinking:

- > 14 drinks/wk or 4 drinks per occasion for men
- > 7 drinks/wk or 3 drinks per occasion for women

Compared with lesser amounts, these amounts are associated with increased risk of a wide variety of medical and psychosocial complications.

Etiology

The maladaptive pattern of drinking that constitutes alcohol abuse may begin with a desire to reach a state of feeling high. Some drinkers who find the feeling rewarding then focus on repeatedly reaching that state. Many who abuse alcohol chronically have certain personality traits: feelings of isolation, loneliness, shyness, depression, dependency, hostile and self-destructive impulsivity, and sexual immaturity.

Alcoholics may come from a broken home and have a disturbed relationship with their family. Societal factors—attitudes transmitted through the culture or child rearing—affect patterns of drinking and consequent behavior. However, such generalizations should not obscure the fact that alcohol use disorders can occur in anyone, regardless of their age, sex, background, ethnicity, or social situation. Thus, clinicians should screen for alcohol problems in all patients.

Genetic factors: As much as 40 to 60% of risk variance is thought to be due to genetic factors. The incidence of alcohol abuse and dependence is higher in biologic children of people with alcohol problems than in adoptive children, and the percentage of biologic children of alcoholics who are problem drinkers is greater than that of the general population. There is evidence of genetic or biochemical predisposition, including data that suggest some people who become alcoholics are less easily intoxicated; ie, they have a higher threshold for CNS effects.

Symptoms and Signs

Serious social consequences usually occur. Frequent intoxication is obvious and destructive; it interferes with the ability to socialize and work. Injuries are common. Eventually, failed relationships and job loss due to absenteeism may result.

People may be arrested because of alcohol-related behavior or be apprehended for driving while intoxicated, often losing driving privileges for repeated offenses; in most US states, the maximum legal blood alcohol concentration (BAC) while driving is 80 mg/dL (0.08%), and this level is likely to be reduced in the future.

Diagnosis

- Clinical evaluation
- Screening

The *Diagnostic and Statistical Manual of Mental Disorders,* Fifth Edition (DSM-5) considers alcohol use disorder to be present if patients have clinically significant impairment or distress as manifested by the presence of ≥ 2 of the following over a 12-mo period:

- Taking alcohol in larger amounts or for a longer time than intended
- Persistently desiring or unsuccessfully attempting to decrease alcohol use
- Spending a great deal of time obtaining, using, or recovering from alcohol
- Craving alcohol
- Failing repeatedly to meet obligations at work, home, or school because of alcohol
- Continuing to use alcohol despite having recurrent social or interpersonal problems because of alcohol
- Giving up important social, work, or recreational activities because of alcohol
- Using alcohol in physically hazardous situations
- Continuing to use alcohol despite having a physical (eg, liver disease) or mental disorder (eg, depression) caused or worsened by alcohol
- Having tolerance to alcohol
- Having alcohol withdrawal symptoms or drinking alcohol because of withdrawal

Screening: Some alcohol-related problems are diagnosed when people seek medical treatment for their drinking or for obvious alcohol-related illness (eg, DT, cirrhosis). However, many of these people remain unrecognized for a long time. Female alcoholics are, in general, more likely to drink alone and are less likely to manifest some of the social signs. Therefore, many governmental and professional organizations recommend alcohol screening during routine health care visits.

A scaled approach (see Table 387–1) can help identify patients who require more detailed questioning. Several validated detailed questionnaires are available, including the AUDIT (Alcohol Use Disorders Identification Test) and the CAGE questionnaire.

Treatment

- Rehabilitation programs
- Outpatient counseling
- Self-help groups
- Consideration of drugs (eg, naltrexone, disulfiram, acamprosate)

All patients should be counseled to decrease their alcohol use to below at-risk levels.

For patients identified as at-risk drinkers, treatment may begin with a brief discussion of the medical and social consequences and a recommendation to reduce or cease drinking, with follow-up regarding compliance (see Table 387–2).

For patients with more serious problems, particularly after less intensive measures have been unsuccessful, a rehabilitation program is often the best approach. Rehabilitation programs combine psychotherapy, including one-on-one and group therapy, with medical supervision. For most patients, outpatient rehabilitation is sufficient; how long patients remain enrolled in programs varies, typically weeks to months, but longer if needed.

Inpatient rehabilitation programs are reserved for patients with more severe alcohol dependence and those with significant and comorbid medical, psychoactive, and substance abuse problems. Treatment duration is usually briefer (typically days to weeks) than that of outpatient programs and may be dictated in part by patients' insurance.

Table 387–1. LEVELS OF SCREENING FOR ALCOHOL PROBLEMS

SCREENING LEVEL	CRITERIA FOR USE	SCREENING TECHNIQUE
1	If only one question is possible	On any single occasion during the past 3 mo, have you had > 5 drinks* containing alcohol?
2	For all patients who report drinking alcohol if time allows *or* For patients who respond "yes" to a level 1 screening question	On average, how many days per week do you drink alcohol? On a typical day when you drink, how many drinks do you have? What is the maximum number of drinks you had on any given day in the past month?
3	If level 2 screening identifies risk of alcohol-related problems (ie, for men, > 14 drinks/wk or 4 drinks/day; for women, > 7 drinks/wk or 3 drinks/day) *or* If the clinician suspects that patients are minimizing their alcohol use	The 10-question Alcohol Use Disorders Identification Test (AUDIT)

*A drink is defined as 12 oz of beer, 5 oz of wine, or 1.5 oz of distilled spirits.

Adapted from Fleming MF: Screening and brief intervention in primary care settings. Available at the National Institute on Alcohol Abuse and Alcoholism (NIAAA) web site.

Table 387–2. BRIEF INTERVENTIONS FOR ALCOHOL PROBLEMS

INTERVENTION LEVEL	CRITERIA FOR USE	BRIEF INTERVENTION TECHNIQUE
1	If screening results determine that intervention is necessary but time is limited	Simply stating concern that the patient's drinking exceeds recommended limits and could lead to alcohol-related problems; recommending that the patient minimize or stop drinking
2	If referral to a specialist is not necessary; if abstinence is not necessarily the goal	Project TrEAT (Trial for Early Alcohol Treatment) protocol: 2 brief face-to-face sessions scheduled 1 mo apart, with a follow-up telephone call 2 wk after each session
3	If the patient has symptoms of alcohol abuse or dependence; if abstinence is the primary goal	Motivational enhancement; referral to a specialist

Psychotherapy involves techniques that enhance motivation and teach patients to avoid circumstances that precipitate drinking. Social support of abstinence, including the support of family and friends, is important.

Maintenance: Maintaining sobriety is difficult. Patients should be warned that after a few weeks, when they have recovered from their last bout, they are likely to find an excuse to drink. They should also be told that although they may be able to practice controlled drinking for a few days or, rarely, a few weeks, they will most likely lose control eventually.

In addition to the counseling provided in outpatient and inpatient alcohol treatment programs, self-help groups and certain drugs may help prevent relapse in some patients.

Alcoholics Anonymous (AA) is the most common self-help group. Patients must find an AA group they feel comfortable in. AA provides patients with nondrinking friends who are always available and a nondrinking environment in which to socialize. Patients also hear others discuss every rationalization they have ever used for their own drinking. The help they give other alcoholics may give them the self-regard and confidence formerly found only in alcohol. Many alcoholics are reluctant to go to AA and find individual counseling or group or family treatment more acceptable. Alternative organizations, such as LifeRing Secular Recovery (Secular Organizations for Sobriety), exist for patients seeking another approach.

Drug therapy should be used with counseling rather than as sole treatment. The National Institute on Alcohol Abuse and Alcoholism (NIAAA) provides a guide for clinicians on medical management and pharmacotherapy for alcohol dependence along with a number of other publications and resources for both health care practitioners and patients.

Disulfiram, the first drug available to prevent relapse in alcohol dependence, interferes with the metabolism of acetaldehyde (an intermediary product in the oxidation of alcohol) so that acetaldehyde accumulates. Drinking alcohol within 12 h of taking disulfiram causes facial flushing in 5 to 15 min, then intense vasodilation of the face and neck with suffusion of the conjunctivae, throbbing headache, tachycardia, hyperpnea, and sweating. With high doses of alcohol, nausea and vomiting may follow in 30 to 60 min and may lead to hypotension, dizziness, and sometimes fainting and collapse. The reaction can last up to 3 h. Few patients risk drinking alcohol while taking disulfiram because of the intense discomfort. Drugs that contain alcohol (eg, tinctures; elixirs; some OTC liquid cough and cold preparations, which contain as much as 40% alcohol) must also be avoided.

Disulfiram is contraindicated during pregnancy and in patients with cardiac decompensation. It may be given on an outpatient basis after 4 or 5 days of abstinence. The initial dosage is 0.5 g po once/day for 1 to 3 wk, followed by a maintenance dosage of 0.25 g once/day. Effects may persist for 3 to 7 days after the last dose. Periodic physician visits are needed to encourage continuation of disulfiram as part of an abstinence program.

Disulfiram's general usefulness has not been established, and many patients are nonadherent. Adherence usually requires adequate social support, such as observation of drinking. For these reasons, use of disulfiram is now limited. Disulfiram is most effective when given under close supervision to highly motivated patients.

Naltrexone, an opioid antagonist, decreases the relapse rate and number of drinking days in most patients who take it consistently. Naltrexone 50 mg po once/day is typically given, although there is evidence that higher doses (eg, 100 mg once/day) may be more effective in some patients. Even with counseling, adherence rates with oral naltrexone are modest. A long-acting depot form is also available: 380 mg IM once/mo. Naltrexone is contraindicated in patients with acute hepatitis or liver failure and in those who are opioid dependent.

Acamprosate, a synthetic analogue of GABA, is given as 2 g po once/day. Acamprosate may decrease the relapse rate and number of drinking days in patients who relapse.

Nalmefene, an opioid antagonist, and **topiramate** are under study for their ability to decrease alcohol craving.

AMPHETAMINES

(Methamphetamine)

Amphetamines are sympathomimetic drugs with CNS stimulant and euphoriant properties whose toxic adverse effects include delirium, hypertension, seizures, and hyperthermia (which can cause rhabdomyolysis and renal failure). Toxicity is managed with supportive care, including IV benzodiazepines (for agitation, hypertension, and seizures) and cooling techniques (for hyperthermia). There is no stereotypical withdrawal syndrome.

The original drug in this class, amphetamine, has been modified by various substitutions on its phenyl ring, resulting in many variations, including methamphetamine, methylenedioxymethamphetamine (Ecstasy, MDMA), methylenedioxyethylamphetamine (MDEA), and numerous others.

Some amphetamines, including dextroamphetamine, methamphetamine, and the related methylphenidate, are widely used medically to treat attention-deficit hyperactivity disorder, obesity, and narcolepsy, thus creating a supply subject to diversion for illicit use. Methamphetamine is easily manufactured illicitly.

Pathophysiology

Amphetamines enhance release of catecholamines, increasing intrasynaptic levels of norepinephrine, dopamine, and serotonin. The resulting marked alpha- and beta-receptor stimulation and general CNS excitation account for the "desired" effects of increased alertness, euphoria, and anorexia, as well as the adverse effects of delirium, hypertension, hyperthermia, and seizures.

Effects of amphetamines are similar, varying in intensity and duration of psychoactive effects; MDMA and its relatives have more mood-enhancing properties, perhaps related to a greater effect on serotonin. Amphetamines can be taken orally as pills or capsules, nasally by inhaling or smoking, or by injection.

Chronic effects: Repeated use of amphetamines induces dependence. Tolerance develops slowly, but amounts several 100-fold greater than the amount originally used may eventually be ingested or injected. Tolerance to various effects develops unequally. Tachycardia and increased alertness diminish, but hallucinations and delusions may occur.

Amphetamines typically cause erectile dysfunction in men but enhance sexual desire. Use is associated with unsafe sex practices, and users are at increased risk of sexually transmitted infections, including HIV infection. Amphetamine abusers are prone to injury because the drug produces excitation and grandiosity followed by excess fatigue and sleepiness.

Necrotizing vasculitis that involves multiple organ systems can occur.

Use of certain amphetamine-related appetite suppressants (dexfenfluramine, fenfluramine, phentermine) has been associated with valvular heart disease. Dexfenfluramine and fenfluramine were removed from the US market in 1997. Phentermine-fenfluramine (Phen-fen) products were similarly withdrawn from the US market, but phentermine alone and in combination with topiramate is available as an anorectic.

Symptoms and Signs

Acute effects: Many psychologic effects of amphetamines are similar to those of cocaine; they include increased alertness and concentration, euphoria, and feelings of well-being and grandiosity. Palpitations, tremor, diaphoresis, and mydriasis may also occur during intoxication.

Binges (perhaps over several days) lead to an exhaustion syndrome, involving intense fatigue and need for sleep after the stimulation phase.

Toxicity or overdose: Tachycardia, arrhythmias, chest pain, hypertension, dizziness, nausea, vomiting, and diarrhea can occur. CNS effects include acute delirium and toxic psychosis. Overdose can also cause stroke (usually hemorrhagic), seizures, muscle rigidity, and hyperthermia (> 40° C); all of these effects may precipitate rhabdomyolysis, which can lead to renal failure.

Chronic effects: A paranoid psychosis may result from long-term use; rarely, the psychosis is precipitated by a single high dose or by repeated moderate doses. Typical features include delusions of persecution, ideas of reference (notions that everyday occurrences have special meaning or significance personally meant for or directed to the patient), and feelings of omnipotence. Some users experience a prolonged depression, during which suicide is possible.

Recovery from even prolonged amphetamine psychosis is usual but is slow. The more florid symptoms fade within a few days or weeks, but some confusion, memory loss, and delusional ideas commonly persist for months.

Users have a high rate of severe tooth decay affecting multiple teeth; causes include decreased salivation, acidic combustion products, and poor oral hygiene.

Withdrawal: Although no stereotypical withdrawal syndrome occurs when amphetamines are stopped, EEG changes occur, considered by some experts to fulfill the physical criteria for dependence. Abruptly stopping use may uncover or exacerbate underlying depression or precipitate a serious depressive reaction. Withdrawal is often followed by 2 or 3 days of intense fatigue or sleepiness and depression.

Diagnosis

- Clinical evaluation
- Testing as needed to exclude serious nondrug-related disorders (eg, causing altered mental status)

Diagnosis is usually made clinically, although when history of drug use and the diagnosis are unclear, tests are done as indicated for the undifferentiated patient with altered mental status, hyperpyrexia, or seizures. Evaluation then typically includes CT, lumbar puncture, and laboratory tests to identify infections and metabolic abnormalities.

Amphetamines are usually part of routine urine drug screens, which are done unless history of ingestion is clear; specific drug levels are not measured. Immunoassay urine screening tests for amphetamines may produce false-positive results and may not detect methamphetamine and methylphenidate.

Treatment

- IV benzodiazepines
- IV nitrates for hypertension unresponsive to benzodiazepines as needed
- Cooling for hyperthermia as needed

Toxicity or overdose: When a significant amount has recently been taken orally (eg, < 1 to 2 h), activated charcoal may be given to limit absorption, although this intervention has not been shown to reduce morbidity or mortality. Urinary acidification hastens amphetamine excretion, but it does not decrease toxicity and may worsen myoglobin precipitation in the renal tubules and thus is not recommended.

Benzodiazepines are the preferred initial treatment for CNS excitation, seizures, tachycardia, and hypertension. Lorazepam 2 to 3 mg IV q 5 min titrated to effect may be used. High doses or a continuous infusion may be required. Propofol, with mechanical ventilation, may be required for severe agitation. Hypertension that does not respond to benzodiazepines is treated with nitrates (occasionally nitroprusside) or other antihypertensives as needed, depending on the severity of the hypertension. Beta-blockers (eg, metoprolol 2 to 5 mg IV) may be used for severe ventricular arrhythmias or tachycardia.

Hyperthermia can be life threatening and should be managed aggressively with sedation plus evaporative cooling, ice packs, and maintenance of intravascular volume and urine flow with IV normal saline solution.

Phenothiazines lower seizure threshold, and their anticholinergic effects can interfere with cooling; thus, they are not preferred for sedation.

Withdrawal and rehabilitation: No specific treatment is needed. BP and mood should be monitored initially. Patients whose depression persists for more than a brief period after amphetamines are stopped may respond to antidepressants.

Cognitive-behavioral therapy (a form of psychotherapy) is effective in some patients. There are no other proven treatments for rehabilitation and maintenance after detoxification.

ANABOLIC STEROIDS

Anabolic steroids are often used to enhance physical performance and promote muscle growth. When used inappropriately, chronically at high doses and without medical supervision, they can cause erratic and irrational behavior and a wide range of physical adverse effects.

Anabolic steroids include testosterone and any drugs chemically and pharmacologically related to testosterone that promote muscle growth; numerous drugs are available. Anabolic steroids are used clinically to treat low testosterone levels in male hypogonadism. Additionally, because anabolic steroids are anticatabolic and improve protein utilization, they are sometimes given to burn, bedbound, or other debilitated patients to prevent muscle wasting.

Some physicians prescribe anabolic steroids to patients with AIDS-related wasting or with cancer. However, there are few data to recommend such therapy and little guidance on how supplemental androgens may affect underlying disorders. Testosterone has been reputed to benefit wound healing and muscle injury, although few data support these claims.

Anabolic steroids are used illicitly to increase lean muscle mass and strength; resistance training and a certain diet can enhance these effects. There is no direct evidence that anabolic steroids increase endurance or speed, but substantial anecdotal evidence suggests that athletes taking them can perform more frequent high-intensity workouts. Muscle hypertrophy is unequivocal.

Estimates of lifetime incidence of anabolic steroid abuse range from 0.5 to 5% of the population, but subpopulations vary significantly (eg, higher rates for bodybuilders and competitive athletes). In the US, the reported rate of use is 6 to 11% among high school–aged males, including an unexpected number of nonathletes, and about 2.5% among high school–aged females.

Pathophysiology

Anabolic steroids have androgenic effects (eg, changes in hair or in libido, aggressiveness) and anabolic effects (eg, increased protein utilization, increased muscle mass). Androgenic effects cannot be separated from the anabolic, but some anabolic steroids have been synthesized to minimize the androgenic effects.

Testosterone is rapidly degraded by the liver; oral testosterone is inactivated too rapidly to be effective, and injectable testosterone must be modified (eg, by esterification) to retard absorption or delay breakdown. Analogs modified by 17-alpha-alkylation are often effective orally, but adverse effects may be increased. Transdermal preparations are also available.

Chronic effects: Adverse effects vary significantly by dose and drug. There are few adverse effects at physiologic replacement doses (eg, methyltestosterone 10 to 50 mg/day or its equivalent). Athletes may use doses 10 to 50 times this range. At high doses, some effects are clear; others are equivocal (see Table 387–3). Uncertainties exist because most studies involve abusers who may not report doses accurately and who also use black market drugs, many of which are counterfeit and contain (despite labeling) varying doses and substances.

Athletes may take steroids for a certain period, stop, then start again (cycling) several times a year. Intermittently stopping the drugs is believed to allow endogenous testosterone levels, sperm count, and the hypothalamic-pituitary-gonadal axis to return to normal. Anecdotal evidence suggests that cycling may decrease harmful effects and the need for increasing drug doses to attain the desired effect.

Table 387–3. ADVERSE EFFECTS OF ANABOLIC STEROIDS

Clearly shown
Erythrocytosis
Abnormal lipid profile (decreased HDL, increased LDL)
Liver abnormalities: Peliosis hepatitis, adenoma
Mood disorders (with high doses)
Androgenic effects: Acne, baldness, virilization and hirsutism in females
Gonadal suppression (decreased sperm count, testicular atrophy)
Gynecomastia
Premature closure of epiphyses
Equivocal
Hypertension and LVH
Worsening of prostatic hypertrophy or preexisting carcinoma
Hepatic carcinoma
Poorly shown*
Increased risk of sudden death in athletes
Significant mood disorder with low doses

*Predominantly with 17-alpha-alkylated analogs.

HDL = high-density lipoprotein; LDL = low-density lipoprotein; LVH = left ventricular hypertrophy.

Athletes frequently use many drugs simultaneously (a practice called stacking) and alternate routes of administration (oral, IM, or transdermal). Increasing the dose through a cycle (pyramiding) may result in doses 5 to 100 times the physiologic dose. Stacking and pyramiding are intended to increase receptor binding and minimize adverse effects, but these benefits have not been proved.

Symptoms and Signs

The most characteristic sign is a rapid increase in muscle mass. The rate and extent of increase are directly related to the doses taken. Patients taking physiologic doses have slow and often unnoticeable growth; those taking megadoses may increase lean body weight by several pounds per month. Increases in energy level and libido (in men) occur but are more difficult to identify.

Psychologic effects (usually only with very high doses) are often noticed by family members:

- Wide and erratic mood swings
- Irrational behavior
- Increased aggressiveness ("roid rage")
- Irritability
- Increased libido
- Depression

Increased acne is common in both sexes; libido may increase or, less commonly, decrease; aggressiveness and appetite may increase. Gynecomastia, testicular atrophy, and decreased fertility may occur in males. Virilizing effects (eg, alopecia, enlarged clitoris, hirsutism, deepened voice) are common among females. Also, breast size may decrease; vaginal mucosa may atrophy; and menstruation may change or stop. Virilization and gynecomastia may be irreversible.

Diagnosis

- Urine testing

A urine screen usually identifies users of anabolic steroids. Metabolites of anabolic steroids can be detected in urine up to 6 mo (even longer for some types of anabolic steroids) after the drugs are stopped.

Testosterone taken exogenously is indistinguishable from endogenous testosterone. However, if high levels of testosterone are detected, the ratio between testosterone and epitestosterone (an endogenous steroid that chemically is nearly identical to testosterone) is measured. Normally, the ratio is < 6:1; if exogenous testosteroneis being used, the ratio is higher.

Treatment

- Cessation of use

The main treatment is cessation of use. Although physical dependence does not occur, psychologic dependence, particularly in competitive bodybuilders, may exist. Gynecomastia may require surgical reduction.

Prevention

Physicians caring for adolescents and young adults should be alert to the signs of steroid abuse and teach patients about its risks. Education about anabolic steroids should start by the beginning of middle school. Use of programs that teach alternative, healthy ways to increase muscle size and improve performance through good nutrition and weight training techniques may help. Presenting both risks and benefits of anabolic steroid use seems to be a more effective way to educate adolescents about the negative effects of illicit steroid use.

ANXIOLYTICS AND SEDATIVES

(Hypnotics)

Anxiolytics and sedatives include benzodiazepines, barbiturates, and related drugs. High doses can cause stupor and respiratory depression, which is managed with intubation and mechanical ventilation. Chronic users may have a withdrawal syndrome of agitation and seizures, so dependence is managed by slow tapering with or without substitution (ie, with pentobarbital or phenobarbital).

The therapeutic benefit of anxiolytics and sedatives is well-established, but their value in alleviating stress and anxiety is also probably the reason that they are abused so frequently. Abused anxiolytics and sedatives include benzodiazepines, barbiturates, and other drugs taken to promote sleep.

Pathophysiology

Benzodiazepines and barbiturates potentiate GABA at specific receptors thought to be located near GABA receptors. The exact mechanism of this potentiation process remains unclear but may be related to opening of chloride channels, producing a hyperpolarized state within the postsynaptic neuron which inhibits cellular excitation.

Chronic effects: Patients taking high doses of sedatives frequently have difficulty thinking, slow speech and comprehension (with some dysarthria), poor memory, faulty judgment, narrowed attention span, and emotional lability. In susceptible patients, psychologic dependence on the drug may develop rapidly. The extent of physical dependence is related to dose and duration of use; eg, pentobarbital 200 mg/day taken for many months may not induce significant tolerance, but 300 mg/day for > 3 mo or 500 to 600 mg/day for 1 mo may induce a withdrawal syndrome when the drug is stopped.

Tolerance and tachyphylaxis develop irregularly and incompletely; thus, considerable behavioral, mood, and cognitive disturbances persist, even in regular users, depending on the dosage and the drug's pharmacodynamic effects. Some cross-tolerance exists between alcohol and barbiturates and nonbarbiturate anxiolytics and sedatives, including benzodiazepines. (Barbiturates and alcohol are strikingly similar in the dependence, withdrawal symptoms, and chronic intoxication they cause.)

Pregnancy: Prolonged use of barbiturates during pregnancy can cause barbiturate withdrawal in the neonate. Perinatal use of benzodiazepines also may cause neonatal withdrawal syndrome or toxicity (eg, apnea, hypothermia, hypotonia).

Symptoms and Signs

Toxicity or overdose: The signs of progressive anxiolytic and sedative intoxication are depression of superficial reflexes, fine lateral-gaze nystagmus, slightly decreased alertness with coarse or rapid nystagmus, ataxia, slurred speech, and postural unsteadiness.

Increasing toxicity can cause nystagmus on forward gaze, miosis, somnolence, marked ataxia with falling, confusion, stupor, respiratory depression, and, ultimately, death. Overdose of a benzodiazepine rarely causes hypotension, and these drugs do not cause arrhythmias.

Withdrawal: When intake of therapeutic doses of anxiolytics and sedatives is stopped or reduced below a critical level, a self-limited mild withdrawal syndrome can ensue. After only a few weeks, attempts to stop using the drug can exacerbate insomnia and result in restlessness, disturbing dreams, frequent awakening, and feelings of tension in the early morning.

Withdrawal from benzodiazepines is rarely life threatening. Symptoms can include tachypnea, tachycardia, tremulousness, hyperreflexia, confusion, and seizures. Onset may be slow because the drugs remain in the body a long time. Withdrawal may be most severe in patients who used drugs with rapid absorption and a quick decline in serum levels (eg, alprazolam, lorazepam, triazolam). Many people who misuse benzodiazepines have been or are heavy users of alcohol, and a delayed benzodiazepine withdrawal syndrome may complicate alcohol withdrawal.

Withdrawal from barbiturates taken in large doses causes an abrupt, potentially life-threatening withdrawal syndrome similar to DT. Occasionally, even after properly managed withdrawal over 1 to 2 wk, a seizure occurs. Without treatment, withdrawal of a short-acting barbiturate causes the following:

- Within the first 12 to 20 h: Increasing restlessness, tremulousness, and weakness
- By the 2nd day: More prominent tremulousness, sometimes increased deep tendon reflexes, and increased weakness
- During the 2nd and 3rd days: Seizures (in 75% of patients who were taking ≥ 800 mg/day), sometimes progressing to status epilepticus and death
- From the 2nd to the 5th day: Delirium, insomnia, confusion, frightening visual and auditory hallucinations, and often hyperpyrexia and dehydration

Diagnosis

- Clinical evaluation

Diagnosis is usually made clinically. Drug levels can be measured for some drugs (eg, phenobarbital), but typically hospital laboratories cannot measure levels of most hypnotics and sedatives. Benzodiazepines and barbiturates are usually included in routine immunoassay-based qualitative urine drug screens. However, detecting drugs on such screening tests usually does not alter clinical management; even if the results are positive, if patients do not have a clear history of sedative-hypnotic ingestion, other causes should be ruled out.

Treatment

- Supportive care
- Rarely flumazenil for benzodiazepines
- Sometimes urine alkalinization and/or activated charcoal for barbiturates

Toxicity or overdose: Acute intoxication generally requires nothing more than observation, although the airway and respirations should be carefully assessed. If ingestion was within 1 h, the gag reflex is preserved, and the patient can protect the airway, 50 g of activated charcoal may be given to reduce further absorption; however, this intervention has not been shown to reduce morbidity or mortality. Occasionally, intubation and mechanical ventilation are required.

The benzodiazepine receptor antagonist flumazenil can reverse severe sedation and respiratory depression secondary to benzodiazepine overdose. Dose is 0.2 mg IV given over 30 sec; 0.3 mg may be given after 30 sec, followed by 0.5 mg q 1 min to total 3 mg. However, its clinical usefulness is not well-defined because most people who overdose on benzodiazepines recover with only supportive care, and occasionally flumazenil precipitates seizures.

Contraindications to flumazenil include long-term benzodiazepine use (because flumazenil may precipitate withdrawal), an underlying seizure disorder, presence of twitching or other motor abnormalities, a concomitant epileptogenic drug overdose (especially of tricyclic antidepressants), and cardiac arrhythmias. Thus, because many of these contraindications are usually unknown in street overdoses, flumazenil is best reserved for patients with respiratory depression during a medical procedure (ie, when medical history is clearly known).

If phenobarbital overdose is diagnosed, urine alkalinization with sodium bicarbonate dose may enhance excretion. Administration of multidose activated charcoal is also considered in case of life-threatening amount of phenobarbital overdose.

Urinary alkalinization is accomplished by adding 150 mEq sodium bicarbonate diluted in 1 liter D5W and infused at a rate of 1 to 1.5 liters per hour. Urinary pH should be maintained as close to 8 as possible for effective alkalinization.

Withdrawal and detoxification: Severe acute withdrawal requires hospitalization, preferably in an ICU, and use of appropriate doses of IV benzodiazepines.

One approach for managing sedative dependence is to withdraw the drug on a strict schedule while monitoring signs of withdrawal. Often, switching to a long-acting drug, which is easier to taper, is better.

As for alcohol withdrawal, patients going through anxiolytic or sedative withdrawal require close monitoring, preferably in an inpatient setting if a moderate to severe withdrawal reaction is expected.

CANNABINOIDS, SYNTHETIC

Synthetic cannabinoids are man-made drugs that are tetrahydrocannabinol (THC) receptor agonists. They are typically applied to dried plant material and smoked.

THC is the primary active ingredient in marijuana (cannabis). There are many chemical families of synthetic cannabinoids, including HU-210, JWH-073, JWH-018, JWH-200, AM-2201, UR-144, and XLR-11; new compounds are being reported regularly.

Effects vary greatly depending on the specific cannabinoid, and many of the acute and chronic effects remain unknown. However, stimulation of the THC receptor causes altered mental status with agitation, hallucinations, and psychosis (that may be irreversible). Cardiovascular effects include hypertension, tachycardia and myocardial infarction. Neurologic effects include seizures and blurred vision. Additional reported effects include vomiting, hyperthermia, rhabdomyolysis, and renal failure.

Symptoms and Signs

Patients may have severe agitation, hallucinations, tachycardia, hypertension, diaphoresis, and seizures.

Diagnosis

- Clinical evaluation

Synthetic cannabinoids are not detected on routine urine screening.

Patients with severe acute intoxication should typically have blood tests (CBC, electrolytes, BUN, creatinine, CK), urine testing for myoglobinuria, and ECG.

Treatment

- IV sedation with benzodiazepines

Sedation with IV benzodiazepines, IV fluids, and supportive care are typically adequate. Patients with hyperthermia, persistent tachycardia or agitation, and elevated serum creatinine should be admitted for further monitoring for rhabdomyolysis and cardiac and renal injury.

CATHINONES

Cathinones are compounds related to the stimulant alkaloid derived from the plant *Catha edulis* (khat).

The khat plant is native to the Horn of Africa and Arabian peninsula. Its leaves contain cathinone, an amphetamine-like alkaloid. For centuries, inhabitants of the plant's native area have chewed the leaves for a mild euphoriant and stimulant effect. In those regions, chewing khat is often a social activity, similar to coffee drinking in other societies. Recently, khat use has spread to other countries and more recently a number of derivatives of the base alkaloid have been synthesized and become drugs of abuse.

Derivatives include the drugs known as bath salts, often containing the substituted cathinones mephedrone or methylenedioxypyrovalerone. However, the actual structures change frequently. The products have been termed "bath salts" and labeled "not for human consumption" to avoid legal challenge. Reported use of substituted cathinones increased several thousand-fold from 2010–2011.

The physiologic effects of the substituted cathinones are similar to those of amphetamines and include the potential to cause myocardial infarction, rhabdomyolysis, renal failure, and liver failure. However, the exact mechanism responsible for organ damage is unknown.

Patients may present with headache, tachycardia and palpitations, hallucinations, agitation, an increased endurance and tolerance for pain, and propensity for violent behavior.

Diagnosis is made by clinical evaluation; substituted cathinones are not detected with routine urine or blood testing. Patients with severe acute intoxication should typically have blood tests (CBC, electrolytes, BUN, creatinine, CK), urine testing for myoglobinuria, and ECG.

Sedation with IV benzodiazepines, IV fluids, and supportive care are typically adequate. Patients with hyperthermia, persistent tachycardia or agitation, and elevated serum creatinine should be admitted for further monitoring for rhabdomyolysis and cardiac and renal injury.

COCAINE

(Crack)

Cocaine is a sympathomimetic drug with CNS stimulant and euphoriant properties. High doses can cause panic, schizophrenic-like symptoms, seizures, hyperthermia, hypertension, arrhythmias, stroke, aortic dissection, intestinal ischemia, and MI. Toxicity is managed with supportive care, including IV benzodiazepines (for agitation, hypertension, and seizures) and cooling techniques (for hyperthermia). Withdrawal manifests primarily as depression, difficulty concentrating, and somnolence (cocaine washout syndrome).

Most cocaine users are episodic recreational users. However, about 25% (or more) of users meet criteria for abuse or dependence. Use among adolescents has declined recently. Availability of highly biologically active forms, such as crack cocaine, has worsened the problem of cocaine dependence. Most cocaine in the US is about 45 to 60% pure; it may contain a wide array of fillers, adulterants, and contaminants.

Most cocaine in the US is volatilized and inhaled, but it may be snorted, or injected IV. For inhalation, the powdered hydrochloride salt is converted into a more volatile form, usually by adding $NaHCO_3$, water, and heat. The resultant precipitate (crack cocaine) is volatilized by heating (it is not burned) and inhaled. Onset of effect is quick, and intensity of the high rivals that associated with IV injection. Tolerance to cocaine occurs, and withdrawal from heavy use is characterized by somnolence, difficulty concentrating, increased appetite, and depression. The tendency to continue taking the drug is strong after a period of withdrawal.

Pathophysiology

Cocaine, an alkaloid present in the leaves of the coca plant, enhances norepinephrine, dopamine, and serotonin activity in the central and peripheral nervous systems.

Enhancement of dopamine activity is the likely cause of the drug's intended effects and thus of the reinforcement that contributes to developing abuse and dependence.

Norepinephrine activity accounts for the sympathomimetic effects: tachycardia, hypertension, mydriasis, diaphoresis, and hyperthermia.

Cocaine also blocks sodium channels, accounting for its action as a local anesthetic. Cocaine causes vasoconstriction and thus can affect almost any organ. MI, cerebral ischemia and hemorrhage, aortic dissection, intestinal ischemia, and renal ischemia are possible sequelae.

Onset of cocaine's effects depends on mode of use:

- IV injection and smoking: Immediate onset, peak effect after about 3 to 5 min, and duration of about 15 to 20 min
- Intranasal use: Onset after about 3 to 5 min, peak effect at 20 to 30 min, and duration of about 45 to 90 min
- Oral use: Onset after about 10 min, peak effect at about 60 min, and duration of about 90 min

Because cocaine is such a short-acting drug, heavy users may inject it or smoke it repeatedly every 10 to 15 min.

Pregnancy: Cocaine use during pregnancy can affect the fetus; the rate of placental abruption and spontaneous abortion is higher.

Symptoms and Signs

Acute effects: Effects may differ depending on mode of use. When injected or smoked, cocaine causes hyperstimulation, alertness, euphoria, a sense of increased energy, and feelings of competence and power. The excitation and high are similar to those produced by injecting amphetamines. These feelings are less intense and disruptive in users who snort cocaine powder.

Users who smoke the drug may develop pneumothorax or pneumomediastinum, causing chest pain, dyspnea, or both. Myocardial ischemia due to cocaine use may also cause chest pain ("cocaine chest pain"), but cocaine can also cause chest pain in the absence of myocardial ischemia; the mechanism is unclear. Arrhythmias and conduction abnormalities may occur. Cardiac effects may result in sudden death. Binges, often over several days, lead to an exhaustion syndrome or "washed out" syndrome, involving intense fatigue and need for sleep.

Toxicity or overdose: An overdose may cause severe anxiety, panic, agitation, aggression, sleeplessness, hallucinations, paranoid delusions, impaired judgment, tremors, seizures, and delirium. Mydriasis and diaphoresis are apparent, and heart rate and BP are increased. Death may result from MI or arrhythmias.

Severe overdose causes a syndrome of acute psychosis (eg, schizophrenic-like symptoms), hypertension, hyperthermia, rhabdomyolysis, coagulopathy, renal failure, and seizures. Patients with extreme clinical toxicity may, on a genetic basis, have decreased (atypical) serum cholinesterase, an enzyme needed for clearance of cocaine.

Patients who inhale cocaine may develop an acute pulmonary syndrome (crack lung) with fever, hemoptysis, and hypoxia, that may progress to respiratory failure.

The concurrent use of cocaine and alcohol produces a condensation product, cocaethylene, which has stimulant properties and may contribute to toxicity.

Chronic effects: Severe toxic effects occur in compulsive heavy users. Myocardial fibrosis, left ventricular hypertrophy, and cardiomyopathy can develop. Rarely, repeated snorting causes nasal septal perforation due to local ischemia. Cognitive impairment, including impaired attention and verbal memory, occurs in some heavy users. Users who inject cocaine are subject to the typical infectious complications.

Withdrawal: The main symptoms are depression, difficulty concentrating, and somnolence (cocaine washout syndrome). Appetite is increased.

Diagnosis

- Clinical evaluation

Diagnosis is usually made clinically. Drug levels are not measured. The cocaine metabolite, benzoylecgonine, is part of most routine urine drug screens.

Treatment

- IV benzodiazepines
- Avoidance of beta-blockers
- Cooling for hyperthermia as needed

Toxicity or overdose: Treatment of mild cocaine intoxication is generally unnecessary because the drug is extremely short-acting. Benzodiazepines are the preferred initial treatment for most toxic effects, including CNS excitation and seizures, tachycardia, and hypertension. Lorazepam 2 to 3 mg IV q 5 min titrated to effect may be used. High doses and a continuous infusion may be required. Propofol infusion, with mechanical ventilation, may be used for resistant cases.

Hypertension that does not respond to benzodiazepines is treated with IV nitrates (eg, nitroprusside) or phentolamine; beta-blockers are not recommended because they allow continued alpha-adrenergic stimulation.

Hyperthermia can be life threatening and should be managed aggressively with sedation plus evaporative cooling, ice packs, and maintenance of intravascular volume and urine flow with IV normal saline solution.

Phenothiazines lower seizure threshold, and their anticholinergic effects can interfere with cooling; thus, they are not preferred for sedation.

Occasionally, severely agitated patients must be pharmacologically paralyzed and mechanically ventilated to ameliorate acidosis, rhabdomyolysis, or multisystem dysfunction.

Cocaine-related chest pain is evaluated as for any other patient with potential myocardial ischemia or aortic dissection, with chest x-ray, serial ECG, and serum cardiac markers. As discussed, beta-blockers are contraindicated, and benzodiazepines are a first-line drug. If coronary vasodilation is required after benzodiazepines are given, nitrates are used, or phentolamine 1 to 5 mg IV given slowly can be considered.

Abuse: Heavy users and people who inject the drug IV or smoke it are most likely to become dependent. Light users and people who take the drug nasally or orally are at lower risk of becoming dependent. Stopping sustained use requires considerable assistance, and the depression that may result requires close supervision and treatment.

Many outpatient therapies, including support and self-help groups and cocaine hotlines, exist. Inpatient therapy is used primarily when it is required by physical or mental comorbidity or when outpatient therapy has repeatedly been unsuccessful.

For treatment of infants born to cocaine-addicted mothers, see p. 2734.

GAMMA HYDROXYBUTYRATE

("G")

Gamma hydroxybutyrate (GHB) causes intoxication resembling alcohol intoxication or ketamine intoxication and, especially when combined with alcohol, can lead to respiratory depression, seizures, and rarely death.

Gamma hydroxybutyrate is similar to the neurotransmitter GABA, but it can cross the blood-brain barrier and so can be taken by mouth. It is similar to ketamine in its effects but lasts longer and is far more dangerous.

GHB produces feelings of relaxation and tranquility. It may also cause fatigue and disinhibition. At higher doses, GHB may cause dizziness, loss of coordination, nausea, and vomiting. Coma and respiratory depression may also occur. Combining GHB and any other sedative, especially alcohol, is extremely dangerous. Most deaths have occurred when GHB was taken with alcohol.

Withdrawal symptoms occur if GHB is not taken for several days after previous frequent use of large amounts. Symptoms are similar to those of alcohol withdrawal and benzodiazepine withdrawal and can be life-threatening.

Treatment is directed at symptoms. Mechanical ventilation may be needed if breathing is affected. Most people recover rapidly, although effects may not fade for 1 to 2 h.

HALLUCINOGENS

(LSD; Lysergic Acid Diethylamide; Mescaline; Psilocybin)

Hallucinogens are a diverse group of drugs that can cause highly unpredictable, idiosyncratic reactions. Intoxication typically causes hallucinations, with altered perception, impaired judgment, ideas of reference, and depersonalization. There is no stereotypical withdrawal syndrome. Diagnosis is clinical. Treatment is supportive.

Traditional hallucinogens include LSD, psilocybin, and mescaline. All are derived from natural products:

- LSD from a fungus that often contaminates wheat and rye flour
- Psilocybin from several types of mushrooms
- Mescaline from the peyote cactus

Many of the newer synthetic compounds ("designer drugs") have been produced, usually based on tryptamine or phenylethylamine molecules. Tryptamines include *N,N*-dimethyltryptamine (DMT) and 5-methoxy-*N, N*-diisopropyltryptamine (5-MeO-DIPT).

To complicate matters, many illicit drugs sold under one name actually contain another drug of abuse—often ketamine or phencyclidine (PCP), anesthetic drugs, dextromethorphan, or other drugs.

Some other drugs, including marijuana, also have hallucinogenic properties. The term hallucinogen persists, although use of these drugs may not cause hallucinations. Alternative terms, such as psychedelic and psychotomimetic, are even less appropriate.

Pathophysiology

LSD, psilocybin, and many designer hallucinogens are serotonin receptor agonists. For mescaline, a phenylethylamine similar to amphetamines, the exact mechanism has not been determined.

Mode of use and effects vary:

- LSD is taken orally from drug-impregnated blotter paper or as tablets. Onset of action is usually 30 to 60 min after ingestion; duration of effects can be 12 to 24 h.
- Psilocybin is taken orally; effects usually last about 4 to 6 h.
- Mescaline is taken orally as peyote buttons. Onset of effects is usually 30 to 90 min after ingestion; duration of effects is about 12 h.
- DMT, when smoked, has onset in 2 to 5 min; duration of effects is 20 to 60 min (accounting for its street name, "businessman's lunch").

A high degree of tolerance to LSD develops and disappears rapidly. Users tolerant to any of these drugs are cross-tolerant to the other drugs. Psychologic dependence varies greatly; there is no evidence of physical dependence or a withdrawal syndrome.

Symptoms and Signs

Intoxication results in altered perceptions, including synesthesias (eg, seeing sounds, hearing colors), intensification of sensations, enhanced empathy, depersonalization (feeling the self is not real), a distorted sense of the environment's reality, and changes in mood (usually euphoric, sometimes depressive). Users often refer to the combination of these effects as a trip. Periods of intense psychologic effects may alternate with periods of lucidity.

LSD may also have several physical effects, including mydriasis, blurred vision, sweating, palpitations, and impaired coordination. Many other hallucinogens cause nausea and vomiting. With all, judgment is impaired.

Responses to hallucinogens depend on several factors, including the user's expectations, ability to cope with perceptual distortions, and the setting. With LSD, delusions and true hallucinations occur but are rare, as are anxiety attacks, extreme apprehensiveness, and panic states.

Psilocybin and mescaline are more likely to cause hallucinations. When hallucinogenic reactions occur, they usually subside quickly if treated appropriately in a secure setting. However, some people (especially after using LSD) remain disturbed and may have a persistent psychotic state. Whether drug use has precipitated or uncovered preexisting psychotic potential or can cause this state in previously stable people is unclear.

Chronic effects: Some people, especially long-term or repeat users (particularly of LSD), experience apparent drug effects long after they have stopped drug use. These recurrent episodes (flashbacks, hallucinogen persisting perception disorder) are usually visual illusions but can include distortions of virtually any sensation (including self-image or perceptions of time or space) and hallucinations.

Flashbacks can be precipitated by use of marijuana, alcohol, or barbiturates or by stress or fatigue or can occur without apparent reason. Mechanisms are not known. Flashbacks tend to subside within 6 to 12 mo, but can recur for years.

Diagnosis

- Clinical evaluation

Diagnosis is usually made clinically. Drug levels are not measured. Except for PCP, most hallucinogens are not included in routine urine drug screens.

Treatment

- For acute intoxication, supportive measures and relief of anxiety and agitation
- For persistent psychosis, psychiatric care

A quiet, calming environment with reassurance that the bizarre thoughts, visions, and sounds are due to the drug and will go away soon usually suffices. Anxiolytics (eg, lorazepam, diazepam) may help reduce severe anxiety.

Persistent psychotic states or other mental disorders require appropriate psychiatric care. Flashbacks that are transient or not unduly distressing to the patient require no special treatment. However, flashbacks associated with anxiety and depression may require anxiolytics as for acute adverse reactions.

KETAMINE AND PHENCYCLIDINE

Ketamine and phencyclidine (PCP) are dissociative anesthetics that can cause intoxication, sometimes with confusion or a catatonic state. Overdose can cause coma and, rarely, death.

Ketamine and PCP are chemically related anesthetics. These drugs are often used to adulterate or pass for other hallucinogens such as LSD.

Ketamine is available in liquid or powder form. When used illicitly, the powder form is typically snorted but can be taken orally. The liquid form is taken IV, IM, or sc.

PCP, once common, is no longer being legally manufactured. It is illegally manufactured and sold on the street under names such as angel dust; it is sometimes sold in combination with herbs, marijuana, and tobacco.

Symptoms and Signs

Intoxication, characterized by a giddy euphoria, occurs with lower doses; euphoria is often followed by bursts of anxiety or mood lability.

Overdose causes a withdrawn state of depersonalization and disassociation; when doses are higher still, disassociation can become severe and response to external stimuli is impaired, with combativeness, ataxia, dysarthria, muscular hypertonicity, nystagmus, hyperreflexia, and myoclonic jerks. With very high doses, acidosis, hyperthermia, tachycardia, severe hypertension, seizures, and coma may occur; deaths are unusual.

Acute effects generally fade rapidly and many patients regain normal consciousness in 45 minutes to several hours.

Diagnosis

- Clinical evaluation

Diagnosis is usually clinical. Ketamine is not detected by routine urine drug screens; gas chromatography and mass spectroscopy testing can be requested when ketamine use must be confirmed.

Treatment

- Supportive measures

Patients should be kept in a quiet, calming environment and closely observed. Benzodiazepines can be used to manage agitation and seizures. Further treatment is rarely needed.

KORSAKOFF PSYCHOSIS

(Korsakoff Amnestic Syndrome)

Korsakoff psychosis is a late complication of persistent Wernicke encephalopathy and results in memory deficits, confusion, and behavioral changes.

Korsakoff psychosis occurs in 80% of untreated patients with Wernicke encephalopathy; severe alcoholism is a common underlying condition. Why Korsakoff psychosis develops in only some patients with Wernicke encephalopathy is unclear. A severe or repeated attack of postalcoholic DT can trigger Korsakoff psychosis whether or not a typical attack of Wernicke encephalopathy has occurred first.

Other triggers include head injury, subarachnoid hemorrhage, thalamic hemorrhage, thalamic ischemic stroke, and, infrequently, tumors affecting the paramedian posterior thalamic region (see p. 3117).

Symptoms and Signs

Immediate memory is severely affected; retrograde and anterograde amnesia occur in varying degrees. Patients tend to draw on memory of remote events, which appears to be less affected than memory of recent events. Disorientation to time is common. Emotional changes are common; they include apathy, blandness, or mild euphoria with little or no response to events, even frightening ones. Spontaneity and initiative may be decreased.

Confabulation is often a striking early feature. Bewildered patients unconsciously fabricate imaginary or confused accounts of events they cannot recall; these fabrications may be so convincing that the underlying disorder is not detected.

Diagnosis

- Clinical evaluation

Diagnosis is based on typical symptoms in patients with a history of severe chronic alcohol dependence. Other causes of symptoms (eg, CNS injury or infection) must be ruled out.

Treatment

- Thiamin and supportive care

Treatment consists of thiamin and adequate hydration.

MARCHIAFAVA-BIGNAMI DISEASE

Marchiafava-Bignami disease is a rare demyelination of the corpus callosum that occurs in chronic alcoholics, predominantly men.

(See also Alcohol Toxicity on p. 3231 and Withdrawal as well as Alcohol Use Disorder and Rehabilitation on p. 3233.)

Pathology and circumstances link this disorder to osmotic demyelination syndrome (previously called central pontine myelinolysis), of which it may be a variant. In Marchiafava Bignami disease, the speed of onset and the degree of physical findings vary.

Patients can present with acute, subacute, or chronic onset of mental status change varying from lethargy to coma, seizure, ocular movement dysfunction, memory loss, and gait disturbance.

Some patients recover over several months. Patients who present in coma and stupor have a mortality rate of about 20%.

There is no specific treatment, but supportive care typically includes vitamin supplementation (particularly of thiamin, folate, and other B vitamins) and correction of malnutrition.

MARIJUANA

(Cannabis)

Marijuana is a euphoriant that can cause sedation or dysphoria in some users. Overdose does not occur. Psychologic dependence can develop with chronic use, but very little physical dependence is clinically apparent. Withdrawal is uncomfortable but requires only supportive treatment.

(See also Cannabinoids, Synthetic on p. 3239.)

Marijuana is the most commonly used illicit drug; it is typically used episodically without evidence of social or psychologic dysfunction.

In the US, marijuana is commonly smoked in cigarettes, made from the flowering tops and leaves of the dried plant, or as hashish, the pressed resin of the plant. The legalization of recreational marijuana in 2010 in certain states in the US created a large market for marijuana products that are ingested, insufflated, vaporized, applied topically in tincture, lotion and spray form.

Dronabinol, a synthetic oral form of the active ingredient, Δ-9-tetrahydrocannabinol (THC), is used to treat nausea and vomiting associated with cancer chemotherapy and to enhance appetite in AIDS patients.

Pathophysiology

Δ-9-THC binds at cannabinoid receptors, which are present throughout the brain.

Chronic effects: Any drug that causes euphoria and diminishes anxiety can cause dependence, and marijuana is no exception. High-dose smokers can develop pulmonary symptoms (episodes of acute bronchitis, wheezing, coughing, and increased phlegm), and pulmonary function may be altered, manifested as large airway changes of unknown significance. However, even daily smokers do not develop obstructive airway disease.

Recent data suggest that heavy marijuana use is associated with significant cognitive impairment and anatomic changes in the hippocampus, particularly if marijuana use begins in adolescence.

There is no evidence of increased risk of head and neck or airway cancers, as there is with tobacco. A sense of diminished ambition and energy is often described.

The effect of prenatal marijuana use on neonates is not clear. Decreased fetal weight has been reported, but when all factors (eg, maternal alcohol and tobacco use) are accounted for, the effect on fetal weight appears less. However, because safety has not clearly been proved, marijuana should be avoided by pregnant women and those who are trying to become pregnant. THC is secreted in breast milk. Although harm to breastfed infants has not been shown, breastfeeding mothers, like pregnant women, should avoid using marijuana.

Symptoms and Signs

Intoxication and withdrawal are not life threatening.

Acute effects: Within minutes, smoking marijuana produces a dreamy state of consciousness in which ideas seem disconnected, unanticipated, and free-flowing. Time, color, and spatial perceptions may be altered. In general, intoxication consists of a feeling of euphoria and relaxation (a high). These effects last 4 to 6 h after inhalation.

Many of the other reported psychologic effects seem to be related to the setting in which the drug is taken. Anxiety, panic reactions, and paranoia have occurred, particularly in naive users. Marijuana may exacerbate or even precipitate psychotic symptoms in schizophrenics, even those being treated with antipsychotics.

Physical effects are mild in most patients. Tachycardia, conjunctival injection, and dry mouth occur regularly. Concentration, sense of time, fine coordination, depth perception, tracking, and reaction time can be impaired for up to 24 h—all hazardous in certain situations (eg, driving, operating heavy equipment). Appetite often increases.

Withdrawal: Cessation in frequent, heavy users can cause a mild withdrawal syndrome; the time of onset of withdrawal symptoms is variable but often begins about 12 h after the last use. Symptoms consist of insomnia, irritability, depression, nausea, and anorexia; symptoms peak at 2 to 3 days and last up to 7 days.

Cannabinoid hyperemesis syndrome is a recently described syndrome of cyclic episodes of nausea and vomiting in chronic cannabis users; symptoms usually resolve spontaneously within 48 h. Hot bathing ameliorates these symptoms and is a clinical clue to the diagnosis.

Diagnosis

- Clinical evaluation

Diagnosis is usually made clinically. Drug levels are not typically measured. Most routine urine drug screens include marijuana, but they may give false-positive or false-negative results.

Treatment

- Supportive measures

Treatment is usually unnecessary; for patients experiencing significant discomfort, treatment is supportive. Patients with cannabinoid hyperemesis syndrome may require IV fluids and antiemetics (anecdotal reports suggest haloperidol is effective).

Management of abuse typically consists of behavioral therapy in an outpatient drug treatment program.

METHYLENEDIOXYMETHAMPHETAMINE

(Ecstasy)

Methylenedioxymethamphetamine (MDMA; 3,4-methylene dioxymethamphetamine) is an amphetamine analog with stimulant and hallucinogenic effects.

MDMA acts primarily on neurons that produce and release serotonin, but it also affects dopaminergic neurons. MDMA is usually taken as a pill; effects begin 30 to 60 min after ingestion and typically last 4 to 6 h. MDMA is often used at dance clubs, concerts, and rave parties.

Symptoms and Signs

MDMA causes a state of excitement and disinhibition and accentuates physical sensation, empathy, and feelings of interpersonal closeness. Toxic effects are similar to those of the other amphetamines but are less common, perhaps because use is more likely to be intermittent. However, even with casual use, significant problems such as hyperthermia and centrally mediated hyponatremia may occur. The effects of intermittent, occasional use are uncertain. Rarely, fulminant hepatic failure occurs.

Chronic, repeated use may cause problems similar to those of amphetamines, including dependence. Some users develop paranoid psychosis. Cognitive decline may also occur with repeated, frequent use.

Diagnosis

- Clinical evaluation

MDMA may not be detected by routine urine immunoassay drug screens.

Treatment

- Symptomatic treatment for acute toxicities and dependency

Treatment for acute toxicity and dependency is similar to treatment for amphetamines, although treatment for acute overdose is less commonly needed.

OPIOID TOXICITY AND WITHDRAWAL

Opioids are euphoriants that, in high doses, cause sedation and respiratory depression. Respiratory depression can be managed with specific antidotes (eg, naloxone) or with endotracheal intubation and mechanical ventilation. Withdrawal manifests initially as anxiety and drug craving, followed by increased respiratory rate, diaphoresis, yawning, lacrimation, rhinorrhea, mydriasis, and stomach cramps and later by piloerection, tremors, muscle twitches, tachycardia, hypertension, fever, chills, anorexia, nausea, vomiting, and diarrhea. Diagnosis is clinical plus with urine tests. Withdrawal can be treated by substitution with a long-acting opioid (eg, methadone) or buprenorphine (a mixed opioid agonist-antagonist).

"Opioid" is a term for a number of natural substances (originally derived from the opium poppy) and their semisynthetic and synthetic analogues that bind to specific opioid receptors. Opioids, which are potent analgesics with a limited role in management of cough and diarrhea, are also common drugs of abuse because of their wide availability and euphoriant properties; see also Opioid Analgesics on p. 1969 and Opioid Use Disorder and Rehabilitation on p. 3246.

Pathophysiology

There are 3 main opioid receptors: delta, kappa, and mu. They occur throughout the CNS but particularly in areas and tracts associated with pain perception. Receptors are also located in some sensory nerves, on mast cells, and in some cells of the GI tract.

Opioid receptors are stimulated by endogenous endorphins, which generally produce analgesia and a sense of well-being. Opioids are used therapeutically, primarily as analgesics. Opioids vary in their receptor activity, and some (eg, buprenorphine) have combined agonist and antagonist actions. Compounds with pure antagonist activity (eg, naloxone, naltrexone) are available.

Exogenous opioids can be taken by almost any route: orally, intravenously, subcutaneously, rectally, through the nasal membranes, or inhaled as smoke. Peak effects are reached about 10 min after IV injection, 10 to 15 min after nasal insufflation, and 90 to 120 min after oral ingestion, although time to peak effects and duration of effect vary considerably depending on the specific drug.

Chronic effects: Tolerance develops quickly, with escalating dose requirements. Tolerance to the various effects of opioids frequently develops unevenly. Heroin users, for example, may become relatively tolerant to the drug's euphoric and respiratory depression effects but continue to have constricted pupils and constipation.

A minor opioid withdrawal syndrome may occur after only several days' use. Severity of the syndrome increases with the size of the opioid dose and the duration of dependence.

Long-term effects of the opioids themselves are minimal; even decades of methadone use appear to be well tolerated physiologically, although some long-term opioid users experience chronic constipation, excessive sweating, peripheral edema, drowsiness, and decreased libido. However, many long-term users who inject opioids have adverse effects from contaminants (eg, talc) and adulterants (eg, nonprescription stimulant drugs) and cardiac, pulmonary, and hepatic damage due to infections such as HIV infection and hepatitis B or C, which are spread by needle sharing and nonsterile injection techniques (see p. 3230).

Pregnancy: Use of opioids during pregnancy can result in opioid dependence in the fetus.

Symptoms and Signs

Acute effects: Acute opioid intoxication is characterized by euphoria and drowsiness. Mast cell effects (eg, flushing, itching) are common, particularly with morphine. GI effects include nausea, vomiting, decreased bowel sounds, and constipation.

Toxicity or overdose: The main toxic effect is decreased respiratory rate and depth, which can progress to apnea. Other complications (eg, pulmonary edema, which usually develops within minutes to a few hours after opioid overdose) and death result primarily from hypoxia. Pupils are miotic. Delirium, hypotension, bradycardia, decreased body temperature, and urinary retention may also occur.

Normeperidine, a metabolite of meperidine, accumulates with repeated use (including therapeutic); it stimulates the CNS and may cause seizure activity.

Serotonin syndrome occasionally occurs when fentanyl, meperidine, tramadol, or oxycodone is taken concomitantly with other drugs that have serotonergic effects (eg, SSRIs, MAOIs). This syndrome consists of one or more of the following:

- Hypertonia
- Tremor and hyperreflexia
- Spontaneous clonus
- Inducible clonus plus agitation or diaphoresis
- Ocular clonus plus agitation or diaphoresis
- Temperature > 38° plus ocular or inducible clonus

Withdrawal: The opioid withdrawal syndrome usually includes symptoms and signs of CNS hyperactivity. Onset and duration of the syndrome depend on the specific drug and its half-life. Symptoms may appear as early as 4 h after the last dose of heroin, peak within 48 to 72 h, and subside after about a week. Anxiety and a craving for the drug are followed by increased resting respiratory rate (> 16 breaths/min), usually with diaphoresis, yawning, lacrimation, rhinorrhea, mydriasis, and stomach cramps. Later, piloerection (gooseflesh), tremors, muscle twitching, tachycardia, hypertension, fever and chills, anorexia, nausea, vomiting, and diarrhea may develop.

Opioid withdrawal does not cause fever, seizures, or altered mental status. Although it may be distressingly symptomatic, opioid withdrawal is not fatal.

The withdrawal syndrome in people who were taking methadone (which has a long half-life) develops more slowly and may be less acutely severe than heroin withdrawal, although users may describe it as worse. Even after the withdrawal syndrome remits, lethargy, malaise, anxiety, and disturbed sleep may persist up to several months. Drug craving may persist for years.

Diagnosis

- Clinically determined

Diagnosis of opioid use is usually made clinically and sometimes with urine drug testing; laboratory tests are done as needed to identify drug-related complications. Drug levels are not measured.

Treatment

- Supportive therapy
- For opioid withdrawal, sometimes drug therapy (eg, with an opioid agonist, opioid agonist-antagonist, opioid antagonist, or clonidine)

Toxicity or overdose: Treatment to maintain the airway and support breathing is the first priority.

- Naloxone 0.4 mg IV
- Sometimes endotracheal intubation

Patients with spontaneous respirations can be treated with an opioid antagonist, typically naloxone 0.4 mg IV (for children < 20 kg, 0.1 mg/kg); naloxone has no agonist activity and a very short half-life (see Table 366–8 on p. 3069). Naloxone rapidly reverses unconsciousness and apnea due to an opioid in most patients. If IV access is not immediately available, IM, sc, or intranasal administration is also effective. A 2nd or 3rd dose can be given if there is no response within 2 min. Almost all patients respond to three 0.4-mg doses (nasal spray is a single dose inhaler with 4 mg). If they do not, the patient's condition is unlikely to be due to an opioid overdose, although massive opioid overdose may require higher doses of naloxone.

Because some patients become agitated, delirious, and combative as consciousness returns and because naloxone precipitates acute withdrawal, soft physical restraints should be applied before naloxone is given. To ameliorate withdrawal in long-term users, some experts suggest titrating very small doses of naloxone (0.1 mg) when the clinical situation does not require emergency total reversal.

Apneic patients can initially be treated with naloxone 2 mg IV if it can be given without delay; note that the dose is higher than for patients who are only somnolent. In some parts of the US and some countries, naloxone is available without a prescription so apneic patients can be rescued by friends or family. When naloxone is available and given quickly, endotracheal intubation is rarely required.

Patients should be observed for several hours after they regain spontaneous respirations. Because the duration of action of naloxone is less than that of some opioids, respiratory depression can recur within several hours of an overdose of methadone or sustained-released oxycodone or morphine tablets. Thus, the duration of observation should vary depending on the half-life of the opioid involved. Typically, patients who took longer-acting opioids should be admitted for observation; patients who took short-acting opioids may be discharged after several hours.

If respiratory depression recurs, naloxone should be readministered at an appropriate dose. The best dosing regimen is unclear. Many clinicians use repeat bolus doses of the same dose that was effective initially. Others use continuous naloxone infusion; they typically begin with about two thirds of the initially effective dose per hour. In theory, the continuous infusion should allow the dose to be titrated to maintain respiratory rate without triggering withdrawal; however, in practice this can be difficult to do and the patient's life is dependent on the security of the IV line—respiratory depression will quickly recur if the infusion is interrupted (eg, by the patient pulling out the IV). Both regimens require close monitoring, typically in an ICU.

Patients should be observed until no naloxone pharmacologic activity is present and they have no opioid-related symptoms. The serum half-life of naloxone is about 1 h, so an observation period of 2 to 3 h after use of naloxone should clarify disposition. The half-life of IV heroin is relatively short, and recurrent respiratory depression after naloxone reversal of IV heroin is rare.

Acute pulmonary edema is treated with supplemental oxygen and often noninvasive or invasive modalities of breathing support (eg, bilevel positive airway pressure [BiPAP], endotracheal intubation).

Withdrawal and detoxification: Treatment may involve several strategies:

- No treatment ("cold turkey")
- Substitution with methadone or buprenorphine
- Clonidine to relieve symptoms
- Long-term support and possibly naltrexone

The opioid withdrawal syndrome is self-limited and, although severely uncomfortable, is not life threatening. Minor metabolic and physical withdrawal effects may persist up to 6 mo. Withdrawal is typically managed in outpatient settings, unless patients require hospitalization for concurrent medical or mental health problems.

Options for management of withdrawal include allowing the process to run its course ("cold turkey") after the patient's last opioid dose and giving another opioid (substitution) that can be tapered on a controlled schedule. Clonidine can provide some symptom relief during withdrawal. The US Substance Abuse and Mental Health Services Administration (SAMHSA) provides information on medication-assisted treatment (see www.samhsa.gov).

Methadone substitution is the preferred method of managing opioid withdrawal for more seriously addicted patients because at appropriate doses, it has a long half-life and less profound sedation and euphoria. Any physician can initiate methadone substitution during hospitalization or for 3 days in an outpatient setting, but further treatment is continued in a licensed methadone treatment program. Methadone is given orally in the smallest amount that prevents severe but not necessarily all symptoms of withdrawal. Typical dose range is 15 to 30 mg once/day; doses ≥ 25 mg can result in dangerous levels of sedation in patients who have not developed tolerance.

Symptom scales are available for estimating the appropriate dose. Higher doses should be given when evidence of withdrawal is observed. After the appropriate dose has been established, it should be reduced progressively by 10 to 20%/day unless the decision is made to continue the drug at a stable dose (methadone maintenance). During tapering of the drug, patients commonly become anxious and request more of the drug.

Methadone withdrawal for addicts who have been in a methadone maintenance program may be particularly difficult because their dose of methadone may be as high as 100 mg once/day; in these patients, the dose should be gradually reduced to 60 mg once/day over several weeks before attempting complete detoxification.

Methadone has been reported to be associated with QTc prolongation and serious arrhythmias including torsades de pointes (see p. 644). Thus, it should be used very carefully with appropriate patient evaluation and monitoring during initiation and dose titration.

Buprenorphine, a mixed opioid agonist-antagonist usually given sublingually, also has been successfully used in withdrawal. It is available in a combination formulation with naloxone to prevent diversion to IV use. The first dose is given when the first signs of withdrawal appear. The dose needed to effectively control severe symptoms is titrated as quickly as possible; sublingual doses of 8 to 16 mg/day are typically used. Buprenorphine is then tapered over several weeks. The SAMHSA website provides additional information on buprenorphine and the training required to qualify for a waiver to prescribe the drug. Protocols for using buprenorphine for detoxification or maintenance therapy are available for download at the US Department of Health and Human Services web site (www.hhs.gov).

Clonidine, a centrally acting adrenergic drug, can suppress autonomic symptoms and signs of opioid withdrawal. Starting dosages are 0.1 mg po q 4 to 6 h and may be increased to 0.2 mg po q 4 to 6 h as tolerated. Clonidine can cause hypotension and drowsiness, and its withdrawal may precipitate restlessness, insomnia, irritability, tachycardia, and headache.

Rapid and ultrarapid protocols have been evaluated for managing withdrawal and detoxification. In rapid protocols, combinations of naloxone, nalmefene, and naltrexone are used to induce withdrawal, and clonidine and various adjuvant drugs are used to suppress withdrawal symptoms. Some rapid protocols use buprenorphine to suppress opioid withdrawal symptoms. Ultrarapid protocols may use large boluses of naloxone and diuretics to enhance excretion of the opioids while patients are under general anesthesia; these ultrarapid protocols are not recommended because they have a high risk of complications and no substantial additional benefit.

Clinicians must understand that detoxification is not treatment per se. It is only the first step and must be followed by an ongoing treatment program, which may involve various kinds of counseling and possibly nonopioid antagonists (eg, naltrexone).

OPIOID USE DISORDER AND REHABILITATION

"Opioid" is a term for a number of natural substances (originally derived from the opium poppy) and their semisynthetic and synthetic analogues that bind to specific opioid receptors. Opioids are potent analgesics that are also common drugs of abuse because of their wide availability and euphoriant properties. See also Opioid Analgesics on p. 1969 and Opioid Toxicity and Withdrawal on p. 3244.

Heroin is commonly abused, and abuse of prescription analgesic opioids (eg, morphine, oxycodone, hydrocodone, fentanyl) is increasing; some of the increase is due to people who began taking them for legitimate medical purposes. Patients with chronic pain requiring long-term use should not be routinely labeled addicts, although they commonly have tolerance and physical dependence. People who take opioids parenterally are at risk of all the complications of injection drug use.

Opioid use disorder: Opioid use disorder involves compulsive, long-term self-administration of opioids for nonmedical purposes. The *Diagnostic and Statistical Manual of Mental Disorders,* Fifth Edition (DSM-5) considers opioid use disorder to be present if the pattern of use causes clinically significant impairment or distress as manifested by the presence of ≥ 2 of the following over a 12-mo period:

- Taking opioids in larger amounts or for a longer time than intended
- Persistently desiring or unsuccessfully attempting to decrease opioid use
- Spending a great deal of time obtaining, using, or recovering from opioids
- Craving opioids
- Failing repeatedly to meet obligations at work, home, or school because of opioids
- Continuing to use opioids despite having recurrent social or interpersonal problems because of opioids
- Giving up important social, work, or recreational activities because of opioids
- Using opioids in physically hazardous situations
- Continuing to use opioids despite having a physical or mental disorder caused or worsened by opioids
- Having tolerance to opioids (not a criterion when use is medically appropriate)
- Having opioid withdrawal symptoms or taking opioids because of withdrawal

Treatment

- For severe, relapsing dependence, maintenance preferred to opioid withdrawal and detoxification

- For maintenance, buprenorphine or methadone
- Ongoing counseling and support

Physicians must be fully aware of federal, state, and local regulations concerning use of an opioid drug to treat an addict. To comply, physicians must establish the existence of physical opioid dependence. In the US, treatment is further complicated by negative societal attitudes toward addicts (including the attitudes of law enforcement officers, physicians, and other health care practitioners) and toward treatment programs, which some view as abetting drug consumption. In most cases, physicians should refer opioid-dependent patients to specialized treatment centers. If trained to do so, physicians may provide office-based treatment for selected patients.

In European countries, access to methadone or buprenorphine maintenance programs and alternative maintenance strategies is easier, and the stigma attached to prescribing psychoactive drugs is less.

Maintenance: Long-term maintenance using an oral opioid such as methadone or buprenorphine (an opioid agonist-antagonist) is an alternative to opioid substitution with tapering. Oral opioids suppress withdrawal symptoms and drug craving without providing a significant high or oversedation and, by eliminating the supply problems of addicts, enable them to be socially productive.

In the US, thousands of opioid addicts are in licensed methadone maintenance programs. For many, such programs work. However, because the participants continue to take an opioid, many people in society disapprove of these programs.

Eligibility criteria include the following:

- A positive drug screen for opioids
- Physical dependence for > 1 yr of continuous opioid use or intermittent use for even longer
- Evidence of withdrawal or physical findings confirming drug use

Clinicians and patients need to decide whether a withdrawal (detoxification) or opioid maintenance approach is indicated. Generally, patients with severe, chronic, relapsing dependence do much better with opioid maintenance. Withdrawal and detoxification, although effective in the short term, have poor outcomes in patients with severe opioid dependence. Whichever course is chosen, it must be accompanied by ongoing counseling and supportive measures.

Methadone is commonly used. Physicians can begin the substitution, but then use of methadone must be supervised in a licensed methadone treatment program.

Buprenorphine is being used increasingly for maintenance. Its effectiveness is comparable to that of methadone, and because it blocks receptors, it inhibits concomitant illicit use of heroin or other opioids. Buprenorphine can be prescribed for office-based treatment by specially trained physicians, including primary care physicians, who have received the required training and have been certified by the federal government.

The typical dosage of buprenorphine is an 8- or 16-mg sublingual tablet once/day. Many patients prefer this option because it eliminates the need for attending a methadone clinic. Buprenorphine is also available in combination with naloxone; the addition of naloxone may further discourage illicit opioid use. The combination formulation is used in office-based treatment.

The SAMHSA web site (www.samhsa.gov) provides additional information on buprenorphine and the training required to qualify for a waiver to prescribe the drug. Protocols for using buprenorphine for detoxification or maintenance therapy are available for download at the US Department of Health and Human Services web site.

Naltrexone, an opioid antagonist, blocks the effects of heroin. The usual dosage is 50 mg po once/day or 350 mg/wk po in 2 or 3 divided doses. A once-monthly depot IM formulation is also available. Because naltrexone is an opioid antagonist and has no direct agonist effects on opioid receptors, naltrexone is often unacceptable to opioid-dependent patients, especially those who have chronic, relapsing opioid dependence. For such patients, opioid maintenance treatment is much more effective.

Naltrexone may be useful for patients with less severe dependence, early-stage opioid dependence, and strong motivation to remain abstinent. For example, opioid-dependent health care practitioners whose future employment is at risk if opioid use persists may be excellent candidates for naltrexone.

Levomethadyl acetate (LAAM), a longer-acting opioid related to methadone, is no longer used because it causes QT-interval abnormalities in some patients. LAAM could be used only 3 times/wk, thereby reducing the expense and problems of daily client visits or take-home drugs. A dose of 100 mg 3 times/wk is comparable to methadone 80 mg once/day.

Support: Most treatment of opioid dependence occurs in outpatient settings, typically in licensed opioid maintenance programs but increasingly in physician offices.

The therapeutic community concept, pioneered by Daytop Village and Phoenix House, involves nondrug treatment in communal residential centers, where drug users receive training, education, and redirection to help them build new lives. Residency is usually 15 mo. These communities have helped, even transformed, some users. However, initial dropout rates are extremely high. Questions of how well these communities work, how many will be opened, and how much funding society will give remain unanswered.

VOLATILE NITRITES

Nitrites (poppers, as amyl, butyl, or isobutyl nitrite, sold with street names such as Locker Room and Rush) may be inhaled to enhance sexual pleasure. There is little evidence of significant risk, although nitrites and nitrates cause vasodilation, with brief hypotension, dizziness, and flushing, followed by reflex tachycardia (see Table 366–8 on p. 3069). Nitrites may cause methemoglobinemia. However, they are dangerous when combined with phosphodiesterase-inhibiting drugs used for erectile enhancement; the combination can lead to severe hypotension and death.

VOLATILE SOLVENTS

Inhalation of volatile industrial solvents and solvents from aerosol sprays can cause a state of intoxication. Chronic use can result in neuropathies and hepatotoxicity.

Use of volatile solvents (eg, acetates, alcohol, chloroform, ether, aliphatic and aromatic hydrocarbons, chlorinated hydrocarbons, ketones) continues to be an endemic problem among adolescents. Common commercial products (eg, glues and adhesives, paints, paint strippers, cleaning fluids) contain these substances; thus, children and adolescents can easily obtain them. About 10% of adolescents in the US have reportedly inhaled volatile solvents. Typically, a solvent-soaked rag is placed in a bag or container that is held to the mouth and nose; the naturally volatilized vapors are then inhaled (huffing, sniffing).

Volatile solvents temporarily stimulate the CNS before depressing it. Partial tolerance and psychologic dependence develop with frequent use, but a withdrawal syndrome does not occur.

Symptoms and Signs

Acute effects: Acute symptoms of dizziness, drowsiness, slurred speech, and unsteady gait occur early. Impulsiveness, excitement, and irritability may occur. As effects on the CNS increase, illusions, hallucinations, and delusions develop. Users experience a euphoric, dreamy high, culminating in a short period of sleep. Delirium with confusion, psychomotor clumsiness, emotional lability, and impaired thinking develop. The intoxicated state may last from minutes to > 1 h.

Sudden death can result from respiratory arrest or airway occlusion due to CNS depression or arrhythmias ("sudden sniffing death," perhaps due to myocardial sensitization).

Methylene chloride (dichlormethane) is metabolized to carbon monoxide and inhalation of this product can cause delayed onset of symptoms of carbon monoxide poisoning; symptoms may persist for a prolonged period.

Methanol inhalation may cause metabolic acidosis and retinal injury.

Chronic effects: Chronic inhalation of volatile hydrocarbons may irritate the skin around the mouth and nose (huffer's eczema).

Complications of chronic use may result from the effect of the solvent or from other toxic ingredients (eg, lead in gasoline). Carbon tetrachloride may cause a syndrome of hepatic and renal failure. Toluene may cause degeneration of CNS white matter, renal tubular acidosis and hypokalemia. Injuries to brain, peripheral nerves, liver, kidneys, and bone marrow may result from heavy exposure or hypersensitivity.

Inhalant abuse during pregnancy can cause premature birth and fetal solvent syndrome, which has features similar to those of fetal alcohol syndrome.

Diagnosis

- Clinical evaluation

Volatile solvents are not detected by routine drug screens. Many of them and their metabolites can be detected by gas chromatography at specialized laboratories, but such testing is rarely necessary or indicated except for forensic purposes.

Treatment

- Supportive care

Treatment for acute toxicity is supportive. Use of catecholamines (eg, for hypotension) should be avoided because of possible solvent-induced myocardial sensitization. Treatment of dysrhythmias is challenging and there is no specific treatment guideline. Beta blockers may have some benefit.

Treatment of solvent-dependent adolescents is difficult, and relapse is frequent. However, most users stop solvent use by the end of adolescence. Intensive attempts to broadly improve patients' social skills and status in family, school, and society may help. For symptoms and treatment of poisoning with specific solvents, see Table 366–8 on p. 3069.

WERNICKE ENCEPHALOPATHY

Wernicke encephalopathy is characterized by acute onset of confusion, nystagmus, partial ophthalmoplegia, and ataxia due to thiamin deficiency. Diagnosis is primarily clinical. The disorder may remit with treatment, persist, or degenerate into Korsakoff psychosis. Treatment consists of thiamin and supportive measures.

Wernicke encephalopathy results from inadequate intake or absorption of thiamin plus continued carbohydrate ingestion. Severe alcoholism is a common underlying condition. Excessive alcohol intake interferes with thiamin absorption from the GI tract and hepatic storage of thiamin; the poor nutrition associated with alcoholism often precludes adequate thiamin intake.

Wernicke encephalopathy may also result from other conditions that cause prolonged undernutrition or vitamin deficiency (eg, recurrent dialysis, hyperemesis, starvation, gastric plication, cancer, AIDS). Loading carbohydrates in patients with thiamin deficiency (ie, refeeding after starvation or giving IV dextrose-containing solutions to high-risk patients) can trigger Wernicke encephalopathy.

Not all thiamin-deficient alcohol abusers develop Wernicke encephalopathy, suggesting that other factors may be involved. Genetic abnormalities that result in a defective form of transketolase, an enzyme that processes thiamin, may be involved.

Characteristically, CNS lesions are symmetrically distributed around the 3rd ventricle, aqueduct, and 4th ventricle. Changes in the mamillary bodies, dorsomedial thalamus, locus ceruleus, periaqueductal gray matter, ocular motor nuclei, and vestibular nuclei are common.

Symptoms and Signs

Clinical changes occur suddenly. Oculomotor abnormalities, including horizontal and vertical nystagmus and partial ophthalmoplegias (eg, lateral rectus palsy, conjugate gaze palsies), are common. Pupils may be abnormal; they are usually sluggish or unequal.

Vestibular dysfunction without hearing loss is common, and the oculovestibular reflex may be impaired. Gait ataxia may result from vestibular disturbances, cerebellar dysfunction, and/or polyneuropathy; gait is wide-based and slow, with short-spaced steps.

Global confusion is often present; it is characterized by profound disorientation, indifference, inattention, drowsiness, or stupor. Peripheral nerve pain thresholds are often elevated, and many patients develop severe autonomic dysfunction characterized by sympathetic hyperactivity (eg, tremor, agitation) or hypoactivity (eg, hypothermia, postural hypotension, syncope). In untreated patients, stupor may progress to coma, then to death.

Diagnosis

- Clinical evaluation

There are no specific diagnostic studies. Diagnosis is clinical and depends on recognition of underlying undernutrition or vitamin deficiency. There are no characteristic abnormalities in CSF, evoked potentials, brain imaging, or EEG. However, these tests, as well as laboratory tests (eg, blood tests, glucose, CBC, liver function tests, ABG measurements, toxicology screening), should typically be done to rule out other etiologies. Thiamin levels are not routinely measured, because serum thiamin levels do not always reflect CSF levels and normal serum levels do not exclude the diagnosis.

Prognosis

Prognosis depends on timely diagnosis. If begun in time, treatment may correct all abnormalities. Ocular symptoms usually begin to abate within 24 h after early thiamin administration. Ataxia and confusion may persist days to months. Memory and learning impairment may not resolve completely. Untreated, the disorder progresses; mortality is 10 to 20%. Of surviving patients, 80% develop Korsakoff psychosis; the combination is called Wernicke-Korsakoff syndrome.

Treatment

- Parenteral thiamin
- Parenteral magnesium

Treatment consists of immediate administration of thiamin 100 mg IV or IM, continued daily for at least 3 to 5 days. Magnesium is a necessary cofactor in thiamin-dependent metabolism, and hypomagnesemia should be corrected using magnesium sulfate 1 to 2 g IM or IV q 6 to 8 h or magnesium oxide 400 to 800 mg po once/day. Supportive treatment includes rehydration, correction of electrolyte abnormalities, and general nutritional therapy, including multivitamins. Patients with advanced disease require hospitalization. Alcohol cessation is mandatory.

Because Wernicke encephalopathy is preventable, all undernourished patients should be treated with parenteral thiamin (typically 100 mg IM followed by 50 mg po once/day) plus vitamin B_{12} and folate (1 mg po once/day for both), particularly if IV dextrose is necessary. Thiamin is also prudent before any treatment is begun in patients who present with a reduced level of consciousness. Patients who are undernourished should continue to receive thiamin as outpatients.

388 Rehabilitation

Rehabilitation aims to facilitate recovery from loss of function. Loss may be due to fracture, amputation, stroke or another neurologic disorder, arthritis, cardiac impairment, or prolonged deconditioning (eg, after some disorders and surgical procedures). Rehabilitation may involve physical, occupational, and speech therapy; psychologic counseling; and social services. For some patients, the goal is complete recovery with full, unrestricted function; for others, it is recovery of the ability to do as many activities of daily living (ADLs) as possible. Results of rehabilitation depend on the nature of the loss and the patient's motivation. Progress may be slow for elderly patients and for patients who lack muscle strength or motivation.

Rehabilitation may begin in an acute care hospital. Rehabilitation hospitals or units usually provide the most extensive and intensive care; they should be considered for patients who have good potential for recovery and can participate in and tolerate aggressive therapy (generally, ≥ 3 h/day). Many nursing homes have less intensive programs (generally, 1 to 3 h/day, up to 5 days/wk) that last longer and thus are better suited to patients less able to tolerate therapy (eg, frail or elderly patients). Less varied and less frequent rehabilitation programs may be offered in outpatient settings or at home and are appropriate for many patients. However, outpatient rehabilitation can be relatively intensive (several hours/day up to 5 days/wk).

An interdisciplinary approach is best because disability can lead to various problems (eg, depression, lack of motivation to regain lost function, financial problems). Thus, patients may require psychologic intervention and help from social workers or mental health practitioners. Also, family members may need help learning how to adjust to the patient's disability and how to help the patient.

Referral: To initiate formal rehabilitation therapy, a physician must write a referral/prescription to a physiatrist, therapist, or rehabilitation center. The referral/prescription should state the diagnosis and goal of therapy. The diagnosis may be specific (eg, after left-sided stroke, residual right-sided deficits in upper and lower extremities) or functional (eg, generalized weakness due to bed rest). Goals should be as specific as possible (eg, training to use a prosthetic limb, maximizing general muscle strength and overall endurance). Although vague instructions (eg, physical therapy to evaluate and treat) are sometimes accepted, they are not in the patients' best interests and may be rejected with a request for more specific instructions. Physicians unfamiliar with writing referrals for rehabilitation can consult a physiatrist.

Goals of therapy: Initial evaluation sets goals for restoring mobility and functions needed to do ADLs, which include caring for self (eg, grooming, bathing, dressing, feeding, toileting), cooking, cleaning, shopping, managing drugs, managing finances, using the telephone, and traveling. The referring physician and rehabilitation team determine which activities are achievable and which are essential for the patient's independence. Once ADL function is maximized, goals that can help improve quality of life are added.

Patients improve at different rates. Some courses of therapy last only a few weeks; others last longer. Some patients who have completed initial therapy need additional therapy.

Patient and caregiver issues: Patient and family education is an important part of the rehabilitation process, particularly when the patient is discharged into the community. Often, the nurse is the team member primarily responsible for this education. Patients arc taught how to maintain newly regained functions and how to reduce the risk of accidents (eg, falls, cuts, burns) and secondary disabilities. Family members are taught how to help the patient be as independent as possible, so that they do not overprotect the patient (leading to decreased functional status and increased dependence) or neglect the patient's primary needs (leading to feelings of rejection, which may cause depression or interfere with physical functioning).

Emotional support from family members and friends is essential. It may take many forms. Spiritual support and counseling by peers or by religious advisors can be indispensable for some patients.

Geriatric Rehabilitation

Disorders requiring rehabilitation (eg, stroke, MI, hip fracture, limb amputation) are common among elderly patients. The elderly are also more likely to have become deconditioned before the acute problem that necessitates rehabilitation.

The elderly, even if cognitively impaired, can benefit from rehabilitation. Age alone is not a reason to postpone or deny rehabilitation. However, the elderly may recover more slowly because of a reduced ability to adapt to a changing environment, including

- Physical inactivity
- Lack of endurance
- Depression or dementia

- Decreased muscle strength, joint mobility, coordination, or agility
- Impaired balance

Programs designed specifically for the elderly are preferable because the elderly often have different goals, require less intensive rehabilitation, and need different types of care than do younger patients. In age-segregated programs, elderly patients are less likely to compare their progress with that of younger patients and to become discouraged, and the social work aspects of postdischarge care can be more readily integrated. Some programs are designed for specific clinical situations (eg, recovery from hip fracture surgery); patients with similar conditions can work together toward common goals by encouraging each other and reinforcing the rehabilitation training.

PHYSICAL THERAPY

Physical therapy (PT) aims to improve joint and muscle function (eg, range of motion, strength) and thus improve the patient's ability to stand, balance, walk, and climb stairs. For example, physical therapy is usually used to train lower-extremity amputees. On the other hand, occupational therapy focuses on self-care activities and improvement of fine motor coordination of muscles and joints, particularly in the upper extremities.

Range of motion: Limited range of motion impairs function and tends to cause pain and to predispose patients to pressure ulcers. Range of motion should be evaluated with a goniometer before therapy and regularly thereafter (for normal values, see Table 388–1).

Range-of-motion exercises stretch stiff joints. Stretching is usually most effective and least painful when tissue temperature is raised to about 43° C (see p. 3255). There are several types:

- **Active:** This type is used when patients can exercise without assistance; patients must move their limbs themselves.
- **Active assistive:** This type is used when muscles are weak or when joint movement causes discomfort; patients must move their limbs, but a therapist helps them do so.
- **Passive:** This type is used when patients cannot actively participate in exercise; no effort is required from them.

Strength and conditioning: Many exercises aim to improve muscle strength (for grading muscle strength, see Table 388–2). Muscle strength may be increased with progressive resistive exercise. When a muscle is very weak, gravity alone is sufficient resistance. When muscle strength becomes fair, additional manual or mechanical resistance (eg, weights, spring tension) is added.

General conditioning exercises combine various exercises to treat the effects of debilitation, prolonged bed rest, or immobilization. The goals are to reestablish hemodynamic balance, increase cardiorespiratory capacity and endurance, and maintain range of motion and muscle strength.

For the elderly, the purpose of these exercises is both to strengthen muscles enough to function normally and possibly to regain normal strength for age.

Proprioceptive neuromuscular facilitation: This technique helps promote neuromuscular activity in patients who have upper motor neuron damage with spasticity; it enables them to feel muscle contraction and helps maintain the affected joint's range of motion. For example, applying strong resistance to the left elbow flexor (biceps) of patients with right hemiplegia causes the hemiplegic biceps to contract, flexing the right elbow.

Table 388–1. NORMAL VALUES FOR RANGE OF MOTION OF JOINTS*

JOINT	MOTION	RANGE (°)
Hip	Flexion	0–125
	Extension	115–0
	Hyperextension†	0–15
	Abduction	0–45
	Adduction	45–0
	Lateral rotation	0–45
	Medial rotation	0–45
Knee	Flexion	0–130
	Extension	120–0
Ankle	Plantar flexion	0–50
	Dorsiflexion	0–20
Foot	Inversion	0–35
	Eversion	0–25
Metatarsophalangeal joints	Flexion	0–30
	Extension	0–80
Interphalangeal joints of toes	Flexion	0–50
	Extension	50–0
Shoulder	Flexion to 90°	0–90
	Extension	0–50
	Abduction to 90°	0–90
	Adduction	90–0
	Lateral rotation	0–90
	Medial rotation	0–90
Elbow	Flexion	0–160
	Extension	145–0
	Pronation	0–90
	Supination	0–90
Wrist	Flexion	0–90
	Extension	0–70
	Abduction	0–25
	Adduction	0–65
Metacarpophalangeal joints	Abduction	0–25
	Adduction	20–0
	Flexion	0–90
	Extension	0–30
Interphalangeal proximal joints of fingers	Flexion	0–120
	Extension	120–0
Interphalangeal distal joints of fingers	Flexion	0–80
	Extension	80–0
Metacarpophalangeal joint of thumb	Abduction	0–50
	Adduction	40–0
	Flexion	0–70
	Extension	60–0
Interphalangeal joint of thumb	Flexion	0–90
	Extension	90–0

*Ranges are for people of all ages. Age-specific ranges have not been established; however, values are typically lower in fully functional elderly people than in younger people.

†Extension beyond midline.

Table 388–2. GRADES OF MUSCLE STRENGTH

GRADE	DESCRIPTION
5 or N	Full range of motion against gravity and full resistance for the patient's size, age, and sex
N–	Slight weakness
G+	Moderate weakness
4 or G	Movement against gravity and moderate resistance at least 10 times without fatigue
F+	Movement against gravity several times or mild resistance one time
3 or F	Full range against gravity
F–	Movement against gravity and complete range of motion one time
P+	Full range of motion with gravity eliminated but some resistance applied
2 or P	Full range of motion with gravity eliminated
P–	Incomplete range of motion with gravity eliminated
1 or T	Evidence of contraction (visible or palpable) but no joint movement
0	No palpable or visible contraction and no joint movement

N = normal; G = good; F = fair; P = poor; T = trace.

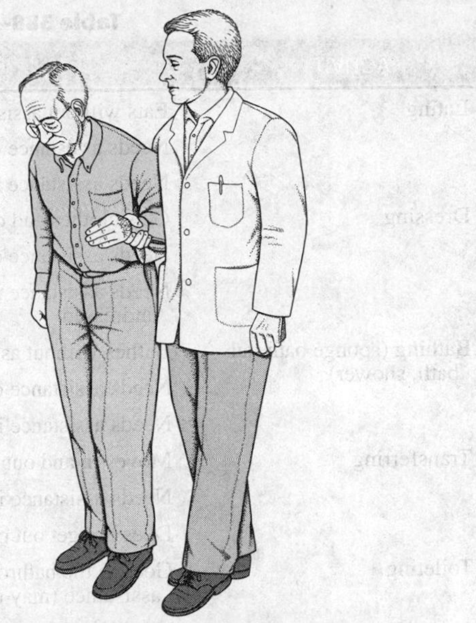

Fig. 388–1. Supporting a patient during ambulation. Aides should place one arm under that of the patient, gently grasp the patient's forearm, and lock their arm firmly under the patient's axilla. Thus, if the patient starts to fall, aides can provide support at the patient's shoulder. If a patient is wearing a waist belt, aides use their free hand to grasp the belt.

Coordination exercises: These task-oriented exercises improve motor skills by repeating a movement that works more than one joint and muscle simultaneously (eg, picking up an object, touching a body part).

Ambulation exercises: Before proceeding to ambulation exercises, patients must be able to balance in a standing position. Balancing exercise is usually done using parallel bars with a therapist standing in front of or directly behind a patient. While holding the bars, patients shift weight from side to side and from forward to backward. Once patients can balance safely, they can proceed to ambulation exercises.

Ambulation is often a major goal of rehabilitation. If individual muscles are weak or spastic, an orthosis (eg, a brace) may be used. Ambulation exercises are commonly started using parallel bars; as patients progress, they use a walker, crutches, or cane and then walk without devices. Some patients wear an assistive belt used by the therapist to help prevent falls. Anyone assisting patients with ambulation should know how to correctly support them (see Fig. 388–1).

As soon as patients can walk safely on level surfaces, they can start training to climb stairs or to step over curbs if either skill is needed. Patients who use walkers must learn special techniques for climbing stairs and stepping over curbs. When climbing stairs, ascent starts with the better leg, and descent starts with the affected leg (ie, good leads up; bad leads down). Before patients are discharged, the social worker or physical therapist should arrange to have secure handrails installed along all stairs in the patients' home.

Transfer training: Patients who cannot transfer independently from bed to chair, chair to commode, or chair to a standing position usually require attendants 24 h/day. Adjusting the heights of commodes and chairs may help. Sometimes assistive devices are useful; eg, people who have difficulty standing from a seated position may benefit from a chair with a raised seat or a self-lifting chair.

OCCUPATIONAL THERAPY

Occupational therapy (OT) focuses on self-care activities and improvement of fine motor coordination of muscles and joints, particularly in the upper extremities. Unlike physical therapy, which focuses on muscle strength and joint range of motion, OT focuses on activities of daily living (ADLs) because they are the cornerstone of independent living. Basic ADLs (BADLs) include eating, dressing, bathing, grooming, toileting, and transferring (ie, moving between surfaces such as the bed, chair, and bathtub or shower). Instrumental ADLs (IADLs) require more complex cognitive functioning than BADLs. IADLs include preparing meals; communicating by telephone, writing, or computer; managing finances and daily drug regimens; cleaning; doing laundry, food shopping, and other errands; traveling as a pedestrian or by public transportation; and driving. Driving is particularly complex, requiring integration of visual, physical, and cognitive tasks.

Evaluation: OT can be initiated when a physician writes a referral for rehabilitation, which is similar to writing a prescription. The referral should be detailed, including a brief history of the problem (eg, type and duration of the disorder or injury) and establishing the goals of therapy (eg, training in IADLs). Lists of occupational therapists may be obtained from a patient's insurance carrier, a local hospital, the telephone book, state occupational training organizations, or the web site of the American Occupational Therapy Association (www.aota.org).

Patients are evaluated for limitations that require intervention and for strengths that can be used to compensate for weaknesses. Limitations may involve motor function, sensation, cognition, or psychosocial function. Examiners determine which activities (eg, work, leisure, social, learning) patients want or need help with. Patients may need help with a general type of activity (eg, social) or a specific activity (eg, attending church), or they may

Table 388–3. KATZ ACTIVITIES OF DAILY LIVING SCALE

ACTIVITY	ITEM	SCORE
Eating	Eats without assistance	2
	Needs assistance only in cutting meat or buttering bread	1
	Needs assistance in eating or is fed intravenously	0
Dressing	Gets clothes and dresses without assistance	2
	Needs assistance only in tying shoes	1
	Needs assistance in getting clothes or in getting dressed or stays partly or completely undressed	0
Bathing (sponge bath, tub bath, shower)	Bathes without assistance	2
	Needs assistance only in bathing one part of the body (eg, back)	1
	Needs assistance in bathing more than one part of the body or does not bathe	0
Transferring	Moves in and out of bed and chair without assistance (may use cane or walker)	2
	Needs assistance in moving in and out of bed or chair	1
	Does not get out of bed	0
Toileting	Goes to the bathroom, uses toilet, cleans self, arranges clothes, and returns without assistance (may use cane or walker for support and may use bedpan or urinal at night)	2
	Needs assistance in going to the bathroom, using toilet, cleaning self, arranging clothes, or returning	1
	Does not go to the bathroom to relieve bladder or bowel	0
Continence	Controls bladder and bowel completely (without occasional accidents)	2
	Occasionally loses control of bladder and bowel	1
	Needs supervision to control bladder or bowel, requires use of a catheter, or is incontinent	0

Modified from Katz S, Downs TD, Cash HR, et al: Progress in the development of the index of ADL. *Gerontologist* 10:20–30, 1970. Copyright The Gerontological Society of America.

need to be motivated to do an activity. Therapists may use an assessment instrument to help in the evaluation. One of the many functional assessment instruments is described in Table 388–3. Patients are asked about their social and family roles, habits, and social support systems. The availability of resources (eg, community programs and services, private attendants) should be determined.

Occupational therapists may also assess the home for hazards and make recommendations to ensure home safety (eg, removing throw rugs, increasing hallway and kitchen lighting, moving a night table within reach of the bed, placing a family picture on a door to help patients recognize their room).

Determining when driving is a risk and whether driver retraining is indicated is best done by occupational therapists with specialized training. Information that can help elderly drivers and their caregivers in coping with changing driving abilities is available from the American Occupational Therapy Association and the American Association for Retired Persons.

Interventions: OT may consist of one consultation or frequent sessions of varying intensity. Sessions may occur in various settings:

- Acute care, rehabilitation, outpatient, adult day care, skilled nursing, or long-term care facilities
- The home (as part of home health care)
- Senior housing developments
- Life-care or assisted-living communities

Occupational therapists develop an individualized program to enhance patients' motor, cognitive, communication, and interaction capabilities. The goal is not only to help patients do ADLs but also to do appropriate preferred leisure activities and to foster and maintain social integration and participation.

Before developing a program, a therapist observes patients doing each activity of the daily routine to learn what is needed to ensure safe, successful completion of the activities. Therapists can then recommend ways to eliminate or reduce maladaptive patterns and to establish routines that promote function and health. Specific performance-oriented exercises are also recommended. Therapists emphasize that exercises must be practiced and motivate patients to do so by focusing on exercise as a means of becoming more active at home and in the community.

Patients are taught creative ways to facilitate social activities (eg, how to get to museums or church without driving, how to use hearing aids or other assistive communication devices in different settings, how to travel safely with or without a cane or walker). Therapists may suggest new activities (eg, volunteering in foster grandparent programs, schools, or hospitals).

Patients are taught strategies to compensate for their limitations (eg, to sit when gardening). The therapist may identify various assistive devices that can help patients do many activities of daily living (see Table 388–4). Most occupational therapists can select wheelchairs appropriate for patients' needs and

Table 388–4. ASSISTIVE DEVICES

PROBLEM	DEVICE
Balance problems or weak legs	Grab bars on the side and back of the bathtub or toilet
Inability to stand for a long time because of weakness or dizziness	Shower chairs
Balance problems or difficulty getting in and out of the bathtub because of pain or weakness in the legs	Bathtub benches
Difficulty standing up	Raised toilet seats and chair leg extenders (which make the chair's seat higher)
Weak grip	Eating utensils, shoehorns, and other tools with large, built-up handles
Tremors	Weighted eating utensils, cups with lids, and swivel spoons
Coordination problems	Plates with rims and rubber grips (to prevent slipping)
Difficulty reaching or limited movement	Grabbers that can pick items off the floor or from a shelf
Hand problems	Tools with spring-loaded or electronic controls
Limited movement or coordination	Devices that turn electrical appliances (eg, lamps, radios, fans) on or off at the sound of the voice
Paralysis of arms or legs or other disorders that greatly limit function	Computer-assisted devices
Impaired vision	Larger dials on telephones and large-print or audio books
Hearing loss	Telephones and doorbells that display a flashing light when they ring
Difficulty remembering	Automatic dialing on a telephone, devices that remind people when to take a drug, and pocket devices that record and play back messages (reminders, instructions, lists) at the appropriate time

provide training for upper-extremity amputees. Occupational therapists may construct and fit devices to prevent contractures and treat other functional disorders.

SPEECH THERAPY

Speech therapists can identify the most effective methods of communication for patients who have aphasia, dysarthria, or verbal apraxia or who have had a laryngectomy:

- Expressive aphasia: A letter or picture board
- Mild to moderate dysarthria or apraxia: Breathing and muscle control plus repetition exercises
- Severe dysarthria or apraxia: An electronic device with a keyboard and message display (print or screen)
- Postlaryngectomy: A new way to produce a voice (eg, by an electrolarynx—see p. 850)

Speech therapists may also assist in the diagnosis and treatment of swallowing disorders.

THERAPEUTIC AND ASSISTIVE DEVICES

Orthoses provide support for damaged joints, ligaments, tendons, muscles, and bones. Most are customized to a patient's needs and anatomy. Orthoses designed to fit into shoes may shift the patient's weight to different parts of the foot to compensate for lost function, prevent deformity or injury, help bear weight, or relieve pain, as well as provide support. Orthoses are often very expensive and not covered by insurance.

Walking aids include walkers, crutches, and canes (see Fig. 388–2). They help with weight bearing, balance, or both. Each device has advantages and disadvantages, and each is available in many models. After evaluation, a therapist should choose the one that provides the best combi-

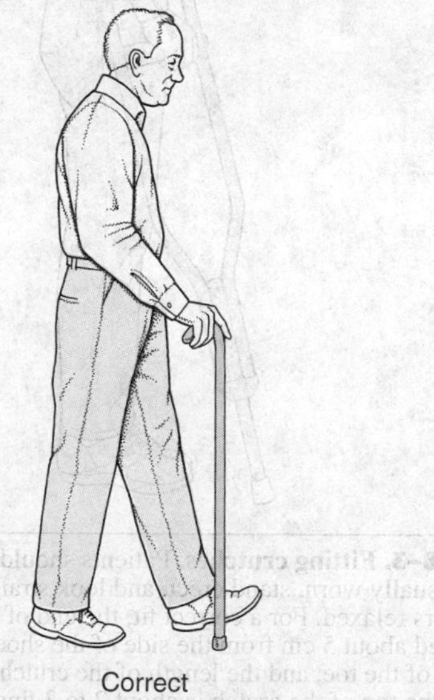

Fig. 388–2. Correct cane height. The patient's elbow should be bent at slightly < 45° when maximum force is applied.

Table 388–5. AMBULATION AIDS

CHARACTERISTIC	WALKER	CRUTCHES	CANES
Stability	Very good	Good	Least stable
Walking speed	Slowest	Slow	Can be fast
Use on steps	None	Training needed	Easy
Strength of arms required for use	Normal	Moderate strength	Normal
Number of hands required for use	2	Usually 2	Usually 1
Possibility of carrying objects	Requires attachment of basket	None	Possible
Cost	Most expensive	Relatively inexpensive	Least expensive

nation of stability and freedom for the patient (see Table 388–5). Physicians should know how to fit crutches (see Fig. 388–3). Prescriptions for assistive devices should be as specific as possible.

Wheelchairs provide mobility to patients who cannot walk. Some models are designed to be self-propelled and to provide stability for traveling over uneven ground and up and down curbs. Other models are designed to be pushed by an assistant; they provide less stability and speed. Wheelchairs are available with various features. For athletic patients with impaired lower extremities but good upper body strength, racing wheelchairs are available. A one-arm–drive or hemi-height wheelchair may be suitable for hemiplegic patients with good coordination. If patients have little or no arm function, a motorized wheelchair is prescribed. Wheelchairs for quadriplegics may have chin or mouth (sip and puff) controls and built-in ventilators.

Mobility scooters are battery-powered, wheeled carts with a steering wheel or tiller, speed control, and ability to move forward and in reverse. They are used on firm, level surfaces inside and outside buildings but cannot negotiate curbs or stairs. Scooters are helpful for people who can stand and walk short distances (ie, to transfer to and from the scooter) but who lack the strength and/or stamina to walk longer distances.

Prostheses are artificial body parts, most commonly limbs designed to replace lower or upper extremities after amputation (see p. 3258). Technical innovations have greatly improved the comfort and functionality of prostheses. Many prostheses can be cosmetically altered to appear natural. A prosthetist should be involved early to help patients understand the many options in prosthetic design, which should meet the patients' needs and safety requirements. Many patients can expect to regain considerable function. Physical therapy should be started even before the prosthesis is fitted; therapy should continue until patients can function with the new limb. Some patients seem unable to tolerate a prosthesis or complete the physical rehabilitation required to successfully use it.

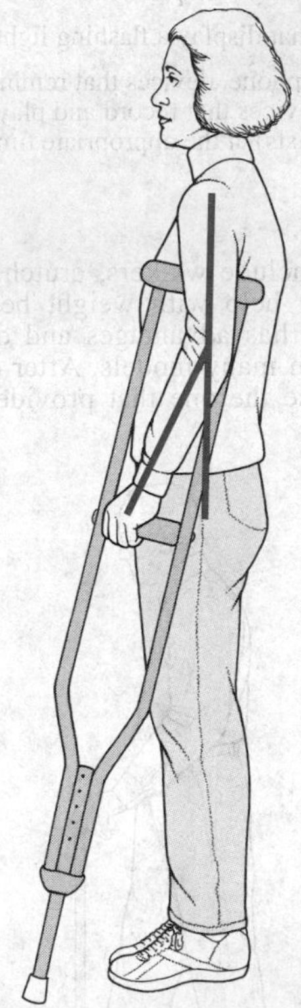

Fig. 388–3. Fitting crutches. Patients should wear the type of shoes usually worn, stand erect, and look straight ahead with the shoulders relaxed. For a correct fit, the end of each crutch should be placed about 5 cm from the side of the shoe and about 15 cm in front of the toe, and the length of the crutch should be adjusted so that the top of the crutch is about 2 to 3 finger widths (about 5 cm) below the axilla. The hand grip should be adjusted so that the elbow bends 20 to 30°.

REHABILITATIVE MEASURES FOR TREATMENT OF PAIN AND INFLAMMATION

Treatment of pain and inflammation aims to facilitate movement and improve coordination of muscles and joints. Nondrug treatments include therapeutic exercise, heat, cold, electrical stimulation, cervical traction, massage, and acupuncture. These treatments are used for many disorders of muscles, tendons, and ligaments (see Table 388–6). Prescribers should include the following:

- Diagnosis
- Type of treatment (eg, ultrasound, hot pack)
- Location of application (eg, right shoulder, low back)
- Frequency (eg, once/day, every other day)
- Duration (eg, 10 days, 1 wk)

Table 388–6. INDICATIONS FOR NONDRUG PAIN TREATMENTS

TREATMENT	INDICATIONS
Heat (eg, infrared heat, hot packs, paraffin bath, hydrotherapy)	Arthralgia Arthritis (various forms) Back pain Fibromyalgia Muscle spasm Myalgia Neuralgia Sprains Strains Tenosynovitis Whiplash injuries
Ultrasound	Bone injuries Bursitis Complex regional pain syndrome Contractures Osteoarthritis Tendinitis
Cold	Inflammation (acute) Low back pain (acute) Muscle spasm Myofascial pain Traumatic pain
Transcutaneous electrical nerve stimulation (TENS)	Musculoskeletal pain Neuralgia Peripheral vascular disease
Cervical traction	Disk prolapse pain Neck pain (chronic) due to cervical spondylosis Torticollis Whiplash injuries
Massage	Amputation Arthritis* Bruises Bursitis* Cancer (certain types) Cerebral palsy* Contracted tissues Fibromyalgia Fibrositis* Fractures Hemiplegia* Joint injuries Low back pain* Multiple sclerosis* Neuritis* Paraplegia* Periarthritis* Peripheral nerve injuries Quadriplegia* Sprain Strain
Acupuncture†	Pain (chronic) Acute and chronic musculoskeletal injuries Inflammatory and degenerative arthritides

*Massage should be considered.
†Acupuncture is used with other treatments.

Heat: Heat provides temporary relief in subacute and chronic traumatic and inflammatory disorders (eg, sprains, strains, fibrositis, tenosynovitis, muscle spasm, myositis, back pain, whiplash injuries, various forms of arthritis, arthralgia, neuralgia). Heat increases blood flow and the extensibility of connective tissue; heat also decreases joint stiffness, pain, and muscle spasm and helps relieve inflammation, edema, and exudates. Heat application may be superficial (infrared heat, hot packs, paraffin bath, hydrotherapy) or deep (ultrasound). Intensity and duration of the physiologic effects depend mainly on tissue temperature, rate of temperature elevation, and area treated.

Infrared heat is applied with a heat lamp, usually for 20 min/day. Contraindications include any advanced heart disorder, peripheral vascular disease, impaired skin sensation (particularly to temperature and pain), and significant hepatic or renal insufficiency. Precautions must be taken to avoid burns.

Hot packs are cotton cloth containers filled with silicate gel; they are boiled in water or warmed in a microwave oven, then applied to the skin. The packs must not be too hot. Wrapping the packs in several layers of towels helps protect the skin from burns. Contraindications are the same as those for infrared heat.

For a **paraffin bath,** the affected area is dipped in, immersed in, or painted with melted wax that has been heated to 49° C. The heat can be retained by wrapping the affected area with towels for 20 min. Paraffin is usually applied to small joints—typically, by dipping or immersion for a hand and by painting for a knee or an elbow. Paraffin should not be applied to open wounds or used on patients allergic to it. A paraffin bath is particularly useful for finger arthritis.

Hydrotherapy may be used to enhance wound healing. Agitated warm water stimulates blood flow and debrides burns and wounds. This treatment is often given in a Hubbard tank (a large industrial whirlpool) with water heated to 35.5 to 37.7° C. Total immersion in water heated to 37.7 to 40° C may also help relax muscles and relieve pain. Hydrotherapy is particularly useful with range-of-motion exercises.

Diathermy is therapeutic heating of tissues using oscillating high-frequency electromagnetic fields, either short-wave or microwave. These modalities do not seem superior to simpler forms of heating and are now seldom used.

Ultrasound uses high-frequency sound waves to penetrate deep (4 to 10 cm) into the tissue; its effects are thermal, mechanical, chemical, and biologic. It is indicated for tendinitis, bursitis, contractures, osteoarthritis, bone injuries, and complex regional pain syndrome. Ultrasound should not be applied to ischemic tissue, anesthetized areas, or areas of acute infection nor be used to treat hemorrhagic diathesis or cancer. Also, it should not be applied over the eyes, brain, spinal cord, ears, heart, reproductive organs, brachial plexus, or bones that are healing.

Cold: The choice between heat and cold therapies is often empiric. When heat does not work, cold is applied. However, for acute injury or pain, cold seems to be better than heat. Cold may help relieve muscle spasm, myofascial or traumatic pain, acute low back pain, and acute inflammation; cold may also help induce some local anesthesia. Cold is usually used during the first few hours or the day after an injury; consequently, it is seldom used in physical therapy.

Cold may be applied locally using an ice bag, a cold pack, or volatile fluids (eg, ethyl chloride, vapocoolant spray), which cool by evaporation. Spread of cold on the skin depends on the thickness of the epidermis, underlying fat and muscle, water content of the tissue, and rate of blood flow. Care must be taken to avoid tissue damage and hypothermia. Cold should not be applied over poorly perfused areas.

Electrical stimulation: Transcutaneous electrical nerve stimulation (TENS) uses low current at low-frequency oscillation to relieve pain. Patients feel a gentle tingling sensation without increased muscle tension. Depending on the severity of pain, 20 min to a few hours of stimulation may be applied several times daily. Often, patients are taught to use the TENS device and decide when to apply treatment. Because TENS may cause arrhythmia, it is contraindicated in patients with any advanced heart disorder or a pacemaker. It should not be applied over the eyes.

Cervical traction: Cervical traction is often indicated for chronic neck pain due to cervical spondylosis, disk prolapse, whiplash injuries, or torticollis. Vertical traction (with patients in a sitting position) is more effective than horizontal traction (with patients lying in bed). Motorized intermittent rhythmic traction with 7.5 to 10 kg is most effective. For best results, traction should be applied with the patient's neck flexed 15 to 20°. Generally, hyperextension of the neck should be avoided because it may increase nerve root compression in the intervertebral foramina. Traction is usually combined with other physical therapy, including exercises and manual stretching.

Massage: Massage may mobilize contracted tissues, relieve pain, and reduce swelling and induration associated with trauma (eg, fracture, joint injury, sprain, strain, bruise, peripheral nerve injury). Massage should be considered for low back pain, arthritis, periarthritis, bursitis, neuritis, fibromyalgia, hemiplegia, paraplegia, quadriplegia, multiple sclerosis, cerebral palsy, certain types of cancer, and amputation. Massage should not be used to treat infections or thrombophlebitis. It is not advised for patients with severe allergies because it causes histamine to be released throughout the body. Only a licensed or certified massage therapist should use massage for treatment of an injury because of variability in therapists' training and skills.

Acupuncture: Thin needles are inserted through the skin at specific body sites, frequently far from the site of pain. Acupuncture is sometimes used with other treatments to manage acute and chronic pain.

CARDIOVASCULAR REHABILITATION

Rehabilitation may benefit some patients who have coronary artery disease or heart failure or who have had a recent MI or coronary artery bypass surgery, particularly those who could do ADLs independently and walk before the event. Cardiac rehabilitation aims to help patients maintain or regain independence (see p. 681).

Typically, rehabilitation begins with light activities and progresses on an individualized basis; ECG monitoring is often used. High-risk patients should exercise only in a well-equipped cardiovascular rehabilitation facility under the supervision of a trained attendant.

When patients are able, they are taken by wheelchair to a physical therapy gym in the hospital. Exercise may involve walking, a treadmill, or a stationary bicycle. When patients tolerate these exercises well, they progress to stair-climbing. If shortness of breath, light-headedness, or chest pain occurs during exercise, the exercise should be stopped immediately, and cardiac status should be reassessed. Before hospital discharge, patients are assessed so that an appropriate postdischarge rehabilitation program or exercise regimen can be recommended.

Physical activity is measured in metabolic equivalents (METs), which are multiples of the resting rate of O_2 consumption; 1 MET (the resting rate) equals about 3.5 mL/kg/min of O_2 (see Table 388–7). Normal working and living activities (excluding recreational activities) rarely exceed 6 METs. Light to moderate housework is about 2 to 4 METs; heavy housework or yard work is about 5 to 6 METs.

For hospitalized patients, physical activity should be controlled so that heart rate remains < 60% of maximum for that age (eg, about 160 beats/min for people aged 60); for patients recovering at home, heart rate should remain < 70% of maximum.

For patients who have had an uncomplicated MI, a 2-MET exercise test may be done to evaluate responses as soon as patients are stable. A 4- to 5-MET exercise test done before discharge helps guide physical activity at home. Patients who

Table 388–7. ENDURANCE EXERCISES AND THEIR METABOLIC REQUIREMENT

ACTIVITY	METABOLIC REQUIREMENT		
	INTENSITY LEVEL	METS*	KCAL/H
Walking at 3–5 km/h (2–3 miles/h) Cycling on level terrain at 10 km/h (6 miles/h) Light stretching exercises Swimming (using a float board) Light to moderate housework	Low	2–4	180–300
Walking at 6 km/h (4 miles/h) Cycling at 13 km/h (8 miles/h) Golf (walking or pulling a cart) Light calisthenics Swimming (treading water) Heavy housework or yard work	Moderate	5–6	300–360
Walking or jogging at 8 km/h (5 miles/h) Cycling at 18–19 km/h (11–12 miles/h) Swimming (0.8 km [1/2 mile] in 30 min) Recreational tennis Hiking	High	7–8	420–480

*The oxygen expenditure at rest (> 3.5 mL/min/kg body weight).
METs = metabolic equivalents.
Adapted from Hanson PG, et al: Clinical guidelines for exercise training. *Postgraduate Medicine* 67(1):120–138, 1980. Copyright McGraw-Hill, Inc.

can tolerate a 5-MET exercise test for 6 min can safely do low-intensity activities (eg, light housework) after discharge if they rest sufficiently between each activity.

Unnecessary restriction of activity is detrimental to recovery. The physician and other members of the rehabilitation team should explain which activities can be done and which cannot and should provide psychologic support. When discharged, patients can be given a detailed home activity program. Most elderly patients can be encouraged to resume sexual activity, but they need to stop and rest if necessary to avoid overexertion. Young couples expend 5 to 6 METs during intercourse; whether elderly couples expend more or less is unknown.

STROKE REHABILITATION

Rehabilitation after stroke aims to preserve or improve range of motion, muscle strength, bowel and bladder function, and functional and cognitive abilities. Specific programs are based on the patient's social situation (eg, prospects of returning to home or work), ability to participate in a rehabilitation program supervised by nurses and therapists, learning ability, motivation, and coping skills. A stroke that impairs comprehension often makes rehabilitation very difficult.

To prevent secondary disabilities (eg, contractures) and help prevent depression, rehabilitation should begin as soon as patients are medically stable. Preventive measures for pressure ulcers must be started even before patients are medically stable. Patients can safely begin sitting up once they are fully conscious and neurologic deficits are no longer progressing, usually ≤ 48 h after the stroke. Early in the rehabilitation period, when the affected extremities are flaccid, each joint is passively exercised through the normal range of motion (see Table 388–1) 3 to 4 times/day.

Regaining the ability to get out of bed and to transfer to a chair or wheelchair safely and independently is important for the patient's psychologic and physical well-being. Ambulation problems, spasticity, visual field defects (eg, hemianopia), incoordination, and aphasia require specific therapy.

Hemiplegia: For patients with hemiplegia, placing 1 or 2 pillows under the affected arm can prevent dislocation of the shoulder. If the arm is flaccid, a well-constructed sling can prevent the weight of the arm and hand from overstretching the deltoid muscle and subluxating the shoulder. A posterior foot splint applied with the ankle in a 90° position can prevent equinus deformity (talipes equinus) and footdrop.

Resistive exercise for hemiplegic extremities may increase spasticity and thus is controversial. However, reeducation and coordination exercises of the affected extremities are added as soon as tolerated, often within 1 wk. Active and active-assistive range-of-motion exercises are started shortly afterward to maintain range of motion. Active exercise of the unaffected extremities must be encouraged, as long as it does not cause fatigue. Various ADLs (eg, moving in bed, turning, changing position, sitting up) should be practiced. For hemiplegic patients, the most important muscle for ambulation is the unaffected quadriceps. If weak, this muscle must be strengthened to assist the hemiplegic side.

A gait abnormality in hemiplegic patients is caused by many factors (eg, muscle weakness, spasticity, distorted body image) and is thus difficult to correct. Also, attempts to correct gait often increase spasticity, may result in muscle fatigue, and may increase the already high risk of falls, which often result in a hip fracture; functional prognosis of hemiplegic patients with a hip fracture is very poor. Consequently, as long as hemiplegic patients can walk safely and comfortably, gait correction should not be tried.

Novel treatments for hemiplegia include the following:

- **Constraint-induced movement therapy:** The functional limb is restrained during waking hours, except during specific activities, and patients are forced to do tasks mainly with the affected extremity.
- **Robotic therapy:** Robotic devices are used to provide intensive repetition of the therapeutic movement, guide an affected extremity in executing the movement, provide feedback (eg, on a computer screen) for patients, and measure patient progress.
- **Partial weight–supported ambulation:** A device (eg, treadmill) that bears part of a patient's weight is used during ambulation. The amount of weight borne and speed of ambulation can be adjusted. This approach is often used with robotics, which allows patients to contribute to ambulation but provides force as needed for ambulation.
- **Total body vibration:** Patients stand on an exercise machine with a platform that vibrates by rapidly shifting weight from one foot to the other. The movement stimulates reflexive muscle contraction.

Ambulation problems: Before ambulation exercises can be started, patients must be able to stand. Patients first learn to stand from the sitting position. The height of the seat may need to be adjusted. Patients must stand with the hips and knees fully extended, leaning slightly forward and toward the unaffected side. Using the parallel bars is the safest way to practice standing.

The goal of ambulation exercises is to establish and maintain a safe gait, not to restore a normal gait. Most hemiplegic patients have a gait abnormality, which is caused by many factors (eg, muscle weakness, spasticity, distorted body image) and is thus difficult to correct. Also, attempts to correct gait often increase spasticity, may result in muscle fatigue, and may increase the already high risk of falls.

During ambulation exercises, patients place the feet > 15 cm (> 6 in) apart and grasp the parallel bars with the unaffected hand. Patients take a shorter step with the hemiplegic leg and a longer step with the unaffected leg. Patients who begin walking without the parallel bars may need physical assistance from and later close supervision by the therapist. Generally, patients use a cane or walker when first walking without the parallel bars. The diameter of the cane handle should be large enough to accommodate an arthritic hand.

For stair-climbing, ascent starts with the better leg, and descent starts with the affected leg (good leads up; bad leads down). If possible, patients ascend and descend with the railing on the unaffected side, so that they can grasp the railing. Looking up the staircase may cause vertigo and should be avoided. During descent, patients should use a cane. The cane should be moved to the lower step shortly before descending with the bad leg.

Patients must learn to prevent falls, which are the most common accident among stroke patients and which often result in hip fracture. Usually, patients explain the fall by saying that their knees gave way. For hemiplegic patients, who almost always fall on their hemiplegic side, leaning their affected side against a railing (when standing or climbing stairs) can help prevent falls. Doing strengthening exercises for weak muscles, particularly in the trunk and legs, can also help.

For patients with symptomatic orthostatic hypotension, treatment includes support stockings, drugs, and tilt table training.

Because hemiplegic patients are prone to vertigo, they should change body position slowly and take a moment after standing to establish equilibrium before walking. Comfortable, supportive shoes with rubber soles and with heels ≤ 2 cm (3/4 in) should be worn.

Spasticity: In some stroke patients, spasticity develops. Spasticity may be painful and debilitating. Slightly spastic knee extensors can lock the knee during standing or cause hyperextension (genu recurvatum), which may require a knee brace with an extension stop. Resistance applied to spastic plantar flexors causes ankle clonus; a short leg brace without a spring mechanism minimizes this problem.

Flexor spasticity develops in most hemiplegic hands and wrists. Unless patients with flexor spasticity do range-of-motion exercises several times a day, flexion contracture may develop rapidly, resulting in pain and difficulty maintaining personal hygiene. Patients and family members are taught to do these exercises, which are strongly encouraged. A hand or wrist splint may also be useful, particularly at night. One that is easy to apply and clean is best.

Heat or cold therapy can temporarily decrease spasticity and allow the muscle to be stretched. Hemiplegic patients may be given benzodiazepines to minimize apprehension and anxiety, particularly during the initial stage of rehabilitation, but not to reduce spasticity. The effectiveness of long-term benzodiazepine therapy for reducing spasticity is questionable. Methocarbamol has limited value in relieving spasticity and causes sedation.

Hemianopia: Patients with hemianopia (defective vision or blindness in half the visual field of one or both eyes) should be made aware of it and taught to move their heads toward the hemiplegic side when scanning. Family members can help by placing important objects and by approaching the patient on the patient's unaffected side. Repositioning the bed so that patients can see a person entering the room through the doorway may be useful. While walking, patients with hemianopia tend to bump into the door frame or obstacles on the hemiplegic side; they may need special training to avoid this problem.

When reading, patients who have difficulty looking to the left may benefit from drawing a red line on the left side of the newspaper column. When they reach the end of a line of text, they scan to the left of the column until they see the red line, cueing them to begin reading the next line. Using a rule to keep focused on each line of text may also help.

Occupational therapy: After a stroke, fine coordination may be absent, causing patients to become frustrated. Occupational therapists may need to modify patients' activities and recommend assistive devices (see Table 388–4).

Occupational therapists should also evaluate the home for safety and determine the extent of social support. They can help obtain any necessary devices and equipment (eg, bathtub bench, grab bars by the bathtub or toilet). Occupational therapists can also recommend modifications that enable patients to do ADLs as safely and independently as possible—for example, rearranging the furniture in living areas and removing clutter. Patients and caregivers are taught how to transfer between surfaces (eg, shower, toilet, bed, chair) and, if necessary, how to modify ways of doing ADLs. For example, patients may be taught to dress or shave using only one hand and to eliminate unnecessary motion while preparing food or shopping for groceries. Therapists may suggest using clothing and shoes with touch fasteners (eg, Velcro) or dinner plates with rims and rubber grips (to facilitate handling). Patients with impairments in cognition and perception are taught ways to compensate. For example, they can use drug organizers (eg, containers marked for each day of the week).

LEG AMPUTATION REHABILITATION

Before amputation, the physician describes to the patient the extensive postsurgical rehabilitation program that is needed. Psychologic counseling may be indicated. The rehabilitation team and the patient decide whether a prosthesis (see p. 3197) or a wheelchair is needed.

Rehabilitation teaches ambulation skills; it includes exercises to improve general conditioning and balance, to stretch the hip and knee, to strengthen all extremities, and to help patients tolerate the prosthesis. Because ambulation requires a 10 to 40% increase in energy expenditure after below-the-knee amputation and a 60 to 100% increase after above-the-knee amputation, endurance exercises may be indicated. As soon as patients are medically stable, rehabilitation should be started to help prevent secondary disabilities. Elderly patients should begin standing and doing balancing exercises with parallel bars as soon as possible.

Flexion contracture of the hip or knee may develop rapidly, making fitting and using the prosthesis difficult; contractures can be prevented with extension braces made by occupational therapists.

Physical therapists teach patients how to care for the stump and how to recognize the earliest signs of skin breakdown.

Stump Conditioning and Prostheses

Stump (residual limb) conditioning promotes the natural process of shrinking that must occur before a prosthesis can be used. After only a few days of conditioning, the stump may have shrunk greatly. An elastic shrinker or elastic bandages worn 24 h/day can help taper the stump and prevent edema. The shrinker is easy to apply, but bandages may be preferred because they better control the amount and location of pressure. However, application of elastic bandages requires skill, and bandages must be reapplied whenever they become loose.

Early ambulation with a temporary prosthesis helps in the following ways:

- Enables the amputee to be active
- Accelerates stump shrinkage
- Prevents flexion contracture
- Reduces phantom limb pain

The socket of the pylon (the internal framework or skeleton of a prosthesis) should fit the stump snugly—made possible by modern computerized design and manufacturing processes. Various temporary prostheses with adjustable sockets are available. Patients with a temporary prosthesis can start ambulation exercises on the parallel bars and progress to walking with crutches or canes until a permanent prosthesis is made.

The permanent prosthesis should be lightweight and meet the needs and safety requirements of the patient. If the prosthesis is made before the stump stops shrinking, adjustments may be needed. Therefore, manufacture of a permanent prosthesis is generally delayed a few weeks until shrinkage stops. For most elderly patients with a below-the-knee amputation, a patellar tendon-bearing prosthesis with a solid-ankle, cushion-heel foot, and suprapatellar cuff suspension is best. Unless patients have special needs, a below-the-knee prosthesis with thigh corset and waist belt is not prescribed because it is heavy and bulky. For above-the-knee amputees, several knee-locking options are available according to the patient's skills and activity level. Some newer technologies include microprocessor-controlled knee and ankle joints that enable patients to adjust movement as needed.

Care of the stump and prosthesis: Patients must learn to care for their stump (see also p. 3201). Because a leg prosthesis is intended only for ambulation, patients should remove it before going to sleep. At bedtime, the stump should be inspected thoroughly (with a mirror if inspected by the patient), washed with mild soap and warm water, dried thoroughly, then dusted with talcum powder. Patients should treat the following possible problems:

- Dry skin: Lanolin or petrolatum may be applied to the stump.
- Excessive sweating: An unscented antiperspirant may be applied.
- Inflamed skin: The irritant must be removed immediately, and talcum powder or a low-potency corticosteroid cream or ointment should be applied.
- Broken skin: The prosthesis should not be worn until the wound has healed.

The stump sock should be changed daily, and mild soap may be used to clean the inside of the socket. Standard prostheses are neither waterproof nor water-resistant. Therefore, if even part of the prosthesis becomes wet, it must be dried immediately and thoroughly; heat should not be applied. For patients who swim or prefer to shower with a prosthesis, a prosthesis that can tolerate immersion can be made.

Complications

Stump pain is the most common complaint. Common causes include

- A poorly fitted prosthetic socket: This cause is the most common.
- Neuroma: An amputation neuroma is usually palpable. Daily ultrasound treatment for 5 to 10 sessions may be most effective. Other treatments include injection of corticosteroids or analgesics into the neuroma or the surrounding area, cryotherapy, and continuous tight bandaging of the stump. Surgical resection often has disappointing results.
- Spur formation at the amputated end of the bone: Spurs may be diagnosed by palpation and x-ray. The only effective treatment is surgical resection.

Phantom limb sensation (a painless awareness of the amputated limb possibly accompanied by tingling) is experienced by some new amputees. This sensation may last several months or years but usually disappears without treatment. Frequently, patients sense only part of the missing limb, often the foot, which is the last phantom sensation to disappear. Phantom limb sensation is not harmful; however, patients, without thinking, commonly attempt to stand with both legs and fall, particularly when they wake at night to go to the bathroom.

Phantom limb pain is less common and can be severe and difficult to control. Some experts think it is more likely to occur if patients had a painful condition before amputation or if pain was not adequately controlled intraoperatively and postoperatively. Various treatments, such as simultaneous exercise of amputated and contralateral limbs, massage of the stump, finger percussion of the stump, use of mechanical devices (eg, a vibrator), and ultrasound, are reportedly effective. Drugs (eg, gabapentin) may help.

Skin breakdown tends to occur because the prosthesis presses on and rubs the skin and because moisture collects between the stump and prosthetic socket. Skin breakdown may be the first indication that the prosthesis needs adjustment and needs to be managed immediately. The first sign of skin breakdown is redness; then cuts, blisters, and sores may develop, the prosthesis is often painful or impossible to wear for long periods of time, and infection can develop. Several measures can help prevent or delay skin breakdown:

- Having an interface that fits well
- Maintaining a stable body weight (even small changes in weight can affect fit)
- Eating a healthy diet and drinking lots of water (to control body weight and maintain healthy skin)
- For patients with diabetes, monitoring and controlling their blood sugar level (to help prevent vascular disease and thus maintain blood flow to the skin)
- For patients with a lower-limb prosthesis, maintaining body alignment (eg, wearing only shoes with a similar heel height)

However, even with a good fit, problems can occur. The stump changes in shape and size throughout a day, depending on activity level, diet, and the weather. Thus, there are times when the interface fits well and times when it fits less well. In response to such ongoing changes, people can help maintain a good fit by switching to a thicker or thinner liner or sock, by using a liner and a sock, or by adding or removing thin-ply socks. But even so, the stump's size may vary enough to cause skin breakdown. If there are signs of skin breakdown, patients should promptly see a health care practitioner and a prosthetist; when possible they should also avoid wearing the prosthesis until it can be adjusted.

HIP SURGERY REHABILITATION

Rehabilitation is started as soon as possible after hip fracture surgery. The first goals may be to increase strength and to prevent atrophy on the unaffected side. Initially, only isometric exercise of the affected limb while it is fully extended is permitted. Placement of a pillow under the knee is contraindicated because it may lead to flexion contracture of the hip and knee.

Gradual mobilization of the affected limb usually results in full ambulation. Speed of rehabilitation depends partly on the type of surgery done. For example, after prosthetic hip replacement, rehabilitation usually progresses more rapidly, less rehabilitation is needed, and the functional outcome is better than that after nail-and-plate or pin-and-plate fixation. Ideally, full weight bearing starts on the 2nd day after surgery. Ambulation exercises are started after 4 to 8 days (assuming that patients can bear their full weight and can balance), and stair-climbing exercises are started after about 11 days.

Patients are taught to do daily exercises to strengthen the trunk muscles and quadriceps of the affected leg. Prolonged lifting or pushing of heavy items, stooping, reaching, or jumping can be harmful. During ambulation, the amount of mechanical stress is about the same whether patients use 1 or 2 canes, but using 2 may interfere with certain ADLs. Patients should not sit on a chair, particularly a low one, for a long period and should use the chair arm for support when standing up. While sitting, they should keep their legs uncrossed.

Occupational therapists teach patients how to modify ways of doing basic ADLs (BADLs) and instrumental ADLs (IADLs) safely after hip replacement, thus promoting healing and improving mobility. For example, patients may learn the following:

- To keep their hip correctly aligned
- To wash dishes and iron while sitting on a high stool
- To use a pillow to raise the seat of the car while transferring in and out
- To use long-handled devices (eg, reachers, shoe horns) to minimize bending over

This instruction may occur in the hospital, in longer-term rehabilitation settings, in the patient's home immediately after discharge, or in outpatient settings.

REHABILITATION FOR OTHER DISORDERS

Arthritis: Patients with arthritis can benefit from activities and exercises to increase joint range of motion and strength and from strategies to protect the joints. For example, patients may be advised

- To slide a pot of boiling water containing pasta rather than carry it from the stove to the sink (to avoid undue pain and strain to joints)
- How to get in and out of the bathtub safely
- To get a raised toilet seat, a bathtub bench, or both (to reduce pain and stress on the lower-extremity joints)
- To wrap foam, cloth, or tape around the handles of objects (eg, knives, cooking pots and pans) to cushion the grip
- To use tools with larger, ergonomically designed handles

Such instruction may occur in outpatient settings, in the home via a home health care agency, or in private practice.

Blindness: Patients are taught to rely more on the other senses, to develop specific skills, and to use devices for the blind (eg, Braille, cane, reading machine). Therapy aims to help patients function to their maximum and become independent, to restore psychologic security, and to help patients deal with and influence the attitudes of other people. Therapy varies depending on the way vision was lost (suddenly or slowly and progressively), extent of vision loss, the patient's functional needs, and coexisting deficits. For example, patients with peripheral neuropathy and diminished tactile sensation in the fingers may have difficulty reading Braille. Many blind people need psychologic counseling (usually cognitive-behavioral therapy) to help them better cope with their condition.

For ambulation, therapy may involve learning to use a cane; canes used by the blind are usually white and longer and thinner than ordinary canes. People who use a wheelchair are taught to use one arm to operate the wheelchair and the other to use a cane. People who prefer to use a trained dog instead of a cane are taught to handle and care for the dog. When walking with a sighted person, a blind person can hold onto the bent elbow of the sighted person, rather than use an ambulation aid. The sighted person should not lead the blind person by the hand because some blind people perceive this action as dominant and controlling.

COPD: Patients with COPD can benefit from exercises to increase endurance and from strategies to simplify activities and thus conserve energy. Activities and exercises that encourage use of the upper and lower extremities are used to increase muscle aerobic capacity, which decreases overall oxygen requirement and eases breathing. Supervising patients while they engage in activity helps motivate them and makes them feel more secure. Such instruction may occur in medical facilities or in the patient's home.

Head injury: The term head injury is often used interchangeably with traumatic brain injury. Abnormalities vary and may include muscle weakness, spasticity, incoordination, and ataxia; cognitive dysfunction (eg, memory loss, loss of problem-solving skills, language and visual disturbances) is common.

Early intervention by rehabilitation specialists is indispensable for maximal functional recovery. Such intervention includes prevention of secondary disabilities (eg, pressure ulcers, joint contractures), prevention of pneumonia, and family education. As early as possible, rehabilitation specialists should evaluate patients to establish baseline findings. Later, before starting rehabilitation therapy, patients should be reevaluated; these findings are compared with baseline findings to help prioritize treatment. Patients with severe cognitive dysfunction require extensive cognitive therapy, which is often begun immediately after injury and continued for months or years.

Spinal cord injury: Specific rehabilitation therapy varies depending on the patient's abnormalities, which depend on the level and extent (partial or complete) of the injury (see p. 3098, particularly Table 368–1 on p. 3099). Complete transsection causes flaccid paralysis; partial transsection causes spastic paralysis of muscles innervated by the affected segment. A patient's functional capacity depends on the level of injury (see p. 2027) and the development of complications (eg, joint contractures, pressure ulcers, pneumonia).

The affected area must be immobilized surgically or nonsurgically as soon as possible and throughout the acute phase. During the acute phase, daily routine care should include measures to prevent contractures, pressure ulcers, and pneumonia; all measures needed to prevent other complications (eg, orthostatic hypotension, atelectasis, deep venous thrombosis, pulmonary embolism) should also be taken. Placing patients on a tilt table and increasing the angle gradually toward the upright position may help reestablish hemodynamic balance. Compression stockings, an elastic bandage, or an abdominal binder may prevent orthostatic hypotension.

389 Tobacco Use

Tobacco use is a major individual and public health problem. Dependence develops rapidly. Major consequences include premature death and morbidity caused by coronary artery disease, lung cancer, COPD, and other disorders. Smokers should be offered smoking cessation interventions.

Tobacco use, although declining in the US, remains quite common. Tobacco is used because of the pleasurable effects of its main active ingredient, nicotine. Nicotine can be toxic, and the combustion products of tobacco contain other substances that can cause significant morbidity and mortality.

Epidemiology

Tobacco is nearly always smoked, primarily as cigarettes. Cigarette smoking is the most harmful form of tobacco use. However, all tobacco products contain toxins and possible carcinogens; even smokeless tobacco products are not safe alternatives to smoking.

Cigarettes: The percentage of people in the US who smoke cigarettes has declined since 1964, when the Surgeon General first publicized the link between smoking and ill health.

Nevertheless, about 20% of adults still smoke. Smoking is more prevalent among men, people with less than a high school education, people living at or below the poverty income level, people with psychiatric disorders (including alcohol and substance use), American Indians, and Alaska natives. Smoking is less common among Hispanics and least common among Asian Americans.

Most smokers start during childhood. Children as young as 5 yr may experiment with cigarettes. About 31% become dependent before age 16 and over half before age 18, and age of initiation continues to decrease. The younger the age at which smoking starts, the more likely smoking is to continue. Risk factors for childhood initiation include

- Parental, peer, and role model (eg, celebrity) smoking
- Poor school performance
- A poor relationship with parents or a single-parent home
- High-risk behavior (eg, excessive dieting, particularly among girls; physical fighting and drunk driving, particularly among boys)
- Availability of cigarettes
- Poor problem-solving abilities

Other kinds of tobacco use: Exclusive **pipe smoking** is relatively rare in the US (< 1% of people ≥ 12 yr), although it has increased among middle and high school students since 1999. In 2008, about 5.3% of people > 12 yr smoked **cigars**; this percentage has declined since 2000. People < 18 yr comprise the largest group of new cigar smokers. Risks of pipe and cigar smoking include cardiovascular disease; COPD; cancers of the oral cavity, lung, larynx, esophagus, colon, and pancreas; and periodontal disease and tooth loss.

E-cigarettes deliver vaporized liquid of which nicotine may be a desired component. There is no combustion involved in using e-cigarettes, as the "smoke" emitted from the device is water vapor and may or may not contain nicotine and flavorings; thus many of the toxic products found in conventional cigarette smoke are not produced in e-cigarettes. E-cigarette use among middle and high school students has tripled from 4.5% in 2013 to 13.4% in 2014, according to the Centers for Disease Control and Prevention (CDC). Long-term risks of e-cigarettes are unknown.

Smokeless tobacco (chewing tobacco and snuff) is used by about 3.3% of people ≥ 18 yr and about 7.9% of high school students. Toxicity of smokeless tobacco varies by brand. Risks include cardiovascular disease, oral disorders (eg, cancers, gum recession, gingivitis, periodontitis and its consequences), and teratogenicity.

Inadvertent oral exposure to tobacco is uncommon but may cause serious toxicity. Young children occasionally ingest cigarettes from unguarded packs, cigarette butts from ashtrays, or nicotine gum. For example, from 2006 to 2008, > 13,700 cases of potentially toxic exposure to tobacco products in children < 6 yr were reported to the American Association of Poison Control Centers (AAPCC); the most common source was cigarettes and the most commonly affected age group was < 1 yr.

Cutaneous exposure to tobacco can be toxic. Tobacco harvesters and processors who handle raw tobacco (especially if wet) without protection may absorb nicotine through the skin and develop symptoms of nicotine toxicity, a syndrome termed green tobacco sickness.

Passive exposure to tobacco smoke occurs when people inhale smoke from a nearby smoker. The amount inhaled (and thus its effects) varies with the proximity and duration of exposure as well as the environment (eg, closed space) and ventilation.

Pathophysiology

Nicotine is a highly addictive drug present in tobacco and is a major component of cigarette smoke. Cravings can begin within days of first use. Nicotine stimulates brain nicotinic cholinergic receptors, releasing dopamine and other neurotransmitters, which activate the brain reward system during pleasurable activities in a manner similar to that of many other addictive drugs (see on p. 1810). Dopamine, glutamate, and gamma-aminobutyric acid (GABA) are important mediators of nicotine dependence.

Psychologic dependence exists when people smoke to affect their mood or avoid withdrawal symptoms; it can develop within 2 wk after starting smoking and occurs in up to about 25% of adolescents who try smoking. Physical dependence (ie, occurrence of withdrawal symptoms with cessation) also develops within 2 wk. People smoke to feed their nicotine dependence but simultaneously inhale thousands of other components, including carcinogens, noxious gases, and chemical additives that are a part of cigarette smoke. These toxic components, rather than nicotine, are responsible for the multiple health consequences of smoking. Nicotine induces its metabolizing enzyme, CYP2A6, leading to multiple potential drug interactions.

Chronic effects of smoking: Smoking harms nearly every organ in the body. Smoking is the leading cause of preventable mortality in the US, accounting for an estimated 435,000 deaths/yr, or about 20% of all deaths. About half of all current smokers die prematurely of a disease directly caused by smoking, losing 10 to 14 yr of life (7 min/cigarette) on average.

The **major chronic effects** are an increased likelihood of the following:

- Coronary artery disease
- Lung cancer
- COPD

Coronary artery disease accounts for about 30 to 40% of all tobacco-related deaths. Risk of MI is increased by probably > 200% if smoking < 1 pack/day and risk of cardiovascular mortality is increased by > 50% over a 35-yr period. Mechanisms may include endothelial cell damage, transient increases in BP and heart rate, induction of a prothrombotic state, and adverse effects on serum lipids.

Lung cancer accounts for about 15 to 20% of tobacco-related deaths. Tobacco is the most common cause of lung cancer in North America and Europe. Inhaled carcinogens are directly exposed to lung tissue.

COPD accounts for roughly 20% of tobacco-related deaths. Smoking impairs local respiratory tract defense mechanisms and, particularly in genetically susceptible people, tends to accelerate decline in pulmonary functions. Coughing and dyspnea on exertion are common.

Less common serious smoking-related disorders include noncardiac vascular diseases (eg, stroke, aortic aneurysm), other cancers (eg, bladder, cervical, esophageal, kidney, laryngeal, oropharyngeal, pancreatic, stomach, throat, acute myelocytic leukemia), and pneumonia.

In addition, smoking is a risk factor for other conditions that convey significant morbidity and disability, such as frequent URIs, cataracts, infertility, premature menopause, peptic ulcer disease, osteoporosis, and periodontitis.

Passive exposure to smoke: Passive exposure to cigarette smoke (secondhand smoke, environmental tobacco smoke) has grave health effects. For adults, passive exposure is linked to the same neoplastic, respiratory, and cardiovascular diseases that threaten active smokers. The risk of illness is less than that of active smokers and is related to dose. For example, between spouses, average risk is increased by about 20% for lung cancer and by about 20 to 30% for coronary artery disease.

Children exposed to cigarette smoke lose more school days because of illness than nonexposed children. Treating children for smoking-related illnesses is estimated to cost $4.6 billion/yr.

Overall, secondhand smoke is estimated to cause 50,000 to 60,000 deaths each year in the US (between 2% and 3% of all deaths). These findings have led states and municipalities across the US to ban smoking within workplaces in an effort to protect the health of workers and others from the substantive risks of environmental tobacco smoke. Currently, > 50% of the US population lives in a state that has implemented a comprehensive indoor smoke-free ordinance.

Smoking during pregnancy is a particularly risky form of passive exposure, potentially causing spontaneous abortion, ectopic pregnancy, and preterm birth (see p. 2365). Infants born of mothers who smoke tend to have a lower birth weight and are at increased risk of

- SIDS
- Asthma and related respiratory illnesses
- Otitis media

Indirect effects of smoking: Indirect effects of smoking can be serious.

Smoking-related fires kill probably > 350 people each year and injure > 900; such fires are the leading cause of deaths resulting from unintentional fires in the US. In addition, each year, 43,000 children lose one or more caregivers who die from smoking-related diseases.

Drug interactions with nicotine are common. Levels and sometimes clinical effects of the following drugs are decreased by chronic smoking, in most cases by induction of CYP2A6 enzymes:

- Antiarrhythmics (some): Flecainide, lidocaine, mexiletine
- Antidepressants (some): Clomipramine, fluvoxamine, imipramine, trazodone
- Antipsychotics (some): Chlorpromazine, clozapine, fluphenazine, haloperidol, olanzapine, thiothixene
- Benzodiazepines
- Beta-blockers
- Caffeine
- Estrogens (oral)
- Insulin (delayed absorption caused by skin vasoconstriction)
- Pentazocine
- Theophylline

Symptoms and Signs

Acute effects: Nicotine slightly increases heart rate, BP, and respiratory rate. Smokers may feel increased energy, increased ability to concentrate, ability to overcome fatigue, and a sense of well-being. Nausea is common on a person's first exposure to nicotine. Nicotine reduces appetite and can be a behavioral substitute for eating. Exercise tolerance tends to decrease because of respiratory tract irritation. Low-grade carbon monoxide toxicity can also limit exercise tolerance, but this is probably only a factor in elite athletes.

Toxicity or overdose: Acute nicotine poisoning is usually caused by oral (eg, children eating a cigarette or nicotine gum) or dermal exposure, rather than smoking.

Mild toxicity, as is common with green tobacco sickness and minor ingestions by children (eg, < 1 cigarette or 3 butts), typically manifests with nausea, vomiting, headache, and weakness. Symptoms spontaneously resolve, usually in 1 to 2 h after ingestion if poisoning is mild; however, symptoms can persist for 24 h if poisoning is severe.

Severe nicotine poisoning causes a cholinergic toxidrome with nausea, vomiting, salivation, lacrimation, diarrhea, urination, fasciculations, and muscle weakness. Patients usually have crampy abdominal pain and, if poisoning is very severe, arrhythmias, hypotension, seizures, and coma. The fatal dose of nicotine is about 60 mg in adult nonsmokers, 120 mg in adult smokers, and as little as 10 mg in young children. Each cigarette contains about 8 mg of nicotine (only about 1 mg is absorbed by smoking). However, the amount ingested by children is usually difficult to ascertain by history because ingestion is rarely observed; any ingestion should be considered potentially dangerous.

Chronic effects: Findings due to smoking itself include yellow stains of teeth and fingers and, in comparison to age-matched controls, weight is slightly lower (≤ 5 kg difference), skin is drier and more wrinkled, and hair is thinner.

Other symptoms are those of smoking-related lung and cardiovascular disease. Chronic cough and dyspnea on exertion are common. Circulatory and respiratory impairments decrease exercise tolerance, often resulting in a more sedentary lifestyle and thus further lowering of exercise tolerance.

Withdrawal: Smoking cessation often causes intense nicotine withdrawal symptoms, primarily a craving for cigarettes but also other symptoms (eg, anxiety, difficulty concentrating, sleep disruption, depression—see p. 3264) and eventual weight gain.

Diagnosis

- Direct questioning

Acute toxicity is not always apparent on history. Children may not have been observed ingesting tobacco or nicotine gum, and patients with green tobacco sickness may not think to mention that they handle tobacco. Thus, children and agricultural workers presenting with typical symptoms, particularly cholinergic manifestations, should be queried about possible tobacco exposure. Testing is not necessary.

Of the > 70% of smokers who present in a primary care setting every year, only a minority receive counseling and drugs to help them quit. To maximize identification of smokers and thus the public health benefit of smoking cessation, all patients should be asked about smoking during medical visits regardless of presenting symptoms and all patients should be asked about smoking, particularly during visits for symptoms possibly related to smoking (eg, circulatory or respiratory symptoms).

Treatment

- Symptomatic treatment for acute poisoning
- Smoking cessation measures

Skin exposed to nicotine should be irrigated. Otherwise, treatment for acute nicotine poisoning is supportive. Gastric emptying is not recommended. In patients with mild symptoms or who have vomited, charcoal is not given; some clinicians would recommend charcoal for patients who have severe symptoms or have ingested large quantities and have not vomited. Airway protection and assisted ventilation may be needed for patients who are obtunded, have excessive respiratory secretions, or have respiratory muscle weakness. Seizures are treated with benzodiazepines. Shock is treated with IV fluids and, if fluids are ineffective, pressors. Atropine can be considered for patients who have excessive respiratory secretions or bradycardia; otherwise, anticholinergics are not recommended.

Smoking-related disorders are treated. All smokers should be advised to stop smoking and helped to quit by smoking cessation counseling and typically drug treatment (see Table 389–1). Pregnant women who smoke should be advised to

Table 389–1. DRUGS FOR SMOKING CESSATION

DRUG	DOSAGE	DURATION	ADVERSE EFFECTS	COMMENTS
Bupropion SR	150 mg every morning for 3 days (beginning 1–2 wk before quitting), then 150 mg twice/day	7–12 wk initially (may continue up to 6 mo)	Insomnia Dry mouth Possibly serious neuropsychiatric symptoms* (eg, behavior changes, agitation, depressed mood, suicidal ideation and behavior)	Prescription only Contraindicated by history of seizure, eating disorder, or MAOI use within the past 2 wk
Nicotine gum	If smoking > 30 min after waking: 2 mg If smoking < 30 min after waking: 4 mg Schedule for both dosage strengths: 1 q 1–2 h for wk 1–6 1 q 2–4 h for wk 7–9 1 q 4–8 h for wk 10–12	Up to 6 mo	Mouth soreness Dyspepsia	OTC only Slow chewing recommended to maximize blood levels and minimize gastric and esophageal irritation
Nicotine lozenge	If smoking > 30 min after waking: 2 mg If smoking < 30 min after waking: 4 mg Schedule for both dosage strengths: 1 q 1–2 h for wk 1–6 1 q 2–4 h for wk 7–9 1 q 4–8 h for wk 10–12	Up to 6 mo	Nausea Insomnia	OTC only
Nicotine inhaler	6–16 cartridges/day for the first 6–12 wk, then tapered down over the next 6–12 wk	3–6 mo	Local irritation of mouth and throat	Prescription only
Nicotine nasal spray	8–40 doses/day (1 dose = 1 spray in each nostril)	14 wk	Nasal and pharyngeal irritation	Prescription only Reaches peak blood levels earlier (in 10 min) than other nicotine replacement products
Nicotine patch	21 mg/24 h for 6 wk, then 14 mg/24 h for 2 wk, then 7 mg/24 h for 2 wk If smoking > 10 cigarettes/day: 21 mg as starting dose If smoking < 10 cigarettes/day: 14 mg as starting dose	10 wk	Local skin reaction Insomnia	OTC and prescription Local skin reactions possibly less likely if location of patch is rotated
Varenicline	0.5 mg po once/day for 3 days, then 0.5 mg bid for 4 days, then 1 mg bid	12–24 wk†	Most commonly, nausea and sleep disturbances Possibly serious neuropsychiatric symptoms* (eg, behavior changes, agitation, depressed mood, suicidal ideation and behavior)	Prescription only

*Neuropsychiatric symptoms have been reported, but clinical trial data have not confirmed a causal relationship; detecting such an association may be confounded by the presence of nicotine withdrawal.

†The longer duration of treatment may increase the likelihood of long-term abstinence among patients who have stopped smoking after 12 wk of varenicline use.

MAOI = monoamine oxidase inhibitor.

stop smoking and helped to quit by intensive smoking cessation counseling. However, the 2015 US Preventive Services Task Force concluded that the evidence was insufficient to assess the benefits and harms of drug therapy for tobacco cessation in pregnant women (see Tobacco Smoking Cessation in Adults, Including Pregnant Women: Behavioral and Pharmacotherapy Interventions at www.uspreventiveservicestaskforce.org).

KEY POINTS

- Cigarette smoking, the leading cause of preventable mortality in the US, tends to begin early in life, with about 31% of smokers becoming dependent before age 16 and over half before age 18.
- Cravings can begin within days of first use.

- Components of cigarette smoke other than nicotine (eg, carcinogens, noxious gases, chemical additives) are responsible for most of the adverse health effects that cigarettes cause.
- Harmful effects include increased risk of fatal disorders (eg, lung cancer, COPD, coronary artery disease), indirect effects (eg, fires), and drug interactions.
- Nicotine acts as a mild stimulant acutely in the usual doses but can cause a cholinergic toxidrome in acute overdose (usually due to oral or dermal exposure).
- Ask all patients about smoking, regardless of presenting symptom.

SMOKING CESSATION

Most smokers want to quit and have tried doing so with limited success. Effective interventions include cessation counseling and drug treatment, such as varenicline, bupropion, or a nicotine replacement product.

About 70% of US smokers say they want to quit and have already tried to quit at least once. Among the barriers are withdrawal symptoms.

Withdrawal

Withdrawal symptoms are often powerful enough that even with knowledge of the health risks, many smokers are unwilling to try quitting. Smoking cessation can cause intense symptoms, including strong cravings for cigarettes, but also often anxiety, depression (mostly mild, sometimes major), inability to concentrate, irritability, restlessness, insomnia, hunger, headaches, GI disturbances, and sleep disruption. These symptoms are worst in the first week (when most smokers trying to quit relapse) and most subside within 2 wk in most smokers, but some symptoms may continue for months. Weight gain is common; quitters gain an average of 4 to 5 kg, and weight gain is another reason for recidivism. Temporary cough and oral ulcers may develop after quitting.

Prognosis

About 20 million smokers in the US try to quit each year (almost half of all smokers), usually by using a cold turkey or other non-evidence-based approach, resulting in relapse within days, weeks, or months. Many cycle through multiple periods of relapse and remission. The long-term success rate for unassisted quitting is about 5%. In contrast, 1-yr success rates of up to 20 to 30% are achieved among smokers who use evidence-based cessation counseling and recommended drugs.

Among smokers < 18 yr, most believe they will not be smoking in 5 yr, and 40 to 50% report having tried to quit in the previous year. However, longitudinal studies show that overall, 73% of daily smokers in high school remain daily smokers 5 to 6 yr later.

Interventions

Evidence-based counseling and drug treatment are both effective treatments for tobacco dependence; combining counseling and drug treatment is more effective than either intervention alone.

Smoking has many characteristics of a chronic disorder. Thus, the optimal evidence-based approach to smokers, particularly those unwilling to quit or those who have not yet considered quitting, should be guided by the same principles that guide chronic disease management, namely

- Continually assessing and monitoring smoking status
- Using different evidence-based interventions (or combinations) for different patients and building on their prior experiences and treatment preferences
- Encouraging temporary abstinence and reduction in consumption for patients who fall short of total smoking cessation while emphasizing that abstinence is the ultimate goal

Although reduction in consumption can increase motivation to quit (particularly when combined with nicotine replacement therapy), smokers should be reminded that reducing the number of cigarettes smoked may not improve health because smokers often inhale more smoke (and thus more toxins) per cigarette to maintain nicotine intake when they reduce the number of cigarettes smoked per day.

Evidence-based counseling: Counseling efforts begin with the 5 A's:

- Ask at every visit whether a patient smokes and document the response.
- Advise all smokers to quit in clear, strong, personalized language they will understand.
- Assess a smoker's willingness to try quitting within the next 30 days.
- Assist smokers willing to make a quit attempt by providing brief counseling and drug treatment.
- Arrange a follow-up, preferably within the first week of the quit date.

For smokers willing to quit, clinicians should establish a quit date, preferably within 2 wk, and stress that total abstinence is better than reduction. Past quitting experiences can be reviewed to identify what helped and what did not, and smoking triggers or challenges to quitting should be planned for in advance. For example, alcohol use is associated with relapse, so alcohol restriction or abstinence should be discussed. In addition, quitting is more difficult with another smoker in the household; spouses and housemates can be encouraged to quit together. In general, smokers should be instructed to develop social support among family and friends for their quit attempt, and clinicians should reinforce their availability and assistance in support of the attempt.

In addition to the brief counseling provided by the smoker's clinician, counseling programs can help. They usually use cognitive-behavioral techniques and are offered by various commercial and voluntary health programs. Success rates are higher than with self-help programs. All states in the US have telephone quit lines that can provide counseling support (and sometimes nicotine replacement therapy) to smokers trying to quit. People can call 1-800-QUIT-NOW (1-800-784-8669) toll-free anywhere in the US. Quit lines appear to be at least as effective as in-person counseling.

Drugs for smoking cessation: Effective and safe drugs for smoking cessation include varenicline, bupropion SR, and 5 types of nicotine replacement therapy (in the form of gum, lozenge, patch, inhaler, and nasal spray—Table 389–1). Bupropion's mechanism may be to increase the brain's release of norepinephrine and dopamine. Varenicline works at the nicotinic acetylcholine receptor (the α-4β-2 subunit), where it acts as a partial agonist, having some nicotinic effects, and as a partial antagonist, blocking the effects of nicotine. Some evidence suggests varenicline is the most effective monotherapy available for smoking cessation.

Research suggests that combinations of different nicotine replacement products are more effective than single products. For example, combining the nicotine patch with a shorter-acting nicotine drug (eg, lozenge, gum, nasal spray, inhaler) is more effective than monotherapy. When used in combination, the patch helps maintain continuous levels, and use of gum, lozenge, inhaler, or nasal spray enables the patient to rapidly increase nicotine levels in response to immediate cravings.

Smokers may worry that they may remain dependent on nicotine after using nicotine products for smoking cessation; however, such dependence rarely persists. Drug choice is guided by the clinician's familiarity with the drug, the smoker's preference and previous experience (positive or negative), and contraindications.

Despite their proven efficacy, smoking cessation drugs are used by < 25% of smokers attempting to quit. Reasons include low rates of insurance coverage, clinicians' concerns about the side effects of centrally acting medications (serious neuropsychiatric events including depression, suicidal ideation, and suicide attempt) and the safety of simultaneous smoking and nicotine replacement, and patient discouragement because of past unsuccessful quit attempts.

Therapies under investigation for smoking cessation include the drugs cytisine, bromocriptine, and topiramate. Vaccine therapy was studied and found ineffective.

Drug safety: Contraindications to bupropion include a history of seizures, an eating disorder, and monoamine oxidase inhibitor use within 2 wk.

Whether bupropion and varenicline increase risk of suicide is not clear. Varenicline and bupropion may increase risk of serious neuropsychiatric effects and accidents. In 2009, the FDA released a boxed warning for both drugs regarding these possible adverse effects. However, most experts recommend varenicline for most smokers because risks of smoking substantially exceed any possible risks of taking the drug. But varenicline should be avoided in smokers with suicidal risk, unstable psychiatric disorders, and possibly major depression.

Nicotine replacement should be used cautiously in smokers with certain cardiovascular risks (those within 2 wk of an MI, with serious arrhythmias, or with serious angina); however, most data suggest that such use is safe. Nicotine gum is contraindicated in smokers with temporomandibular joint syndrome, and nicotine patches are contraindicated in smokers with severe topical sensitization.

Because of safety concerns, inadequate efficacy data, or both, drugs are not recommended for the following:

- Pregnant smokers
- Light smokers (< 10 cigarettes/day)
- Adolescents (< age 18)
- Users of smokeless tobacco

Cessation in children: The counseling approach for children is similar to that for adults; however, drugs are not recommended for smokers under the age of 18.

Children should be screened for smoking and risk factors by age 10. Parents should be advised to maintain smoke-free households and to communicate the expectation to their children that the children will remain nonsmokers.

For children who smoke, cognitive-behavioral therapy that involves establishing awareness of tobacco use, providing motivations to quit, preparing to quit, and providing strategies to maintain abstinence after cessation are effective in treating nicotine dependence. Alternative approaches to smoking cessation, such as hypnosis and acupuncture, have not proved to be effective and cannot be recommended for routine use.

Cessation of non-cigarette tobacco products: Cessation counseling for smokeless tobacco users, as for cigarette smokers, has been shown to be effective. However, drugs have not proved effective among smokeless tobacco users.

Effectiveness of cessation treatments for pipe and cigar smokers is not well documented. Also, cessation may be affected by whether cigarettes are smoked concurrently and whether smokers inhale.

KEY POINTS

- About half of smokers try to quit each year, but few fully succeed.
- Evidence-based methods of smoking cessation increase the 1-yr success rate from about 5% to 20 to 30%.
- Use evidence-based counseling methods, including physician counseling and referral to support programs, for patients interested in quitting.
- Consider drug treatment (eg, with varenicline or combinations of nicotine replacement products).

APPENDIXES

APPENDIX I

Ready Reference Guides

In the US, most laboratory test results are reported in what are termed conventional units; the rest of the world reports results in *Système International d'Unités* (SI) or international units (IU). The unit basis for SI is updated periodically by a panel.

Many SI units are the same as units used in the US system; however, SI units for concentrations are not. SI concentrations are reported as moles (mol) or decimal fractions of a mole (eg, millimole, micromole) per unit volume in liters (L). Conventional units are reported as mass (eg, grams, milligrams) or chemical equivalency (eg, milliequivalents) per unit volume, which may be in liters or decimal fractions of liters (eg, deciliters, milliliters). Results reported in amount per 100 mL (1 dL) are sometimes expressed as percent (eg, 10 mg/dL may be written as 10 mg%).

Moles, milligrams, and milliequivalents: A mole is an Avogadro's number (6.023×10^{23}) of elementary entities (eg, atoms, ions, molecules); the mass of 1 mole of a substance is its atomic weight in grams (eg, 1 mole of sodium = 23 g, 1 mole of calcium = 40 g). Similarly, the mass of a given quantity of substance divided by its atomic weight gives the number of moles (eg, 20 g sodium = 20/23, or 0.87, mol).

An equivalent is a unit that integrates charge and moles; 1 equivalent represents one mole of charges and is calculated by multiplying the number of moles of charged particles in a

METRIC SYSTEM

UNIT	EQUIVALENT SUBUNIT
Mass	
1 kilogram (kg)	1000 grams (10^3 g)
1 gram (g)	1000 milligrams (10^3 mg)
1 milligram (mg)	1000 micrograms (10^{-3} g)
1 microgram (µg)	1000 nanograms (10^{-6} g)
1 nanogram (ng)	1000 picograms (pg; 10^{-9} g)
Volume	
1 liter (L)	1000 milliliters (mL)
1 liter (L)	1000 cubic centimeters (cc)

METRIC–NONMETRIC EQUIVALENTS

METRIC UNIT	EQUIVALENT NONMETRIC UNIT*
Liquid	
30 milliliters (mL)	1 fluid ounce (oz)
250 mL	8 + fluid oz
500 mL	1+ pint
1000 mL (1 liter)	1+ quart
Weight	
65 mg	1 grain (gr)
28.35 g	1 oz
1 kg	2.2 pounds (lb)
Linear	
1 millimeter (mm)	0.04 inch (in)
1 centimeter (cm)	0.4 in
2.54 cm	1 in
1 meter (m)	39.37 in
Household	
4 mL	1 teaspoon (tsp)
5 mL	1 teaspoon, medical
8 mL	1 dessert spoon
15 mL	1 tablespoon (tbsp—½ fluid oz)
240 mL	1 cup (8 fluid oz)

*Approximate.

ATOMIC WEIGHT OF SOME ELEMENTS IMPORTANT IN MEDICINE

ELEMENT	SYMBOL	ATOMIC WEIGHT*
Hydrogen	H	1
Carbon	C	12
Nitrogen	N	14
Oxygen	O	16
Sodium	Na	23
Magnesium	Mg	24
Phosphorus	P	31
Chlorine	Cl	35.5
Potassium	K	39
Calcium	Ca	40

*Approximate.

substance times the valence of that substance. Thus, for ions with a +1 or −1 charge (eg, Na^+, K^+, Cl^-), 1 mole is 1 equivalent (1 × 1 = 1); for ions with a +2 or −2 charge (eg, Ca^{2+}), ½ mole is 1 equivalent (½ × 2 = 1), and so forth for other valence values. A milliequivalent (mEq) is 1/1000 of an equivalent.

The following can be used to convert between mEq, mg, and mmol:

$$\text{mEq} = \text{mg/formula wt} \times \text{valence} = \text{mmol} \times \text{valence}$$

$$\text{mg} = \text{mEq} \times \text{formula wt/valence} = \text{mmol} \times \text{formula wt}$$

$$\text{mmol} = \text{mg/formula wt} = \text{mEq/valence}$$

(Note: Formula wt = atomic or molecular wt.)

Alternatively, conversion tables are available in print and on the Internet.

CENTIGRADE–FAHRENHEIT EQUIVALENTS*

APPLICATION	°C	°F
Freezing for water at sea level	0	32
Clinical range	36.0	96.8
	36.5	97.7
	37.0	98.6
	37.5	99.5
	38.0	100.4
	38.5	101.3
	39.0	102.2
	39.5	103.1
	40.0	104.0
	40.5	104.9
	41.0	105.8
	41.5	106.7
	42.0	107.6
Pasteurization (holding),† 30 min at	62.8	145.0
Pasteurization (flash),† 15 sec at	71.7	161.0
Boiling for water at sea level	100.0	212.0

*Conversion:
To convert °F to °C, subtract 32, then multiply by 5/9 or 0.555.
To convert °C to °F, multiply by 9/5 or 1.8, then add 32.

†According to the FDA Code of Federal Regulations, 1991.

APPENDIX II
Normal Laboratory Values

Reference values (intervals) for blood, urine, CSF, stool, and other fluids (eg, gastric acid) and commonly used panels are included. (NOTE: The reference values provided in these tables should be used as guidelines only.) Reference values vary based on several factors, including the demographics of the healthy population from which specimens were obtained and the specific methods and/or instruments used to assay these specimens. Laboratories that are accredited by the College of American Pathologists (CAP) are required to establish and/or validate their own reference values at least annually. Thus, any given result should be interpreted based on the reference value of the laboratory in which the test was done; the laboratory typically provides these values with the test result.

Table 1. NORMAL LABORATORY VALUES: BLOOD, PLASMA, AND SERUM

TEST	SPECIMEN	CONVENTIONAL UNITS	SI UNITS
Acetoacetate	Plasma	< 1 mg/dL	< 0.1 mmol/L
Acetylcholinesterase (ACE), RBC	Blood	26.7–49.2 U/g Hb	—
Acid phosphatase	Serum	0.5–5.5 U/L	0–0.9 µkat/L
Activated partial thromboplastin time (aPTT)	Plasma	25–35 sec	—
Adrenocorticotropic hormone (ACTH)	Serum	9–52 pg/mL	2–11 pmol/L
Albumin	Serum	3.5–5.5 g/dL	35–55 g/L

Table 1. NORMAL LABORATORY VALUES: BLOOD, PLASMA, AND SERUM (*Continued*)

TEST	SPECIMEN	CONVENTIONAL UNITS	SI UNITS
Aldosterone:			
Standing	Serum	7–20 ng/dL	194–554 pmol/L
Supine	Serum	2–5 ng/dL	55–138 pmol/L
Alkaline phosphatase (ALP)	Serum	36–92 U/L	0.5–1.5 μkat/L
Alpha$_1$-antitrypsin (AAT)	Serum	83–199 mg/dL	—
Alpha fetoprotein (AFP)	Serum	0–20 ng/dL	0–20 pg/L
δ-Aminolevulinic acid (ALA)	Serum	15–23 μg/L	1.14–1.75 μmol/L
Aminotransferase, alanine (ALT)	Serum	0–35 U/L	0–0.58 pkat/L
Aminotransferase, aspartate (AST)	Serum	0–35 U/L	0–0.58 pkat/L
Ammonia	Plasma	40–80 μg/dL	23–47 μmol/L
Amylase	Serum	0–130 U/L	0–2.17 μkat/L
Antibodies to extractable nuclear antigen (AENA)	Serum	< 20.0 units	—
Anti–cyclic citrullinated peptide (anti-CCP) antibodies	Serum	≤ 5.0 units	—
Antidiuretic hormone (ADH; arginine vasopressin)	Plasma	< 1.7 pg/mL	< 1.57 pmol/L
Anti–double-stranded DNA (dsDNA) antibodies, IgG	Serum	< 25 IU	—
Antimitochondrial M2 antibodies	Serum	< 0.1 units	—
Antineutrophil cytoplasmic antibodies (cANCA)	Serum	Negative	—
Antinuclear antibodies (ANA)	Serum	≤ 1.0 units	—
Anti–smooth muscle antibodies (ASMA) titer	Serum	≤ 1:80	—
Antistreptolysin O titer	Serum	< 150 units	—
Antithyroid microsomal antibody titer	Serum	< 1:100	—
α_1-Antitrypsin (AAT)	Serum	83–199 mg/dL	15.3–36.6 μmol/L
Apolipoproteins:			
A-I, females	Serum	98–210 mg/dL	0.98–2.1 g/L
A-I, males	Serum	88–180 mg/dL	0.88–1.8 g/L
B-100, females	Serum	44–148 mg/dL	0.44–1.48 g/L
B-100, males	Serum	55–151 mg/dL	0.55–1.51 g/L
Bicarbonate	Serum	23–28 mEq/L	23–28 mmol/L
Bilirubin:			
Direct	Serum	0–0.3 mg/dL	0–5.1 μmol/L
Total	Serum	0.3–1.2 mg/dL	5.1–20.5 μmol/L
Blood volume:			
Plasma, females	Blood	28–43 mL/kg body wt	0.028–0.043 L/kg body wt
Plasma, males	Blood	25–44 mL/kg body wt	0.025–0.044 L/kg body wt
RBCs, females	Blood	20–30 mL/kg body wt	0.02–0.03 L/kg body wt
RBCs, males	Blood	25–35 mL/kg body wt	0.025–0.035 L/kg body wt
Brain (B-type) natriuretic peptide (BNP)	Plasma	< 100 pg/mL	—
Calcitonin, age ≥ 16 yr:			
Females	Serum	< 8 pg/mL	—
Males	Serum	< 16 pg/mL	—
Calcium	Serum	9–10.5 mg/dL	2.2–2.6 mmol/L

Table continues on the following page.

Table 1. NORMAL LABORATORY VALUES: BLOOD, PLASMA, AND SERUM (*Continued*)

TEST	SPECIMEN	CONVENTIONAL UNITS	SI UNITS
Cancer antigen (CA):			
CA 125	Serum	< 35 U/mL	—
CA 15-3	Serum	< 30 U/mL	—
Carbon dioxide (CO_2) content	Serum	23–28 mEq/L	23–28 mmol/L
Carbon dioxide partial pressure (PCO_2)	Blood	35–45 mm Hg	—
Carboxyhemoglobin	Plasma	0.5–5%	—
Carcinoembryonic antigen (CEA)	Serum	< 2 ng/mL	< 2 μg/L
Carotene	Serum	75–300 μg/L	1.4–5.6 μmol/L
CBC with differential count:			
WBC	Blood	4.5–11 x 10^3 cells/μL	4.5 - 11 x 10^9 cells/L
Differential:			
Segmented neutrophils	Blood	2.6–8.5 x 10^3 cells/μL	2.6 - 8.5 x 10^9 cells/L
Band neutrophils	Blood	0–1.2 x 10^3 cells/μL	0 - 1.2 x 10^9 cells/L
Lymphocytes	Blood	0.77–4.5 x 10^3 cells/μL	0.77 - 4.5 x 10^9 cells/L
Monocytes	Blood	0.14–1.3 x 10^3 cells/μL	0.14 - 1.3 x 10^9 cells/L
Eosinophils	Blood	0–0.55 x 10^3 cells/μL	0 - 0.55 x 10^9 cells/L
Basophils	Blood	0–0.22 x 10^3 cells/μL	0 - 0.22 x 10^9 cells/L
CD4:CD8 ratio	Blood	1–4	—
CD4+ T-cell count	Blood	640–1175/μL	0.64–1.18 x 10^9/L
CD8+ T-cell count	Blood	335–875/μL	0.34–0.88 x 10^9/L
Ceruloplasmin	Serum	25–43 mg/dL	250–430 mg/L
Chloride	Serum	98–106 mEq/L	98–106 mmol/L
Cholesterol, desirable level:			
High-density lipoprotein (HDL-C)	Plasma	≥ 40 mg/dL	≥ 1.04 mmol/L
Low-density lipoprotein (LDL-C)	Plasma	≤ 130 mg/dL	≤ 3.36 mmol/L
Total (TC)	Plasma	150–199 mg/dL	3.88–5.15 mmol/L
Coagulation factors:			
Factor I	Plasma	150–300 mg/dL	1.5–3.5 g/L
Factor II	Plasma	60–150% of normal	—
Factor IX	Plasma	60–150% of normal	—
Factor V	Plasma	60–150% of normal	—
Factor VII	Plasma	60–150% of normal	—
Factor VIII	Plasma	60–150% of normal	—
Factor X	Plasma	60–150% of normal	—
Factor XI	Plasma	60–150% of normal	—
Factor XII	Plasma	60–150% of normal	—
Complement:			
C3	Serum	55–120 mg/dL	0.55–1.20 g/L
C4	Serum	20–59 mg/dL	0.20–0.59 g/L
Total	Serum	37–55 U/mL	37–55 kU/L
Copper	Serum	70–155 μg/L	11–24.3 μmol/L

Table 1. NORMAL LABORATORY VALUES: BLOOD, PLASMA, AND SERUM (*Continued*)

TEST	SPECIMEN	CONVENTIONAL UNITS	SI UNITS
Cortisol:			
1 h after cosyntropin	Serum	> 18 µg/dL and usually ≥ 8 µg/dL above baseline	> 498 nmol/L and usually ≥ 221 nmol/L above baseline
At 5 PM	Serum	3–13 µg/dL	83–359 nmol/L
At 8 AM	Serum	8–20 µg/dL	251–552 nmol/L
After overnight suppression test	Serum	< 5 µg/dL	< 138 nmol/L
C-peptide	Serum	0.9–4.3 ng/mL	297–1419 pmol/L
C-reactive protein (CRP)	Serum	< 0.5 mg/dL	< 0.005 g/L
C-reactive protein, highly sensitive (hsCRP)	Serum	< 1.1 mg/L	< 0.0011 g/L
Creatine kinase (CK)	Serum	30–170 U/L	0.5–2.83 µkat/L
Creatinine	Serum	0.7–1.3 mg/dL	61.9–115 µmol/L
D-Dimer	Plasma	≤ 300 ng/mL	≤ 300 µg/L
Dehydroepiandrosterone sulfate (DHEA-S):			
Females	Plasma	0.6–3.3 mg/mL	1.6–8.9 µmol/L
Males	Plasma	1.3–5.5 mg/mL	3.5–14.9 µmol/L
δ-Aminolevulinic acid (ALA)	Serum	15–23 µg/L	1.14–1.75 µmol/L
11-Deoxycortisol (DOC):			
After metyrapone	Plasma	> 7 µg/dL	> 203 nmol/L
Basal	Plasma	< 5 µg/dL	< 145 nmol/L
D-Xylose level 2 h after ingestion of 25 g of D-xylose	Serum	> 20 mg/dL	> 1.3 nmol/L
Epinephrine, supine	Plasma	< 75 ng/L	< 410 pmol/L
Erythrocyte sedimentation rate (ESR):			
Females	Blood	0–20 mm/h	0–20 mm/h
Males	Blood	0–15 mm/h	0–20 mm/h
Erythropoietin	Serum	4.0–18.5 mIU/mL	4.0–18.5 IU/L
Estradiol, females:			
Day 1–10 of menstrual cycle	Serum	14–27 pg/mL	50–100 pmol/L
Day 11–20 of menstrual cycle	Serum	14–54 pg/mL	50–200 pmol/L
Day 21–30 of menstrual cycle	Serum	19–40 pg/mL	70–150 pmol/L
Estradiol, males	Serum	10–30 pg/mL	37–110 pmol/L
Ferritin	Serum	15–200 ng/mL	15–200 µg/L
α-Fetoprotein (AFP)	Serum	0–20 ng/dL	0–20 pg/L
Fibrinogen	Plasma	150–350 mg/dL	1.5–3.5 g/L
Folate (folic acid):			
RBC	Blood	160–855 ng/mL	362–1937 nmol/L
Serum	Serum	2.5–20 ng/mL	5.7–45.3 nmol/L
Follicle-stimulating hormone (FSH), females:			
Follicular or luteal phase	Serum	5–20 mU/mL	5–20 U/L
Midcycle peak	Serum	30–50 mU/mL	30–50 U/L
Postmenopausal	Serum	> 35 mU/mL	> 35 U/L
Follicle-stimulating hormone (FSH), adult males	Serum	5–15 mU/mL	5–15 U/L
Fructosamine	Plasma	200–285 mol/L	—

Table continues on the following page.

Table 1. NORMAL LABORATORY VALUES: BLOOD, PLASMA, AND SERUM (*Continued*)

TEST	SPECIMEN	CONVENTIONAL UNITS	SI UNITS
Gamma-glutamyl transpeptidase (GGT)	Serum	8–78 U/L	—
Gastrin	Serum	0–180 pg/mL	0–180 ng/L
Globulins:	Serum	2.5–3.5 g/dL	25–35 g/L
α_1-Globulins	Serum	0.2–0.4 g/dL	2–4 g/L
α_2-Globulins	Serum	0.5–0.9 g/dL	5–9 g/L
β-Globulins	Serum	0.6–1.1 g/dL	6–11 g/L
γ-Globulins	Serum	0.7–1.7 g/dL	7–17 g/L
β_2-Microglobulin	Serum	0.7–1.8 µg/mL	—
Glucose:			
2-h postprandial	Plasma	< 140 mg/dL	< 7.8 mmol/L
Fasting	Plasma	70–105 mg/dL	3.9–5.8 mmol/L
Glucose-6-phosphate dehydrogenase (G6PD)	Blood	5–15 U/g Hb	0.32–0.97 mU/ mol Hb
γ-Glutamyl transpeptidase (GGT)	Serum	8–78 U/L	—
Growth hormone:			
After oral glucose	Plasma	< 2 ng/mL	< 2 µg/L
In response to provocative stimuli	Plasma	> 7 ng/mL	> 7 µg/L
Haptoglobin	Serum	30–200 mg/dL	300–2000 mg/L
Hematocrit:			
Females	Blood	36–47%	—
Males	Blood	41–51%	—
Hemoglobin:			
Females	Blood	12–16 g/dL	120–160 g/L
Males	Blood	14–17 g/dL	140–170 g/L
Hemoglobin A_{1c}	Blood	4.7–8.5%	—
Hemoglobin electrophoresis, adults:			
Hb A_1	Blood	95–98%	—
Hb A_2	Blood	2–3%	—
Hb C	Blood	0%	—
Hb F	Blood	0.8–2.0%	—
Hb S	Blood	0%	—
Hemoglobin electrophoresis, Hb F in children:			
Neonate	Blood	50–80%	—
1–6 mo	Blood	8%	—
> 6 mo	Blood	1–2%	—
Homocysteine:			
Females	Plasma	0.40–1.89 mg/L	3–14 µmol/L
Males	Plasma	0.54–2.16 mg/L	4–16 µmol/L
Human chorionic gonadotropin (hCG), quantitative	Serum	< 5 mIU/mL	—
Immunoglobulins:			
IgA	Serum	70–300 mg/dL	0.7–3.0 g/L
IgD	Serum	< 8 mg/dL	< 80 mg/L
IgE	Serum	0.01–0.04 mg/dL	0.1–0.4 mg/L
IgG	Serum	640–1430 mg/dL	6.4–14.3 g/L

Table 1. NORMAL LABORATORY VALUES: BLOOD, PLASMA, AND SERUM (*Continued*)

TEST	SPECIMEN	CONVENTIONAL UNITS	SI UNITS
IgG_1	Serum	280–1020 mg/dL	2.8–10.2 g/L
IgG_2	Serum	60–790 mg/dL	0.6–7.9 g/L
IgG_3	Serum	14–240 mg/dL	0.14–2.4 g/L
IgG_4	Serum	11–330 mg/dL	0.11–3.3 g/L
IgM	Serum	20–140 mg/dL	0.2–1.4 g/L
Insulin, fasting	Serum	1.4–14 μIU/mL	10–104 pmol/L
International normalized ratio (INR):			
Therapeutic range (standard intensity therapy)	Plasma	2.0–3.0	—
Therapeutic range in patients at higher risk (eg, patients with prosthetic heart valves)	Plasma	2.5–3.5	
Therapeutic range in patients with lupus anticoagulant	Plasma	3.0–3.5	—
Iron	Serum	60–160 μg/dL	11–29 μmol/L
Iron-binding capacity, total (TIBC)	Serum	250–460 μg/dL	45–82 μmol/L
Lactate dehydrogenase (LDH)	Serum	60–160 U/L	1–1.67 μkat/L
Lactic acid, venous	Blood	6–16 mg/dL	0.67–1.8 mmol/L
Lactose tolerance test	Plasma	> 15 mg/dL increase in plasma glucose level	> 0.83 mmol/L increase in plasma glucose level
Lead	Blood	< 40 μg/dL	< 1.9 μmol/L
Leukocyte alkaline phosphatase (LAP) score	Peripheral blood smear	13–130/100/ polymorphonuclear (PMN) leukocyte neutrophils and bands	—
Lipase	Serum	< 95 U/L	< 1.58 μkat/L
Lipoprotein (a) [Lp(a)]	Serum	≤ 30 mg/dL	< 1.1 μmol/L
Luteinizing hormone (LH), females:			
Follicular or luteal phase	Serum	5–22 mU/mL	5–22 U/L
Midcycle peak	Serum	30–250 mU/mL	30–250 U/L
Postmenopausal	Serum	> 30 mU/mL	> 30 U/L
Luteinizing hormone, males	Serum	3–15 mU/mL	3–15 U/L
Magnesium	Serum	1.5–2.4 mg/dL	0.62–0.99 mmol/L
Manganese	Serum	0.3–0.9 ng/mL	5.5–16.4 nmol/L
Mean corpuscular hemoglobin (MCH)	Blood	28–32 pg	—
Mean corpuscular hemoglobin concentration (MCHC)	Blood	32–36 g/dL	320–360 g/L
Mean corpuscular volume (MCV)	Blood	80–100 fL	—
Metanephrines, fractionated:			
Metanephrines, free	Plasma	< 0.50 nmol/L	—
Normetanephrines, free	Plasma	< 0.90 nmol/L	—
Methemoglobin	Blood	< 1.0%	—
Methylmalonic acid (MMA)	Serum	150–370 nmol/L	—
Myeloperoxidase (MPO) antibodies	Serum	< 6.0 U/mL	—
Myoglobin:			
Females	Serum	25–58 μg/L	1.4–3.5 nmol/L
Males	Serum	28–72 μg/L	1.6–4.1 nmol/L
Norepinephrine, supine	Plasma	50–440 pg/mL	0.3–2.6 nmol/L

Table continues on the following page.

Table 1. NORMAL LABORATORY VALUES: BLOOD, PLASMA, AND SERUM (*Continued*)

TEST	SPECIMEN	CONVENTIONAL UNITS	SI UNITS
N-Terminal propeptide of BNP (NT-proBNP)	Plasma	< 125 pg/mL	—
5'-Nucleotidase (5'NT)	Serum	4–11.5 U/L	—
Osmolality	Plasma	275–295 mOsm/kg H_2O	275–295 mmol/ kg H_2O
Osmotic fragility test	Blood	Increased fragility if hemolysis occurs in > 0.5% NaCl Decreased fragility if hemolysis is incomplete in 0.3% NaCl	—
Oxygen partial pressure (PO_2)	Blood	80–100 mm Hg	
Parathyroid hormone (PTH)	Serum	10–65 pg/mL	10–65 ng/L
Parathyroid hormone–related peptide (PTHrP)	Plasma	< 2.0 pmol/L	—
Partial thromboplastin time, activated (aPTT)	Plasma	25–35 sec	—
pH	Blood	7.38–7.44	—
Phosphorus, inorganic	Serum	3.0–4.5 mg/dL	0.97–1.45 mmol/L
Platelet count	Blood	150–350 x 10^3/μL	150–350 x 10^9/L
Platelet life span, using chromium-51 (^{51}Cr)	—	8–12 days	—
Porphyrins	Plasma	≤ 1.0 μg/dL	—
Potassium	Serum	3.5–5 mEq/L	3.5–5 mmol/L
Prealbumin (transthyretin)	Serum	18–45 mg/dL	
Progesterone:			
Follicular phase	Serum	< 1 ng/mL	< 0.03 nmol/L
Luteal phase	Serum	3–30 ng/mL	0.1–0.95 nmol/L
Prolactin:			
Females	Serum	< 20 μg/L	< 870 pmol/L
Males	Serum	< 15 μg/L	< 652 pmol/L
Prostate-specific antigen, total (PSA-T)	Serum	0–4 ng/mL	—
Prostate-specific antigen, ratio of free to total (PSA-F:PSA-T)	Serum	> 0.25	—
Protein C activity	Plasma	67–131%	—
Protein C resistance, activated ratio (APC-R)	Plasma	2.2–2.6	—
Protein S activity	Plasma	82–144%	—
Protein, total	Serum	6–7.8 g/dL	60–78 g/L
Prothrombin time (PT)	Plasma	11–13 sec	—
Pyruvate	Blood	0.08–0.16 mmol/L	
RBC count	Blood	4.2–5.9 x 10^6 cells/μL	4.2–5.9 x 10^{12} cells/L
RBC survival rate, using ^{51}Cr	Blood	$T_{1/2}$ = 28 days	—
Renin activity, plasma (PRA), upright, in males and females aged 18–39 yr:			
Sodium-depleted	Plasma	2.9–24 ng/mL/h	—
Sodium-repleted	Plasma	0.6 (or lower)–4.3 ng/mL/h	—
Reticulocyte count:			
Percentage	Blood	0.5–1.5%	—
Absolute	Blood	23–90 x 10^3/μL	23–90 x 10^9/L
Rheumatoid factor (RF)	Serum	< 40 U/mL	< 40 kU/L

Table 1. NORMAL LABORATORY VALUES: BLOOD, PLASMA, AND SERUM (*Continued*)

TEST	SPECIMEN	CONVENTIONAL UNITS	SI UNITS
Sodium	Serum	136–145 mEq/L	136–145 mmol/L
Testosterone, adults:			
Females	Serum	20–75 ng/dL	0.7–2.6 nmol/L
Males	Serum	300–1200 ng/dL	10–42 nmol/L
Thrombin time	Plasma	18.5–24 sec	—
Thyroid iodine-123 (^{123}I) uptake	—	5–30% of administered dose at 24 h	—
Thyroid-stimulating hormone (TSH)	Serum	0.5–5.0 μIU/mL	0.5–5.0 mIU/L
Thyroxine (T_4):			
Free	Serum	0.9–2.4 ng/dL	12–31 pmol/L
Free index	—	4–11 μg/dL	—
Total	Serum	5–12 μg/dL	64–155 nmol/L
Transferrin	Serum	212–360 mg/dL	2.1–3.6 g/L
Transferrin saturation	Serum	20–50%	—
Triglycerides (desirable level)	Serum	< 250 mg/dL	< 2.82 mmol/L
Triiodothyronine (T_3):			
Uptake	Serum	25–35%	—
Total	Serum	70–195 ng/dL	1.1–3.0 nmol/L
Troponin I	Plasma	< 0.1 ng/mL	< 0.1 μg/L
Troponin T	Serum	≤ 0.03 ng/mL	≤ 0.03 μg/L
Urea nitrogen (BUN)	Serum	8–20 mg/dL	2.9–7.1 mmol/L
Uric acid	Serum	2.5–8 mg/dL	0.15–0.47 mmol/L
Vitamin B_{12}	Serum	200–800 pg/mL	148–590 pmol/L
Vitamin C (ascorbic acid):			
Leukocyte	Blood	< 20 mg/dL	< 1136 μmol/L
Total	Blood	0.4–1.5 mg/dL	23–85 μmol/L
Vitamin D:			
1,25-Dihydroxycholecalciferol (calcitriol)	Serum	25–65 pg/mL	65–169 pmol/L
25-Hydroxycholecalciferol	Serum	15–80 ng/mL	37–200 nmol/L
WBC count	Blood	3.9–10.7 x 10^3 cells/μL	3.9–10.7 x 10^9 cells/L
Zinc	Serum	66–110 μg/dL	10.1–16.8 μmol/L

μkat = microkatal; pkat = picokatal.

Table 2. NORMAL LABORATORY VALUES: URINE

TEST	SPECIMEN	CONVENTIONAL UNITS	SI UNITS
Aldosterone	Urine, 24 h	5–19 μg/24 h	13.9–52.6 nmol/24 h
Amino acids, total	Urine, 24 h	200–400 mg/24 h	14–29 nmol/24 h
Amylase	Urine, timed	6.5–48.1 U/h	—
Calcium, with patients on an unrestricted diet	Urine, timed	100–300 mg/day	2.5–7.5 mmol/day
Catecholamines, total	Urine, 24 h	< 100 μg/m^2/24 h	< 591 nmol/m^2/24 h
Chloride	Urine, timed	80–250 mEq/day	80–250 mmol/day

Table continues on the following page.

Table 2. NORMAL LABORATORY VALUES: URINE (*Continued*)

TEST	SPECIMEN	CONVENTIONAL UNITS	SI UNITS
Copper	Urine, 24 h	0–100 μg/24 h	0–1.6 μmol/24 h
Coproporphyrin	Urine, 24 h	50–250 μg/24 h	76–382 nmol/24 h
Cortisol, free	Urine, 24 h	< 90 μg/24 h	< 248 nmol/24 h
Creatine:			
Females	Urine, 24 h	0–100 mg/24 h	0–763 mmol/24 h
Males	Urine, 24 h	4–40 mg/24 h	30–305 mmol/24 h
Creatinine, weight-based	Urine, 24 h	15–25 mg/kg/24 h	133–221 mmol/kg/ 24 h
D-Xylose excretion 5 h after ingestion of 25 g of D-xylose	Urine, 5 h collection	5–8 g	33–53 mmol
Estriol, females	Urine, 24 h	> 12 mg/24 h	> 42 μmol/24 h
17-Hydroxycorticosteroids, fractionated, adults ≥ 18 yr:			
Cortisol	Urine, 24 h	3.5–4.5 μg/24 h	9.7–12.4 nmol/24 h
Cortisone	Urine, 24 h	17–129 μg/24 h	47–359 nmol/24 h
5-Hydroxyindoleacetic acid (5-HIAA)	Urine, 24 h	2–9 mg/24 h	10.4–46.8 μmol/24 h
17-Ketosteroid, fractionated, females > 12 yr:			
Androsterone	Urine, 24 h	55–1589 μg/24 h	—
Pregnanetriol	Urine, 24 h	59–1391 μg/24 h	—
17-Ketosteroid, fractionated, males > 12 yr:			
Androsterone	Urine, 24 h	234–2703 μg/24 h	—
Etiocholanolone	Urine, 24 h	151–3198 μg/24 h	—
11-Hydroxyandrosterone	Urine, 24 h	66–1032 μg/24 h	—
11-Hydroxyetiocholanolone	Urine, 24 h	17–1006 μg/24 h	—
11-Ketoandrosterone	Urine, 24 h	4–55 μg/24 h	—
11-Ketoetiocholanolone	Urine, 24 h	51–1016 μg/24 h	—
Pregnanetriol	Urine, 24 h	245–1701 μg/24 h	—
Metanephrines, fractionated, normotensive patients ≥ 18 yr:			
Females, metanephrine	Urine, 24 h	30–180 μg/24 h	—
Females, total metanephrines	Urine, 24 h	142–510 μg/24 h	—
Males, metanephrine	Urine, 24 h	44–261 μg/24 h	—
Males, total metanephrines	Urine, 24 h	190–583 μg/24 h	—
Metanephrines, fractionated, normotensive males and females aged 18–29 yr:			
Normetanephrine	Urine, 24 h	103–390 μg/24 h	—
Metanephrines, fractionated, hypertensive males and females:			
Metanephrine	Urine, 24 h	< 400 μg/24 h	—
Normetanephrine	Urine, 24 h	< 900 μg/24 h	—
Total metanephrines	Urine, 24 h	< 1300 μg/24 h	—
Microalbumin	Urine, 24 h	< 30 mg/24 h	—
Microalbumin, albumin/ creatinine ratio	Urine, random	< 20 μg/mg	—
Osmolality	Urine, random	38–1400 mOsm/kg H_2O	—

Table 2. NORMAL LABORATORY VALUES: URINE (*Continued*)

TEST	SPECIMEN	CONVENTIONAL UNITS	SI UNITS
Oxalate	Urine, 24 h	0.11–0.46 mmol/ specimen*	—
Phosphate, tubular reabsorption	Urine, random	79–94% of filtered load	—
Porphobilinogens	Urine, random	0–0.5 mg/g creatinine	—
Potassium	Urine, 24 h	25–100 mEq/24 h	25–100 mmol/24 h
Protein, total	Urine, 24 h	< 100 mg/24 h	—
Sodium	Urine, 24 h	100–260 mEq/24 h	100–260 mmol/24 h
Uric acid	Urine, 24 h	250–750 mg/24 h	1.48–4.43 mmol/24 h
Urinalysis, routine†			
pH	Urine, random	5–7	—
Urinalysis, routine, dipstick testing†:			
Bilirubin	Urine, random	Negative	—
Blood	Urine, random	Negative	—
Glucose	Urine, random	Negative	—
Ketones	Urine, random	Negative	—
Leukocyte esterase	Urine, random	Negative	—
Nitrites	Urine, random	Negative	—
Protein	Urine, random	Negative	—
Urobilinogen	Urine, random	0.2–1.0 EU	—
Urobilinogen	Urine, 24 h	0.05–2.5 mg/24 h	0.08–4.22 μmol/24 h
Vanillylmandelic acid (VMA)	Urine, 24 h	< 8 mg/24 h	< 40.4 mol/24 h

*Value is based on 24-h collection.

†Normal findings detected by microscopic examination can include a few RBCs (especially in menstruating women), WBCs, epithelial cells, bacteria, yeast cells, crystals (eg, Ca oxalate, triple phosphate, amorphous phosphates and urates), sperm, and unidentifiable materials. Large amounts of these substances or the presence of certain other materials may be abnormal.

EU = Ehrlich units.

Table 3. NORMAL LABORATORY VALUES: CSF

TEST	CONVENTIONAL UNITS	SI UNITS
Cell count	0–5 cells/μL	0–0.5 x 10^6 cells/L
Differential (see Table 221–1 on p. 1843)	—	—
Glucose	40–80 mg/dL (< 40% of simultaneously measured plasma level if that plasma level is abnormal)	2.5–4.4 mmol/L (< 40% of simultaneously measured plasma level if that plasma level is abnormal)
Myelin basic protein	< 1.5 ng/mL	—
Protein, total	15–60 mg/dL	150–600 mg/L

Table 4. NORMAL LABORATORY VALUES: STOOL

TEST	CONVENTIONAL UNITS	SI UNITS
Fat	< 5 g/day in patients on a 100-g fat diet	—
Nitrogen	< 2 g/day	—
Urobilinogen	40–280 mg/24 h	68–473 mg/24 h
Weight	< 200 g/day	—

Table 393–5. NORMAL LABORATORY VALUES: OTHER

TEST	SPECIMEN	CONVENTIONAL UNITS	SI UNITS
Gastric acid secretion:			
Basal, females	Gastric fluid	36.6–38.2 mEq HCl/h	36.6–38.2 mmol/h
Basal, males	Gastric fluid	3.8–4.2 mEq HCl/h	3.8–4.2 mmol/h
Peak, females	Gastric fluid	23.9–25.9 mEq HCl/h	23.9–25.9 mmol/h
Peak, males	Gastric fluid	1.9–2.3 mEq HCl/h	1.9–2.3 mmol/h
Lipase	Ascitic fluid	< 200 U/L	< 3.33 μkat/L
Sperm concentration	Semen	20–150 x 10^6/mL	20–150 x 10^9/mL

μkat = microkatal.

Table 6. COMMONLY USED PANELS

TEST	PANELS						
	CMP	RFP	BMP	ELEC	HFPA	LPP	AHP
Albumin	X	X			X		
Alkaline phosphatase	X				X		
Aminotransferase, alanine (ALT, formerly SGPT)	X				X		
Aminotransferase, aspartate (AST, formerly SGOT)	X				X		
Bilirubin, direct					X		
Bilirubin, total	X				X		
Calcium	X	X	X				
Carbon dioxide	X	X	X	X			
Chloride	X	X	X	X			
Cholesterol, total						X	
Cholesterol, HDL						X	
Creatinine	X	X	X				
Glucose	X	X	X				
Hepatitis A, IgM antibody							X
Hepatitis B core, IgM antibody							X
Hepatitis B surface antigen							X
Hepatitis C antibody							X
Phosphorus		X					
Potassium	X	X	X	X			
Protein, total	X				X		
Sodium	X	X	X	X			
Triglycerides*						X	
Urea nitrogen (BUN)	X	X	X	X			

*Includes calculations of risk ratios and low-density lipoprotein (LDL).

AHP = acute hepatitis panel; BMP = basic metabolic panel; CMP = comprehensive metabolic panel; ELEC = electrolyte panel; HDL = high-density lipoprotein; HFPA = hepatic function panel; LPP = lipid panel; RFP = renal function panel; SGOT = serum glutamic-oxaloacetic transaminase; SGPT = serum glutamatic-pyruvic transaminase.

APPENDIX III
Brand Names of Some Commonly Used Drugs

Throughout The Manual, generic (nonproprietary) names for drugs are used whenever possible. Most prescription drugs have brand names (also called proprietary, trademark [or sometimes mistakenly, trade], or specialty names) to distinguish them as being produced and marketed by a particular manufacturer. In the US, these names are usually registered as trademarks with the Patent Office, which confers certain legal rights with respect to their use. A brand name may be registered for a product containing a single active ingredient (with or without additives) or ≥ 2 active ingredients (combination drugs). A chemical substance marketed by several manufacturers may have several brand names. A drug may be marketed under different brand names in different countries.

Brand names are found in many publications and are used extensively in clinical medicine. For convenience, the following table lists brand names for most drugs mentioned in The Manual, primarily those marketed in the US. The table is not all-inclusive and does not list every brand name for each drug. A few drugs in the table are investigational and may subsequently be approved by the FDA. Inclusion of a drug does not indicate approval of its use for any indication, nor does it imply efficacy or safety of its action. Inclusion of a brand name indicates neither endorsement nor preference by The Manual.

BRAND NAMES OF SOME COMMONLY USED DRUGS

GENERIC NAME	BRAND NAMES	GENERIC NAME	BRAND NAMES
Abacavir	ZIAGEN	Alefacept	AMEVIVE
Abatacept	ORENCIA	Alemtuzumab	CAMPATH
Abciximab	REOPRO	Alendronate	FOSAMAX
Acamprosate	CAMPRAL	Alfuzosin	UROXATRAL
Acarbose	PRECOSE	Alirocumab	PRALUENT
Acebutolol	SECTRAL	Aliskiren	TEKTURNA
Acetaminophen	TYLENOL	Allopurinol	ZYLOPRIM
Acetazolamide	DIAMOX	All-*trans*-retinoic acid	See Tretonin
Acetohydroxamic acid	LITHOSTAT	Almotriptan	AXERT
Acetylcysteine	ACETADOTE	Alogliptin	NESINA
Acitretin	SORIATANE	Alosetron	LOTRONEX
ACTH	See Corticotropin	Alprazolam	XANAX
Actinomycin	See Dactinomycin	Alprostadil	CAVERJECT, EDEX, MUSE
Aclidinium	TUDORZA PRESSAIR	Alteplase	ACTIVASE
Acyclovir	ZOVIRAX	Amantadine	No US brand name
Adalimumab	HUMIRA	Ambrisentan	LETAIRIS
Adapalene	DIFFERIN	Amifostine	ETHYOL
Adefovir	HEPSERA	Amikacin	No US brand name
Adenosine	ADENOCARD	Amiloride	MIDAMOR
Agalsidase beta	FABRAZYME	Aminocaproic acid	AMICAR
Albendazole	ALBENZA	Aminophylline	No US brand name
Albiglutide	TANZEUM	Amiodarone	CORDARONE
Albuterol	PROVENTIL-HFA, VENTOLIN-HFA	Amitriptyline	No US brand name
Alcaftadine	LASTACAFT	Amlodipine	NORVASC
Aldesleukin	PROLEUKIN	Amobarbital	No US brand name
Alectinib	ALECENSA		

Table continues on the following page.

BRAND NAMES OF SOME COMMONLY USED DRUGS (*Continued*)

GENERIC NAME	BRAND NAMES	GENERIC NAME	BRAND NAMES
Amoxapine	No US brand name	Azacitidine	VIDAZA
Amoxicillin	AMOXIL	Azathioprine	IMURAN
Amoxicillin/clavulanate	AUGMENTIN	Azelaic acid	AZELEX, FINACEA
Amphotericin B	ABELCET, AMBISOME, AMPHOTEC	Azelastine	ASTELIN, OPTIVAR
Ampicillin	No US brand name	Azilsartan	EDARBI
Ampicillin/sulbactam	No US brand name	Azithromycin	ZITHROMAX
Anagrelide	AGRYLIN	Aztreonam	AZACTAM
Anakinra	KINERET	Bacitracin	BACIIM
Anastrozole	ARIMIDEX	Bacitracin/neomycin/polymyxin B	NEOSPORIN
Anidulafungin	ERAXIS	Baclofen	LIORESAL
Anthralin	No US brand name	Balsalazide	COLAZAL
Antihemophilic factor (human)	MONOCLATE-P	Basiliximab	SIMULECT
Antihemophilic factor (recombinant)	RECOMBINATE	Beclomethasone	BECONASE
Antihemophilic factor/von Willebrand factor complex (human)	ALPHANATE	Benazepril	LOTENSIN
Apixaban	ELIQUIS	Bendamustine	TREANDA
Apomorphine	APOKYN	Benzocaine	ANBESOL
Apraclonidine	IOPIDINE	Benzonatate	TESSALON
Apremilast	OTEZLA	Benzoyl peroxide	No US brand name
Aprepitant	EMEND	Benztropine	COGENTIN
Aprotinin	No US brand name	Beractant	SURVANTA
Arformoterol	BROVANA	Betaine	CYSTADANE
Argatroban	No US brand name	Betamethasone	CELESTONE SOLUSPAN, DIPROLENE, LUXIQ
Arginine	R-GENE 10	Betaxolol	BETOPTIC
Aripiprazole	ABILIFY	Bethanechol	DUVOID, URECHOLINE
Armodafinil	NUVIGIL	Bevacizumab	AVASTIN
Artemether/lumefantrine	COARTEM	Bezafibrate	No US brand name
Artesunate	No US brand name	Bicalutamide	CASODEX
Asparaginase	ELSPAR	Bimatoprost	LUMIGAN
Aspirin	No US brand name	Bisacodyl	DULCOLAX
Atazanavir	REYATAZ	Bisoprolol	ZEBETA
Atenolol	TENORMIN	Bivalirudin	ANGIOMAX
Atomoxetine	STRATTERA	Bleomycin	No US brand name
Atorvastatin	LIPITOR	Boceprevir	VICTRELIS
Atovaquone	MEPRON	Bortezomib	VELCADE
Atovaquone/proguanil	MALARONE	Bosentan	TRACLEER
Atracurium	No US brand name	Botulism antitoxin, heptavalent	BAT
Atropine	ATROPEN	Botulism immune globulin (intravenous-human)	Baby BIG
Auranofin	RIDAURA	Botulinum toxin type A (onabotulinumtoxin A)	BOTOX COSMETIC, BOTOX
Avanafil	STENDRA	Botulinum toxin type B (rimabotulinumtoxin B)	MYOBLOC

BRAND NAMES OF SOME COMMONLY USED DRUGS (*Continued*)

GENERIC NAME	BRAND NAMES	GENERIC NAME	BRAND NAMES
Brexpiprazole	REXULTI	Carvedilol	COREG
Brimonidine	ALPHAGAN P	Caspofungin	CANCIDAS
Brinzolamide	AZOPT	Cefaclor	No US brand name
Bromocriptine	PARLODEL	Cefadroxil	No US brand name
Brompheniramine	VELTANE	Cefazolin	ANCEF, KEFZOL
Budesonide	PULMICORT, RHINOCORT	Cefdinir	No US brand name
		Cefditoren	SPECTRACEF
Bumetanide	No US brand name	Cefepime	MAXIPIME
Bupivacaine	MARCAINE	Cefixime	SUPRAX
Buprenorphine	BUPRENEX	Cefotaxime	CLAFORAN
Bupropion	WELLBUTRIN, ZYBAN	Cefotetan	No US brand name
Buserelin	No US brand name	Cefoxitin	MEFOXIN
Buspirone	No US brand name	Cefpodoxime	No US brand name
Busulfan	MYLERAN	Cefprozil	No US brand name
Butenafine	MENTAX	Ceftaroline fosamil	TEFLARO
Butoconazole	FEMSTAT 3	Ceftazidime	FORTAZ, TAZICEF
Butorphanol	No US brand name	Ceftibuten	CEDAX
C1 inhibitor (human)	Berinert	Ceftriaxone	ROCEPHIN
Cabergoline	No US brand name	Cefuroxime	CEFTIN, ZINACEF
Cabozantinib	COMETRIQ	Celecoxib	CELEBREX
Calcipotriene	DOVONEX	Cephalexin	KEFLEX
Calcitonin	MIACALCIN	Ceritinib	ZYKADIA
Calcitriol	ROCALTROL	Cetirizine	ZYRTEC
Calcium chloride	No US brand name	Cetuximab	ERBITUX
Calcium gluconate	No US brand name	Cevimeline	EVOXAC
Calfactant	INFASURF	Chlorambucil	LEUKERAN
Candesartan	ATACAND	Chloramphenicol	No US brand name
Cantharidin	No US brand name	Chlordiazepoxide	LIBRIUM
Capecitabine	XELODA	Chloroquine	ARALEN
Capreomycin	CAPASTAT	Chlorothiazide	DIURIL
Capsaicin	QUTENZA	Chlorpheniramine	CHLOR-TRIMETON
Captopril	CAPOTEN	Chlorpromazine	No US brand name
Carbachol	MIOSTAT	Chlorpropamide	DIABINESE
Carbamazepine	TEGRETOL	Chlorthalidone	THALITONE
Carbidopa	LODOSYN	Chlorzoxazone	PARAFON FORTE DSC
Carbidopa/levodopa	SINEMET	Cholecalciferol	No US brand name
Carboplatin	No US brand name	Cholestyramine resin	PREVALITE
Carfilzomib	KYPROLIS	Choline magnesium trisalicylate	No US brand name
Carisoprodol	SOMA	Ciclopirox	LOPROX, PENLAC
Carmustine	BICNU, GLIADEL	Cidofovir	VISTIDE
Carteolol	OCUPRESS	Cilostazol	PLETAL

Table continues on the following page.

BRAND NAMES OF SOME COMMONLY USED DRUGS (*Continued*)

GENERIC NAME	BRAND NAMES	GENERIC NAME	BRAND NAMES
Cimetidine	TAGAMET	Cyproterone	No US brand name
Cinacalcet	SENSIPAR	Cysteine	See Acetylcysteine
Ciprofloxacin	CILOXAN, CIPRO	Cytarabine	CYTOSAR-U
Cisapride	PROPULSID	Cytomegalovirus immune globulin (intravenous-human)	Cytogam
Cisplatin	PLATINOL	Dabigatran	PRADAXA
Citalopram	CELEXA	Dabrafenib	TAFINLAR
Cladribine	No US brand name	Dacarbazine	DTIC-DOME
Clarithromycin	BIAXIN	Dactinomycin	COSMEGEN
Clemastine	TAVIST-1	Dalfopristin	See Quinupristin
Clevidipine	CLEVIPREX	Dalbavancin	DALVANCE
Clindamycin	CLEOCIN	Dalteparin	FRAGMIN
CloBAZam	ONFI	Danazol	No US brand name
Clobetasol	CLOBEX, TEMOVATE	Dantrolene	DANTRIUM
Clomiphene	CLOMID	Dapagliflozin	FARXIGA
Clomipramine	ANAFRANIL	Dapsone	ACZONE
Clonazepam	KLONOPIN	Daptomycin	CUBICIN
Clonidine	CATAPRES	Darbepoetin alfa	ARANESP
Clopidogrel	PLAVIX	Darifenacin	ENABLEX
Clorazepate	TRANXENE	Darunavir	PREZISTA
Clotrimazole	MYCELEX	Dasatinib	SPRYCEL
Clozapine	CLOZARIL	Daunorubicin	CERUBIDINE
Codeine	No US brand name	Deferasirox	EXJADE
Colchicine	COLCRYS	Deferiprone	FERRIPROX
Colesevelam	WELCHOL	Deferoxamine	DESFERAL
Colestipol	COLESTID	Delavirdine	RESCRIPTOR
Colistimethate	COLY-MYCIN M	Demeclocycline	No US brand name
Conivaptan	VAPRISOL	Desipramine	NORPRAMIN
Corticotropin	H.P. ACTHAR GEL	Desirudin	IPRIVASK
Crizotinib	XALKORI	Desloratadine	CLARINEX
Cromolyn	CROLOM	Desmopressin	DDAVP, STIMATE
Crotalidae polyvalent immune FAB (ovine)	CroFab	Desoximetasone	TOPICORT
Crotamiton	EURAX	Desvenlafaxine	PRISTIQ
Cyclizine	No US brand name	Dexamethasone	OZURDEX
Cyclobenzaprine	AMRIX	Dexchlorpheniramine	No US brand name
Cyclopentolate	AKPENTOLATE, CYCLOGYL	Dexlansoprazole	DEXILANT
Cyclophosphamide	CYTOXAN (LYOPHILIZED)	Dexmedetomidine	PRECEDEX
Cycloserine	SEROMYCIN	Dextroamphetamine	DEXEDRINE
Cyclosporine	NEORAL, SANDIMMUNE	Dextromethorphan	DELSYM
Cyproheptadine	No US brand name	Diazepam	VALIUM
		Diazoxide	PROGLYCEM

BRAND NAMES OF SOME COMMONLY USED DRUGS (*Continued*)

GENERIC NAME	BRAND NAMES
Diclofenac	CATAFLAM, VOLTAREN
Dicloxacillin	No US brand name
Dicyclomine	BENTYL
Didanosine	VIDEX
Dienogest	NATAZIA
Diethylpropion	TENUATE
Diflunisal	No US brand name
Digoxin	LANOXIN
Digoxin immune Fab	DigiFab
Dihydroergotamine	D.H.E. 45, MIGRANAL
Diltiazem	CARDIZEM, CARTIA XT, DILACOR XR
Dimenhydrinate	No US brand name
Dimercaprol	BAL
Dimethyl sulfoxide	RIMSO-50
Dinoprostone	CERVIDIL, PREPIDIL, PROSTIN E2
Diphenhydramine	No US trade name
Diphenoxylate/atropine	LOMOTIL
Dipyridamole	PERSANTINE
Disopyramide	NORPACE
Disulfiram	ANTABUSE
Dobutamine	No US brand name
Docetaxel	TAXOTERE
Docosanol	ABREVA
Dofetilide	TIKOSYN
Dolasetron	ANZEMET
Donepezil	ARICEPT
Dopamine	No US brand name
Doripenem	DORIBAX
Dornase alfa	PULMOZYME
Dorzolamide	TRUSOPT
Doxazosin	CARDURA
Doxepin	ZONALON
Doxercalciferol	HECTOROL
Doxorubicin	No US brand name
Doxorubicin (liposomal)	DOXIL (LIPOSOMAL)
Doxycycline	PERIOSTAT, VIBRAMYCIN
Doxylamine	UNISOM
Dronabinol	MARINOL
Dronedarone	MULTAQ
Droperidol	INAPSINE
Dulaglutide	TRULICITY
Duloxetine	CYMBALTA
Dutasteride	AVODART
Dyclonine	No US brand name
Ecallantide	KALBITOR
Echothiophate iodide	PHOSPHOLINE IODIDE
Econazole	ECOZA
Eculizumab	SOLIRIS
Edetate calcium disodium	CALCIUM DISODIUM VERSENATE
Edoxaban	SAVAYSA
Edrophonium	TENSILON
Efavirenz	SUSTIVA
Eflornithine	VANIQA
Elbasvir and grazoprevir	ZEPATIER
Eletriptan	RELPAX
Eliglustat	CERDELGA
Eltrombopag	PROMACTA
Eluxadoline	VIBERZI
Emedastine	EMADINE
Empagliflozin	JARDIANCE
Emtricitabine	EMTRIVA
Enalapril	VASOTEC
Enalaprilat	No US brand name
Enfuvirtide	FUZEON
Enoxaparin	LOVENOX
Entacapone	COMTAN
Entecavir	BARACLUDE
Enzalutamide	XTANDI
Epinephrine	ADRENALIN
Epirubicin	ELLENCE
Eplerenone	INSPRA
Epoetin alfa	EPOGEN/PROCRIT
Epoprostenol	FLOLAN
Eprosartan	TEVETEN
Eptifibatide	INTEGRILIN
Ergocalciferol	DRISDOL
Ergoloid mesylates	HYDERGINE
Ergonovine	No US brand name
Ergotamine	ERGOMAR

Table continues on the following page.

BRAND NAMES OF SOME COMMONLY USED DRUGS (*Continued*)

GENERIC NAME	BRAND NAMES
Erlotinib	TARCEVA
Ertapenem	INVANZ
Erythromycin	ERY-TAB, ERYTHROCIN
Erythromycin/sulfisoxazole	No US brand name
Escitalopram	LEXAPRO
Eslicarbazepine	APTIOM
Esmolol	BREVIBLOC
Esomeprazole	NEXIUM
Estradiol	ESTRADERM, ESTROGEL, VIVELLE
Estrogens	PREMARIN
Eszopiclone	LUNESTA
Etanercept	ENBREL
Ethacrynic acid	EDECRIN
Ethambutol	MYAMBUTOL
Ethionamide	TRECATOR
Ethosuximide	ZARONTIN
Etidronate	DIDRONEL
Etodolac	No US brand name
Etomidate	AMIDATE
Etonogestrel	IMPLANON
Etoposide	ETOPOPHOS
Etravirine	INTELENCE
Everolimus	AFINITOR
Evolocumab	REPATHA
Exemestane	AROMASIN
Exenatide	BYETTA
Ezetimibe	ZETIA
Ezogabine	POTIGA
Factor IX (human)	MONONINE
Factor IX (recombinant)	RIXUBIS
Factor IX complex (human) [(factors II, IX, X)]	Bebulin
Factor VIIa (recombinant)	NovoSeven
Factor XIII concentrate (human)	Corifact
Famciclovir	FAMVIR
Famotidine	PEPCID
Febuxostat	ULORIC
Felbamate	FELBATOL
Felodipine	PLENDIL
Fenofibrate	ANTARA, LIPOFEN, TRICOR, TRIGLIDE
Fenoldopam	CORLOPAM
Fenoprofen	NALFON
Fentanyl	ACTIQ, DURAGESIC, SUBLIMAZE
Ferric gluconate	FERRLECIT
Ferrous fumarate	No US brand name
Ferrous gluconate	No US brand name
Ferrous sulfate	No US brand name
Fesoterodine	TOVIAZ
Fexofenadine	ALLEGRA
Fidaxomicin	DIFICID
Filgrastim	NEUPOGEN
Finasteride	PROPECIA, PROSCAR
Flavocoxid	LIMBREL
Flavoxate	No US brand name
Flecainide	No US brand name
Floxuridine	No US brand name
Fluconazole	DIFLUCAN
Flucytosine	ANCOBON
Fludarabine	No US brand name
Fludrocortisone	No US brand name
Flumazenil	No US brand name
Flunisolide	AEROSPAN HFA
Fluocinolone (topical)	CAPEX
Fluocinonide	VANOS
Fluorouracil	CARAC
Fluoxetine	PROZAC, SARAFEM
Fluphenazine	No US brand names
Flurandrenolide	CORDRAN
Flurazepam	No US brand name
Flurbiprofen	ANSAID, OCUFEN
Flutamide	No US brand name
Fluticasone	CUTIVATE, FLONASE
Fluvastatin	LESCOL
Fluvoxamine	LUVOX
Fomepizole	ANTIZOL
Fondaparinux	ARIXTRA
Formoterol	FORADIL AEROLIZER, PERFOROMIST
Fosamprenavir	LEXIVA
Foscarnet	FOSCAVIR
Fosfomycin	MONUROL
Fosinopril	No US brand name

BRAND NAMES OF SOME COMMONLY USED DRUGS (*Continued*)

GENERIC NAME	BRAND NAMES	GENERIC NAME	BRAND NAMES
Fosphenytoin	CEREBYX	Hydromorphone	DILAUDID
Frovatriptan	FROVA	Hydroquinone	TRI-LUMA
Fulvestrant	FASLODEX	Hydroxocobalamin	CYANOKIT
Furosemide	LASIX	Hydroxychloroquine	PLAQUENIL
Fusidic acid	No US brand name	Hydroxyurea	HYDREA
Gabapentin	NEURONTIN	Hydroxyzine	VISTARIL
Galantamine	RAZADYNE	Hyoscyamine	No US brand name
Ganciclovir	CYTOVENE	Ibandronate	BONIVA
Gatifloxacin	ZYMAR	Ibritumomab	ZEVALIN
Gefitinib	No US brand name	Ibuprofen	ADVIL, MOTRIN IB
Gemcitabine	GEMZAR	Ibutilide	CORVERT
Gemfibrozil	LOPID	Icatibant	FIRAZYR
Gemifloxacin	FACTIVE	Idarubicin	IDAMYCIN PFS
Gentamicin	GENOPTIC	Idarucizumab	PRAXBIND
Glatiramer acetate	COPAXONE	Ifosfamide	IFEX
Glimepiride	AMARYL	Iloperidone	FANAPT
Glipizide	GLUCOTROL	Iloprost	VENTAVIS
Glucagon	No US brand name	Imatinib	GLEEVEC
Glucarpidase	VORAXAZE	Imipenem/cilastatin	PRIMAXIN
Glyburide	DIABETA, GLYNASE	Imipramine	TOFRANIL
Glycopyrrolate	ROBINUL FORTE, ROBINUL	Imiquimod	ALDARA
Gold/gold sodium thiomalate	See Auranofin	Immune globulin	GAMMAGARD S/D
Golimumab	SIMPONI	Indacaterol	ARCAPTA NEOHALER
Gonadorelin	No US brand name	Indapamide	No US brand name
Goserelin	ZOLADEX	Indinavir	CRIXIVAN
Granisetron	SANCUSO	Indomethacin	INDOCIN
Griseofulvin	GRIFULVIN V	Infliximab	REMICADE
Guanfacine	TENEX	Interferon alfa-2A	ROFERON A
Guanidine	No US brand name	Interferon alfa-2B	INTRON A
Haloperidol	HALDOL	Interferon alfa-N3	ALFERON
Hemin	PANHEMATIN	Iodoquinol	YODOXIN
Heparin	PANHEPRIN	Ipratropium	ATROVENT
Hepatitis B immune globulin	HEPAGAM B	Irbesartan	AVAPRO
Histrelin	VANTAS	Irinotecan	CAMPTOSAR
Homatropine	TUSSIGON	Isocarboxazid	MARPLAN
Hydralazine	No US brand name	Isoniazid	LANIAZID
Hydrochlorothiazide	MICROZIDE	Isoproterenol	ISUPREL
Hydrocodone/acetaminophen	ANEXSIA 5/325	Isosorbide dinitrate	ISORDIL
Hydrocodone/ibuprofen	REPREXAIN	Isosorbide mononitrate	MONOKET
Hydrocortisone (systemic)	CORTEF, SOLU-CORTEF	Isotretinoin	SOTRET

Table continues on the following page.

BRAND NAMES OF SOME COMMONLY USED DRUGS (*Continued*)

GENERIC NAME	BRAND NAMES	GENERIC NAME	BRAND NAMES
Isoxsuprine	VASODILAN	Lindane	No US brand name
Isradipine	No US brand name	Linezolid	ZYVOX
Itraconazole	SPORANOX	Liothyronine	CYTOMEL
Ivacaftor	KALYDECO	Liraglutide	VICTOZA
Ivermectin	STROMECTOL	Lisinopril	PRINIVIL, ZESTRIL
Kanamycin	No US brand name	Lithium	LITHOBID
Ketamine	KETALAR	Lodoxamide	ALOMIDE
Ketoconazole	NIZORAL	Lomitapide	JUXTAPID
Ketoprofen	NEXCEDE	Lomustine	CEENU
Ketorolac	SPRIX	Loperamide	IMODIUM
Ketotifen	ALAWAY, ZADITOR	Lopinavir/ritonavir	KALETRA
Labetalol	No US brand name	Loratadine	ALAVERT, CLARITIN
Lacosamide	VIMPAT	Lorazepam	ATIVAN
Lactulose	CHOLAC	Lorcaserin	BELVIQ
Lamivudine	EPIVIR	Losartan	COZAAR
Lamotrigine	LAMICTAL	Loteprednol	ALREX, LOTEMAX
Lanreotide	SOMATULINE DEPOT	Lovastatin	ALTOPREV
Lansoprazole	PREVACID	Loxapine	ADASUVE
Lanthanum	FOSRENOL	Lubiprostone	AMITIZA
Lapatinib	TYKERB	Lurasidone	LATUDA
Latanoprost	XALATAN	Mafenide	SULFAMYLON
Leflunomide	ARAVA	Magnesium salicylate	DOAN'S EXTRA STRENGTH
Lenalidomide	REVLIMID	Magnesium sulfate	No US brand name
Lepirudin	No US brand name	Mannitol	OSMITROL, RESECTISOL
Letrozole	FEMARA	Maprotiline	No US brand name
Leucovorin calcium	No US brand name	Maraviroc	SELZENTRY
Leuprolide	LUPRON	Mebendazole	No US brand name
Levalbuterol	XOPENEX	Mechlorethamine	MUSTARGEN
Levarternol	See Norepinephrine	Meclizine	ANTIVERT
Levetiracetam	KEPPRA	Meclofenamate	No US brand name
Levobunolol	BETAGAN	Medroxyprogesterone	PROVERA
Levocabastine	No US brand name	Mefenamic acid	PONSTEL
Levocetirizine	XYZAL	Mefloquine	No US brand name
Levofloxacin	IQUIX, LEVAQUIN, QUIXIN	Megestrol	MEGACE
Levomilnacipran	FETZIMA	Meloxicam	MOBIC
Levonorgestrel	MIRENA, PLAN B	Melphalan	ALKERAN
Levorphanol	No US brand name	Memantine	NAMENDA
Levothyroxine	LEVOXYL, SYNTHROID	Meperidine	DEMEROL
Lidocaine	XYLOCAINE	Mercaptopurine	PURINETHOL
Linaclotide	LINZESS	Meropenem	MERREM
Linagliptin	TRADJENTA	Mesalamine	ASACOL, ROWASA

BRAND NAMES OF SOME COMMONLY USED DRUGS (*Continued*)

GENERIC NAME	BRAND NAMES	GENERIC NAME	BRAND NAMES
Mesna	MESNEX	Mirtazapine	REMERON
Metaxalone	SKELAXIN	Misoprostol	CYTOTEC
Metformin	GLUCOPHAGE	Mitomycin	MITOSOL
Methadone	DOLOPHINE	Mitotane	LYSODREN
Methamphetamine	DESOXYN	Mitoxantrone	No US brand name
Methazolamide	No US brand name	Moclobemide	No US brand name
Methenamine	HIPREX, UREX	Modafinil	PROVIGIL
Methimazole	TAPAZOLE	Moexipril	UNIVASC
Methocarbamol	ROBAXIN	Mometasone	ELOCON, NASONEX
Methohexital	BREVITAL SODIUM	Montelukast	SINGULAIR
Methotrexate	OTREXUP	Morphine	DURAMORPH PF, MS CONTIN
Methoxsalen	OXSORALEN, UVADEX	Moxifloxacin	AVELOX
Methsuximide	CELONTIN	Mupirocin	BACTROBAN
Methyclothiazide	No US brand name	Mycophenolate mofetil	CELLCEPT
Methyldopa	No US brand name	Nabumetone	No US brand name
Methylene blue	No US brand name	Nadolol	CORGARD
Methylergonovine	METHERGINE	Nadroparin	No US brand name
Methylphenidate	CONCERTA, RITALIN	Nafarelin	SYNAREL
Methylprednisolone	MEDROL	Nafcillin	NALLPEN IN PLASTIC CONTAINER
Methyltestosterone	TESTRED	Naloxone	EVZIO
Metipranolol	OPTIPRANOLOL	Naltrexone	REVIA
Metoclopramide	REGLAN	Naphazoline	ALBALON
Metolazone	ZAROXOLYN	Naproxen	ALEVE, NAPROSYN
Metoprolol	LOPRESSOR, TOPROL-XL	Naratriptan	AMERGE
Metronidazole	FLAGYL	Natalizumab	TYSABRI
Metyrapone	METOPIRONE	Natamycin	NATACYN
Metyrosine	DEMSER	Nateglinide	STARLIX
Mexiletine	No US brand name	Nebivolol	BYSTOLIC
Micafungin	MYCAMINE	Necitumumab	PORTRAZZA
Miconazole	MONISTAT 3	Nedocromil	ALOCRIL
Midazolam	No US brand name	Nefazodone	No US brand name
Midodrine	ORVATEN	Nelarabine	ARRANON
Mifepristone	MIFEPREX	Nelfinavir	VIRACEPT
Miglitol	GLYSET	Neomycin	NEO-FRADIN
Miglustat	ZAVESCA	Neostigmine	BLOXIVERZ
Milnacipran	SAVELLA	Nesiritide	NATRECOR
Milrinone	No US brand name	Nevirapine	VIRAMUNE
Minocycline	MINOCIN	Niacin	NIACOR, NIASPAN
Minoxidil	ROGAINE	Niacinamide	No US brand name
Mipomersen	KYNAMRO	Nicardipine	CARDENE
Mirabegron	MYRBETRIQ		

Table continues on the following page.

BRAND NAMES OF SOME COMMONLY USED DRUGS (*Continued*)

GENERIC NAME	BRAND NAMES
Nicotine	COMMIT, NICORETTE, NICOTROL
Nicotinic acid	See Niacin
Nifedipine	ADALAT CC, PROCARDIA
Nilotinib	TASIGNA
Nilutamide	NILANDRON
Nimodipine	NIMOTOP
Nintedanib	OFEV
Nisoldipine	SULAR
Nitazoxanide	ALINIA
Nitrofurantoin	FURADANTIN, MACROBID, MACRODANTIN
Nitrogen mustard	See Mechlorethamine
Nitroglycerin	NITRO-DUR
Nitroprusside	NITROPRESS
Nivolumab	OPDIVO
Nizatidine	AXID
Norepinephrine	LEVOPHED
Norethindrone	AYGESTIN, CAMILA
Norfloxacin	NOROXIN
Nortriptyline	AVENTYL
Nystatin	NYSTOP
Octreotide	SANDOSTATIN
Ofloxacin	FLOXIN OTIC
Olanzapine	ZYPREXA
Olmesartan	BENICAR
Olopatadine	PATANOL
Olsalazine	DIPENTUM
Omalizumab	XOLAIR
Ombitasvir, paritaprevir, and ritonavir	TECHNIVIE
Ombitasvir, paritaprevir, ritonavir, and dasabuvir	VIEKIRA PAK
Omeprazole	PRILOSEC
Ondansetron	ZOFRAN
Opium tincture	No US brand name
Oprelvekin	NEUMEGA
Oritavancin	ORBACTIV
Orlistat	ALLI, XENICAL
Orphenadrine	NORFLEX
Oseltamivir	TAMIFLU
Oxacillin	BACTOCILL IN PLASTIC CONTAINER
Oxaliplatin	ELOXATIN
Oxaprozin	DAYPRO
Oxazepam	No US brand name
Oxcarbazepine	TRILEPTAL
Oxiconazole	OXISTAT
Oxybutynin	DITROPAN XL
Oxycodone	OXYCONTIN
Oxycodone/acetaminophen	PERCOCET
Oxymetholone	ANADROL-50
Oxytocin	PITOCIN
Paclitaxel	TAXOL
Paliperidone	INVEGA
Palivizumab	SYNAGIS
Palonosetron	ALOXI
Pamidronate	AREDIA
Pancrelipase	PANCREAZE
Pancuronium	No US brand name
Panitumumab	VECTIBIX
Pantoprazole	PROTONIX
Papaverine	No US brand name
Paregoric	No US brand name
Paromomycin	No US brand name
Paroxetine	PAXIL
Pasireotide	SIGNIFOR
Patiromer	VELTASSA
Pegaptanib	MACUGEN
Pegfilgrastim	NEULASTA
Peginterferon alfa-2a	PEGASYS
Peginterferon alfa-2b	PEGINTRON
Pegloticase	KRYSTEXXA
Pegvisomant	SOMAVERT
Pembrolizumab	KEYTRUDA
Pemetrexed	ALIMTA
Penciclovir	DENAVIR
Penicillamine	CUPRIMINE
Penicillin G (parenteral/aqueous)	No US brand name
Penicillin G benzathine	BICILLIN L-A
Penicillin G procaine	No US brand name
Penicillin V potassium	PENICILLIN-VK
Pentamidine	NEBUPENT
Pentazocine	TALWIN

BRAND NAMES OF SOME COMMONLY USED DRUGS (*Continued*)

GENERIC NAME	BRAND NAMES	GENERIC NAME	BRAND NAMES
Pentobarbital	NEMBUTAL SODIUM	Pramlintide	SYMLIN
Pentosan polysulfate sodium	ELMIRON	Pramoxine	EPIFOAM
Pentostatin	NIPENT	Prasugrel	EFFIENT
Pentoxifylline	TRENTAL	Pravastatin	PRAVACHOL
Perindopril erbumine	ACEON	Praziquantel	BILTRICIDE
Permethrin	ELIMITE, NIX	Prazosin	MINIPRESS
Perphenazine	No US brand name	Prednisolone	ORAPRED, PRELONE
Pertuzumab	PERJETA	Prednisone	RAYOS
Phenazopyridine	No US brand name	Pregabalin	LYRICA
Phenelzine	NARDIL	Primaquine	No US brand name
Phenobarbital	No US brand name	Primidone	MYSOLINE
Phenoxybenzamine	DIBENZYLINE	Probenecid	No US brand name
Phentermine	ADIPEX-P	Procainamide	No US brand name
Phentolamine	No US brand name	Procarbazine	MATULANE
Phenylephrine	No US brand name	Prochlorperazine	COMPRO
Phenytoin	DILANTIN	Procyclidine	No US brand name
Phosphomycin	See Fosfomycin	Progesterone	CRINONE
Phospholipid surfactant	See Beractant, Calfactant, Poractant alfa	Promethazine	PROMETHEGAN
		Propafenone	RYTHMOL
Physostigmine	No US brand name	Propantheline	No US brand name
Phytonadione	MEPHYTON	Proparacaine	ALCAINE, OPHTHETIC
Pilocarpine	ISOPTO CARPINE, PILOPINE HS, SALAGEN	Propofol	DIPRIVAN
Pimecrolimus	ELIDEL	Propranolol	INDERAL
Pimozide	ORAP	Propylthiouracil	No US brand name
Pindolol	No US brand name	Prostaglandin E_1 (PGE_1)	See Alprostadil
Pioglitazone	ACTOS	Protamine	No US brand name
Piperacillin/tazobactam	ZOSYN	Protein C concentrate (human)	CEPROTIN
Pirbuterol	MAXAIR	Prothrombin complex concentrate (human) ([factors II, VII, IX, X], protein C, and protein S)	KCENTRA
Pirfenidone	ESBRIET		
Piroxicam	FELDENE		
Pitavastatin	LIVALO	Protriptyline	VIVACTIL
Podophyllum resin	No US brand name	Pseudoephedrine	AFRINOL, SUDAFED
Polidocanol	ASCLERA	Pyrantel pamoate	PIN-X
Polymyxin B	No US brand name	Pyrazinamide	No US brand name
Poractant alfa	CUROSURF	Pyrethrins/piperonyl butoxide	RID MOUSSE
Posaconazole	NOXAFIL	Pyridostigmine	MESTINON
Potassium chloride	K-TAB, KLOR-CON	Pyrimethamine	DARAPRIM
Potassium iodide	THYROSHIELD	Quazepam	DORAL
Povidone-iodine	BETADINE	Quetiapine	SEROQUEL
Pralidoxime	PROTOPAM CHLORIDE	Quinagolide	No US brand name
Pramipexole	MIRAPEX	Quinapril	ACCUPRIL

Table continues on the following page.

BRAND NAMES OF SOME COMMONLY USED DRUGS (*Continued*)

GENERIC NAME	BRAND NAMES	GENERIC NAME	BRAND NAMES
Quinidine	No US brand name	Rotigotine	NEUPRO
Quinine	QUALAQUIN	Ruxolitinib	JAKAFI
Quinupristin/dalfopristin	SYNERCID	Salicylic acid	No US brand name
Rabeprazole	ACIPHEX	Salmeterol	SEREVENT
Raloxifene	EVISTA	Salsalate	No US brand name
Raltegravir	ISENTRESS	Sapropterin	KUVAN
Ramelteon	ROZEREM	Saquinavir	INVIRASE
Ramipril	ALTACE	Sargramostim	LEUKINE
Ramucirumab	CYRAMZA	Saxagliptin	ONGLYZA
Ranibizumab	LUCENTIS	Scopolamine	TRANSDERM SCOP
Ranitidine	ZANTAC	Secobarbital	SECONAL
Rasagiline	AZILECT	Selegiline	ELDEPRYL
Rasburicase	ELITEK	Selenium sulfide	SELSUN
Raxibacumab	RAXIBACUMAB	Sertraline	ZOLOFT
Repaglinide	PRANDIN	Sevelamer	RENAGEL
Reserpine	No US brand name	Sildenafil	VIAGRA
Reteplase	RETAVASE	Silver sulfadiazine	SILVADENE
Retinoic acid	See Tretinoin	Simethicone	No US brand name
Rho(D) immune globulin	RhoGAM	Simvastatin	ZOCOR
Ribavirin	VIRAZOLE	Sipuleucel-T	PROVENGE
Rifabutin	MYCOBUTIN	Sirolimus	RAPAMUNE
Rifampin	RIFADIN, RIMACTANE	Sitagliptin	JANUVIA
Rifapentine	PRIFTIN	Sodium bicarbonate	No US brand name
Rifaximin	XIFAXAN	Sodium oxybate	XYREM
Rilonacept	ARCALYST	Sodium phosphates	No US brand name
Rilpivirine	EDURANT	Sodium polystyrene sulfonate	KALEXATE
Riluzole	RILUTEK	Sodium tetradecyl	SOTRADECOL
Rimantadine	FLUMADINE	Sodium thiosulfate	NITHIODOTE
Risedronate	ACTONEL	Solifenacin	VESICARE
Risperidone	RISPERDAL	Somatropin	HUMATROPE
Ritonavir	NORVIR	Sorafenib	NEXAVAR
Rituximab	RITUXAN	Sotalol	BETAPACE
Rivaroxaban	XARELTO	Spiramycin	No US brand name
Rivastigmine	EXELON	Spironolactone	ALDACTONE
Rizatriptan	MAXALT	Stavudine	ZERIT
Rocuronium	ZEMURON	Streptokinase	STREPTASE
Roflumilast	DALIRESP	Streptomycin	No US brand name
Romiplostim	NPLATE	Streptozocin	ZANOSAR
Ropinirole	REQUIP	Succimer	CHEMET
Rosiglitazone	AVANDIA	Succinylcholine	ANECTINE, QUELICIN
Rosuvastatin	CRESTOR	Sucralfate	CARAFATE

BRAND NAMES OF SOME COMMONLY USED DRUGS (*Continued*)

GENERIC NAME	BRAND NAMES	GENERIC NAME	BRAND NAMES
Sulconazole	EXELDERM	Thiopental	No US brand name
Sulfacetamide	BLEPH-10	Thioridazine	No US brand name
Sulfadiazine	No US brand name	Thiotepa	No US brand name
Sulfadoxine/pyrimethamine	No US brand name	Thiothixene	NAVANE
Sulfamethoxazole	See Trimethoprim/ sulfamethoxazole	Thyroid hormone, synthetic	See Levothyroxine
Sulfasalazine	AZULFIDINE	L-Thyroxine	See Levothyroxine
Sulindac	CLINORIL	Thyrotropin alfa	THYROGEN
Sumatriptan	IMITREX	Tiagabine	GABITRIL
Sunitinib	SUTENT	Ticagrelor	BRILINTA
Suramin	No US brand name	Ticarcillin/clavulanate potassium	TIMENTIN
Tacrolimus	PROGRAF	Ticlopidine	No US brand name
Tadalafil	CIALIS	Tigecycline	TYGACIL
Tafluprost	ZIOPTAN	Tiludronate	No US brand name
Tamoxifen	NOLVADEX	Timolol	TIMOPTIC
Tamsulosin	FLOMAX	Tinidazole	TINDAMAX
Tazarotene	AVAGE, TAZORAC	Tinzaparin	No US brand name
Tedizolid	SIVEXTRO	Tioconazole	VAGISTAT-1
Tegaserod	No US brand name	Tiopronin	THIOLA
Telavancin	VIBATIV	Tiotropium	SPIRIVA
Telbivudine	TYZEKA	Tipranavir	APTIVUS
Telithromycin	KETEK	Tirofiban	AGGRASTAT
Telmisartan	MICARDIS	Tizanidine	ZANAFLEX
Temazepam	RESTORIL	Tobramycin	TOBI, TOBREX
Temozolomide	TEMODAR	Tocilizumab	ACTEMRA
Temsirolimus	TORISEL	Tofacitinib	XELJANZ
Tenecteplase	TNKASE	Tolazamide	No US brand name
Teniposide	VUMON	Tolbutamide	No US brand name
Tenofovir disoproxil fumarate	VIREAD	Tolmetin	No US brand name
Terazosin	HYTRIN	Tolnaftate 1%	No US brand name
Terbinafine	LAMISIL	Tolterodine	DETROL
Terbutaline	No US brand name	Tolvaptan	SAMSCA
Terconazole	TERAZOL 3	Topiramate	TOPAMAX
Teriparatide	FORTEO	Topotecan	HYCAMTIN
Testosterone	DELATESTRYL	Torsemide	DEMADEX
Tetracaine/lidocaine	SYNERAN	Tositumomab and iodine I 131	BEXXAR
Tetracycline	ACHROMYCIN V	Tramadol	ULTRAM
Tetrahydrozoline	TYZINE	Trandolapril	MAVIK
Thalidomide	THALOMID	Tranexamic acid	CYKLOKAPRON
Theophylline	ELIXOPHYLLIN	Tranylcypromine	PARNATE
Thioguanine	No US brand name	Trastuzumab	HERCEPTIN

Table continues on the following page.

BRAND NAMES OF SOME COMMONLY USED DRUGS (*Continued*)

GENERIC NAME	BRAND NAMES
Travoprost	TRAVATAN Z
Trazodone	OLEPTRO
Treprostinil	REMODULIN
Tretinoin	RETIN-A
Triamcinolone	KENALOG
Triamterene	DYRENIUM
Triazolam	HALCION
Trientine	SYPRINE
Trifluridine	VIROPTIC
Trihexyphenidyl	No US brand name
Trimethadione	TRIDIONE
Trimethobenzamide	TIGAN
Trimethoprim	No US brand name
Trimethoprim/polymixin B	POLYTRIM
Trimethoprim/ sulfamethoxazole	BACTRIM, SEPTRA
Tromethamine	THAM
Tropicamide	MYDRIACYL, TROPICACYL
Trospium	SANCTURA
Ulipristal	ELLA
Undecylenic acid and derivatives	No US brand name
Unoprostone	RESCULA
Ursodiol	ACTIGALL
Ustekinumab	STELARA
Vaccinia immune globulin (intravenous)	CNJ-016
Valacyclovir	VALTREX
Valganciclovir	VALCYTE
Valproate	DEPACON
Valsartan	DIOVAN
Vancomycin	VANCOCIN
Vandetanib	CAPRELSA
Vardenafil	LEVITRA
Varenicline	CHANTIX
Varicella-zoster immune globulin (human)	VariZIG
Vasopressin	VASOSTRICT
Vecuronium	No US brand name
Vedolizumab	ENTYVIO
Vemurafenib	ZELBORAF
Venlafaxine	EFFEXOR XR
Verapamil	CALAN
Vigabatrin	SABRIL
Vinblastine	No US brand name
Vincristine	MARQIBO KIT
Vindesine	No US brand name
Vinorelbine	NAVELBINE
Vismodegib	ERIVEDGE
Voriconazole	VFEND
Warfarin	COUMADIN
Zafirlukast	ACCOLATE
Zaleplon	SONATA
Zanamivir	RELENZA
Ziconotide	PRIALT
Zidovudine	RETROVIR
Zileuton	ZYFLO
Ziprasidone	GEODON
Zoledronic acid	ZOMETA
Zolmitriptan	ZOMIG
Zolpidem	AMBIEN
Zonisamide	ZONEGRAN

GASTROINTESTINAL DISORDERS

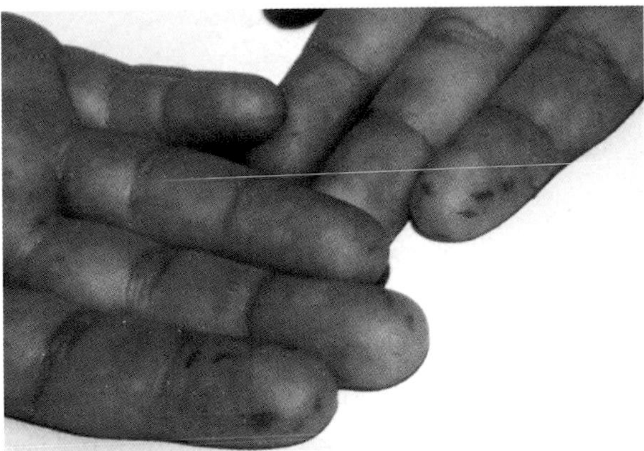

Plate 1. Peutz-Jeghers Syndrome (hand lesions—see p. 169).

MUSCULOSKELETAL AND CONNECTIVE TISSUE DISORDERS

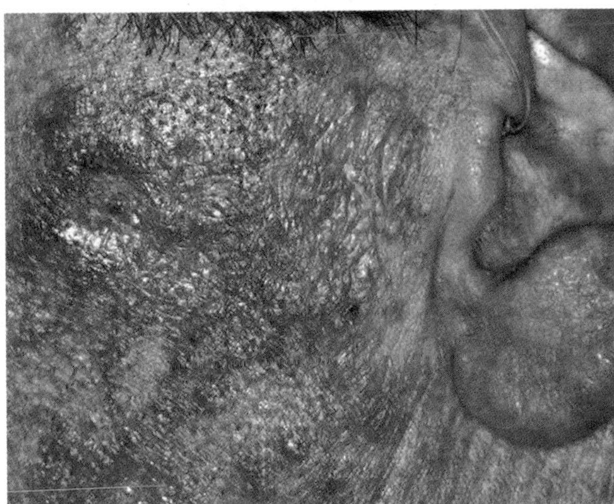

Plate 2. Chronic discoid lupus (see p. 265). This photo shows chronic discoid lupus erythematosus with characteristic hyperkeratotic and erythematous plaques.

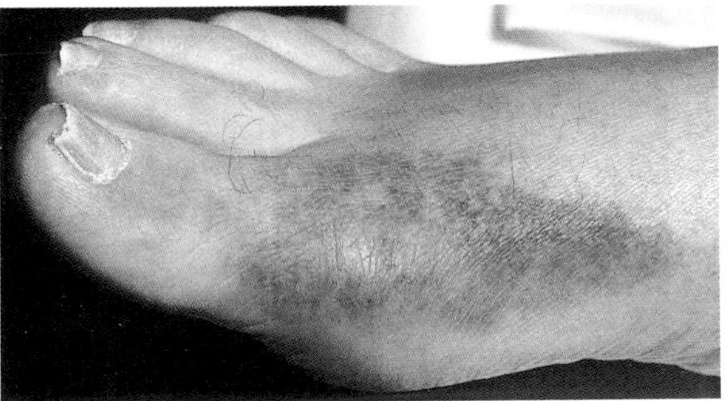

Plate 3. Podagra (see p. 272). Podagra, or acute pain in the 1st metatarsophalangeal joint that is accompanied by redness, tenderness, and swelling, is a common manifestation of acute gout.

CARDIOVASCULAR DISORDERS

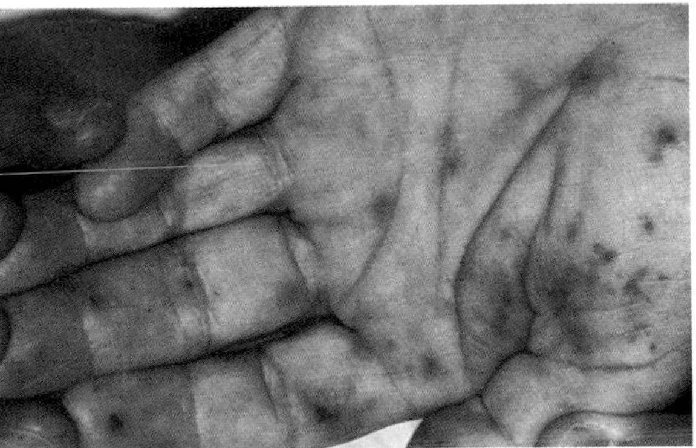

Plate 4. Infective endocarditis (Janeway lesions—see p. 708). This patient with infective endocarditis has multiple Janeway lesions (nontender, erythematous papules) on the palms. The patient also has some Osler nodes (tender, erythematous nodules on the fingers).

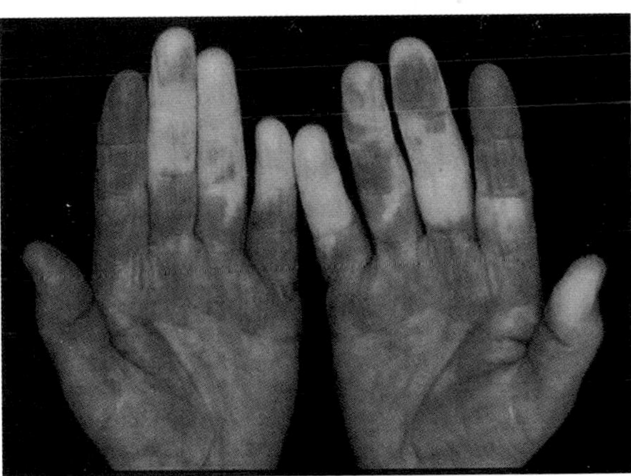

Plate 5. Raynaud syndrome with pallor (see p. 753). Pallor develops irregularly in the fingers.

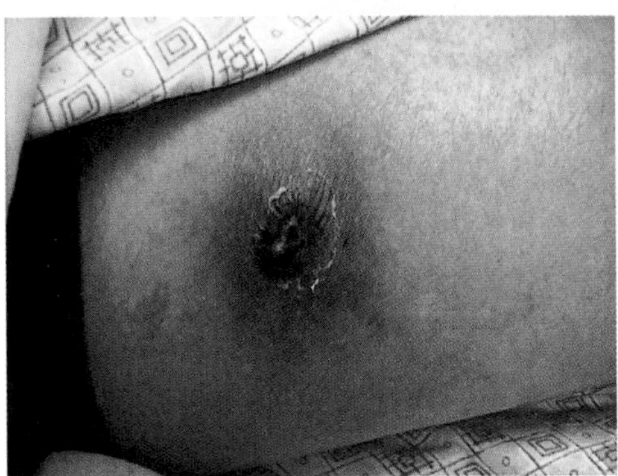

Plate 95. Brown recluse spider bite (see p. 2951). This photo shows a necrotic lesion on the inner thigh resulting from brown recluse spider bite.

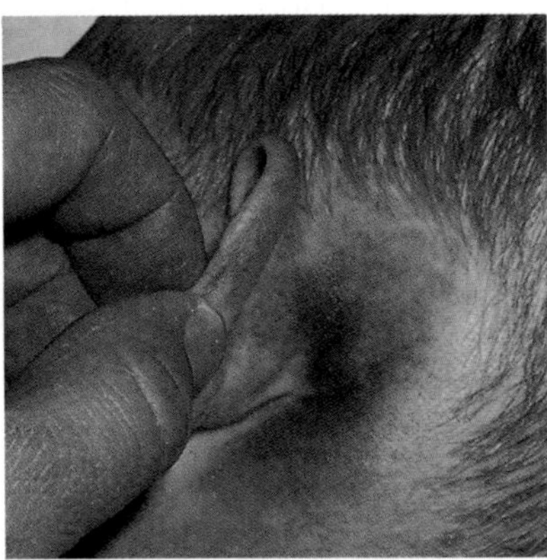

Plate 96. Findings in basilar skull fracture (Battle sign—see p. 3120). This photo shows Battle's sign or mastoid ecchymosis.

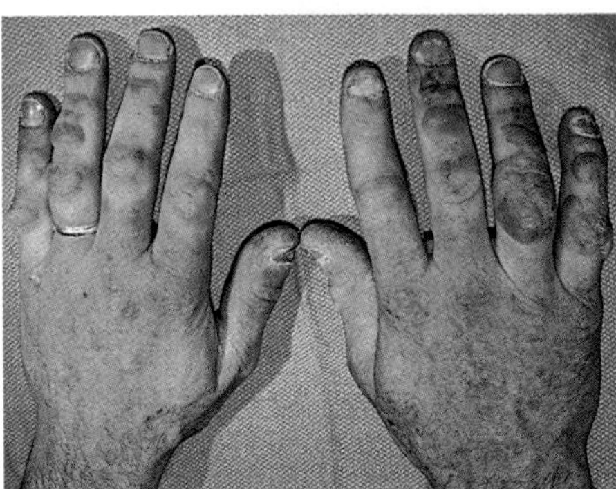

Plate 97. Frostbite of the hands (see p. 2959). This photo shows frostbite of the hands. Blisters (hemorrhagic at right ring and small fingers) are evident, and cyanotic fingertips may portend necrosis. The ring should be removed before swelling occurs.

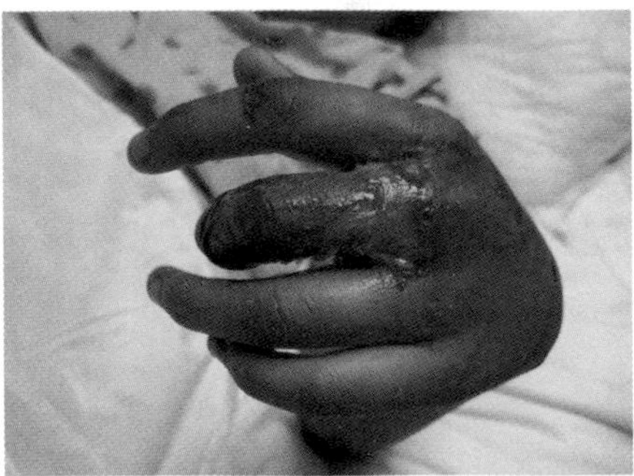

Plate 98. Full-thickness (3rd-degree) burn (see p. 2955). Most of the 3rd finger has a full-thickness burn, where the skin is dark and leathery. The blisters and redness at the finger's base indicate a partial-thickness burn.

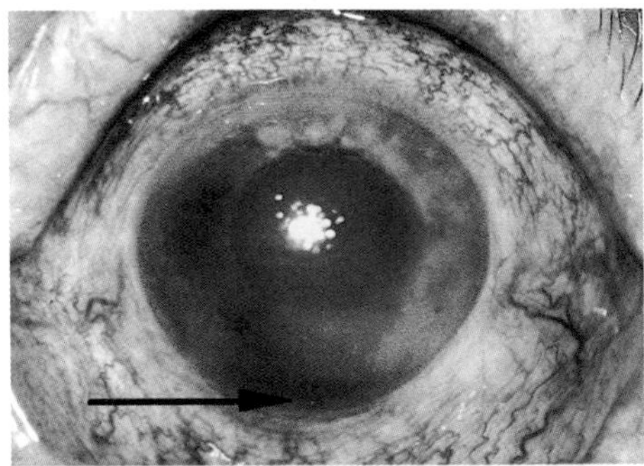

Plate 99. Anterior Chamber Hemorrhage (Hyphema—see p. 2970). This patient has a traumatic hyphema and conjunctival erythema (arrow) after a traumatic injury to the eye.

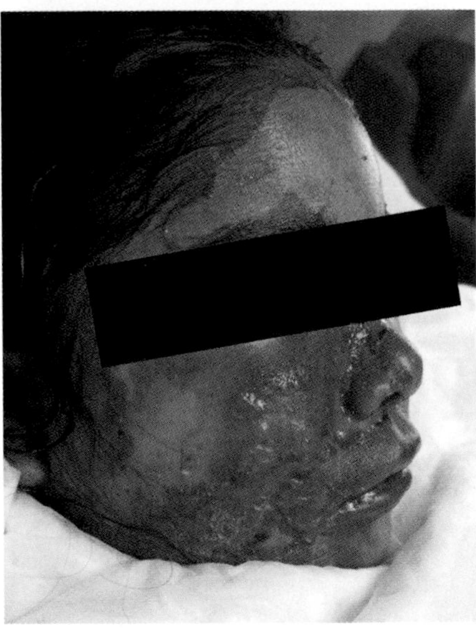

Plate 100. Partial-thickness (2nd-degree) burn (see p. 2955). Blisters on the cheek and some redness are present. Redness is particulary obvious on the forehead, where a large blister has opened and drained.

INDEX

Note: Page numbers in *italics* refer to illustrations, tables, or sidebars. Color plates are indexed with a p followed by the plate number.

A

C

D

E

F

G

H

I

J

K

L

M

N

O

Q

R

S

T

U

V

W

X

Y

Z

NOTES

NOTES

NOTES

NOTES

NOTES

NOTES

NOTES

NOTES

NOTES

NOTES

NOTES

NOTES

NOTES

NOTES

NOTES

NOTES

NOTES

NOTES

NOTES

NOTES

NOTES

NOTES

NOTES

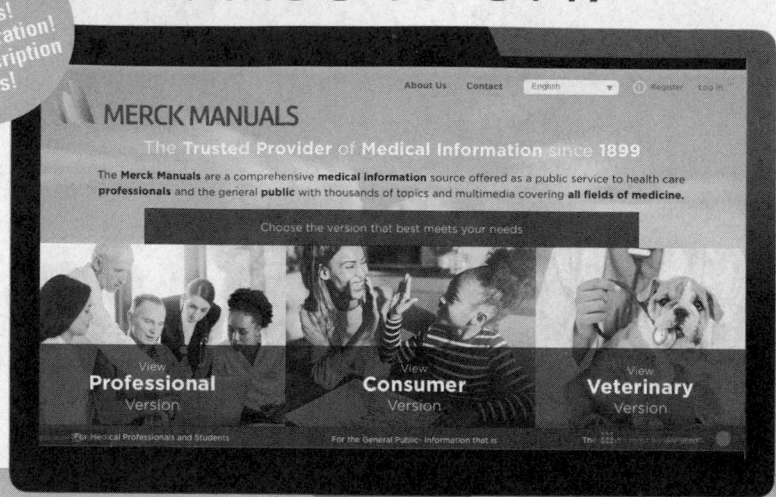

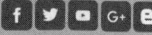

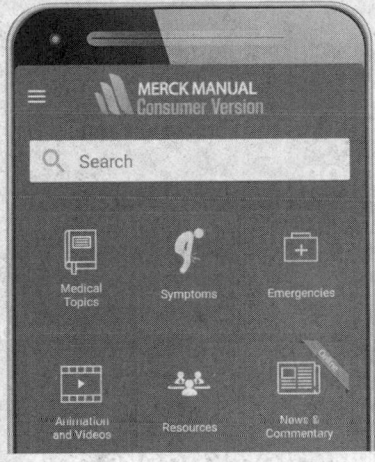

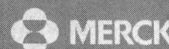